Clinical Bone Marrow and Blood Stem Cell Transplantation, Third Edition

The third edition of this authoritative and highly acclaimed text is entirely revised and updated by the addition of five distinguished new editors and 18 completely new chapters on important topics such as plasticity of stem cells, embryonic stem cells, and nonmyeloablative conditioning regimens. In total there are a comprehensive 124 chapters balancing scientific explanations with practical information on patient care for all aspects of autologous, syngeneic, and allogeneic transplantation. Thoroughly referenced and up-to-the-minute, the chapters are divided into 15 sections covering biological background and practical procedures, clinical results, transplant-related and organ-specific complications, laboratory aspects, and developing areas, with a final "breaking news" chapter from this rapidly evolving field. More than 200 internationally recognized experts contributed to this authoritative and practical text. It is an essential resource for hematologists, oncologists, and transplant specialists.

Kerry Atkinson, MD, is Vice President of Clinical Affairs and Medical Director at Osiris Therapeutics in Baltimore and Courtesy Professor of Medicine at Weill School of Medicine, Cornell University, New York.

Richard Champlin, MD, is Professor of Medicine and Chairman of the Department of Blood and Marrow Transplantation, The University of Texas M. D. Anderson Cancer Center, Houston.

Jerome Ritz, MD, is Professor of Medicine at the Dana-Farber Cancer Institute, Brigham and Women's Hospital, Harvard Medical School, Boston, Massachusetts.

Willem Fibbe, MD, PhD, is Professor in the Department of Hematology, Leiden University Medical Center, Leiden, The Netherlands.

Per Ljungman, MD, PhD, is Professor of Hematology in the Division of Hematology, Department of Medicine, Huddinge University Hospital, Stockholm, Sweden.

Malcom K. Brenner, MD, PhD, is Director of the Center for Cell and Gene Therapy and Professor of Medicine and of Pediatrics at Baylor College of Medicine, Houston, Texas.

Praise for the previous editions:

"The book is a masterpiece and serves as an authoritative background for any reading to be done in the area. This is the book that the reader who will buy only one book on bone marrow transplantation needs to buy."

—*Bloodline* (on second edition)

"The strength of this work lies in its capacity to provide information in two formats: extended textual discussion of the background . . . in clinical and basic science research and brief, practical tables summarizing patient care."

—*The New England Journal of Medicine* (on first edition)

Clinical Bone Marrow and Blood Stem Cell Transplantation
Third Edition

EDITED BY

Kerry Atkinson

Osiris Therapeutics Inc.
Baltimore, Maryland

Richard Champlin

Department of Blood and Marrow Transplantation
The University of Texas-M.D. Anderson Cancer Center
Houston, Texas

Jerome Ritz

Dana-Farber Cancer Institute
Brigham and Women's Hospital
Harvard Medical School
Boston, Massachusetts

Willem E. Fibbe

Department of Hematology
Leiden University Medical Center
Leiden, The Netherlands

Per Ljungman

Division of Hematology, Department of Medicine
Huddinge University Hospital
Stockholm, Sweden

Malcom K. Brenner

Center for Cell and Gene Therapy
Baylor College of Medicine
Houston, Texas

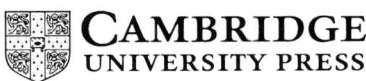
CAMBRIDGE
UNIVERSITY PRESS

PUBLISHED BY THE PRESS SYNDICATE OF THE UNIVERSITY OF CAMBRIDGE
The Pitt Building, Trumpington Street, Cambridge, United Kingdom

CAMBRIDGE UNIVERSITY PRESS
The Edinburgh Building, Cambridge CB2 2RU, UK
40 West 20th Street, New York, NY 10011-4211, USA
477 Williamstown Road, Port Melbourne, VIC 3207, Australia
Ruiz de Alarcón 13, 28014 Madrid, Spain
Dock House, The Waterfront, Cape Town 8001, South Africa

http://www.cambridge.org

First published 2004

Printed in the United States of America

Typeface Times Roman 9.5/12pt   *System* QuarkXPress™   [HT]

A catalog record for this book is available from the British Library.

Library of Congress Cataloging in Publication Data

Clinical bone marrow and blood stem cell transplantation / edited by Kerry Atkinson . . . [et al.].—3rd ed.
       p. ; cm.
    Includes bibliographical references and index.
    ISBN 0 521 82912 7 (HB)
       1. Bone marrow—Transplantation.   I. Atkinson, Kerry.
    [DNLM: 1. Bone Marrow Transplantation.   2. Hematopoietic Stem Cell Transplantation.
    WH 380 C575 2003]
    RD123.5.C54 2003
    617.4′4—dc21
                                                                            2003043806

ISBN 0 521 82912 7 hardback

Contents

Color plates appear after page 928

Contributors List

Claudio Anasetti
Fred Hutchinson Cancer Research Center and
University of Washington
Seattle, Washington, USA

Martin Andreansky
Departments of Hematology-Oncology and Pathology
St. Jude Children's Research Hospital and
University of Tennessee College of Medicine
Memphis, Tennessee, USA

Michael A. Andrykowski
University of Kentucky College of Medicine
Lexington, Kentucky, USA

Paolo Anderlini
The University of Texas M.D. Anderson Cancer Center
Houston, Texas, USA

Emanuele Angelucci
Ospedale di Pesaro
Pesaro, Italy

Joseph H. Antin
Dana-Farber Cancer Institute and
Brigham and Women's Hospital
Harvard University
Boston, Massachusetts, USA

Karen Antman
Columbia University College of Physicians and Surgeons
New York, New York, USA

Jane Apperley
Imperial College School of Medicine
London, United Kingdom

Kerry Atkinson
Osiris Therapeutics Inc.
Baltimore, Maryland, and
Weill School of Medicine
Cornell University
New York, New York, USA

Marcus D. Atlas
Sir Charles Gairdner Hospital
Perth, Australia

Franco Aversa
University of Perugia
Perugia, Italy

Irit Avivi
University College London Hospitals
London, United Kingdom

Norihiro Awaya
Fred Hutchinson Cancer Research Center and
Department of Medicine
University of Washington
Seattle, Washington, USA

Andrea Bacigalupo
Ospendale San Martino
Genova, Italy

J.N.A. Bakker
Department of Immunohematology and Blood Transfusion
Leiden University Medical Center and
Europdonor Foundation
Leiden, The Netherlands

Giuseppe Bandini
Institute of Haematology and Clinical Oncology
"L.A. Seragnoli"
St. Orsola Hospital
University of Bologna
Bologna, Italy

A. John Barrett
National Heart, Lung, and Blood Institute
Bethesda, Maryland, USA

Scott I. Bearman
University of Colorado Health Sciences Center
Denver, Colorado, USA

C. Glenn Begley
Amgen
Thousand Oaks, California, USA

Martin Benesch
Fred Hutchinson Cancer Research Center and
University of Washington
Seattle, Washington, USA

William I. Bensinger
Fred Hutchinson Cancer Research Center and
Department of Medicine
University of Washington
Seattle, Washington, USA

Christophe Bergeron
Centre Léon Berard
Lyon, France

Barbara E. Bierer
Dana-Farber Cancer Institute
Boston, Massachusetts, USA

Philip J. Bierman
University of Nebraska Medical Center
Omaha, Nebraska, USA

Michael R. Bishop
National Cancer Insitute
Bethesda, Maryland, USA

Marie Bleakley
The Children's Hospital at Westmead
Sydney, Australia

Catherine M. Bollard
Baylor College of Medicine
Houston, Texas, USA

Marc A. Boogaerts
University Hospital
Leuven, Belgium

Chiara Bonini
Cancer Immunotherapy and Gene Therapy Program
Milan, Italy

Claudio Bordignon
Cancer Immunotherapy and Gene Therapy Program
Milan, Italy

Christopher Bradbury
St. Vincent's Hospital
Sydney, Australia

Kenneth F. Bradstock
Westmead Hospital
Sydney, Australia

Christopher N. Bredeson
International Bone Marrow Transplant Registry
Milwaukee, Wisconsin, USA

Malcolm Brenner
Baylor College of Medicine
Houston, Texas, USA

David Bryant
St. Vincent's Hospital and
University of New South Wales
Sydney, Australia

Alan K. Burnett
University of Wales College of Medicine and
University Hospital of Wales
Cardiff, United Kingdom

Anna Butturini
Children's Hospital of Los Angeles
Los Angeles, California, USA

Mitchell S. Cairo
Columbia University College of Physicians and Surgeons
New York, New York, USA

Dario Campana
St. Jude Children's Research Hospital and
University of Tennessee College of Medicine
Memphis, Tennessee, USA

Richard E. Champlin
The University of Texas M.D. Anderson Cancer Center
Houston, Texas, USA

Phillip Chang
St. Vincent's Hospital
Sydney, Australia

Richard Childs
National Heart, Lung, and Blood Institute
Bethesda, Maryland, USA

Donald J. Chisholm
St. Vincent's Hospital and
University of New South Wales
Sydney, Australia

Fabio Ciceri
Cancer Immunotherapy and Gene Therapy Program
Milan, Italy

Curt I. Civin
Sidney Kimmel Comprehensive Cancer Center
Johns Hopkins University
Baltimore, Maryland, USA

F.H.J. Claas
Department of Immunohematology and Blood Transfusion
Leiden University Medical Center and
Europdonor Foundation
Leiden, The Netherlands

Milton L. Cohen
St. Vincent's Hospital and
University of New South Wales
Sidney, Australia

Catherine Cordonnier
Henri Mondor Hospital
Creteil, France

Jan J. Cornelissen
University Hospital Rotterdam
Daniel den Hoed Cancer Center
Rotterdam, The Netherlands

Gay Crooks
Children's Hospital Los Angeles and
University of Southern California School of Medicine
Los Angeles, California, USA

M. Reza Dana
Schepens Eye Research Institute
Massachusetts Eye and Ear Infirmary and
Harvard Medical School
Boston, Massachusetts, USA

Virginia Davenport
Herbert Irving Comprehensive Cancer Center
Columbia University College of Physicians and Surgeons
New York, New York, USA

H. Joachim Deeg
Fred Hutchinson Cancer Research Center and
University of Washington
Seattle, Washington, USA

Adrian Dekker
University Medical Center
Utrecht, The Netherlands

Michel Delforge
University Hospital
Leuven, Belgium

Theo De Witte
University Hospital
Nijmegen, The Netherlands

Anthony J. Dodds
St. Vincent's Hospital and
University of New South Wales
Sydney, Australia

Hermann Einsele
University of Tübingen
Tübingen, Germany

Anthony Elias
University of Colorado Cancer Institute and
University of Colorado
Denver, Colorado, USA

Dan Engelhard
Hadassah University Hospital
Jerusalem, Israel

Michael P. Feneley
St. Vincent's Hospital and
University of New South Wales
Sydney, Australia

James L.M. Ferrara
University of Michigan
Ann Arbor, Michigan, USA

Willem E. Fibbe
Leiden University Medical Center
Leiden, The Netherlands

Andrew Field
St. Vincent's Hospital
Sydney, Australia

Jonathan Finlay
Stephen D. Hassenfeld Cancer Center
New York University Cancer Institute
New York, New York, USA

Meri T. Firpo
University of California
San Francisco, California, USA

Alain Fischer
Hôpital Necker-Enfants Malades
Paris, France

Mary E.D. Flowers
Fred Hutchinson Cancer Research Center
Seattle, Washington, USA

Francesco Frassoni
Ospendale San Martino
Genova, Italy

Arnold S. Freedman
Dana-Farber Cancer Institute and
Harvard University
Boston, Massachusetts, USA

Jonathan W. Friedberg
University of Rochester
Rochester, New York, USA

Gösta Gahrton
Karolinska Institute and
Huddinge University Hospital
Stockholm, Sweden

V. Galbusera
Ospendale San Martino
Genova, Italy

Robert Peter Gale
Center for Advanced Studies in Leukemia
Los Angeles, California, USA

Kimberly L. Gandy
Duke University Medical Center
Durham, North Carolina, USA

Sharon Gardner
Stephen D. Hassenfeld Cancer Center
New York University Cancer Institute
New York, New York, USA

Raymond Garrick
St. Vincent's Hospital and
University of New South Wales
Sydney, Australia

Adrian P. Gee
Baylor College of Medicine
Houston, Texas, USA

George Georges
Fred Hutchinson Cancer Research Center and
University of Washington
Seattle, Washington, USA

Sergio A. Giralt
The University of Texas M.D. Anderson Cancer Center
Houston, Texas, USA

Eliane Gluckman
Hôpital Saint Louis
Paris, France

John M. Goldman
Imperial College School of Medicine
London, United Kingdom

Anthony H. Goldstone
University College London Hospitals
London, United Kingdom

Els Goulmy
Leiden University Medical Center
Leiden, The Netherlands

Alois Gratwohl
University Hospital
Basle, Switzerland

John G. Gribben
Dana-Farber Cancer Institute and
Harvard University
Boston, Massachusetts, USA

Andrew P. Grigg
Royal Melbourne Hospital
Melbourne, Australia

Philippe Guardiola
Hôpital Saint Louis
Paris, France

Eva Guinan
Dana-Farber Cancer Institute and
Harvard Medical School
Boston, Massachusetts, USA

Abha Gulati
Schepens Eye Research Institute
Massachusetts Eye and Ear Infirmary and
Harvard Medical School
Boston, Massachusetts, USA

Sridharan Gururangan
Duke University Medical Center
Durham, North Carolina, USA

Geoff Hale
University of Oxford
Oxford, United Kingdom

Gregory Hale
St. Jude Children's Research Hospital
Memphis, Tennessee, USA

Rupert Handgretinger
St. Jude Children's Research Hospital
Memphis, Tennessee, USA

Lauren Harrison
Herbert Irving Comprehensive Cancer Center
Columbia University College of Physicians and Surgeons
New York, New York, USA

Derek N.J. Hart
Mater Medical Research Institute and
Mater Misericordiae Hospitals
Brisbane, Australia

Brandon Hayes-Lattin
Oregon Health Sciences University
Portland, Oregon, USA

P. Jean Henslee-Downey
University of South Carolina
Columbia, South Carolina, USA

Helen E. Heslop
Baylor College of Medicine
Houston, Texas, USA

Ephraim P. Hochberg
Dana-Farber Cancer Institute and
Brigham and Women's Hospital
Harvard University
Boston, Massachusetts, USA

Mary M. Horowitz
International Bone Marrow Transplant Registry
Milwaukee, Wisconsin, USA

Chitra Hosing
The University of Texas M.D. Anderson Cancer Center
Houston, Texas, USA

Harry J. Iland
Royal Prince Alfred Hospital
Sydney, Australia

David Izon
Center for Child Health Research and
Western Australian Institute of Medical Research
University of West Australia
Australia

F. Leonard Johnson
Oregon Health and Science University
Portland, Oregon, USA

Michael Kalos
Corixa Corporation
Seattle, Washington, USA

Neena Kapoor
Children's Hospital Los Angeles and
University of Southern California School of Medicine
Los Angeles, California, USA

Dan S. Kaufman
University of Minnesota
Minneapolis, Minnesota, USA

Armand Keating
Princess Margaret Hospital
Ontario Cancer Institute
Toronto, Canada

John H. Kersey
University of Minnesota Cancer Center
Minneapolis, Minnesota, USA

Issa Khouri
The University of Texas M.D. Anderson Cancer Center
Houston, Texas, USA

John P. Klein
Medical College of Wisconsin
Milwaukee, Wisconsin, USA

Donald B. Kohn
Children's Hospital Los Angeles and
University of Southern California School of Medicine
Los Angeles, California, USA

Hans-Jochem Kolb
Klinikum Grosshadern
Ludwig Maximilians Universität
Munich, Germany

Martin Körbling
The University of Texas M.D. Anderson Cancer Center
Houston, Texas, USA

Steven Kossard
Skin and Cancer Foundation and
University of New South Wales
Sydney, Australia

Scott A. Lanum
University of Washington Medical Center
Seattle Cancer Care Alliance
Seattle, Washington, USA

Hillard M. Lazarus
Comprehensive Cancer Center of
Case Western Reserve University
Cleveland, Ohio, USA

Stephanie J. Lee
Dana-Farber Cancer Center and
Harvard University
Boston, Massachusetts, USA

J.L.W.T. Lie
Department of Immunohematology and Blood Transfusion
Leiden University Medical Center and
Europdonor Foundation
Leiden, The Netherlands

Yiming Lit
Harvard University
Boston, Massachusetts, USA

Per Ljungman
Huddinge University Hospital
Stockholm, Sweden

Guido Lucarelli
Ospedale di Pesaro
Pesaro, Italy

Steven Mackinnon
University College Hospital
London, United Kingdom

Raymond McCrudden
St. Vincent's Hospital and
University of New South Wales
Sydney, Australia

Michael A. McGrath
St. Vincent's Hospital and
University of New South Wales
Sydney, Australia

Ian McNiece
University of Colorado Health Science Center
Denver, Colorado, USA

Richard P. McQuellon
Wake Forest University School of Medicine
Winston-Salem, North Carolina, USA

Peter McSweeney
Colorado Health Sciences Center
Denver, Colorado, USA

Amy R. McWilliams
University of Washington Medical Center
Seattle Cancer Care Alliance
Seattle, Washington, USA

Stephanie B. Magdanz
University of Washington Medical Center
Seattle Cancer Care Alliance
Seattle, Washington, USA

Massimo F. Martelli
University of Perugia
Perugia, Italy

Paul Martin
The Fred Hutchinson Cancer Research Center
Seattle, Washington, USA

Rodrigo Martino
Hospital la Santa Creu i Sant Pau,
Barcelona, Spain

Dana C. Matthews
Fred Hutchinson Cancer Research Center and
University of Washington
Seattle, Washington, USA

Jeffrey A. Medin
Ontario Cancer Institute
Toronto, Canada

Jayesh Mehta
Northwestern University
Chicago, Illinois, USA

Marco Mielcarek
Fred Hutchinson Cancer Research Center and
University of Washington
Seattle, Washington, USA

Sam Milliken
St. Vincent's Hospital
Sydney, Australia

Alessandro Moretta
University of Genoa
Genoa, Italy

Adrienne Morey
St. Vincent's Hospital
Sydney, Australia

Tariq I. Mughal
Imperial College School of Medicine
London, United Kingdom

Vincent Munro
St. Vincent's Hospital
Sydney, Australia

Joyce L. Murata-Collins
City of Hope National Medical Center
Duarte, California, USA

Robert S. Negrin
Stanford University
Stanford, California, USA

Craig R. Nichols
Oregon Health Sciences University
Portland, Oregon, USA

S.K. Nilsson
Peter MacCallum Cancer Institute
Melbourne, Australia

Terrence O'Connor
St. Vincent's Hospital and
University of New South Wales
Sydney, Australia

Ifeyinwa Osunkwo
Herbert Irving Comprehensive Cancer Center
Columbia University College of Physicians and Surgeons
New York, New York, USA

M. Oudshoorn
Department of Immunohematology and Blood Transfusion
Leiden University Medical Center and
Europdonor Foundation
Leiden, The Netherlands

Robertson Parkman
Children's Hospital Los Angeles and
University of Southern California School of Medicine
Los Angeles, California, USA

Thierry Philip
Centre Léon Berard
Lyon, France

Gordon L. Phillips
University of Rochester
Rochester, New York, USA

Anne Poon
University of Washington Medical Center
Seattle Cancer Care Alliance
Seattle, Washington, USA

Ray Powles
Royal Marsden Hospital
Sutton, United Kingdom

Raymond Powles
Dana-Farber Cancer Center and
Harvard Medical School
Boston, Massachusetts, USA

Donna Przepiorka
Baylor College of Medicine
Houston, Texas, USA

Stephen Rainer
St. Vincent's Hospital
Sydney, Australia

Noopur Raje
Royal Marsden Hospital
Sutton, United Kingdom

Donna E. Reece
Princess Margaret Hospital
Toronto, Canada

David Rees
St. Vincent's Hospital and
University of New South Wales
Sydney, Australia

Yair Reisner
Weizmann Institute of Science
Rehovot, Israel

Morayma Reyes
Stem Cell Institute
University of Minnesota
Minneapolis, Minnesota, USA

Alison M. Rice
Mater Medical Research Institute and
Mater Misericordiae Hospitals
Brisbane, Australia

Paul Richardson
Dana-Farber Cancer Institute and
Harvard Medical School
Boston, Massachusetts, USA

David S. Ritchie
Royal Melbourne Hospital
Melbourne, Australia

Jerome Ritz
Dana-Farber Cancer Institute and
Harvard Medical School
Boston, Massachusetts, USA

Vanderson Rocha
Hospital Saint Louis
Paris, France

Cliona M. Rooney
Baylor College of Medicine
Houston, Texas, USA

Claude Roy
Maisonneuve-Rosemont Hospital
Montreal, Canada

Katherine L. Ruffner
Vanderbilt University Medical Center
Nashville, Tennessee, USA

David G. Savage
Columbia University College of Physicians and Surgeons
New York, New York, USA

Matthias Schell
Centre Léon Berard
Lyon, France

Norbert Schmitz
AK St. Georg University Hospital
Hamburg, Germany

G.M. Th. Schreuder
Department of Immunohematology and Blood Transfusion
Leiden University Medical Center
Leiden, The Netherlands

Mark M. Schubert
Fred Hutchinson Cancer Research Center
Seattle Cancer Care Alliance and
University of Washington
Seattle, Washington, USA

Julian Seifter
Harvard University
Boston, Massachusetts, USA

Ami Shah
Children's Hospital Los Angeles and
University of Southern California School of Medicine
Los Angeles, California, USA

Peter J. Shaw
The Children's Hospital at Westmead
Sydney, Australia

P.J. Simmons
Peter MacCallum Cancer Institute
Melbourne, Australia

Bhawna Sirohi
Royal Marsden Hospital
Sutton, United Kingdom

Shimon Slavin
Hadassah University Hospital
Jerusalem, Israel

Marilyn L. Slovak
City of Hope National Medical Center
Duarte, California, USA

Robert J. Soiffer
Dana-Farber Cancer Institute and
Harvard Medical School
Boston, Massachusetts, USA

Scott R. Solomon
National Heart, Lung, and Blood Institute
Bethesda, Maryland, USA

Gerald J. Spangrude
University of Utah
Salt Lake City, Utah, USA

Eric Spierings
Leiden University Medical Center
Leiden, The Netherlands

Ram Srinivasan
National Heart, Lung, and Blood Institute
Bethesda, Maryland, USA

Rainer Storb
Fred Hutchinson Cancer Research Center and
University of Washington
Seattle, Washington, USA

Jan Storek
Fred Hutchinson Cancer Research Center and
University of Washington
Seattle, Washington, USA

Keith M. Sullivan
Duke University Medical Center
Durham, North Carolina, USA

Ania U. Sweet
University of Washington Medical Center
Seattle Cancer Care Alliance
Seattle, Washington, USA

Jeffrey Szer
Royal Melbourne Hospital
Melbourne, Australia

Takanori Teshima
University of Michigan
Ann Arbor, Michigan, USA

Susan Tett
The University of Queensland
Brisbane, Australia

Amy Tiersten
Columbia University College of Physicians and Surgeons
New York, New York, USA

Jan Tollemar
The Karolinska Institute and
Huddinge University Hospital
Stockholm, Sweden

Beverly Torok-Storb
Fred Hutchinson Cancer Research Center and
University of Washington
Seattle, Washington, USA

Hai Tran
The University of Texas M.D. Anderson Cancer Center
Houston, Texas, USA

Robert L. Truitt
Medical College of Wisconsin
Milwaukee, Wisconsin, USA

Sante Tura
Institute of Haematology and Clinical Oncology
"L.A. Seragnoli"
St. Orsola Hospital
University of Bologna
Bologna, Italy

Jennifer Turner
St. Vincent's Hospital
Sydney, Australia

Alan Tyndall
University Hospital
Basel, Switzerland

Nobuko Uchida
Stem Cells Inc.
Sunnyvale, California, USA

Alvaro Urbano-Ispizua
Hospital Clinic of Barcelona
Barcelona, Spain

H.G.M. Van Der Zanden
Leiden University Medical Center and
Europdonor Foundation
Leiden, The Netherlands

Jacob M. Van Laar
Leiden University Medical Center
Leiden, The Netherlands

Andrea Velardi
University of Perugia
Perugia, Italy

Catherine M. Verfaillie
Stem Cell Institute
University of Minnesota
Minneapolis, Minnesota, USA

Michael R. Verneris
Stanford University
Stanford, California, USA

Christopher R. Vickers
St. Vincent's Hospital and
University of New South Wales
Sydney, Australia

Shyan Vijayasekaran
Sir Charles Gairdner Hospital
Perth, Australia

Herman Waldmann
University of Oxford
Oxford, United Kingdom

Kenneth Weinberg
Children's Hospital Los Angeles
University of Southern California School of Medicine
Los Angeles, California, USA

Daniel J. Weisdorf
University of Minnesota
Minneapolis, Minnesota, USA

Irving L. Weissman
Stanford University
Palo Alto, California USA

David B. Williams
St. Vincent's Hospital and
University of New South Wales
Sydney, Australia

Robert P. Witherspoon
Fred Hutchinson Cancer Research Center and
University of Washington
Seattle, Washington, USA

James W. Young
Memorial Sloan-Kettering Cancer Center and
The Weill Medical College of Cornell University
New York, New York, USA

Preface to Third Edition

This third edition is notable for the addition of five new editors – Richard Champlin of M.D. Anderson Cancer Center, Houston, USA; Jerome Ritz of Dana-Farber Cancer Institute, Boston, USA; Malcom Brenner of Baylor College of Medicine, Houston, USA; Per Ljungman of Huddinge University Hospital, Stockholm, Sweden; and Willem Fibbe of Leiden University Medical Centre, Leiden, The Netherlands. This has resulted in a significant improvement in strategic design and content. This edition is some 20% larger than the second edition, has 124 chapters, including 19 new, and more than 200 authors from the United States, Europe, and Australasia. Hematopoietic stem cell transplantation has become a truly international effort, and our goal has been to utilize the very broad base of expertise that has developed in this field in recent years.

The new chapters include those on plasticity of stem cells, embryonic stem cells, mesenchymal stem cells, stem cell homing, biology of nonmyeloablative conditioning regimens, antigen-specific T cells, T/NK cells, improving posttransplant thymopoiesis, role of natural killer cells in hematopoietic stem cell (HSC) transplantation, impact of good tissue practices (GTPs) and good manufacturing practices (GMPs), donor management, monitoring hematopoietic chimerism, autotransplants for myelodysplasia, autotransplants for soft tissue sarcoma and nephroblastoma, myelodysplasia occurring after autotransplant, posttransplant lymphoproliferative disease, allogeneic transplants for solid tumors, and transplantation for HIV disease.

In addition to the new chapters we have attempted to keep the book current by revising and updating all the chapters previously included, referencing through June 2003, and introducing a new final chapter entitled "Breaking News…"

in which the editors have attempted to highlight specific areas of interest presenting in the literature that have emerged or been re-emphasized in the 12 months prior to publication.

The field of hematopoietic stem cell transplantation continues to evolve apace: reduced intensity conditioning regimens with emphasis on graft-versus-tumor effect, the increasing use of allogeneic peripheral blood stem cells, new methods of both in vivo and in vitro T-cell depletion, increasingly sophisticated methods for monitoring minimal residual disease and hematopoietic chimerism posttransplant, new antibiotic, antifungal, and antiviral agents, as well as new methods and agents for minimizing graft-versus-host disease are just some of the elements contributing to both greater patient safety and improved outcomes. The rapid development and incorporation of new concepts and methods place increasing demands on the transplant team to utilize the best therapeutic option or to tailor a therapeutic approach to an individual patient in a risk-adapted manner.

Additionally, stem cell therapy is being increasingly and rapidly applied to therapeutic areas outside hematology/oncology, be it with hematopoietic stem cells, mesenchymal stem cells, organ-specific stem cells, or – in the future – embryonic stem cells. Cardiac, neurological and orthopedic applications represent some of the most potentially interesting approaches. In many institutions it is the HSC transplant physician, as the bone fide practicing cell therapist, who is being approached by his or her colleagues from other disciplines for help in these areas. The future is indeed bright for our field.

Kerry Atkinson, Richard Champlin, Jerome Ritz,
Per Ljungman, Willem Fibbe, and Malcom Brenner

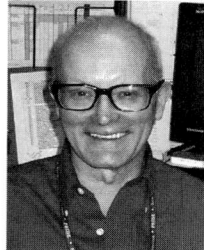 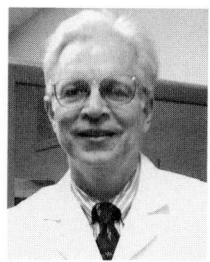 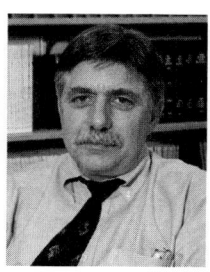 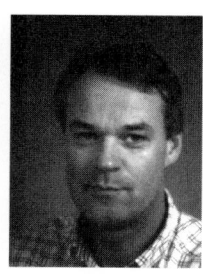 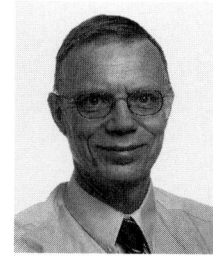 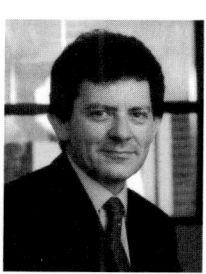

Kerry Atkinson   Richard Champlin   Jerome Ritz   Willem Fibbe   Per Ljungman   Malcom Brenner

Acknowledgments

The editors would first like to acknowledge the contribution of all the chapter authors: the book is truly the result of a huge team effort. In addition, it is again a pleasure to thank the staff at Cambridge University Press, particularly Richard Barling, Pauline Graham, Heidi Lovett, Alice Ra, and Cathy Felgar for their continuing encouragement, help, and hard work from inception to publication and marketing. Larry Meyer and his colleagues at Hermitage Publishing Services once again demonstrated their professionalism and skill in the production of the book. Finally, all of us must acknowledge the support given to us by our partners and families during the long hours involved in the development of the manuscript and in the production of the book itself. In my own case I must single out my wife, Pauline, for her continuing support and tolerance of the time I spent on it.

Kerry Atkinson
New York
August 2003

Preface to Second Edition

The field of bone marrow and, increasingly, blood stem cell transplantation has continued to evolve rapidly since the publication of the first edition of this book. Blood stem cell transplantation is making the same sort of strides into allogeneic grafting as it did in autologous transplantation in the early 1990's. Results are improving with unrelated donor transplantation and there is an increasing interest in the use of haploidentical family member transplantation to the extent that it appears that graft rejection and graft-versus-host disease are no longer the main hurdles to this approach, but rather persistent severe immune cellular deficiencies leading to serious and often fatal opportunistic infections. Interestingly, in this regard is an ever-increasing focus on the use of cellular immune therapy as evidenced by the eight chapters in the last section of the book "Developing areas: posttransplant". Our understanding of the biology and clinical use of the hematopoietic stem cells is increasing, and with it the use of both positive and negative cell selection technology to transplant defined doses of defined cell populations at defined times in the transplant process. Since the first edition was published clinically useful gene therapy has been demonstrated. Finally, at the end of 1998 the first description of the cloning and growth in culture of human embryonic stem cells was published. This has multiple implications for the future transplantation of many different cell types and their potential modification by gene transfer. It is clear that the field will continue to develop over the next decade as rapidly as it has over the last one.

Preface to First Edition

The hematology, oncology and immunology disciplines have perhaps derived the greatest benefit from the biotechnological revolution of the 1970s, '80s and '90s, both in terms of a wide array of new diagnostic and therapeutic reagents, and in terms of the elucidation of disease pathogenesis. Examples of the former include convenient T cell-depletion technology, the use of both cytokines and cytokine antagonists, the introduction of blood stem cell transplants, and, more recently, gene transfer and recombinant immunotoxins. Examples of the latter include the molecular pathogenesis of chronic myeloid leukemia and the pathogenesis of graft-versus-host disease at least at the cell and protein level. Taken together, these advances have put bone marrow transplant practitioners into a unique and astonishingly privileged position in health care at the end of the 20th century. We can carry out therapeutic maneuvers (for example, outpatient marrow transplants) undreamt of 20 years ago. We can barely glimpse what our successors will be doing 20 years hence in this field.

This uniquely privileged position mandates that we embrace in parallel the two concepts of minimization of risk, and full exploitation of biotechnological advance. The bone marrow transplant community is still relatively small worldwide but is very well integrated and well informed. This textbook is written as a postgraduate reference work, and I hope it will be found accessible not only by marrow transplant physicians but by physicians in other disciplines whose clinical practice brings them into contact with marrow transplant recipients, as well as by the nursing profession and by the many allied health disciplines that are involved in the optimal running of a marrow transplant program. I have aimed to present a précis of the sciences underlying marrow transplantation (predominantly hematology and immunology) as well as to give the current results using the various forms of stem cell transplantation, together with the specific problems encountered in the wide array of clinical areas on which marrow transplant medicine impacts. The book ends with a review of the large number of scientific and therapeutic areas in which biotechnology developments, referred to at the beginning of this preface, are already changing the way we approach and manage the marrow transplant recipient.

1 Historical background to hematopoietic stem cell transplantation

JOHN H. KERSEY

University of Minnesota Cancer Center, Minneapolis, USA

Introduction

The use of blood and bone marrow hematopoietic stem cells (HSC) for treatment of human disease has a long and fascinating history, beginning with a series of important animal studies as early as the 1920s. These animal studies, combined with advances in understanding of the histocompatibility antigens and developments in novel therapeutic agents and radiation therapy, permitted the development of clinical blood and bone marrow transplantation. The successful clinical application of HSC transplantation has followed from the early clinical efforts of Robert Good, Don Thomas, and George Santos and their colleagues in the late 1960s and early 1970s. This introductory historical chapter is dedicated to these three pioneers.

Early history

In 1922, a Danish investigator, Fabricious-Moeller, noted that when the legs of guinea pigs were shielded during exposure to total body irradiation (TBI), the usual depression of platelet counts and postirradiation hemorrhagic diathesis was prevented (Fabricious-Moeller, 1922). These important observations were largely ignored or forgotten for 25 years when, in 1949, Jacobson and colleagues (1951) rediscovered these observations. They reported that mice exposed to doses of radiation that caused fatal marrow aplasia could be protected from death by shielding of the spleen, a hematopoietic organ in the mouse. With remarkable insight they also showed that protection from the lethal effects could be accomplished by the intraperitoneal injection of spleen cells following TBI. In the same year, Lorenz et al. showed that lethally irradiated mice and guinea pigs could be protected by the intravenous injection of syngeneic bone marrow (Lorenz et al., 1951). Initially, some consideration was given to the notion that the radiation protection factor might be humoral. However, a number of reports, using a variety of histochemical (Nowell et al., 1956) and genetic markers (Lindsley, Odell, & Tausche, 1955; Ford et al., 1956; Mitchison, 1956), demonstrated that the protection from the lethal effects of TBI was due to the colonization of the recipient by donor cells. Ford et al. (1956) used the

term radiation chimera for an animal that carried a foreign hematopoietic system as a result of TBI followed by transplantation of hematopoietic cells. Subsequently, transplantation of hematopoietic tissue with resulting chimerism was demonstrated in pigeons, mice, rabbits, dogs, monkeys, and humans. Furthermore, transplantation could be demonstrated with non-TBI containing preparative regimens.

It was initially established that the number of allogeneic cells required for optimal hematopoietic reconstitution was 10 to 80 times that required by syngeneic marrow cells (Van Bekkum & de Vries, 1967). Later, it was suggested that, although this was true for radiation, it was not necessarily true for other forms of immune suppressive marrow-ablative regimens (Santos & Owens, 1968; Santos & Haghshenass, 1968). Thus, TBI was not completely immune suppressive even at maximally tolerated doses.

Graft-versus-host disease and graft-host tolerance

The first to report a difference in survival of animals that received syngeneic compared to allogeneic cells were Barnes & Loutit (1957), who reported that carcinoma-bearing mice exposed to lethal-dose TBI and given syngeneic spleen cells were afforded long-lived protection, but that 9 of 16 lethally irradiated carcinoma-bearing mice infused with allogeneic spleen cells died before 100 days. These observations were soon confirmed by many laboratories (Van Bekkum & de Vries, 1967). Cohen, Vos, and van Bekkum noted in 1957 that severe diarrhea, severe weight loss, and skin lesions occurred as part of "secondary disease." This conclusion was given additional support by the observations of Billingham and colleagues (reviewed in 1966–1967). They observed a runting syndrome in newborn mice that had been transplanted with allogeneic spleen cells. Retarded growth, diarrhea, hypoplasia of the lymphatic system, skin lesions, and focal necrosis of liver cells were prominent features. The histologic findings of runt disease were also found in animals with secondary disease following allogeneic marrow transplantation. It became apparent that lymphocytes (Santos & Cole, 1958; Gowans, 1962; Medawar,

1963) initiated this disease, and that the target organs were the lymphoid system, gut, liver, and skin.

By the mid 1960s enough was known from observations in animal models and humans (Kadowaki *et al.,* 1965; Hathaway *et al.,* 1967; Naiman *et al.,* 1969) for Billingham to list the essential requirements for graft-versus-host disease (GVHD) (Billingham, 1966–1967). These were (1) the graft must contain immunologically competent cells; (2) the host must possess important transplantation antigens that are lacking in the graft donor, so that the host appears foreign; (3) the host itself must be incapable of mounting an effective immunologic reaction against the graft, at least for sufficient time to allow the latter to manifest its immunologic capabilities.

Details of the pathophysiology of human GVHD became apparent following the first engraftment of human marrow by Mathé and colleagues in the early 1960s (Mathé, 1968). Kersey and colleagues (1971) further defined the multiorgan pathophysiology from the early transplants for patients with immunodeficiency syndromes transplanted in Minnesota (Kersey *et al.,* 1971). This experience was later expanded (Gatti *et al.,* 1973). The Seattle group provided the first comprehensive clinical grading system for human GVHD (Thomas *et al.,* 1975). This system allowed grading of each of the major organs. The clinical syndrome of GVHD was later shown to often be a consequence of a synergy between the immunologic damage due to major histocompatibility (MHC) antigen mismatch and tissue damage from irradiation or viral infection (Fenyk *et al.,* 1978).

Tolerance to foreign tissue was first described from studies injecting spleen cells into fetal mice (Billingham & Brent, 1957). A similar tolerance was later found in mice that had been neonatally thymectomized (Miller, 1961; Martinez *et al.,* 1962). Main and Prehn in 1955 reported that mice given allogeneic marrow following TBI permanently accepted a skin graft from the donor strain.

Graft-versus-leukemia effect in animal systems

In early studies, Barnes and Loutit (1957) reported cures in mice with a transplantable lymphoid tumor. A remarkable antileukemic effect was observed when allogeneic marrow was used. However, most of the mice died of GVHD (Barnes & Loutit, 1957). A number of studies using allogeneic marrow in the treatment of hematologic tumors following TBI (Van Bekkum & de Vries, 1967), or cyclophosphamide (CY) (Owens, 1970) subsequently appeared. There was a marked antitumor effect in most reports and a few animals survived free of tumor, while the majority died of GVHD. With more effective treatment of GVHD, the number of tumor-free survivors increased (Boranic, 1968; Owens, 1970). However, severe GVHD did not produce a therapeutic effect in a fibrosarcoma (Fefer, 1970) or an adenocarcinoma (Santos, 1970) model. The reasons for the difference between responses in the lymphohematopoietic tumors versus those in the fibrosarcoma and adenocarcinoma tumors are probably complex, but may be due to differences in the type and level of expression of transplantation antigens and/or responses of T and NK lymphoid cells.

Pathophysiology of marrow failure in animal systems

Many of the important concepts and principles of genetic or acquired marrow failure were formulated in the mid to late 1960s. Studies in the ww^v mouse (Russell, 1963; McCulloch, Siminovitch, & Till, 1964), which was shown to have a hematopoietic stem cell defect, and in the S1/S1^d mouse (Russell, 1963; McCulloch *et al.,* 1965), which was shown to have normal hematopoietic stem cells but defects in the microenvironment, were key to our present understanding of marrow failure. Krantz and Kao suggested the possibility in 1967 that some cases of clinical aplastic anemia might have an autoimmune basis. They reported the presence of immunoglobulin in patients with erythroid aplasia that specifically inhibited the development of the patients' erythroid series in vitro. Furthermore, they demonstrated an improvement in erythropoiesis when the immunoglobulin was decreased with immune suppression. The majority of the early animal studies were performed in murine systems. The Seattle group chose the dog as an example of an outbred animal model for marrow transplantation. Among their important studies was the predictive value of histocompatibility testing on outcome of the transplant (Storb, Epstein, & Thomas, 1968). In addition, the dog has been a useful model in the study of hemophilia, cyclic neutropenia, congenital pyruvate kinase deficiency and malignant disease (Thomas *et al.,* 1975).

Histocompatibility

In the late 1930s Gorer (1936, 1937) elucidated the serology of alloantigens belonging to the major histocompatibility complex of the mouse. These alloantigens were closely involved with tissue rejection and identified a genetic histocompatibility system in the mouse that was named H2. This represented a major breakthrough for transplantation. Analogous systems exist in the dog, monkey, and humans (Festenstein & Demant, 1978) and in all mammalian systems studied to date.

Dausset (1958) described the first HLA antigen and named it Mac (now HLA-A2). Later, through the collaboration of a number of investigators in frequently held workshops (the first in 1964), the present knowledge of the HLA system evolved (Festenstein & Demant, 1978). By 1968 the closely linked loci of HLA-A and HLA-B were established. By 1971 the HLA-C locus was identified. Finally, the separate locus (HLA-D) that controls the degree of reactivity seen in the mixed lymphocyte culture (MLC) was established (Dupont, 1980).

The demonstration that there were antigens of the HLA-A and HLA-B locus linked to the locus that defined the mixed leukocyte culture response was an important observation in the late 1960s. This system of genetically linked antigens defined the major histocompatibility complex (MHC). This MHC permitted the identification of siblings who shared both chromosomes of the MHC. Cepellini and van Rood (1974) introduced the term *haplotype* to indicate the products of the MHC in haploid form. These developments in the late 1960s and early 1970s set the stage for a more logical way of choosing a marrow donor than was previously possible.

Major blood group incompatibilities were an impediment to marrow transplantation in the early years and complicated the first successful immunodeficiency transplant (Gatti *et al.*, 1968). Graw *et al.* (1974) were the first to attempt a marrow transplant from a donor with blood group A into a recipient who was blood group O. First, plasmapheresis was performed, then the patient was given Witebsky's A substance to lower the anti-A antibody titer.

Early clinical studies

In 1957 Thomas, and colleagues reported that large amounts of marrow could be infused safely and described a transient marrow graft in humans (Thomas *et al.*, 1957). In 1959 Mathé *et al.* attempted to treat six human victims of a radiation accident from Vinca, Yugoslavia. It was considered that the marrow grafts functioned and produced blood cells for about a month (Mathé, 1968). Beilby and colleagues in London (1960) described a patient with acute bone marrow failure due to chemotherapy for Hodgkin's disease who received a marrow infusion from her sister without additional treatment. The patient improved rapidly and red blood cells of donor origin were detectable 10 months later. Mathé and his group were the most active clinical group during this early period. In 1963 they reported the first case of complete engraftment with survival beyond a year (Mathé *et al.*, 1963). This patient with leukemia developed acute and chronic GVHD, and eventually died free of leukemia 20 months later of varicella encephalitis. In 1968 Mathé summarized some early experience with bone marrow transplantation in 21 patients (Mathe, 1968). Six patients had graft failure. Eight of 15 patients who engrafted died of severe GVHD without evidence of leukemia. Two died

with a less severe form of GVHD without evidence of leukemia, and 1 survived for 20 months, as noted above. Minimal GVHD was seen in 4 patients who died of recurrent leukemia. Mathé and his colleagues provided a clinical description and pathology of acute GVHD as well as the types of fungal and viral infections to which these patients are susceptible (Mathé, 1968; Mathé *et al.*, 1974). The decade of the late 1950s to the late 1960s, despite some encouraging results, was fraught with frustration and disappointment. Most of the transplants were performed in end-stage leukemic patients who often died before adequate evaluation, and when apparent successful engraftment occurred, patients often died of GVHD or fungal or viral infections (Bortin, 1970). It should be noted that many of these patients received marrow from individuals that were either not tissue-typed or were tissue-typed with methods found later to be unreliable.

From these early studies, the number of blood and marrow transplants has increased in patients with lethal human diseases with at least 40,000 cases reported in the year 2002 to the IBMTR/ABMTR (Fig. 1.1)

Genetic diseases

The identification of the MHC set the stage for the use of sibling donors for the first successfully engrafted human bone marrow. The logical candidates for these early human studies were children with genetically defined immunodeficiencies who would be at minimal risk for immunologic rejection of a foreign graft. In 1968 two children with genetically determined immunodeficiencies were successfully transplanted: one infant with an X-linked immunodeficiency was treated in Minnesota by Robert Good and colleagues (Gatti *et al.*, 1968), and a child with the Wiskott-Aldrich syndrome was successfully engrafted in Wisconsin (Bach *et al.*, 1968). The lessons learned from these early cases were several: (1) cellular engraftment would largely correct the underlying disease; (2) while MHC-matched sibling marrow could be successfully and endurably engrafted in the absence of additional immunosuppression and myelo-

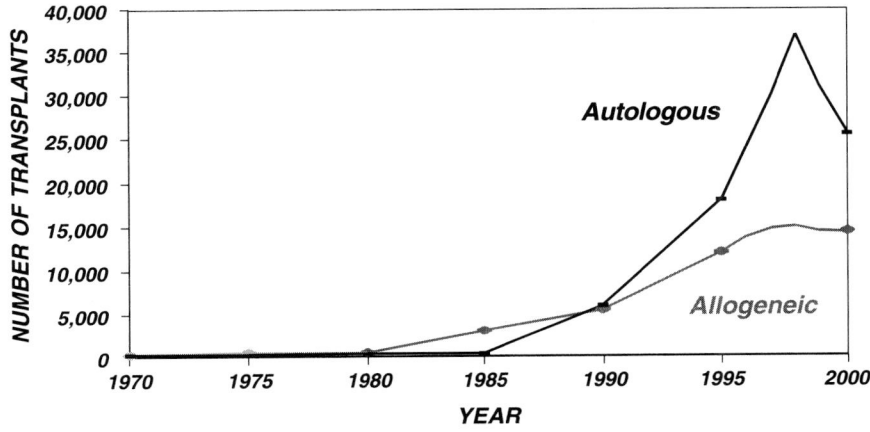

Fig. 1.1. Annual numbers of blood and marrow transplants worldwide; 1970–2000. Reproduced by permission of the IBMTR/ABMTR.

suppression, mixed engraftment (mixed chimerism) was likely to occur; (3) GVHD, while it could occur, was not likely to be severe when sibling donors were used and both the donor and recipient were young. Based on these pioneering stem cell transplants, the use of allogeneic stem cell transplantation has become the treatment of choice for infants and children with life-threatening immunodeficiency syndromes.

The success in transplanting children with immunodeficiencies provided direct evidence that transplantation of HSC from marrow could provide cells and cellular products, such as enzymes and growth factors, that were known or suspected to be absent from humans with a wide spectrum of genetic disorders. In studies in the 1970s and 1980s, diseases with known metabolic defects, including the mucopolysaccharidoses (Hobbs, 1981; Krivit et al., 1984) were corrected with blood or marrow transplants. Additional diseases with undefined genetic defects, such as osteopetrosis, have been successfully transplanted with HSC (Coccia et al., 1980). Currently, a large number of genetic disorders, including congenital marrow failure diseases and metabolic diseases, are treated with allogeneic blood or marrow transplants.

Aplastic anemia

In 1972 Thomas et al. reported the first successful allogeneic marrow transplant for severe aplastic anemia using a genotypically HLA-identical sibling donor. The Seattle group later reported on 37 additional cases (Storb et al., 1974). The majority of patients were prepared with cyclophosphamide, using a regimen modified from the original regimen proposed by Santos and colleagues in Baltimore (1970). Failure to show sustained engraftment was soon recognized as a major problem. Prior studies in mice (Santos & Sensenbrenner, 1971) and dogs (Storb et al., 1971) suggested that such failure was related to the development of sensitization of the host to minor histocompatibility antigens of the donor. The report by Storb et al. (1977) of the sustained engraftment in nontransfused patients with severe aplastic anemia provided clinical data to support the conclusions cited above. However, since most patients were transfused at their time of arrival at the transplant center, additional immunosuppression was needed in many patients. Animal studies by Kersey and colleagues demonstrated that total lymphoid irradiation significantly enhanced the probability of long-term engraftment (Kersey et al., 1979). Subsequently, the Minnesota group pioneered the use of total lymphoid irradiation combined with cyclophosphamide for transfused patients (Ramsay et al., 1983). The Paris group developed a similar thoracoabdominal irradiation approach for these patients (Gluckman et al., 1991). In 1976 Camitta et al. reported the first prospective randomized international trial comparing bone marrow transplantation to more conventional therapy. Survival was significantly better in those receiving transplants.

Transplant regimens for leukemia

TBI at a low-dose rate from a single cobalt source was employed for the initial series of Seattle patients transplanted with end-

stage acute leukemia (Thomas et al., 1971). Subsequently, the Johns Hopkins group developed the rationale for the use of CY for transplantation in acute leukemia (Santos et al., 1970). Because of the high relapse rate, regimens for transplantation with CY alone were abandoned, as were regimens containing TBI alone. The Seattle group reported the use of CY given as 60 mg/kg for 2 days followed on the third day by 1,000 cGy of single-dose TBI using a cobalt 60 radiation source (Thomas et al., 1977). The Minnesota group introduced a linear accelerator as an alternative radiation source to cobalt 60 and this has been adopted by many transplant centers (Kim et al., 1977).

The 1970s and 1980s were characterized by new methods for delivering TBI, particularly the move from single dose to fractionated radiation. Radiobiologic studies had demonstrated that fractionated TBI resulted in enhanced repair of normal compared to leukemia cells, with less damage to normal tissues (Peters et al., 1979; Song et al., 1981; Shank et al., 1981). Most, but not all, transplant centers currently use fractionated rather than single dose radiation if radiation is a component of the conditioning regimen.

While several non-radiation containing regimens were developed, the most popular has combined busulfan with CY. Beginning with studies in rodents in 1968 (Santos & Haghshenass, 1968), the Baltimore group developed the rationale for the use of busulfan and CY for marrow transplantation in acute myeloid leukemia (Santos et al., 1983). Tutschka and colleagues (1987) utilized a modification of this regimen by reducing the CY dose to 60 mg/kg given on 2 successive days.

Acute leukemia: patient selection

In the 1970s most transplants were carried out in patients with highly resistant disease. It was during this period that most of the regimens employing TBI or chemotherapy were developed. In 1977 the Seattle group reported the results of HLA-identical sibling transplants in 100 patients with end-stage leukemia (Thomas et al., 1977). This now classical study illustrated the potential curative effect of allogeneic marrow transplantation in acute leukemia with 13 long-term disease-free survivors. The enthusiasm over this remarkable result was tempered by the actuarial relapse rate of 70% and the high incidence of non-leukemic deaths. A number of investigators reasoned that transplants performed in early remission should fare better since these patients would have a smaller tumor burden and be in better clinical condition than end-stage patients. A report by the Seattle group of transplantation of patients with acute myeloid leukemia in first remission demonstrated this principle (Thomas, 1983). Other centers, including City of Hope, Royal Marsden Hospital, and Minnesota reported success with acute leukemia transplants, particularly early in the course of disease (Blume et al., 1980; Powles et al., 1982; Kersey et al., 1983).

Advances in first remission transplantation invited comparison with the continuing improving chemotherapy regimens of the 1980s. The first "biologically randomized" comparison was carried out by the Children's Cancer Group in the United States and demonstrated significantly better disease-free survival in young patients who received HLA-identical sibling transplants compared to controls (Nesbit *et al.,* 1994).

Non-Hodgkin's lymphoma and multiple myeloma

The successful application of allogeneic transplantation to acute leukemia inspired the evaluation of the procedure to high-risk malignant lymphoma. The Minnesota group began to transplant young patients with high-risk lymphoma; the earliest long-term survivor was transplanted in 1975 (O'Leary *et al.,* 1981). Other groups showed promising results in larger series of patients, primarily in adults (Phillips *et al.,* 1986; Appelbaum *et al.,* 1987).

Most HSC transplants for malignant lymphoma, however, have utilized autologous donation (see below).

Nonrelapse complications following HSC transplantation

In addition to organ toxicities caused by the various preparative regimens and the leukemia recurrences that were seen in studies of end-stage patients, posttransplant infections, interstitial pneumonitis, and acute and chronic GVHD were recognized as major impediments to the successful outcome of allogeneic marrow transplantation (Thomas *et al.,* 1975). Infections with life-threatening viruses, including cytomegalovirus, and bacterial infections have resulted in major disabilities in transplant recipients. Recent advances in supportive care including the use of newer antibacterial and antifungal antibiotics, antiviral agents (such as the use of ganciclovir to minimize the impact of cytomegalovirus disease), hematopoietic growth factors, and methods to prevent and control serious acute and chronic GVHD, have resulted in improved outcomes following allogeneic transplantation.

Alternative allogeneic donors

Only 30% to 35% of patients who are candidates for allogeneic HSC transplantation will have an HLA-identical or one antigen mismatched family member available to act as a donor. Survival for patients who receive a two or three antigen mismatched transplant is significantly worse than that in those receiving a matched graft (Horowitz *et al.,* 1989). Reports of closely matched but unrelated donors have indicated reasonable results with phenotypically matched donors, but poorer results with mismatched donors (Hows *et al.,* 1986; Beatty *et al.,* 1989; Ash *et al.,* 1990). Hobbs and colleagues (1981) were probably the first to successfully employ a haploidentical family member donor (father to son), and the first to employ marrow from an unrelated donor (Hughes-Jones *et al.,* 1991).

There are now over 8 million HLA-typed volunteer donors worldwide, and the number of unrelated transplants as a proportion of total allografts is increasing with a total of more than 2,000 cases reported to the IBMTR in the year 2000 (Horowitz *et al.,* 2002).

Stem cell sources beyond bone marrow

Peripheral blood

Sites other than the bone marrow have long been known to be sources of stem cells (Storb, Epstein, & Thomas, 1968). The peripheral blood was not utilized as a source in the early years of clinical transplantation for several reasons, including concern about the number of stem cells present (low in nonmobilized blood) and concern for the number of lymphocytes present (high), since T lymphocytes were known from many experimental studies to be mediators of GVHD. Also, in the early years of human transplantation methods for mobilization and collection of large numbers of cells were not available. However, beginning in the 1980s, case reports began appearing demonstrating that durable engraftment was possible with peripheral blood (Kessinger *et al.,* 1989), and since then transplantation of peripheral blood stem cells has also been shown to be a satisfactory means of reconstituting the hematopoietic system after marrow-ablative chemotherapy or chemoradiotherapy (To *et al.,* 1984). Transplantation of autologous peripheral blood stem cells results in faster marrow reconstitution than autologous marrow stem cells, with a shorter period of absolute neutropenia and thrombocytopenia (Sheridan *et al.,* 1992). Allogeneic blood stem cell transplantation has also been shown to produce faster hematopoietic reconstitution compared to allogeneic bone marrow transplantation (Bensinger *et al.,* 1995), but may be associated with a higher incidence of chronic GVHD. Allogeneic transplantation using peripheral blood continues to increase in frequency and by the 1998–2000 period there were almost as many peripheral blood transplants as marrow transplants reported to the IBMTR (Horowitz *et al.,* 2002) (Fig. 1.2). The use of peripheral blood has now extended to a large number of centers and studies are under way comparing blood and marrow transplantation relative to engraftment, GHVD, and antitumor effects.

Collection of CD34$^+$ stem and progenitor cells has been utilized to deplete autologous blood or marrow of contaminating tumor cells and allogeneic stem cells of T cells. Selection of stem cells by various physical and immunologic methods has become increasingly important in HSC transplantation. Large numbers of transplanted CD34$^+$ cells (with stringent T-cell depletion) has enabled the utilization of haploidentical family members as donors, with some success (Aversa *et al.,* 1994), especially in pediatric recipients (Handgretinger *et al.,* 2001).

Cord blood

Cord blood as a source of stem cells was proposed as an alternative stem cell source in the late 1980s (Broxmeyer *et al.,* 1989). The use of umbilical cord blood was proposed to have potential advantages over either bone marrow or peripheral blood including (1) an otherwise discarded source of stem cells that can be banked for long periods from a large number of donors; (2) the cord blood is derived at a time when there is a possibility that the lymphocytes are "young" and potentially more easily tolerated, possibly resulting in less GVHD; (3) the cord blood is derived from a source with minimal exposure to infectious disease. The first report of the successful use of cord blood in humans was from Paris in a patient with Fanconi anemia (Gluckman *et al.,* 1989). Cord blood transplantation was subsequently reported for patients with leukemia (Wagner *et al.,* 1992). To date, both unrelated and family member cord blood transplants have been carried out in many patients at multiple transplant centers. While the results are still preliminary, it appears that cord blood can be used with a greater degree of HLA disparity between donor and recipient with less serious GVHD than when marrow is used as the stem cell source. Cord blood transplantation still supplies only a small proportion of allogeneic donations, but is of growing importance particularly in pediatric patients (Fig. 1.2).

Autologous transplants

Autologous transplants are an alternative for patients with malignant diseases who do not have genetically defective stem cells, lack a suitable HLA-compatible donor, and are at high risk for GVHD because of age. Experience in acute leukemia has demonstrated that autologous transplantation results in a tradeoff, with reduced nonrelapse mortality but increased relapse when compared to allogeneic transplantation (Kersey *et al.,* 1987). Autologous transplants now exceed allogeneic transplants in number, largely because of the predominance of autologous grafts in non-Hodgkin lymphoma, Hodgkin's disease, and (until recently) breast cancer (Horowitz *et al.,* 2002) (Fig. 1.3). Notable in Figure 1.1 is the drop in number of autologous transplants from 1998 to 2000. This drop is largely the result of a decrease in the use of autologous transplantion for breast cancer. Similar data have been reported from the European Bone Marrow Transplant Registry (Gratwohl *et al.,*

2002) (see Chapter 124, "Breaking News..."). Autologous HSC transplant studies for lymphoma had their origin at the National Institutes of Health (NIH) in Bethesda. The group at the NIH demonstrated successful engraftment of autologous cryopreserved marrow (Appelbaum *et al.,* 1978). High-dose chemotherapy followed by autologous transplantation has become widely utilized for patients with high-risk malignant lymphoma. As of the year 2000, autologous transplantation for non-Hodgkin lymphoma is the widest indication for blood or marrow transplantation, with more than 3,500 North American cases reported to the IBMTR/ABMTR (Figure 1.3). There are many long-term survivors worldwide.

Transplantation for multiple myeloma began in the 1980s with early studies by McElwain and Powles (1983) in London and Barlogie and colleagues in the United States (1986). In recent years there has been a significant increase in transplantation for myeloma; autologous transplantation for multiple myeloma is currently the second widest indication for transplantation in North America (Fig. 1.3).

Other recent developments

Adoptive allogeneic cellular immunotherapy in the form of donor lymphocyte infusions (DLI) shows promise for the prevention and treatment of many of the complications currently associated with HSC transplantation. Cellular therapy has demonstrated efficacy in the prevention of cytomegalovirus disease in allogeneic HSC transplant recipients (Walter *et al.,* 1995), and in the treatment of Epstein-Barr-associated lymphoproliferative disease after allogeneic transplantation (Papadopoulos *et al.,* 1994). This approach has also become important in the treatment of hematologic malignancy, especially chronic myeloid leukemia, relapsing after an allogeneic transplant (Kolb *et al.,* 1995). Additionally, gene modification of the T cells in such a DLI with, for example a suicide gene such as the herpes simplex virus thymidine kinase

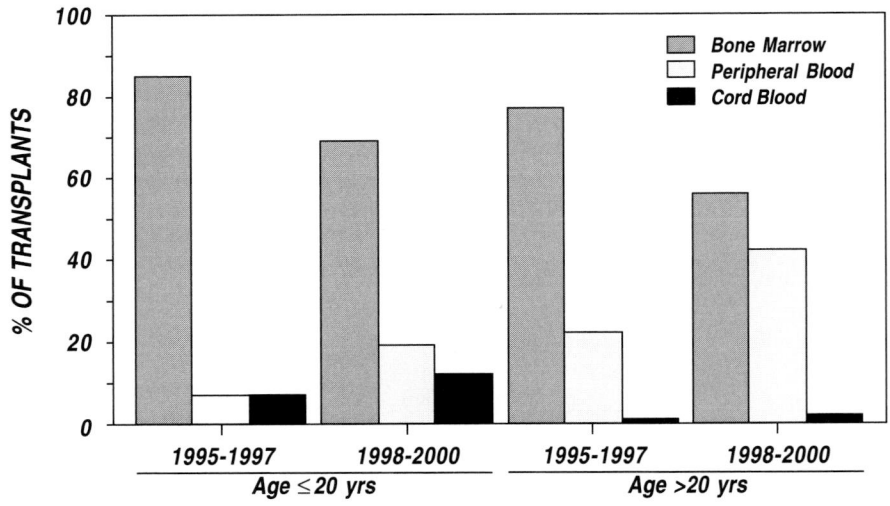

Fig. 1.2. Allogeneic stem cell sources by age: 1995–2000. Reproduced by permission of the IBMTR/ABMTR.

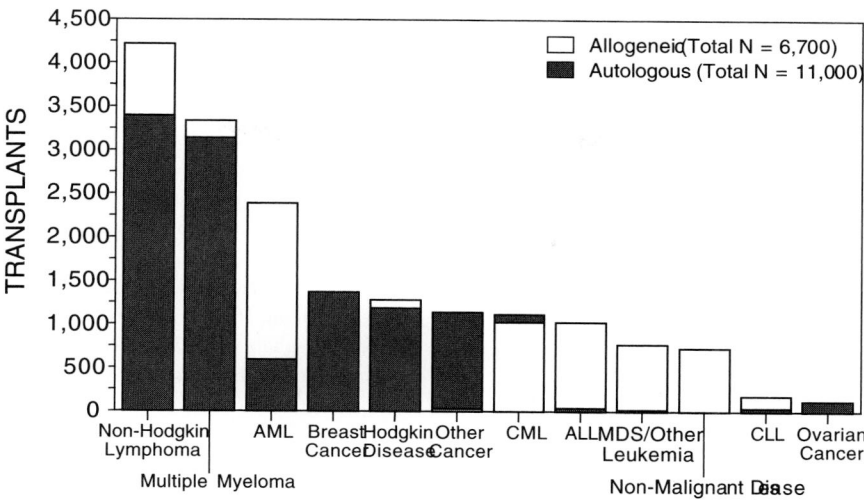

Fig. 1.3. Indications for blood and marrow transplantation in North America in 2000. Reproduced by permission of the IBMTR/ABMTR.

gene, has provided a way to enable the transplant physician to electively and selectively destroy infused T cells should they cause unwanted side effects such as GVHD (Bonini *et al.*, 1997). The use of reduced intensity conditioning (also known as non-myeloablative) regimens allows sufficient cytoreduction to obtain at least partial allo-engraftment, with subsequent reliance on a donor T-cell-mediated graft-versus-tumor effect. This approach, based on animal studies (Storb *et al.*, 1997), is currently under study in a number of institutions.

Conclusions

Since its experimental beginnings in the 1920s, and rapid acceleration from the 1960s, to its current extensive use in patients in many parts of the world, HSC transplantation has been a vigorous scientific and clinical journey. Blood and marrow stem cell transplantation, once a last-resort therapeutic option, has become a viable therapeutic option, or often the treatment of choice for a number of otherwise incurable diseases. A variety of allogeneic HSC donors, including unrelated and partially matched family members, are currently being utilized. Alternative stem cell sources, including peripheral blood and cord blood, as well as stem cell enrichment and expansion are now under study. The challenges for this new century are many. Reduction in transplant-related morbidity and extension of the benefits of HSC transplantion to patients in underserved areas of the world should be high on the priority list.

Acknowledgment

The author is honored to be invited by the editors to update this chapter on the history of hematopoietic stem cell transplantation, excellently written by the late Dr. George Santos in previous editions. Since I could not improve on his writing, I have liberally copied from George, introducing a few of my historical biases and updating where appropriate.

References

Appelbaum, F.R., Herzig, G.P., Ziegler, J.L. *et al.* (1978). Successful engraftment of cryopreserved autologous bone marrow in patients with malignant lymphoma. *Blood,* **52,** 85–95.

Appelbaum, F.R., Sullivan, K.M., Buckner, C.D. *et al.* (1987). Treatment of malignant lymphoma in 100 patients with chemotherapy, total body irradiation and marrow transplantation. *Journal of Clinical Oncology,* **5,** 1340–47.

Ash, R., Casper, J.T., Chitambar, C.R. *et al.* (1990). Successful allogeneic transplantation of T-cell-depleted bone marrow from closely HLA-matched unrelated donors. *New England Journal of Medicine,* **322,** 485–94.

Aversa, F., Tabilo, A., Terenzi, A. *et al.* (1994). Successful engraftment of T-cell-depleted haploidentical "three loci" incompatible transplants in leukemia patients by addition of recombinant human granulocyte colony-stimulating factor-mobilized peripheral blood progenitor cells to bone marrow inoculum. *Blood,* **84,** 3948–55.

Bach, F.H., Albertini, R.J., Anderson, J.L. *et al.* (1968). Bone marrow transplantation in a patient with the Wiskott-Aldrich syndrome. *Lancet,* **2,** 1364.

Barlogie, B., Hall, R., Zander, A. *et al.* (1986). High dose melphalan with autologous bone marrow transplantation for multiple myeloma. *Blood,* **67,** 1298–1301.

Barnes, D.W.H., & Loutit, J.F. (1957). Treatment of murine leukemia with x-rays and homologous bone marrow. II. *British Journal of Haematology,* **3,** 241–52.

Beatty, P.G., Ash, R., Hows, J.M. *et al.* (1989). The use of unrelated bone marrow donors in the treatment of patients with chronic myelogenous leukemia: experience of four marrow transplant centers. *Bone Marrow Transplantation,* **4,** 287–90.

Beilby, J.O.W., Cade, I.S., Jelliffe, A.M., Parkin, D.M., & Stewart, J.W. (1960). Prolonged survival of a bone-marrow graft resulting in a blood-group chimera. *British Medical Journal*, **i**, 96–9.

Bensinger, W.I., Weaver, C.H., Applebaum, F.R. *et al.* (1995). Transplantation of allogeneic peripheral blood stem cells mobilized by recombinant human granulocyte colony-stimulating factor. *Blood*, **85**, 1655–8.

Billingham, R.E. (1966–67). The biology of graft-versus-host reactions. *Harvey Lectures*, **62**, 21–78.

Billingham, R.E. & Brent, L. (1957). A simple method for inducing tolerance of skin grafts in mice. *Transplantation Bulletin*, **4**, 67–71.

Blume, K.G., Beutler, E., Bross, K.J. *et al.* (1980). Bone-marrow ablation and allogeneic marrow transplantation in acute leukemia. *New England Journal of Medicine*, **302**, 1041–6.

Bonini, C., Ferrari, G., Verzeletti, S. *et al.* (1997). HSV-TK gene transfer into donor lymphocytes for control of allogeneic graft-versus–leukemia. *Science*, **276**, 1719–24.

Boranic, M. (1968). Transient graft-versus-host reaction in the treatment of leukemia in mice. *Journal of the National Cancer Institute*, **41**, 421–37.

Bortin, M. (1970). A compendium of reported human bone marrow transplants. *Transplantation*, **9**, 571–87.

Broxmeyer, H.E., Douglas, G.W., Hangoc, G. *et al.* (1989). Human umbilical cord blood as a potential source of transplantable hematopoietic stem/progenitor cells. *Proceedings of the National Academy of Science (USA)*, **86**, 3828–32.

Camitta, B.M., Thomas, E.D., Nathan, D.G. *et al.* (1976). Severe aplastic anemia: a prospective study of the effect of early marrow transplantation on acute mortality. *Blood*, **48**, 63–70.

Ceppellini, R. & van Rood, J.J. (1974). The HLA system. I. Genetics and molecular biology. *Seminars in Hematology*, **11**, 233–51.

Coccia, P.F., Krivit, W., Cervenka, J. *et al.* (1980). Successful bone-marrow transplantation for infantile malignant osteopetrosis. *New England Journal of Medicine*, **301**, 701.

Cohen, J.A., Vos, O., & van Bekkum, D.W. (1957). The present status of radiation protection by chemical and biological agents in mammals. In *Advances in Radiobiology*, ed. G.C. de Hevesy, A.G. Forssberg, & J.D. Abbott, pp. 134–44. Edinburgh: Oliver and Boyd.

Dausset, J. (1958). Iso-leuco-anticorps. *Acta Haematologica (Basel)*, **20**, 156–66.

Dupont, B. (1980). HLA factors and bone marrow grafting. In *Cancer: Achievements, Challenges and Prospects for the 1980's*, ed. J.H. Burchenal & H.F. Oettgen, pp. 683–93. New York: Grune & Stratton.

Fabricious-Moeller, J. (1922). *Experimental Studies of Hemorrhagic Diathesis from X-ray Sickness*. Copenhagen: Levin and Munksgaard.

Fefer, A. (1970). Immunotherapy of primary Moloney sarcoma-virus-induced tumors. *International Journal of Cancer*, **5**, 327–37.

Fenyk, J.R., Jr, Smith, C.M., Warkentin, P.I. *et al.* (1978). Sclerodermatous graft-versus-host disease limited to an area of measles exanthem. *Lancet*, **1**, 472–3.

Festenstein, H. & Demant, P. (1978). HLA and H-2 basic immunogenetics, biology and clinical relevance. In *Current Topics in Immunology*, ed. J. Turk, p. 212. London: Edward Arnold.

Ford, C.E., Hamerton, J.L., Barnes, D.W.H., & Loutit, J.F. (1956). Cytological identification of radiation chimaeras. *Nature*, **177**, 239–47.

Gatti, R.A., Kersey, J.H., Yunis, E.J., Good, R.A. (1973). Graft-versus-host disease. *Progress in Clinical Pathology*, **5**, 1.

Gatti, R.A., Meuwissen, H.J., & Allen, H.D. (1968). Immunological reconstitution of sex-linked lymphopenic immunological deficiency. *Lancet*, **2**, 1366–9.

Gluckman, E., Broxmeyer, H.E., Aurebach, A.D. *et al.* (1989). Hematopoietic reconstitution in a patient with Fanconi's anemia by means of umbilical cord blood from an HLA identical sibling. *New England Journal of Medicine*, **321**, 174–8.

Gluckman, E., Socie, G., Devergie *et al.* (1991). Bone marrow transplantation in 107 patients with severe aplastic anemia using cyclophosphamide and thoraco-abdominal irradiation for conditioning: long-term followup. *Blood*, **78**, 2451.

Gorer, R.A. (1936). The detection of antigenic differences in mouse erythrocytes by the employment of immune sera. *British Journal of Experimental Pathology*, **17**, 42–50.

Gorer, R.A. (1937). The genetic and antigenic basis of tumor transplantation. *Journal of Pathology and Bacteriology*, **44**, 691–7.

Gowans, J.L. (1962). The fate of parental strain small lymphocytes in F1 hybrid rats. *Annals of the New York Academy of Science*, **99**, 432–55.

Gratwohl, A., Baldomero, H., Horisberger, B., *et al.* (2002). Current trends in hematopoietic stem cell transplantation in Europe. *Blood*, **100**, 2374–86.

Graw, R.G. Jr., Lohrmann, H.P., Bull, M.I. *et al.* (1974). Bone marrow transplantation following combination chemotherapy immunosuppression (BACT) in patients with acute leukemia. *Transplantation Proceedings*, **6**, 349–54.

Guttman, R.D., Santos, G.W., & Lindquist, R.R. (1971). Acceptance of renal allografts in rat bone marrow chimeras. *Transplantation*, **12**, 408–9.

Handgretinger, R., Klingbiel, T., Lang, P. *et al.* (2001). Megadose transplantation of purified peripheral blood CD34+ progenitor cells from HLA-mismatched parental donors in children. *Bone Marrow Transplantation*, **27**, 777–83.

Hathaway, W.E., Fulginiti, V.A., Pierce, C.W. *et al.* (1967). Graft-versus-host reaction following a single blood transfusion. *Journal of the American Medical Association*, **201**, 1015–20.

Hobbs, J.E. (1981). The Westminster bone marrow transplantation team: bone marrow transplantation for inborn errors. *Lancet*, **2**, 735.

Horowitz, M.M., Ash, R.C., Bach, F.H. *et al.* (1989). Outcome of bone marrow transplantation using related donors other than HLA-identical siblings. *Bone Marrow Transplantation*, **4**, 38.

Horowitz, M.M. *et al.* (2002). *IBMTR ABMTR Newsletter*, **9**, Issue 1, February.

Hows, J.M., Yin, J.L., Marsh, J. *et al.* (1986). Histocompatible unrelated volunteer donors compared with HLA non-identical family donors in marrow transplantation for aplastic anemia and leukemia. *Blood*, **68**, 1322–8.

Hughes-Jones, K., Selwyn, S., & Riches, P.G. (1991). Who pioneered the use of alternative donors (and stem cells from peripheral blood) in bone marrow transplantation? Letter to Editor. *Archives of Diseases in Children*, **66**, 1102.

Jacobson, L.O., Marks, E.K., Gaston, E.O., & Zirkle, R.E. (1949). Effect of spleen protection on mortality following x-irradiation. *Journal of Laboratory and Clinical Medicine*, **34**, 1538–43.

Jacobson, L.O., Simmons, E.L., Marks, E.K., & Eldredge, J.H. (1951). Recovery from radiation injury. *Science*, **113**, 510–11.

Kadowaki, J.I., Zuelzer, W.W., Brough, A.J. *et al.* (1965). Lymphoid chimerism in congenital immunological deficiency syndrome with thymic alymphoplasia. *Lancet*, **2**, 1152–6.

Kersey, J.H., Krivit, W., Nesbit, M.E. *et al.* (1979). Combined cyclophosphamide–total lymphoid irradiation compared to other forms of immunosuppression for human marrow transplantation. In *Experimental Hematology Today*, ed. S.J. Baum and G.D. Ledney, pp. 179–84. New York: Springer-Verlag.

Kersey, J.H., Meuwissen, J.H., & Good, R.A. (1971). Graft-versus-host reactions following transplantation of allogeneic hematopoietic cells. *Human Pathology*, **2**, 389–402.

Kersey, J., Ramsay, N., Kim, T. *et al.* (1983). Allogeneic bone marrow transplantation in acute nonlymphocytic leukemia: a pilot study. *Blood*, **60**, 400.

Kersey, J.H., Weisdorf, D., Nesbit, M.E. *et al.* (1987). Comparison of autologous and allogeneic bone marrow transplantation for treatment of high risk refractory acute lymphoblastic leukemia. *New England Journal of Medicine*, **319**, 461–7.

Kessinger, A., Smith, D.M., Strandjord, S.E. *et al.* (1989). Allogeneic transplantation of blood-derived T-cell depleted hematopoietic stem cells in a patient with acute lymphoblastic leuekmia. *Bone Marrow Transplantation*, **4**, 643–6.

Kim, T.H., Kersey, J., Sewchand, W. *et al.* (1977). Total body irradiation with a high-dose-rate linear accelerator for bone marrow transplantation in aplastic anemia and neoplastic disease. *Radiology*, **122**, 523–5.

Kolb, H.J., Schattenberg, A., Goldman, J.M. *et al.* (1995). Graft-versus-leukemia effect of donor lymphocyte transfusions in marrow grafted patients. *Blood*, **86**, 2041–50.

Krantz, S.B. & Kao, V. (1967). Studies on red cell aplasia. I. Demonstration of a plasma inhibitor to heme synthesis and an antibody to erythroblast nuclei. *Proceedings of the National Academy of Science (USA)*, **58**, 493–500.

Krivit, W., Pierpont, M.E., Ayaz, K. *et al.* (1984). Bone marrow transplantation in the Maroteaux-Lamy syndrome (mucopolysaccharidosis type VI). *New England Journal of Medicine*, **311**, 1606.

Lindsley, D.L., Odell, Jr. T.T., & Tausche, F.G. (1955). Implantation of functional erythropoietic elements following total-body irradiation. *Proceedings of the Society of Experimental Biology and Medicine*, **90**, 512–15.

Lorenz, E., Uphoff, D.E., Reid, T.R., & Shelton, E. (1951). Modification of acute irradiation injury in mice and guinea pigs by bone marrow injection. *Radiology*, **58**, 863–77.

Lucarelli, G., Galimberti, M., Polchi, P. *et al.* (1990). Bone marrow transplantation in patients with thalassemia. *New England Journal of Medicine*, **322**, 417–21.

Main, J.M. & Prehn, R.T. (1955). Successful skin homografts after the administration of high dosage x-radiation and homologous bone marrow. *Journal of the National Cancer Institute*, **15**, 1023–9.

Martinez, C., Kersey, J., Papermaster, B.W., & Good, R.A. (1962). Skin graft homograft survival in thymectomized mice. *Proceedings of the Society of Experimental Biology and Medicine*, **109**, 193.

Mathé, G. (1968). Bone marrow transplantation. In *Transplantation*, ed. F.T. Rappaport & J. Dausset, pp. 284–303. New York: Grune & Stratton.

Mathé, G., Amiel, J.L., Schwarzenberg, L. *et al.* (1963). Hematopoietic chimera in man after allogeneic (homologous) bone marrow transplantation. *British Medical Journal*, **2**, 1633–5.

Mathé, G., Schwarzenberg, L., Kiger, N. *et al.* (1974). Bone marrow transplantation for aplasias and leukemias. In *Clinical Immunobiology*, ed. F.H. Back & R.A. Good, pp. 33–62. New York: Academic Press.

McCulloch, E.A., Siminovitch, L., & Till, J.E. (1964). Spleen-colony formation in anemic mice of genotype WW^v. *Science*, **144**, 844–6.

McCulloch, E.A., Siminovitch, L., Till, J.E. *et al.* (1965). The cellular basis of the genetically determined hematopoietic defect in anemic mice of genotype S1/S1^d. *Blood*, **26**, 399–410.

McElwain, T. & Powles, R. (1983). High dose intravenous melphalan for plasma-cell leukemia and myeloma. *Lancet*, **2**, 822–4.

Medawar, P.B. (1963). Introduction: definition of the immunologically competent cell. *Ciba Foundation Study Group*, **16**, 1–5.

Miller, J.F. (1961). Immunological function of the thymus. *Lancet*, **2**, 748.

Mitchison, N.A. (1956). The colonization of irradiated tissue by transplanted spleen cells. *British Journal of Experimental Pathology*, **37**, 239–47.

Naiman, J.L., Punnett, H.H., Lischner, W.H. *et al.* (1969). Possible graft-versus-host reaction after intrauterine transfusion for Rh erythroblastosis fetalis. *New England Journal of Medicine*, **281**, 697–701.

Nesbit, M.E., Buckley, J.D., Feig, S.A. *et al.* (1994). Chemotherapy for induction of remission of childhood acute myeloid leukemia followed by marrow transplantation or multiagent chemotherapy: a report from the Childrens Cancer Group. *Journal of Clinical Oncology*, **12**, 127–35.

Nowell, P.C., Cole, L.J., Habermeyer, J.G., & Roan, P.L. (1956). Growth and continued function of rat marrow cells in x-irradiated mice. *Cancer Research*, **16**, 258–61.

O'Leary, M., Ramsay, N.K.C., Nesbit, M.E. *et al.* (1981). Bone marrow transplantation for hematologic malignancy. In *Graft-Versus-Leukemia in Man and Animal Models*, ed. J.P. Okunewick & R.F. Meredith, pp. 53–66. Boca Raton: CRC Press Inc.

O'Leary, M., Ramsay, N.K.C., Nesbit, M.E. *et al.* (1983). Bone marrow transplantation for non-Hodgkin's lymphoma in childhood and young adults: a pilot study. *American Journal of Medicine*, **74**, 497–501.

Owens Jr., A.H. (1970). Effect of graft-versus-host disease on the course of L1210 leukemia. *Experimental Hematology*, **20**, 43–44.

Papadopoulos, E.B., Ladanyi, M., Emanuel, D. *et al.* (1994). Infusions of donor leukocytes to treat Epstein-Barr virus-associated lymphoproliferative disorders after allogeneic BMT. *New England Journal of Medicine*, **330**, 1185–91.

Peters, L.J., Withers, H.R., Cundiff, J.H. *et al.* (1979). Radiobiologic considerations in the use of total-body irradiation for bone marrow transplantation. *Radiology*, **131**, 243–7.

Phillips, G.L., Herzig, R.H., Lazzrus, H.M. *et al.* (1986). High-dose chemotherapy, fractionated total body irradiation and allogeneic marrow transplantation for malignant lymphoma. *Journal of Clinical Oncology*, **4**, 480–8.

Powles, R.L., Watson, J.G., Morgenstern, G.R., & Kay, H.E. (1982). Bone-marrow transplantation in leukemia remission. *Lancet*, **1**, 336–7.

Ramsay, N.K., Kim, T.H., McGlave, P. *et al.* (1983). Total lymphoid irradiation and cyclophosphamide conditioning prior to bone marrow transplantation for patients with severe aplastic anemia. *Blood,* **62,** 622.

Russell, E.S. (1963). Problems and potentialities in the study of genetic action in the mouse. In *Methodology in Mammalian Genetics,* ed. W.J. Burdette, pp. 217–32. San Francisco: Holden-Day.

Santos, G.W. (1970). Effect of graft-versus-host disease on a spontaneous adenocarcinoma in mice. *Experimental Hematology,* **20,** 46–9.

Santos, G.W. & Cole, L.J. (1958). Effect of donor and host lymphoid and myeloid tissue injections in lethally x-irradiated mice treated with rat bone marrow. *Journal of the National Cancer Institute,* **21,** 279–93.

Santos, G.W. & Haghshenass, M. (1968). Cloning of syngeneic hematopoietic cells in the spleens of mice and rats pretreated with cytotoxic drugs. *Blood,* **32,** 629–37.

Santos, G.W. & Owens Jr., A.H. (1968). Syngeneic and allogeneic marrow transplants in the cyclophosphamide pretreated rat. In *Advances in Transplantation,* ed. J. Dausset, J. Hamberger, & G. Mathé, pp. 431–6. Copenhagen: Munksgaard.

Santos, G.W. & Sensenbrenner, L.L. (1971). A sensitive and quantitative assay for non H-2 histocompatibility antigens. *Experimental Hematology,* **21,** 19–20.

Santos, G.W., Burke, P.J., Sensenbrenner, L.L. *et al.* (1970). Rationale for the use of cyclophosphamide as an immunosuppressant for marrow transplants in man. In *Proceedings of the International Symposium on Pharmacological Treatment in Organ and Tissue Transplantation,* ed. A. Bertelli & A.P. Monaco, pp. 24–31. Amsterdam: Excerpta Medica.

Santos, G.W., Sensenbrenner, L.L., Burke, P.J. *et al.* (1971). Marrow transplantation in man following cyclophosphamide. *Transplantation Proceedings,* **3,** 400–4.

Santos, G.W., Tutschka, P.J., Brookmeyer, R. *et al.* (1983). Marrow transplantation for acute non-lymphocytic leukemia after treatment with busulfan and cyclophosphamide. *New England Journal of Medicine,* **309,** 1347–53.

Shank, B., Hopfan, S., Kim, J.H. *et al.* (1981). Hyper-fractionalized total body irradiation for bone marrow transplantation 1. Early results in leukemia patients. *International Journal of Radiation Oncology Biology and Physics,* **7,** 1109–15.

Sheridan, W.P., Begley, C.G., Juttner, C.A. *et al.* (1992). Effect of peripheral blood progenitor cells mobilized by filgrastim (G-CSF) on platelet recovery after high dose chemotherapy. *Lancet,* **339,** 640–4.

Song, C.W., Kim, T.H., Khan, F.M. *et al.* (1981). Radiobiological basis of total body irradiation with different dose rate and fractionation: repair capacity of hematopoietic cells. *International Journal of Radiation Oncology Biology and Physics,* **7,** 1695–1701.

Storb, R., Epstein, R.B., & Thomas, E.D. (1968). Marrow repopulating ability of peripheral blood cells compared to thoracic duct cells. *Blood,* **32,** 662–7.

Storb, R., Rudolph, R.H., Graham, T.C., & Thomas, E.D. (1971). The influence of transfusions from unrelated donors upon marrow grafts between histocompatible canine siblings. *Journal of Immunology,* **107,** 409–13.

Storb, R., Thomas, E.D., Buckner, C.D. *et al.* (1974). Allogeneic marrow grafting for treatment of aplastic anemia. *Blood,* **43,** 157–80.

Storb, R., Thomas, E.D., Buckner, C.D. *et al.* (1977). Marrow transplantation in untransfused patients with severe aplastic anemia. *Blood,* **50,** 316.

Storb, R., Yu, C., Wagner, J. *et al.* (1997). Stable mixed hematopoietic chimerism in DLA-identical dogs given sublethal total body irradiation before and pharmacologic immunosuppression after transplantation. *Blood,* **89,** 3048–54.

Thomas, E.D. (1983). Marrow transplantation for acute nonlymphoblastic leukemia in first remission. *New England Journal of Medicine,* **309,** 1539 (letter).

Thomas, E.D., Buckner, C.D., Banaji, M. *et al.* (1977). One-hundred patients with acute leukemia treated by chemotherapy, total body irradiation, and allogeneic marrow transplantation. *Blood,* **49,** 511–33.

Thomas, E.D., Buckner, C.D., Clift, R.A. *et al.* (1979). Marrow transplantation for acute nonlymphoblastic leukemia in first remission. *New England Journal of Medicine,* **301,** 597–9.

Thomas, E.D., Buckner, C.D., Rudolph, P.H. *et al.* (1971). Allogeneic marrow grafting for hematological malignancy using HLA matched donor-recipient sibling pairs. *Blood,* **38,** 267–87.

Thomas, E.D., Buckner, C.D., Storb, R. *et al.* (1972). Aplastic anemia treated by marrow transplantation. *Lancet,* **1,** 284–9.

Thomas, E.D., Lochte, H.L. Jr., & Lu, W.C. (1975). Intravenous infusion of bone marrow in patients receiving radiation and chemotherapy. *New England Journal of Medicine,* **257,** 491–6.

Thomas, E.D., Storb, R., Clift, R.A. *et al.* (1975). Bone marrow transplantation. *New England Journal of Medicine,* **292,** 832–43, 895–902.

To, L.B., Haylock, D.N., Kimber, R.J., & Juttner, C.A. (1984). High levels of circulating hematopoietic stem cells in very early remission from acute nonlymphoblastic leukemia and their collection and cryopreservation. *British Journal of Haematology,* **58,** 399–410.

Tutschka, P.J., Copelan, E.A., & Klein, J.P. (1987). Bone marrow transplantation for leukemia following a new busulfan and cyclophosphamide regimen. *Blood,* **70,** 1382–8.

Van Bekkum, D.W. & de Vries, J.J. (1967). *Radiation Chimaeras,* p. 277. London: Logos.

Wagner, J.E., Broxmeyer, H.E., Byrd, R.L. *et al.* (1992). Transplantation of umbilical cord blood after myeloablative therapy. Analysis of engraftment. *Blood,* **79,** 1874–81.

Walter, E.A., Greenberg, P.D., Gilbert, M.J. *et al.* (1995). Reconstitution of cellular immunity against cytomegalovirus in recipients of allogeneic bone marrow by transfer of T-cell clones from the donor. *New England Journal of Medicine,* **333,** 1038–44.

PART I   BIOLOGICAL BASIS OF HEMATOPOIETIC STEM CELL TRANSPLANTATION

2 Hematopoietic stem cells: biological targets and therapeutic tools

GERALD J. SPANGRUDE, NOBUKO UCHIDA, AND IRVING L. WEISSMAN

University of Utah, Salt Lake City, StemCells Inc., Sunnyvale, and Stanford University, Palo Alto, USA

Overview

Bone marrow transplantation began as the first serious effort to treat human disease using nucleated cells as the therapeutic tools (Thomas *et al.*, 1957; Juttner & To, 1994; Thomas, 1995). The principal objective was to treat cancer patients with supralethal levels of radiation and/or chemotherapy with curative intent, and to regenerate their hematopoietic and lymphoid (hereafter lymphohematopoietic) systems with a salvage dose of bone marrow (Thomas, 1995). Arguably, the principles of bone marrow (BM) transplantation derived from several critical factors: (1) that BM cells could save lethally irradiated recipients from the radiation syndrome by reconstituting their lymphohematopoietic systems with donor derived cells (Till & McCulloch, 1961; Becker *et al.*, 1963; McCulloch & Till, 1963; Siminovitch *et al.*, 1963; Siminovitch *et al.*, 1964; Till *et al.*, 1964; Wu *et al.*, 1967; Wu *et al.*, 1968; Worton *et al.*, 1969); (2) the emerging understanding of major and minor histocompatibility transplantation antigens, especially in mouse, dog, and humans (Gorer *et al.*, 1948; Vallera *et al.*, 1981; von Melchner & Bartlett, 1983; Ferrara *et al.*, 1985; Bennett, 1987; Bennett *et al.*, 1995); (3) the beginnings of an understanding of stem cells (Till & McCulloch, 1961; Becker *et al.*, 1963; McCulloch & Till, 1963; Siminovitch *et al.*, 1963; Till *et al.*, 1964; Wu *et al.*, 1967; Metcalf & Moore, 1971; Dexter *et al.*, 1977; Hodgson & Bradley, 1979; Harrison & Astle, 1982; Micklem *et al.*, 1983; Ogawa *et al.*, 1983); and (4) the commitment, boldness, and wisdom of a few early champions of experimental and clinical BM transplantation (Thomas *et al.*, 1957; Juttner & To, 1994; Thomas, 1995). In essence, BM transplantation is a method to re'generate the deliberately ablated lymphohematopoietic system. We have proposed that the cells specialized to regenerate an organ or tissue system are most likely descendants of the cells that first committed to generate these systems. Therefore, it was reasonable to seek to identify those cell types in lymphohematopoietic tissues in ontogeny and in adult BM that were capable of regenerating the lymphohematopoietic system.

The first clue that stem cells of the lymphohematopoietic system [hereafter called hematopoietic stem cells (HSC)] would be the operative elements in both generation and regeneration of the lymphohematopoietic system came from the groundbreaking experiments of Till and McCulloch (Till & McCulloch, 1961) and their colleagues (Becker *et al.*, 1963; McCulloch & Till, 1963; Siminovitch *et al.*, 1963; Till *et al.*, 1964; Wu *et al.*, 1967; Wu *et al.*, 1968; Worton *et al.*, 1969). Till and McCulloch first noted that there was a dose-response curve to BM transplantation, and that this quantitative relationship between dose of BM cells injected and the degree of radioprotection afforded could be a quantitative assay for the radiosensitivity of these normal BM regenerative cells (Till & McCulloch, 1961). During the course of their experiments they noted that at subradioprotective doses, mice that died of hematopoietic failure 10 to 15 days later contained in their spleens large colonies of myeloerythroid and megakaryocytic cells (Till & McCulloch, 1961; Siminovitch *et al.*, 1963). The number of colonies found in the spleen 10 days later was a linear function of the dose of BM cells injected (Till & McCulloch, 1961; Siminovitch *et al.*, 1963; Siminovitch *et al.*, 1964; Till *et al.*, 1964). Till, Backer, McCulloch, Wu, and Siminovitch developed an ingenious method to test whether each colony was in fact the product of a clonogenic cell; they irradiated the donor BM at doses that would kill most of the cells, knowing that the surviving cells would often have nonlethal chromosomal anomalies, each anomaly unique to the particular cell that suffered double strand breaks of its DNA (Becker *et al.*, 1963; Wu *et al.*, 1967). By examining the karyotype of each colony derived from the irradiated BM, they were able to conclude that all of the dividing cells in a single colony carried the same anomalous karyotype, and that it was different from each other colony's karyotype. Thus, they proved that there exist clonogenic progenitors that are multipotent for differentiation to myeloerythroid and megakaryocytic populations (Becker *et al.*, 1963; Wu *et al.*, 1967). They also showed that some spleen colonies contained cells that could protect and reconstitute lethally irradiated hosts, demonstrating that the colonies could self-renew or regenerate the essential multipotent elements that formed them (Wu *et al.*, 1967). Secondary transfers of the clonal reconstitution products of these colonies provided donor-derived chromosomally marked cells that also reconstituted cells of the lymphoid system (Wu *et al.*, 1968). They correctly surmised that they were looking at the most primitive BM cell—the HSC—and made what is now the operative definition of that cell population.

Each HSC is a clonogenic progenitor for multiple differentiated cell lineages, and also possesses the capacity for self-renewal (Visser & Van Bekkum, 1990; Ikuta *et al.*, 1992; Morrison, 1995; Aguila *et al.*, 1997). The search for HSC, therefore, required the establishment of clonogenic assays for each of the major lymphohematopoietic outcomes, including the spleen colony assay (Till & McCulloch, 1961), a thymus colony forming assay (Ezine *et al.*, 1984), and a B-lymphocyte lineage clonogenic assay (Müller-Sieburg *et al.*, 1986). The B-lymphocyte lineage clonogenic assay turned out to be the precursor of the current BM stroma-based assays for long-term culture (Müller-Sieburg *et al.*, 1986; Ploemacher *et al.*, 1991), including long-term colony-initiating cells (LTC-IC) (Sutherland *et al.*, 1996) and cobblestone area-forming cells (CAFC) (Müller-Sieburg *et al.*, 1986; Ploemacher *et al.*, 1991; Weilbaecher *et al.*, 1991). Radioprotection was also used as an assay to measure HSC dose quantitatively (Bertoncello *et al.*, 1988; Ploemacher & Brons, 1988; Uchida & Weissman, 1992). Many groups used bulk separation techniques, based on cell size and density (Jones *et al.*, 1990; Orlic *et al.*, 1994; Uchida *et al.*, 1996), cell surface markers, and metabolic properties (Bertoncello *et al.*, 1985; Visser & Van Bekkum, 1990; Udomsakdi *et al.*, 1991; Uchida *et al.*, 1993). Such BM fractionations revealed that a subset of BM cells were capable of spleen colony formation and radioprotection as well as long-term donor-derived blood reconstitution (Aguila *et al.*, 1997). In 1984 Visser and colleagues utilized the newly developed fluorescent activated cell sorter (FACS) to isolate an HSC-enriched population based on lectin binding (WGA+) and high level expression of the H-2K molecule (Visser *et al.*, 1984). In 1988, Spangrude *et al.* used all of the above clonogenic assays in concert to isolate candidate HSC based on the cell surface antigen phenotype Thy $1.1^{lo}Lin^{-/lo}Sca-1^+$ (TLS) (Spangrude *et al.*, 1988). In order to test whether a single clonogenic cell could undergo both multilineage differentiation as well as at least some degree of self-renewal, a competitive reconstitution assay was developed (Smith *et al.*, 1991; Uchida, 1992). Lethally irradiated mice were reconstituted with 100 purified Thy $1.1^{lo}Lin^{-/lo}Sca-1^+$ HSC or 200,000 unfractionated BM cells—the dose that radioprotects 95% to 100% of mice (PD95). Candidate HSC expressing a distinct allele of CD45 were added to these transplants at increasing numbers (1, 5, 10, 15, 20, etc.) (Smith *et al.*, 1991; Uchida, 1992; Morrison & Weissman, 1994). In all but a few cases transplantation of these mixtures led to multilineage (lymphomyeloid) reconstituted animals, demonstrating regeneration of over 10^4 TLS cells that themselves possessed clonogenic multilineage activities (Morrison *et al.*, 1997).

In clinical medicine the need for tissue and organ regeneration is not limited to the lymphohematopoietic system. For example, tissue destruction in vital organs such as the liver, the central nervous system, and other tissues are common when these tissues are treated to eradicate malignant cells. It is our thesis that many of these organ and tissue systems are generated from tissue type-specific stem cells, and therefore, they might be able to be regenerated from stem cells, if such cells could be found. Conceptually it might be useful to use organ or tissue-specific stem cell therapies to regenerate organ systems that need replacement following localized therapy, or to replace pathologic organs. Autologous or allogeneic stem cells for particular organ systems might be appropriate in place of organ or tissue transplants. As we discuss below, allotransplantation of cells, organs, or tissues in mouse models are specifically tolerated if the donor transplants are from the donor of HSC transplanted in a fashion that allows engraftment (Shizuru *et al.*, 1996; Gandy & Weissman, 1998; Uchida *et al.*, 1998; Shizuru *et al.*, 2000).

There are currently a number of major uses for HSC transplantation. First, autologous transplantation allows patients to be given myeloablative doses of chemo- or radiotherapy with the intention of destroying their endogenous malignant disease. Second, allogeneic HSC transplantation can also be used following myelo- and lymphoablative chemo/radiotherapy in patients with malignant disease. As well as providing a source of HSC uncontaminated with tumor cells, this approach has the potential benefit of the well-documented graft-versus-leukemia (GVL) activity of donor T cells. However, such allogeneic transplantation of HSC inclusive of T cells produces not only a graft-versus-tumor effect, but also a major complication of allogeneic transplantation, graft-versus-host disease (GVHD). It has been shown that a megadose of T-cell-depleted bone marrow overcomes major histocompatibility complex (MHC) barriers in sublethally irradiated mice (Bachar-Lustig *et al.*, 1995; Rachamim *et al.*, 1998) and HLA barriers in human transplantation for genetic disease (Elhasid *et al.*, 2000) and leukemia (Reisner & Martelli, 2000). A third major use of HSC transplantation is the use of normal allogeneic HSC to replace host marrow that has an acquired or congenital deficiency of the lymphohematopoietic system. Why would one use purified HSC instead of BM or mobilized peripheral blood (MPB) cells in these situations? In the autologous setting, purified HSC would be free of contaminating tumor cells shown to contribute to recurrence of the underlying malignant disease when autologous BM is used for transplantation (Deisseroth *et al.*, 1994; Brenner, 1998). In the allogeneic setting, purified HSC would be free of alloreactive T cells that cause GVHD, although some T cells would likely have to be added back with the HSC to provide graft facilitation and GVL effects (see below).

In addition to the current major uses of hematopoietic cell transplantation, there are a number of laboratory experiments, and high hopes by investigators, that HSC transplantation can open up new therapies for otherwise intractable diseases. One of these new therapies is gene therapy. Here the hope is to replace a defective gene by transducing the corresponding normal gene into the patient's own HSC; HSC are the only cellular element capable of long-term multilineage reconstitution and self-renewal (Aguila et al., 1997). Although genetic defects are relatively rare, there are important diseases that are much more common in which it is likely that gene-modified HSC could give rise to useful cells that could protect the patient against his or her disease. A success in this arena was realized with the apparent cure of one form of X-linked severe combined immunodeficiency disease by retroviral transduction of a normal copy of the defective gene into HSC prior to autologous transplant (Hacein-Bey-Abina et al., 2002). Another important concept is "intracellular immunization"—the supply of genes to HSC from an infected patient [e.g., with human immunodeficiency virus (HIV)] that block the replication and/or spread of the pathogen (Bonyhadi et al., 1997; Plavec et al., 1997). Acquired immunodeficiency syndrome (AIDS) is a particularly interesting target, because HIV itself is not a lethal infection; the patients succumb when HIV has eliminated T-cell immunity so that opportunistic infections and neoplasms can develop unchecked. Intracellular immunization should allow the emergence of HIV-resistant T cells, and these resistant T cells might provide sufficient immunity to protect against these pathogenic consequences.

Another clinical goal is to render HSC and their progeny resistant to therapies that destroy tumors at the cost of lymphohematopoietic failure. In these cases one would target HSC with drug and/or radiation-resistant genes such as MDR-1 (Sorrentino et al., 1992; Bodine et al., 1994) and BCL-2 (Domen et al., 1998) that provide relative chemo- and radiotherapy resistance. This approach must be taken with caution, however, given the oncogenic potential of such modifications (Bunting et al., 1998).

A third target for gene transfer is to provide patients with enhanced adaptive immunity and appropriate immune response to their tumors and/or infections. In one such example it might be useful to target HSC, common lymphocyte progenitors (CLP), or pre-T cells with transgenic T-cell receptor α/β chain genes that are involved in the recognition of cancer (or viral) peptides in the context of their HLA class I (or class II) molecule. While the high degree of polymorphism of HLA might seem to make this a daunting task, in fact both HLA class I and class II have many alleles of high frequency in defined populations that would make such an approach available to a large proportion of recipients.

A well-documented effect of HSC transplantation is the induction of transplantation tolerance to organs and tissues of the HSC donor (Gandy & Weissman, 1998; Shizuru et al., 2000). The use of HSC transplants as a method of inducing specific immunologic tolerance has been known since the late 1950s (Main & Prehn, 1955). There are at least two reasons that HSC transplantation is not used for this purpose in current medical practice. First, the morbidity and mortality caused by the myeloablative conditioning regimen prior to allogeneic transplantation poses a greater risk than current methods of lifelong immunosuppression. Second, GVHD is a severe and common complication of transplanting human BM or MPB that contain mature T cells. Transplantation of purified HSC in mouse models allows concurrent or subsequent transplantation

of tissues or organs from the HSC donor with no immunosuppression other than that which allows the establishment of the HSC graft (Shizuru et al., 1996; Uchida et al., 1998). Furthermore, methods have been developed that provide sublethal conditioning regimens for both BM and HSC transplantation (Sykes & Sachs, 1990; Colson et al., 1995; Shizuru et al., 1996; Quesenberry et al., 1997). Thus we believe that clinical HSC transplantation to create immunologic tolerance for subsequent solid organ transplantation will emerge as an effective and one-time treatment approach.

Many of the major autoimmune diseases in mice and humans include as a risk factor altered or rare MHC molecules allowing the emergence (from the thymus) of uncensored, potentially autoimmune T cells. HSC transplants might be useful in the treatment of these diseases. One could lymphoablate (and perhaps myeloablate) the patient and subsequently rescue them with autologous HSC. In theory the immune disorder would be eliminated, and "the immunologic clock" reset to zero, allowing a prolonged remission. In some murine models these remissions following autologous BM transplantation are not permanent (Shizuru et al., 1995). Allogeneic HSC transplants contain the potential for permanent remissions. In the 1980s and 1990s BM transplants from murine donor strains that lacked the susceptible MHC allele or haplotype to recipients possessing the autoimmune susceptibility were shown to prevent the development of the autoimmune disease (Ikehara, Good et al., 1985; Ikehara, Ohtsoki et al., 1985; Todd et al., 1987; LaFace & Peck, 1989). For example, HSC from non-diabetogenic AKR mice can not only reconstitute diabetes-prone NOD mice, but can prevent the diabetes. These mice have a mutant MHC gene called I-A^{g7} and lack I-E, which results in their high susceptibility to the generation of autoimmune T cells (Acha-Orbea & McDevitt, 1987; Erlich, 1991; Wicker et al., 1995; Slattery & Miller, 1996). While the autoimmunity is multisystem, the primary targets are the pancreatic islets. Transplantation of AKR (I-A^{k}I-E^k) HSC completely prevents the generation of autoimmune diabetes, whether the HSC are given in a myeloablative or myelosuppressive setting (Shizuru et al., 1996). More preclinical research needs to be carried out in relevant models of human HLA-linked autoimmune disorders such as Type I diabetes (Ikehara, 1998), rheumatoid arthritis (Marmont, 1997), ankylosing spondylitis (Libich et al., 1975), multiple sclerosis (Burt et al., 2002), sarcoidosis (Rizzato & Montemurro, 1998), severe allergy (Denburg, 1999), and systemic lupus erythematosus (SLE) (Tyndall, 1997). Already autologous and allogeneic HSC transplants in humans are being attempted in these diseases. We hope that progress in this area of human HSC transplantation proceeds to the point that issues of relatedness of donor and host, requirement or not for facilitation, dose of HSC required to overcome allogeneic barriers, and sublethal conditioning regimens for successful transplants can emerge, so that one can consider not only the rapidly lethal, but also the more frequent chronic and morbidity-causing autoimmune diseases.

Biology and transplantation of HSC

Although the history of the application of BM transplants to humans involved the use of a large number of animal preclinical models, including the dog, pig, and nonhuman primates (Abrams *et al.,* 1981; Bodine *et al.,* 1993; Sachs *et al.,* 1995; Donahue *et al.,* 1996; Dunbar *et al.,* 1996), it is our view that many if not most of the relevant experiments leading to the isolation and transplantation of HSC were derived from studies using mice. Thus, we pay special attention in this chapter to principles of HSC isolation, characterization, and transplantation in the mouse, and provide—where available—correlative experiments in humans.

Properties of mouse HSC/progenitor subsets

Limit dilution reconstitution experiments in congenic mice using inbred strains that differed only at the CD45 molecule by two known alleles, CD45.1 and CD45.2, led to the observation that multilineage reconstitution followed two distinct patterns: rapid but unsustained multilineage reconstitution, and later sustained reconstitution (Smith *et al.,* 1991; Uchida, 1992; Morrison & Weissman, 1994; Uchida *et al.,* 1997). These properties reflected the productive lifespans of different HSC and/or multipotent progenitor clones (Fig. 2.1). These lifespan differences could have been stochastic or determined. We showed that the lifespan of each clone was predetermined (Fig. 2.1) by demonstrating that long-term reconstituting HSC (LT-HSC) and short-term HSC (ST-HSC) could be separated on the basis of surface phenotypic markers (Morrison & Weissman, 1994). The total population of mouse multipotent progenitors is contained within cells that are c-kit$^+$ Thy 1.1^{lo}, Lin$^{-/lo}$, Sca-1$^+$ (KTLS) (Spangrude *et al.,* 1988; Morrison & Weissman, 1994;

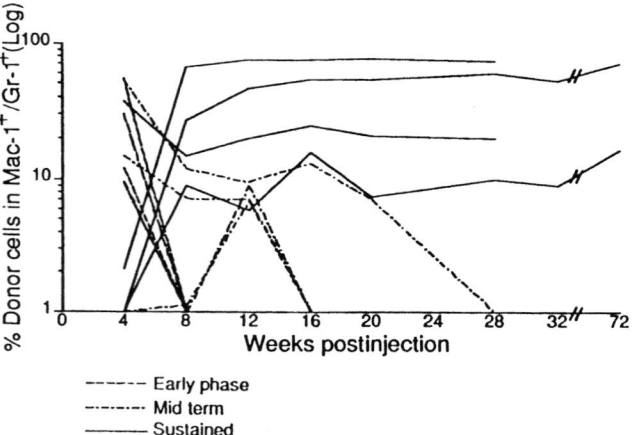

Fig. 2.1. Productive lifespan difference of different HSC and/or multipotent progenitor clones: the production of blood myelomonocytic cells. Limiting dilution doses of donor TLS cells were injected into CD45 congenic recipients. The chimeras were bled at about 4-week intervals and the levels of donor Mac-1$^+$/Gr-1$^+$ cells are shown.

Uchida *et al.,* 1997). Mouse HSC can also be enriched in CD38^{hi} (Randall *et al.,* 1996) or rhodamine (Rh) 123^{lo} (Bertoncello *et al.,* 1985; Spangrude & Johnson, 1990) fraction of BM for the mouse strains that do not express the relevant alleles of Thy-1 and Sca-1 (Spangrude & Brooks, 1992; Spangrude & Brooks, 1993). The Lin designation is for markers found on the surface of blood cells of known committed lineages, such as T cells, B cells, granulocytes, monocytes, erythrocytes, and natural killer cells; a cocktail of antibodies to these markers enabled isolation of Lin$^-$ and Lin^{lo} subsets (Müller-Sieburg *et al.,* 1986; Spangrude *et al.,* 1988; Morrison & Weissman, 1994). Of the Lin markers, two are important for the separation of the different multipotent progenitor populations that differ in productive lifespans—Mac-1 and CD4 (Morrison & Weissman, 1994). As shown in Figure 2.2, the most primitive population of long-term reconstituting HSC are contained in the Mac-1$^-$ and CD4$^-$ subset of KTLS cells, while their immediate descendants are the ST-HSC, which are Mac-1^{lo} and CD4$^-$ (Morrison & Weissman, 1994). A third, more abundant and less completely characterized population of multipotent progenitors (MPPs) are Mac-1^{lo}, CD4^{lo} (Morrison & Weissman, 1994); they include multipotent cells of limited productive lifespan, and a population of progenitors that in the context of transplantation only give rise to B-lineage cells (Morrison & Weissman, 1994). The three classes of cells are arranged in a lineage from LT-HSC to ST-HSC, which in turn give rise to MPP (Morrison *et al.,* 1997). ST-HSC and MPP do not produce LT-HSC and MPP do not produce ST-HSC (Morrison *et al.,* 1997). The difference between these three subsets is primarily in their ability to self-renew; recipients reconstituted with a single clonogenic functional LT-HSC can generate during their lifespan a progeny of 10^4–10^5 KTLS cells; recipients of ST-HSC self-renew only during the time of their production of myelomonocytic cells (Morrison *et al.,* 1997). The BM from mice reconstituted with the Mac-1^{lo} CD4^{lo} subset of MPP do not have detectable BM secondary-transfer reconstituting activity, perhaps because their period of self-renewal is brief, or perhaps because it is absent. Therefore, by these experimental findings we can verify that LT-HSC follow the definition of Till and McCulloch completely; that ST-HSC also follow it, but for a limited time; and that the population we designate MPP do not (yet) have demonstrable self-renewal, although they are multipotent progenitors. The phenotype of HSC in mice appears to be constant throughout the adult life of the animal. Fetal liver HSC and BM after treatment with 5-fluorouracil (5-FU) are Mac-1 positive (Ikuta *et al.,* 1990; Morrison *et al.,* 1995; Randall & Weissman, 1997). The 5-FU situation is interesting, because it implies that the regenerating BM system in this case recapitulates the marker profile of HSC found during ontogeny (Randall & Weissman, 1997). Mobilized peripheral blood & spleen HSC are of the KTLS phenotype, as is BM from extremely old mice (Morrison *et al.,* 1997; Uchida *et al.,* 1997). A murine clonogenic CLP has been found that is represented at about 0.02% of mouse BM, as Lin$^-$ IL-7R$^+$ Thy-1$^-$ Sca-1^{lo} c-kit^{lo} (Kondo *et al.,* 1997).

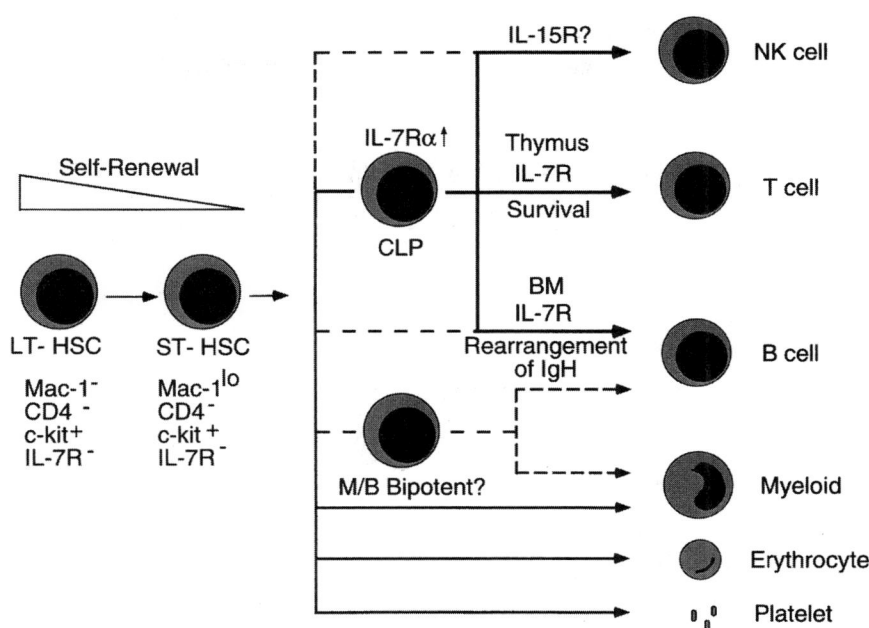

Fig. 2.2. A model of the differentiation pathway from HSC. The KTLS cells can be purified based on Mac-1 and CD4 expression. These populations form a lineage, from long-term self-renewing Mac-1⁻CD4⁻ c-kit⁺ (LT-HSC), to transiently self-renewing Mac-1lo CD4⁻ (ST-LSC), to non-self-renewing Mac-1lo CD4lo (MPP, not shown) cells. Unlike CLP, both LT-HSC and ST-HSC do not express IL-7 receptor (IL-7R). Modified, with permission, from Kondo *et al.* (1997).

This population produced rapid T, B, and NK reconstitution, but completely lacked myeloid differentiation capacity (Kondo *et al.*, 1997). Additional novel oligolineage myeloid progenitors have been described in the mouse, including the common myeloid progenitor (CMP), the granulocyte-myelomonocytic progenitor (GMP), and the myeloid-erythroid progenitor (MEP) (Akashi *et al.*, 2000). Similar cell populations have also been identified in human bone marrow (Manz *et al.*, 2002). In the mouse, HSCs have been shown to coexpress multiple non-hematopoietic genes as well as hematopoietic genes; MPPs coexpress myeloid and lymphoid genes; CMPs coexpress myeloerythroid, but not lymphoid, genes, whereas CLPs coexpress T, B, and natural killer (lymphoid but not myeloid) genes (Akashi *et al.*, 2003). This stepwise decrease in transcriptional accessibility for multilineage-affiliated genes may represent progressive restriction of developmental potential in early hematopoietic cell types. In a murine transplant model, cotransplantation of CMPs and GMPs with HSCs protected against death following an otherwise lethal challenge with two pathogens associated with neutropenia—*Aspergillus fumigatus* and *Pseudomonas aeruginosa* (BitMansour *et al.*, 2002).

Biology of human HSC

As with isolation of mouse HSC, human HSC and progenitor isolation has been characterized by enriching a rare cell population with a combination of monoclonal antibodies. Over the past decade, various cell surface and metabolic markers have been identified and used to isolate human HSC and progenitors (summarized in Table 2.1). Among them, CD34, originally

identified by the My 10 monoclonal antibody (Civin *et al.*, 1984), became the most critical cell surface marker for positively selecting a rare cell population (Strauss *et al.*, 1986). Within the CD34⁺ cell population, HSC can be further enriched into a Thy-1⁺ fraction (Baum *et al.*, 1992; Craig *et al.*, 1993; Humeau *et al.*, 1996; Cashman *et al.*, 1997), a CD38⁻/lo fraction (Terstappen *et al.*, 1991; Petzer *et al.*, 1996; Prosper *et al.*, 1996), or a combination of both (Uchida *et al.*, 1998). The CD34⁺ Thy-1⁺ Lin⁻ designation identifies human HSC in fetal liver and BM, umbilical cord blood, adult bone, and mobilized peripheral blood (MPB) (Baum *et al.*, 1992; Tsukamoto *et al.*, 1995; Murray *et al.*, 1995; DiGiusto *et al.*, 1996; Young *et al.*, 1996). Examples of isolation, as well as post sort and phenotypic analyses, are shown in Figure 2.3.

Human HSC functional activity can be analyzed quantitatively by in vitro and in vivo assays. In vitro assays include the identification of clonogenic primitive cell proliferation on long-term BM stroma co-culture, described as long-term colony initiating cells (LTC-IC) (Sutherland *et al.*, 1990; Eaves *et al.*, 1991) and cobblestone area-forming cells (CAFC) (Baum *et al.*, 1992). In these long-term in vitro assays, primitive human HSC/progenitor cells are enriched in the CD34⁺, but not in the CD34⁻, fraction of fetal and adult tissues (Andrews *et al.*, 1986; Strauss *et al.*, 1986; Andrews *et al.*, 1989; Baum *et al.*, 1992; DiGiusto *et al.*, 1994). When CD34⁺ Lin-MPB cells are further separated into Thy-1⁺ CD38⁻/lo and Thy-1⁺ CD38lo/⁺ and Thy-1⁻ CD38⁺⁺ subsets (Fig. 2.3), Thy-1⁻ CD38⁺⁺ cells are virtually devoid of CAFC activity. Both Thy-1⁺ subsets were highly enriched for CAFC activity. The Thy-1⁺ CD38⁻/lo subset showed slightly higher

Table 2.1.   *Cell surface and metabolic markers associated with human HSC and progenitor cells*

Marker	Expression	Remark	Reference
CD34	Positive		Civin *et al.*, 1984; Andrews *et al.*, 1986; Strauss *et al.*, 1986
Thy-1	Positive		Baum *et al.*, 1992; Craig *et al.*, 1993
CD38	Negative/low		Terstappen *et al.*, 1991; Peter *et al.*, 1996
AC133	Positive		Miraglia *et al.*, 1997; Yin *et al.*, 1997
CD45 RO	Positive		Landsdorp *et al.*, 1990
CD45 RA	Negative		Landsdorp *et al.*, 1990
CD59	Positive		Hill *et al.*, 1996
CD109	Positive		Sutherland *et al.*, 1996
CD117 (c-kit)	Low[a]		Gunji *et al.*, 1993
CD166 (HCA)	Positive		Uchida *et al.*, 1997
HLA DR	Negative to low	ABM HSC	Srour *et al.*, 1992; Brandt *et al.*, 1992
	Positive	FBM, MPB HSC	Tsukamoto *et al.*, 1995; Walker *et al.*, 1995
T-cell markers	Negative	CD2,3,4,8	Baum *et al.*, 1992
B-cell markers	Negative	CD10, 19	Baum *et al.*, 1992
NK marker	Negative	CD16	Baum *et al.*, 1992
Myeloid markers	Negative	CD14, 15	Baum *et al.*, 1992
Erythroid markers	Negative	Glycophorin A	Baum *et al.*, 1992

Metabolic marker[b]

Rhodamine 123[c]	Low	Mitochondria binding dye	Udomsakdi *et al.*, 1991; Uchida *et al.*, 1996
Hoechst 33342[c]	Low	DNA binding dye	Ladd *et al.*, 1997; Gothot *et al.*, 1997
Pyronin Y	Low	RNA binding dye	Ladd *et al.*, 1997; Gothot *et al.*, 1997

Abbreviations: FBM, fetal bone marrow; MPB, mobilized peripheral blood; ABM, adult bone marrow; HSC, hematopoietic stem cells.
[a] c-kit expression can be downregulated on some MPB HSC.
[b] To isolate quiescent HSC.
[c] Substrates for p-glycoprotein, encoded by MDR-1. HSC possess high levels of p-glycoprotein efflux activity.

CAFC activity in later time points than Thy-1$^+$ CD38$^{lo/+}$ subset (Uchida *et al.*, 1998).

An in vivo model for human HSC/progenitor cell engraftment was developed using xenogeneic transplantation of human cells into immunodeficient mice such as SCID (Kamel-Reid & Dick, 1988; McCune *et al.*, 1988; Peault *et al.*, 1991; Lapidot *et al.*, 1992), NOD/SCID (Larochelle *et al.*, 1996; Bhatia *et al.*, 1997; Cashman *et al.*, 1997; Conneally *et al.*, 1998), or beige/nude/xid mice (Nolta *et al.*, 1996). In the SCID-hu bone model, candidates for human HSC populations can be examined for their ability to reconstitute allogeneic human fetal bone giving rise to B-, myeloid, and CD34$^+$ progenitor cells (McCune *et al.*, 1988; Kyoizumi, 1992). The T-cell potential of such candidate populations can be characterized in the SCID-hu thymus model (Peault *et al.*, 1991; Baum *et al.*, 1992; Bonyhadi *et al.*, 1997). Human HSC/progenitors can engraft and differentiate into myeloid and CD3$^+$ cells in beige/nude/xid mice BM (Nolta *et al.*, 1996). Experiments using as recipients NOD-SCID mice that have, in addition to full T- and B-cell deficiency, a partial NK cell deficiency, have allowed human candidate HSC to be identified by their ability to reconstitute lymphohematopoietic cells in marrow and spleen (Larochelle *et al.*, 1996; Bhatia *et al.*, 1997; Cashman *et al.*, 1997; Conneally *et al.*, 1998). One

problem with both types of reconstitution is that all the immune-deficient mice examined so far are able to clear injected human cells from the blood stream with great effectiveness, presumably via a lectin-mediated phagocytic process. Higher doses than one would normally require if one injects candidate HSC i.v. or i.p. into xenogeneic recipients are needed in these model systems. Thus, these in vivo experiments are not easily adapted to clonogenic analysis. Hopefully, the human/mouse difference that leads to rapid elimination of all injected human blood cells from the blood stream of mice can be solved so that a more relevant preclinical model of transplantation can be achieved. In utero transplantation of human hematopoietic cells has also been used to characterize homing and engraftment of candidate HSC populations (Srour *et al.*, 1992; Zanjani *et al.*, 1992; Civin *et al.*, 1996; Sutherland *et al.*, 1996; Uchida *et al.*, 1996). In this model, human HSC/progenitor cells home to appropriate hematopoietic microenvironments and differentiate into mature blood lineages including T-cell subsets, B cells, and myeloid cells (Fig. 2.4). In addition, expanded human CD34$^+$ progenitors can be harvested from the sheep chimera, which are capable of generating further hematopoiesis (Uchida *et al.*, 1996).

In clinical autologous transplantation MPB cells can accelerate early neutrophil and platelet recovery, typically 7 to 10 days

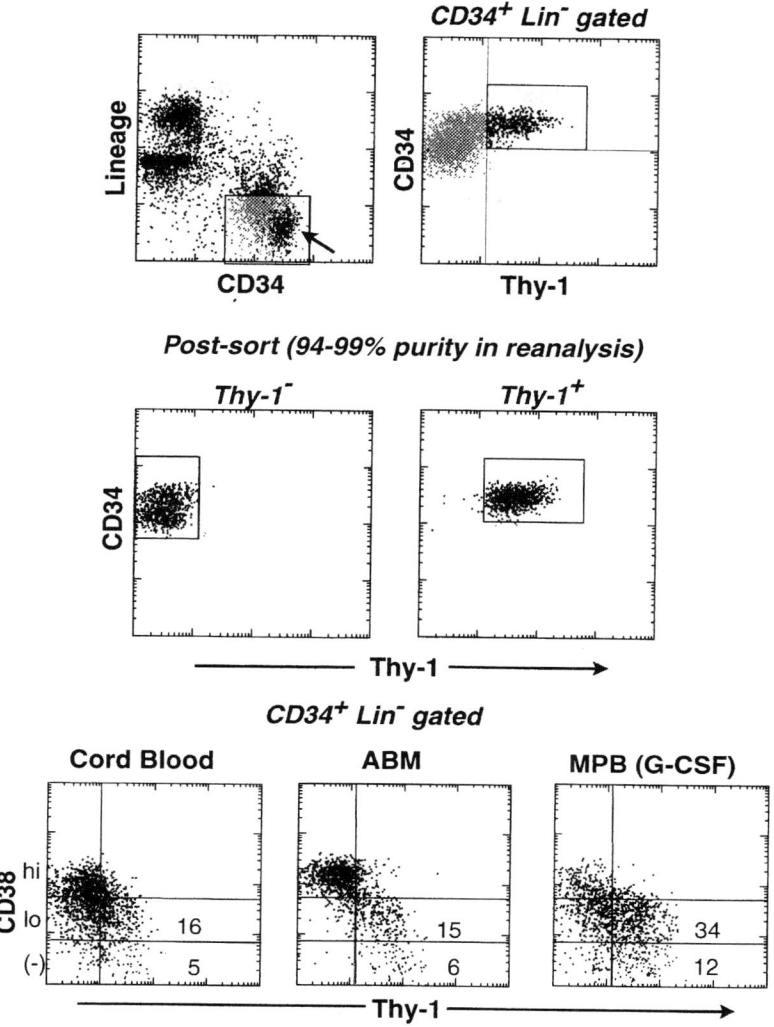

Fig. 2.3. Isolation of human HSC. The human HSC is enriched in CD34+ Lin− fraction. CD34+ Lin− cells are further separated into Thy-1− and Thy-1+ subset. The Thy-1+ CD34+ Lin− cells from cord blood, adult BM, and MPB are CD38−/lo.

faster than autologous BM transplants (Richman *et al.,* 1976; Juttner *et al.,* 1985; Appelbaum *et al.,* 1986; Kessinger *et al.,* 1988). As a result, MPB transplants have largely replaced BM transplants in the autologous setting. The accelerated hematopoietic recovery after transplanting MPB cells could be due to an increased number of CD34+ progenitors in the MPB apheresis collection. Alternatively, HSC and progenitors may be "activated" by cytokines when released into the circulation. These activated MPB HSC/progenitors could have greater proliferative capacity, and thus constitute a better source for gene transduction. However, the cell cycle status of MPB CD34+ cells is exclusively the G0/G1 phases of the cell cycle (Uchida *et al.,* 1997). In addition, CD34+ cord blood cells, another possible source for gene transduction, are also in the G0/G1 phase of the cell cycle (Traycoff *et al.,* 1994). When CD34+ Thy-1+ Lin− HSC from cord blood and MPB were cultured in the presence of multiple cytokines, both cord blood and MPB CD34+ Thy-1+

Lin− cells displayed delayed cell cycle progression (>24 hours) into S phase (Fig. 2.5) (Uchida *et al.,* 1997). The G0/G1 CD34+ Thy-1− progenitors can enter active cell cycle within 24 hours (Fig. 2.5) (Uchida *et al.,* 1997). The use of murine leukemia virus (MLV) vectors requires that cells go through M phase of the cell cycle with breakdown of the nuclear membrane in order to integrate MLV into host chromatin (Roe *et al.,* 1993). Therefore, it is not surprising that MLV-based gene transfer cannot transduce freshly isolated G0/G1 HSC from cord blood or MPB without prior stimulation of the cells with cytokines (Fig. 2.6). In contrast, lentiviruses (such as HIV type 1)-based vectors can transduce nondividing cells including terminally differentiated neurons (Naldini *et al.,* 1996; Blomer *et al.,* 1997; Kafri *et al.,* 1997; Miyoshi *et al.,* 1997). Lentiviral vectors can transduce freshly isolated G0/G1 MPB CD34+ Thy-1+ CD38−/lo Lin− cells with high efficiency, maintain their primitive phenotype, and maintain long-term in vitro transgene expression (Uchida *et al.,*

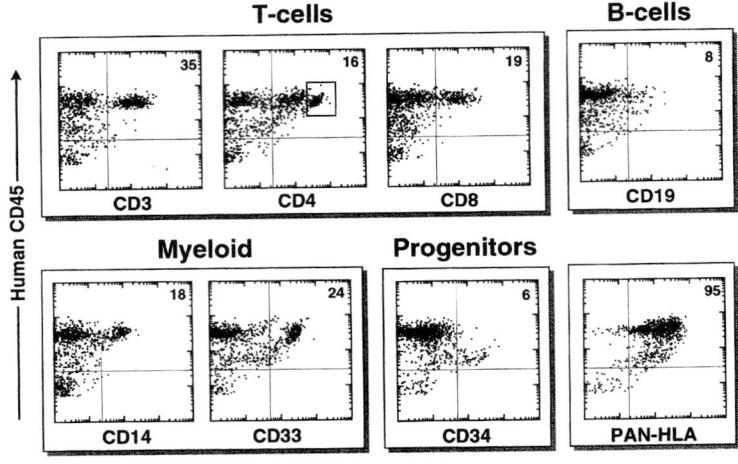

Analysis performed on CD45+ gated cells

Fig. 2.4. In utero transplantation of human HSC into fetal sheep. MPB CD34+ Thy-1+ Lin− HSC engrafted and detectable in sheep BM after birth. About 1% of human CD45+ cells were detected in this sample. FACS plots show the expression of lineage-specific markers compared with the expression of human CD45.

1998). Further development of lentiviral-based vectors may allow highly efficient gene transfer into quiescent HSC without losing primitive characteristics of freshly isolated HSC. Clinical studies of autologous transplantation of positively selected CD34+ cells or purified CD34+ Thy-1+ HSC confirmed that HSC, but not committed progenitors, contribute to the early phase of engraftment (see discussion below). Dose-response studies of human CD34+ cell-enriched transplants indicated that rapid engraftment can be regularly achieved if greater than 2×10^6 CD34+ cells/kg are transplanted (Brugger *et al.*, 1994; Cottler-Fox *et al.*, 1995; Gorin *et al.*, 1995; Bensinger *et al.*, 1996; Civin *et al.*, 1996; Handgretinger *et al.*, 1998). Additionally, human purified MPB CD34+ Thy 1+ cells have been used in autologous transplantation. Rapid and consistent

neutrophil and platelet recovery was achieved when patients were transplanted with greater than 0.8×10^6 CD34+ Thy-1+ HSC/kg (Table 2.2) (Michallet *et al.*, 2000; Negrin *et al.*, 2000). In addition, patients receiving higher doses of purified HSC did not suffer opportunistic infection such as cytomegalovirus (CMV) or aspergillus.

CD34 expression on HSC in humans and mice

How similar are mouse and human HSC in terms of phenotypic markers such as CD34? CD34 is a heavily *O*-glycosylated membrane-bound sialomucin-like phosphoglycoprotein (Steen & Egeland, 1998). CD34 is also present on blood vessels and is the ligand for L-selectin. In humans, a large number of mono-

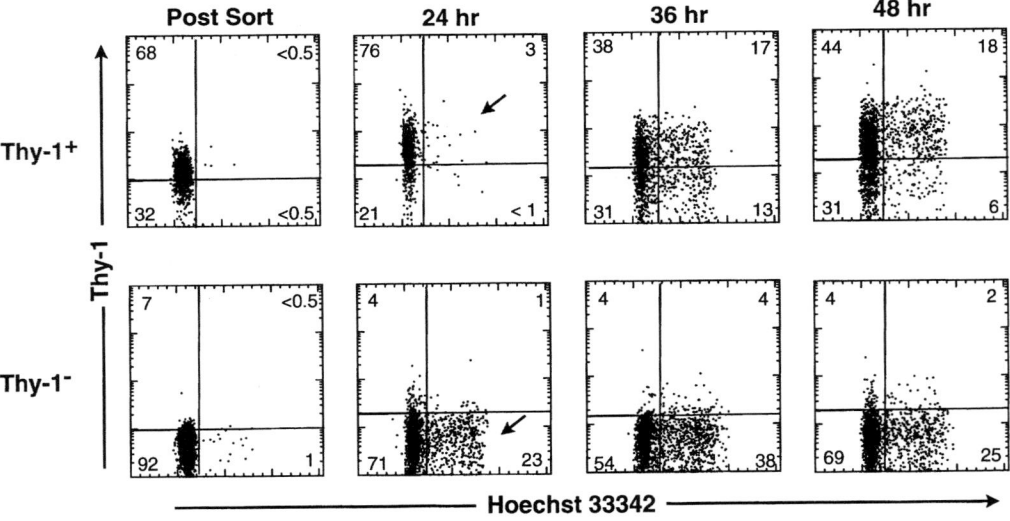

Fig. 2.5. In vitro cell cycle entry of cord blood CD34+ Lin− cells. Cord blood CD34+ Thy-1+ Lin− and CD34+ Thy-1− Lin− cells were cultured in the presence of multiple cytokines. The G_0/G_1 Thy-1− progenitor cells can enter active cell cycle within 24 hours, while Thy-1+ cells displayed delayed cell cycle progression.

Freshly Isolated CD34⁺ Thy-1⁺ CD38⁻/lo Lin⁻ MPB

% G0/G1 >99%

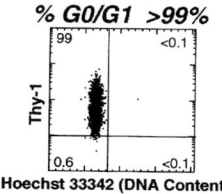

Hoechst 33342 (DNA Content)

Transduced with either HIV (VSV-G) or MuLV

HIV (VSV-G)　　　**MuLV**
GFP⁺ 40%　　　　**GFP⁺ <0.1%**

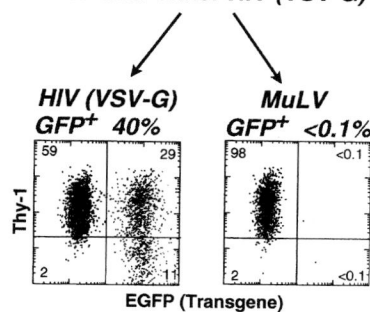

EGFP (Transgene)

Fig. 2.6. Transgene expression of CD34⁺ Lin⁻ Thy-1⁺ CD38⁻/lo cells transduced immediately after isolation by cell sorting. CD34⁺Lin⁻ Thy-1⁺ CD38⁻/lo cells were sorted and analyzed for cell cycle status Hoechst 33342 (DNA content) and Thy-1 profile. These cells were transduced with either HIV-eGFP (VSV-G) or MuLV-eGFP (A-Mo-MLV) by spinoculation for 4 hours without preculture; cells were cultured for 4 days. Adapted, with permission, from Uchida, Sutton *et al.* (1998).

clonal antibodies have been developed to different epitopes on CD34 antigen (Baumhueter *et al.*, 1993; Baumhueter *et al.*, 1994). In contrast, the CD34 molecule in the mouse has been characterized only by one rabbit polyclonal antiserum that is monospecific, and one monoclonal antibody directed against a CD34 epitope (Krause *et al.*, 1994; Osawa *et al.*, 1996). These reagents provide contrasting results: the CD34 positive, but not the CD34 negative cells in mouse bone marrow contained HSC based on the polyclonal serum, whereas the mouse-specific monoclonal antibody RAM34 showed variable expression on the c-kit⁺ Sca-1⁺ Lin⁻(Osawa *et al.*, 1996) or TLS cells (Morel *et al.*,

Table 2.2. *Engraftment rate of autologous transplants of peripheral blood CD34⁺ Thy-1⁺ HSC[a]*

Cell dose (× 10⁶/kg)	Days to reach		
	ANC > 500	Platelets >20k	Platelets >50K
All doses	12 (10–14) n=37	14 (8–73) n=35	25 (11–91) n=35
Dose < 0.8	12.5 (11–14) n=22	18 (10–36) n=20	28 (16–57) n=20
Dose > 0.8	11 (10–12) n=15	11 (8–73) n=15	15 (12–91) n=15

[a] Values represent medians (range).

1996; Morel *et al.*, 1998). Critical evaluation of CD34 subsets in the mouse showed that the c-kit⁺ Sca-1⁺ Lin⁻ population that is CD34ʰⁱ is most like the ST-HSC and MPP by being radioprotective but not long-term reconstitutive (Osawa *et al.*, 1996). The population that is CD34ˡᵒ (but not negative) contains long-term reconstitution activity, as does the CD34⁻ subset of the c-kit⁺ Sca-1⁺ Lin⁻ BM population (Osawa *et al.*, 1996; Krause *et al.*, 1999). The full radioprotective capacity of CD34⁻ and CD34ˡᵒ cells has not been fully investigated. Due to the detection of HSC in the mouse CD34⁻ BM subset as defined by the RAM34 monoclonal antibody, the question arises as to whether the CD34 molecule is not a marker of all long-term reconstitutive cells but rather a marker of a subset (CD34ˡᵒ) of long-term reconstitutive cells in the mouse. This issue was addressed in a series of experiments by Ogawa and colleagues, in which the expression of mouse CD34 was shown to be modulated from negative to positive, depending on the proliferative state of the HSC population under analysis. Thus, while the majority of HSC found under normal steady-state conditions in adult mouse bone marrow lack CD34 expression, stimulation in vivo by 5-FU injection or in vitro by cytokine stimulation resulted in recovery of most HSC activity among CD34⁺ cells (Ogawa *et al.*, 2001). The expression of CD34 was again lost as the cells engrafted in marrow and returned to steady-state conditions. Similar observations were reported in an analysis of mouse ontogeny (Ogawa *et al.*, 2001). Further experiments showed that CD38, which is absent from human HSC but present on mouse HSC under steady-state conditions, also modulates during recovery from 5-FU or during mobilization induced by granulocyte colony-stimulating factor (G-CSF) (Tajima *et al.*, 2001). Thus, in the mouse the expression of CD34 and CD38 reflect the activation state of the HSC. Interestingly, an analysis of the expression of human CD34 in a transgenic mouse model demonstrated that the human and mouse genes are differentially regulated, suggesting that the current practice of human bone marrow transplantation using only CD34⁺ cells is justified in spite of the mouse data (Okuno *et al.*, 2002). This is an important issue, since the initial data from the mouse model could be interpreted to indicate that patients receiving CD34⁺ cell transplants are missing an important subset of human multipotent progenitors. It should be pointed out that in each of the clonogenic and SCID-hu mouse models, human CD34⁻ cells had no activity (Tsukamoto *et al.*, 1995). The question of lineage marker fidelity between mouse and humans is an interesting one biologically, as it might imply important functions for these molecules in the behavior of HSC subsets (Goodell *et al.*, 1996; Goodell *et al.*, 1997; Zanjani *et al.*, 1998). As noted above, CD38 expression is found at very high levels on steady-state mouse HSC subsets (Randall *et al.*, 1996), whereas in human fetal and adult populations CD38 is either low or absent (Terstappen *et al.*, 1991; Petzer *et al.*, 1996; Prosper *et al.*, 1996). What about Sca-1? Sca-1 is one isoform of the CD59 family of LY6A/E molecules (van de Rijn *et al.*, 1989). It was shown that human CD34⁺ CD59⁺ cells were highly enriched for human HSC as measured by CAFC and SCID-hu reconstitution (Hill *et al.*, 1996). It is interesting that two major markers of

HSC in mice and humans, Thy 1 and CD59, are members of the immunoglobulin supergene family held in the cell membrane via a glycophosphatide inositol linkage rather than a transmembrane protein. It will be important to begin to determine the functions of these molecules in mice and humans so that one might gain a better understanding of the gene program that specifies HSC and their functions.

Ontogeny of mouse HSC

The first cells capable of hematopoietic long-term multilineage transplantation are found in the mouse yolk sac blood islands (Moore & Metcalf, 1970; Metcalf & Moore, 1971), and the para-aortic splanchnoderm (Godin et al., 1993; Medivinsky et al., 1993); these appear at about 7.5 to 8.5 days postconception (dpc) in mice, which have a 19 to 21 day gestation. At about dpc 8.5 to 9.5 the vasculogenic activity within the embryo and the yolk sac lead to the formation of the umbilical vein, which connects the yolk sac to the fetal liver (Russell & Bernstein, 1966; Barker, 1968). At that time hematopoietic activity can first be found in the aortal-gonadal-mesonephros (AGM) region (Medivinsky et al., 1993; Medvinsky & Dzierzak, 1996; Sanchez et al., 1996) and fetal liver (Godin et al., 1993; Medivinsky et al., 1993; Sanchez et al., 1996). There are two schools of thought as to the ontogeny of HSC. One group proposes that all long-term hematopoiesis, called definitive hematopoiesis, derives only from intraembryonic origins (Dieterlen-Lievre, 1992), while the other group proposes that the yolk sac blood islands are not only sites of primitive hematopoiesis, but contain HSC that are the progenitors of HSC that inhabit the adult, definitive lymphohematopoietic system (Weissman et al., 1978; Huang & Auerbach, 1993). Experiments in the frog and the mouse tend to substantiate a dual localization of HSC involved in both primitive and definitive hematopoiesis (Yoder et al., 1997), and it remains to be determined whether in the interval between blastula and neurula, earlier HSC origins can be found. However developed, fetal liver HSC numbers increase logarithmically as do fetal liver hematolymphoid cells from roughly dpc 9 to dpc 14.5 (Morrison et al., 1995). While hematolymphoid cell numbers in the fetal liver continue to double from dpc 14.5 onward during gestation, HSC content tends to remain level and decline from dpc 14.5 onward (Morrison et al., 1995); significant numbers of liver HSC are retained for the first several days after birth (Morrison et al., 1995), and can be found in adult livers as well (Morrison et al., 1995). During the exponential phase of increase of HSC in the fetal liver from dpc 9 to 14.5 virtually all HSC are Mac-1+ and dividing (Morrison et al., 1995). By limit dilution analysis over 80% of these dividing HSC cells are, by in vivo clonal analysis, LT-HSC. These fetal HSC are more efficient at engraftment (1 in 5 cells read out in clonal assays, compared to 1 in 10 to 20 KTLS cells in adults), and the relative burst size per injected fetal cell is increased relative to adult HSC, although this could be a reflection of their homing capacity rather than their intrinsic burst size per cell (Morrison et al., 1995). During early hematopoiesis fetal liver HSC are fully multipotent not only in terms of the different cell types that can be produced, but also by the fact that in the lymphoid lineage early fetal liver HSC can give rise to the fullest variety of "fetal" as well as adult T and B lymphocytes (Ikuta et al., 1990). Between dpc 14 and birth the fetal liver HSC gradually lose their capacity first to produce skin-resident T cells that express TCR Vγ3, then female reproductive epithelium-resident, and male and female tongue epithelium-resident TCRVγ4 T cells (Ikuta et al., 1990). Thereafter, all HSCs are restricted to develop, whether in the adult or fetal thymus, only adult T-cell outcomes, including intestine-homing Vγ5 positive and lymphoid-homing Vγ2 positive and all TCR α/β cells (Ikuta et al., 1990). If this is true in humans as well, there may be some conditions, especially in the treatment of fetal recipients, wherein same age fetal donors that have some degree of HLA match might be preferred to the use of a parental or sibling HSC population. However, the ontogeny of human fetal T cells and B cells is far from understood. The time course for development of T cells from HSC is mirrored by the development of B cells, especially the B-1 population of mainly peritoneal-resident CD5+ Mac-1+ B cells that have particular immune functions (Hardy & Hayakawa, 1992), as compared to the classical B cells that express both IgM and IgD as surface receptors (Herzenberg et al., 1992).

Aging of HSC in mice

As mice age the HSC population becomes altered: at about 5 months of age (about 20% to 25% of a mouse's lifespan) the number and percent of cells that have the LT-HSC (Mac-1−) phenotype start to increase, and by 2 years of age—virtually the full mouse lifespan—these cells have increased 10-fold, while the MPP population is virtually absent (Morrison et al., 1996). The Mac-1− HSC in 2-year-old mice appears mainly to be in cell cycle. As in many other situations when these cells are in cycle, their long-term reconstitutive efficiency on intravenous transplantation may be altered, while their in vitro biological activity and their in vivo radioprotective efficiency are not (Morrison et al., 1996) (see below). The loss of the Mac-1lo CD4lo population mirrors the drop in B-lymphocyte levels with age, consistent with the inclusion of B-lineage progenitors in this phenotypically defined subset. It will be important to determine the lineage relationships of MPP B lineage precursors, and to determine whether the CLP population also declines with age. Nevertheless, even in the oldest mice there are enough HSC present for them to be stem cell donors. Because there has been some hesitation in using older humans to be BM or MPB donors for self or others, it will be important to study the phenotype and function of human stem cell subsets with age in the absence of chemotherapy and radiotherapy treatment.

Mobilization of mouse HSC

In the previous section we described two phases of mobilization of HSC during ontogeny: the first from yolk sac to the embryo, and the second, at dpc 14.5, from fetal liver to developing spleen and newly emergent BM medullary cavities (Russell & Bernstein, 1966; Barker, 1968; Godin *et al.,* 1993; Medivinsky *et al.,* 1993). In both of these cases just prior to mobilization the HSC pool was expanding by cell division. In the 1950s and 1960s, it was shown that mouse CFU-S and hematopoietic precursors could be found in the adult spleen at ~10% the level of mouse BM, and in blood at about 1% the level of mouse BM. In the 1970s and 1980s BM transplant clinicians noted that in dogs and humans chemotherapy treatment led to the appearance of hematopoietic progenitors in the blood (Goodman, 1970). In the mid- to late 1980s this led to the use of MPB in autologous transplants, first in myelosuppressed, then in myeloablated patients (Juttner *et al.,* 1985). The efficiency of MPB for autologous transplantation increased dramatically when the mobilization protocols included not only a cytoreductive agent such as cyclophosphamide, but also subsequent treatment with hematopoietic cytokines such as granulocyte-macrophage colony-stimulating factor (GM-CSF), G-CSF, interleukin (IL)-1, IL-3, FLK-2/FLT-3 ligand, or stem cell factor (SCF) (Juttner & To, 1994). This led to the concept that HSC could be mobilized from BM to blood by means of these protocols. It seems reasonable to propose that such mobilization involves the de-adhesion of HSC from BM stroma, release into the circulation, and their homing to secondary hematopoietic sites (Papayannopoulou & Craddock, 1997). It was shown that HSC and early hematolymphoid progenitors express the adhesive molecule integrin $\alpha 4\beta 1$ (VLA4), and that the hematopoietic BM stroma used to isolate mouse and human candidate HSC expresses the integrin $\alpha 4\beta 1$ counter receptor V-CAM1 (Papayannopoulou *et al.,* 1995). Administration of antibodies to integrin $\alpha 4\beta 1$ in mice causes the rapid release of early hematopoietic stem and progenitor cells into the blood stream after a few days of administration (Papayannopoulou *et al.,* 1995). Furthermore, treatment of mice with the chemokine IL-8 led to rapid release (within 20 minutes) of HSC into the mouse blood stream (Laterveer *et al.,* 1995). However, the number of cells released by IL-8 is only a fraction of the number of HSC that can be mobilized by cyclophosphamide plus G-CSF (Morrison *et al.,* 1997) or G-CSF alone (Uchida *et al.,* 1997). Mobilization in response to IL-8 requires in vivo activation of circulating neutrophils (Pruijt *et al.,* 2002), and it is likely that mobilization in response to G-CSF is also mediated by neutrophils accumulating in the marrow in response to the cytokine. Other studies implicate neutrophil-derived proteases that target V-CAM1 as a mechanistic component of G-CSF-induced mobilization (Lévesque *et al.,* 2001).

Cyclophosphamide plus G-CSF (Cy/G) mobilization in the mouse has four phases: (1) a 10- to 15-fold expansion of HSC by cell division in BM; (2) the appearance of HSC in blood; (3) the collection of these HSC by the spleen; and (4) a second exponential expansion of HSC in the spleen (Morrison *et al.,* 1997). These findings are instructive in two ways: first the primary action of Cy/G appears to be a massive endogenous expansion of HSC, and second that "mobilization" occurs best and most frequently in those situations wherein the HSC popu-

lation is dramatically expanding. Oddly, while most BM HSC 1 to 3 days following initiation of Cy/G are in cycle (>2N DNA/cell), the mobilized HSC found in the blood (in both mice and humans) only have 2N amount of DNA/cell, the amount found in G0 or G1 cells (Morrison *et al.,* 1997). To test whether the 2N DNA HSC found in blood in the late phases of expansion under mobilization conditions are derived from dividing precursors, bromodeoxyuridine (BrdU) was made available on days 1 to 3 following initiation of Cy/G, and the next day the blood was examined. A total of 98% to 99% of the BM and blood HSC had incorporated BrdU during the period of exposure to BrDU (Wright, Cheshier *et al.,* 2001). Thus, mobilization is complex, involving cell expansion and cell movement of a subset of the massively expanded HSC pool selectively after the M phase of the cell cycle. It is conceivable that during M phase, HSC are less adherent to each other and to the stroma, and this would explain why the blood HSC appeared to be synchronized in G1 (Wright, Wagers *et al.,* 2001). This is similar to the classical method cell biologists used in the 1960s to synchronize fibroblasts or other adherent cell cultures by shaking the dish, releasing M phase cells only. It will be important to test whether one can improve the frequency of Cy/G expanding HSC in BM that are mobilized to peripheral blood by treatment with agents such as antibodies to VLA-4, to its counter receptor V-CAM1, or treatment with chemokines such as IL-8.

Self-renewal kinetics of mouse HSC

With the single exception to date of fetal liver, isolated HSC that have greater than 2N amount of DNA show poorer per cell reconstitution capacity than 2N HSC. For example, separating Thy-1.1^{lo} Lin$^{-/lo}$ Sca-1$^+$ (TLS) BM cells on the basis of Hoechst 33342 DNA staining showed that the S/G2/M cells were, on a per cell basis, less able to radioprotect and less able to reconstitute by a factor of 2- or 3-fold than the 2N cells (Fleming *et al.,* 1993). Increasing the number of these S/G2/M cells (from 100 to 300 per host) resulted in reconstitution activity similar to 100 2N HSC (Fleming *et al.,* 1993). At that time we proposed that not all of the TLS S/G2/M cells that were dividing were giving rise to HSC (Fleming *et al.,* 1993). When one looks at the cell cycle characteristics of the three KTLS BM subsets, there is a significant difference in their cell cycle characteristics. The Mac-1$^-$ KTLS cells (mainly LT-HSC) representing .007% of all BM cells and roughly 15% of BM KTLS cells are mainly in G0 or G1 with only 4% of the cells in S/G2/M. The Mac-1^{lo} CD4$^-$ KTLS cells represent .01% of BM and about 20% of KTLS cells; they have ~7% S/G2/M amount of DNA. The poorly self-renewing Mac-1^{lo} CD4^{lo} subset of KTLS BM cells are 60% MPP that represent a little over 60% of the BM KTLS population; they have on the order of 20% of cells in S/G2/M (Morrison & Weissman, 1994). Because the relative proportions of these 3 KTLS subsets are stable in young adult mice, and because only KTLS cells have HSC and pre-HSC activity, it is reasonable to assume that on average

50% or less of the progeny of these subsets remain in that subset, and 50% or more are less primitive than the S/G2/M cell from which they derive. Thus for every 100 S/G2/M KTLS cells transferred, only 4 are LT-HSC, 10 ST-HSC, 52 MPP, and ~34 nonmultipotent cells. Given this analysis, it is not surprising that these cells are less radioprotective and reconstitutive.

A more detailed analysis has been carried out of the relative biological functions of cells of the KTLS subsets found under the conditions of mobilization and in aging mice (Morrison et al., 1996). At the single cell level both the S/G2/M and the 2N DNA subsets of all three populations are capable of responding to multiple hematopoietic cytokines by giving rise to in vitro colonies (about 85% of the cells are multipotent by this test). A little over 50% of both populations can respond to mouse BM stroma in a CAFC assay (Morrison et al., 1996). Furthermore, for in vivo radioprotection experiments the PD50 is about 40 cells for each of the populations (Morrison et al., 1996). The major difference comes about when one analyzes at limit dilution the long-term reconstitution activity of these cells: between 1 in 10 and 1 in 20 of the 2N HSC subsets can read out in the in vivo limit dilution assay, and fully 20% to 80% of these are long term, according to the Mac-1 defined subset described previously (Morrison & Weissman, 1994). On the other hand, long-term reconstitution by the S/G2/M subset only occurred with a 1 in 100 limit dilution (Morrison & Weissman, 1994). Several factors make these calculations even more complex. Most, if not all, dividing HSC are resident in tissues, and when transplanted, are more likely to be picked up by spleen than marrow in irradiated hosts. However, marrow is the primary long-term reconstitutive hematopoietic microenvironment. In fact, the postradiation spleen is a highly hematopoietic microenvironment for only about 3 weeks postreconstitution, after which time hematopoietic activity decreases as blood cell levels rise. This opens the possibility that a radioprotective dose of spleen-seeding HSC (perhaps mainly S/G2/M) gets trapped in the spleen, and only a small percentage of HSC that are 2N may land selectively in BM. It is the latter population that may be primarily responsible for long-term reconstitution.

Nevertheless, it is clear from all of the above experiments that the dividing populations include both long-term and short-term HSC subsets, as well as MPP. The low frequency of S/G2/M cells in the LT-HSC appeared at first to be consistent with the clonal succession model of hematopoiesis (Kay, 1965). In that model it was proposed that 1 or 2 HSC at a time are active in hematopoiesis, and the rest are quiescent, much in the way that oocytes are believed to be cell cycle-arrested until fertilized (Kay, 1965). This is consistent with studies using retroviral marking in vitro of BM cells from 5-FU treated donors that were cultured in the presence of IL-3 and used for transplantation (Lemischka et al., 1986). Initially multiple clones, and later only one or two clones, could be found to be responsible for hematopoiesis in irradiated hosts. However, we have shown, using BrdU available in the drinking water of normal mice at levels that did not affect hematopoiesis or the activity of hematopoietic HSC, that about 20% of all KTLS

cells and 7% to 9% of the Mac-1⁻ LT-HSC subset enter cycle every day (Morrison & Weissman, 1994). By 30 days virtually all LT-HSC have undergone at least one cell division. Because the relative frequency and distribution of KTLS defined subsets remains constant over this period, it is inescapable that at last half the products of the LT-HSC cell divisions are LT-HSC, that is, they are undergoing self-renewal (Cheshier et al., 1999). An independent study using BrdU labeling technique was reported with consistent results (Bradford et al., 1997). In addition, retroviral transduction of purified LT-HSC during their first cell division in vitro in response to SCF, IL-6, and leukemia inhibitory factor (LIF) leads to ~10% of cells in cycle that can be retrovirally transduced, and transplantation of large numbers (200 to 400) of these transduced HSC shows that even long after reconstitution large numbers of different clones (as measured by viral integration sites) are present in T cells, B cells, and myeloerythroid cells (Klug et al., 2000). Although only a small percentage of these mature cells that possess the transgene continue to express it, donor-derived HSC in these mice continue to express the transgene (Klug et al., 2000). Thus, one can consider that hematopoiesis is not arranged according to the clonal succession model, but rather is characterized by a more evenly distributed entry into and out of cell cycle by all HSC subsets. It will be important to try to understand whether this process is stochastic or depends on microenvironmental factors.

However this occurs, the fact that over time a large number of LT-HSC enter a division cycle opens the possibility that one might be able to accumulate LT-HSC in cycle by attempting to use agents that are not toxic but that can slow progression of cells through cell cycle. One such agent is hydroxyurea (HU), which acts by blocking DNA S phase progression (Maurer-Schultze et al., 1988; Yarbro, 1992). Administration of HU to mice at the appropriate concentration leads to a dramatic increase in the KTLS population that is in cycle, increasing from 7% to over 20% to 30% S/G2/M. These cells, unlike expanding HSC in other circumstances, have a limit dilution reconstitution activity of 1 in 7 cells injected, of which 20% are the long-term type (Uchida et al., 1997). Unexpectedly, at a dose of 100 mg/kg at day 3 the actual number of HSC increased, as if a fraction of LT-HSC in cell cycle completed cell cycle and retained the LT-HSC characteristics (Uchida et al., 1997). The anomalous action of HU needs to be investigated more thoroughly; studies in humans are also needed.

Genes regulating HSC self-renewal

The self-renewal of most cell populations requires many factors, including the complete replication of telomeric DNA at each cell division. Telomeres consist of many repeats of a hexameric sequence (Moyzis et al., 1988; Meyne et al., 1989). DNA polymerase in all species requires RNA priming, and the 5′ RNA segment is degraded as a function of the DNA synthesis mechanism. As pointed out by J.D. Watson (1972), this is not a problem for most internal DNA, in which the degraded

RNA primer is replaced by an extending fragment, later linked by Okazaki-type ligation; but the 5′ most RNA on the telomeres would be degraded without chance of classic DNA replication, resulting in the end replication problem (Watson, 1972). A number of investigators, using species as broadly divergent as yeast and humans, have shown that telomere replication requires a special RNA/protein complex. High levels of this telomerase complex are detectable in cancer cells and spermatogineal cells, but were not detectable in differentiating tissues (Counter *et al.*, 1994; Kim *et al.*, 1994; Counter, 1996). The continued function of telomerase in primary fibroblast cell lines is correlated with the number of cell doublings (the Hayflick limit) that cells can undergo prior to senescence (Hayflick, 1965). Although in humans there is evidence of a gradual, albeit slow, decline of human telomere lengths in a population of BM cells highly enriched for HSC (Morrison *et al.*, 1996; Lansdorp *et al.*, 1997; Yui *et al.*, 1998), it has also been shown in mice that the LT-HSC contain telomerase levels equivalent to tumor cells, while ST-HSC have slightly less, and MPPs much, much less (Morrison *et al.*, 1996). Looking at all hematolymphoid populations in general, telomerase activity correlates with self-renewal capacity of the tested populations, and so we regard the telomerase complex as one of the gene sets necessary for self-renewal, at least in mice.

A compelling case has been presented supporting the role of a homeobox gene, HOXB4, in regulating the self-renewal of HSC (Sauvageau *et al.*, 1995). These studies demonstrate that expression of HOXB4 from a retroviral vector leads to an enhancement of HSC function in both culture and transplant models (Antonchuk *et al.*, 2002). Importantly, serial transplantation studies have shown that cells overexpressing HOXB4 are effective at reconstituting the numbers of BM HSC to normal levels following transplantation, while control cells expressing an irrelevant gene are not (Antonchuk *et al.*, 2001). Overexpression of HOXB4 has also been implicated in conferring hematopoietic transplantation potential to embryonic stem cells and yolk sac hematopoietic progenitors, populations that do not normally function to reconstitute hematopoiesis when transplanted into irradiated adult recipients (Kyba *et al.*, 2002). These studies establish the role of a development gene family in the regulation of primitive and definitive hematopoiesis, and point the way toward a definition of the genetic regulation of HSC functions.

Lineage infidelity and hematopoietic stem cells

The concept of trans-differentiation by HSC has been the subject of much attention in recent years. The initial observations, in which neural stem cells and muscle tissue differentiated to produce blood cells in transplant models (Bjornson *et al.*, 1999; Jackson *et al.*, 1999; Gussoni *et al.*, 1999), were followed by a flurry of publications showing lineage plasticity of stem cells in general and HSC in particular. Unfortunately, many of the lessons learned from years of research in hematopoiesis have largely been ignored in most studies of stem cell plasticity.

Problems with initial studies within this field are numerous (Anderson *et al.*, 2001). First and foremost, plasticity has primarily been inferred from the behavior of undefined or partially purified mixtures of cells. In general, lineage plasticity studies published to date have failed to utilize a clonal approach to the analysis of multilineage development by the stem cells responsible for trans-differentiation. It is therefore unclear what cells within these mixtures produce the cells that give rise to the original and new phenotypes, and whether separate cell lineages arise from the same cell. A clonal analysis of transplanted HSC showed no contribution of these cells to lineages other than blood (Wagers *et al.*, 2002). Second, in many cases cell populations have been transplanted following a period of time in tissue culture, and it is unclear whether the stem cells as originally isolated had the ability to produce heterologous tissue, or whether epigenetic modification occurred because of the culture period (Terada *et al.*, 2002). Third, most studies have not demonstrated the ability of trans-differentiating stem cells to self-renew. Finally, most studies have not demonstrated functionality of the progeny of trans-differentiated stem cells. These criteria are the measure by which all further studies that claim to demonstrate stem cell plasticity should be evaluated. Hematopoietic stem cell biologists have developed a number of clonal approaches to identify and characterize the behavior of putative stem cells, and by using modifications of these approaches, many of the controversial questions within this field will be resolved. The science that has been performed to date suggesting stem cell plasticity has not clearly established that adult stem cells are plastic. In fact, some of the initial reported studies have proven difficult to reproduce (Morshead *et al.*, 2002; Wagers *et al.*, 2002) or have been attributed to the unexpected presence of HSC in peripheral tissues (Kawada & Ogawa, 2001; Wright *et al.*, 2001). Additional issues are the sensitivity and specificity of assays utilized to detect donor-derived cells in transplant recipients, the often limited degree of donor contributions to recipient tissues, and the problem of distinguishing the rare labeled tissue cells from donor-derived passenger leukocytes within those same tissues. These problems have not prevented the appearance of studies in the literature that describe putative trans-differentiation of HSC in human recipients of sex-mismatched BM transplants (Korbling *et al.*, 2002). At the present time, and given the caveats outlined above, these human studies can be interpreted as suggestive at best (Abkowitz, 2002).

Radioprotection and reconstitution: lessons from mice

BM transplantation in mice and humans has led to hematopoietic engraftment and appearance of white blood cells (> 500/μl) and platelets (>50,000/μl for human) usually in the range of 17 to 30 days (Juttner & To, 1994; Uchida *et al.*, 1994). With the advent of mobilized peripheral blood (MPB) transplantation in humans, autologous transplants have engrafted much earlier (9 to 12 days following transplant)

(Juttner & To, 1994). This leads to the question of whether more rapid engraftment is due to increased numbers of HSC or of HSC plus other oligolineage committed progenitors. In mice, when HSC were given in doses that ranged from the minimal radioprotective dose for 95% of the mice (PD95 = 100 cells) (Uchida et al., 1994) to doses 5-fold that level (500 cells), very little difference could be seen in terms of more rapid or more sustained engraftment from BM (containing all of the oligolineage committed progenitors as well as HSC), and the HSC dose contained within that BM (containing none of the oligolineage committed progenitors) (Uchida et al., 1994). Attempts have been made in both mice and humans to supplement HSC with the massively increased numbers of oligolineage progenitors one can achieve by ex vivo expansion of HSC or CD34-enriched cells with hematopoietic cytokines such as SCF, IL-6, and IL-3 (Alcorn & Holyoake, 1996; Brugger & Kanz, 1996). Populations of cells generated from 1,000 Thy 1.1^{lo} Lin$^{-/lo}$ Sca-1$^+$ (TLS) cells after 7 days under optimized culture conditions contained more than an 80-fold expansion of hematopoietic progenitors (CFCs). However, these expanded populations performed exactly the same as 1,000 freshly isolated TLS cells when transplanted into lethally irradiated mice (Szilvassy et al., 1996). Thus, in that circumstance there was no benefit seen with expanded cells, and so far this has been mirrored by the clinical experience (Alcorn & Holyoake, 1996). The good news about these expansion protocols is that HSC are retained in the culture, and in those cases where a single stem cell began the culture, self-renewal had to involve division of HSC (J. Friedman, L. Jerabek, & I. Weissman, unpublished data). The bad news is that, at least for myeloerythroid and megakaryocytic oligolineage progenitors, one could not improve upon the engraftment time that the same number of HSC could offer. This led to the possibility that the shortened engraftment times using MPB instead of BM might be due to increased stem cell numbers rather than the transplantation of more, or more effective, oligolineage progenitors. When syngeneic (congenic) HSC were transplanted in doses from 100 to 10,000 cells, engraftment times dropped from approximately 23 days down to approximately 11 days (Fig. 2.7). This was true even if the putatively more primitive subset of KTLS cells that are Rh123^{lo} are transplanted at this high cell number (Uchida, Tsukamoto et al., 1998). Thus, the primary determinant of engraftment times of white blood cells and platelets in the context of BM transplantation are the numbers of KTLS cells, and not other oligolineage progenitors. Additional studies also showed that HSC play a major role in early engraftment (Zijlmans et al., 1995; Nibley & Spangrude, 1998; Zijlmans et al., 1998). This might not be the case for T- and B-lymphocyte reconstitution. Injection of 1,000 CLPs gave rise to more rapid engraftment of T and B cells in blood and spleen than injection of 1,000 KTLS HSC (Kondo et al., 1997). [The potential functional utility of the CLP population, which has a counterpart in humans (Galy et al., 1995) will be discussed below.]

Can one use these dose-response profiles generated in mouse models to predict dose-response characteristics of human autologous HSC transplants? The initial problem with doing so is not only the comparison between species, but the comparison between postpubertal healthy mice that had received no previous treatment or had no disease with humans, largely in their 40s to 60s, who have had considerable previous chemotherapy, and also who have malignancies that could alter the physiology of hematopoiesis. Nevertheless, the dose-response data generated using mouse BM HSC and mouse MPB HSC are shown in Figure 2.7 in terms of KTLS transplanted per kg body weight, and are compared with a human MPB transplant trial (Uchida et al., 1998). It should be noted that in the human clinical transplant situation, mobilized peripheral blood CD34$^+$ Thy-1$^+$ cells were transplanted, and not the CD34$^+$ Thy$^+$ Lin$^-$ population; this followed from the demonstration that the CD34$^+$ Thy-1$^+$ population in MPB lacks detectable tumor cells in myeloma patients (using PCR for patient-specific CDR III rearrangements), breast cancer patients (using immune cytochemistry for cytokeratin positive cells), and in non-Hodgkin's lymphoma (using PCR for the bcl-2 rearrangement) (Gazitt et al., 1995; Reading, 1996). Thus, the purity of the population that was used was probably only 50% of that in the mouse, and the corresponding numbers ought to be halved. What is remarkable is that one still achieves a dose-response effect for engraftment rate within the same range of magnitude shown by the mouse studies; thus, to a first-degree approximation, the mouse predicts the human outcome.

One should note that lymphocyte reconstitution in these patients is slow and abnormal, reflecting previous studies with older patients receiving high-dose chemotherapy and/or BM transplantation (Bacigalupo et al., 1997; Bomberger et al., 1998). Because the thymus is smaller in both mice and humans as a function of time following the initiation of puberty, and also because B-lymphocyte levels fall gradually with age, these lymphocyte reconstitution profiles need better study in the mouse model. Furthermore, the effect of previous rounds of chemotherapy and relative age also need to be followed.

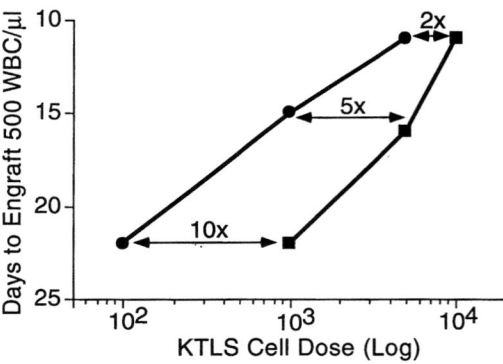

Fig. 2.7. Effect of stem cell dose on syngeneic and allogeneic transplants. Syngeneic or allogeneic mice were transplanted with purified KTLS cells. The dose of HSC and time that was required to achieve blood levels of 500 WBC/µl were compared in syngeneic (circles) and allogeneic (squares) hosts. Adapted, with permission, from Uchida, Tsukomoto et al. (1998).

Finally, as outlined in more detail below, one needs to look at thymus-dependent versus thymus-independent development of T cells from HSC.

The problem of immune reconstitution after HSC transplantation

Autologous HSC transplants in humans result in a prolonged lymphopenia, and specifically a CD4$^+$ T-cell deficiency relative to CD8$^+$ levels, that lasts for years (Archimbaud, 1997; Parrado et al., 1997). Allotransplants of BM from HLA-identical sibling donors also result in prolonged lymphopenia and a relative immune deficiency. Immune deficiency in these allotransplants cannot be explained by poor thymic education, as there is no HLA mismatch between donor and host.

Because most autologous HSC transplants have been carried out in patients ages 40 to 60, a time when most pathologists think that the thymus is minimal or absent, the question arises as to how T cells can redevelop at all, and why they redevelop with a CD8$^+$ skew. There are three likely explanations that come to mind. First, the thymus is in fact not absent in even the most aged populations, but its size and function is dramatically decreased compared to the prepubertal thymus (Hadden et al., 1992; Mackall & Gress, 1997). Second, it is conceivable that the myeloablative chemoradiotherapy preparation is not completely lymphoablative, and that one is simply seeing the regeneration of T cells from pre-existing mature T cells, without a change in the repertoire. Third, a well-described phenomenon (in the mouse) of thymic-independent maturation in BM (Dejbakhsh-Jones et al., 1995) or in epithelial tissues such as the liver (Makino et al., 1993) and intestine (Makino et al., 1993; Leclercq & Plum, 1996) could be responsible for the generation of these unusual T cells. Although one might think that one could distinguish between de novo generation of T cells (in a thymus-dependent and/or thymus-independent fashion) from expansion of mature T cells using surface markers characteristic of naive versus activated and/or memory T cells, the marker systems have not been fully validated. For example, in humans it is commonly believed that CD45 RA$^+$ RO$^-$ CD62 L$^+$ cells are naive T cells indicating recent emigration from the thymus and/or lack of antigen stimulation following emigration from the thymus (Kanegane et al., 1996; Dutton et al., 1998). CD45 RA$^-$ CD45 RO$^+$ CD62 L$^-$ cells are believed to be activated and/or memory T cells (Kanegane et al., 1996; Dutton et al., 1998). More extensive marker studies, including incorporation of CD27 and CD95, make the analysis cleaner, and allow separation of cells that can or cannot respond to recall antigens rapidly in vitro by producing Th1 or Th2 cytokines (Bulfone-Paus et al., 1997; Hamann et al., 1997). Nevertheless, the separation of each T-cell subset into naive, activated, and nonactivated but memory, subsets is difficult in humans, and it is important in the future to provide a more solid basis for T-cell subset designation, perhaps using comparisons with the mouse model wherein migrants, activated cells, and memory cells can be defined more rigorously, and the correlative phenotypes

tested. There are at least two other ways that this information could be obtained: first, allotransplantation of purified HSC, or autologous transplantation of retrovirus-marked HSC should reveal the progression of appearance of transplant-derived T cells and their subsets in a definitive fashion, and might be combined with studies of thymic size by computed tomography (CT) scanning. A second method draws on the fact that thymus cells and recent thymic migrants retain DNA circles that result from the rearrangement and excision of T-cell receptor DNA, especially of the last TCR rearrangement subset; the defined DNA sequence of such circles should allow single cell DNA polymerase chain reaction (PCR)-mediated analysis of phenotypically separated human T-cell subsets.

Nevertheless, it seems to us that the most likely and important source of T cells and B cells in patients who are undergoing autologous HSC transplants are their own purified T and B cells isolated prior to the initiation of any chemotherapy, or at least the chemoradiotherapy associated with the transplant. These cells should represent the immune repertoire for the life of the host, including whatever antitumor immunity the patient might have mustered. It should be straightforward to separate these cells from cells expressing malignancy markers, although one probably requires a high fidelity cell separation technology to do so. If this technology succeeds in facilitating immune reconstitution of the host, one might consider preimmunizing the patient before chemotherapy with antigens from infectious agents, and perhaps even from their own tumor prior to isolation of T and B cells, preparation for transplant, and transplant. The utility of each of these attempts could be tested first in the relevant mouse models.

Another possible mode of immune reconstitution would be to isolate the clonal CLP (Galy et al., 1995; Kondo et al., 1997) from the patient along with HSC, and cotransplant these populations. While it seems unlikely that this would provide an advantage over autotransplantation of already mature T and B cells in large numbers, there are a few circumstances wherein this might prove useful. In the mouse (Kondo et al., 1997), the CLP population appears to be in cell cycle (Kondo et al., 1997). It is unclear at this point if a human CLP subset is also in cycle. Retrovirus-mediated gene insertion cycling CLP might be useful for circumstances wherein a particular transgene in lymphoid cells would be advantageous.

Allotransplantation of HSC

The allotransplantation of hematolymphoid cells differs fundamentally from the transplantation of solid organs or tissues. A classic set of studies beginning in the 1960s in the laboratories of Cudkowicz and of Till demonstrated that lethally irradiated (A×B) F$_1$ mice can reject A or B but not F$_1$ BM grafts (McCulloch & Till, 1963; Cudkowicz & Stimpfling, 1964). Unirradiated F$_1$ mice always accept solid organ transplants from the same parental donors (Bennett, 1987). Cudkowicz and Stimpfling later showed that the relevant antigenic determinants were encoded, for the most part, in the mouse MHC (H-

2) and called them HH (for hybrid histocompatibility) antigens (Cudkowicz & Stimpfling, 1964). They thought that these antigens were recessive in nature, expressed in the parental strains but not in F_1 animals (Bennett et al., 1995). While this is still possible, several groups, including Cudkowicz's student Bennett, have shown that the barrier to allotransplantation and parent-to-F1 transplantation of hematolymphoid cells resides in a population of cells that express natural killer (NK) cell receptors (Yokoyama, 1995; Yu et al., 1996). NK cells have receptors largely specific for MHC class I molecules, and these receptors can deliver either positive or negative signals to the NK cell that expresses them (Trinchieri, 1989; Yokoyama, 1995). The receptors belong to two classes of molecules—C type lectins and immunoglobulin gene superfamily members (Yokoyama et al., 1997). Their ability to transmit positive versus negative signals depends on cytoplasmic domain sequences of these transmembrane proteins that contain T-cell activation motifs (ITAMs) and T-cell inhibition motifs (ITIMs); the latter act by recruiting tyrosine phosphatases that inhibit activation by the tyrosine kinase pathways (Yokoyama et al., 1997). The receptor species that contain ITIM motifs are expressed on NK cells in an oligoclonal fashion, in that one cell may bear a significant fraction of, but not all, inhibitory receptors (Yokoyama et al., 1997). Thus, in an F_1 offspring from strain A and strain B, it is reasonable to propose that many NK cells will have ITIM-containing receptors for class I molecules from both A and B strains, but that subsets of NK cells will have either only anti-A or anti-B MHC class I ITIMs (Yokoyama et al., 1997). An NK cell that has only an anti-A ITIM should be able to inhibit hematolymphoid cells from strain B, while those with only anti-B ITIMs should be able to inhibit hematolymphoid cells of strain A. An NK-mediated recognition phenomenon could result in rejection of parental hematolymphoid cells by F_1 hosts, and of course, rejection of allogeneic hematolymphoid cells. In contrast, conventional T-cell immunity in the F_1-versus-parent setting should not be active, as all histocompatibility antigens of the parental strains ought to be expressed in the F_1, and therefore the F_1 T cell should be tolerant of them. In the fully allogeneic situation, however, radioresistant and/or chemotherapy-resistant T cells might play a role in rejecting allogeneic hematolymphoid transplants. Clinical studies correlate donor-versus-recipient NK activity with the absence of leukemic relapse and graft rejection in human transplants (Ruggeri et al., 2002). It should be pointed out that other studies have indicated that the NK-mediated resistance to hematolymphoid transplants does not appear to require NK killing by either the granule-mediated (Aguila et al., 1995) or the FAS ligand-mediated (Aguila & Weissman, 1996) pathways, and therefore activities other than direct cell killing by these pathways might be involved in cytostasis or cytoelimination of hematolymphoid cells.

Overcoming the allogeneic barriers

The simplest way to overcome allogeneic barriers, at least in mice, is to increase the dose of HSC that are transplanted. The PD95 for congenic transplants is 100 cells, and for parent/F_1 or minor histocompatibility mismatched donor-recipient combinations, somewhere between 500 and 1,000 HSC (Shizuru et al., 1996). The PD95 for fully allogeneic MHC-mismatched combinations is between 1,000 and 6,000 HSC (Shizuru et al., 1996; Uchida et al., 1998). The variability of cell doses even within the same mouse strain combinations seems to relate to the dose of irradiation one can deliver, and the purity of HSC that one can transfer (Uchida, unpublished observations). In those situations where the PD95 is 1,000 cells, like the PD95 of 100 cells in the congenic setting, engraftment of WBCs and platelets takes on the order of 20 to 25 days (Uchida et al., 1998). However, when the dose is increased from 1,000 to 5,000 or 10,000 HSC, engraftment times of 14 and 11 days, respectively, are achieved (Uchida et al., 1998). Thus, once a dose of HSC is achieved to just overcome the allogeneic barrier (the PD95), the difference in the number of cells required to achieve rapid engraftment is much less for allogeneic than congenic combinations (Uchida et al., 1998). In these allotransplanted hosts there is no evidence of GVH or HVG reactions, and in many circumstances MLR and Simonsen's spleen assay also fail to demonstrate this. The most important point from these studies is that transplantation of purified HSC in a fully MHC-mismatched situation at doses that in the congenic setting can give rise to rapid engraftment also gives rise to rapid and sustained engraftment, without either HVG or GVH reactions, with consequently little risk of transplant-related mortality. Because high doses of HSC capable of contributing to rapid engraftment of autologous transplants have already been achieved in humans (Michallet et al., 2000), it is reasonable to propose clinical trials of HLA-matched sibling transplants using purified HSC.

If for some reason the use of purified, high-dose human HSC allotransplants in the HLA-matched sibling setting, the haplotype-mismatched setting, or the unrelated donor setting does not result in rapid and sustained engraftment, one must consider other methods of enabling these transplants to succeed, because the potential benefit of decreased GVHD and/or graft rejection is considerable. One method of lowering the HSC dose barrier in mice is to treat the irradiated host with monoclonal antibodies that eliminate or inactivate NK cells and/or T cells (Shizuru et al., 1996). Such antibodies can lower the PD95 in fully allogeneic mouse combinations dramatically (Shizuru et al., 1996), and even enable engraftment in the most difficult circumstance—from AKR/J to the autoimmune NOD mouse (Shizuru et al., 1996). Using whole BM transplants, these kinds of treatments in mouse and in monkey models have enabled allogeneic transplants using lethal and even sublethal conditioning regimens (Sykes & Sachs, 1990).

Another approach would be to add a defined dose of "graft-facilitating" T cells to the HSC inoculum. In animal models such cells bear T-cell markers and are CD8+ (Ildstad et al., 1986; Sykes et al., 1988; Sykes et al., 1989; Martin, 1993; Kaufman et al., 1994; Gandy et al., 1996). Three cell populations have been shown to have "facilitator cell" activity: classical CD8+, TCR α/β+, CD3+ T cells (Gandy et al., 1996), although these cells can also cause GVHD; a second subset of CD8[+], TCR α/β[-], CD3[+] cells have been reported to have graft-facilitating activity without GVHD (Kaufman *et al.*, 1994; Gaines *et al.*, 1996), as does a third subset CD8[+], TCR α/β[-], CD3[-] cells (Gandy & Weissman, 1997). These latter facilitator cells in particular might be useful in cases where purified stem cell transplants alone do not succeed because of inadequate dose.

There are special problems of immune reconstitution after allogeneic transplants. It may be difficult to use mature T and B cells from either donor or host, as these would have GVH and HVG activity, respectively. It is conceivable that one could use CLP cells; if so, then the proviso that T-cell reconstitution from those progenitors can occur in the absence of an adequate thymus needs to be validated. Finally, in the case of CLP and HSC transplants, at least one MHC haplotype must be matched in order to provide self-relevant T-cell education (Aversa *et al.*, 1994; Aversa *et al.*, 1997; Peters *et al.*, 1998).

Perhaps the greatest use for allogeneic HSC transplantation in the future will be for induction of tolerance to alloantigens. In that situation, optimizing stem cell dose and lymphoablative conditioning regimens that allow transplantation in a nonlethal setting might enable grafting of organs, tissues, and cells. This brings up an interesting issue. When and if liver stem cells, or pancreatic stem cells, or CNS or peripheral nervous system stem cells become available, it is unclear who will perform transplants of these cells. If cotransplantation with HSC becomes the preferred modus operandi, it seems reasonable that BM transplant physicians will supervise transplantation of diverse types of stem cells. If, however, HSC are not cotransplanted, but classical organ transplant immunosuppression is used, then surgeons and internists involved in the perioperative care of organ transplantation will perform these procedures.

Finally, we believe that another future role for HSC transplants will be in the treatment of autoimmune diseases. The primary basis for mouse and human autoimmune diseases appears to be the possession of MHC (H2 and HLA) haplotypes that cannot eliminate emerging T cells that are autoimmune (Ikehara *et al.*, 1985; Shizuru *et al.*, 1995; Ikehara, 1998). Transplantation of autologous HSC into fully lymphoablated and partially myeloablated recipients should enable a return of the immune system to the status of prethymic development, given that mature immune T cells can be eliminated. However, as long as the HLA susceptibility haplotype is the same, and the microenvironments that permit autoimmune disease remain, one should expect that such treatment would lead to important temporary, but not permanent remissions. Therefore, we believe that in the long term the provision of at least a one HLA haplotype mismatched transplant will be required for permanent transformation of the autoimmune-susceptible host to disease resistance. Unfortunately, these diseases produce considerable organ and tissue damage, which may be to some extent irreversible. In these cases it seems likely that the provision of an HLA mismatched HSC and CLP transplant from an HSC and solid organ donor could create a nonautoimmune microenvironment as well as an immunologically tolerant envi-ronment for the cotransplantation or subsequent transplantation of solid organ or solid organ stem cells designed to regenerate these damaged tissues and organs.

References

Abkowitz, J.L. (2002). Can human hematopoietic stem cells become skin, gut, or liver cells? *New England Journal of Medicine*, **346**, 770–2.

Abrams, R., McCormack, K., Bowles, C., & Deisseroth, A.B. (1981). Cyclophosphamide treatment expands the circulating hematopoietic stem cell pool in dogs. *Journal of Clinical Investigation*, **67**, 1392–9.

Acha-Orbea, H. & McDevitt, H. (1987). The first external domain of the nonobese diabetic mouse class II I-Aβ chain is unique. *Proceedings of the National Academy of Sciences USA*, **84**, 2435–9.

Aguila, H., Akashi, K., Domen, J. *et al.* (1997). From stem cells to lymphocytes: biology and transplantation. *Immunological Reviews*, **157**, 13–40.

Aguila, H.L., Hershberger, R.J., & Weissman, I.L. (1995). Transgenic mice carrying the diphtheria toxin A chain gene under the control of the granzyme A promoter: expected depletion of cytotoxic cells and unexpected depletion of CD8 T cells. *Proceedings of the National Academy of Sciences USA*, **92**, 10192–6.

Aguila, H.L. & Weissman, I.L. (1996). Hematopoietic stem cells are not direct targets of natural killer cells. *Blood*, **87**, 1225–31.

Alcorn, M.J. & Holyoake, T.L. (1996). Ex vivo expansion of haemopoietic progenitor cells. *Blood Reviews*, **10**, 167–76.

Akashi, K., Traver, D., Miyamoto, T., & Weissman, I.L. (2000). A clonogenic common myeloid progenitor that gives rise to all myeloid lineages. *Nature*, **404**, 193–7.

Akashi, K., He, X., Chen, J., *et al.* (2003). Transcriptional accessibility for genes of multiple tissues and hematopoietic lineages is hierarchically controlled during early hematopoiesis. *Blood*, **101**, 383–90.

Anderson, D.J., Gage, F.H., & Weissman, I.L. (2001). Can stem cells cross lineage boundaries? *Nature Medicine*, **7**, 393–5.

Andrews, R.G., Singer, J.W., & Bernstein, I.D. (1986). Monoclonal antibody 12–8 recognizes a 115-kd molecule present on both unipotent and multipotent hematopoietic colony-forming cells and their precursors. *Blood*, **67**, 842–5.

Andrews, R.G., Singer, J.W., & Bernstein, I.D. (1989). Precursors of colony-forming cells in humans can be distinguished from colony-forming cells by expression of the CD33 and CD34 antigens and light scatter properties. *Journal of Experimental Medicine*, **169**, 1721–31.

Antonchuk, J., Sauvageau, G., & Humphries, R.K. (2001). HOXB4 overexpression mediates very rapid stem cell regeneration and competitive hematopoietic repopulation. *Experimental Hematology*, **29**, 1125–34.

Antonchuk, J., Sauvageau, G., & Humphries, R.K. (2002). HOXB4-induced expansion of adult hematopoietic stem cells ex vivo. *Cell*, **109**, 39–45.

Appelbaum, F., Deeg, H., Storb, R. *et al.* (1986). Cure of malignant lymphoma in dogs with peripheral blood stem cell transplantation. *Transplantation*, **42**, 19–22.

Archimbaud, E. (1997). Immune reconstitution following transplantation of selected hematopoietic stem cells. *Hematology and Cell Therapy,* **39,** 264–8.

Aversa, F., Martelli, M.M., & Reisner, Y. (1997). Use of stem cells from mismatched related donors. *Current Opinions in Hematology,* **4,** 419–22.

Aversa, F., Tabilio, A., Terenzi, A. *et al.* (1994). Successful engraftment of T-cell-depleted haploidentical "three-loci" incompatible transplants in leukemia patients by addition of recombinant human granulocyte colony-stimulating factor-mobilized peripheral blood progenitor cells to bone marrow inoculum. *Blood,* **84,** 3948–55.

Bachar-Lustig, E., Rachamim, N., Li, H.W. *et al.* (1995). Megadose of T cell-depleted bone marrow overcomes MHC barriers in sublethally irradiated mice. *Nature Medicine,* **1,** 1268–73.

Bacigalupo, A., Mordini, N., Pitto, A. *et al.* (1997). Transplantation of HLA-mismatched CD34+ selected cells in patients with advanced malignancies: severe immunodeficiency and related complications. *British Journal of Haematology,* **98,** 760–6.

Barker, J.E. (1968). Development of the mouse hematopoietic system. I. Types of hemoglobin produced in embryonic yolk sac and liver. *Developmental Biology,* **18,** 14–29.

Baum, C.M., Weissman, I.L., Tsukamoto, A.S. *et al.* (1992). Isolation of a candidate human hematopoietic stem-cell population. *Proceedings of the National Academy of Sciences USA,* **89,** 2804–8.

Baumhueter, S., Dybdal, N., Kyle, C., & Lasky, L.A. (1994). Global vascular expression of murine CD34, a sialomucin-like endothelial ligand for L-selectin. *Blood,* **84,** 2554–65.

Baumhueter, S., Singer, M.S., Henzel, W. *et al.* (1993). Binding of L-selectin to the vascular sialomucin CD34. *Science,* **262,** 436–8.

Becker, A.J., McCulloch, E.A., & Till, J.E. (1963). Cytological demonstration of the clonal nature of spleen colonies derived from transplanted mouse marrow cells. *Nature,* **197,** 452–4.

Bennett, M. (1987). Biology and genetics of hybrid resistance. *Advances in Immunology,* **41,** 333–445.

Bennett, M., Yu, Y.Y., Stoneman, E. *et al.* (1995). Hybrid resistance: 'negative' and 'positive' signaling of murine natural killer cells. *Seminars in Immunology,* **7,** 121–7.

Bensinger, W.I., Buckner, C.D., Shannon-Dorcy, K. *et al.* (1996). Transplantation of allogeneic CD34+ peripheral blood stem cells in patients with advanced hematologic malignancy. *Blood,* **88,** 4132–8.

Bertoncello, I., Hodgson, G.S., & Bradley, T.R. (1985). Multiparameter analysis of transplantable hemopoietic stem cells: I. The separation and enrichment of stem cells homing to marrow and spleen on the basis of rhodamine-123 fluorescence. *Experimental Hematology,* **13,** 999–1006.

Bertoncello, I., Hodgson, G.S., & Bradley, T.R. (1988). Multiparameter analysis of transplantable hemopoietic stem cells. II. Stem cells of long-term bone marrow-reconstituted recipients. *Experimental Hematology,* **16,** 245–9.

Bhatia, M., Wang, J.C.Y., Kapp, U. *et al.* (1997). Purification of primitive human hematopoietic cells capable of repopulating immune-deficient mice. *Proceedings of the National Academy of Sciences USA,* **94,** 5320–5.

BitMansour, A., Burns, S.M., Traver, D. *et al.* (2002). Myeloid progenitors protect against invasive aspergillosis and Pseudomonas aeruginosa infection following hematopoietic stem cell transplantation. *Blood,* **100,** 4660–7.

Bjornson, C.R., Rietze, R.L., Reynolds, B.A. *et al.* (1999). Turning brain into blood: a hematopoietic fate adopted by adult neural stem cells in vivo. *Science,* **283,** 534–7.

Blomer, U., Naldini, L., Kafri, T. *et al.* (1997). Highly efficient and sustained gene transfer in adult neurons with a lentivirus vector. *Journal of Virology,* **71,** 6641–9.

Bodine, D.M., Moritz, T., Donahue, R.E. *et al.* (1993). Long-term in vivo expression of a murine adenosine deaminase gene in rhesus monkey hematopoietic cells of multiple lineages after retroviral mediated gene transfer into CD34+ bone marrow cells. *Blood,* **82,** 1975–80.

Bodine, D.M., Seidel, N.E., Gale, M.S. *et al.* (1994). Efficient retrovirus transduction of mouse pluripotent hematopoietic stem cells mobilized into the peripheral blood by treatment with granulocyte colony-stimulating factor and stem cell factor. *Blood,* **84,** 1482–91.

Bomberger, C., Singh-Jairam, M., Rodey, G. *et al.* (1998). Lymphoid reconstitution after autologous PBSC transplantation with FACS-sorted CD34+ hematopoietic progenitors. *Blood,* **91,** 2588–600.

Bonyhadi, M.L., Moss, K., Voytovich, A. *et al.* (1997). RevM10-expressing T cells derived in vivo from transduced human hematopoietic stem-progenitor cells inhibit human immunodeficiency virus replication. *Journal of Virology,* **71,** 4707–16.

Bradford, G.B., Williams, B., Rossi, R., & Bertoncello, I. (1997). Quiescence, cycling, and turnover in the primitive hematopoietic stem cell compartment. *Experimental Hematology,* **25,** 445–53.

Brenner, M.K. (1998). Applications of gene transfer in hematologic malignancy. *Recent Results in Cancer Research,* **144,** 60–9.

Brugger, W., Henschler, R., Heimfeld, S. *et al.* (1994). Positively selected autologous blood CD34+ cells and unseparated peripheral blood progenitor cells mediate identical hematopoietic engraftment after high-dose VP16, ifosfamide, carboplatin, and epirubicin. *Blood,* **84,** 1421–6.

Brugger, W. & Kanz, L. (1996). Ex vivo expansion of hematopoietic precursor cells. *Current Opinions in Hematology,* **3,** 235–40.

Bulfone-Paus, S., Durkop, H., Paus, R. *et al.* (1997). Differential regulation of human T lymphoblast functions by IL-2 and IL-15. *Cytokine,* **9,** 507–13.

Bunting, K.D., Galipeau, J., Topham, D. *et al.* (1998). Transduction of murine bone marrow cells with an MDR1 vector enables ex vivo stem cell expansion, but these expanded grafts cause a myeloproliferative syndrome in transplanted mice. *Blood,* **92,** 2269–79.

Burt, R.K., Slavin, S., Burns, W.H., & Marmont, A.M. (2002). Induction of tolerance in autoimmune diseases by hematopoietic stem cell transplantation: getting closer to a cure? *Blood,* **99,** 768–84.

Cashman, J.D., Lapidot, T., Wang, J.C. *et al.* (1997). Kinetic evidence of the regeneration of multilineage hematopoiesis from primitive cells in normal human bone marrow transplanted into immunodeficient mice. *Blood,* **89,** 4307–16.

Cheshier, S.H., Morrison, S.J., Liao, X., & Weissman, I.L. (1999). In vivo proliferation and cell cycle kinetics of long-term self-renewing hematopoietic stem cells. *Proceedings of the National Academy of Sciences USA,* **96,** 3120–5.

Civin, C.I., Almeida-Porada, G., Lee, M.J. *et al.* (1996). Sustained, retransplantable, multilineage engraftment of highly purified adult human bone marrow stem cells in vivo. *Blood*, **88**, 4102–9.

Civin, C.I., Strauss, L.C., Brovall, C. *et al.* (1984). Antigenic analysis of hematopoiesis. III. A hematopoietic progenitor cell surface antigen defined by a monoclonal antibody raised against KG-1a cells. *Journal of Immunology*, **133**, 157–65.

Civin, C.I., Trischmann, T., Kadan, N.S. *et al.* (1996). Highly purified CD34-positive cells reconstitute hematopoiesis. *Journal of Clinical Oncology*, **14**, 2224–33.

Colson, Y.L., Wren, S.M., Schuchert, M.J. *et al.* (1995). A nonlethal conditioning approach to achieve durable multilineage mixed chimerism and tolerance across major, minor, and hematopoietic histocompatibility barriers. *Journal of Immunology*, **155**, 4179–88.

Conneally, E., Eaves, C.J., & Humphries, R.K. (1998). Efficient retroviral-mediated gene transfer to human cord blood stem cells with in vivo repopulating potential. *Blood*, **91**, 3487–93.

Cottler-Fox, M., Cipolone, K., Yu, M. *et al.* (1995). Positive selection of CD34+ hematopoietic cells using an immunoaffinity column results in T cell-depletion equivalent to elutriation. *Experimental Hematology*, **23**, 320–2.

Counter, C.M. (1996). The roles of telomeres and telomerase in cell life span. *Mutation Research*, **366**, 45–63.

Counter, C.M., Hirte, H.W., Bacchetti, S., & Harley, C.B. (1994). Telomerase activity in human ovarian carcinoma. *Proceedings of the National Academy of Sciences USA*, **91**, 2882–5.

Craig, W., Kay, R., Cutler, R.L., & Lansdorp, P.M. (1993). Expression of Thy-1 on human hematopoietic progenitor cells. *Journal of Experimental Medicine*, **177**, 1331–42.

Cudkowicz, G. & Stimpfling, J.H. (1964). Deficient growth of C57BL marrow cells transplanted in F1 hybrid mice. Association with the histocompatibility-2 locus. *Immunology*, **7**, 291–306.

Deisseroth, A.B., Zu, Z., Claxton, D. *et al.* (1994). Genetic marking shows that Ph+ cells present in autologous transplants of chronic myelogenous leukemia (CML) contribute to relapse after autologous bone marrow in CML. *Blood*, **83**, 3068–76.

Dejbakhsh-Jones, S., Jerabek, L., Weissman, I.L., & Strober, S. (1995). Extrathymic maturation of alpha beta T cells from hemopoietic stem cells. *Journal of Immunology*, **155**, 3338–44.

Denburg, J.A. (1999). Bone marrow in atopy and asthma: hematopoietic mechanisms in allergic inflammation. *Immunol Today*, **20**, 111–13.

Dexter, T.M., Allen, T.D., & Lajtha, L.G. (1977). Conditions controlling the proliferation of haematopoietic stem cells in vitro. *Journal of Cellular Physiology*, **91**, 335–44.

Dieterlen-Lievre, F. (1992). Embryonic chimeras and hemopoietic system development. *Bone Marrow Transplantation*, **9**, (Suppl), 30–5.

DiGiusto, D., Chen, S., Combs, J. *et al.* (1994). Human fetal bone marrow early progenitors for T, B, and myeloid cells are found exclusively in the population expressing high levels of CD34. *Blood*, **84**, 421–32.

DiGiusto, D.L., Lee, R., Moon, J. *et al.* (1996). Hematopoietic potential of cryopreserved and ex vivo manipulated umbilical cord blood progenitor cells evaluated in vitro and in vivo. *Blood*, **87**, 1261–71.

Domen, J., Gandy, K.L., & Weissman, I.L. (1998). Systemic overexpression of BCL-2 in the hematopoietic system protects transgenic mice from the consequences of lethal irradiation. *Blood*, **91**, 2272–82.

Donahue, R.E., Kirby, M.R., Metzger, M.E. *et al.* (1996). Peripheral blood CD34+ cells differ from bone marrow CD34+ cells in Thy-1 expression and cell cycle status in nonhuman primates mobilized with granulocyte colony-stimulating factor and/or stem cell factor. *Blood*, **87**, 1644–53.

Dunbar, C.E., Seidel, N.E., Doren, S. *et al.* (1996). Improved retroviral gene transfer into murine and Rhesus peripheral blood or bone marrow repopulating cells primed in vivo with stem cell factor and granulocyte colony-stimulating factor. *Proceedings of the National Academy of Sciences USA*, **93**, 11871–6.

Dutton, R.W., Bradley, L.M., & Swain, S.L. (1998). T cell memory. *Annual Review of Immunology*, **16**, 201–23.

Eaves, C., Cashman, J. *et al.* (1991). Methodology of long-term culture of human hemopoietic cells. *Journal of Tissue Culture Methods*, **13**, 55–62.

Elhasid, R., Ben Arush, M.W., Katz, T. *et al.* (2000). Successful haploidentical bone marrow transplantation in Fanconi anemia. *Bone Marrow Transplantation*, **26**, 1221–3.

Erlich, H.A. (1991). HLA class II sequences and genetic susceptibility to insulin dependent diabetes mellitus. *Baillieres Clinical Endocrinology and Metabolism*, **5**, 395–411.

Ezine, S., Weissman, I.L., & Rouse, R.V. (1984). Bone marrow cells give rise to distinct cell clones within the thymus. *Nature*, **309**, 629–31.

Ferrara, J., Mauch, P., Murphy, G., & Burakoff, S.J. (1985). Bone marrow transplantation: the genetic and cellular basis of resistance to engraftment and acute graft-versus-host disease. *Survey of Immunological Research*, **4**, 253–63.

Fleming, W.H., Alpern, E.J., Uchida, N. *et al.* (1993). Functional heterogeneity is associated with the cell cycle status of murine hematopoietic stem cells. *Journal of Cellular Biology*, **122**, 897–902.

Gaines, B.A., Colson, Y.L., Kaufman, C.L., & Ildstad, S. (1996). Facilitating cells enable engraftment of purified fetal liver stem cells in allogeneic recipients. *Experimental Hematology*, **24**, 902–13.

Galy, A., Travis, M., Cen, D., & Chen, B. (1995). Human T, B, natural killer, and dendritic cells arise from a common bone marrow progenitor cell subset. *Immunity*, **3**, 459–73.

Gandy, K. & Weissman, I.L. (1997). Characterization of the mechanism of CD8+ facilitation of HSC engraftment across allogeneic barriers. *Blood*, **90**, 253a (Abstract).

Gandy, K.L., Mebius, R. *et al.* (1996). The facilitation of stem cell transplantation across allogeneic barriers in the rodent. 87th Annual Meeting of the American Association for Cancer Research, Washington, DC.

Gandy, K.L. & Weissman, I.L. (1998). Tolerance of allogeneic heart grafts in mice simultaneously reconstituted with purified allogeneic hematopoietic stem cells. *Transplantation*, **65**, 295–304.

Gazitt, Y., Reading, C.C., Hoffman, R. *et al.* (1995). Purified CD34+ Lin– Thy+ stem cells do not contain clonal myeloma cells. *Blood*, **86**, 381–9.

Godin, I., Garcia-Porrero, J., Coutinho, A. *et al.* (1993). Para-aortic splanchnopleura from early mouse embryos contains B1a progenitors. *Nature*, **364**, 67–70.

Goodell, M.A., Brose, K., Paradis, G. *et al.* (1996). Isolation and functional properties of murine hematopoietic stem cells that are replicating in vivo. *Journal of Experimental Medicine,* **183,** 1797–806.

Goodell, M.A., Rosenzweig, M., Kim, H. *et al.* (1997). Dye efflux studies suggest that hematopoietic stem cells expressing low or undetectable levels of CD34 antigen exist in multiple species. *Nature Medicine,* **3,** 1337–45.

Goodman, J. (1970). Stem cells circulating in the blood. *Revue Europeen D'Etudes Cliniques et Biologique,* **15,** 149–50.

Gorer, P.A., Lyman, S. *et al.* (1948). Studies on the genetic and antigenic basis of tumour transplantation. Linkage between a histocompatibility gene and "fuged" in mice. *Proceedings of the Royal Society of London,* **135,** 499.

Gorin, N.C., Lopez, M., Laporte, J.P. *et al.* (1995). Preparation and successful engraftment of purified CD34+ bone marrow progenitor cells in patients with non-Hodgkin's lymphoma. *Blood,* **85,** 1647–54.

Gothot, A., Pyatt, R., McMahel, J. *et al.* (1997). Functional heterogeneity of human CD34(+) cells isolated in subcompartments of the G0/G1 phase of the cell cycle. *Blood,* **90,** 4384–93.

Gunji, Y., Nakamura, M., Osawa, H. *et al.* (1993). Human primitive hematopoietic progenitor cells are more enriched in KITlow cells than in KIThigh cells. *Blood,* **82,** 3283–9.

Gussoni, E., Soneoka, Y., Strickland, C.D. *et al.* (1999). Dystrophin expression in the mdx mouse restored by stem cell transplantation. *Nature,* **401,** 390–4.

Hacein-Bey-Abina, S., Le Deist, F., Carlier, F. *et al.* (2002). Sustained correction of X-linked severe combined immunodeficiency by ex vivo gene therapy. *New England Journal of Medicine,* **346,** 1241–3.

Hadden, J.W., Malec, P.H., Coto, J., & Hadden, E.M. (1992). Thymic involution in aging. Prospects for correction. *Annals of the New York Academy of Sciences,* **673,** 231–9.

Hamann, D., Baars, P.A., Rep, M.H. *et al.* (1997). Phenotypic and functional separation of memory and effector human CD8+ T cells. *Journal of Experimental Medicine,* **186,** 1407–18.

Handgretinger, R., Lang, P., Schumm, M. *et al.* (1998). Isolation and transplantation of autologous peripheral CD34+ progenitor cells highly purified by magnetic-activated cell sorting. *Bone Marrow Transplantation,* **21,** 987–93.

Hardy, R.R. & Hayakawa, K. (1992). Generation of Ly-1 B cells from developmentally distinct precursors: enrichment by stromal cell culture or cell sorting. CD5 B cells in development and disease. *Annals of the New York Academy of Sciences,* **651,** 99–111.

Harrison, D.E. & Astle, C.M. (1982). Loss of stem cell repopulating ability upon transplantation: effects of donor age, cell number, and transplantation procedure. *Journal of Experimental Medicine,* **156,** 1767–79.

Hayflick, L. (1965). The limited in vitro lifetime of human diploid cell strains. *Experimental Cell Research,* **37,** 614–36.

Herzenberg, L.A., Kantor, A.B., & Herzenberg, L.A. (1992). Layered evolution in the immune system: a model for the ontogeny and development of multiple lymphocyte lineages. *Annals of the New York Academy of Sciences,* **651,** 1–9.

Hill, B., Rozler, E., Travis, M. *et al.* (1996). High-level expression of a novel epitope of CD59 identifies a subset of CD34+ bone marrow cells highly enriched for pluripotent stem cells. *Experimental Hematology,* **24,** 936–43.

Hodgson, G.S. & Bradley, T.R. (1979). Properties of haematopoietic stem cells surviving 5-fluorouracil treatment: evidence for a pre-CFU-S cell? *Nature,* **281,** 381–2.

Huang, H. & Auerbach, R. (1993). Identification and characterization of hematopoietic stem cells from the yolk sac of the early mouse embryo. *Proceedings of the National Academy of Sciences USA,* **90,** 10110–14.

Humeau, L., Bardin, F., Maroc, C. *et al.* (1996). Phenotypic, molecular, and functional characterization of human peripheral blood CD34+/THY1+ cells. *Blood,* **87,** 949–55.

Ikehara, S. (1998). Bone marrow transplantation for autoimmune diseases. *Acta Haematologica,* **99,** 116–32.

Ikehara, S., Good, R., Nakamura, T. *et al.* (1985). Rationale for bone marrow transplantation in the treatment of autoimmune disease. *Proceedings of the National Academy of Sciences USA,* **82,** 2483–6.

Ikehara, S., Ohtsuki, H., Good, R.A. *et al.* (1985). Prevention of type I diabetes in nonobese diabetic mice by allogeneic bone marrow transplantation. *Proceedings of the National Academy of Sciences USA,* **82,** 7743.

Ikuta, K., Kina, T., MacNeil, I. *et al.* (1990). A developmental switch in thymic lymphocyte maturation potential occurs at the level of hematopoietic stem cells. *Cell,* **62,** 863–74.

Ikuta, K., Uchida, N., Friedman, J., & Weissman, I.L. (1992). Lymphocyte development from stem cells. *Annual Review of Immunology,* **10,** 759–83.

Ildstad, S.T., Wren, S.M., Bluestone, J.A. *et al.* (1986). Effect of selective T cell depletion of host and/or donor bone marrow on lymphopoietic repopulation, tolerance, and graft-vs-host disease in mixed allogeneic chimeras (B10+B10.D2—B10). *Journal of Immunology,* **136,** 28–33.

Jackson, K.A., Mi, T., & Goodell, M.A. (1999). Hematopoietic potential of stem cells isolated from murine skeletal muscle. *Proceedings of the National Academy of Sciences USA,* **96,** 14482–6.

Jones, R.J., Wagner, J.E., Celano, P. *et al.* (1990). Separation of pluripotent haematopoietic stem cells from spleen colony-forming cells. *Nature,* **347,** 188–9.

Juttner, C. & To, L. (1994). Autologous peripheral blood stem cell transplantation: potential advantages, practical considerations and initial clinical results. In *Clinical Bone Marrow Transplantation,* ed. K. Atkinson, pp. 142–152. Cambridge: Cambridge University Press.

Juttner, C., To, L., Haylock, D.N., Branford, A., & Kimber, R.J. (1985). Circulating autologous stem cells collected in very early remission from acute non-lymphoblastic leukaemia produce prompt but incomplete haemopoietic reconstitution after high dose melphalan or supralethal chemoradiotherapy. *British Journal of Haematology,* **61,** 739–45.

Kafri, T., Blomer, U., Peterson, D.A. *et al.* (1997). Sustained expression of genes delivered directly into liver and muscle by lentiviral vectors. *Nature Genetics,* **17,** 314–17.

Kamel-Reid, S. & Dick, J. (1988). Engraftment of immune-deficient mice with human hematopoietic cells. *Science,* **241,** 1706–9.

Kanegane, H., Kasahara, Y., Niida, Y. *et al.* (1996). Expression of L-selectin (CD62L) discriminates Th1-and Th2-like cytokine-producing memory CD4+ T cells. *Immunology,* **87,** 186–90.

Kaufman, C.L., Colson, Y.L., Wren, S.M. *et al.* (1994). Phenotypic characterization of a novel bone marrow-derived cell that facilitates engraftment of allogeneic bone marrow stem cells. *Blood,* **84,** 2436–46.

Kawada, H. & Ogawa, M. (2001). Bone marrow origin of hematopoietic progenitors and stem cells in murine muscle. *Blood,* **98,** 2008–13.

Kay, H.E.M. (1965). How many cell-generations? *Lancet,* **2,** 418–19.

Kessinger, A., Armitage, J.O., Landmark, J.D. *et al.* (1988). Autologous peripheral hematopoietic stem cell transplantation restores hematopoietic function following marrow ablative therapy. *Blood,* **71,** 723–7.

Kim, N.W., Piatyszek, M.A., Prowse, K.R. *et al.* (1994). Specific association of human telomerase activity with immortal cells and cancer. *Science,* **266,** 2011–15.

Klug, C.A., Cheshier, S., & Weissman, I.L. (2000). Inactivation of a GFP retrovirus occurs at multiple levels in long-term repopulating stem cells and their differentiated progeny. *Blood,* **96,** 894–901.

Kondo, M., Weissman, I.L., & Akashi, K. (1997). Identification of clonogenic common lymphoid progenitor in mouse bone marrow. *Cell,* **91,** 661–72.

Korbling, M., Katz, R.L., Khanna, A. *et al.* (2002). Hepatocytes and epithelial cells of donor origin in recipients of peripheral-blood stem cells. *New England Journal of Medicine,* **346,** 738–746.

Krause, D.S., Donnelly, D.S., Sharkis, S., & Zelterman, D. (1999). Functional activity of murine CD34+ and CD34– hematopoietic stem cell populations. *Experimental Hematology,* **27,** 788–96.

Krause, D.S., Ito, T., Fackler, M.J. *et al.* (1994). Characterization of murine CD34, a marker for hematopoietic progenitor and stem cells. *Blood,* **84,** 691–701.

Kyba, M., Perlingeiro, R.C., & Daley, G.Q. (2002). HoxB4 confers definitive lymphoid-myeloid engraftment potential on embryonic stem cell and yolk sac hematopoietic progenitors. *Cell,* **109,** 29–37.

Kyoizumi, S., Baum, C.M., Kaneshima, H. *et al.* (1992). Implantation and maintenance of functional human bone marrow in SCID-hu mice. *Blood,* **79,** 1704.

Ladd, A.C., Pyatt, R., Gothot, A. *et al.* (1997). Orderly process of sequential cytokine stimulation is required for activation and maximal proliferation of primitive human bone marrow CD34+ hematopoietic progenitor cells residing in G_0. *Blood,* **90,** 658–68.

LaFace, D.M. & Peck, A.B. (1989). Reciprocal allogeneic bone marrow transplantation between NOD mice and diabetes-nonsusceptible mice associated with transfer and prevention of autoimmune diabetes. *Diabetes,* **38,** 894–901.

Lansdorp, P.M., Sutherland, H.J., & Eaves, C.J. (1990). Selective expression of CD45 isoforms on functional subpopulations of CD34+ hemopoietic cells from human bone marrow. *Journal of Experimental Medicine,* **172,** 363–6.

Lansdorp, P.M., Poon, S., Chavez, E. *et al.* (1997). Telomeres in the haemopoietic system. *Ciba Foundation Symposium,* **211,** 209–18; discussion 219–22.

Lapidot, T., Pflumio, F., Doedens, M. *et al.* (1992). Cytokine stimulation of multilineage hematopoiesis from immature human cells engrafted in SCID mice. *Science,* **255,** 1137–41.

Larochelle, A., Vormoor, J., Hanenberg, H. *et al.* (1996). Identification of primitive human hematopoietic cells capable of repopulating NOD/SCID mouse bone marrow: implications for gene therapy. *Nature Medicine,* **2,** 1329–37.

Laterveer, L., Lindley, I.J., Hamilton, M.S. *et al.* (1995). Interleukin-8 induces rapid mobilization of hematopoietic stem cells with radioprotective capacity and long-term myelolymphoid repopulating ability. *Blood,* **85,** 2269–75.

Leclercq, G. & Plum, J. (1996). Thymic and extrathymic T cell development. *Leukemia,* **10,** 1853–9.

Lemischka, I.R., Raulet, D.H., & Mulligan, R.C. (1986). Developmental potential and dynamic behavior of hematopoietic stem cells. *Cell,* **45,** 917–27.

Lévesque, J.P., Takamatsu, Y., Nilsson, S.K. *et al.* (2001). Vascular cell adhesion molecule-1 (CD106) is cleaved by neutrophil proteases in the bone marrow following hematopoietic progenitor cell mobilization by granulocyte colony-stimulating factor. *Blood,* **98,** 1289–97.

Libich, M., Majsky, A., & Bartsch, D. (1975). HLA-B 27 (W 27) antigen and other immunological factors in ankylosing spondylarthritis. *Casopis Lekaru Ceskych,* **114,** 1521–3.

Mackall, C.L. & Gress, R.E. (1997). Thymic aging and T-cell regeneration. *Immunological Reviews,* **160,** 91–102.

Main, J.M. & Prehn, R.T. (1955). Successful skin homografts after the administration of high dosage x-radiation and homologous bone marrow. *Journal of the National Cancer Institute,* **15,** 1023–9.

Makino, Y., Yamagata, N., Sasho, T. *et al.* (1993). Extrathymic development of V alpha 14-positive T cells. *Journal of Experimental Medicine,* **177,** 1399–408.

Manz, M.G., Miyamoto, T., Akashi, K., & Weissman, I.L. (2002). Prospective isolation of human clonogenic common myeloid progenitors. *Proceedings of the National Academy of Sciences USA,* **99,** 11872–7.

Marmont, A.M. (1997). Stem cell transplantation for severe autoimmune disorders, with special reference to rheumatic diseases. *Journal of Rheumatology,* **48**(Suppl), 13–18.

Martin, P.J. (1993). Donor CD8 cells prevent allogeneic marrow graft rejection in mice: potential implications for marrow transplantation in humans. *Journal of Experimental Medicine,* **178,** 703–12.

Maurer-Schultze, B., Siebert, M., & Bassukas, I.D. (1988). An in vivo study on the synchronizing effect of hydroxyurea. *Experimental Cellular Research,* **174,** 230–43.

McCulloch, E.A. & Till, J.E. (1963). Repression of colony-forming ability of C57BL hematopoietic cells transplanted into non-isologous hosts. *Journal of Cellular and Comparative Physiology,* **61,** 301–8.

McCune, J.M., Namikawa, R., Kaneshima, H. *et al.* (1988). The SCID-hu mouse: murine model for the analysis of human hematolymphoid differentiation and function. *Science,* **241,** 1632–9.

Medvinsky, A. & Dzierzak, E. (1996). Definitive hematopoiesis is autonomous initiated by the AGM region. *Cell,* **86,** 897–906.

Medvinsky, A.L., Samoylina, N.L., Muller, A.M., & Dzierzak, E.A. (1993). An early pre-liver intra-embryonic source of CFU-S in the developing mouse. *Nature,* **364,** 64–7.

Metcalf, D. & Moore, M. (1971). *Haemopoietic Cells.* New York: North-Holland Publishing.

Meyne, J., Ratliff, R.L., & Moyzis, R.K. (1989). Conservation of the human telomere sequence (TTAGGG)n among vertebrates. *Proceedings of the National Academy of Sciences USA,* **86,** 7049–53.

Michallet, M., Philip, T., Philip, I. *et al.* (2000). Transplantation with selected autologous peripheral blood CD34+Thy1+ hematopoietic stem cells (HSCs) in multiple myeloma: impact of HSC dose on engraftment, safety, and immune reconstitution. *Experimental Hematology*, **28**, 858–870.

Micklem, H.S., Ansell, J.D., Wayman, J.E., & Forrester, L. (1983). The clonal organization of hematopoiesis in the mouse. In *Progress in Immunology*, ed. V.Y. Yamamura & T. Tada, pp. 633–44. Tokyo: Academic Press Japan.

Miraglia, S., Godfrey, W., Yin, A.H. *et al.* (1997). A novel five-transmembrane hematopoietic stem cell antigen: isolation, characterization, and molecular cloning. *Blood*, **90**, 5013–21.

Miyoshi, H., Takahashi, M., Gaga, F.H., & Verma, I.M. (1997). Stable and efficient gene transfer into the retina using an HIV-based lentiviral vector. *Proceedings of the National Academy of Sciences USA*, **94**, 10319–23.

Moore, M.A.S. & Metcalf, D. (1970). Ontogeny of the haemopoietic system: yolk sac origin of in vivo and in vitro colony forming cells in the developing mouse embryo. *British Journal of Haematology*, **18**, 279–96.

Morel, F., Galy, A., Chen, B., & Szilvassy, S.J. (1998). Equal distribution of competitive long-term repopulating stem cells in the CD34+ and CD34– fractions of Thy-1lowLin-/lowSca-1+ bone marrow cells. *Experimental Hematology*, **26**, 440–8.

Morel, F., Szilvassy, S.J., Travis, M. *et al.* (1996). Primitive hematopoietic cells in murine bone marrow express the CD34 antigen. *Blood*, **88**, 3774–84.

Morrison, S.J., Prowse, K.R., Ho, P., & Weissman, I.L. (1996). Telomerase activity in hematopoietic cells is associated with self-renewal potential. *Immunity*, **5**, 207–16.

Morrison, S.J., Uchida, N., & Weissman, I.L. (1995). The biology of hematopoietic stem cells. *Annual Review of Cellular and Developmental Biology*, **11**, 35–71.

Morrison, S.J., Hemmati, H.D., Wandycz, A.M., & Weissman, I.L. (1995). The purification and characterization of fetal liver hematopoietic stem cells. *Proceedings of the National Academy of Sciences USA*, **92**, 10302–6.

Morrison, S.J., Wandycz, A.M., Akashi, K. *et al.* (1996). The aging of hematopoietic stem cells. *Nature Medicine*, **2**, 1011–16.

Morrison, S.J., Wandycz, A.M., Hemmati, H.D. *et al.* (1997). Identification of a lineage of multipotent hematopoietic progenitors. *Development*, **124**, 1929–39.

Morrison, S.J. & Weissman, I.L. (1994). The long-term repopulating subset of hematopoietic stem cells is deterministic and isolatable by phenotype. *Immunity*, **1**, 661–73.

Morrison, S.J., Wright, D.E., & Weissman, I.L. (1997). Cyclophosphamide/G-CSF induces hematopoietic stem cells to proliferate prior to mobilization. *Proceedings of the National Academy of Sciences USA*, **94**, 1908–13.

Morshead, C.M., Benveniste, P., Iscove, N.N., & van der Kooy, D. (2002). Hematopoietic competence is a rare property of neural stem cells that may depend on genetic and epigenetic alterations. *Nature Medicine*, **8**, 268–273.

Moyzis, R.K., Buckingham, J.M., Cram, L.S. *et al.* (1988). A highly conserved repetitive DNA sequence, (TTAGGG)n, present at the telomeres of human chromosomes. *Proceedings of the National Academy of Sciences USA*, **85**, 6622–6.

Müller-Sieburg, C.E., Whitlock, C.A., & Weissman, I.L. (1986). Isolation of two early B lymphocyte progenitors from mouse marrow: a committed pre-pre-B cell and a clonogenic Thy-1lo hematopoietic stem cell. *Cell*, **44**, 653–62.

Murray, L., Chen, B., Galy, A. *et al.* (1995). Enrichment of human hematopoietic stem cell activity in the CD34+Thy-1+Lin-subpopulation from mobilized peripheral blood. *Blood*, **85**, 368–78.

Naldini, L., Blomer, U., Gallay, P. *et al.* (1996). In vivo gene delivery and stable transduction of nondividing cells by a lentiviral vector. *Science*, **272**, 263–7.

Negrin, R.S., Atkinson, K., Leemhuis, T. *et al.* (2000). Transplantation of highly purified CD34+Thy-1+ hematopoietic stem cells in patients with metastatic breast cancer. *Biology of Blood and Marrow Transplantation*, **6**, 262–71.

Nibley, W.E. & Spangrude, G.J. (1998). Primitive stem cells alone mediate rapid marrow recovery and multilineage engraftment after transplantation. *Bone Marrow Transplantation*, **21**, 345–54.

Nolta, J.A., Dao, M.A., Wells, S. *et al.* (1996). Transduction of pluripotent human hematopoietic stem cells demonstrated by clonal analysis after engraftment in immune-deficient mice. *Proceedings of the National Academy of Sciences USA*, **93**, 2414–19.

Ogawa, M., Porter, P.N., & Nakahata, T. (1983). Renewal and commitment to differentiation of hemopoietic stem cells. *Blood*, **61**, 823–7.

Ogawa, M., Tajima, F., Ito, T. *et al.* (2001). CD34 expression by murine hematopoietic stem cells. Developmental changes and kinetic alterations. *Annals of the New York Academy of Sciences*, **938**, 139–45.

Okuno, Y., Iwasaki, H., Huettner, C.S. *et al.* (2002). Differential regulation of the human and murine CD34 genes in hematopoietic stem cells. *Proceedings of the National Academy of Sciences USA*, **99**, 6246–51.

Orlic, D., Anderson, S., & Bodine, D.M. (1994). Biological properties of subpopulations of pluripotent hematopoietic stem cells enriched by elutriation and flow cytometry. *Blood Cells*, **20**, 107–17; discussion 118–20.

Osawa, M., Hanada, K., Hamada, H., & Nakauchi, H. (1996). Long-term lymphohematopoietic reconstitution by a single CD34-low/negative hematopoietic stem cell. *Science*, **273**, 242–5.

Papayannopoulou, T. & Craddock, C. (1997). Homing and trafficking of hemopoietic progenitor cells. *Acta Haematologica*, **97**, 97–104.

Papayannopoulou, T., Craddock, C., Nakamoto, B. *et al.* (1995). The VLA4/VCAM-1 adhesion pathway defines contrasting mechanisms of lodgement of transplanted murine hemopoietic progenitors between bone marrow and spleen. *Proceedings of the National Academy of Sciences USA*, **92**, 9647–51.

Parrado, A., Casares, S., Prieto, J. *et al.* (1997). Repopulation of circulating T, B and NK lymphocytes following bone marrow and blood stem cell transplantation. *Hematology and Cell Therapy*, **39**, 301–6.

Peault, B., Weissman, I.L., Baum, C. *et al.* (1991). Lymphoid reconstitution of the human fetal thymus in SCID mice with CD34+ precursor cells. *Journal of Experimental Medicine*, **174**, 1283.

Peters, C., Shapiro, E.G., Anderson, J. *et al.* (1998). Hurler syndrome: II. Outcome of HLA-genotypically identical sibling and HLA-haploidentical related donor bone marrow transplantation in fifty-four children. The Storage Disease Collaborative Study Group. *Blood*, **91**, 2601–8.

Petzer, A.L., Zandstra, P.W., Piret, J.M., & Eaves, C.J. (1996). Differential cytokine effects on primitive (CD34+CD38–) human hematopoietic cells: novel responses to Flt3-ligand and thrombopoietin. *Journal of Experimental Medicine*, **183**, 2551–8.

Plavec, I., Agarwal, M., Ho, K.E. *et al.* (1997). High transdominant RevM10 protein levels are required to inhibit HIV-1 replication in cell lines and primary T cells: implication for gene therapy of AIDS. *Gene Therapy, 4, 128–39.

Ploemacher, R.E. & Brons, N.H. (1988). Isolation of hemopoietic stem cell subsets from murine bone marrow: II. Evidence for an early precursor of day-12 CFU-S and cells associated with radio-protective ability. *Experimental Hematology, 16, 27–32.

Ploemacher, R.E., van der Sluijs, J.P., van Beurden, C.A. *et al.* (1991). Use of limiting-dilution type long-term marrow cultures in frequency analysis of marrow-repopulating and spleen colony-forming hematopoietic stem cell in the mouse. *Blood, 78, 2527–33.

Prosper, F., Stroncek, D., & Verfaillie, C.M. (1996). Phenotypic and functional characterization of long-term culture-initiating cells present in peripheral blood progenitor collections of normal donors treated with granulocyte colony-stimulating factor. *Blood, 88, 2033–42.

Pruijt, J.F.M., Verzaal, P., van Os, R. *et al.* (2002). Neutrophils are indispensable for hematopoietic stem cell mobilization induced by interleukin-8 in mice. *Proceedings of the National Academy of Sciences USA, 99, 6228–33.

Quesenberry, P.J., Stewart, M.F., Peters, S. *et al.* (1997). Engraftment of hematopoietic stem cells in nonmyeloablated and myeloablated hosts. *Stem Cells, 15(Suppl 1), 167–9; discussion 169–70.

Rachamim, N., Gan, J., Segall, H. *et al.* (1998). Tolerance induction by "megadose" hematopoietic transplants: donor-type human CD34 stem cells induce potent specific reduction of host anti-donor cytotoxic T lymphocyte precursors in mixed lymphocyte culture. *Transplantation, 65, 1386–93.

Randall, T., Lund, F., Howard, M.C., & Weissman, I.L. (1996). Expression of murine CD38 defines a population of long-term reconstituting hematopoietic stem cells. *Blood, 87, 4057–67.

Randall, T.D. & Weissman, I.L. (1997). Phenotypic and functional changes induced at the clonal level in hematopoietic stem cells after 5-fluorouracil treatment. *Blood, 89, 3596–606.

Reading, C.L. (1996). Does CD34+ cell selection enrich malignant stem cells in B cell (and other) malignancies? [letter]. *Journal of Hematotherapy, 5, 97–8.

Reisner, Y. & Martelli, M.F. (2000). Transplantation tolerance induced by "mega dose" CD34+ cell transplants. *Experimental Hematology, 28, 119–27.

Richman, C., Weiner, R., & Yankee, R.A. (1976). Increase in circulating stem cells following chemotherapy in man. *Blood, 47, 1031–9.

Rizzato, G. & Montemurro, L. (1998). Clinical spectrum of extrapulmonary sarcoidosis. From the onset to organ transplantation [editorial]. *Recent Progress in Medicine, 89, 82–6.

Roe, T., Reynolds, T.C., Yu, G., & Brown, P.O. (1993). Integration of murine leukemia virus DNA depends on mitosis. *Embo Journal, 12, 2099–108.

Ruggeri, L., Capanni, M., Urbani, E. *et al.* (2002). Effectiveness of donor natural killer cell alloreactivity in mismatched hematopoietic transplants. *Science, 295, 2029–31.

Russell, E. & Bernstein, S. (1966). Blood and blood formation. In *Biology of the Laboratory Mouse,* ed. E. Green, pp. 88–120. New York: McGraw-Hill.

Sachs, D.H., Sykes, M., Greenstein, J.L., & Cosimi, A.B. (1995). Tolerance and xenograft survival. *Nature Medicine, 1, 969.

Sanchez, M.-J., Holmes, A., Miles, C., & Dzierzak, E. (1996). Characterization of the first definitive hematopoietic stem cells in the AGM and liver of the mouse embryo. *Immunity, 5, 513–25.

Sauvageau, G., Thorsteinsdottir, U., Eaves, C.J. *et al.* (1995). Overexpression of HOXB4 in hematopoietic cells causes the selective expansion of more primitive populations in vitro and in vivo. *Genes and Development, 9, 1753–1765.

Shizuru, J., Edwards, C. *et al.* (1995). Transplantation of purified hematopoietic stem cells across allogeneic barriers in spontaneous autoimmune diabetic (NOD) mice. *Blood, 86, 573a (abstract).

Shizuru, J., Weissman, I.L., Kernoff, R. *et al.* (2000). Purified hematopoietic stem cell grafts induce tolerance to alloantigens and can mediate positive and negative T cell selection. *Proceedings of the National Academy of Sciences USA, 97, 9555–60.

Shizuru, J.A., Jerabek, L., Edwards, C.T., & Weissman, I.L. (1996). Transplantation of purified hematopoietic stem cells: requirements for overcoming the barriers of allogeneic engraftment. *Biology of Blood and Marrow Transplantation, 2, 3–14.

Siena, S., Bregni, M., Brando, B. *et al.* (1989). Circulation of CD34+ hematopoietic stem cells in the peripheral blood of high-dose cyclophosphamide-treated patients: enhancement by intravenous recombinant human granulocyte-macrophage colony-stimulating factor. *Blood, 74, 1905–14.

Siminovitch, L., McCulloch, E.A., & Till, J.E. (1963). The distribution of colony-forming cells among spleen colonies. *Journal of Cellular Comparative Physiology, 62, 327–36.

Siminovitch, L., Till, J., & McCulloch, E.A. (1964). Decline in colony forming ability of marrow cells subjected to serial transplantation into irradiated mice. *Journal of Cellular Comparative Physiology, 64, 23.

Slattery, R.M. & Miller, J.F. (1996). Influence of T lymphocytes and major histocompatibility complex class II genes on diabetes susceptibility in the NOD mouse. *Current Topics in Microbiology and Immunology, 206, 51–66.

Smith, L.G., Weissman, I., & Heimfeld, S. (1991). Clonal analysis of hematopoietic stem-cell differentiation in vivo. *Proceedings of the National Academy of Sciences USA, 88, 2788–92.

Sorrentino, B.P., Brandt, S.J., Bodine, D. *et al.* (1992). Selection of drug-resistant bone marrow cells in vivo after retroviral transfer of human MDR1. *Science, 257, 99–103.

Spangrude, G.J. & Brooks, D.M. (1992). Phenotypic analysis of mouse hematopoietic stem cells shows a Thy-1-negative subset. *Blood, 80, 1957–64.

Spangrude, G.J. & Brooks, D.M. (1993). Mouse strain variability in the expression of the hematopoietic stem cell antigen Ly-6A/E by bone marrow cells. *Blood, 82, 3327–32.

Spangrude, G.J., Heimfeld, S., & Weissman, I.L. (1988). Purification and characterization of mouse hematopoietic stem cells. *Science* (Washington DC), 241, 58–62.

Spangrude, G.J. & Johnson, G.R. (1990). Resting and activated subsets of mouse multipotent hematopoietic stem cells. *Proceedings of the National Academy of Sciences USA, 87, 7433–7.

Srour, E.F., Brandt, J.E., Leemhuis, T. *et al.* (1992). Relationship between cytokine-dependent cell cycle progression and MHC class II antigen expression by human CD34+ HLA-DR-bone marrow cells. *Journal of Immunology, 148, 815–20.

Srour, E., Zanjani, E., Brandt, J.E. *et al.* (1992). Sustained human hematopoiesis in sheep transplanted in utero during early gestation with fractionated adult human bone marrow cells. *Blood,* **79,** 1404–12.

Steen, R. & Egeland, T. (1998). CD34 molecule epitope distribution on cells of haematopoietic origin. *Leukemia and Lymphoma,* **30,** 23–30.

Strauss, L.C., Rowley, S.D. *et al.* (1986). Antigenic analysis of hematopoiesis. V. Characterization of My-10 antigen expression by normal lymphohematopoietic progenitor cells. *Experimental Hematology,* **14,** 878–86.

Sutherland, H.J., Lansdorp, P.M., Henkelman, D.H. *et al.* (1990). Functional characterization of individual human hematopoietic stem cells cultured at limiting dilution on supportive marrow stromal layers. *Proceedings of the National Academy of Sciences USA,* **87,** 3584–8.

Sutherland, D.R., Yeo, E.L., Stewart, A.K. *et al.* (1996). Identification of CD34+ subsets after glycoprotease selection: engraftment of CD34+Thy-1+Lin-stem cells in fetal sheep. *Experimental Hematology,* **24,** 795–806.

Sykes, M., Chester, C.H., Sundt, T.M. *et al.* (1989). Effects of T cell depletion in radiation bone marrow chimeras. III. Characterization of allogeneic bone marrow cell populations that increase allogeneic chimerism independently of graft-vs-host disease in mixed marrow recipients. *Journal of Immunology,* **143,** 3503–11.

Sykes, M. & Sachs, D.H. (1990). Bone marrow transplantation as a means of inducing tolerance. *Seminars in Immunology,* **2,** 401–17.

Sykes, M., Sheard, M., & Sachs, D.H. (1988). Effects of T cell depletion in radiation bone marrow chimeras. I. Evidence for a donor cell population which increases allogeneic chimerism but which lacks the potential to produce GVHD. *Journal of Immunology,* **141,** 2282–8.

Szilvassy, S.J., Weller, K.P., Chen, B. *et al.* (1996). Partially differentiated ex vivo expanded cells accelerate hematologic recovery in myeloablated mice transplanted with highly enriched long-term repopulating stem cells. *Blood,* **88,** 3642–53.

Tajima, F., Deguchi, T., Laver, J.H. *et al.* (2001). Reciprocal expression of CD38 and CD34 by adult murine hematopoietic stem cells. *Blood,* **97,** 2618–24.

Terada, N., Hamazaki, T., Oka, M. *et al.* (2002). Bone marrow cells adopt the phenotype of other cells by spontaneous cell fusion. *Nature,* **416,** 542–545.

Terstappen, L.W., Huang, S., Safford, M. *et al.* (1991). Sequential generations of hematopoietic colonies derived from single non-lineage-committed CD34+CD38- progenitor cells. *Blood,* **77,** 1218–27.

Thomas, E.D. (1995). Bone marrow transplantation from bench to bedside. *Annals of the New York Academy of Sciences,* **770,** 34–41.

Thomas, E.D., Lochte, H.L. Jr., Lu, W.C., & Ferrebee, J.W. (1957). Intravenous infusion of bone marrow in patients receiving radiation and chemotherapy. *New England Journal of Medicine,* **257,** 491–6.

Till, J.E. & McCulloch, E.A. (1961). A direct measurement of the radiation sensitivity of normal mouse bone marrow cells. *Radiation Research,* **14,** 213–23.

Till, J.E., McCulloch, E.A., & Siminovitch, L. (1964). A stochastic model of stem cell proliferation based on the growth of colony-forming cells. *Proceedings of the National Academy of Sciences USA,* **51,** 29–36.

Todd, J.A., Bell, J.I., & McDevitt, H.O. (1987). HLA DQ β gene contributes to suceptibility and resistance to insulin dependent diabetes. *Nature,* **329,** 599.

Traycoff, C.M., Abboud, M.R., Laver, J. *et al.* (1994). Rapid exit from G0/G1 phases of cell cycle in response to stem cell factor confers on umbilical cord blood CD34+ cells an enhanced ex vivo expansion potential. *Experimental Hematology,* **22,** 1264–72.

Trinchieri, G. (1989). Biology of natural killer cells. *Advances in Immunology,* **47,** 187–376.

Tsukamoto, A., Weissman, I. *et al.* (1995). Phenotypic and functional analysis of hematopoietic stem cells in mouse and human. In *Hematopoietic Stem Cells: Biology and Therapeutic Applications,* ed. D. Levitt & R. Mertelsmann, pp. 85–124. Marcel Dekker, New York.

Tyndall, A. (1997). Hematopoietic stem cell transplantation in rheumatic diseases other than systemic sclerosis and systemic lupus erythematosus. *Journal of Rheumatology,* **48**(Suppl), 94–7.

Uchida, N. (1992). Characterization of mouse hematopoietic stem cells. Ph.D. Thesis, Stanford University.

Uchida, N., Aguila, H.L., Fleming, W.H., Jerebek, L., & Weissman, I.L. (1994). Rapid and sustained hematopoietic recovery in lethally irradiated mice transplanted with purified Thy-1.1lo Lin-Sca-1+ hematopoietic stem cells. *Blood,* **83,** 3758–79.

Uchida, N., Combs, J., Chen, S. *et al.* (1996). Primitive human hematopoietic cells displaying differential efflux of the rhodamine 123 dye have distinct biological activities. *Blood,* **88,** 1297–305.

Uchida, N., Fleming, W.H., Alpern, E.J., & Weissman, I.L. (1993). Heterogeneity of hematopoietic stem cells. *Current Opinions in Immunology,* **5,** 177–84.

Uchida, N., Friera, A.M., He, D. *et al.* (1997). Hydroxyurea can be used to increase mouse c-kit+Thy-1. 1(lo)Lin-/loSca- 1(+) hematopoietic cell number and frequency in cell cycle in vivo. *Blood,* **90,** 4354–62.

Uchida, N., He, D., Friera, A.M. *et al.* (1997). The unexpected G0/G1 cell cycle status of mobilized hematopoietic stem cells from peripheral blood. *Blood,* **89,** 465–72.

Uchida, N., Jerabek, L., & Weissman, I.L. (1996). Searching for hematopoietic stem cells. II. The heterogeneity of Thy-1.1(lo)Lin(–/lo)Sca-1+ mouse hematopoietic stem cells separated by counterflow centrifugal elutriation. *Experimental Hematology,* **24,** 649–59.

Uchida, N., Sutton, R.E., Friera, A.M. *et al.* (1998). HIV, but not murine leukemia virus vectors mediate high efficiency gene transfer into freshly isolated G0/G1 human hematopoietic stem cells. *Proceedings of the National Academy of Sciences USA,* **95,** 11939–44.

Uchida, N., Tsukamoto, A., He, D. *et al.* (1998). High doses of purified stem cells cause early hematopoietic recovery in syngeneic and allogeneic hosts. *Journal of Clinical Investigation,* **101,** 961–6.

Uchida, N., Yang, Z., Combs, J. *et al.* (1997). The characterization, molecular cloning, and expression of a novel hematopoietic cell antigen from CD34+ human bone marrow cells. *Blood,* **89,** 2706–16.

Uchida, N. & Weissman, I.L. (1992). Searching for hematopoietic stem cells: evidence that Thy-1. 1lo Lin- Sca-1+ cells are the only stem cells in C57BL/Ka-Thy-1.1 bone marrow. *Journal of Experimental Medicine*, **175**, 175–84.

Udomsakdi, C., Eaves, C.J., Sutherland, H.J., & Lansdorp, P.M. (1991). Separation of functionally distinct subpopulations of primitive human hematopoietic cells using rhodamine-123. *Experimental Hematology*, **19**, 338–42.

Vallera, D.A., Soderling, C.C., Carlson, G.J., & Kersey, J.H. (1981). Bone marrow transplantation across major histocompatibility barriers in mice. Effect of elimination of T cells from donor grafts by treatment with monoclonal Thy-1.2 plus complement or antibody alone. *Transplantation*, **31**, 218–22.

van de Rijn, M., Heimfeld, S., Spangrude, G.J., & Weissman, I.L. (1989). Mouse hematopoietic stem-cell antigen Sca-1 is a member of the Ly-6 antigen family. *Proceedings of the National Academy of Sciences USA*, **86**, 4634–8.

Visser, J.W., Bauman, J.G.J., Mulder, A.H. *et al.* (1984). Isolation of murine pluripotent hemopoietic stem cells. *Journal of Experimental Medicine*, **159**, 1576–90.

Visser, J.W.M. & Van Bekkum, D.W. (1990). Purification of pluripotent hemopoietic stem cells. *Experimental Hematology*, **18**, 248–56.

von Melchner, H. & Barlett, P.F. (1983). Mechanisms of early allogeneic marrow graft rejection. *Immunological Reviews*, **71**, 31–56.

Wagers, A.J., Sherwood, R.I., Christensen, J.L., & Weissman, I.L. (2002). Cell fate potential of single, transplanted adult c-kit+Thy-1.1loLin-Sca-1+ hematopoietic stem cells: little evidence for lineage plasticity (submitted).

Waller, E.K., Huang, S., & Terstappen, L. (1995). Changes in the growth properties of CD34+, CD38– bone marrow progenitors during human fetal development. *Blood*, **86**, 710–18.

Watson, J.D. (1972). Origin of concatameric T4 DNA. *Nature New Biology*, **239**, 197–201.

Weilbaecher, K., Weissman, I., Blume, K., & Heimfeld, S. (1991). Culture of phenotypically defined hematopoietic stem cells and other progenitors at limiting dilution on Dexter monolayers. *Blood*, **78**, 945–52.

Weissman, I., Papaioannou, V., & Gardner, R. (1978). Fetal hematopoietic orgins of the adult hematolymphoid system. In *Cold Spring Harbor Conferences on Cell Proliferation. Vol 5: Differentiation of Normal and Neoplastic Hematopoietic Cells*, ed. B. Clarkson, P. Mark, & J. Till, pp. 33–47. New York: Cold Spring Harbor Lab.

Wicker, L.S., Todd, J.A., & Peterson, L.B. (1995). Genetic control of autoimmune diabetes in the NOD mouse. *Annual Review of Immunology*, **13**, 179–200.

Worton, R.G., McCulloch, E.A., & Till, J.E. (1969). Physical separation of hematopoietic stem cells from cells forming colonies in culture. *Journal for Cellular Physiology*, **74**, 171–81.

Wright, D.E., Cheshier, S.H., Wagers, A.J. *et al.* (2001). Cyclophosphamide/granulocyte colony-stimulating factor causes selective mobilization of bone marrow hematopoietic stem cells into the blood after M phase of the cell cycle. *Blood*, **97**, 2278–85.

Wright, D.E., Wagers, A.J., Gulati, A.P. *et al.* (2001). Physiological migration of hematopoietic stem and progenitor cells. *Science*, **294**, 1933–6.

Wu, A.M., Till, J.E., Siminovitch, L., & McCulloch, E.A. (1967). A cytological study of the capacity for differentiation of normal hemotopoietic colony-forming cells. *Journal of Cell Physiology*, **69**, 177–84.

Wu, A.M., Till, J.E., Siminovitch, L., & McCulloch, E.A. (1968). Cytological evidence for a relationship between normal hematopoietic colony-forming cells and cells of the lymphoid system. *Journal of Experimental Medicine*, **127**, 455–64.

Yarbro, J.W. (1992). Mechanism of action of hydroxyurea. *Seminars in Oncology*, **19**,(3 Suppl 9), 1–10.

Yin, A.H. *et al.* (1997). AC133, a novel marker for human hematopoietic stem and progenitor cells. *Blood*, **90**, 5002–12.

Yoder, M., Hiatt, K., & Mukherjee, P. (1997). In vivo repopulating hematopoietic stem cells are present in the murine yolk sac at day 9.0 postcoitus. *Proceedings of the National Academy of Sciences USA*, **94**, 6776–80.

Yokoyama, W.M. (1995). Hybrid resistance and the Ly-49 family of natural killer cell receptors. *Journal of Experimental Medicine*, **182**, 273–7.

Yokoyama, W.M. (1995). Natural killer cell receptors specific for major histocompatibility complex class I molecules. *Proceedings of the National Academy of Sciences USA*, **92**, 3081–5.

Yokoyama, W.M., Matsumoto, K., Scalzo, A.A., & Brown, M.G. (1997). Molecular genetics of the natural killer gene complex and innate immunity. *Biochemistry Society Transactions*, **25**, 691–5.

Young, J.C., Varma, A., DiGusto, D., & Backer, M.P. (1996). Retention of quiescent hematopoietic cells with high proliferative potential during ex vivo stem cell culture. *Blood*, **87**, 545–56.

Yu, Y.Y., George, T., Dorfman, J.R. *et al.* (1996). The role of Ly49A and 5E6(Ly49C) molecules in hybrid resistance mediated by murine natural killer cells against normal T cell blasts. *Immunity*, **4**, 67–76.

Yui, J., Chiu, C.P., & Lansdorp, P.M. (1998). Telomerase activity in candidate stem cells from fetal liver and adult bone marrow. *Blood*, **91**, 3255–62.

Zanjani, E.D., Almeida-Porada, G., Livingston, A.G. *et al.* (1998). Human bone marrow CD34– cells engraft in vivo and undergo multilineage expression that includes giving rise to CD34+ cells. *Experimental Hematology*, **26**, 353–60.

Zanjani, E.D., Pallavicini, M.G., Ascensao, J.L. *et al.* (1992). Engraftment and long-term expression of human fetal hemopoietic stem cell in sheep following transplantation in utero. *Journal of Clinical Investigation*, **89**, 1178–88.

Zijlmans, J.M., Visser, J.W., Kleiverda, K. *et al.* (1995). Modification of rhodamine staining allows identification of hematopoietic stem cells with preferential short-term or long-term bone marrow-repopulating ability. *Proceedings of the National Academy of Sciences USA*, **92**, 8901–5.

Zijlmans, J.M., Visser, J.W., Laterveer, L. *et al.* (1998). The early phase of engraftment after murine blood cell transplantation is mediated by hematopoietic stem cells. *Proceedings of the National Academy of Sciences USA*, **95**, 725–9.

3 Molecular control of hematopoiesis

DAVID IZON AND C. GLENN BEGLEY

*Center for Child Health Research and Western Australian Institute
of Medical Research, University of Western Australia, Australia
and Amgen Inc., Thousand Oaks, USA*

Introduction

Hematopoiesis requires the sustained generation of large quantities of mature cells of distinct lineages from a relatively small number of progenitor cells and stem cells. While the steady-state production of cells needs to be tightly regulated, the system also needs to respond, often urgently, to situations of increased demand. Equally, negative feedback mechanisms are required to restore equilibrium after the emergency situation has passed. The hematopoietic growth factors play a crucial role in mediating these processes. The regulators with known proliferative effects exceed more than 20 in number. In addition, although less well-defined, there are factors with inhibitory effects. It is thus apparent that there are more hematopoietic regulators with similar or overlapping actions than would seem necessary to maintain homeostasis. There is an added layer of complexity: the effect of individual growth factors is not restricted to a single lineage and for some factors their action is not restricted to hematopoietic cells. For example, the interleukin (IL)-6 family of growth factors not only influences multiple hematopoietic lineages, but also exhibits myriad effects on numerous nonhematopoietic organs.

In addition to the extracellular growth factors, it is evident that critical steps in development of hematopoiesis are regulated by transcription factors. This chapter describes the influence of some of the more recently described growth factors on hematopoiesis, the target cell populations responding to these factors, and briefly overviews the current knowledge regarding the important role played by transcription factors in hematopoietic development.

Hematopoietic cell populations

Hematopoietic cells can be broadly classified as transiting through three compartments: (1) the stem cell compartment, (2) committed progenitor cells, and (3) mature functional end-cells (see Fig. 3.1). The cells in each succeeding compartment are the progeny of, and more numerous than, the cells of the preceding compartment (Metcalf & Nicola, 1995).

The concept of a hematopoietic stem cell began to evolve in the late 1950s after it was demonstrated unequivocally that reconstitution of irradiated mice by transplantation of syngeneic bone marrow cells occurred through the proliferation of donor cells (Ford *et al.*, 1956; Micklem *et al.*, 1966). Prior to these experiments controversy existed as to whether bone marrow transplantation led to hematopoietic recovery through the transfer of cells or factors. It was soon recognized that the majority of cells of the hematopoietic system are short-lived and must be continuously produced by differentiation of immature progenitors. The properties of the primitive stem cell were therefore predicted to include capability of self-renewal, extensive proliferative capacity, ability to differentiate into cells of different lineages, and ability to respond to external regulatory signals (Siminovitch, McCulloch, & Till, 1963). Although the issue of self-renewal remains controversial, these characteristics have been confirmed in vivo by studies of hematopoietic reconstitution following myeloablative therapy.

In addition to their biological properties, stem cells can be distinguished on the basis of expression of particular surface antigens and physical properties, for example the handling of specific fluorescent dyes. However, within the stem cell compartment there is a hierarchy of cells and heterogeneity in each of these characteristics. Thus, "primitive" stem cells are more likely to be quiescent (i.e., stem cells capable of long-term hematopoietic reconstitution) while more mature stem cells may be in cell cycle (i.e., the "stem cell" that forms the day-8 colony-forming unit-spleen, d8 CFU-S). Even within the d12 CFU-S cell population there is heterogeneity based on labeling by rhodamine-123 dye. Two limitations have hampered a direct analysis of hematopoietic stem cell behavior. First, the frequency of such cells is extremely low: in the order of 1 in 10,000–100,000 (Boggs *et al.*, 1982; Harrison, Astle, & Lerner, 1988). Second, no well-defined culture system permitting the in vitro clonal expansion of stem cells has been established. Existing long-term culture systems, which support various aspects of hematopoiesis or lymphopoiesis, suffer from the complexity and heterogeneity of the hematopoietic and stromal cell population present in culture (Dexter, Allen, & Lajtha, 1977; Dexter, 1984; Dexter & Spooncer, 1987; Pietrangeli, Hayashi, & Kincade, 1988; Williams *et al.*, 1988). As a result, the most rigorous functional definition of a stem cell remains its ability to reconstitute the hematopoietic system.

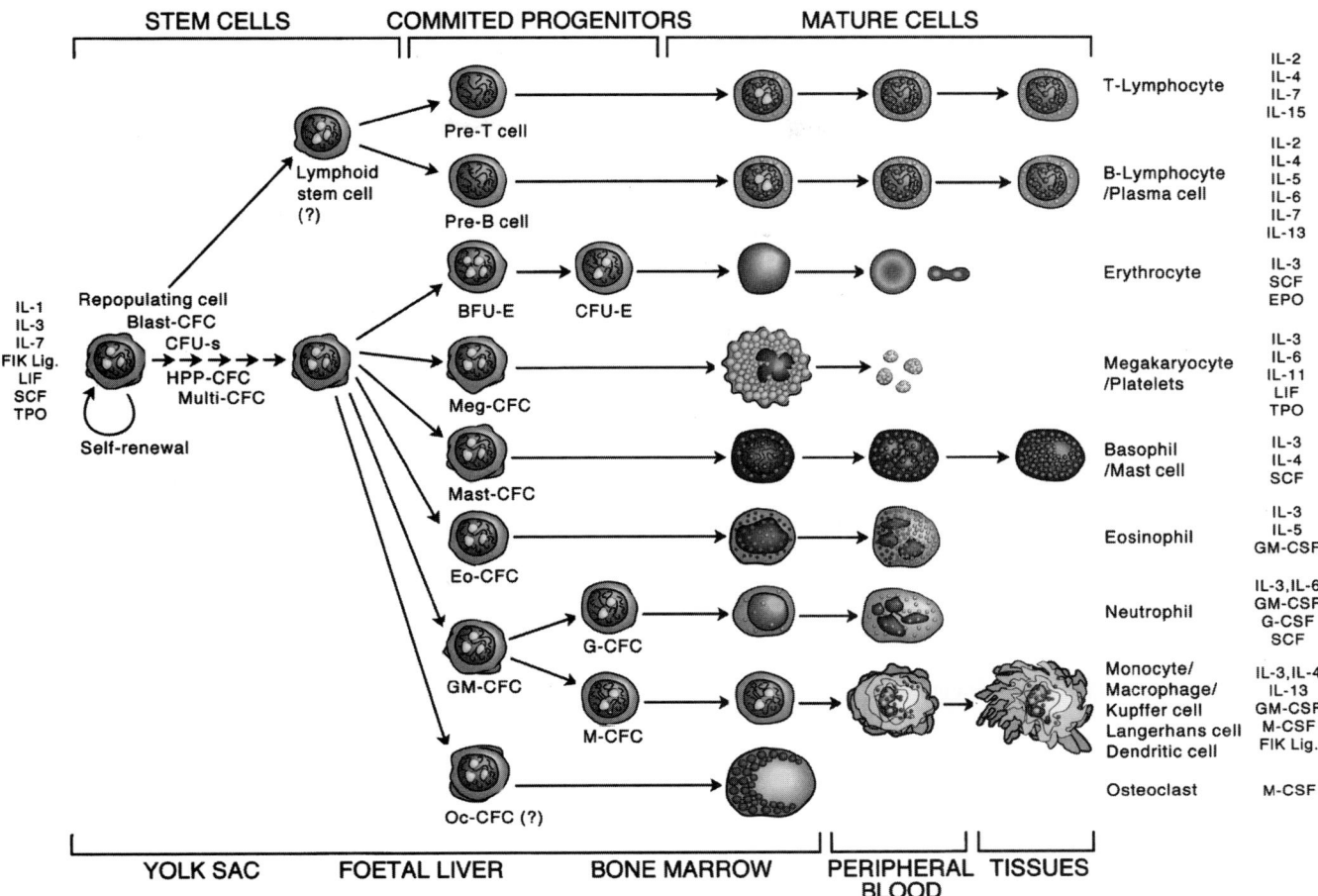

Fig. 3.1. Proliferation and differentiation of hematopoietic lineages is influenced by various growth factors, including interleukins (IL) and colony-stimulating factors (CSF). See text for additional details.

While the analysis of stem cells has required the use of cumbersome in vivo assays, in vitro semisolid culture techniques have permitted analysis of progenitor cells (Pluznik & Sachs, 1965; Bradley & Metcalf, 1966; Ichikawa, Pluznik, & Sachs, 1966). In this system, progenitor cells are characterized by their capacity to form colonies of maturing progeny in response to stimulation by hematopoietic growth factors, thus colony forming cells or CFC (Metcalf, 1984; Metcalf & Nicola, 1995). The majority of progenitor cells within the bone marrow display restricted differentiation potential and give rise to colonies of either myeloid or erythroid cells. However, again there is heterogeneity within the progenitor cell populations. For example, Bradley and Hodgson (1979) described a population of macrophage progenitor cells with high proliferative potential (HPP-CFC). These cells form large colonies of over 50,000 cells and are resistant to cytotoxic treatment in vivo, indicating their normally quiescent status. The HPP-CFC include cells that differ in their physical characteristics, surface markers, and response to growth factors (McNiece et al., 1986; McNiece et al., 1987; Rennick et al., 1989; Kriegler et al., 1990).

A relatively "primitive" progenitor cell population is the CFC-blast (Nakahata & Ogawa, 1982). Colonies derived from these cells contain cells of blast-like morphology and high recloning or replating efficiency, and reside predominantly in the G_0 phase of the cell cycle (Suda, Suda, & Ogawa, 1983). In contrast, CFC-mix are multipotential cells that generate colonies of erythroid cells, neutrophils, macrophages, eosinophils, and megakaryocytes, but have little self-generation potential (Johnson & Metcalf, 1977; Hara & Ogawa, 1978; Fauser & Messner, 1979).

Within the progenitor cell compartment, there is a predominance of cells committed to a single lineage (Bradley & Metcalf, 1966; Ichikawa, Pluznik, & Sachs, 1966). This includes the more primitive erythroid progenitors, BFU-E, and more mature erythroid progenitors CFU-E (Stephenson et al., 1971), megakaryocyte progenitors (MK-CFC) (Metcalf et al., 1975; Long, Heffner, & Gragowski, 1986), lymphocytic lineage CFU-B and CFU-T (Rozenszajn, Shoham, & Kalechman, 1975; Metcalf et al., 1975b); GM-, G-, M-, Eo-, Baso-, and Mast-CFC in the granulocyte lineage (Johnson & Metcalf, 1977; Schrader et al., 1981), fibroblast-CFC (Metcalf et al., 1985), and cells of the osteoclast lineage (Lee, Lottsfeldt, &

Fevold, 1992). Thus the in vitro culture system has allowed the definition of diverse populations of progenitor cells. However, its most important contribution has been to allow the identification and characterization of the extracellular growth factors that are critical in regulating these processes.

Regulation of hematopoiesis by growth factors

It is beyond the scope of this chapter to describe the activity of each hematopoietic growth factor in detail. Several recent reviews have focused on the clinical utility of molecules such as G-CSF, GM-CSF, and erythropoietin (EPO). Each of these three molecules has been used clinically for over 15 years, and second-generation forms of G-CSF and EPO are now available. These second-generation molecules offer greater clinical benefit as a result of prolonged in vivo half-life and therefore require less frequent administration. This is achieved as a result of pegylation of the G-CSF molecule and hyperglycosylation of EPO.

This chapter will focus on some of the more recent developments involving IL-11, stem cell factor (SCF), flt3 ligand (FL), and thrombopoietin (TPO). These factors have been the subject of considerable interest because of their hematopoietic actions in vitro and preclinical and early clinical data.

Interleukin-11

IL-11 was originally identified as a factor produced by stromal cells (Paul et al., 1991) that stimulated the proliferation of a murine plasmacytoma cell line (Paul et al., 1990). It was also independently cloned based on the ability to inhibit adipogenesis in 3T3-L1 cells (Kawashima et al., 1991) and, like other members of the IL-6 family of growth factors, is a pleiotropic cytokine. For example, IL-11 mRNA expression has been demonstrated in thymus, spleen, bone marrow, fibroblasts, bronchial epithelial cells, blood vessels and endothelial cells, endometrial tissues, melanoma cell lines, normal skin, glioblastoma cells, osteoblasts, developing spermatids, and in certain regions of the brain and spinal cord (Du & Williams, 1997).

The most prominent action of IL-11 in the hematopoietic compartment is on the megakaryocyte lineage. While IL-11 acting alone has no MK-CFC activity in vitro, it can augment the activity of cytokines such as IL-3, SCF, and TPO (Paul et al., 1990; Bruno et al., 1991; Burstein et al., 1992; Teramura et al., 1992; Yonemura et al., 1992; Broudy, Lin, & Kaushansky, 1995; Kaushansky et al., 1995a). It also induces features of megakaryocyte maturation (increased ploidy, size, and production of acetylcholinesterase) in synergy with IL-3 (Burstein et al., 1992; Yonemura et al., 1992) and acting alone (Burstein et al., 1992). Additional support for the action of IL-11 in megakaryocytopoiesis has also come from in vivo studies. Administration of IL-11 alone to normal and splenectomized mice results in a dose-related increase in platelet count (1.5–1.7-fold), and is associated with an increment in the number of megakaryocytes and megakaryocyte progenitors in bone marrow and spleen (Cairo et

al., 1993; Neben et al., 1993; Yonemura et al., 1993). A similar effect has also been observed in monkeys (Schlerman et al., 1996) and dogs (Nash et al., 1995). Administration of IL-11 to humans also results in an elevation of platelet count, increased megakaryocyte numbers in the marrow with a higher fraction of cycling cells, and shift to higher megakaryocyte ploidy (Gordon et al., 1996; Orazi et al., 1996; Tepler et al., 1996). This action can be exploited for therapeutic advantage since IL-11 hastens platelet recovery in patients with a known history of chemotherapy-induced thrombocytopenia. In a phase I trial, women with advanced breast cancer and with a prior episode of treatment-related thrombocytopenia requiring platelet transfusion were treated with IL-11 at various doses (25–100 µg/kg/day) before and after chemotherapy (Gordon et al., 1996). Doses above 25 µg/kg/day showed attenuation of posttreatment thrombocytopenia. There was an increase in the number of marrow megakaryocytes and in their ploidy content, as well as in megakaryocyte progenitors. A similar benefit in decreasing the need for platelet transfusion was also noted in other trials evaluating IL-11 during chemotherapy treatment (Tepler et al., 1996; Issacs et al., 1997). However, there was no benefit when IL-11 was administered in conjunction with high-dose chemotherapy with marrow or blood stem cell support (Vredenburgh et al., 1998). IL-11 when used clinically has demonstrated a reasonable safety profile. Reversible side effects such as myalgia and arthralgia were seen at doses of 50 µg/kg/day, but fever was not noted. Plasma concentrations of acute-phase reactants were elevated at all doses, and there was associated fluid retention and volume expansion (Berl & Schwertschlag, 2000; Dykstra et al., 2000.). Treatment with IL-11 in humans was not found to induce platelet hyperaggregability (Gordon et al., 1996).

IL-11 has also been shown to influence multiple stages of erythropoiesis; it stimulates growth of BFU-E when combined with IL-3 (even in the absence of EPO) (Quesniaux et al., 1992; Rodriguez, Arnaud, & Blanchet, 1995) and with other growth factors such as SCF and GM-CSF (Lemoli et al., 1993). IL-11 can also support the maturation of CFU-E (Quesniaux et al., 1992). In contrast to the stimulatory activity of IL-11 on all less mature erythroid parameters, IL-11 induced a mild anemia in mice (de Haan et al., 1995). Such an effect has also been seen in dogs (Nash et al., 1995), monkeys (Schlerman et al., 1996), and humans (Gordon et al., 1996), and is thought to be due to volume expansion, as mentioned above.

Several investigators have shown that IL-11 alone supports the growth of few myeloid colonies, but enhances the growth of a range of multipotential and committed myeloid progenitors when combined with other growth factors such as IL-3, SCF, G-CSF, GM-CSF (Musashi et al., 1991a; Musashi et al., 1991b; Tsuji et al., 1992; Cairo et al., 1993; Keller et al., 1993; Ariyama, Misawa, & Sonoda, 1995; Tanaka et al., 1995; van de Ven et al., 1995), IL-4 (Musashi et al., 1991b; Jacobsen et al., 1994), IL-7 and IL-12 (Ploemacher et al., 1993a; Ploemacher et al., 1993b; Hirayama et al., 1994), IL-13 (Jacobsen et al., 1994), FL (Lemieux et al., 1997), and TPO (Ku et al., 1996). Expansion of myeloid progenitors and an associated peripheral blood neutrophilia also occurs with in vivo administration (Du et al., 1993; Hangoc et al., 1993; Schlerman et al., 1996). However, a neutrophilic response is not consistently seen in all experimental models. For example, mice enforced to overproduce IL-11 showed a greater than 20-fold elevation in myeloid progenitors, but had unchanged leukocyte levels (Hawley et al., 1993). Neutrophilia was not noted in canine studies (Nash et al., 1995), nor in the human phase I trial (Gordon et al., 1996). Administration of IL-11 with G-CSF resulted in mobilization of CD34-positive cells in heavily pretreated patients (Goldman et al., 2001).

With regard to primitive hematopoietic stem cells, IL-11 appears to regulate both stem cell self-renewal and commitment. Addition of IL-11 to long-term marrow cultures was reported to increase the number of multilineage and committed progenitors such as d12 CFU-S, CFC-mix, GM-CFC, and BFU-E (Keller et al., 1993; Du et al., 1995). This action was due to the entry of a quiescent (G_0) population into active cell cycle and the shortening of cell cycle time (Leary et al., 1992; Tanaka e· al., 1995). However, there was, if anything, a decrease in the frequency of more primitive cells (Neben et al., 1994; Du et al., 1995). This implied that the increased commitment of stem cells into a multipotential progenitor compartment occurred at the expense of stem cell renewal. Other experimental systems have also attempted to delineate the role of IL-11 in the stem cell compartment. IL-11 in combination with other cytokines resulted in a 50-fold amplification of multipotential progenitors in short-term cultures (Holyoake et al., 1996). However, this observation is at variance with reports that showed that ex vivo expansion with IL-11, IL-3, IL-6, and SCF resulted in cells that showed a significant engraftment defect (Peters et al., 1995; Peters et al., 1996). Chronic IL-11 overexposure models have also been generated (Hawley et al., 1993; Paul et al., 1994; Hawley et al., 1996) and bone marrow cells from these animals produced accelerated engraftment in serial transplantation experiments and showed no evidence of stem cells becoming extinguished.

Despite these findings, and despite its utility in treating patients with thrombocytopenia, IL-11 does not appear to play a physiologic role in regulating hematopoiesis. For example, there is no consistent inverse relationship between platelet/megakaryocyte mass and circulating levels of IL-11, suggesting, that unlike TPO, IL-11 is not regulated by total mass of the megakaryocyte lineage (Heits et al., 1997). Of greater significance, mice in which IL-11 signaling is ablated have normal blood counts and normal responses to thrombopoietic stresses (Nandurkar et al., 1997; Nandurkar et al., 1998). In fact, in these animals the principal defect is in female fertility: in mice that lack the IL-11 receptor, normal decidualization does not occur following implantation of the embryo (Bilinski et al., 1998; Robb et al., 1998). Moreover, IL-11 does not appear to be responsible for maintaining platelet counts, even in the absence of the key platelet regulator, TPO (Gainsford et al., 2000).

Stem cell factor

Stem cell factor (SCF, also known as kit ligand, mast cell growth factor, or Steel factor) is a hematopoietic growth factor for which the receptor is the tyrosine kinase c-kit (Flanagan & Leder, 1990; Huang et al., 1990; Williams et al., 1990; Zsebo et al., 1990a). The importance of this factor in hematopoiesis, as well as in the development of other organs, is demonstrated by the numerous abnormalities observed in mice bearing naturally occurring mutations of the SCF gene (SI mutation) or of the c-kit gene (W mutation) (Besmer et al., 1993). While complete absence of SCF or its receptor is associated with embryonic death or perinatal mortality from severe macrocytic anemia, less severe abnormalities are associated with reduced levels or function of these proteins. Thus there is a spectrum in disease phenotype, the severity of which correlates with the severity of the deficit in the ligand or the receptor (Reith et al., 1990; Blouin & Bernstein, 1993). The predominant abnormalities include macrocytic anemia, diminished fertility, decrease in coat color, lymphocyte abnormalities, reduced number of tissue mast cells, and a defect in intestinal pacemaker activity (Blouin & Bernstein, 1993; Huizinga et al., 1995).

SCF occurs naturally in two active forms, a membrane-anchored form and a soluble form, that results from proteolytic cleavage (Flanagan, Chan, & Leder, 1991). The membrane-anchored form is a consequence of an alternative splicing event that excludes the proteolytic cleavage site (Flanagan, Chan, & Leder, 1991; Huang et al., 1992). Animal models have demonstrated that the phenotypic consequences resulting from the absence of the transmembrane form cannot be completely ameliorated by soluble SCF: the SI/SI[d] mice, which produce only a functional soluble SCF protein, continue to display anemia and the germ cell and pigmentation defects (McCulloch et al., 1965; Barker, 1994).

SCF also plays an important role in adult murine hematopoiesis (Brannan et al., 1991; Flanagan, Chan, & Leder, 1991). Administration of an SCF-neutralizing antibody (ACK2) results in pancytopenia (Ogawa et al., 1991), abnormalities of gut motility (Maeda et al., 1992), intestinal infection with helminths (Donaldson et al., 1996), and defects in spermatogenesis. Despite the multiorgan phenotype seen in mice with the SI or W mutation, the analogous human condition piebaldism, which is caused by a mutation of c-kit (Spritz, 1994; Ezoe et al., 1995), results in only altered pigmentation but with no hematopoietic or fertility defects.

The role of SCF within the hematopoietic stem cell compartment is less clear. For example, the use of SCF as a component of cytokine cocktails for ex vivo expansion of cells has shown inconsistent results. In combination with IL-11, SCF has been shown to enhance long-term reconstitution potential (Holyoake et al., 1996); however, in combination with IL-3, IL-6, and IL-11 there was impairment of engraftment (Peters et al., 1995; Peters et al., 1996). Equally, SCF may not be required for the maintenance of stem cell numbers: fibroblasts from SI/SI mice show similar ability to wild-type fibroblasts to support long-term bone marrow culture-initiating cells (LTBMC-IC) (Sutherland *et al.*, 1993), and exposure of stromal cells to the ACK2 antibody does not diminish stem cell survival (Kodama *et al.*, 1992; Wineman, Nishikawa, & Muller-Sieburg, 1993). In human studies, combination of SCF with other growth factors causes an impressive expansion of progenitor cells, but such an augmentation in LTBMC-IC has not been consistently observed (Henschler *et al.*, 1994; Petzer *et al.*, 1996b). Also, the cells capable of long-term reconstitution display heterogeneity in their expression of c-kit. Both long-term reconstituting stem cells that are c-kit positive (Ikuta & Weissman, 1992; Orlic *et al.*, 1993; Wineman, Nishikawa, & Muller-Sieburg, 1993; Li & Johnson, 1995; de Jong *et al.*, 1996), as well as those that are c-kit negative (or c-kit low), have been described (Jones *et al.*, 1996; Doi *et al.*, 1997). SCF has demonstrated a potent mobilizing effect on progenitor cells in humans: adding SCF to an optimal dose of G-CSF increases the number of progenitors that can be harvested (Begley *et al.*, 1997; reviewed in Lacerna *et al.*, 1998). It is because of this effect that SCF is available clinically in Australia and Canada.

While the action of SCF within the stem cell compartment remains controversial, its action within the progenitor compartment is well defined. Within this compartment it displays dramatic synergy with cytokines such as EPO, IL-3, GM-CSF, and G-CSF, resulting in an increase in number and size of colonies (Nocka *et al.*, 1990; Andrews *et al.*, 1991; Bernstein, Andrews, & Zsebo, 1991; Broxmeyer *et al.*, 1991; Migliaccio *et al.*, 1991; Metcalf & Nicola, 1991; Brandt *et al.*, 1992). This effect is seen in myeloid, erythroid, and multipotential cells. Similarly, while SCF acting alone has little potential to support MK-CFC, it promotes MK-CFC in combination with TPO, IL-3, and EPO and IL-11 (Briddell *et al.*, 1991; Broudy, Lin, & Kaushansky, 1995). However, the normal platelet and leukocyte numbers in the Sl or W mutant mice argue against a pivotal role for SCF in these lineages.

A prominent feature of mutations of SCF or c-kit is the marked reduction in the number of tissue mast cells (Kitamura, Go, & Hatanaka, 1978). Consistent with this, in vivo administration of SCF results in an increase in mast cells (Zsebo *et al.*, 1990b; Galli *et al.*, 1995; Costa *et al.*, 1996), and SCF promotes the in vitro development of mast cells from a variety of cell sources including peripheral blood mononuclear cells (Valent *et al.*, 1992), CD34$^+$ cells (Kirshenbaum *et al.*, 1992), and cord blood cells (Durand *et al.*, 1994). The activity of SCF on mast cells also extends to mature cells where, at concentrations vastly lower than those required for mast cell colony-stimulating activity, SCF stimulates histamine and leukotriene release. This activity contributes to the toxicity associated with in vivo use of SCF (Table 3.1).

Flt3-ligand

The fms-like tyrosine kinase 3 receptor (flt3; also cloned as the fetal liver kinase 2 receptor) bears similarity to the M-CSF receptor (c-fms), c-kit, and to the platelet-derived growth factor receptors. The cognate ligand for flt3 (FL) is structurally simi-

Table 3.1. *Effects of SCF on mast cells*

Survival
Proliferation
Maturation
Mediator release
Chemotaxis
Adhesion to fibroblasts or extracellular matrix
Survival
Proliferation
Locally at injection site
Systemically
Mediator release
Histamine
α Tryptase
Migration of mast cell precursors

Reproduced, with permission, from Broudy (1997).

lar to SCF (Lyman *et al.*, 1993; Hannum *et al.*, 1994) and M-CSF (Bazan, 1991), and the genomic structures for the FL, SCF, and M-CSF genes share conserved features (Lyman *et al.*, 1995), suggesting a probable common origin. The flt3 receptor is expressed on human myeloid and monocytic cell lines (DaSilva *et al.*, 1994; Brasel *et al.*, 1995; Meierhoff *et al.*, 1995), as well as pre-B-cell lines (DaSilva *et al.*, 1994; Meierhoff *et al.*, 1995), but has not been found on T-cell lines (Rossner *et al.*, 1994; Brasel *et al.*, 1995), nor on erythroid cell lines (Brasel *et al.*, 1995; Meierhoff *et al.*, 1995). While the receptor is generally not expressed in murine myeloid cell lines (Rossner *et al.*, 1994; Brasel *et al.*, 1995), it has been observed on the CD34-positive M1 leukemic cell line (Brasel *et al.*, 1995; Begley *et al.*, 1996), in which FL inhibits the macrophage differentiation induced by LIF (Begley *et al.*, 1996). The receptor is expressed in many cases of human adult myeloid leukemia, as well as in B-lineage acute lymphoblastic leukemia (ALL), but rarely in T-lineage ALL, or in lymphomas (Birg *et al.*, 1994; DaSilva *et al.*, 1994; Brasel *et al.*, 1995; Meierhoff *et al.*, 1995). Human CD34-positive bone marrow cells and myeloid progenitors express flt3 receptor, and it appears to be downregulated during myeloid differentiation (Gabbianelli *et al.*, 1995; Rappold *et al.*, 1997). While human (Rappold *et al.*, 1997) and murine (Rasko *et al.*, 1995) pro-B cells display the receptor on their surface, it is not seen on immature or mature murine B cells (Rasko *et al.*, 1995).

In vitro, FL, in combination with other agents including IL-7, primarily promotes B-cell commitment and differentiation of uncommitted progenitors from yolk sac, fetal liver, and bone marrow (Ray *et al.*, 1996; Veiby, Lyman, & Jacobsen, 1996). FL influences primitive murine B-cell progenitors (CD43$^+$, B220^{low}, CD24$^-$), but not the more differentiated CD24$^+$ cells (Hunte *et al.*, 1996). Combination of FL with growth factors results in improved retroviral transduction efficiency of human progenitor cells (Elwood *et al.*, 1996). Multiple growth factor combinations containing FL can not only expand murine and human myeloid progenitors, but also the more primitive LTBMC-IC (Petzer *et al.*, 1996a; Shah *et al.*, 1996).

However, probably the most important effect of FL is on dendritic cells. FL expands and regulates dendritic cells (McKenna, 2001). In vivo administration of FL results in an impressive increase in dendritic cells in mouse bone marrow, spleen, and nonhematopoietic organs (Maraskovsky et al., 1996). There is also an increment in peripheral blood lymphocytes, neutrophils, and monocytes (Brasel et al., 1996). This is associated with an augmentation of committed and multipotential progenitors in bone marrow and spleen, as well as in d12 CFU-S stem cells (Brasel et al., 1996). When FL is given to humans, there is a similar dramatic increase in dendritic cells (Maraskovsky et al., 2000). This striking action on dendritic cells raises the possibility that FL will find application as an agent promoting immune responses to neoplastic cells (Lynch et al., 1997). To this end, studies have been performed to address the possible role of FL as an adjuvant to heighten the immune response in cancer (Disis et al, 2002; Merad et al., 2002). FL is also being examined as an agent that might improve engraftment in the context of lower-dose conditioning regimens for HSC transplantation (Noach et al., 2002).

Gene targeting studies of the flt3 receptor (Mackarehtschian et al., 1995), as well as analysis of FL$^-$ mutant mice (McKenna et al., 2000), have helped delineate the influence of this growth factor on the various hematopoietic lineages. Flt3-deficient mice have normal numbers of peripheral blood cells, but display a reduction in B-cell progenitor numbers, as well as in long-term reconstituting stem cells (Mackarehtschian et al., 1995). This defect is exaggerated in mice made doubly mutant for the flt3 and the c-kit receptors (Mackarehtschian et al., 1995). Consistent with its in vivo effects, there is also a defect in dendritic cells in the FL null mice (McKenna et al., 2000).

Thrombopoietin

The term "thrombopoietin" was first coined in 1958 to parallel erythropoietin and to describe a natural activity that promoted platelet production (Kelemen, Cserháti, & Tanos, 1958). However, it was characterization of the viral oncogene v-Mpl that provided the molecular catalyst for the cloning of thrombopoietin (TPO).

In a series of experiments in the 1980s, murine myeloproliferative leukemia virus (MPLV) was identified. In inoculated mice, MPLV induces an acute myeloproliferative leukemia with expansion of maturing cells of multiple hematopoietic lineages (Wendling et al., 1986; Wendling et al., 1989). Genetic analysis showed that part of a novel gene, v-Mpl, had rearranged with the virus, and that this new gene encoded a member of the cytokine receptor superfamily (Souyri et al., 1990; Vigon et al., 1992). Evidence that the new receptor displayed a restricted pattern of expression confined to the megakaryocyte lineage, and that anti-sense oligonucleotides specifically reduced megakaryocyte colony formation, served to heighten interest in the normal receptor c-Mpl and its unknown ligand (Methia et al., 1993).

The ligand for c-Mpl was cloned by five independent laboratories utilizing several different approaches. One approach took advantage of the specific interaction between the receptor and its ligand (Bartley et al., 1994; de Sauvage et al., 1994). A second procedure involved a daunting purification from serum (Kuter, Beeler, & Rosenberg, 1994; Kato et al., 1995). Others used chemical mutagenesis to render cells growth-factor independent as a consequence of autocrine production of TPO (Kaushansky et al., 1994; Lok et al., 1994). The ligand for c-Mpl is variously known as thrombopoietin, megakaryocyte growth and development factor (MGDF), megapoietin, and c-Mpl ligand. These differing names reflect in part the realization that some of the activities of the newly isolated Mpl-ligand differ from those previously attributed to thrombopoietin. However, the cDNA molecules identified by all groups appear identical. The native protein consists of an amino-terminal domain that shows homology to erythropoietin, interacts with the c-Mpl receptor, and is sufficient for full biological activity. In addition, the endogenous molecule has a unique, carbohydrate-rich carboxyl domain that is probably important in maintaining in vivo stability (Kaushansky, 1995).

The action of TPO in vitro has been documented by many groups. Consistent with the distribution of its receptor, TPO acts throughout megakaryocytopoiesis. Alone, it stimulates formation of small colonies of megakaryocytes. This action can be significantly enhanced by the addition of other cytokines, for example, IL-3, IL-11, SCF, and erythropoietin (Kaushansky et al., 1994; Broudy, Lin, & Kaushansky, 1995; Hunt et al., 1995). TPO also stimulates increases in megakaryocyte ploidy and expression of megakaryocyte surface markers (Bartley et al., 1994; de Sauvage et al., 1994). However, TPO does not act as a platelet release factor, and at high concentrations it may even inhibit proplatelet formation (Choi et al., 1996). Although mature platelets express c-Mpl, TPO does not appear to directly induce platelet activation, but it does "prime" platelets for aggregation induced by several agonists (Toombs et al., 1995; Harker et al., 1996; Montrucchio et al., 1996; Oda et al., 1996).

In addition to its action on cells of the megakaryocyte lineage, TPO acts on other hematopoietic lineages and on stem cells. It promotes survival and proliferation of erythroid progenitors and, in synergy with other factors, stimulates granulocyte-macrophage progenitors and multipotential precursors (Kobayashi et al., 1995; Kobayashi et al., 1996; Rasko, O'Flaherty, & Begley, 1997). Similar effects have been established for its action on populations of stem cells (Stinicka et al., 1996). TPO in combination with FL allows dramatic expansion of primitive hematopoietic cells ex vivo (Piacibello et al., 1997).

Animal models have documented that TPO and its receptor are the major physiologic regulators of platelet production. Mice that lack the ligand or the receptor show platelet counts that are less than 20% of normal and a reduction in megakaryocytes (Gurney et al., 1994; Alexander et al., 1996; Carver-Moore et al., 1996; de Sauvage et al., 1996). The residual platelets are not due to compensation, for example by IL-3, IL-6, or IL-11 (Gainsford et al., 1998; Gainsford et al., 2000).

Although blood erythroid and myeloid parameters are normal in these mice, the number of progenitor cells for these lineages and the number of stem cells is reduced (Alexander *et al.*, 1996; Kimura *et al.*, 1997).

TPO has been administered to mice (Bartley *et al.*, 1994; de Sauvage *et al.*, 1994; Lok *et al.*, 1994), dogs (Peng *et al.*, 1996), monkeys (Farese *et al.*, 1995), and baboons (Harker *et al.*, 1996). These studies demonstrated a dose-related increase in the platelet count, but with differences in the kinetics of response in different species. The increase in platelet count was associated with an increase in frequency of bone marrow megakaryocytes, megakaryocyte size, and megakaryocyte ploidy. The action of TPO was lineage-specific or lineage-restricted with little change in other blood parameters.

Many studies have also examined the action of TPO following chemotherapy and/or radiotherapy and shown the anticipated enhancement of platelet recovery (Farese *et al.*, 1995; Farese *et al.*, 1996; Ulich *et al.*, 1996; Grossman *et al.*, 1996a; Grossman *et al.*, 1996b). In some of these studies TPO was combined with G-CSF with no adverse effect, and, if anything, a further enhancement of neutrophil and platelet recovery (Farese *et al.*, 1996; Grossman *et al.*, 1996a). Although the action of administered TPO is predominantly evident on platelets, its effect is not restricted to this lineage. In mice there is an expansion of all classes of progenitor cells and an acceleration of erythroid recovery after myelosuppression (Kaushansky *et al.*, 1995b; Kaushansky *et al.*, 1996).

The clinical evaluation of this molecule commenced with two recombinant preparations. Scientists at Genentech prepared a full-length recombinant human molecule (recombinant human thrombopoietin, rHuTPO). Scientists at Amgen replaced the carbohydrate-rich carboxy terminus with a poly (ethylene glycol) moiety to improve in vivo stability. This material is known as pegylated recombinant human megakaryocyte growth and development factor (PEG-rHuMGDF).

The first clinical studies showed that, as predicted from the animal studies, there was a dose-related increase in the platelet count (Basser *et al.*, 1996). However, the rise in the platelet count occurred later than anticipated, with maximum counts occurring between 12 and 18 days after the commencement of PEG-rHuMGDF. Platelets generated in response to PEG-rHuMGDF were of normal appearance, functioned normally in in vitro assays, and showed no evidence of activation in vivo (O'Malley *et al.*, 1996). As with other growth factors, PEG-rHuMGDF stimulated the release of progenitor cells of multiple hematopoietic lineages into the blood (Rasko *et al.*, 1997; Somlo *et al.*, 1999). PEG-rHuMGDF reduced the severity of chemotherapy-induced thrombocytopenia (Basser *et al.*, 1997; Fanucchi *et al.*, 1997; Basser *et al.*, 2000). It was also used successfully to increase platelet yields in healthy platelet donors (Kuter *et al.*, 2001). However it was not of benefit in the context of leukemia (Archimbaud *et al.*, 1999; Schiffer *et al.*, 2000). Although the molecule was associated with minimal side effects, its use was associated with the development of antibodies (Li *et al.*, 2001; Basser *et al.*, 2002). A similar series of studies was performed with rHuTPO, which was also well tolerated and caused a dose-related increase in the platelet count (Vadhan-Raj *et al.*, 1997; Nash *et al.*, 2000; Vadhan-Raj *et al.*, 2000). Despite the early enthusiasm that surrounded identification of TPO, its role in the clinic remains uncertain.

Growth factors and receptors: lessons from Drosophila, Notch, and Wnt

In addition to the growth factors discussed above that have an established or emerging role in clinical medicine, there are newer classes of growth factors of importance in hematopoiesis. Although much still remains to be learned, these molecules are likely to be significant given the key role they play in development and differentiation events in lower organisms such as Drosophila, where their function has been well defined. Once such molecule is Notch.

Notch was originally identified in mutant flies with "notches" in their wings. Subsequently, the Notch signaling pathway has been demonstrated to be vitally important for the cell fate decisions in the development of a number of tissues. It appears that Notch exerts its effect by inhibiting or suppressing certain differentiation pathways in Drosophila and C. elegans, thereby allowing cells to differentiate along an alternative path, or to undergo self-renewal (Varnum-Finney *et al.*, 2000). It is perhaps not surprising therefore that Notch expression can also influence lineage commitment and stem cell function throughout hematopoiesis (Varnum-Finney *et al.*, 1998; Karanu *et al.*, 2001; Walker *et al.*, 2001).

The Notch molecules are transmembrane receptors that effect cell fate decisions by regulating downstream helix-loop-helix (HLH) transcription factor proteins (see below) including the transcription factor E2A (Ordentlich *et al.*, 1998), that is critical in the development of pre-B ALL. Notch signaling is initiated by binding of its extracellular domain to a Notch ligand. At present, two Notch ligand families, Delta and Serrate/Jagged, have been described. As mentioned above, Notch signaling determines the developmental fates of progeny derived from bipotential precursors. Interactions between cells expressing Notch receptors and ligands induce lineage commitment and determine cell fate.

Notch has been implicated in hematopoietic stem cell self-renewal (Varnum-Finney *et al.*, 2000) and constitutive Notch signaling was able to generate immortalized cytokine-dependent cell lines. However, further studies will be required to ascertain if these Notch-transduced bone marrow cell lines can be used to elucidate events involved in normal cell lineage commitment of hematopoietic stem cells. Consistent with these findings, expression of Jagged-1 on the cell surface of fibroblast cells elicited an increase in the formation of c-kit+, Sca-1+, lineage-negative, precursors. In addition, soluble Delta-1 and Delta-4 proteins were able to enhance the proliferation of CD34+, CD38−, lineage-negative progenitors in vitro. Thus these results imply that Notch ligands could be used to expand hematopoietic stem cells in vitro.

As well as its function in normal hematopoiesis, Notch signaling has been demonstrated to cause malignant transformation of human T cells and Notch itself is involved in recurrent chromosomal translocations (Ellisen *et al.,* 1991). Removal of Notch from developing T cells blocks their differentiation at a very immature stage while concomitantly inducing ectopic intrathymic B-cell development (Radtke *et al.,* 1999). Similarly, experiments that overexpressed molecules involved in inhibiting Notch function or altering its spatial localization demonstrated induction of ectopic B cells within a thymic environment. Notch signaling therefore appears to determine lineage commitment during consecutive phases of hematopoietic and T-cell development. Its frequent involvement in these cellular decisions parallels the frequent use of this pathway throughout Drosophila development. Elucidation of the multiple functions of Notch signaling in hematopoiesis and lymphoid development may lead to unique approaches to stem cell manipulation and cancer treatment.

Another signaling pathway of emerging importance for hematopoiesis is the Wnt gene pathway. Like Notch, Wnt signaling regulates cell proliferation and differentiation in species as divergent as flies and mammals. The incredible conservation of this pathway also suggests that Wnt signal transduction is an important mechanism for directing lineage commitment in developing tissues. The Wnt genes encode a family of secreted glycoproteins that involve a spectrum of activities during development. The Wnt proteins are thought to be associated with the cell surface or the extracellular matrix of the secreting cells. They act through their cell-surface receptors (Frizzled and Disheveled) to influence a critical intracellular pathway, the β-catenin pathway.

The mRNAs of both Wnt10a and Wnt10b genes have been found in the thymus and spleen. Additionally, Wnt10a is also expressed in the fetal liver (Wang & Shackleford, 1996). The Wnt genes have also been found to be expressed in adult bone marrow (Austin *et al.,* 1997; Van Den Berg *et al.,* 1998). Specifically, Wnt-5a and Wnt-10b were expressed in day-11 murine yolk sac and day-14 fetal liver (Austin *et al.,* 1997). The function of the Wnt proteins has been examined by using culture supernatants: the addition of conditioned media from cells transfected with Wnt-1, Wnt-5a, or Wnt-10b to cultures of ckit+, Sca-1+, fetal liver cells led to a significant expansion in cell number. Similarly, transduction of ckit+, Sca-1+ fetal liver cells with a Wnt-5a retrovirus also enhanced cellular proliferation.

Wnt-3a conditioned media has been shown to significantly reduce B-lineage and myeloid cells in long-term bone marrow cultures in the presence of stromal cells. Surprisingly, Wnt-3a conditioned media did not produce this effect in stromal cell-free conditions. It was therefore concluded that Wnt proteins exert their function by modulating stromal cell activity (Yamane *et al.,* 2001).

Further evidence of a critical role for Wnt function in lymphoid development has been provided by mice deficient in components of the Wnt signaling pathway (Reya *et al.,* 2000; Staal & Clevers, 2000). TCF-1/LEF-1 proteins are downstream effectors of the Wnt signaling pathway. LEF-1-deficient mice display reduced proliferation and survival of pro-B cells, while TCF-1 deficient mice show significant impairment of T-cell development. LEF-1 deficient pro-B cells exhibit increased levels of fas and c-myc transcription, providing a potential mechanism for their increased apoptosis. It was discovered that Wnt proteins were mitogenic for pro-B cells and that this was mediated by LEF-1 (Reya *et al.,* 2000). Therefore, this conclusion is in direct contrast to the previous results that demonstrated a Wnt-dependent inhibition of B-cell development.

These apparent contradictory results may be explained based on differences in developmental context. Previously, it has been demonstrated that Notch's effects are sensitive to developmental context. Wnt function in hematopoiesis may be similarly sensitive. Therefore, the challenge for the future is to more carefully document Wnt function in hematopoiesis with this in mind. These results have identified a role in lymphoid development, but perhaps more importantly may provide a basis for future expansion of hematopoietic stem cells for use in transplantation.

Transcriptional regulation of hematopoiesis

While the extracellular growth factors have a clear role in modulating hematopoiesis (both in vitro and in vivo), it has become increasingly clear that transcription factors play a central role in hematopoietic development, differentiation, and oncogenesis. In addition, the application of gene targeting techniques has provided further evidence for the important role of these molecules. For example, the generation of mice unable to elaborate GM-CSF revealed that the principal physiologic function of the molecule is to maintain pulmonary homeostasis (Dranoff *et al.,* 1994; Stanley *et al.,* 1994). This was confirmed using mice in which the GM-CSF receptor was ablated; these animals also developed an alveolar-proteinosis-like syndrome (Nishinakamura *et al.,* 1995; Robb *et al.,* 1995c; Nishinakamura *et al.,* 1996). This role for GM-CSF was not suspected from analyses of GM-CSF action in vitro, nor from its clinical application. The loss of GM-CSF signalling had only modest consequences within the hematopoietic compartment, with a decrease in eosinophils as a result of ablation of the shared receptor for GM-CSF, IL-3, and IL-5 (Nishinakamura *et al.,* 1995; Robb *et al.,* 1995c; Nishinakamura *et al.,* 1996). In contrast, ablation of genes encoding hematopoietic transcription factors has revealed dramatic consequences within the hematopoietic compartment. Some of these findings are briefly discussed below.

SCL and LMO2

The transcription factor SCL (Begley & Green 1999) was first identified because of its involvement in a chromosomal translocation in a unique, multipotential leukemia (Begley *et al.,* 1989a; Begley *et al.,* 1989b). These leukemic cells displayed an early T-cell phenotype and differentiated into myeloid cells in vivo and in vitro (Hershfield *et al.,* 1984; Kurtzberg, Bigner, & Hershfield, 1985). The t(1;14) chromosomal translocation was molecularly cloned to reveal the involvement of SCL, a previously unknown member of the helix-loop-helix (HLH) family of transcription factors. It was subsequently realized that the majority of leukemias that harbor an abnormality of SCL show a more typical T-cell phenotype, hence the alternative name Tal1 (Brown *et al.*, 1990a; Robb & Begley, 1996). The oncogenic action of SCL has been documented in murine models (Elwood *et al.*, 1993), and the requirement for additional genetic events established. In these in vivo models, SCL can cooperate with ABL, casein kinase II, LMO2 (RBTN2/TTG2), RAS, and p53 deficiency (Robb *et al.*, 1995b; Condorelli *et al.*, 1996; Larson *et al.*, 1996; Curtis *et al.*, 1997).

Studies of the expression pattern of SCL first suggested it might play an important role in normal hematopoietic differentiation (Begley *et al.*, 1989b). Expression is readily detected in mast cells, megakaryocytes, and erythroid cells (Green, Salvaris, & Begley, 1991; Green *et al.*, 1992; Chiba *et al.*, 1993; Cross *et al.*, 1994), an expression pattern very similar to that of GATA 1, a hematopoietic transcription factor of the Zinc-finger class (Pevny *et al.*, 1991). SCL expression is not normally detected in T cells but is evident in, for example, developing brain and endothelial cells. Gene transfer experiments demonstrated that, while enforced SCL expression enhanced erythroid differentiation (Aplan *et al.*, 1992), macrophage differentiation was inhibited (Tanigawa *et al.*, 1993; Tanigawa *et al.*, 1995). Experiments in the zebrafish system demonstrated that enforced expression of SCL could expand both hematopoietic and endothelial cell compartments, implying a function in the putative hemangioblast (Gering *et al.*, 1998).

The results of the gene targeting experiments were unexpectedly dramatic. Loss of SCL function results in the complete absence of hematopoietic cells, an absence of blood vessels in the yolk sac, and death of the embryo (Robb *et al.*, 1995a; Shivdasani, Mayer, & Orkin, 1995). These findings, established a crucial role for SCL in the development of all yolk sac or "primitive" hematopoietic cells. Experiments to address the function of SCL during adult hematopoiesis were equally dramatic. While SCL-null embryonic stem cells contributed to all nonhematopoietic tissues, these cells failed to generate any hematopoietic elements (Porcher *et al.*, 1996; Robb *et al.*, 1996). Moreover, these cells are incapable of hematopoietic differentiation in vitro (Elefanty *et al.*, 1997), thus establishing a central role for SCL in adult, "definitive" hematopoiesis.

The results described above for SCL show striking parallels with the Zinc-finger containing protein LMO2. As with SCL, LMO2 was first identified because of its involvement in a chromosome translocation in human T-cell acute lymphoblastic leukemia (Boehm *et al.*, 1991; Royer-Pokora, Loos, & Ludwig, 1991). Again, like SCL, its expression is not normally detected in T cells, but is readily evident in erythroid cells and hematopoietic precursors (Warren *et al.*, 1994). Moreover, both genes cooperate in models of leukemogenesis (Larson *et al.*, 1996). The remarkable similarity between these two genes is probably explicable given their ability to form a protein com-

plex, whereas part of a larger multiprotein complex, LMO2, forms a molecular bridge between SCL and GATA 1 (Osada *et al.*, 1995; Wadman *et al.*, 1997). One member of this multiprotein complex is the SCL-partner protein, the product of the E2A gene that is involved in the t(1;19) chromosome translocation and is also downstream of Notch signaling (Mellentin *et al.*, 1989; McWhirter *et al.*, 1999; Engel & Murre, 2001).

The GATA family

The GATA proteins bind a specific DNA sequence via a highly conserved Zinc-finger domain (Evans & Felsenfeld, 1989; Tsai *et al.*, 1989). Several family members show a predominantly hematopoietic expression. GATA-1 is primarily expressed in erythroid cells, mast cells, and megakaryocytes, but is also detected in the testis (Weiss & Orkin, 1995). Within hematopoietic cells GATA-2 is expressed in populations of hematopoietic progenitor/stem cells, megakaryocytes, and mast cells, while GATA-3 is detected in T lymphocytes. Functionally important GATA-binding sites are present in the *cis*-regulatory elements of many hematopoietic-restricted genes, suggesting an important role for family members in modulating gene expression (Shivdasani & Orkin, 1996). Gene targeting studies have confirmed the important role played by GATA family members in hematopoiesis. GATA-1 deficient embryos die from anemia (Fujiwara *et al.*, 1996) and GATA-1 deficient embryonic stem cells generate erythroid precursors that are arrested at the proerythroblast stage (Weiss, Keller, & Orkin, 1994; Pevny *et al.*, 1995). In addition, these embryonic stem cells are also unable to generate mature erythroid cells in adult mice (Pevny *et al.*, 1991). Together these demonstrate a crucial role for GATA-1 in erythroid development. In addition, it is also important in ensuring normal megakaryocyte development (Shivdasani *et al.*, 1997). Mice that are deficient in GATA-2 have a more severe defect in embryonic hematopoiesis than occurs with GATA-1, but less than that seen with LMO2 or SCL. These animals also die in utero with marked anemia and reduction in progenitor cells within the yolk sac. GATA-2 deficient embryonic stem cells fail to generate fetal liver-derived blood cells and contribute only poorly to primitive yolk sac hematopoiesis. In keeping with these findings, hematopoietic differentiation of GATA-2 deficient embryonic stem cells results in a reduced frequency of hematopoietic precursors of all lineages and a complete absence of mast cells (Tsai *et al.*, 1994; Tsai & Orkin, 1997). These results suggest that GATA-2 is vital at a stage of hematopoietic development between SCL/LMO2 and GATA-1, and is required for the expansion of the multipotential stem cell compartment. GATA-3 null animals show a complex phenotype, reflecting the wider expression of this family member. However, within the hematopoietic compartment GATA-3 is required for the normal development of T lymphocytes (Pandolfi *et al.*, 1995; Ting *et al.*, 1996).

Analysis of numerous other transcription factors has provided important insights into their critical role in hematopoietic development. For example, AML-1, one of the genes most frequently involved in human leukemia, is crucial for the development of fetal-liver derived hematopoiesis, but yolk sac-derived hematopoiesis occurs normally in mice that lack its function (Okuda *et al.*, 1996; Wang *et al.*, 1996). A similar defect is seen in mice that lack function of MYB; primitive yolk-sac hematopoiesis occurs normally, but fetal liver hematopoiesis is defective (Mucenski *et al.*, 1991). In comparison, the defect in mice that lack p45 NFE2 is far more restricted. These mice die neonatally of hemorrhage, since megakaryocytic differentiation fails to proceed normally and platelets are not generated (Shivdasani & Orkin, 1995; Shivdasani *et al.*, 1995). Thus, analysis of the role of transcription factors in hematopoietic development and differentiation has confirmed the vital role of these molecules in regulating these processes.

Conclusions

Over recent years much has been learned about the hematopoietic growth factors, with several of these having clearly established roles in a clinical environment. In addition, promising new growth factors are currently undergoing clinical development and second-generation, longer acting versions of G-CSF and EPO are now available. While the task of clinical evaluation has been relatively simple for the growth factors that are "lineage-restricted" in their predominant action, it will be more difficult to evaluate many of the pleiotropic molecules whose clinical role remains to be more broadly defined. In addition, the development of gene targeting has demonstrated that the current clinical utility of some of these molecules bears little relationship to their physiologic function in the intact animal. In contrast, some of the key regulators for establishing hematopoiesis have been revealed by their involvement in leukemogenic events and their importance confirmed by gene ablation techniques. The future challenge will be to marry these two lines of research and to determine how extrinsic signals and intrinsic mechanisms are balanced in order to determine the fate of hematopoietic cells in a clinically useful manner.

References

Alexander, W.S., Roberts, A.W., Nicola, N.A. *et al.* (1996). Deficiencies in progenitor cells of multiple hematopoietic lineages and defective megakaryocytopoiesis in mice lacking the thrombopoietic receptor c-Mpl. *Blood,* **87,** 2162–70.

Andrews, R.G., Knitter, G.H., Bartelmez, S.H. *et al.* (1991). Recombinant human stem cell factor, a c-kit ligand, stimulates hematopoiesis in primates. *Blood,* **78,** 1975–80.

Aplan, P.D., Nakahara, K., Orkin, S.H. *et al.* (1992). The SCL gene product: a positive regulator of erythroid differentiation. *EMBO Journal,* **11,** 4073–81.

Archimbaud, E., Ottmann, O.G., Yin, J.A. *et al.* (1999). A randomized, double-blind, placebo-controlled study with pegylated recombinant human megakaryocyte growth and development factor (PEG-rHuMGDF) as an adjunct to chemotherapy for adults with de novo acute myeloid leukemia. *Blood,* **94,** 3694–701.

Ariyama, Y., Misawa, S., & Sonoda, Y. (1995). Synergistic effects of stem cell factor and interleukin 6 or interleukin-11 on the expansion of murine hematopoietic progenitors in liquid suspension culture. *Stem Cells,* **13,** 404–13.

Austin, T.W., Solar, G.P., Ziegler, F.C. *et al.* (1997). A role for the Wnt gene family in hematopoiesis: expansion of multilineage progenitor cells. *Blood,* **89,** 3624.

Barker, J.E. (1994). Sl/Sld hematopoietic progenitors are deficient in situ. *Experimental Hematology,* **22,** 174–7.

Bartley, T.D., Bogenberger, J., Hunt, P. *et al.* (1994). Identification and cloning of a megakaryocyte growth and development factor that is a ligand for the cytokine receptor Mpl. *Cell,* **77,** 1117–24.

Basser, R.L., O'Flaherty, E., Green, M. *et al.* (2002). Development of pancytopenia with neutralizing antibodies to thrombopoietin after multicycle chemotherapy supported by megakaryocyte growth and development factor. *Blood,* **99,** 2599–602.

Basser, R.L., Rasko, J.E.J., Clarke, K. *et al.* (1996). Thrombopoietic effects of pegylated recombinant human megakaryocyte growth and development factor (PEG-rHuMGDF) in patients with advanced cancer. *Lancet,* **348,** 1279–81.

Basser, R.L., Rasko, J.E.J., Clarke, K. *et al.* (1997). Randomised, blinded, placebo-controlled phase 1 trial of pegylated recombinant human megakaryocyte growth and development factor (PEG-rHuMGDF) with filgrastim after dose intensive chemotherapy in patients with advanced cancer. *Blood,* **89,** 3118–28.

Basser, R.L., Underhill, C., Davis, I. *et al.* (2000). Enhancement of platelet recovery after myelosuppressive chemotherapy by recombinant human megakaryocyte growth and development factor in patients with advanced cancer. *Journal of Clinical Oncology,* **18,** 2852–61.

Bazan, J.F. (1991). Genetic and structural homology of stem cell factor and macrophage colony-stimulating factor. *Cell,* **65,** 9–10.

Begley, C.G. & Green, A.R. (1999). The SCL gene: from case report to critical hematopoietic regulator. *Blood,* **93,** 2760–70.

Begley, C.G., Aplan, P.D., Davey, M.P. *et al.* (1989a). Chromosomal translocation in a human leukemic stem-cell line disrupts the T-cell antigen receptor delta-chain diversity region and results in a previously unreported fusion transcript. *Proceedings of the National Academy of Sciences USA,* **86,** 2031–5.

Begley, C.G., Aplan, P.D., Denning, S.M. *et al.* (1989b). The gene SCL is expressed during early hematopoiesis and encodes a differentiation-related DNA-binding motif. *Proceedings of the National Academy of Sciences USA,* **86,** 10128–32.

Begley, C.G., Basser, R.L., Mansfield, R. *et al.* (1997). Enhanced levels and enhanced clonogenic capacity of blood progenitor cells following administration of SCF plus G-CSF to humans. *Blood,* **90,** 3378–89.

Begley, C.G., Rasko, J.E., Curtis, D. *et al.* (1996). Murine flt3 ligand protects M1 leukemic cells from LIF-induced differentiation and suppression of self-renewal. *Experimental Hematology,* **24,** 1247–57.

Berl, T. & Schwertschlag, U. (2000). Preclinical pharmacologic basis for clinical use of rhIL-11 as an effective platelet-support agent. *Oncology,* **14**(Suppl 8), 12–20.

Bernstein, I.D., Andrews, R.G., & Zsebo, K.M. (1991). Recombinant human stem cell factor enhances the formation of colonies by CD34+ and CD34+lin- cells, and the generation of colony-forming cell progeny from CD34+lin- cells cultured with interleukin-3, granulocyte colony-stimulating factor, or granulocyte-macrophage colony-stimulating factor. *Blood*, **77**, 2316–21.

Besmer, P., Manova, K., Duttlinger, R. *et al.* (1993). The kit-ligand (steel factor) and its receptor c-kit/W: pleiotropic roles in gametogenesis and melanogenesis. *Development Supplement*, 125–37.

Bilinski, P., Roopenian, D., & Gossler, A. (1998). Maternal IL-11Ralpha function is required for normal decidua and fetoplacental development in mice. *Genes and Development*, **15;12**, 2234–43.

Birg, F., Rosnet, O., Carbuccia, N. *et al.* (1994). The expression of FMS, KIT and FLT3 in hematopoietic malignancies. *Leukemia & Lymphoma*, **13**, 223–7.

Blouin, R. & Bernstein, A. (1993). The white spotting and hereditary anemias of the mouse. In *Clinical Disorders and Experimental Models of Erythropoietic Failure*. p. 157. Boca Raton, FL: CRC Press.

Boehm, T., Foroni, L., Kaneko, Y. *et al.* (1991). The rhombotin family of cysteine-rich LIM-domain oncogenes: distinct members are involved in T-cell translocations to human chromosomes 11p15 and 11p13. *Proceedings of the National Academy of Sciences USA*, **88**, 4367–71.

Boggs, D.R., Boggs, S.S., Saxe, D.F. *et al.* (1982). Hematopoietic stem cells with high proliferative potential. Assay of their concentration in marrow by the frequency and duration of cure of W/Wv mice. *Journal of Clinical Investigation*, **70**, 242–53.

Bradley, T.R. & Hodgson, G.S. (1979). Detection of primitive macrophage progenitor cells in mouse bone marrow. *Blood*, **54**, 1446–50.

Bradley, T.R. & Metcalf, D. (1966). The growth of mouse bone marrow cells in vitro. *Australian Journal of Experimental Biology & Medical Science*, **44**, 287–99.

Brandt, J., Briddell, R.A., Srour, E.F. *et al.* (1992). Role of c-kit ligand in the expansion of human hematopoietic progenitor cells. *Blood*, **79**, 634–41.

Brannan, C.I., Lyman, S.D., Williams, D.E. *et al.* (1991). Steel-Dickie mutation encodes a c-kit ligand lacking transmembrane and cytoplasmic domains. *Proceedings of the National Academy of Sciences USA*, **88**, 4671–4.

Brasel, K., Escobar, S., Anderberg, R. *et al.* (1995). Expression of the flt3 receptor and its ligand on hematopoietic cells. *Leukemia*, **9**, 1212–18.

Brasel, K., Mckenna, H.J., Morrissey, P.J. *et al.* (1996). Hematologic effects of flt3 ligand in vivo in mice. *Blood*, **88**, 2004–12.

Briddell, R.A., Bruno, E., Cooper, R.J. *et al.* (1991). Effect of c-kit ligand on in vitro human megakaryocytopoiesis. *Blood*, **78**, 2854–9.

Broudy, V.C. (1997). Stem cell factor and hematopoiesis. *Blood*, **90**, 1345–64.

Broudy, V.C., Lin, N.L., & Kaushansky, K. (1995). Thrombopoietin (c-mpl ligand) acts synergistically with erythropoietin, stem cell factor, and interleukin-11 to enhance murine megakaryocyte colony growth and increases megakaryocyte ploidy in vitro. *Blood*, **85**, 1719–26.

Brown, L., Cheng, J.T., Chen, Q. *et al.* (1990). Site-specific recombination of the tal-1 gene is a common occurrence in human T cell leukemia. *EMBO Journal*, **9**, 3343–51.

Broxmeyer, H.E., Hangoc, G., Cooper, S. *et al.* (1991). Influence of murine mast cell growth factor (c-kit ligand) on colony formation by mouse marrow hematopoietic progenitor cells. *Experimental Hematology*, **19**, 143–6.

Bruno, E., Briddell, R.A., Cooper, R.J. *et al.* (1991). Effects of recombinant interleukin-11 on human megakaryocyte progenitor cells. *Experimental Hematology*, **19**, 378–81.

Burstein, S.A., Mei, R.L., Henthorn, J. *et al.* (1992). Leukemia inhibitory factor and interleukin-11 promote maturation of murine and human megakaryocytes in vitro. *Journal of Cellular Physiology*, **153**, 305–12.

Cairo, M.S., Plunkett, J.M., Nguyen, A. *et al.* (1993). Effect of interleukin-11 with and without granulocyte colony-stimulating factor on in vivo neonatal rat hematopoiesis: induction of neonatal thrombocytosis by interleukin-11 and synergistic enhancement of neutrophilia by interleukin-11 plus granulocyte colony-stimulating factor. *Pediatric Research*, **34**, 56–61.

Carver-Moore, K., Broxmeyer, H.E., Luoh, S.M. *et al.* (1996). Low levels of erythroid and myeloid progenitors in thrombopoietin- and c-mpl-deficient mice. *Blood*, **88**, 803–8.

Chiba, T., Nagata, Y., Kishi, A. *et al.* (1993). Induction of erythroid-specific gene expression in lymphoid cells. *Proceedings of the National Academy of Sciences USA*, **90**, 11593–7.

Choi, E.S., Hokom, M.M., Chen, J.L. *et al.* (1996). The role of megakaryocyte growth and development factor in terminal stages of thrombopoiesis. *British Journal of Haematology*, **95**, 227–33.

Condorelli, G.L., Facchiano, F., Valtieri, M. *et al.* (1996). T-cell-directed TAL-1 expression induces T-cell malignancies in transgenic mice. *Cancer Research*, **56**, 5113–19.

Costa, J.J., Demetri, G.D., Harrist, T.J. *et al.* (1996). Recombinant human stem cell factor (kit ligand) promotes human mast cell and melanocyte hyperplasia and functional activation in vivo. *Journal of Experimental Medicine*, **183**, 2681–6.

Cross, M.A., Heyworth, C.M., Murrell, A.M. *et al.* (1994). Expression of lineage restricted transcription factors precedes lineage specific differentiation in a multipotent haemopoietic progenitor cell line. *Oncogene*, **9**, 3013–16.

Curtis, D., Robb, L., Strasser, A. *et al.* (1997). The CD2-SCL transgene alters the phenotype and the frequency of T-lymphomas in N-ras transgenic or p53 deficient mice. *Oncogene*, **15**, 2975–83.

Dasilva, N., Hu, Z.B., Ma, W. *et al.* (1994). Expression of the FLT3 gene in human leukemia-lymphoma cell lines. *Leukemia*, **8**, 885–8.

De Haan, G., Dontje, B., Engel, C. *et al.* (1995). In vivo effects of interleukin-11 and stem cell factor in combination with erythropoietin in the regulation of erythropoiesis. *British Journal of Haematology*, **90**, 783–90.

de Jong, M.O., Rozemuller, H., Kieboom, D. *et al.* (1996). Purification of repopulating hemopoietic cells based on binding of biotinylated Kit ligand. *Leukemia*, **10**, 1813–22.

de Sauvage, F.J., Carver-Moore, K., Luoh, S.M. *et al.* (1996). Physiological regulation of early and late stages of megakaryocytopoiesis by thrombopoietin. *Journal of Experimental Medicine*, **183**, 651–6.

de Sauvage, F.J., Hass, P.E., Spencer, S.D. *et al.* (1994). Stimulation of megakaryocytopoiesis and thrombopoiesis by the c-Mpl ligand. *Nature,* **369,** 533–8.

Dexter, T.M. (1984). Long-Term Marrow Cultures: An Overview of Techniques and Experience. In *Long-Term Marrow Cultures.* pp. 57–96. New York: Alan R Liss.

Dexter, T.M., Allen, T.D., & Lajtha, L.G. (1977). Conditions controlling the proliferation of haemopoietic stem cells in vitro. *Journal of Cellular Physiology,* **91,** 335–44.

Dexter, T.M. & Spooncer, E. (1987). Growth and differentiation in the hemopoietic system. *Annual Review of Cell Biology,* **3,** 423–41.

Disis, M.L., Rinn, K., Knutson, K.L. *et al.* (2002). Flt3 ligand as a vaccine adjuvant in association with HER-2/neu peptide-based vaccines in patients with HER-2/neu-overexpressing cancers. *Blood,* **99,** 2845–50.

Doi, H., Inaba, M., Yamamoto, Y. *et al.* (1997). Pluripotent hemopoietic stem cells are c-kit low. *Proceedings of the National Academy of Sciences USA,* **94,** 2513–17.

Donaldson, L.E., Schmitt, E., Huntley, J.F. *et al.* (1996). A critical role for stem cell factor and c-kit in host protective immunity to an intestinal helminth. *International Immunology,* **8,** 559–67.

Dranoff, G., Crawford, A.D., Sadelain, M. *et al.* (1994). Involvement of granulocyte-macrophage colony-stimulating factor in pulmonary homeostasis. *Science,* **264,** 713–16.

Du, X. & Williams, D.A. (1997). Interleukin-11: review of molecular, cell biology, and clinical use. *Blood,* **89,** 3897–908.

Du, X.X., Neben, T., Goldman, S. *et al.* (1993). Effects of recombinant human interleukin-11 on hematopoietic reconstitution in transplant mice: acceleration of recovery of peripheral blood neutrophils and platelets. *Blood,* **81,** 27–34.

Du, X.X., Scott, D., Yang, Z.X. *et al.* (1995). Interleukin-11 stimulates multilineage progenitors, but not stem cells, in murine and human long-term marrow cultures. *Blood,* **86,** 128–34.

Durand, B., Migliaccio, G., Yee, N.S. *et al.* (1994). Long-term generation of human mast cells in serum-free cultures of CD34+ cord blood cells stimulated with stem cell factor and interleukin-3. *Blood,* **84,** 3667–74.

Dykstra, K.H., Rogge, H., Stone, A. *et al.* (2000). Mechanism and amelioration of recombinant human interleukin-11 (rhIL-11)-induced anemia in healthy subjects. *Journal of Clinical Pharmacology,* **40,** 880–8.

Elefanty, A., Robb, L., Birner, R. *et al.* (1997). Hematopoietic-specific genes are not induced during in-vitro differentiation of SCL-null embryonic stem cells. *Blood,* **90,** 1435–47.

Ellisen, L.W., Bird, J., West, D.C. *et al.* (1991). TAN-1, the human homolog of the Drosophila notch gene, is broken by chromosomal translocations in T lymphoblastic neoplasms. *Cell,* **66,** 649.

Elwood, N.J., Cook, W.D., Metcalf, D. *et al.* (1993). SCL, the gene implicated in human T-cell leukaemia, is oncogenic in a murine T-lymphocyte cell line. *Oncogene,* **8,** 3093–101.

Elwood, N.J., Zogos, H., Willson, T. *et al.* (1996). Retroviral transduction of human progenitor cells: use of granulocyte colony-stimulating factor plus stem cell factor to mobilize progenitor cells in vivo and stimulation by Flt3/Flk-2 ligand in vitro. *Blood,* **88,** 4452–62.

Engel, I. & Murre, C. (2001). The function of E- and Id proteins in lymphocyte development. *Nature Reviews in Immunology,* **1,** 193–9.

Evans, T. & Felsenfeld, G. (1989). The erythroid-specific transcription factor Eryf1: a new finger protein. *Cell,* **58,** 877–85.

Ezoe, K., Holmes, S.A., Ho, L. *et al.* (1995). Novel mutations and deletions of the KIT (steel factor receptor) gene in human piebaldism. *American Journal of Human Genetics,* **56,** 58–66.

Fanucchi, M., Glaspy, J., Crawford, J. *et al.* (1997). Effects of polyethylene glycol-conjugated recombinant megakaryocyte growth and development factor on platelet counts after chemotherapy for lung cancer. *New England Journal of Medicine,* **366,** 404–9.

Farese, A.M., Hunt, P., Boone, T. *et al.* (1995). Recombinant human megakaryocyte growth and development factor stimulates thrombocytopoiesis in normal nonhuman primates. *Blood,* **86,** 54–9.

Farese, A.M., Hunt, P., Grab, L.B. *et al.* (1996). Combined administration of recombinant human megakaryocyte growth and development factor and granulocyte colony-stimulating factor enhances multilineage hematopoietic reconstitution in nonhuman primates after radiation-induced marrow aplasia. *Journal of Clinical Investigation,* **97,** 2145–51.

Fauser, A.A. & Messner, H.A. (1979). Proliferative state of human pluripotent hemopoietic progenitors (CFU-GEMM) in normal individuals and under regenerative conditions after bone marrow transplantation. *Blood,* **54,** 1197–200.

Flanagan, J.G., Chan, D.C., & Leder, P. (1991). Transmembrane form of the kit ligand growth factor is determined by alternative splicing and is missing in the Sld mutant. *Cell,* **64,** 1025–35.

Flanagan, J.G. & Leder, P. (1990). The kit ligand: a cell surface molecule altered in steel mutant fibroblasts. *Cell,* **63,** 185–94.

Ford, C.E., Hamerton, J.H., Barnes, W.H. *et al.* (1956). Cytological identification of radiation chimeras. *Nature,* **177,** 452–4.

Fujiwara, Y., Browne, C.P., Cunniff, K. *et al.* (1996). Arrested development of embryonic red cell precursors in mouse embryos lacking transcription factor GATA-1. *Proceedings of the National Academy of Sciences USA,* **93,** 12355–8.

Gabbianelli, M., Pelosi, E., Montesoro, E. *et al.* (1995). Multi-level effects of flt3 ligand on human hematopoiesis: expansion of putative stem cells and proliferation of granulomonocytic progenitors/monocytic precursors. *Blood,* **86,** 1661–70.

Gainsford, T., Roberts, A.W., Kimura, S. *et al.* (1998). Cytokine production and function in c-mpl-deficient mice: no physiological role for interleukin-3 in residual megakaryocyte and platelet production. *Blood,* **91,** 2745–52.

Gainsford, T., Nandurkar, H., Metcalf, D. *et al.* (2000). The residual megakaryocyte and platelet production in c-Mpl-deficient mice is not dependent on the actions of interleukin-6, interleukin-11 or leukemia inhibitory factor. *Blood,* **95,** 528–34.

Galli, S.J., Tsai, M., Wershil, B.K. *et al.* (1995). Regulation of mouse and human mast cell development, survival and function by stem cell factor, the ligand for the c-kit receptor. *International Archives of Allergy & Immunology,* **107,** 51–3.

Gering, M., Rodaway, A.R., Gottgens, B. *et al.* (1998). The SCL gene specifies haemangioblast development from early mesoderm. *EMBO Journal,* **17,** 4029–45.

Goldman, S.C., Bracho, F., Davenport, V. *et al.* (2001). Feasibility study of IL-11 and granulocyte colony-stimulating factor after myelosuppressive chemotherapy to mobilize peripheral blood stem cells from heavily pretreated patients. *Journal of Pediatric Hematology and Oncology,* **23,** 300–5.

Gordon, M.S., McCaskill-Stevens, W.J., Battiato, L.A. *et al.* (1996). A phase I trial of recombinant human interleukin-11 (neumega rhIL 11 growth factor) in women with breast cancer receiving chemotherapy. *Blood,* **87,** 3615–24.

Green, A.R., DeLuca, E., & Begley, C.G. (1991). Antisense SCL suppresses self-renewal and enhances spontaneous erythroid differentiation of the human leukaemic cell line K562. *EMBO Journal,* **10,** 4153–8.

Green, A.R., Lints, T., Visvader, J. *et al.* (1992). SCL is coexpressed with GATA-1 in hemopoietic cells but is also expressed in developing brain [published erratum appears in *Oncogene* 1992, **7,** 1459]. *Oncogene,* **7,** 653–60.

Green, A.R., Salvaris, E., & Begley, C.G. (1991). Erythroid expression of the 'helix-loop-helix' gene, SCL. *Oncogene,* **6,** 475–9.

Grossmann, A., Lenox, J., Deisher, T.A. *et al.* (1996a). Synergistic effects of thrombopoietin and granulocyte colony-stimulating factor on neutrophic recovery in myelosuppressed mice. *Blood,* **88,** 3363–70.

Grossmann, A., Lenox, J., Ren, H.P. *et al.* (1996b). Thrombopoietin accelerates platelet, red blood cell and neutrophil recovery in myelosuppressed mice. *Experimental Hematology,* **24,** 1238–46.

Gurney, A.L., Carver-Moore, K., De Sauvage, F.J. *et al.* (1994). Thrombocytopenia in c-mpl-deficient mice. *Science,* **265,** 1445–7.

Hangoc, G., Yin, T., Cooper, S. *et al.* (1993). In vivo effects of recombinant interleukin-11 on myelopoiesis in mice. *Blood,* **81,** 965–72.

Hannum, C., Culpepper, J., Campbell, D. *et al.* (1994). Ligand for FLT3/FLK2 receptor tyrosine kinase regulates growth of haematopoietic stem cells and is encoded by variant RNAs. *Nature,* **368,** 643–8.

Hara, H. & Ogawa, M. (1978). Murine hemopoietic colonies in culture containing normoblasts, macrophages, and megakaryocytes. *American Journal of Hematology,* **4,** 23–34.

Harker, L.A., Hunt, P., Marzec, U.M. *et al.* (1996). Regulation of platelet production and function by megakaryocyte growth and development factor in nonhuman primates. *Blood,* 1833–44.

Harrison, D.E., Astle, C.M., & Lerner, C. (1988). Number and continuous proliferative pattern of transplanted primitive immunohematopoietic stem cells. *Proceedings of the National Academy of Sciences USA,* **85,** 822–6.

Hawley, R.G., Fong, A.Z., Ngan, B.Y. *et al.* (1993). Progenitor cell hyperplasia with rare development of myeloid leukemia in interleukin-11 bone marrow chimeras. *Journal of Experimental Medicine,* **178,** 1175–88.

Hawley, R.G., Hawley, T.S., Fong, A.Z. *et al.* (1996). Thrombopoietic potential and serial repopulating ability of murine hematopoietic stem cells constitutively expressing interleukin-11. *Proceedings of the National Academy of Sciences USA,* **93,** 10297–302.

Heits, F., Katschinski, D.M., Wilmsen, U. *et al.* (1997). Serum thrombopoietin and interleukin 6 concentrations in tumour patients and response to chemotherapy-induced thrombocytopenia. *European Journal of Haematology,* **59,** 53–8.

Henschler, R., Brugger, W., Luft, T. *et al.* (1994). Maintenance of transplantation potential in ex vivo expanded CD34(+)-selected human peripheral blood progenitor cells. *Blood,* **84,** 2898–903.

Hershfield, M.S., Kurtzberg, J., Harden, E. *et al.* (1984). Conversion of a stem cell leukemia from a T-lymphoid to a myeloid pheno-type induced by the adenosine deaminase inhibitor 2'-deoxycoformycin. *Proceedings of the National Academy of Sciences USA,* **81,** 253–7.

Hirayama, F., Katayama, N., Neben, S. *et al.* (1994). Synergistic interaction between interleukin-12 and steel factor in support of proliferation of murine lymphohematopoietic progenitors in culture. *Blood,* **83,** 92–8.

Holyoake, T.L., Freshney, M.G., McNair, L. *et al.* (1996). Ex vivo expansion with stem cell factor and interleukin-11 augments both short-term recovery posttransplant and the ability to serially transplant marrow. *Blood,* **87,** 4589–95.

Huang, E., Nocka, K., Beier, D.R. *et al.* (1990). The hematopoietic growth factor KL is encoded by the S1 locus and is the ligand of the c-kit receptor, the gene product of the W locus. *Cell,* **63,** 225–33.

Huang, E.J., Nocka, K.H., Buck, J. *et al.* (1992). Differential expression and processing of two cell associated forms of the kit-ligand: KL-1 and KL-2. *Molecular Biology of the Cell,* **3,** 349–62.

Huizinga, J.D., Thuneberg, L., Kluppel, M. *et al.* (1995). W/kit gene required for interstitial cells of Cajal and for intestinal pacemaker activity. *Nature,* **373,** 347–9.

Hunt, P., Li, Y.S., Nichol, J.L. *et al.* (1995). Purification and biologic characterization of plasma-derived megakaryocyte growth and development factor. *Blood,* **86,** 540–7.

Hunte, B.E., Hudak, S., Campbell, D. *et al.* (1996). flk2/flt3 ligand is a potent cofactor for the growth of primitive B cell progenitors. *Journal of Immunology,* **156,** 489–96.

Ichikawa, Y., Pluznik, D.H., & Sachs, L. (1966). In vitro control of the development of macrophage and granulocyte colonies. *Proceedings of the National Academy of Sciences USA,* **56,** 488–95.

Ikuta, K. & Weissman, I.L. (1992). Evidence that hematopoietic stem cells express mouse c-kit but do not depend on steel factor for their generation. *Proceedings of the National Academy of Sciences USA,* **89,** 1502–6.

Isaacs, C., Robert, N.J., Bailey, F.A. *et al.* (1997). Randomized placebo-controlled study of recombinant human interleukin-11 to prevent chemotherapy-induced thrombocytopenia in patients with breast cancer receiving dose-intensive cyclophosphamide and doxorubicin. *Journal of Clinical Oncology,* **15,** 3368–77.

Jacobsen, S.E., Okkenhaug, C., Veiby, O.P. *et al.* (1994). Interleukin 13: novel role in direct regulation of proliferation and differentiation of primitive hematopoietic progenitor cells. *Journal of Experimental Medicine,* **180,** 75–82.

Johnson, G.R. & Metcalf, D. (1977). Pure and mixed erythroid colony formation in vitro stimulated by spleen conditioned medium with no detectable erythropoietin. *Proceedings of the National Academy of Sciences USA,* **74,** 3879–82.

Jones, R.J., Collector, M.I., Barber, J.P. *et al.* (1996). Characterization of mouse lymphohematopoietic stem cells lacking spleen colony-forming activity. *Blood,* **88,** 487–91.

Karanu, F.N., Murdoch, B., Miyabayashi, T. *et al.* (2001). Human homologues of Delta-1 and Delta-4 function as mitogenic regulators of primitive human hematopoietic cells. *Blood,* **97,** 1960.

Kato, T., Ogami, K., Shimada, Y. *et al.* (1995). Purification and characterization of thrombopoietin. *Journal of Biochemistry,* **118,** 229–36.

Kaushansky, K. (1995). Thrombopoietin: the primary regulator of platelet production. *Blood,* **86,** 419–31.

Kaushansky, K., Broudy, V.C., Grossmann, A. *et al.* (1995b). Thrombopoietin expands erythroid progenitors, increases red cell production, and enhances erythroid recovery after myelosuppressive therapy. *Journal of Clinical Investigation,* **96,** 1683–7.

Kaushansky, K., Broudy, V.C., Lin, N. *et al.* (1995a). Thrombopoietin, the Mp1 ligand, is essential for full megakaryocyte development. *Proceedings of the National Academy of Sciences USA,* **92,** 3234–8.

Kaushansky, K., Lin, N., Grossmann, A. *et al.* (1996). Thrombopoietin expands erythroid, granulocyte-macrophage, and megakaryocytic progenitor cells in normal and myelosuppressed mice. *Experimental Hematology,* **24,** 265–9.

Kaushansky, K., Lok, S., Holly, R.D. *et al.* (1994). Promotion of megakaryocyte progenitor expansion and differentiation by the c-Mpl ligand thrombopoietin. *Nature,* **369,** 568–71.

Kawashima, I., Ohsumi, J., Mita-Honjo, K. *et al.* (1991). Molecular cloning of cDNA encoding adipogenesis inhibitory factor and identity with interleukin-11. *FEBS Letters,* **283,** 199–202.

Kelemen, E., Cserháti, I., & Tanos, B. (1958). Demonstration of some properties of human thrombopoietin in thrombocythaemic serum. *Acta Haematologica,* **20,** 350–5.

Keller, D.C., Du, X.X., Srour, E.F. *et al.* (1993). Interleukin-11 inhibits adipogenesis and stimulates myelopoiesis in human long-term marrow cultures. *Blood,* **82,** 1428–35.

Kimura, S., Roberts, A.W., Metcalf, D. *et al.* (1998). Hematopoietic stem cell deficiencies in mice lacking c-Mpl, the receptor for thrombopoietin. *Proceedings of the National Academy of Sciences USA,* **95,** 1195–200.

Kirshenbaum, A.S., Goff, J.P., Kessler, S.W. *et al.* (1992). Effect of IL-3 and stem cell factor on the appearance of human basophils and mast cells from CD34+ pluripotent progenitor cells. *Journal of Immunology,* **148,** 772–7.

Kitamura, Y., Go, S., & Hatanaka, K. (1978). Decrease of mast cells in W/Wv mice and their increase by bone marrow transplantation. *Blood,* **52,** 447–52.

Kobayashi, M., Laver, J.H., Kato, T. *et al.* (1995). Recombinant human thombopoietin (Mpl ligand) enhances proliferation of erythroid progenitors. *Blood,* **86,** 2494–9.

Kobayashi, M., Laver, J.H., Kato, T. *et al.* (1996). Thrombopoietin supports proliferation of human primitive hematopoietic cells in synergy with steel factor and/or interleukin-3. *Blood,* **88,** 429–36.

Kodama, H., Nose, M., Yamaguchi, Y. *et al.* (1992). In vitro proliferation of primitive hemopoietic stem cells supported by stromal cells: evidence for the presence of a mechanism(s) other than that involving c-kit receptor and its ligand. *Journal of Experimental Medicine,* **176,** 351–61.

Kriegler, A.B., Bradley, T.R., Bertoncello, I. *et al.* (1990). Progenitor cells in murine bone marrow stimulated by growth factors produced by the AF1-19T rat cell line. *Experimental Hematology,* **18,** 372–8.

Ku, H., Yonemura, Y., Kaushansky, K. *et al.* (1996). Thrombopoietin, the ligand for the Mpl receptor, synergizes with steel factor and other early acting cytokines in supporting proliferation of primitive hematopoietic progenitors of mice. *Blood,* **87,** 4544–51.

Kurtzberg, J., Binger, S.H., & Hershfield, M.S. (1985). Establishment of the DU.528 human lymphohemopoietic stem cell line. *Journal of Experimental Medicine,* **162,** 1561–78.

Kuter, D.J., Beeler, D.L., & Rosenberg, R.D. (1994). The purification of megapoietin: a physiological regulator of megakaryocyte growth and platelet production. *Proceedings of the National Academy of Sciences USA,* **91,** 11104–8.

Kuter, D.J., Goodnough, L.T., Romo, J. *et al.* (2001). Thrombopoietin therapy increases platelet yields in healthy platelet donors. *Blood,* **98,** 1339–45.

Lacerna, L., Basser, B., Begley, C.G. *et al.* (1998). Stem cell factor. In *Hematopoietic Stem Cell Therapy,* ed. A.D. Ho & R.E. Champlin. Cambridge: Cambridge University Press.

Larson, R.C., Lavenir, I., Larson, T.A. *et al.* (1996). Protein dimerization between Lmo2 (Rbtn2) and Tal1 alters thymocyte development and potentiates T cell tumorigenesis in transgenic mice. *EMBO Journal,* **15,** 1021–7.

Leary, A.G., Zeng, H.Q., Clark, S.C. *et al.* (1992). Growth factor requirements for survival in G_0 and entry into the cell cycle of primitive human hemopoietic progenitors. *Proceedings of the National Academy of Sciences USA,* **89,** 4013–17.

Lee, M.Y., Lottsfeldt, J.L., & Fevold, K.L. (1992). Identification and characterization of osteoclast progenitors by clonal analysis of hematopoietic cells. *Blood,* **80,** 1710–16.

Lemieux, M.E., Chappel, S.M., Miller, C.L. *et al.* (1997). Differential ability of flt3-ligand, interleukin-11, and Steel factor to support the generation of B cell progenitors and myeloid cells from primitive murine fetal liver cells. *Experimental Hematology,* **25,** 951–7.

Lemoli, R.M., Fogli, M., Fortuna, A. *et al.* (1993). Interleukin-11 stimulates the proliferation of human hematopoietic CD34+ and CD34+CD33-DR- cells and synergizes with stem cell factor, interleukin-3, and granulocyte-macrophage colony-stimulating factor. *Experimental Hematology,* **21,** 1668–72.

Li, C.L. & Johnson, G.R. (1995). Murine hematopoietic stem and progenitor cells: I. Enrichment and biologic characterization. *Blood,* **85,** 1472–9.

Li, J., Yang, C., Xia, Y. *et al.* (2001). Thrombocytopenia caused by the development of antibodies to thrombopoietin. *Blood,* **98,** 3241–8.

Lok, S., Kaushansky, K., Holly, R.D. *et al.* (1994). Cloning and expression of murine thrombopoietin cDNA and stimulation of platelet production in vivo. *Nature,* **369,** 565–8.

Long, M.W., Heffner, C.H., & Gragowski, L.L. (1986). In vitro differences in responsiveness of early (BFU-Mk) and late (CFU-Mk) murine megakaryocyte progenitor cells. *Progress in Clinical & Biological Research,* **215,** 179–86.

Lyman, S.D., James, L., Vanden Bos, T. *et al.* (1993). Molecular cloning of a ligand for the flt3/flk-2 tyrosine kinase receptor: a proliferative factor for primitive hematopoietic cells. *Cell,* **75,** 1157–67.

Lyman, S.D., Stocking, K., Davison, B. *et al.* (1995). Structural analysis of human and murine flt3 ligand genomic loci. *Oncogene,* **11,** 1165–72.

Lynch, D.H., Andreasen, A., Maraskovsky, E. *et al.* (1997). Flt3 ligand induces tumor regression and antitumor immune responses in vivo. *Nature Medicine,* **3,** 625–31.

Mackarehtschian, K., Hardin, J.D., Moore, K.A. *et al.* (1995). Targeted disruption of the flk2/flt3 gene leads to deficiencies in primitive hematopoietic progenitors. *Immunity,* **3,** 147–61.

Maeda, H., Yamagata, A., Nishikawa, S. *et al.* (1992). Requirement of c-kit for development of intestinal pacemaker system. *Development,* **116,** 369–75.

Maraskovsky, E., Brasel, K., Teepe, M. *et al.* (1996). Dramatic increase in the numbers of functionally mature dendritic cells in Flt3 ligand-treated mice: multiple dendritic cell subpopulations identified. *Journal of Experimental Medicine,* **184,** 1953–62.

Maraskovsky, E., Daro, E., Roux, E. *et al.* (2000). In vivo generation of human dendritic cell subsets by Flt3 ligand. *Blood,* **96,** 878–84.

McCulloch, E.A., Siminovitch, L., Till, J.E. *et al.* (1965). The cellular basis of the genetically determined hemopoietic defect in anemic mice of genotype Sl-Sld. *Blood,* **26,** 399–410.

McKenna, H.J. (2001). Role of hematopoietic growth factors/flt3 ligand in expansion and regulation of dendritic cells. *Current Opinion in Hematology,* **8,** 149–54.

McKenna, H.J., Stocking, K.L., Miller, R.E. *et al.* (2000). Mice lacking flt3 ligand have deficient hematopoiesis affecting hematopoietic progenitor cells, dendritic cells, and natural killer cells. *Blood,* **95,** 3489–97.

McNiece, I.K., Bradley, T.R., Kriegler, A.B. *et al.* (1986). Subpopulations of mouse bone marrow high-proliferative-potential colony-forming cells. *Experimental Hematology,* **14,** 856–60.

McNiece, I.K., Williams, N.T., Johnson, G.R. *et al.* (1987). Generation of murine hematopoietic precursor cells from macrophage high-proliferative-potential colony-forming cells. *Experimental Hematology,* **15,** 972–7.

McWhirter, J.R., Neuteboom, S.T., Wancewicz, E.V. *et al.* (1999). Oncogenic homeodomain transcription factor E2A-Pbx1 activates a novel WNT gene in pre-B acute lymphoblastoid leukemia. *Proceedings of the National Academy of Science USA,* **96,** 11464–9.

Meierhoff, G., Dehmel, U., Gruss, H.J. *et al.* (1995). Expression of FLT3 receptor and FLT3-ligand in human leukemia-lymphoma cell lines. *Leukemia,* **9,** 1368–72.

Mellentin, J.D., Murre, C., Donlon, T.A. *et al.* (1989). The gene for enhancer binding proteins E12/E47 lies at the t(1;19) breakpoint in acute leukemias. *Science,* **246,** 379–82.

Merad, M., Sugie, T., Engleman, E.G. *et al.* (2002). In vivo manipulation of dendritic cells to induce therapeutic immunity. *Blood,* **99,** 1676–82.

Metcalf, D. (1984). *Clonal Cultures of Hemopoietic Cells: Techniques and Applications.* Amsterdam: Elsevier.

Metcalf, D. & Nicola, N.A. (1991). Direct proliferative actions of stem cell factor on murine bone marrow cells in vitro: effects of combination with colony-stimulating factors. *Proceedings of the National Academy of Sciences USA,* **88,** 6239–43.

Metcalf, D. & Nicola, N.A. (1995). *The Haemopoietic Colony-Stimulating Factors. From Biology to Clinical Applications.* Cambridge: Cambridge University Press.

Metcalf, D., Begley, C.G., Nicola, N.A. (1985). The proliferative effects of human GM-CSF-α and β and murine G-CSF in microwell cultures of fractionated human marrow cells. *Leukemia. Research,* **9,** 521–7.

Metcalf, D., Macdonald, H.R., Odartchenko, N. *et al.* (1975). Growth of mouse megakaryocyte colonies in vitro. *Proceedings of the National Academy of Sciences USA,* **72,** 1744–8.

Metcalf, D., Nossal, G.J., Warner, N.L. *et al.* (1975b). Growth of B-lymphocyte colonies in vitro. *Journal of Experimental Medicine,* **142,** 1534–49.

Methia, N., Louache, F., Vainchenker, W. *et al.* (1993). Oligodeoxynucleotides antisense to the proto-oncogene c-mpl specifically inhibit in vitro megakaryocytopoiesis. *Blood,* **82,** 1395–401.

Micklem, H.S., Ford, C.E., Evans, E.P. *et al.* (1966). Interrelationships of myeloid and lymphoid cells: studies with chromosome-marked cells transfused into lethally irradiated mice. *Proceedings of the Royal Society of London Series B: Biological Sciences,* **165,** 78–102.

Migliaccio, G., Migliaccio, A.R., Valinsky, J. *et al.* (1991). Stem cell factor induces proliferation and differentiation of highly enriched murine hematopoietic cells. *Proceedings of the National Academy of Sciences USA,* **88,** 7420–4.

Montrucchio, G., Brizzi, M.F., Calosso, G. *et al.* (1996). Effects of recombinant human megakaryocyte growth and development factor on platelet activation. *Blood,* **87,** 2762–8.

Mucenski, M.L., McLain, K., Kier, A.B. *et al.* (1991). A functional c-myb gene is required for normal murine fetal hepatic hematopoiesis. *Cell,* **65,** 677–89.

Musashi, M., Clark, S.C., Sudo, T. *et al.* (1991b). Synergistic interactions between interleukin-11 and interleukin-4 in support of proliferation of primitive hematopoietic progenitors of mice. *Blood,* **78,** 1448–51.

Musashi, M., Yang, Y.C., Paul, S.R. *et al.* (1991a). Direct and synergistic effects of interleukin-11 on murine hemopoiesis in culture. *Proceedings of the National Academy of Sciences USA,* **88,** 765–9.

Nakahata, T. & Ogawa, M. (1982). Identification in culture of a class of hemopoietic colony-forming units with extensive capability to self-renew and generate multipotential hemopoietic colonies. *Proceedings of the National Academy of Sciences USA,* **79,** 3843–7.

Nandurkar, H.H., Robb, L., & Begley, C.G. (1998). The role of IL-11 in hematopoiesis as revealed by a targeted mutation of its receptor. *Stem Cells,* **16**(Suppl 2), 53–65.

Nandurkar, H.H., Robb, L., Tarlinton, D. *et al.* (1997). Adult mice with targeted mutation of the interleukin-11 receptor (IL11Ra) display normal hematopoiesis. *Blood,* **90,** 2148–59.

Nash, R.A., Kurzrock, R., DiPersio, J. *et al.* (2000). A phase I trial of recombinant human thrombopoietin in patients with delayed platelet recovery after hematopoietic stem cell transplantation. *Biology of Blood and Marrow Transplantation,* **6,** 25–34.

Nash, R.A., Seidel, K., Storb, R. *et al.* (1995). Effects of rhIL 11 on normal dogs and after sublethal radiation. *Experimental Hematology,* **23,** 389–96.

Neben, S., Donaldson, D., Sieff, C. *et al.* (1994). Synergistic effects of interleukin-11 with other growth factors on the expansion of murine hematopoietic progenitors and maintenance of stem cells in liquid culture. *Experimental Hematology,* **22,** 353–9.

Neben, T.Y., Loebelenz, J., Hayes, L. *et al.* (1993). Recombinant human interleukin-11 stimulates megakaryocytopoiesis and increases peripheral platelets in normal and splenectomized mice. *Blood,* **81,** 901–8.

Nishinakamura, R., Miyajima, A., Mee, P.J. *et al.* (1996). Hematopoiesis in mice lacking the entire granulocyte-macrophage colony-stimulating factor/interleukin-3/interleukin-5 functions. *Blood,* **88,** 2458–64.

Nishinakamura, R., Nakayama, N., Hirabayashi, Y. *et al.* (1995). Mice deficient for the IL-3/GM-CSF/IL-5 beta c receptor exhibit lung pathology and impaired immune response, while beta IL3 receptor-deficient mice are normal. *Immunity,* **2,** 211–22.

Noach, E.J., Ausema, A., Dillingh, J.H. *et al.* (2002). Growth factor treatment prior to low-dose total body irradiation increases donor cell engraftment after bone marrow transplantation in mice. *Blood,* **100,** 312–7.

Nocka, K., Buck, J., Levi, E. *et al.* (1990). Candidate ligand for the c-kit transmembrane kinase receptor: KL, a fibroblast derived growth factor stimulates mast cells and erythroid progenitors. *EMBO Journal,* **9,** 3287–94.

Oda, A., Miyakawa, Y., Druker, B.J. *et al.* (1996). Thrombopoietin primes human platelet aggregation induced by shear stress and by multiple agonists. *Blood,* **87,** 4664–70.

Ogawa, M., Matsuzaki, Y., Nishikawa, S. *et al.* (1991). Expression and function of c-kit in hemopoietic progenitor cells. *Journal of Experimental Medicine,* **174,** 63–71.

Okuda, T., Van Deursen, J., Hiebert, S.W. *et al.* (1996). AML1, the target of multiple chromosomal translocations in human leukemia, is essential for normal fetal liver hematopoiesis. *Cell,* **84,** 321–30.

O'Malley, C.J., Rasko, J.E.J., Basser, R.L. *et al.* (1996). Administration of pegylated recombinant human megakaryocyte growth and development factor to humans stimulates the production of functional platelets that show no evidence of in vivo activation. *Blood,* **88,** 3288–98.

Orazi, A., Cooper, R.J., Tong, J. *et al.* (1996). Effects of recombinant human interleukin-11 (Neumega rhIL 11 growth factor) on megakaryocytopoiesis in human bone marrow. *Experimental Hematology,* **24,** 1289–97.

Ordentlich, P.A., Lin, C.P., Shen, C. *et al.* (1998). Notch inhibition of E47 supports the existence of a novel signaling pathway. *Molecular and Cellular Biology,* **6,** 18, 2230.

Orlic, D., Fischer, R., Nishikawa, S. *et al.* (1993). Purification and characterization of heterogeneous pluripotent hematopoietic stem cell populations expressing high levels of c-kit receptor. *Blood,* **82,** 762–70.

Osada, H., Grutz, G., Axelson, H. *et al.* (1995). Association of erythroid transcription factors: complexes involving the LIM protein RBTN2 and the zinc-finger protein GATA1. *Proceedings of the National Academy of Sciences USA,* **92,** 9585–9.

Pandolfi, P.P., Roth, M.E., Karis, A. *et al.* (1995). Targeted disruption of the GATA3 gene causes severe abnormalities in the nervous system and in fetal liver hematopoiesis. *Nature Genetics,* **11,** 40–4.

Paul, S.R., Bennett, F., Calvetti, J.A. *et al.* (1990). Molecular cloning of a cDNA encoding interleukin-11, a stromal cell-derived lymphopoietic and hematopoietic cytokine. *Proceedings of the National Academy of Sciences USA,* **87,** 7512–16.

Paul, S.R., Hayes, L.L., Palmer, R. *et al.* (1994). Interleukin-11 expression in donor bone marrow cells improves hematological reconstitution in lethally irradiated recipient mice. *Experimental Hematology,* **22,** 295–301.

Paul, S.R., Yang, Y.C., Donahue, R.E. *et al.* (1991). Stromal cell-associated hematopoiesis: immortalization and characteriza-

tion of a primate bone marrow-derived stromal cell line. *Blood,* **77,** 1723–33.

Peng, J., Friese, P., Wolf, R.F. *et al.* (1996). Relative reactivity of platelets from thrombopoietin- and interleukin-6-treated dogs. *Blood,* **87,** 4158–63.

Peters, S.O., Kittler, E.L., Ramshaw, H.S. *et al.* (1995). Murine marrow cells expanded in culture with IL-3, IL-6, IL-11, and SCF acquire an engraftment defect in normal hosts. *Experimental Hematology,* **23,** 461–9.

Peters, S.O., Kittler, E.L., Ramshaw, H.S. *et al.* (1996). Ex vivo expansion of murine marrow cells with interleukin-3 (IL-3), IL-6, IL-11, and stem cell factor leads to impaired engraftment in irradiated hosts. *Blood,* **87,** 30–7.

Petzer, A.L., Hogge, D.E., Landsdorp, P.M. *et al.* (1996b). Self-renewal of primitive human hematopoietic cells (long-term-culture-initiating cells) in vitro and their expansion in defined medium. *Proceedings of the National Academy of Sciences USA,* **93,** 1470–4.

Petzer, A.L., Zandstra, P.W., Piret, J.M. *et al.* (1996a). Differential cytokine effects on primitive (CD34+CD38–) human hematopoietic cells: novel responses to Flt3-ligand and thrombopoietin. *Journal of Experimental Medicine,* **183,** 2551–8.

Pevny, L., Lin, C.S., D'agati, V. *et al.* (1995). Development of hematopoietic cells lacking transcription factor GATA-1. *Development,* **121,** 163–72.

Pevny, L., Simon, M.C., Robertson, E. *et al.* (1991). Erythroid differentiation in chimaeric mice blocked by a targeted mutation in the gene for transcription factor GATA-1. *Nature,* **349,** 257–60.

Piacibello, W., Sanavio, F., Garetto, L. *et al.* (1997). Extensive amplification and self-renewal of human primitive hematopoietic stem cells from cord blood. *Blood,* **89,** 2644–53.

Pietrangeli, C.E., Hayashi, S., & Kincade, P.W. (1988). Stromal cell lines which support lymphocyte growth: characterization, sensitivity to radiation and responsiveness to growth factors. *European Journal of Immunology,* **18,** 863–72.

Ploemacher, R.E., Van Soest, P.L., Boudewijn, A. *et al.* (1993b). Interleukin-12 enhances interleukin-3 dependent multilineage hematopoietic colony formation stimulated by interleukin-11 or steel factor. *Leukemia,* **7,** 1374–80.

Ploemacher, R.E., Van Soest, P.L., Voorwinden, H. *et al.* (1993a). Interleukin-12 synergizes with interleukin-3 and steel factor to enhance recovery of murine hemopoietic stem cells in liquid culture. *Leukemia,* **7,** 1381–8.

Pluznik, D.H. & Sachs, L. (1965). The cloning of normal "mast" cells in tissue culture. *Journal of Cellular Physiology,* **66,** 319–24.

Porcher, C., Swat, W., Rockwell, K. *et al.* (1996). The T cell leukemia oncoprotein SCL/tal-1 is essential for development of all hematopoietic lineages. *Cell,* **86,** 47–57.

Quesniaux, V.F., Clark, S.C., Turner, K. *et al.* (1992). Interleukin-11 stimulates multiple phases of erythropoiesis in vitro. *Blood,* **80,** 1218–23.

Radtke, F., Wilson, A., Stark, G. *et al.* (1999). Deficient T cell fate specification in mice with an induced inactivation of Notch 1. *Immunity,* **10,** 547.

Rappold, I., Ziegler, B.L., Kohler, I. *et al.* (1997). Functional and phenotypic characterization of cord blood and bone marrow subsets expressing FLT3 (CD135) receptor tyrosine kinase. *Blood,* **90,** 111–25.

Rasko, J.E., Basser, R.L., Boyd, J. *et al.* (1997). Multilineage mobilization of peripheral blood progenitor cells in humans following administration of PEG-rHuMGDF. *British Journal of Haematology,* **97,** 871–80.

Rasko, J.E., Metcalf, D., Rossner, M.T. *et al.* (1995). The flt3/flk-2 ligand: receptor distribution and action on murine haemopoietic cell survival and proliferation. *Leukemia,* **9,** 2058–66.

Rasko, J.E., O'Flaherty, E., & Begley, C.G. (1997). Mpl ligand (MGDF) alone and in combination with stem cell factor (SCF) promotes proliferation and survival of human megakaryocyte, erythroid and granulocyte/macrophage progenitors. *Stem Cells,* **15,** 33–42.

Ray, R.J., Paige, C.J., Furlonger, C. *et al.* (1996). Flt3 ligand supports the differentiation of early B cell progenitors in the presence of interleukin-11 and interleukin-7. *European Journal of Immunology,* **26,** 1504–10.

Reith, A.D., Rottapel, R., Giddens, E. *et al.* (1990). W mutant mice with mild or severe developmental defects contain distinct point mutations in the kinase domain of the c-kit receptor. *Genes & Development,* **4,** 390–400.

Rennick, D., Jackson, J., Yang, G. *et al.* (1989). Interleukin-6 interacts with interleukin-4 and other hematopoietic growth factors to selectively enhance the growth of megakaryocytic, erythroid, myeloid, and multipotential progenitor cells. *Blood,* **73,** 1828–35.

Reya, T., O'Riordan, M., Okamura, R. *et al.* (2000). Wnt signaling regulates B lymphocyte proliferation through a LEF-1 dependent mechanism. *Immunity,* **13,** 15–24.

Robb, L. & Begley, C.G. (1996). The helix-loop-helix gene SCL: implicated in T-cell acute lymphoblastic leukaemia and in normal haematopoietic development. *International Journal of Biochemistry & Cell Biology,* **28,** 609–18.

Robb, L., Drinkwater, C.C., Metcalf, D. *et al.* (1995c). Hematopoietic and lung abnormalities in mice with a null mutation of the common beta subunit of the receptors for granulocyte-macrophage colony-stimulating factor and interleukins 3 and 5. *Proceedings of the National Academy of Sciences USA,* **92,** 9565–9.

Robb, L., Elwood, N.J., Elefanty, A.G. *et al.* (1996). The scl gene product is required for the generation of all hematopoietic lineages in the adult mouse. *EMBO Journal,* **15,** 4123–9.

Robb, L., Li, R., Hartley, L. *et al.* (1998). Female mice lacking the receptor for interleukin 11 are infertile due to a defective uterine response to implantation. *Nature Medicine,* **4,** 303–8.

Robb, L., Lyons, I., Li, R. *et al.* (1995a). Absence of yolk sac hematopoiesis from mice with a targeted disruption of the scl gene. *Proceedings of the National Academy of Sciences USA,* **92,** 7075–9.

Robb, L., Rasko, J.E., Bath, M.L. *et al.* (1995b). scl, a gene frequently activated in human T cell leukaemia, does not induce lymphomas in transgenic mice. *Oncogene,* **10,** 205–9.

Rodriguez, M.H., Arnaud, S., & Blanchet, J.P. (1995). IL-11 directly stimulates murine and human erythroid burst formation in semi-solid cultures. *Experimental Hematology,* **23,** 545–50.

Rossner, M.T., Mcarthur, G.A., Allen, J.D. *et al.* (1994). Fms-like tyrosine kinase 3 catalytic domain can transduce a proliferative signal in FDC-P1 cells that is qualitatively similar to the signal delivered by c-fms. *Cell Growth & Differentiation,* **5,** 549–55.

Royer-Pokora, B., Loos, U., & Ludwig, W.D. (1991). TTG-2, a new gene encoding a cysteine-rich protein with the LIM motif, is overexpressed in acute T-cell leukaemia with the t(11;14)(p13;q11). *Oncogene,* **6,** 1887–93.

Rozenszajn, L.A., Shoham, D., & Kalechman, I. (1975). Clonal proliferation of PHA-stimulated human lymphocytes in soft agar culture. *Immunology,* **29,** 1041–55.

Schiffer, C.A., Miller, K., Larson, R.A. *et al.* (2000). A double-blind, placebo-controlled trial of pegylated recombinant human megakaryocyte growth and development factor as an adjunct to induction and consolidation therapy for patients with acute myeloid leukemia. *Blood,* **95,** 2530–5.

Schlerman, F.J., Bree, A.G., Kaviani, M. *et al.* (1996). Thrombopoietic activity of recombinant human IL-11 (rhuIL 11) in normal and myelosuppressed nonhuman primates. *Stem Cells,* **14,** 517–32.

Schrader, J.W., Lewis, S.J., Clark-Lewis, I. *et al.* (1981). The persisting (P) cell: histamine content, regulation by a T cell-derived factor, origin from a bone marrow precursor, and relationship to mast cells. *Proceedings of the National Academy of Sciences USA,* **78,** 323–7.

Shah, A.J., Smogorzewska, E.M., Hannum, C. *et al.* (1996). Flt3 ligand induces proliferation of quiescent human bone marrow CD34+CD38– cells and maintains progenitor cells in vitro. *Blood,* **87,** 3563–70.

Shivdasani, R.A., Fujiwara, Y., Mcdevitt, M.A. *et al.* (1997). A lineage-selective knockout establishes the critical role of transcription factor GATA-1 in megakaryocyte growth and platelet development. *EMBO Journal,* **16,** 3965–73.

Shivdasani, R.A., Mayer, E.L., & Orkin, S.H. (1995). Absence of blood formation in mice lacking the T-cell leukemia oncoprotein tal-1/SCL. *Nature,* **373,** 432–4.

Shivdasani, R.A. & Orkin, S.H. (1995). Erythropoiesis and globin gene expression in mice lacking the transcription factor NF-E2. *Proceedings of the National Academy of Sciences USA,* **92,** 8690–4.

Shivdasani, R.A. & Orkin, S.H. (1996). The transcriptional control of hematopoiesis. *Blood,* **87,** 4025–39.

Shivdasani, R.A., Rosenblatt, M.F., Zucker-Franklin, D. *et al.* (1995). Transcription factor NF-E2 is required for platelet formation independent of the actions of thrombopoietin/MGDF in megakaryocyte development. *Cell,* **81,** 695–704.

Siminovitch, L., McCulloch, E.A., & Till, J.E. (1963). The distribution of colony-forming cells among spleen colonies. *Journal of Cellular Comparative Physiology,* **62,** 327–36.

Somlo, G., Sniecinski, I., ter Veer, A. *et al.* (1999). Recombinant human thrombopoietin in combination with granulocyte colony-stimulating factor enhances mobilization of peripheral blood progenitor cells, increases peripheral blood platelet concentration, and accelerates hematopoietic recovery following high-dose chemotherapy. *Blood,* **93,** 2798–806.

Souyri, M., Vigon, I., Penciolelli, J.F. *et al.* (1990). A putative truncated cytokine receptor gene transduced by the myeloproliferative leukemia virus immortalizes hematopoietic progenitors. *Cell,* **63,** 1137–47.

Spritz, R.A. (1994). Molecular basis of human piebaldism. *Journal of Investigative Dermatology,* **103,** 137S–40S.

Staal, F.J. & Clevers, H. (2000). Tcf/Lef transcription factors during T-cell development: unique and overlapping functions. *Hematology Journal,* **1,** 3–6.

Stanley, E., Lieschke, G.J., Grail, D. *et al.* (1994). Granulocyte/macrophage colony-stimulating factor-deficient mice show no major perturbation of hematopoiesis but develop a characteristic pulmonary pathology. *Proceedings of the National Academy of Sciences USA,* **91,** 5592–6.

Stephenson, J.R., Axelrad, A.A., McLeod, D.L. *et al.* (1971). Induction of colonies of hemoglobin-synthesizing cells by erythropoietin in vitro. *Proceedings of the National Academy of Sciences USA,* **68,** 1542–6.

Stinicka, E., Lin, N., Priestley, G.V. *et al.* (1996). The effect of thrombopoietin on the proliferation and differentiation of murine hematopoietic stem cells. *Blood,* **87,** 4998–5005.

Suda, T., Suda, J., & Ogawa, M. (1983). Proliferative kinetics and differentiation of murine blast cell colonies in culture: evidence for variable G_0 periods and constant doubling rates of early pluripotent hemopoietic progenitors. *Journal of Cellular Physiology,* **117,** 308–18.

Sutherland, H.J., Hogge, D.E., Cook, D. *et al.* (1993). Alternative mechanisms with and without steel factor support primitive human hematopoiesis. *Blood,* **81,** 1465–70.

Tanaka, R., Katayama, N., Ohishi, K. *et al.* (1995). Accelerated cell-cycling of hematopoietic progenitor cells by growth factors. *Blood,* **86,** 73–9.

Tanigawa, T., Elwood, N., Metcalf, D. *et al.* (1993). The SCL gene product is regulated by and differentially regulates cytokine responses during myeloid leukemic cell differentiation. *Proceedings of the National Academy of Sciences USA,* **90,** 7864–8.

Tanigawa, T., Nicola, N., Mcarthur, G.A. *et al.* (1995). Differential regulation of macrophage differentiation in response to leukemia inhibitory factor/oncostatin-M/interleukin-6: the effect of enforced expression of the SCL transcription factor. *Blood,* **85,** 379–90.

Tepler, I., Elias, L., Smith, J. *et al.* (1996). A randomized placebo-controlled trial of recombinant human interleukin-11 in cancer patients with severe thrombocytopenia due to chemotherapy. *Blood,* **87,** 3607–14.

Teramura, M., Kobayashi, S., Hoshino, S. *et al.* (1992). Interleukin-11 enhances human megakaryocytopoiesis in vitro. *Blood,* **79,** 327–31.

Ting, C.N., Olson, M.C., Barton, K.P. *et al.* (1996). Transcription factor GATA-3 is required for development of the T-cell lineage. *Nature,* **384,** 474–8.

Toombs, C.F., Young, C.H., Glaspy, J.A. *et al.* (1995). Megakaryocyte growth and development factor (MGDF) moderately enhances in vitro platelet aggregation. *Thrombosis Research,* **80,** 23–33.

Tsai, F.Y., Keller, G., Kuo, F.C. *et al.* (1994). An early haematopoietic defect in mice lacking the transcription factor GATA-2. *Nature,* **371,** 221–6.

Tsai, F.Y. & Orkin, S.H. (1997). Transcription factor GATA-2 is required for proliferation/survival of early hematopoietic cells and mast cell formation, but not for erythroid and myeloid terminal differentiation. *Blood,* **89,** 3636–43.

Tsai, S.F., Martin, D.I., Zon, L.I. *et al.* (1989). Cloning of cDNA for the major DNA-binding protein of the erythroid lineage through expression in mammalian cells. *Nature,* **339,** 446–51.

Tsuji, K., Lyman, S.D., Sudo, T. *et al.* (1992). Enhancement of murine hematopoiesis by synergistic interactions between steel factor (ligand for c-kit), interleukin-11, and other early acting factors in culture. *Blood,* **79,** 2855–60.

Ulich, T.F., Del Castillo, J., Senaldi, G. *et al.* (1996). Systemic hematologic effects of PEG-rHuMGDF-induced megakaryocyte hyperplasia in mice. *Blood,* **87,** 5006–15.

Vadhan-Raj, S., Murray, L.J., Bueso-Ramos, C. *et al.* (1997). Stimulation of megakaryocyte and platelet production by a single dose of recombinant human thrombopoietin in patients with cancer. *Annals of Internal Medicine,* **126,** 673–81.

Vadhan-Raj, S., Verschraegen, C.F., Bueso-Ramos, C. *et al.* (2000). Recombinant human thrombopoietin attenuates carboplatin-induced severe thrombocytopenia and the need for platelet transfusions in patients with gynecologic cancer. *Annals of Internal Medicine,* **132,** 364–8.

Valent, P., Spanblochl, E., Sperr, W.R. *et al.* (1992). Induction of differentiation of human mast cells from bone marrow and peripheral blood mononuclear cells by recombinant human stem cell factor/kit-ligand in long-term culture. *Blood,* **80,** 2237–45.

Van Den Berg, D.J., Sharma, A.K., Bruno, E., & R. Hoffman. (1998). Role of members of the Wnt gene family in human hematopoiesis. *Blood,* **92,** 3189.

van De Ven, C., Ishizawa, L., Law, P. *et al.* (1995). IL-11 in combination with SLF and G-CSF or GM-CSF significantly increases expansion of isolated CD34+ cell population from cord blood vs. adult bone marrow. *Experimental Hematology,* **23,** 1289–95.

Varnum-Finney, B., Purton, L.E., Yu, M. *et al.* (1998). The Notch ligand, Jagged-1, influences the development of primitive hematopoietic precursor cells. *Blood,* **91,** 4084.

Varnum-Finney, B., Xu, C. *et al.* (2000). Pluripotent, cytokine-dependent, hematopoietic stem cells are immortalized by constitutive Notch 1 signaling. *Nature Medicine,* **6,** 1278.

Veiby, O.P., Lyman, S.D., & Jacobsen, S.E. (1996). Combined signaling through interleukin-7 receptors and flt3 but not c-kit potently and selectively promotes B-cell commitment and differentiation from uncommitted murine bone marrow progenitor cells. *Blood,* **88,** 1256–65.

Vigon, I., Mornon, J.P., Cocault, L. *et al.* (1992). Molecular cloning and characterization of MPL, the human homolog of the v-mpl oncogene: identification of a member of the hematopoietic growth factor receptor superfamily. *Proceedings of the National Academy of Sciences USA,* **89,** 5640–4.

Vredenburgh, J.J., Hussein, A., Fisher, D. *et al.* (1998). A randomized trial of recombinant human interleukin-11 following autologous bone marrow transplantation with peripheral blood progenitor cell support in patients with breast cancer. *Biology of Blood and Marrow Transplantation.* 4(3), 134–41.

Wadman, I.A., Osada, H., Grutz, G.G. *et al.* (1997). The LIM-only protein Lmo2 is a bridging molecule assembling an erythroid, DNA-binding complex which includes the TAL1,E47,GATA-1 and Ldb1/NLI proteins. *EMBO Journal,* **16,** 3145–57.

Walker, L., Carlson, A., Tan-Pertel, H.T. *et al.* (2001). The notch receptor and its ligands are selectively expressed during hematopoietic development in the mouse. *Stem Cells,* **19,** 543.

Wang, J. & Shackleford, G.M. (1996). Murine Wnt10a and Wnt10b: cloning and expression in developing limbs, face and skin of embryos and in adults. *Oncogene,* **13,** 1537.

Wang, Q., Stacy, T., Binder, M. *et al.* (1996). Disruption of the Cbfa2 gene causes necrosis and hemorrhaging in the central nervous system and blocks definitive hematopoiesis. *Proceedings of the National Academy of Sciences USA,* **93,** 3444–9.

Warren, A.J., Colledge, W.H., Carlton, M.B. *et al.* (1994). The oncogenic cysteine-rich LIM domain protein rbtn2 is essential for erythroid development. *Cell,* **78,** 45–57.

Weiss, M.J., Keller, G., & Orkin, S.H. (1994). Novel insights into erythroid development revealed through in vitro differentiation of GATA-1 embryonic stem cells. *Genes & Development,* **8,** 1184–97.

Weiss, M.J. & Orkin, S.H. (1995). GATA transcription factors: key regulators of hematopoiesis. *Experimental Hematology,* **23,** 99–107.

Wendling, F., Varlet, P., Charon, M. *et al.* (1986). MPLV: a retrovirus complex inducing an acute myeloproliferative leukemic disorder in adult mice. *Virology,* **149,** 242–6.

Wendling, F., Vigon, I., Souyri, M. *et al.* (1989). Myeloid progenitor cells transformed by the myeloproliferative leukemia virus proliferate and differentiate in vitro without the addition of growth factors. *Leukemia,* **3,** 475–80.

Williams, D.A., Rosenblatt, M.F., Beier, D.R. *et al.* (1988). Generation of murine stromal cell lines supporting hematopoietic stem cell proliferation by use of recombinant retrovirus vectors encoding simian virus 40 large T antigen. *Molecular & Cellular Biology,* **8,** 3864–71.

Williams, D.E., Eisenman, J., Baird, A. *et al.* (1990). Identification of a ligand for the c-kit protooncogene. *Cell,* **63,** 167–74.

Wineman, J.P., Nishikawa, S., & Muller-Sieburg, C.E. (1993). Maintenance of high levels of pluripotent hematopoietic stem cells in vitro: effect of stromal cells and c-kit. *Blood,* **81,** 365–72.

Yamane, T., Kunisada, T., Tsukamoto, H. *et al.* (2001). Wnt signaling regulates hemopoiesis through stromal cells. *Journal of Immunology,* **167,** 765.

Yonemura, Y., Kawakita, M., Masuda, T. *et al.* (1992). Synergistic effects of interleukin-3 and interleukin-11 on murine megakaryopoiesis in serum-free culture. *Experimental Hematology,* **20,** 1011–16.

Yonemura, Y., Kawakita, M., Masuda, T. *et al.* (1993). Effect of recombinant human interleukin-11 on rat megakaryopoiesis and thrombopoiesis in vivo: comparative study with interleukin-6. *British Journal of Haematology,* **84,** 16–23.

Zsebo, K.M., Williams, D.A., Geissler, E.N. *et al.* (1990a). Stem cell factor is encoded at the SI locus of the mouse and is the ligand for the c-kit tyrosine kinase receptor. *Cell,* **63,** 213–24.

Zsebo, K.M., Wypych, J., McNiece, I.K. *et al.* (1990b). Identification, purification, and biological characterization of hematopoietic stem cell factor from buffalo rat liver–conditioned medium. *Cell,* **63,** 195–201.

4 Hematopoietic stem cell homing and the marrow microenvironment

S.K. NILSSON AND P.J. SIMMONS

Peter MacCallum Cancer Institute, Melbourne, Australia

Stem cell transplantation

Under normal adult steady-state conditions, hematopoiesis takes place within the bone marrow, where hematopoietic stem cells (HSC) and their progeny, hematopoietic progenitor cells (HPC), reside in intimate association with a complex cellular milieu collectively termed the *hematopoietic microenvironment* (HM). Reconstitution of hematopoietic cell development within the bone marrow following intravenous infusion of a source of HSC from bone marrow or cytokine-mobilized peripheral blood (PBSC), involves a complex series of coordinated events comprising the selective recruitment of circulating HSC by the microvasculature of the marrow, extravasation into the extravascular compartment of the bone marrow, and lodgement at defined anatomical sites within the marrow. Herein we review recent insights into the molecular mechanisms that regulate the process of HSC homing to the bone marrow and the subsequent events that culminate in the lodgement of HSC in stem cell "niches."

The microenvironment of the bone marrow

During ontogeny, the development of the hematopoietic system is marked by the sequential migration of blood-borne HSC from one supportive microenvironment to the next. The mechanisms that govern this ordered pattern of migration of primordial HSC are only partially understood but ultimately result in the lodgement of definitive HSC in the bone marrow, which in the adult human represents a tissue with a unique capacity to support hematopoiesis. Although, in the steady state, the majority of adult HSC reside within the bone marrow, hematopoietic precursors do circulate within the peripheral blood. Studies using parabiotic mice suggest that circulating HSC in fact rapidly migrate through the circulation and play a functional role through engraftment of nonablated bone marrow (Wright *et al.*, 2001). HSC within the marrow together with their immediate progeny develop in intimate association with a heterogeneous population of marrow stromal cells (Dexter, 1982; Simmons, Zannettino, Gronthos, & Leavesley, 1994). Numerous reports have documented the complex cellular composition of marrow stromal tissue in vivo and in vitro (Weiss, 1976; Dexter, Allen, & Lajtha,

1977; Lichtman, 1981; Allen, Dexter, & Simmons, 1990). Anatomically, the stromal tissue of mammalian bone marrow (BM) is a three-dimensional continuum of cell surfaces comprising cells commonly referred to as "reticular" cells, adipocytes, osteogenic cells near bone surfaces, vascular endothelial cells, smooth muscle cells in vessel walls, and macrophages (Weiss, 1976; Weston & Bainton, 1979; Lichtman, 1981; Galmiche *et al.*, 1993; Bianco & Riminucci, 1998). This complex tissue, together with its associated biosynthetic products including extracellular matrix components (ECM) and hematopoietic growth factors, as a collective, constitutes the unique HM of the bone marrow (Weiss, 1976; Simmons, Levesque, & Zannettino, 1997; Bianco & Riminucci, 1998). ECM proteins produced by the stromal tissue of the marrow include fibronectin; collagen types I, III, and IV; laminin; thrombospondin; vitronectin; hemonectin; hyaluronan; and various proteoglycans. Many of these have been shown to be expressed at indistinct locations within the HM (Nilsson *et al.*, 1998).

Hematopoietic cell interactions with the hematopoietic microenvironment

Considerable evidence supports the proposal that the localization of hematopoiesis to the BM involves developmentally regulated adhesive interactions between primitive HSC and the stromal cell-mediated hematopoietic microenvironment of the marrow (Trentin, 1970; Tavassoli, 1975; Dexter, 1982; Simmons *et al.*, 1997). The picture emerging from cell adhesion studies in many diverse cellular systems demonstrates a coupling between physical adhesion and developmental signaling that serves as a mechanism to tightly integrate the localization of cells within a given microenvironment with signals responsible for survival, growth, and differentiation. It is therefore likely, although as yet unproven, that the adhesive interactions that occur in the HM serve multiple functions, including not only the homing and subsequent lodgement of HSC to the bone marrow during ontogeny or following transplantation, but also participation directly in the regulation of the proliferation and differentiation of primitive hematopoietic cells (Levesque *et al.*, 1995; Simmons *et al.*, 1997).

A wide variety of cell surface molecules participate in hematopoietic regulation within the BM. Of these, cell adhesion molecules (CAMs) play a critical role in mediating interactions between HPC and the various components of the marrow stroma, as well as their associated biosynthetic products. Based on structure and function, these CAMs can be divided into six main groups; the immunoglobulin (Ig) super-family (IgSF), integrin, cadherin, selectin, CD44, and mucin-like families. Primitive hematopoietic cells exhibit a broad repertoire of CAMs including various members of the integrin, sialomucin, Ig super family, and CD44 families (reviewed in Simmons et al., 1994) (Fig. 4.1A). Marrow stromal cells have also been shown to express multiple CAMs including CD54, CD56, CD106, CD58, CD51/CD61, and CD90 (Zukerman & Wicha, 1983; Gallagher, 1989; Kincade et al., 1989; Campbell, Long, & Wicha, 1990; Long & Dixit, 1990; Simmons et al., 1992; Teixido, Hemler, Greenberger, & Anklessaria, 1992; Yoder & Williams, 1995). The importance of the role of the β$_1$ integrin VLA-4 and its counter-receptor VCAM-1 on marrow stromal tissue is particularly noteworthy. VCAM-1 is constitutively expressed by BM stromal cells in vivo and in vitro and supports the VLA-4-mediated adhesion of hematopoietic progenitor cells (Miyake, Weissman, Greenberger, &

Kincade, 1991b; Simmons et al., 1992). In vitro, the addition of function-blocking anti-VCAM-1 and/or anti-VLA-4 antibodies inhibits both B-lymphopoiesis and myelopoiesis in long-term marrow cultures (Miyake et al., 1991a, 1991b). In vivo, VCAM-1 is constitutively expressed on both sinusoidal endothelial cells and reticular cells (Jacobsen, Kravitz, Kincade, & Osmond, 1996). Injection of anti-VCAM-1 antibody in mice was shown to both disrupt native associations between stromal cells and HSC (Funk, Kincade, & Witte, 1994) and to induce mobilization of HPC into the peripheral blood, similar to the effect of systemically administered anti-VLA-4 antibody (Papayannopoulou et al., 1995; Papayannopoulou & Nakamoto, 1993).

Within the bone marrow, cytokines also play an important role in mediating cell to microenvironment interactions. Cytokines act both locally by cell-to-cell contact or alternatively by binding to the ECM at sites where stem and progenitor cells adhere (Nugent & Newman, 1989; Nathan & Sporn, 1991). Some cytokines, for example, macrophage colony-stimulating factor (M-CSF) and stem cell factor (SCF), can exist in both a soluble and/or membrane-bound form, allowing them to mediate the adhesion of cells possessing the relevant receptors (Rettenmier et al., 1987; Massague, 1990;

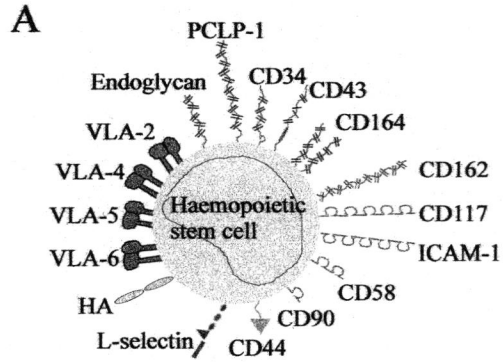

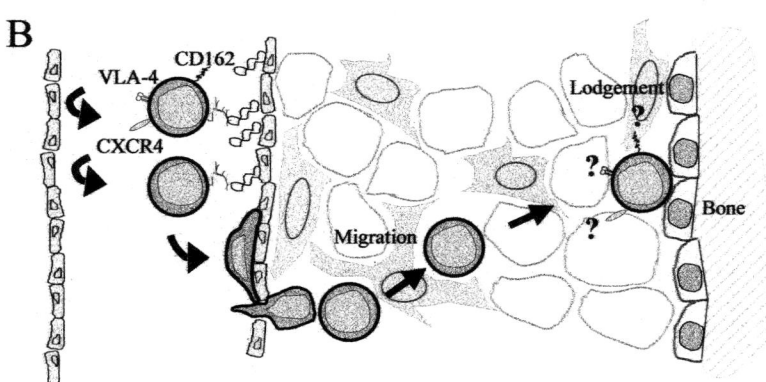

Fig. 4.1. **(A)** Primitive human HPCs exhibit an extensive array of CAMs, each of which interacts with specific receptors. These CAMs include members of the integrin, selectin, sialomucin, immunoglobulin, and CD44 families. **(B)** Homing of HSC to the marrow following transplantation. Cells roll within the marrow microvasculature, strongly adhere, extravasate, and migrate through the extravascular space of the bone marrow to lodge within a microenvironmental "niche."

Rathjen *et al.*, 1990; Flanagan, Chan, & Leder, 1991; Long *et al.*, 1992).

Furthermore, a number of cytokines including SCF, thrombopoietin (TPO), Flt3-ligand, interleukin-3 (IL-3), and granulocyte-macrophage colony-stimulating factor (GM-CSF) have been shown to mediate interactions between hematopoietic cells and their microenvironment as a consequence of their ability to modulate the affinity state of adhesion receptors on cytokine-responsive cells (Kinashi & Springer, 1994). For example, the integrins VLA-4 and VLA-5 are expressed on primitive (CD34+) human hematopoietic cells in a low affinity state, allowing only weak adhesion to their cognate ligands fibronectin and VCAM-1. However, exposure of these cells to a range of cytokines (including SCF, IL-3, and GM-CSF) results in a rapid, transient, dose-dependent specific cytokine stimulation of adhesion to fibronectin through the activation of VLA-4 and VLA-5 function (Levesque *et al.*, 1995). This is followed by a secondary stimulatory signal (outside-in signaling) resulting from the binding of HSC to fibronectin through VLA-4 and VLA-5 (Levesque, Haylock, & Simmons, 1996).

Homing and transendothelial migration of transplanted cells

The initial event in the engraftment process, homing, is defined as the specific recruitment of circulating HSC to the BM and involves the selective recognition of HSC by the microvascular endothelium of the marrow and transendothelial cell migration into the extravascular hematopoietic space. No single adhesion receptor is responsible for the recruitment of HSC to the BM. Rather, a unique *combination* of CAMs expressed in a *constitutive* manner by BM endothelial cells represent a marrow addressin. Accordingly, current data suggest that homing involves the combined action of CAMs, cytokines, and chemotactic factors.

Cell adhesion molecules

Considerable evidence suggests that the specific recruitment of HSC to the BM reflects the paradigm defined for lymphocyte recirculation (Springer, 1990) and the extravasation of mature leukocytes into tissues (Carlos & Harlan, 1994; Frenette & Wagner, 1996). Current data suggest key roles for the sialomucin receptor for P-selectin, PSGL-1 (Frenette *et al.*, 1998; Ma *et al.*, 1998), the β_1 integrin VLA-4 (Papayannopoulou *et al.*, 2001), and the receptor for SDF-1, CXCR4 (Lapidot, 2001), in the homing of HSC to the BM. Both E- and P-selectin are constitutively expressed on marrow endothelial cells (Schweitzer *et al.*, 1996; Mazo *et al.*, 1998). Previous studies have shown that primitive progenitor cells are capable of rolling and adhering on both E- and P-selectin in vivo and in vitro (Zannettino, Berndt, Butcher, & Vadas, 1995; Frenette *et al.*, 1996; Mazo *et al.*, 1998; Greenberg, Kerr, & Hammer, 2000), a critical step in the process of homing to the bone marrow (Frenette *et al.*, 1998). PSGL-1 is the only P-selectin ligand expressed by HSC, while the identity

of E-selectin receptors has not been firmly established. VLA-4 is also critical in cell homing to the bone marrow through its role in progenitor cell attachment to marrow stromal cells (Miyake *et al.*, 1991b). In addition, the injection of blocking antibodies against VLA-4 or its cellular ligand VCAM-1 was shown to block the initial homing of progenitor cells to the marrow (Papayannopoulou *et al.*, 1995).

Evidence for the involvement of SDF-1 and its ligand CXCR4 comes from in vitro studies, which identify SDF-1 as a potent chemoattractant for primitive BM CD34+CD38− cells that include HSC that express the SDF-1 receptor CXCR4 (Aiuti *et al.*, 1997; Jo, Rafii, Hamada, & Moore, 2000; Peled *et al.*, 2000). SDF-1 produced by the marrow stroma and bone tissue forms a decreasing gradient from the marrow extravascular compartment toward the lumen of infiltrating vessels (Ponomaryov *et al.*, 2000). This SDF-1 gradient has been shown to be essential in the process of HSC migration from the liver to the BM during fetal development (Ma *et al.*, 1998; Zou *et al.*, 1998), as well as in promoting engraftment of transplanted HSC to the marrow and the subsequent hematopoietic reconstitution (Peled *et al.*, 1999). The SDF-1-dependent attraction is due to the chemotactic role of CXCR4, which, when bound to SDF-1, activates integrin-mediated firm adhesion and transendothelial migration (Aiuti *et al.*, 1997; Jo *et al.*, 2000). CXCR4 is synthesized and expressed on marrow vascular endothelial cells as well as bone cells. The treatment of HSC with blocking antibodies to CXCR4 also results in the disruption of homing (Peled *et al.*, 1999).

Lodgement of transplanted cells in the bone marrow

In contrast to the homing process, HSC lodgement encompasses events following extravasation and is defined as the selective migration of cells to suitable hematopoietic microenvironment "niches" in the extravascular compartment of the BM. Very little is known about the molecules that influence the site of HSC lodgement following homing to the BM.

Histological examination of the BM demonstrates that hematopoiesis is restricted to the extravascular compartment by a single layer of endothelial cells that form a series of arborized venous sinuses that emerge from the capillary bed along the endosteal surface of the bone (Weiss, 1976). The apparent random organization of hematopoietic cells within these compact extravascular cords, upon closer examination reveals consistent cellular associations such as those occurring between developing erythroblasts and stromal macrophages (Bessis, 1958), megakaryocytes and vascular endothelial cells (Weston & Bainton, 1979) and between developing myeloid, B-lymphoid cells and stromal fibroblast-like cells (Hermans, Hartsniker, & Opstelten, 1989). Similarly, previous studies in the mouse have established that lineage-restricted clonogenic HPC conform to a well-defined spatial distribution across the axis of the femur, with greatest numbers near the central longitudinal vein (Lord,

Testa, & Hendry, 1975; Mason, Lord, & Hendry, 1989). Furthermore, hierarchically more primitive progenitors, colony-forming units spleen (CFU-S) exhibit the converse distribution with low numbers in the central region of the marrow and greatest enrichment in a region adjacent to bone, the endosteum (Gong, 1978; Schoeters & Vanderborght, 1980; Lambertsen & Weiss, 1984; Lord, 1990). Such observations foster the widely held belief that the distinct spatial organization exhibited by these various cell populations within the BM is a manifestation of specific adhesive interactions occurring with the underlying stromal tissue of the BM.

As initially demonstrated by Croizat, Frindel, and Tubiana (1970) and Gidali and Lajtha (1972), the control of HSC proliferation and differentiation is affected by the location of the cells themselves. Encapsulating this concept of very specific local interactions regulating hematopoiesis, Schofield (1978) formulated the "niche hypothesis" suggesting that true HSC are in essence fixed tissue cells, existing in association with one or more other supporting cells. It is these microenvironmental cells that were postulated to form the "niche" that enable HSC to indefinitely self-renew, while effectively inhibiting differentiation and maturation. Supporting evidence comes from multiple studies showing interactions between BM microenvironmental elements and HPC. Examples include thrombospondin alone acting as a cytoadhesion molecule for human HPC (Long & Dixit, 1990), and together with c-kit ligand in a signal complex regulating HSC in vitro, and heparan sulfate proteoglycan mediating HPC adhesion to cytokines in vitro (Bruno, Luikart, Long, & Hoffman, 1995). Within the marrow microenvironment, the distinct locations of ECM proteins further support the hypothesis that they also play an important role in the lodgement of HSC in a "niche" (Nilsson et al., 1998).

Immediately following BM transplantation, although the majority of cells enter the BM from the central marrow vessels, the subsequent redistribution within the extravascular spaces is not random but varies according to their phenotype. Candidate murine stem cells preferentially trans-marrow migrate to the endosteal region, whereas mature terminally differentiated and lineage-committed cells selectively redistribute away from the endosteal region into the central marrow region (Nilsson et al., 1997; Nilsson, Johnston, & Coverdale, 2001) (Fig. 4.1B). These data add to accumulating evidence that HSC "niches" are in very close association to bone (Lord et al., 1975; Taichman, Reilly, & Emerson, 1996). The ECM components found within this region include fibronectin, collagen type I, and laminin (Nilsson et al., 1998). Furthermore, murine HSC have been shown to express receptors and adhere to these proteins in vitro (Berrios et al., 2001). The development of methodology allowing the tracking of transplanted cells at the single cell level as they lodge within the marrow microenvironment for the first time provides opportunities to identify molecules in situ that are important in HSC lodgement within the hematopoietic microenvironment.

Cell cycle dependent adhesive properties of primitive hematopoietic cells

Several studies demonstrate that the engraftment of primitive hematopoietic cells within the bone marrow is also dependent on their position in the cell cycle, with those cells providing long-term engraftment in murine models being predominantly quiescent, while cells in S-G_2-M phases of the cell cycle exhibit an engraftment defect (Peters, Kittler, Ramshaw & Quesenberry, 1995; Peters, Kittler, Ramshaw & Quesenberry, 1996; Orschell-Traycoff et al., 2000). In accord with these data, ex vivo culture of murine HSC in combinations of cytokines that recruit these cells into cycle markedly alters their cell adhesion receptor expression and significantly reduces their binding to ECM proteins in vitro (Berrios et al., 2001). This engraftment defect is reversible when the cell exit the cell cycle (Habibian et al., 1998). Furthermore, this cell-cycle defect also occurs with human HPC, with a significant loss in the ability of CD34+ cells to repopulate NOD/SCID recipients following cell cycle progression from G_0 to G_1 either in situ, or following ex vivo cytokine stimulation (Gothot et al., 1998). Studies by Jetmore et al. (2002) suggest that proliferation inhibition in the marrow of preconditioned recipients inhibits cycling of transplanted HSC and may trigger apoptosis of transplanted cycling cells. Furthermore, these studies also suggest that trafficking of transplanted cells to the marrow is in fact not selective as traditionally believed, but it is the lodgment of BM homed cells that is specific.

Summary

Our understanding of the process of homing and lodgement within the BM microenvironment has rapidly expanded over the past decade. From simple descriptive studies that initially focused on defining the expression and role of particular CAM-ligand pairs in vitro, the field has now moved to a stage at which there is consensus regarding the identity of some of the key molecules involved in homing of HSC to the bone marrow in vivo. As with recruitment of mature leukocytes to inflammatory sites, no single adhesion molecule is responsible for recruitment of primitive hematopoietic cells to the bone marrow. Rather, a bone marrow addressin comprises a unique combination of CAMs expressed in a constitutive manner by BM endothelial cells.

Less is known about the lodgement of HSC, a process that involves the directed migration of cells to microanatomical sites within the marrow that represent unique stem cell niches. Identifying the precise location of these niches within the BM and defining their precise cellular and molecular constituents remains one of the fundamental objectives of future studies. Such knowledge will not only provide valuable insights into the precise mechanisms that contribute to homing and engraftment of HSC in conditioned recipients, but will also yield important clues to the processes involved in stem cell engraftment in the nonmyeloablated setting. The latter issue is of great significance given the potential application of HSC transplantation as a therapy for nonmalignant diseases.

References

Aiuti, A., Webb, I.J., Bleul, C. *et al.* (1997). The chemokine SDF-1 is a chemoattractant for human CD34+ hematopoietic progenitor cells and provides a new mechanism to explain the mobilization of CD34+ progenitors to peripheral blood. *Journal of Experimental Medicine,* **185,** 111–20.

Allen, T.D., Dexter, T.M., & Simmons, P.J. (1990). Marrow biology and stem cells. In *Colony Stimulating Factors: Molecular and Cellular Biology,* ed. T.M. Dexter, J.M. Garland, & N.G. Testa, pp. 1–38. New York: Marcel Dekker.

Berrios, V., Dooner, G.J., Nowakowski, G. *et al.* (2001). The molecular basis for the cytokine-induced defect in homing and engraftment of hematopoietic stem cells. *Experimental Hematology,* **29,** 1326–35.

Bessis, M. (1958). Erythoblastic island, functional unity of bone marrow. *Reviews in Hematology,* **13,** 8–11.

Bianco, P. & Riminucci, M. (1998). The bone marrow stroma in vivo: ontogeny, structure, cellular composition and changes in disease. In *Marrow Stromal Cell Culture. Handbooks in Practical Animal Cell Biology,* ed. J.N. Beresford & M.E. Owen, pp. 10–25. Cambridge: Cambridge University Press.

Bruno, E., Luikart, S.D., Long, M.W., & Hoffman, R. (1995). Marrow-derived heparan sulfate proteoglycan mediates the adhesion of hematopoietic progenitor cells to cytokines. *Experimental Hematology,* **23,** 1212–17.

Campbell, A.D., Long, M.W., & Wicha, M.S. (1990). Developmental regulation of granulocytic cell binding to haemonectin. *Blood,* **75,** 1758–64.

Carlos, T.M. & Harlan, J.M. (1994). Leukocyte-endothelial adhesion molecules. *Blood,* **84,** 2068–101.

Croizat, H., Frindel, E., & Tubiana, M. (1970). Proliferative activity of the stem cells in the bone-marrow of mice after single and multiple irradiations (total- or partial-body exposure). *International Journal of Radiation Oncology, Biology, Physics,* **18,** 347–58.

Dexter, T.M. (1982). Stromal cell-associate hematopoiesis. *Journal of Cellular Physiology,* **1,** 87–94.

Dexter, T.M., Allen, T.D., & Lajtha, L.G. (1977). Conditions controlling the proliferation of haemopoietic stem cells in vitro. *Journal of Cellular Physiology,* **91,** 335–44.

Flanagan, J.G., Chan, D.C., & Leder, P. (1991). Transmembrane form of the kit ligand growth factor is determined by alternative splicing and is missing in the Sl^d mutant. *Cell,* **64,** 1025–35.

Frenette, P.S., Mayadas, T.N., Rayburn, H. *et al.* (1996). Susceptibility to infection and altered hematopoiesis in mice deficient in both P- and E-selectins. *Cell,* **84,** 563–74.

Frenette, P.S. & Wagner, D.D. (1996). Adhesion molecules. *New England Journal of Medicine,* **334,** 1526–9.

Frenette, P.S., Subbarao, S., Mazo, I.B. *et al.* (1998). Endothelial selectins and vascular cell adhesion molecule-1 promote hematopoietic progenitor homing to bone marrow. *Proceedings of the National Academy of Sciences USA,* **95,** 14423–8.

Funk, P.E., Kincade, P.W., & Witte, P.L. (1994). Native associations of early hematopoietic stem cells and stromal cells isolated in bone marrow cell aggregates. *Blood,* **83,** 361–9.

Gallagher, J.T. (1989). The extended family of proteoglycans: social residents of the pericellular zone. *Current Opinions in Cell Biology,* **1,** 1201–18.

Galmiche, M.C., Kotelianski, V.E., Herve, P., & Charbord, P. (1993). Stromal cells from human long-term marrow cultures are mesenchymal cells that differentiate following a vascular smooth muscle pathway. *Blood,* **82,** 66–74.

Gidali, J. & Lajtha, L.G. (1972). Regulation of haemopoietic stem cell turnover in partially irradiated mice. *Cell and Tissue Kinetics,* **5,** 147–57.

Gong, J.K. (1978). Endosteal marrow: a rich source of hematopoietic stem cells. *Science,* **199,** 1443–5.

Gothot, A., Pyatt, R., McMahel, J. *et al.* (1998). Assessment of proliferative and colony-forming capacity after successive in vitro divisions of single human CD34+ cells initially isolated in G0. *Experimental Hematology,* **26,** 562–70.

Greenberg, A.W., Kerr, W.G., & Hammer, D.A. (2000). Relationship between selectin-mediated rolling of hematopoietic stem and progenitor cells and progression in hematopoietic development. *Blood,* **95,** 478–86.

Habibian, H.K., Peters, S.O., Hsieh, C.C. *et al.* (1998). The fluctuating phenotype of the lymphohematopoietic stem cell with cell cycle transit. *Journal of Experimental Medicine,* **188,** 393–8.

Hermans, M.H.A., Hartsniker, H., & Opstelten, D. (1989). An in situ study of B-lymphocytopoiesis in rat bone marrow. *Journal of Immunology,* **142,** 67–73.

Jacobsen, K., Kravitz, J., Kincade, P.W., & Osmond, D.G. (1996). Adhesion receptors on bone marrow stromal cells: in vivo expression of vascular cell adhesion molecule-1 by reticular cells and sinusoidal endothelium in normal and gamma-irradiated mice. *Blood,* **87,** 73–82.

Jetmore, A., Plett, P.A., Tong, X. *et al.* (2002). Homing efficiency, cell cycle kinetics, and survival of quiescent and cycling human CD34(+) cells transplanted into conditioned NOD/SCID recipients. *Blood,* **99,** 1585–93.

Jo, D.Y., Rafii, S., Hamada, T., & Moore, M.A. (2000). Chemotaxis of primitive hematopoietic cells in response to stromal cell-derived factor-1. *Journal of Clinical Investigation,* **105,** 101–11.

Kinashi, T. & Springer, T.A. (1994). Steel factor and c-kit regulate cell-matrix adhesion. *Blood,* **83,** 1033–8.

Kincade, P.W., Lee, G., Pietrangeli, C.E. *et al.* (1989). Cells and molecules that regulate B-lymphopoiesis in bone marrow. *Annual Review of Immunology,* **7,** 111–43.

Lambertsen, R.H. & Weiss, L. (1984). A model of intramedullary hematopoietic microenvironments based on stereologic study of the distribution of endocloned marrow colonies. *Blood,* **63,** 287–97.

Lapidot, T. (2001). Mechanism of human stem cell migration and repopulation of NOD/SCID and B2mnull NOD/SCID mice. The role of SDF-1/CXCR4 interactions. *Annals of the New York Academy of Sciences,* **938,** 83–95.

Levesque, J.P., Haylock, D.N., & Simmons, P.J. (1996). Cytokine regulation of proliferation and cell adhesion are correlated events in human CD34+ haemopoietic progenitors. *Blood,* **88,** 1168–76.

Levesque, J.P., Leavesley, D.I., Niutta, S. *et al.* (1995). Cytokines increase human haemopoietic cell adhesiveness by activation of very late antigen (VLA)-4 and VLA-5 integrins. *Journal of Experimental Medicine,* **181,** 1805–15.

Lichtman, M.A. (1981). The ultrastructure of the hemopoietic environment of the marrow: a review. *Experimental Hematology,* **9,** 391–410.

Long, M.W. & Dixit, V.M. (1990). Thrombospondin functions as a cytoadhesion molecule for human hematopoietic progenitor cells. *Blood,* **75,** 2311–18.

Long, M.W., Briddell, R., Walter, A.W. *et al.* (1992). Human hematopoietic stem cell adherence to cytokines and matrix molecules. *Journal of Clinical Investigation,* **90,** 251–5.

Lord, B.I. (1990). The architecture of bone marrow cell populations. *International Journal of Cell Cloning,* **8,** 317–31.

Lord, B.I., Testa, N.G., & Hendry, J.H. (1975). The relative spatial distribution of CFUs and CFUc in the normal mouse femur. *Blood,* **46,** 65–72.

Ma, Q., Jones, D., Borghesani, P.R. *et al.* (1998). Impaired B-lymphopoiesis, myelopoiesis, and derailed cerebellar neuron migration in CXCR4- and SDF-1-deficient mice. *Proceedings of the National Academy of Sciences USA,* **95,** 9448–53.

Mason, T.M., Lord, B.I., & Hendry, J.H. (1989). The development of spatial distributions of CFU-S and in-vitro CFC in femora of mice of different ages. *British Journal of Hematology,* **73,** 455–61.

Massague, J. (1990). Transforming growth factor β. A model for membrane-anchored growth factors. *Journal of Biological Chemistry,* **265,** 21393–6.

Mazo, I.B., Gutierrez-Ramos, J.C., Frenette, P.S. *et al.* (1998). Hematopoietic progenitor cell rolling in bone marrow microvessels: parallel contributions by endothelial selectins and vascular cell adhesion molecule 1. *Journal of Experimental Medicine,* **188,** 465–74.

Miyake, K., Medina, K.L., Ishihara, K. *et al.* (1991a). A VCAM-like adhesion molecule on murine bone marrow stromal cells mediates binding of lymphocytic precursors in culture. *Journal of Cell Biology,* **114,** 557–65.

Miyake, K., Weissman, I.L., Greenberger, J.S., & Kincade, P.W. (1991b). Evidence for a role of the integrin VLA-4 in lymphohemopoiesis. *Journal of Experimental Medicine,* **173,** 599–607.

Nathan, C. & Sporn, M. (1991). Cytokines in context. *Journal of Cell Biology,* **113,** 981–6.

Nilsson, S.K., Debatis, M.E., Dooner, M.S. *et al.* (1998). Immunofluorescence characterization of key extracellular matrix proteins in murine bone marrow in situ. *Journal of Histochemistry and Cytochemistry,* **46,** 371–7.

Nilsson, S.K., Dooner, M.S., Tiarks, C.Y. *et al.* (1997). Potential and distribution of transplanted hematopoietic stem cells in a nonablated mouse model. *Blood,* **89,** 4013–20.

Nilsson, S.K., Johnston, H.M., & Coverdale, J.A. (2001). Spatial localization of transplanted haemopoietic stem cells: inferences for the localization of stem cell niches. *Blood,* **97,** 2293–9.

Nugent, M.A. & Newman, M.J. (1989). Inhibition of normal rat kidney cell growth by transforming growth factor-beta is mediated by collagen. *Journal of Biological Chemistry,* **264,** 18060–7.

Orschell-Traycoff, C.M., Hiatt, K., Dagher, R.N. *et al.* (2000). Homing and engraftment potential of Sca-1(+)lin(–) cells fractionated on the basis of adhesion molecule expression and position in cell cycle. *Blood,* **96,** 1380–7.

Papayannopoulou, T., Craddock, C., Nakamoto, B. *et al.* (1995). The VLA4/VCAM-1 adhesion pathway defines contrasting mechanisms of lodgement of transplanted murine hemopoietic progenitors between bone marrow and spleen. *Proceedings of the National Academy of Sciences USA,* **92,** 9647–51.

Papayannopoulou, T. & Nakamoto, B. (1993). Peripheralization of hemopoietic progenitors in primates treated with anti-VLA4 integrin. *Proceedings of the National Academy of Sciences USA,* **90,** 9374–8.

Papayannopoulou, T., Priestley, G.V., Nakamoto, B. *et al.* (2001). Molecular pathways in bone marrow homing: dominant role of alpha (4)beta(1) over beta(2)-integrins and selectins. *Blood,* **98,** 2403–11.

Peled, A., Kollet, O., Ponomaryov, T. *et al.* (2000). The chemokine SDF-1 activates the integrins LFA-1, VLA-4, and VLA-5 on immature human CD34(+) cells: role in transendothelial/stromal migration and engraftment of NOD/SCID mice. *Blood,* **95,** 3289–96.

Peled, A., Petit, I., Kollet, O. *et al.* (1999). Dependence of human stem cell engraftment and repopulation of NOD/SCID mice on CXCR4. *Science,* **283,** 845–8

Peters, S.O., Kittler, E.L., Ramshaw, H.S., & Quesenberry, P.J. (1995). Murine marrow cells expanded in culture with IL-3, IL-6, IL-11, and SCF acquire an engraftment defect in normal hosts. *Experimental Hematology,* **23,** 461–9.

Peters, S.O., Kittler, E.L., Ramshaw, H.S., & Quesenberry, P.J. (1996). Ex vivo expansion of murine marrow cells with interleukin-3 (IL-3), IL-6, IL-11, and stem cell factor leads to impaired engraftment in irradiated hosts. *Blood,* **87,** 30–7.

Ponomaryov, T., Peled, A., Petit, I. *et al.* (2000). Induction of the chemokine stromal-derived factor-1 following DNA damage improves human stem cell function. *Journal of Clinical Investigation,* **106,** 1331–9.

Rathjen, P.D., Toth, S., Willis, A. *et al.* (1990). Differentiation inhibiting activity is produced in matrix-associated and diffusible forms that are generated by alternate promoter usage. *Cell,* **62,** 1105–14.

Rettenmier, C.W., Roussel, M.F., Ashmun, R.A. *et al.* (1987). Synthesis of membrane-bound colony-stimulating factor-1 (CSF-1) and downmodulation of CSF-1 receptors in NIH 3T3 cells transformed by cotransfection of the human CSF-1 and c-fms (CSF-1 receptor) genes. *Molecular and Cellular Biology,* **7,** 2378–87.

Schoeters, G.E. & Vanderborght, O.L. (1980). Haemopoietic stem cell concentration and CFUs in DNA synthesis in bone marrow from different bone regions. *Experientia* **36,** 459–61.

Schofield, R. (1978). The relationship between the CFU-S and the hemopoietic stem cell. *Blood Cells,* **4,** 7–25.

Schweitzer, C.M., Dräger, A.M., van der Valk, P. *et al.* (1996). Constitutive expression of E-selectin and VCAM-1 on endothelial cells of haemopoietic tissues. *American Journal of Pathology,* **148,** 165–75.

Simmons, P.J., Levesque, J-P., & Zannettino, A. (1997). Adhesion molecules in hematopoiesis. *Bailliere's Clinical Haematology,* **10,** 485–505.

Simmons, P.J., Masinovsky, B., Longenecker, B.M. *et al.* (1992). Vascular cell adhesion molecule-1 expressed by bone marrow stromal cells mediates the binding of hematopoietic progenitor cells. *Blood,* **80,** 388–95.

Simmons, P.J., Zannettino, A.C.W., Gronthos, S., & Leavesley, D. (1994). Potential adhesion mechanisms for localisation of haemopoietic progenitors to bone marrow stroma. *Leukaemia and Lymphoma,* **12,** 353–63.

Springer, T.A. (1990). Adhesion receptors of the immune system. *Nature,* **346,** 425–34.

Taichman, R.S., Reilly, M.J., & Emerson, S.G. (1996). Human osteoblasts support human hematopoietic progenitor cells in in vitro bone marrow cultures. *Blood,* **87,** 518–24.

Tavassoli, M. (1975). Studies in hemopoietic microenvironments. *Experimental Hematology,* **3,** 213–26.

Teixido, J., Hemler, M.E., Greenberger, J.S., & Anklessaria, P. (1992). Role of β1 and β2 integrins in the adhesion of human CD34^{hi} cells to bone marrow stroma. *Journal of Clinical Investigations,* **90,** 358–67.

Trentin, J.J. (1970). Influence of hematopoietic organ stroma (hematopoietic inductive microenvironments) on stem cell differentiation. In *Regulation of Hematopoiesis,* ed. A.S. Gordon, Vol, 1, pp. 161–86. New York : Appleton-Century-Crofts.

Weiss, L. (1976). The hematopoietic microenvironment of the bone marrow: an ultrastructural study of the stroma in rats. *Anatomical Record,* **186,** 161–84.

Weston, H. & Bainton, D.F. (1979). Association of alkaline-phosphatase-positive reticulum cells in bone marrow with granulocytic precursors. *Journal of Experimental Medicine,* **150,** 919–37.

Wolf, N.S. (1979). The haemopoietic microenvironment. *Clinical Hematology,* **8,** 469–500.

Wright, D.E., Wagers, A.J., Gulati, A.P. *et al.* (2001). Physiological migration of hematopoietic stem and progenitor cells. *Science,* **294,** 1933–6.

Yoder, M. & Williams, D.A. (1995). Matrix molecule interactions with hematopoietic stem cells. *Experimental Hematology,* **23,** 961–7.

Zannettino, A.C., Berndt, M.C., Butcher, E.C., & Vadas, M.A. (1995). Primitive human hematopoietic progenitors adhere to P-selectin (CD62P). *Blood,* **85,** 3466–77.

Zou, Y.R., Kottmann, A.H., Kuroda, M. *et al.* (1998). Function of the chemokine receptor CXCR4 in haematopoiesis and in cerebellar development. *Nature,* **393,** 595–9.

Zuckerman, K.S. & Wicha, M.S. (1983). Extracellular matrix production by the adherent cells in long-term murine bone marrow cultures. *Blood,* **61,** 540–7.

5 Mesenchymal stem cells and hematopoietic stem cell transplantation

WILLEM E. FIBBE AND HILLARD M. LAZARUS

Leiden University Medical Center, Leiden, The Netherlands, and Comprehensive Cancer Center of Case Western Reserve University, Cleveland, USA

Introduction

Allogeneic hematopoietic stem cell transplantation (HSCT) is increasingly used in the treatment of hematologic and nonhematologic diseases of neoplastic and non-neoplastic origin. The transplant procedure involves infusion of hematopoietic stem cells (HSC) into the circulation, employing the capacity of these cells to home to the marrow and to dock at specific sites in the marrow microenvironment (Torok-Storb & Holmberg, 1994). Maintenance of hematopoiesis depends on the self-renewal and multilineage differentiation capacity of HSC that is thought to be regulated and controlled by the bone marrow microenvironment (Uchida *et al.*, 1993). The spatial organization of stem cells in the marrow, mediated by the hematopoietic microenvironment and extracellular matrix, may be crucial for hematopoietic regeneration following HSCT (Nilsson *et al.*, 2001).

The bone marrow serves as a reservoir for different classes of stem cells. In addition to HSC the bone marrow comprises a population of marrow stromal cells or mesenchymal stem cells (MSCs). Stromal cells exhibit multilineage differentiation capacity, and are able to generate progenitors with restricted developmental potential, including fibroblasts, osteoblasts, adipocytes, and chondrocyte progenitors (Caplan, 1994; Pittenger *et al.*, 1999; Deans & Moseley, 2000). MSCs might be used either to replace host cells in the marrow microenvironment that have been damaged by chemotherapy or irradiation, or as vehicles for gene therapy.

Techniques are now available to isolate and grow mesenchymal progenitors and to manipulate their growth under defined in vitro culture conditions. As a result MSCs can be rapidly expanded to numbers that are required for clinical application. This advance has allowed the clinical testing of culture-expanded MSCs in the context of hematopoietic stem cell transplantation. Here, we discuss the role of MSC in hematopoietic engraftment following stem cell transplantation.

Marrow stromal cells

Marrow stromal cells comprise a heterogeneous population of cells, including reticular endothelial cells, fibroblasts, adipocytes, and osteogenic precursor cells that provide hematopoietic growth factors, facilitate cell to cell interactions, and elaborate matrix proteins that play a role in the regulation of hematopoiesis (Tavassoli & Friedenstein, 1983; Lichtman, 1981; Allen *et al.*, 1990; Conget & Minguell, 1999). The notion that a stromal microenvironment could support hematopoiesis was followed by the development of the long-term bone marrow culture (LTBMC) technique by Dexter. In this system an adherent bone marrow derived stromal culture could support the production of hematopoietic progenitor cells over a period of several weeks to months. Friedenstein and colleagues (Friedenstein *et al.*, 1974) had already described a population of adherent cells from the bone marrow that were nonphagocytic and exhibited a fibroblast-like appearance. Upon culture at low density, either as whole bone marrow or following separation over a density gradient, the cells formed characteristic colonies derived from a single precursor, referred to as colony-forming-unit fibroblastic or CFU-F. After ectopic transplantation under the kidney capsule these cells gave rise to a broad spectrum of differentiated connective tissues including bone, cartilage, adipose tissue, and myelosupportive stroma (Freidenstein *et al.*, 1974; Owen, 1988) Majumdar and colleagues utilized culture-expanded stromal cells to support hematopoietic progenitors ex vivo in a manner similar to the Dexter technique (Majumdar *et al.*, 2000; Majumdar *et al.*, 1998). Based on these observations it was proposed that these tissues were derived from a common precursor cell residing in the bone marrow, termed the stromal stem cell, the bone marrow stromal stem cell, the mesenchymal stem cell, or the skeletal stem cell (Prockop, 1997; Gerson, 1999).

MSCs are present in postnatal bone marrow and also in the bone marrow of adults, and there is evidence that the frequency declines with age. For instance the frequency in the newborn is about 1 MSC per 10^4 nucleated marrow cells and decreases to approximately 1 per 2×10^6 in an individual 80 years of age. After allogeneic stem cell transplantation the frequency of CFU-F is transiently reduced in children and recovers over a period of several years, while the defect is permanent in adult recipients of stem cell grafts (Galotto *et al.*, 1999). These observations formed the basis for the clinical application of culture-expanded MSCs in the context of allogeneic stem cell transplantation.

Sources and phenotype of MSCs

Although the bone marrow serves as the primary reservoir for MSCs, their presence has been detected in a variety of other tissues including periosteum and muscle connective tissue (Nathanson, 1985; Nakahara et al., 1991), fetal bone marrow, liver, and blood (Campagnoli, et al., 2001). Although an ongoing debate, their presence in steady state peripheral blood is likely to be of extremely low frequency, according to reports by several groups who have described circulating MSC-like populations (Zvaifler et al., 2000; Ferrari et al., 1998; Chesney et al., 1997). Using functional and immunologic assays, MSCs have not been identified in cytokine [granulocyte colony-stimulating factor (G-CSF)]-mobilized peripheral blood stem cell collections (Lazarus et al., 1997); however, one group did report the presence of adherent cells that could be cultured and expressed CD106 (VCAM), CD54 (ICAM), SH-2 (CD105), and SH-3 (CD73) but did not express CD34, CD14, and CD45 (Fernandez et al., 1997). MSCs have been identified in fetal blood (Campagnoli et al., 2001); although some laboratories have been able to grow MSCs from umbilical cord blood (Erices et al., 2000; Gutierrez-Rodriguez et al., 2000), other laboratories have been unable to do so (Mareschi et al., 2001). The frequency of MSCs in these sources is very low. In fetal blood the frequency has been reported to decline with gestational age, from about 1 per 10^6 mononuclear cells in first-trimester fetal blood to 0.3 per 10^6 in term umbilical cord blood (Campagnoli et al., 2001).

At present no unique phenotype has been identified that allows the reproducible isolation of MSC precursors with predictable developmental potential. The isolation and characterization of stromal cell function therefore still relies primarily on their ability to adhere to plastic and their expansion potential, which is at least a factor of 10^5 (Pittenger et al., 1999). Standard conditions for expansion of MSCs require the presence of as yet unidentified factors present in serum, and in most instances prescreened fetal bovine serum is used (Lennon et al., 1996). Cell density is a critical factor affecting the growth of cells and culture attempts below a critical cell density are usually unsuccessful. The cells can be grown directly (i.e., unmanipulated following collection) or after density gradient separation. The CFU-F limiting dilution assay has been used to determine the frequency in bone marrow.

MSCs express many surface markers and some of these epitopes have been used to enrich MSCs from populations of adherent bone marrow stromal cells. For instance, CFU-F enrichment has been accomplished using the STRO-1 antibody (Gronthos & Simmons, 1996). The CFU-F precursor cell was in the CD34,[neg/low] (Deans & Moseley, 2000) CD45[neg], Glycophorin-A[neg] fraction and expressed the markers Thy-1 (CD90), CD106 (VCAM), the beta-1 integrin CD29/CD49, as well as CD10, CD13, and receptors for PDGF, EGF, NGF, and IGF-1 (Gronthos & Simmons, 1996).

The immunophenotypical characterization is usually applied to culture-expanded cells and not to primary cells. In some fetal tissues, such as fetal lung, the frequency is considerably higher, thus allowing the characterization of primary cells. The CD34 marker is not expressed on culture-expanded MSCs, but on primary fetal lung–derived MSCs the frequency of MSC precursors is higher in the CD34[pos] than in the CD34[neg] cell fraction (Noort et al., 2001). These data suggest that CD34 may be present on primary cells and may be lost during expansion. Characteristic markers for expanded MSCs have been reported and designated SH-2, SH-3, and SH-4. The SH-2 antibody raised against human bone marrow–derived MSCs recognizes an epitope of endoglin (CD105), the TGF-beta receptor III present on endothelial cells, syncytiotrophoblasts, macrophages, and connective tissue stromal cells (Barry et al., 1999). The SH-3 and SH-4 antibodies recognize epitopes on human MSCs, the antigens now being identified as distinct epitopes of CD73, an antigen also involved in the activation of B lymphocytes (Barry et al., 2001). However, none of these markers are specific for MSCs, thus hampering the isolation of pure populations of MSCs. In addition, expanded MSCs express HLA class I but not HLA class II antigens and lack expression of costimulatory molecules. The immune phenotype of MSCs is detailed in Table 5.1, and in Figures 5.1 and 5.2, and properties are summarized in Table 5.2.

Multilineage potential of MSCs

The differentiation potential of MSCs into multiple mesenchymal lineages (i.e., bone, cartilage, and adipose tissue) is most commonly used as a functional criterion defining MSC precursor cells. (Fig. 5.3). Following culture expansion in vitro, human MSCs exhibit a spindle shape fibroblastic morphology. It has been reported that a proportion of the initial adherent bone marrow–derived stromal colonies are multipotent and maintain multilineage potential into osteogenic, condrogenic, and adipogenic lineages (Pittenger et al., 1999). These results suggest that the progeny of MSCs following culture expansion retain multipotentiality. Human MSCs derived from bone marrow have been reported to maintain their differentiation capacity into the osteogenic lineages for over 40 cell doublings (Reyes et al., 2001).

When cultured in the presence of dexamethasone and ascorbic acid, purified MSCs undergo a development characterized by the transient induction of alkaline phosphatase, expression of bone matrix protein mRNAses, and deposition of calcium. In vivo bone formation occurs following loading on a hydroxy apatite-tricalcium phosphate matrix and in vivo implantation into NOD-SCID mice (Krebsbach et al., 1997). These observations suggest that the osteogenic potential of bone marrow–derived MSCs may be applied clinically to correct or reconstruct local bone defects in a variety of disorders.

To promote adipogenic differentiation expanded MSCs are cultured in the presence of dexamethasone, methyl-isobutylxanthine, insulin, and indomethacin (Pittenger et al., 1999). Following induction, cells accumulate lipid-rich vacuoles that can be stained with Oil Red O. MSCs can also be promoted to

Table 5.1. *Immune phenotype of culture-expanded MSC*

Antigens	CD number	Expression
VLA-2	CD49b	+
VLA-4	CD49d	–
VLA-5	CD49e	+
LFA-1	CD11a	–
E-selectins	CD62E	–
P-selectins	CD62P	–
L-selectins	CD62L	– or +
PECAM	CD31	–
VWF		–
LFA-3	CD58	+ or ±
ICAM-1	CD54	+
ICAM-2	CD102	+ or –
ICAM-3	CD50	+ or –
VCAM-1	CD106	+ or –
SB10 / ALCAM	CD166	+
B7.1	CD80	–
B7.2	CD86	–
HCAM-1	CD44	+
	CD34	–
	CD13	+
	CD14	–
	CD45	–
Transferrin receptor	CD71	+ or ±
Thy-1	CD90	+
Endoglin, SH2	CD105	+
SH3	CD73	+
SH4	CD73	+
HLA ABC		+ or –
HLA DR		– or +
IL-2 receptor	CD25	–
IL-3 receptor	CD123	+ or ±
IL-7 receptor	CD127	+ or –
TNF-a1 receptor	CD120a	+ or –
TNF-a2 receptor	CD120b	+ or –

Expression: +, positive, –, negative, ±, weakly positive.
[a] Depending on culture conditions.

differentiate into the chondrogenic lineage when cultured without serum in the presence of transforming growth factor (Mackay *et al.*, 1998). Cells can be stained for type 2 collagen, which is characteristic for articular cartilage. Repair of articular cartilage has been undertaken in animal models with full thickness defects of the weight-bearing surface of the medial femoral condyles (Wakitani *et al.*, 1994). Several weeks after injection of expanded MSCs, remodeling of subchondral bone was observed with repair of the overlying cartilage (Mackay *et al.*, 1998). In other studies MSCs have been applied in a collagen matrix for tendon repair and improvement of biomechanical function (Young *et al.*, 1998).

Bone marrow–derived stromal cells have also been shown to be able to differentiate into cardiomyocytes (Makino *et al.*, 1999). Murine bone marrow stromal cells were immortalized and, following treatment with 5-azacytidine, could be induced to express cardiomyocyte-specific genes similar to in vivo developing cardiomyocytes. The cells formed myotubes and ultimately developed into contracting cardiomyocytes. Human bone marrow–derived lacZ labeled MSCs have been injected into the left ventricular wall of immune-deficient CB17 SCID beige adult mice (Toma *et al.*, 2002). Over time a proportion of the cells morphologically resembled the surrounding host cardiomyocytes and also exhibited de novo expression of myogenic markers such as desmin and cardiac troponin T (Toma *et al.*, 2002). Other reports have demonstrated the ability of rat or mouse bone marrow–derived cells to engraft in infarcted myocardium and to form cardiomyocytes and vascular structures (Tomita *et al.*, 1999; Orlic *et al.*, 2001). These studies form the basis for the clinical use of MSCs for cellular cardiomyoplasty.

Verfaillie's group described a population of mesodermal progenitor cells (MPCs) or multipotent adult progenitor cells (MAPCs), isolated from postnatal bone marrow, that copurifies with MSCs (Reyes *et al.*, 2001; Schwartz *et al.*, 2002; Reyes *et al.*, 2002; Jiang *et al.*, 2002). MAPCs have been isolated from normal human, mouse, and rat postnatal bone marrow and can be expanded in culture for over 80 population doublings (Schwartz *et al.*, 2002; Reyes *et al.*, 2002). When cultured in serum-free medium on Matrigel with FGF-4 and HGF, the cells differentiated into epithelioid cells expressing hepatocyte nuclear factor 3β (HNF-3β), cytokeratin-19, and α-fetoprotein (Schwartz *et al.*, 2002). They also acquired the functional characteristics of hepatocytes and secreted urea and albumin, showing that MAPCs are able to differentiate in vitro to cells with a hepatocyte phenotype and function (Schwartz *et al.*, 2002). MAPCs are derived from an adherent CD45⁻ glycophorin A⁻, AC133+, Flk-1+ population and are able to differentiate into lineages belonging to the limb-bud mesoderm (i.e., osteoblasts, chondrocytes, adipocytes, and skeletal muscle), but also to visceral mesoderm (i.e. endothelial cells) (Reyes *et al.*, 2002). Following injection into blastocysts, they contribute to most somatic tissues, and after infusion into NOD-SCID recipient mice they engrafted in hematopoietic tissues and epithelium of lung, liver, and intestine (Jiang *et al.*, 2002). Using retroviral marking the clonal origin of the cells was demonstrated (Reyes *et al.*, 2001; Jiang *et al.*, 2002). Altogether these studies indicate that MAPCs have a broad developmental potential, both in vitro and in vivo at the single cell level, that resembles that of embryonic stem cells (Jiang *et al.*, 2002; Orkin & Zon, 2002).

Table 5.2. *Properties of MSCs*

Mitotically quiescent
Long lived in vivo
Expandable in vitro
Differentiation into multiple mesenchymal lineages
Clonally derived cells remain multipotent
Residing in bone marrow
Noncirculating in steady-state peripheral blood
Isolation by adherence to plastic

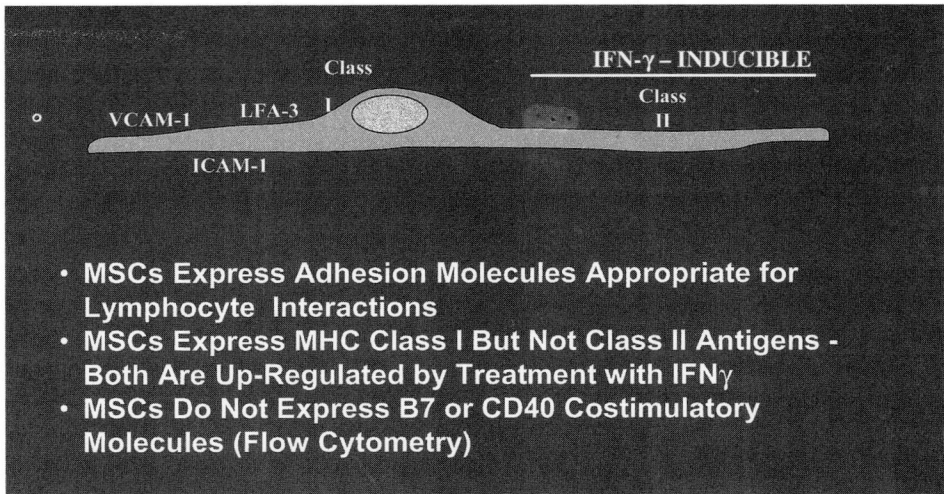

Fig. 5.1. A cartoon representation of MSC surface molecules involved in immune interactions: MHC class I antigens are expressed, but not class II molecules or co-stimulatory molecules.

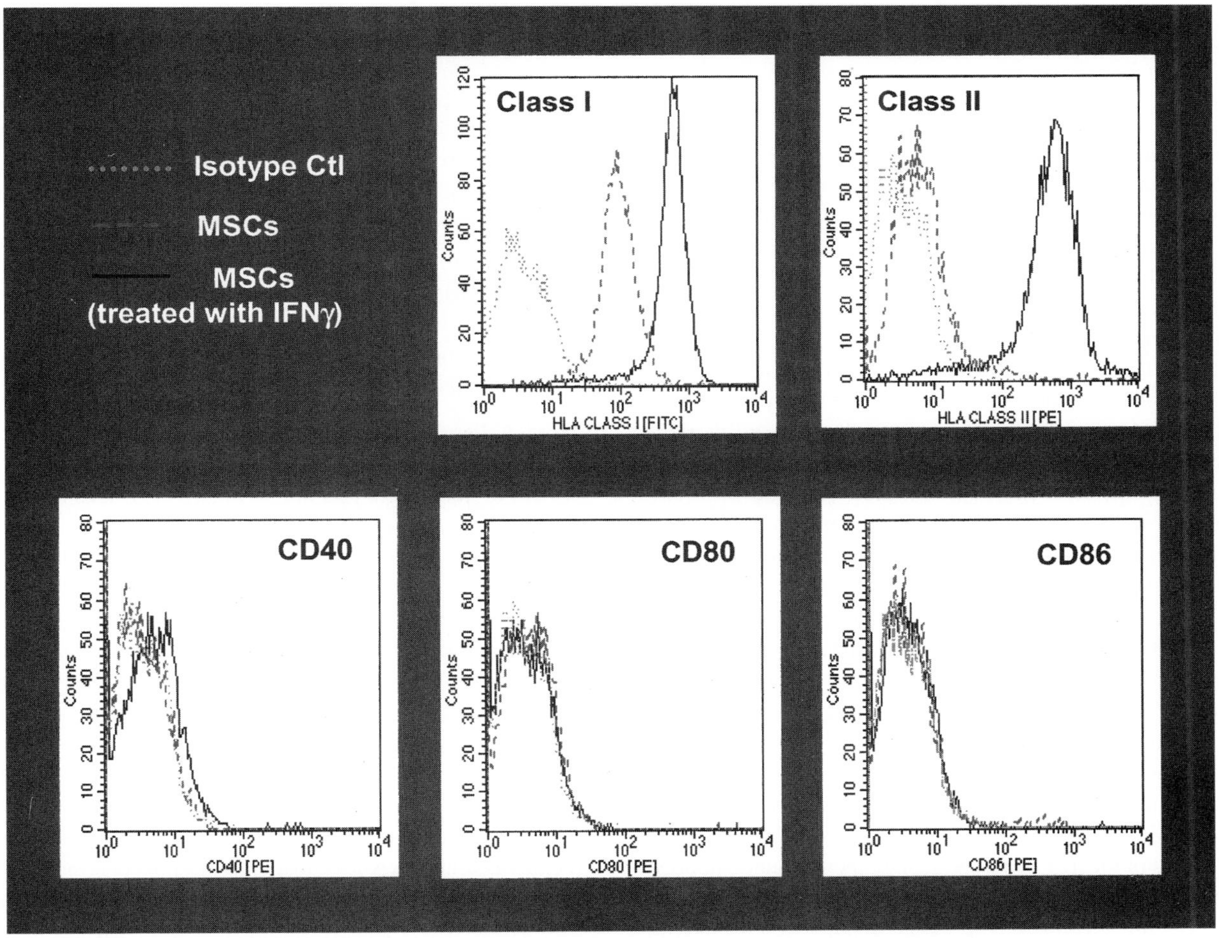

Fig. 5.2. Treatment with interferon-γ upregulates MHC class I antigens on the MSC surface and enables expression of MHC class II molecules, but the co-stimulatory molecules CD40, CD80, and CD86 are not expressed even after treatment with interferon-γ.

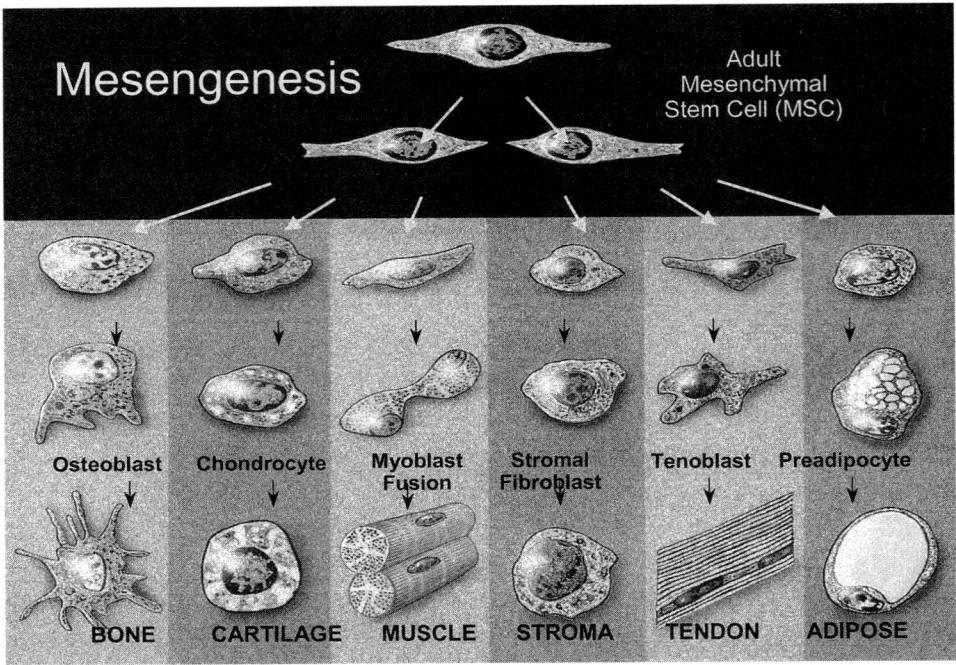

Fig. 5.3. The process of mesengenesis: mesenchymal stem cells are capable of differentiating into bone, cartilage, muscle, stroma (including marrow stroma), tendon, and adipose tissue.

Immunomodulation by MSCs

Several studies suggest that MSCs may play a role in modulation of immune responses. MSCs are poor antigen-presenting cells and do not express major histocompatibility complex (MHC) class II or costimulatory molecules. Expanded MSCs do not stimulate T-cell proliferation in mixed lymphocyte reactions (MLR), yet are able to downregulate alloreactive T-cell responses when added to mixed lymphocyte cultures (Fig. 5.4) (Klyushnenkova et al., 1998). At present the mechanism underlying this suppressive effect is unknown, but it may involve the production of soluble factors. DiNicola and co-workers (DiNicola et al., 2002) reported that MSCs can provide a global, dose-dependent in vitro inhibition of T-cell proliferation. Furthermore, transwell experiments supported the belief that this effect is mediated by both direct interaction as well as by soluble factors. Blocking experiments using neutralizing monoclonal antibodies directed against transforming growth factor β1 (TGF-β1) and hepatocyte growth factor (HGF) indicated restoration of T-cell proliferation, suggesting that these factors were in part responsible for the observed inhibition by MSCs (DiNicola et al., 2002). T lymphocytes inhibited by MSCs are not apoptotic and could be induced to proliferate when restimulated with cellular or humoral stimuli in the absence of MSCs (DiNicola et al., 2002). Animal experiments support the notion that MSCs also mediate immune suppression in vivo. In a baboon skin graft rejection model, in vivo infusion of MSCs resulted in prolonged skin graft survival in comparison to control animals not treated with MSCs (Bartholomew et al., 2002). The suppression of immune responses appears to be nonspecific and there is as yet no evidence for antigen specificity of this effect. These immunosuppressive properties provide a rationale for use of this cellular product in clinical settings including allogeneic HSCT, as well as solid organ transplantation (see below).

Transplantability of MSCs

Repopulation of the recipient microenvironment by stromal cells in the bone marrow graft

Most studies that have explored the question have reported that in patients undergoing allogeneic HSCT, mesenchymal tissues remain of host origin (Galotto et al., 1999; Erices et al., 2002; Gutierrez-Rodriguez et al., 2000; Mareschi et al., 2001; Laver et al., 1987; Agematsu & Nakahori, 1991; Santucci et al., 1992; Keating et al., 1982; Koc et al., 1999; Simmons et al., 1987; Horwitz et al., 1999; Horwitz et al., 2001). Possible exceptions were reported by Horwitz and colleagues (Horwitz et al., 1999; Horwitz et al., 2001), Mareschi and co-workers (Mareschi et al., 2001), and Keating et al (Keating et al., 1982). In the two Horwitz studies, 1% to 2% of the osteoblasts recovered after culture were of donor origin (Horwitz et al., 1999). The report by Mareschi and associates (Mareschi et al., 2001) detected donor osteoblasts in osteogenesis imperfecta (OI) recipients after HLA-identical sibling allogeneic bone marrow transplantation. It is unclear if this observation indicates if osteoblasts were passively transferred to the recipient, or whether MSCs present in the marrow graft traveled to bone and differentiated into osteoblasts. In the communication by Keating

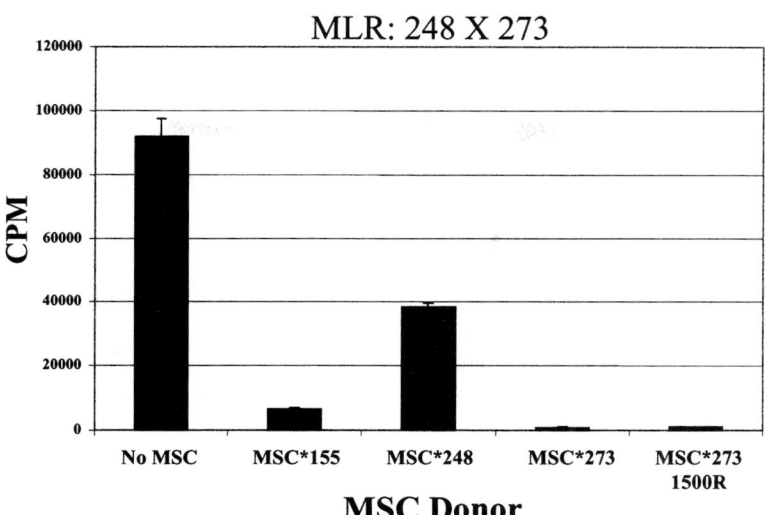

Fig. 5.4. MSCs downregulate an ongoing mixed lymphocyte reaction when added on day 4, regardless of whether the MSCs are derived from the MLR responder, the MLR stimulator, or a third party.

et al., (Keating *et al.*, 1982), the question has been raised as to whether macrophage contamination accounted for the results. The finding that stroma remains host in origin after an allograft is attributed to the inability of the conditioning regimen to ablate host marrow stroma, the inability of stromal progenitors to engraft, or the combination. In addition, the number of MSCs is estimated to be too few in an average bone marrow graft (2 to 5 MSCs per 1×10^6 mononuclear cells, suggesting that a bone marrow graft composed of 2×10^8 MNC/kg contains 400 to 1,000 MSCs/kg). Nevertheless, these data suggest that osteoblasts may be transplanted successfully in certain conditions and diseases, although the optimal approach has not yet been established. Most patients undergoing allogeneic HSCT have hematologic malignancies and exhibit a relatively slow turnover of their mesenchymal tissues, even after the conditioning regimen. In contrast, OI patients may have much faster turnover of their osteoid tissue. As a result, it may be possible to detect donor-derived osteoblasts, MSCs, or both cells participating in this process, especially since normal osteoblasts have a competitive survival advantage compared to endogenous OI osteoblasts.

The allogeneic HSC transplant field has noted a trend toward the increased use of alternative stem cell sources such as mobilized peripheral blood progenitor cells (PBPC) rather than bone marrow as well as umbilical cord blood (UCB) units. We and others have been unable to detect or culture-expand MSCs from hematopoietic growth factor and/or chemotherapy-mobilized peripheral blood, or from UCB (Noort *et al.*, 2001). Since PBPC grafts usually contain at least a log more hematopoietic stem and progenitor cells than marrow grafts, the lack of an MSC component may not be deleterious to engraftment in most patients. On the other hand, Cilloni *et al.* (Cilloni *et al.*, 2000) reported that marrow stromal progenitors re-infused into patients receiving T-cell-depleted allografts have a limited capacity to reconstitute MSC; the authors suggested that HSC

grafts be augmented with ex vivo generated MSC. Furthermore, hematopoietic recovery after UCB transplants, especially in adult recipients, is exceedingly slow (Laughlin *et al.*, 2001) and the need to supplement these types of grafts with marrow-derived MSCs may be important. The question still remains whether the bone marrow microenvironment can be repopulated by allogeneic bone marrow or culture-expanded MSCs in patients who have no intrinsic mesenchymal defect. Furthermore, it remains to be shown if this cellular therapy improves engraftment rates, particularly if UCB grafts containing a marginal number of stem cells are utilized.

Transplantability of expanded MSCs

Although most of the current evidence from conventional HSC allografts performed for malignant disorders indicates that marrow stromal cells are host-derived (Galotto *et al.*, 1999; Erices *et al.*, 2002; Gutierrez-Rodriguez *et al.*, 2000; Laver *et al.*, 1987; Agematsu & Nakahori, 1991; Santucci *et al.*, 1992; Keating *et al.*, 1982; Koc *et al.*, 1999; Simmons *et al.*, 1987) data derived from allogeneic bone marrow transplantation in OI patients showed approximately 2% of osteoblasts to be of donor origin, suggesting that donor-derived MSC precursors in the marrow were capable of homing to, and engrafting and differentiating within, bone marrow (Horwitz *et al.*, 1999; Horwitz *et al.*, 2001). These conflicting data sets indicate the ability of donor-derived stromal cell progenitors to engraft, as well as the fact that host-derived marrow stromal cells may be able to survive the conditioning regimen. As discussed above, the numbers of MSCs in an "average" bone marrow graft may be below the level required for engraftment. From these observations, in vivo studies in animals and humans have been undertaken in an attempt to promote engraftment of HSC by cotransplantation of MSCs. Pereira *et al.* (1998) infused normal mouse bone marrow–derived stromal cells into irradiated transgenic recipient mice with an OI phenotype. Several months after transplantation they demonstrated the presence of donor-derived MSCs in various organs of recipient mice, including bone, cartilage, lung, and spleen. MSCs that homed to the bones differentiated into osteocytes, and produced normal levels of collagen type I with partial restoration of the OI phenotype.

In the absence of a "mesenchymal" defect in the recipient bone or bone marrow, it has been more difficult to demonstrate donor engraftment of MSCs following transplantation. Mosca and co-workers (Mosca et al., 1998) reported their results in dogs given total body irradiation (TBI) and canine G-CSF-mobilized autologous blood stem cells along with ex vivo–expanded canine MSCs retrovirally transduced with the green fluorescent protein (GFP) gene. Hematopoietic recovery was prompt and GFP-positive cells were detected using DNA PCR and RT-PCR at 6 months after transplant. Sandmaier and colleagues (Sandmaier et al., 1998) transplanted dogs with DLA-matched allogeneic bone marrow and ex vivo–expanded, canine GFP retrovirally transduced MSCs following 920 cGy TBI. The mean time to platelet engraftment was 20 days, transfusions were not required, and marked cells were noted using DNA PCR at 40 days after transplant. Almeida-Porada and associates (Almeida-Porada et al., 2000) employed DNA analysis to detect the presence of human MSCs in the bone marrow and spleen of sheep that had been injected in utero with stromal cells alone, indicating that these cells are capable of low-level engraftment in the bone marrow. Preclinical, nonhuman primate data indicate that ex vivo–expanded MSCs are capable of homing to the marrow and establishing residence for an extended period after systemic administration (Devine et al., 2001). Using ex vivo–expanded MSCs transduced with a green fluorescent retroviral construct, the same group found baboon MSCs to distribute to a wide range of tissues including the gastrointestinal tract, kidney, lung, liver, thymus, and skin (Devine et al., 2003). In a single NOD-SCID mouse, Noort et al. (Noort et al., 2001) observed a PCR signal in the bone marrow following intravenous injection of fetal lung–derived MSCs. Additional experiments using infusion of MSCs alone or co-infusion of gene-marked MSCs and UCB-derived CD34+ cells indicated the differential homing of CD34+ cells to the marrow while MSCs traveled to recipient lung. Rombouts and Ploemacher (2003) systematically studied MSC homing of both primary and cultured MSCs in a syngeneic mouse model. They found that primary bone marrow-derived MSCs were able to home efficiently to the bone marrow and spleen, while culture-expanded MSCs had lost this capacity after being cultured for 24–48 hours. These data suggest that in vitro propagation of BM-derived MSCs dramatically decreases their homing to BM and spleen.

Preclinical results

Almeida-Porada et al. (Almeida-Porada et al., 2000) observed that cotransplantation of human stromal cells into pre-immune fetal sheep resulted in an enhancement of long-term engraftment of human cells in the bone marrow and higher levels of donor cells in the circulation, both during gestation as well as after birth. El-Badri and colleagues (El-Badri et al., 1998; El-Badri, 2001) demonstrated that infusion of bone marrow–derived osteoblasts facilitated the engraftment of allogeneic hematopoietic stem cells across major histoincompatibility barriers in mice. Other studies in NOD/SCID mice indicate that cotransplantation of MSCs enhances engraftment of human hematopoietic cells in the bone marrow of NOD/SCID mice (Noort et al., 2001; Novelli et al., 1998). Co-infusion of fetal lung–derived MSCs and umbilical cord blood–derived CD34+ cells promoted the engraftment of both myeloid and B-lymphoid cells in the marrow of recipient mice, showing that the engraftment-promoting effect of MSCs was not lineage-specific. The latter studies also found engraftment enhancement to be independent of the homing of MSCs to the marrow and that it might be mediated by the release of cytokines that promote either the homing or proliferation of HSCs. Indeed, MSCs produce a variety of cytokines that are involved in homing (SDF-1) or proliferation and differentiation of hematopoietic cells [granulocyte-macrophage colony-stimulating factor (GM-CSF), G-CSF, stem cell factor (SCF), interleukin (IL)-6]. The engraftment-promoting effect was most pronounced after transplantation using relatively low numbers of CD34+ cells, suggesting that the engraftment delay associated with clinical UCB transplantation might be accelerated by cotransplantation of MSCs.

MSCs of fetal origin have been identified in second trimester amniotic fluid and could be expanded in three to four weeks to about 180×10^6, suggesting that a small aliquot of amniotic fluid can potentially be used to generate MSCs to supplement cord blood grafts in the setting of family cord blood transplantation (Anker et al., 2003).

Clinical results

Application of MSCs in autologous stem cell transplantation

A number of studies have shown that chemotherapy and radiation therapy damage the bone marrow microenvironment, and this may result in diminished hematopoiesis (O'Flaherty et al., 1995; McMannus & Weiss, 1984; Uhlman et al., 1991; Domenech et al., 1994). The damaged marrow stroma must reconstitute itself to provide the optimal environment for hematopoietic regeneration. Thus, studies designed to restore the microenvironment using MSCs were initiated. In initial phase I studies involving bone marrow–derived MSCs, Lazarus and co-workers (Lazarus et al., 1995) showed that MSCs could be collected, ex vivo culture–expanded for 4 to 7 weeks, and safely administered to patients with hematologic malignancy who were in complete remission. The infusions contained up to 50×10^6 MSCs and were well-tolerated without adverse reactions. This group subsequently conducted a phase I–II autotransplant clinical trial in 28 breast cancer patients. Autologous MSCs were generated from 20 to 25 ml bone marrow aspirates and expanded ex vivo over 20 to 50 days (Koc *et al.*, 2000). A total of 1.0 to 2.2 × 10⁶ MSCs per kg were co-infused with autologous PBPCs after the STAMP V high-dose chemotherapy regimen. Clonogenic MSCs could be detected in venous blood up to 1 hour after infusion in the majority of patients. Again, MSC infusion-related toxicities were not observed and hematopoietic reconstitution was more rapid compared to an autotransplant breast cancer patient cohort treated during a similar time period at the same center, suggesting efficacy of MSC infusion in accelerating hematopoietic reconstitution. However, while this study shows the feasibility and safety of MSC infusion, an appropriate control group was lacking and therefore the clinical efficacy remains uncertain.

Application of MSCs in allogeneic stem cell transplantation

Malignant hematological disorders

In a multicenter, phase I–II study, donor bone marrow–derived MSCs (1.0 to 2.5 × 10⁶ per kg recipient weight) were co-infused into 36 patients with hematological malignancies undergoing HLA-identical sibling HSC transplantation (Lazarus *et al.*, 2000). Seventeen patients received donor bone marrow while 19 subjects were given G-CSF-mobilized PBPC as the HSC source; graft-versus-host disease (GVHD) prophylaxis consisted of cyclosporine and three doses of methotrexate. Preliminary data suggest rapid engraftment and a low incidence of GVHD in comparison to historic controls; only three patients developed grade III–IV acute GVHD and only two patients had extensive chronic GVHD. In a matched-pair analysis, 14 recipients of unmanipulated bone marrow and 17 recipients of mobilized peripheral blood in this same study were compared with matched controls selected from the EBMT Registry (Frassoni *et al.*, 2002). Both the incidence of acute and chronic GVHD were significantly reduced in patients cotransplanted with MSCs. Patients receiving MSC infusion also had better survival at 6 months (Frassoni *et al.*, 2002). These intriguing results warrant prospective, controlled clinical trials in order to determine the efficacy of this approach.

Inborn errors of metabolism

Allogeneic bone marrow transplantation has been applied in children with OI as a form of MSC transplantation (Horwitz *et al.*, 1999; Horwitz *et al.*, 2001). In 3 out of 5 patients with documented osteoblast engraftment following transplantation, an increase in bone mineral content and in body length was observed in comparison with age-matched controls (Horwitz *et al.*, 2001). In these studies osteoblast engraftment may have resulted from the passive transfer of residual osteoblasts in the marrow graft. These data indicate that osteoblasts may be newly formed or may be transplanted successfully in patients with OI. However, it remains to be determined to what extent the cells contributed to the clinical improvement reported for these patients.

Future directions

Transplantation of MSCs represents an attractive new form of cellular therapy for clinical application in the transplantation area. The potential for clinical use relates to facilitation of hematopoietic engraftment, immunomodulation, and correction of disorders of mesenchymal cells.

Allogeneic MSCs in the autologous transplant setting

Although initial studies appear promising, randomized studies are required to show the potential of cotransplantation of MSCs given systemically with HSC in order to accelerate hematopoietic reconstitution after stem cell transplantation. This maneuver may be useful for those types of transplants that are associated with delayed engraftment, for example, autografts for acute myeloid leukemia or extensively pretreated lymphoma and multiple myeloma (Table 5.3). A number of groups have used a variety of expansion systems to shorten the obligate period of neutropenia and thrombocytopenia during autologous hematopoietic stem cell transplantion (Paquette *et al.*, 2000; Reiffers *et al.*, 1999; McNiece *et al.*, 2000; Stiff *et al.*, 2000; Engelhardt *et al.*, 2001). In theory, MSCs could also be used to facilitate expansion of autologous stem cells ex vivo as MSCs have been reported to retard the differentiation of CD34+CD38low/neg cells exposed to cytokines (Bennaceur-Griscelle *et al.*, 2001).

Allogeneic MSCs in the allogeneic transplant setting

In the allogeneic setting, cotransplantation of donor-derived MSCs may prevent or ameliorate GVHD by exerting their immunosuppressive effect. MSCs transferred in a bone marrow

Table 5.3. *Potential clinical uses for MSCs*

Hematopoietic support
    Facilitate hematopoietic engraftment in patients undergoing autografts for leukemia, lymphoma, and myeloma
    Facilitate hematopoietic engraftment in patients undergoing allografts using umbilical cord blood grafts, unrelated donor marrow grafts, and haploidentical family member donor grafts
Immune modulation
    Reduce or prevent GVHD after allogeneic HSC transplantation
    Induce tolerance for solid organ allografting
Delivery of corrective genes
    Correction of mesenchymal genetic disorders such as osteogenesis imperfecta
    In vivo production of secreted proteins for diseases such as hemophilia
Cardiology
    Cardiac muscle repair
Orthopedics
    Repair of bone fractures, cartilage repair, meniscal regeneration
    Osteoporosis therapy
    Repair of bone metastases

graft may play a potential therapeutic role in the correction of OI. However, controlled studies are required to further substantiate this effect. MSCs may also serve as vehicles for gene therapy in the correction of inborn errors of metabolism.

MSC for use with UCB Transplantation

Wagner and co-workers infused UCB units along with culture-expanded MSCs obtained from a "third party" (i.e., parents) in an attempt to enhance hematopoietic recovery after allograft (Wagner, personal communication). Use of third party MSCs was a consideration in view of the favorable immunologic properties of MSCs and the unavailability of corresponding marrow samples from the same donor for ex vivo expansion. Preliminary results in a small patient population suggested no improvement in tempo to blood count recovery but overall survival appeared improved. MSCs also have been used in vitro as a means to expand UCB units for clinical use and clinical trials are planned (Kozik *et al.*, 2002).

MSCs as vehicles for gene therapy

MSCs may have significant advantages for gene therapy when compared to HSC. As reported above, MSCs can be isolated and expanded in in vitro culture at a significantly greater rate compared to HSC (Gronthos *et al.*, 1994; Phinney *et al.*, 1999; Keating *et al.*, 1984; Otsuka *et al.*, 1991; Gordon *et al.*, 1996). Furthermore, MSCs possess the ability to self-renew at a high proliferative rate. Adherent stromal cells can be transduced efficiently providing a stable, long-term gene expression (Li *et al.*, 1995; Drize *et al.*, 1992). In various small animal systems, gene-transduced MSCs secreted cytokines such as IL-3 and human factor IX for long periods (Dao & Nolta, 1998; Brouard *et al.*, 1998; Gordon *et al.*, 1997). Human MSCs also could be cotransfected successfully and expressed both a marker gene LacZ and secreted a protein (IL-3) (Allay *et al.*, 1997). Furthermore, mesenchymal progenitor cells maintained the cell phenotype as evidenced by forming bone in vivo in an osteogenic assay. Other investigators have demonstrated that this approach can be reproduced in larger animals. Hurwitz and co-workers (Hurwitz *et al.*, 1997) showed that both human growth hormone and human factor IX can be detected in the serum of dogs undergoing transplantation with genetically modified autologous bone marrow stroma.

Unresolved issues

A number of fundamental questions relating to the biology of MSC are still unanswered, such as survival and homing capacity to populate host tissues after transplantation. What is the relationship between immunophenotype and function? Should MSC therapy be applied systemically or does implantation at local sites make more sense? Several investigators have developed strategies for targeting cells specifically to bone marrow and these techniques could be applied to improve systemic

Table 5.4. *Potential advantages for "universal donor" MSCs*

Off-the-shelf availability
Multiple dosing potential
Defined MSC potency
Higher infusion doses possible
Reduced costs of product

administration (Blair & Thomas, 1997; Peled *et al.*, 1999). Are MSCs derived from different sources functionally similar and do culture-expanded cells retain their self-renewal and multilineage differentiation potential after transplantation? Ex vivo culture of MSCs is an expensive, labor-intense, and very lengthy process, and the properties of each expansion product appear to vary from individual to individual. New approaches for expansion must address the development of a more homogeneous product. Given the significant property of being nonimmunogenic while retaining immunosuppressive potential, one group has begun to advance the concept for use of a "universal donor" MSC. In this regard, healthy volunteers can provide bone marrow samples for culture expansion for use in clinical investigation Some of the advantages of this approach are listed in Table 5.4. Some data suggest that marrow stromal cells may help provide a more suitable marrow environment for tumor cells (Hombauer & Minguell, 2000). Clinical investigations in cancer patients that employ MSCs must be designed to monitor for the possibility of tumor progression. Clearly, continued fundamental and clinical studies are required to turn a distant hope into a therapeutic reality.

References

Agematsu, K. & Nakahori, Y. (1991). Recipient origin of bone marrow-derived fibroblastic stromal cells during all periods following bone marrow transplantation in humans. *British Journal of Haematology*, **79**, 359–65.

Allay, J.A., Dennis, J.E., Haynesworth, S.E. *et al.* (1997). LacZ and interleukin-3 expression in vivo after retroviral transduction of marrow-derived human osteogeneic mesenchymal progenitors. *Human Gene Therapy*, **8**, 1417–27.

Allen, T.D., Dexter, T.M., & Simmons, P.J. (1990). Marrow biology and stem cells. *Immunology Series*, **49**, 1–38.

Almeida-Porada, G., Porada, C.D., Tran, N., & Zanjani, E.D. (2000). Cotransplantation of human stromal cell progenitors into preimmune fetal sheep results in early appearance of human donor cells in circulation and boosts cell levels in bone marrow at later time points after transplantation. *Blood*, **95**, 3620–7.

Barry, F.P., Boynton, R.E., Haynesworth, S. *et al.* (1999). The monoclonal antibody SH-2, raised against human mesenchymal stem cells, recognizes an epitope on endoglin (CD105). *Biochemical and Biophysical Research Communications*, **265**, 134–9.

Barry, F.P., Boynton, R., Murphy, M., & Zaia, J. (2001). The SH-3 and SH-4 antibodies recognize distinct epitopes on CD73 from human mesenchymal stem cells. *Biochemical and Biophysical Research Communications*, **289**, 519–24.

Bartholomew, A., Sturgeon, C., Siatskas, M. *et al.* (2002). Mesenchymal stem cells suppress lymphocyte proliferation in vitro and prolong skin graft survival in vivo. *Experimental Hematology*, **30**, 42–8.

Bennaceur-Griscelli, A., Pondarre, C., Schiavon, V. *et al.* (2001). Stromal cells retard the differentiation of CD34(+)CD38(low/neg) human primitive progenitors exposed to cytokines independent of their mitotic history. *Blood*, **97**, 435–41.

Blair, A. & Thomas, D.B. (1997). Preferential adhesion of fetal liver derived primitive haematopoietic progenitor cells to bone marrow stroma. *British Journal of Hematology*, **99**, 726–31.

Brouard, N., Chapel, A., Neildez-Nguyen, T.M. *et al.* (1998). Transplantation of stromal cells transduced with the human IL3 gene to stimulate hematopoiesis in human fetal bone grafts in non-obese, diabetic-severe combined immunodeficiency mice. *Leukemia*, **12**, 1128–35.

Campagnoli, C., Roberts, I.A., Kumar, S. *et al.* (2001). Identification of mesenchymal stem/progenitor cells in human first-trimester fetal blood, liver, and bone marrow. *Blood*, **98**, 2396–402.

Caplan, A.I. (1994). The mesengenic process. *Clinics in Plastic Surgery*, **21**, 429–35.

Chesney, J., Bacher, M., Bender, A., & Bucala, R. (1997). The periperal blood fibrocyte is a potent antigen-processing cell capable of priming naïve T cells in situ. *Proceedings of the National Academy of Science USA*, **94**, 6307–12.

Cilloni, D., Carlo-Stella, C., Falzetti, F. *et al.* (2000). Limited engraftment capacity of bone marrow-derived mesenchymal cells following T-cell-depleted hematopoietic stem cell transplantation. *Blood*, **96**, 3637–43.

Conget, P.A. & Minguell, J.J. (1999). Phenotypical and functional properties of human bone marrow mesenchymal progenitor cells. *Journal of Cellular Physiology*, **181**, 67–73.

Dao, M.A., Nolta, J.A. (1998). Use of the bnx/bu xenograft model of human hematopoiesis to optimize methods for retrovirally-mediated stem cell transduction. *International Journal of Molecular Medicine*, **1**, 257–64.

Deans, R.J. & Moseley, A.B. (2000). Mesenchymal stem cells: biology and potential clinical uses. *Experimental Hematology*, **28**, 875–84.

Devine, S.M., Bartholomew, A.M., Mahmud, N. *et al.* (2001). Mesenchymal stem cells are capable of homing to the bone marrow of non-human primates following systemic infusion. *Experimental Hematology*, **29**, 244–55.

Devine, S.M., Cobbs, C., Jennings, M., Bartholomew, A., & Hoffman, R. (2003). Mesenchymal stem cells distribute to a wide range of tissues following systemic infusion into nonhuman primates. *Blood*, **102**, 2999–3001.

DiNicola, M., Carlo-Stella, C., Magni, M. *et al.* (2002). Human bone marrow stromal cells suppress T-lymphocyte proliferation induced by cellular or nonspecific mitogenic stimuli. *Blood*, **99**, 3838–43.

Domenech, J., Gihana, E., Dayan, A. *et al.* (1994). Haemopoiesis of transplanted patients with autologous marrows assessed by long-term marrow culture. *British Journal of Haematology*, **88**, 488–96.

Drize, N.J., Surin, V.L., Gan, O.I. *et al.* (1992). Gene therapy model for stromal precursors cells of hematopoietic microenvironment. *Leukemia*, **3**, 174S.

El-Badri, N.S. (2001). The role of osteoblasts in experimental and clinical transplantation. *Graft*, **3**, 307–10.

El-Badri, N.S., Wang, B.Y., Cherry, Good, R.A. (1998). Osteoblasts promote engraftment of allogeneic hematopoietic stem cells. *Experimental Hematology*, **26**, 110–16.

Engelhardt, M., Douville, J., Behringer, D. *et al.* (2001). Hematopoietic recovery of ex vivo perfusion culture expanded bone marrow and unexpanded peripheral blood progenitors after myeloablative chemotherapy. *Bone Marrow Transplantation*, **27**, 249–59.

Erices, A., Conget, P., & Minguell, J.J. (2000). Mesenchymal progenitor cells in human umbilical cord blood. *British Journal of Haematology*, **109**, 235–42.

Fernandez, M., Simon, V., Herrera, G. *et al.* (1997). Detection of stromal cells in peripheral blood progenitor cell collections from breast cancer patients. *Bone Marrow Transplantation*, **20**, 265–71.

Ferrari, G., Cusella-DeAngelis, G., Coletta, M., & Paolucci, E. (1998). Muscle regeneration by bone marrow-derived myogenic progenitors. *Science*, **279**, 1528–30.

Frassoni, F., Labopin, M., Bacigalupo, A. *et al.* (2002). Expanded mesenchymal stem cells (MSC), co-infused with HLA identical hemopoietic stem cell transplants, reduce acute and chronic graft versus host disease: a matched pair analysis. *Bone Marrow Transplantation*, **29**, (Suppl), 2 (Abstract 75).

Friedenstein, A.J., Deriglasova, U.F., Kulagina, N.N. *et al.* (1974). Precursors for fibroblasts in different populations of hematopoietic cells as detected by the in vitro colony assay method. *Experimental Hematology*, **2**, 83–92.

Galotto, M., Berisso, G. Delfino, L. *et al.* (1999). Stromal damage as consequence of high-dose chemo/radiotherapy in bone marrow transplant recipients. *Experimental Hematology*, **27**, 1460–6.

Gerson, S.L. (1999). Mesenchymal stem cells: no longer second class marrow citizens. *Nature Medicine*, **5**, 262–4.

Gordon, E.M., Skotzko, M., Kundu, R.K. *et al.* (1997). Capture and expansion of bone marrow-derived mesenchymal progenitor cells with a transforming growth factor-betal-von Willebrand's factor fusion protein for retrovirus-mediated delivery of coagulation factor IX. *Human Gene Therapy*, **8**, 1385–94.

Gordon, M.Y., Lewis, J.L., Grand, E.H. *et al.* (1996). Phenotype and progeny of primitive adherent human haematopoietic progenitors. *Leukemia*, **10**, 1347–53.

Gronthos, S. & Simmons, P.J. (1996). The biology and application of human bone marrow stromal cell precursors. *Journal of Hematotherapy*, **5**, 15–23.

Gronthos, S., Graves, S.E., Ohta, S., & Simmons, P.J. (1994). The STRO-1+ fraction of adult human bone marrow contains the osteogenic precursors. *Blood*, **84**, 4164–73.

Gutierrez-Rodriguez, M., Reyes-Maldonado, E., & Mayani, H. (2000). Characterization of the adherent cells developed in Dexter-type long-term cultures from human umbilical cord blood. *Stem Cells*, **18**, 46–52.

Hombauer, H. & Minguell, J.J. (2000). Selective interactions between epithelial tumor cells and bone marrow mesenchymal stem cells. *British Journal of Cancer*, **82**, 1290–6.

Horwitz, E.M., Prockop, D.J., Fitzpatrick, L.A. *et al.* (1999). Transplantability and therapeutic effects of bone marrow-derived mesenchymal cells in children with osteogenesis imperfecta. *Nature Medicine*, **5**, 309–13.

Horwitz, E.M., Prockop, D.J., Gordon, P.L. *et al.* (2001). Clinical responses to bone marrow transplantation in children with severe osteogenesis imperfecta. *Blood*, **97**, 1227–33.

Hurwitz, D.R., Kirchgesser, M., Merrill, W. *et al.* (1997). Systemic delivery of human growth hormone or human factor IX in dogs by reintroduced genetically modified autologous bone marrow stromal cells. *Human Gene Therapy,* **8,** 137–56.

in 't Anker, P.S., Scherjon, S.A., Kleijburg-van der Keur C., *et al.* (2003). Amniotic fluid as a novel source of mesenchymal stem cells for therapeutic application. *Blood,* in press.

Jiang, Y., Jahagirdar, B.N., Reinhardt, R.L. *et al.* (2002). Pluripotency of mesenchymal stem cells derived from adult marrow. *Nature,* **418,** 41–9.

Keating, A., Powell, J., Takahashi, M., & Singer, J.W. (1984). The generation of human long-term bone marrow cultures from marrow depleted of Ia (HLA-DR) positive cells. *Blood,* **64,** 1159–62.

Keating, A., Singer, J.W., Killen, P.D. *et al.* (1982). Donor origin of the in vitro haematopoietic microenvironment after marrow transplantation in man. *Nature,* **298,** 280–2.

Klyushnenkova, E., Mosca, J.D., & McIntosh, K.R. (1998). Human mesenchymal stem cells suppress allogeneic T cell responses in vitro: implications for allogeneic transplantation. *Blood,* **92,** 642a.

Koc, O.N., Gerson, S.L., Cooper, B.W. *et al.* (2000). Rapid hematopoietic recovery after coinfusion of autologous-blood stem cells and culture-expanded marrow mesenchymal stem cells in advanced breast cancer patients receiving high-dose chemotherapy. *Journal of Clinical Oncology,* **18,** 307–16.

Koc, O.N., Peters, C., Aubourg, P. *et al.* (1999). Bone marrow-derived mesenchymal stem cells remain host-derived despite successful hematopoietic engraftment after allogeneic transplantation in patients with lysosomal and peroxisomal storage diseases. *Experimental Hematology,* **27,** 1675–81.

Kozik, M.M., Bos, L., Kadereit, S. *et al.* (2002). Effects of mesenchymal stem cell stromal layer on umbilical cord blood LTC-IC and CD34 populations during short term expansion. *Blood,* **92** (Supp1), 86a (abstract 360).

Krebsbach, P.H., Kuznetsov, S.A., Satomura, K. *et al.* (1997). Bone formation in vivo: comparison of osteogenesis by transplanted mouse and human marrow stromal fibroblasts. *Transplantation,* **63,** 1059–69.

Laughlin, M.J., Barker, J., Bambach, B. *et al.* (2001). Hematologic engraftment and survival after unrelated placental cord transplant in adult recipients. *New England Journal of Medicine,* **344,** 1815–22.

Laver, J., Jhanwar, S.C., O'Reilly, R.J., & Castro-Malaspina, H. (1987). Host origin of the human hematopoietic microenvironment following allogeneic bone marrow transplantation. *Blood,* **70,** 1966–8.

Lazarus, H.M., Curtin, P., Devine, S. *et al.* (2000). Role of mesenchymal stem cells in allogeneic transplantation: early phase I clinical results. *Blood,* **96,** 1691a.

Lazarus, H.M., Haynesworth, S.E., Gerson, S.L. *et al.* (1995). Ex vivo expansion and subsequent infusion of human bone marrow-derived stromal progenitor cells (mesenchymal progenitor cells): implications for therapeutic use. *Bone Marrow Transplantation,* **16,** 557–64.

Lazarus, H.M., Haynesworth, S.E., Gerson, S.L., & Caplan, A.I. (1997). Human bone marrow-derived mesenchymal (stromal) progenitor cells (MPCs) cannot be recovered from peripheral blood progenitor cell collections. *Journal of Hematotherapy,* **6,** 447–55.

Lennon, D.P., Haynesworth, S.E., Bruder, S.P. *et al.* (1996). Development of a serum screen for mesenchymal progenitor cells from bone marrow. *In Vitro Cellular and Developmental Biology,* **32,** 602–11.

Li, K.J., Dilber, M.S., Abedi, M.R. *et al.* (1995). Retroviral-mediated gene transfer into human bone marrow stromal cells; studies of efficiency and in vivo survival in SCID mice. *European Journal of Haematology,* **55,** 302–6.

Lichtman, M.A. (1981). The ultrastructure of the hemopoietic environment of the marrow: a review. *Experimental Hematology,* **9,** 391–410.

Mackay, A.M., Beck, S.C., Murphy, J.M. *et al.* (1998). Chondrogenic differentiation of cultured human mesenchymal stem cells from marrow. *Tissue Engineering,* **4,** 415–28.

Majumdar, M.K., Thiede, M.A., Haynesworth, S.E. *et al.* (2000). Human marrow-derived mesenchymal stem cells (MSCs) express hematopoietic cytokines and support long-term hematopoiesis when differentiated toward stromal and osteogenic lineages. *Journal of Hematotherapy Stem Cell Research,* **9,** 841–8.

Majumdar, M.K., Thiede, M.A., Mosca, J.D. *et al.* (1998). Phenotypic and functional comparison of cultures of marrow-derived mesenchymal stem cells (MSCs) and stromal cells. *Journal of Cellular Physiology,* **176,** 57–66.

Makino, S., Fukuda, K., Miyoshi, S. *et al.* (1999). Cardiomyocytes can be generated from adult marrow stromal cells in vitro. *Journal of Clinical Investigation,* **103,** 697–705.

Mareschi, K., Biasin, E., Piacibello, W. *et al.* (2001). Isolation of human mesenchymal stem cells: bone marrow versus umbilical cord blood. *Haematologica,* **86,** 1099–100.

McMannus, P.M. & Weiss, L. (1984). Busulfan-induced chronic bone marrow failure: changes in cortical bone, marrow stromal cells, and adherent cell colonies. *Blood,* **64,** 1036–41.

McNiece, I., Jones, R., Bearman, S.I. *et al.* (2000). Ex vivo expanded peripheral blood progenitor cells provide rapid neutrophil recovery after high-dose chemotherapy in patients with breast cancer. *Blood,* **96,** 3001–7.

Mosca, J., Buyaner, D., & Kniley, J. (1998). Biodistribution and bone marrow 'homing' of canine mesenchymal stem cells after culture expansion and re-infusion into a canine transplantation model. *Blood,* **92**(Suppl), 664a.

Nakahara, H., Dennis, J.E., Bruder, S.P. *et al.* (1991). In vitro differentiation of bone and hypertrophic cartilage from periosteal-derived cells. *Experimental Cell Research,* **195,** 492–503.

Nathanson, M.A. (1985). Bone matrix-directed chondrogenesis of muscle in vitro. *Clinical Orthopedics,* **200,** 142–58.

Nilsson, S.K., Johnston, H.M., & Coverdale, J.A. (2001). Spatial localization of transplanted hemopoietic stem cells: inferences for the localization of stem cell niches. *Blood,* **97,** 2293–9.

Noort, W.A., Kruisselbrink, de Paus, R.A. *et al.* (2001). Co-transplantation of mesenchymal stem cells (MSC) and UCB CD34+ cells results in enhanced hematopoietic engraftment in NOD/SCID mice without homing of MSC to the bone marrow. *Blood,* **98,** 295a.

Novelli, E. Buyner, D., & Chopra, R. (1998). Human mesenchymal stem cells can enhance human CD34+ cell repopulation of NOD/SCID mice. *Blood,* **92,** 117a.

O'Flaherty, E., Sparrow, R., & Szer, J. (1995). Bone marrow stromal function from patients after bone marrow transplantation. *Bone Marrow Transplantation, 15,* 207–12.

Orkin, S.H. & Zon, L. (2002). Hematopoiesis and stem cells: plasticity versus developmental heterogeneity. *Nature Immunology, 3,* 323–8.

Orlic, D., Kajstura, J., Chimenti, S. *et al.* (2001). Bone marrow cells regenerate infarcted myocardium. *Nature, 410,* 701–5.

Otsuka, T., Humphries, R.K., Hogge, D.E. *et al.* (1991). Continuous activation of primitive haematopoietic cells in long-term human marrow cultures containing irradiated tumour cells. *Journal of Cellular Physiology, 148,* 370–9.

Owen, M. (1988). Marrow stromal stem cells. *Journal of Cell Science Supplement, 10,* 63–76.

Paquette, R.L., Dergham, S.T., Karpf, E. *et al.* (2000). Ex vivo expanded unselected peripheral blood: progenitor cells reduce posttransplantation neutropenia, thrombocytopenia, and anemia in patients with breast cancer. *Blood, 96,* 2385–90.

Peled, A., Petit, I., Kollet, O. *et al.* (1999). Dependence of human stem cell engraftment and repopulation of NOD/SCID mice on CXCR4. *Science, 283,* 845–8.

Pereira, R.F., O'Hara, M.D., Laptev, A.V. *et al.* (1998). Marrow stromal cells as a source of progenitor cells for nonhematopoietic tissues in transgenic mice with a phenotype of osteogenesis imperfecta. *Proceedings of the National Academy of Sciences USA, 95,* 1142–7.

Phinney, D.G., Kopen, G., Isaacson, R.L., & Prockop, D.J. (1999). Plastic adherent stromal cells from the bone marrow of commonly used strains of inbred mice: variations in yield, growth, and differentiation. *Journal of Cellular Biochemistry, 72,* 570–85.

Pittenger, M.F., Mackay, A.M., Beck, S.C. *et al.* (1999). Multilineage potential of adult human mesenchymal stem cells. *Science, 284,* 143–7.

Prockop, D.J. (1997). Marrow stromal cells as stem cells for nonhematopoietic tissues. *Science, 276,* 71–4.

Reiffers, J., Cailliot, C., Dazey, B. *et al.* (1999). Abrogation of postmyeloablative chemotherapy neutropenia by ex-vivo expanded autologous CD34-positive cells. *Lancet, 354,* 1092–3.

Reyes, M., Dudek, A., Jahagirdar, B. *et al.* (2002). Origin of endothelial progenitors in human postnatal bone marrow. *Journal of Clinical Investigation, 109,* 337–46.

Reyes, M., Lund, T., Lenvik, T. *et al.* (2001). Purification and ex vivo expansion of postnatal human marrow mesodermal progenitor cells. *Blood, 98,* 2615–25.

Rombouts, W.J. & Ploemacher, R.E. (2003). Primary murine MSC show highly efficient homing to the bone marrow but lose homing ability following culture. *Leukemia, 17,* 160–70.

Sandmaier, B.M., Storb, R., Kniley, J. *et al.* (1998). Evidence of allogeneic stromal engraftment in bone marrow using canine mesenchymal stem cells (abstract # 473). *Blood, 92*(Suppl), 116a.

Santucci, M.A., Trabetti, E., Martinelli, G. *et al.* (1992). Host origin of bone marrow fibroblasts following allogeneic bone marrow transplantation for chronic myeloid leukemia. *Bone Marrow Transplantation, 10,* 255–9.

Schwartz, R.E., Reyes, M., Koodie, L. *et al.* (2002). Multipotent adult progenitor cells from bone marrow differentiate into functional hepatocyte-like cells. *Journal of Clinical Investigation, 109,* 1291–302.

Simmons, P.J., Przepiorka, D., Thomas, E.D., & Torok-Storb, B. (1987). Host origin of marrow stromal cells following allogeneic bone marrow transplantation. *Nature, 328,* 429–32.

Stiff, P., Chen, B., Franklin, W. *et al.* (2000). Autologous transplantation of ex vivo expanded bone marrow cells grown from small aliquots after high-dose chemotherapy for breast cancer. *Blood, 95,* 2169–74.

Tavassoli, M. & Friedenstein, A. (1983). Hemopoietic stromal microenvironment. *American Journal of Hematology, 15,* 195–203.

Toma, C., Pittenger, M.E., Cahill, K.S. *et al.* (2002). Human mesenchymal stem cells differentiate to a cardiomyocyte phenotype in the adult murine heart. *Circulation, 105,* 93–8.

Tomita, S., Li, R.K., Weisel, R.D. *et al.* (1999). Autologous transplantation of bone marrow cells improves damaged heart function. *Circulation, 100* (Suppl II), II-247–II-256.

Torok-Storb, B. & Holmberg, L. (1994). Role of marrow microenvironment in engraftment and maintenance of allogeneic hematopoietic stem cells. *Bone Marrow Transplantation, 14*(Suppl 4), S71.

Uchida, N., Fleming, W.H., Alpern, E.J., & Weissman, I.L. (1993). Heterogeneity of hematopoietic stem cells. *Current Opinion in Immunology, 5,* 177–84.

Uhlman, D.L., Verfaillie, C., Jones, R.B., & Luikart, S.D. (1991). BCNU treatment of marrow stromal monolayers reversibly alters haematopoiesis. *British Journal of Haematology, 78,* 3304–9.

Wagner, J. Personal communication.

Wakitani, S., Goto, T., Pineda, S.J. *et al.* (1994). Mesenchymal cell based repair of large, full-thickness defects of articular cartilage. *Journal of Bone and Joint Surgery (American), 76,* 579–92.

Young, R.G., Butler, D.L., Weber, W. *et al.* (1998). Use of mesenchymal stem cells in a collagen matrix for Achilles tendon repair. *Journal of Orthopaedic Research, 16,* 406–13.

Zvaifler, N.J., Marinova-Mutafchieva, L., Adams, G. *et al.* (2000). Mesenchymal precursor cells in the blood of normal individuals. *Arthritis Research, 2,* 477–88.

6 Embryonic stem cells in the field of hematopoietic stem cells and immune therapy

MERI T. FIRPO AND DAN S. KAUFMAN

University of California, San Francisco and University of Minnesota, Minneapolis, USA

Introduction

Stem cells have been studied and utilized by hematologists for over 40 years. Pioneering studies to demonstrate spleen colony-forming cells were derived from a clonal population of hematopoietic cells that could generate a variety of differentiated blood cell types paved the way to better understanding of hematopoietic stem cells (HSCs) (Becker *et al.,* 1963; Till & McCullough, 1961). Many other clinical fields have now recognized the power that stem cell biology can bring to understanding various aspects of developmental biology and potential utility for cellular therapies. Stem cells are defined as cells that are able to both self-renew as undifferentiated cells and still retain the capacity to differentiate into two or more cell types. In general, stem cells can be divided into two broad categories: embryonic and adult. Embryonic stem (ES) cells are derived from early precursor cells that normally exist only during the blastocyst stage of development. These cells can be cultured long-term (perhaps indefinitely) in an undifferentiated state yet preserve their ability to differentiate into any cell type within the body. In contrast, adult stem cells are derived from postnatal tissue, and are generally considered more limited in their developmental potential. It is important to note that under this standard terminology, HSCs isolated from umbilical cord blood are still considered an adult stem cell, even though the cells come from a newborn baby. Therefore, HSCs are a type of adult stem cell that gives rise to all differentiated blood cells (lymphocytes, granulocytes, megakaryocytes, erythrocytes, etc.). Neural stem cells, another adult stem cell, give rise to a variety of neurons and glial cells (astrocytes, oligodendrocytes). Other lineage-specific stem cells for tissues such as liver, muscle, and skin have been at least partially characterized. However, by definition, ES cells are able to differentiate into cells of all three embryonic germ layers: ectoderm, endoderm, and mesoderm. This vast developmental potential has made mouse ES cells a standard resource to understand mammalian genetics and developmental biology (Keller, 1995). The more recent derivation of human ES cells has important implications to studies of human development and potential novel cell-based therapies.

Mouse embryonic stem cells

ES cells are cell lines derived by culturing the inner cell mass (ICM) of mammalian preimplantation blastocyts under conditions that support self-renewal and inhibit differentiation to allow maintenance of a pluripotent population of cells. The ICM is a cluster of approximately a dozen cells that appear only transiently in the early developing embryo. During normal embryonic development these cells of the ICM derive all the cells of the fetal and adult body; cells of the outer cell layer (trophectoderm) develop into the outer layers of the placenta. By careful isolation of the ICM cells, they can be propagated and maintained in culture where they are described as ES cells (Evans & Kaufman, 1981; Martin, 1981) (Fig. 6.1a). Like the cells of the ICM, ES cells are pluripotent. Initially, ICM outgrowths were established and grown on monolayers of mouse embryonic fibroblasts. Later, leukemia inhibitory factor (LIF) or other agonists of the gp130-STAT3 signaling pathway were found to be necessary and sufficient to establish and maintain self-renewal of mouse ES cells (Williams *et al.,* 1988; Pease *et al.,* 1990; Niwa *et al.,* 1998). However, at least one report suggests a gp130-independent mechanism to support self-renewal of mouse ES cells (Dani *et al.,* 1997). Currently, LIF is widely used to culture mouse ES cells in an undifferentiated state, with full differentiation potential. In addition to their pluripotency, mouse ES cells share a characteristic morphology (Fig. 6.2A). The cells are small, with a high nulear/cytoplasmic ratio, tight cell-cell adhesion, and express the transcription factor oct 4 (Rosner *et al.,* 1990; Scholer *et al.,* 1990), alkaline phosphatase, telomerase (Kim, 1991), and embryonic antigen SSEA-1 (Solter & Knowles, 1978).

Embryonic stem cell lines are characterized at least in part by the following criteria: (1) derivation from preimplantation embryo, (2) prolonged undifferentiated proliferation, (3) ability to differentiate into cells representative of all three embryonic gem layers (endoderm, ectoderm, and mesoderm) and germ cells, and (4) maintenance of normal karyotype. The pluripotency of mouse ES cells is best demonstrated by studies that found that mouse ES cells contribute to all cell types of the mouse, including germ cells (Bradley *et al.,* 1984) when

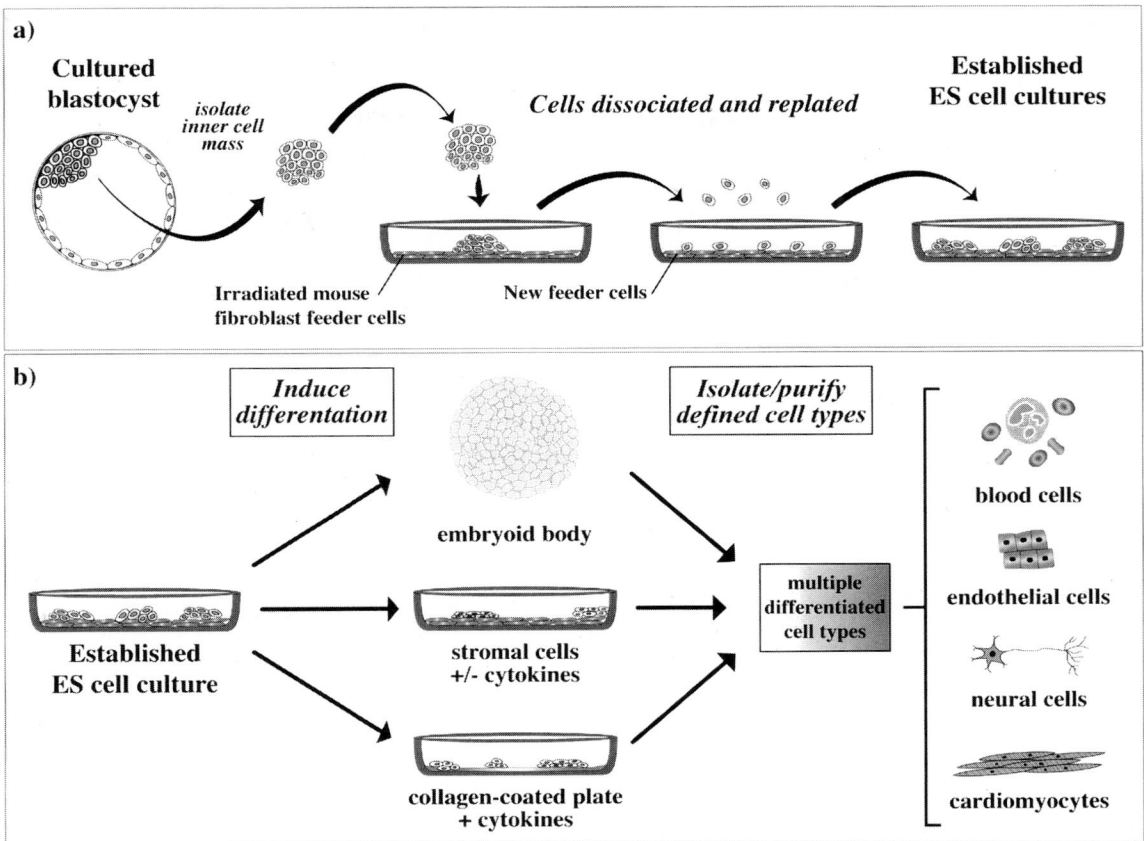

Fig. 6.1. ES cell growth and differentiation. (a) Lines of mammalian ES cells are derived by isolation of the ICM and culture on irradiated fibroblast cells. Cell lines can be propagated and expanded in serial cultures. (b) Established ES cell lines can be induced to differentiate with various methods including embryoid body formation, co-culture of specific stromal lines, or culture on tissue culture plates coated with proteins such as collagen. Addition of specific cytokines or growth factors can impact differentiation or survival of specific cell types. Varying methods can identify, purify, and characterize defined differentiated cell types.

injected into an intact blastocyst stage embryo. The cells can be genetically modified without loss of differentiation potential, allowing the generation of strains of mice with specific mutations. Transgenic and genetic "knock-out" mice have been used to identify roles for individual genes and combinations of genes in mouse development and physiology.

Derivation of ES cells from species other than mice have met with varying success. Cell lines have been isolated from cultured ICM cells in the hamster (Doetschman *et al.,* 1988), sheep (Handyside *et al.,* 1987), pig (Notarianni *et al.,* 1990; Strojek *et al.,* 1990; Evans *et al.,* 1990; Wheeler, 1994), cow (Evans *et al.,* 1990; Saito *et al.,* 1992; van Stekelenburg-Hamers *et al.,* 1995), mink (Sukoyan *et al.,* 1992), rabbit (Giles *et al.,* 1993; Graves & Moreadith, 1993), and chicken (Pain *et al.,* 1996). Most of these cell lines are similar in morphology to mouse ES cells. Some have the capacity to differentiate in vitro to multiple cell types. Lines from the sheep and pig have also yielded chimeric offspring when injected into the developing embryo (Wheeler, 1994; Schoonjans *et al.,* 1996), although these offspring had no germline contribution from the injected

cells. Stable cell lines from medakafish have been established that can contribute to embryonic and extraembryonic tissues when injected into intact blastocysts (Hong *et al.,* 1998). These medakafish embryonic cells have not been shown to contribute to the germline, or to differentiate in vitro.

In addition to the extensive work on mouse ES cells that has been accomplished in the past 20 years, other research models of multipotent embryonic cells have been developed. Work on embryonal carcinoma (EC) cell lines derived from mouse and human teratomas and teratocarcinomas preceded the isolation of mouse ES cells (Solter, 1970; Stevens, 1970; and Hogan *et al.,* 1977; reviewed in Andrews *et al.,* 2001). Indeed, these studies on EC cells were crucial to defining the culture conditions that would permit long-term undifferentiated growth of nonmalignant mouse and human ES cells. EC cells, while having a transformed phenotype and typically containing multiple cytogenetic abnormalities, actually have many similarities to ES cells. Like ES cells, EC cells can be maintained in long-term culture without evidence of differentiation; yet EC cells retain the ability to produce derivatives of all three embryonic germ cell layers (Andrews *et al.,*

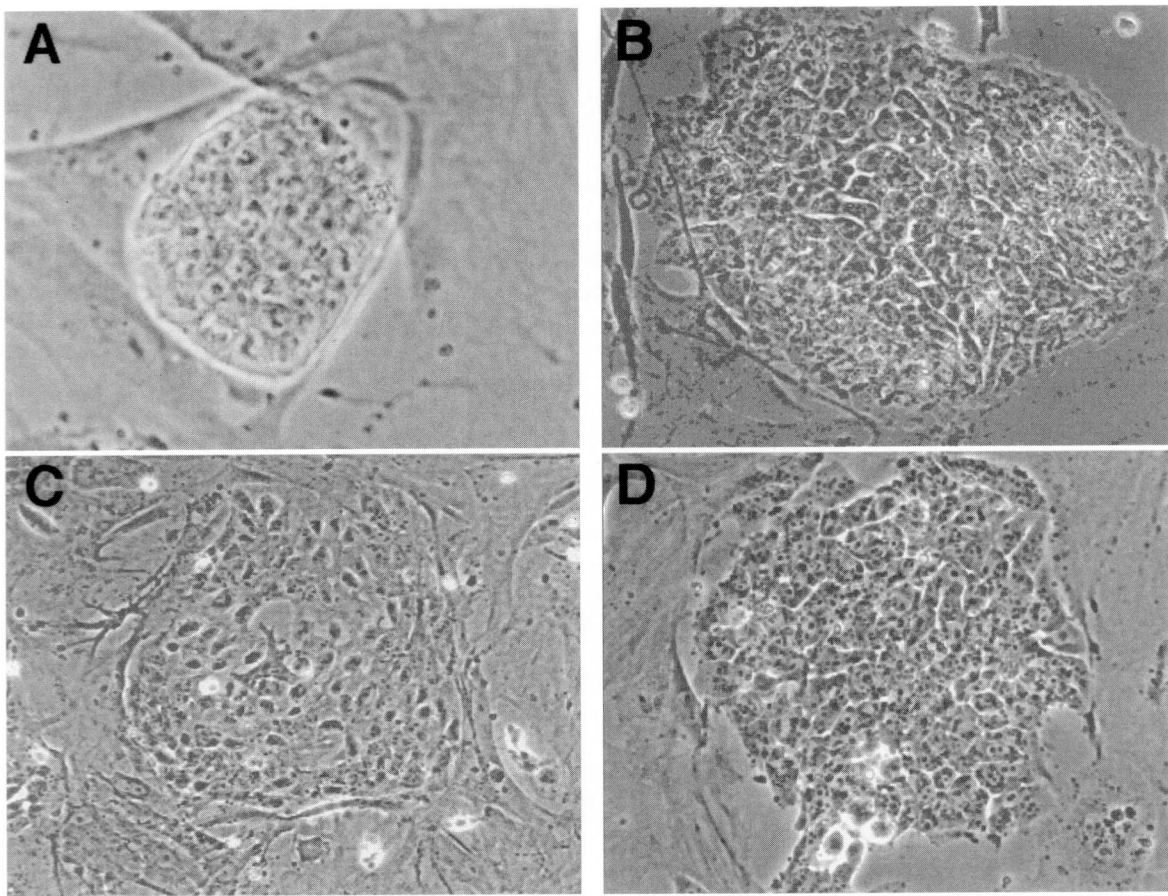

Fig. 6.2. Photomicrographs of mammalian embryonic cell lines all grown on MEF feeder cells. Colonies of mouse ES cells (**A**), human ES cells (**B**), rhesus monkey ES cells (**C**), and the human embryonic carcinoma cell lines Ntera-2 (**D**). The mouse ES cell form small compact colonies of cells, whereas the human and rhesus monkey cells are typically less compact. Human ES cells and human EC cells have a similar morphology. Origianl magnification 200× for all panels. Ntera-2 cells courtesy of P.W. Andrews, Sheffield University, Sheffield, England. Human and rhesus monkey ES cells courtesy of J.A. Thomson, University of Wisconsin, Madison.

2001). EC cell differentiation can be accomplished either in vitro by addition of specific agents (such as retinoic acid to induce neural differentiation) or by transplantation into immunodeficient animals leading to development of teratocarcinomas composed of multiple cell lineages. However, the developmental potential of EC cells is typically limited. Pertaining to hematopoiesis, no specific means to induce EC cells to form hematopoietic cells have been characterized. However, these cells do have clinical relevance since malignant human germ cell tumors (GCT) can evolve into leukemia, often not becoming evident until years after treatment of the original germ cell tumor, with potentially fatal consequences (Hartmann *et al.*, 2000). Therefore, EC cells and GCT could serve as a model to better understand pathogenesis of some hematologic malignancies.

When LIF or other agents that stimulate self-renewal are removed from cultures of mouse ES cells, the cells will continue to proliferate but be induced toward differentiation. Since the use of ES cells in vitro provides virtually unlimited numbers of differentiating cells in an environment that can be easily altered,

in vitro differentiation of ES cells has been exploited as a model of mouse development. In vitro studies have characterized many defined cell types including hematopoietic cells (Doetschman *et al.*, 1985; Wiles & Keller, 1991; Nakano *et al.*, 1994), vascular tissue (Doetschman *et al.*, 1985; Risau *et al.*, 1988), adipocytes (Dani *et al.*, 1997), bone and cartilage (Kramer *et al.*, 2000; Buttery *et al.*, 2001), pancreas (Lumelsky *et al.*, 2001), neural cells (Bain *et al.*, 1995; Fraichard *et al.*, 1995; Brustle *et al.*, 1999), skin (Bagutti *et al.*, 1996), and muscle tissue (Wobus *et al.*, 1991; Sanchez *et al.*, 1991; Robbins *et al.*, 1990).

Models of ES cell differentiation allow the study of rare cell types, even at stages of development that are difficult to access in a developing embryo. In vitro differentiation of ES cells can also be used to elucidate the role of mutations that cause embryonic lethal phenotypes in vivo. Furthermore, mature cells generated from differentiated ES cells can be used to assay biologically active agents, and can theoretically be used for transplantation in vivo, although few transplantation studies have been carried out successfully.

ES cell differentiation as a model of hematopoiesis

Of all medical specialties, hematology may have the greatest affinity for cellular medicine. Hematologic malignancies are typically derived from a single aberrant clonal cell that becomes transformed (for example, a chromosome 9:22 translocation leading to chronic myelogenous leukemia). If the abnormal cell population can be eliminated and replaced with normal HSCs, the disease can be cured. These normal HSCs can either be of the patient's own population, or from an allogeneic donor. Indeed, hematopoietic stem cell transplantation (HSCT), which has been in practice for over 30 years, offers the only routine "stem cell therapy" in use today (Thomas, 1999). In fact, whereas "stem cells" are now widely touted as a new medical advance that will serve as a source to treat and cure a host of degenerative and malignant diseases, hematologists should remind the public of their long history of successful "stem cell therapy." This knowledge of the power and potential for HSCT to cure otherwise fatal illnesses, and the current deficiencies in HSCT, makes human ES cells a very tantalizing prospective source of HSCs to overcome some of the existing limits.

In vitro differentiation of ES cells has been achieved using at least three basic strategies (Fig. 6.1b). With the first method, undifferentiated ES cells are removed from the feeder cells or soluble factors that maintain them in an undifferentiated state. Individual cells or clusters of cells are then allowed to proliferate in suspension or in semisolid medium to form tight colonies of cells known as embryoid bodies (EBs) (Evans & Kaufman, 1981; Martin, 1981; Doetschman et al., 1985). Under appropriate conditions, the various hematopoietic lineages develop within the EB in a defined temporal pattern, similar to development of hematopoiesis in the intact embryo (Burkert et al., 1991; Wiles & Keller, 1991; Keller et al., 1993). Hematopoietic development in the EB can be determined by the detection of lineage-specific mRNAs (Lindenbaum & Grosveld, 1990; Schmitt et al., 1991; Keller et al., 1993; McClanahan et al., 1993) or by the detection of hematopoietic precursors based on their capacity to form colonies of mature hematopoietic cells in the colony-forming cell (CFC) assay (Keller et al., 1993). Within the embryoid bodies, precursors for the embryonic erythroid lineage can be detected 4 to 5 days after the removal of differentiation inhibitors. Shortly after the appearance of these embryonic erythroid CFCs, precursors for the adult erythroid and myeloid lineages can be detected within the EBs (Burkert et al., 1991; Wiles & Keller, 1991; Chen, 1992; Keller et al., 1993; Lieschke & Dunn, 1995). Precursors of megakaryocyte and lymphoid lineages are detected after 10 days of culture (Potocnik et al., 1994; Berthier et al., 1997). Although these lineage-committed precursors are detected only after day 3 of differentiation using standard hematopoietic colony assays, EBs also contain multilineage precursors prior to the development of committed embryonic or adult precursors (Kennedy et al., 1997). These primitive cells give rise to precursors of all hematopoietic lineages. Structures similar to embryonic blood islands have been observed in developing EBs, which contain endothelial cells with associated hematopoietic precursors that have the potential to differentiate into erythroid and myeloid lineages (Burkert et al., 1991; Bautch et al., 1996; Risau et al., 1988). EBs have also been used to derive putative hemangioblast cells, a common precursor to both blood and endothelial cell lineages (Choi et al., 1998).

The second strategy for in vitro differentiation subjects undifferentiated ES cells to proliferate in contact with specific feeder cells that are permissive for differentiation. While ES cells differentiating in adherent cultures look different than EBs, temporal regulation of hematopoietic differentiation is maintained (Nakano et al., 1994). Precursors of erythroid, myeloid, and lymphoid lineages have all been identified during the differentiation of ES cells in this manner (Nakano et al., 1994, 1996; Berthier et al., 1997). Other laboratories developed multistep differentiation methods, culturing EB cells with adherent cells that support hematopoietic differentiation to enrich hematopoietic cells from the whole population of EB cells (Bigas et al., 1995; Perkins, 1998). Thus, both strategies of differentiating ES cells provide in vitro models of hematopoiesis. One study (Dang et al., 2002) reported that the numbers of hematopoietic precursors were significantly higher in EBs than in colonies differentiated on adherent cultures. However, others (Berthier et al., 1997), found that co-culture in the presence of the cell line MS-5 supported the differentiation of a greater number of myeloid precursors than a combination of cytokines in day 12 embryoid bodies in suspension culture.

A third strategy directly cultured ES cells on collagen-coated plates, thereby eliminating the unknown effects of feeder cells. Growth of ES cells on type IV collagen-coated plates in the absence of LIF leads to differentiation into a Flk-1$^+$ cell population that can then be induced to form blood or endothelial cells depending on the specific culture conditions (Nishikawa et al., 1998). Notably, this collagen-based method has also been used to demonstrate that a single Flk-1+ cell can derive from either endothelial cells (by culture with vascular endothelial growth factor, VEGF) or smooth muscle cells (by culture with platelet-derived growth factor-BB). Most remarkably, these cells can be combined to form vascular-type structures (Yamashita et al., 2000).

Manipulation of hematopoiesis in vitro

The establishment of the differentiation of ES cells as a viable in vitro model led to the manipulation of the system to identify genes that regulate hematopoiesis. Keller and colleagues initially demonstrated that the addition of exogenous cytokines to differentiating EBs did not affect the number of hematopoietic precursors when added before day 10, although later addition of stem cell factor (SCF) and interleukin 11 (IL-11) did increase hematopoietic precursors in EBs (Keller et al., 1993). Other groups have altered differentiation patterns in EBs using agents such as retinoic acid (Bain et al., 1995), IL-6 (Biesecker & Emerson, 1993), basic fibroblast growth factor (Faloon et al., 2000), Mpl ligand (Mitjavila et al., 1998) and low oxygen tension (Potocnik *et al.*, 1994). The specific timing and effect that these agents have when added to the culture of ES cells varies between groups. Wiles and Johansson identified a role for activin and bone morphogenetic protein-4 (BMP-4) in the differentiation of early mesoderm and hematopoiesis from ES cells in chemically defined medium, suggesting that in vitro differentiation of ES cells may be a model of germ layer formation in addition to lineage commitment in vitro, and that the presence of serum influences the activities of added factors to differentiating ES cells (Johansson & Wiles, 1995; Wiles & Johansson, 1997). A later study found vascular endothelial growth factor to be a synergistic factor in BMP-4-induced hematopoiesis (Nakayama *et al.*, 1998).

Ectopic expression of genes suspected of having a role in hematopoiesis has been used to increase differentiation to specific cell types and to elucidate the role of these genes in hematopoiesis. For example, expression of the erythropoietin receptor in undifferentiated ES cells resulted in an increase in precursors of erythroid and mixed colonies, and the expression of genes expressed during erythropoiesis (Dai *et al.*, 2000). Expression of transcription factors c-myb or GATA-2 enhanced hematopoietic differentiation in the absence of added cytokines, and c-myb increased the expression of receptors of hematopoietic cytokines in vitro (Bielenska *et al.*, 1996). Dramatic increases in early hematopoietic precursors were observed when homeobox genes LH2 (Pinto *et al.*, 1998), HOX11 (Keller *et al.*, 1998), and HOXB4 (Savageau *et al.*, 1995; Helgason *et al.*, 1996) were expressed in ES cells. Further, expression of HOX11 and LH2 resulted in the immortalization of early hematopoietic precursors that could be differentiated with the addition of hematopoietic cytokines. Hematopoietic precursors derived from ES lines expressing LH2 or HOXB4 were able to engraft and contribute to hematopoiesis in adult mice (Pinto *et al.*, 2002; Rideout *et al.*, 2002).

Homologous recombination to create targeted mutagenesis is widely used to eliminate one or both copies of a gene in mouse ES cells. This powerful method can be used to create mouse strains deficient in a single gene in order to better identify regulatory pathways requiring expression of specific genes. However, some of these knockout mutations have an early embryonic lethal phenotype, preventing observation of the embryo at stages that are affected by the loss of the targeted gene (Tsai *et al.*, 1994; Weiss *et al.*, 1994). In other cases (Zhang *et al.*, 1994; Hirsch *et al.*, 1996), the early lethality of the mutation prevents observation of a function of the gene later in development. Analysis of in vitro differentiation is a valuable tool to supplement information obtained from knockout mice in vivo. A series of experiments focused on erythropoiesis identified specific stages at which GATA-1 and GATA-2 mutations were damaging erythroid precursor differentiation and survival. Loss of GATA-1 leads to lethality at day 12.5 (E12.5) of development. In vitro differentiation of GATA-1$^{-/-}$ ES cells revealed that embryonic (primitive) erythroid precursors do not develop, although adult (definitive) precursors appear, but are arrested and die at the proerythroblast stage

(Weiss *et al.*, 1994). Mice deficient for GATA-2 expression die at E10-11, due to severe anemia. In vitro differentiation of GATA-2$^{-/-}$ ES cells revealed a lack of primitive and definitive, as well as myeloid, precursors (Tsai *et al.*, 1994). In vitro differentiation of myb$^{-/-}$ ES cells identified that a block in definitive erythropoiesis at the stage of a multilineage precursor is likely responsible for the severe anemia that kills myb-deficient mice at E15 (Clarke *et al.*, 2000).

Targeted mutagenesis of the vav oncogene leads to lethality of implantation-stage embryos (Zmuidzinas *et al.*, 1995). Because of its expression during early ES differentiation (Keller, 1993) and in hematopoietic cells (Zmuidzinas *et al.*, 1995), the loss of vav expression was expected to impair hematopoiesis. However, in vitro differentiation of vav$^{-/-}$ ES cells revealed normal erythropoiesis and myelopoiesis, with a defect limited to lymphoid cells (Zhang *et al.*, 1994). Similar studies revealed the effect of targeted mutations of β-1-integrin (Hirsch *et al.*, 1996), Shp-2 (Qu *et al.*, 1997), Flk-1 (Hidaka *et al.*, 1999), AML-1 (Okuda *et al.*, 2000), Huntingtin (Metzler *et al.*, 2000), CD 105 (Cho *et al.*, 2001), core-binding factor β (Miller *et al.*, 2001), and phospholipase C-α1 (Shirane *et al.*, 2001). Studies of mouse ES cells to identify novel genes and other agents that regulate hematopoiesis will continue to be crucial to further define pathways that control this model developmental system.

Engraftment of ES cell-derived cells

While many laboratories have identified hematopoietic progenitors in the embryoid body, little progress has been made in long-term transplantation of ES cell-derived cells. To date, two approaches have been used to differentiate HSC from ES cell lines in vitro. The first approach is to inject unfractionated cells from embryoid bodies intravenously in irradiated adult mice. The second method is to differentiate ES cells adhering to stromal cells that have been shown to support the growth of in vivo–derived hematopoietic precursors. Both approaches have yielded limited success. One group reported that transient engraftment of lymphocytic lineages was observed in some mice injected with day 9–13 EB cells (Muller & Dzierzak, 1993). This study showed that cells from earlier EBs yielded tumors in the injected recipients. Lymphoid engraftment has also been observed by other groups at low levels (Nisitani *et al.*, 1994; Potocnik *et al.*, 1997). Others reported higher levels of engraftment in two studies after injecting cells from EBs grown adhering to hematopoietic stromal cell lines (Gutierrez-Ramos & Palacios, 1992; Palacios *et al.*, 1995). Another study injected unfractionated day 25 EB cells into the circulation or directly into hematopoietic organs of sublethally irradiated mice (Gutierrez-Ramos & Palacios, 1992). Again, a subset of the injected mice developed tumors. Some mice, however, had evidence of lymphoid engraftment 10 to 16 weeks after injection. A later study using 21 day EB cells cultured on stromal cultures and enriched for hematopoietic precursors reported reconstitution of lymphoid and myeloid lineages in injected SCID mice (Palacios *et al.*, 1995). Yet another report showed that variable levels of engraftment of lymphoid and myeloid cells could be found in lethally irradiated mice injected with unseparated day 4 EB cells and spleen carrier cells (Hole *et al.,* 1996).

Studies by Daley and colleagues demonstrate significant progress toward establishing long-term hematopoietic engraftment of ES cell-derived blood cells. First, expression of the bcr/abl fusion protein in ES cells led to derivation of clonal HSCs that sustained multilineage engraftment, although not unexpectedly these cells had a leukemogenic phenotype (Perlingeiro *et al.,* 2001). Subsequently, ES cells that expressed the homeobox protein HOXB4 known to be important for hematopoietic development were established (Kyba *et al.,* 2002). HSCs capable of long-term, multilineage engraftment could be established from these cells. Moreover, bone marrow cells containing these ES cell-derived HSCs could be serially transplanted into secondary recipients. Notably, hematopoiesis is not completely normal in these mice since granulocytes are produced to a much greater extent than lymphocytes. However, this model was successfully combined with a nuclear reprogramming strategy to repair a Rag2 genetic defect to demonstrate the potential of combined cell and gene therapy to treat and cure immunodeficiencies (Rideout *et al.,* 2002).

Derivation and characterization of nonhuman primate and human ES cells

Isolation and characterization of ES cells from nonhuman primates paved the way for the derivation of human ES cells. Work by Thomson and colleagues produced ES cells from rhesus monkeys *(Macaca mulatta)* and common marmosets *(Callithrix jacchus)* (Thomson *et al.,* 1995; Thomson *et al.,* 1996). These nonhuman primate ES cells share much of the same morphology and growth characteristics of human EC cells and have proved to be very similar to human ES cells (Fig. 6.2B,C, & D). Interestingly, while human and nonhuman primate ES cells appear quite similar, these cells have important differences when compared with mouse ES cells. While it is trite to point out that mice and humans are not the same, their developmental equivalency is often implied when using murine systems as a development model. The earliest stages of embryonic development are actually quite distinct between these species. For example, mouse embryos can be maintained in diapause, a state of suspended embryo growth prior to uterine implantation. Diapause requires LIF to be present in the uterine environment (Nichols *et al.,* 2001). Most mouse ES cell lines are derived from mouse embryos that have been maintained in diapause and as previously mentioned, mouse ES cells have a strict requirement for LIF or other agonists of the gp130-STAT3 signaling pathway to maintain growth as undifferentiated cells (Smith, 2001). However, human and nonhuman primate embryos do not have the capacity to undergo diapause, and therefore lack the requirement for LIF to regulate embryogenesis. Understanding these developmental species differences makes recognition of the fact that human ES cells do not require LIF for undifferentiated growth a reflection of the embryonic milieu from which these cell lines are derived.

Another example of an important species difference perhaps more directly relevant to studies of hematopoiesis, is the developmental biology of the yolk sac, site of the earliest stages of primitive hematopoiesis. Whereas the yolk sac exists as a single structure during mouse embryogenesis, human embryos produce both a primary and secondary yolk sac (Palis & Yoder, 2001). Therefore, lessons derived from studies of mouse ES cells may not directly correspond to normal human development.

Lessons obtained from the derivation of ES cells of nonhuman primates proved essential for the eventual isolation and characterization of human ES cells. As with mouse and nonhuman primate ES cells, human ES cells are derived from the inner cell mass (ICM) of early blastocysts. The ICM is isolated by "immunosurgery" to remove the outer cell layer and co-cultured with irradiated mouse embryonic fibroblasts that serve as "feeder" cells. (Again, use of MEF feeder cells were originally used for propagation of undifferentiated EC cells.) Under these conditions, the cells of the ICM divide, grow, and can be serially passed in culture without evidence of differentiation, eventually producing lines of what are recognized as ES cells (Thomson *et al.,* 1998). Human ES cells are defined by the same criteria given for mouse ES cells earlier in this chapter with the exception that for ethical reasons, human ES cells cannot be tested for the ability to contribute to germ line cells in vivo. Nevertheless, human ES cells have now been grown in continuous culture for well over a year without evidence of differentiation and without obvious genetic abnormalities. However, when placed in the appropriate environment, these cells retain the ability to differentiate into a host of cell types. The most efficient means of inducing multilineage differentiation is by injection of cells into immunodeficient mice. Here, teratomas are formed that display derivatives of all three embryonic lineages (endoderm, ectoderm, and mesoderm) (Thomson *et al.,* 1998).

Since the initial description of human ES cells, several improvements in the methods of culture of these cells have been made. Most important, clonally derived human ES cell lines have been produced, and these clonal lines retain all the same characteristics and developmental potential of the original cell lines (Amit *et al.,* 2000). The ability to now use clonally derived ES cells eliminates the possibility that differentiation of the human ES cells can only be achieved with a heterogeneous group of cells, or that development is only possible from a fraction of the originally isolated cell population. Also, human ES cells can now be grown as "feeder-independent" cells without direct contact with MEFs and in media that does not contain fetal bovine serum (FBS) (Xu *et al.,* 2001). However, even under these slightly better defined growth conditions, MEF-conditioned media is still required and the serum-free media still contains animal-derived proteins such as albumin that may be heterogeneous and poorly characterized. Therefore, several advances remain before culture conditions for human ES cells are fully "defined." Achieving the goal of a chemically defined culture system is likely to be essential if human ES cells are to one day serve as the basis for cellular therapies.

Initial studies to demonstrate the multilineage developmental potential of human ES cells used nonspecific methods to induce differentiation such as teratoma formation or embryoid body formation (Thomson *et al.,* 1998; Itskovitz-Eldor *et al.,* 2000). An interesting, more thorough, and controlled analysis of differentiation characterized the unique effects of eight different cytokines or growth factors to regulate human ES cell development (Schuldiner *et al.,* 2000). However, all of these results are mainly a descriptive summary of varying means to induce differentiated progeny from the human ES cells.

The next goal for human ES cell research becomes to produce defined cell types that have the potential to serve as the basis of a novel source of cell replacement therapy. Research groups have focused on the cell lineages that reflect the interest of a specific medical specialty: neurology, hematology, cardiology, etc. For the most part, as with initial studies with mouse ES cells, these early studies with human ES cells have used relatively nonspecific means to support growth of differentiated cell types. Using feeder cells, serum, or growth factors to skew development, mixed cell populations that contain a few percent of the cell type of interest can be identified (for example, blood, cardiomyocyte, or pancreatic beta cell) (Assady *et al.,* 2001; Kaufman *et al.,* 2001b; Kehat *et al.,* 2001; Odorico *et al.,* 2001). One notable exception involves derivation of neural cells or neural percursors that can be produced more uniformly such that they make up greater then 90% of the differentiated cell population (Zhang *et al.,* 2001). These studies will serve as the basis to use human ES cells both to understand better the mechanistic basis of the earliest stages of human development and conceivably as a source for new cell-based therapies.

Human ES cells as a model to study hematopoiesis

Initial studies to induce hematopoietic differentiation of human ES cells have used a co-culture system with stromal cells isolated from hematopoietic microenvironments to serve as "feeder" cells. S17 cells derived from mouse bone marrow, C166 cells derived from mouse yolk sac, OP9 cells from mouse calvaria, and human bone marrow stroma have all been used to support hematopoiesis from human ES cells (Kaufman *et al.,* 2001b, and unpublished observations). Here, the human ES cells are taken out of the conditions that support their undifferentiated growth, and instead co-cultured with one of the irradiated stromal cell lines in media that contains FBS but no other specific cytokines or growth factors. The ES cells rapidly differentiate under these conditions. After 2 to 3 weeks, approximately 2% to 5% of the differentiated cell population are CD34+ (undifferentiated human ES cells are CD34−). When replated in a methylcellulose-based media containing requisite hematopoietic cytokines, these differentiated ES cells form stereotypical hematopoietic colonies that appear identical to those colonies derived from normal human bone marrow or cord blood. Also, enrichment for CD34+ cells derived from the human ES cells dramatically increases the yield of hematopoietic colony-forming cells

(CFCs). Co-culture of the ES cells on fibroblasts (non-hematopoietic stromal cells) or in serum-free media, does not lead to generation of CFCs. However, the specific elements within the FBS, or produced by the feeder cells, that leads to recognizable hematopoietic differentiation remain unknown.

The data described above clearly demonstrate the hematopoietic potential of human ES cells. Since human ES cells can be grown in essentially unlimited numbers in well-defined conditions, these cells become an ideal starting population to define better the phenotype (and genotype) of human HSCs. However, HSCs produced from human ES cells have not yet been identified. While numerous surrogate assays exist to characterize human HSCs (Chang *et al.,* 2000), demonstration of long-term engraftment with multilineage differentiation in vivo currently seems to be the standard method. Typically, prospective human HSC populations are injected intravenously into immunodeficient mice (typically NOD/SCID or related strain), and blood or bone marrow is analyzed at appropriate intervals for presence of human blood cells (Dao & Nolta, 1999; Lapidot *et al.,* 1997). Identification of human-derived cells approximately 12 weeks postinjection is considered evidence of a long-term repopulating cell, in this case called a SCID-repopulating cell (SRC). Experiments to induce in vitro differentiation of human ES cells, then transplant the whole population or varying subpopulations (for example CD34− vs. CD34+ cells) into NOD/SCID mice will be the first step to identify human HSCs within this population. Whether or not many of the same hurdles described above regarding engraftment of mouse ES cell-derived HSCs will also present barriers to transplantation of human ES cell-derived HSCs remains to be determined.

Human ES cells, hematopoiesis, and immunity

Research on hematopoietic development from human ES cells has at least three important implications for studies of immunity and HSC transplantation. First, development and education of human blood cells, including lymphocytes from truly naive precursors, can be analyzed in a prospective manner. Recent studies clearly show derivation of lymphocytes from human ES cells in vitro (M. Firpo, unpublished observations). More comprehensive studies are obviously needed, but these methods may be used to define both the cell-bound and soluble factors required for production of antigen-independent and antigen-dependent immune effector cells. Using the controlled environment afforded by in vitro studies, individual variables that may influence development of B cells, T cells, NK cells as well as nonlymphoid effectors such as granulocytes and monocytes, can be regulated. For example, elegant studies using fractionated mouse bone marrow or fetal liver shows that lineage-specific precursors can be identified in part by surface receptors for specific cytokines such as IL-7 and thrombopoietin (Kondo *et al.,* 1997; Akashi *et al.,* 2000). Moreover, developmental "decisions" can be regulated by specific soluble factors (Kondo *et al.,* 2000; Traver *et al.,* 2001). How closely the human hematopoietic developmental system recapitulates this mouse remains to be defined. Moreover, human ES cells can also be used for genetic analysis of developing lymphocytes and other effector cells. Genetic modification of ES cells (Pfeifer *et al.*, 2002) to permit programming down desired developmental pathways will permit a more reductionistic view. For example, the studies showing overexpression of HoxB4 in murine ES cells leads to production of transplantable hematopoietic progenitors capable of long-term engraftment in vivo is of considerable interest (Kyba *et al.*, 2002). However, while granulocytes are robustly produced from these precursors, few lymphocytes are seen. How this cellular repertoire becomes skewed is unknown, but points to the unique pathways these studies can open.

Second, human ES cells are obviously poised to become a potential new source of transplantable HSCs for patients who would benefit from HSCT but do not have an HLA-matched donor. However, the novel characteristics and potential plasticity of the undifferentiated ES cells raise the possibility of deriving HSCs or other blood cells with unique characteristics. In this way, human ES cell-derived HSCs suitable for clinical transplantation will not only increase the number of patients with a potential source of donor cells, but these cells should also qualitatively improve the known benefits of HSCT. For example, it may be possible to modify the ES cells such that lymphocytes that are derived after transplantation overexpress T-cell receptors specific for tumor antigens in order to target specific areas of disease. In regards to immunodeficiencies due to known genetic defects such as severe combined immunodeficiency-X1 (SCID-X1), studies clearly show that retroviral-based transduction of the absent γc cytokine receptor subunit in CD34-selected bone marrow leads to functional T-cell expression and improved immunity (Cavazzana-Calvo *et al.*, 2000; Hacein-Bey-Abina *et al.*, 2002). However, transduction of HSCs is notoriously difficult and similar results have not been demonstrated for other genetic diseases. Human ES cells present an attractive target as a starting point for combined gene and cell therapy. Stable genetic modification of mouse ES cells is now routine, and similar methods seem suitable for human ES cells (Pfeifer *et al.*, 2002; J. Thomson, unpublished results).

Genetic modification of human ES cell-derived blood cells can be applied to areas of hematology beyond HSCT. For example, transfusion medicine could be markedly improved by derivation of platelets with a longer "shelf-life," by expression of genes for "antifreeze proteins" that permit long-term storage (Tomczak *et al.*, 2002). Erythrocytes could be produced from cells that have the genes for specific glycosyltransferases deleted to prevent expression of A and B blood group antigens, thus creating a greater source of "universal donor" blood type O red blood cells. Many hurdles must be surmounted before these speculative therapies become a reality. The vast potential of these cells emphasizes the importance of permitting a wide variety of research groups to work on human ES cells.

A third potential use of human ES cell-derived blood cells is to create a state of hematopoietic chimerism to facilitate transplantation of other human ES cell-derived cells and tissues without immunosuppressive drugs. The clinical utility of hematopoietic chimerism to induce tolerance is demonstrated by multiple patients who have received bone marrow and a second organ (typically a kidney) from the same donor. In these cases, since the developing lymphocytes from the HSCT share the same HLA expression as the solid organ, they are tolerant to the graft and immunosuppression can be weaned off (Dey *et al.*, 1998). Current, prospective clinical studies that apply this principle in the setting of renal transplants appear promising (Spitzer *et al.*, 1999; Millan *et al.*, 2002). In these studies, patients with or without an underlying hematologic problem that would benefit from HSCT (such as multiple myeloma) have demonstrated graft tolerance when given CD34-selected hematopoietic cells from the same donor as the kidney. In some cases, all immunosuppressive drugs have been weaned off. Since human ES cells can be induced to differentiate into any tissue, the potential to derive both HSCs and a second cell type (for example, pancreatic beta cell, hepatocyte, cardiomyocyte) from the same parental cell line is particularly attractive. Here, human ES cell-derived HSCs would be transplanted, possibly using a minimally myeloblative condition regimen since full donor cell chimerism is not required. Subsequently, a second cell type derived from the same parental ES cell line could be transplanted without need for further immune suppression since the ES cell-derived HLA-identical lymphocytes should render the host tolerant to the second tissue type. One study using rat ES cell-like cells found that intraportal injection of these cells led to hematopoietic mixed chimerism and prolonged graft survival of cardiac allografts matched to the ES cells (Fandrich *et al.*, 2002). This strategy is particularly attractive for treatment of autoimmune diseases such as Type 1 diabetes mellitus. If pancreatic islets are derived from ES cells that are precisely matched to the patient (for example, by substitution of self-HLA genes or via nuclear transfer technology), it would be expected that the donor beta cells would be rejected by the host due to the underlying autoimmune process. This is unfortunately seen in cases of diabetics who receive and subsequently reject pancreas transplants from identical twins (Sutherland *et al.*, 1989). Multiple other means to modify human ES cells to permit transplantation tolerance have also been proposed (Kaufman *et al.*, 2000; Odorico *et al.*, 2001). Obviously, considerably more research is needed before clinical trials involving cellular therapies based on human ES cells are contemplated. The availability of rhesus monkey ES cells (Thomson *et al.*, 1995), and the ability to induce differentiation of these cells much like human ES cells (Kaufman *et al.*, 2001a; Li *et al.*, 2001), makes this an attractive model for preclinical studies.

Conclusions

Several recent studies purport to demonstrate that adult stem cells may be less restricted in their developmental potential and may be able to "transdifferentiate" into other tissue types (reviewed in Fuchs & Segre, 2000; Blau *et al.*, 2001; Lagasse *et al.*, 2001). These results have been interpreted by some to suggest that adult stem cells may have the same developmental potential as ES cells. However, these data have not been sufficiently corroborated to draw any definitive conclusions (McKinney-Freeman *et al.*, 2002; Morshead *et al.*, 2002). Other studies suggest that cell-fusion events may play a role in apparent transdifferentiation of adult stem cells (Terada *et al.*, 2002; Ying *et al.*, 2002). Therefore, while there remains significant confusion and controversy regarding the capabilities of adult stem cells, ES cells are better able to serve as a model for cellular development and differentiation. Perhaps most important, ES cells maintain a unique capacity to sustain prolonged (perhaps indefinite) self-renewal without evidence of genetic changes. Since self-renewal is a common characteristic of all stem cells, it is now vital to pursue further research to understand how these cells maintain perpetual self-renewal without differentiation or senescence.

Research on human ES cells is in its infancy. On the basis of the voluminous work accomplished from mouse ES cells in the past 20 years, human ES cells will profoundly impact our understanding of human developmental biology. Whether (or when) human ES cell-based therapies can be directly applied to treat a host of currently incurable diseases brought on by degenerative, malignant, or otherwise damaging processes remains promising but speculative at this point. Most likely, the impact of human ES cells will at least initially be more indirect. For example, in the field of HSCT, the ability to expand transplantable HSCs ex vivo remains a long sought goal. While methods to permit this expansion are under study, this is not currently a routinely available process. The ability to use human ES cells to analyze the earliest stages of hematopoiesis in a human system should permit identification of genes and proteins that function to maintain HSCs capable of long-term engraftment. It may be then possible to add these "factors" to improve existing means of HSC expansion to make this process more clinically feasible. Human ES cells will serve as the basis in a new era of cell-based therapies, although the specific impact of these cells remains to be determined.

References

Akashi, K., Traver, D., Miyamoto, T., & Weissman, I.L. (2000). A clonogenic common myeloid progenitor that gives rise to all myeloid lineages. *Nature*, **404**, 193–7.

Amit, M., Carpenter, M.K., Inokuma, M.S. *et al.* (2000). Clonally derived human embryonic stem cell lines maintain pluripotency and proliferative potential for prolonged periods of in vitro culture. *Developmental Biology*, **227**, 271–8.

Andrews, P.W., Przyborski, S.A., & Thomson, J.A. (2001). Embryonal carcinoma cells as embryonic stem cells. In *Stem Cell Biology*, ed. D.R. Marshak, R. Gardner, & D. Gottlieb, pp. 231–65. Cold Spring Harbor, NY: Cold Spring Harbor Laboratory Press.

Assady, S., Maor, G., Amit, M. *et al.* (2001). Insulin production by human embryonic stem cells. *Diabetes*, **50**, 1691–7.

Axelrod, H.R. (1984). Embryonic stem cell lines derived from blastocysts by a simplified technique. *Developmental Biology*, **101**, 225–8.

Bagutti, C., Wobus, A.M., Fassler, R., & Watt, F.M. (1996). Differentiation of embryonal stem cells into keratinocytes: comparison of wild-type and beta 1 integrin-deficient cells. *Developmental Biology*, **179**, 184–96.

Bain, G., Kitchens, D., Yao, M. *et al.* (1995). Embryonic stem cells express neuronal properties in vitro. *Developmental Biology*, **168**, 342–57.

Bautch, V.L., Stanford, W.L., Rapoport, R. *et al.* (1996). Blood island formation in attached cultures of murine embryonic stem cells. *Developmental Dynamics*, **205**, 1–12.

Becker, A.J., McCulloch, E.A., & Till, J.E. (1963). Cytological demonstration of the clonal nature of spleen colonies derived from transplanted mouse marrow cells. *Nature*, **197**, 452–4.

Berthier, R., Prandini, M.H., Schweitzer, A. *et al.* (1997). The MS-5 murine stromal cell line and hematopoietic growth factors synergize to support the megakaryocytic differentiation of embryonic stem cells. *Experimental Hematology*, **25**, 481–90.

Bielinska, M., Narita, N., Heikinheimo, M. *et al.* (1996). Erythropoiesis and vasculogenesis in embryoid bodies lacking visceral yolk sac endoderm. *Blood*, **88**, 3720–30.

Biesecker, L.G. & Emerson, S.G. (1993). Interleukin-6 is a component of human umbilical cord serum and stimulates hematopoiesis in embryonic stem cells in vitro. *Experimental Hematology*, **21**, 774–8.

Bigas, A., Martin, D.I., & Bernstein, I.D. (1995). Generation of hematopoietic colony-forming cells from embryonic stem cells: synergy between a soluble factor from NIH-3T3 cells and hematopoietic growth factors. *Blood*, **85**, 3127–33.

Blau, H.M., Brazelton, T.R., & Weimann, J.M. (2001). The evolving concept of a stem cell: entity or function? *Cell*, **105**, 829–41.

Bloch, W., Forsberg, E., Lentini, S. *et al.* (1997). Beta 1 integrin is essential for teratoma growth and angiogenesis. *Journal of Cellular Biology*, **139**, 265–78.

Bradley, A., Evans, M., Kaufman, M., & Robertson, E. (1984). Formation of germ-line chimaeras from embryo-derived teratocarcinoma cell lines. *Nature*, **309**, 255–6.

Brinster, R. (1993). Stem cells and transgenic mice in the study of development. *International Journal of Developmental Biology*, **37**, 89–99.

Brustle, O., Jones, K.N., Learish, R.D. *et al.* (1999). Embryonic stem cell-derived glial precursors: a source of myelinating transplants. *Science*, **285**, 754–6.

Burkert, U., von, R.T., & Wagner, E.F. (1991). Early fetal hematopoietic development from in vitro differentiated embryonic stem cells. *New Biology*, **3**, 698–708.

Buttery, L.D., Bourne, S., Xynos, J.D. *et al.* (2001). Differentiation of osteoblasts and in vitro bone formation from murine embryonic stem cells. *Tissue Engineering*, **7**, 89–99.

Calabretta, B. & Gewirtz, A.M. (1991). Functional requirements of c-myb during normal and leukemic hematopoiesis. *Critical Reviews Oncogenetics*, **2**, 187–94.

Cavazzana-Calvo, M., Hacein-Bey, S., de Saint Basile, G. *et al.* (2000). Gene therapy of human severe combined immunodeficiency (SCID)-X1 disease. *Science*, **288**, 669–72.

Chang, H., Jensen, L., Quesenberry, P., & Bertoncello, I. (2000). Standardization of hematopoietic stem cell assays: a summary of a workshop and working group meeting sponsored by the

National Heart, Lung, and Blood Institute held at the National Institutes of Health, Bethesda, MD on September 8–9, 1998 and July 30, 1999. *Experimental Hematology, 28,* 743–52.

Chen, U. (1992). Differentiation of mouse embryonic stem cells to lympho-hematopoietic lineages in vitro. *Developmental Immunology, 2,* 29–50.

Cherny, R., Stokes, T., Merei, J. *et al.* (1994). Strategies for the isolation and characterization of bovine embryonic stem cells. *Reproduction, Fertility, and Development, 6,* 569–75.

Cho, S.K., Webber, T.D., Carlyle, J.R. *et al.* (1999). Functional characterization of B lymphocytes generated in vitro from embryonic stem cells. *Proceedings of the National Academy of Sciences USA, 96,* 9797–802.

Choi, K., Kennedy, M., Kazarov, A. *et al.* (1998). A common precursor for hematopoietic and endothelial cells. *Development, 125,* 725–32.

Clarke, D., Vegiopoulos, A., Crawford, A. *et al.* (2000). In vitro differentiation of c-myb(−/−) ES cells reveals that the colony forming capacity of unilineage macrophage precursors and myeloid progenitor commitment are c-Myb independent. *Oncogene, 19,* 3343–51.

Dai, M.S., Ge, Y., Xia, Z.B. *et al.* (2000). Introduction of human erythropoietin receptor complementary DNA by retrovirus-mediated gene transfer into murine embryonic stem cells enhances erythropoiesis in developing embryoid bodies. *Biology of Blood Marrow Transplantation, 6,* 395–407.

Dang, S.M., Kyba, M., Perlingeiro, R. *et al.* (2002). Efficiency of embryoid body formation and hematopoietic development from embryonic stem cells in different culture systems. *Biotechnology Bioengineering, 78,* 442–53.

Dani, C., Smith, A.G., Dessolin, S. *et al.* (1997). Differentiation of embryonic stem cells into adipocytes in vitro. *Journal of Cell Science, 110,* 1279–85.

Dey, B., Sykes, M., & Spitzer, T.R. (1998). Outcomes of recipients of both bone marrow and solid organ transplants. A review. *Medicine (Baltimore), 77,* 355–69.

Doetschman, T., Eistetter, H., Katz, M. *et al.* (1985). The in vitro development of blastocyst-derived embryonic stem cell lines: formation of visceral yolk sac, blood islands and myocardium. *Journal of Embryology and Experimental Morphology, 87,* 27–45.

Doetschman, T., Williams, P., & Maeda, N. (1988). Establishment of hamster blastocyst-derived embryonic stem (ES) cells. *Developmental Biology, 127,* 224–7.

Evans, M. & Kaufman, M. (1981). Establishment in culture of pluripotential cells from mouse embryos. *Nature, 292,* 154–6.

Evans, M., Notarianni, E., Laurie, S., & Moor, R. (1990). Derivation and preliminary characterization of pluripotent cell lines from porcine and bovine blastocysts. *Theriogenology, 33,* 125–8.

Faloon, P., Arentson, E., Kazarov, A. *et al.* (2000). Basic fibroblast growth factor positively regulates hematopoietic development. *Development, 127,* 1931–41.

Fandrich, F., Lin, X., Chai, G.X. *et al.* (2002). Preimplantation-stage stem cells induce long-term allogeneic graft acceptance without supplementary host conditioning. *Nature Medicine, 8,* 171–8.

Field, S.J., Johnson, R.S., Mortensen, R.M. *et al.* (1992). Growth and differentiation of embryonic stem cells that lack an intact c-fos gene. *Proceedings of the National Academy of Sciences USA, 89,* 9306–10.

Fraichard, A., Chassande, O., Bilbaut, G. *et al.* (1995). In vitro differentiation of embryonic stem cells into glial cells and functional neurons. *Journal of Cell Science, 108,* (Pt 10), 3181–8.

Fuchs, E. & Segre, J.A. (2000). Stem cells: a new lease on life. *Cell, 100,* 143–55.

Gajovic, S., St-Onge, L., Yokota, Y., & Gruss P. (1997). Retinoic acid mediates Pax6 expression during in vitro differentiation of embryonic stem cells. *Differentiation, 62,* 187–92.

Giles, J., Yang, X., Mark, W., & Foote, R. (1993). Pluripotency of cultured rabbit inner cell mass cells detected by isozyme analysis and eye pigmentation of fetuses following injection into blastocysts or morulae. *Molecular Reproduction and Development, 36,* 130–8.

Graves, K. & Moreadith, R. (1993). Derivation and characterization of putative pluripotential embryonic stem cells from preimplantation rabbit embryos. *Molecular Reproduction and Development, 36,* 424–33.

Gutierrez-Ramos, J.C. & Palacios, R. (1992). In vitro differentiation of embryonic stem cells into lymphocyte precursors able to generate T and B lymphocytes in vivo. *Proceedings of the National Academy of Sciences USA, 89,* 9171–5.

Hacein-Bey-Abina, S., Le Deist, F., Carlier, F. *et al.* (2002). Sustained correction of X-linked severe combined immunodeficiency by ex vivo gene therapy. *New England Journal of Medicine, 346,* 1185–93.

Handyside, A., Hooper, M., Kaufman, M., & Wilmut, I. (1987). Towards the isolation of embryonal stem cell lines from the sheep. *Roux's Archives of Developmental Biology, 196,* 185–90.

Hartmann, J.T., Nichols, C.R., Droz, J.P. *et al.* (2000). Hematologic disorders associated with primary mediastinal nonseminomatous germ cell tumors. *Journal of the National Cancer Institute, 92,* 54–61.

Helgason, C.D., Sauvageau, G., Lawrence, H.J. *et al.* (1996). Overexpression of HOXB4 enhances the hematopoietic potential of embryonic stem cells differentiated in vitro. *Blood, 87,* 2740–9.

Hidaka, M., Stanford, W.L., & Bernstein, A. (1999). Conditional requirement for the Flk-1 receptor in the in vitro generation of early hematopoietic cells. *Proceedings of the National Academy of Sciences USA, 96,* 7370–5.

Hilberg, F. & Wagner, E.F. (1992). Embryonic stem (ES) cells lacking functional c-jun: consequences for growth and differentiation, AP-1 activity and tumorigenicity. *Oncogene, 7,* 2371–80.

Hirsch, E., Iglesias, A., Potocnik, A.J. *et al.* (1996). Impaired migration but not differentiation of haematopoietic stem cells in the absence of beta1 integrins. *Nature, 380,* 171–5.

Hogan, B., Fellous, M., Avner, P., & Jacob, F. (1977). Isolation of a human teratoma cell line which expresses F9 antigen. *Nature, 270,* 515–8.

Hole, N., Graham, G.J., Menzel, U., & Ansell, J.D. (1996). A limited temporal window for the derivation of multilineage repopulating hematopoietic progenitors during embryonal stem cell differentiation in vitro. *Blood, 88,* 1266–76.

Hong, Y., Winkler, C., & Schartl, M. (1998). Production of medakafish chimeras from a stable embryonic stem cell line. *Proceedings of the National Academy of Sciences USA, 95,* 3679–84.

Itskovitz-Eldor, J., Schuldiner, M., Karsenti, D. *et al.* (2000). Differentiation of human embryonic stem cells into embryoid bodies comprising the three embryonic germ layers. *Molecular Medicine, 6,* 88–95.

Johansson, B.M. & Wiles, M.V. (1995). Evidence for involvement of activin A and bone morphogenetic protein 4 in mammalian mesoderm and hematopoietic development. *Molecular and Cell Biology,* **15,** 141–51.

Kabrun, N., Buhring, H.J., Choi, K. *et al.* (1997). Flk-1 expression defines a population of early embryonic hematopoietic precursors. *Development,* **124,** 2039–48.

Kaufman, D.S., Lewis, R.L., Hanson, E.T. *et al.* (2001a). Functional endothelial cells derived from rhesus monkey embryonic stem cells. *Blood,* **98,** 822a.

Kaufman, D.S., Lewis, R.L., Hanson, E.T. *et al.* (2001b). Hematopoietic colony-forming cells derived from human embryonic stem cells. *Proceedings of the National Academy of Sciences USA,* **98,** 10716–21.

Kaufman, D.S., Odorico, J.S., & Thomson, J.A. (2000). Transplantation therapies from human embryonic stem cells— Circumventing immune rejection. *e-biomed: Journal of Regenerative Medicine,* **1,** 11–15.

Kehat, I., Kenyagin-Karsenti, D. *et al.* (2001). Human embryonic stem cells can differentiate into myocytes with structural and functional properties of cardiomyocytes. *Journal of Clinical Investigation,* **108,** 407–14.

Keller, G., Kennedy, M., Papayannopoulou, T., & Wiles, M.V. (1993). Hematopoietic commitment during embryonic stem cell differentiation in culture. *Molecular & Cellular Biology,* **13,** 473–86.

Keller, G., Wall, C., Fong, A.Z. *et al.* (1998). Overexpression of HOX11 leads to the immortalization of embryonic precursors with both primitive and definitive hematopoietic potential. *Blood,* **92,** 877–87.

Keller, G.M. (1995). In vitro differentiation of embryonic stem cells. *Current Opinion in Cell Biology,* **7,** 862–9.

Kennedy, M., Firpo, M., Choi, K. *et al.* (1997). A common precursor for primitive erythropoiesis and definitive haematopoiesis. *Nature,* **386,** 488–93.

Kim, N., Piatyszek, M., Prowse, K. *et al.* (1994). Specific association of human telomerase activity with immortal cells and cancer. *Science,* **266,** 2011–4.

Kondo, M., Scherer, D.C., Miyamoto, T. *et al.* (2000). Cell-fate conversion of lymphoid-committed progenitors by instructive actions of cytokines. *Nature,* **407,** 383–6.

Kondo, M., Weissman, I.L., & Akashi, K. (1997). Identification of clonogenic common lymphoid progenitors in mouse bone marrow. *Cell,* **91,** 661–72.

Kramer, J., Hegert, C., Guan, K. *et al.* (2000). Embryonic stem cell-derived chondrogenic differentiation in vitro: activation by BMP-2 and BMP-4. *Mechanisms of Development,* **92,** 193–205.

Kyba, M., Perlingeiro, R.C., & Daley, G.Q. (2002). HoxB4 confers definitive lymphoid-myeloid engraftment potential on embryonic stem cell and yolk sac hematopoietic progenitors. *Cell,* **109,** 29–37.

Lagasse, E., Shizuru, J.A., Uchida, N. *et al.* (2001). Toward regenerative medicine. *Immunity,* **14,** 425–36.

Lee, S.H., Lumelsky, N., Studer, L. *et al.* (2000). Efficient generation of midbrain and hindbrain neurons from mouse embryonic stem cells. *Nature Biotechnology,* **18,** 675–9.

Li, F., Lu, S., Vida, L. *et al.* (2001). Bone morphogenetic protein 4 induces efficient hematopoietic differentiation of rhesus monkey embryonic stem cells in vitro. *Blood,* **98,** 335–42.

Lian, R.H., Maeda, M., Lohwasser, S. *et al.* (2002). Orderly and nonstochastic acquisition of CD94/NKG2 receptors by developing NK cells derived from embryonic stem cells in vitro. *Journal of Immunology,* **168,** 4980–7.

Lieschke, G.J. & Dunn, A.R. (1995). Development of functional macrophages from embryonal stem cells in vitro. *Experimental Hematology,* **23,** 328–34.

Lindenbaum, M.H. & Grosveld, F. (1990). An in vitro globin gene switching model based on differentiated embryonic stem cells. *Genes and Development,* **4,** 2075–85.

Liu, S., Qu, Y., Stewart, T.J. *et al.* (2000). Embryonic stem cells differentiate into oligodendrocytes and myelinate in culture and after spinal cord transplantation. *Proceedings of the National Academy of Sciences USA,* **97,** 6126–31.

Lumelsky, N., Blondel, O., Laeng, P. *et al.* (2001). Differentiation of embryonic stem cells to insulin-secreting structures similar to pancreatic islets. *Science,* **292,** 1389–94.

Maltsev, V.A., Rohwedel, J., Hescheler, J., & Wobus, A.M. (1993). Embryonic stem cells differentiate in vitro into cardiomyocytes representing sinus, nodal, atrial and ventricular cell types. *Mechanisms of Development,* **44,** 41–50.

Maltsev, V.A., Wobus, A.M., Rohwedel, J. *et al.* (1994). Cardiomyocytes differentiated in vitro from embryonic stem cells developmentally express cardiac-specific genes and ionic currents. *Circulation Research,* **75,** 233–44.

Martin, G.R. (1981). Isolation of a pluripotent cell line from early mouse embryos cultured in medium conditioned by teratocarcinoma stem cells. *Proceedings of the National Academy of Sciences USA,* **78,** 7634–8.

McClanahan, T., Dalrymple, S., Barkett, M., & Lee, F. (1993). Hematopoietic growth factor receptor genes as markers of lineage commitment during in vitro development of hematopoietic cells. *Blood,* **81,** 2903–15.

McKinney-Freeman, S.L., Jackson, K.A., Camargo, F.D. *et al.* (2002). Muscle-derived hematopoietic stem cells are hematopoietic in origin. *Proceedings of the National Academy of Sciences USA,* **99,** 1341–6.

Metzler, M., Helgason, C.D., Dragatsis, I. *et al.* (2000). Huntingtin is required for normal hematopoiesis. *Human Molecular Genetics,* **9,** 387–94.

Millan, M.T., Shizuru, J.A., Hoffmann, P. *et al.* (2002). Mixed chimerism and immunosuppressive drug withdrawal after HLA-mismatched kidney and hematopoietic progenitor transplantation. *Transplantation,* **73,** 1386–91.

Miller, J.D., Stacy, T., Liu, P.P., & Speck, N.A. (2001). Core-binding factor beta (CBFbeta), but not CBFbeta-smooth muscle myosin heavy chain, rescues definitive hematopoiesis in CBFbeta-deficient embryonic stem cells. *Blood,* **97,** 2248–56.

Miller-Hancet, W.C., LaCorbiere, M., Fuller, S.J. *et al.* (1993). In vitro chamber specification during embryonic stem cell cardiogenesis. *Journal of Biological Chemistry,* **268,** 25244–52.

Mitjavila, M.T., Filippi, M.D., Cohen-Solal, K. *et al.* (1998). The Mpl-ligand is involved in the growth-promoting activity of the murine stromal cell line MS-5 on ES cell-derived hematopoiesis. *Experimental Hematology,* **26,** 124–34.

Morshead, C.M., Benveniste, P., Iscove, N.N., & van der Kooy, D. (2002). Hematopoietic competence is a rare property of neural stem cells that may depend on genetic and epigenetic alterations. *Nature Medicine,* **8,** 268–73.

Muller, A.M. & Dzierzak, E.A. (1993). ES cells have only a limited lymphopoietic potential after adoptive transfer into mouse recipients. *Development,* **118,** 1343–51.

Muthuchamy, M., Pajak, L., Howles, P. *et al.* (1993). Development analysis of tropomyosin gene expression in embryonic stem cells and mouse embryos. *Molecular Cell Biology,* **13,** 3311–23.

Nakano, T., Kodama, H., & Honjo, T. (1994). Generation of lymphohematopoietic cells from embryonic stem cells in culture. *Science,* **265,** 1098–101.

Nakayama, N., Fang, I., & Elliott, G. (1998). Natural killer and B-lymphoid potential in CD34+ cells derived from embryonic stem cells differentiated in the presence of vascular endothelial growth factor. *Blood,* **91,** 2283–95.

Nakayama, N., Lee, J., Chiu, L. (2000). Vascular endothelial growth factor synergistically enhances bone morphogenetic protein-4-dependent lymphohematopoietic cell generation from embryonic stem cells in vitro. *Blood,* **95,** 2275–83.

Nichols, J., Chambers, I., Taga, T., & Smith, A. (2001). Physiological rationale for responsiveness of mouse embryonic stem cells to gp130 cytokines. *Development,* **128,** 2333–9.

Nishikawa, S.I., Nishikawa, S., Hirashima, M. *et al.* (1998). Progressive lineage analysis by cell sorting and culture identifies FLK1+VE-cadherin+ cells at a diverging point of endothelial and hemopoietic lineages. *Development,* **125,** 1747–57.

Nisitani, S., Tsubata, T., & Honjo, T. (1994). Lineage marker-negative lymphocyte precursors derived from embryonic stem cells in vitro differentiate into mature lymphocytes in vivo. *International Immunology,* **6,** 909–16.

Niwa, H., Burdon, T., Chambers, I., & Smith, A. (1998). Self-renewal of pluripotent embryonic stem cells is mediated via activation of STAT3. *Genes and Development,* **12,** 2048–60.

Nogueira, M.M., Mitjavila-Garcia, M.T., Le Pesteur, F. *et al.* (2000). Regulation of Id gene expression during embryonic stem cell-derived hematopoietic differentiation. *Biochemical and Biophysical Research Communications,* **276,** 803–12.

Notarianni, E., Laurie, S., Moor, R.M., & Evans, M.J. (1990). Maintenance and differentiation in culture of pluripotential embryonic cell lines from pig blastocysts. *Journal of Reproduction and Fertility,* **41** (Suppl), 51–6.

Odorico, J.A., Kaufman, D.S., & Thomson, J.A. (2001). Multilineage differentiation from human embryonic stem cell lines. *Stem Cells,* **19,** 193–204.

Okuda, T., Takeda, K., Fujita, Y. *et al.* (2000). Biological characteristics of the leukemia-associated transcriptional factor AML1 disclosed by hematopoietic rescue of AML1-deficient embryonic stem cells by using a knock-in strategy. *Molecular Cell Biology,* **20,** 319–28.

Pain, B., Clark, M., Nakazawa, H. *et al.* (1996). Long-term in vitro culture and characterization of avian embryonic stem cells with multiple morphogenetic potentialities. *Development,* **122,** 2339–48.

Palacios, R., Golunski, E., & Samaridis, J. (1995). In vitro generation of hematopoietic stem cells from an embryonic stem cell line. *Proceedings of the National Academy of Sciences USA,* **92,** 7530–4.

Palis, J. & Yoder, M.C. (2001). Yolk-sac hematopoiesis: the first blood cells of mouse and man. *Experimental Hematology,* **29,** 927–36.

Papaioannou, V., Evans, E., Gardner, R., & Graham C. (1979). Growth and differentiation of an embryonal carcinoma cell line (CL45b). *Journal of Embryology and Experimental Morphology,* **54,** 277–95.

Pease, S., Braghetta, P., Gearing, D. *et al.* (1990). Isolation of embryonic stem (ES) cells in media supplemented with recombinant leukemia inhibitory factor (LIF). *Developmental Biology,* **141,** 344–52.

Perkins, A.C. (1998). Enrichment of blood from embryonic stem cells in vitro. *Reproduction, Fertility, and Development,* **10,** 563–72.

Perlingeiro, R.C., Kyba, M., & Daley, G.Q. (2001). Clonal analysis of differentiating embryonic stem cells reveals a hematopoietic progenitor with primitive erythroid and adult lymphoid-myeloid potential. *Development,* **128,** 4597–604.

Pfeifer, A., Ikawa, M., Dayn, Y., & Verma, I.M. (2002). Transgenesis by lentiviral vectors: lack of gene silencing in mammalian embryonic stem cells and preimplantation embryos. *Proceedings of the National Academy of Sciences USA,* **99,** 2140–5.

Pineault, N., Helgason, C.D., Lawrence, H.J., & Humphries, R.K. (2002). Differential expression of Hox, Meis1, and Pbx1 genes in primitive cells throughout murine hematopoietic ontogeny. *Experimental Hematology,* **30,** 49–57.

Pinto do, O.P., Kolterud, A., & Carlsson, L. (1998). Expression of the LIM-homeobox gene LH2 generates immortalized steel factor-dependent multipotent hematopoietic precursors. *EMBO Journal,* **17,** 5744–56.

Pinto do, O.P., Richter, K., & Carlsson, L. (2002). Hematopoietic progenitor/stem cells immortalized by Lhx2 generate functional hematopoietic cells in vivo. *Blood,* **99,** 3939–46.

Pinto do, O.P., Wandzioch, E., Kolterud, A., & Carlsson, L. (2001). Multipotent hematopoietic progenitor cells immortalized by Lhx2 self-renew by a cell nonautonomous mechanism. *Experimental Hematology,* **29,** 1019–28.

Potocnik, A.J., Kohler, H., & Eichmann, K. (1997). Hemato-lymphoid in vivo reconstitution potential of subpopulations derived from in vitro differentiated embryonic stem cells. *Proceedings of the National Academy of Sciences USA,* **94,** 10295–300.

Potocnik, A.J., Nielsen, P.J., & Eichmann, K. (1994). In vitro generation of lymphoid precursors from embryonic stem cells. *EMBO Journal,* **13,** 5274–83.

Qu, C.K., Shi, Z.O., Shen, R. *et al.* (1997). A deletion mutation in the SH2-N domain of Shp-2 severely suppresses hematopoietic cell development. *Molecular Cell Biology,* **17,** 5499–507.

Ray, W.J., Bain, G., Yao, M., & Gottlieb, D.I. (1997). CYP26, a novel mammalian cytochrome P450, is induced by retinoic acid and defines a new family. *Journal of Biological Chemistry,* **272,** 18702–8.

Robbins, J., Gulick, J., Sanchez, A. *et al.* (1990). Mouse embryonic stem cells express the cardiac myosin heavy chain genes during development in vitro. *Journal of Biological Chemistry,* **265,** 11905–9.

Reubinoff, B.E., Pera, M.E., Fong, C.Y. *et al.* (2000). Embryonic stem cell lines from human blastocysts: somatic differentiation in vitro. *Nature Biotechnology,* **18,** 399–404.

Rideout, W.M., 3rd, Hochedlinger, K., Kyba, M. *et al.* (2002). Correction of a genetic defect by nuclear transplantation and combined cell and gene therapy. *Cell,* **109,** 17–27.

Risau, W., Sariola, H., Zerwes, H.G. *et al.* (1988). Vasculogenesis and angiogenesis in embryonic-stem-cell-derived embryoid bodies. *Development,* **102,** 471–8.

Robertson, S.M., Kennedy, M., Shannon, J.M., & Keller, G. (2000). A transitional stage in the commitment of mesoderm to hematopoiesis requiring the transcription factor SCL/tal-1. *Development,* **127,** 2447–59.

Rohwedel, J., Maltsev, V., & Bober, E. *et al.* (1994). Muscle cell differentiation of embryonic stem cells reflects myogenesis in vivo: developmentally regulated expression of myogenic determination genes and functional expression of ionic currents. *Developmental Biology,* **164,** 87–101.

Rosner, M., Vigano, M., Ozato, K. *et al.* (1990). A POU-domain transcription factor in early stem cells and germ cells of the mammalian embryo. *Nature,* **345,** 686–92.

Rossant, J. & Papaioannou, V. (1984). The relationship between embryonic, embryonal carcinoma and embryo-derived stem cells. *Cell Differentiation,* **15,** 155–61.

Saito, S., Strelchenko, N., & Niemann, H. (1992). Bovine embryonic stem cell-like cell lines cultured over several passages. *Roux's Archives of Developmental Biology,* **201,** 134–41.

Sanchez, A., Jones, W.K., Gulick, J. *et al.* (1991). Myosin heavy chain gene expression in mouse embryoid bodies. An in vitro developmental study. *Journal of Biological Chemistry,* **266,** 22419–26.

Sauvageau, G., Thorsteinsdottir, U., Eaves, C.J. *et al.* (1995). Overexpression of HOXB4 in hematopoietic cells causes the selective expansion of more primitive populations in vitro and in vivo. *Genes and Development,* **9,** 1753–65.

Schmitt, R.M., Bruyns, E., & Snodgrass, H.R. (1991). Hematopoietic development of embryonic stem cells in vitro: cytokine and receptor gene expression. *Genes and Development,* **5,** 728–40.

Schöler, H., Dressler, G., Balling, R. *et al.* (1990). Oct-4: a germline-specific transcription factor mapping to the mouse t-complex. *EMBO Journal,* **9,** 2185–95.

Schoonjans, L., Albright, G., Li, J-L. *et al.* (1996). Pluripotential rabbit embryonic stem (ES) cells are capable of forming overt coat color chimeras following injection into blastocysts. *Molecular Reproduction and Development,* **45,** 439–43.

Schuldiner, M., Yanuka, O., Itskovitz-Eldor, J. *et al.* (2000). Effects of eight growth factors on the differentiation of cells derived from human embryonic stem cells. *Proceedings of the National Academy of Sciences USA,* **97,** 11307–12.

Shaw-White, J.R., Denko, N., Albers, L. *et al.* (1993). Expression of the lacZ gene targeted to the HPRT locus in embryonic stem cells and their derivatives. *Transgenic Research,* **2,** 1–13.

Shirane, M., Sawa, H., Kobayashi, Y. *et al.* (2001). Deficiency of phospholipase C-gammal impairs renal development and hematopoiesis. *Development,* **128,** 5173–80.

Smith, A.G. (2001). Embryo-derived stem cells: Of Mice and Men. *Annual Review of Cell Development and Biology,* **17,** 435–503.

Solter & Knowles, B.B. (1978). Monoclonal antibody defining a stage-specific mouse embryonic antigen (SSEA-1). *Proceedings of the National Academy of Sciences USA,* **75,** 5565–9.

Spitzer, T.R., Delmonico, F., Tolkoff-Rubin, N. *et al.* (1999). Combined histocompatibility leukocyte antigen-matched donor bone marrow and renal transplantation for multiple myeloma with end stage renal disease: the induction of allograft tolerance through mixed lymphohematopoietic chimerism. *Transplantation,* **68,** 480–4.

Stewart, T. & Mintz, B. (1981). Successive generations of mice produced from an established culture line of euploid teratocarcinoma cells. *Proceedings of the National Academy of Sciences USA,* **78,** 6314–8.

Stice, S., Strelchenko, N., Keefer, C., & Matthews, L. (1996). Pluripotent bovine embryonic cell lines direct embryonic development following nuclear transfer. *Biology of Reproduction,* **54,** 100–10.

Strojek, R.M., Reed, M.A., Hoover, J., & Wagner, T. (1990). A method for cultivating morphologically undifferentiated embryonic stem cells from porcine blastocysts. *Theriogenology,* **33,** 901–13.

Suemori, H., Tada, T., Torii, R. *et al.* (2001). Establishment of embryonic stem cell lines from cynomolgus monkey blastocysts produced by IVF or ICSI. *Developmental Dynamics,* **222,** 273–9.

Sukoyan, M., Golubitsa, A., Zhelezova, A. *et al.* (1992). Isolation and cultivation of blastocyst-derived stem cell lines from american mink (mustela vison). *Molecular Reproductive Development,* **33,** 418–31.

Sukoyan, M., Vatolin, S., Golubitsa, A. *et al.* (1993). Embryonic stem cells derived from morulae, inner cell mass, and blastocysts of mink: comparisons of their pluripotencies. *Molecular Reproduction and Development,* **36,** 148–58.

Sutherland, D.E., Goetz, F.C., & Sibley, R.K. (1989). Recurrence of disease in pancreas transplants. *Diabetes,* **38,** 85–7.

Suwabe, N., Takahashi, S., Nakano, T., & Yamamoto, M. (1998). GATA-1 regulates growth and differentiation of definitive erythroid lineage cells during in vitro ES cell differentiation. *Blood,* **92,** 4108–18.

Talbot, N., Rexroad, C., Pursel, V., & Powell, A. (1993). Alkaline phosphatase staining of pig and sheep epiblast cells in culture. *Molecular Reproduction and Development,* **36,** 139–47.

Terada, N., Hamazaki, T., Oka, M. *et al.* (2002). Bone marrow cells adopt the phenotype of other cells by spontaneous cell fusion. *Nature,* **416,** 542–5.

Thomas, E.D. (1999). Bone marrow transplantation: a review. *Seminars in Hematology,* **36,** 95–103.

Thomson, J.A., Itskovitz-Eldor, J., Shapiro, S.S. *et al.* (1998). Embryonic stem cell lines derived from human blastocysts. *Science,* **282,** 1145–7.

Thomson, J.A., Kalishman, J., Golos, T.G. *et al.* (1995). Isolation of a primate embryonic stem cell line. *Proceedings of the National Academy of Sciences USA,* **92,** 7844–8.

Thomson, J.A., Kalishman, J., Golos, T.G. *et al.* (1996). Pluripotent cell lines derived from common marmoset (Callithrix jacchus) blastocysts. *Biology of Reproduction,* **55,** 254–9.

Till, J.E., & McCullough, E.A. (1961). A direct measurement of the radiation sensitivity of normal mouse bone marrow cells. *Radiation Research,* **14,** 213–22.

Tomczak, M.M., Hincha, D.K., Estrada, S.D. *et al.* (2002). A mechanism for stabilization of membranes at low temperatures by an antifreeze protein. *Biophysical Journal,* **82,** 874–81.

Traver, D., Miyamoto, T., Christensen, J. *et al.* (2001). Fetal liver myelopoiesis occurs through distinct, prospectively isolatable progenitor subsets. *Blood,* **98,** 627–35.

Tronik-Le Roux, D., Roullot, V., Schweitzer, A. *et al.* (1995). Suppression of erythro-megakaryocytopoiesis and the induction of reversible thrombocytopenia in mice transgenic for the thymidine kinase gene targeted by the platelet glycoprotein alpha IIb promoter. *Journal of Experimental Medicine,* **181,** 2141–51.

Tsai, F.Y., Keller, G., Kuo, F.C. *et al.* (1994). An early haematopoietic defect in mice lacking the transcription factor GATA-2. *Nature,* **371,** 221–6.

Uzan, G., Prandini, M.H., Rosa, J.P., & Berthier, R. (1996). Hematopoietic differentiation of embryonic stem cells: an in vitro model to study gene regulation during megakaryocytopoiesis. *Stem Cells,* **14** (Suppl 1), 194–9.

van Stekelenburg-Hamers, A., van Achterberg, T., Rebel, H. *et al.* (1995). Isolation and characterization of permanent cell lines from inner cell mass cells of bovine blastocysts. *Molecular Reproduction and Development,* **40,** 444–54.

Wang, Z.O., Ovitt, C., Grigoriadis, A.E. *et al.* (1992). Bone and haematopoietic defects in mice lacking c-fos. *Nature,* **360,** 741–5.

Weiss, M.J., Keller, G., & Orkin, S.H. (1994). Novel insights into erythroid development revealed through in vitro differentiation of GATA-1 embryonic stem cells. *Genes and Development,* **8,** 1184–97.

Wheeler, M. (1994). Development and validation of swine embryonic stem cells: a review. *Reproduction, Fertility and Development,* **6,** 563–8.

Wiles, M.V. (1993). Embryonic stem cell differentiation in vitro. *Methods in Enzymology,* **225,** 900–18.

Wiles, M.V. & Johansson, B.M. (1997). Analysis of factors controlling primary germ layer formation and early hematopoiesis using embryonic stem cell in vitro differentiation. *Leukemia,* **11** (Suppl 3), 454–6.

Wiles, M.V. & Keller, G. (1991). Multiple hematopoietic lineages develop from embryonic stem (ES) cells in culture. *Development,* **111,** 259–67.

Williams, R., Hilton, D., Pease, S. *et al.* (1988). Myeloid leukaemia inhibitory factor maintains the developmental potential of embryonic stem cells. *Nature,* **336,** 684–7.

Wobus, A.M., Kaomei, G., Shan, J. *et al.* (1997). Retinoic acid accelerates embryonic stem cell-derived cardiac differentiation and enhances development of ventricular cardiomyocytes. *Journal of Molecular and Cellular Cardiology,* **29,** 1525–39.

Wobus, A.M., Rohwedel, J., Maltsey, V., & Hescheler, J. (1995). Development of cardiomyocytes expressing cardiac-specific genes action potentials, and ionic channels during embryonic stem cell-derived cardiogenesis. *Annals of the New York Academy of Sciences,* **752,** 460–9.

Wobus, A.M., Wallukat, G., & Hescheler, J. (1991). Pluripotent mouse embryonic stem cells are able to differentiate into cardiomyocytes expressing chronotropic responses to adrenergic and cholinergic agents and Ca2+ channel blockers. *Differentiation,* **48,** 173–82.

Wright, W.E., Piatyszek, M.A., Rainey, W.E. *et al.* (1996). Telomerase activity in human germline and embryonic tissues and cells. *Developmental Genetics,* **18,** 173–9.

Xu, C., Inokuma, M.S., Denham, J. *et al.* (2001). Feeder-free growth of undifferentiated human embryonic stem cells. *Nature Biotechnology,* **19,** 971–4.

Yamashita, J., Itoh, H., Hirashima, M. *et al.* (2000). Flk1-positive cells derived from embryonic stem cells serve as vascular progenitors. *Nature,* **408,** 92–6.

Yanai, J., Doetchman, T., Laufer, N. *et al.* (1995). Embryonic cultures but not embryos transplanted to the mouse's brain grow rapidly without immunosuppression. *International Journal of Neuroscience,* **81,** 21–6.

Ying, Q.L., Nichols, J., Evans, E.P., & Smith, A.G. (2002). Changing potency by spontaneous fusion. *Nature,* **416,** 545–8.

Zhang, R., Tsai, F.Y., & Orkin, S.H. (1994). Hematopoietic development of vav–/– mouse embryonic stem cells. *Proceedings of the National Academy of Sciences USA,* **91,** 12755–9.

Zhang, S.-C., Wernig, M., Duncan, I.D. *et al.* (2001). In vitro differentiation of transplantable neural precursors from human embryonic stem cells. *Nature Biotechnology,* **19,** 1129–33.

Zmuidzinas, A., Fischer, K.D., Lira, S.A. *et al.* (1995). The vav proto-oncogene is required early in embryogenesis but not for hematopoietic development in vitro. *EMBO Journal,* **14,** 1–11.

7   Adult stem cell plasticity

MORAYMA REYES AND CATHERINE M. VERFAILLIE

Stem Cell Institute, University of Minnesota, Minneapolis, USA

Pluripotent embryonic stem cells

The study of stem cells is important because they promise to be very useful for the understanding and treatment of all diseases. Embryonic stem (ES) cells are derived from the inner cell mass of a blastocyst. Mouse ES cells have been studied for more than three decades. Mouse ES cells can be maintained in culture indefinitely in an undifferentiated state, and can differentiate in vivo and in vitro into all intraembryonic tissues (Smith, 2001). Therefore, ES cells are considered pluripotent. Human ES cells were first described in 1998 (Trounson & Pera, 2001). Human ES cells have been maintained in culture for more than 300 population doublings. Like mouse ES cells, human ES cells form teratomas, indicating their pluripotent nature. A series of studies since has shown that human ES cells can be induced to differentiate into neural cells, cardiac myocytes, pancreatic beta cells, hepatocytes, hematopoietic cells, and endothelium (Pera *et al.*, 2000; Reubinoff *et al.*, 2000; Trounson & Pera, 2001). Thus, human ES cells hold great promise for regenerative medicine. However, there are ethical issues that may prevent the use of ES cells for clinical purposes, as creation of ES cell lines requires that the blastocyst is destroyed. In addition, the very nature of ES cells, namely their ability to differentiate into many cell types and form teratomas, will make ES cell-based therapies challenging, as undifferentiated ES cells will need to be fully eliminated from clinical products. Also, using a limited genetic pool of donor ES cells for cellular therapies will require immunosuppression of the host to avoid immune rejection. Such a limited number of ES cells may also not include cells with the correct genetic background to study, understand, and eventually treat some diseases that are more prevalent in certain ethnic groups. To circumvent immune problems, ES cells could be created from the patient him/herself by transferring the nucleus from a somatic cell of the patient (e.g., skin) into a human oocyte to generate a blastocyst, from which ES cells can be obtained. This is called therapeutic cloning. However, therapeutic cloning is even more ethically controversial because of fear that this will lead to creation of whole human beings (reproductive cloning).

Adult stem cells: does pluripotency exist?

When a sperm cell fertilizes an oocyte, a zygote is formed (Fig. 7.1). Cells derived from the zygote (a fertilized egg) are totipotent, because they can generate both extra- and intraembryonic tissue. The zygote develops to the blastocyst stage, where cells in the inner cell mass give rise to the embryo. These cells are considered pluripotent because they can give rise to all intra- but not extraembryonic tissues. Cells in the inner cell mass become specified to the three embryonic layers (ectoderm, mesoderm, and endoderm) during gastrulation. Ectoderm gives rise to eyes, skin, and central and peripheral nervous system. Mesoderm gives rise to the skeleton, muscle, heart, vasculature, kidneys, and reproductive organs. Endoderm gives rise to lungs, thyroid, and gastrointestinal (GI) organs. As the embryo develops, somatic stem cells become more restricted and differentiate only into cells of the organ in which they reside or, at the most, cells from the same embryonic layer. Hematopoietic stem cells (HSC), for instance, can regenerate all cells of the hematopoietic system. Neural stem cells (NSC) differentiate into neurons, oligodendrocytes, and astrocytes.

Over the past 5 years, a series of publications has suggested that adult stem cells from different organs are more plastic than what was previously thought (Table 7.1). A number of studies reported that NSC differentiate into blood (Bjornson *et al.*, 1999), skeletal myoblasts (Galli *et al.*, 2000), and many other tissues, when injected into blastocysts (Clarke *et al.*, 2000). Cells from liver differentiate into cardiomyocytes (Malouf *et al.*, 2001). Bone marrow (BM) cells differentiate into hepatocytes (Lagasse *et al.*, 2000) and other epithelial cells (lung, skin, GI) (Krause *et al.*, 2001), neurons (Brazelton *et al.*, 2000; Mezey *et al.*, 2000), skeletal myoblasts (Ferrari *et al.*, 1998), or cardiac myoblasts (Toma *et al.*, 2002). Other studies have shown that cells within muscle reconstitute the hematopoietic system. Mesenchymal stem cell (MSC), known to differentiate into osteoblasts, adipocytes, chondrocytes, and skeletal myocytes, may give rise to cardiomyocytes (Toma *et al.*, 2002), astrocytes (Kopen *et al.*, 1999), and neurons. Another cell in BM, termed multipotent adult progenitor cell (MAPC), differentiates into osteoblasts, chondrocytes, adipocytes, skeletal myoblasts, endothelial cells, hepatocytes, and neurons.

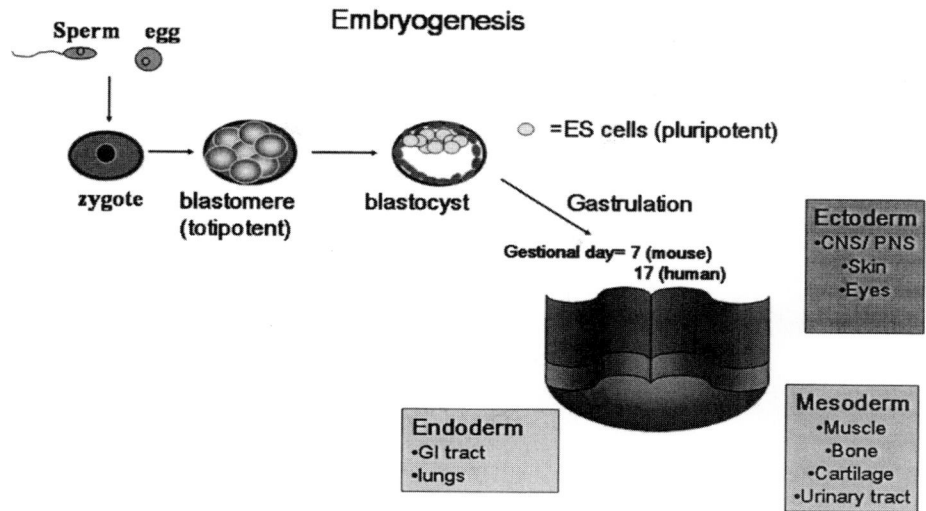

Fig. 7.1. Origin of embryonic stem cells and adult stem cells. A zygote is formed when a sperm cell fertilizes an oocyte, which develops into a blastocyst. Cells in the inner cell mass give rise to the embryo. Cells in the inner cell mass become specified to the three embryonic layers (ectoderm, mesoderm, and endoderm) during gastrulation.

Possible mechanism underlying plasticity

These recent studies have led to the novel hypothesis that adult stem cells can adapt to new environments and differentiate to cell types that they were not destined to become, even cell types from different embryonic layers. There are three possible explanations for this unexpected behavior of organ stem cells (see Fig. 7.2): (1) multiple different tissue stem cells exist in different organs, (2) stem cells undergo trans- or de-differentiation and re-differentiation, or (3) multipotent, perhaps, pluripotent stem cells persist in adulthood. Yet another explanation recently emerged that may explain the trans-differentiation phenomenon: (4) somatic stem cells may fuse with other somatic cells.

Multiple stem cells exist in multiple organs

There is a large body of evidence from HSC that adult stem cells leave their usual environment, circulate, and home into another organ(s). Indeed, "mobilization" of HSC from BM is seen in response to stress, infections, chemotherapy, or growth factor administration (Fu & Liesveld, 2000). Another example is represented by the studies demonstrating hematopoietic engraftment from muscle cells. It was originally thought that a muscle cell could trans-differentiate into hematopoietic stem cells that could repopulate the hematopoietic system upon transplantation (see below). Subsequent studies have shown that the "muscle" cells with hematopoietic reconstitution ability are BM-derived HSC (Jackson *et al.,* 1999; McKinney-Freeman *et al.,* 2002). A recent study showed that cells with oval cell characteristics (CK19 and α-fetoprotein positive) exist in the BM, presumably derived from the liver (Peterson *et al.,* 1999; Theise *et al.,* 2000; Mitaka, 2001). These studies support the thesis that some "plasticity" may be due to circulating stem cells that migrate from one tissue to another hematogenously.

De-differentiation and trans-differentiation

De-differentiation (Fig. 7.3) is a phenomenon classically associated with malignant transformation. However, a number of studies have suggested that primary differentiated, nontumorigenic cells can de- and re-differentiate into another lineage (Table 7.2). For instance, oligodendrocyte progenitor cells (OPC), which are phenotypically and morphologically well defined, were thought to only give rise to oligodendrocytes. Kondo & Raff (2000) documented that OPC isolated from the optic nerve can de-differentiate when cultured in vitro in the absence of serum. These de-differentiated OPC acquired extensive proliferative capacity and could make neurospheres. When induced with basic fibroblast growth factor (bFGF), single de-differentiated OPC differentiated into oligodendrocytes, type I astrocytes, and neurons.

Two separate studies have identified astrocytes as central nervous system (CNS) stem cells: ependymal cells of the ventricular zone (VZ) and astrocytes of the subventricular zone (SVZ). Ependymal cells are ciliated cells that reside in the luminal lining of the ventricles. Ependymal cells use their cilia to move spinal fluid within the ventricles. Johansson *et al.* (1999) labeled ependymal cells with the the fluorescent label, DiI, injected them into the ventricle, and followed their track through the rostral migratory stream. After 10 days DiI[+] cells that co-stained with neuronal markers were seen. Because DiI could have been taken up by nonastrocytes, single DiI[+] ependymal cells that displayed multiple beating cilia were cultured in vitro. After 1 day cilia did not beat any longer and more than 50% of the cells began to divide. Approximately 6% of cells could subsequently differentiate into astrocytes, oligodendrocytes, and neurons. Concomitantly, Doetsch *et al.* (1999) showed that glial cells from the SVZ, which express the glial acidic fibrillary protein (GFAP), might be stem cells for the CNS. Doetsch used a trans-

Table 7.1. *Stem cell plasticity studies*

Progenitor cell	Derivative	Purification	In vitro expansion	Clonality	Reference
BM	Muscle	No	No	No	Ferrari *et al.*, 1998
BM	Hepatocyte	No	No	No	Peterson *et al.*, 1999
HSC	Hepatocyte	Yes	No	No	Lagasse *et al.*, 2000
BM stem cell	Epithelial cell of lung, liver, skin	Enriched	No	Yes	Krause *et al.*, 2001
BM SP	Muscle	Enriched	No	No	Gussoni *et al.*, 1999
BM SP	Heart muscle and endothelium	Enriched	No	No	Goodell *et al.*, 2001
Lin⁻/c-Kit⁺ BM cells	Heart muscle, endothelium, and smooth muscle	Enriched	No	No	Orlic *et al.*, 2001
Hoechst-excluding muscle	Blood cells	Enriched	Yes	No	Jackson *et al.*, 1999
Mesenchymal stem cell	Cardiomyocytes	Yes	Yes	No	Toma *et al.*, 2002
MSC	Astrocytes	Enriched	Yes	No	Kopen *et al.*, 1999
BM	Neurons	No	No	No	Mezey *et al.*, 2000
BM	Neurons	No	No	No	Brazelton *et al.*, 2000
Neurospheres	Blood cells	No	Yes	In vitro "clonal" differentiation	Bjornson *et al.*, 1999
Neurospheres	Muscle	No	Yes	In vitro "clonal" differentiation	Galli *et al.*, 2000
Neurospheres	Chimeric embryo	No	Yes	In vitro "clonal" differentiation	Clarke *et al.*, 2000
Stem cell from dermis	Neurons, glia, smooth muscle cells, and adipocytes	No	Yes	In vitro "clonal" differentiation	Toma *et al.*, 2001
Endothelial cells	Cardiomyocytes	No	Yes	No	Condorelli *et al.*, 2001
Muscle satellite cells	Osteoblasts, adipocytes	No	Yes	No	Asakura *et al.*, 2001
Hepatic stem cells	Cardiomyocytes	Yes	Yes	No	Malouf *et al.*, 2001
Oligodendrocytes precursors	Neurons	Yes	Yes	No	Kondo *et al.*, 2000
MAPC	Bone, cartilage, adipocytes, chondrocytes, skeletal muscle, and endothelial cells	Yes	Yes	Yes	Reyes *et al.*, 2001
MAPC	Endothelial cells	Yes	Yes	Yes	Reyes *et al.*, 2002
MAPC	Hepatocyte-like cells	Yes	Yes	Yes	Schwartz *et al.*, 2002
MAPC	All somatic cell types	Yes	Yes	Yes	Jiang *et al.*, 2002

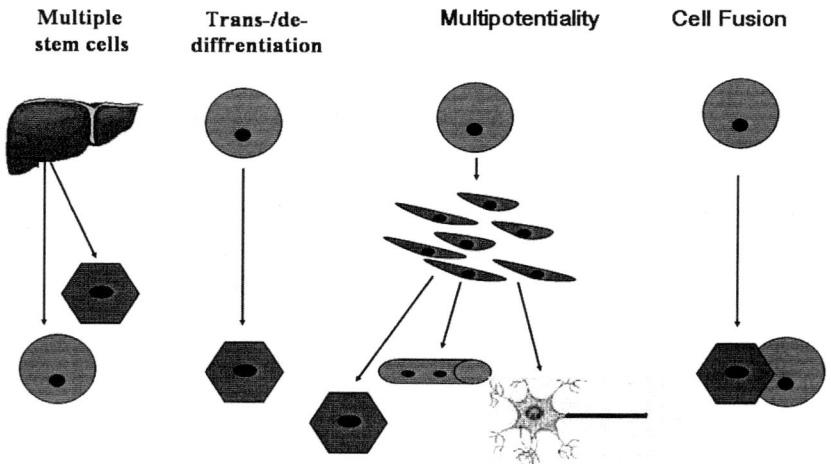

Fig. 7.2. Explanations for stem cell plasticity. **(A)** Multiple stem cells exists in multiple organs. There is evidence that multiple tissue-specific stem cells may exist in several organs. For instance muscle and liver contain aside from muscle and hepatic stem cells, respectively, also hematopoietic stem cells. **(B)** De-differentiation and *trans*-differentiation. Dedifferentiation is cellular reprogramming that results in change of the former differentiated state and allows redirection of cell fate. In contrast, *trans*-differentiation involves a direct change in cell fate without cell division. **(C)** Multipotent adult stem cells. Aside from germ cells, there may be other multipotent stem cells residing in adult tissues that retain the potential to different not just into cells of that tissue but also other tissue cells. **(D)** Cell fusion. As suggested by studies from Ying *et al.* (Ying *et al.* 2002) and Terada *et al.*, (Terada *et al.*, 2002), cell fusion may occur between two adult cells.

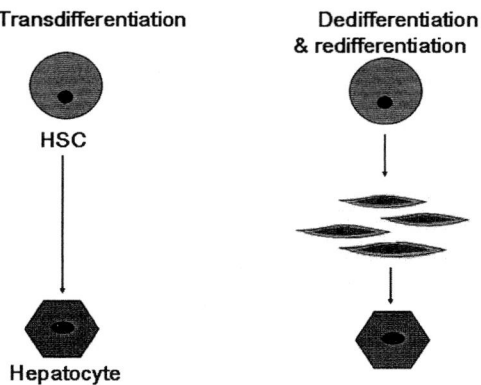

Fig. 7.3. Trans- versus de- and re-dedifferentiation. Dedifferentiation is cellular reprogramming that results in change of the former differentiation state and allows redirection of cell fate. In contrast, *trans*-differentiation involves a direct change in cell fate without cell division.

genic mouse engineered to express the avian leukosis virus (ALV) receptor driven by the GFAP promoter. Thus, GFAP-expressing cells that express the ALV receptor can be selectively infected by AVL. Alkaline phosphatase (AP) cDNA-encoding AVL was injected in the ventricles. Through following the fate of AP+ cells, this study showed that SVZ astrocytes gave rise to olfactory bulb neurons. When such SVZ astrocytes were plated in vitro, they also gave rise to neurospheres that differentiated into astrocytes, oligodendrocytes, and neurons.

Trans-differentiation (Fig. 7.3), in contrast to de-differentiation, involves a direct change in phenotype without cell division. A recent study demonstrated trans-differentiation of the exocrine pancreatic cell line, AR42J-B13, into hepatocyte-like cells when induced with dexamethasone. Shen *et al.* (2000) tracked the fate of exocrine pancreatic cells transfected with a green fluorescence protein (GFP)-reporter gene driven by the elastase promoter. After 5 days of exposure to dexamethasone, some GFP+ cells expressed hepatic markers. Bromo-deoxy-uridine (BrdU) labeling was used to demonstrate that the switch in fate occurred without cell division. Similar results were seen with E 11.5 amylase pancreatic cells

that could be induced to express albumin and other hepatic proteins.

One limitation of some of these studies is that the terminal differentiated stage of the mature cells is questionable, because this was defined based on the expression of a single protein specific for differentiated cells. However, stem cells can express proteins thought to be expressed only in differentiated cells. For instance, keratinocyte stem cells express proteins, K5 and K14, which are expressed in mature keratinocytes (Li *et al.*, 1998).

The mechanism underlying the perceived de-differentiation is not clear. De-differentiation is common in nonmammals, such as amphibians. Amphibians such as Urodeles can regenerate whole limbs. Msx1 is expressed in the regenerating blastema. Odelberg and colleagues (2001) demonstrated that mouse myotubes could undergo de-differentiation when the nuclear transcription factor msx1 is expressed. Msx1, transcribed from a tetracycline-inducible promoter, was introduced in C2C12 myotubes. Myotubes regressed into multiple mononuclear myoblasts, which, in turn, proliferated and could be induced to differentiate into osteoblasts, chondrocytes, and adipocytes. Studies were done using very low-density cultures and following lysis of mononuclear cells by injecting water. As these studies were performed with the embryonic cell line, C2C12, it is not known whether the embryonic nature, or the "immortalization" required to generate the cell line, contributed to this phenomenon.

In another study by Condorelli *et al.* (2001), endothelial cells derived from embryonic vessels or umbilical vein (HUVEC) were transduced with GFP and co-cultured with embryonic cardiomyocytes. Some endothelial cells "transformed" into binucleated cells that expressed myosin heavy chain and troponin, and had sarcomeric banding by electron microscopy (EM). This transformation was not seen when endothelial cells and myocytes were cultured in a trans-well culture system, leaving the door open that the "trans-differentiation" was due to fusion with cardiomyocytes.

All studies quoted above used embryonic or early postnatal progenitor cells. It remains to be seen if these studies can be reproduced with cells from adult tissue. De-differentiation/re-differentiation or trans-differentiation phenomena were also

Table 7.2. *De-differentiation and trans-differentiation studies*

Progenitor cell	Unexpected derivative	Purification	Developmental stage	Clonality	Occurs in vivo?	Reference
Oligodendrocyte	Neurons/astro/oli	Sequential immunopanning	P6 rat	Dilution	Unknown	Kondo & Raff, 2000
Pancreatic	Hepatocytes	Dorsal pancreatic buds No purification	11.5-day mouse embryo	Yes	Hepatic foci in pancreas	Shen *et al.*, 2000
Myotubes	Bone/cartilage/ adipocytes	C2C12	Mouse embryonic cell line	No	Unknown	Odelberg *et al.*, 2000
Astrocytes	Neurons			No	Unknown	Doetsch *et al.*, 1999; Johansson *et al.*, 1999
Melanocytes	Glial cells	FACS-sorted pigmented cells	E7.5 quail	Micromanipulation	Unknown	Dupin *et al.*, 2000
Endothelial cells	Cardiomyocytes		Embryonic, newborn	No	Yes	Condorelli *et al.*, 2001
Smooth muscle	Skeletal muscle		Fetal	No	Yes	Stratton *et al.*, 2000

shown between very closely related cells derived from the same embryonic layer. Therefore, one wonders if these de- or trans-differentiation phenomena represent a "normal" organogenesis. For instance, a recent study indicated that trans-differentiation of smooth muscle into skeletal muscle of the esophagus occurs. The origin of skeletal muscle during esophageal organogenesis was unknown until recently. Stratton *et al.* (2000) studied the transformation from E17 to P4 in mouse embryos, and clearly demonstrated that smooth muscle cells trans-differentiate into skeletal muscle by undergoing changes in morphology, cytoskeleton, sarcomere assembly, and protein production, remarkably different from changes seen for differentiation of skeletal muscle from splanchnic mesoderm.

Multipotent adult stem cells

The only known relative of the pluripotent stem cells, the ES cells, that resides in the adult organism is the germ cell. Germ cells are established very early in development, even before gastrulation, and are directly derived from embryonic stem cells. Their origin is independent of germinal layers, as they are found in different layers among different species. In Drosophila and C. elegans germ cells first appear at the posterior end of the blastula (Lehmann & Ephrussi, 1994; Ellis & Kimble, 1994), in Xenopus in the endoderm (Kamimura *et al.,* 1980; Turner *et al.,* 1989), in the chicken in the epiblast (Kagami *et al.,* 1997), and in mouse in the mesoderm (Matsui, 1998). Even in simple animals, such as Hydra and Volvox, that lack germinal layers, germ cells are set apart from other cells very early in development (Burnett *et al.,* 1966; Wei & Mahowald, 1994). This suggests that the specification of germ cells is much conserved through evolution and precedes the evolution of three primary germinal layers. Primordial germ cells can be isolated from the developing embryo, and when cultured ex vivo, may have the ability to differentiate to multiple somatic cells (Shamblott *et al.,* 2001).

Aside from germ cells, other more multipotent cells may also exist after gastrulation. For instance, cells can be isolated from the fetal liver that reconstitute not only liver and biliary epithelial cells, but also epithelium of the pancreas and the GI tract (Suzuki *et al.,* 2002). Muscle contains cells with a Hoechst-excluding side population (SP) phenotype, that, depending on the activation of the transcription factor Pax-7, differentiate into either muscle cells or HSCs. These studies suggest, therefore, that cells that precede the known somatic stem cells may persist and, depending on the milieu, differentiate to cells different from those of the organ of origin.

Fusion

Another possible explanation for plasticity was recently suggested to be fusion. Terada *et al.* (2002) used co-cultured mononuclear BM cells from male GFP/puromicin-resistant[R] transgene mice with female murine ES cells in the presence of leukemia inhibitory factor (LIF) and interleukin (IL)-3. After day 7 puromicin was added to remove ES cells. After 14 days, multiple GFP+ clones were seen that could be maintained for

more than 6 months ex vivo and expressed markers of undifferentiated ES cells: Oct3/4 and UTF1. After removal of LIF, GFP+ cells differentiated into different cell types that expressed markers of mesoderm, endoderm, and ectoderm. When injected into NOD/SCID mice, the cells formed teratomas, but no chimerism was seen following injection of the GFP+ cultured cells into a blastocyst. Surprisingly, GFP+ cells were tetraploid and were XXXY. This demonstrates that the GFP+ cultured cells were the result of spontaneous cell fusion between the BM cells and the ES cells. The frequency with which BM cells fused with ES cells was 2–11/10^6 BM cells. The nature of the BM cell responsible for this fusion is unknown.

Ying *et al.* (2002) generated neurospheres from the forebrain of fetuses from female mice transgenic for the β-galactosidase (β-gal) gene and the neomycin-resistance (NEO^R) gene (Rosa26 mice) or Oct4 promoter-GFP. Neurospheres were co-cultured with male mouse hygromicin^R HT2 ES cells. After 4 days, mixtures were cultured with G418 or puromicin to eliminate the HT2 ES cells. After 2 to 4 weeks colonies of LacZ+ or GFP+ cells that expressed Oct4 with characteristics of undifferentiated ES cells were seen. However, cells were also resistant to hygromicin, indicating that cells were hybrids. As shown by Terada *et al.* (2002), cells in the study by Ying were tetraploid, XXXY. These hybrids differentiated into neurons and cardiomyocytes, formed embryoid bodies, and when injected into a blastocyst, chimerism was observed in 30% of the embryos, with minor contributions to intestine, kidney, heart, and most notably liver. Similar results were seen when neurospheres from adult mouse brain were used. The frequency of hybrids was 10^-4–10^-5 per neural cell plated.

The concept that cellular fusion can change the fate of a cell is not new. Heterokaryon studies were performed early in the 20th century and a number of studies have shown that cell fate can be changed upon heterokaryon formation. For instance, myoblast fusion with fibroblasts induces expression of muscle proteins in the fibroblasts. This indicates that cytoplasm of myoblasts contains factors that induce muscle differentiation of nonmuscle cells. Does fusion shown in the experiments from Ying *et al.* (2002) and Terada *et al.* (2002) explain all phenomena of plasticity seen with adult stem cells? This is not likely. First, fusion required significant drug-electable pressure to select for the tetraploid cells. This likely helped the tetraploid cells outgrow the euploid adult stem cells. However, a number of studies describing stem cell plasticity were not done under conditions of selectable pressure (Ferrari *et al.,* 1998; Gussoni *et al.,* 1999; Kopen *et al.,* 1999; Brazelton *et al.,* 2000; Goodell *et al.,* 2001; Krause *et al.,* 2001; Orlic *et al.,* 2001; Toma *et al.,* 2002). Second, these two studies demonstrate fusion between ES cells and tissue-specific cells but not tissue-specific stem cells and differentiated cells. Third, fusion was only documented in vitro, not in vivo.

Tissue specific stem cell plasticity: critical evaluation

The definition of a stem cell includes three criteria (Fig. 7.4): (1) self-renewal, (2) clonal multilineage differentiation, and (3) reconstitution of the differentiated tissue for the life of a recipient. Thus a stem cell with "plasticity" should have self-renewal ability (i.e., give rise to daughter cells with similar plasticity), clonal multilineage differentiation ability (i.e., a single cell gives rise to cells of the tissue of origin and additional tissues), and functionally reconstitute two tissues in vivo. In vivo engraftment and differentiation from stem cells with plasticity would recapitulate tissue-specific stem cell engraftment: engraftment of a stem cell in the liver would result in replacement of some of the hepatic cords irradiating from the portal tracts. Engraftment in the gut would be seen in the crypts, where stem cells reside, leading to replacement of epithelial cells on the adjacent villi. In addition, engrafted cells should replace the function of the tissue in which they engraft.

We will now review the studies published in the field of stem cell plasticity with these criteria in mind (Table 7.3).

Hematopoietic stem cells

HSC are the best-studied adult stem cell. HSC give rise to all blood cells. The cell surface phenotype of mouse HSC, and to a lesser extent human HSC, is known (see Chapter 2), allowing purification to homogeneity. Serial transplantation has proven that HSC can self-renew, and single mouse HSC studies have shown that single HSC can reconstitute the hematopoietic system of a lethally irradiated recipient. A number of recent studies have suggested that HSC may be capable of differentiating into other mesodermal, ectodermal, and endodermal lineages.

Peterson *et al.* (1999) showed that following a sex-mismatched HSC transplantat, BM-derived cells (Y-chromosome+ cells) contributed to oval cell proliferation when rats underwent partial hepatectomy and were treated with 2 acetylaminofluorene to block mature hepatocyte proliferation. The identity of the BM cell responsible for hepatic cell regeneration was

unknown. Also not shown was whether a single cell reconstituted the hematopoietic system and gave rise to oval cells, or whether oval cells differentiated into functional hepatocytes.

Lagasse *et al.* (2000) transplanted cells highly enriched for HSC (c-kit+Thy1lowLin-Sca1+ [KTLS]) from Rosa26 donors into fumarylacetoacetate hydrolase (FAH)−/− mice, a model of hereditary tyrosinemia type I. When maintained on 2-(2-nitro-4-fluoromethylbenzoyl)-1,3-cyclohexanedione (NTBC), animals survive, but when NTBC is withdrawn, liver cell necrosis occurs and animals die. After transplantation of β-Gal+ KTLS cells, Lagasse withdrew NTBC and found regeneration of the liver with BM-derived cells, and with significant contribution of BM donor-derived cells to the hepatocytes in the liver. This indicates that KTLS cells differentiated into functioning hepatocytes. Whether the same cell that gave rise to hematopoiesis also gave rise to the hepatocyte population was not tested.

Krause *et al.* (2001) showed that HSC may give rise to liver, lung, gut, and skin epithelium. They transplanted male Lin− BM cells into female recipients. After 48 hours donor cells were recovered from the BM and single cells transplanted into second female recipients. They found hematopoietic reconstitution with some Y-chromosome+ donor cells, in the liver, lung, gut, and skin epithelia that stained positive for epithelial markers, such as cytokeratins. The study by Krause *et al.* (2001) demonstrated that a single cell gives rise to hematopoietic and epithelial-like cells. Unlike the studies by Lagasse and Peterson, in which donor stem cells regenerated whole liver nodules or an oval cell population, only isolated, scattered donor cells were seen in the different epithelia, some in areas where stem cells are not likely to be found. No functional analysis of the epithelial cells was done.

Jackson *et al.* (2001) injected Hoechst-excluding, SP BM cells from Rosa26 mice into syngeneic mice. Ten weeks after transplantation, a myocardial infarction was induced by coro-

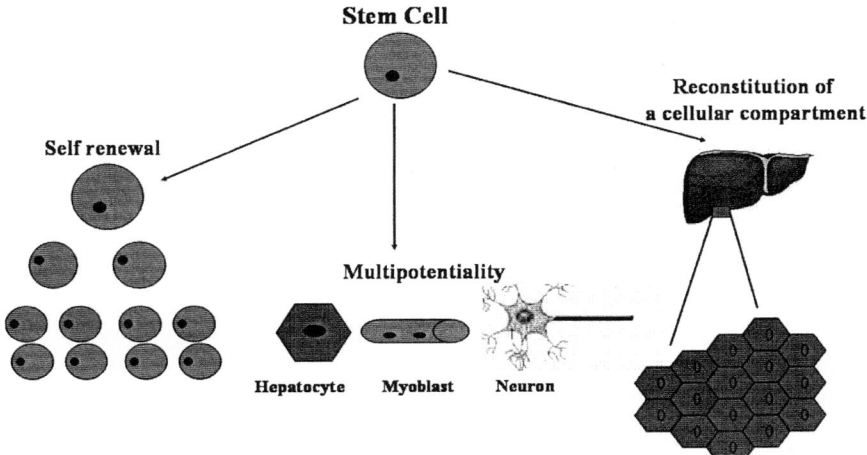

Fig. 7.4. Stem cell definition. The definition of a stem cell includes three criteria: (1) self renewal, in each cellular division at least one daughter cell is identical to the mother cell and retains the same multi-lineage differentiation capacity; (2) clonal multi-lineage differentiation, a single stem cell should give rise to more than one type of differentiated progeny; and (3) reconstitution of the differentiated tissue for the life of a recipient, stem cell should be able to engraft, repopulate and restore the function of the organ.

Table 7.3. *Review of the stem cell plasticity studies based on the stem cell criteria*

Tissue stem cells	Stem cell plasticity studies	Self-renewal	Clonal multilineage differentiation	Reconstitution of cellular compartment
BM	Muscle	No	No	No
	Neuroectoderm	No	No	No
	Liver, oval cells	No	No	No
"HSC" SP (Gussoni *et al.*)	SK muscle	No	No	No
SP (Goodell *et al.*)	Cardiac muscle	No	No	No
Lin-/c-kit+ (Orlic *et al.*)	Cardiac muscle	No	No	Yes
KTLS (Lagasse *et al.*)	Liver	No	No	Yes
Lin-(Krause *et al.*)	Lung, liver, gut, skin	Yes	Yes	No
NSC	Blastocyst	Yes	No	Yes
	Blood	No	Yes	N/A
	SK myoblasts	No	Yes	N/A
Skin cells	Neurons, glial, smooth muscle cells and adipocytes	No	Yes	N/A
MSC	Astrocytes	No	No	No
	Cardiomyocytes	No	No	No
MAPC	Blastocyst	Yes	Yes	Yes
	Liver, lung, gut	Yes	No	No

nary artery occlusion. After 2 weeks, animals were sacrificed and necropsy demonstrated that 0.02% of cells in the heart muscle were β-gal$^+$ and co-labeled with β-actinin, and 3% of the endothelium of small vessels adjacent to the infarct were β-gal+. The clonal origin of the cardiac and endothelial cells, or the function of the trans-differentiated cells, was not tested.

Orlic *et al.* (2001) also studied the use of BM cells to repair myocardial infarction. They injected Lin$^-$c-kit$^+$ BM cells from GFP-transgenic mice directly into the myocardium of syngeneic mice 3 to 5 hours after the infarct. In 40% of mice transplanted, Orlic and colleagues detected GFP or Y-chromosome$^+$ BM cells that co-labeled with myocardial, endothelial, and smooth muscle markers. Approximately 50% of cells found in the infarct zone were GFP$^+$. Hemodynamic evaluation 9 days after transplant showed an improvement in the hemodynamic function compared to infarcted, but not mock-transplanted, mice. The clonal origin of these cells and the exact phenotype of the cell contributing to cardiac and arterial structures were not fully defined.

Gussoni *et al.* (1999) injected male SP BM cells into female mdx mice, a model for muscular dystrophy. Up to 10% of the skeletal muscle cells were derived from the SP population, determined by labeling for Y-chromosome and dystrophin. Again, no clonal analysis was done.

A final set of studies showed that cells from the BM may be found in the brain, where they express neuronal markers. Mezey and colleagues (2000) used newborn PU.1$^{-/-}$ mice, which have defective myelo- and lymphopoiesis, as recipients for BM transplantation. Newborn animals underwent a sex-mismatched transplant and were analyzed 4 months later for the presence of Y-chromosome$^+$ cells in the brain. Between 0.3% and 2% of donor cells co-staining with NeuN were seen, without accumulation of donor cells in neurogenic regions. In a second paper

from this group, Brazelton *et al.* (2000) transplanted BM from GFP-transgenic mice into adult lethally irradiated recipients. Animals were sacrificed several months later. Twenty percent of GFP$^+$ cells in the brain were CD45$^-$ and CD11b$^-$, and 0.2% to 0.3% of GFP$^+$ cells co-labeled with NeuN, TuJ1, and neurofilament 200. The nature of the BM population responsible for the neuroectodermal phenotype is unknown; the investigators did not assess the clonal origin of cells with neuroectodermal phenotype, and no functional studies were done.

In light of the studies by Terada *et al.* (2002) and Ying *et al.* (2002) some of the findings described above may be explained by spontaneous cell fusion. For instance, the low level contribution seen by the Mezey, Brazelton, Krause, and Jackson groups is in the same range as the frequency of fusion seen in vitro. The studies by Lagasse, in which significant selectable pressure existed for wild-type cells, could be consistent with fusion. Studies are likely ongoing in a number of laboratories to rule in or out that the observed plasticity is due to fusion.

Neural stem cells

A second cell population that may have greater therapeutic potential than previously thought are NSC. Bjornson *et al.* (1999) isolated neurospheres from Rosa26 mice and showed that progeny of primary and secondary cultures differentiated into neurons, astrocytes, and oligodendrocytes. Neurospheres were then injected into lethally irradiated mice and β-gal$^+$ multilineage hematopoiesis was seen in blood, BM, and spleen. A similar contribution was seen from embryonic and adult neurospheres. However, a study by Morshead *et al.* (2002) could not confirm these results.

Galli and colleagues (2000) used the same "clonal" neurospheres to prove myogenic differentiation from NSC through co-culture with the embryonic myoblast cell line C2C12. They found that NSC could be induced to form myotubes and express muscle proteins, and that some myotubes were generated from β-gal+ cells only. However, heterokaryon studies have previously shown that myoblast cytoplasm can be instructive of muscle differentiation. Exclusion of NSC-C2C12 fusion will therefore be required to prove that NSC trans-differentiated to skeletal muscle.

Toma et al. (2001) isolated stem cells from the dermis of newborn mice that could differentiate in vitro into neurons, astrocytes, smooth muscle cells, and adipocytes at the single cell level. However, as adipocyte differentiation was short-lived it is possible that they isolated neural crest stem cells that are known to give rise to neurons, glia, and smooth muscle cells.

Finally Clarke et al. (2000) showed that NSC injected into blastocysts contribute to several tissues. Neurospheres were generated from adult Rosa26 mouse brain and injected into blastocysts. When embryos were analyzed, chimerism was detected in some tissues outside the neuroectoderm. However, in no animal was balanced chimerism noted, and no data are available regarding the impact of the donor cells in tissue function as all animals were evaluated prior to birth. The partial chimerism noted here is reminiscent of the studies done by Ying et al. (2002), leaving the possibility that fusion of NSC with cells of the inner cell mass is responsible for the phenomenon.

Liver

One study reported that liver stem cells may differentiate into cardiomyocytes. Malouf et al. (2001) used a clonal cell line (WB-F344) derived from adult male rat liver. This clonal cell line could differentiate into hepatocytes in vivo and in vitro and, surprisingly, also into troponin-I positive cells when injected in the ventricular wall, where they displayed sarcomeric structures by EM. The frequency of this event or functional data were not provided. Furthermore, the possibility of fusion between two cell populations that are often tetraploid was not addressed.

Muscle

Jackson et al. reported in 1999 that a population of muscle satellite cells could contribute, after ex vivo culture, to the hematopoietic system. The initial report did not identify the cell responsible for hematopoietic differentiation. Since then, three reports have shed light on this phenomenon. First, Kawada and Ogawa (2001) cleverly used a BM chimeric mouse model to identify the nature of the muscle cell with hematopoietic capacity. A chimeric model was generated by transplantation of BM cells from Ly-5.1 mice into Ly-5.2 mice. They found that in mice that were 60% chimeric, 60% of the hematopoietic cells generated in vitro from muscle cells were of donor origin, suggesting that the muscle cells with hematopoietic differentiation capacity were derived from BM. They then confirmed this by transplanting muscle cells from chimeric mice into secondary Ly-5.2 mice, finding hematopoi-

etic engraftment only by Ly-5.1 cells, demonstrating the BM origin of these cells. In a second study by McKinney-Freeman and colleagues (2002), it was conclusively demonstrated that the hematopoietic cells derived from muscle were hematopoietic in origin, as they were Sca-1+ and CD45+, generated hematopoietic but not myogenic colonies in vitro, and were responsible for the hematopoietic repopulation in vivo. However, another study suggests that muscle may harbor cells capable of muscle, as well as hematopoietic, differentiation. Seale et al. (2000) demonstrated that a rare population of muscle cells that has an SP phenotype is the progenitor of satellite cells. The transcription factor Pax7 is needed for the commitment of SP cells into satellite cells and thus myogenic lineage. However, in the absence of Pax7, these progenitors differentiate into hematopoietic cells, suggesting that this SP cell may be a mesodermal stem cell.

Mesenchymal stem cells

MSCs can be obtained from bone marrow (Caplan et al., 1991; Lennon et al., 1995) and adipose tissue (Zuk et al., 2001). Caplan's group demonstrated that MSCs differentiate into osteoblasts, chondroblasts, adipocytes, and skeletal myoblasts (Wakitani et al., 1995). Other studies have reported that MSCs, transplanted in mouse brain, may differentiate into cells expressing astrocyte markers. More recently two groups have shown that MSCs may differentiate in vitro into cells expressing neuronal markers (Sanchez-Ramos et al., 2000; Woodbury et al., 2000). However, no functional assessment was performed. A recent study by Toma et al. (2002) also showed that MSCs transplanted into an infarcted heart may express cardiomyocyte proteins. Again, no functional studies were performed.

Multipotential adult progenitor cells

We have recently identified a MAPC in cultures of human and rodent BM. When human BM mononuclear cells depleted of CD45+ and glycophorin (Gly)A+ cells are cultured in vitro on fibronectin, low concentrations of fetal calf serum, platelet derived growth factor (PDGF)-BB, and epidermal growth factor (EGF), populations of small adherent cells that can be culture-expanded for greater than 80 PDs can be generated. MAPC express telomerase, and have long telomeres (9–15 kb) that do not shorten in culture. MAPC are euploid. These cultured cell populations are CD34−, CD44−, CD45−, HLA-class I− and II, ckit−, but Thy-1low and Flk-1low. MAPC differentiate into osteoblasts, chondroblasts, adipocytes, and skeletal myoblasts (Reyes et al., 2001), all cells that are part of the limb bud mesoderm, but also into endothelium, part of visceral mesoderm (Reyes et al., 2002). In addition, these cells can differentiate into cells that express markers of astrocytes, oligodendrocytes, and neurons, cells that also have voltage-gated sodium channels. Finally these cells differentiate into cells with morphological, phenotypic, and functional characteristics of hepatocytes (Schwartz et al., 2002). Using retroviral marking, it was demonstrated that single cells were capable of differentiating into cells of limb-bud mesoderm, visceral mesoderm, neuroectoderm, and endoderm. Moreover, differentiation in vitro could be induced at multiple time points after initiation of the culture, consistent with the notion that the cells can undergo self-renewing cell divisions in vitro. These cells have been termed multipotent adult progenitor cells or MAPC. When attempting to generate MAPC from rodent marrow, cultures could not be established unless leukemia inhibitory factor (LIF) was added to the cultures. LIke human MAPC, mouse and rat MAPC differentiate in vitro at the single cell level into cells with endothelial, neuroectodermal, and hepatocyte characteristics. Furthermore, when single mouse MAPC are introduced in the blastocyst, 1 of 3 animals born are chimeric, and chimerism is detected in all somatic tissues. When mouse MAPC are infused into postnatal recipients, 2% to 4% engraftment is seen in the hematopoietic system, liver, intestine, and lung, where cells acquire phenotypic characteristics of the organ they engraft in. When transplants are done in minimally irradiated recipients (250 cGy), increased levels of engraftment are seen in the hematopoietic system and the intestinal system. Of note, donor cells could be detected in the crypts of the intestine, and could sometimes be seen covering half of villi, consistent with the notion that engraftment occured in one of two crypts contributing epithelial cells to a villus (Jiang *et al.*, 2002). MAPC therefore fulfill almost all criteria for "stem cell plasticity": self-renewal, clonal differentiation into cells of multiple germ layers that have functional characteristics of the tissues they differentiate in, and engraftment. However, functional repopulation has yet to be shown.

Clinical relevance and future directions

Before adult stem cells can be used as therapy for genetic or degenerative diseases, many questions will need to be answered. We are at the early stages of the stem cell plasticity field. Skepticism regarding the occurrence of plasticity persists, caused in part by the lack of consistency and reproducibility of many plasticity studies. Further, as described above, no study has fully met the criteria of "stem cells." Therefore, it remains to be determined if some of the plasticity seen is the result of in vitro culture artifact—even though this might not preclude their clinical usefulness, cell fusion—which also may not preclude their clinical usefulness for therapy, or in vivo detection artifact. There is no doubt that adult stem cells exist, exemplified by HSC that have been studied for almost a century. What is less clear is why plasticity has only now been detected. Obviously this phenomenon, if real, must have existed before the last decade. However, it is likely that in the era of "Dolly the sheep," scientists are now looking in places they never looked before, and may accept the notion of cellular reprogramming. Possibly, irrespective of the nature of the stem cell plasticity, be it the result of cell fusion, existence of multiple progenitor cells in different tissues, or true multi/pluripotency of adult stem cells, adult stem cells may prove to be suitable for clinical therapies of genetic and/or degenerative diseases. As mentioned before, one of the major potential constraints for ES cell therapy is their tendency to develop teratomas. In none of the adult stem cell plasticity studies has teratoma formation been reported. Nonetheless, most studies had relatively short-term follow-up and further studies to exclude tumor formation will be needed.

References

Asakura, A., Komaki, M., & Rudnicki, M. (2001). Muscle satellite cells are multipotential stem cells that exhibit myogenic, osteogenic, and adipogenic differentiation. *Differentiation; Research in Biological Diversity*, **68**, 245–53.

Bjornson, C.R., Rietze, R.L., Reynolds, B.A. *et al.* (1999). Turning brain into blood: a hematopoietic fate adopted by adult neural stem cells in vivo. *Science*, **283**, 534–7.

Brazelton, T.R., Rossi, F.M., Keshet, G.I., & Blau, H.M. (2000). From marrow to brain: expression of neuronal phenotypes in adult mice. *Science*, **290**, 1775–9.

Brook, F.A. & Gardner, R.L. (1997). The origin and efficient derivation of embryonic stem cells in the mouse. *Proceedings of the National Academy of Sciences USA*, **94**, 5709–12.

Burnett, A.L., Davis, L.E., & Ruffing, F.E. (1966). A histological and ultrastructural study of germinal differentiation of interstitial cells arising from gland cells in Hydra viridis. *Journal of Morphology*, **120**, 1–8.

Clarke, D.L., Johansson, C.B., Wilbertz, J. *et al.* (2000). Generalized potential of adult neural stem cells. *Science*, **288**, 1660–3.

Condorelli, G., Borello, U., De Angelis, L. *et al.* (2001). Cardiomyocytes induce endothelial cells to trans-differentiate into cardiac muscle: implications for myocardium regeneration. *Proceedings of the National Academy of Sciences USA*, **98**, 10733–8.

Doetsch, F., Caille, I., Lim, D.A. *et al.* (1999). Subventricular zone astrocytes are neural stem cells in the adult mammalian brain. *Cell*, **97**, 703–16.

Ellis, R.E. & Kimble, J. (1994). Control of germ cell differentiation in Caenorhabditis elegans. *Ciba Foundation Symposium*, **182**, 179–88.

Fu, S. & Liesveld, J. (2000). Mobilization of hematopoietic stem cells. *Blood Reviews*, **14**, 205–18.

Galli, R., Borello, U., Gritti, A. *et al.* (2000). Skeletal myogenic potential of human and mouse neural stem cells. *Nature Neuroscience*, **3**, 986–91.

Gussoni, E., Soneoka, Y., Strickland, C.D. *et al.* (1999). Dystrophin expression in the mdx mouse restored by stem cell transplantation. *Nature*, **401**, 390–4.

Jackson, K.A., Majka, S.M., Wang, H. *et al.* (2001). Regeneration of ischemic cardiac muscle and vascular endothelium by adult stem cells. *The Journal of Clinical Investigation*, **107**, 1395–402.

Jackson, K.A., Mi, T., & Goodell, M.A. (1999). Hematopoietic potential of stem cells isolated from murine skeletal muscle. *Proceedings of the National Academy of Sciences USA*, **96**, 14482–6.

Jiang, Y., Jahagirdar, B., Schwartz, R.E. *et al.* (2002). Pluripotent nature of adult marrow derived mesenchymal stem cells. *Nature*, **418**, 41–9.

Johansson, C.B., Momma, S., Clarke, D.L. *et al.* (1999). Identification of a neural stem cell in the adult mammalian central nervous system. *Cell,* **96,** 25–34.

Johansson, C.B., Svensson, M., Wallstedt, L. *et al.* (1999). Neural stem cells in the adult human brain. *Experimental Cell Research,* **253,** 733–6.

Kagami, H., Tagami, T., Matsubara, Y. *et al.* (1997). The developmental origin of primordial germ cells and the transmission of the donor-derived gametes in mixed-sex germline chimeras to the offspring in the chicken. *Molecular Reproduction and Development,* **48,** 501–10.

Kamimura, M., Kotani, M., & Yamagata, K. (1980). The migration of presumptive primordial germ cells through the endodermal cell mass in Xenopus laevis: a light and electron microscopic study. *Journal of Embryology and Experimental Morphology,* **59,** 1–17.

Kawada, H. & Ogawa, M. (2001). Bone marrow origin of hematopoietic progenitors and stem cells in murine muscle. *Blood,* **98,** 2008–13.

Kondo, T. & Raff, M. (2000). Oligodendrocyte precursor cells reprogrammed to become multipotential CNS stem cells. *Science,* **289,** 1754–7.

Kopen, G.C., Prockop, D.J., & Phinney, D.G. (1999). Marrow stromal cells migrate throughout forebrain and cerebellum, and they differentiate into astrocytes after injection into neonatal mouse brains. *Proceedings of the National Academy of Sciences USA,* **96,** 10711–6.

Krause, D.S., Theise, N.D., Collector, M.I. *et al.* (2001). Multiorgan, multi-lineage engraftment by a single bone marrow-derived stem cell. *Cell,* **105,** 369–77.

Lagasse, E., Connors, H., Al-Dhalimy, M. *et al.* (2000). Purified hematopoietic stem cells can differentiate into hepatocytes in vivo. *Nature Medicine,* **6,** 1229–34.

Lehmann, R. & Ephrussi, A. (1994). Germ plasm formation and germ cell determination in Drosophila. *Ciba Foundation Symposium,* **182,** 282–96.

Lennon, D.P., Haynesworth, S.E., Young, R.G. *et al.* (1995). A chemically defined medium supports in vitro proliferation and maintains the osteochondral potential of rat marrow-derived mesenchymal stem cells. *Experimental Cell Research,* **219,** 211–22.

Li, A., Simmons, P.J., & Kaur, P. (1998). Identification and isolation of candidate human keratinocyte stem cells based on cell surface phenotype. *Proceedings of the National Academy of Sciences USA,* **95,** 3902–7.

Malouf, N.N., Coleman, W.B., Grisham, J.W. *et al.* (2001). Adult-derived stem cells from the liver become myocytes in the heart in vivo. *American journal of Pathology,* **158,** 1929–35.

Matsui, Y. (1998). Developmental fates of the mouse germ cell line. *International Journal of Developmental Biology,* **42,** 1037–42.

McKinney-Freeman, S.L., Jackson, K.A., Camargo, F.D. *et al.* (2002). Muscle-derived hematopoietic stem cells are hematopoietic in origin. *Proceedings of the National Academy of Sciences USA,* **99,** 1341–6.

Mezey, E., Chandross, K.J., Harta, G. *et al.* (2000). Turning blood into brain: cells bearing neuronal antigens generated in vivo from bone marrow. *Science,* **290,** 1779–82.

Mitaka, T. (2001). Hepatic stem cells: from bone marrow cells to hepatocytes. *Biochemical and Biophysical Research Communications,* **281,** 1–5.

Morshead, C.M., Benveniste, P., Iscove, N.N., & van der Kooy, D. (2002). Hematopoietic competence is a rare property of neural stem cells that may depend on genetic and epigenetic alterations. *Nature Medicine,* **8,** 268–73.

Odelberg, S.J., Kollhoff, A., & Keating, M.T. (2000). Dedifferentiation of mammalian myotubes induced by msx1. *Cell,* **103,** 1099–109.

Orlic, D., Kajstura, J., Chimenti, S. *et al.* (2001). Bone marrow cells regenerate infarcted myocardium. *Nature,* **410,** 701–5.

Patapoutian, A., Wold, B.J., & Wagner, R.A. (1995). Evidence for developmentally programmed transdifferentiation in mouse esophageal muscle. *Science,* **270,** 1818–21.

Pera, M.F., Reubinoff, B., & Trounson, A. (2000). Human embryonic stem cells. *Journal of Cell Science,* **113,** 5–10.

Petersen, B.E., Bowen, W.C., Patrene, K.D. *et al.* (1999). Bone marrow as a potential source of hepatic oval cells. *Science,* **284,** 1168–70.

Reubinoff, B.E., Pera, M.F., Fong, C.Y. *et al.* (2000). Embryonic stem cell lines from human blastocysts: somatic differentiation in vitro. *Nature Biotechnology,* **18,** 399–404.

Reyes, M., Dudek, A., Jahagirdar, B. *et al.* (2002). Origin of endothelial progenitors in human postnatal bone marrow. *The Journal of Clinical Investigation,* **109,** 337–46.

Reyes, M., Lund, T., Lenvik, T. *et al.* (2001). Purification and ex vivo expansion of postnatal human marrow mesodermal progenitor cells. *Blood,* **98,** 2615–25.

Sanchez-Ramos, J., Song, S., Cardozo-Pelaez, F. *et al.* (2000). Adult bone marrow stromal cells differentiate into neural cells in vitro. *Experimental Neurology,* **164,** 247–56.

Schwartz, R.E., Reyes, M., Koodie, L. *et al.* (2002). Multipotent adult progenitor cells from bone marrow differentiate into functional hepatocyte-like cells. *The Journal of Clinical Investigation,* **109,** 1291–302.

Seale, P., Sabourin, L.A., Girgis-Gabardo, A. *et al.* (2000). Pax7 is required for the specification of myogenic satellite cells. *Cell,* **102,** 777–86.

Shamblott, M.J., Axelman, J., Littlefield, J.W. *et al.* (2001). Human embryonic germ cell derivatives express a broad range of developmentally distinct markers and proliferate extensively in vitro. *Proceedings of the National Academy of Sciences USA,* **2,** 113–8.

Shen, C.N., Slack, J.M., & Tosh, D. (2000). Molecular basis of transdifferentiation of pancreas to liver. *National Cellular Biology,* **2,** 879–87.

Smith, A.G. (2001). Embryo-derived stem cells: of mice and men. *Annual Review of Cell and Developmental Biology,* **17,** 435–62.

Stratton, C.J., Bayguinov, Y., Sanders, K.M., & Ward, S.M. (2000). Ultrastructural analysis of the transdifferentiation of smooth muscle to skeletal muscle in the murine esophagus. *Cell and Tissue Research,* **301,** 283–98.

Suzuki, A., Zheng, Y.W., Kaneko, S. *et al.* (2002). Clonal identification and characterization of self-renewing pluripotent stem cells in the developing liver. *The Journal of Cell Biology,* **156,** 173–84.

Terada, N., Hamazaki, T., Oka, M. *et al.* (2002). Bone marrow cells adopt the phenotype of other cells by spontaneous cell fusion. *Nature,* **416,** 542–5.

Theise, N.D., Badve, S., Saxena, R. *et al.* (2000). Derivation of hepatocytes from bone marrow cells in mice after radiation-induced myeloablation. *Hepatology (Baltimore, Md.),* **31,** 235–40.

Toma, C., Pittenger, M.F., Cahill, K.S. *et al.* (2002). Human mesenchymal stem cells differentiate to a cardiomyocyte phenotype in the adult murine heart. *Circulation,* **105,** 93–8.

Toma, J.G., Akhavan, M., Fernandes, K.J. *et al.* (2001). Isolation of multipotent adult stem cells from the dermis of mammalian skin. *Nature Cell Biology,* **3,** 778–84.

Trounson, A. (2002). The genesis of embryonic stem cells. *Nature Biotechnology,* **20,** 237–8.

Trounson, A. & Pera, M. (2001). Human embryonic stem cells. *Fertility and Sterility,* **76,** 660–1.

Trounson, A.O. (2001). The derivation and potential use of human embryonic stem cells. *Reproduction, Fertility and Development,* **13,** 523–32.

Turner, A., Snape, A.M., Wylie, C.C., & Heasman, J. (1989). Regional identity is established before gastrulation in the Xenopus embryo. *The Journal of Experimental Zoology,* **251,** 245–52.

Wakitani, S., Saito, T., & Caplan, A.I. (1995). Myogenic cells derived from rat bone marrow mesenchymal stem cells exposed to 5-azacytidine. *Muscle & Nerve,* **18,** 1417–26.

Wei, G. & Mahowald, A.P. (1994). The germline: familiar and newly uncovered properties. *Annual Review of Genetics,* **28,** 309–24.

Woodbury, D., Schwarz, E.J., Prockop, D.J., & Black, I.B. (2000). Adult rat and human bone marrow stromal cells differentiate into neurons. *Journal of Neuroscience Research,* **61,** 364–70.

Ying, Q.L., Nichols, J., Evans, E.P., & Smith, A.G. (2002). Changing potency by spontaneous fusion. *Nature,* **416,** 545–8.

Zuk, P.A., Zhu, M., Mizuno, H. *et al.* (2001). Multilineage cells from human adipose tissue: implications for cell-based therapies. *Tissue Engineering,* **7,** 211–28.

8 Histocompatibility typing procedures for stem cell transplantation

G.M.TH. SCHREUDER, M. OUDSHOORN, AND F.H.J. CLAAS

Department of Immunohematology and Blood Transfusion, Leiden University Medical Centre and Europdonor Foundation, Leiden, The Netherlands

Introduction

Histocompatibility between the donor and the recipient plays an important role in the field of allogeneic bone marrow or blood stem cell transplantation. Over the past decade new techniques and approaches have been developed to improve histocompatibility testing in order to find the best matching donor. This chapter reviews the major histocompatibility complex (MHC), its structure, its polymorphism, and the typing techniques that are presently used.

The major histocompatibility complex

The human MHC consists of a cluster of genes located on the short arm of chromosome 6 (Figs. 8.1 and 8.2). The MHC consists of three classes of genes. The molecules encoded by the class I and class II genes are known to be highly polymorphic and are called the human leukocyte antigens (HLA). The HLA class I antigens are expressed on the cell surface of virtually all nucleated cells, whereas HLA class II antigens have a more restricted tissue distribution.

The primary function of these HLA molecules is to present foreign antigens or peptides to CD4[+] helper T cells (class II gene products) or CD8[+] cytotoxic T cells (class I gene products). This important role in the immune response has a major impact on the outcome of stem cell transplantation. Allogeneic MHC molecules are likely to be recognized as foreign and initiate a rejection or graft-versus-host reaction.

The class III region contains "non-HLA genes" such as the 21-hydroxylase gene and a number of others with immune response function, like C2, C4, BF, and TNF, and is located in between the class I and II regions. In this review, we will focus on class I and class II alleles and gene products (antigens) only.

HLA nomenclature

The WHO Nomenclature Committee for Factors of the HLA System provides the names of antigens (or HLA specificities), the alleles, the genes, and the loci at which the genes are located (Bodmer *et al.*, 1997; Marsh *et al.*, 2002). Updates are

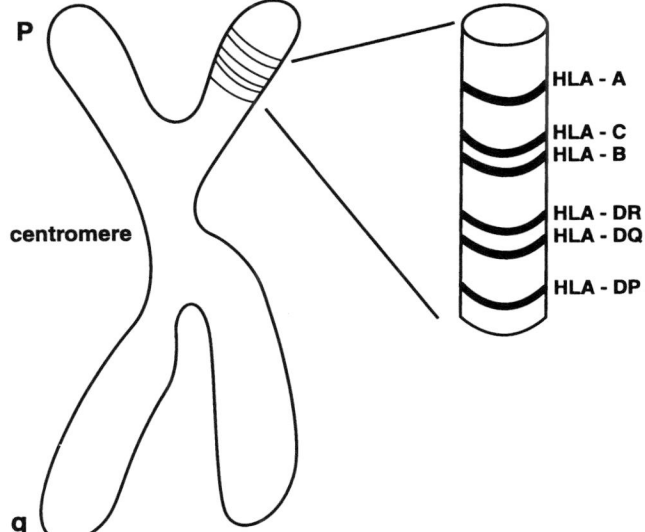

Fig. 8.1. Human chromosome 6 in metaphase.

published regularly, which provide names for newly identified genes and alleles. Originally, the HLA antigens were identified by serological methods, but now their encoding alleles are identified by molecular techniques that determine the nucleotide sequence of an HLA gene, while serology defines antigenic determinants (epitopes) on the HLA gene product (i.e., the HLA glycoprotein molecule) (see below).

The following nomenclature system is used (Table 8.1)

1. HLA class I loci are indicated by capital letters: HLA-A, -B, -C, -E, -F, etc. The HLA class I antigens or specificities, as defined by serological methods, are identified by a number after the locus designation (e.g., HLA-A2, HLA-B7, HLA-Cwl) (Table 8.2). The "w" from "workshop" in the C locus names originally indicated a provisional name but has been retained to distinguish the C locus products from complement factors. For transplantation purposes only the HLA-A, -B, and -C class I loci are taken into account.

2. The HLA class II region contains a number of similar genes, some of which are pseudo-genes. For historical reasons

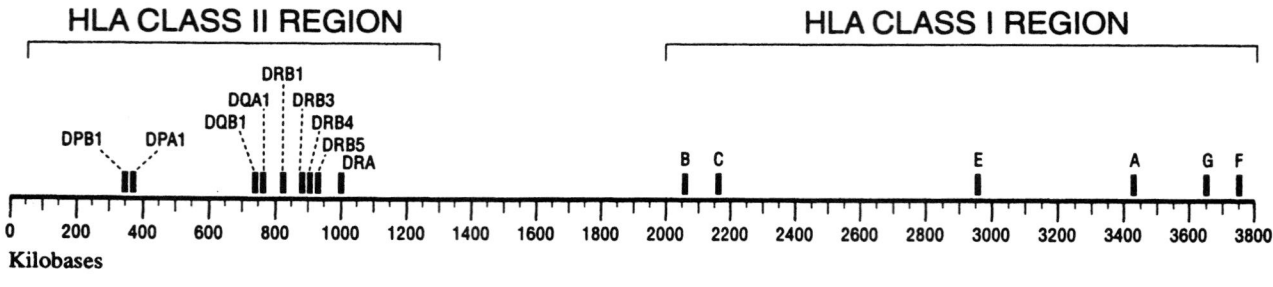

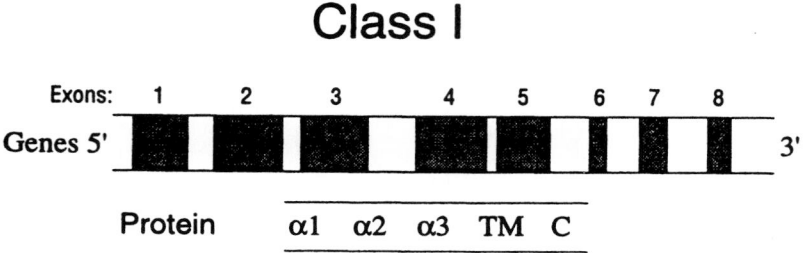

Fig. 8.2. The HLA system indicating the relative location of the class I and class II genes (**A**), the exon-intron organization of a class I gene (panel *1B*), and the protein encoded by a class I gene (**B**). TM indicates transmembrane domain; C indicates intracytoplasmic domain; and α1, α2, α3 indicate the extracellular domains of the class I protein. Reproduced, with permission, from O'Reilly *et al.* (1996).

the HLA class II region was called HLA-D and its products DR (D-related), hence the prefix "D" for the name of the class II region loci: DRA, DRB1, DRB3, DQA1, DQB1, DPB1, etc., where A or B indicates whether the gene encodes an alpha or a beta chain, respectively, and 1, 2, and 3 etc. indicate high similarity. The class II antigens are indicated by a two-letter code followed by a number: DR1, DR2, DR3, DQ1, DQ2, DR51, DR52, etc. (see Table 8.2).

3. HLA genes are highly polymorphic and each gene has many different alleles in a population. Alleles are designated by an asterisk (*) followed by a two-digit number indicating the most closely associated serologic specificity, followed by another two-digit number that defines a unique allele (identified by molecular techniques). For example, the serologically defined HLA-A2 specificity can be encoded by over 58 distinct alleles. These alleles are defined as HLA-A*0201 through HLA-A*0258. Therefore, HLA-A2 is a broad serologic specificity, but HLA-A*0201 is a unique allele whose protein product reacts with the antibody that is used to identify HLA-A2.

4. If alleles differ by a single nucleotide substitution but the amino acid sequence remains the same (silent substitution), two more digits (previously one digit) can be added as in HLA-Cw*020201 and HLA-Cw*020202.

5. For some alleles polymorphism is identified outside exon-2 and -3 (see below). This is indicated by adding a seventh and eighth digit (B*15170101 and B*15170102).

6. Some alleles contain mutations, which cause abnormal expression of the antigenic molecules. This is indicated by, respectively, N (nonexpressed or Null alleles: e.g., A*2409N, A*29020102N), L (low expression: e.g., A*24020102L), S

Table 8.1. *Rules for HLA nomenclature*

Nomenclature	Indication
HLA	Human leukocyte antigens: prefix for all HLA loci, genes, alleles, and antigens
HLA-A	A particular HLA locus: i.e., A
HLA-A9, A23(9)	The HLA-A9 broad antigen and its A23 split antigen
HLA-A*02	A group of HLA-A alleles that encode the A2 antigen
HLA-A*0201	A specific allele name
HLA-A*0215N	A null allele
HLA-A*020101, A*020102	A*0201 alleles that differ only by silent substitution and encode the same A2 antigen
HLA-A*24020102L	A*2402 allele that contains a mutation outside exon-2 and -3, causing low expression of the A24 antigen; may also be written as A*2402L
HLA-B*44020102S	B*4402 allele with a mutation, which prevents expression on the cell surface and causing only a soluble B44 molecule; may also be written as B*4402S

Table 8.2. *Complete listing of recognized serological and cellular HLA specificities*

A	B	C	D	DR	DQ	DP
A1	B5	Cw1	Dw1	DR1	DQ1	DPw1
A2	B7	Cw2	Dw2	DR103	DQ2	DPw2
A203	B703	Cw3	Dw3	DR2	DQ3	DPw3
A210	B8	Cw4	Dw4	DR3	DQ4	DPw4
A3	B12	Cw5	Dw5	DR4	DQ5(1)	DPw5
A9	B13	Cw6	Dw6	DR5	DQ6(1)	DPw6
A10	B14	Cw7	Dw7	DR6	DQ7(3)	
A11	B15	Cw8	Dw8	DR7	DQ8(3)	
A19	B16	Cw9(w3)	Dw9	DR8	DQ9(3)	
A23(9)	B17	Cw10(w3)	Dw10	DR9		
A24(9)	B18		Dw11(w7)	DR10		
A2403	B21		Dw12	DR11(5)		
A25(10)	B22		Dw13	DR12(5)		
A26(10)	B27		Dw14	DR13(6)		
A28	B2708		Dw15	DR14(6)		
A29(19)	B35		Dw16	DR1403		
A30(19)	B37		Dw17(w7)	DR1404		
A31(19)	B38(16)		Dw18(w6)	DR15(2)		
A32(19)	B39(16)		Dw19(w6)	DR16(2)		
A33(19)	B3901		Dw20	DR17(3)		
A34(10)	B3902		Dw21	DR18(3)		
A36	B40		Dw22			
A43	B4005		Dw23	DR51		
A66(10)	B41		Dw24	DR52		
A68(28)	B42		Dw25	DR53		
A69(28)	B44(12)		Dw26			
A74(19)	B45(12)					
A80	B46					
	B47					
	B48					
	B49(21)					
	B50(21)					
	B51(5)					
	B5102					
	B5103					
	B52(5)					
	B53					
	B54(22)					
	B55(22)					
	B56(22)					
	B57(17)					
	B58(17)					
	B59					
	B60(40)					
	B61(40)					
	B62(15)					
	B63(15)					
	B64(14)					
	B65(14)					
	B67					
	B70					
	B71(70)					
	B72(70)					
	B73					
	B75(15)					
	B76(15)					
	B77(15)					
	B78					
	B81					
	Bw4					
	Bw6					

Reproduced, with permission, from Bodmer *et al.* (1997).

(soluble antigen, lacking the cell membrane bound form: e.g., B*44020102S), and A (aberrant, where absence or presence of the molecule has not yet been defined). For practical reasons groups of alleles can be designated by two digits (low resolution, e.g., A*02), and 4 digits (high resolution, e.g., Cw*0401), if needed, extended by an expression indicator (e.g., A*2402L, DRB4*0103N). Guidelines for nomenclature usage have been published recently (Tiercy *et al.*, 2002).

7. Several broad serologic specificities were split on the basis of the reactivity of more specific antibodies: for example, the A9 broad specificity was split into A23 and A24, and B5 into B51 and B52. The name of the broad antigen can be included in parentheses after the name of the split (e.g., A23(9), B51(5)). Later, associated antigens were defined by serological patterns that were thought to be expressed by single allelic products [e.g., A203 encoded by A*0203, A2403 by A*2403, DR103 encoded by DRB1*0103 (Table 8.3)]. As only a few laboratories were able to distinguish these associated antigens from their broad specificities, these names have hardly been used.

The region on an HLA molecule that an antibody recognizes is termed an *epitope*. There are two general types of HLA epitopes, private epitopes and public epitopes. Private epitopes occur only on a single gene product, for example, HLA-A1, and thus distinguish the HLA specificities. Public epitopes are common to more than one gene product. Examples are the high-frequency public epitopes Bw4 and Bw6, which are present on almost all HLA-B specificities, and similar sequences can also be found on some HLA-A specificities.

Antibodies that bind or cross-react with more than one HLA specificity have been used to place HLA gene products into major cross-reactive groups (CREGs). A list of cross-reacting groups at HLA-A and -B loci is given in Table 8.4.

Table 8.3. *Examples of HLA-A and-B broad specificities, splits, and associated antigens*

Broad specificities	Splits	Associated antigens
A2		A203, A210
A9	A23, A24	A2403
A10	A25, A26, A34, A66	
A19	A29, A30, A31, A32, A33, A74	
A28	A68, A69	
B5	B51, B52	B5102, B5103
B7		B703
B12	B44, B45	
B14	B64, B65	
B15	B62, B63, B75, B76, B77	
B16	B38, B39	B3901, B3902
B17	B57, B58	
B21	B49, B50	
B22	B54, B55, B56	
B27		B2708
B40	B60, B61	B4005
B70	B71, B72	

Table 8.4. *Examples of cross-reacting groups (CREGs) at HLA-A and HLA-B loci*

A locus

1.	A1	A3	A11	A36		
2.	A9	A23	A24			
3.	A10	A25	A26	A34	A66	A43
4.	A19	A29	A30	A31	A32	A33 A74
5.	A2	A28	A68	A69		

B locus

1.	B5	B18	B35	B51	B52	B53	B70	B71	B72
2.	B12	B21	B44	B45	B49	B50			
3.	B14	B64	B65						
4.	B8	B59							
5.	B15	B17	B46	B57	B58	B62	B63	B70	B71 B72
	B75	B76	B77						
6.	B16	B38	B39	B67					
7.	B37								
8.	B7	B27	B42	B73					
9.	B7	B22	B54	B55	B56	B67			
10.	B7	B40	B41	B48	B60	B61			
11.	B13	B47							

Genetics of the HLA system

HLA class I genes and molecules (Table 8.5)

The class I region contains between 20 and 30 genes, many of them being pseudo-genes (genes for which no mRNA or protein product has been detected). HLA-A, HLA-B, and HLA-C genes are the only class I genes so far identified as having an expressed product on virtually all nucleated cells. These products are glycoprotein molecules expressed on the cell surface membrane in association with β2-microglobulin, a nonpolymorphic invariant chain encoded by a gene located on chromosome 15. Figure 8.3 shows the organization of a class I gene and its relationship to the expressed product. The gene's exons correspond to distinct regions of the glycoprotein molecule, such as the extracellular, transmembrane, and intracellular domains. The hypervariable (or polymorphic) region of the class I molecule is largely restricted to the first two domains of the extracellular region. Parts of the domains form two alpha helices that, together with a beta-pleated sheet, form a cleft of an appropriate size to bind a 9 to 11 amino acid fragment (peptide) of a foreign antigen for presentation to cytotoxic T cells. The three-dimensional structure of a class I molecule (HLA-A2) was first elucidated by Bjorkman *et al.* (1987) using X-ray crystallography (Fig. 8.4).

HLA class II genes and molecules (Table 8.6)

HLA class II molecules are expressed only on B lymphocytes, activated T lymphocytes, endothelial cells, macrophages, dendritic cells, and a few other cell types. Class II molecules comprise two glycosylated polypeptide chains that are noncovalently bound. These heterodimers consist of an alpha chain and a beta chain. The DRA, DQA1, or DPA1 genes, of which DRA

is not polymorphic, encode the alpha chain. The beta chain is encoded by DRB, DQB1, or DPB1 genes, which are all highly polymorphic (Fig. 8.5). Both classes of HLA molecules have a similar three-dimensional structure with a similar typical cleft (Brown *et al.*, 1993). The cleft of the class II molecules is able to bind peptides for presentation to CD4+ helper T cells. It is open ended, which enables binding of peptides longer than 11 amino acids (Fig. 8.6). Other genes in the class II region, such as TAP1, TAP2, PSMB8 (previously LMP7), and PSMB9 (previously LMP2), play an important role in the processing and expression of HLA class I molecules.

Polymorphism of the HLA system

Polymorphism refers to the presence of more than one allele of a gene. Based on nucleotide sequences, an ever-increasing number of alleles is being identified (Fig. 8.7), the names of which are regularly published in the HLA Nomenclature Reports (Marsh *et al.*, 2002) and updates of DNA nucleotide sequences and corresponding amino acid sequences of all alleles are available every 3 months at the IMGT/HLA database (Robinson & Marsh, 2001; www.ebi.ac.uk/imgt/hla/). Many different alleles can express the same serologic equivalent of HLA specificities. For instance, the product of most HLA-A*02 alleles reacts with anti-HLA-A2 specific antibodies including monoclonal antibodies. All officially known HLA antigens were listed in the 1996 HLA Nomenclature report (Bodmer *et al.*, 1997), and are shown in Table 8.2. For all frequently occurring alleles the serologic equivalents are known, but for many rare and newly identified alleles these equivalents are not available. The HLA dictionary for serology to DNA equivalents presents all alleles with their expressed antigen if at all known, and is regularly updated (Schreuder *et al.*, 2001). For some alleles the expressed antigens are known to be clearly different from any of the well-defined antigens. This complicates the search for a suitable donor once such an allele has been identified in a potential transplant recipient. Disparities between HLA sequence polymorphisms that are serologically detectable are termed *antigen mismatches,* whereas those that can be identified only by DNA-based typing methods are termed *allele mismatches.*

Allelic products with the same serologic specificity do not always have the same effect in functional tests. For example, DRB1*0401 and DRB1*0404 alleles, encoding the serologically defined DR4 specificity, will result in a reactive mixed lymphocyte culture (MLC) indicating a class II mismatch, if expressed on stimulator and responder cell populations. On the other hand, different alleles encoding molecules with the same serologic reactivity can be functionally identical, for example, CTL precursors were not detectable in combinations that only differed for Cw*0303 and Cw*0304 (Oudshoorn *et al.*, 2002). Probably these allelic differences do not affect the three-dimensional structure of the peptide-binding region of the HLA molecule. To test the hypothesis that allele mismatches that are detectable only at the DNA level are less immunogenic than those that are serologically detectable, Petersdorf *et al.* (2001)

Table 8.5. *Full list of HLA Class I alleles assigned as of October 2002 (from Marsh et al., 2002)*

HLA-A

A*010101	A*021701	A*0253N	A*2303	A*2429	A*2906	A*3404	A*7402
A*010102	A*021702	A*0254	A*2304	A*2430	A*2907	A*3601	A*7403
A*0102	A*0218	A*0255	A*2305	A*2431	A*3001	A*3602	A*7404
A*0103	A*0219	A*0256	A*2306	A*2432	A*3002	A*3603	A*7405
A*0104N	A*022001	A*0257	A*2307N	A*2433	A*3003	A*3604	A*7406
A*0106	A*022002	A*0258	A*2308N	A*2434	A*3004	A*4301	A*7407
A*0107	A*0221	A*0259	A*2309	A*2435	A*3006	A*6601	A*7408
A*0108	A*0222	A*0260	A*24020101	A*2436N	A*3007	A*6602	A*7409
A*0109	A*0224	A*030101	A*24020102L	A*2437	A*3008	A*6603	A*8001
A*020101	A*0225	A*030102	A*240202	A*2501	A*3009	A*6604	
A*020102	A*0226	A*030103	A*240203	A*2502	A*3010	A*680101	
A*020103	A*0227	A*0302	A*240204	A*2503	A*3011	A*680102	
A*020104	A*0228	A*0303N	A*240301	A*2504	A*3012	A*6802	
A*020105	A*0229	A*0304	A*240302	A*2601	A*310102	A*680301	
A*020106	A*0230	A*0305	A*2404	A*2602	A*3102	A*680302	
A*020107	A*0231	A*0306	A*2405	A*2603	A*3103	A*6804	
A*020108	A*0232N	A*0307	A*2406	A*2604	A*3104	A*6805	
A*0202	A*0233	A*0308	A*2407	A*2605	A*3105	A*6806	
A*0203	A*0234	A*0309	A*2408	A*2606	A*3106	A*6807	
A*0204	A*0235	A*0310	A*2409N	A*2607	A*3107	A*6808	
A*0205	A*0236	A*110101	A*2410	A*2608	A*3108	A*6809	
A*0206	A*0237	A*110102	A*2411N	A*2609	A*3109	A*6810	
A*0207	A*0238	A*1102	A*2413	A*2610	A*3201	A*6811N	
A*0208	A*0239	A*1103	A*2414	A*2611N	A*3202	A*6812	
A*0209	A*0240	A*1104	A*2415	A*2612	A*3203	A*6813	
A*0210	A*0241	A*1105	A*2417	A*2613	A*3204	A*6814	
A*0211	A*0242	A*1106	A*2418	A*2614	A*3205	A*6815	
A*0212	A*0243N	A*1107	A*2419	A*2615	A*3206	A*6816	
A*0213	A*0244	A*1108	A*2420	A*2616	A*3207	A*6817	
A*0214	A*0245	A*1109	A*2421	A*2617	A*3208	A*6818N	
A*0215N	A*0246	A*1110	A*2422	A*2618	A*3209	A*6819	
A*0216	A*0247	A*1111	A*2423	A*29010101	A*3301	A*6820	
	A*0248	A*1112	A*2424	A*29010102	A*3303	A*6821	
	A*0249	A*1113	A*2425	A*2902	A*3304	A*6822	
	A*0250	A*1114	A*2426	A*2903	A*3305	A*6823	
	A*0251	A*2301	A*2427	A*2904	A*3306	A*6901	
	A*0252	A*2302	A*2428	A*2905	A*3401	A*7401	
					A*3402		
					A*3403		

HLA-B

B*070201	B*0801	B*150103	B*1536	B*180102
B*070202	B*0802	B*150104	B*1537	B*1802
B*070203	B*0803	B*1502	B*1538	B*1803
B*0703	B*0804	B*1503	B*1539	B*1804
B*0704	B*0805	B*1504	B*1540	B*1805
B*0705	B*0806	B*1505	B*1542	B*1806
B*0706	B*0807	B*1506	B*1543	B*1807
B*0707	B*0808N	B*1507	B*1544	B*1808
B*0708	B*0809	B*1508	B*1545	B*1809
B*0709	B*0810	B*1509	B*1546	B*1810
B*0710	B*0811	B*1510	B*1547	B*1811
B*0711	B*0812	B*151101	B*1548	B*1812
B*0712	B*0813	B*151102	B*1549	B*1813
B*0713	B*0814	B*1512	B*1550	B*1814
B*0714	B*0815	B*1513	B*1551	B*1815
B*0715	B*0816	B*1514	B*1552	B*1817N
B*0716	B*0817	B*1515	B*1553	B*1818
B*0717	B*1301	B*1516	B*1554	B*2701
B*0718	B*1302	B*15170101	B*1555	B*2702
B*0719	B*1303	B*15170102	B*1556	B*2703
B*0720	B*1304	B*1518	B*1557	B*2704
B*0721	B*1306	B*1519	B*1558	B*270502
B*0722	B*1307N	B*1520	B*1560	B*270503
B*0723	B*1308	B*1521	B*1561	B*270504
B*0724	B*1309	B*1523	B*1562	B*270505
B*0725	B*1310	B*1524	B*1563	B*270506
B*0726	B*1311	B*1525	B*1564	B*2706
B*0727	B*1401	B*1526N	B*1565	B*2707
B*0728	B*1402	B*1527	B*1566	B*2708
B*0729	B*1403	B*1528	B*1567	B*2709
B*0730	B*1404	B*1529	B*1568	B*2710
B*0731	B*1405	B*1530	B*1569	B*2711
	B*140601	B*1531	B*1570	B*2712
	B*140602	B*1532	B*1571	B*2713
	B*15010101	B*1533	B*1572	B*2714
	B*15010102N	B*1534	B*1573	B*2715
	B*150102	B*1535	B*180101	B*2716

B*2717	B*3528	B*3903	B*4010	B*4105	B*4430	B*5104	B*5302	B*5705
B*2718	B*3529	B*3904	B*4011	B*4106	B*4431	B*5105	B*5303	B*5706
B*2719	B*3530	B*3905	B*4012	B*4201	B*4432	B*5106	B*5304	B*5707
B*2720	B*3531	B*390601	B*4013	B*4202	B*4501	B*5107	B*5305	B*5708
B*2721	B*3532	B*390602	B*4014	B*4204	B*4502	B*5108	B*5306	B*5709
B*2723	B*3533	B*3907	B*4015	B*44020101	B*4503	B*5109	B*5307	B*5801
B*2724	B*3534	B*3908	B*4016	B*44020102S	B*4504	B*5110	B*5308	B*5802
B*2725	B*3535	B*3909	B*4018	B*440202	B*4505	B*5111N	B*5309	B*5804
B*350101	B*3536	B*3910	B*4019	B*440203	B*4506	B*5112	B*5401	B*5805
B*350102	B*3537	B*3911	B*4020	B*440301	B*4601	B*511301	B*5402	B*5806
B*3502	B*3538	B*3912	B*4021	B*440302	B*4602	B*511302	B*5501	B*5901
B*3503	B*3539	B*3913	B*4022N	B*4404	B*47010101	B*5114	B*5502	B*670101
B*3504	B*3540N	B*3914	B*4023	B*4405	B*47010102	B*5115	B*5503	B*670102
B*3505	B*3541	B*3915	B*4024	B*4406	B*4702	B*5116	B*5504	B*6702
B*3506	B*3542	B*3916	B*4025	B*4407	B*4703	B*5117	B*5505	B*7301
B*3507	B*3543	B*3917	B*4026	B*4408	B*4704	B*5118	B*5507	B*7801
B*3508	B*3544	B*3918	B*4027	B*4409	B*4801	B*5119	B*5508	B*780201
B*350901	B*3701	B*3919	B*4028	B*4410	B*4803	B*5120	B*5509	B*780202
B*350902	B*3702	B*3920	B*4029	B*4411	B*4804	B*5121	B*5510	B*7803
B*3510	B*3703N	B*3922	B*4030	B*4412	B*4805	B*5122	B*5511	B*7804
B*3511	B*3704	B*3923	B*4031	B*4413	B*4806	B*5123	B*5512	B*7805
B*3512	B*3705	B*3924	B*4032	B*4414	B*4807	B*5124	B*5601	B*8101
B*3513	B*3801	B*3925N	B*4033	B*4415	B*4901	B*5126	B*5602	B*8201
B*3514	B*380201	B*3926	B*4034	B*4416	B*4902	B*5127N	B*5603	B*8202
B*3515	B*380202	B*3927	B*4035	B*4417	B*4903	B*5128	B*5604	B*8301
B*3516	B*3803	B*400101	B*4036	B*4418	B*5001	B*5129	B*5605	
B*3517	B*3804	B*400102	B*4037	B*4419N	B*5002	B*5130	B*5606	
B*3518	B*3805	B*400103	B*4038	B*4420	B*5004	B*5131	B*5607	
B*3519	B*3806	B*4002	B*4039	B*4421	B*510101	B*5132	B*5608	
B*3520	B*3807	B*4003	B*4040	B*4422	B*510102	B*520101	B*5609	
B*3521	B*3808	B*4004	B*4042	B*4423N	B*510103	B*520102	B*5610	
B*3522	B*3809	B*4005	B*4043	B*4424	B*510104	B*520103	B*570101	
B*3523	B*390101	B*40060101	B*4044	B*4425	B*510105	B*5202	B*570102	
B*3524	B*390103	B*40060102	B*4101	B*4426	B*510201	B*5203	B*5702	
B*3525	B*390104	B*4007	B*4102	B*4427	B*510202	B*5204	B*570301	
B*3526	B*390201	B*4008	B*4103	B*4428	B*5103	B*5205	B*570302	
B*3527	B*390202	B*4009	B*4104	B*4429		B*5301	B*5704	

HLA-C

Cw*0102	Cw*0314	Cw*0708	Cw*150202
Cw*0103	Cw*0315	Cw*0709	Cw*1503
Cw*0104	Cw*0316	Cw*0710	Cw*1504
Cw*0105	Cw*04010101	Cw*0711	Cw*150501
Cw*0106	Cw*04010102	Cw*0712	Cw*150502
Cw*0107	Cw*040102	Cw*0713	Cw*1506
Cw*0108	Cw*0403	Cw*0714	Cw*1507
Cw*0109	Cw*0404	Cw*0715	Cw*1508
Cw*020201	Cw*0405	Cw*0716	Cw*1509
Cw*020202	Cw*0406	Cw*0717	Cw*1510
Cw*020203	Cw*0407	Cw*080101	Cw*1511
Cw*020204	Cw*0408	Cw*080102	Cw*1601
Cw*020205	Cw*0409N	Cw*0802	Cw*160401
Cw*0203	Cw*0410	Cw*0803	Cw*1701
Cw*0204	Cw*0501	Cw*0804	Cw*1702
Cw*0205	Cw*0502	Cw*0805	Cw*1703
Cw*030201	Cw*0503	Cw*0806	Cw*1801
Cw*030202	Cw*0504	Cw*0807	Cw*1802
Cw*030301	Cw*0505	Cw*0808	
Cw*030302	Cw*0506	Cw*0809	
Cw*030303	Cw*0602	Cw*120201	
Cw*030401	Cw*0603	Cw*120202	
Cw*030402	Cw*0604	Cw*120203	
Cw*0305	Cw*0605	Cw*120301	
Cw*0306	Cw*0606	Cw*120302	
Cw*0307	Cw*0607	Cw*120401	
Cw*0308	Cw*0608	Cw*120402	
Cw*0309	Cw*070101	Cw*1205	
Cw*0310	Cw*070102	Cw*1206	
Cw*0311	Cw*07020101	Cw*1207	
Cw*0312	Cw*07020102	Cw*1208	
Cw*0313	Cw*0703	Cw*140201	
	Cw*070401	Cw*140202	
	Cw*070402	Cw*1403	
	Cw*0705	Cw*1404	
	Cw*0706	Cw*1405	
	Cw*0707	Cw*150201	

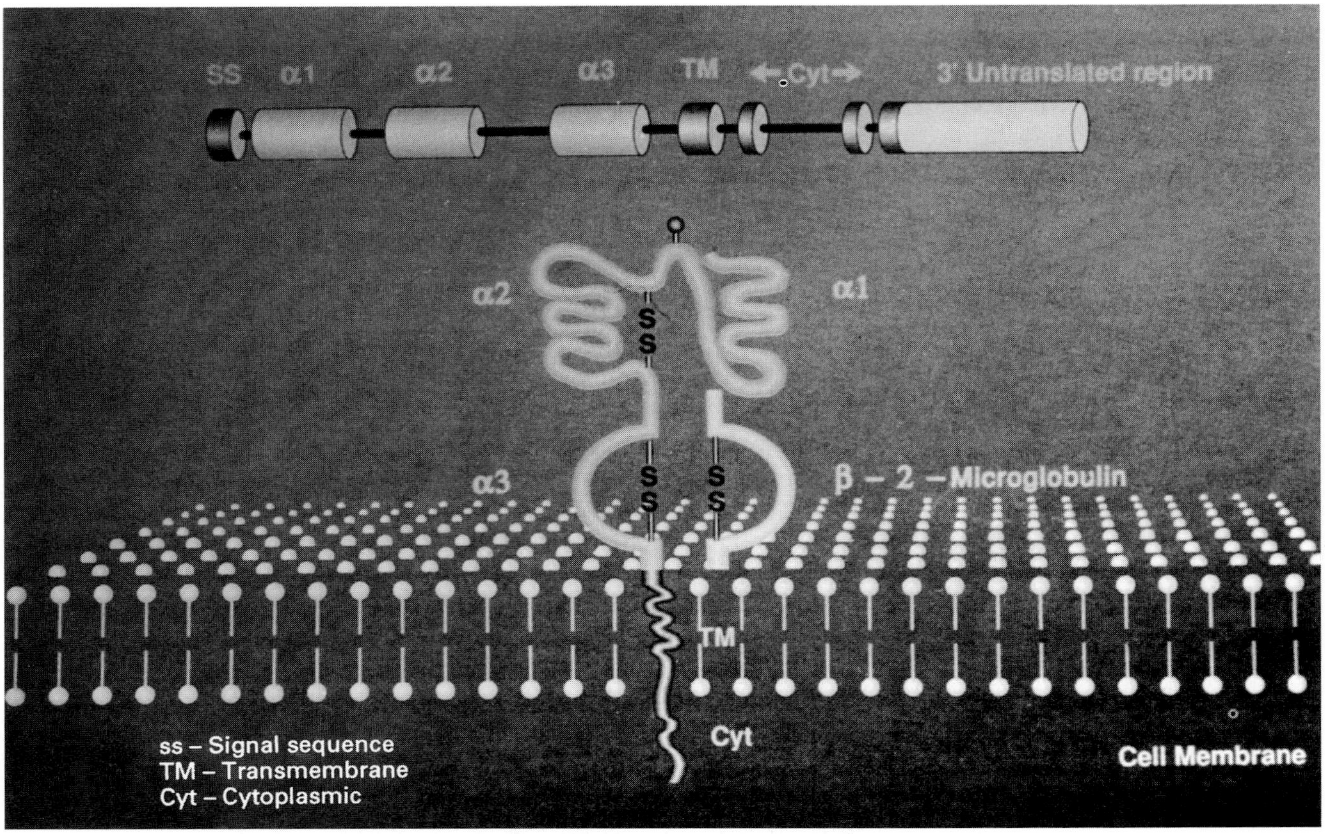

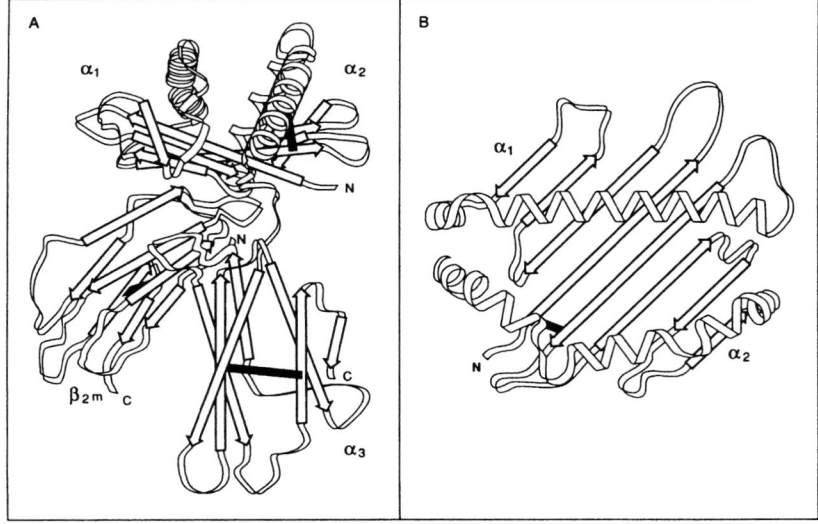

Fig. 8.3. Organization of class I genes and corresponding domains on class I molecules. Reproduced, with permission, from Tait (1990).

Fig. 8.4. Polypeptide folding pattern of a human class I MHC molecule. Panel **A** shows a side view and Panel **B** depicts a top view, revealing the peptide-binding cleft. The white arrows represent polypeptide folded as β-pleated sheet, the white coils represent polypeptide folded as α-helix, and the black bars represent disulfide bonds. Adapted, with permission, from Bjorkman *et al.* (1987).

Table 8.6. *Full list of HLA Class II alleles assigned as of October 2002 (from Marsh et al., 2002)*

HLA-DRA	HLA-DRB1						
DRA*0101	DRB1*010101	DRB1*0319	DRB1*0427	DRB1*0807	DRB1*1111	DRB1*120201	DRB1*1325
DRA*010201	DRB1*010102	DRB1*0320	DRB1*0428	DRB1*0808	DRB1*111201	DRB1*120202	DRB1*1326
DRA*010202	DRB1*010201	DRB1*0321	DRB1*0429	DRB1*0809	DRB1*111202	DRB1*120302	DRB1*1327
	DRB1*010202	DRB1*0322	DRB1*0430	DRB1*0810	DRB1*1113	DRB1*1204	DRB1*1328
	DRB1*0103	DRB1*0323	DRB1*0431	DRB1*0811	DRB1*1114	DRB1*1205	DRB1*1329
	DRB1*0104	DRB1*040101	DRB1*0432	DRB1*0812	DRB1*1115	DRB1*1206	DRB1*1330
	DRB1*0105	DRB1*040102	DRB1*0433	DRB1*0813	DRB1*1116	DRB1*1207	DRB1*1331
	DRB1*0106	DRB1*0402	DRB1*0434	DRB1*0814	DRB1*1117	DRB1*1208	DRB1*1332
	DRB1*0107	DRB1*040301	DRB1*0435	DRB1*0815	DRB1*1118	DRB1*130101	DRB1*1333
	DRB1*0108	DRB1*040302	DRB1*0436	DRB1*0816	DRB1*1119	DRB1*130102	DRB1*1334
	DRB1*0109	DRB1*0404	DRB1*0437	DRB1*0817	DRB1*1120	DRB1*130201	DRB1*1335
	DRB1*030101	DRB1*040501	DRB1*0438	DRB1*0818	DRB1*1121	DRB1*130202	DRB1*1336
	DRB1*030102	DRB1*040502	DRB1*0439	DRB1*0819	DRB1*1122	DRB1*130301	DRB1*1337
	DRB1*030201	DRB1*040503	DRB1*0440	DRB1*0820	DRB1*1123	DRB1*130302	DRB1*1338
	DRB1*030202	DRB1*040504	DRB1*0441	DRB1*0821	DRB1*1124	DRB1*1304	DRB1*1339
	DRB1*0303	DRB1*0406	DRB1*0442	DRB1*0822	DRB1*1125	DRB1*1305	DRB1*1340
	DRB1*0304	DRB1*040701	DRB1*0443	DRB1*0823	DRB1*1126	DRB1*1306	DRB1*1341
	DRB1*030501	DRB1*040702	DRB1*0444	DRB1*0824	DRB1*112701	DRB1*130701	DRB1*1342
	DRB1*030502	DRB1*0408	DRB1*070101	DRB1*090102	DRB1*112702	DRB1*130702	DRB1*1343
	DRB1*0306	DRB1*0409	DRB1*070102	DRB1*0902	DRB1*1128	DRB1*1308	DRB1*1344
	DRB1*0307	DRB1*0410	DRB1*0703	DRB1*100101	DRB1*1129	DRB1*1309	DRB1*1345
	DRB1*0308	DRB1*0411	DRB1*0704	DRB1*100102	DRB1*1130	DRB1*1310	DRB1*1346
	DRB1*0309	DRB1*0412	DRB1*0705	DRB1*110101	DRB1*1131	DRB1*1311	DRB1*1347
	DRB1*0310	DRB1*0413	DRB1*0706	DRB1*110102	DRB1*1132	DRB1*1312	DRB1*1348
	DRB1*0311	DRB1*0414	DRB1*0707	DRB1*110103	DRB1*1133	DRB1*1313	DRB1*1349
	DRB1*0312	DRB1*0415	DRB1*080101	DRB1*110104	DRB1*1134	DRB1*13140	DRB1*1350
	DRB1*0313	DRB1*0416	DRB1*080102	DRB1*1102	DRB1*1135	DRB1*13140	DRB1*1351
	DRB1*0314	DRB1*0417	DRB1*080201	DRB1*1103	DRB1*1136	DRB1*1315	DRB1*1352
	DRB1*0315	DRB1*0418	DRB1*080202	DRB1*110401	DRB1*1137	DRB1*1316	DRB1*1353
	DRB1*0316	DRB1*0419	DRB1*080203	DRB1*110402	DRB1*1138	DRB1*1317	DRB1*1354
	DRB1*0317	DRB1*0420	DRB1*080302	DRB1*1105	DRB1*1139	DRB1*1318	DRB1*140101
	DRB1*0318	DRB1*0421	DRB1*080401	DRB1*1106	DRB1*1140	DRB1*1319	DRB1*140102
		DRB1*0422	DRB1*080402	DRB1*1107	DRB1*1141	DRB1*1320	DRB1*1402
		DRB1*0423	DRB1*080403	DRB1*110801	DRB1*1142	DRB1*1321	DRB1*1403
		DRB1*0424	DRB1*080404	DRB1*110802	DRB1*1143	DRB1*1322	DRB1*1404
		DRB1*0425	DRB1*0805	DRB1*1109	DRB1*120101	DRB1*1323	DRB1*140501
		DRB1*0426	DRB1*0806	DRB1*1110	DRB1*120102	DRB1*1324	DRB1*140502

		HLA-DRB2-9		HLA-DQA1		HLA-DQB1	HLA-DPA1
DRB1*1406	DRB1*1442	DRB2*0101	DRB3*0215	DQA1*010101	DQB1*0603	DQB1*0201	DPA1*010301
DRB1*140701	DRB1*1443	DRB3*010101	DRB3*0216	DQA1*010102	DQB1*060401	DQB1*0202	DPA1*010302
DRB1*140702	DRB1*1444	DRB3*01010201	DRB3*0217	DQA1*010201	DQB1*060402	DQB1*0203	DPA1*0104
DRB1*1408	DRB1*1445	DRB3*01010202	DRB3*030101	DQA1*010202	DQB1*060501	DQB1*030101	DPA1*0105
DRB1*1409	DRB1*150101	DRB3*010103	DRB3*030102	DQA1*0103	DQB1*060502	DQB1*030102	DPA1*0106
DRB1*1410	DRB1*150102	DRB3*010104	DRB3*0302	DQA1*010401	DQB1*0606	DQB1*0302	DPA1*0107
DRB1*1411	DRB1*150103	DRB3*0102	DRB3*0303	DQA1*010402	DQB1*0607	DQB1*030302	DPA1*0108
DRB1*1412	DRB1*150104	DRB3*0103	DRB4*010101	DQA1*0105	DQB1*0608	DQB1*030303	DPA1*020101
DRB1*1413	DRB1*150201	DRB3*0104	DRB4*010102	DQA1*0106	DQB1*0609	DQB1*0304	DPA1*020102
DRB1*1414	DRB1*150202	DRB3*0105	DRB4*01030101	DQA1*0201	DQB1*0610	DQB1*030501	DPA1*020103
DRB1*1415	DRB1*150203	DRB3*0106	DRB4*01030102N	DQA1*030101	DQB1*061101	DQB1*030502	DPA1*020104
DRB1*1416	DRB1*1503	DRB3*0107	DRB4*010302	DQA1*0302	DQB1*061102	DQB1*0306	DPA1*020105
DRB1*1417	DRB1*1504	DRB3*0108	DRB4*010303	DQA1*0303	DQB1*0612	DQB1*0307	DPA1*020106
DRB1*1418	DRB1*1505	DRB3*0109	DRB4*010304	DQA1*0401	DQB1*0613	DQB1*0308	DPA1*020201
DRB1*1419	DRB1*1506	DRB3*0110	DRB4*0104	DQA1*050101	DQB1*0614	DQB1*0309	DPA1*020202
DRB1*1420	DRB1*1507	DRB3*0201	DRB4*0105	DQA1*050102	DQB1*0615	DQB1*0310	DPA1*020203
DRB1*1421	DRB1*1508	DRB3*020201	DRB4*0106	DQA1*0502	DQB1*0616	DQB1*0311	DPA1*0203
DRB1*1422	DRB1*1509	DRB3*020202	DRB4*0201N	DQA1*0503	DQB1*0617	DQB1*0312	DPA1*0301
DRB1*1423	DRB1*1510	DRB3*020203	DRB4*0301N	DQA1*0504	DQB1*0618	DQB1*0313	DPA1*0302
DRB1*1424	DRB1*1511	DRB3*020204	DRB5*010101	DQA1*0505	DQB1*0619	DQB1*0401	DPA1*0401
DRB1*1425	DRB1*1512	DRB3*0203	DRB5*010102	DQA1*060101	DQB1*0620	DQB1*0402	
DRB1*1426	DRB1*1513	DRB3*0204	DRB5*0102	DQA1*060102		DQB1*050101	
DRB1*1427	DRB1*160101	DRB3*0205	DRB5*0103			DQB1*050102	
DRB1*1428	DRB1*160102	DRB3*0206	DRB5*0104			DQB1*050201	
DRB1*1429	DRB1*160201	DRB3*0207	DRB5*0105			DQB1*050202	
DRB1*1430	DRB1*160202	DRB3*0208	DRB5*0106			DQB1*050301	
DRB1*1431	DRB1*1603	DRB3*0209	DRB5*0107			DQB1*050302	
DRB1*1432	DRB1*1604	DRB3*0210	DRB5*0108N			DQB1*0504	
DRB1*1433	DRB1*1605	DRB3*0211	DRB5*0109			DQB1*060101	
DRB1*1434	DRB1*1607	DRB3*0212	DRB5*0110N			DQB1*060102	
DRB1*1435	DRB1*1608	DRB3*0213	DRB5*0111			DQB1*060103	
DRB1*1436		DRB3*0214	DRB5*0112			DQB1*0602	
DRB1*1437			DRB5*0202				
DRB1*1438			DRB5*0203				
DRB1*1439			DRB5*0204				
DRB1*1440			DRB5*0205				
DRB1*1441			DRB6*0101				

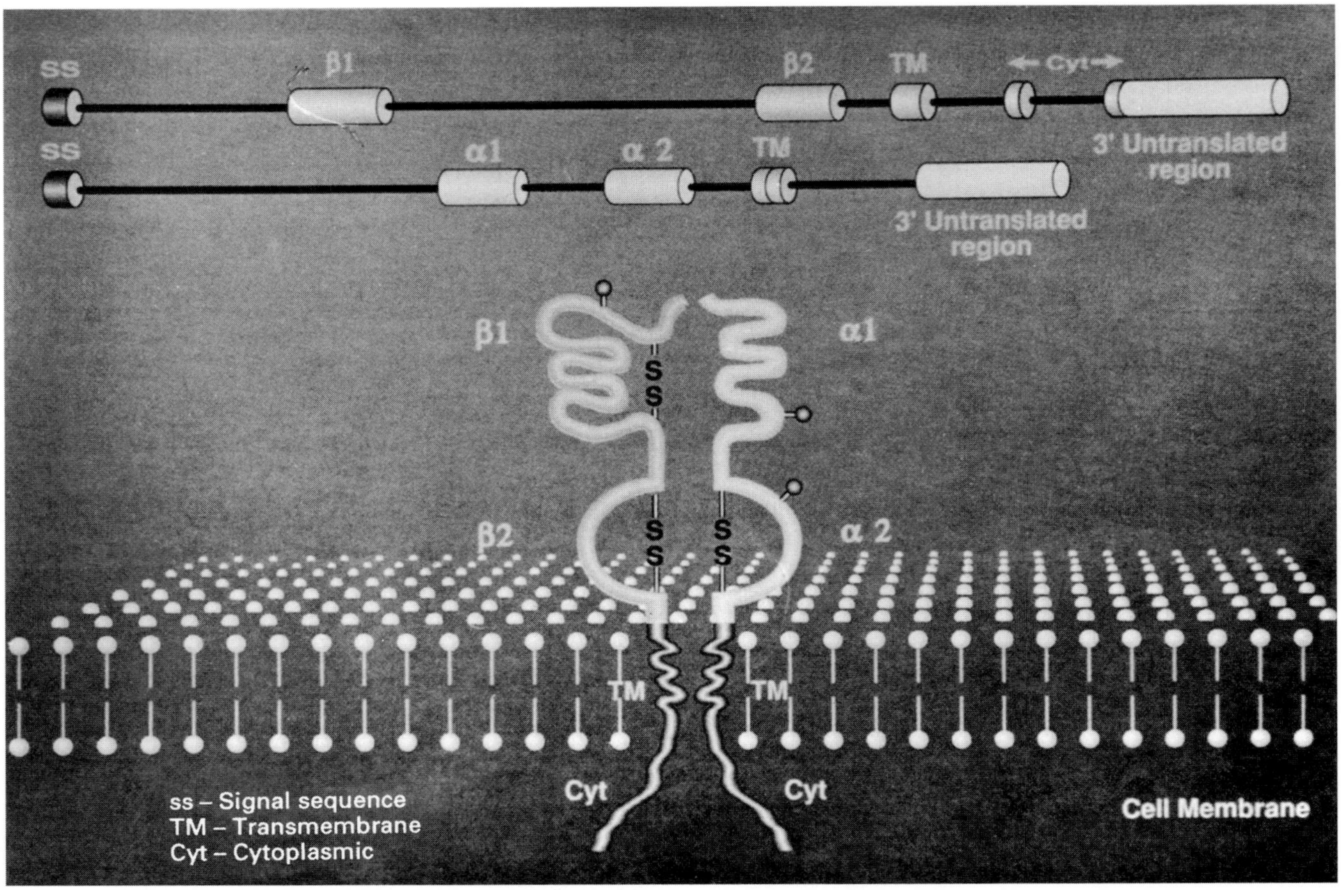

Fig. 8.5. Organization of class II genes and corresponding domains on class II molecules. Reproduced, with permission, from Tait (1990).

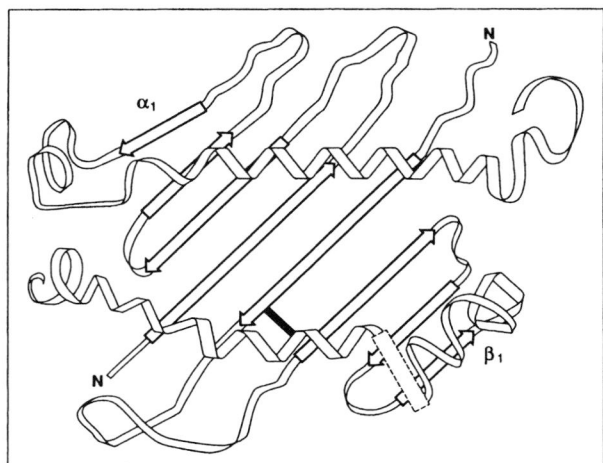

Fig. 8.6. Polypeptide folding pattern proposed for the peptide-binding cleft of class II MHC molecule. Note the similarities to the class I peptide-binding cleft. The white arrows represent polypeptide folded as β-pleated sheet, the white coils represent polypeptide folded as α-helix, and the black bar represents a disulfide bond. Adapted, with permission, from Brown *et al.* (1988).

DNA-sequenced the HLA-A, -B, and -C alleles in 471 patients who received bone marrow transplants from unrelated donors as treatment for chronic myeloid leukemia. A single antigen mismatch significantly increased the risk of graft failure, while a single HLA allele mismatch did not.

Linkage disequilibrium and haplotype frequencies

Since all relevant HLA loci are within a range of 4,000 kilobases on chromosome 6, HLA alleles are usually inherited en bloc. The combined alleles on a single chromosome are known as a haplotype. An individual inherits one set of HLA alleles from each parent, the paternal and maternal haplotypes. In a certain number of cases, crossing-over can occur within the HLA complex, resulting in a haplotype with a recombination of HLA genes. No more than two alleles per locus can be present in one individual.

Given the extensive polymorphism of HLA genes, an enormous number of phenotypes can in theory be derived from any possible combination of the HLA-A, HLA-B, and HLA-DR alleles (for reasons of clarity it is common to identify a haplotype by its three most important loci). However, some allelic combinations appear in a considerably higher fre-

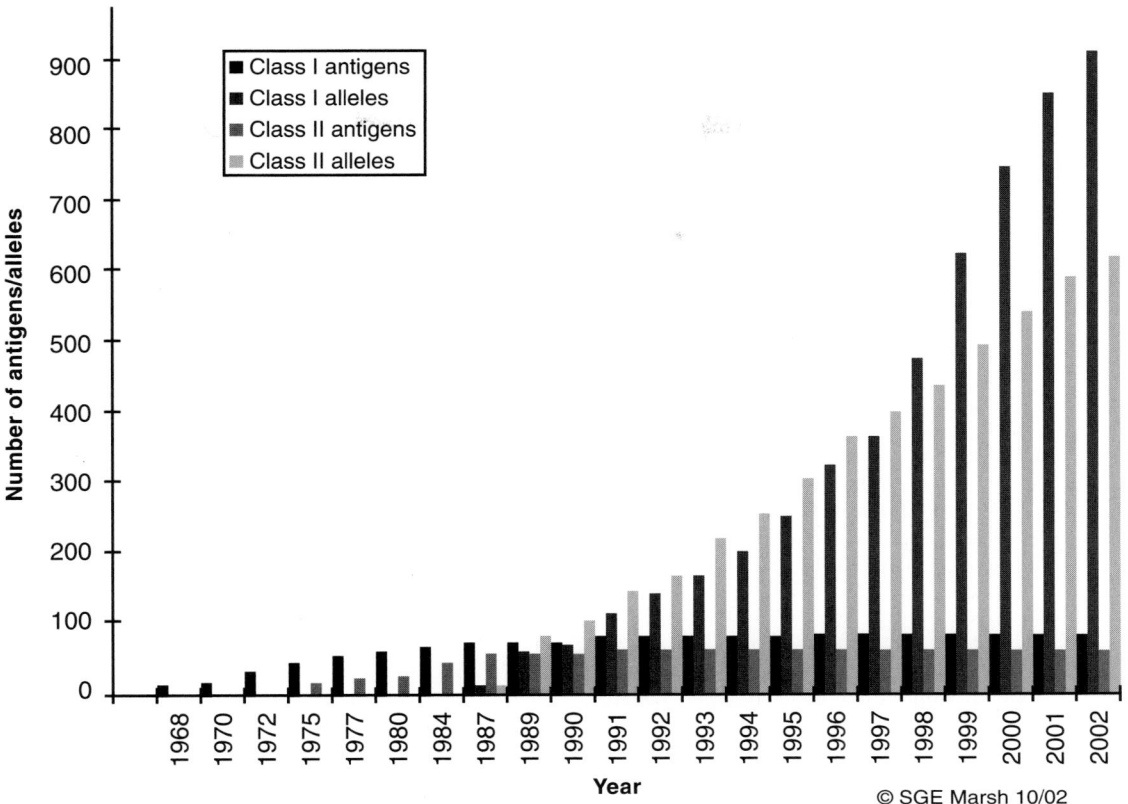

Fig. 8.7. The increasing degree of HLA polymorphism (from Marsh at: www.anthonynolan.org.uk/hig/)

quency in the population than one might expect based on their individual allele frequencies. This phenomenon is called *linkage disequilibrium.*

In the class II region further polymorphism is introduced because one or two different functional polymorphic DRB gene products can be expressed on one haplotype. For example (Table 8.7) a DR11 haplotype does express DR11 molecules (encoded by DRA and DRB1*11) and DR52 molecules (encoded by DRA and DRB*02). DR1 haplotypes generally carry only a DRB1 gene with the DRB1*01 allele, but on rare occasions a DRB5 gene has been observed to be present as well.

Another phenomenon is that combinations of HLA alleles appear in different frequencies in different ethnic groups. Table 8.8 shows the most frequent haplotypes among several ethnic groups in North America, demonstrating clearly that different ethnic backgrounds have different haplotypes.

Technical aspects of tissue typing and matching

Currently two methods of tissue typing are routinely used: serologic typing and molecular typing. In the past cellular and biochemical typing techniques have been used but these techniques are now abandoned. Cellular techniques may be used for further characterization of functionally important polymorphism.

Serologic typing techniques

The HLA antigens were originally defined by serologic techniques using sets of highly selected human allo-antisera (mostly generated by pregnancy) and, later on, also monoclonal antibodies. Originally, the technique of choice was an agglutination technique; later, almost exclusively, complement-dependent lymphocyte microcytotoxicity assays were used. Reliability of the test depends largely on the quality of the typing sera, viability of the test cells, and expression of the HLA molecules. The technique is

Table 8.7. *HLA DR haplotypes have different arrangements of functional DRB genes. Rare exceptions to the scheme below may be found.*

Gene	DRB1	DRB3	DRB4	DRB5	DRA
DR1, DR10	+	–	–	–	+
DR2 (15, 16)	+	–	–	DR51	+
DR3, (17, 18), DR5 (11, 12), DR6 (13, 14)	+	DR52	–	–	+
DR4, DR7, DR9	+	–	DR53[a]	–	+
DR8	+	–	–	–	+

[a] DR7 DQ2 haplotypes express DR53, but the majority of DR7 DQ9 haplotypes carry a DRB4-Null allele, which does not express DR53.

Table 8.8. *Fifteen most common Caucasian American, African American, Asian American and Latin American HLA-A, -B, -DR haplotypes with their estimated frequencies (HF) in the National Marrow Donor Program file (adapted from Mori et al., 1997).*

Caucasian American	HF	African American	HF	Asian American	HF	Latin American	HF
A1;B8;DR3	5.1812	A30;B42;DR3	1.6759	A33;B58;DR3	1.5859	A2;B35;DR8	1.7641
A3;B7;DR2	2.6285	A1;B8;DR3	1.2491	A33;B44;DR6	1.4687	A29;B44;DR7	1.7057
A2;B44;DR4	2.1507	A3;B7;DR2	0.7596	A24;B52;DR2	1.3832	A1;B8;DR3	1.6733
A2;B7;DR2	1.7900	A2;B44;DR4	0.6506	A2;B46;DR9	1.3481	A2;B35;DR4	1.2858
A29;B44;DR7	1.4702	A33;B53;DR8	0.6294	A33;B44;DR7	1.3468	A3;B7;DR2	1.1986
A2;B62;DR4	1.2503	A2;B7;DR2	0.5747	A30;B13;DR7	1.0929	A28;B39;DR4	0.9717
A3;B35;DR1	1.0224	A28;B58;DR12	0.5511	A24;B7;DR1	1.0747	A2;B39;DR4	0.8834
A1;B57;DR7	0.9998	A2;B45;DR6	0.5181	A33;B58;DR6	1.0052	A24;B39;DR6	0.8566
A2;B60;DR6	0.8688	A30;B42;DR8	0.4946	A11;B62;DR4	0.9299	A33;B14;DR1	0.7834
A2;B8;DR3	0.7674	A34;B44;DR2	0.4913	A1;B57;DR7	0.7996	A24;B35;DR4	0.7398
A24;B7;DR2	0.7157	A30;B57;DR6	0.4829	A11;B13;DR2	0.7785	A30;B18;DR3	0.7196
A2;B57;DR7	0.6348	A2;B53;DR6	0.4587	A11;B62;DR12	0.7543	A2;B44;DR4	0.6906
A30;B13;DR7	0.6172	A28;B70;DR3	0.4458	A2;B38;DR2	0.6742	A2;B7;DR2	0.6688
A2;B44;DR7	0.6081	A29;B44;DR7	0.4415	A2;B46;DR8	0.6740	A24;B61;DR4	0.6454
A2;B44;DR2	0.5920	A28;B7;DR2	0.4086	A24;B60;DR4	0.6532	A2;B51;DR6	0.5924

Abbreviations: HF, haplotype frequency (%).

fast and can be performed within a day. Leukemic patients are often difficult to type because some of the HLA molecules are not, or only weakly, expressed on leukemic blast cells. Some HLA specificities are difficult to type serologically due to lack of proper allosera or low expression of the molecules on the cell surface (i.e., HLA-C and HLA-DP molecules). Class II typing techniques were further complicated by the fact that class II antigens are primarily expressed only on B cells, monocytes, and dendritic cells. All these complications resulted in great variability of typing accuracy between laboratories. At present serologic typing is still performed for class I, predominantly using sets of commercially available allo antisera and/or monoclonal antibodies. Serological class II typing is hardly performed anymore. Interpretation of the serologic testing depends on the quality of the human allosera used, cross-reactive patterns, and known linkages. Cross-reactivity can sometimes make it impossible to distinguish whether an individual is homo- or heterozygous, for example, to detect an A30 next to A31, B70 or B75 next to B62. It also requires special reagents to type for the B17 splits in a B62 positive individual, or for the A28 splits next to A2. This results in donor registry HLA typings that combine broad and split antigens. Moreover the presence of only one serological specificity on a locus does not per definition mean that this person is homozygous for that specificity.

Molecular typing techniques

The polymorphism of the HLA system is often determined at the DNA level. All common alleles have been sequenced and this knowledge is used for routine typing. Target regions for typing are the second and third exons of class I genes and the second exon of class II genes, because most of the polymorphism is found in those regions. Once polymerase chain reaction (PCR)

technology became available for the amplification of specific DNA fragments, many different typing methods were developed (Erlich, 1999). They can be classified according to three major principles: (1) the PCR-SSP technique in which genomic DNA is PCR-amplified with a number of sequence-specific primer pairs, (2) PCR-SSOP, in which locus-specific exon-2 and/or exon-3 PCR-amplified DNA is hybridized with sequence specific oligonucleotide probes, and (3) SBT (sequencing based typing) in which a whole stretch of PCR-amplified DNA is sequenced (Bidwell, 1994; Middleton, 1999).

The techniques differ in other ways, including duration (from a few hours to several days), degree of resolution (low, intermediate, or high), ambiguities, and costs. Most laboratories combine several methods in order to fulfill the needs for reliable typing results for the clinic. The increasing number of laboratories that are able to sequence donors and patients worldwide has led to a tremendous increase in the number of alleles identified per locus. Many of these are extremely rare or have a restricted distribution in small populations. With each release of new sequences in the IMGT/HLA database, typing kits will have to be updated for their ability to recognize such new alleles. To understand the problem of typing ambiguities, one has to realize that heterozygosity will be detected at a number of nucleotide positions in an individual who carries two different alleles of a certain gene. It then has to be decided if these heterozygous positions are found on the same chromosome or not (in *cis* or in *trans* position). This may result in two or more possible allele combinations. Even with low resolution typing it can be difficult to distinguish, for example, the common combination B*51, B*35 from the less frequent combination B*53, B*78. One also has to realize that high resolution typing by current methods may in the future contain ambiguities (once new alleles are detected that cannot be distinguished by current typing methods).

Ambiguities sometimes involve combinations of normally expressed and nonexpressed alleles. Typing should then be extended to recognize the chromosomal region that causes the nonexpression of the allele. Alternatively, serological typing can be performed to determine if the corresponding antigen is indeed expressed at the cell surface.

The World Marrow Donor Association has published recommended guidelines for the histocompatibility testing of unrelated donors (Hurley et al., 1999). These include the required use of DNA-based testing for HLA-DR and for HLA-A and -B. Further, if serology is used for HLA- and -B, then a DNA-based method must be used to define antigens in the population tested that are frequently missed and/or misassigned. In terms of the resolution of testing, at a minimum, serologic split/low-level DNA-based resolution was recommended.

Cellular techniques

In addition to the typing techniques discussed above, several cellular tests can be used for functional matching and can give an indication of subsequent clinical outcome.

Although it has been reported that the results of MLC between prospective donor-recipient pairs do not correlate with outcome after unrelated bone marrow transplantation (Mickelson et al., 1996; Segall et al., 1996), the test can be used as an additional technique to confirm HLA class II typing results.

The cytotoxic T-lymphocyte precursor (CTLp) frequency assay is based on limiting dilution analysis and estimates the frequency of alloreactive CTL precursors. It has been demonstrated that CTLp frequencies in responder/stimulator pairs correlate with the number of HLA class I mismatches (Kaminski et al., 1989; Spencer et al., 1995; van der Meer et al., 2000; Oudshoorn et al., 2002). Significant correlations between the CTLp test outcome and graft-versus-host disease (GVHD) or survival have been described (Speiser et al., 1996). However, lack of correlation has also been described between CTLp frequencies and GVHD after T-depleted bone marrow transplantation (Fussel et al., 1994), suggesting that the usefulness of CTLp testing in donor selection is still debatable (Montagna et al., 1996). Whether the reported discrepancies are due to technical differences or to the T-cell content of the marrow inoculum remains to be established.

The helper T-lymphocyte precursor frequency (HTLp) analysis is based on a limiting dilution test defining the frequencies of T-helper precursor cells and may be helpful in determining minor histocompatibility differences between HLA-identical siblings (Theobald et al., 1992), or in selecting unrelated stem cell donors (Schwarer et al., 1994; Keever-Taylor et al., 1997).

References

Bidwell, J. (1994). Advances in DNA-based HLA-typing methods. *Immunology Today*, **15**, 303–7.

Bjorkman, P.J., Saper, M.A., Samraoui, B. *et al.* (1987). Structure of the human class I histocompatibility antigen HLA-A2. *Nature*, **329**, 506–12.

Bodmer, J.G., Marsh, S.G.E., Albert, E.D. *et al.* (1997). Nomenclature for factors of the HLA system, 1996. *Tissue Antigens*, **49**, 297–321.

Brown, J.H., Jardetsky, T., Saper, M.A. *et al.* (1988). A hypothetical model of the foreign antigen binding site of class II histocompatibility molecules. *Nature*, **332**, 845–50.

Brown, J.H., Jardetzky, T.S., Gorga, J.C. *et al.* (1993). Three-dimensional structure of the human class II histocompatibility antigen HLA-DR1. *Nature*, **364**, 33–9.

Erlich, H.A. (1999). Principles and applications of the polymerase chain reaction. *Reviews in Immunogenetics*, **1**, 127–34.

Fussel, S.T., Donnellan, M., Cooley, M.A., & Farrell, C. (1994). Cytotoxic T lymphocyte precursor frequency does not correlate with either the incidence or severity of graft-versus-host disease after matched unrelated donor bone marrow transplantation. *Transplantation*, **57**, 673–6.

Hurley, C.K., Wade, J.A., Oudshoorn, M. *et al.* (1999). Histocompatibility testing guidelines for hematopoietic stem cell transplantation using voluteer donors: report from The World Marrow Donor Association. *Bone Marrow Transplantation*, **24**, 119–21.

Kaminski, E., Hows, J., Man, S. *et al.* (1989). Prediction of graft versus host disease by frequency analysis of cytotoxic T-cells after unrelated donor bone marrow transplantation. *Transplantation*, **48**, 608–13.

Keever-Taylor, C.A., Passweg, J., Kawanishi, Y. *et al.* (1997). Association of donor-derived host-reactive cytolytic and helper T cells with outcome following alternative donor T cell-depleted bone marrow transplantation. *Bone Marrow Transplantation*, **19**, 1001–9.

Marsh, S.G.E., Albert, E.D., Bodmer, W.F. *et al.* (2002). Nomenclature for factors of the HLA system, 2002. *Human Immunology*, **63**, 1213–68.

Meer, A.van der, Joosten, I., Schattenberg, A.V. *et al.* (2000). Cytotoxic T-lymphocyte precursor frequency (CTLp-f) as a tool for distiguishing permissible from non-permissible class I mismatches in T-cell-depleted allogeneic bone marrow transplantation. *British Journal of Haematology*, **111**, 685–94.

Mickelson, E.M., Longton, G., Anasetti, C. *et al.* (1996). Evaluation of the mixed lymphocyte culture (MLC) assay as a method for selecting unrelated donors for marrow transplantation. *Tissue Antigens*, **47**, 27–36.

Middleton, D. (1999). History of DNA typing for the human MHC. *Reviews in Immunogenetics*, **1**, 135–56.

Montagna, D., Maccario, R., Comoli, P. *et al.* (1996). Frequency of donor cytotoxic T cell precursors does not correlate with occurrence of acute graft-versus-host disease in children transplanted using unrelated donors. *Journal of Clinical Immunology*, **16**, 107–14.

Mori, M., Beatty, P., Graves, M. *et al.* (1997). HLA gene and haplotype frequencies in the North American population: the National Marrow Donor Program Donor Registry. *Transplantation*, **64**, 1017–27.

O'Reilly, R.J., Hansen, J.A., Kurtzberg, J. *et al.* (1996). Allogeneic marrow transplants: approaches for the patient lacking a donor. *Hematology 1996. American Society of Hematology Education Program*, 132–46.

Oudshoorn, M., Doxiadis, I.I.N., Van den Berg-Loonen, P.M. *et al.* (2002). Functional versus structural matching: can the CTLp test be replaced by HLA allele typing? *Human Immunology*, **63**, 176–84.

Petersdorf, E.W., Hansen, J.A., Martin, P.J. *et al.* (2001). Major-histocompatibility-complex class I alleles and antigens in hematopoietic-cell transplantation. *New England Journal of Medicine, 345,* 1794–1800.

Robinson, J. & Marsh, S.G.E. (2001). The IMGT/HLA Sequence Database. *Reviews in Immunogenetics, 4,* 518–31.

Schreuder, G.M.T., Hurley, C.K., Marsh, S.G.E. *et al.* (2001). The HLA dictionary 2001: a summary of HLA-A, -B, -C, -DRB1/3/4/5, -DQB1 alleles and their association with serologically defined HLA-A, -B, -C, -DR and -DQ antigens. *Tissue Antigens, 58,* 109–40.

Schwarer, A.P., Jiang, Y.Z., Deacock, S. *et al.* (1994). Comparison of helper and cytotoxic antirecipient T cell frequencies in unrelated bone marrow transplantation. *Transplantation, 58,* 1198–203.

Segall, M., Noreen, H., Edwins, L. *et al.* (1996). Lack of correlation of MLC reactivity with acute graft-versus-host disease and mortality in unrelated bone marrow transplantation. *Human Immunology, 49,* 49–55.

Speiser, D.E., Löliger, C.-C., Siren, M.-K., & Jeannet, M. (1996). Pretransplant cytotoxic donor T-cell activity specific to patient HLA class I antigens correlating with mortality after unrelated BMT. *British Journal of Haematology, 93,* 935–9.

Spencer, A., Brookes, P.A., Kaminski, E. *et al.* (1995). Cytotoxic T lymphocyte precursor frequency analysis in bone marrow transplantation with volunteer unrelated donors. *Transplantation, 59,* 1302–8.

Tait, B. (1990). *Today's Life Science, 2,* 30–9.

Theobald, M., Nierle, T., Bunjes, D. *et al.* (1992). Host-specific interleukin-2-secreting donor T-cell precursors as predictors of acute graft-versus-host disease in bone marrow transplantation between HLA-identical siblings. *New England Journal of Medicine, 327,* 1613–17.

Tiercy, J.M., Marsh, S.G.E., Schreuder, G.M.T. *et al.* (2002). Guidelines for nomenclature usage in HLA reports: ambiguities and conversion to serotypes. *European Journal of Immunogenetics, 29,* 273–4.

9 Human minor histocompatibility antigens: recognition and application for hematopoietic stem cell transplantation

ERIC SPIERINGS AND ELS GOULMY

Leiden University Medical Center, Leiden, The Netherlands

Introduction

Minor histocompatibility antigens (mHags) or non-HLA antigens are capable of eliciting alloimmune cellular responses in vivo. mHags are peptides from polymorphic intracellular proteins that are encoded by genes on the Y chromosome and autosomal genes. Their immunogenicity arises as a result of their expression on the plasma membrane where they are recognized by alloreactive MHC-restricted T cells (Goulmy, 1996). The development of graft-versus-host-disease (GVHD) in recipients of HLA-identical, yet mHags-disparate, sibling hematopoietic stem cell transplants (HSCT) reflects the role of mHags in transplantation (Beatty & Hervé, 1990; Bortin *et al.,* 1991). Moderate to severe acute GVHD occurs, depending on the age of the recipient and the amount of T-cell depletion of the graft, in 15% to 35% HLA genotypically identical recipient transplants. mHag disparities between donor and recipient may also induce alloresponses participating in graft-versus-leukemia (GVL) reactivities. In vivo data underline this notion. Several clinical studies indicate a direct relationship between the GVL effect and acute and chronic GVHD (Weiden *et al.,* 1979, 1981; Butturini, Bortin, & Gale, 1987). In syngeneic hematopoietic stem cell (HSC) transplantation (between identical twins), where no major or minor H antigen disparity exists and thus no alloreactivity can be induced, relapse rates are high (Horowitz *et al.,* 1990). Recipients of autologous transplants also have a high risk of developing recurrent leukemia (Champlin, 1992). In recipients of allogeneic HSCT, the relapse rates vary according to the degree of acute and/or chronic GVHD that develops (Horowitz *et al.,* 1990). Another indication of the involvement of mHags in the GVL effect is the successful use of donor lymphocyte infusions (DLI) as immunotherapy for relapse of chronic myeloid leukemia after HLA-identical HSCT (Kolb *et al.* 1990, 1995; Slavin *et al.* 1996). The therapeutic effect of DLI is mediated to a large extent by donor-derived alloimmune T cells that recognize patient-specific mHags that are expressed on the patient's blood cells, including the patient's leukemic cells (Mutis & Goulmy, 2000).

Assuming that the human genome has an abundance of mH loci resulting in various mHag incompatibilities between an HLA-identical HSC donor and recipient, one may conclude that mHags are key players in both GVH and GVL activities.

This chapter reflects a summary of our current knowledge on human mHag characteristics and discusses these data in relation to their relative clinical importance.

Cellular minor H antigen recognition

mHags have been defined by MHC-restricted T cells obtained from individuals primed in vivo. In humans, mHag studies have predominantly been performed in the HLA-identical HSCT setting.

Generation of minor H antigen specific T-cell lines and clones

The basic idea of generating anti-host cytotoxic T lymphocytes (CTLs) and T helper (Th) cells with specific activity for mHag is based on the following assumption: posttransplant (i.e., donor) cells, when sensitized against the patient's own pretransplant cells, are directed against host-specific target structures, such as mHags, which are absent from the donor cells. Our studies have been carried out with material obtained from HLA genotypically identical bone marrow donor-recipient pairs. The protocol that we commonly use enables the generation of anti-host mHag specific T-cell lines and clones. A flow chart for the induction and effector phases of host-specific CTL (protocol 1) and Th cells (protocol 2) is outlined in Table 9.1. For detailed protocols the reader is referred to Van Els *et al.* (1990).

Generation of host-specific T-cell lines

The generation of host-specific T-cell lines is essentially based on the protocol described in Goulmy *et al.* (1983). A total of 4×10^6 posttransplant peripheral blood lymphocytes (PBLs) from the recipient (i.e., of donor origin) are stimulated with different host-specific lymphocytes as antigen presenting cells (APCs)—either with 4×10^6 30 Gy-irradiated PBLs or with 0.8×10^6 50 Gy-irradiated EBV-LCLs, both derived from the patient before transplantation (host origin) (Table 9.1). After 6 days 0.1×10^6 responder cells are specifically restimulated either with host

PBLs at a responder-to-stimulator cell ratio (R:S) of 1:10 or with host EBV-LCL at an R:S ratio of 1:2, both in the presence of 2% highly purified interleukin-2 (IL-2). Thereafter, posttransplant, T-cell lines are maintained in culture by weekly addition of a mixture of irradiated host EBV-LCLs and (autologous) donor PBLs in medium containing 1% Leuco A, alternating with fresh medium containing 15% IL-2. To limit experimental variation, posttransplant T-cell lines induced with either PBLs or EBV-LCLs are established and functionally tested in the same experiments. Not only mHag-specific responses but also autoreactive (Rosenkrantz, Dupont, & Flomenberg, 1985; Tilkin *et al.*, 1986), as well as EBV antigen-specific (Rickinson, Wallace, & Epstein, 1980), T cells might be generated when using EBV-LCLs as APCs, especially if recipients and/or their donors are EBV-seropositive prior to transplant, To identify the latter possibilities, the CTL and Th cell activities are assessed against different target cells and stimulator cells including EBV-LCLs of both host and donor origin.

Cell-mediated lympholysis assay (CML)
Cytotoxic activity of the host-sensitized T-cell lines is assessed against host T-cell blasts, host EBV-LCLs, and, as negative controls, donor T-cell blasts and donor EBV-LCLs in a chromium release assay (Table 9.1).

Proliferation assay
Proliferative activity of the host-sensitized T-cell lines is assessed against host PBLs, host EBV-LCLs, and, as negative controls, donor PBLs and donor EBV-LCLs in a primed lymphocyte test (PLT) (Table 9.1).

Generation of host-specific T-cell clones
Once host specificity is established, the T-cell lines undergo cloning (Van Els *et al.*, 1992). Briefly, the T-cell lines are suspended at 1.5 cells/ml in a feeder cell mixture and plated at 0.2 ml/well (i.e., 0.3 cells/well) in 96-well round bottom microtiter plates. This feeder cell mixture contains (1) allogeneic PBLs (10^6 cells/ml from two or three randomly selected donors, irradiated with 30 Gy); (2) patient's pretransplant EBV-LCLs; 5×10^5 cells/ml irradiated with 50 Gy; (3) 1 µg/ml Leuco A (Pharmacia, Uppsala, Sweden); and (4) 20 U/ml recombinant IL-2 (Ortho, Braintree, MA). After 9 to 10 days, 0.1 ml aliquots from each well are transferred into replicate wells and are tested for host-specific activity.

Expansion of CTL clones
Large scale expansion (30- to 60-fold) of these clones for extensive panel typing can be performed as follows: 1×10^6 CTLs are cultured together with 10 ml of the above-mentioned feeder cell mixture and with 20 U/ml (final concentration) of IL-2 in an upright 75 cm^2 tissue culture flask (45° angle) in a total volume of 80 ml of medium for 5 days. Then fresh medium containing 20 U IL-2/ml is added for 1 to 3 more days.

Using these culture protocols, the first series of human mHag was recognized cellularly (Goulmy, 1997). From the data gathered so far by us and other investigators, it is clear that both CTL and Th cell clones recognize mHags encoded by genes on the Y chromosome and by autosomal genes in the context of various class I and class II MHC molecules; all of them are recognized in a classical MHC-restricted fashion.

Generation of anti-host T-cell reactivities

The skin-explant model (Vogelsang *et al.*, 1985; Dickinson *et al.*, 1988) and mixed epidermal cell-lymphocyte cultures can also be used to detect anti-host T-cell activities between HLA-identical sibling pairs (Bagot *et al.*, 1986). The skin-explant model involves the use of donor lymphocytes that have been sensitized against recipient's lymphocytes in vitro and then co-cultured with the recipient's skin. The mixed epidermal cell-lymphocyte reaction involves the use of donor lymphocytes as responder cells and epidermal cells from trypsin-treated suction blisters of the recipient as stimulator cells.

Table 9.1. *Flow chart of the induction and effector phase of host-specific CTL and Th cell lines*

	Induction phase		Effector phase	
Responder cells	APC added on days 0 and 6	Feeder cells for maintenance of the culture	Target cells in the cell-mediated lympholysis assay	Stimulator cells in primed lymphocyte tests
Protocol 1 post-BMT PBLs	Host[a] PBLs	Host EBV-LCLs and donor PBLs	Host PHA-blasts Host EBV-LCLs Donor PHA-blasts Donor EBV-LCLs	Host PBLs Host EBV-LCLs Donor PBLs Donor EBV-LCLs
Protocol 2 post-BMT PBLs	Host EBV-LCLs	Host EBV-LCLs and donor PBLs	Host PHA-blasts Host EBV-LCLs Donor PHA-blasts Donor EBV-LCLs	Host PBLs Host EBV-LCLs Donor PBLs Donor EBV-LCLs

Abbreviations: APC, antigen-presenting cell; CTL, cytotoxic T cells; Th, helper T cells; PBL, peripheral blood lymphocytes; EBV-LCL, Epstein-Barr virus lymphoblastoid cell line; PHA, phytohemagglutinin. Protocol 1 is used for the induction of CTLs; protocol 2 for the induction of Th cells.
[a]Derived from the patient before transplantation.

T-cell precursor frequency analyses assays have been reported to detect mHag differences between HLA genotypically identical BM donors and recipients (Theobald *et al.*, 1992; Schwarer *et al.*, 1993). The respective target structures recognized in the skin-explant models and T-cell precursor tests remain to be identified.

Molecular minor H antigen recognition

Peptide and gene identification and chromosomal location

Since mHags are recognized by T cells in association with MHC molecules, an obvious but cumbersome approach is to isolate these antigens from their respective MHC molecules. The application of a microcapillary high-performance liquid chromatography (HPLC)-electrospray ionization tandem mass spectrometry enables the detection of nonabundant peptides among a pool of MHC-bound peptides and was successfully applied for the first identification of a human mHag, the HLA-A2 restricted mHag HA-2 (Den Haan *et al.*, 1995); the same technique was used to identify the HLA-B7 restricted mHag H-Y, abbreviated as B7HY, and mHags A2HY, A2HA-1, A1HY A2HA-8, A1HA-3 (Wang *et al.*, 1995; Meadows *et al.*, 1997; Den Haan *et al.*, 1998; Pierce *et al.*, 1999; Brickner *et al.*, 2001; Spierings *et al.*, 2003). Besides the latter technology, cDNA expression systems have been successfully applied to identify the mHags B44HB-1, B8H-Y, B60 HY, A1HY, DQ5HY, and DRB3*0301HY (Dolstra *et al.*, 1999; Warren *et al.*, 2000; Vogt *et al.*, 2000a, 2000b, 2002; Spierings, 2002). Genetic linkage analysis making use of large pedigrees of families can be applied to identify the genes encoding the T-cell defined mHags (Warren *et al.*, 2002). Table 9.2A lists the human mHags chemically analyzed to date. Their characteristics can be summarized as follows. mHags are naturally processed peptides of cellular polymorphic "self" proteins that associate with MHC molecules. mHags are derived from evolutionarily conserved genes with important biological function (Goulmy, 1997). In a transplantation setting, however, these peptides can be immunogenic and can induce cellular immune responses. Which peptides from polymorphic "self" proteins can give rise to alloreactivity, albeit in the nonphysiologic setting of transplantation, can be analyzed by gathering information on issues such as mHag processing and presentation. Examples of such studies are the identification of a novel HLA-B60 T cell epitope of the mHag HA-1 locus and in the characterization of the mHag HA-3 (Mommaas *et al.*, 2002; Spierings *et al.*, 2003). Naturally, "reverse immunology" can be applied to identify candidate mHags. Here, products of known polymorphic genes are analyzed as risk factors for survival and occurrence of GVHD in HLA-identical HSCT settings. The presence of alloimmune T cells specific for the latter allelic peptides is as yet unclear. Table 9.2B lists examples of these candidate mHags such as CD31 (Behar *et al.*, 1996), CD62L (Maruya *et al.*, 1998), and human platelet antigens (Maruya *et al.*, 1998; Balduini *et al.*, 1999; Juji *et al.*, 1999).

Minor H antigen characteristics

Population frequencies and Mendelian segregation

The phenotype frequencies for the human mHags known to date are listed in Table 9.3. The studies reveal that in general mHags appear with relatively high phenotype frequencies. The polymorphic loci encoding the mH peptides have so far limited (i.e. di-allelic or tri-allelic) variation of which often solely one allele leads to a functional T-cell epitope.

Analysis of the genetic traits of some mHags was studied with mHag-specific CTL clones (Schreuder *et al.*, 1993) and for some mHags (i.e., HA-1, HA-2, HA-3) confirmed on the DNA level (Wilke *et al.*, 1998, 2002; Spierings *et al.*, 2003). Analysis of distribution of the mHags in the parent population among the mating types, together with their inheritance patterns in the families, demonstrated that the mHags behaved as Mendelian traits. Each can be considered a product of a gene with two alleles, one expressing and one not expressing the detected specificity. Mendelian segregation of mHags has also been clearly demonstrated for other mHags (for review see Goulmy, 1997).

Tissue distribution

Information on the tissue distribution of the mHags is crucial; their mode of tissue expression (i.e., hematopoietic restricted or ubiquitous) evidently determines their role as target molecules in GVHD and/or GVL. We anticipate that the mHags particularly relevant in the development of GVHD, namely the mHags with expression on GVHD target organs, are the mHags with broad tissue distribution. mHags with tissue expression limited to cells of the hematopoietic system are especially relevant for GVL activity (Mutis & Goulmy, 2000). With regard to the possible influence of mHags on HSC graft rejection, expression of mHags on stem cells might be relevant in presensitized patients receiving a mHag-positive T-cell-depleted stem cell graft. Analysis of the membrane expression of mHags can be performed by functional assays such as cell-mediated lympholysis and growth inhibition of clonogenic normal and leukemic precursor cells (as reviewed in Goulmy, 1997, 1998). The Taqman real-time RT-PCR is a sensitive method that can be used for the quantitation of gene expression. Examples of quantification of RNA levels of mHags have so far been executed for the mHags HB-1 and HA-1 (Dolstra *et al.*, 1999; Wilke *et al.*, 2002). It is not only a simple question as to whether the mHag allele is present or absent: the quantity of RNA expression of a particular mHag allele may provide additional important information for HSCT-related GVHD or GVL activities. Table 9.3 lists the information on the tissue distribution of the human mHags analyzed to date.

Applications for hematopoietic stem cell transplantation

Minor H antigen typing

To date, the clinical usefulness of typing for the cellular and/or chemically identified mHags is evident in the area of

Table 9.2. *Identification of human mHags*

A

Restriction molecule	mHag	Peptide	Chromosomal location	Gene	Reference
HLA-A1	H-Y	IVDCLTEMY	Y	DFFRY	Pierce et al., 1999 Vogt *et al.*, 2000b
HLA-A2	H-Y	FIDSYICQV	Y	SMCY	Meadows *et al.*, 1997
HLA-B7	H-Y	SPSVDKARAEL	Y	SMCY	Wang *et al.*, 1995
HLA-B8	H-Y	LPHNHTDL	Y	UTY	Warren *et al.*, 2000
HLA-B60	H-Y	RESEEESVSL	Y	UTY	Vogt *et al.*, 2000a
HLA-DQ5	H-Y	HIENFSDIDMGE	Y	DBY	Vogt *et al.*, 2002
HLA-DRB3*0301	H-Y	VIKVNDTVQI	Y	RPS4Y	Spierings *et al.*, 2002
HLA-A2	HA-1	VLHDDLLEA	19	KIAA0023	Den Haan *et al.*, 1998
HLA-B60	HA-1	KECVLHDDLL	19	KIAA0023	Mommaas *et al.*, 2002
HLA-A2	HA-2	YIGEVLVSV	7	Myosin I G	Den Haan *et al.*, 1995
HLA-A1	HA-3	VTEPGTAQY	15	AKAP-13	Spierings *et al.*, 2003
HLA-A2	HA-8	RTLDKVLEV	9	KIAA0020	Brickner *et al.*, 2001
HLA-B44	HB-1	EEKRGSLHVW	5	Unknown	Dolstra *et al.*, 1999

B

Candidate mHag	Identification level	Chromosomal location	Gene	
CD31	cDNA	17	PECAM-1: adhesion molecule	Behar et al., 1996
CD42 (HPA-2)	cDNA	17	GPAIb?	Maruya *et al.*, 1998
CD49b (HPA-5 and -13)	cDNA	5	VLA-2, GPIa	Maruya *et al.*, 1998
CD61 (HPA-1, -4, -6, -7, -8, -10, -11)	cDNA	17	GPIIIa	Kuijpers *et al.*, 1992
CD62L	cDNA	1	LECAM-1: adhesion molecule	Maruya *et al.*, 1998

HSCT. mHag typing in the HLA-matched transplant setting will increase in value when it can be combined with information on cytokine genotypes, immunization status (e.g., pregnancies and blood transfusions), viral status, and gender of donor and recipient prior to transplant. As outlined above, except for graft rejection, there are two clinically related issues that justify mHag typing in HSCT—GVHD and GVL. The need for mHag typing for the latter clinical manifestation depends on the particular mHag characteristics, such as

population frequency and tissue distribution. HA-1 is especially relevant for GVL activity. Nonetheless, we and others determined that HA-1 incompatibility is associated with the development of GVHD after HLA-identical HSCT (Goulmy *et al.*, 1996; Tseng *et al.*, 1999; Gallardo *et al.*, 2001; Socié *et al.*, 2001). It should be noted, however, that other studies found no statistically significant correlation between disparity for HA-1 and a range of transplant outcomes including acute and chronic GVHD, relapse, nonrelapse mortality, and

Table 9.3. *Characteristics of the identified human mHags*

Restriction molecule/mHag	Phenotype frequency of immunogenic peptide	Tissue distribution	Reference
HLA-A1/H-Y	Male restricted	Ubiquitous	de Bueger *et al.*, 1992
HLA-A2/H-Y	Male restricted	Ubiquitous	de Bueger *et al.*, 1992
HLA-B7/H-Y	Male restricted	Ubiquitous	de Bueger *et al.*, 1992
HLA-B8/H-Y	Male restricted	Hematopoietic cells	Warren *et al.*, 1998
HLA-B60/H-Y	Male restricted	Ubiquitous	de Bueger *et al.*, 1992
HLA-DQ5/H-Y	Male restricted	Ubiquitous	Vogt *et al.*, 2002
HLA-DRB3*0301/H-Y	Male restricted	Unknown	Spierings *et al.*, 2002
HLA-A2/HA-1	69%	Hematopoietic cells	de Bueger *et al.*, 1992
HLA-B60/HA-1	69%	Hematopoietic cells	de Bueger *et al.*, 1992
HLA-A2/HA-2	95%	Hematopoietic cells	de Bueger *et al.*, 1992
HLA-A1/HA-3	88%	Ubiquitous	de Bueger *et al.*, 1992
HLA-A2/HA-8	65%	Ubiquitous	
HLA-B44/HB-1	79%	Hematopoietic cells	Dolstra *et al.*, 1999

survival (Murata *et al.,* 2000; Lin *et al.,* 2001; Tait *et al.,* 2001). We currently ascribe the association between HA-1 mismatch and the development of GVHD to the significant expression of HA-1 on the patient's professional APCs; HA-1 presentation on the remaining patient DCs early after HSCT induces strong donor anti-host alloimmune HA-1-specific CTLs. Subsequent production of cytokines (Ferrara, 1993) would lead to activation of "bystander" alloimmune T cells specific for ubiquitously expressed mHags, such as the mHag H-Y (de Bueger *et al.,* 1992). The latter notion is in accordance with a study on the role of hematopoietic APCs in GVHD in an MHC-identical, mHag-mismatched murine model (Shlomchik *et al.,* 1999). This study showed that depleting host APCs before conditioning abrogates GVHD, that replacement of host with donor APCs abrogates T-cell activation, and cross-presentation of host antigens by donor APCs does not cause GVHD. With regard to the role of the "candidate" mHag CD31 in the outcome of HSC transplantation, reports are also controversial (Nichols *et al.,* 1996; Maruya *et al.,* 1998; Balduini *et al.,* 1999; Behar *et al.,* 2000; Grumet *et al.,* 2001). For information on the molecular typing of the various mHag systems discussed herein, the reader is referred to Wilke and Goulmy (2002).

In situ ex vivo analysis to study GVH activities

Direct effects of mHag specific T-cell populations can be read out using a skin-explant assay. To gain insight into the migration patterns of mHag-specific CTLs, we investigated their in situ localization in human skin tissues. Skin sections were incubated with CTLs specific for the ubiquitously expressed mHag H-Y or for the hematopoietic system-restricted mHags HA-1 and HA-2, and visualized by tetrameric HLA-mHag peptide complexes. CTLs specific for the ubiquitously expressed mHags induced severe GVH reactions of grade III–IV; CTLs specific for the hematopoietic system-restricted mHags HA-1 and HA-2 induced

no or low GVH reactions (Dickinson *et al.,* 2002). This in situ ex vivo readout system allows evaluation of mHag T-cell populations relevant for GVHD and for immunotherapeutic GVL applications (see below).

Immunotherapy of leukemia

mHag disparities between donor and recipient may induce alloresponses participating not only in GVHD, but also in GVL reactivities. Therefore, a logical application of mHags is the use of CTLs specific for mHag peptides for the treatment of refractory, residual, or relapsed leukemia. As mentioned earlier, mHags are clearly expressed on circulating leukemic cells and clonogenic leukemic precursor cells of both myeloid and lymphoid origin; thus both types of leukemias can be targeted. Clearly, mHags restricted to the hematopoietic cell system (Table 9.3) are candidates for adoptive immunotherapy of leukemia (Goulmy, 1997). This strategy is similar in principle to the adoptive immunotherapy of donor buffy coat cells, whereby remission in chronic myeloid patients relapsed after allogeneic HSCT is often induced (Kolb *et al.,* 1995; Giralt & Champlin, 1994). However, donor leukocyte therapy is often associated with GVHD. In addition, donor leukocyte infusions for relapsed ALL and AML patients are far less effective than for CML patients (Kolb *et al.,* 1995). As exemplified in Figure 9.1, mHag peptide-specific CTLs can be generated ex vivo from mHag-negative HSC donors for mHag-positive patients at high risk of relapse (Mutis *et al.,* 1999). Upon infusion (either pre-HSCT as part of the conditioning regimen or post-HSCT as adjuvant therapy), the mHag peptide-specific CTLs may eliminate the mHag-positive patient's leukemic cells and leukemic progenitor cells. Because of the use of mHags with expression restricted to the hematopoietic cell lineage, the patient's non-hematopoietic cells, as well as the cells of the mHag-negative HSC donor cells, will be spared. A universal option would be to generate "prefabricated" mHag peptide-specific CTLs by using

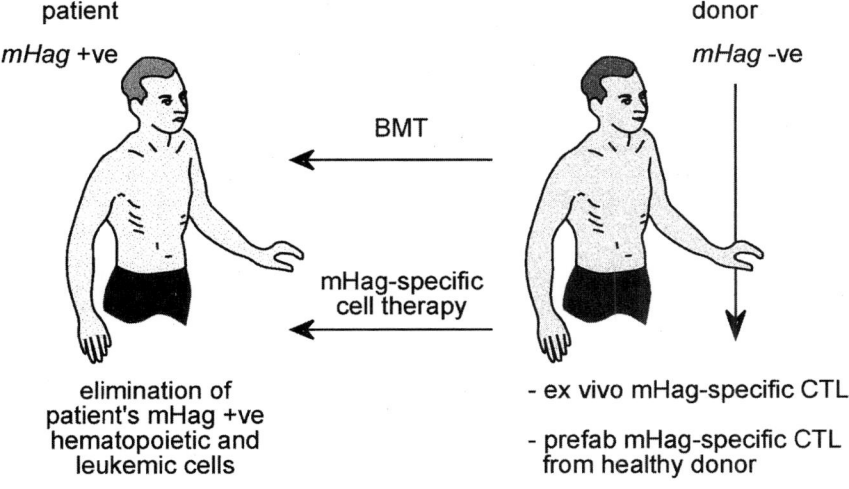

Fig. 9.1. mHag peptide-specific adoptive cellular immunotherapy for HLA-identical, mHag-mismatched HSC transplantation.

mHag-negative healthy blood donors with common homozygous HLA haplotypes. Patients who are HA-1 or HA-2-positive (and their HSC donors HA-1- or HA-2-negative), and who match the HLA type of the CTL donor, could be treated with these "ready for use" allo HA-1 or HA-2 peptide-specific CTLs. Transduction of these CTLs with a suicide gene would render elimination of the CTLs possible, should adverse effects (such as GVHD) occur. Future studies should also focus on vaccination strategies with hematopoietic system specific mHags. Either vaccination of the HSC donor with the relevant mHags or boosting of the HSCT recipient posttransplant are relevant approaches. The timing of the latter boost (i.e., the chimeric status of the patient) is crucial (see Mutis & Goulmy, 2002).

References

Bagot, H., Cordonnier, C., Tilkin, A.F. et al. (1986). A possible predictive test for graft-versus-host disease in bone marrow graft recipients: the mixed epidermal cell-lymphocyte reaction. *Transplantation*, **41**, 316–9.

Balduini, C.L., Noris, P., Giorgiani, G. et al. (1999). Incompatibility for CD31 and human platelet antigens and acute graft-versus-host disease after bone marrow transplantation. *British Journal of Haematology*, **106**, 723–9.

Beatty, P.G. & Hervé, P. (1990). Immunogenetic factors relevant to acute graft-versus-host disease. In *Graft-versus-Host Disease: Immunology, Pathophysiology and Treatment*, ed. S.J. Burakoff, H.J., Deeg, S., Ferrara, & K. Atkinson, pp. 415–423. New York: Marcel Dekker.

Behar, E., Chao, N.J., Hiraki, D.D. et al. (1996). Polymorphism of adhesion molecule CD31 and its role in acute graft-versus-host disease. *New England Journal of Medicine*, **334**, 286–91.

Bortin, M.M., Horowitz, M.M., Mrsic, M. et al. (1991). Progress in bone marrow transplantation for leukemia: a preliminary report from the Advisory Committee of the International Bone Marrow Transplant Registry. *Transplantation Proceedings*, **23**, 61–2.

Brickner, A.G., Warren, E.H., Caldwell, J.A. et al. (2001). *Journal of Experimental Medicine*, **193**, 195–205.

Butturini, A., Bortin, M.M., & Gale, R.P. (1987). Graft-versus-leukemia following bone marrow transplantation. *Bone Marrow Transplantation, 2*, 233–42.

Champlin, R. (1992). Graft-versus-leukemia without graft-versus-host disease: an elusive goal of bone marrow transplantation. *Seminars in Hematology, 29*, 46–52.

de Bueger, M., Bakker, A., Van Rood, J.J. et al. (1992). Tissue distribution of human minor histocompatibility antigens. Ubiquitous versus restricted tissue distribution indicates heterogeneity among human cytotoxic T lymphocyte-defined non-MHC antigens. *Journal of Immunology, 149*, 1788–94.

Den, Haan, J.M.M., Sherman, N.E., Blokland, E. et al. (1995). Identification of graft-versus-host disease associated human minor histocompatibility antigen. *Science*, **268**, 1478–80.

Den Haan, J.M.M., Meadows, L.M., Wang, W. et al. (1998). The minor histocompatibility antigen HA-1: a diallelic gene with a single amino acid polymorphism. *Science*, **279**, 1054–7.

Dickinson, A.M., Sviland, L., Carey, P. et al. (1988). Skin explant culture as a model for cutaneous graft versus host disease in humans. *Bone Marrow Transplantation*, **3**, 323–9.

Dickinson, A.M., Wang, X.N., Sviland, L. et al. (2002). In situ dissection of the graft-versus-host activities of cytotoxic T cells specific for minor histocompatibility antigens. *Nature Medicine*, **8**, 410–4.

Dolstra, H., Fredrix, H., Maas, F. et al. (1999). A human minor histocompatibility antigen specific for B cell acute lymphoblastic leukemia. *Journal of Experimental Medicine*, **189**, 301–8.

Ferrara, J.L. (1993). Cytokine dysregulation as a mechanism of graft versus host disease. *Current Opinion in Immunology*, **5**, 794–9.

Gallardo, D., Arostegui, J.I., Balas, A. et al. (2001). Disparity for the minor histocompatibility antigen HA-1 is associated with an increased risk of acute graft-versus-host disease (GVHD) but it does not affect chronic GVHD incidence, disease-free survival or overall survival after allogeneic human leucocyte antigen-identical sibling donor transplantation. *British Journal of Haematology*, **114**, 931–6.

Giralt, S.A. & Champlin, R.E. (1994). Leukemia relapse after allogeneic bone marrow transplantation. *Blood*, **84**, 3603–12.

Goulmy, E. (1996). Human minor histocompatibility antigens. *Current Opinion in Immunology*, **8**, 75–81.

Goulmy, E. (1997). Human minor histocompatibility antigens: new concepts for marrow transplantation and adoptive immunotherapy. *Immunological Reviews*, **157**, 125–40.

Goulmy, E., Schipper, R., Pool, J. et al. (1996). Mismatches of minor histocompatibility antigen between HLA-identical donor and recipients and the development of graft-versus-host disease after bone marrow transplantation. *New England Journal of Medicine*, **334**, 281–5.

Grumet, F.C., Hiraki, D.D., Brown, B.W.M. et al. (2001). CD31 mismatching affects marrow transplantation outcome. *Biology of Blood and Marrow Transplantation*, **7**, 503–12.

Horowitz, M.M., Gale, R.P., Sondel, P.M. et al. (1990). Graft-versus-leukemia reactions after bone marrow transplantation. *Blood*, **75**, 555–62.

Juji, T.Y., Watanabe, Y., Ishikawa, K. et al. (1999). Human platelet alloantigen (HPA)-5a/b mismatch, decreases free survival in unrelated bone marrow transplantation. *Tissue Antigens*, **54**, 229–34.

Kolb, H.J., Mittermuller, J., Clemm, C. et al. (1990). Donor leukocyte transfusions for treatment of recurrent chronic myelogenous leukemia in marrow transplant patients. *Blood*, **76**, 2462.

Kolb, H.J., Schattenberg, A., Goldman, J.M. et al. (1995). Graft-versus-leukemia effect of donor lymphocyte transfusions in marrow grafted patients. *Blood, 86*, 2041–50.

Kuijpers, R.W., von dem Borne, A.E., Kiefel, V. et al. (1992). Leucine33-proline33 substitution in human platelet glycoprotein IIIa determines HLA-DRw52a (Dw24) association of the immune response against HPA-1a (Zwa/PlA1) and HPA-1b (Zwb/PlA2). *Human Immunology*, **34**, 253–256.

Lin, M-T., Gooley, T., Hansen, J.A. et al. (2001). Absence of statistically significant correlation between disparity for the minor histocompatibility antigen HA-1 and outcome after allogeneic hematopoietic cell transplantation. *Blood*, **98**, 3172–3.

Maruya, E., Saji, H., Seki, S. et al. (1998). Evidence that CD31, CD49b and CD62L are immunodominant minor histocompatibility antigens in HLA identical sibling bone marrow transplants. *Blood,* **92,** 2169–76.

Meadows, L., Wang, W., den Haan, J.M. *et al.* (1997). The HLA-A *0201-restricted H-Y antigen contains a posttranslationally modified cysteine that significantly affects T cell recognition. *Immunity,* **6,** 273–81.

Mommaas, B., Kamp, J., Drijfhout, J.W. *et al.* (2002). Identification of a novel HLA-B60-restricted T cell epitope of the minor histocompatibility antigen HA-1 locus. *Journal of Immunology,* **169,** 3131–6.

Murata, M., Emi, N., Hirabayashi, N. *et al.* (2000). No significant association between HA-1 incompatibility and incidence of acute graft-versus-host disease after HLA-identical sibling bone marrow transplantation in Japanese patients. *International Journal of Hematology,* **72,** 371–5.

Mutis, T. & Goulmy, E. (2000). Minor histocompatibility antigens in graft versus leukemia. In *The Graft versus Leukemia Effect in Allogeneic Stem Cell Transplantation,* ed. J. Barret & J.Z. Jiang, pp. 119–33. New York: Marcel Dekker, Inc.

Mutis, T. & Goulmy, E. (2002). Hematopoietic system-specific antigens as targets for cellular immunotherapy of hematological malignancies. *Seminars in Hematology,* **39,** 23–31.

Mutis, T., Verdijk, R., Schrama, E. *et al.* (1999). Feasibility of immunotherapy of relapsed leukemia with ex vivo-generated cytotoxic T lymphocytes specific for hematopoietic system-restricted minor histocompatibility antigens. *Blood,* **93,** 2336–41.

Nichols, W.C., Antin, J.H., Lunetta, K.L. *et al.* (1996). Polymorphism of adhesion molecule CD31 is not a significant risk factor for graft-versus-host disease. *Blood,* **88,** 4429–34.

Pierce, R.A., Field, E.D., den Haan, J.M.M. *et al.* (1999). The HLA-A*0101-restricted HY minor histocompatibility antigen originates from DFFRY and contains a cysteinylated cysteine residue as identified by a novel mass spectrometric technique. *Journal of Immunology,* **163,** 6360–4.

Pierce, R.A., Field, E.D., Mutis, T. *et al.* (2001). The HA-2 minor histocompatibility antigen is derived from a diallelic gene encoding a novel human class I myosin protein. *Journal of Immunology,* **167,** 3223–30.

Rickinson, A.B., Wallace, L.E., & Epstein, M.A. (1980). HLA-restricted T cell recognition of Epstein-Barr virus-infected B cells. *Nature,* **283,** 865–7.

Rosenkrantz, K., Dupont, B., & Flomenberg, N. (1985). Generation and regulation of autocytotoxicity in mixed lymphocyte cultures: evidence for active suppression of autocytotoxic cells. *Proceedings of the National Academy of Science USA,* **82,** 4508–12.

Schreuder, G.M., Pool, J., Blokland, E. *et al.* (1993). A genetic analysis of human minor histocompatibility antigens demonstrates Mendelian segregation independent from HLA. *Immunogenetics,* **38,** 98–105.

Schwarer, A.P., Jiang, J.Z., Barrett, J.M. *et al.* (1993). Helper T-lymphocyte precursor (HTLp) frequency predicts the occurence and severity of acute GVHD and survival after allogeneic BMT in both recipients of genotypically HLA-identical sibling (SIB) and phenotypically HLA-matched unrelated donor (MUD) marrow. *Lancet,* **341,** 203–5.

Shlomchik, W.D., Couzens, M.S., Tang, C.B. *et al.* (1999). Prevention of graft versus host disease by inactivation of host antigen-presenting cells. *Science,* **285,** 412–5.

Slavin, S., Naparstek, E., Nagler, A. *et al.* (1996). Allogeneic cell therapy with donor peripheral blood cells and recombinant human interleukin-2 to treat leukemia relapse after allogeneic bone marrow transplantation. *Blood,* **87,** 2195.

Socié, G., Loiseau, P., Tamouza, R. *et al.* (2001). Both genetic and clinical factors predict the development of graft-versus-host disease after allogeneic hematopoietic stem cell transplantation. *Transplantation,* **72,** 699–706.

Spierings, E., Brickner, A.G., Caldwell, J.A. *et al.* (2003). The minor histocompatibility antigen HA-3 arises from differential proteasome-mediated cleavage of the lymphoid blast crisis (Lbc) oncoprotein. *Blood,* in press.

Spierings, E., Vermeulen, C.J., Vogt, M.H. *et al.* (2002). Identification of an HLA class II-restricted H-Y-specific T-helper epitope leading to genuine CD4+ T-helper cells in the event of a male-to-female transplantation (submitted for publication).

Tait, B.D., Maddison, R., McCluskey, J. *et al.* (2001). Clinical relevance of the minor histocompatibility antigen HA-1 in allogeneic bone marrow transplantation between HLA identical siblings. *Transplantation Proceedings,* **33,** 1760–1.

Theobald, M., Nierle, T., Bunjes, D. *et al.* (1992). Host specific interleukin-2 secreting donor T cell precursors as predictors of acute graft-versus-host disease in bone marrow transplantation between HLA-identical siblings. *New England Journal of Medicine,* **327,** 1613–7.

Tilkin, A.F., Bagot, M., Kayibanda, M. *et al.* (1986). A human autoreactive T cell line specific for minor histocompatibility antigen isolated from a bone marrow-grafted patient. *Journal of Immunology,* **137,** 3772–6.

Tseng, L.-H., Lin, M.-T., Hansen, J.A. *et al.* (1999). Correlation between disparity for the minor histocompatibility antigen HA-1 and the development of acute graft-versus-host disease after allogeneic marrow transplantation. *Blood,* **94,** 2911–4.

Van Els, C.A., Bakker, A., Van Rood, J.J., & Goulmy, E. (1990). Induction of minor histocompatibility antigen-specific T-helper but not T-cytotoxic response is dependent on the source of antigen-presenting cell. *Human Immunology,* **28,** 39–50.

Van Els, C.A., D'Amaro, J., Pool, J. *et al.* (1992). Immunogenetics of human minor histocompatibility antigen: their polymorphism and immunodominance. *Immunogenetics,* **35,** 161–5.

Vogelsang, G.B., Hess, A.D., Berkman, A.W. *et al.* (1985). An in vitro predictive test for graft-versus-host disease in patients with genotypic HLA-identical bone marrow transplants. *New England Journal of Medicine,* **312,** 645–50.

Vogt, M.H., Goulmy, E., Kloosterboer, F.M. *et al.* (2000a). UTY gene codes for an HLA-B60-restricted human male-specific minor histocompatibility antigen involved in stem cell graft rejection: characterization of the critical polymorphic amino acid residues for T-cell recognition. *Blood,* **96,** 3126–32.

Vogt, M.H.J., de Paus, R.A., Voogt, P.J. *et al.* (2000b). DFFRY codes for a new human male-specific minor transplantation antigen involved in bone marrow graft rejection. *Blood,* **95,** 1100–5.

Vogt, M.H.J., van den Muijsenberg, J.W., Goulmy, E. *et al.* (2002). The DBY gene codes for an HLA-DQ5 restricted human male-specific minor histocompatibility antigen involved in graft versus host disease. *Blood,* **99,** 3027–32.

Wang, W., Meadows, L.R., den Haan, J.M. *et al.* (1995). Human H-Y: a male-specific histocompatibility antigen derived from the SMCY protein. *Science,* **269,** 1588–90.

Warren, E.H., Gavin, M.A., Simpson, E. *et al.* (2000). The human UTY gene encodes a novel HLA-B8 restricted H-Y antigen. *The Journal of Immunology,* **164,** 2807–14.

Warren, E.H., Greenberg, P.D., & Riddell, S.R. (1998). Cytotoxic T-lymphocyte-defined human minor histocompatibility antigens with a restricted tissue distribution. *Blood,* **91,** 2197–207.

Warren, E.H., Otterud, B.E., Linterman, R.W. *et al.* (2002). Feasibility of using genetic linkage analysis to identify the genes encoding T cell-defined minor histocompatibility antigens. *Tissue Antigens,* **59,** 293–303.

Weiden, P.L., Flournoy, N., Thomas, E.D. *et al.* (1979). Antileukemic effect of graft-versus-host disease in human recipients of allogeneic marrow grafts. *New England Journal of Medicine,* **300,** 1068–73.

Weiden, P.L., Sullivan, K.M., Flournoy, N. *et al.* (1981). Antileukemic effect of chronic graft-versus-host disease. Contribution to improved survival after allogeneic marrow transplantation. *New England Journal of Medicine,* **304,** 1529–32.

Wilke, M., Dolstra, H., Maas, F. *et al.* (2002). Quantification of the HA-1 gene product at the RNA level; relevance for immunotherapy of hematological malignancies (submitted for publication).

Wilke, M. & Goulmy, E.J. (2002). Minor histocompatibility antigens. In *Manual of Clinical Laboratory Immunology, 6th edition,* ed. N.R. Rose, R.G., Hamilton, & B., Detrick, pp. 1201–7. Washington DC: ASM Press.

Wilke, M., Pool, J., Den Haan, J.M.M., & Goulmy, E. (1998). Genomic identification of the minor histocompatibility antigen HA-1 locus by allele-specific PCR. *Tissue Antigens,* **52,** 312–7.

Wilke, M., Pool, J., & Goulmy, E. (2002). Allele specific PCR for the minor histocompatibility antigen HA-2. *Tissue Antigens,* **59,** 304–7.

10 Biology of reduced intensity conditioning regimens

SHIMON SLAVIN

Hadassah University Hospital, Jerusalem, Israel

Introduction

Considering the lack of specific treatment modalities against cancer, and the well-established dose-response effects in treating tumor cells in vitro and in vivo, the dogma over the past years in treating cancer with available anticancer modalities has been "the more the better," attempting to eradicate all malignant cells with aggressive chemoradiotherapy. These concepts led to the development of myeloablative chemoradiotherapy, followed by rescue with stem cell transplantation as a means for elimination of a maximal possible number of tumor cells. Over the years it became apparent that none of the available anticancer modalities or even combinations thereof could accomplish such a goal, since relapse continued to be the single major obstacle in treatment of hematologic malignancies, especially in patients with advanced or primary resistant disease. On the other hand, as the intensity of the regimen used for bone marrow or blood stem cell (hematopoietic stem cell) transplantation (HSCT) was escalated, procedure-related toxicity and mortality increased accordingly (Passweg *et al.*, 1996; Gratwohl *et al.*, 1998). In addition, the increased incidence and severity of late complications became an important issue in the quality of life of long-term survivors. It became apparent that newer modalities needed to be introduced, focusing on reduced intensity conditioning, in order to improve the cure rate of patients with hematologic malignancies and metastatic solid tumors, as well as to improve the quality of life of successfully treated patients. For patients resistant to available chemotherapy, immunotherapy became a rational alternative, especially if carried out in conjunction with stem cell transplantation as a means to induce host-versus-graft transplantation tolerance. Unfortunately, no tumor-specific antigens could be identified in patients with hematologic malignancies. Likewise, experiments in animal models of human disease never featured effective humoral control of disease, neither were there any clinical trials documenting efficacy of tumor cell vaccines (Bast, 1985). Spontaneous murine leukemias, like the human disease, were considered "nonimmunogenic." Clearly, the major obstacles in developing effective immunotherapy programs for patients with hematologic malignancies as replacement for myeloablative regimens, stemmed from either lack of tumor-specific antigens or from failure to recognize weak antigens, or alternatively from failure to recognize the existing tolerance against ubiquitous tumor antigens and failure to induce an "autoimmune" response against tumor cells that were recognized as "self" (Weiss *et al.*, 1994). Even to date, when tumor-associated antigens are available, antibodies, such as anti-CD20 in patients with B-cell non-Hodgkin's lymphoma, that can effectively debulk the number of tumor cells in responding patients, are not sufficient for eradication of the disease (Grillo-Lopez *et al.*, 2000).

In this chapter evidence for induction of graft-versus-malignancy (GVM) effects mediated by donor lymphocytes following induction of tolerance in recipients with leukemia, and in preclinical animal models, will be presented. The use of alloreactive lymphocytes following adoptive immunotherapy is based on the exquisite antitumor effects inducible by donor lymphocyte infusion (DLI) following induction of transplantation tolerance to donor alloantigens by engraftment of donor stem cells, thus ensuring durable engraftment of donor lymphocytes, as a means to treat or prevent relapse following maximally tolerated doses of chemoradiotherapy in HSCT recipients considered incurable by any of the existing anticancer modalities. The development of the concept of nonmyeloablative conditioning as potential replacement of conventional myeloablative HSCT as a safer and more practical means to exploit the use of alloreactive donor lymphocytes as the main therapeutic tool against malignant cells of hematopoietic origin, and possibly also nonhematopoietic metastatic solid tumors, will be reviewed. A future goal is to maximize the therapeutic potential of alloreactive donor lymphocytes while restricting their reactivity against normal host tissues, using tumor- or tissue-specific effector cells introduced into recipients immunosuppressed by transient lymphoablation. Finally, the scientific basis suggesting the feasibility of innovative approaches for immunotherapy of malignant and nonmalignant diseases will be presented.

Maternal-fetal tolerance, spontaneous mixed chimerism, and bilateral transplantation tolerance as Mother Nature's models of reduced intensity conditioning

Transplantation tolerance across the major histocompatibility complex (MHC) occurs spontaneously in nature, as evidenced by the fact that pregnant females do not reject their class I and class II- (with multiple additional "minor" loci) mismatched conceptus. In fact, male cells can be easily identified in pregnant mothers carrying a male fetus, suggesting that microchimerism may be a normal phenomenon, thus indicating that chimerism may participate in the state of unresponsiveness induced during the advanced stages of pregnancy. Important along these lines is the observation of Owen in the 1940s, documenting that placental parabiosis in utero led to permanent mixed chimerism and bilateral transplantation tolerance (Owen, 1945). These observations instigated one of the most exciting experiments carried out in the 1950s by Billingham et al., (Billingham et al., 1953) who documented that infusion of parental hematopoietic stem cells into neonates shortly after birth resulted in microchimerism and induction of life-long unresponsiveness to donor alloantigens, with no conditioning and no exogenous immunosuppressive agents. This phenomenon, known as neonatal tolerance, suggested that there is a window of opportunity, shortly after delivery, during which tolerance can be induced without the need for any conditioning. Tolerant recipients were shown to be chimeras with only a small proportion of donor cells. However, important as this observation was, this approach could not be applied in clinical practice for successful induction of transplantation tolerance in immunocompetent recipients. Nonetheless, these experiments suggested that stable mixed chimerism could be induced when uncommitted hematopoietic cells mature in contact with an allogeneic environment. In addition, these observations indicated that, if antigen-specific unresponsiveness can be achieved without myeloablative immunosuppression, it should be possible to accomplish the same goal with minimal or no conditioning (i.e., by immune regulation rather than myeloablative immunosuppression), analogous to the mechanism of unresponsiveness that operates at the stage of "self/non-self" discrimination and during pregnancy. Since transplantation tolerance is induced by engraftment of hematopoietic stem cells, mixed chimerism, or another source of donor alloantigens, may be required, and may be sufficient, for induction of host-versus-graft (HVG) and graft-versus-host (GVH) unresponsiveness. Thus, protocols resulting in mixed chimerism, rather than full donor chimerism, may be the safest method for induction of transplantation using donor stem cells.

Induction of transplantation tolerance by nonmyeloablative conditioning

The feasibility of establishing bilateral transplantation tolerance by induction of mixed chimerism following nonmyeloablative conditioning in immunologically mature recipients across the MHC was established in the 1970s (Slavin et al., 1976; Slavin et al., 1977; Slavin et al., 1978a; Slavin et al., 1978b; Howard et al., 1981; Slavin, 1987; Prigozhina et al., 1999). Lymphoablative conditioning was based on the use of total lymphoid irradiation (TLI). Experiments in mice (Slavin et al., 1976; Slavin et al., 1977; Slavin et al., 1978a), rats (Slavin et al., 1978b), and dogs (Howard et al., 1981) indicated that, following nonmyeloablative conditioning with well-tolerated TLI, recipients experienced durable engraftment of donor bone marrow and skin or perfused organ allografts, with no clinically overt graft-versus-host disease (GVHD). However, the mechanisms responsible for this balanced equilibrium in mixed chimeras were not understood. After TLI, circulating and tissue-bound T cells were eliminated and newly formed T cells acquired tolerance to protein antigens (Zan-Bar et al., 1978) and alloantigens (Weigensberg et al., 1984; Slavin & Seidel, 1982; Morecki et al., 1985; Morecki et al., 1987; Slavin & Strober, 1979). Circulating cells and spleen cells were large cells carrying the null phenotype (Weigensberg et al., 1984). As T cells reappeared in the circulation, the proportion of this large cell subpopulation with null phenotype decreased, suggesting that the latter played some role in the development of the unresponsive state. These large cells consisted of enriched hematopoietic progenitor cells, indicating that, after intensive immunosuppression and maturation of newly derived lymphocytes in the thymus, new antigens encountered would be regarded as "self," thus resulting in apoptosis of self. Following TLI, without transplantation of stem cells, enrichment with such immature cells (Slavin & Seidel, 1982) enabled the recipients to develop tolerance, mainly as a result of clonal deletion (Morecki et al., 1987). Similarly, following TLI and infusion of allogeneic bone marrow stem cells, newly developing host T cells from uncommitted immature progenitor cells acquired unresponsiveness to donor alloantigens by a similar mechanism of thymic clonal deletion (Morecki et al., 1985; Morecki et al., 1987).

In support of clonal deletion as the primary mechanism of unresponsiveness in mixed chimeras, we documented that spleen cells from chimeras with intact skin allografts did not cause GVHD in sublethally irradiated secondary adoptive recipients, and could transfer their specific tolerance for skin allografts to secondary recipients. Although suppressor cells could also be documented in chimeras (Slavin & Strober, 1979), specific unresponsiveness could not be induced in vitro or in vivo by adoptive transfer experiments. Likewise, mixing of tolerant with alloreactive spleen cells failed to reduce the frequency of cytotoxic T-lymphocyte precursor activity (Morecki et al., 1985), thus supporting the concept that clonal deletion, and possibly anergy of residual alloreactive T cells, might be the primary mechanism explaining antigen-specific unresponsiveness.

Ildstad and Sachs (Ildstad & Sachs, 1984) and subsequently Sykes and Sachs (Sykes et al., 1988; Sykes & Sachs, 1983; Sykes & Sachs, 1990), showed similar results, except that they initially used myeloablative TBI and concomitantly infused host as well as donor hematopoietic cells, rather than protecting the recipient's own stem cell compartment. More recently, tolerance has been induced using truly minimal conditioning following infusion of donor stem cells in combination with co-stimulatory blockade (Werkerle *et al.*, 2000). In clinical HSCT, there are two ways to achieve consistent engraftment without GVHD. The first is complete T-cell depletion in both the graft and the host, leading to no GVHD and no rejection, although this requires aggressive and hazardous myeloablative conditioning (Bachar-Lustig *et al.*, 1995; Reisner & Martelli, 1995). Second is balancing immunocompetent T cells present in the graft and residual hematopoietic cells and T cells in the host (Prigozhina *et al.*, 1997; Prigozhina *et al.*, 1999). We have previously documented that donor T cells can downregulate host anti-donor alloreactivity, and host T cells, predominantly CD8+, can downregulate donor anti-host alloreactivity, most likely by a veto mechanism (Weiss & Slavin, 1999). However, theoretically, the optimal way to achieve engraftment without GVHD would be to selectively deplete the relevant donor-alloreactive host T cells, while in parallel, depleting host-alloreactive donor T cells. Such a protocol represents the ideal nonmyeloablative procedure.

In general, the more effective the conditioning regimen, resulting in either effective nonspecific depletion of alloreactive T cells, or deletion of alloantigen-specific T-cell clones, the better the engraftment of donor stem cells and tolerance induction. Consequently, fewer donor hematopoietic cells are required for durable engraftment of donor stem cells following effective depletion of HVG alloreactive T cells (Prigozhina *et al.*, 1997; Prigozhina *et al.*, 1999), whereas megadoses of donor stem cells are required for sustained engraftment of donor hematopoietic stem cells following very mild and ineffective depletion of HVG alloreactive T cells (Bachar-Lustig *et al.*, 1995; Reisner & Martelli, 1995; Prigozhina *et al.*, 1997; Prigozhina *et al.*, 1999). Similarly, due to the graft facilitating effect of donor alloreactive T cells, smaller amounts of unmodified stem cells containing donor T cells are sufficient following nonmyeloablative conditioning. In contrast, very large numbers of purified donor stem cells, lacking any T-cell-mediated graft facilitation, are mandatory for durable engraftment, especially as the intensity of the conditioning is reduced. In parallel, the more intensive the pregrafting immunosuppression, the more aggressive the GVHD, suggesting some possible downregulation between host and donor immunohematopoietic cells, probably mediated by bilateral veto effects (Weiss & Slavin, 1999).

Induction of transplantation tolerance and mixed chimerism by TLI was also accomplished in dogs by adding pharmacological immunosuppression after marrow transplantation (Storb *et al.*, 1999). Chimerism could also be accomplished in mice by using monoclonal antibodies for immunosuppression of allograft rejection, supported by generation of CD4+ suppressor cells (Waldmann & Cobbold 1998). In summary, mildly immunosuppressed hosts required either higher numbers of donor stem cells or induction of effective donor-specific clonal deletion. These considerations imply that all the components in the process of stem cell transplantation may be crucial for successful and safe engraftment.

The role of allogeneic lymphocytes in conjunction with HSCT in the treatment of hematologic malignancies and solid tumors

Until recently the use of high-dose, myeloablative chemoradiotherapy supported by autologous or allogeneic HSCT, was considered the treatment of choice for patients resistant to conventional doses of chemotherapy, for patients relapsing following conventional chemotherapy, and subsequently for patients at high risk for relapse. Subsequently, HSCT was successfully utilized for the treatment of genetic diseases and other life-threatening nonmalignant indications using the same therapeutic principles for replacement of abnormal host hematopoietic cells with donor hematopoietic cells. Traditionally, it was considered that high-dose chemoradiotherapy was the main component of the HSC transplant procedure and that transplantation of genotypically or phenotypically matched stem cells was indicated for rescue of the lethally treated recipient. Hence, much attention was given to maximizing tumor cell kill by maximally tolerated doses of chemotherapy (single agents and combinations of non-cross-reactive agents) and total body irradiation (Thomas, 1963). However, it was recognized following many years of experience that the incidence of relapse was higher among recipients of autologous as well as syngeneic grafts, compared with recipients of allogeneic grafts who developed GVHD, suggesting that immune-mediated graft-versus-leukemia (GVL) effects played a major role in elimination of residual tumor cells escaping chemoradiotherapy (Weiden *et al.*, 1981; Weiden *et al.*, 1981; Sullivan *et al.*, 1989; Horowitz *et al.*, 1990). The possibility that allogeneic lymphocytes administered in the course of HSCT eliminate leukemia through immune-mediated GVL effects has been suggested since the earliest days of experimental (Sinkovics *et al.*, 1965; Boranic & Tonkovic, 1971; Bortin *et al.*, 1979; Slavin *et al.*, 1981; Truitt *et al.*, 1983; Meredith & O'Kunewick, 1983; Weiss *et al.*, 1990; Truitt & Atasoylu, 1991) and clinical HSCT (Weiden *et al.*, 1981; Weiden *et al.*, 1981; Sullivan *et al.*, 1989; Horowitz *et al.*, 1990). A convincing direct correlation between acute and chronic GVHD and a reduced rate of relapse of leukemia in clinical BMT practice was first reported by Weiden *et al.* (Weiden *et al.*, 1981; Weiden *et al.*, 1981). Similarly, in analogy to GVL effects, graft-versus-tumor (GVT) effects were also described in a murine model of spontaneous sarcoma (Moscovitch & Slavin, 1984), and more recently in one of metastatic breast cancer (Morecki *et al.*, 1997; Morecki *et al.*, 1998), as well as in preliminary trials in humans (Eibl *et al.*, 1996; Ueno *et al.*, 1998; Or *et al.*, 1998). The role of immune-mediated GVL effects in the course of HSCT was further supported by observations suggesting that relapse while patients were on immunosuppressive treatment with cyclosporine (CSP) was occasionally reversed by discontinuing immunosuppression (Higano *et al.*, 1990). Likewise, it has been documented that the incidence of relapse is lower in patients treated with suboptimal doses of CSP (Bacigalupo *et al.*, 1991). In support, data in mice inoculated with murine leukemia and treated by HSCT indicated that GVL effects mediated by mismatched bone marrow cells were totally abrogated by concomitant administration of CSP for 10 days (Weiss *et al.*, 1990a). All of the above suggested that allogeneic HSCT provided immunocompetent allogeneic donor T lymphocytes, which could react against residual tumor cells of host origin. Hence, the advantage of HSCT over conventional chemotherapy lies in the combined effects of the myeloablative dose of chemoradiotherapy given pretransplant and the ability of immunocompetent allogeneic donor T lymphocytes to eliminate residual tumor cells of host origin, giving rise to GVL and GVT effects, or, in fact, graft versus any undesirable hematopoietic cells of host origin, including genetically abnormal stem cells or their progeny (Kapelushnik *et al.*, 1996; Kapelushnik *et al.*, 1997; Aker *et al.*, 1998; Slavin *et al.*, 1999). Interestingly, similar to the data first reported in mice (Bortin *et al.*, 1979; Slavin *et al.*, 1981; Truitt *et al.*, 1983), GVL effects independent of GVHD were confirmed in clinical practice, both following HSCT (Horowitz *et al.*, 1990) and following DLI given posttransplant to induce GVL effects to treat or prevent relapse when patients were off posttransplant immunosuppressive agents (Slavin *et al.*, 1988; Slavin *et al.*, 1995; Slavin *et al.*, 1996).

Based on the murine data that suggested the feasibility of induction of posttransplant GVL effects induced by T cells present in the allografts, we hypothesized that cell therapy with donor lymphocytes given postgrafting, especially in patients with no spontaneous GVHD following discontinuation of posttransplant GVHD prophylaxis, might induce effective antitumor responses (Slavin *et al.*, 1995; Slavin *et al.*, 1996; Kolb *et al.*, 1990; Kolb *et al.*, 1995; Collins *et al.*, 1997; Porter *et al.*, 1994; Mackinnon *et al.*, 1995). We hypothesized that allogeneic lymphocytes of donor origin could be given postgrafting for treatment, as well as for prevention of relapse in high-risk cases. Below is documented the first successful case in which GVL effects were induced by DLI in a patient with resistant acute lymphoblastic leukemia (ALL) who relapsed shortly after HSCT, and the cumulative international experience in a variety of malignant hematologic diseases.

Induction of GVL effects by DLI for treatment of relapse after HSCT

The first patient successfully treated by DLI for relapse following HSCT was a 2-year-old boy that was referred for HSCT at the Hadassah University Hospital in Jerusalem in November 1986 (Slavin *et al.*, 1988; Slavin *et al.*, 1995; Slavin *et al.*, 1996). He had been diagnosed with pre-B ALL with greater than 90% circulating blast cells, and splenomegaly. Cytogenetic analysis indicated abnormal clonal translocation in all blasts. The patient entered first complete remission but relapsed on therapy. Second remission was short and the patient was admitted for HSCT with resistant relapse. In December 1986, allogeneic HSCT was carried out from a fully HLA-matched sister. Conditioning included total body irradiation 1,200 cGy (2 daily fractions of 200 cGy at high dose rate on days -6, -5, and -4) followed by 2 doses of cyclophosphamide 60 mg/kg (days -3

and -2) and melphalan 60 mg/m^2 (day -1), and CNS prophylaxis with 2 intrathecal injections of cytosine arabinoside and methotrexate. Following transplantation the patient showed prompt engraftment with no signs of acute GVHD. At 1 month post-HSCT, the patient presented with massive infiltration of lymphoblasts in the marrow and blood, splenomegaly, and several bulky masses confirmed as extramedullary disease with a retrotracheal mass that necessitated emergency tracheotomy. Starting on day +92 after HSCT, the patient received increments of donor (sister) lymphocyte infusions equivalent to 5×10^5–1×10^6 T cells/kg to induce GVL effects after failure of maximally tolerated doses of chemoradiotherapy. On day +102 post-HSCT, the patient developed mild grade I acute cutaneous GVHD, which gradually increased within 2 weeks to grade II with involvement of the skin and liver. He responded to a short course of corticosteroids. Surprisingly, within 2 weeks the visible masses decreased in size, and within the next few weeks peripheral blood and bone marrow morphology normalized and cytogenetic analysis confirmed 100% normal female karyotype in all 50 metaphases investigated. To date, more than 15 years post-HSCT and DLI, no residual male cells can be detected in the blood or marrow by polymerase chain reaction (PCR) analysis and molecular remission persists with no clinical evidence of chronic GVHD. On the basis of the success in this patient, the first ever treated with DLI, similar treatment was given to additional patients and the therapeutic role of alloreactive donor lymphocytes was soon confirmed.

These data, now confirmed in many transplant centers, provided for the first time a second chance for cure for patients failing all known anticancer modalities (Slavin *et al.*, 1995; Slavin *et al.*, 1996; Kolb *et al.*, 1990; Kolb *et al.*, 1995; Collins *et al.*, 1997; Porter *et al.*, 1994; Mackinnon *et al.*, 1995; De witte *et al.*, 1992; Bar *et al.*, 1993; Leber *et al.*, 1993). The cumulative international data document a total incidence of clinically significant GVHD in at least 60% of patients treated with DLI. However, in some reports the frequency of GVHD was much higher among responders, and seemed to correlate with induction of remission. Documentation of response to DLI in up to 40% of patients with no clinically significant GVHD, mostly in patients treated at a stage of minimal residual disease (which may require lower doses of donor lymphocytes) confirmed the possible existence of GVL effects independent of GVHD, although admittedly only in a small minority of patients (Slavin *et al.*, 1995; Slavin *et al.*, 1996; Kolb *et al.*, 1990; Kolb *et al.*, 1995; Collins *et al.*, 1997; Porter *et al.*, 1994; Mackinnon *et al.*, 1995). Unfortunately, some patients developed severe, occasionally fatal complications. In addition, DLI was frequently associated with depression of bone marrow function. Mild to severe marrow aplasia often reversed spontaneously but in a few cases bone marrow aplasia was severe and occasionally fatal. An update of the European experience based on the European Bone Marrow Transplant Registry database using DLI for the treatment of relapse post-HSCT is shown in Table 10.1 (courtesy of Dr. Hans Kolb). Of particular interest were patients with sec-

Table 10.1. *GVL effects induced with donor lymphocyte infusions—EBMT database*

Diagnosis	No. of patients studied	No. of patients evaluable[a]	CR(%)
CML: Cytogenetic relapse	57	50	40 (80%)
Hematologic relapse	124	114	88 (77%)
Transformed phase	42	36	13 (36%)
Polycythemia vera/MPS	2	1	1
AML/MDS	97	58	15 (26%)
ALL	55	20	3 (15%)
MMy	25	17	5 (29%)

Abbreviations: CR, complete remission; CML, chronic myeloid leukemia; MPS, myeloproliferative syndrome; AML/MDS, acute myeloid leukemia/myelodysplasia; ALL, acute lymphoblastic leukemia; MMy, multiple myeloma.
[a] > 30-day survival.

ondary EBV-positive lymphoma. Posttransplant lymphoma induced by EBV is highly malignant and rarely responds to any of the available antilymphoma modalities. As reported first by Papadopoulos *et al.,* (Papadopoulos *et al.,* 1994) patients with posttransplant lymphoma also responded to DLI. Posttransplant lymphoma induced by EBV can now be eradicated by EBV-specific cytotoxic cells generated in vitro from donor lymphocytes (Kuzushima *et al.,* 1996).

Along the same lines, it was previously shown that effective post-HSCT immunosuppression by agents such as cyclosporine may increase the incidence of relapse in experimental animals (Weiss *et al.,* 1990) and humans (Bacigalupo *et al.,* 1991). It was also shown that discontinuation of cyclosporine as soon as relapse is diagnosed may lead to reinduction of remission (Stockschlaeder *et al.,* 1992; Odom *et al.,* 1978). Antileukemic effects induced by DLI are mediated by immunocompetent donor T lymphocytes recognizing minor histocompatibility determinants on the surface of tumor cells of host origin, an effect that may most likely depend on the alloreactive capacity of donor lymphocytes. Based on earlier animal data suggesting that the incidence of GVHD decreased as the time interval from HSCT to DLI was prolonged (Slavin *et al.,* 1978a; Weiss *et al.,* 1992; Johnson *et al.,* 1993), a simple and cost-effective way to control the incidence, intensity, and severity of GVHD may be based on administration of graded increments of donor lymphocytes, because different doses of T cells may be required for each patient. Thus, DLI may be initiated with a low, suboptimal T-cell dose such as 10^5 T cells/kg, which can be escalated at 2 to 4 week intervals 10-fold for patients receiving no anti-GVHD prophylaxis. Most patients with minimal residual disease following HSCT, especially patients with CML with cytogenetic or molecular relapse treated with pre-emptive DLI, respond favorably to DLI, with no marrow aplasia, in response to small increments with donor peripheral blood lymphocytes (Naparstek *et al.,* 1995; Naparstek *et al.,*

1996). However, further modifications may be required to improve the benefit-to-risk ratio following DLI.

The feasibility of inducing long-term remission or cure in many patients considered incurable by available anticancer modalities, paved the road to the hypothesis that adoptive allogeneic cell-mediated immunotherapy, rather than myeloablative conditioning, is the most important component of the transplant procedure. These observations established the basis for replacement of the hazardous myeloablative conditioning with better tolerated reduced intensity regimens, or nonmyeloablative stem cell transplantation (NST) (also termed "mini transplants"). This is based on the need for immune-mediated cell therapy rather than increased myeloablation, in order to eliminate chemoradiotherapy-resistant tumor cells. The main problem associated with DLI, as with HSCT, is acute and chronic GVHD, which tend to be more severe if donor lymphocytes are given earlier following HSCT. Taken together, although relapse following myeloablative HSCT was always considered incurable, the cumulative international experience has confirmed the efficacy of immunotherapy by donor lymphocytes after induction of HVG transplantation tolerance induced by engraftment of donor hematopoietic stem cells (Slavin *et al.,* 2001; Slavin, 2001).

Experiments with a murine model of B-cell lymphocytic leukemia/lymphoma showed that GVL effects mediated by DLI could be initiated after initial reconstitution of tumor-bearing mice with T-cell-depleted bone marrow allografts (Weiss *et al.,* 1992), suggesting that pre-emptive DLI may be initiated late following HSCT, in hosts with full hematopoietic reconstitution and no GVHD. Theoretically, tumor-specific GVL effects in the absence of GVHD could be mediated by donor-derived tumor-infiltrating lymphocyte (TIL)-like cells reacting exclusively or predominantly against tumor cells (Rosenberg, 1992), or tumor-reactive cytotoxic T lymphocytes (CTL) induced in vitro (Van Lochem *et al.,* 1992; Falkenburg *et al.,* 1993). Additional activation of donor effector cells, for treatment of patients with residual or resistant disease and no GVHD, may be accomplished by adding cytokines such as interleukin-2 (IL-2) or α-interferon (α-IFN) or both, which should be considered for patients who do not respond to DLI alone (Slavin *et al.,* 1996).

Induction of GVL effects by immune donor lymphocytes in a preclinical animal model

Since treatment of minimal residual resistant disease with DLI can be optimized by using activated lymphocytes (Leshem *et al.,* 2000), in correlation with an increased frequency of CTLp, it seemed reasonable to try to amplify the antitumor potential of donor lymphocytes by using specifically immune, rather than naive or polyclonally activated, lymphocytes. Hence, we attempted induction of GVL effects with allogeneic T cells obtained from immune donors in recipients of HSCT in mice inoculated with BCL1, the equivalent of human B-cell leukemia/lymphoma. GVL effects were induced with donor spleen cells derived from C57BL/6 mice immunized across major or minor histocompatibility barriers with BCL1-cells from the spleens of BALB/c mice inoculated with either tumor or normal BALB/c spleen cells (Ji *et al.*, manuscript submitted for publication; Prigozhina *et al.*, 2000). Our data suggested that spleen cells from donor mice immunized against both BCL1, or to lesser extent against normal host alloantigens, induced better therapeutic GVL effects with less GVHD across both minor histocompatibility antigens (mHag) and the MHC. A preferential upregulation of IL-10 secretion and downregulation of α-IFN, α-TNF, and IL-2 was detected in donor spleen cells from mice immunized with allogeneic tumor cells compared with normal cells of the same strain. This suggested that antihost responses might be downregulated in parallel with amplification of antitumor effects by a shift of the cytokine profile from Th1 to Th2, thereby reducing GVHD while enhancing GVL. This type of immunotherapy involving the use of specifically immune donor lymphocytes may lead to new approaches for eradicating leukemia, while at the same time reducing procedure-related morbidity and mortality due, primarily, to uncontrolled GVHD.

NST for treatment of malignant and nonmalignant diseases

Although the HSCT procedure offers a most important advantage in the form of alloreactivity against malignant cells of host origin, it seems unlikely that a substantial improvement in the outcome of patients with high-risk hematologic malignancies may be accomplished merely by increasing the intensity of the conditioning based on the well-known "log-dose" relationship between the dose of cytoreductive agents and the degree of tumor cell kill. Moreover, by comparing numerous protocols comprising a wide range of intensities for each of the cytoreductive components used for over 20,000 transplants reported to the International Bone Marrow Transplant Registry, no clear advantage could be documented for any of the different regimens administered as preparation for autologous or allogeneic HSCT, including or excluding TBI. It appears that the intensity of the conditioning in the course of allogeneic bone marrow or blood stem cell transplantation plays a relatively minor role in the overall outcome. As indicated earlier, the importance of immune-mediated antitumor effects can be best documented by comparing the rate of relapse following allogeneic as compared with autologous HSCT and syngeneic allografts (Horowitz *et al.*, 1990), and mostly, by documentation of the remarkable therapeutic potential of GVL effects induced by DLI.

Documentation of the feasibility of eradicating tumor cells (hematologic malignancies and to a lesser extent metastatic solid tumors) by adoptive allogeneic cell therapy in preclinical animal models and in patients relapsing following DLI suggested that alloreactive T lymphocytes may provide the strongest, possibly the only, tool available against tumor cells of hematopoietic origin resistant to chemoradiotherapy. Hence, we have developed a working hypothesis suggesting that the main role of the transplant procedure may involve induction of a state of HVG unre-

sponsiveness for accomplishing durable engraftment of donor-derived T lymphocytes, thus providing alloreactive T cells of donor origin the opportunity to recognize and eradicate host-derived tumor cells, or otherwise abnormal stem cells, provided the recipient is off immunosuppressive treatment. This hypothesis prompted us and others to develop a new approach for the treatment of both malignant and nonmalignant hematologic diseases, avoiding the use of myeloablative conditioning, in order to improve the immediate outcome of the HSCT procedure by preventing or minimizing procedure-related toxicity and mortality. Thus, a number of protocols have been developed with minimization of the intensity of the conditioning regimen to the range of nonmyeloablative levels, followed by infusion of donor stem cells—preferably granulocyte colony-stimulating factor (G-CSF)-mobilized blood stem cells enriched with circulating T lymphocytes collected by apheresis. The main component of most of the new regimens has been the use of fludarabine pregrafting, as a well-tolerated antilymphocyte agent.

As reported (Carella *et al.*, 2000a; Carella *et al.*, 2000b), the nonmyeloablative approaches can be roughly divided into three categories:

1. Focusing on lymphoablative conditioning with fludarabine and an alkylating agent
2. Focusing on low-dose total body irradiation (TBI) with intensive posttransplant immunosuppression
3. Combining high-dose chemotherapy and an autograft for maximal tumor debulking, followed by an allogeneic NST for eradication of tumor cells escaping chemoradiotherapy, hopefully in a minimal residual disease situation.

In each of these settings, NST served as a platform for subsequent adoptive cell-mediated immunotherapy (by DLI) for residual tumor cells postgrafting or for recurrence of malignancy.

At the Hadassah University Hospital in Jerusalem we focused on induction of a window of immunosuppression (step 1) followed by induction of HVG tolerance accompanied by GVL effects, mediated by donor lymphocytes infused with the mobilized blood stem cells (step 2) or DLI given later as an outpatient procedure (step 3), reasoning that this approach may offer the prospect of safer treatment of malignant and nonmalignant diseases at all age groups with minimal and controllable early and late procedure-related toxicity and minimal mortality (Slavin *et al.*, 1998; Slavin *et al.*, 2001; Slavin, 2001). Intensive pretransplant immunosuppressive therapy was accomplished with a combination of fludarabine 30 mg/m²/day for 6 days, busulfan 4 mg/kg/day for 2 days or cyclophosphamide for 2 days (60 mg/kg for aplastic anemia and other indications; 5–10 mg/kg for patients with Fanconi anemia), without or with anti-T-lymphocyte globulin (ATG, Fresenius) 5 or 10 mg/kg/day for 4 days to control residual host T cells and/or partially control donor T cells capable of causing GVHD. Following the conditioning, each patient received one or two infusions of G-CSF-mobilized blood stem cell collections. Low-dose CSP (3 mg/kg/day) was used as the sole GVHD prophylactic agent for less than 100 days posttransplant.

Our preliminary data in patients with standard indications for allogeneic HSCT, including acute leukemia, chronic leukemia, non-Hodgkin's lymphoma, myelodysplastic syndrome, multiple myeloma, and a variety of nonmalignant indications (Slavin et al., 1996; Nagler et al., 2000) including genetic diseases (Kapelushnik et al., 1998; Nagler et al., 1999), severe aplastic anemia (Slavin et al., 1996), Fanconi anemia (Kapelushnik et al., 1997; Aker et al., 1999), and other diseases, suggest that nonmyeloablative conditioning based on the use of fludarabine was extremely well tolerated. Engraftment of allografts obtained from matched siblings and matched unrelated donors (MUD) following infusion of G-CSF-mobilized blood stem cells was consistent and durable (Nagler et al., 2001). Analysis of host and donor markers using VNTR-PCR or amelogenine gene-based PCR suggested a transient stage of mixed chimerism and full replacement of host with donor hematopoietic cells. The only problem encountered using low-dose cyclosporine as the sole anti-GVHD prophylaxis was acute and chronic GVHD, which was occasionally severe. The absolute neutrophil count (ANC) did not decrease below $0.1 \times 10^9/l$ and several patients never experienced an ANC less than $0.5 \times 10^9/l$. Platelet counts did not decrease below $20 \times 10^9/l$, thus requiring no platelet transfusions in 10% to 20% of the patients. The incidence of relapse did not appear to be higher than that following conventional myeloablative HSCT, and relapse could be reversed by DLI. To date with an observation period extending over 5 years, it can be confirmed that successful eradication of malignant and genetically abnormal host hematopoietic cells can be accomplished by alloreactive donor peripheral blood lymphocytes, under conditions of HVG transplantation tolerance in patients with acute and chronic leukemia, non-Hodgkin's lymphoma, as well as in patients with life-threatening nonmalignant diseases.

The most effective outcome of NST can be anticipated in patients with CML because they respond best to DLI. The first cohort of patients with CML was treated with fludarabine, low-dose busulfan, and ATG, employed in 24 patients with CML in first chronic phase aged 3 to 63 years (Or et al., 2003). Prophylaxis against GVHD consisted of low-dose CSP. Early discontinuation of CSP was attempted in cases of mixed chimerism in an attempt to amplify GVL effects. All 24 patients showed rapid trilineage engraftment, mostly without complete aplasia; 6 patients did not require transfusion of any blood products. NST was associated with minimal procedure-related toxicity. The incidence of acute GVHD grade I was 54%; however, this increased following CSP withdrawal. After a follow-up of up to 70 (median 42) months, 21 of 24 patients remain alive and free of disease. The GVL effects induced by donor immunocompetent lymphocytes eradicated all host hematopoietic cells, as evidenced by molecular testing. The Kaplan-Meier probability of survival and disease-free survival at 5 years is 85% (confidence interval 70% to 100%). We conclude that NST may successfully replace myeloablative HSCT, thus providing a safer, better-tolerated therapeutic procedure for all patients with CML in first chronic phase with a matched

donor; however, this conclusion must be tested in a prospective randomized clinical trial. Likewise, it remains to be seen if similar results can be accomplished with the specific tyrosine kinase inhibitor imatinib (Glivec) alone, and whether similar results can be accomplished in patients failing imatinib.

Because of minimal pancytopenia and lack of mucositis, the fact that most patients do not require hyperalimentation, and the low incidence of acute toxicity and other complications (febrile neutropenia, bleeding, veno-occlusive disease of the liver, interstitial pneumonitis, and multiorgan failure), we anticipate that allogeneic nonmyeloablative stem cell transplantation may eventually become an outpatient procedure of choice for a large number of patients. Perhaps even more important, the state of transient mixed chimerism that results from the nonmyeloablative conditioning helps in accomplishing a reduced rate of severe acute GVHD.

The use of NST may also help reduce the incidence of late complications, which may result from the combined effects of high-dose chemoradiotherapy in addition to prior conventional treatments, especially in the lower and upper age groups. In the low age group, in contrast to myeloablative HSCT, NST may eliminate growth retardation and infertility. In elderly individuals, who normally may not qualify for a standard HSCT procedure, NST may allow a relatively safe clinical application of a potentially curative procedure. In the long run, induction of a transient state of mixed chimerism may help reduce the incidence and severity of GVHD. Based on animal data, mixed chimerism seems to be protective against GVHD, probably due to the regulatory effects mediated by residual hematopoietic cells of host origin, predominantly CD8$^+$ T cells, as indicated above (Weiss & Slavin, 1999). Apparently, as suggested by experimental data in mice, host hematopoietic cells can veto donor antihost alloreactivity while donor hematopoietic cells can veto residual alloreactive host cells, thus explaining the possible induction of bilateral transplantation tolerance that can be accomplished in mixed chimeras (Ildstad & Sachs, 1984; Sykes et al., 1988; Sykes & Sachs, 1983; Sykes & Sachs, 1990; Werkle et al., 2000; Slavin, 1987).

In Seattle and several other transplant centers, conditioning focused on the use of low-dose TBI. The protocol was based on canine studies designed to achieve engraftment across minor and major histocompatibility barriers and for the prevention of GVHD. The feasibility of using TBI as the main component of the conditioning was supported by the following studies: TBI delivered in a single fraction at a dose rate of 7 cGy per minute in dogs given intensive supportive care but no stem cell grafts invariably caused lethal marrow failure at >400 cGy whereas at doses <200 cGy dogs spontaneously recovered after a period of myelosuppression (Storb et al., 1989; Storb et al., 1997). Additional experiments evaluated whether immunosuppressive agents given posttransplant could facilitate engraftment. CSP alone was effective at a dose of 450 cGy with stable engraftment in 7 of 7 dogs, and the combination of CSP and mycophenolate mofetil (MMF) allowed for stable engraftment in 10 of 11 dogs after a nonmyeloablative dose of only 200 cGy TBI

(Storb et al., 1997). Engraftment was achieved as stable mixed chimerism with the donor component comprising 45% to 80% of hematopoietic cells. Dogs were followed for up to several years and continued to show stable donor engraftment. These results supported the hypothesis that marrow grafts could create their own space and that myelosuppressive therapy was not necessary to establish allogeneic engraftment.

The safety and efficacy of the canine preclinical studies helped develop a conceptual scheme of studies in patients with hematologic malignancy. Accordingly, immunosuppression was divided into two components, one directed at host cells before the transplant, and the other at both donor and host cells after the transplant to provide simultaneous control of both GVH and HVG reactions. The goal was to establish bidirectional graft-host tolerance as manifested by stable mixed donor-host hematopoietic chimerism. The goal of these studies was to evaluate whether allogeneic hematopoietic cell engraftment could be established in patients with malignancies using peripheral blood stem cell grafts from HLA-identical donors using an immunosuppressive conditioning regimen consisting of 200 cGy TBI pretransplant and postgrafting immunosuppression with MMF and CSP (McSweeney et al., 1998). CSP was given at 6.25 mg/kg orally twice daily from day −1 through day +35 or day +56 and targeted to blood levels at the upper end of the therapeutic range, with supratherapeutic levels tolerated in the absence of CSP toxicities. MMF was given at a dose of 15 mg orally twice daily from day 0 to day +27 and discontinued without tapering. Eligibility for the study required a contraindication to the use of conventional allografting because of age, prior high-dose therapy, or organ dysfunction. A number of patients from several American and European centers over the age of 50 years (range of 31–72) or with other high-risk features have been treated. Diagnoses were acute and chronic leukemias, multiple myeloma, Hodgkin's disease, non-Hodgkin's lymphoma, myelodysplastic syndromes, breast cancer, and amyloidosis. Many patients were transplanted in an outpatient setting; the median number of days of subsequent hospitalization during the initial 60 days posttransplant was 0 (range 0–26). Transplants were very well tolerated with mild myelosuppression with no development of mucositis and no alopecia. However, nonfatal graft rejection occurred in nearly 20% of patients. Spontaneous acute GVHD requiring treatment occurred in 36% of patients. Transplant-related deaths occurred in 6.5%. Significant disease responses have been observed in the majority of patients with sustained engraftment after transplant. This has included molecular remissions in CML patients and in CLL patients and disappearance of paraprotein in myeloma patients. Responses have frequently been gradual in onset, occurring over a period of 4 to 12 months. This is an important difference from conventional allografting in which detection of disease posttransplant usually represents treatment failure. Following HSCT, DLI can be used for elimination of residual hematopoietic cells of host origin.

The MD Anderson group in Houston reported several NST protocols, initially combining melphalan (140–180 mg/m^2) and either fludarabine (125 mg/m^2) or cladribine (60 mg/m^2) for treatment of advanced acute leukemia. Whereas in patients with refractory relapse disease usually recurred rapidly, 56% of patients with chemotherapy-sensitive disease remained in continuous remission beyond 1 year (Giralt et al., 1997a; Giralt et al., 1997b). Indolent lymphoid malignancies also appear to be amenable to a similar strategy. Heavily pretreated patients with CLL or low-grade lymphoma were treated with a well-tolerated regimen consisting of fludarabine 30 mg/m^2/day × 3 days with cyclophosphamide 300 mg/m^2/day × 3 days or fludarabine, cytarabine, and cisplatin (Khouri et al., 1998). All patients had failed to respond to, or had relapsed after, primary chemotherapy. Nine patients had CLL in relapse after prior fludarabine treatment and 6 had lymphoma. Eleven of the 15 patients had durable engraftment, with 50% to 100% donor cells at 1 month posttransplant, typically converting to 100% over the next 2 months, either spontaneously or after infusion of additional donor lymphocytes. Hematopoietic recovery was prompt and, with the exception of a patient with hepatitis C infection, no patient had nonhematologic toxicity of greater than grade 2. The patients failing to engraft recovered endogenous hematopoiesis promptly and had no serious adverse effects. All 11 patients with engraftment responded and 8 achieved complete remission. Maximal responses were slow to develop and gradually occurred over a period of several months to 1 year.

The strategy of a nonablative preparative regimen was applied also to multiple myeloma, harnessing a graft-versus-myeloma effect while reducing regimen-related toxicities. The team in Houston explored a regimen of melphalan (140–180 mg/m^2) and fludarabine (30 mg/m^2 for 4 days). This appeared to be a promising strategy since 7 of 13 patients with advanced myeloma achieved complete remissions. Use of less toxic, non-myeloablative preparative regimens produced engraftment and generated graft-versus-malignancy effects. This approach allowed the use of stem cell transplantation for older patients and those with comorbidities, which precluded high-dose chemoradiotherapy. A regimen comparable to the one reported from Houston and consisting of cyclophosphamide and fludarabine was used with a similar success rate by investigators in Bethesda (Childs et al., 1999; Childs et al., 2000) and elsewhere.

Investigators in Boston used cyclophosphamide 150 to 200 mg/kg along with ATG and thymic irradiation before HLA-identical sibling HSCT in 21 patients with advanced, refractory hematologic malignancies. Grade II–IV acute GVHD was seen in only 1 of 21 patients not receiving DLI. Prophylactic DLI was given to patients in whom no GVHD was present by day 35. Seven patients were alive and free of disease progression 105 to 548 (median 445) days after transplantation. Durable chimerism has been seen in about 90% of patients receiving HLA-identical and mismatched transplants with this protocol, and lasting mixed chimerism has been demonstrated greater than 1.5 years in an extensively mismatched transplant recipient (Sykes et al., 1999). The sustained remissions obtained in this group of patients with advanced and refractory disease suggest that this is a promising approach for achieving disease eradication, possibly with less GVHD than seen with conventional transplants.

Investigators in Genoa designed a combined protocol consisting of autografting with myeloablative chemotherapy followed by allogeneic NST for patients with advanced hematologic neoplasia and metastatic breast cancer (Carella *et al.*, 2000a; Carella *et al.*, 2000b; Carella *et al.*, 1998). Patients with high-risk Hodgkin's disease, non-Hodgkin's lymphoma, blastic or accelerated phase CML, or metastatic breast cancer entered various modifications of this combined approach. After engraftment of autologous stem cells, all patients were conditioned for allografting with fludarabine 30 mg/m^2/day × 3 days and cyclophosphamide 300 mg/m^2/day × 3 days. Peripheral blood stem cells (PBSC) from HLA-matched donors were mobilized with G-CSF. GVHD prophylaxis consisted of CSP and methotrexate. After autografting, the results in the different diseases were encouraging, with many patients achieving complete response after NST and others only after DLI. Most patients did not develop severe neutropenia. In summary, these observations confirmed the efficacy of immunosuppressive therapy with reduced intensity conditioning for engraftment of hematopoietic progenitor cells from HLA-matched donors with minimal toxicity and low mortality rate. This approach was recently adopted by several centers, following successful application of a similar protocol for the treatment of patients with multiple myeloma by Seattle and the Nonmyeloablative Transplant Consortium, using high-dose melphalan and autologous HSCT for optimal tumor cytoreduction followed by allogeneic NST for elimination of minimal residual disease. Cytoreduction and autologous PBSC transplantation was accomplished by mobilization of stem cells with cyclophosphamide, paclitaxel, and G-CSF, followed by high-dose melphalan of 200 mg/m^2 supported by autologous PBSC transplantation. Transplantation of mobilized blood stem cells from HLA-matched allogeneic donors was performed after conditioning with TBI 200 cGy, followed by GVHD prophylaxis with a combination of MMF and CSP. This protocol was extremely well tolerated. With a median follow-up of 399 days (range, 266–916 days) after autologous SCT and a median 330 (range, 198–793) days after allogeneic NST, 17 of a total of 21 patients enrolled in the pilot study (now confirmed in a larger cohort of patients from several centers), remain alive after beginning the two-step procedure. The causes of death were infection and grade IV acute GVHD in two patients who died 136 and 136 days after NST. In addition, one patient died 91 days after allografting from disease progression and one patient died after autologous HSCT from CMV-related lung infection. The day 100 mortality was 9.5% with one of two patients dying of disease progression. Overall survival was 81% and disease-free survival was 48% (Molina *et al.*, 2000).

In summary, availability of a relatively safe protocol for adoptive cell therapy based on well-tolerated reduced intensity conditioning may offer physicians an effective therapeutic tool for a larger number of patients at an early, thus optimal, stage of their disease. Many clinicians would agree that as far as utilizing chemotherapy and other available cytoreductive anticancer agents, whatever cannot be achieved at an early stage of conventional chemotherapy is unlikely to be accomplished later on by additional doses of chemotherapy, since tumor cells usually acquire resistance to subsequent chemotherapy. In addition to preventing the development of resistant tumor cell clones by continuous courses of conventional doses of chemotherapy, clinical application of a curative modality at an earlier stage of disease may avoid the need for repeated courses of chemotherapy, each accompanied by a risk of pancytopenia and sensitization against blood products. Also avoided are cumulative multiorgan toxicity and development of resistant strains of various infective agents, which frequently develop in the course of antimicrobial protocols given for treatment or prevention of infections that may be unavoidable during repeated courses of conventional anticancer modalities. Hopefully, immunotherapy mediated by allogeneic lymphocytes in tolerant hosts at an early stage of the disease, mediated by NST for every patient with a fully matched sibling not expected to be cured with conventional chemotherapy, may result in a significant improvement of disease-free survival, quality of life, and cost effectiveness. Once such a hypothesis is confirmed, this approach may open new avenues for the treatment of hematologic malignancies and a long list of genetic diseases.

In the future, it seems reasonable to assume that even safer approaches will be available for engraftment of donor stem cells while more effective and more selective immunotherapy may be accomplished with specifically immune T cells, including natural killer (NK) and NK/T cells, that may not cause GVHD while reacting against tumor cells, thus enabling gradual elimination of all host-type hematopoiesis over time, while controlling for GVHD (Ruggieri *et al.*, 1999). It remains to be seen whether a similar therapeutic approach can be developed for patients with partially matched allografts. Furthermore, the induction of mixed chimerism using mismatched stem cells may allow the use of similar technology for induction of unresponsiveness to perfused living related or cadaveric organ allografts. Since complete prevention of GVHD can be easily accomplished by negative selection of T cells or positive selection of CD34$^+$ stem cells, the future application of mismatched stem cells must await development of safer methods for more effective deletion of donor-reactive T cells and cytotoxic T-lymphocyte precursor cells.

Immunotherapy of metastatic solid tumors with alloreactive lymphocytes in conjunction with NST

Tumor cells are uniformly rejected when implanted in immunocompetent allogeneic recipients. Therefore, it seems reasonable to assume that the mirror image is also true, that is, that donor lymphocytes may also react against tumor cells of host origin, by a mechanism that resembles allograft rejection, or rather "reversed" allograft rejection. Indeed, we documented in the early 1980s the existence of GVT effects following induction of HVG transplantation tolerance in female (NZBxNZW)F$_1$ recipients, susceptible to spontaneously developing systemic lupus erythematosus as well as sarcomas (Moscovitch & Slavin, 1984). Following induction of BALB/c into (NZBxNZW)F$_1$ mixed chimerism by NST using TLI, complete prevention of development of spontaneous sarcomas occurred, as compared with lethal sarcomas in 24% of untreated controls. The data suggested induction of GVT effects following nonmyeloablative conditioning independently of clinically overt GVHD (Moscovitch & Slavin, 1984).

Recently, we demonstrated the efficacy of allogeneic cell therapy in a murine mammary carcinoma model (4T1) of BALB/c mice, using naive MHC-mismatched splenocytes (Morecki et al., 1997; Morecki et al., 1998; Prigozhina et al., 2002). The encouraging clinical results with cell therapy in hematologic malignancies using MHC-identical donor cells that differ from the phenotype of the tumor by minor histocompatibility antigens (mHag) only, led us to test the feasibility of induction of GVT effects across mHag barriers in a murine model of mammary carcinoma. Cell therapy in this setting was investigated in BALB/c mice inoculated with 4T1 treated with DBA/2-derived splenocytes. GVT effects were assayed in secondary recipients of adoptively transferred lung cells derived from primary hosts, previously inoculated intravenously with 4T1 cells and injected with either (1) naive BALB/c splenocytes (2) naive DBA/2 splenocytes, (3) 4T1-immune DBA/2 splenocytes, or (4) DBA/2 splenocytes immunized with host-derived BABL/c spleen cells.

Naive DBA/2 splenocytes inhibited tumor growth only slightly and hardly prolonged the survival of secondary recipients, in comparison with fully matched tumor/host BALB/c spleen cells. Much more efficient GVT reaction was demonstrated in vitro and in vivo using DBA/2 splenocytes from mice presensitized by multiple injections of irradiated tumor or BALB/c-derived spleen cells. All 30 mice adoptively inoculated with lung cells from primary hosts that had previously been treated with these presensitized effector cells were tumor-free for more than 250 days. Secondary recipients inoculated with lung cells from mice given naive BALB/c or DBA/2 spleen cells died of metastatic tumors within 33 to 46 days. Pre-immunization with mHag-mismatched splenocytes sensitized against tumor or spleen cells of host origin can therefore upregulate antitumor responses while not enhancing clinical manifestations of antihost reactivity. Taken together, our data provided the background for considering the possibility of using donor lymphocytes activated against tumor antigens or host type alloantigens as a new clinical tool for overcoming residual disease in patients with resistant cancer cells. A measurable response against liver metastases that disappeared transiently following administration of fully matched donor lymphocytes was documented in a patient who developed hepatic lesions following myeloablative combination chemotherapy supported by autologous stem cell transplantation (Or et al., 1998). The data suggested that, analogous to GVL effects, GVT effects may occur against solid tumors, as long as the host accepts the donor lymphocytes. GVT effects following standard myeloablative conditioning were reported in patients with metastatic breast cancer. However, the cell therapy procedure proved toxic in conjunction with the myeloablative conditioning used for the HSCT procedure; hence, widespread clinical application of cell therapy for patients with metastatic cancer has not been recommended (Eibl et al., 1996; Ueno et al., 1998).

It was recently documented by Childs et al. that cell therapy may be applied following NST for elimination of metastatic renal cell cancer, including patients fully resistant to all available anticancer modalities (Childs et al., 1999; Childs et al., 2000). These observations are most promising, and should encourage similar investigations for other metastatic tumors on an experimental basis, since the clinical benefits were limited to 10% to 20% of the patients and acute and chronic GVHD, which correlated with response to allogeneic cell-mediated immunotherapy, still remained problematic. The association between GVT and the occurrence of GVHD in most of the patients with renal cell cancer studied suggests that the antitumor effect of donor lymphocytes is mediated at least in part by an immune reaction against tumor cells that display the recipient's histocompatibility antigens. Nevertheless, preclinical and early clinical studies indicate that both GVL and GVT effects may occur in the absence of clinically significant GVHD. Indeed, in several of the patients with renal cell cancer, a GVT effect was observed in the absence of GVHD at the time of disease regression (Childs et al., 1999). Likewise, regression of metastases was often delayed by months from the onset of GVHD, again suggesting that the antitumor effector mechanisms may be distinct from those that cause antihost responses.

The clinical responses observed in patients with renal cell cancer have not yet been documented in any other large series of metastatic solid tumors. Indeed, several patients with metastatic malignant melanoma failed to respond; however, all had advanced disease state and since the time to response may take several months up to 1 year, it is possible that failure to observe response was due to the short life expectancy. Clearly, once the principle can be confirmed in clinical practice, several newer approaches may enhance the efficacy and reduce the risks of immunotherapy with donor lymphocytes. One such approach, based on murine data, is the use of immune T cells generated in vitro against tumor-specific peptides or the patient's own tumor cell suspension, as long as tumor antigens are presented by antigen-presenting cells. It may also be possible to manipulate the donor lymphocytes in vitro by insertion of a suicide gene, such as the herpes simplex virus thymidine kinase gene, which provides an option for limiting the lifespan of donor T cells, thus reducing the risk of uncontrolled GVHD. Clearly, targeting donor anticancer effector cells to the tumor by using immune specific donor lymphocytes, or by targeting killer cells to cell surface tumor markers not shared by normal somatic cells may be the next step for inducing GVT independently of GVHD. An alternative approach to amplify GVL while avoiding or minimizing GVHD may involve the use of allogeneic NK and NK/T cells with potent antitumor activity, yet devoid of antihost reactivity.

Induction of GVL effects by immune donor lymphocytes in clinical practice

Based on successful experiments in preclinical animal models of human disease, showing that adoptive immunotherapy of leukemia with DLI is much more efficient when donor lymphocytes are obtained from specifically immunized donors, we described a successful clinical attempt to treat DLI-resistant replase with donor lymphocytes pulsed in vitro against host alloantigens (Slavin et al., 2001). A 7-year-old girl with Philadelphia-positive CML underwent HSCT from a fully matched 6-month-old sibling (male) following conditioning with standard doses of busulfan and cyclophosphamide; she relapsed 9 months after HSCT (95% of the marrow cells 46XX t(9:22)) and failed to respond to DLI, including to donor lymphocytes activated with IL-2 both in vivo and in vitro (four attempts). The patient never developed any clinical signs of GVHD. Donor lymphocytes were subsequently pulsed in vitro with a mixture of irradiated PBL obtained from both parents in order to trigger alloactivation of donor lymphocytes against host alloantigens presented by parental cells, using as stimulating cells maternal PBL expressing the shared maternal haplotype and paternal PBL expressing the shared paternal haplotype of the patient. Alpha-interferon was administered to the patient in an attempt to increase the immunogenicity of tumor cells by upregulating cell surface expression of MHC antigens. Subsequently, hematologic, cytogenetic, and molecular remission (negative RT-PCR for bcr/abl) was induced for the first time and maintained since 1992 with a normal karyotype consisting of 100% 46XY cells in both blood and marrow. Using immune rather than naive donor lymphocytes may open new horizons for cancer immunotherapy by adoptively transferred donor lymphocytes.

Summary and conclusions

Alloreactive donor lymphocytes given at the time of allogeneic hematopoietic stem cell infusion, or DLI given later post-HSCT, represent the main therapeutic weapon of the transplant procedure. Hence, future investigations should focus on new approaches for improving the NST procedure as a platform for cell-mediated immunotherapy with donor lymphocytes. The next goal should be maximizing tumor-specific responses while protecting normal host cells from such an attack. Future HSCT protocols are likely to focus on reducing the intensity of the conditioning and improving the immune effects mediated by allogeneic donor lymphocytes. NST is relatively safe even in heavily treated, high-risk patients, in a range of malignant and nonmalignant indications for stem cell transplantation. NST is associated with minimal procedure-related toxicity and mortality, shorter periods of pancytopenia with minimal or no aplasia and hence reduced consumption of blood products and antimicrobial therapy. Therefore, NST is well tolerated by all patients, including those considered ineligible for HSCT because of older age or poor performance status. With currently available approaches, stable complete or mixed chimerism can be induced consistently for patients with a matched sibling or matched unrelated donor. Early complete engraftment is observed in most patients but in cases of mixed chimerism, conversion to 100% donor cells can be accomplished by discontinuation of CSP or by DLI. Thus, NST may become the allotransplant procedure of choice for elderly patients, as well as for infants and younger patients, in whom it may reduce the risk of sterility and other late complications including endocrine adenopathies and growth retardation. Once proven safe, NST may provide clinicians a tool for curative, rather than palliative, treatment of otherwise incurable disease at an early stage of disease for both malignant and nonmalignant indications.

We believe that the aforementioned goals can be accomplished by better understanding of the mechanism of transplantation tolerance and of the mechanisms of target-specific anticancer immunotherapy by cells and biologic response modifying agents. Meanwhile, successful phase I and II clinical trials are needed to define optimal NST protocols (dose and schedule of fludarabine; type and dose of alkylating agents or TBI; role of monoclonal or polyclonal antilymphocyte antibodies given as part of the conditioning; optimal posttransplant immunosuppression for prevention of GVHD. Finally, phase III clinical trials may be required in different disease categories to compare the overall responses of NST in comparison with conventional HSCT based on myeloablative conditioning.

References

Aker, A., Varadi, G., Slavin, S., & Nagler, A. (1999). A fludarabine based nonmyeloablative protocol for human umbilical cord blood transplantation in Fanconi's anemia. Fludarabine-based protocol for human umbilical cord blood transplantation in children with Fanconi's anemia. *Journal of Pediatric Hematology and Oncology*, **21**, 237–9.

Aker, M., Kapelushnik, J., Pugatsch, T. *et al.* (1998). Donor lymphocyte infusions to displace residual host hematopoietic cells after allogeneic HSCT for beta thalassemia major. *Journal of Pediatric Hematology and Oncology*, **20**, 145–8.

Bachar-Lustig, E., Rachamin, N., Li, H.W. *et al.* (1995). Megadose of T cell-depleted bone marrow overcomes MHC barriers in sublethally irradiated mice. *Nature Medicine*, **1**, 1268–73.

Bacigalupo, A., Van Lint, M.T., Occhini, D. *et al.* (1991) Increased risk of leukemia relapse with high dose cyclosporine A after allogeneic marrow transplantation for acute leukemia. *Blood*, **77**, 1423.

Bar, B.M., Schattenberg, A., Mensink, E.J. *et al.* (1993). Donor leukocyte infusions for chronic myeloid leukemia relapsed after allogeneic bone marrow transplantation. *Journal of Clinical Oncology*, **11**, 513–19.

Bast, C.R. (1985). Principles of cancer biology: tumor immunology. In *Cancer; Principles & Practice of Oncology*, ed. V.T. DeVitta, S. Hellman, & S.A. Rosenberg pp. 125–41. Philadelphia: J.B. Lippincott.

Billingham, R.E., Brent, I., & Medawar, P.B. (1953). Actively acquired tolerance to foreign cells. *Nature*, **172**, 606.

Boranic, M. & Tonkovic, I. (1971). Time pattern of the antileukemia effect of graft-versus-host reaction in mice, I. Cellular events. *Cancer Research*, **31**, 1140–7.

Bortin, M.M., Truitt, R.L., Rimm, A.A., & Bach, F.H. (1979). Graft-versus-leukaemia reactivity induced by alloimmunization without augmentation of graft-versus-host reactivity. *Nature,* **281,** 490–1.

Carella, A.M., Champlin, R., Slavin, S. *et al.* (2000a). "Mini-allografts": ongoing trials in humans. *Bone Marrow Transplantation,* **25,** 345–50.

Carella, A.M., Giralt, S., & Slavin, S. (2000b). Low intensity regimens with allogeneic hematopoietic stem cell transplantation as treatment of hematologic neoplasia. *Haematologica,* **85,** 304–13.

Carella, A.M., Lerma, E., Corsetti, M.T. *et al.* (1998). Evidence of cytogenetic and molecular remission by allogeneic cells after immunosuppressive therapy alone. *British Journal of Haematology,* **103,** 565–7.

Childs, R., Chernoff, A., Contentin, N. *et al.* (2000). Regression of metastatic renal-cell carcinoma after nonmyeloablative allogeneic peripheral-blood stem-cell transplantation. *New England Journal of Medicine,* **14,** 750–8.

Childs, R.W., Clave, E., Tisdale, J. *et al.* (1999). Successful treatment of metastatic renal cell carcinoma with a nonmyeloablative allogeneic peripheral-blood progenitor-cell transplant: evidence for a graft-versus-tumor effect. *Journal of Clinical Oncology,* **17,** 2044–50.

Collins, R.H., Shpilberg, O., Drobyski, W.R. (1997). Donor leukocyte infusions in 140 patients with relapsed malignancy after allogeneic bone marrow transplantation. *Journal of Clinical Oncology,* **15,** 433–44.

De Witte, T., Schattenberg, A., Preijers, F., & Mensink, E. (1992). Treatment of relapse in recipients of lymphocyte depleted grafts with infusion of lymphocytes of the original bone marrow donor. *Experimental Hematology,* **20,** 723.

Eibl, B., Schwaighofer, H., Nachbaur, D. *et al.* (1996). Evidence for a graft-versus-tumor effect in a patient treated with marrow ablative chemotherapy and allogeneic bone marrow transplantation for breast cancer. *Blood,* **88,** 1501–8.

Falkenburg, J.H.F., Faber, L.M., van den Elshout, M. *et al.* (1993). Generation of donor derived antileukemic cytotoxic T lymphocyte responses for treatment of relapsed leukemia after allogeneic HLA identical bone marrow transplantation. *Journal of Immunotherapy,* **14,** 305.

Giralt, S., Cohen, A., Mehra, R. *et al.* (1997a). Preliminary results of fludarabine/melphalan or 2CDA/melphalan as preparative regimens for allogeneic progenitor cell transplantation in poor candidates for conventional myeloablative conditioning. *Blood,* **90** (Suppl 1), 1853a.

Giralt, S., Gajewski, J., Khouri, I. *et al.* (1997b). Induction of graft-versus-leukemia as primary treatment of chronic myelogenous leukemia. *Blood,* **90** (Suppl. 1), 1857a.

Gratwohl, A., Hermans, J., Goldman, J.M. *et al.* (1998). For the chronic leukemia Working Party of the EHSCT. *Lancet,* **352,** 1087.

Grillo-Lopez, A.J., White, C.A., Dallaire, B.K. *et al.* (2000). Rituximab: the first monoclonal antibody approved for the treatment of lymphoma. Review. *Current Pharmaceutical Biotechnology,* **1,** 1–9.

Higano, C.S., Brixey, M., & Bryant, E.M. (1990). Durable complete remission of acute nonlymphocytic leukemia associated with dis-continuation of immunosuppression following relapse after allogeneic bone marrow transplantation. A case report of a probable graft-versus-leukemia effect. *Transfusion,* **50,** 175–8.

Horowitz, M., Gale, R.P., Sondel, P.M. *et al.* (1990). Graft-versus-leukemia reactions after bone marrow transplantation. *Blood,* **75,** 555–62.

Howard, R.J., Sutherland, D.E.P., Lum, C.T. *et al.* (1981). Kidney allograft survival in dogs treated with total lymphoid irradiation. *Annals of Surgery,* **193,** 196–200.

Ildstad, S.T. & Sachs, D.H. (1984). Reconstitution with syngeneic plus allogeneic or xenogeneic bone marrow leads to specific acceptance of allografts or xenografts. *Nature,* **307,** 168–70.

Ji, Y.H., Weiss, L., Zeira, M. *et al.* Allogeneic cell-mediated immunotherapy of leukemia with immune donor lymphocytes to up-regulate anti-tumor effects and down-regulate anti-host responses. (Submitted for publication).

Johnson, B.D., Drobyski, W.R., & Truitt, R.L. (1993). Delayed infusion of normal donor cells after MHC-matched bone marrow transplantation provides an antileukemia reaction without graft-versus-host disease. *Bone Marrow Transplantation,* **11,** 329–36.

Kapelushnik, J., Aker, M., Or, R. *et al.* (1997). Allogeneic cell therapy as a new modality for displacement of genetically abnormal stem cells as part of the conditioning for allogeneic bone marrow transplantation. In *Correction of Genetic Diseases by Transplantation IV,* pp. 111–9. Cogent Press.

Kapelushnik, J., Aker, M., Pugatsch, T. *et al.* (1998). Bone marrow transplantation from a cadaveric donor. *Bone Marrow Transplantation,* **21,** 857–8.

Kapelushnik, J., Or, R., Aker, M. *et al.* (1996). Allogeneic cell therapy of severe beta thalassemia major by displacement of host stem cells in mixed chimera by donor blood lymphocytes. *Bone Marrow Transplantation,* **19,** 96–98.

Kapelushnik, J., Or, R., Slavin, S., & Nagler, A. (1997). Fludarabine based protocol for HSCT in Fanconi anemia. *Bone Marrow Transplantation,* **29,** 1109–10.

Khouri, I.F., Keating, M., Korbling, M. *et al.* (1998). Transplant-lite: induction of graft-versus-malignancy using fludarabine-based nonablative chemotherapy and allogeneic blood progenitor-cell transplantation as treatment for lymphoid malignancies. *Journal of Clinical Oncology,* **16,** 2817–24.

Kolb, H.J., Mittermuller, J., Clemm, C. *et al.* (1990). Donor leukocyte transfusions for treatment of recurrent chronic myelogenous leukemia in marrow transplant patients. *Blood,* **76,** 2462–5.

Kolb, H.J., Schattenberg, A., Goldman, J.M. *et al.* (1995). Graft-versus-leukemia effect of donor lymphocyte transfusions in marrow grafted patients: European Group for Blood and Marrow Transplantation Working Party Chronic Leukemia. *Blood,* **86,** 2041–50.

Kuzushima, K., Yamamoto, M., Kimura, H. *et al.* (1996). Establishment of anti-Epstein-Barr virus (EBV) cellular immunity by adoptive transfer of virus specific cytotoxic T lymphocytes from an HLA matched sibling to a patient with severe chronic active EBV infection. *Clinical and Experimental Immunology,* **103,** 192–8.

Leber, B., Walker, I.R., Rodrigues, A. *et al.* (1993). Reinduction of remission of chronic myeloid leukemia by donor leukocyte transfusion following relapse after bone marrow transplantation:

recovery complicated by initial pancytopenia and late dermatomyositis. *Bone Marrow Transplantation*, **12**, 405–7.

Leshem, B., Vourka Karussis, U., & Slavin, S. (2000). Correlation between enhancement of graft vs leukemia effects following allogeneic bone marrow transplantation by rIL-2 and increased frequency of cytotoxic t-lymphocyte precursors in murine myeloid leukemia. *Cytokines, Cellular and Molecular Therapy*, **6**, 141–7.

Mackinnon, S., Papadopoulos, E.B., Carabassi, M.H. *et al.* (1995). Adoptive immunotherapy evaluating escalating doses of donor leukocytes for relapse of chronic myeloid leukemia after bone marrow transplantation: separation of graft-versus-leukemia responses from graft-versus-host disease. *Blood*, **86**, 1261–8.

McSweeney, P.A., Wagner, J.L., Maloney, D.G. *et al.* (1998). Outpatient PBSC allografts using immunosuppression with low-dose TBI before, and cyclosporine (CSP) and mycophenolate mofetil (MMF) after transplant. *Blood*, **92** (Suppl 1), 519a (abstr. 2133).

Meredith, R.F. & O'Kunewick, J.P. (1983). Possibility of graft-vs-leukemia determinants independent of the major histocompatibility complex in allogeneic marrow transplantation. *Transplantation*, **35**, 378–85.

Molina, A.S.F., Maloney, D.G., Sandmaier, B.M. *et al.* (2000). Nonmyeloablative peripheral blood stem cell (PBSC) allografts following cytoreductive autotransplants in the treatment of multiple myeloma. *Blood*, **96** (Suppl. 1), 480a (abstract).

Morecki, S., Leshem, B., Eid, A., & Slavin, S. (1987). Alloantigen persistence in induction and maintenance of transplantation tolerance. *Journal of Experimental Medicine*, **165**, 1468–80.

Morecki, S., Leshem, B., Weigensberg, M. *et al.* (1985). Functional clonal deletion verus active suppression in transplantation tolerance induced by total lymphoid irradiation (TLI). *Transplantation*, **40**, 201–10.

Morecki, S., Moshel, Y., Gelfend, Y. *et al.* (1997). Induction of graft vs tumor effect in a murine model of mammary adenocarcinoma. *International Journal of Cancer*, **71**, 59–63.

Morecki, S., Yacovlev, E., Diab, A., & Slavin, S. (1998). Allogeneic cell therapy for a murine mammary carcinoma. *Cancer Research*, **58**, 3891–5.

Moscovitch, M. & Slavin, S. (1984). Anti-tumor effects of allogeneic bone marrow transplantation in (NZB × NZW)F1 hybrids with spontaneous lymphosarcoma. *Journal of Immunology*, **132**, 997–1000.

Nagler, A., Ackerstein, A., Kapelushnik, J. *et al.* (1999). Donor lymphocyte infusion post nonmyeloablative allogeneic peripheral blood stem cell transplantation for chronic granulomatous disease. *Bone Marrow Transplantation, ,* **24**, 339–42.

Nagler, A., Aker, M., Or, R. *et al.* (2001). Low-intensity conditioning is sufficient to ensure engraftment in matched unrelated bone marrow transplantation. *Experimental Hematology*, **29**, 362–70.

Nagler, A., Slavin, S., Varadi, G. *et al.* (2000). Allogeneic peripheral blood stem cell transplantation using a fludarabine-based low intensity conditioning regimen for a malignant lymphoma. *Bone Marrow Transplantation*, **25**, 1021–8.

Naparstek, E., Nagler, A., Or, R., & Slavin, S. (1996). Allogeneic cell mediated immunotherapy using donor lymphocytes for prevention of relapse in patients treated with allogeneic HSCT for hematological malignancies. North America. *Clinical Transplants, 1995,* ed. J.M. Cecka & P.I. Terasaki, pp. 281–90. Angeles: UCLA Tissue Typing Laboratory.

Naparstek, E., Or, R., Nagler, A. *et al.* (1995). T-cell-depleted allogeneic bone marrow transplantation for acute leukaemia using Campath-1 antibodies and post-transplant administration of donor's peripheral blood lymphocytes for prevention of relapse. *British Journal of Haematology*, **89**, 506–15.

Odom, L.F., August, C.S., Githens, J.H. *et al.* (1978). Remmission of relapsed leukaemia during a graft-versus-host reaction. A "graft-versus-leukaemia reaction" in man? *Lancet*, **2**, 537–8.

Or, R., Ackerstein, A., Nagler, A. *et al.* (1998). Allogeneic cell-mediated and cytokine-activated immunotherapy for malignant lymphoma at the stage of minimal residual disease after autologous stem cell transplantation. *Journal of Immunotherapy*, **21**, 447–53.

Or, R., Shapira, M.Y., Amar, A. *et al.* (2003). Nonmyeloablative allogeneic stem cell transplantation for the treatment of chronic myeloid leukemia in first chronic phase. *Blood*, **101**, 441–5.

Owen, R.D. (1945). Immunogenetic consequences of vascular anastomoses between bovine twins. *Science*, **102**, 400.

Papadopoulos, E.B., Ladanyi, M., Emanual, D. *et al.* (1994). Infusions of donor leukocytes to treat Epstein-Barr virus-associated lympho-proliferative disorders after allogeneic bone marrow transplantation. *New England Journal of Medicine*, **330**, 1185–91.

Passweg, J.R., Rowlings, P.A., Armitage, J.O. *et al.* (1996). Report from the International Bone Marrow Transplant Registry and Autologous Blood and Marrow Transplant Registry—North America. *Clinical Transplants, 1995,* ed. J.M. Cecka & P.I. Terasaki, pp. 117–27, Los Angeles: UCLA Tissue Typing Laboratory.

Porter, D.L., Roth, M.S., McGarigle, C. *et al.* (1994). Induction of graft-versus-host disease as immunotherapy for relapsed chronic myeloid leukemia. *New England Journal of Medicine*, **330**, 100–6.

Prigozhina, T., Gurevitch, O., & Slavin, S. (1999). Nonmyeloablative conditioning to induce bilateral tolerance after allogeneic bone marrow transplantation in mice. *Experimental Hematology*, **27**, 1503–10.

Prigozhina, T., Gurevitch, O., Morecki, S. *et al.* (2002). Nonmyeloablative allogeneic bone marrow transplantation as immunotherapy for hematologic malignancies and metastatic solid tumors in preclinical models. *Experimental Hematology*, **30**, 89–96.

Prigozhina, T., Gurevitch, O., Zhu, J., & Slavin, S. (1997). Permanent and specific transplantation tolerance induced by a nonmyeloablative treatment to a wide variety of allogeneic tissues. *Transplantation*, **63**, 1394–9.

Reisner, Y. & Martelli, M.F. (1995). Bone marrow transplantation across HLA barriers by increasing the number of transplanted cells. *Immunology Today*, **16**, 437–40.

Rosenberg, S.A. (1992). The immunotherapy and gene therapy of cancer. *Journal of Clinical Oncology*, **10**, 180–92.

Ruggeri, L., Capanni, M., Casucci, M. *et al.* (1999). Role of natural killer cell alloreactivity in HLA-mismatched hematopoietic stem cell transplantation. *Blood*, **94**, 333–9.

Sinkovics, J.G., Shullenberger, C.C., & Howe, C.D. (1965). Prolongation and prevention of Rauscher virus mouse leukemia by spleen cells of naturally resistant or actively immunized mice. *Clinical Research*, **13**, 36–9.

Slavin, S. & Seidel, H.J. (1982). Hematopoietic activity in bone marrow chimeras prepared with total lymphoid irradiation (TLI). *Experimental Hematology*, **10**, 206–16.

Slavin, S. & Strober, S. (1979). Induction of allograft tolerance after total lymphoid irradiation (TLI): development of suppressor cells of the mixed leukocyte reaction MLR. *Journal of Immunology*, **123**, 942–6.

Slavin, S. (1987). Total lymphoid irradiation (TLI). *Immunology Today*, **8**, 88–92.

Slavin, S. (1987). Total lymphoid irradiation. *Immunology Today*, **3**, 88.

Slavin, S. (2001). Immunotherapy of cancer with alloreactive lymphocytes (Review). *Lancet Oncology*, **2**, 491–8.

Slavin, S., Fuks, Z., Kaplan, H.S., & Strober, S. (1978). Transplantation of allogeneic bone marrow without graft vs host disease using total lymphoid irradiation. *Journal of Experimental Medicine*, **147**, 963–72.

Slavin, S., Nagler, A., Aker, M. *et al.* (2001). Nonmyeloablative stem cell transplantation and donor lymphocyte infusion for the treatment of cancer and life-threatening non-malignant disorders. *Review of Clinical and Experimental Hematology*, 135–46.

Slavin, S., Nagler, A., Naparstek, E. *et al.* (1998). Nonmyeloablative stem cell transplantation and cell therapy as an alternative to conventional bone marrow transplantation with lethal cytoreduction for the treatment of malignant and non malignant hematologic diseases. *Blood*, **91**, 756–63.

Slavin, S., Nagler, A., Naparstek, E. *et al.* (1999). Minitransplants and cell-based therapies for malignant and non-malignant disorders. *Current Opinion in Organ Transplantation*, **4**, 184–8.

Slavin, S., Naparstek, E., Nagler, A. *et al.* (1995). Allogeneic cell therapy for relapsed leukemia following bone marrow transplantation with donor peripheral blood lymphocytes. *Experimental Hematology*, **23**, 1553–62.

Slavin, S., Naparstek, E., Nagler, A. *et al.* (1996). Allogeneic cell therapy with donor peripheral blood cells and recombinant human interleukin-2 to treat leukemia relapse post allogeneic bone marrow transplantation. *Blood*, **87**, 2195–204.

Slavin, S., Or, R., Naparstek, E. *et al.* (1988). Cellular-mediated immunotherapy of leukemia in conjunction with autologous and allogeneic bone marrow transplantation in experimental animals and man. *Blood*, **72** (Suppl 1), 407a.

Slavin, S., Reitz, B., Bieber, C.P. *et al.* (1978). Transplantation tolerance in adult rats using total lymphoid irradiation (TLI): permanent survival of skin, heart and marrow allografts. *Journal of Experimental Medicine*, **147**, 700–7.

Slavin, S., Strober, S., Fuks, Z., & Kaplan, H.S. (1976). Long-term survival of skin allografts in mice treated with fractionated total lymphoid irradiation. *Science*, **193**, 1252–4.

Slavin, S., Strober, S., Fuks, Z., & Kaplan, H.S. (1977). Induction of specific tissue transplantation tolerance using fractionated total lymphoid irradiation in adult mice: long-term survival of allogeneic bone marrow and skin grafts. *Journal of Experimental Medicine*, **146**, 34–48.

Slavin, S., Weiss, L., Morecki, S., & Weingensberg, M. (1981). Eradication of murine leukemia with histoincompatible marrow grafts in mice conditioned with total lymphoid irradiation (TLI). *Cancer Immunology and Immunotherapy*, **11**, 155–61.

Slavin, S., Ackerstein, A., Morecki, S., *et al.* (2001). Immunotherapy of relapsed resistant chronic myelogenous leukemia post allogeneic bone marrow transplantation with alloantigen pulsed donor lymphocytes. *Bone Marrow Transplantation*, **28**, 795–8.

Stockschlaeder, M., Storb, R., Pepe, M. *et al.* (1992). A pilot study of low-dose cyclosporin for graft-versus-host prophylaxis in marrow transplantation. *British Journal of Haematology*, **80**, 49–54.

Storb, R., Raff, R.F., Appelbaum, F.R. *et al.* (1989). Comparison of fractionated to single-dose total body irradiation in conditioning canine littermates for DLA-identical marrow grafts. *Blood*, **74**, 1139.

Storb, R., Yu, C., Barnett, T. *et al.* (1999). Stable mixed hematopoietic chimerism in dog leukocyte antigen-identical littermate dogs given lymph node irradiation before and pharmacological immunosuppression after marrow transplantation. *Blood*, **94**, 1131–6.

Storb, R., Yu, C., Wagner, J.L. *et al.* (1997). Stable mixed hematopoietic chimerism in DLA-identical littermate dogs given sublethal total body irradiation before and pharmacological immunosuppression after marrow transplantation. *Blood*, **89**, 3048.

Sullivan, K.M., Weiden, P.L., Storb, R. *et al.* (1989). Influence of acute and chronic graft-versus-host disease on relapse and survival after bone marrow transplantation from HLA-identical siblings as treatment of acute and chronic leukemia. *Blood*, **73**, 1720–6.

Sykes, M. & Sachs, D.H. (1988). Mixed allogeneic chimerism as an approach to transplantation tolerance. *Immunology Today*, **9**, 23–27.

Sykes, M. & Sachs, D.H. (1990). Bone marrow transplantation as a means of inducing tolerance. *Seminars in Immunology*, **2**, 401–17.

Sykes, M., Chester, C.H., & Sachs, D.H. (1988). Protection from graft-vs-host disease in fully allogeneic chimeras by prior administration of T cell-depleted syngeneic bone marrow. *Transplantation*, **46**, 327–30.

Sykes, M., Preffer, F., McAfee, S. *et al.* (1999). Mixed lymphohematopoietic chimerism and graft versus lymphoma effect are achievable in adult recipients following nonmyeloablative therapy and HLA-mismatched donor bone marrow transplantation. *Lancet*, **353**, 1755–9.

Thomas, E.D. (1963). The role of marrow transplantation in the eradication of malignant disease. *Cancer*, **49**, 1963–8.

Truitt, R.L. & Atasoylu, A.A. (1991). Impact of pretransplant conditioning and donor T cells on chimerism, graft-versus-host disease, graft-vs-leukemia reactivity, and tolerance after bone marrow transplantation. *Blood*, **77**, 2515–23.

Truitt, R.L., Shih, F.-H., LeFever, A.V. *et al.* (1983). Characterization of alloimmunization-induced T lymphocytes reactivated against AKR leukemia in vitro and correlation with graft-vs-leukemia activity in vivo. *Journal of Immunology*, **131**, 2050–8.

Ueno, N.T., Rondón, G., Mirza, N.O. *et al.* (1998). Allogeneic peripheral-blood progenitor-cell transplantation for poor-risk patients with metastatic breast cancer. *Journal of Clinical Oncology*, **16**, 986–93.

Van Lochem, E., De Gast, B., Goulmy, E. (1992). In vitro separation of host specific graft-versus-host and graft-versus-leukemia cytotoxic-T cell activities. *Bone Marrow Transplantation*, **10**, 181–3.

Waldmann, H. & Cobbold, S. (1998). How do monoclonal antibodies induce tolerance? A role for infectious tolerance? *Annual Review of Immunology*, **16**, 619–44.

Weiden, P.L., Fluornoy, N., Sanders, J.E. *et al.* (1981a). Antileukemic effect of graft-versus-host disease contributes to improved survival after allogeneic marrow transplantation. *Transplantation*, **13**, 248–51.

Weiden, P.L., Sullivan, K.M., Fluornoy, N. *et al.* (1981b). Antileukemic effect of chronic graft-versus-host disease: contribution to improved survival after allogeneic marrow transplantation. *New England Journal of Medicine*, **304**, 1529–33.

Weigensberg, M., Morecki, S., Weiss, L. *et al.* (1984). Suppression of cell mediated immune responses following total lymphoid irradiation (TLI). 1. Characterization of suppresor cell of mixed lymphocyte reaction. *Journal of Immunology*, **132**, 971–8.

Weiss, L., Lubin, I., Factorowich, Y. *et al.* (1994). Effective graft vs leukemia effects independent of graft vs host disease after T-cell depleted allogeneic bone marrow transplantation in a murine model of B cell leukemia/lymphoma. Role of cell therapy and rIL-2. *Journal of Immunology*, **153**, 2562–67.

Weiss, L. & Slavin, S. (1999). Prevention and treatment of graft vs host disease by down-regulation of anti-host reactivity with veto cells of host origin. *Bone Marrow Transplantation*, **3**, 1139–43.

Weiss, L., Reich, S., & Slavin, S. (1990a). Effect of cyclosporine A and methylprednisolone on the GVL effect across major histocompatibility barriers in mice following allogeneic bone marrow transplantation. *Bone Marrow Transplantation*, **6**, 229–33.

Weiss, L., Reich, S., & Slavin, S. (1992). Use of recombinant human interleukin-2 in conjunction with bone marrow transplantation as a model for control of minimal residual disease in malignant hematological disorders. I. Treatment of murine leukemia in conjunction with allogeneic bone marrow transplantation and IL2-activated cell-mediated immunotherapy. *Cancer Investigation*, **10**, 19–26.

Weiss, L., Weigensberg, M., Morecki, S. *et al.* (1990b). Characterization of effector cells of graft vs leukemia (GVL) following allogeneic bone marrow transplantation in mice inoculated with murine B-cell leukemia (BCL1). *Cancer Immunology and Immunotherapy*, **31**, 236–42.

Werkerle, T., Kurtz, J., Ito, H. *et al.* (2000). Allogeneic bone marrow transplantation with co-stimulatory blockade induces macrochimerism and tolerance without cytoreductive host treatment. *Nature Medicine*, **4**, 464–9.

Zan-Bar, I., Slavin, S., & Strober, S. (1978). Induction and mechanism of tolerance to bovine serum albumin after total lymphoid irradiation (TLI). *Journal of Immunology*, **121**, 1400–4.

11 Blood compared to marrow as a source of allogeneic hematopoietic stem cells for transplantation

WILLIAM I. BENSINGER AND NORBERT SCHMITZ

Fred Hutchinson Cancer Research Center and the Department of Medicine, University of Washington, Seattle, USA, and AK St. Georg University Hospital, Hamburg, Germany

Introduction

It has long been known that hematopoietic precursors circulate in the peripheral blood and could potentially be utilized for autologous or allogeneic transplantation (Goodman & Hodgson, 1962; McCredie *et al.*, 1971). The steady state concentration of these cells is usually less than 0.1% of all nucleated cells, which precludes harvesting of useful numbers within a practical number of apheresis procedures. The administration of recombinant growth factors increases the concentration of, or "mobilizes", peripheral blood progenitor cells (PBSC), which can then be collected by apheresis. PBSC produce rapid and durable autologous hematopoietic reconstitution when infused after myeloablative therapy (Bensinger *et al.*, 1993a; Bensinger *et al.*, 1994; Bensinger *et al.*, 1995a). These observations led to the demonstration that the administration of granulocyte-colony stimulating factor (G-CSF) to normal individuals increased the number of hematopoietic precursors in the peripheral blood where they could be collected in large quantities and used for syngeneic and potentially for allogeneic transplantation (Schwinger, 1993; Weaver *et al.*, 1993; Dreger *et al.*, 1994). Syngeneic transplants were ideal for initial trials of PBSC collected from normal donors, as the infusion of large numbers of syngeneic T-cells should not cause severe graft-versus-host-disease (GVHD). Successful syngeneic PBSC transplants have been performed with durable engraftment and follow-up extending beyond 5 years (Weaver *et al.*, 1993). The administration of relatively high doses of G-CSF to normal syngeneic PBSC and allogeneic granulocyte donors was well tolerated and without measurable effects over up to 6 years of follow-up (Bensinger *et al.*, 1993b; Casper *et al.*, 1993; Weaver *et al.*, 1993). For donors, PBSC harvest in lieu of marrow has the advantages of avoiding an anesthetic procedure, surgery, possible blood transfusion, or hospitalization.

The first primary allogeneic transplant utilizing PBSC collected after G-CSF was reported by Russell *et al.*, in 1993 (Russell *et al.*, 1993). PBSC were used in this case because the donor was at high risk for anesthetic complications due to morbid obesity. The recipient had acute lymphocytic leukemia in second remission and was treated with cyclophosphamide and total body irradiation followed by unmodified PBSC and GVHD prophylaxis with cyclosporine and methotrexate. He engrafted promptly and did not develop acute or chronic GVHD. PBSC were also used for a second transplant following an allogeneic bone marrow graft failure (Dreger *et al.*, 1993). These initial observations led to the rapid application of this technology (Russell & Hunter, 1994; Azevedo *et al.*, 1995; Bensinger *et al.*, 1995a; Bensinger *et al.*, 1995b; Goldman, 1995; Körbling *et al.*, 1995b; Majolino *et al.*, 1995; Schmitz *et al.*, 1995; Anderlini *et al.*, 1996; Anderlini *et al.*, 1996a; Bensinger *et al.*, 1996a, 1996b; Bensinger *et al.*, 1996c; Korbling & Champlin, 1996; Russell *et al.*, 1996; Przepiorka *et al.*, 1997; Champlin *et al.*, 2000).

Results of allogeneic PBSC transplantation to date, including large retrospective surveys (Ringden et al., 2002), suggest that this technique can produce substantially more rapid engraftment than observed with BM. Acute GVHD has been tolerable, even with unmanipulated PBSC containing many more T cells than are present in a normal BM graft. Phase II studies of patients receiving PBSC, when compared to historical patients who have received BM, suggest that chronic GVHD may be more prevalent. This disadvantage could be offset, however, by potential advantages of PBSC over BM for the patient, which would include faster immune reconstitution, reduced early mortality and the possibility of an enhanced anti-leukemic (GVL) effects.

Characteristics of growth factor mobilized PBSC

Phenotypic and functional characteristics

PBSC collected after growth factor administration have been shown to contain a mixture of primitive and committed hematopoietic precursors in which the quantities of CD34+ cells are twofold to fivefold greater than BM, while T cells are 10-fold greater (Rice & Reiffers, 1992). Antigenic analysis of CD34+ PBSC revealed that these cells co-expressed a variety of differentiation antigens with properties that were similar to BM derived CD34+ cells including subpopulations that were CD34+/CD33−, CD34+/HLADR−, CD34+/HLADR+ and CD34+/CD33+ (Bender *et al.*, 1991; To *et al.*, 1994). Further work has indicated that there are important differences between

CD34+ cells purified from steady state BM compared to mobilized PBSC including high co-expression of CD13 antigens and low co-expression of CD7, CD10, CD19, CD71, c-kit and rhodamine uptake (Gyger et al., 2000). CD34+ cells collected from the peripheral blood after G-CSF differ from those in BM in terms of adhesion molecule expression, proliferative potential and cytokine response (McQuaker et al., 1995; To et al., 1997). Comparisons of PBSC and BM cell harvests indicate that PBSC contain 24-fold greater numbers of monocytes (CD45+CD14+) and 13-fold greater numbers of NK cells (CD16+CD56+CD3−) (Ottinger et al., 1996). These data show that the numbers of T-cells infused with a PBSC transplant will be directly related to the number of apheresis collections infused. Thus, efforts to maximize the CD34+ content of each collection to achieve the desired number with the fewest collections will reduce the number of T-cells infused in the graft.

The exact mechanism by which G-CSF mobilizes stem cells is unknown, but recently it was shown in patients that proteolytic cleavage of vascular intercellular adhesion molecule (VCAM-1) on CD34+ cells plays an important role in the egress of stem cells from marrow to blood (Levesque et al., 2000). This agrees with data in primates showing excellent mobilization of PBSC using antibodies to VCAM-1 and very late antigen-4 (VLA-4) showing potent synergy with G-CSF (Papayannopoulou et al., 1997). Additional studies are needed to define qualitative or quantitative differences between BM and PBSC that influence engraftment kinetics and determine if these differences are dependent on the specific growth factor or combination of growth factors used for mobilization.

Rapid engraftment of PBSC may not be due entirely to increased numbers but rather to the presence of accessory cells that are increased in number or qualitatively more capable of enhancing the milieu of the hematopoietic microenvironment. Initial studies designed to test this hypothesis evaluated the generation of cytokines by stromal cells cocultured with BM mononuclear cells or mononuclear cells collected from the blood after the administration of G-CSF or with BM mononuclear cells. IL-6 and G-CSF levels were increased when BM or G-CSF-stimulated peripheral blood mononuclear cells were added to stroma but the increase was 10-fold greater with the latter (Mielcarek et al., 1996).

Immunologic characteristics of PBSC

Data concerning the risk of acute GVHD are inconclusive. While the largest study indicates an increased risk of acute GVHD with PBSC (Schmitz et al., 2002) the majority of studies indicate that acute GVHD is not increased after PBSC transplantation despite the infusion of 1-2 logs more of T cells as compared to BM. In a meta-analysis that examined 15 trials, a small, but statistically significant increase in the relative risk (RR 1.13, 95% confidence interval 1.01–1.26) of acute GVHD was noted (Cutler et al., 2001). There are at least three possible explanations for this observation. First, it is possible that the number of T cells in a BM graft is sufficient to produce the maximum possible severity of GVHD for the degrees of genetic disparities between donors and recipients and that further increases in T-cell doses have no additive effect. Support for this hypothesis comes from clinical studies of T-depleted allogeneic BM, in which a threshold dose of approximately 10^5 residual CD3+ cells/kg was identified, below which acute GVHD was significantly reduced (Kernan et al., 1986; Verdonck et al., 1994). The second explanation is that the T cells are functionally altered in G-CSF-mobilized PBSC. G-CSF could alter the function of the lymphocytes infused or could alter cytokine production by infused accessory cells. Support for this hypothesis comes from studies in mice, where G-CSF pretreatment was found to polarize CD4+ cells toward a T-helper type-2 (Th2) response with a decrease in IL-2 and interferon production and a corresponding reduction in acute GVHD and improved survival (Pan et al., 1995). In vitro studies of patient samples have identified increased suppressor cell activity of CD14+ cells in G-CSF-mobilized PBSC from patients (Mielcarek et al., 1997). Other work has shown a fourfold to fivefold increase in CD4−CD8−αβ T-cells in the blood of normal donors receiving G-CSF (Kusnierz-Glaz et al., 1997). These cells were shown to have in vitro suppressor activity. In vitro G-CSF has been shown to directly downregulate responder cells via inhibition of tumor necrosis factor α production (Kitabayashi et al., 1995). The third possibility may be due to a differential risk of acute GVHD depending on whether patients have good risk or poor risk hematologic malignancies. The studies that have reported an increased incidence of GVHD enrolled mainly good risk patients.

Allogeneic PBSC transplantation in humans

Safety of G-CSF in normal donors

Administration of G-CSF in doses up to 16 μg/kg/day has been well tolerated in normal donors, with bone pain, flulike symptoms and myalgias being the major side effects; this subject has been reviewed (Anderlini et al., 1996a; Anderlini et al., 1996b; Bensinger et al., 1996b). There are no reports of discontinuation of G-CSF due to immediate side effects in normal PBSC donors. Both the side effects and the granulocytosis are, in general, reversed within 48 hours of discontinuing the drug.

In donors undergoing daily administration of G-CSF and daily granulocyte collections for 7 to 14 days there were significant decrements in platelet levels when compared to patients undergoing the same collection procedures without the administration of G-CSF (Bensinger et al., 1993b). In patients undergoing one or two apheresis procedures for the collection of PBSC, platelet decrements to levels below 100×10^9/L usually are not observed. It is known from phase I studies of G-CSF administration to patients who were not apheresed that platelet levels decrease (Lindemann et al., 1989). Similar findings of platelet decrements have also been observed following human or canine GM-CSF administration in a dog model (Nash et al.,

1995). The exact mechanisms of thrombocytopenia following cytokine-facilitated PBSC or granulocyte harvests are unknown but may be related to the secondary induction of cytokines by G-CSF, which can affect platelet turnover.

Self-limited laboratory abnormalities including elevated alkaline phosphatase, lactate dehydrogenase, uric acid, alanine aminotransferase and/or-glutamyl transpeptidase and decreases in potassium and magnesium have been reported (Fossa et al., 1992; Dreger et al., 1993; Dreger et al., 1994; Anderlini et al., 1997b; Stroneck et al., 1997). Several reports have demonstrated that G-CSF administration induces a transient, mild hypercoagulable state as shown by shortening of the in vitro bleeding test, increase in fibrinogen and factor VIII levels with a reduction in proteins C and S (Söhngen et al., 1998) or increases in prothrombin fragment, thrombin-antithrombin complex, and D-dimer (LeBlanc et al., 1999; Falanga et al., 1999). Case reports have described rare events such as myocardial infarction (Cavallaro et al., 2000) or stroke in association with G-CSF administration (Anderlini et al., 1997c). Although these thrombotic complications are distinctly uncommon in normal donors given G-CSF, these findings should engender caution when considering donors with a history of peripheral vascular disease, myocardial infarction or stroke. In an IBMTR/EBMT survey of 1488 PBSC donors, 20% required placement of a central venous catheter (Anderlini et al., 2001). Donation-related complications were reported in 1.1% (Table 11.1). One third of the reported complications were related to the central venous catheter; the incidence of complications was 3.6% in those with a central venous catheter versus 1.1% in those without ($P = 0.04$). There was a linear correlation between increasing complication rates and increasing numbers of collections. No donor fatalities were reported.

Spontaneous splenic rupture (Becker et al., 1997; Falzetti et al., 1999) acute iritis (Parkkali et al., 1996) severe pyogenic infections (Hilbe et al., 2000) cutaneous papular, erythematous eruption (Torrelo et al., 2000), acute gouty arthritis (Spitzer et

Table 11.1. *Peripheral blood donor complications as reported verbatim in report forms*

Bleeding around catheter site during apheresis
Capillary leak syndrome
Episode of pericarditis 1 month after collection
Hematoma from catheter placement
Hemothorax (related to) catheter placement
Hypercalcemia, anxiety requiring hospitalization
Hypertension
Hypotension, hypoxia, dyspnea
Nausea, diarrhea
Platelet count drop
Thrombocytopenia
Subclavian vein thrombosis
Back pain, hypertension
Catheter replacement twice (kinks)
Decreased platelet count

al., 1998), and an anaphylactoid reaction (Adkins, 1998) constitute unusual and rare adverse effects following G-CSF administration for PBSC collection from normal donors. Splenic rupture has been reported in a 22-year-old male donor without prior medical problems who received G-CSF at 10 µg/kg/daily for 6 days (Becker et al., 1997) and in a 33-year-old male donor with a significant history of smoking who received G-CSF at 16 µg/kg/daily for 6 days (Falzetti et al., 1999). A 44-year-old male donor with a prior history of dermatitis herpetiformis developed acute iritis while receiving G-CSF at 10 µg/kg/daily for 5 days (Parkkali et al., 1996). A 33-year-old woman who received G-CSF at 5 µg/kg/twice daily for 4 days developed an apical tooth abscess requiring surgical incision (Hilbe et al., 2000). A 42-year-old man receiving the same dose and schedule of G-CSF developed a perianal abscess, which required surgical incision (Hilbe et al., 2000). An episode of acute gouty arthritis occurred in a 65-year-old man receiving G-CSF at 10 µg/kg for 5 days. This donor had a history of several diseases including asthma, coronary artery disease with two previous angioplastic procedures, degenerative arthritis of the right knee, and hypercholesterolemia. The baseline uric acid level was 8.2 mg/dl (range 3.6 to 8.5) (Spitzer et al., 1998). A 16-year-old woman without prior medical problems developed an anaphylactoid reaction within 1 hour of G-CSF therapy given at 10 µg/kg/d but rapidly responded to directed therapy (Adkins, 1998).

The only case report of an adverse effect occurring in healthy pediatric donors after the administration of G-CSF for PBSC collection was in a 10-month-old boy who developed a cutaneous papular, erythematous eruption 3 weeks after G-CSF given at 16 µg/kg/ for 5 days. A skin biopsy showed irregularly shaped lymphocytes with mitoses, suggesting an activation of lymphocytes by G-CSF as a possible etiology (Torrelo et al., 2000).

Comparison of the risks of bone marrow vs. PBSC harvests

There is concern that the administration of G-CSF to normal individuals could result in future disorders of hematopoiesis including leukemic transformation. Although myelodysplasia and acute leukemia have been reported to occur in patients with aplastic anemia and congenital neutropenia given G-CSF (Imashuku et al., 1995), these potential complications of G-CSF administration would be difficult or impossible to detect after autologous transplantation where myelodysplastic syndromes are relatively common (Stone et al., 1994). G-CSF has been given to over 4000 normal individuals to facilitate the collection of granulocytes or PBSC, with the longest follow-up being 6 years without obvious long-term effects (Bensinger et al., 1993b; Dreger et al., 1993; Weaver et al., 1993; Bensinger et al., 1995b; Anderlini et al., 1996c; Bensinger et al., 1996a, 1996c; Majolino et al., 1997; Stroncek et al., 1997; Basara et al., 2000; Cavallaro et al., 2000; Dreger et al., 1993; Anderlini et al., 1996; Majolino et al., 1997; Stroncek et al., 1997).

Although there is genuine concern about the long-term effects of administering recombinant G-CSF to normal individuals, the existence and frequency of such effects will not be confidently known until very large numbers of donors are evaluated over a long period of time. It has been estimated that more than 6000 donors would have to be followed for 10 years to detect nine cases of excess leukemia due to G-CSF (Hasenclever & Sextro, 1996). It is relevant to reflect that it took many donations and many years for the risks of BM harvesting to be assessed.

The advantages to the donor of PBSC rather than BM harvesting include avoidance of general anesthesia, blood transfusions and other complications. In a review of 1549 BM harvests at the FHCRC, 27% had "significant" complications including 3% which were considered major (more than five units of blood administered, more than 21 days of hip pain requiring hospitalization or severe hypotension) and 0.4% which were considered life threatening complications (cardiac arrest, severe hypotension, septicemia, and osteomyelitis) (Buckner et al., 1994). Elsewhere, there have been two unreported postoperative deaths following BM harvest, both occurring in elderly donors. Thus, any consideration of the risks to normal individuals from G-CSF administration and PBSC harvest needs to be weighed against the relatively well-defined and significant risks of BM harvest. Recently, two studies that have prospectively examined donor well-being after PBSC or BM donation have reported similar levels of both pain and anxiety with both procedures (Lochte et al., 1942; Rowley et al., 2001; Stuart et al., 2001; Fortanier et al., 2002). PBSC donors, however, appeared to have faster resolution of their symptoms after the procedures compared to BM donors.

PBSC dose for allogeneic transplantation

The first consideration in evaluating the dose of PBSC is to determine what benchmark should be used for judging the adequacy of harvests for allogeneic transplantation. A dose of 5.0×10^6/kg is probably the best target CD34$^+$ cell dose for consistent and prompt engraftment of allogeneic PBSC (Brown et al., 1997). In a randomized study of PBSC vs. BM a target dose of 5.0×10^6 CD34$^+$ cells/kg recipient weight was established (Bensinger et al., 2001). Using a G-CSF dose of 16 μg/kg/day, 67% of donors achieved this target in a single collection while an additional 30% achieved it in two collection with only 3% of donors requiring more than two collections. Successful allogeneic PBSC transplants have been achieved with doses as low as 1 to 2×10^6/kg CD34$^+$ cells in several patients but the minimum CD34$^+$ cell dose needed for rapid and complete allogeneic engraftment of all patients is unknown. The administration of myelosuppressive agents after PBSC infusion also affects CD34$^+$ cell dose requirements. In 68 consecutive allogeneic PBSC transplants, the median time to achieve 500 neutrophils/μl was 3 days longer ($P = 0.0001$) and the median time to achieve platelet independence was 4 days longer ($P < 0.02$) for the 40 patients who received methotrexate + cyclosporine as their GVHD prophylaxis com-

pared to the 28 patients receiving cyclosporine ± prednisone (Bensinger et al., 1996b). Other reports have confirmed that methotrexate delays the recovery of neutrophils and platelets (Urbano-Ispizua et al., 1996). Thus, to achieve the benefit of earlier engraftment, larger CD34$^+$ cell doses may be required in patients receiving methotrexate than for patients receiving immunosuppressive anti-GVHD prophylaxis regimens that are not myelosuppressive.

G-CSF has been administered as single or twice daily subcutaneous doses ranging from 3.5 to 30 μg/kg mainly for patients rather than normal donors (Bensinger et al., 1993b; Dreger et al., 1993; Russell et al., 1995; Korbling et al., 1995a; Anderlini et al., 1996c; Stroncek et al., 1996; Waller et al., 1996; Anderlini et al., 1997b; Majolino et al., 1997; Stroncek et al., 1997; Arbona et al., 1998; Anderlini et al., 1999; de la Rubia et al., 1999; Martínez et al., 1999a, 1999b; Anderlini et al., 1999; McCullough et al., 1999; Murata et al., 1999; Stroncek et al., 1999; Anderlini et al., 2000; Carlo-Stella et al., 2000; Lee S et al., 2000; Lee V et al., 2000; Waller et al., 1996). Continuous intravenous infusion, a far less convenient method, has been described (Lee et al., 2000). The rationale of single dose administration is based on mobilization kinetic studies (Bensinger et al., 1993b; de Haas et al., 1994; Russell et al., 1995; Stroncek et al., 1997; de Haas et al., 1994). It is known that 48 to 72 hours following the G-CSF administration the number of progenitor cells in the peripheral blood increases, reaching the highest levels between days 4 and 6 (de Haas et al., 1994; Russell et al., 1995; Stroncek et al., 1997). Efforts to identify both the best dose and schedule of G-CSF continue (Stroncek et al., 1999; Martínez et al., 1999a, 1999b; Anderlini et al., 2000; Basara et al., 2000; Carlo-Stella et al., 2000; Lee S. et al., 2000; Lee V. et al., 2000). Several studies have examined dose and schedules of G-CSF given either at 10 to 12 μg/kg/once daily or 5 to 10 μg/kg twice daily (Stroncek et al., 1999; Martínez Urbano-Ispizua et al., 1999; Martínez et al., 1999a, 1999b; Anderlini et al., 2000; Basara et al., 2000; Carlo-Stella et al., 2000; Lee S. et al., 2000; Lee V. et al., 2000). Twice-daily schedules have also been evaluated because of the relatively short (only 3 to 4 hours) half-life of G-CSF after subcutaneous or intravenous administration (de Haas et al., 1994). A higher number of progenitor cells as measured by CD34$^+$ cells and CFU-GM was collected after administration of split dosing G-CSF at 5 to 10 μg/kg/12 h in normal donors in four of five studies (Anderlini et al., 2000; Basara et al., 2000; Carlo-Stella et al., 2000; Lee S. et al., 2000; Lee V. et al., 2000). One of these directly compared 10μg/kg given twice a day (20 μg/kg/day, total dose) or once a day (10 μg/kg/day, total dose) in 40 normal donors (Martínez et al., 1999b). The yield of CD34$^+$ cells/kg in the first collection was almost twice as great for patients receiving the twice daily dosing. In contrast one study comparing 12 μg/kg/day in single or split dosing found no differences in the apheresis yield (Anderlini et al., 2000).

Peripheral blood stem cells have been collected from normal donors after administration of G-CSF in doses of 2 to 16 µg/kg/day and this subject has been reviewed (Anderlini *et al.,* 1996; Anderlini *et al.,* 1996a; Bensinger *et al.,* 1996b). There is, in general, an increase in the number of CD34$^+$ cells collected with increasing doses of G-CSF, but variations in CD34$^+$ cell yield also could be influenced by the timing of apheresis, centrifugation characteristics, or the duration of apheresis. A small study compared mobilizing doses of 3, 5, or 10 µg/kg of G-CSF in normal donors (Grigg *et al.,* 1995). Although there was considerable overlap of CD34$^+$ cells and CFU-GM in peripheral blood among the different dose cohorts, significantly higher median levels of CD34$^+$ cells and CFU-GM were found at the 10 µg/kg dose level.

Very limited information exists on the effects of G-CSF in doses higher than 16 µg/kg for PBSC mobilization. For autologous patients the optimal dose of G-CSF for mobilization and collection of CD34$^+$ cells appears to be approximately 30 µg/kg/day (Weaver *et al.,* 1996). A study that compared 10 µg/kg/day with two injections of 10 to 12 µg/kg in healthy donors found significantly higher yields of CD34$^+$ cells in leukapheresis products without an increase in side effects (Waller *et al.,* 1996). Another split dosing study found 15 µg/kg/day total dose to be superior to 8 or 11 µg/kg/day as measured by CD34$^+$ cell yield (Basara *et al.,* 2000). It will be important to determine the optimal dose and schedule of G-CSF to maximize collections of CD34$^+$ cells and to provide background data for future studies of combinations of growth factors. In all the series of PBSC mobilization in normal donors, there is an approximate 1 log variation in PBSC yield among a particular group. One study of fixed dose G-CSF found a twofold difference in day 5 peripheral blood CFU-GM between young (20 to 30 years) and old (70 to 80 years) normal volunteers (Chatta *et al.,* 1994). In a small study of 14 normal donors more than 60 years old a target dose of 4.0×10^6 CD34$^+$ cells/kg was achieved in 57% with one apheresis using G-CSF 6 µg/kg twice a day (Anderlini *et al.,* 1997a). Other reports have found an inverse relationship between peak CD34$^+$ peripheral blood cell concentration and age (Dreger *et al.,* 1994). This variation, however, is only partially explained by donor size and age. Thus any study designed to evaluate the optimum dose of G-CSF for mobilization will require relatively large numbers of subjects to account for the intersubject variability.

Most investigators agree that the optimal collection days for PBSC are on the fourth and fifth day of G-CSF administration and 10 to 20 liters of blood are processed in most studies (Schwinger, 1993; Anderlini *et al.,* 1996b). In one study 77 normal donors mobilized with 12 µg/kg/day of G-CSF were collected beginning on day 4 or day 5. Day 5 collections yielded a higher number of CD34$^+$ cells in one apheresis (Anderlini *et al.,* 1996). In a detailed time course study of low dose (2 µg/kg) G-CSF given to normal donors, an additional rise in CFU-GM, Mix, and BFU-E were noted 4 to 6 hours after the day 3 and day 5 doses of cytokine (Sato *et al.,* 1994).

If this observation holds true for higher doses of G-CSF, optimum scheduling for mobilization would include administration of the days 4 and 5 G-CSF 4 to 6 hours before collection.

The only other growth factor evaluated in normal individuals for PBSC harvesting has been GM-CSF, which was given to five normal donors resulting in relatively poor collections (Lane *et al.,* 1995). Recently, it was reported that GM-CSF could be combined with G-CSF to successfully mobilize PBSC from normal donors in whom the stem cell products contained higher numbers of dendritic cells. When used for allogeneic transplants, a lower incidence of acute GVHD was reported (Brown *et al.,* 2001). Further work will be required to confirm this report.

T-cell depletion studies

As with BM, investigators have been interested in T-cell depletion approaches as a means of reducing GVHD. The main advantage of T depletion in PBSC is that larger numbers of stem and progenitor cells can be harvested to offset the inevitable losses when cells are manipulated. The major disadvantage of PBSC is the very large total cell number that create technical problems with classic T-depletion methods. Dreger *et al.* (1995). compared three other approaches to T-cell depletion of PBSC; CAMPATH-1 plus autologous complement, immunomagnetic CD34$^+$ selection and biotin-avidin-mediated CD34$^+$ selection. They found the immunomagnetic CD34$^+$ selection technique to be the most effective with the elimination of four logs of T cells. Suzue *et al.* (1994) reported three different techniques for T-cell depletion of PBSCs, all of which were associated with a large loss of hematopoietic progenitor cells. Aversa *et al.* (1994) reduced the number of CD3$^+$ cells in PBSCs to 1.24×10^5/kg with good recovery of CD34$^+$ cells using a soybean agglutination and E-rosetting technique.

Several reports have documented the experience of using CD34-enriched PBSC from HLA matched sibling donors. In one study of 10 patients a median of 1.2×10^6 CD3 cells/kg were infused (Link *et al.,* 1996). Engraftment was rapid but grade 3 to 4 acute GVHD occurred in 80% recipients given cyclosporine prophylaxis and in 20% recipients given cyclosporine and methotrexate. These results were confirmed in another study of 16 patients with advanced hematologic malignancies transplanted with HLA-identical PBSC which were enriched for CD34$^+$ cells by the same avidin-biotin immunoadsorption technique (Bensinger *et al.,* 1996c). A median of 18.64 (6.74–34.97) $\times 10^6$/kg were collected and a median of 8.96 (2.62–17.34) $\times 10^6$ CD34$^+$ cells/kg were recovered after avidin-biotin adsorption, which represented a median CD34$^+$ cell yield of 53% with a median purity of 62%. There was a 2.8 log reduction in T cells resulting in the infusion of 0.73, 0.40 and 0.32 $\times 10^6$ CD3$^+$, CD4$^+$ and CD8$^+$ cells/kg, respectively. The median day to achieve neutrophils of 0.5×10^9/L and platelets of 20×10^9/L were 15 and 11 days. Grades 2 to 4 acute GVHD occurred in 87% and grade 3 to 4 in 40% of evaluable patients. These studies demonstrated the feasibility of allogeneic transplantation using CD34[+] selected PBSC with prompt and sustained engraftment in all patients. The high incidence of acute and chronic GVHD that occurred despite significant T-cell depletion may partly be explained by the older age of patients studied, which was a median of 48 years (range 37–66), but it is also possible that populations of cells capable of downregulating GVHD are removed by this technique of CD34[+] selection (Bensinger et al., 1996c). In a more recent study of 20 older allograft recipients of HLA-identical sibling, CD34[+] enriched PBSC, there was only a 10% incidence of grade 3 or 4 acute GVHD (Bensinger et al., 1996). CD34 selection in this study was accomplished using the immunomagnetic bead technique, which resulted in a 3.9 log T-cell reduction. The lower incidence of severe GVHD in that study may have been due to fewer infused T cells, which were on the order of 10^5 CD3[+] cells/kg. The largest multicenter study enrolled 62 patients who had allogeneic PBSC from HLA-matched sibling donors, which were CD34-enriched using immunomagnetic beads or avidin-biotin (Urbano-Ispizua et al., 1998). In that study engraftment was rapid and GVHD was virtually eliminated with cyclosporine prophylaxis. Only short-term outcomes were available, making the questions of relapse and chronic GVHD in further follow-up important. It is not clear why these later studies reported such a low incidence of GVHD compared to the earlier trials. One theoretical advantage of CD34[+] cell enrichment over complement lysis techniques is that a second stage selection technique could be utilized to select other cell populations such as CD56[+] or CD8[+] cells that could be added back to the graft. This approach would potentially allow the selective infusion of cells able to enhance immune reconstitution against infectious agents or antileukemic effects without the development of GVHD.

Addition of PBSC to marrow for allografting in HLA-mismatched allografts

Resistance to allogeneic grafts is affected by cell dose, the degree of genetic disparity between host and donor (Anasetti et al., 1989), transfusion-induced immunity in the patient (Storb et al., 1994), and by depletion of T cells from the graft (Kernan, 1994). Experimental animal data have indicated that increasing the number of donor hematopoietic progenitor cells in the graft improves the probability of engraftment across an allogeneic mismatched barrier (Kernan, 1994). There are also data from patients with aplastic anemia receiving HLA-identical transplants demonstrating a decrease in rejection and an improved survival with the infusion of high BM cell doses (Niederwieser et al., 1988). The number of donor hematopoietic cells available from BM harvesting is limited and often suboptimal. The ability to collect PBSC after the administration of G-CSF has made it possible to test the hypothesis that increasing the dose of donor hematopoietic cells results in more consistent engraftment.

The incidence of graft rejection has exceeded 50% in recipients of T-cell depleted BM transplants from donors incompatible for two or three antigens using a soybean-lectin technique

(O'Reilly et al., 1988). Using the same technique for T-cell depletion not only of BM but also of PBSC collected after G-CSF, Aversa et al. (1998) reported engraftment in 41 of 43 patients transplanted from HLA-haploidentical donors, of whom 15 received T-depleted PBSC. Patients received a mean of 30,000 CD3[+] cells/kg and none developed acute or chronic GVHD. Survival was poor, however, with only 28% alive at 18 months. Deaths occurred predominantly from infections, relapse and toxicity related to the very intense conditioning regimen that included cyclophosphamide, thiotepa, anti-thymocyte globulin, and single dose total body irradiation given at a high dose rate. Results of this study suggest that the addition of T-cell depleted PBSC assisted the establishment of allogeneic engraftment. However, T-cell depletion of both BM and PBSC requires a complicated, labor-intensive, and error-prone laboratory separation procedure, and Aversa has shown that BM is unnecessary when PBSC are used.

Allogeneic PBSC transplants using PBSCs alone

Several thousand allogeneic transplants have been performed using G-CSF mobilized PBSC. The European Group for Blood and Bone Marrow Transplantation (EBMT) has published the results of a recent survey in which the activity of transplant centers was assessed (Gratwohl et al., 1999). In 1996, out of 4,400 allogeneic transplants, PBSC were used in 30%, a doubling of the activity over the previous 2 years. PBSC accounted for 36% of a total of 5308 EBMT allografts by 1998 (Gratwohl et al., 2000). Unpublished data of the EBMT show that 50% of all allogeneic transplants in 2000 were done with PBSC.

In almost all the phase II studies of allogeneic PBSC, the tempo of recovery of neutrophils and platelets to self-supporting levels has been superior to historical patients who received BM. The role of posttransplant growth factors in allogeneic PBSC transplants was addressed in a randomized study comparing the use of G-CSF or placebo after allogeneic stem cells (Bishop et al., 2000). Patients receiving G-CSF experienced a 4-day earlier neutrophil recovery without differences in platelet recovery. It should be noted that at least 3.0×10^6 CD34[+] cells/kg recipient weight were required for study entry. These findings were confirmed in a subsequent study (Przieporka et al., 2001).

Studies of donor engraftment after allogeneic PBSC have demonstrated chimerism equivalent to BM. In a study comparing chimerism in patients receiving allografts from BM or PBSC, there was a higher level of donor engraftment observed within the first 30 days after transplant and lower levels of donor chimerism observed at 1 to 6 months after transplant in BM recipients (Miflin et al., 1999). Beyond 6 months none of nine PBSC recipients showed low-level mixed chimerism compared with four of nine BM recipients.

In phase I-II studies, GVHD prophylaxis has consisted of either cyclosporine or tacrolimus combined with either methotrexate or prednisone. Severe (grades 3 to 4) acute GVHD occurred in 5% to 21% of patients. In general, the estimated risks for developing acute GVHD after PBSC were not greater than would be expected after BM grafts. The EBMT survey reported a 24% incidence of severe acute GVHD and did not report differences in GVHD incidence among patients given different prophylaxis regimens (Schmitz *et al.*, 1996). Chronic GVHD has been reported in 24% to 71% of allogeneic PBSC recipients, but due to large differences in patient population and follow-up, the accuracy of these estimates is incomplete. In some early reports the estimated risks of chronic GVHD appeared to be higher with allogeneic PBSC (Majolino *et al.*, 1996; Storek *et al.*, 1997; Majolino *et al.*, 1996). However, in other studies this was not the case (Miflin *et al.*, 1997). In the EBMT/IBMTR registry analysis the 1-year probability of chronic GVHD was 65% for PBSC recipients compared to 53% for patients who received BM, $P = 0.02$ (Champlin *et al.*, 2000). Most patients given allogeneic PBSC have had advanced and often refractory hematologic malignancies making evaluation of outcomes difficult. Most trials that have retrospectively analyzed patients receiving allogeneic PBSC or BM have indicated lower transplant-related mortality with PBSC but no differences in overall survival. The EBMT/IBMTR registry analysis, which compared 288 recipients of PBSC to 536 BM recipients, demonstrated lower treatment-related mortality and better leukemia-free survival among PBSC patients with more advanced leukemias (Champlin *et al.*, 2000). In an update, the risk of chronic GVHD was increased (Schmitz *et al.*, 2001). A retrospective comparison of HLA-identical sibling PBSC transplantation versus marrow transplantation found a lower two year transplant-related mortality rate in the PBSC recipients and improved 2 year event-free survival rate in all groups except those with refractory anemia or high-risk cytogenetics (Guardiola et al., 2002).

There is mounting evidence of an increased risk of immune hemolysis when PBSC, as opposed to bone marrow, grafts are used (Lapierre *et al.*, 2001). This may be due to the increased numbers of lymphoid cells present in the PBSC inoculum capable of producing isohemagglutinins against recipient red cell antigens. This propensity may be enhanced by the use of non-myeloablative regimens (see Chapter 22), possibly due to the utilization of cyclosporine alone as GVHD prophylaxis after such procedures. Vigilant monitoring during the first 2 weeks posttransplant (to include daily LDH estimation, daily direct antiglobulin test and twice daily blood counts on days 5 to 12) has been recommended. Additionally, increased presence of anti-HLA antibodies early posttransplant has been described after HLA-identical sibling PBSC transplantation compared to BM transplantation (Lapierre et al., 2002). This was observed despite a reduction in the median number of platelet transfusion episodes per patient in the PBSC recipients compared to the BM recipients and is further evidence that PBSC transplantation alters alloimmune responses.

A study by Trenschel *et al.* (2000). suggested a lower risk of persistent CMV pp65 antigenemia (Fig. 11.1) and CMV interstitial pneumonitis in recipients of allogeneic PBSC compared to allogeneic BMT recipients.

A study by Elmaagacli *et al.* (1999) described a lower risk of residual cytogenetic and molecular disease in patients with Ph-

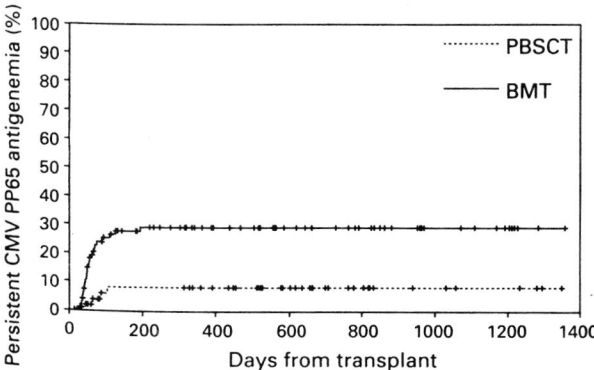

Fig. 11.1. Cumulative incidence of persistent pp65 antigenemia after BMT and PBSCT (log rank test: $P < 0.01$). Reproduced, with permission, from Trenschel *et al.* (2000).

positive CML given family member blood stem cell transplants in first chronic phase compared to those given marrow grafts.

Trial of G-CSF-stimulated marrow

Based on the hypothesis that G-CSF may improve yield of BM from normal donors, several small studies have examined engraftment and GVHD for patients receiving allogeneic BM from donors who received 3 to 4 days of G-CSF immediately before harvest (Couban *et al.*, 2000; Isola *et al.*, 2000; Serody *et al.*, 2000; Ji et al., 2002a and 2002b). When compared to G-CSF-mobilized PBSC, recipients of G-CSF-stimulated allogeneic BM experienced similar neutrophil engraftment, but slower platelet recovery, significantly lower incidences of acute and chronic GVHD, and similar survival (Serody *et al.*, 2000). Two studies that compared G-CSF-stimulated BM to historical BM patients showed earlier neutrophil and platelet recovery in patients given stimulated BM with similar rates of GVHD, relapse, and survival (Couban *et al.*, 2000; Isola *et al.*, 2000). In a small, prospective randomized trial of G-CSF-stimulated BM versus PBSC, similar engraftment times were noted, but patients receiving PBSC developed more steroid-resistant GVHD (Morton *et al.*, 2001). Ji and colleagues (2002b) have applied this approach to haploidentical family member transplantation with encouraging results. These preliminary studies provide data suggesting that G-CSF-stimulated allogeneic BM may confer early engraftment similar to mobilized PBSC but possibly without the increased risk of GVHD. It is unknown whether immune reconstitution and the potential for greater antileukemic effects will be found with G-CSF-stimulated BM. Prospective randomized studies will be needed for definitive conclusions.

Prospective randomized comparisons of PBSC and BM

Results of eight randomized studies comparing mobilized PBSC and unstimulated BM for allogeneic transplantation have been reported in abstracts or full manuscripts. (Table 11.2). These studies enrolled 30 to 350 patients each and in total contain nearly 1200 patients. All studies utilized the combination

Table 11.2. *Randomized comparisons of allogeneic PBSC vs. BM*

| Reference | Total no. pts | % Patients with advanced disease[a] | Stem cell source | Engraftment: median day to: | | Acute GVHD % | | Chronic GVHD % | DFS[b] % | Survival % |
				Neutrophils 500 µl	Platelets 20,000 µl	Grade 2–4	Grade 3–4			
Blaise et al., 2000	101	5	PBSC	15*	13*	44	17	50*	58	61
			BM	21	21	42	23	28	62	61
Heldal *et al.,* 2000	61[c]	28	PBSC	17*	13*	25	NR	55	85	82
			BM	23	21	10		26	65	75
Vigorito *et al.,* 1998	37	30	PBSC	16	12*	27	13	100*	58	47
			BM	18	17	19	13	50	52	51
Mahmoud *et al.,* 1999	30	NR[d]	PBSC	9*	10*	7	7	NR	NR	NR
			BM	25	30	40	40			
Schmitz *et al.,* in press	350	14	PBSC	12*	15*	52*	28*	74*	60	NR
			BM	15	20	39*	16	53	68	
Powles *et al.,* 2000	39	46	PBSC	17*	11*	50	NR	44	NR	70
			BM	23	19	47		40		63
Simpson *et al.,* 2000	228	27	PBSC	19*	16*	40	NR	71	NR	68*
			BM	22	22	40		55		55
Bensinger *et al.,* 2001	172	47	PBSC	16*	13*	64	15	46	65*	66
			BM	21	19	57	12	35	45	54

[a] Advanced disease = CML >CP, Acute leukemias >1st CR, Lymphomas >2nd CR, RAEB(T), multiple myeloma
[b] DFS = disease-free survival
[c] 6 donor-recipients were 5/6 antigen matches
[d] NR = not reported
*P < 0.05

of cyclosporine and methotrexate for GVHD prevention (Storb *et al.,* 1987); however, in three studies the day 11 methotrexate dose was omitted. Posttransplant myeloid growth factors were not used with the exception of the 350 patient European Group for Blood and Bone Marrow Transplantation (EBMT) study. Neutrophil engraftment occurred significantly earlier with PBSC in seven studies and all studies showed significantly earlier platelet recovery with PBSC. The risks of acute GVHD grades 2 to 4 were similar in all studies except for the multicenter EBMT trial, which noted a 13% greater incidence of grades 2 to 4 GVHD and a 12% greater incidence of grade 3–4 acute GVHD in the PBSC group. An important difference in the design of this study compared to the others was the omission of day 11 methotrexate from GVHD prophylaxis. In prior studies of BM transplant recipients, omission of day 11 methotrexate increased the risks of GVHD (Nash *et al.,* 1992). Although these were randomized studies, this omission may have further predisposed recipients of PBSC to develop GVHD.

All studies showed a trend toward more chronic GVHD with PBSC, and in three studies the trend became statistically significant (Fig. 11.2). It is interesting that the day 11 dose of methotrexate was omitted in the three studies that reported a statistically higher incidence of chronic GVHD with PBSC. While this observation does not directly explain a higher incidence of chronic GVHD, patients who have acute GVHD are more likely to develop chronic GVHD. It is also possible that higher proportions of good risk patients may have played a role in the differences in incidence of chronic GVHD.

Two large studies of 172 and 228 patients reported statistically better survival or disease-free survival among patients who were randomized to receive PBSC. In the U.S. study, disease-free survival was better but overall survival was not. Survival differences were greatest among patients with more advanced hematologic malignancies, and this was due to both reduced transplant-related mortality and relapse (Bensinger *et al.,* 2001). In comparison to the other published, randomized clinical trials, the U.S. study enrolled a larger number of patients with more advanced hematologic malignancies, the patients in whom the benefit of peripheral blood cells was most apparent. Patients with more advanced hematologic malignancies tend to have a higher nonrelapse mortality and higher relapse rates after transplant. That study was not large enough to determine whether the use of peripheral blood cells improved survival for patients with less advanced hematologic malignancies. The Canadian intergroup trial was composed mainly of patients with less advanced leukemias, but due to larger patient numbers, the survival differences were significant (Simpson *et al.,* 2000). This trial showed that overall survival was better with PBSC primarily due to reduced non-relapse mortality without significant differences in relapse. In contrast the larger EBMT trial, which was also composed almost exclusively of less advanced patients, showed no differences in disease-free survival or overall survival (Schmitz *et al.,* 2002). This trial had important differences from the Canadian study, including omission of the day 11 methotrexate and the use of posttransplant G-CSF. This study also had the shortest follow-

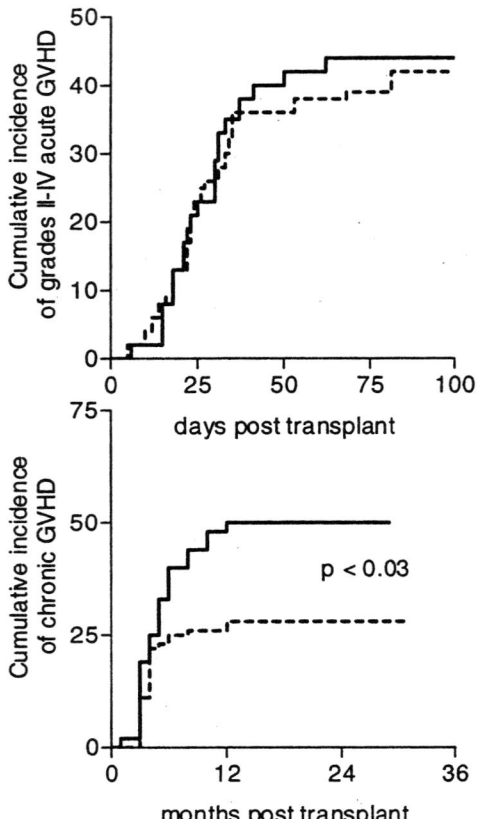

Fig. 11.2. GVHD. BCT = solid line; BMT = dotted line. Reproduced, with permission, from Blaise *et al.* (2000).

up time, making these findings very preliminary. A follow-up of the study by Blaise and colleagues (median follow-up 45 months) found a 3-year cumulative incidence of chronic GVHD of 65% in the PBSC recipients and 36% in the marrow recipients (Mohty et al., 2002). The incidence of extensive chronic GVHD was 44% and 17%, respectively ($p = 0.004$).

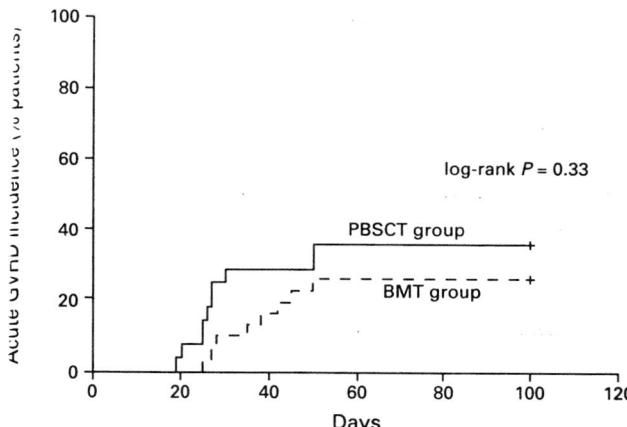

Fig. 11.4. Time to and incidence of grades II to IV acute GVHD after hematopoietic stem cell transplantation with unmanipulated HLA-identical PBSC ($n = 27$) or BM ($n = 30$). PBSCT group versus BM group (HLA-identical) $P = 0.33$. Reproduced, with permission, from Blau *et al.* (2001).

Prevalence of chronic GVHD was always higher in the PBSC group, ocular involvement was more common and the PBSC group required more hospitalization. In the long-term follow-up of another randomized trial, the incidence of chronic GVHD was similar in the two arms, but the number of successive treatments needed to control chronic GVHD was higher after PBSC tranplantation and the duration of corticosteroid treatment was longer (Flowers et al., 2002).

In one of the prospective, randomized trials of PBSC versus BM immune reconstitution was monitored between 30 and 365 days after transplant in a subset of 115 patients (Storek et al., 2001). The most important differences were a fourfold increase in $CD4^+$ $CD45RA^+$ and twofold increase in $CD4^+$ $CD45RA^-$ cells of PBSC recipients compared to BM recipients. There was also noted to be a 1.7-fold increase in definite infections in the BM recipients compared to BM recipients.

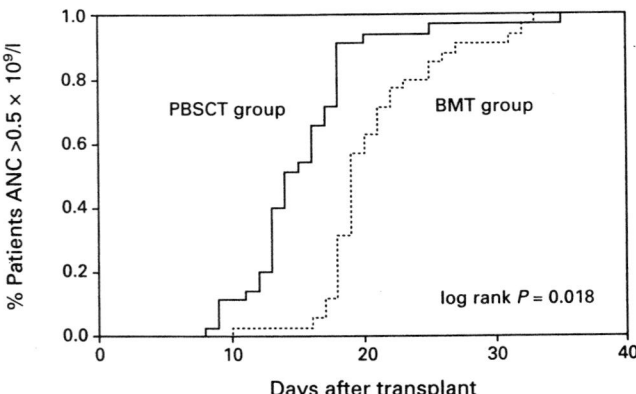

Fig. 11.3. Days to an ANC recovery $> 0.5 \times 10^9/l$ after hematopoietic stem cell transplantation with unmanipulated PBSC or BM. PBSCT group versus BMT group $P < 0.02$. Reproduced, with permission, from Blau *et al.* (2001).

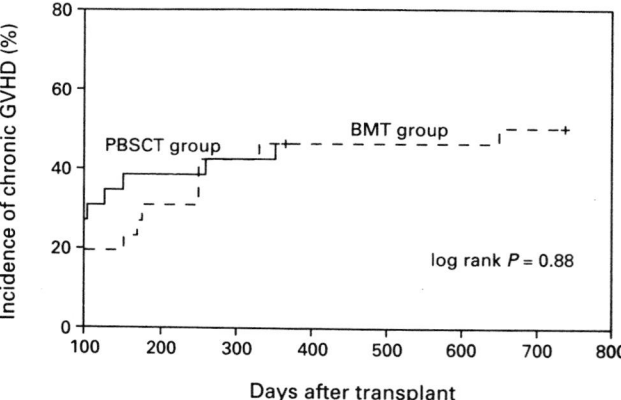

Fig. 11.5. Time to and incidence of chronic GVHD after hematopoietic stem cell transplantation with unmanipulated PBSC or BM. PBSCT group versus BM group $P = 0.88$. Reproduced, with permission, from Blau *et al.* (2001).

Experience with unrelated donors

Due in part to concerns about exposure of normal volunteer donors to G-CSF during the mobilization process, fewer allogeneic transplants have been performed using unrelated donor PBSC. In a limited study of the experience from four European centers, 45 patients received unmanipulated, G-CSF mobilized PBSC from volunteer unrelated donors, and the results were retrospectively compared to those who received BM (Ringden *et al.*, 1999). Engraftment of neutrophils and platelets was more rapid with PBSC, with similar incidences of acute and chronic GVHD, transplant-related mortality, and overall survival. In a larger study, 107 patients receiving allogeneic PBSC from matched, unrelated donors were compared to control subjects who were matched for important prognostic variables (Remberger *et al.*, 2001). Faster engraftment of neutrophils and platelets was observed with similar degrees of chimerism, acute and chronic GVHD, mortality, relapse, and overall survival. In a case-controlled study involving 37 recipients of unrelated donor PBSC, Blau *et al.* (2001) found faster neutrophil (but not platelet) engraftment compared to those receiving unrelated donor marrow (Fig. 11.3), but no difference in the HLA-identical recipients in incidence of grade II-IV acute GVHD (Fig. 11.4) nor in the time to, and incidence of, chronic GVHD (Fig. 11.5). The use of CD34-megadose PBSC transplants T-cell depleted using the CliniMACS device has resulted in prompt hematopoietic recovery in children (Schwinger *et al.*, 2000).

Current and future studies

The rapid application of allogeneic PBSC for transplantation in the past 6 years has raised legitimate concerns about the relative benefits of this source of stem cells compared to BM. It is clear that engraftment is more rapid with PBSC than BM and that this is often associated with a reduced transplant-related mortality. Most comparison trials using the optimum GVHD prophylaxis regimen of cyclosporine and methotrexate have demonstrated equivalent rates of acute GVHD. It is likely that the incidence of chronic GVHD can be expected to be 15% to 20% higher with PBSC than with BM. This chronic GVHD, however, is associated with a significant antileukemic effect, which in turn confers a major survival benefit to patients with more advanced hematologic malignancies. Further follow-up studies are needed to define the relative benefits of PBSC for patients with less advanced disease. Small, preliminary studies indicate that pretreatment of BM donors with G-CSF may confer some of the benefits of mobilized PBSC. Further, randomized comparison studies will be required to be certain of this. Early phase II data using allogeneic PBSC from phenotypically matched unrelated donors indicate more rapid engraftment than with BM with similar rates of acute GVHD. More studies, especially randomized trials, will be needed to define the value of allogeneic PBSC from unrelated donors compared to BM. The very large quantities of stem and progenitor cells made available from mobilized PBSC will allow future trials of graft engineering in which highly purified stem and progenitor cells will be transplanted along with purified or manipulated T-cell subsets capable of ensuring engraftment, immune reconstitution, and antileukemic effects without GVHD.

References

Adkins, D.R. (1998). Anaphylactoid reaction in a normal donor given granulocyte colony-stimulating factor (Letter to the Editor). *Journal of Clinical Oncology*, **16**, 812–3.

Anasetti, C., Amos, D., Beatty, P.G. *et al.* (1989). Effect of HLA compatibility on engraftment of bone marrow transplants in patients with leukemia or lymphoma. *The New England Journal of Medicine*, **320**, 197–204.

Anderlini, P., Donato, M., Chan, K-W. *et al.* (1999). Allogeneic blood progenitor cell collection in normal donors after mobilization with filgrastim: the M.D. Anderson Cancer Center experience. *Transfusion*, **39**, 555–60.

Anderlini, P., Donato, M., Lauppe, M.I. *et al.* (2000). A comparative study of once-daily versus twice-daily filgrastim administration for the mobilization and collection of CD34+ peripheral blood progenitor cells in normal donors. *British Journal of Haematology*, **109**, 770–2.

Anderlini, P., Körbling, M., Dale, D. *et al.* (1997c). Allogeneic blood stem cell transplantation: considerations for donors (Editorial). *Blood*, **90**, 903–8.

Anderlini, P., Przepiorka, D., Champlin, R. *et al.* (1996a). Biologic and clinical effects of granulocyte colony-stimulating factor in normal individuals (Review). *Blood*, **88**, 2819–25.

Anderlini, P., Przepiorka, D., Huh, Y. *et al.* (1996b). Duration of filgrastim mobilization and apheresis yield of CD34+ progenitor cells and lymphoid subsets in normal donors for allogeneic transplantation. *British Journal of Haematology*, **93**, 940–2.

Anderlini, P., Przepiorka, D., Lauppe, J. *et al.* (1997a). Collection of peripheral blood stem cells from normal donors 60 years of age or older. *British Journal of Haematology*, **97**, 485–7.

Anderlini, P., Przepiorka, D., Seong, C. *et al.* (1997b). Factors affecting mobilization of CD34+ cells in normal donors treated with filgrastim. *Transfusion*, **37**, 507–12.

Anderlini, P., Przepiorka, D., Seong, D. *et al.* (1996). Clinical toxicity and laboratory effects of granulocyte-colony-stimulating factor (filgrastim) mobilization and blood stem cell apheresis from normal donors, and analysis of charges for the procedures. *Transfusion*, **36**, 590–5.

Anderlini, P., Przepiorka, D., Seong, D. *et al.* (1996c). Clinical toxicity and laboratory effects of granulocyte-colony-stimulating factor (filgrastim) mobilization and blood stem cell apheresis from normal donors, and analysis of charges for the procedures. *Transfusion*, **36**, 590–5.

Anderlini, P., Rizzo, J.D., Nugent, M.L. *et al.* (2001). Peripheral blood stem cell donation: an analysis from the International Bone Marrow Transplant Registry (IBMTR) and European Group for Blood and Marrow Transplant (EBMT) databases. *Bone Marrow Transplantation*, **27**, 689–92.

Arbona, C., Prosper, F., Benet, I. *et al.* (1998). Comparison between once a day vs twice a day G-CSF for mobilization of peripheral blood progenitor cells (PBPC) in normal donors for allogeneic PBPC transplantation. *Bone Marrow Transplantation*, **22**, 39–45.

Aversa, F., Tabilio, A., Terenzi, A. *et al.* (1994). Successful engraftment of T-cell-depleted halpoidentical "Three-Loci" incompatible transplants in leukemia patients by addition of recombinant human granulocyte colony-stimulating factor-mobilized peripheral blood progenitor cells to bone marrow inoculum. *Blood,* **11,** 3948–55.

Aversa, F., Tabilio, A., Velardi, A. *et al.* (1998). Treatment of high-risk acute leukemia with T-cell-depleted stem cells from related donors with one fully mismatched HLA haplotype. *The New England Journal of Medicine,* **339,** 1186–93.

Azevedo, W.M., Aranha, F.J.P., Gouvea, J.V. *et al.* (1995). Allogeneic transplantation with blood stem cells mobilized by rhG-CSF for hematologic malignances. *Bone Marrow Transplantation,* **16,** 647–53.

Basara, N., Schmetzer, B., Blau, I.W. *et al.* (2000). Lenograstim-mobilized peripheral blood progenitor cells in volunteer donors: an open label randomized split dose escalating study. *Bone Marrow Transplantation,* **25,** 371–6.

Becker, P.S., Wagle, M., Matous, S. *et al.* (1997). Spontaneous splenic rupture following administration of granulocyte colony-stimulating factor (G-CSF): occurrence in an allogeneic donor of peripheral blood stem cells. *Biology of Blood and Marrow Transplantation,* **3,** 45–9.

Bender, J.G., Unverzagt, K.L., Walker, D.E. *et al.* (1991). Identification and comparison of CD34-positive cells and their subpopulations from normal peripheral blood and bone marrow using multicolor flow cytometry. *Blood,* **77,** 2591–6.

Bensinger, W., Appelbaum, F., Rowley, S. *et al.* (1995a). Factors that influence collection and engraftment of autologous peripheral-blood stem cells. *Journal of Clinical Oncology,* **13,** 2547–55.

Bensinger, W., Singer, J., Appelbaum, F. *et al.* (1993a). Autologous transplantation with peripheral blood mononuclear cells collected after administration of recombinant granulocyte stimulating factor. *Blood,* **81,** 3158–63.

Bensinger, W.I., Buckner, C.D., Shannon-Dorcy, K. *et al.* (1996c). Transplantation of allogeneic CD34+ peripheral blood stem cells in patients with advanced hematologic malignancy. *Blood,* **88,** 4132–8.

Bensinger, W.I., Clift, R., Martin, P. *et al.* (1996a). Allogeneic peripheral blood stem cell transplantation in patients with advanced hematologic malignancies: A retrospective comparison with marrow transplantation. *Blood,* **88,** 2794–800.

Bensinger, W.I., Clift, R.A., Anasetti, C. *et al.* (1996b). Transplantation of allogeneic peripheral blood stem cells mobilized by recombinant human granulocyte colony-stimulating factor. *Stem Cells* **14,** 90–105.

Bensinger, W.I., Longin, K., Appelbaum, F. *et al.* (1994). Peripheral blood stem cells (PBSCs) collected after recombinant granulocyte colony stimulating factor (rhG-CSF): an analysis of factors correlating with the tempo of engraftment after transplantation. *British Journal of Haematology,* **87,** 825–31.

Bensinger, W.I., Martin, P.J., Storer, B. *et al.* (2001). Transplantation of bone marrow as compared with peripheral-blood cells from HLA-identical relatives in patients with hematologic cancers. *The New England Journal of Medicine,* **344,** 175–181.

Bensinger, W.I., Price, T.H., Dale, D.C. *et al.* (1993b). The effects of daily recombinant human granulocyte colony stimulating factor

administration on normal granulocyte donors undergoing leukapheresis. *Blood,* **81,** 1883–8.

Bensinger, W.I., Rowley, S., Lilleby, K. *et al.* (1996). Reduction in graft-versus-host-disease (GVHD) after transplantation of CD34 selected, allogeneic peripheral blood stem cells (PBSC) in older patients with advanced hematologic malignancies. *Blood,* **88,** (Suppl. 1), 421a, #1672, (Abstract).

Bensinger, W.I., Weaver, C.H., Appelbaum, F.R. *et al.* (1995b). Transplantation of allogeneic peripheral blood stem cells mobilized by recombinant human granulocyte colony-stimulating factor. *Blood,* **85,** 1655–8.

Bishop, M.R., Tarantolo, S.R., Geller, R.B. *et al.* (2000). A randomized, double-blind trial of filgrastim (granulocyte colony-stimulating factor) versus placebo following allogeneic blood stem cell transplantation. *Blood,* **96,** 80–5.

Blaise, D., Kuentz, M., Fortanier, C. *et al.* (2000). Randomized trial of bone marrow versus lenograstim-primed blood cell allogeneic transplantation in patients with early-stage leukemia: a report from the Société Française de Greffe de Moelle. *Journal of Clinical Oncology,* **18,** 537–46.

Blau, I.W., Basara, N., Lentini, G. *et al.* (2001). Feasibility and safety of peripheral blood stem cell transplantation from unrelated donors: results of a single-center study. *Bone Marrow Transplantation,* **27,** 27–33.

Brown, R.A., Adkins, D., Goodnough, L.T. *et al.* (1997). Factors that influence the collection and engraftment of allogeneic peripheral-blood stem cells in patients with hematologic malignancies. *Journal of Clinical Oncology,* **15,** 3067–74.

Brown, R.A., Adkins, D.R., Khoury, H. *et al.* (2001). Mobilization of allogeneic PBSC with GM-CSF instead of G-CSF is associated with a reduced risk of acute graft-vs-host disease (GVHD). *Blood,* **98,** (Part I), 737a, #3074, (Abstract).

Buckner, C.D., Petersen, F.B., & Bolonesi, B.A. (1994). Bone marrow donors, in Forman S.J., Blume K.G., Thomas, E.D. (eds): *Bone Marrow Transplantation,* Boston, MA, Blackwell Scientific Publications, pp. 259–270.

Carlo-Stella, C., Cesana, C., Regazzi, E. *et al.* (2000). Peripheral blood progenitor cell mobilization in healthy donors receiving recombinant human granulocyte colony-stimulating factor. *Experimental Hematology,* **28,** 216–224.

Casper, C.B., Seger, R.A., & Berger, J. (1993). Effective stimulation of donors in granulocyte transfusions with recombinant methionyl granulocyte colony-stimulating factor. *Blood,* **81,** 2866–71.

Cavallaro, A.M., Lilleby, K., Majolino, I. *et al.* (2000). Three to six year follow-up of normal donors who received recombinant human granulocyte colony stimulating factor. *Bone Marrow Transplantation,* **25,** 85–9.

Champlin, R.E., Schmitz, N., Horowitz, M.M. *et al.* (2000). Blood stem cells compared with bone marrow as a source of hematopoietic cells for allogeneic transplantation. *Blood,* **95,** 3702–9.

Chatta, G.S., Price, T.H., Allen, R.C. *et al.* (1994). Effects of in vivo recombinant methionyl human granulocyte colony-stimulating factor on the neutrophil response and peripheral blood colony-forming cells in healthy young and elderly adult volunteers. *Blood,* **84,** 2923–9.

Couban, S., Messner, H.A., Andreou, P. *et al.* (2000). Bone marrow mobilized with granulocyte colony-stimulating factor in related allogeneic transplant recipients: a study of 29 patients. *Biology of Blood and Marrow Transplantation, 6,* 422–7.

Cutler, C., Giri, S., Jeyapalan, S. *et al.* (2001). Acute and chronic graft-versus-host disease after allogeneic peripheral-blood stem-cell and bone marrow transplantation: a meta-analysis. *Journal of Clinical Oncology, 19,* 3685–91.

de Haas, M., Kerst, J.M., van der Schoot, C.E. *et al.* (1994). Granulocyte colony-stimulating factor administration to healthy volunteers: analysis of the immediate activating effects on circulating neutrophils. *Blood, 84,* 3885–94.

de la Rubia, J., Martínez, C., Solano, C. *et al.* (1999). Administration of recombinant human granulocyte colony-stimulating factor to normal donors: results of the Spanish National Donor Registry. *Bone Marrow Transplantation, 24,* 723–8.

Dreger, P., Haferlach, T., Eckstein, V. *et al.* (1994). G-CSF-mobilized peripheral blood progenitor cells for allogeneic transplantation: safety, kinetics of mobilization, and composition of the graft. *British Journal of Haematology, 87,* 609–13.

Dreger, P., Suttorp, M., Haferlach, T. *et al.* (1993). Allogeneic granulocyte colony-stimulating factor-mobilized peripheral blood progenitor cells for treatment of engraftment failure after bone marrow transplantation (Correspondence). *Blood, 81,* 1404–9.

Dreger, P., Viehmann, K., Steinmann, J. *et al.* (1995). G-CSF-mobilized peripheral blood progenitor cells for allogeneic transplantation: Comparison of T cell depletion strategies using different CD34+ selection systems or CAMPATH-1. *Experimental Hematology, 23,* 147–54.

Elmaagacli, A.H., Beelen, D.W., Opalka, B. *et al.* (1999). The risk of residual molecular and cytogenetic disease in patients with Philadelphia-chromosome positive first chronic phase chronic myelogenous leukemia is reduced after transplantation of allogeneic peripheral blood stem cells compared with bone marrow. *Blood, 94,* 384–9.

Falanga, A., Marchetti, M., Evangelista, V. *et al.* (1999). Neutrophil activation and hemostatic changes in healthy donors receiving granulocyte colony-stimulating factor. *Blood, 93,* 2506–14.

Falzetti, F., Aversa, F., Minelli, O. *et al.* (1999). Spontaneous rupture of spleen during peripheral blood stem-cell mobilisation in a healthy donor (Research Letter). *Lancet, 353,* 555.

Flowers, M.E.D., Parker, P.M., Johnston, L.J. et al. (2002). Comparison of chronic graft-versus-host disease after transplantation of peripheral blood stem cells versus bone marrow in allogeneic recipients: long-term follow-up of a randomized trial. *Blood, 100,* 415–9.

Fortanier, C., Kuentz, M., Sutton, L. *et al.* (2002). Healthy sibling donor anxiety and pain during bone marrow or peripheral blood stem cell harvesting for allogeneic transplantation: results of a randomised study. *Bone Marrow Transplantation, 29,* 145–9.

Fossa, S.D., Poulsen, J.P., & Aaserud, A. (1992). Alkaline phosphatase and lactate dehydrogenase changes during leucocytosis induced by G-CSF in testicular cancer (Letter). *Lancet, 340,* 1544.

Goldman, J. (1995). Peripheral blood stem cells for allografting. *Blood, 85,* 1413–5.

Goodman, J.W. & Hodgson, G.S. (1962). Evidence for stem cells in the peripheral blood of mice. *Blood, 19,* 702–14.

Gratwohl, A., Passweg, J., Baldomero, H. *et al.* (1999). Blood and marrow transplantation activity in Europe 1997 (Special Report). *Bone Marrow Transplantation, 24,* 231–45.

Gratwohl, A., Passweg, J., Baldomero, H. *et al.* (2000). Hematopoietic stem cell transplantation in Europe 1998. *The Hematology Journal, 1,* 333–50.

Grigg, A.P., Roberts, A.W., Raunow, H. *et al.* (1995). Optimizing dose and scheduling of filgrastim (granulocyte colony-stimulating factor) for mobilization and collection of peripheral blood progenitor cells in normal volunteers. *Blood, 86,* 4437–45.

Gyger, M., Stuart, R.K., & Perreault, C. (2000). Immunobiology of allogeneic peripheral blood mononuclear cells mobilized with granulocyte-colony stimulating factor (Review). *Bone Marrow Transplantation, 26,* 1–16.

Hasenclever, D. & Sextro, M. (1996). Safety of AlloPBPCT donors: biometrical considerations on monitoring long term risks (Review). *Bone Marrow Transplantation, 17,* S28–30.

Heldal, D., Tjonnfjord, G.E., Brinch, L. *et al.* (2000). A randomised study of allogeneic transplantation with stem cells from blood or bone marrow. *Bone Marrow Transplantation, 25,* 1129–36.

Hilbe, W., Nussbaumer, W., Bonatti, H. *et al.* (2000). Unusual adverse events following peripheral blood stem cell (PBSC) mobilisation using granulocyte colony stimulating factor (G-CSF) in healthy donors (Case Report). *Bone Marrow Transplantation, 26,* 811–3.

Imashuku, S., Hibi, S., Kataoka-Morimoto, Y. *et al.* (1995). Myelodysplasia and acute myeloid leukaemia in cases of aplastic anaemia and congenital neutropenia following G-CSF administration. *British Journal of Haematology, 89,* 188–90.

Isola, L., Scigliano, E., & Fruchtman, S. (2000). Long-term follow-up after allogeneic granulocyte colony-stimulating factor-primed bone marrow transplantation. *Biology of Blood and Marrow Transplantation, 6,* 428–33.

Ji, S.Q., Chen, H.R., Wang, H.X. *et al.* (2002a). Comparison outcome of allogeneic bone marrow transplantation with and without granulocyte colony-stimulating factor (G-CSF) (lenograstim) donor marrow priming in patients with chronic myeloid leukemia (CML). *Biology of Blood and Marrow Transplantation, 8,* 261–7.

Ji, S.Q., Chen, H.R., Wang, H.X. *et al.* (2002b). G-CSF primed haploidentical marrow transplantation without ex vivo T cell depletion: an excellent alternative for high-risk leukemia. *Bone Marrow Transplantation, 30,* 861–6.

Kernan, N.A. (1994). T-cell depletion for prevention of graft-versus-host disease, in Forman S.J., Blume, K.G., Thomas, E.D. (eds): *Bone Marrow Transplantation*. Boston, MA, Blackwell Scientific Publications, pp. 124–35.

Kernan, N.A., Collins, N.M., Juliano, L. *et al.* (1986). Clonable T lymphocytes in T cell-depleted bone marrow transplants correlate with development of graft-v-host disease. *Blood, 68,* 770–3.

Kitabayashi, A., Hirokawa, M., Hatano, Y. *et al.* (1995). Granulocyte colony-stimulating factor downregulates allogeneic immune responses by posttranscriptional inhibition of tumor necrosis factor-α, production. *Blood, 86,* 2220–7.

Korbling, M. & Champlin, R. (1996). Peripheral blood progenitor cell transplantation: a replacement for marrow auto- or allografts (Review). *Stem Cells 14,* 185–195.

Korbling, M., Huh, Y.O., Durett, A. *et al.* (1995a). Allogeneic blood stem cell transplantation: peripheralization and yield of donor-derived primitive hematopoietic progenitor cells (CD34+ Thy-1 dim) and lymphoid subsets, and possible predictors of engraftment and graft-versus-host disease. *Blood, 86,* 2842–8.

Körbling, M., Przepiorka, D., Huh, Y.O. *et al.* (1995b). Allogeneic blood stem cell transplantation for refractory leukemia and lymphoma: potential advantage of blood over marrow allografts. *Blood*, **85**, 1659–65.

Kusnierz-Glaz, C.R., Still, B.J., Amano, M. *et al.* (1997). Granulocyte colony-stimulating factor-induced comobilization of CD4⁻CD8⁻ T cells and hematopoietic progenitor cells (CD34⁺) in the blood of normal donors. *Blood*, **89**, 2586–95.

Lane, T.A., Law, P., Maruyama, M. *et al.* (1995). Harvesting and enrichment of hematopoietic progenitor cells mobilized into the peripheral blood of normal donors by granulocyte-macrophage colony-stimulating factor (GM-CSF) or G-CSF; potential role in allogeneic marrow transplantation. *Blood*, **85**, 275–82.

Lapierre, V., Oubouzar, N., Auperin, A. *et al.* (2001). Influence of the hematopoietic stem cell source on early immunohematologic reconstitution after allogeneic transplantation. *Blood*, **97**, 2580–6.

Lapierre, V., Auperin, A., Tayebi, H. *et al.* (2002). Increased presence of anti-HLA antibodies early after granulocyte colony-stimulating factor-mobilized peripheral blood hematopoietic stem cell transplantation compared with bone marrow transplantation. *Blood*, **100**, 1484–9.

LeBlanc, R., Roy, J., Demers, C. *et al.* (1999). A prospective study of G-CSF effects on hemostasis in allogeneic blood stem cell donors. *Bone Marrow Transplantation*, **23**, 991–6.

Lee, S., Im, S-A., Yoo, E-S. *et al.* (2000). Mobilization kinetics of CD34⁺ cells in association with modulation of CD44 and CD31 expression during continuous intravenous administration of G-CSF in normal donors. *Stem Cells*, **18**, 281–6.

Lee, V., Li, C.K., Shing, M.M. *et al.* (2000). Single vs twice daily G-CSF dose for peripheral blood stem cells harvest in normal donors and children with non-malignant diseases. *Bone Marrow Transplantation*, **25**, 931–5.

Levesque, J.P., Takamatsu, Y., Nilsson, S.K. *et al.* (2000). Mobilization of hemopoietic progenitor cells into peripheral blood is associated with VCAM-1 proteolytic cleavage in the bone marrow. *Blood*, **96** (Part 1), 221a, #945, (abstr).

Lindemann, A., Herrmann, F., Oster, W. *et al.* (1989). Hematologic effects of recombinant human granulocyte colony-stimulating factor in patients with malignancy. *Blood*, **74**, 2644–51.

Link, H., Arseniev, L., Bahre, O. *et al.* (1996). Transplantation of allogeneic CD34+ blood cells. *Blood*, **87**, 4903–9.

Lochte, H.L., Crouch, W.W., & Thomas, E.D. (1942). The nitrogen compounds in petroleum distillates. XXIV. Isolation and identification of $C_{11}H_{17}N$ base from California petroleum. *Journal of the American Chemical Society*, **64**, 2753–5.

Mahmoud, H.K., Fahmy, O.A., Kamel, A. *et al.* (1999). Peripheral blood vs bone marrow as a source for allogeneic hematopoietic stem cell transplantation. *Bone Marrow Transplantation*, **24**, 355–8.

Majolino, I., Aversa, F., Bacigalupo, A. *et al.* (1995). Allogeneic transplants of rhG-CSF-mobilized peripheral blood stem cells (PBSC) from normal donors. *Haematologica*, **80**, 40–3.

Majolino, I., Cavallaro, A.M., Bacigalupo, A. *et al.* (1997). Mobilization and collection of PBSC in healthy donors: a retrospective analysis of the Italian bone marrow transplantation group (GITMO). *Haematologica*, **82**, 47–52.

Majolino, I., Saglio, G., Scime, R. *et al.* (1996). High incidence of chronic GVHD after primary allogeneic peripheral blood stem

cell transplantation in patients with hematologic malignancies. *Bone Marrow Transplantation*, **17**, 555–60.

Martínez, C., Urbano-Ispizua, A., Marín, P. *et al.* (1999b). Efficacy and toxicity of a high-dose G-CSF schedule for peripheral blood progenitor cell mobilization in healthy donors. *Bone Marrow Transplantation*, **24**, 1273–8.

Martínez, C., Urbano-Ispizua, A., Rozman, M. *et al.* (1999a). Effects of short-term administration of G-CSF (filgrastim) on bone marrow progenitor cells: analysis of serial marrow samples from normal donors. *Bone Marrow Transplantation*, **23**, 15–19.

McCredie, K.B., Hersh, E.M., & Freireich, E.J. (1971). Cells capable of colony formation in the peripheral blood of man. *Science*, **171**, 293–4.

McCullough, J., Clay, M., Herr, G. *et al.* (1999). Effects of granulocyte-colony-stimulating factor on potential normal granulocyte donors. *Transfusion*, **39**, 1136–40.

McQuaker, G., Haynes, A.P., Long, S.G. *et al.* (1995). Study of the release of CD34 cells and colony forming cells in healthy subjects using G-CSF. *Bone Marrow Transplantation*, **15** (Supp2), S27, (Abstract)(abstr).

Mielcarek, M., Martin, P., & Torok-Storb, B. (1997). Suppression of alloantigen-induced T-cell proliferation by CD14+ cells derived from granulocyte colony-stimulating factor (G-CSF)-mobilized peripheral blood mononuclear cells. *Blood*, **89**, 1629–34.

Mielcarek, M., Roecklein, B.A., & Torok-Storb, B. (1996). CD14+ cells in granulocyte colony-stimulating factor (G-CSF)-mobilized peripheral blood mononuclear cells induce secretion of interleukin-6 and G-CSF by marrow stroma. *Blood*, **87**, 574–80.

Miflin, G., Russell, N.H., Hutchinson, R.M. *et al.* (1997). Allogeneic peripheral blood stem cell transplantation for haematological malignancies – an analysis of kinetics of engraftment and GVHD risk. *Bone Marrow Transplantation*, **19**, 9–13.

Miflin, G., Stainer, C.J., Carter, G.I. *et al.* (1999). Comparative serial quantitative measurements of chimaerism following unmanipulated allogeneic transplantation of peripheral blood stem cells and bone marrow. *British Journal of Haematology*, **107**, 429–40.

Mohty, M., Kuentz, M., Michallet, M. *et al.* (2002). Chronic graft-versus-host disease after allogeneic blood stem cell transplantation: long-term results of a randomized study. *Blood*, **100**, 3128–34.

Morton, J., Hutchins, C., & Durrant, S. (2001). Granulocyte-colony-stimulating factor (G-CSF)-primed allogeneic bone marrow: significantly less graft-versus-host disease and comparable engraftment to G-CSF-mobilized peripheral blood stem cells. *Blood*, **98**, 3186–91.

Murata, M., Harada, M., Kato, S. *et al.* (1999). Peripheral blood stem cell mobilization and apheresis: analysis of adverse events in 94 normal donors. *Bone Marrow Transplantation*, **24**, 1065–71.

Nash, R.A., Burstein, S.A., Storb, R. *et al.* (1995). Thrombocytopenia in dogs induced by granulocyte-macrophage colony-stimulating factor: increased destruction of circulating platelets. *Blood*, **86**, 1765–75.

Nash, R.A., Pepe, M.S., Storb, R. *et al.* (1992). Acute graft-versus-host disease: analysis of risk factors after allogeneic marrow transplantation and prophylaxis with cyclosporine and methotrexate. *Blood*, **80**, 1838–45.

Niederwieser, D., Pepe, M., Storb, R. *et al.* (1988). Improvement in rejection, engraftment rate and survival without increase in graft-versus-host disease by high marrow cell dose in patients transplanted for aplastic anemia. *British Journal of Haematology,* **69,** 23–8.

O'Reilly, R.J., Kernan, N., Cunningham, I. *et al.* (1988). Soybean lectin agglutination and E-rosette depletion for removal of T-cells from HLA-identical and non-identical marrow grafts administered for the treatment of leukemia, in Martelli M.F., Grignani F., Reisner Y. (eds): T-Cell Depletion in Allogeneic Bone-Marrow Transplantation. Rome, *Ares-Serono Symposia,* pp. 123–9.

Ottinger, H.D., Beelen, D.W., Scheulen, B. *et al.* (1996). Improved immune reconstitution after allotransplantation of peripheral blood stem cells instead of bone marrow. *Blood,* **88,** 2775–9.

Pan, L., Delmonte, J., Jr., Jalonen, C.K. *et al.* (1995). Pretreatment of donor mice with granulocyte colony-stimulating factor polarizes donor T lymphocytes toward type-2 cytokine production and reduces severity of experimental graft versus host disease. *Blood,* **86** (12), 4422–9.

Papayannopoulou, T., Nakamoto, B., Andrews, R.G. *et al.* (1997). In vivo effects of Flt3/Flk2 ligand on mobilization of hemopoietic progenitors in primates and potent synergistic enhancement with granulocyte colony-stimulating factor. *Blood,* **90,** 620–9.

Parkkali, T., Volin, L., Sirèn, M-K. *et al.* (1996). Acute iritis induced by granulocyte colony-stimulating factor used for mobilization in a volunteer unrelated peripheral blood progenitor cell donor (Case report). *Bone Marrow Transplantation,* **17,** 433–4.

Powles, R., Mehta, J., Kulkarni, S. *et al.* (2000). Allogeneic blood and bone-marrow stem-cell transplantation in haematological malignant diseases: a randomised trial. *Lancet,* **355,** 1231–7.

Przepiorka, D., Anderlini, P., Ippoliti, C. *et al.* (1997). Allogeneic blood stem cell transplantation in advanced hematologic cancers. *Bone Marrow Transplantation,* **19,** 455–60.

Przieporka, D., Smith, T.L., Folloder, J. *et al.* (2001). Controlled trial of filgrastim for acceleration of neutrophil recovery after allogeneic blood stem cell transplantation from human leukocyte antigen-matched related donors. *Blood,* **97,** 3405–10.

Remberger, M., Ringden, O., Blau, I.W. *et al.* (2001). No difference in graft-versus-host disease, relapse, and survival comparing peripheral stem cells to bone marrow using unrelated donors. *Blood,* **98,** 1739–45.

Rice, A. & Reiffers, J. (1992). Mobilized blood stem cells, Immunophenotyyping and functional characteristics. *Journal of Hematotherapy & Stem Cell Research,* **1,** 19–26.

Ringden, O., Remberger, M., Runde, V. *et al.* (1999). Peripheral blood stem cell transplantation from unrelated donors: a comparison with marrow transplantation. *Blood,* **94,** 455–64.

Ringden, O., Labopin, M., Bacigalupo, A. *et al.* (2003). Transplantation of peripheral blood stem cells as compared with bone marrow from HLA-identical siblings in adult patients with acute myeloid leukemia and acute lymphoblastic leukemia. *Journal of Clinical Oncology,* **20,** 4655–64.

Rowley, S.D., Donaldson, G., Lilleby, K. *et al.* (2001). Experiences of donors enrolled in a randomized study of allogeneic bone marrow or peripheral blood stem cell transplantation. *Blood,* **97,** 2541–8.

Russell, J.A., Bowen, T., Brown, C. *et al.* (1996). Allogeneic blood cell transplants for haematological malignancy: Comparison of engraftment and graft-versus-host disease with bone marrow transplantation. *Bone Marrow Transplantation,* **17,** 703–8.

Russell, J.A., Luider, J., Weaver, M. *et al.* (1995). Collection of progenitor cells for allogeneic transplantation from peripheral blood of normal donors. *Bone Marrow Transplantation,* **15,** 111–5.

Russell, N.H., Hunter, A., Rogers, S. *et al.* (1993). Peripheral blood stem cells as an alternative to marrow for allogeneic transplantation. *Lancet,* **341,** 1482.

Russell, N.H. & Hunter, A.E. (1994). Peripheral blood stem cells for allogeneic transplantation. *Bone Marrow Transplantation,* **13,** 353–5.

Sato, N., Sawada, K., Takahashi, T.A. *et al.* (1994). A time course study for optimal harvest of peripheral blood progenitor cells by granulocyte colony-stimulating factor in healthy volunteers. *Experimental Hematology,* **22,** 973–8.

Schmitz, N., Bacigalupo, A., Labopin, M. *et al.* (1996). Transplantation of peripheral blood progenitor cells from HLA-identical sibling donors. *British Journal of Haematology,* **95,** 715–23.

Schmitz, N., Champlin, R.E., Loberiza, F.R., Jr. *et al.* (2001). Long term follow-up of allogeneic blood stem cell and bone marrow transplantation: a collaborative study of EBMT and IBMTR. *Blood,* **98** (Part 1), 744a, #3099, (abstr).

Schmitz, N., Dreger, P., Suttorp, M. *et al.* (1995). Primary transplantation of allogeneic peripheral blood progenitor cells mobilized by filgrastim (granulocyte colony-stimulating factor). *Blood,* **85,** 1666–72.

Schmitz, N., Beksac, M., Hasenclever, D. *et al.* (2002). Transplantation of mobilized peripheral blood cells to HLA-identical siblings with standard-risk leukemia. *Blood,* **100,** 761–7.

Schwinger, W. (1993). Single dose of filgrastim (rhG-CSF) increases the number of hematopoietic progenitors in the peripheral blood of adult volunteers. *Bone Marrow Transplantation,* **11,** 489–92.

Schwinger, W., Urban, Ch., Lackner, H. *et al.* (2000). Unrelated peripheral blood stem cell transplantation with "megadoses" of purified CD34+ cells in three children with refractory severe aplastic anemia. *Bone Marrow Transplantation,* **25,** 513–7.

Serody, J.S., Sparks, S.D., Lin, Y. *et al.* (2000). Comparison of granulocyte colony-stimulating factor (G-CSF)-mobilized peripheral blood progenitor cells and G-CSF-stimulated bone marrow as a source of stem cells in HLA-matched sibling transplantation. *Biology of Blood and Marrow Transplantation,* **6,** 434–40.

Simpson, D.R., Couban, S., Bredeson, C. *et al.* (2000). A Canadian randomized study comparing peripheral blood (PB) and bone marrow (BM) in patients undergoing matched sibling transplants for myeloid malignancies. *Blood,* **96** (Part 1), 481a, #2067, (abstr).

Söhngen, D., Wienen, S., Siebler, M. *et al.* (1998). Analysis of rhG-CSF-effects on platelets by in vitro bleeding test and transcranial Doppler ultrasound examination. *Bone Marrow Transplantation,* **22,** 1087–90.

Spitzer, T., McAfee, S., Poliquin, C. *et al.* (1998). Acute gouty arthritis following recombinant human granulocyte colony-stimulating factor therapy in an allogeneic blood stem cell donor (Correspondence). *Bone Marrow Transplantation,* **21,** 966–7.

Stone, R.M., Neuberg, D., Soiffer, R. *et al.* (1994). Myelodysplastic syndrome as a late complication following autologous bone marrow transplantation for non-Hodgkin's lymphoma. *Journal of Clinical Oncology,* **12,** 2535–42.

Storb, R., Deeg, H.J., Whitehead, J. *et al.* (1987). Marrow transplantation for leukemia and aplastic anemia: Two controlled trials of a combination of methotrexate and cyclosporine versus cyclosporine alone or methotrexate alone for prophylaxis of acute graft-versus-host disease. *Transplantation Proceedings, 19,* 2608–13.

Storb, R., Etzioni, R., Anasetti, C. *et al.* (1994). Cyclophosphamide combined with antithymocyte globulin in preparation for allogeneic marrow transplants in patients with aplastic anemia. *Blood,* **84,** 941–9.

Storek, J., Dawson, M.A., Storer, B. *et al.* (2001). Immune reconstitution after allogeneic marrow transplantation compared with blood stem cell transplantation. *Blood, 97,* 3380–9.

Storek, J., Gooley, T., Siadak, M. *et al.* (1997). Allogeneic peripheral blood stem cell transplantation may be associated with a high risk of chronic graft-versus-host disease. *Blood, 90,* 4705–9.

Stroncek, D.F., Clay, M.E., Herr, G. *et al.* (1997). The kinetics of G-CSF mobilization of CD34+ cells in healthy people. *Transfusion Medicine, 7,* 19–24.

Stroncek, D.F., Clay, M.E., Jascz, W. *et al.* (1999). Collection of two peripheral blood stem cell concentrates from healthy donors. *Transfusion Medicine, 9,* 37–50.

Stroncek, D.F., Clay, M.E., Petzoldt, M.L. *et al.* (1996). Treatment of normal individuals with granulocyte-colony-stimulating factor: donor experiences and the effects on peripheral blood CD34+ cell counts and on the collection of peripheral blood stem cells. *Transfusion, 36,* 601–10.

Stuart, M.J., Chao, N.S., Horning, S.J. *et al.* (2001). Efficacy and toxicity of a CCNU-containing high-dose chemotherapy regimen followed by autologous hematopoietic cell transplantation in relapsed or refractory Hodgkin's disease. *Biology of Blood and Marrow Transplantation, 7,* 552–60.

Suzue, T., Kawano, Y., Takaue, Y. *et al.* (1994). Cell processing protocol for allogeneic peripheral blood stem cells mobilized by granulocyte colony-stimulating factor. *Experimental Hematology, 22,* 888–92.

To, L.B., Haylock, D.N., Dowse, T. *et al.* (1994). A comparative study of the phenotype and proliferative capacity of peripheral blood (PB) CD34+ cells mobilized by four different protocols and those of steady-phase PB and bone marrow CD34+ cells. *Blood, 84,* 2930–9.

To, L.B., Haylock, D.N., Simmons, P.J. *et al.* (1997). The biology and clinical uses of blood stem cells (Review). *Blood, 89,* 2233–58.

Torrelo, A., Madero, L., Mediero, I.G. *et al.* (2000). A cutaneous eruption from G-CSF in a healthy donor. *Pediatric Dermatology,* **17,** 205–7.

Trenschel, R., Ross, S., Husing, J. *et al.* (2000). Reduced risk of persisting cytomegalvirus pp65 antigenemia and cytomegalovirus interstitial pneumonia following allogeneic PBSCT. *Bone Marrow Transplantation,* **25,** 665–72.

Urbano-Ispizua, A., Solano, C., Brunet, S. *et al.* (1996). Allogeneic peripheral blood progenitor cell transplantation: analysis of short-term engraftment and acute GVHD incidence in 33 cases. *Bone Marrow Transplantation,* **18,** 35–40.

Urbano-Ispizua, A., Solano, C., Brunet S. *et al.* (1998). Allogeneic transplantation of selected CD34+ cells from peripheral blood: experience of 62 cases using immunoadsorption or immunomagnetic technique. Spanish Group of Allo-PBT. *Bone Marrow Transplantation,* **22,** 519–25.

Verdonck, L.F., Dekker, A.W., de Gast, G.C. *et al.* (1994). Allogeneic bone marrow transplantation with a fixed low number of T cells in the marrow graft. *Blood,* **83** (10), 3090–3096.

Vigorito, A.C., Azevedo, W.M., Marques, J.F. *et al.* (1998). A randomised, prospective comparison of allogeneic bone marrow and peripheral blood progenitor cell transplantation in the treatment of haematological malignancies. *Bone Marrow Transplantation,* **22,** 1145–51.

Waller, C.F., Bertz, H., Wenger, M.K. *et al.* (1996). Mobilization of peripheral blood progenitor cells for allogeneic transplantation: efficacy and toxicity of a high-dose rhG-CSF regimen. *Bone Marrow Transplantation,* **18,** 279–83.

Weaver, C.H., Buckner, C.D., Longin, K. *et al.* (1993). Syngeneic transplantation with peripheral blood mononuclear cells collected after the administration of recombinant human granulocyte colony-stimulating factor. *Blood,* **82,** 1981–4.

Weaver, C.H., Hazelton, B., Palmer, P.A. *et al.* (1996). A randomized dose finding study of filgrastim for mobilization of peripheral blood progenitor cells (PBPCs). *ASCO Annual Meeting,* (Abstract).

12 Mechanisms of failure of sustained engraftment

MARCO MIELCAREK, NORIHIRO AWAYA, AND BEVERLY TOROK-STORB

Fred Hutchinson Cancer Research Center and Department of Medicine, University of Washington, Seattle, USA

Introduction

Hematopoietic stem cell transplantation (HSCT) has proven to be a successful treatment modality for a variety of hematologic malignancies, certain solid tumors, and nonmalignant disorders; however, a number of problems still remain. Included among these is poor graft function or its extreme, graft failure, which still occurs in a proportion of patients. In myeloablative HSCT, the initial recovery of peripheral counts after transplantation may be ascribed to homing, proliferation, and differentiation of committed hematopoietic progenitors, whereas long-term hematopoiesis requires homing and appropriate regulation of primitive totipotent stem cells. Unfortunately, little is known about the mechanisms that control this process. It is generally agreed that stromal elements of the marrow microenvironment are required to continuously regulate hematopoiesis, but it is only recently that we have come to realize the considerable number of cells and cell products that may be involved. Given the complexity of the system, there are by definition many ways for it to fail.

The recent introduction of nonmyeloablative HSCT into clinical practice has further complicated the evaluation and study of donor-graft function due to the potential development of a mixed chimeric state, which is the transient or permanent coexistence of donor and host hematopoietic systems. Thus, autologous reconstitution may mask donor-graft failure after this type of HSCT, and specific strategies are required to distinguish donor from host hematopoiesis.

A number of clinical variables have been associated with poor marrow function or failure of sustained engraftment. These variables may influence the likelihood of rejection; may directly affect the homing ability and function of stem cells, progenitor cells, and accessory cells; or may impact on the function of the marrow microenvironment. In this chapter some of the more obvious variables associated with poor graft function are discussed.

Conditioning regimens

Pretransplant conditioning therapy in myeloablative allogeneic HSCT has been used to serve two important purposes. First,

high-dose cytotoxic therapy kills tumor cells and, in addition to donor T-cell-mediated graft-versus-tumor effects, which become established after transplant, appears to contribute to eradication of the malignancy in the recipient. Second, the conditioning regimen must provide sufficient host immunosuppression to prevent rejection of donor cells as a prerequisite for sustained engraftment.

Inadequate conditioning regimens have been associated with failure to maintain donor hematopoiesis. Anasetti *et al.* (1989) showed that conditioning with cyclophosphamide (60 mg/kg × 2 days), and 6 doses of 200 cGy radiation was specifically associated with late graft failure in human leukocyte antigen (HLA)-mismatched allogeneic bone marrow transplantations. In some cases the loss of donor cells was associated with the appearance of host lymphocytes exhibiting antidonor activities indicative of immune-mediated graft rejection.

Historically, graft failure was a problem for patients with severe aplastic anemia transplanted with HLA-identical marrow after conditioning with high doses of cyclophosphamide only. In the early 1970s, between 30% and 60% of aplastic anemia patients so treated experienced a recurrence of aplastic anemia. Two factors predicted graft failure: a low number of transplanted marrow cells (less than 3×10^8 nucleated cells/kg) and in vitro tests indicative of allosensitization pretransplant (Storb, 1989), which were interpreted to indicate transfusion-induced sensitization of patient lymphocytes against minor non-HLA antigens on donor cells. Apparently this allosensitization was not suppressed by the cyclophosphamide conditioning regimen. However, a change in the conditioning regimen at Fred Hutchinson Cancer Research Center to add antithymocyte globulin and infuse viable donor buffy coat cells increased survival to 80% in multiply transfused patients with aplastic anemia (Storb *et al.*, 1994). Patients with sickle cell anemia and thalassemia are still at an increased risk of graft rejection due to transfusion-related allosensitization (Walters *et al.*, 1996).

The dogma of high-dose cytotoxic therapy as being a crucial element to achieving disease eradication after HSCT has been recently challenged by the demonstration of excellent tumor responses observed in patients transplanted with allogeneic peripheral blood stem cells (PBSC) after conditioning with only minimally toxic and nonmyeloablative regimens (Storb *et al.*, 1999b; McSweeney *et al.*, 2001; Storb *et al.*, 2001; Mielcarek *et al.*, 2002). Disease responses observed in these patients were presumably mediated by allogeneic graft-versus-tumor effects rather than significant cytoreduction by the pre-transplant conditioning regimen. The nonmyeloablative pre-transplant conditioning regimen used for HLA-matched HSCT from related and unrelated donors at the Fred Hutchinson Cancer Research Center consists of fludarabine (90 mg/m²) and low-dose (200 cGy) total body irradiation and provides suffi-cient immunosuppression to ensure donor cell engraftment when cyclosporine and mycophenolate mofetil are given for immunosuppression over several weeks after HSCT. These results in conjunction with observations made in the preclinical canine HSCT model also demonstrate that donor cells are capa-ble of creating marrow space by immunologic means making a high-dose conditioning regimens obsolete for this pupose (Storb *et al.*, 1999a and 1999b).

In the beginning era of nonmyeloablative HSCT, however, the term *poor marrow function* may require a new definition because marrow aplasia and ensuing peripheral blood cytope-nias, which are powerful indicators of graft function and rejec-tion after myeloablative HSCT, are less useful markers in the nonmyeloablative setting. Because graft rejection is usually accompanied by autologous reconstitution by normal and malignant hematopoiesis, it may not be associated with abnor-mal marrow morphology or decreasing peripheral blood counts. Thus, monitoring of donor marrow function after non-myeloablative HSCT requires laboratory techniques able to distinguish donor from host hematopoietic cells in marrow and blood. For this purpose, fluorescence in situ hybridization (FISH) using sex chromosome-specific probes has been used in sex-mismatched HSCT (van Dekken *et al.*, 1989; Crescenzi *et al.*, 2000), whereas variable number tandem repeat (VNTR) analysis has proven to be a valuable tool in sex-matched HSCT (Leclair *et al.*, 1995; Rothberg *et al.*, 1997; Antin *et al.*, 2001).

A state of mixed donor-host chimerism may persist for weeks or even months after nonmyeloablative HSCT and may eventually result in full donor chimerism, persistent mixed donor-host chimerism or graft rejection. Based on the trans-plant protocol used at the FHCRC, a high degree of donor chimerism in the peripheral blood T-cell compartment by post-transplant day 28 has proven to be a positive predictor for sus-tained engraftment after HLA-matched nonmyeloablative HSCT from unrelated donors (Maris *et al.*, 2001).

Finally, given that the nonhematopoietic elements of the marrow microenvironment are not replaced by donor cells, even decades after myeloablative HSCT (Simmons *et al.*, 1987; Koc *et al.*, 1999; Awaya *et al.*, 2002), there is the potential for some conditioning regimens to compromise the resident microenvironment resulting in poor graft function. Agents such as doxorubicine and 5-fluorouracil (5-FU), as well as ionizing radiation have been associated with injuries to the marrow microenvironment (Greenberger 1991; Gibson *et al.*, 1997; Galotto *et al.*, 1999; Schwartz *et al.*, 2000; Banfi *et al.*, 2001). It is conceivable therefore that patients receiving conditioning for HSCT after multiple rounds of chemotherapy may have problems establishing a robust and stable graft.

Graft composition

The number and function of hematopoietic stem cells (HSC) and progenitor cells contained in a graft, and donor cells in addition to HSC, the so-called accessory cells, may influence marrow function after HSCT (Table 12.1). Tempo of engraft-ment, graft failure rates, and graft function have been associ-ated with the number of CD34+ cells transplanted in the autolo-gous and allogeneic HSCT setting. In clinical practice, a CD34+ cell number of greater than $2.5–5.0 \times 10^6$/kg recipient body weight is considered to be a critical threshold to ensure timely hematopoietic recovery and sustained graft function (Bensinger *et al.*, 1995; Weaver *et al.*, 1995). At least in theory, the replicative stress imposed on HSC during reconstitution of the hematopoietic system after HSCT could pose a potential risk for stem cell exhaustion due to critical telomere shorten-ing. However, although some degree of telomere shortening has been described in CD34+ cells and their progeny obtained from HSCT recipients (Mathioudakis *et al.*, 2000; de Pauw *et*

Table 12.1. *Hematopoietic stem cell sources and graft composition*

	BM	G-PBMC	UCB
$TNC \times 10^8$kg	3.1 (1.6–4.5)[a]	7.0 (2.6–14)[a]	0.2 (0.1–0.63)[b]
$CD34^+ \times 10^6$kg	1.4 (0.3–4.2)[a]	4.2 (1.4–19)[a]	0.12(0.02–1.7)[b]
$CD3^+ \times 10^8$kg	0.3 (0.1–1.6)[a]	1.8 (0.7–3.7)[a]	0.05 (0.009–0.09)[b]
$CD14^+ \times 10^8$/kg	0.083 (0.004–0.67)[c]	2.9 (0.6–7.6)[d]	0.008 (0.004–0.012)[e]

Median dose (range) for allograft recipients
Numbers derived from:
[a] Singhal *et al.*, 2000.
[b] Rocha *et al.*, 2000; Laughlin *et al.*, 2001.
[c] Unpublished own data (n = 412).
[d] Mielcarek *et al.*, 1997; Zaucha *et al.*, 2001a.
[e] Sorg *et al.*, 2001.

al., 2002; Thornley *et al.,* 2002), there is currently no convincing evidence linking this proposed mechanism to cases of graft failure or poor marrow function.

The importance of accessory cells for engraftment and graft function is probably different in autologous and allogeneic HSCT. Donor T cells play a pivotal role in overcoming donor-directed host immunity, thereby facilitating engraftment across histocompatibility barriers. This is supported by increasing rates of rejections seen with increasing efficiencies of T-cell depletion in allogeneic HSCT (Martin *et al.,* 1988; Mauch *et al.,* 1989; Bunjes *et al.,* 1990; Martin, 1990; Martin, 1996; Urbano-Ispizua *et al.,* 2001) (Fig. 12.1).

Based on the current knowledge of the role of T cells in graft-versus-host disease (GVHD), investigators have developed a variety of physical and biologic strategies to remove T cells for the prevention of clinical GVHD. These include CD34-selection, immunotoxin treatment, immune absorption, lectin agglutination, antibody and complement depletion, or elutriation. The current consensus is that although pan-T-cell depletion reduces the severity of GVHD, it increases the incidence of graft failure. In HLA-matched transplants, the rejection rate is reported as 2% to 3% with unmanipulated marrow versus 10% to 30% with pan-T-cell depleted marrow (Vallera & Blazar, 1989). In histoincompatible transplants, the rejection rate is 10% to 15% with unmanipulated marrow versus 40% to 75% with pan-T-cell-depleted marrow (Vallera & Blazar, 1989). Some graft failures in this setting can be clearly attributed to immune-mediated graft rejection involving host lymphocytes with anti-donor activities. In such instances it has been suggested that T-cell depletion has compromised the ability of donor marrow to overcome residual host immunity. This is supported by the observation that increasing the radiation dose, and thereby increasing the immunosuppression of the patient, improved the engraftment rate (Martin *et al.,* 1985).

In some patients, however, persisting host cells are not detected, raising the issue that mechanisms other than rejection can mediate failure in this setting. Such patients may have donor lymphocytes with abnormal phenotypes and limited function (Voltarelli *et al.,* 1989; Bunjes *et al.,* 1990). The mechanisms responsible for this kind of failure are unknown; however, it has been speculated that T-cell depletion may compromise accessory cell function either because T cells themselves serve an important accessory function to augment engraftment, or other accessory cells, like macrophages, are lost during the depletion procedures. As mentioned previously, a considerable amount of experimental data suggests macrophages can play an important role in microenvironmental function. Whether T cells also play a role is less clear. T cells have been shown to synthesize many cytokines, including IL-3, and it is possible that by migrating to the damaged microenvironment they could contribute to production of the localized concentration of cytokines needed for stem cell proliferation.

In the autologous setting it is conceivable that accessory cells may be required to facilitate engraftment in ways unrelated to overcoming host resistance. How this is accomplished is not precisely defined; however, it is known that donor macrophages become a part of the marrow microenvironment and that activities produced by macrophages have an important role in modulating cytokine production by other microenvironmental components (Mielcarek *et al.,* 1996). Therefore, a critical mass of functional donor accessory cells may be required to establish the appropriate milieu in the microenvironment needed for the support and regulation of donor stem cells. It is reasonable to hypothesize that both the size and function of this compartment of cells could influence graft function.

In addition to numbers of HSC and accessory cells provided with a graft, their quality may impact on graft function. It has been hypothesized that HSC may have a limited self-renewal potential (Mauch *et al.,* 1989) that in the autologous setting, may have been further compromised by preceding therapy with cytotoxic agents such as busulfan, BCNU, methyl-CCNU, cisplatinum, and chlorambucil, which are known to damage human stem cells. In mice, busulfan and BCNU treatment of bone marrow causes a loss in self-renewal capacity (Mauch *et al.,* 1989). Therefore, the use of autologous bone marrow transplantation in an increasing number of patients with advanced lymphoma, leukemia, and solid tumors who have had extensive prior exposures to chemotherapy may lead to an increased incidence of late graft failure. The failure of chemically purged autologous bone marrow transplantations to respond to growth factor therapy such as GM-CSF (Nemunaitis *et al.,* 1990) is also in keeping with the damaged compartment of progenitor or stem cells.

Quality and quantity of HSC and accessory cells may vary greatly among different sources of stem cells used for clinical HSCT. In comparison to bone marrow, which has been the standard HSC source over decades, G-CSF-mobilized peripheral blood mononuclear cells (G-PBMC) contain larger numbers of CD34+ cells, T cells, and monocytes (Mielcarek & Torok-Storb, 1997). Although CD34+ cells in G-PBMC are non-cycling, cytokine stimulation induces rapid transition into

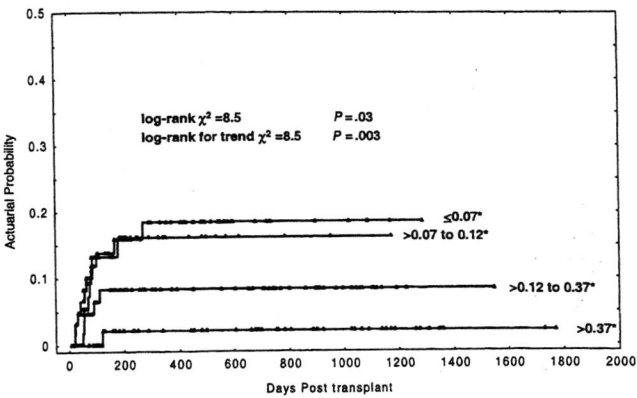

Fig. 12.1. Actuarial probability of graft failure by grouping the number of CD3+ cells infused to patients in quartiles. *indicates × 10⁶/kg. Reproduced, with permission, from Urbano-Ispizua *et al.* (2001).

cell cycle (Roberts & Metcalf, 1995). G-PBMC show faster engraftment kinetics than marrow and appear to be a superior product when histocompatibility barriers have to be overcome in allogeneic transplantation (Bensinger et al., 2001). This is supported by the fact that sustained donor engraftment was observed more consistently when G-PBMC were used instead of marrow in a preclinical canine transplantation model (Zaucha et al., 2001b) as well as in clinical HLA-matched nonmyeloablative HSCT from unrelated donors (Maris et al., 2001). A possible mechanism may be the 10-fold greater number of functionally distinct T cells (Pan et al., 1995; Zaucha et al., 2001a) or the 50-fold increased number of monocytes in G-PBMC compared to marrow (Mielcarek et al., 1997a; Mielcarek et al., 1998).

In comparison, umbilical cord blood blood (UCB) has been used as a source of HSC in young patients with sibling donors where successful sustained engraftment has only been documented in 91% of cases (Wagner et al., 1995; Wagner & Kurtzberg, 1997; Barker & Wagner, 2002). Further results suggest that UCB transplants may also be feasible in unrelated donor settings (Barker et al., 2001; Laughlin et al., 2001). However, considerably delayed neutrophil and platelet recoveries confer greater transplant-related risks to UCB compared to marrow and G-PBMC transplants (Rubinstein et al., 1998). The delayed platelet recovery appears to be associated with a decrease in the number of CD34+ CD41+ megakaryocytic progenitor cells found in UCB (Drygalski et al., 2000; Kanamaru et al., 2000), suggesting that stem cell and progenitor cell numbers may be limiting. In addition, the adhesion receptor repertoire on UCB-derived CD34+ cells is distinct from the repertoire found on CD34+ cells in G-PBMC, which may impair their ability to efficiently home to the marrow (Asosingh et al., 1998). Despite the obvious advantage the presence of naïve T cells in UCB products may have with regard to acceptable severity of GVHD in HLA-mismatched transplants, decreased graft-versus-host reactivity of UCB-derived T cells may also influence their ability to control host-versus-graft reactions and thereby compromise engraftment, particularly in the HLA-mismatched and unrelated donor setting.

Ex vivo culture of harvested marrow, mobilized blood, or cord blood in the presence of growth factors has become an attractive experimental strategy aimed at accelerating hematopoietic recovery by increasing the number of colony forming units (CFU) in the graft (Piacibello et al., 1999; Reiffers et al., 1999; Kobari et al., 2000; McNiece et al., 2000; Paquette et al., 2000). While CFU assays performed postexpansion can estimate the number of clonogenic progenitors, and assays of long-term culture-initiating cells (LTC-IC) may estimate long-term repopulating ability, a functional assay to predict the ability of progenitors to home to the marrow microenvironment postexpansion has not yet been developed. However, it is conceivable that critical homing receptors might be downregulated or functionally altered during this growth factor driven culture period. This is supported by evidence in animal models which suggest that reconstituting ability may be lost

following ex vivo culture of progenitor cells in certain growth factor conditions (Yonemura et al., 1996; Holyoake et al., 1997; Glimm et al., 2000). Therefore, an increase in CFU number does not necessarily mean a more rapid or sustained engraftment if the ability of these cells to migrate to the marrow has been compromised.

The homing mechanisms of progenitor cells are only marginally understood. In analogy to the better characterized mechanisms of leukocyte homing to peripheral lymphoid tissues, investigators have proposed that the same or similar adhesion mechanisms might be involved in progenitor cell homing (Papayannopoulou & Craddock 1997; Yong et al., 1998; Mohle et al., 2001). According to this hypothesis, progenitor cells must bind to receptors on endothelial cells lining the marrow microvasculature and then transmigrate this layer to gain access to niches in the marrow microenvironment.

We have found that during ex vivo culture of CD34-enriched progenitor cells from G-PBMC and UCB, adhesion receptors such as VLA-4, LFA-1, PECAM-1, CD44, and L-selectin can be considerably downregulated or even lost depending on the growth factor combination used (Mielcarek et al., 1997b; Reems et al., 1997). Future studies combining different expansion protocols with gene marking and subsequent transplantation into animals are needed to define molecules critical for homing of hematopoietic progenitor and stem cells.

In autologous transplantation, relapse may occur due to graft contamination with tumor cells, residual tumor cells in the patient, and/or the absence of graft-versus-tumor effects. Investigators have applied different strategies aimed at reducing numbers of tumor cells that are potentially contaminating marrow or peripheral blood cell grafts. Ex vivo treatment of marrow or mobilized blood with cytotoxic agents (e.g., cyclophosphamide derivatives) or immunotoxins with presumed preferential activity against tumor cells have been used in hematologic and nonhematologic malignancies. More recently, CD34-selection has been applied in autologous transplantation to achieve tumor cell depletion by positive selection for nonmalignant hematopoietic progenitors.

In acute myeloid leukemia in first or second remission, for example, marrow purging with 4-hydroxycyclophosphamide significantly reduced relapse rates but also led to delayed leukocyte recovery in the purged group (Gorin et al., 1990; Gorin, 2002). In chronic myeloid leukemia, ex vivo marrow purging with γ-interferon (McGlave et al., 1990) or ex vivo marrow culture, which also depletes for Philadelphia chromosome-positive progenitors (Barnett et al., 1994), led to partial or even complete cytogenetic responses in a significant proportion of patients. However, 15 of 44 patients transplanted after γ-interferon-purging and 5 of 22 patients transplanted after ex vivo marrow culture experienced delayed or partial engraftment requiring infusion of untreated back-up cells. This illustrates that the purging process may be associated with damage or loss of viable stem cells and/or accessory cells or, alternatively, the process may interfere with their ability to home to the marrow. In summary, delayed or failure of sustained engraftment seen after ex vivo purging might not only be attributable to numeric losses or damage to the progenitor cell compartment, but also to changes in composition or function of accessory cells.

Underlying disease

Clinical observations suggest that the type of the underlying malignant or non-malignant disease may influence graft function after transplant. As discussed above in more detail, patients with aplastic anemia experienced a relatively high incidence of graft failure due to transfusion-related allosensitization causing rejection before intensification of the conditioning regimen with improved host-immunosuppression ameliorated this problem (Storb, 1989). The type of the underlying disease may also determine whether patients have been exposed to multiple cycles of potentially immunosuppressive chemotherapy prior to HSCT, or whether their disease has required no or only minimal prior therapy. In HLA-matched nonmyeloablative HSCT from unrelated donors, for example, patients with chronic myelogenous leukemia (CML) and myelodysplasia (MDS) experienced greater rejection rates compared to patients with other hematologic malignancies (Maris et al., 2001). These findings can be interpreted to suggest mechanisms such as allosensitization due to increased pretransplant transfusion requirements in the MDS group, and minimal host-immunosuppression due to usually minimal pretransplant chemotherapy in chronic phase CML patients. Alternatively it needs to be considered that in nonmyeloablative HSCT for CML and MDS, macrophages belonging to the malignant clone remain vital components of the recipient's hematopoietic microenvironment even after transplant (Bhatia et al., 1995). Therefore, it is conceivable that a functionally deficient host marrow microenvironment may not provide the optimal array of signals required for successful engraftment of donor HSC in this population.

HLA disparity

Because HLA-matched related or unrelated HSC donors are frequently not available, indications for HSCT have been broadened to include donor-recipient combinations that are not genetically matched for HLA. However, an unequivocal correlation between donor-recipient HLA disparities and increasing risks of graft failure have been demonstrated in early studies (Anasetti et al., 1989; Ash et al., 1990). As high-resolution HLA-matching techniques based on DNA sequencing became available and it has been shown that multiple HLA class I allele mismatches, or one antigen mismatches significantly increased the risk of graft failure (Petersdorf et al., 2001). In contrast, a correlation between HLA class II allele mismatches (HLA-DR, DQ, and DP) and graft failure could not be detected (Petersdorf et al., 2001).

In many graft failure cases studied, residual host lymphocytes could be detected suggesting host-mediated graft rejection was responsible for marrow failure. In some cases, however, the presence of antidonor antibodies in patient serum was associated with graft failure, suggesting the antibody-dependent destruction of donor cells (Barge et al., 1989). A substantial number of studies have shown that graft rejection after HLA-identical marrow transplantation can be mediated by multiple cytotoxic T-lymphocyte clones that specifically recognize minor histocompatibility peptides that differ between donor and recipient (Marijt et al., 1995). In addition, evidence that natural killer (NK) cells may be involved in graft rejection is based on experience from severe combined immunodeficiency (SCID) patients, who are lacking T-cell function but have retained NK function and are able to reject HLA-mismatched HSC grafts (Fischer et al., 1986).

However, not all graft failures in recipients of HLA-mismatched marrow were associated with donor-directed immune reactions. In some cases graft failure was associated with GVHD. Peralvo et al. (1987) summarized a retrospective analysis of 171 recipients of HLA-matched bone marrow transplantations, in which 14% of the patients experienced late graft failure with leukopenia and thrombocytopenia occurring more than 2 months after transplantation. Multivariate analysis showed that acute GVHD ($\geq$ grade II) was a major risk factor for developing late graft failure in this study.

These observations were interpreted by several investigators to suggest that donor lymphocytes involved in GVH reactions may adversely affect the host components in the microenvironment. This hypothesis was supported by the observation that alloactivated blood mononuclear cells could lyse stromal cells in vitro (Torok-Storb, 1990). Given these observations it is reasonable to hypothesize that in some instances of donor-recipient HLA-disparity, the host stromal cells become targets of GVH reactions. If completely destroyed, graft failure ensues because the supportive microenvironment does not exist. Given that donor stromal cells are not readily transplantable and not replaced by donor-derived marrow stem cells, as evidenced by studies in long-term survivors of transplantation (Awaya et al., 2002), it is unlikely that a patient with GVH-mediated stromal destruction can be rescued.

Stromal cell damage

Hematopoietic reconstitution following allogeneic bone marrow transplantationation requires donor-derived stem cells to come under the influence of the microenvironment that consists of host stromal cells and donor accessory cells. Stromal cells provide an important matrix for hematopoietic cellular communication through either direct cell-cell contact or through elaboration of hematopoietic growth factors presented in the context of an extracellular matrix. As mentioned above, stromal cells are not readily transplantable, therefore, it is imperative that they remain functional to provide the appropriate milieu for the incoming marrow. Since various forms of chemotherapy, conditioning therapy, and GVHD have been associated with injury to the hemopoietic microenvironment (discussed above), it is reasonable to assume that some combinations of therapy may compromise the resident microenvironment. It is also reasonable to assume that infectious agents, such as cytomegalovirus (CMV), that target the marrow stroma may contribute to marrow failure.

Infection

Even in non-immunocompromised hosts, certain bacterial, fungal, protozoal, and viral infections have all been associated with suppression of hematopoiesis. Historically, CMV has been the most common cause of death in HSCT recipients; but with the advent of antiviral agents, such as ganciclovir, the incidence of fatal CMV disease has substantially decreased. Nevertheless, CMV still causes significant morbidity and mortality in the population.

In vitro studies revealed that maturation and growth of hematopoietic progenitor cells generated in CMV-infected marrow cultures were decreased (Apperley et al., 1989; Simmons et al., 1990) and that certain CMV clinical isolates appeared to preferentially affect stromal rather than hematopoietic cells (Simmons et al., 1990). In addition, the presence of CMV-associated antigens in stromal cells correlated with decreased production of cytokine mRNA (Simmons et al., 1990). These data suggest that CMV may affect hematopoietic cells directly or indirectly by disturbing marrow stromal function. Furthermore, CMV infection may cause myelosuppression by triggering immune reactions in which the release of IL-2 stimulates the production of lymphokine-activated killer (LAK) cells which are able to lyse CMV-infected marrow fibroblasts in an MHC-unrestricted fashion (Duncombe et al., 1991).

More recently, death attributed to infectious complications of myelosuppression in CMV-infected patients was found to be associated with specific CMV strains distinguishable by genetic differences in envelope glycoproteins. This observation may explain in part why only a subset of patients with CMV infections experience poor marrow function (Torok-Storb et al., 1997). In addition to the direct infection-mediated disturbances of the marrow microenvironment, which may result in poor graft function, certain drugs used to treat infections, such as ganciclovir used in the setting of CMV reactivation and disease, are known to cause myelosuppression (Goodrich et al., 1991).

The potential of CMV-mediated marrow failure in non-myeloablative HSCT recipients is unknown. One matched-pair control study showed that among cases at high risk for CMV reactivation (seropositive recipients), CMV-reactivation and the onset of CMV disease were significantly delayed compared to myeloablative HSCT recipients (Junghanss et al., 2002). Nevertheless, the overall 1-year incidence of CMV disease was similar to myeloablative HSCT recipients, suggesting the possibility of late CMV-mediated marrow failure after nonmyeloablative HSCT. Further investigations are warranted on CMV-mediated marrow failure in nonmyeloablative HSCT patients.

References

Anasetti, C., Amos, D., Beatty, P.G. et al. (1989). Effect of HLA compatibility on engraftment of bone marrow transplantations in patients with leukemia or lymphoma. New England Journal of Medicine, 320(4), 197–204.

Antin, J.H., Childs, R., Filipovich, A.H. et al. (2001). Establishment of complete and mixed donor chimerism after allogeneic lymphohematopoietic transplantation: recommendations from a workshop at the 2001 Tandem Meetings of the International Bone Marrow Transplantation Registry and the American Society of Blood and Marrow Transplantation. Biology of Blood and Marrow Transplantation, 7(9), 473–85.

Apperley, J.F., Dowding, C., Hibbin, J. et al. (1989). The effect of cytomegalovirus on hemopoiesis: in vitro evidence for selective infection of marrow stromal cells. Experimental Hematology, 17(1), 38–45.

Ash, R.C., Casper, J.T., Chitambar, C.R. et al. (1990). Successful allogeneic transplantation of T-cell-depleted bone marrow from closely HLA-matched unrelated donors. New England Journal of Medicine, 322(8), 485–94.

Asosingh, K., Renmans, W., Van der Gucht, K. et al. (1998). Circulating CD34+ cells in cord blood and mobilized blood have a different profile of adhesion molecules than bone marrow CD34+ cells. European Journal of Haematology, 60(3), 153–60.

Awaya, N., Rupert, K., Bryant, E., Torok-Storb, B. (2002). Failure of adult marrow-derived stem cells to generate marrow stroma after successful hematopoietic stem cell transplantation. Experimental Hematology, 30, 937–42.

Banfi, A., Bianchi, G., Galotto, M. et al. (2001). Bone marrow stromal damage after chemo/radiotherapy: occurrence, consequences and possibilities of treatment. Leukemia and Lymphoma, 42(5), 863–70.

Barge, A.J., Johnson, G., Witherspoon, R. et al. (1989). Antibody-mediated marrow failure after allogeneic bone marrow transplantationation. Blood, 74(5), 1477–80.

Barker, J.N., Davies, S.M., DeFor, T. et al. (2001). Survival after transplantation of unrelated donor umbilical cord blood is comparable to that of human leukocyte antigen-matched unrelated donor bone marrow: results of a matched-pair analysis. Blood, 97(10), 2957–61.

Barker, J.N., Wagner, J.E. (2002). Umbilical cord blood transplantation: current state of the art. Current Opinion in Oncology, 14(2), 160–4.

Barnett, M.J., Eaves, C.J., Phillips, G.L. et al. (1994). Autografting with cultured marrow in chronic myeloid leukemia: results of a pilot study. Blood, 84(3), 724–32.

Bensinger, W., Appelbaum, F., Rowley, S. et al. (1995). Factors that influence collection and engraftment of autologous peripheral-blood stem cells. Journal of Clinical Oncology, 13(10), 2547–55.

Bensinger, W.I., Martin, P.J., Storer, B. et al. (2001). Transplantation of bone marrow as compared with peripheral-blood cells from HLA-identical relatives in patients with hematologic cancers. New England Journal of Medicine, 344(3), 175–81.

Bhatia, R., McGlave, P.B., Dewald, G.W. et al. (1995). Abnormal function of the bone marrow microenvironment in chronic myelogenous leukemia: role of malignant stromal macrophages. Blood, 85(12), 3636–45.

Bunjes, D., Wiesneth, M., Hertenstein, B. *et al.* (1990). Graft failure after T cell-depleted bone marrow transplantationation: clinical and immunological characteristics and response to immunosuppressive therapy. *Bone Marrow Transplantation,* **6**(5), 309–14.

Crescenzi, B., Fizzotti, M., Piattoni, S. *et al.* (2000). Interphase FISH for Y chromosome, VNTR polymorphisms, and RT-PCR for BCR-ABL in the monitoring of HLA-matched and mismatched transplants. *Cancer Genetics and Cytogenetics,* **120**(1), 25–9.

de Pauw, E.S., Otto, S.A., Wijnen, J.T. *et al.* (2002). Long-term follow-up of recipients of allogeneic bone marrow grafts reveals no progressive telomere shortening and provides no evidence for haematopoietic stem cell exhaustion. *British Journal of Haematology,* **116**(2), 491–6.

Drygalski, A., Xu, G., Constantinescu, D. *et al.* (2000). The frequency and proliferative potential of megakaryocytic colony-forming cells (Meg-CFC) in cord blood, cytokine-mobilized peripheral blood and bone marrow, and their correlation with total CFC numbers: implications for the quantitation of Meg-CFC to predict platelet engraftment following cord blood transplantation. *Bone Marrow Transplantation,* **25**(10), 1029–34.

Duncombe, A.S., Grundy, J.E., Prentice, H.G. *et al.* (1991). IL2 activated killer cells may contribute to cytomegalovirus induced marrow hypoplasia after bone marrow transplantationation. *Bone Marrow Transplantation,* **7**(2), 81–7.

Fischer, A., Griscelli, C., Friedrich, W. *et al.* (1986). Bone-marrow transplantation for immunodeficiencies and osteopetrosis: European survey, 1968–1985. *Lancet,* **2**(8515), 1080–4.

Galotto, M., Berisso, G., Delfino, L. *et al.* (1999). Stromal damage as consequence of high-dose chemo/radiotherapy in bone marrow transplantation recipients. *Experimental Hematology,* **27**(9), 1460–6.

Gibson, L.F., Fortney, J., Landreth, K.S. *et al.* (1997). Disruption of bone marrow stromal cell function by etoposide. *Biology of Blood and Marrow Transplantation,* **3**(3), 122–32.

Glimm, H., Oh, I.H., & Eaves, C.J. (2000). Human hematopoietic stem cells stimulated to proliferate in vitro lose engraftment potential during their S/G(2)/M transit and do not reenter G(0). *Blood,* **96**(13), 4185–93.

Goodrich, J.M., Mori, M., Gleaves, C.A. *et al.* (1991). Early treatment with ganciclovir to prevent cytomegalovirus disease after allogeneic bone marrow transplantationation. *New England Journal of Medicine,* **325**(23), 1601–7.

Gorin, N.C. (2002). Autologous stem cell transplantation for adult acute leukemia. *Current Opinion in Oncology,* **14**(2), 152–9.

Gorin, N.C., Aegerter, P., Auvert, B. *et al.* (1990). Autologous bone marrow transplantationation for acute myelocytic leukemia in first remission: a European survey of the role of marrow purging. *Blood,* **75**(8), 1606–14.

Greenberger, J.S. (1991). Toxic effects on the hematopoietic microenvironment. *Experimental Hematology,* **19**(11), 1101–9.

Holyoake, T.L., Alcorn, M.J., Richmond, L. *et al.* (1997). CD34 positive PBPC expanded ex vivo may not provide durable engraftment following myeloablative chemoradiotherapy regimens. *Bone Marrow Transplantation,* **19**(11), 1095–101.

Junghanss, C., Boeckh, M., Carter, R.A. *et al.* (2002). Incidence and outcome of cytomegalovirus infections following nonmyeloabla-

tive compared with myeloablative allogeneic stem cell transplantation, a matched control study. *Blood,* **99**(6), 1978–85.

Kanamaru, S., Kawano, Y., Watanabe, T. *et al.* (2000). Low numbers of megakaryocyte progenitors in grafts of cord blood cells may result in delayed platelet recovery after cord blood cell transplant. *Stem Cells,* **18**(3), 190–5.

Kobari, L., Pflumio, F., Giarratana, M. *et al.* (2000). In vitro and in vivo evidence for the long-term multilineage (myeloid, B, NK, and T) reconstitution capacity of ex vivo expanded human CD34(+) cord blood cells. *Experimental Hematology,* **28**(12), 1470–80.

Koc, O.N., Peters, C., Aubourg, P. *et al.* (1999). Bone marrow-derived mesenchymal stem cells remain host-derived despite successful hematopoietic engraftment after allogeneic transplantation in patients with lysosomal and peroxisomal storage diseases. *Experimental Hematology,* **27**(11), 1675–81.

Laughlin, M.J., Barker, J., Bambach, B. *et al.* (2001). Hematopoietic engraftment and survival in adult recipients of umbilical-cord blood from unrelated donors. *New England Journal of Medicine,* **344**(24), 1815–22.

Leclair, B., Fregeau, C.J., Aye, M.T. *et al.* (1995). DNA typing for bone marrow engraftment follow-up after allogeneic transplant: a comparative study of current technologies. *Bone Marrow Transplantation,* **16**(1), 43–55.

Marijt, W.A., Kernan, N.A., Diaz-Barrientos, T. *et al.* (1995). Multiple minor histocompatibility antigen-specific cytotoxic T lymphocyte clones can be generated during graft rejection after HLA-identical bone marrow transplantationation. *Bone Marrow Transplantation,* **16**(1), 125–32.

Maris, M., Niederwieser, D., Sandmaier, B.M. *et al.* (2001). Nonmyeloablative hematopoietic stem cell transplantation (HSCT) using 10/10 HLA antigen matched unrelated donors (URDs) for patients with advanced hematologic malignancies ineligible for conventional HSCT. *Blood,* **98**(11), 858a (abstract #3563).

Martin, P.J. (1990). The role of donor lymphoid cells in allogeneic marrow engraftment. *Bone Marrow Transplantation,* **6**(5), 283–9.

Martin, P.J. (1996). Prevention of allogeneic marrow graft rejection by donor T cells that do not recognize recipient alloantigens: potential role of a veto mechanism. *Blood,* **88**(3), 962–9.

Martin, P.J., Hansen, J.A., Buckner, C.D. *et al.* (1985). Effects of in vitro depletion of T cells in HLA-identical allogeneic marrow grafts. *Blood,* **66**(3), 664–72.

Martin, P.J., Hansen, J.A., Torok-Storb, B. *et al.* (1988). Graft failure in patients receiving T cell-depleted HLA-identical allogeneic marrow transplants. *Bone Marrow Transplantation,* **3**(5), 445–56.

Mathioudakis, G., Storb, R., McSweeney, P.A. *et al.* (2000). Polyclonal hematopoiesis with variable telomere shortening in human long-term allogeneic marrow graft recipients. *Blood,* **96**(12), 3991–4.

Mauch, P., Ferrara, J., & Hellman, S. (1989). Stem cell self-renewal considerations in bone marrow transplantationation. *Bone Marrow Transplantation,* **4**(6), 601–7.

McGlave, P.B., Arthur, D., Miller, W.J. *et al.* (1990). Autologous transplantation for CML using marrow treated ex vivo with recombinant human interferon gamma. *Bone Marrow Transplantation,* **6**(2), 115–20.

McNiece, I., Jones, R., Bearman, S.I. *et al.* (2000). Ex vivo expanded peripheral blood progenitor cells provide rapid neutrophil recovery after high-dose chemotherapy in patients with breast cancer. *Blood,* **96**(9), 3001–7.

McSweeney, P.A., Niederwieser, D., Shizuru, J.A. *et al.* (2001). Hematopoietic cell transplantation in older patients with hematologic malignancies: replacing high-dose cytotoxic therapy with graft-versus-tumor effects. *Blood,* **97**(11), 3390–400.

Mielcarek, M., Graf, L., Johnson, G. *et al.* (1998). Production of interleukin-10 by granulocyte colony-stimulating factor-mobilized blood products: a mechanism for monocyte-mediated suppression of T-cell proliferation. *Blood,* **92**(1), 215–22.

Mielcarek, M., Martin, P.J., & Torok-Storb, B. (1997a). Suppression of alloantigen-induced T-cell proliferation by CD14+ cells derived from granulocyte colony-stimulating factor-mobilized peripheral blood mononuclear cells. *Blood,* **89**(5), 1629–34.

Mielcarek, M., Reems, J., & Torok-Storb, B. (1997b). Extrinsic control of stem cell fate: practical considerations. *Stem Cells,* **15** Suppl 1, 229–32; discussion 233–6.

Mielcarek, M., Roecklein, B.A., & Torok-Storb, B. (1996). CD14+ cells in granulocyte colony-stimulating factor (G-CSF)-mobilized peripheral blood mononuclear cells induce secretion of interleukin-6 and G-CSF by marrow stroma. *Blood,* **87**(2), 574–80.

Mielcarek, M., Sandmaier, B., Maloney, D.G. *et al.* (2002). Nonmyeloablative hematopoietic cell transplantation: status quo and future perspectives. *Journal of Clinical Immunology,* **22**(2), 70–74.

Mielcarek, M. & Torok-Storb, B. (1997). Phenotype and engraftment potential of cytokine-mobilized peripheral blood mononuclear cells. *Current Opinion in Hematology,* **4**(3), 176–82.

Mohle, R., Bautz, F., Denzlinger, C. *et al.* (2001). Transendothelial migration of hematopoietic progenitor cells. Role of chemotactic factors. *Annals of the New York Academy of Science,* **938**, 26–34; discussion 34–5.

Nemunaitis, J., Singer, J.W., Buckner, C.D. *et al.* (1990). Use of recombinant human granulocyte-macrophage colony-stimulating factor in graft failure after bone marrow transplantation. *Blood,* **76**(1), 245–53.

Pan, L., Delmonte, J., Jr., Jalonen, C.K. *et al.* (1995). Pretreatment of donor mice with granulocyte colony-stimulating factor polarizes donor T lymphocytes toward type-2 cytokine production and reduces severity of experimental graft-versus-host disease. *Blood,* **86**(12), 4422–9.

Papayannopoulou, T. & Craddock, C. (1997). Homing and trafficking of hemopoietic progenitor cells. *Acta Haematologica,* **97**(1–2), 97–104.

Paquette, R.L., Dergham, S.T., Karpf, E. *et al.* (2000). Ex vivo expanded unselected peripheral blood: progenitor cells reduce posttransplantation neutropenia, thrombocytopenia, and anemia in patients with breast cancer. *Blood,* **96**(7), 2385–90.

Peralvo, J., Bacigalupo, A., Pittaluga, P.A. *et al.* (1987). Poor graft function associated with graft-versus-host disease after allogeneic marrow transplantation. *Bone Marrow Transplantation,* **2**(3), 279–85.

Petersdorf, E.W., Hansen, J.A., Martin, P.J. *et al.* (2001). Major-histocompatibility-complex class I alleles and antigens in hematopoietic-cell transplantation. *New England Journal of Medicine,* **345**(25), 1794–800.

Petersdorf, E.W., Kollman, C., Hurley, C.K. *et al.* (2001). Effect of HLA class II gene disparity on clinical outcome in unrelated donor hematopoietic cell transplantation for chronic myeloid leukemia: the US National Marrow Donor Program Experience. *Blood,* **98**(10), 2922–9.

Piacibello, W., Sanavio, F., Severino, A. *et al.* (1999). Engraftment in nonobese diabetic severe combined immunodeficient mice of human CD34(+) cord blood cells after ex vivo expansion: evidence for the amplification and self-renewal of repopulating stem cells. *Blood,* **93**(11), 3736–49.

Reems, J.A., Mielcarek, M., & Torok-Storb, B. (1997). Differential modulation of adhesion markers with ex vivo expansion of human umbilical CD34+ progenitor cells. *Biology of Blood and Marrow Transplantation,* **3**(3), 133–41.

Reiffers, J., Cailliot, C., Dazey, B. *et al.* (1999). Abrogation of postmyeloablative chemotherapy neutropenia by ex-vivo expanded autologous CD34-positive cells. *Lancet,* **354**(9184), 1092–3.

Roberts, A.W. & Metcalf, D. (1995). Noncycling state of peripheral blood progenitor cells mobilized by granulocyte colony-stimulating factor and other cytokines. *Blood,* **86**(4), 1600–5.

Rocha, V., Wagner, J.E., Jr., Sobocinski, K.A. *et al.* (2000). Graft-versus-host disease in children who have received a cord-blood or bone marrow transplantation from an HLA-identical sibling. Eurocord and International Bone Marrow Transplant Registry Working Committee on Alternative Donor and Stem Cell Sources. *New England Journal of Medicine,* **342**(25), 1846–54.

Rothberg, P.G., Gamis, A.S., & Baker, D. (1997). Use of DNA polymorphisms to monitor engraftment after allogeneic bone marrow transplantationation. *Clinical and Laboratory Medicine,* **17**(1), 109–18.

Rubinstein, P., Carrier, C., Scaradavou, A. *et al.* (1998). Outcomes among 562 recipients of placental-blood transplants from unrelated donors. *New England Journal of Medicine,* **339**(22), 1565–77.

Schwartz, G.N., Kammula, U., Warren, M.K. *et al.* (2000). Thrombopoietin and chemokine mRNA expression in patient post-chemotherapy and in vitro cytokine-treated marrow stromal cell layers. *Stem Cells,* **18**(5), 331–42.

Simmons, P., Kaushansky, K., & Torok-Storb, B. (1990). Mechanisms of cytomegalovirus-mediated myelosuppression: perturbation of stromal cell function versus direct infection of myeloid cells. *Proceedings of the National Academy of Science USA,* **87**(4), 1386–90.

Simmons, P.J., Przepiorka, D., Thomas, E.D. *et al.* (1987). Host origin of marrow stromal cells following allogeneic bone marrow transplantationation. *Nature,* **328**(6129), 429–32.

Singhal, S., Powles, R., Kulkarni, S. *et al.* (2000). Comparison of marrow and blood cell yields from the same donors in a double-blind, randomized study of allogeneic marrow vs blood stem cell transplantation. *Bone Marrow Transplantation,* **25**(5), 501–5.

Sorg, R.V., Andres, S., Kogler, G. *et al.* (2001). Phenotypic and functional comparison of monocytes from cord blood and granulocyte colony-stimulating factor-mobilized apheresis products. *Experimental Hematology,* **29**(11), 1289–94.

Storb, R. (1989). Graft rejection and graft-versus-host disease in marrow transplantation. *Transplantation Proceedings,* **21**(1 Pt 3), 2915–8.

Storb, R., Etzioni, R., Anasetti, C. *et al.* (1994). Cyclophosphamide combined with antithymocyte globulin in preparation for allogeneic marrow transplants in patients with aplastic anemia. *Blood,* **84**(3), 941–9.

Storb, R., Yu, C., Barnett, T. *et al.* (1999a). Stable mixed hematopoietic chimerism in dog leukocyte antigen-identical littermate dogs given lymph node irradiation before and pharmacologic immunosuppression after marrow transplantation. *Blood,* **94**(3), 1131–6.

Storb, R., Yu, C., Sandmaier, B.M. *et al.* (1999b). Mixed hematopoietic chimerism after marrow allografts. Transplantation in the ambulatory care setting. *Annals of the New York Academy of Science,* **872**, 372–5; discussion 375–6.

Storb, R.F., Champlin, R., Riddell, S.R. *et al.* (2001). Non-myeloablative transplants for malignant disease. *Hematology (Am Soc Hematol Educ Program),* 375–91.

Thornley, I., Sutherland, R., Wynn, R. *et al.* (2002). Early hematopoietic reconstitution after clinical stem cell transplantation: evidence for stochastic stem cell behavior and limited acceleration in telomere loss. *Blood,* **99**(7), 2387–96.

Torok-Storb, B., Boeckh, M., Hoy, C. *et al.* (1997). Association of specific cytomegalovirus genotypes with death from myelosuppression after marrow transplantation. *Blood,* **90**(5), 2097–102.

Torok-Storb, B., Simmons, P., Barge, A. (1990). Mechanisms of marrow graft failure. *Molecular Biology of Haematopoiesis.* L. Sachs, Abraham, N.G., Wiedermann, C.J., Levine, A.S., Konwalinka, G. Andover, Hampshire, Intercept, 589–596.

Urbano-Ispizua, A., Rozman, C., Pimentel, P. *et al.* (2001). The number of donor CD3+ cells is the most important factor for graft failure after allogeneic transplantation of CD34+ selected cells from peripheral blood from HLA-identical siblings. *Blood,* **97**, 383–7.

Vallera, D.A. & Blazar, B.R. (1989). T cell depletion for graft-versus-host-disease prophylaxis. A perspective on engraftment in mice and humans. *Transplantation,* **47**(5), 751–60.

van Dekken, H., Hagenbeek, A., & Bauman, J.G. (1989). Detection of host cells following sex-mismatched bone marrow transplantation by fluorescent in situ hybridization with a Y-chromosome specific probe. *Leukemia,* **3**(10), 724–8.

Voltarelli, J.C., Przepiorka, D., Shankar, P. *et al.* (1989). CD8+/DR+/CD25—T-lymphocytes associated with marrow graft failure. *Bone Marrow Transplantation,* **4**(6), 647–52.

Wagner, J.E., Kernan, N.A., Steinbuch, M. *et al.* (1995). Allogeneic sibling umbilical-cord-blood transplantation in children with malignant and non-malignant disease. *Lancet,* **346**(8969), 214–9.

Wagner, J.E. & Kurtzberg, J. (1997). Cord blood stem cells. *Current Opinion in Hematology,* **4**(6), 413–8.

Walters, M.C., Patience, M., Leisenring, W. *et al.* (1996). Bone marrow transplantationation for sickle cell disease. *New England Journal of Medicine,* **335**(6), 369–76.

Weaver, C.H., Hazelton, B., Birch, R. *et al.* (1995). An analysis of engraftment kinetics as a function of the CD34 content of peripheral blood progenitor cell collections in 692 patients after the administration of myeloablative chemotherapy. *Blood,* **86**(10), 3961–9.

Yonemura, Y., Ku, H., Hirayama, F. *et al.* (1996). Interleukin 3 or interleukin 1 abrogates the reconstituting ability of hematopoietic stem cells. *Proceedings of the National Academy of Science U S A,* **93**(9), 4040–4.

Yong, K.L., Watts, M., Shaun Thomas, N. *et al.* (1998). Transmigration of CD34+ cells across specialized and nonspecialized endothelium requires prior activation by growth factors and is mediated by PECAM-1 (CD31). *Blood,* **91**(4), 1196–205.

Zaucha, J.M., Gooley, T., Bensinger, W.I. *et al.* (2001a). CD34 cell dose in granulocyte colony-stimulating factor-mobilized peripheral blood mononuclear cell grafts affects engraftment kinetics and development of extensive chronic graft-versus-host disease after human leukocyte antigen-identical sibling transplantation. *Blood,* **98**(12), 3221–7.

Zaucha, J.M., Zellmer, E., Georges, G. *et al.* (2001b). G-CSF-mobilized peripheral blood mononuclear cells added to marrow facilitates engraftment in nonmyeloablated canine recipients, CD3 cells are required. *Biology of Blood and Marrow Transplantation,* **7**(11), 613–9.

13 Hematopoietic reconstitution after hematopoietic stem cell transplantation

JAN J. CORNELISSEN

University Hospital Rotterdam, Daniel den Hoed Cancer Center, Rotterdam, The Netherlands

Introduction

The main objective of chemoradiotherapy given immediately pretransplant to prepare recipients for allogeneic hematopoietic stem cell (HSC) transplantation is to eradicate or inhibit the recipient's immune system so that the incoming donor graft will be accepted. In addition, eradication of the recipient's diseased marrow is also a major goal of high-dose chemoradiotherapy in myeloablative allo-SCT. Alternatively, non-myeloablative approaches have been developed with the aim of reducing toxicity and establishing a platform for immunotherapy (Maris & Storb, 2002). Those approaches depend largely on the graft-versus-leukemia (GVL) effect to eradicate the underlying disease. Provision of "space" in the recipients' marrow cavity by high-dose chemoradiotherapy has long been considered a prerequisite for allogeneic stem cell transplantation. However, the high percentage of engraftment following non-myeloablative allo-SCT in CML demonstrates that donor stem cells may easily engraft even in an environment packed with recipient hematopoiesis.

The pluripotent hematopoietic stem cells present in the infused donor marrow give rise in the recipient to both a new hematopoietic system and a new immune system. The first detectable sign of proliferation of the pluripotent hematopoietic stem cells that occupy the marrow cavity (and possibly sites of extramedullary hematopoiesis as well) is a rise in the recipient's peripheral blood leukocyte count; within several days most of these white cells are neutrophils. The newly derived neutrophils, as well as platelets and erythrocytes, are able to carry out their most important respective functions as soon as they are generated. Such acquisition of full normal function, however, does not apply to T and B lymphocytes, some of whose functional activity is depressed long-term posttransplant.

There are three main reasons for this delay in acquisition of lymphocyte function; first, it simply takes time for full functional development of lymphocytes to take place. These cells are undergoing ontogeny in a relatively adult, (often) allogeneic environment where, not only may there be minor or major histocompatibility differences between donor and recipient, but the amount of thymic epithelial tissue available for T-lymphocyte education is markedly reduced compared with the situation obtaining during fetal lymphocyte development (Broers *et al.,* 2002). A second reason for the suppression of lymphocyte function is the administration of immune suppressive drugs to the recipient posttransplant with the primary aim of minimizing the severity of graft-versus-host disease (GVHD). Cyclosporine, prednisone, and antithymocyte globulin are all inhibitory or destructive of lymphocytes, and methotrexate will adversely affect any cell in the DNA synthesis phase of the cell cycle. Third, GVHD selects the lymphoid system (besides the skin, liver, and gut) as a target organ. Lymphoid hypocellularity and atrophy are characteristic histologic hallmarks of moderate or severe GVHD. Thus, GVHD per se is immune suppressive.

These deficits of the hematopoietic and immune systems are responsible for the marked susceptibility of marrow transplant recipients to infection (Atkinson *et al.,* 1979; Winston *et al.,* 1979; Atkinson *et al.,* 1980; Meyers & Atkinson, 1983, Storek *et al.,* 2001; Broers *et al.,* 2002). During periods of neutropenia, bacterial (and to a lesser extent fungal) infections are common. Defects of T-cell function contribute to susceptibility to viral infection particularly with cytomegalovirus (CMV) (Meyers *et al.,* 1982; Gratama & Cornelissen, 2001), herpes simplex, and varicella zoster (Atkinson *et al.,* 1980; Locksley *et al.,* 1985).

Reconstruction of the hematopoietic and immune systems should be considered together since hematopoietic stem cells give rise to all the circulating cells of both systems; additionally, lymphocytes are an integral part of both systems, and T cells are intimately involved in hematopoiesis (Nathan *et al.,* 1978). For clarity, however, the kinetics of ontogeny and the defects in the two systems will be described separately. Hematopoietic reconstruction is described below. Reconstruction of the immune system posttransplant is described in Chapter 14.

The hematopoietic system

The mature cells of the hematopoietic system comprise erythrocytes, neutrophils, eosinophils, basophils, lymphocytes, monocytes, and platelets. Through the use of semisolid agar systems a

Table 13.1. *Hematopoietic regulatory proteins*

Colony-stimulating factors (CSFs)
  G-CSF
  GM-CSF
  M-CSF
  IL-3
  Erythropoietin (EPO)
  Thrombopoietin (TPO)
  IL-5
Stem cell factors
  kit ligand (stem cell factor)
  flk ligand
Synergistic factors
  Interleukin-1 (IL-1)
  Interleukin-6 (IL 6)
  Interleukin-7 (IL 7)
  Interleukin-9 (IL 9)
  Interleukin-10 (IL 10)
  Interleukin-11 (IL 11)
  Interleukin-12 (IL 12)
Leukemia inhibitory factor (LIF)
Inhibitors/bidirectional regulators
  Tumor necrosis factor α (TNF-α)
  Transforming growth factor β (TFG-β)
  Macrophage inhibitory protein 1α (MIP-1α)
  Gamma-interferon (IFN-γ)

lineage of progenitor cells has been identified for each of these end cells; consequent upon the development of these culture systems has been the discovery and characterization of soluble regulatory glycoproteins (Table 13.1) that control the proliferation, differentiation, and function of cells in the different lineages. An overview of the regulation of the hematopoietic system is shown in Fig. 13.1 (also see Chapter 3).

Disappearance of host (recipient) peripheral blood cells

With the initiation of the conditioning regimen pretransplant, a rapid decline in peripheral blood white cells of host (recipient) origin begins. The rate of decline depends to some extent on the preparatory regimen utilized. Regimens employing busulfan are associated with a slower rate of decline than those utilizing total body irradiation (Atkinson *et al.*, 1987b). Hematopoietic cells are extremely sensitive to damage by ionizing radiation: the 50% lethal dose (LD50) to human bone marrow is estimated to be 3 to 4Gy, and damage to hematopoietic stem cells after doses exceeding 8Gy is usually considered irreversible. The sensitivity is further underscored by the strong immunosuppressive effect of the conditioning regimen developed by Storb *et al.*,

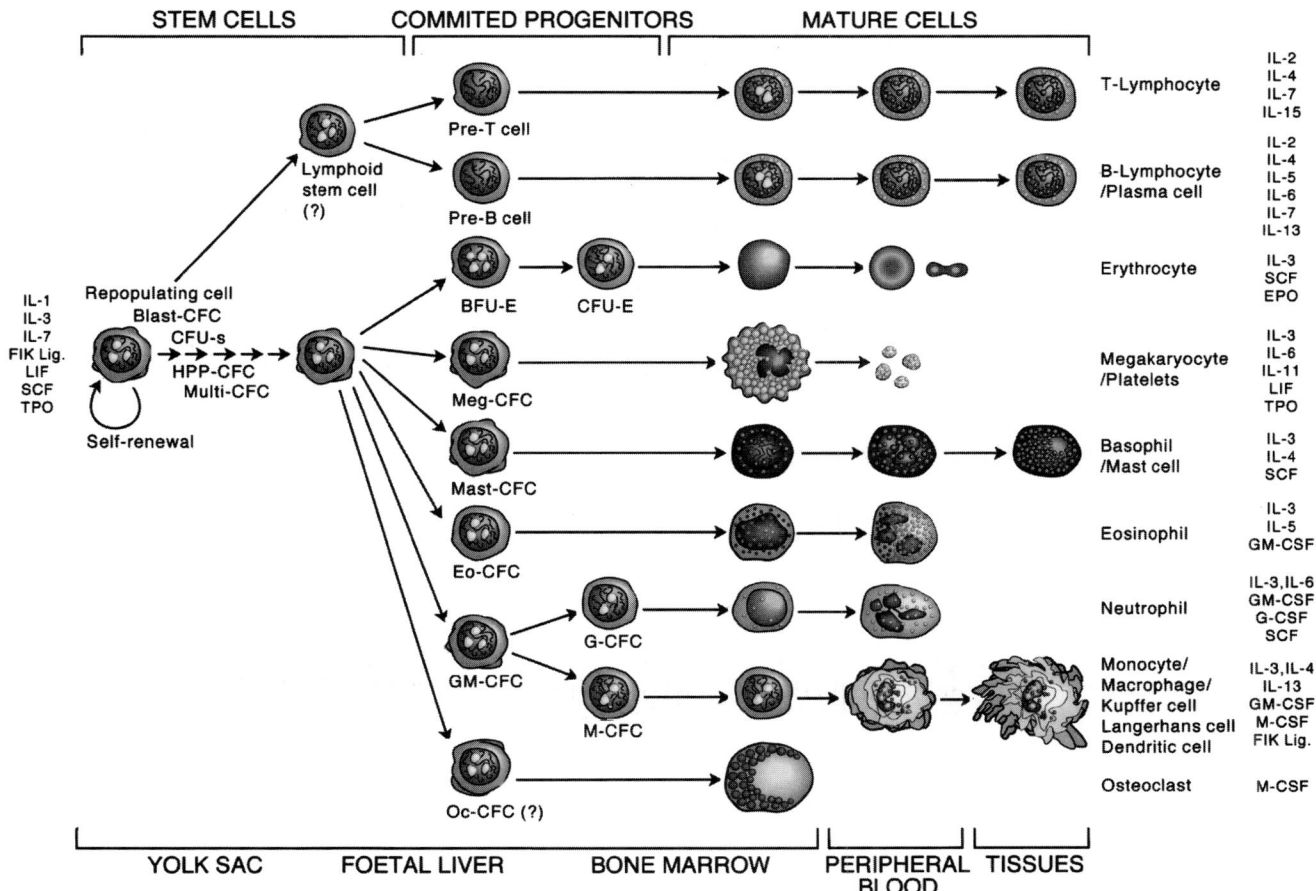

Fig. 13.1. The human hematopoietic system and its control by regulatory glycoproteins: stimulation of proliferation, differentiation, and function are included.

who showed that dosages of 2 × 2 Gy (combined with cyclosporine and mycofenolate mofetil [MMF] is sufficient for durable engraftment of DLA-identical stem cells in littermate dogs (Storb *et al.,* 1997; Storb *et al.,* 1999).

The duration of the nadir of the white blood cell count after completion of the conditioning regimen is dependent on both the rate of disappearance of host cells and the rate of appearance of mature cells newly generated from the infused stem cell inoculum. Neutrophils (and platelets) present in the stem cell inoculum normally have little impact on circulating cell numbers in the recipient, but when G-CSF-primed, HLA-identical sibling bone marrow was used, a marked increase in the circulating white blood count was seen on day 1 posttransplant (up to 40 × 10⁹/l and almost entirely all neutrophils) (Atkinson *et al.,* 1997) (Fig. 13.2). Mature lymphocytes present in the donor inoculum after allogeneic transplantation have been shown to contribute func-

tionally to recipient immunity posttransplant (Donnenberg *et al.,* 1984; Lum *et al.,* 1986; Wimperis *et al.,* 1986, Gratama *et al.,* 2001).

Reconstitution of peripheral blood cells

Leukocytes usually begin to reappear in the blood during the second or third week posttransplant. The rate of reappearance of leukocytes, neutrophils, lymphocytes, monocytes, platelets, and reticulocytes is shown in Fig. 13.3. The duration of severe neutropenia and the risk of transplant-related mortality (TRM) are correlated: a study of 2,276 recipients of allogeneic or autologous marrow grafts demonstrated consistently higher risks of mortality in patients with severe prolonged neutropenia (Offner *et al.,* 1996). Prolonged neutropenia after initial engraftment may be associated with several factors including GVHD, CMV

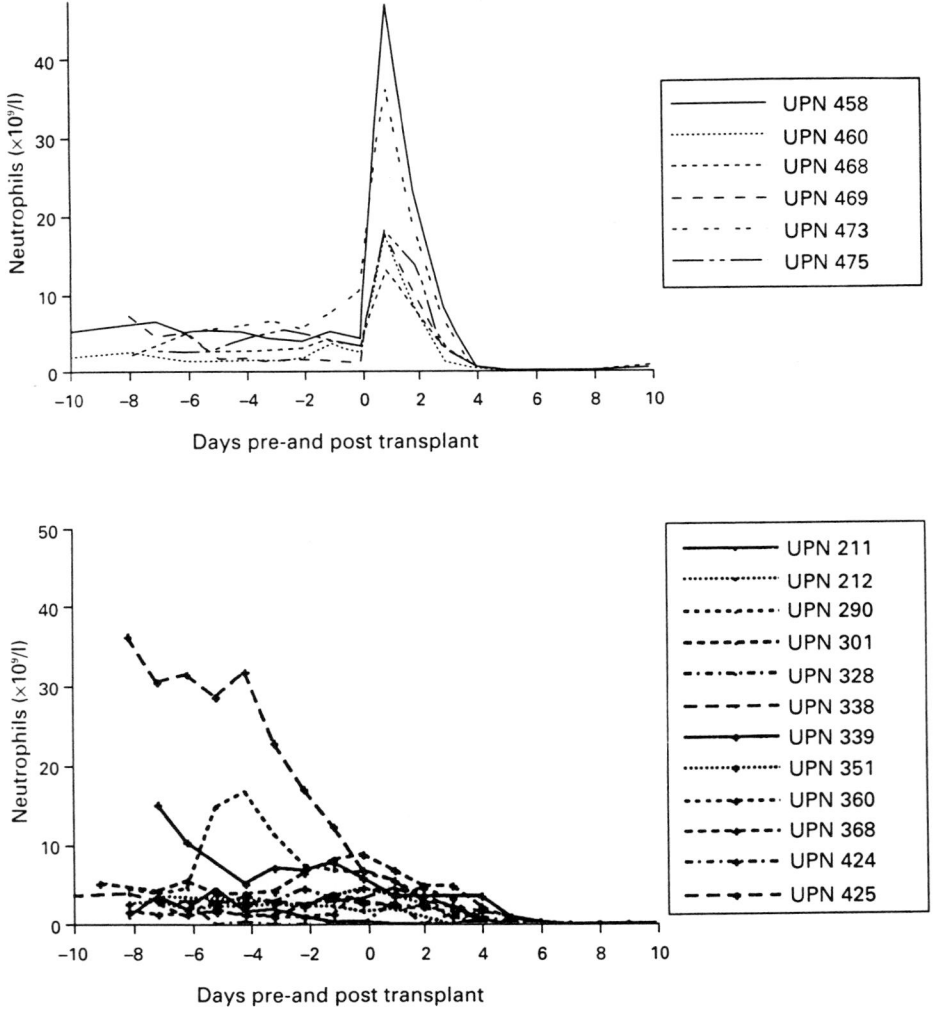

Fig. 13.2. *Top panel:* Peripheral blood neutrophil counts in 6 recipients of G-CSF primed, T-replete, HLA-identical sibling bone marrow after conditioning with busulfan and cyclophosphamide. *Bottom panel:* Peripheral blood neutrophil counts in 12 control patients given normal, T-replete, HLA-identical sibling bone marrow after conditioning with busulfan and cyclophosphamide. *Abbreviation:* UPN, unique patient number. Reproduced, with permission, from Atkinson *et al.* (1997).

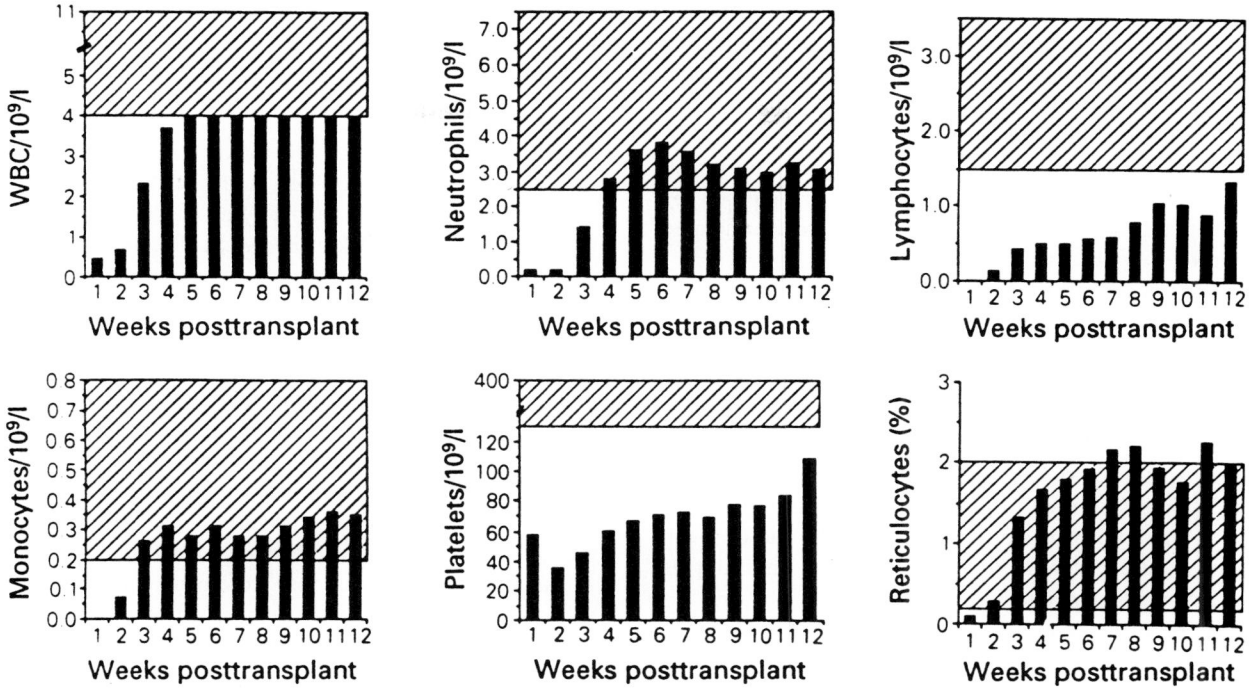

Fig. 13.3. Reconstitution of leukocytes, neutrophils, lymphocytes, monocytes, platelets, and reticulocytes after HLA-identical sibling marrow transplantation. The data are derived from 79 recipients of HLA-identical sibling marrow transplants for hematologic malignancy who were prepared with cyclophosphamide 120 mg/kg and fractionated total body irradiation 12–14 Gy and immune suppressed with cyclosporine. They received non-T-cell-depleted bone marrow. Reproduced, with permission, from Atkinson, *Bone Marrow Transplantation,* **5,** 209–26 (1990).

infection, myelosuppressive effects of medications such as cotrimoxazole and/or ganciclovir and autoimmune reactivity. Neutropenia posttransplant is sometimes related to the presence of antibodies reactive to neutrophils. In one prospective study, 16 of 36 evaluable marrow graft recipients (44%) showed detectable antineutrophil antibodies posttransplant. In patients with detectable antibodies in the posttransplant period, an absolute neutrophil count (ANC) of $0.5 \times 10^9/l$ was reached a median of 3.5 days later than in patients without such antibodies (Klumpp et al., 1996). Four of the 16 patients with detectable antibodies showed a subsequent fall in the ANC to $<0.5 \times 10^9/l$ for at least 2 consecutive days following initial engraftment. In contrast, none of 20 patients without detectable antineutrophil antibodies posttransplant developed postengraftment neutropenia. Multivariate analysis revealed that only the presence of such antibodies was independently predictive of postengraftment neutropenia. All four patients with antibody-associated postengraftment neutropenia responded to steroid-based treatment.

There is an increased amount of fetal hemoglobin circulating for up to 6 months posttransplant (Alter et al., 1976). Additionally, nucleated red cells are frequently seen in the blood film until 3 to 6 months posttransplant. Usually, erythroid engraftment as assessed by the appearance of immature reticulocytes precedes neutrophil engraftment. Torres et al. (2001) showed that immature reticulocytes may appear in the peripheral blood as early as 9 days after SCT.

Hematopoiesis is normally polyclonal after both allogeneic and autologous transplantation (Saunders et al., 1995a). Peripheral blood cell counts and marrow cellularity are usually sustained satisfactorily long term after both autologous (Nieboer et al., 2001) (Fig. 13.4) and allogeneic bone marrow

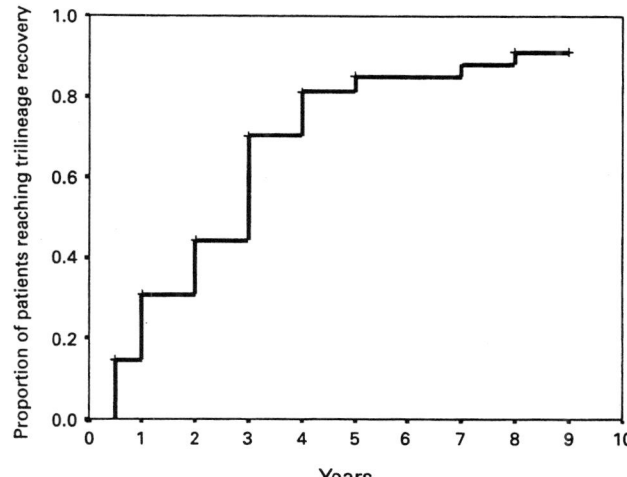

Fig. 13.4. Cumulative proportion of patients reaching trilineage recovery in 10 years following HDC and ABMT/PSCT. Reproduced, with permission, from Nieboer et al. (2001).

or blood stem cell transplantation. In Nieboer's study of patients with solid tumors given autologous bone marrow or blood stem cell transplants, 91% had normal white blood cell counts, 94% had normal hemoglobin values and 75% had normal platelet counts at 3 years posttransplant. Trilineage recovery in the blood was complete in 85% by 5 years posttransplant (Fig. 13.4). Marrow hematopoiesis as assessed by progenitor cell numbers, however, is considerably impaired (see below).

A number of factors affect the rate of reappearance of cells in the blood and, consequently, blood product transfusion requirements during the early posttransplant period. Almost all patients require both packed cells and platelet transfusions during the first month after myeloblative conditioning. A major factor influencing these requirements is one under the control of the transplant physician, namely the type of prophylactic immune suppression used to minimize GVHD. As seen from Fig. 13.5, engraftment is slower when methotrexate or T-cell depletion is used compared to cyclosporine, and this is reflected in transfusion requirements.

A decrease or delay in hematopoietic reconstitution can be caused by a number of the common complications that occur especially after allogeneic transplantation, including acute GVHD, sepsis, and viral infection. Cytomegalovirus is the pathogen most often associated with this complication (Salzberger *et al.*, 1997; Broers *et al.*, 2000). More recently, human herpes virus 6 (HHV-6) has been incriminated. One recent study showed that bone marrow samples from allogeneic transplant recipients demonstrating bone marrow suppression of unknown etiology were more likely to test positive for HHV-6 than those from patients whose bone marrow suppression had been definitively diagnosed (Carrigan & Knox, 1994).

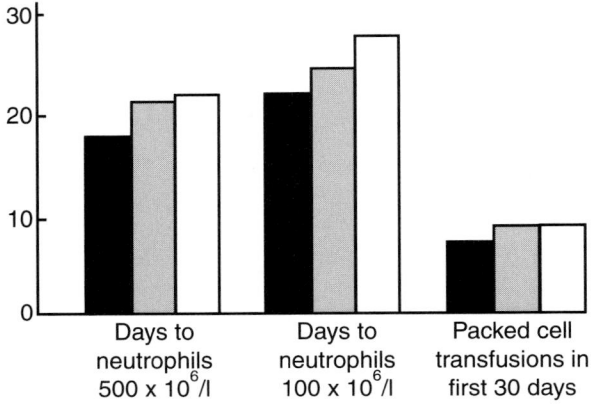

Fig. 13.5. Duration of neutropenia and packed cell transfusion requirements in recipients of HLA-identical sibling marrow transplants for hematologic malignancy who were prepared with cyclophosphamide 120mg/kg and fractionated total body irradiation 12–14 Gy. For GVHD prophylaxis patient received cyclosporine (*n* = 79) (■) or methotrexate (*n* = 16) (▦) or T-cell depletion of the donor marrow with monoclonal anti-T-cell antibody and complement incubation together with cyclosporine (*n* = 16) (□).

Factors affecting the rate of hematopoietic reconstitution

Graft characteristics

Nucleated cells

The total number of nucleated marrow cells infused into the allogeneic recipient may favorably affect the engraftment rate (Thomas *et al.*, 1977; Atkinson *et al.*, 1985; Sierra *et al.*, 1997; Cornelissen *et al.*, 2001; Dominietto *et al.*, 2001 and 2002). A large retrospective EBMT study showed lower nonrelapse mortality, improved leukemia-free survival, and a decreased relapse rate in patients with AML in first remission receiving allografts with $> 2.6 \times 10^8$ nucleated bone marrow cells/kg (Rocha *et al.*, 2002). Also, a higher number of infused total nucleated marrow cells ($>3 \times 10^8$/kg recipient weight) has been shown to decrease the risk of graft rejection in patients with severe aplastic anemia conditioned with cyclophosphamide and given HLA-identical sibling marrow grafts (Storb *et al.*, 1977).

The total nucleated cell dose from bone marrow harvests in patients with acute myeloid leukemia (AML) undergoing autologous marrow transplantation had a significant impact on outcome (Demirer *et al.*, 1995). Patients whose marrow harvest yielded $< 2 \times 10^8$ total nucleated cells (TNC)/kg had a 100-day mortality of 50%, and only 54% achieved a posttransplant granulocyte count of $>0.5 \times 10^9$/l. In contrast, patients whose marrow harvest yielded $2–4 \times 10^8$ TNC/kg had a 20% mortality by day 100, and 91% recovered granulocytes to 0.5×10^9/l. Autologous transplantation in AML with bone marrow as the source of stem cells has consistently been associated with delayed recovery, whereas peripheral blood derived stem cells has brought marked improvement. In a study of 240 patients given unpurged marrow autografts (*n* = 210) or unpurged blood autografts (*n* = 30) with AML (*n* = 128) or acute lymphoblastic leukemia (ALL) (*n* = 112), multivariate analysis showed that blood stem cell autografts and a nucleated cell dose of $>2 \times 10^8$/kg were associated with faster neutrophil recovery. There was a strong correlation between blood cell autografts and higher cell doses and between marrow autografts and lower cell doses. The authors also showed that hematologic recovery after autografting was faster in patients with ALL, probably due to the nature and amount of prior chemotherapy (Mehta *et al.*, 1996). In a study of 100 recipients of syngeneic bone marrow transplants reported to the IBMTR, a nucleated cell dose $>3 \times 10^8$/kg was associated with a lower incidence of treatment failure (relapse or death) in those patients surviving in remission at 9 months or later posttransplant (Barrett *et al.*, 2000) (Fig. 13.6).

Progenitor cells

The influence of the number of infused allogeneic progenitor (e.g., CFU-GM) cells on the rate of engraftment is controversial, with some reports showing no relationship (Atkinson *et al.*, 1985) but others documenting a correlation, at least for some parameters of engraftment rate (Faille *et al.*, 1981; Arnold *et al.*, 1986). One study suggested that numbers of CFU-GM infused in allogeneic marrow had no effect on the speed of engraftment but did affect

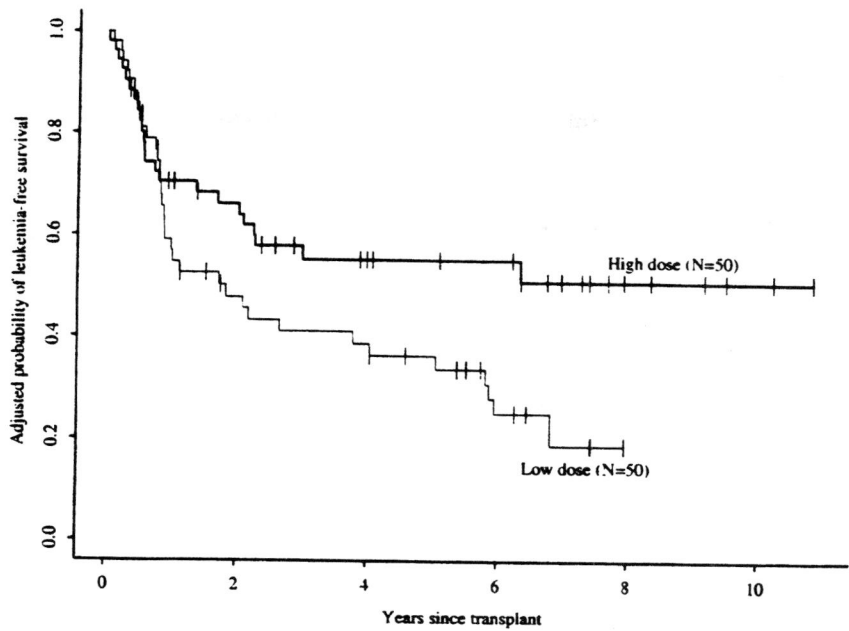

Fig. 13.6. Adjusted probabilities of leukemia-free survival rates after identical twin bone marrow transplantation with high (more than 3×10^8 cells/kg) versus low (less than or equal to 3×10^8 cells/kg) cell doses. Reproduced, with permission, from Barrett *et al.* (2000).

the quality of hematologic recovery, as well as transplant-related mortality. Patients who received less than the median value of 2.4 $\times 10^4$ CFU-GM/kg had a transplant-related mortality rate of 53% versus 5% for patients receiving a CFU-GM dose greater than this. While neutrophil counts were comparable at all time intervals and there was no difference in platelet counts between the two groups on days +7 and +50 posttransplant, those who received higher numbers of CFU-GM cells had significantly higher platelet counts on day 80, day 100, and day 150 posttransplant (Bacigalupo *et al.*, 1995). Another study used limiting dilution assay of mafosfamide-resistant progenitors as an assay of pre-CFU cells (ancestral to committed progenitors such as CFU-GM) to analyze the kinetics of myeloid engraftment posttransplant, and found that in patients given allografts from unrelated or family member donors, the rate of neutrophil engraftment correlated strongly with the number of pre-CFU transfused cells/kg recipient weight in the donor inoculum, while there was no such relationship with CFU-GM content (Kirkland *et al.*, 1996).

For autologous transplantation, a number of studies, including that of Haas *et al.* (1995), have shown a correlation between the number of infused CFU-GM in autologous marrow or autologous peripheral blood stem cell inoculum and the rate of engraftment of neutrophils and platelets posttransplant. Furthermore, the long-term culture colony-forming cell (LTC-CFC) assay may represent a reliable prediction for poor engraftment and graft failure following autologous stem cell transplantation, as was shown in a recent study by Van Hennik *et al.* (2000).

CD34+ cells

For autologous peripheral blood progenitor cell transplantation, it is generally agreed that an infusion containing more than

2.0×10^6 CD34+ cells/kg recipient weight is generally associated with rapid engraftment of both neutrophils and platelets, while infusions containing less than this number are often associated with delayed recovery (Haas *et al.*, 1995) (Fig. 13.7). In a study of 95 patients with myeloma treated at a single center with high-dose melphalan and autologous blood stem cell transplantation, platelet recovery to >25, 50, and $100 \times 10^9/l$ was delayed in all patients who received $<2 \times 10^6$ CD34+ cells/kg (Millar *et al.*, 1996).

In several studies of autologous peripheral blood stem cell transplantation, the number of CD34+ cells expressing the L-selectin adhesion molecule predicted rapid platelet recovery (Fig. 13.8); the number of L-selection positive CD34+ cells also correlated better with time to neutrophil recovery than did the total number of reinfused CD34+ cells, although this did not reach statistical significance (Dercksen *et al.*, 1995; Pratt *et al.*, 2001). In contrast, other studies have found that CD34+ cell numbers predicted engraftment better than any CD34+ subset, including CD34+/41+, CD34+/33+, CD34+/38+ and CD34+/90+ (Stewart *et al.*, 2000). In addition to the rate of neutrophil and platelet recovery, the dose of CD34+ cells infused has been shown to influence later engraftment-related parameters including transfusion requirements, febrile episodes, days of hospitalization, and antibiotic requirements throughout the first year posttransplant (Perez-Simon *et al.*, 1999).

As with autologous blood stem cell transplantation, a relationship has been reported between the dose of CD34+ cells in HLA-identical sibling bone marrow and the rate of hematologic recovery posttransplant (Mavroudis *et al.*, 1996). Eighty-eight patients with hematologic malignancies received a T-

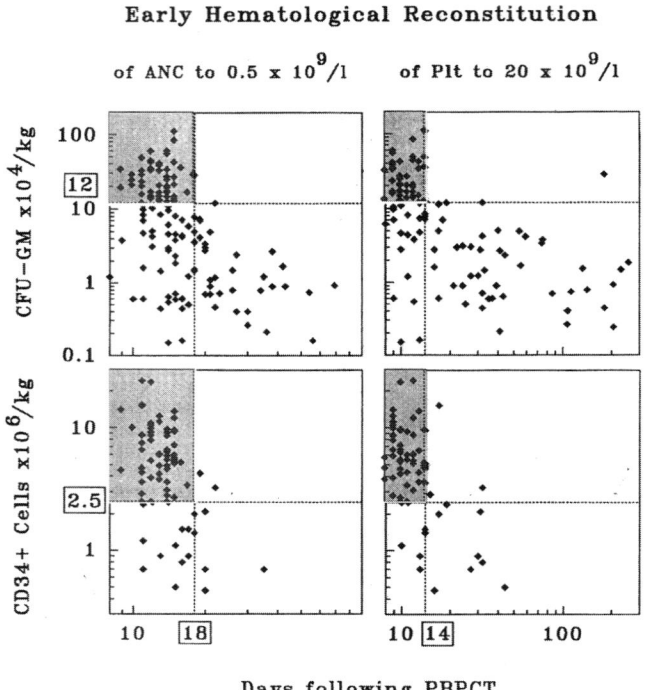

Early Hematological Reconstitution

Fig. 13.7. Comparison of CFU-GM and CD34+ cells autografted per kilogram body weight with days to recovery of neutrophil counts to $0.5 \times 10^9/l$ and of platelet counts (Plt) to $20 \times 10^9/l$. For CFU-GM, the evaluation is based on a total of 123 patients autografted between May 1985 and December 1993, while the number of CD34+ cells transplanted is available for 78 patients. As indicated by the shaded areas, threshold quantities of 2.5×10^6 CD34+ cells per kilogram or 12.0×10^4 CFU-GM per kilogram became evident and were associated with rapid neutrophil and platelet recovery within less than 18 and 14 days, respectively. Abbreviation: PBPCT, peripheral blood progenitor cell transplantation. Reproduced, with permission, from Haas *et al.* (1995).

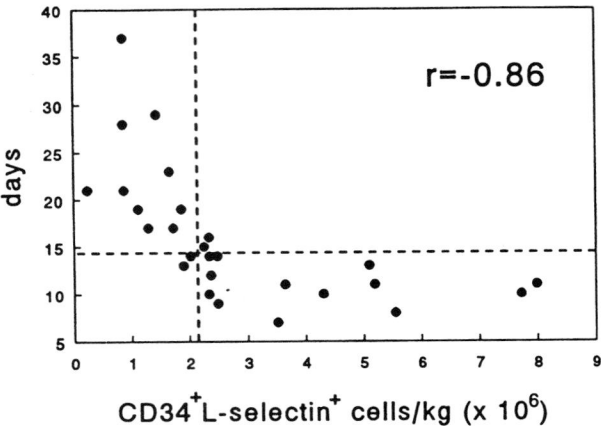

Fig. 13.8. Correlation between reinfusion of CD34+ L-selectin+ cells and time to platelet transfusion independence. Calculated threshold of reinfused CD34+ L-selectin+ cells (2.1×10^6 CD34+ L-selectin+ cells/kg) for rapid platelet recovery and the time for rapid recovery (arbitrarily set as the time to platelet transfusion independence within 14 days after PBSC transplantation) are depicted as dashed lines. Reproduced, with permission, from Dercksen *et al.* (1995).

cell-depleted, HLA-identical sibling marrow transplant, and cyclosporine was used for GVHD prophylaxis posttransplant. Patients receiving more than 2×10^6 CD34+ cells/kg showed significantly earlier recovery of monocytes and a trend to earlier recovery of lymphocytes. They achieved platelet and red blood cell transfusion independence earlier, required less G-CSF support during ganciclovir treatment, and spent fewer days in hospital posttransplant. They had less treatment-related mortality (primarily due to infections and cytopenias) and better survival at a median of 1 year posttransplant than a group receiving $<1 \times 10^6$ CD34+ cells/kg (confirmed by Bahceci *et al.*, 2000 and Morariu-Zamfir *et al.*, 2001) (Fig. 13.9). Subsequently, the same group reported that CD34-selected, G-CSF primed, HLA-identical sibling grafts were associated with delayed pancytopenia occurring between days 55 and 130 posttransplant (Mavroudis *et al.*, 1998). In a series of 546 recipients of related and unrelated, T-cell-depleted allografts (48% of which were HLA-mismatched), CD34+ cell

dose $>5.0 \times 10^6$/kg and hematopoietic growth factor administration were independently associated with a faster rate of neutrophil recovery (Keever-Taylor *et al.*, 2001). Faster platelet recovery was associated with a CD34+ cell dose $>2.0 \times 10^6$/kg, transplantation for chronic leukemia, an HLA-matched donor and the absence of growth factor use. Nakamura *et al.* (2001) reported that a CD34+ cell dose $<4.6 \times 10^6$/kg was one risk factor for lower disease-free survival and overall survival in recipients of T-cell-depleted, HLA-identical sibling PBSC transplants. Other studies, however, have suggested that a higher number of CD34+ cells in allogeneic PBSC transplants is associated with a higher incidence of acute GVHD (Przieporka *et al.*, 1999) or extensive chronic GVHD (Zaucha *et al.*, 2001) or a higher incidence of transplant-related mortality (Urbano-Ispizua *et al.*, 2001).

Marrow stromal cell growth characteristics

In a study of the impact of Dexter long-term bone marrow culture characteristics as a prognostic factor for hematopoietic reconstitution after autologous marrow transplantation, the absence of a stromal layer defined a group with very poor hematologic recovery posttransplant. Only one of nine cases in this group had recovery of granulocytes and platelets posttransplant compared to 90% of patients whose pretransplant long-term culture displayed normal adherent cell behavior (Gilbert & Ayats, 1994). In the special circumstance of patients receiving high-dose chemotherapy and autologous marrow rescue for malignant brain tumors, the exposure to pretransplant craniospinal irradiation had a significant impact on delaying engraftment (Faulkner *et al.*, 1996).

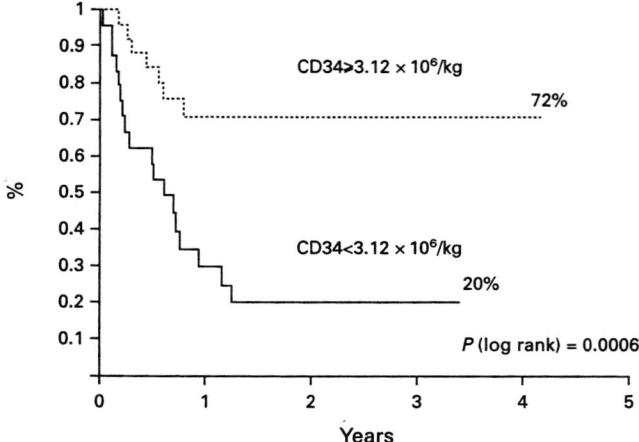

Fig. 13.9. Influence of number of bone marrow CD34+ cells infused on survival after HLA-identical BMT for patients with CML. Reproduced, with permission, from Morariu-Zamfir *et al.* (2001).

Genetic disparity of sources of allogeneic stem cells

Matched unrelated donor (MUD) SCT

A number of studies have indicated that engraftment after unrelated donor transplantation is slower than that after HLA-identical family member transplantation given equivalent posttransplant immune suppression to minimize GVHD risk (Fig. 13.10) (Davies *et al.*, 1994; Davies *et al.*, 2000; Dominietto *et al.*, 2001; and see Chapter 67). In one large retrospective series comparing patients given an HLA-matched unrelated donor transplant (*n* = 40) or a partially HLA-matched unrelated donor transplant (*n* = 68) with 236 patients given an HLA-matched sibling transplant over the same period of time, the median day on which the ANC exceeded 0.5×10^9/l was day 25 for patients with a sibling donor and day 26 for those given an unrelated donor transplant (*P* = .02). In this series, the incidence of both early and late (primary and secondary) graft failure was significantly higher in the recipients of unrelated donor transplants (see below) (Davies *et al.*, 1994). As observed following sibling allo-SCT, the use of peripheral blood stem cells significantly improves the rate of engraftment of both neutrophils and platelets. Ringden *et al.* (1999) performed a retrospective study comparing 63 recipients of MUD PBSC versus 45 recipients of

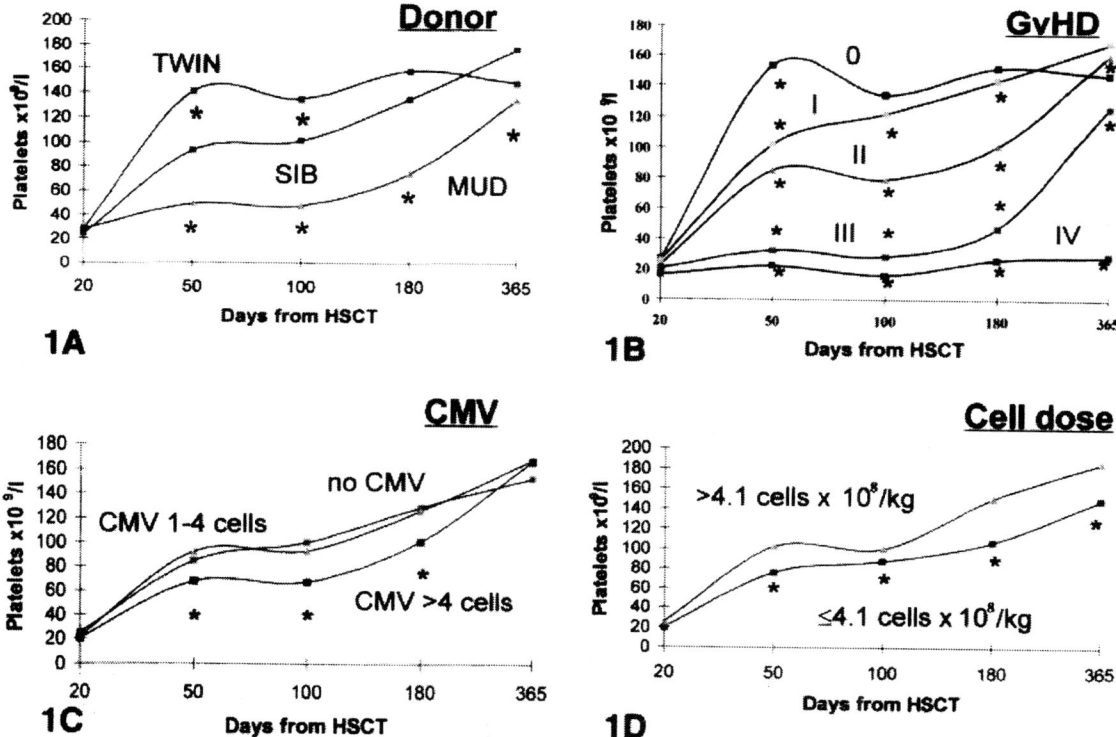

Fig. 13.10. Factors influencing hematological recovery after allogeneic hematopoietic stem cell transplantation (HSCT). (A) Donor type: significantly lower platelet counts were recorded in recipients of unrelated (MUD) grafts than in HLA-identical sibling (SIB) and twin (TWIN) grafts. (B) GvHD: the effect of acute graft-versus-host disease (GvHD) is clearly seen at all time intervals and correlated with the severity of the disease. (C) CMV: patients with absent (no cells) cytomegalovirus (CMV) antigenaemia or low numbers of CMV antigen-positive cells (1–4) have significantly higher platelet counts than patients with a greater CMV load (> 4 cells). D. Cell dose: patients grafted with a larger number of cells (> 4.1×10^8/kg) have higher platelet counts throughout the transplant (*P* > 0.01). Reproduced, with permission, from Dominietto *et al.* (2001).

MUD BMT. They showed faster engraftment with a median time to reach ANC > 0.5 × 10⁹/l of 16 days in the PBSC group versus 20 days in the BM group. In addition, the median time to reach platelets > 50 × 10⁹/l was 23 days in the PBSC group versus 29 days in the BM group. The difference was most likely explained by the higher number of CD34⁺ progenitor cells infused with the PB graft (median 6.3 versus 3.2 × 10⁶ CD34⁺ MNC/kg, $P < 0.001$). As MUD PBSCT may also be associated with a better recovery of T and B cells (Ottinger *et al.*, 1996) and the risks and benefits for the donor also seem better, it is expected that the use of MUD-PBSCT will largely replace MUD-BMT in the future.

Unrelated cord blood transplantation

Since the first unrelated donor UCB transplant in 1993, several thousands of UCB transplants have been performed worldwide (Wagner *et al.*, 1995; Kurtzberg *et al.*, 1996, Gluckman *et al.*, 1997; Rubinstein *et al.*, 1998). It has been shown that 0 to 3 HLA-A, B, DRB-l mismatched donors may contain sufficient stem cells to engraft most pediatric patients. Experience has indicated that UCB-SCT is generally associated with a slower rate of hematopoietic recovery with a median number of approximately 4 weeks to achieve neutrophil recovery (> 0.5 × 10⁹/l) (Fig. 13.11). The number of nucleated cells in the umbilical cord blood before it was frozen appeared critically associated with the rate of engraftment in several studies. However, recent studies in pediatric patients show that the UCB cell dose is sufficient to achieve survival in children similar to that seen with unrelated donor BMT (Barker *et al.*, 2001; Davies, 2000), despite more HLA-disparity. Studies in adults showed encouraging results with engraftment rates comparable to those seen in pediatric series, but survival seems not as good as can be obtained with MUD-BMT. One of the factors critically associated with survival was the number of CD34⁺ cells (Laughlin *et al.*, 2001) which number is significantly lower than that obtained with bone marrow or peripheral blood-derived stem cells.

Haploidentical, 3-loci mismatched transplantation

The probability of identifying a matched unrelated donor through one of the international registries is up to 80–90% for Caucasians, but far less for ethnic minorities. As an alternative, a haploidentical familydonor (either parent or sibling) is available for almost every patient. Allogeneic haploidentical SCT using peripheral blood stem cells has been developed over the last decade, both in pediatric patients and in adults (Handgretinger *et al.*, 1998; Handgretinger, 2001; Aversa *et al.*, 1994, 1998). It appears that a combination of ablative high-dose chemoradiotherapy, rigorous T-cell depletion of the graft and a high number of CD34⁺ cells/kg are required for effective engraftment and prevention of GVHD. The number of progenitor cells is especially critical and preferably more than 10 × 10⁶ CD34⁺ cells/kg should be obtained. These numbers are readily achieved in pediatric patients. Handgretinger

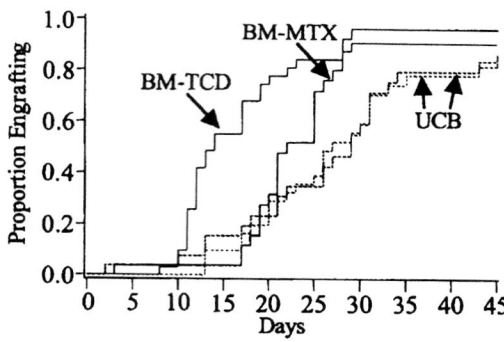

Fig. 13.11. Neutrophil recovery. Cumulative incidence of neutrophil recovery in recipients of unrelated donor UCB versus HLA-matched BM who received GVHD prophylaxis with MTX (BM-MTX) and UCB versus HLA-matched BMwhor received GVHD prophylaxis with TCD (BM-TCD). UCB versus BM-MTX: engraftment rate, p = .03; engraftment without at day 45, $P = .41$. UCB versus BM-TCD: engraftment rate, $P < .01$; engraftment at day 45, $P = .32$. Reproduced, with permission from Barker *et al.*, 2001.

et al showed that when the number exceeded 20 × 10⁶ CD34⁺ cells/kg, all (pediatric) patients engrafted and the time to recover normal numbers of CD3⁺ T cells was relatively short (80 to 90 days).

Prophylactic regimen for graft-versus-host disease

As indicated above, the use of cyclosporine has clearly been associated with a faster rate of engraftment than the use of methotrexate (MTX) for GVHD prophylaxis (Hows *et al.*, 1982; Atkinson *et al.*, 1983; Deeg *et al.*, 1985). Impairment of renal function delays excretion of MTX, and raised plasma MTX levels have been associated with delayed engraftment.

Graft-versus-host disease

Although acute GVHD may affect initial recovery of neutrophils and platelets, its effect is limited. In contrast, the quality or durability of hematological recovery is strongly affected by GVHD. Both acute and chronic GVHD have been associated with thrombocytopenia. Sullivan *et al.* (1988) showed a correlation of (extensive) chronic GVHD with prolonged thrombocytopenia, and the subset of patients with GVHD and a reduced platelet count beyond day 100 appeared to be at high risk of treatment-related mortality (TRM). Comparible findings with respect to acute GVHD have been made by others (Dominietto *et al.*, 2001; Bruno *et al.*, 2001). Dominietto *et al.* (2001) showed that patients experiencing acute GVHD II-IV were at higher risk for prolonged thrombocytopenia, and the subset of patients with acute GVHD grade II with thrombocytopenia experienced significantly more TRM compared to patients with GVHD grade II without a low platelet count beyond day 50 and 100 (Figure 13.12). These findings may be explained by reduced platelet production and/or increased consumption. Experimentally, reduced production as well as a decrease of donor stem cells has been shown to occur in mice with acute GVHD (Van Dijken *et al.,* 1991). Apart from cytokines that may suppress hematopoiesis, GVHD itself may attack the stromal compartment of the bone marrow, thereby inhibiting progenitor cell function. Furthermore, increased platelet consumption may be explained by autoimmune thrombocytopenia or the TTP/HUS syndrome, which are associated with severe GVHD (Roy *et al.,* 2001).

Cytomegalovirus infection

Several clinical studies have shown that CMV infection post-transplant, as evidenced by antigenemia or DNA-emia, may adversely affect long-term hematopoietic recovery (Salzberger *et al.,* 1997; Broers *et al.,* 2000). Both its treatment and the infection itself suppress growth of hematopoietic progenitor cells. Treatment with ganciclovir is associated with neutropenia, which may give rise to opportunistic infections. The virus itself may infect hematopoietic progenitor cells and stromal cells growth, thereby inhibiting their growth. Furthermore, subtypes of CMV have been described, which are especially implicated in bone marrow failure (Torok-Storb *et al.,* 1992, 1997).

ABO incompatibility

Major ABO incompatibility between donor and recipient has little or no effect on the rate of leukocyte and platelet engraftment, but erythrocyte reconstitution is delayed for up to 9 to 12 months in exceptional cases, and packed cell transfusion requirement increased in such recipients (Brain *et al.,* 1982;

Hows *et al.,* 1983; Sniecinski *et al.,* 1985). This also occurs after T-depleted transplantation (Bär *et al.,* 1995). Pure red cell aplasia can develop posttransplant. For example, six patients with blood group O developed this complication in the latter study; in five patients, it resolved without therapeutic intervention: anti-A antibody titers were persistently high during the first 3 months posttransplant. This was in contrast to 22 patients with timely recovery of erythropoiesis in whom anti-A and anti-B antibody titers showed a steady decrease after marrow transplantation (Bär *et al.,* 1995). A number of cases of such red cell aplasia have been shown to be resistant to the use of intravenous gamma globulin, but such cases may respond to antithymocyte globulin and methylprednisolone (Roychowdhury & Linker, 1995), or to erythropoietin and methylprednisolone (Ohashi *et al.,* 1994). Additional cases have responded to erythropoietin alone (Heyll *et al.,* 1991; Paltiel *et al.,* 1993), as well as to plasmapheresis (Or *et al.,* 1991). Occasionally, the red cell aplasia may be of long duration (Gmur *et al.,* 1990; Volin & Ruutu, 1990).

Marrow fibrosis

It has been suggested that the presence of marrow fibrosis results in delayed engraftment after allogeneic transplantation (Rajantie *et al.,* 1986; Thiele *et al.,* 2000). In a retrospective study of 203 patients with marrow fibrosis compared to 203 matched controls without, there was no significant difference in the time distributions for reaching an ANC of 0.5 or $1 \times 10^9/l$, but the time to platelet transfusion independence was 3 days longer in those with marrow fibrosis. In the subgroup of 33 patients with severe fibrosis, there was a 7-day delay in the time to reach platelet transfusion independence and a 2-day delay in the time to reach red blood cell transfusion independence, although these differences were not statistically significant (Soll *et al.,* 1995).

Peripheral blood progenitor cell transplantation

Hematopoietic progenitor cells can be detected in very limited numbers (< 1%) in the peripheral blood under physiological conditions, but the number increases rapidly upon mobilization by colony-stimulating factors. There are important differences between BM-derived progenitors and peripheral blood stem cells (PBSC). PBSC may express more lineage-specific differentiation antigens and have a lower proportion of cells in S phase (Gyger *et al.,* 2000), but may exert higher in vitro and in vivo clonogeneic capacity. PBSC transplantation has become standard in the autologous setting, while the use of PBSC in allogeneic transplantation (related and unrelated donors) is still increasing. A significantly shorter time to neutrophil and platelet engraftment has been demonstrated after autologous PBSCT and allogeneic PBSCT. Champlin *et al.* (2000) performed a large retrospective study demonstrating a reduction of 5 days to neutrophil engraftment and a reduction of 7 days to platelet engraftment ($P < 0.001$) after allogeneic PBSCT as

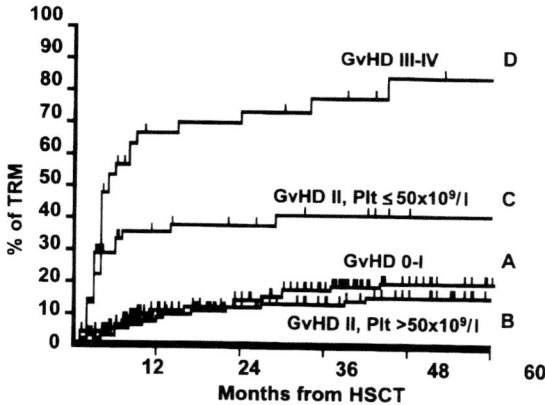

Fig. 13.12. Actuarial transplant-related mortality (TRM) of patients with actue GvHD grade 0–1 (A) (*n* = 151, 18%), grade II and platelets > 50 × 10^9/l (B) (*n* = 106, 16%), grade II and platelets < 50 × 10^9/l (C) (*n* = 44, 43%), and grade III-IV (D) (*n* = 41, 86%). *P*-values in the log-rank test are: A vs. B P=0.9; A vs. C P<0.00001; A vs. D P=0.001; B vs. D P=0.0001; B vs. C P=0.001; C vs. D P=0.004. Reproduced, with permission from Dominietto *et al.,* 2001.

compared to conventional BMT. These differences are most likely explained by the greater number of CD34+ progenitor cells transplanted with PBSCT. Lymphocyte recovery may also improve upon PBSCT, as was suggested by a Spanish study (Martinez *et al.*, 1999). As PBSC grafts may contain 10–100 times more CD3+ T cells, the incidence of acute and chronic GVHD has been a concern. Recently, a meta-analysis of 15 trials was performed and significantly higher relative risks for acute and chronic GVHD were observed following allogeneic PBSCT (1.13 and 1.58 respectively) (Cutler *et al.*, 2000). Patients with high-risk underlying disease may experience a lower relapse rate and better survival (Champlin *et al.*, 2000; Bensinger *et al.*, 2001).

Use of mesenchymal stem cells in addition to hematopoietic stem cells (see Chapter 5)

Multipotential mesenchymal stem cells (MSC) are found in human bone marrow and can secrete hematopoietic cytokines and support hematopoietic progenitors in vitro. Purified and culture-expanded MSCs differentiate along the osteogenic, chondrogenic, and adipogenic lineages (Deans & Mosely, 2000; Koc & Lazarus, 2001). In unstimulated cultures MSCs appear as fusiform fibroblasts with expression of surface proteins (SH2, SH3, SH4) that are not found on hematopoietic precursors. MSCs lack expression of hematopoietic markers such as CD45, CD14 and CD34. They constitutively secrete interleukins 6, 7, 8, 11, 12, 14, and 15, M-CSF, Flt-3 ligand and SCF, and have immunomodulatory properties, being suppressive of T cell function (Di Nicola *et al.*, 2002). In an in utero model of human-sheep hematopoietic stem cell (HSC) transplantation, the co-transplantation of human stormal cell progenitors simultaneiously with human HSC enhanced long-term engraftment of human cells in the bone marrow of the chimeric animals and in earlier and higher levels of donor cells in the circulation, both during gestation and after birth (Almeida-Porada *et al.*, 2000). In a phase I/II study Koc *et al.* (2000) infused 1–2.2 × 10⁶ MSCs/kg (Fig. 13.13), along with a median of 13.9 × 10⁶ CD34+ cells/kg, into women undergoing high-dose chemotherapy and autologous stem cell transplantation for breast cancer. The median days to reach ANC of 500/μl and platelets 20,000/μl were 8 and 8.5, respectively. Additionally, it should be noted that allogeneic mesenchymal stem cells, delivered with an HSC allograft, have been shown to help correct the defect in osteogenesis imperfecta (Horwitz *et al.*, 1999, 2001).

Reconstitution of marrow hematopoietic cells

Bone marrow cellularity is normally decreased for the first 2 to 3 months posttransplant (Fig. 13.14). Indeed, in patients given HLA-identical sibling bone marrow grafts and immune suppressed with MTX alone, engraftment was often bilineage (no detectable megakaryocytes) at day 14 posttransplant, although all three cell lineages were usually represented in marrow aspi-

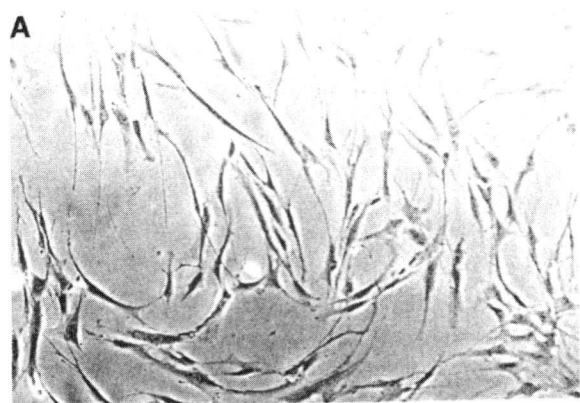

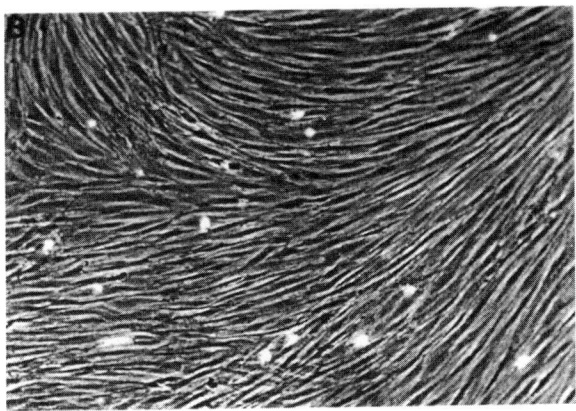

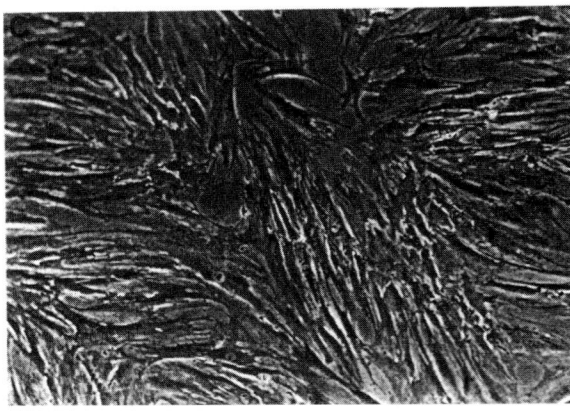

Fig. 13.13. Phase contrast photomicrograph of cultured MSCs (magnification × 100). (**A**) Single fusiform adherent cells early in the primary culture. (**B**) Late (day 13) in the primary culture, showing confluent patches of MSCs immediately before first passage. (**C**) Confluent layer of fifth-passage MSCs. Reproduced, with permission, from Koc *et al.* (2000).

rate samples by day 21 posttransplant (Atkinson *et al.*, 1986). Marrow cells can look considerably dysplastic, particularly in the first 3 months posttransplant: one report of three patients correlated dysplastic changes after allogeneic transplantation with moderate to severe anemia, leukopenia, and/or thrombocytopenia between days 40 and 68 posttransplant. A ferroki-

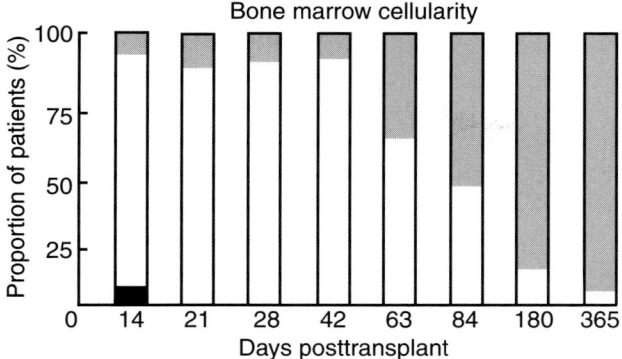

Fig. 13.14. Bone marrow cellularity posttransplant. The data were derived from 31 recipients of T-replete HLA-identical sibling marrow for hematologic malignancy who were prepared with cyclophosphamide 120 mg/kg and fractionated total body irradiation 12–14 Gy. Immune suppression was with cyclosporine. (■) Hypocellular with bilineage engraftment. (▨) Hypocellular with trilineage engraftment. (□) Normocellular. Reproduced, with permission, from Atkinson, *Bone Marrow Transplantation* **5**, 209–26 (1990).

netic study showed ineffective erythropoiesis in one patient. Hematopoietic cells were shown to be of donor origin in all three cases (Okamoto *et al.*, 1996). These changes usually resolve with time.

In contrast to the normalization of numbers of most morphologically recognizable cellular components of the blood and marrow by 3 to 6 months posttransplant, numbers of committed progenitor cells (CFU-GM, CFU-E, BFU-E, CFU-Mix) in both blood and marrow remain abnormally low in the long term in most stud-

ies (Arnold *et al.*, 1986; Atkinson *et al.*, 1986; Ma *et al.*, 1987), particularly in recipients of autologous transplants (Vellenga *et al.*, 1987; Domenech *et al.*, 1995). Podesta and colleagues (1997) found markedly low levels of early progenitor cells (measured as LTC-IC) long term postallografting (Fig. 13.15).

In the study by Domenech and colleagues (1995), the values for CFU-GM, CFU-E, BFU-E, and CFU-Meg remained low for several years after autologous bone marrow transplantation, although peripheral blood counts nearly normalized within a few weeks of transplant. Pregraft values were reached after 2 years for CFU-GM and BFU-E and after 4 years for CFU-E, while CFU-Meg failed to reach pregraft values after this time. Normal levels were reached after 4 years only for CFU-GM. On univariate and multivariate analysis the following factors appeared to delay marrow progenitor cell reconstitution: the underlying disease (particularly AML), graft characteristics such as a low stem cell content and in vitro purging, conditioning regimens with total body irradiation or busulfan, and a lack of postgraft administration of growth factors. Additionally, the mean number of pre-CFU in the marrow in 25 patients studied 6 to 66 months after allotransplant was $3.1/10^5$ mononuclear cells compared with a value of $24.7/10^5$ mononuclear cells for normal individuals (Kirkland *et al.*, 1996). It would thus appear that marrow reserve capacity is considerably diminished in HSC transplant recipients.

Reconstitution of marrow stromal cells

In one study the number of marrow stromal cells as determined by the CFU-F assay was low at 3 weeks posttransplant, but returned to the normal range thereafter (Da *et al.*, 1986). Another study of allogeneic bone marrow transplantation used a two-

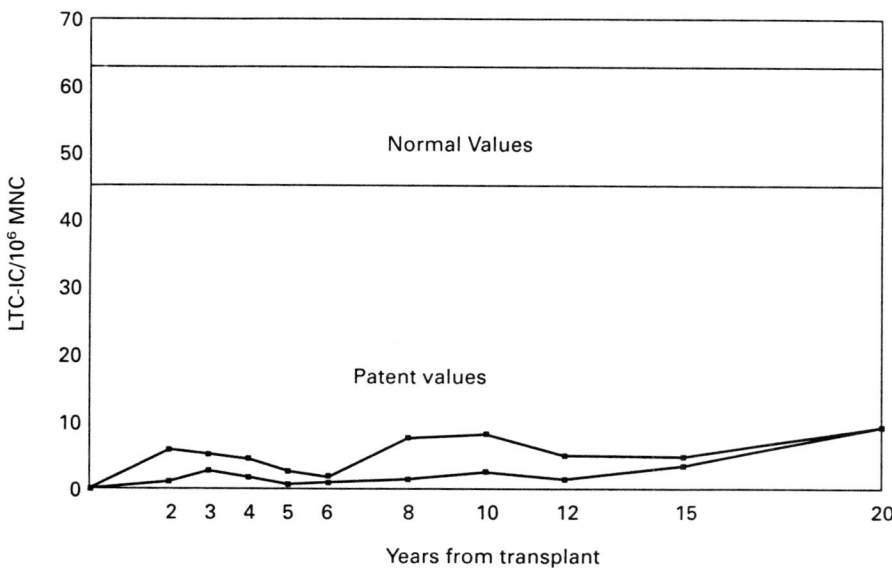

Fig. 13.15. Hematopoietic reconstitution in long-term survivors: LTC-IC frequency. Limited area defines the range of LTC-IC frequencies/10^6 MNC per patients analyzed at each time point. Normal range is depicted at the top of the figure as the areas between the two horizontal lines ($n = 30$ samples). Reproduced, with permission, from Podesta *et al.* (1997).

stage long-term bone marrow culture (LTBMC) assay in which irradiated confluent marrow stromal cells derived from recipients posttransplant were recharged with flow cytometry-sorted CD34+/CD38− cells from normal marrow donors. In 58% of patients, the marrow stroma was considerably compromised in its ability to support early uncommitted hematopoietic cells contained within the CD34+/CD38− cells. Bone marrow stroma from recipients exhibited severe deficits in its ability to support primitive hematopoietic cells, and in some patients this defect lasted for several years. While the growth of stroma from these patients was severely delayed and often incomplete, characterization of cell types did not show significant differences proportionally when compared with normal cultures (O'Flaherty, 1995). The origin of marrow stromal cells posttransplant is controversial, with some reports indicating predominantly host origin (Hollings et al., 1984; Lennon & Micklem, 1986), some predominantly donor origin (Keating et al., 1982), and some mixed (Piersma et al., 1983; Marshall et al., 1984; Cilloni et al., 2000). One study using in situ hybridization technology showed marrow-derived stromal cells proliferating in long-term marrow cultures from recipients of allogeneic transplant to be exclusively of host genotype, whereas the macrophage component of the adherent layer in these cultures originated from the donor (Simmons et al., 1987).

Reconstitution of neutrophil function

Neutrophil oxidative killing function returns to normal early posttransplant (Sosa et al., 1980). This is mirrored clinically by the rapid resolution of fever (presumed infectious), and the healing of chemoradiation-induced oropharyngeal mucositis coincident with the early rise in neutrophil numbers. Neutrophil chemotaxis, however, may remain impaired for several months posttransplant (Clark et al., 1976; Territo et al., 1977). The effect of the administration of recombinant human GM-CSF after autologous marrow transplantation has been studied. While there was no difference in neutrophil margination, neutrophil phagocytosis of Cryptococcus neoformans, or neutrophil production of hydrogen peroxide before or during GM-CSF infusion, there was a marked reduction in neutrophil migration to a sterile inflammatory site during its infusion (Peters et al., 1988).

Additional factors that contribute to neutropenia subsequent to engraftment are the occurrence of GVHD, infection (particularly viral), and the use of myelosuppressive medications including MTX, cotrimoxazole (Deeg et al., 1979), and ganciclovir (Atkinson et al., 1991).

Production of hematopoietic growth factors posttransplant

Bone marrow (adherent cells, Fc receptor positive natural killer-like cells, and T cells) and blood (T cells and mononuclear cells) from allogeneic marrow transplant recipients produce less GM-CSF and interleukin-3 (both at messenger RNA and protein levels) than normal cells (Emerson et al., 1987; Thomas et al.,

1990; Atkinson et al., 1992). In the case of T cells this defect of production is likely due to a markedly reduced precursor frequency of T cells able to respond to activation stimuli. Defective production of growth factors by marrow stromal cells in the marrow microenvironment may be caused by damage to the stromal cells by the pretransplant chemoradiotherapy, viral infections (especially cytomegalovirus), or by GVHD. Additionally, in HLA-nonidentical transplants, genetic restriction in the interaction of marrow stromal cells (of host origin) with cooperating hematopoietic cells (of donor origin) may further limit stromal cell production of these factors (Torok-Storb et al., 1987).

Serum concentrations of hematopoietic growth factors have been assessed before, during, and after autologous and allogeneic stem cell transplantation. Testa and colleagues (1994) evaluated the kinetics in serum of stem cell factor (SCF), leukemia inhibitory factor (LIF), and IL-3 (Fig. 13.17), and IL-6, G-CSF, and IL-8 (Fig. 13.16) in patients undergoing autologous marrow or blood stem cell transplantation for leukemia, lymphoma, or ovarian cancer. SCF, a cytokine present at relatively high levels in the serum of normal subjects, exhibited only slight fluctuations before and after transplant (Fig. 13.17). Plasma LIF concentrations exhibited a unique pattern. Before chemotherapy LIF was present at high levels and then declined rapidly and subsequently remained stable. IL-3 serum levels were low before transplant but markedly increased during marrow-ablative chemotherapy, peaked on day 0 and then progressively returned to baseline levels posttransplant. Serum IL-6 levels were low before and during chemotherapy and in the first few days posttransplant (Fig. 13.16). A sharp increase was observed at day 6 with subsequent decline. All patients exhibited a pronounced increase in both G-CSF and IL-8 levels at day 6 posttransplant (i.e., 5 to 6 days before neutrophil recovery). Levels subsequently declined. There seemed to be a coordinate pattern of cytokine release during hematopoietic ablation and recovery following autologous transplant; the fluctuations of LIF and IL-3 during chemotherapy may have been related to stem cell recruitment, whereas the posttransplant increases in IL-6, G-CSF, and IL-8 likely underlay neutrophil recovery.

Similar results for elevations of G-CSF (Cairo et al., 1992; Ho et al., 1994; Busch et al., 1997) have been reported. In the study by Busch et al., delayed engraftment was associated with elevated plasma G-CSF levels at days 7 to 10 posttransplant. Reports on endogenous IL-3 levels after high-dose chemotherapy and autologous transplantation are contradictory. While Mangan et al. (1993) detected a burst of IL-3 in the immediate posttransplant period between day 0 and day 14, the report by Ho and colleagues (1994) and that by Kawano and colleagues (1993) described no significant change in IL-3 levels. Significant increases of endogenous GM-CSF levels were not found in the studies by Ho et al. or Kawano et al. In a study of T-cell-depleted allogeneic transplantation, an inverse relationship between serial G-CSF levels and the concomitant circulating absolute neutrophil count was documented (Papadakis et al., 1995). Serum thrombopoietin (TPO) levels after autologous

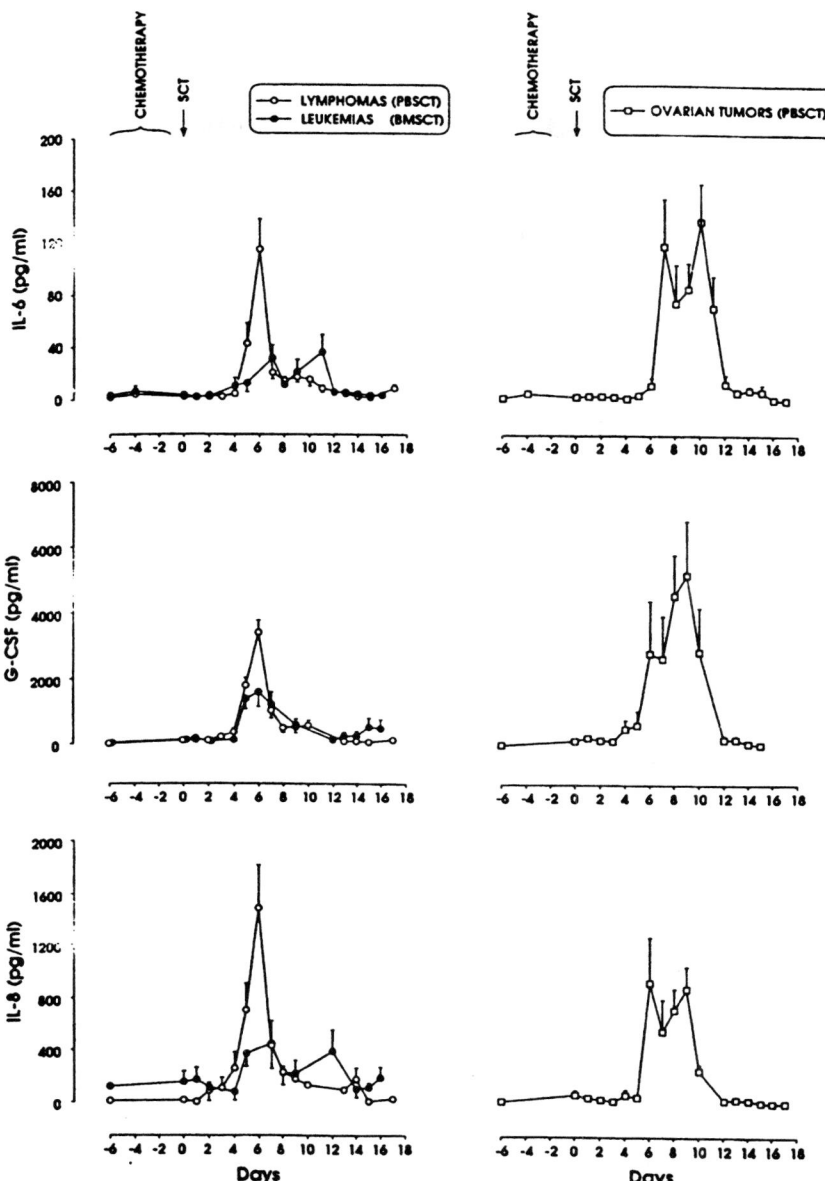

Fig. 13.16. Kinetics of IL-6, G-CSF, and IL-8 serum concentrations in 10 lymphoma, 5 leukemia, and 6 ovarian cancer patients undergoing autologous transplantation after high-dose chemotherapy. Mean ± SEM values are presented. Reproduced, with permission, from Testa *et al.* (1994).

blood stem cell (Shimazaki *et al.,* 1997) or allogeneic bone marrow transplantation showed a reciprocal relationship with the platelet count: the TPO level increased proportionately with the decrease in platelet mass after myeloablative therapy and peaked during the platelet nadir, but then decreased with subsequent normalization of the platelet mass (Figs. 13.18 and 13.19). Interestingly, the TPO level decreased during acute GVHD in several patients and was significantly lower in patients with hepatic veno-occlusive disease (VOD) than in patients without GVHD and VOD (Hamaguchi *et al.,* 1996). In another study, circulating endogenous TPO, IL-3, IL-6, and IL-

11 levels were measured in patients undergoing allogeneic bone marrow transplantation (Ishida *et al.,* 1996); again, serum TPO levels and platelet counts showed a strong inverse relationship in all patients examined. In contrast, serum levels of IL-3 had no apparent correlation with platelet count, and serum levels of IL-11 remained below the level of detection. Serum levels of IL-6 were high during the period of aplasia posttransplant and were additionally upregulated during episodes of fever.

When IL-1 production by endotoxin-stimulated cultured monocytes from 31 recipients of grafts of marrow depleted of mature cellular elements by treatment with soybean agglu-

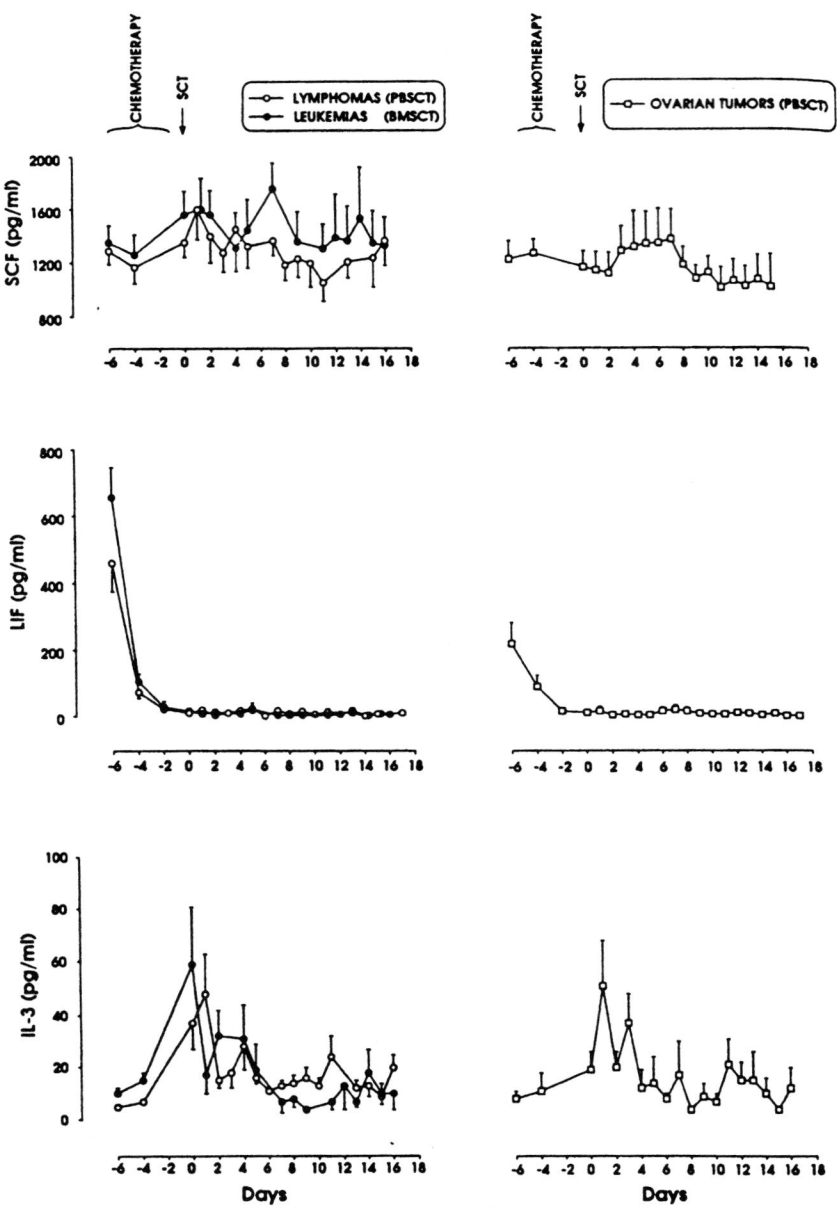

Fig. 13.17. Kinetics of SCF, LIF, and IL-3 serum levels in 10 lymphoma, 5 leukemia, and 6 ovarian cancer patients undergoing autologous transplantation after high-dose chemotherapy. Chemotherapy days correspond to –6 to –1 in leukemia/lymphoma patients and –5 to –3 in ovarian cancer cases, transplant to day 0, and the posttransplantation period to days +1 to +17. Mean ± SEM values are presented. Reproduced, with permission, from Testa *et al.* (1994).

tinin and sheep red blood cells (SBA-E-) and 12 recipients of unfractionated bone marrow were studied, deficiencies in IL-1 production (< 50 units) were detected in both transplant groups prior to and at 1 month after BMT. From 2 to 4 months posttransplant, 67% of the recipients of unmodified marrow and 45% of the recipients of SBA-E-marrow grafts produced a normal level of IL-1. By 5 to 6 months posttransplant and thereafter, the proportions of patients exhibiting deficiencies in IL-1 production in each group were equally low (Sahdev *et al.*, 1996).

IL-10 production by anti-CD3 stimulated mononuclear cells was reduced in one-third of patients after allogeneic BMT (and this appeared associated with an increased risk of GVHD; Körholz *et al.*, 1996; Körholz *et al.*, 1997), although, in contrast, another study described a correlation between high serum levels of IL-10 and a fatal outcome posttransplant (Hempel *et al.*, 1997). Serum levels of IL-12 were found to be relatively low (140 to 300 pg/ml by radioimmunoassay) after allogeneic BMT compared to autologous BMT (350 pg/ml). Normal donor levels were around 180 pg/ml. No correlations with

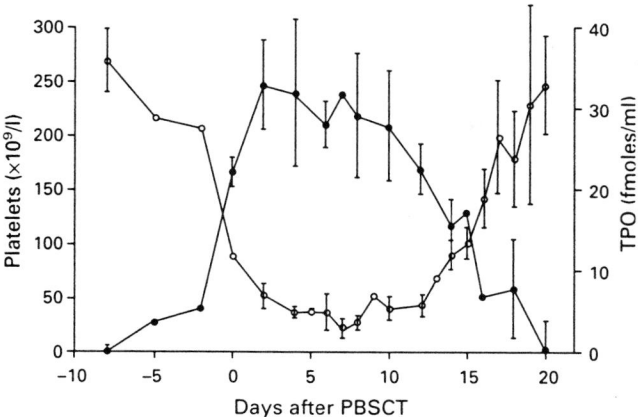

Fig. 13.18. Relationship between serum TPO level (●) and absolute platelet count (○) in seven patients undergoing peripheral blood stem cell transplantation (PBSCT). Serum TPO levels rose immediately after PBSCT, reaching a peak between days 0 and 10. TPO levels decreased as the platelet counts rose. Error bars indicate the standard error of the mean. Reproduced, with permission, from Shimazaki *et al.* (1997).

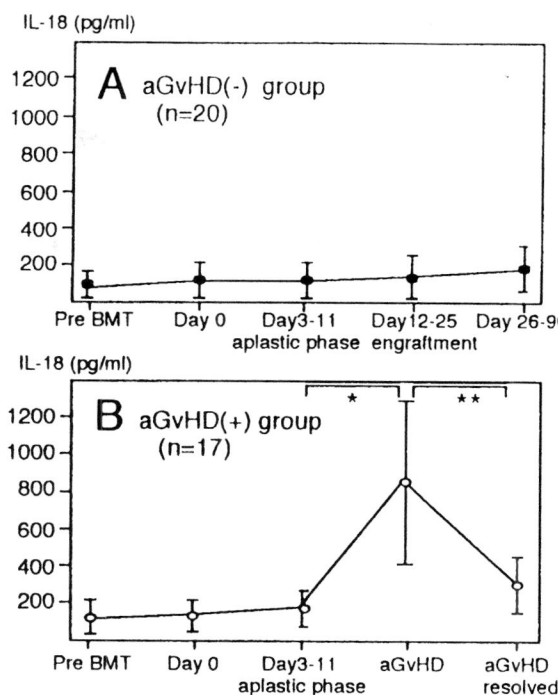

Fig. 13.20. Serial serum IL-18 levels in patients with haematological malignancy undergoing BMT. (**A**) aGVHD (–) group (*n* = 20); (**B**) grade I-IV aGVHD (+) group (*n* = 17). Values are given as means +/– SD. *P < 0.0002. **P < 0.02. Reproduced, with permission, from Fujimori *et al.* (2000).

GVHD or infection were noted (Bonnotte *et al.*, 1996). Another study found no defect of either production of endogenous IL-12 by *S. aureus* Cowan-stimulated PBMC, or of responsiveness of PBMC to exogenous IL-12 in recipients of autologous grafts (Guillaume *et al.*, 1996). IL-18, a cytokine produced by macrophages which induces IFN-γ production from Th1 cells, especially in collaboration with IL-12, is elevated in the serum during acute GVHD (Fujimori *et al.*, 2000) (Figs. 13.20 and 13.21).

Engraftment syndrome

The occurrence of a potentially lethal syndrome accompanying prompt hematologic recovery after autologous or (less com-

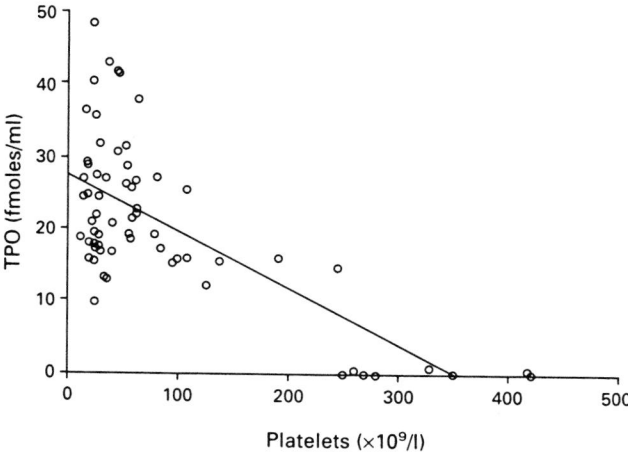

Fig. 13.19. Inverse correlation between serum level of TPO and absolute platelet count (r = –0.70, P < .001). Reproduced, with permission, from Shimazaki *et al.* (1997).

monly) allogeneic marrow or blood stem cell transplantation has been reported and is known as the engraftment syndrome (Lee *et al.*, 1995; Moreb *et al.*, 1997; Nurnberger *et al.*, 1997; reviewed in Spitzer, 2001). Characteristic clinical findings include noninfectious fever, skin rash, capillary leak, and pulmonary infiltrates (Ravenel *et al.*, 2000) occurring during the early engraftment period soon after infusion of the stem cells (Cahill *et al.*, 1996). Neutrophil recovery occurred earlier and more steeply in patients with the syndrome than in those without (Fig. 13.22) (Edenfield *et al.*, 2000). Distinction from GVHD in the allogeneic setting can be difficult. It can occur after non-myeloablative conditioning regimens. A proposal for a uniform definition of engraftment syndrome (Spitzer, 2001) included the following as major criteria: temperature >38.5°C with no identifiable infectious etiology; erythrodermatous rash involving >25% of body surface area and not attributable to medication; and non-cardiogenic pulmonary edema manifested by diffuse pulmonary infiltrates consistent with this diagnosis, and hypoxia. The incidence of the syndrome varies widely in different reports at the present time. In one study of 248 patients, 59% had both skin rash and noninfectious neutropenic fever, and were thought to have the syndrome. In this series, posttransplant G-CSF administration increased the incidence to 79%. The median time of onset was 7 (range 4 to 22) days posttransplant with a median duration of 11 (range 4 to 28) days

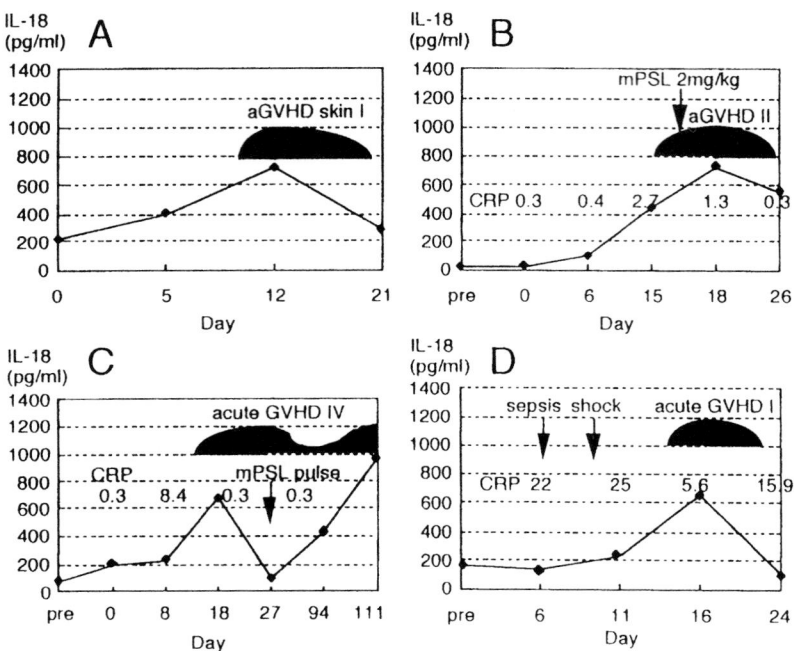

Fig. 13.21. Typical examples of the changes in serum IL-18 levels in BMT patients with acute GVHD. (A) IL-18 levels during grade I acute skin GVHD. (B) IL-18 levels during grade II aGVHD. (C) IL-18 levels during grade IV aGVHD. (D) IL-18 levels during sepsis and grade I aGVHD. Reproduced, with permission, from Fujimori *et al.* (2000).

(Lee *et al.*, 1995). In another series of 61 patients, only 6 developed a syndrome of noninfectious fever, fluid retention, and pulmonary infiltrates during the early phase of neutrophil recovery (Ravoet *et al.*, 1996). The clinical condition of one patient improved spontaneously while the syndrome resolved within 48 hours after initiation of corticosteroid therapy in four others. In Lee's series, prompt defervescence of fever occurred in > 90% patients within a median of 1 day after initiating corticosteroid

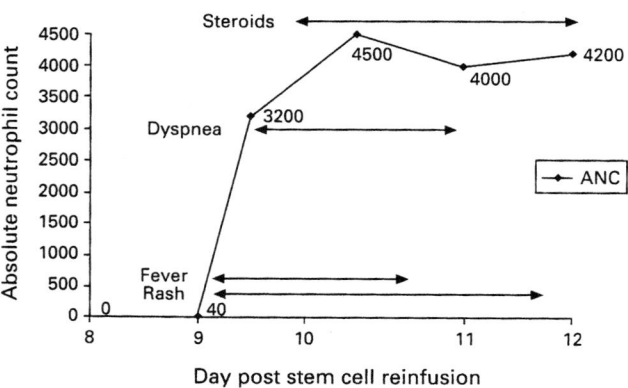

Fig. 13.22. Time course of neutrophil recovery in a patient with engraftment syndrome. Neutrophil recovery in relation to clinical features of the engraftment syndrome. A two log increment in absolute neutrophil count (ANC) occurred over the span of 12h and coincided with clinical deterioration. Reproduced, with permission, from Edenfield *et al.* (2000).

treatment. The reported mortality rate after autologous transplantation has also been variable, but is higher in those with a capillary leak component. Most deaths have occurred as a result of respiratory failure (Capizzi *et al.*, 2001). Engraftment syndrome (defined in this report as unexplained erythematous rash, non-infectious fever and generalized non-focal and transiently increased weakness within 60 days of transplant) was described in 5/19 (26%) patients undergoing autologous HSC transplant for multiple sclerosis (Oyama *et al.*, 2002). Clinically and histologicaly, the rash was very similar to that of acute GVHD. Pulmonary symptoms including rhinorrhea, dry cough, and transient oxygen desaturation occurred in two patients and eosinophilia in three. The duration of fever and rash varied from 5 to 14 days. In this study the authors did not distinguish between engraftment syndrome and autologous GVHD.

Hematopoietic chimerism (and see Chapter 30)

After allogeneic HSC transplantation the recipient's hematopoietic system may be entirely of donor-origin (donor chimerism), entirely of recipient-origin (graft rejection with autologous recovery), or a mixture of donor and recipient (host) elements (mixed chimerism). While mixed chimerism is the term used to describe the detection of host (recipient) cells in a given cellular compartment (for example 10% of circulating lymphocytes), the term split chimerism is used when one (or more) whole lineage is of host origin and one (or more) is of donor origin. Examples are shown in Fig.

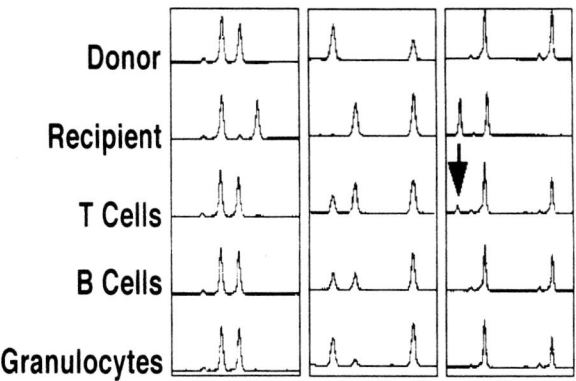

Fig. 13.23. Analysis of fluorescent polymerase chain reaction (PCR) products using the ABI 310 sequencer: lineage-specific chimerism analyses from three separate patients following nonmyeloablative transplantation using microsatellite PCR. The arrow indicates persistence of recipient cells. Three separate patterns of chimerism are shown. The left panel shows full donor chimerism following transplantation, the center panel indicates mixed chimerism in all lineages, and the right panel shows mixed chimerism in the T-cell lineage alone. Stutter peaks can be seen in the donor and recipient alleles in the left and right panels. Reproduced, with permission, from Antin *et al.* (2001).

13.23. *Microchimerism* is a term used to describe a situation in which highly sensitive techniques detect <1% host cells. Recent studies have shown that persistence or reappearance of recipient hematopoietic elements is not uncommon. It can be, but is not necessarily, associated with graft rejection or disease relapse; in many instances mixed chimerism may coexist with clinical remission.

Guidelines developed under the sponsorship of the National Marrow Donor Program and the International Bone Marrow Transplant Registry (Antin *et al.,* 2001) have suggested the following:

1. Chimerism analysis should use sensitive, informative techniques such as short tandem repeats (STRs) or variable number tandem repeats (VNTRs).
2. Periperal blood cells are generally more useful than marrow cells for chimerism analysis.
3. Lineage-specific chimerism should be considered the assay of choice in the setting of non-myeloablative and reduced-intensity conditioning (Fig. 13.23).
4. The use of T-cell depletion, nonmyeloablative or reduced intensity conditioning, or novel GVHD prophylactic regimens warrants chimerism analysis at 1, 3, 6, and 12 months posttransplant, because interventions such as donor lymphocyte infusions may depend on chimerism status.
5. After nonmyeloablative conditioning regimens, the early patterns of chimerism may predict either GVHD (increasing donor chimerism) or graft loss (T-cell chimerism declining to <20% donor cells). Therefore, more frequent (every 2 to 4 weeks) peripheral blood analysis may be warranted.

6. For nonmalignant disorders, chimerism status should generally be evaluated 1, 2, and 3 months after transplantation. Interventions to enhance donor engraftment must be considered on a disease-specific basis in relation to concurrent GVHD and clinical rationale.

Numerous methods have been used to evaluate the origin of hematopoietic engraftment following allogeneic transplantation including red blood cell phenotyping, immunoglobulin allotyping, cytogenetic analysis, fluorescence in situ hybridization, restriction fragment length polymorphisms (usually with Southern blotting techniques), and mini-satellite or micro-satellite analysis [often employing polymerase chain reaction (PCR)] techniques. Each of these techniques has one or more limitations such as intensity of labor, sensitivity of detection, or degree of informativeness.

Comparison of molecular methodologies

DNA typing is now widely used to document engraftment and degree of chimerism after allogeneic hematopoietic stem cell transplantation. Most DNA typing procedures discriminate allogeneic engraftment on the basis of DNA length polymorphisms or sequence variations found in a variable number of tandem repeat (VNTR) loci, or the presence of Y chromosome-specific DNA. In some sex-mismatched transplant situations Y-specific DNA probing has been shown to be an efficient way to assess chimerism. In other situations, the analysis of highly polymorphic regions found in the human genome ("mini-satellites" and " micro-satellites") has proved useful. VNTR alleles are highly variable and inherited in a Mendelian fashion, making them excellent markers for the generation of specific DNA typing profiles. Such highly polymorphic tandemly repeated "mini-satellite" or "micro-satellite" loci are abundant in the human genome. The core size of repeating units can range from 2 to 5 bases for the latter and from 8 to 70 bases for the former. The discrimination potential for each locus depends on the number of observable alleles present in any given population and on the capacity to resolve alleles by gel electrophoresis. Some of these polymorphic loci are amenable to PCR amplification and are sometimes referred to as amplified fragment length polymorphisms (AmpFLPs) and short tandem repeats (STRs). One study compared three types of VNTR analysis and Y chromosome DNA detection to assess the strengths and limitations of each approach after allografting (Leclair *et al.,* 1995). In this study, chimerism was assessed in eight recipients posttransplant. Samples were subjected to 6 RFLP loci analysis using radioactivity, 2 AmpFLP loci analysis using a silver stain mode of detection, 12 STR loci analysis using fluorescence detection, and Y chromosome analysis. In sex-mismatched transplants with a female donor, Y chromosome probing proved most efficient. In all other cases, AmpFLPs proved to be a rapid and efficient procedure with sufficient discriminating capability and sensitivity to warrant its use in clinical settings. STRs were found to be a rapid procedure as well, but required a large loci complement to discriminate efficiently under the conditions of the study, and did not detect all cases of mixed chimerism. RFLPs were clearly superior at discriminating siblings but were found to be time-consuming and served best in cases where AmpFLP and STR analyses failed. The value of Y chromosome-specific probing was confirmed in another study by Petit and colleagues (1994). In this study, 24 male patients who had received marrow from a female donor and who demonstrated completed donor chimerism when analyzed by PCR amplification of mini-satellite sequences were also studied by PCR amplification of the Y chromosome-specific DYZ 1 sequence. Residual recipient male cells were detected in all peripheral blood samples collected within 1 year posttransplant. These residual cells were present in both the lymphocyte and polymorphonuclear fractions. Sensitivity of the technique was 0.01%. The sensitivity limit for the detection of residual recipient cells using PCR amplification of mini-satellite sequences is of the order of 0.1% to 1%. A PCR-based assay that can detect one male cell in one million female cells has recently been described (Pugatsch et al., 1996).

Another study also compared VNTR PCR analysis and RFLP using Southern blotting (Sreenan et al., 1997). VNTR analysis showed complete chimerism in 68 samples, mixed chimerism in 9 samples, and recurrence of the original malignancy in 2. This agreed with the RFLP results in 80% of the samples. Cost analysis revealed approximately 50% savings with the use of VNTR. VNTR was considered a viable alternative to RFLP in the detection of chimerism posttransplant and offered substantial cost savings, a fast turnaround time, easier preparation of the DNA, smaller DNA requirements, and the elimination of radioisotopes and cumbersome restriction enzymes. Using a single PCR that simultaneously amplified four micro-satellites, Oberkircher and colleagues (1995) were able to identify an informative locus in 48 of 50 consecutive recipient-donor pairs. Donor chimerism of as little as 0.5% could be detected, and donor chimerism of 10% could be detected in as few as 100 cells.

Another useful technique is fluorescence in situ hybridization (FISH) using probes for X and Y chromosomes or for disease-related rearrangements such as BCR-ABL. FISH can detect minimal residual disease or chromosome rearrangements even in interface nuclei. This has an advantage over conventional cytogenetic techniques that do not provide any information about G_0 cells or in patients who are severely pancytopenic or transfusion-dependent, or in sex-matched cases when a chromosome marker is not present. One study of 33 patients showed that recipient cells were invariably present posttransplant and that stable minimal residual disease was associated with clinical and hematologic remission while a progressive increase of host cells was related to disease relapse (Pilka et al., 1996). FISH can be combined with immune phenotyping in order to examine specific cell types (Hessel et al., 1996) (and see Chapter 103).

Finally, restriction endonuclease in situ digestion (REISD) has been described for analysis of chimerism posttransplant.

This technique can analyze polymorphisms of metaphase chromosomes and interphase nuclei (Buno et al., 1996; Diez-Martin et al., 1996; Gosalvez et al., 1996).

Kinetics and incidence of mixed chimerism

Using FISH with X and Y probes indirectly labeled with rhodamine and fluorescine isothiocyanate, respectively, Lapointe and colleagues (1996) detected the presence of donor neutrophils as early as 24 hours after allogeneic marrow infusion followed by a significant expansion at 48 hours. At 96 hours posttransplant, the median percentage of donor neutrophils was greater than 90%. During this time, however, most of the lymphocytes present were of recipient origin. Starting at day 5 posttransplant, a significant expansion in the number of donor lymphocytes occurred in most patients. Almost complete chimerism for the myeloid and lymphoid lineages was established at days 10 and 25 posttransplant, respectively. Thus, there appeared to be a distinct biphasic pattern of myeloid and lymphoid engraftment after HLA-identical family member transplantation. Using PCR for STRs, Frankel and colleagues (1996) demonstrated full donor chimerism between day 9 and 14 in HLA-matched allogeneic blood stem cell recipients and between day 14 and 16 in HLA-matched allogeneic bone marrow transplant recipients. The initial rise in the white blood count occurred within 3 days of the onset of full chimerism. Kögler and colleagues (1995), using in situ hybridization (for X and Y chromosomes) combined with simultaneous immunophenotypic analysis for CD3+, CD4+, CD8+, CD20+, CD34+, and CD10+ cells found mixed chimerism in the T-cell populations (median 26% host cells) and in the myelomonocytic cell population (median 16% host cells) from day 7 posttransplant. By days 14 to 18 posttransplant this mixed chimerism had reduced to 18% host T cells and 7% host myelomonocytic cells. Beyond day 21, stable donor chimerism for T cells, myelomonocytic cells, and granulocytes was observed in 7 of the 8 patients, although 0.5 to 1% host cells of different lineages were detectable in 5 of the 8 patients at later time points (beyond day 100). Another study using FISH and immunophenotyping described the appearance of donor-type Langerhans cells and the persistence of host-type Langerhans cells at various times posttransplant (36 to 1,395 days). Complete donor chimerism of Langerhans cells could not be detected in any case. The frequency of host Langerhans cells ranged from 7% to 92% and showed no correlation with time posttransplant (Hessel et al., 1996).

Using a quantitative, nonisotopic method involving VNTR and STR markers, Scharf et al. (1995) found 7 of 32 allograft recipients to be informative for some degree of mixed chimerism, and again found different degrees of engraftment in myeloid and T-cell populations.

For patients prepared with cyclophosphamide and total body irradiation, early studies using red cell antigen and enzyme testing, immunoglobulin allotype testing, direct marrow metaphase karyotyping analysis, and karyotyping of mitogen-stimulated mononuclear cell preparations showed that, by 3 months posttransplant, the majority of erythrocytes, B cells, dividing marrow cells, and blood T cells, respectively, are predominantly of donor origin. Additionally, alveolar macrophages (Thomas et al., 1976), hepatic Kupffer cells (Gale et al., 1978), cutaneous Langerhans cells (Volc-Platzer et al., 1984), circulating endothelial progenitor cells (positive for von Willebrand factor, CD31 and Flk-1/KDR) (Ikpeazu et al., 2000; Hebbel et al., 2000) and mast cells (Fodinger et al., 1994) have been shown to be of donor origin posttransplant.

In another early report, a minority of patients with leukemia were shown to be mixed chimeras with residual cells of host origin present (Branch et al., 1982). Interestingly, this appeared to have conferred a survival advantage, with a lower than expected incidence of recurrent leukemia. Again in earlier studies, in patients with severe aplastic anemia conditioned with cyclophosphamide, the incidence of mixed chimerism was high in some (Hill et al., 1986) but not all (Keable et al., 1989) reports. With the advent of the molecular era for chimerism testing, some of these data have been revised, and are reviewed below.

Hibi and colleagues (1997) found mononuclear cells in the cerebrospinal fluid to be of donor origin 19 to 97 days posttransplant when hematopoiesis was entirely of donor origin.

Biological correlates of mixed chimerism

The first reports of the use of molecular technology for assessing chimerism status after allogeneic transplant were by Ginsburg et al. (1985), and Blazar et al. (1985). Using flow cytometry and PCR amplification of VNTRs, van Leeuwen et al. (1994) studied 46 recipients of HLA-identical, T-replete transplants and 7 recipients of HLA-non-identical T-cell-depleted transplants. Those recipients who were children showed either stable mixed chimerism ($n = 14$), transient mixed T-lymphoid chimerism ($n = 9$), or complete chimerism ($n = 30$) in peripheral blood studies. In bone marrow studies only donor-type cells were found in children with either complete chimerism or transient mixed T-lymphoid chimerism. Persistence of host-type hematopoiesis was significantly related to a lower age of the recipient, the type of conditioning regimen used, a lower total body irradiation dose, T-cell depletion of the bone marrow, and the use of cyclosporine for GVHD prophylaxis. No significant differences were found between patients with stable mixed chimerism and those without persistent host-type hematopoiesis with respect to leukemia or survival, and the authors concluded that ablation of host-type hematopoiesis was not compulsory for survival long-term after allogeneic transplantation. Fishleder et al. (1992) reported an incidence of mixed chimerism in 15% of recipients of T-replete, HLA-identical transplant recipients prepared with busulfan and cyclophosphamide. In contrast, Yamaguchi et al. (1995) reported three recipients of allogeneic transplants conditioned with busulfan and cyclophosphamide in whom early recovery of host-derived hematopoiesis ensued.

In recipients given a fixed low number of T cells in partially T-cell-depleted marrow grafts (1×10^5 donor T cells/kg recipient weight), all T cells in all 45 patients studied from 6 months posttransplant (by PCR amplification of VNTR) were exclusively of donor origin. Furthermore, the T cells of 15 patients who relapsed posttransplant were also exclusively of donor origin (Verdonck et al., 1996). In contrast, Hamblin et al. (1996) studied 14 patients given the panleukocyte antibody CAMPATH 1G for up to 9 days pretransplant as part of the conditioning regimen (to minimize the risk of graft rejection) (Group 1), and 9 patients in whom CAMPATH 1G was continued posttransplant until day +5 (to reduce the risk of GVHD) (Group 2). Three patients developed late graft failure in Group 1, and 2 patients had early graft failure in Group 2. PCR of STRs showed that of 11 patients with initial neutrophil engraftment, only 1 had 100% donor hematopoiesis at all times, and the remaining patients had either transient mixed chimerism or persistence of recipient cells. It was concluded that in vivo CAMPATH-1G administration was associated with a high incidence of mixed chimerism that tipped the balance away from GVHD and toward graft rejection. A case report of a 21-year-old adult with AML given a haplo-identical, T-cell-depleted marrow transplant after conditioning with TBI, thiotepa, ATG, and cyclophosphamide showed by DNA polymorphism analysis that granulocytes and monocytes were of donor origin but that T and B cells were of host origin. The patient suffered from serious recurrent CMV infections until this mixed chimerism converted to full donor chimerism 2 years posttransplant (Terenzi et al., 1996).

The association of mixed chimerism with GVHD, graft rejection, disease recurrence, and survival was investigated in 116 patients with aplastic anemia and 197 patients with CML transplanted with T-replete marrow from an HLA-identical sibling donor of the opposite sex (Huss et al., 1996). The patients with aplastic anemia were conditioned with cyclophosphamide while those with CML were conditioned with a combination of cyclophosphamide and TBI or busulfan. Fifty-four percent of the patients with aplastic anemia and 51% of those with CML were categorized as having mixed chimerism 14 days or later posttransplant. The dose of TBI was inversely correlated with the development of mixed chimerism among the CML patients. No other patient or transplant-related parameter was identified that contributed significantly to the development of mixed chimerism. The incidence of rejection was higher, but not significantly so, in patients with aplastic anemia who were mixed chimeras. The incidence of leukemic relapse in patients with CML who were mixed chimeras was increased only if mixed chimerism occurred after day 100. The incidence of acute GVHD grades II–IV was lower in mixed chimeras than in complete chimeras, but this difference was statistically significant only for patients with aplastic anemia given single-agent GVHD prophylaxis. Mixed chimeras in that group also had better survival than complete chimeras. Among patients with CML, both overall survival and leukemia-free survival was significantly superior in mixed compared to complete chimeras. These authors concluded that mixed chimerism was frequent among patients with aplastic anemia and with CML and was not uniformly associated with graft failure or leukemic relapse. It is clear that the interaction between the conditioning regimen, GVHD prophylaxis regimen, and the degree of chimerism is complex.

A child with severe combined immune deficiency given a paternal, T-cell-depleted marrow transplant had recipient metaphases only by marrow karyotyping at 1 year posttransplant, but subsequent karyotyping of PHA-stimulated peripheral blood mononuclear cells showed donor metaphases only. Molecular analysis, however, confirmed mixed chimerism in the blood. Granulocytes were of recipient origin and mononuclear cells of mixed origin; T cells were of donor origin, whereas B cells and myeloid cells were mainly of recipient origin (Lau *et al.*, 1995). The following reports have also shown an apparent increase in mixed chimerism following T-cell-depleted allogeneic marrow transplants: Bretagne *et al.*, 1987; Schattenberg *et al.*, 1989; Roy *et al.*, 1990; Lawler *et al.*, 1991; Roux *et al.*, 1992 and 1993.

Recently, mixed chimerism received renewed interest, as non-myeloablative conditioning regimens were developed with a goal of establishing mixed chimerism (Storb *et al.*, 1997; Storb *et al.*, 1999; Sykes *et al.*, 1999; McSweeney & Storb, 1999). However, mixed chimerism proved transient in most patients, resulting either in rejection or in complete chimerism (McSweeney *et al.*, 2001). The development of intensified immunosuppressive conditioning using fludarabine seems to result in complete chimerism in the majority of patients.

Reports in specific diseases

Leukemia

Mixed T-cell chimerism has been associated with the persistence of minimal residual disease and leukemia relapse after HLA-identical sibling marrow transplantation for CML (MacKinnon *et al.*, 1994). Molloy *et al.* (1996) studied 23 children given unrelated donor transplants for ALL. Of these, two had evidence (by PCR STR) of complete donor engraftment at all times and eight showed stable low-level mixed chimerism (less than 1% recipient hematopoiesis). All 10 of these patients remained in remission with a minimum follow-up of 24 months at the time of the report. In contrast, 13 patients in this study demonstrated a progressive return of recipient hematopoiesis and 5 of these relapsed 4 to 9 months posttransplant. These findings of a high level of mixed chimerism in some patients were similar to those in recipients of HLA-identical sibling transplants receiving T-cell-depleted marrow grafts, and in contrast to findings after T-replete sibling grafts. Stable donor engraftment or low level mixed chimerism correlated with continued remission; detection of a progressive return of host cells did not universally correlate with relapse but highlighted those at greatest risk. It appears that the clinical impact of mixed chimerism depends to some extent on the underlying hematologic malig-

nancy and the influence of any GVL effect in mediating remission posttransplant of that malignancy. A slightly different pattern, however, was found in another study of pediatric recipients of allogeneic transplants for ALL, in whom donor chimerism or transient mixed chimerism was also associated with long-term leukemia-free survival, but relapse was always associated with progressive increase in host hematopoiesis (Ramirez *et al.*, 1996).

One study has reported DNA-based chimerism studies in three patients given HLA-identical sibling transplants for chronic lymphatic leukemia (Martino *et al.*, 1995). One patient in continuous complete remission demonstrated complete donor chimerism for 110 months posttransplant; another showed mixed chimerism with minimal residual disease at 3 months posttransplant, but with conversion to complete remission and complete donor chimerism at 6 months, suggesting an ongoing GVL effect. The third patient showed persistent mixed chimerism up to 24 months posttransplant, although the patient remained in complete remission with no evidence of minimal residual CLL.

Severe aplastic anemia

Seventeen patients who received allogeneic transplants for severe aplastic anemia had chimerism studies performed using PCR and Southern blotting for VNTR loci. At a median of 4 years posttransplant, all patients had normal blood counts, and those conditioned with radiation-based regimens showed full donor chimerism. Conversely, of five patients who received only cyclophosphamide for conditioning, two had late graft failure at 2.4 and 3 years posttransplant, and one of these had mixed chimerism, first detected 1 month posttransplant (Casado *et al.*, 1996).

Fanconi anemia

Nineteen patients given allogeneic transplants after low-dose cyclophosphamide and thoracoabdominal irradiation were analyzed for chimerism posttransplant. All but one engrafted successfully, and engraftment was complete early after transplant in 12 of the 18. A persistence of a small proportion of host cells was detected in 6 (using PCR for mini-satellite loci). This mixed chimerism was transient in 5 of the 6 (Socie *et al.*, 1993).

Thalassemia

Of 55 patients given an allogeneic transplant for beta thalassemia major, graft rejection occurred in 20 patients, evidence of host hematopoiesis disappeared in a further 20, and mixed chimerism without the need for packed cell transfusion persisted for 1 to 7 years in the remaining 15. In three patients with stable mixed chimerism for 4, 5, and 7 years, respectively, host hematopoiesis fluctuated between 25% and 75%. Despite this, donor pattern betaglobin chain synthesis maintained hemoglobin levels between 10 and 13.5 g/dl without transfusion. In these three patients, PCR for VNTR and FISH analysis revealed the coexistence of donor and host cells in different blood cell populations (CD2$^+$, CD4$^+$, CD8$^+$, CD19$^+$, granulocytes, glycophorin-A$^+$ cells, CD33$^+$ cells, and BFU-E; (Andreani *et al.*, 1996).

Early graft failure

The transplanted stem cells may fail to establish themselves permanently. Two distinct mechanisms can lead to graft failure after allogeneic transplantation (see also Chapters 12 and 70). Both represent the action of host immunity surviving the pretransplant chemotherapy or chemoradiotherapy. One mechanism involves sensitization of recipients to minor and/or major histocompatibility antigens of the stem cell donor before transplantation, usually by transfusions of blood products. Preceding transfusions jeopardize a subsequent allograft through the action of specifically sensitized T cells. Once sensitized, host T cells are less likely to be destroyed by high doses of chemotherapy or chemoradiotherapy, enabling them to reject the transplanted stem cells.

The second mechanism, termed graft resistance or allogeneic resistance, does not require prior sensitization to donor histocompatibility antigens in order to destroy the foreign stem cell graft. Host cells involved in resistance may not be typical T cells. They recognize codominantly inherited donor antigens associated with the major histocompatibility complex. In recipients of HLA-identical sibling marrow transplants for hematologic malignancy who are conditioned with cyclophosphamide and total body irradiation, the incidence of early graft failure is less than 1% (Thomas *et al.*, 1977). In contrast, patients with severe aplastic anemia conditioned with cyclophosphamide alone, reconstituted with HLA-identical sibling marrow and immune suppressed with MTX, had an initial graft failure rate of 16% (Storb *et al.*, 1974). This appeared to be due to recipient sensitization to the marrow donor by preceding random blood transfusions. Different marrow transplant centers have utilized different maneuvers to overcome this. Such maneuvers have included the addition of donor buffy coat cells (as a source of both stem cells and T lymphocytes) (Storb *et al.*, 1982), the substitution of cyclosporine for MTX as pre-and posttransplant immune suppression (Hows *et al.*, 1982), and the addition of total lymphoid (Ramsay *et al.*, 1984), thoracoabdominal (Devergie & Gluckman, 1982), or low-dose total body (UCLA BMT Team, 1981) irradiation to cyclophosphamide. With each, the graft rejection rate has fallen to approximately 10%. More recently the combination of cyclosporine and antithymocyte globulin as the pretransplant preparative regimen has been associated with an even lower rate of early graft failure (see Chapter 58).

T-cell depletion of donor marrow results not only in a slower rate of engraftment, but in an appreciable graft failure rate in recipients of HLA-identical sibling marrow, even when employed with preparatory regimens that include high-dose total body irradiation (Trigg *et al.*, 1985; Martin *et al.*, 1988). Partial (in stead of complete) T-cell depletion, however, has consistently been associated with favorable engraftment, comparing well to T-cell-replete BMT (Verdonck *et al.*, 1994; Urbano-Isipizua *et al.*, 2001). A lower threshold of 1–3×10^5 CD3$^+$ T-cells/kg seems required to prevent graft failure in those studies (Figure 13.24).

In recipients of HLA-nonidentical family member transplants (Powles *et al.*, 1983; Beatty *et al.*, 1985) or matched unrelated donor transplants receiving non-T-cell-depleted marrow after preparation with cyclophosphamide and total body irradiation, the incidence of graft failure has been significantly higher than with non-T-cell-depleted HLA-identical sibling transplantation. The incidence of graft failure seems related to

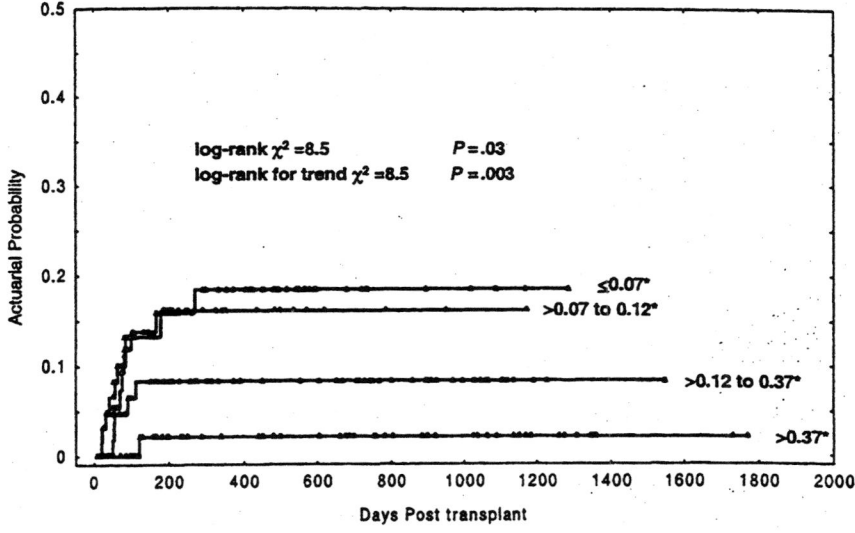

Fig. 13.24. Actuarial probability of graft failure by grouping the number of CD3+ cells infused to the patients in quarties. *indicates x 10^6/kg. (Reproduced, with permission, Urbano-Ispizua, 2001).

the degree of HLA disparity (Anasetti *et al.*, 1989). It is likely that allogeneic resistance to mismatched marrow cells plays an etiologic role. Additionally, the presence of cytotoxic antibodies to donor HLA antigens has also been associated with graft rejection in such patients (Anasetti *et al.*, 1989). The incidence of graft failure when non-HLA-identical marrow is depleted of T cells prior to infusion is even higher, reaching an incidence of approximately 50% in one study (Trigg *et al.*, 1985). In a retrospective analysis the incidence of primary graft failure in recipients of HLA-matched sibling transplants, HLA-matched unrelated donor transplants, and partially HLA-matched unrelated donor transplants was 5%, 6%, and 15%, respectively ($P =. 06$) (Davies *et al.*, 1994). Multivariate analysis of factors relating to primary graft failure showed the only significant variable to be full or partial serologic HLA-matching in the unrelated donor group.

Finally, the degree of marrow fibrosis pretransplant has shown a positive correlation with the incidence of graft failure. GM-CSF has been reported to be useful in the treatment of neutropenia associated with graft failure after autologous or allogeneic transplantation (see Chapters 32 and 70). G-CSF has occasionally been reported to be useful in cases that have initially responded to GM-CSF but subsequently lost this response (Boulad *et al.*, 1994).

Late graft failure

Late graft failure has been described in recipients of HLA-identical sibling marrow transplants prepared with cyclophosphamide and immune suppressed with cyclosporine for severe aplastic anemia (Hows *et al.*, 1985). This was thought to be associated with too rapid a taper in the cyclosporine dosage, since in some cases it was reversible with reintroduction of an increased immune suppressive regimen. Late graft failure has also been reported in patients with hematologic malignancy who were given T-cell-depleted HLA-identical sibling marrow after preparation with cyclophosphamide and total body irradiation (Waldmann *et al.*, 1984), and in recipients of T-depleted and T-replete allogeneic marrow from donors other than HLA-identical siblings. The incidence of secondary graft failure in recipients of HLA-identical sibling transplants, in recipients of HLA-identical unrelated donor transplants, and in recipients of partially HLA-identical unrelated donor transplants was 0.7%, 15%, and 25%, respectively ($P < .0001$) (Davies *et al.*, 1994). Multivariate analysis of secondary graft failure in this study showed the only significant variable to be a related or unrelated donor.

Aplasia associated with donor lymphocyte infusions

With the increasing use of donor lymphocyte infusions to treat recurrence of hematologic malignancy relapsed postallografting (see Chapter 65), pancytopenia and aplasia have been seen posttransplant more commonly than previously; they are assumed to represent a GVHD attack by mature donor T cells on the bone marrow. This development may occur a number of months after the donor lymphocyte infusion (Garicochea *et al.*, 1994). It may require reinfusion of donor hematopoietic stem cells.

Hypersplenism

The most common causes of cytopenia after hematopoietic stem cell transplantation are sepsis, viral infection, GVHD, drug-induced marrow suppression, and recurrence of the underlying disease. The role of the spleen and delayed engraftment after allografting has been noted, and Grigg and colleagues (1992) first reported three patients with progressive pancytopenia, normocellular marrow, and progressive splenomegaly who improved after splenectomy. An additional four patients who responded to splenectomy have also been reported (von Bueltzingsloewen *et al.*, 1994). All four received marrow from an HLA-compatible sibling for CML in three cases and thalassemia in one case. Conditioning utilized either cyclophosphamide and total body irradiation or busulfan/cyclophosphamide. Platelet recovery above $20 \times 10^9/l$ was delayed or did not occur in all four, and the ANC prior to splenectomy ranged between 0.18 and $0.5 \times 10^9/l$. Bone marrow cellularity was normal in all four, and splenomegaly was present in two posttransplant. Splenectomy was carried out at days 114, 140, 168, and 220, respectively; 2 weeks postsplenectomy the ANC ranged between 1.3 and $19.8 \times 10^9/l$. Three of the four remained in remission at 36 to 51 months posttransplant, although it should be noted that one patient died suddenly at 29 months, possibly as a result of fulminant postsplenectomy septicemia. Confirmatory reports have been published (Richard *et al.*, 1996).

Telomere length of blood cells posttransplant

Telomeres are the non-encoding regions of DNA at each end of eukaryotic chromosomes. They consist of oligonucleotide repeats and associated protein. They mediate important chromosome/nuclear matrix interactions, protect encoding DNA from enzymatic breakdown, prevent dicentric fusion and other aberrations and interact with cell cycle regulatory mechanisms. Telomeres normally shorten during cell replication and they have been likenened to a "mitotic clock" – their length being a marker of replication history and a measure of remaining replicative potential.

Most studies of telomere length of circulating blood cells after autologous and allogeneic HSC transplantation have revealed significant shortening (Akiyama *et al.*, 1998; Nataro *et al.*, 1998; Wynn *et al.*, 1998; Shay, 1998; Wynn *et al.*, 1999), with donor age being a factor in the allogeneic recipients. In the study by Wynn (1999), telomere length in both neutrophils and T cells was shortened compared to that of the donor (by 0.6 and 0.5 kb, respectively). In another study 9 of 17 recipients of HLA-identical sibling marrow transplants exhibited a less than 1.0 kb shortening of granulocyte telomere length compared with their respective donors (Mathioudakis *et al.*, 2000). The biological significance of these findings is unclear. No difference was found in a study comparing allogeneic PBSC with marrow transplants (Robertson *et al.*, 2001). In this study telomere shortening occurred in the first year posttransplant. Furthermore, although reduced telomere length has been observed in several studies, progressive shortening during long-term follow-up probably does not occur and stem cell exhaustion is highly unlikely (De Pauw *et al.*, 2002).

Acceleration of hematopoietic reconstitution by hematopoietic growth factors

The existence of a series of glycoprotein hormones that regulate the proliferation and differentiation of hematopoietic progenitor cells has been known for some years (Fig. 13.1). Currently there are at least 20 molecularly cloned agents with regulatory activity on human hematopoiesis (including lymphopoiesis) (see Chapters 3 and 14). These include G-CSF, GM-CSF, M-CSF, IL-3 or multi-CSF, and erythropoietin. The cloning of the genes for these glycoproteins has enabled the confirmation (with the use of recombinant DNA-derived reagents) of studies previously performed using purified native molecules. Additional studies indicate that these molecules have a dramatic stimulatory effect on hematopoiesis in some in vivo models, as predicted from the in vitro experiments. For example, GM-CSF has been shown to elevate the circulating granulocyte count in primates (Donahue *et al.*, 1986) and in mice (Metcalf *et al.*, 1987). IL-3 has been shown to have panhematopoietic stimulatory activity in vivo in mice (Metcalf *et al.*, 1986). G-CSF has been shown to have hematopoietic stimulatory activity in mice (Moore & Warren, 1987), and erythropoietin has been shown to have marked erythropoietic stimulatory activity in humans (Eschbach *et al.*, 1987).

Studies utilizing these recombinant reagents after human stem cell transplantation have been reported (Sheridan *et al.*, 1989; Bensinger *et al.*, 1994). When compared to historical controls, both G-CSF and GM-CSF accelerated the rate of neutrophil recovery after autologous transplant. This translated into a lower incidence of fever, a decreased usage of antibiotics, and a shortened hospital stay.

G-CSF, GM-CSF, and M-CSF have likewise been shown to accelerate leukocyte recovery after allogeneic transplantation, and they do not appear to have an adverse effect on incidence of GVHD or leukemic relapse. Because of their high cost, cost-effectiveness analysis will be a required parameter for examination in prospectively controlled randomized trials.

The use of hematopoietic growth factors in autologous transplantation is more widely discussed in Chapter 31, and in allogeneic transplantation in Chapter 32.

References

Akiyama, M., Hoshi, Y., Sakurai, S. *et al.* (1998). Changes of tolomere length in children after hematopoietic stem cell transplantation. *Bone Marrow Transplantation*, **21**, 167–71.

Almeida-Porada, G., Porada, C.D., Tran, N., & Zanjani, E.D. (2000). Cotransplantation of human stromal cell progenitors into preimmune fetal sheep results in early appearance of human donor cells in circulation and boosts cell levels in bone marrow at later time points after transplantation. *Blood*, **95**, 3620–7.

Alter, B.P., Rappeport, J.M., Huisman, T.H. *et al.* (1976). Fetal erythropoiesis following bone marrow transplantation. *Blood*, **48**, 843–53.

Anasetti, C., Amos, D, Beatty, P.G. *et al.* (1989). Effect of HLA histocompatibility on engraftment of bone marrow transplants in patients with leukemia or lymphoma. *New England Journal of Medicine*, **320**, 197–204.

Andreani, M., Manna, M., Lucarelli, G. *et al.* (1996). Persistence of mixed chimerism in patients transplanted for the treatment of thalassemia. *Blood*, **87**, 3494–9.

Antin, J.H., Childs, R., Filipovich, A.H. *et al.* (2001). Establishment of complete and mixed donor chimerism after allogeneic lymphohematopoietic transplantation: recommendations from a workshop at the 2001 Tandem Meetings. *Biology of Blood and Marrow Transplantation*, **7**, 473–85.

Arnold, R., Schmeiser, T., Heit, W. *et al.* (1986). Hemopoietic reconstitution after bone marrow transplantation. *Experimental Hematology*, **14**, 271–7.

Atkinson, K., Biggs, J., Cooley, M. *et al.* (1987a). A comparative study of T cell depleted and non-depleted marrow transplantation for haematological malignancy. *Australian and New Zealand Journal of Medicine*, **17**, 16–23.

Atkinson, K., Biggs, J., Noble, G.S. *et al.* (1987). Preparative regimes for marrow transplantation containing busulphan are associated with haemorrhagic cystitis and hepatic veno-occlusive disease but a short duration of leukopenia and little oro-pharyngeal mucositis. *Bone Marrow Transplantation*, **2**, 385–94.

Atkinson, K., Biggs, J.C., Ting, A. *et al.* (1983). Cyclosporin A is associated with faster engraftment and less mucositis than methotrexate after allogeneic bone marrow transplantation. *British Journal of Haematology*, **53**, 265–70.

Atkinson, K., Downs, K., Ashby, M. *et al.* (1989). Recipients of HLA-identical sibling marrow transplants with severe aplastic anemia engraft more quickly, and those with chronic myeloid leukemia more slowly, than those with acute leukemia. *Bone Marrow Transplantation*, **4**, 23–7.

Atkinson, K., Downs, K., Golenia, M. *et al.* (1991). Prophylactic use of ganciclovir in allogeneic bone marrow transplantation: absence of clinical cytomegalovirus infection. *British Journal of Haematology*, **79**, 57–62.

Atkinson, K., Fay, K., Nivison-Smith, I., & Downs, K. (1997). Lenograstim administration to HLA-identical donor-recipient pairs to accelerate marrow recovery posttransplant. *Bone Marrow Transplantation*, **19**, 15–21.

Atkinson, K., Meyers, J.D., Storb, R. *et al.* (1980). Varicella-zoster virus infection after marrow transplantation for aplastic anemia or leukemia. *Transplantation*, **29**, 47–50.

Atkinson, K., Norrie, S., Chan, P. *et al.* (1985). Lack of correlation between nucleated bone marrow cell dose, marrow CFU-GM dose or marrow CFU-E dose and the rate of HLA-identical sibling marrow engraftment. *British Journal of Haematology*, **60**, 245–51.

Atkinson, K., Norrie, S., Chan, P. *et al.* (1986). Haemopoietic progenitor cell function after HLA-identical sibling bone marrow transplantation: influence of chronic graft-versus-host disease. *International Journal of Cell Cloning,* **4**, 203–20.

Atkinson, K., Seymour, R., Altavilla, N. *et al.* (1992). Cytokine activity after allogeneic bone marrow transplantation. IV. Production of mRNA for IL-3 and GM-CSF by mitogen-stimulated circulating mononuclear cells. *Bone Marrow Transplantation,* **9**, 175–83.

Atkinson, K., Storb, R., Prentice, R.L. *et al.* (1979). Analysis of late infections in 89 long-term survivors of bone marrow transplantation. *Blood,* **53**, 720–31.

Aversa, F., Tabilio, A., Terenzi, A. *et al.* (1994). Successful engraftment of T cell-depleted haploidentical "three-loci" incompatible transplants in leukemia patients by addition of recombinant human granulocyte colony-stimulating factor-mobilized peripheral blood progenitor cells to bone marrow inoculum. *Blood,* **84**, 3948–55.

Aversa, F., Tabilio, A., Velardi, A. *et al.* (1998). Treatment of high-risk acute leukemia with T cell-depleted stem cells from related donors with one fully mismatched HLA haplotype. *New England Journal of Medicine,* **339**, 1186–93.

Bacigalupo, A., Piaggio, G., Podesta, M. *et al.* (1995). Influence of marrow CFU-GM content on engraftment and survival after allogeneic bone marrow transplantation. *Bone Marrow Transplantation,* **15**, 221–6.

Bahceci, E., Read, E.J., Leitman, S. *et al.* (2000). CD34+ cell dose predicts relapse and survival after T-cell-depleted HLA-identical haematopoietic stem cell transplantation (HSCT) for haematologic malignancies. *British Journal of Haematology,* **108**, 408–14.

Bär, B.M.A.M., Van Dijk, V.A., Schattenberg, A. *et al.* (1995). Erythrocyte repopulation after major ABO incompatible transplantation with lymphocyte-depleted bone marrow. *Bone Marrow Transplantation,* **16**, 793–9.

Baranov, A.E., Selidovkin, G.D., Butturini, A., Gale, R.P. (1994). Hematopoietic recovery after 10-Gy acute total body radiation. *Blood,* **83**, 596–9.

Barker, J.N., Davies, S.M., DeFor, T. *et al.* (2001). Survival after transplantation of unrelated donor umbilical cord blood is comparable to that of human leukocyte antigen-matched unrelated donor bone marrow: results of a matched-pair analysis. *Blood,* **97**, 2957–61.

Barrett, A.J., Ringden, O., Zhang, M-J. *et al.* (2000). Effect of nucleated marrow cell dose on relapse and survival in identical twin bone marrow transplants for leukemia. *Blood,* **95**, 3323–7.

Beatty, P.G., Clift, R.A., Mickelson, E.M. *et al.* (1985). Marrow transplantation from related donors other than HLA-identical siblings. *New England Journal of Medicine,* **313**, 765–71.

Beguin, Y., Collignon, J., Laurent, C., & Fillet, G. (1996). Spontaneous complete remission and recovery of donor haemopoiesis without GVHD after relapse and apparent marrow graft rejection in poor-prognosis myelodysplastic syndrome. *British Journal of Haematology,* **94**, 507–9.

Bensinger, W.I., Longin, K., Appelbaum, F. *et al.* (1994). Peripheral blood stem cells collected after recombinant granulocyte colony-stimulating factor (rh G-CSF): an analysis of factors correlating with the tempo of engraftment after transplantation. *British Journal of Haematology,* **87**, 825–31.

Bensinger, W.I., Martin, P.J., Storer, B. *et al.* (2001). Transplantation of bone marrow as compared with peripheral-blood cells from HLA-identical relatives in patients with hematologic cancers. *New England Journal of Medicine,* **344**, 175–81.

Blazar, B.R., Orr, H.T., Arthur, D.C. *et al.* (1985). Restriction fragment length polymorphisms as markers of engraftment in allogeneic marrow transplantation. *Blood,* **66**, 1436–44.

Bonnotte, B., Burdiles, A.M., Chehimi, J. *et al.* (1996). Serum interleukin-12 levels in patients undergoing allogeneic or autologous bone marrow transplantation. *European Cytokine Network,* **7**, 389–94.

Boulad, F., Gillio, A., Small, T.N. (1994). Correction of neutropenia with rHuG-CSF after loss of response to rHuGM-CSF following autologous bone marrow transplant. *Bone Marrow Transplantation,* **13**, 661–3.

Brain, H.G., Sensenbrenner, L.L., Wright, S.K. *et al.* (1982). Bone marrow transplantation with major ABO blood group incompatibility using erythrocyte depletion of marrow prior to infusion. *Blood,* **60**, 420–5.

Branch, D.R., Gallagher, M.T., Forman, S.J. *et al.* (1982). Endogenous stem cell repopulation resulting in mixed hematopoietic chimerism following total body irradiation and marrow transplantation for acute leukemia. *Transplantation,* **34**, 226–8.

Bretagne, S., Vidaud, M., Kuentz, M. *et al.* (1987). Mixed blood chimerism in T-cell-depleted bone marrow transplant recipients: evaluation using DNA polymorphisms. *Blood,* **70**, 1692–5.

Broers, A.E.C., Gratama, J.W., Löwenberg, B. *et al.* (2002). Lymphocyte recovery following allogeneic stem cell transplantation: new possibilities for improvement. *Clinical and Applied Immunological Reviews,* in press.

Broers, A.E.C., Van der Holt, R., Van Esser, J.W.J. *et al.* (2000). Increased transplant-related morbidity and mortality in CMV-seropositive patients despite highly effective prevention of CMV disease after allogeneic T-cell-depleted stem cell transplantation. *Blood,* **95**, 2240–45.

Buno, I., Lopez-Fernandez, C., Fernandez, J.L. *et al.* (1996). Improving chimaerism quantification in bone marrow transplant recipients by image processing and analysis after restriction endonuclease in situ digestion (IPA-REISD). *Leukemia,* **10**, 1232–6.

Busch, F.W., Pilgrim, T.B., Krämer, A., & Ehninger, G. (1997). Plasma levels of granulocyte colony-stimulating factor in patients after allogeneic bone marrow transplantation for chronic myeloid leukemia correlate with engraftment of transplanted marrow. *Bone Marrow Transplantation,* **19**, 653–9.

Cahill, R.A., Spitzer, T.R., & Mazumder, A. (1996). Marrow engraftment and clinical manifestations of capillary leak syndrome. *Bone Marrow Transplantation,* **18**, 177–84.

Cairo, M.S., Suen, Y., Sender, L. *et al.* (1992). Circulating granulocyte colony-stimulating factor (G-CSF) levels after allogeneic and autologous bone marrow transplantation: endogenous G-CSF production correlates with myeloid engraftment. *Blood,* **79**, 1869–73.

Cao, T.M., Kusnierz-Glaz, C., Valone, F. *et al.* (2001). Rapid engraftment after allogeneic transplantation of density-enriched peripheral blood CD34+ cells in patients with advanced hematologic malignancies. *Cancer,* **91,** 2205–13.

Capizzi, S.S., Kumar, S., Huneke, N.E. *et al.* (2001). Peri-engraftment respiratory distress syndrome during autologous hematopoietic stem cell transplantation. *Bone Marrow Transplantation,* **27,** 1299–1303.

Carrigan, D.R. & Knox K.K. (1994). Human herpesvirus 6 (HHV-6) isolation from bone marrow: HHV-6 associated bone marrow suppression in bone marrow transplant patients. *Blood,* **84,** 3307–10.

Casado, L.F., Steegman, J.L., Pico, M. *et al.* (1996). A study of chimerism in long-term survivors after bone marrow transplantation for severe acquired aplastic anemia. *Bone Marrow Transplantation,* **18,** 405–9.

Champlin, R.E., Schmitz, N, Horowitz, M.M. *et al.* (2000). Blood stem cells compared with bone marrow as a source of hematopoietic cells for allogeneic transplantation. *Blood,* **95,** 3702–09.

Cilloni, D., Carlo-Stella, C., Falzetti, F. *et al.* (2000). Limited engraftment capacity of bone marrow-derived mesenchymal stem cell following T-cell-depleted hematopoietic stem cell transplantation. *Blood,* **96,** 3637–43.

Clark, R.A., Johnson, F.L., Klebanoff, S.I., & Thomas, E.D.(1976). Defective neutrophil chemotaxis in bone marrow transplant patients. *Journal of Clinical Investigation,* **58,** 22–31.

Cornelissen, J.J., Carston, M., Kollman, C. *et al.* (2001). Unrelated marrow transplantation for adult patients with poor-risk acute lymphoblastic leukemia: strong graft-versus-leukemia effect and risk factors determining outcome. *Blood,* **97,** 1572–77.

Cornelissen, J.J., Löwenberg, B. (2000). Develpments in T-cell depletion of allogeneic stem cell grafts. *Current Opinions in Haematology,* **7,** 348–52.

Cutler, C., Antin, J.H. (2001). Peripheral blood stem cells for allogeneic transplantation: a review. *Stem cells,* **19,** 108–17.

Cutler, C., Giri, S., Jeyapalan, S. *et al.* (2000). Incidence of acute and chronic graft-versus-host disease after allogeneic peripheral blood stem cell and bone marrow transplantation: a meta-analysis. *Blood,* **96,** 205a.

Da, W.M., Ma, D.D., Biggs, J.C. (1986). Studies of hemopoietic stromal fibroblastic colonies in patients undergoing bone marrow transplantation. *Experimental Hematology,* **14,** 266–70.

Davies, S.M., Kollman, C., Anasetti, C. *et al.* (2000). Engraftment and survival after unrelated-donor bone marrow transplantation: a report from the National Marrow Donor Program. *Blood,* **96,** 4096–4102.

Davies, S.M, Ramsay, N.K.C., Haake, R.J. *et al.* (1994). Comparison of engraftment in recipients of matched sibling or unrelated donor marrow allografts. *Bone Marrow Transplantation,* **13,** 51–7.

De Pauw, E.S., Otta, S.A., Wijnen, J.T. *et al.* (2002). Long-term follow-up of recipients of allogeneic bone marrow grafts reveals no progressive telemore shortening and provides no evidence for haematopoietic stem cell exhaustion. *British Journal of Haematology,* **116,** 491–6.

Deans, R.J & Mosely, A.B. (2000). Mesenchymal stem cells: biology and potential clinical uses. *Experimental Hematology,* **28,** 875–84.

Deeg, H.J., Meyers, J.D., Storb, R. *et al.* (1979). Effect of trimethoprim-sulfamethoxazole on hematological recovery after total body irradiation and autologous marrow infusion in dogs. *Transplantation,* **28,** 243–6.

Deeg, H.J., Storb, R., & Thomas, E.D. (1985). Cyclosporin as prophylaxis for graft-versus-host disease; a randomized study in patients undergoing bone marrow transplantation for acute non-lymphoblastic leukemia. *Blood,* **6,** 1325–34.

Demirer, T., Gooley, T., Buckner, C.D. *et al.* (1995). Influence of total nucleated cell dose from marrow harvest on outcome in patients with acute myelogenous leukemia undergoing autologous transplantation. *Bone Marrow Transplantation,* **15,** 907–13.

Dercksen, M.W., Gerritsen, W.R., Rodenhuis, S. *et al.* (1995). Expression of adhesion molecules on CD34$^+$ cells: CD34$^+$ L-selectin$^+$ cells predict a rapid platelet recovery after peripheral blood stem cell transplantation. *Blood,* **85,** 3313–19.

Devergie, A. & Gluckman, E. (1982). Bone marrow transplantation in severe aplastic anemia following cytoxan and thoraco-abdominal irradiation. *Experimental Hematology,* **10** (Suppl 10), 17–18.

Diez-Martin, J.L., Buno, I., Lopez-Fernandez, C. *et al.* (1996). Restriction endonuclease in situ digestions (REISD): a novel quantitative sex-independent method to analyze chimerism after bone marrow transplantation. *Experimental Hematology,* **24,** 1333–9.

Domenech, J., Linassier, C., Gihana, E. *et al.* (1995). Prolonged impairment of hematopoiesis after high-dose therapy followed by autologous bone marrow transplantation. *Blood,* **85,** 3320–7.

Di Nicola, M., Carlo-Stella, C., Magni *et al.* (2002). Human bone marrow stromal cells suppress T-lymphocyte proliferation induced by cellular or nonspecific mitogenic stimuli. *Blood,* **99,** 3838–43.

Dominietto, A., Raiola, A.M., van Lint, M.T. *et al.* (2001). Factors influencing haematological recovery after allogeneic haematopoietic stem cell transplants: graft-versus-host disease, donor type, cytomegalovirus infections and cell dose. *British Journal of Haematology,* **112,** 219–27.

Dominietto, A., Lamparelli, T., Raiola, A.M. *et al.* (2002). Transplant-related mortality and long-term graft function are significanly influenced by cell dose in patients undergoing marrow transplantation. *Blood,* **100,** 3930–4.

Donahue, R.E., Wang, E.A., Stone, D.K. *et al.* (1986). Stimulation of haematopoiesis in primates by continuous infusion of recombinant human GM-CSF. *Nature,* **321,** 872–5.

Donnenberg, A.D., Hess, A.D., Saral, R., & Santos, G.W. (1984). Adoptive transfer of immunity after allogeneic bone marrow transplant in man: role of immunization immediately after marrow infusion. *Experimental Hematology,* **12,** 390 (Abstract).

Edenfield, W.J., Moores, L.K., Goodwin, G. & Lee, N. (2000). An engraftment syndrome in autologous stem cell transplantation related to mononuclear cell dose. *Bone Marrow Transplantation,* **25,** 405–9.

Emerson, S.G., Sieff, C.A., Gross, R.G. *et al.* (1987). Decreased hematopoietic accessory cell function following bone marrow transplantation. *Experimental Hematology,* **15,** 1013–21.

Eschbach, J.W., Egrie, J.C., Downing, M.R. *et al.* (1987). Correction of the anemia of end-stage renal disease with recombinant human erythropoietin. Results of a phase I and II clinical trial. *New England Journal of Medicine,* **316,** 73–8.

Faille, A., Maraninchi, D., & Gluckman, E. (1981). Granulocyte progenitor compartments after allogeneic bone marrow grafts. *Scandinavian Journal of Haematology,* **26,** 202–14.

Faulkner, L.B., Lindsley, K.L., Kher, U. *et al.* (1996). High-dose chemotherapy with autologous marrow rescue for malignant brain tumors: analysis of the impact of prior chemotherapy and cranio-spinal irradiation on hematopoietic recovery. *Bone Marrow Transplantation,* **17,** 389–94.

Fishleder, A.J., Bolwell, B., & Lichten, A.E. (1992). Incidence of mixed chimerism using busulphan/cyclophosphamine containing regimens in allogeneic bone marrow transplantation. *Bone Marrow Transplantation,* **9,** 293–7.

Flowers, M.E.D., Leisering, W., Beach, K. *et al.* (2000). Granulocyte colony-stimulating factor given to donors before apheresis does not prevent aplasia in patients treated with donor leukocyte insuions for recurrent chronic myeloid leukemia after bone marrow transplantation. *Biology of Blood Marrow Transplantation,* **6,** 321–26.

Fodinger, M., Fritsch, G., Winkler, K. *et al.* (1994). Origin of human mast cells: development from transplanted hematopoietic stem cells after allogeneic bone marrow transplantation. *Blood,* **84,** 2954–9.

Frankel, W., Chan, A., Corringham R.E. *et al.* (1996). Detection of chimerism and early engraftment after allogeneic peripheral blood stem cell or bone marrow transplantation by short tandem repeats. *American Journal of Hematology,* **52,** 281–7.

Fujimori, Y., Takatsuka, H., Takemoto, Y. *et al.* (2000). Elevated interleukin (IL)-18 levels during acute graft-versus-host disease after allogeneic bone marrow transplantation. *British Journal of Haematology,* **109,** 652–7.

Gale, R.P., Sparkes, R.S., & Golde, D.W. (1978). Bone marrow origin of hepatic macrophages (Kupffer cells) in humans. *Nature,* **201,** 937–8.

Garicochea, B., van Rhee, F., Spencer, A. *et al.* (1994). Aplasia after donor lymphocyte infusion (DLI) for CML in relapse after sex-mismatched BMT: recovery of donor-type haempoiesis predicted by non-isotopic in situ hybridization (ISH). *British Journal of Haematology,* **88,** 400–2.

Gilabert R. & Ayats R. (1994). Human long-term bone marrow culture as a prognostic factor for hematopoietic reconstitution in autologous transplantation. *Bone Marrow Transplantation,* **13,** 635–40.

Ginsburg, D., Antin, J.H., Smith, B.R. *et al.* (1985). Origin of cell populations after bone marrow transplantation. Analysis using DNA sequence polymorphisms. *Journal of Clinical Investigation,* **75,** 596–603.

Giralt, S., Estey, E., Albitar, M. *et al.* (1997). Engraftment of allogeneic hematopoietic progenitor cells with purine analog-containing chemotherapy: harnessing graft-versus-leukemia without myeloablative therapy. *Blood,* **89,** 4531–36.

Gluckman, E, Rocha, V., Boyer-Chammard, A. *et al.* (1997a). Outcome of cord-blood transplantation from related and unrelated donors. *New England Journal of Medicine,* **337,** 373–81.

Gluckman, E., Rocha, V., Boyer-Chammard, A. *et al.* (1997b). Outcome of cord-blood transplantation from related and unrelated donors. Eurocord Transplant Group and Marrow Transplantation Group. *New England Journal of Medicine,* **337,** 373–81.

Gmur, J.P., Burger, J., Schaffner, A. *et al.* (1990). Pure red cell aplasia of long duration complicating major ABO-incompatible bone marrow transplantation. *Blood,* **75,** 290–5.

Gooley, B.B., Sullivan, K.M., Davis, C. *et al.* (2001). Secondary failure of platelet recovery after hematopoietic stem cell transplantation. *Biology of Blood and Marrow Transplantation,* **7,** 154–62.

Gosalvez, J., Lopez-Fernandez, C., Buno I. *et al.* (1996). Restriction endonuclease in situ digestion (REISD) and fluorescence in situ hybridization (FISH) as complementary methods to analyze chimerism and residual disease after bone marrow transplantation. *Cancer, Genetics and Cytogenetics,* **89,** 141–5.

Gratama, J.W. & Cornelissen J.J. (2001). Potential clinical utility of monitoring cytomegalovirus-specific T lymphocytes in allogeneic stem cell transplantation. *Clinical and Applied Immunology Reviews,* **2,** 17–32.

Gratama, J.W., Van Esser, J.W.J, Lamers, C.H.J *et al.* (2001). Tetramer-based quantification of cytomegalovirus (CMV)-specific CD8+ T lymphocytes in T-cell-depleted stem cell grafts and after transplantation may identify patients at risk for progressive CMV infection. *Blood,* **98,** 1358–64.

Greinix, H.T., Linkesch, W., Keil F. *et al.* (1994). Early detection of hematopoietic engraftment after bone marrow and peripheral blood stem cell transplantation by highly fluorescent reticulocyte counts. *Bone Marrow Transplantation,* **14,** 307–13.

Grigg, A.P., Bearean, K., Shore, T., & Phillips, G.L. (1992). Pancytopenia due to hypersplenism after allogeneic bone marrow transplantation. *Bone Marrow Transplantation,* **10,** 177–9.

Guillaume, T., Kubin, M., Sekhavat, M. *et al.* (1996). Peripheral blood mononuclear cells from autologous hematopoietic stem cell transplantation recipients produce and respond to IL-12. *Bone Marrow Transplantation,* **18,** 733–9.

Gyger, M., Stuart, R.K., Perreault, C. (2000). Immunobiology of allogeneic peripheral blood mononuclear cells mobilized with granulocyte-colony stimulating factor. *Bone Marrow Transplantation,* **26,** 1–16.

Haas, R., Witt, B., Möhler, R. *et al.* (1995). Sustained long-term hematopoiesis after myeloablative therapy with peripheral blood progenitor support. *Blood,* **85,** 3754–61.

Hamaguchi, M., Yamada, H., Morishima, Y. *et al.* (1996). Serum thrombopoietin levels after allogeneic bone marrow transplantation: possible correlations with platelet recovery, acute graft-versus-host disease and hepatic veno-occlusive disease. *International Journal of Hematology,* **64,** 241–8.

Hamblin, M., Marsh, J.C., Lawler, M. *et al.* (1996). CAMPATH-1G in vivo confers a low incidence of graft-versus-host disease associated with a high incidence of mixed chimaerism after bone marrow transplantation for severe aplastic anaemia using HLA-identical sibling donors. *Bone Marrow Transplantation,* **17,** 819–24.

Hanania, E.G., Giles, R.E., Kavanagh, J. *et al.* (1996). Results of MDR-1 vector modification trial indicate that granulocyte/macrophage colony-forming unit cells do not contribute to post-transplant hematopoietic recovery following intensive systemic therapy. *Proceedings of the National Academy of Science USA,* **93,** 15346–51.

Handgretinger, R., Klingebiel, T., Lang, P. *et al.* (2001). Megadose transplantation of purified peripheral blood CD34+ progenitor cells from HLA-mismatched parental donors in children. *Bone Marrow Transplantation,* **27,** 777–83.

Handgretinger, R., Lang, P., Schumm, M. *et al.* (1998). Isolation and transplantation of autologous peripheral CD34+ progenitor cells highly purified by magnetic-activated cell sorting. *Bone Marrow Transplantation,* **21,** 987–93.

Hebbel, R.P., Lin, Yi., Solovey, A., & Weisdorf, D.J. (2000). Origins of circulating endothelial cells and endothelial outgrowth from blood. *Journal of Clinical Investigation,* **105,** 71–7.

Hempel, L., Körholz, D., Nussbaum, P. *et al.* (1997). High inter-leukin-10 serum levels are associated with fatal outcome in patients after bone marrow transplantation. *Bone Marrow Transplantation,* **20,** 365–8.

Henon, P.H., Sovalat, H., Bourderont, D. (2001). Importance of CD34+ cell subsets in autologous PBSC transplantation: the mul-houde experience using CD34+CD38- cells as predictive tool for hematopoietic engraftment. *The Journal of Biological Regulation of Homeostatic Agents,* **15,** 62–7.

Hessel, H., Mittermuller, J., Zitzelsberger, H. *et al.* (1996). Combined immunophenotyping and FISH with sex chromosome-specific DNA probes for the detection of chimerism in epidermal Langerhans cells after sex-mismatched bone marrow transplanta-tion. *Histochemistry and Cell Biology,* **106,** 481–5.

Heyll, A., Aul, C., Runde, V. *et al.* (1991). Treatment of pure red cell aplasia after major ABO-incompatible bone marrow transplanta-tion with recombinant erythropoietin. *Blood,* **77,** 906.

Hibi, S.K., Tsunamoto, S., Todo, S. *et al.* (1997). Chimerism analy-sis on mononuclear cells in the CSF after allogeneic bone mar-row transplantation. *Bone Marrow Transplantation,* **20,** 503–6.

Hill, R.S., Petersen, F.B., Storb, R. *et al.* (1986). Mixed hematologic chimerism after allogeneic marrow transplantation for severe aplastic anemia is associated with a higher risk of graft rejection and a lessened incidence of acute graft-versus-host disease. *Blood,* **67,** 811–16.

Ho, A.D., Maruyama, M., Maghazachi, A. *et al.* (1994). Soluble CD4, soluble CD8, soluble CD25, lymphopoietic recovery, and indigenous cytokines after high-dose chemotherapy and blood stem cell transplantation. *Blood,* **84,** 3550–7.

Hollings, P.E., Fitzgerald, P.H., Heaton, D.E. *et al.* (1984). Host ori-gin of in vitro bone marrow fibroblasts after bone marrow trans-plantation in man. *Internal Journal of Cell Cloning,* **2,** 348–55.

Horwitz, E.M., Prockop, D.J., Fitzpatrick, L.A. *et al.* (1999). Transplantability and therapeutic effects of bone marrow-derived mesenchymal cells in children with osteogenesis imperfecta. *Nature Medicine,* **5,** 309–13.

Horwitz, E.M., Prockop, D.J., Gordon, P.L. *et al.* (2001). Clinical responses to bone marrow transplantation in children with severe osteogenesis imperfecta. *Blood,* **97,** 1227–31.

Hows, J., Palmer, S., & Gordon-Smith, E.C. (1982). Use of cyclosporin A in allogeneic bone marrow transplantation for severe aplastic anemia. *Transplantation,* **33,** 382–6.

Hows, J., Palmer, S., & Gordon-Smith, E.C. (1985). Cyclosporin and graft failure following bone marrow transplantation for severe aplastic anemia. *British Journal of Haematology,* **60,** 611–17.

Hows, J.M., Chipping, P.M., Palmer, S. *et al.* (1983). Regeneration of peripheral blood cells following ABO-incompatible allogeneic bone marrow transplantation for severe aplastic anaemia. *British Journal of Haematology,* **53,** 145–51.

Hows, J.M., Kaffaf, S., Palmer, S. *et al.* (1982). Regeneration of peripheral blood cells following allogeneic bone marrow trans-plantation for severe aplastic anaemia. *British Journal of Haematology,* **52,** 551–8.

Huss, R., Deeg, H.J., Gooley, T. *et al.* (1996). Effect of mixed chimerism on graft-versus-host disease, disease recurrence and survival after HLA-identical marrow transplantation for aplastic anemia or chronic myelogenous leukemia. *Bone Marrow Transplantation,* **18,** 767–76.

Ikpeazu, C., Davidson, M.K., Halteman, D. *et al.* (2000). Donor ori-gin of circulating endothelial progenitors after allogeneic bone marrow transplantation. *Biology of Blood and Marrow Transplantation,* **6,** 301–8.

Imrie, K.R., Prince, H.M., Couture, F. *et al.* (1995). Effect of anti-microbial prophylaxis on hematopoietic recovery following autologous bone marrow transplantation: ciprofloxacin versus cotrimoxazole. *Bone Marrow Transplantation,* **15,** 267–70.

Ishida, A., Miyakawa, Y., Tanosaki *et al.* (1996). Circulating endoge-nous thrombopoietin, interleukin-3, interleukin-6 and inter-leukin-11 levels in patients undergoing allogeneic bone marrow transplantation. *International Journal of Hematology,* **65,** 61–9.

Kanold, J., Bezou, M.J., Coulet, M. *et al.* (1993). Evaluation of ery-thropoietic/hematopoietic reconstitution after BMT by highly fluorescent reticulocyte counts compares favorably with tradi-tional peripheral blood cell counting. *Bone Marrow Transplantation,* **11,** 313–18.

Kawano, Y., Takaue, Y., Saito, S. *et al.* (1993). Granulocyte colony-stimulating factor (CSF), macrophage-CSF, granulocyte-macrophage CSF, interleukin-3, and interleukin-6 levels in sera from children undergoing blood stem cell autografts. *Blood,* **81,** 856–60.

Keable, H., Bourhis, J.H., Brison, O. *et al.* (1989). Long-term study of chimaerism in bone marrow transplantation recipients for severe aplastic anaemia. *British Journal of Haematology,* **71,** 525–33.

Keating, A., Singer, J.W., Killen, P.D. *et al.* (1982). Donor origin of the in vitro haemopoietic micro-environment after bone marrow transplantation in man. *Nature,* **298,** 280–3.

Keever-Taylor, C.A., Klein, J.P., Eastwood, D. *et al.* (2001). Factors affecting neutrophil and platelet reconstitution following T cell-depleted bone marrow transplantation: differential effects of growth factor type and role of CD34+ cell dose. *Bone Marrow Transplantation,* **27,** 791–800.

Khouri, I.F., Keating, M., Körbling, M. *et al.* (1998). Transplant-lite: induction of graft-versus-malignancy using fludarabine-based nonablative chemotherapy and allogeneic blood progenitor-cell transplantation as treatment for lymphoid malignancies. *Journal of Clinical Oncology,* **16,** 2817–24.

Kirkland, M.A., Spencer, A., Davidson, R.J. *et al.* (1996). Quantitation of mafosfamide-resistant pre-colony-forming units in allogeneic bone marrow transplantation: relationship with rate of engraftment and evidence for long-lasting reduction in stem cell numbers. *Blood,* **87,** 3963–9.

Klumpp, T.R., Herman, J.H., Schnel, M.K. *et al.* (1996). Association between antibodies reactive with neutrophils, rate of neutrophil engraftment, and incidence of post-engraftment neutropenia fol-lowing BMT. *Bone Marrow Transplantation,* **18,** 559–64.

Koc, O.N. & Lazarus, H.M. (2001). Mesenchymal stem cells: head-ing into the clinic. *Bone Marrow Transplantation,* **27,** 235–9.

Koc, O.N., Gerson, S/L., Cooper, B.W. *et al.* (2000). Rapid hematopoietic recovery after coinfusion of autologous blood stem cells and culture-expanded marrow mesenchymal stem cells in advanced breast cancer patients receiving high-dose chemotherapy. *Journal of Clinical Oncology,* **18,** 307–16.

Kögler, G., Wolf, H.H., Heyll, A. *et al.* (1995). Detection of mixed chimerism and leukemic relapse after allogeneic bone marrow transplantation in cell populations of leukocytes by fluorescent in situ hybridization in combination with the simultaneous immunophenotypic analysis of interphase cells. *Bone Marrow Transplantation*, **15**, 41–8.

Körholz, D., Hempel, L., Packeisen, J. *et al.* (1996). Significance of interleukin 10 for acute graft versus host disease in children and adolescents after allogenic bone marrow transplantation. *Klinische Padiatrie*, **208**, 141–4.

Körholz, D., Kunst, D., Hempel, L. *et al.* (1997). Decreased interleukin 10 and increased interferon production in patients with chronic graft-versus-host disease after allogeneic bone marrow transplantation. *Bone Marrow Transplantation*, **19**, 691–5.

Kurtzberg, J., Laughlin, M., Graham, M.L. *et al.* (1996). Placental blood as a source of hematopoietic stem cells for transplantation into unrelated recipients. *New England Journal of Medicine*, **335**, 157–66.

Lanza, F., Campioni, D., Moretti, S. *et al.* (2001). CD34+ cell subsets and long-term culture colony-forming cells evaluated on both autologous and normal bone marrow stroma predict long-term hematopoietic engraftment in patients undergoing autologous peripheral blood stem cell transplantation. *Experimental Hematology*, **29**, 1484–93.

Lapierre, V., Oubouzar, N., Auperin, A. *et al.* (2001). Influence of the hematopoietic stem cell source on early immunohematologic reconstitution after allogeneic transplantation. *Blood*, **97**, 2580–86.

Lapointe, C., Forest, L., Lussier, P. *et al.* (1996). Sequential analysis of early hematopoietic reconstitution following allogeneic bone marrow transplantation with fluorescence in situ hybridization (FISH). *Bone Marrow Transplantation*, **17**, 1143–8.

Lau, Y.L., Kwong, Y.L., Lee, A.C.W. *et al.* (1995). Mixed chimerism following bone marrow transplantation for severe combined immunodeficiency: a study by DNA fingerprinting and simultaneous immunophenotyping and fluorescence in situ hybridization. *Bone Marrow Transplantation*, **15**, 971–6.

Laughlin, M.J., Barker, J., Bambach, B. *et al.* (2001). Hematopoietic engraftment and survival in adult recipient of umbilical-cord blood from unrelated donors. *New England Journal of Medicine* **344**, 1815–22.

Lawler, M., Humphries, T., & McCann, S.R. (1991). Evaluation of mixed chimerism by in vitro amplification of dinucleotide repeat sequences using the polymerase chain reaction. *Blood*, **77**, 2504–14.

Leclair, B., Fregeau C.J., Aye, M.T., & Fourney R.M. (1995). DNA typing for bone marrow engraftment follow-up after allogeneic transplant: a comparative study of current technologies. *Bone Marrow Transplantation*, **15**, 43–55.

Lee, C.-K., Gingrich, R.D., Hohl, R.I., & Ajram, K.A. (1995). Engraftment syndrome in autologous bone marrow and peripheral stem cell transplantation. *Bone Marrow Transplantation*, **16**, 175–82.

Lennon, J.E. & Micklem, H.S. (1986). Stromal cells in long term murine bone marrow culture: FACS studies and origin of stromal cells in radiation chimeras. *Experimental Hematology*, **14**, 287–92.

Locksley, R.M., Flournoy, N., Sullivan, K.M., & Meyers, J.D. (1985). Infection with varicella-zoster virus after marrow transplantation. *Journal of Infectious Diseases*, **152**, 1172–81.

Lum, L.G., Noges, J.E., Culbertson, N.J. *et al.* (1986). Transfer of specific immunity in marrow recipients who received T cell depleted marrow. *Experimental Hematology*, **14**, 447 (Abstract).

Ma, D.D.F., Varga, D.E., & Biggs, J.C. (1987). Haemopoietic reconstitution after allogeneic bone marrow transplantation in man: recovery of haemopoietic progenitors (CFU-Mix, BFU-E and CFU-GM). *British Journal of Haematology*, **65**, 5–10.

MacKinnon, S., Barnett, L., Heller, G., & O'Reilly, R.J. (1994). Minimal residual disease is more common in patients who have mixed T cell chimerism after bone marrow transplantation for chronic myelogenous leukemia. *Blood*, **83**, 3409–16.

Mangan, K.F., Mullaney, M.T., Barrientos T.D., Kernan, N.A. (1993). Serum interleukin-3 levels following autologous or allogeneic bone marrow transplantation: effects of T-cell depletion, blood stem cell infusion, and hematopoietic growth factor treatment. *Blood*, **81**, 1915–22.

Maris, M., Storb, R. Outpatient allografting in hematologic malignancies and nonmalignant disorders-applying lessons learned in the canine model to humans. (2002). *Cancer Treatment Research*, **110**, 149–75.

Marshall, M.J., Nisbet, N.W., & Evans, S. (1984). Donor origin of the in vitro haemopoietic micro-environment after bone marrow transplantation in mice. *Experientia*, **40**, 385–6.

Martin, P.J., Hansen, J.A., Buckner, C.D. *et al.* (1985). Effects of in vitro depletion of T cells in HLA-identical allogeneic marrow grafts. *Blood*, **66**, 664–72.

Martin, P.J., Hansen, J.A., Torok-Storb, B. *et al.* (1988). Graft failure in patients receiving T cell-depleted HLA-identical allogeneic marrow transplants. *Bone Marrow Transplantation*, **3**, 445–56.

Martinez, C., Urbano-Ispizua, A., Rozman, C. *et al.* (1999). Immune reconstitution following allogeneic peripheral blood progenitor cell transplantation: Comparison of recipients of positive CD34+ selected grafts with recipients of unmanipulated grafts. *Experimental Hematology*, **27**, 561–68.

Martino, R., Brunet, S., Garcia A. *et al.* (1995). Various patterns of chimerism after allogeneic bone marrow transplantation for advanced chronic lymphocytic leukemia. *Bone Marrow Transplantation*, **16**, 783–6.

Martino, R., Caballero, M.D., Canals, C. *et al.* (2001). Allogeneic peripheral blood stem cell transplantation with reduced-intensity conditioning: results of a prospective multicentre study. *British Journal of Haematology*, **115**, 653–59.

Mathioudakis, G., Storb, R., McSweeney, P.A. *et al.* (2000). Polyclonal hematopoiesis with variable telomere shortening in human long-term allogeneic marrow graft recipients. *Blood*, **96**, 3991–4.

Mavroudis, D., Read, E., Cottler-Fox, M. *et al.* (1996). CD34+ cell dose predict survival, posttransplant morbidity, and rate of hematologic recovery after allogeneic marrow transplants for hematologic malignancies. *Blood*, **88**, 3223–9.

Mavroudis, D.A., Read, E.J., Molldrem, J. *et al.* (1998). T-cell-depleted granulocyte colony-stimulating factor (G-CSF) modified allogeneic bone marrow transplantation for hematological malignancy improves graft CD34+ cell content but is associated with delayed pancytopenia. *Bone Marrow Transplantation*, **21**, 431–40.

McSweeney, P.A., Niederwieser, D., Shizuru, J.A. *et al.* (2001). Hematopoietic cell transplantation in older patients with hematologic malignancies: replacing high-dose cytotoxic therapy with graft-versus-tumor effects. *Blood, 97,* 3390–3400.

McSweeney, P.A., Storb, R. (1999). Mixed chimerism: preclinical studies and clinical applications [review]. *Biology of Blood and Marrow Transplantation, 5,* 192–203.

Mehta, J., Powles, R., Horton C. *et al.* (1996). Factors affecting engraftment and hematopoietic recovery after unpurged autografting in acute leukemia. *Bone Marrow Transplantation, 18,* 319–24.

Mehta, J., Powles, R., Singhal, S. *et al.* (1997). Early identification of patients at risk of death due to infections, hemorrhage, or graft failure after allogeneic bone marrow transplantation on the basis of the leukocyte counts. *Bone Marrow Transplantation, 19,* 349–55.

Metcalf, D., Begley, C.G., & Williamson, D.J. (1987). Hemopoietic responses in mice injected with purified recombinant murine GM-CSF. *Experimental Hematology, 15,* 1–9.

Metcalf, D., Begley, C.G., Johnson, G.R. *et al.* (1986). Effects of purified bacterially synthesized murine multi-CSF (IL-3) on hematopoiesis in normal adult mice. *Blood, 68,* 46–57.

Meyers, J.D. & Atkinson, K. (1983). Infection in bone marrow transplantation. In Clinics in Haematology. *Bone Marrow Transplantation,* ed. D. Nathan. London:WB Saunders. pp 791–812.

Meyers, J.D., Flournory, N., Thomas, E.D. (1982). Non-bacterial pneumonia after allogeneic bone marrow transplantation: a review of ten years' experience. *Review of Infectious Diseases, 4,* 1119–32.

Mielcarek, M., Zaucha, J.M., Sandmaier, B. *et al.* (2002). Type of post-grafting immunosuppression after non-myeloablative blood cell transplantation may influence risk of delayed haemolysis due to minor ABO incompatibility. *British Journal of Haematology, 116,* 500–1.

Millar, B.C., Millar, J.L., Bell, J.B.G. *et al.* (1996). Role of CD34+ cells and engraftment after high-dose melphalan in multiple myeloma patients given peripheral blood stem cell autografts. *Bone Marrow Transplantation, 18,* 871–8.

Min, C.K., Kim, D.W., Lee, J.W. *et al.* (2001). Hematopoietic stem cell transplantation for high-risk adult patients with severe aplastic anemia; reduction of graft failure by enhancing stem cell dose. *Haematologica, 86,* 303–10.

Mitsuyasu, R.T., Champlin, R. E., & Ho, W.G. (1985). Prospective randomised controlled trial of ex vivo treatment of donor bone marrow with monoclonal anti-T cell antibody and complement for prevention of graft-versus-host disease: a preliminary report. *Transplantation Proceedings, 17,* 482–5.

Molloy, K., Goulden, N., Lawler, M. *et al.* (1996). Patterns of hematopoietic chimerism following bone marrow transplantation for childhood acute lymphoblastic leukemia from volunteer unrelated donors. *Blood, 87,* 3027–31.

Moore, M.A.S. & Warren, D.J. (1987). Synergy of interleukin 1 and granulocyte colony-stimulating factor: in vivo stimulation of stem cell recovery and hematopoietic regeneration following 5-fluorouracil treatment of mice. *Proceedings of the National Academy of Science USA, 84,* 7134.

Morariu-Zamfir, R., Rocha, V., Devergie, A. *et al.* (2001). Influence of CD34+ marrow cell dose on outcome of HLA-identical sibling allogeneic bone marrow transplants in patients with chronic myeloid leukaemia. *Bone Marrow transplantation, 27,* 575–80.

Moreb, J., Kubilis, P.S., Mullins, D.L. *et al.* (1997). Increased frequency of auto aggression syndrome associated with autologous stem cell transplantation in breast cancer patients. *Bone Marrow Transplantation, 19,* 101–6.

Nakamura, R., Bahceci, E., Read, E.J. *et al.* (2001). Transplant dose of CD34+ and CD3+ cells predicts outcome in patients with haematological malignancies undergoing T-cell-depleted peripheral blood stem cell transplants with delayed donor lymphocyte add-back. *British Journal of Haematology, 115,* 95–104.

Nataro, R., Cimmino, A., Tabanni, D. *et al.* (1998). In vivo telomere dynamics of human hematpoietic stem cells. *Proceedings of the National Academy of Science USA, 94,* 13782–5.

Nathan, D.G., Chess, L., Hillman, D.G. *et al.* (1978). Human erythroid burst forming unit: T cell requirement for proliferation in vitro. *Journal of Experimental Medicine, 147,* 324–39.

Nicholls, M.D., Atkinson, K., Biggs, J.C. *et al.* (1984). Pyridoxine-responsive sideroblastic anaemia after allogeneic bone marrow transplantation: a treatable cause of late transfusion dependence. *British Journal of Haematology, 56,* 153–6.

Nieboer, P., de Vries, E.G.E., Mulder, N.H. *et al.* (2001). Long-term haematological recovery following high-dose chemotherapy with autologous bone marrow transplantation or peripheral stem cell transplantation in patients with solid tumors. *Bone Marrow Transplantation, 27,* 959–66.

Nollet, F., Billiet, J., Selleslag, D., & Criel, A. (2001). Standardization of multiplex fluorescent short tandem repeat analysis for chimerism testing. *Bone Marrow Transplantation, 28,* 511–8.

Nurnberger, W., Willers, R., Burdach, S., & Gobel, U. (1997). Risk factors for capillary leakage syndrome after bone marrow transplantation. *Annals of Hematology, 74,* 221–4.

Oberkircher, A.R., Strout, M.P., Herzig, G.P. *et al.* (1995). Description of an efficient and highly informative method for the evaluation of hematopoietic chimerism following allogeneic bone marrow transplantation. *Bone Marrow Transplantation, 16,* 695–702.

Offner, F., Schoch, G., Fisher, L.D. *et al.* (1996). Mortality hazard functions as related to neutropenia at different times after marrow transplantation. *Blood, 88,* 4058–62.

O'Flaherty, E., Sparrow, R., & Szer, J. (1995). Bone marrow stromal function from patients after bone marrow transplantation. *Bone Marrow Transplantation, 15,* 207–12.

Ohashi, K., Akiyama, H., Takamoto, S. *et al.* (1994). Treatment of pure red cell aplasia after major ABO-incompatible bone marrow transplantation resistant to erythropoietin. *Bone Marrow Transplantation, 13,* 335–6.

Okamoto, T., Kanamaru, A., Okada, M. *et al.* (1996). Myelodysplastic changes in 3 cases within 100 days after allogeneic bone marrow transplantation. *International Journal of Hematology, 63,* 155–60.

Okamato, T., Kanamaru, A., Wada, H. *et al.* (1993). Hematopoietic recovery from host progenitors with normal karyotype devoid of Philadelphia chromosomes in a patient with CML after allogeneic BMT. *Bone Marrow Transplantation, 12,* 89–92.

Or, R., Naparstek, E., Mani, N., & Slavin, S. (1991). Treatment of pure red cell aplasia following major ABO-mismatched T cell-depleted bone marrow transplantation: 2 case reports with successful response to plasmapheresis. *Transplantation International*, **4**, 99–102.

Ottinger, H.D., Beelen, D.W., Scheulen, B. *et al.* (1996) Improved immune reconstitution after allotransplantation of peripheral blood stem cells instead of bone marrow. *Blood*, **88**, 2775–79.

Oyama, Y., Cohen, B., Traynor, A. *et al.* (2002). Engraftment syndrome: a common cause for rash and fever following autologous hematopoietic stem cell transplantation for multiple sclerosis. Bone Marrow *Transplantation*, **29**, 81–5.

Paltiel, O., Cournoyer, D., & Ribka, W. (1993). Pure red cell aplasia following ABO-incompatible bone marrow transplantation: response to erythropoietin. *Transfusion*, **33**, 418–21.

Papadakis, V., Diaz-Barrientos, T., Heller, G. *et al.* (1995). Serum granulocyte-colony stimulating factor (G-CSF) levels after allogeneic T cell-depleted marrow transplantation. *Bone Marrow Transplantation*, **15**, 955–61.

Perez-Simon, J.A., Martin, A., Caballero, D. *et al.* (1999). Clinical significance of CD34+ cell dose in long-term engraftment following autologous peripheral blood stem cell engraftment. *Bone Marrow Transplantation*, **24**, 1279–83.

Peters, W.P., Stuart, A., Affranti, M.L. *et al.* (1988). Neutrophil migration is defective during recombinant human granulocyte-macrophage colony-stimulating factor infusion after autologous bone marrow transplantation in humans. *Blood*, **72**, 1310–15.

Petit, T., Raynal, B., Socié, G. *et al.* (1994). Highly sensitive polymerase chain reaction methods showed the frequent survival of residual recipient multipotent progenitors after non-T-cell depleted bone marrow transplantation. *Blood*, **84**, 3575–83.

Piersma, A.H., Ploemacher, R.E., & Brockbank, K.G.M. (1983). Transplantation of bone marrow fibroblastoid stromal cells in mice via the intravenous route. *British Journal of Haematology*, **54**, 285–90.

Pilka, G., Stuppia, L., Di Bartolomeo, P. *et al.* (1996). FISH detection of mixed chimerism in 33 patients submitted to bone marrow transplantation. *Bone Marrow Transplantation*, **17**, 231–6.

Podesta, M., Piaggio, G., Frassoni, F. *et al.* (1997). Deficient reconstitution of early progenitors after allogeneic bone marrow transplantation. *Bone Marrow Transplantation*, **19**, 1011–17.

Powles, R.L., Morgenstern, G.R., Kay, H. *et al.* (1983). Mismatched family donors for bone marrow transplantation as treatment for acute leukaemia. *Lancet*, **1**, 612–15.

Pratt, G., Rawstron, A.C., English, A.E. *et al.* (2001). Analysis of CD34+ cell subsets in stem cell harvests can more reliably predict rapidity and durability of engraftment than total CD34+ cell dose, but steady state levels do not correlate with bone marrow reserve. *British Journal of Haematology*, **114**, 937–43.

Przepiorka, D., Smith, T.L., Folloder, J. *et al.*(1999). Risk factors for acute graft-versus-host disease after allogeneic blood stem cell transplantation. *Blood*, **94**, 1465–70.

Pugatsch, T., Oppenheim, A., & Slavin, S. (1996). Improved single-step PCR assay for sex identification post-allogeneic sex-mismatched BMT. *Bone Marrow Transplantation*, **17**, 273–5.

Rajantie, J., Sale, G.E., Deeg, H.J. *et al.* (1986). Adverse effect of severe marrow fibrosis on hematologic recovery after chemoradiotherapy and allogeneic bone marrow transplantation. *Blood*, **67**, 1693–7.

Ramirez, M., Diaz, M.A., Garcia-Sanchez, F. *et al.* (1996). Chimerism after allogeneic hematopoietic cell transplantation in childhood acute lymphoblastic leukemia. *Bone Marrow Transplantation*, **18**, 1161–5.

Ramsay, N.K.C., & Kersey, J.H. (1984). Conditioning of bone marrow recipients with cyclophosphamide and total lymphoid irradiation. In Tolerance in Bone Marrow and Organ Transplantation, ed. S. Slavin. Amsterdam:Elsevier Science Publishers BV.

Ravenel, J.G., Scalzetti, E.M. & Zamkoff, K.W. (2000). Chest raduographic features of engraftment syndrome. *Journal of Thoracic Imaging*, **15**, 56–60.

Ravoet, C., Feremans, W., Husson, B. *et al.* (1996). Clinical evidence for an engraftment syndrome associated with early and steep neutrophil recovery after autologous blood stem cell transplantation. *Bone Marrow Transplantation*, **18**, 943–7.

Reisner, Y., Martelli, M.F. (1995). Bone marrow transplantation across HLA barriers by increasing the number of transplanted cells. *Immunology Today*, **16**, 437–40.

Richard, C., Romon, I., Perez-Encinas, M. *et al.* (1996). Splenectomy for poor graft function after allogeneic bone marrow transplantation in patients with chronic myeloid leukemia. *Leukemia*, **10**, 1615–18.

Ringden, O., Remberger, M., Runde, V. *et al.* (1999). Peripheral blood stem cell transplantation from unrelated donors: a comparison with marrow transplantation. *Blood*, **94**, 455–64.

Robertson, J.D., Testa, N.G., Russell, N.H. *et al.* (2001). Accelerated telomere shortening following allogeneic transplantation is independent of the cell source and occurs within the first year post transplant. *Bone Marrow Transplantation*, **27**, 1283–6.

Rocha,V., Labopin, M., Gluckman, E. *et al.* (2002). Relevance of bone marrow cell dose on allogeneic transplantation outcomes for patients with acute myeloid leukemia in first remission: results of European survey. *Journal of Clinical Oncology*, **20**, 4324–30.

Roux, E., Abdi, K., Speiser, D. *et al.* (1993). Characterization of mixed chimerism in patients with chronic myeloid leukemia transplanted with T-cell-depleted bone marrow: involvement of different lineages before and after relapse. *Blood*, **81**, 243–8.

Roux, E., Helg, C., Chapuis, B. *et al.* (1992). Evolution of mixed chimerism after allogeneic bone marrow transplantation as determined on granulocytes and mononuclear cells by the polymerase chain reaction. *Blood*, **79**, 2775–83.

Roy, D.C., Tantravahi, R., Murray, C. *et al.* (1990). Natural history of mixed chimerism after bone marrow transplantation with CD6-depleted allogeneic marrow. A stable equilibrium. *Blood*, **75**, 296–304.

Roy, V., Rizvi, M.A., Vesely, S.K., and George, J.N. (2001). Thrombotic thrombocytopenic purpura-like syndromes following bone marrow transplantation: an analysis of associated conditions and clinical outcomes. *Bone Marrow Transplantation*, **27**, 641–6.

Roychowdhury, D.F., & Linker, C.A. (1995). Pure red cell aplasia complicating an ABO-compatible allogeneic bone marrow transplantation, treated successfully with anti-thymocyte globulin. *Bone Marrow Transplantation*, **16**, 471–2.

Rubinstein, P., Carrier, C., Scaradavou, A. *et al.* (1998). Outcomes among 562 recipients of placental-blood transplants from unrelated donors. *New England Journal of Medicine*, **339**, 1565–77.

Sahdev, I., O'Reilly, R., Black, P. *et al.* (1996). Interleukin-1 production following T-cell depleted and unmodified marrow grafts. *Pediatric Hematology and Oncology*, **13**, 55–67.

Salzberger, B., Bowden, R.A., Hackman, R.C. *et al.* (1997) Neutropenia in allogeneic marrow transplant recipients receiving ganciclovir for prevention of cytomegalovirus disease: risk factors and outcome. *Blood,* **90,** 2502.

Saunders, M.J., Jowitt, S.N., & Liu Yin, J.A. (1995a). Clonality studies in patients undergoing allogeneic and autologous bone marrow transplantation for hematological malignancies. *Bone Marrow Transplantation,* **15,** 81–5.

Scharf, S.J., Smith, A.G., Hansen, J.A. *et al.* (1995b). Quantitative determination of bone marrow transplant engraftment using fluorescent polymerase chain reaction primers for human identity markers. *Blood,* **85,** 1954–63.

Schattenberg, A., DeWitte, T., Salden, M. *et al.* (1989). Mixed hematopoietic chimerism after allogeneic transplantation with lymphocyte- depleted bone marrow is not associated with a high incidence of relapse. *Blood,* **73,** 1367–72.

Schick, F., Einsele, H., Kost, R. *et al.* (1994). Hematopoietic reconstitution after bone marrow transplantation: assessment with MR imaging and H-1 localized spectroscopy. *Journal of Magnetic Resonance Imaging,* **4,** 71–8.

Shay, J.W. (1998). Accelerated telomere shortening in bone marrow recipients. *Lancet,* **351,** 153–4.

Sheridan, W.P., Morstyn, G., Wolf, M. *et al.* (1989). Granulocyte colony-stimulating factor and neutrophil recovery after high-dose chemotherapy and autologous marrow transplantation. *Lancet,* **2,** 891–5.

Shimazaki, C., Inaba, T., Uchiyama, H. *et al.* (1997). Serum thrombopoietin levels in patients undergoing autologous peripheral blood stem cell transplantation. *Bone Marrow Transplantation,* **19,** 771–5.

Siena, S., Schiavo, R., Pedrazzoli, P. *et al.* (2000). Therapeutic relevance of CD34 cell dose in blood cell transplantation for cancer therapy. *Journal of Clinical Oncology,* **18,** 3319–20.

Sierra, J., Storer, B., Hansen, J.A. *et al.* (1997). Transplantation of marrow cells from unrelated donors for treatment of high-risk acute leukemia: the effect of leukemic burden, donor HLA-matching, and marrow cell dose. *Blood,* **89,** 4226–35.

Sill, H., Rule, S.A., Joske, D.J. *et al.* (1996). Reconstitution with Philadelphia chromosome-negative recipient hematopoiesis early after allogeneic BMT for CML. *Bone Marrow Transplantation,* **17,** 453–5.

Simmons, P.J., Przepiorka, D., Thomas, E.D., & Torok-Storb, B. (1987). Host origin of marrow stromal cells following allogeneic bone marrow transplantation. *Nature,* **328,** 429–32.

Slavin, S., Nagler, A., Naparstek, E. *et al.* (1998). Nonmyeloablative stem cell transplantation and cell therapy as an alternative to conventional bone marrow transplantation with lethal cytoreduction for the treatment of malignant and nonmalignant hematologic diseases. *Blood,* **91,** 756–63.

Sniecinski, I., Henry, S., Richey, B. *et al.* (1985). Erythrocyte depletion of ABO-incompatible bone marrow. *Journal of Clinical Apheresis,* **2,** 231–4.

Socie, G., Gluckman, E., Raynal, B. *et al.* (1993). Bone marrow transplantation for Fanconi anemia using low-dose cyclophosphamide/thoracoabdominal irradiation as conditioning regimen: chimerism studied by the polymerase chain reaction. *Blood,* **82,** 2249–56.

Soll, E., Massumoto, C., Clift, R.A. *et al.* (1995). Relevance of marrow fibrosis in bone marrow transplantation: a retrospective analysis of engraftment. *Blood,* **86,** 4667–73.

Sosa, R., Weiden, P.L., Storb, R. *et al.* (1980). Granulocyte function in human allogeneic marrow graft recipients. *Experimental Hematology,* **8,** 1183–9.

Spitzer, T.R. (2001). Engraftment syndrome following hematopoietic stem cell transplantation. *Bone Marrow Transplantation,* **27,** 893–8.

Sreenan, J.J., Pettay, J.D., Tpakhi, A. *et al.* (1997). The use of amplified variable number of tandem repeats (VNTR) in the detection of chimerism following bone marrow transplantation. A comparison with restriction fragment length polymorphism (RFLP) by Southern blotting. *American Journal of Clinical Pathology,* **107,** 292–8.

Stewart, D.A., Guo, D., Luider, J. *et al.* (1999). Factors predicting engraftment of autologous blood stem cells: CD34+ subsets inferior to the total CD34+ cell dose. *Bone Marrow Transplantation,* **23,** 1237–43.

Stewart, D.A., Guo, D., Luider, J. *et al.* (2000). The CD34+90+ cell dose does not predict early engraftment of autologous blood stem cells as well as the total CD34+ cell dose. *Bone Marrow Transplantation,* **25,** 435–40.

Storb, R., Doney, K.C., Thomas, E.D. *et al.* (1982). Marrow transplantation with or without donor buffy coat cells for 65 transfused aplastic anemia patients. *Blood,* **59,** 236–46.

Storb, R., Prentice, R.L., & Thomas, E.D. (1997a). Marrow transplantation for treatment of aplastic anemia. An analysis of factors associated with graft rejection. *New England Journal of Medicine,* **296,** 61–6.

Storb, R., Thomas, E.D., & Buckner, C.D. (1974). Allogeneic marrow grafting for treatment of aplastic anemia. *Blood,* **43,** 157–180.

Storb, R., Yu, C., Wagner, J.L. *et al.* (1997b). Stable mixed hematopoietic chimerism in DLA-identical littermate dogs given sublethal total body irradiation before and pharmalogical immunosuppression after bone marrow transplantation. *Blood,* **89,** 3048–54.

Storb, R., Yu, C., Zaucha, J.M. *et al.* (1999). Stable mixed hematopoietic chimerism in dogs given donor antigen, CTLA4lg, and 100 cGy total body irradiation before and pharmacologic immunosuppression after marrow transplant. *Blood,* **94,** 2523–29.

Storek J, Dawson, M.A., Storer, B. *et al.* (2001). Immune reconstitution after allogeneic marrow transplantation compared with blood stem cell transplantation. *Blood,* **97,** 3380–89.

Sullivan, K.M., Whiterspoon, R.P., Storb, R. *et al.* (1988). Prednisone and azathioprine compared with prednisone and placebo for treatment of chronic graft-versus-host disease: prognostic incluence of prolonged thrombocytopenia after allogeneic marrow transplantation. *Blood,* **72,** 546–54.

Sykes, M., Preffer, F., McAfee, S. *et al.* (1999). Mixed lympho-haematopoietic chimerism and graft-versus-lymphoma effects after non- myeloablative therapy and HLA-mismatched bone-marrow transplantation. *Lancet,* **353,** 1755–59.

Terenzi, A., Aversa, F., Mencarelli, A. *et al.* (1996). Unusual split chimaerism after mismatched T-depleted BMT. *Bone Marrow Transplantation,* **18,** 465–7.

Territo, M.C., Gale, R.P., & Cline, M.J. (The UCLA Bone Marrow Transplantation Team) (1977). Neutrophil function in bone marrow transplant recipients. *British Journal of Haematology,* **35,** 245–50.

Testa, U., Martucci, R., Rutella, S. *et al.* (1994). Autologous stem cell transplantation: release of early and late acting growth factors relates with hematopoietic ablation and recovery. *Blood,* **84,** 3532–9.

Thiele, J., Kvasnicka, H.M., Beelen, D.W. *et al.* (2000). Relevance and dynamics of myelofibrosis regarding hematopoietic reconstitution after allogeneic bone marrow transplantation in chronic myelogenous leukemia – a single center experience on 160 patients. *Bone Marrow Transplantation,* **26,** 275–81.

Thomas, E.D., Buckner, C.D., Banaji, M. *et al.* (1977). One hundred patients with acute leukemia treated by chemotherapy, total body irradiation and allogeneic marrow transplantation. *Blood,* **49,** 511–33.

Thomas, E.D., Ramberg, R.E., Sale, G.E. *et al.* (1976). Direct evidence for a bone marrow origin of the alveolar macrophage in man. *Science,* **192,** 1016–18.

Thomas, S., Clark, S.C., Rappeport, J.M. *et al.* (1990). Deficient T cell granulocyte-macrophage colony stimulating factor production in allogeneic bone marrow transplant recipients. *Transplantation,* **49,** 703–7.

Thomson, B.G., Robertson, K.A., Gowan D. *et al.* (2000). Analaysis of engraftment, graft-versus-host disease, and immune recovery following unrelated donor cord blood transplantation. *Blood,* **96,** 2703–11.

Thornley, I., Sutherland, R., Wynn, R. *et al.* (2002). Early hematopoietic reconstitution after clinical stem cell transplantation: evidence for stochastic stem cell behaviour and limited acceleration in telomere loss. *Blood,* **99,** 2387–96.

To, L.B., Dyson, P.G., Branford, AL. *et al.* (1987). Peripheral blood stem cells collected in very early remission produce rapid and sustained autologous haemopoietic reconstitution in acute nonlymphoblastic leukemia. *Bone Marrow Transplantation,* **2,** 103–8.

Torok-Storb, B., Boeckh, M., Hoy, C. *et al.* (1997). Association of specific cytomegalovirus genotypes with death from myelosuppresion after marrow transplantation. *Blood,* **90,** 2097–2102.

Torok-Storb, B., Simmons, P., Khaira, D. *et al.* (1992). Cytomegalovirus and marrow function. *Annals of Hematology,* **64,** 128–31.

Torok-Storb, B., Simmons, P., Przepio, R.K.A., & Deeg, H.J. (1987). Impairment of hemopoiesis in human allografts. *Transplantation Proceedings,* **19,** Suppl 7, 33–7.

Torres, A., Sanchez, J., Lakomsky, D. *et al.* (2001). Assessment of hematologic progenitor engraftment by complete reticulocyte maturation parameters after autologous and allogeneic hematopoietic stem cell transplantation. *Haematologica,* **86,** 24–9.

Trigg, M.E., Billing, R., Sondel, P.M. *et al.* (1985). Clinical trial depleting T lymphocytes from donor marrow for matched and mismatched allogeneic bone marrow transplants. *Cancer Treatment Reports,* **69,** 377–86.

UCLA Bone Marrow Transplant Team (1981). Prevention of graft rejection following bone marrow transplantation. *Blood,* **57,** 9–12.

Urbano-Ispizua, A., Carreras, E., Marin, P. *et al.* (2001a). Allogeneic transplantation of CD34+ selected cells from peripheral blood from human leukocyte antigen-identical siblings: detrimental effect of a high number of donor CD34+ cells? *Blood,* **98,** 2352–7.

Urbano-Ispizua, A., Rozman, C., Pimentel, P. *et al.* (2001b). The number of donor CD3+ cells is the most important factor for graft failure after allogeneic transplantation of CD34+ selected cells from peripheral blood from HLA-identical siblings. *Blood,* **97,** 383–87.

Van Hennik, P.B., Breems, D., Kusadasi, N. *et al.* (2000). Stroma-supported progenitor production as a prognostic tool for graft failure following autologous stem cell transplantation. *British Journal of Haematology,* **111,** 674–84.

van Leeuwen, J.E. M., van Tolm, J.D., Joosten, A.M. *et al.* (1994). Persistence of host-type hematopoiesis after allogeneic bone marrow transplantation for leukemia is significantly related to the recipients age and/or the conditioning regimen, but it is not associated with an increased risk of relapse. *Blood,* **83,** 3059–67.

Vellenga, E., Sizoo, W., Hagenbeek, A., & Lowenberg, B. (1987). Different repopulation kinetics of erythroid (BFU-E), myeloid (CFU-GM) and T lymphocyte (TL-CFU) progenitor cells after autologous and allogeneic bone marrow transplantation. *British Journal of Haematology,* **65,** 137–42.

Verdonck, L.F., Dekker, A.W., De Gast, G.C. *et al.* (1994). Allogeneic bone marrow transplantation with a fixed low number of T-cells in the marrow graft. *Blood,* **15,** 3090–6.

Verdonck, L.F., van Blokland, W.T.M., Bosboom-Kalsbeek, E.K. *et al.* (1996). Complete donor T cell chimerism is accomplished in patients transplanted with bone marrow grafts containing a fixed low number of T cells. *Bone Marrow Transplantation,* **18,** 389–95.

Vincent, P.C., Young, G.A.R., Singh, S. *et al.* (1986). Ph[1] negative haematological chimerism after marrow transplantation in Ph[1] positive chronic granulocytic leukemia. *British Journal of Haematology,* **63,** 181–5.

Visani, G., Lemoli, R., Tosi, P. *et al.* (1999). Use of peripheral blood stem cells for autologous transplantation in acute myeloid leukemia patients allows faster engraftment and equivalent disease-free survival compared with bone marrow cells. *Bone Marrow Transplantation,* **24,** 467–72.

Volc-Platzer, B., Stingl, G., Wolff, K. *et al.* (1984). Cytogenetic identification of allogeneic epidermal Langerhans cells in a bone marrow graft recipient. *New England Journal of Medicine,* **310,** 1123.

Volin, L. & Ruutu T. (1990). Pure red cell aplasia of long duration after major ABO-incompatible bone marrow transplantation. *Acta Haematologica,* **84,** 195–7.

Wagner, J.E., Kernan, N.A., Steinbuch, M. *et al.* (1995). Allogeneic sibling umbilical cord-blood transplantation in children with malignant and non-malignant disease. *Lancet,* **346,** 214–19.

Wagner, J.E., Rosenthal, J., Sweetman, R. *et al.* (1996). Succesful transplantation of HLA-matched and HLA-mismatched umbilical cord blood from unrelated donors: analysis of engraftment and acute graft-versus-host disease. *Blood,* **88,** 795–802.

Waldmann, H., Polliak, A., Hale, G. *et al.* (1984). Elimination of graft-versus-host disease by in vitro depletion of alloreactive lymphocytes with a monoclonal rat antihuman lymphocyte antibody (Campath-1). *Lancet,* **2,** 483–5.

Weissinger F., Sandmaier B.M., Maloney, D.G. *et al.* (2001). Decreased transfusion requirements for patients receiving non-myeloablative compared with conventional peripheral blood stem cell transplants from HLA-identical siblings. *Blood,* **98,** 3584–88.

Wimperis, J.Z., Brenner, M.K., Prentice, H.G. *et al.* (1986). Transfer of a functioning humoral immune system in transplantation of T lymphocyte-depleted bone marrow. *Lancet,* **1,** 339–43.

Winston, D.J., Schiffman, G., Wang, D.C. *et al.* (1979). Pneumococcal infections after human bone marrow transplantation. *Annals of Internal Medicine,* **91,** 835–41.

Wynn, R., Thornley, I., Freedman, M., & Saunders, E.F. (1999). Telomere shortening in leucocyte subsets of long-term survivors of allogeneic bone marrow transplantation. *British Journal of Haematology,* **105,** 997–1001.

Wynn, R.F., Cross, M.A. Hatton, C. *et al.* (1998). Accelerated telomere shortening in young recipients of allogeneic bone marrow transplants. *Lancet,* **351,** 178–81.

Yamaguchi, M., Nakao, S., Ueda, M. *et al.* (1995). Early recovery of host-derived hematopoiesis in transplant recipients conditioned with high-dose busulphan and cyclophosphamide. *Bone Marrow Transplantation,* **15,** 787–9.

Zaucha, J.M., Gooley, T., Bensinger, W.I. *et al.* (2001). CD34 cell dose in granulocyte colony-stimulating factor-mobilized peripheral blood mononuclear cell grafts affects engraftment kinetics and development of extensive chronic graft-versus-host disease after human leukocyte antigen-identical sibling transplantation. *Blood,* **98,** 3221–7.

14 Immunological reconstitution after hemopoietic stem cell transplantation

JAN STOREK AND ROBERT P. WITHERSPOON

Fred Hutchinson Cancer Research Center and University of Washington, Seattle, USA

Introduction

Infections resulting from immune deficiency are an unfortunate side effect of hematopoietic stem cell grafting (Fig. 14.1) (Meyers, 1986). Almost all the components of both the innate immune system (e.g., epithelial barriers, granulocytes) as well as the adaptive immune system (e.g., T and B cells) are deficient. Granulocyte deficiency may be the primary cause of the infections occurring during the first month, whereas CD4+ T cell and B lymphocyte deficiency may be the primary cause of the infections occurring later after transplant (Storek *et al.*, 1997a; Storek *et al.*, 2000). Lymphocyte deficiency might also contribute to posttransplant relapses of the primary malignancy or the development of secondary malignancies (Lucas *et al.*,

1996; Porrata *et al.*, 2001a; Porrata *et al.*, 2001b; Porrata *et al.*, 2002a; Porrata *et al.*, 2002b). The following factors influence the degree of the immune deficiency: time posttransplant (Fig. 14.1), donor/host histocompatibility, and graft-versus-host disease (GVHD) and/or its treatment (Atkinson *et al.*, 1982a; Sullivan *et al.*, 1992; Ochs *et al.*, 1995; Hakim & Mackall, 1997).

Throughout this chapter, "early posttransplant" refers to the first 3 months whereas "late posttransplant" refers to the period between 6 months and several years after grafting. Supranormal/subnormal values of an immune test refer to values higher/lower than the normal adult (age 18–60) range. Post-bone marrow transplant (BMT) immune recovery has been studied most extensively and, therefore, is the primary focus of this chapter. Whenever known, we also point out the distinct features of

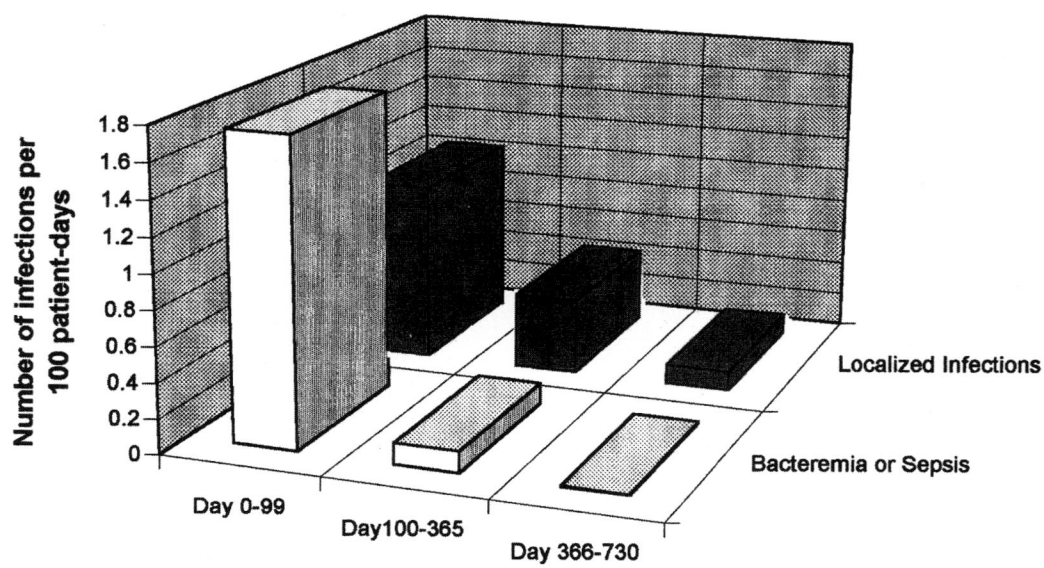

Fig. 14.1. The incidence of bacteremias (including fungemias) and localized infections (excluding infections of mouth and upper airways) in BMT recipients (80% allogeneic) transplanted in Seattle between 1986 and 1988, showing the decreased propensity to develop infections in long versus short-term transplant survivors. Infection prophylaxis included laminar air-flow rooms in ~40% patients, CMV-negative blood products in all CMV-seronegative patients with CMV-seronegative donors, and trimethoprim-sulfamethoxazole till day 120 in all and beyond day 120 in 19% patients; no other prophylactic antiviral/bacterial/fungal drugs, no intravenous immunoglobulin and no pathogen-specific T cells were given. Reproduced, with permission, from Sullivan *et al.* (1996).

immune reconstitution following cytokine-mobilized peripheral blood stem cell transplantation (PBSCT) or cord blood transplantation (CBT). Little is known about the impact of low-intensity conditioning regimens; our preliminary data suggest that compared to the immunity of patients receiving high intensity regimens the immunity of patients receiving low intensity regimens is better early, but not late, posttransplant.

Innate Immunity

Epithelial barriers

The radiation, chemotherapy or acute GVHD-induced damage to the skin and the respiratory and digestive mucosa increases the chance of pathogen penetration into the organism early posttransplant. Late posttransplant, the epithelium is healed; the volume of protective secretions (e.g., saliva) and their IgA content become gradually normal in patients without chronic GVHD, but continue to be subnormal in those with chronic GVHD (Fig. 14.2) (Beschorner et al., 1981; Izutsu et al., 1983; Chaushu et al., 1995).

Neutrophils

The quantity of circulating neutrophils usually becomes normal by 1 month, earlier after PBSC than marrow grafting (Ma et al., 1987; Atkinson 1991; DeWitte et al., 1992; VanDer Wall et al., 1994; Bensinger et al., 1996). However, neutrophil function (e.g., chemotaxis, phagocytosis, superoxide production, and killing of bacteria) early posttransplant is often subnormal. Late posttransplant, neutrophil function gradually becomes normal, except in patients with chronic GVHD (Clark et al., 1976; Territo et al., 1977; Sosa et al., 1980; Zimmerli et al., 1989; Zimmerli et al., 1991).

Natural killer cells

The quantity of circulating natural killer (NK) cells usually becomes normal by 1 month posttransplant (Atkinson et al., 1990b; Leino et al., 1991; Ericson et al., 1992; Storek et al., 1992; Keever et al., 1993; Roberts et al., 1993; Scambia et al.,

1993; Ashihara et al., 1994; Ottinger et al., 1996; Talmadge et al., 1997; Storek et al., 2001a). The recovery is faster, and the early posttransplant NK cell counts tend to be higher in cytomegalovirus (CMV)-seropositive than CMV-seronegative patients (Hokland et al., 1988; Kook et al., 1996). This is not surprising since an important role of NK cells in human beings is defense against herpes viruses (Biron et al., 1989; Whiteside & Heberman, 1994).

When tested in vitro for their ability to kill NK-sensitive malignant cells (e.g., K562 cell line), NK cells from transplant recipients appear fully functional (Niederwieser et al., 1987; Hokland et al., 1988; Reittie et al., 1989).

Complement

After BMT, C3 and C4 are not deficient (Noel et al., 1978). Mannose binding lectin, a serum molecule binding to repeating carbohydrate moieties on pathogens and opsonizing phagocytosis, may be deficient in some transplant recipients, who have high rates of infections (Mullighan et al., 2002).

B Cells

Quantity

Blood B cell counts are low to undetectable during the first 2 months after marrow grafting (Baumgartner et al., 1988; Bengtsson et al., 1989b; Pedrazzini et al., 1989; Champlin et al., 1990; Small et al., 1990; Leino et al., 1991; Ericson et al., 1992; Foot et al., 1993; Scambia et al., 1993; Storek et al., 1993; Ashihara et al., 1994; Koehne et al., 1997; Storek et al., 2001a). Then they rise and usually become supranormal by 1–2 years after grafting. The rise is faster in autologous than allogeneic marrow recipients. It is faster in patients without chronic GVHD than in those with chronic GVHD (Fig. 14.3) (Small et al., 1990; Storek et al., 1993; Kook et al., 1996), probably because chronic GVHD and/or its treatment hamper B-cell generation in the marrow (Storek et al., 1996; Storek et al., 2001c).

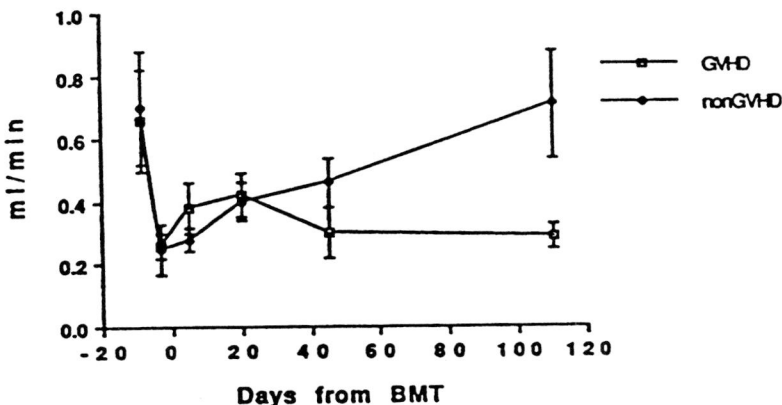

Fig. 14.2. Parotid salivary flow rate in BMT recipients (73% allogeneic), showing the drop soon after conditioning and the gradual normalization in patients without, but not those with, GVHD. Normal volunteers' flow rate was 0.68 ± 0.11 ml/min. Reproduced, with permission, from Chaushu et al. (1995).

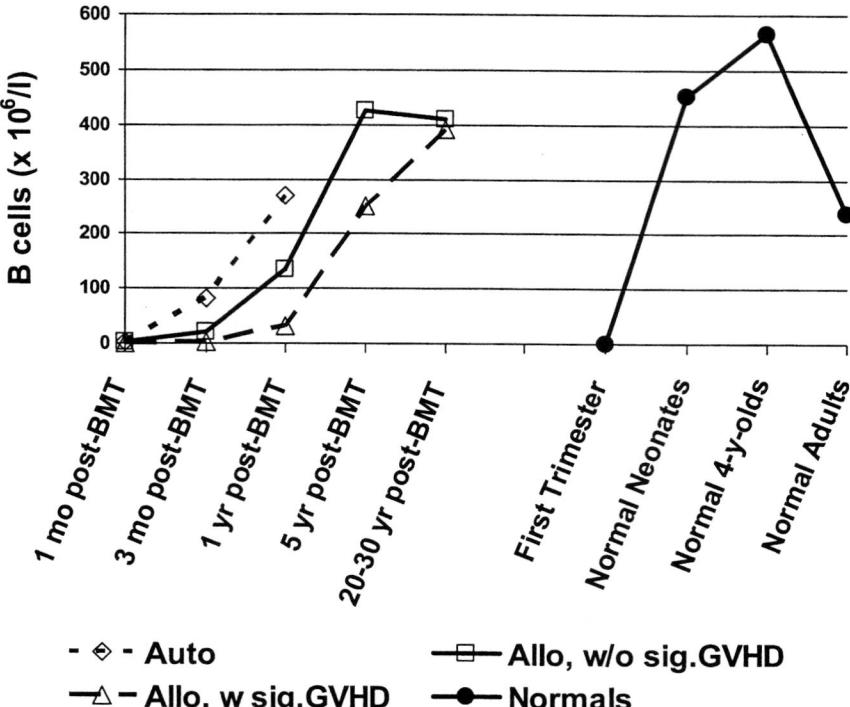

Fig. 14.3. Circulating B cell counts after BMT (left) and in normal ontogeny (right). In early ontogeny, there is a rapid rise leading to supranormal (higher than in normal adults) counts at 0 and 4 years of age, followed by a decline. After BMT, the trend is similar, though the initial rise is less steep, particularly in allograft recipients with significant GVHD (grade 2–4 acute GVHD or clinical extensive chronic GVHD). Each data point represents the median of typically >7 individuals. The B-cell count in the first trimester of pregnancy was arbitrarily assigned a value of zero as B-lymphopoiesis starts in the third month of gestation.

The rising B cells are largely composed of naive B cells; the recovery of memory B-cell counts lags behind (Fig. 14.4) (Storek et al., 1997d). Both the relatively fast rise of naive B cells above the normal adult range and the relatively slow rise of memory B cells are reminiscent of normal B-cell development in early ontogeny. In early ontogeny, naive B-cell counts rise from zero in the first trimester of pregnancy to supranormal levels by birth, whereas memory B-cell counts rise from zero in the first trimester to subnormal levels at birth and to supranormal levels only by the age of 4 (Fig. 14.4).

After PBSCT compared to BMT (Fig. 14.5), B cells are more abundant early posttransplant. This is true for the allogeneic but not for the autologous setting (Roberts et al., 1993; Ottinger et al., 1996; Rosillo et al., 1996; Storek et al., 1997c; Talmadge et al., 1997; Storek et al., 2001a). It may be related to the high content of B cells in PBSC allografts (10- to 20-fold higher than in marrow) (Ottinger et al., 1996; Storek et al., 1997c; Storek et al., 2001a). Late posttransplant, B-cell counts are similar or higher after BMT than PBSCT (Roberts et al., 1993; Ottinger et al., 1996; Rosillo et al., 1996; Storek et al., 2001a).

After CBT, the rise from very low to supranormal B-cell counts may occur earlier than after BMT (at 2–6 months after CBT) (Locatelli et al., 1996; Thomson et al., 2000).

Phenotype

Early posttransplant, phenotyping of B cells is difficult due to their scarcity. Late posttransplant, compared to normal adults, B cells from transplant recipients are larger (Fig. 14.6) (Storek et al., 1993). A lower percentage express CD25 and CD62L (Antin et al., 1987; Kagan et al., 1989; Storek et al., 1993). A greater percentage express CD1c, CD38, membrane IgM (mIgM), and membrane IgD (mIgD) (Velardi et al., 1988a; Small et al., 1990; Storek et al., 1993). Moreover, the amount of CD38, mIgM and mIgD molecules per CD38+/mIgM+/mIgD+ cell is greater (Elfenbein et al., 1982; Velardi et al., 1988a; Storek et al., 1993). This phenotype is remarkably similar to that of neonatal B cells.

Also, supranormal percents of CD5+ B cells are present both in infancy as well as during the first 6 months after autologous BMT (Small et al., 1990; Storek et al., 1993; Parra et al., 1996). After allogeneic BMT, the percent of CD5+ B cells is variable; they may be lower in patients with GVHD than in those without GVHD (Antin et al., 1987; Drexler et al., 1987; Storek et al., 1993).

Repertoire

Host defenses against infections require diverse B cells, i.e., B cells that use diverse combinations of variable (V), diversity

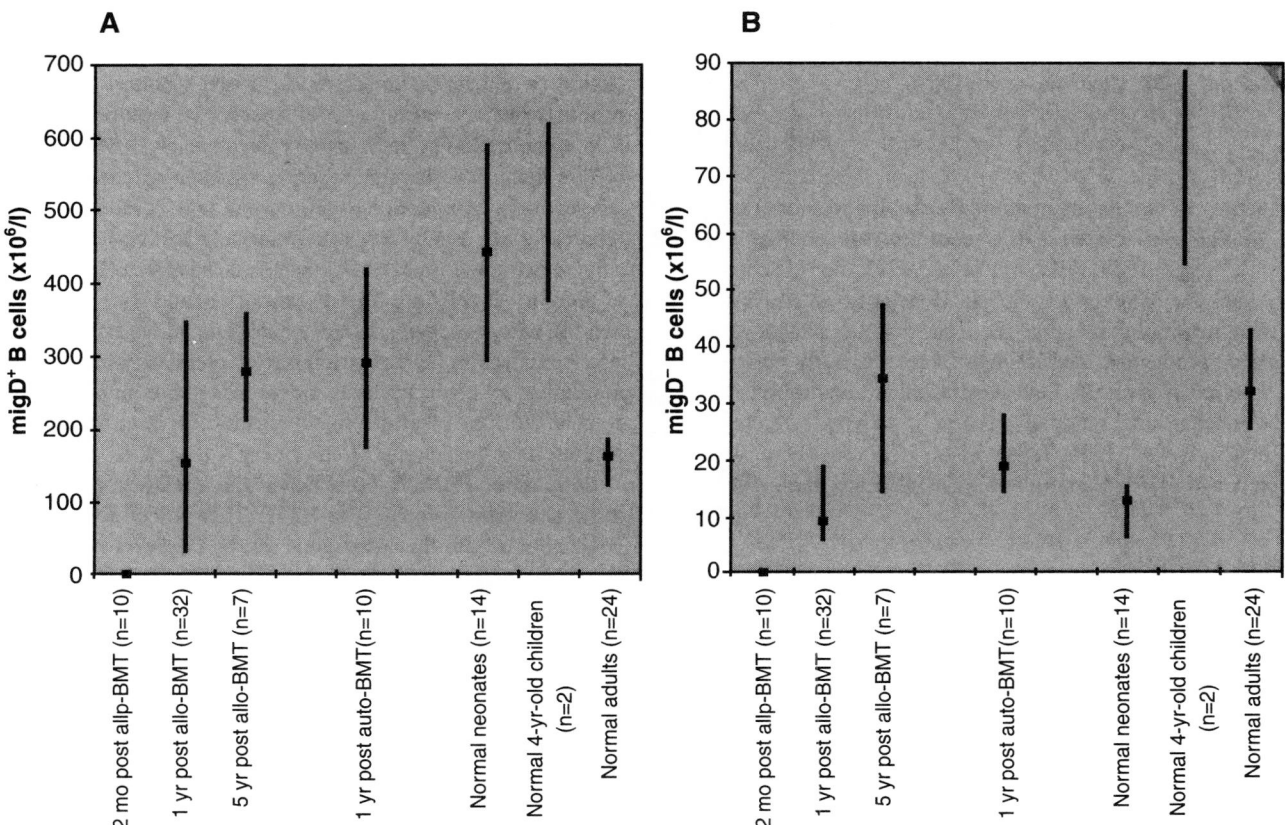

Fig. 14.4. The reconstitution of naive (mIgD+) (A) and memory (mIgD−) (B) B-cell counts in patients after BMT and in normal ontogeny. In early ontogeny, naive B cell counts rise from zero in the first trimester of pregnancy (not shown) to supranormal levels by birth, whereas memory B cells rise from zero in the first trimester (not shown) to subnormal levels at birth and supranormal levels only by the age of 4. Following allogeneic BMT, naive B cell counts are zero to subnormal early posttransplant, normal by 1 year and supranormal by 5 years posttransplant, whereas memory B-cell counts are zero to subnormal early posttransplant, subnormal at 1 year and normal by 5 years posttransplant. The recovery of B-cell counts after autologous BMT proceeds faster: the naive B-cell count is already supranormal at 1 year, and the memory B-cell count is close to normal at 1 year posttransplant. Reproduced, with permission, from Storek et al. (1997d).

(D) and joint (J) gene segments and junctional (N and P) nucleotides. To further enhance the immunity, B cells with somatically mutated VDJ genes are required that have been selected because the antibodies encoded by the mutated genes had higher affinity for the infectious agent than the antibodies encoded by the nonmutated B cells. After transplant, the percent B cells with somatically mutated VDJ genes is subnormal for at least 1 year (Fig. 14.7) (Fumoux et al., 1993; Storek et al., 1994b; Minegishi et al., 1995; Nasman & Lundkvist, 1996; Suzuki et al., 1996; Gokmen et al., 1998; Glas et al., 2000).

The restricted repertoire of B cells with different VDJ genes translates into the restricted repertoire of antibodies: The electrophoretic heterogeneity of tetanus-specific antibodies in BMT recipient sera is subnormal (Gerritsen et al., 1994).

Function in vitro

Early posttransplant, blood B cells are scarce and therefore difficult to obtain and study in vitro. Late posttransplant, B cell activation, proliferation and IgM production after polyclonal stimulation (e.g., with anti-Ig, cytokines, *Staphylococcus aureus* Cowan, Epstein-Barr virus [EBV]) are normal or only slightly abnormal (Anderson et al., 1987; Kiesel et al., 1988; Kagan et al., 1989; Storek et al., 1994a). However, IgG and IgA production is abnormal until about 2 years post-BMT, as it is in normal newborns (Fig. 14.8) (Matsue et al., 1987; Wimperis et al., 1987a; Pedrazzini et al., 1989; Small et al., 1990; Storek et al., 1995a). This may be because both patient and neonatal B cells contain few memory (isotype-switched, somatically mutated) B cells (Figs. 14.4 and 14.7) (i.e., B cells programmed to produce IgG or IgA upon activation). In vitro function of B cells may be worse in patients with than without chronic GVHD (Matsue et al., 1987; Korholz et al., 1996).

Function in vivo

There is no in vivo test for B cells only. In the following paragraphs, we review the results of tests that assess the function of

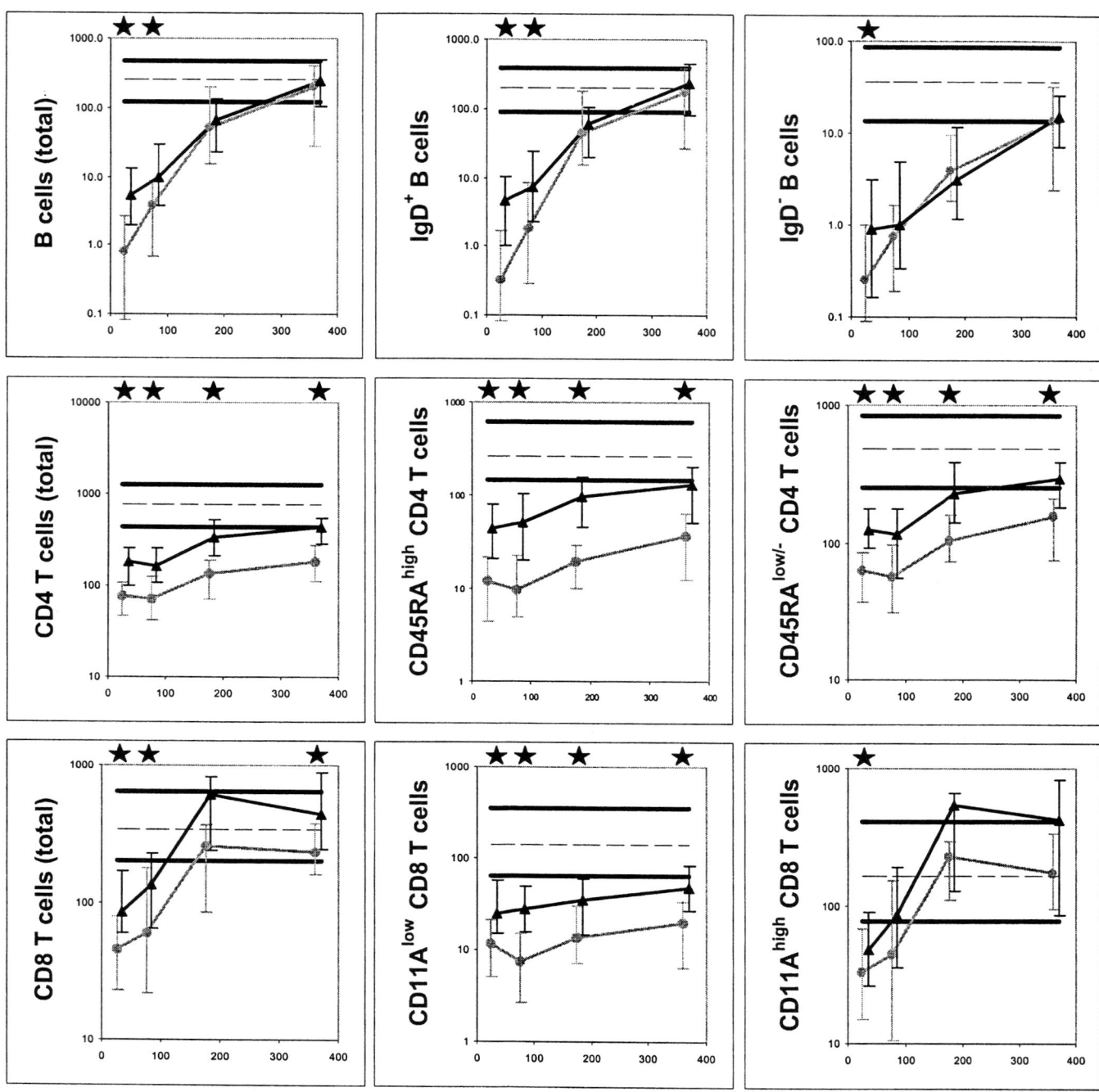

Fig. 14.5. Reconstitution of B cells (top), CD4[+] T cells (middle) and CD8[+] T cells (bottom) after allogeneic PBSCT (black triangles) versus BMT (grey circles) at approximately 30, 80, 180 and 365 days posttransplant (x-axes). On all y-axes, values for cell counts are per microliter of blood. Stars indicate a significant difference ($P < .05$). Error bars indicate the 25th to 75th percentiles. Normal values are shown as horizontal lines (thick solid lines for the 10th and 90th percentiles and thin broken lines for the medians). Reproduced, with permission, from Storek et al. (2001a).

B cells together with other components of the humoral immune system (e.g., CD4[+] T cells, follicular dendritic cells).

Antibody levels

Humoral immunity has been indirectly assessed by serial measurements of serum antibodies. After an initial fall early post-

transplant, serum total isotype levels recover in the same sequence as in small children: IgM, IgG$_1$ and IgG$_3$ become normal or even supranormal within months whereas IgG$_2$, IgG$_4$ and IgA become normal within years after BMT (Fig. 14.9) (Velardi et al., 1988a; Zintl et al., 1989; Abedi et al., 1990; Sheridan et al., 1990; Norhagen et al., 1994; Sullivan et al.,

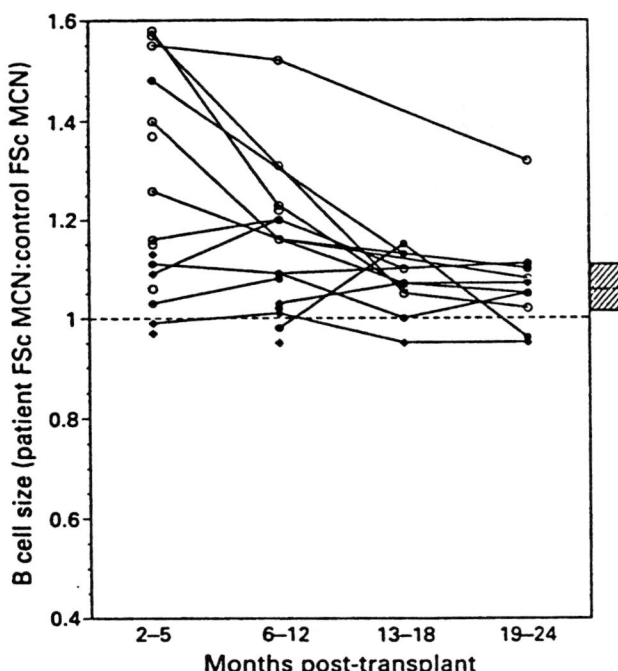

Fig. 14.6. Relative B cell size expressed as the ratio of the patient or new-born forward scatter mean channel number (FSc MCN) to the normal adult control FSc MCN, showing that posttransplant, as well as neonatal, B cells are generally larger (relative size >1). Closed diamonds represent auto-BMT recipients, closed circles allo-BMT recipients without chronic GVHD, and open circles allo-BMT recipients with chronic GVHD. The diagonally striped box and the dashed line inside the box represent the 10th to 90th percentiles and the median for normal neonates. Reproduced, with permission, from Storek et al. (1996).

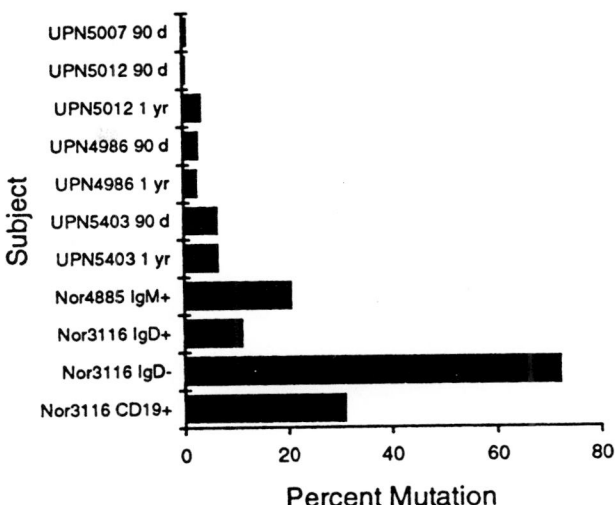

Fig. 14.7. Percent somatically mutated B cells among B cells utilizing VH3–23 gene. In a normal individual (Nor3116 CD19+), approximately 30% VH3–23-utilizing B cells have accumulated somatic mutations, whereas in patients (UPN…) at 90 days or 1 year post-allo-BMT, <10% VH3–23-utilizing B cells have accumulated somatic mutations. When mIgD+ or mIgD− B cells rather than total B cells from the normal individual were used for the assay of VH3–23 mutations, as expected, the mIgD− but not the mIgD+ subset was shown to contain the vast majority of the somatically mutated cells (2nd and 3rd bars from the bottom). Therefore, long-term transplant survivors lack memory B cells (somatically mutated and isotype-switched B cells) as shown here and in Fig. 1 to 4. Reproduced, with permission, from Suzuki et al. (1996).

1996; Storek et al., 2001b). However, total isotype levels are imperfect markers of humoral immunity since posttransplant immunoglobulins are frequently composed of autoantibodies (Smith et al., 1985; Holmes et al., 1989; Kier et al., 1990; Sanmarco et al., 1991; Lortan et al., 1992a; Hebart et al., 1996; Soderberg et al., 1996a; Soderberg et al., 1996b) and mono/oligoclonal antibodies of irrelevant specificity (not against the antigens of infectious agents) (VanDenBerg et al., 1976; Mink et al., 1979; Mitus et al., 1989; Fischer et al., 1990; Radl et al., 1991; Tissot et al., 1992; Gerritsen et al., 1996; Hebart et al., 1996).

Antibodies with a relevant specificity also fall early posttransplant. Subsequent to that, their levels depend on posttransplant encounter with the antigen (Fig. 14.10). If the encounter with the antigen does not occur, the levels of specific antibodies may become undetectable within 10 to 15 years post-BMT (earlier if the donor or the recipient have not encountered the antigen pretransplant) (Wahren et al., 1984; Ljungman et al., 1990; LiVolti et al., 1994; Ljungman et al., 1994; Parkkali et al., 1996b; Storek et al., 2001b; Machado et al., 2002). If the encounter with the antigen occurs (e.g., CMV in patients that were CMV-seropositive pretransplant), the levels of specific antibodies nor-

malize within about 1 year—earlier in patients with, and later in patients without, immune donors (Engelhard et al., 1991b; Lutz et al., 1996). This applies to protein antigens. In the case of polysaccharide antigens (e.g., pneumococcal capsular polysaccharides), the levels of specific antibodies may only normalize very late (2 to 20 years after transplant) even if the encounter with antigen is likely (Giebink et al., 1986; Aucouturier et al., 1987; Lortan et al., 1992b; Storek et al., 2001b).

Transient rise of IgE early after BMT has been reported repeatedly (Ringden et al., 1983; Saryan et al., 1983; Walker et al., 1984; Brenner et al., 1986; Heyd et al., 1988; Norhagen-Engstrom et al., 1988; Bengtsson et al., 1989a). The cause is unknown. In one study, monomeric IgM (an ontogenetically less mature form of IgM) was frequently detected during the first 9 months post-BMT (Jol-v.d. Zijde et al., 1983).

After PBSCT, total serum IgG levels as well as pathogen-specific IgG levels do not appear to be higher than after BMT (Chan et al., 1997; Storek et al., 1997c; Storek et al., 2003). It is unclear why this is the case in view of the quantities of circulating CD4+ T cells and, in some patients early posttransplant, higher B cells numbers in PBSC recipients (Fig. 14.5).

After CBT, serum total isotype levels appear to follow the same pattern of reconstitution as after BMT (Locatelli et al., 1996).

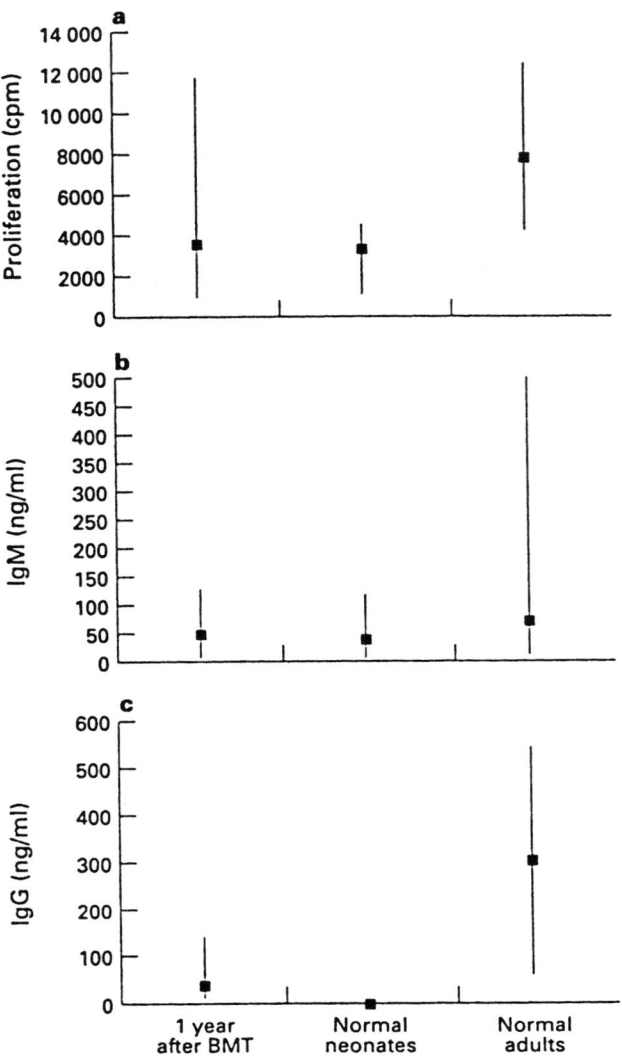

Fig. 14.8. In comparison with normal adults, proliferation of B cells (a) and IgM production by B cells (b) from patients at 1 year after transplant (79% allogeneic) or from normal neonates are only slightly reduced (43–67% of normal), whereas IgG production (c) is markedly reduced (≤13% of normal). Highly purified B cells were stimulated with anti-μ plus CD40 ligand plus interleukin-10. Similar results were obtained when only CD40 ligand plus interleukin-10 were used for stimulation. Proliferation was measured by ³H-thymidine incorporation on day 4; counts per minute (cpm) shown here are the resulting cpm after the background cpm (of unstimulated B cells) had been subtracted. The amount of IgM and IgG in supernatants was measured by ELISA on day 9. Results are expressed as medians (closed squares) and 25th–75th percentiles (horizontal lines). Reproduced, with permission, from Storek et al. (1995a).

Antibody responses to immunization

Antibody response refers to the increase of antigen-specific serum antibody levels after immunization. It is usually defined as the 1 month post-immunization level/the pre-immunization level. Early posttransplant responses to any antigen are subnormal. Responses to protein antigens recover faster (usually

within 1 to 2 years, Fig. 14.10) than responses to polysaccharide antigens (usually at ≥2 years posttransplant). Responses to protein recall antigens (e.g., poliovirus or tetanus toxoid) tend to recover faster than responses to protein neoantigens (e.g., keyhole limpet hemocyanin). The recovery of antibody responses to any antigen is delayed in patients with chronic GVHD (Noel et al., 1978; Witherspoon et al., 1981; Witherspoon et al., 1982; Winston et al., 1983; Amlot et al., 1986; Giebink et al., 1986; Ljungman et al., 1989; Ljungman et al., 1990; Otsuka et al., 1990; Quinti et al., 1990; Engelhard et al., 1991a; Engelhard et al., 1991b; Ljungman et al., 1991; Barra et al., 1992; Lortan et al., 1992b; Pauksen et al., 1992; Engelhard et al., 1993; Guinan et al., 1994; LiVolti et al., 1994; Nagler et al., 1995; King et al., 1996; Parkkali et al., 1996a; Parkkali et al., 1996b; Parkkali et al., 1997). T-cell depletion of the graft or posttransplant treatment with anti-T-cell antibodies may delay the recovery of antibody responses (Witherspoon et al., 1981; Guinan et al., 1994). Also, the responses may recover faster in young versus old individuals (Guinan et al., 1994), which could be related to the faster recovery of CD4+ T cells in younger patients (Storek et al., 1995b; Weinberg et al., 1995). The conditioning regimen may also play a role: in a mouse model, 9.5 Gy total body irradiation was associated with lower antibody responses than 8.0 Gy (Ishii et al., 1991). The responses to Haemophilus influenzae capsular polysaccharide conjugated to a protein are better than the responses to the polysaccharide alone (Barra et al., 1992). It remains to be determined whether this is also true for Streptococcus pneumoniae-conjugated capsular polysaccharides (Storek et al., 1997b; Molrine & Hibberd 2001).

Little is known about antibody responses after allogeneic PBSCT or CBT. One study suggests improved antibody responses after autologous PBSCT compared to autologous BMT (Chan et al., 1997). After allogeneic PBSCT, antibody responses do not appear to be superior compared to allogeneic BMT (Storek et al., 2003).

Origin

From the donor or the recipient?

Most or all circulating lymphocytes are of donor origin by 1 to 2 months after T-cell-replete transplantation with high intensity conditioning (Fig. 14.11). After T-cell-depleted transplantation and after transplantation with low intensity conditioning, a variable degree of incomplete chimerism is frequently established (Roux et al., 1992; Wessman et al., 1993; VanLeeuwen et al., 1994b; Lapointe et al., 1996; McSweeney et al., 2001; Auffermann-Gretzinger et al., 2002).

Virtually all circulating B cells are of donor origin after T-cell-replete grafting with high intensity conditioning (Sadamori et al., 1983; Ault et al., 1985; Korver et al., 1987a; Korver et al., 1987b; Auffermann-Gretzinger et al., 2002; Storek et al., 2002b). By Ig allotyping (Gm, Inv), serum antibodies are primarily of recipient origin early posttransplant. This may be due to the relative radioresistance of recipient plasma cells (Miller &

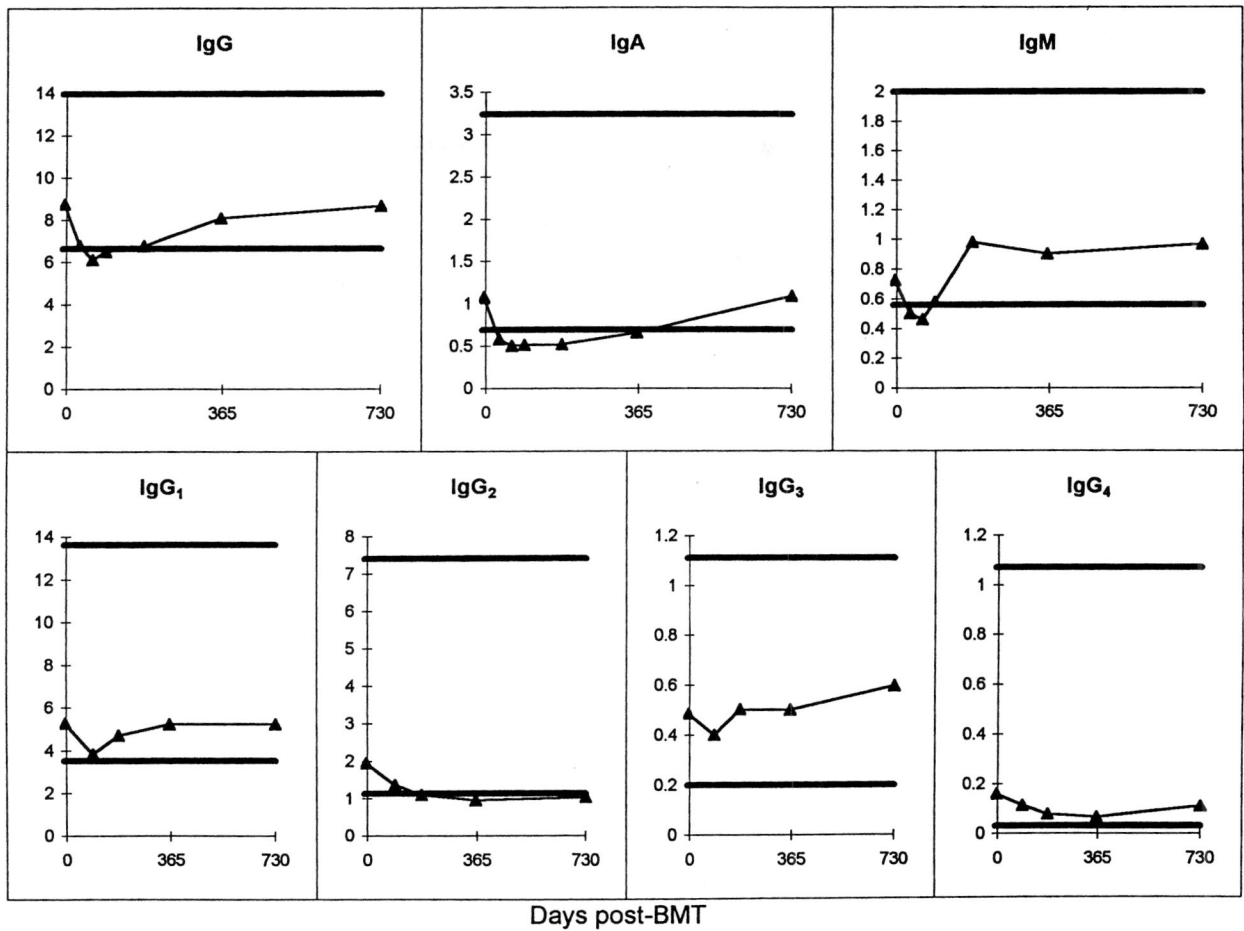

Fig. 14.9. Serum total Ig isotype levels (g/l) in BMT recipients (80% allogeneic) transplanted in Seattle between 1986 and 1988, showing that IgM, IgG_1, and IgG_2 recover faster than IgA, IgG_2, and IgG_4. Patient data are expressed as geometric means. Normal range (thick horizontal lines) is given as the 5th–95th percentiles based on 315 (IgG, IgA, IgM) or 170 (IgG subclasses) primarily adult marrow donors. The following numbers of patients were studied: 127 pretransplant, 125 on day 30, 123 on day 60, 122 on day 90, 76 on day 180, 68 at 1 year, and 17 at 2 years posttransplant. Patients were not receiving IVIG, except for 3 patients—one of them as part of CMV pneumonia therapy and two of them because of very low serum IgG (<4 g/l) with infections. Reproduced, with permission, from Sullivan *et al.* (1996).

Cole, 1967) and the lack of B cells early posttransplant. Late posttransplant, recipient antibodies tend to disappear and be replaced by donor-type antibodies. Nevertheless, a small amount of recipient Ig has been detected up to 8 years, even after T-cell-replete BMT (Fig. 14.12), which may be due to a relatively long life span of plasma cells (Witherspoon *et al.*, 1978; Sparkes *et al.*, 1979; Petz *et al.*, 1987; Schouten *et al.*, 1988; Sniecinski *et al.*, 1988; Barge *et al.*, 1989; Bar *et al.*, 1990; Bar *et al.*, 1995; Slifka *et al.*, 1995; Van Tol *et al.*, 1996; Slifka *et al.*, 1998).

An interesting insight into the kinetics of the gradual replacement of recipient with donor humoral immunity can be obtained from one patient who acquired IgA deficiency from his marrow donor, and one patient whose IgA deficiency was corrected by allogeneic BMT. In the former case, serum IgA fell from normal levels during the first month to below the detection limit on day 100 posttransplant and remained undetectable thereafter (Hammarstrom *et al.*, 1985). In the latter case, a steady rise of serum and salivary IgA from barely detectable to normal levels occurred between day 50 and 150 (Kurobane *et al.*, 1991). The former case may illustrate the gradual disappearance of host plasma cells, since the half-life of IgA is short (3 to 4 days). The latter case illustrates the gradual emergence of donor humoral immunity, despite the fact that normalization of IgA levels occurred earlier that usual.

Patients transplanted for severe combined immunodeficiency (SCID), frequently using T-cell-depleted grafts and no conditioning, behave differently. They typically reconstitute recipient-type B cells (and recipient-type myeloid cells and donor-type T cells) (Wijnaendts *et al.*, 1989; Dror *et al.*, 1993; Vossen *et al.*, 1993; O'Reilly *et al.*, 1994; VanLeeuwen *et al.*, 1994a; Flake *et al.*, 1996; Stiehm *et al.*, 1996; Haddad *et al.*, 1999).

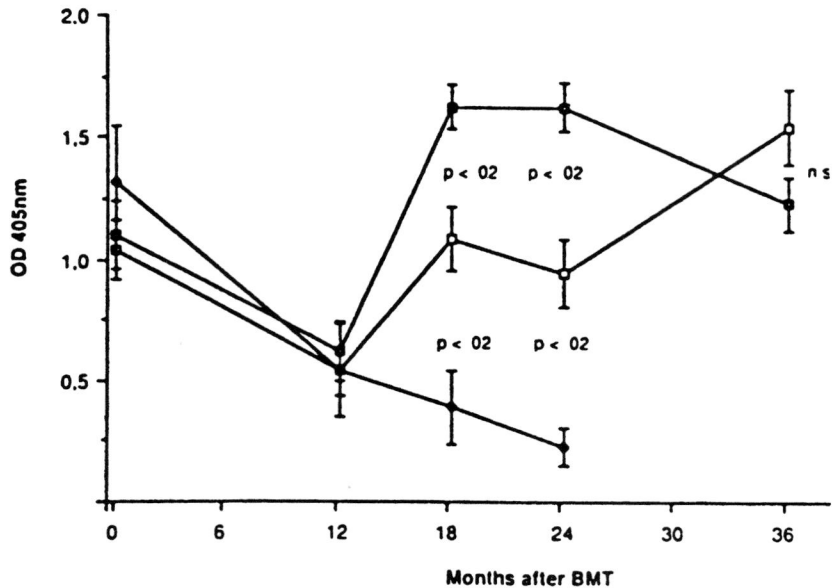

Fig. 14.10. Serum tetanus-specific Ig levels (expressed as OD 405 nm) in 48 allo-BMT recipients, showing the gradual decline in patients that were not vaccinated posttransplant (diamonds), and the postvaccination rise in patients that were vaccinated with tetanus toxoid posttransplant. The latter group is split into those who received 3 doses of the vaccine at 12, 13, and 14 months (closed squares with a white dot) and those who received 1 dose at 12 months and 2 doses between 24 and 36 months posttransplant (open squares with a black dot). OD 405 nm of 0.5 was regarded as representative of seropositivity. Reproduced, with permission, from Ljungman *et al.* (1990).

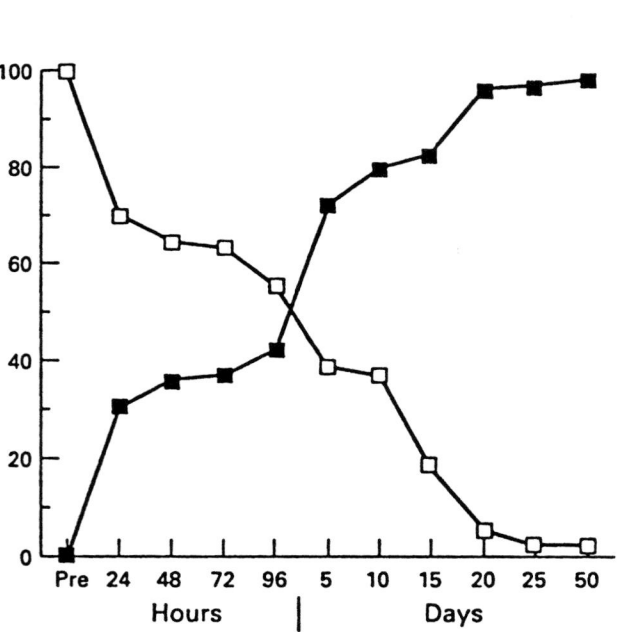

Fig. 14.11. Median proportion of donor and recipient lymphocytes (by X/Y-chromosome in situ hybridization) in 10 recipients of T cell-replete and sex-mismatched BMT with high intensity conditioning, showing that by 1 month posttransplant most circulating lymphocytes are of donor (closed squares), and not recipient (open squares), origin. Reproduced, with permission, from Lapointe *et al.* (1996).

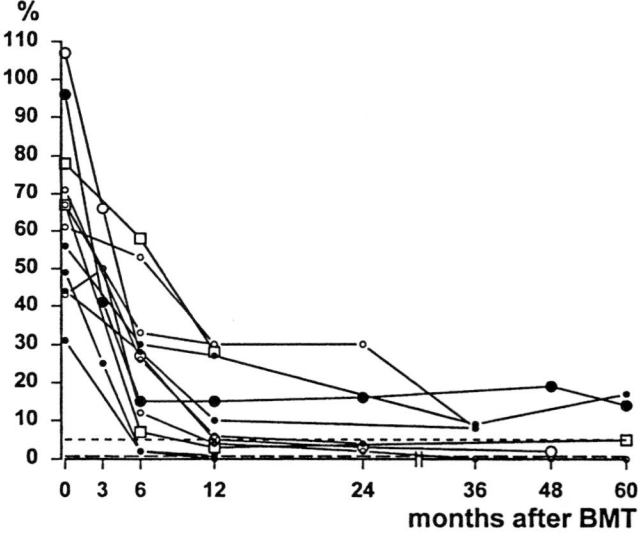

Fig. 14.12. Persistence of recipient-type IgG_1 in the serum of allogeneic BMT patients. Data are expressed as the percents of IgG_1 with the relevant G_1m allotype relative to the total amount of IgG_1. Symbols represent recipients homozygous (large closed circles) or heterozygous (small closed circles) for $G_1m(a)$ with a $G_1m(a)$-negative donor, recipients homozygous (large open circles) or heterozygous (small open circles) for $G_1m(f)$ with a $G_1m(f)$-negative donor, and recipients heterozygous for $G_1m(z)$ with a $G_1m(z)$-negative donor. The upper normal limit for individuals negative for $G_1m(a)$ or $G_1m(f)$ is indicated by the dashed line with long segments, and the upper normal limit for individuals negative for $G_1m(z)$ is indicated by the dashed line with short segments. Reproduced, with permission, from VanTol *et al.* (1996).

In summary, except for SCID patients and some non-SCID patients receiving T-cell-depleted grafts, B-cell immunity is primarily of donor origin by several months posttransplant.

From B cells or de novo from stem cells?

Are the donor-type B cells derived from the B cells infused with the graft, from the infused stem cells, or both? Support for the origin of B cells infused with the graft comes from studies showing that memory-type humoral immunity can be adoptively transferred from immune donors, even with T-cell-depleted grafts (reviewed below). Support for the origin from stem cells comes from the following indirect evidence:

1. Supranormal amounts of B-cell precursors are frequently found in the marrow at 2 to 12 months after transplant, i.e., prior to the overshoot of circulating B-cell counts above the normal adult range (Asma *et al.*, 1987; Uckun *et al.*, 1992; Leitenberg *et al.*, 1994; Storek *et al.*, 1996).
2. In recipients of B cell purged autologous marrow, the tempo of B-cell reconstitution is not slower than in recipients of unmanipulated marrow (Baumgartner *et al.*, 1988; Bengtsson *et al.*, 1989b; Pedrazzini *et al.*, 1989; Bomberger *et al.*, 1998).
3. The phenotype of the posttransplant B cells is conspicuously similar to the phenotype of B cells in early life (reviewed above).

In summary, it is likely that both B-cell-derived and stem cell-derived B cells coexist after grafting. However, whereas the former ones may predominate early, the latter ones probably predominate late posttransplant.

Adoptive transfer

Antigen-specific humoral immunity can be transferred with marrow grafting. This could be due to the transfer of antigen-primed B cells, T cells, or pre-plasma/plasma cells. B cells may play an important role in this transfer, because not only are ongoing antibody responses transferred, but specific antibody responses can be elicited upon immunizing the patient early posttransplant (presumably before a significant number of B cells have been generated from stem cells) (Saxon *et al.*, 1986), even if the graft was depleted of T cells (Wimperis *et al.*, 1987b).

Host exposure to the antigen pretransplant or early posttransplant influences the success of the adoptive transfer (Fig. 14.13). The transfer of humoral immunity to antigens that were encountered by both the donor and the recipient occurs regularly and the resultant immunity is relatively long-lasting (months to years) (Lum *et al.*, 1986; Shiobara *et al.*, 1986; Lum *et al.*, 1988; Bar *et al.*, 1990; Ljungman *et al.*, 1994; Lutz *et al.*, 1996; Molrine *et al.*, 1996a; Molrine *et al.*, 1996b). This is true provided the first encounter of the donor with the antigen happened more than 1 to 2 weeks pretransplant, presumably because the antigen-specific B cells expand sufficiently only after 1 to 2 weeks (Wimperis *et al.*, 1990). In contrast, no antibody production or antibody production lasting only weeks to

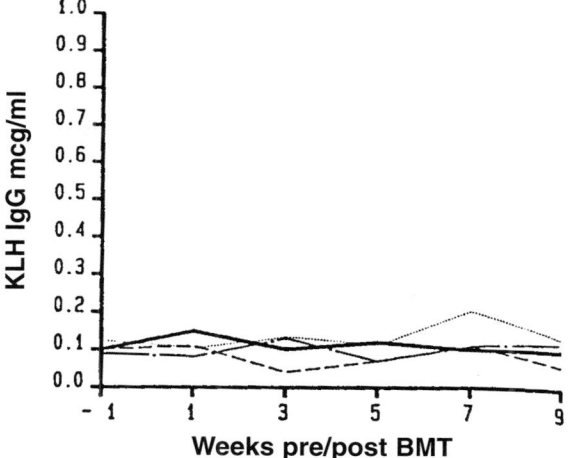

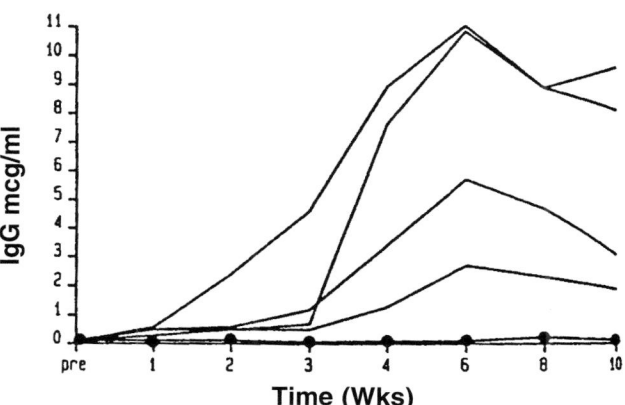

Fig. 14.13. Serum anti-keyhole limpet hemocyanin (KLH) IgG levels in the recipients of T-cell-depleted allogeneic marrow, showing that both donor exposure to KLH at 3 weeks (not at 1 week) pretransplant and recipient exposure to KLH peritransplant are essential for the success of the adoptive transfer of humoral immunity. The top graph shows the mean anti-KLH levels in the following groups of patients: neither donor nor recipient immunized (solid line), donor immunized at 1 week pretransplant and recipient not immunized (dashed line), both donor and recipient immunized at 1 week pretransplant (dotted line), and donor not immunized and recipient immunized at 1 week pretransplant (dashed and dotted line). The bottom graph shows the mean anti-KLH levels in the group of donors immunized at 3 weeks pretransplant and recipients not immunized (closed circles), and the anti-KLH levels in four patients whose donors were immunized at 3 weeks pretransplant and who were immunized at 1 week pretransplant (solid lines). In both graphs, the x-axis shows weeks posttransplant, and the y-axis shows anti-KLH IgG levels, however, using different scales. Reproduced, with permission, from Wimperis *et al.* (1990).

months is detected in the host if the antigen was encountered only by the donor and not by the recipient pretransplant or early posttransplant (Wimperis *et al.*, 1986; Donnenberg *et al.*, 1987; Gottlieb *et al.*, 1990; Cryz *et al.*, 1991; Labadie *et al.*,

1992; Chen et al., 1994), presumably because the life span of memory B cell clones is short in the absence of the antigen (Gray & Skarvall, 1988; Markham & Donnenberg, 1992; Gallucci et al., 1999) (Fig. 14.13).

Humoral immunity not only to microbial antigens but also to autoantigens can be transferred with the marrow. Thus, autoimmune diseases like myasthenia gravis, IgE-mediated allergies, Hashimoto's thyroiditis or immune thrombocytopenia have been transferred (Minchinton et al., 1982; Smith et al., 1983; Saarinen, 1984; Smith et al., 1985; Tucker & Barnetson, 1985; Agosti et al., 1988; Wyatt et al., 1990).

As expected, transfer of humoral immunity with blood mononuclear cells does occur (Ilan et al., 1994). Whether cytokine-mobilized PBSCs are a better graft than marrow for the adoptive transfer of B-cell immunity remains to be documented; our preliminary data do not suggest so. Transfer of humoral immunity to recall antigens with cord blood has not been studied. Theoretically, it should not be feasible because newborns are generally immunologically naive and vaccination in utero would be unethical.

CD4$^+$ T cells

Quantity

Blood CD4$^+$ T cell counts are very low (usually $<200 \times 10^6$/l) during the first 1 to 3 months after marrow grafting (Atkinson et al., 1982b; Friedrich et al., 1982; DeGast et al., 1985; Janossy et al., 1986; Bengtsson et al., 1989c; Keever et al., 1989; Atkinson et al., 1990a; Leino et al., 1991; Ericson et al., 1992; Storek et al., 1992; Foot et al., 1993; Scambia et al., 1993; Ashihara et al., 1994; DeSouza et al., 1994; Storek et al., 1995b; Kook et al., 1996; Bacigalupo et al., 1997; Koehne et al., 1997; Small et al., 1997; Small et al., 1999; Mackall et al., 2000; Storek et al., 2001a). They then rise slowly to around 300×10^6/l at 1 year and around 450×10^6/l at 5 years and become normal by 20 years after marrow grafting into adults (Storek et al., 2001b). (The reference range in our laboratory is 545-1257×10^6/l.) The CD4$^+$ T-cell counts early posttransplant are primarily influenced by the number of T cells given with the graft. For example, they are very low after T-cell-depleted grafting (using depletion ex vivo or in vivo [e.g., with the infusion of anti-T-cell antibody]), and only mildly low if grafts enriched for T cells (e.g., allogeneic PBSCs, Fig. 14.5) are used, or if donor lymphocytes are infused after grafting. The tempo of recovery is faster in pediatric than adult patients. The tempo may be similar in recipients of autologous and allogeneic grafts. However, in allograft recipients with severe GVHD, the tempo may be hampered, possibly due to inhibiting both de novo generation and peripheral expansion of T cells (Dulude et al., 1999). The above phenotypic studies enumerating CD4-expressing T cells are in agreement with the limiting dilution studies enumerating helper cells (the precursors of interleukin-2-producing cells upon polyclonal activation) (Daley et al., 1987; Miller et al., 1991), as they also show very slow recovery of helper T cells.

Phenotypic studies published prior to 1995 tend to report higher CD4 counts at all time points after grafting than later phenotypic studies. This may be related to differences in techniques. For example, in the older studies CD4$^+$ T cells were usually identified as cells expressing CD4 whereas in the more recent studies as cells expressing both CD3 and CD4 to minimize the error of counting monocytes as CD4$^+$ T cells.

In contrast to B cells, the rising CD4$^+$ T cells are largely composed of memory CD4$^+$ T cells and the recovery of naive CD4$^+$ T-cell counts in adult patients is extremely slow (Fig. 14.14) (Storek et al., 1995b; Weinberg et al., 1995; Small et al., 1997; Dumont-Girard et al., 1998; Small et al., 1999). This is probably related to the natural involution of the thymus and the thymic damage due to chemo/radiotherapy and GVHD (Chung et al., 2001; Weinberg et al., 2001; Storek et al., 2002a). Therefore, it is not surprising that the pattern of CD4$^+$ T-cell reconstitution posttransplant differs from the pattern in normal ontogeny, which is marked by a tremendous expansion of naive CD4$^+$ T cells from zero in the first trimester of pregnancy to supranormal levels by birth (Fig. 14.14).

After allogeneic PBSCT compared to BMT, both naive and memory CD4$^+$ T cells are more abundant (Fig. 14.5) (Bacigalupo et al., 1996; Ottinger et al., 1996; Storek et al., 1997c; Storek et al., 2001a; Elmaagacli et al., 2002). This may be related to the high content of CD4$^+$ T cells in the allogeneic PBSC grafts (~ 10-fold higher compared to marrow grafts) (Ottinger et al., 1996; Storek et al., 2001a). In the autologous setting, there is only a minor or no difference in CD4$^+$ T-cell counts between PBSC and marrow recipients (Roberts et al., 1993; Rosillo et al., 1996; Talmadge et al., 1997).

After CBT, the tempo of CD4$^+$ T-cell regeneration appears comparable to that after BMT (Locatelli et al., 1996; Takahashi et al., 1997; Thomson et al., 2000).

Phenotype

Both early and late post-BMT, the following antigens are more frequently expressed by CD4$^+$ T cells from transplant recipients than by those from normal adults: CD11a, CD29, CD45RO, and HLA-DR. The following antigens are less frequently expressed: CD28, CD45RA, and CD62L (Bengtsson et al., 1989c; Gorla et al., 1993; Sugita et al., 1994b; Storek et al., 1995b; Weinberg et al., 1995). Also, CD4$^+$ T cells from transplant recipients are larger than those from normal adults (Fig. 14.15) (Storek et al., 1992). This phenotype is markedly different from that of CD4$^+$ T cells from normal neonates and children, whose cells express CD11a, CD29 and CD45RO less frequently and CD28, CD45RA and CD62L more frequently than CD4$^+$ T cells from normal adults (Hannet et al., 1992; Storek et al., 1995b). Moreover, neonatal CD4$^+$ T cells are as large as CD4$^+$ T cells from normal adults (Fig. 14.15) (Storek et al., 1992). The phenotype of posttransplant CD4$^+$ T cells suggests the preponderance of antigen-primed cells as opposed to the preponderance of naive cells in normal early ontogeny. Interestingly, the phenotype of CD4$^+$ T cells from posttrans-

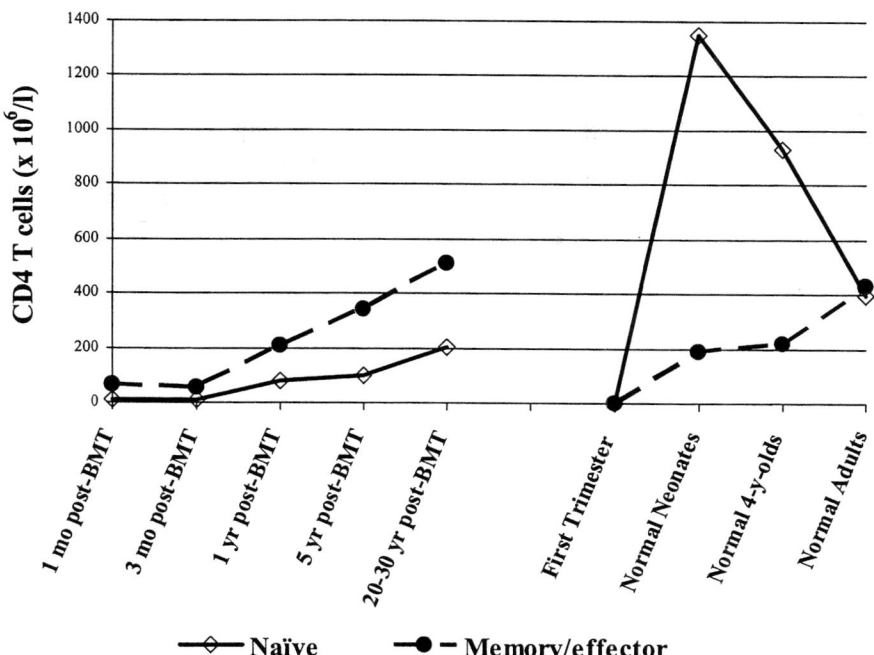

Fig. 14.14. Circulating CD4[+] T cell counts after BMT (left) and in normal ontogeny (right). In early ontogeny, there is a rapid increase in naïve (CD45RA[high]) CD4[+] T cells leading to supranormal (higher than in normal adults) counts at birth, followed by a decline. In contrast, after BMT into adults, the reconstitution of naïve CD4[+] T cells is extremely slow, and most posttransplant CD4[+] T cells are memory/effector cells (CD45RA[low/−], likely derived from T cells infused with the graft). Each data points represents the median of typically >7 individuals. The CD4[+] T-cell count in the first trimester of pregnancy was arbitrarily assigned a value of zero as T lymphopoiesis starts in the third month of gestation.

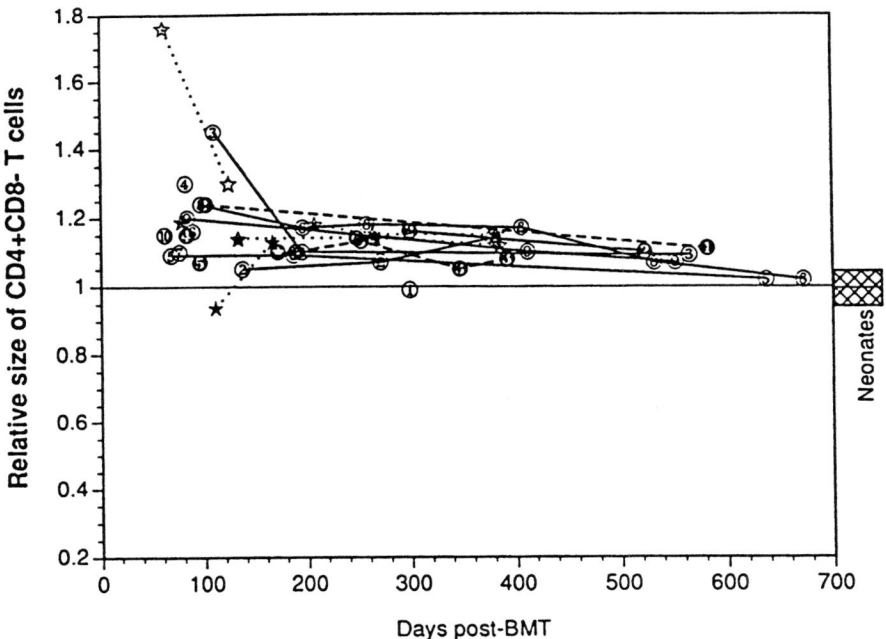

Fig. 14.15. Relative CD4[+] T cell size expressed as the ratio of the patient or newborn forward scatter mean channel number (FSc MCN) to the normal adult control FSc MCN, showing that posttransplant but not neonatal CD4[+] T cells are generally larger than normal adult CD4[+] T cells. Stars represent auto-BMT recipients, closed circles allo-BMT recipients without chronic GVHD and open circles allo-BMT recipients with chronic GVHD. The bidirectionally diagonally striped box and the horizontal line inside the box represent the 10th to 90th percentiles and the median for normal neonates. Reproduced, with permission, from Storek *et al.* (1992).

plant patients is similar to the phenotype of CD4+ T cells from SCID mice that have received human T cells. The "SCID mouse, human lymphocyte" chimeras do not develop GVHD (perhaps due to being kept in a germ-free environment) and the human T cells appear anergic (Tary-Lehmann & Saxton, 1992; Tary-Lehmann *et al.*, 1994).

Repertoire

The heterogeneity of posttransplant circulating T cells has been studied either by the flow cytometric detection of various T cell receptor families (with variable region-specific monoclonal antibodies), or by molecular detection of the length or the sequence of various VDJ DNA or RNA segments (Gorochov *et al.*, 1994; Gorski *et al.*, 1994; Villers *et al.*, 1994; Gaschet *et al.*, 1995; Gorski *et al.*, 1995; Smith *et al.*, 1995; Akatsuka *et al.*, 1996; Kubo *et al.*, 1996; Liu *et al.*, 1996; Masuko *et al.*, 1996; Roux *et al.*, 1996a; Roux *et al.*, 1996b; Vavassori *et al.*, 1996; Bomberger *et al.*, 1998; Godthelp *et al.*, 1999; Verfuerth *et al.*, 2000; Wu *et al.*, 2000; Bellucci *et al.*, 2002). Most studies did not separate T cells into subsets. With both techniques, the repertoire of total T cells appears skewed; compared to T cells from normal donors, some clones appear overrepresented while other clones are underrepresented or even absent. The overrepresentation of certain clones appears particularly frequent among CD8+ T cells and particularly in patients with GVHD. The undetectability (presumed absence) of clones appears particularly frequent in patients having received T-cell-depleted grafts (Fig. 14.16). Diversification of the repertoire occurs late posttransplant, with the advent of de novo generated T cells (Knobloch & Friedrich, 1991; Dumont-Girard *et al.*, 1998; Roux *et al.*, 2000; Talvensaari *et al.*, 2002).

Function in vitro

The following responses of posttransplant T cells to antigens or to polyclonal stimuli like anti-CD3 or lectins have been studied in vitro: signal transduction (e.g., Ca++ flux), upregulation of activation markers (e.g., CD25), proliferation and cytokine production (Quinnan *et al.*, 1982; Shiobara *et al.*, 1982; Brkic *et al.*, 1985; Cayeux *et al.*, 1989b; Cayeux *et al.*, 1989a; Cooley *et al.*, 1989; DeGast *et al.*, 1989; Izquierdo *et al.*, 1989; Keever *et al.*, 1989; Soiffer *et al.*, 1990; Yamagami *et al.*, 1990; Cooley *et al.*, 1991; Reusser *et al.*, 1991; Balboa *et al.*, 1992; Tollemar *et al.*, 1992; Lum *et al.*, 1993; Guillaume *et al.*, 1994; Lum *et al.*, 1994; Sugita *et al.*, 1994a; Tanaka *et al.*, 1994; Jin *et al.*, 1995; Kameoka *et al.*, 1995; Pauksen *et al.*, 1995; Guillaume *et al.*, 1996; Ottinger *et al.*, 1996; Pignata *et al.*, 1996; Vavassori *et al.*, 1996; Storek *et al.*, 1999; Heitger *et al.*, 2002). Anti-CD3 or lectin-induced responses are subnormal both early and late post-BMT. However, most studies measured the responses using total mononuclear cells. The results of the few studies on purified CD4+ T cells suggest that their responses to polyclonal stimuli are subnormal early and normal late post-BMT (Storek *et al.*, 1999) (Fig. 14.17), except for anti-

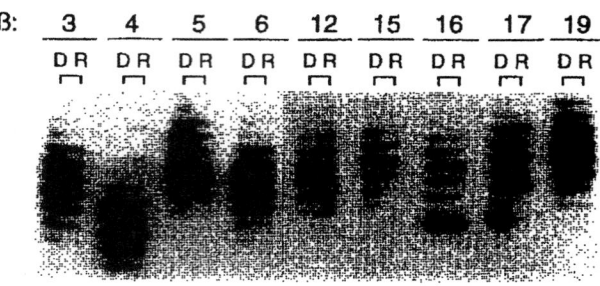

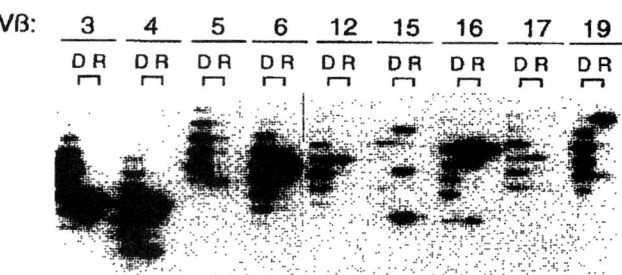

Fig. 14.16. T-cell receptor repertoire complexity in a recipient of an unmanipulated marrow graft (top) and in a recipient of a T-cell-depleted marrow graft (bottom), showing that the heterogeneity of T cells after T-depleted grafting is restricted. Spectratypes of nine Vβ families of the donors (D) and the recipients (R) are displayed. Both patients were studied at approximately 1 month posttransplant. Reproduced, with permission, from Roux *et al.* (1996b).

CD3-induced Ca++ flux which may be normal even early post-BMT. Antigen-induced proliferative responses of mononuclear cells (which reflect the proliferation of primarily CD4+ T cells) using antigens that are not likely encountered after grafting (e.g., tetanus) are subnormal both early and late post-BMT. This may be due to the low frequency of antigen-specific CD4+ T cells among mononuclear cells rather than the poor function of the antigen-specific CD4+ T cells, at least late posttransplant (Vavassori *et al.*, 1996). Antigen-induced mononuclear cell proliferative responses using antigens that are likely encountered after grafting (e.g., *Candida*) are usually subnormal early and usually normal late post-BMT. The proliferative responses to specific antigens have not been measured among purified CD4+ T cells.

Lum *et al.* (1982, 1985) evaluated the ability of purified CD4+ T cells from patients late posttransplant to provide help for normal B cells. In patients without chronic GVHD, the helper function was normal or only slightly subnormal. In patients with chronic GVHD it was subnormal.

The decreased function early posttransplant may be due to the suppression of T cells by monocytes/macrophages (Bobe *et al.*, 1999; Heitger *et al.*, 2002).

In summary, the responsiveness of CD4+ T cells to a polyclonal stimulus appears subnormal early and subnormal or normal late post-BMT, possibly depending on the presence or absence of chronic GVHD. The responsiveness to an antigen has been hard to assess. Even if purified CD4[+] T cells were used in a standard assay, one could not distinguish between low response due to the decreased number (percent) versus decreased function of the CD4[+] T cells specific for the antigen. This problem may be overcome by limiting dilution analysis or flow cytometric assays detecting cytokine production by single T cells. At present, the functional status of antigen-specific CD4[+] T cells after grafting is not known.

Function in vivo

The in vivo function of CD4[+] T cells has been assessed in two ways:

1. By skin testing for delayed-type hypersensitivity
2. By detecting an increase in antigen-specific proliferative response among blood mononuclear cells upon encountering an antigen (e.g., a herpesvirus antigen). Neither test evaluates only CD4[+] T cells since other cells like dendritic cells may play a role in the responses.

The former assessment (skin testing) showed subnormal responses to both neo-antigens (dinitrochlorobenzene and keyhole limpet hemocyanin) and recall antigens (trichophytin, streptokinase-streptodornase, *Candida* dermatophytin or a mumps virus antigen) for 2 to 3 years after marrow grafting (Witherspoon *et al.*, 1984).

The later studies of the increase in proliferative response suggest that the number or function of circulating antigen-specific CD4[+] T cells do increase upon encountering the antigen both early and late post-BMT, except in some patients with GVHD (DeGast *et al.*, 1985; Ljungman *et al.*, 1986; Kato *et al.*, 1990; Li *et al.*, 1994; Ottinger *et al.*, 1996). Comparison of the magnitude of the increase in transplant recipients versus healthy individuals has not been made.

Origin

From the donor or the recipient?
As reviewed above (B cells, Origin), most or all circulating lymphocytes are of donor origin by 1 to 2 months post-BMT (Fig. 14.11), unless the graft is depleted of T cells or the conditioning is of low intensity. The same probably applies to CD4[+] T cells (Gratama *et al.*, 1984).

From T cells or de novo from stem cells?
Are the donor-type CD4[+] T cells derived from the CD4[+] T cells infused with the graft, from the infused stem cells, or both? The following data support origin from T cells infused with the graft:

1. CD4[+] T cell memory can be adoptively transferred from immune donors (reviewed below).
2. The quantitative recovery of memory CD4[+] T cells is not preceded by the tremendous expansion of naive CD4[+] T cells seen in normal ontogeny (Fig. 14.17) (Storek *et al.*, 1995b).

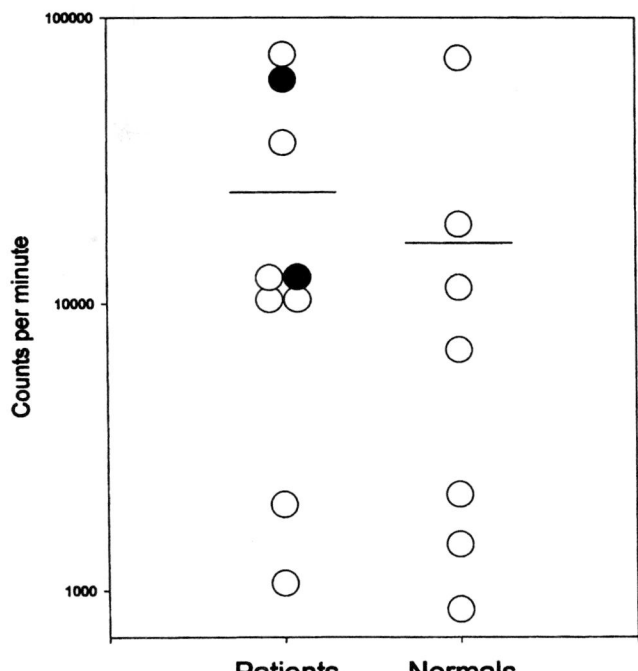

Fig. 14.17. Similar proliferation of anti-CD3-stimulated CD4[+] T cells from allogeneic BMT recipients at one year posttransplant and normal individuals. The horizontal lines denote the mean. Full circles denote two patients on immunosuppressive drugs (for chronic GVHD) at the time of evaluation. Reproduced, with permission, from Storek *et al.* (1999).

3. There appears to be a correlation between the number of CD4[+] T cells in the graft and the number of circulating CD4[+] T cells after grafting (Tayebi *et al.*, 2000; Storek, unpublished).
4. In a mouse model where T-cell origin can be easily distinguished from stem cell origin, most CD4[+] T cells in thymectomized, irradiated and marrow-grafted animals originated from the memory CD4[+] T cells infused with the graft, provided the marrow inoculum contained > 3×10^7/kg T cells (similar to the number of T cells in a regular human marrow graft) (Mackall *et al.*, 1993; Mackall *et al.*, 1996). This model is probably applicable to adult patients whose thymuses are involuted and severely damaged by transplant conditioning and GVHD (Muller-Hermelink *et al.*, 1987; Fukushi *et al.*, 1990; Chung *et al.*, 2001).
5. The recipients of allogeneic PBSC grafts, which contain more CD4[+] T cells than marrow grafts, have higher counts of circulating CD4[+] T cells than recipients of marrow (Fig. 14.5) (Ottinger *et al.*, 1996; Storek *et al.*, 1997c; Storek *et al.*, 2001a; Elmaagacli *et al.*, 2002).
6. Slower quantitative reconstitution of CD4[+] T cells after T-depleted compared to T-replete BMT was described in one study (Janossy *et al.*, 1986), although not in another study (Keever *et al.*, 1989).
7. Phytohemagglutinin, anti-CD3 or specific antigen-induced proliferative responses among mononuclear cells are higher

in patients with T-replete than those with T-depleted grafts (DeGast *et al.*, 1989; Comoli *et al.*, 1994; Small 1996). The repertoire of T cells appears less restricted in patients with T-replete than those with T-depleted grafts (Fig. 14.16) (Roux *et al.*, 1996a; Roux *et al.*, 1996b).

8. The phenotype of the bulk of the posttransplant CD4[+] T cells differs markedly from the phenotype of early life CD4[+] T cells (reviewed above).

The support for at least some CD4[+] T cells originating from the grafted hematopoietic stem cells comes from the observation that the number of phenotypically naïve or T-cell receptor excision circle-containing (TREC[+]) CD4[+] T cells increases, usually between 3 and 12 months after grafting. The slope of increase appears to be inversely proportional to patient age (Fig. 14.18) (Storek *et al.*, 1995b; Weinberg *et al.*, 1995; Brugnoni *et al.*, 1998; Douek *et al.*, 2000; Hazenberg *et al.*, 2002; Myers *et al.*, 2002; Storek *et al.*, 2002a). This suggests that patients with less involuted thymuses are more likely to produce CD4[+] T cells from stem cells than patients with more involuted thymuses. The thymus appears essential for the generation of CD4[+] T cells from stem cells (Ma *et al.*, 1987; Kennedy *et al.*, 1992; Mackall *et al.*, 1993; Mackall *et al.*, 1995; Mackall *et al.*, 1996; Dulude *et al.*, 1997; Heitger *et al.*, 1997). Thus, the generation of CD4[+] T cells de novo from stem cells appears to play a significant role in pediatric patients. It is inefficient in adult patients, who generally have subnormal CD4[+] T-cell counts for >5 years and subnormal counts of TREC[+] CD4[+] T cells for >20 years post-BMT (Storek *et al.*, 1995b; Storek *et al.*, 2001b). Within the pediatric group, there is one exception: after transplantation for SCID (typically using T-depleted grafts and no conditioning), de novo generation of T cells ceases after ~14 years posttransplant, most likely due to the lack of long-term

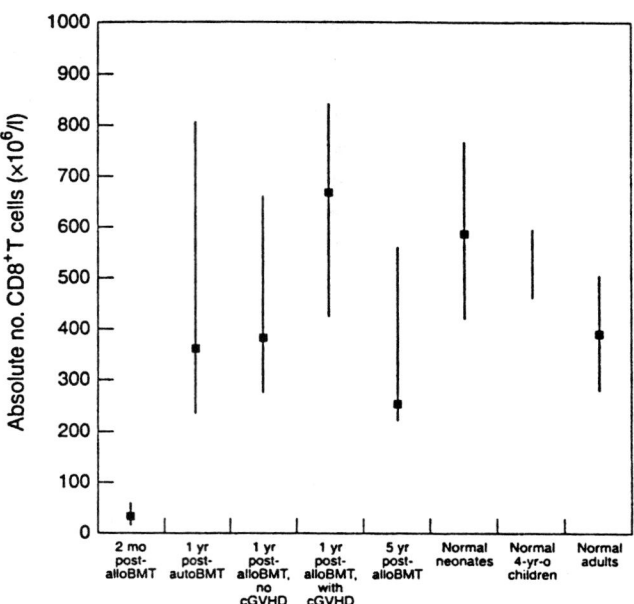

Fig. 14.19. The reconstitution of blood CD8[+] T-cell counts after BMT and in normal ontogeny, showing that while supranormal counts are typical for early life, subnormal counts are typical for the early and normal to supranormal counts for the late posttransplant periods. Data are expressed as medians (squares) and 25th–75th percentiles (vertical lines), with the exception of the two 4-year-old children in which case the vertical line represents the range. Number of individuals (n) tested in each group: 10 allogeneic graft recipients at 2 months after BMT, 8 autograft recipients at 1 year after BMT, 13 allograft recipients without clinical chronic GVHD at 1 year after BMT, 13 allograft recipients with clinical chronic GVHD at 1 year after BMT, 8 allograft recipients at 5 years after BMT, 14 normal neonates, 2 normal 4-year-old children, and 22 normal adults. Reproduced, with permission, from Storek *et al.* (1995b).

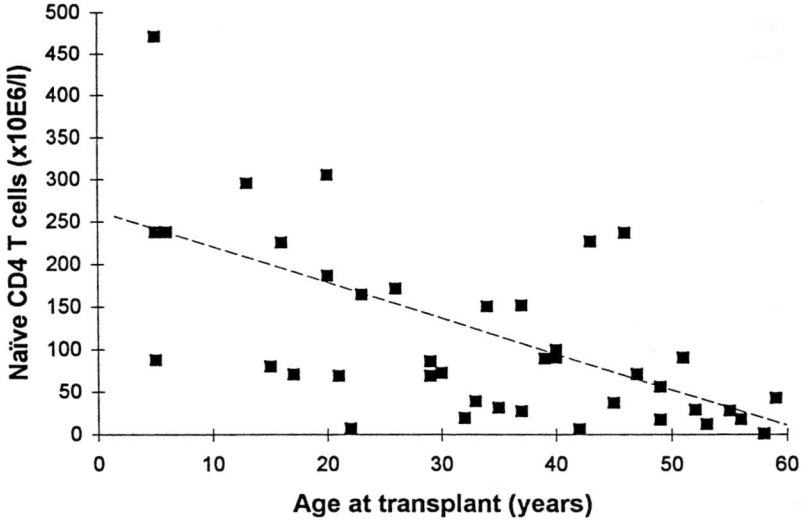

Fig. 14.18. Naïve (CD45RA[high]) CD4[+] T-cell count at 1 year after BMT inversely correlates with patient age at transplant, suggesting diminished ability of CD4[+] T cell production de novo (from stem cells) with increasing age. The Spearman rank correlation coefficient is –0.68 ($P < 0.001$). Thirty-three allograft and seven autograft recipients were studied. Reproduced, with permission, from Storek *et al.* (1995b).

engraftment of donor-derived stem cells (Tjonnfjord *et al.*, 1994; Müller *et al.*, 2000; Patel *et al.*, 2000).

In summary, both CD4+ T cell-derived and stem cell-derived CD4+ T cells probably coexist after grafting. The CD4+ T cell-derived ones predominate early posttransplant. Late posttransplant, the stem cell-derived CD4+ T cells may predominate in most pediatric transplant recipients, whereas the CD4+ T-cell-derived CD4+ T cells probably predominate in adult transplant recipients. This contrasts with B cells and myeloid cells that are predominantly stem cell-derived.

Adoptive transfer

The transfer of antigen-primed CD4+ T cells with marrow was documented by Kwak *et al.* (1995) who immunized the marrow donor of a myeloma patient with the myeloma immunoglobulin. The myeloma immunoglobulin-specific proliferative response of the patient's mononuclear cells, which was negative pretransplant, became positive posttransplant. A cell line established from the responding mononuclear cells expressed CD3 and CD4 and was of donor origin.

The transfer of functional CD4+ T cells may have also occured in the study of Grob *et al.* (1987) showing that CMV-seropositive recipients of marrow from CMV-seropositive donors had substantially lower mortality due to CMV infection than CMV-seropositive recipients of marrow from CMV-seronegative donors. In this study the marrow grafts were partially CD4 T-cell depleted and vigorously CD8 T-cell depleted.

The conditions for a successful transfer (e.g., the need for the presence of the antigen in the host) remain to be worked out.

CD8+ T cells

Quantity

Circulating CD8+ T-cell counts are subnormal (usually <200 × 10⁶/l) during the first 3 months after marrow grafting (Atkinson *et al.*, 1982b; Friedrich *et al.*, 1982; DeGast *et al.*, 1985; Janossy *et al.*, 1986; Bengtsson *et al.*, 1989c; Keever *et al.*, 1989; Atkinson *et al.*, 1990a; Leino *et al.*, 1991; Ericson *et al.*, 1992; Storek *et al.*, 1992; Foot *et al.*, 1993; Scambia *et al.*, 1993; Ashihara *et al.*, 1994; DeSouza *et al.*, 1994; Storek *et al.*, 1995b; Kook *et al.*, 1996; Koehne *et al.*, 1997; Storek *et al.*, 2001a; Storek *et al.*, 2001b). They then rise quickly, and reach normal or transiently supranormal levels by 1 year posttransplant (Fig. 14.19). The rapid rise could be due to the expansion of CD8+ T cells specific for herpesviruses present in the host (Marshall *et al.*, 2000; Cwynarski *et al.*, 2001; Hebart *et al.*, 2002). Patient age does not appear to influence the tempo of the quantitative CD8+ T-cell recovery. The CD8+ T-cell content of the graft appears to influence the tempo to a mild degree. The tempo appears faster and a marked transient overshoot to supranormal levels occurs more frequently in patients with GVHD and/or CMV seropositivity than those without GVHD and/or CMV seropositivity (Soiffer *et al.*, 1993; Fukuda *et al.*, 1994; Storek *et al.*, 1995b; Kook *et al.*, 1996). Phenotypic studies published in the 1980s or early 1990s tend to report higher early posttransplant CD8 counts than studies published in mid-1990s. This may be related to differences in techniques. For example, in the older studies CD8+ T cells were usually identified as cells expressing CD8 whereas in the more recent studies as cells expressing both CD3 and CD8, in order to minimize the error of counting natural killer (NK) cells (that are abundant early posttransplant) as CD8+ T cells.

The rising CD8+ T cells are largely composed of memory cells. The recovery of naive or TREC+ CD8+ T-cell counts is slow – much slower than the development of naive CD8+ T cell counts in normal ontogeny (from zero in the first trimester of pregnancy to supranormal levels by birth) (Fig. 14.20) (Storek *et al.*, 1995b; Weinberg *et al.*, 2001; Storek *et al.*, 2002a). Nevertheless, it appears faster than the reconstitution of de novo generated CD4+ T-cell counts posttransplant as TREC+ CD8+ T cell, but not TREC+ CD4+ T-cell counts, become normal by 20 years posttransplant. (Storek *et al.*, 2001b)

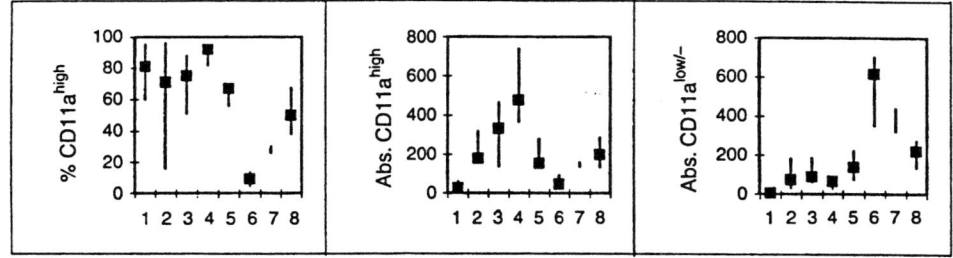

Fig. 14.20. Percent memory/effector (CD11a^high) CD8+ T cells of total circulating CD8+ T cells (left panel), the absolute number (x10⁶/l) of memory CD8+ T cells (middle panel) and the absolute number (x10⁶/l) of naive (CD11a^low/−) CD8+ T cells (right panel) after BMT and in normal ontogeny, showing the deficiency of naive CD8+ T cells posttransplant in contrast to the abundance of naive cells in early life. The patient and control groups are as follows: 1, allograft recipients at 2 months after BMT (*n* = 10); 2, autograft recipients at 1 year after BMT (*n* = 8); 3, allograft recipients without clinical chronic GVHD at 1 year after BMT (*n* = 13); 4, allograft recipients with clinical chronic GVHD at 1 year after BMT (*n* = 13); 5, allograft recipients at 5 years after BMT (*n* = 8); 6, normal newborns (*n* = 14); 7, normal 4-year-old children (*n* = 2); and 8, normal adults (*n* = 22). Data are expressed as medians (squares) and 25th–75th percentiles (vertical lines), with the exception of the two 4-year-old children in which case the vertical line represents the range. Reproduced, with permission, from Storek *et al.* (1995b).

After allogeneic PBSCT compared to allogeneic BMT, as well as after autologous PBSCT compared to autologous BMT, CD8+ T cell counts are similar or mildly higher after PBSCT (Fig. 14.5) (Roberts *et al.*, 1993; Ottinger *et al.*, 1996; Rosillo *et al.*, 1996; Storek *et al.*, 1997c; Talmadge *et al.*, 1997; Storek *et al.*, 2001a). Allogeneic PBSC grafts contain ~10-fold more CD8+ T cells than allogeneic marrow grafts.

After CBT, the tempo of CD8+ T-cell regeneration appears similar to, or mildly delayed, compared to BMT (Locatelli *et al.*, 1996; Takahashi *et al.*, 1997; Thomson *et al.*, 2000).

Phenotype

Both early and late post-BMT, the following antigens are more frequently or more "brightly" expressed by CD8+ T cells from transplant recipients than by those from normal adults: CD11a, CD11b, CD29, CD57, HLA-DR and, to a lesser degree, CD45RO. The following antigens are less frequently or less "brightly" expressed: CD28 and, to a lesser degree, CD45RA and CD62L (Bengtsson *et al.*, 1988; Velardi *et al.*, 1988b; Yabe *et al.*, 1990; Fukuda *et al.*, 1994; Sugita *et al.*, 1994b; Garin *et al.*, 1995; Storek *et al.*, 1995b; Weinberg *et al.*, 1995; Storek *et al.*, 2001a). The CD11a+, CD11b+, CD28– and CD57+ cells are particularly frequent in patients with chronic GVHD. CD8+ T cells from transplant recipients are larger than those from normal adults (Storek *et al.*, 1992). The phenotype of posttransplant CD8+ T cells appears different from that of CD8+ T cells from normal neonates and children: these cells express CD11a, CD29, and CD45RO less frequently/brightly and CD28, CD45RA, and CD62L more frequently/brightly than CD8+ T cells from normal adults (Hannet *et al.*, 1992; Storek *et al.*, 1995b). The phenotype of posttransplant CD8+ T cells suggests a preponderance of antigen-primed cells as opposed to the preponderance of naive cells in normal early ontogeny (Okumura *et al.*, 1993a; Okumura *et al.*, 1993b). The preponderance of CD11b+/CD28–/CD57+ cells suggests that a high percent of CD8+ T cells may be suppressive, anergic, or terminally differentiated (effectors with short telomeres) (Klingemann *et al.*, 1987; Izquierdo *et al.*, 1990; Leroy *et al.*, 1990; Madariaga *et al.*, 1990; Autran *et al.*, 1991; Azuma *et al.*, 1993; Lake *et al.*, 1993; Lombardi *et al.*, 1994; Boussiotis *et al.*, 1996; Effros *et al.*, 1996).

Repertoire

Repertoire is discussed in the section "CD4+ T cells, Repertoire."

Function in vitro

The results of in vitro assays testing both CD4+ and CD8+ T cells (e.g., anti-CD3-induced proliferation) are discussed under "CD4+ T cells, Function in vitro," (page 206). Here we discuss the two functions attributed primarily to CD8+ T cells (i.e., cytotoxicity and suppression).

HLA-restricted cytotoxicity toward antigens that are likely encountered posttransplant (e.g., CMV in CMV-seropositive patients) is frequently subnormal early post-BMT (Quinnan *et al.*, 1981; Quinnan *et al.*, 1982; Reusser *et al.*, 1991; Riddell *et al.*, 1992; Walter *et al.*, 1995). However, the responses were measured among total mononuclear cells, which makes the distinction between quantitative versus qualitative deficiency of antigen-specific cytotoxic T cells early posttransplant impossible. Limiting dilution analyses and flow cytometric detection of virus peptide-specific T cells suggest that the subnormal cytotoxicity responses of mononuclear cells early posttransplant are due at least in part to the quantitative deficiency of virus-specific cytotoxic CD8+ T cells (Lucas *et al.*, 1996; Gratama *et al.*, 2001). By 3 to 6 months posttransplant, the number of virus-specific T cells typically becomes normal, except for patients that do not harbor the virus (e.g., CMV-seronegative patients) and for patients that develop viral disease (e.g., CMV pneumonia) (Lucas *et al.*, 1996; Gratama *et al.*, 2001) (Fig. 14.21).

Nonspecific suppressive activity of mononuclear cells appears supranormal early post-BMT. Late post-BMT, it is usually normal in patients without, and usually supranormal in patients with, chronic GVHD (Tsoi *et al.*, 1979; DeBruin *et al.*, 1981; Azogui *et al.*, 1983; Autran *et al.*, 1991). One study suggested that the nonspecific suppression could be mediated via a soluble factor produced by the relatively abundant CD57+ CD8+ T cells (Autran *et al.*, 1991). Specific donor-anti-host

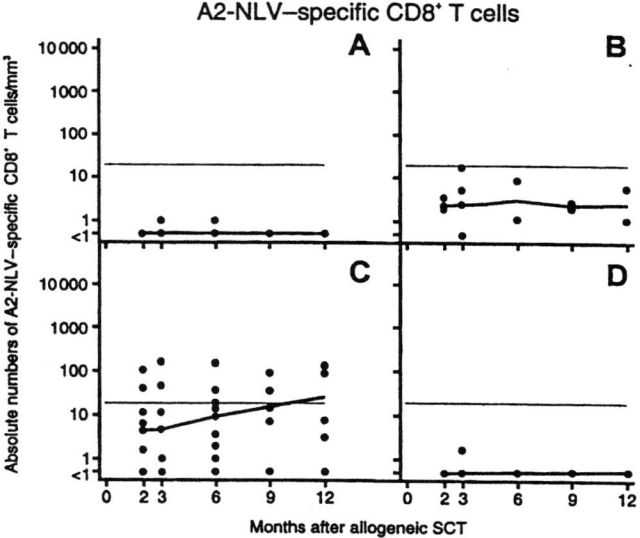

Fig. 14.21. Counts of circulating CMV immunodominant peptide-specific CD8+ T cells in the recipients of partially T-depleted allografts. (**A**) Undetectable or barely detectable specific CD8+ T cells in CMV seronegative patients with CMV seropositive (*n* = 3) or seronegative (*n* = 6) donors. (**B-D**) Variable counts of specific CD8+ T cells in CMV seropositive patients with CMV seropositive (*n* = 13) or seronegative (*n* = 5) donors. The counts were normal in patients without CMV antigenemia (**B**), normal to supranormal in patients with antigenemia who did not develop CMV disease (**C**), and usually undetectable in patients with antigenemia who developed CMV disease (**D**). Upper normal limit (95th percentile of 29 healthy CMV seropositive individuals) is denoted by the horizontal lines. Reproduced, with permission, from Gratama *et al.* (2001).

suppressive activity may be higher in patients without, than those with, chronic GVHD (Tsoi *et al.*, 1981).

Function in vivo

Quinnan *et al.* prospectively monitored 58 recipients of allogeneic or syngeneic marrow for CMV infection as well as for CMV-specific and HLA-restricted cytotoxicity of blood mononuclear cells (Quinnan *et al.*, 1982). Fifteen patients did not develop CMV infection; of the remaining 43 patients who developed CMV infection, 23 survived, 12 died of the CMV infection, and 8 died of another cause. The patients who survived the infection significantly increased the cytotoxicity index by 2 weeks from the onset of the infection, whereas no significant increase in the cytotoxicity index was detected among the patients who died of the infection or who did not develop the infection. This suggested poor in vivo function of CD8+ T cells in one third (12/35) of the actively infected patients. Similarly, in 14 patients who developed CMV antigenemia, CMV peptide-specific CD8+ T cells were measured (Gratama *et al.*, 2001). Counts of these cells were typically normal or supranormal in the 10 patients who did not develop CMV disease and were usually undetectable in the 4 patients who developed CMV disease (Fig. 14.21, C and D). This study also suggested poor in vivo function of CD8+ T cells in one third (4/14) of the actively infected patients.

Origin

From the donor or the recipient?

As discussed above, most or all circulating lymphocytes are of donor origin by 1 to 2 months post-BMT (Fig. 14.11), unless the graft is depleted of T cells or the conditioning is of low intensity. The same probably applies to CD8+ T cells (Gratama *et al.*, 1984; Auffermann-Gretzinger *et al.*, 2002).

From T cells or de novo from stem cells?

The following data support the origin from the CD8+ T cells transferred with the graft:

1. The quantitative recovery of memory CD8+ T cells is not preceded by the tremendous expansion of naive CD8+ T cells seen in normal ontogeny (Fig. 14.20) (Storek *et al.*, 1995b).
2. The repertoire of total T cells is less restricted in patients with T-replete than those with T-depleted grafts (Roux *et al.*, 1996a; Roux *et al.*, 1996b).
3. The phenotype of the bulk of the posttransplant CD8+ T cells does not resemble the phenotype of CD8+ T cells in early life (reviewed above).
4. Recipients of allogeneic PBSC grafts, that contain more CD8+ T cells than marrow grafts, tend to have higher posttransplant CD8+ T-cell counts than marrow recipients (Storek *et al.*, 2001a).

In contrast, the following data support the origin from the hematopoietic stem cells in the graft:

1. Recipients of CD8+ T cell-depleted marrow from HLA-identical related donors increased their CD8+ T-cell counts to normal levels by 6 months and to supranormal levels by 1 year posttransplant (Champlin *et al.*, 1990), which is not delayed compared to the rate seen in recipients of unmodified marrow from HLA-identical related donors (Storek *et al.*, 2001a).
2. TREC+ CD8+ T cells are readily detectable late posttransplant (Storek *et al.*, 2002a).
3. In the mouse model where the T-cell origin can be easily distinguished from the stem cell origin, stem cell-derived CD8+ T cells were frequently detected (Mackall *et al.*, 1993; Mackall *et al.*, 1996).
4. In contrast to CD4+ T cells, that can be generated only in the thymus, de novo generation of CD8+ T cells appears less thymus-dependent (Kennedy *et al.*, 1992; Sato *et al.*, 1995).

In summary, the coexistence of both the CD8+ T-cell-derived and stem cell-derived CD8+ T cells after grafting is likely. The TREC data suggest that T-cell-derived CD8+ T cells may predominate early posttransplant (TREC+ CD8+ T cells are rarely detectable early posttransplant) and that stem cell-derived CD8+ T cells are present late posttransplant.

Adoptive transfer

The transfer of antigen-specific CD8+ T cells with marrow probably occurs because CMV-seropositive patients with CMV-seropositive donors have a higher likelihood of developing detectable CMV-specific and HLA class I-restricted cytotoxicity early posttransplant than CMV-seropositive patients with CMV-seronegative donors (Li *et al.*, 1994). Successful posttransplant transfer of CMV as well as EBV-specific CD8+ T-cell clones and their persistence for at least 2 years has been documented (Riddell *et al.*, 1992; Walter *et al.*, 1995; Heslop *et al.*, 1996a; Heslop *et al.*, 1996b; Heslop & Rooney, 1997).

Antigen-specific CD8+ T cells or their progeny may persist in the adoptive host for a prolonged period of time (perhaps lifetime), even in the absence of the antigen and in the absence of CD4+ T cells (Hou *et al.*, 1994; Lau *et al.*, 1994). However, in the absence of the antigen or of the CD4+ T cells specific for the antigen, the number or function of the CD8+ T cells declines possibly to levels lower than those needed for controlling infection (Li *et al.*, 1994; Matloubian *et al.*, 1994; Walter *et al.*, 1995; Gratama *et al.*, 2001).

Other T Cells

CD4−CD8− T cells

Circulating CD4−CD8− T-cell counts are usually subnormal early and normal to supranormal late post-BMT (Gratama *et al.*, 1989; Storek *et al.*, 1992; Storek *et al.*, 2001a). The function of this T-cell subset is not known. This subset may be composed primarily of γ/δ T cells. Supranormal counts of γ/δ T cells late posttransplant have been associated with a low relapse rate (Lamb *et al.*, 1996) and with viral or fungal infections (Cela *et al.*, 1996).

CD4+CD8+ T cells

These cells are barely detectable in the blood of normal adults whereas supranormal counts of CD4+CD8+ T cells are detected in some patients late posttransplant and in normal neonates (Storek *et al.*, 1992; Storek *et al.*, 2001a). It is not known whether these cells represent T-cell precursors or a subset of, perhaps activated, mature T cells (Griffiths-Chu *et al.*, 1984; Blue *et al.*, 1985; Kay *et al.*, 1990; Ebisawa *et al.*, 1991; Schauer *et al.*, 1992).

Antigen-presenting cells

Dendritic cells in the blood, epithelium, and extrafollicular areas of peripheral lymphatic tissues

The primary role of these cells, which originate from hematopoietic stem cells, is to present the antigenic peptide-HLA complex to T cells and provide the T cells with co-stimulatory signals (e.g., through CD80-CD28 interaction). Immunohistological studies of the skin suggest that the number of Langerhans cells is subnormal early and near-normal by 6 months posttransplant (Fig. 14.22) (Perreault *et al.*, 1984; Murphy *et al.*, 1985; Sviland *et al.*, 1991; Walsh *et al.*, 1996). Dendritic cells in the extrafollicular areas of lymph nodes from autopsies were found in about one third of transplant recipi-

ents, more frequently late than early posttransplant (Dilly *et al.*, 1986; Dilly & Sloane 1988; Horny *et al.*, 1990). The counts of dendritic cells or their precursors in the blood are low in the first 3 months posttransplant; subsequently, DC1 counts tend to normalize whereas DC2 counts are low even at 1 year posttransplant (Fearnley *et al.*, 1999; Klangsinsirikul *et al.*, 2002).

Thymic dendritic cells

These cells, which originate from hematopoietic stem cells, play a role in the negative selection of de novo generated T cells (Brocker *et al.*, 1997). Their reconstitution after human marrow grafting has not been studied. In mice, these cells appear in the thymus within weeks after stem cell transplantation (Wu *et al.*, 1996).

Follicular dendritic cells

These cells play a role in the germinal center reaction, during which IgD/IgM/IgG/IgA/IgE-switched and somatically mutated memory B cells are generated from naive B cells. The origin of these cells (possibly hematopoietic stem cells or fibroblasts?) is not known. Immunohistologic studies of lymph nodes and spleen suggest that the quantitative reconstitution of follicular dendritic cells is extremely slow—even at 1 year after grafting these cells appear sparse (Dilly & Sloane, 1988; Sale *et al.*, 1992). This could explain why germinal centers appear only late posttransplant (Dilly *et al.*, 1986; Dilly & Sloane, 1988; Horny *et al.*, 1988; Horny *et al.*, 1990; Sale *et al.*, 1992)

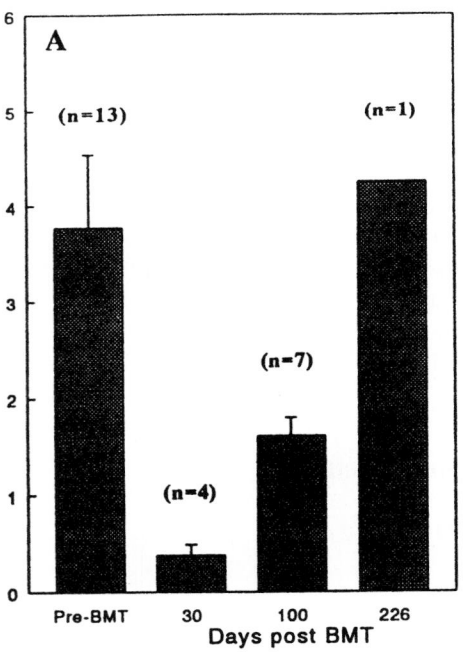
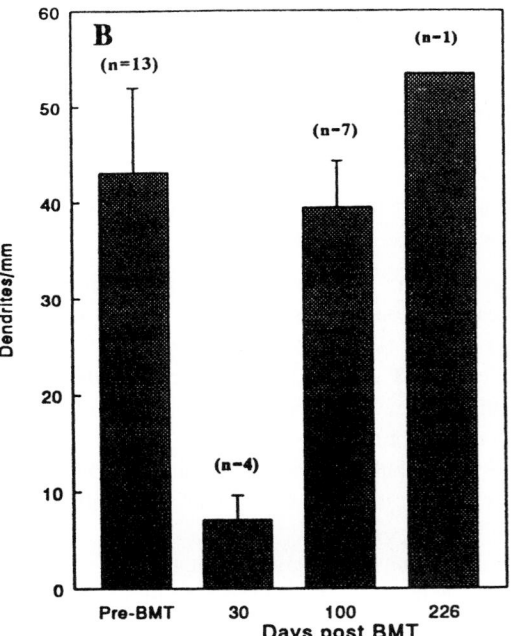

Fig. 14.22. Quantitative immunohistological analysis of Langerhans (CD1a+) cells in the skin of allogeneic marrow recipients, showing the deficiency of Langerhans cells early posttransplant and the subsequent recovery. The y-axes show the frequencies of Langerhans cell bodies (**A**) or Langerhans cell dendrites (**B**) per mm epidermal length. Means ± SEM are displayed. Reproduced, with permission, from Walsh *et al.* (1996).

and the reconstitution of memory B cells is slow (Suzuki *et al.,* 1996; Storek *et. al.,* 1997d).

Monocytes/Macrophages

The quantity of circulating monocytes becomes normal by 1 month post-BMT (Atkinson *et al.,* 1991; DeWitte *et al.,* 1992; Ericson *et al.,* 1992; Storek *et al.,* 1992; Ottinger *et al.,* 1996; Talmadge *et al.,* 1997; Storek *et al.,* 2001a). Macrophages/ microglia become regularly detected in tissues by 1 to 3 months post-BMT (Beschorner *et al.,* 1981; Dilly *et al.,* 1986; Dilly & Sloane, 1988; Horny *et al.,* 1988; Horny *et al.,* 1990; Bowden *et al.,* 1993; Krall *et al.,* 1994; Nakata *et al.,* 1999). The function (e.g., IL-1 production or antigen presentation) of the recovering monocytes may be subnormal for approximately 1 year (Cayeux *et al.,* 1989a; Sahdev *et al.,* 1996), although some studies suggest normal function early after BMT (Tsoi *et al.,* 1982; Shiobara *et al.,* 1984; Brkic *et al.,* 1985). Chemotaxis of pulmonary macrophages may be abnormal throughout the first year post-BMT (Winston *et al.,* 1982).

G-CSF- or GM-CSF-mobilized PBSC grafts contain a large number of monocytes (~2 logs more than marrow grafts), which suppress some T-cell functions (e.g., proliferative response to alloantigens) (Ino *et al.,* 1997; Kusnierz-Glaz *et al.,* 1997; Mielcarek *et al.,* 1997; Mielcarek *et al.,* 1998). This may explain why allogeneic PBSC recipients do not have a greater incidence of acute GVHD than BMT recipients despite the higher content of T cells in the PBSC grafts. Most of the monocytes infused with PBSCs probably either die or become tissue macrophages within days, because monocytes in the blood of PBSC recipients become virtually undetectable by day 7 (Storek, unpublished data).

Strategies to improve posttransplant immunity

Examples of attempts to improve the innate immunity include glutamine or keratinocyte growth factor (KGF) to reduce the conditioning-induced damage to mucosa (MacBurney *et al.,* 1994; MacDonald & Hill, 2002), infusion of in vivo cytokine-expanded donor granulocytes during the first week posttransplant to shorten the period of absolute neutropenia (Brown *et al.,* 1996), or G-CSF to enhance the function of recovering neutrophils (Ericson *et al.,* 1995). So far, none of these strategies has gained acceptance.

The following strategies to improve adaptive immunity have been tried.

Vaccines

Posttransplant immunization of patients is feasible (see B Cells, Function in vivo, Antibody responses to immunization), and is recommended (Dykewicz *et al.,* 2000) (see Chapters 73 and 74). However, its clinical benefit is relatively minor because most existing vaccines are against diseases that do not commonly develop in transplant recipients (e.g., tetanus, diphteria, pertussis, hepatitis A, hepatitis B, polio, influenza A/B, typhoid, measles, mumps, and rubella) and because one can

effectively immunize only after patient immunity has recovered to the point of responding to the vaccines (6 to 12 months posttransplant). Pretransplant immunization of the donor and the patient combined with multiple posttransplant immunizations of the patient appears more efficacious than immunizing only the patient at >6 months posttransplant, because high antibody levels can be achieved already early posttransplant (see B cells, Adoptive transfer). This vaccination strategy has the potential of becoming accepted for *Haemophilus influenzae* polysaccharide-protein conjugate vaccine (e.g., HibTiter, ProHibit, or PedvaxHib), second-generation *Streptococcus pneumoniae* polysaccharide-protein conjugate vaccine (Prevnar), and varicella-zoster live attenuated virus vaccine (Molrine *et al.,* 1996b; Molrine & Hibberd, 2001; Hata *et al.,* 2002).

Immunoglobulins

Intravenous immunoglobulin has a minor to moderate effect in preventing posttransplant infections (Bass *et al.,* 1993; Sullivan *et al.,* 1996). However, its high cost as well as its apparently negative effect on the reconstitution of humoral immunity (Sullivan *et al.,* 1996) limit its use only to patients with very low IgG levels or active infections.

Donor lymphocytes

Ex vivo expanded CMV- or EBV-specific donor T-cell clones have been successfully used for both treatment and prophylaxis (Walter *et al.,* 1995; O'Reilly *et al.,* 1996; Rooney *et al.,* 1997; Einsele *et al.,* 2002). They have the advantage of not causing GVHD; however, they cannot react against escape mutants of viruses. Their efficacy is limited in the setting of GVHD and its treatment with immunosuppressive drugs. Total (polyclonal) lymphocytes from immune donors also appear efficacious, as evidenced by their ability to induce a complete remission of EBV lymphoma (Papadopoulos *et al.,* 1994) and prevent a variety of other infections (Storek *et al.,* 2001a). Theoretically, fresh lymphocytes should have the advantage of being effective against a broad spectrum of pathogens. However, to avoid the risk of GVHD, fresh lymphocytes may need to be purged of alloreactive T cells, if feasible in the future. An initial attempt at this (by purging donor lymphocyte infusions of CD8[+] cells) resulted in increased numbers of CD20[+] B cells, a more rapid improvement in TCR V beta repertoire, and increased numbers of TRECs in CD3[+] T cells (Bellucci *et al.,* 2002).

Thymus grafts

Because the deficiency of CD4[+] T cells, probably due to the involution and damage to the thymus in adult transplant recipients (Muller-Hermelink *et al.,* 1987), may be the major cause of the long-lasting posttransplant immunodeficiency, and the thymus is the only site of generating CD4[+] T cells from hematopoietic stem cells (Kennedy *et al.,* 1992; Mackall *et al.,* 1993; Mackall *et al.,* 1995; Mackall *et al.,* 1996), thymus grafting is an appealing idea. It is feasible and does hasten immune reconstitution in animal models, where a thymus from a young animal syngeneic to the donor of hematopoietic stem cells is readily available (Astle *et al.*, 1984). Human studies, using thymuses from partially HLA-matched donors unrelated to either the marrow donor or the recipient, failed to hasten immune recovery, probably due to the rejection of the thymus grafts (Atkinson *et al.*, 1982c; Witherspoon *et al.*, 1988). Banks of human cadaveric thymuses have not been established; theoretically, this would allow thymic transplantation from a young donor, HLA-matched to the donor of hematopoietic stem cells. An "artificial thymus" (Poznansky *et al.*, 2000), derived from epithelial cells of the recipient, is being developed.

Cytokines promoting thymopoiesis

Interleukin-7 (IL-7) and insulin-like growth factor-I (IGF-I) appear to stimulate the reconstitution of T cells in mice, possibly by inducing a transient hypertrophy of the thymus (Robbins *et al.*, 1994; Boerman *et al.*, 1995; Mathur *et al.*, 1995; Abdul-Hai *et al.*, 1996; Bolotin *et al.*, 1996; Alpdogan *et al.*, 2001; Mackall *et al.*, 2001; Okamoto *et al.*, 2002). KGF appears to protect mouse thymic stroma from radiation or GVHD-induced damage (Min *et al.*, 2002; Rossi *et al.*, 2002). Currently, it is unknown whether IL-7, IGF-I, KGF, or other cytokines elicit the same effect in humans.

Conclusions

In the 1970s, the characteristics of posttransplant immune deficiency were described. In the 1980s, it was postulated that the posttransplant immune deficiency is analogous to the immune deficiency of normal neonates or infants because of the similarities between the reconstitution of immunity after BMT and the development of immunity in early life. In the 1990s, dissimilarities between the reconstitution of T cells (primarily CD4$^+$ T cells) in adult transplant recipients and the development of T cells in early life were described. It was postulated that while B cells reconstitute primarily from the grafted stem cells (similar to early life), T cells in adult transplant recipients reconstitute primarily from the grafted mature T cells (in contrast to early life), probably because the production of T cells from stem cells in the involuted and radiation/chemotherapy/GVHD-damaged thymus is insufficient or absent. The transfer of additional T cells from the donor to the recipient has become a standard approach for the treatment or prophylaxis of certain infections (CMV, EBV) and certain malignancies (relapse of chronic myeloid leukemia). In the 2000s, we need to learn how to use the whole repertoire of donor lymphocytes against infectious agents and malignant cells without causing GVHD, how to enhance T-cell production de novo from stem cells, how to hasten B cell reconstitution, particularly the differentiation from naive to memory B cells, and how to hasten the recovery of innate immunity.

References

Abdul-Hai, A., Or, R. *et al.* (1996). Stimulation of immune reconstitution by IL-7 after syngeneic BMT in mice. *Experimental Hematology,* **24,** 1416–22.

Abedi, M. R., Hammarstrom, L. *et al.* (1990). Development of IgA deficiency after bone marrow transplantation. *Transplantation,* **50,** 415–21.

Agosti, J. M., Sprenger, J. D. *et al.* (1988). Transfer of allergen-specific IgE-mediated hypersensitivity with allogeneic bone marrow transplantation. *The New England Journal of Medicine,* **319,** 1623–8.

Akatsuka, Y., Cerveny, C. *et al.* (1996). T cell receptor clonal diversity following allogeneic marrow grafting. *Human Immunology,* **48,** 125–34.

Alpdogan, O., Schmaltz, C. *et al.* (2001). Administration of interleukin-7 after allogeneic bone marrow transplantation improves immune reconstitution without aggravating graft-versus-host disease. *Blood,* **98**(7), 2256–65.

Amlot, P. L., Hayes, A. E. *et al.* (1986). Human immune responses in vivo to protein (KLH) and polysaccharide (DNP-Ficoll) neoantigens: normal subjects compared with bone marrow transplant patients on cyclosporine. *Clinical and Experimental Immunology,* **64,** 125–35.

Anderson, K. C., Ritz, J. *et al.* (1987). Hematologic engraftment and immune reconstitution posttransplantation with anti-B1 purged autologous bone marrow. *Blood,* **69,** 597–604.

Antin, J. H., Ault, K. A. *et al.* (1987). B lymphocyte reconstitution after human marrow transplantation: Leu-1 antigen defines a distinct population of B lymphocytes. *The Journal of Clinical Investigation,* **80,** 325–32.

Ashihara, E., Shimazaki, C. *et al.* (1994). Reconstitution of lymphocyte subsets after peripheral blood stem cell transplantation: two-color flow cytometric analysis. *Bone Marrow Transplantation,* **13,** 377–81.

Asma, G.E.M., Langois, R. *et al.* (1987). Regeneration of TdT+, pre-B and B cells in bone marrow after allogeneic bone marrow transplantation. *Transplantation,* **43,** 865–70.

Astle, C. M., Harrison, D. E. (1984). Effects of marrow donor and recipient age on immune responses. *Journal of Immunology,* **132,** 673–7.

Atkinson, K. (1990a). Reconstitution of the haematopoietic and immune systems after marrow transplantation. *Bone Marrow Transplantation,* **5,** 209–26.

Atkinson, K., Bradstock, K. *et al.* (1991). GM-CSF after allogeneic BMT: accelerated recovery of neutrophils, monocytes and lymphocytes. *The Australian and New Zealand Journal of Medicine,* **21,** 686–92.

Atkinson, K., Farewell, V. *et al.* (1982a). Analysis of late infections after human bone marrow transplantation: role of genotypic nonidentity between marrow donor and recipient and of nonspecific suppressor cells in patients with chronic graft-versus-host disease. *Blood,* **60**(3), 714–20.

Atkinson, K., Hansen, J. A. *et al.* (1982b). T cell subpopulations identified by monoclonal antibodies after human marrow transplantation. I. Helper-inducer and cytotoxic-suppressor subsets. *Blood,* **59,** 1292–97.

Atkinson, K., Horowitz, M. M. *et al.* (1990b). Risk factors for chronic graft-versus-host disease after HLA-identical sibling bone marrow transplantation. *Blood,* **75**(12), 2459–64.

Atkinson, K., Storb, R. *et al.* (1982c). Thymus transplantation after allogeneic bone marrow graft to prevent chronic GVHD in humans. *Transplantation,* **33,** 168–73.

Aucouturier, P., Barra, A. et al. (1987). Long lasting IgG subclass and antibacterial polysaccharide antibody deficiency after allogeneic bone marrow transplantation. Blood, 70(3), 779–85.

Auffermann-Gretzinger, S., Lossos, I. S. et al. (2002). Rapid establishment of dendritic cell chimerism in allogeneic hematopoietic cell transplant recipients. Blood, 99(4), 1442–8.

Ault, K. A., Antin, J. H. et al. (1985). Phenotype of recovering lymphoid cell populations after marrow transplantation. The Journal of Experimental Medicine, 161, 1483–1502.

Autran, B., Leblond, V. et al. (1991). A soluble factor released by CD8+CD57+ lymphocytes from bone marrow transplanted patients inhibits cell-mediated cytolysis. Blood, 77, 2237–41.

Azogui, O., Gluckman, E. et al. (1983). Inhibition of IL2 production after human allogeneic bone marrow transplantation. Journal of Immunology, 131, 1205–8.

Azuma, M., Phillips, J. H. et al. (1993). CD28-T lymphocytes. Antigenic and functional properties. Journal of Immunology, 150(4), 1147–59.

Bacigalupo, A., Mordini, N. et al. (1997). Transplantation of HLA-mismatched CD34+ selected cells in patients with advanced malignancies: severe immunodeficiency and related complications. British Journal of Haematology, 98(3), 760–6.

Bacigalupo, A., VanLint, M. T. et al. (1996). Thiotepa cyclophosphamice followed by granulocyte colony-stimulating factor mobilized allogeneic peripheral blood stem cells in adults with advanced leukemia. Blood, 88, 353–7.

Balboa, M. A., Izquierdo, M. et al. (1992). Analysis of different protein kinase C-dependent events in T cells from allogeneic BMT recipients. Clinical and Experimental Immunology, 87, 478–84.

Bar, B.M.A.M., Santos, G. W. et al. (1990). Reconstitution of antibody response after allogeneic bone marrow transplantation: effect of lymphocyte depletion by conterflow centrifugal elutriation on the expression of hemagglutinins. Blood, 76, 1410–8.

Bar, B.M.A.M., VanDijk, B. A. et al. (1995). Erythrocyte repopulation after major ABO incompatible transplantation with lymphocyte-depleted bone marrow. Bone Marrow Transplantation, 16, 793–9.

Barge, A. J., Johnson, G. et al. (1989). Antibody-mediated marrow failure after allogeneic bone marrow transplantation. Blood, 74, 1477–80.

Barra, A., Cordonnier, C. et al. (1992). Immunogenicity of Haemophilus influenzae type b conjugate vaccine in allogeneic bone marrow recipients. The Journal of Infectious Diseases, 166(5), 1021–8.

Bass, E. B., Powe, N. R. et al. (1993). Efficacy of immune globulin in preventing complications of BMT: a meta-analysis. Bone Marrow Transplantation, 12, 273–82.

Baumgartner, C., Morell, A. et al. (1988). Humoral immune function in pediatric patients treated with autologous bone marrow transplantation for B cell non-Hodgkin's lymphoma: The influence of ex vivo marrow decontamination with anti-Y29/55 monoclonal antibody and complement. Blood, 71, 1211–7.

Bellucci, R., Alyea, E. P. et al. (2002). Immunologic effects of prophylactic donor lymphocyte infusion after allogeneic marrow transplantation for multiple myeloma. Blood, 99(12), 4610–7.

Bengtsson, M., Gordon, J. et al. (1989a). B cell reconstitution after autologous bone marrow transplantation: increase in serum CD23 (IgE binding factor) precedes IgE and B cell regeneration. Blood, 73, 2139–44.

Bengtsson, M., Smedmyr, B. et al. (1989b). B lymphocyte regeneration in marrow and blood after autologous bone marrow transplantation: increased numbers of B cells carrying activation and progression markers. Leukemia Research, 13(9), 791–7.

Bengtsson, M., Totterman, T. H. et al. (1988). Regeneration of functional and activated NK and T sub-subset cells in the marrow and blood after autologous BMT: a prospective phenotypic study with 2/3-color FACS analysis. Leukemia, 3, 68–75.

Bengtsson, M., Totterman, T. H. et al. (1989c). Regeneration of functional and activated NK and T sub-subset cells in the marrow and blood after autologous bone marrow transplantation: a prospective phenotypic study with 2/3-color FACS analysis. Leukemia, 3(1), 68–75.

Bensinger, W. I., Clift, R. et al. (1996). Allogeneic peripheral blood stem cell transplantation in patients with advanced hematologic malignancies: a retrospective comparison with marrow transplantation. Blood, 88, 2794–800.

Beschorner, W. E., Yardley, J. H. et al. (1981). Deficiency of intestinal immunity with GVHD in humans. The Journal of Infectious Diseases, 144, 38–46.

Biron, C. A., Byron, K. S. et al. (1989). Severe herpesvirus infections in an adolescent without natural killer cells. The New England Journal of Medicine, 320, 1731–5.

Blue, M. L., Daley, J. F. et al. (1985). Coexpression of T4 and T8 on peripheral blood T cells demonstrated by 2-color flow cytometry. Journal of Immunology, 134, 2281–4.

Bobe, P., Benihoud, K. et al. (1999). Nitric oxide mediation of active immunosuppression associated with graft-versus-host reaction. Blood, 94(3), 1028–37.

Boerman, O. C., Gregorio, T. A. et al. (1995). Recombinant human IL-7 administration in mice affects colony-forming units-spleen and lymphoid precursor cell localization and accelerates engraftment of bone marrow transplants. Journal of Leukocyte Biology, 58, 151–8.

Bolotin, E., Smogorzewska, M. et al. (1996). Enhancement of thymopoiesis after BMT by in vivo interleukin-7. Blood, 88, 1887–94.

Bomberger, C., Singh-Jairam, M. et al. (1998). Lymphoid reconstitution after autologous PBSC transplantation with FACS-sorted CD34+ hematopoietic progenitors. Blood, 91, 2588–600.

Boussiotis, V. A., Freeman, G. J. et al. (1996). The role of B7-1/B7-2-CD28/CTLA-4 pathways in the prevention of anergy, induction of productive immunity and down-regulation of the immune response. Immunological Reviews, 153, 5–26.

Bowden, R. A., Mori, M. et al. (1993). Mononuclear cell reconstitution in the lung after marrow transplantation. Transplantation, 55, 557–61.

Brenner, M. K., Wimperis, J. Z. et al. (1986). Recovery of Ig isotypes following T cell depleted allogeneic bone marrow transplantation. British Journal of Haematology, 64, 125–32.

Brkic, S., Tsoi, M. S. et al. (1985). Cellular interactions in marrow-grafted patients. III. Normal interleukin-1 and defective interleukin-2 production in short-term patients and in those with chronic GVHD. Transplantation, 39, 30–5.

Brocker, T., Riedinger, M. et al. (1997). Targeted expression of major histocompatibility complex (MHC) class II molecules demonstrates that dendritic cells can induce negative but not positive selection of thymocytes in vivo. *The Journal of Experimental Medicine,* **185,** 541–50.

Brown, R. A., Adkins, D. R. *et al.* (1996). Infusion of granulocytes collected from HLA-identical sibling donors reduces the duration of neutropenia following allogeneic PBSC transplant (abstract). *Blood,* **88** (Suppl 1), 261b.

Brugnoni, D., Airo, P. *et al.* (1998). Rapid regeneration of normally functional naive CD4(+) T cells after bone marrow transplantation from unrelated donors for combined immunodeficiency. *Blood,* **92**(9), 3484–6.

Cayeux, S., Meuer, S. *et al.* (1989a). Allogeneic mixed lymphocyte reactions during a second round of ontogeny: normal accessory cells did not restore defective IL-2 synthesis in T cells but induced responsiveness to exogenous IL-2. *Blood,* **74,** 2278–84.

Cayeux, S., Meuer, S. *et al.* (1989b). T-cell ontogeny after autologous bone marrow transplantation: failure to synthesize interleukin-2 (IL-2) and lack of CD2– and CD3-mediated proliferation by both CD4– and CD8+ cells even in the presence of exogenous IL-2. *Blood,* **74**(6), 2270–7.

Cela, M. E., Holladay, M. S. *et al.* (1996). Gamma delta T lymphocyte regeneration after T lymphocyte-depleted bone marrow transplantation from mismatched family members or matched unrelated donors. *Bone Marrow Transplantation,* **17**(2), 243–7.

Champlin, R., Ho, W. *et al.* (1990). Selective depletion of CD8 T lymphocytes for prevention of GVHD after allogeneic bone marrow transplantation. *Blood,* **76,** 418–23.

Chan, C. Y., Molrine, D. C. *et al.* (1997). Antibody responses to tetanus toxoid and Haemophilus influenzae type b conjugate vaccines following autologous peripheral blood stem cell transplantation (PBSCT). *Bone Marrow Transplantation,* **20**(1), 33–8.

Chaushu, G., Itzkovitz-Chaushu, S. *et al.* (1995). A longitudinal follow-up of salivary secretion in bone marrow transplant patients. *Oral Surgery, Oral Medicine, Oral Pathology, Oral Radiology, and Endodontics,* **79,** 164–9.

Chen, Y. C., Lin, K. H. *et al.* (1994). Bone marrow transplantation in Taiwan: an overview (with special emphasis on immunity to hepatitis B). *Bone Marrow Transplantation,* **13,** 705–8.

Chung, B., Barbara-Burnham, L. *et al.* (2001). Radiosensitivity of thymic interleukin-7 production and thymopoiesis after bone marrow transplantation. *Blood,* **98**(5), 1601–6.

Clark, R. A., Johnson, F. L. *et al.* (1976). Defective neutrophil chemotaxis in bone marrow transplant patients. *The Journal of Clinical Investigation,* **58,** 22–31.

Comoli, P., Maccario, R. *et al.* (1994). Expression of p75 chain of IL-2 receptor in the early immunological reconstitution after allogeneic BMT. *Clinical and Experimental Immunology,* **97,** 510–6.

Cooley, M. A., Atkinson, K. *et al.* (1991). In vitro function of CD4+ cells of naive and memory phenotype in bone marrow transplant recipients. *Transplantation Proceedings,* **23,** 165–6.

Cooley, M. A., McLachtan, K. *et al.* (1989). Cytokine activity after human BMT. III. Defect in IL-2 production by peripheral blood mononuclear cells is not corrected by stimulation with Ca++ ionophore plus phorbol ester. *British Journal of Haematology,* **73,** 341–7.

Cryz, S.J.J., Furer, E. *et al.* (1991). Clinical evaluation of an octavalent Pseudomonas aeruginosa conjugate vaccine in plasma donors and in bone marrow transplant and cystic fibrosis patients. *Psedomonas aeruginosa in Human Diseases. Antibiotic Chemotherapy,* J. Y. Homma, H. Tanimoto, I. A. holder, N. Hoiby and G. Doring. Basel, Karger. **44,** 157–62.

Cwynarski, K., Ainsworth, J. *et al.* (2001). Direct visualization of cytomegalovirus-specific T-cell reconstitution after allogeneic stem cell transplantation. *Blood,* **97**(5), 1232–40.

Daley, J. P., Rozans, M. K. *et al.* (1987). Retarded recovery of functional T cell frequencies in T cell-depleted bone marrow transplant recipients. *Blood,* **70,** 960–4.

DeBruin, H. G., Astaldi, A. *et al.* (1981). T lymphocyte characteristics in bone marrow-transplanted patients. II. Analysis with monoclonal antibodies. *Journal of Immunology,* **127,** 244–51.

DeGast, G. C., Gratama, J. W. *et al.* (1989). The influence of T cell depletion on recovery of T cell proliferation to herpesviruses and Candida after allogeneic BMT. *Transplantation,* **48,** 111–5.

DeGast, G. C., Verdonck, L. F. *et al.* (1985). Recovery of T cell subsets after autologous bone marrow transplantation is mainly due to proliferation of mature T cells in the graft. *Blood,* **66,** 428–31.

DeSouza, M.H.O., Diamond, H. R. *et al.* (1994). Immunological recovery after BMT for severe aplastic anemia: a Brazilian experience. *European Journal of Haematology,* **53,** 150–5.

DeWitte, T., Gratwohl, A. *et al.* (1992). Recombinant human granulocyte-macrophage colony-stimulating factor accelerates neutrophil and monocyte recovery after allogeneic T cell-depleted BMT. *Blood,* **79,** 1359–65.

Dilly, S. A. & Sloane, J. P. (1988). Cellular composition of the spleen after human allogeneic bone marrow transplantation. *The Journal of Pathology,* **155,** 151–60.

Dilly, S. A., Sloane, J. P. *et al.* (1986). The cellular composition of human lymph nodes after allogeneic bone marrow transplantation: an immunohistological study. *The Journal of Pathology,* **150,** 213–21.

Donnenberg, A. D., Hess, A. D. *et al.* (1987). Regeneration of genetically restricted immune functions after human bone marrow transplantation: influence of four different strategies for GVHD prophylaxis. *Transplantation Proceedings,* **19** (Suppl 7), 144–52.

Douek, D. C., Vescio, R. A. *et al.* (2000). Assessment of thymic output in adults after haematopoietic stem-cell transplantation and prediction of T-cell reconstitution [see comments]. *Lancet,* **355**(9218), 1875–81.

Drexler, H. G., Brenner, M. K. *et al.* (1987). CD5 positive B cells after T cell depleted bone marrow transplantation. *Clinical and Experimental Immunology,* **68,** 662–8.

Dror, Y., Gallagher, R. *et al.* (1993). Immune reconstitution in severe combined immunodeficiency disease after lectin-treated, T cell-depleted haplocompatible bone marrow transplantation. *Blood,* **81,** 2021–30.

Dulude, G., Brochu, S. *et al.* (1997). Thymic and extrathymic differentiation and expansion of T lymphocytes following bone marrow transplantation in irradiated recipients. *Experimental Hematology,* **25**(9), 992–1004.

Dulude, G., Roy, D. C. *et al.* (1999). The effect of graft-versus-host disease on T cell production and homeostasis. *The Journal of Experimental Medicine,* **189**(8), 1329–42.

Dumont-Girard, F., Roux, E. *et al.* (1998). Reconstitution of the T-cell compartment after bone marrow transplantation: restoration of the repertoire by thymic emigrants. *Blood,* **92**(11), 4464–71.

Dykewicz, C. A., Jaffe, H. W. *et al.* (2000). Guidelines for preventing opportunistic infections among hematopoietic stem cell transplant recipients. *Biology of Blood Marrow Transplantation,* **6**(6a), 659–713; 715; 717–27; quiz 729–33.

Ebisawa, M., Reason, D. C. *et al.* (1991). IL-4-mediated inductions of CD4+CD8+ T cells during infancy. *Annals of Allergy, Asthma & Immunology,* **67**, 612–7.

Effros, R. B., Allsopp, R. *et al.* (1996). Shortened telomeres in the expanded CD28-CD8+ cell subset in HIV disease implicate replicative senescence in HIV pathogenesis. *AIDS (London, England),* **10**(8), F17–22.

Einsele, H., Roosnek, E. *et al.* (2002). Infusion of cytomegalovirus (CMV)-specific T cells for the treatment of CMV infection not responding to antiviral chemotherapy. *Blood,* **99**(11), 3916–22.

Elfenbein, G. J., Bellis, M. M. *et al.* (1982). Phenotypically immature Bm cells in the peripheral blood after bone marrow grafting in man. *Experimental Hematology,* **10**, 551–9.

Elmaagacli, A. H., Basoglu, S. *et al.* (2002). Improved disease-free-survival after transplantation of peripheral blood stem cells as compared with bone marrow from HLA-identical unrelated donors in patients with first chronic phase chronic myeloid leukemia. *Blood,* **99**(4), 1130–5.

Engelhard, D., Handsher, R. *et al.* (1991a). Immune response to polio vaccination in bone marrow transplant recipients. *Bone Marrow Transplantation,* **8**(4), 295–300.

Engelhard, D., Nagler, A. *et al.* (1993). Antibody response to a two-dose regimen of influenza vaccine in allogeneic T cell-depleted and autologous BMT recipients. *Bone Marrow Transplantation,* **11**(1), 1–5.

Engelhard, D., Weinberg, M. *et al.* (1991b). Immunoglobulins A, G, and M to cytomegalovirus during recurrent infection in recipients of allogeneic bone marrow transplantation. *The Journal of Infectious Diseases,* **163**, 628–30.

Ericson, S. G., Colby, E. *et al.* (1992). Engraftment of leukocyte subsets following autologous bone marrow transplantation in acute myeloid leukemia using anti-myeloid (CD14 and CD15) monoclonal antibody-purged bone marrow. *Bone Marrow Transplantation,* **9**, 129–37.

Ericson, S. G., Guyre, C. A. *et al.* (1995). Antibody-dependent cellular cytotoxicity (ADCC) function of peripheral blood polymorphonuclear neutrophils (PMN) after autologous bone marrow transplantation (ABMT). *Bone Marrow Transplantation,* **16**, 787–91.

Fearnley, D. B., Whyte, L. F. *et al.* (1999). Monitoring human blood dendritic cell numbers in normal individuals and in stem cell transplantation. *Blood,* **93**(2), 728–36.

Fischer, A. M., Simon, F. *et al.* (1990). Prospective study of the occurrence of monoclonal gammapathies following bone marrow transplantation in young children. *Transplantation,* **49**, 731–5.

Flake, A. W., Roncarolo, M. G. *et al.* (1996). Treatment of X-linked severe combined immunodeficiency by in utero transplantation of paternal bone marrow. *The New England Journal of Medicine,* **335**, 1806–10.

Foot, A.B.M., Potter, M. N. *et al.* (1993). Immune reconstitution after BMT in children. *Bone Marrow Transplantation,* **11**, 7–13.

Friedrich, W., O'Reilly, R. J. *et al.* (1982). T-lymphocyte reconstitution in recipients of bone marrow transplants with and without GVHD: imbalances of T cell subpopulations having unique regulatory and cognitive functions. *Blood,* **59**, 696–70.

Fukuda, H., Nakamura, H. *et al.* (1994). Marked increase of CD8+S6F1+ and CD8+CD57+ cells in patients with GVHD after allogeneic BMT. *Bone Marrow Transplantation,* **13**, 181–5.

Fukushi, N., Arase, H. *et al.* (1990). Thymus: a direct target tissue in graft-versus-host reaction after allogeneic bone marrow transplantation that results in abrogation of induction of self-tolerance. *Proceedings of the National Academy of Sciences of the United States of America,* **87**(16), 6301–5.

Fumoux, F., Guigou, V. *et al.* (1993). Reconstitution of human immunoglobulin VH repertoire after bone marrow transplantation mimics B cell ontogeny. *Blood,* **81**, 3153–7.

Gallucci, S., Lolkema, M. *et al.* (1999). Natural adjuvants: endogenous activators of dendritic cells. *Nature Medicine,* **5**(11), 1249–55.

Garin, L., Rigal, D. *et al.* (1995). Allogeneic BMT in children: differential lymphocyte subset reconstitution according to the occurrence of acute GVHD. *Clinical Immunology and Immunopathology,* **77**, 139–48.

Gaschet, J., Denis, C. *et al.* (1995). Alterations of T cell repertoire after bone marrow transplantation: characterization of over-represented subsets. *Bone Marrow Transplantation,* **16**, 427–35.

Gerritsen, E. J., Van Tol, M. J. *et al.* (1994). Clonal dysregulation of the antibody response to tetanus-toxoid after bone marrow transplantation. *Blood,* **84**(12), 4374–82.

Gerritsen, E.J.A., VanTol, M.J.D. *et al.* (1996). Search for the antigen specificity of homogeneous IgG components (H-IgG) after allogeneic bone marrow transplantation. *Bone Marrow Transplantation,* **17**, 825–33.

Giebink, G. S., Warkentin, P. I. *et al.* (1986). Titers of antibody to pneumococci in allogeneic bone marrow transplant recipients before and after vaccination with pneumococcal vaccine. *The Journal of Infectious Diseases,* **154**, 590–6.

Glas, A. M., van Montfort, E. H. *et al.* (2000). B-cell-autonomous somatic mutation deficit following bone marrow transplant. *Blood,* **96**(3), 1064–9.

Godthelp, B. C., van Tol, M. J. *et al.* (1999). T-Cell immune reconstitution in pediatric leukemia patients after allogeneic bone marrow transplantation with T-cell-depleted or unmanipulated grafts: evaluation of overall and antigen-specific T-cell repertoires. *Blood,* **94**(12), 4358–69.

Gokmen, E., Raaphorst, F. M. *et al.* (1998). Ig heavy chain third complementarity determining regions (H CDR3s) after stem cell transplantation do not resemble the developing human fetal H CDR3s in size distribution and Ig gene utilization. *Blood,* **92**(8), 2802–14.

Gorla, R., Airo, P. *et al.* (1993). Predominance of "memory" phenotype within CD4+ and CD8+ lymphocytes subsets after allogeneic BMT. *Bone Marrow Transplantation,* **11**, 346–7.

Gorochov, G., Debre, P. *et al.* (1994). Oligoclonal expansion of CD8+CD57+ T cells with restricted T cell receptor beta chain variability after bone marrow transplantation. *Blood,* **83**, 587–95.

Gorski, J., Yassai, M. *et al.* (1994). Circulating T cell repertoire complexity in normal individuals and bone marrow recipients analyzed by CDR3 spectratyping. Correlation with immune status. *The Journal of Immunology,* **152**, 5109–19.

Gorski, J., Yassai, M. *et al.* (1995). Analysis of reconstitution T cell receptor repertoires in bone marrow transplant recipients. *Archivum Immunologiae et Therapie Experimentalis,* **43**, 93–7.

Gottlieb, D. J., Cryz, Jr., S. J. et al. (1990). Immunity against Pseudomonas aeruginosa adoptively transferred to bone marrow transplant recipients. *Blood,* **76**(12), 2470–5.

Gratama, J. W., Fibbe, W. E. et al. (1989). Different repopulation kinetics of CD3+, 4+ and/or 8+ T cells and CD3+, 4-, 8- T cells after allogeneic BMT. *Transplantation Proceedings,* **21**, 2978–9.

Gratama, J. W., Naipal, A. et al. (1984). T lymphocyte repopulation and differentiation after bone marrow transplantation. Early shifts in the ratio between T4+ and T8+ T lymphocytes correlate with the occurrence of acute GVHD. *Blood,* **63**, 1416–23.

Gratama, J. W., van Esser, J. W. et al. (2001). Tetramer-based quantification of cytomegalovirus (CMV)-specific CD8+ T lymphocytes in T-cell-depleted stem cell grafts and after transplantation may identify patients at risk for progressive CMV infection. *Blood,* **98**(5), 1358–64.

Gray, D. & Skarvall, H. (1988). B-cell memory is short-lived in the absence of antigen. *Nature,* **336**(6194), 70–3.

Griffiths-Chu, S., Patterson, J.A.K. et al. (1984). Characterization of immature T cell subpopulations in neonatal blood. *Blood,* **64**, 296–70.

Grob, J. P., Prentice, H. G. et al. (1987). Immune donors can protect marrow transplant recipients from severe cytomegalovirus infections. *Lancet,* **i**, 774–6.

Guillaume, T., Kubin, M. et al. (1996). Peripheral blood mononuclear cells from autologous hematopoietic stem cell transplantation recipients produce and response to IL-12. *Bone Marrow Transplantation,* **18**, 733–9.

Guillaume, T., Sekhavat, M. et al. (1994). Defective cytokine production following autologous stem cell transplantation for solid tumors and hematologic malignancies regardless of bone marrow or peripheral blood origin and lack of evidence for a role for IL-10 in delayed immune reconstitution. *Cancer Research,* **54**, 3800–97.

Guinan, E. C., Molrine, D. C. et al. (1994). Polysaccharide conjugate vaccine responses in bone marrow transplant patients. *Transplantation,* **57**, 677–84.

Haddad, E., Le Deist, F. et al. (1999). Long-term chimerism and B-cell function after bone marrow transplantation in patients with severe combined immunodeficiency with B cells: A single-center study of 22 patients. *Blood,* **94**(8), 2923–30.

Hakim, F. T. & Mackall, C. L. (1997). The immune system: effector and target of GVHD. *Graft-vs.-Host Disease.* J.L.M. Ferrara, H.J. Deeg and S. J. Burakoff. New York, Marcel Dekker: 257–89.

Hammarstrom, L., Lonnqvist, B. et al. (1985). Transfer of IgA deficiency to a bone marrow-grafted patient with aplastic anemia. *Lancet,* **i**, 778–81.

Hannet, I., Erkeller-Yuksel, F. et al. (1992). Developmental and maturational changes in human blood lymphocyte subpopulations. *Immunology Today,* **13**, 215–8.

Hata, A., Asanuma, H. et al. (2002). Use of an inactivated varicella vaccine in recipients of hematopoietic-cell transplants. *The New England Journal of Medicine,* **347**(1), 26–34.

Hazenberg, M. D., Otto, S. A. et al. (2002). T-cell receptor excision circle and T-cell dynamics after allogeneic stem cell transplantation are related to clinical events. *Blood,* **99**(9), 3449–53.

Hebart, H., Daginik, S. et al. (2002). Sensitive detection of human cytomegalovirus peptide-specific cytotoxic T-lymphocyte responses by interferon-gamma-enzyme-linked immunospot assay and flow cytometry in healthy individuals and in patients after allogeneic stem cell transplantation. *Blood,* **99**(10), 3830–7.

Hebart, H., Einsele, H. et al. (1996). CMV infection after allogeneic bone marrow transplantation is associated with the occurence of various autoantibodies and monoclonal gammopathies. *British Journal of Haematology,* **95**, 138–44.

Heitger, A., Neu, N. et al. (1997). Essential role of the thymus to reconstitute naive (CD45RA+) T-helper cells after human allogeneic bone marrow transplantation. *Blood,* **90**(2), 850–7.

Heitger, A., Winklehner, P. et al. (2002). Defective T-helper cell function after T-cell-depleting therapy affecting naive and memory populations. *Blood,* **99**(11), 4053–62.

Heslop, H. E., Ng, C. Y. et al. (1996a). Long-term restoration of immunity against EBV infection by adoptive transfer of gene-modified virus-specific T lymphocytes. *Nature Medicine,* **2**, 551–5.

Heslop, H. E. & Rooney, C. M. (1997). Adoptive cellular immunotherapy for EBV lymphoproliferative disease. *Immunological Reviews,* **157**, 217–22.

Heslop, H. E., Rooney, C. M. et al. (1996b). Use of gene marking in bone marrow transplantation. *Cancer Detection Prevention,* **20**, 108–13.

Heyd, J., Donnenberg, A. D. et al. (1988). IgE levels following allogeneic, autologous, and syngeneic bone marrow transplantation: an indirect association between hyperproduction and acute GVHD in allogeneic BMT. *Blood,* **72**, 442–6.

Hokland, M., Jacobsen, N. et al. (1988). Natural killer function following allogeneic bone marrow transplantation. *Transplantation,* **45**, 1080–4.

Holmes, J. A., Livesey, S. J. et al. (1989). Autoantibody analysis in chronic GVHD. *Bone Marrow Transplantation,* **4**, 529–31.

Horny, H. P., Horst, H. A. et al. (1988). Lymph node morphology after allogeneic BMT for chronic myeloid leukemia: a histological and immunohistological study focusing on the phenotype of the recovering lymphoid cells. *Blut,* **57**, 31–40.

Horny, H. P., Ruck, M. et al. (1990). Immunohistology of the human spleen after bone marrow transplantation for leukemia with special reference to the early post-transplantation period. *Pathology, Research and Practice,* **186**, 775–83.

Hou, S., Hyland, L. et al. (1994). Virus-specific CD8+ T-cell memory determined by clonal burst size. *Nature,* **369**(6482), 652–4.

Ilan, Y., Nagler, A. et al. (1994). Development of antibodies to hepatitis B virus surface antigen in bone marrow transplant recipient following treatment with peripheral blood lymphocytes from immunized donors. *Clinical and Experimental Immunology,* **97**, 299–302.

Ino, K., Singh, R. K. et al. (1997). CD14+ suppressor cells in mobilized stem cell products. *Journal Leukocyte Biology,* **61**, 583–91.

Ishii, E., Gengozian, N. et al. (1991). Influence of dimethyl myleran on tolerance induction and immune function in major histocompatibility complex-haploidentical murine bone marrow transplantation. *Proceedings of the National Academy of Sciences of the United States of America,* **88**, 8435–9.

Izquierdo, M., Balboa, M. A. et al. (1990). Relation between the increase of circulating CD3+CD57+ lymphocytes and T cell dysfunction in recipients of bone marrow transplantation. *Clinical and Experimental Immunology,* **82**, 145–50.

Izquierdo, M., Redondo, J. M. et al. (1989). Deficient protein kinase C-dependent Na+/H+ exchanger activity in T cells from BMT recipients. Journal of Immunology, 143, 2185–92.

Izutsu, K. T., Sullivan, K. M. et al. (1983). disordered salivary Ig secretion and sodium transport in human chronic GVHD. Transplantation, 35, 441–5.

Janossy, G., Prentice, H. G. et al. (1986). T lymphocyte regeneration after transplantation of T cell depleted allogeneic bone marrow. Clinical and Experimental Immunology, 63, 577–86.

Jin, N. R., Lum, L. G. et al. (1995). Signal transduction by B and T cells early after bone marrow transplantation: B cell calcium flux responses are intact whereas lack of CD4 cells accounts for impaired T cell responses. Bone Marrow Transplantation, 16, 103–9.

Jol-vd Zijde, C. M., Vossen, J. M. et al. (1983). Low molecular weight IgM in sera of children following bone marrow transplantation for severe aplastic anaemia and acute leukemia. Clinical and Experimental Immunology, 53, 151–8.

Kagan, J. M., Champlin, R. E. et al. (1989). B cell dysfunction following human BMT: functional-phenotypic dissociation in the early posttransplant period. Blood, 74, 777–85.

Kameoka, J., Sato, T. et al. (1995). Differential CD26-mediated activation of the CD3 and CD2 pathways after CD6-depleted allogeneic bone marrow transplantation. Blood, 85, 1132–7.

Kato, S., Yabe, H. et al. (1990). Studies on transfer of varicella-zoster-virus specific T cell immunity from bone marrow donor to recipient. Blood, 75, 806–9.

Kay, N. E., Bone, N. et al. (1990). Expansion of a lymphocyte population co-expressing CD4 and CD8 antigens in the peripheral blood of a normal adult male. Blood, 75, 2024–7.

Keever, C. A., Klein, J. et al. (1993). Effect of GVHD on the recovery of NK cell activity and LAK precursors following BMT. Bone Marrow Transplantation, 12, 289–95.

Keever, C. A., Small, T. N. et al. (1989). Immune reconstitution following bone marrow transplantation: comparison of recipients of T-cell depleted marrow with recipients of conventional marrow grafts. Blood, 73, 1340–50.

Kennedy, J. D., Pierce, C. W. et al. (1992). Extrathymic T cell maturation. Phenotypic analysis of T cell subsets in nude mice as a function of age. Journal of Immunology, 148(6), 1620–9.

Kier, P., Penner, E. et al. (1990). Autoantibodies in chronic GVHD: high prevalence of antinucleolar antibodies. Bone Marrow Transplantation, 6, 93–6.

Kiesel, S., Pezzutto, A. et al. (1988). B cell proliferative and differentiative responses after autologous peripheral blood stem cell or bone marrow transplantation. Blood, 72, 672–8.

King, S. M., Saunders, E. F. et al. (1996). Response to measles, mumps and rubella vaccine in paediatric bone marrow transplant recipients. Bone Marrow Transplantation, 17, 633–6.

Klangsinsirikul, P., Carter, G. I. et al. (2002). Campath-1G causes rapid depletion of circulating host dendritic cells (DCs) before allogeneic transplantation but does not delay donor DC reconstitution. Blood, 99(7), 2586–91.

Klingemann, H. G., Lum, L. G. et al. (1987). Phenotypical and functional studies on a subtype of suppressor cells (CD8+/CD11+) in patients after vone marrow transplantation. Transplantation, 44, 381–6.

Knobloch, C. & Friedrich, W. (1991). T cell receptor diversity in severe combined immunodeficiency following HLA-haploidentical bone marrow transplantation. Bone Marrow Transplantation, 8, 383–7.

Koehne, g., Zeller, W. et al. (1997). Phenotype of lymphocyte subsets after autologous peripheral blood stem cell transplantation. Bone Marrow Transplantation, 19, 149–56.

Kook, H., Goldman, F. et al. (1996). Reconstitution of the immune system after unrelated or partially matched T cell-depleted bone marrow transplantation in children: immunophenotypic analysis and factors affecting the speed of recovery. Blood, 88, 1089–97.

Korholz, D., Kunst, D. et al. (1996). Humoral immunodeficiency in patients after bone marrow transplantation. Bone Marrow Transplantation, 18, 1123–30.

Korver, K., Boeschoten, E. W. et al. (1987a). Dose-response effects in immunizations with keyhole limpet haemocyanin and rabies vaccine: shift in some immunodeficiency states. Clinical and Experimental Immunology, 70(2), 328–35.

Korver, K., DeLange, G. G. et al. (1987b). Lymphoid chimerism after allogeneic bone marrow transplantation. Transplantation, 44, 643–50.

Krall, W. J., Challita, P. M. et al. (1994). Cells expressing human glucocerebrosidase from a retroviral vector repopulate macrophages and central nervous system microglia after murine bone marrow transplantation. Blood, 83, 2737–48.

Kubo, K., Yamanaka, K. et al. (1996). Different T cell receptor repertoires between lesions and peripheral blood in acute GVHD after allogeneic bone marrow transplantation. Blood, 87, 3019–26.

Kurobane, I., Riches, P. G. et al. (1991). Incidental correction of severe IgA deficiency by displacement bone marrow transplantation (letter). Bone Marrow Transplantation, 7, 494–5.

Kusnierz-Glaz, C. R., Still, B. J. et al. (1997). Granulocyte conlony-stimulating factor-induced comobilization of CD4-CD8-T cells and hematopoietic progenitor cells (CD34+) in the blood of normal donors. Blood, 89, 2586–95.

Kwak, L. W., Taub, D. D. et al. (1995). Transfer of myeloma idiotype-specific immunity from an actively immunised marrow donor. Lancet, 345, 1016–20.

Labadie, J., VanTol, J. D. et al. (1992). Transfer of specific immunity from donor to recipient of an allogeneic bone marrow graft: effect of conditioning on the specific immune response of the graft recipient. British Journal of Haematology, 80, 381–90.

Lake, R. A., O'Hehir, R. E. et al. (1993). CD28 mRNA rapidly decays when activated T cells are functionally anergized with specific peptide. International Immunology, 5, 461–6.

Lamb, L. S., Henslee-Downey, P. J. et al. (1996). Increased frequency of TCR gamma delta + T cells in disease-free survivors following T cell-depleted, partially mismatched, related donor bone marrow transplantation for leukemia. Journal of Hemathotherapy and Stem Cell Research, 5, 503–9.

Lapointe, C., Forest, L. et al. (1996). Sequential analysis of early hematopoietic reconstitution following allogenic bone marrow transplantation with fluorescence in situ hybridization. Bone Marrow Transplantation, 17, 1143–8.

Lau, L. L., Jamieson, B. D. et al. (1994). Cytotoxic T-cell memory without antigen. Nature, 369(6482), 648–52.

Leino, L., Lilius, E. M. *et al.* (1991). The reappearance of 10 differentiation antigens on peripheral blood lymphocuytes after allogeneic bone marrow transplantation. *Bone Marrow Transplantation*, **8**, 339–44.

Leitenberg, D., Rapport, J. M. *et al.* (1994). B cell precursor bone marrow reconstitution after bone marrow transplantation. *American Journal of Clinical Pathology*, **102**, 231–6.

Leroy, E., Madariaga, L. *et al.* (1990). Abnormally expanded CD8+/CD57+ lymphocytes persisting in long-term bone marrow-transplanted patients are resting pre-cytotoxic T-lymphocytes. *Experimental Hematology*, **18**, 770–4.

Li, C. R., Greenberg, P. D. *et al.* (1994). Recovery of HLA-restricted cytomegalovirus (CMV)-specific T-cell responses after allogeneic bone marrow transplant: correlation with CMV disease and effect of ganciclovir prophylaxis. *Blood*, **83**(7), 1971–9.

Liu, X., Chesnokova, V. *et al.* (1996). Molecular analysis of T cell receptor repertoire in bone marrow transplant recipients: evidence of oligoclonal T cell expansion in GVHD lesions. *Blood*, **87**, 3032–44.

LiVolti, S., Mauro, L. *et al.* (1994). Immune status and immune response to diphteria-tetanus and polio vaccines in allogeneic bone marrow-transplanted thalassemic patients. *Bone Marrow Transplantation*, **14**, 225–7.

Ljungman, P., Duraj, V. *et al.* (1991). Response to immunization against polio after allogeneic marrow transplantation. *Bone Marrow Transplantation*, **7**(2), 89–93.

Ljungman, P., Fridell, E. *et al.* (1989). Efficacy and safety of vaccination of marrow transplant recipients with a live attenuated measles, mumps and rubella vaccine. *Journal of Infectious Diseases*, **159**, 610–5.

Ljungman, P., Lewensohn-Fuchs, I. *et al.* (1994). Long-term immunity to measles, mumps and rubella after allogeneic bone marrow transplantation. *Blood*, **84**, 657–63.

Ljungman, P., Lonnqvist, B. *et al.* (1986). Cytomegalovirus-specific lymphocyte proliferation and in vitro cytomegalovirus IgG synthesis for diagnosis of cytomegalovirus infections after BMT. *Blood*, **68**, 108–12.

Ljungman, P., Wiklund-Hammarsten, M. *et al.* (1990). Response to tetanus toxoid immunization after allogeneic bone marrow transplantation. *Journal of Infectious Diseases*, **162**(2), 496–500.

Locatelli, F., Maccario, R. *et al.* (1996). Hematopoietic and immune recovery after transplantation of cord blood progenitor cells in children. *Bone Marrow Transplantation*, **18**, 1095–101.

Lombardi, G., Sidhu, S. *et al.* (1994). Anergic T cells as suppressor cells in vitro. *Science*, **264**, 1587–9.

Lortan, J. E., Rochfort, N. C. *et al.* (1992a). Autoantibodies after bone marrow transplantation in children with genetic disorders: relation to chronic graft-versus-host disease. *Bone Marrow Transplantation*, **9**(5), 325–30.

Lortan, J. E., Vellodi, A. *et al.* (1992b). Class- and subclass-specific pneumococcal antibody levels and response to immunization after bone marrow transplantation. *Clinical and Experimental Immunology*, **88**, 512–9.

Lucas, K. G., Small, T. N. *et al.* (1996). The development of cellular immunity to EBV after allogeneic bone marrow transplantation. *Blood*, **87**, 2594–603.

Lum, L. G., Joshsi, I. D. *et al.* (1993). Coactivation with anti-CD28 monoclonal antibody enhances anti-CD3 monoclonal antibody-induced proliferation and IL-2 synthesis in T cells from autologous bone marrow transplant recipients. *Bone Marrow Transplantation*, **12**, 565–71.

Lum, L. G., Joshi, I. D. *et al.* (1994). Constitutive and mitogen-stimulated cytokine mRNA expression by peripheral blood mononuclear cells from most autologous and allogeneic bone marrow transplant recipients is intact. *Bone Marrow Transplantation*, **13**, 187–95.

Lum, L. G., Munn, N. A. *et al.* (1986). The detection of specific antibody formation to recall antigens after human bone marrow transplantation. *Blood*, **67**, 582–7.

Lum, L. G., Noges, J. E. *et al.* (1988). Transfer of specific immunity in marrow recipients given HLA-mismatched, T cell-depleted, or HLA-identical marrow grafts. *Bone Marrow Transplantation*, **3**, 399–406.

Lum, L. G., Orcutt-Thordarson, N. *et al.* (1982). The regulation of Ig synthesis after marrow transplantation: IV. T4 and T8 subset function in patients with chronic graft-versus-host disease. *Journal of Immunology*, **129**, 113–9.

Lum, L. G., Seigneuret, M. C. *et al.* (1985). The regulation of Ig synthesis after HLA-identical BMT: VI. Differential rates of maturation of distinct functional groups within lymphoid subpopulations in patients after human marrow grafting. *Blood*, **65**, 1422–33.

Lutz, E., Ward, K. N. *et al.* (1996). Cytomegalovirus antibody avidity in allogeneic bone marrow recipients: evidence for primary or secondary humoral responses depending on donor immune status. *Journal of Medical Virology*, **49**, 61–5.

Ma, D.D.F., Varga, D. E. *et al.* (1987). Haemopoietic reconstitution after allogeneic bone marrow transplantation in man: recovery of haemopoietic progenitors (CFU-Mix, BFU-E and CFU-GM). *British Journal of Haematology*, **65**, 5–10.

MacBurney, M., Young, L. S. *et al.* (1994). Nutrition support of glutamine-supplemented parenteral nutrition in adult bone marrow transplant patients. *Journal of the American Dietetic Association*, **94**, 1263–6.

MacDonald, K. P. & Hill, G. R. (2002). Keratinocyte Growth Factor (KGF) in hematology and oncology. *Current Pharmaceutical Design*, **8**(5), 395–403.

Machado, C. M., Goncalves, F. B. *et al.* (2002). Measles in bone marrow transplant recipients during an outbreak in Sao Paulo, Brazil. *Blood*, **99**(1), 83–7.

Mackall, C. L., Bare, C. V. *et al.* (1996). Thymic-independent T cell regeneration occurs via antigen-driven expansion of peripheral T cells resulting in a repertoire that is limited in diversity and prone to skewing. *Journal of Immunology*, **156**, 4609–16.

Mackall, C. L., Fleisher, T. A. *et al.* (1995). Age, thymopoiesis, and CD4+ T-lymphocyte regeneration after intensive chemotherapy. *The New England Journal of Medicine*, **332**(3), 143–9.

Mackall, C. L., Fry, T. J. *et al.* (2001). IL-7 increases both thymic-dependent and thymic-independent T-cell regeneration after bone marrow transplantation. *Blood*, **97**(5), 1491–7.

Mackall, C. L., Granger, L. *et al.* (1993). T-cell regeneration after bone marrow transplantation: differential CD45 isoform expression on thymic-derived versus thymic-independent progeny. *Blood*, **82**(8), 2585–94.

Mackall, C. L., Stein, D. *et al.* (2000). Prolonged CD4 depletion after sequential autologous peripheral blood progenitor cell infusions in children and young adults. *Blood*, **96**(2), 754–62.

Madariaga, L., Leroy, E. *et al.* (1990). Induction of cytolytic function in resting peripheral blood CD8+/Leu-7+ T cells through IL2/p75 IL2-receptor interaction: a study in the allogeneic human bone marrow transplantation model. *Cellular Immunology*, **130**, 291–302.

Markham, R. B. & Donnenberg, A. D. (1992). Effect of donor and recipient immunization protocols on primary and secondary human antibody responses in SCID mice reconstituted with human peripheral blood mononuclear cells. *Infection and Immunity*, **60**, 2305–8.

Marshall, N. A., Howe, J. G. *et al.* (2000). Rapid reconstitution of Epstein-Barr virus-specific T lymphocytes following allogeneic stem cell transplantation. *Blood*, **96**(8), 2814–21.

Masuko, K., Kato, S. *et al.* (1996). Stable clonal expansion of T cells induced by bone marrow transplantation. *Blood*, **87**, 789–99.

Mathur, A., Vallera, D. A. *et al.* (1995). Effect of IL-7 or IL-4 on reconstitution of donor lymphoid cells in congenic murine BMT. *Bone Marrow Transplantation*, **16**, 119–24.

Matloubian, M., Concepcion, R. J. *et al.* (1994). CD4+ T cells are required to sustain CD8+ cytotoxic T cell responses during chronic viral infection. *Journal Virology*, **68**, 8056–63.

Matsue, K., Lum, L. G. *et al.* (1987). Proliferative and differentiative responses of B cells from human marrow graft recipients to T cell-derived factors. *Blood*, **69**(1), 308–15.

McSweeney, P. A., Niederwieser, D. *et al.* (2001). Hematopoietic cell transplantation in older patients with hematologic malignancies: replacing high-dose cytotoxic therapy with graft-versus-tumor effects. *Blood*, **97**(11), 3390–400.

Meyers, J. D. (1986). Infection in bone marrow transplant recipients. *The American Journal of Medicine*, **81** (Suppl 1A), 27–38.

Mielcarek, M., Graf, L. *et al.* (1998). Production of interleukin-10 by granulocyte colony-stimulating factor-mobilized blood products: a mechanism for monocyte-mediated suppression of T-cell proliferation. *Blood*, **92**(1), 215–22.

Mielcarek, M., Martin, P. J. *et al.* (1997). Suppression of alloantigen-induced T cell proliferation by CD14+ cells derived from granulocyte colony-stimulating factor-mobilized peripheral blood mononuclear cells. *Blood*, **89**, 1629–34.

Miller, J. J. & Cole, L. J. (1967). The radiation resistance of long-lived lymphocytes and plasma cells in mouse and rat lymph nodes. *Journal of Immunology*, **98**, 982–90.

Miller, R. A., Daley, J. *et al.* (1991). Clonal analysis of T cell deficiencies in autotransplant recipients. *Blood*, **77**, 1845–50.

Min, D., Taylor, P. A. *et al.* (2002). Protection from thymic epithelial cell injury by keratinocyte growth factor: a new approach to improve thymic and peripheral T-cell reconstitution after bone marrow transplantation. *Blood*, **99**(12), 4592–600.

Minchinton, R. M., Waters, A. H. *et al.* (1982). Autoimmune thrombocytopenia acquired from an allogeneic bone marrow graft. *Lancet*, **ii**, 627–9.

Minegishi, Y., Ishii, N. *et al.* (1995). T cell reconstitution by haploidentical BMT does not restore the diversification of the Ig heavy chain gene in patients with X-linked SCID. *Bone Marrow Transplantation*, **16**, 801–6.

Mink, J. G., Radl, J. *et al.* (1979). Homogenous Igs in the serum of irradiated and bone marrow reconstituted mice: the role of thymus and spleen. *Immunology*, **37**, 889–94.

Mitus, A. J., Stein, R. *et al.* (1989). Monoclonal and oligoclonal gammopathy after bone marrow transplantation. *Blood*, **74**(8), 2764–8.

Molrine, D. C., Guinan, E. C. *et al.* (1996a). Donor Immunization With Haemophilus Influenzae Type B (Hib)-Conjugate Vaccine In Allogeneic Bone Marrow Transplantation. *Blood*, **87**(7), 3012–8.

Molrine, D. C., Guinan, E. C. *et al.* (1996b). Haemophilus influenzae type b (HIB)-conjugate immunization before bone marrow harvest in autologous bone marrow transplantation. *Bone Marrow Transplantation*, **17**, 1149–55.

Molrine, D. C. & Hibberd, P. L. (2001). Vaccines for transplant recipients. *Infectious Disease Clinics of North America*, **15**(1), 273–305, xii.

Muller, S. M., Kohn, T. *et al.* (2000). Similar pattern of thymic-dependent T-cell reconstitution in infants with severe combined immunodeficiency after human leukocyte antigen (HLA)-identical and HLA-nonidentical stem cell transplantation. *Blood*, **96**(13), 4344–9.

Muller-Hermelink, H. K., Sale, G. E. *et al.* (1987). Pathology of the thymus after allogeneic bone marrow transplantation in man. *American Journal Pathology*, **129**, 242–56.

Mulligan, C. G., Heatley, S. *et al.* (2002). Mannose-binding lectin gene polymorphisms are associated with major infection following allogeneic hemopoietic stem cell transplantation. *Blood*, **99**(10), 3524–9.

Murphy, G. F., Merot, Y. *et al.* (1985). Depletion and repopulation of epidermal dendritic cells after allogeneic BMT in humans. *The Journal of Investigative Dermatology*, **84**, 210–4.

Myers, L. A., Patel, D. D. *et al.* (2002). Hematopoietic stem cell transplantation for severe combined immunodeficiency in the neonatal period leads to superior thymic output and improved survival. *Blood*, **99**(3), 872–8.

Nagler, A., Ilan, Y. *et al.* (1995). Successful immunization of autologous bone marrow transplantation recipients against hepatitis B virus by active vaccination. *Bone Marrow Transplantation*, **15**, 475–8.

Nakata, K., Gotoh, H. *et al.* (1999). Augmented proliferation of human alveolar macrophages after allogeneic bone marrow transplantation. *Blood*, **93**(2), 667–73.

Nasman, I. & Lundkvist, I. (1996). Evidence for oligoclonal diversification of the VH6-containing Ig repertoire during reconstitution after bone marrow transplantation. *Blood*, **87**, 2795–804.

Niederwieser, D., Gastl, G. *et al.* (1987). Rapid reappearance of large granular lymphocytes (LGL) with concomitant reconstitution of natural killer (NK) activity after human bone marrow transplantation (BMT). *British Journal of Haematology*, **65**, 301–5.

Noel, D. R., Witherspoon, R. P. *et al.* (1978). Does graft-versus-host disease influence the tempo of immunologic recovery after allogeneic human marrow transplantation? An observation on 56 long-term survivors. *Blood*, **51**(6), 1087–105.

Norhagen, G., Engstrom, P. E. *et al.* (1994). Salivary and serum immunoglobulins in recipients of transplanted allogeneic and autologous bone marrow. *Bone Marrow Transplantation,* **14,** 229–34.

Norhagen-Engstrom, G., Hammarstrom, L. *et al.* (1988). Ontogeny of immunoglobulins in bone marrow-transplanted individuals. *Transplantation,* **46,** 710–5.

Ochs, L., Shu, X. O. *et al.* (1995). Late infections after allogeneic bone marrow transplantation: comparison of incidence in related and unrelated donor transplant recipients. *Blood,* **86,** 3979–86.

Okamoto, Y., Douek, D. C. *et al.* (2002). Effects of exogenous interleukin-7 on human thymus function. *Blood,* **99**(8), 2851–8.

Okumura, M., Fujii, Y. *et al.* (1993a). Both CD45RA+ and CD45RA- subpopulations of CD8+ T cells contain cells with high levels of lymphocyte function-associated antigen-1 expression, a phenotype of primed T cells. *Journal of Immunology,* **150**(2), 429–37.

Okumura, M., Fujii, Y. *et al.* (1993b). Age-related accumulation of LFA-1high cells in a CD8+CD45RAhigh T cell population. *European Journal of Immunology,* **23,** 1057–63.

O'Reilly, R. J., Friedrich, W. *et al.* (1994). Transplantation approaches for severe combined immunodeficiency disease, Wiskott-Aldrich syndrome, and other lethal genetic, combined immunodeficiency disorders. *Bone Marrow Transplantation.* S. J. Forman, K. G. Blume and E. D. Thomas. Boston, Blackwell: 849–73.

O'Reilly, R. J., Lacerda, J. F. *et al.* (1996). Adoptive cell therapy with donor lymphocytes for EBV-associated lymphomas developing after allogeneic marrow transplants. *Important Advances in Oncology,* **i,** 149–66.

Otsuka, M., Shiobara, S. *et al.* (1990). Antigen-specific antibody response in allogeneic bone marrow transplantation patients: in vivo and in vitro antibody production after the primary immunization with tetanus toxoid. *Japanese Journal of Clinical Hematology,* **31,** 301–7.

Ottinger, H. D., Beelen, D. W. *et al.* (1996). Improved immune reconstitution after allotransplantation of peripheral blood stem cells instead of bone marrow. *Blood,* **88,** 2775–9.

Papadopoulos, E. B., Ladanyi, M. *et al.* (1994). Infusions of donor leukocytes to treat Epstein-BArr virus-associated lymphoproliferative disorders after allogeneic BMT. *The New England Journal of Medicine,* **330,** 1185–91.

Parkkali, T., Kayhty, H. *et al.* (1996a). A comparison of early and late vaccination with haemophilus influenzae type b conjugate and pneumococcal polysaccharide vaccines after allogeneic BMT. *Bone Marrow Transplantation,* **18,** 961–7.

Parkkali, T., Olander, R. M. *et al.* (1997). A randomized comparison between early and late vaccination with tetanus toxoid vaccine after allogeneic BMT. *Bone Marrow Transplantation,* **19**(9), 933–8.

Parkkali, T., Ruutu, T. *et al.* (1996b). Loss of protective immunity to polio, diphteria and Haemophilus influenzae type b after allogeneic bone marrow transplantation. *APMIS: Acta Pathologica, et microbiologica, et immunologica Scandinavica,* **104,** 383–8.

Parra, C., Roldan, E. *et al.* (1996). Deficient expression of adhesion molecules by human CD5-B lymphocytes both after bone marrow transplantation and during normal ontogeny. *Blood,* **88,** 1733–40.

Patel, D. D., Gooding, M. E. *et al.* (2000). Thymic function after hematopoietic stem-cell transplantation for the treatment of severe combined immunodeficiency. *The New England Journal of Medicine,* **342**(18), 1325–32.

Pauksen, K., Duraj, V. *et al.* (1992). Immunity to and immunization against measles, rubella and mumps in patients after autologous bone marrow transplantation. *Bone Marrow Transplantation,* **9,** 427–32.

Pauksen, K., Linde, A. *et al.* (1995). Specific T and B cell immunity to measles after allogeneic and autologous bone marrow transplantation. *Bone Marrow Transplantation,* **16,** 807–13.

Pedrazzini, A., Freedman, A. S. *et al.* (1989). Anti-B cell monoclonal antibody-purged autologous BMT for B cell non-Hodgkin's lymphoma: Phenotypic reconstitution and B cell function. *Blood,* **74,** 2203–11.

Perreault, C., Pelletier, M. *et al.* (1984). Study of Langerhans cells after allogeneic BMT. *Blood,* **63,** 807–11.

Petz, L. D., Yam, P. *et al.* (1987). Mixed hematopoietic chimerism following bone marrow transplantation for hematologic malignancies. *Blood,* **70,** 1331–7.

Pignata, C., Sanghera, J. S. *et al.* (1996). Defective activation of mitogen-activated protein kinase after allogeneic bone marrow transplantation. *Blood,* **88,** 2334–41.

Porrata, L. F., Gertz, M. A. *et al.* (2001a). Early lymphocyte recovery predicts superior survival after autologous hematopoietic stem cell transplantation in multiple myeloma or non-Hodgkin lymphoma. *Blood,* **98**(3), 579–85.

Porrata, L. F., Ingle, J. N. *et al.* (2001b). Prolonged survival associated with early lymphocyte recovery after autologous hematopoietic stem cell transplantation for patients with metastatic breast cancer. *Bone Marrow Transplantation,* **28**(9), 865–71.

Porrata, L. F., Inwards, D. J. *et al.* (2002a). Early lymphocyte recovery post-autologous haematopoietic stem cell transplantation is associated with better survival in Hodgkin's disease. *British Journal of Haematology,* **117**(3), 629–33.

Porrata, L. F., Litzow, M. R. *et al.* (2002b). Early lymphocyte recovery is a predictive factor for prolonged survival after autologous hematopoietic stem cell transplantation for acute myelogenous leukemia. *Leukemia,* **16**(7), 1311–8.

Poznansky, M. C., Evans, R. H. *et al.* (2000). Efficient generation of human T cells from a tissue-engineered thymic organoid. *Nature Biotechnology,* **18**(7), 729–34.

Quinnan, G. V., Kirmani, N. *et al.* (1981). HLA-restricted cytotoxic T lymphocyte and non-thymic cytotoxic lymphocyte responses to cytomegalovirus infection of bone marrow transplant recipients. *Journal of Immunology,* **126,** 2036–41.

Quinnan, G.V.J., Kirmani, N. *et al.* (1982). HLA-restricted T-lymphocyte and non-T-lymphocyte cytotoxic responses correlate with recovery from CMV infection in BMT recipients. *The New England Journal of Medicine,* **307,** 6–13.

Quinti, I., Velardi, A. *et al.* (1990). Antibacterial polysaccharide antibody deficiency after allogeneic bone marrow transplantation. *Journal of Clinical Immunology,* **10,** 160–6.

Radl, J., Liu, M. *et al.* (1991). Monoclonal gammapathies in long-term surviving rhesus monkeys after lethal irradiation and bone marrow transplantation. *Clinical Immunology and Immunopathology,* **60,** 305–9.

Reittie, J. E., Gottlieb, D. *et al.* (1989). Endogenously generated activated killer cells circulate after autologous and allogeneic marrow transplantation but not after chemotherapy. *Blood,* **73,** 1351–8.

Reusser, P., Riddell, S. R. et al. (1991). Cytotoxic T-lymphocyte response to CMV after human allogeneic BMT: pattern of recovery and correlation with CMV infection and disease. Blood, 78, 1373–80.

Riddell, S. R., Watanabe, K. S. et al. (1992). Restoration of viral immunity in immunodeficient humans by the adoptive transfer of T cell clones. Science, 257, 238–41.

Ringden, O., Persson, U. et al. (1983). Markedly elevated serum IgE levels following allogeneic and syngeneic bone marrow transplantation. Blood, 61, 1190–5.

Robbins, K., McCabe, S. et al. (1994). Immunological effects of insulin-like growth factor-I – enhancement of immunoglobulin synthesis. Clinical and Experimental Immunology, 95, 337–42.

Roberts, M. M., To, L. B. et al. (1993). Immune reconstitution following peripheral blood stem cell transplantation, autologous bone marrow transplantation and allogeneic bone marrow transplantation. Bone Marrow Transplantation, 12, 469–75.

Rooney, C. M., Smith, C. A. et al. (1997). Control of virus-induced lymphoproliferation – EBV-induced lymphoproliferation and host immunity. Molecular Medicine Today, 3, 24–30.

Rosillo, M. C., Ortuno, F. et al. (1996). Immune recovery after autologous or ghG-CSF primed PBSC transplantation. European Journal of Haematology, 56, 301–7.

Rossi, S., Blazar, B. R. et al. (2002). Keratinocyte growth factor preserves normal thymopoiesis and thymic microenvironment during experimental graft-versus-host disease. Blood, 100(2), 682–91.

Roux, E., Dumont-Girard, F. et al. (2000). Recovery of immune reactivity after T-cell-depleted bone marrow transplantation depends on thymic activity. Blood, 96(6), 2299–303.

Roux, E., Helg, C. et al. (1992). Evolution of mixed chimerism after allogeneic bone marrow transplantation as determined on granulocytes and mononuclear cells by the polymerase chain reaction. Blood, 79, 2775–83.

Roux, E., Helg, C. et al. (1996a). T cell repertoire complexity after allogeneic bone marrow transplantation. Human Immunology, 48, 135–8.

Roux, E., Helg, C. et al. (1996b). Analysis of T cell repopulation after bone marrow transplantation: Significant differences between recipients of T cell depleted and unmanipulated grafts. Blood, 87, 3984–92.

Saarinen, U. M. (1984). Transfer of latent atropy by bone marrow transplantation? A case report. The Journal of Allergy and Clinical Immunology, 74, 196–200.

Sadamori, N., Ozer, H. et al. (1983). Chromosomal evidence of donor B-lymphocyte engraftment after bone marrow transplantation in a patient with multiple myeloma (letter). The New England Journal of Medicine, 308, 1423.

Sahdev, I., O'Reilly, R. et al. (1996). Interleukin-1 production following T cell depleted and unmodified marrow grafts. Pediatric Hematology and Oncology, 13, 55–67.

Sale, G. E., Alavaikko, M. et al. (1992). Abnormal CD4:CD8 rations and delayed germinal center reconstitution in lymph nodes of human graft recipients with graft-versus-host disease: an immunohistological study. Experimental Hematology, 20, 1017–21.

Sanmarco, M., Vialettes, B. et al. (1991). Autoantibody formation after bone marrow transplantation: a comparison between autologous and allogeneic grafts. Autoimmunity, 11, 7–12.

Saryan, J. A., Rappeport, J. et al. (1983). Regulation of human IgE synthesis in acute GVHD. The Journal of Clinical Investigation, 71, 556–64.

Sato, K., Ohtsuka, K. et al. (1995). Evidence of extrathymic generation of intermediate T cell receptor cells in the liver revealed in thymectomized, irradiated mice subjected to bone marrow transplantation. The Journal of Experimental Medicine, 182, 759–67.

Saxon, A., Mitsuyasu, R. et al. (1986). Designed transfer of specific immune responses with bone marrow transplantation. The Journal of Clinical Investigation, 78(4), 959–67.

Scambia, G., Panici, P. B. et al. (1993). Immunological reconstitution after high-dose chemotherapy and autologous blood stem cell transplantation for advanced ovarian cancer. European Journal of Cancer, 29A, 1518–22.

Schauer, U., Kohl, I. et al. (1992). Coexpression of CD4 and CD8 on mitogen-activated peripheral blood T cells from children with asthma: possible involvement of IL-4. Annals of Allergy, Asthma & Immunology, 68, 354–9.

Schouten, H. C., V. t., Sizoo, M. B. et al. (1988). Incomplete chimerism in erythroid, myeloid and B lymphocyte lineage after T cell depleted allogeneic bone marrow transplantation. Bone Marrow Transplantation, 3, 407–12.

Sheridan, J. F. (1990). Immunoglobulin G subclass deficiency and pneumococcal infection after allogeneic BMT. Blood, 75, 1583–6.

Shiobara, S., Harada, M. et al. (1982). Difference in posttransplant recovery of immune reactivity between allogeneic and autologous bone marrow transplantation. Transplantation Proceedings, 14, 429–33.

Shiobara, S., Lum, L. G. et al. (1986). Antigen-specific antibody responses of lymphocytes to tetansu toxoid after human marrow transplantation. Transplantation, 41, 587–92.

Shiobara, S., Witherspoon, R. P. et al. (1984). Immunoglobulin synthesis after HLA-identical marrow grafting. V. The role of peripheral blood monocytes in the regulation of in vitro immunoglobulin secretion stimulated by pokeweed mitogen. Journal of Immunology, 132, 2850–6.

Slifka, M. K., Antia, R. et al. (1998). Humoral immunity due to long-lived plasma cells. Immunity, 8(3), 363–72.

Slifka, M. K., Matloubian, M. et al. (1995). Bone marrow is a major site of long-term antibody production after acute viral infection. Journal of Virology, 69, 1895–902.

Small, T. N. (1996). Immunologic reconstitution following stem cell transplantation. Current Opinion in Hematology, 3, 461–5.

Small, T. N., Avigan, D. et al. (1997). Immune reconstitution following T-cell depleted bone marrow transplantation: effect of age and posttransplant graft rejection prophylaxis. Biology of Blood and Marrow Transplantation, 3(2), 65–75.

Small, T. N., Keever, C. A. et al. (1990). B-cell differentiation following autologous, conventional, or T-cell depleted bone marrow transplantation: a recapitulation of normal B-cell ontogeny. Blood, 76(8), 1647–56.

Small, T. N., Papadopoulos, E. B. et al. (1999). Comparison of immune reconstitution after unrelated and related T-cell-depleted bone marrow transplantation: effect of patient age and donor leukocyte infusions [In Process Citation]. Blood, 93(2), 467–80.

Smith, C.I.E., Aarli, J. A. et al. (1983). Myasthenia gravis after bone marrow transplantation. Evidence for donor origin. The New England Journal of Medicine, 309, 1565–8.

Smith, C.I.E., Hammarstrom, L. *et al.* (1985). Bone marrow grafting induces acetylcholine receptor antibody formation (letter). *Lancet,* **i,** 978.

Smith, F. S., Rencher, S. D. *et al.* (1995). T cell receptor repertoire of CD4+ and CD8+ T cell subsets in the allogeneic bone marrow transplant recipients. *Cancer and Immunology Immunotherapy: CII,* **41,** 104–10.

Sniecinski, I. J., Oien, L. *et al.* (1988). Immunohematologic consequences of major ABO-mismatched bone marrow transplantation. *Transplantation, 45,* 530–4.

Soderberg, C., Larsson, S. *et al.* (1996a). Cytomegalovirus-induced CD13-specific autoimmunity–a possible cause of chronic GVHD. *Transplantation,* **61,** 600–9.

Soderberg, C., Sumitran-Karuppan, S. *et al.* (1996b). CD13-specific autoimmunity in cytomegalovirus-infected immunocompromised patients. *Transplantation,* **61,** 594–600.

Soiffer, R. J., Bosserman, L. *et al.* (1990). Reconstitution of T cell function after CD6-depleted allogeneic bone marrow transplantation. *Blood, 75,* 2076–84.

Soiffer, R. J., Gonin, R. *et al.* (1993). Prediction of GVHD by phenotypic analysis of early immune reconstitution after CD6-depleted allogeneic BMT. *Blood, 82,* 2216–23.

Sosa, R., Weiden, P. L. *et al.* (1980). Granulocyte function in human allogeneic marrow graft recipients. *Experimental Hematology, 8,* 1183–9.

Sparkes, R. S., Sparkes, M. C. *et al.* (1979). Immunoglobulin synthesis following allogeneic bone marrow transplantation in man. Conversion to donor allotype. *Transplantation,* **27**(3), 212–3.

Stiehm, E. R., Roberts, R. L. *et al.* (1996). Bone marrow transplantation in severe combined immunodeficiency from a sibling who had received a paternal bone marrow transplant. *The New England Journal of Medicine, 335,* 1811–4.

Storek, J., Dawson, M. A. *et al.* (1999). Normal anti-CD3-stimulated proliferation of CD4+ T cells at one year after allogeneic marrow transplantation. *Transplantation Immunology, 7*(2), 123–5.

Storek, J., Dawson, M. A. *et al.* (2001a). Immune reconstitution after allogeneic marrow transplantation compared with blood stem cell transplantation. *Blood, 97*(11), 3380–9.

Storek, J., Espino, G. *et al.* (2000). Low B cell and monocyte counts on day 80 are associated with high infection rates between day 100 and 365 after allogeneic marrow transplantation. *Blood, 96*(9), 3290–3.

Storek, J., Ferrara, S. *et al.* (1992). Recovery of mononuclear cell subsets after bone marrow transplantation: overabundance of CD4+CD8+ dual-positive T cells reminiscent of ontogeny. *Journal of Hematotherapy & Stem Cell Research, 1*(4), 303–16.

Storek, J., Ferrara, S. *et al.* (1993). B cell reconstitution after human bone marrow transplantation: recapitulation of ontogeny? *Bone Marrow Transplantation, 12*(4), 387–98.

Storek, J., Gooley, T. *et al.* (1997a). Infectious morbidity in long-term survivors of allogeneic marrow transplantation is associated with low CD4 T cell counts. *American Journal of Hematology,* **54,** 131–8.

Storek, J., Hultin, L. E. *et al.* (1994a). B cell dysfunction after bone marrow transplantation is associated with decreased Ca2+ flux upon membrane Ig crosslinking. *Clinical Immunology and Immunopathology, 72*(2), 210–6.

Storek, J., Joseph, A. *et al.* (2001b). Immunity of patients surviving 20 to 30 years after allogeneic or syngeneic bone marrow transplantation. *Blood,* **98**(13), 3505–12.

Storek, J., Joseph, A. *et al.* (2002a). Factors influencing T lymphopoiesis after allogeneic hematopoietic cell transplantation. *Transplantation,* **73**(7), 1154–8.

Storek, J., King, L. *et al.* (1994b). Abundance of a restricted fetal B cell repertoire in marrow transplant recipients. *Bone Marrow Transplantation, 14*(5), 783–90.

Storek, J., Lalovic, B. B. *et al.* (2002b). Kinetics of B, CD4 T, and CD8+ T cells infused into humans: estimates of intravascular:extravascular ratios and total body counts. *Clinical Immunology,* **102**(3), 249–57.

Storek, J., Mendelman, P. M. *et al.* (1997b). IgG response to pneumococcal polysaccharide-protein conjugate appears similar to IgG response to polysaccharide in marrow transplant recipients and in normal adults. *Clinical Infectious Diseases, 25,* 1253–5.

Storek, J., Wells, D. *et al.* (2001c). Factors influencing B lymphopoiesis after allogeneic hematopoietic cell transplantation. *Blood,* **98**(2), 489–91.

Storek, J., Witherspoon, R. P. *et al.* (1995a). Low IgG Production By Mononuclear Cells From Marrow Transplant Survivors and From Normal Neonates Is Due to a Defect of B Cells. *Bone Marrow Transplantation, 15*(5), 679–84.

Storek, J., Witherspoon, R. P. *et al.* (1995b). T cell reconstitution after bone marrow transplantation into adult patients does not resemble T cell development in early life. *Bone Marrow Transplantation, 16*(3), 413–25.

Storek, J., Witherspoon, R. P. *et al.* (1997c). Improved reconstitution of CD4+ T cells and B cells but worsened reconstitution of serum IgG levels after allogeneic transplantation of blood stem cells instead of marrow (letter). *Blood, 89,* 3891–93.

Storek, J., Witherspoon, R. P. *et al.* (1997d). Reconstitution of membrane IgD– (mIgD–) B cells after marrow transplantation lags behind the reconstitution of mIgD+ B cells (letter). *Blood,* **89,** 350–51.

Storek, J., Witherspoon, R. P. *et al.* (1996). Lack of B cell precursors in marrow transplant recipients with chronic GVHD. *American Journal of Hematology, 52,* 82–9.

Storek, J., Viganego, F., Dawson, M. A. *et al.* (2003). Factors affecting antibody levels after allogeneic hematopoietic cell transplantation. *Blood, 101,* 3319–24.

Sugita, K., Nojima, Y. *et al.* (1994a). Prolonged impairment of very late activating antigen-mediated T cell proliferation via the CD3 pathway after T cell-depleted allogeneic bone marrow transplantation. *Journal of Clinical Investigation,* **94,** 481–8.

Sugita, K., Soiffer, R. J. *et al.* (1994b). The phenotype and reconstitution of immunoregulatory T cell subsets after T cell-depleted allogeneic and autologous BMT. *Transplantation, 57,* 1465–73.

Sullivan, K. M., Mori, M. *et al.* (1992). Late complications of allogeneic and autologous marrow transplantation. *Bone Marrow Transplantation, 10* (Suppl 1), 127–34.

Sullivan, K. M., Storek, J. *et al.* (1996). A controlled trial of long-term administration of intravenous immunoglobulin to prevent late infection and chronic GVHD following marrow transplantation: Clinical outcome and effect on subsequent immune recovery. *Biol Blood Marrow Transplantation, 2,* 44–53.

Suzuki, I., Milner, E.C.B. *et al.* (1996). Immunoglobulin heavy chain variable region gene usage in bone marrow transplant recipients: Lack of somatic mutation indicates a maturational arrest. *Blood,* **87,** 1873–80.

Sviland, L., Pearson, A.D.J. *et al.* (1991). Immunopathology of early GVHD – a prospective study of skin, rectum, and peripheral blood in allogeneic and autologous bone marrow transplant recipients. *Transplantation,* **52,** 1029–36.

Takahashi, M., Komiya, T. *et al.* (1997). A comparison of young and aged populations for the diphtheria and tetanus antitoxin titers in Japan. *Japanese Journal of Medicine, Science & Biology,* **50**(2), 87–95.

Talmadge, J. E., Reed, E. *et al.* (1997). Rapid immunologic reconstitution following transplantation with mobilized peripheral blood stem cells as compared to bone marrow. *Bone Marrow Transplantation,* **19,** 161–72.

Talvensaari, K., Clave, E. *et al.* (2002). A broad T-cell repertoire diversity and an efficient thymic function indicate a favorable long-term immune reconstitution after cord blood stem cell transplantation. *Blood,* **99**(4), 1458–64.

Tanaka, J., Imamura, M. *et al.* (1994). Cytokine gene expression by concavalin A-stimulated peripheral mononuclear cells after bone marrow transplantation: an indicator of immunological abnormality due to chronic GVHD. *Bone Marrow Transplantation,* **14,** 695–701.

Tary-Lehmann, M., Lehmann, P. V. *et al.* (1994). Anti-SCID mouse reactivity shapes the human CD4+ T cell repertoire in hu-PBL-SCID chimeras. *The Journal of Experimental Medicine,* **180,** 1817–27.

Tary-Lehmann, M. & Saxon, A. (1992). human mature T cells that are anergic in vivo prevail in SCID mice reconstituted with human peripheral blood. *The Journal of Experimental Medicine,* **175,** 503–16.

Tayebi, H., Tiberghien, P. *et al.* (2001). Allogeneic peripheral blood stem cell transplantation results in less alteration of early T cell compartment homeostasis than bone marrow transplantation. *Bone Marrow Transplantation,* **27**(2), 167–75.

Territo, M. C., Gale, R. P. *et al.* (1977). Neutrophil function in bone marrow transplant recipients. *British Journal of Haematology,* **35,** 245–50.

Thomson, B. G., Robertson, K. A. *et al.* (2000). Analysis of engraftment, graft-versus-host disease, and immune recovery following unrelated donor cord blood transplantation. *Blood,* **96**(8), 2703–11.

Tissot, J. D., Helg, C. *et al.* (1992). Clonal imbalances of serum Igs after allogeneic bone marrow transplantation: an analysis by high-resolution two-dimensional gel electrophoresis. *Bone Marrow Transplantation,* **10,** 347–53.

Tjonnfjord, G. E., Steen, R. *et al.* (1994). Evidence for engraftment of donor-type multipotent CD34+ cells in a patient with selective T-lymphocyte reconstitution after bone marrow transplantation for B-SCID. *Blood,* **84**(10), 3584–9.

Tollemar, J., Sundberg, B. *et al.* (1992). Immune response to Candida before and 5 years after allogeneic bone marrow transplantation. *Transplantation Proceedings,* **24,** 378–9.

Tsoi, M. S., Storb, R. *et al.* (1979). Nonspecific suppressor cells in patients with chronic GVHD after marrow grafting. *Journal of Immunology,* **123,** 1970–5.

Tsoi, M. S., Storb, R. *et al.* (1981). Specific suppressor cells in graft-host tolerance of HLA-identical marrow transplantation. *Nature,* **292,** 355–7.

Tsoi, M. S., Storb, R. *et al.* (1982). Cellular interactions in marrow-grafted patients. II. Normal monocyte antigen-presenting and defective T cell proliferative function early after grafting and during chronic graft-versus-host disease. *Transplantation,* **37,** 556–61.

Tucker, J. & Barnetson, R. S. C. (1985). Atopy after bone marrow transplantation. *British Medical Journal,* **290,** 116–7.

Uckun, F. M., Haissig, S. *et al.* (1992). Developmental hierarchy during early human B cell ontogeny after autologous bone marrow transplantation using autografts depleted of CD19+ B cell precursors by an anti-CD19 pan-B-cell immunotoxin containing pokeweed antiviral protein. *Blood,* **79,** 3369–79.

VanDenBerg, P., Radl, J. *et al.* (1976). Homogeneous antibodies in lethally irradiated and autologous bone marrow reconstituted Rhesus monkeys. *Clinical and Experimental Immunology,* **23,** 355–9.

VanDerWall, E., Richel, D. J. *et al.* (1994). Bone marrow reconstitution after high-dose chemotherapy and autologous peripheral blood progenitor cell transplantation: effect of graft size. *Annals of Oncology,* **5,** 795–802.

VanLeeuwen, J.E.M., VanTol, M.J.D. *et al.* (1994a). Relationship between patterns of engraftment in peripheral blood and immune reconstitution after allogeneic bone marrow transplantation for severe combined immunodeficiency. *Blood,* **84,** 3936–47.

VanLeeuwen, J.E.M., VanTol, M.J.D. *et al.* (1994b). Persistence of host-type hematopoiesis after allogeneic bone marrow transplantation for leukemia is significantly related to the recipient's age and/or conditioning regimen, but it is not associated with an increased relapse. *Blood,* **83,** 3059–67.

VanTol, M.J.D., Gerritsen, E.J.A. *et al.* (1996). The origin of IgG production and homogenous IgG components after allogeneic bone marrow transplantation. *Blood,* **87,** 818–26.

Vavassori, M., Maccario, R. *et al.* (1996). Restricted TCR repertoire and lont-term persistence of donor-derived antigen-experienced CD4+ T cells in allogeneic bone marrow transplantation recipients1. *Journal of Immunology,* **157,** 5739–47.

Velardi, A., Cucciaioni, S. *et al.* (1988a). Acquisition of Ig isotype diversity after bone marrow transplantation in adults. A recapitulation of normal B cell ontogeny. *Journal of Immunology,* **141**(3), 815–20.

Velardi, A., Terenzi, A. *et al.* (1988b). Imbalances within the peripheral blood T-helper (CD4+) and T-suppressor (CD8+) cell populations in the reconstitution phase after human bone marrow transplantation. *Blood,* **71**(5), 1196–200.

Verfuerth, S., Peggs, K. *et al.* (2000). Longitudinal monitoring of immune reconstitution by CDR3 size spectratyping after T-cell-depleted allogeneic bone marrow transplant and the effect of donor lymphocyte infusions on T-cell repertoire. *Blood,* **95**(12), 3990–5.

Villers, D., Milpied, N. *et al.* (1994). Alteration of the T cell repertoire after bone marrow transplantation. *Bone Marrow Transplantation,* **13,** 19–26.

Vossen, J. M., VanLeeuwen, J.E.M. *et al.* (1993). Chimerism and immune reconstitution following allogeneic bone marrow transplantation for severe combined immunodeficiency disease. *Immunodeficiency,* **4,** 311–3.

Wahren, B., Gahrton, G. *et al.* (1984). Transfer and persistence of viral antibody-producing cells in bone marrow transplantation. *Journal of Infectious Diseases,* **150,** 358–65.

Walker, S. A., Rogers, t. R. *et al.* (1984). Increased serum IgE concentrations during infection and GVHD after bone marrow transplantation. *Journal of Clinical Pathology,* **37,** 460–2.

Walsh, L. J., Athanasas-Platsis, S. *et al.* (1996). Reconstitution of cutaneous neural-immunological networks following bone marrow transplantation. *Transplantation,* **61,** 413–7.

Walter, E. A., Greenberg, P. D. *et al.* (1995). Reconstitution of cellular immunity against cytomegalovirus in recipients of allogeneic bone marrow by transfer of T-cell clones from the donor [see comments]. *The New England Journal of Medicine,* **333**(16), 1038–44.

Weinberg, K., Annett, G. *et al.* (1995). The effect of thymic function on immunocompetence following bone marrow transplantation. *Biology of Blood and Marrow Transplantation,* **1,** 18–23.

Weinberg, K., Blazar, B. R. *et al.* (2001). Factors affecting thymic function after allogeneic hematopoietic stem cell transplantation. *Blood,* **97**(5), 1458–66.

Wessman, M., Popp, S. *et al.* (1993). Detection of residual host cells after bone marrow transplantation using non-isotopic in situ hybridization and karyotype analysis. *Bone Marrow Transplantation,* **11,** 179–284.

Whiteside, T. L. & Herberman, R. B. (1994). Role of human natural killer cells in health and disease. *Clinical Diagnosis and Lab Immunology,* **1,** 125–33.

Wijnaendts, L., Le Deist, F. *et al.* (1989). Development of immunologic functions after bone marrow transplantation in 33 patients with severe combined immunodeficiency. *Blood,* **74**(6), 2212–9.

Wimperis, J. Z., Brenner, M. K. *et al.* (1987a). Rapid recovery of helper activity following T cell depleted allogeneic marrow transplant. *Clinical and Experimental Immunology,* **69,** 601–10.

Wimperis, J. Z., Brenner, M. K. *et al.* (1987b). B cell development and regulation after T cell depleted marrow transplantation. *Journal of Immunology,* **138,** 2445–50.

Wimperis, J. Z., Gottlieb, D. *et al.* (1990). Requirements for the adoptive transfer of antibody responses to a priming antigen in man. *Journal of Immunology,* **144**(2), 541–7.

Wimperis, J. Z., Prentice, H. G. *et al.* (1986). Transfer of functional humoral immune system in transplantation of T-lymphocyte depleted bone marrow. *Lancet,* **8477,** 339–43.

Winston, D. J., Ho, W. G. *et al.* (1983). Pneumococcal vaccination of recipients of bone marrow transplants. *Archives of Internal Medicine,* **143,** 1735–7.

Winston, D. J., Territo, M. C. *et al.* (1982). Alveolar macrophage dysfunction in human BMT recipients. *American Journal of Medicine,* **73,** 859–65.

Witherspoon, R. P., Kopecky, K. *et al.* (1982). Immunological recovery in 48 patients following syngeneic marrow transplantation for hematological malignancy. *Transplantation,* **33,** 143–9.

Witherspoon, R. P., Matthews, D. *et al.* (1984). Recovery of in vivo cellular immunity after human marrow grafting. *Transplantation,* **37,** 145–50.

Witherspoon, R. P., Schanfield, M. S. *et al.* (1978). Immunoglobulin production of donor origin after marrow transplantation for acute leukemia or aplastic anemia. *Transplantation,* **26**(6), 407–8.

Witherspoon, R. P., Storb, R. *et al.* (1981). Recovery of antibody production in human allogeneic marrow graft recipients: influence of time posttransplantation, the presence or absence of chronic graft-versus-host disease, and antithymocyte globulin treatment. *Blood,* **58**(2), 360–8.

Witherspoon, R. P., Sullivan, K. M. *et al.* (1988). Use of thymic grafts of thymic factors to augment immunologic recovery after BMT: brief report with 2 to 12 years' follow-up. *Bone Marrow Transplantation,* **3,** 425–35.

Wu, C. J., Chillemi, A. *et al.* (2000). Reconstitution of T-cell receptor repertoire diversity following T-cell depleted allogeneic bone marrow transplantation is related to hematopoietic chimerism. *Blood,* **95**(1), 352–9.

Wu, L., Li, C. L. *et al.* (1996). Thymic dendritic cell precursors: relationship to the T lymphocyte lineage and phenotype of the dendritic cell progeny. *Journal of Experimental Medicine,* **184,** 903–11.

Wyatt, D. T., Lum, L. G. *et al.* (1990). Autoimmune thyroiditis after BMT. *Bone Marrow Transplantation,* **5,** 357–61.

Yabe, H., Yabe, M. *et al.* (1990). Increased numbers of CD8+CD11+, CD8+CD11– and CD8+Leu7+ cells in patients with chronic GVHD after allogeneic bone marrow transplantation. *Bone Marrow Transplantation,* **5,** 295–300.

Yamagami, M., McFadden, P. W. *et al.* (1990). Failure of T cell receptor-anti-CD3 monoclonal antibody interaction in T cells from marrow recipients to induce increases in intracellular ionized calcium. *Journal of Clinical Investigation,* **86,** 1347–51.

Zimmerli, W., Zarth, A. *et al.* (1989). Granulocyte-macrophage colony-stimulating factor for granulocyte defects of bone marrow transplant patients (letter). *Lancet,* **i,** 494.

Zimmerli, W., Zarth, A. *et al.* (1991). Neutroophil function and pyogenic infections in BMT recipients. *Blood,* **77,** 393–9.

Zintl, F., Prager, J. *et al.* (1989). Immune reconstitution after human bone marrow transplantation. *Folia Haematology,* **3–4,** 519–26.

15 Pathogenesis of acute and chronic graft-versus-host disease

TAKANORI TESHIMA AND JAMES L.M. FERRARA

University of Michigan, Ann Arbor, USA

Definition and etiology

Graft-versus-host disease (GVHD) is the major complication of allogeneic hematopoietic stem cell (HSC) transplantation. The transfer of tissues between normal individuals usually results in the recognition and destruction (rejection) of the foreign tissue in a host-versus-graft reaction. Immunologically competent cells contained in the transplanted graft can result in immunologic recognition in the other direction, initiating a graft-versus-host (GVH) reaction. This GVH phenomenon was first noted when irradiated mice were infused with normal spleen cells. Although mice given allogeneic marrow recovered from radiation injury and marrow aplasia, they subsequently died with "secondary disease," a syndrome consisting of diarrhea, weight loss, skin changes, and liver abnormalities (van Bekkum & De Vries, 1967). This phenomenon was subsequently recognized as GVHD and was shown to be the same as runt disease in mice infused at birth with allogeneic cells.

In 1966, these observations led Billingham to formulate the requirements for the development of GVHD (Billingham, 1966). First, the graft must contain immunologically competent cells; second, the recipient must be incapable of mounting an effective response to destroy the transplanted cells; third, the recipient must express tissue antigens that are not present in the transplant donor. According to these criteria, GVHD can develop in various clinical settings when tissues containing immunocompetent cells (blood products, bone marrow, solid organs) are transferred between individuals (Table 15.1).

The first requirement of a GVHD reaction, immunocompetent cells, is now recognized to be the presence of mature T cells in the stem cell inoculum (Korngold & Sprent, 1990). Clinical studies confirm extensive experimental data that demonstrate that the severity of GVHD correlates with the number of donor T cells transfused (Kernan *et al.*, 1986). The ability of marrow T cells to induce GVHD is much less potent than blood T cells (Zeng *et al.*, 1999); therefore, contamination of bone marrow with peripheral blood at the time of harvest may be causally related to the development of GVHD.

The second requirement stipulates that the recipient must be immunocompromised with respect to the graft. A patient with a normal immune system will usually reject T cells from a foreign donor and thus prevent GVHD. This requirement is most commonly met in allogeneic HSC transplantation, where recipients have usually received very immunosuppressive doses of chemotherapy and/or radiation before stem cell infusion, but it may also be met in other situations (Table 15.1). Recipients of solid organ grafts are also treated with immunosuppressive drugs to prevent rejection of the transplanted organ and thereby become susceptible to the attack of donor T cells that are present in the donor graft. Many reported cases of GVHD in this setting involve liver transplant recipients and the incidence of GVHD appeared to be the highest after small bowel transplant, approximately 5% (Triulzi & Nalesnik, 2001); both organs are rich in T cells. T cells in blood products can induce GVHD in patients receiving blood transfusion (Anderson, 1997). Less obviously immunocompromised hosts who are susceptible to GVH reactions include fetuses who have received maternofetal transfusions in utero and neonates who are given exchange transfusions. GVHD can also occur in an immunocompetent recipient if genetic factors are permissive. Normal recipients, who are heterozygous for HLA proteins will not reject lymphocytes that are transfused from a donor who is homozygous for one of the recipient's haplotypes (since the donor HLA antigens are already codominantly expressed on the recipient's cells). On this basis, patients undergoing surgery who receive genetically permissive, directed blood transfusions (e.g., trans-

Table 15.1. *Procedures associated with a high risk of GVHD*

Procedure	Risk factors
Hematopoietic stem cell transplantation	No GVHD prophylaxis; HLA mismatch; Unrelated donor
Donor leukocyte infusion (DLI)	Larger dose of DLI
Solid organ transplantation	Small bowel transplants
Blood transfusion	Unirradiated blood products; neonates; immunosuppressed patients; blood donation from relatives

fusion of blood from an HLA homozygous child to a heterozygous parent) may develop GVHD, even though they are not immunocompromised (Anderson, 1997). Thus, blood transfusion from first degree relatives should be irradiated prior to transfusion to prevent a possible GVH reaction.

The third requirement, the expression of recipient tissue antigens not present in the donor, became the focus of intensive research with the discovery of the major histocompatibility complex (MHC). Human leukocyte antigen (HLA) proteins are the products of the MHC genes that are expressed on the cell surfaces of all nucleated cells in the human body, and they are essential to the activation of allogeneic T cells (Krensky et al., 1990). MHC differences between donor and recipient are the most important risk factor for the induction of GVHD. In addition, there are minor histocompatibility antigens (MiHA) encoded by other genetic loci (many as yet undefined) that also can be recognized as foreign. Surprisingly, experimental models have demonstrated that GVH reactions can occur between genetically identical strains and individuals (Hess & Fischer, 1989). These observation have necessitated a revision of Billingham's third postulate to include, in addition to the recognition of foreign host antigens, the inappropriate recognition of host self-antigens (i.e., an autoimmune process).

Pathology

Acute GVHD

Without prophylactic immunosuppression, most allogeneic HSC transplants will be complicated by GVHD. Acute GVHD can occur within days (in HLA-nonidentical recipients or in patients not given any prophylaxis) or as late as several months after donor leukocyte infusions. The principal target organs include the immune system, skin, liver, intestine, and possibly the lung. In cases of transfusion-associated GVHD, bone marrow aplasia is often observed because the host's hematopoietic system is targeted. Likewise, marrow aplasia is a serious complication of donor leukocyte infusions given to treat hematologic malignancy in cases involving relapse after an HSC allograft, and results from a GVH reaction against residual host hematopoietic system.

The pathologic findings of acute GVHD characteristically include epithelial damage of selective target organs; this damage is usually apoptotic in nature (Crawford, 1997). In the skin, the epidermis and hair follicles are often destroyed. In the liver, small bile ducts are profoundly affected, and segmental disruption is common. Intestinal crypt destruction results in mucosal ulcerations that may be either patchy or diffuse. A prominent pathologic feature of acute GVHD is the disparity between the severity of tissue destruction and the paucity of the lymphocytic infiltrate. During GVHD, MHC class II molecules are aberrantly expressed on epithelial and endothelial target cells (Lampert et al., 1981; Mason et al., 1981; Barclay & Mason, 1982), and it has been generally assumed that this aberrant MHC expression is essential for target cell damage in GVHD.

However, a recent murine study demonstrated that the aberrant MHC class II expression is the result of tissue inflammation rather than the cause of GVHD (Teshima et al., 2002a). This study also demonstrated that direct contact between target cell and lymphocyte is often not required for target cell destruction, and that soluble mediators of GVHD such as interleukin-1 (IL-1) and tumor necrosis factor (TNF)-α can mediate target injury (Teshima et al., 2002a).

Chronic GVHD

Chronic GVHD was initially defined as a GVHD syndrome presenting more than 100 days posttransplant either as an extension of acute GVHD (progressive onset), after a disease-free interval (quiescent), or without preceding acute GVHD (de novo) (Sullivan et al., 1981). Any grade of acute GVHD increases the probability of chronic GVHD, although no single pathologic feature is predictive of its development. As with acute GVHD, the immune system appears to be affected in all patients, and they are highly susceptible to bacterial, viral, fungal, and opportunistic infections. The skin can show erythema with macules and plaques, desquamation, dyspigmentation, lichen planus, atrophy, and, in severe cases, chronic skin ulcers. Chronic cholestatic liver disease can occur, as can involvement of the gastrointestinal tract resulting in weight loss and malnutrition. Chronic GVHD commonly produces a sicca syndrome, caused by lymphocytic destruction of exocrine glands, most frequently affecting the eyes and mouth. The pathologic findings of chronic GVHD in the immune system include involution of thymic epithelium, lymphocyte depletion, and absence of secondary germinal centers in lymph nodes (Ghayur et al., 1990). The skin shows epidermal atrophy, dermal fibrosis, and sclerosis. Gastrointestinal lesions include inflammation, and rarely stenosis and stricture formation, particularly in the esophagus. Histologic finding in the liver are often intensified versions of acute GVHD, with chronic changes such as fibrosis, hyalinization of portal triads, and obliteration of bile ducts. The glands of the skin and digestive tract show destruction focused on centrally draining ducts with secondary involvement of alveolar components. Pulmonary tissue can also be involved, although histologic distinctions from bacterial and viral infections have been difficult. Nevertheless bronchiolitis obliterans, similar to those observed in the rejection of lung transplants, is now generally considered a manifestation of chronic GVHD. It has become apparent that clinical and histologic changes considered characteristic for chronic GVHD can develop as early as 40 or 50 days posttransplant and thus overlap with acute GVHD. Hence, the time of onset is an increasingly arbitrary criterion, and it is more meaningful to define the disease on the basis of clinical, histologic, and immunologic findings.

Immunopathophysiology

The development of acute GVHD is proposed to consist of a three-step process where mononuclear phagocytes and other accessory cells are responsible for both initiation of a GVH reaction and for the subsequent injury to host tissues after complex interactions with cytokines secreted by activated donor type 1 T cells (Fig. 15.1). In step 1, the conditioning regimen (irradiation and/or chemotherapy) leads to the damage and activation of host tissues, including intestinal mucosa, liver, and other tissues, and induces the secretion of inflammatory cytokines TNF-α and IL-1. The consequences of the action of these cytokines are the increased expression of MHC antigens and adhesion molecules, thus enhancing the recognition of host alloantigens by donor T cells. Donor T-cell activation in step 2 is characterized by proliferation of donor T cells and secretion of cytokines including IL-2 and IFN-γ. The host antigen-presenting cell (APC) presents antigen in the form of a peptide-HLA complex (alloantigen) to the resting donor T cells. Costimulatory signals, required for T-cell activation and signaling, also activate APCs, thus further promoting donor T-cell activation. IL-2 and IFN-γ enhance T-cell expansion, induce cytotoxic T cells (CTL) and natural killer (NK) cell responses, and prime additional mononuclear phagocytes to produce TNF-α and IL-1. These inflammatory cytokines in turn stimulate production of inflammatory chemokines, thus recruiting effector cells into target organs. In step 3, effector functions of mononuclear phagocytes are triggered via a secondary signal

provided by lipopolysaccharide (LPS) that leaks through the intestinal mucosa damaged during step 1. This mechanism may result in the amplification of local tissue injury and further promotion of an inflammatory response, which, together with the CTL and NK components, leads to target tissue destruction in the transplant host. There is now substantial evidence to implicate the inappropriate production of cytokines, which are the central regulatory molecules of the immune system, as a primary cause for the induction and maintenance of experimental and clinical GVHD (Antin & Ferrara, 1992; Teshima *et al.*, 2002a). Dysregulation of this complex cytokine cascade can occur at various steps in the sequence and eventually is thought to be responsible for the manifestations of this disease.

Conditioning

The first step involves the transplant conditioning regimen, which includes total body irradiation (TBI) and/or chemotherapy. Donor T cells are infused into a host that has been profoundly damaged by underlying disease, infection, and conditioning, all of which result in substantial proinflammatory changes in endothelial and epithelial cells. Activated host cells then secrete inflammatory cytokines, such as TNF-α and IL-1 (Xun *et al.*, 1994). The presence of inflammatory cytokines

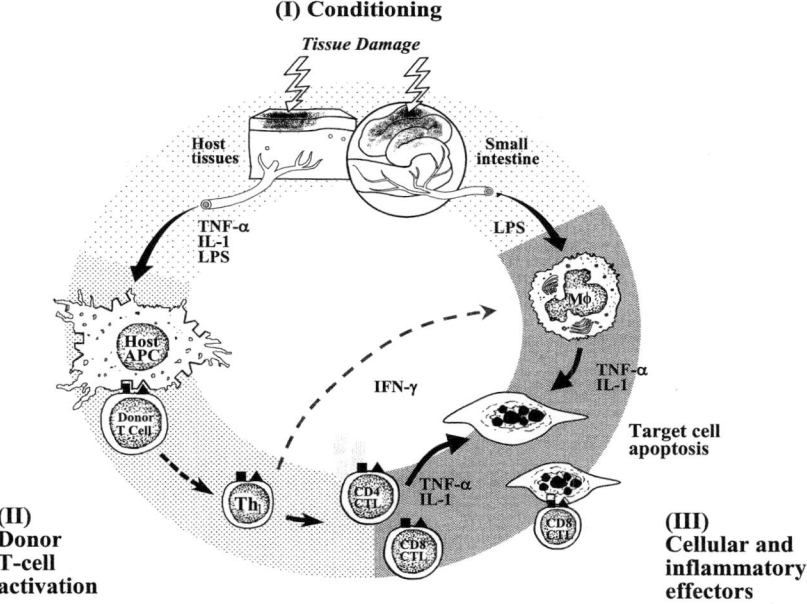

Fig. 15.1. The immunopathology of GVHD. GVHD pathophysiology can be summarized in a three-step process. In phase 1, the conditioning regimen (irradiation, chemotherapy, or both) leads to the damage and activation of host tissues, especially the intestinal mucosa. This allows the translocation of LPS from the intestinal lumen to the circulation, stimulating the secretion of the inflammatory cytokines TNF-α and IL-1 from host tissues, particularly macrophages. These cytokines increase the expression of MHC antigens and adhesion molecules on host tissues, enhancing the recognition of MHC and minor histocompatability antigens by mature donor T cells. Donor T-cell activation in phase 2 is characterized by the proliferation of Th1 cells and the secretion IFN-γ, which activates mononuclear phagocytes. The CTL damages tissue by perforin/granzyme, FasL, and TNF-α. In phase 3, effector functions of activated mononuclear phagocytes are triggered by the secondary signal provided by LPS and other stimulatory molecules that leak through the intestinal mucosa damaged during phases 1 and 2. This damage results in the amplification of local tissue injury, and it further promotes an inflammatory response. Damage to the GI tract in this phase, principally by inflammatory cytokines, amplifies LPS release and leads to the "cytokine storm" characteristic of severe acute GVHD.

during this phase may upregulate adhesion molecules, costimulatory molecules, and MHC antigens (Cavender et al., 1986; Chang & Lee, 1986; Pober et al., 1986; Leeuwenberg et al., 1988; Thornhill et al., 1991). Such "danger signals" (Matzinger, 2002) expressed by injured host tissues are critical for the activation of host dendritic cells (DCs), necessary for the initiation of primary and secondary immune responses. This concept explains a number of unique and seemingly unrelated aspects of GVHD. For example, a number of analyses of clinical transplants have noted increased risks of GVHD associated with advanced stage leukemia, certain intensive conditioning regimens, and histories of viral infections (Gale et al., 1987; Clift et al., 1990; Ringden, 1990). TBI is particularly important because it also induces endothelial apoptosis in gastrointestinal tract followed by epithelial cell damage (Paris et al., 2001), allowing immunostimulatory microbial products such as LPS to enter into systemic circulation, leading to further amplification of GVHD. The relationship between conditioning intensity, inflammatory cytokine, and GVHD severity was further supported by animal models (Hill et al., 1997) and clinical observation (Gale et al., 1987; Clift et al., 1990).

T-cell activation

Donor T-cell activation occurs during the second step of the afferent phase of acute GVHD, and it includes antigen presentation by host APCs and subsequent activation, proliferation, and differentiation of donor T cells. Murine studies demonstrated that host APCs alone are sufficient to activate donor T cells (Teshima et al., 2002a), and thus this process appears to occur within secondary lymphoid organs (Lakkis et al., 2000). In murine models of BMT across MHC disparities, robust proliferation of donor T cells is observed in spleen as early as day 3, preceding the engraftment of donor BM cells (Yang et al., 1998; Reddy et al., 2001; Teshima et al., 2002a; Teshima et al., 2002a). Although alloantigens can be directly presented by host-derived APCs and indirectly by donor-derived APCs that cross-present host antigens, host-derived APCs appear to be critical in inducing GVHD across MiHA mismatch (Shlomchik et al., 1999) and MHC mismatch (Teshima et al., 2002a). In humans, most cases of acute GVHD develop when host DCs are still present, although host DCs are rapidly replaced by donor DCs in peripheral blood after BMT (Auffermann-Gretzinger et al., 2002). Advanced age of the BMT recipient is an important determinant of GVHD severity (Sullivan et al., 1989). A recent murine study identified the enhanced allostimulatory activity of host APCs in aged mice as one of the important factors for this association (Ordemann et al., 2002).

The initial binding of T cells with APCs is mediated by the interaction of adhesion molecules (Fig. 15.2). When a T cell recognizes a specific ligand on an APC, signaling through the T-cell receptor (TCR) induces a conformational change in adhesion molecules, resulted in higher affinity binding (Dustin & Springer, 1989). In allogeneic interactions such as GVHD, donor T cells recognize recipient peptide HLA complexes in which both the HLA molecules and the bound peptides are seen as foreign. T-cell activation further requires costimulatory signals provided by APCs. There are four known CD28 superfamily members expressed on T cells: CD28, cytotoxic T lymphocyte antigen 4 (CTLA-4), inducible costimulator (ICOS), and programmed death (PD)-1; and four TNF receptor families: CD40 ligand (CD154), 4-1BB (CD137), and OX40 (Fig. 15.2). The best-characterized costimulatory molecules, CD80 and CD86, deliver positive signals through CD28 that lower the threshold for T-cell activation and promote T-cell differentiation and survival, while CTLA-4 delivers an inhibitory signal. Changes in phase 1 dramatically augment these processes.

The most potent APCs are dendritic cells (DCs), although the relative contribution of DCs and other semiprofessional APCs such as monocytes/macrophages and B cells in inducing GVHD remains to be elucidated. DCs can be matured and activated by 1) inflammatory cytokines such as TNF-α and IL-1, 2) microbial products such as LPS and CpG entering systemic circulation from intestinal mucosa damaged by conditioning, and 3) necrotic cells that were damaged by recipient conditioning (Gallucci et al., 1999). These effects are extremely important because mature DCs induce a T-cell response, whereas immature DCs can induce tolerance (Roncarolo et al., 2001). In addition, T-cell proliferation, migration, and survival are dramatically enhanced in vivo when T cells are exposed to antigens in the presence of adjuvant such as LPS (Reinhardt et al., 2001).

The alloantigen composition of the host determines which T-cell subset proliferates and differentiates. MHC class II (HLA-DR,DP,DQ) differences stimulate CD4$^+$ T cells; MHC class I (HLA-A, B, C) differences stimulate CD8$^+$ T cells. CD4 and CD8 proteins are coreceptors for constant portions of MHC class II and MHC class I molecules, respectively. In mouse models of GVHD, where genetic differences between multiple strain combinations can be controlled, CD4$^+$ cells induce GVHD to MHC class II differences, and CD8$^+$ cells induce GVHD to MHC class I differences (Korngold & Sprent, 1990). In the majority of HLA-identical HSC transplants, GVHD may be induced by either subset or by both subsets in response to MiHA, which are derived from the expression of polymorphic genes that distinguish host from donor. While the number of MiHA in humans is not defined, the actual number of so called "major minor" antigens that can potentially induce GVHD are likely to be limited.

The role of NK cells on GVHD is controversial. NK cells are negatively regulated by MHC class I-specific inhibitory receptors; thus, HLA mismatched transplants may trigger donor NK-mediated alloreactivity. In murine models of BMT, infusion of donor NK cells can reduce GVHD, probably through the elimination of host APCs (Ruggeri et al., 2002) or through their secretion of TGF-β (Asai et al., 1998). Interestingly, HLA class I disparity driving donor NK-mediated alloreactions in the GVH direction mediates strong GVL effects and produces higher engraftment rates without causing acute GVHD (Ruggeri et al., 2001; Ruggeri et al., 2002). NK cells also pro-

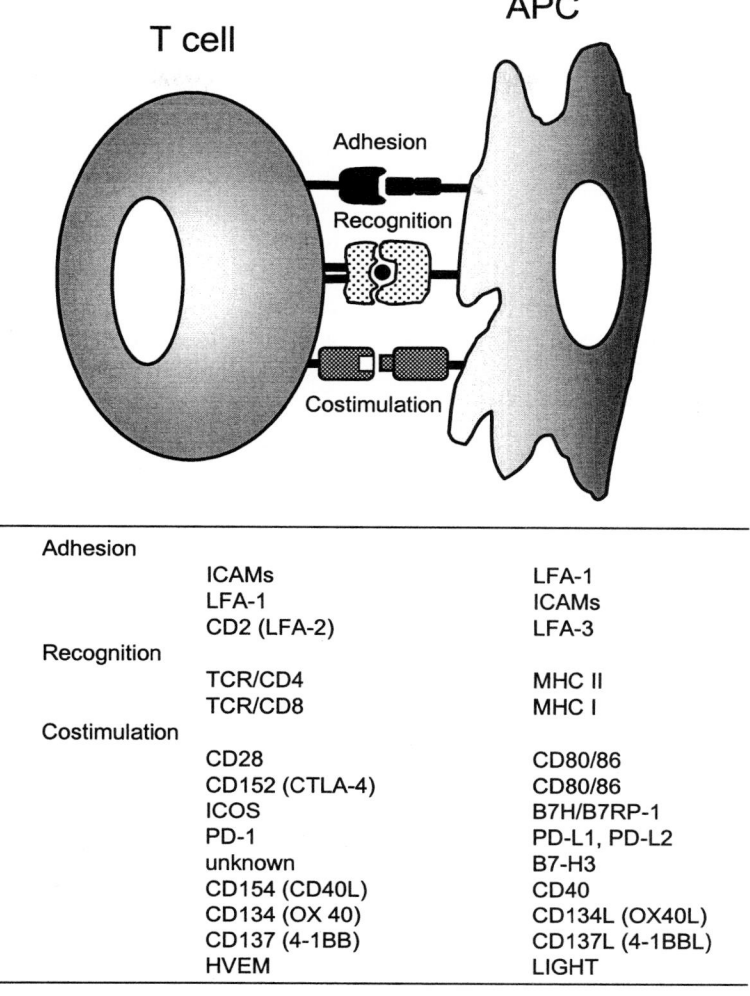

Adhesion		
	ICAMs	LFA-1
	LFA-1	ICAMs
	CD2 (LFA-2)	LFA-3
Recognition		
	TCR/CD4	MHC II
	TCR/CD8	MHC I
Costimulation		
	CD28	CD80/86
	CD152 (CTLA-4)	CD80/86
	ICOS	B7H/B7RP-1
	PD-1	PD-L1, PD-L2
	unknown	B7-H3
	CD154 (CD40L)	CD40
	CD134 (OX 40)	CD134L (OX40L)
	CD137 (4-1BB)	CD137L (4-1BBL)
	HVEM	LIGHT

Fig. 15.2. T-cell and APC interactions. Antigen-specific interactions between T cells and APCs are mediated by three successive events: adhesion, recognition, and costimulation.

duce IFN-γ and TNF-α after stimulation with IL-12 and IL-18, and can thus also participate in the development of GVHD. A murine BMT study using mice lacking SH2-containing inositol phosphatase (SHIP), in which the NK compartment is dominated by cells that express two inhibitory receptors capable of binding either self or allogeneic MHC ligands, suggested that host NK cells may play a role in the initiation of GVHD (Wang *et al.,* 2002).

Cytokines

Antigen presentation induces the activation of individual T cells. This involves multiple, rapidly occurring intracellular biochemical changes, including the rise of cytoplasmic free calcium and activation of protein kinase C and tyrosine kinases (Nishizuka, 1986; Samelson *et al.,* 1986). These pathways in turn activate transcription of genes for cytokines, such as IL-2, IFN-γ, and their receptors. These cytokines are preferentially

produced by the T-helper 1 (Th1) subset of T cells (Mosmann *et al.,* 1986). Both IL-2 and IFN-γ have long been implicated in the pathophysiology of acute GVHD; they play central roles in further T-cell activation, induction of CTL responses, and in the priming of additional donor and residual host mononuclear phagocytes to produce IL-1 and TNF-α. The T-cell activation phase is followed by clonal expansion and differentiation. Activated T cells produce proteins required for specific effector functions, such as the protein esterases that are required by CTLs (Weiss, 1989). The expression of many cell surface molecules is also altered such as adhesion molecules and chemokines, thus altering the ability of T cells to traffic in vivo (Forster *et al.,* 1999).

Th1 cells producing IL-2 have a pivotal role in controlling and amplifying the immune response against alloantigens, representing step two of the cytokine cascade that initiates acute GVHD (Fig. 15.1). Experimental data show that IL-2 is secreted primarily by donor CD4+ T cells in the first several days after GVHD induction (Via & Finkelman, 1993). IL-2 induces the expression of its own receptor (autocrine effect) and stimulates proliferation of other cells expressing the receptor (paracrine effect). The addition of low doses of IL-2 during the first week after allogeneic BMT enhanced the severity and mortality of GVHD except when GVHD was induced to MHC class II antigens (Jadus & Peck, 1983; Malkovsky et al., 1986). The precursor frequency of host-specific IL-2 producing cells (pHTL) predicts the occurrence of GVHD after transplantation between HLA-identical siblings (Theobald et al., 1992; Nierle et al., 1993; Schwarer et al., 1993). pHTL cells were detectable as early as day 20 after transplant, often preceding the onset of acute GVHD by approximately 2 weeks, and persisted until the GVHD resolved. Because of their apparent importance in initiating acute GVHD, IL-2 producing donor T cells have been the target of many experimental approaches to control GVHD. Cyclosporine (CSP) and tacrolimus (FK506), inhibitors of IL-2 production, are effective prophylactic agents against GVHD.

The importance of IL-2 is further underscored by experiments showing that monoclonal antibodies (mAbs) against the IL-2 receptor are efficient in preventing GVHD in animals or in clinical GVHD when administered shortly after the infusion of T cells (Ferrara et al., 1986; Herve et al., 1990). It should be noted, however, that in two clinical trials, the addition of an anti-IL-2 receptor mAb was only moderately successful in reducing the incidence of severe GVHD (Anasetti et al., 1990; Belanger et al., 1993). The cytokines IL-2 and IL-15 are redundant in stimulating T cell proliferation. A recent kinetics study of T-cell division and expression of IL-2 and IL-15 receptor subunits demonstrated that IL-15 is a critical cytokine in initiating allogeneic T-cell division in vivo (Li et al., 2001), and elevated serum levels of IL-15 are associated with acute GVHD in humans (Kumaki et al., 1998). IL-15 may therefore be a critical factor in initiating GVHD.

IFN-γ is another crucial cytokine that can be implicated in the second step of the pathophysiology of acute GVHD. Using a method to enumerate cytokine mRNA-containing cells that combined limiting dilution analysis (LDA) and RT-PCR, IFN-γ levels are significantly higher in mice with GVHD than those without it (Troutt & Kelso, 1992; Szebeni et al., 1994; Wang et al., 1995; Hill et al., 1997). The release of IFN-γ is also an early event in the cascade leading to GVHD because IFN-γ production in animals with GVHD peaks at day 7 posttransplant before clinical manifestations are apparent. In several models of experimental acute GVHD, T cells produce large amounts of IFN-γ when restimulated in vitro (Wall et al., 1988; Kelso, 1990; Smith et al., 1991; Troutt et al., 1992). A large proportion of T-cell clones isolated from GVHD patients also produce IFN-γ (Velardi et al., 1989). Increased serum levels of IFN-γ have also been found in humans, but the increase was not dramatic, and in a small number of patients studied, there were no significant differences between groups (Niederwieser et al., 1990).

Experimental data suggest that IFN-γ is involved in several aspects of the pathophysiology of acute GVHD. First, IFN-γ upregulates numerous molecules such as adhesion molecules, chemokines, and MHC; and its associated machinery molecules, important for antigen presentation, thus facilitating antigen presentation and effector recruitment. Second, IFN-γ can mediate the development of pathologic processes in the gastrointestinal tract and skin during GVHD; the administration of anti-IFN-γ mAbs prevents gastrointestinal GVHD (Mowat, 1989) and high levels of both IFN-γ and TNF-α correlate with the most intense cellular damage in skin (Dickinson et al., 1991). Third, IFN-γ mediates GVHD-associated immunosuppression in several experimental GVHD systems through the induction of nitric oxide (NO) and Fas (Holda et al., 1988; Wall et al., 1988; Klimpel et al., 1990; Huchet et al., 1993; Wall & Sheehan, 1994; Brochu et al., 1999). Fourth, exposure to IFN-γ results in a significant reduction in the amount of LPS needed to trigger macrophages to produce proinflammatory cytokines and NO (Gifford & Lohmann-Matthes, 1987; Nestel et al., 1992). Additional data have confirmed these observations and demonstrated that the inhibition of IFN-γ production after MHC class I or II disparate transplantation by injection of polarized donor T cells (which secrete IL-4 but not IFN-γ) resulted in the downregulation of LPS-triggered TNF-α production and reduced GVHD-related mortality (Krenger et al., 1995). Lastly, IFN-γ plays an important role in regulating the death of activated donor T cells by enhancing Fas-mediated apoptosis, thus regulating GVHD (Liu & Janeway, 1990; Yang et al., 1998; Reddy et al., 2001).

Cytokines secreted by activated T cells are generally classified as Th1 (secreting IL-2 and IFN-γ) or Th2 (secreting IL-4, IL-5, IL-10, and IL-13) (Mosmann et al., 1986). Several factors influence the ability of DCs to instruct naive CD4+ T cells to secrete Th1 or Th2 cytokines, including the type of signal that activate DCs, the duration of DC activation, the ratio of DCs to T cells, as well as subsets of DCs (Rissoan et al., 1999; Reid et al., 2000). Differential activation of Th1 or Th2 cells has been evoked in the immunopathogenesis of GVHD. There is now considerable evidence that the GVHD cascade is inhibited if donor T cells are activated to produce a Th2 cytokine profile after allogeneic HSC transplantation. The downregulation of both cell-mediated immune responses and the secretion of inflammatory cytokines is associated with decreased GVHD-related tissue destruction and mortality. Transplantation of polarized Th2 donor cells inhibited the secretion of TNF-α and protected mice from LPS-induced, TNF-α-mediated mortality and these Th2 donor cells suppressed LPS-induced lethality mediated by donor naive T cells (Fowler et al., 1994). Similarly, ex vivo polarized donor Th2 cells in the presence of IL-4 during a MLR to host alloantigens failed to induce acute GVHD to MHC class I or class II antigens (Krenger et al., 1995). NK1.1+ T (NK/T) cells in bone marrow (Zeng et al., 1999) and peripheral blood (Lan et al., 2001) can suppress GVHD induced by peripheral blood T cells through their IL-4 production. Pretreatment of BMT donors with granulocyte colony-stimulating factor (G-CSF) can polarize donor T cells towards Th2, resulting in less GVHD (Pan et al., 1995). Pretreatment of donors with the G-CSF and Flt-3 receptor agonist, progenipoietin-1, is superior to G-SCF in this regard (MacDonald *et al.,* 2003). Recruitment of CCR5+ T cells that usually secrete Th1 cytokines is associated with the development of hepatic GVHD (Murai *et al.,* 1999). Other studies have shown that GVHD can still occur using donor mice deficient in signal transducer and activator of transcription (STAT) 4 which is crucial to Th1 responses, although GVHD induced by STAT4 deficient donors was less severe than GVHD induced by donor cells deficient in STAT6, a molecule critical for Th2 polarization (Nikolic *et al.,* 2000). These experiments support the concept that the balance of Th1 and Th2 cytokines is critical for the development of acute GVHD and that Th1 cells can cause more severe GVHD than Th2 cells, and that Th2 cells can sometimes suppress acute GVHD.

The Th1/Th2 cytokine balance in acute GVHD remains controversial. A brief administration of high doses of exogenous IL-2 early after BMT protects animals from GVHD mortality (Sykes *et al.,* 1990). The injection of IFN-γ twice weekly from day 0 to week 6 prevents the development of experimental GVHD in lethally irradiated recipients (Brok *et al.,* 1993), and neutralization of IFN-γ results in accelerated GVHD (Wall & Sheehan, 1994). The use of IFN-γ-deficient donor cells results in accelerated GVHD in lethally irradiated recipients (Murphy *et al.,* 1998; Yang *et al.,* 1998), but reduces GVHD in sublethally irradiated or unirradiated recipients (Ellison *et al.,* 1998; Welniak *et al.,* 2000). Administration of IFN-γ-inducing cytokines such as IL-12 or IL-18 early after BMT protects lethally irradiated recipients from GVHD (Sykes *et al.,* 1995; Reddy *et al.,* 2001). (With IL-18 administration a perforin-dependent graft-versus-leukemia effect was preserved [Reddy *et al.,* 2002].) These paradoxes related to IFN-γ may be explained by complex dynamics of the activation, expansion, and contraction of donor T cells. IL-12 and IL-18 induce IFN-γ production, resulting in the contraction of alloreactive T cells via Fas-mediated activation-induced cell death (AICD) (Dey *et al.,* 1998; Yang *et al.,* 1998; Reddy *et al.,* 2001). IL-2 primes activated T cells susceptible to AICD. Thus, a physiologic and adequate amount of Th1 cytokine production is critical for GVHD induction, while inadequate production (extremely low or high) could modulate GVHD through a breakdown of negative feedback mechanisms for activated donor T cells.

Cellular effectors

The efferent phase of acute GVHD is a complex cascade of multiple effectors. Regulation of effector cell migration into target tissues occurs in a complex milieu of chemotactic signals where several receptors may be triggered simultaneously or successively. Inflammatory chemokines expressed in inflamed tissues upon stimulation by proinflammatory cytokines are specialized for the recruitment of effector cells, including T cells, neutrophils, and monocytes (Moser & Loetscher, 2001). The unusual cluster of GVHD target organs (skin, gut, and liver) may be explained by the differential migration of effector cells into different organs. Studies have demonstrated that naive T cells differentiate into CCR7+ CD62L+ central memory T (T_{CM})

cells and CCR7- effector memory T (T_{EM}) cells following antigenic stimulation in vivo (Sallusto *et al.,* 1999). T_{CM} cells, which reside in secondary lymphoid organs, lack immediate effector function, but efficiently differentiate into T_{EM} cells upon secondary stimulation (Sallusto *et al.,* 1999; Reinhardt *et al.,* 2001). The involvement of inflammatory chemokines and their receptors in GVHD has been investigated in mouse models. Macrophage inflammatory protein-1α (MIP-1α) recruits CCR5+ CD8+ T cells into the liver, lung, and spleen during GVHD (Murai *et al.,* 1999; Serody *et al.,* 2000), and levels of several chemokines are elevated in GVHD-associated lung injury (Panoskaltsis-Mortari *et al.,* 2000). Chemokines and their receptors are thus potential targets for modulation of GVHD.

Effector mechanisms of acute GVHD can be divided into cellular effectors such as CTLs and NK cells, and inflammatory effectors such as TNF-γ, IL-1 and NO. The Fas/Fas ligand (FasL) and the perforin/granzyme (or granule exocytosis) pathways are the classic effector mechanisms that CTLs and NK cells utilize to lyse target cells (Kagi *et al.,* 1994; Lowin *et al.,* 1994). CTL-mediated cytotoxicity is thought to contribute to the destruction of GVHD target tissues (Fig.15.3). Following secretion of granules by CTLs, the polymerization of perforin upon binding to the target membrane is crucial to optimize penetration of granule contents, including granzymes A and B, into the targeted cells (Shresta *et al.,* 1998). Apoptosis of target cells occurs, rapidly induced by the activation of the caspase cascade. This cascade ultimately results in the release of an inhibitor (ICAD) bound to a caspase-associated DNase molecule (CAD) which is followed by fragmentation of target cell DNA. FasL also triggers activation of caspases. A number of ligands have been identified on T cells which possess the ability to trimerize TNFR-like death receptors (DR), such as TNF-related apoptosis-inducing ligand (TRAIL: DR4,5 ligand) and TNF-like weak inducer of apoptosis (TWEAK: DR3 ligand) (Chinnaiyan *et al.,* 1996; Chicheportiche *et al.,* 1997; Pan *et al.,* 1997) (Fig. 15.3).

During the past several years, a number of experimental allogeneic BMT studies have utilized donor inocula that are unable to mediate either perforin/granzyme or Fas/FasL-dependent killing. Transplantation of perforin-deficient T cells resulted in a marked delay in the onset of GVHD in transplants across MiHA disparities, but mortality and histological signs of GVHD were induced in the *absence* of perforin dependent killing (Baker *et al.,* 1996). The importance of the perforin/granzyme pathway for GVHD induction has been evident in studies employing donor T-cell subsets. Perforin or granzyme B deficient CD8+ T cells induced significantly less mortality compared to wild type T cells in experimental transplants across a single MHC class I mismatch, while this pathway seems to be less important compared to Fas/FasL pathway in CD4-mediated GVHD (Graubert *et al.,* 1996; Graubert *et al.,* 1997). Thus, it has been thought that CD4+ CTLs preferentially use the Fas/FasL pathway, while CD8+ CTLs mostly use the perforin/granzyme pathways. Most studies failed to detect a role for the perforin/granzyme pathway in target organ pathology.

In contrast, FasL-mediated cytotoxicity may be a particularly important effector pathway in target organ GVHD. FasL-

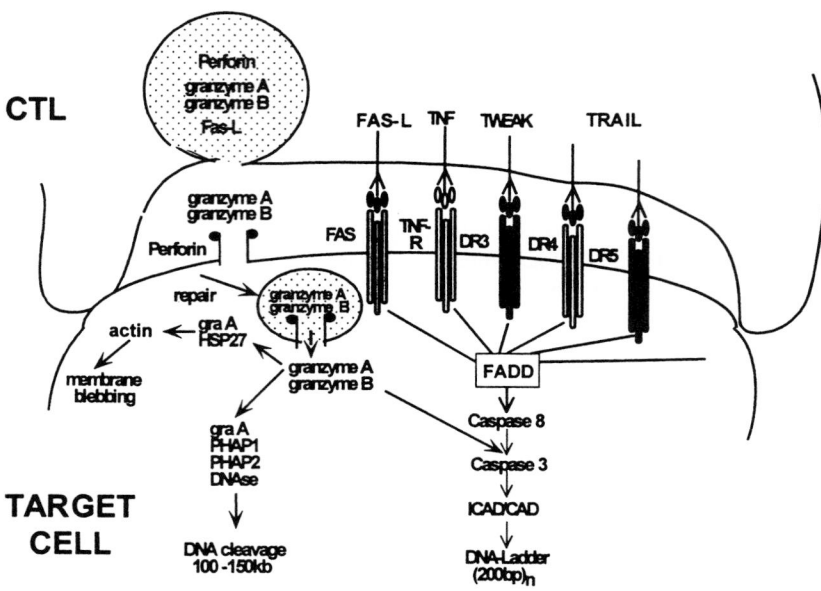

Fig. 15.3. CTL effector pathways. The various components of the molecular pathways of CTL-mediated lysis. Reproduced, with permission, from Ferrara, Levy & Chao (1999).

defective T cells markedly diminish GVHD in liver, skin, and lymphoid organs (Baker *et al.*, 1996; Via *et al.*, 1996; Baker *et al.*, 1997). This pathway is particularly important in hepatic GVHD, which is in agreement with keen sensitivity of hepatocytes to Fas-mediated cytotoxicity in experimental models of murine hepatitis (Kondo *et al.*, 1997). During GVHD, Fas expression on bile duct epithelial cells, one of major targets in hepatic GVHD, is upregulated (Ueno *et al.*, 2000). Fas deficient recipients are protected from hepatic GVHD, but not from other organ GVHD (van Den Brink *et al.*, 2000) and administration of anti-FasL (but not anti-TNF mAbs) significantly blocked the hepatic damage occurring in murine models of GVHD (Hattori *et al.*, 1998). Elevated serum levels of soluble FasL and Fas have been observed in at least some patients with acute GVHD (Kanda *et al.*, 1998; Liem *et al.*, 1998; Das *et al.*, 1999; Kayaba *et al.*, 2000).

The utilization of a perforin/granzyme and FasL cytotoxic double deficient (cdd) mouse provides the opportunity to address whether other effector pathways are capable of inducing GVHD target organ pathology. An initial study demonstrated that cdd T cells were unable to induce GVHD lethality in recipients transplanted with cells from donors mismatched at MHC class I and class II after sublethal irradiation (Braun *et al.*, 1996). However, two subsequent studies demonstrated that cytotoxic effector mechanisms of donor T cells are critical in preventing host resistance to GVHD (Martin *et al.*, 1998; Jiang *et al.*, 2001). Thus, when recipients were conditioned with a lethal dose of irradiation, cdd CD4$^+$ T cells produced similar mortality to wild type CD4$^+$ T cells in a murine model of GVHD across MHC class I and class II differences (Jiang *et al.*, 2001). These results demonstrate that other effector molecules

are sufficient to induce GVHD mediated by CD4$^+$ T cells in the absence of perforin/granzyme and FasL dependent functions.

Inflammatory effectors

Macrophages, which had been primed with IFN-γ during step two produce inflammatory cytokines TNF-α and IL-1 when stimulated by a secondary, triggering signal. This stimulus may be provided through Toll-like receptors (TLRs) by microbial products such as LPS, peptidoglycan, lipoteichoic acid and other components of microbial agents, which can leak through the intestinal mucosa or skin damaged by the conditioning regimen and GVHD. The role of LPS and TNF-α in GVHD was elucidated using an experimental murine GVHD model with unirradiated recipients, where macrophages in animals with GVHD were primed to release TNF-α after stimulation with LPS (Nestel *et al.*, 1992). Injection of normally nonlethal amounts of LPS caused elevated TNF-α serum levels and death in animals with GVHD; this mortality could be prevented with anti-TNF-α antiserum. These experiments strongly supported the role of mononuclear phagocytes as sources of inflammatory cytokines during the effector phase of acute GVHD. Subsequent murine studies further demonstrated that TNF-α production by donor cells in response to LPS predicts the severity of GVHD (Cooke *et al.*, 1998) and that direct antagonism of LPS reduces GVHD (Cooke *et al.*, 2001). It has long been known that pathogen-free mice are protected from GVHD after allogeneic transplantation, and recolonization of Gram-negative bacteria in the gut leads to increased GVHD severity (Jones *et al.*, 1971; van Bekkum *et al.*, 1974). A clinical study of GVHD suggested the possible association with

Table 15.2. *Effector mechanisms of GVHD*

Effector	Target tissue damage	Systemic toxicity
Fas ligand	Liver, skin, lymphoid tissue	±
Perforin/granzyme	±	+
Cytokines	Intestine, skin, lymphoid tissue	++
Nitric oxide	Lymphoid tissue	±
Myeloid cells	+	±

mutation of TLR genes in either donors or recipients and reduced severity of GVHD (Lorenz *et al.*, 2001). Thus, the gastrointestinal tract plays a major role in the amplification of systemic GVHD and is critical in the propagation of the "cytokine storm" characteristics of acute GVHD (Hill & Ferrara, 2000) (Fig. 15.1).

The cytokines TNF-α and IL-1 have often synergistic, pleiotrophic, and redundant effects on both the afferent and efferent phases of GVHD. A critical role for TNF-α in the pathophysiology of acute GVHD was first suggested almost 15 years ago when mice transplanted with mixtures of allogeneic bone marrow and T cells developed severe skin, gut and lung lesions that were associated with high levels of TNF-α mRNA in these tissues (Piguet *et al.*, 1987; Piguet *et al.*, 1989; McCarthy *et al.*, 1991). Target organ damage could be inhibited by infusion of anti-TNF-α mAbs, and mortality could be reduced from 100% to 50% by the administration of the soluble form of the TNF-α receptor (sTNFR), an antagonist of TNF-α (Xun *et al.*, 1994). Subsequent experiments suggest that TNF-α may be involved in a multistep process of GVHD pathophysiology. First, TNF-α activates DCs and enhances alloantigen presentation. Second, TNF-α recruits effector T cells, neutrophils, and monocytes into target organs via the induction of inflammatory chemokines. Third, TNF-α causes direct tissue damage by inducing apoptosis and necrosis (Laster *et al.*, 1988). Lastly, TNF-α may regulate donor T-cell expansion by inducing AICD on CD8+ T cells (Zheng *et al.*, 1995).

TNF-α plays a central role in intestinal GVHD in murine and human studies (Piguet *et al.*, 1987; Herve *et al.*, 1992; Hattori *et al.*, 1998). TNF-α also seems to be an important effector molecule in GVHD in skin and lymphoid tissue (Piguet *et al.*, 1987; Gilliam *et al.*, 1996; Hattori *et al.*, 1998). A role for TNF-α in clinical acute GVHD has been suggested by studies demonstrating elevated levels of TNF-α in the serum of patients with acute GVHD and other endothelial complications, such as hepatic veno-occlusive disease (VOD) (Holler *et al.*, 1990; Holler *et al.*, 1993; Tanaka *et al.*, 1993).

The second major proinflammatory cytokine that appears to play an important role in the effector phase of acute GVHD is IL-1. Secretion of IL-1 appears to occur predominantly during the effector phase of GVHD of the spleen and skin, two major GVHD target organs (Abhyankar *et al.*, 1993). At 4 weeks posttransplant, when the majority of animals had died of GVHD and where surviving animals clearly had active disease, a striking increase in IL-1 mRNA (by at least 200 times above controls) in both organs was observed. A similar increase in mononuclear cell IL-1 mRNA has been shown during acute GVHD in humans (Tanaka *et al.*, 1993). Indirect evidence of a role for IL-1 in GVHD was obtained with administration of this cytokine to recipients in an allogeneic murine BMT model (Atkinson *et al.*, 1991). Mice receiving IL-1 displayed a wasting syndrome and increased mortality that appeared to be an accelerated form of disease. Investigations of the role of IL-1 in GVHD intensified after the discovery of IL-1 receptor antagonist (IL-1ra) (Eisenberg *et al.*, 1990; Hannum *et al.*, 1990). Administration of IL-1ra, an anti-IL-1 receptor, to recipients reduces GVHD mortality in animal models (McCarthy *et al.*, 1991; Hill *et al.*, 1999).

As a result of activation during GVHD, macrophages also produce NO and induce the release of iron from target cells, resulting in a inhibition of the recovery of injured target tissues by inhibiting proliferation of epithelial stem cells in the gut and skin (Nestel *et al.*, 2000). NO also contributes to the deleterious effects on GVHD target tissues, particularly immunosuppression (Falzarano *et al.*, 1996; Krenger *et al.*, 1996). In humans and rats, development of GVHD is preceded by an increase in serum levels of NO oxidation products (Langrehr *et al.*, 1992; Weiss *et al.*, 1995). These inflammatory effectors may synergize with the lytic component provided by CTLs, resulting in the amplification of local tissue injury and further promotion of an inflammatory response, which ultimately leads to the observed target tissue destruction in the transplant recipient.

The central role of inflammatory cytokines in acute GVHD was confirmed in a murine study by using bone marrow chimeras in which either MHC class I or MHC class II alloantigens were not expressed on target epithelium but on APCs alone (Teshima *et al.*, 2002a). GVHD target organ injury was induced in these chimeras even in the absence of epithelial alloantigens and mortality and target organ injury was prevented by the neutralization of TNF-α and IL-1. These observations were particularly true for CD4-mediated acute GVHD but also applied, at least in part, to CD8-mediated disease. In this study, lymphocytic infiltration to target organs occurred even in the absence of alloantigen expression on target cells, and this infiltration was prevented by the neutralization of TNF-γ and IL-1, suggesting a central role for inflammatory cytokines in recruiting effector T cells into target organs, probably via the induction of inflammatory chemokines.

Chronic GVHD

Chronic GVHD is sometimes thought of as an autoimmune disease because of distinctive similarities to various autoimmune disorders, especially collagen-vascular disease. The relationship is difficult to prove clinically, but experimental studies have confirmed the autoimmune pathophysiology of chronic GVHD (Parkman, 1986). In contrast to T cells from animals with acute GVHD that are specific for host alloantigens, T cells from animals with chronic GVHD are specific for a public (common) determinant of MHC class II molecules. These T cells produce unusual patterns of cytokines, such as IL-4 and IFN-γ in the absence of IL-2. These cytokines can stimulate collagen production by fibroblasts, and this stimulation can be further amplified by the secretion of IL-4. These autoreactive cells help to explain the strong association between chronic GVHD and a damaged thymus. The thymus may be injured by acute GVHD, the conditioning regimen, or it may be subject to age-related involution and atrophy. The normal ability of the thymus to delete autoreactive T cells and to induce tolerance may thus be impaired. There is now considerable evidence that the preferential expansion of Th2 T cells after allogeneic transplantation is associated with the development of a chronic GVHD in both murine models and humans (Doutrelepont et al., 1991; Umland et al., 1992; Allen et al., 1993; De Wit et al., 1993; Garlisi et al., 1993; Tanaka et al., 1997). Consistent with this notion, chronic GVHD is associated with a high prevalence of autoantibidies. A recent analysis of the outcome of BMT in humans suggested that increased numbers of type 2 DC progenitors (pDC2) in the graft, which promote Th2 responses, were associated with less chronic GVHD (Waller et al., 2001). Murine studies of chronic GVHD suggested that donor derived monocyte/macrophage play an important role in chronic GVHD by producing transforming growth factor (TGF)-β that induces collagen synthesis in the skin and lung (McCormick et al., 1999; Zhang et al., 2002). Administration of anti-TGF-β mAb prevents chronic GVHD. In some patients with chronic GVHD, serum level of TGF-β is elevated (Liem et al., 1999). IL-1 and TNF-γ mRNA expression are also upregulated in peripheral blood mononuclear cells in patients with chronic GVHD, suggesting the involvement of inflammatory cytokines in chronic GVHD (Tanaka et al., 1995).

Syngeneic GVHD

A GVHD-like syndrome can also develop after autologous or syngeneic BMT. In experimental models, pathologic changes of GVHD have been observed in animals transplanted with bone marrow from genetically identical donors (or even with autologous marrow); findings that substantiated reports of GVHD between identical twins have been described (Rappeport et al., 1979). This form of GVHD occurred when irradiated rat recipients were given CSP for several weeks. GVHD occurred after the cessation of CSP administration. Syngeneic GVHD is usually limited to the skin. Although grades II–III have been observed, the disease generally resolves promptly without treatment or with administration of corticosteroids, and is not a life-threatening entity. Experimental models suggest that administration of CSP, conditioning, and an intact thymus are essential for the development of the disease. Effector mechanisms involve CD8+ T cells that promiscuously recognize a peptide from MHC class II invariant chain (CLIP) presented in the context of MHC class II (Hess et al., 1998). Autoreactive T cells are thought to develop in a severely damaged thymic medulla where MHC class II expres-

sion is decreased. T cells thus escape negative selection (clonal deletion) within the thymus and migrate to the periphery where they can trigger or mediate target organ damage. Peripheral regulatory mechanisms by CD4+ CD25+ T cells (Wu & Goldschneider, 2001), which would normally inactivate or eliminate such autoreactive cells, have themselves been eliminated by conditioning. The experimental transfer of normal lymphocytes to these irradiated hosts restores the regulatory mechanism and prevents the autoaggressive process. The effects of CSP are important in these models, both in preventing the reestablishment of regulatory cells and in allowing the development of autoreactive cells; these two processes seem related to the damage that CSP inflicts on the thymic medulla (Fischer et al., 1989).

Syngeneic GVHD can thus be seen as an imbalance between autoreactive and autoregulatory lymphocytes, an imbalance that results from thymic dysfunction. In experimental animals, cutaneous pathologic findings of syngeneic and chronic GVHD are similar, and it appears that the efferent arms of syngeneic and chronic GVHD are similar if not identical. These observations further strengthen the perception of chronic GVHD as an autoimmune disorder.

Graft-host tolerance

The prevention of antihost alloreactivity by immunologically competent donor cells is termed immunologic tolerance. Several mechanisms have been proposed and these mechanisms can be considered in two categories: deletion and nondeletional immunoregulation (Li et al., 2001).

Clonal deletion, in which host-reactive donor T cells are eliminated, primarily occurs in the thymus (central tolerance). The presence of donor APCs, particularly DCs, in the thymus is critical for this process (Sykes, 1996). It is now clear that such deletion also occurs for mature T cells in the periphery (Sprent et al., 1993; Li et al., 1999; Wells et al., 1999). The chief mechanism of clonal deletion is apoptosis by AICD and passive cell death. This mechanism is largely responsible for the rapid contraction of donor T cells following an initial massive expansion. Destruction of effector cells at the end of the primary response is a rapid and highly efficient process; activation of T cells induces dissociation of FLIP from Fas and converts Fas to a death-inducing molecule, with the result that ligation of FasL triggers activation of caspases (Irmler et al., 1997). Although AICD is largely mediated through Fas and through related members of TNF receptor family such as death receptor (DR)3, DR4, and DR5 (Van Parijs & Abbas, 1998), priming of T cells to undergo AICD appears to require IL-2 (Refaeli et al., 1998). Many different molecules seem to be involved in the elimination of activated T cells, since unrestrained T-cell proliferation is observed in mice with deletion or mutation of Fas, FasL, PD-1, CTLA-4, CD25 (IL-2Rβ), CD45, CD122 (IL-2Rα), and TGF-β.

The second mechanism of tolerance induction is nondeletional immunoregulation, where alloreactive T cells no longer respond to an antigenic stimulus but are not physically deleted.

This unresponsiveness includes clonal anergy, immune deviation, and active suppression. Such anergy or "paralysis" has been demonstrated clearly in many in vitro systems by blocking critical co-stimulatory pathways such as B7/CD28 interactions. It should be noted that in vivo such anergy appears to be flexible, dynamic, and reversible rather than static. During active suppression, alloreactive T cells are present and functional but are actively suppressed or modified by a second cell population. Although many cell types have been shown to have regulatory properties, much attention has focused on CD4$^+$ 25$^+$ regulatory T (T$_r$) cells (Maloy & Powrie, 2001). Suppression by CD25$^+$ regulatory T cells is primarily contact-dependent and cytokine-independent (Shevach et al., 2001). Interestingly, repeated stimulation of CD4$^+$ T cells with alloantigens in vitro results in the emergence of a population of T-cell clones (T$_r$1 cells) that secretes high amounts of IL-10 and TGF-~β The immunosuppressive properties of these cytokines are explained by their ability to inhibit APC function and to regulate proliferation of T cells directly. Similarly, Th3 cells that produce large amount of TGF-β can be regulatory T cells. Nonspecific suppression in the form of NO can also be invoked, particularly during a GVHD reaction (Krenger et al., 1996). Studies suggest that immature DCs may control peripheral tolerance by inducing Tr cells (Roncarolo et al., 2001).

Other types of cells may also have regulatory functions. CD8$^+$ suppressor cells have been identified in both murine and humans (Tsoi et al., 1979; Hurtenbach & Shearer, 1983; Rolink & Gleichmann, 1983; Autran et al., 1991). A specific subpopulation of CD8$^+$ T cells that expresses CD57 has been identified as having suppressor function in patients with acute and chronic GVHD (Autran et al., 1991; Fukuda et al., 1994). Natural suppressor (NS) cells suppress GVHD in a variety of host and donor combinations (Strober, 1984). It is now suggested that NK/T cells possess such a NS cell function (Lan et al., 2001). Peripheral blood NK/T cells that are rapidly reconstituted from bone marrow cells after BMT (Eberl & MacDonald, 1998), as well as marrow NK/T cells, are both able to suppress GVHD by secretion of IL-4 (Zeng et al., 1999; Lan et al., 2001). Activated NK cells can also suppress GVHD via their TGF-β secretion (Asai et al., 1998).

Evidence for these mechanisms of graft-host tolerance following HSC transplantation have been extensively documented in both experimental and clinical models. Patients with chronic GVHD have cells of donor origin with specific antihost activity, while patients without GHVD do not (Tsoi et al., 1980). Similarly, a large portion of T-cell clones obtained from animals with acute GVHD are specific for host alloantigens, while very few such clones were detectable from animals without GVHD (Parkman, 1986). Active suppression has also been observed after clinical HSC transplantation. Antigen-specific suppressor cells have been identified in patients with no evidence of GVHD (Tsoi et al., 1981), whereas only nonspecific suppressor cells were present in patients with GVHD (Tsoi et al., 1979). Transplantation of HLA-mismatched HSC in patients with

severe combined immunodeficiency (SCID) can result in a selective engraftment of donor T cells with complete immunologic reconstitution and tolerance. This tolerance induction is associated with the development of donor-derived regulatory T cells that produce large amounts of IL-10 (Bacchetta et al., 1994). The details of how these three tolerance mechanisms interact with each other after allogeneic HSC transplantation is an area of active research that will likely yield future novel therapeutic strategies.

Therapeutic interventions

Blockade of inflammatory arm

As discussed above, conditioning is an important risk factor for GVHD. A reduced intensity (nonmyeloablative) conditioning has been increasingly used by many BMT centers (Feinstein & Storb, 2001). In animal models, all cytotoxic conditioning can be eliminated by giving a very large dose of MHC-mismatched bone marrow cells followed by costimulatory blockade (Durham et al., 2000; Wekerle et al., 2000). Anintriguing study suggests that alloreactive NK cells can also obviate the need for high-intensity conditioning and reduce GVHD (Ruggeri et al., 2002). The ability to replace host T-cell depletion with costimulatory blockade or alloreactive NK cells is encouraging and is an active area of investigation.

Studies of inflammatory pathways involved in GVHD in mice have shown that the gastrointestinal tract is critical to the propagation of the "cytokine storm" characteristic of acute GVHD (Hill & Ferrara, 2000). Experimental approaches to prevent GVHD thus include reducing the damage to the GI tract by protection of the GI mucosal barrier through novel "cytokine shields." Growth factors, IL-11, keratinocyte growth factor (KGF), and hepatocyte growth factor (HGF) have direct protective effects on the GI tract epithelium in various models of gut injury. In experimental mouse models of GVHD, the protective effect of these growth factors on the GI tract resulted in improved survival (Hill et al., 1998; Panoskaltsis-Mortari et al., 1998; Krijanovski et al., 1999; Kuroiwa et al., 2001). In this regard, blockade of LPS by administrating LPS antagonist intraperitoneally from day 0 to day 6 posttransplant reduces serum TNF-α levels and prevents experimental GVHD (Cooke et al., 2001). Such strategies to protect the GI tract have reduced GVHD while preserving a T-cell mediated GVL effect (Krijanovski et al., 1999; Teshima et al., 1999; Cooke et al., 2001).

Suppression of donor T cells

Current strategies for GVHD prevention or treatment are primarily targeted at donor T cells. These have included pretreatment of the stem cell donor, in vitro manipulation of the stem cell products, and treatment of the patient posttransplant. Immunophilin-binding agents, such as CSP and tacrolimus (FK506), are the most commonly used drugs for GVHD prophylaxis. CSP and tacrolimus bind to cyclophilin and FKBP-12, respectively, and inhibit calcineurin, resulting in inhibition of IL-2 gene expression. Thus, the combined use of CSP/tacrolimus and costimulatory blockade in mice prevents tolerance induction by inhibiting cell cycle-dependent T-cell apoptosis triggered by IL-2 and the development of Tr cells (Li et al., 1999). In contrast rapamycin, which does not inhibit IL-2-triggered apoptotic signals, provides strong synergy to costimulatory blockade (Li et al., 1999). Animal studies show an emergence of Tr cells following high-dose rapamycin treatment after BMT (Blazar et al., 1993; Chen et al., 2000). Glucocorticoids are also widely used as both prophylaxis and treatment of GVHD. Although the effects of steroids have been attributed primarily to their influence on T cells and monocytes/macrophages, recent studies suggest that they can also affect DC functions (Piemonti et al., 1999; Rea et al., 2000) and allow the generation of IL-10 producing Tr cells (Barrat et al., 2002). These different sites of action provide the rationale for the use of drug combinations, and indeed, the use of any pairwise combination of these agents is more effective prophylaxis against GVHD than any single agent, although they also cause substantial drug-induced toxicity.

The most effective prophylaxis is the removal of all T cells from the stem cell inoculum. This can be accomplished either by physical separation (lectin agglutination) or by treatment with mAbs directed at T cells. With the latter approach, T cells can be destroyed by a toxin (e.g., ricin A chain) that has been attached to the antibody, or by complement, which lyses antibody-coated T cells. Alternatively, antibodies can be linked to magnetic beads, which remove T cells expressing the appropriate specificities by passage over a magnet. These procedures usually achieve 90% to 99.9% reduction in T-cell content of the inoculum and result in substantial reductions in the incidence and severity of GVHD (Ho & Soiffer, 2001). Unfortunately, the use of T-cell-depleted stem cells is associated with a higher rate of graft failure, which has dire clinical consequences and is frequently fatal. Although the removal of T cells may cause an unintentional loss of stem cells, T cells themselves probably mediate a graft-enhancing effect (Martin, 1993). This effect may be due to the suppression of radioresistant, alloreactive host immune cells (Gale & Reisner, 1986) or to the release by T cells of hematopoietic growth factors (Vallera & Blazar, 1989). Protocols that increase the immunosuppression of the conditioning regimen or remove only subsets of T cells reduce the risk of graft failure.

Another concern is the increased incidence of relapse among recipients of T-cell-depleted marrow grafts with certain types of leukemia, particularly chronic myeloid leukemia (Goldman et al., 1988). This phenomenon appears related to a GVL effect associated with GVHD in experimental systems (Truitt et al., 1990). Although some data suggest that certain T cells from transplanted patients may recognize tumor-specific antigens (Sosman et al., 1990), it has been difficult to achieve separation of GVHD and GVL effects in humans. In fact, data from Seattle suggest that only clinical GVHD was associated with a GVL effect, whereas subclinical disease showed no benefit (Sullivan et al., 1988). Thus, although T-cell depletion reduces

mortality from GVHD, problems with engraftment and increased leukemic relapse have resulted in survival rates similar to those of patients who receive conventional prophylaxis after T-replete transplants.

The induction of anergy in donor T cells that are specific to host antigens is an attractive strategy, since it would theoretically preserve the functional capacity of the remaining T cells to respond to infectious agents or leukemia cells. The presentation of antigens in the absence of costimulation not only fails to prime T cells but can also delete them (Critchfield et al., 1994) and blockade of costimulatory pathways has shown great promise in preclinical studies (Fig. 15.2). A soluble form of CD152, CTLA4-Ig, inhibits the interaction of CD80/CD86 with CD28 and partially suppresses GVHD in animal models (Blazar et al., 1994). The blockade of this pathway by combined administration of anti-CD80 mAbs and anti-CD86 mAbs is more effective than either agent alone (Blazar et al., 1996). Blockade of other costimulatory pathways has been shown to be effective in animal models, but so far these strategies seem to be partially effective, perhaps because CD4$^+$ and CD8$^+$ T cells require distinct costimulatory pathways for activation (Whitmire & Ahmed, 2000). Costimulation is also essential for the survival of Tr cells (Salomon et al., 2000); thus combined blockade of several costimulatory pathways may be an attractive strategy (Tamada et al., 2002).

Ex vivo blockade of costimulatory pathways prior to infusion of T cells is an alternative approach. The first clinical study of this approach used CTLA4-Ig with partial success (Guinan et al., 1999). In mice, ex vivo treatment of donor T cells with anti-CD154 mAbs also prevented GVHD, but donor T cells retained responses to nominal antigens (Blazar et al., 1998). Interestingly, this effect is associated with the emergence of CD4$^+$ CD25$^+$ Tr cells (Taylor et al., 2000). Tolerance induction can also be achieved ex vivo by the addition of IL-10 or TGF-β to mixed lymphocyte reaction (MLR) cultures (Zeller et al., 1999), which induces alterations in biochemical signaling similar to costimulatory blockade (Boussiotis et al., 2001). Suppression of donor T-cell activation can be achieved by the modulation of host DCs (Shlomchik et al., 1999). This concept was recently proved by murine studies; administration of alloreactive NK cells reduce GVHD by ablating host APCs (Ruggeri et al., 2002), and administration of Flt3 ligand to recipients prior to BMT alters host DCs and reduces acute GVHD (Teshima et al., 2002).

As mentioned above, Th1 cytokines interact to mediate the deleterious effects observed after allogeneic transplantation. The fact that Th2-cell-derived cytokines can downregulate cell-mediated immunity provided a rationale to test their therapeutic potential in GVHD. Thus one potential strategy to prevent GVHD might be the inhibition of Th1 cytokine production by the administration of Th2 cytokines such as IL-10 and IL-4. Several murine studies, however, demonstrated direct administration of Th2 cytokines to be either ineffective or toxic (Atkinson et al., 1991; Krenger et al., 1994; Blazar et al., 1995).

Infusion of polarized donor T cells is an alternative approach. Fowler and co-workers (Fowler *et al.*, 1994) generated Th2 cells by treating donor mice in vivo with a combination of IL-2 and IL-4. Subsequent transplantation of these cells into nonirradiated F$_1$ recipients inhibited the secretion of TNF-α and protected recipient mice from LPS-induced, TNF-α-mediated lethality. Cell mixtures of Th2 donor cells with otherwise lethal inocula also protected recipient mice from LPS-induced lethality, demonstrating the ability of Th2 cells to modulate Th1 responses after allogeneic transplantation without the impairment of allogeneic engraftment (Fowler *et al.*, 1994). Similarly, ex vivo polarized donor Th2 cells in the presence of IL-4 during a MLR to host alloantigens failed to induce acute GVHD (Krenger *et al.*, 1995).

A final opportunity to inhibit donor T-cell function resides at the level of effector mechanisms. In mice, inhibition of CTL lysis by Fas blockade prevents the development of hepatic, skin, and GVHD-associated lymphoid hypoplasia (Hattori *et al.*, 1998), whereas neutralization of TNF-α prevents GVHD of gut, skin, and lymphoid organ (Hattori *et al.*, 1998). Administration of a metalloproteinase inhibitor inhibits the release of both FasL and TNF-α and effectively prevents hepatic and gut GVHD (Hattori *et al.*, 1997). Since donor T cells mediate both GVHD and GVL activity, assessment of the relative contributions from each to the cytotoxic pathways in individual T-cell subsets may help to disassociate GVHD from GVL effects (Pan *et al.*, 1999; Teshima *et al.*, 1999; Tsukada *et al.*, 1999; Hsieh & Korngold, 2000; Schmaltz *et al.*, 2001). A phase I/II trial using TNF-α receptor mAbs during the conditioning regimen as prophylaxis in patients at high risk for severe acute GVHD showed reduction in lesions of the intestine, skin, and liver (Herve *et al.*, 1992). In the majority of patients, GVHD flared after discontinuation of treatment. These preliminary data, as well as animal and laboratory studies, suggest that approaches to limit TNF-α secretion will be a very important avenue of investigation in allogeneic HSC transplantation. A final strategy in this regard is the genetic alteration of donor T cells with a conditional suicide mechanism that can be triggered when needed. Donor lymphocyte infusion (DLI) is the treatment of choice in patients with recurrent leukemia after allogeneic HSC transplantation, but DLI may be complicated by GVHD. In an attempt to avoid GVHD, several centers have initiated DLI trials in which the infused lymphocytes carry suicide genes such as herpes simplex virus thymidine kinase, which confers sensitivity to ganciclovir (Burt *et al.*, 1999), or a chimeric human protein consisting of the intracellular domain of Fas and FKBP, which is activated by FKBP ligand (Thomis *et al.*, 2001). Such novel strategies to eliminate specific T-cell responses in vivo will likely open important avenues for further modulation of GVHD.

Conclusions

Complications of allogeneic HSC transplantation, particularly GVHD, remain major barriers to the wider application of allografting for a variety of diseases. Advances in the understanding of cytokine networks have led to improved understanding of this complex disease process. Cytokine dysregulation can now be analyzed at both the cellular and molecular levels in vitro and in vivo. Insights from these systems are currently being tested in animal models of GVHD, and clinical trials to modulate cytokines are currently in progress.

References

Abhyankar, S., Gilliland, D. G., & Ferrara, J. L. M. (1993). Interleukin 1 is a critical effector molecule during cytokine dysregulation in graft-versus-host disease to minor histocompatibility antigens. *Transplantation,* **56,** 1518–23.

Allen, R. D., Staley, T. A., & Sidman, C. L. (1993). Differential cytokine expression in acute and chronic murine graft-versus-host disease. *European Journal of Immunology,* **23,** 333–7.

Anasetti, C., Martin, P. M., Hansen, J. A. *et al.* (1990). A phase I–II study evaluating the murine anti-IL-2 receptor antibody 2A3 for treatment of acute graft-versus-host disease. *Transplantation,* **50,** 49–54.

Anderson, K. C. (1997). Transfusion-associated graft-versus-host disease. *In Graft-vs.-Host Disease,* ed. J. L. M. Ferrara, H. J. Deeg & S. J. Burakoff, pp. 587–605. New York: Marcel Dekker.

Antin, J. H. & Ferrara, J. L. M. (1992). Cytokine dysregulation and acute graft-versus-host disease. *Blood,* **80,** 2964–8.

Asai, O., Longo, D. L., Tian, Z. G. *et al.* (1998). Suppression of graft-versus-host disease and amplification of graft-versus-tumor effects by activated natural killer cells after allogeneic bone marrow transplantation. *Journal of Clinical Investigation,* **101,** 1835–42.

Atkinson, K., Matias, C., Guiffre, A. *et al.* (1991). In vivo administration of granulocyte colony-stimulating factor (G-CSF), granulocyte-macrophage CSF, interleukin-1 (IL-1), and IL-4, alone and in combination, after allogeneic murine hematopoietic stem cell transplantation. *Blood,* **77,** 1376–82.

Auffermann-Gretzinger, S., Lossos, I. S., Vayntrub, T. A. *et al.* (2002). Rapid establishment of dendritic cell chimerism in allogeneic hematopoietic cell transplant recipients. *Blood,* **99,** 1442–8.

Autran, B., Leblond, V., & Sadat-Sowti, B. E. A. (1991). A soluble factor released by CD8+CD57+ lymphocytes from bone marrow transplanted patients inhibits cell-mediated cytolysis. *Blood,* **77,** 2237–41.

Bacchetta, R., Bigler, M., Touraine, J. L. *et al.* (1994). High levels of interleukin 10 production in vivo are associated with tolerance in SCID patients transplanted with HLA mismatched hematopoietic stem cells. *Journal of Experimental Medicine,* **179,** 493–502.

Baker, M. B., Altman, N. H., Podack, E. R., & Levy, R. B. (1996). The role of cell-mediated cytotoxicity in acute GVHD after MHC-matched allogeneic bone marrow transplantation in mice. *Journal of Experimental Medicine,* **183,** 2645–56.

Baker, M. B., Riley, R. L., Podack, E. R., & Levy, R. B. (1997). Graft-versus-host-disease-associated lymphoid hypoplasia and B cell dysfunction is dependent upon donor T cell-mediated Fas-ligand function, but not perforin function. *Proceedings of the National Academy of Science USA,* **94,** 1366–71.

Barclay, A. N. & Mason, D. W. (1982). Induction of Ia antigen in rat epidermal cells and gut epithelium by immunological stimuli. *Journal of Experimental Medicine,* **156,** 1665–76.

Barrat, F. J., Cua, D. J., Boonstra, A. *et al.* (2002). In vitro generation of interleukin 10-producing regulatory CD4(+) T cells is induced by immunosuppressive drugs and inhibited by T helper type 1 (Th1)- and Th2-inducing cytokines. *Journal of Experimental Medicine,* **195,** 603–16.

Belanger, C., Esperou-Bourdeau, H., Bordigoni, P. *et al.* (1993). Use of an anti-interleukin-2 receptor monoclonal antibody for GVHD prophylaxis in unrelated donor BMT. *Bone Marrow Transplantation,* **11,** 293–7.

Billingham, R. E. (1966). The biology of graft-versus-host reactions. *Harvey Lectures,* **62,** 21–78.

Blazar, B. R., Sharpe, A. H., Taylor, P. A. *et al.* (1996). Infusion of anti-B7.1 (CD80) and anti-B7.2 (CD86) monoclonal antibodies inhibit murine graft-versus-host disease lethality in part via direct effects on CD4+ and CD8+ T cells. *Journal of Immunology,* **157,** 3250–9.

Blazar, B. R., Taylor, P. A., Linsley, P. S., & Vallera, D. A. (1994). In vivo blockade of CD28/CTLA4: B7/BB1 interaction with CTLA4-Ig reduces lethal murine graft-versus-host disease across the major histocompatibility complex barrier in mice. *Blood,* **83,** 3815–25.

Blazar, B. R., Taylor, P. A., Noelle, R. J., & Vallera, D. A. (1998). CD4(+) T cells tolerized ex vivo to host alloantigen by anti-CD40 ligand (CD40L:CD154) antibody lose their graft-versus-host disease lethality capacity but retain nominal antigen responses. *Journal of Clinical Investigation,* **102,** 473–82.

Blazar, B. R., Taylor, P. A., Smith, S., & Vallera, D. A. (1995). Interleukin-10 administration decreases survival in murine recipients of major histocompatibility complex disparate donor bone marrow grafts. *Blood,* **85,** 842–51.

Blazar, B. R., Taylor, P. A., Snover, D. C. *et al.* (1993). Murine recipients of fully mismatched donor marrow are protected from lethal graft-versus-host disease by the in vivo administration of rapamycin but develop an autoimmune-like syndrome. *Journal of Immunology,* **151,** 5726–41.

Boussiotis, V. A., Chen, Z. M., Zeller, J. C. *et al.* (2001). Altered T-cell receptor + CD28-mediated signaling and blocked cell cycle progression in interleukin 10 and transforming growth factor-beta-treated alloreactive T cells that do not induce graft-versus-host disease. *Blood,* **97,** 565–71.

Braun, Y. M., Lowin, B., French, L. *et al.* (1996). Cytotoxic T cells deficient in both functional Fas ligand and perforin show residual cytolytic activity yet lose their capacity to induce lethal acute graft-versus-host disease. *Journal of Experimental Medicine,* **183,** 657–61.

Brochu, S., Rioux-Masse, B., Roy, J. *et al.* (1999). Massive activation-induced cell death of alloreactive T cells with apoptosis of bystander postthymic T cells prevents immune reconstitution in mice with graft-versus-host disease. *Blood,* **94,** 390–400.

Brok, H. P. M., Heidt, P. J., van der Meide, P. H. *et al.* (1993). Interferon-g prevents graft-versus-host disease after allogeneic bone marrow transplantation in mice. *Journal of Immunology,* **151,** 6451–9.

Burt, R., Drobyski, W., Traynor, A., & Jr, C. L. (1999). Herpes simplex thymidine kinase (HStk) transgenic donor lymphocytes. *Bone Marrow Transplantation,* **24,** 1043–51.

Cavender, D. E., Haskard, D. O., Joseph, B., & Ziff, M. (1986). Interleukin-1 increases the binding of human B and T lympho-cytes to endothelial cell monolayers. *Journal of Immunology,* **136,** 203–7.

Chang, R. J. & Lee, S. H. (1986). Effects of interferon-gamma and tumor necrosis factor-alpha on the expression of an Ia antigen on a murine macrophage cell line. *Journal of Immunology,* **137,** 2853–6.

Chen, B. J., Morris, R. E., & Chao, N. J. (2000). Graft-versus-host disease prevention by rapamycin: cellular mechanisms. *Biology of Blood Marrow Transplantation,* **6,** 529–36.

Chicheportiche, Y., Bourdon, P. R., Xu, H. *et al.* (1997). TWEAK, a new secreted ligand in the tumor necrosis factor family that weakly induces apoptosis. *The Journal of Biological Chemistry,* **272,** 32401–10.

Chinnaiyan, A. M., O'Rourke, K., Yu, G. L. *et al.* (1996). Signal transduction by DR3, a death domain-containing receptor related to TNFR-1 and CD95. *Science,* **274,** 990–2.

Clift, R. A., Buckner, C. D., Appelbaum, F. R. *et al.* (1990). Allogeneic marrow transplantation in patients with acute myeloid leukemia in first remission: a randomized trial of two irradiation regimens. *Blood,* **76,** 1867–71.

Cooke, K. R., Gerbitz, A., Crawford, J. M. *et al.* (2001). LPS antagonism reduces graft-versus-host disease and preserves graft-versus-leukemia activity after experimental bone marrow transplantation. *Journal of Clinical Investigation,* **107,** 1581–9.

Cooke, K. R., Hill, G. R., Crawford, J. M. *et al.* (1998). TNFa production to LPS stimulation by donor cells predicts the severity of experimental acute graft-versus-host disease. *Journal of Clinical Investigation,* **102,** 1882–91.

Crawford, J. M. (1997). Graft-versus-host disease of the liver. In *Graft-versus-Host Disease,* eds. J. L. M. Ferrara, H. J. Deeg, & S. J. Burakoff, pp. 315–336. New York: Marcel Dekker.

Critchfield, J. M., Racke, M. K., Zuniga-Pflucker, J. C. *et al.* (1994). T cell deletion in high antigen dose therapy of autoimmune encephalomyelitis. *Science,* **263,** 1139–43.

Das, H., Imoto, S., Murayama, T. *et al.* (1999). Levels of soluble FasL and FasL gene expression during the development of graft-versus-host disease in DLT-treated patients. *British Journal of Haematology,* **104,** 795–800.

De Wit, D., Van Mechelen, M., Zanin, C. *et al.* (1993). Preferential activation of Th2 cells in chronic graft-versus-host disease. *Journal of Immunology,* **150,** 361–6.

Dey, B. R., Yang, Y. G., Szot, G. L. *et al.* (1998). Interleukin-12 inhibits graft-versus-host disease through an Fas-mediated mechanism associated with alterations in donor T-cell activation and expansion. *Blood,* **91,** 3315–22.

Dickinson, A. M., Sviland, L., Dunn, J. *et al.* (1991). Demonstration of direct involvement of cytokines in graft-versus-host reactions using an in vitro skin explant model. *Bone Marrow Transplantation,* **7,** 209–16.

Doutrelepont, J. M., Moser, M., Leo, O. *et al.* (1991). HyperIgE in stimulatory graft-versus-host disease: role of Interleukin-4. *Clinical and Experimental Immunology,* **83,** 133–6.

Durham, M. M., Bingaman, A. W., Adams, A. B. *et al.* (2000). Cutting edge: administration of anti-CD40 ligand and donor bone marrow leads to hemopoietic chimerism and donor-specific tolerance without cytoreductive conditioning. *Journal of Immunology,* **165,** 1–4.

Dustin, M. L. & Springer, T. A. (1989). T-cell receptor cross-linking transiently stimulates adhesiveness through LFA-1. *Nature*, **341**, 619–24.

Eberl, G. & MacDonald, H. R. (1998). Rapid death and regeneration of NKT cells in anti-CD3epsilon- or IL-12-treated mice: a major role for bone marrow in NKT cell homeostasis. *Immunity*, **9**, 345–53.

Eisenberg, S. P., Evans, R. J., Arend, W. P. *et al.* (1990). Primary structure and functional expression from complementary DNA of a human interleukin-1 receptor antagonist. *Nature*, **343**, 341.

Ellison, C. A., Fischer, J. M., HayGlass, K. T., & Gartner, J. G. (1998). Murine graft-versus-host disease in an F1-hybrid model using IFN-gamma gene knockout donors. *Journal of Immunology*, **161**, 631–40.

Falzarano, G., Krenger, W., Snyder, K. M. *et al.* (1996). Suppression of B cell proliferation to lipopolysaccharide is mediated through induction of the nitric oxide pathway by tumor necrosis factor-a in mice with acute graft-versus-host disease. *Blood*, **87**, 2853–60.

Feinstein, L. & Storb, R. (2001). Nonmyeloablative hematopoietic cell transplantation. *Current Opinions in Oncology*, **13**, 95–100.

Ferrara, J. L. M., Marion, A., McIntyre, J. F. *et al.* (1986). Amelioration of acute graft-versus-host disease due to minor histocompatibility antigens by in vivo administration of anti-interleukin 2 receptor antibody. *Journal of Immunology*, **137**, 1874–7.

Fischer, A. C., Laulis, M. K., Horwitz, L. *et al.* (1989). Host resistance to cyclosporine induced syngeneic graft-versus-host disease. Requirement for two distinct lymphocyte subsets. *Journal of Immunology*, **143**, 827–32.

Forster, R., Schubel, A., Breitfeld, D. *et al.* (1999). CCR7 coordinates the primary immune response by establishing functional microenvironments in secondary lymphoid organs. *Cell*, **99**, 23–33.

Fowler, D. H., Kurasawa, K., Husebekk, A. *et al.* (1994). Cells of the Th2 cytokine phenotype prevent LPS-induced lethality during murine graft-versus-host reaction. *Journal of Immunology*, **152**, 1004–11.

Fowler, D. H., Kurasawa, K., Smith, R. *et al.* (1994). Donor CD4-enriched cells of Th2 cytokine phenotype regulate graft-versus-host disease without impairing allogeneic engraftment in sublethally irradiated mice. *Blood*, **84**, 3540–9.

Fowler, D. H., Kurasawa, K., Smith, R., & Gress, R. E. (1994). Donor lymphoid cells of Th2 cytokine phenotype reduce lethal graft versus host disease and facilitate fully allogeneic cell transfers in sublethally irradiated mice. *Progress in Clinical & Biological Research*, **389**, 533–40.

Fukuda, H., Nakamura, H., Tominaga, N. *et al.* (1994). Marked increase of CD8+S6F1+ and CD8+CD57+ cells in patients with graft-versus-host disease after allogeneic bone marrow transplantation. *Bone Marrow Transplantation*, **13**, 181–5.

Gale, R. P., Bortin, M. M., van Bekkum, D. W. *et al.* (1987). Risk factors for acute graft-versus-host disease. *British Journal of Haematology*, **67**, 397–406.

Gale, R. P. & Reisner, Y. (1986). Graft rejection and graft-versus-host disease: mirror images. *Lancet*, **1**, 1468–70.

Gallucci, S., Lolkema, M., & Matzinger, P. (1999). Natural adjuvants: endogenous activators of dendritic cells. *Nature Medicine*, **5**, 1249–55.

Garlisi, C. G., Pennline, K. J., Smith, S. R. *et al.* (1993). Cytokine gene expression in mice undergoing chronic graft-versus-host disease. *Molecular Immunology*, **30**, 669–77.

Ghayur, T., Seemayer, T., & Lapp, W. S. (1990). Histologic correlates of immune functional deficits in graft-vs-host disease. In *Graft-vs.-Host Disease: Immunology, Pathophysiology, and Treatment*, eds. S. J. Burakoff, H. J. Deeg, J. Ferrara & K. Atkinson, pp. 109–32. New York: Marcel Dekker.

Gifford, G. E. & Lohmann-Matthes, M.-L. (1987). Gamma interferon priming of mouse and human macrophages for induction of tumor necrosis factor production by bacterial lipopolysaccharide. *Journal of the National Cancer Institute*, **78**, 121–4.

Gilliam, A. C., Whitaker-Menezes, D., Korngold, R., & Murphy, G. F. (1996). Apoptosis is the predominant form of epithelial target cell injury in acute experimental graft-versus-host disease. *Journal of Investigative Dermatology*, **107**, 377–83.

Goldman, J. M., Gale, R. P., Horowitz, M. M. *et al.* (1988). Bone marrow transplantation for chronic myelogenous leukemia in chronic phase. Increased risk for relapse associated with T-cell depletion. *Annals of Internal Medicine*, **108**, 806–14.

Graubert, T. A., DiPersio, J. F., Russell, J. H., & Ley, T. J. (1997). Perforin/granzyme-dependent and independent mechanisms are both important for the development of graft-versus-host disease after murine bone marrow transplantation. *Journal of Clinical Investigation*, **100**, 904–11.

Graubert, T. A., Russell, J. H., & Ley, T. (1996). The role of granzyme B in murine models of acute graft-versus-host disease and graft rejection. *Blood*, **87**, 1232–7.

Guinan, E. C., Boussiotis, V. A., Neuberg, D. *et al.* (1999). Transplantation of anergic histoincompatible bone marrow allografts. *New England Journal of Medicine*, **340**, 1704–14.

Hannum, C. H., Wilcox, C. J., Arend, W. P. *et al.* (1990). Interleukin-1 receptor antagonist activity of a human interleukin-1 inhibitor. *Nature*, **343**, 336–40.

Hattori, K., Hirano, T., Miyajima, H. *et al.* (1998). Differential effects of anti-Fas ligand and anti-tumor necrosis factor-a antibodies on acute graft-versus-host disease pathologies. *Blood*, **91**, 4051–5.

Hattori, K., Hirano, T., Ushiyama, C. *et al.* (1997). A metalloproteinase inhibitor prevents lethal acute graft-versus-host disease in mice. *Blood*, **90**, 542–8.

Herve, P., Flesch, M., Tiberghien, P. *et al.* (1992). Phase I–II trial of a monoclonal anti-tumor necrosis factor alpha antibody for the treatment of refractory severe acute graft-versus-host disease. *Blood*, **81**, 1993–9.

Herve, P., Wijdenes, J., Bergerat, J. P. *et al.* (1990). Treatment of corticosteroid-resistant acute graft-versus-host disease by in vivo administration of anti-interleukin-2 receptor monoclonal antibody (B-B10). *Blood*, **75**, 1017–23.

Hess, A. D. & Fischer, A. C. (1989). Immune mechanisms in cyclosporine-induced syngeneic graft-versus-host disease. *Transplantation*, **48**, 895–900.

Hess, A. D., Thoburn, C., & Horwitz, L. (1998). Promiscuous recognition of major histocompatibility complex class II determinants in cyclosporine-induced syngeneic graft-versus-host disease: specificity of cytolytic effector T cells. *Transplantation*, **65**, 785–92.

Hill, G. R., Cooke, K. R., Teshima, T. *et al.* (1998). Interleukin-11 promotes T cell polarization and prevents acute graft-versus-host disease after allogeneic bone marrow transplantation. *Journal of Clinical Investigation,* **102,** 115–23.

Hill, G. R., Crawford, J. M., Cooke, K. J. *et al.* (1997). Total body irradiation and acute graft versus host disease. The role of gastrointestinal damage and inflammatory cytokines. *Blood,* **90,** 3204–13.

Hill, G. R. & Ferrara, J. L. (2000). The primacy of the gastrointestinal tract as a target organ of acute graft-versus-host disease: rationale for the use of cytokine shields in allogeneic bone marrow transplantation. *Blood,* **95,** 2754–9.

Hill, G. R., Teshima, T., Gerbitz, A. *et al.* (1999). Differential roles of IL-1 and TNF-alpha on graft-versus-host disease and graft versus leukemia. *Journal of Clinical Investigation,* **104,** 459–67.

Ho, V. T. & Soiffer, R. J. (2001). The history and future of T-cell depletion as graft-versus-host disease prophylaxis for allogeneic hematopoietic stem cell transplantation. *Blood,* **98,** 3192–204.

Holda, J. H., Maier, T., & Claman, N. H. (1988). Evidence that IFN-g is responsible for natural suppressor activity in GVHD spleen and normal bone marrow. *Transplantation,* **45,** 772–7.

Holler, E., Kolb, H. J., Hintermeier-Knabe, R. *et al.* (1993). The role of tumor necrosis factor alpha in acute graft-versus-host disease and complications following allogeneic bone marrow transplantation. *Transplantation Proceedings,* **25,** 1234–6.

Holler, E., Kolb, H. J., Moller, A. *et al.* (1990). Increased serum levels of tumor necrosis factor alpha precede major complications of bone marrow transplantation. *Blood,* **75,** 1011–6.

Hsieh, M. H. & Korngold, R. (2000). Differential use of FasL- and perforin-mediated cytolytic mechanisms by T-cell subsets involved in graft-versus-myeloid leukemia responses. *Blood,* **96,** 1047–55.

Huchet, R., Bruley-Rosset, M., Mathiot, C. *et al.* (1993). Involvement of IFN-gamma and transforming growth factor-beta in graft-vs-host reaction-associated immunosuppression. *Journal of Immunology,* **150,** 2517–24.

Hurtenbach, U. & Shearer, G. M. (1983). Analysis of murine T lymphocyte markers during the early phases of GvH-associated suppression of cytotoxic T lymphocyte responses. *Journal of Immunology,* **130,** 1561–6.

Irmler, M., Thome, M., Hahne, M. *et al.* (1997). Inhibition of death receptor signals by cellular FLIP. *Nature,* **388,** 190–5.

Jadus, M. R. & Peck, A. B. (1983). Lethal murine graft-versus-host disease in the absence of detectable cytotoxic T lymphocytes. *Transplantion,* **36,** 281–9.

Jiang, Z., Podack, E., & Levy, R. B. (2001). Major histocompatibility complex-mismatched allogeneic bone marrow transplantation using perforin and/or Fas ligand double-defective CD4(+) donor T cells: involvement of cytotoxic function by donor lymphocytes prior to graft-versus-host disease pathogenesis. *Blood,* **98,** 390–7.

Jones, J. M., Wison, R., & Bealmear, P. M. (1971). Mortality and gross pathology of secondary disease in germfree mouse radiation chimeras. *Radiation Research,* **45,** 577.

Kagi, D., Vignaux, F., Ledermann, B. *et al.* (1994). Fas and perforin pathways as major mechanisms of T cell-mediated cytotoxicity. *Science,* **265,** 528–30.

Kanda, Y., Tanaka, Y., Shirakawa, K. *et al.* (1998). Increased soluble Fas-ligand in sera of bone marrow transplant recipients with acute graft-versus-host disease. *Bone Marrow Transplantation,* **22,** 751–4.

Kayaba, H., Hirokawa, M., Watanabe, A. *et al.* (2000). Serum markers of graft-versus-host disease after bone marrow transplantation. *Journal of Allergy and Clinical Immunology,* **106,** S40–4.

Kelso, A. (1990). Frequency analysis of lymphokine-secreting CD4+ and CD8+ T cells activated in a graft-versus-host reaction. *Journal of Immunology,* **145,** 2167–76.

Kernan, N. A., Collins, N. H., Juliano, L. *et al.* (1986). Clonable T lymphocytes in T cell-depleted bone marrow transplants correlate with development of graft-vs-host disease. *Blood,* **68,** 770–3.

Klimpel, G. R., Annable, C. R., Cleveland, M. G. *et al.* (1990). Immunosuppression and lymphoid hypoplasia associated with chronic graft-versus-host disease is dependent upon IFN-g production. *Journal of Immunology,* **144,** 84–93.

Kondo, T., Suda, T., Fukuyama, H. *et al.* (1997). Essential roles of the Fas ligand in the development of hepatitis. *Nature Medicine,* **3,** 409–13.

Korngold, R. & Sprent, J. (1990). T cell subsets in graft-vs.-host disease. In *Graft-vs.-Host Disease: Immunology, Pathophysiology, and Treatment,* eds. S. J. Burakoff, H. J. Deeg, J. Ferrara and K. Atkinson, pp. 31–50. New York: Marcel Dekker.

Krenger, W., Falzarano, G., Delmonte, J. *et al.* (1996). Interferon-g suppresses T-cell proliferation to mitogen via the nitric oxide pathway during experimental acute graft-versus-host disease. *Blood,* **88,** 1113–21.

Krenger, W., Snyder, K., Smith, S., & Ferrara, J.L.M. (1994). Effects of exogenous interleukin-10 in a murine model of graft-versus-host disease to minor histocompatibility antigens. *Transplantation,* **58,** 1251–7.

Krenger, W., Snyder, K. M., Byon, C. H. *et al.* (1995). Polarized type 2 alloreactive CD4+ and CD8+ donor T cells fail to induce experimental acute graft-versus-host disease. *Journal of Immunology,* **155,** 585–93.

Krensky, A. M., Weiss, A., Crabtree, G. *et al.* (1990). T-lymphocyte-antigen interactions in transplant rejection. *New England Journal of Medicine,* **322,** 510–7.

Krijanovski, O. I., Hill, G. R., Cooke, K. R. *et al.* (1999). Keratinocyte growth factor separates graft-versus-leukemia effects from graft-versus-host disease. *Blood,* **94,** 825–31.

Kumaki, S., Minegishi, M., Fujie, H. *et al.* (1998). Prolonged secretion of IL-15 in patients with severe forms of acute graft-versus-host disease after allogeneic bone marrow transplantation in children. *International Journal of Hematology,* **67,** 307–12.

Kuroiwa, T., Kakishita, E., Hamano, T. *et al.* (2001). Hepatocyte growth factor ameliorates acute graft-versus-host disease and promotes hematopoietic function. *Journal of Clinical Investigation,* **107,** 1365–73.

Lakkis, F. G., Arakelov, A., Konieczny, B. T., & Inoue, Y. (2000). Immunologic 'ignorance' of vascularized organ transplants in the absence of secondary lymphoid tissue. *Nature Medicine,* **6,** 686–8.

Lampert, I. A., Suitters, A. J., & Chisholm, P. M. (1981). Expression of Ia antigen on epidermal keratinocytes in graft-versus-host disease. *Nature* **293,** 149–50.

Lan, F., Zeng, D., Higuchi, M. *et al.* (2001). Predominance of NK1.1+TCR alpha beta+ or DX5+TCR alpha beta+ T cells in mice conditioned with fractionated lymphoid irradiation protects against graft-versus-host disease: "natural suppressor" cells. *Journal of Immunology, 167,* 2087–96.

Langrehr, J. M., Murase, N., Markus, P. M. *et al.* (1992). Nitric oxide production in host-versus-graft and graft-versus-host reactions in the rat. *Journal of Clinical Investigation, 90,* 679–83.

Laster, S. M., Wood, J. G., & Gooding, L. R. (1988). Tumor necrosis factor can induce both apoptotic and necrotic forms of cell lysis. *Journal of Immunology, 141,* 2629.

Leeuwenberg, J. F., Van Damme, J., Maeger, T. *et al.* (1988). Effects of tumor necrosis factor on the interferon-gamma-induced major histocompatibility complex class II antigen expression by human endothelial cells. *European Journal of Immunology, 18,* 1469–72.

Li, X. C., Demirci, G., Ferrari-Lacraz, S. *et al.* (2001). IL-15 and IL-2: a matter of life and death for T cells in vivo. *Nature Medicine, 7,* 114–8.

Li, X. C., Strom, T. B., Turka, L. A., & Wells, A. D. (2001). T cell death and transplantation tolerance. *Immunity, 14,* 407–16.

Li, Y., Li, X. C., Zheng, X. X. *et al.* (1999). Blocking both signal 1 and signal 2 of T-cell activation prevents apoptosis of alloreactive T cells and induction of peripheral allograft tolerance. *Nature Medicine, 5,* 1298–302.

Liem, L. M., Fibbe, W. E., van Houwelingen, H. C., & Goulmy, E. (1999). Serum transforming growth factor-beta1 levels in bone marrow transplant recipients correlate with blood cell counts and chronic graft-versus-host disease. *Transplantation, 67,* 59–65.

Liem, L. M., van Lopik, T., van Nieuwenhuijze, A. E. *et al.* (1998). Soluble Fas levels in sera of bone marrow transplantation recipients are increased during acute graft-versus-host disease but not during infections. *Blood, 91,* 1464–8.

Liu, Y. & Janeway, C. A., Jr. (1990). Interferon gamma plays a critical role in induced cell death of effector T cell: a possible third mechanism of self-tolerance. *Journal of Experimental Medicine, 172,* 1735–9.

Lorenz, E., Schwartz, D. A., Martin, P. J. *et al.* (2001). Association of TLR4 mutations and the risk for acute GVHD after HLA-matched-sibling hematopoietic stem cell transplantation. *Biology of Blood and Marrow Transplantation, 7,* 384–7.

Lowin, B., Hahne, M., Mattmann, C., & Tschopp, J. (1994). Cytolytic T-cell cytotoxicity is mediated through perforin and Fas lytic pathways. *Nature, 370,* 650–620.

MacDonald, K. P. A., Rowe, V., Filippich, C. *et al.* (2003). Donor pretreatment with progenipoietin-1 is superior to granulocyte colony-stimulating factor in preventing graft-versus-host disease after allogeneic stem cell transplantation. *Blood, 101,* 2033–42.

Malkovsky, M., Brenner, M. K., Hunt, R. *et al.* (1986). T cell-depletion of allogeneic bone marrow prevents acceleration of graft-versus-host disease induced by exogenous interleukin-2. *Cellular Immunology, 103,* 476–80.

Maloy, K. J. & Powrie, F. (2001). Regulatory T cells in the control of immune pathology. *Nature Immunology, 2,* 816–22.

Martin, P. J. (1993). Donor CD8 cells prevent allogeneic marrow graft rejection in mice: potential implications for marrow transplantation in humans. *Journal of Experimental Medicine, 178,* 703–12.

Martin, P. J., Akatsuka, Y., Hahne, M., & Sale, G. (1998). Involvement of donor T-cell cytotoxic effector mechanisms in preventing allogeneic marrow graft rejection. *Blood, 92,* 2177–81.

Mason, D. W., Dallman, M., & Barclay, A. N. (1981). Graft-versus-host disease induces expression of Ia antigen in rat epidermal cells and gut epithelium. *Nature, 293,* 150–1.

Matzinger, P. (2002). The Danger Model: A Renewed Sense of Self. *Science, 296,* 301–5.

McCarthy, P. L., Abhyankar, S., Neben, S. *et al.* (1991). Inhibition of interleukin-1 by an interleukin-1 receptor antagonist prevents graft-versus-host disease. *Blood, 78,* 1915–8.

McCormick, L. L., Zhang, Y., Tootell, E., & Gilliam, A. C. (1999). Anti-TGF-beta treatment prevents skin and lung fibrosis in murine sclerodermatous graft-versus-host disease: a model for human scleroderma. *Journal of Immunology, 163,* 5693–9.

Moser, B. & Loetscher, P. (2001). Lymphocyte traffic control by chemokines. *Nature Immunology, 2,* 123–8.

Mosmann, T. R., Cherwinski, H., Bond, M. W. *et al.* (1986). Two types of murine helper T cell clone. I. Definition according to profiles of lymphokine activities and secreted proteins. *Journal of Immunology, 136,* 2348–57.

Mowat, A. (1989). Antibodies to IFN-gamma prevent immunological mediated intestinal damage in murine graft-versus-host reactions. *Immunology, 68,* 18–24.

Murai, M., Yoneyama, H., Harada, A. *et al.* (1999). Active participation of CCR5(+)CD8(+) T lymphocytes in the pathogenesis of liver injury in graft-versus-host disease. *Journal of Clinical Investigation, 104,* 49–57.

Murphy, W. J., Welniak, L. A., Taub, D. D. *et al.* (1998). Differential effects of the absence of interferon-gamma and IL-4 in acute graft-versus-host disease after allogeneic bone marrow transplantation in mice. *Journal of Clinical Investigation, 102,* 1742–8.

Nestel, F. P., Greene, R. N., Kichian, K. *et al.* (2000). Activation of macrophage cytostatic effector mechanisms during acute graft-versus-host disease: release of intracellular iron and nitric oxide-mediated cytostasis. *Blood, 96,* 1836–43.

Nestel, F. P., Price, K. S., Seemayer, T. A., & Lapp, W. S. (1992). Macrophage priming and lipopolysaccharide-triggered release of tumor necrosis factor alpha during graft-versus-host disease. *Journal of Experimental Medicine, 175,* 405–13.

Niederwieser, D., Herold, M., Woloszczuk, W. *et al.* (1990). Endogenous IFN-gamma during human bone marrow transplantation. *Transplantation, 50,* 620–5.

Nierle, T., Bunjes, D., Arnold, R. *et al.* (1993). Quantitative assessment of posttransplant host-specific interleukin-2-secreting T-helper cell precursors in patients with and without acute graft-versus-host disease after allogeneic HLA-identical sibling bone marrow transplantation. *Blood, 81,* 841–8.

Nikolic, B., Lee, S., Bronson, R. T. *et al.* (2000). Th1 and Th2 mediate acute graft-versus-host disease, each with distinct end-organ targets. *Journal of Clinical Investigation, 105,* 1289–98.

Nishizuka, Y. (1986). Studies and perspectives of protein kinase C. *Science, 233,* 305–12.

Ordemann, R., Hutchinson, R., Friedman, J. *et al.* (2002). Enhanced allostimulatory activity of host antigen-presenting cells in old mice intensifies acute graft-versus-host disease. *Journal of Clinical Investigation, 109,* 1249–56.

Pan, L., Delmonte, J., Jalonen, C. K., Ferrara, J. L. (1995). Pretreatment of donor mice with granulocyte colony-stimulating factor polarizes donor T lymphocytes towards type-2 cytokine production and reduces severity of experimental graft-versus-host disease. *Blood,* **86,** 4422–9.

Pan, G., O'Rourke, K., Chinnaiyan, A. M. *et al.* (1997). The receptor for the cytotoxic ligand TRAIL. *Science,* **276,** 111–3.

Pan, L., Teshima, T., Hill, G. R. *et al.* (1999). Granulocyte colony-stimulating factor-mobilized allogeneic stem cell transplantation maintains graft-versus-leukemia effects through a perforin-dependent pathway while preventing graft-versus-host disease. *Blood,* **93,** 4071–8.

Panoskaltsis-Mortari, A., Lacey, D. L., Vallera, D. A., & Blazer, B. R. (1998). Keratinocyte Growth Factor administered before conditioning ameliorates graft-versus-host disease after allogeneic bone marrow transplantation in mice. *Blood,* **92,** 3960–7.

Panoskaltsis-Mortari, A., Strieter, R. M., Hermanson, J. R. *et al.* (2000). Induction of monocyte- and T-cell-attracting chemokines in the lung during the generation of idiopathic pneumonia syndrome following allogeneic murine bone marrow transplantation. *Blood,* **96,** 834–9.

Paris, F., Fuks, Z., Kang, A. *et al.* (2001). Endothelial apoptosis as the primary lesion initiating intestinal radiation damage in mice. *Science,* **293,** 293–7.

Parkman, R. (1986). Clonal analysis of murine graft-vs.-host disease. I. Phenotypic and functional analysis of T lymphocyte clones. *Journal of Immunology,* **136,** 3543–8.

Piemonti, L., Monti, P., Allavena, P. *et al.* (1999). Glucocorticoids affect human dendritic cell differentiation and maturation. *Journal of Immunology,* **162,** 6473–81.

Piguet, P. F., Grau, G. E., Allet, B., & Vassalli, P. J. (1987). Tumor necrosis factor/cachectin is an effector of skin and gut lesions of the acute phase of graft-versus-host disease. *Journal of Experimental Medicine,* **166,** 1280–9.

Piguet, P. F., Grau, G. E., Collart, M. A. *et al.* (1989). Pneumopathies of the graft-versus-host reaction. Alveolitis associated with an increased level of tumor necrosis factor MRNA and chronic interstitial pneumonitis. *Laboratory Investigation,* **61,** 37–45.

Pober, J. S., Gimbrone, M. A., Lapierre, L. A. *et al.* (1986). Overlapping patterns of activation of human endothelial cells by interleukin-1, tumor necrosis factor, and immune interferon. *Journal of Immunology,* **137,** 1893.

Rappeport, J., Reinherz, E., Mihin, M. *et al.* (1979). Acute graft-versus-host disease in recipients of bone marrow transplantation from identical two donors. *Lancet,* **2,** 717–20.

Rea, D., van Kooten, C., van Meijgaarden, K. E. *et al.* (2000). Glucocorticoids transform CD40-triggering of dendritic cells into an alternative activation pathway resulting in antigen-presenting cells that secrete IL-10. *Blood,* **95,** 3162–7.

Reddy, P., Teshima, T., Kukuruga, M. *et al.* (2001). Interleukin-18 Regulates Acute Graft-Versus-Host Disease by Enhancing Fas-mediated Donor T Cell Apoptosis. *Journal of Experimental Medicine,* **194,** 1433–40.

Reddy, P., Teshima, T., Hildebrandt, G. *et al.* (2002). Interleukin 18 preserves a perforin-dependent graft-versus-leukemia effect after allogeneic bone marrow transplantation. *Blood,* **100,** 3429–31.

Refaeli, Y., Van Parijs, L., London, C. A. *et al.* (1998). Biochemical mechanisms of IL-2-regulated Fas-mediated T cell apoptosis. *Immunity,* **8,** 615–23.

Reid, S. D., Penna, G., & Adorini, L. (2000). The control of T cell responses by dendritic cell subsets. *Current Opinions in Immunology,* **12,** 114–21.

Reinhardt, R. L., Khoruts, A., Merica, R. *et al.* (2001). Visualizing the generation of memory CD4 T cells in the whole body. *Nature,* **410,** 101–5.

Ringden, O. (1990). Viral infections and graft-vs.-host disease. In Graft-vs.-Host Disease, S. J. Burakoff, H. J. Deeg, J. Ferrara & K. Atkinson, eds. (New York: Marcel Dekker), pp. 467.

Rissoan, M. C., Soumelis, V., Kadowaki, N. *et al.* (1999). Reciprocal control of T helper cell and dendritic cell differentiation. *Science,* **283,** 1183–6.

Rolink, A. G. & Gleichmann, E. (1983). Allosuppressor- and allo-helper-T cells in acute and chronic graft-versus-host (GVH) disease. III. Different Lyt subsets of donor T cells induce different pathological syndromes. *Journal of Experimental Medicine,* **158,** 546–58.

Roncarolo, M. G., Levings, M. K., & Traversari, C. (2001). Differentiation of T Regulatory Cells by Immature Dendritic Cells. *Journal of Experimental Medicine,* **193,** F5–F10.

Ruggeri, L., Capanni, M., Martelli, M. F., & Velardi, A. (2001). Cellular therapy: exploiting NK cell alloreactivity in transplantation. *Current Opinions in Hematology,* **8,** 355–9.

Ruggeri, L., Capanni, M., Urbani, E. *et al.* (2002). Effectiveness of Donor Natural Killer Cell Alloreactivity in Mismatched Hematopoietic Transplants. *Science,* **295,** 2097–100.

Sallusto, F., Lenig, D., Forster, R. *et al.* (1999). Two subsets of memory T lymphocytes with distinct homing potentials and effector functions. *Nature,* **401,** 708–12.

Salomon, B., Lenschow, D. J., Rhee, L. *et al.* (2000). B7/CD28 costimulation is essential for the homeostasis of the CD4+CD25+ immunoregulatory T cells that control autoimmune diabetes. *Immunity,* **12,** 431–40.

Samelson, L. E., Patel, M. D., Weissman, A. M. *et al.* (1986). Antigen activation of murine T cell induces tyrosine phosphorylation of a polypeptide associated with the T cell antigen receptor. *Cell,* **46,** 1083–90.

Schmaltz, C., Alpdogan, O., Horndasch, K. J. *et al.* (2001). Differential use of Fas ligand and perforin cytotoxic pathways by donor T cells in graft-versus-host disease and graft-versus-leukemia effect. *Blood,* **97,** 2886–95.

Schwarer, A. P., Jiang, Y. Z., Brookes, P. A. *et al.* (1993). Frequency of anti-recipient alloreactive helper T-cell precursors in donor blood and graft-versus-host disease after HLA-identical sibling bone-marrow transplantation. *Lancet,* **341,** 203–5.

Serody, J. S., Burkett, S. E., Panoskaltsis-Mortari, A. *et al.* (2000). T-lymphocyte production of macrophage inflammatory protein-1alpha is critical to the recruitment of CD8(+) T cells to the liver, lung, and spleen during graft-versus-host disease. *Blood,* **96,** 2973–80.

Shevach, E. M., McHugh, R. S., Piccirillo, C. A., & Thornton, A. M. (2001). Control of T-cell activation by CD4+ CD25+ suppressor T cells. *Immunology Reviews,* **182,** 58–67.

Shlomchik, W. D., Couzens, M. S., Tang, C. B. *et al.* (1999). Prevention of graft versus host disease by inactivation of host antigen-presenting cells. *Science,* **285,** 412–5.

Shresta, S., Pham, C. T., Thomas, D. A. *et al.* (1998). How do cytotoxic lymphocytes kill their targets? *Current Opinion in Immunology,* **10,** 581–7.

Smith, S. R., Terminelli, C., Kenworthy-Bott, L., & Phillips, D. L. (1991). A study of cytokine production in acute graft-vs-host disease. *Cellular Immunology,* **134,** 336–48.

Sosman, J. A., Oettel, K. R., Smith, S. D. et al. (1990). Specific recognition of human leukemic cells by allogeneic T cells. II. Evidence for HLA-D restricted determinants on leukemic cells that are crossreactive with determinants present on unrelated nonleukemic cells. Blood, 75, 2005–16.

Sprent, J., Kosaka, H., Gao, E. K. et al. (1993). Intrathymic and extrathymic tolerance in bone marrow chimeras. Immunology Review, 133, 151–76.

Strober, S. (1984). Natural suppressor (NS) cells, neonatal tolerance, and total lymphoid irradiation: exploring obscure relationships. Annual Review of Immunology, 2, 219–37.

Sullivan, K., Storb, R., Buckner, D., & Fefer, A. (1989). Graft-versus-Host Disease as Adoptive Immunotherapy in Patients with Advanced Hematologic Neoplasms. New England Journal of Medicine, 320, 828–34.

Sullivan, K. M., Shulman, H. M., Storb, R. et al. (1981). Chronic graft-versus-host disease in 52 patients: Adverse natural course and successful treatment with combination immunosuppression. Blood, 57, 267–76.

Sullivan, K. M., Witherspoon, R. P., Storb, R. et al. (1988). Prednisone and azathioprine compared to prednisone and placebo for treatment of chronic graft-versus-host disease: prognostic influence of prolonged thrombocytopenia after allogeneic marrow transplantation. Blood, 72, 546–54.

Sykes, M., Romick, M. L., Hoyles, K. A., & Sachs, D. H. (1990). In vivo administration of interleukin 2 plus T cell-depleted syngeneic marrow prevents graft-versus-host disease mortality and permits alloengraftment. Journal of Experimental Medicine, 171, 645–58.

Sykes, M., Szot, G. L., Nguyen, P. L., & Pearson, D. A. (1995). Interleukin-12 inhibits murine graft-versus-host disease. Blood, 86, 2429–38.

Szebeni, J., Wang, M. G., Pearson, D. A. et al. (1994). IL-2 inhibits early increases in serum gamma interferon levels associated with graft-versus-host disease. Transplantation, 58, 1385–93.

Tamada, K., Tamura, H., Flies, D. et al. (2002). Blockade of LIGHT/LTbeta and CD40 signaling induces allospecific T cell anergy, preventing graft-versus-host disease. Journal of Clinical Investigation, 109, 549–57.

Tanaka, J., Imamura, M., Kasai, M. et al. (1993). Cytokine gene expression in peripheral blood mononuclear cells during graft-versus-host disease after allogeneic bone marrow transplantation. British Journal of Haematology, 85, 558–65.

Tanaka, J., Imamura, M., Kasai, M. et al. (1995). Cytokine gene expression after allogeneic bone marrow transplantation. Leukemia & Lymphoma, 16, 413–8.

Tanaka, J., Imamura, M., Kasai, M. et al. (1997). The important balance between cytokines derived from type 1 and type 2 helper T cells in the control of graft-versus-host disease. Bone Marrow Transplantation, 19, 571–6.

Taylor, P. A., Panoskaltsis-Mortari, A., Noelle, R. J., & Blazar, B. R. (2000). Analysis of the requirements for the induction of CD4+ T cell alloantigen hyporesponsiveness by ex vivo anti-CD40 ligand antibody. Journal of Immunology, 164, 612–22.

Teshima, T., Hill, G. R., Pan, L. et al. (1999). IL-11 separates graft-versus-leukemia effects from graft-versus-host disease after bone marrow transplantation. Journal of Clinical Investigation, 104, 317–25.

Teshima, T., Ordemann, R., Reddy, P. et al. (2002a). Acute graft-versus-host disease does not require alloantigen expression on host epithelium. Nature Medicine, 8, 575–81.

Teshima, T., Reddy, P., Lowler, K. P. et al. (2002b). Flt3 ligand therapy for recipients of allogeneic bone marrow transplants expands host CD8 alpha(+) dendritic cells and reduces experimental acute graft-versus-host disease. Blood, 99, 1825–32.

Theobald, M., Nierle, T., Bunjes, D. et al. (1992). Host-specific interleukin-2-secreting donor T-cell precursors as predictors of acute graft-versus-host disease in bone marrow transplantation between HLA-identical siblings. New England Journal of Medicine, 327, 1613–17.

Thomis, D. C., Marktel, S., Bonini, C. et al. (2001). A Fas-based suicide switch in human T cells for the treatment of graft-versus-host disease. Blood, 97, 1249–57.

Thornhill, M. H., Wellicome, S. M., Mahiouz, D. L. et al. (1991). Tumor necrosis factor combines with IL-4 or IFN-g to selectively enhance endothelial cell adhesiveness for T cells. Journal of Immunology, 146, 592–8.

Triulzi, D. J. & Nalesnik, M. A. (2001). Microchimerism, GVHD, and tolerance in solid organ transplantation. Transfusion, 41, 419–26.

Troutt, A. B. & Kelso, A. (1992). Enumeration of lymphokine mRNA-containing cells in vivo in a murine graft-versus-host reaction using the PCR. Proceedings of the Natural Academy of Sciences of the USA, 89, 5276–80.

Troutt, A. B., Maraskovsky, E., Rogers, L. A. et al. (1992). Quantitative analysis of lymphokine expression in vivo and in vitro. Immunology and Cell Biology, 70, 51–57.

Truitt, R. L., LeFever, A. V., Shih, C. C. Y. et al. (1990). Graft-vs.-leukemia effect. In Graft-vs.-Host Disease: Immunology, Pathophysiology, and Treatment, S. J. Burakoff, H. J. Deeg, J. Ferrara & K. Atkinson, eds. (New York: Marcel Dekker, Inc.), pp. 177–204.

Tsoi, M. S., Storb, R., Dobbs, S. et al. (1979). Non-specific suppressor cells in patients with chronic graft-versus-host disease after marrow grafting. Journal of Immunology, 123, 1970–3.

Tsoi, M. S., Storb, R., Dobbs, S. et al. (1980). Cell mediated immunity to non-HLA antigens of the host by donor lymphocytes in patients with chronic graft-versus-host disease. Journal of Immunology, 125, 2258.

Tsoi, M. S., Storb, R., Dobbs, S., & Thomas, E. D. (1981). Specific suppressor cells in graft-versus-host tolerance of HLA-identical marrow transplantation. Nature, 292, 355–7.

Tsukada, N., Kobata, T., Aizawa, Y. et al. (1999). Graft-versus-leukemia effect and graft-versus-host disease can be differentiated by cytotoxic mechanisms in a murine model of allogeneic bone marrow transplantation. Blood, 93, 2738–47.

Ueno, Y., Ishii, M., Yahagi, K. et al. (2000). Fas-mediated cholangiopathy in the murine model of graft versus host disease. Hepatology, 31, 966–74.

Umland, S. P., Razac, S., Nahrebne, D. K., & Seymour, B. W. (1992). Effects of in vivo administration of interferon (IFN)-gamma, anti-IFN-gamma, or anti-interleukin-4 monoclonal antibodies in chronic autoimmune graft-versus-host disease. Clinics in Immunology and Immunopathology, 63, 66–73.

Vallera, D. A. & Blazar, B. R. (1989). T cell depletion for graft-versus-host disease prophylaxis. A perspective on engraftment in mice and humans. Transplantation, 47, 751–60.

van Bekkum, D. W. & De Vries, M. J. (1967). *Radiation chimaeras* (London: Logos Press).

van Bekkum, D. W., Roodenburg, J., Heidt, P. J., & van der Waaij, D. (1974). Mitigation of secondary disease of allogeneic mouse radiation chimeras by modification of the intestinal microflora. *Journal of the National Cancer Institute, 52*, 401–4.

van Den Brink, M. R., Moore, E., Horndasch, K. J. *et al.* (2000). Fas-deficient 1pr mice are more susceptible to graft-versus-host disease. *Journal of Immunology,* **164,** 469–80.

Van Parijs, L. & Abbas, A. K. (1998). Homeostasis and self-tolerance in the immune system: turning lymphocytes off. *Science,* **280,** 243–8.

Velardi, A., Varese, P., Terenzi, A. *et al.* (1989). Lymphokine production by T-cell clones after human bone marrow transplantation. *Blood,* **74,** 1665–72.

Via, C. S. & Finkelman, F. D. (1993). Critical role of interleukin-2 in the development of acute graft-versus-host disease. *International Immunology,* **5,** 565–72.

Via, C. S., Nguyen, P., Shustov, A. *et al.* (1996). A major role for the Fas pathway in acute graft-versus-host disease. *Journal of Immunology,* **157,** 5387–93.

Wall, D. A., Hamberg, S. D., Reynolds, D. S. *et al.* (1988). Immunodeficiency in graft-versus-host reaction. I. Mechanism of immune suppression. *Journal of Immunology,* **140,** 2970–6.

Wall, D. A. & Sheehan, K. C. (1994). The role of tumor necrosis factor-alpha and interferon gamma in graft-versus-host disease and related immunodeficiency. *Transplantation,* **57,** 273–9.

Waller, E. K., Rosenthal, H., Jones, T. W. *et al.* (2001). Larger numbers of CD4(bright) dendritic cells in donor bone marrow are associated with increased relapse after allogeneic bone marrow transplantation. *Blood,* **97,** 2948–56.

Wang, J. W., Howson, J. M., Ghansah, T. *et al.* (2002). Influence of SHIP on the NK Repertoire and Allogeneic Bone Marrow Transplantation. *Science,* **295,** 2094–7.

Wang, M. G., Szebeni, J., Pearson, D. A. *et al.* (1995). Inhibition of graft-versus-host disease by interleukin-2 treatment is associated with altered cytokine production by expanded graft-versus-host-reactive CD4+ helper cells. *Transplantation,* **60,** 481–90.

Weiss, A. (1989). T lymphocyte activation. In *Fundamental Immunology,* ed. W. E. Paul, pp. 359–84. New York: Raven Press.

Weiss, G., Schwaighofer, H., & Herold, M. (1995). Nitric oxide formation as predictive parameter for acute graft-versus-host dis-ease after human allogeneic bone marrow transplantation. *Transplantation,* **60,** 1239–44.

Wekerle, T., Kurtz, J., Ito, H. *et al.* (2000). Allogeneic bone marrow transplantation with co-stimulatory blockade induces macrochimerism and tolerance without cytoreductive host treatment. *Nature Medicine,* **6,** 464–9.

Wells, A. D., Li, X. C., Li, Y. *et al.* (1999). Requirement for T-cell apoptosis in the induction of peripheral transplantation tolerance. *Nature Medicine,* **5,** 1303–7.

Welniak, L. A., Blazar, B. R., Anver, M. R. *et al.* (2000). Opposing roles of interferon-gamma on CD4+ T cell-mediated graft-versus-host disease: effects of conditioning. *Biology of Blood and Marrow Transplantation,* **6,** 604–12.

Whitmire, J. K. & Ahmed, R. (2000). Costimulation in antiviral immunity: differential requirements for CD4(+) and CD8(+) T cell responses. *Current Opinions in Immunology,* **12,** 448–55.

Wu, D. Y. & Goldschneider, I. (2001). Tolerance to cyclosporin A-induced autologous graft-versus-host disease is mediated by a CD4+CD25+ subset of recent thymic emigrants. *Journal of Immunology,* **166,** 7158–64.

Xun, C. Q., Thompson, J. S., Jennings, C. D. *et al.* (1994). Effect of total body irradiation, busulfan-cyclophosphamide, or cyclophosphamide conditioning on inflammatory cytokine release and development of acute and chronic graft-versus-host disease in H-2-incompatible transplanted SCID mice. *Blood,* **83,** 2360–7.

Yang, Y. G., Dey, B. R., Sergio, J. J. *et al.* (1998). Donor-derived interferon gamma is required for inhibition of acute graft-versus-host disease by interleukin 12. *Journal of Clinical Investigation,* **102,** 2126–35.

Zeller, J. C., Panoskaltsis-Mortari, A., Murphy, W. J. *et al.* (1999). Induction of CD4+ T cell alloantigen-specific hyporesponsiveness by IL-10 and TGF-beta. *Journal of Immunology,* **163,** 3684–91.

Zeng, D., Lewis, D., Dejbakhsh-Jones, S. *et al.* (1999). Bone marrow NK1.1(–) and NK1.1(+) T cells reciprocally regulate acute graft versus host disease. *Journal of Experimental Medicine,* **189,** 1073–81.

Zhang, Y., McCormick, L. L., Desai, S. R. *et al.* (2002). Murine sclerodermatous graft-versus-host disease, a model for human scleroderma: cutaneous cytokines, chemokines, and immune cell activation. *Journal of Immunology,* **168,** 3088–98.

Zheng, L., Fisher, G., Miller, R. E. *et al.* (1995). Induction of apoptosis in mature T cells by tumour necrosis factor. *Nature,* **377,** 348–51.

16 Role of natural killer cell alloreactivity in hematopoietic stem cell transplantation

ANDREA VELARDI AND ALESSANDRO MORETTA

University of Perugia and University of Genoa, Italy

Introduction

Natural killer (NK) cells are lymphocytes of innate immunity that kill cells and produce cytokines. They contribute to early defense against viral infections and mediate allogeneic responses in human leukocyte antigen (HLA)-disparate hematopoietic stem cell (HSC) transplants. Mismatched transplants have been developed over the past 10 years because not all patients have matched sibling or unrelated donors, and even fewer make it to transplant because of delays due to the donor search and bone marrow harvesting. However, virtually every patient has a family member who is identical for one HLA haplotype and fully mismatched for the other, and who could immediately serve as a donor. The use of such donors has presented a major challenge during the past three decades as a result of lethal GVHD and graft rejection.

During the early 1980s, effective T-cell depletion was shown to completely prevent GVHD in severe combined immune deficiency patients even when haploidentical 3-loci HLA-mismatched bone marrow was used (Reisner *et al.*, 1983). In leukemia patients, however, the benefit of GVHD prevention was offset by a markedly increased rate of graft rejection. Subsequent experimental data highlighted the crucial role of high numbers of hematopoietic stem cells for engraftment (Bachar-Lustig *et al.*, 1995). In leukemia patients, high-intensity immune and myeloablative conditioning regimens were combined with the transplantation of very large doses of T-cell-depleted, G-CSF-mobilized peripheral blood hematopoietic stem cells and hematopoietic transplantation across full HLA barriers became a clinical reality. The conditioning protocols, as well as the stem cell purification systems, evolved over time to reduce toxicity, improve engraftment, and reduce GVHD (Aversa *et al.*, 1994; Aversa *et al.*, 1998; Reisner *et al.*, 1999).

In mismatched transplants, the high frequency of alloreactive donor T cells recognizing major histocompatibility antigens causes lethal GVHD, and so extensive T-cell depletion is essential, as it is the only way to prevent GVHD. One unique feature of major HLA-disparate transplants is their ability to trigger another form of immune reaction directed from the donor to the recipient, which is mediated by NK cells.

Research in mice originally established the concepts of MHC class I recognition by NK cells (Kärre *et al.*, 1986). In humans NK cell lysis is negatively regulated by receptors (termed killer cell Ig-like receptors, or KIRs), which recognize epitopes ("KIR ligands") shared by certain major histocompatibility complex (MHC) class I alleles (Moretta A. *et al.*, 1997; Valiante *et al.*, 1997; Lanier 1998). Although KIRs and other inhibitory class I receptors, such as CD94/NKG2A, are broadly expressed on NK cells, in any given individual's repertoire there may be cells expressing a single KIR which are, therefore, blocked only by a specific (self) class I allele group. Missing expression of the correct inhibitory class I KIR ligand on mismatched allogeneic cells triggers NK cell alloreactivity (Ciccone *et al.*, 1988; Ciccone *et al.*, 1992a; Ciccone *et al.*, 1992b; Colonna *et al.*, 1993a; Colonna *et al.*, 1993b). It is well established that MHC class I molecules control rejection of bone marrow grafts by host NK cells in mice (Öhlén *et al.*, 1998).

This chapter describes the biology underlying NK cell alloreactivity and focuses on its role in hematopoietic stem cell transplantation (Ruggieri *et al.*, 2002; Farag *et al.*, 2002).

Natural killer cell biology and alloreactivity

Natural killer cells are lymphoid cells that play an important role in innate immune responses by killing a variety of tumor and virus-infected cells and by secreting cytokines, such as TNF-α and IFN-γ and chemokines, especially MIP-1 and RANTES (Kiessling *et al.*, 1975; Trincheri 1990; Biron, 1998).

Unlike T or B lymphocytes, NK cells do not require a specialized gene rearrangement to create a receptor repertoire capable of discriminating different targets. Thus, NK cells kill tumors or virally infected cells expressing decreased levels of self-MHC class I molecules and certain allogeneic cells, but spare normal autologous cells (Heberman *et al.*, 1975; Kärre *et al.*, 1986; Moretta L. *et al.*, 1992). Based on this evidence, Ljunggren and Kärre (1990) formulated the "missing self" hypothesis: NK cells ignore autologous cells which express adequate levels of major histocompatibility complex (MHC) class I molecules. On the contrary, cells not expressing self class I molecules promote an NK cell-mediated immune response. It was also suggested MHC-specific receptors are expressed on NK cells. Upon recognition of their (self) HLA class I ligands, these receptors may deliver inhibitory signals to downregulate NK cell functions.

Pioneering studies using human NK cell clones (Ferrini et al., 1987) indicated that the NK cell function is regulated by recognition of HLA on target cells. These studies demonstrated (1) human NK clones may kill allogeneic targets, (2) clonal heterogeneity in killing allogeneic cells, and (3) different NK specificities within a given individual's repertoire (Ciccone et al., 1988; Moretta L. et al., 1994), that is, NK clones discriminated in killing one or more types of allogeneic targets from a representative panel (Ciccone et al., 1992a). Genetic analysis demonstrated the genes governing resistance/susceptibility to lysis were located on chromosome 6 (Ciccone et al., 1990). Further studies provided proof that NK cells spare autologous cells expressing normal levels of HLA class I but kill HLA defective autologous cell variants. All these data, together with the analysis of HLA class I negative target cells transfected with different HLA molecules, demonstrated that HLA-C alleles have a pivotal role in the mechanism of target cell protection from NK cell-mediated-cytotoxicity (Ciccone et al., 1992b; Colonna et al., 1992).

Two distinct allelic groups of HLA-C molecules protect target cells from lysis mediated by different groups of NK clones (Colonna et al., 1993; Ciccone et al., 1994). Group 1 contains the Cw1, 3, 7, and 9 alleles, while Group 2 includes Cw2, 4, 5, and 6. The two groups of alleles can be distinguished on the basis of alternative amino acid sequence motifs at position 77 and 80 of the α helix (Biassoni et al., 1995; Winter et al., 1997). Thus, a group of NK cell clones is cytolytic against cell transfectants expressing Group 2 HLA-C alleles (characterized by Asn 77, Lys 80), but not against those expressing Group 2 HLA-C alleles (Ser 77, Asp 80). These data suggested the existence of different inhibitory receptors for HLA-C alleles expressed by the two groups of NK clones.

In 1990, two monoclonal antibodies (GL183 and EB6) were found to react with distinct, partially overlapping subsets of human NK cells (Moretta A. et al., 1990a; Moretta A. et al., 1990b). The surface molecules recognized by EB6 (termed P58.1 molecules) or by GLI83 (P58.2 molecules) were clonally distributed and expressed by CD16+ but not by CD16−, CD56+ NK cells. Expression of these molecules correlated with the ability of NK cells to mediate specific recognition of allogeneic targets. Thus, EB6+ GLI83− (P58.1+, P58.2−) cells corresponded to NK cells displaying specificity 1 and EB6−, GLI83+ (P58.1−, P58.2+) NK cells displayed specificity 2, while double-positive NK cells were unable to kill normal allogeneic target cells (Moretta A. et al., 1990a; Vitale et al., 1995). Antibodies against P58 molecules strongly inhibited NK-mediated cytotoxicity in redirected killing assays against murine P815 target cells, while anti-P58 mAb strongly enhanced the NK-mediated lysis of HLA class I+ human tumors (Moretta A. et al., 1990a; Moretta A. et al., 1990b). These data first suggested that P58 molecules represented the inhibitory receptors involved in NK alloreactivity.

In 1993, the P58 molecules were identified as the NK receptors for HLA-C molecules (Moretta A. et al., 1993), as it was shown that P58.1 and P58.2 molecules were specifically involved in the recognition of HLA-Cw4 (group 2) and HLA-Cw3 (group 1) alleles. MAb blocking of the interaction between P58 receptors and HLA-C molecules reconstituted lysis of HLA "protected" target cells (Moretta A. et al., 1996).

These studies demonstrated that HLA-specific inhibitory receptors exist on human NK cells and that they regulate NK-mediated cytotoxicity against allogeneic cells and against tumors.

One year later additional inhibitory receptors were found to be involved in HLA recognition. The NKB1 (or P70) receptor recognizes HLA-B alleles of the Bw4 supertype (Litwin et al., 1994), and the CD94 receptor recognizes cells transfected with Bw6, but not with Bw4, alleles (Moretta A. et al., 1994).

In 1995 molecular variants of the HLA-C receptors were discovered. The EB6 and the GLI83 mAb, in addition to the P58 molecules, also recognized shorter (P50) molecular variants mediating activation rather than inhibition (Moretta A. et al., 1995).

Molecular cloning of HLA-C (Colonna et al., 1995; Wagtmann et al., 1995) and HLA-B (D'Andrea et al., 1995) specific receptors demonstrated that they belong to the Ig superfamily and are encoded by nonrearranging genes located on chromosome 19. They were subsequently termed killer Ig-like receptors or KIR. The difference in molecular size between inhibitory (P58) and activating (P50) HLA-C receptors was found to be due to the different length of their cytoplasmic tails. The cytoplasmic tail of the inhibitory receptors contains "Immune receptor Tyrosine-based Inhibition Motives" (ITIM) which, once phosphorylated (upon engagement of the receptor with its ligands), bind the SH2 domains of phosphatases such as SHP.1 and SHP.2 (reviewed in Long, 1999). When inhibitory KIR bind their HLA ligand, src family kinases phosphorylate the ITIM, allowing binding of the tyrosine phosphatase SHP-1 (and possibly SHP-2) through its SH2 domain. SHP-1 is able to dephosphorylate multiple targets in the immune receptor tyrosine-based activating motives (ITAM) activating pathway, thereby mediating its negative signal. Since the activation of NK cytotoxicity requires the activity of tyrosine kinases, the inhibitory receptors block NK cell effector functions (cytotoxicity and cytokine secretion) by recruiting tyrosine phosphatases which counteract the kinase activity.

The activating (P50) receptors for HLA-C do not contain ITIM in their short cytoplasmic tail. However, they display characteristic transmembrane regions (Biassoni et al., 1996; Bottino et al., 1996; Bottino et al., 2000) that allow association with signaling polypeptides (KARAP/DAP12) (Olcese et al., 1997; Lanier et al., 1998), which contain ITAM.

The CD94 receptors also mediate activating and inhibiting functions (Pérez-Villar et al., 1995). The CD94 molecules form a series of heterodimers with different members of the NKG2 family (Lazetic et al., 1996; Carretero et al., 1997; Cantoni et al., 1998). Association between CD94 and NKG2A results in a receptor displaying inhibitory functions (Sivori et al., 1996), whereas the CD94/NKG2C heterodimer induces triggering signals (Cantoni *et al.*, 1998). Like the HLA-C specific receptors, the inhibitory NKG2 molecules (NKG2A) are characterized by ITIM sequences, and the activating NKG2 chains (NKG2C) associate with ITAM-containing signaling polypeptides (Houchins *et al.*, 1991; Houchins *et al.*, 1997). It is now well established that the various CD94/NKG2 receptors recognize nonclassical HLA class Ib molecules. They bind HLA-E molecules complexed with peptides derived from the leader sequences of certain HLA class I alleles (Braud *et al.*, 1998; Borrego *et al.*, 1998; Lee *et al.*, 1998). The HLA-E binding to leader sequences of Bw6 alleles, but not of Bw4 alleles, is in line with the original observation that the CD94/NKG2 receptors distinguish between Bw4 and Bw6-transfected cells (Moretta A. *et al.*, 1994).

Each NK cell may express multiple inhibitory receptors (Vitale *et al.*, 1995; Vitale *et al.*, 1996), so the human NK cell repertoire in every single individual is the consequence of the NK cell gene expression of different combinations of the various KIRs and of the CD94/NKG2 molecules. Importantly, every NK cell in the repertoire expresses at least one receptor that is specific for self HLA class I molecules, so the individual's HLA selects the self-tolerant repertoire.

KIR are encoded by a compact family of genes on chromosome 19, which exhibits extensive haplotypic variation in gene number and content as well as allelic polymorphism for individual genes (Uhrberg *et al.*, 1997; Wilson *et al.*, 2000; Vilches *et al.*, 2002). Variations in KIR gene expression are due to polymorphism of the gene rather than to differential regulation of gene expression. Indeed, in no instance does an individual possess a KIR gene not found to be expressed by some NK cell. Importantly the KIR repertoire is defined and stable over time and cannot be perturbed by infection or other environmental agents (Vilches *et al.*, 2002). Genes encoding CD94 and NKG2 family members are conserved in the population and are encoded on chromosome 12 in the human natural killer complex (NKC). Since the genes for KIR, HLA and CD94/NKG2 are located on different chromosomes, both ligands and receptors can segregate independently in human pedigrees. As a consequence, a substantial fraction of the population has genes for KIR for which they have no HLA class I ligands. The number of KIR ligands varies from one to three depending on a person's HLA type (whereas every person can be expected to express HLA molecules that engage CD94/NKG2A). The number of KIR ligands determines the extent of KIR usage as inhibitory receptors; the CD94/NKG2A may compensate for lack of KIR usage (Uhrberg *et al.*, 1997; Valiante *et al.*, 1997b).

In molecular terms, the human NK cell receptor repertoire is highly diverse. This was directly demonstrated by the extensive analysis of NK cell clones which indicated that at least 30 different receptor phenotypes (KIR and CD94/NKG2) can be identified on a panel of 100 NK clones (Valiante *et al.*, 1997a). Using the RT-PCR based typing system, over 20 different phenotypes were detected in a panel of 68 donors (Uhrberg *et al.*, 1997). The most common, found in 33% of the donors, were expression of the four major inhibitory KIRs (KIR2DL1, KIR2DL3, KIR3DL1, and

KIR3DL2), the activating KIR2DS4, and the HLA-G specific KIR2DL4. All the individuals expressed KIR2DL1, KIR2DL2, and KIR2DL4. Importantly, KIR2DL1, which is specific for one HLA-C allele group, and either KIR2DL2 or KIR2DL3, which are specific for the other, were present in all. The P70/KIR3DL1 receptor for Bw4 was expressed in all but four.

As stated above, in humans the NK tolerance to self is related to the expression of at least one inhibitory receptor for self HLA class I by every NK cell in the repertoire, indicating that the HLA class I type influences the repertoire of NK cells expressing inhibitory HLA class I receptors for self. A study focused on this issue (Shilling *et al.*, 2002) and demonstrated that KIR genes dominate over HLA class I genes in determining the KIR repertoire expressed by mature NK cells. The study also showed the HLA class I genotype modifies the relative frequencies of NK cells expressing particular KIRs. Thus, the HLA class I genotype imposes selection during development of the NK cell receptor repertoire by dictating which KIRs are to be used as inhibitory receptors for self-HLA class I. However, since KIRs are expressed stochastically, a proportion of NK cell clones will express the CD94/NKG2A receptor in order to be tolerant to self. Indeed, a coordinate expression of the two types of genes appears to exist, since virtually all KIR-negative NK cells express CD94/NKG2A, while KIR+ cells may be predominantly CD94/NKG2A−.

NK cell-mediated alloreactivity

Thus, alloreactive NK clones may be restricted to cells that use KIRs as a source of inhibitory receptors for self HLA class I molecules. Indeed, KIR−/CD94:NKG2A+ cells may not be alloreactive since all individuals express its ligand, HLA-E. On the other hand, among KIR+ NK cells the high diversity in terms of KIR expression may ensure that in individuals mismatched for the two subgroups of HLA-C alleles, the KIR repertoire (dictated by the KIR genotype but controlled by the HLA genotype), will allow the generation of alloreactive NK cells. Thus NK cells expressing the KIR2DL1 (P58.1) receptor specific for group 2 HLA-C alleles will be able to kill cells expressing group 1 (but not group 2) HLA-C alleles (Moretta A. *et al.*, 1990a). Vice versa, NK cells expressing either one of the two inhibitory receptors (KIR2DL2 or KIR2DL3) specific for group 1 HLA-C alleles will be able to kill target cells expressing group 2 (but not group 1) HLA-C alleles (Moretta A. *et al.*, 1993). Obviously, NK cells coexpressing inhibitory receptors for both HLA-C groups are not alloreactive, because every individual expresses alleles from either one or both HLA-C groups.

Cells expressing the Bw4-specific KIR3DL1 receptor are also alloreactive effectors, as they kill Bw4− (Bw6+) cells but not, of course, cells expressing Bw4+ alleles.

Triggering NK receptors

It is now generally accepted that the regulation of human NK cell function is controlled by the recognition of HLA class I molecules by appropriate inhibitory receptors. When a target cell does not express HLA class I ligands for the inhibitory receptors (for example allogeneic cells, infected or transformed cells) (Moretta A. *et al.*, 1996; Garrido *et al.*, 1997; Pende *et al.*, 1998), the effector function of NK cells may be induced by a series of NK receptors that are involved in triggering of NK-mediated cytotoxicity and cytokine/chemokine release. Such receptors are specific for non-HLA ligands expressed at the cell surface of potential target cells and their function is normally counterbalanced by that of the inhibitory receptors (Moretta A. *et al.*, 2001). This balance, however, is rapidly altered as soon as the magnitude of the inhibitory signals is decreased by an insufficient engagement of the HLA-specific inhibitory receptors.

The nature of the triggering NK receptors has been identified as a heterogeneous family of NK-specific Ig-like molecules termed natural cytotoxicity receptors (including NKp30, NKp46, and NKp44) (Sivori *et al.*, 1997; Pessino *et al.*, 1998; Vitale *et al.*, 1998; Cantoni *et al.*, 1999; Pende *et al.*, 1999; Moretta A. *et al.*, 2000; Moretta A. *et al.*, 2001) and by NKG2D, a member of the lectin superfamily which is shared by NK and cytolytic T cells (Moretta A. *et al.*, 2001; Cerwenka *et al.*, 2001; Diefenbach *et al.*, 2001). The NKp44 and NKp30 receptors are encoded on chromosome 6, while NKp46 and NKG2D receptors are on chromosomes 19 and 12, respectively. The cellular ligands for NCR still remain to be determined while those for NKG2D are the class I-like molecules MICA/B (Bauer *et al.*, 1999) and ULBP (Sutherland *et al.*, 2001). Functional studies indicate that the ligands recognized by NCR and NKG2D are expressed on most tumor target cells analyzed (Pende *et al.*, 1998; Sivori *et al.*, 1999; Sivori *et al.*, 2000a; Sivori *et al.*, 2000b; Sivori *et al.*, 2001; Pende *et al.*, 2001; Moretta A. *et al.*, 2001; Costello *et al.*, 2002). Both NCR and NKG2D transduce activating signals because of their physical association with ITAM-containing polypeptides. These are DAP12 that associates to NKp44, CD3β that associates to NKp30 and NKp46 (Moretta A. *et al.*, 2000; Moretta A. *et al.*, 2001) and DAP10 in the case of NKG2D (Cerwenka *et al.*, 2001; Diefenbach *et al.*, 2001). Similar to the activating forms of the triggering receptors specific for HLA class I (KIR2DS and CD94/NKG2C), the association of these non-HLA specific receptors with ITAM-containing polypeptides requires the presence of charged residues in the transmembrane region of the receptors. Additional molecules have been implicated in NK cell activation possibly acting as coreceptors able to enhance the function of NCR and NKG2D. These molecules are 2B4 (Sivori *et al.*, 2000a), NTB-A (Bottino *et al.*, 2001), and CD2 (Lanier *et al.*, 1997) that are members of the so-called CD2-like molecular superfamily encoded on chromosome 1, and the NKp80 molecule (Vitale *et al.*, 2001) encoded on the NK gene complex on chromosome 12 together with NKG2D and CD94/NKG2A.

As receptors and ligands involved in NK cell activation are continuously being identified, our perception of the rules governing NK cell function is changing accordingly. For example, under normal conditions NK cells were once believed to be tonically activated by ligands expressed on normal tissues and a continuous inhibition via the HLA class I-specific receptors was required to prevent normal cell damage. Now it is quite clear that this concept is only partially correct and that a number of exceptions to this rule exist (Raulet *et al.*, 2001). Thus, a target cell may become NK-susceptible by upregulating one or another ligand for the triggering receptors while remaining substantially normal in terms of HLA class I expression (Lanier *et al.*, 1997; Raulet *et al.*, 2001). Conversely, certain tissues, even when they fail to express inhibitory HLA class I molecules, display no susceptibility to NK-mediated cytotoxicity (Ruggeri *et al.*, 1998; Ruggeri *et al.*, 2002; Costello *et al.*, 2002). In this case the level of expression of adhesion molecules and/or ligands recognized by the triggering receptors may be insufficient to induce NK-cell activation. In other situations, the low surface density of the triggering receptors has been implicated in the inability of NK lymphocytes to kill autologous tumor cells (Costello *et al.*, 2002). It has been speculated that the ability of NK cells to discriminate among target cells expressing high or low surface density of the triggering ligands may have represented the original principle utilized by primordial NK cells during evolution, even before the expression of MHC-specific inhibitory receptors (Khakoo *et al.*, 2000; Diefemback *et al.*, 2001).

Role in haploidentical HSC transplants

Allogeneic hematopoietic transplantation may cure leukemia through two sequential mechanisms: (1) a myeloablative and immune suppressive radiotherapy- and/or chemotherapy-based conditioning regimen, and (2) T lymphocytes in the graft recognizing and eliminating residual leukemic cells, which survive the conditioning regimen and have the potential to cause relapse of the underlying malignancy (reviewed in Thomas *et al.*, 1999). Donor T lymphocytes react against host alloantigens expressed by normal lymphohematopoietic and/or leukemic cells (Molldrem *et al.*, 2000; Mutis *et al.*, 2002). As a consequence, they also mediate graft-versus-host disease (GVHD). The immunosuppression required to prevent or treat GVHD, in turn, is responsible for infections or leukemic relapses, which are frequent causes of transplant failure and patient death.

For the many leukemic patients who could not find a suitable matched donor (see introduction), hematopoietic transplantation across HLA barriers became a clinical reality when high-intensity immune and myeloablative conditioning regimens were combined with the transplantation of very large numbers of highly purified peripheral blood hematopoietic stem cells (Aversa *et al.*, 1994; Aversa *et al.*, 1998). In mismatched transplants, lethal GVHD develops as a consequence of the high frequencies of alloreactive donor T cells recognizing major histocompatibility antigens. Therefore, the alloreactivity of T lymphocytes cannot be exploited to clear leukemic cells and, indeed, extensive T-cell depletion of the graft is mandatory to prevent GVHD. As a consequence, a major question arose: is there any chance, in mismatched transplants, of obtaining a graft-versus-leukemia (GVL) effect? The discovery of NK cell alloreactivity (see above) offered an important clue.

Indeed, a unique feature of major HLA-disparate transplants is their ability to trigger NK cell alloreactions (Ruggeri et al., 1998; Ruggeri et al., 2002). In full haplotype-mismatched hematopoietic stem cell transplantation, in which donors and recipient pairs are identical for one HLA haplotype and incompatible at the HLA class I and II loci of the unshared haplotype, all cases are at high risk of T-cell mediated alloreactions in the host-versus-graft (HVG), as well as in the graft-versus-host (GVH) direction. These T-cell-mediated responses can be controlled to a large extent by (1) an appropriate immunosuppressive intensity of the conditioning regimen to prevent graft rejection, and (2) extensive T-cell depletion of the graft to prevent GVHD. However, another type of alloreactivity is provided by mismatches at the epitopes expressed by HLA class I alleles that are recognized by KIRs expressed by NK cells (Table 16.1 and Fig. 16.1). For example, individuals who are homozygous for Group 2 HLA-C alleles generate NK cells that express KIR specific for Group 2 HLA-C alleles (e.g., KIR2DL1) (Table 16.1), while individuals who are homozygous for Group 1 HLA-C alleles generate NK cells with KIR specific for Group 1 HLA-C alleles (e.g., KIR2DL2/3). Thus, since NK cells distinguish groups of HLA-class I molecules and not single allelic variants (Table 16.1), haploidentical transplants can be classified in two categories on the basis of HLA typing: (1) "NK matched" donor-recipient combinations in which NK alloreactivity does not occur because KIR of the graft recognize HLA class I alleles of the host; (2) "NK mismatched" donor-recipient combinations, in which NK cells in the graft express KIR that do not recognize HLA class I molecules expressed in the host. In this case, grafted NK cells are alloreactive in the GVH direction.

In HLA haplotype-mismatched hematopoietic transplantation with a potential for graft-versus-host NK reactions, Ruggeri et al. (1998) observed that the engrafted stem cells gave rise to an NK cell wave of donor origin containing high-frequency donor-versus-recipient alloreactive NK clones which killed pretransplant cryopreserved host lymphocytes, and which could only be blocked by targets expressing the donor class I allele group missing in the recipient. Remarkably, alloreactive NK clones killed 100% acute and chronic myeloid leukemias, but only a minority of acute lymphoblastic leukemias (ALL). Interestingly, ALL resistance to killing was associated with no expression of LFA-1 on tumor cells.

These data suggested, for the first time, that donor-versus-recipient NK cell alloreactivity could result in improved transplant outcomes.

Animal transplant models

Experimental evidence suggests that NK cells predominantly attack the hematopoietic cells of the host while sparing other tissues which are common targets for T-cell-mediated GVH disease. For example, in the hybrid resistance murine model, alloreactive NK cells cause rejection of bone marrow grafts, but do not appear to attack other tissues. Indeed, the hybrid mouse readily tolerates organ grafts (reviewed in Murphy et al., 2001). Studies in mice suggested that allogeneic NK cells can mediate a GVL effect in the absence of GVHD (Glass et al., 1996; Zeis et al., 1997; Asai et al., 1998; Hyraiama et al., 1998).

Table 16.1. *HLA-class I allele specificity of the main KIR expressed by human NK cells*

KIR genes	Encoded protein	HLA specificity
1. KIR 2DL1	P58.1 receptor	HLA-C group 2 (-Cw2, -Cw4, -Cw5, -Cw6) (Asn77, Lys80)[a]
2. KIR 2DL2/3	P58.2 receptor	HLA-C group 1 (-Cw1, -Cw3, -Cw7, -Cw8) (Ser77, Asn80)[a]
3. KIR 3DL1	P70/NKB1 receptor	all Bw4 alleles (e.g., HLA-B27)
4. KIR 3DL2	P140 receptor	HLA-A3 and A11 alleles

Each KIR group comprises one to six alleles, which differ by 1–9 nucleotide substitutions (Uhrberg et al., 1997). KIR 2D refer to receptor molecules with two Ig-like a domains whereas KIR 3D refer to those displaying 3 Ig-like domains. Receptors having a long (inhibitory) cytoplasmic tail are designated as L (long), whereas those having an activating short tail are termed S.

[a] Note that the two groups of HLA-C alleles can be distinguished on the basis of alternative aminoacid sequence motif at position 77 and 80 of the α 1 helix. Site-directed mutagenesis unequivocally demonstrated that these residues are crucial for KIR-mediated recognition.

N.B. Additional KIR genes are KIR2DL4 that codes for an HLA-G specific receptor, and various genes which code for activating receptors (including P50.1/KIR2DS1, P50.2/KIR2DS2, and P50.3/KIR2DS4).

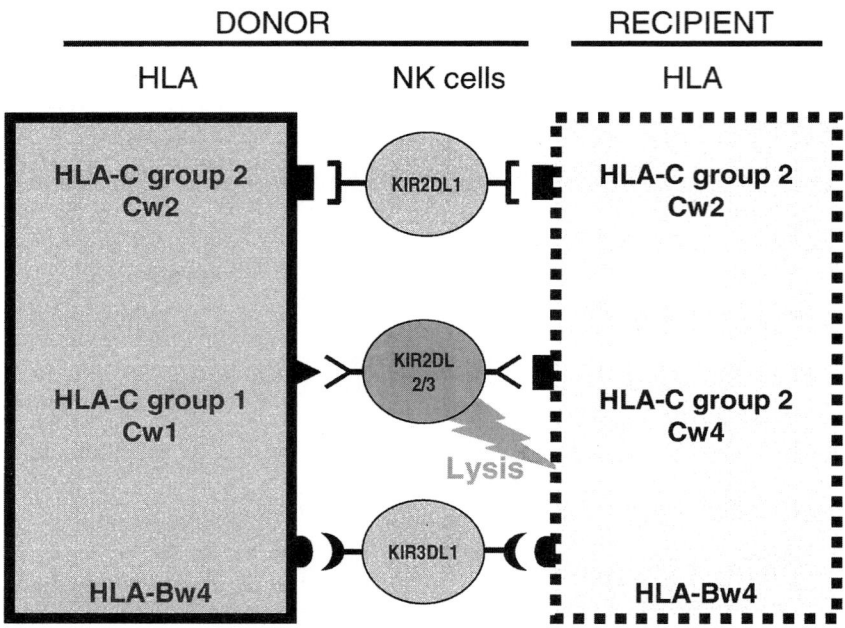

Fig. 16.1. Donor-versus-recipient NK cell alloreactivity in HLA haplotype-mismatched transplants. This figure illustrates one example of several possible HLA haplotype-mismatched transplants with NK cell alloreactivity in the GVH direction. Besides being HLA haplotype-mismatched, this transplant is also KIR ligand-mismatched in the GVH direction. In this example, the NK cell in the donor repertoire (expressing KIR2DL2/3) is blocked by self HLA-Cw1 (a "Group 1" HLA-C allele), but not by the recipient HLA-Cw4 (a "Group 2" HLA-C allele). Consequently, this NK cell is alloreactive and lyses recipient's cells (lightning bolt). Remarkably, when donor-recipient haplo-mismatched pairs are also KIR ligand mismatched in the GVH direction (as in this example), 100% of the donors tested had alloreactive NK cells in their repertoires. On the other hand, in the haplo-mismatched pairs that were not KIR ligand-mismatched in the GVH direction no donor alloreactive NK cells were found (Ruggeri et al., 2002).

In a series of experiments (Ruggeri et al., 2002), human alloreactive NK clones were infused into human AML-engrafted NOD-SCID mice. Mice infused with human AML developed advanced disease in 5 to 6 weeks. If left untreated, or given non-alloreactive human NK clones, mice died over the following 3 weeks. In contrast, much fewer human alloreactive NK cells cleared leukemia, and mice survived until sacrifice (120 days).

Ruggeri et al. (2002) next tested whether alloreactive NK cells ablate the host immune system, thereby allowing engraftment of haploidentical hematopoietic transplants in an MHC mismatched F_1 parent mouse bone marrow transplant (BMT) model. In F_1 H-$2^{d/b}$ to parent H-2^b transplants, donor T cells are tolerant of the recipient MHC, but donor NK cells not expressing H-2^b-specific Ly49C/I inhibitory receptor, and bearing instead H-2^d-specific Ly49A/G2 receptors, are activated to kill the recipient's targets. Alloreactive NK cells did not cause GVHD even when infused in high numbers into lethally irradiated recipients. However, in nonlethally irradiated recipients, alloreactive NK cells, but not control non-alloreactive NK cells, reduced recipient-type T cell and granulocyte counts in marrow and spleen to levels observed after lethal irradiation.

Mice conditioned with nonlethal (<7 Gy) total body irradiation (TBI) alone rejected donor marrow grafts. In contrast, all recipients conditioned with non-lethal irradiation and alloreactive NK cells engrafted with durable, donor-type hematopoietic chimerism. Notably, as few as 2×10^5 alloreactive NK cells resulted in major donor hematopoiesis; nonalloreactive NK cells had no effect. Similar results were obtained in F_1 H-$2^{d/b}$ to parent H-2^d transplants. In this case, donor NK cells used for conditioning did not express H-2^d-specific Ly49A/G2 receptors, and expressed instead the H-2^b-specific Ly49C/I receptor. Alloreactive NK cells allowed mismatched BMT even when combined with reduced-intensity conditioning regimens adopted from HLA-matched human transplant practice (reviewed in Giralt et al., 2000). Thus, mice given these regimens plus low doses of alloreactive NK cells achieved >80% donor chimerism, unlike controls receiving nonalloreactive NK cells (Fig. 16.2). Even after milder immune suppression, fludarabine alone, followed by the infusion of alloreactive NK cells, recipients achieved a substantial degree of donor chimerism (30%). The infusion of alloreactive NK cells 6 weeks posttransplant was able to convert mixed chimeras to stable full-donor chimerism.

Ruggeri et al. (2002) next tested whether NK conditioning could reduce the need for extensive T-cell depletion. Lethally irradiated H-2^b mice transplanted with H-2^d bone marrow containing 10^6 T cells died from GVHD in 2 to 4 weeks. After conditioning with TBI plus alloreactive NK cells, cohorts of transplanted mice were given escalating doses of H-2^d T-cells. Even with as many as 2×10^7 T cells, 100% of mice survived until sacrifice (120 days) with no signs of GVHD. In contrast, adminis-

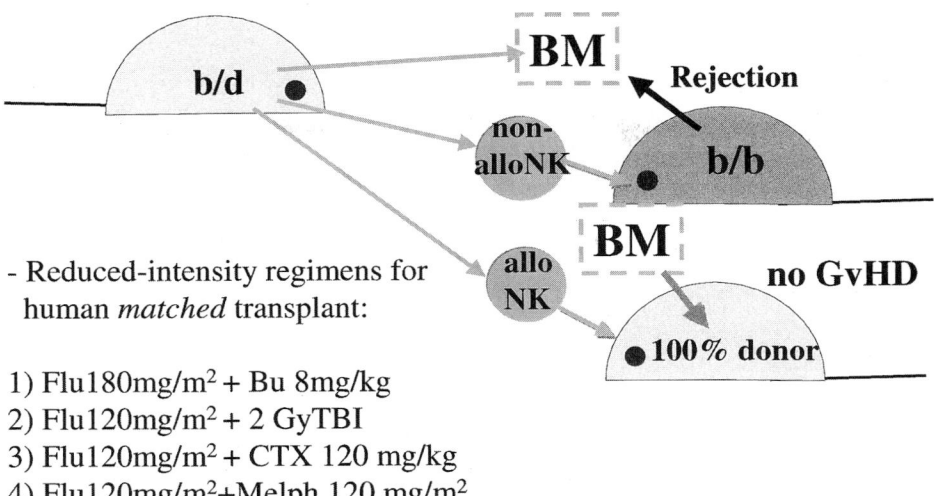

- Reduced-intensity regimens for human *matched* transplant:

1) Flu180mg/m² + Bu 8mg/kg
2) Flu120mg/m² + 2 GyTBI
3) Flu120mg/m² + CTX 120 mg/kg
4) Flu120mg/m²+Melph 120 mg/m²

Fig. 16.2. Alloreactive NK cells ablate the host immune system thereby allowing engraftment of haploidentical hematopoietic stem cell transplants in an MHC mismatched F_1 parent mouse bone marrow transplant model (Ruggeri *et al.,* 2002). In F_1 H-$2^{d/b}$ parent H-2^b transplants, donor T cells are tolerant of the recipient MHC, but donor NK cells not expressing H-2^b-specific Ly49C/I inhibitory receptor, and bearing instead H-2^d-specific Ly49A/G2 receptors, are activated to kill the recipient's targets. The pretransplant infusion of alloreactive NK cells enables mismatched BMT, even when performed with reduced-intensity conditioning regimens adopted from HLA-matched human transplant practice (reviewed in Giralt *et al.,* 2000). Thus, mice given these regimens plus low doses of alloreactive NK cells achieve >80% donor chimerism with no GVHD, unlike controls receiving the drugs alone or followed by non-alloreactive NK cells (top right).

tration of nonalloreactive NK cells, even in very high numbers, provided no protection. It could be hypothesized that this protection might be mediated by alloreactive NK cells attacking recipient antigen-presenting cells (APCs), shown to be responsible for initiating GVHD (Shlomchik *et al.,* 1999) and that, consequently, mice with APCs that are resistant to alloreactive NK killing might not be protected from GVHD. Ruggeri *et al.* (2002) therefore made B6xBALB/c to B6 bone marrow chimeras to replace the alloreactive NK cell-sensitive H-2^b mouse hematopoietic cells, including APCs, with H-$2^{d/b}$ cells that

would be resistant to NK cell killing (H-$2^{d/b}$ H-2^b chimeras). While the H-2^d allele protects against alloreactive NK cells, the H-2^b molecules can still present antigen to donor H-2^d T cells, thus priming GVH reactions. When analyzed 4 months posttransplant, > 90% of bone marrow, spleen, and gut dendritic cells in these chimeras were of H-$2^{d/b}$ origin. When these chimeras were reconditioned with TBI plus alloreactive NK cells and reconstituted with H-2^d BMT containing 10^6 T cells, 100% died from GVHD. Control H-2^b H-2^b chimeras given 2×10^7 T cells survived with no signs of GVHD (Fig. 16.3). It was also found

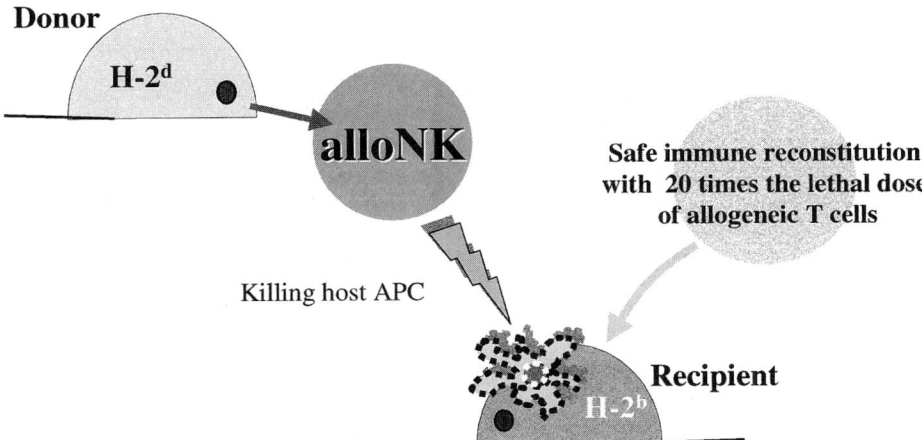

Fig. 16.3. NK conditioning reduces the need for extensive T cell depletion (Ruggeri *et al.,* 2002). Lethally-irradiated H-2^b mice transplanted with H-2^d bone marrow containing 10^6 T cells die from GVHD in 2 to 4 weeks. After conditioning with TBI plus alloreactive NK cells, transplanted mice can be given as many as 2×10^7 T cells and survive with no signs of GVHD. Alloreactive NK cells ablated bone marrow, spleen, and gut APCs, indicating that alloreactive NK cells prevent GVHD via elimination of recipient APCs.

that alloreactive NK cells accelerated the loss of bone marrow, spleen, and gut APCs, as compared to mice conditioned with either TBI or TBI plus nonalloreactive NK cells. Taken together, these data indicate that alloreactive NK cells prevent GVHD via elimination of recipient APCs. Therefore, in the mouse model, alloreactive NK cells not only fail to cause GVHD, but can also block the T-cell-mediated GVHD which is initiated by DC. In addition, alloreactive NK cells used in the pretransplant conditioning regimen protected from GVHD to such an extent as to allow a safe infusion of otherwise lethal doses of allogeneic T cells (Ruggeri et al., 2002).

Impact on clinical HSC transplantation

Ruggeri et al. (2002) next determined the impact of donor-versus-recipient NK cell alloreactivity on clinical relapse, rejection, GVHD, and survival. One hundred and twelve high-risk acute leukemia patients received hematopoietic stem cell transplants from HLA haplotype-mismatched family donors (Aversa et al., 1994; Aversa et al., 1998; Martelli et al., 2002). Typing of the HLA-C locus was available in 92 of these individuals (57 with acute myeloid leukemia (AML) and 35 with acute lymphoblastic leukemia (ALL) (Table 16.2). Overall, primary engraftment was achieved in 90.2%, GVHD occurred in 8.6%, event-free survival was 26% in AML and 8% in ALL.

To evaluate the role of donor-versus-recipient NK alloreactivity in transplantation outcomes, donor-recipient pairs were divided into two groups: the first without, and the second with, KIR ligand incompatibility in the GVH direction (Table 16.3). Donors were evaluated for NK alloreactivity by screening >200 NK clones (>100 on each of two separate occasions), and were scored positive when the frequency of lytic clones was <1 in 50 (as a rule, frequencies of positive clones were either high, 1 in 2 to 1 in 20, or nondetectable, < 1 in 200). KIR ligand incompatibility correlated closely with detection of donor NK clones killing recipient targets. Transplantation from NK alloreactive

donors totally protected from rejection, and GVHD (Table 16.3). As predicted by the in vitro ALL resistance to alloreactive NK killing, GVH KIR ligand incompatibility had no effect on ALL relapse (Table 16.3 and Fig. 16.4). Most impressively, again as predicted by the in vitro killing assays and by the alloreactive NK cell rescue of AML bearing mice, transplantation from NK alloreactive donors totally controlled AML relapse (Table 16.3 and Fig. 16.4). In AML, the probability of event-free survival at 5 years was 5% in the first group versus 60% in the second ($P < 0.0005$) (Fig. 16.5). Multivariate analysis which considered crucial variables affecting transplantation outcome, such as conditioning regimens, number of stem cells and T cells in the graft, and status of disease at transplant, showed GVH KIR ligand incompatibility to be the only independent predictor of survival in AML. Conversely, absence of GVH KIR ligand incompatibility was the only independent factor predicting poor outcome (hazard ratio 0.33, 95% confidence interval 0.11–0.94, $P < 0.04$).

These data show that spontaneously generated NK cell alloreactions from stem cell grafts are associated with a remarkable GVL effect and complete control of rejection and GVHD. This impacts dramatically on survival of AML patients (5% in the absence versus 60% in the presence of NK alloreactivity). This is far better than survival after matched unrelated-donor transplant (reviewed in Thomas et al., 1999), which is 34% in 1st complete remission, 27% in 2nd complete remission, and 7% in ≥ 3rd complete remission or in relapse (see insert in Fig. 16.5). This survival rate is striking, as most of our AML patients were in ≥ 3rd complete remission or in relapse (Table 16.2).

The haploidentical transplant study provided direct evidence that KIR ligand incompatibility in the GVH direction is, without exception, predictive of donor-versus-recipient NK cell alloreactivity. Furthermore, analyses to date of 32 unrelated normal donor pairs indicate KIR ligand mismatches are predictive of NK cell alloreactivity also among genetically unrelated individuals (Velardi et al., unpublished observations). NK cell alloreactivity, whether between related or unrelated individuals, can be explained by the following observations. As stated above, almost everyone in the general population possesses major KIR genes. In particular, the study by Uhberg et al. (1997) shows KIR2DL1, which is specific for one HLA-C allele group, and either KIR2DL2 or KIR2DL3, which are specific for the other, are present in all individuals. The P70/KIR3DL1 receptor for Bw4 is expressed in > 90% of people. In other words, almost everybody can generate different NK cell clones expressing an inhibitory receptor for each of the self HLA class I ligands. Although KIRs and CD94/NKG2A inhibitory receptors may be coexpressed by NK cells, in any given individual's NK repertoire there may be cells which express a single KIR and are blocked only by a specific class I allele group. Missing expression of the KIR ligand on mismatched allogeneic cells can therefore trigger NK cell alloreactivity.

Susceptibility to NK alloreactivity is limited by the recipient's HLA type. Approximately 30% of the population express all major HLA class I KIR ligands (HLA-C group 1, HLA-C

Table 16.2. *Disease status at transplant and graft composition in 92 HLA haplotype-mismatched transplants with and without KIR ligand incompatibility in the GVH direction*

KIR ligand incompatibility in GVH direction	No	Yes
	(n = 58)	(n = 34)
ALL[a]	21	14
AML[a]	37	20
Graft composition (mean ± s.d.):		
CD34+ × 10^6/kg	15 ± 5.1	14.5 ± 5.1[b]
CD3+ × 10^4/kg	3.5 ± 4.3	3.9 ± 4.6[b]

[a] 85% of patients were in ≥3rd complete remission or relapse; the others were in high-risk 1st or 2nd complete remission (bulky disease; first-line induction therapy failure; myelodysplasia; unfavorable cytogenetics).

[b] N.S. by two-tailed Student's t-test.

Table 16.3. *Clinical data and transplantation outcomes in HLA haplotype-mismatched transplants with and without KIR ligand incompatibility in the GVH direction*

KIR ligand incompatibility in GVH direction	No	Yes
Donor NK cell alloreactivity	No	Yes
Transplantation outcomes:		
Better engraftment	No (rejection = 15.5%)	Yes (no rejection)
Protection from GVHD	No (GVHD = 13.7%)	Yes (no GVHD)
Control of leukemia relapse		
ALL at high risk of relapse	No (5-year probability of relapse = 90%)	No (5-year probability of relapse = 85%)
AML at high risk of relapse	No (5-year probability of relapse = 75%)	Yes (5-year probability of relapse = 0%)
Impact on event-free survival	No (5-year probability of survival = 5%)	Yes (5-year probability of survival = 60%)

group 2, and HLA-Bw4 alleles) that engage NK cells of any allospecificity. These individuals are not therefore susceptible to NK cell alloreactivity by any donor.

Workup for NK alloreactive donor selection

A remarkable consequence of these studies is the need to rapidly exploit these results by revising the current criteria for donor selection for haploidentical transplants. At least in the case of high-risk AML, donor selection may now involve, not only standard donor inclusion criteria, but also a deliberate

search for the "perfect mismatch" (Kärre, 2002) at certain HLA loci; that is, for the mismatch that drives donor-versus-recipient NK cell alloreactivity. Haploidentical donors can be selected for KIR ligand mismatches (on the unshared haplotype) in the graft-versus-host direction. Selection for KIR mismatching is based on HLA typing as performed by serological and high-resolution molecular techniques. The search for NK alloreactive donors may require extension from the immediate family (parents and siblings) to other family members such as aunts, uncles, and cousins. Such an extended search raises the chance of finding an NK alloreactive donor from the random 30% to >

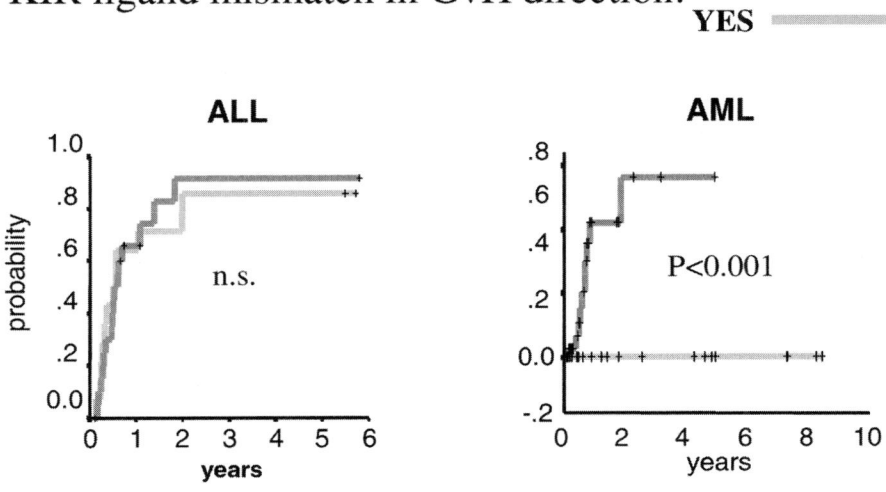

Fig. 16.4. Control of AML relapse by haploidentical transplants from NK alloreactive donors (Ruggeri *et al.,* 2002). Transplantation from NK alloreactive donors (■) did not have an impact on the high relapse rate of these ALL patients. The AML patients were also at high risk of relapse. Indeed, when transplanted from donors who were not able to mount NK alloreactions, the Kaplan-Meier curve (■) projects a high probability of relapse. However, the probability of relapse is 0% in patients transplanted from donors able to mount NK alloreactions (■).

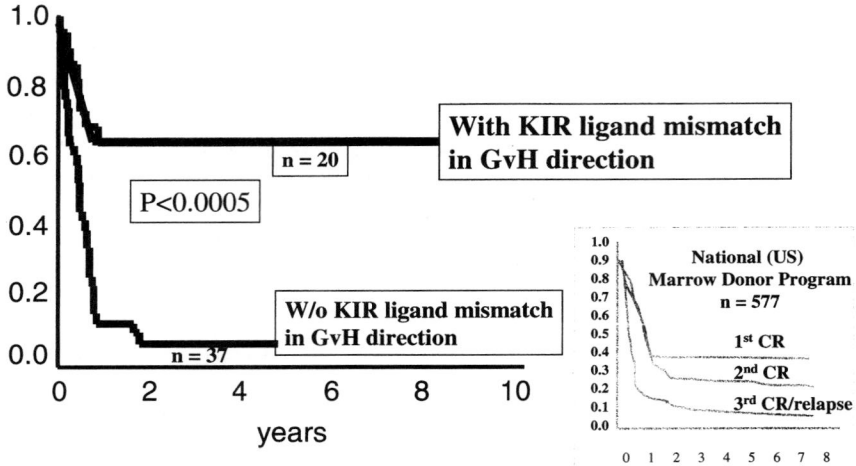

Fig. 16.5. Event-free survival of AML patients (Ruggeri *et al.*, 2002). Most patients were transplanted in ≥3rd complete remission or in relapse. The expected survival for this risk category when transplanted from HLA-matched unrelated donors is 7% (Insert) (Thomas *et al.*, 1999). Survival of patients transplanted from haploidentical donors who could not mount NK reactions is 5%. Transplantation from NK alloreactive donors had a dramatic impact on survival, which rose to 60%.

Table 16.4. *List of group 1 and group 2 HLA-C and HLA-Bw4 alleles*

Group 1 HLA-C alleles (Ser 77, Asn 80)	Group 2 HLA-C alleles (Asn 77, Lys 80)	HLA-Bw4 alleles
Cw1 (all)[a]	Cw2 (all)	B5 (all)
Cw3 (all except C*0307, C*0310 and C*0315)	C*0307	B13 (all)
Cw7 (all except C*0707 and C*0709)	C*0315	B17 (all)
Cw8 (all)	Cw4 (all)	B27 (all)
Cw12 (all except C*1205, C*12041, C*12042)	Cw5 (all)	B37 (all)
Cw13 (all)	Cw6 (all)	B38 (all)
Cw14 (all, except C*1404)	C*0707	B44 (all)
C*1507	C*0709	B47 (all)
Cw16 (all except C*1602)	C*1205	B49 (all)
	C*12041	B51 (all)
	C*12042	B52 (all)
	Cw15 (all except C*1507)	B53 (all)
	C*1602	B57 (all)
	Cw17 (all)	B58 (all)
	Cw18 (all)	B59 (all)
		B63 (all)
		B77 (all)
		B*1513
		B*1516
		B*1517
		B*1523
		B*1524

[a] "all" = all molecular types within a serologically-defined group of alleles.

N.B. C*0310 (Ser77, Lys80) behaves as if it belonged to Group 1 and to Group 2 HLA-C (Biassoni *et al.*, 1995). If a patient expresses this allele, he or she should be considered to express both allele groups. In other words, C*0310 blocks NK cells expressing any HLA-C-specific receptor; it does not block clones expressing the Bw4 receptor.

C*1404 (Asn77, Asn80) is the opposite. It does not belong to Group 1 or to Group 2 HLA-C (Biassoni *et al.*, 1995). In other words, it does not block NK cells expressing HLA-C specific receptors. So, expression of C*1404 may be ignored in a patient, because it is as if the patient did not express HLA-C alleles at all. Of course one has to consider the other allele.

C*1207 Gly77, Asn80, cannot be assigned to either group based on its amino acid sequence, and still needs to be tested functionally.

60% (which is close to the maximum, bearing in mind that the HLA type of about 30% of the population makes them resistant to alloreactive NK killing; see above).

For NK alloreactive donor selection, first type the recipient. Recipients who express class I alleles belonging to the three major class I groups (HLA-C group 1, HLA-C group 2, and HLA-Bw4 alleles) will block all NK cells from every donor. Recipients who express alleles belonging to only one or two of these three class I groups, have a chance of finding NK alloreactive donors. Donor typing will then proceed to find the relative who expresses the allele in the class I group that is not expressed by the patient. Table 16.4 shows HLA-C group 1, and HLA-C group 2 alleles, along with the amino acid sequences which is the basis of the group classification. As new alleles are discovered, they are grouped according to their amino acid sequence. Table 16.4 also includes HLA-B alleles sharing the Bw4 supertypic specificity.

Several donor-recipient combinations are possible which, based on current knowledge, are reported in Table 16.5. When, for example, the recipient's HLA type contains HLA-C group 1, HLA-C group 2, and HLA-Bw4 alleles, no NK alloreactive donor can be found. If the recipient expresses Group 1 and Group 2 HLA-C alleles (but not Bw4 alleles), the donor must have a Bw4 allele (in addition to whatever other allele groups) in order to provide NK alloreactivity. Should the recipient express Group 1 HLA-C alleles and HLA-Bw4 alleles, the donor must have a Group 2 HLA-C allele to be NK-alloreactive. When the recipient expresses Group 2 HLA-C and HLA-Bw4 alleles, the donor needs to have a Group 1 HLA-C allele. If the recipient expresses Group 1 HLA-C alleles only, the donor must have a Group 2 HLA-C allele, and/or an HLA-Bw4 allele to ensure NK alloreactions. Finally, if the recipient has a Group 2 HLA-C allele only, the donor must have a Group 1 HLA-C and/or an HLA-Bw4 allele. One very rare additional mismatch is the HLA-A3/11 negative recipient and HLA-A3/A11 positive donor. In the Ruggeri *et al.* study (2002), the HLA-A3/A11 mismatch was never found alone but only in conjunction with HLA-C group mismatches. Therefore, no prediction as to the efficacy of this mismatch combination can be made.

Conclusions

Over the last 10 years, we have seen an explosion in our understanding of NK cell receptors. We now know that NK cell responses are regulated by competing signals mediated through inhibitory and activating receptors. The inhibitory signals result from the interaction of KIRs and CD94/NKG2A receptors with MHC class I molecules. Appreciation of this concept has already led to the successful use of the antileukemic potential of donor NK cells through KIR-epitope mismatches in the setting of haplotype-mismatched HSC transplantation. Spontaneously generated NK cell alloreactions from stem cell grafts are associated with a remarkable GVL effect and complete control of rejection and GVHD. This impacts dramatically on survival of advanced stage AML patients, which is similar to that reported in patients transplanted in first complete remission from HLA-identical siblings. NK cell alloreactivity is, therefore, a powerful tool which enhances the efficacy and safety of allogeneic HSC transplantation.

Moreover, as preclinical studies show, pretransplant alloreactive NK cell infusions have the potential to improve outcomes of KIR ligand-mismatched transplants even further and are therefore of great therapeutic interest. In mice, they were successfully combined with reduced intensity conditioning to achieve durable full-donor engraftment. Even alone, alloreactive NK cells converted mixed to full-donor chimerism and eradicated leukemia. NK conditioning even protected from GVHD sufficiently efficiently as to allow the safe infusion of otherwise lethal doses of allogeneic T cells for immune reconstitution.

Table 16.5. *Donor/recipient combinations predicting NK cell alloreactivity in the GVH direction*

Recipient HLA type	HLA type of NK alloreactive donor[a]
Group 1 HLA-C, Group 2 HLA-C, HLA-Bw4	No NK alloreactive donor
Group 1 HLA-C, Group 2 HLA-C	HLA-Bw4
Group 1 HLA-C, HLA-Bw4	Group 2 HLA-C
Group 2 HLA-C, HLA-Bw4	Group 1 HLA-C
Group 1 HLA-C	Group 2 HLA-C and/or HLA-Bw4
Group 2 HLA-C	Group 1 HLA-C and/or HLA-Bw4

[a] In each recipient/donor combination the donor has an NK repertoire which contains NK cells that are specifically blocked by the allele group(s) indicated in the donor column. These NK cells will be alloreactive because the corresponding recipient does not express this allele group.

N.B. One very rare additional mismatch is the HLA-A3/11 negative recipient and HLA-A3/A11 positive donor. In the Ruggeri *et al.* study (2002) the HLA-A3/A11 mismatch was never found alone, but only in conjunction with HLA-C group mismatches. Therefore, no prediction as to the efficacy of this mismatch combination can be made.

Whatever other alleles are present in the donor's HLA type, the ones listed here predict NK cell alloreactions against the specific HLA type of the recipient

Alloreactive NK cells are emerging as a form of cell therapy which might be used in conditioning regimens for host immune suppression and leukemia ablation. Their ability to prevent GVHD could allow a greater T-cell content in the graft and consequently reduce the infection-related morbidity and mortality which is associated with extensive T-cell depletion. With this approach, mismatched transplants can be envisaged for the elderly and heavily pretreated patients.

References

Albi, N., Ruggeri, L., Aversa, F. *et al.* (1996). Natural killer (NK)-cell function and anti-leukemic activity of a large population of CD3+/CD8+ T cells expressing NK receptors for MHC class I after "three-loci" HLA-incompatible bone marrow transplantation. *Blood,* **87,** 3993–9.

Asai, O., Longo, D.L., Tian, Z. *et al.* (1998). Suppression of graft-versus-host disease and amplification of graft-versus-tumor effects by activated natural killer cells after allogeneic bone marrow transplantation. *Journal of Clinical Investigation,* **101,** 1835–42.

Aversa, F., Tabilio, A., Terenzi, A. *et al.* (1994). Successful engraftment of T-cell-depleted haploidentical "three-loci" incompatible transplants in leukemia patients by addition of recombinant human granulocyte colony-stimulating factor-mobilized peripheral blood progenitor cells to bone marrow inoculum. *Blood,* **84,** 3948–55.

Aversa, F., Tabilio, A., Velardi, A. *et al.* (1998). Transplantation for high-risk acute leukemia with high doses of T cell-depleted hematopoietic stem cells from haploidentical "three loci" incompatible donors. *The New England Journal of Medicine,* **339,** 1186–93.

Bachar-Lustig, E., Rachamim, N., Li, H.W. *et al.* (1995). Megadose of T cell-depleted bone marrow overcomes MHC barriers in sublethally irradiated mice. *Nature Medicine,* **1,** 1268–73.

Bauer, S. *et al.* (1999). Activation of NK cells and T cells by NKG2D, a receptor for stress-inducible MICA. *Science,* **285,** 727–9.

Biassoni, R. *et al.* (1995). Amino acid substitution can influence the NK-mediated recognition of HLA-C molecules. Role of serine-77 and lysine-80 in the target cell protection from lysis mediated by "group 2" or "group 1" NK clones. *Journal of Experimental Medicine,* **182,** 605–9.

Biassoni, R., Cantoni, C., Falco, M. *et al.* (1996). The HLA.C specific "activatory" and "inhibitory" Natural Killer cell receptors display highly homologous extracellular domains but differ in their transmembrane and intracytoplasmic portions. *Journal of Experimental Medicine,* **183,** 645–50.

Biron, C.A. (1998). Role of early cytokines, including alpha and beta interferons (IFN-alpha/beta), in innate and adaptive immune responses to viral infections. *Seminars in Immunology,* **10,** 383–90.

Bonnet, D., Warren, E.H., Greenberg, P.D. *et al.* (1999). CD8+ minor histocompatibility antigen-specific cytotoxic T lymphocyte clones eliminate human acute myeloid leukemia stem cells. *Proceedings of the National Academy of Science USA,* **96,** 8639–44.

Borrego, F., Ulbrecht, M., Wiess, E.H. *et al.* (1998). Recognition of human histocompatibility leucocyte antigen (HLA)-E complexed with HKLA class I signal sequence-derived peptides by CD94/NKG2 confers protection from natural killer cell-mediated lysis. *Journal of Experimental Medicine,* **187,** 813–8.

Bottino, C., Sivori, S., Vitale, M. *et al.* (1996). A novel surface molecule homologous to the p58/p50 family of receptors is selectively expressed on a subset of human Natural Killer cells and induces both triggering of cell functions and proliferation. *European Journal of Immunology,* **26,** 1816–24.

Bottino, C., Falco, M., Parolini, S. *et al.* (2001). NTB-A, a Novel SH2D1A-associated Surface Molecule Contributing to the Inability of natural Killer Cells to Kill Epstein-Barr Virus-infected B Cells in X-linked Lymphoproliferative Diseases. *Journal of Experimental Medicine,* **194,** 235–46.

Bottino, C., Falco, M., Sivori *et al.* (2000). Identification and molecular characterization of a natural mutant of the p50.2/KIR2DS2 activating NK receptor that fails to mediate NK cell triggering. *European Journal of Immunology,* **30,** 3569–74.

Braud, V.M. *et al.* (1998). HLA-E binds to natural killer cell receptors CD94/NKG2A, B and C. *Nature,* **391,** 795–9.

Cantoni, C., Biassoni, R., Pende, D. *et al.* (1998). The activating form of CD94 receptor complex. CD94 covalently associates with the Kp39 protein that represents the product of the NKG2-C gene. *European Journal of Immunology,* **28,** 327–38.

Cantoni, C., Bottino, C., Vitale, M. *et al.* (1999). NKp44, a triggering receptor involved in tumor cell lysis by activated human Natural Killer cells, is a novel member of the immunoglobulin superfamily. *Journal of Experimental Medicine,* **189,** 787–96.

Carretero, M., Cantoni, C., Bellon, T. *et al.* (1997). The CD94 and NKG2-A C-type lectins covalently assamble to form a NK cell inhibitory receptor for HLA class I molecules. *European Journal of Immunology,* **27,** 563–7.

Cerwenka, A. & Lanier, L.L. (2001). Ligands for natural killer cell receptors: redundancy or specifity. *Immunology Reviews,* **181,** 158–69.

Ciccone, E., Colonna, M., Viale, O. *et al.* (1990). Susceptibility or resistance to lysis by alloreactive NK cells is governed by a gene in the human major histocompatibility complex between Bf and HLA-B. *Proceedings of the National Academy of Science of the USA,* **87,** 9794–7.

Ciccone, E., Pende, D., Viale, O. *et al.* (1992a). Evidence of a natural killer (NK) cell repertoire for (allo) antigen recognition: definition of five distinct NK-determined allospecificities in humans. *Journal of Experimental Medicine,* **175,** 709–18

Ciccone, E., Pende, D., Viale, O. *et al.* (1992b). Involvement of HLA class I alleles in natural killer (NK) cell-specific functions: expression of HLA-Cw3 confers selective protection from lysis by alloreactive NK clones displaying a defined specificity (specificity 2). *Journal of Experimental Medicine,* **176,** 963–71

Ciccone, E., Pende, D., Vitale, M. *et al.* (1994). Self Class I molecules protect normal cells from lysis mediated by autologous Natural Killer Cells. *European Journal of Immunology,* **24,** 1003–6.

Ciccone, E., Viale, O., Pende, D. *et al.* (1988). Specific lysis of allogeneic cells after activation of CD3- lymphocytes in mixed lymphocyte culture. *Journal of Experimental Medicine,* **168,** 2403–8.

Colonna, M., Spies, T., Strominger, J.L. *et al.* (1992). Alloantigen recognition by two human Natural Killer cells is associated with HLA-C or a closely linked gene. *Proceedings of the National Academy of Science USA,* **89,** 7983–5.

Colonna, M., Brooks, E.G., Falco, M. *et al.* (1993). Generation of allospecific natural killer cells by stimulation across a polymorphism of HLA-C. *Science,* **260,** 1121–4.

Colonna, M., Borsellino, G., Falco *et al.* (1993). HLA-C is the inhibitory ligand that determines dominant resistance to lysis by NK1- and NK2-specific natural killer cells. *Proceedings of the National Academy of Science of the USA,* **90,** 1200–4.

Colonna, M. & Samaridis, J. (1995). Cloning of immunoglobulin-superfamily members associated with HLA-C and HLA-B recognition by human natural killer cells. *Science,* **268,** 405–8.

Costello, R., Sivori, S., Marcenaro, E. *et al.* (2002). Defective expression and function of natural killer cell-triggering receptors in patients with acute myeloid leukemia. *Blood,* **99,** 3661–7.

D'Andrea, A., Chang, C., Franz-Bacon, K. *et al.* (1995). Molecular cloning of NKB1. A natural killer cell receptor for HLA-B allotypes. *Journal of Immunology,* **155,** 2306–10.

Diefenbach, A. & Raulet, D.H. (2001). Strategies for target cell recognition by natural killer cells. *Immunology Reviews,* **181,** 170–84.

Farag, S.S., Fehniger, T.A., Ruggeri, L. *et al.* (2002). Natural Killer Cell Receptors: New Biology and Insights into the Graft versus Leukemia Effect. *Blood,* **100,** 1935–47.

Ferrini, S., Miescher, S., Zocchi, M.R. *et al.* (1987). Phenotypic and functional characterization of recombinant interleukin-2 (rIL-2)-induced killer cells: analysis at the population and the clonal level. *Journal of Immunology,* **138,** 1297–302.

Garrido, F. *et al.* (1997). Implications for immunosurveillance of altered HLA-class I phenotypes in human tumors. *Immunology Today,* **18,** 89–95.

Giralt, S. & Slavin, S. (2000). *Non-myeloablative Stem Cell Transplantation (NST).* Abingdon, UK: Darwin Scientific Publishing.

Glass, B., Uharek, L., Zeis, M. *et al.* (1996). Gaft-versus-leukemia activity can be predicted by natural cytotoxicity against leukemia cells. *British Journal of Haematology,* **93,** 412–20.

Herberman, R.B., Nunn, M.E., & Lavrin, D.H. (1975). Natural cytotoxic reactivity of mouse lymphoid cells against syngeneic and allogeneic tumors. I. Distribution of reactivity and specificity. *International Journal of Cancer,* **16,** 216–29.

Hirayama, M., Genyea, C., Brownell, A. *et al.* (1998). IL-2-activated murine newborn liver NK cells enhance engraftment of hematopoietic stem cells in MHC-mismatched recipients. *Bone Marrow Transplantation,* **21,** 1245–52.

Houchins, J.P., Lanier, L.L., Niemi, E. *et al.* (1997). Natural killer cell cytolytic activity is inhibited by NKG2-A and activated by NKG2-C. *Journal of Immunology,* **158,** 3603–9.

Houchins, J.P., Yabe, T., Mc Sherry, C. *et al.* (1991). DNA sequence analysis of NKG2, a family of related cDNA clonesencoding type II integral membrane proteins on human natural killer cells. *Journal of Experimental Medicine,* **173,** 1017–20.

Kärre, K. (2002). A perfect mismatch. *Science,* **295,** 2029–31.

Kärre, K., Ljunggren, H.G., Piontek, G. *et al.* (1986). Selective rejection of H-2 deficient lymphoma variants suggests alternative immune defence strategy. *Nature,* **319,** 675–8.

Khakoo, S. *et al.* (2000). Rapid Evolution of NK cell receptor systems demonstrated by comparison of chimpanzees and humans. *Immunity,* **12,** 687–98.

Kiessling, R., Klein, E., & Wigzell, H. (1975). "Natural" killer cells in the mouse. I. Citotoxic cells with specificity for mouse Moloney leukemia cells. Specificity and distribution according to genotype. *The European Journal of Immunology,* **5,** 112–7.

Lanier, L.L. (1998). NK receptors. *Annual Reviews in Immunology,* **16,** 359–93.

Lanier, L.L., Corliss, B., & Phillips, J.H. (1997). Arousal and inhibition of human NK cells. *Immunology Reviews,* **155,** 145–54.

Lanier, L.L., Corliss, B.C., Jun, W. *et al.* (1998). Immunoreceptor DAP12 bearing a tyrosine-based activation motifs is involved in activating NK cells. *Nature,* **391,** 703–7.

Lazetic, S., Chang, C., Houchins, J.P., Lanier, L.L., & Phillipa, J.H. (1996). Human natural killer cell receptors involved in MHC class I recognition are disulphide-linked heterodimers of CD94 and NKG2 subunits. *Journal of Immunology,* **157,** 4741–5.

Lee, N. *et al.* (1998). HLA-E is a major ligand for the natural killer inhibitory receptor CD94/NKG2A. *Proceedings of the National Academy of the USA,* **95,** 5199–204.

Litwin, V., Gumperz, J.E., Parham, P. *et al.* (1994). NKB1: a natural killer cell receptor involved in the recognition of polymorphic HLA-B molecules. *Journal of Experimental Medicine,* **180,** 537–43.

Ljunggren, H.G. & Karre, K. (1990). In search of the "missing self". MHC molecules and NK cell recognition. *Immunology Today,* **11,** 237–44.

Long, E.O. (1999). Regulation of immune responses through inhibitory receptors. *Annual Reviews in Immunology,* **17,** 875–904.

Martelli, M.F., Aversa, F., Bachar-Lustig, E. *et al.* (2002). Transplants across human leukocyte antigen barriers. *Seminars in Hematology,* **39,** 48–56.

Molldrem, J.J., Lee, P.P., Wang, C. *et al.* (2000). Evidence that specific T lymphocytes may participate in the elimination of chronic myelogenous leukemia. *Nature Medicine,* **6,** 1018–23

Moretta, A. *et al.* (2001). Activating receptors and coreceptors involved in human natural killer cell-mediated cytolysis. *Annual Reviews in Immunology,* **19,** 197–223.

Moretta, A., Biassoni, R., Bottino, C. *et al.* (2000). Natural Cytotoxicity Receptors that trigger human NK-mediated cytolysis. *Immunology Today,* **21,** 228–34.

Moretta, A., Bottino, C., Pende, D. *et al.* (1990b). Identification of four subset of human CD3-CD16+ NK cells by the expression of clonally distributed functional surface molecules. Correlation between subset assignment of NK clones and ability to mediate specific alloantigen recognition. *Journal of Experimental Medicine,* **172,** 1589–98.

Moretta, A., Bottino, C., Vitale, M. *et al.* (1996). Receptors for HLA-class I molecules in human Natural Killer cells. *Annual Review of Immunology,* **14,** 619–48.

Moretta, A. & Moretta, L. (1997). HLA class I specific inhibitory receptors. *Current Opinion in Immunology,* **9,** 964–701.

Moretta, A., Sivori, S., Vitale, M. *et al.* (1995). Existence of both inhibitory (p58) and activatory (p50) receptors for HLA.C molecules in human Natural Killer cells. *Journal of Experimental Medicine,* **182,** 875–84.

Moretta, A., Tambussi, G., Bottino, C. *et al.* (1990a). A novel surface antigen expressed by a subset of human CD3-CD16+ Natural Killer cells. Role in cell activation and regulation of cytolytic function. *Journal of Experimental Medicine,* **171,** 695–714.

Moretta, A., Vitale, M., Bottino, C. *et al.* (1993). P58 molecules as putative receptors for MHC class I molecules in human Natural Killer (NK) cells. Anti-p58 antibodies reconstitute lysis of MHC class I-protected cells in NK clones displaying different specificities. *Journal of Experimental Medicine,* **178,** 597–604.

Moretta, A., Vitale, M., Sivori, S. *et al.* (1994). Human NK receptors for HLA-class I molecules. Evidence that the KP43 (CD94) molecule functions as receptor for HLA-B alleles. *Journal of Experimental Medicine,* **180,** 545–55.

Moretta, L., Ciccone, E., Moretta, A. *et al.* (1992). Allorecognition by NK cells: nonself or no self? *Immunology Today,* **13,** 300–6.

Moretta, L., Ciccone, E., Mingari, M.C. *et al.* (1994). Human NK cells: origin, clonality, specificity and receptors. *Advances in Immunology,* **55,** 341–80.

Murphy, W.J., Koh, C.Y., Raziuddin, A. *et al.* (2001). Immunobiology of natural killer cells and bone marrow transplantation: merging of basic and preclinical studies. *Immunology Reviews,* **181,** 279–89.

Mutis, T. & Goulmy, E. (2002). Hematopoietic system-specific antigens as targets for cellular immunotherapy of hematological malignancies. *Seminars in Hematology,* **39,** 23–31.

Öhlén, C., Kling, G., Höglund, P. *et al.* (1989). Prevention of allogeneic bone marrow graft rejection by H-2 transgene in donor mice. *Science,* **246,** 666–68

Olcese, L., Cambiaggi, A., Semenzato, G. *et al.* (1997). Human killer cell activatory receptors for MHC class I molecules are included in a multimeric complex expressed by Natural Killer cells. *Journal of Immunology,* **158,** 5083–6.

Pende, D., Accame, L., Pareti, L. *et al.* (1998). The susceptibility to Natural Killer cell-mediated lysis of HLA class I-positive melanomas reflects the expression of insufficient amounts of HLA class I alleles. *European Journal of Immunology,* **28,** 2384–94.

Pende, D., Parolinin, S., Pessino, A. *et al.* (1999). Identification and molecular characterization of NKp30, a novel triggering receptor involved in natural cytotoxicity mediated by human natural killer cells. *Journal of Experimental Medicine,* **190,** 1505–16.

Pende, D., Cantoni, C., Rivera, P. *et al.* (2001). Role of NKG2D in tumor cell lysis mediated by human NK cells: cooperation with natural cytotoxicity receptors and capability of recognizing tumors of non epithelial origin. *European Journal of Immunology,* **31,** 1076–86.

Pérez-Villar, J.J., Melero, I., Rodriguez, A. *et al.* (1995). Functional ambivalence of the Kp43 (CD94) NK cell-associated surface antigen. *Journal of Immunology,* **154,** 5779–5778.

Pessino, A., Sivori, S., Bottino, C. *et al.* (1998). Molecular cloning of NKp46: a novel member of the immunoglobulin superfamily involved in triggering of natural cytotoxicity. *Journal of Experimental Medicine,* **188,** 953–60.

Raulet, D.H., Vance, R.E., & McMahon, C.W. (2001). Regulation of the natural killer cell receptor repertoire. *Annual Reviews in Immunology,* **19,** 291–330.

Reisner, Y., Kapoor, N., Kirkpatrick, D. *et al.* (1983). Transplantation for severe combined immunodeficiency with HLA-A, B, D, DR incompatible parental marrow cells fractionated by soybean agglutinin and sheep red blood cells. *Blood,* **61,** 341–8.

Reisner, Y. & Martelli, M.F. (1999). Stem cell escalation enables HLA-disparate haematopoietic transplants in leukaemia patients. *Immunology Today,* **20,** 343–7.

Ruggeri, L., Capanni, M., Casacci, M. *et al.* (1999). Role of natural killer cell alloreactivity in HLA-mismatched hematopoietic stem cell transplantation. *Blood,* **94,** 333–9.

Ruggeri, L., Capanni, M., Urbani, E. *et al.* (2002). Effectiveness of Donor Natural Killer Cell Alloreactivity in Mismatched Hematopoietic Transplants. *Science,* **295,** 2097–100.

Shilling, H., Young, N., Guethlein, L.A. *et al.* (2002). Genetic Control of human NK cell repertoire. *Journal of Immunology,* **169,** 239–47.

Shlomchik, W.D., Couzens, M.S., Tang, C.B. *et al.* (1999). Prevention of graft versus host disease by inactivation of host antigen-presenting cells. *Science,* **285,** 412–5.

Sivori, S., Vitale, M., Bottino, C. *et al.* (1996). CD94 functions as a natural killer cell inhibitory receptor for different HLA class I alleles: identification of the inhibitory form of CD94 by the use of novel monoclonal antibodies. *European Journal of Immunology,* **26,** 2487–92.

Sivori, S., Vitale, M., Morelli, L. *et al.* (1997). p46, a novel Natural Killer cell-specific surface molecule which mediates cell activation. *Journal of Experimental Medicine,* **186,** 1129–36.

Sivori, S., Pende, D., Bottino, C. *et al.* (1999). NKp46 is the major triggering receptor involved in the natural cytotoxicity of fresh or cultured human natural killer cells. Correlation between surface density of NKp46 and natural cytotoxicity against autologous, allogeneic or xenogeneic target cells. *European Journal of Immunology,* **29,** 1656–66.

Sivori, S., Parolini, S., Marcenaro, E. *et al.* (2000a). Involvement of Natural Cytotoxicity Receptors in human Natural Killer cell mediated lysis of neuroblastoma and glyoblastoma cell lines. *Journal of Neuroimmunology,* **107,** 220–5.

Sivori, S., Parolini, S., Marcenaro, E. *et al.* (2000b). Triggering receptors involved in Natural Killer cell mediated cytotoxicity against choriocarcinoma cell lines. *Human Immunology,* **61,** 1055–8.

Sivori, S., Parolini, S., Falco, M. *et al.* (2000c). 2B4 functions as a co-receptor in human natural killer cell activation. *European Journal of Immunology,* **30,** 787–93.

Sutherland, C.L., Chalupny, N.J., & Cosman, D. (2001). The UL16-binding proteins, a novel family of MHC class I-related ligands for NKG2D, activate natural killer cell functions. *Immunology Reviews,* **181,** 185–92.

Thomas, E.D., Blume, K.G., & Forman, S.J. (1999). Hematopoietic Cell Transplantation. *Blackwell Science,* Inc.

Trincheri, G. (1990). Biology of Natural Killer cells. *Advances in Immunology,* **47,** 187–76.

Valiante, N.M., Lienert, K., Shilling, H.G. *et al.* (1997a). Killer cell receptors: keeping pace with MHC class I evolution. *Immunology Reviews,* **155,** 155–64.

Valiante, N.M. *et al.* (1997b). Functionally and structurally distinct NK cell receptor repertoires in the peripheral blood of two human donors. *Immunity,* **7,** 739–51.

Uhrberg, M., Valiante, N.M., Shum, B.P. *et al.* (1997). Human diversity in killer cell inhibitory receptor genes. *Immunity,* **7,** 753–60.

Vilches, C. & Parham, P. (2002). KIR: diverse, rapidly evolving receptors of innate and adaptive immunity. *Annual Review of Immunology,* **20,** 217–51.

Vitale, M., Bottino, C., Sivori, S. *et al.* (1998). NKp44, a novel triggering surface molecule specifically expressed by activated Natural Killer cells is involved in non-MHC restricted tumor cell lysis. *Journal of Experimental Medicine,* **187,** 2065–72.

Vitale, M., Falco, M., Castriconi, R. *et al.* (2001). Identification of NKp80, a novel triggering molecule expressed by human natural killer cells. *European Journal of Immunology,* **31,** 233–42.

Vitale, M., Sivori, S., Pende, D. *et al.* (1995). Coexpression of two functionallly indipendent p58 inhibitory receptors in human NK cell clones results in the inability to kill normal allogeneic target cells. *Proceedings of the National Academy of Science USA,* **95,** 3536–40.

Vitale, M., Sivori, S., Pende, D. *et al.* (1996). Physical and functional independency of p70 and p58 NK cell receptors for HLA-class I. Their role in the definition of different groups of alloreactive NK cell clones. *Proceedings of the National Academy of Science of the USA,* **93,** 1453–7.

Wagtmann, N., Biassoni, R., Cantoni, C. *et al.* (1995). Molecular clones of the p58 Natural Killer cell receptor reveal Ig-related molecules with diversity in both the extra- and intracellular domains. *Immunity,* **2,** 439–49.

Wilson, M.J., Torkar, M., Haode, A. *et al.* (2000). Plasticity in the organization and sequences of human KIR/ILT gene families. *Proceedings of the National Academy of Science USA,* **97,** 4778–84.

Winter, C.C. & Long, E.O. (1997). A single amino acid in the p58 killer cell inhibitory receptor controls the ability of natural killer cells to discriminate between the two groups of HLA-C allotypes. *The Journal of Immunology,* **158,** 4026–8.

Zeis, M., Uharek, L., Lass, B. *et al.* (1997). Allogeneic MHC-mismatched activated natural killer cells administered after bone marrow transplantation provide a strong graft-versus-leukemia effect in mice. *British Journal of Haematology,* **96,** 757–61.

17 The role of tumor cell purging in autologous hematopoietic stem cell transplantation for malignant disease: laboratory basis and clinical results

KENNETH F. BRADSTOCK AND DENIS CLAUDE ROY

Westmead Hospital, Sydney, Australia, and Maisonneuve-Rosemont Hospital, Montreal, Canada

Introduction

The concept behind purging of autologous bone marrow or blood stem cells is simple and elegant. Autologous marrow and blood stem cells are able to reconstitute hematopoiesis after myeloablative therapy for malignant disease, resulting in cure in a substantial proportion of patients (Dicke *et al.*, 1984). Disease relapse, however, is a common occurrence, and it has been hypothesized that, in some cases, this is due to reinfusion of small numbers of viable clonogenic tumor cells contaminating the stem cell inoculum (Jansen *et al.*, 1984). Peripheral blood stem cell grafts generally contain a lower tumor burden than bone marrow grafts, although the stem cell mobilization procedure may itself recruit tumor cells into the peripheral circulation (Gee, 1995). Effective techniques for removal, or purging, of viable tumor cells from autologous harvests would theoretically circumvent this problem (O'Reilly, 1986).

For this strategy to be successful in practice, several problems must be overcome. As with all forms of autologous hematopoietic stem cell (HSC) transplantation, effective conditioning regimens must be available to eradicate residual disease in the patient pretransplant. Second, it is necessary to have access to relatively normal autologous HSC with the least possible contamination with malignant cells. Finally, a highly selective purging process must be devised, capable of removing clonogenic tumor cells while sparing normal hematopoietic cells required for marrow engraftment. Because the cellular properties of the tumor cells in bone-marrow-derived diseases such as acute myeloid leukemia (AML) closely resemble those of normal stem cells, the selectivity of the purging process is a difficult and critical issue.

The effectiveness of the purging procedure required in clinical practice is uncertain. First, it is clear that autografting with unpurged marrow can be curative in some patients with acute leukemia and lymphoma (Burnett *et al.*, 1984; Lowenberg *et al.*, 1984; Gorin *et al.*, 1990; Philip *et al.*, 1987). This could be explained on the basis of fortuitous selection of patients already cured by preceding therapy. Equally, it can be argued that, in some patients with low tumor burden, the process of stem cell collection and subsequent manipulation during cryopreservation and thawing may reduce the number of viable tumor cells reinfused to such low levels that the disease process is not reinitiated (Hagenbeek & Martens, 1989), aided possibly by concurrent activation of host immune defenses such as natural cytotoxic cells (Reittie *et al.*, 1989). In patients with lymphoma, distinct cell surface adhesion properties may result in selective homing of malignant cells to lymph nodes, with minimum numbers of cells in the venous circulation and bone marrow (Freedman *et al.*, 1990). Unfortunately, however, this is not the case for a large number of patients with non-Hodgkin's lymphoma and particularly acute and chronic leukemias. Indeed, the total number of malignant cells remaining in patients with acute leukemia in remission may be as high as 10^8, implying that 10^6 may contaminate a typical harvest. If in vitro models of leukemia growth are correct, the proportion of proliferative or clonogenic cells is approximately 3 logs lower than this (Griffin & Lowenberg, 1986). Therefore, to effectively render such a marrow leukemia-free, purging techniques capable of at least a 3 log reduction of clonogenic cells would be necessary. With autologous blood stem cell harvests, there is some evidence to suggest that these products may have less tumor contamination than marrow, either in the steady state (Kessinger *et al.*, 1989) or after mobilization with chemotherapy and cytokines (Vescio *et al.*, 1996).

Similarly, quantitative polymerase chain reaction (PCR) evaluation demonstrated that bone marrow samples were infiltrated by approximately 10-fold higher numbers of bcl-2/immunoglobulin heavy chain (IgH)-rearranged lymphoma cells than unmobilized peripheral blood (Leonard *et al.*, 1998) (Figure 17.1). However, other groups found that peripheral blood samples were infiltrated by bcl-2/IgH-rearranged cells as frequently as bone marrow (Berinstein *et al.*, 1993; Negrin & Pesando, 1994). In addition, the mobilization procedure has also been shown to release malignant cells into the circulation, resulting in the presence of a proportion of malignant cells similar to that of marrow (Ross *et al.*, 1993; Brugger *et al.*, 1994; Leonard *et al.*, 1998). The nature of the stem cell mobilization strategy may represent a determining factor in allowing tumor cells to permeate the blood-marrow barrier. Indeed, chemotherapy, such as cyclophosphamide, has been shown to damage

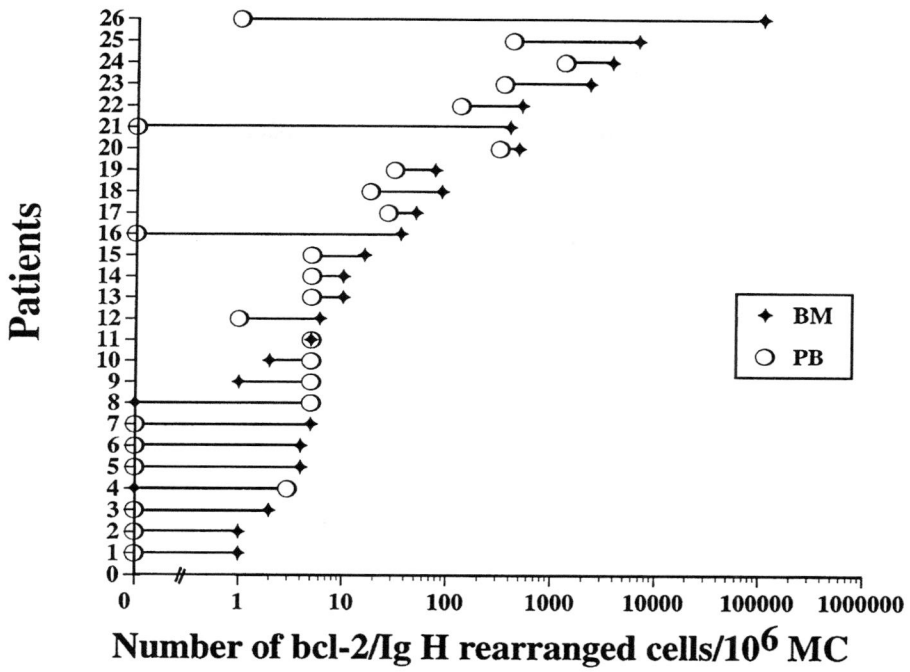

Fig. 17.1. When levels of contamination by bcl-2/IgH-rearranged lymphoma cells are compared in bone marrow (BM) and peripheral blood (PB), BM samples demonstrate greater infiltration than PB. However, the difference is only of 1 logarithm (10-fold). Reproduced, with permission, from Leonard *et al.* (1998).

marrow endothelial cells (Shirota & Tavassoli, 1991), and growth factors to alter the regulation of adhesion molecules (Levesque *et al.*, 1996). Moreover, since peripheral blood stem cell grafts usually contain larger numbers of cells than marrow grafts, the absolute number of tumor cells in these grafts may actually be higher than in marrow.

A variety of ingenious techniques have been devised for this purpose (Table 17.1). First, the immunologic approach exploits the ability of murine monoclonal antibodies (Mabs) to bind preferentially to antigens expressed on tumor cells but not on normal marrow stem cells (Jansen *et al.*, 1984). The removal of antibody-coated cells can be achieved by direct killing, using complement-mediated cytotoxicity or specifically constructed immunotoxins (Mab coupled to drugs or naturally occurring toxins such as ricin), or, alternatively, by coupling Mabs to magnetic microspheres, antibody-coated cells can be physically removed from marrow suspensions by placement in a strong magnetic field (Jansen *et al.*, 1984) (Figure 17.2A).

The other major purging approach has been the use of pharmacologic agents to treat marrow ex vivo (Herve *et al.*, 1986). The most extensively investigated drugs have been the cyclophosphamide analogs, 4-hydroperoxycyclophosphamide (4HC) and mafosfamide, which are cytotoxic in vitro. Pharmacologic purging is less selective than immunologic methods, and relies upon the relative insensitivity of resting marrow stem cells to doses of cytotoxic drugs that are capable of eliminating clonogenic tumor cells (Gordon, Goldman, & Gordon-Smith, 1985).

Purging has also been attempted by positive selection of CD34+ stem and progenitor cells, as opposed to negative selection of tumor cells. Advantages and disadvantages can be identified for either positive or negative selection strategies, but it has been difficult, if not impossible, to clearly compare these approaches, primarily because of limited accessibility and concentration of efforts to optimize individual methodologies (Table 17.2). Interestingly, the two approaches are now being combined within the same device (see Chapter 27).

Preclinical evaluation of purging techniques

Purging with monoclonal antibodies

The immunologic approach to bone marrow purging has been most extensively used in acute lymphoblastic leukemia (ALL) and B-cell non-Hodgkin's lymphoma (NHL). Several investigators have shown that, using murine Mabs to B-cell differentiation antigens such as CD9, CD10, CD19, CD20, and CD24, cell killing of up to 5 logs could be achieved with malignant B-cell lines, thus approaching levels of cytoreduction that could render marrow from patients with precursor B-cell ALL or B-cell NHL disease-free (Bast *et al.*, 1985; Le Bien *et al.*, 1985; Bradstock *et al.*, 1986). Investigating the effect of Mab purging on clinical samples has proved more difficult. Janossy *et al.* (1988) showed a greater than 3 log reduction in precursor B ALL blast cells with anti-CD10 and CD19 Mabs using a sensitive immunofluorescence technique. Other investigators have

Table 17.1. *Hematopoietic stem cell purging techniques*

Immunological
  Negative selection of malignant cells:
    Complement-mediated lysis
    Magnetic microsphere separation
    Immunotoxins
    High-density microparticles
    High-speed flow cytometry
Pharmacological
  Cyclophosphamide analogues
    4-Hydroperoxycyclophosphamide
    Mafosfamide
  Other drugs
    Etoposide
    Vincristine
    Methylprednisolone
Photosensitizing agents
  Merocyanine 540
  Dibromorhodamine
Physical and membrane-active agents
  Alkyl-lysophospholipids
  Taurolidine
  Pulsed electric fields
Molecular biological and gene transduction approaches
  Anti-sense oligonucleotides against:
    Mutated oncogenes
    Critical proteins of short half-life
    Gene rearrangements
  Ribozymes
  Enzymes for prodrug activation
Immune effector cells
  Cytokine-activated T and NK cells
  Peptide-specific T-cell clones
Long-term bone marrow culture
Positive selection of hematopoietic cells
  CD34+ stem cells
  CD4+ or CD8+ T cells or NK cells

used clonogenic assays capable of detecting small numbers of residual proliferative ALL cells after purging, and have established that, while individual Mabs can reduce the number of clonogenic leukemic cells by up to 3 logs, cocktails of two or more antibodies are generally more effective because of the problem of heterogeneity of antigen expression of the clonogenic population (Uckun *et al.*, 1986; Marie *et al.*, 1987; Hudson *et al.*, 1989).

Similarly, in T-cell ALL, antibodies to T-lymphocyte differentiation antigens have been used to establish the potential efficacy of purging. Janossy *et al.* (1988) demonstrated a greater than 3 log reduction in 74% of cases of T ALL using a complement-fixing anti-CD7 Mab. Casellas *et al.* (1985) and Preijers *et al.* (1989) used CD5 and CD7 ricin immunotoxins, and showed over 6 log inhibition of T leukemic cell line growth. Uckun *et al.* (1987) evaluated similar immunotoxins in a clonogenic assay on 12 cases of T ALL, and showed much more variable effectiveness of purging. The reduction in clonogenic cells ranged from 0.7 to over 3 logs, with residual leukemic colonies being detected in eight cases. Addition of the pharma-

cologic agent 4HC to the purging cocktail, however, greatly enhanced the effect of immunotoxins.

In follicular NHL, the effect of purging with Mabs and complement has been monitored by PCR amplification of the t(14;18) translocation involving bcl-2. A Stanford University study of 15 cases that had PCR-positive marrow showed a reduction in PCR signal in two-thirds of cases after Mab purging (Negrin & Pesando, 1994). Similar results have been reported from the Dana-Farber group (Gribben *et al.*, 1991). This group demonstrated that immunomagnetic bead purging was superior in this setting to complement lysis, and that cocktails of three or four antibodies with three rounds of bead purging were necessary to produce PCR-negative marrows in all cases (Gribben *et al.*, 1992). Real-time quantitative PCR now enables easy and rapid measurement of the pre- and post-purging tumor loads (Ladettto *et al.*, 2001). This tool promises to help identify the efficacy of purging strategies and select more intensive strategies to eliminate high tumor loads. In addition, it should provide a unique opportunity to determine graft conditions in which purging may represent a determining factor for clinical outcome.

In contrast to the lymphoid malignancies, immunologic purging approaches in AML are more difficult, because of the similarity of immunophenotypic profiles of myeloid leukemic blast cells to normal bone marrow precursor cells. However, subtle antigenic differences between leukemic clonogenic cells and marrow stem cells have been exploited for purging. Sabbath *et al.* (1985) showed a reduction in AML clonogenic cells after treatment with Mabs to CD14, CD15, and CD33. Similar results were achieved with immunotoxins prepared from CD33 (Roy *et al.*, 1991), or CD13, and CD14 (Myers *et al.*, 1988) antibodies. However, when Bonnet & Dick (1997) evaluated clonogenic leukemic progenitors in the severe combined immunodeficiency (SCID)-repopulating assay, they identified these cells as highly immature, with a CD34+ CD38− phenotype. This finding raised significant concern about the nature of targeted antigens, such as CD33, CD13, and CD14, in acute leukemia, that one would not expect to be expressed on the surface of such early clonogenic CD34+CD38− cell subsets. Interestingly, the in vivo administration of an anti-CD33 immunotoxin alone was able to induce complete and durable remissions in patients with relapsed AML (Sievers *et al.*, 2001). The activity of anti-CD33 immunotoxins against AML, in addition to the clinical purging results presented below, suggests that the immunophenotypic profile of AML cells does not correspond to the ontogeny of normal progenitors, and that surface antigens normally present on more mature progenitor subsets are aberrantly expressed on the leukemic stem cells. Moreover, data from long-term marrow cultures indicate that these myeloid antigens, which are expressed on normal progenitor cells, are absent from early stem cells required for prolonged hematopoiesis (Andrews *et al.*, 1986). Thus, while graft function could be expected to be delayed by myeloid antibody purging because of loss of committed progenitors, long-term engraftment would not necessarily be impaired.

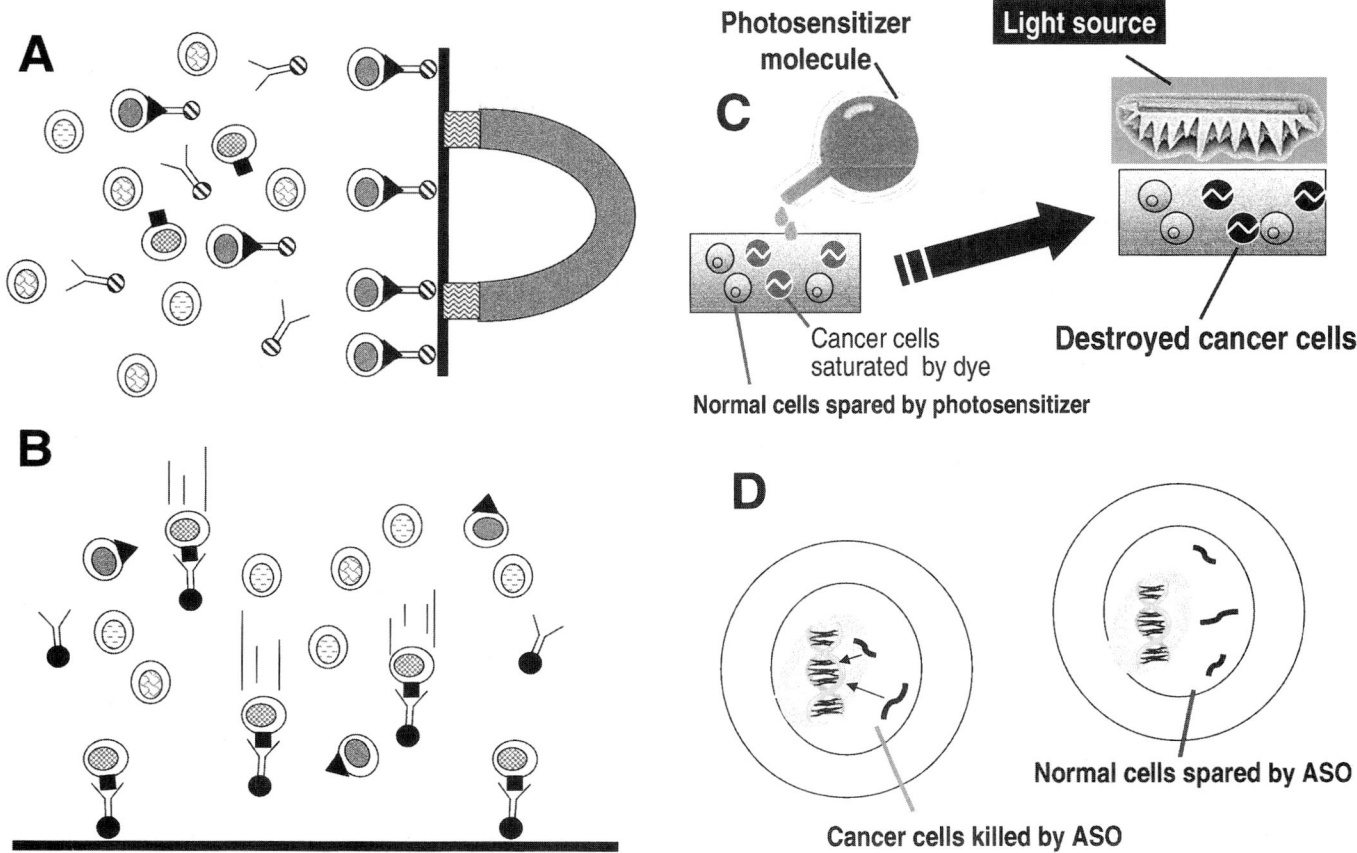

Fig. 17.2. Schema of various purging strategies: (A) Immunomagnetic labeling of cells harboring defined antigens (triangles) enables either negative or positive selection of target cells. (B) High-density microparticles use the simple principle of gravity to deplete target cells coated with monoclonal antibodies. (C) Photodynamic therapy takes advantage of the selective retention of the photosensitizing dye in malignant cells for their eradication after light exposure. (D) Anti-sense oligonucleotides (ASO) rather target molecular rearrangements or preferential pathways of malignant cells to inhibit their proliferation and induce cell death.

Purging with pharmacologic agents

Pharmacologic purging, despite its relative unselectivity, has gained acceptance in clinical practice, and has been extensively used in AML (Gorin *et al.*, 1991). This purging modality was initially investigated in rodent leukemia models. In human leukemia studies, Gorin *et al.* (1986) assessed the effect of mafosfamide, and showed little difference in sensitivity between

Table 17.2. *Negative versus positive selection[a]*

	Negative selection	Positive selection
Advantages:	Selective eradication of malignant cells.	Only need to select for normal cells.
	Spares immune cell populations for activity against infection and disease relapse.	Same methodology for different malignant disorders.
	High levels of efficacy (3–6 logs).	Non-specific elimination of stem cells is limited and constant.
Disadvantages:	Difficult to identify targets present on malignant cells only.	Antigenic or biologic characteristics of normal cells can be shared by malignant cells.
	Non-specific toxicity varies according to purging method and disease.	Trapping of malignant cells among normal progenitors.
	Usually requires individual reagents for different diseases.	Early stem cells (CD34$^-$) are eliminated. Elimination of immune cells.

[a] Note, both approaches can be combined.

AML clonogenic cells and normal myeloid progenitors. Considerable interpatient variation in drug sensitivity has also been observed, leading to the use of dose individualization at some transplant centers (Mangoni et al., 1990). In general, the dose of 4HC or mafosfamide used for clinical purging is sufficient to eradicate most, if not all, myeloid progenitor growth, inevitably leading to slower engraftment. However, a direct correlation has been demonstrated between the efficiency of killing of myeloid progenitors in vitro by 4HC and the subsequent rate of leukemic relapse, implying that effective purging reduces the risk of AML regrowth (Rowley et al., 1989). This remains true for patients with AML transplanted in second or subsequent remission between 1987 and 1997, where age and sensitivity to 4HC of clonogenic leukemia (CFU-L) were identified as predictors of event-free-survival in a multivariate analysis, and superseded even cytogenetics and duration of first remission, which were not retained in the final model (Smith et al., 2002). In addition, it has been shown that the phosphorylated aminothiol, amifostine, is able to protect normal hematopoietic progenitor cells from the effect of mafosfamide, while enhancing its effects on AML clonogenic cells (Douay et al., 1995). Amifostine may therefore prove to be a useful agent for pharmacologic purging. Other pharmacologic agents, such as etoposide, vincristine, and methylprednisolone, have also been investigated for marrow purging in AML (Ciobanu et al., 1986; Auber et al., 1988). Efforts at increasing selectivity have also resulted in the development of an adenovirus to deliver cDNA that encodes an enzyme activating the prodrug irinotecan, the virus preferentially infecting malignant cells (Meck et al., 2001).

The efficacy of pharmacologic purging in ALL and lymphoma is less clear. Uckun et al. (1985) showed a greater than 4 log kill of a B-lymphoma line with mafosfamide. Jones et al. (1990) reported a 6 log kill of a pre-B ALL cell line with 4HC, an effect potentiated by addition of vincristine and methylprednisolone. This drug combination also had some effect on ALL clonogenic cells. However, when the activity of 4HC alone was assessed in 10 cases of ALL and 43 cases of AML, ALL clonogenic cells were considerably less sensitive to 4HC than AML cells (Miller et al., 1991). Similarly, Makrynikola, Kabral, and Bradstock (1991) showed that clonogenic cells in precursor B ALL were less sensitive to mafosfamide than normal progenitors.

Other purging techniques

Several other interesting approaches to marrow purging have been investigated at the preclinical level, with autografts also being performed in pilot studies in some instances. The sensitivity of some tumor cells, including leukemias, to light exposure after photosensitization with agents such as merocyanine 540 has been exploited for marrow purging, in view of the resistance of normal marrow cells to photolysis (Atzpodien et al., 1987; Sieber & Krueger, 1989). Photodynamic therapy had fallen into obscurity for several years, but successes in the selective elimination of alloreactive T cells (Guimond et al., 2002) and treatment of graft rejection and graft-versus-host

disease (GVHD) have rejuvenated interest in this approach (Barr et al., 1998; Greinix et al., 2000). Indeed, the preferential accumulation of photosensitizers such as dibromorhodamine methyl ester, not only in immunoreactive T cells but also in malignant cells, resulted in the eradication of 3 to 6 logs of NHL and chronic myeloid leukemia (CML) cells with preservation of normal hematopoietic progenitors for engraftment of autologous purged stem cell grafts (Roy et al., 2000; Dallaire et al., 2001) (Figure 17.2C). This photodynamic approach is currently being investigated in clinical studies for the purging of NHL and CML cells. In both settings, the extent of tumor cell elimination from peripheral blood stem cell grafts reflects preclinical results. Other membrane-active agents such as alkyl-lysophospholipids have been investigated because of relative selectivity for tumor cells (Okamoto et al., 1988; Vogler et al., 1992). The broad spectrum antibiotic taurolidine also demonstrates important cytotoxic activity against a variety of leukemia and solid tumor cells (Ribizzi et al., 2002).

Molecular biological approaches to purging include targeting the mRNA of mutated oncogenes (e.g., p53) (Hirai et al., 2000), critical proteins of short half-life such as c-myb (Luger et al., 2002), or gene rearrangements resulting from chromosomal translocations that produce biologically altered fusion proteins [e.g., bcr-abl in CML]. CML has provided a unique model to test this approach, and in vitro studies have been carried out using anti-sense oligonucleotides (Szczylik et al., 1991) or ribozymes (Leopold et al., 1995) directed at bcr-abl mRNA (Figure 17.2D). Such anti-proliferative activity may be potentiated by transducing cells with retroviral vectors expressing high levels of ribozymes in either nucleus or cytoplasm (Mendoza-Maldonado et al., 2002). Pulsed electric fields are also being used to increase the potential difference across the cell membrane and induce pore formation, an event leading to a fatal alteration of cell physiology. Thus, threshold electric fields can be applied to eliminate malignant cells, which are usually found in the large cell subsets, and spare the smaller $CD34^+CD38^-$ cells (Eppich et al., 2000).

Another form of negative depletion technology is the use of high-density microparticles (approximately 40 microns in diameter) coated with a monoclonal antibody to a surface antigen on the target cell. This approach utilizes sedimentation under gravity to effect the depletion and appears associated with a high degree of depletion with >80% recovery of non-target cells (Kenyon et al., 1998) (Figure 17.2B). Clinical studies using these particles coated with anti-CD19 and anti-CD20 antibodies demonstrated the capacity to eradicate B cells from 5 out of 6 autografts from patients with non-Hodgkin's lymphoma, resulting in a median of greater than 2 logs depletion of target cells (Webb et al., 2002). Studies are also in progress with particles coated with anti-CD8-coated particles to remove $CD8^+$ cells from HSC or lymphocyte inocula, in an attempt to minimize GVHD while retaining a graft-versus-tumor effect.

A different approach to reducing malignant contamination is short- or long-term marrow culture. Short-term incubation of autologous marrow with cytotoxic immune effector cells, generated by exposure to cytokines such as interleukin-2, has been used for removal of residual blast cells in ALL (Beaujean et al., 1995). The specificity of immune cell populations for specific peptides can even be harnessed to eliminate malignant cells from autologous stem cell grafts. Indeed, the Wilm's tumor gene transcription factor (WT1) is highly expressed in acute and chronic myeloid leukemia, but not by normal CD34$^+$ progenitors, and can be targeted by cytotoxic T lymphocytes (Gao et al., 2000). Although this reaction is HLA-A0201-restricted, one can surmise that it will be possible to derive T cell clones directed at other HLA molecules. Long-term bone marrow culture has also been used as a method for selective removal of leukemic cells, following the demonstration that acute and chronic myeloid leukemias may fail to grow for extended periods under conditions that allow growth of normal myeloid stem cells (Chang et al., 1986; Chang et al., 1989; Turhan et al., 1990).

Finally, there has been interest in positive selection of normal marrow stem cells for autotransplantation, particularly in solid tumors, using immunoaffinity columns constructed with anti-CD34 antibodies that select CD34$^+$ stem and progenitor cells for later use (Berenson et al., 1991) (see also Chapter 27). These approaches can be combined with negative selection strategies, with ensuing increased purging of malignant cells (Straka et al., 1995; Dreger et al., 2000). In addition, improvements in the automated CD34 selection process have improved CD34$^+$ cell yield and engraftment is not delayed (Mohr et al., 2001).

Immunomagnetic selection can also be used to positively select for cell populations involved in immune responses. For example, grafts can be enriched in CD4$^+$ cells by first performing immunomagnetic positive selection of these cells, and then purging contaminating cells by negative selection (Dettke et al., 2002). The administration of CD4$^+$ cells at the time of transplant could help prevent the development of T-cell immunodeficiency. Such an approach could also be used to select for natural killer (NK) cells, CD8$^+$, and other cell populations for the prevention of infectious complications and disease relapse.

Clinical results of purged autografts

Acute myeloid leukemia

Many patients with AML have received marrow autografts purged with 4HC or mafosfamide. Initial transplants were carried out for patients after first remission (Kaizer et al., 1985; Yeager et al., 1986, Gorin et al., 1986). Although no randomized trial has been conducted to evaluate the effect of purging compared to the use of unpurged marrow, the European Bone Marrow Transplant Group (EBMT) has collated data from 59 transplant centers on 919 autografts for AML, 671 in first complete remission (CR) and 196 in second (Gorin et al., 1991). Of the first remission cases, 26% were purged with mafosfamide, while 41% of second remission marrows were purged. The leukemia-free survival for all remission patients was projected

to be 48% ± 3%. The relapse rate for those patients receiving purged marrow (35%) was significantly lower than for those treated with an unpurged graft (47%), although there was no difference in relapse risk for second remission cases. An analysis encompassing 1393 patients with AML registered with the EBMT confirmed the advantage in terms of leukemia-free survival and relapse incidence for the purged transplant group (Reiffers et al., 2000) (Figure 17.3A). Interestingly, this advantage for purging is sustained when grafts consist of mobilized peripheral blood. Similar trends have been reported for smaller series using nonrandomized or historical controls (Chao et al., 1993; Linker et al., 1993; Linker et al, 1998). A multicenter North American analysis of the use of 4HC for marrow purging in first remission AML reached the same conclusion, with a 56% (range 47–64%) leukemia-free survival for purged versus 31% (range 18–45%) for unpurged autografts (Miller et al, 2001) (Figure 17.3B). Improved results with purging were also observed in patients in second CR.

Experience with immunologic purging in AML has been more limited. Ball et al. (1990) treated remission marrow of 30 patients (6 in first remission, 18 in second, 6 in third) with anti-CD14 and anti-CD15 antibodies. Four of the first remission patients, and 6 of the group beyond first remission, survived leukemia-free. Follow-up on 46 AML patients autografted beyond first remission showed a 3-year leukemia-free survival of 31% for CR2/3 patients and 45% for first relapse cases (Selvaggi et al., 1994). Purging with an anti-CD33 immunotoxin has also resulted in 4-year EFS of 62% for CR1 patients and 33% for CR2/3 patients (Robertson et al., 1994). These results appear comparable with those reported for pharmacologic purging, and it is noteworthy that the pattern of engraftment was also similar. Outcome from a subsequent follow-up report of 110 patients with AML transplanted in first to third remission has been reported (Ball et al., 2000). For patients in first remission 5 year leukemia-free survival ranged from 45 to 57%, depending on the type of conditioning therapy used, while, for patients in subsequent remission, corresponding results were from 23 to 28%.

Strong evidence for the contribution of tumor contamination of unpurged marrow in AML to postautograft relapse has come from gene marking studies (Brenner et al., 1993). Eight children with AML at the St. Jude Children's Hospital received marrow autografts in first remission after marking of the marrow cells with the neomycin-resistance gene. In two cases of posttransplant relapse, the leukemic cells contained the marker gene, indicating that leukemia cells in the infused marrow at least contributed to the relapse. Similar findings have been reported in CML following autologous transplants with genetically marked marrow (Deisseroth et al., 1994). Studies directly comparing 4HC purged versus immunologically purged remission marrows in AML using two different retroviral vectors have also been carried out by the St. Jude's group. So far, 4 of the 15 patients have relapsed, but marked leukemic cells have not been detected (H. Heslop, personal communication).

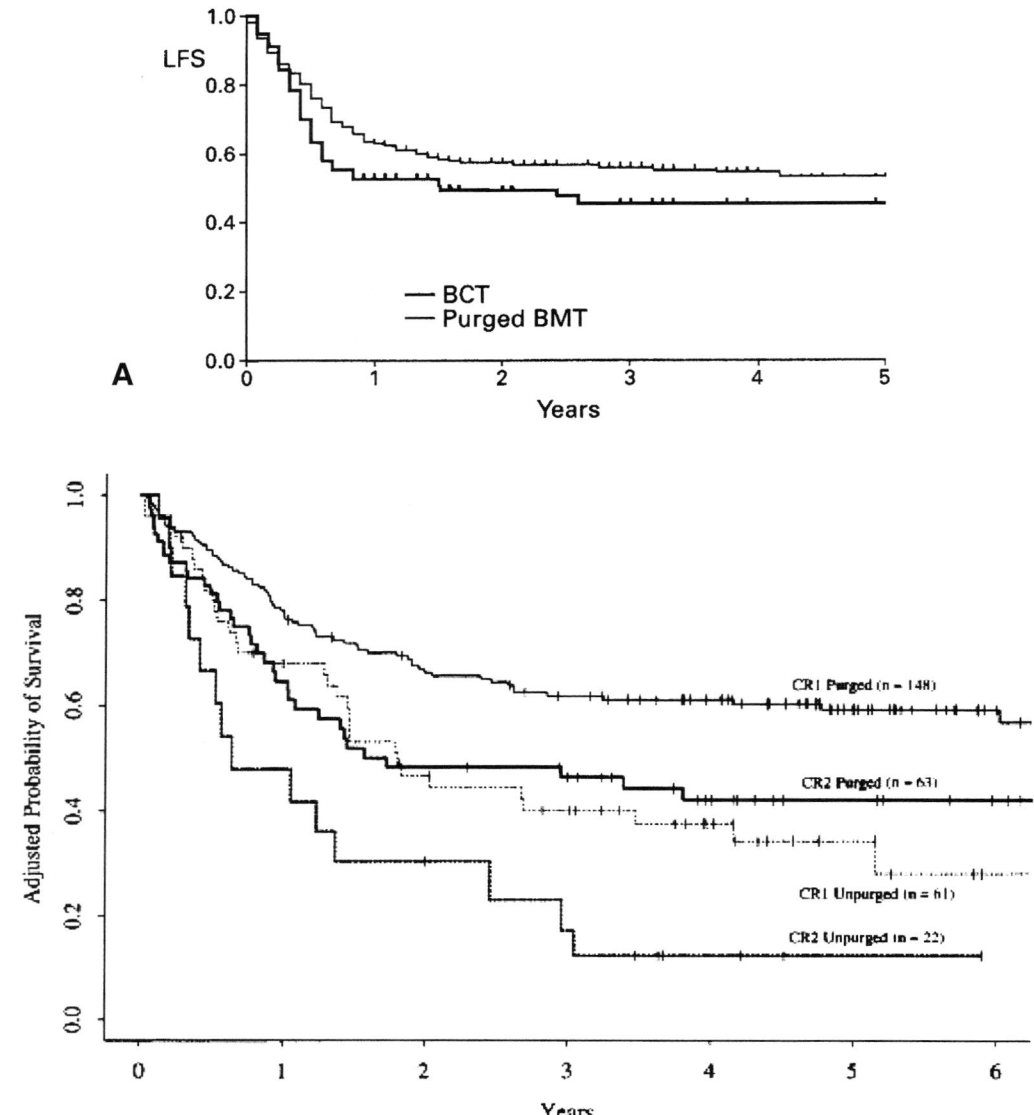

Fig. 17.3. **(A)** In this EBMT analysis, Reiffers showed that autologous stem cell transplantation for patients with AML resulted in better leukemia-free survival when grafts were purged of contaminating leukemia cells, even when unpurged cells were obtained from the peripheral blood. Reproduced, with permission, from Reiffers *et al.* (2000). **(B)** The contribution of purging to improved leukemia-free survival was corroborated in this single center (Johns Hopkins University) study. The benefit of purging was present whether patients were transplanted in their first or second CR. Reproduced, with permission, from Miller *et al.* (2001).

Acute lymphoblastic leukemia

In contrast to AML, interest in marrow purging for ALL has predominantly been with immunologic approaches. The first report of autografts for patients with ALL was in 1980, when two patients with precursor B ALL in third relapse received marrows purged with a heteroantiserum to the common acute lymphoblastic leukemia antigen (Netzel *et al.,* 1980). Ritz *et al.* (1982) subsequently reported autografts for four relapsed ALL patients using marrow treated with anti-CD10 Mab. Since that time, the Dana-Farber Cancer Institute has described its experience of CD10 (ICD19)-purged autografts for 80 precursor B

ALL patients in second or subsequent remission (Soiffer *et al.,* 1990). The leukemia-free survival for the pediatric patients was 36% ± 7%, and for adults 34% ± 13%. Among the larger pediatric group, the length of initial remission was a predictive factor for relapse posttransplant, with patients with initial remission of over 2 years having a lower relapse rate.

The University of Minnesota transplant group used a cocktail of Mabs (anti-CD9, anti-CD10, anti-CD24) for marrow purging in 45 precursor B ALL patients in second or third remission (Kersey *et al.,* 1987). The relapse rate was high (79%), but the overall leukemia-free survival of 20% did not differ significantly from the outcome of a concurrent group of patients receiving allogeneic transplants, owing to the considerably higher procedure-related death rate in the latter group. In a retrospective analysis, the Barcelona group described a benefit in disease-free survival for purging of high-risk ALL patients transplanted in first remission (Granena et al., 1999). A Spanish pediatric study of 55 cases of ALL in second remission reported a 46% event-free survival after antibody-purged autograft (Maldonado et al, 1998).

The clinical value of pharmacologic purging in ALL has not been critically evaluated. The EBMT described 74 high-risk ALL patients autografted in first remission (Gorin, Aegerter, & Auvert, 1989). No significant difference in outcome was observed for patients receiving marrow purged with either mafosfamide or Mabs compared to unpurged marrow.

The Minnesota group has investigated combined purging with Mabs and 4HC. In 14 T ALL patients, marrows were treated with 4HC plus CD5 and CD7 immunotoxins, but only two patients survived in remission (Uckun et al., 1990). As measured by a sensitive leukemia clonogenic assay, the efficiency of purging was not predictive of posttransplant relapse; rather, the estimated total leukemic burden in the patient pretransplant was a more accurate indication of outcome, suggesting that failure of eradication of disease in the patient was more important than the efficiency of purging, or the number of viable clonogenic cells reinfused into the patient. Similar findings have been reported by the same group in a study of 14 precursor B ALL patients autografted with Mabs and 4HC (Uckun et al., 1992), as well as in a Dutch study of pediatric precursor B ALL patients in second remission, where purging efficiency was measured by PCR amplification of immunoglobulin gene rearrangements (Vervoordeldonk et al., 1997). The latter study also demonstrated a relationship between PCR detection of residual leukemia after purging and posttransplant relapse; all 9 patients with PCR-positive marrows relapsed, compared to 6 of 14 transplanted with PCR-negative marrow.

Purging has also been described in BCR-ABL-positive-ALL (Atta et al., 1996). These investigators evaluated the degree of residual leukemia in autologous bone marrow grafts harvested in first or second complete remission from 14 patients with BCR-ABL-positive-ALL. A limiting dilution reverse transcriptase PCR was used to semiquantify BCR-ABL-positive cells. All autografts appeared to be severely contaminated with residual leukemia cells. The BCR-ABL-specific titers ranged from 1 in 10^3 to 1 in 10^6 (median 1 in 10^4) above the level of detection. The grafts were then purged using two cycles of immunomagnetic beads coated with anti-CD10, anti-CD19, and the AB4 monoclonal antibody. Purging resulted in a median of 3 (range 2–4) log tumor depletion.

Non-Hodgkin's lymphoma

Due to frequent involvement of the bone marrow in NHL, increasing attention has been paid to the issue of marrow purging for patients receiving autografts for this disease. Although most common in follicular lymphoma, up to 50% of patients with diffuse large cell lymphoma have tumor cell contamination detectable by DNA PCR of mobilized peripheral blood stem cell collections, although the clinical significance of this remains uncertain (Jacquy et al., 2000).

Takvorian et al. (1987) reported 49 patients with poor prognosis NHL who were autografted with marrows treated with a B-cell Mab (anti-CD20). Thirteen patients relapsed, and 34 remained disease-free. In an update of 69 patients with low-grade NHL treated with the same protocol, over 80% of patients transplanted in complete remission remained disease-free (Freedman et al., 1991). Similar results have been reported from St. Bartholomew's Hospital (Rohatiner et al., 1990).

The Dana-Farber group evaluated the effectiveness of Mab purging in NHL by PCR amplification of the t(14;18) abnormality in 113 informative autografted patients (Freedman et al., 1999) (Figure 17.4A). The relapse rate was very low with only 6 relapses in the 48 patients in whom no residual disease could be detected in the marrow by PCR after purging, whereas 49 of 65 cases with positive PCR results subsequently relapsed. Although patients autografted in clinical complete remission also had a lower risk of relapse than patients with detectable disease, complete eradication of lymphoma cells on PCR analysis remained an independent predictive factor for (lack of) posttransplant recurrence. These findings were not confirmed in a study reported from St. Bartholomew's Hospital (Apostolidis et al., 2000). Of 43 marrow samples demonstrating the presence of a t(14;18) by PCR in the graft and evaluable after purging with anti-CD20 antibody alone or with anti-CD10, anti-CD19, and anti-B5 and complement for low-grade NHL, only 14 became PCR-negative for t(14;18). Post-BMT relapse occurred in 4 of 14 PCR-negative patients and in 13 of 29 PCR-positive patients, but the presence of bcl-2 rearranged cells posttransplant correlated with disease relapse.

Similar findings have been reported by the University of Nebraska Medical Center (Sharp, Kessinger, & Mann, 1996), who used tumor cell culture techniques and/or Southern analysis to detect minimal residual disease in the stem cell harvest. In this nonrandomized study the actuarial relapse-free survival rate at 5 years posttransplant was 64% for those who received a tumor-negative apheresis product, 57% for those who received a tumor-negative marrow harvest, and 17% for those who received a histologically negative, but minimally contaminated bone marrow harvest.

A single case report from the Fred Hutchinson Cancer Research Center described a patient who died of massive pulmonary involvement with Ki-1 antigen (CD30)-positive immunoblastic lymphoma 2 months after transplantation with unpurged autologous marrow. The lungs had not been previously involved in this individual and resectioning of the prestorage marrow biopsy resulted in identification of one small aggregate of lymphoma cells (Rossetti, Deeg, & Hackman, 1995).

In contrast, the outcome of marrow purging with either mafosfamide or Mabs in a large EBMT survey appeared nega-

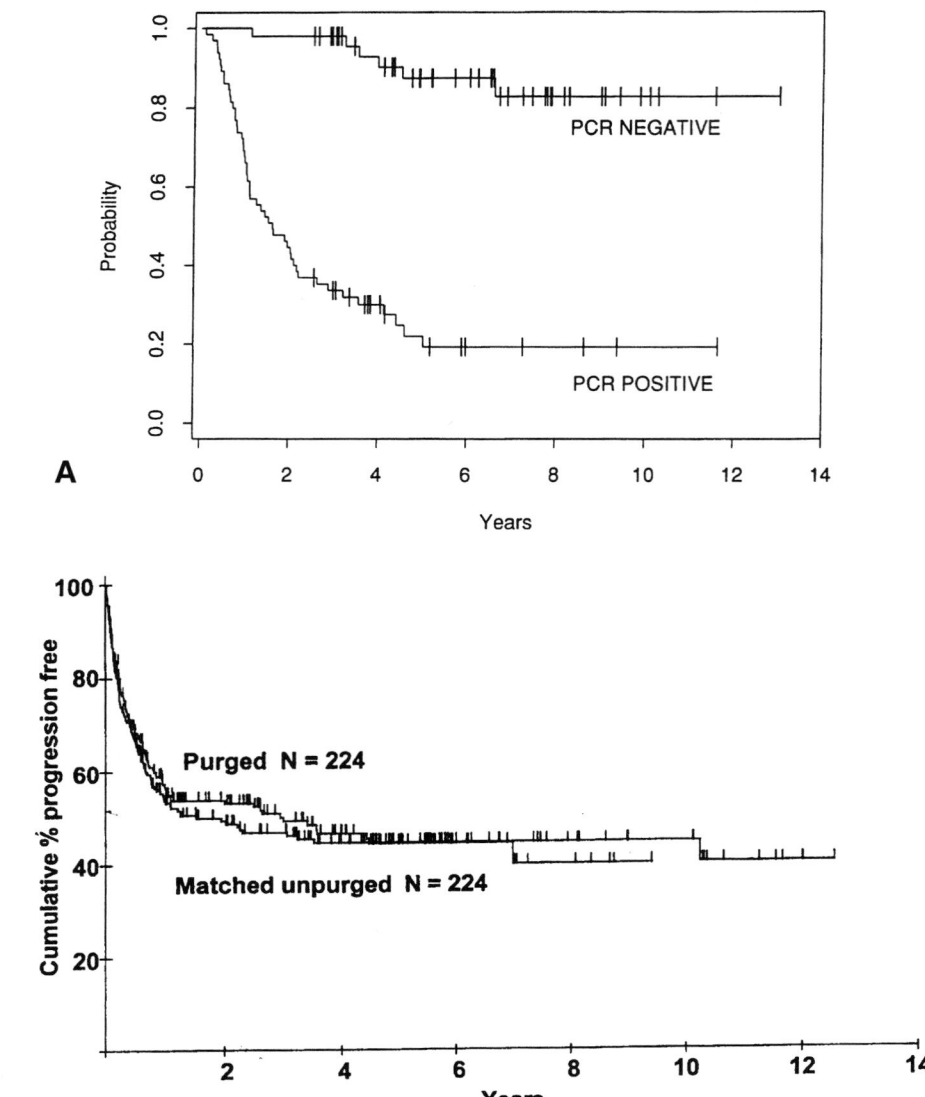

Fig. 17.4. **(A)** Within the group of patients receiving autologous purged bone marrow transplantation, the probability of remaining relapse-free after transplantation was significantly better for patients receiving grafts where bcl-2/IgH rearranged lymphoma cells could be eliminated. Reproduced, with permission, from Freedman *et al.* (1999). **(B)** In a case-matched but non-randomized study, Williams *et al.* failed to identify a survival advantage for patients receiving purged over unpurged grafts (*P* = .1961). This study assessed the total population of patients with non-Hodgkin's lymphoma regardless of the efficacy of treatment. Reproduced, with permission, from Williams *et al.* (1996).

tive. In a case control study, 224 cases of autografts with purged marrow (chemically purged in 109, antibody purged in 104) were retrospectively compared with matched cases receiving unpurged grafts. No differences in relapse rates or progression-free survival were observed between the two groups, although better overall survival was observed in a subset of low-grade lymphoma patients receiving purged grafts (Williams *et al.,* 1996) (Figure 17.4B). The clinical benefit of marrow purging in NHL therefore remains controversial.

Magni and colleagues (2000) have used the chimeric anti-CD20 monoclonal antibody rituximab to effectively purge in vivo peripheral blood stem autografts from patients with

CD20+ follicular or mantle cell lymphoma. The Mab was administered together with hematopoietic growth factor immediately after the chemotherapy used to mobilize PBSC. CD34+ cells harvested from rituximab recipients were PCR-negative for tumor markers in 93% of cases compared to 40% of controls who did not receive rituximab. Additionally, clinical and molecular remission was obtained in all 14 evaluable rituximab recipients compared to 70% of controls. Others have performed quantitative evaluation of lymphoma cells using real-time PCR to measure the effect of anti-CD20 in vivo purging. They also reported significant decreases in PCR-detectable bcl-2/IgH rearranged cells following the administration of such Mabs

(Voso *et al.*, 2000) (Figure 17.5). This approach may represent a useful adjunct to *in vitro* depletion strategies.

Only one randomized study, the CUP trial, has attempted to evaluate the role of autologous transplantation and purging for patients with low-grade NHL (Schouten *et al.*, 2000). In this trial, in which 140 patients from 26 European institutions were registered, patients received three cycles of chemotherapy and those demonstrating chemosensitivity were randomized to 3 additional cycles of the same chemotherapy, or autologous transplantation with either a Mab purged or non-purged graft. Preliminary results demonstrated improved relapse-free survival for patients undergoing autologous transplantation, with a trend favoring the purged arm. Although promising, this clinical trial was closed prematurely due to limited accrual.

Use of CD34⁺ cell selection as a purging technique

The combination of CD34 antigen expression on hematopoietic stem/progenitor cells, with lack of expression on most types of solid tumors and on many types of hematologic malignancies, renders CD34⁺ cell selection a de facto method of tumor cell

purging. Berenson *et al.* (1991) demonstrated that hematopoiesis was reconstituted after transplantation of autologous CD34⁺ cells in patients with breast cancer or neuroblastoma who had received myeloablative chemoradiotherapy. This approach has been widely applied over the past several years in breast cancer (Shpall *et al.*, 1994), NHL (Gorin *et al.*, 1995), and myeloma (Schiller *et al.*, 1995; Vescio *et al.*, 1999; Lemoli *et al.*, 2000; Michallet *et al.*, 2000). The degree of depletion of contaminating tumor cells is closely related to the purity of the CD34⁺ cells obtained, but a several log reduction can be obtained. For example, utilizing PCR technology with patient-specific complementarity determining region immunoglobulin primers in patients with myeloma, a 2.7 to 4.5 log reduction in contaminating myeloma cells was achieved (Schiller *et al.*, 1995). No survival or disease-free survival benefit has yet been demonstrated with this approach. A randomized phase III trial comparing unpurged peripheral blood stem cells with CD34⁺ cells selected with the CEPRATE SC device showed no difference in relapse rate or survival post-autograft (Stewart *et al.*, 2001). These results probably underline the profound resistance of multiple myeloma cells to in vivo chemotherapy. In addition,

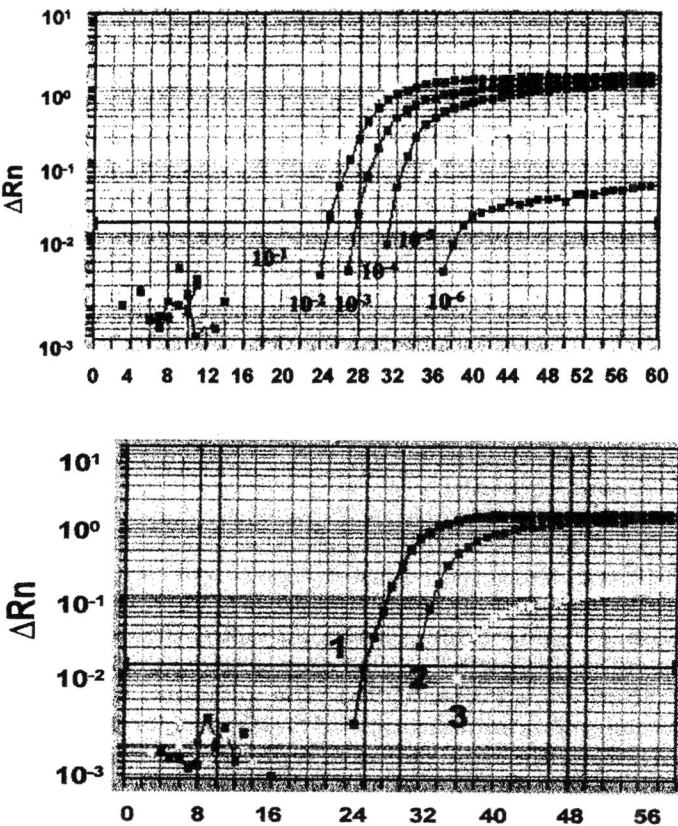

Fig. 17.5. **(A)** Using conditions of linear amplification and optimal probe hybridization, the "real-time" PCR ensures rapid and reproducible quantification of t(14;18)-positive cells. Amplification of the t(14;18) translocation and of the reference gene *bcl-2* of DNA samples extracted from a dilution of the K422 cell line among normal PB mononuclear cells. Increasing cell numbers are associated with fluorescent signals after a lower number of cycles of amplification. **(B)** Amplification curves of samples from one patient demonstrate decreasing numbers of t(14;18) rearranged cells from before (1) to after CHOP chemotherapy (2) and after exposure to rituximab and chemotherapy (3). Reproduced, with permission, from Voso *et al.* (2000).

the identification of hyperdiploid B cells expressing CD34 and CD19, and demonstrating clonotypic immunoglobulin heavy chain transcripts raises questions about the usefulness of positive selection of CD34+ cells in multiple myeloma (Pilarski *et al.*, 2000). Moreover, these patients usually present with very high levels of tumor cell infiltration of their grafts, a crucial factor that could contribute to the very low numbers of PCR negative grafts after CD34 selection in some studies (Voena *et al.*, 2002; Barbui *et al.*, 2002; Rasmussen *et al.*, 2002). Additionally, the incidence of cytomegalovirus disease and associated mortality may be higher after CD34-selected autografts compared to unpurged autografts (Holmberg *et al.*, 1999; Michallet *et al.*, 2000), although other studies have not reported this (Yanovich *et al.*, 2000).

Conclusions

While the concept of autologous hematopoietic stem cell purging remains intuitively attractive, its value is still scientifically uncertain, since no randomized clinical trial evaluating the relative merits of purged versus unpurged autografts has conclusively demonstrated the clinical benefit of purging. Although in vitro studies with cell lines have indicated levels of purging efficiency capable of totally cleansing stem cell collections of contaminating tumor cells, biological assays on clinical samples have revealed a more uncertain picture, with incomplete purging detectable in a significant proportion of cases, even with combined immunologic and pharmacologic techniques. The predictive value of purging efficiency is also unclear. Clonal assays and PCR data in ALL strongly suggest that the pretransplant tumor burden in the patient (a direct reflection of the quality of the remission) is a more important prognostic factor than the efficiency of purging. In contrast, PCR studies in lymphoma indicate that the completeness of purging is an independent prognostic indicator. Further studies are clearly required.

Pooled retrospective data on mafosfamide-purged autografts for AML in first remission have shown an advantage over unpurged autologous transplants, but no randomized trial has yet been reported. Retrospective data from the EMBT have not reported any substantial benefit for purging in NHL. Clearly, further carefully conducted multicenter studies comparing purged autografts directly with unpurged autografts are necessary to resolve this issue.

At the laboratory level, there is considerable scope for further refinements and innovations to improve the efficiency and selectivity of purging. Such improvements and simplification of the purging process will be crucial to the feasibility and success of large multicenter randomized studies.

References

Andrews, R. G., Takahashi, M., Segal, G. M. *et al.* (1986). The L4F3 antigen is expressed by unipotent and multipotent colony-forming cells but not by their precursors. *Blood,* **68,** 1030–5.

Apostolidis, J., Gupta, R. K., Grenzelias, D. *et al.* (2000). High-dose therapy with autologous bone marrow support as consolidation of remission in follicular lymphoma: long-term clinical and molecular follow-up. *Journal of Clinical Oncology,* **18,** 527–36.

Atta, J., Martin, H., Bruecker, J. *et al.* (1996). Residual leukemia and immunomagnetic bead purging in patients with BCR-ABL-positive acute lymphoblastic leukemia. *Bone Marrow Transplantation,* **18,** 541–8.

Atzpodien, J., Gulati, S. C., Strife, A., & Clarkson, B. D. (1987). Photoradiation models for the clinical ex vivo treatment of autologous bone marrow grafts. *Blood,* **70,** 484–9.

Auber, M. L., Horwitz, L. J., Blaauw, A. *et al.* (1988). Evaluation of drugs for elimination of leukemic cells from the bone marrow of patients with acute leukemia. *Blood,* **71,** 166–72.

Ball, E. D., Mills, L. E., Cornwell, G. G. *et al.* (1990). Autologous bone marrow transplantation for acute myeloid leukemia using monoclonal antibody-purged bone marrow. *Blood,* **79,** 1199–206.

Ball, E. D., Wilson, J., Phelps, V. & Neudorf, S. (2000). Autologous bone marrow transplantation for acute myeloid leukemia in remission or first relapse using monoclonal antibody-purged marrow: results of phase II studies with long-term follow-up. *Bone Marrow Transplantation,* **25,** 823–9.

Barbui, A. M., Galli, M., Dotti, G. *et al.* (2002). Negative selection of peripheral blood stem cells to support a tandem autologous transplantation programme in multiple myeloma. *British Journal of Haematology,* **116,** 202–10.

Barr, M. L., Meiser, B. M., Eisen, H. J. *et al.* (1998). Photopheresis for the prevention of rejection in cardiac transplantation. Photopheresis Transplantation Study Group. *New England Journal of Medicine,* **339,** 1744–51.

Bast, R. C., Defabritis, P., Lipton, J. *et al.* (1985). Elimination of malignant clonogenic cells from human bone marrow using multiple monoclonal antibodies and complement. *Cancer Research,* **45,** 499–503.

Beaujean, F., Bernaudin, F., Kuentz, M. *et al.* (1995). Successful engraftment after autologous transplantation of 10-day cultured bone marrow activated by interleukin 2 in patients with acute lymphoblastic leukemia. *Bone Marrow Transplantation,* **15,** 691–6.

Berenson, R. J., Bensinger, W. I., Hill, R. S. *et al.* (1991). Engraftment after infusion of CD-34+ marrow cells in patients with breast cancer or neuroblastoma. *Blood,* **77,** 1717–22.

Berinstein, N. L., Reis, M. D., Ngan, B. Y. *et al.* (1993). Detection of occult lymphoma in the peripheral blood and bone marrow of patients with untreated early-stage and advanced-stage follicular lymphoma. *Journal of Clinical Oncology,* **11,** 1344–52.

Bonnet, D. & Dick, J. E. (1997) Human acute myeloid leukemia is organized as a hierarchy that originates from a primitive hematopoietic cell. *Nature Medicine,* **3,** 730–7.

Bradstock, K. F., Favaloro, E. J., Kabral, A. *et al.* (1986). Standardization of monoclonal antibodies for use in autologous bone marrow transplantation for common acute lymphoblastic leukemia. *Pathology,* **18,** 197–205.

Brenner, M. K., Rill, D. R., Moen, R. C. *et al.* (1993). Gene marking to trace origin of relapse after autologous bone marrow transplantation. *Lancet,* **341,** 85–6.

Brugger, W., Bross, K. J., Glatt, M. *et al.* (1994). Mobilization of tumor cells and hematopoietic progenitor cells into peripheral blood of patients with solid tumors. *Blood,* **83,** 636–40.

Burnett, A. K., Watkins, R., Maharaj, D. *et al.* (1984). Transplantation of unpurged autologous bone marrow in acute myeloid leukemia in first remission. *Lancet, 2*, 1068–70.

Casellas, P., Canat, X., Fauser, A. A. *et al.* (1985). Optimal elimination of leukemic T cells from bone marrow with T-101-ricin A chain immunotoxin. *Blood, 65*, 289–97.

Chang, J., Morgenstern, G., Coutinho, L. H. *et al.* (1989). The use of bone marrow cells grown in long-term culture for autologous BMT in acute myeloid leukemia: an update. *Bone Marrow Transplantation, 4*, 5–9.

Chang, J., Morgenstern, G., Deakin, D. *et al.* (1986). Reconstitution of hematopoietic system with autologous marrow taken during relapse of acute myeloblastic leukemia and growth in long-term culture. *Lancet, 1*, 294–5.

Chao, N. J., Stein, A. S., Long, G. D. *et al.* (1993). Busulfan/etoposide—initial experience with a new preparatory regimen for autologous bone marrow transplantation in patients with acute non-lymphoblastic leukemia. *Blood, 81*, 319–23.

Ciobanu, N., Paietta, E., Andreeff, M. *et al.* (1986). Etoposide as an in vitro purging agent for the treatment of acute leukemias and lymphomas in conjunction with autologous bone marrow transplantation. *Experimental Hematology, 14*, 626–35.

Dallaire, N., Leonard, B., Moreau, B. *et al.* (2001). Preferential eradication of B-lineage lymphoma cells over T cells using TH9402 photodynamic cell therapy, and hierarchical preservation of myeloid and erythroid progenitors. *Blood, 98*, 391a.

Deisseroth, A. B., Zu, Z., Claxton, D. *et al.* (1994). Genetic marking shows that Ph+ cells present in autologous transplants of chronic myelogenous leukemia (CML) contribute to relapse after autologous bone marrow in CML. *Blood, 83*, 3068–76.

Dettke, M., Berger, R., Jurko, S. *et al.* (2002) Selection of autologous CD4+ T-cells for adoptive T-cell substitution in patients with CD23+ B-cell CLL. *Cytotherapy, 4*, 119–25.

Dicke, K. A., Jagannath, S., Spitzer, G. *et al.* (1984). The role of autologous bone marrow transplantation in various malignancies. *Seminars in Hematology, 21*, 109–22.

Dreger, P., Viehmann, K., von Neuhoff, N. *et al.* (2000). A prospective study of positive/negative ex vivo B-cell depletion in patients with chronic lymphocytic leukemia. *Experimental Hematology, 28*, 1187–96.

Douay, L., Hu, C., Giarratana, M. C. *et al.* (1995). Amifostine improves the antileukemic therapeutic index of mafosfamide: implications for bone marrow purging. *Blood, 86*, 2849–55.

Eppich, H. M., Foxall, R., Gaynor, K. *et al.* (2000). Pulsed electric fields for selection of hematopoietic cells and depletion of tumor cell contaminants. *Nature Biotechnology, 18*, 882–7.

Freedman, A. S., Munro, J. M., Rice, G. E. *et al.* (1990). Adhesion of human B cells to germinal centers in vitro involves VLA-4 and INCAM-110. *Science, 249*, 1030–3.

Freedman, A. S., Ritz, J., Neuberg, D. *et al.* (1991). Autologous bone marrow transplantation in 69 patients with a history of low grade B cell non Hodgkin's lymphoma. *Blood, 77*, 2524–9.

Freedman, A. S., Neuberg, D., Mauch, P. *et al* (1999). Long-term follow-up of autologous bone marrow transplantation in patients with relapsed follicular lymphoma. *Blood, 94*, 3325–33.

Gao, L., Bellantuono, I., Elsasser, A. *et al.* (2000). Selective elimination of leukemic CD34(+) progenitor cells by cytotoxic T lymphocytes specific for WT1. *Blood, 95*, 2198–2203.

Gee, A., (1995). Purging of peripheral blood stem cell grafts. *Stem Cells, 13* (Suppl 3), 52–65.

Gordon, M. Y., Goldman, J. M., & Gordon-Smith, E. C. (1985). 4-hydroperoxycyclophosphamide inhibits proliferation by human granulocyte-macrophage colony-forming cells (GM-CFC) but spares more primitive progenitor cells. *Leukemia Research, 9*, 1017–21.

Gorin, N. C., Aegerter, P., & Auvert, B. (1989). Autologous bone marrow transplantation for acute leukemia in remission: an analysis on 1322 cases. *Bone Marrow Transplantation, 4* (Suppl 2), 3–5.

Gorin, N. C., Aegerter, P., Auvert, B. *et al.* (1990). Autologous bone marrow transplantation for acute myelocytic leukemia in first remission. A European survey of the value of marrow purging. *Blood, 75*, 1606–14.

Gorin, N. C., Douay, L., Laporte, J. P. *et al.* (1986). Autologous bone marrow transplantation using marrow incubated with ASTA Z 7557 in adult acute leukemia. *Blood, 67*, 1367–76.

Gorin, N. C., Labopin, M., Meloni, G. *et al.* (1991). Autologous bone marrow transplantation for acute myeloblastic leukemia in Europe: further evidence for the role of marrow purging by mafosfamide. *Leukemia, 5*, 896–904.

Gorin, N. C., Lopez, M., Laporte, J. P. *et al.* (1995). Preparation and successful engraftment of purified CD34+ bone marrow progenitor cells in patients with non-Hodgkin's lymphoma. *Blood, 85*, 1647–54.

Granena, A., Castellsague, X., Badell, I. *et al* (1999). Autologous bone marrow transplantation for high risk acute lymphoblastic leukemia: clinical relevance of ex vivo bone marrow purging with monoclonal antibodies and complement. *Bone Marrow Transplantation, 24*, 621–7.

Greinix, H. T., Volc-Platzer, B., Kalhs, P. *et al.* (2000). Extracorporeal photochemotherapy in the treatment of severe steroid-refractory acute graft-versus-host disease: a pilot study. *Blood, 96*, 2426–31.

Gribben, J. G., Freedman, A. S., Neuberg, D. *et al.* (1991). Immunologic purging of marrow assessed by PCR before autologous bone marrow transplantation for B cell lymphoma. *New England Journal of Medicine, 325*, 1525–33.

Gribben, J. G., Saporito, L., Barber, M. *et al.* (1992). Bone marrow of non-Hodgkin's lymphoma patients with bcl-2 translocation can be purged of polymerase chain reaction-detectable lymphoma cells using monoclonal antibodies and immunomagnetic bead depletion. *Blood, 80*, 1083–9.

Griffin, J. D. & Lowenberg, B. (1986). Clonogenic cells in acute myeloblastic leukemia. *Blood, 68*, 1185–95.

Guimond, M., Balassy, A., Barrette, M. *et al.* (2002). P-Glycoprotein targeting : a unique strategy to selectively eliminate immunoreactive T cells. *Blood, 100*, 375–82.

Hagenbeek, A. & Martens, A. C. M. (1989). Cryopreservation of autologous marrow grafts in acute leukemia: survival of in vivo clonogenic cells and normal hemopoietic stem cells. *Leukemia, 3*, 535–7.

Herve, P., Tamayo, E., Cahn, J. Y. *et al.* (1986). Attempts to eliminate residual acute myeloid leukemia from autologous bone marrow grafts through in vitro chemotherapy—a review. In *Minimal Residual Disease in Acute Leukemia*, ed. A. Hagenbeek & B.

Lowenberg, pp. 248–265. Dordrecht, the Netherlands: Martinus Nijhoff.

Hirai, M., Kelsey, L. S., Vaillancourt, M. *et al.* (2000). Purging of human breast cancer cells from stem cell products with an adenovirus containing p53. *Cancer Gene Therapy,* **7,** 197–206.

Holmberg, L., Boeckh, M., Hooper, H. *et al.* (1999). Increased incidence of cytomegalovirus disease after autologous CD34-selected peripheral blood stem cell transplantation. *Blood,* **94,** 4029–35.

Hudson, A. M., Makrynikola, V., Kabral, A., & Bradstock, K. F. (1989). Immunophenotypic analysis of clonogenic cells in acute lymphoblastic leukemia using an in vitro colony assay. *Blood,* **74,** 2112–20.

Jacquy, C., Soree, A., Lambert, F. *et al.* (2000). A quantitative study of peripheral blood stem cell contamination in diffuse large-cell non-Hodgkin's lymphoma: one-half of patients significantly mobilize malignant cells. *British Journal of Haematology,* **110,** 631–7.

Janossy, G., Campana, D., Burnett, A. *et al.* (1988). Autologous bone marrow transplantation in acute lymphoblastic leukemia—preclinical studies. *Leukemia,* **2,** 485–95.

Jansen, J., Falkenburg, J. H. F., Stepan, D. E., & Le Bien, T. W. (1984). Removal of neoplastic cells from autologous bone marrow grafts with monoclonal antibodies. *Seminars in Hematology,* **21,** 164–81.

Jones, R. J., Miller, C. B., Zehnbauer, B. A. *et al.* (1990). In vitro evaluation of combination drug purging for autologous bone marrow transplantation. *Bone Marrow Transplantation,* **5,** 301–8.

Kaizer, H., Stuart, R. K., Brookmeyer, R. *et al.* (1985). Autologous bone marrow transplantation in acute leukemia: a phase 1 study of in vitro treatment of marrow with 4-hydroperoxycyclophosphamide to purge tumor cells. *Blood,* **65,** 1504–10.

Kenyon, N. S., Ricordi, C., Gribben, J. G. *et al.* (1998). High-density particles: a novel, highly efficient cell separation technology. In *Cell Separation Methods and Applications,* eds. D., Recktenwald, & A., Radbruch, pp. 103–32 New York: Marcel Dekker, Inc.

Kersey, J. H., Weisdorf, M. D., Nesbit, M. E. *et al.* (1987). Comparison of autologous and allogeneic bone marrow transplantation for treatment of high-risk refractory acute lymphoblastic leukemia. *New England Journal of Medicine,* **317,** 461–7.

Kessinger, A., Armitage, J. A., Smith, D. M. *et al.* (1989). High dose therapy and autologous peripheral blood stem cell transplantation for patients with lymphoma. *Blood,* **74,** 1260–5.

Ladetto, M., Sametti, S., Donovan, J. W. *et al.* (2001). A validated real-time quantitative PCR approach shows a correlation between tumor burden and successful ex vivo purging in follicular lymphoma patients. *Experimental Hematology,* **29,** 183–193.

Le Bien, T. W., Stepan, D. E., Bartholomew, R. M. *et al.* (1985). Utilization of a colony assay to assess the variables influencing elimination of leukemic cells from human bone marrow with monoclonal antibodies and complement. *Blood,* **65,** 945–50.

Lemoli, R. M., Martinelli, G., Zamagni, E. *et al.* (2000). Engraftment, clinical, and molecular follow-up of patients with multiple myeloma who were reinfused with highly purified CD34+ cells to support single or tandem high-dose chemotherapy. *Blood,* **95,** 2234–9.

Leonard, B. M., Hetu, F., Busque, L. *et al.* (1998). Lymphoma cell burden in progenitor cell grafts measured by competitive polymerase chain reaction: less than one log difference between bone marrow and peripheral blood sources. *Blood,* **91,** 331–9.

Leopold, L. H., Shore, S. K., Newkirk, T. A. *et al.* (1995). Multi-unit ribozyme-mediated cleavage of bcr-abl mRNA in myeloid leukemias. *Blood,* **85,** 2162–70.

Levesque, J. P., Haylock, D. N. & Simmons, P. J. (1996). Cytokine regulation of proliferation and cell adhesion are correlated events in human CD34+ hemopoietic progenitors. *Blood,* **88,** 1168–76.

Linker, C. A., Ries, C. A., Damon, L. E. *et al.* (1993). Autologous bone marrow transplantation for acute myeloid leukemia using busulfan plus etoposide as a conditioning regimen. *Blood,* **81,** 311–8.

Linker, C. A., Ries, C. A., Damon, L. E., Rugo, H. S., and Wolf, J. L. (1998). Autologous bone marrow transplantation for acute myeloid leukemia using 4-hydroperoxycyclophosphamide-purged marrow and the busulfan/etoposide preparative regimen: a follow-up report. *Bone Marrow Transplantation.* **22,** 865–72.

Lowenberg, B., Abels, J., Van Bekkum, D. W. *et al.* (1984). Transplantation of nonpurified autologous bone marrow in patients with AML in first remission. *Cancer,* **54,** 2840–5.

Luger, S. M., O'Brien, S. G., Ratajczak, J. *et al.* (2002). Oligodeoxynucleotide-mediated inhibition of c-myb gene expression in autografted bone marrow: a pilot study. *Blood,* **99,** 1150–8.

Magni, M., Di Nicola, M., Devizzi, L. *et al.* (2000). Successful in vivo purging of CD34-containing peripheral blood harvests in mantle cell and indolent lymphoma: evidence for a role of both chemotherapy and rituximab infusion. *Blood,* **96,** 864–9.

Makrynikola, V., Kabral, A., & Bradstock, K. F. (1991). Effect of mafosfamide (ASTA-Z-7654) on the clonogenic cells in precursor-B acute lymphoblastic leukemia: significance for ex vivo purging of bone marrow for autologous transplantation. *Bone Marrow Transplantation,* **8,** 351–5.

Maldonado, M. S., Diaz-Heredia, C., Badell, I. *et al* (1998). Autologous bone marrow transplantation with monoclonal antibody purged marrow for children with acute lymphoblastic leukemia in second remission. Spanish Working party for BMT in Children. *Bone Marrow Transplantation,* **22,** 1043–7.

Mangoni, L., Carlo-Stella, C., Caffo, O. *et al.* (1990). Autologous bone marrow transplantation in acute non-lymphoid leukemia in first remission: effect of mafosfamide purging with standard versus adjusted dose. In *Autologous Bone Marrow Transplantation. Proceedings of the Fifth International Symposium,* ed. K. A. Dicke, J. O. Armitage, & M. J. Dicke-Evinger, pp. 43–54. Omaha: The University of Nebraska Medical Center.

Marie, J. P., Choquet, C., Perrot, J. Y. *et al.* (1987). In vitro depletion of clonogenic cells in adult acute lymphoblastic leukemia with a CD10 (anti-CALLA) monoclonal antibody. *European Journal of Cancer and Clinical Oncology,* **23,** 1181–7.

Meck, M. M., Wierdl, M., Wagner, L. M. *et al.* (2001). A virus-directed enzyme prodrug therapy approach to purging neuroblastoma cells from hematopoietic cells using adenovirus encoding rabbit carboxylesterase and CPT-11. *Cancer Research,* **61,** 5083–9.

Mendoza-Maldonado, R., Zentilin, L., Fanin, R. & Giacca, M. (2002). Purging of chronic myelogenous leukemia cells by retrovirally expressed anti-bcr-abl ribozymes with specific cellular compartmentalization. *Cancer Gene Therapy,* **9,** 71–86.

Michallet., M., Philip, T., Philip, I. *et al.* (2000). Transplantation with selected autologous peripheral blood CD34+ Thy1+

hematopoietic stem cells (HSCs) in multiple myeloma: impact of HSC dose on engraftment, safety, and immune reconstitution. *Experimental Hematology,* **28,** 858–70.

Miller, C. B., Rowlings, P. A., Zhang, M. J. *et al.* (2001). The effect of graft purging with 4-hydroperoxycyclophosphamide in autologous bone marrow transplantation for acute myelogenous leukemia. *Experimental Hematology,* **29,** 1336–46.

Miller, C. B., Zehnbauer, B. A., Piantadosi, S. *et al.* (1991). Correlation of occult clonogenic leukemia drug sensitivity with relapse after autologous bone marrow transplantation. *Blood,* **78,** 1125–31.

Mohr, M., Dalmis, F., Hilgenfeld, E. *et al.* (2001). Simultaneous immunomagnetic CD34+ cell selection and B-cell depletion in peripheral blood progenitor cell samples of patients suffering from B-cell non-Hodgkin's lymphoma. *Clinical Cancer Research,* **7,** 51–7.

Myers, D. E., Uckun, F. M., Ball, E. D., & Vallera, D. A. (1988). Immunotoxins for ex vivo marrow purging in autologous bone marrow transplantation for acute nonlymphocytic leukemia. *Transplantation,* **46,** 240–5.

Negrin, R. S. & Pesando, J. (1994). Detection of tumor cells in purged bone marrow and peripheral- blood mononuclear cells by polymerase chain reaction amplification of bcl-2 translocations. *Journal of Clinical Oncology,* **12,** 1021–7.

Netzel, B., Haas, R. J., Rodt, H. *et al.* (1980). Immunological conditioning of bone marrow for autotransplantation in childhood acute lymphoblastic leukemia. *Lancet,* **1,** 1330–2.

Okamoto, S., Olson, A. C., Berdel, W. E., & Vogler, W. R. (1988). Purging of acute myeloid leukemic cells by ether lipids and hyperthermia. *Blood,* **72,** 1777–83.

O'Reilly, R. J. (1986). New promise for autologous marrow transplants in leukemia. *New England Journal of Medicine,* **315,** 186–8.

Philip, T., Armitage, J. O., Spitzer, G. *et al.* (1987). High dose therapy and autologous bone marrow transplantation after failure of conventional chemotherapy in adults with intermediate-grade or high-grade non-Hodgkin's lymphoma. *New England Journal of Medicine,* **316,** 1493–8.

Pilarski, L. M., Hipperson, G., Seeburger, K. *et al.* (2000). Myeloma progenitors in the blood of patients with aggressive or minimal disease: engraftment and self-renewal of primary human myeloma in the bone marrow of NOD SCID mice. *Blood,* **95,** 1056–65.

Preijers, F. W. M. B., De Witte, T., Wessels, J. M. C. *et al.* (1989). Cytotoxic potential of anti-CD-7 immunotoxin (WT1-ricin A) to purge ex vivo malignant T cells in bone marrow. *British Journal of Haematology,* **71,** 195–202.

Rasmussen, T., Bjorkstrand, B., Andersen, H., Gaarsdal, E. & Johnsen, H. E. (2002). Efficacy and safety of CD34-selected and CD19-depleted autografting in multiple myeloma patients: a pilot study. *Experimental Hematology,* **30,** 82–8.

Reiffers, J., Labopin, M., Sanz, M. *et al.* (2000). Autologous blood cell vs marrow transplantation for acute myeloid leukemia in complete remission: an EBMT retrospective analysis. *Bone Marrow Transplantation,* **25,** 1115–1119.

Reittie, J. E., Gottlieb, D. J., Heslop, H. E. *et al.* (1989). Endogenously generated activated killer cells circulate after autologous and allogeneic marrow transplantation but not after chemotherapy. *Blood,* **73,** 1351–8.

Ribizzi, I., Darnowski, J. W., Goulette, F. A. *et al.* (2002). Taurolidine: preclinical evaluation of a novel, highly selective, agent for bone marrow purging. *Bone Marrow Transplantation,* **29,** 313–9.

Ritz, J., Sallan, S. E., Bast, R. C. *et al.* (1982). Autologous bone marrow transplantation in CALLA-positive acute lymphoblastic leukemia after in-vitro treatment with J5 monoclonal antibody and complement. *Lancet,* **2,** 60–3.

Robertson, M. J., Roy, D. C., Stone, R. M. & Ritz, J. (1994). Use of CD33 monoclonal antibodies in bone marrow transplantation for acute myeloid leukemia. *Progress in Clinical & Biological Research,* **389,** 47–63.

Rohatiner, A. Z. S., Price, C. G. A., Arnott, S. *et al.* (1990). Ablative therapy with autologous bone marrow transplantation as consolidation of remission in patients with follicular lymphoma. In *Autologous Bone Marrow Transplantation. Proceedings of the Fifth International Symposium,* ed K. A. Dicke, J. O. Armitage, & M. J. Dicke-Evinger, pp. 465–471. Omaha: The University of Nebraska Medical Center.

Ross, A. A., Cooper, B. W., Lazarus, H. M., Mackay, W., Moss, T. J. (1993). Detection and viability of tumor cells in peripheral blood stem cell collections from breast cancer patients using immunocytochemical and clonogenic assay techniques. *Blood,* **10,** 936–41.

Rossetti, F., Deeg, H. J., & Hackman, R. C. (1995). Early pulmonary recurrence of non-Hodgkins' lymphoma after autologous marrow transplantation; evidence for reinfusion of lymphoma cells? *Bone Marrow Transplantation,* **15,** 429–32.

Rowley, S. D., Jones, R. J., Piantadosi, S. *et al.* (1989). Efficacy of ex vivo purging for autologous bone marrow transplantation in the treatment of acute non lymphoblastic leukemia. *Blood,* **74,** 501–6.

Roy, D. C., Boileau, J., Laplante, J. *et al.* (2000). Phase I study of autologous progenitor cell transplantation purged with a photodynamic approach for patients with chronic myeloid leukemia. *Blood,* **96,** 2504.

Roy, D. C., Griffin, J. D., Belvin, M. *et al.* (1991). Anti-MY9-blocked-ricin: an immunotoxin for selective targeting of acute myeloid leukemia cells. *Blood,* **77,** 2404–12.

Sabbath, K. D., Ball, E. D., Larcom, P. *et al.* (1985). Heterogeneity of clonogenic cells in acute myeloblastic leukemia. *Journal of Clinical Investigation,* **75,** 746–53.

Schiller, G., Vescio, R., Freytes, C. *et al.* (1995). Transplantation of CD34+ peripheral blood progenitor cells after high dose chemotherapy for patients with advanced multiple myeloma. *Blood,* **86,** 390–7.

Schouten, H. C., Kvaloy, S., Sydes, M., Qian, W. & Fayers, P. M. (2000). The CUP trial: a randomized study analyzing the efficacy of high dose therapy and purging in low-grade non-Hodgkin's lymphoma (NHL). *Annals of Oncology,* **11** (Suppl 1), 91–4.

Selvaggi, K. J., Wilson, J. W., Mills, I. E. *et al.* (1994). Improved outcome for high-risk acute myeloid leukemia patients using autologous bone marrow transplantation and monoclonal antibody-purged bone marrow. *Blood,* **83,** 1698–705.

Sharp, J. G., Kessinger, R. A. & Mann, S. (1996). Outcome of high-dose therapy and autologous transplantation in non-Hodgkins' lymphoma based on the presence of tumor in the marrow or infused hematopoietic harvest. *Journal of Clinical Oncology,* **14,** 214–9.

Shirota, T. & Tavassoli, M. (1991). Cyclophosphamide-induced alterations of bone marrow endothelium: implications in homing of marrow cells after transplantation. *Experimental Hematology,* **19,** 369–73.

Shpall, E. J., Jones, R. B., Bearman, S. I. *et al.* (1994). Transplantation of enriched CD34-positive autologous marrow into breast cancer patients following high-dose chemotherapy: influence of CD34-positive peripheral blood progenitors and growth factors on engraftment. *Journal of Clinical Oncology,* **12,** 28–36.

Sieber, F. & Krueger, G. J. (1989). Photodynamic therapy and bone marrow transplantation. *Seminars in Hematology,* **26,** 35–9.

Sievers, E. L., Larson, R. A., Stadtmauer, E. A. *et al.* (2001). Efficacy and safety of gemtuzumab ozogamicin in patients with CD33-positive acute myeloid leukemia in first relapse. *Journal of Clinical Oncology,* **19,** 3244–54.

Smith, B. D., Jones, R. J., Lee, S. M. *et al.* (2002). Autologous bone marrow transplantation with 4-hydroperoxycyclophosphamide purging for acute myeloid leukaemia beyond first remission: a 10-year experience. *British Journal of Haematology,* **117,** 907–13.

Soiffer, R. J., Billett, A. L., Roy, D. C. *et al.* (1990). Autologous bone marrow transplantation for acute lymphoblastic in second or subsequent complete remission: ten years experience at Dana-Farber Cancer Institute. In *Autologous Bone Marrow Transplantation. Proceedings of the Fifth International Symposium,* ed. K. A. Dicke, J. O. Armitage, & M. J. Dicke-Evinger, pp. 167–176, Omaha: The University of Nebraska Medical Center.

Stewart, A. K., Vescio, R., Schiller, G. *et al.* (2001). Purging of autologous peripheral blood stem cells using CD34 selection does not improve overall or progression-free survival after high dose chemotherapy for multiple myeloma: a multicenter randomized controlled trial. *Journal of Clinical Oncology,* **19,** 3771–9.

Straka, C., Drexler, E., Mitterer, M. *et al.* (1995). Autotransplantation of B-cell purged peripheral blood progenitor cells in B-cell lymphoma. *Lancet,* **345,** 797–8.

Szczylik, C., Skorski, T., Nicolaides, N. C. *et al.* (1991). Selective inhibition of leukemic cell proliferation by BCR-ABL antisense oligonucleotides. *Science,* **253,** 562–5.

Takvorian, T., Canellos, G. P., Ritz, J. *et al.* (1987). Prolonged disease-free survival after autologous bone marrow transplantation in patients with non-Hodgkin's lymphoma with a poor prognosis. *New England Journal of Medicine,* **316,** 1499–505.

Turhan, A. G., Humphries, R. K., Eaves, C. J. *et al.* (1990). Detection of breakpoint cluster region negative and nonclonal hematopoiesis in vitro and in vivo after transplantation of cells selected in cultures of chronic myeloid leukemia marrow. *Blood,* **76,** 2404–10.

Uckun, F. M., Gajl-Peczalska, K. J., Kersey, J. H. *et al.* (1986). Use of a novel colony assay to evaluate the cytotoxicity of an immunotoxin containing pokeweed antiviral protein against blast progenitor cells freshly obtained from common B-lineage acute lymphoblastic leukemia. *Journal of Experimental Medicine,* **163,** 347–68.

Uckun, F. M., Kersey, J. H., Vallera, D. A. *et al.* (1990). Autologous bone marrow transplantation in high risk remission T-lineage acute lymphoblastic leukemia using immunotoxins plus 4-hydroperoxy-cyclophosphamide for marrow purging. *Blood,* **76,** 1723–33.

Uckun, F. M., Kersey, J. H., Haake, R. *et al.* (1992). Autologous bone marrow transplantation in high-risk remission B-lineage acute lymphoblastic leukemia using a cocktail of three mono-

clonal antibodies (BA-1/CD24, BA-2/CD9, BA-3/CD10) plus complement and 4-hydroperoxycyclophosphamide for ex vivo bone marrow purging. *Blood,* **79,** 1094–1104.

Uckun, F. M., Gajl-Peczalska, K., Meyers, D. E. *et al.* (1987). Marrow purging in autologous bone marrow transplantation for T-lineage acute lymphoblastic leukemia: efficacy of ex vivo treatment with immunotoxins and 4-hydroperoxycyclophosphamide against fresh leukemic marrow progenitor cells. *Blood,* **69,** 361–6.

Uckun, F. M., Ramakrishnan, S., Haag, D., & Houston, L. L. (1985). Ex vivo elimination of lymphoblastic leukemia cells from human marrow by mafosfamide. *Leukemia Research,* **9,** 83–95.

Vervoordeldonk, S. F., Merle, P. A., Behrendt, H. *et al.* (1997). PCR-positivity in harvested bone marrow predicts relapse after transplantation with autologous purged bone marrow in children in second remission of precursor-B-cell acute leukemia. *British Journal of Haematology,* **96,** 395–402.

Vescio, R., Schiller, G., Stewart, A. K. *et al.* (1999). Multicenter phase III trial to evaluate CD34+ selected versus unselected autologous peripheral blood progenitor cell transplantation in multiple myeloma. *Blood,* **93,** 1858–68.

Vescio, R. A., Han, E. J., Schiller, G. J. *et al.* (1996). Quantitative comparison of multiple myeloma tumor contamination in bone marrow harvest and leukapheresis autografts. *Bone Marrow Transplantation,* **18,** 103–10.

Voena, C., Locatelli, G., Castellino, C. *et al.* (2002). Qualitative and quantitative polymerase chain reaction detection of the residual myeloma cell contamination after positive selection of CD34+ cells with small- and large-scale Miltenyi cell sorting system. *British Journal Haematology,* **117,** 642–5.

Vogler, W. R., Berdel, W. E., Olson, A. C. *et al.* (1992). Autologous bone marrow transplantation in acute leukemia with marrow purged with alkyl-lysophospholipid. *Blood,* **80,** 1423–9.

Voso, M. T., Pantel, G., Weis, M. *et al.* (2000). In vivo depletion of B cells using a combination of high-dose cytosine arabinoside/mitoxantrone and rituximab for autografting in patients with non-Hodgkin's lymphoma. *British Journal of Haematology,* **109,** 729–35.

Webb, I. J., Friedberg, J. W., Gribben, J. G. *et al.* (2002). Effective purging of autologous hematopoietic stem cells prior to high dose therapy for patients with non-Hodgkin's lymphoma using anti-B cell monoclonal antibody coated high density microparticles. *Biology of Blood and Marrow Transplantation,* **8,** 429–34.

Williams, C. D., Goldstone, A. H., Pearce, R. M. *et al.* (1996). Purging of bone marrow in autologous bone marrow transplantation for non-Hodgkin's lymphoma: a case-matched comparison with unpurged cases by the European Blood and Marrow Transplant Lymphoma Registry. *Journal of Clinical Oncology,* **14,** 2454–64.

Yanovich, S., Mitsky, P., Cornetta, K. *et al.* (2000). Transplantation of CD34+ peripheral blood cells selected using a fully automated immunomagnetic system in patients with high-risk breast cancer: results of a prospective randomized multicenter clinical trial. *Bone Marrow Transplantation,* **25,** 1165–74.

Yeager, A. M., Kaizer, H., Santos, G. W. *et al.* (1986). Autologous bone marrow transplantation in patients with acute nonlymphocytic leukemia, using ex-vivo marrow treatment with 4-hydroperoxycyclophosphamide. *New England Journal of Medicine,* **315,** 141–7.

18 Cellular component therapy: stem cells, graft-facilitating cells, and graft-versus-tumor cells

SCOTT R. SOLOMON AND A. JOHN BARRETT

National Heart, Lung and Blood Institute, Bethesda, USA

Introduction

Almost 50 years of experimentation and clinical practice have provided ample evidence that bone marrow cells can reconstitute the entire hematopoietic and lymphoid system of a myeloablated and immunoablated individual. It has long been known that the hematopoietic stem cell (HSC) is the functional unit transplanted. The HSC is necessary and sufficient for the restoration of lifelong hematopoiesis and re-establishment of immune function in the recipient. In clinical practice, other cell types are transferred to the recipient, together with the HSC. Only recently have techniques for the transplantation of highly purified HSC been developed. Concurrently, with the introduction of peripheral blood and umbilical cord blood transplants, there is growing experience in the use of stem cells from sources other than bone marrow. This new ability to modify the composition of the transplant heightens the interest in determining the optimum cellular composition and source for specific types of transplant. Just as blood product component therapy revolutionized blood banking over 20 years ago, so the time has come to reconsider the issues of cell composition, quality, and dose in order to deliver an optimized transplant to the recipient. In this chapter, we identify clinical outcomes that are determined by the composition of the transplant in the allogeneic setting and review current and future approaches to select the dose and types of cells for transplantation.

Objectives of bone marrow and blood stem cell transplantation

Allogeneic HSC transplantation has several functionally distinct aims:

1. To restore hematopoiesis following high-dose chemotherapy and radiation
2. To reconstitute immunity without GVHD
3. To provide immunity against the tumor in the case of malignant disease
4. To establish engraftment in the allogeneic recipient

Establishment of sustained hematopoiesis requires stem cells capable of rapidly restoring marrow production of granulocytes, platelets, and red cells, as well as stem cells with much greater capacity for self-replication to provide lifelong marrow cell production. Full immune recovery requires the transfer of post-thymic lymphocytes in the transplant, as well as the repopulation of the lymphoid compartment from stem cell–derived pre-thymic lymphocyte precursors. Lymphocytes, natural killer cells, and specialized "facilitator" cells are also involved in the establishment of the graft. Donor cells with antigen presentation properties such as dendritic cells and their precursors, monocytes, and B cells transferred to the recipient have a less well-understood effect on the outcome of the transplant, but may be important accessory cells in establishing donor immune responsiveness (Table 18.1, Fig. 18.1). As the contribution of the different cell types to the risks and benefits of the transplant is better understood, the opportunity arises to improve the transplant outcome by selecting and modifying the quantity and the quality of the transplanted cells.

Restoring hematopoiesis following high-dose chemotherapy and radiation

Defining stem cell quantity and quality

In a balanced state stem cells divide to form two cells, one with the ability to differentiate while losing self-renewal ability, and the other remaining stem cell–like and replenishing the stem cell pool (Ratajczak & Gewirtz, 1995). Although theoretically, a single pluripotent HSC should be able to reconstitute hematopoiesis following transplantation, many factors such as homing and stem cell kinetics significantly increase the number of stem cells required for clinical engraftment (Gordon & Blackett, 1995). Furthermore, one study suggested that, even for engrafted patients, there is a permanent reduction of the stem cell reservoir after allogeneic bone marrow transplantation (BMT) (Podesta *et al.,* 1997). Some experimental data and clinical observations indicate that early engraftment occurs from committed progenitor cells contained in the graft, although there is currently controversy regarding this. Sustained engraftment requires the presence of undifferentiated stem cells with unlimited self-renewal capacity.

Table 18.1. *Contribution of transplant cell types to functional transplant outcome*

Cell type	Time posttransplant	Functional outcome
Committed progenitor (CFU-GM, BFU-E, CFU-E, CFU-MK); late pluripotent stem cell	Early[a]	Hematopoietic recovery
Primitive rare HSC with high proliferative potential	Late	
Primed CD4+ and CD8+ T cells (post-thymic CD45 RO+); NK cells	Early	Immunologic recovery
Prethymic T-cell precursors derived from donor CD34+ cells; pre-B cells derived from donor CD34+ cells	Late	
Monocytes; dendritic cell precursors		Antigen presentation
CD4+ and CD8+ cells; NK cells; veto cells; facilitator cells		Engraftment
CD4+, CD8+ T cells; NK cells		Graft-versus-host disease
Virus-specific CD8+ T cells; monocytes and dendritic cells		Immunity to DNA viruses
T cells recognizing tissue- or leukemia-restricted minor histocompatibility antigens; T cells recognizing normal but overexpressed proteins on leukemia cells; monocytes and dendritic cells		Graft-versus-leukemia/antitumor immunity

[a] Controversy exists in this area: some data indicate committed progenitor cells may have little impact on early hematopoietic recovery.

Abbreviations: CFU-GM, granulocyte-macrophage colony-forming units; BFU-E, erythrocyte burst-forming units; CFU-E; erythrocyte colony-forming units; CFU-MK, megakaryocyte colony-forming units; NK, natural killer.

The number of nucleated cells in bone marrow harvests has been used for decades as a surrogate for graft quality, in order to predict engraftment potential. Although subject to many inaccuracies, a number of studies have clearly shown that the bone marrow cell dose correlates with transplant outcome (Ringden & Nilsson, 1985; Paulin, 1992; Sierra *et al.*, 1997). However, this approach cannot be applied with any equivalence to peripheral blood stem cell (PBSC) allografts, because these products are strongly dominated by differentiated cells with variable numbers of hematopoietic progenitors. Although stem cells were initially enumerated using colony-forming cell assays

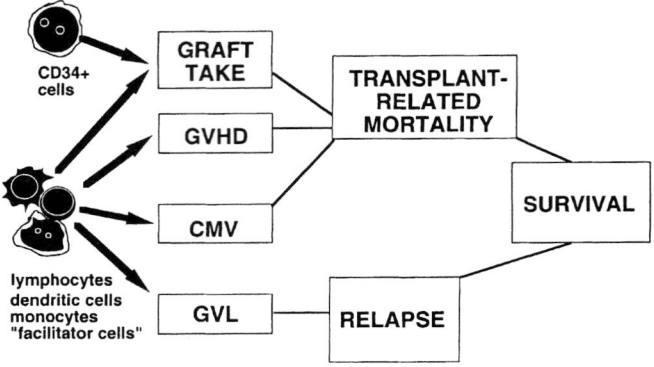

Fig. 18.1. Composition of the transplant affects outcome.

(Moore *et al.*, 1973), such measurements are tedious and poorly reproducible. As a consequence, in humans data correlating the granulocyte-macrophage colony-forming units (CFU-GM) content of the graft with the speed of hematopoietic recovery are conflicting. Only two studies have demonstrated a relationship between CFU-GM dose and neutrophil recovery (Atkinson *et al.*, 1985; To *et al.*, 1992). In the 1990s, a series of clinical studies began to define the impact of stem cell dose on transplant outcomes, aided by the identification of the CD34 antigen as a reliable marker of hematopoietic progenitor cells (Krause *et al.*, 1996) and the ability to collect very large numbers of stem cells using growth factors to mobilize stem cells into the peripheral blood. The CD34+ cell dose of granulocyte colony-stimulating factor (G-CSF)-mobilized PBSC transplants has been correlated with the kinetics of trilineage engraftment in the autologous (Weaver *et al.*, 1995) and the allogeneic setting (Korbling *et al.*, 1995). However, evidence closely correlating CD34+ cell dose with speed of recovery in the allograft setting is scanty (Miflin *et al.*, 1997; Siena *et al.*, 2000; Soiffer *et al.*, 2001). Because so many factors impact on engraftment, the critical stem cell dose required to ensure engraftment will depend upon the genetic disparity of donor and recipient as well as the specific conditions of the transplant and have not been defined for all transplant conditions.

Determining the optimal stem cell dose

Distinct from effects on speed and completeness of engraftment, there is evidence that the CD34+ cell dose can strongly influence transplant-related mortality (TRM) and survival. We found that in marrow depleted of T cells by elutriation, the TRM was significantly higher in patients receiving <1 × 10^6 CD34 cells/kg (65% vs. 7%, respectively) (Mavroudis *et al.*, 1996a). The high TRM in the low stem cell dose group was due almost entirely to fatal viral reactivation from cytomeaglovirus or adenovirus. Patients receiving more than 2 × 10^6 CD34+ cells/kg showed a faster recovery of monocytes and lymphocytes, achieved platelet and red cell transfusion independence earlier, required less G-CSF support during ganciclovir therapy, and spent fewer days in the hospital after transplantation.

In a second analysis, now extended to 78 recipients of T cell-depleted BMT ($n = 50$) or peripheral blood stem cell transplantation (PBSCT) ($n = 28$) and cyclosporine, followed by delayed add-back of donor lymphocytes, we again found that stem cell doses above 2×10^6/kg optimized the TRM and leukemia-free survival (LFS) (Figure 18.2). The overall actuarial survival in patients given >3, 2–2.99, 1–1.99 or <1×10^6 CD34$^+$ cells/kg was 68%, 52%, 35%, and 10%, respectively (Bahceci et al., 2000). Higher CD34$^+$ cell doses were also associated with a decreased risk of relapse (Figure 18.3). This effect was seen both in standard risk (chronic phase chronic myeloid leukemia [CML] and acute myeloid leukemia [AML] in first remission) and high relapse risk patients (multiple myeloma, advanced CML, acute leukemia, and myelodysplastic syndrome). However, because stem cell dose and stem cell source were strongly correlated, it was not clear whether the beneficial effect came from the use of PBSCT or the stem cell dose. A further analysis of stem cell dose in 51 PBSCT recipients was therefore carried out (Nakamura et al., 2001). Recipients received a standardized T lymphocyte dose at transplant with a fixed and timed T cell add-back at day 45 posttransplant. Thus although CD34$^+$ dose varied, the T cell dose was kept constant. Reflecting efforts to increase CD34$^+$ dose to optimize transplant outcome, the median stem cell dose for this group was 4.6×10^6/kg. Again recipients of higher stem cell doses had a significantly better TRM, overall survival (OS) and LFS than those receiving doses below the median (Nakamura et al., 2001).

These results indicate that stem cell dose is a strong independent factor for low TRM and high leukemia-free survival in

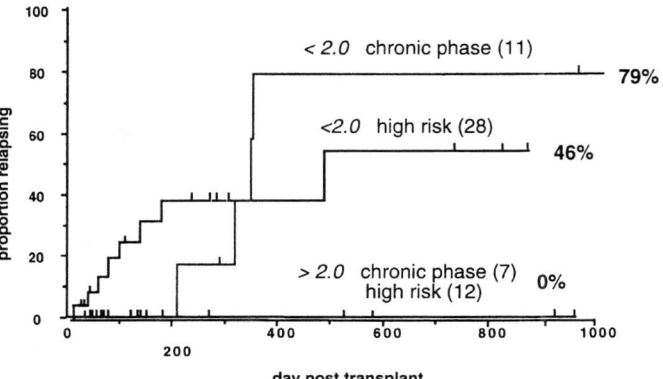

Fig. 18.3. CD34$^+$ cell dose and relapse. Actuarial probability of disease relapse for 78 patients with hematologic malignancies receiving T-cell-depleted HSC transplants of marrow or peripheral blood. CD34$^+$ cell doses (in million/kg recipient weight) in italics, patient numbers in brackets. In patients with high relapse-risk malignancies, relapse rates were significantly higher in patients receiving <3.0 million CD34$^+$ cells/kg (75.8% vs. 20%, $P = .028$). For standard relapse-risk patients, a significant difference in relapse risk was found in patients receiving <1 or ≥1 million CD34$^+$ cells/kg (80% vs. 10%, $P = .0005$). Reproduced, with permission, from Schmitz & Barrett (2002).

both BM and PBSCT T cell-depleted transplants. Other studies also support a beneficial effect of higher stem cell doses on TRM and OS (Noga et al., 1998; Singhal et al.,2000; Morariu-Zamfir et al., 2001). A beneficial effect of higher doses of transplanted cells has also been reported for recipients of unrelated donor (Sierra et al., 1997, 2000), cord blood (Gluckman et al., 1997), and haploidentical related transplants (Aversa et al., 1994). While it appears that a higher CD34$^+$ cell dose is favorable for transplant outcome, the possibility has been raised that very high stem cell doses could be harmful by provoking more GVHD. Higher CD34$^+$ cell doses have been associated with an increased risk of both acute GVHD (Przepiorka et al., 1999) and extensive chronic GVHD (Zaucha et al., 2001) after PBSCT. An additional study showed an association between higher CD34$^+$ cell doses and decreased survival (Urbano-Izpizua et al., 2001). These studies question the safety of very high CD34$^+$ cell doses. Some light has been shed on this issue by a retrospective study performed by the International Bone Marrow Transplant Registry (IBMTR). Ringden et al. (in press) studied transplant outcomes in recipients of T cell-replete BM ($n = 359$) or PBSC ($n = 511$), performed between 1995 and 1998. PBSC recipients on average received twice the CD34 dose as BM recipients (median CD34 dose of 6×10^6/kg and 3×10^6/kg, respectively). A favorable impact of high CD34 dose on LFS was seen in both BM and PBSC recipients. No relationship was found between high CD34 doses and acute GVHD in this large patient population. There was some evidence that chronic GVHD may be more frequent in PBSC recipients receiving high CD34 doses; however, the magnitude of the effect was small. High CD34 dose was correlated with an improved TRM only in BM recipients,

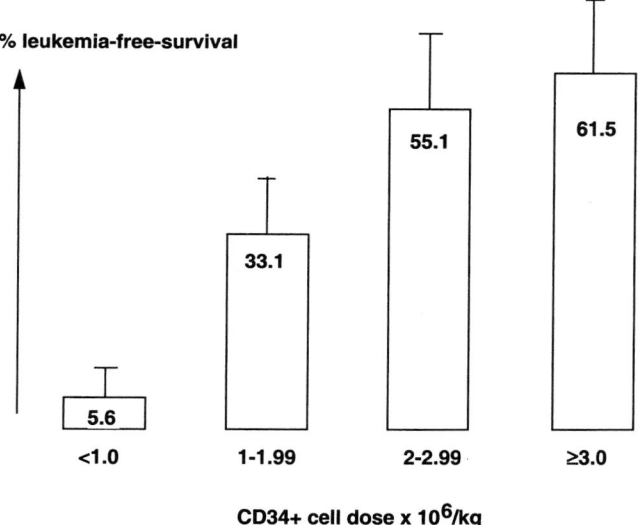

% leukemia-free-survival

CD34+ cell dose x 10^6/kg

Fig. 18.2. Stem cell dose and LFS. Actuarial probability of leukemia-free survival (LFS) for 78 patients with hematologic malignancies receiving T-cell-depleted HSC transplants of marrow or peripheral blood. CD34$^+$ cell doses are in million/kg recipient weight. Difference in LFS between patients receiving >2.0 and <2.0 million CD34$^+$ cell/kg is significant ($P < .05$). Reproduced, with permission, from Schmitz & Barrett (2002).

and this effect was not seen in the PBSC group. In summary, this study defined the optimal CD34$^+$ cell dose range which minimizes TRM in unmanipulated transplants as 3×10^6/kg for bone marrow and around 6×10^6/kg for peripheral blood. However, since the negative effect of very high CD34$^+$ cell doses may be due to an increased risk of chronic GVHD, it is possible that higher doses of stem cells may be more advantageous in the setting of T cell depleted transplants. In addition, a favorable effect of high CD34 dose on relapse was seen only in PBSC recipients receiving >6×10^6/kg CD34$^+$ cells, posing the as yet unanswered question of whether the beneficial effect of high CD34 dose on relapse is due to qualitative or quantitative differences between BM and PBSC.

Role of the stem cell source

There are currently three sources of hematopoietic stem cells used in allogeneic stem cell transplantation—marrow harvests, growth-factor-mobilized peripheral blood collections, and umbilical cord blood (UCB) cells. With modern cell separation techniques and the ability to collect large numbers of stem cells from peripheral blood transplants, we now have enormous flexibility in the choice of stem cell and lymphocyte doses to transplant. Given the inherent differences between the cellular constituents of the various stem cell sources, it is important to understand the impact of the transplant cell source, in addition to dose, on transplant outcomes.

Quantitative and qualitative differences among the three stem cell sources have been evaluated according to CD34$^+$ cell phenotype, clonogenic progenitor assays, proliferative capacity in long-term culture, and ability to repopulate in SCID mice. The CD34$^+$ compartment is heterogeneous and consists of a major fraction of committed progenitor cells (CD34$^+$ CD38$^+$) and a minor fraction of pluripotent HSCs (CD34$^+$ CD38$^-$). The percentage of CD34$^+$ CD38$^-$ HSCs is highest in UCB and lowest in PBSC allografts. However, UCB contains significantly lower absolute numbers of CD34$^+$ and CD34$^+$ CD38$^-$ than either PBSC or bone marrow harvests. Both PBSC and UCB cells contain more differentiated CD34$^+$ cells co-expressing CD33 and CD13, and a higher proportion of CFU-GM. In contrast, BM CD34$^+$ cells have the highest proportion of B-lineage committed HSCs (CD34$^+$CD19$^+$) (Steen et al., 1994). Functionally much bigger differences are seen: UCB has a superior ability to proliferate in long term culture, contains higher numbers of long-term culture initiating cells, and possesses a greater ability to engraft in SCID mice (Wang et al., 1997). The more rapid recovery of platelet and neutrophil counts after PBSC transplants has been attributed to the much larger population of more mature stem cells in the transplant compared to bone marrow (Bensinger et al., 1996; Miflin et al., 1997). There is controversy surrounding this issue, with some data suggesting that early hematopoietic recovery is predominantly due to early stem cells. However, both BM and PBSC transplants appear to ensure sustained engraftment, indicating that long-lived stem cells are present in both transplant sources. Hematopoietic recovery after

UCB transplantation, however, is often very delayed, probably because stem cell numbers are limiting (Kurtzberg, 1996).

Lymphocytes contained in BM, UCB, and PBSC allografts also vary significantly. Compared to BM, PBSC grafts contain approximately 10-fold more T-cells and NK cells. Lymphocytes from G-CSF–mobilized PBSCs contain higher proportions of T-helper-2 (Th2) cells producing interleukin (IL)-4 and IL-10. These cytokines are protective for GVHD (Pan et al., 1995). The high content of CD14$^+$ cells in PBSCT may also suppress alloantigen-induced T-cell proliferation (Mielcarek et al., 1997). These facts may help explain the finding of similar acute GVHD rates in PBSCT and BMT, despite 10-fold more mature T cells in the PBSC product. UCB, on the other hand, has approximately one log less lymphocytes than BM with a higher percentage of immunologically naive CD45RA$^+$) cells (Theilgaard-Mönch et al., 2001). Functionally, UCB lymphocytes also appear immature as shown by minimal responses to stimulation with IL-2, phytohemagglutinin, or alloantigens (Harris et al., 1992), although frequencies of both alloreactive T helper cell precursors (HTLp) and cytotoxic T lymphocyte precursors (CTLp), determined by limiting dilution analysis, have been shown to be similar (Deacock et al., 1992). Clinically, UCB transplants are associated with less GVHD than predicted for the degree of HLA matching (Rocha et al., 2000), highlighting the functional immaturity of transplanted immune cells. Thus, differences in lymphocyte properties can lead to major differences between BMT, PBSCT, and UCBT in the quality of immune recovery.

Establishing immunity without GVHD

Immune function is restored after allogeneic HSC transplants either by the direct transfer of post-thymic (CD45 RO$^+$) T cells in the transplant or by the later generation of prethymic naive (CD45 RA$^+$) T cells that mature in thymic remnants and possibly extrathymic sites. In children and young adults (<25 years), the recipient thymus can function sufficiently well to ensure immune recovery from thymically tolerized, HSC-derived donor cells. However, this process is at best slow to establish immunity and may not occur to any great extent in older patients (Heitger et al., 1997). Thymic function may be significantly impaired in the adult recipient of an allogeneic HSCT as a result of age-dependent thymic involution, radiation damage, and GVHD. Thus, at least in the first few months after transplantation and sometimes permanently, immune function depends almost entirely on the T cells given at the time of transplant. The immune repertoire transferred with marrow or blood transplants represent post-thymic T cells, the majority of which possess a memory phenotype (CD45 RO$^+$). They confer a broad spectrum of immune function that is both beneficial (e.g., immunity against infective agents) and harmful (e.g., causing GVHD). In turn, the development of acute GVHD has an adverse effect on the speed and quality of immune recovery. In addition, the immunosuppressive agents cyclosporine and corticosteroids, commonly used to prevent or treat GVHD, further compromise immune function.

Although the effector cells mediating GVHD and graft-versus-leukemia (GVL) remain incompletely characterized (Barrett, 1997), the primary importance of donor-derived alloreactive T lymphocytes has been clearly demonstrated. Evidence for this includes the higher relapse rates seen in recipients of TCD or syngeneic grafts (Horowitz et al., 1990) and the successful use of donor lymphocyte infusions (DLI) as adoptive therapy for CML patients relapsing after allogeneic HSCT (Kolb et al., 1990). The GVL effect is closely but not inseparably linked with the development of GVHD. The occurrence of GVL without evidence of GVHD in some patients indicates that at least clinically, GVHD is separable from GVL. It would, therefore, be advantageous to separate out the effector cells that cause GVHD from others that generate GVL and provide protective immunity against infection. Harnessing the anti-leukemic properties of allogeneic lymphocytes remains the major challenge for improving the success of allogeneic SCT.

T-cell dose and GVHD

To date, ex vivo T-cell depletion (TCD) is the most effective strategy for reducing GVHD. T-cell depletion has also allowed the expansion of the donor pool by permitting allogeneic HSCT to be performed using HLA-mismatched donors. Murine transplant studies have shown a clear relationship between the number of T cells added to the marrow graft and the incidence and severity of acute GHVD (Truitt & Atasoylu, 1991). Several clinical studies show that GVHD can be prevented almost totally, provided a threshold of CD3$^+$ cells in the transplant is not surpassed. In HLA-matched sibling transplants, the threshold is approximately 10^5 CD3$^+$ cells/kg (Kernan et al., 1986; Lowenberg et al., 1986). In HLA-mismatched transplants, it is in the region of 10^4 CD3$^+$ cells/kg (Muller et al., 1999). Above this CD3 dose, the relationship between T-cell dose and acute GVHD is less clear, with some studies showing an association (Rocha et al., 2001), while others do not (Przepiorka et al., 1999) suggesting that once this initial threshold of clonogenic T cells has been exceeded, a further increase in T cell numbers does not necessarily translate into more GVHD. In addition to the number of T cells present in the graft, other variables such as genetic disparity, inherent immune reactivity, conditioning regimen toxicity, and concurrent viral infections are all factors independently determining the risk of GVHD. It is also clear that the T cell threshold dose for generation of acute GVHD is directly related to the degree of posttransplant immunosuppression. We have demonstrated that PBSC allografts containing a low, fixed dose of T cells (5 × 10^4 CD3$^+$/kg) can still elicit significant acute GVHD when no posttransplant immunosuppression is given (Solomon et al., 2001). In 24 evaluable patients, 12 developed evidence of early acute GVHD before day +45 (grade I [5], grade II [3], grade III [3], grade IV [1]). In contrast, in a cohort receiving the same T-cell dose with low-dose cyclosporine, only three patients (16%) developed acute GVHD (grade I [1], grade II [2]) Therefore, it is highly probable that for the same number of T lymphocytes

present in an allograft, posttransplant alloreactivity will vary from patient to patient and from study to study.

The relationship between T-cell dose and chronic GVHD is less clear. The main risk factor for chronic GVHD is the prior occurrence of acute GVHD. T-cell depletion reduces, but does not universally prevent, the occurrence of chronic GVHD. We have shown a strong correlation between residual CD3 dose following TCD PBSCT and the incidence and severity of chronic GVHD (an incidence of 70% vs. 29% in recipients of allografts containing above and below a median CD3 dose of 0.83 × 10^5 CD3$^+$ cells/kg, respectively, $P = 0.02$) (Nakamura et al., 2001). The high incidence of chronic GVHD in unmanipulated PBSC transplants (where very high T-cell doses are infused) also suggests that chronic GVHD risk is in some way related to the T-cell dose.

Delayed add-back of donor T cells

While T-cell depletion can almost completely prevent clinically significant acute GVHD, it increases the risk of relapse, infection, and graft failure after transplant (Marmont et al., 1991; Couriel et al., 1996; and reviewed in Butturini & Gale, 1988). "Hybrid" strategies have therefore been developed where T-cell depletion is followed after a delay by prophylactic DLI. In these approaches, T-cell depletion is used to allow hematopoietic recovery in the absence of GVHD and the need for its associated immunosuppressive prophylaxis. Subsequently, carefully dosed and selected T cells can be added back in a more hospitable environment to restore useful donor immunity. Both experimental (Johnson & Truitt, 1995) and clinical studies (Lee et al., 1999; Barrett et al., 1998) indicate that the longer the interval between transplant and T-cell add-back, the lower the risk of GVHD. However, without GVHD prophylaxis, even small T-cell doses, received months after transplant, are capable of causing acute GVHD (Naparstek et al., 1995). In a trial of 44 HLA-matched sibling transplants for hematologic malignancies, we demonstrated that large T-cell doses of up to 5 × 10^7 CD3$^+$ cells/kg could be safely added back 45 days after a T-cell depleted transplant in conjunction with cyclosporine prophylaxis (Barrett et al., 1998). Doses of 1 × 10^7 CD3$^+$ cells/kg given earlier posttransplant (for example at day 30) can cause severe GVHD (de Lima et al., 2001). In our current transplant protocol, a TCD PBSCT (CD3 dose fixed at 5×10^4/kg) is followed by two DLIs on days +45 and +100 at doses of 1 × 10^7 and 5 × 10^7 CD3$^+$ cells/kg, respectively. The associated rates of acute GVHD (39% grade II-IV, 8% grade III-IV) and chronic GVHD (54% total, 18% extensive) have been acceptable, and no patient has died from GVHD or its consequences. Furthermore, the probability of relapse (12% for the standard-risk patients and 66% for high-risk patients) is similar to what can be expected with T cell-replete transplants (Nakamura et al., 2001). Although the GVHD reduction with this approach is arguably modest, such a strategy allows the transplant physician considerably more control and flexibility over donor immune reconstitution posttransplant.

Selective T cell depletion techniques

Although T cells in the donor graft initiate both GVL and GVHD effects, evidence suggests that different subsets of T lymphocytes may be preferentially involved in these processes. In animal models, both donor CD4+ and CD8+ cells play a significant role in GVHD, but donor CD4+ cells in the absence of CD8+ cells can still mediate GVL activity (Korngold & Sprent, 1987). Based in part on these observations, Champlin and colleagues have shown that CD8+ depletion followed by posttransplant cyclosporine can reduce the incidence and severity of GVHD without compromising GVL activity. In their initial study of 36 leukemia patients given CD8-depleted matched sibling grafts, 2 (8%) developed grade III to IV GVHD, and only 3 (11%) had leukemia relapse at 2 years (Champlin et al., 1990). In a follow-up double-blind randomized trial, the cyclosporine plus CD8-depletion arm experienced significantly less grade II to IV GVHD compared to the control arm receiving cyclosporine alone (20% versus 80%, $P < .004$), and the leukemia relapse rates were similar between the two groups (Nimer et al., 1994). In CML patients that relapse following an allogeneic transplant, CD8-depleted DLIs have been shown to possess similar efficacy to that of unmanipulated lymphocytes, with a significantly reduced incidence of GVHD (Giralt et al., 1995; Alyea et al., 1998) Although studies of CD8+ depletion have been encouraging, the pathophysiologic differences between GVHD and GVL are inevitably determined by antigen specific responses which transcend these crude attempts at cell selection. Both CD4+ and CD8+ T cells with cytotoxicity against leukemia cells can be detected after BMT (Jiang et al., 1991; Hoffmann et al., 1993) and after successful therapy of leukemic relapse with DLI (Jiang et al., 1993; Bunjes et al., 1995). Therefore, it appears that both CD4+ and CD8+ T cells are important for an optimal GVL effect. Definitive dissection of the anatomic subsets underlying GVHD and GVL remains a crucial but elusive goal for investigators hoping to reduce disease relapse after TCD BMT.

Instead of focusing on removal of anatomic subsets, some investigators have turned their attention to TCD techniques in which only alloreactive T cells are removed from the graft. In one such system, donor T cells are co-incubated with recipient mononuclear cells in vitro. After 2–4 days, alloreactive cells are identified by expression of activation markers, such as CD25 or CD69, and are physically separated from the remaining cells using either an immunotoxin (Cavazzana-Calvo et al., 1990; Mavroudis et al., 1996b) or immunomagnetic cell sorting (Koh et al., 1999 and 2002). Another strategy is to exploit the downregulation of the P glycoprotein pump in activated T cells which renders them more susceptible to damage by toxic agents. By incubation with a photosensitizing rhodamine dye, activated T cells can be selectively killed by exposure to light (Guimond et al., 2002). The hypothesis underpinning all these approaches is that alloreactive lymphocytes responsible for GVHD can be removed from the graft, while retaining T cells responsible for immune reconstitution, including immunity to

viruses and residual malignant disease. This strategy has been used successfully to decrease the incidence and severity of acute GVHD in MHC-mismatched murine transplant models (Cavazzana-Calvo et al., 1994, Hartwig et al., 2002). Furthermore, a CD25 immunotoxin-based selective depletion technique has been applied clinically to augment immune reconstitution following haploidentical PBSC transplantation in young children. Thirteen patients (median age of 18 months) with non-malignant diseases were treated with a TCD PBSCT transplant from an HLA-mismatched related donor. Two weeks following the transplant, they received escalating doses of donor lymphocytes (doses of 1 to 8×10^5 CD3+ cells/kg) that had been selectively depleted ex vivo utilizing an anti-CD25 ricin-conjugated immunotoxin. No posttransplant immunosuppressive therapy was given. Only 4 of 13 patients developed mild or moderate (grade I or II) acute GVHD. All but one of the 13 patients engrafted, and all patients demonstrated accelerated immune reconstitution (Cavazzana-Calvo et al., 2002). We have begun a clinical trial to examine the utility of this approach in the HLA-identical transplant setting. Older individuals with hematologic malignancies will be treated with a low intensity preparative regimen followed by a PBSC allograft in which host-reactive donor lymphocytes have been selectively depleted ex vivo (Solomon et al., 2002). Other investigators have attempted to induce anergy in donor T cells prior to transplantation as a means of reducing GVHD. Murine BMT studies have shown that GVHD can be reduced even across major genetic barriers by treating the recipient with CTLA4-Ig, an agent that blocks CD28-B7 interaction between T lymphocytes and antigen-presenting cells (Blazar et al., 1994). A study in pediatric patients has suggested that ex vivo co-stimulatory signal blockade using CTLA-Ig may reduce GVHD after HLA-mismatched BMT (Guinan et al., 1999).

Antigen-specific T cell therapy (and see Chapter 113)

Infusions of unmanipulated donor lymphocytes posttransplant can successfully reconstitute immunity against viral pathogens and malignancies, but often at the expense of GVHD. Furthermore, any requirement for subsequent immunosuppressive drug therapy can further limit the proliferative and cytotoxic capacity of the infused lymphocytes. Thus, adoptive transfer of antigen-specific cytotoxic T lymphocytes (CTLs) has become an attractive strategy for the treatment of viral diseases and malignancy following allogeneic SCT. Major obstacles to such a therapy are the identification of appropriate antigen targets, the development of reliable and efficient methods for ex vivo activation and expansion of antigen-specific donor lymphocytes, and the elimination of residual alloreactivity.

After allogeneic transplantation, the reactivation of DNA viruses normally controlled by the host's T-cell immune function represents the most common serious infectious problems encountered after allografts. Cytomegalovirus (CMV), Epstein-Barr virus (EBV), and adenovirus have a high mortality and antiviral agents are only partially effective in controlling reactivation. After HSC transplants, donor T cells gradually restore immune competence against infectious agents, but the speed and completeness of the response varies widely. Clinical results and measurement of the immune response necessary for effective immunosurveillance against DNA viruses show that the first 6 months is the period of greatest risk.

Riddell's group (Li *et al.*, 1994) correlated the establishment of effective donor immunity against CMV with an increase in precursor frequency of CMV-specific CTLs. These findings support the idea of preventing CMV reactivation after transplant, by the adoptive transfer of a protective dose of donor CMV-specific CTLs. Initial "proof-of-principle" studies demonstrated that CMV-specific CD8+ clones could indeed restore immunity to CMV and prevent virus reactivation (Walter *et al.*, 1995). However, maintenance of CD8+ T cell immunity required a concurrent CD4+ T helper response, and, although transferred CTLs remained detectable for more than 3 months, a strong CTL response persisted only in patients that recovered CD4+ CMV-specific T cells. A follow-up study in which both CD4 and CD8 clones were transferred to patients has shown long-term persistence of transferred immunity (Greenberg & Riddell, 1999). The importance of both a CD4- and a CD8-specfic immune response in the maintenance of long-term immunity has been confirmed by several groups. In a similar approach, adoptive immunotherapy with EBV-specific CTLs has been utilized successfully to prevent and treat post-transplant EBV lymphoproliferative disease (Papadopoulos *et al.*, 1994; Riddell & Greenberg, 1994; reviewed by Rooney *et al.*, 1995). Gene marking studies have demonstrated long-term persistence of CTLs that retain the ability to respond to re-challenge with virus (Heslop *et al.*, 1996). Generation of these virus-specific CTLs required costly and labor-intensive in vitro culture systems and live virus; however, these pioneering trials showed that adoptive immunotherapy for viral disease is feasible, effective, and safe in the HSC allograft recipient. A number of differing approaches to generate virus-specific CTLs have been described, focusing on reducing the time required for culture, eliminating the need for live virus, and optimizing antigen presentation. These methods include the use of viral lysates (Peggs *et al.*, 2001), recombinant proteins (Vaz-Santiago *et al.*, 2001), or peptides (Szmania *et al.*, 2001), in conjunction with monocytes and DCs as antigen-presenting cells (APCs). The next few years should reveal which of the currently available approaches provide the best balance of efficacy, toxicity, and cost. In the future, such technologies could be applied to other viruses that cause postransplant complications (varicella-zoster virus, herpes simplex virus, adenovirus, and viruses responsible for hemorrhagic cystitis), and secondly serve as a model for the generation of tumor-specific T cells as useful tumor-specific antigens are identified.

The limiting factor for the generation of leukemia-specific T-cell therapy has been the identification of appropriate target antigens. In the HLA-matched transplant setting, donor T cells generate GVL through the recognition of minor histocompatibility antigens (mHAs) presented by MHC class I and II molecules on leukemic cells and/or neighboring APCs. By definition, mHAs represent polymorphic peptides derived from intracellular proteins, which give rise to antigenic differences between MHC-matched donor-recipient pairs. Although several of these antigens are expressed ubiquitously on all host tissues (e.g., HA-3, H-Y), the expression of others is restricted to the hematopoietic system (e.g., HA-1, HA-2, HB-1) (de Bueger *et al.*, 1992; Dolstra *et al.*, 1997), which may help explain the occurrence of GVL without GVHD, and makes them exciting candidates for adoptive immunotherapy. Goulmy and colleagues have published an ex vivo, good manufacturing practice (GMP) grade protocol for generating HA-1- and HA-2-specific CTLs for adoptive immunotherapy using peptide-pulsed dendritic cells (Mutis *et al.*, 1999), and a phase I/II study has been initiated for patients with relapsed leukemias following allogeneic SCT. Other promising target antigens for adoptive immunotherapy include overexpressed nonpolymorphic proteins, such as the Wilms tumor antigen, WT1, and the neutrophil primary granule protein, proteinase-3. The WT1 transcription factor is normally expressed at low-levels in immature CD34+ progenitor cells and is downregulated during differentiation. Elevated levels of WT1 expression have been observed in the majority of patients with acute myeloid or lymphoid leukemias and blast crisis CML (Menssen *et al.*, 1995), and it is overexpressed in CD34+ cells in patients with chronic phase CML. CTLs generated against a WT1 peptide have been shown to selectively kill CML cells in vitro (Gao *et al.*, 2000). Proteinase-3 is a myeloid tissue-restricted protease that is abundantly expressed in azurophilic granules in normal myeloid cells and is over-expressed by two- to five-fold in some myeloid leukemia cells. CTL lines specific for PR1, an HLA-A2.1-restricted peptide, preferentially inhibit CML progenitors over normal marrow cells, and there appears to be a strong correlation between the presence of PR1-specific T cells and clinical responses after interferon (IFN) treatment and allogeneic BMT (Molldrem *et al.*, 2000).

In addition to T cells, donor NK cells may also contribute to the antileukemic effect of allogeneic BMT (Hercend *et al.*, 1986). NK cells recover early after the transplant and can be selectively cytotoxic to leukemia cells but not to normal tissues (Niederwieser *et al.*, 1987; Silla *et al.*, 1996). In rodents, administration of mismatched NK cells after BMT can eradicate residual leukemia without causing severe GVHD (Zeis *et al.*, 1997). Indirect evidence for a GVL effect of NK cells in humans includes an association of NK cell recovery posttransplant with a GVL effect independent of GVHD (Jiang *et al.*, 1997). Increased NK activity has also been associated with a GVL effect after donor buffy coat transfusions to treat CML relapse (Jiang *et al.*, 1993). In the HLA haplotype-mismatched transplant setting, Velardi and colleagues (Ruggeri *et al.*, 2001) have demonstrated a strong association between the presence of NK alloreactivity, generated by killer inhibitory receptor epitope incompatibility, and improved leukemic control in AML patients.

Establishing engraftment in the allogeneic recipient

Prior to the advent of TCD, graft failure after allogeneic BMT was uncommon, occurring in 1% to 5% of patients. In contrast, most TCD BMT series in the 1980s and early 1990s reported higher rates of graft failure (Maraninchi *et al.*, 1987; Mitsuyasu *et al.*, 1986). In some of these studies, the incidence of graft failure was as high as 50% to 70% (Patterson *et al.*, 1986; Martin *et al.*, 1988), seen in patients receiving lower radiation doses during conditioning. In an analysis from the IBMTR of more than 3,000 patients who received TCD or non-TCD BMT for leukemia, TCD was associated with a nine-fold increased risk for graft failure compared to unmanipulated marrow transplantation (Marmont *et al.*, 1991). In addition to TCD, many factors are known to influence engraftment, including the intensity of pretransplant conditioning and posttransplant immunosuppression, recipient sensitization through preceding blood product transfusion, and HLA disparity between the patient and donor, which may increase rejection rates by 5- to 10-fold (Anasetti *et al.*, 1989). Recipient CD8+ and CD4+ T cells with specific anti-donor cytotoxic activity have been isolated in cases of graft failure after TCD BMT (Bunjes *et al.*, 1987; Donohue *et al.*, 1993). It has been clearly shown that the negative effects of HLA disparity and TCD on engraftment can be successfully overcome by combining an increased number of donor stem cells in the graft and a more immunosuppressive preparative regimen (Reisner & Martelli, 1995). In two to three HLA-antigen-mismatched related donor transplants, such an approach has resulted in early and sustained engraftment without the development of severe acute GVHD (Aversa *et al.*, 1994).

The existence of graft-facility cells

In the process of TCD, ancillary marrow elements are also removed that may be necessary for sustained engraftment. It has been postulated that selective purging of T cells using narrow-specificitiy antibodies, but sparing NK cells and other graft-facilitating lymphocyte populations, could maintain the protective effects against GVHD without increasing the risk for graft failure. Several selective antibody-purging methods have been successfully used. Studies using anti-CD5 immunotoxins, anti-CD6, and anti-TCR (T10B9) antibodies have all demonstrated low graft failure rates without compromising GVHD prophylaxis. An IBMTR study analyzing 870 patients with leukemia undergoing alternative donor TCD BMT (Champlin *et al.*, 2000) demonstrated that recipients of BM allografts depleted with narrow specificity antibodies (targeting T cell and/or T-cell subsets) had significantly less graft failure and improved leukemia-free survival than recipients of BM allografts depleted with broad specificity antibodies (targeting other immune cells as well).

In murine BMT models, the depletion of donor T cells from the graft increases the risk of graft rejection, while the addition of donor T cells can prevent it (Murphy *et al.*, 1990). In two different strain combinations, donor CD8+ T cells were more effective in preventing graft rejection than donor CD4+ T cells (Martin, 1993). In human BMT, CD8+ T-cell depletion of bone marrow grafts has resulted in a decreased incidence of acute GVHD, but also in a higher risk of graft rejection (Nimer *et al.*, 1994). This finding underscores the importance of CD8+ donor T cells in facilitating engraftment. Work by Ildstad and coworkers (Gaines *et al.*, 1996) has drawn attention to a powerful facilitatory effect on engraftment of a rare subset of CD3+ CD8lo TCRαβ− T cells. Only 10^3 to 10^4 of such cells are required to confer engraftment across major histocompatibility barriers in mice. Murine studies have demonstrated reduced GVHD after TCD using antibodies against TCRαβ without affecting engraftment, and current studies using selected facilitator cells with purified HSC transplants are ongoing. The mechanism by which these cells facilitate engraftment is not known; however, the process is clearly MHC-restricted as the facilitator cell and HSC must be genetically matched for the facilitating effect to be mediated (Kaufman *et al.*, 1994). In addition, donor CD8+ cells may recognize alloantigens on residual host T cells and destroy them via a cytolytic mechanism before they can mediate graft rejection, although the importance of such a graft-versus-host immunosuppressive effect of donor T cells has been questioned (Uharek *et al.*, 1994). In this regard, it has been shown that the presence of T cells void of graft-versus-host reactivity can enhance marrow engraftment (Lapidot *et al.*, 1990). This may be due to the production of cytokines from donor T cells, which promote hematopoietic engraftment. Alternatively, the presence of donor T cells may result in a veto inactivation of the host T cells involved in graft rejection (Martin, 1993). The veto cell inhibits CTL responses only against its own antigens and results in the clonal deletion of CTL precursors (Hiruma *et al.*, 1992). Work by Reisner and colleagues have shown that anti-third party donor CTLs, depleted of alloreactivity, can provide potent veto activity, an effect mediated by the simultaneous expression of both CD8 and FasL (Reich-Zeliger *et al.*, 2000).

Optimizing the components of the graft—current developments

It is now possible not only to better define the ideal HSC transplant, but also, with new technologies, to deliver with increasing precision the cell types required in a given circumstance. To restore hematopoiesis, a transplant containing early and late repopulating CD34+ cells is required. This can readily be achieved by a G-CSF-mobilized PBSC transplant containing at least 3×10^6 CD34+ cells/kg for HLA-matched family member recipients and around 10×10^6/kg for other transplants. To prevent acute and chronic GVHD from PBSC transplants, T-cell depletion below the threshold of 10^5 CD3+ cells/kg in HLA-matched recipients (Kernan *et al.*, 1986) and below 10^4 CD3+ cells/kg in mismatched recipients (Aversa *et al.*, 1994; Henslee-Downey *et al.*, 1997) should be effective in most cases. Current technology permits the collection of a very high number of CD34+ cells from the peripheral blood of normal donors. In cases of poor mobilization, repeated apheresis procedures after stimulation with G-CSF can be performed and the product cryopreserved until sufficient cells are collected. Alternatively, more stem cells can be obtained from the bone marrow (Link *et al.,* 1995). Achieving a high stem cell dose can enhance engraftment across the HLA barrier despite a low number of T cells present in the graft (Reisner & Martelli, 1995). A further potential advantage of high stem cell dose transplants is the possibility of achieving engraftment with reduced intensity preparative regimens. In conjunction with immunosuppressive, but nonmyeloablative agents such as fludarabine, engraftment can be achieved without increased toxicity (Giralt *et al.,* 1997; Khouri *et al.,* 1998).

Engraftment may be facilitated by the inclusion of selected facilitator cell populations. Broad immune reconstitution without GVHD may be achieved by delayed add-back of T cells selected to remove GVHD-reactive cells. Immunity to EBV, CMV, and adenovirus may be able to be further boosted by the adoptive transfer of ex vivo manipulated virus-specific lymphocytes. To prevent leukemic relapse, adoptively selected T cells with antileukemia activity could be given. Alternatively, lymphocytes with specific antitumor activity could be obtained from an actively immunized donor for adoptive immunotherapy (Kwak *et al.,* 1995). Genetically engineered T-cell clones

expressing a suicide gene could also be used to induce a GVL reaction, with the safeguard of their pharmaceutical elimination should severe GVHD develop (Gallot *et al.,* 1996).

Future prospects

In the future, it is reasonable to anticipate that, by a component therapy approach, allogeneic HSC transplantation could be made not only much safer, but also more effective as a treatment for malignant diseases. It is reasonable to expect TRM from allografts to fall below 5% (the level seen after autologous HSC transplants today). The precise approach will depend on the specifics of the disease treated and the degree of histocompatibility between patient and donor. Stem cell mobilization may be enhanced with the use of additional growth factors such as Flt-3 ligand, preferentially mobilizing stem cells and early hematopoietic progenitors. After selection and administration of a stem cell-rich transplant, T cells and antigen-presenting cells separated from the stem cells could be subjected to ex vivo manipulation. Engraftment-facilitating cells and T cells without GVHD potential could be given concurrently with the transplant. The remaining material could be used to generate large numbers of T-cell clones against leukemia-associated

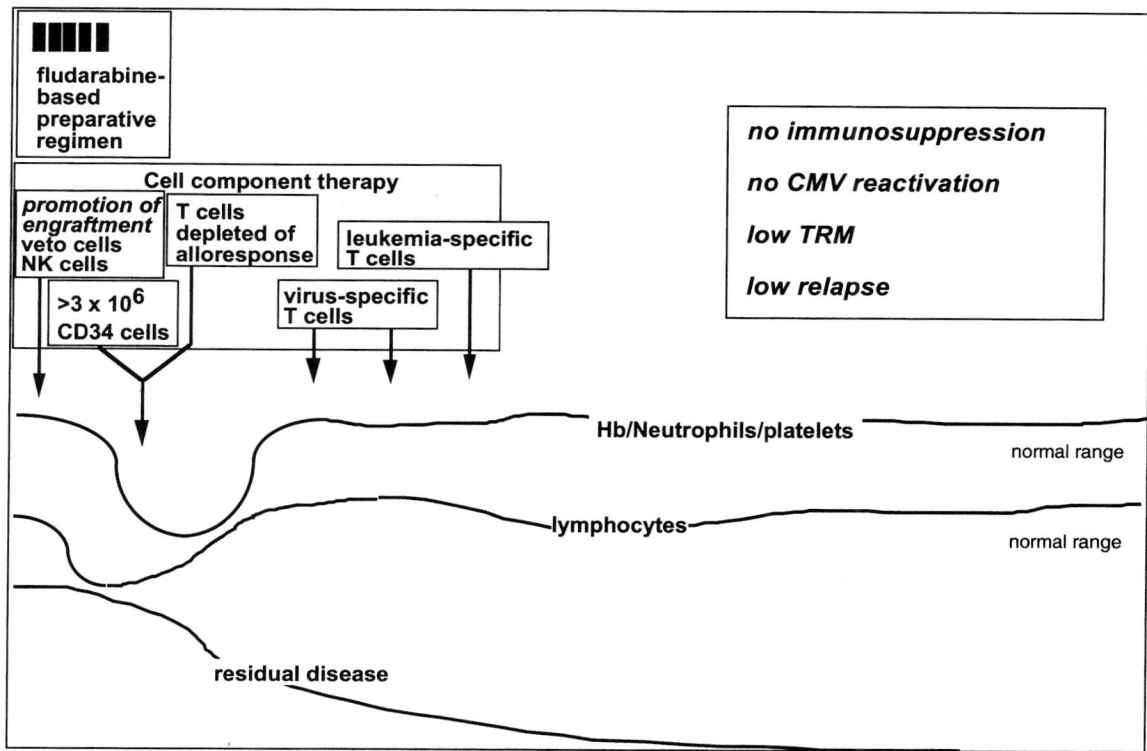

Fig. 18.4. Application of cell component therapy in a hypothetical transplant of the future. Engraftment-facilitating cells (CD8$^+\alpha\beta^-$ cells, veto cells, NK cells) are utilized in combination with a reduced intensity-conditioning regimen to establish rapid hematological recovery and immune reconstitution in the absence of posttransplant immunosuppressive treatment. Stem cells are positively selected for transplantation, while the lymphocyte fraction is selectively depleted of host-reactive T cells to provide broad-based immune reconstitution without GVHD. Further lymphocytes are put aside for expansion and selection of antigen-specific T cells with potent cytotoxic activity against the recipient's malignancy and against viruses such as CMV and EBV. Anticipated morbidity is low while a strong anti-malignancy effect is achieved.

and viral antigens using advanced bioreactors to rapidly expand cells. Figure 18.4 shows the potential application of the component therapy approach to SCT for malignant disease in a transplant of the future. Such regulation of the different components of the graft should lead to swift and stable engraftment with controlled immune reconstitution. Further improvements of HSC transplantation will derive from our increased ability to manipulate the reactivity of the immune system against tumor cells.

References

Alyea, E. P., Soiffer, R. J., Canning, C. et al. (1998). Toxicity and efficacy of defined doses of CD4(+) donor lymphocytes for treatment of relapse after allogeneic bone marrow transplant. *Blood*, **91**, 3671–80.

Anasetti, C., Amos, D., Beatty, P. G. et al. (1989). Effect of HLA compatibility on engraftment of bone marrow transplants in patients with leukemia or lymphoma. *New England Journal of Medicine*, **320**, 197–204.

Atkinson, K., Norrie, S., Chan, P. et al. (1985). Lack of correlation between nucleated bone marrow cell dose, marrow CFU- GM dose or marrow CFU-E dose and the rate of HLA-identical sibling marrow engraftment. *British Journal of Haematology*, **60**, 245–51.

Aversa, F., Tabilio, A., Terenzi, A. et al. (1994). Successful engraftment of T-cell-depleted haploidentical "three-loci" incompatible transplants in leukemia patients by addition of recombinant human granulocyte colony-stimulating factor-mobilized peripheral blood progenitor cells to bone marrow inoculum. *Blood*, **84**, 3948–55.

Bahceci, E., Read, E. J., Leitman, S. et al. (2000). CD34+ cell dose predicts relapse and survival after T-cell-depleted HLA-identical haematopoietic stem cell transplantation (HSCT) for haematological malignancies. *British Journal of Haematology*, **108**, 408–14.

Barrett, A. J. (1997). Mechanisms of the graft-versus-leukemia reaction. *Stem Cells*, **15**, 248–58.

Barrett, A. J., Mavroudis, D., Tisdale, J. et al. (1998). T cell-depleted bone marrow transplantation and delayed T cell add-back to control acute GVHD and conserve a graft-versus-leukemia effect. *Bone Marrow Transplantation*, **21**, 543–51.

Bensinger, W. I., Clift, R., Martin, P. et al. (1996). Allogeneic peripheral blood stem cell transplantation in patients with advanced hematologic malignancies: a retrospective comparison with marrow transplantation. *Blood*, **88**, 2794–800.

Blazar, B R., Taylor, P. A., Linsley, P. S., & Vallera, D. A. (1994). In vivo blockade of CD28/CTLA4: b7/BB1 interaction with CTLA4-Ig reduces lethal muringe graft-versus-host diseases across the major histocompatibility complex barrier in mice. *Blood*, **83**, 3815–3825.

Bunjes, D., Heit, W., Arnold, R. et al. (1987). Evidence for the involvement of host-derived OKT8-positive T cells in the rejection of T-depleted, HLA-identical bone marrow grafts. *Transplantation*, **43**, 501–5.

Bunjes, D., Theobald, M., Hertenstein, B. et al. (1995). Successful therapy with donor buffy coat transfusions in patients with

relapsed chronic myeloid leukemia after bone marrow transplantation is associated with high frequencies of host-reactive interleukin 2-secreting T helper cells. *Bone Marrow Transplantation*, **15**, 713–9.

Butturini, A. & Gale, R. P. (1988). T cell depletion in bone marrow transplantation for leukemia: current results and future directions. *Bone Marrow Transplantation*, **3**, 185–92.

Cavazzana-Calvo, M., Andre-Schmutz, I., Hacein-Bey-Abina, S. et al. (2002). Improving immune reconstitution while preventing graft-versus-host disease in allogeneic stem cell transplantation. *Seminars in Hematology*, **39**, 32–40.

Cavazzana-Calvo, M., Fromont, C., Le Deist, F. et al. (1990). Specific elimination of alloreactive T cells by an anti-interleukin-2 receptor B chain-specific immunotoxin. *Transplantation*, **50**, 1–7.

Cavazzana-Calvo, M., Stephan, J. L., Sarnacki, S. et al. (1994). Attenuation of graft-versus-host disease and graft rejection by ex vivo immunotoxin elimination of alloreactive T cells in an H-2 haplotype disparate mouse combination. *Blood*, **83**, 288–98.

Champlin, R., Ho, W., Gajewski, J. et al. (1990). Selective depletion of CD8+ T lymphocytes for prevention of graft-versus-host disease after allogeneic bone marrow transplantation. *Blood*, **76**, 418–23.

Champlin, R. E., Passweg, J. R., Zhang, M. J. et al. (2000). T-cell depletion of bone marrow transplants for leukemia from donors other than HLA-identical siblings: advantage of T-cell antibodies with narrow specificities. *Blood*, **95**, 3996–4003.

Couriel, D., Canosa, J., Engler, H. et al. (1996). Early reactivation of cytomegalovirus and high risk of interstitial pneumonitis following T-depleted BMT for adults with hematological malignancies. *Bone Marrow Transplantation*, **18**, 347–53.

de Bueger, M., Bakker, A., Van Rood, J .J. et al. (1992). Tissue distribution of human minor histocompatibility antigens. Ubiquitous versus restricted tissue distribution indicates heterogeneity among human cytotoxic T lymphocyte-defined non-MHC antigens. *Journal of Immunology*, **149**, 1788–94.

de Lima, M., Bonamino, M., Vasconcelos, Z. et al. (2001). Prophylactic donor lymphocyte infusions after moderately ablative chemotherapy and stem cell transplantation for hematological malignancies: high remission rate among poor prognosis patients at the expense of graft-versus-host disease. *Bone Marrow Transplantation*, **27**, 73–8.

Deacock, S. J., Schwarer, A. P., Bridge, J. et al. (1992). Evidence that umbilical cord blood contains a higher frequency of HLA class II-specific alloreactive T cells than adult peripheral blood. A limiting dilution analysis. *Transplantation*, **53**, 1128–34.

Dolstra, H., Fredrix, H., Preijers, F. et al. (1997). Recognition of a B cell leukemia-associated minor histocompatibility antigen by CTL. *Journal of Immunology*, **158**, 560–5.

Donohue, J., Homge, M., & Kernan, N. A. (1993). Characterization of cells emerging at the time of graft failure after bone marrow transplantation from an unrelated marrow donor. *Blood*, **82**, 1023–9.

Gaines, B. A., Colson, Y. L., Kaufman, C. L. et al. (1996). Facilitating cells enable engraftment of purified fetal liver stem cells in allogeneic recipients. *Experimental Hematology*, **24**, 902–13.

Gallot, G., Hallet, M. M., Gaschet, J. *et al.* (1996). Human HLA-specific T-cell clones with stable expression of a suicide gene: a possible tool to drive and control a graft-versus-host- graft-versus-leukemia reaction? *Blood,* **88,** 1098–103.

Gao, L., Bellantuono, I., Elsasser, A. *et al.* (2000). Selective elimination of leukemic CD34(+) progenitor cells by cytotoxic T lymphocytes specific for WT1. *Blood,* **95,** 2198–203.

Giralt, S., Estey, E., Albitar, M. *et al.* (1997). Engraftment of allogeneic hematopoietic progenitor cells with purine analog-containing chemotherapy: harnessing graft-versus-leukemia without myeloablative therapy. *Blood,* **89,** 4531–6.

Giralt, S., Hester, J., Huh, Y. *et al.* (1995). CD8-depleted donor lymphocyte infusion as treatment for relapsed chronic myelogenous leukemia after allogeneic bone marrow transplantation. *Blood,* **86,** 4337–43.

Gluckman, E., Rocha, V., Boyer-Chammard, A. *et al.* (1997). Outcome of cord-blood transplantation from related and unrelated donors. Eurocord Transplant Group and the European Blood and Marrow Transplantation Group. *The New England Journal of Medicine,* **337,** 373–81.

Gordon, M. Y. & Blackett, N. M. (1995). Some factors determining the minimum number of cells required for successful clinical engraftment. *Bone Marrow Transplantation,* **15,** 659–62.

Greenberg, P. D. & Riddell, S. R. (1999). Deficient cellular immunity—finding and fixing the defects. *Science,* **285,** 546–51.

Guimond, M., Balass, A., Barrette, M. *et al.* (2002). P-Glycoprotein targeting: a unique strategy to selectively eliminate immunoreactive T cells. *Blood,* **100,** 375–82.

Guinan, E. C., Boussiotis, V. A., Neuberg, D. *et al.* (1999). Transplantation of anergic histoincompatible bone marrow allografts. *The New England Journal of Medicine,* **340,** 1704–14.

Harris, D. T., Schumacher, M. J., Locascio, J. *et al.* (1992). Phenotypic and functional immaturity of human umbilical cord blood T lymphocytes. *Proceedings of the National Academy of Sciences in the USA,* **89,** 10006–10010.

Hartwig, U. F., Robbers, M., Wickenhauser, C., & Huber, C. (2002). Murine acute graft-versus-host disease can be prevented by depletion of alloreactive T lymphocytes using activation-induced cell death. *Blood,* **99,** 3041–9.

Heitger, A., Neu, N., Kern, H. *et al.* (1997). Essential role of the thymus to reconstitute naive (CD45RA+) T-helper cells after human allogeneic bone marrow transplantation. *Blood,* **90,** 850–7.

Henslee-Downey, P. J., Abhyankar, S. H., Parrish, R. S. *et al.* (1997). Use of partially mismatched related donors extends access to allogeneic marrow transplant . *Blood,* **89,** 3864–72.

Hercend, T., Takvorian, T., Nowill, A. *et al.* (1986). Characterization of natural killer cells with antileukemia activity following allogeneic bone marrow transplantation. *Blood,* **6,** 722–8.

Heslop, H. E., Ng, C. Y., Li, C. *et al.* (1996). Long-term restoration of immunity against Epstein-Barr virus infection by adoptive transfer of gene-modified virus-specific T lymphocytes. *Nature Medicine,* **2,** 551–5.

Hiruma, K., Nakamura, H., Henkart, P. A. *et al.* (1992). Clonal deletion of postthymic T cells: veto cells kill precursor cytotoxic T lymphocytes. *Journal of Experimental Medicine,* **175,** 863–8.

Hoffmann, T., Theobald, M., Bunjes, D. *et al.* (1993). Frequency of bone marrow T cells responding to HLA-identical non-leukemic and leukemic stimulator cells. *Bone Marrow Transplantation,* **12,** 1–8.

Horowitz, M. M., Gale, R. P., Sondel, P. M. *et al.* (1990). Graft-versus-leukemia reactions after bone marrow transplantation. *Blood,* **75,** 555–62.

Jiang, Y. Z., Barrett, A. J., Goldman, J. M. *et al.* (1997). Association of natural killer cell immune recovery with a graft-versus-leukemia effect independent of graft-versus-host disease following allogeneic bone marrow transplantation. *Annals of Hematology,* **74,** 1–6.

Jiang, Y. Z., Cullis, J. O., Kanfer, E. J. *et al.* (1993). T cell and NK cell mediated graft-versus-leukaemia reactivity following donor buffy coat transfusion to treat relapse after marrow transplantation for chronic myeloid leukaemia. *Bone Marrow Transplantation,* **11,** 133–8.

Jiang, Y. Z., Kanfer, E. J., Macdonald, D. *et al.* (1991). Graft-versus-leukaemia following allogeneic bone marrow transplantation: emergence of cytotoxic T lymphocytes reacting to host leukaemia cells. *Bone Marrow Transplantation,* **8,** 253–8.

Johnson, B. D. & Truitt, R. L. (1995). Delayed infusion of immunocompetent donor cells after bone marrow transplantation breaks graft-host tolerance allows for persistent antileukemic reactivity without severe graft-versus-host disease *Blood,* **85,** 3302–12.

Kaufman, C. L., Colson, Y. L., Wren, S. M. *et al.* (1994). Phenotypic characterization of a novel bone marrow-derived cell that facilitates engraftment of allogeneic bone marrow stem cells. *Blood,* **84,** 2436–46.

Kernan, N. A., Collins, N. H., Juliano, L. *et al.* (1986). Clonable T lymphocytes in T cell-depleted bone marrow transplants correlate with development of graft-v-host disease. *Blood,* **68,** 770–3.

Khouri, I. F., Keating, M., Korbling, M. *et al.* (1998). Transplant-lite: induction of graft-versus-malignancy using fludarabine-based nonablative chemotherapy and allogeneic blood progenitor-cell transplantation as treatment for lymphoid malignancies. *Journal of Clinical Oncology,* **16,** 2817–24.

Koh, M. B., Prentice, H. G., & Lowdell, M. W. (1999). Selective removal of alloreactive cells from haematopoietic stem cell grafts: graft engineering for GVHD prophylaxis. *Bone Marrow Transplantation,* **23,** 1071–9.

Koh, M. B. C., Prentice, H. G., Corbo, M. *et al.* (2002). Alloantigen-specific T-cell depletion in a major histocompatibility complex fully mismatched murine model provides effective graft-versus-host disease prophylaxis in the presence of lymphoid engraftment. *British Journal of Haematology,* **118,** 108–16.

Kolb, H. J., Mittermuller, J., Clemm, C. *et al.* (1990). Donor leukocyte transfusions for treatment of recurrent chronic myelogenous leukemia in marrow transplant patients. *Blood,* **76,** 2462–5.

Korbling, M., Huh, Y. O., Durett, A. *et al.* (1995). Allogeneic blood stem cell transplantation: peripheralization and yield of donor-derived primitive hematopoietic progenitor cells (CD34+ Thy-1 dim) and lymphoid subsets, and possible predictors of engraftment and graft-versus-host disease. *Blood,* **86,** 2842–8.

Korngold, R. & Sprent, J. (1987). T cell subsets and graft-versus-host disease. *Transplantation,* **44,** 335–9.

Krause, D. S., Fackler, M. J., Civin, C. I. *et al.* (1996). CD34: structure, biology, and clinical utility. *Blood,* **87,** 1–13.

Kurtzberg, J. (1996). Umbilical cord blood: a novel alternative source of hematopoietic stem cells for bone marrow transplantation. *Journal of Hematotherapy*, **5**, 95–6.

Kwak, L. W., Taub, D. D., Duffey, P. L. *et al.* (1995). Transfer of myeloma idiotype-specific immunity from an actively immunised marrow donor. *Lancet*, **345**, 1016–20.

Lapidot, T., Lubin, I., Terenzi, A. *et al.* (1990). Enhancement of bone marrow allografts from nude mice into mismatched recipients by T cells void of graft-versus-host activity. *Proceedings of the National Academy of Sciences USA*, **87**, 4595–9.

Lee, C. K., Gingrich, R. D., deMagalhaes-Silverman, M. *et al.* (1999). Prophylactic reinfusion of T cells for T cell-depleted allogeneic bone marrow transplantation. *Biology of Blood and Marrow Transplantation*, **5**, 15–27.

Li, C. R., Greenberg, P. D., Gilbert, M. J. *et al.* (1994). Recovery of HLA-restricted cytomegalovirus (CMV)-specific T-cell responses after allogeneic bone marrow transplant: correlation with CMV disease and effect of ganciclovir prophylaxis. *Blood*, **83**, 1971–9.

Link, H., Arseniev, L., Bahre, O. *et al.* (1995). Combined transplantation of allogeneic bone marrow and CD34+ blood cells. *Blood*, **86**, 2500–8.

Lowenberg, B., Wagemaker, G., van Bekkum, D. W. *et al.* (1986). Graft-versus-host disease following transplantation of 'one log' versus 'two log' T-lymphocyte-depleted bone marrow from HLA-identical donors. *Bone Marrow Transplantation*, **1**, 133–40.

Maraninchi, D., Gluckman, E., Blaise, D. *et al.* (1987). Impact of T-cell depletion on outcome of allogeneic bone-marrow transplantation for standard-risk leukaemias. *Lancet*, **2**, 175–8.

Marmont, A. M., Horowitz, M. M., Gale, R. P. *et al.* (1991). T-cell depletion of HLA-identical transplants in leukemia. *Blood*, **78**, 2120–30.

Martin, P. J. (1993). Donor CD8 cells prevent allogeneic marrow graft rejection in mice: potential implications for marrow transplantation in humans. *Journal of Experimental Medicine*, **178**, 703–12.

Martin, P. J., Hansen, J. A., Torok-Storb, B. *et al.* (1988). Graft failure in patients receiving T cell-depleted HLA-identical allogeneic marrow transplants. *Bone Marrow Transplantation*, **3**, 445–56.

Mavroudis, D., Read, E., Cottler-Fox, M. *et al.* (1996a). CD34+ cell dose predicts survival, posttransplant morbidity, and rate of hematologic recovery after allogeneic marrow transplants for hematologic malignancies. *Blood*, **88**, 3223–9.

Mavroudis, D. A., Jiang, Y. Z., Hensel, N. *et al.* (1996b). Specific depletion of alloreactivity against haplotype mismatched related individuals by a recombinant immunotoxin: a new approach to graft-versus-host disease prophylaxis in haploidentical bone marrow transplantation. *Bone Marrow Transplantation*, **17**, 793–9.

Menssen, H. D., Renkl, H. J., Rodeck, U. *et al.* (1995). Presence of Wilms' tumor gene (*wt1*) transcripts and the WT1 nuclear protein in the majority of human acute leukemias. *Leukemia*, **9**, 1060–7.

Mielcarek, M., Martin, P. J., & Torok-Storb, B. (1997). Suppression of alloantigen-induced T-cell proliferation by CD14+ cells derived from granulocyte colony-stimulating factor-mobilized peripheral blood mononuclear cells. *Blood*, **89**, 1629–34.

Miflin, G., Russell, N. H., Hutchinson, R. M. *et al.* (1997). Allogeneic peripheral blood stem cell transplantation for haematological malignancies—an analysis of kinetics of engraftment and GVHD risk. *Bone Marrow Transplantation*, **19**, 9–13.

Mitsuyasu, R. T., Champlin, R. E., Gale, R. P. *et al.* (1986). Treatment of donor bone marrow with monoclonal anti-T-cell antibody and complement for the prevention of graft-versus-host disease. A prospective, randomized, double-blind trial. *Annals of Internal Medicine*, **105**, 20–6.

Molldrem, J. J., Lee, P. P., Wang, C. *et al.* (2000). Evidence that specific T lymphocytes may participate in the elimination of chronic myelogenous leukemia. *Nature Medicine*, **6**, 1018–23.

Moore, M. A., Williams, N., & Metcalf, D. (1973). In vitro colony formation by normal and leukemic human hematopoietic cells: characterization of the colony-forming cells. *Journal of the National Cancer Institute*, **50**, 603–23.

Morariu-Zamfir, R., Rocha, V., Devergie, A. *et al.* (2001). Influence of CD34(+) marrow cell dose on outcome of HLA-identical sibling allogeneic bone marrow transplants in patients with chronic myeloid leukaemia. *Bone Marrow Transplantation*, **27**, 575–80.

Muller, S., Schulz, A., Reiss, U. *et al.* (1999). Definition of a critical T cell threshold for prevention of GVHD after HLA non-identical PBPC transplantation in children. *Bone Marrow Transplantation*, **24**, 575–81.

Murphy, W. J., Kumar, V., Cope, J. C. *et al.* (1990). An absence of T cells in murine bone marrow allografts leads to an increased susceptibility to rejection by natural killer cells and T cells. *Journal of Immunology*, **144**, 3305–11.

Mutis, T., Verdijk, R., Schrama, E. *et al.* (1999). Feasibility of immunotherapy of relapsed leukemia with ex vivo–generated cytotoxic T lymphocytes specific for hematopoietic system–restricted minor histocompatibility antigens. *Blood*, **93**, 2336–41.

Nakamura, R., Bahceci, E., Read, E. J. *et al.* (2001). Transplant dose of CD34(+) and CD3(+) cells predicts outcome in patients with haematological malignancies undergoing T cell-depleted peripheral blood stem cell transplants with delayed donor lymphocyte add-back. *British Journal of Haematology*, **115**, 95–104.

Naparstek, E., Or, R., Nagler, A. *et al.* (1995). T-cell-depleted allogeneic bone marrow transplantation for acute leukaemia using Campath-1 antibodies and postransplant administration of donor's peripheral blood lymphocytes for prevention of relapse. *British Journal of Haematology*, **89**, 506–15.

Niederwieser, D., Gastl, G., Rumpold, H. *et al.* (1987). Rapid reappearance of large granular lymphocytes (LGL) with concomitant reconstitution of natural killer (NK) activity after human bone marrow transplantation (BMT). *British Journal of Haematology*, **65**, 301–5.

Nimer, S. D., Giorgi, J., Gajewski, J. L. *et al.* (1994). Selective depletion of CD8+ cells for prevention of graft-versus-host disease after bone marrow transplantation. A randomized controlled trial. *Transplantation*, **57**, 82–7.

Noga, S. J., Seber, A., Davis, J. M. *et al.* (1998). CD34 augmentation improves allogeneic T cell-depleted bone marrow engraftment. *Journal of Hematotherapy*, **7**, 151–7.

Pan, L., Delmonte, J., Jr., Jalonen, C. K. *et al.* (1995). Pretreatment of donor mice with granulocyte colony-stimulating factor polarizes donor T lymphocytes toward type-2 cytokine production and reduces severity of experimental graft-versus-host disease. *Blood*, **86**, 4422–29.

Papadopoulos, E. B., Ladanyi, M., Emanuel, D. *et al.* (1994). Infusions of donor leukocytes to treat Epstein-Barr virus–associated lymphoproliferative disorders after allogeneic bone marrow transplantation. *The New England Journal of Medicine, 330,* 1185–91.

Patterson, J., Prentice, H. G., Brenner, M. K. *et al.* (1986). Graft rejection following HLA matched T-lymphocyte depleted bone marrow transplantation. *British Journal of Haematology, 63,* 221–30.

Paulin, T. (1992). Importance of bone marrow cell dose in bone marrow transplantation. *Clinical Transplantation, 6,* 48–54.

Peggs, K., Verfuerth, S., and Mackinnon, S. (2001). Induction of cytomegalovirus (CMV)-specific T-cell responses using dendritic cells pulsed with CMV antigen: a novel culture system free of live CMV virions. *Blood, 97,* 994–1000.

Podesta, M., Piaggio, G., Frassoni, F. *et al.* (1997). Deficient reconstitution of early progenitors after allogeneic bone marrow transplantation. *Bone Marrow Transplantation, 19,* 1011–7.

Przepiorka, D., Smith, T. L., Folloder, J. *et al.* (1999). Risk factors for acute graft-versus-host disease after allogeneic blood stem cell transplantation. *Blood, 94,* 1465–70.

Ratajczak, M. Z. & Gewirtz, A. M. (1995). The biology of hematopoietic stem cells. *Seminars in Oncology, 22,* 210–7.

Reich-Zeliger, S., Zhao, Y., Krauthgamer, R. *et al.* (2000). Anti-third party CD8+ CTLs as potent veto cells: coexpression of CD8 and FasL is a prerequisite. *Immunity, 13,* 507–15.

Reisner, Y. & Martelli, M. F. (1995). Bone marrow transplantation across HLA barriers by increasing the number of transplanted cells. *Immunology Today, 16,* 437–40.

Riddell, S. R. & Greenberg, P. D. (1994). Therapeutic reconstitution of human viral immunity by adoptive transfer of cytotoxic T lymphocyte clones. *Current Topics in Microbiology and Immunology, 189,* 9–34.

Ringden, O. & Nilsson, B. (1985). Death by graft-versus-host disease associated with HLA mismatch, high recipient age, low marrow cell dose, and splenectomy. *Transplantation, 40,* 39–44.

Ringden, O., Barrett, A. J., Zhang, M. J., Loberiza, F., and Horowitz, M. M. Improved leukemia-free survival in recipients of HLA-identical bone marrow or peripheral blood stem cells is associated with a high CD34 cell dose. *Blood,* in press.

Rocha, V., Carmagnat, M. V., Chevret, S. *et al.* (2001). Influence of bone marrow graft lymphocyte subsets on outcome after HLA-identical sibling transplants. *Experimental Hematology, 29,* 1347–52.

Rocha, V., Wagner, J. E., Jr., Sobocinski, K. A. *et al.* (2000). Graft-versus-host disease in children who have received a cord-blood or bone marrow transplant from an HLA-identical sibling. Eurocord and International Bone Marrow Transplant Registry Working Committee on Alternative Donor and Stem Cell Sources. *The New England Journal of Medicine, 342,* 1846–54.

Rooney, C. M., Smith, C. A., Ng, C. Y. *et al.* (1995). Use of gene-modified virus-specific T lymphocytes to control Epstein-Barr-virus–related lymphoproliferation. *Lancet, 345,* 9–13.

Ruggeri, L., Capanni, M., Martelli, M. F. *et al.* (2001). Cellular therapy: exploiting NK cell alloreactivity in transplantation. *Current Opinion in Hematology, 8,* 355–9.

Schmitz, N. & Barrett, J. (2002). Optimizing engraftment-source and dose of stem cells. *Seminars in Hematology, 39,* 3–14.

Siena, S., Schiavo, R., Pedrazzoli, P. *et al.* (2000). Therapeutic relevance of CD34 cell dose in blood cell transplantation for cancer therapy. *Journal of Clinical Oncology, 18,* 1360–77.

Sierra, J., Storer, B., Hansen, J. A. *et al.* (1997). Transplantation of marrow cells from unrelated donors for treatment of high-risk acute leukemia: the effect of leukemic burden, donor HLA-matching, and marrow cell dose. *Blood, 89,* 4226–35.

Sierra, J., Storer, B., Hansen, J. A. *et al.* (2000). Unrelated donor marrow transplantation for acute myeloid leukemia: an update of the Seattle experience. *Bone Marrow Transplantation, 26,* 397–04.

Silla, L. M., Pincus, S. M., Locker, J. D. *et al.* (1996). Generation of activated natural killer (A-NK) cells in patients with chronic myelogenous leukaemia and their role in the in vitro disappearance of BCR/abl-positive targets. *British Journal of Haematology, 93,* 375–85.

Singhal, S., Powles, R., Treleaven, J. *et al.* (2000). A low CD34+ cell dose results in higher mortality and poorer survival after blood or marrow stem cell transplantation from HLA-identical siblings: should 2 × 10(6) CD34+ cells/kg be considered the minimum threshold? *Bone Marrow Transplantation, 26,* 489–96.

Soiffer, R. J., Weller, E., Alyea, E. P. *et al.* (2001). CD6+ donor marrow T-cell depletion as the sole form of graft-versus-host disease prophylaxis in patients undergoing allogeneic bone marrow transplant from unrelated donors. *Journal of Clinical Oncology, 19,* 1152–9.

Solomon, S. R., Nakamura, R., Read, E. *et al.* (2001). Is cyclosporine necessary to prevent graft-versus-host-disease after T cell depleted peripheral blood stem cell transplantation? *Blood, 98,* 416a.

Solomon, S. R., Tran, T., Carter, C. S. *et al.* (2002). Optimized clinical-scale culture conditions for ex vivo selective depletion of host-reactive donor lymphocytes: a strategy for gvhd prophylaxis in allogeneic peripheral blood stem cell transplantation. *Cytotherapy, 4,* 395–400.

Steen, R., Tjonnfjord, G. E., and Egeland, T. (1994). Comparison of the phenotype and clonogenicity of normal CD34+ cells from umbilical cord blood, granulocyte colony-stimulating factor–mobilized peripheral blood, and adult human bone marrow. *Journal of Hematotherapy, 3,* 253–62.

Szmania, S., Galloway, A., Bruorton, M. *et al.* (2001). Isolation and expansion of cytomegalovirus-specific cytotoxic T lymphocytes to clinical scale from a single blood draw using dendritic cells and HLA-tetramers. *Blood, 98,* 505–12.

Theilgaard-Mönch, K., Raaschou-Jensen, K., Palm, H. *et al.* (2001). Flow cytometric assessment of lymphocyte subsets, lymphoid progenitors, and hematopoietic stem cells in allogeneic stem cell grafts. *Bone Marrow Transplantation, 28,* 1073–82.

To, L. B., Roberts, M. M., Haylock, D. N. *et al.* (1992). Comparison of haematological recovery times and supportive care requirements of autologous recovery phase peripheral blood stem cell transplants, autologous bone marrow transplants and allogeneic bone marrow transplants. *Bone Marrow Transplantation, 9,* 277–84.

Truitt, R. L. & Atasoylu, A. A. (1991). Impact of pretransplant conditioning and donor T cells on chimerism, graft-versus-host disease, graft-versus-leukemia reactivity, and tolerance after bone marrow transplantation. *Blood, 77,* 2515–23.

Uharek, L., Glass, B., Gaska, T. *et al.* (1994). Influence of donor lymphocytes on the incidence of primary graft failure after allogeneic bone marrow transplantation in a murine model. *British Journal of Haematology*, **88,** 79–87.

Urbano-Ispizua, A., Carreras, E., Marin, P. *et al.* (2001). Allogeneic transplantation of CD34(+) selected cells from peripheral blood from human leukocyte antigen-identical siblings: detrimental effect of a high number of donor CD34(+) cells? *Blood*, **98,** 2352–7.

Vaz-Santiago, J., Lule, J., Rohrlich, P. *et al.* (2001). Ex vivo stimulation and expansion of both CD4(+) and CD8(+) T cells from peripheral blood mononuclear cells of human cytomegalovirus-seropositive blood donors by using a soluble recombinant chimeric protein, IE1-pp65. *Journal of Virology,* **75,** 7840–7.

Walter, E. A., Greenberg, P. D., Gilbert, M. J. *et al.* (1995). Reconstitution of cellular immunity against cytomegalovirus in recipients of allogeneic bone marrow by transfer of T-cell clones from the donor. *The New England Journal of Medicine,* **333,** 1038–44.

Wang, J. C., Doedens, M., and Dick, J. E. (1997). Primitive human hematopoietic cells are enriched in cord blood compared with adult bone marrow or mobilized peripheral blood as measured by the quantitative in vivo SCID-repopulating cell assay. *Blood,* **89,** 3919–24.

Weaver, C. H., Hazelton, B., Birch, R. *et al.* (1995). An analysis of engraftment kinetics as a function of the CD34 content of peripheral blood progenitor cell collections in 692 patients after the administration of myeloablative chemotherapy. *Blood,* **86,** 3961–9.

Zaucha, J. M., Gooley, T., Bensinger, W. I. *et al.* (2001). CD34 cell dose in granulocyte colony-stimulating factor-mobilized peripheral blood mononuclear cell grafts affects engraftment kinetics and development of extensive chronic graft-versus-host disease after human leukocyte antigen-identical sibling transplantation. *Blood,* **98,** 3221–7.

Zeis, M., Uharek, L., Glass, B. *et al.* (1997). Allogeneic MHC-mismatched activated natural killer cells administered after bone marrow transplantation provide a strong graft-versus-leukaemia effect in mice. *British Journal of Haematology,* **96,** 757–61.

19 Graft-versus-leukemia effects of hematopoietic stem cell transplantation

CHRISTOPHER N. BREDESON, MARY M. HOROWITZ, AND ROBERT L. TRUITT

International Bone Marrow Transplant Registry and Department of Pediatrics, Medical College of Wisconsin, Milwaukee, USA

Introduction

Allogeneic blood and bone marrow transplantation is an effective and widely used therapy for acute myeloid leukemia (AML), acute lymphoblastic leukemia (ALL), chronic myeloid leukemia (CML), and other hematologic malignancies. Fewer than 20% of patients relapse when transplants are performed early in the course of these diseases (Barrett et al., 1989; Gale et al., 1989; Goldman et al., 1993). Relapse rates after allogeneic transplants are substantially lower than conventional chemotherapy. It is often assumed that the antileukemia efficacy of transplants results chiefly from high-dose chemotherapy and radiation given pretransplant. However, both experimental and clinical data suggest that graft-mediated effects are at least as important as high-dose therapy.

In 1956, Barnes and colleagues proposed that allogeneic bone marrow transplantation had an antitumor effect not explained by pretransplant chemotherapy or radiation. They studied leukemic mice treated with high-dose total body radiation (TBI) and compared those receiving syngeneic and allogeneic bone marrow infusions. The mice receiving syngeneic marrow died of leukemia. Those receiving allogeneic cells survived longer although they eventually developed fatal graft-versus-host disease (GVHD). Importantly, they had no evidence of leukemia at death. Mathé and colleagues (1965) proposed the term "adoptive immunotherapy" for the antitumor effect of allogeneic cells. Antitumor effects could be specific, that is, after sensitization of the donor (Woodruff, 1980) or the donor's cells (Cheever, Greenberg, & Fefer, 1981) to antigens present on malignant cells, or nonspecific, that is, associated with GVHD, which targets normal as well as malignant cells. The term graft-versus-leukemia (GVL) was coined by Bortin and co-workers (1973a, 1973b, 1974) to indicate the adoptive immunotherapeutic effect of transplanted allogeneic bone marrow cells against leukemia cells. In recent years, with realization that immune-mediated antitumor reactivity is clinically important, other terms have been coined, including graft-versus-lymphoma, graft-versus-myeloma, and the more generic graft-versus-tumor and graft-versus-malignancy effect, to describe antitumor immune responses following allogeneic (and in some cases autologous) hematopoietic stem cell transplantation.

In some animal models, the GVL effect could not be distinguished from GVHD, while in others the two were separable (e.g., Bortin et al., 1979; Truitt et al., 1983; Truitt, LeFever, & Shih, 1986; Sykes et al., 1993, 1994; Pelot et al., 1999). For decades, the biological basis for separation of GVL and GVH reactions remained obscure (Slavin, 1990). It was postulated that either distinct and, therefore, separable effector cells were responsible for GVL and GVH reactions and/or that the same effector cells with differing thresholds of reactivity against leukemia and normal host cells mediated preferential killing of leukemia. Recent work indicates that even when the target antigen for alloreactive T cells is expressed on both normal (antihost, GVH) and leukemic (antileukemia, GVL) host cells, the immune reaction can be manipulated to separate the GVHD syndrome from the GVL effect. For example, delayed infusion of donor T cells can produce a "lymphohematopoietic" GVH reaction that effectively eliminates leukemia without inducing systemic GVHD (Johnson & Truitt, 1995; Johnson, Becker, & Truitt, 1999; Pelot et al., 1999). Co-stimulatory blockade of alloreactive T cells can mimimize GVHD while preserving the antiviral and GVL effector cells (Guinan et al., 1999; Comoli et al., 2001). Administration of T cells that recognize host antigens with limited tissue distribution may reduce the severity of GVHD (Bonnet et al., 1999). Separation of the GVL effect from GVHD can also be achieved by selective blockade or inhibition of cytokines that are responsible for many of the pathophysiological manifestations of GVHD (Hill & Ferrara, 2000) and by the use of alloreactive natural killer (NK) cells (Ruggeri et al., 2002). However, clinical experience with reduced-intensity conditioning regimens has not borne out the idea that lower cytokine levels at the time of presentation of alloreactive cells will result in decreased GVHD. Initial experiences with non-myeloablative transplants have not always been associated with a decreased incidence of GVHD (Slavin et al., 1998; McSweeney et al., 2001).

GVHD and GVL effector mechanisms

Histocompatibility antigens

In historical context, histocompatibility antigens were discovered during the course of studies on rejection of skin and tumor grafts. Studies elucidating the major histocompatibility complex (MHC; HLA in man and H-2 in mouse) paralleled studies on immunological mechanisms contributing to the GVHD syndrome. Molecules encoded by the MHC are the primary targets of T-cell-mediated GVHD; however, GVHD occurs even when donor and recipient are MHC-matched. In such cases, targets for alloactivated T cells are non-MHC-encoded minor histocompatibility molecules (see Chapter 9). Several studies demonstrate the importance of such antigens (mHA) in eliciting GVH reactions (de Haan et al., 1995; Scott, Ehrmann, & Ellis, 1995; Behar et al., 1996; Goulmy et al., 1996; Pion et al., 1997). A significant advance in our understanding of the role of host MHC molecules in triggering GVH reactive T cells in vivo came from studies using MHC class I–deficient bone marrow (BM) chimeras as hosts (Shlomckhik et al., 1999). These investigators found that GVHD failed to develop when the host antigen-presenting cells (APC) were deficient in MHC class I molecules, regardless of MHC expression on other host tissues.

T cells

Both CD4[+] and CD8[+] T cells are involved in GVHD (Korngold & Sprent, 1987a; Theobald, 1995). Immunogenetic factors dictate their relative importance (Parkman, 1986; Korngold & Sprent, 1987a, 1987b; O'Kunewick et al., 1990; Shlomchik & Emerson, 1996). In mice that are identical at the MHC, but mismatched at multiple mHA loci, depletion of CD8[+] T cells is sufficient to reduce or prevent GVHD in some, but not all, combinations of donor and host (Korngold & Sprent, 1987b). CD8[+] T cells are activated primarily by mHA presented in the context of MHC class I molecules, while CD4[+] T cells recognize peptide in the context of class II MHC molecules. Alloactivated CD4[+] T cells are an important source of immunoregulatory lymphokines such as interleukin (IL)-2 and gamma-interferon (IFN-γ), which drive clonal expansion of T cells and activate NK cells and macrophages involved in GVH reactions. Pan-T-cell depletion eliminates GVHD in both clinical and experimental settings (Marmont et al., 1991) (see Chapter 26); however, T cells are not the only cells that exert GVHD effects. Other cells contribute through direct or indirect damage to host tissues or by modulating immunologic reactivity.

Cytokines

In recent years attention has been focused on the role of T cells and inflammatory cytokines in GVH pathophysiology (Antin & Ferrara, 1992; Jadus & Wepsic, 1992) (see Chapter 15). Proinflammatory cytokines are initially produced by host tissues in response to irradiation and other conditioning agents

used to prepare the recipient for transplantation (Holler et al., 1997). Conditioning-related inflammation represents the first crucial step in induction of GVHD and efforts to block cytokine release offer a novel approach to avoiding GVHD. Donor T cells, regardless of their CD4[+] or CD8[+] phenotype, are also activated during a GVH reaction to produce specific cytokines that trigger the production of additional cytokines by other cell types. Triggering of this "cytokine cascade" contributes significantly to the pathophysiology of GVHD (Ferrara, 1994). Macrophages, activated by T-cell lymphokines such as IFN-γ, secrete a variety of factors affecting hemostasis and immunologic reactivity. Tumor necrosis factor (TNF) (Nedwin et al., 1985; Piguet et al., 1987), IL-1 (Gerrard et al., 1987; McCarthy et al., 1991), and IL-12 (Williamson et al., 1996), in particular, play an important role in GVHD. Release of these cytokines in response to tissue injury from pretransplant preparative regimens may significantly augment severity and mortality of acute GVHD (Antin & Ferrara, 1992; Jadus & Wepsic, 1992).

Several groups have had some success in decreasing the pathophysiologic effects of various cytokines in animal models of GVHD (Hill & Ferrara, 2000). Such maneuvers are promising approaches to "separating" the pathologic effects of GVHD from effector cell-mediated GVL reactivity, but they have not translated readily to the clinical setting. A direct role of cytokines in elimination of residual leukemia remains to be clearly established.

Separation of GVHD from GVL

T cell subsets

Recognition of type 1 (Th1) and type 2 (Th2) T-helper cells has led to development of strategies to avoid GVHD by polarizing the cytokine response away from proinflammatory type 1 cytokines and toward type 2 cytokines (Krenger et al., 1995). Allospecific CD8[+] cytotoxic T lymphocytes (CTLs) can also be biased toward type 1 and type 2 cytokine-secreting subsets. In a murine model of allogeneic BMT, CTLs with a type 2 cytokine phenotype (Tc2) failed to cause detectable GVHD, whereas CTLs with a type 1 cytokine profile (Tc1) did (Fowler et al., 1996). Differential induction of Th2 and Tc2 cells ex vivo offers a novel cytokine-based approach to separation of GVL from GVH reactivity (Fowler & Gress, 2000).

Both CD4[+] and CD8[+] T cells can exert GVL effects (Truitt et al., 1990; Truitt & Atasoylu, 1991a, 1991b; Korngold, Leighton, & Manser, 1994; Palathumpat et al., 1995). Under experimental conditions, cloned alloantigen-specific CD8[+] cytotoxic T lymphocytes can engraft in vivo without causing GVHD (Gao et al., 1999) and can mediate a GVL effect in the absence of CD4[+] T cells or exogenous growth factors (Truitt et al., 1990). CD4[+] T cells may enhance the GVL reaction by inducing clonal expansion of CD8[+] T cells through secretion of IL-2. Falkenburg and colleagues observed that, in general, CD8[+] and CD4[+] mHA-specific CTL clones do not differentially recognize leukemic versus normal hematopoietic progenitor cells (Faber *et al.*, 1995). They suggested that differences in susceptibility to lysis of malignant versus normal cells contributed to a differential GVL effect. Human CTL clones specific for histocompatibility antigens with a restricted tissue distribution may be appropriate targets for a preferential GVL effect without unacceptable GVHD (Warren *et al.*, 1998). In mice, LeFever *et al.* (1985) found that the differentially expressed MHC class Ib molecule Qa-1 was a preferential target for a GVL effect without associated GVHD. However, the degree of the preferential GVL versus GVH effect varied with different CD8+ T-cell clones, suggesting that functional properties of the effector clone rather than the nature of the leukemia target antigen may be more important. Human T cell clones specific for mHA have been shown to mediate a GVL reaction in a murine non-obese diabetic/severe combined immunodeficiency (NOD/SCID) model (Bonnet *et al.*, 1999). Cytotoxic CD4+ T cells may play a role in the killing of leukemias and lymphomas that express class II MHC molecules, or may act through Fas/Fas ligand (FasL) interactions (Jiang *et al.*, 1996). In a murine model of tumor antigen-specific syngeneic GVL, CD4+ cells employed both a FasL-mediated mechanism and a perforin-utilizing mechanism, while CD8+ T cells used a perforin mechanism predominantly (Hsieh & Korngold, 2000). In a murine model for allogeneic BMT, donor T cells mediated GVHD primarily through the Fas/FasL effector pathway and GVL activity through the perforin pathway, suggesting that specific blockade of one cytotoxic pathway may be used to prevent GVHD without diminishing the GVL effect (Schmaltz *et al.*, 2001). In humans, CD4+ T cells play an important role in the GVL effect (Jiang *et al.*, 1991, 1996), and transplantation of CD8-depleted peripheral blood cells is associated with a decreased rate of leukemia relapse and GVHD (Nimer *et al.*, 1994; Shimoni *et al.*, 2001).

Delayed administration of T cells

Delayed administration of GVH-reactive donor T cells (i.e., donor leukocyte infusion or DLI therapy) can also result in a decrease in the adverse effects of GVHD while preserving GVL activity in both humans and animal models (e.g., Johnson & Truitt, 1995; Kolb *et al.*, 1995; Johnson, Becker, & Truitt, 1999; Porter *et al.*, 2000). Several overlapping mechanisms are likely to contribute to decreased GVH reactivity after DLI therapy. First, delayed infusion of donor T cells is associated with a temporal separation from the initial "cytokine storm" induced by the transplant-conditioning regimen (Ferrara, 1994). Second, with time, the host antigen-presenting cells (APCs) that are potent triggers of alloreactive T cells are replaced with less immunogenic donor APCs (Shlomchik *et al.*, 1999), without affecting the antileukemia reactivity of the infused T cells. Third, donor-derived CD4+ regulatory T cells eventually emerge from the repopulating host thymus and preferentially suppress the alloreactivity of infused CD4+ T cells, but they have less effect on the CD8+ effector cells that kill leukemia (Johnson *et al.*, 1999).

NK cells, LAK cells, and CIK cells

NK cells are throught to play an important role in the development and control of hematologic malignancies through "immune surveillance" mechanisms (Delman *et al.*, 1986). NK cells rapidly regenerate after hematopoietic stem cell transplantation. They contribute to both GVH and GVL reactivity, with several studies clearly identifying donor NK cells as an effector population (Hercend *et al.*, 1986; Ghayur *et al.*, 1988; Johnson & Truitt 1992; O'Kunewick *et al.*, 1995; Weiss, Resch, & Slavin, 1995; Glass *et al.*, 1996). In a murine model of matched BMT, NK 1.1+ cells contributed to early, but not late, phases of GVL reactivity (Truitt *et al.*, 1997). NK cells that contribute to GVHD appear to be dependent on T cells for activation, but paradoxically, very early posttransplant administration of IL-2 or IL-12 (potent activators of NK cells) results in protection from GVHD (Sykes *et al.*, 1990; Sykes & Abraham, 1992; Yang *et al.*, 1997). In a landmark paper, Velardi and colleagues described human and murine alloreactive NK cells that eliminated leukemia and faciliated engraftment of MHC-mismatched marrow while protecting against GVHD (Ruggeri *et al.*, 2002). It is of note that these investigators found that the alloreactive NK cells prevented GVHD in a mouse model of MHC-mismatched BMT by eliminating host APCs.

Lymphokine-activated or cytokine-induced killer (LAK and CIK) cells also are important GVL effector cells (e.g., Weiss *et al.*, 1994; Vourka-Karussis *et al.*, 1995; Margolin *et al.*, 1997). Although precursors of IL-2-activated killer cells derive primarily from large granular lymphocytes of the NK lineage, activated non-MHC-restricted killer cells of both T (CD3+) and NK (CD56+) lineages may participate in the antitumor effect after allogeneic transplantation. Precursor and fully activated LAK cells have been isolated from peripheral blood following autologous and allogeneic bone marrow transplants (Hercend *et al.*, 1986; Heslop *et al.*, 1989). The antitumor effect of LAK or CIK cells may be mediated by direct lytic activity as well as by release of lymphokines such as IL-2, tumor necrosis factor (TNF), and IFN-γ, which act directly or indirectly on tumor cells. LAK cells increase the GVL reactivity of T-cell-deficient allogeneic bone marrow in animal studies (Truitt *et al.*, 1990).

The relative importance of T versus non-T effector cells in antileukemia reactivity following allogeneic stem cell transplantation is still not clear. Furthermore, certain leukemias, such as acute lymphoblastic leukemia, are highly resistant to both T cell and NK cell-mediated killing (Horowitz *et al.*, 1990; Weiden & Horowitz, 1990; Ruggeri *et al.*, 2002). Posttransplant clonal evolution of myeloid leukemia to a T cell- or NK cell-resistant phenotype may also limit the GVL effect of DLI therapy (Dermime *et al.*, 1997). In both humans and mice, several immune effector cells may act independently or in association with antihost or GVH-reactive cells to mediate a GVL effect. The relationship between GVL-reactive cytotoxic T cells and GVHD has been examined on a clonal level with multiple GVL effector populations identified (Truitt *et al.*, 1990). Some antileukemic cytotoxic T cells that are specific for mHA cause lethal GVHD, while others do not. Cytotoxicity alone does not correlate with ability to cause GVHD; other factors, such as ability to secrete lymphokines, may be important. Separation of antihost- and antileukemia-reactive cytotoxic cells has also been described in humans using in vitro lytic assays (Hercend et al., 1986; van Rood et al., 1987; Sosman et al., 1989, 1990). Analysis of the T cell receptor Vβ repertoire may identify T cell families that mediate GVL and/or GVH responses after stem cell transplantation and allow for selection of effector T cells with preference for leukemia (Margolis et al., 2000; Orsini et al., 2000; Epperson et al., 2001; Patterson & Korngold, 2001).

Cord blood transplantation

Cord blood, despite its immunological naïveté, also contains potent GVL effector populations (Keever et al., 1995), and cord blood transplantation can be used to minimize GVHD without loss of a GVL effect (Howrey et al., 2000).

Co-stimulatory blockade

Another novel approach to the separation of GVH and GVL reactivity is the use of co-stimulatory blockade to induce anergy in alloreactive T cells (Guinan et al., 1999; Comoli et al., 2001). Importantly, anergy induction by co-stimulatory blockade in vitro preserves the T cell precursors that respond to virus, such as EBV and CMV, as well as those that recognize leukemia (Comoli et al., 2001). An important caveat to this approach is that if the GVL effect is mediated exclusively through T cells specific for host alloantigens present on the leukemia cell (i.e., an allo-specific GVL rather than a leukemia-specific GVL reaction), then the antileukemia benefit may be lost or decreased after anergy induction. This is similar to the loss of allo-specific GVL reactivity against a murine acute T-cell leukemia (AKR-L) that occurs after tolerance induction with T cell-specific anti-CD3ε F(ab')$_2$ monoclonal antibody (Mab) in the early post-BMT period (Johnson et al., 1995). In this model, delaying administration of the tolerance-inducing Mab for at least 8 days after BMT resulted in a curative lymphohematopoietic GVL effect with significantly diminished GVH mortality.

Leukemia antigens

In addition to normal histocompatibility antigens expressed on allogeneic leukemia cells, leukemia-specific or leukemia-associated antigens are also potential targets for immune effector cells in the GVL reaction. The precise nature of such antigens in human leukemia is not known. Possible targets include novel fusion proteins like those produced by the bcr-abl translocation in CML, the PML/RARA hybrid protein in acute promyelocytic leukemia (FAB M3), mutations in the Ras protein commonly detected in several human tumors, immunoglobulin idiotypes expressed on leukemia cells of B-cell origin, and, in animal models, retrovirus-associated glycoproteins. While leukemia-specific T cells have been shown to exist in experimental systems, their role in GVL reactivity following clinical allogeneic bone marrow transplants remains unclear. However, one cannot exclude the possibility that GVL reactivity in the absence of GVHD may be directed against unique leukemia-associated antigens (Claret et al., 1997). The immunogenicity of leukemia-specific antigens may depend on how they are presented and techniques to enhance antigen presentation are receiving considerable attention, including upregulation of co-stimulatory molecules and use of "professional" APCs such as dendritic cells (Kovacsovics-Bankowski et al., 1993; Pardoll, 1993; Guinan et al., 1994; Troy & Hart, 1997). While introduction of co-stimulatory molecules may enhance the immunogenicity of leukemia cells, in some instances co-stimulator molecules (e.g., B7.1) preferentially interact with negative regulatory molecules (e.g., CTLA-4) to turn off a T cell-mediated immune response (LaBelle et al., 2002).

GVL effects in clinical HSC transplants

Evidence for an antileukemia effect of transplanted allogeneic cells includes the following clinical observations:

1. Lower incidence of leukemia relapse in allograft recipients with acute and/or chronic GVHD compared to those without GVHD
2. Higher relapse rates after identical twin versus allogeneic bone marrow transplants
3. High relapse rates after T-cell-depleted transplants
4. Durable cytogenetic and molecular remissions induced after posttransplant relapse by infusion of donor leukocytes without other antileukemia therapy
5. Durable responses including complete remissions that are gradually achieved many months after non-myeloablative or reduced intensity conditioning allogeneic blood or marrow transplants in which the conditioning regimen has little or no significant anti-tumor activity.

The antileukemia effect of GVHD

Numerous single and multi-institution reports in the late 1970s and 1980s demonstrated an inverse correlation between development of GVHD and risk of leukemia recurrence. These studies are summarized in Table 19.1. In 1979, Weiden and colleagues reported that the risk of relapse was 2.5 times less in 79 allograft recipients with moderate-to-severe acute or chronic GVHD than in 117 with no or minimal GVHD. Patients included those transplanted for ALL or AML with a variety of disease states prior to transplant. Survival was similar with and without GVHD. A 1981 report from the same group described an association between chronic GVHD and relapse in 163 patients with ALL and AML transplanted in remission or relapse and surviving in remission at least 150 days after transplant (Weiden et al., 1981). Actuarial probability of relapse was

Table 19.1. *Associations between GVHD and relapse after allogeneic bone marrow transplants*

Institution	Reference	*n*	Acute GVHD	Chronic GVHD	Acute and/or chronic GVHD	Comments
FHCRC	Weiden *et al.*, 1979	196	NE	NE	↓[a]	ALL, AML in remission or relapse
FHCRC	Weiden *et al.*, 1981	163	↓		↓	ALL, AML in remission or relapse; surviving ≥ 150 days
UCLA	McIntyre & Gale, 1981	46	↓	NE	NE	Acute leukemia in relapse
EBMTG	Zwaan *et al.*, 1984	229	–	↓	NE	AML in remission
Genoa	Bacigalupo *et al.*, 1985	78	–	↓	NE	ALL, AML, CML
FHCRC	Sanders *et al.*, 1985	114	–	–	↓	Children; ALL in remission or relapse
U Minn	Weisdorf *et al.*, 1987	40	↓	NE	NE	ALL in remission or relapse
U Minn	Kersey *et al.*, 1987	46	NE	NE	↓	ALL in remission or relapse
MSK	Brochstein *et al.*, 1987	97	–	↓	NE	ALL in remission or relapse
FHCRC	Sullivan *et al.*, 1989	481	↓	–	–	Early ALL, AML, CML
		263	↓	–	–	Intermediate ALL, AML, CML
		458	–	–	↓	Advanced ALL, AML, CML
IBMTR	Horowitz *et al.*, 1990	1,783	↓	↓	↓	Early ALL, AML, CML
EBMTG	Ringden *et al.*, 1996	1,634	↓	↓	NE	AML; all pts CSP/MTX
NMPD	Castro-Malaspina *et al.*, 2002	510	↓	–	–	MDS with half being poor risk (RAEB, RAEBt, AML); Unrelated donors

Abbreviations: CSP, cyclosporine; FHCRC, Fred Hutchinson Cancer Research Center; EBMTG, European Bone Marrow Transplant Group; IBMTR, International Bone Marrow Transplant Registry; MDS, myelodysplastic syndromes; MSK, Memorial Sloan-Kettering; MTX, methotrexate; NMDP, National Marrow Donor Program (USA); RAEB, refractory anemia with excess blasts; RAEBt, refractory anemia with excess blasts in transformation; UCLA, University of California, Los Angeles; U Minn, University of Minnesota.

[a] ↓ indicates decreased relapse; – indicates no association with relapse; NE indicates association with relapse not evaluated.

62% among patients without acute or chronic GVHD, 43% among those with only acute GVHD, 34% among those with only chronic GVHD, and 12% among those with both acute and chronic GVHD. In multivariate analysis, chronic GVHD was significantly associated with decreased relapse, with a rate 0.31 to 0.36 times the rate in patients without GVHD ($P <$ .005). In this study, restricted to patients already surviving 150 days posttransplant, subsequent survival was significantly higher in patients with chronic GVHD. However, this does not give an accurate estimate of the impact of GVHD on survival of transplant recipients in general, since more than 80% of all GVHD-related deaths occur before 150 days posttransplant (Bortin *et al.*, 1989).

A 1981 study from UCLA examined relapse rates in 46 allograft recipients surviving 30 days or more posttransplant (McIntyre & Gale, 1981). All were in relapse at the time of transplant; 10 had never achieved remission. Actuarial relapse rates were 62% in 22 patients with grade 0–I acute GVHD and 20% in 24 with grade II–IV acute GVHD ($P =$ .05). There was no difference in survival.

A 1984 study from the European Bone Marrow Transplant Group (EBMT) including 229 patients with AML in first or second remission from 27 centers reported decreased relapse with chronic, but not acute, GVHD (Zwaan *et al.*, 1984). Similarly, a report from Genoa of 78 patients with ALL, AML, or CML reported probabilities of relapse of 13% and 63% for patients with and without chronic GVHD, respectively ($P =$ .00004) (Bacigalupo *et al.*, 1985).

A 1985 report from Seattle of 114 children with ALL (5 in first marrow remission, 46 in second or subsequent remission, and 63 in relapse) showed a decreased risk of relapse among patients with acute and/or chronic GVHD (relative risk 0.26, $P =$ .002) (Sanders *et al.*, 1985). In this study development of chronic GVHD was associated with improved survival ($P =$ .005).

A 1987 study at the University of Minnesota of 40 patients with high-risk ALL reported decreased relapse risk in patients with grade II–IV acute GVHD (73% versus 57%, $P =$ .04) (Weisdorf *et al.*, 1987). There was a trend toward improved relapse-free survival among patients with GVHD, but this was not statistically significant ($P =$ .11) (Weisdorf *et al.*, 1987). Comparison of allogeneic and autologous transplants for high-risk, refractory ALL at the same institution showed a higher relapse risk after autologous (79%) than allogeneic (56%) transplants (Kersey *et al.*, 1987). Relapses after autotransplants tended to occur earlier than after allogeneic transplants. Some recurrences after autologous transplants may have been due to re-infusion of leukemia cells in the autologous graft, as suggested by data from gene-marking studies (Brenner *et al.*, 1993, 1994). However, the relapse rate with autologous transplants was similar to that after allografts without GVHD (73%), suggesting that the absence of GVHD-mediated antileukemia activity was an important factor. Transplant-related mortality was higher after allogeneic than autologous transplants. Leukemia-free survival was similar.

A 1987 study from Memorial Sloan-Kettering Cancer Center of 97 children with ALL or AML reported an antileukemia effect of chronic, but not acute, GVHD after adjustment for other risk factors (Brochstein *et al.*, 1987).

Sullivan and colleagues (1989b) studied 1,202 recipients of allografts for AML, ALL, and CML. Four hundred and eighty-one patients had early leukemia (acute leukemia in first remission or CML in chronic phase); 263, intermediate leukemia (acute leukemia in second or subsequent remission or CML in accelerated phase); and the remainder, advanced disease. Using multivariate analyses, they were unable to show an effect of acute or chronic GVHD upon relapse in patients with early leukemia, except in ALL. Acute GVHD was associated with decreased relapse in patients with intermediate ALL and AML. Development of acute or chronic GVHD was associated with decreased relapse in advanced acute leukemia and CML.

A large study of GVL effects in clinical bone marrow transplantation was published by the International Bone Marrow Transplant Registry (IBMTR) in 1990. It included 2,254 recipients of allogeneic transplants for early leukemia (first remission acute leukemia or CML in first chronic phase) and demonstrated a statistically significant reduction in relapse risk among patients developing GVHD (Fig. 19.1) (Horowitz *et al.*, 1990). In this study, recipients of non-T-cell-depleted allografts not developing GVHD had a 3-year probability of relapse of 25% ± 6% (95% confidence interval). Recipients with acute GVHD only, chronic GVHD only, or both had 3-year probabilities of relapse of 22% ± 5%, 10% ± 7%, and 7% ± 3%, respectively. In multivariate analyses adjusting for other variables affecting relapse, patients developing only acute GVHD had a relative risk of relapse of 0.68 (P = .03) compared to patients without acute or chronic GVHD; those with only chronic GVHD had a relative risk of 0.43 (P = .01); and those with both acute and chronic GVHD had a relative risk of 0.33 (P = .0001). GVHD was associated with decreased relapse in ALL, AML, and CML, although the relative importance of acute and chronic GVHD differed for the three types of leukemia (Table 19.2). Chronic GVHD had a stronger

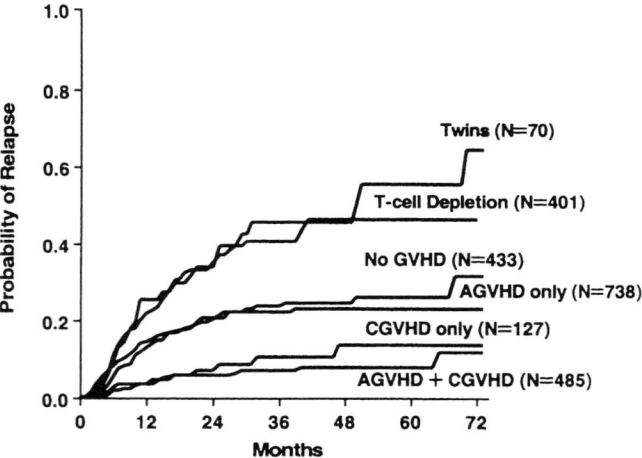

Fig. 19.1. Actuarial probability of relapse after bone marrow transplantation for early leukemia according to type of graft and development of GVHD. Reproduced, with permission, from Horowitz *et al.* (1990).

antileukemia effect in AML and CML and acute GVHD a stronger effect in ALL. Patients with both acute and chronic GVHD had the lowest risk of relapse in all cases. Relapse correlated inversely with severity of GVHD. One hundred and forty-one patients with mild acute and chronic GVHD had a relative risk of relapse of 0.50 (P = .02) or a two-fold decrease in relapse risk as compared to those without GVHD; 72 patients with moderate GVHD had a relative risk of 0.22 (P = .009) or a 4.5-fold decrease in risk; none of 49 patients with severe acute and chronic GVHD relapsed (P = .04).

In a study of 1,634 recipients of HLA-identical sibling bone marrow transplants with acute leukemia reported from the EBMT (Ringden *et al.*, 1996), a GVL effect was maintained both by acute and chronic GVHD; all the patients in this study received cyclosporine and methotrexate as GVHD prophylaxis (Table 19.1).

In a subsequent EBMT study comparing relapse risk in 5,200 autograft recipients, 1,039 HLA-identical allograft recipients, who never showed clinical evidence of acute or chronic GVHD, and 67 syngeneic recipients transplanted for AML or ALL in first remission, the HLA-identical sibling recipients had a lower risk of relapse (Fig. 19.2) and a better leukemia-free survival (Fig. 19.3) (Ringden *et al.*, 2000). This suggests the existence of a GVL effect in the absence of clinical GVHD. A similar benefit was not seen in a recent report of the NMDP experience with unrelated bone marrow transplantation (Castro-Malaspina *et al.*, 2002). Lower relapse rates in patients developing GVHD after transplants from unrelated or HLA-mismatched related donors have been reported (Ash *et al.*, 1991; Davies *et al.*, 1996). The GVL effect has been less well examined in studies comprised solely of recipients of unrelated donor transplants. In a Swedish study of 214 patients, 86% of whom were HLA-A, -B and -DRβ1 identical with their donors, risk factors for relapse included absence of grade II-IV acute GVHD and absence of chronic GVHD (Remberger *et al.*, 2002).

Besides a GVL effect in AML, ALL, and CML, allogeneic transplantation appears to mediate a GVL effect in chronic lymphatic leukemia and prolymphocytic leukemia (Mehta *et al.*, 1996), in myeloma (Tricot *et al.*, 1996; Verdonck *et al.*, 1996), renal cell cancer (Childs *et al.*, 2000), Hodgkin's lymphoma (Phillips *et al.*, 1989; Akpek *et al.*, 2001), and non-Hodgkin's lymphoma (Bierman, 2000). Additionally, there are reports of a graft-versus-tumor effect after allogeneic transplantation for breast cancer (Ben-Yosef *et al.*, 1996; Eibl *et al.*, 1996; Ueno *et al.*, 1998), non-small-cell lung cancer (Moscardo *et al.*, 2000), and ovarian cancer (Bay *et al.*, 2000).

While there is increasing evidence for a graft-versus-tumor effect against a variety of diseases, this effect is not always associated with improved survival due to the inherent toxicity of allogeneic transplant conditioning regimens and graft-versus-host disease. Non-myeloablative or reduced intensity conditioning allogeneic transplants have been developed in an attempt to harness the graft-versus-tumor effect of allogeneic transplants without the early high mortality (Champlin *et al.*, 2000a).

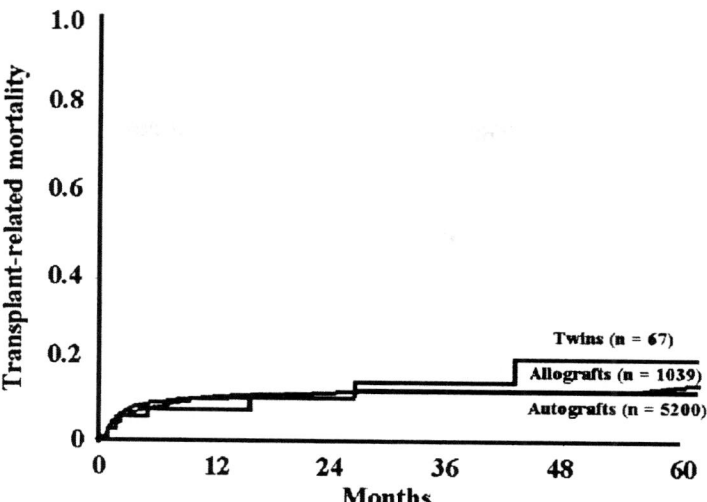

Fig. 19.2. Probability of relapse in patients with acute leukemia undergoing autologous bone marrow transplantation, transplantation from an identical twin, or receiving an allograft from an HLA-identical sibling without developing acute or chronic graft-versus-host disease. Reproduced, with permission, from Ringden *et al.* (2000).

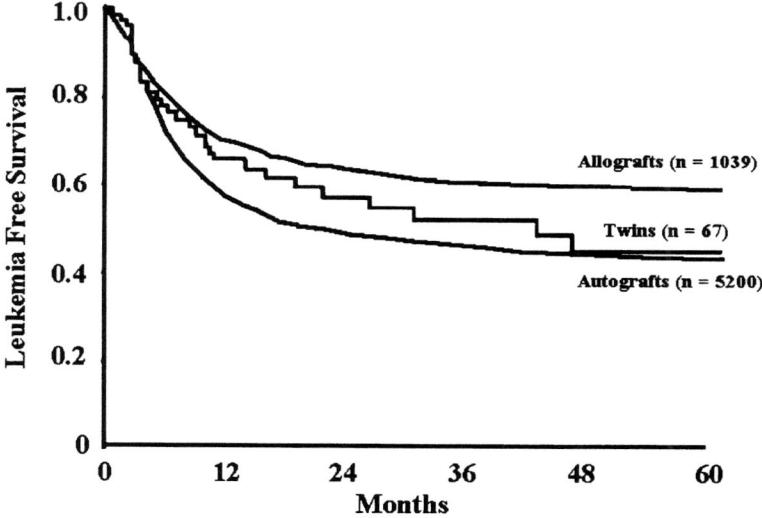

Fig. 19.3. Leukemia-free survival in patients with acute leukemia undergoing autologous bone marrow transplantation, transplantation from an identical twin, or receiving an allograft from an HLA-identical sibling without developing acute or chronic graft--versus-host disease. Reproduced, with permission, from Ringden *et al.* (2000).

Another development has been the use of mobilized allogeneic peripheral blood stem cell (PBSC) grafts instead of BM. The different composition of the two graft sources and initial results of clinical trials and analyses (Champlin *et al.,* 2000c) include interesting, but inconclusive, observations related to GVHD and GVL as reviewed by Korbling & Anderlini (2001) and discussed in the more recent Canadian National Trial publication (Couban *et al.,* 2002). PBSC grafts contain approximately one log more T-cells than BM grafts. Despite this, the cumulative incidence of acute GVHD in most reports is not increased. This may be due to a threshold effect of T-cells that is exceeded by both unmanipulated BM and PBSC grafts, or

immunomodulation of the T-cells by the hematopoietic growth factors used in their mobilization, or by currently undetermined factors. Only one study has reported increased acute GVHD with PBSC versus BM grafting (Schmitz *et al.,* 2000). The data regarding chronic GVHD after PBSC transplants is also mixed, with reports equally split between an increased risk with PBSC and no difference (Korbling & Anderlini, 2001; Couban *et al.,* 2002). The largest study, a retrospective analysis by the IBMTR, indicates an increased risk of chronic GVHD with PBSC (65%) versus BM (53%) ($P = .02$) (Champlin *et al.,* 2000c). The completed randomized trials are either not powered for, or require longer follow-up regarding, chronic GVHD. It is also unclear whether there is an enhanced GVL effect with PBSC grafts. In all but one study (Powles *et al.*, 2000) overall relapse rates have been similar between BM and PBSC grafts. Post-hoc subgroup analyses, however, have identified patients with advanced disease (e.g., CML beyond first chronic phase and AML in second remission) as having lower relapse rates with PBSC than BM (Champlin *et al.*, 2000c; Bensinger *et al.*, 2001; Couban *et al.*, 2002). Confirmation will require larger disease-specific trials or a meta-analysis of primary data from the existing completed trials to more fully address this possibility.

Leukemia relapse after identical twin transplants

The importance of allogeneic cells in eradicating leukemia after bone marrow transplants can be studied by comparing relapse rates after allogeneic and identical twin transplants.

Weiden *et al.* (1979) compared the relapse rate in 46 recipients of identical twin transplants for AML or ALL with the relapse rate in 117 recipients of allogeneic transplants with grade 0 or I acute GVHD and no chronic GVHD and with that in 79 recipients of allografts with grade II–IV acute or any chronic GVHD. The relapse rate after syngeneic transplants was about 1.5 times higher than after allogeneic transplants ($P < .10$). The rate was similar after identical twin transplants and allogeneic transplants without GVHD (relative risk 1.2, $P = $ NS), but it was significantly higher after identical twin transplants than after allogeneic transplants associated with grade II–IV acute or any chronic GVHD (relative risk 2.7, $P = .0003$), suggesting that the increased antileukemia efficacy of allografts was due to GVHD-mediated antileukemia effects. Most of the twin recipients in this study were in relapse at the time of transplant.

In 1984, Gale and Champlin summarized results of 31 identical twin transplants for AML in first remission reported by five centers and one cooperative group, and compared these to results of HLA-identical sibling transplants for AML in first remission at the same centers. The actuarial relapse rate was $59\% \pm 20\%$ for twins compared to $18\% \pm 4\%$ for HLA-identical siblings. Allogeneic transplants with and without GVHD were not examined separately, so the extent to which the difference in relapse rates was explained by GVHD could not be evaluated.

A 1987 update of the Seattle twin transplant data compared the probability of relapse in 53 recipients of twin transplants for AML or ALL with 785 recipients of allogeneic transplants for AML or ALL (Fefer *et al.*, 1987). The probability of relapse was 75% after twin transplants and 62% after allogeneic transplants ($P < .0001$).

The 1990 IBMTR study of GVL effect in 2,254 recipients of bone marrow transplants for early leukemia included 70 identical twin transplants (Fig. 19.1, Table 19.2) (Horowitz *et al.*, 1990). The relative risks of relapse for recipients of identical twin transplants compared to recipients of allogeneic transplants without acute or chronic GVHD was 2.09 ($P = .005$). When different leukemias were analyzed separately, a significant increase in relapse risk with identical twin transplants was observed only in AML, with a trend toward increased relapse in CML.

A subsequent IBMTR analysis of 103 identical twin transplants for ALL, AML, and CML confirmed these results (Gale *et al.*, 1994). Relative risks for relapse after identical twin versus HLA-identical sibling transplants, after adjustment for GVHD effects, were 1.4 for ALL ($P > .2$), 3.8 for AML ($P < .001$), and 5.5 for CML ($P < .001$). These data suggest that allogeneic cells have an antileukemia effect independent of clinically detectable GVHD. It may be that leukemia-associated antigens, not recognized by genetically identical immune cells, are recognized by allogeneic immune cells. Alternatively, the different relapse rates may reflect nonspecific effects of subclinical GVHD directed against mHA preferentially expressed on hematopoietic cells (Mutis *et al.*, 1997).

Table 19.2. *Relative risk of relapse after bone marrow transplantation for early leukemia*[a]

Study group	ALL 1st CR			AML 1st CR			CML CP			All patients		
	n	RR	*P*	*n*	RR	*P*	*n*	RR	*P*	*n*	RR	*P*
Allogeneic, non-T-depleted												
No GVHD[b]	90	1.00	–	228	1.00	–	115	1.00	–	433	1.00	–
Acute GVHD only	141	0.36	.004	330	0.78	.26	267	1.15	.75	738	0.68	.03
Chronic GVHD only	28	0.44	.16	54	0.48	.12	45	0.28	.16	127	0.43	.01
Acute and chronic GVHD	84	0.38	.02	237	0.34	.0003	164	0.24	.03	485	0.33	.0001
Syngeneic	12	0.99	.99	34	2.58	.008	24	2.95	.08	70	2.09	.005
Allogeneic, T-depleted												
All patients	84	1.20	.61	163	1.30	.33	154	5.14	.0001	401	1.76	.002
No GVHD	43	1.48	.33	83	1.57	.12	74	6.91	.0001	200	2.14	.0001
Acute and/or chronic GVHD	41	0.98	.97	80	0.80	.60	80	4.45	.003	201	1.32	.25

Abbreviations: ALL, acute lymphoblastic leukemia; AML, acute myeloid leukemia; CML, chronic myeloid leukemia; CP, chronic phase; CR, complete remission; GVHD, graft-versus-host disease; RR, relative risk in comparison to reference group.

[a] Relative risks are derived from multivariate Cox regression adjusting for leukocyte count at diagnosis, recipient age, organ impairment pretransplant, donor-recipient sex match, and drug(s) used to prevent GVHD.

[b] Reference group.

Data from Horowitz *et al.* (1990).

Table 19.3.   *Adjusted 2-year probabilities and relative risks of relapse following T-cell-depleted bone marrow transplantation*[a]

Disease	Status	Non-T-cell-depleted		T-cell-depleted		Relative risk	P
		Number at risk	Probability of relapse	Number at risk	Probability of relapse		
ALL	1st remission	260	17%	89	29%	1.83	< .05
AML	1st remission	560	17%	159	30%	1.94	< .007
CML	Chronic phase	452	10%	172	44%	5.61	< .0001
All patients	**Early leukemia**	**1,272**	**15%**	**420**	**37%**	**2.75**	**< .0001**
ALL	2nd remission	312	39%	61	59%	1.79	< .03
AML	2nd remission	105	41%	28	26%	0.57	NS
CML	Accelerated phase	219	24%	73	51%	2.65	< .002
All patients	**Intermediate leukemia**	**636**	**34%**	**162**	**51%**	**1.71**	**< .003**
ALL	Relapse	171	55%	35	75%	1.73	< .03
AML	Relapse	205	45%	43	66%	1.79	< .03
CML	Blast phase	81	57%	31	63%	1.17	NS
All patients	**Advanced leukemia**	**457**	**51%**	**109**	**70%**	**1.70**	**< .002**

[a] Probabilities adjusted for age of patient, infection present in the week pretransplant, performance score pretransplant, donor age, and year of transplant, using Cox proportional hazard regression.
Data from Marmont *et al.* (1991).

In a subsequent IBMTR study of cell dose in identical twin transplants, a higher nucleated cell dose ($>3.0 \times 10^8$ cells/kg) was associated with a decreased relative risk of late relapse 0.28 ($P = .003$) compared to the low cell dose group, suggesting again the possibility of a graft-versus-leukemia effect that is dependent on graft content and separate from clinical graft-versus-host disease (Barrett *et al.*, 2000).

Leukemia relapse after T-cell-depleted transplants

Another way of determining whether the bone marrow graft has antileukemia activity is to observe whether manipulating the graft affects relapse. This situation occurs with T-cell-depleted transplants.

Removing T cells from the donor marrow decreases the incidence and severity of acute and chronic GVHD regardless of the method of T-cell depletion (Martin *et al.*, 1985; Sondel *et al.*, 1985; Apperley *et al.*, 1986; Cobbold *et al.*, 1986; de Witte *et al.*, 1986; Kernan *et al.*, 1986; Butturini & Gale, 1987; Herve *et al.*, 1987; Maraninchi *et al.*, 1987; Prentice, 1987; O'Reilly *et al.*, 1988; Poynton, 1988; Prentice *et al.*, 1988; Marmont *et al.*, 1991; Goldman *et al.*, 1993). Because GVHD is a major cause of mortality and morbidity after allogeneic transplantation, some centers deplete T cells from the donor stem cell inoculum prior to infusion. Generally, pretransplant preparative regimens are similar whether or not the donor stem cells are T-cell depleted, except that some centers use higher doses of radiation or chemotherapy for T-cell-depleted transplants (Sondel *et al.*, 1985; Apperley *et al.*, 1986; Cobbold *et al.*, 1986). Despite similar or more intense conditioning, the risk of leukemia relapse is substantially higher after T-cell-depleted than non-T-cell-depleted transplants, indicating that an important mediator of antileukemia activity is removed during the process of T-cell

depletion. This increased leukemia relapse rate has been observed after HLA-identical sibling transplants in multiple centers using a variety of methods for T-cell depletion (Marmont *et al.*, 1991).

Since GVHD has an antileukemia effect, increased relapses observed with T-cell depletion may result completely, or in part, from removal of cells responsible for GVHD. However, in the 1990 IBMTR study of GVL effects in early leukemia, 154 CML patients receiving T-cell-depleted transplants, with or without GVHD, had higher probabilities of relapse with or without the occurrence of GVHD (relative risks 4.45 and 6.91, respectively, $P = .0001$) than 115 recipients of non-T-cell-depleted allografts without GVHD (Table 19.2) (Horowitz *et al.*, 1990). These data suggest that T-cell depletion alters the antileukemia effect of transplants in CML by a mechanism separate from GVHD.

The IBMTR analyzed results of 731 HLA-identical sibling T-cell-depleted transplants for all stages of leukemia performed between January 1982 and December 1987 (Marmont *et al.*, 1991). Results were compared to 2,480 non-T-cell-depleted transplants performed during the same time period. The likelihood of leukemia relapse after T-cell-depleted and non-T-cell-depleted transplants was compared after stratifying for type of leukemia and disease state (Table 19.3). There was significantly increased leukemia relapse in all T-cell-depleted recipients except for those with AML beyond second remission and CML in blast phase. The adverse effect on relapse in early leukemia was greatest in CML (relative risk 5.61, $P < .0001$), intermediate in AML (relative risk 1.94, $P < .007$), and least in ALL (relative risk 1.83, $P < .05$) (Table 19.3). After adjusting for the incidence and severity of acute and chronic GVHD, the relative relapse risks for AML and ALL in first remission and CML in chronic phase were 1.66 ($P = $ NS), 1.55 ($P = $ NS), and 4.87 ($P < .0001$), respectively.

The increased relapse rate after T-cell-depleted transplants for ALL and AML appears to be wholly explained by the decreased incidence of GVHD and, presumably, of GVHD-associated antileukemia effects. Other mechanisms appear to operate in CML. This effect is presumably mediated by T cells, but could result from some other cells or factor affected by T-cell depletion. T cells might interact with leukemia cells directly, or by facilitating engraftment or producing lymphokines that affect growth of leukemia cells. In ALL and AML, the risks of relapse with T-cell depletion were similar to non-T-cell depleted transplants without GVHD, suggesting that increased relapse in this setting is due primarily to decreased GVHD-associated antileukemia activity.

T-cell depletion (TCD) has also been employed in unrelated and alternate donor transplants where the risk of GVHD is known to be much higher. Some data suggest that TCD may not abrogate GVL effects after unrelated donor transplants to the same degree as observed with HLA-identical sibling transplants (Drobyski *et al.*, 1994). More recently, an IBMTR report found that the incidence of acute GVHD and 5-year leukemia-free survival (LFS) rate after transplants from donors other than HLA-matched siblings were in part dependent on the particular technique used for TCD of the unrelated donor marrow, with techniques employing narrow specificity antibodies more likely to preserve GVL effects (Champlin *et al.*, 2000b). Although LFS was not improved over T-cell replete transplants utilizing conventional GVHD prophylaxis, the retention of a GVL effect while decreasing GVHD supports further the notion that GVL and GVHD can be separated clinically. Further studies of novel selective approaches to TCD (e.g., Nimer *et al.*, 1994; Chen *et al.*, 2002), or T-cell inhibition (Guinan *et al.*, 1999) will be required to determine whether this potential can be realized. Further complicating this area is the coupling of TCD to strategies for the reinfusion of alloreactive cell populations of differing composition, at various times and for various different indications posttransplant.

While TCD has been shown to reduce GVHD and with some methodologies to retain GVL, a prospective phase III trial is required to define the role of TCD as GVHD prophylaxis in allogeneic transplantation.

Re-infusion of donor cells to treat posttransplant relapse

A report from Kolb *et al.* (1990) demonstrated the importance of donor cells in maintaining remission after transplants for CML. This paper described three patients with hematologic relapse 1.5 to 3 years after HLA-identical sibling transplants for CML in chronic phase who received unmanipulated leukocyte transfusions from their original donors. Between 4.4 and 7.4×10^8 mononuclear cells/kg were administered. Prior therapy with IFN-α, administered daily for 3 months or more, had failed to induce clinical or cytogenetic remission. Two of the three patients developed clinically significant GVHD that responded to immune suppression. All achieved complete clinical and cytogenetic remission with re-establishment of full hematopoietic chimerism. Similar results were reported by Cullis *et al.* (1992) in two CML patients.

Drobyski *et al.* (1993) reported similar results with donor lymphocyte infusions in 8 patients relapsing after transplant for CML. Six patients in accelerated phase achieved remissions in association with GVHD while 2 patients in blast crisis died, one of fatal GVHD and one of disease progression. Thus, disease status is important in predicting response to DLI therapy, and nearly all patients receiving high doses of DLI ($>1 \times 10^8$/kg) develop some GVHD. This successful application of adoptive cellular immunotherapy, without the use of cytotoxic chemotherapy, provides strong evidence for an important role of immune cells in maintaining remission after transplantation. It led to the widespread use of DLI to treat posttransplant relapse of CML and other hematologic malignancies (Kolb *et al.*, 1995; Naparstek *et al.*, 1995; Collins *et al.*, 1997).

Recent results have been reviewed by Kolb *et al.* (1995), who summarized data from 27 European centers, and by Collins *et al.* (1997), who summarized results from 25 North American centers. Forty-one percent and 46% of patients in these two series developed grade II–IV acute GVHD. Twelve percent in each group died of nonleukemia causes. Overall response rates in 109 and 124 evaluable patients were 56% and 46%, respectively; however, response rates varied by disease. The approach seemed most effective in CML where response rates of 75% to 80% were seen in patients with cytogenetic or chronic phase relapses. Much lower response rates of 12%–28% were observed in patients with more advanced CML. Disease status at the time of DLI has been the only consistent predictor of response or maintenance of response following DLI for CML (Kolb *et al.*, 1995; Collins *et al.*, 1997; Porter *et al.*, 1999a; Dazzi *et al.*, 2000b).

Porter and colleagues undertook to exploit the graft-versus-tumor effect of DLI as primary therapy for patients with a variety of relapsed malignancies (Porter *et al.*, 1999b). Initial therapy was 4 weeks of IFN-α followed by 4 DLIs over 2 weeks. The median dose of DLI delivered at level 1 was 3.6×10^8 mononuclear cells/kg. Three of 18 patients had transient graft-versus-tumor responses. Low level donor chimerism was detected 4 weeks later in 4 patients who had had previous autologous stem cell transplants, but not in any other patients. Six patients went on to receive additional DLI with a median dose of 2.14×10^8 mononuclear cells/kg. Interestingly, one patient had a delayed response at a time when no donor lymphocytes were detectable in the patient (sensitivity 0.5%–1.0%). It was apparent that more profound prior immunosuppression (prior autotransplant) was associated with a higher likelihood of donor chimerism, GVHD and graft-versus-tumor effect, an observation that is now being exploited with non-myeloablative stem cell allotransplants (NST) and in tandem strategies of autologous transplantation followed by non-myeloablative allotransplantation.

Results with DLI for AML or MDS are much more modest with complete responses observed in only 25% to 30% of patients with AML or myelodysplasia in the European and

North American series (Kolb *et al.*, 1995; Kolb, 1998; Collins *et al.*, 1997). Responses have also been less stable with 3-year LFS of only 20% in a follow up report of the EBMT series. (Kolb, 1998). Attempts to improve results through a strategy of chemotherapy debulking followed by DLI for AML relapsed post-allograft met with improved short-term but similar long-term results. While 56% achieved a complete response (CR), the 2-year survival was only 19% (Levine *et al.*, 2002).

None of 12 evaluable patients with ALL in the European series had a complete response and only 2 of 11 in the North American series had a complete response (Kolb *et al.*, 1995; Collins *et al.*, 1997). Responses were more likely in patients whose initial transplant had been T-cell depleted and who developed GVHD after donor lymphocyte infusion. However, responses were observed in some patients without GVHD. A subsequent report by Levine *et al.* (2002) of 44 patients was equally disappointing with a 3-year survival rate of 13%.

There have been a number of case reports or small series identifying a graft-versus-myeloma effect (Tricot *et al.*, 1996; Mehta & Singhal, 1998; Lokhorst *et al.*, 2000; Salama *et al.*, 2000). In one of the larger series, 25 patients were treated in a heterogeneous fashion, some with chemotherapy before DLI, others not (Salama *et al.*, 2000). The initial DLI dose varied with a median of approximately 1×10^8/kg; 9 patients received additional higher doses of DLI. There were 7 complete responders: 3 of 3 who had received chemotherapy for debulking prior to the DLI and 4 of 22 who had not. Three other patients experienced a partial response. All responses were associated with GVHD.

Another series of similar size, but primarily including patients with partially T-cell depleted HLA-matched sibling grafts given DLI later posttransplant (median 30 months), resulted in a somewhat higher response rate (14 out of 27) but a similar CR rate of 22% (Lokhorst *et al.*, 2000). As in the previous study, responses were seen in patients given cell doses greater or equal to 1×10^8 mononuclear cells/kg. Responding patients had minimal disease before DLI, analogous to those with a successful outcome in the previous study of patients who received chemotherapy prior to DLI.

There have been numerous case reports or small series of patients receiving DLI for CLL and follicular, mantle cell, large B-cell and lymphoblastic lymphoma (van Besien *et al.*, 1997, 1998; Khouri *et al.*, 1998, 1999; Sohn *et al.*, 2000; McSweeney *et al.*, 2001). Childs and colleagues (2000) tested DLI as part of an NST strategy in renal cell cancer with some success, while the same approach had a dismal outcome in malignant melanoma (Childs, personal communication, 2002).

Response to DLI in most reported series is associated with GVHD independent of indication. In some series, such as the North American series reported by Collins *et al.* (1997), a very high concordance between response and GVHD was found. Other reports showed more variability with high response rates in the presence of GVHD, but also responses in patients not experiencing clinical GVHD (Kolb *et al.*, 1995; MacKinnon *et al.*, 1995; Collins *et al.*, 1997; Kolb, 1998; Dazzi *et al.*, 2000b;

de Lima *et al.*, 2001). Predictors of GVHD have varied depending on the report, but they include the use of interferon with the DLI, high cell dose, the preceding HSC transplant being T-cell depleted and prior GVHD posttransplant. GVHD-related mortality after DLI remains second only to relapse or progression as a cause of death.

There have been a variety of strategies undertaken to try and improve the results of DLI. Illustrative with regards to GVL and GVHD are studies of prophylactic administration, dose escalation and timing variations, and manipulation of the DLI.

Prevention of relapse by prophylactic infusion of donor cells posttransplant

Deliberate induction of GVHD by employing either no, or abbreviated, posttransplant immune suppression, with or without infusion of donor buffy coat cells immediately posttransplant was attempted in the 1980s to decrease leukemia recurrence in patients at high risk of relapse (Sullivan *et al.*, 1986, 1989a). The incidence of acute, but not chronic, GVHD was increased by these maneuvers, but the results were disappointing with no significant decrease in relapse observed and overall survival decreased due to higher transplant-related mortality. Animal studies have since shown that GVHD may be decreased by delaying the reinfusion of T-cells until later posttransplant (Johnson & Truitt, 1995; Johnson *et al.*, 1999). Several groups have revisited the strategy of delayed prophylactic DLI (Naparstek *et al.*, 1995; Barrett *et al.*, 1998; Lee *et al.*, 1999; Spitzer *et al.*, 2000; de Lima *et al.*, 2001; de Lima *et al.*, 2001; Ferra *et al.*, 2001). Lee *et al.* (1999), with the largest reported experience ($n = 144$), found that even low doses of DLI ($1-2.5 \times 10^5$ CD3+ T cells/kg) early after related ($n = 90$) or unrelated ($n = 54$) T-cell depleted transplants (first dose on day 0) resulted in GVHD comparable to that after T-cell replete grafts, and was unable to demonstrate with this approach that GVL was separable from GVHD. This confirmed the observation of others that such low T-cell doses are capable of inducing GVHD when given on the day of transplant (Kernan *et al.*, 1989). Ferra *et al.* (2001) reached similar conclusions in 12 patients receiving low-dose DLI (2×10^5 CD3+ T cells/kg) starting on day +28 and repeated approximately monthly for a total of 2 or 3 infusions, as tolerated based on relapse and GVHD risk, for a total of 2 or 3 infusions (Ferra 2001). They concluded, however, that the GVHD following this approach was easily controlled, particularly in patients at high risk of GVHD. Prophylactic DLI initiated early posttransplant has not clearly resulted in evidence of GVL being separable from GVHD, nor does it appear that it will allow for dose escalation and an enhanced GVL effect. Although there are numerous permutations of prophylactic dose, timing, and concomitant GVHD prophylaxis treatments, it is unlikely that one approach will be applicable to all recipients of T-cell depleted transplants in an attempt to couple the low GVHD risk of these transplants with the reintroduction of the GVL activity that is requisite for cure.

Dose Escalation of DLI

Initial DLI strategies involved the delivery of one (large) dose of T-cells generally on the order of $> 1 \times 10^8$ CD3+ T cells/kg. Several groups have attempted to decrease the high GVHD rate while maintaining the GVL effect by giving the DLI in smaller aliquots, spread out over time based on clinical response and/or the development of GVHD (Mackinnon *et al.*, 1995; Dazzi *et al.*, 2000a).

Mackinnon *et al.* (1995) reported on 22 patients with CML who relapsed following a T-cell depleted allograft. Dose-escalated DLIs were administered a median of every 6 weeks beginning as low as 1×10^5 CD3+ T cells/kg in the first 11 patients and then 1×10^7 CD3+ T cells/kg in the remainder. Nineteen of 22 patients achieved a CR, 8 following a single infusion of 1×10^7 CD3+ T cells/kg, with only one of the 8 developing GVHD (chronic) at this cell dose. No GVL effect or GVHD was seen below this dose. As the cell dose was escalated, the proportion of patients developing GVHD rose (Table 19.4). A separate but equally important observation was that a GVL effect was coincident with the development of complete donor T-cell chimerism in 16 of 17 responders, while nonresponders remained mixed chimeras. Again, there was the impression (although insufficient numbers for statistical verification) that disease status correlated with response with 2 of 4 accelerated phase patients, 9 of 10 chronic-phase patients, and 8 of 8 patients with cytogenetic or molecular relapse patients responding.

Dazzi *et al.* (2000a) analyzed two consecutive cohorts of patients, the first receiving a bulk dose regimen (BDR) and the other an escalated dose regimen (EDR) following relapse from T-cell depleted ($n = 30$) or T-cell replete ($n = 18$) allogeneic transplants. The BDR group ($n = 28$) received a median of 1×10^8 CD3+ T cells/kg, i.e., more than a log above the 1×10^7 CD3+ T cells/kg that Mackinnon *et al.* (1995) demonstrated was sufficient for a GVL effect. The EDR group ($n = 20$) received a median of 1.9×10^8 CD3+ T cells/kg in aliquots starting at 1×10^7 CD3+ T cells/kg for HLA-matched sibling

donors and 1×10^6 CD3+ T cells/kg for unrelated donors. The median interval between DLIs was 20 weeks. The probability of cytogenetic remission at 2 years was 67% in the BDR and 91% in the EDR group (not significantly statistically different). The grade II–IV acute GVHD rates, however, were significantly higher in the BDR group (45% versus 10%) ($P = .011$). A subgroup analysis looked at only those patients in the EDR group who received the same total dose of CD3+ T cells ($n = 12$) as the BDR group to determine if the difference was due to different numbers of CD3+ T+ cells or the timing of administration. The complete remission rate was the same (68% for BDR and 67% for EDR groups), but again the BDR group had more GVHD, highlighting that GVL can be separated from GVHD in many patients with this type of strategy (Table 19.4). The mechanisms for the improved results following dose-escalated DLI delivered over a protracted period of time in the reports by Dazzi *et al.* (2000a) and Mackinnon *et al.* (1995) are unknown.

Manipulation of DLI by CD8+ T-cell depletion

There are a number of approaches to manipulating the DLI itself beyond controlling the total T-cell number. Of these, CD8+ T-cell depletion has received the most extensive clinical testing to date. A previous clinical trial suggested that CD8+ depletion of bone marrow could reduce the incidence of GVHD without decreasing the GVL effect (Champlin *et al.*,1990; Nimer *et al.*,1994). Two groups have have extended this approach to DLI, and have demonstrated what appears to be some reduction in GVHD with retention of GVL (Giralt *et al.*, 1995; Alyea *et al.*, 1998). Alyea *et al.* (1998) observed 18% grade III–IV acute GVHD in 40 patients while retaining GVL activity (79% CR in early-phase CML relapse and 83% in 5 of 6 patients with relapsed multiple myeloma). The GVHD incidence was related to the dose of CD4+ T-cells. Of more interest, while all patients developing GVHD responded, approximately half of the patients responding to the CD8-depleted DLI did not develop GVHD. Whether these initial results will be superior to unselected DLI is unknown.

Non-myeloablative stem cell transplants (NST)

Reduced intensity conditioning or non-myeloablative allogeneic stem cell transplants (NST) have been developed as an extension of the GVL effect for carrying out allogeneic transplants in older or less robust transplant candidates. Building on animal models (Storb *et al.*, 1997) and the highly immunosuppressive nature of purine analogues, several groups have performed allogeneic transplants following less intensive conditioning regimens (Giralt *et al.*, 1997; Khouri *et al.*, 1998; Slavin *et al.*, 1998; Childs *et al.*, 1999; McSweeney *et al.*, 2001). While some have been nearly myeloablative (Slavin *et al.*, 1998), others are of very low intensity, resulting in little to no myelosuppression (Khouri *et al.*, 1998; McSweeney *et al.*, 2001). The very low intensity regimens are combined with potent postgrafting immunosuppression to facilitate engraft-

Table 19.4. *Incidence of GVHD and leukemia response rate in CML patients treated with bulk-dose versus escalating-dose DLI*[a]

	Bulk-dose (n = 25)	Escalating-dose (n = 12)
Incidence of acute GVHD		
Grade 0–I	52% (13)	92% (11)
Grade II	20% (5)	8% (1)
Grade III–IV	28% (7)	0% (0)
Incidence of chronic GVHD		
None or limited	56% (14)	92% (11)
Extensive	44% (11)	8% (1)
Leukemia response rate (CR)	68% (17)	67% (8)

[a] Lymphocyte doses = 0.4 to 3.3×10^8/kg.
Data taken from Dazzi et al. (2000a).

ment and prevent GVHD. The majority of NST regimens, as reported to the IBMTR, have used mobilized PBSC grafts.

Several observations can be made regarding GVHD and GVL following NST. One of the initial hopes was that NST approaches would result in less GVHD by resulting in less tissue injury and less of the cytokine storm that has been proposed as central to the pathogenesis of GVHD (Ferrara, 1994). Unfortunately, this has not been the case to date. Acute GVHD and chronic GVHD rates approximate those seen with traditional myeloablative transplants, despite the lack of mucositis and other regimen-related toxicities. In addition, although initially targeting mixed chimerism as a platform for subsequent DLI, most NST approaches have resulted in complete or near complete T-cell chimerism by 2 to 3 months posttransplant. Conversion to complete T-cell chimerism appears to be a requirement prior to development of either GVHD or GVL (Childs et al., 1999; McSweeney et al., 2001). When donor T cells are below approximately 40%, DLI therapy in the NST setting has generally been unsuccessful in reversing graft rejection as measured by declining donor T cell chimerism in peripheral blood (P.A. McSweeney, personal communication).

Existence of GVL activity is supported by the observation of clinical responses following NST in which the conditioning regimen would not have been expected to result in disease control. Continued response despite treatment of GVHD further suggests that these responses are robust and may be separable from GVHD. As the GVL effect can be very gradual, taking up to 1 year for some patients to achieve a CR, the best responses have been observed in indolent diseases that are known to be immunologically sensitive (CML, CLL, low-grade lymphoma). Results in more aggressive diseases (acute leukemia, myelodysplasia) have been less encouraging. Similarly, although responses have been reported in patients with bulky disease, it is expected that long-term disease control is more likely in patients with minimal disease at the time of transplant. In addition, NST has been carried out for diseases not previously considered as target candidates for allogeneic transplants such as renal cell carcinoma (Childs et al., 2000) and melanoma (R. Childs, personal communication). Results are mixed, promising in renal cell carcinoma and disappointing for melanoma. More recently, promising results have been reported for multiple myeloma with a strategy that combines a traditionally dose-intensive autologous transplant to decrease tumor bulk with a subsequent NST to exploit the graft-versus-myeloma effect in a state of minimal residual disease (Maloney et al., 2001). Multicenter clinical trials will be required to refine NST approaches and clarify the role of NST versus traditional ablative allogeneic HSC transplants or non-transplant therapies.

Summary

Considerable data exist supporting the notion of an antileukemia effect of allogeneic HSC transplants not fully explained by pretransplant cytotoxic therapy and attributable to transplantation of immune competent donor cells. This GVL activity may be mediated through a variety of mechanisms and is not always associated with clinically significant GVHD. These observations have led to the development of DLI as a curative therapy for some patient populations and to the advent of NSTs, which have the potential to greatly expand patient eligiblility for allogeneic transplantation. Further advances in characterization and control of the GVL effect are needed, both to improve the results of clinical HSC transplantation and to determine how to use this effect to treat leukemia and other malignancies outside the transplant setting.

References

Akpek, G., Ambinder, R. F., Piantadosi, S. et al. (2001). Long-term results of blood and marrow transplantation for Hodgkin's lymphoma. Journal of Clinical Oncology, 19, 4314–21.

Alyea, E. P., Soiffer, R. J., Canning, C. et al. (1998). Toxicity and efficacy of defined doses of CD4+ donor lymphocytes for treatment of relapse after allogeneic bone marrow transplant. Blood, 91, 3671–80.

Antin, J. H. & Ferrara, J.L.M. (1992). Cytokine dysregulation and acute graft-versus-host disease. Blood, 80, 2964–70.

Apperley, J. F., Jones, L., Hale, G. et al. (1986). Bone marrow transplantation for patients with chronic myeloid leukemia: T-cell depletion with Campath-1 reduces the incidence of graft-versus-host disease but may increase the risk of leukemic relapse. Bone Marrow Transplantation, 1, 53–66.

Ash, R. C., Horowitz, M. M., Gale, R. P. et al. (1991). Bone marrow transplantation from related donors other than HLA-identical siblings: effect of T-cell depletion. Bone Marrow Transplantation, 7, 443–52.

Bacigalupo, A., Van Lint, M. T., Frassini, F., & Marmont, A. (1985). Graft-versus-leukemia effect following allogeneic bone marrow transplantation. British Journal of Haematology, 61, 749–51.

Barnes, D.W.H., Corp, M. J., Loutit, J. F. et al. (1956). Treatment of murine leukemia with x-rays and homologous bone marrow. British Medical Journal, 2, 626–7.

Barrett, A. J., Horowitz, M. M., Gale, R. P. et al. (1989). Marrow transplantation for acute lymphoblastic leukemia: factors affecting relapse and survival. Blood, 74, 862–71.

Barrett, A. J., Mavroudis, D., Tisdale, J. et al. (1998). T cell-depleted bone marrow transplantation and delayed T cell add-back to control acute GVHD and conserve a graft-versus-leukemia effect. Bone Marrow Transplantation, 21, 543–51.

Barrett, A. J., Ringden, O., Zhang, M. J. et al. (2000). Effect of nucleated marrow cell dose on relapse and survival in identical twin bone marrow transplants for leukemia. Blood, 95, 3323–7.

Bay, J. O., Choufi, B., Pomel, C. et al. (2000). Potential allogeneic graft-versus-tumor effect in a patient with ovarian cancer. Bone Marrow Transplantation, 25, 681–2.

Behar, E., Chao, N. H., Hiraki, D. D. et al. (1996). Polymorphism of adhesion molecule CD31 and its role in acute graft-versus-host disease. New England Journal of Medicine, 334, 286–91.

Bensinger, W. I., Martin, P. J., Storer, B. et al. (2001). Transplantation of bone marrow as compared with peripheral-blood cells from

HLA-identical relatives in patients with hematologic cancers. *New England Journal of Medicine*, **344**, 175–81.

Ben-Yosef, R., Or, R., Nagler, A., & Slavin, S. (1996). Graft-versus-tumor and graft-versus-leukaemia effect in patient with concurrent breast cancer and acute myelocytic leukaemia. *Lancet*, **348**, 1242–3.

Bierman, P. J. (2000). Allogeneic bone marrow transplantation for lymphoma. *Blood Reviews*, **14**, 1–13.

Bonnet, D., Warren, E. H., Greenberg, P. D., Dick, J. E., & Riddell, S. R. (1999). CD8+ minor histocompatibility antigen-specific cytotoxic T lymphocyte clones eliminate human acute myeloid leukemia stem cells. *Proceedings of the National Academy of Sciences USA*, **96**, 8639–44.

Bortin, M. M. (1974). Graft-versus-leukemia. In *Clinical Immunobiology*, eds. F. H. Bach & R. A. Good, pp. 287–306. New York: Academic Press.

Bortin, M. M., Rimm, A. A., Saltzstein, E. C. *et al.* (1973a). Graft-versus-leukemia III. Apparent independent antihost and antileukemia activity of transplanted immunocompetent cells. *Transplantation*, **16**, 182–8.

Bortin, M. M., Rimm, A. A., & Saltzstein, E. C. (1973b). Graft-versus-leukemia: quantification of adoptive immunotherapy in murine leukemia. *Science*, **179**, 811–3.

Bortin, M. M., Ringdén, O., Horowitz, M. M. *et al.* (1989). Temporal relationship between the major complications of bone marrow transplantation for leukemia. *Bone Marrow Transplantation*, **4**, 339–44.

Bortin, M. M., Truitt, R. L., Rimm, A. A. *et al.* (1979). Graft-versus-leukemia reactivity induced by alloimmunization without augmentation of graft-versus-host reactivity. *Nature*, **281**, 490–1.

Brenner, M. K., Rill, D. R., Holladay, M. S. *et al.* (1993). Gene marking to determine whether autologous marrow infusion restores long-term hemapoiesis in cancer patients. *Lancet*, **342**, 1134–7.

Brenner, M. K., Rill, D. R., Moen, R. C. *et al.* (1994). Gene marking and autologous bone marrow transplantation. *Annals of the New York Academy of Sciences*, **716**, 204–15, 225–7.

Brochstein, J. A., Kernan, N. A., Groshen, S. *et al.* (1987). Allogeneic bone marrow transplantation after hyperfractionated total-body irradiation and cyclophosphamide in children with acute leukemia. *New England Journal of Medicine*, **317**, 1618–24.

Butturini, A. & Gale, R. P. (1987). The role of T-cells in preventing relapse in chronic myelogenous leukemia. *Bone Marrow Transplantation*, **2**, 351–4.

Castro-Malaspina, H., Harris, R. E., Gajewski, J. *et al.* (2002). Unrelated donor marrow transplantation for myelodysplastic syndromes: outcome analysis in 510 transplants facilitated by the National Marrow Donor Program. *Blood*, **99**, 1943–51.

Champlin, R., Ho, W., Gajewski, J. *et al.* (1990). Selective depletion of CD8+ T lymphocytes for prevention of graft-versus-host disease after allogeneic bone marrow transplantation. *Blood*, **76**, 418–23.

Champlin, R., Khouri, I., Shimoni, A. *et al.* (2000a). Harnessing graft-versus-malignancy: non-myeloablative preparative regimens for allogeneic haematopoietic transplantation, an evolving strategy for adoptive immunotherapy. *British Journal of Haematology*, **111**, 18–29.

Champlin, R. E., Passweg, J. R., Zhang, M. J. *et al.* (2000b). T-cell depletion of bone marrow transplants for leukemia from donors other than HLA-identical siblings: advantage of T-cell antibodies with narrow specificities. *Blood*, **95**, 3996–4003.

Champlin, R. E., Schmitz, N., Horowitz, M. M. *et al.* (2000c). Blood stem cells compared with bone marrow as a source of hematopoietic cells for allogeneic transplantation. IBMTR Histocompatibility and Stem Cell Sources Working Committee and the European Group for Blood and Marrow Transplantation (EBMT). *Blood*, **95**, 3702–9.

Cheever, M. A., Greenberg, P. D., & Fefer, A. (1981). Specific adoptive therapy of established leukemia with syngeneic lymphocytes sequentially immunized in vivo and in vitro and nonspecifically expanded by culture with interleukin 2. *Journal of Immunology*, **126**, 1318–22.

Chen, B. J., Cui, X., Liu, C., & Chao, N. J. (2002). Prevention of graft-versus-host disease while preserving graft-versus-leukemia effect after selective depletion of host-reactive T cells by photodynamic cell purging process. *Blood*, **99**, 3083–8.

Childs, R., Chernoff, A., Contentin, N. *et al.* (2000). Regression of metastatic renal-cell carcinoma after nonmyeloablative allogeneic peripheral-blood stem-cell transplantation. *New England Journal of Medicine*, **343**, 750–8.

Childs, R., Clave, E., Contentin, N. *et al.* (1999). Engraftment kinetics after nonmyeloablative allogeneic peripheral blood stem cell transplantation: full donor T-cell chimerism precedes alloimmune responses. *Blood*, **94**, 3234–41.

Claret, E. J., Alyea, E. P., Orsini, E. *et al.* (1997). Characterization of T cell repertoire in patients with graft-versus-leukemia after donor lymphocyte infusion. *Journal of Clinical Investigation*, **100**, 855–66.

Cobbold, S., Martin, G., & Waldmann, H. (1986). Monoclonal antibodies for the prevention of graft-versus-host disease and marrow graft rejection: the depletion of T-cell subsets in vitro and in vivo. *Transplantation*, **42**, 239–47.

Collins, R. H. Jr., Shpilberg, O., Drobyski, W. R. *et al.* (1997). Donor leukocyte infusions in 140 patients with relapsed malignancy after allogeneic bone marrow transplantation. *Journal of Clinical Oncology*, **15**, 433–44.

Comoli, P., Locatelli, F., Moretta, A. *et al.* (2001). Human alloantigen-specific anergic cells induced by a combination of CTLA4-Ig and CsA maintain anti-leukemia and anti-viral cytotoxic responses. *Bone Marrow Transplantation*, **27**, 1263–73.

Couban, S., Simpson, D. R., Barnett, M. J. *et al.* (2002). A randomized multicentre comparison of bone marrow and peripheral blood in recipients of matched sibling allogeneic transplants for myeloid malignancies. *Blood*, **100**, 1525–31.

Cullis, J. O., Jiang, Y. Z., Schwarzer, A. P. *et al.* (1992). Donor leukocyte infusions for chronic myeloid leukemia in relapse after allogeneic bone marrow transplantation. *Blood*, **79**, 1379–81.

Davies, S. M., Wagner, J. E., Weisdorf, D. J. *et al.* (1996). Unrelated donor bone marrow transplantation for hematological malignancies—current status. *Leukemia & Lymphoma*, **23**, 221–6.

Dazzi, F., Szydlo, R. M., Craddock, C. *et al.* (2000a). Comparison of single-dose and escalating-dose regimens of donor lymphocyte infusion for relapse after allografting for chronic myeloid leukemia. *Blood*, **95**, 67–71.

Dazzi, F., Szydlo, R. M., Cross, N. C. *et al.* (2000b). Durability of responses following donor lymphocyte infusions for patients who relapse after allogeneic stem cell transplantation for chronic myeloid leukemia. *Blood,* **96,** 2712–6.

de Haan, J.M.M., Sherman, N. E., Blokland, E. *et al.* (1995). Identification of a graft-versus-host disease-associated minor histocompatibility antigen. *Science,* **268,** 1476–9.

de Lima, M., Bonamino, M., Vasconcelos, Z. *et al.* (2001). Prophylactic donor lymphocyte infusions after moderately ablative chemotherapy and stem cell transplantation for hematological malignancies: high remission rate among poor prognosis patients at the expense of graft-versus-host disease. *Bone Marrow Transplantation,* **27,** 73–8.

de Witte, T., Hoogenhout, J., de Pauw, B. *et al.* (1986). Depletion of donor lymphocytes by counterflow centrifugation successfully prevents acute graft-versus-host disease in matched allogeneic marrow transplantation. *Blood,* **67,** 1302–8.

Delman, L., Ythier, P., Moingeon, P. *et al.* (1986). Characterization of antileukemia cells' cytotoxic effector function: implications for monitoring natural killer responses following allogeneic bone marrow transplantation. *Transplantation,* **42,** 252–6.

Dermime, S., Mavroudis, D., Jiang, Y. Z., Hensel, N., Molldrem, J., & Barrett, A. J. (1997). Immune escape from a graft-versus-leukemia effect may play a role in the relapse of myeloid leukemias following allogeneic bone marrow transplantation. *Bone Marrow Transplantation,* **19,** 989–99.

Drobyski, W. R., Ash, R. C., Casper, J. T. *et al.* (1994). Effect of T-cell depletion as graft-versus-host disease prophylaxis on engraftment, relapse, and disease-free survival in unrelated marrow transplantation for chronic myelogenous leukemia. *Blood,* **83,** 1980–7.

Drobyski, W. R., Keever, C. A., Roth, M. S. *et al.* (1993). Salvage immunotherapy using donor leukocyte infusions as treatment for relapsed chronic myelogenous leukemia after allogeneic bone marrow transplantation: efficacy and toxicity of a defined T-cell dose. *Blood,* **82,** 2310–8.

Eibl, B., Schwaighofer, H., Nachbaur, D. *et al.* (1996). Evidence for a graft-versus-tumor effect in a patient treated with marrow ablative chemotherapy and allogeneic bone marrow transplantation for breast cancer. *Blood,* **88,** 1501–8.

Epperson, D. E., Margolis, D. A., McOlash, L., Janczac, T., & Barrett, A. J. (2001). In vitro T cell receptor Vβ repertoire analysis may identify which T cell Vβ families mediate graft-versus-leukaemia and graft-versus-host responses after human leucocyte antigen-matched sibling stem cell transplantation. *British Journal of Haematology,* **114,** 57–62.

Faber, L. M., van der Hoeven, J., Goulmy, E. *et al.* (1995). Recognition of clonogenic leukemic cells, remission bone marrow and HLA-identical donor bone marrow by CD8+ or CD4+ minor histocompatibility antigen-specific cytotoxic T lymphocytes. *Journal of Clinical Investigation,* **96,** 877–83.

Fefer, A., Sullivan, K. M., Weiden, P. *et al.* (1987). Graft-versus-leukemia effect in man: the relapse rate of acute leukemia is lower after allogeneic than after syngeneic marrow transplantation. In *Cellular Immunotherapy of Cancer,* eds. R. L. Truitt, R. P. Gale, & M. M. Bortin, pp. 401–8. New York: Alan R. Liss, Inc.

Ferra, C., Rodriguez-Luaces, M., Gallardo, D. *et al.* (2001). Individually adjusted prophylactic donor lymphocyte infusions after CD34-selected allogeneic peripheral blood stem cell transplantation. *Bone Marrow Transplantation,* **28,** 963–8.

Ferrara, J. L. (1994). Cytokines other than growth factors in bone marrow transplantation. *Current Opinion in Oncology,* **6,** 127–34.

Fowler, D. H., Breglio, J., Nagel, G. *et al.* (1996). Allospecific CD8+ Tc1 and Tc2 populations in graft-versus-leukemia effect and graft-versus-host disease. *Journal of Immunology,* **157,** 4811–21.

Fowler, D. H. & Gress, R. E.. (2000). Th2 and Tc2 cells in the regulation of GVHD, GVL, and graft rejection: considerations for the allogeneic transplantation therapy of leukemia and lymphoma. *Leukemia & Lymphoma,* **38,** 221–34.

Gale, R. P. & Champlin, R. E. (1984). How do bone marrow transplants cure leukemia? *Lancet,* **2,** 28–30.

Gale, R. P., Horowitz, M. M., Ash, R. C. *et al.* (1994). Identical twin bone marrow transplants for leukemia. *Annals of Internal Medicine,* **120,** 646–52.

Gale, R. P., Horowitz, M. M., Biggs, J. C. *et al.* (1989). Transplant or chemotherapy in acute myelogenous leukemia. *Lancet,* **1,** 1119–22.

Gao, L., Yang, T. H., Tourdot, S. *et al.* (1999). Allo-major histocompatibility complex-restricted cytotoxic T lymphocytes engraft in bone marrow transplant recipients without causing graft-versus-host disease. *Blood,* **94,** 2999–3006.

Gerrard, T. L., Siegel, J. P., Dyer, D. R., & Zoon, K. C. (1987). Differential effects of interferon-alpha and interferon-gamma on interleukin-1 secretion by monocytes. *Journal of Immunology,* **138,** 2535–40.

Ghayur, T., Seemayer, T. A., & Lapp, W. S. (1988). Prevention of murine graft-versus-host disease by inducing and eliminating ASGM1+ cells of donor origin. *Transplantation,* **45,** 586–9.

Giralt, S., Estey, E., Albitar, M. *et al.* (1997). Engraftment of allogeneic hematopoietic progenitor cells with purine analog-containing chemotherapy: harnessing graft-versus-leukemia without myeloablative therapy. *Blood,* **89,** 4531–6

Giralt, S., Hester, J., Huh, Y. *et al.* (1995). CD8-depleted donor lymphocyte infusion as treatment for relapsed chronic myelogenous leukemia after allogeneic bone marrow transplantation. *Blood,* **86,** 4337–43.

Glass, B., Uharek, L., Zeis, M. *et al.* (1996). Graft-versus-leukaemia activity can be predicted by natural cytotoxicity against leukaemia cells. *British Journal of Haematology,* **93,** 412–20.

Goldman, J. M., Szydlo, R., Horowitz, M. M. *et al.* (1993). Choice of pretransplant treatment and timing of transplants for chronic myelogenous leukemia in chronic phase. *Blood,* **82,** 2235–8.

Goulmy, E., Schipper, R., Pool, J. *et al.* (1996). Mismatches of minor histocompatibility antigens between HLA-identical donors and recipients and the development of graft-versus-host disease after bone marrow transplantation. *New England Journal of Medicine,* **334,** 281–5.

Guinan, E. C., Boussiotis, V. A., Neuberg, D. *et al.* (1999). Transplantation of anergic histoincompatible bone marrow allografts. *New England Journal of Medicine,* **340,** 1704–14.

Guinan, E. C., Gribben, J. G., Boussioti, V. A. *et al.* (1994). Pivotal role of the B7:CD28 pathway in transplantation tolerance and tumor immunity. *Blood,* **84,** 3261–82.

Hercend, T., Takvorian, T., Nowill, A. *et al.* (1986). Characterization of NK cells with antileukemia activity following allogeneic bone marrow transplantation. *Blood,* **67,** 722–8.

Herve, P., Cahn, J. Y., Flesch, M. *et al.* (1987). Successful graft-versus-host disease prevention without graft failure in 32 HLA-identical allogeneic bone marrow transplantations with marrow depleted of T-cells by monoclonal antibodies and complement. *Blood,* **69,** 388–93.

Heslop, H. E., Gottlieb, D. J., Reittie, J. E. *et al.* (1989). Spontaneous and interleukin-2 induced secretion of tumor necrosis factor and gamma interferon following autologous marrow transplantation or chemotherapy. *British Journal of Haematology,* **72,** 122–6.

Hill, G. R. & Ferrara, J. L. (2000). The primacy of the gastrointestinal tract as a target organ of acute graft-versus-host disease: rationale for the use of cytokine shields in allogeneic bone marrow transplantation. *Blood,* **95,** 2754–9.

Holler, E., Ertl, B., Hintermeier-Knabe, R. *et al.* (1997). Inflammatory reactions induced by pretransplant conditioning—an alternative target for modulation of acute GvHD and complications following allogeneic bone marrow transplantation? *Leukemia & Lymphoma,* **25,** 217–24.

Horowitz, M. M., Gale, R. P., Sondel, P. M. *et al.* (1990). Graft-versus-leukemia reactions after bone marrow transplantation. *Blood,* **75,** 555–62.

Howrey, R. P., Martin, P. L., Driscoll, T. *et al.* (2000). Graft-versus-leukemia-induced complete remission following unrelated umbilical cord blood transplantation for acute leukemia. *Bone Marrow Transplantation,* **26,** 1251–4.

Hsieh, M. H. & Korngold, R. (2000). Differential use of FasL- and perforin-mediated cytolytic mechanisms by T-cell subsets involved in graft-versus-myeloid leukemia responses. *Blood,* **96,** 1047–55.

Jadus, M. R. & Wepsic, H. T. (1992). The role of cytokines in graft-versus-host reactions and disease. *Bone Marrow Transplantation,* **10,** 1–14.

Jiang, Y. Z., Knafr, E. J., MacDonald, D. *et al.* (1991). Graft-versus-leukaemia following allogeneic bone marrow transplantation: emergence of cytotoxic T-lymphocytes reacting to host leukaemia cells. *Bone Marrow Transplantation,* **8,** 253–8.

Jiang, Y. Z., Mavroudis, D., Dermime, S. *et al.* (1996). Alloreactive CD4+ T lymphocytes can exert cytotoxicity to chronic myeloid leukaemia cells processing and presenting exogenous antigen. *British Journal of Haematology,* **93,** 606–12.

Johnson, B. D., Becker, E. E., LaBelle, J. L., & Truitt, R. L. (1999). Role of immunoregulatory donor T cells in suppression of graft-versus-host disease following donor leukocyte infusion therapy. *Journal of Immunology,* **163,** 6479–87.

Johnson, B. D., Becker, E. E., & Truitt, R. L. (1999). Graft-versus-host and graft-versus-leukemia reactions after delayed infusions of donor T-subsets. *Biology of Blood and Marrow Transplantation,* **5,** 123–32.

Johnson, B. D., McCabe, C., Hanke, C. A., & Truitt, R. L. (1995). Use of anti-CD3ε F(ab′)2 fragments in vivo to modulate graft-versus-host disease without loss of graft-versus-leukemia reactivity after MHC-matched bone marrow transplantation. *Journal of Immunology,* **154,** 5542–54.

Johnson, B. D. & Truitt, R. L., (1992). A decrease in graft-versus-host disease without loss of graft-versus-leukemia reactivity after MHC-matched bone marrow transplantation by selective depletion of donor NK cells in vivo. *Transplantation,* **54,** 104–12.

Johnson, B. D. & Truitt, R. L. (1995). Delayed infusion of immunocompetent donor cells after bone marrow transplantation breaks graft-host tolerance and allows for persistent antileukemic reactivity without severe graft-versus-host disease. *Blood,* **85,** 3302–12.

Keever, C. A., Abu-Hajir, M., Graf, W. *et al.* (1995). Characterization of the alloreactivity and anti-leukemia reactivity of cord blood mononuclear cells. *Bone Marrow Transplantation,* **15,** 407–19.

Kernan, N. A., Collins, N. H., Juliana, L. *et al.* (1986). Clonable T lymphocytes in T-cell depleted bone marrow transplants correlate with development of graft-versus-host disease. *Blood,* **68,** 770–3.

Kersey, J. H., Weisdorf, D., Nesbit, M. E. *et al.* (1987). Comparison of autologous and allogeneic bone marrow transplantation for treatment of high-risk refractory acute lymphoblastic leukemia. *New England Journal of Medicine,* **317,** 461–7.

Khouri, I. F., Keating, M., Korbling, M. *et al.* (1998). Transplant-lite: induction of graft-versus-malignancy using fludarabine-based nonablative and allogeneic blood progenitor-cell transplantation as treatment for lymphoid malignancies. *Journal of Clinical Oncology,* **16,** 2817–24.

Khouri, I. F., Lee, M. S., Romaguera, J. *et al.* (1999). Allogeneic hematopoietic transplantation for mantle-cell lymphoma: molecular remissions and evidence of graft-versus-malignancy. *Annals of Oncology,* **10,** 1293–9.

Kolb, H. J. (1998). Donor leukocyte transfusions for treatment of leukemic relapse after bone marrow transplantation. EBMT Immunology and Chronic Leukemia Working Parties. *Vox Sanguinis,* **74** (Suppl2), 321–9.

Kolb, H. J., Mittermüller, J., Clemin, C. H. *et al.* (1990). Donor leukocyte transfusions for treatment of recurrent chronic myelogenous leukemia in marrow transplant patients. *Blood,* **76,** 462–5.

Kolb, H.-J., Schattenberg, A., Goldman, J. M. *et al.* (1995). Graft-versus-leukemia effect of donor lymphocyte transfusions in marrow grafted patients. *Blood,* **86,** 2041–50.

Korbling, M. & Anderlini, P. (2001). Peripheral blood stem cell versus bone marrow allotransplantation: does the source of hematopoietic stem cells matter? *Blood,* **98,** 2900–8.

Korngold, R., Leighton, C., & Manser, T. (1994). Graft-versus-myeloid responses following syngeneic and allogeneic bone marrow transplantation. *Transplantation,* **15,** 278–87.

Korngold, R. & Sprent, J. (1987a). T-cell subsets and graft-versus-host disease. *Transplantation,* **44,** 335–9.

Korngold, R. & Sprent, J. (1987b). Variable capacity of L3T4+ T-cells to cause lethal graft-versus-host disease across minor histocompatibility barriers in mice. *Journal of Experimental Medicine,* **165,** 1552–64.

Kovacsovics-Bankowski, M., Clark, K., Benacerraf, B., & Rock, K. L. (1993). Efficient major histocompatibility complex class I presentation of exogenous antigen upon phagocytosis by macrophages. *Proceedings of the National Academy of Sciences USA,* **90,** 4942–6.

Krenger, W., Snyder, K. M., Byon, J.C.H. *et al.* (1995). Polarized type 2 alloreactive CD4+ and CD8+ donor T cells fail to induce experimental graft-versus-host disease. *Journal of Immunology,* **155,** 585–93.

LaBelle, J. L., Hanke, C. A., Blazar, B. R., & Truitt, R. L. (2002). Negative effect of CTLA-4 on induction of T-cell immunity in vivo to B7-1+, but not B7-2+, murine myelogenous leukemia. *Blood*, **99**, 2146–53.

Lee, C. K., Gingrich, R. D., deMagalhaes-Silverman, M. *et al.* (1999). Prophylactic reinfusion of T cells for T cell-depleted allogeneic bone marrow transplantation. *Biology of Blood and Marrow Transplantation*, **5**, 15–27.

LeFever, A. V., Truitt, R. L., & Shih, C. C. (1985). Reactivity of in-vitro-expanded alloimmune cytotoxic T lymphocytes and Qa-1-specific cytotoxic T lymphocytes against AKR leukemia in vivo. *Transplantation*, **40**, 531–7.

Levine, J. E., Braun, T., Penza, S. L. *et al.* (2002). Prospective trial of chemotherapy and donor leukocyte infusions for relapse of advanced myeloid malignancies after allogeneic stem-cell transplantation. *Journal of Clinical Oncology*, **20**, 405–12.

Lokhorst, H. M., Schattenberg, A., Cornelissen, J. J. *et al.* (2000). Donor lymphocyte infusions for relapsed multiple myeloma after allogeneic stem-cell transplantation: predictive factors for response and long-term outcome. *Journal of Clinical Oncology*, **18**, 3031–7.

Mackinnon, S., Papadopoulos, E. B., Carabasi, M. H. *et al.* (1995). Adoptive immunotherapy evaluating escalating doses of donor leukocytes for relapse of chronic myeloid leukemia after bone marrow transplantation: separation of graft-versus-leukemia responses from graft-versus-host disease. *Blood*, **86**, 1261–8.

Maloney, D. G., Sahebi, F., Stockeri-Goldstein, K. E. *et al.* (2001). Combining an allogeneic graft-versus-myeloma effect with high-dose autologous stem cell rescue in the treatment of multiple myeloma. *Blood*, **98**, 1822a (Abstract).

Maraninchi, D., Gluckman, E., Blaise, D. *et al.* (1987). Impact of T-cell depletion on outcome of allogeneic bone-marrow transplantation for standard-risk leukemias. *Lancet*, **2**, 175–8.

Margolin, K. A., Negrin, R. S., Wong, K. K. *et al.* (1997). Cellular immunotherapy and autologous transplantation for hematologic malignancy. *Immunological Reviews*, **157**, 231–40.

Margolis, D. A., Casper, J. T., Segura, A. D. *et al.* (2000). Infiltrating T cells during liver graft-versus-host disease show a restricted T-cell repertoire. *Biology of Blood and Marrow Transplantation*, **6**, 408–15.

Marmont, A. M., Horowitz, M. M., Gale, R. P. *et al.* (1991). T-cell depletion of HLA-identical transplants in leukemia. *Blood*, **78**, 2120–30.

Martin, P. J., Hansen, J. A., Buckner, C. D. *et al.* (1985). Effect of in vitro depletion of T-cells in HLA-identical allogeneic marrow grafts. *Blood*, **66**, 664–72.

Mathé, G., Amiel, J. L., Schwarzenberg, L. *et al.* (1965). Adoptive immunotherapy of acute leukemia: experimental and clinical results. *Cancer Research*, **25**, 1525–31.

McCarthy, P. L., Abhyankar, S., Neben, S. *et al.* (1991). Inhibition of interleukin-1 by an interleukin-1 receptor antagonist prevents graft-versus-host disease. *Blood*, **78**, 1915–18.

McIntyre, R. & Gale, R. P. (1981). Relationship between graft-versus-leukemia and graft-versus-host in man—UCLA experience. In *Graft-versus-Leukemia in Man and Animal Models*, eds. J. P. O'Kunewick & R. F. Meredith, pp. 1–9. Boca Raton, FL: CRC Press.

McSweeney, P. A., Niederwieser, D., Shizuru, J. A. *et al.* (2001). Hematopoietic cell transplantation in older patients with hemato-logic malignancies: replacing high-dose cytotoxic therapy with graft-versus-tumor effects. *Blood*, **97**, 3390–400.

Mehta, J., Powles, R., Singhal, S. *et al.* (1996). Clinical and hematologic response of chronic lymphocytic and prolymphocytic leukemia persisting after allogeneic bone marrow transplantation with the onset of acute graft-versus-host disease: possible role of graft-versus-leukemia. *Bone Marrow Transplantation*, **17**, 371–5.

Mehta, J. & Singhal, S. (1998). Graft-versus-myeloma. *Bone Marrow Transplantation*, **22**, 835–43.

Moscardo, F., Martinez, J. A., Sanz, G. F., *et al.* (2000). Graft-versus-tumour effect in non-small-cell lung cancer after allogeneic peripheral blood stem cell transplantation. *British Journal of Haematology*, **111**, 708–10.

Mutis, T., Schrama, E., van Luxemburg-Heijs, S.A.P. *et al.* (1997). HLA class II restricted T-cell reactivity to a developmentally regulated antigen shared by leukemia cells and CD34+ early progenitor cells. *Blood*, **90**, 1083–90.

Naparstek, E., Or, R., Nagler, A. *et al.* (1995). T-cell-depleted allogeneic bone marrow transplantation for acute leukemia using Campath-1 antibodies and post-transplant administration of donor's peripheral blood lymphocytes for prevention of relapse. *British Journal of Haematology*, **89**, 506–15.

Nedwin, G. E., Suedersky, L. P., Bringman, T. S. *et al.* (1985). Effect of IL-2, IFN, and mitogens on the production of tumor necrosis factors alpha and beta. *Journal of Immunology*, **135**, 2492–9.

Nimer, S. D., Giorgi, J., & Gajewski, J. L. (1994). Selective depletion of CD8+ cells for prevention of graft-versus-host disease after bone marrow transplantation. *Transplantation*, **57**, 82–7.

O'Kunewick, J. P., Kochiban, D. L., & Buffo, M. J. (1990). Comparative effects of various T-cell subtypes on GVHD in a murine model for MHC-matched unrelated donor transplant. *Bone Marrow Transplantation*, **5**, 145–52.

O'Kunewick, J. P., Kociban, D. L., Machen, L. L., & Buffo, M. J. (1995). Evidence for a possible role of asialo-GM1-positive cells in the graft-versus-leukemia repression of a murine type-C retroviral leukemia. *Bone Marrow Transplantation*, **16**, 451–6.

O'Reilly, R. J., Kernan, N. A., Cunningham, I. *et al.* (1988). Allogeneic transplants depleted of T-cells by soybean lectin agglutination and E rosette depletion. *Bone Marrow Transplantation*, **3** (Suppl 1), 3–6.

Orsini, E., Alyea, E. P., Schlossman, R. *et al.* (2000). Changes in T cell receptor repertoire associated with graft-versus-tumor effect and graft-versus-host disease in patients with relapsed multiple myeloma after donor lymphocyte infusion. *Bone Marrow Transplantation*, **25**, 623–32.

Palathumpat, S., Dejbakhsh-Jones, S., & Strober, S. (1995). The role of purified CD8+ T cells in graft-versus-leukemia activity and engraftment after allogeneic bone marrow transplantation. *Transplantation*, **60**, 355–61.

Pardoll, D. M. (1993). New strategies for enhancing the immunogenicity of tumors. *Current Opinion in Immunology*, **5**, 719–25.

Parkman, R. (1986). Clonal analysis of murine graft-versus-host disease. I. phenotype and functional analysis of T lymphocyte clones. *Journal of Immunology*, **136**, 3543–8.

Patterson, A. E. & Korngold, R. (2001). Infusion of select leukemia-reactive TCR Vβ+ T cells provides graft-versus-leukemia responses with minimization of graft-versus-host disease following murine hematopoietic stem cell transplantation. *Biology of Blood and Marrow Transplantation*, **7**, 187–96.

Pelot, M. R., Pearson, D. A., Swenson, K. *et al.* (1999). Lymphohematopoietic graft-versus-host reactions can be induced without graft-versus-host disease in murine mixed chimeras established with a cyclophosphamide-based nonmyeloablative conditioning regimen. *Biology of Blood and Marrow Transplantation*, **5**, 133–43.

Phillips, G. L., Reece, D. E., Barnett, M. J. *et al.* (1989). Allogeneic marrow transplantation for refractory Hodgkin's disease. *Journal of Clinical Oncology*, **7**, 1039–45.

Piguet, P. F., Grau, G. E., Allet, B., & Vasalli, P. (1987). Tumor necrosis factor/cachectin is an effector of skin and gut lesions of the acute phase of graft versus host disease. *Journal of Experimental Medicine*, **166**, 1280–9.

Pion, S., Fontaine, P., Desaulniers, M. *et al.* (1997). On the mechanism of immunodominance in cytotoxic T-lymphocyte responses to minor histocompatibility antigens. *European Journal of Immunology*, **27**, 421–30.

Porter, D. L., Collins, R. H. Jr, Hardy, C. *et al.* (2000). Treatment of relapsed leukemia after unrelated donor marrow transplantation with unrelated donor leukocyte infusions. *Blood*, **95**, 1214–21.

Porter, D. L., Collins, R. H. Jr., Shpilberg, O. *et al.* (1999a). Long-term follow-up of patients who achieved complete remission after donor leukocyte infusions. *Biology of Blood and Marrow Transplantation*, **5**, 253–61.

Porter, D. L., Connors, J. M., Van Deerlin, V. M. *et al.* (1999b). Graft-versus-tumor induction with donor leukocyte infusions as primary therapy for patients with malignancies. *Journal of Clinical Oncology*, **17**, 1234–43.

Powles, R., Mehta, J., Kulkarni, S. *et al.* (2000). Allogeneic blood and bone-marrow stem-cell transplantation in haematological malignant diseases: a randomised trial. *Lancet*, **355**, 1231–7.

Poynton, C. H. (1988). T-cell depletion in bone marrow transplantation. *Bone Marrow Transplantation*, **3**, 265–79.

Prentice, H. G. (1987). T-cell depletion in allogeneic bone marrow transplantation. *Transplantation Proceedings*, **19**, 155–6.

Prentice, H. G., Hermans, J., & Zwaan, F.E . (1988). Relapse risk in allogeneic BMT with T-cell depletion of donor marrow. *Bone Marrow Transplantation*, **3**(S1), 30–2.

Ratanatharathorn, V., Uberti, J., Karanes, C. *et al.* (1994). Prospective comparative trial of autologous versus allogeneic bone marrow transplantation in patients with non-Hodgkin's lymphoma. *Blood*, **84**, 1050–5.

Remberger, M., Mattsson, J., Hentschke, P. *et al.*, (2002). The graft-versus-leukemia effect in haematopoietic stem cell transplantation using unrelated donors. *Bone Marrow Transplantation*, **30**, 761–8.

Ringden, O., Labopin, M., Gluckman, E. *et al.* (1996). Graft-versus-leukemia effect in allogeneic marrow transplant recipients with acute leukemia is maintained using cyclosporin A combined with methotrexate as prophylaxis. *Bone Marrow Transplantation*, **18**, 921–9.

Ringden, O., Labopin, M., Gorin, N. C. *et al.* (2000). Is there a graft-versus-leukemia effect in the absence of graft-versus-host disease in patients undergoing bone marrow transplantation for acute leukemia? *British Journal of Haematology*, **111**, 1130–7.

Ruggeri, L., Capanni, M., Urbani, E. *et al.* (2002). Effectiveness of donor natural killer cell alloreactivity in mismatched hematopoietic transplants. *Science*, **295**, 2097–2100.

Salama, M., Nevill, T., Marcellus, D. *et al.* (2000). Donor leukocyte infusions for multiple myeloma. *Bone Marrow Transplantation*, **26**, 1179–84.

Sanders, J. E., Flournoy, N., Thomas, E. D. *et al.* (1985). Marrow transplant experience in children with acute lymphoblastic leukemia: an analysis of factors associated with survival, relapse and graft-versus-host disease. *Medical and Pediatric Oncology*, **13**, 165–72.

Schmaltz, C., Alpdogan, O., Horndasch, K. J. *et al.* (2001). Differential use of Fas ligand and perforin cytotoxic pathways by donor T cells in graft-versus-host disease and graft-versus-leukemia effect. *Blood*, **97**, 2886–95.

Schmitz, N., Beksac, M., Hasenclever, D. *et al.* (2000). A randomized study from the European Group for Blood and Marrow Transplantation comparing allogeneic transplantation of filgrastim-mobilized peripheral blood progenitor cells with bone marrow transplantation in 350 patients with leukemia. *Blood*, **96**, 481 (Abstract).

Scott, D. M., Ehrmann, I. E., & Ellis, P. S. (1995). Identification of a mouse male-specific transplantation antigen, H-Y. *Nature*, **376**, 695–8.

Shimoni, A., Gajewski, J. A., Donato, M. *et al.* (2001). Long-term follow-up of recipients of CD8-depleted donor lymphocyte infusions for the treatment of chronic myelogenous leukemia relapsing after allogeneic progenitor cell transplantation. *Biology of Blood and Marrow Transplantation*, **7**, 568–75.

Shlomchik, W. D., Couzens, M. S., Tang, C. B. *et al.* (1999). Prevention of graft versus host disease by inactivation of host antigen-presenting cells. *Science*, **285**, 412–5.

Shlomchik, W. D. & Emerson, S. G. (1996). The immunobiology of T-cell therapies for leukemia. *Acta Haematologica*, **96**, 189–213.

Slavin, S. (1990). The graft-versus-leukemia (GVL) phenomenon: is GVL separable from GVHD? *Bone Marrow Transplantation*, **6**, 155–61.

Slavin, S., Nagler, A., Naparstek, E. *et al.* (1998). Nonmyeloablative stem cell transplantation and cell therapy as an alternative to conventional bone marrow transplantation with lethal cytoreduction for the treatment of malignant and nonmalignant hematologic diseases. *Blood*, **91**, 756–63.

Sohn, S. K., Baek, J. H., Kim, D. H. *et al.* (2000). Successful allogeneic stem-cell transplantation with prophylactic stepwise G-CSF primed-DLIs for relapse after autologous transplantation in mantle cell lymphoma: a case report and literature review on the evidence of GVL effects in MCL. *American Journal of Hematology*, **65**, 75–80.

Sondel, P. M., Bozdech, M. J., Trigg, M. E. *et al.* (1985). Additional immunosuppression allows engraftment following HLA-mismatched T-cell depleted bone marrow transplantation for leukemia. *Transplantation Proceedings*, **17**, 460–1.

Sosman, J. A., Oettel, K. R., Hank, J. A. *et al.* (1989). Specific recognition of human leukemic cells by allogeneic T-cell lines. *Transplantation*, **48**, 486–95.

Sosman, J. A., Oettel, K. R., Smith, S. D. *et al.* (1990). Specific recognition of human leukemic cells by allogeneic T-cell. II. Evidence for HLA-D restricted determinants on leukemic cells which are crossreactive with determinants present on unrelated non-leukemic cells. *Blood*, **75**, 2005–16.

Spitzer, T. R., McAfee, S., Sackstein, R. et al. (2000). Intentional induction of mixed chimerism and achievement of antitumor responses after nonmyeloablative conditioning therapy and HLA-matched donor bone marrow transplantation for refractory hematologic malignancies. *Biology of Blood and Marrow Transplantation,* **6,** 309–20.

Storb, R., Yu, C., Wagner, J. L. et al. (1997). Stable mixed hematopoietic chimerism in DLA-identical littermate dogs given sublethal total body irradiation before and pharmacological immunosuppression after marrow transplantation. *Blood,* **89,** 3048–54.

Sullivan, K. M., Deeg, H. J., Sanders, J. et al. (1986). Hyperacute graft-versus-host disease in patients not given immunosuppression after allogeneic marrow transplantation. *Blood,* **4,** 1172–5.

Sullivan, K. M., Storb, R., Buckner, C. D. et al. (1989a). Graft-versus-host disease as adoptive immunotherapy in patients with advanced hematologic neoplasms. *New England Journal of Medicine,* **320,** 828–34.

Sullivan, K. M., Weiden, P. L., Storb, R. et al. (1989b). Influence of acute and chronic graft-versus-host disease on relapse and survival after bone marrow transplantation from HLA-identical siblings as treatment of acute and chronic leukemia. *Blood,* **73,** 1720–8.

Sykes, M. & Abraham, V. S. (1992). The mechanism of IL-2-mediated protection against GVHD in mice. II. Protection occurs independently of NK/LAK cells. *Transplantation,* **53,** 1063–70.

Sykes, M., Abraham, V. S., Harty, M. W. et al. (1993). IL-2 reduces graft-versus-host disease and preserves a graft-versus-leukemia effect by selectively inhibiting CD4+ T cell activity. *Journal of Immunology,* **150,** 197–205.

Sykes, M., Harty, M. W., Szot, G. L. et al. (1994). Interleukin-2 inhibits graft-versus-host disease-promoting activity of CD4+ cells while preserving CD4- and CD8-mediated graft-versus-leukemia effects. *Blood,* **83,** 2560–9.

Sykes, M., Romick, M. L., & Sachs, D. H. (1990). Interleukin-2 prevents graft-versus-host disease without diminishing the graft-versus-leukemia effect of allogeneic lymphocytes. *Proceedings of the National Academy of Sciences USA,* **87,** 5633–7.

Theobald, M. (1995). Allorecognition and graft-versus-host disease. *Bone Marrow Transplantation,* **15,** 489–98.

Tricot, G., Vesole, D. H., Jagannath, S. et al. (1996). Graft-versus-myeloma effect: proof of principle. *Blood,* **87,** 1196–8.

Troy, A. J. & Hart, D.N.J. (1997). Dendritic cells and cancer: progress toward a new cellular therapy. *Journal of Hematotherapy,* **6,** 523–34.

Truitt, R. L. & Atasoylu, A. A. (1991a). Contribution of CD4+ and CD8+ T-cells to graft-versus-host disease and graft-versus-leukemia reactivity after transplantation of MHC-compatible bone marrow. *Bone Marrow Transplantation,* **8,** 51–8.

Truitt. R. L. & Atasoylu, A. A. (1991b). Impact of pretransplant conditioning and donor T-cells on chimerism, graft-versus-host disease, graft-versus-leukemia reactivity, and tolerance after bone marrow transplantation. *Blood,* **77,** 2515–23.

Truitt, R. L., Johnson, B. D., McCabe, C. M., & Weiler, M. B. (1997). Graft versus leukemia. In *Graft-versus-Host Disease,* second edition, eds. J.L.M. Ferrara, H. J., Deeg, & S. J. Burakoff, pp. 385–423. New York: Marcel Dekker, Inc.

Truitt, R. L., LeFever, A. V., & Shih, C. C.-Y. (1986). Manipulation of graft-versus-host disease for a graft-versus-leukemia effect after allogeneic bone marrow transplantation in AKR mice with spontaneous leukemia/lymphoma. *Transplantation,* **41,** 301–10.

Truitt, R. L., LeFever, A. V., Shih, C. C.-Y. et al. (1990). Graft-versus-leukemia effect. In *Graft-versus-Host Disease: Immunology, Pathophysiology and Treatment,* eds. S. J. Burakoff, H. J., Deeg, J. Ferrara, & K. Atkinson, pp. 177–204. New York: Marcel Dekker, Inc.

Truitt, R. L., Shih, C.-Y., Lefever, A. V. et al. (1983). Characterization of alloimmunization-induced T lymphocytes reactive against AKR leukemia in vitro and correlation with graft-versus-leukemia activity in vivo. *Journal of Immunology,* **131,** 2050–8.

Ueno, N. T., Rondon, G., Mirza, N. Q. et al. (1998). Allogeneic peripheral-blood progenitor-cell transplantation for poor-risk patients with metastatic breast cancer. *Journal of Clinical Oncology,* **16,** 986–93.

van Besien, K., Sobocinski, K. A., Rowlings, P. A. et al. (1998). Allogeneic bone marrow transplantation for low-grade lymphoma. *Blood,* **92,** 1832–6.

van Besien, K. W., de Lima, M., Giralt, S. A. et al. (1997). Management of lymphoma recurrence after allogeneic transplantation: the relevance of graft-versus-lymphoma effect. *Bone Marrow Transplantation,* **19,** 977–82.

van Rood, J. J., Goulmy, E., & van Leeuwen, A. (1987). The immunogenetics of chronic graft-versus-host disease and its relevance to the graft-versus-leukemia effect. In *Cellular Immunotherapy of Cancer,* eds. R. L. Truitt, R. P. Gale, & M. M. Bortin, p. 433. New York: Alan R. Liss, Inc.

Verdonck, L. F., Lokhorst, H. M., Dekker, A. W. et al. (1996). Graft-versus-myeloma effect in two cases. *Lancet,* **347,** 800–1.

Vourka-Karussis, V., Karussis, D., Acherstein, A., & Slavin, S. (1995). Enhancement of a GVL effect with rhIL-2 following BMT in a murine model for acute myeloid leukemia. *Experimental Hematology,* **23,** 196–201.

Warren, E. H., Greenberg, P. D., & Riddell, S. R.. (1998). Cytotoxic T-lymphocyte-defined human minor histocompatibility antigens with a restricted tissue distribution. *Blood,* **91,** 2197–207.

Weiden, P. L., Flournoy, N., Thomas, E. D. et al. (1979). Antileukemic effect of graft-versus-host disease in human recipients of allogeneic-marrow grafts. *New England Journal of Medicine,* **300,** 1068–73.

Weiden, P. L. & Horowitz, M. M. (1990). Graft-versus-leukemia effects in clinical bone marrow transplantation. In *Graft-versus-Host Disease: Immunology, Pathophysiology, and Treatment,* eds. S. J. Burakoff, H. J. Deeg, J. Ferrara, & K. Atkinson, pp. 691–708. New York: Marcel Dekker, Inc.

Weiden, P. L., Sullivan, K. M., Flournoy, N. et al. (1981). Antileukemic effect of chronic graft-versus-host disease: contribution to improved survival after allogeneic marrow transplantation. *New England Journal of Medicine,* **304,** 1529–33.

Weisdorf, D. J., Nesbit, M. E., Ramsay, N.K.C. et al. (1987). Allogeneic bone marrow transplantation for acute lymphoblastic leukemia in remission: prolonged survival associated with acute graft-versus-host disease. *Journal of Clinical Oncology,* **5,** 1348–55.

Weiss, L., Lubin, I., Factorowich, I. et al. (1994). Effective graft-versus-leukemia effects independent of graft-versus-host disease after T-cell depleted allogeneic bone marrow transplantation in a murine model of B cell leukemia/lymphoma: role of cell therapy and IL-2. *Journal of Immunology,* **153,** 2562–7.

Weiss, L., Reich, S., & Slavin, S. (1995). The role of antibodies to IL-2 receptor and asialo GM1 on graft-versus-leukemia effects induced by bone marrow allografts in murine B cell leukemia. *Bone Marrow Transplantation,* **16,** 457–61.

Williamson, E., Garside, P., Bradley, J. A., & Mowat, A. M. (1996). IL-12 is a central mediator of acute graft-versus-host disease in mice. *Journal of Immunology,* **157,** 689–99.

Woodruff, M.F.A. (1980). The experimental basis of immunotherapy. In *The Interaction of Cancer and Host: Its Therapeutic Significance,* ed. M.F.A. Woodruff, pp. 164–233. New York: Grune & Stratton.

Yang, Y. G., Sergio, J. J., Pearson, D. A., Szot, G. L., Shimizu, A., & Sykes, M. (1997). Interleukin-12 preserves the graft-versus-leukemia effect of allogeneic CD8 T cells while inhibiting CD4-dependent graft-versus-host disease in mice. *Blood,* **90,** 4651–60.

Zwaan, F. E., Hermans, J., Barrett, A. J., & Speck, B. (1984). Bone marrow transplantation for acute nonlymphoblastic leukemia: a survey of the European Group for Bone Marrow Transplantation. *British Journal of Haematology,* **56,** 645–53.

PART 2   METHODS AND PROCEDURES IN HEMATOPOIETIC STEM CELL TRANSPLANTATION

20 Management of patients undergoing marrow or blood stem cell transplantation

MARY E.D. FLOWERS AND KEITH M. SULLIVAN

Fred Hutchinson Cancer Research Center, Seattle, and Duke University Medical Center, Durham, USA

Introduction

Blood stem cell and marrow transplantation can be carried out safely and with less cost in a specialized ambulatory facility (Meisenberg *et al.,* 1998; Smith *et al.,* 1997; Weaver *et al.,* 1997; Anonymous, 1997) (Table 20.1). In the autologous setting, transplantation has been practiced even in the patient's home (Herrmann *et al.,* 1999). Additionally, HLA-matched related and unrelated blood stem cell transplants have been carried out as home procedures after completion of the myeloablative-conditioning regimen, with encouraging results (Svahn *et al.,* 2000). In the allogeneic non-myeloablative setting, transplantation has been carried out entirely as an outpatient procedure (McSweeney *et al.,* 2001; Gomez-Almaguer *et al.,* 2000). We describe here management and procedures used at the Fred Hutchinson Cancer Research Center and the Seattle Cancer Care Alliance for donors and patients undergoing allogeneic and autologous hematopoietic stem cell transplantation. We acknowledge that other centers may use different approaches, and where possible we will outline these practice differences.

Ambulatory clinics

The major factors that contributed to the shift of transplant care from a hospital setting to the ambulatory facility were the availability of hematopoietic growth factors, greater efficacy of antimicrobial prophylaxis and antiemetics, specialized ambulatory clinics (AC) supporting patient recovery and, more recently, the use of non-myeloablative pretransplant regimens. AC include a structure and organization for multidisciplinary patient care provided by physicians, nurses, middle level practitioners (or fellows), pharmacists, dietitians, dentists, social workers, psychologists, and support staff. Also part of this team are subspecialties including infectious disease, respiratory disease, gastroenterology, clinical pathology laboratories, pharmacology, histocompatibility, blood banking, cell processing and cryopreservation facilities, radiology, and radiation-oncological services.

Facility and services provided at AC include:

1. Infusion of fluids and other treatments 7 days a week
2. Administration of myeloablative chemotherapy and radiotherapy including total body irradiation (TBI)
3. Isolation of patients with contagious disease
4. Monitoring of early and late transplant-related toxicities
5. Surveillance and treatment of infections
6. Diagnosis and treatment of acute and chronic graft-versus-host disease (GVHD)
7. Monitoring of engraftment, relapse of malignancy, and other medical complications
8. Administration of growth factors to, monitoring of, and support of stem cell donors
9. Placement and removal of intravenous central lines
10. Diagnostic procedures including radiologically guided fine needle aspirations, bronchoalveolar lavage, upper and lower gastrointestinal endoscopic biopsies, etc.
11. Provision of clinical pathology laboratory services
12. Provision of apheresis facility to collect peripheral blood stem cells, lymphocytes, and other blood cell products

Table 20.1. *Inpatient and outpatient charges and costs (in US dollars) of HSC transplantation*

	Inpatient (*n* = 20)	Subtotal outpatient (*n* = 46)	Total outpatient (*n* = 28)
Charges (US$)			
mean	$74,417	$60,447	$48,874
s.d.	19,695	29,069	26,782
minimum	45,805	34,452	29,697
maximum	124,681	166,564	172,145
f value	6.57	–	–
P value	0.002	–	–
Costs			
mean	$39,703	83,618	82,937
s.d.	10,652	13,143	16,336
minimum	27,316	23,758	18,569
maximum	75,037	94,597	105,967
f value	3.7	–	–
P value	0.029	–	–

Reproduced with permission from Meisenberg *et al.*(Meisenberg *et al.,* 1998)

13. Provision of education to patients, families, and caregivers regarding home care procedures
14. Standardization of cost-effective medical practices
15. Provision of infrastructure, medical records, and data management to conduct clinical investigations.

Pretransplant procedures

Referral for transplantation

The clinical coordinator is an experienced transplant physician whose job is to discuss with referring doctors and with patients alternative treatment options including transplants and non-transplant protocols. Medical records, including HLA typing, are reviewed and, where applicable, a search for an unrelated donor through the National Marrow Donor Program is initiated. Patients are offered consultation at the transplant center to review treatment options in detail and discuss the risks and benefits of transplantation and other available therapies. Consultation is particularly important to identify suitable candidates for transplantation at an early stage of disease (Berman et al., 1992) and to facilitate education and informed consent (Singer et al., 1990; Levine, 1986; Prentice et al., 1997). In vitro fertilization (IVF) counseling and arrangements for sperm banking, oocyte storage, or embryo storage are necessary, especially in patients with early stage of disease.

The age limit for transplantation has been increasing in the past decade as a result of less toxic pretransplant regimens and continued improvement in treatment support. In Seattle, the age limits for myeloablative transplantation are as follows: HLA-identical sibling transplantation, ≤65 years; HLA-identi-cal unrelated transplantation, ≤55 years; autologous blood stem cell transplantation, ≤70 years; allogeneic non-myeloablative transplantation, ≤75 years. Age greater than 50 years has been associated with inferior outcome after myeloablative autologous transplantation (Kusnierz-Glaz et al., 1997). However, another study comparing outcome of recipients of autologous or allogeneic bone marrow transplants aged 40 years and above or less than 40 years found no difference in outcome after autotransplant (Fig. 20.1) and indeed a trend for better survival for those aged over 40 years after allogeneic transplantation, although the difference was mainly due to a higher proportion of patients with good risk for leukemia in the older age group (Fig. 20.2) (Rappoport et al., 1995). Similar data have been published by other investigators using myeloablative transplant regimens (Ringden et al., 1993; Ringdén et al., 1998; Miller et al., 1996; Guba et al., 1997). Early results of non-myeloablative transplantation in older patients (60–75 years) are encouraging with <10% transplant-related mortality (McSweeney et al., 2001). At the other end of the age spectrum, outcome of transplantation in infants appears similar to that in older patients (Woolfrey et al., 1998; Pirich et al., 1999; Marco et al., 2000; Leung et al., 2001). Another recipient factor reported by some, but not all, to impact adversely on transplant-related mortality and disease-free survival is obesity at time of transplant (Dickson et al., 1999; Meloni et al., 2001). Obese individuals have altered pharmacokinetics for many medications including chemotherapeutic agents and potentially longer drug exposure may be responsible for the observed increase in treatment-related toxicity. Dose adjustment and weight normalization should be considered if possible.

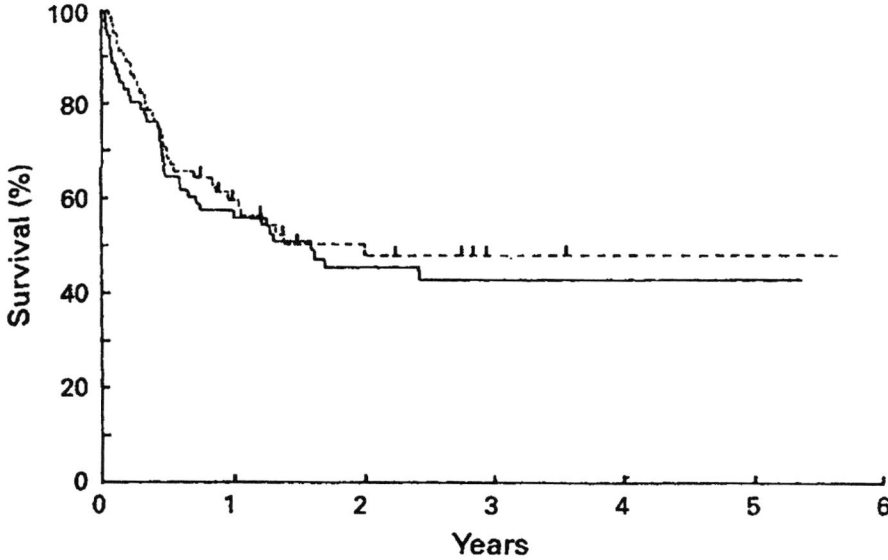

Fig. 20.1. Actuarial (Kaplan-Meier) event-free survival (EFS) curves for the autotransplant patients according to age group. Among the 78 patients aged ≥40 years (—), there were 41 alive and event-free (48%). Tick marks indicate the length of follow-up for the 11 patients ≥60 years at the time of transplantation who remain alive and free of disease relapse or progression. Among 70 patients age <40 years (—), there were 32 censored observations; EFS = 43%. P = .56. Reproduced, with permission, from Rappoport et al.(Rappoport et al., 1995)

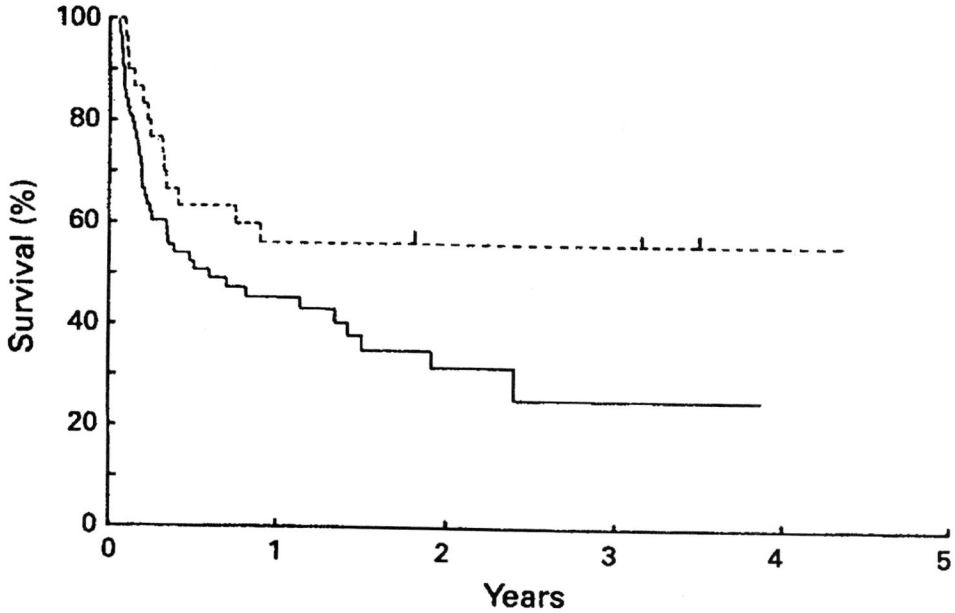

Fig. 20.2. Actuarial (Kaplan-Meier) EFS curves for the allotransplantation patients according to age group. Among the 30 patients age ≥40 years (—) there were 17 alive and event-free (56%). The tick marks indicate the length of follow-up for the 3 patients age ≥50 years at the time of transplantation who remain alive and free of disease relapse. Among the 62 patients age <40 years (—), there were 23 censored observations; EFS = 26%. These curves were marginally different (P = .57, log rank) but this difference was even less significant after adjustment for prognostic factors. Reproduced, with permission, from Rappoport *et al.*(Rappoport *et al.,* 1995)

Prior to the patient and the donor arrival at the transplant center, a book with information about the transplant, housing, and other logistics regarding their stay is mailed to them by the clinical coordinator's office.

The volunteer service, located in the reception areas of the AC, assists the patient, donor, and family with transition to local housing and facilities and provides other support during the transplantation treatment.

On arrival, patients and donors undergo a comprehensive pretransplant evaluation by one of the multidisciplinary medical teams specialized in allogeneic, autologous, or pediatric care. Each of the transplant teams consists of a senior attending physician, two oncology-hematology fellows (or middle level practitioners), two nurses, a dietitian, a social worker, a pharmacist, and a scheduler/records assistant. Each team cares for, on average, 30 to 40 pre- and posttransplant patients.

Family conferences and informed consent

The attending physician conducts the arrival conference with the patient and the donor (if applicable) to review in detail the natural history of the underlying disease, alternative therapies, the results of these treatments, and the risks involved with marrow or blood stem cell transplantation. Consent forms for standard diagnostic studies are reviewed and signed by the patient and donor. In addition, available phase I, II, or III clinical protocols are discussed, and consent forms given to the patient and donor for review. Issues are discussed and presented again separately by social workers. Approximately one week later, a second informed consent conference is conducted by the attending physician to review the results of the pretransplant evaluations. Questions concerning the research studies, treatment protocols, and consent information are answered and informed consent is obtained prior to the transplant. Written consents are filed in the patient's and donor's medical records. Patient (and donors) may be enrolled in several clinical trials regarding conditioning regimens, graft-versus-host disease prevention and treatment, infection prevention or treatment, long-term follow up studies, or others.

Selection of transplant regimen

The attending physician and the clinical coordinator select the treatment strategy, donor, and source of cells for the transplant (i.e., marrow or blood stem cell; myeloablative or non-myeloablative regimen) taking into account a number of factors including diagnosis and stage of disease, medical condition and age of the patient, donor availability, and availability of clinical trials.

Pretransplant evaluation

Table 20.2 outlines the pretransplant work-up studies for the patient. Special attention is given to determination of organ dysfunction that could increase regimen-related toxicity or exclude patients from myeloablative transplantation [for example, in many programs, a serum creatinine >0.25 mmol/l, a serum bilirubin >40 mmol/l, a left ventricular ejection fraction

Table 20.2. *Pretransplant patient evaluation*

Review of records and history and physical (H&P) exam by
    primary provider
Conference with attending physician to review the natural history
    of disease, provide information about available treatments,
    review results and complications related to transplantation, and
    review informed consent forms.
Review original diagnostic slides to confirm the primary disease
Laboratory tests[a]. CBC with platelet and reticulocyte counts;
    chemistry panel including creatinine, BUN, electrolytes, glu-
    cose, alkaline phosphatase, ALT, AST, bilirubin, LDH, choles-
    terol, triglycerides, immunoglobulin levels; ABO, Rh typing;
    direct Coombs; FSH, LH, estradiol and HCG (females) and
    testosterone total and free (males), hepatitis screening; anti-
    HIV, CMV, HSV, VZV, EBV, HTLV 1 and 2, syphilis serology
Blood specific disease makers
HLA typing including DNA studies and leukocyte cross match
Bone marrow aspiration and biopsy,[b] cell surface markers
Chest x-ray and dental x-rays; other specific disease staging (i.e.,
    bone marrow MRI, CT scans, skeletal survey, bone scans, etc.)
Lumbar puncture[c]
Electrocardiogram
Cardiac ejection studies
Pulmonary function tests including DLCO and arterial blood gas
Social worker assessment
Gynecological, oral medicine, nutrition evaluations
Other subspecialty consultant evaluation as indicated

Abbreviations: CBC, complete blood cell count; FSH, follicle-
stimulating hormone; LH, luteinizing hormone; HCG, human
chorionic gonadotropin; HIV, human immunodeficiency virus;
CMV, cytomegalovirus: HSV, herpes simplex virus: VZV,
varicella zoster virus; EBV, Epstein-Barr Virus; HTLV, human T-
lymphotropic virus; HLA, human leukocyte antigen; CNS, central
nervous system; DLCO, diffusing lung capacity of carbon
monoxide; MRI, magnetic resonance imaging; CT, computed
tomography.

[a] Other centers may include serological screening for toxoplasma.
Chagas disease, and others as appropriate.

[b] Morphology, cytogenetics, immunophenotyping and other
disease-specific tests (e.g., polymerase chain reaction for *bcr/abl*
in CML patients).

[c] Diagnostic spinal tap with instillation of intrathecal methotrexate
in patients at risk for CNS disease (ALL, history of prior CNS
involvement).

[d] Other testing may include creatinine clearance rate (24 hour
urine collection) or microbiology screening e.g., throat swab, nose
swab, Hickman catheter exit site swab (to detect antibiotic-
resistant organisms such as methicillin-resistant *Staphylococcus
aureus* (MRSA) methicillin-resistant *S. epidermidis* (MRSE),
Pseudomonas).

<50%, or a poor performance status (e.g., <70% Karnofsky
score)] (Bearman *et al.,* 1988; Bearman *et al.,* 1990; Crawford
& Fisher, 1992). In a study of 383 consecutive HSC transplants,
factors predictive of early transplant-related mortality in multivariate analysis included FEV_1 less than 78% of predicted,
serum creatinine greater than 1.1 mg/dl and serum bilirubin
greater than 1.1mg/dl (Goldberg *et al.,* 1998). An FEV_1/FVC
less than 70% pretransplant, male gender, increasing patient

age, and cigarette smoking are pretransplant risk factors for airway obstruction in recipients of bone marrow transplants
(Clark *et al.,* 1987).

In summary, the aims of the pretransplant evaluation are to:

1. Confirm diagnosis and status of the underlying disease.
2. Assess patient and donor physical and psychological condition and organ function.
3. Confirm HLA typing and establish the transplant type
   (autologous, allogeneic, or syngeneic)
4. Treat coexisting medical disorders.
5. Assign appropriate transplant protocols including stem cell
   source (blood or bone marrow) and other therapies.
6. Educate and train the patient and family about home care
   procedures.

Selection and evaluation of allogeneic transplant donors are
described in Table 20.3 (and see Chapters 23 and 25).

Pretransplant supportive care

Venous access

To provide adequate venous access in the patient, a double-lumen
right atrial catheter (Hickman or similar) is inserted by a vascular
surgeon. For donors without adequate peripheral vein access for
apheresis, a temporary central line is placed (i.e., Quinton-
Mahurkar or similar catheter). For recipients of autologous transplants a multi-purpose, silastic, dual-lumen catheter, such as the
Bard-Hickman hemodialysis/apheresis catheter or the Quinton-
Raaf PermCath, is suitable for the apheresis procedure and
chemotherapy administration, stem cell infusion, and supportive
care during and after transplant (Lazarus *et al.,* 2000). An important aspect of catheter placement is to use a dedicated vascular
surgeon with expertise in immunocompromised patients.

Transfusion support (and see Chapter 69)

With the exception of the hematopoietic stem cells used for
transplant and donor lymphocytes used posttransplant, all cellular blood products (pre- and posttransplant) are irradiated with
25 Gy irradiation to prevent transfusion-associated graft-versus-
host disease (GVHD). For allogeneic marrow donors, one unit of
autologous blood is stored about 30 days prior to marrow harvest. A similar unit is stored prior to autologous marrow harvesting, unless anemia is present. Donors of peripheral blood stem
cells do not need autologous blood storage because of minimal
blood cell loss during apheresis. Recombinant human erythropo-
etin (rh-EPO) 100 units/kg s.c. daily for 14 days before marrow
donation, or 600 units/kg s.c. weekly for three weeks prior to
marrow harvest, along with iron supplementation, may be used
in pediatric donors who weight less than 45 kg or less than the
marrow recipient, who will donate 10–20 ml/kg of marrow, and
who have normal iron studies.

When transplantation is carried out across major ABO blood
group incompatibilities, red cell depletion from the donor mar-

Table 20.3. *Selection and evaluation of allogeneic donors*

Donor selection

1. If there is a choice of HLA-identical sibling donors:
   use a nontransfused male or nulliparous, nontransfused female donor (less risk for GVHD)
   use a younger donor (less risk for GVHD)
   use a CMV-seronegative donor (less risk for CMV disease)
   use an ABO-compatible donor (less risk of hemolysis)
2. If there is a choice between an HLA-identical sibling donor and an identical twin donor:
   use the identical twin donor for nonmalignant disease (e.g. severe aplastic anemia)
   consider using the HLA-identical sibling for malignant disease, especially if the patient is less than 30 years of age and/or patient has advanced malignant disease

Donor evaluation

1. History and physical examination
   History of serious or chronic illnesses
   History of hematologic problems including bleeding tendencies
   Cancer history
   Transfusion history
   Adverse anesthesia reactions
   Current medications
   Allergies
   Risk factors for HIV or viral hepatitis infection
   Pregnancy history for females
2. Confirmation of HLA typing, ABO/Rh typing
3. Complete blood cell count; blood chemistry screen, including urea, electrolytes, creatinine, blood sugar, calcium, phosphate, liver function tests
4. Serology for CMV, HIV, HBV, HCV, HTLV-1 and 2[a]; as appropriate, HSV, VZV, EBV, toxoplasma
5. Coagulation tests (PTT, APTT)
6. Electrocardiogram, and chest x-ray as appropriate
7. Pregnancy test for female donors

Abbreviations: CMV, cytomegalovirus; HIV, human immunodeficiency virus; HBV, hepatitis B virus; HCV, hepatitis C virus; HTLV, human T-lymphotropic virus; HSV, herpes simplex virus; VZV, varicella zoster virus; EBV, Epstein-Barr virus; PTT, partial thromboplastin time; APTT, activated partial thromboplastin time.

[a] HIV (and HTLV) positivity is an absolute contraindication to marrow donation. HBV or HCV positivity is a relative contraindication to donation.

row product and/or reduction of isohemagglutinin titers in the recipient or transplant product may be required to prevent hemolytic reactions (Bensinger *et al.*, 1987). Hemagglutinin titers and reticulocyte counts should be followed to monitor the change from recipient to donor blood type. Type O red cells should be used for patients who have isoagglutinins against donor red blood cell antigens until the donor blood group type is fully established in the recipient.

Platelet transfusions are indicated to maintain a platelet count equal to or above $20 \times 10^9/l$ (depending on patient status) to decrease the risk of bleeding complications. Higher platelet counts ($50 \times 10^9/l$) are necessary for invasive procedures, such as lumbar puncture, catheter placement, or other

surgical procedures. Donor-type platelets should be used for transfusions.

Patients who are cytomegalovirus (CMV)-seronegative pretransplant should be transfused with CMV-seronegative blood products. Leukocyte-depleted blood product should be used if CMV-negative blood products are unavailable.

Infection prophylaxis (and see Chapters 73–76)

To reduce the number and severity of opportunistic infections in HSC transplant recipients, antibiotic prophylaxis, hospital infection control, vaccination, and other measures in preventing disease and exposure are used. In 2000, the Centers for Disease Control (CDC), the Infectious Diseases Society for America (IDSA), and the American Society for Blood and Marrow Transplantation (ASBMT) issued guidelines for preventing opportunistic infections among hematopoietic stem cell transplant (HSCT) recipients (Centers for Disease Control and Prevention *et al.*, 2000; Bowden *et al.*, 1995). Infection prophylaxis currently used in Seattle is described in Tables 20.4 and 20.5.

Pneumocystis carinii pneumonia (PCP) prophylaxis

Trimethoprim-sulfamethoxazole (TMP-SMX) (cotrimoxazole) is administered b.i.d. (twice) daily for prophylaxis of PCP starting two weeks before starting the conditioning regimen. Adults are given one double strength (DS) (160 mg TMP and 800 mg SMX) tablet po b.i.d. and patients between 20 and 35 kg are given one single strength (SS) (80 mg TMP and 400 mg SMX) tablet po b.i.d. Pediatric patients <20 kg receive 5mg/kg/day TMP component po b.i.d. Prophylaxis is discontinued in all patients 48 hours prior to the infusion of hematopoietic cells. When the absolute neutrophil count reaches >500/mm^3 for three days posttransplant, TMP-SMX (DS or SS or suspension according to patient weight) is reinstituted po b.i.d. twice weekly on two consecutive days, until day 180 posttransplant or until 2–6 months after cessation of immunosuppressive therapy, whichever is longer. A TMP-SMX desensitization program is strongly recommended in patients with a drug allergy history (see Chapter 78 for details). Dapsone (50 mg po b.i.d. or 1 mg/kg/day up to 100 mg/day for children) is an alternative regimen for patients unable to tolerate TMP-SMX, but it may be less effective against PCP (Souza *et al.*, 1999). Patients should be tested for G6PD deficiency before starting dapsone. Atovaquone is a possible alternative drug for PCP prophylaxis among dapsone-intolerant patients (Chan *et al.*, 1999). Use of aerosolized pentamidime is associated with the poorest PCP prevention rates (Link *et al.*, 1993) and should only be used if other agents cannot be tolerated.

Cytomegalovirus (CMV) prevention

CMV-seronegative blood products are given to all CMV-seronegative patients. Leukocyte-depleted blood products are

Table 20.4. *Cytomegalovirus (CMV) pre-emptive therapy for prophylaxis of disease*

Recipient CMV serostatus	Donor CMV serostatus	Risk of antigenemia	CMV-seronegative filtered blood products[a]	Antiviral therapy
Allogeneic recipients				
Positive	Positive or negative	Before day 100: 80% any level	No	Day 0–100: Start ganciclovir for antigenemia at any level (or viremia) 5 mg/kg b.i.d. for 7 days followed by 5 mg/kg daily dosing until day 100[b,c] After day 100: Start ganciclovir for antigenemia (if >5 positive cells/slide or 2 consecutive positive PCR results or viremia) at 5 mg/kg b.i.d. for 7 days followed by 5 mg/kg daily for 2 additional weeks[b]
Negative	Positive	30%	Yes	As above
Autologous recipients (unmodified)				
Positive	N/A	17%	Yes	Day 0–100: Start ganciclovir for antigenemia at any level (or viremia) 5 mg/kg b.i.d. for 5 days followed by 5 mg/kg daily dose until day 100[b,c]
Autologous recipients (CD34-selected)				
Positive	N/A	26%		Pre-transplant to day –3: Start ganciclovir (if >5 positive cells/slide or PCR DNA >100 copies/ml or viremia) at 5 mg/kg b.i.d. for 7 days followed by 5 mg/kg daily for 5 days per week. Ganciclovir **should not** be given beyond day –3 pretransplant. Day 0 to engraftment: Foscarnet for PCR DNA >100 copies/ml, at 60 mg/kg b.i.d. for 7 days (or longer[b]) followed by 90 mg/kg/day 7 days week i.v. until absolute neutrophil count 750/mm^3 × 2 days). Between engraftment and day 100, and after day 100: same as for allogeneic recipients
Negative	N/A	1–2%	Yes	As for seropositive autograft recipient

[a] Patients receive blood products from seronegative donors, or filtered blood products if no seronegative blood products are available. 1–2% of patients are still at risk for early CMV infection/disease because of insensitivity of pretransplant serologic screening method (Bowden *et al.*, 1995).

[b] Continue twice daily dosing if antigenemia or DNA levels by PCR are more than 2 times baseline level at day 7 of treatment until the levels start to decline (minimum one additional week); if subsequent level is declining or in case of moderate increase (i.e., less than 2 times baseline), continue once a day dosing (7 days a week) until day 100 or for two weeks or for negative antigenemia or PCR, whichever occurs later.

[c] A minimum of three weeks treatment (or until negative antigenemia or PCR) is recommended for allogeneic patients who become antigen positive.

recommended if seronegative products are unavailable (Bowden *et al.*, 1991; Bowden *et al.*, 1991). Table 20.4 presents current guidelines used in Seattle for preemptive treatment with ganciclovir for prevention of CMV disease in HSCT recipients. The decision for initiating ganciclovir for prevention of CMV disease is based on detection of CMV pp65 antigen in leukocytes (antigenemia) or direct detection of CMV DNA (deoxyribonucleic acid) by polymerase chain reaction (PCR), as described in Table 20.4. Ganciclovir dose

adjustment is recommended for cytopenia and renal dysfunction (see Chapter 83). Ganciclovir is discontinued when (1) the absolute neutrophil count falls below 1.0×10^9/l for 2 consecutive days; (2) high-dose acyclovir (500 mg/m^2 q 8 hours) is started; or (3) CMV viremia is present after 4 weeks of ganciclovir, which indicates a need to switch treatment to foscarnet (180 mg/kg/day divided into 2 doses for 7 days followed by 90 mg/kg/day until day 100). The dose of foscarnet needs to be adjusted for renal function (Chapter 83). Anti-

Table 20.5. *Prophylaxis of infectious diseases – current regimen at FHCRC/SCCA (adults)*

Drug	Timing	Purpose
1. Cotrimoxazole, 1 double strength (DS) tablet b.i.d. (800 mg sulfamethoxazole, 160 mg trimethoprim) or, (if unable to tolerate cotrimoxazole):	Daily for 2 weeks before transplant until day –1; then twice weekly from day +28 until 6 months posttransplant or until 2–6 months after cessation of immunosuppressive medications	*Pneumocystis carinii* pneumonia (PCP) prophylaxis
Dapsone, 150 mg po daily (G6PD deficiency must be ruled out prior to start of therapy)	As for cotrimoxazole	PCP prophylaxis if patients cannot tolerate cotrimoxazole
2. Ganciclovir or, if unable to tolerate ganciclovir:	(see Table 20.4)	CMV prophylaxis
Foscarnet	(see Table 20.4)	CMV prophylaxis if patient cannot tolerate ganciclovir
3. Fluconazole, 200 mg (allogeneic) or 100 mg (autologous) b.i.d., po or i.v.	Start with conditioning; through day 75 (allogeneic) or 30 (autologous or syngeneic)	*Candida* prophylaxis
4. Acyclovir, 800 mg b.i.d. po or valaciclovir 500 mg b.i.d. or 250 mg/m^2 iv q 12 hours if unable to tolerate oral	Day 0 to day +30 (VZV seronegative) or day +365 (VZV) seropositive)	HSV and VZV prophylaxis
5. Levofloxacin,[a] 750 mg b.i.d. po, or	When absolute neurophil count <500/mm^3	Gram-negative bacterial prophylaxis
Ceftazidime 2 g i.v. q 8 hrs	If extensive use of quinolones or documented, or colonization of, Gram-negative organism known to be resistant to levofloxacin or a prior history of quinolone allergy	Gram-negative bacterial prophylaxis
6. Abelcet 3 mg/kg/day i.v.	If fever persists >72 hours or if patient is colonized with yeast (fluconazole is stopped)	Fungal prophylaxis

[a] Other similar agents available.

CMV specific lymphocyte clones, generated in vitro from the donor's blood, have been shown to be safe and to prevent CMV disease; they may be more commonly employed in the future (Riddell *et al.,* 1992).

Herpes simplex virus (HSV) prophylaxis

To decrease the morbidity associated with oral HSV infection, especially during the time of peritransplant oral mucositis, HSV-seropositive patients are given acyclovir prophylaxis. High-dose oral acyclovir (800 mg po b.i.d. or 600 mg/m^2 po b.i.d. for individuals <35 kg) or valaciclovir (500 mg po b.i.d. or 250 mg/m^2 for individuals <35 kg) is used for prophylaxis of both HSV and varicella zoster virus (VZV). Acyclovir is started on the first day of conditioning and discontinued on day 30 or upon resolution of mucositis, whichever occurs first (HSV-seropositive patients only). If the recipient is also VZV-seropositive pretransplant, prophylaxis with acyclovir or valaciclovir is extended to one year after transplant (see VZV prophylaxis below). If oral acyclovir or valaciclovir is not tolerated, intravenous acyclovir is administered (250 mg/m^2 q 12 hours). Close monitoring of renal function is necessary during treatment with acyclovir (or valaciclovir). Dose adjustments are recommended according to renal function. Prophylactic acyclovir (or valaciclovir) is withheld during ganciclovir for CMV prophylaxis or treatment, because the latter is also an adequate prophylactic therapy for all herpesviruses. Acyclovir (or valaciclovir) prophylaxis should be resumed upon discontinuation of ganciclovir.

Varicella zoster virus (VZV) prophylaxis

Prevention of VZV infection depends upon the serologic status of the pretransplant recipient. The greatest risk for infection with exogenous virus occurs in the seronegative patient, but reinfection with VZV can occur even in the seropositive patient. Eliminating or limiting exposure to varicella is recommended for all HSCT recipients. This includes recommending that children who will be in direct contact with the HSCT recipient be vaccinated for VZV before coming to the transplant center if they have not already had chickenpox. In addition, antiviral treatment is recommended for individuals in close contact with the HSCT recipient if they develop varicella infection. If the transplant recipient has direct exposure to persons with known chickenpox or shingles, valaciclovir (1 g po t.i.d., *or* 500 mg po t.i.d. for individuals < 35 kg, *or* acyclovir suspension 600 mg/m^2 for pediatric patients <35 kg), is administered from day 3 after VZV exposure to day 22, unless the recipient is already receiving suppressive doses of acyclovir at the time of exposure. In VZV-seronegative patients who are not receiving acyclovir prophylaxis at the time of VZV exposure, varicella zoster immunoglobulin (VZIG) is administered within 96 hours of the exposure. In patients unable to take antiviral medications orally, intravenous acyclovir (500 mg/m^2 q 8 hours) is given (with i.v. fluids to decrease renal toxicity associated with this therapy). Prophylactic oral acyclovir (or valaciclovir) is given to VZV-seropositive transplant recipients or those with a prior history of chickenpox or shingles, using the same dose regimen for HSV prophylaxis described above. VZV prophylaxis is started on the first day of the conditioning regimen and continued for one year after transplant, or longer for those requiring systemic corticosteroids ($\geq$ 0.5 g/kg/day). If oral acyclovir or valaciclovir is not tolerated, intravenous acyclovir is administered (250 mg/m^2 q 12 hours). Close monitoring of renal function is necessary during treatment with acyclovir (or valaciclovir). Dose adjustments are recommended according to renal function.

Respiratory virus (RV) prevention

Healthcare workers and visitors with symptoms of an upper respiratory tract infection should be restricted from contact with HSCT recipients and those undergoing conditioning treatment, in order to minimize the risk of transmission of community respiratory virus (CRV) infections. Active clinical surveillance for CRV disease should be conducted on all hospitalized HSC patients undergoing conditioning (Centers for Disease Control and Prevention et al., 2000; Bowden et al., 1995). This includes daily checking for signs and symptoms of CRV infection. In some centers, transplants may be postponed if patients are symptomatic or if respiratory syncytial virus (RSV) is positive on rapid assay.

Influenza vaccination of family members and close or household contacts is strongly recommended for each influenza season (i.e., October–May in the United States), starting the season before the patient undergoes transplantation and continuing for >24 months posttransplant. Seasonal influenza vaccination is strongly recommended for all healthcare workers in contact with HSCT recipients. All family members and all close and household contacts of patients who remain immunocompromised >24 months posttransplant should continue to be vaccinated annually as long as the patient's immunocompromised state persists. Lifelong seasonal influenza vaccination is recommended for all HSC transplant recipients, beginning with the influenza season before transplant and resuming >6 months posttransplant. During influenza type A or type B outbreaks, chemoprophylaxis represents an alternative means of providing protection to immunocompromised patients who are unlikely to respond to vaccination. During influenza outbreaks, the Fred Hutchinson Cancer Research Center/Seattle Cancer Care Alliance (FHCRC/SCCA) infectious control committee strongly recommends starting prophylaxis against influenza type A (rimantadine) or type B (neuraminidase inhibitors such as oseltamivir or zanamir) in immunocompromised HSCT recipients.

Antibacterial and antifungal agents

Prophylactic systemic antibiotics are started when the absolute neutrophil count falls below 0.5 × 10^9/l. A quinolone antibiotic (levofloxacin) is currently the standard oral prophylactic antibiotic used at FHCRC/SCCA for neutropenic patients with or without fever. If fever develops or persists on levofloxacin for more than 48 hours, ceftazidime is started. If fever persists for more than 72 hours, a lipid formulation of amphotericin B such as Abelcet is added if the patient is colonized with yeast; gentamycin is added if the patient is colonized with Gram-negative bacilli. Vancomycin is not employed unless there is documented infection with coagulase-negative staphylococcus or other methicillin-resistant staphylococcus species.

Prophylaxis of fungal infection

With increasingly effective antibiotic and antiviral prophylaxis, fungal infections have emerged as an important cause of morbidity and mortality. Results of a randomized, placebo-controlled trial showed fluconazole prophylaxis to be associated with persistent protection against candidiasis-related death in allogeneic marrow transplant recipients (Marr et al., 2000). Table 12.5 describes the antifungal prophylaxis with triazoles (fluconazole) which is started at the beginning of myeloablative therapy and continued through day +75 posttransplant (allogeneic) or day +30 (autologous or syngenic) in HSCT recipients (Goodman et al., 1992). Fluconazole is stopped during treatment with Abelcet or other amphotericin B formulations. For hospitalized patients, the CDC recommends that allograft recipients be placed in rooms with greater than 12 air exchanges per hour and point-of-use high-efficiency (>99%) particulate air (HEPA) filters that are capable of removing particles >0.3 μm in diameter (Centers for Disease Control and Prevention et al., 2000; Bowden et al., 1995). This is particularly important during times of hospital construction and renovation due to increase risk of aspergillosis. Use of HEPA-filtered rooms should be also considered for autologous HSC transplant recipients with prolonged neutropenia, which is the main risk factor for nosocomial aspergillosis. Additionally, hospital rooms for HSC transplant recipients should have positive room-air pressure when compared to adjoining hallways, toilets, and anterooms. A consistent pressure differential should be maintained at <2.5 pascals or 0.01 inch by water gauge.

Although exposure to plants, fresh or dried flowers has not conclusively been shown to increase the risk of fungal infections in immunocompromised patients, most physicians strongly recommend that plants and flowers not be allowed in the rooms of hospitalized HSC recipients or candidates.

Immunoglobulin (IVIG) prophylaxis

Passive antibody prophylaxis with IVIG is used in some centers to prevent and or treat infections following HSC transplantation. In a randomized trial, the incidence of acute graft-versus-host disease (GVHD) in adult allogeneic transplant recipients was reduced from 51% in untreated controls to 32% in IVIG recipients, and transplant-related mortality was reduced (Sullivan *et al.*, 1990). The doses studied in Seattle were 400 to 500 mg/kg i.v. weekly from day 0 or 7 to approximately day 100, although smaller doses have also been shown to be effective (100 mg/kg and 250 mg/kg weekly) (Nims & Strom, 1988). IVIG should be considered in patients with chronic GVHD, especially if hypogammaglobulinemia is present (<400 mg/dl), to decrease bacterial infections (IVIG 400 mg/kg monthly). IVIG (400–500 mg/kg) administered every second day for a total of 7 doses) is recommended for the treatment of CMV pneumonia in combination with ganciclovir. The role of IVIG for infection prophylaxis has not been demonstrated in autologous transplant recipients.

Hematopoietic growth factors

Several studies have shown faster granulocyte recovery after myeloablative therapy in patients given hematopoietic growth factors after autologous or allogeneic HSC transplantation (Sheridan *et al.*, 1989; Nemunaitis *et al.*, 1991; Nemunaitis *et al.*, 1991; Bensinger *et al.*, 1994; Schmitz *et al.*, 1995). Because of the faster engraftment with peripheral blood stem cell transplants (PBSC) in comparison to bone marrow transplants, use of recombinant human granulocyte colony-stimulating factor (rh-G-CSF) has declined in patients after transplant.

The dose of G-CSF given to the donor for mobilization of PBSC in Seattle is 16 μg/kg/d s.c. for 4 to 6 days prior to the apheresis. The dose of rh-G-CSF given for delayed neutrophil recovery after transplant ranges from 5 to 10 μg/kg/day.

Other aspects of supportive care

To avoid menorrhagia during the thrombocytopenia period, women are given progesterone (Provera 10 mg/day) prior to starting the myeloablative regimen. Once sustained platelet engraftment is achieved posttransplant, patients are placed on combined estrogen-progesterone hormone replacement to prevent late effects of gonadal failure and bone loss, unless contraindicated (i.e., history or increased risk of breast cancer, hypercoagulability status, etc.).

Pretransplant prophylaxis and treatment of central nervous system (CNS) leukemia

Prophylaxis

Patients at risk of involvement of CNS malignancy (i.e., acute lymphoblastic leukemia, lymphoid blast crisis of chronic myeloid leukemia, etc.) or with a history of prior CNS involvement should undergo lumbar puncture for cerebrospinal fluid (CSF) examination pretransplant. Intrathecal chemotherapy (usually methotrexate) should be injected after the CSF sample is obtained. Such patients may be at risk for CNS complications posttransplant (van Besien *et al.*, 1996). A total of 6 intrathecal methotrexate doses are administered for prophylaxis of CNS leukemia or lymphoma in patients at risk (i.e., 1–2

doses pretransplant and 4–5 doses after transplant, usually starting at week 6 or later, as clinical status allows).

Treatment

The CSF should be cleared of malignant cells prior to initiating the conditioning regimen, although active CNS malignancy pretransplant may not be an absolute contraindication to transplant. This can be done using intrathecal methotrexate (MTX), intrathecal cytosine arabinoside, or both in combination with hydrocortisone (to reduce the risk of chemical arachnoiditis) (Table 20.6). Intrathecal chemotherapy (MTX is the most commonly used) should be reinitiated at 5 weeks posttransplant, and be given every second week until day 100 posttransplant. One approach then administers a dose every second month for a total of 8 doses.

Pretransplant conditioning

Conventional hematopoietic stem cell transplantation utilizes high-dose chemotherapy with or without total body irradiation (TBI) with the aim of eradicating the underlying disease and/or suppressing the recipient's immune system (Thomas *et al.*, 1975). Several components of the regimens can now be carried out safely in an ambulatory setting (Meisenberg *et al.*, 1997). TBI-containing conditioning regimens are not favored for infants and children because of the effect of TBI on growth, endocrine development, cataracts, dentition, aortic arch dysgenesis and agenesis of the female breast. The following measures are used to prevent, or minimize, regimen-related toxicities associated with myeloablative and non-myeloablative conditioning.

Chemotherapy dose and adjustments

To ensure accuracy of chemotherapy dosing and schedule, verification of medical orders is required by two physicians, two pharmacists, and two nurses. Details of these procedures are given in Table 20.7. Drug dosing is based on either body surface area or body weight, according to specific protocols. The ideal body weight (IBW) is calculated using standard charts per

Table 20.6.   *Intrathecal therapy for leukemia/lymphoma—adult dosages*[a]

	Methotrexate	Cytosine arabinoside[b]	Hydro-cortisone[c]
As single agent	15 mg	50–70 mg	–
In combination	15 mg	30 mg	15–50 mg

[a] All drugs should be in preservative-free diluent. Extreme care is needed to ensure that drugs and doses are correct. Fatalities have been reported from administration of the wrong drug or dose intrathecally.

[b] Use cytarabine powder with preservative-free diluent, not cytarabine liquid, which is hypertonic. Avoid giving at same time as systemic cytosine arabinoside, which may increase toxicity.

[c] Dissolve in preservative-free normal saline.

Table 20.7. *Guidelines for high-dose chemotherapy administration*

Physician orders
    Use preprinted orders.
    Specify protocol number and name of study on the orders.
    Specify daily drug dose and specific chemotherapy dates for all drugs.
Physician procedures
    Physician verifies that two staff members independently confirm the patient's height and weight.
    Attending physician verifies the name and protocol number and recalculates the drug dose.
    Attending physician co-signs all chemotherapy orders.
Pharmacist procedures
    Pharmacist verifies the name and protocol and recalculates the drug dose.
    Cumulative dose is recalculated and compared to the protocol maximum total cumulative dose.
Nursing procedures
    Two nurses establish the patient's identity and the drug for administration.
    Nurse verifies drug doses against both the order sheet and the protocol.
Institutional Procedures
    Multidisciplinary review of new or revised protocols and preprinted orders.
    Continuing staff education of chemotherapy safeguards.

age and sex. If the patient's weight is <100% of IBW, the actual weight is used for all drug dosing. If weight is >125% of IBW, an adjusted IBW is utilized for drug dosing. Adjusted IBW is calculated according to the following formula: Adjusted IBW = IBW + 0.25 [actual weight – IBW].

Busulfan targeted blood levels have been shown to decrease toxicity and optimize the therapeutic index in transplantation (Slattery *et al.*, 1997). To ensure adequate dosing of oral busulfan, antiemetics are given 1 hour prior to treatment, and the patient remains "nil by mouth" 1 hour before and after dosing. If any dose is vomited, the number of tablets is readministered. Subsequent dosing is adjusted on blood steady-state concentration values.

Total body irradiation (TBI)

Outpatient total body irradiation can be safely administered and patients can go home between each treatment dose. A regimen of four fractions of 3 Gy over 4 consecutive days has been described (Algara *et al.*, 1994; Dagher *et al.*, 1997; Applegate *et al.*, 1998), as has one of 6 fractions of 2 Gy over 3 days (Bredeson *et al.*, 2002). Ondansetron is effective for prevention of nausea.

Fluid administration

During irradiation, 1 to 1.5 times maintenance i.v. hydration (1,500 ml/m^2/24 hours) is started. A 16-hour infusion is administered at home through an infusion pump. To prevent dehydration and to decrease organ toxicity, i.v. hydration is also started in patients receiving i.v. chemotherapy in the AC. Patients

receiving busulfan treatment do not routinely receive i.v. fluids unless clinically indicated.

Alkalinization and allopurinol administration

To prevent crystallization of uric acid and to prevent obstructive nephropathy in patients at risk for tumor lysis (leukocytosis >20 × 10^9/l or bulky tumor), sodium bicarbonate (50 mEq/l) is added to i.v. dextrose-saline (DSW 1/4 NS) solution, also containing KCl (20 mEq/l). This is not a universal practice at other transplant centers. Allopurinol (200 mg/m^2/day) is given to patients with malignant disorders until 24 hours before the HSC infusion.

Mesna administration

To decrease the risk of cyclophosphamide-induced hemorrhagic cystitis, patients are treated with mesna. The total dose of mesna in milligrams equals the total cyclophosphamide dose, and it is administered in three divided doses daily during cyclophosphamide administration.

Anticonvulsants

To prevent seizures in patients receiving busulfan, phenytoin prophylaxis is administered. A loading dose of 15 mg/kg is given in three divided doses. The loading dose should be started the day before starting busulfan. A daily phenytoin maintenance dose is started 12 hours after the loading dose and continued for 2 days after the last busulfan dose. The dose is adjusted according to blood levels. It should be noted that phenytoin reduces cyclosporine (CSP) and tacrolimus (FK-506) blood levels. Other centers use clonazepam (1 mg i.v. b.i.d. daily) starting 2 hours before the initial dose of busulfan and stopping 4 days posttransplant. Other benzodiazepines have also been used including diazepam, clobezam, and lorazepam (Chan *et al.*, 2002).

Antiemetics

Several antiemetics are effective for controlling emesis induced by chemotherapy and TBI. Ondansetron has become one of the most common oral antiemetics used. Its antiemetic effect is mediated by antagonizing type 3 serotonin receptors (5-HT$_3$) in the brain and gastrointestinal tract. Ondansetron is given 1 to 2 hours po or 30 minutes i.v. prior to chemotherapy. The oral dose is 8 mg t.i.d. (adult) and 4 mg t.i.d. (4–11 years old). Ondansetron is continued for 24 hours after the last dose of cyclophosphamide because of delayed nausea/vomiting with this agent. Oral dosing has approximately 56% bioequivalency of i.v. dosing and is 4 times less expensive. The i.v. dose (0.15 mg/kg) is rounded to the nearest 10 mg/dose (adult) or to the nearest 1 mg (4–11 years old); for adults > 90 kg, round to 15 mg/dose. It is used in combination with dexamethasone in patients receiving cisplatin if the serotonin antagonist is not effective alone. Anxiolytic drugs (e.g., lorazepam) may also be appropriate in combination with ondansetron. Considering its cost, ondansetron is not recommended on an "as needed" basis, or for prolonged nausea and vomiting not responding after 24 hours of treatment.

Oral mucositis and treatment guidelines

Oral mucositis is the most common indication for analgesia after transplantation, especially after myeloablative TBI conditioning (Chapko *et al.,* 1989). In hospital, patient-controlled analgesia pumps decrease the total amount of analgesia (e.g., morphine) administered, while providing maximum pain relief (Hill *et al.,* 1990). Topical measures include oral rinsing with 0.9% saline every 30 to 60 minutes to prevent opportunistic infection and to wash out cellular debris. If mucous membranes are intact, viscous lidocaine or Dyclone every 30 to 60 minutes may be helpful in controlling pain. Recently, oral mucosal fentanyl citrate has been reported to relieve breakthrough cancer pain via mucosal absorption (Cleary, 1997; Simmonds, 1997). A new fentanyl transmucosal formulation is now being reviewed by the U.S. Food and Drug Administration. If efficacy and safety are also established in transplant recipients, short-acting lozenges may represent an ideal oral analgesic option for mucositis (and see Chapter 80).

One grading system is the World Health Organization oral mucosal toxicity scale:

Grade 0	Mucositis absent
Grade 1	Erythema and sore throat
Grade II	Ulcerations present but can eat
Grade III	Ulcerations present but cannot eat
Grade IV	Total parenteral nutrition needed

Total parenteral nutrition (TPN)

Most patients will require parenteral (PN), or total parenteral nutrition (TPN) for some period after transplant (Lenssen *et al.,* 1983). The indication for initiating PN or TPN depends on several factors: patient nutritional status, inability of oral intake for several days, and degree of gastrointestinal toxicity. A standard central venous TPN solution consisting of dextrose and amino acids with electrolytes, minerals, and vitamin additives is used (Table 20.8). TPN has been associated with improved survival when compared with i.v. hydration (Weisdorf *et al.,* 1987); however, results of a double-blind randomized trial found a delay in the resumption of oral intake in patients given TPN compared to i.v. hydration, and without significant differences in hospital readmission rate or survival between the two treatment groups (Charuhas *et al.,* 1997). The cost, duration, and benefits of TPN need to be carefully assessed in each patient (Klein & Koretz, 1994).

Procurement of hematopoietic stem cells and donor safety issues (and see Chapters 24 and 25)

Bone marrow

Leukapheresis of mobilized peripheral blood stem cells (PBSC) has now largely replaced use of autologous bone mar-

Table 20.8. *Total parenteral nutrition (TPN)*

Indication depends on
    Patient pretransplant nutritional status,
    Inability to eat for several days, and
    Degree of gastrointestinal toxicity

TPN guidelines
1. The dextrose load should not exceed 5 mg/kg/min over 24 hours (adults), 7–10 mg/kg/min (adolescent) and 12–14 mg/kg/min (children).
2. If a situation requiring salt restriction arises (pulmonary edema, hepatic VOD, fluid retention), the same TPN preparation, but without electrolytes, can be used. Potassium, magnesium and calcium supplementation may be required.
3. If hyperglycemia occurs (common with prednisone treatment for acute GVHD) Actrapid insulin, 10 units, may be added to each liter bag of glucose/amino acid TPN solution if the blood sugar level is 10 or higher. Increase the Actrapid dose by 10 units/bag daily, until the BSL is less than 10.
4. TPN solutions should only be infused through a central venous catheter.
5. TPN supplements
    Twice weekly: fat supplement (e.g., 20% Intralipid, 500 ml)
    Weekly: vitamin K, 10 mg s.c.
    Daily: multivitamin preparation; folic acid 5 mg i.v. or po
6. Laboratory monitoring
    Daily: biochemistry screen, including BSL
    Weekly: serum zinc; ionized calcium
    Twice weekly: coagulation screen (PTT, APTT)
    Thrice weekly: liver function tests

Abbreviations: VOD, veno-occlusive disease; BSL, blood sugar level; PTT, partial thromboplastin time; APTT, activated partial thromboplastin time.

row cells, and these cells are routinely collected on an outpatient basis. In a prospective randomized study of the two types of collection, more anxiety before the procedure was experienced by the bone marrow harvested patients (Auquier *et al.,* 1995). The marrow harvested patients also had more inconvenience with the procedure and significantly more pain. If autologous marrow harvesting needs to be performed it can be done as an ambulatory procedure with a very low postanesthesia complication rate, and postoperative pain is generally easily controlled (Bolwell *et al.,* 1995; Kovacs *et al.,* 1995; Thorne *et al.,* 1996). As an alternative to general anesthesia with endotracheal intubation, the use of local anesthesia and patient-controlled analgesia with fentanyl has been described for marrow harvesting (Sim *et al.,* 1996).

Bone marrow is still the commonest source of stem cells for allogeneic transplantation, although its use has been decreasing in the past few years because of increasing use of PBSC. The harvesting of bone marrow is not without risk. In a National Marrow Donor Program survey of 5,505 donors, the following non-life-threatening adverse events (AE) were noted: fatigue 79%, pain at the collection site 74%, pain on walking 68%, back pain 63%, sore throat 57%, pain on sitting 55%, nausea 52%, pain on climbing stairs 48%, light-headedness 46%, headache 34%, pain at i.v. site 31%, vomiting 29%, fever 27%, bandage pain 23%, prolonged bleeding 8%, and fainting 5%. Sciatic pain due to compression of the sciatic nerve by hematoma formation can be severe (Irving et al., 2000). Analgesic infiltration at the site of harvest can significantly reduce donor morbidity (Chern et al., 1999). In an IBMTR survey of 8,296 allogeneic donations, 24 life-threatening or incapacitating complications were identified (0.29%): three myocardial infarction, three severe anemia, two anaphylaxis, two prolonged paralysis during anesthesia, two pulmonary embolism, two severe back pain, one acute renal failure from incompatible blood transfusion, one anaphylaxis from incompatible blood transfusion, one hepatitis B infection, one intervertebral disk collapse, one malignant hypothermia, one paroxysmal tachycardia, one pulmonary edema, one retroperitoneal hemorrhage, one severe hypotension, and one severe vasovagal reaction. There are six known deaths reported following marrow donation. The causes of death reported included: two cardiac arrests prior to donation, one ventricular fibrillation during the marrow harvest, one anaphylaxis due to anesthetic, one cardiac arrest during the marrow harvest, and one pulmonary embolism after marrow harvest. Only four of the six deaths were clearly related to donation. Since the denominator was an estimated 60,000 marrow allografts at the time of the report, the risk was approximately 1 in 15,000 or 0.005%.

Bone marrow primed with G-CSF is being explored. In one study, hematopoietic reconstitution was faster with G-CSF primed marrow compared to unprimed marrow, but was not as fast as G-CSF mobilized PBSC (Lowenthal et al., 1999). A prospective, randomized clinical study found that the use of G-CSF primed, HLA-identical sibling bone marrow was associated with a comparable engraftment rate to that of G-CSF mobilized PBSC, a reduced incidence of severe acute GVHD and a reduced incidence of extensive chronic GVHD (Morton et al., 2001). The cumulative incidence of prednisone-refractory acute GVHD was 18% and 47% respectively ($P < .002$), and the cumulative incidence of extensive chronic GVHD was 22% and 80% respectively ($P < .003$).

Minors and even infants as young as 6 months of age can be used as allogeneic marrow donors (Chan et al., 1996). G-CSF was used in one 11-month-old HLA-matched sibling donor in order to obtain an adequate number of mononuclear cells in a limited volume of bone marrow (Pession et al., 1996).

In a study of the effect of short-term in vivo administration of G-CSF on autologous bone marrow prior to harvesting, 57 patients with solid tumors had approximately 500 ml of steady-state marrow harvested as outpatients under local anesthesia. Each patient then received 5 µg/kg of G-CSF every 12 hours for either 24 hours, 36 hours, or 48 hours prior to harvesting 500 ml of activated bone marrow. Marrow cellularity increased after G-CSF administration, and although the percentage of CD34+ cells did not significantly change in stimulated marrow, the total number of CD34+ cells collected increased from 34×10^6 to 52×10^6 after two injections of G-CSF and from 28 to 75 $\times 10^6$ after four injections of G-CSF. Further phenotyping

demonstrated a significant increase in CD34+ HLA-DR+ cells with all three G-CSF schedules. Reinfusion of the median of 1.6×10^6 activated CD34+ cells/kg resulted in recovery of 0.1×10^9/l neutrophils and more than 20×10^9/l platelets by days 9 and 19, respectively (Dicke et al., 1997).

Peripheral blood stem cells

The use of PBSC transplantation has been increasing rapidly for HLA-identical sibling transplantation and is being explored for unrelated donor transplantation. Allogeneic PBSCT has emerged as an alternative to bone marrow transplantation (BMT) for the treatment of advance hematologic malignant diseases. Nearly all studies have shown earlier hematopoietic recovery with PBSCT than with BMT and similar rates of acute GVHD (Bensinger et al., 2001; Champlin et al., 2000; Powles et al., 2000; Schmitz et al., 1998). In some studies, the incidence of clinical extensive chronic GVHD in allogeneic recipients was higher with PBSCT than with BMT (Vigorito et al., 1998; Solano et al., 1998), but others have not confirmed these findings (Bensinger et al., 2001; Champlin et al., 2000). Results of a meta-analysis showed that chronic GVHD occurred more frequently after PBSCT compared to BMT, with a trend towards a protective effect of PBSCT in preventing relapse (Ito et al., 2001). In a multi-center phase III trial comparing PBSCT to BMT from HLA-matched related donors, we found no statistically significant difference in the cumulative incidence of acute or clinical extensive chronic GVHD in the 2 groups (Bensinger et al., 2001). However, in a recent study, we found that the number of successive treatments needed to control chronic GVHD was higher after PBSCT than after BMT ($P = .03$), and the duration of glucocorticoid treatment was longer after PBSCT compared to BMT ($P = .03$) (Flowers et al., 2002). These results suggest that chronic GVHD after PBSCT may be more protracted and less responsive to current treatment than chronic GVHD after BMT. Assessment of the overall benefits of PBSCT compared to BMT will require continued long-term evaluation of quality of life and follow up of morbidity associated with chronic GVHD in long-term survivors.

In a survey of donors enrolled in a randomized study of marrow versus PBSC transplants, the levels of physical discomfort were similar between the two groups, but a quicker resolution of symptoms occurred in the PBSC donors: all PBSC donors, as opposed to 79% of marrow donors, reported good physical status by 14 days after the harvest procedure (Rowley et al., 2001). In an NMDP study of unrelated donors whose first donation was marrow and whose second donation was either peripheral blood stem cells or marrow, PBSC donation was associated with fewer donation-related side-effects, was less physically difficult, time-consuming and inconvenient, and was considered preferable by the donors (Switzer et al., 2001) (Fig. 20.3). Adverse events also occur with the use of PBSC as a source of stem cells for transplantation: non-life-threatening AEs due to G-CSF include bone pain in the majority (80–90%), headache in 30–40%, myalgia (~20%), fatigue (~15%), nausea and vomiting (~10%), injection

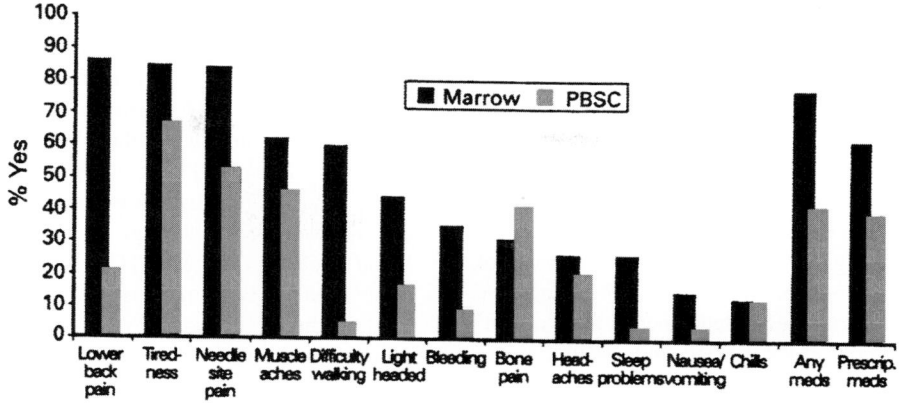

Fig. 20.3. Physical side-effects of second donation. Reproduced, with permission, from Switzer *et al.* (2001)

site reactions (rare), a rise in liver enzymes (common), a rise in white blood cell count (universal), and mild thrombocytopenia (common) (Fig. 20.4). Non-life-threatening AEs due to the apheresis procedure include bruising around the antecubital veins (common), symptoms of hypocalcemia due to use of acid citrate dextrose as anticoagulant (fairly common), thrombocytopenia (common), and mild lymphopenia (common). Pyogenic infection (dental and perianal abscesses) immediately following mobilization with G-CSF have been described (Hilbe *et al.*, 2000). Several major and life-threatening complications have been reported with PBSC donation, including flares of rheumatoid arthritis, ankylos-

ing spondylitis and iritis/episcleritis. One case of ruptured spleen and one of myocardial infarction have been reported. Two deaths are known to have been associated with PBSC donation. One donor had a stroke several days after donation, and one had a cardiac arrest several days after apheresis.

Pediatric PBSC donors have been also utilized (González *et al.*, 1999; Pahys *et al.*, 2000). The smallest donor reported (Pahys *et al.*, 2000) weighed 6.1 kg and was 7 months old. Since a very slow flow rate was expected, the donor was given 80 mg of aspirin on the night before the apheresis. A 7-French double-lumen dialysis catheter inserted in the right femoral

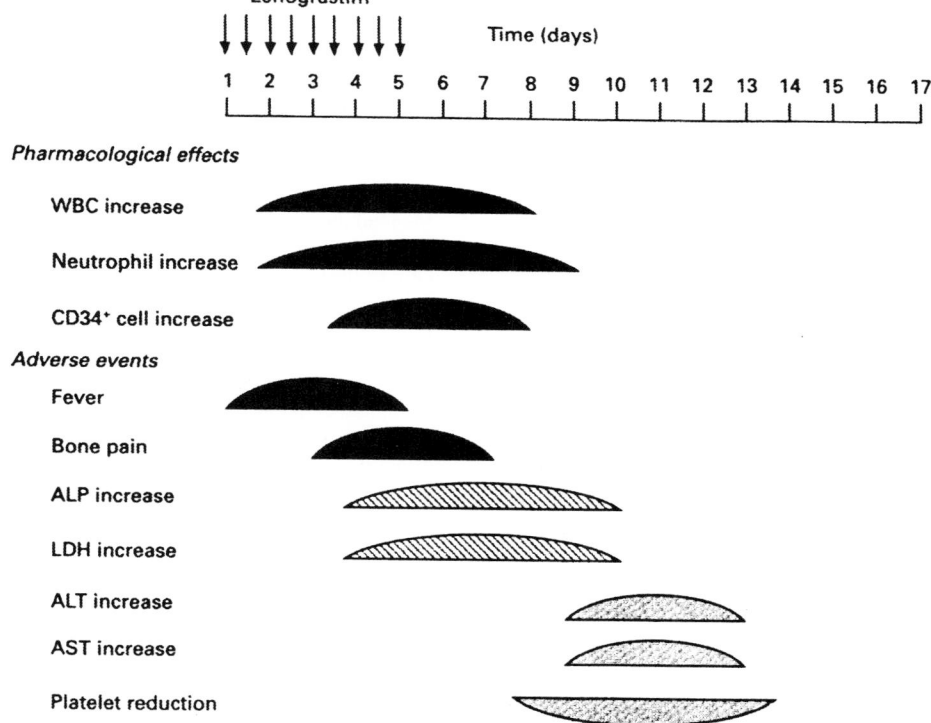

Fig. 20.4. Adverse events after rhG-CSF administration. Pharmacological effects and adverse events including abnormal clinical laboratory test results during and after repeated-dose administration of rh-G-CSF (lenograstim). Reproduced, with permission, from Akizuki *et al.* (2000).

vein was used for access and the right leg was subsequently immobilized in a buttock-to-ankle splint. Heparin and ACD-A were used for anticoagulation. After approximately 6 hours and processing 2,972 ml of the donor's blood, a total of 4.4×10^6 CD34+ cells/kg recipient weight were collected.

Other donor issues

The likelihood of requiring central line placement because of poor venous access in normal donors is up to 10% and adverse events associated with central lines include pneumothorax, hemorrhage and infection—both of the exit site and systemic infection (line sepsis). Only a single needle pass was required in 95% of cases when ultrasound guidance was used for placement of a central venous catheter by the transjugular route in a series of 91 allogeneic donors (Sadler et al., 2000). Guidelines for donor workup have been published (Cleaver et al., 1997). A number of studies have reported on microbial contamination of both bone marrow and peripheral blood stem cell preparations (Prince et al., 1995; Attarian et al., 1996; Cohen et al., 1996; Padley et al., 1996; Smith et al., 1996). Isolates were predominantly skin contaminants (Gram-positive cocci) or Gram-negative rods. There was a 6% rate of positivity in marrow compared to a 0.5% rate of positivity in peripheral blood preparations in one study (Padley et al., 1996). No adverse clinical sequelae were noted following infusion of any contaminated products.

Occasionally donors have been reported who themselves have had an illness, including one receiving prednisone, azathioprine, and cyclosporine after a renal allograft (Adams et al., 1994), one with the Fragile X syndrome of mental retardation (Morton et al., 1995), one with systemic lupus erythematosu (Sturfelt et al., 1996), and one with Hunter syndrome (Meyer et al., 2000). No untoward effects were noted in either recipient or donor. In contrast, there have been several instances of donors being diagnosed retrospectively with hematological malignancies, with subsequent transmission of the disease to the recipient. Inadvertent transmission of a donor's acute myeloid leukemia has been described in a patient transplanted for CML (Niederwieser et al., 1990). A patient with refractory Hodgkin's disease received bone marrow and peripheral blood stem cells from her sister who was subsequently found to have early asymptomatic myelodysplasia (refractory anemia with [del(20q)]. Engraftment was prompt, and was of donor origin, but throughout the period of observation, the percentage of cells with this abnormality was comparable to that in the donor (Mielcarek et al., 1999). T-cell lymphoma has been transmitted by allogeneic marrow transplantation (Berg et al., 2001): subcutaneous panniculitic T-cell lymphoma occurred three and five years respectively after the procedure in both donor and recipient. The finding of identical T cell clones in the tumors of both sisters implicated the transfer of neoplastic T cells during the marrow transplant as the cause of the recipient's lymphoma.

Graft-versus-host disease (GVHD) prophylaxis

Cyclosporine (CSP) and methotrexate (MTX) comprise the standard method of acute GVHD prophylaxis at FHCRC (Storb et al., 1986). CSP is started the day before the transplant and continued through day 180 posttransplant (1.5 mg/kg i.v. b.i.d. or 6 mg/kg po b.i.d.). MTX is given i.v. on day +1 posttransplant (15 mg/m^2) and then at 10 mg/m^2 on days +3, +6, and +11. Other regimens, including tacrolimus plus MTX, and prednisone plus CSP (Chao et al., 1993), have not been shown to be superior to the CSP/MTX combination. Blood levels of CSP and tacrolimus are followed weekly through day +100. In Seattle, therapeutic blood levels for CSP using TDX assay are between 150 and 250 ng/ml, and for tacrolimus using IMX, 10 to 15 ng/ml. Criteria used to adjust CSP and tacrolimus dose are based on renal function, risk and severity of GVHD, and blood levels. For instance, CSP and tacrolimus are withheld if the serum creatinine value exceeds double the patient's baseline value or exceeds 2.0 mg/dl. Dose adjustment is recommended for tacrolimus blood levels >15 ng/ml. Tacrolimus blood levels ≥ 20 ng/dl are associated with increased toxicity (Ratanatharathorn et al., 1996) (see Chapter 83).

Two retrospective analyses reported no difference in the incidence of acute GVHD grade II-IV in patients in whom the day +11 MTX was omitted for clinical reasons (Atkinson & Downs, 1995; Kumar et al., 2002), although the incidence of grade III-IV was increased in one (Kumar et al., 2002). Guidelines used in some programs for withholding MTX are as follows: Methotrexate dose may be withheld in the following circumstance: (a) Presence of Grade IV oral mucositis; Methotrexate dose should be withheld in the following circumstances: (b) Development of significant collections of ascitic or pleural fluid. (c) Increase in serum creatinine of >50% above baseline; Methotrexate dose should be reduced by 50% in the

Table 20.9. *Chronic GVHD screening studies*

Complete skin examination with percent of body surface area recorded using the rule of nine
Medical photographs recommended if abnormal skin exam
Skin biopsy (sun-exposed area if normal exam)
Oral examination (look for lichen-planus, pseudomembrane, hyerkeratosis, ulcers, lip and buccal mucosa atrophy, erythema)
Pulmonary function tests[a] (obstructive or restrictive defect)
Schirmer's test (abnormal if median value of both eyes <10 mm with symptoms)
Complete blood count (thrombocytopenia; eosinophilia)
Liver function tests (alkaline phosphatase, AST, bilirubin)
Renal function (serum creatinine, urea)
Serum IgG, IgA, IgM
Range of motion (ROM) of joints (if fasciitis, scleroderma suspected)
CPK, aldolase (if myopathy suspected); autoantibodies such as AMA, ASMA, ANA, RA (if joint or myofascial involvement suspected but without other manifestation of chronic GVHD)
Clinical performance (Karnofsky, ECOG, SWOG or Lansky Play scales)[b]

[a] Including: FEV1, FEV1/FVC, FEF 25–75%, RV, TLC & DLCO corrected
[b] See Tables 20.12–20.15.

Table 20.10.   *Criteria for hospital re-admission*

1. Shaking chills and/or fever ≥ 38.5°C in neutropenic patient
2. Septicemia
3. Gram-negative bacteremia or fungemia
4. Uncontrolled GVHD
5. Graft failure
6. Interstitial pneumonia
7. Varicella zoster infection (some cases)
8. Medical emergencies/acute organ failure
9. Failure to thrive
   weight loss [>10% of discharge weight (adult) or >5% of
     discharge weight (child)]
   fluid losses exceeding what can be replaced with maximal
     ambulatory support

following circumstance: (d) Increase in serum creatinine of 25-50% above baseline.

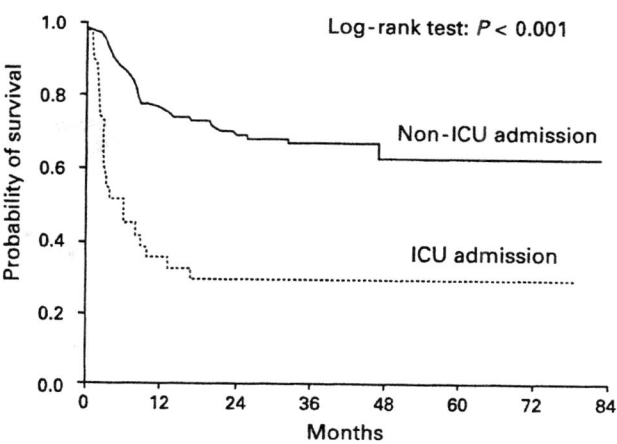

Fig. 20.7. Probabilities of survival for bone marrow transplanted patients according to ICU admission or non-admission. Reproduced, with permission, from Diaz de Heredia *et al.* (1999)

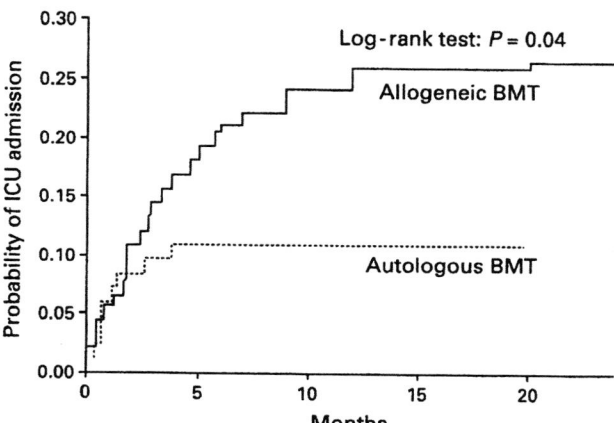

Fig. 20.5. Probabilities of presenting a complication requiring ICU admission in patients undergoing allogeneic BMT and autologous BMT. Reproduced, with permission, from Diaz de Heredia *et al.* (1999).

Acute graft-versus-host disease treatment

Corticosteroids (for example methylprednisolone, 2 mg/kg/day for 14 days or longer) are the mainstay of acute GVHD therapy. Complete responses occur in 20%, and useful responses overall in about 40% to 50% of patients with grades II to IV acute GVHD. A prospective randomized study comparing 2 mg/kg/day of methylprednisolone to 10 mg/kg/day failed to show any advantage of the higher dose for any end point studied (Van Lint *et al.*, 1998). Steroid-refractory acute GVHD is a serious development with no adequate therapy, although ATG has been a commonly used approach (Arai *et al.*, 2002) (and see Chapter 71). A definition of steroid-refractory acute GVHD used by some programs is as follows: (a) acute GVHD grade II-IV progressive after 3 days of treatment with methylprednisolone at a dose of 2 mg/kg/day; (b) persistent actue GVHD grade III-IV after 7 days of treatment with methylprednisolone at a dose of 2 mg/kg/day; and (c) persistent acute GVHD grade II after 14 days treatment with methylprednisolone 2 mg/kg/day.

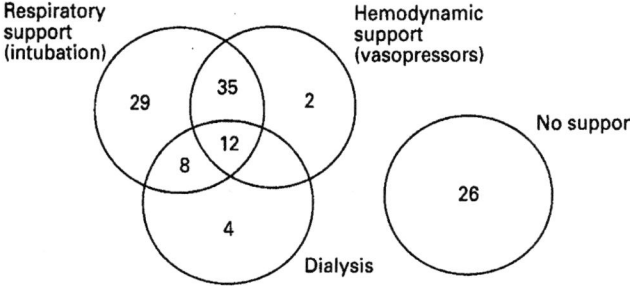

Fig. 20.6. Number of patients requiring different types of supportive care during their initial ICU admission. Reproduced, with permission, from Jackson *et al.* (1998).

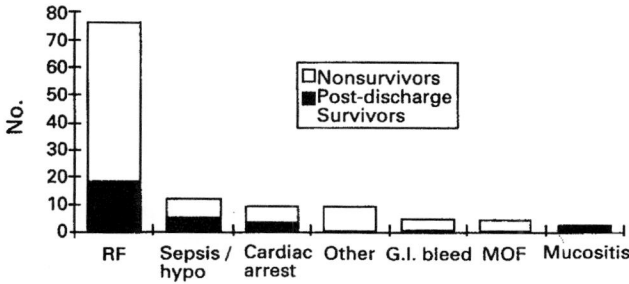

Fig. 20.8. Post-discharge survival of patients by ICU admission diagnosis. RF = respiratory failure; Hypo = hypotension; MOF = multiorgan failure. Reproduced, with permission, from Jackson *et al.* (1998).

Table 20.11. *Indications for mechanical ventilation and post-ventilation survival*

Reasons for mechanical ventilation	n	Numbers of patients	
		Survival to ICU discharge	Survival to hospital discharge
Pulmonary			
Pneumonia/infection	26	11	2
Idiopathic pneumonitis	4	1	1
ARDS	5	4	1
Post-bronchoscopy/OLB	11	2	0
Hemorrhage	14	7	3
Total	60	25	8
Nonpulmonary			
Sepsis/metabolic acidosis	8	2	1
Cardiac arrest	9	3	3
CNS depression	10	1	0
Postoperative	3	2	0
Fluid overload	10	5	4
Total	40	13	8

Abbreviations: ARDS, acute respiratory distress syndrome; OLB, open lung biopsy; CNS, central nervous system.
Reproduced with permission from Jackson *et al.* (1998)

Chronic GVHD screening

Chronic GVHD screening (Table 20.9) and assessment of GVHD morbidity are obtained in allogeneic patients transplanted in Seattle between days 80 and 100, when the diagnosis of chronic GVHD is suspected or documented, at one year after transplant and when treatment response is assessed.

Hospital admission and discharge criteria

The most frequent reasons for hospital admission during conditioning are inability to tolerate oral medications, neutropenic fever, infection, and diarrhea. Criteria for hospital readmission are listed in Table 20.10.

The probability of admission of transplant patients to the intensive care unit (ICU) is shown in Fig. 20.5 and the proportion of patients admitted to ICU according to the different type of supportive care needed are shown in Fig. 20.6. For patients requiring ICU the outlook historically has been relatively poor (Jackson *et al.*, 1998; Díaz de Heredia *et al.*, 1999) (Figs. 20.7 and 20.8). Indications for, and survival of, patients requiring mechanical ventilation are shown in Table 20.11.

Hospital discharge is facilitated by a transition nurse, who plays an essential role in discharge planning. Clinical parameters used at FHCRC/SCCA for hospital discharge to the AC facility include:

1. Sufficient ambulation to maintain daily clinic visits
2. Adequate training of caregivers for continuing monitoring and treatment at home

3. Ability to take oral fluids
4. Tolerance of oral medications
5. IV medication deliverable in minibag preparation (e.g., cyclosporine, ganciclovir, etc.)
6. No need for i.v. narcotics
7. Manageable amounts of i.v. fluids for home delivery
8. Successful transfer from i.v. to po medications 48 hours prior to discharge
9. Platelets $\geq 10 \times 10^9/l$ supportable with <2 platelet transfusions/day
10. Absence of fever and active infection

Ambulatory follow-up care

Rounds

Daily rounds are carried out by the ambulatory health care team daily during regular week days. Primary physicians or middle level practitioners review the results of diagnostic tests and medical history for discussion with the attending physician, primary care nurse, pharmacist, dietitian, and social worker.

Clinic visits

Patients are seen daily for clinic visits during the conditioning regimen. After engraftment, comprehensive patient examination is continued with weekly clinic visits by the primary physician and by the attending physician. Drop-in clinic visits are triaged by the ambulatory nurse.

Laboratory and ambulatory follow-up monitoring

General guidelines for frequency of routine blood tests and other evaluations are described below:

- Daily complete blood counts (CBC) if white blood cell count $< 1.0 \times 10^9/l$ or platelets $<20 \times 10^9/l$. After counts stabilize, CBC frequency is reduced to 1 to 3 times per week. Patients on ganciclovir or mycophenolate mofetil need at least twice weekly CBC. After day 100, weekly CBC for the first two months is performed, and if stable, twice monthly thereafter, unless receiving immunosuppressive mediations, when weekly CBC is recommended.
- Daily creatinine, BUN, electrolytes, and glucose measurements usually required during conditioning until day 7 post-transplant; then, if stable, 2 to 3 times per week if on CSP, tacrolimus, TPN, or MTX. A score based on day 7 blood urea nitrogen and creatinine values has been used to predict risk of transplant-related mortality (Bacigalupo *et al.*, 1999). Calcium, magnesium, phosphorus, and albumin measurements twice weekly; then, if stable, weekly until off TPN. If CSP or tacrolimus result in magnesium wasting, twice weekly magnesium serum levels are obtained. Alkaline phosphatase, transaminases, and bilirubin measurements initially 3 times weekly; then, if stable, 1 to 2 times weekly.
- Weekly CSP or tacrolimus blood levels until day 100 and monthly thereafter if levels stable.

Table 20.12. *Karnofsky performance score*

	Score %	
Able to carry on normal activity; no special care is needed	100	Normal; no complaints; no evidence of disease
	90	Able to carry on normal activity; minor signs or symptoms of disease
	80	Normal activity with effort; some signs or symptoms of disease
Unable to work; able to live at home and care for most personal needs; varying amounts of assistance are needed	70	Cares for self; unable to carry on normal activity or to do active work
	60	Requires occasional assistance but is able to care for most needs
	50	Requires considerable assistance and frequent medical care
Unable to care for self; requires equivalent of institutional or hospital care; disease may be progressing rapidly	40	Disabled; requires special care and assistance
	30	Severely disabled; hospitalization indicated, although death not imminent
	20	Very sick; hospitalization necessary
	10	Moribund; fatal processes progressing rapidly
	0	Dead

Table 20.13. *ECOG/WHO Performance Status*

Score	Description
0	Fully active; able to carry out all predisease activities without restriction and without the aid of analgesia
1	Restricted in strenuous activity, but ambulatory and able to carry out light work or pursue a sedentary occupation; patients who are fully active but require analgesia
2	Ambulatory and capable of all self-care, but unable to carry out any work; up and about more than 50% of waking hours
3	Capable of only limited self-care, confined to bed or chair more than 50% of waking hours
4	Completely disabled; unable to carry out any self-care, confined totally to bed or chair
5	Dead
Summary:	
0	Normal activity
1	Symptoms, but ambulatory
2	In bed <50% of time
3	In bed >50% of time
4	100% bedridden
5	Dead

Table 20.14. *SWOG patient performance status grading scale*

Grade	Scale
0	Fully active; able to carry on all predisease activities without restriction. (Karnofsky 90% to 100%)
1	Restricted in physically strenuous activity but ambulatory and able to perform work of a light or sedentary nature, e.g., light housework or office work. (Karnofsky 70% to 80%)
2	Ambulatory and capable of all self-care but unable to perform any work activities. Up and about more than 50% of waking hours. (Karnofsky 50% to 60%)
3	Capable of only limited self-care; confined to bed or chair more than 50% of waking hours. (Karnofsky 40% to 50%)
4	Completely disabled. Cannot perform any self-care. Totally confined to bed or chair. (Karnofsky 10% to 20%)
5	Dead

- Blood cultures for fevers, and weekly if receiving corticosteroids >1.0 mg/kg/day.
- CMV blood surveillance (using CMV DNA by PCR or hybrid capture, pp67 mRNA or pp65 antigenemia) is recommended weekly for seropositive patients until day 100. For CMV-seronegative allogeneic recipients and CD34-selected autologous transplant patients, CMV in blood should be monitored weekly until day 60 after transplant. After day 60 or 100 posttransplant, CMV monitoring should continue, initially weekly, until 1 year after transplant for allogeneic patients at risk of late CMV disease which include:

Table 20.15. *Lansky play scale (for children ages 1–16 years)*

The Lansky play-performance scale is designed to provide a standardized measure of the performance status of the child with cancer. Parents are asked to select the description that best describes the child's play during the past week, averaging out good days and bad days:

Score %	Description
100	Fully active, normal
90	Minor restrictions in physically strenuous activity
80	Active, but tires more quickly
70	Both greater restriction of, and less time spent in, play activity
60	Up and around, but minimal active play; keeps busy with quieter activities
50	Gets dressed, but lies around much of the day; no active play; able to participate in all quiet play and activities
40	Mostly in bed; participates in quiet activities
30	In bed; needs assistance even for quiet play
20	Often sleeping; play entirely limited to very passive activities
10	No play; does not get out of bed
0	Unresponsive

CMV-seropositive recipients receiving steroids for chronic GVHD

Patients who were treated for CMV early after transplant.

- Frequency of CMV blood surveillance after day 100 posttransplant is outlined in more detail below under long-term follow-up recommendations.
- Bone marrow aspiration/biopsy on day +28 and between days +75 and 100 posttransplant
- Chimerism tests on peripheral blood (CD3+ and CD33+ cells) using sex chromosome probes, in situ hybridization or DNA fingerprinting between days +75 and +100
- Chest x-ray twice monthly through day 100 for patients at high risk of fungal infection: absolute neutrophil count $<0.5 \times 10^9$/l; acute GVHD grade $\geq$ 2; on corticosteroid treatment >0.5 mg/kg/day; thereafter once a month or as clinically indicated.
- Daily caloric and fluid intake records until stable.

Departure evaluation and chronic GVHD screening

Between days 75 and 100 posttransplant, recipients undergo a complete evaluation including disease-specific staging, engraftment status with assessment of donor chimerism, organ toxicity assessment, clinical performance assessment, chronic GVHD screening for allograft recipients (Loughran et al., 1990), and other protocol-specific evaluations as indicated. Chronic GHVD screening is described in Table 20.9. Patient's clinical performance is recorded using validated methods such as the Karnofsky (Table 20.12), ECOG (Table 20.13) or SWOG (Table 20.14) performance scores or the Lansky play scale (Table 20.15). Based on the results of the departure evaluation and patient eligibility, patients will be enrolled in protocols for GVHD prevention or treatment (Sullivan et al., 1991), late infection (Marr et al., 2000; Boeckh et al., 1996), or recurrent disease prevention studies (Radich et al., 2001). The aim of these clinical trials is to decrease the morbidity and mortality associated with late transplant complications.

In preparation for return to the care of the primary physician, patients transplanted in Seattle and their families attend classes by the long-term follow-up (LTFU) team. These LTFU classes focus on management of medications, recognition of side effects, nutrition, guidelines for daily activities, manifestations of chronic GVHD, and monitoring of signs of late transplant complications. Referring physicians are contacted by telephone and receive a LTFU guidelines brochure to help with the continued care of the transplant patient. Prior to discharge, patients are asked to complete the LTFU patient heath questionnaire which includes:

1. contact information
2. self-assessment performance score
3. review of systems
4. interval events and complications
5. medications list
6. SF-12 Quality of Life assessment.

In addition, a GVHD morbidity assessment (Table 20.16) by the LTFU middle level practitioner and medical photographs

are taken of all allogeneic recipients prior to their discharge from our center.

Long-term follow-up recommendations

Prior to departure from the transplant center, the attending physician conducts a discharge conference with the patient and his or her family and team nurse. The physician reviews the results of the departure evaluation and discusses in detail the treatment plan and monitoring to be continued at home. These recommendations are discussed by telephone with the primary physician before the patient is discharged home. In addition, a discharge letter and medical summaries are sent by the attending and the primary physician detailing the patient's transplant course, treatment, and long-term follow-up recommendations. Printed schedules of immunosuppression, antibiotic prophylaxis, and frequency of blood drawings and clinic visits are provided. CMV blood surveillance after day 100 posttransplant should be continued weekly for at least one year posttransplant for patients at risk of late CMV disease (Boeckh et al., 1996; Boeckh et al., 1996) (i.e., prior history of CMV infection or seropositive patients receiving treatment with corticosteroids $\geq$1 mg/kg/day for GVHD). CMV monitoring every other week may be sufficient for patients receiving lower dose of corticosteroids and who have had three consecutive negative surveillance tests after day 100. If treatment with corticosteroids is increased or if additional systemic immunosuppressive treatment for chronic GVHD is added, weekly CMV monitoring should be resumed for as long as is clinically indicated.

Complete blood cell counts should be monitored at least weekly in patients treated with ganciclovir (see Table 20.4) because of the 40% incidence of cytopenia observed with this medication (Atkinson et al., 1991; Goodrich et al., 1993). Patients receiving immunosuppressive medications for chronic GVHD should receive daily TMP-SMX or a combination of daily penicillin-VK and twice weekly TMP-SMX for prevention of encapsulated bacterial and PCP infections. IVIG replacement (400 mg/kg/monthly) is recommended for patients with serum IgG levels <400 mg/dl until levels become self-sustaining. Vaccination should be deferred at least until one year after transplantation (Chapters 73 and 74).

Table 20.17 describes a fact sheet with additional general LTFU guidelines sent to the referring physicians for patients transplanted in Seattle. The referring physician is asked to complete a diagnostic checklist yearly after transplant which includes the following:

1. sites affected by chronic GVHD
2. disabling complications due to chronic GVHD
3. infections listed by organism
4. other organ system problems
5. new and recurrent malignancy
6. discontinuation of immunosuppressive medications
7. patient clinical performance scale.

Referring physicians are also encouraged to contact the LTFU office if there are any new medical developments. Patients are asked to complete the patient health questionnaire at 6-month

Table 20.16. *Chronic GVHD morbidity assessment scale after allogeneic transplantation[a]*

Performance score: PS:___	☐ asymptomatic and fully active (ECOG 0; KPS/Lansky 100%) ☐ symptomatic, fully ambulatory, restricted only in physically strenuous activity (ECOG 1, KPS 80–90%) ☐ symptomatic, ambulatory, capable of self-care, > 50% of waking hours out of bed (ECOG 2, KPS 60–70%) ☐ symptomatic, limited self care, > 50% of waking hours in bed (ECOG 3–4, KPS <60%)

Skin:	☐ no cutaneous changes caused by chronic GVHD
	☐ <18% BSA rash (erythema, pigment change, ichthyosis or lichenoid) *or* any scleroderma (pockets of normal skin)
	☐ 18–50% BSA rash *or* any scleroderma (no pockets of normal skin but not hidebound)
	☐ >50% BSA rash, *or* any scleroderma (hidebound, unable to pinch) *or* interference with ADL due to impaired
	   mobility or ulceration
	☐ abnormality present but not thought to represent GVHD
	Clinical features: ☐ erythematous macular papular ☐ lichenoid changes ☐ hyperpigmentation ☐ erythema
	                    ☐ pruritus ☐ hypopigmentation ☐ ichthyosis, ☐ scleroderma
	                 % BSA involved:_____ Rodnan Score:_____

Mouth:	☐ asymptomatic, no physical manifestations of chronic GVHD ☐ oral symptoms (dryness, food sensitivity or oral pain) *or* physical manifestations (erythema, hyperkeratosis, lichenoid or ulceration), no interference with oral intake ☐ oral symptoms or physical manifestations with partial limitation of oral intake ☐ oral symptoms or physical manifestations with major limitation of oral intake ☐ abnormality present but not thought to represent GVHD

Eyes:
 	
Tear test:
 	
OD___
OS___
	☐ asymptomatic, no keratitis, Schirmer's test >10 mm (mean of both eyes)
	☐ asymptomatic keratitis *or* symptomatic ocular sicca (Schirmer's 5–10 mm, mean of both eyes) not affecting ADL
	☐ symptoms caused by keratoconjunctivitis ocular sicca without vision impairment but requiring frequent use of
	   moisturizers (>3 × day)
	
	☐ loss of vision caused by pseudomembranes, corneal ulceration *or* needing special glasses (i.e., goggles) to relieve
	   pain/discomfort despite punctual ligation *or* unable to work due only to ocular symptoms
	☐ abnormality present but not thought to represent GVHD

Gut:	☐ no GI symptoms (anorexia, nausea, vomiting or diarrhea), weight stable ☐ GI symptoms, not requiring parenteral fluids or nutrition, weight stable ☐ GI symptoms requiring partial support with parenteral fluids or nutrition, weight stable ☐ GI symptoms requiring virtually complete parenteral nutrition *or* weight loss ≥ 15% not due to other causes ☐ abnormality present but not thought to represent GVHD
Liver:	☐ total bilirubin < 1.6, AP < 130 ☐ total bilirubin 1.6–3.0, AP 130–260 ☐ total bilirubin 3.1–6.0, AP 261–520 ☐ abnormal liver function tests not due to other causes with total bilirubin >6.0, AP >5 × normal, AST or ALT >3 × normal ☐ abnormality present but not thought to represent GVHD
Lungs:	☐ asymptomatic ☐ 51–75% FEV_1, <65% FEV_1/FVC *or* decrease of DLCO by >12% within <1 year *or* dyspnea with moderate exertion ☐ 25–50% FEV_1 *or* dyspnea with mild exertion *or* desaturation with exercise ☐ <25% FEV_1 *or* dyspnea at rest *or* requirement for supplemental oxygen during exercise or rest ☐ abnormality present but not thought to represent GVHD
Joints and fasciae:	☐ full range of motion ☐ tightness limited to arms *or* tightness limited to legs ☐ contractures that do not affect ADL *or* tightness involving both upper and lower extremities ☐ contractures that interfere with ADL ☐ abnormality present but not thought to represent GVHD
Genital tract:	☐ asymptomatic ☐ physical manifestations (atrophy, erythema, lichenoid changes or edema) with no effect on coitus or ADL ☐ physical manifestations causing coital symptoms without affecting any other ADL ☐ physical manifestations affecting ADL ☐ abnormality present but not thought to represent GVHD

Clinical manifestations or severe complications related to chronic GVHD (Check all that apply):

☐ Weight loss	☐ Bronchiolitis obliterans	☐ Bronchiolitis obliterans organizing pneumonia (BOOP)		
☐ Eosinophilia (>0.4 × 10³/µl)	☐ Malabsorption	☐ Esophageal stricture or web	☐ Fasciitis	☐ Serositis
Platelets <100,000	☐ Yes☐ No	☐ Myositis	☐ Other:_____	☐ None

Abbreviations: KPS, Karnofsky performance score; BSA, body surface area; AP, alkaline phosphatase; ADL, activities of daily living.

[a] Baseline at days 80–100, at the time of GVHD diagnosis, at one year and at time of treatment assessments

Table 20.17. *General long-term follow-up recommendations for adult patients*

These long-term follow-up guidelines describe generally accepted practices for medical care after hematopoietic stem cell transplantation. Recommendations in these guidelines must be implemented in a way that accounts for the specific situation of each individual patient. Recommendations for patients who are enrolled in specific protocols may be different and will be communicated separately.

1. Oncologic screening evaluation at yearly intervals should include an interval history and complete physical examination, Pap smears and mammogram (women), prostate exam (men), and testing for occult blood in stool. Oral examination should be done by a dentist at 6 month intervals. The skin and head and neck are the most common sites of secondary malignancies.

2. The detection of *bcr/abl* transcripts by PCR at 6–12 months after transplant for treatment of CML is associated with a 40% increase in the risk of relapse. A positive test result at >18 months after transplant is associated with a 20% increase in the risk of relapse. We recommend routine monitoring for *bcr/abl* transcripts by PCR testing of a blood sample every 6 months for the first 2 years after transplant and yearly thereafter if results of the PCR test remain negative. We would prefer that all the follow-up testing be done in our laboratory. The LTFU office will send you the results of PCR testing with further recommendations as applicable.

3. Measures should be taken to prevent osteoporosis in patients receiving long-term treatment with corticosteroids:
   Calcium 1500 mg/day in the diet or in supplements to meet daily requirements
   Vitamin D of 800 IU/day in the diet or in supplements to meet daily requirements
   Daily weight bearing exercise for 20–60 minutes
   Bone density test annually
   Sex hormone replacement therapy if levels are low
   The safety of bisphosphonates for prevention of bone loss after hematopoetic transplantation has not been studied in a systematic fashion.

4. Antibiotic prophylaxis should be maintained for 6 months after discontinuing all immunosuppressive medications in patients who have had chronic GVHD. Herbal medications and naturopathic remedies should not be administered to immunocompromised patients.

5. Pulmonary function should be tested at 1 year and at 5 years after transplant and annually in patients receiving treatment for chronic GVHD.

6. Thyroid function should be tested at annual intervals.

7. Ophthalmologic examination, Schirmer's test, and slit lamp exam should be performed at annual intervals.

8. Immunizations should be deferred until one year after transplant (see Chapters 73 and 74).

and yearly intervals to update the LTFU database. Data received by the LTFU are entered immediately in the data base if they are major data items:

1. death of the patient
2. diagnosis or change in therapy of chronic GVHD
3. diagnosis of recurrent malignancy
4. diagnosis of secondary malignancy or myelodysplasia
5. surgery or biopsy planned for secondary malignancy

6. change of referring physician
7. change of patient's name or address and
8. request from patients that we not contact them.

The remaining clinical research data on long-term survivors transplanted in Seattle are entered at the yearly audited process.

Allogeneic transplant recipients are encouraged to return to the transplant center for assessment of chronic GVHD activity, immunologic recovery, hematopoietic function, growth and development assessment (children and adolescents) (Sanders *et al.*, 1988), and disease status at 1, 5, and 10 years posttransplant (Sullivan *et al.*, 1992).

Conclusions

Marrow and blood stem cell transplantation has become a worldwide clinical activity. Thousands of long-term survivors are leading productive lives, and patients are now surviving more than 20 years after transplantation. Excellent results can be obtained without protective isolation facilities to minimize infection risk (Russell *et al.*, 1992). Since the number of days spent in the hospital is a major determinant of the cost of care (Welch & Larson, 1989), much effort has been put into developing ambulatory care for the stem cell transplant recipient (Corcoran-Buchsel & Parchem, 1988; New *et al.*, 1991). Home care is likely to be explored further and embraced in the future (criteria for home care in the study by Svahn and colleagues (Svahn *et al.*, 2000) included water temperature >50°C, no plants in pots (because of the risk of *Aspergillus* in the soil), no animals, sheets changed three times weekly, home cleaned once weekly, and caregiver availability. Results were encouraging: 36 patients, 30 of whom received a full myeloablative conditioning regimen prior to a family member or unrelated allograft, elected to be treated at home after the graft was infused. Compared to patients who chose to be treated in the hospital and to a matched control group of patients, those electing home care had fewer days on TPN, less acute GVHD grades II-IV, lower transplant-related mortality, and lower costs. The 2-year survival rates were 70% in the home care group versus 51% and 57% (NS) in the control group (Suahn *et al.*, 2002). Methods developed to lessen GHVD and to prevent infectious complications have contributed to a reduction in the morbidity and mortality of transplantation. Key to this success is the formation of the multidisciplinary transplant team of the ambulatory facility.

References

Adams, G. B., Lipton, J. H., Jamal, N. & Messner, H. A. (1994). Allogeneic bone marrow transplantation from a related donor undergoing long-term immunosuppressive and cytotoxic therapy. *Bone Marrow Transplantation*, **13,** 831–3.

Akizuki, S., Mizorogi, F., Inoue T, Sudo, K., Ohnishi, A. (2000). Pharmacokinetics and adverse events following 5-day repeated administratic lenograstim, a recombinant human granulocyte colony-stimulating factor, in healthy subjects. *Bone Marrow Transplantation*, **26,** 936–46.

Algara, M., Valls, A., Vivancos, P. & Granena, A. (1994). Outpatient total body irradiation for bone marrow transplantation. *Bone Marrow Transplantation*, **14,** 381–2.

Anonymous (1997). Shift to outpatient care dramatically lowers transplantation cost in NHL. *Oncology News International,* **6** (Suppl 2), 30–1.

Applegate, G. L., Mittal, B. B., Kletzel, M. *et al.* (1998). Outpatient total body irradiation prior to bone marrow transplantation in pediatric patients: a feasibility analysis. *Bone Marrow Transplantation,* **21**, 651–2.

Arai, S., Margolis, J., Zaburak, M. *et al.* (2002). Poor outcome in steroid-refractory graft-versus-host disease with antithymocyte globulin treatment. *Biology of Blood and Marrow Transplantation,* **8**, 155–60.

Atkinson, K., Downs, K., Golenia, M. *et al.* (1991). Prophylactic use of ganciclovir in allogeneic bone marrow transplantation: absence of clinical cytomegalovirus infection. *British Journal of Haematology,* **79**, 57–62.

Atkinson, K. & Downs, K. (1995). Omission of day +11 methotrexate does not appear to influence the incidence of moderate to severe graft-versus-host disease, chronic graft-versus-host disease, relapse rate or survival after HLA-identical sibling bone marrow transplantation. *Bone Marrow Transplantation,* **16**, 755–8.

Attarian, H., Bensinger, W. I., Buckner, C. D. *et al.* (1996). Microbial contamination of peripheral blood stem cell collections. *Bone Marrow Transplantation,* **17**, 699–702.

Auquier, P., Macquart-Moulin, G., Moatti, J. P. *et al.* (1995). Comparison of anxiety, pain and discomfort in two procedures of hematopoietic stem cell collection: leukacytapheresis and bone marrow harvest. *Bone Marrow Transplantation,* **16**, 541–7.

Bacigalupo, A., Oneto, R., Bruno, B. *et al.* (1999). Early predictors of transplant-related mortality (TRM) after allogeneic bone marrow transplants (BMT): blood urea nitrogen (BUN) and bilirubin. *Bone Marrow Transplantation,* **24**, 653–9.

Bearman, S. I., Appelbaum, F. R., Buckner, C. D. *et al.* (1988). Regimen-related toxicity in patients undergoing bone marrow transplantation. *Journal of Clinical Oncology,* **6**, 1562–8.

Bearman, S. I., Petersen, F. B., Schor, R. A. *et al.* (1990). Radionuclide ejection fractions in the evaluation of patients being considered for bone marrow transplantation: Risk for cardiac toxicity. *Bone Marrow Transplantation,* **5**, 173–7.

Bensinger, W. I., Buckner, C. D., Clift, R. A. & Thomas, E. D. (1987). Plasma exchange and plasma modification for the removal of anti-red cell antibodies prior to ABO-incompatible marrow transplant. *Journal of Clinical Apheresis,* **3**, 174–7.

Bensinger, W. I., Longin, K., Appelbaum, F. *et al.* (1994). Peripheral blood stem cells (PBSCs) collected after recombinant granulocyte colony stimulating factor (rhG-CSF): an analysis of factors correlating with the tempo of engraftment after transplantation. *British Journal of Haematology,* **87**, 825–31.

Bensinger, W. I., Martin, P. J., Storer, B. *et al.* (2001). Transplantation of bone marrow as compared with peripheral-blood cells from HLA-identical relatives in patients with hematologic cancers. *New England Journal of Medicine,* **344**, 175–81.

Berg, K. D., Brinster, N. K., Huhn, K. M. *et al.* (2001). Transmission of a T-cell lymphoma by allogeneic bone marrow transplantation. *New England Journal of Medicine,* **345**, 1458–63.

Berman, E., Little, C., Gee, T. *et al.* (1992). Reasons that patients with acute myelogenous leukemia do not undergo allogeneic bone marrow transplantation. *New England Journal of Medicine,* **326**, 156–60.

Boeckh, M., Gooley, T. A., Myerson, D. *et al.* (1996). Cytomegalovirus pp65 antigenemia-guided early treatment with ganciclovir versus ganciclovir at engraftment after allogeneic marrow transplantation: a randomized double-blind study. *Blood,* **88**, 4063–71.

Boeckh, M., Riddell, S. R., Cunningham, T. *et al.* (1996). Increased risk of late CMV infection and disease in allogeneic marrow transplant recipients after ganciclovir prophylaxis is due to a lack of CMV-specific T cell responses. *Blood,* **88** (Suppl 1), 1195a (Abstract).

Bolwell, B. J., Maurer, W., Anderson, J. *et al.* (1995). Outpatient bone marrow harvest: the Cleveland Clinic experience. *Bone Marrow Transplantation,* **16**, 703–5.

Bowden, R. A., Sayers, M., Flournoy, N. *et al.* (1986). Cytomegalovirus immune globulin and seronegative blood products to prevent primary cytomegalovirus infection after marrow transplantation. *New England Journal of Medicine,* **314**, 1006–10.

Bowden, R. A., Slichter, S. J., Sayers, M. *et al.* (1995). A comparison of filtered leukocyte-reduced and cytomegalovirus (CMV) seronegative blood products for the prevention of transfusion-associated CMV infection after marrow transplant (see comments). *Blood,* **86**, 3598–603.

Bowden, R. A., Slichter, S. J., Sayers, M. H. *et al.* (1991). Use of leukocyte-depleted platelets and cytomegalovirus-seronegative red blood cells for prevention of primary cytomegalovirus infection after marrow transplant. *Blood,* **78**, 246–50.

Bredeson, C., Perry, G., Martens, C. *et al.* (2002). Outpatient total body irradiation as a component of a comprehensive outpatient transplant program. *Bone Marrow Transplantation,* **29**, 667–71.

Centers for Disease Control and Prevention, Infectious Disease Society of America & American Society of Blood and Marrow Transplantation. (2000). Guidelines for preventing opportunistic infections among hematopoietic stem cell transplant recipients. *MMWR – Morbidity & Mortality Weekly Report,* **49**, 1–125.

Champlin, R. E., Schmitz, N., Horowitz, M. M. *et al.* (2000). Blood stem cells compared with bone marrow as a source of hematopoietic cells for allogeneic transplantation. *Blood,* **95**, 3702–9.

Chan, C., Montaner, J., Lefebvre, E.-A. *et al.* (1999). Atovaquone suspension compared with aerosolized pentamidine for prevention of *Pneumocystis carinii* pneumonia in human immunodeficiency virus-infected subjects intolerant of trimethoprim or sulfonamides. *Journal of Infectious Diseases,* **180**, 369–76.

Chan, K. W., Gajewski, J. L., Supkis, D. J. *et al.* (1996). Use of minors as bone marrow donors: current attitude and management. A survey of 56 pediatric transplantation centers. *Journal of Pediatrics,* **128**, 644–8.

Chan, K. W., Mullen, C. A., Worth, L. L. *et al.* (2002). Lorazepam for seizure prophylaxis during high-dose busulfan administration. *Bone Marrow Transplantation,* **29**, 963–5.

Chao, N. J., Schmidt, G. M., Niland, J. C. *et al.* (1993). Cyclosporine, methotrexate, and prednisone compared with cyclosporine and prednisone for prophylaxis of acute graft-versus-host disease. *New England Journal of Medicine,* **329**, 1225–30.

Chapko, M. K., Syrjala, K. L., Schilter, L. *et al.* (1989). Chemoradiotherapy toxicity during bone marrow transplantation: Time course and variation in pain and nausea. *Bone Marrow Transplantation,* **4**, 181–6.

Charuhas, P. M., Fosberg, K. L., Bruemmer, B. *et al.* (1997). A double-blind randomized trial comparing outpatient parenteral nutrition with intravenous hydration: effect on resumption of oral intake after marrow transplantation. *Journal of Parenteral and Enteral Nutrition*, **21**, 157–61.

Chern, B., McCarthy, N., Hutchins, C. & Durrant, S. T. (1999). Analgesic infiltration at the site of bone marrow harvest significantly reduces donor morbidity. *Bone Marrow Transplantation*, **23**, 947–9.

Clark, J. G., Schwartz, D. A., Flournoy, N. *et al.* (1987). Risk factors for airflow obstruction in recipients of bone marrow transplants. *Annals of Internal Medicine*, **107**, 648–56.

Cleary, J. (1997). Double blind randomized study of the treatment of breakthrough pain in cancer patients: oral transmucosal fentanyl citrate versus placebo. *Program/Proceedings American Society of Clinical Oncology*, **16**, 179a (Abstract).

Cleaver, S. A., Warren, P., Kern, M. *et al.* (1997). Donor work-up and transport of bone marrow—recommendations and requirements for a standardized practice throughout the world from the Donor Registries and Quality Assurance Working Groups of the World Marrow Donor Association (WMDA). *Bone Marrow Transplantation*, **20**, 621–9.

Cohen, A., Tepperberg, M., Waters-Pick, B. *et al.* (1996). The significance of microbial cultures of the hematopietic support for patients receiving high-dose chemotherapy. *Journal of Hematotherapy*, **5**, 289–94.

Corcoran-Buchsel, P. & Parchem, C. (1988). Ambulatory care of the bone marrow transplant patient. *Seminars in Oncology Nursing*, **4**, 41–6.

Crawford, S. W. & Fisher, L. (1992). Predictive value of pulmonary function tests before marrow transplantation. *Chest*, **101**, 1257–64.

Dagher, R., Robertson, K. A., Lucas, K. G. *et al.* (1997). Outpatient total body irradiation for pediatric patients undergoing stem cell transplantation. *Bone Marrow Transplantation*, **19**, 1065–67.

Díaz de Heredia, C., Moreno, A., Olive, T. *et al.* (1999). Role of the intensive care unit in children undergoing bone marrow transplantation with life-threatening complications. *Bone Marrow Transplantation*, **24**, 163–8.

Dicke, K. A., Hood, D. L., Arneson, M. *et al.* (1997). Effects of short-term in vivo administration of G-CSF on bone marrow prior to harvesting. *Experimental Hematology*, **25**, 34–8.

Dickson, T. M., Kusnierz-Glaz, C. R., Blume, K. G. *et al.* (1999). Impact of admission body weight and chemotherapy dose adjustment on the outcome of autologous bone marrow transplantation. *Biology of Blood & Marrow Transplantation*, **5**, 299–305.

Flowers, M. E. D., Parker, P., Johnston, L. *et al.* (2002). Comparison of chronic graft-versus-host disease after transplantation of peripheral blood stem cells versus bone marrow in allogeneic recipients: long term follow up of a randomized trial. *Blood*, **100**, 415–9.

Goldberg, S. L., Klumpp, T. R., Magdalinski, A. J. & Mangan, K. F. (1998). Value of the pretransplant evaluation in predicting toxic day-100 mortality among blood stem-cell and bone marrow transplant recipients. *Journal of Clinical Oncology*, **16**, 3796–802.

Gomez-Almaguer, D., Ruiz-Arguelles, G. J., Ruiz-Arguelles, A. *et al.* (2000). Hematopoietic stem cell allografts using a nonmyeloablative conditioning regimen can be safely performed on an outpatient basis: report of four cases. *Bone Marrow Transplantation*, **25**, 131–3.

González, M., Benito, A., Diaz, M. A. & Madero, L. (1999). Peripheral blood progenitor cell (PBPC) collection by large-volume leukapheresis from pediatric donors. *Bone Marrow Transplantation*, **23**, 631–2.

Goodman, J. L., Winston, D. J., Greenfield, R. A. *et al.* (1992). A controlled trial of fluconazole to prevent fungal infections in patients undergoing bone marrow transplantation. *New England Journal of Medicine*, **326**, 845–51.

Goodrich, J. M., Bowden, R. A., Fisher, L. *et al.* (1993). Ganciclovir prophylaxis to prevent cytomegalovirus disease after allogeneic marrow transplant. *Annals of Internal Medicine*, **118**, 173–8.

Guba, S. C., Vesole, D. H., Jagannath, S. *et al.* (1997). Peripheral stem cell mobilization and engraftment in patients over age 60. *Bone Marrow Transplantation*, **20**, 1–3.

Herrmann, R. P., Trent, M., Cooney, J. & Cannell, P. K. (1999). Infections in patients managed at home during autologous stem cell transplantation for lymphoma and multiple myeloma. *Bone Marrow Transplantation*, **24**, 1213–7.

Hilbe, W., Nussbaumer, W., Bonatti, H. *et al.* (2000). Unusual adverse events following peripheral blood stem cell (PBSC) mobilisation using granulocyte colony stimulating factor (G-CSF) in healthy donors (Case Report). *Bone Marrow Transplantation*, **26**, 811–3.

Hill, H. F., Chapman, C. R., Kornell, J. A. *et al.* (1990). Self-administration of morphine in bone Marrow transplant patients reduces drug requirement. *Pain*, **40**, 121–9.

Irving, I., Cooper, M. & Durrant, S. (2000). Sciatic nerve compression following bone marrow harvest. *Bone Marrow Transplantation*, **26**, 705–6.

Ito, H., Kurtz, J., Shaffer, J. & Sykes, M. (2001). CD4 T cell-mediated alloresistance to fully MHC-mismatched allogeneic bone marrow engraftment is dependent on CD40–CD40 ligand interactions, and lasting T cell tolerance is induced by bone marrow transplantation with initial blockade of this pathway. *Journal of Immunology*, **166**, 2970–81.

Jackson, S. R., Tweeddale, M. G., Barnett, M. J. *et al.* (1998). Admission of bone marrow transplant recipients to the intensive care unit: outcome, survival and prognostic factors. *Bone Marrow Transplantation*, **21**, 697–704.

Klein, S. & Koretz, R. L. (1994). Nutrition support in patients with cancer: what do the data really show? (Review). *Nutrition in Clinical Practice*, **9**, 91–100.

Kovacs, M. J., Crump, M. & Keating, A. (1995). Outpatient bone marrow harvesting: an update. *Bone Marrow Transplantation*, **15**, 125–7.

Kumar, S., Wolf, R. C., Chen, M.G. *et al.* (2002). Omission of day +11 methotrexate after allogeneic bone marrow transplantation is associated with increased risk of severe graft-versus-host disease. *Bone Marrow Transplantation*, **30**, 161–5.

Kusnierz-Glaz, C. R., Schlegel, P. G., Wong, R. M. *et al.* (1997). Influence of age on the outcome of 500 autologous bone marrow transplant procedures for hematologic malignancies. *Journal of Clinical Oncology*, **15**, 18–25.

Lazarus, H. M., Trehan, S., Miller, R. *et al.* (2000). Multi-purpose silastic dual-lumen central venous catheters for both collection and transplantation of hematopoietic progenitor cells. *Bone Marrow Transplantation*, **25**, 779–85.

Lenssen, P., Moe, G. L., Cheney, C. L. *et al.* (1983). Parenteral nutrition in marrow transplant recipients after discharge from the hospital. *Experimental Hematology*, **11**, 974–81.

Leung, W., Pitts, N., Burnette, K. *et al.* (2001). Allogeneic bone marrow transplantation for infants with acute leukemia or myelodysplastic syndrome. *Bone Marrow Transplantation*, **27**, 717–22.

Levine, R. J. (1986). Referral of patients with cancer for participation in randomized clinical trials: Ethical considerations. CA: *A Cancer Journal for Clinicians*, **36**, 95–9.

Link, H., Vöhringer, H.-F., Wingen, F. *et al.* (1993). Preliminary report: pentamidine aerosol for prophylaxis of *Pneumocystis carinii* pneumonia after BMT. *Bone Marrow Transplantation*, **11**, 403–6.

Loughran, T. P., Jr., Sullivan, K., Morton, T. *et al.* (1990). Value of day 100 screenign studies for predicting the development of chronic graft-versus-host disease after allogeneic bone marrow transplantation. *Blood*, **76**, 228–34.

Lowenthal, R. M., Tuck, D., Tegg, E. *et al.* (1999). Hemopoietic stem-cell harvesting and transplantation using G-CSF-primed BM: comparison with unprimed BM and G-CSF-primed PBSC. *Cytotherapy*, **1**, 409–16.

Marco, F., Bureo, E., Ortega, J. J. *et al.* (2000). High survival rate in infant acute leukemia treated with early high-dose chemotherapy and stem-cell support. Groupo Espanol de Trasplante de Medula Osea en Ninos. *Journal of Clinical Oncology*, **18**, 3256–61.

Marr, K. A., Seidel, K., Slavin, M. *et al.* (2000). Prolonged fluconazole prophylaxis is associated with persistent protection against candidiasis-related death in allogeneic marrow transplant recipients: long-term follow-up of a randomized, placebo-controlled trial. *Blood*, **96**, 2055–61.

McSweeney, P. A., Niederwieser, D., Shizuru, J. A. *et al.* (2001). Hematopoietic cell transplantation in older patients with hematologic malignancies: replacing high-dose cytotoxic therapy with graft-versus-tumor effects. *Blood*, **97**, 3390–3400.

Meisenberg, B. R., Ferran, K., Hollenbach, K. *et al.* (1998). Reduced charges and costs associated with outpatient autologous stem cell transplantation. *Bone Marrow Transplantation*, **21**, 927–32.

Meisenberg, B. R., Miller, W. E., McMillan, R. *et al.* (1997). Outpatient high-dose chemotherapy with autologous stem-cell rescue for hematologic and nonhematologic malignancies. *Journal of Clinical Oncology*, **15**, 11–7.

Meloni, G., Proia, A., Capria, S. *et al.* (2001). Obesity and autologous stem cell transplantation in acute myeloid leukemia. *Bone Marrow Transplantation*, **28**, 365–7.

Meyer, S., Thornley, M., Wynn, R. F. *et al.* (2000). Donor bone marrow from a sibling with inborn error of metabolism for treatment of acute leukaemia—clinical and biochemical consequences in the non-affected recipient. *Bone Marrow Transplantation*, **25**, 909–11.

Mielcarek, M., Bryant, E., Loken, M. *et al.* (1999). Haemopoietic reconstitution by donor-derived myelodysplastic progenitor cells after haemopoietic stem cell transplantation. *British Journal of Haematology*, **105**, 361–5.

Miller, C. B., Piantadosi, S., Vogelsang, G. B. *et al.* (1996). Impact of age on outcome of patients with cancer undergoing autologous bone marrow transplant. *Journal of Clinical Oncology*, **14**, 1327–32.

Morton, J., Arnold, L., Fletcher, B. *et al.* (1995). Allogeneic BMT from a donor with Fragile X syndrome: cytogenetic and molecular evaluation. *Bone Marrow Transplantation*, **16**, 625–6.

Morton, J., Hutchins, C., & Durrant, S. (2001). Granulocyte-colony-stimulating factor (G-CSF)-primed allogeneic bone marrow: significantly less graft-versus-host disease and comparable engraftment to G-CSF-mobilized peripheral blood stem cells. *Blood*, **98**, 3186–91.

Nemunaitis, J., Buckner, C. D., Appelbaum, F. R. *et al.* (1991). Phase I/II trial of recombinant human granulocyte-macrophage colony-stimulating factor following allogeneic bone marrow transplantation. *Blood*, **77**, 2065–71.

Nemunaitis, J., Rabinowe, S. N., Singer, J. W. *et al.* (1991). Recombinant granulocyte-macrophage colony-stimulating factor after autologous bone marrow transplantation for lymphoid cancer. *New England Journal of Medicine*, **324**, 1773–8.

New, P. B., Swanson, G. F., Bullich, R. G. & Taplin, G. C. (1991). Ambulatory antibiotic infusion devices: extending the spectrum of outpatient therapies. *American Journal of Medicine*, **91**, 455–61.

Niederwieser, D. W., Appelbaum, F. R., Gastl, G. *et al.* (1990). Inadvertent transmission of a donor's acute myeloid leukemia in bone marrow transplantation for chronic myelocytic leukemia. *New England Journal of Medicine*, **322**, 1794–6.

Nims, J. W. & Strom, S. (1988). Late complications of bone marrow transplant recipients: Nursing care issues. *Seminars in Oncology Nursing*, **4**, 47–54.

Padley, D., Koontz, F., Trigg, M. E. *et al.* (1996). Bacterial contamination rates following processing of bone marrow and peripheral blood progenitor cell preparations. *Transfusion*, **36**, 53–6.

Pahys, J., Fisher, V., Carneval, M. *et al.* (2000). Successful large volume leukapheresis on a small infant allogeneic donor. *Bone Marrow Transplantation*, **26**, 339–41.

Pession, A., Locatelli, F., Prete, A. *et al.* (1996). G-CSF in an infant donor: a method of reducing harvest volume in bone marrow transplantation. *Bone Marrow Transplantation*, **17**, 431–2.

Pirich, L., Haut, P., Morgan, E. *et al.* (1999). Total body irradiation, cyclophosphamide, and etoposide with stem cell transplant as treatment for infants with acute lymphocytic leukemia. *Medical & Pediatric Oncology*, **32**, 1–6.

Powles, R., Mehta, J., Kulkarni, S. *et al.* (2000). Allogeneic blood and bone-marrow stem-cell transplantation in haematological malignant diseases: a randomised trial. *Lancet*, **355**, 1231–7.

Prentice, E. D., Gordon, B. G., Oki, G. S. F. & Zaia, J. A. (1997). Informed consent in oncology clinical trials. *Cancer Management*, **2**, 6–71.

Prince, H. M., Page, S. R., Keating, A. *et al.* (1995). Microbial contamination of harvested bone marrow and peripheral blood. *Bone Marrow Transplantation*, **15**, 87–91.

Radich, J. P., Gooley, T., Bryant, E. *et al.* (2001). The significance of *bcr-abl* molecular detection in chronic myeloid leukemia patients "late," 18 months or more after transplantation. *Blood*, **98**, 1701–7.

Rappoport, A. P., DiPersio, J. F., Martin, B. A. *et al.* (1995). Patients ≥age 40 years undergoing autologous or allogeneic BMT have regimen-related mortality rates and event-free survivals comparable to patients < age 40 years. *Bone Marrow Transplantation*, **15**, 523–30.

Ratanatharathorn, V., Nash, R. A., Devine, S. M. *et al.* (1996). Phase III study comparing tacrolimus (Prograf FK506) with cyclosporine for graft-versus-host disease (GVHD) prophylaxis after HLA-identical sibling bone marrow transplantation (BMT). *Blood*, **88** (Suppl 1), 1826a (Abstract).

Riddell, S. R., Watanabe, K. S., Goodrich, J. M. *et al.* (1992). Restoration of viral immunity in immunodeficient humans by the adoptive transfer of T cell clones. *Science*, **257**, 238–41.

Ringden, O., Horowitz, M. M., Gale, R. P. *et al.* (1993). Outcome after allogeneic bone marrow transplant for leukemia in older adults. *Journal of the American Medical Association*, **270**, 57–60.

Ringden, O., Remberger, M., Mattsson, J. *et al.* (1998). Transplantation with unrelated bone marrow in leukaemic patients above 40 years of age. *Bone Marrow Transplantation*, **21**, 43–49.

Rowley, S. D., Donaldson, G., Lilleby, K. *et al.* (2001). Experiences of donors enrolled in a randomized study of allogeneic bone marrow or peripheral blood stem cell transplantation. *Blood,* **97,** 2541–8.

Russell, J. A., Poon, M.-C., Jones, A. R. *et al.* (1992). Allogeneic bone-marrow transplantation without protective isolation in adults with malignant disease. *Lancet,* **339,** 38–40.

Sadler, D. J., McCarthy, M., Saliken, J. C. *et al.* (2000). Image-guided central venous catheter placement for apheresis in allogeneic stem cell donors. *Journal of Clincial Apheresis,* **15,** 173–5.

Sanders, J. E., Buckner, C. D., Sullivan, K. M. *et al.* (1988). Growth and development in children after bone marrow transplantation. *Hormone Research,* **30,** 92–7.

Schmitz, N., Bacigalupo, A., Hasenclever, D. *et al.* (1998). Allogeneic bone marrow transplantation vs filgrastim-mobilised peripheral blood progenitor cell transplantation in patients with early leukaemia: first results of a randomised multicentre trial of the European Group for Blood and Marrow Transplantation. *Bone Marrow Transplantation,* **21,** 995–1003.

Schmitz, N., Dreger, P., Suttorp, M. *et al.* (1995). Primary transplantation of allogeneic peripheral blood progenitor cells mobilized by filgrastim (granulocyte colony-stimulating factor). *Blood,* **85,** 1666–72.

Sheridan, W. P., Morstyn, G., Wolf, M. *et al.* (1989). Granulocyte colony-stimulating factor and neutrophil recovery after high-dose chemotherapy and autologous bone marrow transplantation. *Lancet,* **ii,** 891–5.

Sim, K. M., Boey, S. K. & Wong, L. T. (1996). Bone marrow harvesting using local anaesthesia and PCA-alfentanil: a feasible alternative to general or regional anaesthesia. *Bone Marrow Transplantation,* **18,** 787–90.

Simmonds, M. A. (1997). Oral transmucosal fentanyl citrate produces pain relief faster than medication typically used for breakthrough pain in cancer patients. *Program/Proceedings American Society of Clinical Oncology,* **16,** 180a (Abstract).

Singer, D. A., Donnelly, M. B. & Messerschmidt, G. L. (1990). Informed consent for bone marrow transplantation: identification of relevant information by referring physicians. *Bone Marrow Transplantation,* **6,** 431–7.

Slattery, J. T., Clift, R. A., Buckner, C. D. *et al.* (1997). Marrow transplantation for chronic myeloid leukemia: the influence of plasma busulfan levels on the outcome of transplantation. *Blood,* **89,** 3055–60.

Smith, D., Bradley, S. J. & Scott, G. M. (1996). Bacterial contamination of autologous bone marrow during processing. *Journal of Hospital Infection,* **33,** 71–6.

Smith, T. J., Hillner, B. E., Schmitz, N. *et al.* (1997). Economic analysis of a randomized clinical trial to compare filgrastim-mobilized peripheral-blood progenitor-cell transplantation and autologous bone marrow transplantation in patients with Hodgkin's and non-Hodgkin's lymphoma. *Journal of Clinical Oncology,* **15,** 5–10.

Solano, C., Martinez, C., Brunet, S. *et al.* (1998). Chronic graft-versus-host disease after allogeneic peripheral blood progenitor cell or bone marrow transplantation from matched related donors. A case-control study. *Bone Marrow Transplantation,* **22,** 1129–35.

Souza, J. P., Boeckh, M., Gooley, T. A. *et al.* (1999). High rates of *Pneumocystis carinii* pneumonia in allogeneic blood and marrow transplant recipients receiving Dapsone prophylaxis. *Clinical Infectious Diseases,* **29,** 1467–71.

Storb, R., Deeg, H. J., Whitehead, J. *et al.* (1986). Methotrexate and cyclosporine compared with cyclosporine alone for prophylaxis of acute graft versus host disease after marrow transplantation for leukemia. *New England Journal of Medicine,* **314,** 729–35.

Sturfelt, G., Lenhoff, S., Sallerfors, B. *et al.* (1996). Transplantation with allogenic bone marrow from a donor with systemic lupus erythematosus (SLE): successful outcome in the recipient and induction of an SLE flare in the donor. *Annals of the Rheumatic Diseases,* **55,** 638–41.

Sullivan, K. M., Agura, E., Anasetti, C. *et al.* (1991). Chronic graft-versus-host disease and other late complications of bone marrow transplantation. *Seminars in Hematology,* **28,** 250–9.

Sullivan, K. M., Kopecky, K. J., Jocom, J. *et al.* (1990). Immunomodulatory and antimicrobial efficacy of intravenous immunoglobulin in bone marrow transplantation. *New England Journal of Medicine,* **323,** 705–12.

Sullivan, K. M., Mori, M., Sanders, J. *et al.* (1992). Late complications of allogeneic and autologous marrow transplantation (Review). *Bone Marrow Transplantation,* **10,** 127–134.

Svahn, B. M., Bjurman, B., Myrback, K. E. *et al.* (2000). Is it safe to treat allogeneic stem cell transplant recipients at home during the pancytopenic phase? A pilot trial. *Bone Marrow Transplantation,* **26,** 1057–60.

Svahn, B-M, Remberger, M., Myrbäck, K.-E. *et al.* (1998). Early treatment of acute graft-versus-host disease with high- or low-dose 6-methylprednisolone: a multicenter randomized trial from the Italian Group for Bone Marrow Transplantation. *Blood,* **92,** 2288–2293.

Switzer, G. E., Goycoolea, J. M., Dew, M. A. *et al.* (2001). Donating stimulated peripheral blood stem cells vs bone marrow: do donors experience the procedures differently? *Bone Marrow Transplantation,* **27,** 917–23.

Thomas, E. D., Storb, R., Clift, R. A. *et al.* (1975). Bone-marrow transplantation. *New England Journal of Medicine,* **292,** 832–43, 895–902.

Thorne, A. C., Malbin, K. F., Jain, M. *et al.* (1996). Autologous bone marrow harvesting in outpatients. *Journal of Clinical Anesthesia,* **8,** 551–6.

van Besien, K., Przepiorka, D., Mehra, R. *et al.* (1996). Impact of preexisting CNS involvement on the outcome of bone marrow transplantation in adult hematologic malignancies. *Journal of Clinical Oncology,* **14,** 3036–42.

Vigorito, A. C., Azevedo, W. M., Marques, J. F. *et al.* (1998). A randomised, prospective comparison of allogeneic bone marrow and peripheral blood progenitor cell transplantation in the treatment of haematological malignancies. *Bone Marrow Transplantation,* **22,** 1145–51.

Weaver, C. H., Schwartzberg, L. S., Hainsworth, J. *et al.* (1997). Treatment related mortality in 1,000 consecutive patients receiving high-dose chemotherapy and peripheral blood progenitor cell transplantation in community cancer centers. *Bone Marrow Transplantation,* **19,** 671–8.

Weisdorf, S. A., Lysne, J., Wind, D. *et al.* (1987). Positive effect of prophylactic total parenteral nutrition on long-term outcome of bone marrow transplantation. *Transplantation,* **43,** 833–8.

Welch, H. G. & Larson, E. B. (1989). Cost effectiveness of bone marrow transplantation in acute nonlymphocytic leukemia. *New England Journal of Medicine,* **321,** 807–12.

Woolfrey, A. E., Gooley, T. A., Sievers, E. L. *et al.* (1998). Bone marrow transplantation for children less than 2 years of age with acute myelogenous leukemia or myelodysplastic syndrome. *Blood,* **92,** 3546–56.

21 High-dose chemotherapy and chemoradiotherapy preparative regimens

WILLIAM I. BENSINGER

Fred Hutchinson Cancer Research Center and University of Washington, Seattle, USA

Introduction

This chapter reviews high-dose chemotherapy and chemoradiotherapy regimens administered prior to autologous, syngeneic, or allogeneic hematopoietic stem cell (HSC) infusion. Most of the high-dose regimens described have been utilized in patients with hematologic malignancies. However, many of the newer high-dose regimens have been developed specifically for patients with solid tumors, especially breast cancer. The overall results of stem cell transplantation utilizing these high-dose treatment regimens are discussed in more detail in chapters dealing with specific diseases.

High-dose regimens are primarily designed to provide maximum tumor cytoreduction without encountering dose-limiting organ toxicities exclusive of bone marrow. The success of this approach as curative therapy for patients with malignancy is limited, in part, by transplant-related morbidity and mortality. However, even if all transplant-related problems were solved, approximately 50% (range 10%–90% according to disease status at time of grafting) of patients receiving transplants for various stages of various malignant diseases would die due to the inability of high-dose regimens to eradicate the malignancy. This has led to intensive efforts to develop more effective high-dose regimens.

Evaluation of new treatment regimens

The development of new treatment regimens has mostly been empirical with the evaluation of a variety of drug and radiation doses and schedules. Attempts have been made to systematize the development of new treatment regimens by performing phase I dose escalation trials followed by phase II potential efficacy trials. Promising new regimens should then be compared to established treatment regimens in randomized phase III trials, but in practice this has happened rarely.

Regimen-related toxicity (RRT) grading system

In order to carry out phase I and II studies of new high-dose treatment regimens in transplant patients, a new toxicity grad-

ing system, excluding hematologic toxicities, was designed. This grading system estimates the nonhematologic toxicities directly caused by a given transplant treatment regimen (Bearman, Appelbaum, & Buckner 1988, and see Chapter 64). Morbidity is assessed in nine organ systems: heart, bladder, kidneys, lungs, liver, mucosa, central nervous system (CNS), gastrointestinal (GI) tract, and skin. Toxicity is graded on a 0 to 4 scale with grade 3 being life-threatening and grade 4 being fatal. Toxicities due to graft-versus-host-disease (GVHD), infection, and drugs administered posttransplant are excluded from this grading system. Utilizing this grading system, one can begin to estimate the specific contribution the treatment regimen makes to the overall morbidity and mortality of the transplant procedure (Bearman *et al.,* 1989, 1994; Petersen & Bearman 1994).

Phase I studies

Dose escalation trials to define maximum tolerated doses (MTD) and phase II trials to define potential efficacy are, in general, performed in patients with advanced disease incurable by conventional therapy. Once a tolerable regimen is developed, it can be evaluated in phase II and III trials in patients with less-advanced disease. Conventional phase I trials of chemotherapeutic agents have starting doses that are known to be nontoxic and are escalated to mild or moderate toxicity, which is usually hematologic. In the transplant setting this is not an appropriate strategy as only nonhematologic toxicities are considered. An alternative approach is to make an estimate of the likely MTD, based on nonhematologic toxicities, for a combination of agents given in high doses. This estimated MTD is then used as the starting dose with subsequent escalation and de-escalation depending on observed toxicities. The RRT grading system parameters, described above, are used as the criteria for escalation or de-escalation of doses. In phase I studies, attempts are made to keep observed grade 3–4 toxicities to less than 25% and patients are studied in groups of four in the following scheme:

Severe RRT/total	Dose level for next 4 patients
0/4	Next higher
1/4	Same
2/4	Next lower

With this scheme, a maximum of 16 to 20 patients is required to determine the MTD of most new treatment regimens. Using the above methodology, several phase I trials have been successfully performed (Petersen *et al.*, 1988, 1989a, 1992a, 1992b; Weaver *et al.*, 1994; Demirer *et al.*, 1995).

Marrow-ablative single agents—maximum tolerated dose and toxicities when administered with stem cell support

A number of marrow-ablative agents have been used alone and at high dosage followed by stem cell support (Table 21.1).

Total body irradiation

Total body irradiation (TBI) has been the primary therapeutic modality for autologous and allogeneic stem cell transplantation for patients with hematologic malignancies. TBI has retained wide usage over the past 30 years because of excellent immunosuppressive properties, activity against a wide variety of malignancies (even if resistant to chemotherapy), penetration of sanctuary sites such as the CNS and testicles, and the relative lack of nonmarrow toxicities when given at high doses. There has been concern, however, about potential long-term adverse effects of TBI, which include the development of myelodysplasia (Friedberg *et al.*, 1999; Wheeler *et al.*, 2001).

Only one early study evaluated TBI alone (Thomas *et al.*, 1971) while all other trials have involved the concomitant administration of cytotoxic agents, usually cyclophosphamide (CY). Extensive experience has been accumulated with 10 to 16 Gy[1] of TBI given as a single dose or fractionated, following or preceding high doses of CY.

A large body of experimental data has been developed concerning methods to improve the therapeutic index of TBI and this subject has been reviewed (Vriesendorp, 1990; Appelbaum *et al.*, 1992a). Larger doses of TBI that might reduce the likelihood of relapse can be limited early after administration by GI and pulmonary toxicity and long-term by impaired growth and development, chronic pulmonary insufficiency, and second malignancies. In addition to the total dose, many factors, including radiation exposure rate, dose per fraction, interval between fractions, and radiation source (^{60}Co or linear acceler-

ator[2]), can have an effect on efficacy and toxicity (Vriesendorp, 1990). Experimental studies and clinical trials indicate that TBI administered in fractions is more tolerable than single-dose administration and that fractionation, if compensated for by increased total dose, can be given without compromising anti-tumor effects. Based on this principle, the use of fractionated TBI regimens has been explored in several centers, but there is a paucity of controlled studies of acute and delayed toxicities or of clinical efficacy as compared to single-dose TBI. Only one prospective randomized study of fractionated versus single-dose TBI (both with the same dose of CY) has been performed that demonstrated clear superiority in event-free survival (EFS) following a fractionated regimen in patients with acute myeloid leukemia (AML) transplanted in first remission (Thomas *et al.*, 1982; Deeg *et al.*, 1986). Other studies suggest that fractionation decreases the incidence of idiopathic interstitial pneumonitis syndrome (IPS) and cataracts (Storb, 1994). In a survey of TBI administration at 15 transplant centers it was found that 13 utilized some form of fractionation (Vriesendorp, 1990).

In most TBI regimens used at the Fred Hutchinson Cancer Research Center, radiation has been delivered from dual opposing ^{60}Co sources (Storb, 1994). This approach has the advantage of providing highly homogeneous radiation exposure and allows the patient some freedom of movement. However, it is difficult to shield organs and radiation can be delivered only at relatively low exposure rates. Because of the costs associated with dedicated ^{60}Co units and the difficulties with organ shielding, most marrow transplant teams use linear accelerators to deliver TBI. With a linear accelerator, dose rates of 40 cGy/min or higher can be administered. The use of linear accelerators may have additional benefits as the radiation field can be shaped with the use of lung shielding, which may reduce pulmonary toxicity (Brochstein *et al.*, 1987). Electron beam radiation can also be delivered to the chest wall and spine to compensate for the lower dose of TBI to these shielded areas (Brochstein *et al.*, 1987; Bensinger *et al.*, 1993). Shielding of other organs, such as the liver, may be useful if specific organ toxicity limits further increase in TBI dose (Bensinger *et al.*, 1993). Delivery of TBI with shielding of both lung and liver may be useful in patients with disease limited to bone, such as multiple myeloma, breast cancer, and Ewing's sarcoma (Bensinger *et al.*, 1993).

Busulfan

Busulfan (BU) is an alkylating agent with profound myeloablative properties and marked activity against nondividing bone marrow cells and possibly nondividing malignant cells as well.

---

[1] The basic unit for absorbed radiation dose is the gray (Gy). A previously used term was the rad (radiation absorbed dose). 1 rad = 0.01 Gy [i.e., 100 rad = 1 Gy = 100 centi Gy (cGy)].

[2] Linear accelerators produce X-rays through high-energy electrons bombarding a target. A ^{60}Co source produces gamma rays that originate from the nuclear decay of radioactive material. X-rays and gamma rays have identical photon radiations.

Table 21.1. *Marrow-ablative single agents used at high dosage with stem cell support*

Agent	MTD	Dose-limiting toxicities	Reference
Total body irradiation	10–16 Gy	GI, hepatic, pulmonary	Vriesendorp, 1990
Busulfan	20 mg/kg	GI, hepatic, pulmonary	Peters *et al.*, 1987
Carmustine	1,200 mg/m^2	Pulmonary, hepatic	Phillips *et al.*, 1983
Melphalan	200 mg/m^2	GI	Corringham *et al.*, 1983
Thiotepa	1,135 mg/m^2	CNS, GI	Wolff *et al.*, 1990
Etoposide	2,400 mg/m^2	GI	Wolff *et al.*, 1983
Carboplatin	2,000 mg/m^2	Hepatic, renal	Shea *et al.*, 1989

Abbreviations: MTD, maximum tolerated dose; GI, gastrointestinal; CNS, central nervous system.

The maximum tolerated dose of BU, given as a single agent over 4 days followed by stem cell support, is approximately 20 mg/kg (Peters *et al.*, 1987) (Table 21.1). Single agent testing to determine the spectrum of activity in patients with malignant disease has not been extensive (Peters *et al.*, 1987; Kanfer *et al.*, 1987b; Mansi *et al.*, 1992). However, BU is probably active in a variety of malignancies including multiple myeloma (Bensinger *et al.*, 1992; Mansi *et al.*, 1992; Schiller *et al.*, 1994; Cavo *et al.*, 1998), lymphoma (Copelan & Deeg, 1992), ALL (Copelan & Deeg, 1992), testicular tumors (Kanfer *et al.*, 1987a), Ewing's sarcoma (Kanfer *et al.*, 1987a), myeloid metaplasia (Anderson *et al.*, 2001), and breast cancer (Demirer *et al.*, 1996a). The Hammersmith Hospital group has used BU alone as the conditioning regimen prior to first autologous transplants, and for second allogeneic transplants, in patients with CML (Olivarria *et al.*, 2000). The probability of survival of 14 allograft recipients was 78% at 5 years. For patients autografted for CML in chronic phase, the actuarial 3-year survival was 76% for those transplanted in chronic phase and 30% for those transplanted with advanced phase disease. Except for mild mucositis, little toxicity was experienced. No patients developed hepatic veno-occlusive disease (VOD).

One of the problems with optimal utilization of BU is availability of, until recently, only the oral form. Pharmacokinetic variability between patients is high with a two- to threefold difference in plasma levels between patients (Grochow, 1993). Children have lower mean plasma levels of BU (650 ng/ml) than adults (1,050 ng/ml) (Grochow *et al.*, 1990; Slattery *et al.*, 1995), which may be partially compensated for by dosing children by body surface area rather than weight (Slattery *et al.*, 1995). Variation in BU plasma levels between individuals probably contributes to the significant differences observed in toxicity and clinical response in patients receiving the same mg/kg or mg/m^2 dose. Slattery *et al.* (1995) demonstrated a relationship between low BU steady-state plasma concentrations and graft rejection in children. There are also data that suggest a direct relationship between the severity of RRT, especially VOD of the liver, and high BU plasma levels (Grochow *et al.*, 1989; Grochow, 1993). Slattery and colleagues (1997) demonstrated a relationship between steady-state BU concentration

and relapse in patients receiving HLA-compatible transplants for chronic myeloid leukemia (CML) in chronic phase. In that study there were seven relapses among the 22 patients with BU state concentrations below the median value of 918 ng/ml and none among the 23 patients at or above the median ($P = .0003$).

Thus, the average steady-state concentration of BU over a 4-day period may be a more important determinant of toxicity and efficacy than the exact mg/kg or mg/m^2 dose administered. Fortunately, in a given patient, BU is a pharmacokinetically predictable drug and its absorption and elimination rate remain linear over a wide dose range and constant with time (Slattery *et al.*, 1995). With repeated oral administration, steady-state BU plasma concentrations are achieved rapidly and can be predicted from first dose kinetics. Others have used a similar approach in children receiving BU and reported less toxicity and improved engraftment (Bleyzac *et al.*, 2001). Following determination of first dose kinetics, oral doses can be adjusted up or down to achieve the desired plasma levels. The strategy of targeted steady-state BU dosing has been used successfully to perform a dose escalation trial in patients receiving fixed doses of CY and TBI (Demirer *et al.*, 1996b). Theoretically, targeting of the steady-state plasma level of BU should increase the therapeutic index. A prospective trial in patients with CML is currently being carried out to test this hypothesis.

Recently, an intravenous preparation of BU has become available and initial phamacokinetic data indicate considerably less individual variation in area under the curve (AUC) values than seen with the oral preparation (Andersson *et al.*, 1998). In preliminary studies, intravenous BU could be given as a single daily dose over 3 hours rather than the usual 4 oral doses per day (Schuler *et al.*, 2001).

In a patient accidentally overdosed with busulfan, hemodialysis resulted in accelerated clearance of the drug (Stein *et al.*, 2001).

Carmustine

Carmustine is a commonly used marrow-ablative agent active against a variety of tumors (Phillips *et al.*, 1983). The MTD, as a single agent, is 1,200 mg/m^2 when given with autologous stem cell infusions. The dose-limiting toxicities are pulmonary and hepatic (Phillips *et al.*, 1983) (Table 21.1).

Melphalan

The administration of high doses of melphalan has been reviewed (Sarosy *et al.*, 1988). Single doses of melphalan, 150 to 240 mg/m^2, followed by autologous stem cell infusion have been evaluated in patients with multiple myeloma, acute myeloid leukemia, and breast cancer, with the dose-limiting toxicities being GI and hepatic (Corringham, Gilmore, & Prentice, 1983; Cesaro *et al.*, 2001) (Table 21.1). Melphalan 240 mg/m^2 has been utilized alone as a conditioning regimen for patients with hematologic malignancies receiving allogeneic transplants from HLA-matched siblings (Singhal *et al.*, 1996). Melphalan 100 mg/m^2 has been reported to result in allogeneic engraftment in 29 of 31 patients who had failed a prior autologous transplant (Badros *et al.*, 2002).

Thiotepa

The MTD for thiotepa, as a single agent with stem cell support, is approximately 1,100 mg/m^2. Dose-limiting toxicities are CNS, GI, hepatic, and skin (Wolff *et al.*, 1990) (Table 21.1).

Etoposide

The MTD for etoposide, as a single agent with stem cell support, is approximately 2,400 mg/m^2 with the dose-limiting toxicity being GI (Wolff *et al.*, 1983) (Table 21.1). Etoposide exposure has been implicated as a risk factor for the development of secondary myelodysplasia after high-dose therapy and autologous transplantation (Krishnan *et al.*, 2000).

Carboplatin

The MTD for carboplatin with stem cell support is approximately 2,000 mg/m^2 with the dose-limiting toxicities being hepatic and renal (Shea *et al.*, 1989) (Table 21.1). Carboplatin in conventional doses is usually dosed on a formula based on renal function (Calvert *et al.*, 1989). However, Shea administered carboplatin in doses of 375 to 2,400 mg/m^2 and found a direct correlation between mg/m^2 and measured AUC, suggesting that high doses could be based on body surface area (Shea *et al.*, 1989). In one study, carboplatin was administered at doses of 1,000 to 1,600 mg/m^2 in conjunction with high doses of melphalan and mitoxantrone (Weaver *et al.*, 1997a). In a retrospective analysis of this study, dosing by the Calvert formula was more predictive of grade 3–4 toxicities than dosing by body surface area (Weaver *et al.*, 1997a). These data suggested that dosing of carboplatin to an AUC of 20 mg/ml/min rather than 1,400 mg/m^2 would decrease grade 3–4 RRT in patients receiving melphalan (160 mg/m^2) and mitoxantrone (50 mg/m^2) followed by autologous PBSC infusion.

Non–marrow-ablative single agents used at high dosage with stem cell support

Cyclophosphamide

CY alone was originally used to achieve allogeneic engraftment in patients with aplastic anemia and hematologic malignancies, but was abandoned in patients with malignant disease in favor of TBI-based regimens or combinations of chemotherapeutic agents. However, CY, with or without antithymocyte globulin, is still the most commonly used regimen for immunosuppression of patients with aplastic anemia prior to allogeneic transplantation (Storb, 1994). CY is very immunosuppressive but is not marrow ablative, with the dose-limiting toxicity being cardiac (hemorrhagic myocarditis) (Storb *et al.*, 1970). The maximum tolerated dose, as a single agent, is approximately 200 mg/kg and infusion of stem cells has no impact on survival at this or higher doses (Buckner *et al.*, 1972) (Table 21.2). The major side effect, at doses of 120 to 200 mg/kg, is hemorrhagic cystitis, which can probably be diminished by bladder irrigation or the administration of mesna.

Ifosfamide

Ifosfamide has been evaluated in high-dose regimens followed by autologous stem cells as a substitute for CY. However, as with CY, hematopoietic toxicity is not dose-limiting when high doses of ifosfamide are administered (Elias *et al.*, 1990). The MTD is 18 to 20 g/m^2 with the dose-limiting toxicities being renal and bladder (Table 21.2). Ifosfamide is always given with mesna for bladder protection.

Single agents used at high dosage with stem cell support but without MTD determination

Anthracyclines

Anthracyclines have not been widely employed in high-dose regimens because their primary dose-limiting toxicity is cardiac. The potential use of mitoxantrone in high-dose regimens has been reviewed (LeMaistre & Herzig 1990). However, the

Table 21.2. *Non–marrow-ablative single agents used at high dosage with stem cell support*

Agent	MTD	Dose-limiting toxicities	Reference
Cyclophosphamide	200 mg/kg	Cardiac	Buckner *et al.*, 1972
Ifosfamide	10–20 g/m^2	Renal and bladder	Elias *et al.*, 1990

Abbreviation: MTD, maximum tolerated dose.

Table 21.3. *Single agents used at high dosage with stem cell support but without MTD determination*

Agent	MTD[a]	Dose-limiting toxicities	Reference
Mitoxantrone	90 mg/m^2	Cardiac	Fields *et al.*, 1993
Cisplatin	250 mg/m^2	Renal	Somlo *et al.*, 1994
Cytosine arabinoside	36 g/m^2	CNS	Coccia *et al.*, 1988
Paclitaxel	1,400 mg/m^2	CNS	Stiff *et al.*, 1997

[a] *Maximum dose given in combination with other agents.*

MTD as a single agent with stem cell support has not been reported. The highest dose of mitoxantrone administered in a high-dose combination regimen has been 90 mg/m^2, given with 1,200 mg/m^2 of thiotepa (Fields *et al.*, 1993; Stiff *et al.*, 1997) (Table 21.3). Idarubicin 42 mg/m^2 has been combined with BU and melphalan without apparent cardiotoxicity (See Table 21.8) (Meloni *et al.*, 2000).

Cisplatin

The MTD for cisplatin as a single agent with stem cell support has not been reported and the highest dose given in combination regimens has been 250 mg/m^2, administered with etoposide 60 mg/kg and CY 100 mg/kg (Somlo *et al.*, 1994) (Table 21.3).

Cytosine arabinoside

The MTD for cytosine arabinoside administered as a single agent with stem cell support has not been determined. However, in combination with other agents also given in high doses, cytosine arabinoside is usually administered in doses of 3 g/m^2 for 4 to 12 doses at 12-hour intervals (Coccia *et al.*, 1988; Matulonis, Griffin, & Canellos, 1994) (Table 21.3).

Paclitaxel

The MTD for paclitaxel administered as a single agent with stem cell support has not been determined. The highest dose of paclitaxel administered was 350 mg/m^2/day for 4 days in a reg-

imen that included melphalan 180 mg/kg and mitoxantrone 90 mg/m^2 (Stiff *et al.*, 1997) (Table 21.3).

High-dose regimens with TBI

TBI with CY

The use of CY with TBI was based on empirical observations. CY (120 mg/kg) was originally given prior to TBI to a patient undergoing a syngeneic marrow transplant for advanced lymphoma in 1971 (Fefer *et al.*, 1974). The purpose of giving the CY was to avoid tumor lysis and acute renal failure that had been previously observed with TBI given in a single dose of 10 Gy. This patient is alive without disease more than 20 years posttransplant. Subsequently, CY was commonly administered prior to TBI in patients receiving allogeneic or syngeneic marrow transplants with no apparent excess toxicity over that observed using TBI alone, and thus, this has become a "standard regimen" widely used in many transplant centers. Although several agents have been added to, or substituted for CY, most of the TBI regimens tested over the past 20 years have included CY before or after TBI. A variety of TBI regimens have been evaluated in attempts to define an optimal dose and schedule. Table 21.4 summarizes the MTD for several different schedules of TBI (delivered by ^{60}Co sources at dose rates of 5 to 10 cGy/min) given after CY 120 mg/kg (Deeg *et al.*, 1986; Clift *et al.*, 1990, 1991).

Randomized trials involving different TBI regimens

There has been a paucity of randomized controlled trials evaluating different TBI regimens. Three trials reported by the Seattle Marrow Transplant Team are summarized in Table 21.5 (Thomas *et al.*, 1982; Deeg *et al.*, 1986; Clift *et al.*, 1990, 1991).

The first study demonstrated that 12.0 Gy of TBI given in 2.0 Gy daily fractions was superior to 10.0 Gy TBI delivered as a single dose (Thomas *et al.*, 1982; Deeg *et al.*, 1986). The second and third trials evaluated a higher dose of TBI (15.75 Gy) in patients with AML in first remission or CML in chronic phase (Clift *et al.*, 1990, 1991). Both studies showed a decrease in the probability of relapse following the higher dose of TBI, but no improvement in survival due to increased transplant-related mortality. Methods to decrease the toxicity of TBI or the use of an intermediate dose of TBI could possibly improve survival in

Table 21.4. *Maximum tolerated doses of total body irradiation given with cyclophosphamide 120 mg/kg*

Total dose (Gy)	Fraction size (Gy)	Fractionation interval (hrs)	Fraction number	Days of TBI	Reference
10.00	10	–	1	1	Thomas *et al.*, 1982
15.75	2.25	24	7	7	Clift *et al.*, 1990
16.00	2	24	8	8	Clift *et al.*, 1990
16.00	2	6–8	8	4	Petersen *et al.*, 1992b
14.40 (child)	1.2	4–6	12	4	Brochstein *et al.*, 1987
13.20 (adult)	1.2	4–6	11	4	Demirer *et al.*, 1995

Table 21.5. *Randomized trials of total body irradiation regimens given with cyclophosphamide 120 mg/kg*

Diagnosis (reference)	Number of patients	Fraction size (Gy)	Number of daily fractions	Total dose (Gy)	Probability of relapse	Probability of EFS
AML—first remission	27	10.0	1	10.0	.55	.33
(Thomas *et al.,* 1982)	26	2.0	6	12.0	.20	.54
AML—first remission	34	2.0	6	12.0	.35	.60
(Clift *et al.,* 1990)	37	2.25	7	15.75	.12	.60
CML—chronic phase	57	2.0	6	12.0	.19	.73
(Clift *et al.,* 1991)	59	2.25	7	15.75	0	.66

Abbreviations: EFS, event-free survival; AML, acute myeloid leukemia; CML, chronic myeloid leukemia.

these patients. Nonrandomized comparisons of TBI dose and fractionation schedule have also been reported. One such study, performed in lymphoma patients, compared 1.7 Gy for 6 fractions over 3 days to 3 Gy, 4 fractions over 4 days; total doses 10.2 Gy vs. 12 Gy, combined with CY and etoposide (Gopal *et al.,* 2001). There were no differences in acute or late toxicities and overall survival. There was a significantly lower rate of progression for patients given 3 Gy single daily fractions.

TBI with drugs other than CY

Drugs other than CY have been administered with TBI, as shown in Table 21.6 (Blume *et al.,* 1987; Coccia *et al.,* 1988; Riddell *et al.,* 1988; Powles *et al.,* 1989; Mehta *et al.,* 1996). At the present time there is no evidence that any of these agents are superior to CY when given with TBI, but randomized controlled trials have not been reported.

CY and TBI with other drugs

Other agents have been combined with CY and TBI, as shown in Table 21.7 (Riddell *et al.,* 1988; Petersen *et al.,* 1989b; Horning *et al.,* 1991; Kantarjian *et al.,* 1994; Lynch *et al.,* 1995). Phase II trials suggest that some of these combinations may have better therapeutic efficacy than CY/TBI; however, none of these regimens has been subjected to randomized controlled trials.

Table 21.6. *Total body irradiation (TBI) with chemotherapeutic agents other than cyclophosphamide*

Total dose TBI (Gy)	Chemothera-peutic agent	Total dose	Reference
10–12	Cytosine arabinoside	36 g/m^2	Coccia *et al.,* 1988
13.2	Etoposide	60 mg/kg	Blume *et al.,* 1987
9.5–11.5	Melphalan	110 mg/m^2	Powles *et al.,* 1989
5 or 12 Gy[a]	Melphalan Etoposide	140–180 mg/m^2 60 mg/kg	Keating & Brandwein, 1990

[a] 5 Gy at 50 cGy/min × 1 or 12 Gy in 6 fractions.

High-dose chemotherapy regimens

There have been extensive efforts to develop non-TBI-containing transplant regimens. There are several reasons for pursuing this. Many patients have received prior dose-limiting radiotherapy, especially to the mediastinum, which results in a high incidence of fatal IPS following TBI (Pecego *et al.,* 1986). Chemotherapy regimens may also avoid or diminish the long-term sequelae of TBI including cataracts, sterility, second malignancies, and growth and development problems in children. There is also an advantage in convenience, and possibly in expense, in that TBI utilizes already-crowded radiation facilities, often for prolonged periods of time and requires the skills of physicists and radiotherapists. Finally, it may be possible to develop chemotherapy regimens that are more effective than those containing TBI.

Busulfan-based regimens (Table 21.8)

A regimen of BU combined with CY has been developed that has had a wide application for the treatment of a variety of malignant and nonmalignant diseases using autologous and allogeneic stem cell support (Santos, Tutschka, & Brookmeyer, 1983). The original regimen included BU 4 mg/kg/day for 4 days followed by CY 50 mg/kg/day for 4 days (Santos, Tutschka, & Brookmeyer, 1983). This regimen was subsequently modified by lowering the dose of CY to 120 mg/kg with an apparent decrease in toxicity without an increase in relapse rate (Tutschka, Copeland, & Klein 1987). It has been reported that 16 mg/kg combined with 120 mg/kg of CY results in prohibitive toxicity in older patients with multiple myeloma and breast cancer undergoing autologous or allogeneic transplantation (Bensinger *et al.,* 1992, 1996; Demirer *et al.,* 1996a). Lowering the dose of BU to 14 mg/kg decreased toxicity and allowed for an increase in the dose of CY to 150 mg/kg (Bensinger *et al.,* 1992).

Etoposide (60 mg/kg) has been substituted for CY in the treatment of patients with AML undergoing autologous bone marrow transplantation (Chao *et al.,* 1993; Linker *et al.,* 1993a, 1993b, 1995). Etoposide has also been added to BU and CY as a preparative regimen for patients with lymphoma (Tutschka *et al.,* 2001).

Table 21.7. *Chemotherapeutic agents given with cyclophosphamide and total body irradiation*

Cyclophosphamide (mg/kg)	TBI (Gy)	Chemotherapeutic agent	Total dose of chemotherapy	Reference
60–120	5–12	Cytosine arabinoside	36 g/m^2	Riddell *et al.*, 1988
50	12	Busulfan	7 mg/kg (allo)	Petersen *et al.*, 1989b
60	12	Busulfan	8 mg/kg (auto)	
50	12	Busulfan	7 mg/kg	Lynch *et al.*, 1995
100	12	Etoposide	60 mg/kg × 1	Horning *et al.*, 1991
120	10.2	Etoposide	1,500 mg/m^2	Kantarjian *et al.*, 1994

A regimen of BU (16 mg/kg) and melphalan (140 mg/m^2) followed by autologous or allogeneic stem cell infusion has been evaluated in patients with a variety of hematologic malignancies (Srivastava *et al.*, 1993; Alegre *et al.*, 1995; Cony-Makhoul *et al.*, 1995; Martino *et al.*, 1995; van Besien *et al.*, 1995a; Vey *et al.*, 1996).

A regimen of BU (12 mg/kg), melphalan (100 mg/m^2), and thiotepa (500 mg/m^2) followed by autologous stem cell support has been evaluated in patients with a variety of malignant diseases (Weaver *et al.*, 1994; Schiffman *et al.*, 1996; Gutierrez-Delgado *et al.*, 2000, 2001). This regimen produces profound marrow ablation with significant mucositis and is associated

Table 21.8. *Busulfan-based high-dose chemotherapy regimens*

Regimen	Chemotherapeutic agents	Total dose	Reference
BU/CY	Busulfan	16 mg/kg	Santos *et al.*, 1983
	Cyclophosphamide	120–200 mg/kg	
BU/CY	Busulfan	16 mg/kg	Tutschka *et al.*, 1987
	Cyclophosphamide	120 mg/kg	
BU/CY	Busulfan	14 mg/kg	Bensinger *et al.*, 1992
	Cyclophosphamide	150 mg/kg	
BU/Mel	Busulfan	16 mg/kg	Martino *et al.*, 1995
	Melphalan	140 mg/m^2	
BU/Mel/Ida	Busulfan	16 mg/kg	Meloni *et al.*, 2000
	Melphalan	60 mg/kg	
	Idarubicin	42 mg/m^2	
BU/E	Busulfan	16 mg/kg	Chao *et al.*, 1993
	Etoposide	60 mg/kg	Linker *et al.*, 1993b
Bu/Mel/TT	Busulfan	12 mg/kg	Weaver *et al.*, 1994
	Melphalan	100 mg/m^2	
	Thiotepa	500 mg/m2	
BU/CY/Mel	Busulfan	16 mg/kg	Phillips *et al.*, 1991
	Cyclophosphamide	120 mg/kg	Locatelli *et al.*, 1994
	Melphalan	90–130 mg/m^2	
BU/CY/TT (autografts)	Busulfan	10 mg/kg	Dimopoulos *et al.*, 1993
	Cyclophosphamide	120 mg/kg	
	Thiotepa	750 mg/m^2	
BU/CY/TT (allografts)	Busulfan	12 mg/kg	Przepiorka *et al.*, 1993
	Cyclophosphamide	120 mg/kg	
	Thiotepa	750 mg/m^2	
BU/CY/E	Busulfan	16 mg/kg	Jones & Santos, 1989
	Cyclophosphamide	150 mg/kg	
	Etoposide	30 mg/kg	
BU/CY/E	Busulfan	16 mg/kg	Crilley *et al.*, 1993, 1995
	Cyclophosphamide	120mg/kg	
	Etoposide	5–40 mg/kg	
BU/A/Mel	Busulfan	21 mg/kg (480 mg/m^2)	Rubie *et al.*, 1994
	Cytosine arabinoside	24 g/m^2	
	Melphalan	140 mg/m^2	
BU/Mito	Busulfan	16 mg/kg	Khalil *et al.*, 1995
	Mitoxantrone	45 mg/m^2	

with an approximate 5% treatment-related mortality due to interstitial pneumonitis.

Regimens involving BU, thiotepa, and CY have been utilized for both autologous (Dimopoulos *et al.*, 1993) and allogeneic (Przepiorka *et al.*, 1994) transplantation. Phase II studies of this regimen have been reported in patients with myeloma (Shimoni *et al.*, 2001), myelodysplasia, and acute leukemia (Bibawi *et al.*, 2001).

A regimen involving BU, CY, and etoposide has been utilized prior to auto- and allografting (Jones & Santos, 1989; Crilley *et al.*, 1993, 1995). A regimen of BU, cytosine arabinoside, and melphalan has been used prior to allografting in children in order to avoid the long-term sequelae of TBI (Rubie *et al.*, 1994). A regimen of BU and mitoxantrone resulted in a high incidence of RRT (Khalil *et al.*, 1995).

Carmustine-based regimens

Carmustine (BCNU) and CY are often combined and may have synergistic activity. The first combination chemotherapy transplant regimen consisted of a combination of carmustine, cytosine arabinoside, CY, and thioguanine (BACT) (Graw *et al.*, 1974). Variations of this combination have evolved into the three- and four-drug combinations involving carmustine in common use today.

Regimens involving various doses of CY, carmustine (BCNU), and etoposide (e.g., CBV) have been evaluated extensively in patients with malignant lymphoma receiving autologous transplants (Phillips & Reece, 1986; Ahmed *et al.*, 1989; Gribben *et al.*, 1989). The doses of drugs and the schedules are shown in Table 21.9. Although not extensively evaluated, all of these regimens are probably sufficiently immunosuppressive to

Table 21.9. *Carmustine-based high-dose chemotherapy regimens*

Regimen	Chemotherapeutic agents	Total dose	Reference
CBV[a]	Carmustine	300–600 mg/m^2	Gulati *et al.*, 1988
	Cyclophosphamide	6–7.2 g/m^2	Ahmed *et al.*, 1989
	Etoposide	600–2,400 mg/m^2	
CBV[b]	Carmustine	15 mg/kg	Horning *et al.*, 1991
	Cyclophosphamide	100 mg/kg	
	Etoposide	60 mg/kg	
CBV plus cisplatin	Carmustine	500 mg/m^2	Reece *et al.*, 1994
	Cyclophosphamide	7.2 g/m^2	
	Etoposide	2.4 g/m^2	
	Cisplatin	150 mg/m^2	
	Lomustine	15 mg/kg	Chao *et al.*, 1995
	Cyclophosphamide	100 mg/kg	
	Etoposide	60 mg/kg	
BEAM	Carmustine	300–600 mg/m^2	Gaspard *et al.*, 1988
	Etoposide	400–800 mg/m^2	Chopra *et al.*, 1992
	Cytosine arabinoside	800–1,600 mg/m^2	Mills *et al.*, 1995
	Melphalan	140 mg/m^2	van Besien *et al.*, 1995
BEAC	Carmustine	300 mg/m^2	Philip *et al.*, 1986
	Etoposide	300 mg/m^2	Philip *et al.*, 1995
	Cytosine arabinoside	800 mg/m^2	
	Cyclophosphamide	6 g/m^2	
STAMP-1	Carmustine	600 mg/m^2	Peters *et al.*, 1988
	Cyclophosphamide	5.6 g/m^2	
	Cisplatin	165 mg/m^2	
BAVC	Carmustine	800 mg/m^2	Meloni *et al.*, 1990
	Amsacrine	450 mg/m^2	
	Cytosine arabinoside	900 mg/m^2	
	Etoposide	450 mg/m^2	
CME	Carmustine	300–600 mg/m^2	Zulian *et al.*, 1989
	Melphalan	80–140 mg/m^2	Ager *et al.*, 1996
	Etoposide	300–2,000 mg/m^2	
CM	Carmustine	500 mg/m^2	Zulian *et al.*, 1989
	Melphalan	140 mg/m^2	
CEC	Carmustine	60–100 mg/m^2	Lazarus *et al.*, 1992
	Etoposide	2,400–3,000 mg/m^2	
	Cisplatin	200 mg/m^2	

[a] Drugs given simultaneously over 3 days.

[b] Each drug given on a separate day with a day's rest in between.

enable allogeneic engraftment (Blume & Buckner, 1995; Cull *et al.*, 2000). Regimens that involve carmustine doses above 400 to 500 mg/m^2 are associated with excessive pulmonary toxicity. Lomustine has been substituted for carmustine in an attempt to decrease pulmonary toxicities, but without success (Chao *et al.*, 1995; Stuart *et al.*, 2001).

Various doses of carmustine, etoposide, cytosine arabinoside, and cyclophosphamide (BEAC) have been extensively evaluated and this is considered a "standard regimen" for patients with malignant lymphoma (Philip *et al.*, 1986, 1995), although some studies have reported a high incidence of RRT, particularly pulmonary and cardiac toxicity with it, especially in patients who had received prior chest radiotherapy (van Besien *et al.*, 1995b).

Melphalan has been substituted for CY in the BEAC regimen to create BEAM and has also been extensively evaluated in patients with malignant lymphoma (Gaspard *et al.*, 1988; Chopra *et al.*, 1992; Mills *et al.*, 1995; van Besien *et al.*, 1995a). Since currently the majority of patients with malignant lymphoma have blood stem cells mobilized with CY-containing regimens, the BEAM regimen is more attractive than the BEAC regimen. Furthermore, the substitution of melphalan for CY obviates the problem of hemorrhagic cystitis and thus the need for mesna and/or bladder irrigation, making this a preferred outpatient regimen for patients with malignant lymphoma. Allogeneic marrow transplants have been performed following administration of BEAM (van Besien *et al.*, 1995a).

A regimen of carmustine, cisplatin, and CY (STAMP I) was commonly used for patients with breast cancer (Peters *et al.*, 1988). However, even in patients with stage II–III breast cancer, treatment-related mortality was 12%, predominantly due to pulmonary toxicity associated with the high dose of carmustine (600 mg/m^2) (Peters *et al.*, 1993). Pharmacokinetic studies have found an association between patients who had faster CY clearance (higher cytotoxic metabolites) and acute cardiac toxicity (Petros *et al.*, 2002). There was no correlation of carmustine clearance with pulmonary toxicity.

Melphalan-based regimens

Melphalan is included in several of the BU and carmustine-based regimens in Tables 21.8 and 21.9; Table 21.10 summarizes additional regimens that have included melphalan for myeloablation.

Thiotepa-based regimens

Thiotepa is included in several of the above BU, carmustine, and melphalan-based regimens outlined in Tables 21.8 to 21.10 and Table 21.11 summarizes additional regimens that include high doses of thiotepa. The most frequently used regimen for women with breast cancer has been the combination of thiotepa, CY, and carboplatin (STAMP V) (Antman *et al.*, 1992). Some investigators administered all three drugs by continuous infusion over 3 days (Antman *et al.*, 1992), others by bolus injection on 3 consecutive days (Weaver *et al.*, 1997b), and others gave CY and thiotepa by bolus injection and carboplatin by continuous infusion. Although STAMP V was widely used for patients with breast cancer, recently published negative results of high-dose chemotherapy in breast cancer using the STAMP V regimen have impacted the use of this regimen (Stadtmauer *et al.*, 2000). The superiority of any one of these methods of administration has not been documented. Bacigalupo and colleagues (1996) have described the successful use of thiotepa and CY prior to allogeneic blood stem cell transplantation for adults with advanced leukemia.

Etoposide-based regimens

The use of etoposide in high-dose regimens has been reviewed (Blume & Buckner, 1995). Etoposide is commonly used in the

Table 21.10. *Melphalan-based high-dose chemotherapy regimens*

Regimen	Chemotherapeutic agents	Total dose	Reference
Mel/E	Melphalan	140–180 mg/m^2	Blume & Buckner, 1995
	Etoposide	60 mg/kg or 1,200–3,600 mg/m^2	Lazarus *et al.*, 1994
Mel/A	Melphalan	140 mg/m^2	Matulonis *et al.*, 1994
	Cytosine arabinoside	12 g/m^2	
Mel/Mito	Melphalan	180 mg/m^2	Mulder *et al.*, 1989
	Mitoxantrone	60 mg/m^2	
Mel/Mito/Carbo	Melphalan	160 mg/m^2	Weaver *et al.*, 1997a
	Mitoxantrone	50 mg/m^2	
	Carboplatin	1,400 mg/m^2	
Mel/CY/P	Melphalan	80 mg/m^2	Peters *et al.*, 1989
	Cyclophosphamide	5.6 g/m^2	
	Cisplatin	180 mg/m^2	
Mel/Mito/Tax	Melphalan	180 mg/m^2	Stiff *et al.*, 1997
	Mitoxantrone	60–90 mg/m^2	
	Paclitaxel	1,000–1,400 mg/m^2	

Table 21.11. *Thiotepa-based high-dose chemotherapy regimens*

Regimen	Chemotherapeutic agents	Total dose	Reference
STAMP-V (CTCb)	Thiotepa	500 mg/m^2	Antman *et al.*, 1992
	Cyclophosphamide	6 g/m^2	Holland *et al.*, 1996
	Carboplatin	800 mg/m^2	
TT/CY Mito	Thiotepa	675 mg/m^2	Ellis *et al.*, 1990
	Cyclophosphamide	7.5 g/m^2	
	Mitoxantrone	60 mg/m^2	
TT/Mit	Thiotepa	1.2 g/m^2	Fields *et al.*, 1993
	Mitoxantrone	90 mg/m^2	
CY/TT	Thiotepa	700 mg/m^2	Williams *et al.*, 1987
	Cyclophosphamide	7 g/m^2	
CY/TT/P	Thiotepa	600 mg/m^2	Shpall *et al.*, 1990
	Cisplatin	40 mg/m^2	Stiff *et al.*, 1997
	Cyclophosphamide	3.75 g/m^2	
CY/TT/H	Thiotepa	600 mg/m^2	Vaughan *et al.*, 1994
	Cyclophosphamide	6 g/m^2	
	Hydroxyurea	18 g/m^2	

regimens listed in Tables 21.8 to 21.10 and additional regimens are outlined in Table 21.12.

Carboplatin

High-dose combination alkylating agent chemotherapy with carboplatin has been reviewed (Eder *et al.*, 1990). High-dose chemotherapy regimens including carboplatin are outlined in Tables 21.10 to 21.12. The MTD for carboplatin and CY administered together are 1.8 and 6.0 g/m^2, respectively (Spitzer *et al.*, 1995). Carboplatin (1,500 mg/m^2) with CY (120 mg/m^2) and mitoxantrone (75 mg/m^2) appeared to be an active regimen for the treatment of patients with ovarian cancer (Stiff *et al.*, 1994). Carboplatin has been substituted for BU given with melphalan and thiotepa in a phase I study (Demirer *et al.*, 2000). The maximum tolerable doses of carboplatin with this regimen were 1,350 mg/m^2 with dose-limiting toxicities being mucositis and colitis.

Cisplatin

Regimens including cisplatin are outlined in Tables 21.9 to 21.12.

Paclitaxel

Paclitaxel 775 mg/m^2 has been substituted for carmustine in a regimen including 5.6 mg/m^2 of CY and 165 mg/m^2 of cisplatin (Cagnoni *et al.*, 1996; Stemmer *et al.*, 1996). Paclitaxel

Table 21.12. *Etoposide-based high-dose chemotherapy regimens*

Regimen	Chemotherapeutic agents	Total dose	Reference
ICE	Ifosfamide	16 g/m^2	Wilson *et al.*, 1992
	Carboplatin	1.8 g/m^2	Elias *et al.*, 1995
	Etoposide	1.2–1.5 g/m^2	
ICE	Ifosfamide	20 g/m^2	Fields *et al.*, 1993
	Carboplatin	1.8 g/m^2	
	Etoposide	3 g/m^2	
ECC	Etoposide	650 mg/m^2	Pierelli *et al.*, 1991
	Cisplatin	100 mg/m^2	
	Carboplatin	1.8 g/m^2	
CEP	Etoposide	30 mg/kg	Somlo *et al.*, 1994
	Cyclophosphamide	100 mg/kg	
	Carboplatin	250 mg/m^2	
CEP	Cyclophosphamide	4.5–5.25 g/m^2	Dunphy *et al.*, 1990
	Etoposide	750–1,200 mg/m^2	
	Cisplatin	120–180 mg/m^2	
EC	Etoposide	2,250 mg/m^2	Broun *et al.*, 1995a, 1995b
	Carboplatin	2,100 mg/m^2	

1,400 mg/m^2 has been administered with mitoxantrone (90 mg/m^2) and melphalan 180 mg/kg to patients with advanced ovarian cancer (Table 21.10) (Stiff et al., 1997).

Mitoxantrone

Regimens including mitoxantrone are included in Tables 21.10 and 21.11. In one study, CY 7 g/m^2 and escalating doses of mitoxantrone led to unacceptable hemorrhagic cystitis, despite the use of mesna, inducing the investigators to substitute melphalan for CY (Mulder et al., 1989).

Cytosine arabinoside

Cytosine arabinoside 12 to 36 g/m^2 has been included in several regimens utilized for the treatment of patients with hematologic malignancies, as outlined in Tables 21.9 and 21.10.

High-dose chemotherapy versus high-dose TBI-based regimens

Two randomized trials have demonstrated equivalency of BU/CY and CY/TBI in patients with CML in chronic phase receiving HLA-matched allografts (Clift et al., 1994; Devergie et al., 1995). Two studies in patients receiving HLA-compatible transplants for AML or CML (one study) showed superiority for the CY/TBI regimen due to a lower relapse rate (Blaise et al., 1992; Ringden et al., 1994) (Table 21.13). In a long-term follow-up of these four randomized trials, there were no statistically significant differences for survival between either BU or TBI regimens, although patients with acute leukemia had a 10% lower survival with BU, which was not significantly different (Socié et al., 2001).

Ringden and colleagues (1996) retrospectively compared the outcome of patients in the EBMT database transplanted for acute leukemia from January 1987 to January 1994 who received either BU/CY versus those who received CY/TBI. Patients were matched for the type of transplant (autologous versus allogeneic), diagnosis (ALL or AML), and disease status at the time of transplant (early first complete remission or intermediate second or later remission or first relapse), as well as age and other parameters. For the allogeneic recipients treatment-related mortality, relapse rate, and leukemia-free survival rate did not differ significantly between the two treatments. For the autologous transplant recipients with ALL intermediate disease, the probability of relapse was higher and the 2-year leukemia-free survival lower in those treated with BU/CY. Interestingly, hepatic VOD and hemorrhagic cystitis were both more common in the BU/CY group compared to the CY/TBI group for both autologous and allogeneic recipients. An IBMTR study found the use of CY and TBI to be associated with better leukemia-free survival and lower treatment-related mortality compared to busulfan and CY in children with ALL (Davies et al., 2000). A study in patients with multiple myeloma compared melphalan 200 mg/m^2 with melphalan 140 mg/m^2 and TBI 8 Gy (Moreau et al., 2002). The median event-free survival was similar in both arms (21 versus 20.5 months), but overall survival at 45 months was better with melphalan alone (65.8% versus 45.5%), presumably due to better salvage therapy. Finally, Horning et al. (1991) have reported equivalency, in nonrandomized trials, between patients with lymphoma receiving TBI and etoposide or CBV.

Marrow ablation using radioisotopes

Alternatives to external beam delivery of radiation have been reviewed (Appelbaum et al., 1992a). One approach to improving the curative ability of transplant conditioning regimens, while simultaneously decreasing toxicity to normal organs, is to replace or augment nonspecific, external beam TBI with targeted radiotherapy. Bone-seeking isotopes or radiolabeled monoclonal antibodies have the potential to focus higher doses of radiation on tumor sites than is possible with external beam TBI and expose normal organs to lower doses of radiation. Evaluations of these techniques have been performed in patients with multiple myeloma, malignant lymphoma, and AML.

Table 21.13. *Randomized trials of high-dose chemotherapy versus Cy/TBI*

Diagnosis	Regimen	Number	Survival	Relapse	EFS	Reference
AML	BU/Cy	51	.51	.34	.47	Blaise et al., 1992
	Cy/TBI	50	.75	.14	.72	
CML	BU/CY	65	.61	.44	.59	Devergie et al., 1995
	CY/TBI	55	.63	.11	.55	
CML	BU/CY	73	.80	.13	.68	Clift et al., 1994
	Cy/TBI	69	.80	.13	.71	
AML & CML	BU/CY	88	.62	–	–	Ringden et al., 1994
	CY/TBI	79	.76	–	–	
Multiple myeloma	MEL	140	.66	–	.30	Moreau et al., 2001
	MEL/TBI	142	.46	–	.20	

Abbreviations: BU, busulfan; CY, cyclophosphamide; MEL, melphalan; TBI, total body irradiation; AML, acute myeloid leukemia; EFS, event-free survival.

Radioisotopes alone

Few studies have utilized radioisotopes alone for marrow ablation. Bayouth *et al.* (1995) performed a phase I trial of [166]Holmium complexed to the bone-seeking isotope-1,4,7,10 tetraazacyclododecane-1,4,7,10-tetramethylene-phosphonic acid ([166]H-DOTMP) in patients with multiple myeloma. The total radiation adsorbed dose delivered to the marrow in six patients ranged from 7.9 to 41.4 Gy, and marrow ablation requiring the infusion of stem cells was achieved in two patients. Several phase I–II studies of [166]H-DOTMP combined with melphalan or with melphalan plus 8 Gy TBI have shown promise with complete response rates higher than reported with melphalan alone or with TBI. The role of bone-seeking isotopes should be expanded over the next several years and may become a major therapeutic approach to the treatment of malignancies involving the bone marrow. A phase II trial of ^{131}I-CD20 antibody followed by autologous bone marrow infusion was performed in patients with low-grade lymphoma who had failed conventional treatment (Press *et al.*, 1993, 1995). Estimated radiation delivered to normal organs was 1,000 to 3,075 cGy with 1,010 to 9,150 cGy to tumor sites. One patient died of infection but 15 of 17 patients were alive and disease-free at the time of publication.

Radiolabeled monoclonal antibody studies

Twelve patients with advanced Hodgkin's disease were treated with an [90]Yttrium-labeled antiferritin monoclonal antibody followed by the CBV regimen and autologous bone marrow transplantation (Bierman *et al.*, 1993). Three of the 12 patients were alive and disease-free at 24 to 28 months.

[131]I-tositumomab (anti-CD20) was given with etoposide and CY to 52 patients with relapsed B-cell lymphomas, escalating the doses of isotope, followed by autologous stem cell transplantation (Press *et al.*, 2000). The maximum tolerable dose to critical normal organs (nonmarrow) was 25 Gy. At 2 years the estimated overall survival and event-free survival were 83% and 68%, respectively, which compared favorably to a historical control group receiving external beam TBI. This approach was used to treat 16 patients with relapsed mantle cell lymphoma (Gopal *et al.*, 2002). Estimated survival and progression-free survival at 3 years were 93% and 61%, respectively, a result that may be considerably improved over standard high-dose regimens for this disease.

Anti-CD33 monoclonal antibody therapy for patients with AML has been reviewed (Jurcic *et al.*, 1995). Initial studies utilizing a ^{131}I labeled anti-CD33 monoclonal antibody, p67, were relatively unsuccessful with only 4 of 9 patients achieving a favorable biodistribution (Appelbaum *et al.*, 1992b). Scheinberg and colleagues (1991) have reported better biodistribution, with longer marrow retention, of a ^{131}I labeled anti-CD33 monoclonal antibody, M195, in patients with AML. The same antibody-isotope combination has been given to patients with advanced AML before undergoing conditioning for allo-geneic transplantation with a BU/CY regimen (Papadopoulos *et al.*, 1993). In that study, the delivery of up to 160 mCi/m^2 of ^{131}I was well tolerated.

[131]I labeled anti-CD45 antibody achieved a favorable biodistribution in 37 of 44 patients with advanced AML or myelodysplasia (Matthews *et al.*, 1999). In that study 34 patients received ^{131}I labeled anti-CD45 monoclonal antibody prior to receiving CY and TBI. Patients received up to 12.3 Gy to the liver and 24 to 28 Gy to bone marrow in addition to the 12.0 Gy of TBI. Seven of 25 patients with AML or RAEB were alive and disease-free at 15 to 89 months. Preliminary studies suggest that the same approach can be utilized in patients with AML in first complete remission receiving a BU/CY regimen (Matthews *et al.*, 1996).

The above studies are exciting and promise to add a new approach to the eradication of malignancy in selected patients with AML or lymphoma. However, these studies are labor intensive, involve a few, highly selected patients (less than 1 patient per month being treated in most studies), and have been carried out only in large research institutions. Recently, a low dose ^{90}Y-CD20 antibody (Zevalin) has been approved by the FDA and could be utilized for high-dose studies (Wiseman *et al.*, 2002).

Treatment regimens that are not marrow-ablative

Sequential regimens with peripheral blood stem cell (PBSC) support

Tandem cycles of high-dose therapy have been advocated as a strategy to reduce the high rates of relapse associated with autologous transplantation. This approach has been especially attractive for disease such as multiple myeloma, which is not cured with conventional therapy or high-dose chemotherapy and autologous HSC transplantation. Tandem cycles of melphalan or melphalan and TBI followed by autologous stem cell transplantation have been reported to produce better outcomes than historical controls (Barlogie *et al.*, 1997, 1999). Prospective, randomized trials are underway to examine this question, but only preliminary incomplete data are available.

The concept of administering less intensive treatments more frequently as an alternative to single high-dose marrow ablative therapy has been explored (Fennelly *et al.*, 1994). Sequential cycles of high-dose carboplatin have been administered with hematopoietic growth factor and repeated PBSC infusions (Shea *et al.*, 1992). Tandem cycles of high-dose therapy have also been utilized for patients with metastatic breast cancer (Broun *et al.*, 1995b). Long *et al.* (1995) administered 4 cycles of mitoxantrone (18 mg/m^2), thiotepa (150–200 mg/m^2), and CY (4.5–5.0 g/m^2) each followed by infusion of PBSC. It remains to be determined whether or not this approach will be superior to single high-dose ablative regimens.

Agents that may protect from regimen-related toxicities

At the present time it is not possible to further increase the doses of currently available chemotherapeutic agents used with a single regimen because of nonmarrow toxicities. Drugs that have the potential to protect normal tissues from toxicity without compromising tumor cell kill are thus very attractive to study. In addition, decreasing RRT associated with current high-dose treatment regimens would allow more transplants to be performed in an outpatient setting, making this therapy available to more patients at lower cost.

Amifostine is an organic thiophosphate that has been shown to protect animals from doses of radiation, nitrogen mustard, melphalan, and cisplatin that would otherwise be lethal. A randomized trial in 242 patients with advanced ovarian cancer receiving cisplatin and CY was carried out (Rose, 1996). Pretreatment with amifostine reduced renal toxicity, neurologic toxicity, febrile neutropenia, hospitalization, and transfusion therapy. Moreover, during 6 cycles of chemotherapy significantly fewer patents treated with amifostine discontinued chemotherapy. A phase II trial of amifostine, cisplatin, and vinblastine was found to be a highly active regimen in patients with non–small-cell lung cancer (Schiller et al., 1996). Current clinical trials are evaluating the effects of amifostine in patients receiving autologous PBSC transplants. One study examined the potential benefit of amifostine given during 4 days of oral BU as part of a regimen of BU, melphalan, and thiotepa (Chauncey et al., 2000). There was less nephrotoxicity but no salutory effect on mucositis or serious toxicities. A phase II study of amifostine given prior to melphalan demonstrated significantly less mucositis when compared to a group of historical patients.

Two cytokines, interleukin-11 (IL-11) and keratinocyte growth factor (KGF) are currently being evaluated for their ability to decrease mucositis and GI toxicity associated with the administration of conventional and high-dose chemotherapy. In animal models IL-11 has been shown to enhance hematopoietic and gastrointestinal recovery following chemoradiotherapy (Du & Williams, 1994; Du et al., 1994). In a phase I study in patients with breast cancer, IL-11 appeared to have a dose-related effect on platelet recovery at doses ≥ 25 μg/day given before and after conventional dose chemotherapy (Gordon et al., 1996). In a randomized study of IL-11 for prevention of mucositis after allogeneic transplantation, IL-11 was associated with severe fluid retention and early mortality which made it impossible to evaluate (Antin et al., 2002).

KGF has been shown in animal studies to stimulate growth of GI epithelium (Rubin et al., 1989). These properties, as well as results of unpublished studies conducted in animal models of radiation and chemotherapeutic damage to the GI epithelium, make KGF a promising drug for ameliorating mucositis and GI toxicity associated with high-dose chemotherapy or chemoradiotherapy. In a phase II randomized study of KGF for patients receiving a TBI, CY, and etoposide regimen, there was a significant reduction in incidence and severity of mucositis (Spielberger et al., 2001).

Summary

Because of the relatively high probability of relapse in most patients receiving HSC transplants, further development of new treatment regimens is warranted. However, one can predict that it will continue to be difficult to identify more effective treatment regimens. Incremental improvements in treatment regimens are expected to be small, difficult to measure, and will require the study of large numbers of patients. As stem cell transplantation becomes more widely used, there will be a great need for controlled trials to evaluate the effectiveness of specific treatment regimens for specific groups of patients. Only centers with large numbers of patients or cooperative groups can successfully perform the trials necessary to substantiate the effectiveness of a given treatment regimen. In order to make high-dose therapies and PBSC support generally available, the procedure will have to be performed with low mortality and minimal morbidity in an outpatient setting. To achieve this goal without sacrificing efficacy, agents that protect from RRT will have to be utilized.

References

Ager, S., Mahendra, P., Richards, E.M. et al. (1996). High dose carmustine, etoposide and melphalan ("BEM") with autologous stem cell transplantation: a dose-toxicity study. Bone Marrow Transplantation, 17, 335–40.

Ahmed, M.T., Ciavarella, D., & Feldman, E. (1989). High-dose, potentially, myeloablative chemotherapy and autologous bone marrow transplantation for patients with advanced Hodgkin's disease. Leukemia, 3, 19–22.

Alegre, A., Lamana, M., Arranz, R. et al. (1995). Busulfan and melphalan as conditioning regimen for autologous peripheral blood stem cell transplantation in multiple myeloma. British Journal of Haematology, 91, 380–6.

Anderson, J.E., Tefferi, A., Craig, F. et al. (2001). Myeloblation and autologous peripheral blood stem cell rescue results in hematological and clinical responses in patients with myeloid metaplasia with myelofibrosis. Blood, 98, 586–93.

Andersson, B.S., McWilliams, K., Tran, H. et al. (1998). IV busulfan, cyclophosphamide (BuCy) and allogeneic hemopoietic stem cells (BMT) for chronic myeloid leukemia (CML). Blood, 92, 285a (Abstract).

Antin, J.H., Lee, S.J., Neuberg, D. et al. (2002). A phase I/II double-blind, placebo-controlled study of recombinant human interleukin-11 for mucositis and acute GVHD prevention in allogeneic stem cell transplantation. Bone Marrow Transplantation, 29, 373–7.

Antman, K., Ayash, L., Elias, A. et al. (1992). A phase II study of high-dose cyclophosphamide, thiotepa, and carboplatin with autologous marrow support in women with measurable advanced breast cancer responding to standard-dose therapy. Journal of Clinical Oncology, 10, 102–10.

Appelbaum, F.R., Badger, C.C., Bernstein, I.D. *et al.* (1992a). Is there a better way to deliver total body irradiation? *Bone Marrow Transplantation,* **10,** (Suppl 1): 77–81.

Appelbaum, F.R., Matthews, D.C., Eary, J.F. *et al.* (1992b). Use of radiolabeled anti-CD33 antibody to augment marrow irradiation prior to marrow transplantation for acute myelogenous leukemia. *Transplantation,* **54,** 829–33.

Bacigalupo, A., Van Lint, M.T., Valbonesi, M. *et al.* (1996). Thiotepa cyclophosphamide followed by granulocyte colony-stimulating factor mobilized allogeneic peripheral blood cells in adults with advanced leukemia. *Blood,* **88,** 353–7.

Badros, A., Barlogie, B., Siegel, E. *et al.* (2002). Improved outcome of allogeneic transplantation in high-risk multiple myeloma patients after nonmyeloablative conditioning. *Journal of Clinical Oncology,* **20,** 1295–303.

Barlogie, B., Jagannath, S., Desikan, K.R. *et al.* (1999). Total therapy with tandem transplants for newly diagnosed multiple myeloma. *Blood,* **93,** 55–65.

Barlogie, B., Jagannath, S., Vesole, D.H. *et al.* (1997). Superiority of tandem autologous transplantation over standard therapy for previously untreated multiple myeloma. *Blood,* **89,** 789–93.

Bayouth, J.E., Macey, D.J., Kasi, L.P. *et al.* (1995). Pharmacokinetics, dosimetry and toxicity of holmium-166-DOTMP for bone marrow ablation in multiple myeloma. *Journal of Nuclear Medicine,* **36,** 730–7.

Bearman, S.I., Appelbaum, F.R., & Buckner, C.D. (1988). Regimen-related toxicity in patients undergoing bone marrow transplantation. *Journal of Clinical Oncology,* **6,** 1562–8.

Bearman, S.I., Appelbaum, F.R., Back, A. *et al.* (1989). Regimen-related toxicity and early posttransplant survival in patients undergoing marrow transplantation for lymphoma. *Journal of Clinical Oncology,* **7,** 1288–94.

Bearman, S.I., Mori, M., Beatty, P.G. *et al.* (1994). Comparison of morbidity and mortality after marrow transplantation from HLA-genotypically identical siblings and HLA-phenotypically identical unrelated donors. *Bone Marrow Transplantation,* **13,** 31–5.

Bensinger, W., Tesh, D., Appelbaum, F. *et al.* (1993). A phase I study of total body irradiation with liver and lung shielding, busulfan (BU) and cyclophosphamide (CY) in preparation for marrow transplant for multiple myeloma (MM). *Experimental Hematology,* **21,** 1110.

Bensinger, W.I., Buckner, C.D., Clift, R.A. *et al.* (1992). Phase I study of busulfan and cyclophosphamide in preparation for allogeneic marrow transplant for patients with multiple myeloma. *Journal of Clinical Oncology,* **10,** 1492–7.

Bensinger, W.I., Rowley, S.D., Demirer, T. *et al.* (1996). High-dose therapy followed by autologous hematopoietic stem cell infusion for patients with multiple myeloma. *Journal of Clinical Oncology,* **14,** 1447–56.

Bibawi, S., Abi-Said, D., Fayad, L. *et al.* (2001). Thiotepa, busulfan, and cyclophosphamide as a preparative regimen for allogeneic transplantation for advanced myelodysplastic syndrome and acute myelogenous leukemia. *American Journal of Hematology,* **67,** 227–33.

Bierman, P.J., Vose, J.M., Leichner, P.K. *et al.* (1993). Yttrium 90-labeled antiferritin followed by high-dose chemotherapy and autologous bone marrow transplantation for poor-prognosis Hodgkin's disease. *Journal of Clinical Oncology,* **11,** 698–703.

Blaise, D., Maraninchi, D., Archimbaud, E. *et al.* (1992). Allogeneic bone marrow transplantation for acute myeloid leukemia in first remission, a randomized trial of a busulfan-cytoxan versus cytoxan-total body irradiation as preparative regimen: a report from the Group d'Etudes de la Greffe de Moelle Osseuse. *Blood,* **79,** 2578–82.

Bleyzac, N., Souillet, G., Magron, P. *et al.* (2001). Improved clinical outcome of paediatric bone marrow recipients using a test dose and Bayesian pharmacokinetic individualization of busulfan dosage regimens. *Bone Marrow Transplantation,* **28,** 743–51.

Blume, K. & Buckner, D. (1995). Workshop: high dose etoposide containing regimens. *Bone Marrow Transplantation,* **15,** S207–S212.

Blume, K., Forman, S., O'Donnell, M. *et al.* (1987). Total body irradiation and high-dose etoposide: a new preparatory regimen for bone marrow in patients with advanced hematologic malignancies. *Blood,* **69,** 1015–20.

Brochstein, J., Kernan, N., Groshen, S. *et al.* (1987). Allogeneic bone marrow transplantation after hyperfractionated total-body irradiation and cyclophosphamide in children with acute leukemia. *New England Journal of Medicine,* **317,** 1618–24.

Broun, E.R., Nichols, C.R., Mandanas, R. *et al.* (1995a). Dose escalation study of high dose carboplatin and etoposide with autologous bone marrow support in patients with recurrent and refractory germ cell tumors. *Bone Marrow Transplantation,* **16,** 353–8.

Broun, E.R., Sridhara, R., Sledge, G.W. *et al.* (1995b). Tandem autotransplantation for the treatment of metastatic breast cancer. *Journal of Clinical Oncology,* **13,** 2050–5.

Buckner, C.D., Rudolph, R.H., Fefer, A. *et al.* (1972). High-dose cyclophosphamide therapy for malignant disease. Toxicity, tumor response, and the effects of stored autologous marrow. *Cancer,* **29,** 357–65.

Cagnoni, P., Shpall, E., Bearman, S., & Al, E. (1996). Paclitaxel-containing high-dose chemotherapy: the University of Colorado experience. *Seminars in Oncology,* **23,** 43–8.

Calvert, A.H., Newell, D.R., Gumbrell, L.A. *et al.* (1989). Carboplatin dosage: prospective evaluation of a simple formula based on renal function. *Journal of Clinical Oncology,* **7,** 1748–56.

Cavo, M., Bandini, G., Benni, M. *et al.* (1998). High-dose busulfan and cyclophosphamide are an effective conditioning regimen for allogeneic bone marrow transplantation in chemosensitive multiple myeloma. *Bone Marrow Transplantation,* **22,** 27–32.

Cesaro, S., Meloni, G., Messina, C. *et al.* (2001). High-dose melphalan with autologous hematopoietic stem cell transplantation for acute myeloid leukemia: results of a retrospective analysis of the Italian Pediatric Group for Bone Marrow Transplantation. *Bone Marrow Transplantation,* **28,** 131–6.

Chao, N., Kastrissios, H., Long, G. *et al.* (1995). A new preparatory regimen for autologous bone marrow transplantation for patients with lymphoma. *Cancer,* **75,** 1354–9.

Chao, N.J., Stein, A.S., Long, G.D. *et al.* (1993). Busulfan/etoposide-initial experience with a new preparatory regimen for autologous bone marrow transplantation in patients with acute non-lymphoblastic leukemia. *Blood,* **81,** 319–23.

Chauncey, T.R., Gooley, T.A., Lloid, M.E. *et al.* (2000). Pilot trial of cytoprotection with amifostine given with high-dose chemotherapy and autologous peripheral blood stem cell transplantation. *American Journal of Clinical, Oncology,* **23,** 406–11.

Chopra, R., Goldstone, A.H., Pearce, R. *et al.* (1992). Autologous versus allogeneic bone marrow transplantation for non-Hodgkin's lymphoma: a case-controlled analysis of the European Bone Marrow Transplant Group registry data. *Journal of Clinical Oncology,* **10,** 1690–5.

Clift, R., Buckner, C., Appelbaum, F. *et al.* (1990). Allogeneic marrow transplantation in patients with acute myeloid leukemia in first remission: a randomized trial of two irradiation regimens. *Blood,* **76,** 1867–71.

Clift, R., Buckner, C., Appelbaum, F. *et al.* (1991). Allogeneic marrow transplantation in patients with chronic myeloid leukemia in the chronic phase: a randomized trial of two irradiation regimens. *Blood,* **77,** 1660–5.

Clift, R.A., Buckner, C.D., Thomas, E.D. *et al.* (1982). Allogeneic marrow transplantation for acute lymphoblastic leukemia in remission using fractionated total body irradiation. *Leukemia Research,* **6,** 409–12.

Clift, R.A., Buckner, C.D., Thomas, E.D. *et al.* (1994). Marrow transplantation for chronic myeloid leukemia: a randomized study comparing cyclophosphamide and total body irradiation with busulfan and cyclophosphamide. *Blood,* **84,** 2036–43.

Coccia, P., Strandjord, S., Warkentin, P. *et al.* (1988). High-dose cytosine arabinoside and fractionated total-body irradiation: an improved preparative regimen for bone marrow transplantation of children with acute lymphoblastic leukemia in remission. *Blood,* **77,** 888–93.

Cony-Makhoul, P., Marit, G., Boiron, J. *et al.* (1995). Busulphan and melphalan prior to autologous transplantation for myeloid malignancies. *Bone Marrow Transplantation,* **16,** 69–70.

Copelan, E.A. & Deeg, H.J. (1992). Conditioning for allogeneic marrow transplantation in patients with lymphohematopoietic malignancies without the use of total body irradiation. *Blood,* **80,** 1648–58.

Corringham, R., Gilmore, M., & Prentice, H. (1983). High-dose melphalan with autologous bone marrow transplant: treatment of poor prognosis tumors. *Cancer,* **52,** 1783–7.

Crilley, P., Lazarus, H., Topolsky, D. *et al.* (1993). Comparison of preparative transplantation regimens using carmustine/etoposide/cisplatin or busulfan/etoposide/cyclophosphamide in lymphoid malignancies. *Seminars in Oncology,* **20,** 50–4.

Crilley, P., Topolsky, D., & Styler, M.J. (1995). Extramedullary toxicity of a conditioning regimen containing busulphan, cyclophosphamide and etoposide in 84 patients undergoing autologous and allogeneic bone marrow transplantation. *Bone Marrow Transplantation,* **15,** 361–5.

Cull, G.M., Haynes, A.P., Byrne, J.L. *et al.* (2000). Preliminary experience of allogeneic stem cell transplantation for lymphoproliferative disorders using BEAM-CAMPATH conditioning: an effective regimen with low procedure-related toxicity. *British Journal of Haematology,* **108,** 754–60.

Davies, S.M., Ramsay, N.K.C., Klein, J.P. *et al.* (2000). Comparison of preparative regimens in transplants for children with acute lymphoblastic leukemia. *Journal of Clinical Oncology,* **18,** 340.

Deeg, H.J., Sullivan, K.M., Buckner, C.D. *et al.* (1986). Marrow transplantation for acute nonlymphoblastic leukemia in first remission: toxicity and long-term follow-up of patients conditioned with single dose or fractionated total body irradiation. *Bone Marrow Transplantation,* **1,** 151–7.

Demirer, T., Buckner, C.D., Appelbaum, F.R. *et al.* (1996a). High-dose busulfan and cyclophosphamide followed by autologous transplantation in patients with advanced breast cancer. *Bone Marrow Transplantation,* **17,** 769–74.

Demirer, T., Buckner, C.D., Appelbaum, F.R. *et al.* (1996b). Busulfan, cyclophosphamide and fractionated total body irradiation for allogeneic marrow transplantation for advanced acute and chronic myelogenous leukemia: phase I dose escalation of busulfan based on targeted plasma levels. *Bone Marrow Transplantation,* **17,** 341–6.

Demirer, T., Ilhan, O., Mandel, N.M. *et al.* (2000). A phase I dose escalation study of high-dose thiotepa, melphalan and carboplatin (TMCb) followed by autologous peripheral blood stem cell transplantation (PBSCT) in patients with solid tumors and hematologic malignancies. *Bone Marrow Transplantation,* **25,** 697–703.

Demirer, T., Petersen, F.B., Appelbaum, F.R. *et al.* (1995). Allogeneic marrow transplantation following cyclophosphamide and escalating doses of hyperfractionated total body irradiation in patients with advanced lymphoid malignancies: a phase I/II trial. *International Journal of Radiation Oncology, Biology, and Physics,* **32,** 1103–9.

Devergie, A., Blaise, D., Attal, M. *et al.* (1995). Allogeneic bone marrow transplantation for chronic myeloid leukemia in first chronic phase: a randomized trial of busulfan-cytoxan versus cytoxan-total body irradiation as preparative regimen: a report from the French society of bone marrow graft (SFGM). *Blood,* **85,** 2263–8.

Dimopoulos, M.A., Alexanian, R., Przepiorka, D. *et al.* (1993). Thiotepa, busulfan, and cyclophosphamide: a new preparative regimen for autologous marrow or blood stem cell transplantation in high-risk multiple myeloma. *Blood,* **82,** 2324–8.

Du, X. & Williams, D. (1994). Interleukin-11: a multifunctional growth factor derived from the hematopoietic microenvironment. *Blood,* **83,** 2023–30.

Du, X., Doerschuk, C., Orazi, A., & Williams, D.A. (1994). A bone marrow stromal-derived growth factor, interleukin-11, stimulates recovery of small intestinal mucosal cells after cytoablative therapy. *Blood,* **83,** 33–7.

Dunphy, F.R., Spitzer, G., Buzdar, A.U. *et al.* (1990). Treatment of estrogen receptor-negative or hormonally refractory breast cancer with double high-dose chemotherapy intensification and bone marrow support. *Journal of Clinical Oncology,* **8,** 1207–16.

Eder, J., Shea, T., Henner, W. *et al.* (1990). In *Carboplatin (JM-8); Current Perspectives and Future Directions,* ed. P. Bunn, R. Canetta, R. Ozols, & M. Rozecweig, pp. 353–60. Philadelphia: W.B Saunders.

Elias, A., Eder, J., Shea, T. *et al.* (1990). High-dose ifosfamide with mesna uroprotection: a phase I study. *Journal of Clinical Oncology,* **8,** 170–8.

Elias, A.D., Ayash, L.J., Wheeler, C. *et al.* (1995). Phase I study of high-dose ifosfamide, carboplatin and etoposide with autologous hematopoietic stem cell support. *Bone Marrow Transplantation,* **15,** 373–9.

Ellis, E.D., Williams, S.F., Moormeier, J.A. *et al.* (1990). A phase I-II study of high-dose cyclophosphamide, thiotepa and escalating doses of mitoxantrone with autologous stem cell rescue in patients with refractory malignancies. *Bone Marrow Transplantation,* **6,** 439–42.

Fefer, A., Einstein, A.B., Thomas, E.D. *et al.* (1974). Bone-marrow transplantation for hematologic neoplasia in 16 patients with identical twins. *New England Journal of Medicine, 290,* 1389–93.

Fennelly, D., Wasserheit, C., Schneider, J. *et al.* (1994). Simultaneous dose escalation and schedule intensification of carboplatin-based chemotherapy using peripheral blood progenitor cells and filgrastim: a phase I trial. *Cancer Research,* **54,** 6137–42.

Fields, K.K., Elfinbein, G.J., Perkins, J.B. *et al.* (1993). Two novel high-dose treatment regimens for metastatic breast cancer—ifosfamide, carboplatin, plus etoposide and mitoxantrone plus thiotepa: outcomes and toxicities. *Seminars in Oncology,* **20,** 59–66.

Friedberg, J.W., Neuberg, D., Stone, R.M. *et al.* (1999). Outcome in patients with myelodysplastic syndrome after autologous bone marrow transplantation for non-Hodgkin's lymphoma. *Journal of Clinical Oncology,* **17,** 3128–35.

Gaspard, M., Maraninchi, D., Stoppa, A. *et al.* (1988). Intensive chemotherapy with high doses of BCNU, etoposide, cytosine arabinoside and melphalan (BEAM) followed by autologous bone marrow transplantation: toxicity and antitumor activity in 26 patients with poor-risk malignancies. *Cancer Chemotherapy and Pharmacology,* **22,** 256–62.

Giralt, S., Estey, E., Albitar, M. *et al.* (1997). Engraftment of allogeneic hematopoietic progenitor cells with purine analog-containing chemotherapy: harnessing graft-versus-leukemia without myeloablative therapy. *Blood,* **89,** 4531–6.

Gopal, A.K., Rajendran, J.G., Pedersdorf, S.H. *et al.* (2002). High-dose chemo-radioimmunotherapy with autologous stem cell support for relapsed mantle cell lymphoma. *Blood,* **99,** 3158–62.

Gopal, R., Ha C.S., Tucker, S.L. *et al.* (2001). Comparison of two total body irradiation fractionation regimens with respect to acute and late pulmonary toxicity. *Cancer,* **92,** 1949–58.

Gordon, M., McCaskill-Stevens, W., Battiato, L. *et al.* (1996). A phase I trial of recombinant human interleukin-11 (neumega rhIL-11 growth factor) in women with breast cancer receiving chemotherapy. *Blood,* **87,** 3615–24.

Graw, R.G.J., Lohrmann, H., Bull, M.I. *et al.* (1974). Bone-marrow transplantation following combination chemotherapy immunosuppression (B.A.C.T.) in patients with acute leukemia. *Transplantation Proceedings,* **6,** 349–54.

Gribben, J.G., Linch, D.C., & Singer, C.R.J. (1989). Successful treatment of refractory Hodgkin's disease by high-dose combination chemotherapy and autologous bone marrow transplantation. *Blood,* **73,** 340–4.

Grochow, L. (1993). Busulfan disposition: the role of therapeutic monitoring in bone marrow transplantation induction regimens. *Seminars in Oncology,* **20,** 18–25.

Grochow, L., Jones, R., Brundrett, R. *et al.* (1989). Pharmacokinetics of busulfan: correlation with veno-occlusive disease in patients undergoing bone marrow transplantation. *Cancer Chemotherapy and Pharmacology,* **25,** 55–61.

Grochow, L.B., Krivit, W., Whitley, C.B., & Blazar, B. (1990). Busulfan disposition in children. *Blood,* **75,** 1723–7.

Gulati, S.C., Shank, B., Black, P. *et al.* (1988). Autologous bone marrow transplantation for patients with poor-prognosis lymphoma. *Journal of Clinical Oncology,* **6,** 1303–13.

Gutierrez-Delgado, F., Holmberg, L.A., Hooper, H. *et al.* (2000). High-dose busulfan, melphalan and thiotepa as consolidation for non-inflammatory high risk breast cancer. *Bone Marrow Transplantation,* **26,** 51–9.

Gutierrez-Delgado, F., Maloney, D.G., Press, O.W. *et al.* (2001). Autologous stem cell transplantation for non-Hodgkin's lymphoma: comparison of radiation-based and chemotherapy-only preparative regimens. *Bone Marrow Transplantation,* **28,** 455–61.

Holland, H.K., Dix, S.P., Geller, R.B. *et al.* (1996). Minimal toxicity and mortality in high risk breast cancer patients receiving high dose cyclophosphamide, thiotepa, and carboplatin plus autologous marrow/stem cell transplantation and comprehensive supportive care. *Journal of Clinical Oncology,* **14,** 1156–64.

Horning, S., Chao, N., Negrin, R. *et al.* (1991). The Stanford experience with high-dose etoposide cytoreductive regimens and autologous bone marrow transplantation in Hodgkin's disease and non-Hodgkin's lymphoma: preliminary data. *Annals of Oncology,* **2,** 47–50.

Jones, R. & Santos, G. (1989). New conditioning regimens for high risk marrow transplants. *Bone Marrow Transplantation,* **4,** 15–7.

Jurcic, J., Caron, P., Nikula, T. *et al.* (1995). Radiolabeled anti-CD33 monoclonal antibody M195 for myeloid malignancies. *Cancer Research,* **55,** 5908s–10s.

Kanfer, E.J., Buckner, C.D., Fefer, A. *et al.* (1987a). Allogeneic and syngeneic marrow transplantation following high dose dimethylbusulfan, cyclophosphamide and total body irradiation. *Bone Marrow Transplantation,* **1,** 339–46.

Kanfer, E.J., Petersen, F.B., Buckner, C.D. *et al.* (1987b). Phase I study of high-dose dimethylbusulfan followed by autologous bone marrow transplantation in patients with advanced malignancy. *Cancer Treatment Reports,* **71,** 101–2.

Kantarjian, H.M., Talpaz, M., Andersson, B. *et al.* (1994). High doses of cyclophosphamide, etoposide and total body irradiation followed by autologous stem cell transplantation in the management of patients with chronic myelogenous leukemia. *Bone Marrow Transplantation,* **14,** 57–61.

Keating, A. & Brandwein, J. (1990). In *Autologous Bone Marrow Transplantation: Proceedings of the Fifth International Symposium,* ed. K. Dicke, J. Armitage, & M. Dicke-Evinger, pp. 427–31. Omaha: University of Nebraska Medical Center.

Khalil, A., Ciobanu, N., & Sparano, J.A. (1995). Pilot study of high dose mitoxantrone and busulfan plus autologous bone marrow transplantation in patients with advanced malignancies. *Bone Marrow Transplantation,* **15,** 93–7.

Krishnan, A., Bhatia, S., Slovak, M.L. *et al.* (2000). Predictors of therapy-related leukemia and myelodysplasia following autologous transplantation for lymphoma: an assessment of risk factors. *Blood,* **95,** 1588–93.

Lazarus, H.M., Crilley, P., Ciobanu, N. *et al.* (1992). High-dose carmustine, etoposide, and cisplatin and autologous bone marrow transplantation for relapsed and refractory lymphoma. *Journal of Clinical Oncology,* **10,** 1682–9.

Lazarus, H.M., Gray, R., Ciobanu, N. *et al.* (1994). Phase I trial of high dose melphalan, high dose etoposide and autologous bone marrow reinfusion in solid tumors: an Eastern Cooperative Oncology Group (ECOG) study. *Bone Marrow Transplantation*, **14**, 443–8.

LeMaistre, C.F. & Herzig, R. (1990). Mitoxantrone: potential for use in intensive therapy. *Seminars in Oncology*, **17**, 43–8.

Linker, C., Ries, C., Damon, L. *et al.* (1993a). Autologous bone marrow transplantation for acute myeloid leukemia using busulfan plus etoposide as a preparative regimen. *Blood*, **81**, 311–8.

Linker, C.A., Damon, L.E., Ries, C.A. *et al.* (1993b). Busulfan plus etoposide as a preparative regimen for autologous bone marrow transplantation for acute myelogenous leukemia: an update. *Seminars in Hematology*, **20** (Suppl 4), 40–8.

Linker, C.A., Ries, C.A., Damon, L.E. *et al.* (1995). Autologous stem cell transplantation for acute myeloid leukemia in first remission. *Blood*, **86**, 384 (Abstract).

Locatelli, F., Pession, A., Bonetti, F. *et al.* (1994). Busulfan, cyclophosphamide and melphalan as conditioning regimen for bone marrow transplantation in children with myelodysplastic syndromes. *Leukemia*, **8**, 844–9.

Long, G.D., Negrin, R.S., Hoyle, C.F., & Kusnierz-Glaz, C.R. (1995). Multiple cycles of high dose chemotherapy supported by hematopoietic progenitor cells as treatment for patients with advanced malignancies. *Cancer*, **76**, 860–8.

Lynch, M.H., Petersen, F.B., Appelbaum, F.R. *et al.* (1995). Phase II study of busulfan, cyclophosphamide and fractionated total body irradiation as a preparatory regimen for allogeneic bone marrow transplantation in patients with advanced myeloid malignancies. *Bone Marrow Transplantation*, **15**, 59–64.

Mansi, J., De Costa, F., Viner, C. *et al.* (1992). High-dose busulfan in patients with myeloma. *Journal of Clinical Oncology*, **10**, 1569–73.

Martino, R., Badell, I., Brunet, S. *et al.* (1995). High-dose busulfan and melphalan before bone marrow transplantation for acute non-lymphoblastic leukemia. *Bone Marrow Transplantation*, **16**, 209–12.

Matthews, D., Appelbaum, F., Eary, J. *et al.* (1996). ^{131}I-anti-CD45 antibody plus busulfan/cyclophosphamide in matched related transplants for AML in first remission. *Blood*, **88**, 142a (Abstract).

Matthews, D.C., Appelbaum, F.R., Eary, J.F. *et al.* (1999). Phase I study of ^{131}I-Anti-CD45 antibody plus cyclophosphamide and total body irradiation for advanced acute leukemia and myelodysplastic syndrome. *Blood*, **94**, 1237–47.

Matulonis, U.A., Griffin, J.D., & Canellos, G.P. (1994). Autologous peripheral blood stem cell transplantation of the blastic phase of chronic myeloid leukemia following sequential high-dose cytosine arabinoside and melphalan. *American Journal of Hematology*, **45**, 283–7.

Mehta, J., Powles, R., Singhal, S. *et al.* (1996). Melphalan-total body irradiation and autologous bone marrow transplantation for adult acute leukemia beyond first remission. *Bone Marrow Transplantation*, **18**, 119–23.

Meloni, G., Capria, S., Trasarti, S. *et al.* (2000). High-dose idarubicine, busulphan and melphalan as conditioning for autologous blood stem cell transplantation in multiple myeloma. A feasibility study. *Bone Marrow Transplantation*, **26**, 1045–49.

Meloni, G., De Fabritiis, P., Petti, M., & Mandelli, F. (1990). BAVC regimen and autologous bone marrow transplantation in patients

with acute myelogenous leukemia in second remission. *Blood*, **75**, 2282–5.

Mills, W., Chopra, R., McMillan, A. *et al.* (1995). BEAC chemotherapy and autologous bone marrow transplantation for patients with relapsed or refractory non-Hodgkin's lymphoma. *Journal of Clinical Oncology*, **13**, 588–95.

Moreau, P., Facon, T., Attal, M. *et al.* (2002). Comparison of 200 mg/m[2] melphalan and 8 Gy total body irradiation plus 140 mg/m[2] melphalan as conditioning regimens for peripheral blood stem cell transplantation in patients with newly diagnosed multiple myeloma: final analysis of the Intergroupe Francophone du Myélome 9502 randomized trial. *Blood*, **99**, 731–5.

Mulder, P.O., Sleijfer, D.T., Willemse, P.H. *et al.* (1989). High-dose cyclophosphamide or melphalan with escalating doses of mitoxantrone and autologous bone marrow transplantation for refractory solid tumors. *Cancer Research*, **49**, 4654–8.

Olivarria, E., Kanfer, E., Szydlo, R. *et al.* (2000). High-dose busulphan alone as cytoreduction before allogeneic or autologous stem cell transplantation for chronic myeloid leukaemia: a single-centre experience. *British Journal of Haematology*, **108**, 769–77.

Papadopoulos, E., Caron, P., Castro-Malaspina, H. *et al.* (1993). Results of allogeneic bone marrow transplant following ^{131}I/M195/busulfan/cyclophosphamide (BY/CY) in patients with advanced/refractory myeloid malignancies. *Blood*, **82**, 80a (Abstract).

Pecego, R., Hill, R., Appelbaum, F.R. *et al.* (1986). Interstitial pneumonitis following autologous bone marrow transplantation. *Transplantation*, **42**, 515–7.

Peters, W., Henner, W., Grochow, L. *et al.* (1987). Clinical and pharmacologic effects of high dose single agent busulfan with autologous bone marrow support in the treatment of solid tumors. *Cancer Research*, **47**, 6402–6.

Peters, W., Stuart, A., Klotman, M. *et al.* (1989). High-dose combination cyclophosphamide, cisplatin, and melphalan with autologous bone marrow support. A clinical and pharmacologic study. *Cancer Chemotherapy and Pharmacology*, **23**, 377–83.

Peters, W.P., Ross, M., Vredenburgh, J.J. *et al.* (1993). High-dose chemotherapy and autologous bone marrow support as consolidation after standard-dose adjuvant therapy for high-risk primary breast cancer. *Journal of Clinical Oncology*, **11**, 1132–43.

Peters, W.P., Shpall, E.J., Jones, R.B. *et al.* (1988). High-dose combination alkylating agents with bone marrow support as initial treatment for metastatic breast cancer. *Journal of Clinical Oncology*, **6**, 1368–76.

Petersen, F.B. & Bearman, S.I. (1994). In *Bone Marrow Transplantation*, ed. S.J. Forman, K.G. Blume, & E.D. Thomas, pp. 79–95. Boston: Blackwell Scientific Publications.

Petersen, F.B., Appelbaum, F.R., & Bigelow, C.L. (1989a). High-dose cytosine arabinoside, total body irradiation and marrow transplantation for advanced malignant lymphoma. *Bone Marrow Transplantation*, **4**, 483–8.

Petersen, F.B., Appelbaum, F.R., Buckner, C.D. *et al.* (1988). Simultaneous infusion of high-dose cytosine arabinoside with cyclophosphamide followed by total body irradiation and marrow infusion for the treatment of patients with advanced hematological malignancies. *Bone Marrow Transplantation*, **3**, 619–24.

Petersen, F.B., Buckner, C.D., Appelbaum, F.R. *et al.* (1989b). Busulfan, cyclophosphamide, and fractionated total body irradiation as a preparatory regimen for marrow transplantation in patients with advanced hematological malignancies: a phase I study. *Bone Marrow Transplantation*, **4**, 617–23.

Petersen, F.B., Buckner, C.D., Appelbaum, F.R. *et al.* (1992a). Etoposide, cyclophosphamide and fractionated total body irradiation as a preparative regimen for marrow transplantation in patients with advanced hematological malignancies: a phase I study. *Bone Marrow Transplantation*, **10**, 83–8.

Petersen, F.B., Deeg, H.J., Buckner, C.D. *et al.* (1992b). Marrow transplantation following escalating doses of fractionated total body irradiation and cyclophosphamide—a phase I trial. *International Journal of Radiation Oncology, Biology and Physics*, **23**, 1027–32.

Petros, W.P., Broadwater, G., Berry, D. *et al.* (2002). Association of high-dose cyclophosphamide, cisplatin, and carmustine pharmacokinetics with survival, toxicity, and dosing weight in patients with primary breast cancer. *Clinical Cancer Research*, **8**, 698–705.

Philip, T., Dumont, J., & Teillet, F. (1986). High-dose chemotherapy and autologous bone marrow transplantation in refractory Hodgkin's disease. *British Journal of Cancer*, **53**, 737–42.

Philip, T., Guglielmi, C., Hagenbeek, A. *et al.* (1995). Autologous bone marrow transplantation as compared with salvage chemotherapy in relapses of chemotherapy-sensitive non-Hodgkin's lymphoma. *New England Journal of Medicine*, **333**, 1540–5.

Phillips, G. & Reece, D. (1986). In *Clinics in Hematology. Autologous Bone Marrow Transplantation*, ed. A. Goldstone, pp. 151–66. Philadelphia: W.B. Saunders.

Phillips, G., Fay, J., Herzig, G. *et al.* (1983). Intensive 1,3-bis(2-chloroethyl)-1-nitrosourea (BCNU), NSC #4366650 and cryopreserved autologous marrow transplantation for refractory cancer. A phase I–II study. *Cancer*, **52**, 1792–802.

Phillips, G., Shepherd, J., Barnett, M. *et al.* (1991). Busulfan, cyclophosphamide and melphalan conditioning for autologous bone marrow transplantation in hematologic malignancy. *Journal of Clinical Oncology*, **9**, 1880–8.

Pierelli, L., Menichella, G., Foddai, M. *et al.* (1991). High dose chemotherapy with cisplatin, VP16 and carboplatin with stem cell support in patients with advanced ovarian cancer. *Haematologica*, **76** (Suppl 1), 63–5.

Powles, R., Milliken, S., Helenglass, G. *et al.* (1989). The use of melphalan in conjunction with total body irradiation as treatment for acute leukaemia. *Transplantation Proceedings*, **21**, 2955–7.

Press, O.W., Eary, J.F., Appelbaum, F.R. *et al.* (1993). Radiolabeled-antibody therapy of B-cell lymphoma with autologous bone marrow support. *New England Journal of Medicine*, **329**, 1219–24.

Press, O.W., Eary, J.F., Appelbaum, F.R., & Bernstein, I.D. (1995). In *Technical and Biological Components of Marrow Transplantation*, ed. C.D. Buckner & R. Clift, pp. 281–97. Boston: Kluwer Academic.

Press, O.W., Eary, J.F., Gooley, T. *et al.* (2000). A phase I/II trial of iodine-131-tositumomab (anti-CD20), etoposide, cyclophosphamide, and autologous stem cell transplantation for relapsed B-cell lymphomas (Plenary paper). *Blood*, **96**, 2934–42.

Przepiorka, D., Ippoliti, C., Giralt, S. *et al.* (1994). Phase I-II study of high-dose thiotepa, busulfan and cyclophosphamide as a preparative regimen for allogeneic marrow transplantation. *Bone Marrow Transplantation*, **14**, 449–53.

Reece, D.E., Connors, J.M., Spinelli, J.J. *et al.* (1994). Intensive therapy with cyclophosphamide, carmustine, etoposide, cisplatin, and autologous bone marrow transplantation for Hodgkin's disease in first relapse after combination chemotherapy. *Blood*, **83**, 1193–9.

Riddell, S., Appelbaum, F.R., Buckner, C.D. *et al.* (1988). High-dose cytarabine and total body irradiation with or without cyclophosphamide as a preparative regimen for marrow transplantation for acute leukemia. *Journal of Clinical Oncology*, **6**, 576–82.

Ringden, O., Labopin, M., Tura, S. *et al.* (1996). A comparison of busulphan versus total body irradiation combined with cyclophosphamide as conditioning for autograft or allograft bone marrow transplantation in patients with acute leukaemia. *British Journal of Haematology*, **93**, 637–45.

Ringden, O., Ruutu, T., Remberger, M. *et al.* (1994). A randomized trial comparing busulfan with total body irradiation as conditioning in allogeneic marrow transplant recipients with leukemia: a report from the Nordic bone marrow transplantation group. *Blood*, **83**, 2723–30.

Rose, P. (1996). Amifostine cytoprotection with chemotherapy for advanced ovarian carcinoma. *Seminars in Oncology*, **23**, 83–9.

Rubie, H., Attal, M., Dumur, C. *et al.* (1994). Intensified conditioning regimen with busulfan followed by allogeneic BMT in children with myelodysplastic syndromes. *Bone Marrow Transplantation*, **13**, 759–62.

Rubin, J., Osada, H., Finch, P. *et al.* (1989). Purification and characterization of a newly identified growth factor specific for epithelial cells. *Proceedings of the National Academy of Sciences USA*, **86**, 802–6.

Santos, G.W., Tutschka, P.J., & Brookmeyer, R. (1983). Marrow transplantation for acute nonlymphocytic leukemia after treatment with busulfan and cyclophosphamide. *New England Journal of Medicine*, **309**, 1347–53.

Sarosy, G., Leyland-Jones, B., Soochan, P., & Cheson, B. (1988). The systemic administration of intravenous melphalan. *Journal of Clinical Oncology*, **6**, 1768–82.

Scheinberg, D., Lovett, D., Divgi, C. *et al.* (1991). A phase I trial of monoclonal antibody M195 in acute myelogenous leukemia: specific bone marrow targeting and internalization of radionuclide. *Journal of Clinical Oncology*, **9**, 478–90.

Schiffman, K.S., Bensinger, W.I., Appelbaum, F.R. *et al.* (1996). Phase II study of high-dose busulfan, melphalan and thiotepa with autologous peripheral blood stem cell support in patients with malignant disease. *Bone Marrow Transplantation*, **17**, 943–50.

Schiller, G., Nimer, S., Vescio, R. *et al.* (1994). Phase I–II study of busulfan and cyclophosphamide conditioning for transplantation in advanced multiple myeloma. *Bone Marrow Transplantation*, **14**, 131–6.

Schiller, J., Storer, B., Berlin, J. *et al.* (1996). Amifostine, cisplatin, and vinblastine in metastatic non-small-cell lung cancer: a report of high response rates and prolonged survival. *Journal of Clinical Oncology*, **14**, 1913–21.

Schuler, U.S., Renner, U., Kroschinsky, F. *et al.* (2001). Intravenous busulfan for conditioning before autologous or allogeneic human blood stem cell transplantation. *British Journal of Haematology*, **114**, 944–50.

Shea, T.C., Flaherty, M., Elias, A. *et al.* (1989). A phase I clinical and pharmacokinetic study of carboplatin and autologous bone marrow support. *Journal of Clinical Oncology*, **7**, 651–61.

Shea, T.C., Mason, J.R., Storniolo, A.M. *et al.* (1992). Sequential cycles of high-dose carboplatin administered with recombinant human granulocyte-macrophage colony-stimulating factor and repeated infusions of autologous peripheral-blood progenitor cells: a novel and effective method for delivering multiple courses of dose-intensive therapy. *Journal of Clinical Oncology,* **10,** 464–73.

Shimoni, A., Smith, T.L., Aleman, A. *et al.* (2001). Thiotepa, busulfan, cyclophosphamide (TBC) and autologous hematopoietic transplantation: an intensive regimen for the treatment of multiple myeloma. *Bone Marrow Transplantation,* **27,** 821–8.

Shpall, E.J., Clarke-Pearson, D., Soper, J.T. *et al.* (1990). High-dose alkylating agent chemotherapy with autologous bone marrow support in patients with stage III/IV epithelial ovarian cancer. *Gynecological Oncology,* **38,** 386–91.

Singhal, S., Powles, R., Treleaven, J. *et al.* (1996). Melphalan alone prior to allogeneic bone marrow transplantation from HLA-identical sibling donors for hematologic malignancies: alloengraftment with potential preservation of fertility in women. *Bone Marrow Transplantation,* **18,** 1049–55.

Slattery, J.T., Clift, R.A., Buckner, C.D. *et al.* (1997). Marrow transplantation for chronic myeloid leukemia: the influence of plasma busulfan levels on the outcome of transplantation. *Blood,* **89,** 3055–60.

Slattery, J.T., Sanders, J.E., Buckner, C.D. *et al.* (1995). Graft rejection and toxicity following bone marrow transplantation in relation to busulfan pharmacokinetics. *Bone Marrow Transplantation,* **16,** 31–42.

Socié, G., Clift, R.A., Blaise, D. *et al.* (2001). Busulfan plus cyclophosphamide compared with total-body irradiation plus cyclophosphamide before marrow transplantation for myeloid leukemia: long-term follow-up of the 4 randomized studies. *Blood,* **98,** 3569–74.

Somlo, G., Doroshow, J.J., Forman, S.J. *et al.* (1994). High-dose cisplatin, etoposide, and cyclophosphamide with autologous stem cell reinfusion in patients with responsive metastatic or high-risk primary breast cancer. *Cancer,* **73,** 125–34.

Spielberger, R.T., Stiff, P., Emmanouilides, C. *et al.* (2001). Efficacy of recombinant human keratinocyte growth factor (RHUKGF) in reducing mucositis in patients with hematologic malignancies undergoing autologous peripheral blood progenitor cell transplantation (Auto-PBPCT) after radiation-based conditioning—results of a Phase 2 trial. ASCO Annual Meeting (Abstract).

Spitzer, T., Cirenza, E., McAfee, S., & Al, E. (1995). Phase I–II trial of high-dose cyclophosphamide, carboplatin and autologous bone marrow or peripheral blood stem cell rescue. *Bone Marrow Transplantation,* **15,** 537–42.

Srivastava, A., Bradstock, K.F., Szer, J. *et al.* (1993). Busulphan and melphalan prior to autologous bone marrow transplantation. *Bone Marrow Transplantation,,* **12,** 323–9.

Stadtmauer, E.A., O'Neill, A., Goldstein, L.J. *et al.* (2000). Conventional-dose chemotherapy compared with high-dose chemotherapy plus autologous hematopoietic stem-cell transplantation for metastatic breast cancer. *New England Journal of Medicine,* **342,** 1069–76.

Stein, J., Davidovitz, M., Yaniv, I. *et al.* (2001). Accidental busulfan overdose: enhanced drug clearance with hemodialysis in a child with Wiskott-Aldrich syndrome. *Bone Marrow Transplantation,* **27,** 551–3.

Stemmer, S.M., Cagnoni, P.J., & Shpall, E.J. (1996). High dose paclitaxel, cyclophosphamide, and cisplatin with autologous hematopoietic progenitor cell support: a phase I trial. *Journal of Clinical Oncology,* **14,** 1463–72.

Stiff, P., Bayer, R., Kerger, C. *et al.* (1997). High-dose chemotherapy with autologous transplantation for persistent/relapsed ovarian cancer: a multivariate analysis of survival for 100 consecutively treated patients. *Journal of Clinical Oncology,* **15,** 1309–17.

Stiff, P.J., McKenzie, R.S., Alberts, D.S. *et al.* (1994). Phase I clinical and pharmacokinetic study of high-dose mitoxantrone combined with carboplatin, cyclophosphamide, and autologous bone marrow rescue: high response rate for refractory ovarian carcinoma. *Journal of Clinical Oncology,* **12,** 176–83.

Storb, R. (1994). Preparative regimens for patients with leukemias and severe aplastic anemia (overview)—biological basis, experimental animal studies and clinical trials at the Fred Hutchinson Cancer Research Center. *Bone Marrow Transplantation,* **14,** (Suppl 4), S1–S3.

Storb, R., Buckner, C.D., Dillingham, L.A., & Thomas, E.D. (1970). Cyclophosphamide regimens in rhesus monkeys with and without marrow infusion. *Cancer Research,* **30,** 2195–203.

Stuart, M.J., Chao, N.S., Horning, S.J. *et al.* (2001). Efficacy and toxicity of a CCNU-containing high-dose chemotherapy regimen followed by autologous hematopoietic cell transplantation in relapsed or refractory Hodgkin's disease. *Biology of Blood and Marrow Transplantation,* **7,** 552–60.

Thomas, E.D., Buckner, C.D., Rudolph, R.H. *et al.* (1971). Allogeneic marrow grafting for hematologic malignancy using HLA-matched donor-recipient sibling pairs. *Blood,* **38,** 267–87.

Thomas, E.D., Clift, R.A., Hersman, J. *et al.* (1982). Marrow transplantation for acute nonlymphoblastic leukemia in first remission using fractionated or single-dose irradiation. *International Journal of Radiation Oncology, Biology, and Physics,* **8,** 817–21.

Thomas, E.D., Motulsky, A.G., & Walters, D.H. (1955). Homozygous hemoglobin C disease. Report of a case with studies on the pathophysiology and neonatal formation of hemoglobin C. *American Journal of Medicine,* **18,** 832–8.

Tutschka, P.J., Bilgrami, S.A., Feingold, J.M. *et al.* (2001). Cytoreduction and stem cell mobilization with a regimen of paclitaxel, etoposide and cyclophosphamide followed by autologous transplantation using a preparative regimen of busulfan, etoposide and cyclophosphamide for patients with advanced lymphoma. *Acta Haematologica,* **105,** 222–32.

Tutschka, P.J., Copeland, E.A., & Klein, J.P. (1987). Bone marrow transplantation for leukemia following a new busulfan and cyclophosphamide regimen. *Blood,* **70,** 1382–8.

van Besien, K., Demuynck, H., Lemaistre, C. *et al.* (1995a). High-dose melphalan allows durable engraftment of allogeneic bone marrow. *Bone Marrow Transplantation,* **15,** 321–3.

van Besien, K., Tabocoff, J., Rodriguez, M. *et al.* (1995b). High dose chemotherapy with BEAC regimen and autologous bone marrow transplantation for intermediate grade and immunoblastic lymphoma: durable complete remissions, but a high rate of regimen-related toxicity. *Bone Marrow Transplantation,* **15,** 549–55.

Vaughan, W.P., Reed, E.C., Edwards, B., & Kessinger, A. (1994). High dose cyclophosphamide, thiotepa and hydroxyurea with autologous hematopoietic stem cell rescue: an effective consolidation chemotherapy regimen for early metastatic breast cancer. *Bone Marrow Transplantation*, **13,** 619–24.

Vey, N., Deprijck, B., Faucher, C. *et al.* (1996). A pilot study of busulfan and melphalan as preparatory regimen prior to allogeneic bone marrow transplantation in refractory or relapsed hematological malignancies. *Bone Marrow Transplantation*, **18,** 495–9.

Vriesendorp, H. (1990). Radiobiological speculations on therapeutic total body irradiation. *Critical Reviews in Oncology Hematology*, **10,** 211–24.

Weaver, C.H., Bensinger, W.I., Appelbaum, K. *et al.* (1994). Phase I study of high-dose busulfan, melphalan, thiotepa with autologous stem cell support in patients with refractory malignancies. *Bone Marrow Transplantation*, **14,** 813–19.

Weaver, C.H., Greco, F.A., Hainsworth, J. *et al.* (1997a). A phase I–II study of high-dose melphalan, mitoxantrone and carboplatin with peripheral blood stem cell support in patients with advanced ovarian or breast carcinoma. *Bone Marrow Transplantation*, **10,** 847–53.

Weaver, C.H., West, W.H., Schwartzberg, L.S. *et al.* (1997b). Induction, mobilization of peripheral blood stem cells (PBSC), high-dose chemotherapy and PBSC infusion in patients with untreated stage IV breast cancer: outcomes by intent to treat analyses. *Bone Marrow Transplantation*, **19,** 661–70.

Wheeler, C., Khurshid, A., Ibrahim, J. *et al.* (2001). Incidence of post transplant myelodysplasia/acute leukemia in non-Hodgkin's lymphoma patients compared with Hodgkin's disease patients undergoing autologous transplantation following cyclophosphamide, carmustine, and etoposide (CBV). *Leukemia and Lymphoma*, **40,** 499–509.

Wiseman, G.A., Leigh, B., Erwin, W.D. *et al.* (2002). Radiation dosimetry results for Zevalin radioimmunotherapy of rituximab-refractory non-Hodgkin lymphoma. *Cancer,* **94,** (Suppl 4), 1349–1357.

22 Non-myeloablative conditioning: induction of graft-versus-disease effect as a therapeutic modality

SERGIO GIRALT, ISSA KHOURI, AND RICHARD CHAMPLIN

University of Texas MD Anderson Cancer Center, Houston, USA

Introduction

High-dose chemoradiotherapy with allogeneic hematopoietic stem cell (HSC) transplantation is an effective therapy for patients with hematologic malignancies (Gale & Champlin, 1984; Bortin *et al.*, 1992). The curative potential of allogeneic transplantation is mediated in part by an immune graft-versus-leukemia effect. Evidence of a graft-versus-leukemia effect is demonstrated by the lower relapse rate in patients with graft-versus-host disease (GVHD) and the higher risk of relapse after syngeneic or T-cell-depleted transplants (Weiden *et al.*, 1981; Goldman *et al.*, 1988; Sullivan *et al.*, 1989a, 1989b; Horowitz *et al.*, 1990; Gale *et al.*, 1994). The most direct evidence for this effect is the reinduction of remission obtained with infusions of donor lymphocytes in patients relapsing after an allogeneic transplant (Antin, 1993; Drobyski *et al.*, 1993; Van Rhea *et al.*, 1994; Kolb *et al.*, 1995; Mackinnon *et al.*, 1995). This effect is more pronounced in patients with chronic myeloid leukemia (CML), but has also been observed in patients with acute leukemia, chronic lymphatic leukemia (CLL), myeloma, and lymphoma relapsing after allogeneic bone marrow transplantation (BMT) (Rondón *et al.*, 1996; Tricot *et al.*, 1996; Collins *et al.*, 1997). These observations suggest that in certain situations the induction of graft-versus-leukemia may be sufficient for cure and that intense myeloablative therapy may not be needed. However, due to the toxicities traditionally associated with myeloablative therapy and allogeneic transplantation, this immune effect has not been effectively explored, for example, in elderly or debilitated patients, since they have generally been excluded from allogeneic transplant programs.

Many investigators have shown that inflammatory cytokines are essential for triggering and maintaining GVHD (Ferrara & Deeg, 1991). Holler *et al.* (1990) have demonstrated that higher levels of tumor necrosis factor (TNF)-α predict for regimen-related toxicities and GVHD. Hill and collaborators (1997) showed in an animal model that lower doses of total body irradiation (TBI) (900 cGy versus 1,300 cGy) were associated with a reduced incidence of GVHD mortality and morbidity in a variety of murine donor-recipient strain combinations. This report also demonstrated significant increases in TNF-α and interleukin (IL)-1β at day 7 posttransplant for the mice receiving the higher TBI dose. Thus, a strategy of utilizing a less intensive, non-myelosuppressive preparative regimen that was sufficiently immunosuppressive to prevent graft rejection and allow engraftment of allogeneic stem cells, and which could then be used to induce a graft-versus-malignancy against susceptible malignancies, was suggested. This strategy could in theory be used in patients ineligible for high-dose chemotherapy or TBI because of their age or concurrent medical conditions. If successful, it could then be extended to all transplant candidates.

The hypothesis underlying this treatment strategy is that a less intensive preparative regimen would be associated with lower production of inflammatory cytokines and, therefore, less regimen-related toxicity and less GVHD (Fig. 22.1). In contrast to the significant increase in intestinal permeability that occurs after conventional, myeloablative conditioning regimens, it has been demonstrated that after non-myeloablative regimens the integrity of the mucosal barrier in the intestine is preserved (Johansson, Brune, & Ekman, 2001). In this chapter we summarize the current experience with allogeneic progenitor cell transplantation after non-myeloablative or reduced intensity conditioning therapies (also known as "mini-transplants").

Development of non-myeloablative conditioning regimens

To explore the graft-versus-leukemia effect as primary therapy it seemed necessary to first achieve stable engraftment of allogeneic stem cells (Fig. 22.1). To accomplish this it was necessary to provide sufficient immune suppression to prevent graft rejection and also possibly to provide myelosuppression in order to create "space" and allow engraftment. Therefore, harnessing the graft-versus-leukemia effect without myeloablative therapy depends on the development of preparative regimens that are sufficiently immunosuppressive to allow durable engraftment, yet have little, if any, nonhematologic toxicity (i.e., which are myelosuppressive but not myeloablative). TBI and cyclophosphamide have been the best studied immune

Induction of GVL as primary therapy

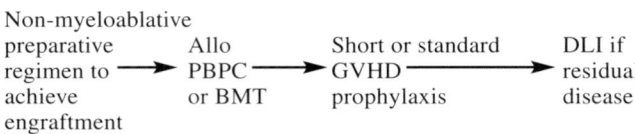

Fig. 22.1.   Induction of the graft-versus-malignancy effect as primary therapy. Abbreviations: GVL, graft-versus-leukemia effect; PBPC, peripheral blood progenitor cells; BMT, bone marrow transplantation; GVHD, graft-versus-host disease; DLI, donor lymphocyte infusion

suppressive regimens used to achieve engraftment. However, neither the minimum nor the optimum dose of this regimen required to establish HSC engraftment in humans has been well defined (van Bekkum, 1984). In a canine model, Yu *et al.* (1995) showed that transient, but prolonged, donor hematopoietic chimerism could be obtained with a TBI dose of 450 cGy, if followed by posttransplant cyclosporine, and that donor cell engraftment was enhanced by posttransplant methotrexate. In a subsequent study, durable sustained allogeneic hematopoietic engraftment was achieved by combining a TBI dose of 200 cGy with posttransplant immune suppression using cyclosporine and mycophenolate mofetil. Dogs receiving 100 cGy TBI, or less intense posttransplant immune suppressive therapy, either failed to engraft or had late graft failure post-transplant (Storb *et al.*, 1997). However, in this latter setting, prolonging the duration of posttransplant immunosuppression with cyclosporine (but not substituting blood for marrow stem cells) favorably influenced stable donor engraftment (Zaucha *et al.*, 2001).

The same regimen has been explored in clinical studies (McSweeney *et al.*, 2001). Forty-five patients with a wide range of hematologic malignancies (median age 56 years) received an HLA-identical sibling PBSC transplant followed by immune suppression with cyclosporine and mycophenolate mofetil. Regimen-related toxicity and myelosuppression were mild, allowing 53% of eligible patients to have an outpatient transplant. However, nonfatal graft rejection occurred in 20% of patients. The incidence of grade II to III acute GVHD was 47% in patients with sustained engraftment. With a median follow-up of 417 days, the overall survival was 66%, nonrelapse mortality was 6%, and mortality due to relapse was 26%.

In mice given 200 cGy TBI engraftment of allogeneic bone marrow has been enhanced by treatment with anti-CD154 (anti CD40 ligand) (Taylor *et al.*, 2001).

In humans, cyclophosphamide doses of 200 mg/kg have been associated with a graft rejection rate of 30% in transfusion-sensitized aplastic anemia patients (Storb *et al.*, 1983). Engraftment depends not only on the immune suppressive regimen, but also on features such as the degree of HLA disparity between donor and recipient, T-cell depletion of the stem cell inoculum, pretransplant transfusions, infused cell dose, and other host and donor factors (Champlin, Feig, & Gale, 1984; Deeg *et al.*, 1986).

The purine analogues fludarabine and 2-chlorodeoxyadenosine (2-CDA) have been shown to be active against a variety of hematologic malignancies (Plunkett & Sanders, 1991). These compounds are also immunosuppressive, effectively inhibiting the mixed lymphocyte reaction in vitro (Goodman *et al.*, 1995). They have also been shown to inhibit the mechanisms of DNA repair from alkylator-induced damage and may therefore potentiate the antitumor effect of alkylating agents (Li *et al.*, 1997). Thus, purine analogue-conditioning, non-myeloablative regimens appeared an appropriate way of exploring induction of a graft-versus-malignancy effect without myeloablative therapy. Examples of such regimens are shown in Table 22.1. Engraftment has been rapid after such regimens as fludarabine, melphalan, and carmustine with a median time to an absolute neutrophil count of $1.0 \times 10^9/l$ of 11 days and a time to a platelet count of $> 20 \times 10^9/l$ of 13 days (Wäsch *et al.*, 2000). In a study by Kottaridis and colleagues (2000), CAMPATH-1H at a dose of 20 mg/kg/day from day -8 to day -4 was added to the combination of fludarabine and melphalan. Nineteen of the 44 patients had had a prior transplant. The incidence of acute GVHD grade II or higher was low, occurring in only 2 patients. The estimated probability of treatment-related mortality was 11% (Fig. 22.2).

In a study using thiotepa 10 mg/kg, cyclophosphamide 60 mg/kg, and fludarabine 30 mg/m² daily for for 2 days prior to T-replete, HLA-identical sibling PBSC or marrow, Corradini and colleagues (2002) reported a 13% nonrelapse mortality and a 57% progression-free survival in a cohort of 45 patients with poor-risk hematological malignancies, 26 of whom had failed a prior autograft and 18 of whom had refractory disease at the time of transplantation. In another study of 76 patients, fludarabine 150 mg/m² plus melphalan 140 mg/m² was used for lymphoid malignancies while fludarabine and busulfan 10 mg/kg was used for myeloid malignancies prior to a T-replete, HLA-identical sibling PBSC transplant (Martino *et al.*, 2001). With a median follow-up of 283 days, the 1 year probability of trans-

Table 22.1.   *Reduced-intensity non-myeloablative conditioning regimens used in treatment of malignancy*

Regimen

1. Fludarabine 30 mg/m² × 4, cytosine arabinoside 2 g/m² × 4, idarubicin 12 mg/m² × 3
2. Fludarabine 30 mg/m² × 4, melphalan 140 mg/m² × 1
3. 2-Chlorodeoxyadenosine 12 mg/m²/d × 5, cytosine arabinoside 1 g/m² × 5
4. Fludarabine 30 mg/m² × 3–5, cyclophosphamide 300 mg/m² to 1,000 mg/m² × 1–2
5. Fludarabine 30 mg/m² × 2, cytosine arabinoside 500 mg/m² × 2, cisplatin 25 mg/m² × 4
6. Fludarabine 30 mg/m² × 6, busulfan 4 mg/kg/d × 2, antithymocyte globulin 10 mg/kg/d × 4
7. Cyclophosphamide 50 mg/kg × 4, ATG × 3 or 4 pre- and post-transplant, thymic irradiation 7 Gy × I
8. Fludarabine 25 mg/m² × 4, cyclophosphamide 60 mg/kg × 2

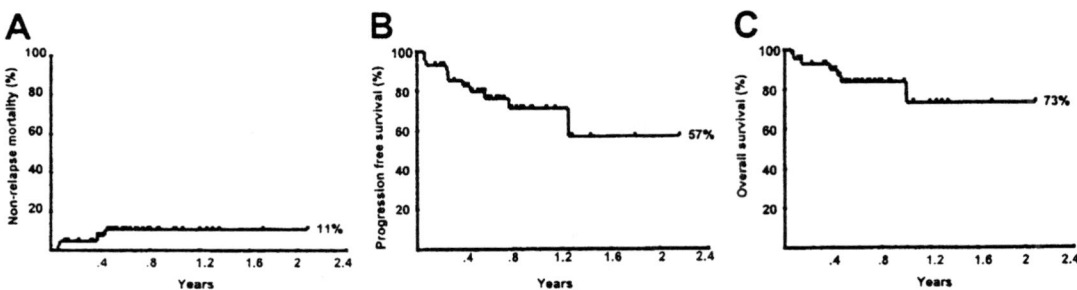

Fig. 22.2. Kaplan-Meier curves. (**A**) Nonrelapse mortality; (**B**) progression-free survival; and (**C**) overall survival for the entire group of 44 patients. Reproduced, with permission, from Kottaridis *et al.* (2000).

plant-related mortality was 20% and progression-free survival was 55%. Michallet and colleagues (2001) found diagnosis and disease status at the the time of transplant to significantly influence survival in 92 patients with predominantly hematologic malignancies. Age and type of GVHD prophylaxis significantly influenced transplant-related mortality.

In animal systems the use of other immunosuppressive, noncytotoxic agents, such as those that induce transient blockade of the CD40-CD154 co-stimulatory pathway using an anti-CD154 (CD40 ligand) antibody appears promising (Seung *et al.*, 2000).

After non-myeloablative conditioning regimens, the early patterns of chimerism may predict either GVHD (increasing donor T-cell chimerism) or graft loss (T-cell chimerism declining to <20% donor cells) (Childs *et al.*, 1999). Therefore, more frequent (every 2 to 4 weeks) peripheral blood analysis may be warranted (Antin *et al.*, 2001). Additionally, the degree of donor engraftment (chimerism), particularly of T cells, can be analyzed to guide the need for further therapy, such as the infusion of donor lymphocytes in patients transplanted for hematologic malignancy (Fig. 22.3) (Spitzer *et al.*, 2000; Marks *et al.*,

2002). Donor chimerism levels desirable for functional correction of various genetic disorders are shown in Table 22.2.

In a matched control study comparing non-myeloablative HSC transplantation, the incidence of early bacteremia was reduced in the non-myeloablative group due to the shorter period of severe neutropenia (Junghanss *et al.*, 2002b). A high incidence of CMV antigenemia and late bacterial infection have been reported in some series (Mohty *et al.*, 2000; Mossad *et al.*, 2001; Chakrabarti *et al.*, 2002; Perez-Simon *et al.*, 2002). while a reduced incidence of CMV disease was reported in a retrospective, historically controlled study (Martino *et al.*, 2001). In a case-matched controlled study, the onset of CMV disease was significantly delayed in recipients of non-myeloablative conditioning compared to the controls who received conventional myeloablative conditioning (Fig. 22.4) (Junghanss *et al.*, 2002), although the overall 1-year incidences were similar. It was concluded that CMV surveillance and pre-emptive ganciclovir treatment should extend beyond day 100, at least in recipients of this specific non-myeloablative conditioning regimen (TBI 200 cGy with or without fludarabine).

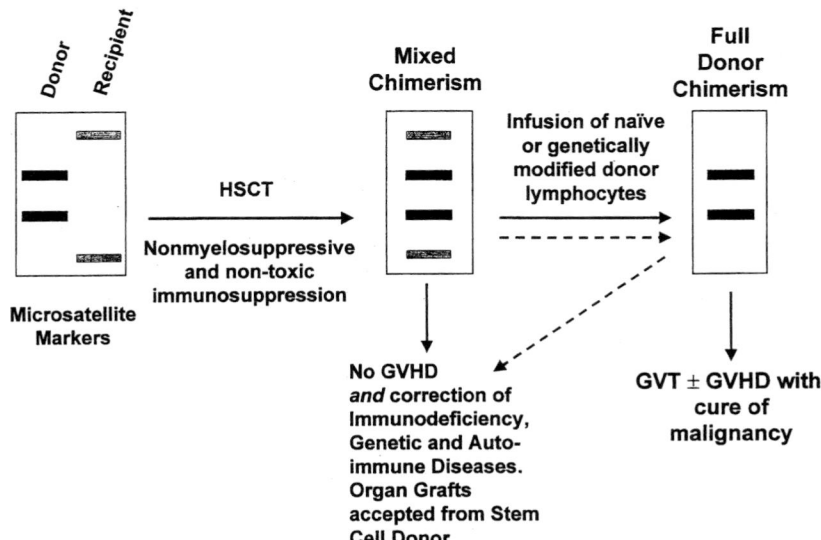

Fig. 22.3. Conceptual approach to clinical application of mixed chimerism. Microsatellite markers represent chimerism analysis of hematopoietic cell DNA using PCR and gel electrophoresis to identify donor and recipient specific bands. Reproduced, with permission, from McSweeney & Storb (1999).

Table 22.2. *Donor chimerism levels desirable for functional correction of genetic disorders*

Percentage donor cells[a]	Diseases	Comments
3–10	Sickle cell anemia	RBC graft required
	Chronic granulomatous disease	PMN graft required
	Leukocyte adhesion deficiency	PMN, lymphoid graft required
> 10	Severe combined immunodeficiency	Usually T cells[b]
	Wiskott-Aldrich syndrome	Platelet graft required
	CD40 ligand deficiency	
	Hemophagocytic lymphohistiocytosis	NK-cell, CTL graft required
100	Autoimmune lymphoproliferative syndrome	
	Fanconi's anemia	

Abbreviations: RBC, red blood cells; PMN, polymorphonucleocytes; NK, natural killer; CTL, cytotoxic T lymphocyte.

[a] Peripheral blood nucleated cells.

[b] Many patients required lifetime intravenous immunoglobulin G because of lack of B-cell engraftment.

The use of non-myeloablative conditioning regimens in patients who have a major ABO incompatibility with their donor appears to enhance the delay of donor erythropoiesis: initial detection of donor-origin red cells was later after nonablative conditioning compared to that after ablative conditioning and the decline of anti-donor isohemagglutinins was slower (Bolan *et al.*, 2001). Pure red cell aplasia occurred in 29% of the patients in this study receiving nonablative conditioning versus none of 12 given an ablative regmen.

In a comparison of patients given non-myeloablative versus conventional conditioning regimens, platelet transfusion requirements were reduced in the former group (23% versus 100%), as were red blood cell requirements (63% versus 96%) (Weissinger *et al.*, 2001). Using T-cell-receptor Vβ spectratype analysis to examine the distribution of complementarity-determining region 3 (CDR3)-size bands as a measure of the complexity of the redeveloping T-cell repertoire, Friedman and colleagues (2001) found more rapid repertoire reconstitution after non-myeloablative, than after myeloablative, conditioning.

Posttransplant EBV-associated lymphoproliferative disease has been described after non-myeloablative conditioning (Ho *et al.*, 2002).

The decreased toxicity associated with this approach has enabled the transplants to be carried out as outpatient procedures in many patients (Ruiz-Argüelles *et al.*, 2001).

The 2001 EBMT activity survey indicated an increase in reduced intensity conditioning for allografts from less than 1% in 1998 to 27% of all allogeneic transplants in 2001 (Gratwohl *et al.*, 2003).

Non-myeloablative regimens for acute leukemia or myelodysplasia

Non-myeloablative regimens for acute leukemia or myelodysplasia are described in Chapters 50, 51, and 54.

Non-myeloablative regimens for chronic myeloid leukemia

Non-myeloablative regimens for chronic myeloid leukemia are described in Chapter 52.

Non-myeloablative regimens for lymphoid malignancies (and see Chapter 51, 56, and 57)

Lymphoid malignancies appear very sensitive to graft-versus-tumor (GVL) effects. Allogeneic transplants are associated with a substantially lower relapse rate than purged autologous transplants. Other evidence to support the GVL effect comes from the observation that patients with progressive disease after allogeneic transplantation who undergo withdrawal of immunosuppression, develop GVHD, which is often accompanied by a simultaneous regression of their lymphomas. Van Besien *et al.* (1997) demonstrated that of 9 patients who relapsed after allogeneic transplantation, 4 responded to withdrawal of immunosuppression (2 complete remissions, 2 partial remissions), with responses that lasted nearly 2 years.

Success of non-myeloablative stem cell transplantation (NST) requires engraftment of donor cells. It also requires the development of an effective GVL effect before the underlying disease can progress. Therefore the pretransplant regimen must also suppress the lymphoma sufficiently to prevent any marked early progression.

At M.D. Anderson Cancer Center, fludarabine-based chemotherapy was used at conventional doses. In the initial studies the combination of cisplatin, fludarabine, and cytarabine (PFA) was used as a non-myeloablative preparative regimen for patients with aggressive lymphoma (Fig. 22.5). This was based on the well-established activity of this combination in these diseases. Patients with indolent lymphoma received fludarabine, 25 mg/m^2 administered intravenously (i.v.) daily on days −6 to −2 before transplantation and cyclophosphamide, 1,000 mg/m^2 given i.v.

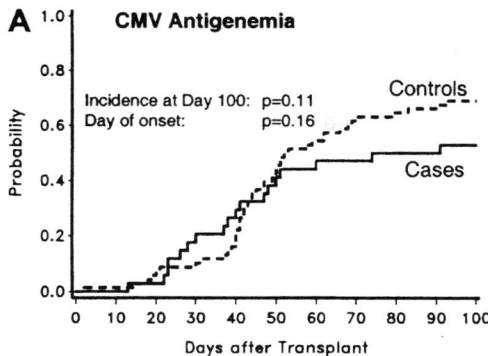

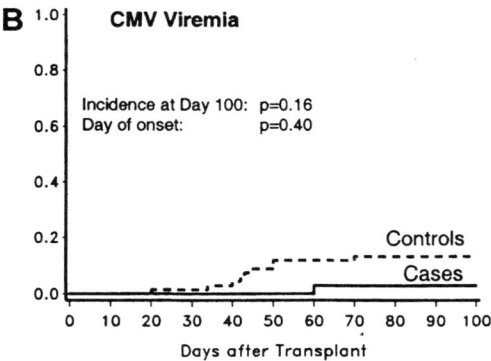

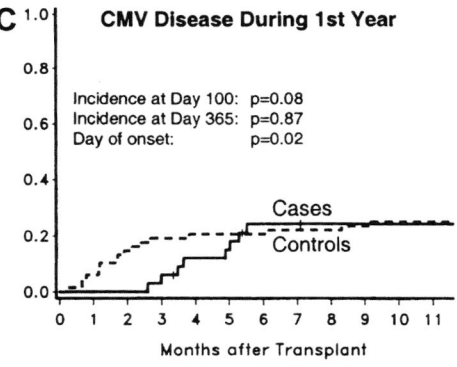

Fig. 22.4. CMV antigenemia, viremia, and disease in CMV high-risk patients. The probabilities of CMV antigenemia (**A**), CMV viremia (**B**), and CMV disease (**C**) are displayed. The probability for CMV disease was analyzed for the first year after transplantation; for other events, the analyses were done for the first 100 days after transplantation. Reproduced, with permission, from Junghanss *et al.* (2002).

daily on days −3 and −2 before transplantation. In 1999, the schedule of fludarabine/cyclophosphamide was changed to be given sequentially at 4-hour intervals in order to maximize inhibition of DNA repair and subsequent tumor kill. Rituximab was also added to our treatment protocol with the consideration that it might be synergistic with chemotherapy and produce no overlapping toxicity. The dose of rituximab was based on studies from our institution, demonstrating a dose-response relationship in patients with chronic lymphatic leukemia. This regimen was later used as an NST preparative regimen for all CD20+ B-cell lymphomas including those with aggressive histologies.

We studied adult patients who had recurrent indolent, mantle cell, discordant, or transformed lymphoma after a prior response to conventional treatment. Patients with de novo diffuse large cell lymphoma were included only if they were not eligible for autologous transplantation or if they had failed a prior autotransplant.

Posttransplantation, patients received immunosuppressive therapy with tacrolimus in combination with 5 mg of methotrexate per square meter of body surface area on days 1, 3, and 6. The dose of tacrolimus was tapered by day 60 to 90 if there were signs of residual disease; otherwise it was continued for 6 months.

Filgrastim was administered as a subcutaneous injection of 5 μg per kilogram of body weight daily from day 0 until recovery of the granulocyte count to greater than 1×10^9 per liter of blood. Infection prophylaxis during the peritransplantation period consisted of 400 mg of norfloxacin given orally twice daily; 500 mg of penicillin VK given orally every 6 hours; and 200 mg of fluconazole given orally every 12 hours. Patients also received 500 mg of valacyclovir given orally daily and were screened biweekly for cytomegalovirus antigenemia.

Seventy-two patients were studied. The patients ranged in age from 21 to 68 years (median, 52 years). Twenty-nine patients had follicular lymphoma, 29 had transformed, or de novo diffuse large cell lymphoma, and 14 patients had mantle cell lymphoma. All patients had advanced recurrent disease and were previously pretreated. The number of prior chemotherapy regimens received by each patient ranged from 1 to 8 (median, 3). Nineteen patients (26%) had failed a prior autologous transplant. At the time of transplantation, 57 (71%) had chemosensitive and 15 (21%) had chemorefractory disease. Each patient had an HLA-identical sibling donor.

All patients had prompt hematopoietic recovery. Neutrophil counts recovered to more than $0.5 \times 10^9/l$ at a median of 11 days after transplantation (range, 7–18 days). Thirty-four patients never required any platelet transfusion. The median percentage of donor cells at 1 month after transplantation was 80% (range, 0%–100%). Two patients had a primary graft failure and recovered autologous hematopoiesis promptly.

Six patients had a secondary graft failure. Two of these patients were still in complete remission (CR) at the time of this analysis, at 12+, and 39+ months posttransplant. These two patients never had CR with any form of conventional chemotherapy prior to transplantation. Two other patients achieved CR with rituximab that was durable at 3+ and 35+ months, respectively.

Five patients received donor lymphocyte infusion of 1×10^7 to 1×10^8 CD3+ cells per kilogram after transplantation due to persistent or progressive disease. These patients also received rituximab with their immunomanipulation. Rituximab was given weekly × 4, with a first dose at 375 mg/m^2 body surface area and subsequent doses at 1,000 mg/m^2 body surface area. Three of these five patients were reinduced into durable CR.

The median follow-up period of all patients who were alive was 16 months (range, 3–63 months). Actuarial overall survival at 2 years was 80% (95% CI, 66%–89%) (Fig. 22.6). Lymphoma-free-survival was 76% (standard error +/− 10%).

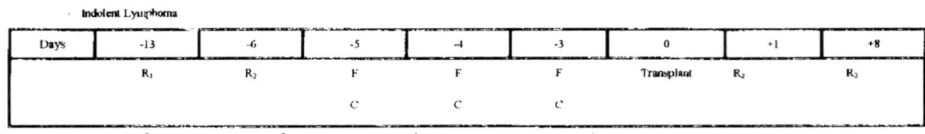

Fig. 22.5. Non-myeloablative preparative regimens for lymphoma.

The cumulative incidence of acute grade II–IV and III–IV GVHD was 19% and 7%, respectively. The cumulative incidence of extensive chronic GVHD was 35% (95% CI, 21%–58%). Three patients (4%) died within 100 days. Eight other patients died secondary to relapse (three patients), chronic GVHD (two patients), infection (two patients), and secondary malignancy (one patient). One additional patient died in CR secondary to a cerebral infarct.

Several other groups have explored different drug combinations to develop reduced-intensity regimens. Slavin *et al.* (1998) pioneered the use of fludarabine in combination with 8 mg/kg busulfan. Kottaridis *et al.* (2000) have employed a fludarabine/melphalan regimen in combination with Campath-1H antibody. The results of these and other studies were recently addressed by the EBMT group (Robinson *et al.,* 2000). In their analysis, treatment-related mortality at 1 year was 39% for patients with low-grade and high-grade histologies. Acute and chronic GVHD contributed to 55% of the mortality rate. This difference in outcome with our study is probably related to their use of more intense preparative regimens, a shorter duration of GVHD prophylaxis, and their indication for donor lymphocyte infusion (DLI). DLI has been used in several centers to convert mixed chimerism into complete chimerism irrespective of the disease status. In our studies, we were cautious about the use of DLI because we have not observed a correlation between the percentage of donor cells and the ultimate response. Patients who engraft tend to spontaneously move toward complete chimerism and

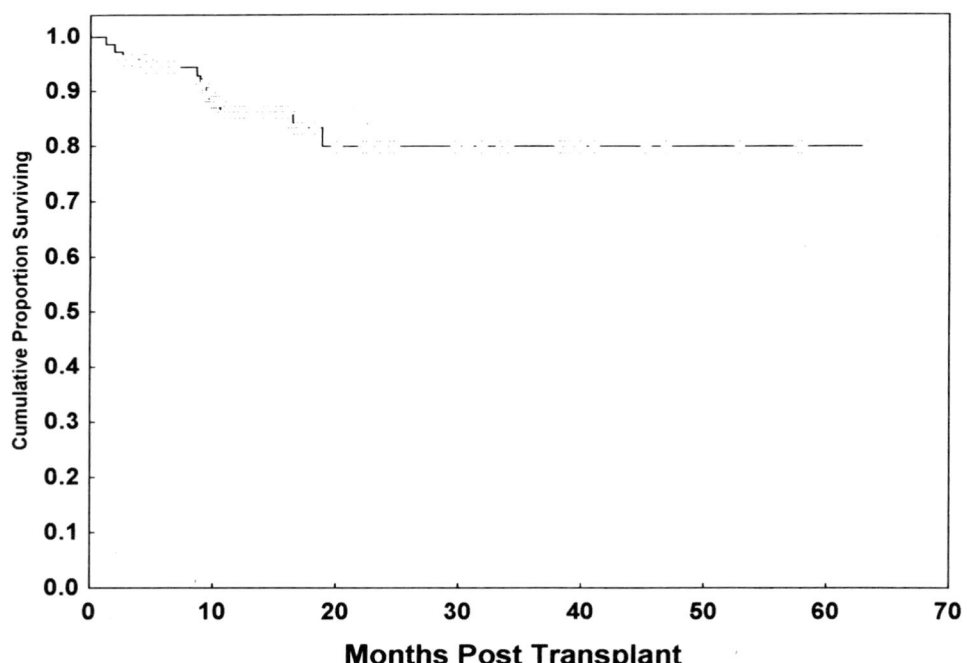

Fig. 22.6. Kaplan-Meier survival curve of 72 patients with lymphoma after NST.

DLI was not required in most cases. Controlled studies comparing various NST strategies and alternative standard treatment for relapsed lymphoma are needed.

Non-myeloablative regimens for multiple myeloma

Non-myeloablative regimens for multiple myeloma are described in Chapter 55.

Autologous HSC transplantation followed by elective reduced intensity conditioning and allografting for myeloma

A new approach involves the use of a standard autograft for tumor debulking purposes followed by an elective allograft (using reduced intensity conditioning) and an allograft to exploit the graft-versus-myeloma effect (Maloney *et al.*, 2001; Kröger *et al.*, 2002). Kröger and colleagues (2002) treated 17 patients with advanced stage II/III myeloma with melphalan 200 mg/m² and an autologous transplant. After a median interval of 119 days, a reduced intensity conditioning regimen of fludarabine 180 mg/m², melphalan 100 mg/m², and ATG 10 mg/kg for 3 doses was administered prior to an allogeneic transplant from an HLA-matched related donor in 7 patients, an HLA-mismatched related donor in 2 patients, and an unrelated donor in 8 patients. Complete donor chimerism was detected after a median of 30 days. The 100 day mortality rate postallograft was 11%. The complete remission rate with negative immunofixation increased from 0% after induction or salvage chemotherapy to 18% after autologous transplantation to 73% after allografting. At a median follow-up of 13 months postallografting, the 2 year estimated event-free survival was 56% (see also Chapter 124).

Non-myeloablative regimens for solid tumors (and see Chapter 120)

Renal cell carcinoma

Because of their well-known response to immune therapeutic maneuvers, malignant melanoma and renal cell carcinoma were solid tumors initially targeted for allogeneic treansplants after nonablative conditioning. The early results in renal cell carcinoma have been particularly gratifying, with complete resolution occurring in some patients with metastatic disease (Childs *et al.*, 1999, 2000): These patients had refractory disease and almost all had failed previous cytokine immunotherapy with interleukin-2 or interferon-α or both. The patients were prepared with cyclophosphamide 120 mg/kg and fludarabine 25 mg/kg daily for 5 days prior to receipt of a T-replete peripheral blood stem cell transplant containing a median of 8×10^6 CD34⁺ cells/kg. Cyclosporine was used as posttransplant immune suppression, and was withdrawn early in patients with mixed T-cell chimerism or disease progression. Three patients had a complete response and seven a partial response. Regression of metastases was delayed, occurring at a median of 129 days posttransplant.,

and often following withdrawal of cyclosporine and the establishment of donor T-cell chimerism. Responses were much more frequent in those with GVHD than in those without.

Breast cancer

Five patients with metastatic breast cancer were treated at MD Anderson Hospital in Houston with mini-allogeneic transplantation with a conditioning regimen of fludarabine 30 mg/m2 iv daily from day -6 to -2 and melphalan 70 mg/m2 iv daily from day -3 to -2 and tacrolimus and mini-methotrexate GVHD prophylaxis. Tacrolimus was tapered for disease progression at 100 days after transplant. On day 30 all patients had 100% donor myelo- and lympho-chimerism. One patient who presented with metastatic disease is in complete response. Three additional patients have had prolonged stable disease (Ueno *et al.*, 2002). Two of 6 patients given a nonmyeloablative conditioning regimen of thiotepa, cyclophosphamide, and fludarabine prior to an HLA-identical sibling PBSC transplant showed a partial response after posttransplant donor lymphocyte infusions with or without interferon (Bregni *et al.*, 2002).

Non-myeloablative regimens for nonmalignant diseases

Non-myeloablative preparative regimens that could consistently result in donor cell engraftment have potential applications in nonmalignant disorders, such as the hemoglobinopathies (Slavin *et al.*, 1998; Sykora *et al.*, 2001), congenital immune deficiency disorders, and inborn errors of metabolism. However, it is possible that regimens that are capable of achieving allogeneic progenitor cell engraftment in a severely immune compromised patient (such as a patient with CLL who has received prior fludarabine) may not be immune suppressive enough for a patient with, for example, sickle cell disease, although two adults with the latter disease, who were conditioned with fludarabine, melphalan, and ATG, engrafted quickly and demonstrated 100% donor chimerism (van Besien *et al.*, 2000). (While free of pain crises posttransplant, both subsequently died of GVHD.)

Preliminary results in patients with congenital immune deficiencies are encouraging, however: eight patients who all had severe organ dysfunction pretransplant were conditioned with fludarabine, melphalan, and anti-thymocyte globulin prior to a T-replete, HLA-matched unrelated (six) or sibling (two) donor BMT (Amrolia *et al.*, 2000). All eight patients engrafted with predominantly donor hematopoiesis. One died of disease recurrence and three showed stable mixed chimerism. At a median of 1 year posttransplant, all patients showed good recovery of CD3⁺ T cells and six of seven evaluable had normal phytohemagglutinin stimulation indices. Two patients who had CD40 ligand deficiency showed significant expression posttransplant and one patient with adenosine deaminase deficiency showed improved deoxy adenosine triphosphate metabolites. Additionally, the use of non-myeloablative conditioning (with cyclophosphamide, fludarabine, and ATG) followed by a T-cell depleted, HLA-identical sibling PBSC transplant has been described in five children and five adults with chronic granulomatous disease (Horwitz et al., 2001). After a median follow-up of 17 months, the proportion of donor neutrophils in the circulation in 8 of the 10 patients ranged from 33% to 100%. Graft failure occurred in two patients; three patients died—of graft failure, pneumococcal pneumonia, and GVHD. Preexisting granulomatous lesions resolved in the patients in whom transplantation was successful.

Non-myeloablative regimens as preparation for second transplants

Non-myeloablative regimens have been utilized successfully as preparative regimens for second transplants, for example after rejection of the first transplant (Byrne et al., 2001), and in patients who relapsed or developed secondary malignancies following autologous transplantation (Nagler et al., 2000; Kottaridis et al., 2000; Badros et al., 2001; Dey et al., 2001; Vesole, Simic, & Lazarus, 2001).

Non-ablative regimens and the use of T-cell depletion

Theoretically, the use of a non-ablative regimen and T-cell depletion of the stem cell inoculum might lead to a high incidence of nonengraftment, since both are risk factors for graft rejection. On the other hand the use of PBSC may counter such a risk. In practice, varying results have been obtained. Lack of engraftment was not a major problem in two studies utilizing in vivo T-cell depletion of the recipient at the time of transplant, with ATG (Slavin et al., 1998) or Campath I (Kottarides et al., 2000) as part of the conditioning regimen. It was problematic, however, in one study (Kreiter et al., 2001), but not another (Craddock et al., 2000) using CD34 selection, and in patients given Campath 1 in the stem cell bag (Chakrabati et al., 2001). It should be noted that in the study by Kottarides et al. there was a significant incidence of viral reactivation posttransplant, particularly CMV, and it was postulated that this was due to Campath administration causing delay of immune reconstitution (Chakrabarti et al., 2002; Perez-Simon et al., 2002).

Non-myeloablative regimens and the use of alternate donors

Again, the concern here is the possibility of an increased risk of nonengraftment. This did not appear to be a major problem in a small series of patients with congenital immune deficiencies given HLA-identical unrelated donor transplants (Amrolia et al., 2000). Boulad and colleagues (2000) reported successful outcomes in two patients with Fanconi anemia given HLA-DRB1-disparate family member PBSC grafts that were T-cell-depleted by CD34 selection followed by E-rosetting. Chan and colleagues (2001) reported three patients with severe aplastic anemia given a T-replete, 1 HLA antigen-mismatched family member transplant and two patients given an HLA-matched unrelated donor transplant after conditioning with fludarabine,

cyclophosphamide, and ATG. With a median follow-up of 9 months, all five were alive with complete donor chimerism.

A regimen of Campath-1H 20 mg on days –8 to –4, fludarabine 30 mg/m^2 on days –7 to –3, and melphalan 140 mg/m^2 on day –2 was administered prior to an unrelated bone marrow transplant in 46 patients (and an unrelated PBSC transplant in 1) with hematological malignancies (Chakraverty et al., 2002). Twenty-nine patients had failed a prior autologous transplant. Twenty of the transplants were mismatched for HLA class I and/or class II alleles. Cyclosporine was used for GVHD prophylaxis. Primary graft failure occurred in 2 of 44 evaluable patients (4.5%). Only 3 patients developed grade III to IV acute GVHD, and at the time of the report no patients had developed extensive chronic GVHD. The estimated probability of nonrelapse mortality at day 100 was 14.9%. With a median follow-up of 344 (range 79–830) days, progression-free survival at 1 year was 61.5%. Serious infective complications occurred in 62% and were the cause of death in 5 patients. Nine patients relapsed or died of progressive disease. None of 4 patients with refractory disease showed a response. All 5 patients with CML entered molecular remission. Five patients failed to establish full donor chimerism.

Using fludarabine 30 mg/m^2/day from day -4 to day -2 together with TBI 2 Gy on day 0, Niederwieser and colleagues (2003) reported 25% of patients alive and in remission with a median follow-up of 19 months. Cyclosporine and mycophenolate mofetil were used for GVHD prophylaxis in this series of 52 patients receiving HLA-matched or mismatched grafts. Most patients (88%) had a preceding conventional transplant or had refractory/advanced disease. These results indicate that certain low-intensity conditioning regimens without high dose total body irradiation can ensure stable engraftment of unrelated donor HSC grafts.

Summary and conclusions

The success of donor lymphocyte infusions to induce remission in patients relapsing after allogeneic transplantation for CML and other hematologic malignancies suggests an alternative approach to conventional myeloablative conditioning, namely a low-dose non-myeloablative conditioning regimen followed by allogeneic marrow or peripheral blood progenitor cell transplantation to obtain engraftment. Subsequently, donor lymphocyte infusions are used to induce complete remission (Marks et al., 2002; Perez-Simon et al., 2002). One study of engraftment kinetics after non-ablative conditioning demonstrated that full donor T-cell engraftment preceded myeloid engraftment, acute GVHD, and disease regression, consistent with a requirement for 100% donor chimerism for full expression of the alloresponse (Childs et al., 1999). This strategy could be used to offer the benefits of allogeneic progenitor cell transplantation to older or more infirm patients, as, for example, demonstrated by its success in enabling a transplant in a patient with progressive pulmonary aspergillosis (Xun et al., 1999).

The major problems with non-myeloablative regimens thus far have been disease eradication, engraftment, and GVHD.

More intense non-myeloablative regimens using intermediate doses of busulfan or melphalan may produce adequate leukemia control to allow time for establishment of a graft-versus-leukemia effect, as well as allowing engraftment of T-cell-depleted marrow or peripheral blood stem cells, which may not engraft with less intense non-myeloablative regimens.

A major challenge continues to be the separation of the graft-versus-leukemia effect from the adverse effects of GVHD. We have evaluated selective depletion of CD8$^+$ cells from allogeneic donor marrow. This procedure has been documented to reduce the incidence of GVHD to approximately 20% without increasing the risk of relapse in CML (Champlin et al., 1990; Nimer et al., 1994). We have demonstrated that donor lymphocyte infusions using CD8$^+$ depleted cells can reliably reinduce remission in patients with CML with a low rate of GVHD (Giralt et al., 1995). CD8$^+$ depleted lymphocyte infusions have also been successful in selected cases of multiple myeloma (Alyea et al., 1995). Although less intense preparative regimens should decrease regimen-related toxicity (possibly by decreasing inflammatory cytokine production), GVHD will remain the major obstacle. Elimination of alloreactive donor T lymphocytes would be expected to abrogate development of GVHD. A novel approach to achieve this is transduction of donor T cells with the herpes simplex virus thymidine kinase (HSV-TK) gene, which renders human cells sensitive to ganciclovir treatment. Lymphocytes have been used successfully as targets for retroviral vector-mediated gene transfer. In preliminary studies lymphocytes transduced with the HSV-TK gene are capable of alloreactivity resulting in graft-versus-leukemia effects; when GVHD develops, it can be abrogated by administration of ganciclovir (Bonini et al., 1997). This approach requires further evaluation and testing. If successful, use of these suicidal lymphocytes could markedly improve the safety of donor lymphocyte infusion therapy and broaden its potential application to a wide range of clinical settings (see Chapter 117).

Such novel therapies may provide a safety cushion for allogeneic transplantation by enabling effective treatment (or indeed prophylaxis) of GVHD, thus abrogating the need for corticosteroid treatment with its considerable side effects. Likewise, identification, cloning, and expansion of lymphocyte clones with preferential antileukemia reactivity to hematopoietic host targets could also dramatically improve the potential application of this type of therapy by promoting graft-versus-leukemia over GVHD.

Use of non-ablative preparative regimens is a promising approach to reduce the morbidity and mortality associated with allogeneic blood and marrow transplantation. It appears possible to carry out such allografts on an outpatient basis (Gomez-Almaguer et al., 2000). The potent graft-versus-leukemia effect against susceptible malignancies suggests that strategies to induce a graft-versus-leukemia effect could emerge as a major new modality for treatment of such diseases.

References

Alyea, E., Soiffer, R., Murray, C. et al. (1995). Adoptive immunotherapy following allogeneic bone marrow transplantation (BMT) with donor lymphocytes depleted of CD8$^+$ cells. Blood, 86, 293a (Abstract).

Amrolia, P., Gasspar, H.B., Hassan, A. et al. (2000). Nonmyelablative stem cell transplantation for congenital immunodeficiencies. Blood, 96, 1239–46.

Anderlini, P., Giralt, S., Andersson, B. et al. (2000). Allogeneic stem cell transplantation with fludarabine-based, less intensive conditioning regimens as adoptive immunotherapy in advanced Hodgkin's disease. Bone Marrow Transplantation, 26, 615–20.

Antin, J.H. (1993). Graft-versus-leukemia: no longer an epiphenomenon. Blood, 82, 2273–7.

Antin, J.H., Childs, R., Filipovich, A.H. et al. (2001). Establishment of complete and mixed donor chimerism after allogeneic lymphohematopoietic transplantation: recommendations from a workshop at the 2001 Tandem Meetings. Biology of Blood and Marrow Transplantation, 7, 473–85.

Auffermann-Gretzinger, S., Lossos, I.S., Vayntrub, T.A. et al. (2002). Rapid establishment of dendritic cell chimerism in allogeneic hematopoietic cell transplant recipients. Blood, 99, 1442–8.

Badros, A., Barlogie, B., Morris, C. et al. (2001). High response rate in refractory and high-risk multiple myeloma after allotransplantation using a nonmyeloablative conditioning regimen and donor lymphocyte infusions. Blood, 97, 2574–9.

Bjorkstrand, B., Ljungman, P., Svensson, H. et al. (1996). Allogeneic bone marrow transplantation versus autologous stem cell transplantation in multiple myeloma: a retrospective case-matched study from the European Group for Blood and Marrow Transplantation. Blood, 88, 4711–18.

Bolan, C.D., Leitman, S.F., Griffith, L.M. et al. (2001). Delayed donor red cell chimerism and pure red cell aplasia following major ABO-incompatible nonmyeloablative hematopoietic stem cell transplantation. Blood, 98, 1687–94.

Bonini, C., Ferrari, G., Verzeletti, S. et al. (1997). HSV-tk gene transfer into donor lymphocytes for control of allogeneic graft-versus-leukemia. Science, 276, 1719–24.

Bortin, M., Horowitz, M., Gale, R. et al. (1992). Changing trends in allogeneic bone marrow transplantation for leukemia in the 1980's. Journal of the American Medical Association, 268, 607–12.

Boulad, F., Gillio, A., Small, T.N. et al. (2000). Stem cell transplantation for the treatment of Fanconi anaemia using a fludarabine-based regimen and T-cell-depleted related HLA-mismatched peripheral blood stem cell grafts. British Journal of Haematology, 111, 1153–7.

Bregni, M., Dodero, A., Peccatori, J. et al. (2002). Nonmyeloablative conditioning followed by hematopoietic cell allografting and donor lymphocyte infusions for patients with metastati renal and breast cancer. Blood, 99, 4234–6.

Byrne , J.L. Musuka, C., Davy, B. et al. (2001). Successful engraftment of a second transplant using non-myeloablative conditioning as treatment for graft failure following unrelated donor BMT. Bone Marrow Transplantation, 27, 547–9.

Chakrabati, S., McDonald, D., & Milligan, D.W. (2001). T cell-depleted nonmyeloablative stem cell transplantation: what is the optimum balance between the intensity of host conditioning and the degree of T cell depletion of the graft? Bone Marrow Transplantation, 28, 313–4 (Letter).

Chakrabarti, S., Mackinnon, S., Chopra, R. *et al.* (2002). High incidence of CMV infection after nonmyeloablative stem cell transplantation: potential role of Campath-1H in delaying immune reconstitution. *Blood,* **99,** 4357–63.

Chakraverty, R., Peggs, K., Chopra, R. *et al.* (2002). Limiting transplant-related mortality following unrelated donor stem cell transplantation by using a non-myeloablative conditioning regimen. *Blood,* **99,** 1071–8.

Champlin, R., Feig, S., & Gale, R. (1984). Case problems in bone marrow transplantation. I. Graft failure in aplastic anemia: its biology and treatment. *Experimental Hematology,* **12,** 728–33.

Champlin, R., Ho, W., Gajewski, J. *et al.* (1990). Selective depletion of CD8⁺ T lymphocytes for prevention of graft-versus-host disease after allogeneic bone marrow transplantation. *Blood,* **76,** 418–23.

Chan, K.W., Li, C.K., Worth, L.L. *et al.* (2001). A fludarabine-based conditioning regimen for severe aplastic anemia. *Bone Marrow Transplantation,* **27,** 125–8.

Childs, R., Clave, E., Contentin, N. *et al.* (1999). Engraftment kinetics after nonmyeloablative allogeneic peripheral blood stem cell transplantation: full donor T-cell chimerism precedes alloimmune response. *Blood,* **94,** 3234–41.

Childs, R.W., Clave, E., Tisdale, J. *et al.* (1999). Successful treatment of metastatic renal cell carcinoma with a nonmyeloablative allogeneic peripheral blood progenitor-cell transplant: evidence for a graft-versus-tumor effect. *Journal of Clinical Oncology,* **17,** 2044–9.

Childs, R., Chernoff, A., Contentin, A. *et al.* (2000). Regression of metastatic renal-cell carcinoma after nonmyeloablative allogeneic peripheral blood stem cell transplantation. *New England Journal of Medicine,* **343,** 750–8.

Collins, R., Shpilberg, O., Drobyski, W. *et al.* (1997). Donor leukocyte infusions in 140 patients with relapsed malignancy after allogeneic bone marrow transplant. *Journal of Clinical Oncology,* **15,** 433–44.

Corradini, P., Tarella, C., Olivieri, A. *et al.* (2002). Reduced-intensity conditioning followed by allografting of hematopoietic cells can produce clinical and molecular remissions in patients with poor-risk hematologic malignancies. *Blood,* **99,** 75–82.

Craddock, C., Bardy, P., Kreiter, S. *et al.* (2000). Engraftment of T cell-depleted allogeneic hematopoietic stem cells using a reduced intensity conditioning regimen. *British Journal of Haematology,* **111,** 797–800.

Deeg, H., Self, S., Storb, R. *et al.* (1986). Decreased incidence of marrow graft rejection in patients with severe aplastic anemia: changing impact of risk factors. *Blood,* **68,** 1363–8.

Dey, B.R., McAfee, S., Sackstein, R. *et al.* (2001). Successful allogeneic stem cell transplantation with nonmyeloablative conditioning in patients with relapsed hematologic malignancy following autologous stem cell transplantation. *Biology of Blood and Marrow Transplantation,* **7,** 604–12.

Drobyski, W.R., Keever, C.A., Roth, M.S. *et al.* (1993). Salvage immunotherapy using donor leukocyte infusions as treatment for relapsed chronic myelogenous leukemia after allogeneic bone marrow transplantation: efficacy and toxicity of a defined T cell dose. *Blood,* **82,** 2310–18.

Ferrara, J.L.M. & Deeg, H.J. (1991). Mechanisms of disease: graft-versus-host disease. *New England Journal of Medicine,* **324,** 667–74.

Friedman, T.M., Varadi, G., Hopely, D.D. *et al.* (2001). Non-myeloablative conditioning allows for more rapid T-cell repertoire reconstitution following allogeneic matched unrelated bone marrow transplantation compared to myeloablative approaches. *Biology of Blood and Marrow Transplantation,* **7,** 656–64.

Gale, R.P. & Champlin, R.E. (1984). How does bone marrow transplantation cure leukemia? *Lancet,* **2,** 28–30.

Gale, R.P., Horowitz, M.M., Ash, R.C. *et al.* (1994). Identical-twin bone marrow transplants for leukemia. *Annals of Internal Medicine,* **120,** 646–52.

Gandhi, V., Kemena, A., Keating, M.J., & Plunkett, W. (1993). Cellular pharmacology of fludarabine triphosphate in chronic lymphocytic leukemia cells during fludarabine therapy. *Leukemia Lymphoma,* **10,** 49–56.

Giralt, S., Estey, E., Albitar, M. *et al.* (1997). Engraftment of allogeneic hematopoietic progenitor cells with purine analog-containing chemotherapy: harnessing graft-versus-leukemia therapy. *Blood,* **89,** 4531–6.

Giralt, S., Hester, J., Huh, Y. *et al.* (1995). CD8⁺ depleted donor lymphocyte infusion as treatment for relapsed chronic myelogenous leukemia after allogeneic bone marrow transplantation: graft-versus-leukemia without graft-versus-host disease. *Blood,* **86,** 4337–43.

Goldman, J.M., Gale, R.P., Bortin, M.M. *et al.* (1988). Bone marrow transplantation for chronic myelogenous leukemia in chronic phase: increased risk of relapse associated with T cell depletion. *Annals of Internal Medicine,* **108,** 806–14.

Gomez-Almaguer, D., Ruiz-Arguelles, G.J., Ruiz-Arguelles, A. *et al.* (2000). Hematopoietic stem cell allografts using a non-myeloablative conditioning regimen can be safely performed on an outpatient basis: report of four cases. *Bone Marrow Transplantation,* **25,** 131–3.

Goodman, E., Fiedor, P., Fein, S. *et al.* (1995). Fludarabine phosphate and 2-chlorodeoxyadenosine: immunosuppressive DNA synthesis inhibitors with potential application in islet allo-xeno-transplantation. *Transplantation Proceedings,* **27,** 3293.

Gratwohl, A., Baldomero, H., Passweg, J. *et al.* (2003). Increasing use of reduced intensity conditioning transplants: report of the 2001 EBMT activity survey. *Bone Marrow Transplantation,* **30,** 813–31.

Hill, G., Crawford, J., Cooke, K. *et al.* (1997). Total body irradiation and acute graft-versus-host disease: the role of gastrointestinal damage and inflammatory cytokines. *Blood,* **90,** 3204–13.

Ho, A.Y.L., Adams, S., Shaikh, H. *et al.* (2002). Fatal donor-derived Epstein-Barr virus-associated posttransplant lymphoproliferative disorder following reduced intensity volunteer-unrelated bone marrow transplant for myelodysplastic syndrome. *Bone Marrow Transplantation,* **29,** 867–9.

Holler, E., Kolb, H., Moller, A. *et al.* (1990). Increased serum levels of tumor necrosis factor α precede major complications of bone marrow transplantation. *Blood,* **75,** 1011–6.

Horwitz, M.E., Barrett, A.J., Brown, M.R. *et al.* (2001). Treatment of chronic granulomatous disease with nonmyeloablative conditioning and a T-cell-depleted hematopoietic allograft. *New England Journal of Medicine,* **344,** 881–8.

Horowitz, M.M., Gale, R.P.O., Sondel, P.M. *et al.* (1990). Graft-versus-leukemia reactions after bone marrow transplantation. *Blood,* **75,** 555–62.

Johansson, J-E., Brune, M., & Ekman, T. (2001). The gut mucosa barrier is preserved during allogeneic, haemopoietic stem cell transplantation with reduced intensity conditioning. *Bone Marrow Transplantation*, **28**, 737–42.

Junghanss, C., Boeckh, M., Carter, R.A. et al. (2002a). Incidence and outcome of cytomegalovirus infections following nonmyeloablative compared with myeloablative allogeneic stem cell transplantation, a matched control study. *Blood*, **99**, 1978–85.

Junghanss, C., Marr, K. A., Carter, R. A. et al. (2002b). Incidence and outcome of bacterial and fungal infections following nonmyeloablative compared with myeloablative allogeneic hematopoietic stem cell transplantation: a matched control study. *Biology of Blood and Marrow Transplantation*, **8**, 512–20.

Khouri, I.F., Keating, M., Körbling, M. et al. (1998). Transplant-lite: induction of graft-versus-malignancy using fludarabine-based nonablative chemotherapy and allogeneic blood progenitor-cell transplantation as treatment for lymphoid malignancies. *Journal of Clinical Oncology*, **16**, 2817–24.

Khouri, I.F., Keating, M.J., Vriesendorp, H.M. et al. (1994). Autologous and allogeneic bone marrow transplantation for chronic lymphocytic leukemia: preliminary results. *Journal of Clinical Oncology*, **12**, 748–58.

Khouri, I.F., Saliba, R.M., Giralt, S.A. et al. (2001). Nonablative allogeneic hematopoietic transplantation as adoptive immunotherapy for indolent lymphoma: low incidence of toxicity, acute graft-versus-host disease, and treatment-related mortality. *Blood*, **98**, 3595–9.

Kolb, H.J., Schattenberg, A., Goldman, J.M. et al. (1995). Graft-versus-leukemia effect of donor lymphocyte transfusions in narrow grafted patients. *Blood*, **86**, 2041–50.

Kottaridis, P.D., Milligan, D.W., Chopra, R. et al. In vivo CAM-PATH-1H prevents graft-versus-host disease following nonmyeloablative stem cell transplantation. *Blood*, **96**, 2419–25.

Kreiter, S., Winkelmann, N., Schneider, P.M. et al. (2001). Failure of sustained engraftment after non-myeloablative conditioning with low-dose TBI and T cell-reduced allogeneic peripheral stem cell transplantation. *Bone Marrow Transplantation*, **28**, 157–61.

Kröger, N., Schwerdtfeger, R., Kiehl, M. et al. (2002). Autologous stem cell transplantation followed by a reduced-dose allograft induces high complete remission rate in multiple myeloma. *Blood*, **100**, 755–60.

Li, L., Glassman, A., Keating, M. et al. (1997). Fludarabine triphosphate inhibits nucleotide excision repair of cisplatin-induced DNA adducts in vitro. *Cancer Research*, **57**, 1487–94.

Mackinnon, S., Papadopoulos, E.B., Carabasi, M.H. et al. (1995). Adoptive immunotherapy evaluating escalating doses of donor leukocytes for relapse of chronic myeloid leukemia after bone marrow transplantation: separation of graft-versus-leukemia responses from graft-versus-host disease. *Blood*, **86**, 1261–8.

Maloney, D.G., Sahebi, F., Stockerl-Goldstein, K. E. et al. (2001). Combining an allogeneic graft-vs-myeloma effect with high-dose autologous stem cell rescue in the treatment of multiple myeloma. *Blood*, **98**, 434–51 (abstract).

Marks, D.I., Lush, R., Cavenagh, J. et al. (2002). The toxicity and efficacy of donor lymphocyte infusions given after reduced-intensity conditioning allogeneic stem cell transplantation. *Blood*, **100**, 3108–14.

McSweeney, P.A., Niederwieser, D., Shizuru, J.A. et al. (2001). Hematopoietic cell transplantation in older patients with hematologic malignancies: replacing high-dose cytotoxic therapy with graft-versus-tumor effects. *Blood*, **97**, 3390–400.

McSweeney, P.A. & Storb, R. (1999). Mixed chimerism: preclinical studies and clinical applications. *Biology of Blood and Marrow Transplantation*, **5**, 192–203.

McSweeney, P.A., Niederwieser, D., Shizuru, J.A. et al (2001). Hematopoietic cell transplantation in older patients with hematologic malignancies: replacing high-dose cytotoxic therapy with graft-versus-tumor effect. *Blood*, **97**, 3390–400.

Martino, R., Caballero, M.D., Canals, C. et al. (2001). Reduced-intensity conditioning reduces the risk of severe infections after allogeneic peripheral blood stem cell transplantation. *Bone Marrow Transplantation*, **28**, 341–7.

Martino, R., Caballero, M.D., Canals, C. et al. (2001). Allogeneic peripheral blood stem cell transplantation with reduced-intensity conditioning: results of a prospective multicentre study. *British Journal of Haematology*, **115**, 653–9.

Michallet, M., Bilger, K., Garban, F. et al. (2001). Allogeneic hematopoietic stem cell transplantation after non-myeloablative preparative regimens: impact of pretransplantation and posttransplantation factors on outcome. *Journal of Clinical Oncology*, **19**, 3340–9.

Mohty, M., Faucher, C., Vey, N. et al. (2000). High rate of secondary viral and bacterial infections in patients undergoing allogeneic bone marrow mini-transplantation. *Bone Marrow Transplantation*, **26**, 251–5.

Mossad, S.B., Avery, R.K., Longworth, D.L. et al. (2001). Infectious complications within the first year after nonmyeloablative allogeneic peripheral blood stem cell transplantation. *Bone Marrow Transplantation*, **28**, 491–5.

Nagler, A., Or, R., Naparstek, E. et al. (2000). Second allogeneic stem cell transplantation using nonmyeloablative conditioning for patients who relapsed or developed secondary malignancies following autologous transplantation. *Experimental Hematology*, **28**, 1096–1104.

Niederwieser, D., Maris, M., Shizuru, J.A. et al. (2003). Low-dose total body irradiation (TBI) and fludarabine followed by hematopoietic cell transplantation (HCT) from HLA-matched or mismatched unrelated donors and postgrafting immunosuppression with cyclosporine and mycophenolate mofetil (MMF) can induce durable complete chimerism and sustained remissions in patients with hematological diseases. *Blood*, **101**, 1620–9.

Nimer, S.D., Giorgi, J., Gajewski, J.L. et al. (1994). Selective depletion of CD8$^+$ cells for prevention of graft-versus-host disease after bone marrow transplantation: a randomized controlled trial. *Transplantation*, **57**, 82–7.

O'Brien, S.M., Kantarjian, H., Thomas, D. et al. (2001). Rituximab dose-escalation trial in chronic lymphocytic leukemia. *Journal of Clinical Oncology*, **19**, 2165–70.

Perez-Simon, J.A., Kottaridis, P.D., Martino, R. et al. (2002). Nonmyeloablative transplantation with or without alemtuzumab: comparison between 2 prospective studies in patients with lymphoproliferative disorders. *Blood*, **100**, 3121–7.

Plunkett, W. & Sanders, P. (1991). Metabolism and action of purine nucleoside analogs. *Pharmacological Therapy*, **49**, 239–45.

Robinson, S.P., Mackinnon, S., Goldstone, A.H. *et al.* (2000). Higher than expected transplant-related mortality and relapse following non-myeloablative stem cell transplantation for lymphoma adversely effects progression free survival. *Blood,* **96**, 554a.

Rondón, G., Giralt, S., Huh, Y. *et al.* (1996). Graft-versus-leukemia effect after allogeneic bone marrow transplantation for chronic lymphocytic leukemia. *Bone Marrow Transplantation,* **18**, 669–72.

Ruiz-Argüelles, G.J., Gomez-Almaguer, D., & Ruiz-Argüelles, A. (2001). Results of an outpatient-based stem cell allotransplant program using nonmyeloablative conditioning regimens. *American Journal of Hematology,* **66**, 241–4.

Seung, E., Iwakoshi, N., Woda, B.A. *et al.* (2000). Allogeneic hematopoietic chimerism in mice treated with sublethal myeloablation and anti-CD154 antibody: absence of graft-versus-host disease, induction of skin graft tolerance, and prevention of recurrent autoimmunity in islet-allografted NOD/Lt mice. *Blood,* **95**, 2175–82.

Singhal, S., Powles, R., Treleaven, J. *et al.* (1996). Melphalan alone prior to allogeneic bone marrow transplantation from HLA-identical sibling donors for hematologic malignancies: allo engraftment with potential preservation of fertility in women. *Bone Marrow Transplantation,* **18**, 1049–55.

Slavin, S., Nagler, A., Naparstek, E. *et al.* (1998). Nonmyeloablative stem cell transplantation and cell therapy as an alternative to conventional bone marrow transplantation with lethal cytoreduction for the treatment of malignant and nonmalignant hematologic diseases. *Blood,* **91**, 756–63.

Spitzer, T.R., McAfee, S., Sackstein, R. *et al.* (2000). Intentional induction of mixed chimerism and achievement of antitumor responses after nonmyeloablative conditioning therapy and HLA-matched donor bone marrow transplantation for refractory hematologic malignancies. *Biology of Blood and Marrow Transplantation,* **6**, 309–20.

Storb, R., Prentice, R., Thomas, E. *et al.* (1983). Factors associated with graft rejection after HLA-identical marrow transplantation for aplastic anemia. *British Journal of Haematology,* **55**, 573–85.

Storb, R., Yu, C., Wagner, J. *et al.* (1997). Stable mixed hematopoietic chimerism in DLA-identical littermate dogs given sublethal total body irradiation before and pharmacological immunosuppression after marrow transplantation. *Blood,* **89**, 3048–54.

Sullivan, K.M., Storb, R., Buckner, C.D. *et al.* (1989a). Graft-versus-host disease as adoptive immunotherapy in patients with advanced hematologic neoplasms. *New England Journal of Medicine,* **320**, 828–34.

Sullivan, K.M., Weiden, P.L., Storb, R. *et al.* (1989b). Influence of acute and chronic graft-versus-host disease on relapse and survival after bone marrow transplantation from HLA-identical siblings as treatment of acute and chronic leukemia. *Blood,* **73**, 1720–8.

Sykes, M., Preffer, F., McAfee, S. *et al.* (1999). Mixed lymphohematopoietic chimerism and graft-vs-lymphoma effects after nonmyeloablative therapy and HLA-mismatched donor bone marrow transplantation. *Lancet,* **353**, 1755–9.

Sykora, K-W., Schrauder, A., Beilken, A., & Welte, K. (2001). A fludarabine-based conditioning regimen for patients with thalassemia: report of two cases. *Bone Marrow Transplantation,* **27** (Suppl 1), S193 (abstract).

Taylor, P.A., Lees, C.J., Waldmann, H. *et al.* (2001). Requirements for the promotion of allogeneic engraftment by anti-CD154 (anti-CD40L) monoclonal antibody under nonmyeloablative conditions. *Blood,* **98**, 467–74.

Ueno, N.T., Cheng, Y.C., Giralt, S.A. *et al.* (2002). Complete donor chimerism by fludarabine/melphalan in mini-allogeneic transplantation for metastatic renal cell carcinoma and breast cancer. *Proceedings of American Society of Clinical Oncology,* abstract 1659.

van Bekkum, D. (1984). Conditioning regimens for marrow grafting. *Seminars in Hematology,* **21**, 81–90.

van Besien, K., Bartholomew, A., Stock, W. *et al.* (2000). Fludarabine-based conditioning for allogeneic transplantation in adults with sickle cell disease. *Bone Marrow Transplantation,* **26**, 445–9.

Van Besien, K.W., de Lima, M., Giralt, SA. *et al.* (1997). Management of lymphoma recurrence after allogeneic transplantation: the relevance of graft-versus-lymphoma effect. *Bone Marrow Transplantation,* **19**, 977–82.

Van Rhee, R., Lin, F., Cullis, J.O. *et al.* (1994). Relapse of chronic myeloid leukemia after allogeneic bone marrow transplant: the case for giving donor leukocyte transfusions before the onset of hematologic relapse. *Blood,* **83**, 3377–83.

Verdonck, L.F., Dekker, A.W., Lokhorst, H.M. *et al.* (1997). Allogeneic versus autologous bone marrow transplantation for refractory and recurrent low-grade non-Hodgkin's lymphoma. *Blood,* **90**, 4201–45.

Vesole, D.H., Simic, A., & Lazarus, H.M. (2001). Controversy in multiple myeloma transplants: tandem autotransplants and mini-allografts. *Bone Marrow Transplantation,* **28**, 725–35.

Wäsch, R., Reisser, S., Hahn, J. *et al.* (2000). Rapid achievement of complete donor chimerism and low regimen-related toxicity after reduced conditioning with fludarabine, carmustine, melphalan and allogeneic transplantation. *Bone Marrow Transplantation,* **26**, 243–50.

Weiden, P.L., Sullivan, K.M., Floumoy, N. *et al.* (1981). Antileukemic effect of chronic graft-versus-host disease: contribution to improved survival after allogeneic marrow transplantation. *New England Journal of Medicine,* **304**, 1529–32.

Weissinger, F., Sandmaier, B.M., Maloney, D.G. *et al.* (2001). Decreased transfusion requirements for patients receiving nonmyeloablative compared with conventional peripheral blood stem cell transplants from HLA-identical siblings. *Blood,* **98**, 3584–8.

Xun, C.Q., McSweeney, P.A., Boeckh, M., & Storb, R. (1999). Successful non-myeloablative allogeneic hematopoietic stem cell transplant in an acute leukemia patient with chemotherapy-induced marrow aplasia and progressive pulmonary aspergillosis. *Blood,* **94**, 3271–6.

Yu, C., Storb, R., Mathey, B. *et al.* (1995). DLA-identical bone marrow grafts after low dose total body irradiation: effects of high-dose corticosteroids and cyclosporine on engraftment. *Blood,* **86**, 4376–81.

Zaucha, J.M., Yu, C., Zellmer, E. *et al.* (2001). Effects of extending the duration of postgrafting immunosuppression and substituting granulocyte-colony-stimulating factor-mobilized peripheral blood mononuclear cells for marrow in allogeneic engraftment in a nonmyeloablative canine transplantation model. *Biology of Blood and Marrow Transplantation,* **7**, 513–6.

23 Finding the most suitable allogeneic hematopoietic stem cell donor

M. OUDSHOORN, J.L.W.T. LIE, J.N.A. BAKKER, H.G.M. VAN DER ZANDEN, AND F.H.J. CLAAS

Europdonor Foundation and Leiden University Medical Centre, Leiden, The Netherlands

Introduction

Allogeneic HLA-identical sibling hematopoietic stem cell transplantation is an accepted form of treatment for a number of hematologic malignancies, syndromes of bone marrow failure, and congenital disorders of the lympho-hematopoietic system (Thomas, 1983; Thomas *et al.*, 1984). However, more than 70% of patients who could benefit from allogeneic hematopoietic stem cell transplantation do not have a genotypically identical sibling donor. Phenotypically matched or partly mismatched family members or unrelated donors can provide suitable stem cell transplants for some of the patients lacking an HLA-identical sibling donor.

The first HLA-identical unrelated donor marrow transplant in a patient with severe aplastic anemia was described in 1973 (Speck *et al.*, 1973). This patient subsequently died due to failure of sustained engraftment. The first HLA-matched unrelated donor transplant for a patient with hematologic malignancy was described in 1980 (Hansen *et al.*, 1980) and involved a young woman with acute lymphoblastic leukemia. The posttransplant course was smooth, but the leukemia recurred at 18 months posttransplant. Many reports published since then bear witness that bone marrow transplantation using unrelated donors is possible and gives acceptable results.

Of the many obstacles that can prevent successful hematopoietic stem cell transplantation, one of the most frustrating is difficulty locating a suitable (partially) HLA-identical donor. The steps involved in the search for a donor are shown in Figure 23.1. This scheme maximizes the chance of finding the best matched donor for a patient. Bone marrow donor searches among patient's siblings are standard; depending on the number of siblings, a patient has a 25% to 30% chance of having such an HLA-identical donor. If a genotypically HLA-identical donor is not available, searching for related (partially) HLA-matched donors other than an HLA-identical sibling will increase the likelihood of finding a matched or partly matched donor by well over 10 percent. For patients without a suitable related donor, a search for an unrelated donor or cord blood unit can be started.

The first bone marrow donor registry was started in 1970 (van Rood, 1971), followed in 1974 by the Anthony Nolan Trust, which established a tradition of making unrelated bone marrow donors available not only locally but all over the world (Cleaver, 1992). In 1987 the National Marrow Donor Program (NMDP) of the United States started recruiting donors and, currently, over 49 different registries operate in Europe, Israel, North America, Mexico, South Africa, Australia, New Zealand, Brazil, India, Singapore, Hong Kong, Taiwan, South Korea, and Japan (Bone Marrow Donors Worldwide Annual Report, 2001). In 1988 it was shown that cells from cord blood could be used for transplantation (Gluckman *et al.*, 1989) and the first transplant using cord blood cells from unrelated donors was performed by Kurtzberg and colleagues in 1994. In 1992 the first cord blood registry was set up by Dr. Pablo Rubinstein at the New York Blood Center (Rubinstein *et al.*, 1993). Since then the number of cord blood registries has gradually increased to 26 registries in 17 countries (Bone Marrow Donors Worldwide Annual Report, 2001).

The polymorphism of the human leukocyte antigens (HLA) is extensive but fortunately some of the HLA phenotypes are relatively frequent. This makes the use of unrelated matched marrow or blood stem cell donors or cord blood units a realistic option for patients in need of such a donor, but lacking an HLA-compatible family member.

The combination of the extreme polymorphism of HLA and the ever-increasing number of donor registries creates a logistic problem of its own. The ideal solution would be to link all registries electronically and, although technically feasible, lack of standardization, national restrictions, and lack of funds make it unlikely that this will happen in the next few years. Large-scale computer networks do exist, however, such as STAR (Search, Tracking and Registry) of the National Marrow Donor Program in the United States, and the European Donor Secretariat (EDS) and the European Marrow Donor Information System (EMDIS) in Europe and Netcord (for cord blood units only).

Family donor search

When searching for an HLA-matched sibling donor, some transplant centers HLA type the siblings of the patient but fail to HLA type the parents. It is important to know the HLA typ-

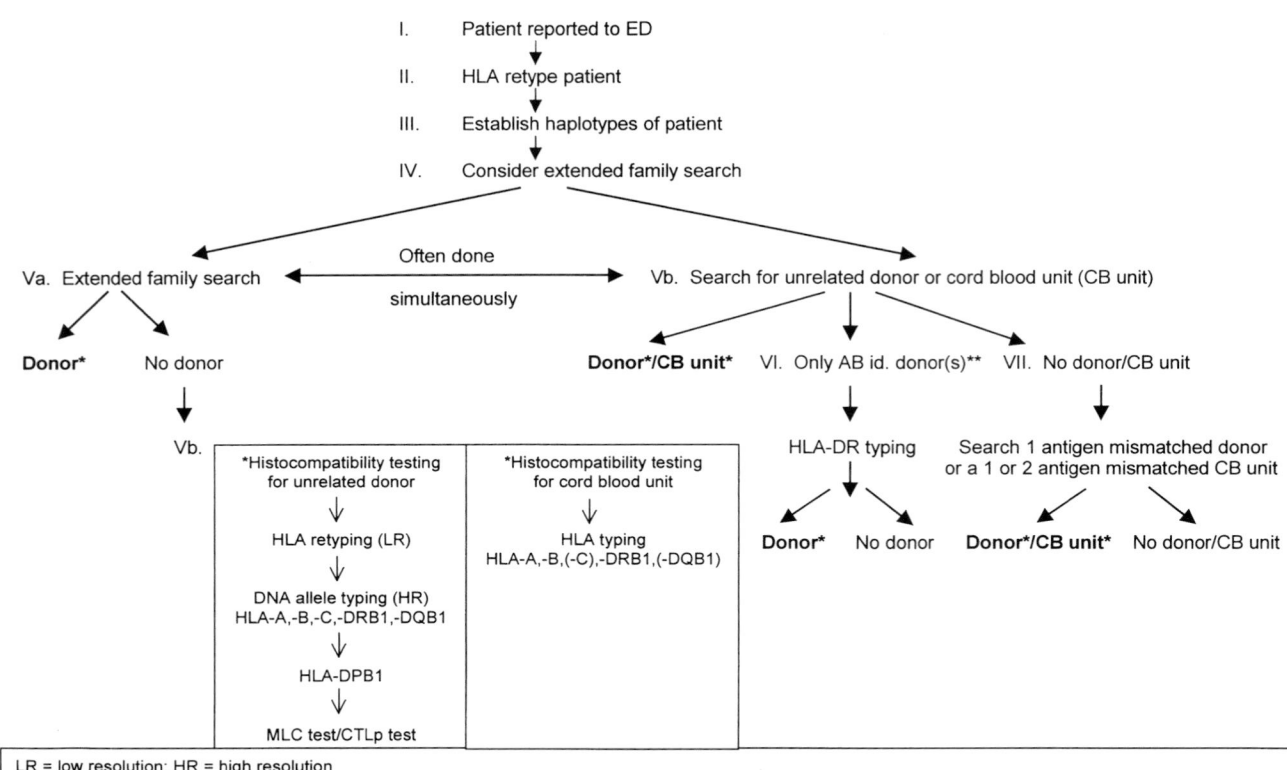

Fig. 23.1. Outline of process for selecting a bone marrow donor. Reproduced, with permission, from Oudshoorn *et al.*, 1997, with adaptations.

ing of the parents in order to determine the patient's haplotype. Homozygosity for one or more alleles of the parent, a recombination of HLA alleles, or sharing of haplotypes among parents, will increase the chance of finding a family donor. Searching for suitable related donors other than HLA-identical siblings will increase the likelihood of finding a matched or partly matched family donor by well over 10 percent.

A distinction should be made between HLA-genotypically identical family donors and family donors who are HLA-phenotypically identical but HLA genotypically haploidentical. The latter category of donor only shares one inherited haplotype with the patient, implying that the noninherited haplotype may contain mismatches for nontested HLA loci. Figure 23.2 illustrates how genotypically identical and phenotypically identical family member donors may be available.

HLA-genotypically identical sibling

The classic strategy for identification of an HLA-genotypically identical donor is to type the available siblings of the patient and the parents. The identical sibling possesses exactly the same two inherited haplotypes (indicated by the letters a and c) with all the same HLA alleles as the patient (Fig. 23.2a).

Donors available due to consanguinity or other interfamily relationships

In cultures where consanguinity is commonplace, family members other than siblings can be HLA genotypically matched donors. A comparable situation can occur when the father and mother of the patient share the same ancestor(s). Figure 23.2b depicts such a family in which an HLA-genotypically identical aunt has been identified. The patient and donor share the same ancestor. Another example of possible genotypically identical family members is shown in Figure 23.2c, depicting the situation of two brothers, sharing one haplotype, from one family who are married to two sisters from another family, also sharing one haplotype. In this unique family setting, the children of one family are as likely potential HLA genotypically identical donors for their cousins as are siblings.

HLA-phenotypically identical, haploidentical sibling

If one parent is serologically homozygous, one should be aware that HLA-identical siblings are only phenotypically identical by serology or low resolution molecular typing, but

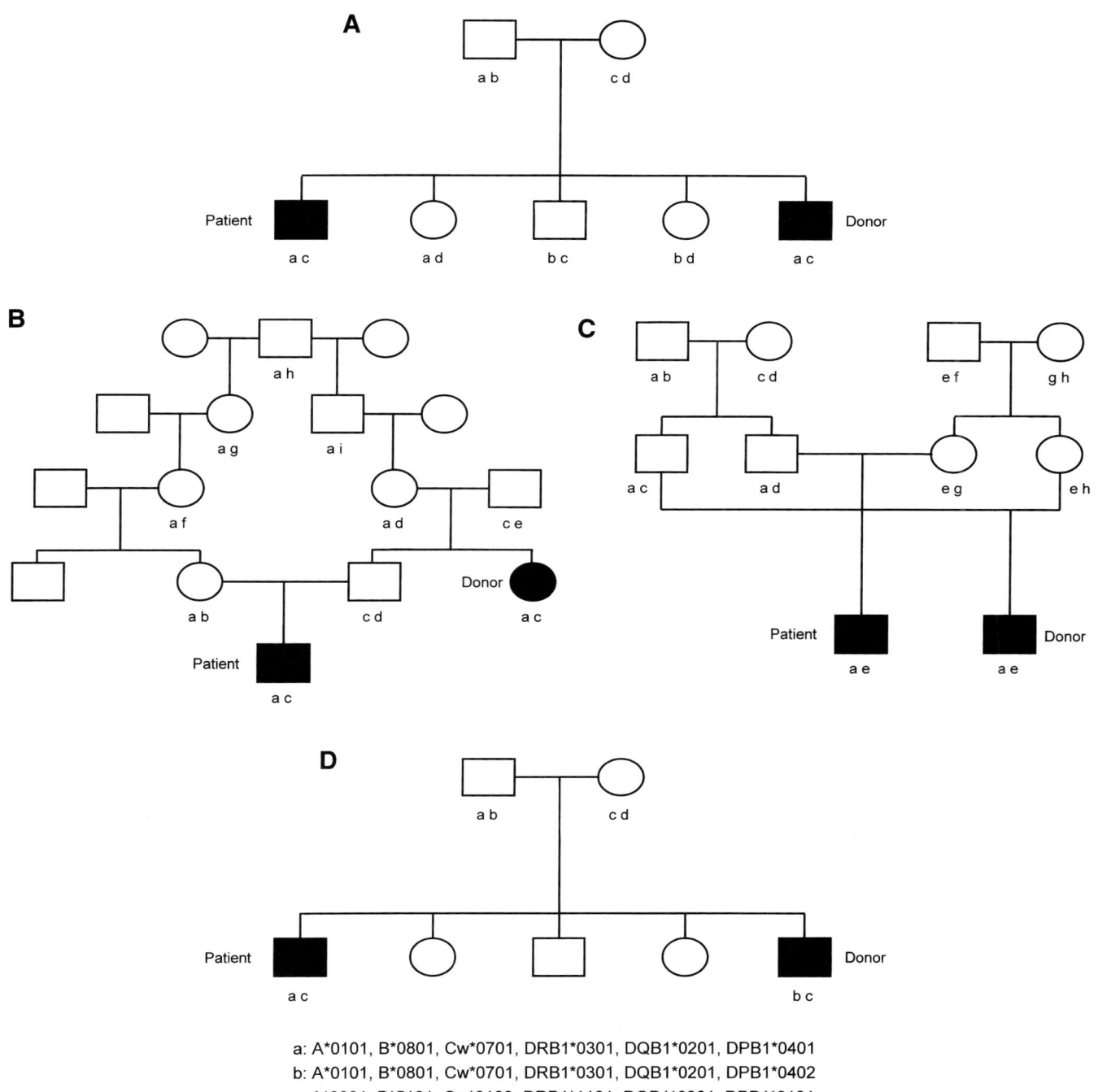

a: A*0101, B*0801, Cw*0701, DRB1*0301, DQB1*0201, DPB1*0401
b: A*0101, B*0801, Cw*0701, DRB1*0301, DQB1*0201, DPB1*0402
c: A*0201, B*5101, Cw*0102, DRB1*1101, DQB1*0301, DPB1*0101

Fig. 23.2. **(a–g)** Examples of family donor search processes. The HLA haplotypes are indicated as the letters a to 1. *(Figure continues.)*

may be mismatched when typed at the allele level. Figure 23.2d depicts the situation in which the father is homozygous for HLA-A, -B, -C, -DR, -DQ. The haplotypes are given the letters a and b. Additional DPB1 testing shows that the donor shares only one genetically identical haplotype with the patient, haplotype c.

HLA-phenotypically identical, haploidentical parent

HLA typing of parents will not only determine the haplotypes of the patient, but also demonstrates that parents can quite often be HLA-phenotypically identical and genotypically haploidentical to the patient (Fig. 23.2e). When haplotypes of both par-

E

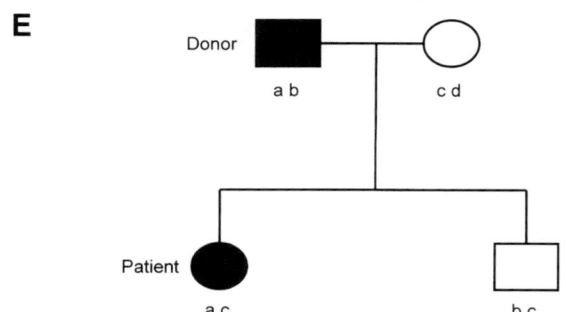

a: A*0201, B*0702, Cw*0702, DRB1*1501, DQB1*0602, DPB1*1501
b: A*0101, B*0801, Cw*0701, DRB1*0301, DQB1*0201, DPB1*0401
c: A*0101, B*0801, Cw*0701, DRB1*0301, DQB1*0201, DPB1*0402

F

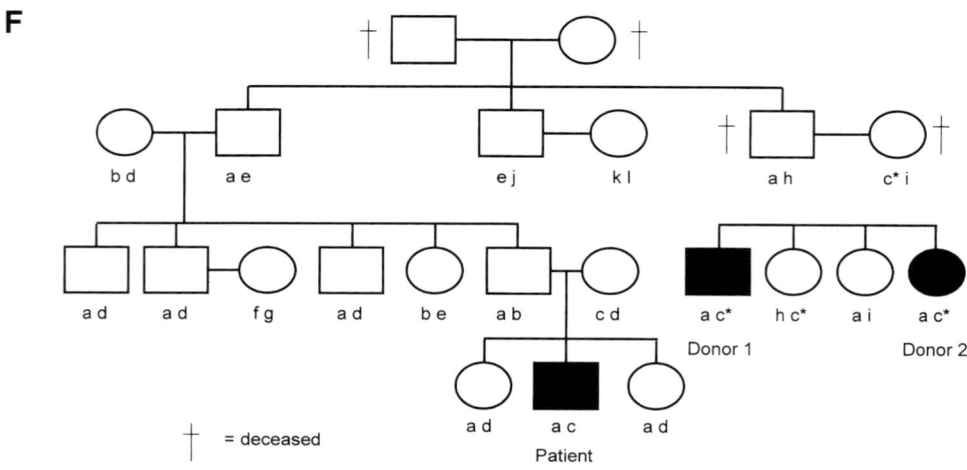

† = deceased

a: A*0301, B*5101, Cw*0702, DRB1*0301, DQB1*0201, DPB1*0201
c: A*0101, B*0801, Cw*0701, DRB1*0301, DQB1*0201, DPB1*0401
c*: A*0101, B*0801, Cw*0701, DRB1*0301, DQB1*0201, DPB1*0401

G

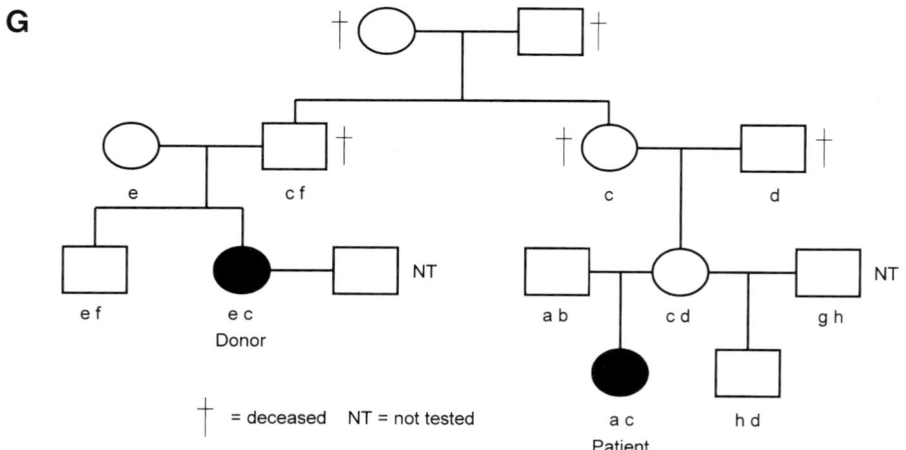

† = deceased   NT = not tested

a: A*2601 B*0702 Cw*0702 DRB1*1501 DQB1*0602 DPB1*0401
c: A*1101 B*5601 Cw*0102 DRB1*0901 DQB1*0303 DPB1*0201
e: A*0201 B*0702 Cw*0702 DRB1*1501 DQB1*0602 DPB1*0501

Fig. 23.2. *(Figure continued.)*

ents (haplotype b of father and haplotype c of mother) are phenotypically identical for HLA-A, -B, -DR, and -DQ ("shared"), especially when a common haplotype is involved, there is a chance that one of them (in this case the father) can be phenotypically identical for HLA-A, -B, -C, -DR, and -DQ, though genotypically haploidentical to the patient. Patient and donor are not identical for HLA-DPB1.

Donor derived from an extended family search

When one of the haplotypes of the patient occurs frequently in the general population, an extended family donor search is often worthwhile. The strategy for such a family search is to explore the side of the family from which the least common haplotype in the patient has been inherited, in the hope that the more common haplotype has been introduced by marriage (Fig. 23.2f). It seems reasonable only to conduct extended family studies on the basis of the five most common haplotypes of the patient's ethnic origin. Computer programs have been developed to calculate the likelihood of finding a related donor by this strategy (Schipper, D'Amaro, & Oudshoorn, 1996; Kaufman, 1996). An extended family search may also be indicated if the patient only has part of a common haplotype and no HLA matched unrelated donors are available (Fig. 23.2g): the patient had the common HLA-B*0702, Cw*0702, DRB1*1501, DQB1*0602 haplotype but with HLA-A*2601 instead of A*0201 or A*0301, which is normally found with this haplotype. The donor found in this family inherited the same c haplotype as the patient and had the expected A*0201 B*0702 Cw*0702 DRB1*1501 DQB1*0602, making this donor an HLA-A mismatched donor.

Unrelated donor search

The decision to carry out a search for an unrelated donor is generally made after finding no suitable matched sibling or extended family donor. The development over the last 10 to 15 years of large national registries of HLA typed unrelated donors has provided an increasingly favorable chance of finding a match for a growing number of patients (Oudshoorn et al., 1997; Tiercy et al., 2000). Currently, 49 different registries operate in Europe, North America, Australia, Asia, South Africa, and Mexico. The total number of donors is approximately 8 million. All donor registries are a member of the World Marrow Donor Association (WMDA). The WMDA was created in 1988 with the aim of facilitating the efficient, timely and reliable transfer of marrow and other forms of hematopoietic stem cells collected from healthy volunteers resident in one country for transplantation of patients resident in another country (Goldman, 1994; http://www.worldmarrow.org).

There are 26 cord blood registries in 17 countries. Together they have over 100,000 unrelated cord blood units available for transplantation. Several of the cord blood registries have joined Netcord, an unrelated cord blood allocation network organization.

The global hematopoietic stem cell donor and cord blood registry network

The problem of searching all registries separately lies not only in making the request but also in getting a reply. A search process can involve a large amoung of unproductive work (there may be no donor) at sizable expense and with considerable time delay.

To facilitate the search process for an international donor, the Immunology Working Party of the European Bone Marrow Transplant (EBMT) Group took the initiative in 1988 to collect and compile an easily accessible listing of all donors worldwide in a four-monthly publication: Bone Marrow Donors Worldwide (van Rood, 1989). If no HLA-matched donor is available in the national or local registry, a quick electronic search in BMDW can determine whether a suitable donor is available in another registry without having to approach all registries individually (Oudshoorn et al., 1994).

The listing entitled Bone Marrow Donors Worldwide (BMDW) is available on the Internet (http://www.bmdw.org). The logistics of the BMDW listing are described below.

Setting up the BMDW computer file: Collecting the unrelated donor and unrelated cord blood unit files

When the word "donors" is referred to in this section, it should be interpreted as referring to unrelated donors or unrelated cord blood units.

Every month a circular letter is sent to the collaborating national registries with a request to send an updated file of their respective donors. All registries have access to, and send their donor files, via the Internet, using e-mail or uploading them to the BMDW Internet server using file transfer protocol (FTP). The majority of donor files are encrypted before they are sent via the Internet, so that they cannot be read if they were to be intercepted. Upon receipt, the donor files are decrypted and inspected for file formatting errors. Errors in the file format are reported to the registries. Files that do not comply with the BMDW file format are rejected. If registries have no other way of sending their data, BMDW will try to assist in this matter.

Quality control

The tissue typing data in each donor file is checked, using the latest nomenclature for factors of the HLA system (www.ebi.ac.uk/imgt/hla). The serologic phenotypes are verified and invalid antigens are rejected. The DNA typings are checked for validity, and their relationship with the serologic antigens is verified. Invalid antigens or DNA typings are any antigens or alleles not listed in the latest HLA Nomenclature Report.

The computer programs

Since 1995 BMDW has gradually transferred its facilities on to the Internet, particularly the world wide web (WWW). The emergence of the WWW opened up possibilities such as accessibility by large numbers of registries, transplant centers, and search coordinators; very frequent updates of the donor file;

and a wide range of match programs not hampered by the problems of distribution on diskette that we experienced in the past.

The core of BMDW's WWW site (http://www.bmdw.org) consists of a number of match programs. These programs present HLA-identical, potentially HLA-identical, and HLA-mismatched donors, and cord blood units. The user enters a patient's identification (ID) and the potential recipient's HLA phenotype (HLA-A, -B, -DR). The donors and cord blood units are shown in categories, with their HLA-A, -B, -DR phenotype including DNA-based typing data if available, and with the identity of the registry from which they can be requested. The results typically reach the user 5 to 10 seconds after starting a match run (Table 23.1).

If no donors are found for a patient, a request for search advice can be submitted to Europdonor. BMDW's medical staff will study the patient's phenotype, ethnic background, the typing of parents and siblings, and other factors, and send advice for the search strategy to the requesting physician (Ebeling *et al.*, 1994). This facility is complemented by a computer program for the calculation of the probability of finding an HLA-identical donor in the patient's extended family (i.e., uncles, aunts, and cousins) (Schipper, D'Amaro & Oudshoorn, 1996). Another program calculates the chance of finding a DR-identical donor after class II typing of HLA-A and -B-typed donors. There is also a program that shows the haplotype frequencies in the different registries.

Security is of the utmost importance. Therefore, BMDW uses a secure protocol for WWW downloads and for the on-line match programs. With this protocol all data transmitted from a browser such as Netscape or Internet Explorer to BMDW, and from BMDW to a browser, are encrypted. This means that passwords and all medical data are protected. BMDW has also

acquired a so-called digital ID. The digital ID allows our web server to operate in a secure mode, and unambiguously identifies and authenticates the BMDW server.

BMDW uses a dedicated server (i.e., functioning for BMDW only). It became active on May 1, 1996. The server is available virtually 24 hours a day, 7 days a week (sometimes maintenance for a few hours occurs).

The growth of the BMDW file

The first edition was distributed during the 1989 EBMT meeting and comprised the phenotypes of eight registries with a total of almost 160,000 donors. Over the last 12 years there has been a steady increase in the number of registries and donors (Figs. 23.3 and 23.4). In 2001, 49 unrelated donor registries from 36 countries participated in the BMDW effort and 26 cord blood registries from 17 countries (BMDW Annual Report, 2001). The unrelated donor total is nearing 8 million. The cord blood units are practically all fully typed for HLA-A, -B, and -DR and over 80% of the units are class II DNA typed and 27% class I DNA typed. Completeness of unrelated donor HLA typing varies among the registries, but has greatly improved over the years. The World Marrow Donor association has published recommended guidelines for the histocompatibility testing of unrelated donors (Hurley *et al.*, 1999). These include the required use of DNA-based testing for HLA-DR and the recommended use of DNA-based testing for HLA-A and -B. Further, if serology is used for HLA- and -B, then a DNA-based method must be used to define antigens in the population tested that are frequently missed and/or misassigned. In terms of the resolution of testing, at a minimum, serologic split/low-level DNA-based resolution is recommended.

Table 23.1. *An excerpt from the August 2002 edition of Bone Marrow Donors Worldwide*

HLA of patient	A 1	A 3	B 13	B 52	DR 15	DR 7	Registries	Number of donors
	HLA	A 1	A 3	B 13	B 52	DR 15	DR 7		
ABDR split	1	3	52	13	15	7	UK-BBMR Cord	1[a]
	–	–	–	–	–	–	Germany	1[a]
	–	–	–	–	–	–	Germany	2[a]
	–	–	–	–	–	–	Germany	1[a]
	–	–	–	–	–	–	UK-Anthony Nolan	2[a]
ABDR broad	1	3	5	13	15	7	Germany	1
	1	3	52	13	2	7	Israel-Hadassah	1[a]
	–	–	–	–	–	–	USA-NMDP	5
ABDR split-mismatch	1	3	51	13	2	7	Cyprus BMDR	1
	–	–	–	–	–	–	UK-BBMR	1
	–	–	–	–	–	–	USA-NMDP	2
	1	3	51	13	15	7	Germany	1[a]
	–	–	–	–	–	–	USA-NMDP	3
	1	3	52	13	16	7	Germany	1

Abbreviations: UK-BBMR Cord: Great Britain—British Bone Marrow Registry Cord Blood; UK-Anthony Nolan: Great Britain—Anthony Nolan Trust; USA-NMDP: United States of America—National Marrow Donor Program; Cyprus BMDR: Cyprus Bone Marrow Donor Registry; UK-BBMR: Great Britain—British Bone Marrow Registry.

[a] DNA typing available; presented after pressing a function key.

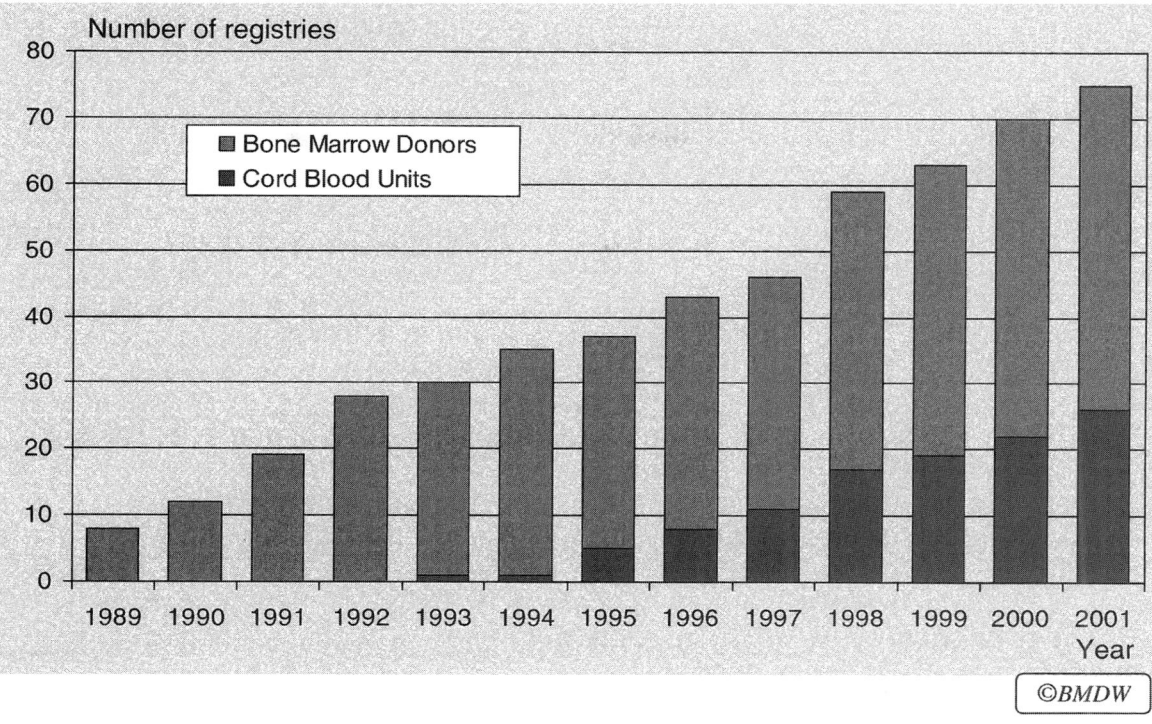

Fig. 23.3. Number of participating stem cell donor and cord blood registries in BMDW.

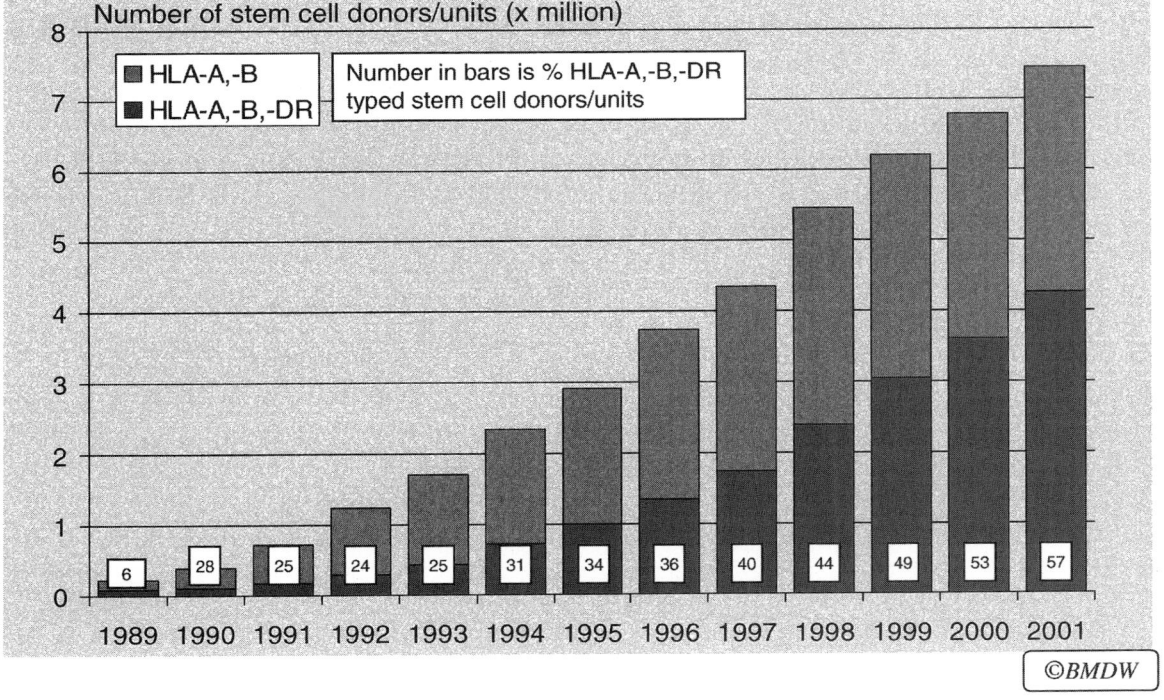

Fig. 23.4. Total number of HLA-A, -B and -A, -B, -DR typed stem cell donors and unrelated cord blood units in BMDW.

The proportion of donors fully typed for HLA-A, -B, and -DR has increased from 6% in 1989 to 57% in 2001, resulting in more than 4.3 million HLA-A, -B, -DR typed donors. This is important as completely typed donors are far more likely to proceed to marrow/PBSC donation than those only HLA-A and -B typed (Confer, 1997; Oudshoorn et al., 1997). Five percent of all donors were HLA class I DNA typed and 16% class II DNA typed.

Table 23.2 compares the number of theoretically possible phenotypes with the number of phenotypes found in 1990, 1995, and 2001. The data for broad and split antigens are given. If HLA-DR is ignored, the percentage of HLA-A and -B phenotypes present in 2001 is already sizable and emphasizes that the polymorphism of HLA is finite, although large. However, if HLA-DR is taken into account, the percentage of phenotypes found in 2001 (with 4,342,380 HLA-A, -B, and -DR typed donors) is well under 10% of the potential total number of possible phenotypes. Analysis of the HLA phenotype of new donors added to the file has shown that registries with almost exclusively North Western European donors, such as those in Scandinavia, have a chance of 1 in 14 donors being an HLA-A, -B, -DR serological split phenotype not already present in the BMDW file. This chance is one in six for registries from the Mediterranean countries; one in seven for registries with some degree of non-Caucasoid donors (such as those in North America); one in 11 for Asian registries; one in five for Mexico, and one in four for South Africa. This clearly indicates the under-representation of non-Caucasoid (with the exception of Asian) donors. To determine how effective the increase of donors (and thus phenotypes) was for an individual patient, 497 consecutive search requests for a matched unrelated donor for Dutch patients received by Europdonor were checked against the BMDW file of 1990, 1994, 1997, and 2001. In 1990 an HLA-A, -B, -DR split-matched donor could be found for only 181 of the 497 patients (36%). In 1994, this had increased to 372 (75%), and in 1997 to 403 (82%) and in 2001 to 434 (87%). A more than twofold increase in the total numbers of HLA-A, -B, -DR split typed donors from 1997 (1.0 million) to 2001 (2.5 million) thus led to an increase of 5% of patients for whom a potentially HLA-matched unrelated donor is available.

Donor selection/degree of matching

Donor selection relies on HLA typing (HLA-A, -B, -C, -DR, -DQ) by serology, molecular typing, and, in some centers, biological assays. The general working strategy is to request blood or DNA samples from several of the selected potential donors or cord blood units for further testing. The best matched potential donor or cord blood unit will then be chosen.

Blood or DNA samples of potential donors or cord blood units can be requested via several computer networks such as the European Donor Secretariat (EDS), the European Marrow Information System (EMDIS), TRANSlink (NMDP) or Netcord. For registries not attached to one of these computer systems, blood samples of donors can be requested by fax.

HLA-DR typing of donors who are only typed for HLA-A and HLA-B can be a feasible option for finding HLA-A, -B, -DR identical donors, depending on the linkage disequilibrium between the class I antigens and the expected DR antigen. Two computer programs are available (Mori et al., 1996; Schipper, D'Amaro, & Oudshoorn, 1997), both calculating the likelihood of finding an HLA-A, -B, -DR matched donor when requesting DR typing of a given number of HLA-A and -B typed unrelated donors. Requests for HLA-DR typing to be performed can be made via the same computer networks described above.

Degree of matching

More than 80% to 90% of the searches for patients from North Western European descent identify at least one HLA-A, -B, -DR phenotypically matched donor and 40% to 50% of patients identify a donor matched for HLA-A, -B, and -DRB1 alleles (Hansen et al., 1997; Tiercy et al., 2000). If it is not possible to find a completely HLA-matched donor for a particular patient, transplant protocols at some centers allow the use of mismatched donors. This will, of course, increase the number of available potential donors, but at the same time introduces the question of which mismatch, or how many mismatches at which loci, are acceptable.

Degree of mismatch

In hematopoietic stem cell transplantation, mismatches due to cross-reacting groups (CREGs) as described by Duquesnoy et

Table 23.2. *Number of HLA phenotypes (theoretically) possible versus the number found*

Phenotypes	A, B broad	A, B split	A, B, DR broad	A, B, DR split
Theoretically possible phenotypes[a]	66,150	367,500	6.0×10^6	56.2×10^6
Phenotypes in 1990	8,563 (12.9%)	18,266 (5.0%)	38,649 (0.6%)	18,273 (0.03%)
Phenotypes in 1995	12,165 (18.3%)	45,062 (12.3%)	163,808 (2.7%)	211,592 (0.4%)
Phenotypes in 2001	18,572 (28.1%)	68,520 (18.6%)	304,030 (5.1%)	558,813 (1.0%)

[a] Based on the WHO HLA Nomenclature Committee Report 2000 (Marsh et al., 2001).

al. (1990), were considered to be minor mismatches, although severe GVHD in the presence of these so-called minor mismatches has been reported. These CREGs only indicate sharing of some, but not all, serologically detectable polymorphisms and give no indication of possible T-cell recognition. Analyses by Wade *et al.* (2001) have shown that there is no advantage of transplanting with a CREG mismatch over a non-CREG mismatch.

Several studies have been performed to determine acceptable mismatches using functional assays to determine donor anti-recipient immune responses by limiting dilution analysis. Limiting dilution assays that quantitate donor cytotoxic or helper T-lymphocyte precursors (CTLp and HTLp) have the potential advantage of detecting minor histocompatibility antigens as well as major histocompatibility complex (MHC) antigens and may identify alloimmunized donors whose T cells could have an increased ability to cause GVHD (Kaminski *et al.*, 1989; Roosnek *et al.*, 1993; Spencer *et al.*, 1995; Speiser *et al.*, 1996; van der Meer *et al.*, 2000; Oudshoorn *et al.*, 2002).

Number and types of mismatches

The fewer the mismatches the better, is a general rule. Disparities between HLA sequence polymorphisms that are serologically detectable are termed *antigen mismatches,* whereas those that can be identified only by DNA-based typing methods are termed *allele mismatches.*

An allele mismatch is preferred over an antigen mismatch (Petersdorf *et al.*, 2001a), but an antigen mismatch may be considered a better option than two allele mismatches, especially if one of the mismatches is class I and the other class II.

Locus of the mismatch

HLA-A and HLA-B

The preferred strategy for a mismatch at the HLA-A or HLA-B loci is to select a mismatch that will lead to a single allele or antigen mismatched donor. There is some preference for an HLA-A locus mismatch over an HLA-B locus mismatch. This is because of the high linkage disequilibrium between HLA-B and HLA-C: an HLA-B locus mismatch will usually be associated with an HLA-C mismatch, thus resulting in two mismatches. Since DNA typing of class I antigens is now becoming available, retrospective studies have been carried out to evaluate possible mismatches of class I antigens and the concept of their permissibility. A study by Petersdorf *et al.* (2001a) demonstrated that HLA class I antigen mismatches that are serologically detectable confer an enhanced risk of graft failure, and that transplants from donors with a single class I allele mismatch, that is not serologically detectable, may be used without an increased risk of graft failure (Petersdorf *et al.*, 1998, 2001a). A large Japanese study on HLA allele compatibility and transplant outcome showed that an HLA-A and/or HLA-B allele mismatch reduced overall survival (Sasazuki *et al.*, 1998; Morishima *et al.*, 2002).

HLA-C

HLA-C locus antigens have until recently not been used for selection of potential donors. Typing for HLA-C has been error-prone and incomplete due to lack of adequate serologic reagents and low expression of the molecule on the cell surface. This problem has now been overcome by molecular typing techniques. Furthermore, data show that HLA-C mismatches are associated with a positive CTLp outcome (Barnardo *et al.*, 1996; Tiercy *et al.*, 2002; Van der Meer *et al.*, 2001; Oudshoorn *et al.*, 2002) and a significantly higher incidence of GVHD (Bishara *et al.*, 1995; Tatari *et al.*, 1996) compared to HLA-C matched transplantations. Additionally, patients with chronic myeloid leukemia (CML) transplanted from HLA-C mismatched unrelated donors are more likely to experience graft failure (Nagler *et al.*, 1996; Petersdorf, 1997; Petersdorf *et al.*, 2001a).

A Japanese study showed a strong synergistic effect of the HLA-C allele mismatch with other HLA allele mismatches on acute GVHD; however, HLA-C mismatches as such did not reduce overall survival (Morishima *et al.*, 2002).

HLA-C molecules have been demonstrated as ligands for receptors expressed on natural killer (NK) cells. A dimorphic epitope at residues 77 and 80 on the alpha-1 domain of HLA-C is recognized by distinct killer inhibitory receptors (KIR) (Colonna *et al.*, 1993), leading to inhibition of NK cell-mediated lysis. Thus, mismatching between donor and patients for this dimorphic motif could affect subsequent NK cell-mediated immune responses and thus have an effect on transplant outcome. Studies of haplotype-mismatched hematopoietic stem cell transplants (Aversa *et al.*, 1998) have shown that choosing donors with KIR epitope incompatibility in the GVHD direction increased survival dramatically (Ruggeri *et al.*, 1999, 2002).

HLA-DRB1

Previous studies showed that HLA-DRB1 allele mismatching between the donor and the recipient is associated with an decreased chance of survival after unrelated marrow transplantation (Tiercy *et al.*, 1991; Petersdorf *et al.*, 1995). A later study confirmed the fact that HLA-DRB1 allele disparity is detrimental to survival and that this effect may be independent of HLA-DQB1 and HLA-DPB1 (Petersdorf *et al.*, 2001b). A large study on 1,298 patient/donor pairs showed that disparity for the HLA-DRB1 allele was a risk factor for acute GVHD (Morishima *et al.*, 2002). The selection of appropriate stem cell donors should thus include DNA allele typing of donor and recipient for HLA-DRB1.

HLA-DRB3/DRB4/DRB5

Single cases of transplantation with an HLA-DRB3 mismatched donor have been reported. No data are currently available on the outcome of HLA-DRB4/B5 mismatched transplants.

HLA-DQB1

Until recently, matching for HLA-DQB1 seemed unimportant for the outcome of transplants from unrelated donors matched for HLA-A, -B, -DR. It was generally assumed that matching for HLA-DRB1 would automatically match for DQ alleles, because of the strong linkage disequilibrium between DRB1 and DQB1. However, a single HLA-DQB1 mismatch can increase GVHD (Petersdorf et al., 1996), although HLA-DQB1 disparity was not associated with significantly poorer survival in patients serologically matched for HLA-A, -B (Petersdorf et al., 2001b; Morishima et al., 2002).

HLA-DPB1

The role of HLA-DPB1 as a transplantation antigen is controversial. Therefore, typing for DPB1 is not routinely performed. Petersdorf et al. (1993) showed in a study of 129 cases that HLA-DPB1 disparity did not significantly influence the risk of acute GVHD after unrelated donor transplantation. Other authors have reported single cases of severe acute GVHD in such a situation or have isolated cytotoxic T cells against mismatched HLA-DPB1 antigens. According to Fleischhauer et al. (2002) HLA-DP can be the target antigen of cytotoxic CD4$^+$ T lymphocytes involved in peripheral blood stem cell allograft rejection. Since the HLA-DPB1 locus does not show strong linkage disequilibrium with the other loci of the HLA region, an unrelated donor matched for HLA-A, -B, -C, -DRB1, -DQB1 is not likely to be matched for DPB1. In current practice, HLA-DPB1 mismatches are not, in general, considered an exclusion criterion for donor selection in unrelated hematopoietic stem cell transplantation. However, recent studies have shown that there may be some merit in matching for DPB1, particularly in otherwise fully identical recipient/donor pairs (Varney et al., 1999; Tate et al., 2002; Shaw et al., 2002).

Choice of stem cell source

Unrelated donor versus family donor

A matched family donor is preferred over a matched unrelated donor. Moreover, studies from Seattle and Düsseldorf could not demonstrate a significant difference in survival rates between transplants from a one locus-mismatched family donor or from a genotypically identical sibling donor (Anasetti et al., 1990, Ottinger et al., 1996), although this was not confirmed by an IBMTR study (Szydlo et al., 1997). With the development of DNA-based methods for high-resolution HLA typing, it is now possible to evaluate matching at the allele level. There are no studies available that compare a fully HLA-A, -B, -C, -DRB1, -DQB1 matched unrelated donor with a one locus-mismatched related donor.

Preference for a mismatched family member donor over a similarly mismatched unrelated donor lies in the fact that a family donor shares at least one complete inherited haplotype with the recipient and may be less disparate for minor histocompatibility antigens.

A clinical protocol has been developed by Aversa et al. (1998) that enables the engraftment of hematopoietic stem cells across a complete HLA haplotype mismatch without the occur-

rence of severe GVHD. The protocol is based on the use of large doses of highly purified CD34$^+$ cells. A haplotype-mismatched transplant may thus be an option for patients without suitable family donors, unrelated donors, or cord blood units (Aversa et al., 1998; Martelli et al., 2002).

Unrelated cord blood units

During the past decade the use of placental blood as a source of hematopoietic stem cells for transplantation has been increasing. Adequate stem cell engraftment can be achieved in patients who receive an adequate dose of nucleated cells ($\geq 2.4 \times 10^7$/kg) (Laughlin et al., 2001). The decreased risk of both acute and chronic GVHD with placental blood allows for less stringent HLA matching criteria (Wagner et al., 1995; Kurtzberg et al., 1996; Gluckman et al., 1997, 1998; Rubinstein et al., 1998; Rocha et al., 2001; Barker et al., 2001). Additionally, there may be a better access to minority HLA phenotypes (Brown et al., 2000). Recent studies have shown that HLA-mismatched cord blood from unrelated donors is a feasible alternative source of hematopoietic stem cells for transplantation, not only in children, but also in adults (Laughlin et al., 2001). Since cord blood units are collected in advance of their use, the units are available for transplant at the time of the search. Routinely, units are made available for patients within 1 to 2 weeks of initiating a donor search. In clinical settings, where timing is critical, HLA matching is problematic, or viral transmission is a concern, cord blood transplants may be the preferred stem cell choice (Cairo & Wagner, 1997; Wall, 2001).

Other non-HLA compatibility factors

The selection of an HLA-compatible related or unrelated HSC donor can be extended to nonhistocompatibility selection criteria such as donor gender and parity/transfusion status, cytomegalovirus (CMV) and Epstein-Barr virus (EBV) status, age, and ABO blood group (Kollman et al., 2001; Dominietto et al., 2001; Gratwohl et al., 2001). The characterization of human minor histocompatibility (mHag) antigens has been an important step forward toward our knowledge of these antigens and offers novel therapeutic approaches (Chapter 9) (Wang et al., 1995; Den Haan et al., 1995, 1998). It is now possible to DNA type the alleles of HA-1, HA-2, and HA-3. Whether to try and match or mismatch for these loci depends on several factors such as diagnosis (leukemia versus nonleukemia), HLA mismatches present, and transplant protocol.

General comments

Successful allogeneic HSC transplantation became a reality through an understanding of the genetics of HLA and a series of clinical, nursing, microbiological, and immunologic advances. The logistics of large HSC donor files and the collection of cord blood units for transplantation are the latest additions to this list of achievements, but a large number of challenges remain (Chapman, Atkinson, & Lapsley, 1990). One of the most important, and a crucial one, is locating a suitable donor. The BMDW file was developed to facilitate the search process. Using the state-of-the-art data transfer mechanisms and computer facilities, we are able to merge donor data from more than 38 countries into a single file that can be easily accessed on the Internet by transplant centers or search coordinating units (Oudshoorn et al., 1997).

Searching the BMDW file provides an immediate answer as to whether a potential unrelated donor is available and where the donor is located. In 1995 at least one HLA-A, -B, -DR volunteer unrelated donor could be identified in the BMDW file for over 70% of Caucasian patients (Oudshoorn et al., 1997). In 2000 this had risen to 80% to 90%, because of the greater number of donors available in registries world-wide (Hansen et al., 1997; Tiercy et al., 2000). After applying high-resolution DRB1 testing, an HLA-A/B/DRB1-matched donor can be found for approximately 40% to 50% of such individuals and an HLA-A/B/Cw/DRB1/DRB5/DQB1-matched donor for about 38% (Tiercy et al., 2000). This figure is lower if the patient is not of Caucasoid origin (Beatty et al., 1995; Freytes & Beatty, 1996; Shaw et al., 1997; Oh et al., 1999; Velickovic & Carter, 1999). Matching for HLA is just one of many factors contributing to successful transplantation. Other factors such as disease stage, conditioning regimen, patient age, and the stem cell manipulation process have great influence on survival, graft rejection, GVHD, or relapse.

In the search process it is important to be aware of the technical problems that may arise when searching for related and unrelated donors (Schreuder et al., 2001) Full comprehension of available and evolving laboratory techniques, and the immunogenetics of HLA and population genetics, is needed in order to find the best matched donor. Websites with useful information on HLA are now available and may be of use in the donor search (www.ebi.ac.uk/imgt/hla and www.allelfrequencies.net). Constant evaluation of the clinical outcome of allogeneic hematopoietic stem cell transplantation is essential for fine-tuning donor selection criteria.

Perspectives

In the summer of 2002 the consensus of most of the major transplant centers was that the availability of a donor HLA-A, -B, -DRB1 identical (or near identical) to the patient was a sine qua non if one wanted to perform an HSC transplantation. Allogeneic HSC transplantation is just over 30 years old and during this time the central role of HLA matchign has been virtually undisputed.

There are, however, new developments that open the possibility that in the near future the need of finding an HLA-matched donor will become less stringent. First is the identification of permissive mismatches, that is, those mismatches that will not jeopardize the transplant outcome (Oudshoorn et al., 2000; Van der Meer et al., 2000; Eljaafari et al., 2001, 2002;

Tiercy et al., 2002). Second, cord blood transplants allow for less stringent HLA matching criteria. For the success of these transplants, HLA matching and obtaining a sufficient number of stem cells are equally important. It should be noted that over 10% of unrelated stem cell transplants use cord blood and that this percentage is increasing (8% in 2000; 12% in 2001) (WMDA Annual Report). If it can be substantiated that two cord blood units can be used for a single recipient, a much larger number of adult patients could be transplanted (Barker et al., 2001a, 2001b). If one is willing to accept two major HLA-A, -B, or -DR mismatches—as a few centers already do—the 100,000 cord bloods now available could cover the need of virtually all present-day patients (Van Rood et al., 1998). Obviously, this would influence the logistics of finding a suitable donor as described in this chapter in a major way.

A third development is the use of haploidentical donors with one fully mismatched haplotype as described by Aversa et al. (1998). Because virtually all patients have a family member who is haploidentical to the patient, this approach could solve the donor availability problem.

References

Anasetti, C., Beatty, P.G., Storb, R. et al. (1990). Effect of HLA incompatibility on graft-versus-host disease, relapse, and survival after marrow transplantation for patients with leukaemia and lymphoma. *Human Immunology, 29,* 79–91.

Aversa, F., Tabilio, A., Velardi, A. et al. (1998). Treatment of high-risk acute leukemia with T-cell-depleted stem cells from related donors with one fully mismatched HLA haplotype. *New England Journal of Medicine, 339,* 1186–93.

Barker, J.N., Davies, S.M., DeFor, T. et al. (2001a). Survival after transplantation of unrelated donor umbilical cord blood is comparable to that of human leukocyte antigen-matched unrelated donor bone marrow: results of a matched-pair analysis. *Blood, 97,* 2957–61.

Barker, J.N., Weisdorf, D.J., & Wagner, J.E. (2001b). Creation of a double chimera after the transplantation of umbilical-cord blood from two partially matched unrelated donors. *New England Journal of Medicine, 344,* 1870–1.

Barker, J.N., Weisdorf, D.J., Defor, T. et al. (2001). Impact of multiple unit unrelated donor umbilical cord blood transplantation in adults: preliminary analysis of safety and efficacy. www.hematology.org

Barnardo, N.C., Davey, M.J., Bunce, M. et al. (1996). A correlation between HLA-C matching and donor anti-recipient CTL precursor frequency in bone marrow transplantation. *Transplantation, 61,* 1420–3.

Beatty, P.G., Mori, M., & Milford, E. (1995). Impact of racial genetic polymorphism on the probability of finding an HLA-matched donor. *Transplantation, 60,* 778–83.

Bishara, A., Amar, A., Brautbar, C. et al. (1995). The putative role of HLA-C recognition in graft versus host disease (GVHD) and graft rejection after unrelated bone marrow transplantation (BMT). *Experimental Hematology, 23,* 1667–75.

Bone Marrow Donors Worldwide Annual Report, 2001, Drukkerij Groen B.V. (2000).

Brown, J., Poles, A., Brown, C.J. *et al.* (2000). HLA-A, -B, and -DR antigens frequencies of the London Cord Blood Bank units differ from those found in established bone marrow donor registries. *Bone Marrow Transplantation, 25,* 475–81.

Cairo, M.S. & Wagner, J.E. (1997). Placental and/or umbilical cord blood: an alternative source of hematopoietic stem cells for transplantation. *Blood, 90,* 4665–78.

Chapman, J.R., Atkinson, K., & Lapsley, H. (1990). Costs of bone marrow transplants using unrelated donors. *Blood Reviews, 5,* 112–6.

Cleaver, S. (1992). The Anthony Nolan Research Centre and other matching registries. In *Bone Marrow Transplantation in Practice,* ed. J. Treleaven & J. Barrett. Edinburgh: Churchill Livingstone.

Colonna, M., Borsellino, G., Falco, M. *et al.* (1993). HLA-C is the inhibitory ligand that determines dominant resistance to lysis by NK- and NK2-specific natural killer cells. *Proceedings of the National Academy of Sciences of the United States of America, 90,* 12000–4.

Confer, D.L. (1997). Unrelated marrow donor registries. *Current Opinions in Hematology, 4,* 408–12.

Den Haan, J.M., Sherman, N.E., Blokland, E. *et al.* (1995). Identification of a graft versus host disease-associated human minor histocompatibility antigen. *Science, 268,* 1476–80.

Den Haan, J.M., Meadows, L.M., Wang, W. *et al.* (1998). The minor histocompatibility antigen HA-1: a diallelic gene with a single amino acid polymorphism. *Science, 279,* 1054–7.

Dominietto, A., Raiola, A.M., van Lint, J.T. *et al.* (2001). Factors influencing haematological recovery after allogeneic haematopoietic stem cell transplants: graft-versus-host disease, donor type, cytomegalovirus infections and cell dose. *British Journal of Haematology, 112,* 219–27.

Duquesnoy, R.J., White, L.T., Fierst, J.W. *et al.* (1990). Multiscreen serum analysis of highly senzitized renal dialysis patients for antibodies toward public and private class I HLA determinants. *Transplantation, 50,* 427–37.

Ebeling, L.J., Oudshoorn, M., van der Zanden, H.G.M. *et al.* (1994). Playing with BMDW (Bone Marrow Donors Worldwide). Don't take no for an answer! *EBMT News,* 4, 3, 10.

Eljaafari, A., Farre, A., Galambrun, C. *et al.* (2001). DRB1*1104 does not stimulate DRB1*1101: from biology to clinic. *European Journal of Immunogenetics, 28,* 251 (Abstract).

Eljaafari, A., Juliard, C., Farre, A., & Gebuhrer, L. (2002). Assessment of cellular permissivity between HLA-A*2403 at the clonal level clones. *Tissue Antigens, 59,* P27.3, 111–2 (Abstract).

Fleischhauer, K., Zino, E., Mazzi, B. *et al.* (2001). Peripheral blood stem cell allograft rejection mediated by CD4+ T lymphocytes recognizing a single mismatch at HLA-DP? 1*0901. *Blood, 98,* 1122–6.

Freytes, C.O. & Beatty, P.G. (1996). Representation of Hispanics in the National Marrow Donor Program. *Bone Marrow Transplantation, 17,* 323–7.

Gluckman, E., Broxmeyer, H.E., Auerback, A.D. *et al.* (1989). Hematopoietic reconstitution in a patient with Fanconi's anemia by means of umbilical cord blood from an HLA-identical sibling *New England Journal of Medicine, 321,* 1174–8.

Gluckman, E., Rocha, V., Boyer-Chammard, A. *et al.* and the Eurocord Transplant Group and the European Blood and Marrow Transplantation Group. (1997). Outcome of cord-blood transplantation from related and unrelated donors. *New England Journal of Medicine, 337,* 373–81.

Gluckman, E., Rocha, V., & Chastang, C. and the Eurocord group. (1998). European results of unrelated cord blood transplants. *Bone Marrow Transplantation, 21* (Suppl 3), S87–S91.

Goldman, J.M. for the WMDA Executive Committee. (1994). A special report: Bone marrow transplants using volunteer donors—Recommendations and requirements for a standardized practice throughout the world—1994 update. *Blood, 84,* 2833–9.

Gratwohl, A., Hermans, J., Niederwieser, D. *et al.* for the Chronic Leukemia Working Party of the European Group for Blood and Marrow Transplantation EBMT. (2001). Female donors influence transplant-related mortality and relapse incidence in male recipients of sibling blood and marrow transplants. *Blood, 2,* 363–70.

Hansen, J.A., Clift, R.A., Thomas, E.D. *et al.* (1980). Transplantation of marrow from an unrelated donor to a patient with acute leukemia. *New England Journal of Medicine, 303,* 565–7.

Hansen, J.A., Petersdorf, E., Martin, P.J., & Anasetti, C. (1997). Hematopoietic stem cell transplants from unrelated donors. *Immunology Reviews, 157,* 141–51.

Hurley, C.K., Wade, J.A., Oudshoorn, M. *et al.* (1999). Histocompatibility testing guidelines for hematopoietic stem cell transplantation using volunteer donors: report from The World Marrow Donor Association. *Bone Marrow Transplantation, 24,* 119–21.

Kaminski, E., Hows, J., Man, S. *et al.* (1989). Prediction of graft versus host disease by frequency analysis of cytotoxic T-cells after unrelated donor bone marrow transplantation. *Transplantation, 48,* 608–13.

Kaufman, R. (1996). A generalized HLA prediction model for related donor matches. *Bone Marrow Transplantation, 17,* 1013–20.

Kollman, C., Howe, C.W.S., Anasetti, C. *et al.* (2001). Donor characteristics as risk factors in recipients after transplantation of bone marrow from unrelated donors: the effect of donor age. *Blood, 98,* 2043–51.

Kurtzberg, J., Graham, M., Casey, J. *et al.* (1994). The use of umbilical cord blood in mismatched related and unrelated hematopoietic stem cell transplantation. *Blood Cells, 20,* 275–84.

Kurtzberg, J., Laughlin, M., Graham, M.L. *et al.* (1996). Placental blood as a source of hematopoietic stem cells for transplantation into unrelated recipients. *New England Journal of Medicine, 335,* 157–66.

Laughlin, M.J., Barker, J., Bambach, M. *et al.* (2001). Hematopoietic engraftment and survival in adult recipients of umbilical cord blood from unrelated donors. *New England Journal of Medicine, 344,* 1815–22.

Marsh, S.G.E., Bodmer, J.G., Albert, E.D. *et al.* (2001). Nomenclature for factors of the HLA system, 2000. *Journal of Immunogenetics, 28,* 377–424.

Martelli, M.F., Aversa, F., Bachar-Lustig, E. *et al.* (2002). Transplants across human leukocyte antigen barriers. *Seminars in Hematology, 39,* 48–56.

Mori, M., Graves, M., Milford, E.L., & Beatty, P.G. (1996). Computer program to predict likelihood of finding an HLA-matched donor: methodology, validation, and application. *Biology of Blood and Marrow Transplantation*, **2**, 134–44.

Morishima, Y., Sasazuki, T., Inoko, H. *et al.* (2002). The clinical significance of human leukocyte antigen (HLA) allele compatibility in patients receiving a marrow transplant from serologically HLA-A, HLA-B and HLA-DR matched unrelated donors. *Blood*, **99**, 4200–6.

Nagler, A., Brautbar, C., Slavin, S., & Bishara, A. (1996). Bone marrow transplantation using unrelated and family related donors: the impact of HLA-C disparity. *Bone Marrow Transplantation*, **18**, 891–7.

Oh, H.B., Kim, S.I., Park, M.H. *et al.* (1999). Probability of finding HLA-matched unrelated marrow donors for Koreans and Japanese from the Korean and Japan Marrow Donor Programs. *Tissue Antigens*, **53**, 347–9.

Ottinger, H., Beelen, D., Sayer, H. *et al.* (1996). Bone marrow transplantation from partially HLA-matched related donors in adults with leukemia: the experience at the University Hospital of Essen. *British Journal of Haematology*, **92**, 913–21.

Oudshoorn, M., Cornelissen, J.J., Fibbe, W.E. *et al.* (1997). Problems and possible solutions in finding an unrelated bone marrow donor. Results of consecutive searches for 240 Dutch patients. *Bone Marrow Transplantation*, **20**, 1011–7.

Oudshoorn, M., Doxiadis, I.I.N., van den Berg-Loonen, P.M. *et al.* (2002). Functional versus structural matching: Can the CTLp test be replaced by HLA allele typing? *Human Immunology*, **63**, 176–84.

Oudshoorn, M., van Leeuwen, A., van der Zanden, H.G.M., & van Rood, J.J. (On behalf of the Editorial Board of BMDW). (1994). Bone Marrow Donors Worldwide. A successful exercise in international co-operation. *Bone Marrow Transplantation*, **14**, 3–8.

Petersdorf, E.W. (1997). Association of HLA-C disparity with graft failure after marrow transplantation from unrelated donors. *Blood*, **89**, 1818–23.

Petersdorf, E.W., Gooley, T.A., Anasetti, C. *et al.* (1998). Optimizing outcome after unrelated marrow transplantation by comprehensive matching of HLA class I and II alleles in the donor and recipient. *Blood*, **92**, 3515–20.

Petersdorf, E.W., Hansen, J.A., Martin, P.J. *et al.* (2001a). Major-histocompatibility-complex class I alleles and antigens in hematopoietic-cell transplantation. *New England Journal of Medicine*, **345**, 1794–1800.

Petersdorf, E.W., Kollman, C., Hurley, C.K. *et al.* (2001b). Effect of HLA class II gene disparity on clinical outcome in unrelated donor hematopoietic cell transplantation for chronic myeloid leukemia: the US National Marrow Donor Program Experience. *Blood*, **98**, 2922–9.

Petersdorf, E.W., Longton, G.M. Anasetti, C. *et al.* (1995). The significance of HLA-DRB1 matching on clinical outcome after HLA-A, B, DR identical unrelated donor marrow transplantation. *Blood*, **86**, 1606–13.

Petersdorf, E.W., Longton, G.M., Anasetti, C. *et al.* (1996). Definition of HLA-DQ as a transplantation antigen. *Proceedings of the National Academy of Sciences of the United States of America*, **93**, 15358–63.

Petersdorf, E.W., Smith, A.G., Mickelson, E.M. *et al.* (1993). The role of HLA-DPB1 disparity in the development of acute graft-versus-host disease following unrelated donor marrow transplantation. *Blood*, **81**, 1923–32.

Rocha, V., Cornish, J., Sievers, E.L. *et al.* (2001). Comparison of outcomes of unrelated bone marrow and umbilical cord blood transplants in children with acute leukemia. *Blood*, **97**, 2962–71.

Roosnek, E., Hogendijk, S., Zawadynski, S. *et al.* (1993). The frequency of pretransplant donor cytotoxic T cell precursors with anti-host specificity predicts survival of patients transplanted with bone marrow from donors other than HLA-identical siblings. *Transplantation*, **56**, 691–6.

Rubinstein, P., Carrier, C., Scaradavou, A. *et al.* (1998). Outcomes among 562 recipients of placental blood transplants from unrelated donors. *New England Journal of Medicine*, **339**, 1565–77.

Rubinstein, P., Rosenfield, R.E., Adamson, J.W., & Stevens, C.E. (1993). Stored placental blood for unrelated bone marrow reconstitution. *Blood*, **81**, 1679–90.

Ruggeri, L., Capanni, M., Casucci, M. *et al.* (1999). Role of natural killer cell alloreactivity in HLA-mismatched hematopoietic stem cell transplantation. *Blood*, **94**, 333–9.

Ruggeri, L., Capanni, M., Urbani, E. *et al.* (2002). Effectiveness of donor natural killer cell alloreactivity in mismatched hematopoietic transplants. *Science*, **295**, 2097–100.

Sasazuki, T., Juji, T., Morishima, Y. *et al.* (1998). Effect of matching of class I HLA alleles on clinical outcome after transplantation of hematopoietic stem cells from an unrelated donor. *New England Journal of Medicine*, **339**, 1177–85.

Schipper, R.F., D'Amaro, J., & Oudshoorn, M. (1996). The probability of finding a suitable related donor for bone marrow transplant in extended families. *Blood*, **87**, 800–4.

Schipper, R.F., D'Amaro, J., & Oudshoorn, M. (1997). The probability of finding a haplotypically identical unrelated bone marrow donor. In *HLA: Genetic Diversity of HLA, Functional and Medical Implication*, Vol. II, ed. D. Charron, pp. 583–5. Sèvres/Paris: EDK Med. & Scient. Int. Publ.

Schreuder, G.M.Th., Hurley, C.K., Marsh, S.G.E. *et al.* (2001). The HLA Dictionary 2001: A summary of HLA-A, -B, -C, -DRB1/3/4/5, -DQB1 alleles and their association with serologically defined HLA-A, -B, -C, -DR, and -DQ antigens. *Human Immunol*, **62**, 826–49.

Shaw, B.E., Pay, A.L., Potter, M.N. *et al.* (2002). HLA-DPB1 plays a role in the outcome of unrelated stem cell transplants in pairs completely matched at the other five transplantation loci. *Bone Marrow Transplantation*, **29** (Suppl 2), S25, O161 (Abstract).

Shaw, C.-K., Chang, T.-K., Chen, S.N., & Wu, S. (1997). HLA polymorphism and probability of finding HLA-matched unrelated marrow donors for Chinese in Taiwan. *Tissue Antigens*, **50**, 610–9.

Speck, B., Zwaan, F.E., van Rood, J.J., & Eernisse, J.G. (1973). Allogeneic boen marrow transplantation in a patient with aplastic anemia using a phenotypically HLA-identical unrelated donor. *Transplantation*, **16**, 24–8.

Speiser, D.E., Löliger, C.-C., Siren, M.-K., & Jeannet, M. (1996). Pretransplant cytotoxic donor T-cell activity specific to patient HLA class I antigens correlating with mortality after unrelated BMT. *British Journal of Haemotology*, **93**, 935–9.

Spencer, A., Brookes, P.A., Kaminski, E. *et al.* (1995). Cytotoxic T lymphocyte precursor frequency analysis in bone marrow transplantation with volunteer unrelated donors. *Transplantation*, **59**, 1302–8.

Szydlo, R., Goldman, J.M., Klein, J.P. *et al.* (1997). Results of allogeneic bone marrow transplants for leukemia using donors other than HLA-identical siblings. *Journal of Clinical Oncology*, **15**, 1767–77.

Tatari, Z., Esperou, H., Chastang, C. *et al.* (1996). Influence of donor/recipient HLA-C disparity in 110 unrelated bone marrow transplantation. *Human Immunology*, **47**, 80 (Abstract).

Tate, D.G., Davidson, J.A., Chopra, R. *et al.* (2002). The optimal unrelated bone marrow donor: HLA-DP matching as an additional selection criteria: *Bone Marrow Transplantation*, **29** (Suppl 2), S109, P486 (Abstract).

Thomas, E.D. (1983). Marrow transplantation for malignant disease. *Journal of Clinical Oncology*, **1**, 517–31.

Thomas, E.D., Clift, R.A., & Storb, R. (1984). Indications for marrow transplantation. *Annual Review Medicine*, **35**, 1–9.

Tiercy, J.M., Morel, C., Freidel, A.C. *et al.* (1991). Selection of unrelated donors for bone marrow transplantation is improved by HLA class II genotyping with oligonucleotide hybridization. *Proceedings of the National Academy of Sciences of the United States of America*, **88**, 7121–5.

Tiercy, J.M., Villard, J., & Roosnek, E. (2002). Selection of unrelated bone marrow donors by serology, molecular typing, and cellular assays. *Transplantation Immunology*, **10**, 215–21.

Tiercy, J-M., Bujan-Lose, M., Chapuis, B. *et al.* (2000). Bone Marrow Transplantation with unrelated donors: what is the probability of identifying an HLA-A/B/Cw DRB1/B3/B5/DQB1-matched donor? *Bone Marrow Transplantation*, **26**, 437–41.

Van der Meer, A., Allebes, W.A., Paardekooper, J. *et al.* (2001). HLA-C mismatches induce strong cytotoxic T-cell reactivity in the presence of an additional DRB/DQB mismatch and affect NK cell-mediated alloreactivity. *Transplantation*, **72**, 923–9.

van der Meer, A., Joosten, I., Schattenberg, A.V. *et al.* (2000). Cytotoxic T-lymphocyte precursor frequency (CTLp-f) as a tool for distinguishing permissible from non-permissible class I mismatches in T-cell-depleted allogeneic bone marrow transplantation. *British Journal of Haematology*, **111**, 685–94.

van Rood, J.J. (1971). Die Bedeutung der Leukozytengruppen für die Transplantationsserologie. *Bibliography in Haematology*, **37**, 53–69.

van Rood, J.J. (1989). Report of the 1989 Immunology Working Party. *Bone Marrow Transplantation*, **4** (Suppl 2), 6.

Van Rood, J.J., Schipper, R.F., Bakker, J.N.A. *et al.* (1998). Bone Marrow Donors Worldwide and cord blood stem cell transplantation. *Bone Marrow Transplantation*, **22** (Suppl 1), S19–S21.

Varney, M.D., Lester, S., McCluskey, J. *et al.* (1999). Matching for HLA-DPA1 and -DPB1 alleles in unrelated bone marrow transplantation. *Human Immunology*, **60**, 532–8.

Velickovic, Z.M. & Carter, J.M. (1999). Feasibility of finding an unrelated bone marrow donor on international registries for New Zealand patients. *Bone Marrow Transplantation*, **23**, 291–4.

Wade, J., Hurley, C.K., Takemoto, S. *et al.* (2001). HLA mismatching for crossreactive groups (CREG) is not a permissive mismatch for unrelated bone marrow transplantation (BMT). *Human Immunology*, **62** (Suppl 1), S17, 6.2 (Abstract).

Wagner, J.E., Kernan, N.A., Steinbuch, M. *et al.* (1995). Allogeneic sibling umbilical-cord-blood transplantation in children with malignant and non-malignant disease. *Lancet*, **346**, 214–9.

Wall, D.A. (2001). The case for umbilical cord blood as the unrelated donor hematopoietic stem cell source of choice. *Blood Therapies in Medicine*, **1**, 81–4.

Wang, W., Meadows, L.R., den Haan, J.M. *et al.* (1995). Human H-Y: a male-specific histocompatibility antigen derived from the SMCY protein. *Science*, **269**, 1588–90.

24 Mobilization regimens for harvesting autologous and allogeneic peripheral blood stem cells

MARTIN KÖRBLING

The University of Texas M.D. Anderson Cancer Center, Houston, USA

Introduction

Under steady-state conditions progenitor cells and—among them—pluripotent and self-renewing stem cells are circulating at a constant concentration. This is explained by the fact that there is a dynamic equilibrium of progenitor cells between extravascular marrow sites and circulating blood. If progenitor cells are removed from the circulating pool (e.g., by apheresis), there is an immediate influx from marrow spaces, and, vice versa, progenitor cells may return to marrow spaces to aid in the reestablishment of local marrow stem cell levels, if necessary (e.g., after local irradiation) (Fliedner & Steinbach, 1988; Wright *et al.*, 2001). The concept of stem cell mobilization or peripheralization is based on a temporary shifting of progenitor cells from extravascular marrow sites toward the circulatory system, rendering them easily accessible by apheresis. How the temporary shift is achieved is not clear, but at least three possibilities have been suggested:

1. Altered expression of cell adhesion molecules (Fig. 24.1).
2. Alterations in the functional integrity of the bone marrow stroma sinusoidal endothelium.
3. Perturbation of the dynamics of the hematopoietic progenitor cell population.

In a murine model, treatment with anti-vascular adhesion molecule-1 (VCAM-1) increased the number of colony-forming cells in the blood more than 11-fold, and CFU-S more than 21-fold (Kikuta *et al.*, 2000). Cotreatment with granulocyte colony-stimulating factor (G-CSF) was synergistic.

An additional mechanism is the secretion of gelatinase B by G-CSF-stimulated neutrophils, which cleaves extracellular matrix molecules and weakens the adhesion between stem cells and stromal cells (Fig. 24.1) (Gyger *et al.*, 2000).

Interleukin-8 (IL-8) a member of the CXC chemokine family, induces a rapid mobilization of stem and progenitor cells, by upregulating matrix metalloproteinase-9 activity. SB-251353 is an N-terminal truncated form of the chemokine GROβ, also a member of the CXC family. A single subcutaneous injection of this molecule rapidly mobilized stem and progenitor cells in both mice and rhesus monkeys (King *et al.*, 2001). In combination with G-CSF, mobilization was augmented five-fold compared to that with G-CSF alone. Its mechanism of action appears similar to that of IL-8.

Levesque and colleagues (2001) presented data suggesting that an essential step in G-CSF-mediated mobilization of stem cells is the proteolytic cleavage of VCAM-1 expressed on marrow stromal cells, an event triggered by the degranulation of neutrophils accumulating in the marrow in response to the administration of G-CSF, and their release of two serine proteases, neutrophil elastase and cathepsin G.

Hematopoietic progenitor cells and stem cells in unperturbed circulating blood

The bone marrow cell compartment contains short- and long-term repopulating stem cells that are identified and quantified for clinical routine purposes by phenotypic analysis of cell surface antigens using flow cytometry.

In unperturbed, steady-state peripheral blood (PB) from normal subjects the percentage of CD34+ cells among circulating nucleated cells is on average 0.06% (Körbling *et al.*, 1995a) (Table 24.1). The absolute number of circulating CD34+ cells in normal individuals has been independently reported to be 3.8 × 10^6/l (Körbling *et al.*, 1995a; Link *et al.*, 1995). The more primitive circulating CD34+ subsets such as CD34+CD90dim and CD34+CD90dim CD38− encompass 30% and 2.5% respectively, of the unperturbed circulating CD34+ cell pool (Körbling *et al.*, 1995a), or approximately 1.1 × 10^6/l and 0.1 × 10^6/l, respectively.

Collection of peripheral blood stem cells from steady-state peripheral blood

Besides initial reports on autologous peripheral blood stem cell (PBSC) transplantation, the largest experience with collecting unmobilized PBSC from patients (with relapsed Hodgkin's disease) has been reported by the University of Nebraska transplant group (Kessinger *et al.*, 1991). Apheresis products containing at least 6.5 × 10^8 mononuclear cells (MNC)/kg and facilitating sustained engraftment after myeloablative or near-ablative treat-

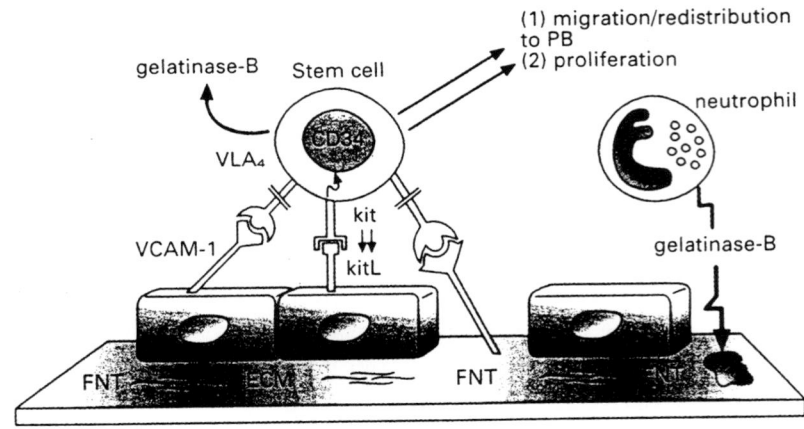

Fig. 24.1. Peripheralization of stem/progenitor cells after G-CSF administration encompasses several mechanisms. Disruption of cytoadhesive interactions with bone marrow stroma is among the leading hypotheses. Analyses of G-PBMNCs reveal a reduced expression of the VLA-4 integrin which normally binds strongly to its ligand VCAM-1. VLA-4 binds also to fibronectin (FNT) fragments in the extracellular matrix (ECM). G-PBMNCs show a significant reduction in the expression of several adhesion molecules, among which is the VLA-4 (CD49d/CD29) alpha integrin. A global reduction and downregulation of *c-kit* on stem/progenitor cells may lessen adhesion to membrane bound kit L on stromal cells. G-CSF may also initiate mobilization through neutrophils, by gelatinase B secretion, cleaving extracellular matrix molecules and weakening the adhesive interactions between stem/progenitor cells and stromal cells. Stem/progenitor cells have also been shown to secrete gelatinase B, a mechanism that could enhance their migration to the PB. Finally, there is experimental evidence that G-CSF might act indirectly with a stem cell factor/receptor ligand and stimulate proliferation of stem cells. Reproduced, with permission, from Gyger *et al.* (2000).

ment, required processing a substantial volume of patient blood (in the range of 40 to 150 litres with a median of 9 four-hour apheresis procedures). Platelet recovery posttransplant was a limiting factor with independence from platelet transfusion reached at a median of 50 days (Kessinger *et al.*, 1993), significantly slower than observed after autologous bone marrow (BM) transplantation. Therefore, the development of transient stem cell mobilization and peripheralization techniques was believed to be a requisite for the clinical feasibility of PBSC transplantation. A clear relationship has since been demonstrated between the number of CD34+ cells infused at the time of autologous transplant and the rate of neutrophil and platelet engraftment posttransplant (Shpall, Champlin, & Glaspy, 1998).

Cytokine administration alone for stem cell mobilization

Cytokine administration is a powerful tool for transiently increasing the circulating stem cell concentration. As shown by Molineux *et al.* (1990) in a sex-mismatched mouse model, the transplantation of 10 μl of recombinant human G-CSF-mobi-

lized PB was equivalent to 3,000 μl of unperturbed PB cells in rescuing 98% or more of leathally irradiated mice. The clinical advantage of using G-CSF mobilized PBSC autografts over nonmobilized autografts has also been clearly documented in a study of 85 patients with relapsed Hodgkin's disease (Chao *et al.*, 1993). The median number of aphereses required to achieve a target progenitor cell dose for engraftment was nine in nonmobilized patients, whereas only four procedures were required when giving patients G-CSF for stem cell mobilization. Also the time to recovery of granulocytes and platelets after autologous transplantation was significantly shortened when using G-CSF-mobilized PBSC.

Cytokine administration for stem cell mobilization is used in the autologous transplant setting in situations in which the patient's condition does not allow additional chemotherapy priming treatment (chemopriming) (see below), and/or to save time: the time to complete chemopriming/cytokine treatment and apheresis is approximately 3 weeks, whereas cytokine treatment alone and stem cell collection takes approximately 1 week. For obvious ethical reasons, mobilization of stem cells from normal donors for allogeneic transplantation cannot uti-

Table 24.1.   *CD34+ cell and subset concentrations in normal peripheral blood at steady state*

Parameters	CD34+ cells	CD34+ Thy-1dim cells	CD34+ Thy-1dim CD38− cells
Cell concentration × 10⁶/l	3.8	1.1	0.095
% of TNC	0.06	0.018	0.0015
% of CD34+ cells		30%	2.5%

Adapted, with permission, from Körbling *et al.* (1995a).

lize chemopriming treatment. Cytokine priming alone, however, has emerged as an acceptable and efficient alternative for stem cell mobilization in normal donors.

Autologous transplant setting—cytokine treatment alone

Recombinant human granulocyte colony-stimulating factor

G-CSF alone or in combination with other cytokines/chemokines is currently considered the cytokine of choice for stem cell mobilization. As first reported by Sheridan et al. (1992), the administration of G-CSF 12 µg/kg/day subcutaneously daily for 6 days to patients with nonmyeloid malignant disorders increased the CFU-GM level in blood by a median of 58-fold over baseline, and the BFU-E level by a median of 24-fold. Using 16 µg/kg/day G-CSF in patients with hematologic malignancies or solid tumors, Bensinger et al. (1993) observed a 10-fold increase of PB CD34+ cell concentration over baseline, reaching peak values at about day 5. G-CSF doses of 24 µg/kg/day (Kroger et al., 1998) up to 32 µg/kg/day (Körbling, 2002) are well tolerated in lymphoma patients. It has been suggested that stem cell mobilization in breast cancer patients is more effective when giving G-CSF in divided doses (Kroger et al., 1999). The same group reported higher CD34+ cell yields in breast cancer patients when harvested on day 5 of G-CSF treatment as compared to day 4 (Kroger et al., 2000). Typical kinetics of the white blood cell

(WBC) and CD34+ cell concentrations in the PB of normal donors given G-CSF are shown in Figures 24.2 and 24.3, and Table 24.2. Hematopoietic stem cells (HSC) (CD34+CD90+) in mobilized blood (both in mice and humans) were found not to be in cell cycle (Uchida et al., 1997). This was surprising because a significant proportion of HSC from bone marrow taken at the same time were actively proliferating. A polyethylene glycol (PEG)-derivatized form of G-CSF has been introduced with a resultant increase in plasma half-life. As reported by Johnston et al. (2000) in patients with non-small-cell lung cancer, a single dose of PEGylated G-CSF resulted in CD34+ cell mobilization comparable or greater than that achieved with daily G-CSF application.

Preclinical and/or clinical experience with other cytokines, with or without G-CSF, is still limited, but arousing much interest as new cytokines/chemokines become available (Table 24.3). The main purposes of using combined cytokine/chemokine regimens are (1) reducing side effects of a single higher dosed cytokine, (2) targeting progenitors at different maturation levels, and (3) mobilizing simultaneously progenitor cells of different hematopoietic cell lineages.

Combined recombinant human granulocyte-macrophage colony-stimulating factor (GM-CSF) and G-CSF

GM-CSF appears to be less effective than G-CSF in mobilizing CD34+ progenitors (Peters et al., 1993; Lane et al., 1995), although comparative data are scarce. In a randomized study in

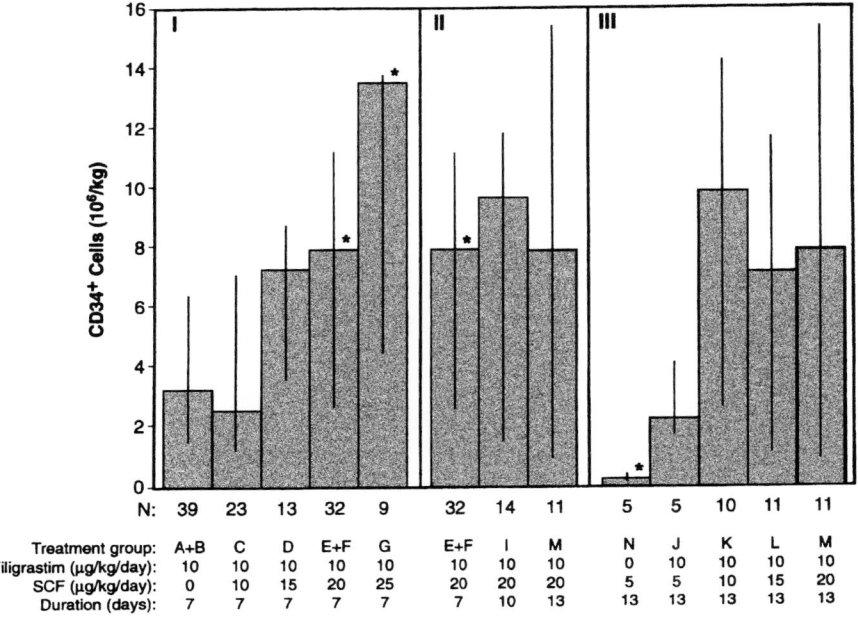

Fig. 24.2. CD34+ cell yields (median, 25th, and 75th percentiles) from 3 days of leukapheresis treatment for each treatment group. Section I includes the 7-day treatment groups, section II the 20 µg/kg/d SCF and filgrastim groups, and section III the 13-day treatment groups. Only 3 patients received 30 µg/kg/d SCF and filgrastim (H); their individual CD34+ cell yields were 1.43, 5.20, and 8.52 × 10⁶/kg. *P <.05, comparing all other treatment groups with the filgrastim alone groups (**A** and **B**). Reproduced, with permission, from Glaspy et al. (1997).

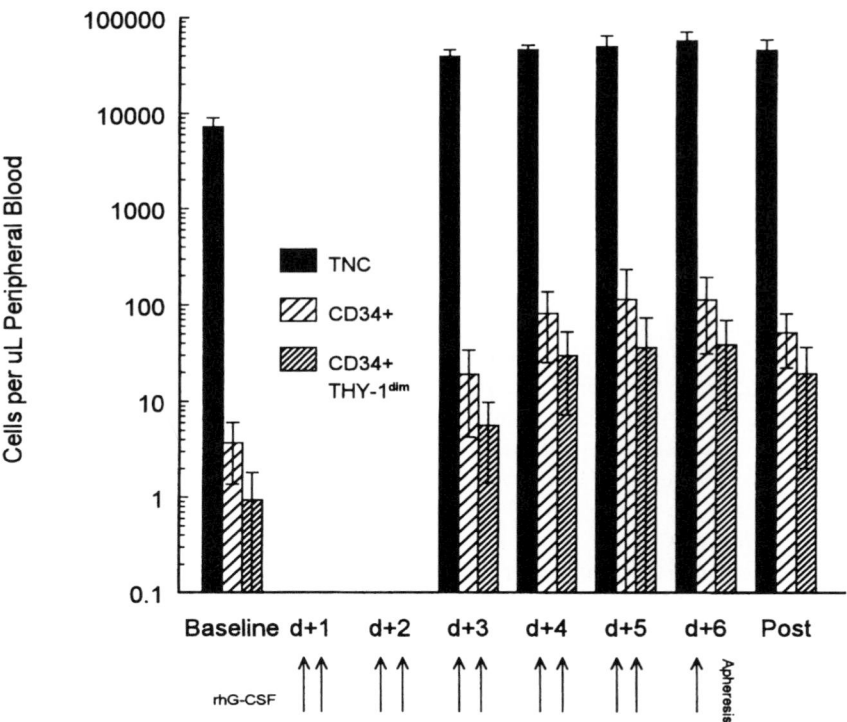

Fig. 24.3. Serial evaluation of peripheral blood concentrations of total nucleated cells (TNC), CD34[+] cells, and CD34[+] Thy-1[dim] subsets prior to and during rhG-CSF treatment, and 1 day after apheresis and completion of rhG-CSF treatment in 10 normal blood stem cell donors. Error bars represent ±SD.

patients with breast cancer and melanoma comparing G-CSF with GM-CSF mobilization, G-CSF treatment resulted in a more rapid increase in leukocyte counts, and a higher yield of nucleated cells and CD34[+] cells collected by apheresis. However, the number of CFU-GM in both G-CSF and GM-CSF primed PBSC autografts was not significantly different, reflecting a higher proportion of CFU-GM in the GM-CSF primed patients (Peters *et al.,* 1993). In another study, administration of G-CSF to patients already receiving GM-CSF caused the number of hematopoietic progenitor cells to surge to nearly 80-fold baseline (Winter *et al.,* 1996). The reverse sequence, that is, the addition of GM-CSF to patients already receiving rhG-CSF, was less effective.

Combined recombinant methionyl human stem cell factor (r-metHuSCF) and G-CSF

SCF further improves stem cell peripheralization, stem cell apheresis yield, and potentially the quality of the stem cell graft when administered together with G-CSF. A murine study demonstrated a 10-fold increase in repopulating ability of marrow collected after administration of stem cell factor (SCF) and G-CSF compared to untreated marrow (Bodine, Seidel, & Orlic, 1996).

As shown by Andrews *et al.* (1995) in nonhuman primates, low-dose r-metHuSCF treatment in combination with G-CSF resulted in a 14-fold higher yield of progenitor cells contained

Table 24.2. *Increase of CD34[+] cell and subset concentrations in the peripheral blood of normal donors after 3 days of rhG-CSF treatment*

	CD34[+] cells × 10[6]/l	CD34[+] Thy-1[dim] cells × 10[6]/l	CD34[+] Thy-1[dim] CD38[-] cells × 10[6]/l
Prior to rhG-CSF treatment at steady state (*n*=14)	3.8	1.1	0.095
Prior to apheresis at day 4 of rhG-CSF treatment (*n*=16)	61.9	26.6	2.2
Fold increase preapheresis over precytokine values	16.3	24.2	23.2

Adapted, with permission, from Körbling *et al.* (1995a).

Table 24.3. *Novel cytokine/chemokine combinations for stem cell mobilization*

Stem cell mobilization regimen	Clinical use	Reference
rhGM-CSF plus rhG-CSF	Yes	Lane *et al.*, 1995
r-metHuSCF plus rhG-CSF	Yes	Shpall *et al.*, 1997
Flt3 ligand plus rhGM-CSF/rhG-CSF	Yes	Lebsack *et al.*, 1997
rhTPO plus rhG-CSF	Yes	Champlin *et al.*, 1997
Interleukin-3 plus rhG-CSF	Yes	Geissler *et al.*, 1996
Human macrophage inflammatory protein-1α (MIP-1α, BB10010)	Yes	Broxmeyer *et al.*, 1995
Interleukin-1	No	Levesque *et al.*, 1995
Interleukin-8	No	Laterveer *et al.*, 1995

in the apheresis product compared with G-CSF administration alone. WBC, PMN, and platelets engrafted significantly faster when using a combined r-metHuSCF and G-CSF treated blood stem cell autograft. A randomized phase III study in patients with high-risk breast cancer compared the number of aphereses required to collect a target dose of 5×10^6 CD34$^+$ cells/kg for autologous transplantation, using either SCF 20 µg/kg/day in combination with G-CSF 10 µg/kg/day, or G-CSF 10 µg/kg/day alone. There was a statistically significant reduction ($P < .01$) in the number of aphereses required to reach the target CD34$^+$ cell dose for patients receiving the combined cytokine treatment (median of three aphereases) compared with those receiving G-CSF alone (median of ≥6 aphereses) (Shpall *et al.*, 1997, 1999). In a similar randomized trial in heavily pretreated patients with non-Hodgkin's lymphoma (NHL) or Hodgkin's disease, the combined SCF and G-CSF treatment was superior to G-CSF treatment alone regarding CD34$^+$ cell yield, the proportion of patients reaching the CD34$^+$ cell target dose, the number of aphereses required to reach the target CD34$^+$ cell dose, and the number of patients failing to reach the minimum collection dose for safe engraftment (Stiff *et al.*, 1997a). In patients with extensive prior chemotherapy, the CD34$^+$ cell apheresis yield was 1.76×10^6/kg in those mobilized with a combination of SCF and G-CSF versus 0.28×10^6/kg when using G-CSF alone. This resulted in a decrease of 10.5 days to reach an unsupported platelet count of 20×10^9/l after autologous PBSC transplantation (Moskowitz *et al.*, 1997). In a study by Glaspy *et al.* (1997), using SCF in combination with G-CSF in breast cancer patients, the optimal dose and schedule was found to be G-CSF 10 µg/kg/day plus 20 µg/kg/day of SCF with apheresis beginning on day 5 (Fig. 24.2). When using the combined G-CSF and SCF treatment, the blood volume required to be processed during the apheresis procedure to obtain a specific target stem cell dose was significantly less (Weaver & Testa, 1998).

One concern about using SCF is mast cell activation with the potential of inducing anaphylactoid reactions. With appropriate premedication, no deaths or life-threatening reactions due to SCF administration have been observed in the above-mentioned multicenter or single institution trials encompassing a total of more than 300 patients.

As per current knowledge, the potential clinical benefits of SCF in combination with G-CSF treatment include:

1. Higher CD34$^+$ cell yield per apheresis
2. Fewer apheresis procedures needed to reach a dose of CD34$^+$ cells targeted for safe engraftment
3. A higher proportion of patients who are considered "poor mobilizers" achieve the minimum number of CD34$^+$ cells required to undergo a PBSC transplant
4. A higher proportion of patients benefit from the rapid hematologic recovery associated with transplantation of higher numbers of PBSC.

Combined flt3 ligand and G-CSF

Flt3 ligand is believed to have similar biological activities on the hematopoietic system as SCF. It is a potent direct stimulator of the growth of both primitive and committed human CD34$^+$ progenitor cells (Rusten *et al.*, 1996). Molineux *et al.*, (1997) studied the effect of combined flt3 ligand and G-CSF administration on circulating CFU-GM in mice. Whereas flt3 ligand alone was a relatively modest mobilizer of CFU-GM (2.3-fold increase over baseline), combined flt3 and G-CSF administration resulted in a 645-fold increase of circulating CFU-GM. Similar data have been reported by Brasel *et al.* (1997) (Fig. 24.4) and by Sudo *et al.* (1997) (Fig. 24.5). In a randomized study in healthy volunteers using flt3 ligand at escalating doses (Lebsack *et al.*, 1997), the following mobilization characteristics were observed:

1. The WBC, especially the monocyte fraction, was elevated after flt3 ligand administration
2. Flt3 ligand-treated subjects exhibited sustained blood levels following subcutaneous administration
3. Flt3 ligand produced sustained mobilization of progenitor cells with elevated circulating levels persisting for up to a week after the last dose of flt3 ligand
4. Circulating dendritic cells were increased up to 30-fold following flt3 ligand administration

In mice, daily treatment with recombinant human flt3 ligand also results in a dramatic increase in the number of dendritic cells: when challenged with a syngeneic methylcholanthrene-induced fibrosarcoma, complete tumor regression was observed in a significant proportion of mice. This suggests that flt3 ligand might augment the generation of specific anti-tumor immune responses in vivo (Lynch *et al.*, 1997). In healthy volunteers flt3 ligand was shown to increase the absolute number of functionally mature circulating dendritic cells by 30-fold over baseline at day 9 of treatment (Maraskovsky *et al.*, 1997). Papayannopoulou and colleagues (1997) explored the in vivo effects of flt 3 ligand in primates on mobilization of hematopoietic progenitors both alone and in combination with G-CSF.

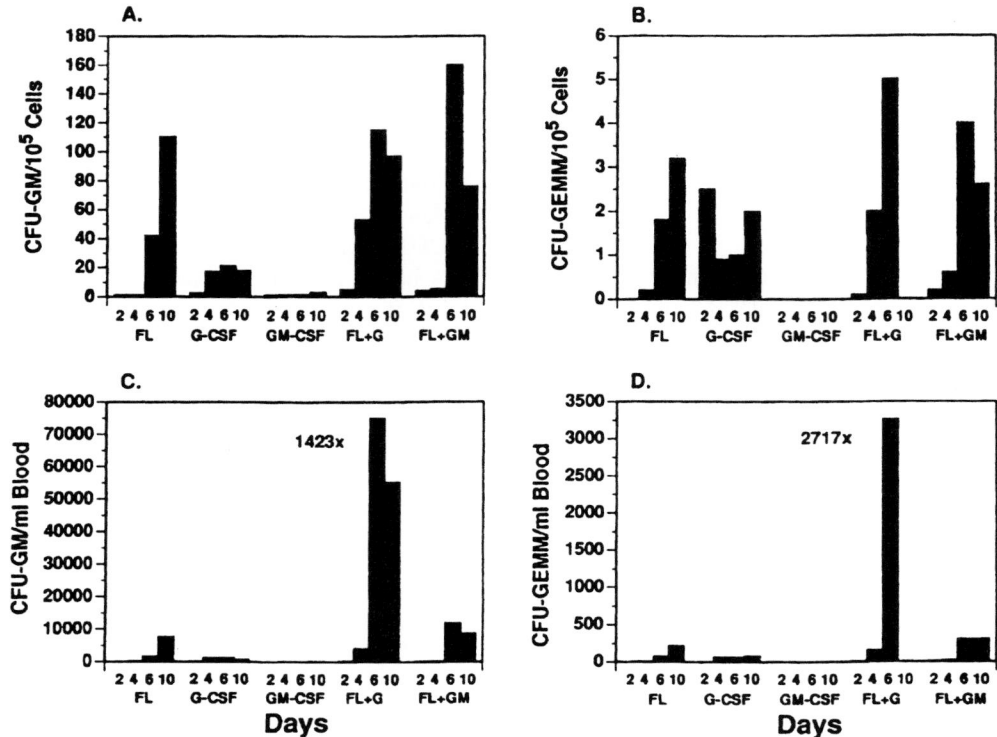

Fig. 24.4. Mobilization of CFU into the PB after growth factor administration. (**A** and **B**) The frequency of CFU-GM and CFU-GEMM (per 10^5 cells) in PB after 2, 4, 6, and 10 days growth factor treatment, respectively. (**C** and **D**) The absolute number of CFU-GM and CFU-GEMM per ml of PB. PBMNC count multiplied by CFU frequency after 2, 4, 6, and 10 days growth factor treatment, respectively. PBMNC from four mice were pooled within each group for CFU. In all growth factor-treated groups, total CFU per ml of PB and CFU frequency per 10^5 cells had almost returned to pretreatment values 1 week postgrowth factor treatment (data not shown). This experiment was performed twice giving very similar results, only differing in the route of injection (i.p.) and dosage of rhG-CSF and rhGM-CSF (5 μg/mouse/d). Reproduced, with permission, from Brasel *et al.* (1997).

Flt3 ligand alone mobilized progenitor cells with slow kinetics, giving a peak effect at the end of 2 weeks of treatment. To assess the possible synergy of flt3 ligand with G-CSF two different schedules were used: one in which G-CSF was given for the last 5 days of a 12-day treatment with flt3 ligand; the other

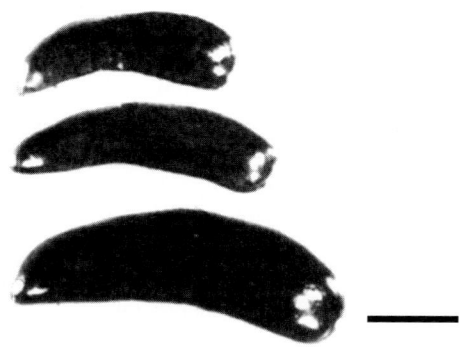

Fig. 24.5. Spleens from a control mouse (top) and from mice treated for 5 days with rhG-CSF (250 μg/kg) alone (middle), or together with FL (20 μg/kg) (bottom). The bar indicates 5 mm. Reproduced, with permission, from Sudo *et al.* (1997).

in which both cytokines were given concurrently for 5 days only. Both protocols yielded much higher progenitor mobilization levels than observed with either flt 3 ligand alone or G-CSF alone at the same doses.

Since flt3 ligand does not share the mast cell degranulation effect with SCF, flt3 ligand might also have a different toxicity profile. Flt3 ligand was well tolerated by healthy volunteers without the need for premedication. Injection site reactions and enlarged lymph nodes appeared to be the only adverse events related to flt3 ligand administration. After discontinuation of flt3 ligand, all adverse events resolved without sequelae.

Combined recombinant human thrombopoietin (rhTPO) and G-CSF

As shown by Molineux *et al.* (1996), irradiated mice that received PBSC mobilized by PEGylated recombinant human megakaryocyte growth and development factor (PEGrHuMGDF) (thrombopoietin) showed a significantly reduced period (4 or 5 days) of thrombocytopenia compared with those that received non-mobilized PBSC transplantation (9 days). This model also provided evidence that PEGrHuMGDF stimulated the mobilization of myeloid progenitor cells. As shown in a phase I clinical trial (Champlin *et al.*, 1997), combined mobilization treatment with G-CSF and rhTPO in patients with stage II/III breast cancer resulted in a higher CD34+ cell apheresis yield compared with G-CSF treatment alone (34.5×10^6/kg versus 15.3×10^6/kg CD34+ cells). One nonrandomized study suggested that combined cytokine treatment enhanced CD34+ cell mobilization and accelerated hematopoietic recovery after autologous transplantation (Somlo *et al.*, 1999).

Combined interleukin-3 (IL-3) and G-CSF

Combined treatment with G-CSF and IL-3 has been reported to further increase circulating progenitor cells in patients with Hodgkin's disease and non-Hodgkin's lymphoma compared with G-CSF alone. G-CSF alone (5 µg/kg/day for 5 days) increased the number of circulating CFU-GM over baseline 21-fold, whereas combined treatment with IL-3 (5 µg/kg/day for 7 days) followed by G-CSF at the same dose level for 5 days increased the circulating CFU-GM level 56-fold over baseline (Geissler *et al.*, 1996). When G-CSF (5 µg/kg/day) was administered for 7 consecutive days either alone or preceded by IL-3 (5 µg/kg/day) for 4 consecutive days in sequential or partially overlapping schedules, the mean circulating CD34+ cell counts on day 3 of cytokine treatment were significantly higher in the sequential treatment group (Huhn *et al.*, 1996).

A genetically engineered agonist of the IL-3 receptor complex (daniplestim) has been introduced. As reported by DiPersio *et al.* (2000) in a phase I/II study, daniplestim given to patients with adenocarcinoma of the breast together with G-CSF may have an additional mobilizing effect on hematopoietic progenitor cells.

Human macrophage inflammatory protein (MIP-1α)

MIP-1α is considered a potential myeloprotective cytokine based on its myelosuppressive and cycle-inhibitory functions (Hunter *et al.*, 1995). As reported by Lord *et al.* (1995), MIP-1α also induces a rapid mobilization effect on early progenitor cells into the circulation in mice. In a phase I clinical trial the administration of BB 10010, a genetically engineered and stable variant of MIP-1α, at 5 or 10 µg/kg significantly reduced cycling rates of bone marrow progenitor cells, as well as their concentration, but modestly increased the number of circulating progenitor cells between 2.6- and 4.1-fold over baseline (Broxmeyer *et al.*, 1995).

Interleukin-1 (IL-1) and IL-8

In studies in mice, IL-1 administration (1 µg) increased the number of circulating CFU-GM 30-fold over baseline. Transplantation of IL-1 mobilized blood progenitor cells resulted in long-term donor chimerism (Levesque *et al.*, 1995). The toxicity of IL-1 most probably precludes it from clinical use. IL-8, a chemotactic cytokine, has been shown to induce rapid (15–30 min) mobilization of hematopoietic progenitor cells (Laterveer *et al.*, 1995). Fifteen minutes after a single intraperitoneal injection of 30 µg of IL-8 into mice, circulating CFU-GM increased by 17-fold over baseline, and returned to almost pretreatment values after 60 minutes. Sex-mismatched transplantation of IL-8 mobilized hematopoietic progenitor cells resulted in complete and permanent hematopoietic reconstitution (Fig. 24.6). It has been suggested that IL-8 induced stem cell mobilization requires the in vivo activation of circulating granulocytes (Fibbe *et al.*, 1999; Pruijt *et al.*, 2002) and, therefore, acts primarily as a granulocyte recruiting agent rather than a stem cell mobilizing agent (Vetillard *et al.*, 1999).

Autologous transplant setting—chemotherapy followed by cytokine treatment

Induction of peripheral blood stem cell rebound by chemotherapy priming (chemopriming)

The previously mentioned dynamic equilibrium between the marrow and circulating stem cell pools can be intentionally perturbed by administering chemotherapy treatment to a patient. A transient posttreatment cytopenia is usually followed by a rebound of WBC and—to a greater extent—by peripheral blood progenitor cells (Fig. 24.7) (Richman *et al.*, 1976; Hahn *et al.*, 1980), which allows collection of an approximately 1 log or higher yield of progenitor cells by apheresis. Since the marrow progenitor cell pool is 60 to 100 times larger than the total number of circulating progenitors at any given time (Fliedner & Steinbach, 1988), relatively small treatment-related changes

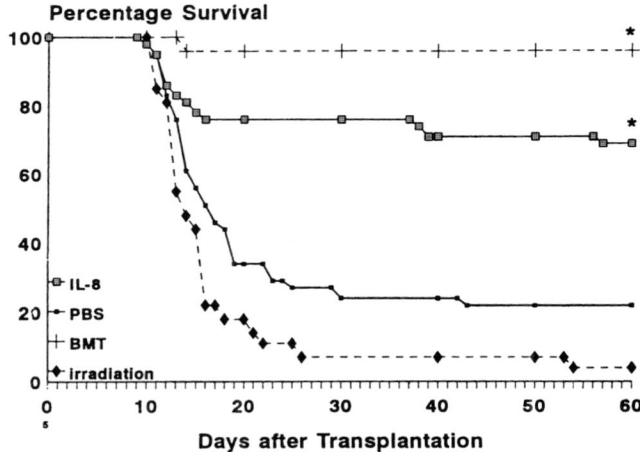

Fig. 24.6. Actual survival of mice transplanted with 5×10^5 blood MNC obtained from animals at 30 minutes after pretreatment with 30 µg IL-8 or saline (PBS). Results are derived from 23 mice [four experiments for bone marrow transplantation controls (BMT)], 27 mice (four experiments for irradiation controls), 42 mice (six experiments for a dose of 30 µg Il-8), or 41 mice (six experiments for PBS controls). *$P < .05$ as compared with recipients of blood MNC obtained from saline-treated donors. Reproduced, with permission, from Laterveer *et al.* (1995).

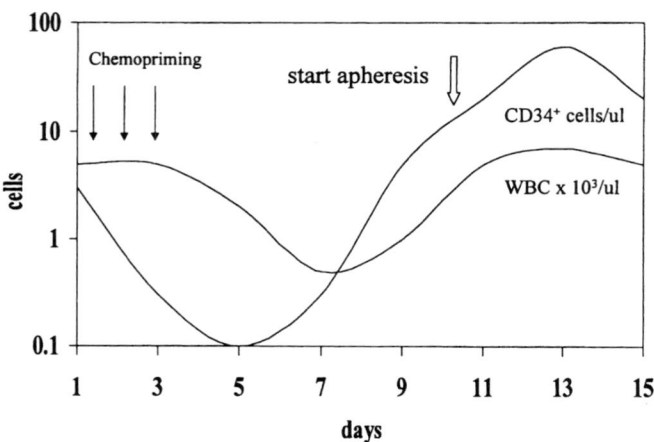

Fig. 24.7. Schematic course of WBC and CD34⁺ cell concentrations following chemopriming. Induction of a CD34⁺ cell rebound.

in marrow cellularity are reflected in the peripheral blood as major oscillations of WBC and progenitor cell concentrations. Since the initial report by Richman *et al.* in 1976, cyclophosphamide is considered a model drug for inducing a rebound of PBSCs because of its lack of significant stem cell toxicity (Korbling *et al.*, 1986; To *et al.*, 1989; Kotasek *et al.*, 1992). Comparative results of different mobilization protocols are shown in Table 24.4 and Figure 24.8.

Since cyclophosphamide alone has only limited antitumor activity, current chemopriming strategies frequently use disease-oriented, intensification treatment regimens in patients with malignant hematologic disorders and selected solid tumors (breast cancer, ovarian cancer). The chemopriming regimens used for stem cell mobilization at our institution are listed in Table 24.5. Other regimens include mini-ICE (idarabine, cytarabine, etoposide) in patients with chronic myelogenous leukemia (Sureda *et al.*, 1999), IVE (ifosfamide, etoposide, epirubicin) in patients with NHL and Hodgkin's disease (McQuaker *et al.*, 1999), TEC (paclitaxel, etoposide, cyclophosphamide) (Bilgrami

Table 24.4. *Comparative results using different protocols for mobilization of peripheral blood stem and progenitor cells*

Mobilization protocol	CD34⁺ cells (× 10⁶/kg)	CFU-GM (× 10⁴/kg)
Cyclophosphamide (CY) 7 g/m²	3.6	44
Chemotherapy + rhGM-CSF	13	152
Chemotherapy + rhG-CSF	7.9	77
rhG-CSF (no prior chemotherapy)	7.3	137
IL 3 → rhGM-CSF	1.5	24
Autologous bone marrow harvest	0.8	11

Adapted from To *et al.* (1996).

et al., 2000), or CP (cyclophosphamide, paclitaxel) (Klein *et al.*, 1999) in patients with metastatic breast cancer, and ICE (ifosfamide, carboplatin, etoposide) in patients with NHL (Moskowitz *et al.*, 1999). The mobilizing efficiency of chemopriming is limited by the following:

1. Major reduction of marrow stem cell pool size due to prior progenitor/stem cell-toxic treatment, particularly with agents such as BCNU and fludarabine (Dreger *et al.*, 1995; Khouri *et al.*, 1998). Factors that impact on this include:
   - number of previous chemotherapy cycles (Chabannon *et al.*, 1995)
   - duration of previous chemotherapy (To *et al.*, 1989; Tricot *et al.*, 1995)
   - cell recovery from previous chemotherapy at the time of starting mobilization treatment (Tarella *et al.*, 1995)
   - previous local irradiation to marrow stem cell-containing compartments (e.g., pelvic bones, spinal column) (Dreger *et al.*, 1995)
2. Extensive tumor cell involvement of the marrow

The induction of a chemotherapy-induced stem cell rebound depends on the critical mass of the marrow stem cell pool. Administering chemopriming treatment to a patient whose residual stem cell pool is below this critical mass impairs cell recovery, causing a prolonged cytopenia without stem cell rebound. In addition, stem cell mobilization by chemopriming imposes potential risks of neutropenic fever and sepsis, and a potential risk of bleeding or even death from the mobilization/apheresis procedures (Kotasek *et al.*, 1992).

Interleukin-2

Besides chemotherapy, IL-2 has also been reported to induce a progenitor cell rebound (Schaafsma *et al.*, 1990). Administration of 3×10^6 U/m²/day by continuous infusion for 5 days resulted in lymphocytopenia and a decline in circulating progenitor cell concentration, followed, after discontinuation of the IL-2 infusion, by lymphocytosis, neutrophilia, and eosinophilia. The numbers of circulating CFU-GM, BFU-E, and CFU-GEMM markedly increased, reaching a maximum 5 days (day 10 from start of IL-2 treatment) after completion of IL-2 treatment. The circulating progenitor cell pool was calculated to expand in the rebound phase 20-fold over the pretreatment level.

Chemopriming plus cytokine treatment

Chemopriming combined with cytokine administration act synergistically and is a widely used and preferred mobilization strategy for collection of autologous stem cells in cancer patients (Elias *et al.*, 1992; Schwartzberg *et al.*, 1992; Pettengell *et al.*, 1993). A potential increase in toxicity may be offset by a higher stem cell yield and a reduced transplant-related toxicity. In an ongoing trial, 85 patients with stage II–IV breast cancer were randomized to receive either G-CSF alone or chemopriming (cyclophosphamide, etoposide, cisplatin) plus G-CSF.

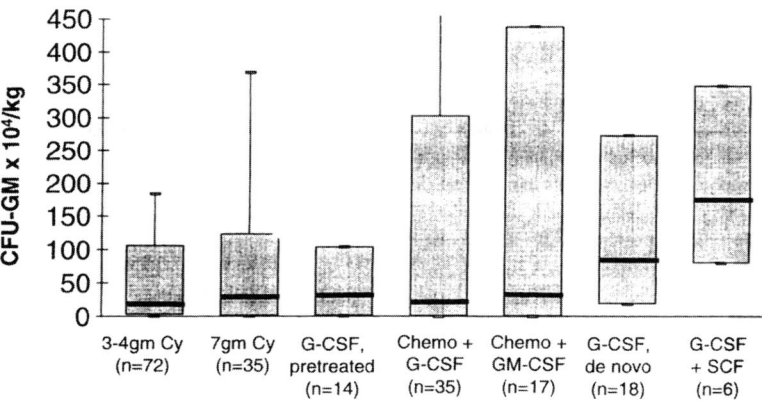

Fig. 24.8. The CFU-GM yield of different mobilization protocols used in the authors' institution. "3–4gm Cy" denotes patients who recyclophosphamide 3 to 4 g/m^2 intravenously and had blood cells harvested during recovery from myelosuppression. "7gm Cy" denotes patient received cyclophosphamide 7 g/m^2 intravenously and had blood cells harvested during recovery from myelosuppression. "G-CSF, pretreated" denotes patients who received G-CSF at 12 µg/kg subcutaneously and had blood cells harvested on days 5, 6, and 7. "Chemo $^+$G-CSF" and "Chemo + GM denote patients who received myelosuppressive chemotherapy and rhG-CSF or rhGM-CSF and had blood cells harvested during recovery from myelosuppression. "G-CSF, de novo" denotes chemotherapy naive patients who received G-CSF at 12 µg/kg subcutaneously daily and had blood cells harvested on days 5, 6, and 7. "G-CSF + SCF" denotes chemotherapy naive patient who received G-CSF at 12 µg/kg subcutaneously daily and SCF at 5 to 15 subcutaneously daily and had blood cells harvested on days 5, 6, and 7 of G-CSF administration. For each group of patients the horizontal bar denotes the median value, the box plot denotes the 5th and the 95th percentiles, and the whiskers denote the maximum and minimum values. Reproduced, with permission, from To *et al.* (1997).

Apheresis started either (chemopriming arm) when the recovering WBC reached >1.5 × 10^9/l or (cytokine alone) at day 4 of G-CSF treatment. The median number of aphereses needed to reach the target CD34$^+$ cell dose of 4 × 10^6/kg was 1 (range 1–5) after chemopriming plus G-CSF versus 3 (range 1–9) after G-CSF alone (P = .0001). The total number of CD34$^+$ cells harvested was 13.4 × 10^6/kg (range 3.3–122) and 9.1 × 10^6/kg, respectively. However, in the chemopriming plus G-CSF arm, there were significantly more infectious complications during mobilization and more deaths after the subsequent high-dose treatment (Gajewski *et al.*, 1998). Another study investigated stem cell mobilization efficiency in patients with advanced breast cancer who underwent chemopriming treatment with cyclophosphamide, etoposide, and cisplatin (CVP) followed by G-CSF (12 µg/kg/day) and escalating doses of TPO. Compared with a historical control group, the study patients receiving G-CSF and TPO had a higher stem cell yield and required less apheresis procedures to reach the stem cell transplant target dose (Gajewski *et al.*, 2002).

Allogeneic transplant setting

The optimal cytokine for stem cell mobilization in normal donors

G-CSF has emerged as the preferred cytokine for stem cell mobilization in normal donors partly based on the positive experience and toxicity profile reported with its administration to granulocyte donors (Bensinger *et al.*, 1993; Casper *et al.*, 1993). Molineux *et al.* (1999) reported promising data on using the PEGylated rhG-GM-CSF for stem cell mobilization in normal individuals with sustained duration of action requiring just a single dose application.

GM-CSF appears to be less effective in mobilizing CD34$^+$ progenitors in normal donors (Lane *et al.*, 1995). In one study, a combined G-CSF and GM-CSF mobilization treatment was well tolerated in normal individuals. However, the combined treatment did not translate into a more efficient mobilization of CD34$^+$ progenitors when compared to G-CSF alone, but did result in a significantly greater peripheralization of CD34$^+$ cells with the early CD34$^+$CD38$^-$ phenotype (Lane *et al.*, 1995). A potential clinical benefit of this finding is unknown.

Combined G-CSF and GM-CSF treatment has also been reported to result in a significantly reduced number of circulating and collected CD3$^+$ cells, CD4$^+$ cells, and CD8$^+$ cells compared to G-CSF treatment alone (DiPersio *et al.*, 2000). These findings suggest that GM-CSF in combination with other

Table 24.5. *Chemopriming regimens commonly used at the University of Texas M.D. Anderson Cancer Center for stem cell mobilization*

Disease	Mobilization treatment
Breast cancer/ovarian cancer	Cyclophosphamide/etoposide/cisplatin [CVP]
	High-dose cyclophosphamide
Non-Hodgkin's lymphoma	Ifosfamide/etoposide
Multiple myeloma	Cyclophosphamide/vincristine/doxorubicin/dexamethasone [HyperCVAD] (Dimopoulos *et al.*, 1996)

cytokines deserves further investigation as a mobilizing agent in normal individuals.

Effect of G-CSF treatment on the peripheralization of WBC, PMN cells, lymphocytes, and CD34⁺ cells and subsets in normal subjects

To assess the effects of G-CSF (12 µg/kg/day) on the peripheralization of HSC and lymphoid subsets, we studied a cohort of 41 normal blood stem cell donors. After 3 days of G-CSF treatment, the WBC, PMN, and lymphocyte concentrations in the donor's PB exceeded baseline by 6.4, 8.0, and 2.2-fold, respectively (Korbling et al., 1995a). A similar increase of T lymphocytes by day 3 of treatment with 16 µg/kg/day G-CSF has been reported by Weaver et al. (1994), namely 1.5 to 2.0 times over baseline. On the other hand, PB CD34⁺ cells and primitive subsets such as CD34⁺CD90^{dim} and CD34⁺CD90^{dim}CD38⁻ cells increased by 16.3-fold, 24.2-fold, and 23.2-fold, respectively, suggesting a selective peripheralization effect by G-CSF on hematopoietic progenitor cells and, in particular, on the more primitive stem cell subsets (Korbling et al., 1995a; Prosper et al., 1995) (Table 24.1). The percentage of CD34⁺ cells among total nucleated cells in normal individuals increases up to almost 1% by the fourth day of G-CSF treatment. The clonogenic potential of G-CSF-mobilized PBSC is also reported to be significantly higher than steady-state PBSC. In a study on PBSC obtained from G-CSF-treated normal individuals, the replating capacity of primary colonies from 5-week-old longterm culture (LTC) initiated a steady state (Fujisaki et al., 1995). In normal donors, a 5-day course of G-CSF increased the frequency of LTC-initiating cells among CD34⁺ cells by ninefold over baseline (Prosper et al., 1995).

Kinetics of CD34⁺ cells and subsets with G-CSF mobilization treatment

The mobilization kinetics of WBC and progenitor cell subsets with G-CSF treatment is quite uniform in an unperturbed, normal hematopoietic system, although an interindividual variability in the degree of progenitor cell mobilization has become evident (Tjønnfjord et al., 1994; Link et al., 1995; Grigg et al., 1995). When we monitored 10 healthy stem cell donors undergoing G-CSF treatment (12 µg/kg/day) for 6 days, the kinetics of circulating CD34⁺ cells and subsets paralleled each other, reaching a plateau from day 4 on (day 1 = first day of cytokine treatment) (Fig. 24.3). Based on these data and data reported by others (Dreger et al., 1994; Tanaka et al., 1994), the most favorable day for stem cell collection (15- to 35-fold increase of circulating CD34⁺ cells at peak level over baseline values) would appear to be day 4 or day 5 of G-CSF administration. Continuation of G-CSF administration beyond a 5-day course leads to a progressive decline in the mobilization efficiency of CD34⁺ progenitors (Stroncek et al., 1994; Grigg et al., 1995). In contrast to expression of CD90, G-CSF mobilized peripheral blood CD34⁺ cells showed a downregulation of c-kit expression (Fig. 24.9).

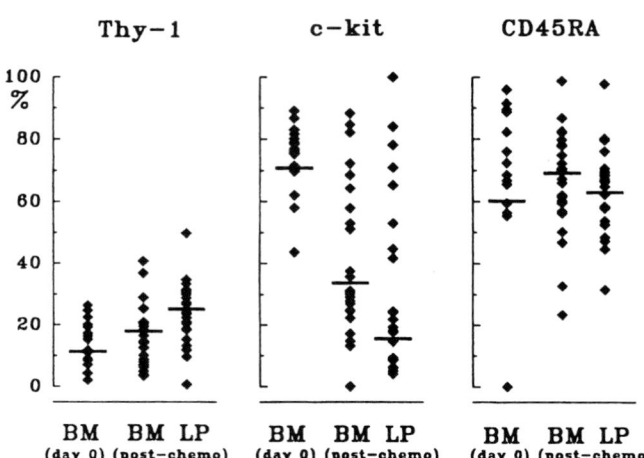

Fig. 24.9. Two-color immunofluorescence analysis of CD34⁺ cells. Twenty-four samples of LPs and BM obtained during filgrastim-supported recovery (postchemotherapy) are shown. BM samples before PBPC mobilization are available for 16 patients (day 0). The horizontal line represents the mean. The differences found for the co-expression of c-kit were statistically significant (P < .01). LPs contained the largest proportion of CD34⁺/Thy-1⁺ hematopoietic progenitor cells. Reproduced, with permission, from Haas et al. (1995).

Dose-dependent mobilization of CD34⁺ progenitor cells

It has been shown that, at least for G-CSF doses between 5 and 10 µg/kg/day, a dose-response relationship exists for the degree of mobilization of CD34⁺ progenitor cells (Höglund et al., 1996; Stroncek et al., 1996) (Fig. 24.10). G-CSF given to normal donors at a dose of 10 to 12 µg/kg twice daily resulted in a higher yield of CD34⁺ cells as compared with 10 µg/kg given once a day (Waller et al., 1996). Nevertheless, bone pain and headache were more severe in the high-dose G-CSF donor cohort, although still tolerable. G-CSF doses of up to 32 µg/kg/day given in two divided doses have been safely employed in patients with advanced ovarian cancer (Stiff et al., 1997b). When compared with standard dose (10 µg/kg/day) G-CSF, the CD34⁺ cell yield was higher. Seventy percent of patients receiving high-dose G-CSF reached a target CD34⁺ cell dose of 4 × 10⁶/kg after two aphereses versus 33% of the standard-dose group.

Factors affecting mobilization of CD34⁺ progenitor cells

In an effort to elucidate factors affecting mobilization in normal donors and stem cell yield by apheresis, the CD34⁺ cell yield from the first day of apheresis in 119 donors who underwent apheresis on days 4 to 6 of G-CSF treatment (12 µg/kg/day) was analyzed. The CD34⁺ cell yield was significantly lower in donors greater than 55 years of age, or who underwent apheresis on day 4 of G-CSF administration. There was also a correlation between CD34⁺ cell yield and baseline WBC, pre-apheresis WBC, and pre-apheresis mononuclear cell (MNC) count. Twenty-one (18%) donors were considered

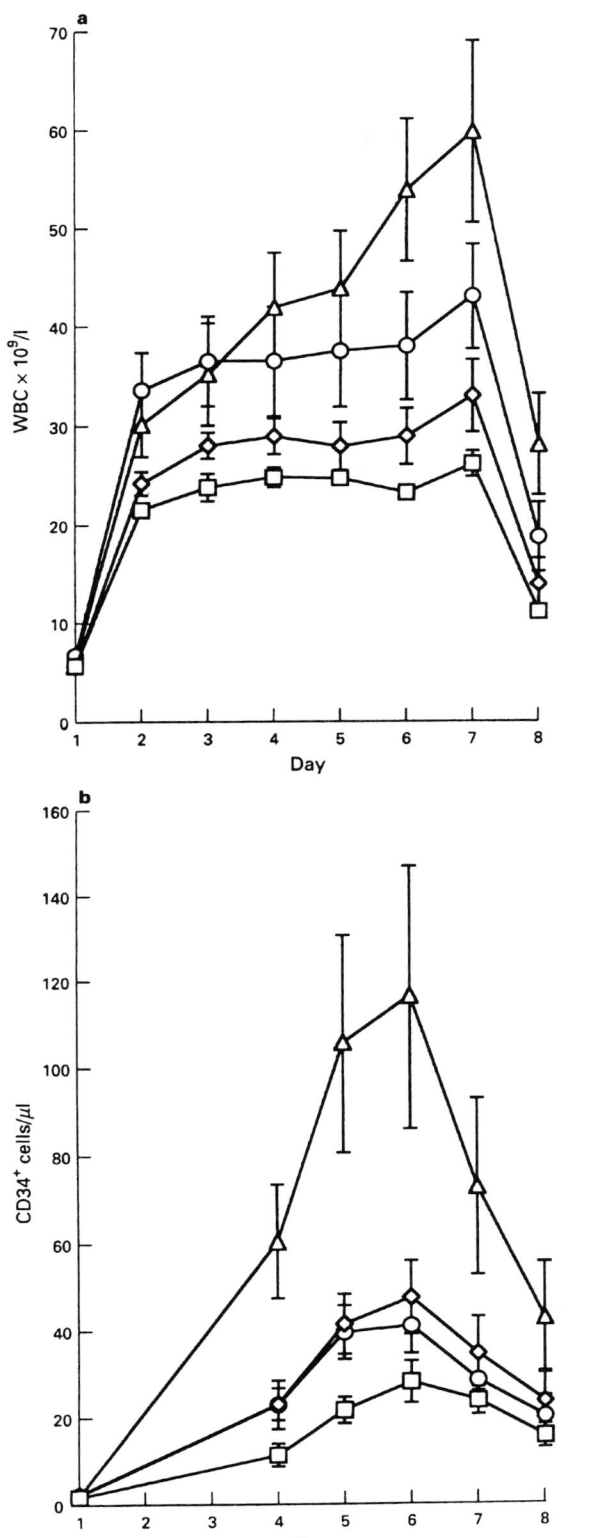

Fig. 24.10. WBC (**a**) and number of CD34[+] cells (**b**) in peripheral blood from 24 healthy volunteers who received lenograstim 3 (□), 5 (◇), 7.5 (○), or 10 (△) µg/kg s.c. once daily for 6 days. Day 1 = day of first injection. Six volunteers in each dose group. Data given as mean ± 1 S.E.M. Reproduced, with permission, from Höglund *et al.* (1996).

"poor mobilizers" yielding less than 20×10^6 cells/l of blood processed. In multivariate analysis, the only significant risk factor for inferior mobilization was age greater than 55 years, which conferred a 3.8-fold increased risk ($P = .04$). As poor mobilizers occurred in all age groups, the predictive value (and clinical usefulness) of the model was limited (Anderlini *et al.*, 1997b).

Side effects of G-CSF administration for stem cell mobilization in normal donors

There are now sufficient data on the short-term safety profile of G-CSF in normal apheresis donors (Anderlini *et al.*, 1996a). The most commonly reported adverse effects, which are partly dose-related, include bone pain, headache, fatigue, and nausea. They ordinarily resolve within a few days of rhG-CSF discontinuation and can be managed successfully in most cases with minor analgesics. Severe adverse events requiring G-CSF discontinuation have been rare. G-CSF-induced laboratory abnormalities include cytopenias and transient increases (about two- to threefold) of serum alkaline phosphatase and lactate dehydrogenase, and less commonly decreases in serum potassium and magnesium (Tables 24.6 and 24.7) These are seemingly related to the expanding myeloid cell mass. One case of splenic rupture 4 days following a 6-day course of G-CSF treatment for stem cell mobilization has been reported, although the etiology of this event was probably multifactorial (Becker *et al.*, 1997). Additionally there have been reports of arterial thrombosis (Conti & Sher, 1992; Kawachi *et al.*, 1996), acute inflammatory eye disease (irtis/episcleritis) (Huhn *et al.*, 1996; Parkkali *et al.*, 1996), marginal keratitis (Esmaeli *et al.*, 2002), and acute gouty arthritis during G-CSF treatment for stem cell mobilization in normal individuals. In two independent reports G-CSF mobilization treatment was shown to have caused a sickle cell crisis and multiorgan dysfunction, in one case with fatal consequences (Adler *et al.*, 2001; Grigg, 2001).

Data on long-term safety of G-CSF administration in PBPC donors are scarce (Gutierrez & Bensinger, 2001). The main theoretical risk is believed to be the possible development of leukemia. We conducted a survey among healthy G-CSF treated sibling donors to determine the incidence of leukemia after PBPC donation. Two hundred and eighty-one PBPC donors were interviewed by phone. The median follow-up after PBPC donation was 39 (range 7–80) months. At the time of the interview, none of the donors had been diagnosed with acute or chronic leukemia (Anderlini *et al.*, 2002).

Safety considerations for normal peripheral blood stem cell donors

Although the short-term G-CSF safety profile seems acceptable (Anderlini *et al.*, 1996a), experience remains limited and the optimal dose and schedule have not been defined. Only limited data exist regarding long-term safety (i.e., the development of

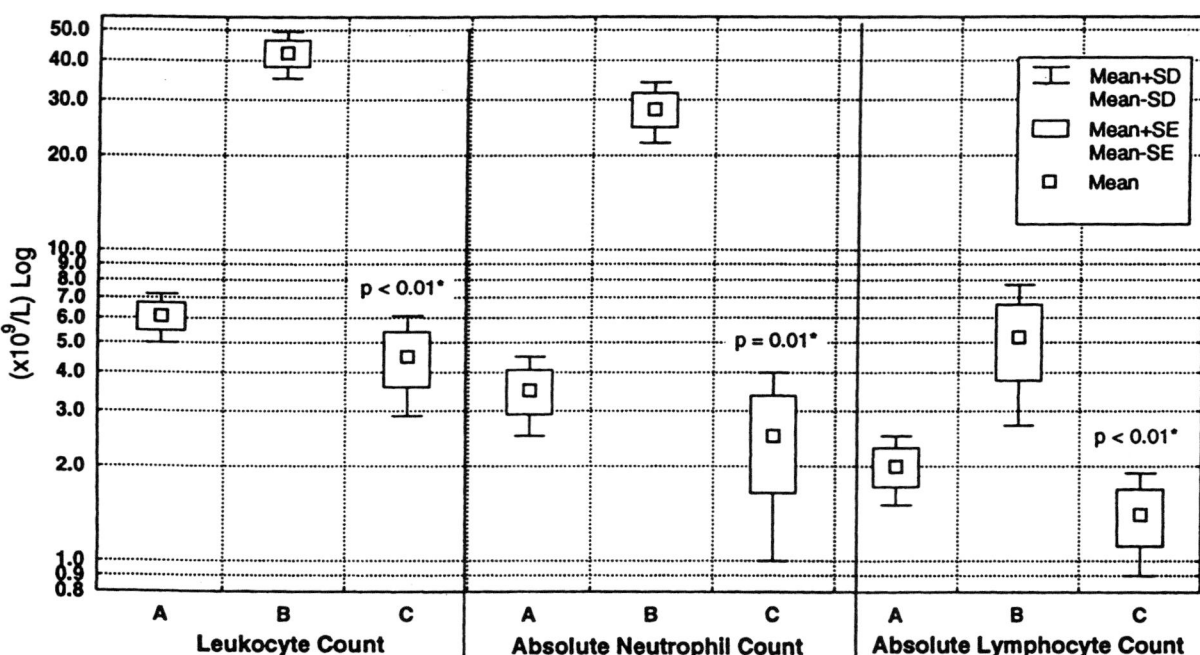

Fig. 24.11. Comparison between baseline leukocyte, neutrophil, and lymphocyte counts and counts measured 7 to 10 day after leukapheresis in normal donors ($n = 13$). Counts expressed as ($\times 10^9$/l) log. A = baseline; B = before leukapheresis; C = 7 to 10 days after leukapheresis. *Comparison between baseline values and values 7 to 10 days after leukapheresis. Reproduced, with permission, from Anderlini *et al.* (1996).

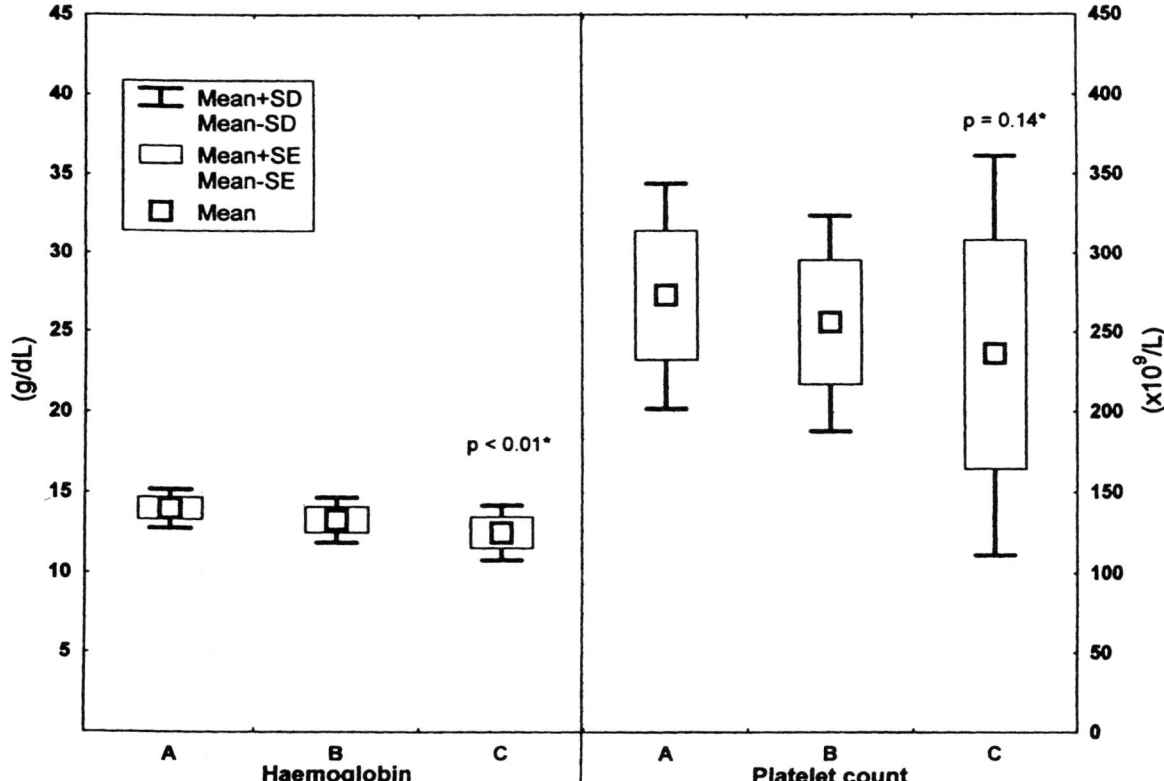

Fig. 24.12. Comparison between hemoglobin level and platelet count as baseline and 7 to 10 days after leukapheresis in normal donors ($n = 13$). A = baseline; B = before leukapheresis; C = 7 to 10 days after leukapheresis. *Comparison between baseline values and values 7 to 10 days after leukapheresis. Reproduced, with permission, from Anderlini *et al.* (1996a).

Table 24.6. *Effect of rhG-CSF mobilization treatment on hematologic values*

	Baseline	Prior to 1st apheresis	*P* value
PMN [$\times 10^9$/l]	4.2	31	<.0001
Lympho [$\times 10^9$/l]	1.9	4.3	<.0001
Monocytes [$\times 10^9$/l]	0.3	2.4	<.0001
Hemoglobin [g/dl]	14.0	13.5	.01
Platelets [$\times 10^9$/l]	241	226	.01

myelodysplasia or myeloid leukemia), primarily derived from experience in patients with chronic neutropenia (Bonilla *et al.,* 1994). Available data are largely limited to isolated case reports (Sakamaki *et al.,* 1995).

It has been estimated, that to detect a 10-fold increase in the leukemia risk (a substantial risk increase), more than 2,000 normal donors would need to be followed for up to 10 years or longer, and the detection of a smaller risk increase would require the follow-up of a comparably larger donor pool (Hasenclever & Sextro, 1996). This can be accomplished only by international registries and will require an intensive cooperative effort with individual transplant teams and centers. The data available on the long-term effects of G-CSF in patients with severe congenital neutropenia and aplastic anemia do not answer these questions, as these diseases have been shown to carry a predisposition to the development of acute leukemia regardless of G-CSF therapy (Gilman, Jackson, & Guild, 1970; de Planque *et al.,* 1989).

Partly related to the long-term effects issue is the issue of PBSC collections from unrelated, HLA-matched donors. A limited number of PBSC allografts from matched unrelated donors have been performed worldwide (Russell, Gratwohl, & Schmitz, 1996). Until recently, the National Marrow Donor Program in the United States has endorsed PBSC collections only for second transplants (i.e., for treatment of relapse following marrow transplantation). Currently many national registries are gradually becoming more amenable to the idea of administering G-CSF to unrelated HLA-matched donors, although some logistical issues and safety concerns remain. PBSC collection seems to be gaining increasing acceptance in the blood banking community as well (Lane, 1996). A more "user-friendly" and possibly safer collection procedure may

Table 24.7. *Effect of rhG-CSF mobilization treatment on chemistry values*

	Baseline	Prior to 1st apheresis	*P* value
AP [U/l]	90	181	<.0001
LDH [U/l]	415	1,089	<.0001
Potassium [mEq/l]	4.2	3.8	.0001
Magnesium [mg/dl]	1.9	1.8	.02
Uric acid [μmol/l]	309	386	<.001

allow a substantial expansion of the unrelated donor pool in national and international registries, particularly among minorities and older individuals (Körbling *et al.,* 1995b).

The current consensus (Anderlini *et al.,* 1997a) regarding safety issues related to G-CSF administration to normal donors can be summarized as follows:

1. G-CSF has an acceptable short-term safety profile.
2. G-CSF doses up to 12 μg/kg/day show a consistent dose-response relationship with the mobilization and collection of CD34$^+$ cells.
3. Transient cytopenias following cytokine treatment and apheresis are generally asymptomatic and self-limited (see below).
4. Donors should meet the eligibility criteria that apply to platelet apheresis donors with the exception of multiple donations on consecutive days and the donor's age. Criteria used at the M.D. Anderson Hospital for stem cell apheresis from normal donors are shown in Table 24.8.
5. The creation of an International PBSC Donor Registry is desirable to assess long-term effects of cytokine treatment for stem cell mobilization.

When to start apheresis

Apheresis following cytokine treatment from steady state

As indicated above, the duration of G-CSF administration predicts the level of circulating progenitor cells and the apheresis yield of CD34$^+$ progenitor cells. We studied 77 normal donors who underwent stem cell apheresis for HLA-matched related recipients beginning on day 4 ($n = 45$) or day 5 ($n = 32$) of G-CSF treatment (12 μg/kg/day). Both cohorts were comparable for age, weight, and blood volume processed by apheresis; the target CD34$^+$ cell dose was 4 $\times$ 10^6/kg recipient weight. Ninety-four percent of all donors on the day 5 G-CSF schedule reached the target CD34$^+$ cell dose with a single apheresis, whereas 67% of donors reached the target with the day 4

Table 24.8. *Stem cell apheresis parameters: normal donors*

Peripheral venous access preferred
rhG-CSF administration 2 hrs prior to start of apheresis
Total blood volume processed per run: 3 times the donor's total
  blood volume
I.V. CaCl$_2$ replacement: (ACD-A flow rate $\times$ 0.5 $\times$ procedure
  time) mg/min
Hb prior to start of rhG-CSF: 11.0 g/dl
Hb prior to start of apheresis: 11.0 g/dl
Drop Hb after apheresis: not >20%
Platelets prior to start of rhG-CSF: 150,000 μl
Platelets prior to start of apheresis: 120,000/μl
Drop platelets after apheresis: not >20%
If platelet count prior to subsequent apheresis <100,000/μl:
  soft spin and autotransfusion

schedule. There was no statistically significant difference in the apheresis yield of lymphoid subsets or natural killer cells (Anderlini *et al.,* 1996b). In normal donors and inpatients, we recommend day 4 or 5 of G-CSF treatment as the first day of apheresis.

Apheresis following chemopriming plus cytokine treatment

Cell recovery from chemopriming is variable. During cell expansion, evaluation of the circulating CD34+ cell concentration has been shown to be helpful in predicting the day of first apheresis that results in collecting a sufficient amount of progenitor cells (Haas *et al.,* 1994; D'Hondt *et al.,* 1997; Hoglund *et al.,* 1996) (Figs. 24.13 and 24.14).

Potential parameters that are predictive of the patient's CD34+ cell yield by apheresis are circulating WBC, MNC, and CD34+ cell concentrations checked either prior to mobilization initiation (steady state), prior to the day of apheresis, or on the day apheresis is to be performed. The relevance of peripheral WBC concentrations as a predictor of the stem cell apheresis yield is controversial. Whereas Pettengell *et al.* (1993) and Jones *et al.* (1994) reported cytokine-mobilized WBC to correlate with CD34+ cell yield, others failed to show such a correlation. On the other hand, peripheral blood CD34+ cell counts have been demonstrated to be predictive of CD34+ cell apheresis yield (Korbling *et al.,* 1995a; Grigg *et al.,* 1995; Schwella *et al.,* 1996). In patients with hematologic malignancies and solid tumors, steady-state peripheral blood concentrations of CD34+ cells correlated with CD34+ cell apheresis yield following chemopriming and G-CSF treatment. A peripheral blood con-

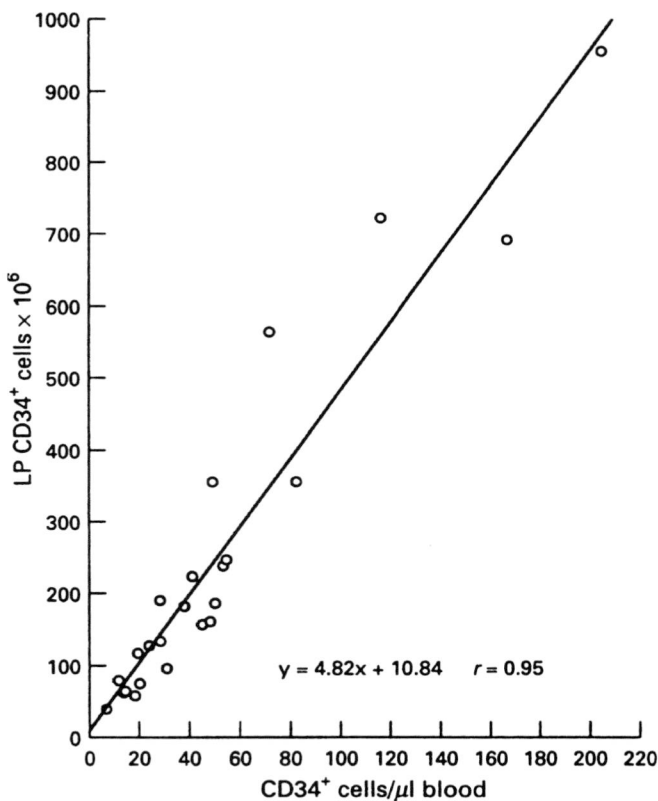

Fig. 24.14. Correlation between the number of CD34+ cells per µl blood (1 hour prior to leukapheresis) and the total number of CD34+ cells collected by a 10 liter leukapheresis; $r = 0.95$, $P = .001$, $n = 24$, y, equals the number of CD34+ cells in the leukapheresis product and x, equals the number of CD34+ cells/µl blood. Reproduced, with permission, from Höglund *et al.* (1996).

centration of 0.4×10^6 CD34+ cells/1 was predictive (with 95% probability) of a yield of 2.5×10^6 CD34+ cells/kg collected by 6 aphereses (Fruehauf *et al.,* 1995). Evaluation by flow cytometry of the CD34+ cell population in the range of 0.01% to 0.1% of total nucleated cells is at the limit of detection with a major potential margin of error. However, CD34+ cell evaluation during early WBC recovery from prior chemopriming seems to predict apheresis outcome satisfactorily. As reported by Schwella *et al.* (1996) a preleukapheresis CD34+ cell concentration of greater than 40×10^3/ml was highly predictive of a CD34+ cell harvest of more than 2.5×10^6/kg by a single apheresis procedure. In our own experience with 84 patients undergoing stem cell apheresis after mobilization with either chemotherapy and/or G-CSF treatment, a peripheral blood CD34+ cell concentration of 16×10^3/ml on the day prior to apheresis was calculated to yield a dose of 2.6×10^6 CD34+ cells/kg (M. Donato & M. Korbling, unpublished data).

The determination of peripheral blood CD34+ cell concentration prior to apheresis is considered a routine procedure to streamline stem cell apheresis efficiency by avoiding unnecessary, low-yield apheresis procedures. The cut-off blood concen-

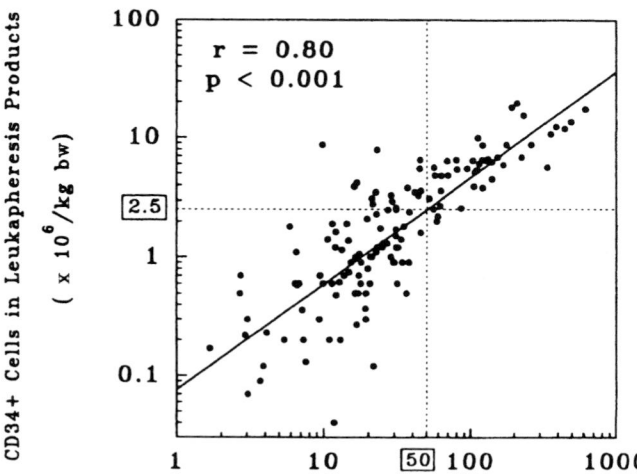

Fig. 24.13. Number of CD34+ cells/µl in the peripheral blood before leukapheresis and yield of CD34+ cells/kg in the respective product. The correlation analysis is based on a total of 142 paired samples and was performed after logarithmic transformation. As reflected by the regression curve, a CD34+ cell count of at least 50/µl is highly predictive for a yield greater than 2.5×10^6 cells/kg, sufficient for grafting with this single product. Reproduced, with permission, from Haas *et al.* (1994).

Table 24.9. *Detection of tumor cells upon VIP+ G-CSF-induced mobilization of PBPCs*

Patient with circulating tumor cells after VIP+ G-CSF

	Patient	Steady state	Between days 1–7	Between days 9–16
BM-positive (n = 8)	Breast 1	–	+	+
	Breast 2	–	–	+
	Breast 3	–	–	+
	Breast 4	+	+	+
	Breast 5	+	–	+
	SCLC 1	+	+	+
	SCLC 2	–	–	+
	SCLC 3	–	–	+
BM-negative (n = 38)	Breast 6	–	+	–
	Breast 7	–	+	–
	NSCLC 1	–	+	–
	SCLC 4	–	+	–
	SCLC 5	+	+	–

Reproduced, with permission, from Brugger *et al.* (1994).

tration of CD34+ cells for predicting a sufficient CD34+ cell yield is widely believed to be between 15 and 40 × 10^3/ml (15–40/µl or 0.015–0.04 × 10^9/1).

Mobilization of tumor cells

Brugger and colleagues (1994) demonstrated that tumor cells were also mobilized into the circulation by chemopriming treatment and G-CSF. They evaluated 358 blood samples from 46 patients with stage IV or high-risk stage II/III breast cancer, small cell or non-small-cell lung cancer, or other advanced malignancies. All stage IV breast cancer patients and 50% of the small cell lung cancer patients were found to mobilize tumor cells concomitantly with peripheral blood progenitor cells. Two patterns of tumor mobilization were found, depending on the presence or absence of bone marrow involvement with tumor: either early after chemotherapy (between days 1 and 7) in those without marrow infiltration, or between days 9 and 16 in patients with marrow infiltration (i.e., within the optimal time period for the collection of PBPCs) (Table 24.9, Fig. 24.15). In patients with stage IV breast cancer mobilized by G-CSF alone, mobilization of tumor cells was similar to that described in patients mobilized with cyclophosphamide and GM-CSF (Passos-Coelho *et al.*, 1996). In patients with myeloma mobilized with cyclophosphamide and GM-CSF there appeared to be a differential mobilization of myeloma cells and stem cells, with the highest proportion of stem cells occurring during the first 2 days of apheresis whereas peak levels of myeloma cells were present on days 5 and 6 of apheresis (Gazitt *et al.*, 1996). The issue of tumor cell contamination in re-infused stem cell autografts has been extensively reviewed by Shimoni and Korbling (2002).

Poor stem cell mobilizers

In a subset of patients (usually those who have been heavily pretreated), CD34+ cells are difficult to mobilize. There are essentially three groups of patients or donors that mobilize stem cells poorly:

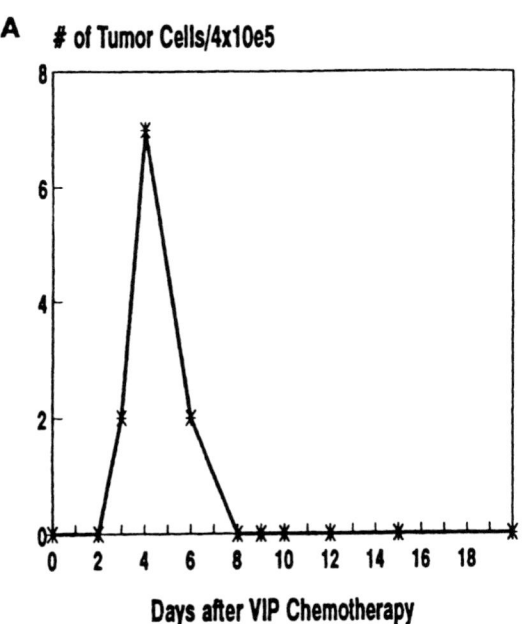

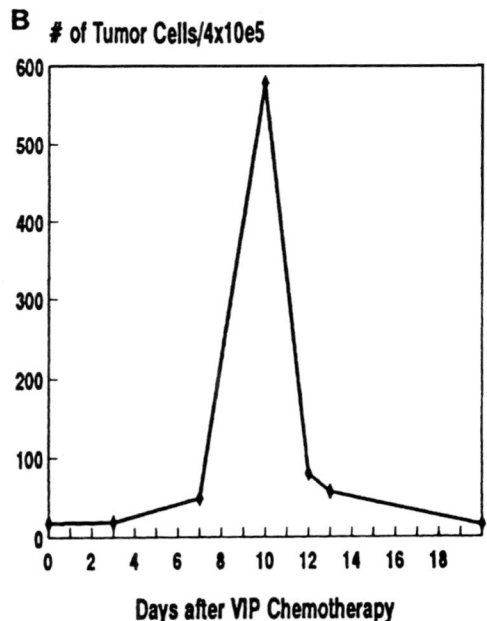

Fig. 24.15. Pattern of recruitment of malignant epithelial tumor cells in patients without (**A**) or with (**B**) BM infiltration. Data are presented as number of HEA and/or cytokeratin-positive tumor cells per 4 × 10^5 mononuclear cells from two patients. Reproduced, with permission, from Brugger *et al.* (1994).

1. Patients whose peripheral blood CD34+ cell concentration stays below 5/μl despite prolonged treatment with high-dose G-CSF (up to 32 μg/kg/day). Those patients when undergoing repeated aphereses do not reach more than 2 × 10⁶/kg CD34+ cells.

2. Patients whose WBC count is in the range of what is expected during G-CSF mobilization treatment (between 30,000/μl and 70,000/μl). However, the peripheral blood CD34+ cell count is low (between 5/μl and 10/μl). In these patients CD34+ cell recovery may be delayed for unknown reasons and keeping those patients on G-CSF for a longer period of time is a promising option.

3. Normal individuals whose peripheral blood CD34+ cell count stays low (between 5/μl and 10/μl) despite appropriate G-CSF treatment. Those individuals, although rare, are usually of young age; a genetic predisposition to a lympho-hematopoietic disorder cannot be excluded.

Several factors are associated with poor stem cell mobilization (Demirer *et al.*, 1996; Moskowitz *et al.*, 1998; Stiff, 1999):

1. The number of previous chemotherapy cycles
2. Prior use of certain chemotherapeutic agents with stem cell toxic characteristics including melphalan, nitrosoureas, nitrogen mustard, platinum compounds, and, in particular, fludarabine
3. Disease category
4. Older age (>60 years)
5. Prior radiotherapy to major bone marrow-containing regions
6. Inadequate chemopriming regimens and/or low dose G-CSF treatment

There are no established mobilization treatment strategies for poorly mobilizing patients or donors. It should be emphasized that in patients whose bone marrow stem cell pool is diminished because of extensive prior chemotherapy, additional chemopriming treatment for stem cell mobilization may result in the opposite effect, namely further reduce the bone marrow stem cell availability.

In our experience the following steps may help to improve the shifting of bone marrow stem cells into the circulating blood:

1. Increasing the dose of G-CSF up to 32 μg/kg/day divided into 2 doses of 16 μg/kg each
2. Adding GM-CSF (Winter *et al.*, 1996; Spitzer *et al.*, 1997) or SCF (Bearman, 1997) to G-CSF
3. When using G-CSF alone, try chemopriming and G-CSF as a second option
4. Waiting until the patient's WBC count has recovered, then mobilize from steady state using high-dose G-CSF
5. Checking for viral infections (which can exert a myelosuppressive effect). If suspected, remobilize the patient/donor 4 weeks later
6. Consider harvesting bone marrow or the use of G-CSF-primed bone marrow (which has equivalent engraftment kinetics to G-CSF mobilized PBPC) (Damiani *et al.*, 1997) (Figs. 24.16 and 24.17).

Even 5% to 10% of healthy blood stem cell donors have difficulty in mobilizing adequately (for unknown reasons). As reported by Bishop *et al.* (1997) in a prospective study, 6 of 53 HLA-matched related donors (11%) were identified as "poor mobilizers," requiring more than two aphereses to reach a minimum dose of 3 × 10⁶ CD34+ cells/kg. A lower lymphocyte percentage, a lower absolute lymphocyte number, a lower monocyte percentage, and low percentages of CD3+ and CD8+ cells predicted for poor mobilization prior to G-CSF administration.

PBSC mobilization in pediatric donors

In the autologous transplant setting, G-CSF at a dose ranging from 5 to 10 μg/kg/day, combined with chemopriming, is well tolerated in small children (Kanold *et al.*, 1994; Takaue *et al.*, 1995).

G-CSF 12 μg/kg/day seems to be a satisfactory dose for normal pediatric donors (Korbling *et al.*, 1996). Compared with cord blood transplantation the use of G-CSF-mobilized PBSCs from HLA-matched related pediatric donors combines the advantages of higher stem cell numbers, even for adult recipients, with rapid cell recovery. For example, one apheresis using G-CSF mobilization was sufficient to collect 4 × 10⁶ CD34+ cells from an 8-year-old boy for successful engraftment of his leukemic father despite the substantial body weight discrepancy between donor (27 kg) and recipient (93 kg) (Korbling *et al.*, 1996).

Blood stem cell collection from normal pediatric donors and pediatric patients seems feasible and safe, providing adequate CD34+ cell doses. This is particularly interesting in a haploidentical transplant setting where large numbers of CD34+ cells are harvested to ensure engraftment of the adult parent recipient (Aversa *et al.*, 1998).

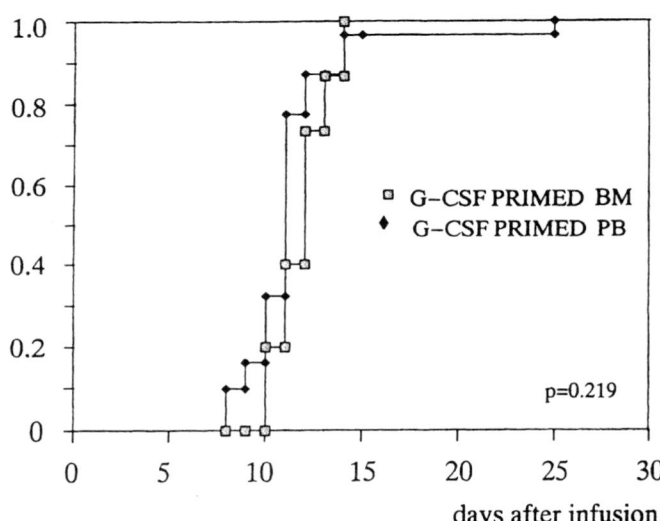

Fig. 24.16. Time to neutrophil recovery ≥ 0.5 × 10⁹/l after G-CSF-primed BM or G-CSF primed PB transplantation. Reproduced, with permission, from Damiani *et al.* (1997).

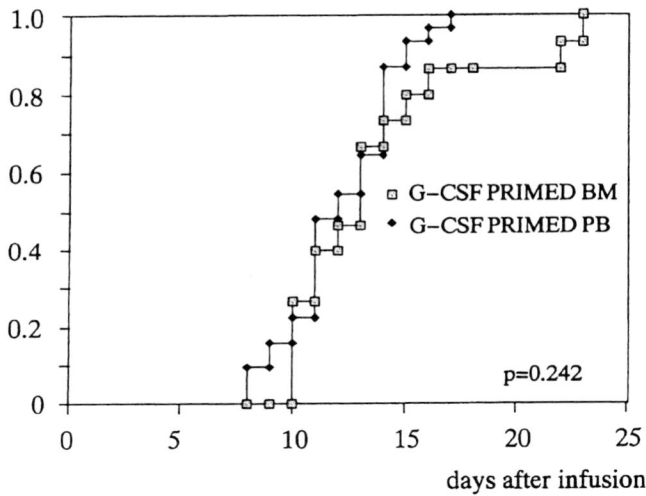

Fig. 24.17. Time to achieve platelets $\geq 20 \times 10^9$/l after G-CSF-primed BM or G-CSF-primed PB transplantation. Reproduced, with permission, from Damiani *et al.* (1997).

Conclusions

New treatment regimens for increasing the circulating stem cell concentration in patients and normal donors are rapidly evolving. The clinical research effort is currently focused on

1. Reducing side effects of cytokine/chemokine treatment
2. Evaluating treatment strategies to peripheralize stem cells in individuals who are considered "poor mobilizers"
3. Evaluating treatment strategies to block adhesion of CD34$^+$ cells to the extracellular matrix
4. Evaluating the effect of cytokine/chemokine treatment on the peripheralization and collection of lymphoid subsets, in particular dendritic cells.

Besides the procurement of hematopoietic progenitor and stem cells, the mobilization and harvest of lymphoid subsets including dendritic cells, mesenchymal stem cells, and endothelial stem cells represent fascinating subjects of ongoing research.

References

Adler, B.K., Salzman, D.E., Carabasi, M.H. *et al.* (2001). Fatal sickle cell crisis after granulocyte colony-stimulating factor administration. *Blood,* **97,** 3313–4.

Ali, S.M., Brown, R.A., Adkins, D.R. *et al.* (1997). Analysis of lymphocyte subsets and peripheral blood progenitor cells (PBPC) in apheresis products from normal donors mobilized with either G-CSF or concurrent G-CSF and GM-CSF. *Blood,* **80,** (Suppl 1) 564a (Abstract).

Anderlini, P., Chan, F.A., Korbling, M. *et al.* (2002). Long-term follow-up of normal peripheral blood progenitor cell donors: no evidence for increased risk of leukemia development. *Bone Marrow Transplantation,* **30,** 661–3.

Anderlini, P., Körbling, M., Dale, D. *et al.* (1997a). Allogeneic blood stem cell transplantation: considerations for donors. *Blood,* **90,** 903–8.

Anderlini, P., Przepiorka, D., Champlin, R., & Körbling, M. (1996a). Biologic and clinical effects of granulocyte colony-stimulating factor in normal individuals. *Blood,* **88,** 2819–25.

Anderlini, P., Przepiorka, D., Huh, Y. *et al.* (1996b). Duration of filgrastim mobilization and apheresis yield of CD34$^+$ progenitor cells and lymphoid subsets in normal donors for allogeneic transplantation. *British Journal of Haematology,* **93,** 940–2.

Anderlini, P., Przepioroka, D., Seong, D. *et al.* (1996c). Transient neutropenia in normal donors after G-CSF mobilization and stem cell apheresis. *British Journal of Haematology,* **94,** 155–8.

Anderlini, P., Przepiorka, D., Seong, D. *et al.* (1997b). Factors affecting mobilization of CD34$^+$ cells in normal donors treated with filgrastim. *Transfusion,* **37,** 507–12.

Andrews, R.G., Briddell, R.A., Knitter, G.H. *et al.* (1995). Rapid engraftment by peripheral blood progenitor cells mobilized by recombinant human stem cell factor and recombinant human granulocyte colony-stimulating factor in nonhuman primates. *Blood,* **85,** 15–20.

Aversa, E., Tabilio, A., Velardi, A. *et al.* (1998). Treatment of highrisk acute leukemia with T-cell-depleted stem cells from related donors with one fully mismatched HLA haplotype. *New England Journal of Medicine,* **339,** 1186–93.

Bearman, S.I. (1997). Use of stem cell factor to mobilize hematopoietic progenitors. *Current Opinions in Hematology,* **4,** 157-62.

Bearman, S.I. (2002). Use of stem cell factor to mobilize hematopoietic progenitors. *Current Opinion in Hematology,* **4,** 157–62.

Becker, P.S., Wagle, M., Matous, S. *et al.* (1997). Spontaneous splenic rupture following administration of granulocyte colony-stimulating factor (G-CSF): occurrence in an allogeneic donor of peripheral blood stem cells. *Biology of Blood and Marrow Transplantation,* **3,** 45–9.

Bensinger, W.I., Price, T.H., Dale, D.C. *et al.* (1993). The effects of daily recombinant human granulocyte colony-stimulating factor administration on normal granulocyte donors undergoing leukapheresis. *Blood,* **81,** 1883–8.

Bilgrami, S., Feingold, J.M., Bona, R.D. *et al.* (2000). Dose-intense paclitaxel, etoposide and cyclophosphamide: a safe and active regimen for tumor cytoreduction and stem cell mobilization in metastatic breast cancer. *Bone Marrow Transplantation,* **25,** 123–30.

Bishop, M.R., Tarantolo, S.R., Bierman, P.J. *et al.* (1997). Predictive factors for the identification of allogeneic blood stem cell donors as "poor mobilizers" prior to stem cell collection. *Blood,* **80,** (Suppl 1) 592a (Abstract).

Bodine, D.M., Seidel, N.E., & Orlic, D. (1996). Bone marrow collected 14 days after in vivo administration of granulocyte colony-stimulating factor and stem cell factor to mice has 10-fold more repopulating ability than untreated bone marrow. *Blood,* **88,** 89–97.

Bonilla, M.A., Dale, D., Zeidler, C. *et al.* (1994). Long-term safety of treatment with recombinant human granulocyte colony-stimulating factor (r-metHuG-CSF) in patients with severe congenital neutropenias. *British Journal of Haematology,* **88,** 723–30.

Brasel, K., McKenna, H.J., Charrier, K. *et al.* (1997). Flt3 ligand synergizes with granulocyte-macrophage colony-stimulating factor or granulocyte colony-stimulating factor to mobilize hematopoietic progenitor cells into the peripheral blood of mice. *Blood,* **90,** 3781–88.

Broxmeyer, H.E., Hague, N.L., Sledge, G.W. *et al.* (1995). Suppression of marrow and mobilization of blood myeloid progenitors in vivo by BB10010, a genetically engineered variant of human macrophage inflammatory protein (MIP-1α), in a phase I clinical trial in patients with relapsed/refractory breast cancer. *Blood,* **86,** (Suppl 1), 12a (Abstract).

Broxmeyer, H.E., Orazi, A., Hague, N.L. *et al.* (1998). Myeloid progenitor cell proliferation and mobilization effects of BB10010, a genetically engineered variant of human macrophage inflammatory protein-1 alpha, in a phase I clinical trial in patients with relapsed/refractory breast cancer. *Blood Cells and Molecular Disease,* **24,** 14–30.

Brugger, W., Bross, K.J., Blatt, M. *et al.* (1994). Mobilization of tumor cells and hematopoietic progenitor cells in peripheral blood of patients with solid tumors. *Blood,* **83,** 636–40.

Caspar, C.B., Seger, R.A., Burger, J., & Gmur, J. (1993). Effective stimulation of donors for granulocyte transfusions with recombinant methionyl granulocyte colony-stimulating factor. *Blood,* **81,** 2866–71.

Chabannon, C., Le Coroller, A-G., Faucher, C. *et al.* (1995). Patient condition affects the collection of peripheral blood progenitors after priming with recombinant granulocyte colony-stimulating factor. *Journal of Hematotherapy,* **4,** 171–9.

Champlin, R., Körbling, M., Donato, M. *et al.* (1997). Recombinant human thrombopoietin (rhTPO) for mobilization of peripheral blood progenitor cells (PBPC) for autologous transplantation in breast cancer: preliminary results of a phase I trial. *Proceedings of the American Society of Clinical Oncology,* **16,** 100a (Abstract).

Chao, N.J., Schriber, J.R., Grimes, K. *et al.* (1993). Granulocyte colony-stimulating factor "mobilized" peripheral blood progenitor cells accelerate granulocyte and platelet recovery after high-dose chemotherapy. *Blood,* **81,** 2031–5.

Conti, J.A., & Sher, H.L. (1992). Acute arterial thrombosis after escalated-dose methotrexate, vincristine, doxorubicin, cisplatin chemotherapy with recombinant human granulocyte colony stimulating factor. *Cancer,* **70,** 2699–702.

Damiani, D., Fanin, R., Silvestri, F. *et al.* (1997). Randomized trial of autologous filgrastim-primed bone marrow transplantation versus filgrastim-mobilized peripheral blood stem cell transplantation in lymphoma patients. *Blood,* **90,** 36–42.

Demirer, T., Buckner, C.D., Gooley, T. *et al.* (1996). Factors influencing collection of peripheral blood stem cells in patients with multiple myeloma. *Bone Marrow Transplantation,* **17,** 937–41.

de Planque, M.M., Bacigalupo, A., Würsch, A. *et al.* (1989). Long-term follow-up of severe aplastic anemia patients treated with antithymocyte globulin. *British Journal of Haematology,* **73,** 121–6.

D'Hondt, L., André, M., Guillaume, T. *et al.* (1997). Quantification of CD34+ cells mobilized into the peripheral blood predicts the yield of leukapheresis product and can replace progenitor assays. *Cytokines, Cellular and Molecular Therapy,* **3,** 21–6.

Dimopoulos, M.A., Weber, D., K'antarjian, H. *et al.* (1996). HperCVAD for VAD-resistant myeloma. *American Journal of Hematology,* 77–81.

DiPersio, J.F., Khoury, H., Haug, J. *et al.* (2000). Innovations in allogeneic stem-cell transplantation. *Seminars in Hematology,* **37,** 33–41.

DiPersio, J.F., Schuster, M.W., Abboud, C.N. *et al.* (2000). Mobilization of peripheral-blood stem cells by concurrent administration of daniplestim and granulocyte colony-stimulating factor in patients with breast cancer or lymphoma. *Journal of Clinical Oncology,* **18,** 2762–71.

Dreger, P., Haferlach, T., Eckstein, V. *et al.* (1994). G-CSF mobilized peripheral blood progenitor cells for allogeneic transplantation:

safety, kinetics and mobilization, and composition of the graft. *British Journal of Haematology,* **87,** 609–13.

Dreger, P., Kloss, M., Petersen, B. *et al.* (1995). Autologous progenitor cell transplantation: prior exposure to stem cell-toxic drugs determines yield and engraftment of peripheral blood progenitor cell but not of bone marrow grafts. *Blood,* **86,** 3970–8.

Elias, A.D., Ayash, L., Anderson, K.C. *et al.* (1992). Mobilization of peripheral blood progenitor cells by chemotherapy and granulocyte macrophage colony stimulating factor for hematologic support after high dose intensification for breast cancer. *Blood,* **79,** 3036–44.

Esmaeli, B., Ahmadi, M.A., Kim, S. *et al.* (2002). Marginal keratitis associated with administration of filgrastim and sargramostim in a healthy peripheral blood progenitor cell donor. *Cornea,* **21,** 621–2.

Fibbe, W.E., Pruijt, J.F., Velders, G.A. *et al.* (1999). Biology of IL-8-induced stem cell mobilization. *Annals of the New York Academy of Science,* **872,** 71–82.

Fliedner, T.M. & Steinbach, K.H. (1988). Repopulating potential of hematopoietic precursor cells. *Blood Cells,* **14,** 393–410.

Fruehauf, S., Haas, R., Conradt, C. *et al.* (1995). Peripheral blood progenitor cell (PBPC) counts during steady state hematopoiesis allow to estimate the yield of mobilized PBPC after filgrastim (R-metHuG-CSF)-supported cytotoxic chemotherapy. *Blood,* **85,** 2619–26.

Fujisaki, T., Otsuka, T., Harada, M. *et al.* (1995). Granulocyte colony-stimulating factor mobilizes primitive hematopoietic stem cells in normal individuals. *Bone Marrow Transplantation,* **16,** 57–62.

Gajewski, J., Rondon, G., Donato, M. *et al.* (2002). Use of thrombopoietin in combination with chemotherapy and granulocyte colony-stimulating factor for peripheral blood progenitor cell mobilization. *Biology of Blood and Marrow Transplantation,* **8,** 550–6.

Gajewski, J., Rondon, G., Mirza, N. *et al.* (1998). Preliminary results of a randomized trial comparing intensive chemotherapy with growth factor (GF) for peripheral blood progenitor cell (PBPC) mobilization to GF alone for hematopoietic rescue after high dose chemotherapy (HDC). *Proceedings of the American Society of Clinical Oncology,* **17,** 80a (Abstract).

Gazitt, Y., Tian, D., Barlogie, B. *et al.* (1996). Differential mobilization of myeloma cells and normal hematopoietic stem cells in multiple myeloma after treatment with cyclophosphamide and granylocyte-macrophage colony-stimulating factor. *Blood,* **87,** 805–11.

Geissler, K., Peschel, C., Niederwieser, D. *et al.* (1996). Potentiation of granulocyte colony-stimulating factor-induced mobilization of circulating progenitor cells by seven-day pretreatment with interleukin-3. *Blood,* **87,** 2732–9.

Gilman, P., Jackson, D., & Guild, H. (1970). Congenital agranulocytosis: prolonged survival and terminal acute leukemia. *Blood,* **36,** 576–85.

Glaspy, J.A., Shpall, E.J., Le Maistre, C.F. *et al.* (1997). Peripheral blood progenitor cell mobilization using stem cell factor in combination with filgrastim in breast cancer patients. *Blood,* **90,** 2939–51.

Grigg, A.P. (2001). Granulocyte colony-stimulating factor-induced sickle cell crisis and multiorgan dysfunction in a patient with compound heterozygous sickle cell/beta+ thalassemia. *Blood,* **97,** 3998–9.

Grigg, A.P., Roberts, A.W., Raunow, H. *et al.* (1995). Optimizing dose and scheduling of filgrastim (granulocyte colony-stimulating factor) for mobilization and collection of peripheral blood progenitor cells in normal volunteers. *Blood,* **86,** 4437–45.

Gutierrez-Delgado, F., & Bensinger, W. (2001). Safety of granulocyte colony-stimulating factor in normal donors. *Current Opinion in Hematology, 8,* 155–60.

Gyger, M. Stuart, R.K. & Perrault, C. (2000). Immunobiology of allogeneic peripheral blood mononuclear cells mobilized with granulocyte colony-stimulating factor. *Bone Marrow Transplantation, 26,* 1-16.

Hähn, M., Grilli, G., Nothdurft, W., & Fliedner, T.M. (1980). Studies on the repopulating ability of blood stem cells of dogs given a single high-dose of cyclophosphamide. *Experimental Hematology, 8,* (Suppl 7), 26.

Hasenclever, D. & Sextro, M. (1996). Safety of alloPBSCT donors: biometrical considerations on monitoring long term risks. *Bone Marrow Transplantation, 17,* (Suppl 2), S28–S30.

Haas, R., Möhle, R., Pförsich, M. *et al.* (1995). Blood derived autografts collected during granulocyte colony-stimulating factor-enhanced recovery are enriched with early Thy-1$^+$ hematopoietic progenitor cells. *Blood, 85,* 1930–43.

Haas, R., Moller, H., Fruhauf, S. *et al.* (1994). Patient characteristics associated with successful mobilising and autografting of peripheral blood progenitor cells in malignant lymphoma. *Blood, 83,* 3787–91.

Höglund, M., Smedmyr, B., Simonsson, B. *et al.* (1996). Dose-dependent mobilization of hematopoietic progenitor cells in healthy volunteers receiving glycosylated rHuG-CSF. *Bone Marrow Transplantation, 18,* 19–27.

Huhn, R.D., Yurkow, E.J., Tushinski, R. *et al.* (1996). Recombinant human interleukin-3 (rhIL-3) enhances the mobilization of peripheral blood progenitor cells by recombinant human granulocyte colony-stimulating factor (G-CSF) in normal volunteers. *Experimental Hematology, 24,* 839–47.

Hunter, M.G., Bawden, L., Brotherton, D. *et al.* (1995). BB-10010: an active variant of human macrophage inflammatory protein-1a with improved pharmaceutical properties. *Blood, 86,* 4400–8.

Johnston, E., Crawford, J., Blackwell, S. *et al.* (2000). Randomized, dose-escalation study of SD/01 compared with daily filgrastim in patients receiving chemotherapy. *Journal of Clinical Oncology, 18,* 2522–8.

Jones, H.M., Jones, S.A., Watts, M.J. *et al.* (1994). Development of a simplified single-apheresis approach for peripheral-blood progenitor-cell transplantation in previously treated patients with lymphoma. *Journal of Clinical Oncology, 12,* 1693–702.

Kanold, J., Rapatel, C., Berger, M. *et al.* (1994). Use of G-CSF alone to mobilize peripheral blood stem cells for collection from children. *British Journal of Haematology, 88,* 633–5.

Kawachi, Y., Watanabe, A., Uchida, T. *et al.* (1996). Acute arterial thrombosis due to platelet aggregation in a patient receiving granulocyte colony-stimulating factor. *British Journal of Haematology, 94,* 413–16.

Kessinger, A., Bierman, P.J., Vose, J.M. *et al.* (1991). High dose cyclophosphamide, carmustine and etoposide followed by autologous peripheral stem cell transplantation for patients with relapsed Hodgkin's disease. *Blood, 77,* 2322–5.

Kessinger, A., Bierman, P., Bishop, M. *et al.* (1993) Effects of GM-CSF used for mobilization and after peripheral stem cell transplant for patients with previously treated low grade non-Hodgkin's lymphoma. *Blood, 82* (Suppl 1) 633a (Abstract).

Khouri, I.F., Romaguera, J., Kantarjian, H. *et al.* (1998). HyperCVAD and high dose methotrexate/cytarabine followed by stem cell transplantation: an active regimen for aggressive mantle cell lymphoma. *Journal of Clinical Oncology, 16,* 3803–9.

King, A.G., Horowitz, D., Dillon, S.B. *et al.* (2001). Rapid mobilization of murine hematopoietic stem cells with enhanced engraftment properties and evaluation of hematopoietic progenitor cell mobilization in rhesus monkeys by a single injection of SB-251353, a specific truncated form of the human CXC chemokine GROβ. *Blood, 97,* 1534-42.

Kikuta, T., Shimazaki, C., Ashihara, E. *et al.* (2000). Mobilization of hematopoietic primitive and committed progenitor cells into blood in mice by anti-vascular adhesion molecule-1 antibody alone or in combination with granulocyte colony-stimulating factor. *Experimental Hematology, 28,* 311-7.

Klein, J.L., Rey, P.M., Dansey, R. *et al.* (1999). Cyclophosphamide and paclitaxel as initial or salvage regimen for the mobilization of peripheral blood progenitor cells. *Bone Marrow Transplantation, 24,* 959–63.

Korbling, M. (2002). Personal observation.

Körbling, M., Chan, K.W., Anderlini, P. *et al.* (1996). Allogeneic peripheral blood stem cell transplantation using normal patient-related pediatric donors. *Bone Marrow Transplantation, 18,* 885–90.

Körbling, M., Dorken, B., Ho, A.D. *et al.* (1986). Autologous transplantation of blood derived hemopoietic stem cells after myeloablative therapy in a patient with Burkitt's lymphoma. *Blood, 67,* 629–32.

Körbling, M., Huh, Y.O., Durett, A. *et al.* (1995a). Allogeneic blood stem cell transplantation: peripheralization and yield of donor-derived primitive hematopoietic progenitor cells (CD34$^+$ Thy-1^{dim}) and lymphoid subsets, and possible predictors of engraftment and GVHD. *Blood, 86,* 2842–8.

Körbling, M., Przepiorka, D., Gajewski, J. *et al.* (1995b). With first successful allogeneic transplantations of apheresis-derived hematopoietic progenitor cells reported; can the recruitment of volunteer matched, unrelated stem cell donors be expanded substantially? *Blood, 86,* 1235 (Letter).

Kotasek, D.D., Shepard, K.M., Sage, R.E. *et al.* (1992). Factors affecting blood stem cell collections following high dose cyclophosphamide mobilization in lymphoma, myeloma and solid tumors. *Bone Marrow Transplantation, 9,* 11–17.

Kroger, N., Kruger, W., Renges, H. *et al.* (2000). Comparison of progenitor cell collection in day 4 or day 5 after steady-state stimulation with G-CSF alone in breast cancer patients: influence on CD34+ cell yield, subpopulation, and breast cancer cell contamination. *Journal of Hematotherapy and Stem Cell Research, 9,* 111–17.

Kroger, N., Zeller, W., Fehse, N. *et al.* (1998). Mobilizing peripheral blood stem cells with high-dose G-CSF alone is as effective as with Dexa-BEAM plus G-CSF in lymphoma patients. *British Journal of Haematology, 102,* 1101–6.

Kroger, N., Zeller, W., Hassan, H.T. *et al.* (1999). Stem cell mobilization with G-CSF alone in breast cancer patients: higher progenitor cell yield by delivering divided doses (2 × 5 microg/kg) compared to a single dose (1 × 10 microg/kg). *Bone Marrow Transplantation, 23,* 125–9.

Lane, T. (1996). Allogeneic marrow reconstitution using peripheral blood stem cells: the dawn of a new era. *Transfusion, 36,* 585–9.

Lane, T.A., Law, P., Maruyama, M. *et al.* (1995). Harvesting and enrichment of hematopoietic progenitor cells mobilized into the peripheral blood of normal donors by granulocyte-macrophage colony-stimulating factor or G-CSF: potential role in allogeneic marrow transplantation. *Blood*, **85**, 275–82.

Laterveer, L., Lindley, I.J.D., Hamilton, M.S. *et al.* (1995). Interleukin-8 induces rapid mobilization of hematopoietic stem cells with radioprotective capacity and long-term myelolymphoid repopulating ability. *Blood*, **85**, 2269–75.

Lebsack, M.E., McKenna, H.J., Hoek, J.A. *et al.* (1997). Safety of FLT3 ligand in healthy volunteers. *Blood*, **90** (Suppl 1), 170a (Abstract).

Levesque, J.P., Leavesley, D.I., Niutta, S. *et al.* (1995). Cytokines increase human hemopoietic cell adhesiveness by activation of very late antigen (VLA)-4 and VLA-5 integrins. *Journal of Experimental Medicine*, **181**, 1805–15.

Levesque, J-P., Takamatsu, Y., Nilsson, S.K., Haylock, D.N. & Simmons, P.J. (2001). Vascular cell adhesion molecule-1 (CD106) is cleaved by neutrophil proteases in the bone marrow following hematopoietic progenitor cell mobilization by granulocyte colony-stimulating factor. *Blood*, **98**, 1289-97.

Link, D.C. (2000). Mechanisms of granulocyte colony-stimulating factor-induced hematopoietic progenitor-cell mobilization. *Seminars in Hematology*, **37**, 25–32.

Link, H., Arseniev, L., Bähre, O. *et al.* (1995). Combined transplantation of allogeneic bone marrow and CD34+ blood cells. *Blood*, **86**, 2500–8.

Lord, B.I., Woolford, L.B., Wood, L.M. *et al.* (1995). Mobilization of early hematopoietic progenitor cells with BB-10010: a genetically engineered variant of human macrophage inflammatory protein -1a. *Blood*, **85**, 3412–15.

Lynch, D.H., Andreasen, A., Maraskovsky E.,. *et al.* (1997). Flt3 ligand induces tumor regression and antitumor immune responses in vivo. *Nature Medicine*, **3**, 625–31.

Maraskovsky, E., Roux, E., Teepe, M. *et al.* (1997). Flt3 ligand increases peripheral blood dendritic cells in healthy volunteers. *Blood*, **90**, (Suppl 1), 581a.

McQuaker, I.G., Haynes, A.P., Stainer, C. *et al.* (1997). Stem cell mobilization in resistant or relapsed lymphoma: superior yield of progenitor cells following salvage regimen comprising ifosfamide, etoposide and epirubicin compared to intermediate-dose cyclophosphamide. *British Journal of Haematology*, **98**, 228–33.

Molineux, G., Hartley, C., McElroy, P. *et al.* (1996). Megakaryocyte growth and development factor accelerates platelet recovery in peripheral blood progenitor cell transplant recipients. *Blood*, **88**, 366–76.

Molineux, G., Kinstler, O., Briddell, B. *et al.* (1999). A new form of filgrastim with sustained duration in vivo and enhanced ability to mobilize PBPC in both mice and humans. *Experimental Hematology*, **27**, 1724–34.

Molineux, G., McCrea, C., Yan, X.Q. *et al.* (1997). Flt-3 ligand synergizes with granulocyte colony-stimulating factor to increase neutrophil numbers and to mobilize peripheral blood stem cells with long-term repopulating potential. *Blood*, **89**, 3998–4004.

Moskowitz, C.H., Bertino, J.R., Glassman, J.R. *et al.* (1999). Ifosfamide, carboplatin, and etoposide: a highly effective cytoreduction and peripheral-blood progenitor-cell mobilization regimen for transplant-eligible patients with non-Hodgkin's lymphoma. *Journal of Clinical Oncology*, **17**, 3776–85.

Moskowitz, C.H., Glassman, J.R., Wuest, D. *et al.* (1998). Factors affecting mobilization of peripheral blood progenitor cells in patients with lymphoma. *Clinical Cancer Research*, **4**, 311–16.

Moskowitz, C.H., Stiff, P., Gordon, M.S. *et al.* (1997). Recombinant methionyl human stem cell factor and filgrastim for peripheral blood progenitor cell mobilization and transplantation in non-Hodgkin's lymphoma patients—results of a phase I/II trial. *Blood*, **89**, 3136–47.

Papayannopoulou, T. & Nakamoto, B. (1993). Peripheralization of hemopoietic progenitors in primates treated with anti-VLA4 integrin. *Proceedings of the National Academy of Science USA*, **90**, 9374–8.

Papayannopoulou, T., Nakamoto, B., Andrews, R.G. *et al.* (1997). In vivo effects of flt 3, flk, 2 ligand on mobilization of hematopoietic progenitors in primates and potent synergistic enhancement with granulocyte colony-stimulating factor. *Blood*, **90**, 620–9.

Parkkali, T., Volin, L., Siren, M.K. *et al.* (1996). Acute iritis induced by granulocyte colony-stimulating factor in a volunteer unrelated peripheral blood progenitor cell donor. *Bone Marrow Transplantation*, **17**, 433–4.

Passos-Coelho, J.L., Ross, A.A., Kahn, D.J. *et al.* (1996). Similar breast cancer contamination of single day peripheral blood progenitor cell collections obtained after priming with hematopoietic growth factor alone or after cyclophosphamide followed by growth factor. *Journal of Clinical Oncology*, **14**, 2569–75.

Peters, W.P., Rosner, G., Ross, M. *et al.* (1993). Comparative effects of granulocyte-macrophage colony-stimulating factor (GM-CSF) and granulocyte colony-stimulating factor (G-CSF) on priming peripheral blood progenitor cells for use with autologous bone marrow after high-dose chemotherapy. *Blood*, **81**, 1709–19.

Pettengell, R., Morgenstern, G.R., Woll, P.J. *et al.* (1993). Peripheral blood progenitor cell transplantation in lymphoma and leukemia using a single leukapheresis. *Blood*, **82**, 3770–7.

Prosper, F., Stroncek, D., & Verfaillie, C.M. (1995). Mobilization of LTC-IC in normal donors treated with G-CSF: phenotypic analysis of mobilized PBSC. *Blood*, **86**, (Suppl 1), 464a (Abstract).

Pruijt, J.F., Verzaal, P., van Os, R. *et al.* (2002). Neutrophils are indispensable for hematopoietic stem cell mobilization induced by interleukin-8 in mice. *Proceedings of the National Academy of Science USA*, **99**, 6228–33.

Richman, C.M., Weiner, R.S., & Yankee, R.A. (1976). Increase in circulating stem cells following chemotherapy in man. *Blood*, **47**, 1031–4.

Russell, N., Gratwohl, A., & Schmitz, N. (1996). The place of blood stem cells in allogeneic transplantation. *British Journal of Haematology*, **93**, 747–53.

Rusten, L.S., Lyman, S.D., Veiby, O.P., & Jacobsen, S.E.W. (1996). The FLT3 ligand is a direct and potent stimulator of the growth of primitive and committed CD34+ bone marrow progenitor cells in vitro. *Blood*, **87**, 1317–25.

Sakamaki, S., Matsunaga, T., Hirayama, Y. *et al.* (1995). Hematological study of healthy volunteers 5 years after G-CSF. *Lancet*, **346**, 1432–3 (Letter).

Schaafsma, M.R., Fibbe, W.E., van der Harst, D. *et al.* (1990). Increased numbers of circulating hematopoietic progenitor cells after treatment with high-dose interleukin-2 in cancer patients. *British Journal of Haematology*, **76**, 180–5.

Schwatzberg, L.S., Birch, R., Hazleton, B. *et al.* (1992). Peripheral blood stem cell mobilization by chemotherapy with and without recombinant human granulocyte colony-stimulating factor. *Journal of Hematotherapy*, **1**, 317–27.

Schwella, N., Beyer, J., Schwaner, I. *et al.* (1996). Impact of preleukapheresis cell counts on collection results and correlation of progenitor-cell dose with engraftment after high-dose chemotherapy in patients with germ cell cancer. *Journal of Clinical Oncology,* **14,** 1114–21.

Sheridan, W.P., Begley, C.G., Juttner, C.A. *et al.* (1992). Effect of peripheral blood progenitor cells mobilized by filgrastim (G-CSF) on platelet recovery after high dose chemotherapy. *Lancet,* **339,** 640–4.

Shimoni, A., & Korbling, M. (2002). Tumor cell contamination in re-infused stem cell autografts: does it have clinical significance? *Critical Reviews in Oncology/Hematology,* **41,** 241–50.

Shpall, E., Champlin, R., & Glaspy, J.A. (1998). Effect of CD34+ peripheral blood progenitor cell dose on hematopoietic recovery. *Biology of Blood and Marrow Transplantation,* **4,** 84–92.

Shpall, E.J., Wheeler, C.A., Turner, S.A. *et al.* (1997). A randomized phase 3 study of PBPC mobilization by stem cell factor (SCF, STEMGEN®) and Filgrastim in patients with high-risk breast cancer. *Blood,* **90,** (Suppl 1), 591a (Abstract).

Shpall, E.J., Wheeler, C.A., Turner, S.A. *et al.* (1999). A randomized phase 3 study of peripheral blood progenitor cell mobilization with stem cell factor and filgrastim in high-risk breast cancer patients. *Blood,* **93,** 2491–501.

Somlo, G., Sniecinski, I., ter Veer, A. *et al.* (1999). Recombinant human thrombopoietin in combination with granulocyte colony-stimulating factor enhances mobilization of peripheral blood progenitor cells, increases peripheral blood platelet concentration, and accelerates hematopoietic recovery following high-dose chemotherapy. *Blood,* **93,** 2798–806.

Spitzer, G., Adkins, D., Mathews, M. *et al.* (1997). Randomized comparison of G-CSF+ GM-CSF vs G-CSF alone for mobilization of peripheral blood stem cells: effects on hematopoietic recovery after high-dose chemotherapy. *Bone Marrow Transplantation,* **20,** 921–30.

Stiff, P., Gingrich, R., Luger, S. *et al.* (1997a). Improved PBPC collection using STEMGEN® (stem cell factor, SCF) and Filgrastim (G-CSF) compared to G-CSF alone in heavily pretreated lymphoma (NHL) and Hodgkin's Disease (HD) patients (pts). *Blood,* **90,** (Suppl 1), 591a (Abstract).

Stiff, P., Malhotra, D., Bayer, R. *et al.* (1997b). High dose G-CSF improves stem cell mobilization and collection compared to standard doses in patients with ovarian cancer which leads to a decrease in delayed platelet engraftment following stem cell transplants. *Blood,* **80,** (Suppl 1), 591a (Abstract).

Stiff, P.J. (1999). Management strategies for the hard-to-mobilize patient. *Bone Marrow Transplantation,* **23,** (Suppl 2), S29–S33.

Stroncek, D., Clay, M., Jaszcz, W. *et al.* (1994). Longer than 5 days of G-CSF mobilization of normal individuals results in lower CD34+ cell counts. *Blood,* **84,** (Suppl 1), 541a (Abstract).

Stroncek, D., Clay, M., Lennon, S. *et al.* (1996). Collection of two blood progenitor cell components from healthy donors. *Blood,* **88,** (Suppl 1), 396a (Abstract).

Sudo, Y., Shimazaki, C., Ashihara, E. *et al.* (1997). Synergistic effect of FLT-3 ligand on the granulocyte colony-stimulating factor-induced mobilization of hematopoietic stem cells and progenitor cells into blood in mice. *Blood,* **89,** 3186–91.

Suehiro, Y., Muta, K., Umemura, T. *et al.* (1999). Macrophage inflammatory protein 1 alpha enhances in a different manner adhesion of hematopoietic progenitor cells from bone marrow, cord blood, and mobilized peripheral blood. *Experimental Hematology,* **27,** 1637–45.

Sureda, A., Petit, J., Brunet *et al.* (1999). Mini-ICE regimen as mobilization therapy for chronic myelogenous leukemia patients at diagnosis. *Bone Marrow Transplantation,* **24,** 1285–90.

Takaue, Y., Kawano, Y., Abe, T. *et al.* (1995). Collection and transplantation of peripheral blood stem cells in very small children weighing 20 kg or less. *Blood,* **86,** 372–80.

Tanaka, R., Matsudaira, T., Tanaka, I. *et al.* (1994). Kinetics and characteristics of peripheral blood progenitor cells mobilized by G-CSF in normal healthy volunteers. *Blood,* **84,** (Suppl 1), 541a (Abstract).

Tarella, C., Caracciolo, D., Gavarotti, P. *et al.* (1995). Circulating progenitors following high-dose sequential (HDS) chemotherapy with G-CSF: short intervals between drug courses severely impair progenitor mobilization. *Bone Marrow Transplantation,* **16,** 223–8.

Tjønnfjord, G.E., Steen, R., Evensen, S.A. *et al.* (1994). Characterization of CD34+ peripheral blood cells from healthy adults mobilized by recombinant human granulocyte-stimulating factor. *Blood,* **84,** 2795–801.

To, L.B., Haylock, D., Dyson, P. *et al.* (1996). Chemotherapy-based approach to mobilization of progenitor cells. In *Cell Therapy,* ed. G. Morstyn & W. Sheridan, pp. 130–145. Cambridge: Cambridge University Press.

To, L.B., Haylock, D.N., Simmons, P.J., & Juttner, C.A. (1997). The biology and clinical use of blood stem cells. *Blood,* **89,** 2233–58.

To, L.B., Sheppard, K.M., Haylock, D.N. *et al.* (1989). Single high doses of cyclophosphamide enable the collection of high numbers of hemopoietic stem cells from the peripheral blood. *Experimental Hematology,* **18,** 442–7.

Tricot, G., Jagannath, S., Vesole, D. *et al.* (1995). Peripheral blood stem cell transplants for multiple myeloma: identification of favorable variables for rapid engraftment in 225 patients. *Blood,* **85,** 588–96.

Uchida, N., He, D., Frefriera, A.M. *et al.* (1997). The unexpected G_0/G_1 cell cycle status of mobilized hematopoietic stem cells from peripheral blood. *Blood,* **89,** 465–72.

Vetillard, J., Drouet, M., Neildez-Nguyen, T.M. *et al.* (1999). Interleukin-8 acts as a strong peripheral blood granulocyte-recruiting agent rather than as a hematopoietic progenitor cell mobilizing factor. *Journal of Hematotherapy and Stem Cell Research,* **8,** 365–79.

Waller, C.F., Bertz, H., Wenger, M.K. *et al.* (1996). Mobilization of peripheral blood progenitor cells for allogeneic transplantation: efficacy and toxicity of a high-dose G-CSF regimen. *Bone Marrow Transplantation,* **18,** 279–83.

Weaver, C.H., Longin, K., Buckner, C.D., & Bensinger, W. (1994). Lymphocyte content in peripheral blood mononuclear cells collected after administration of recombinant human granulocyte colony-stimulating factor. *Bone Marrow Transplantation,* **13,** 411–5.

Weaver, A., & Testa, N.G. (1998). Stem cell factor leads to reduced blood processing during apheresis or the use of whole blood aliquots to support dose-intensive chemotherapy. *Bone Marrow Transplantation,* **22,** 33–8.

Winter, J.N., Lazarus, H.M., Rademaker, A. *et al.* (1996). Phase I/II study of combined granulocyte colony-stimulating factor and granulocyte-macrophage colony-stimulating factor administration for the mobilization of hematopoietic progenitor cells. *Journal of Clinical Oncology,* **14,** 277–86.

Wright, D.E., Wagers, A.J., Gulati, A.P. *et al.* (2001). Physiological migration of hematopoietic stem and progenitor cells. *Science,* **294,** 1933–6.

25 Management of related and unrelated donors

CHITRA HOSING AND PAOLO ANDERLINI

The University of Texas M.D. Anderson Cancer Center, Houston, USA

Introduction

Allogeneic hematopoietic stem cell (HSC) transplantation is a curative option for many patients with relapsed acute leukemia or chronic leukemia and for selected patients with lymphoproliferative disorders. It is also increasingly used to treat various metabolic and immunologic disorders and is being investigated for the treatment of solid malignancies. The stem cells used in allogeneic transplantation are usually derived from healthy donors—either related or unrelated to the recipient. Bone marrow (BM) harvested from the posterior iliac crests has been the traditional source of stem cells. Although marrow harvesting is still widely employed, with the availability of hematopoietic growth factors, peripheral blood stem cells (PBSC) are being increasingly used as the source of hematopoietic stem cells in many related donor transplants (Goldman, 1995; Lane, 1996; Russell, Gratwohl, & Schmitz 1996). To this date, BM remains the source of stem cells for most unrelated donors, although this trend appears to be changing. The reason for this difference has been the concern regarding administration of growth factors to unrelated donors and the technical expertise required for PBSC collections.

Other sources of unrelated HSC such as umbilical cord blood and fetal hematopoietic tissues, although promising, remain largely investigational. Healthy donors continue to provide the vast majority of stem cell products for allogeneic transplants. Each of these sources has distinct characteristics, including time to hematologic recovery, and acute and chronic graft-versus-host disease rates.

This chapter will address the evaluation and management of related and unrelated stem cell donors, with particular attention to the differences in the two groups.

Evaluation of donors

In general, the eligibility criteria for both BM and PBSC donors are largely the same, with the exceptions detailed below. These criteria are also slightly different for related and unrelated donors. According to the guidelines established by the National Marrow Donor Program (NMDP), donors for both BM and PBSC must be healthy and be between the ages of 18 and 55 years. However, for related family donors the criteria are less stringent. For example, donors who are older than 55 or younger than 18 may donate for family members. Also, related donors with certain stable and well-controlled medical illnesses (e.g., hypertension, diabetes mellitus, coronary artery disease) may be considered as donors. Moreover, related donors with certain potentially transmissible illnesses (e.g., chronic hepatitis B or C) may still donate if the recipient is appropriately counseled and no alternative suitable donor is available. In all of these instances, these donors would be otherwise ineligible under NMDP guidelines.

Donor history and physical examination

All potential donors should undergo a full medical evaluation, including psychosocial evaluation before the planned donation procedure to determine their suitability. Whenever possible, this evaluation should be conducted by a physician not involved with the transplant procedure. The interview should include the following:

- Detailed review of past medical history
- Concurrent medical illnesses
- Current medications
- Family history
- Drug allergies

For BM donors special attention should be paid to the following

- Past surgical history and type of anesthesia received
- History of musculoskeletal disorders
- Assessment of oral airways
- Accessibility to the posterior iliac crests

Whenever possible an anesthesiologist should also participate in the evaluation.

For PBSC donors the evaluation should cover the following:

- History of autoimmune diseases
- History of venous thrombosis

- Adequacy of venous access
- Presence or absence of splenomegaly (i.e., a palpable spleen)

Certain potential BM donors determined to be ineligible because of musculoskeletal problems may be considered instead for PBSC donation. Similarly, PBSC donors with history of autoimmune or inflammatory disorders, for whom administration of filgrastim, a recombinant human granulocyte-colony-stimulating factor (rhG-CSF) could pose significant risks for a flare-up of the underlying disease, may be considered for BM harvesting if their disease is well-controlled.

Both related and unrelated donors with a prior history of malignancy are generally excluded from donations because of concern about transmission of the malignancy. Indeed, there have been reports of the transmission of T-cell lymphoma and acute myeloid leukemia by allogeneic bone marrow transplantation (Niederwieser et al., 1990; Berg et al., 2001). In selected cases, however exceptions can be made. These include donors with a past history of localized breast, colon, or prostate cancer who received seemingly curative treatment and have been cancer-free for many years, and selected patients with a past history of successfully treated Hodgkin's disease. In all such cases, the lack of availability of a more suitable donor can play a major role in the decision-making process.

Psychological considerations

Related donors are often under considerable cultural and societal pressures to donate. Unrelated donors, on the other hand, generally donate out of altruism. NMDP policies forbid direct contact between donors and recipients to prevent the recipients or their family members from pressuring the donor. In most cases, this confidentiality is maintained permanently. In certain cases, however, the recipient and donor have been allowed to meet 6 months or later after a successful transplantation if doing so is mutually agreeable. Determining whether the donor is truly committed to donating is also important, and this must be known before the recipient starts his or her preparative regimen. In many cases, this regimen is myeloablative and if the donor backs out at the last minute, the recipient is not likely to survive the procedure.

Very little attention has been paid to the psychological and emotional effects of donating. Most nontransplantation–related surgery patients choose to undergo surgery because the benefits outweigh the risks; this rationale, however, does not apply to stem cells donors since the procedure offers them no benefit. Yet in one study by Nishimori et al. (2002), the authors report that despite considerable pain after BM harvesting, the donors' mental health, general health perception, and vitality remained high. Similarly, in an earlier study of 20 unrelated marrow donors, no serious emotional or physical effects were observed. Moreover, 95% (19 of 20) of the donors interviewed said they would be willing to donate again (Stroncek et al., 1989).

Ethical considerations

All donors are required to sign informed consent forms before donating. In most countries a person can provide this consent legally at the age of 18; thus children younger than 18 generally cannot be enrolled as unrelated donors. However, with parental consent they may be considered for related donations. Since parental involvement has the potential for conflict of interest, a legal guardian (or other third party) is sometimes required to determine whether it is in the child's best interest to donate.

Donors may participate in transplantation research protocols approved by local institutional review boards provided that they are counseled about risks and that they provide written informed consent.

Laboratory evaluation

All donors must have the following laboratory studies performed before donating: a complete blood count; a serum chemistry profile of electrolytes, liver function, serum creatinine, blood urea nitrogen, albumin, and a total protein; and urine analysis. They should also be checked for infectious diseases by testing for the presence of the following: anti-human immunodeficiency virus (HIV) type 1, anti-HIV 2, HIV p24 antigen, hepatitis B virus (HBV) surface antigen, anti-HBV core antigen, anti-hepatitis C virus (HCV) antibody, anti-human T-cell lymphotropic virus (HTLV) I and II. Screening for prior exposure to varicella-zoster virus (VZV), herpes simplex virus (HSV), syphilis, Epstein-Barr virus (EBV), and cytomegalovirus (CMV) is also desirable (Goldman, 1994). Screening for hemoglobin S may also be considered (see below). Chest radiography and electrocardiography should also be done.

Potential donors who are positive for HIV or HTLV-I should not be used. Those who are positive for HCV antibodies should have their viral load checked by polymerase chain reaction (PCR) for HCV RNA. Failure to detect HCV RNA by PCR, however, does not ensure lack of transmission to the recipient. On the other hand, potential donors with prior HBV infection who have seroconverted fully may be used as donors. Whenever possible, CMV-seronegative recipients should be matched with CMV-negative donors.

A pregnancy test must be given to all females of child-bearing age. Pregnant females are not acceptable as donors, although there was one case report (Jones et al., 1995) in which marrow was successfully collected from a pregnant donor at 26 weeks gestation.

Bone marrow aspiration and a biopsy procedure with cytogenetic studies is usually unnecessary and not cost-effective for the evaluation of most healthy donors. It should be performed, however, for donors with a family history of hematologic malignancy or if a significant abnormality is detected in the peripheral blood.

Technique of marrow harvesting

Marrow is usually harvested from the posterior iliac crests while the donor is under general anesthesia. Regional anesthesia can also be used if the donor and medical team performing the harvest procedure agree. In the past, donors required overnight hospitalization, but current practice in most centers is to discharge them the same day. Most donors give two units of autologous packed red cells prior to the harvesting procedure; these are then infused during or after the bone marrow harvesting is complete. Rarely, if the donor is anemic, allogeneic red cells are used, provided the donor understands the risks and consents.

Two physicians generally perform the harvest, one for each iliac crest, which is usually entered via a skin puncture or a small incision. The posterior superior iliac spine is used as the landmark for the harvest. In rare cases the anterior iliac crest or the sternum may also be used (Buckner *et al.*, 1984). Large bore needles with syringes rinsed in heparinized solution are used to aspirate the marrow with a sharp suctioning technique. No more than 5 to 10 ml of marrow is withdrawn with each pull, since pulling more may dilute the marrow with peripheral blood (Batinic *et al.*, 1990; Bacigalupo *et al.*, 1992). The total volume collected depends on the recipient's weight. Usually the aim is to collect a total of 10 to 15 ml of bone marrow, or 2 to 4×10^8 total nucleated cells per kilogram, of the recipient's weight. Obtaining this much marrow may require up to 200 to 300 aspirations, several of which can be performed at the same puncture site (Thomas & Storb, 1970). The contents are collected in a bag or other container, which holds an anticoagulant solution. Donors are given a prescription for oral opioid pain medications when they are discharged, and have a follow-up appointment the next day.

Side effects associated with bone marrow harvesting

BM harvesting from normal donors has been performed since the 1970s and is considered to have a remarkably good safety profile. The reported frequency of major and life-threatening complications following marrow donation is less than 1%.

Commonly reported side effects

Most donors report minor pain or discomfort after donation. Other commonly reported side effects include fatigue, light-headedness, nausea, vomiting, fever, and prolonged bleeding. In a review of 1,270 harvests from 1,160 normal, related donors, almost all donors reported some pain (Buckner *et al.*, 1984).

In the case of unrelated donors in the United States, donation-related side effects and donor recovery are monitored by the NMDP donor center coordinators through regular phone contact with donors. The data obtained are reported to the NMDP National Coordinating Center and analyzed annually. The data now available from almost 5,505 donors indicate that the major side effects are fatigue and pain at the harvest site. Other commonly reported side effects are summarized in Table 25.1 (Confer

Table 25.1. *Side effects reported during the first 72 hours following marrow donation (n = 5,505)*

Side effect	Percentage reporting
Fatigue	79
Pain at collection site	74
Pain on walking	68
Back pain	63
Sore throat	57
Pain on sitting	55
Nausea	52
Pain on climbing stairs	48
Light-headedness	46
Headache	34
Pain at intravenous site	31
Vomiting	29
Fever	27
Bandage pain	23
Prolonged bleeding	8
Fainting	5

Reproduced, with permission, from Confer and Stroncek (1999).

& Stroncek, 1999). Nishimori *et al.* (2002) also found that pain at the harvest site and in the lower back were the most commonly reported problems. They also reported that most patients had to limit their daily activity after the harvest procedure.

Other minor complications reported include hypotension, syncope, postspinal headache (if epidural anesthesia used), minor infections, and problems requiring hospitalization. These have been reported in 6% to 12% of marrow donors and usually resolve within a few days of onset (Buckner *et al.*, 1984; Stroncek *et al.*, 1993).

Life-threatening side effects

Major and sometimes life-threatening complications have occasionally been reported after marrow donation. The estimated frequency of such complications is 0.1% to 0.3%. Bortin and Buckner (1983) reviewed data for 3,290 allogeneic marrow donations performed between 1969 and 1983 and reported to the International Bone Marrow Transplant Registry (IBMTR) as well as some conducted at Seattle. They found nine cases of major complications (0.27%). These included aspiration pneumonia (1 case); deep venous thrombosis (2 cases), one of which was a pulmonary embolism; bacterial infections (3 cases); cardiac arrhythmia (2 cases); and cerebral infarction (1 case). Five of these were attributable to the general anesthetic. There were no deaths related to the donation procedure.

In their review of the first 493 marrow donors reported to the NMDP, Stroncek *et al.* (1993) identified only one (incidence of 0.2%) potentially life-threatening complication: that of apnea and bradycardia. Of 7,857 evaluable bone marrow harvests reported to the IBMTR and to the European Group for Blood and Marrow Transplant (EBMT) between 1994 and 1998, the overall complication rate was 0.5%; and there were 2 fatalities (Anderlini *et al.*, 2001b).

Complications resulting from the administration of anesthetic such as hypotension, bradycardia, laryngospasm, hypoxia, and cardiac arrest, as well as a case of malignant hyperthermia induced by the general anesthesia have been reported. The donor with malignant hyperthermia made a full recovery, but required hospitalization for 3 weeks (Hosoya *et al.*, 1997). Another complication that has been reported is fracture of the ilium (Klumpp, Mangan, MacDonald, & Mesgarzadeh, 1992). Osteomyelitis has also been reported (Riley & Evans, 1992).

Rowley *et al.* (2001) reviewed the records of donors who had participated in a randomized trial of either allogeneic bone marrow or peripheral blood stem cell transplantation. A total of 38 donors had undergone bone marrow harvesting. Most (95%) were given a general anesthetic. The median range of anesthesia duration was 87.5 minutes (range, 48 to 159). The harvest procedures lasted a median of 62.5 minutes (range, 27 to 120). As expected, the most commonly recorded side effect was pain (84%), followed by hypotension (34%), nausea (26%), and hemorrhage (13%). Two donors required overnight hospitalization, and one was hospitalized for 2 days because of postoperative hypotension, nausea, and pain. A fourth donor was hospitalized for 6 days after the harvest because of deep venous thrombosis.

Transfusion-related side effects

In an earlier study of 923 related marrow donors involving 1,008 procedures (Buckner *et al.*, 1984), 12% of the males older than 10, 23% of females older than 10, and 35% of male and female children under 10 required allogeneic blood transfusions. Only in more recent years have the risks related to allogeneic blood transfusions (particularly the transmission of infectious agents) been recognized, and thus autologous blood transfusions have largely replaced allogeneic transfusions for both related and unrelated donors. According to current NMDP standards, all unrelated donors must receive autologous transfusions except in emergencies. In the previously mentioned review of 493 unrelated donors (Stroncek *et al.*, 1993), three (0.6%) required allogeneic blood transfusion.

Age-related side effects

Information on older marrow donors is scarce. Doney, Buckner and Storb (1995) published information about 37 donors who were older than 65 at the time of harvesting. They had donated over a 16-year period. Eight donors (22%) required blood transfusions from random donors. Their overall complication rate was the same as that in 1,160 donors of all ages who had undergone harvesting at the same institution between 1969 and 1983. Thus, it appears that in general marrow harvesting can be carried out safely in older donors without significant comorbidities.

Filgrastim-stimulated bone marrow harvests

In recent years, administration of filgrastim to donors prior to BM harvesting has been reported. In a pilot study of 10 BM donors by Isola *et al.* (1997), stimulated BM infusions contained almost the same number of CD34+ and CD3+ cells as unstimulated marrow, but had more granulocyte-macrophage colony-forming units. Patients who had received stimulated marrow experienced prompt and durable engraftment and had a shorter hospital stay than those who received unstimulated marrow infusions. In addition, no increase was seen in the incidence of chronic graft-versus-host disease (GVHD) although the cases had not been followed for very long after transplantation. Since that 1997 report, others have reported that priming with rhG-CSF allows faster engraftment without any increase in GVHD or mortality (Couban *et al.*, 2000; Isola, Scigliano, & Fruchtman, 2000; Serody *et al.*, 2000; Morton, Hutchins, & Durant, 2001). Couban *et al.* (2000) also found that the median time required for BM aspiration was almost half that of historical controls, suggesting a potential benefit for donors.

One case was reported in 1996 in which rhG-CSF-mobilized allogeneic bone marrow was used for transplantation because of significant differences in the donor's and recipient's weights. A single rather than double BM harvest was then feasible, and the small marrow volume (10% donor volume) made it possible to avoid red cell transfusion in the donor and thus the related risks of transfusion in a normal donor (Pession *et al.*, 1996).

There are still several unanswered questions about filgrastim-mobilized BM harvests. Because of the small number of patients treated so far, the risks for donors are unknown, and the optimal duration of filgrastim administration is uncertain. There is also concern that because of the time it takes to treat the donor with filgrastim, stem cell progenitors may be depleted from a BM harvest. Because these donors are exposed to the risks of both marrow harvesting and cytokine administration, researchers must document a substantial benefit for recipient before the procedure can be more widely endorsed.

Peripheral blood stem cell donation

In the past few years, a dramatic increase has been reported in the use of cytokine-mobilized allogeneic peripheral blood stem cells for allogeneic transplantation. The reason for this rise is that allogeneic PBSC transplants, when compared to BM transplants in HLA-identical siblings, are associated with a more rapid recovery of granulocytes and platelets after transplantation and seemingly, a lower regimen-related and transplant-related mortality (Dreger *et al.*, 1994; Goldman, 1995; Körbling *et al.*, 1995; Schmitz *et al.*, 1995; Champlin, 1996; Lane, 1996; Russell, Gratwohl, & Schmitz, 1996; Przepiorka *et al.*, 1996). Because mobilized PBSC collections contain approximately 1 log more of T lymphocytes than do BM harvests, concern has existed about a potential increase in the incidence of acute and chronic GVHD after transplantation, especially with unrelated donors. However, none of the studies published so far have documented an increase in the incidence of acute GVHD after stem cell transplantation, although some reported an increase in the incidence of chronic GVHD (Schmitz *et al.*, 1998; Scott *et al.*, 1998; Ringden *et al.*, 1999; Levine *et al.*, 2000). For these reasons, several unrelated donor programs also now provide PBSC instead of BM for transplantation.

In most cases, the PBSCs are collected after filgrastim administration. In a study of 1,306 patients, 99% of donors were mobilized with filgrastim (Anderlini *et al.*, 2001a). Some of the other growth factors that have been used are lenograstim (recombinant methionyl human granulocyte colony-stimulating factor), sargramostim (recombinant human granulocyte-macrophage colony-stimulating factor), Flt 3 ligand, and stem cell factor, all either alone or in combination.

Procurement of peripheral blood stem cells

PBSC procurement can be safely carried out on an outpatient basis. Donors are started on filgrastim at a dose of 10 to 16 µg/kg/day, although a wide range of doses has been used (5–24 µg/kg/day) (Sato *et al.*, 1994; Bensinger *et al.*, 1995; Waller *et al.*, 1996; Bishop *et al.*, 1997). The optimal dose of filgrastim needed to collect enough CD34$^+$ stem cells with minimal toxicity to the donors has not been established. For filgrastim doses of up to 10 µg/kg/day, a dose-response relationship exists between the dose of filgrastim and the mobilization of CD34$^+$ progenitor cells (Höglund *et al.*, 1996; Stroncek *et al.*, 1996a). Experience with doses higher than 10 µg/kg/day has been limited. Filgrastim can be administered as a single daily injection or as twice-a-day injection (Grigg *et al.*, 1995; Link *et al.*, 1996). After administration, the total white blood cell count rises within 4 to 6 hours, but a substantial increase in circulating CD34$^+$ progenitor cells does not occur until the third day after the first filgrastim injection (Link *et al.*, 1995). Therefore, stem cell collection is usually not started until the fourth or fifth day after the filgrastim injections begin.

The PBSCs are collected with a continuous flow cell-separation device. The total volume processed is usually two times the donor's total blood volume. Some centers perform large-volume leukapheresis, in which up to three to six times the donor's total blood volume can be processed (Hillyer, Tiegerman, & Berkman, 1991; Malachowski *et al.*, 1992; Passos-Coelho *et al.*, 1995). The collection process usually takes 3 to 5 hours. Approximately 59% of normal donors need only one apheresis procedure to reach the target CD34+ cell dose, while 31% require two procedures and 10% require three procedures (Körbling *et al.*, 2001). Other studies have reported similar results. Overall, more than 85% of donors can complete the apheresis procedure successfully in one or two collections (Majolino *et al.*, 1997).

The target dose to be collected is not established, but most centers collect between 4 and 6 × 10^6 CD 34$^+$ cells/kilogram of the recipient's body weight. Venous access is usually obtained through the antecubital veins. From 5% to 20% of normal donors have inadequate venous access and need a central

venous catheter (Anderlini *et al.*, 1999; Anderlini *et al.*, 2001a). Confer *et al.* (2001) reported that central venous access was required more often for female rather than for male donors (21% versus 2%, $P < .001$).

Acid-citrate-dextrose-A (ACD-A) is usually used for anticoagulation. Some centers combine ACD-A with heparin for large-volume leukapheresis to limit citrate toxicity. However, heparin is not without side effects. A total of 1,000 to 2,000 units per hour infused over several hours for large-volume leukapheresis may result in some systemic anticoagulation. In a randomized study of allogeneic BM versus PBSC donation (Rowley *et al.*, 2001), the only severe side effect of the PBSC collection was a hematoma associated with heparin administration. However, whether this adverse event was solely the result of heparin use is uncertain.

Postdonation cytopenias

Transient postdonation neutropenia and lymphocytopenia have been reported after PBSC collection. (Anderlini *et al.*, 1996c; Körbling *et al.*, 1996a; Martinez *et al.*, 1996; Stroncek *et al.*, 1996b). Platelet counts generally drop 30% to 50% after leukapheresis, especially when two or more blood volumes are processed (Hillyer, Tiegerman, & Berkman, 1991; Malachowski *et al.*, 1992; Bandarenko *et al.*, 1996; Confer *et al.*, 2001). In normal donors, the administration of filgrastim may contribute to thrombocytopenia (Anderlini *et al.*, 1996b; Stroncek *et al.*, 1996c). Major hemorrhagic complications, however, have not yet been reported.

For donors whose postdonation platelet counts are less than 80 to 100 × 10^9/l, reinfusion of autologous platelet-rich plasma has been suggested (Bensinger *et al.*, 1996; Link *et al.*, 1996). Most centers will not perform leukapheresis if the donor's predonation platelet count is less than 70 × 10^9/l, and the NMDP will accept only those donors with a platelet count of at least 100 × 10^9/l. These postdonation values generally return to baseline at day +30 (Körbling *et al.*, 1996a) with no obvious clinical consequences.

Safety profile of filgrastim

Filgrastim has been used extensively in patients with hematological disorders and in those with cancer (Lieschke & Burgess, 1992; Bonilla *et al.*, 1994; Anonymous, 1994; Vose & Armitage, 1995). Some patients with chronic neutropenia tolerated the drug for several years without major side effects (Bonilla *et al.*, 1994). Several publications have documented the safety of filgrastim in allogeneic PBSC donors and in granulocyte donors (Anderlini *et al.*, 1996b). The procedure appears safe even in donors older than 60 (Anderlini *et al.*, 1997c).

Side effects associated with filgrastim

A wide range of side effects have been reported after filgrastim administration. Most of these side effects are minor and not life-threatening. There have been occasional case reports of life-threatening complications after filgrastim administration. In a study of 1,306 patients reported to the IBMTR and the EBMT databases and on whom data were available, the overall complication rate was 1.1% with no reported fatalities (Anderlini *et al.*, 2001b).

Common but minor ("expected") side effects

Almost all patients report some bone pain after growth factor administration. In most cases, the pain can be relieved by acetaminophen, and very rarely narcotics are required. Other commonly reported side effects are headache, fatigue, nausea, and vomiting. Less frequently reported side effects include noncardiac chest pain, dizziness, fluid retention, insomnia, night sweats, and local injection site reactions (Dreger *et al.*, 1994; Anderlini *et al.*, 1996b; Stroncek *et al.*, 1999; Anderlini *et al.*, 1996a; Anderlini *et al.*, 1999). To some extent, the side effects are dose related and resolve within a few days of filgrastim discontinuation (Stroncek *et al.*, 1996a; Anderlini *et al.*, 1996a; Anderlini *et al.*, 1999). The most commonly reported side effects are summarized in Table 25.2.

The pain experienced by donors of PBSC is related to the filgrastim administration and is more pronounced in the days immediately preceding the apheresis procedure. It resolves rapidly after the growth factors have been discontinued. In marrow donors, however, the pain is related to the harvest procedure. After the donation, almost all PBSC donors return to baseline within 2 weeks whereas only about 80% of marrow donors return to baseline during that period and about 20% experience prolonged pain (Stroncek *et al.*, 1993; Rowley *et al.*, 2001). Fewer than 1% of donors require the filgrastim to be discontinued because of side effects (Anderlini *et al.*, 1999).

The NMDP conducted a prospective trial evaluating the feasibility and safety of PBSC donations by volunteer donors. The preliminary analysis of 395 donors with at least 1 month of follow-up indicated that while filgrastim was generally well tolerated, with no significant changes in blood cell counts 1 year after donation, most PBSC donors did experience side effects. The most notable was bone pain, which peaked on day 5 of filgrastim administration, when approximately 85% of the donors reported some bone pain. On these days more than 90% of the donors classified their pain as mild or moderate. A total of 44 donors (11%) reported severe (grade 3 to 4) toxicities. Commonly reported severe toxicities were insomnia, headache, and malaise. One week after donation, all symptoms had returned to baseline (Confer *et al.*, 2001).

Uncommon but severe ("unexpected") side effects

Uncommon but severe side effects requiring discontinuation of filgrastim have been reported in 1% to 3% of donors (Stroncek *et al.*, 1996a; Anderlini *et al.*, 1999). For example, splenic rupture has been reported after filgrastim administration (Falzetti, Aversa, Minelli, & Tabilio 1999; Becker *et al.*, 1997). Also, in one reported case, life-threatening capillary leak syndrome occurred in a sibling donor whose stem cells were being mobilized with filgrastim. In that case, a total of 5 days of filgrastim was administered, and the white blood cell count on the day of collection was 90.5×10^9/l. The donor developed severe hypotension, pallor, pulmonary rales, hypoxemia, cyanosis, and confusion. Computed tomography (CT) scans showed ascites, pericardial fluid, and bilateral pulmonary effusion (de Azevedo & Tabak, 2001). Another case was reported of a donor developing myocardial infarction after apheresis. The donor had a history of coronary artery disease and myocardial infarction (Bensinger *et al.*, 1996). In both of these cases, the donors recovered without any major sequelae. Others have reported chest pain with PBSC donation that has been both cardiac and noncardiac in origin

Table 25.2. *Commonly reported symptoms associated with filgrastim administration*

Reference	Grigg *et al.*, 1995	Anderlini *et al.*, 1999	Bishop *et al.*, 1997	Stroncek *et al.*, 1999	Stroncek *et al.*, 1999
Dose of filgrastim, μg/kg/day	10	12	5	5	10
No. of patients	15	341	41	19	21
Bone pain	87	84	–	53	76
Myalgias/arthralgias	27	–	83	32/11	68/0
Headache	33	54	44	74	67
Fever	7[a]	0	27	–	–
Chills/rigors	–	–	22	5	14
Body aches	–	–	–	–	–
Fatigue	47	31	–	37	43
Nausea/vomiting	–	13	–	16	24
Insomnia	–	–	–	16	24
Paresthesia	–	–	–	16	38
Diarrhea	–	–	–	11	5
Rash	–	–	–	11	5

[a] Flu-like symptoms.

(Stroncek *et al.,* 1996a; Anderlini *et al.,* 1999; Vij *et al.,* 1999). An anaphylactoid reaction (Adkins, 1998) and acute gouty arthritis have also been reported (Spitzer, McAfee, Poliquin, & Colby, 1998).

Other uncommon side effects

Exacerbation of autoimmune disease with growth factor administration has also been reported. Donors with rheumatoid arthritis and ankylosing spondylitis have experienced a flare-up of their disease when filgrastim or sargramostim were administered (De Vries *et al.,* 1991; Storek *et al.,* 1993). One case of iritis and another case of episcleritis have also been reported (Parkkali, Volin, Siren, & Ruutu, 1996; Huhn *et al.,* 1996). A case of thyroid dysfunction and goiter was reported after therapy with sargramostim in a patient with preexisting thyroid antibodies (Hoekman *et al.,* 1991). In one study of autologous transplantation for autoimmune diseases (Snowden *et al.,* 1998), flare-up of rheumatoid arthritis was reported after rhG-CSF administration in some patients. This flare-up was more likely to happen with a dose of 10 µg/kg/day than with a dose of 5 µg/kg/day.

Some of the unusual and/or major adverse events reported during or shortly after rhG-CSF administration are summarized in Table 25.3. Some reports suggest that rhG-CSF in doses of 15 µg/kg/day may lead to a transient hypercoagulable state (Avenarius, Freund, Deinhardt, & Poliwada, 1992; Shimoda *et al.,* 1993; Harada *et al.,* 1996; LeBlanc, Roy, Demers, Vu, & Cantin, 1999). The clinical significance (if any) of this laboratory finding is unclear. To date, only two cases of vascular events have been reported in normal donors. One was a cerebrovascular accident in a 54-year-old donor that occurred 2

days after an uneventful collection, and another was a myocardial infarction after PBSC collection experienced by a 64-year old donor (Bensinger *et al.,* 1996; Anderlini *et al.,* 1997a). A third case was that of a donor who experienced unstable angina during filgrastim administration (Vij *et al.,* 1999).

Finally, filgrastim administration has been reported to precipitate serious and even life-threatening sickle cell crises in donors with hemoglobin SS, hemoglobin S ± beta thalassemia, or hemoglobin SC (Abboud, Laver, & Blau, 1998; Wei & Grigg, 2001; Adler *et al.,* 2001), This complication has not been reported in donors with the sickle cell trait (Kang *et al.,* 2002). In view of these associations, the NMDP is currently excluding participation by donors with any demonstrable amount of hemoglobin S (Confer, D., personal communication, July 2001). It is probably wise to administer filgrastim with great caution (if at all) to normal donors with any demonstrable hemoglobin S.

Laboratory effects of filgrastim administration

In addition to an increase in the white blood cell count, filgrastim administration causes transient alterations in several other blood chemistry values. For example, elevations in the levels of lactate dehydrogenase (LDH), alkaline phosphatase (AP), and alanine aminotransferase (ALT) have been noted after 4 to 5 days of filgrastim administration (Anderlini *et al.,* 1996b; Stroncek *et al.,* 1996a; Körbling *et al.,* 1996a). At the same time the levels of serum potassium, magnesium, and blood urea nitrogen declined minimally (Stroncek *et al.,* 1996a).

The increase in the white blood cell count after filgrastim administration is mostly due to the increase in the absolute neutrophil counts. The total white blood cell count may be as high as 70 or 80 × 10⁹/l after 5 days of administration. Although leukostasis has never been reported in these donors, most physicians decrease the filgrastim dose when the white blood cell count is higher than 70 or 75 × 10⁹/l (Anderlini *et al.,* 1997a; Stroncek & McCullough, 1997). In primates, a filgrastim-induced increase in the leukocyte count was associated with cerebrovascular events because of neutrophilic infiltration of the brain parenchyma.

Long-term safety profile of filgrastim administration

The long-term safety profile of growth factor administration in normal donors is not fully established. Concerns exist regarding an increased risk of acute leukemias and other hematological malignancies. However, the available information for 1 and 5-year follow-up after growth factor administration has revealed no adverse events (Miflin *et al.,* 1996; Sakamaki *et al.,* 1995; Anderlini *et al.,* 1997; Stroncek *et al.,* 1997; Cavallaro *et al.,* 2000). In the largest follow-up study to date (Cavallaro *et al.,* 2000) the authors contacted 101 donors, whose stem cells were mobilized with filgrastim, at a median of 43 months (range, 35–73 months) after collection. No instances of hematological malignancies were reported. In

Table 25.3. *Unusual and/or major adverse events reported during (or shortly after) filgrastim administration in normal donors*

Reference	Side effect
Becker *et al.,* 1997; Falzetti *et al.,* 1999	Splenic rupture
de Azevedo & Tabak, 2001	Capillary leak syndrome
Vij *et al.,* 1999	Unstable angina
Bensinger *et al.,* 1996	Myocardial infarction[a]
Parkkali *et al.,* 1996; Huhn *et al.,* 1996	Iritis, episcleritis
De Vries *et al.,* 1991; Storek *et al.,* 1993;	Flare-up of rheumatoid arthritis; ankylosing spondylitis
Spitzer *et al.,* 1998	Acute gouty arthritis
Anderlini *et al.,* 1997	Cerebrovascular accident
Adkins, 1998	Anaphylactoid reaction
Abboud, Laver, & Blau, 1998; Adler *et al.,* 2001; Wei & Grigg, 2001	Sickle cell crisis in patients with hemoglobin SS, hemoglobin SC, or hemoglobin S± β thalassemia

[a] Donor had a prior history of coronary artery disease and myocardial infarction.

70 donors, the hematological parameters measured at a median follow-up of 40 months (range, 16–70 months) were normal. In another survey, no hematological malignancy was recorded in a cohort of 281 donors after a median follow-up duration of 3 years (Anderlini et al., 2001). However, these are only observations on a small number of cases. It has been estimated that to detect a 10-fold increase (a very substantial and quite unlikely increase in risk) in the incidence of leukemia, more than 2,000 normal donors must be followed for 10 or more years (Hasenclever & Sextro, 1996). This estimate is based on the annual incidence of leukemia in the United States. Since related donors may be at an increased risk for leukemias compared with unrelated donors, a control group of related donors of equal size would be necessary to ensure that the data are statistically significant. To detect a smaller risk, many more donors will be required, and would be a major logistical challenge feasible only with the establishment of international registries.

Second stem cell collections

Second stem cell collections from the same donor have been reported with no adverse effects. In one study (Anderlini et al., 1997b), PBSCs were collected a second time from 13 normal donors after a median interval of 5 months. No differences were found in the pre-apheresis leukocyte count or in the yield of CD34+ cells per liter of blood processed between the two donations. Filgrastim-related adverse events were also comparable. Similar results were reported by Stroncek et al. (1997).

Pediatric donors

Traditionally, the source of HSC in children has been BM with the harvest performed under general anesthesia. With the success of filgrastim-mobilized PBSCs in adults and the recognition of potential benefits to donors, this mobilization strategy has also been studied for pediatric donors. Preliminary clinical data indicate that PBSC collection from pediatric donors, usually for pediatric recipients, is safe and feasible and provides adequate CD34+ cell doses. Filgrastim at a dose of 12 μg/kg/day is considered adequate, and with that dose a pediatric donor may be able to provide enough stem cells for transplantation of an adult recipient. In one reported case, just one apheresis procedure was sufficient to collect 4×10^6 CD34+ cells from an 8-year-old boy after filgrastim administration, and resulted in successful engraftment in his father who had leukemia. This success was achieved despite a significant difference in their weights: the donor weighed 27 kg, and the recipient weighed 93 kg (Körbling et al., 1996b). In very young donors (up to 6 years) vascular access for leukapheresis (and the leukapheresis procedure itself) can be challenging and usually requires a central venous catheter placement under general anesthesia. Under these circumstances, a traditional marrow harvest may be the better choice.

Poor mobilizers

Healthy donors vary widely in their ability to mobilize PBSCs in response to cytokine administration; some are able to shift into the peripheral blood only small numbers of CD34+ cells ("poor mobilizers"). One study has attempted to determine the factors affecting the mobilization of CD34+ cells in normal donors and the stem cell yield by apheresis. Data were analyzed for 119 donors who had undergone apheresis on days 4, 5, or 6 of rhG-CSF treatment. The CD34+ yield was significantly lower in donors older than 55 and in those who had undergone apheresis on day 4 of rhG-CSF administration. A weak but direct correlation was also found between the CD34+ cell yield and baseline white blood cell count, pre-apheresis white blood cell count, and pre-apheresis mononuclear cell counts (Fig. 25.1). Twenty-one of 119 donors (18%) were considered poor mobilizers, who yielded fewer than 20×10^6 cells per liter of blood processed. On multivariate analysis, the only significant risk factor for poor mobilization was age greater than 55 years ($P = 0.04$) (Anderlini et al., 1997d; Fig. 25.2). In another study, de la Rubia et al. (2002) similarly found that age (donors older than 38) and a single daily dose of rhG-CSF predicted a low CD34+ cell yield. In routine clinical practice, however, it is usually impossible to identify in advance those who are poor mobilizers, although closer monitoring may be justified in older donors and donors with very low baseline circulating CD34+ cell counts (when measured). Even in poor mobilizers, a CD34+ cell dose of at least 2 to 3×10^6 per kg of recipient weight can usually be collected, and that amount may be enough for allogeneic engraftment.

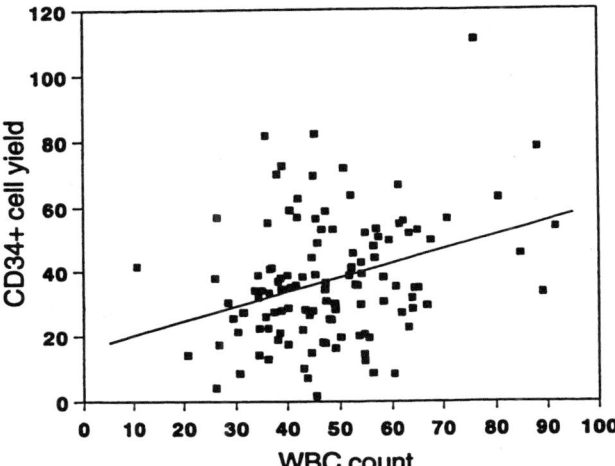

Fig. 25.1. A plot of preapheresis WBC counts ($\times 10^9$/l) versus CD34+ cell yield ($\times 10^6$/l) of blood processed) showing the wide scatter associated with the significant but weak correlation ($r = 0.25$; $P = .007$). Reproduced, with permission, from Anderlini et al. (1997d).

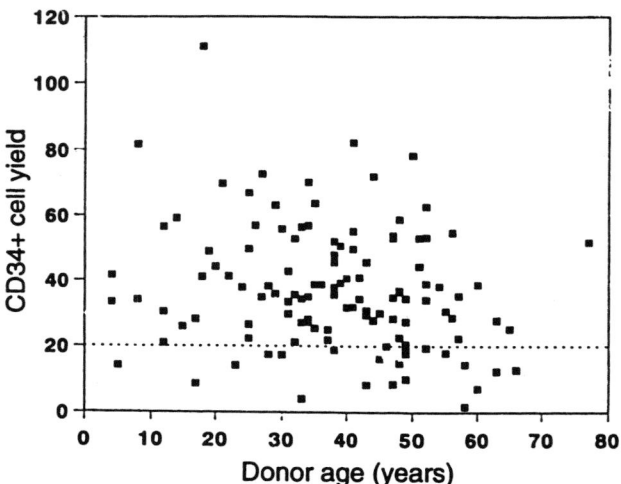

Fig. 25.2. A plot of age versus CD34⁺ cell yield (CD34⁺ cells × 10⁶/l of blood processed) showing donors with poor mobilization (< 20 × 10⁶ CD34⁺ cells/l of blood processed) across the age spectrum. Reproduced, with permission, from Anderlini *et al.* (1997d).

Conclusions

Allogeneic BM donation has an extensive clinical track record and is generally considered safe. Major and life-threatening side effects, although well described, are uncommon. PBSC collection after filgrastim mobilization is a more recently introduced procedure but is also generally well tolerated and considered an acceptable alternative to the more traditional BM harvesting. The primary advantages of PBSC collection are the lack of need for general anesthesia and the lack of need for transfusion of blood products. The procedure is also seemingly more donor-friendly and results in faster donor recovery. However, the long-term safety profile of filgrastim administration to normal donors has not been clearly established and should be further clarified. Such clarification, however, is possible only with the establishment of international donor registries.

The choice between two donation modalities described is ordinarily dictated by a variety of factors, including donor preference, transplantation physician preference, donor-recipient HLA compatibility, donor age and medical history, donation procedure logistics, and the relationship, or lack thereof, of the donor to the recipient. Ultimately, those involved in the decision-making process should make every effort to balance the needs of the different parties and to resolve any potential conflicts of interest.

References

Abboud, M., Laver, J., & Blau, C. A. (1998). Granulocytosis causing sickle-cell crisis. *Lancet*, **351**, 959.

Adkins, D. R. (1998). Anaphylactoid reaction in a normal donor given granulocyte colony-stimulating factor. *Journal of Clinical Oncology*, **16**, 812–3 (Letter).

Adler, B. K., Salzman, D. E., Carabasi, M. H. *et al.* (2001). Fatal sickle cell crisis after granulocyte colony-stimulating factor administration. *Blood*, **97**, 3313–4.

Anderlini, P., Donato, M., Chan, K-W. *et al.* (1999). Allogeneic blood progenitor cell collection in normal donors after mobilization with filgrastim: the M. D. Anderson Cancer Center experience. *Transfusion*, **39**, 555–60.

Anderlini, P., Körbling, M., Chan, K. W. *et al.* (2001a). Long-term follow up and safety of normal peripheral blood progenitor cell (PBPC) donors treated with filgrastim: the MD Anderson Cancer Center experience. *Blood*, **98**, 183a (Abstract #771).

Anderlini, P., Körbling, M., Dale, D. *et al.* (1997a). Allogeneic blood stem cell transplantation: considerations for donors. *Blood*, **90**, 903–8 (Editorial).

Anderlini, P., Lauppe, J., Przepiorka, D. *et al.* (1997b). Peripheral blood stem cell apheresis in normal donors: feasibility and yield of second collections. *British Journal of Haematology*, **96**, 415–7.

Anderlini, P., Przepiorka, D., Champlin, R. E., & Körbling, M. (1996a). Biologic and clinical effects of granulocyte colony-stimulating factor in normal individuals. *Blood*, **88**, 2819–25 (Review).

Anderlini, P., Przepiorka, D., Lauppe, J. *et al.* (1997c). Collection of peripheral blood stem cells from normal donors 60 years of age or older. *British Journal of Haematology*, **97**, 485–7.

Anderlini, P., Przepiorka, D., Seong, D. *et al.* (1996b). Clinical toxicity and laboratory effects of granulocyte colony-stimulating factor (filgrastim) mobilization and blood stem cell apheresis from normal donors, and analysis of charges for the procedures. *Transfusion*, **36**, 590–5.

Anderlini, P., Prezpiorka, D., Seong, D. *et al.* (1997d). Factors affecting mobilization of CD34+ cells in normal donors treated with filgrastim. *Transfusion*, **37**, 507–12.

Anderlini, P., Przepiorka, D., Seong, D., Champlin, R., & Körbling, M. (1996c). Transient neutropenia in normal donors after G-CSF mobilization and stem cell apheresis. *British Journal of Haematology*, **94**, 155–8.

Anderlini, P., Rizzo, J. D., Nugent, M. L. *et al.* (2001b). Peripheral blood stem cell donation: an analysis from the International Bone Marrow Transplant Registry (IBMTR) and the European Group for Blood and Marrow Transplant (EBMT) databases. *Bone Marrow Transplantation*, **27**, 689–92.

Anonymous. (1994). American Society of Clinical Oncology: recommendations for the use of hematopoietic colony-stimulating factors: evidence-based, clinical practice guidelines. *Journal of Clinical Oncology*, **12**, 2471–508.

Avenarius, H. J., Freund, M., Deinhardt, J., & Poliwada, H. (1992). Effect of recombinant human granulocyte colony-stimulating factor (rhG-CSF) on circulating platelets. *Annals of Hematology*, **65**, 6–9.

Bacigalupo, A., Tong, J., Podesta, M. *et al.* (1992). Bone marrow harvest for marrow transplantation: effect of multiple small (2 ml) or large (20 ml) aspirates. *Bone Marrow Transplantation*, **9**, 467–70.

Bandarenko, N., Brecher, M. E., Owen, H. *et al.* (1996). Thrombocytopenia in allogeneic peripheral blood stem cell collections. *Transfusion*, **36**, 668–9 (Letter).

Batinic, D., Marusic, M., Pavletic, Z. *et al.* (1990). Relationship between differing volumes of bone marrow aspirates and their cellular composition. *Bone Marrow Transplantation*, **6**, 103–7.

Becker, P. S., Wagle, M., Matous, S. *et al.* (1997). Spontaneous splenic rupture following administration of granulocyte colony-stimulating factor (G-CSF): occurrence in an allogeneic donor of peripheral blood stem cells. *Biology of Blood and Marrow Transplantation*, **3**, 45–9.

Bensinger, W. I., Buckner, C. D., Rowley, S. *et al.* (1996). Treatment of normal donors with recombinant growth factors for transplantation of allogeneic blood stem cells. *Bone Marrow Transplantation*, **17** (Suppl 2), S19–S21.

Bensinger, W. I., Weaver, C. H., Appelbaum, F. R. *et al.* (1995). Transplantation of allogeneic peripheral blood stem cells mobilized by recombinant human granulocyte colony stimulating factor. *Blood*, **85**, 1655–8.

Berg, K. D., Brinster, N. K., Huhn, K. M. *et al.* (2001). Transmission of a T-cell lymphoma by allogeneic bone marrow transplantation. *New England Journal of Medicine*, **345**, 1458–63.

Bishop, M. R., Tarantolo, S. R., Jackson, J. D. *et al.* (1997). Allogeneic-blood stem cell collection following mobilization with low-dose granulocyte colony-stimulating factor. *Journal of Clinical Oncology*, **15**, 1601–7.

Bonilla, M. A., Dale, D., Zeidler, C. *et al.* (1994). Long-term safety of treatment with recombinant human granulocyte colony-stimulating factor (r-metHuG-CSF) in patients with severe congenital neutropenias. *British Journal of Haematology*, **88**, 723–30.

Bortin, M. M. & Buckner, C. D. (1983). Major complications of marrow harvesting for transplantation. *Experimental Hematology*, **11**, 916–21.

Buckner, C. D., Clift, R. A., Sanders, J. E. *et al.* (1984). Marrow harvesting from normal donors. *Blood*, **64**, 630–4.

Cavallaro, A. M., Lilleby, K., Majolino, I. *et al.* (2000). Three to six year follow-up of normal donors who received recombinant human granulocyte colony-stimulating factor. *Bone Marrow Transplantation*, **25**, 85–9.

Champlin, R. E. (1996). Peripheral blood progenitor cells: a replacement for marrow transplantation? *Seminars in Oncology*, **23** (2 Suppl 4), 15–21 (Review).

Confer, D. L., Haagenson, M., Anderlini, P. *et al.* (2001). Collection of rhG-CSF mobilized blood stem cells from 395 unrelated donors. *Blood*, **98**, 857a (Abstract).

Confer, D. L. & Stroncek, D. F. (1999). Bone marrow and peripheral blood stem cell donors. In *Hematopoietic Cell Transplantation*, eds. E. D. Thomas, K. G. Blume, & S. J. Forman, pp. 421–30. Boston: Blackwell Science, Inc.

Couban, S., Messner, H. A., Andreou, P. *et al.* (2000). Bone marrow mobilized with granulocyte colony-stimulating factor in related allogeneic transplant recipients: A study of 29 patients. *Biology of Blood and Marrow Transplantation*, **6**, 422–7.

de Azevedo, A. M. & Tabak, D. G. (2001). Life-threatening capillary leak syndrome after G-CSF mobilization and collection of peripheral blood progenitor cells for allogeneic transplantation. *Bone Marrow Transplantation*, **28**, 311–2.

de la Rubia, J., Arbona, C., de Arriba, F. *et al.* (2002). Analysis of factors associated with low peripheral blood progenitor cell collection in normal donors. *Transfusion*, **42**, 4–9.

De Vries, E.G.E., Willemse, P.H.B., Biesma, B. *et al.* (1991). Flare-up of rheumatoid arthritis during GM-CSF treatment after chemotherapy. *Lancet*, **338**, 517–8 (Letter).

Doney, K., Buckner, C. D., & Storb, R., for the Seattle Bone Marrow Transplant Team. (1995). Marrow harvesting from donors ≥ 65 years of age. *Experimental Hematology*, **23**, 861a (Abstract #416).

Dreger, P., Haferlach, T., Eckstein, V. *et al.* (1994). GCSF-mobilized peripheral blood progenitor cells for allogeneic transplantation: safety, kinetics of mobilization, and composition of the graft. *British Journal of Haematology*, **87**, 609–13.

Falzetti, F., Aversa, F., Minelli, O., & Tabilio, A. (1999). Spontaneous rupture of spleen during peripheral blood stem-cell mobilization in a healthy donor. *Lancet*, **353**, 555 (Letter).

Goldman, J. (1995). Peripheral blood stem cells for allografting. *Blood*, **85**, 1413–5 (Editorial).

Goldman, J. M. for the WMDA Executive Committee. (1994). A special report: bone marrow transplants using volunteer donors—recommendations and requirements for a standardized practice throughout the world—1994 update. *Blood*, **84**, 2833–9.

Grigg, A. P., Roberts, A. W., Raunow, H. *et al.* (1995). Optimizing dose and scheduling of filgrastim (granulocyte colony stimulating factor) for mobilization and collection of peripheral blood progenitor cells in normal volunteers. *Blood*, **86**, 4437–45.

Harada, M., Nagafuji, K., Fugisaki, T. *et al.* (1996). G-CSF induced mobilization of peripheral blood stem cells from healthy adults for allogeneic transplantation. *Journal of Hematotherapy*, **5**, 63–71.

Hasenclever, D. & Sextro, M. (1996). Safety of alloPBSCT donors: biometrical considerations on monitoring long-term risks. *Bone Marrow Transplantation*, **17** (Suppl 2), S28–S30.

Hillyer, C. D., Tiegerman, K. O., & Berkman, E. M. (1991). Increase in circulating colony-forming units-granulocyte-macrophage during large volume leukapheresis: evaluation of a new cell separator. *Transfusion*, **31**, 327–32.

Hoekman, K., von Blomberg-van der Flier, B. M. E., Wagstaff, J. *et al.* (1991). Reversible thyroid dysfunction during treatment with GM-CSF. *Lancet*, **338**, 541–2.

Höglund, M., Smedmyr, B., Simonsson, B., Tötterman, T., & Bengtsson, M. (1996). Dose-dependent mobilization of hematopoietic progenitor cells in healthy volunteers receiving glycosylated rHuG-CSF. *Bone Marrow Transplantation*, **18**, 19–27.

Hosoya, N., Miyagawa, K., Mimura, T. *et al.* (1997). Malignant hyperthermia induced by general anesthesia for bone marrow harvesting. *Bone Marrow Transplantation*, **19**, 509–11.

Huhn, R. D., Yurkow, E. J., Tushinski, R. *et al.* (1996). Recombinant human interleukin-3 (rhIL-3) enhances the mobilization of peripheral blood progenitor cells by recombinant human granulocyte colony-stimulating factor (rhG-CSF) in normal volunteers. *Experimental Hematology*, **24**, 839–47.

Isola, L., Scigliano, E., & Fruchtman, S. (2000). Long-term follow-up after allogeneic granulocyte colony-stimulating factor-primed bone marrow transplantation. *Biology of Blood and Marrow Transplantation*, **6**, 428–33.

Isola, L. M., Scigliano, E., Skerrett, D. *et al.* (1997). A pilot study of bone marrow transplantation using related donors stimulated with G-CSF. *Bone Marrow Transplantation*, **20**, 1033–7.

Jones, M. D. Petrikovsky, B. M., Sahdev, I., & Prisco, M. (1995). Continuous fetal heart rate monitoring during bone marrow harvesting in pregnancy. *American Journal of Perinatology*, **12**, 243–4.

Kang, E. M., Areman, E. M., David-Ocampo, V. *et al.* (2002). Mobilization, collection, and processing of peripheral blood stem cells in individuals with sickle cell trait. *Blood,* **99,** 850–5.

Klumpp, T. R., Mangan, K. F., MacDonald, J. S., & Mesgarzadeh, M. (1992). Fracture of the ilium: an unusual complication of bone marrow harvesting. *Bone Marrow Transplantation,* **9,** 503–4 (Letter).

Körbling, M., Anderlini, P., Durett, A. *et al.* (1996a). Delayed effects of rhG-CSF mobilization treatment and apheresis on circulating CD34+ and CD34+Thy-1dimCD38- progenitor cells and lymphoid subsets in normal stem cell donors for allogeneic transplantation. *Bone Marrow Transplantation,* **18,** 1073–9.

Körbling, M., Chan, K-W., Anderlini, P. *et al.* (1996b). Allogeneic peripheral blood stem cell transplantation using normal patient-related pediatric donors. *Bone Marrow Transplantation,* **18,** 885–90.

Körbling, M., Giralt, S., Khouri, I. *et al.* (2001). Donor lymphocyte apheresis for adoptive immunotherapy compared with blood stem cell apheresis. *Journal of Clinical Apheresis,* **16,** 82–7.

Körbling, M., Przepiorka, D., Huh, Y. O. *et al.* (1995). Allogeneic blood stem cell transplantation for refractory leukemia and lymphoma: potential advantage of blood over marrow allografts. *Blood,* **85,** 1659–65.

Lane, T. A. (1996). Allogeneic marrow reconstitution using peripheral blood stem cells: the dawn of a new era. *Transfusion,* **36,** 585–9 (Editorial).

LeBlanc, R., Roy, J., Demers, C. *et al.* (1999). A prospective study of G-CSF effects on hemostasis in allogeneic blood stem cell donors. *Bone Marrow Transplantation,* **23,** 991–6.

Levine, J. E., Wiley, J., Kletzel, M. *et al.* (2000). Cytokine-mobilized allogeneic peripheral blood stem cell transplants in children result in rapid engraftment and a high incidence of chronic GVHD. *Bone Marrow Transplantation,* **25,** 13–8.

Lieschke, G. J. & Burgess, A. W. (1992). Granulocyte colony-stimulating factor and granulocyte-macrophage colony-stimulating factor. *New England Journal of Medicine,* **327,** 28–35.

Link, H., Arseniev, L., Bähre, O. *et al.* (1995). Combined transplantation of allogeneic bone marrow and CD34+ blood cells. *Blood,* **86,** 2500–8.

Link, H., Arseniev, L., Bähre, O. *et al.* (1996). Transplantation of allogeneic CD34+ cells. *Blood,* **87,** 4903–9.

Majolino, I., Buscemi, F., Scime, R. *et al.* (1995). Treatment of normal donors with rhG-CSF 16 micrograms/kg for mobilization of peripheral blood stem cells and their apheretic collection for allogeneic transplantation. *Hematologica,* **80,** 219–26.

Majolino, I., Cavallaro, A. M., Bacigalupo, A. *et al.* (1997). Mobilization and collection of PBSC in healthy donors: a retrospective analysis of the Italian Bone Marrow Transplantation Group (GITMO). *Hematologica,* **82,** 47–52.

Malachowski, M. E., Comenzo, R. L., Hillyer, C. D. *et al.* (1992). Large-volume leukapheresis for peripheral blood stem cell collection in patients with hematological malignancies. *Transfusion,* **32,** 732–5.

Martinez, C., Urbano-Ispizua, A., Rozman, C. *et al.* (1996). Effects of G-CSF administration and peripheral blood progenitor cell collection in 20 healthy donors. *Annals of Hematology,* **72,** 269–72.

Miflin, G., Charley, C., Stainer, C. *et al.* (1996). Stem cell mobilization in normal donors for allogeneic transplantation: analysis of safety and factors affecting efficacy. *British Journal of Haematology,* **95,** 345–8.

Morton, J., Hutchins, C., & Durant, S. (2001). Granulocyte-colony-stimulating factor (G-CSF)-primed allogeneic bone marrow: significantly less graft-versus-host disease and comparable engraftment to G-CSF mobilized peripheral blood stem cells. *Blood,* **98,** 3186–91.

Neupogen® Thousand Oaks, CA, Amgen, 1994 (package insert).

Niederwieser, D. W., Appelbaum, F. R., Gastl, G. *et al.* (1990). Inadvertent transmission of a donor's acute myeloid leukemia in bone marrow transplantation for chronic myelocytic leukemia. *New England Journal of Medicine,* **322,** 1794–6.

Nishimori, M., Yamada, Y., Hoshi, K. *et al.* (2002). Health-related quality of life of unrelated bone marrow donors in Japan. *Blood,* **99,** 1995–2001.

Parkkali, T., Volin, L., Sirén, M-K., & Ruutu, T. (1996). Acute iritis induced by granulocyte colony-stimulating factor used for mobilization in a volunteer unrelated peripheral blood progenitor cell donor. *Bone Marrow Transplantation,* **17,** 433–4.

Passos-Coelho, J. L., Braine, H. G., Wright, S. K. *et al.* (1995). Large-volume leukapheresis using regional citrate anticoagulation to collect peripheral blood progenitor cells. *Journal of Hematotherapy,* **4,** 11–9.

Pession, A., Locatelli, F., Prete, A. *et al.* (1996). G-CSF in an infant donor: a method of reducing harvest volume in bone marrow transplantation. *Bone Marrow Transplantation,* **17,** 431–2.

Przepiorka, D., Ippolitti, C., Khouri, I. *et al.* (1996). Allogeneic transplantation for advanced leukemia: improved short-term outcome with blood stem cell grafts and tacrolimus. *Transplantation,* **62,** 1806–10.

Riley, D. & Evans, T. G. (1992). Osteomyelitis complicating bone marrow harvest. *Clinical Infectious Diseases,* **14,** 980–1 (Letter).

Ringdén, O., Remberger, M., Runde, V. *et al.* (1999). Peripheral blood stem cell transplantation from unrelated donors: a comparison with marrow transplantation. *Blood,* **94,** 455–64.

Rowley, S. D., Donaldson, G., Lilleby, K. *et al.* (2001). Experiences of donors enrolled in a randomized study of allogeneic bone marrow or peripheral blood stem cell transplantation. *Blood,* **97,** 2541–8.

Russell, N., Gratwohl, A., & Schmitz, N. (1996). The place of blood stem cells in allogeneic transplantation. *British Journal of Haematology,* **93,** 747–53 (Editorial).

Sakamaki, S., Matsunaga, T., Hirayama, Y. *et al.* (1995). Hematological study of healthy volunteers at 5 years after G-CSF. *Lancet,* **346,** 1432–3 (Letter).

Sato, N., Sawada, K., Takahashi, T. A. *et al.* (1994). A time course study for optimal harvest of peripheral blood progenitor cells by granulocyte colony-stimulating factor in healthy volunteers. *Experimental Hematology,* **22,** 973–8.

Schmitz, N., Bacigalupo, A., Hasenclever, D. *et al.* (1998). Allogeneic bone marrow transplantation vs. filgrastim-mobilized peripheral blood progenitor cell transplantation in patients with early leukemia: first results of a randomized multicenter trial of the European Group for Blood and Marrow Transplantation. *Bone Marrow Transplantation,* **21,** 995–1003.

Schmitz, N., Dreger, P., Suttorp, M. *et al.* (1995). Primary transplantation of allogeneic peripheral blood progenitor cells mobilized by filgrastim (granulocyte colony stimulating factor). *Blood,* **85,** 1666–72.

Scott, M. A., Gandhi, M. K., Jestice, H. K. *et al.* (1998). A trend towards an increased incidence of chronic graft-versus-host disease following allogeneic peripheral blood progenitor cell transplantation: a case controlled study. *Bone Marrow Transplantation,* **22,** 273–6.

Serody, J. S., Sparks, S. D., Lin, Y. *et al.* (2000). Comparison of granulocyte colony-stimulating factor (G-CSF)-mobilized peripheral blood progenitor cells and G-CSF-stimulated bone marrow as a source of stem cells in HLA-matched sibling transplantation. *Biology of Blood and Marrow Transplantation,* **6,** 434–40.

Shimoda, K., Okamura, S., Inaba, S. *et al.* (1993). Granulocyte colony-stimulating factor and platelet aggregation. *Lancet,* **341,** 633 (Letter).

Snowden, J. A., Biggs, J. C., Milliken, S. T. *et al.* (1998). A randomized, blinded, placebo-controlled, dose escalation study of the tolerability and efficacy of filgrastim for hematopoietic stem cell mobilization in patients with severe active rheumatoid arthritis. *Bone Marrow Transplantation,* **22,** 1035–41.

Spitzer, T., McAfee, S., Poliquin, C., & Colby, C. (1998). Acute gouty arthritis following recombinant human granulocyte colony-stimulating factor in an allogeneic blood stem cell donor. *Bone Marrow Transplantation,* **21,** 966–7.

Storek, J., Glaspy, J. A., Grody, W. W. *et al.* (1993). Adult-onset cyclic neutropenia responsive to cyclosporine therapy in a patient with ankylosing spondylitis. *American Journal of Hematology,* **43,** 139–43.

Stroncek, D. F., Clay, M. E., Herr, G. *et al.* (1997). Blood counts in healthy donors 1 year after the collection of granulocyte-colony-stimulating factor-mobilized progenitor cells and the results of a second mobilization and collection. *Transfusion,* **37,** 304–8.

Stroncek, D. F., Clay, M. E., Jaszcz, W. *et al.* (1999). Collection of two peripheral blood stem cell concentrates from healthy donors. *Transfusion Medicine,* **9,** 37–50.

Stroncek, D. F., Clay, M. E., Lennon, S. *et al.* (1996b). Neutropenia following the collection of granulocyte colony-stimulating factor mobilized blood progenitor cell components is due to the collection of progenitor cells. *Blood,* **88,** 396a (Abstract #1573).

Stroncek, D. F., Clay, M. E., Petzoldt, M. L. *et al.* (1996a). Treatment of normal individuals with granulocyte colony-stimulating factor: donor experiences and the effects on peripheral blood CD34+ cell counts and on the collection of peripheral blood stem cells. *Transfusion,* **36,** 601–10.

Stroncek, D. F., Clay, M. E., Smith, J. *et al.* (1996c). Changes in blood counts after the administration of granulocyte-colony-stimulating factor and the collection of peripheral blood stem cells from healthy donors. *Transfusion,* **36,** 596–600.

Stroncek, D. F., Holland, P. V., Bartch, G. *et al.* (1993). Experiences of the first 493 unrelated marrow donors in the National Marrow Donor Program. *Blood,* **81,** 1940–6.

Stroncek, D. F. & McCullough, J. (1997). Policies and procedures for the establishment of an allogeneic blood stem cell collection programme. *Transfusion Medicine,* **7,** 77–87.

Stroncek, D. F., Strand, R., Scott, E. *et al.* (1989). Attitudes and physical condition of unrelated marrow donors immediately after donation. *Transfusion,* **29,** 317–22.

Thomas, E. D. & Storb, R. (1970). Technique for human marrow grafting. *Blood,* **36,** 507–15.

Vij, R., Adkins, D. R., Brown, R. A. *et al.* (1999). Unstable angina in a peripheral blood stem cell and progenitor cell donor given granulocyte-colony stimulating factor. *Transfusion,* **39,** 542–3.

Vose, J. M. & Armitage, J. O. (1995). Clinical applications of hematopoietic growth factors. *Journal of Clinical Oncology,* **13,** 1023–35.

Waller, C. F., Bertz, H., Wenger, M. K. *et al.* (1996). Mobilization of peripheral blood progenitor cells for allogeneic transplantation: efficacy and toxicity of a high-dose rhG-CSF regimen. *Bone Marrow Transplantation,* **18,** 279–83.

Wei, A. & Grigg, A. (2001). Granulocyte colony-stimulating factor-induced sickle cell crisis and multiorgan dysfunction in a patient with compound heterozygous sickle cell/β+ thalassemia. *Blood,* **97,** 3998–9.

26 T-cell depletion of allogeneic hematopoietic stem cell grafts

ROBERT J. SOIFFER AND PAUL MARTIN

Dana-Farber Cancer Institute, Boston USA and Fred Hutchinson Cancer Research Center, Seattle, USA

Introduction

T-cell depletion (TCD) of donor marrow was first introduced into clinical trials during the early 1980s. The impetus for clinical studies of TCD emanated from animal experiments that showed a dramatic reduction in graft-versus-host disease (GVHD) risk when T cells were removed from the graft. Initial human studies confirmed that TCD decreased the incidence and severity of GVHD. However, it soon became clear that some methods of TCD also predisposed to graft failure, Epstein-Barr virus (EBV)-associated lymphoproliferative disorders, delayed immune reconstitution, and disease relapse. Despite the problems associated with T-cell depletion, there continues to be great interest in developing and improving this technology, particularly for recipients of HLA mismatched or unrelated grafts. It is hoped that understanding the immunobiology of hematopoietic stem cell (HSC) transplantation can lead to advances in graft engineering that could prevent GVHD without adversely affecting engraftment, immune competence, and antileukemic activity (reviewed by Ho & Soiffer, 2001).

Methods: extent and specificity of TCD

Aspirated marrow or apheresed peripheral blood cells for allogeneic transplantation in humans provide the stem cells required for hematopoietic reconstitution, but also contain T lymphocytes that can contribute to the development of GVHD. Murine studies have demonstrated that GVHD does not occur when the graft does not contain T lymphocytes. Bone marrow used for human transplantation contains approximately 2 to 4 $\times$ 10^{10} nucleated cells, 10% to 20% of which are mature lymphocytes. An average patient transplanted with unmodified bone marrow would thus receive 2 to 8 $\times$ 10^7 T cells/kg recipient body weight. The number of T cells infused into recipients when mobilized peripheral blood is utilized as a stem cell source may be 10-fold greater.

The extent of T-cell depletion required to prevent GVHD also depends on multiple factors already known to affect the risk of GVHD after transplantation of unmodified HSC. These factors include

1. HLA disparity between the patient and donor
2. use of related versus unrelated stem cells
3. the amount and type of posttransplant immune suppression
4. alloimmunization of the donor caused by prior pregnancy and possibly by transfusions.

In addition, the risk of GVHD varies among donor-recipient pairs as a function of differences in minor histocompatibility antigens. The precise extent of TCD needed to prevent GVHD is not clear. However, most studies suggest that a minimum of 2 log-depletion of functional T cells from the marrow is necessary for effective GVHD prophylaxis with reduced or no posttransplant immune suppression. In general, the more exhaustive the TCD, the lower the risk of GVHD.

Both antibody-based and physical methods have been developed for ex vivo depletion of T cells (for review see Martin & Kernan, 1996) (Table 26.1). The most extensively studied techniques include antigen-specific monoclonal antibody and complement, anti-CD52 Campath antibody without complement, CD34 selection, counterflow centrifugal elutriation, and soybean lectin agglutination. These methods can remove at least 95% of T cells in the graft. Some methods can remove more than 99% of T cells. Antibody-based methods can be further divided into antibodies with narrow specificity, targeting T

Table 26.1. *Common methods of TCD*

Physical methods
  Density gradient fractionation
  Soybean lectin agglutination + E-rosette depletion
  Counterflow centrifugal elutriation
Immunologic methods
  Monoclonal antibody and rabbit complement, e.g., anti-CD6 (T12), anti-TCRαβ ($T_{10}B_9$)
  Campath-1 antibodies ex vivo
  Campath-1 antibodies in vivo
  Immunotoxins (e.g., anti-CD5-ricin)
Combined physical/immunologic methods
  CD34 selection by immuno-absorption columns
  Immunomagnetic beads
  Soybean agglutination + monoclonal antibody

cells or T-cell subsets, and broad specificity antibodies targeting T cells and other immune cells.

Most ex vivo techniques rely on negative selection whereby the targeted cell population is removed from the bone marrow or apheresis product. More recently, there has been considerable interest in positive stem cell selection, utilizing anti-CD34 antibody coated columns to select hematopoietic progenitors (see Chapter 27). By selecting CD34+ stem cells, this technique can reduce the lymphocyte content in the infused product by 4 to 5 logs. Moreover, it may offer practical advantages over traditional negative selection methods for the depletion of PBSCs given the larger volume and 10-fold excess lymphocyte content in mobilized peripheral blood compared to bone marrow (Urbano-Ispizua et al., 1998).

In vivo TCD with anti-thymocyte globulin or humanized anti-T-cell antibodies such as Campath-1H has been used with increasing frequency as a primary or adjunctive method of GVHD prophylaxis (see Chapter 109). These antibodies have been administered both pre and post donor stem cell infusion to facilitate engraftment and as a way to delay recovery of donor T cells that might otherwise cause GVHD or rejection (Hale et al., 2000). It should be noted that Campath-1 antibodies may prevent GVHD not only by depleting T cells, but also by removing monocyte-derived dendritic cells and their precursors (Klaninsirikul et al., 2002; Ratzinger et al., 2003). The use of intravenously administered anti-T-cell antibodies may permit effective TCD without cumbersome and time consuming ex vivo manipulations. The optimal degree and duration of in vivo TCD remains undefined.

During the past several years, new approaches to TCD have been explored. Functional, rather than strictly anatomic, techniques of TCD have been tested. The goal of such strategies has been to remove only those T cells potentially reactive with host alloantigens. After exposure to host cells ex vivo, the stem cell inoculum can be purged of stimulated donor T cells expressing activation antigens such as CD25, CD69, CD71, or HLA-DR (Garderet et al., 1999; Koh, Prentice, & Lowdell, 1999; Harris et al., 1999; van Dijk et al., 1999; Koh et al., 2002). Additionally, advantage can be taken of modulation of ion channel transporter function characteristic of activated T cells such as that of p-glycoprotein (Guimond et al., 2002). An alternative strategy to physical removal of T cells has been induction of anergy (or tolerization) in donor T cells potentially reactive to host alloantigens. Attempts have been made to induce recipient-specific anergy or nonresponsiveness by incubating the donor product with recipient antigen-presenting cells in the presence of costimulatory blockade (Guinan et al., 1999). Initial studies of these approaches have been promising, although longer follow-up and confirmation in larger studies is needed.

Effects on acute and chronic GVHD

As predicted by preclinical data, the earliest trials of TCD in humans confirmed a major reduction in the incidence of GVHD. In patients given no posttransplant immune suppression, the incidence of clinically significant (grades II–IV) acute GVHD decreases from approximately 80% with unmodified marrow to 20% or less when 95% to 99% of T cells are removed. In HLA-mismatched recipients, the incidence of clinically significant acute GVHD can be reduced to 20% or less if at least 99.9% of T cells are removed. It has been estimated that the threshold of infused T cells for the development of acute GVHD grade II–IV after HLA-identical sibling transplantation is approximately 1×10^5/kg (Kernan et al., 1986), and 5×10^4/kg or less after haploidentical family member transplantation (Muller et al., 1999). The threshold of infused T cells leading to GVHD induction may be different with transplantation of mobilized peripheral blood progenitors given the differences in the number and composition of the T-cell compartment in bone marrow and peripheral blood. A very low incidence of GVHD has been reported after transplantation of haploidentical allogeneic stem cells that have been exhaustively depleted of T cells through CD34+ stem cell selection and sebsequently E-rosetting/lectin agglutination (Aversa et al., 1998). In patients transplanted with grafts containing an appreciable number of residual T cells, the risk of GVHD can be reduced by posttransplant immune suppression with methotrexate and cyclosporine. There is relatively little published information concerning the effects of TCD on chronic GVHD, although the incidence in some studies appears to be much lower than usually seen in patients transplanted with unmodified marrow (Atkinson et al., 1990; Marmont et al., 1991; Soiffer et al., 1997).

TCD has also been studied in an attempt to control GVHD after administration of donor lymphocyte infusions (DLI). Based on data that suggested that CD8 depletion of donor bone marrow could reduce GVHD without compromising GVL activity (Champlin et al., 1990), several trials of CD8 depletion of DLI have been undertaken. GVHD rates have been lower than expected without any apparent decrease in antileukemic activity (Giralt et al., 1995; Alyea et al., 1998). A novel approach to GVHD control after DLI has been the insertion of a thymidine kinase gene into infused T cells, which would render them susceptible to destruction by gancyclovir administration in the event of GVHD development (Tiberghien et al., 2001).

Graft failure

Graft failure occurs in 1% to 2% of cases when unmodified HLA-identical sibling bone marrow is used for allogeneic transplantation in patients with a hematologic malignancy, treated with a myeloablative conditioning regimen. With a few notable exceptions, most clinical studies involving TCD have shown an increased incidence of graft failure. Graft failure after TCD marrow transplantation may occur in three distinct patterns:

1. failure of initial engraftment
2. partial or full initial engraftment followed by graft rejection within 2 weeks of HSCT
3. delayed graft failure that can occur months following transplant (Champlin et al., 1989; Martin & Kernan, 1996).

In an analysis from the International Bone Marrow Registry (IBMTR) of more than 3,000 patients who received related donor TCD or non-TCD BMT for leukemia, TCD was associated with a significantly increased risk for graft failure compared to unmanipulated marrow transplantation (relative risk 9.29, $P < .0001$) (Marmont et al., 1991).

Two general explanations that are not mutually exclusive could account for the increased incidence of graft failure after TCD transplantation: (1) stem cell damage or loss during in vitro manipulations, and (2) absence of a graft-enhancing effect mediated by donor T cells. It is less likely that failure of initial engraftment is caused by injury to hematopoietic progenitors or auxiliary cells during marrow manipulation, since autologous marrow processed with monoclonal antibodies and complement engrafts without significant difficulty (Anderson et al., 1990). While stem cell loss or damage cannot be excluded as a contributory cause of graft failure, data from animal experiments and circumstantial evidence from clinical trials have indicated that donor T cells represent an important determinant of allogeneic HSC engraftment. In humans, the risk of graft failure has correlated inversely with the amount and rate of total body irradiation (TBI) exposure (Marmont et al., 1991), suggesting that graft failure is caused by residual host cells that survive the conditioning regimen. This suggestion is consistent with additional observations that the risk of graft failure was decreased in patients who received posttransplant immune suppression (Marmont et al., 1991). As further substantiation of this notion, many studies have shown that host T cells with specific antidonor cytotoxic or suppressive activity can be recovered from the blood of patients with graft failure after T-cell-depleted marrow transplantation. Cytotoxic donor CD8[+] cells that recognize alloantigens on recipient immune effector cells may have important effects in preventing marrow graft rejection (Martin, 1993, 1998). Taken together, these observations indicate that donor T cells prevent rejection primarily by eliminating host effectors that survive the pretransplant conditioning regimen.

Several approaches have been used to avoid the increased risk of graft failure associated with TCD (Table 26.2). Cytosine arabinoside, thiotepa, and T-cell-specific immunotoxins have been added to cyclophosphamide and TBI in order to improve the immunosuppressive efficacy of the pretransplant conditioning regimen, but the benefit of decreased graft failure may be offset by increased regimen-related toxicity. Fludarabine, total lymphoid irradiation, antithymocyte globulin, monoclonal antibodies (Hale & Waldmann, 1996; Soiffer et al., 1997; Jabado et al., 1996) and high-dose glucocorticosteroids have been tested as potentially less toxic alternatives. Many investigators have taken the approach of leaving some T cells in the marrow, with or without the use of posttransplant immunosuppression to control GVHD (Ash et al., 1990; Soiffer et al., 1992; Nimer et al., 1994; Verdonck et al., 1994; van der Stratten et al., 2001). When this approach is used for transplantation from an HLA-identical sibling, the risk of graft failure can be as low as 3% with a 20% risk of clinically significant GVHD. Other studies have evaluated whether the risk of graft failure can be decreased by the use of HSC mobilized into the peripheral blood by treatment of the donor with recombinant human granulocyte colony-stimulating

Table 26.2. *Approaches for improving outcomes of TCD*

Improving graft failure
  Intensifying conditioning regimen
    Additional chemotherapy
    Antithymocyte globulin
    Increased total body irradiation
    Total lymphoid irradiation
  Simultaneous donor/host (in vitro/in vivo) TCD (e.g., Campath-1, ATG)
  Narrow specificity TCD
  Stem cell dose augmentation
    Megadose PBSC transplant
Restoring GVL activity
  Posttransplant immune modulation
    Delayed T-cell add-back, prophylactic DLI
    Low-dose interleukin-2
Prevention of EBV-LPD
  Combined T- and B-cell depletion
  Prophylactic administration of EBV-specific CTLs
  Early detection and administration of rituximab
Reducing GVHD rates
  Induction of host specific alloimmune tolerance
    Co-stimulatory signal blockade
  Functional TCD
    Selective depletion of allo-reactive T cells (e.g., anti-CD25, CD69)
  Elimination of genetically manipulated T cells
    Insertion of HSV-TK suicide gene

factor (G-CSF), granulocyte-macrophage (GM)-CSF, or other similar growth factors (Aversa et al., 1994). In many studies, hematopoietic growth factors have been administered after transplantation. Although such treatment can accelerate myeloid engraftment, effects on the incidence of graft failure remain uncertain. The biological interpretation of many published studies is hampered by the simultaneous incorporation of several approaches for avoiding graft failure. Future assessment of methods for overcoming this problem will require more carefully designed prospective studies.

Leukemic relapse

Associations between TCD and increased risk of posttransplant relapse have been widely recognized and reported both from single institutions and from marrow transplant registries. The most striking effects have been observed with HLA-identical marrow transplantation during the initial phase of chronic myeloid leukemia (CML) (Goldman et al., 1988), where patients transplanted with T-cell-depleted marrow have a fivefold increased risk of relapse compared to those transplanted with unmodified marrow (Marmont et al., 1991). In patients with CML, TCD shows a strong association with increased relapse risk even after adjusting for GVHD (Fig. 26.1). TCD is also associated with increased persistence of recipient myeloid cells in patients with diseases other than CML. Since hematopoiesis in CML origi-

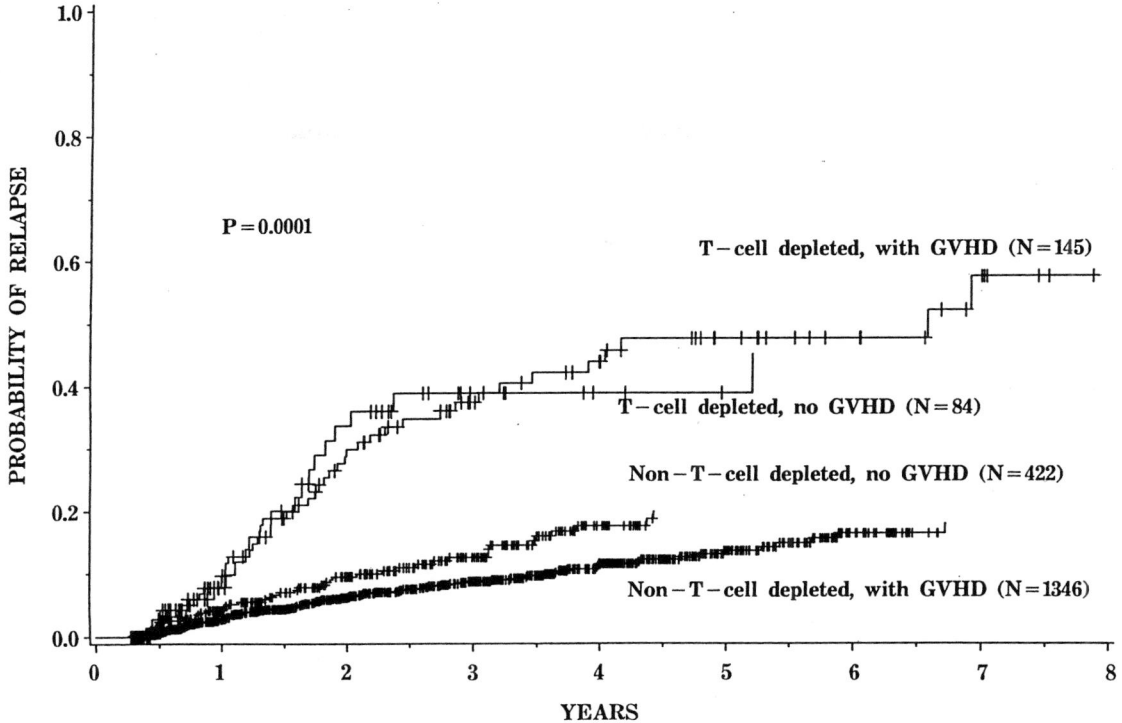

Fig. 26.1. Actuarial probability of relapse after T-cell-depleted and unmodified (i.e., T-replete) HLA-genotypically identical marrow transplantation for patients with stable phase CML who experienced any acute or chronic GVHD or who had no GVHD (IBMTR data).

nates from a clonal population of pluripotent stem cells that have largely replaced the normal population, the increased risk of CML relapse and the increased incidence of myeloid mixed chimerism suggest that malignant and normal HSC are highly susceptible to elimination by donor T cells. This notion is further supported by the observation that both leukemic cells and residual hematopoietic elements can be eliminated by DLI in patients who have relapsed after transplantation (Alyea *et al.*, 1998)

TCD has also been associated with an increased risk of relapse after HLA-identical transplantation in patients with acute leukemia (Horowitz *et al.*, 1990). The strength of this association has been comparable to that seen between GVHD and the reduced relapse risk in patients transplanted with unmodified marrow. Thus, the increased risk of relapse associated with TCD in patients with acute leukemia could simply reflect a decreased incidence of GVHD. Multivariate analyses have shown no association between TCD and relapse risk in patients with acute leukemia when adjustments are made for the development of GVHD (Marmont *et al.*, 1991). In some series of patients with AML, the risk of relapse has been reported to be very low despite a very low incidence of GVHD (Papadopoulos *et al.*, 1998). In contrast to AML, TCD shows a strong association with increased relapse risk even after adjusting for GVHD in patients with CML. In several series of unrelated or HLA-mismatched related transplantation, TCD has not been associated with a significantly

increased risk of relapse (Ash *et al.*, 1991; Hessner *et al.*, 1995; Lee *et al.*, 2002) (Fig. 26.2). This may reflect the increased risk of GVHD in this population compared to that in HLA matched related transplant recipients. GVHD, relapse, and nonrelapse mortality rates are clearly different after unrelated or TCD-BMT than after TCD-related transplantation (Alyea *et al.*, 2002; Fig. 26.3).

Several approaches have been proposed for avoiding the increased risk of recurrent malignancy associated with TCD (Table 26.2). With the use of intensified conditioning regimens, the benefit of decreased posttransplant relapse may be offset by increased regimen-related toxicity. Some investigators have suggested that the risk of GVHD can be decreased without increasing the risks of recurrent malignancy in CML patients by depleting CD8+ cells from the graft (Nimer *et al.*, 1994). It has been noted in several studies that T cells are less liable to cause GVHD when they are administered after inflammatory effects of the pretransplant conditioning regimen have subsided. These observations have led to suggestions that the risk of malignancy might be decreased by delayed (prophylactic) infusions of donor lymphocytes (Naparstek *et al.*, 1995; Lee *et al.*, 1999; Sehn *et al.*, 1999), especially in patients who have molecular-genetic evidence of persistent CML after T-cell-depleted transplantation (Mackinnon *et al.*, 1996). As an alternative approach, IL-2 has been administered after transplantation in order to test whether activation of T cells or natural killer (NK) cells might decrease the risk of relapse (Soiffer *et*

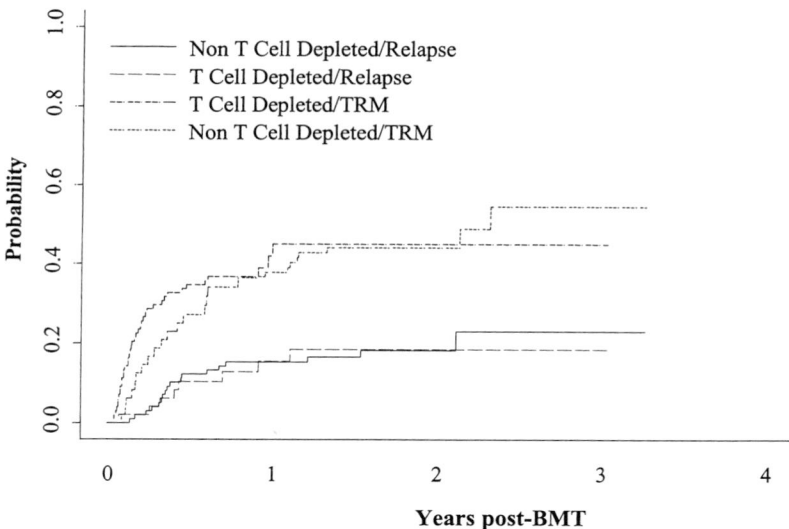

Fig. 26.2. Causes of treatment failure after T-cell-depleted and unmodified marrow transplantation from unrelated donors. The probability of transplant-related mortality and relapse are similar after TCD (anti-CD6 and complement) and non-TCD unrelated transplantation Reproduced, with permission, from Lee *et al.* (2002).

al., 1994). The success of these approaches has not yet been determined.

Immunologic reconstitution

Depletion of mature T cells from the donor marrow appears to have some effect on lymphoid reconstitution after transplantation. For example, the number of CD4+ cells begins to reach normal values at 10 to 12 months after T-cell-depleted transplantation, approximately 3 months later than seen in patients transplanted with unmodified marrow (Keever *et al.,* 1989). Recovery of lymphocyte function as measured by in

vitro assays is also somewhat delayed after T-cell-depleted transplantation. Proliferative responses to phytohemagglutinin begin to reach the normal range at approximately 10 to 12 months after transplantation, as opposed to 4 to 6 months in patients transplanted with unmodified marrow. Similarly, in vitro production of IgG showed recovery at 13 to 15 months as opposed to 7 to 9 months. During the first 6 months, more sensitive limiting dilution assays have shown lower precursor frequencies for cytotoxic and proliferating T cells in patients transplanted with T-cell-depleted marrow compared with those transplanted with unmodified marrow (Daley *et al.,* 1987).

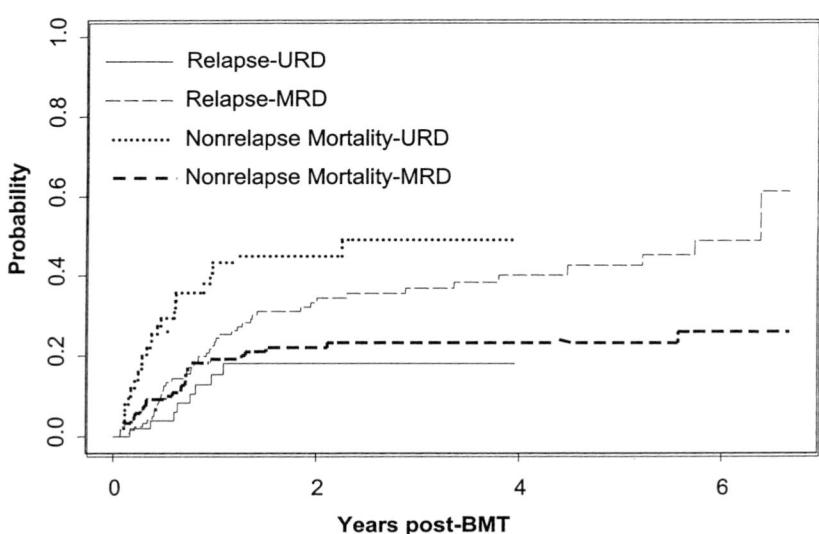

Fig. 26.3. Comparison of treatment failure in recipients of TCD marrow from matched related (MRD) and unrelated (URD) donors. Relapse rates are lower and transplant-related mortality higher after URD TCD (anti-CD6) BMT than after MRD TCD BMT. Reproduced, with permission, from Alyea *et al.* (2002).

TCD does not appear to increase the risk of bacterial or fungal infection after marrow transplantation if patients with graft failure are excluded, although a high incidence of adenoviral infection has been reported in patients given Campath-1H in vivo as part of the conditioning regimen (Chakrabarti *et al.*, 2002). In this study, severe lymphocytopenia (<300/μl) at the time of first detection of adenovirus was a major risk factor for the development of adenovirus disease, as was failure to reduce immune suppression and a positive adenovirus PCR result in blood. TCD does not detectably affect the risk of interstitial pneumonia (Marmont *et al.*, 1991). On the other hand, TCD is associated with an increased risk of lymphoproliferative disorders (LPD) caused by EBV infection (Bhatia *et al.*, 1996). The risk of this usually fatal complication appears to be greatest in patients transplanted with marrow from unrelated donors or from HLA-mismatched relatives. A potential strategy for the treatment of EBV-LPD has been adoptive immunotherapy using DLI. Papadapoulos *et al.* (1994) treated five patients with confirmed posttransplant EBV-LPD using infusions of unirradiated donor leukocytes and observed a 100% response. The therapeutic effect was attributed to the development of EBV-specific immunity mediated by cytotoxic lymphocytes (CTLs) present in the infusion. As an extension of this strategy, it has been demonstrated that administration of EBV-specific CTLs cultivated in vitro from donor lymphocytes is effective treatment of EBV-LPD (Heslop *et al.*, 1994) (see Chapter 88). For patients who are not candidates for DLI or EBV-specific CTL therapy, small case series have reported promising responses with the use of the anti-CD20 monoclonal antibody rituximab (Kuehnle *et al.*, 2000). B-cell depletion of the donor graft has been investigated as a strategy to

decrease the incidence of EBV-LPD after TCD BMT. Cavazzana-Calvo and colleagues. (1998) have shown that combined ex vivo depletion of B and T cells from the graft using monoclonal antibodies effectively prevented EBV-LPD and improved survival compared to control patients who received TCD grafts without B-cell purging. Polymerase chain reaction (PCR) methods to detect EBV DNA may be an effective means of diagnosing patients with EBV-LPD prior to the onset of clinically evident disease (Rooney *et al.*, 1995). As these and other methods of early detection improve, clinicians may now intervene with DLI or anti-CD20 at a stage of low disease burden, and perhaps alter the poor outcome often associated with this condition.

Current approaches for accelerating immune reconstitution after marrow transplantation remain limited. Clinical and experimental studies have indicated that initial reconstitution of T cells after transplantation occurs primarily through proliferation of mature T cells in the graft (Mackall et al., 1993; Storek *et al.*, 1995; Roux *et al.*, 1996). In particular, production of CD4+ cells through intrathymic differentiation of marrow progenitors is severely impaired in adults. For this reason, exhaustive depletion of CD4+ cells in the graft could lead to prolonged deficiency of CD4+ cells after transplantation, thereby increasing the risk of infections (Storek *et al.*, 1997). By the same token, delayed infusion of donor lymphocytes might accelerate immune reconstitution. For example, reconstitution of EBV-specific immunity can be accomplished with a relatively small number of donor lymphocytes (Lucas *et al.*, 1996). If large numbers of donor lymphocytes are administered, however, strategies for selective removal of T cells with specificity for recipient alloantigens might be needed in order to avoid

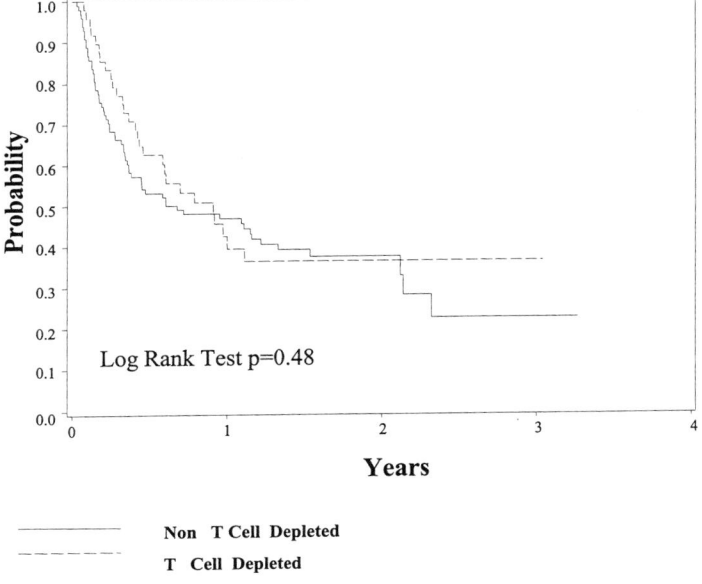

Fig. 26.4. Probability of event-free survival (EFS) after TCD and non-TCD BMT from unrelated donors. No difference in EFS was observed in 148 recipients undergoing TCD (*n* = 50) or non-TCD (*n* = 98) URD BMT between 1997 and 1999 at Dana Farber Cancer Institute. Reproduced, with permission, from Lee *et al.* (2002).

Table 26.3. *Advantages and disadvantages of TCD*

Advantages	Disadvantages
Low incidence of acute and chronic GVHD	Higher incidence of graft failure
Reduced or no requirement for posttransplant immune suppression as GVHD prophylaxis	Loss of GVL activity, leading to higher incidence of disease relapse, especially in CML
Decreased early transplant-related mortality	Delayed immune reconstitution
Decreased pulmonary, hepatic, and renal complications early after transplant	Increased risk for posttransplant EBV-associated lymphoproliferative disorder
Earlier engraftment and shorter duration of hospital stay	Higher incidence of CMV reactivation
Decreased cost	Overall survival not improved compared to non-TCD BMT

GVHD. Alternatively, reconstitution of immune response against specific pathogens can be accomplished through infusion of cloned T cells (Riddell & Greenberg, 1995). Immune reconstitution conceivably might also be accelerated by the administration of cytokines such as IL-7, which might promote thymocyte maturation in vivo.

Relapse-free survival

Originally, it was anticipated that the use of TCD would substantially decrease posttransplant morbidity by making it possible to omit prophylactic immune suppression and avoid the need for immune suppressive treatment in most patients. Indeed, in some series, TCD has been associated with a low incidence of severe organ toxicity, such as hepatic veno-occlu-

sive disease, renal failure, and diffuse alveolar hemorrhage (Soiffer *et al.*, 1991; Ho *et al.*, 2001). Overall, however, there is little or no evidence that TCD has improved relapse-free survival after marrow transplantation (Ash *et al.*, 1991; Marmont *et al.*, 1991; Champlin *et al.*, 2000; Lee *et al.*, 2002; Fig. 26.4). It appears that the increased risks of graft failure and relapse have offset the benefits of decreased GVHD (Table 26.3). The benefits of decreased morbidity afforded by TCD may be negated by the intensified conditioning sometimes used to avoid rejection or posttransplant relapse as well as by delays in immunologic recovery. For these reasons, TCD has not decreased transplant-related mortality in many studies. However, outcome after TCD transplantation is dependent on the method utilized for purging. In an IBMTR study of unrelated donor transplantation, the use of narrow specificity anti-T-cell antibodies was associated with better leukemia-free survival than the use of other techniques to deplete T cells from the stem cell inoculum, such as Campath 1 antibodies, conterflow centrifugal elutriation, and soybean lectin agglutination (Champlin *et al.*, 2000) (Fig. 26.5). In the future, expanded studies of narrow specificity antibodies, administration of immune effector cells to restore GVL activity, and pre-emptive measures to prevent complications from EBV will hopefully greatly improve overall disease-free survival after TCD transplantation.

Conclusions

In the 20 years since the first TCD transplants were performed, there remain no data to prove that TCD can lead to better overall survival compared to conventional BMT using pharmacologic agents for GVHD prophylaxis. Although outcomes after TCD transplantation have improved over the past decade from the use of selective TCD and adoptive immunotherapy, the role of TCD in transplantation remains undefined. Reasonable applications for TCD may include those patients at high risk

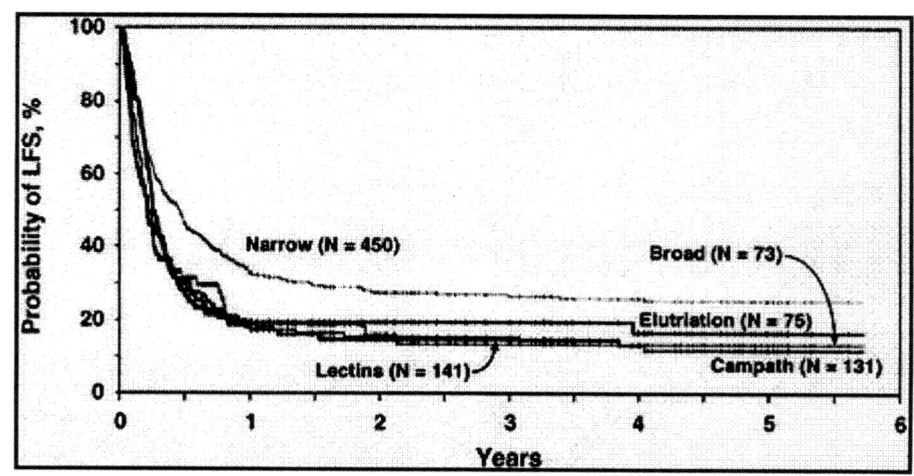

Fig. 26.5. Adjusted 5-year probabilities of leukemia-free survival (LFS) by TCD technique. Adjusted probability of LFS in patients undergoing TCD transplantation using narrow or broad specificity depletion techniques. Survival is superior in patients undergoing URD BMT in recipients of marrow depleted with narrow specificity antibodies. Reproduced, with permission, from Champlin *et al.* (2000).

for GVHD (unrelated or mismatched grafts), or patients with comorbid medical conditions who might have a high risk of complications after conventional HSCT. TCD may be ideal for patients with diseases where GVL activity is less critical, such as first remission acute leukemia. We still do not know what particular patient population would benefit most from TCD or what method should be used for purging. There have been no definitive randomized trials to date to help resolve these issues. In the future, studies will need to assess the potential role of TCD when mobilized peripheral blood stem cells are used for allogeneic transplantation, particularly with respect to their effect on chronic GVHD. It would be ideal to be able to manipulate different lymphoid subgroups responsible for GVHD and GVL, but whether these processes can be effectively separated at a clinical level remains unknown. Hopefully, as new immunologic targets of GVL, graft failure, and GVHD are identified, exciting opportunities will emerge that will enable researchers to tease these processes apart, and engineer grafts that will improve overall outcome after allogeneic HSCT.

References

Alyea, E.P., Soiffer, R.J., Canning, C. et al. (1998). Toxicity and efficacy of defined doses of CD4+ donor lymphocytes for treatment of relapse after allogeneic BMT. Blood, 91, 3671–80.

Anderson, K.C., Soiffer, R., Delage, R. et al. (1990). Monoclonal antibody purged autologous bone marrow transplantation therapy for T cell leukemia and lymphoma. Blood, 76, 235–44.

Ash, R.C., Casper, J.T., Chitambar, C.R. et al. (1990). Successful allogeneic transplantation of T-cell depleted bone marrow from closely HLA-matched unrelated donors. New England Journal of Medicine, 322, 485–94.

Ash, R.C., Horowitz, M.M., Gale, R.P. et al. (1991). Bone marrow transplantation from related donors other than HLA-identical siblings: effect of T cell depletion. Bone Marrow Transplantation, 7, 443–52.

Atkinson, K., Horowitz, M.M., Gale, R.P. et al. (1990). Risk factors for chronic graft-versus-host disease after HLA-identical sibling bone marrow transplantation. Blood, 75, 2459–64.

Aversa, F., Tabilio, A., Terenzi, A. et al. (1994). Successful engraftment of T-cell-depleted haploidentical "three-loci" incompatible transplants in leukemia patients by addition of recombinant human granulocyte colony-stimulating factor-mobilized peripheral blood progenitor cells to bone marrow inoculum. Blood, 84, 3948–55.

Aversa, F., Tabilio, A., Velardi, A. et al. (1998). Treatment of high-risk acute leukemia with T-cell-depleted stem cells from related donors with one fully mismatched HLA haplotype. New England Journal of Medicine, 339, 1186–94.

Bhatia, S., Ramsay, N.K., Steinbuch, M. et al. (1996). Malignant neoplasms following bone marrow transplantation. Blood, 87, 3633–9.

Cavazzana-Calvo, M., Bensoussan, D., Jabado, N. et al. (1998). Prevention of EBV-induced B-lymphoproliferative disorder by ex vivo marrow B-cell depletion in HLA-phenoidentical or non-identical T-depleted bone marrow transplantation. British Journal of Haematology, 103, 543–8.

Chakrabarti, S., Mautner, V., Osman, H. et al. (2002). Adenovirus infections following allogeneic stem cell transplantation: incidence and outcome in relation to graft manipulation, immunosuppression and immune recovery. Blood, 100, 1619–27.

Champlin, R., Ho, W., Gajewski, J. et al. (1990). Selective depletion of CD8+ T lymphocytes for prevention of graft-versus-host disease after allogeneic bone marrow transplantation. Blood, 76, 418.

Champlin, R.E., Horowitz, M.M., van Bekkum, D.W. et al. (1989). Graft failure following bone marrow transplantation for severe aplastic anemia: risk factors and treatment results. Blood, 73, 606–13.

Champlin, R.E., Passweg, J.R., Zhang, M.J. et al. (2000). T cell depletion of bone marrow transplants for leukemia from donors other than HLA-identical siblings: advantages of T-cell antibodies with narrow specificities. Blood, 95, 3996–4003.

Cottler-Fox, M., Cipolone, K., Uyu, M. et al. (1995). Positive selection of CD34+ hematopoietic cells using an immunoaffinity column results in T cell depletion equivalent to elutriation. Experimental Hematology, 23, 320–2.

Daley, J.P., Rozans, M.K., Smith, B.R. et al. (1987). Retarded recovery of functional T cell frequencies in T cell-depleted bone marrow transplant recipients. Blood, 70, 960–4.

Gaderet, L., Snell, V., Przepiorka, D. et al. (1999). Effective depletion of alloreactive lymphocytes from peripheral blood mononuclear cell preparations. Transplantation, 67, 124–30.

Giralt, S., Hester, J., Huh, Y. et al. (1995). CD8-depleted lymphocyte infusion as treatment for relapsed chronic myelogenous leukemia after allogeneic bone marrow transplantation. Blood, 86, 4337–43.

Goldman, J.M., Gale, R.P., Horowitz, M.M. et al. (1988). Bone marrow transplantation for chronic myelogenous leukemia in chronic phase: increased risk of relapse associated with T cell-depletion. Annals of Internal Medicine, 108, 806–14.

Guimond, M., Balassy, A., Barrette, M. et al. (2002). P-glycoprotein targeting: a unique strategy to selectively eliminate immunoreactive T cells. Blood, 100, 375–82.

Guinan, E.A., Boussiotis, V.A., Neuberg, D. et al. (1999). Transplantation of anergic histoincompatible bone marrow allografts. New England Journal of Medicine, 340, 1704–14.

Hale, G. & Waldmann, H. (1994). Control of graft-versus-host disease and graft rejection by T cell depletion of donor and recipient with Campath-1 antibodies. Results of matched sibling transplants for malignant diseases. Bone Marrow Transplantation, 13, 597–611.

Hale, G., Jacobs, P., Wood, L. et al. (2000). CD52 antibodies for prevention of graft-versus-host disease and graft rejection following transplantation of allogeneic peripheral blood stem cells. Bone Marrow Transplantation, 26, 69–75.

Harris, D.T., Sakiestewa, D., Lyons, C. et. al. (1999). Prevention of graft-versus-host disease (GVHD) by elimination of recipient-reactive donor T cells with recombinant toxins that target the interleukin 2 (IL-2) receptor. Bone Marrow Transplantation, 23, 137–44.

Heslop, H.E., Brenner, M.K., Rooney, C. et al. (1994). Administration of neomycin-resistance-gene-marked EBV-specific cytotoxic T lymphocytes to recipients of mismatched-related or phenotypically similar unrelated donor marrow grafts. Human Gene Therapy, 5, 381, 1994.

Hessner, M.J., Endean, D.J., Casper, J.T. *et al.* (1995). Use of unrelated marrow grafts compensates for reduced graft-versus-leukemia reactivity after T-cell-depleted allogeneic marrow transplantation for chronic myelogenous leukemia. *Blood,* **86,** 3987–96.

Ho, V., Weller, E. Lee, S. *et al.* (2001). Prognostic factors for severe pulmonary complications after hematopoietic stem cell transplantation. *Biology of Blood and Marrow Transplantation,* **7,** 223–9.

Ho, V.T. & Soiffer, R.J. (2001). The history and future of T-cell depletion as graft-versus-host disease prophylaxis for allogeneic hematopoietic stem cell transplantation. *Blood,* **98,** 3192–204.

Horowitz, M.M., Gale, R.P., Sondel, P.M. *et al.* (1990). Graft-versus-leukemia reactions after bone marrow transplantation. *Blood,* **75,** 555–62.

Jabado, N., LeDeist, F., Cant, A. *et al.* (1996). Bone marrow transplantation from genetically HLA-nonidentical donors in children with fatal inherited disorders excluding severe combined immunodeficiencies: use of two monoclonal antibodies to prevent graft rejection. *Pediatrics,* **98,** 420–8.

Jansen, J., Hanks, S., Akard, L. *et al.* (1995). Selective T cell depletion with CD8-conjugated magnetic beads in the prevention of graft-versus-host disease after allogeneic bone marrow transplantation. *Leukemia,* **9,** 271–8.

Jansen, J., Hanks, S., Akard, L.P. *et al.* (1996). Immunomagnetic CD4$^+$ and CD8$^+$ cell depletion for patients at high-risk for severe acute GVHD. *Bone Marrow Transplantation,* **17,** 377–8.

Kawanishi, Y., Passweg, J., Drobyski, W.R. *et al.* (1997). Effect of T cell subset dose on outcome of T cell-depleted bone marrow transplantation. *Bone Marrow Transplantation,* **19,** 1069–77.

Keever, C.A., Small, T.N., Flomenberg, N. *et al.* (1989). Immune reconstitution following bone marrow transplantation: comparison of recipients of T cell-depleted marrow with recipients of conventional marrow grafts. *Blood,* **73,** 1340–50.

Kernan, N.A., Collins, N.M., Juliano, L. *et al.* (1986). Clonable T lymphocytes in T cell-depleted bone marrow transplants correlate with development of graft-v-host disease. *Blood,* **68,** 770–3.

Klangsinsirikul, P., Carter, G.I., Byrne, J.L. *et al.* (2002). Campath-1G causes rapid depletion of circulating host dendritic cells (DCs) before allogeneic transplantation but does not delay donor DC reconstruction. *Blood,* **99,** 2586–91.

Koh, M.B.C., Prentice, H.G., & Lowdell, M.W. (1999). Selective removal of alloreactive cells from haematopoietic stem cell grafts: graft engineering for GVHD prophylaxis. *Bone Marrow Transplantation,* **23,** 1071–9.

Koh, M.B.C., Prentice, H.G., Corbo, M. *et al.* (2002). Alloantigen-specific T-cell depletion in a major histocompatibility complex fully mismatched murine model provides effective graft-versus-host disease prophylaxis in the presence of lymphoid engraftment. *British Journal of Haematology,* **118,** 108–16.

Kuehnle, I., Huls, M.H., Liu, Z. *et al.* (2000). CD20 monoclonal antibody (rituximab) for therapy of Epstein-Barr virus lymphoma after hemopoietic stem-cell transplantation. *Blood,* **95,** 1502–8.

Lee, C.-K., Gingrich, R.D., deMagalhaes-Silverman, M. *et al.* (1999). Prophylactic reinfusion of T cells for T cell-depleted allogeneic bone marrow transplantation. *Biology of Blood and Marrow Transplantation,* **5,** 15–27.

Lee, S.J., Zahrieh, D., Alyea, E.P. *et al.* (2002). Comparison of T-cell depleted and non-T-cell depleted unrelated donor transplantation for hematologic diseases: clinical outcomes, quality of life, and costs. *Blood,* **100,** 2697–702.

Lucas, K.G., Small, T.N., Heller, G. *et al.* (1996). The development of cellular immunity to Epstein-Barr virus after allogeneic bone marrow transplantation. *Blood,* **87,** 2594–603.

Mackall, C.L., Granger, L., Sheard, M.A. *et al.* (1993). T-cell regeneration after bone marrow transplantation: differential CD45 isoform expression on thymic-derived versus thymic-independent progeny. *Blood,* **82,** 2585–94.

Mackinnon, S., Barnett, L., & Heller, G. (1996). Polymerase chain reaction is highly predictive of relapse in patients following T cell-depleted allogeneic bone marrow transplantation for chronic myeloid leukemia. *Bone Marrow Transplantation,* **17,** 643–7.

Marmont, A.M., Horowitz, M.M., Gale, R.P. *et al.* (1991). T-cell depletion of HLA-identical transplants in leukemia. *Blood,* **78,** 2120–30.

Martin, P.J. (1993). Donor CD8 cells prevent allogeneic marrow graft rejection in mice: potential implications for marrow transplantation in humans. *Journal of Experimental Medicine,* **178,** 703–12.

Martin, P.J. & Kernan, N.A. (1996). T cell depletion for the prevention of graft-versus-host disease in man. In *Graft Versus Host Disease: Research and Clinical Management,* ed. S. Burakoff, H.J. Deeg, & J. Ferrara, pp. 615–37. New York: Dekker.

Mavroudis, D.A., Jiang, Y.-Z., Hensel, N. *et al.* (1996a). Specific depletion of alloreactivity against haplotype mismatched related individuals with immunotoxin: a new approach to graft-versus-host disease prophylaxis in haploidentical bone marrow transplantation. *Bone Marrow Transplantation,* **17,** 793–9.

Mavroudis, D., Read, D., Cottler-Fox, M. *et al.* (1996b). CD34$^+$ cell dose predicts survival, posttransplant morbidity, and rate of hematologic recovery after allogeneic marrow transplants for hematologic malignancy. *Blood,* **88,** 3223–9.

Muller, S.M., Schulz, A.S., Reiss, U.M. *et al.* (1999). Definition of a critical T cell threshold for prevention of GVHD after HLA nonidentical PBPC transplantation in children. *Bone Marrow Transplantation,* **24,** 575–81.

Nagler, A., Condiotti, R., Nabet, C. *et al.* (1998). Selective CD4$^+$ T-cell depletion does not prevent graft-versus-host disease. *Transplantation,* **66,** 138–41.

Naparstek, E., Or, R., Nagler, A. *et al.* (1995). T-cell-depleted allogeneic bone marrow transplantation for acute leukaemia using Campath-1 antibodies and posttransplant administration of donor's peripheral blood lymphocytes for prevention of relapse. *British Journal of Haematology,* **89,** 506–15.

Nimer, S.D., Giorgi, J., Gajewski, J.L. *et al.* (1994). Selective depletion of CD8+ cells for prevention of graft-versus-host disease after bone marrow transplantation. *Transplantation,* **57,** 82–7.

Papadapoulos, E.B., Ladanyi, M., Emmanuel, D. *et al.* (1994). Infusions of donor leukocytes to treat Epstein-Barr-associated lymphoproliferative disorders after allogeneic bone marrow transplantation. *New England Journal of Medicine,* **330,** 1185–94.

Papadopoulos, E.B., Carabasi, M.H., Castro-Malaspina, H. *et al.* (1998). T-cell-depleted allogeneic bone marrow transplantation as postremission therapy for acute myelogenous leukemia: freedom from relapse in the absence of graft-versus-host disease. *Blood,* **91,** 1083–1190.

Ratzinger, G., Reagan, J.L., Heller, G. et al. (2003). Differential CD52 expression by distinct myeloid dendritic cell subsets: implications for alemtuzumab activity at the level of antigen presentation in allogeneic graft-host interactions in transplantation. Blood, 101, 1422–9.

Riddell, S.R. & Greenberg, P.D. (1995). Principles for adoptive T cell therapy of human viral diseases. Annual Review of Immunology, 13, 545–86.

Rooney, C.M., Loftin, S.K., Holladay, M.S. et al. (1995). Early identification of Epstein-Barr virus-associated post-transplantation lymphoproliferative disease. British Journal of Haematology, 89, 98–104.

Roux, E., Helg, C., Dumont-Girard, R. et al. (1996). Analysis of T-cell repopulation after allogeneic bone marrow transplantation: significant differences between recipients of T-cell depleted and unmanipulated grafts. Blood, 87, 3984–92.

Sehn, L.H., Alyea, E.P., Weller, E. et al. (1999). Comparative outcomes of T-cell-depleted and non-T-cell-depleted allogeneic bone marrow transplantation for chronic myelogenous leukemia: impact of donor lymphocyte infusion. Journal of Clinical Oncology, 17, 561–8.

Soiffer, R.J., Dear, K., Rabinowe, S.N. et al. (1991). Hepatic dysfunction following T cell depleted allogeneic bone marrow transplantation. Transplantation, 52, 1014–19.

Soiffer, R.J., Fairclough, D., Robertson, M. et al. (1997). CD6-depleted allogeneic bone marrow transplantation for acute leukemia in first complete remission. Blood, 89, 3039–47.

Soiffer, R.J., Mauch, P., Fairclough, D. et al. (1997). CD6+ T cell depleted allogeneic bone marrow transplantation from genotypically HLA non-identical related donors. Biology of Blood and Marrow Transplantation, 3, 11–7.

Soiffer, R.J., Murray, C., Gonin, R., & Ritz, J. (1994). Effect of low-dose interleukin-2 on disease relapse after T-cell-depleted allogeneic bone marrow transplantation. Blood, 84, 964–71.

Soiffer, R.J., Murray, C., Mauch, P. et al. (1992). Prevention of graft-versus-host disease by selective depletion of CD6-positive T lymphocytes from donor marrow. Journal of Clinical Oncology, 10, 1191–200.

Storek, J., Gooley, T., Witherspoon, R.P. et al. (1997). Infectious morbidity in long-term survivors of allogeneic marrow transplantation is associated with low CD4 T cell counts. American Journal of Hematology, 54, 131–8.

Storek, J., Witherspoon, R.P., & Storb, R. (1995). T cell reconstitution after bone marrow transplantation into adult patients does not resemble T cell development in early life. Bone Marrow Transplantation, 16, 413–25.

Tiberghien, P., Ferrand, C. et al. (2001). Administration of herpes simplex-thymidine kinase-expressing donor cells with a T-cell depleted allogeneic marrow graft. Blood, 97, 63–72.

Urbano-Ispizua, A., Solano, C., Brunet, S. et al. (1998). Allogeneic transplantation of selected CD34+ cells from peripheral blood: experience of 62 cases using immunoadsorption or immunomagnetic technique. Spanish Group of Allo-PBT. Bone Marrow Transplantation, 22, 519–26.

van der Stratten, H.M., Fijnheer, R., Dekker, A.W. et al. (2001). Relationship between graft-versus-host disease and graft-versus-leukemia in partial T cell-depleted bone marrow transplantation. British Journal of Haematology, 114, 31–5.

Van Dijk, A.M.C., de Gast, G.C., Gijsbert, C. et al. (1999). Selective depletion of major and minor histocompatibility antigen reactive T cells: towards prevention of acute graft-versus-host disease. British Journal of Haematology, 107, 169–75.

Verdonck, L.F., Dekker, A.W., de Gast, G.C. et al. (1994). Allogeneic bone marrow transplantation with a fixed low number of T cells in the marrow graft. Blood, 83, 3090–6.

27 Use of purified stem and progenitor cells for transplantation

CURT I. CIVIN, RUPERT HANDGRETINGER, AND ALVARO URBANO-ISPIZUA

Sidney Kimmel Comprehensive Cancer Center at Johns Hopkins, Baltimore, USA; St. Jude Children's Research Hospital, Memphis, USA; and Hospital Clinic of Barcelona, Barcelona, Spain

Introduction

The availability of new technologies and strategies to engineer the cell content of human lympho-hematopoietic stem-progenitor cell grafts has expanded the use, and potentially the efficacy, of transplantation in the treatment of a spectrum of malignant or hereditary, hematologic and autoimmune diseases. Specifically, clinically applicable technologies for immunoaffinity "positive" selection of CD34+ cells have been developed. CD34 positive selection has been used to deplete tumor cells from grafts for autologous transplantation in cancer, to deplete T cells for allogeneic transplantation, and to enrich stem-progenitor cells for gene therapy and ex vivo expansion strategies. This chapter summarizes the most relevant biology of the CD34 molecule and stem-progenitor cells, then describes clinical results using purified CD34+ stem-progenitor cells for lympho-hematopoietic transplantation.

CD34 molecular structure and monoclonal antibodies

CD34 is the International Workshop cluster designation (CD) for many (over 50) monoclonal antibodies recognizing the human cell membrane molecule detected by the prototype My 10 monoclonal antibody (Civin *et al.*, 1984, 1989; Tindle *et al.*, 1985; Andrews, Singer, & Bernstein, 1986; for review, see Krause *et al.*, 1996; Zhou *et al.*, 2001). These antibodies identify different epitopes of the monomeric integral cell membrane CD34 phosphoglycoprotein (Fig. 27.1.) (Civin *et al.*, 1989). The CD34 molecule is heavily glycosylated, with *N*- and *O*-linked sugars. High sialic acid content confers a strong net negative charge to the CD34 molecule and causes the CD34 molecule to migrate anomalously, with a relative mobility approximately 105 to 115 kilodaltons (kD) on SDS-polyacrylamide gel electrophoresis (Civin *et al.*, 1984). However, based on the CD34 cDNA sequence, the predicted actual molecular weight of the core polypeptide is only approximately 40 kD. The mouse and human CD34 genes have been molecularly cloned and sequenced (Brown, Greaves, & Molgaard, 1991; Simmons *et al.*, 1992; Zhou *et al.*, 2001). The lq32 chromoso-

mal location of the CD34 gene in humans is not a frequent site of alteration in leukemias or solid tumors. These murine and human CD34 cDNA sequences were without significant homology to other already sequenced genes until the identification of two homologs, podocalyxin (Doyonnas *et al.*, 2001) and endoglycan (Sasseti *et al.*, 2000). Each member of this new "CD34 family" of molecules is implicated in cell-cell adhesion (see below).

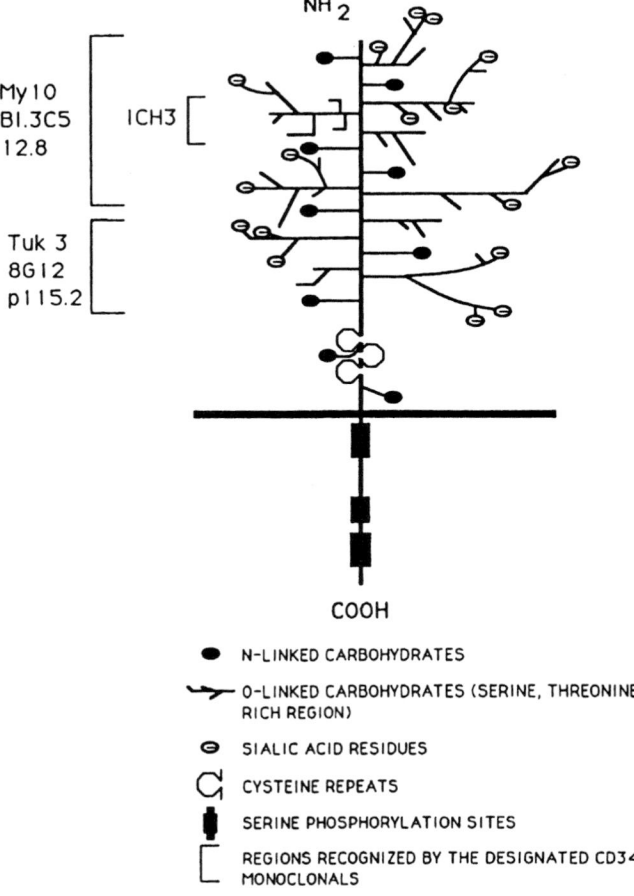

Fig. 27.1. Predicted structure of the human CD34 antigen.

A rat monoclonal antibody against mouse CD34 facilitates study of the CD34 molecule and CD34-defined cell subsets in mouse models (Osawa et al., 1996), and a mouse monoclonal antibody against canine CD34 allows similar studies in dog models (Hagglund et al., 2000). Certain monoclonal antibodies against human CD34 epitopes bind to CD34 of nonhuman primates, permitting transplantation experiments in these species utilizing certain mouse anti-human CD34 monoclonal antibodies. The CD34 molecule is distinct from a new marker for human hematopoietic stem and progenitor cells, CD133, identified by monoclonal antibody AC133 (Miraglia et al., 1997; Yin et al., 1997; Mason et al., 2001) (Figs. 27.2 and 27.3), which has also been used to positively select hematopoietic stem and progenitor cells for transplantation (Koehl et al., 2002).

Function of the CD34 molecule

Attempts to block hematopoietic cell proliferation and differentiation with multiple CD34 antibodies were unrewarding (Civin et al., 1989). The intracellular tail of the molecule is a target for phosphorylation by activated protein kinase C and other protein kinases (Fackler et al., 1990, 1992), suggesting that CD34 plays a role in cellular signal transduction. The highly charged N-terminal extracellular portion of the CD34 molecule shares some biochemical features with the leukosialin family of cell surface glycoproteins. Some determinants on the CD34 molecule are involved in signal transduction and can enhance adhesiveness of CD34$^+$ cell lines (Majdic et al., 1994). Fackler et al. (1995) found that forced expression of full-length mouse CD34 could partially block differentiation of the M1 myeloid leukemic cell line. In additon, an alloantigen-presenting function has been described for human CD34$^+$ cells (Rondelli et al., 1996).

Knockout mice with disrupted CD34 developed normally, although subtle hematopoietic defects were described (Cheng et al., 1996; Suzuki et al., 1996). Perhaps another CD34 family member, endoglycan or podocalyxin, can substitute for CD34 in CD34 knockout mice, or perhaps some other compensatory mechanisms are at play. CD34 and podocalyxin are expressed on endothelial cells of high endothelial venules (HEV), where they can bind to L-selectin on lymphocytes. Thus, both CD34 and podocalyxin function in homing of lymphocytes to HEV (Baumhueter et al., 1993). It also has been suggested that highly negatively charged CD34 and podocalyxin can act like "Teflon™" to allow adjacent endothelial cells to spread apart and permit leukocyte diapedesis (Delia et al., 1993; Doyonnas et al., 2001). Thus, CD34 may be involved in adhesive and/or repellant cell-cell interactions. However, the sugars on the CD34 expressed by non-HEV endothelial cells or hematopoietic stem-progenitor cells do not bind leukocyte L-selectin (Satomaa et al., 2002). In summary, despite the availability of monoclonal antibodies and cDNA clones for CD34 in multiple species, knockout mice, the widespread use of CD34 to identify or isolate stem-progenitor cells in thousands of patients, and over 7,000 publications on CD34, the function of the CD34 molecule remains cryptic. Explication of the exact molecular

interactions may require investigation of cell type-specific CD34 glycoforms.

CD34 expression in normal human tissues

CD34 antigen expression is restricted to approximately 1.5% of aspirated normal human bone marrow mononuclear cells, 0.1% or less of normal adult peripheral blood cells, and approximately 0.5% of cord blood cells or mobilized peripheral blood stem-progenitor cells (PBSC) (Civin et al., 1984; Tindle et al., 1985). The CD34$^+$ cell population, as isolated by fluorescence-activated cell sorting or other methodologies, consists morphologically of blast cells and other immature cellular elements such as "young lymphoid" cells, early promyelocytes, promonocytes, and "young" megakaryocytes (Civin et al., 1984; Ryan et al., 1986; Civin & Loken, 1987). CD34$^+$ cells include essentially all the in vitro assayed human hematopoietic progenitor cells [colony-forming unit (CFU)-blast, CFU-granulocyte-macrophage (GM), CFU-megakaryocyte (MK), CFU-mix, and burst forming unit-erythroid (BFU-E)]. Thus, the CD34 antigen is selectively expressed on progenitor cells of all human lympho-hematopoietic lineages, but not on mature human B- or T-lymphoid cells, natural killer cells, dendritic cells, monocytes, granulocytes, erythrocytes, platelets, basophils, or mast cells (Table 27.1; Fig. 27.4). Human stem-progenitor cells express on average approximately 50,000 CD34 surface molecules per cell, with the highest expression on the earliest CD34$^+$/CD38$^-$/lineage antigen$^-$ cells (Civin et al., 1996a). Endothelial cells and the precursors of osteoclasts and dendritic cells (derived from CFU-GM) also express CD34 (Beschorner et al., 1985; Fina et al., 1990). The CD34$^+$ cell population can be subdivided into functionally distinct progenitor populations, based on expression of other lympho-hematopoietic "lineage" antigens, such as CD33, CD19, CD3, CD7, and CD41. Lineage antigens are co-expressed on about 50% of CD34$^+$ marrow cells (Civin, 1990) (Table 27.2). For example, early CD34$^+$ cells (e.g., CFU-blast and long-term culture initiating cells) are CD34$^+$/CD33$^-$, while more committed granulocytic or monocytic progenitor cells are CD34$^+$/CD33$^+$. Committed B-lymphoid precursors co-express CD34 with CD10, CD19, and intranuclear terminal deoxynucleotidyl transferase (TdT). Committed T lymphoid or megakaryoblastic progenitors co-express CD5/CD7 or CD41/CD61, respectively (Gore, Kastan, & Civin, 1991). CD34$^+$ cells express only low levels of HLA-DR. The cells that provide sustained, retransplantable, multilineage engraftment in immunodeficient animals are CD34$^+$/CD38$^-$ (Civin et al., 1996a). This rare CD34$^+$/CD38$^-$ population accounts for only approximately 1% to 10% of CD34$^+$ cells and does not contain cells expressing lineage antigens. CD34$^+$/CD38$^-$ cells occur at a frequency of approximately 1:10,000 in human marrow, approaching the estimated frequency of the stem cell, but are definitely not a pure population of stem cells. Other markers, such as CD90 (Thy-1) and FLT3, further subdivide the CD34$^+$/CD38$^-$ cell population (Baum et al., 1992; Small et al., 1994).

A

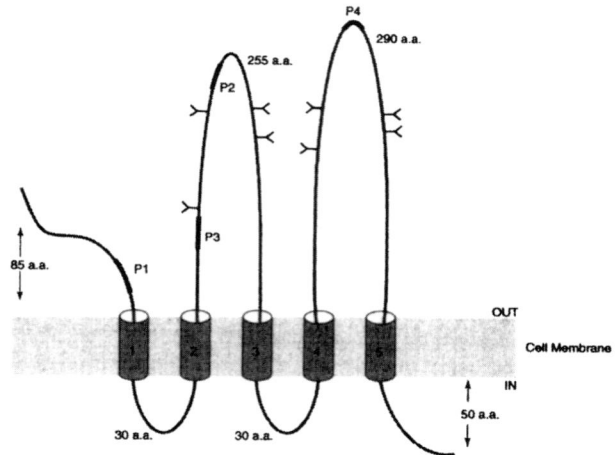

B

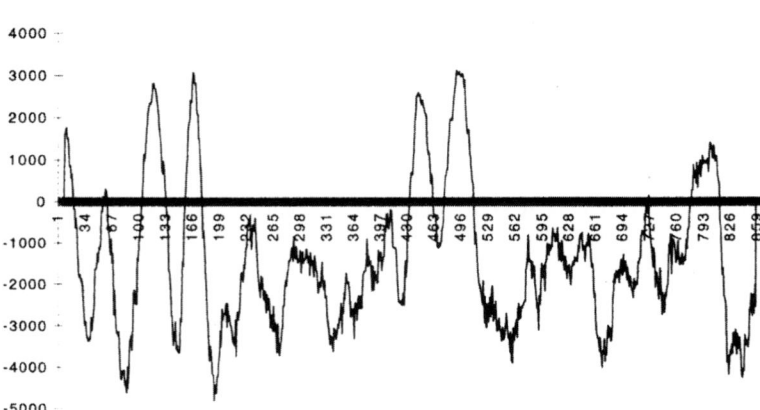

C

Fig. 27.2. Sequence analysis of AC133 antigen. (**A**) Sequence of AC133 antigen cDNA. The 5-TM domains are underlined, the 8 *N*-linked glycosylation sites are in boxes (the seventh and eighth glycosylation sites are in 1 larger box; dashed lines indicate where they overlap), and the polyadenylation signal is in a small box. (**B**) Hydrophobicity analysis of the AC133 antigen protein sequence. The hydrophobic signal peptide is notable along with 5 very hydrophobic TM domains. The last TM domain contains a single lysine in the middle of the TM sequence. (**C**) Graphic of the proposed structural model of AC133 antigen. This protein is modeled as having an extracellular N-terminus, a cytoplasmic C-terminus (containing 5 tyrosine residues), 2 small cysteine-rich cytoplasmic loops, and 2 very large extracellular loops each containing 4 consensus sequences for *N*-linked glycosylation. The position of the 4 original peptides is indicated in bold. Reproduced, with permission, from Miraglia *et al.* (1997).

In humans, the CD34⁻ marrow cell population is severely depleted of progenitor cells, except for the most mature unipotent colony-forming cells, for example CFU-erythroid (CFU-E), which may express low levels of CD34. CD34 expression is lost as cells mature beyond the progenitor cell compartment. Thus, CD34 is a lympho-hematopoietic stem-progenitor stage-specific, leukocyte differentiation antigen. Thus it was surprising when it was found that substantial fractions of engrafting mouse stem cells appeared to express low (or zero) amounts of CD34 (Osawa *et al.*, 1996; Ogawa, 2002). However, fewer than 1% of the human cells with the ability to engraft in nonobese diabetic mice with severe immunodeficiency (NOD/SCID), were CD34⁻ (Bhatia *et al.*, 1997), and the finding of human CD34⁻ stem cells has been questioned by other studies using NOD/SCID mice (Gao *et al.*, 2001), as well as by data from nonhuman primate transplantation models (Andrews *et al.*, 2000). Molecular studies have shown that the regulation of CD34 gene transcription is strikingly different in mice versus humans, potentially explaining much of the above controversy (Okuno *et al.*, 2002). Thus, while there may be a potential reservoir of stem cell capacity in the human CD34- cell subset, this population may be very small; it remains to conclusively isolate these cells and determine their unique phenotype, frequency, precise levels of CD34 expression, and position on the developmental hematopoietic map.

The expression of CD34 on hematopoietic stromal cell progenitors is controversial, and may reflect undefined subsets of stromal cell progenitors. Some mesenchymal stem cells reside in the bone marrow, but these are generally thought to be CD34⁻ cells that are discrete from the population of CD34⁺ hematopoietic stem-progenitor cells (Pittenger *et al.*, 1999). Even more interesting, the cells that we identify as restricted "lympho-hematopoietic" stem cells appear to be far more "plastic" (i.e., flexible in differentiation potential) than we had thought. There are multiple studies in mice and humans that highly purified or even single "lympho-hematopoietic" stem cells can generate cells in tissues as diverse as liver, lung, skin, and gut (e.g., Lagasse *et al.*, 2000; Krause *et al.*, 2001). Still at issue is whether clinically useful numbers of these non-lympho-hematopoeitic cells can be developed from this accessible adult stem cell source (Abkowitz, 2002).

CD34 expression in human malignancies

CD34⁺ malignancies (Table 27.3; for review see Silvestri *et al.*, 1992; Krause *et al.*, 1996) include approximately 40% of acute myeloid leukemias (AML) (many FAB M1 or M2 cases, most cases of AML following myelodysplasia, and most cases of AML with the 8;21 translocation) and approximately 70% of B-lineage acute lymphoblastic leukemias (ALL) (Tindle *et al.*, 1985). However, CD34 is expressed on a minority of T-cell ALL cases (~5–20%). CD34 may be expressed on approximately 5% of the blood cells in chronic phase chronic myeloid leukemia: the number of CD34⁺ blood cells increases with progression from the chronic to the accelerated and blast phases. The cells capable of initiating human AML (except FAB M3 cases) in NOD/SCID mice were exclusively CD34⁺/CD38⁻ (Bonnet & Dick, 1997).

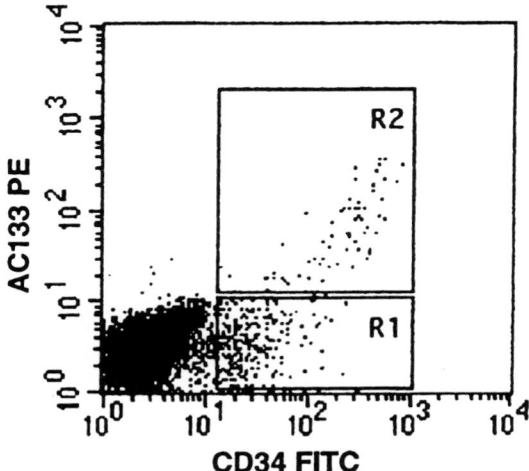

Fig. 27.3. AC133 expression on fetal liver cells. Fetal liver mononuclear cells were stained with AC133PE (vertical axis) and CD34FITC (horizontal axis) as described. CD34^bright/AC133⁺ cells are seen in region R2. The gates R1 and R2 are representative of those used in selection of bone marrow CD34/AC133 subpopulations for in vitro colony assays. Reproduced, with permission, from Yin *et al.* (1997).

Table 27.1. *Normal cells expressing CD34*

Lymphohematopoietic progenitor cells (including pluripotent stem cells, T and B lymphoid, myeloid, erythroid, and megakaryocytic cells, fibroblasts, osteoclasts, and stromal progenitor cells)
Endothelial cells (most highly expressed on small vessel endothelium)
Fetal endothelial cells and fibroblasts
Brain tissue [cell type(s) not yet determined]

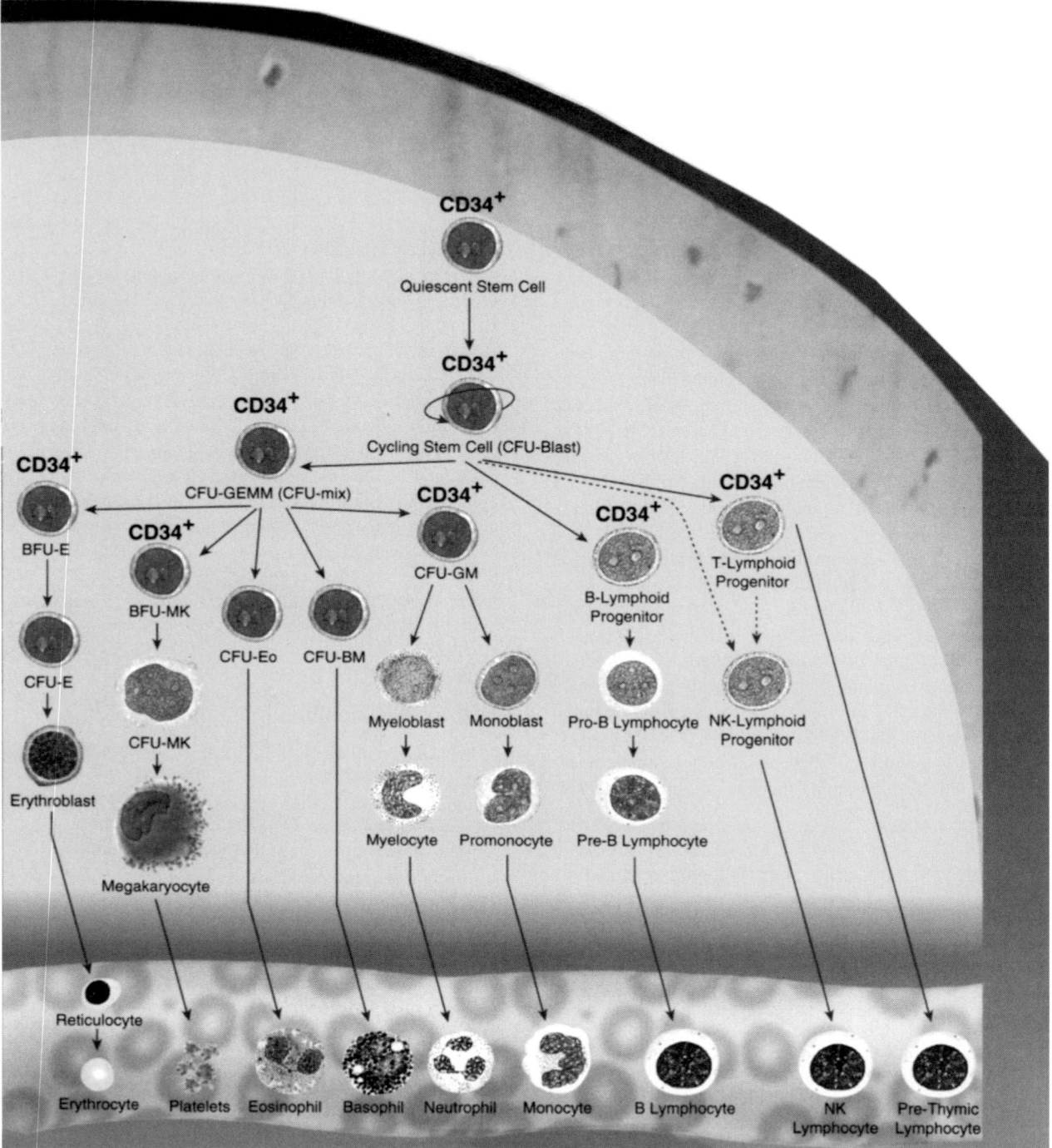

Fig. 27.4. CD34 antigen expression on normal tissues. Abbreviations: BFU-E, burst forming unit-erythroid; BFU-MK, BFU-megakaryocyte; CFU-BM, colony forming unit-basophil/mast cell; CFU-E, CFU-erythroid; CFU-Eo, CFU-eosinophil; CFU-GEMM, CFU-granulocyte/erythroid/macrophage/megakaryocyte; CFU-GM, CFU-granulocyte/macrophage; CFU-MK, CFU-megakaryocyte; →, actual relationship; -→, potential relationship. For color reproduction, see Color Plate 27.4.

Table 27.2. *Immune phenotype of early stem cells and lineage-committed progenitor cells*

Subpopulation	Immune phenotype			
Early stem cell	CD34+	CDW90+	CD33−	CD38−
Myeloid-committed progenitor	CD34+	CD13+ CD33+	CD38+	CD117+
Erythroid-committed progenitor	CD34+	CD71+	CD117+	
Megakaryocyte-committed progenitor	CD34+	CD38+ CD41+	CD61+	CD117+
T-lymphoid-committed progenitor	CD34+	CD5+	CD7+	CD38+
B-lymphoid-committed progenitor	CD34+	CD10+ CD19+	CD38+	

Hodgkin's and non-Hodgkin's lymphomas, chronic lymphatic leukemia (CLL), and multiple myeloma consist predominantly of CD34− cells (Berenson *et al.*, 1989; Vescio *et al.*, 1994). Most cases of CLL, lymphoma, and myeloma appear to arise from transformation of a cell more mature than the CD34+ stem-progenitor cell stage. Angiomas, hemangioendotheliomas, angiosarcomas, Kaposi, and gastrointestinal sarcomas (Kantarjian *et al.*, 2002) are usually CD34+. However, most solid tumors, including neuroblastoma, breast cancer, small cell carcinoma of the lung (tumors with frequent marrow involvement) are generally CD34− (Berenson *et al.*, 1989, Silvestri *et al.*, 1992).

CD34 as a target antigen in clinical applications

The CD34 membrane phosphoglycoprotein is the marker of choice for human lympho-hematopoietic stem-progenitor cells because of its exquisitely specific expression on only the most immature cells within the lympho-hematopoietic system. Additional properties of CD34 facilitate its wide use as a target antigen in research and clinical applications requiring

Table 27.3. *CD34 expression in malignancies*

Neoplasms	CD34 expression (% of cases)
Acute myeloid leukemia	+ (40)
Colony-forming progenitor cells of chronic myeloid leukemia	+
B-lineage acute lymphoblastic leukemia (childhood)	+ (60–70)
T-lineage acute lymphoblastic leukemia	+ (5–20)
Malignancies of vascular origin (angioma, hemangioendothelioma, angiosarcoma, and Kaposi's sarcoma)	+
Squamous cell lung carcinoma	+/−
Hodgkin's disease	−
Non-Hodgkin's lymphoma	−
Chronic lymphatic leukemia	−
Multiple myeloma	−
Most solid tumors (including neuroblastoma, breast cancer, small cell carcinoma of lung)	−

identification and purification of stem-progenitor cells. First, CD34 expression is quite intense on stem-progenitor cells and is not down-modulated by antibody binding (Sutherland & Keating, 1992; Civin & Small, 1995); low level expression, endocytosis, or shedding of targeted CD34 molecules would reduce cell labeling. Second, antibody binding to CD34 does not detectably affect the major functions of stem and progenitor cells: homing, survival, proliferation, and differentiation. Third, multiple, well-characterized CD34 monoclonal antibodies are widely available. More than 50 CD34 monoclonal antibodies have been reported (e.g., Greaves *et al.*, 1995). This allows investigators to choose the best CD34 antibody or cocktails of antibodies for diverse assays, such as for tissue sections or proteomic antibody microarrays. Fourth, these antibodies bind to at least three distinct extracellular domains (epitopes) (Civin, 1990; Sutherland & Keating, 1992; Champagne & Civin, 1994; Greaves *et al.*, 1995). Antigen-antibody binding in one domain of the CD34 molecules does not block binding to another CD34 epitope(s). Likewise, enzymatic cleavage or alteration of a given molecular domain still allows the identification of other CD34 epitopes by antibodies specific for those unaltered epitopes. This provides the ability to enumerate (or repeatedly purify) positively selected hematopoietic stem-progenitor cells (Civin, 1992). Thus, notwithstanding the concern discussed above that CD34 may not be expressed at high levels on small numbers of human hematopoietic stem cells, CD34 will continue to be the molecular target of choice for stem-progenitor cell identification and purification until a better marker is developed. CD34 monoclonal antibodies are used extensively to identify and purify stem-progenitor cells for laboratory research. In addition, CD34 immunostaining is used widely for subclassification of hematologic malignancies, as well as in histopathology for identification of hematopoietic and endothelial cells and tumors. The former International Society of Hematotherapy and Graft Engineering (ISHAGE) (now the International Society for Cellular Therapy) has published guidelines on the determination of CD34+ cell numbers in apheresis and bone marrow samples to assess the hematopoietic potential of blood or marrow grafts (Sutherland *et al.*, 1996). Despite these important uses in research and for cell identification in clinical hematology and pathology, the use of CD34 for isolation of cells for human hematopoietic stem cell transplantation has captured the most attention.

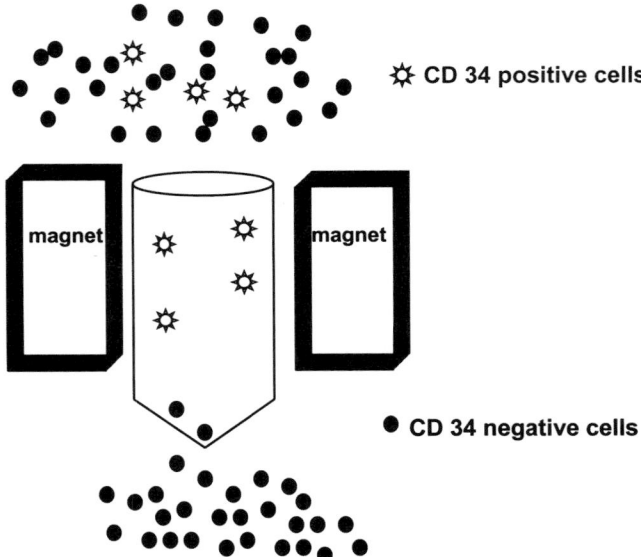

☆ CD 34 positive cells

● CD 34 negative cells

Fig. 27.5. Scheme of the principle of magnetic-activated cell sorting (MACS). Cells are labeled with an anti-CD34 antibody conjugated to magnetic microbeads. Only the CD34+ cells are retained in a column placed in a strong magnetic field, whereas unlabeled cells pass through.

Several clinically applicable immunoaffinity methods for positive selection of CD34+ cells have been developed and published (Fig. 27.5). Automated instruments have been developed to capture CD34+ cells from bone marrow, mobilized blood containing PBSC, or placental/umbilical cord blood on the large scale needed for clinical transplantation. CD34 antibody can be directly (or indirectly) coupled to an affinity matrix, to bind the CD34+ cells. Clinically used capture systems include flow cytometry and fluid/suspension (immunomagnetic beads, ferric colloids, flow cytometry) or solid (columns, tissue culture surfaces) platforms (Civin, 1992; Champagne & Civin, 1994; Civin & Small, 1995; Colter et al., 1996; Leung et al., 1998; McNiece et al., 1997; Schumm et al., 1999). In early studies, purified cell preparations had CD34+ cell purities (i.e., CD34+ cell content) ranging from approximately 40% to 90%, with CD34+ cell recoveries (yields) of approximately 25% to 70% (Champagne & Civin, 1994). In general, the purity of the final product was positively correlated with the concentration of CD34+ cells in the original clinical harvest. For example, if there were 10% CD34+ cells in the starting material (as is occasionally observed in hematopoietic growth factor-treated patients, as opposed to normal marrow, which contains only approximately 1.5% CD34+ cells), it is relatively easy to achieve greater than 90% purity of CD34+ cells in the final product. Unfortunately, PBSC mobilized with granulocyte colony-stimulating factor (G-CSF) or granulocyte-macrophage colony-stimulating factor (GM-CSF) generally contain 0.5% or fewer CD34+ cells. Nevertheless, newer immunomagnetic methods have resulted in improved purities and yields.

Ceprate™ method using avidin-biotin immunoabsorption columns

The separation method called the Ceprate™ SC Stem Cell concentration system was developed by CellPro Inc. (Fig. 27.6). A biotinylated mouse anti-human monoclonal CD34 antibody was used to label low-density marrow or blood mononuclear cells. After washing, labeled cells were captured by passage through a column containing avidin-coated polyacrylamide beads (average diameter 200 μm). The column was flushed to remove unbound cells, and the bound cells were then eluted by mechanical agitation. The reported median purity of CD34+ cells was approximately 75%, and median recovery of CD34+ cells was approximately 35% using this column procedure (Ceprate™ package insert; Colter, Jones, & Heimfeld, 1996). The mean T-cell depletion was approximately 2 to 3 logs, and greater than 3 log depletion of contaminating tumor cells has been reported (Vescio et al., 1999). Selection of CD34+ cells by this method was successfully performed after overnight storage of PBPC at 4°C (to allow pooling of consecutive-day collections) without compromising CD34+ cell yield or purity, or rate of neutrophil or platelet recovery (Lazarus et al., 2000). Unfortunately, this device is no longer commercially available.

Isolex™ method using immunomagnetic microspheres

The selection method called the Isolex™ system was developed by Baxter Inc. (Fig. 27.7). Low-density marrow or blood mononuclear cells are incubated with a mouse anti-human CD34 monoclonal antibody. After washing, the cells are incubated with sheep anti-mouse Ig-coated paramagnetic

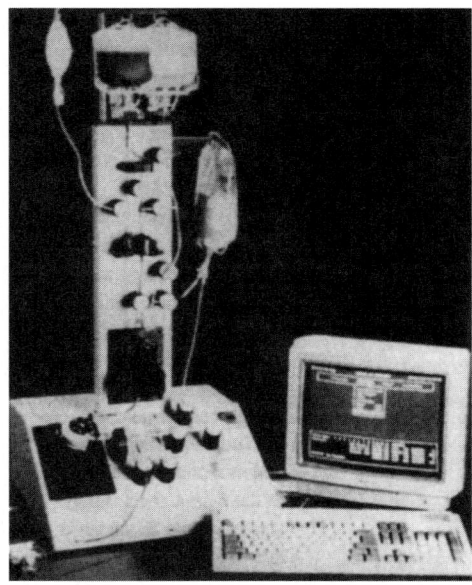

Fig. 27.6. The CellPro Ceprate device.

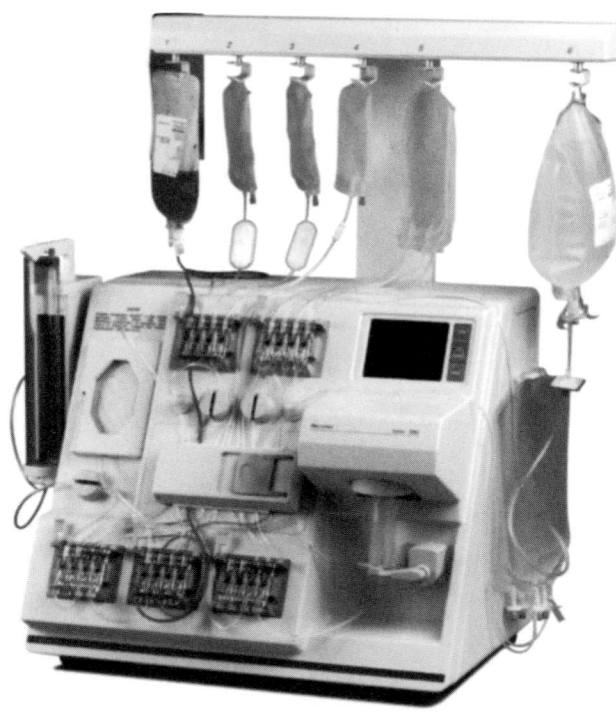

Fig. 27.7. The Baxter Isolex 300i device.

microspheres (diameter 3–4 μm). Unbound CD34⁻ cells are removed by magnetic washes on the Isolex™ Magnetic Cell Separator. In the earlier devices, enzymatic treatment with chymopapain was used to release cells from the immunomagnetic complexes. In the newer procedure, PR34 peptide is used instead of chymopapain to release the microspheres from the bound CD34⁺ cells. PR34, a solubilized octapeptide, binds strongly to CD34 antibody, effectively competing off the CD34 antigen of labeled cells (Hansen *et al.*, 1995; Tseng-Law *et al.*, 1995). The resulting free microsphere/antibody complexes are removed by passage over the magnetic

separator. Using earlier versions of the device, reported purities and recoveries from adult or pediatric patient bone marrow or PBSC were as follows: mean CD34⁺ cell purity 74% to 90%, mean recovery 41% to 69%, and the mean T-cell depletion was approximately 2 to 3 logs. Newer versions of the device have improved purities, yields, and depletions of unwanted cells (Lane *et al.*, 1995; Civin *et al.*, 1996; Williams et al., 1996; Zimmerman *et al.*, 1996; Mapara *et al.*, 1997; Leung *et al.*, 1998).

MACS method using colloidal immunomagnetic particles

The separation system called the MACS™ (magnetic-activated cell sorting) (Miltenyi *et al*, 1990) method was developed by Miltenyi Biotech. Positive selection of CD34⁺ cells is performed via a mouse anti-human CD34 antibody directly conjugated to paramagnetic iron-dextran microbeads with a median diameter of 50 to 100 nm. Antibody-labeled cells thus become magnetic and are retained in a column with a ferromagnetic core placed in a high-density magnetic field, whereas CD34⁻ cells are not labeled and so, not affected by the magnetic field, they pass through the column. The CD34⁺ cells are recovered by removing the column from the magnetic field. No further attempts are made to remove the particles from the cell surface of the CD34 cells after positive selection. The microparticles can only be visualized by electron microscopy (Fig. 27.8), and they do not appear to interfere with the biology of the CD34⁺ cells. After positive selection, the CD34⁺ progenitors are either cryopreserved or injected into the patient. Positive selection with the MACS technology resulted in a median purity of CD34⁺ cells of >96% with high recovery and viability (McNiece *et al*, 1997; Schumm *et al*, 1999). With this one-step positive selection method, a high indirect T-cell depletion of >5 logs was achieved. In addition, B cells were effectively removed from the graft (Fig. 27.9). The method allows the positive selection of CD34⁺ progenitors from bone marrow, PBSC (Schumm

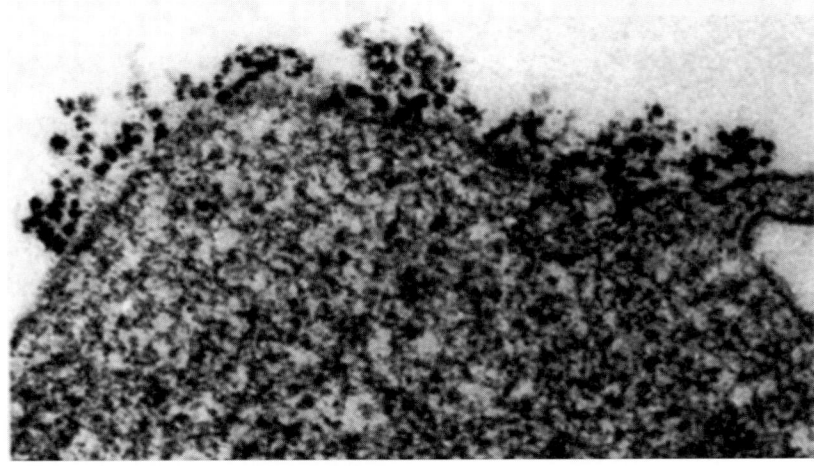

Fig. 27.8. Ultrastructure of the magnetically labeled CD34⁺ cells. The paramagnetic particles are attached to the cell surface (original magnification × 25,000).

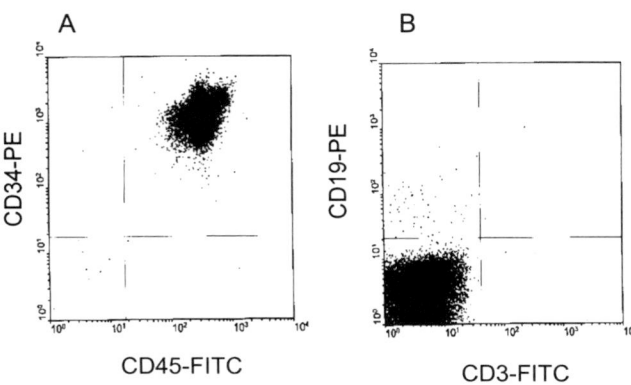

Fig. 27.9. Flow cytometric analysis of cells after positive selection. Almost all cells stain positive for CD45 and CD34 (**A**). The number of contaminating CD3+ T-lymphocytes and CD19+ B-cells is very low (**B**).

et al, 1999), and cord blood (Kogler *et al*, 1999), using a clinical grade semiautomated Clinimacs™ device (Fig. 27.10).

CD34⁺ cell enrichment using high-speed flow cytometry

Initial studies were carried out using high-speed flow cytometry to sort autologous CD34+/CD90+ stem-progenitor cells in a small number of patients with myeloma (Tricot *et al.*, 1998; Michallet *et al.*, 2000), non-Hodgkin's lymphoma (Vose *et al.*, 2001), and breast cancer (Negrin *et al.*, 2000). Gazitt and col-

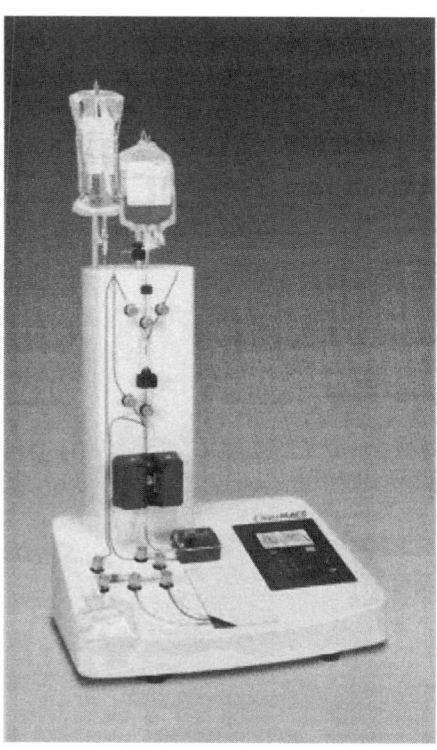

Fig. 27.10. The Miltenyi Biotec Clinimacs device.

leagues (1995), in a preclinical study, described depletion of greater than 2.7 to 7.3 logs of myeloma cells in flow-sorted CD34+/CD90+ cells (Fig. 27.11. Table 27.4). Using polymerase chain reaction (PCR) for the CDRIII region of the immunoglobulin heavy chain of each patient, they showed a reduction in the level of myeloma cell contamination to less than 1 clonal B cell in 100,000 CD34+/CD90+ cells. CD34+ cell purity of 95% or greater was obtained, and yields were 30% to 40%, but the process was labor-intensive, lengthy, and expensive. Of interest, however, was the observation (Archimbaud *et al.*, 1997; Michallet *et al.*, 2000) that engraftment of neutrophils was as rapid as that of unselected mobilized PBPC if a CD34+/CD90+ cell dose of at least 8×10^5/kg was infused. In G-CSF mobilized PBSC from normal donors, a mean T-cell depletion of approximately 4 to 4.5 logs was obtained. A schematic illustration of the detector and illumination assemblies of the clinical high-speed cell sorter developed by Systemix Inc. is shown in Figure 27.12 (Sasaki *et al.*, 1995). Unfortunately, this method is no longer available for clinical use.

Safety and quality control

The processing of clinical grafts should follow the standards published by the American Association of Blood Banks (AABB) and the Foundation for the Accreditation of Hematopoietic Stem Cell Therapy (FAHCT). CD34+ cell purity and recovery, together with other parameters such as sterility, viability, and CFU assays, should be documented for quality assurance. Residual antibody in the final product may theoretically cause a hypersensitivity reaction or induce formation of a human anti-mouse antibody (HAMA) response. This might be of particular concern for patients who may undergo multiple infusions of CD34-selected grafts. Major standardization efforts have been implemented (Sovalat *et al.*, 1994; Brecher *et al.*, 1996; Johnsen & Knudsen, 1996; Sutherland *et al.*, 1996).

Autologous CD34⁺ bone marrow transplantation

Gene marking studies have shown that tumor cells that contaminate hematopoietic transplant grafts can contribute to relapse (Brenner *et al.*, 1993; Rill *et al.*, 1994). The combination of CD34 expression on stem-progenitor cells with lack of expression on most cases of solid tumors suggested that positive selection of CD34+ cells might be used to "reverse purge" autologous hematopoietic grafts of tumor cells for transplantation in a broad range of cancers. Additionally, this approach may be used to deplete autologous grafts of autoreactive T cells for transplantation in autoimmune diseases.

Purified autologous CD34+ cells mediated hematopoietic engraftment in non-human primates (Andrews *et al.*, 1991), whereas CD34⁻ cells did not engraft (Berenson *et al.*, 1988, 1991; Andrews *et al.*, 2000). Positive selection of CD34+ cells in human autologous bone marrow transplantation (BMT) was first reported by Berenson *et al.* (1991), who demonstrated that hematopoiesis was reconstituted after transplantation of autolo-

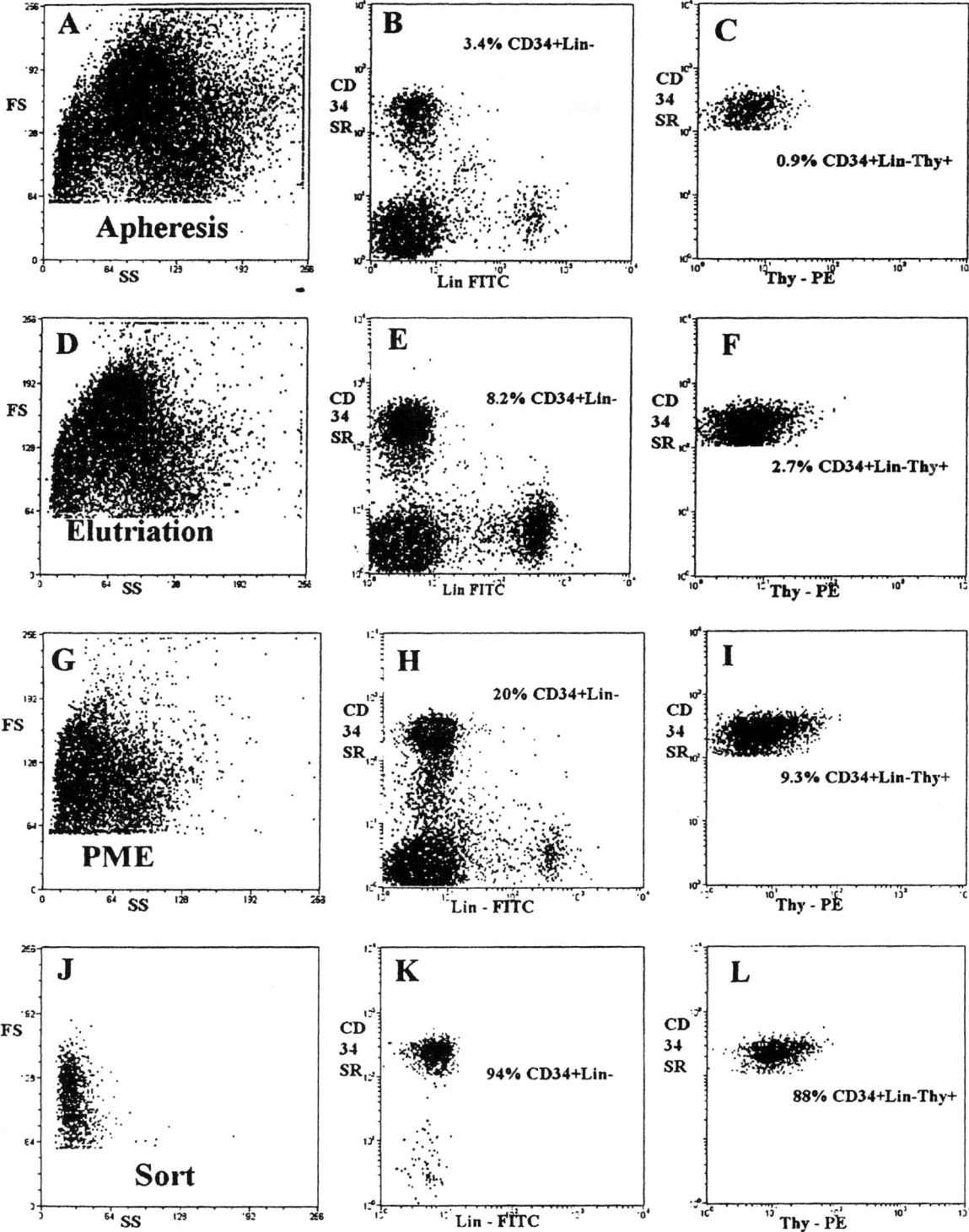

Fig. 27.11. Purification of CD34+ Lin− Thy+ cells by counterflow elutriation centrifugation, treatment with PME, and flow-sorting. (A through C) Apheresis cells. (D through F) After elutriation. (G through I) After PME-treatment. (J through L) Reanalysis after sorting for CD34+ Lin− Thy+ stem cells. Panels A, D, G, and J are light scatter dot plots in the various fractions. Panels B, E, H, and K are two-color immunofluorescence dot plots and show the progressive increase in CD34+ Lin− cells. Panels C, F, I, and L are also two-color dot plots and show the relative enrichment for CD34+ Lin− Thy+ stem cells during the purification process. Reproduced, with permission, from Gazitt et al. (1995).

Table 27.4. *Depletion of myeloma cells from flow-sorted hematopoietic stem cells*

	Pre Sort		CD34+ Lin− Thy+		
Patient	Total cells (× 10⁸)	Myeloma cells (× 10⁴)	Total cells (× 10⁵)	Myeloma cells (× 1)	Log depletion
1	3.6	<0.4	6.8	<7	>2.7
2	4.2	0.8	18	<18	>2.7
3	13.8	1.7	28.2	<28	>2.8
4	3.7	0.4	10.9	<3	>3.0
5	6.3	1.9	12.6	<1	>3.2
6	4.4	26.4	12	<10	>4.4
7	22.3	1,520	106	<100	>5.2
8	89.7	6,370	312	<312	>5.3
9	7.3	1,240	4.1	<4	>6.5
10	8.4	8,400	3.5	<4	>7.3

Reproduced, with permission, from Gazitt *et al.* (1995).

gous CD34+ cells, isolated using CD34 avidin-biotin immunoaffinity columns, in six patients who had received mye-loablative radiochemotherapy. The patients received from 1.2 to 5.2×10^6 CD34+ cells/kg from grafts that were 54% to 92% CD34+. Shpall *et al.* (1994, 1997) and Gorin *et al.* (1995) confirmed this with reports that CD34+ autologous bone marrow cells (12%–85% CD34+), isolated by a modification of the same methodology, produced engraftment in larger series of patients with breast cancer or non-Hodgkins lymphoma, respectively. Details of the number of progenitor cells infused, the kinetics of engraftment, and blood support needed in the study by Gorin and colleagues are shown in Table 27.5. Survival has not been shown to be significantly different from that using unselected autografts (Fig. 27.13). Civin *et al.* (1996a) further demonstrated that highly purified (up to 99%) CD34+ marrow grafts from patients with pediatric solid tumors, selected using immunomagnetic microspheres, reconstituted hematopoiesis. This confirmed that CD34+ cells alone are sufficient to provide autologous hematopoietic reconstitution for

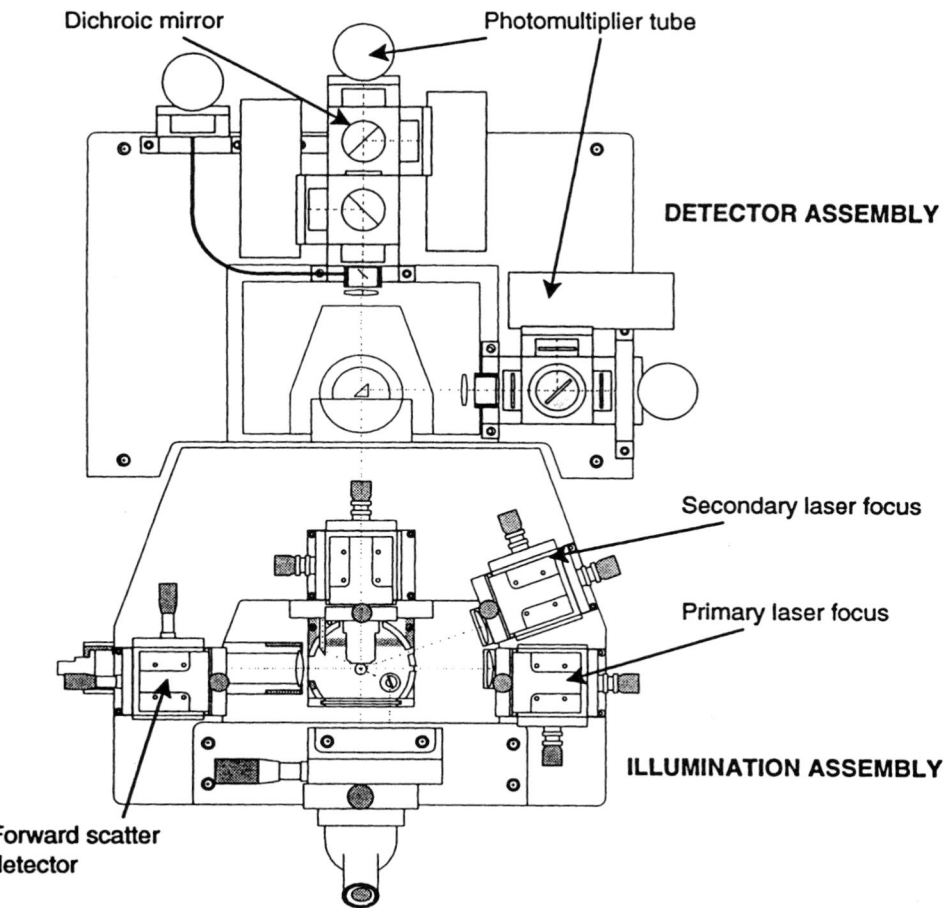

Fig. 27.12. Schematic drawing of the top view of a portion of the clinical high-speed cell sorter. The detector assembly houses the photomultiplier detectors (fluorescence), beam steering optics, and individual bandpass filters. The illumination assembly houses the nozzle drive assembly, laser focusing optics, forward angle scatter detector, and fluorescence collection optics. The sorter can process up to 20,000 cells/second. Reproduced, with permission, from Sasaki *et al.* (1995).

Table 27.5.   *CD34 purified stem cell transplantation: progenitor cells infused, kinetics of engraftment, and blood support (n = 15)*

CD34+ (%)	Concentrated CD34+ graft			Recovery to (d)		Blood support (total no. of)	
	CD34+ (10⁶/kg)	Early CFU-GM (10⁴/kg)	BFU-E (10⁴/kg)	Neutrophils >0.5 (10⁹/l)	Platelets >50 (10⁹/l)	RBC units	Platelet transfusions
66	1.12	–	–	16	23	8	8
59	1.84	19.9	6.63	25	68	10	26
51	0.66	11.2	6.14	12	13	4	4
50	0.58	10.45	3.66	20	42	10	13
68	2.20	16.95	16.62	13	18	6	8
72	2.96	25.55	8.34	12	NE	10	20
72	1.59	10.62	9.17	11	27	8	9
58	1.48	13.17	5.96	10	11	4	3
40	0.55	10.9	3.78	17	40	16	20
30	0.41	9.45	3.74	15	15	4	4
64	1.29	7.79	0.80	17	25	6	5
27	0.30	0.92	0.62	33	NR	19	31+
34	0.69	8.97	1.28	12	20	6	7
52	0.38	3.36	0.90	16	19	4	4
59	0.89	3.46	0.70	14	29	8	7
58	1	10.62	3.76	15	23	8	8
(27–72)[a]	(0.3–2.96)	(0.92–25.55)	(16.62–0.70)	(10–33)	(11–68)	(4–19)	(3–31 +)

Abbreviations: NR, not reached; NE, nonevaluable.
[a] Values shown at the bottom of each column are the median with the range in parentheses.
Reproduced, with permission, from Gorin *et al.* (1995).

myeloablated patients. CD34+ cell selection and subsequent hematopoietic reconstitution were successfully performed in children as young as 1 year of age and as small as 10 kg. However, in the last study, hematopoietic engraftment following transplantation of CD34+ cell grafts required an average of approximately 5 weeks.

In the above early studies, CD34+ cell selection reduced tumor cell levels by approximately 2 to 3 logs (depending on CD34+ cell purity and recovery). For heavily contaminated grafts, complete purging of tumor cells may not be achieved following CD34+ cell selection (Leung *et al.*, 1998). Repeated

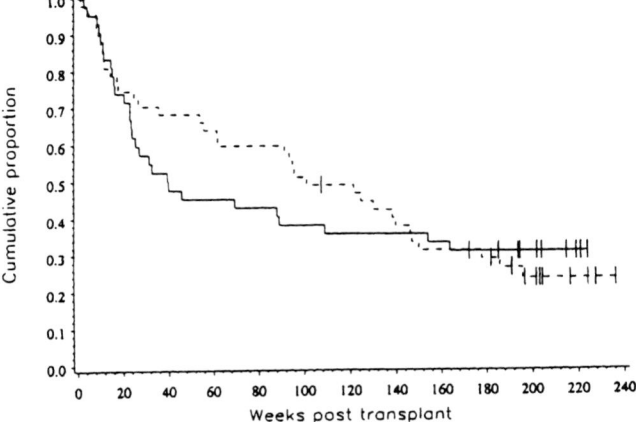

Fig. 27.13. The progression-free survival for patients on both arms of the study was 31% (*P* = .492). Reproduced, with permission, from Shpall *et al.* (1997).

CD34 selection and combination of positive selection of CD34+ cells followed by negative tumor purging procedures are currently being tested, as are newer single-step methodologies that result in higher purities of positively selected CD34+ cells (see below).

In the autologous setting, the MACS™ technology has been used to purge tumor cells from grafts harvested for hematopoietic rescue after high-dose chemotherapy in patients with solid tumors. Highly purified autologous CD34+ cells isolated using this technique provided rapid engraftment following high-dose chemotherapy in breast cancer patients (Richel *et al*, 2000). Since in this setting, positive selection of CD34+ cells is associated not only with tumor cell depletion, but also with an accompanying T-cell depletion, the transplantation of such an autologous graft after myeloablative therapy might result in delayed immunologic reconstitution. In a study in adult patients with hematological malignancies, the delay in the lymphocyte recovery was associated with a higher incidence of viral infections, whereas granulocyte and platelet engraftment was rapid (Laurenti *et al*, 2001). Moreover, reduced diversity of the T-cell repertoire has been described in recipients of highly purified CD34+ cells (Bomberger *et al.*, 1998). In contrast, in a pediatric study in children with high-risk neuroblastoma, positive selection of CD34+ progenitors from mobilized PBSC resulted in a >3 log depletion of neuroblastoma cells (Handgretinger *et al*, 2002); in these pediatric patients, no increased incidence of viral infections was seen.

Autologous CD34+ stem-progenitor cells purified with the immunomagnetic techniques have also been used for hematopoietic reconstitution after immunoablative therapy in patients with severe autoimmune diseases (Rosen *et al.*, 2000). In this setting, CD34 positive selection is used to effect purging of T lymphocytes, which mediate the autoimmune disease.

Autologous CD34⁺ mobilized blood stem cell transplantation

Mobilization and collection of large numbers of stem-progenitor cells from peripheral blood by apheresis is made possible by the administration of human hematopoietic growth factors, such as G-CSF and GM-CSF, with or without chemotherapy. These so-called peripheral blood stem cells (PBSC) have been increasingly used for hematopoietic rescue after myeloablative chemotherapy in patients with solid cancers, including high-risk cases of small cell lung cancer, breast cancer, and neuroblastoma, as well as in patients with hematologic malignancy. Reasons to substitute PBSC for bone marrow include rapid hematopoietic recovery after PBSC rescue (if the requisite numbers of CD34⁺ stem-progenitor cells can be harvested) (Figs. 27.14 and 27.15), ability to collect PBSC without an operative procedure, and ability to collect PBSC in patients with residual marrow disease or fibrotic marrow due to previous radiation. PBSC grafts have been postulated to contain fewer tumor cells than bone marrow grafts. However, with improvement in culture, immunohistochemistry, and reverse transcriptase polymerase chain reaction (RT-PCR) techniques, tumor cells have also been detected in (peripheral blood and) PBSC grafts of breast cancer, lung cancer, lymphoma, and neuroblastoma patients. More than 80% of unprocessed PBSC grafts and marrow grafts from patients with poor-risk neuroblastoma or peripheral primitive neuroectodermal tumor were contaminated with tumor cells, as detected by highly sensitive RT-PCR and/or immunocytochemistry methods (Leung *et al.*, 1998). Unprocessed PBSC grafts and marrow grafts from the same patient contained similar quantities of tumor cells

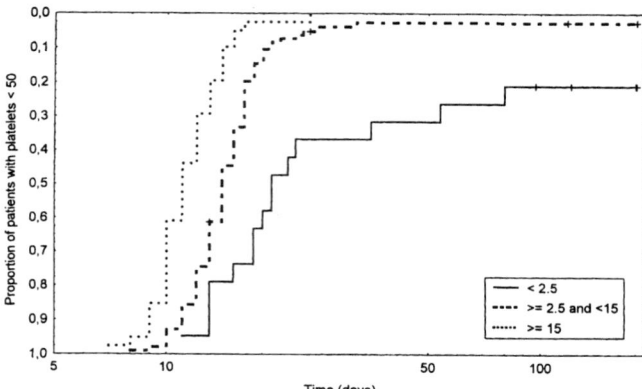

Fig. 27.15. Time to recovery to a platelet count greater than $50 \times 10^9/l$ in intermediate CD34⁺ group patients (dashed line) compared with low CD34⁺ group patients (solid line) ($P < .0001$) and with high CD34⁺ group patients (dotted line) ($P < .0001$). Of note, the time is shown on a logarithmic scale. Reproduced, with permission, from Ketterer *et al.* (1998).

(approximately 200,000 tumor cells/graft). The 0.5 to 1 log higher concentration of tumor cells in marrow grafts was compensated by 0.5 to 1 log lower total number of mononuclear cells in marrow grafts compared to PBSC grafts. Therefore, as with BMT, tumor cell purging appears to be desirable for autologous PBSC transplantation, especially for tumors that carry a high propensity for hematologic metastasis. Schiller *et al.* (1995) and Vescio *et al.* (1999) described a greater than 2.7 to 4.5 log reduction in contaminating multiple myeloma cells after mononuclear cells. They used PCR for patient-specific CDR1 and CDR3 of the patients' monoclonal myeloma protein (Table 27.6). Di Nicola and colleagues (1996) were unable to detect BCL-2⁺ follicular non-Hodgkin's lymphoma cells after CD34 selection of PBSC, which contained such cells prior to selection.

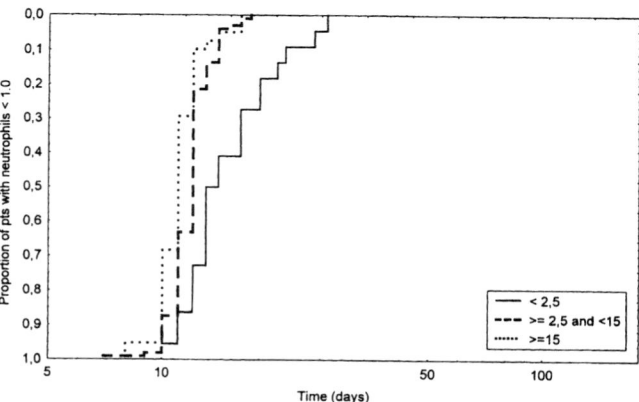

Fig. 27.14. Time to recovery to an ANC greater than $1.0 \times 10^9/l$ in intermediate CD34⁺ group patients (dashed line) compared with low CD34⁺ group patients (solid line) ($P < .0001$) and with high CD34⁺ group patients (dotted line) ($P = .003$). Of note, the time is shown on a logarithmic scale. Reproduced, with permission, from Ketterer *et al.* (1998).

Table 27.6. *Tumor cell reduction by CD34 affinity-cell processing of leukapheresis products*

UPN	Leukapheresis contamination, cells/kg[a]	Adsorbed cell contamination, cells/kg[a]	Tumor cell log reduction by CD34 selection
321	29,550	<20	>3.2
327	480,000	<16	>4.5
339	127,440	83	3.2
419	16,660	<32	>2.7
452	2,139,000	2,090	3.0
461	11,325	<8	>3.2
481	243,380	<14	>4.2
491	90,000	250	2.8

Abbreviation: UPN, unique patient number.
[a] Tumor cell contamination in cells/kg was calculated by multiplying the percentage contamination by the number of mononuclear cells/kg collected.
Reproduced, with permission, from Schiller *et al.* (1995).

Similar to CD34⁺ bone marrow cells, highly purified CD34⁺ PBSC are sufficient to provide hematopoietic reconstitution in myeloablated patients. Retrovirally marked CD34⁺ PBSC and bone marrow cells have both been shown to contribute to long-term (>18 months) engraftment after autologous transplantation (Dunbar *et al.*, 1995). CD34⁺ PBSC grafts generally engraft much faster than do CD34⁺ bone marrow grafts. Recovery from neutropenia (ANC $\geq 0.5 \times 10^9/l$) generally occurs in less than 2 weeks, even in heavily pretreated patients. Recovery from thrombocytopenia (platelet count >20 × 10⁹/l) usually takes less than 2 to 3 weeks. These data indicate that the infusion of CD34⁺ PBSC grafts results in a period of neutropenia and thrombocytopenia comparable to that of unfractionated PBSC transplants (Brugger *et al.*, 1994; Shpall *et al.*, 1994; Schiller *et al.*, 1995, 1998) (Table 27.7). There is a clear correlation between the number of CD34⁺ cells infused and the rate of subsequent recovery of both neutrophils and platelets posttransplant (Shpall, Champlin, & Glaspy, 1998), as well as on later engraftment-related parameters such as transfusion requirements, febrile episodes, days of hospitalization and antibiotic requirements throughout the first year posttransplant (Perez-Simon *et al.*, 1999). The minimum CD34⁺ cell dose at which engraftment is rapid and durable after autologous PBSC transplant is generally recommended to be approximately 1–3 × 10⁶ CD34⁺ PBSC cells/kg (Passos-Coelho *et al.*, 1995). Posttransplant, however, there has been relatively wide variation in reported thresholds for optimal CD34⁺ cell dose. First, in most studies, investigators have given their patients relatively high CD34⁺ cell doses. Since CD34⁺ cell enumeration is not uniform or quantitatively comparable across institutions, major standardization efforts have been made (Siena, Bregni, & Brando, 1991; Sovalat *et al.*, 1993; Brecher *et al.*, 1996; Johnsen & Knudsen, 1996; Sutherland *et al.*, 1996). It is strongly recommended that a validated procedure such as the ISHAGE method (Sutherland *et al.*, 1996) be used. In addition, a single platform approach in which the white cell count and the CD34⁺ cell quantitation are performed on the same machine (Barnett *et al.*, 1999) is advised.

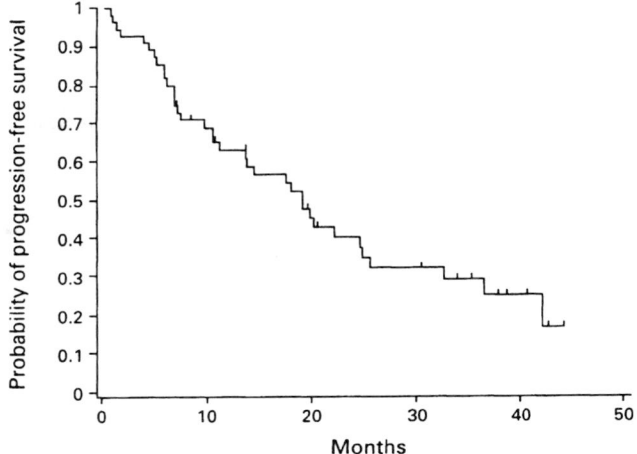

Fig. 27.16. Probability of progression-free survival for patients undergoing CD34-selected peripheral blood progenitor cell transplantation for multiple myeloma, *n* = 55. Reproduced, with permission, from Schiller *et al.* (1998).

Immunomagnetic CD34⁺ cell selection of PBSC reduces tumor cell contamination by approximately 3 to 4 logs. As with autologous marrow, repeated CD34 selection, or a combination of positive selection of CD34⁺ cells followed by negative purging procedures, may be necessary for heavily contaminated PBSC grafts (Mapara *et al.*, 1999). Survival has not yet been shown to be significantly different from that obtained using unselected autologous blood stem cell transplants (Schiller *et al.*, 1998; Lemoli *et al.*, 2000) (Figs. 27.16 and 27.17). An increased incidence of cytomegalovirus disease and associated mortality (Holmberg *et al.*, 1999) (Fig. 27.18 and Table 27.8), more varicella zoster, parainfluenza, and bacterial infections (Crippa *et al.*, 2002), and a greater number of total infectious episodes and bacterial infections (Friedman, Lazarus, & Koc, 2000) have been reported after CD34⁺ transplants compared to unpurged auto-

Table 27.7. *Time to neutrophil and platelet recovery and transfusion requirements as a function of CD34 peripheral blood progenitor cell number infused*

	CD34 PBPC/kg		
	<2 × 10⁶	>2 × 10⁶	*P*
Patients (no.)	6	31	
Time to ANC >500 mm⁻³			
Median (days)	14	12	.05
Time to platelet >20,000 mm⁻³			
Median (days)	21	12	<.001
Red blood cell transfusions (no.)	19	6	.005
Platelet transfusions (no.)	30	2	.002

Reproduced, with permission, from Schiller *et al.* (1995).

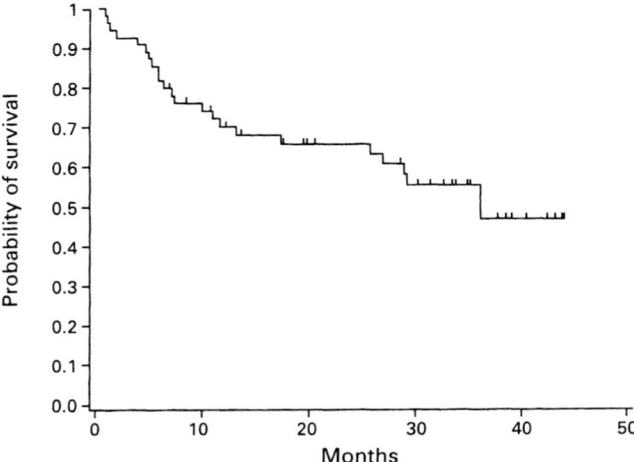

Fig. 27.17. Probability of survival for patients undergoing CD34-selected peripheral blood progenitor cell transplantation for multiple myeloma, *n* = 55. Reproduced, with permission, from Schiller *et al.* (1998).

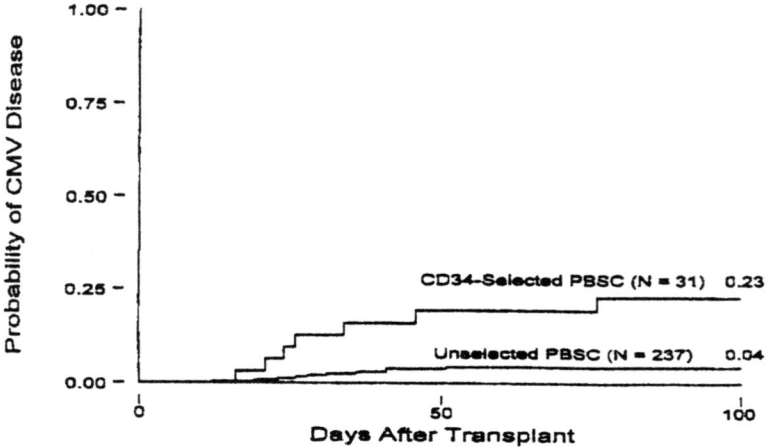

Fig. 27.18. Cumulative incidence curves for CMV disease in CD34-selected and unselected PBSC autologous transplant patients. Reproduced, with permission, from Holmberg *et al.* (1999).

grafts, as well as an increased incidence of both early and late infections in myeloma patients given CD34+/CD90+ grafts (Michallet *et al.*, 2000). However, there are also studies showing no such differences (Blystad *et al.*, 2001).

Allogeneic CD34+ cell transplantation

Technical aspects

Ex vivo T-cell depletion (TCD) of the graft can effectively reduce the incidence and severity of graft-versus-host disease (GVHD) after allogeneic bone marrow transplantation

(O'Reilly, 1992). Compared to harvested bone marrow, G-CSF-mobilized PBSC provide far greater numbers of hematopoietic stem-progenitor cells and accessory cells for graft engineering, and TCD has also been performed in allogeneic transplantation of PBSC (Corringham *et al.*, 1995; Link *et al.*, 1996; Bensinger *et al.*, 1996; Urbano-Ispizua *et al.*, 1997). Several techniques have been developed to deplete T cells from human marrow allografts (O'Reilly *et al.*, 1992), including counterflow centrifugation, lectin agglutination, and the use of any of several monoclonal antibodies directed against T lymphocytes. Most of these methods are time-consuming and difficult to standardize across different transplanta-

Table 27.8. *CMV disease in CD34-selected and unselected PBSC autologous transplant patients*

Disease	Disease site	Day posttransplant symptoms began	Day CMV disease diagnosed	Cause of death
CD34-selected				
MM	Pneumonia	16	46	Pneumonia, D52
NHL	Pneumonia	72	76	Pneumonia, D82
NHL	Pneumonia	23	37	Pneumonia, D60
MM	Pneumonia	15	21	–
MM	Pneumonia	13	16	Pneumonia, D30
NHL	Enteritis	34	34	–
MM	Pneumonia	12	18	–
Unselected				
Breast	Pneumonia	51	51	Pneumonia, D57
NHL	Enteritis	26	26	ARDS, D74
Ovarian	Pneumonia	39	None	Pneumonia, D40
Breast	Enteritis	28	28	–
Breast	Pneumonia	34	36	Pneumonia, D53
Hodgkin's	Pneumonia	18	19	Pneumonia, D31
Sarcoma	Enteritis	30	31	–
Breast	Enteritis	12	12	–
Breast	Enteritis	23	23	–
MM	Pneumonia	41	41	–

Reproduced, with permission, from Holmberg *et al.* (1999).

tion centers. As described above, simple, automated, and reproducible methods of positively selecting CD34+ hematopoietic stem-progenitor cells are available. On this basis, CD34+ cell selection has been used as a single-step procedure to deplete T cells from allogeneic grafts in order to reduce the risk of GVHD (Mavroudis et al., 1996). In addition, a purified CD34+ product will be depleted of antigen-presenting cells.

Approximately 3 logs of T-cell removal was been reported using Ceprate™ CD34+ selection columns for TCD; this corresponds to a median of 0.4×10^6/kg T cells infused to patients (Link et al., 1996; Schreiner et al., 1996; Watts et al., 1997; Urbano-Ispizua et al., 1997; Urbano-Ispizua et al., 1998); 4–5 logs TCD have been reported by the immunomagnetic bead techniques, with a median of 0.1 to 0.01×10^6/kg T cells infused to the patients reported using the Isolex™ or CliniMacs™, respectively (Papadimitriou et al., 1995; Dreger et al., 1995; McNiece et al., 1997; Aversa et al., 1998; Beelen et al., 2000; Handgretinger et al., 2001a; Handgretinger et al., 2001b; Eyrich et al., 2001). Several reports suggest that, in HLA-identical sibling recipients, administration of at least 0.1 to 0.4×10^6/kg T cells results in a certain degree of graft-versus-leukemia (GVL) effect and facilitates engraftment (Schattenberg et al., 1990; Verdonck et al., 1994; Lowenberg et al., 1986) without triggering GVHD (Lowenberg et al., 1986; Wagner et al., 1990; Verdonck et al., 1994; Noga et al., 1997). More efficient TCD is necessary in mismatched or haploidentical transplantation (Aversa et al., 1994), and probably in the unrelated setting (Stockschlader et al., 1995; Aversa et al., 1998; Handgretinger et al., 2001b).

Clinical aspects

Graft failure
TCD results in a high incidence of graft failure. In contrast to recipients of unmodified HLA-identical marrow grafts, in which there is a 0.1% incidence of graft failure (Beatty et al., 1985), the reported incidence of this complication among recipients of TCD HLA-identical transplants ranges from 10% to 30% (O'Reilly et al., 1985; Patterson et al., 1986; Filipovich et al., 1987; Hale et al., 1988; Kernan et al., 1989). Graft failure is usually a fatal complication (Hale et al., 1988; Kernan et al., 1989), since in many patients secondary transplants cause unacceptable toxicity, and a considerable proportion do not result in stable engraftment (Hale et al., 1988; Martin et al., 1988; Kernan et al., 1989; Urbano-Ispizua et al., 2001a, b, c). Gender-pairing between donor and recipient (Kernan et al., 1989), intensity of the conditioning regimen (Patterson et al., 1986; Guyotat et al., 1987; Burnett et al., 1988), marrow cell dose (Uharek et al., 1994), and degree of TCD (Voltarelli et al., 1990) have each been correlated with the risk of graft failure. A strong correlation between the quantity of T cells in the graft and the probability of engraftment has been reported (Urbano-Ispizua et al., 2001a, b, c). Thus, 23 of 155 patients (15%) receiving fewer than 0.2×10^6 T cells/kg experienced graft failure, compared with only one of 102 patients (1%) receiving more than 0.2×10^6 T cells/kg, with the actuarial probability

being 18% vs. 1%, respectively ($P = .0001$). This is in agreement with results in mouse models showing that rejection associated with TCD marrow can be overcome by adding a small quantity of donor CD8+ cells (Martin et al., 1993) or thymocytes to the grafts (Lapidot et al., 1990; Murphy et al., 1990).

GVHD
Whereas it is accepted that TCD of bone marrow decreases the incidence of both acute and chronic GVHD (Marmont et al., 1991), the impact of CD34+ selection of G-CSF mobilized allogeneic PBSC on the incidence of GVHD is controversial (Finke et al., 1996; Link et al., 1996; Bensinger et al., 1996; Urbano-Ispizua et al., 1997). In a comparative study, the actuarial probability of severe acute and extensive chronic GVHD was significantly lower in the group transplanted with CD34+ selected allogeneic PBSC than in the group that received unmanipulated PBSC (Urbano-Ispizua et al., 1998). The actuarial probabilities of acute GVHD grade II–IV were 16% and 43%, respectively ($P = .002$), and the actuarial probabilities for extensive chronic GVHD were 22% and 47%, respectively ($P = .02$). Risk factors for acute GVHD have been identified in 315 patients receiving CD34+ allogeneic PBSC from HLA identical sibling donors: increased CD34+ cell dose, increased CD3+ cell dose, and higher patient age (>42 years) (Urbano-Ispizua et al., 2002). In this study, the rate of acute GVHD stages I–IV increased with increasing doses of CD34+ cells: recipients of ≤2, >2–4, or >4 × 10^6 CD34+ cells/kg had a cumulative acute GVHD incidence of 21%, 35%, or 43%, respectively ($P = .01$). A similar association of the number of CD34+ cells with incidence of acute (Przepiorka et al., 1999) and chronic (Zaucha et al., 2000) GVHD after unmanipulated allogeneic PBSC transplantion has been published. In 315 patients receiving CD34+ allogeneic PBSC, infusion of ≤0.05, >0.05–0.1, or >0.1 × 10^6 CD3+ cells/kg was associated with a cumulative incidence of acute GVHD stages I–IV of 18%, 35%, or 44%, respectively ($P = .007$) (Urbano-Ispizua et al., 2002). Kernan et al. (1986) estimated the number of marrow T cells necessary to initiate clinically detectable acute GVHD in an HLA-identical host to be 0.1 × 10^6/kg, although other groups have reported that infusion of 0.1 × 10^6 CD3+ cells/kg does not totally prevent severe GVHD (Urbano-Ispizua et al., 2002). The rate of acute GVHD in recipients of fewer than 0.1 × 10^6 CD3+ cells/kg is low, but this is associated with a high incidence of graft failure. This observation supports the concept that both complications behave as "mirror images," and suggests that there is no standard quantity of T cells low enough to totally prevent severe GVHD while high enough to totally avoid graft failure. A T cell dose to attenuate both complications might be in the range of 0.1 to 0.3 × 10^6 CD3+ cells/kg, followed by posttransplant immunosuppression.

In the allogeneic setting, the MACS™ device has been used for TCD of either bone marrow or mobilized PBSC in matched sibling (Beelen et al., 2000; Elmaagacli et al., 2003), matched unrelated (Lang et al., 1999 and 2003), or haploidentical transplantion (Handgretinger et al., 2001a). In all these transplant settings, rapid hematopoietic recovery has been obtained. Due to the highly efficient TCD obtained, even three-loci HLA-mismatched haploidentical transplants can be performed with a low incidence of severe acute and extensive chronic GVHD in the absence of posttransplant immunosuppression for GVHD prophylaxis (Handgretinger et al., 2001a). In addition, the incidence of posttransplant EBV-associated lymphoproliferative syndrome is very low, probably due to the effective removal of mature donor B lymphocytes from the graft. In allogeneic transplants with highly purified CD34$^+$ stem-progenitor cells, immunologic reconstitution, especially of T cells, is delayed and a higher rate of posttransplant infections has been seen in some studies. A correlation between the number of transplanted CD34$^+$ cells and the speed of T-cell recovery has been described (Handgretinger et al., 2001a; Eyrich et al., 2001). The importance of the number of transplanted CD34$^+$ cells is further illustrated by the observation that pediatric patients grafted with haploidentical peripheral CD34$^+$ stem-progenitor cells had faster immunologic reconstitution than patients transplanted with CD34$^+$ cells obtained from matched unrelated donor PBSC (Handgretinger et al., 2001b). In this study, the number of transplanted haploidentical CD34$^+$ cells was two times higher than the number of transplanted CD34$^+$ cells obtained from matched unrelated donors. While it is not yet clear whether the use of purified CD34$^+$ cell grafts will improve the overall outcome of patients with hematological malignancies after matched sibling and matched unrelated transplantation, the reliable prevention of severe acute and chronic GVHD in the three-loci haploidentical setting allows this transplantation modality to be offered to patients who otherwise would not have the option of an allogeneic transplant due to the lack of a suitable donor (Aversa et al., 1998).

To minimize the risk of disease relapse after CD34-selected transplants, prophylactic T cell add-back in the form of donor lymphocyte infusions can be employed (Emaagacli et al., 2003). CD34$^+$ cell selection has also been used as an "add-back" procedure after TCD by elutriation (Noga et al., 1997). Elutriation rapidly separates grafts into cell populations with virtually no cell loss. When elutriation was used to deplete small lymphocytes from allogeneic grafts, the incidence and severity of both acute and chronic GVHD were reduced. However, hematopoietic engraftment was slow (>3 weeks) and the incidence of graft failure was 10%. A large proportion of the small-sized CD34$^+$ cells was excluded from the elutriated (T-cell-depleted) grafts. The addition of purified CD34$^+$ cells salvaged from the small-sized lymphocyte-rich fractions shortened the time to neutrophil and platelet recovery by 6 and 11 days, respectively. Using 180 days of cyclosporine for prophylaxis, the incidence of acute GVHD (>stage 1) remained low at 12%, with a chronic GVHD incidence of 3%. Over 150 allogeneic transplants have now been performed using this procedure involving elutriation plus CD34$^+$ cell add-back.

CD34 selection is also increasingly used in the transplantation of (mostly) pediatric patients with nonmalignant acquired or inherited diseases. The advantage in this setting is the almost complete lack of GVHD in these patients. In pediatric patients with severe aplastic anemia transplanted with purified CD34$^+$ cells from matched unrelated, as well as from mismatched family donors, a high engraftment rate and a low incidence of acute and chronic GVHD was seen (Schwinger et al., 2000a; Urban et al., 2001). Highly purified, partially HLA- matched unrelated CD34$^+$ PBSC have also been successfully used for engraftment in a pediatric patient with Wiskott-Aldrich syndrome (Schwinger et al., 2000b). In another series of pediatric patients with various nonmalignant diseases, a low incidence of GVHD and an excellent long-term outcome has been observed after myeloablative therapy and transplantation of purified CD34$^+$ cells obtained from matched unrelated and mismatched family donors (Lang et al., 2000). In this study, 17 patients with various nonmalignant diseases were transplanted with purified CD34$^+$ cells. In 16 patients, no or mild GVHD was seen, and only 1 patient experienced grade II GVHD. Fourteen of the 17 patients are alive with a median follow-up of 1.8 years. Although these data need to be verified in larger studies, it can be envisioned that the use of highly purified CD34$^+$ cells may be advantageous in pediatric patients with nonmalignant diseases, such as imunodeficiencies, severe aplastic anemia, hemoglobinopathies, and inborn errrors of metabolism.

Relapse

A major disadvantage with TCD is that the clinical benefit of decreasing GVHD can be offset by an increased relapse rate (Marmont et al., 1991). This is a significant clinical problem in patients with chronic myeloid leukemia (CML), in whom an increased relapse rate (50% to 70%) has been observed in TCD transplant patients (Marmont et al., 1991). However, in CML, donor lymphocyte infusions (DLI) have a powerful antileukemic effect, and many patients relapsing after a TCD transplant can be successfully rescued with DLI (Kolb et al., 1995; Collins et al., 1997). For patients with acute myeloid leukemia (AML), acute lymphoblastic leukemia (ALL), or myelodysplastic syndrome (MDS), the effect of TCD on disease recurrence is less important clinically (Marmont et al., 1991; Papadopoulos et al., 1997; Soiffer et al., 1997; Urbano-Ispizua et al., 1998). It must be noted that, after allogeneic transplants, the number of donor T cells is not the only immunologic factor affecting leukemia relapse. The use of cyclosporine plus methotrexate, compared with cyclosporine alone, has been associated with a higher incidence of relapse of AML (Storb et al., 1989), and the incidence of relapse decreases when the intensity of the conditioning regimen is increased (Clift et al., 1991; Geller et al., 1992).

Infections, toxicity, and outcome

With CD34-selected T-cell depleted allografts, there is a slow recovery of CD4$^+$ lymphocytes during the first 6 months after the transplant, which is likely a factor in the high probability of severe infections in such patients (Martínez et al., 1999). On the other hand, recipients of unmodified allografts have a higher incidence of GHVD, which necessitates intense immunosuppressive treatment. It is not surprising, therefore, that no differences in the incidence of fatal infections between the two groups (CD34-selected versus unmanipulated) have been observed. However, it must be noted that those patients receiving a CD34-selected graft who develop acute GVHD are at a high risk of infection-related mortality. One concern with CD34 selection of the allograft is the potential increase of CMV infections (Link *et al.*, 1999). CMV reactivation is more frequently observed in patients receiving CD34-selected, T-cell depleted allografts, but CMV disease seems not to be increased (Urbano-Ispizua *et al.*, 1998). In one study, CD34-selected, T-cell depleted allogeneic transplants were associated with less nephrotoxicity, hepatotoxicity and mucositis, a lower incidence of veno-occlusive disease, and better performance status at last follow-up compared with unmanipulated allogeneic transplants (Urbano-Ispizua *et al.*, 1998). This was most likely due to the fact that patients receiving T-cell depleted allografts did not receive methotrexate posttransplant and had a lower incidence of GVHD.

Although there are no randomized trials to demonstrate the effects on outcome of performing CD34 selection of the allograft, a retrospective comparison showed an improved disease-free survival in a group of AML/MDS patients receiving a CD34-selected allograft compared with a similar group of patients receiving an unmanipulated allograft. This difference was mainly due to the low GVHD-related death rate, without an increase in the relapse rate, in the CD34-selected group (Urbano-Ispizua *et al.*, 1998). Mavroudis *et al.* (1996), in a series of T-cell depleted allogeneic bone marrow transplants, found an actuarial probability of survival of 74% for patients receiving 1 to 3×10^6 CD34$^+$ cells/kg. Since that study did not include patients receiving more than 3×10^6 CD34$^+$ cells/kg, the question of whether the clinical outcome could be further improved by increasing the CD34$^+$ cell dose remained unanswered. One study analyzed the association of characteristics of the donor, recipient, and the cell content of the graft with outcome in 84 consecutive adult patients with hematological malignancies who received CD34-selected allogeneic transplants from HLA-identical siblings (Urbano-Ispizua *et al.*, 2001a, b, c). Besides accepted factors influencing the clinical outcome, such as the stage of the disease or CMV serology of donor and recipient (Broers *et al.*, 2000), a strong association between the number of donor CD34$^+$ cells and survival was observed. Patients who received between 1 and 3×10^6 CD34$^+$ cells/kg had improved survival compared to patients receiving over 3×10^6 CD34$^+$ cells/kg (actuarial probability 75% versus 42%, respectively; $P = .01$). The high CD34$^+$ cell dose impaired survival as a result of higher transplant-related mortality. This might be due to the fact that this group of patients had a higher incidence, and earlier appearance, of GVHD.

Future directions

Table 27.9 summarizes current issues in the clinical use of purified stem and progenitor cells for hematopoietic grafting. In addition to autologous and allogeneic bone marrow and blood stem cell transplantation, the use of CD34$^+$ cells is being explored for gene therapy, in utero transplantation, and cord blood transplantation. The use of ex vivo "expanded" CD34$^+$ cells is also under active investigation.

For gene therapy, the low cell numbers in the purified CD34$^+$ cell sample results in higher transduction efficiencies and reduces the volume of retroviral supernatant and other components

Table 27.9. *Positive selection for CD34$^+$ stem and progenitor cells in human transplantation*

Advantages and potential uses	Unknowns and disadvantages
1. Decreases malignant contamination in CD34$^-$ cell neoplasms 2. Provides purified populations that can be submitted to further purging, genetic manipulation, or expansion 3. Minimizes volume of cells to be infused (small amounts of DMSO, important for large volume peripheral blood harvests) 4. Potential for T-cell depletion for allogeneic transplantation (to minimize GVHD) 5. Uniformly applicable for allogeneic and autologous transplantation	1. Limited clinical experience, especially with regard to long-term effects and problems (engraftment, recurrence of cancer, secondary neoplasms) 2. Unproven clinical benefit vs. other methods currently in use 3. Some malignancies, especially leukemias, are CD34$^+$ (need to be combined with other manipulations) 4. Removal of accessory cells may impair engraftment

required, relative to unprocessed marrow or PBSC (Karlsson, 1991; Cassel *et al.*, 1993; Brenner, 1996). Diseases that have been investigated in humans include Fanconi anemia, chronic granulomatous disease, hemoglobinopathies, and severe combined immunodeficiency (SCID); in SCID patients, there has been considerable success (Kohn, 1997; Hacein-Bey-Abina, 2002).

Umbilical cord blood can serve as an alternative source of hematopoietic stem cells for transplantation. Many of the initial problems (adequate sample collection, sample manipulation, cryopreservation) have been solved, and a number of cord blood banks have been established. Allogeneic transplants have demonstrated that cord blood has sufficient hematopoietic precursors for long-term engraftment, and suggest that the incidence of GVHD is low (Wagner *et al.*, 1995, 1996; Kurtzberg *et al.*, 1996; Gluckman *et al.*, 1997). Higher engraftment potential per CD34$^+$ cell of cord blood versus marrow or PBSC may make CD34$^+$ cord blood a better source of cells for expansion and gene therapy (Leung *et al.*, 1999; Wang, Doedens, & Dick, 1997).

Thus, CD34$^+$ cell selection is likely to be a useful therapeutic manipulation in human hematopoietic cell transplantation performed for a spectrum of indications.

References

Abkowitz, J.L. (2002). Can human hematopoietic stem cells become skin, gut, or liver cells? *New England Journal of Medicine*, **346**, 770–2.

Andrews, R.G., Bartelmez, S.H., Knitter, G.H. *et al.* (1991). Isolated allogeneic CD34$^+$ marrow cells engraft and reconstitute hematopoiesis in lethally irradiated baboons. *Blood*, **78** (Suppl 1), 257a (Abstract).

Andrews, R.G., Peterson, L.J., Morris, J. *et al.* (2000). Differential engraftment of genetically modified CD34(+) and CD34(–) hematopoietic cell subsets in lethally irradiated baboons. *Experimental Hematology*, **28**, 508–18.

Andrews, R.G., Singer, J.W., & Bernstein, I.D. (1986). Monoclonal antibody 12.8 recognizes a 115-kD molecule present on both unipotent and multipotent hematopoietic colony-forming cells and their precursors. *Blood*, **67**, 842–5.

Aversa, F., Tabilio, A., Terenzi, A. *et al.* (1994). Successful engraftment of T-cell depleted haploidentical three loci incompatible transpalnts in leukemia patients by addition of recombinant human granulocyte colony-stimulating factor mobilized peripheral blood progenitor cells to bone marrow inoculum. *Blood*, **84**, 3948–55.

Aversa, F., Tabilio, A., Velardi, A. *et al.* (1998). Treatment of high-risk acute leukemia with T-cell-depleted stem cells from related donors with one fully mismatched HLA haplotype. *New England Journal of Medicine*, **339**, 1186–93.

Bambach, B.J., Moser, H.W., Blakemore, K. *et al.* (1997). Engraftment following in utero bone marrow transplantation for globoid cell leukodystrophy. *Bone Marrow Transplantation*, **19**, 399–402.

Barnett, D., Granger, V., Whitby, L. *et al.* (1999). Absolute CD4+ T-lymphocyte and CD34+ stem cell counts by single-platform flow cytometry: the way forward. *British Journal of Haematology*, **106**, 1059–62.

Barnett, M.J., Eaves, C.J., Phillips, G.L. *et al.* (1994). Autografting with cultured marrow in chronic myeloid leukemia: results of a pilot study. *Blood*, **84**, 724–32.

Baum, C.M., Weissman, I.L., Tsukamoto, A.S. *et al.* (1992). Isolation of a candidate human hematopoietic stem-cell population. *Proceedings of the National Academy of Science USA*, **89**, 804–8.

Baumheter, S., Singer, M.S., Henzel, W. *et al.* (1993). Binding of L-selectin to the vascular sialomucin CD34. *Science* **262**, 436–38.

Beatty, P., Clift, R.A., Mickelson, E.M. *et al.* (1985). Marrow transplantation from related donors other than HLA-identical siblings. *New England Journal of Medicine*, **313**, 765–71.

Beelen, D.W., Peceny, R., Elmaagacli, A. *et al.* (2000). Transplantation of highly purified HLA-identical sibling donor peripheral blood CD34+ cells without prophylactic posttransplant immunosuppression in adult patients with first chronic phase chronic myeloid leukemia: results of a phase II study. *Bone Marrow Transplantation*, **26**, 823–9.

Bensinger, W.I., Berenson, R.J., Andrews, R.G. *et al.* (1990). Positive selection of hematopoietic progenitors from marrow and peripheral blood for transplantation. *Journal of Apheresis*, **5**, 74–6.

Bensinger, W.I., Buckner, C.D., Shanon-Dorcy, K. *et al.* (1996). Transplantation of allogeneic CD34+ peripheral blood stem cells in patients with advanced hematologic malignancy. *Blood*, **88**, 4132–38.

Berenson, R.J., Andrews, R.G., Bensinger, W.I. *et al.* (1988). Antigen CD34+ marrow cells engraft lethally irradiated baboons. *Journal of Clinical Investigation*, **81**, 951–60.

Berenson, R.J., Andrews, R.G., Bensinger, W.I. *et al.* (1989). Selection of CD34+ marrow cells for autologous bone marrow transplantation. In *Autologous Bone Marrow Transplantation, Proceedings of the Fourth International Symposium*, ed. K.A. Dicke, G. Spitzer, S. Jagannath, & M.J. Evinder-Hodges, pp. 55–60. Houston: The University of Texas and MD Anderson Cancer Center.

Berenson, R.J., Bensinger, W.I., Hill, R. *et al.* (1991). Engraftment after infusion of CD34+ marrow cells in patients with breast cancer or neuroblastoma. *Blood*, **77**, 1717–22.

Beschorner, W.E., Civin, C.I., & Strauss, L.C. (1985). Localization of hematopoietic progenitor cells in tissue with the anti-My-10 monoclonal antibody. *American Journal of Pathology*, **119**, 1–4.

Bhatia, M., Wang, J.C., Kapp, U. *et al.* (1997). Purification of primitive human hematopoietic cells capable of repopulating immune-deficient mice. *Proceedings of the National Academy of Science*, **94**, 5320–5.

Blystad, A.K., Holte, H., Kvaloy, S. *et al.* (2001). High-dose therapy in patients with Hodgkin's disease: the use of selected CD34(+) cells is as safe as unmanipulated peripheral blood progenitor cells. *Bone Marrow Transplantation*, **28**, 849–57.

Bonnet, D. & Dick, J.E. (1997). Human acute myeloid leukemia is organized as a hierarchy that originates from a primitive hematopoietic cell. *Nature Medicine*, **3**, 730–7.

Brecher, M.E., Sims, L., Schmitz, J.L. *et al.* (1996). North American multicenter study on flow cytometric enumeration of CD34+ hematopoietic stem cells. *Journal of Hematotherapy*, **5**, 227–36.

Brenner, M.K., Rill, D.R., Moen, R.C. *et al.* (1993). Gene-marking to trace origin of relapse after autologous bone-marrow transplantation. *Lancet* **341**, 85–6.

Brenner, M.K. (1996). Gene transfer to hematopoietic cells. *New England Journal of Medicine*, **335**, 337–9.

Broers, A.E., van Der Holt, R., van Esser, J.W. *et al.* (2000). Increased transplant-related morbidity and mortality in CMV-seropositive patients despite highly effective prevention of CMV disease after allogeneic T-cell-depleted stem cell transplantation. *Blood*, **95**, 2240–5.

Brown, J., Greaves, M.F., & Molgaard, H.V. (1991). The gene encoding the stem cell antigen, CD34, is conserved in mouse and expressed in hematopoietic progenitor cell lines, brain, and embryonic fibroblasts. *International Immunology*, **3**, 175–84.

Brugger, W., Heimfeld, S., Berenson, R.J. *et al.* (1995). Reconstitution of hematopoiesis after high-dose chemotherapy by autologous progenitor cells generated ex vivo. *New England Journal of Medicine*, **333**, 283–7.

Brugger, W., Henschler, R., Heimfeld, S. *et al.* (1994). Positively selected autologous blood CD34+ cells and unseparated peripheral blood progenitor cells mediate identical hematopoietic engraftment after high-dose VP16, ifosfamide, carboplatin, and epirubicin. *Blood*, **84**, 1421–6.

Brugger, W., Scheding, S., Subklewe, M. *et al.* (1996). Transplantation of positively selected allogeneic blood CD34+ cells. *Blood*, **88**, (Suppl 1), S599a.

Burnett, A.K., Hann, I.M., Robertson, A.G. *et al.* (1988). Prevention of graft-versus-host disease by ex vivo T cell depletion: reduction in graft failure with augmented total body irradiation. *Leukemia*, **2**, 300–3.

Carbonell, F., Calvo, W., Fliedner, T.M. *et al.* (1984). Cytogenetics studies in dogs after total body irradiation and allogeneic transfusion with cryopreserved blood mononuclear cells: observations in long-term chimeras. *International Cell Cloning* **2**, 81–8.

Cassel, A., Cottler-Fox, M., Doren, S., & Dunbar, C.E. (1993). Retroviral-mediated gene transfer into CD34- enriched human peripheral blood stem cells. *Experimental Hematology*, **21**, 585–91.

Champagne, M.A. & Civin, C.I. (1994). CD34+ progenitor/stem cells for transplantation. *Hematology Review*, **8**, 15–25.

Cheng, J., Baumhueter, S., Cacalano, G. *et al.* (1996). Hematopoietic defects in mice lacking the sialomucin CD34. *Blood*, **87**, 479–90

Civin, C.I. (1990). Human monomyeloid cell membrane antigens. *Experimental Hematology*, **18**, 461–7.

Civin, C.I. (1992). Identification and positive selection of human progenitor/stem cells for bone marrow transplantation. In *Advances in Bone Marrow Purging and Processing*, eds. A.P.

Gee, S. Gross, D.A. & Worthing-White, pp. 461–73. New York: Wiley-Liss.

Civin, C.I., Trischmann, T., Kadan, N.S. *et al.* (1996). Highly purified CD34-positive cells reconstitute hematopoiesis. *Journal of Clinical Oncology*, **14**, 2224–33.

Civin, C.I. & Loken, M.R. (1987). Cell surface antigens on human marrow cells: dissection of hematopoietic development using monoclonal antibodies and multi-parameter flow cytometry. *International Journal of Cell Cloning*, **5**, 267–88.

Civin, C.I., Strauss, L.C., Fackler, M.J. *et al.* (1990). Positive stem cell selection: basic science. In *Bone Marrow Purging and Processing*, ed. S. Gross, A.P. Gee, & D.A. Worthington-White, pp. 387–402. New York: Wiley-Liss.

Civin, C.I., Strauss, L.C., Brovall, C. *et al.* (1984). Antigenic analysis of hematopoiesis III: a hematopoietic progenitor cell surface antigen defined by a monoclonal antibody raised against KG-la cells. *Journal of Immunology*, **133**, 157–65.

Civin, C.I. & Small, D. (1995). Purification and expansion of human hematopoietic stem/progenitor cells. *Annals of New York Academy of Science*, **770**, 91–8.

Civin, C.I., Trischmann, T.M., Fackler, M.J. *et al.* (1989). Summary of CD34 cluster workshop section. In *Leukocyte Typing IV. White Cell Differentiation Antigens*, eds. W. Knapp, B. Dorken, W.R. Gilks *et al.*, pp. 818–25. New York: Oxford University Press.

Civin, C.I., Almeida-Porada, G., Lee, M.J. *et al.* (1996b). Sustained, retransplantable, multilineage engraftment of highly purified adult human bone marrow stem cells in vivo. *Blood*, **88**, 4102–9.

Clift, R.A., Buckner, C.D., Appelbaum, F.R. *et al.* (1991). Allogeneic marrow transplantation in patients with chronic myeloid leukemia in the chronic phase: a randomized trial of two irradiation regimens. *Blood*, **77**, 1660–5.

Collins, R.H. Jr., Shpilberg, O., Drobyski, W.R. *et al.* (1997). Donor leukocyte infusions in 140 patients with relapsed malignancy after allogeneic bone marrow transplantation. *Journal of Clinical Oncology*, **15**, 433–44.

Colter, M., Jones, M., & Heimfeld, S. (1996). CD34⁺ progenitor cell selection: clinical transplantation, tumor cell purging, gene therapy, ex vivo expansion, and cord blood processing. *Journal of Hematotherapy*, **5**, 179–84.

Cornetta, K., Gharpure, V., Hromas, R. *et al.* (1995). Sibling-matched allogeneic bone marrow transplantation using CD34⁺ cells obtained by immunomagnetic bead separation. *Blood*, **86**, 389a (Abstract).

Cornetta, K., Gharpure, V., Mills, B. *et al.* (1998). Rapid engraftment after allogeneic transplantation using CD34⁻ enriched marrow cells. *Bone Marrow Transplantation*, **21**, 65–71.

Corringham, R.E.T. & Ho, A.D. (1995). Rapid and sustained allogeneic transplantation using immunoselected CD34+-selected peripheral blood progenitor cells mobilized by recombinant granulocyte- and granulocyte-macrophage colony-stimulating factors. *Blood*, **86**, 2052–54 (Letter).

Coulombel, L., Kalousek, D.K., Eaves, C.J. *et al.* (1983). Long-term marrow culture reveals chromosomally normal hematopoietic progenitor cells in patients with Philadelphia chromosome positive chronic myelogenous leukemia. *New England Journal of Medicine*, **308**, 1493–8.

Crippa, F., Holmberg, L., Carter, R.A. *et al.* (2002). Infectious complications after autologous CD34-selected peripheral blood stem cell transplantation. *Biology of Blood and Marrow Transplantation*, **8**, 281–9.

Da, W.M., Douay, L., Barbu, V. *et al.* (1991). Serum-free liquid marrow culture in patients with acute lymphoblastic leukemia: a potential application to purge marrow for autologous transplantation. *British Journal of Haematology*, **78**, 42–7.

Delia, D., Lampugnani, M.G., Resnati, M. *et al.* (1993). CD34 expression is regulated reciprocally with adhesion molecules in vascular endothelial cells in vitro. *Blood*, **81**, 1001–8.

Di Nicola, M., Siena, S., Corradini, P. *et al.* (1996). Elimination of bcl-2-IgH-positive follicular lymphoma cells from blood transplants with high recovery of hematopoietic progenitors by the Miltenyi CD34⁺ cell sorting system. *Bone Marrow Transplantation*, **18**, 1117–21.

Doyonnas, R., Kershaw, D.B., Duhme, C. *et al.* (2001). Anuria, omphalocele, and perinatal lethality in mice lacking the CD34-related protein podocalyxin. *Journal of Experimental Medicine*, **194**, 13–27.

Dreger, P., Viehmann, K., Steinmann, J. *et al.* (1995). G-CSF-mobilized peripheral blood progenitor cells for allogeneic transplantation: comparison of T cell depletion strategies using different CD34+ selection systems or CAMPATH-1. *Experimental Hematology*, **23**, 147–54.

Dunbar, G.E., Cottler-Fox, M., O'Shaughnessy, J.A. *et al.* (1995). Retrovirally marked CD34⁻ enriched peripheral blood and bone marrow cells contribute to long-term engraftment after autologous transplantation. *Blood*, **85**, 3048–57.

Elmaagacli, A.H., Peceny, R., Steckel, N. *et al.* (2003). Outcome of transplantation of highly purified blood CD34⁺ cells with T-cell add-back compared with unmanipulated bone marrow or peripheral blood stem cells from HLA-identical sibling donors in patients with first chronic phase chronic myeloid leukemia. *Blood*, **101**, 446–53.

Eyrich, M., Lang, P., Lal, S. *et al.* (2001). A prospective analysis of the pattern of immune reconstitution in a paediatric cohort following transplantation of positively selected human leucocyte antigendisparate haematopoietic stem cells from parental donors. *British Journal of Haematology*, **114**, 422–32.

Fackler, M.J., Civin, C.I., May, W.S., & Stratferd, D.W. (1992). Up-regulation of surface CD34 is associated with protein kinase C-mediated hyperphosphorylation of CD34. *Journal of Biological Chemistry*, **267**, 17540–6.

Fackler, M.J., Civin, C.I., Sutherland, D.R. *et al.* (1990). Activated protein kinase C directly phosphorylates the CD34 antigen on hematopoietic cells. *Journal of Biological Chemistry*, **265**, 11056–61.

Fackler, M.J., Krause, D.S., Smith, O.M. *et al.* (1995). Full-length but not truncated CD34 inhibits hematopoietic cell differentiation of M1 cells. *Blood*, **85**, 3040–7.

Filipovich, A.H., Vallera, D.A., Youle, R.J. *et al.* (1987). Graft versus host disease prevention in allogeneic bone marrow transplantation from histocompatible siblings. *Transplantation*, **44**, 62–9.

Fina, L., Molgaard, H.V., Robertson, D. *et al.* (1990). Expression of the CD34 gene in vascular endothelial cells. *Blood*, **75**, 2417–26.

Finke, J., Brugger, W., Bertz, H. *et al.* (1996). Allogeneic transplantation of positively selected peripheral blood CD34+ progenitor cells from matched related donors. *Bone Marrow Transplantation*, **18**, 1081–6.

Flake, A.W. & Zanjani, E.D. (1997). In utero hematopoietic stem cell transplantation. *Journal of the American Medical Association*, **27**, 932–7.

Friedman, J., Lazarus, H.M., & Koc, O.N. (2000). Autologous CD34⁺ enriched peripheral blood progenitor cell (PBPC) transplantation is associated with higher morbidity in patients with lymphoma when compared to unmanipulated PBPC transplantation. *Bone Marrow Transplantation, 26,* 831–6.

Gahn, B., Schäfer, C., Neef, J. *et al.* (1997). Detection of trisomy 12 and Rb-deletion in CD34⁺ cells of patients with B-cell chronic lymphocytic leukemia. *Blood, 89,* 4275–81.

Gao, Z., Fackler, M.J., Leung, W. *et al.* (2001). Human CD34+ cell preparations contain over 100-fold greater NOD/SCID mouse engrafting capacity than do CD34– cell preparations. *Experimental Hematology, 29,* 910–21.

Gazitt, Y., Reading, C.C., Hoffman, R. *et al.* (1995). Purified CD34+ Lin– Thy+ stem cells do not clone myeloma cells. *Blood, 86,* 381–9.

Geller, R.B., Myers, S., Devine, S. *et al.* (1992). Phase I study of busulfan, cyclophosphamide, and timed sequential escalating doses of cytarabine followed by bone marrow transplantation. *Bone Marrow Transplantation, 9,* 41–7.

Gluckman, E., Rocha, V., Boyer-Chammard, A. *et al.* (1997). Outcome of cord blood transplantation from related and unrelated donors. *New England Journal of Medicine, 337,* 373–81.

Gore, S.D., Kastan, M.B., & Civin, C.I. (1991). Normal human bone marrow precursors that express terminal deoxynucleotidyl transferase include T-cell precursors and possible lymphoid stem cells. *Blood, 77,* 1681–90.

Gorin, N.C., Lopez, M., Laporte, J.P. *et al.* (1995). Preparation and successful engraftment of purified CD34⁺ bone marrow progenitor cells in patients with non-Hodgkin's lymphoma. *Blood, 85,* 1647–54.

Greaves, M.F, Titley, L., Colman, S.M. *et al.* (1995). M10 CD34 cluster workshop report. In *Leukocytes Typing* V, pp. 840–9. Oxford, England: Oxford University Press.

Guyotat, D., Dutou, L., Ehrsam, A. *et al.* (1987). Graft rejection after T-cell depleted marrow transplantation: role of fractionated irradiation. *British Journal of Haematology, 65,* 499.

Hacein-Bey-Abina, S., Le Deist, F., Carlier, F. *et al.* (2002). Sustained correction of X-linked severe combined immunodeficiency by ex vivo gene therapy. *New England Journal of Medicine, 346,* 1185–93.

Hagglund, H.G., McSweeney, P.A., Mathioudakis, G. *et al.* (2000). Ex vivo expansion of canine dendritic cells from CD34+ bone marrow progenitor cells. *Transplantation, 70,* 1437–42.

Hale, G., Cobbold, S., & Waldmann, H. (1988). T-cell depletion with Campath-1 in allogeneic bone marrow transplantion. *Transplantation, 45,* 753–9.

Handgretinger, R., Klingebiel, T., Lang, P. *et al.* (2001a). Megadose transplantation of purified peripheral blood CD34(+) progenitor cells from HLA-mismatched parental donors in children. *Bone Marrow Transplantation, 27,* 777–83.

Handgretinger, R., Lang, P., Ihm, K. *et al.* (2002). Isolation and transplantation of highly purified autologous peripheral CD34+ progenitor cells: purging efficacy, hematopoietic reconstitution and long-term outcome in children with high-risk neuroblastoma. *Bone Marrow Transplantation, 29,* 731–5.

Handgretinger, R., Lang, P., Schumm, M. *et al.* (2001b). Immunological aspects of haploidentical stem cell transplantation in children. *Annals of the New York Academy of Science, 938,* 340–57; discussion 357–8, 340–57.

Handgretinger, R., Schumm, M., Lang, P. *et al.* (1999). Transplantation of megadoses of purified haploidentical stem cells. *Annals of the New York Academy of Science, 872,* 351–62.

Holmberg, L., Boeckh, M., Hooper, H. *et al.* (1999). Increased of cytomegalovirus disease after autologous CD34–selected peripheral blood stem cell transplantation. *Blood, 94,* 4029–35.

Ishizawa, L., Hangoc, G., Van de Ven, C. *et al.* (1993). Immunomagnetic separation of CD34+ cells from human bone marrow, cord blood, and mobilized peripheral blood. *Journal of Hematotherapy, 2,* 333–8.

Johnsen, H.E. & Knudsen, L.M. (1996). Nordic flow cytometry standards for CD34⁺ cell enumeration in blood and leukapheresis products: report from the Second Nordic Workshop. *Journal of Hematotherapy, 5,* 237–45.

Kantarjian, H., Sawyers, C., Hochhaus, A. *et al.* (2002). Hematologic and cytogenetic responses to imatinib mesylate in chronic myelogenous leukemia. *New England Journal of Medicine, 346,* 645–52.

Karlsson, S. (1994). Treatment of genetic defects in hematopoietic cell function by gene transfer. *Blood, 78,* 2481–92.

Kernan, N.A., Bordignon, C., Heller, G. *et al.* (1989). Graft failure after T-cell-depleted human leukocyte antigen identical marrow transplants for leukemia: I. Analysis of risk factors and results of secondary transplants. *Blood, 74,* 2227–36.

Kernan, N.A., Collins, N.H., Juliano, L. *et al.* (1986). T lymphocytes in T-cell depleted bone marrow transplants correlate with development of graft versus host disease. *Blood, 68,* 770–3.

Ketterer, N., Salles, G., Raba, M. *et al.* (1998). High CD34(+) cell counts decrease hematologic toxicity of autologous peripheral blood progenitor cell transplantation. *Blood, 91,* 3148–55.

Klingemann, H.G., Eaves, C.J., Barnett, M.J. *et al.* (1994). Transplantation of patients with high risk acute myeloid leukemia in first remission with autologous marrow cultured in interleukin-2 followed by interleukin-2 administration. *Bone Marrow Transplantation, 14,* 389–96.

Koehl, U., Zimmermann, S., Esser, R. *et al.* (2002). Autologous transplantation of CD133 selected hematopoietic progenitor cells in a pediatric patient with relapsed leukemia. *Bone Marrow Transplantation, 29,* 927–30.

Kogler, G., Nurnberger, W., Fischer, J. *et al.* (1999). Simultaneous cord blood transplantation of ex vivo expanded together with non-expanded cells for high risk leukemia. *Bone Marrow Transplantation, 24,* 397–403.

Kohn, D.B. (1997). Gene therapy for hematopoietic and lymphoid disorders. *Clinical and Experimental Immunology,* (Suppl 1), 54–7.

Kolb, H.-J., Schattenberg, A., Goldman, J.M. *et al.* (1995). European Group for Blood and Marrow Transplantation Working Party Chronic Leukemia: graft-vs.-leukemia effect of donor lymphocyte transfusions in marrow grafted patients. *Blood, 86,* 2041–50.

Krause, D.S., Fackler, M.J., Civin, C.I., & May, W.S. (1996). CD34: structure, biology, and clinical utility. *Blood, 87,* 1–13.

Krause, D.S., Theise, N.D., Collector, M.I. *et al.* (2001). Multi-organ, multi-lineage engraftment by a single bone marrow-derived stem cell. *Cell, 105,* 369–77.

Kurtzberg, J., Laughlin, M., Graham, M.L. *et al.* (1996). Placental blood as a source of hematopoietic stem cells for transplantation into unrelated recipients. *New England Journal of Medicine, 335,* 157–66.

Lagasse, E., Connors, H., Al-Dhalimy, M. *et al.* (2000). Purified hematopoietic stem cells can differentiate into hepatocytes in vivo. *Nature Medicine, 6,* 1229–34.

Lane, T.A., Law, P., Maruyama, M. *et al.* (1995). Harvesting and enrichment of hematopoietic progenitor cells mobilized into the peripheral blood of normal donors by granulocyte-macrophage colony-stimulating factor (GM-CSF) or G-CSF: potential role in allogeneic marrow transplantation. *Blood,* **85,** 275–82.

Lang, P., Handgretinger, R., Niethammer, D. *et al.* (2003). Transplantation of highly purified CD34⁺ progenitor cells from unrelated donors in pediatric leukemia. *Blood,* **101,** 1630–6.

Lang, P., Handgretinger, R., Schlegel, P.G. *et al.* (2000). Transplantation of allogeneic purified peripheral CD34+ stem cells for nonmalignant diseases in children. *Blood,* **56,** 418a (Abstract).

Lang, P., Handgretinger, R., Schumm, M. *et al.* (1999). Transplantation of purified peripheral CD34+ stem cells from unrelated donors in children: effective prevention of GVHD. *Blood,* **94,** 667a (Abstract).

Lapidot, T., Lubin, I., Terenzi, A. *et al.* (1990). Enhancement of bone marrow allografts from nude mice into mismatched recipients by T cells void of graft-versus-host activity. *Proceedings of the National Academy of Science USA,* **87,** 4595–9.

Laurenti, L., Sora, F., Piccirillo, N. *et al.* (2001). Immune reconstitution after autologous selected peripheral blood progenitor cell transplantation: comparison of two CD34+ cell-selection systems. *Transfusion,* **4,** 783–9.

Lemoli, R.M., Martinelli, G., Zamagni, E. *et al.* (2000). Engraftment, clinical, and molecular follow-up of patients with multiple myeloma who were reinfused with highly purified CD34+ cells to support single or tandem high-dose chemotherapy. *Blood,* **95,** 2234–9.

Leung, W., Chen, A.R., Klann, R.C. *et al.* (1998). Frequent detection of tumor cells in hematopoietic grafts in neuroblastoma and peripheral primitive neuroectodermal tumor: purging by immunomagnetic CD34⁺ cell selection. *Blood,* **22,** 971–9.

Leung, W., Ramirez, M., & Civin, C.I. (1999). Quantity and quality of engrafting cells in cord blood and autologous mobilized peripheral blood. *Biology of Blood and Marrow Transplantation,* **5,** 69–76.

Link, H., Arseniev, L., Bähre, O. *et al.* (1996). Transplantation of allogeneic CD34+ blood cells. *Blood,* **87,** 4903–9.

Link, H. (1999). T cell depletion of allogeneic peripheral blood stem cells. *Baillieres Clin Haematol,* ed. C. Gorin, Vol 12, p. 87.

Lowenberg, B., Wagemaker, G., van Bekkum, D.W. *et al.* (1986). Graft-versus-host disease following transplantation of 'one log' versus 'two log' T-lymphocyte-depleted bone marrow from HLA-identical donors. *Bone Marrow Transplantation,* **1,** 133–40.

Majdic, O., Stockl, J., Pickl, W.F. *et al.* (1994). Signaling and induction of enhanced cytoadhesiveness via the hematopoietic progenitor cell surface molecule CD34. *Blood,* **83,** 1226–34.

Mapara, M.Y., Korner, I.J., Lentzsch, S. *et al.* (1999). Combined positive/negative purging and transplantation of peripheral blood progenitor cell autografts in breast cancer patients: a pilot study. *Experimental Hematology,* **27,** 169–75.

Marmont, A., Horowitz, M.M., Gale, R.P. *et al.* (1991). T-cell depletion of HLA-identical transplants in leukemia. *Blood,* **78,** 2120–30.

Martin, P.J. (1993). Donor CD8 cells prevent allogeneic marrow graft rejection in mice: potential implications for marrow transplantation in humans. *Journal of Experimental Medicine,* **178,** 703–12.

Martin, P.J., Hansen, J.A., Torok-Storb, B. *et al.* (1988). Graft failure in patients receiving T cell-depleted HLA-identical allogeneic marrow transplants. *Bone Marrow Transplantation,* **3,** 445–56.

Martínez, C., Urbano-Ispizua, A., Rozman, C. *et al.* (1999). Immune reconstitution following allogeneic peripheral blood progenitor cell transplantation: comparison of recipients of positive CD34+

selected grafts with recipients of unmanipulated grafts. *Experimental Hematology,* **27,** 561–8.

Mason, D.Y., Andre, P., Bensussan, A. *et al.* (2001). CD antigens 2001. *Tissue Antigens,* **58,** 425–30.

Mavroudis, D., Read, E., Cottler-Fox, M. *et al.* (1996). CD34+ cell dose predicts survival, posttransplant morbidity, and rate of hematologic recovery after allogeneic marrow transplants for hematologic malignancies. *Blood,* **88,** 3223–9.

McNiece, J., Briddell, R., Stoney, G. *et al.* (1997). Large-scale isolation of CD34+ cells using the Amgen cell selection device results in high levels of purity and recovery. *Journal of Hematotherapy,* **6,** 5–11.

Michallet, M., Philip, T., Philip, I. *et al.* (2000). Transplantation with selected autologous peripheral blood CD34+ Thy1+ hematopoietic stem cells (HSCs) in multiple myeloma: impact of HSC dose on engraftment, safety, and immune reconstitution. *Experimental Hematology,* **28,** 858–70.

Miltenyi, S., Muller, W., Weichel, W., & Radbruch, A. (1990). High gradient magnetic cell separation with MACS. *Cytometry,* **11,** 231–8.

Miraglia, S., Godfrey, W., Yin, A.H. *et al.* (1997). A novel five-transmembrane hematopoietic stem cell antigen: isolation, characterization, and molecular cloning. *Blood,* **90,** 5013–21.

Murphy, W.J., Kumar, V., Cope, J.C., & Bennett, M. (1990). An absence of T cells in murine bone marrow allografts leads to an increased susceptibility to rejection by natural killer cells and T cells. *Journal of Immunology,* **144,** 3305–11.

Negrin, R.S., Atkinson, K., Leemhuis, T. *et al.* (2000). Transplantation of highly-purified CD34⁺ Thy-1⁺ hematopoietic stem cells in patients with metastatic breast cancer. *Biology of Blood and Marrow Transplantation,* **6,** 262–71.

Noga, S.J., Vogelsang, G.B., Seber, A. *et al.* (1997). CD34+ stem cell augmentation of allogeneic, elutriated marrow grafts improves engraftment but cyclosporine A is still required to reduce GVHD and morbidity. *Transplant Proc,* **29,** 728–32.

O'Reilly, R.J. (1992). T cell depletion and allogeneic bone marrow transplantation. *Semin Hematol,* **29,** (Suppl 1), 20–6.

O'Reilly, R.J., Collins, N.H., Kernan, N.A. *et al.* (1985). Transplantation of marrow-depleted T-cells by soybean lectin agglutination and E-rosette depletion: major histocompatibility complex-related graft resistance in leukemic transplant patients. *Transplantation Proceedings,* **17,** 455–9.

Ogawa, M. (2002). Changing phenotypes of hematopoietic stem cells. *Experimental Hematology,* **30,** 3–6.

Okuno, Y., Iwasaki, H., Huettner, C.S. *et al.* (2002). Differential regulation of the human and murine CD34 genes in hematopoietic stem cells. *Proceedings of the National Academy of Science, USA,* **99,** 9246–51.

Osawa, M., Hanada, K., Hamada, H. *et al.* (1996). Long-term lymphohematopoietic reconstitution by a single CD34-low/negative hematopoietic stem cell. *Science,* **273,** 242–5.

Papadimitriou, C.A., Roots, A., Koenigsmann, M. *et al.* (1995). Immunomagnetic selection of CD34+ cells from fresh peripheral blood mononuclear cell preparations using two different separation techniques. *Journal of Hematotherapy,* **4,** 539–44.

Papadopoulos, E.B., Carabasi, M.H., Castro-Malaspina, H. *et al.* (1998). T-cell-depleted allogeneic bone marrow transplantation as postremission therapy for acute myelogenous leukemia: freedom from relapse in the absence of graft-versus-host disease. *Blood,* **91,** 1083–90.

Passos-Coelho, J.L., Braine, H.G., Davis, J.M. *et al.* (1995). Predictive factors for peripheral-blood progenitor-cell collections using a single large-volume leukapheresis after cyclophosphamide and granulocyte-macrophage colony-stimulating factor mobilization. *Journal of Clinical Oncology,* **13,** 705–14.

Patterson, J., Prentice, H.G., Brenner, M.K. *et al.* (1986). Graft failure following HLA matched T-lymphocyte depleted bone marrow transplantation. *British Journal of Haematology,* **63,** 221–30.

Perez-Simon, J.A., Martin, A., Caballero, D. *et al.* (1999). Clinical significance of CD34+ cell dose in long-term engraftment following autologous peripheral blood stem cell transplantation. *Bone Marrow Transplantation,* **24,** 1279–83.

Petzer, A.L., Eaves, C.J., Barnett, M.J., & Eaves, A.C. (1997). Selective expansion of primitive normal hematopoietic cells in cytokine-supplemented cultures of purified cells from patients with chronic myeloid leukemia. *Blood,* **90,** 64–9.

Pittenger, M.F., Mackay, A.M., Beck, S.C. *et al.* (1999). Multilineage potential of adult human mesenchymal stem cells. *Science,* **284,** 143–7.

Przepiorka, D., Smith, T.L., Folloder, J. *et al.* (1999). Risk factors for acute graft-versus-host disease after allogeneic blood stem cell transplantation. *Blood,* **94,** 1465–70.

Richel, D.J., Johnsen, H.E., Canon, J. *et al.* (2000). Highly purified CD34+ cells isolated using magnetically activated cell selection provide rapid engraftment following high-dose chemotherapy in breast cancer patients. *Bone Marrow Transplantation,* **25,** 243–9.

Rill, D.R., Santana, V.M., Roberts, W.M. *et al.* (1994). Direct demonstration that autologous bone marrow transplantation for solid tumors can return a multiplicity of tumorigenic cells. *Blood,* **84,** 380–3.

Rondelli, D., Andrews, R.G., Hansen, J. *et al.* (1996). Alloantigen presenting function of normal CD34+ hematopoietic cells. *Blood,* **88,** 2619–25.

Rosen, O., Thiel, A., Massenkeil, G. *et al.* (2000). Autologous stem-cell transplantation in refractory autoimmune disease after in vivo immunoablation and ex vivo depletion of mononuclear cells. *Arthritis Research,* **2,** 327–36.

Ryan, D., Kossover, S., Mitchell, S. *et al.* (1986). Subpopulations of common acute lymphoblastic leukemia antigen-positive lymphoid cells in normal bone marrow identified by hematopoietic differentiation antigens. *Blood,* **68,** 417–25.

Sandstrom, C.E., Bender, J.G., Papoutsakis, E.T. *et al.* (1995). Effects of CD34+ cell selection and perfusion on ex vivo expansion of peripheral blood mononuclear cells. *Blood,* **86,** 958–70.

Sasaki, D.T., Tichenor, E.H., Lopez, F. *et al.* (1995). Development of a clinically applicable high-speed flow cytometer for the isolation of transplantable human hematopoietic stem cells. *Journal of Hematotherapy,* **4,** 503–4.

Sassetti, C., Van Zante, A., & Rosen, S.D. (2000). Identification of endoglycan, a member of the CD34/podocalyxin family of sialomucins. *Journal of Biological Chemistry,* **275,** 9001–10.

Satomaa, T., Renkonen, O., Helin, J. *et al.* (2002). O-glycans on human high endothelial CD34 putatively participating in L-selectin recognition. *Blood,* **99,** 2609–11.

Schattenberg, A., De Whitte, T., Preijers, F. *et al.* (1990). Allogeneic bone marrow transplantation for leukemia with marrow grafts depleted of lymphocytes by counterflow centrifugation. *Blood,* **75,** 1356–63.

Schiller, G., Vescio, R., Freytes, C. *et al.* (1995). Transplantation of CD34+ peripheral blood progenitor cells after high-dose chemotherapy for patients with advanced multiple myeloma. *Blood,* **86,** 390–7.

Schiller, G., Vescio, R., Freytes. C. *et al.* (1998). Autologous CD34–selected blood progenitor cell transplants for patients with advanced multiple myeloma. *Bone Marrow Transplantation,* **21,** 141–5.

Schreiner, T., Maccari, B., Erne, E. *et al.* (1996). Highly effective CD34+ selection of granulocyte colony-stimulating factor-mobilized allogeneic peripheral blood progenitor cells. *Blood,* **88,** 1517–8 (Letter).

Schumm, M., Lang, P., Taylor, G. *et al.* (1999). Isolation of highly purified autologous and allogeneic peripheral CD34+ cells using the CliniMACS device. *Journal of Hematotherapy,* **8,** 209–18.

Schwinger, W., Urban, C., Lackner, H. *et al.* (2000a). Unrelated peripheral blood stem cell transplantation with 'megadoses' of purified CD34+ cells in three children with refractory severe aplastic anemia. *Bone Marrow Transplantation,* **25,** 513–7.

Schwinger, W., Urban, C., Lackner, H. *et al.* (2000b). Unrelated partially matched peripheral blood stem cell transplantation with highly purified CD34+ cells in a child with Wiskott-Aldrich syndrome. *Bone Marrow Transplantation,* **26,** 235–7.

Shpall, E., LeMaistre, C.F., Holland, K. *et al.* (1997). A prospective randomized trial of buffy coat versus CD34– selected autologous bone marrow support in high-risk breast cancer patients receiving high-dose chemotherapy *Blood,* **90,** 4313–20.

Shpall, E.J., Champlin, R., & Glaspy, J.A. (1998). Effect of CD34+ peripheral blood progenitor cell dose on hematopoietic recovery. *Biology of Blood and Marrow Transplantation,* **4,** 84–92.

Shpall, E.J., Jones, R.B., Bearman, S.I. *et al.* (1994). Transplantation of enriched CD34– positive autologous marrow into breast cancer patients following high-dose chemotherapy: influence of CD34– positive peripheral-blood progenitors and growth factors on engraftment. *Journal of Clinical Oncology,* **12,** 28–36.

Siena, S., Bregni, M., & Brando, B. (1991). Flow cytometry for clinical estimation of circulating hematopoietic progenitors for autologous transplantation in cancer patients. *Blood,* **77,** 400–9.

Silvestri, F., Banavali, S., Baccarani, M., & Preisler, H.D. (1992). The CD34 hematopoietic progenitor cell associated antigen: biology and clinical applications. *Hematologica,* **77,** 265–73.

Simmons, D.L., Satterth Waite, A.B., Tenen, D.G., & Seed, B. (1992). Molecular cloning of a cDNA encoding CD34, a sialomucin of human hematopoietic stem cells. *Journal of Immunology,* **143,** 267–71.

Small, D., Levenstein, M., Kim, E. *et al.* (1994). STK-1, the human homolog of Flk-2/Flt-3, is selectively expressed in CD34+ human bone marrow cells and is involved in the proliferation of early progenitor/stem cells. *Proceedings of the National Academy of Science USA,* **91,** 459–63.

Soiffer, R.J., Fairclough, D., Robertson, M. *et al.* (1997). CD6-depleted allogeneic bone marrow transplantation for acute leukemia in first complete remission. *Blood,* **89,** 3039–47.

Sovalat, H., Wunder, E., Tienhaara, A. *et al.* (1993). Commentary: prospects for standardization of stem cell determination within Europe. *Journal of Hematotherapy,* **2,** 293–6.

Stockschlader, M., Loliger, C., Kruger, W. *et al.* (1995). Transplantation of allogeneic rh-G-CSF mobilized peripheral CD34+ cells from an HLA-identical unrelated donor. *Bone Marrow Transplantation,* **16,** 719–22.

Storb, R., Deeg, H.J., Pepe, M. *et al.* (1989). Methotrexate and cyclosporine versus cyclosporine alone for prophylaxis of graft-versus-host disease in patients given HLA-identical marrow grafts for leukemia: long-term follow-up of a controlled trial. *Blood,* **73,** 1729–34.

Sutherland, D.R. & Keating, A. (1992). The CD34 antigen: structure, biology, and potential clinical applications. *Journal of Hematotherapy,* **1,** 115–29.

Sutherland, D.R., Anderson, L., Keeney, M. *et al.* (1996). The ISHAGE guidelines for CD34⁺ cell determination by flow cytometry. *Journal of Hematotherapy,* **5,** 213–26.

Suzuki, A., Andrew, D.P., Gonzalo, I.A. *et al.* (1996). CD34-deficient mice have reduced eosinophil accumulation after allergen exposure and show a novel crossreactive 90-kD protein. *Blood,* **87,** 3550–62.

Szczepek, A.J., Bergsagel, P.L., Axelsson, L. *et al.* (1997). CD34⁺ in the blood of patients with multiple myeloma express CD19 and IgH mRNA and have patient-specific IgH VDJ gene rearrangements. *Blood,* **89,** 1824–33.

Tindle, R.W., Nichols, R.A.B., Chen, L. *et al.* (1985). A novel monoclonal antibody BI-3CS recognizes myeloblasts and non-B non-T lymphoblasts in acute leukemias and CGL blast crisis, and reacts with immature cells in normal bone marrow. *Leukemia Research,* **9,** 1–9.

Uharek, L., Glass, B., Gaska, T. *et al.* (1994). Influence of donor lymphocytes on the incidence of primary graft failure after allogeneic bone marrow transplantation in a murine model. *British Journal of Haematology,* **88,** 79–87.

Urban, C., Schwinger, W.E., Sykora, K.W. *et al.* (2001). Unrelated and mismatched family donor SCT with highly purified peripheral CD34+ cells in children with SAA refractory to immunosuppressive therapy. *Blood,* **98,** 675a (Abstract).

Urbano-Ispizua, A., Brunet, S., Solano, C. *et al.* (2001a). Allogeneic transplantation of CD34⁺-selected cells from peripheral blood in patients with myeloid malignancies in early phase: a case control comparison with unmodified peripheral blood transplantation. *Bone Marrow Transplantation,* **28,** 349–54.

Urbano-Ispizua, A., Carrears, E., Marin, P. *et al.* (2001b). Allogeneic transplantation of CD34+ selected cells from peripheral blood from HLA-identical siblings: detrimental effect of a high number of donor CD34+ cells? *Blood,* **98,** 2352–7.

Urbano-Ispizua, A., Rozman, C., Pimentel, P. *et al.* (2001c). The number of donor CD3+ cells is the most important factor for graft failure after allogeneic transplantation of CD34+ selected cells from peripheral blood from HLA-identical siblings. *Blood,* **97,** 383–7.

Urbano-Ispizua, A., Rozman, C., Pimentel, P. *et al.* (2002). Risk factors for acute graft-versus-host disease in patients transplanted with CD34+ selected blood cells from HLA-identical siblings. *Blood,* **100,** 724–7.

Urbano-Ispizua, A., Rozman, C., Martínez, C. *et al.* (1997). Rapid engraftment without significant GVHD after allogeneic transplantation of CD34+ selected cells from peripheral blood. *Blood,* **89,** 3967–73.

Urbano-Ispizua, A., Solano, C., Brunet, S. *et al.* (for the Spanish Group of Allo-PBT). (1998). Allogeneic transplantation of selected CD34+ cells from peripheral blood: experience of 62 cases using immuno-adsorption or immunomagnetic technique. *Bone Marrow Transplantation,* **22,** 519–25.

Verdonck, L.F., Dekker, A.W., de Gast, G.C. *et al.* (1994). Allogeneic bone marrow transplantation with fixed low number of T cells in the marrow graft. *Blood,* **83,** 3090–6.

Vescio, R., Schiller, G., Stewart, A.K. *et al.* (1999). Multicenter phase III trial to evaluate CD34+ selected versus unselected autologous peripheral blood progenitor cell transplantation in multiple myeloma. *Blood,* **93,** 1858–68.

Vescio, R.A., Hong, C.H., Cao, J. *et al.* (1994). The hematopoietic stem cell antigen, CD34, is not expressed on the malignant cells in multiple myeloma. *Blood,* **84,** 3283–90.

Voltarelli, J.C., Corpuz, S. & Martin, P.J. (1990). In vitro comparison of two methods of T cell depletion associated with different rates of graft failure after allogeneic marrow transplantation. *Bone Marrow Transplantation,* **6,** 419–23.

Vose, J.M., Bierman, P.J., Lynch, J.C. *et al.* (2001). Transplantation of highly-purified CD34⁺ Thy-1⁺ hematopoietic stem cells in patients with recurrent indolent non-Hodgkin's lymphoma. *Biology of Blood and Marrow Transplantation,* **7,** 680–7.

Wagner, J.E., Kernan, N.A., Steinbuch, M. *et al.* (1995). Allogeneic sibling umbilical-cord-blood transplantation in children with malignant and non-malignant disease. *Lancet,* **346,** 214–9.

Wagner, J.E., Rosenthal, J., Sweetman, R. *et al.* (1996). Successful transplantation of HLA-matched and HLA-mismatched umbilical cord blood from unrelated donors: analysis of engraftment and acute graft-versus-host disease. *Blood,* **88,** 795–802.

Wagner, J.E., Santos, G.W., Noga, S.J. *et al.* (1990). Bone marrow graft engineering by counterflow centrifugal elutriation: results of a phase I–II clinical trial. *Blood,* **75,** 1370–7.

Wang, J.C., Doedens, M., & Dick, J.E. (1997). Primitive human hematopoietic cells are enriched in cord blood compared with adult bone marrow or mobilized peripheral blood as measured by the quantitative in vivo SCID-repopulating cell assay. *Blood,* **89,** 3919–24.

Watts, M.J., Sullivan, A.M., Ings, S.J. *et al.* (1997). Evaluation of clinical scale CD34+ cell purification: experience of 71 immunoaffinity column procedures. *Bone Marrow Transplantation,* **20,** 157–62.

Williams, S.F., Lee, W.J., Bender, J.G. *et al.* (1996). Selection and expansion of peripheral blood CD34⁺ cells in autologous stem cell transplantation for breast cancer. *Blood,* **87,** 1687–91.

Yin, A.H., Miraglia, S., Zanjani, E.D. *et al.* (1997). AC133, a novel marker for human hematopoietic stem and progenitor cells. *Blood,* **90,** 5002–12.

Zaucha, J.M., Gooley, T., Heimfeld, S. *et al.* (2000). The ratio of CD3:CD14 cells and the number of CD34 cells in G-CSF mobilized peripheral blood mononuclear cell (G-PBMC) products are significantly associated with clinical outcome in HLA-identical sibling transplantation. *Blood,* **96,** (Suppl. 1), 205a.

Zhou, G., Chen, J., Lee, S. *et al.* (2001). The pattern of gene expression in human CD34(+) stem/progenitor cells. *Proceedings of the National Academy of Science, USA,* **98,** 13966–71.

28 Cryopreservation and functional assessment of harvested bone marrow and blood stem cells

JEFFREY SZER

Royal Melbourne Hospital, Melbourne, Australia

Introduction

High-dose anticancer therapy given in marrow-ablative or near-ablative doses is now an accepted or investigational form of therapy for many hematologic and nonhematologic malignant and nonmalignant diseases. A source of "protected" hematopoietic stem cells is required to circumvent the lethal marrow toxicity of many such treatment regimens (Armitage & Gale, 1989).

The aims of cryopreservation are to preserve living tissue (in this case, pluripotent hematopoietic stem cells obtained from the bone marrow or peripheral blood) in a form in which it can be resuscitated with a high degree of viability and functional integrity and in a form suitable for administration without undue toxicity.

Fresh allogeneic bone marrow may be used for transplantation when there is an appropriate donor available, but there are clinical situations in which such a donor cannot be found or where allogeneic transplantation is inadvisable. Under these circumstances, hematopoietic stem calls may be obtained from the patient prior to the institution of therapy, to be reinfused at the completion of the treatment program. If there is a delay of more than 72 hours between the collection and reinfusion of the cells, there is a need to cryopreserve them in a form that preserves viability and engraftment potential (Lasky, McCullough & Zanjani, 1986). In addition, there are occasional situations in which it may be advisable or necessary to cryopreserve allogeneic marrow. This need may arise when delivery to the patient cannot be guaranteed within a reasonable time (under 40 hours) from harvest for reasons of geographic isolation, or where the availability of the donor is time-limited and does not comply with the time required for the patient to complete the conditioning regimen. Additionally, some transplant centers offer cryopreserve allogeneic peripheral blood stem cells,

Stockschläder and colleagues (1995, 1996, 1997) compared the rate of engraftment in recipients of cryopreserved related bone marrow and fresh related bone marrow and found no difference in the time to neutrophil recovery. Additionally they found the same incidence of acute and chronic graft-versus-host disease (GVHD) in each group. Day 100 survival and long-term hematopoiesis did not appear adversely affected by the use of cryopreserved marrow. The same group has also reported on the results of 10 patients given cryopreserved unrelated bone marrow transplants and again found no adverse impact on rate of neutrophil recovery.

Peripheral blood-derived stem cells are usually collected over a period of days by one or multiple leukapheresis procedures, necessitating cryopreservation so that the entire collection may be administered as a single infusion at a later time (To & Juttner, 1987). These cells may be used alone or in association with bone marrow for autotransplantation. Studies utilizing allogeneic peripheral blood-derived stem cell transplantation have demonstrated that this cell product may have utility in patients with diseases at high risk of relapse where the increased rate of GVHD has been offset by a reduced relapse rate (Bensinger *et al.*, 2001).

Collection of marrow and peripheral blood stem cells

The harvesting of bone marrow is performed using standard sterile techniques (Thomas & Storb, 1970), usually from the posterior iliac crests of the pelvis. The marrow is collected into an anticoagulant solution containing acid-citrate-dextrose or heparin in a bag with outlet ports suitable for subsequent processing. It is usual to perform a count of nucleated cells in the final collection mix and a simultaneous nucleated cell count in the blood, so as to correct for the number of contaminating peripheral blood white cells in the final marrow mix. With processing, it can no longer be assumed that the various populations of nucleated cells will remain in the original ratios, making the correction less useful.

Peripheral blood stem cells can be collected by cytapheresis either in the steady state (although this requires multiple leukaphereses and is seldom practical), or, after chemotherapy, hematopoietic growth factors or both have been administered to provoke their release from the bone marrow (see Chapter 24).

The number of cells cryopreserved is expressed as the total number of nucleated cells or CD34+ cells, or mononuclear cells, the latter being used primarily where techniques known to enrich for this population (such as density gradient separation) are utilized.

If bone marrow is to be harvested, one unit of autologous blood should be collected approximately 1 week prior to harvest, for subsequent reinfusion during marrow harvest. Allogeneic blood transfusion should be avoided in this situation. A 3-month course of iron tablets should be given after the harvest.

Volume reduction

Unless the stem cells have been positively selected for CD34 antigen expression, volume reduction of the collection is required. At a very basic level, the amount of storage space available to most transplant units is finite and is most efficiently utilized when the volume of stem cells frozen is least. This approach also leads to the use of lower volumes of cryoprotectant and the lowest final infusion volume, which reduces the risk and severity of toxicity related to the infusion (Davis et al., 1990). The toxicities associated with infusion of cryopreserved cells are summarized in Table 28.1. Some unusual toxicities such as neurological effects have been reported (Hoyt, Szer & Grigg, 2000)

The small volume collection chambers that are now available for some cell separator machines may overcome the need for separate volume reduction. The removal of the majority of red cells (using hydroxyethyl starch sedimentation, manual centrifugation, or a cell washer) makes available autologous red cells for reinfusion after the harvest. In addition, there is evidence that red cells interfere with the action of some reagents, particularly 4-hydroperoxycyclophosphamide, which is sometimes used to treat marrow in vitro, prior to cryopreservation (Santos & Colvin, 1986). The final cell product is either a buffy coat or mononuclear cell preparation, depending on the technique used for processing. The ideal final concentration of cells in the freezing mixture is still uncertain, although some studies suggest that concentrations as high as 200×10^6 nucleated cells/ml are achievable (Villalón et al. 2002).

Addition of cryoprotectant

Dimethylsulfoxide (DMSO) is the most widely used cryoprotectant utilized in the cryopreservation of hematopoietic stem cells. This agent is a universal solvent capable of crossing cell membranes under rapidly changing environmental conditions and so stabilizes the membrane. In this setting, the major effect is to protect the cells from destruction due to the formation of intracellular ice crystals during freezing and the release of heat during the period of phase transition (Fig. 28.1). The toxicity of DMSO to cells at room temperature is well described, and thus freezing protocols have emphasized the need to add DMSO at low temperature (4°C) at a constant rate with immediate transfer to the freezing stage, so as to minimize exposure of stem cells to DMSO in the nonfrozen state. Some investigators have reported the use of hydroxyethyl starch in addition to DMSO to reduce clumping after thawing (Makino et al., 1991). Various concentrations of DMSO have been used, but a typical freezing mixture contains final concentrations of 10% DMSO and 5% human serum albumin.

The final solution is transferred either to vials or more conveniently to plastic (usually polyolefin) bags capable of withstanding the freeze-thaw cycle without damage. Freezing bags with a capacity of approximately 100 to 200 ml are the most convenient since, after thawing, the content may be infused immediately. The use of smaller freezing vials necessitates a number of steps between thawing and infusion, as the thawed material must be transferred to a syringe or bag in a sterile fashion and infused rapidly. A number of small aliquots of the cell mixture are cryopreserved in vials along with the bags for assessment of in vitro colony formation.

If bag storage is employed, a critical step is the exclusion of all air prior to heat sealing. Failure to adhere to this may result in explosion of the bag as it is removed from the nitrogen storage to room temperature. Diligence is required as each bag is thawed, and if it appears that some air has been trapped, it is generally safer to create a small opening with a sterile scalpel blade with subsequent sealing of the affected corner by an appropriately sized clamp.

Freezing technique

Traditionally, freezing has been undertaken in an apparatus in which liquid nitrogen is pumped into the freezing chamber so that the temperature of the cell suspension falls at a constant rate, usually 2°C/min. At phase transition, heat is given off by the solution, and as described above, this may be damaging to the cells. An additional injection of nitrogen is required at this point in order to smooth the freezing curve (arrow in Fig. 28.1). Freezing machines either require manual supplementation by an operator carefully observing the temperature of the solution, or are microprocessor-controlled. The final phase of cooling is usually quicker, with the temperature drop adjusted to 5°C/min (Fig. 28.1). When the mixture has reached a final temperature of approximately −120°C it is transferred to the liquid nitrogen storage container.

Some investigators (Makino et al., 1991; Galmés et al., 1996) have described the use of a simplified freezing technique in which the final freezing mixture (including hydroxyethyl

Table 28.1. *Toxicities associated with infusion of cryopreserved stem cells*

Nausea
Vomiting
Flushing
Fevers
Chills
Encephalopathy
Dyspnea
Reduced forced vital capacity
Bradycardia and other arrhythmias (see Chapter 92)
Hypertension
Coagulopathies

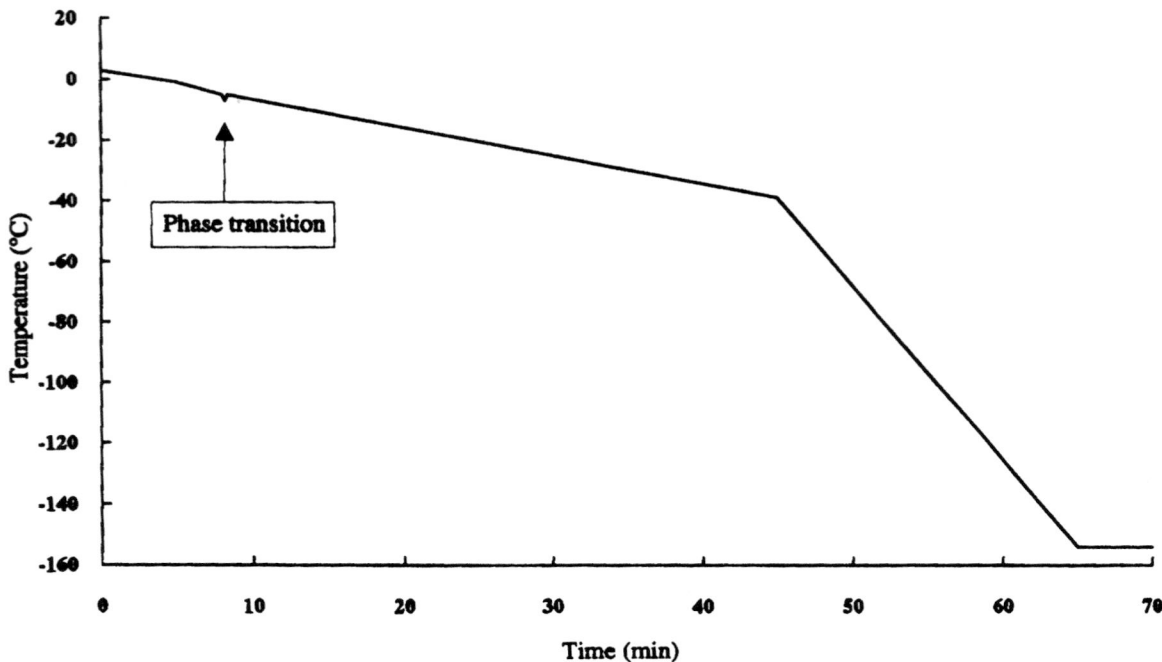

Fig. 28.1. An idealized freezing curve of a bone marrow harvest in a liquid nitrogen-driven, microprocessor-controlled freezer. The point of phase transition (arrow) is where an additional burst of liquid nitrogen is required to prevent a sudden change in temperature of the mixture. The second phase of freezing is at a more rapid rate (5°C/min) than the first (2°C/min).

starch) was placed into a mechanical freezer at −80°C that also served as the storage location. Adequate autologous engraftment in a small number of patients using this technique was described, but this must still be regarded as an experimental approach that may find applicability in some settings.

Additionally there are a number of reports of freezing without a programmed rate freezer, without any apparent adverse impact on rate of hematopoietic recovery postinfusion (Takaue et al., 1994; Hernández-Navarro et al., 1995, 1998; Feremans et al., 1996).

Storage conditions

The majority of centers currently freezing stem cells store the product in the liquid phase of liquid nitrogen (−196°C), although some do so in the vapor phase (−156°C), and as described above, others do so in a mechanical freezer (−80°C). Other reports have described the storage of either apheresis products or even simply venesected blood at 4°C for up to 96 hours and one case for up to 9 days without markedly adverse effects (Jestice et al., 1994; Preti et al., 1994; Ossenkoppele et al., 1996; Pettengell et al., 1995; Ruiz-Arguelles et al. 1995). In some studies a number of parameters such as the granulocyte-macrophage colony-forming unit (CFU-GM) content and the pH of cells stored at 4°C have remained constant for 48 hours, but then began to change (Jestice et al., 1994) (Figs. 28.2 and 28.3). The plasma lactate and glucose levels showed reciprocal changes. The glucose level gradually decreased to

below physiologic levels between 72 and 96 hours of storage (Fig. 28.4). While the lowest possible temperature has been described as producing the best recovery of bone marrow cells after storage (Malini et al., 1970), it is certainly possible that refinements in preparative and storage techniques will make current interpretation of those data obsolete.

In any event, a major aspect of quality control is a system whereby the status of the frozen product is assessed continuously and an alarm system is in operation to preclude the possibility of inadvertent thawing. Ideally, there should be a backup

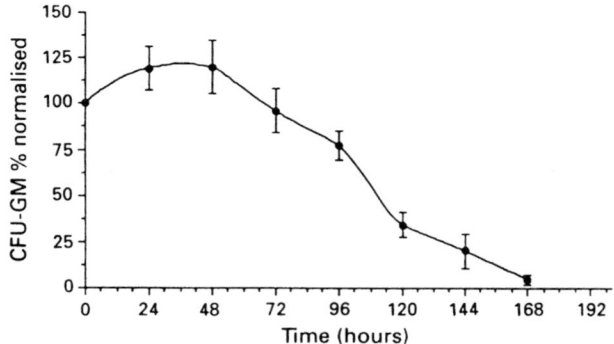

Fig. 28.2. Normalized CFU-GM change at 4°C. Each value is the mean of nine patients ± SEM with the normalized, corrected CFU-GM as a percentage of initial collection values. Reproduced, with permission, from Jestice et al. (1994).

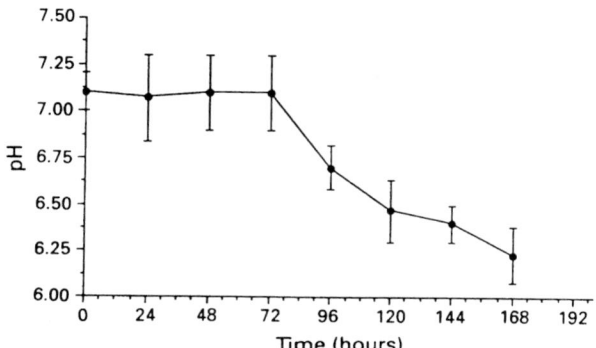

Fig. 28.3. pH change of cells stored at 4°C. Each value is the mean of nine patients ± SEM of the pH change in the stored cell supernatant. Reproduced, with permission, from Jestice *et al.* (1994).

storage facility (either liquid nitrogen or more conventional freezer) available in the event of failure of the primary system.

It is unclear for what period a collection may be stored successfully. At a storage temperature of −196°C, there is no reason for any significant deterioration of viability beyond that caused by the freezing procedure itself. Marrow has resulted in successful engraftment after more than 9 years of storage (Areman, Sacher & Deeg, 1990; Attarian *et al.*, 1996).

Assessment of frozen product

The only absolute evidence of engraftment potential of frozen stem cells (either bone marrow or peripheral blood) is the reconstitution of hematopoiesis by these cells in an individual who has received marrow-ablative therapy. Ideally one wishes to have some indication prior to the delivery of such therapy that an adequate stem cell yield has been obtained. On the basis of allograft data in patients with aplastic anemia, an unfractionated bone marrow cell number of 3×10^8/kg nucleated cells is generally used as a target cell dose. The applicability of this number to autologous

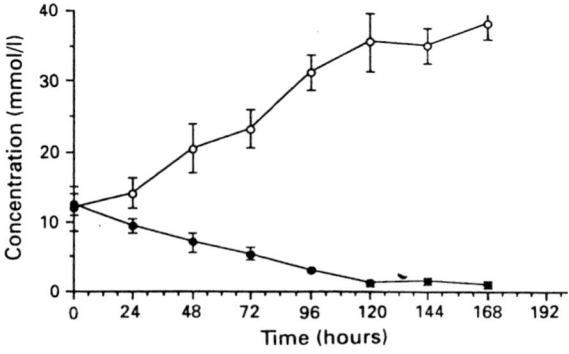

Fig. 28.4. Plasma lactate and glucose. Each value is the mean of nine patients ± SEM. Plasma lactate (○) and glucose (●) concentrations (mmol/l) of the stored cell supernatant. $R = 0.98$, $P < .0001$. Reproduced, with permission, from Jestice *et al.* (1994).

transplantation is unknown, although it is likely that fewer cells than this adequate. This figure is also unlikely to be useful in the context of peripheral blood stem cell transplantation.

Functional assays of in vitro hematopoiesis have been utilized in an attempt to predict the reconstitutive potential of frozen stem cells. The most widely used of these assays initially was the 14-day CFU-GM. While this assay is recognized as measuring a relatively mature progenitor cell, most investigators have chosen to aim at a target number of these cells in the final product of 0.1 to 1×10^4/kg (Gorin, 1986) for bone marrow and 50×10^4/kg (Gianni *et al.*, 1989) for blood stem cells. Unfortunately, there has been little standardization of this assay, so results on the same sample may vary widely in different laboratories. There is also the confounding evidence that after purging with pharmacologic agents, samples with effectively no detectable CFU-GM growth may result in adequate engraftment (Santos & Colvin, 1986). In addition, improvements in the assay conditions over time may make the results of functional assays difficult to compare, even in the same laboratory.

Assays of apparently more primitive progenitor cells such as the granulocyte-erythroid-macrophage-megakaryocyte colony-forming unit (CFU-GEMM or CFU-mix) (Stewart & Kaiser, 1989) and the long-term colony-initiating cell culture (LTC-IC) (Petzer *et al.*, 1996), have been suggested as more reliable, but there is not general agreement on this point, and they have not been widely adopted in routine practice to quantify the engraftment potential of a stem cell collection.

These assays are cumbersome, time-consuming, and operator-dependent. They have the added disadvantage of not providing "real-time evaluation" of the sample being collected. While this is generally not critical with bone marrow collections, it may have a considerable effect on peripheral blood stem cell collections under some circumstances. It is now widely accepted that the majority of cells responsible for engraftment are contained within the fraction of bone marrow (or peripheral blood cells) expressing the CD34 antigen (Siena *et al.*, 1992). Most laboratories now use flow cytometry-based determination of CD34+ cells in the peripheral blood to guide the timing of leukapheresis (Feugier *et al.*, 1995; Zimmerman *et al.*, 1995) and quantitation of CD34+ cells in the leukapheresis product to determine the adequacy of collections (Bensinger *et al.*, 1994). Results of CD34+ cell enumeration can vary widely between centers and it is strongly recommended that a validated procedure such as the ISHAGE method (Sutherland *et al.*, 1996) be used. In addition, a single platform approach in which the white cell count and the CD34+ cell quantitation are performed on the same machine (Barnett *et al.*, 1999) is advised. Standardization of assays across 20 centers in Australia has resulted in the desired reliability of results in that country (Chang & Ma, 1996)

Our center has analyzed engraftment based on the number of CD34+ cells infused and has set a minimum target of 2×10^6 CD34+ cells/kg recipient weight for reliable, rapid engraftment after autologous blood stem cell transplants (Fig. 28.5). Other centers have set a similar target. Slight, albeit significant, accel-

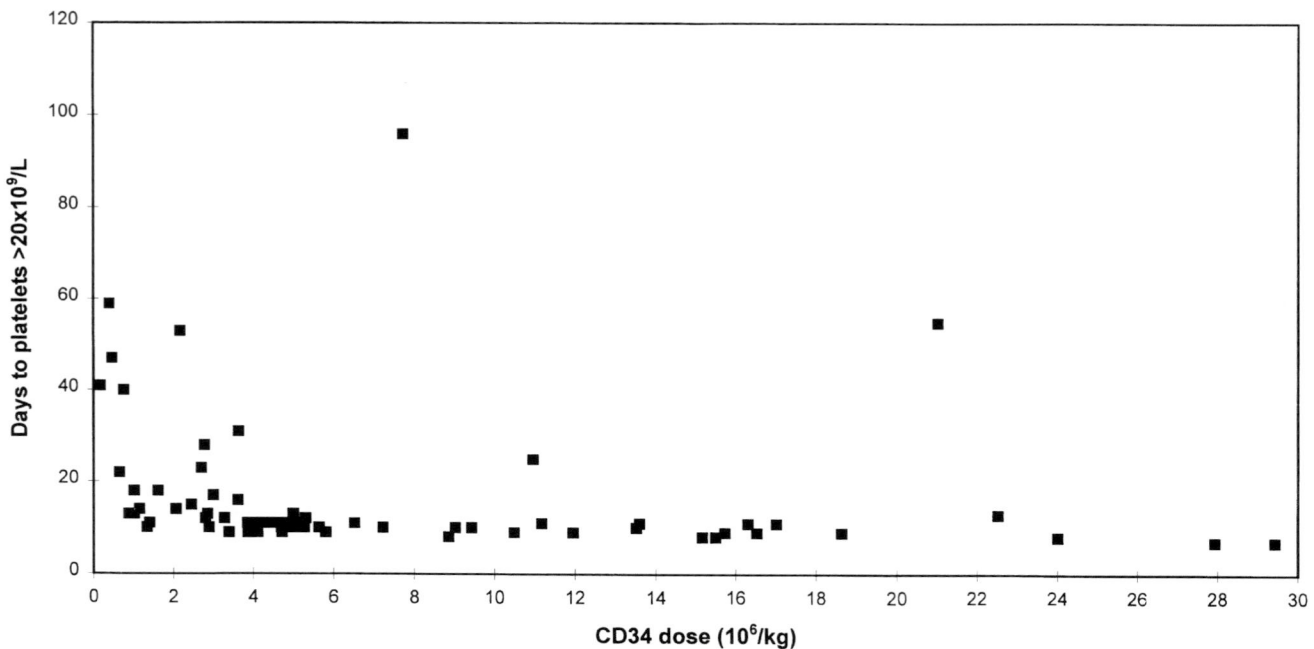

Fig. 28.5. The relationship between CD34+ cell dose and rate of platelet engraftment in an unselected series of patients at the Royal Melbourne Hospital mobilized with hematopoietic growth factor and chemotherapy prior to autografting. The Y axis represents the number of days from transplant to an unsupported platelet count of 20×10^9/l plotted against the number of CD34+ cells infused on the X axis. Points beyond $>30 \times 10^6$ CD34+ cells/kg were not plotted but all days to engraftment for these patients were between 8 and 11 days (Elizabeth O'Flaherty, unpublished data).

eration of both neutrophil and platelet (Figs. 28.6 and 28.7) recovery is obtained by increasing the number of infused CD34+ cells.

Conclusions

Cryopreservation of hematopoietic stem cells has now been practiced for over 25 years. There is, however, no absolute con-

sensus on methods of preparation, cryoprotectant solutions, freezing techniques, concentration of cells, or assays. The determination of CD34+ cells in peripheral blood stem cell collections prior to cryopreservation has become the standard for assessing the adequacy of such collections. It is, however, still the role of each individual center to establish local criteria for, and techniques of, cryopreservation that result in a consistently high-quality stem cell preparation.

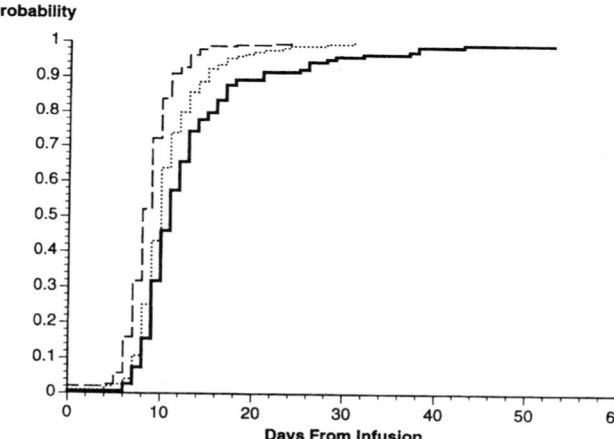

Fig. 28.6. The Kaplan-Meier probability of achieving $\geq 0.5 \times 10^9$ neutrophils/l for $<5.0 \times 10^6$ (—), >5.0 to 10×10^6 (…), and $\geq 10 \times 10^6$ (---) CD34+ cells/kg ($P = .0001$). Reproduced, with permission, from Weaver *et al.* (1995).

Fig. 28.7. The Kaplan-Meier probability of achieving $\geq 20.0 \times 10^9$ platelets/l for $<5.0 \times 10^6$ (—), >5.0 to 10×10^6 (…), and $\geq 10 \times 10^6$ (---) CD34+ cells/kg ($P = .0001$) Reproduced, with permission, from Weaver *et al.* (1995).

References

Areman, E.M., Sacher, R.A., & Deeg, H.J. (1990). Processing and storage of human bone marrow: a survey of current practices in North America. *Bone Marrow Transplantation, 6,* 203–9.

Armitage, J. & Gale, R.P. (1989). Bone marrow autotransplantation. *American Journal of Medicine,* **86,** 203–6.

Attarian, H., Feng, Z., Buckner, C.D. et al. (1996). Long-term cryopreservation of bone marrow for autologous transplantation. *Bone Marrow Transplantation,* **17,** 425–30.

Barnett, D., Granger, V., Whitby, L. et al. (1999). Absolute CD4+ T-lymphocyte and CD34+ stem cell counts by single-platform flow cytometry: the way forward. *British Journal of Haematology,* **106,** 1059–62.

Bensinger, W.I., Longin, K., Appelbaum, F. et al. (1994). Peripheral blood stem cells (PBSCs) collected after recombinant granulocyte colony stimulating factor (rhG-CSF): an analysis of factors correlating with the tempo of engraftment after transplantation. *British Journal of Haematology,* **87,** 835–41.

Bensinger, W.I., Martin, P.J., Storer, B. et al. (2001). Transplantation of bone marrow as compared with peripheral-blood cells from HLA-identical relatives in patients with hematologic cancers. *New England Journal of Medicine,* **344,** 175–81.

Chang, A. & Ma, D.D.F. (1996). The influence of flow cytometric gating strategy in the standardization of CD34+ cell quantitation: an Australian Multicenter Study. *Journal of Hematotherapy,* **5,** 605–16.

Davis, J.M., Rowley, S.D., Braine, H.G. et al. (1990). Clinical toxicity of cryopreserved bone marrow graft infusion. *Blood,* **75,** 781–6.

Feremans, W.W., Bastin, G., Moine, F.L. et al. (1996). Simplification of the blood stem cell transplantation (BSCT) procedure: large volume apheresis and uncontrolled rate cryopreservation at –80°C. *European Journal of Haematology,* **56,** 278–82.

Feugier, P., Schooneman, F., Humbert, J.C. et al. (1995). The number of circulating CD34 positive cells is the best preleukapheresis parameter for predicting the quality of peripheral blood progenitor cell harvest. *Nouvelle Revue Française Hématologie,* **37,** 301–5.

Galmés, A., Besalduch, J., Bargay, N. et al. (1996). Cryopreservation of hematopoietic progenitor cells with 5-percent dimethyl sulfoxide at –80°C without rate-controlled freezing. *Transfusion,* **36,** 794–7.

Gianni, A.M., Siena, S., Bregni, M. et al (1989). Granulocyte-macrophage colony-stimulating factor to harvest circulating haemopoietic stem cells for autotransplantation. *Lancet,* **2,** 580–5.

Gorin, N.C. (1986). Collection, manipulation and freezing of haemopoietic stem cells. *Clinics in Haematology,* **15,** 19–48.

Hernandez-Navarro, F., Ojeda, E., Arrieta, R. et al. (1995). Single center experience of peripheral blood stem cell transplantation using cryopreservation by immersion in a methanol bath. *Bone Marrow Transplantation,* **16,** 71–7.

Hernández-Navarro, E., Ojeda, E., Arrieta, R. et al. (1998). Hematopoietic cell transplantation using plasma and DMSO without HEs, with non-programmed freezing by immersion in a methanol bath: results in 213 cases. *Bone Marrow Transplantation,* **21,** 511–7.

Hoyt, R., Szer, J., & Grigg, A. (2000). Neurological events associated with the infusion of cryopreserved bone marrow and/or peripheral blood progenitor cells. *Bone Marrow Transplantation,* **25,** 1285–7.

Jestice, J.K., Scott, M.A., Ager, S. et al. (1994). Liquid storage of peripheral blood progenitor cells for transplantation. *Bone Marrow Transplantation,* **14,** 991–4.

Lasky, L.C., McCullough, J., & Zanjani, E.D. (1986). Liquid storage of unseparated human bone marrow. Evaluation of hematopoietic progenitors by clonal assay. *Transfusion,* **26,** 331–4.

Makino, S., Harada, M., Akashi, K. et al. (1991). A simplified method for cryopreservation of peripheral blood stem cell at –80°C without rate-controlled freezing. *Bone Marrow Transplantation,* **8,** 239–44.

Malini, T.I., Pegg, D.E., Perry, V.P., & Brodine, V.P. (1970). Long-term storage of bone marrow cells in liquid nitrogen and dry ice temperatures. *Cryobiology,* **7,** 65–9.

Ossenkoppele, G.J., Schuurhuis, G.J., Joukhoff, A.R. et al. (1996). G-CSF (filgrastim)-stimulated whole blood kept unprocessed at 4°C does support a BEAM-like regimen in bad risk lymphoma. *Bone Marrow Transplantation,* **18,** 427–31.

Pettengell, R., Woll, P.J., Thatcher, N. et al. (1995). Multicyclic dose-intensive chemotherapy supported by sequential reinfusion of hematopoietic progenitors in whole blood. *Journal of Clinical Oncology,* **13,** 148–56.

Petzer, A.L., Hogge, D.E., Landsdorp, P.M. et al. (1996). Self-renewal of primitive human hematopoietic cells (long-term-culture-initiating cells) in vitro and their expansion in defined medium. *Proceedings of the National Academy of Sciences USA,* **93,** 1470–4.

Preti, R.A., Razis, E., Ciavarella, D. et al. (1994). Clinical and laboratory comparison study of refrigerated and cryopreserved bone marrow for transplantation. *Bone Marrow Transplantation,* **13,** 253–60.

Ruiz-Arguelles, J.G.J., Ruiz-Arguelles, A., Perez-Romano, B. et al. (1995). Filgrastim-mobilized peripheral blood stem cells can be stored at 4° and used in autografts to rescue high-dose chemotherapy. *American Journal of Hematology,* **48,** 100–3.

Santos, G.W. & Colvin, O.M. (1986). Pharmacologic purging of bone marrow with reference to autografting. *Clinics in Hematology,* **15,** 67–83.

Siena, S., Bregni, M., Belli, N. et al. (1992). Practical aspects of flow cytometry to guide large-scale collections of circulating hemopoietic progenitors for autologous transplantation in cancer patients. *International Journal of Cell Cloning,* **10** (Suppl 1), 26–9.

Stewart, F.M. & Kaiser, D.L. (1989). Progenitor cell numbers (CFU-GM, CFU-D, and CFU-mix) and hemopoietic recovery following autologous marrow transplantation. *Experimental Hematology,* **17,** 974–80.

Stockschläder, M., Hassan, H.T., Krog, C. et al. (1997). Long-term follow-up of leukaemia patients after related cryopreserved allogeneic bone marrow transplantation. *British Journal of Haematology,* **96,** 382–6.

Stockschläder, M., Krüger, W., Kroschke, G. et al. (1995). Use of cryopreserved bone marrow in allogeneic bone marrow transplantation. *Bone Marrow Transplantation,* **15,** 569–72.

Stockschläder, M., Krüger, W., tom Dieck, A. et al. (1996). Use of cryopreserved bone marrow in unrelated allogeneic transplantation. *Bone Marrow Transplantation,* **17,** 197–9.

Sutherland, D.R., Anderson, L., Keeney, M. *et al.* (1996). The ISHAGE guildelines for CD34⁺ cell determination by flow cytometry. *Journal of Hematotherapy,* **5,** 213–26.

Takaue, Y., Abe, T., Kawano, Y. *et al.* (1994). Comparative analysis of engraftment after cryopreservation of peripheral blood stem cell autografts by controlled versus uncontrolled rate methods. *Bone Marrow Transplantation,* **13,** 801–4.

Thomas, E.D. & Storb, R. (1970). Technique for human marrow grafting. *Blood,* **36,** 507–15.

To, L.B. & Juttner, C.A. (1987). Peripheral blood stem cell autografting; a new therapeutic option for AML? *British Journal of Haematology,* **66,** 283–8.

Villalón, L., Odriozola, J., Ramos, P. *et al.* (2002). Cryopreserving with increased cellular concentrations of peripheral blood progenitor cells: clinical results. Haematologica, **87,** ELT06.

Weaver, C.H., Hazelton, B., Birch, R. *et al.* (1995). An analysis of engraftment kinetics as a function of CD34 content of peripheral blood progenitor cell collections in 692 patients after the administration of myeloablative chemotherapy. *Blood,* **86,** 3961–9.

Zimmerman, T.M., Lee, W.J., Bender, J.G. *et al.* (1995). Quantitative CD34 analysis may be used to guide peripheral blood stem cell harvests. *Bone Marrow Transplantation,* **9,** 439–44.

29 The impact of regulation on cellular and gene therapy

ADRIAN P. GEE

Baylor College of Medicine, Houston, USA

Introduction

Cellular therapy (including hematopoietic stem cell [HSC] transplantation and immunotherapy) has undergone a resurgence in recent years, spurred on by new discoveries in stem cell and T-cell biology, the mechanisms of antigen presentation, the use of genetic manipulation of target and effector cells, and the availability of new cytokines and growth factors. In parallel, the numbers and types of cell therapy products have increased, ranging from peripheral and cord blood HSC, multipotent stem cells, allogeneic lymphocytes used for the prevention and/or treatment of disease relapse post–stem cell transplant, through specifically targeted T lymphocytes used to prevent or treat virus-induced tumors, to vaccines composed of genetically manipulated autologous or allogeneic tumor cells (Guermonprez *et al.,* 2002; Mitchell, 2002; Park *et al.,* 2002). The preparation of cellular therapeutic products has been the focus of regulatory interest for a number of years and policies have been developed that address the conditions under which such products must be manufactured (Gee, 2002). The responsibility for the development and enforcement of regulations in this area in the United States falls to the Food and Drug Administration's (FDA) Center for Biological Evaluation and Research (CBER). Recently it has been proposed that, within CBER, an Office of Cellular, Tissue and Gene Therapy will be established, with primary responsibility for these therapies.

In the case of nonmanipulated allogeneic leukocytes or lymphocytes used for donor leukocyte infusions (DLI), preparation, testing, and release criteria currently fall under the practice of medicine and do not require an investigational new drug exemption (IND). The FDA (often referred to as the Agency) has, however indicated that, in the future, it proposes to regulate DLI as cellular and tissue-based products rather than blood products ("Ask the FDA" presentation at the 2001 meeting of the American Association of Blood Banks). The requirement for an IND application is largely predicated upon the perceived risk to the donor and recipient of the cells. Procedures that involve ex vivo culture of the cells and/or their genetic modification are classified as "more than minimal" manipulation and must be performed under an IND (Proposed Approach to Regulation of Cellular and Tissue-Based Products, CBER 1997). This requires that the cell products must be prepared under current Good Manufacturing Practices (cGMP). Similarly, use of cells for other than their normal in vivo function (homologous function) places them into the same classification. In general, products that are prepared for therapeutic use, and do not require an IND, will be regulated under proposed current Good Tissue Practice regulations (cGTP) (Current Good Tissue Practice for Manufacturers of Human Cellular and Tissue-Based Products; Inspection and Enforcement; Proposed Rule, CBER 2001), which incorporate many of the components of cGMP (see Table 29.1).

Current Good Manufacturing Practices

cGMP are defined as a set of current scientifically sound methods, practices, or principles that are implemented during product development and production to ensure consistent manufacture of safe, pure, and potent products. They have their origins in a number of public health and safety problems that arose following the use of toxic and unsafe pharmaceuticals. The components of pharmaceutical cGMP are spelled out in Title 21 of the Code of Federal Regulations (CFR) Parts 210 and 211. Subsequently, the regulations were extended to manufacturers of blood and blood components (Part 606). The regulations provide a detailed infrastructure to be used for manufacturing these types of products. This includes the design and operation of the facility, training and testing of staff, installation, cleaning and calibration of equipment, standard operating procedures for all aspects of operations, labeling, quality assurance and control programs, records, release testing, controls, and complaints files. It is not completely clear at the time of writing how cGMP regulations will be applied to cell therapy products.

The FDA has indicated that it will use a sliding scale of implementation, such that products prepared for phase I trials will not require implementation of full cGMP (Fig. 29.1). For example, full validation of procedures and stability testing data will not be required. By the time the products are in phase III studies, however, full cGMP, as specified in the pharmaceutical regulations (CFR Title 21, Parts 210 and 211) will be required.

The difficulty for establishments manufacturing products that are in transition from phase 1 to phase 3 studies is to know

Table 29.1. *A risk-based approach to regulation of somatic cell therapy*

Product type	Action required	FDA submission
Risk of transmission of communicable diseases		
Autologous that is processed	Follow cGTP	None required
Banked or shipped	Recommend donor screening	
Allogeneic	Follow cGTP	None required
	Require donor screening	
Risk posed by processing		
Autologous or family member that is minimally manipulated ex vivo	Follow cGTP	None required
Unrelated allogeneic OR extensively manipulated	>cGTP (cGTP + cGMP) regulation	IND/IDE – PMA/BLA Compliance with professional standards?
Clinical safety considerations		
Unrelated donor OR Extensively manipulated AND/OR Nonhomologous function AND/OR Combined with nontissue (device)	Generate safety and efficacy date	IND/IDE – PMA/BLA
Labeling and registration		
All products EXCEPT autologous transplanted in single surgical procedures	Clear, accurate, & nonmisleading labeling	Depends on type of product
	Notify FDA of existence of facility & products manufactured	Facility registration and annual listing of products

Abbreviations: PMA, pre-market approval; BLA, biological license application.
Adapted from "Proposed Approach to the Regulation of Cellular and Tissue-Based Products," CBER 1997.

what "level" of cGMP is required. Recently, the FDA has requested from holders of INDs that deal with cell therapy products comprehensive information on manufacturing and quality control systems. The level of detail requested suggests that the bar for full cGMP implementation will not be lowered and that the requirements will become more rigorous.

Academic cGMP

Implementation of cGMP has come as something of a culture shock to most academic cell therapy facilities, unused to

being regarded as product manufacturers. As a result, the interpretation of what is required has varied widely. There has been a particular emphasis on the type of facility that is required. In some cases, manufacturing has been performed in pharmaceutical-grade clean rooms, while in others, modified areas of research laboratories have been used. The reality is that cGMP does not specifically prescribe the precise environmental conditions under which manufacturing occurs. Part 211.46 of Title 21 CFR states that "air filtration systems, including prefilters and particulate matter air filters, shall be used when appropriate on air supplies to production

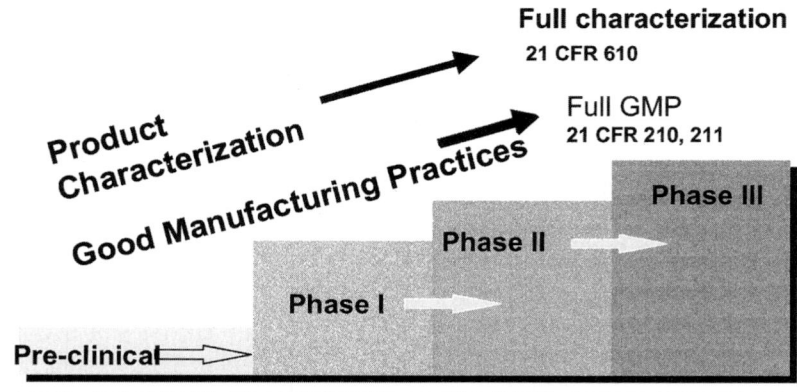

Fig. 29.1. Step-wise approach to application of regulatory requirements adapted from slide shown at an FDA presentation. This figure shows the increasing level of cGMP implementation and product characterization required as a cellular product moves from preclinical to phase III clinical evaluation.

areas." The proposed cGTP regulations indicate that when filtration systems are in use they must be appropriately checked and maintained. The FDA has not indicated that it will require Class 10,000 clean rooms for preparation of cell therapy products, where the drive has already been toward the use of closed handling systems and production in Class 100 biological safety cabinets.

The regulations, instead, provide basic criteria that must be met with respect to adequacy, cleanliness, and organization of space and product flow. This can be achieved in the absence of HEPA-filtered air handling systems. The primary emphasis is therefore on using systems that ensure that there is a consistent, controlled, and auditable manufacturing process that results in a safe and effective product.

From the laboratory to the bedside

In the case of cellular immunotherapy products, efficacy is usually evaluated in the clinical study, so the primary emphasis for manufacturing becomes meeting criteria for functional activity measured ex vivo, and also for ensuring the safety of the cell donor and recipient. This necessitates the involvement of the cell processing facility (CPF) at all stages of development from basic research experiments through to clinical studies. Basic research studies provide the evidence that specific cell populations may have efficacy for a particular clinical application. This information must be generated under good laboratory practice conditions (GLP). These are described in the Code of Federal Regulations (Title 21 CFR, Part 58); however, many basic researchers are unaware of, or poorly understand, GLP. Since many components of GLP resemble those of cGMP (see below), a close interaction between the basic research laboratory and the CPF can facilitate the smooth transition of the research into clinical studies. The CPF staff can also provide useful advice on the selection of cGMP-friendly reagents and methods, as well as expertise on the scale-up of cell preparation to a clinically applicable level. This can eliminate extensive repetition of experiments when procedures move to the CPF.

The next stage in development of protocols that involve more-than-minimal manipulation of the cell product, is the preparation and submission of an IND application. This will require preparation of Standard Operating Procedures (SOPs) that describe the production and testing methods that will be used in the manufacturing process. In addition, the CPF may be asked to provide information on the facility that will be used and the quality program that is in operation. The documentation that is submitted should allow the Agency to clearly understand the manufacturing flowpath and what testing will be used at each stage for monitoring product quality. Release criteria must also be provided to specify what test results must be achieved in order for the product to be administered to the patient.

Usually a sample Certificate of Analysis (C of A) will be provided, which lists each test to be performed and the required results. The selection of tests depends on the particular product; however, the panel that is chosen routinely contains assays that reflect product safety (bacterial and fungal sterility, mycoplasma [all negative] and endotoxin [usually <5 EU/ml]); product potency (a functional assay for product activity, e.g., secretion levels of a product or cytotoxic activity); viability (usually >70%), and purity (usually by flow cytometric analysis). In some cases, HLA typing of the original cell donor and confirmatory typing of the product will be required as an identity check.

The selection of test methods is also an important factor, as many frequently used commercial tests do not meet the requirements specified by the Code of Federal regulations (see below).

The C of A will be reviewed by a representative of the quality program, the production facility, and a physician who is familiar with the study, but is not the holder of the IND, to prevent potential conflict of interest. Additional information on staff training and competency, test methods, and reagent specifications may also be required as a part of the IND submission.

An issue that frequently arises during IND submission is the substitution of clinical grade reagents for research materials that were used in the preclinical studies. In most cases it is possible to find substitutes for media, etc. Growth factors and cytokines, however, present a more difficult problem. There are few FDA-approved factors available, and it is usually necessary to obtain certificates of analysis from the manufacturers of research products and select the source that has been most rigorously tested. In consultation with the regulatory agency, the specifications of these agents can be examined and decisions made as to whether additional testing will be required for clinical use. The assembly of material for the IND provides the foundation for moving a procedure into the CPF.

GMP operation of a cell processing facility

Regardless of the particulars of the procedure, the CPF must have in place SOPs that cover the infrastructure and daily operation of the cGMP facility. These will cover facility management, cleaning procedures, staff training, competency and proficiency testing, quality assurance and control programs, process and equipment validation, materials management, and equipment maintenance and calibration.

Operational SOPs

The foundation for cGMP compliance for a CPF consists of basic systems that show that the facility is in compliance, even when there is no active product manufacturing ongoing. As indicated previously, these cover the daily operation and maintenance of the facility. There must be training files on all the staff. These include their job descriptions, curriculum vitae, documentation of training, details of mandatory training (e.g., safety, bloodborne pathogens, universal precautions, cGMP operations), continuing education, and evaluations. Programs should be developed for testing the proficiency and competency of the staff on an ongoing basis.

There should be a detailed plan of the facility indicating product, waste, and personnel flow, air handling systems, and evacuation routes. The procedures for cleaning the facility must be described and cleaning agents should be validated for their efficacy against potential contaminating organisms. Efficacy of cleaning and air handling systems must be documented, usually by means of an environmental monitoring program. This specifies the cleaning schedule and agents, monitoring of cleaning and contamination (e.g., by use of RODAC plates), and remedial actions when required. There must be procedures to describe cleaning procedures between handling different products (changeover procedures). Specialized air handling systems must be calibrated, maintained, and shown to be within specifications by particulate and viable counts and fall-out plates. SOPs must be developed for ordering, quarantine testing, and release of supplies and reagents and management of inventory. These should include information on the selection and audit of vendors and specifications for product acceptance. Detailed SOPs should cover the installation, qualification, validation, calibration, cleaning, and maintenance of all equipment. Systems should be developed to track each product prepared using a particular piece of equipment, and conversely, all equipment used for the preparation of a particular product. Each facility should also have procedures on file to deal with emergencies, system failures, evacuation, and actions to be taken in case of equipment alarms. Electronic data management systems are also of particular interest to the FDA (Draft Guideline for the Validation of Blood Establishment Computer Systems, CBER, 1993), and the Agency has recently published a Guidance Document on the General Principles of Software Validation (CDER/CBER, 2002). The requirements are detailed and most facilities will struggle to meet them without the aid of an outside consultant. At very least, a plan should be in place to detail how compliance is to be achieved.

Manufacturing SOPs

Facility management procedures are supplemented with specific SOPs that cover each manufacturing procedure and documentation that staff have been trained on that procedure. Since few cell therapy products are highly characterized when introduced into phase 1 studies, it is important to set realistic expectations in the SOP and provide sufficient flexibility in the procedure to address biological variability. The basic structure of all SOPs is, however, the same. There should be a standardized format and numbering system to allow the document and subsequent revisions to be tracked. The format should include title, purpose, materials, reagents and equipment, procedure, expected results, attachments, references, and a sign-off section that shows that the SOP has undergone appropriate review and release. Instructions for the preparation release and annual review of all SOPs should be available in an SOP for SOPs. Effective SOPs are written in a style that provides sufficient information for an appropriately experienced individual to perform the procedure and achieve the expected results. Overly detailed procedures are unhelpful, since they tend to be lengthy, difficult to follow, and can result in the generation of multiple variance documents describing minor and unimportant deviations. The expected results section is important since it provides the user with an indication of when the procedure has been performed successfully. The expected results can be written in a manner that allow for normal biological variability, but set alert limits that will trigger remedial action. Establishment of expected results for a manufacturing procedure is achieved by validation.

Validation

Validation is an important component of the introduction of a new procedure and provides the evidence that the procedure is cable of routinely achieving the required and expected results. For a new procedure validation is prospective. The criteria for acceptable performance of the procedure are established and the procedure is performed multiple times to determine whether these can be routinely met. In the case of manufacturing of cellular products, the validation process can be more complex, due to the variability of biological materials and processes. Selection of the criteria for acceptability can be simplified by use of those specified in the Certificate of Analysis. Criteria such as maintenance of sterility during production can be applied rigidly for validation, whereas others, such as functional activity, must allow for inherent variability and the criteria should be given as a range of acceptable results. These studies should be designed in collaboration with quality assurance/quality control personnel (QA/QC), who will ultimately be responsible for signing off on the validation. Recently, CBER has published a Guidance document titled "Validation of Procedures for Processing Human Tissues for Transplantation" which primarily discusses validation measures intended to prevent contamination during processing (CBER, 2002).

In some cases, procedures have been in use for a long time without formal validation. In these cases a retrospective validation should be performed. This can be accomplished by collating historical results and comparing them to those published in the literature, or by the manufacturer of the equipment used. Ongoing documentation of results can provide a check on the proficiency of specific staff members, as well as a warning of any developing problems.

Documentation

Efficient documentation is at the heart of cGMP. It provides primary evidence that the facility is in routine compliance with the regulations. It is essential to develop a user-friendly system for recording the required data during the manufacturing process. Direct linkage to other associated data (such as environmental monitoring, calibration information, etc.) is also valuable. Manufacturing data are usually assembled in the form of a batch record and the sections that follow describe the system used at the Baylor College of Medicine Center for Cell and Gene Therapy for assembling this document.

Production starts with the generation of a prescription for cell collection. This details the identity of the donor and recipient, the number and type of cells to be collected, the study protocol, and the nature of the product to be manufactured. This is signed by the attending physician and a Laboratory (GMP Facility) Medical Director. Receipt of the prescription by the CPF generates a query on infectious disease testing of the donor, to determine whether this already exists and whether it will be within 30 days of currency at the time of cell collection. Guidance on donor infectious disease can be obtained from the FDA Proposed Rule "Suitability Determination for Donors of Human Cellular and Tissue Based products" published in 1999. This has been recently supplemented by a Guidance document "Preventive Measures to Reduce the Possible Risk of Transmission of Creutzfeld-Jakob Disease (CJD) and Variant Creutzfeld-Jakob Disease (vCJD) by Human Cells, Tissues and Cellular and Tissue-Based products (HCT/Ps)." If required by the IND, HLA typing information will be obtained or requested. This serves as a confirmation of the identity of the cells in the final product.

The next step is accessioning of the cells. Since the Center handles products from multiple hospitals, we have developed our own internal unique identifier system that issues a "P" number to each patient and donor and a "C" to each component that is received by the CPF. The "C" number can be modified as subcomponents are generated from the parent component (e.g., C123.1). The identifiers are generated by QA/QC using a software program. The cells and the rudimentary batch record (Prescription, ID/HLA results, and component numbers) are then transferred with the cells to the technologist who will do the hands-on manufacturing.

Cell handling systems

Culture systems have to be very flexible for most immunotherapy products. In contrast to hematopoietic progenitor cell processing, where a large volume or number of cells is processed, immunotherapy starting materials can come in a variety of forms, ranging from a small volume of blood, to a large tissue sample. In many cases the practice is to start with a relatively small sample, from which the target cell population must be isolated, manipulated, and expanded. While there has been considerable progress in the development of closed handling systems for larger cell numbers, small numbers still often start out in petri dishes, cluster plates, or 96 well plates, and progress through progressively larger open culture systems until sufficient cells have been grown to permit transfer into a bag. Overexpansion at an early stage can result in decreased viability or loss of the culture. The use of open systems obviously increases the risk for contamination, and requires particular attention to aseptic technique and sterility monitoring. Regulatory guidance discourages the routine use of antibiotics in culture media, and when they are used, recommends that they should be assayed for in the final cell product, and/or that a validated system should be used for their removal.

There are incidences where a starting product is irreplaceable and is received contaminated. Antibiotic decontamination should be used with care under these circumstances, and discussed with the regulatory agency before such a product is used clinically. When developing and implementing a new cell handling or culture process it is important to establish a system for checking sterility and functionality during manufacture. This can be used to identify problematic steps in the procedure and also to validate aseptic technique so that some of the in-process testing can be eventually eliminated.

Each stage of cell manipulation is recorded on worksheets that provide step-by-step documentation of cell culture processes (stimulation, cryopreservation, etc.). Each worksheet is accompanied by an Activity Report. This lists all the reagents used, the manufacturer, lot number, and expiration date. It also provides a listing of equipment used, the serial number, and the date of calibration. Although such data can be recorded manually, we have encoded it into barcodes that are scanned during the manufacturing process. Barcodes are applied to reagents at the time of receipt and accessioning into cGMP storage. In order to be released into storage the reagent or supply must also have a certificate of analysis from the manufacturer or supplier on file.

Each worksheet and activity report is signed by the technologist and reviewed by a second staff member. Testing is documented by inclusion of the test request form, the confirmatory e-mail from the test laboratory that provides an accessioning number for tracking the results, and eventually by a summary sheet listing the results generated by the QA/QC Laboratory database system. Labeling during processing is computer-generated in-house, and copies of labels are attached to the worksheets and cross-checked by a second staff member before use. These checks are documented. At the time of cryopreservation and storage, an inventory form is completed listing the products to be stored and the storage locations and providing a copy of the labels used on the storage containers. These data are transcribed into a computer-based inventory system by a designated individual. This system has features that prevent double entry into the same location and that track and archive all entries and changes and the identity of the person making the entries.

Testing and test selection

Testing protocols during, and at the end of, manufacturing can be problematic for some cell therapy products. Some guidance can be found in "Guidance for Human Somatic Cell Therapy and Gene Therapy" published in 1998 by CBER. Often total cell numbers are relatively small and the entire product could be consumed in performing the required tests for release. Under such circumstances, it is often possible, in consultation with the FDA, to develop alternative test systems. For example, final wash supernatants or culture media may be used to monitor sterility rather than using the cell product itself. When the product is cryopreserved before use, testing can usually be completed prior to release for therapeutic use. For some products, storage is not indicated and cells are simply washed and infused. Under these circumstances rapid testing is required, and this usually consists of an immediate Gram stain for sterility, an LAL assay for endotoxin, and a polymerase chain reaction (PCR) assay for mycoplasma. These tests can produce results within hours, but routine test methods should be used in parallel and the results documented retrospectively.

Viability testing can also be problematic. A routine practice has been to test cell viability prior to freezing, rather than monitor the thawed product. One reason for this is that some types of cells lose viability if they sit for any length of time in a medium containing cryoprotectant, and logistically it may be difficult to get a thawed sample back to the laboratory quickly. In addition, widely used dye-exclusion viability assays are of questionable value, since they only measure membrane integrity, which may not correlate directly with functionality or cell death. Nonetheless, viability measurements should be taken after thawing, and data should be collected to measure the stability of the product both during the period of storage and at various times after thawing. This information will be required as the clinical study progresses toward a phase III trial.

Test information is obviously critically important if a product is to be released and it is important in the United States to use methods that are acceptable to the FDA (see 21 CFR Part 610.10–14 and 610.40). For example, many hospital laboratories use automated sterility testing systems that finalize test results at 4 to 5 days. In contrast, the CFR sterility testing methods are based on older technologies and require 14 to 28 day incubation times. Use of automated systems may, therefore, not be acceptable without validation that the methods are of equivalent sensitivity. In contrast, for some cellular products there are not, for example, standardized functional (potency) testing assays and each facility may have its own in-house system for these. Under these circumstances it is important for QA/QC to have reviewed the test system to ensure that it is GLP-compliant.

Once manufacturing is completed, the batch record is transferred to QA. Here it is reviewed for completeness and accuracy. Copies of original testing data are obtained and attached to the summary reports already in the record. Successful review will lead to the generation of the Certificate of Analysis as discussed previously. This becomes a component of the batch record, which is retained by QA.

Release for use

When the cells are required for administration to a patient, a prescription for infusion is generated. This lists the products that are available for that patient. It is usually accompanied by a copy of the protocol flowchart, which provides specific dosing information. The prescription is reviewed by QA, who will also print out an inventory sheet that confirms the existence and location of the stored products. The patient's physician reviews and selects the specific components that are to be administered and signs the prescription. The product is then retrieved from storage and this is documented on an inventory form that also records cross-checking of the product identity by a second staff member. If necessary the product may be manipulated prior to infusion and this is recorded on a worksheet and activity report.

Frozen components are transported in liquid nitrogen to the bedside together with an infusion form that details the patient, component, and dosing information. The identity of the component and patient are cross-checked and documented at the bedside. The identity of the nurse or physician performing the infusion is recorded, as are details and timing of the procedure. The patient is observed for any early adverse events and this information is recorded on the infusion form. An activity report is also generated for all equipment and supplies used for the infusion. The infusion documentation is returned to QA, where it is reviewed and added to the batch record. If an adverse reaction is observed, this will trigger generation of an incident report and an investigation by QA of the possible causes. This information will, in turn be added to the batch record for that product. There should also be procedures on file for dealing with products that do not meet release criteria, or that are returned for some reason to the CPF after issue for use.

Quality program

An active quality program is an essential component of the operation of a cGMP facility. This should be independent of the manufacturing unit and report directly to the Director of the Facility or Program. This can be a problem in smaller academic facilities, where there is no stand-alone quality program or staff. Proposed solutions include quality review by a manufacturing staff member not directly involved with preparation of the particular product, a temporal delay between quality review and processing when both functions are performed by a single individual, and use of institutional quality program staff. As regulatory rigor increases it is likely that some of these solutions will no longer be acceptable to the FDA, and plans should be in place to develop a truly independent quality program.

The quality assurance program has the responsibility for ensuring that manufacturing is designed, implemented, and performed in such a way as to routinely yield products of consistent quality. The responsibilities of the quality unit include (1) ensuring that SOPs exist for all manufacturing procedures including testing, and that these are maintained, followed, archived, and reviewed; (2) reviewing and approving SOPs prior to implementation; (3) ensuring that there are procedures to establish validation; (4) ensuring that there are methods available for proficiency and competency testing; (5) performing quality audits; and (6) developing and maintaining systems for required documentation. The unit is also directly responsible for staff training and education, error/accident reports, complaints and adverse reaction documentation, records management, and lot release procedures.

The design and implementation of such a program can be a daunting task for a smaller facility, but it is a mandatory component of cGMP operations. A manageable way of developing a program is to identify the critical points in procedures performed in the facility, where failure could be catastrophic to manufacturing. These are then initially used as quality indicators for routine review. An example for cell therapy products would be maintenance of sterility. Each contamination can be reviewed for potential source, identity of the organism, and remedial action. Other indicators could include number of variances issued, accidents and errors, failure to meet expected results, and failure to obtain infectious disease testing within the required time frame. The program should formally review these indicators at regular meetings, and determine action to be taken and a follow-up plan. These meetings must be documented and trends in indicators monitored. There should be ongoing audits of cGMP compliance and an annual report by the Quality Program to the Facility Director or Management. Since quality improvement in health care is now a high profile activity, many institutions have quality programs in place or under development. It makes sense, where possible, for the CPF to leverage the expertise within these programs when developing its own quality unit.

Accreditation

In an attempt to improve the quality of cellular therapies, professional organizations, such as the Foundation for the Accreditation of Cellular Therapy, the American Association of Blood Banks, the Joint Accreditation Committee in Europe, and NetCord have published standards for facilities engaged in the preparation of therapeutic cell products. In most cases, these reflect the expectations of the FDA. However, they lack the power of law.

CPFs may apply to the organizations for voluntary accreditation. This involves an on-site inspection visit and correction of any deficiencies that are found. While successful accreditation does not imply compliance with FDA regulations, the Agency has indicated that accredited facilities will find it easier and more cost-effective to come into regulatory conformity.

Good Tissue Practices

In January 2001 the FDA published a proposed rule "Current Good Tissue Practice for Manufacturers of Human Cellular and Tissue-Based Products; Inspection and Enforcement". cGTP would provide core requirements that would be applicable to all human cellular and tissue-based products, regardless of their regulatory category. They would be supplemented by other subparts (A through F) of Part 1271 of Title 21 of the CFR. Subpart A describes the scope and purpose of Part 1271 and provides definitions. Subpart B would cover facility registration. Subpart C would describe the screening and testing of donors in order to determine their suitability. Subpart E describes labeling and reporting requirements, and Subpart F contains inspection and enforcement provisions. cGTP would form Subpart D and provide a new form of cGMP that would be more appropriate to the preparation of cellular and tissue-

based therapeutic products, and aimed primarily at preventing the transmission of communicable diseases. The document calculates the potential risk to a recipient from receiving a contaminated product and the potential cost in terms of providing treatment and lost productivity. The accuracy of these calculations is open to debate, as is the claimed cost of implementing the proposals in an academic environment.

Facilities preparing products that require an IND or IDE application would, in addition, be subject to the provisions of cGTP. Similarly cGTP are considered to supplement rather than supersede existing cGMP regulations (Table 29.2).

The proposals are comprehensive, containing sections on establishment of a quality program (including functions, authority over the program, audits, computers, and procedures); organization and personnel (including competency, training, and records); procedures; facilities, environmental control and monitoring; equipment; supplies and reagents; process controls, changes and validation; labeling controls; storage; receipt and distribution; tracking; and complaint files. The proposal is intended to cover all forms of cellular and tissue-based therapies.

Implementation of cGTP, the proposed regulations on donor screening, and the final rule on facility registration would complete a chapter in the regulation of cellular therapies and move the field into an era in which academic institutions find themselves formally classified as product manufacturers, subject to the same rules as large pharmaceutical companies.

Gene therapy

The controversies surrounding cellular therapies pale by comparison to those swirling around gene therapy in the United States. The death of a patient on a gene therapy study in Philadelphia ignited a storm of concern about the way such studies were being conducted. The regulatory authorities were called to account by the Congress and charged with developing regulations that would safeguard participants in these therapies more effectively. An investigation of the circumstances in Philadelphia highlighted many deficiencies ranging from potential conflicts of interest to poor understanding and compliance with GLP and cGMP. In response, gene therapy centers were requested to provided extensive documentation on vector manufacturing procedures, quality programs, and product testing. There is no doubt that this is resulting in increased regulatory oversight and implementation of more stringent regulations. Vector products facilities will be expected to comply with cGMP and the expectation is likely to be that this must be at a pharmaceutical manufacturing level.

The future

Advances in knowledge have spurred the development of cell-based therapies at a rate that could not have been imagined even 5 years ago. Cells derived from many sources are now being purified, cultured, activated, genetically manipulated, frozen,

Table 29.2. *A comparison of cGMP and cGTP Regulations*[a]

Cell Therapy Products

Establishment Registration ← → Donor Screening
(Final Rule: CFR21, 1271 Subpart B) — *(Proposed Rule: CFR21, 1271 Subpart C)*
Current Good Manufacturing Practices → Current Good Tissue Practices
(More-than-minimally-Manipulated Products) — *(Minimally-Manipulated Products)*
(CFR 21 Parts 210, 211, 606) — *(Proposed Rule: CFR21 1271 Subpart D)*

	cGMP		cGTP
Facilities	Adequate space for all activities Clean, orderly, construction suitable for cleaning & maintenance Adequate lighting & ventilation, bathroom facilities & drains Safe & sanitary disposal of trash, blood, & components	Facilities	As per cGMP Organized to prevent mix-ups and cross-contamination Appropriate cleaning procedures and documentation of cleaning Environment adequate to prevent adverse effects on products; document and maintain
Staff	Adequate number Appropriate training & experience Exclude unauthorized staff from area Qualified & knowledgeable Director for supervision, discipline, & training	Staff	Adequate number Appropriate training & experience Aware of consequences of improper performance Maintain records of education, experience training, & retraining
Supplies & reagents	Safe, orderly & sanitary storage Surface in contact with blood must be sterile, pyrogen-free, & nonreactive Observe containers for damage & contamination before & after filling Use oldest lots first Use sterile disposable materials where possible Written procedures for receipt, identification, storage, handling, sampling, testing, etc. Store off floor & in manner to prevent contamination Record lot numbers & test lots	Supplies & reagents	As per cGMP Procedures for receiving and verifying that supplies meet appropriate specifications Appropriate reagent grade for use, sterile. Validated systems for testing Records manufacturer, lot #, C of A or verification, test results, use Use sterile disposable materials where possible Records of products for which reagents were used; record lot numbers & test lots
Equipment	Maintain in clean, orderly manner & locate to facilitate cleaning & maintenance Regular calibration & cleaning	Equipment	Appropriate design. Maintain in clean orderly manner & locate to facilitate cleaning & maintenance Regular calibration & cleaning. Inspected for cleanliness / calibration / maintenance. Record the above, plus products manufactured using the equipment
Laboratory controls	Establish specifications & test to ensure safety, purity, potency, & effectiveness Monitor test reliability, accuracy, precision, & performance Adequate identification of product & test samples to allow tracking Compatibility testing between donor/product/recipient	Process controls	Control process to ensure products are sterile, meet specifications & maintain function & integrity Procedures for monitoring and removing processing materials that may have adverse effects Do not pool cells or tissue from 2 or more donors Procedures and specifications required for in-process testing
Finished product controls	Separate areas to prevent mix-ups Use labeling controls Provide instruction circular	Process changes & validation	Formal change control procedures with documentation Validate procedures where results cannot be verified by inspection or testing. Document Revalidate after changes and deviations
Records & reports	Maintain concurrently with each step of the procedure Include identity of person performing work, test results & interpretation, product expiration dates, history of work performed, lot numbers, donor records, information on storage & distribution, compatibility testing, infusion reactions, etc.	Records & reports	As per cGMP plus system for upstream and downstream notification & tracking. Use of distinct identification code. Records of disposition. 10 year retention. Records of contracts
		Complaints file	Maintain a record of all complaints with review and evaluation. Report to FDA as required
		Quality program	Establish & maintain appropriate procedures Follow-up mechanisms for tracking possible product contamination & notifying FDA Corrective action mechanisms & documentation Perform audits, document deviations & corrections Appropriate monitoring systems, e.g., of environment

[a] These regulations in their final forms are meant to be complementary and supplementary. Compliance with one does not exclude a CPF from compliance with the other.

Reproduced, with permission, from *Transplant Immunology*.

thawed, and infused to treat a host of diseases. These types of treatments have been regarded by many simply as the practice of medicine that should not be subject to regulatory oversight. It is reasonable to say, however, that this notion has been abused by a minority of practitioners, to the extent that it has caused public anxiety at the highest levels. The FDA, long concerned about certain activities in the field, has re-examined its regulatory approach and developed a comprehensive risk-based strategy anchored around cGMP, cGTP, establishment registration and donor screening. This moves cell processing facilities clearly into the classification of product manufacturers, and, in the case of products covered under INDs, the expectation is that manufacturing will resemble that of pharmaceuticals.

There is, however, a major difference between current types of cell therapy products and pharmaceuticals. In complete contrast to drugs, the vast majority of cellular therapeutics are currently prepared for a single or very restricted number of recipients. Administration is under informed consent where the potential risks and benefits have been explained. Most of these therapies are in phase I or II clinical trials. The FDA has addressed this by indicating that full cGMP compliance and product characterization (CFR Title 21 Part 610) will not be required until phase III. The problem for the field is that the degree of cGMP compliance required at earlier stages has not been elaborated. Recent communications to the field from the FDA, and information conveyed during Agency audits, suggest that there is increasingly less tolerance for incomplete compliance at most stages. While the goals of ensuring safety and efficacy are laudable, the chosen means to this end may endanger progress in the field. Most academic institutions, which remain the incubator for these emerging therapies, will find it prohibitively expensive to implement pharmaceutical-grade cGMP manufacturing to generate products to treat small numbers of patients. Industry support is limited, since, in their present incarnation, most of these products are unlikely to be translatable into commercially viable products. That leaves government as the only viable funding source. Given the controversy surrounding cell and gene therapy at many levels, it is not clear whether such resources will be readily available.

References

Gee, A.P. (2002). Regulatory issues in cellular therapies. *Journal of Cellular Biochemistry,* Suppl **38,** 104–12.

Guermonprez, P., Valladeau, J., Zitvogel, L. *et al.* (2002). Antigen presentation and T cell stimulation by dendritic cells. *Annual Review in Immunology,* **20,** 621–7.

Mitchell, M.S. (2002). Cancer vaccines, a critical review—Part I. *Current Opinion in Investigational Drugs,* **3,** 140–9.

Park, K.I., Ourednik, J., Ourednik, V. *et al.* (2002). Global gene and cell replacement strategies via stem cells. *Gene Therapy,* **9,** 613–24.

30 Hematopoietic chimerism after allogeneic stem cell transplantation

EPHRAIM P. HOCHBERG AND JEROME RITZ

Dana-Farber Cancer Institute and Brigham & Women's Hospital, Harvard University, Boston, USA

Introduction

The success of allogeneic hematopoietic stem cell transplantation (HSCT) is dependent on the successful engraftment of donor hematopoietic stem cells and the long-term reconstitution of donor hematopoiesis and lymphopoiesis. Monitoring engraftment with donor cells is thus an important aspect of allogeneic HSCT and is often used in the evaluation of clinical outcomes. Thus, studies based on measurements of chimerism have shown that persistent recipient cells can mediate graft rejection, resulting in graft failure despite administration of myeloablative therapy (Kernan *et al.*, 1987; Bordignon *et al.*, 1989, Bosserman *et al.*, 1989). Long-term persistence of recipient cells occurs frequently in patients who receive T-cell-depleted donor stem cells (Roy *et al.*, 1990; Schaap *et al.*, 2002). Graft-versus-host disease (GVHD) often results in the establishment of complete donor hematopoiesis, but elimination of residual recipient hematopoietic cells can also occur in the absence of GVHD (Pichert *et al.*, 1995; Mackinnon *et al.*, 1995). Moreover, persistence of mixed hematopoietic chimerism has also been associated with delayed reconstitution of a diverse T-cell repertoire after transplant (Wu *et al.*, 2000). Following administration of nonmyeloablative chemotherapy, assessments of chimerism often demonstrate engraftment of donor stem cells and subsequent establishment of complete donor hematopoiesis without evident changes in the total numbers of circulating white cells or platelets (Orsini *et al.*, 2000; Bellucci *et al.*, 2002). None of these clinically significant observations could have been made without methods for the detection and quantitative assessment of hematopoietic chimerism.

In conjunction with increased awareness of the clinical need to assess chimerism, considerable progress has been made in the development of laboratory methods to detect and quantitate chimerism. This chapter will review various methods that have been used to distinguish recipient from donor cells and summarize the advantages and limitations of different approaches. We will also summarize current clinical recommendations for the assessment of hematopoietic chimerism after different allogeneic transplant procedures.

Methods for assessment of chimerism

Various methods used to measure hematopoietic chimerism are summarized in Table 30.1. Early methods for the assessment of chimerism used distinctions between donor and host proteins to document engraftment of donor cells and quantitate the degree of hematopoietic chimerism after allogeneic bone marrow transplantation. For example, red blood cell (RBC) antigen typing between mismatched patient/donor pairs was used to determine the degree of erythrocyte engraftment and to infer the degree of total marrow engraftment. Other methods utilized HLA disparities, leukocyte enzyme polymorphisms, and immunoglobulin allotype differences to assess engraftment following transplant. These protein-based techniques for assessment of hematopoietic chimerism all share two major limitations. First, the number of potentially informative protein polymorphisms is relatively small and it is therefore likely that an informative marker will not be found for many patient/donor pairs. Second, protein expression in different hematopoietic cell types is regulated to an extent that can limit the assessment of chimerism. For example, RBC antigen typing is limited to the erythrocyte lineage and engraftment of donor red blood cells may not reflect the level of engraftment of other cell types.

More recently, technologies relying on genetic disparities have been used to distinguish recipient and donor cells and to accurately quantitate chimerism in specific cellular populations. Initial methods were based on the assessment of macroscopic differences such as the presence of the Y chromosome in sex-mismatched transplants, disease-specific translocations, and large restriction-fragment length polymorphisms (Knowlton *et al.*, 1986; Yam *et al.*, 1987; Roth *et al.*, 1990). More recently, methods have been developed to detect smaller scale genomic DNA disparities. These include variable number tandem repeats (VNTR), short tandem repeats (STR) (Mackinnon *et al.*, 1992; Oberkircher *et al.*, 1995), and single nucleotide polymorphisms (SNP) (Hochberg *et al.*, 2003; Oliver *et al.*, 2000). These methods are more widely applicable and circumvent the two major limitations of protein-based chimerism assays. The large number of these genomic polymorphisms ensures that an informative marker will be identi-

Table 30.1. *Comparison of different methods of assessing chemerism*

Method	Disadvantages	Advantages
RBC antigens	Limited to erythroid lineage Limited to RBC antigen mismatched pairs	Ease of use Standardized reagents
HLA antigens	Limited to HLA mismatched pairs	Ease of use
Cytogenetics	Limited to sex mismatched pairs Limited to dividing cells Low sensitivity (>5%)	Flow cytometric quantitation Standardized method for clinical use
FISH	Limited to sex mismatched pairs	More quantitative and sensitive than conventional cytogenetics Standardized probes available
Y gene PCR	Limited to sex mismatched pairs	Highly sensitive (~0.0001%)
RFLP	Limited number of informative alleles Difficult to quantify	Ease of use
VNTR/STR	Standardized reagents only available for a limited number of alleles	Standardized assays available Quantitative and sensitive assay (1% to 3%)
SNP	Standardized assays not yet available Limited ability to detect <5% chimerism	Very large number of potentially informative loci Rapid and inexpensive assay Can identify clinically relevant polymorphisms

fied in almost all patient/donor pairs. Moreover, DNA polymorphisms are present in all cells and can be used to assess chimerism in any cellular population. Genetic polymorphisms are also amenable to polymerase chain reaction (PCR) amplification, increasing the ability to detect low levels of chimerism and the ability to quantify chimerism in different cell types.

RBC antigens

Posttransplant analysis of the relative contributions of red blood cells from patient and donors with disparate blood group types has been historically used to determine the degree of engraftment of donor hematopoietic stem cells. Many of the major RBC antigens have been used as markers of chimerism including ABO, Rh, Duffy, and Kidd alleles (Hosoi *et al.,* 1977). Because the HLA locus on chromosome 6 is genetically distant from the ABO locus on chromosome 9 and the Rh locus on chromosome 1, major and minor ABO incompatibility, and hence informative RBC antigens, have been found in up to 40% of HLA-matched related transplants and up to 60% of HLA-matched unrelated donor transplants (Mielcarek *et al.,* 2000). Reagents specific for these RBC antigens are well characterized and the methods to detect RBCs of different origin are relatively rapid and easy to use. Nevertheless, analysis of engraftment using RBC antigens is limited by several factors. The extended lifespan of erythrocytes in the circulation makes it difficult to determine the state of chimerism shortly after transplant or after an intervention such as donor lymphocyte infusion. It is possible to overcome this limitation by using antigens limited to reticulocytes (Zuazu *et al.,* 1988) which reflect the production of new RBCs. However, transfusions administered to almost all ablative allogeneic transplant recipients often confuse the distinction between donor-specific antigens and recipient antigens by introducing numerous other sets of "transfusion

donor" antigens. Importantly, ABO incompatibility between donor and recipient can induce hemolysis. In this setting erythroid chimerism may be completely discrepant from myeloid and lymphoid chimerism. For these reasons RBC antigen typing has been almost completely supplanted by other methods. Interestingly, it is possible to return to RBC antigen polymorphisms as markers of chimerism by targeting the genomic SNPs that encode these protein antigens in molecular assays (Kapelushnik *et al.,* 1995).

HLA antigens

In patients who receive hematopoietic stem cells from HLA disparate donors, the HLA molecules themselves can be used as informative markers for the assessment of chimerism. HLA antigens are expressed on the cell surface and monoclonal antibodies specific for many HLA class I and class II alleles are now available. These reagents can be used in conjunction with cell-type specific monoclonal antibodies and immunofluorescence flow cytometry to determine the extent of chimerism in different cell types (Dahmen *et al.,* 2002). This provides an elegant quantitative method for determining lineage-specific chimerism, but there are also several limitations to this approach. Most importantly, the number of patients who receive HLA-mismatched transplants is limited and this method is therefore only rarely applied. Moreover, the number of HLA alleles is very large, but specific reagents capable of discriminating between different alleles is limited. Thus, reagents to specifically detect many HLA alleles are not yet available. Patients who receive solid organ transplants are often HLA-mismatched with their donors. Hematopoietic chimerism has been demonstrated in many of these individuals (Fontes *et al.,* 1994; Spriewald *et al.,* 1998; Jonsson *et al.,* 1997), but flow cytometric methods are not usually able to accurately detect the low levels of microchimerism that are present after solid organ transplant (Dahmen *et al.*, 2002; Fontes *et al.*, 1994; Spriewald *et al.*, 1988).

Immunoglobulin allotypes and enzyme isotypes

Similar to RBC antigen typing, immunoglobulin allotypes and enzyme isotypes can be used to measure chimerism (Witherspoon *et al.*, 1978; Sparkes *et al.*, 1979; Blume *et al.*, 1980; Witherspoon *et al.*, 1984). Immunoglobulin allotypes have historically been used to infer the presence of B-cell chimerism after transplant. B lymphocytes characteristically appear quite late and in small numbers after myeloablative allo-geneic conditioning regimens (Witherspoon *et al.*, 1984; Lum *et al.*, 1985; Soiffer *et al.*, 1990) and chimerism in this lineage can therefore be difficult to detect by other methods. In cases where informative allotype distinctions are present, semiquantitative estimates of the appearance of donor allotypes over time can be made (van Tol *et al.*, 1996). Several problems arise with this method. Informative allotype disparities are relatively rare and the long half-life of intact immunoglobulin in vivo represent major limitations. Moreover, platelet transfusions often contain significant amounts of donor plasma, which can confound the distinction between donor and recipient. In cases where simultaneous analysis of immunoglobulin allotypes and peripheral blood B-cell chimerism were performed by cytogenetics, the results were inconsistent. This observation suggests that immunoglobulin-secreting cells of recipient origin can persist in the bone marrow for prolonged periods and this further limits the use of immunoglobulin allotypes to assess donor B-cell reconstitution (Korver *et al.*, 1987). Analysis of enzyme isotypes is hampered by the same factors. Considering these significant limitations, immunoglobulin allotypes and enzyme isotypes are now rarely used to assess chimerism.

Cytogenetics

Chromosomal distinctions between donor and patient are well-defined markers that can easily be used to assess chimerism. Analysis of the presence or absence of the Y chromosome in metaphase spreads is frequently used to determine chimerism after sex-mismatched HSCT. In sex-matched transplants, the presence of somatic chromosomal rearrangements has been used to monitor engraftment, although these distinctions are uncommon. Disease-specific rearrangements such as the t(9;22) translocation are often used to monitor residual disease but are not accurate markers of chimerism since normal host hematopoietic tissues do not bear the translocation and are therefore missed by this assay. Many of the limitations of cytogenetic determination of chimerism are a result of technical requirements for cytogenetic analysis. Thus, cytogenetic measurement of chimerism requires both a chromosomal marker and dividing cells capable of generating a metaphase spread. The Y chromosome provides an informative marker for all sex-mismatched donor/recipient pairs, but very few sex-matched transplants will have such an informative marker. The accurate analysis of metaphase spreads

is technically challenging and time-consuming, thus limiting the number of cells that can be practically analyzed. Finally, cytogenetic analysis is limited to dividing cells and these may not be representative of the entire hematopoietic compartment. Taken together, these factors limit the utility as well as the accuracy of cytogenetics-based chimerism evaluation.

Fluorescent in situ hybridization

Fluorescent in situ hybridization (FISH) uses molecular probes to visualize chromosomal differences between patient and donor. The probes consist of large genomic DNA fragments that can be directly labeled with a fluorophore or secondarily labeled through a variety of techniques (Palka *et al.*, 1996; Lau *et al.*, 1995; Rondon *et al.*, 1997; Najfeld *et al.*, 1997). A major advantage of FISH over cytogenetics is that a larger number of cells can be analyzed for the presence of donor-specific genetic material, allowing for more accurate quantitation of the presence of donor chimerism (Crescenzi *et al.*, 2000). A second advantage of FISH is that morphologic characteristics of cells are preserved allowing for simultaneous histologic and genotypic analysis (Diez-Martin *et al.*, 1998). The technique of using FISH in sex-mismatched transplants was first developed in the late 1980s. A single probe specific for Y-chromosome sequences was initially described by several groups (van Dekken *et al.*, 1989; Wessman *et al.*, 1989; Morisaki *et al.*, 1988; Durnam *et al.*, 1989). In laboratory evaluations the sensitivity of this technique was estimated to be approximately 0.5% (1 male cell detected in 200 female cells), but is likely to be lower in routine clinical samples. Addition of a second probe with X chromosome-specific sequences greatly improved the sensitivity and specificity of the method. A large multicenter trial of the ability of clinical laboratories at 26 centers to reliably score metaphases and interphases from normal individuals found only a 0.03% false positive rate (XY cells in normal females or XX cells in normal males) (Dewald *et al.*, 1998). It is important to note that the sensitivity of the technique relies on the evaluation of several hundred cells, which can be time-consuming when low levels of chimerism are clinically suspected. New advances in FISH allow the simultaneous assessment of disease-specific chromosomal rearrangements, such as bcr-abl, simultaneously with chimerism evaluations in appropriate patients (Crescenzi *et al.*, 2000). An important final advantage of FISH over traditional cytogenetics is the ability to analyze non-dividing cells. This allows the analysis of cells that may be difficult or impossible to culture in vitro. Methods for PCR amplification of Y-specific genes have also been developed and further increase the sensitivity of this technique for detecting very small numbers of male cells after transplantation (Orsini *et al.*, 2000; Viard *et al.*, 1993).

Restriction fragment length polymorphisms

Current methods for assessment of chimerism rely primarily on "molecular" distinctions between recipient and donor DNA.

One of the first molecular methods used to assess chimerism was based on detection of restriction fragment length polymorphisms (RFLP) (Roy *et al.*, 1990; Knowlton *et al.*, 1986; Yam *et al.*, 1987; Roth *et al.*, 1990; Ginsburg *et al.*, 1985). Restriction endonucleases cleave genomic DNA at specific sequences resulting in the formation of DNA fragments of different lengths. These DNA fragments are separated by gel electrophoresis and visualized as a distinct pattern of DNA bands of different sizes on Southern blot. Insertions and deletions of varying DNA sequences as well as SNP at the enzyme recognition sites alter the pattern of bands seen on Southern blots. When comparing DNA from different individuals, distinct RFLP patterns can be used to distinguish recipient from donor DNA. Hybridization of a radiolabeled probe to a specific sequence of interest and comparison of signal intensity between known host, donor, and posttransplant patterns can provide estimates of chimerism.

A number of DNA polymorphisms that can be detected by RFLP have been identified and these provide informative markers that can distinguish recipient from donor DNA. Nevertheless, there are several limitations to this technique. The number of RFLPs is relatively small compared to other DNA polymorphisms, and as a result, informative RFLPs are often not available. Since this method does not rely on PCR amplification, relatively large amounts of DNA are needed to assess chimerism. It is also relatively difficult to provide accurate quantitative results. When RFLP analysis has been directly compared to STR/VNTR methods, the sensitivity of the PCR-based techniques has been superior (Nuckols *et al.*, 2000; Sreenan *et al.*, 1997).

Methods using PCR to amplify RFLP fragments improve the sensitivity of this technique. Methods for detection and assessment of RFLP and other DNA polymorphisms are shown schematically in Figure 30.1. For detection of RFLP, PCR primers external to the variable restriction site are used to generate a PCR amplicon containing the RFLP site. The amplicon is then digested with a restriction enzyme and the sizes of the resulting fragments are determined by gel electrophoresis. This technique allows the use of much smaller quantities of starting material than standard RFLP. This method may also be more sensitive than conventional RFLP but it is difficult to provide accurate quantitative measurements of chimerism. Consequently, RFLP is now seldom used for measurement of hematopoietic chimerism after HSCT.

Variable number tandem repeats and short tandem repeats

Repeating genomic DNA sequences are widely dispersed within the genome and are highly polymorphic. These DNA sequences have been termed variable number tandem repeats (VNTR), short tandem repeats (STR), minisatellites, or microsatellites, depending on the number of base pairs that are repeated. The differences between these repeating DNA elements are summarized in Table 30.2. In each of these cases a relatively short genomic sequence known as the "core sequence" is highly conserved, but the number of repeats of these core sequences is highly variable. This variability is felt to be created either by the slippage of DNA polymerase on these long repeated sequences

Table 30.2. *Comparison of repeating DNA sequence elements*

	Size variability	Repeat size
STR/microsatellite	4 to 50 repeats	3 to 7 base pairs
VNTR/minisatellite	2 to 20 repeats	8 to 80 base pairs

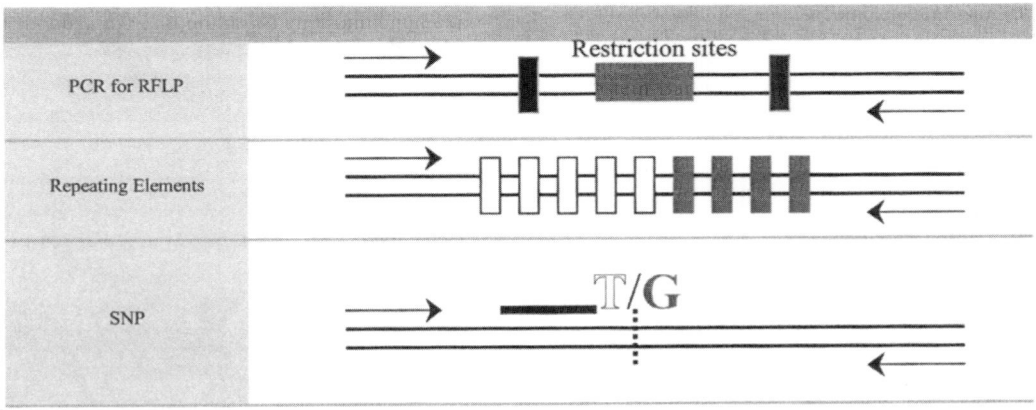

Fig. 30.1. The first row shows a schematic diagram of PCR for RFLP. The presence or absence of the shaded DNA element in the center of the amplicon varies the size of the DNA fragments after they have been digested with restriction enzymes and permits the distinction of two individuals. The diagram in the second row shows the PCR amplification of repeating DNA elements (VNTR/STR/minisatellite/microsatellite). The presence of different numbers of the shaded repeating elements varies the size of the amplicon and permits the distinction of the two individuals. The third row shows a schematic for SNP-based PCR. In this example, the PCR amplicon includes either a thymidine or guanine at the polymorphic position, which is detected by DNA sequencing starting at the dark gray probe. Alternatively, polymorphism specific probes can be used to detect either the thymidine or guanine-containing PCR amplicon.

or by misalignment during recombination. In most cases these repeated sequences are not expressed and each individual has two alleles of each VNTR/STR. Each of these alleles is likely to have a different number of repeated core sequences, which are inherited as co-dominant Mendelian traits. The high variability of these loci and the lack of dependence on levels of expression in various hematopoietic lineages make these markers superior to others previously reviewed for the analysis of chimerism (Roux *et al.,* 1992). Numerous online databases catalog the known STR/VNTRs (http://www.atcc.org/Products/str.cfm; http://www.cstl.nist.gov/biotech/strbase/; http://ystr.charite.de/index_gr.html). As a result, these polymorphisms are now widely used to assess chimerism.

The detection and analysis of VNTR/STR sequences has rapidly been made more accessible. Previous methods of detection used Southern blots (Ginsburg *et al.,* 1985). The area surrounding the highly variable sequence was cleaved with restriction endonucleases and separated by gel electrophoresis. The gel was then stained with a probe for either the core sequence or a short unique flanking sequence. The quantitation of these staining techniques was quite difficult, although the qualitative assessment of "small residual levels of host chimerism" could be relatively easily ascertained. This technique has given way to PCR-based analysis of STR/VNTR that is shown schematically in Figure 30.1. PCR primers external to the repeated sequences are used to generate a PCR amplicon containing the

repeated elements. The size of the amplicon will vary depending on the number of repeated elements and this is determined by either gel or capillary electrophoresis (Roux *et al.,* 1992).

A commercial kit initially developed for forensic testing is now commonly used to measure STR polymorphisms and quantify hematopoietic chimerism in patient samples (AmpFLSTR® Profiler Plus™ PCR Amplification Kit, Applied Biosystems, www.appliedbiosystems.com). This kit includes fluorophore-labeled primers for nine tetra-nucleotide STRs as well as a set of labeled primers for the amelogenin locus. The amelogenin gene is located on both the X and Y chromosomes but the X and Y alleles have slightly different sizes. The size of the PCR-amplified amelogenin band can therefore be used to distinguish between male and female individuals. The reactions have been optimized so that all 10 sets of primers amplify sufficiently in a single well. The mixed PCR products range in size from 100 to 300 base pairs and are analyzed on either a gel-based or capillary-based DNA sequencing instrument. Three different fluorophores are used, two of which amplify 3 loci and the third which amplifies 4 loci. The PCR product sizes have been designed so that each STR is separate from the others and can be independently evaluated regardless of the number of observed repeats. A representative example of the results using this method to assess chimerism in a male patient with a female donor is shown in Figure 30.2. In this sex-mismatched pair, the amelogenin locus as well as an STR locus provide informative

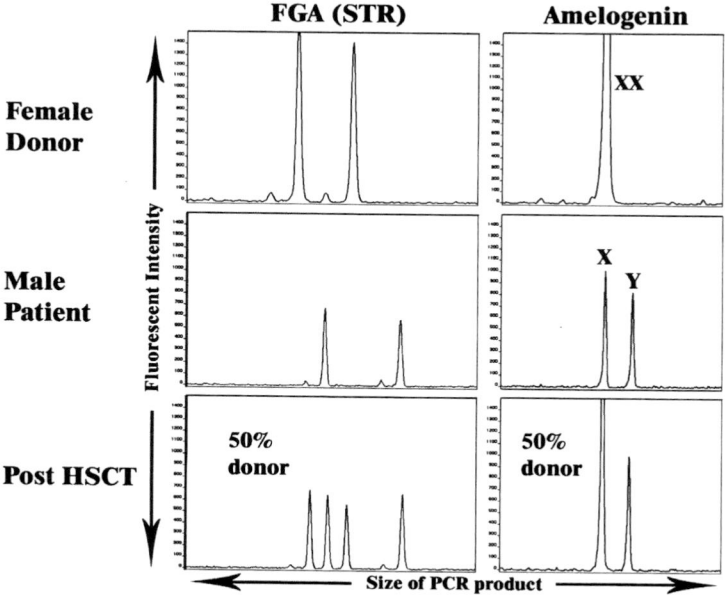

Fig. 30.2. PCR amplification of STR/VNTR from patient and donor samples. In this example, female donor and male recipient DNA can be distinguished by FGA short tandem repeat (STR) locus and amelogenin polymorphisms. The samples on the left show the different lengths of the PCR-amplified products for the FGA locus in donor and recipient. The post-HSCT sample contains equal amounts of donor-specific and patient-specific bands indicating 50% chimerism. The samples on the right from the same donor and recipient show the size analysis of a PCR amplicon. The amelogenin locus is encoded on both the X and Y genes. The X- and Y-specific PCR products have different lengths that can be distinguished by gel electrophoresis. The female donor sample contains only a single size X band in comparison to the male patient sample that contains equal amounts of both X and Y bands. The post-HSCT sample contains both X and Y bands, but the unequal proportions of X and Y bands indicate 50% chimerism. (STR graphics courtesy of Doreen Sese and Jennifer Langley, Brigham and Women's Hospital HLA Laboratory.)

markers. Analysis of the female donor demonstrates 2 distinct STR peaks representing different numbers of repeating elements and a single amelogenin peak representing both X alleles. Male patient cells also contain 2 STR peaks, but these have different sizes compared to the donor peaks indicating that both patient alleles contain different numbers of repeating elements. Male cells also contain 2 amelogenin peaks of similar height representing both the X and Y alleles. A posttransplant patient sample contains 4 distinct STR peaks, demonstrating the presence of both recipient and donor DNA. The observation that both patient-specific and donor-specific STR peaks are of similar height indicates that the sample contains 50% donor and 50% recipient cells. The same sample contains 2 amelogenin peaks indicating the presence of male cells. The increased height of the X-peak compared to the Y-peak indicates the presence of female cells and the ratio of X:Y peak heights reflects the relative contribution of donor and recipient cells.

The sensitivity and specificity of this technique are dependent on three factors. First is the ability of the sequencing instrument to accurately quantitate either the peak height or the area under the curve of the fluorescent signal for each allele. Quantitation of chimerism is also dependent on whether PCR amplification is linear across a wide range of amplicon sizes. The third limitation arises from the mechanism of formation of these STR/VNTRs. Sensitive techniques for analyzing these PCR products also detect small bands that appear at fixed intervals smaller than the main product. These "stutter" peaks represent slippage of DNA polymerase on the repeated sequence. Although further improvements in this method are being developed, these intrinsic problems are likely to continue to limit the sensitivity of STR/VNTR to approximately the current 1% to 3% level.

Single nucleotide polymorphisms

SNPs comprise the major source of human genetic disparity. Estimates of SNP frequency range from one in every 300 to 1,000 nucleotides (Cargill et al., 1999; Halushka et al., 1999; Wang et al., 1998). The genome is therefore estimated to contain $>3 \times 10^6$ SNPs. This represents an effectively unlimited source of markers that can be used to distinguish all individuals except for monozygotic twins. Depending on their position in the codon and their position either within a gene or in extragenic sequences, these SNPs can be classified as either coding or noncoding. Coding polymorphisms play a primary role in determining genetic diversity. Phenomena as diverse as severe combined immune deficiency, sickle cell disease, acute myeloid leukemia (Griffin et al., 2001), resting heart rate (Ranade et al., 2002), susceptibility to asthma (Immervoll et al., 2001), and risk of oral mucositis after HSCT (Ulrich et al., 2001) have been associated with coding SNPs.

Our laboratory has designed an SNP-based chimerism assay using a panel of 9 high allele-frequency SNPs derived from the Human Genome Variation Database (http://hgvbase.cgb.ki.se/) and 5 SNPs that encode putative minor histocompatibility antigens (mHA) (Hochberg et al., 2002; Tseng et al., 1998; Pierce et al., 2001; Grumet et al., 2001; Brickner et al., 2001). As shown in Figure 30.1, PCR primers are designed to amplify a short segment of DNA containing the known SNP. DNA sequencing of the PCR amplicon is then used to determine whether the donor and recipient are disparate for the SNP. If DNA sequencing of the PCR amplicon is quantitative, this method can also be used to provide a measurement of the relative contribution of each SNP allele, and thus the relative quantities of recipient and donor DNA.

The method used to type these SNPs is a short read quantitative sequencing technology called *pyrosequencing* (Pyrosequencing AB, Uppsala, Sweden), which uses the DNA synthesis reaction to sequence DNA (Alderborn et al., 2000). Briefly, a PCR reaction with one biotinylated primer is performed to generate a short amplicon surrounding the SNP of interest. Biotinylated single-strand DNA fragments are generated and an automated pyrosequencing instrument is used to determine DNA sequence. The DNA sequencing protocol utilizes stepwise elongation of the primer strand by sequential addition of deoxynucleoside triphosphates and the simultaneous degradation of residual unincorporated nucleotides. As the sequencing reaction continues, extension of the cDNA strand by successful nucleotide incorporation results in the release of light by conversion of the released pyrophosphate molecules into a substrate for firefly luciferase. As shown in Figure 30.3, the DNA sequence is determined from the peaks in the pyrogram using the pyrosequencing software. The height of each peak is directly related to the quantitative representation of each nucleotide at the indicated position in the DNA sequence. In the example shown in Figure 30.3, pyrosequencing is clearly able to distinguish DNA from individuals who are either homozygous or heterozygous for each SNP.

Prior to assembling our panel of 14 SNPs, we calculated that 7 SNPs of 50% allele frequency would provide a 99% probability of identifying at least a single informative SNP locus for HLA-identical sibling/patient pairs. Similarly, a panel of 7 SNPs with 50% allele frequency would be sufficient to identify a single informative locus in 99.2% of unrelated pairs. These results were confirmed experimentally with our panel of 14 SNPs that were tested on 55 patient/donor pairs. Using this panel we found that either 11 or 6 SNPs were sufficient to provide 99.6% probability of identifying at least one informative locus in related and unrelated pairs, respectively. This is consistent with estimates of the number of SNPs required to generate an informative panel by other investigators (Oliver et al., 2000). The median number of informative disparities seen in a series of 55 patients with either related or unrelated HLA-identical donors using our panel of 14 SNPs was 5 disparities (range 1–9) for related individuals and 8 disparities (range 1–12) for unrelated pairs.

To determine whether SNP pyrosequencing could be used to quantify the degree of mixed chimerism, DNA from two individuals with disparate genotypes at three SNP loci were mixed in different concentrations between 0% and 100% "donor". The mixed genomic DNA was then PCR-amplified as described above and the SNP sequence was determined by pyrosequencing. The percentage of hematopoietic chimerism was deter-

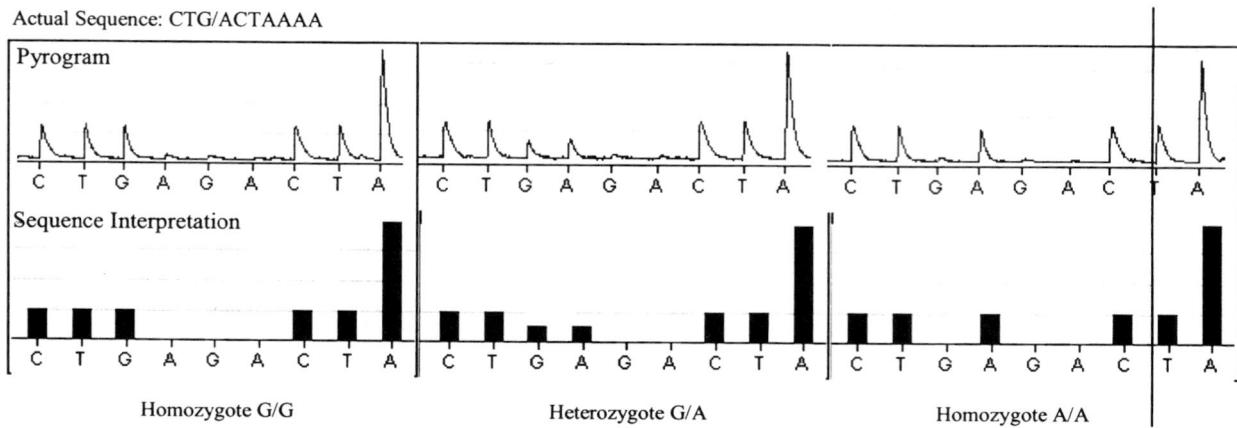

Fig. 30.3. SNP sequence determination by pyrosequencing. The DNA sequence of samples from 3 different donors is shown in the top rows and the DNA sequence interpreted by the pyrosequencing software is shown in the bottom rows. The actual sequence for the SNP is CTG/ACTAAAA. A homozygous G/G sample is shown in the left panel; a heterozygous G/A sample is shown in the middle panel; a homozygous A/A sample is shown in the right panel.

mined by the PSQ96 Allele Discrimination Software (Pyrosequencing AB, Uppsala, Sweden). These experiments demonstrated a reproducible linear relationship between the relative amounts of recipient and donor DNA in the mixture and the quantitative results of pyrosequencing. Levels of 5% donor DNA could be reliably detected in repeated experiments, but lower levels of chimerism were not consistently detected. Finally, this method has been tested on serial samples obtained from patients after allogeneic HSCT. Results for a representative patient who received a non-myeloablative conditioning regimen are shown in Figure 30.4. Early posttransplant, SNP analysis demonstrated substantial donor engraftment in peripheral blood mononuclear cells (PBMC). This was confirmed by separate analysis of both granulocytes and CD3+ T cells demon-

strating donor engraftment in both myeloid and lymphoid lineages. At 6 and 9 months post-HSCT, analysis of PBMC demonstrated persistent and stable mixed chimerism (82% donor and 18% recipient). However, further analysis of granulocytes and T cells in the same samples clearly showed that granulocytes were >95% donor but T cells were only approximately 50% donor. Thus, all myeloid cells appeared to be derived from donor stem cells and mixed chimerism was limited to the lymphoid lineage. Further follow-up in this individual and others will be needed to determine the clinical significance of these types of observations. Nevertheless, it is evident that the SNP-based chimerism assay can provide a rapid and quantitative method for measurement of chimerism in well-defined cellular populations, as well as in either PBMC or bone marrow.

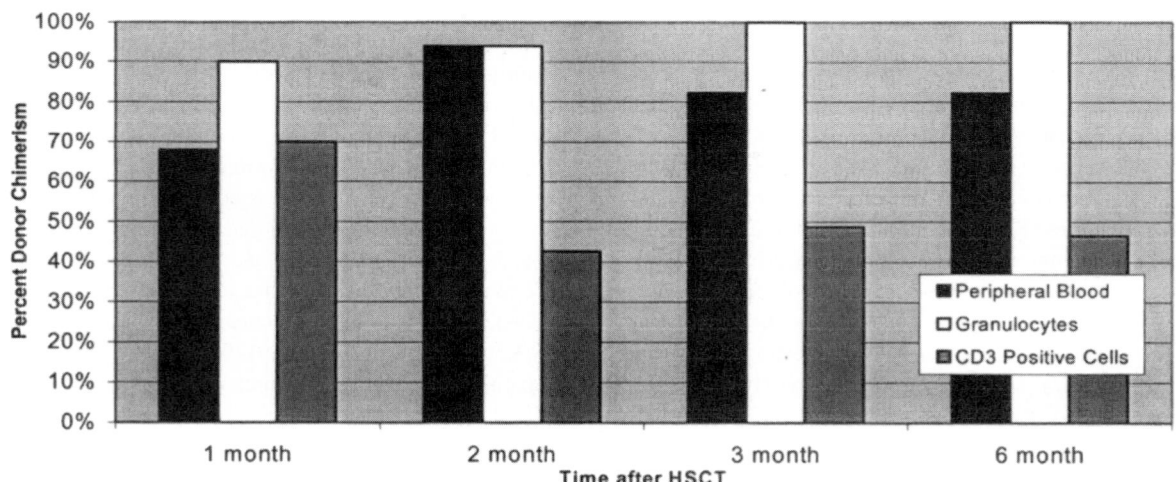

Fig. 30.4. Quantitation of hematopoietic chimerism in peripheral blood samples obtained after allogeneic HSCT. Pyrosequencing was used to quantify hematopoietic chimerism in peripheral blood samples after non-myeloablative conditioning. Analysis of peripheral blood mononuclear cells (PBMC) is compared to results of purified granulocytes and CD3+ T cells. Analysis of PBMC demonstrated persistent mixed chimerism for 6 months post-HSCT. Analysis of purified cell populations demonstrated complete donor hematopoiesis in the granulocyte lineage and approximately 50% chimerism in CD3+ T cells.

SNP-based analysis of chimerism has several advantages over STR/VNTR testing. First, SNP sequencing also provides a genomic "context" for the chimerism analysis. Thus, the DNA sequence that is determined provides additional confirmation that the correct locus has been amplified. This is not possible when evaluating bands on a gel or fluorescent signals in capillary electrophoresis. Second, the vast number of available SNPs in the genome allows the development of large panels of markers and greatly increases the ability to identify an informative marker in almost all patient/donor pairs. The identification of large numbers of informative markers also facilitates the use of multiple SNPs to determine chimerism at each time point. Evaluation of chimerism based on multiple SNPs allows statistical analysis of the results and increases the validity of the result. Last and most importantly, the SNPs that are used for the panel need not be limited to noncoding SNPs. Numerous SNPs have been postulated to be important contributors to various transplant outcomes and additional clinically informative SNPs are likely to be discovered. These range from minor histocompatibility antigens such as HA-1 (Tait *et al.*, 2001; Gallardo *et al.*, 2001) HA-2 (Pierce *et al.*, 2001), and HA-8 (Brickner *et al.*, 2001) to markers of regimen-related toxicity such as MTHFR polymorphisms (Ulrich *et al.*, 2001) and polymorphisms of various cytokines such as interleukin (IL-6) and interferon-gamma (Cavet *et al.*, 2001). These SNPs can be used both as targets for chimerism testing as well as genotyping for prediction of transplant outcomes (Hochberg *et al.*, 2002).

Summary of chimerism methods

The advantages and disadvantages of different methods for determining chimerism are summarized in Table 30.1. The use of protein distinctions (RBC antigens, HLA antigens, or enzyme isotypes) as methods for the assessment of chimerism are now only recommended in specific clinical situations such as HLA-mismatched transplantation where the ease of use of the method outweighs its general inapplicability. In most cases these methods are intrinsically limited by tissue protein expression to a single cell lineage and in the case of HLA mismatching by clinical criteria. Cytogenetics is often used in sex-mismatched pairs to determine chimerism, but the low number of cells examined limits the sensitivity of this method. FISH is capable of analyzing larger numbers of cells in each sample but is nevertheless largely restricted to sex-mismatched pairs. The current mainstay of chimerism analysis in both gender-matched and gender-mismatched transplants is the analysis of VNTR/STR polymorphisms. There are at least 8,000 described STR loci (Center for Medical Genetics), and each locus has a relatively large number of alleles. Thus, there may be as many as 120,000 possible informative STR patterns. Although many of these alleles are rare, this represents a large number of potentially informative alleles that can be used to identify genomic differences between recipient and donor pairs. The availability of commercial kits for VNTR/STR assays is another practical and important advantage that facilitates the validation and reproducibility of results using this technique. However, relatively few VNTR/STR polymorphisms are targeted in these commercial kits. With this limited number of targeted polymorphisms, occasional patient/donor pairs will not have informative markers.

In our assessment, SNP-based analysis of chimerism represents a potentially important new technique (Hochberg *et al.*, 2002). When compared to DNA repeat elements, there are a much larger number of SNPs. Conservative estimates suggest the presence of >3 million SNPs in the human genome. Each of these can be present as either a homozygote or heterozygote resulting in at least 9 million possible informative SNP patterns. With this practically unlimited number of markers, it is likely that multiple informative alleles will be identified in almost all recipient/donor pairs. SNP-based chimerism has the additional significant advantage of simultaneously providing independent information about polymorphisms that may be important in predicting transplant outcomes. The development of large validated SNP panels and standardized reagents and methods for quantitative measurement of SNPs in patient samples, would facilitate the use of SNP-based assessment of chimerism following allogeneic HSCT.

Clinical relevance of hematopoietic chimerism

Initial methods to distinguish recipient from donor cells were used primarily to document engraftment of donor hematopoietic stem cells. In patients who received high-dose conditioning regimens and unmanipulated marrow grafts, the analysis of chimerism confirmed the engraftment of donor stem cells in all hematopoietic lineages. Moreover, complete donor hematopoiesis was established in the great majority of such patients and the presence of significant numbers of recipient cells often suggested leukemia relapse, graft rejection, or graft failure (Bertheas *et al.*, 1991; Fishleder *et al.*, 1992; Huss *et al.*, 1996). In contrast, patients who received high-dose conditioning regimens and T-cell-depleted marrow grafts often developed mixed hematopoietic chimerism. Mixed chimerism was often stable for long periods and the presence of recipient cells in these individuals was therefore not clearly associated with relapse or graft failure (Roy *et al.*, 1990; Roux *et al.*, 1992; Petz *et al.*, 1987). Since these patients had received conventional myeloablative therapy, these chimerism studies also provided evidence that high-dose conditioning regimens were not often truly myeloablative. Taken together with the observation that GVHD was almost always associated with the establishment of complete donor hematopoiesis, these studies provided convincing evidence that donor T cells in the marrow graft played an important role in the elimination of normal recipient hematopoietic cells as well as leukemia cells and the establishment of complete donor hematopoiesis after stem cell transplantation.

In patients who receive reduced intensity conditioning regimens, the success of treatment is largely dependent on immunologic interactions between donor and recipient immune systems after allogeneic HSCT (Mielcarek *et al.*, 2002). In this setting, the assessment of hematopoietic chimerism is an important surrogate marker that is often used to evaluate several transplant outcomes. Early posttransplant, measurement of chimerism is used to document engraftment with donor cells and has been used extensively in the development of effective conditioning regimens. The presence of stable mixed hematopoietic chimerism occurs frequently in such individuals and represents the establishment of immunologic tolerance between recipient and donor immune systems (Spitzer *et al.*, 2000). In such patients, mixed chimerism has been used as an indication for further immunologic interventions such as donor lymphocyte infusions (DLI) (Mielcarek *et al.*, 2002). When successful, DLI results in the conversion to complete donor hematopoiesis, which is also associated with enhanced reconstitution of donor immunity. In patients with both hematologic and nonhematologic malignancies, conversion to complete donor hematopoiesis may also be required for more effective elimination of residual tumor cells and long-lasting remission (Childs *et al.*, 1999; Childs *et al.*, 2000). All of these important transplant outcomes have been associated with hematopoietic chimerism, and the accurate measurement of chimerism after transplant has therefore become increasingly important in the evaluation of these outcomes.

Recommendations for assessment of chimerism

Recent consensus recommendations for the measurement of chimerism have been established by the IBMTR/ABMTR (Antin *et al.*, 2001). These are summarized in Table 30.3. The first section gives the recommendations for the type of chimerism testing. DNA-based methods are the current mainstay of testing. In addition to STR/VNTR or SNP, FISH can often be used in sex-mismatched pairs. In rare cases of transplantation for nonmalignant disease, the presence of cells of normal phenotype is sufficient indication of the presence of donor chimerism. For example, in severe combined immunodeficiency the presence of phenotypically normal T and B cells can provide sufficient evidence of transplant chimerism without additional molecular diagnostics. In general, the measurement of bone marrow chimerism is insufficient to predict the presence or absence of peripheral blood subset chimerism such as T cells. Thus, peripheral blood is the recommended cell source for most chimerism studies. The recommendations for chimerism testing after HSCT vary by both the disease being treated and the type of conditioning regimen that is used. After myeloablative conditioning regimens and conventional GVHD prophylaxis regimens, most patients will establish complete donor hematopoiesis. Unless the clinical situation raises suspicions of graft failure, routine chimerism testing is not warranted in this situation. In contrast the use of T-cell depletion or novel and aggressive GVHD prophylaxis regimens are much more likely to produce a state of mixed hematopoietic chimerism. In these situations the panel recommended chimerism testing at 1, 3, 6, and 12 months and then as clinically indicated. In transplants for aplastic anemia, relatively non-myeloablative regimens are frequently used. These regimens often produce states of mixed hematopoietic chimerism. Chimerism testing is therefore recommended at 1, 3, 6, and 12 months and then as clinically indicated.

Table 30.3. *Recommendations for chimerism testing*

Type of transplant	Recommedation
Sex-matched transplants	STR/VNTR or SNP
Sex-mismatched transplants	STR/VNTR, SNP, or FISH
HLA-mismatched transplants	STR/VNTR, SNP, or flow cytometry
Assessment of lineage specific chimerism	
Peripheral blood	Analyze whole PBMC, myeloid and lymphoid subsets
Bone marrow	Bone marrow chimerism is only used for analysis of myeloid chimerism
Myeloablative HSCT with conventional GVHD prophylaxis	No routine chimerism evaluation required
Myeloablative HSCT with T-cell depletion or novel GVHD prophylaxis regimen	Testing at 1, 3, 6, and 12 months
	Additional testing if clinically indicated
Non-myeloablative HSCT/reduced intensity conditioning	
After transplant	Testing every 2–4 weeks until DLI
After DLI	Testing every 2–4 weeks then every 3–6 months
After full donor chimerism achieved	Testing every 3–6 months and if clinically indicated
HSCT for nonmalignant disease except aplastic anemia	
After transplant	Testing at 1, 2, and 3 months
If donor chimerism is declining	Monthly testing
HSCT for aplastic anemia	
After transplant	Testing at 1, 3, 6, and 12 months
	Additional testing if clinically indicated

Reprinted, with permission, from Antin *et al.* (2001).

Non-myeloablative HSCT regimens are even more likely to produce states of mixed hematopoietic chimerism or donor microchimerism. In many of these patients, the establishment of hematopoietic chimerism is a therapeutic objective and the presence of hematopoietic chimerism can be an indication for DLI (Spitzer *et al.*, 2000). The generation of initial mixed T cell chimerism has been suggested to be critical in the eventual conversion to full donor chimerism and successful implementation of the graft-versus-malignancy effect (Sykes *et al.*, 1999; Sykes & Spitzer, 2000). In these patients, frequent chimerism testing at 2 to 4 week intervals until DLI, followed by slightly less frequent testing until full donor chimerism is established, is the recommended strategy. In HSCT for nonmalignant diseases a lower degree of donor chimerism may be sufficient to treat the clinically significant symptoms of disease (Kapelushnik *et al.*, 1995; Walters *et al.*, 2001). Early chimerism testing at 1, 2, and 3 months should be sufficient to determine the degree of donor mixed chimerism that has developed. Subsequent testing may be necessary to determine the stability of mixed chimerism when clinically indicated.

The future of chimerism testing

With increasing use of reduced intensity conditioning regimens and DLI as immunotherapy for both hematologic and non-hematologic diseases, chimerism testing will continue to be an important measure of treatment outcomes (Mielcarek *et al.*, 2002; Giralt *et al.*, 1997; Khouri *et al.*, 1998; McSweeney *et al.*, 2001). Because of the close association of chimerism endpoints with clinical outcomes, measurement of chimerism will also continue to be an important surrogate endpoint in the development and evaluation of new treatment approaches for allogeneic HSCT. Thus, the establishment of stable chimerism can appropriately be used as an endpoint in the development of non-myeloablative conditioning regimens and in the comparison of different regimens (Sykes *et al.*, 1999; Sykes & Spitzer, 2002). Similarly, the conversion of mixed hematopoietic chimerism to complete donor hematopoiesis can be used as an endpoint following DLI and to compare the effectiveness of different DLI approaches.

Although previous assessments of chimerism were primarily based on the evaluation of mixed populations of white blood cells in marrow or peripheral blood, the emergence of PCR-based methods that target DNA polymorphisms now makes possible the measurement of chimerism in well-defined distinct cellular populations. Indeed, the recent recommendations from IBMTR/ABMTR (Antin *et al.*, 2001) suggest that analysis of peripheral blood chimerism is preferred for most evaluations since this can provide an assessment of both myeloid and lymphoid cells posttransplant. In contrast, lymphoid cells comprise only a small and highly variable fraction of bone marrow, and marrow chimerism is therefore primarily a measurement of the myeloid compartment. Future studies are likely to examine chimerism in different lymphoid subsets including B cells, NK cells, and T cell subsets. These results will be correlated with myeloid chimerism as well as transplant outcomes such as GVHD and relapse. Reconstitution of immune function may also be dependent on the levels of chimerism in different cellular compartments. Assessment of T cell reconstitution can now be measured by analysis of T cell receptor repertoire (Wu *et al.*, 2000) and T cell receptor excision circles (TREC) (Douek *et al.*, 2000; Weinberg *et al.*, 2001; Hochberg *et al.*, 2002). In addition to conventional phenotypic and functional assays, these new quantitative measures of T cell reconstitution provide objective methods for evaluating changes in global T cell immunity. In conjunction with these new assays, future studies will be able to specifically examine the impact of chimerism within well-defined lymphoid and myeloid populations on the reconstitution of T cell, B cell and NK cell immunity post-HSCT.

The increasing emphasis on transplantation of stem cells as therapy for nonmalignant nonhematopoietic diseases such as Parkinson's disease (Arenas, 2002) and the growing recognition of the role of transplanted cells in numerous organs such as heart, liver, and brain (Korbling *et al.*, 2002; Quaini *et al.*, 2002) will inevitably expand the role of chimerism testing outside the conventional bone marrow transplant setting. The recognition that hematopoietic stem cells can develop into numerous and surprisingly diverse types of terminally differentiated cells has led to interest in using these, and other, stem cells therapeutically for nonhematopoietic diseases. For example, a recent trial of embryonic stem cell transplantation in Parkinson's disease relied on clinical and radiologic outcome measures (Freed *et al.*, 2001). Histologic examination of two patients was only completed after their incidental deaths. Chimerism measurements in the cerebrospinal fluid or postmortem microdissection of dopaminergic neurons followed by chimerism analysis would have allowed these investigators to determine another important outcome measure, survival of transplanted stem cells. Measurement of the ability of transplanted cells to survive in an allogeneic donor will always require the distinction of donor from recipient and will bring chimerism testing to a far larger clinical spectrum of diseases.

References

Alderborn, A., Kristofferson, A., Hammerling, U. (2000). Determination of single-nucleotide polymorphisms by real-time pyrophosphate DNA sequencing. *Genome Research,* **10**, 1249–58.

Antin, J.H., Childs, R., Filipovich, A.H. *et al.* (2001). Establishment of complete and mixed donor chimerism after allogeneic lymphohematopoietic transplantation: recommendations from a workshop at the 2001 tandem meetings. *Biology of Blood and Marrow Transplantion,* **7**, 473–85.

Arenas, E. (2002). Stem cells in the treatment of Parkinson's disease. *Brain Research Bulletin,* **57**, 795–808.

Bellucci, R., Alyea, E.P., Weller, E. *et al.* (2002). Immunologic effects of prophylactic donor lymphocyte infusion after allogeneic marrow transplantation for multiple myeloma. *Blood,* **99**, 4610–7.

Bertheas, M.F., Lafage, M., Levy, P. *et al.* (1991). Influence of mixed chimerism on the results of allogeneic bone marrow transplantation for leukemia. *Blood,* **78**, 3103–6.

Blume, K.G., Beutler, E., Bross, K.J. *et al.* (1980). Genetic markers in human bone marrow transplantation. *American Journal of Human Genetics,* **32,** 414–9.

Bordignon, C., Keever, C.A., Small, T.N. *et al.* (1989). Graft failure after T-cell-depleted human leukocyte antigen identical marrow transplants for leukemia: II. In vitro analyses of host effector mechanisms. *Blood,* **74,** 2237–43.

Bosserman, L.D., Murray, C., Takvorian, T. *et al.* (1989). Mechanism of graft failure in HLA-matched and HLA-mismatched bone marrow transplant recipients. *Bone Marrow Transplantion,* **4,** 239–45.

Brickner, A.G., Warren, E.H., Caldwell, J.A. (2001). The immunogenicity of a new human minor histocompatibility antigen results from differential antigen processing. *Journal of Experimental Medicine,* **193,** 195–206.

Cargill, M., Altshuler, D., Ireland, J. *et al.* (1999). Characterization of single-nucleotide polymorphisms in coding regions of human genes. *Nature Genetics,* **22,** 231–8.

Cavet, J., Dickinson, A.M., Norden, J. *et al.* (2001). Interferon-gamma and interleukin-6 gene polymorphisms associate with graft-versus-host disease in HLA-matched sibling bone marrow transplantation. *Blood,* **98,** 1594–600.

Center for Medical Genetics. http://research.marshfieldclinic.org/genetics/Map_Markers/maps/IndexMapFrames.html

Childs, R., Chernoff, A., Contentin, N. *et al.* (2000). Regression of metastatic renal-cell carcinoma after nonmyeloablative allogeneic peripheral-blood stem-cell transplantation. *New England Journal of Medicine,* **343,** 750–8.

Childs, R., Clave, E., Contentin, N. *et al.* (1999). Engraftment kinetics after nonmyeloablative allogeneic peripheral blood stem cell transplantation: full donor T-cell chimerism precedes alloimmune responses. *Blood,* **94,** 3234–41.

Crescenzi, B., Fizzotti, M., Piattoni, S. *et al.* (2000). Interphase FISH for Y chromosome, VNTR polymorphisms, and RT-PCR for BCR-ABL in the monitoring of HLA-matched and mismatched transplants. *Cancer Genetics and Cytogenetics,* **120,** 25–9.

Dahmen, U.M., Boettcher, M., Krawczyk, M., & Broelsch, C.E. *et al.* (2002). Flow cytometric "rare event analysis": a standardized approach to the analysis of donor cell chimerism. *Journal of Immunological Methods,* **262,** 53–69.

Dewald, G., Stallard, R., Al Saadi, A. *et al.* (1998). A multicenter investigation with interphase fluorescence in situ hybridization using X- and Y-chromosome probes. *American Journal of Medical Genetics,* **76,** 318–26.

Diez-Martin, J.L., Llamas, P., Gosalvez, J. *et al.* (1998). Conventional cytogenetics and FISH evaluation of chimerism after sex-mismatched bone marrow transplantation (BMT) and donor leukocyte infusion (DLI). *Haematologica,* **83,** 408–15.

Douek, D.C., Vescio, R.A., Betts, M.R. *et al.* (2000). Assessment of thymic output in adults after haematopoietic stem-cell transplantation and prediction of T-cell reconstitution. *Lancet,* **355,** 1875–81.

Durnam, D.M., Anders, K.R., Fisher, L. *et al.* (1989). Analysis of the origin of marrow cells in bone marrow transplant recipients using a Y-chromosome-specific in situ hybridization assay. *Blood,* **74,** 2220–6.

Fishleder, A.J., Bolwell, B., & Lichtin, A.E. (1992). Incidence of mixed chimerism using busulfan/cyclophosphamide containing regimens in allogeneic bone marrow transplantation. *Bone Marrow Transplantion,* **9,** 293–7.

Fontes, P., Rao, A.S., Demetris, A.J. *et al.* (1994). Bone marrow augmentation of donor-cell chimerism in kidney, liver, heart, and pancreas islet transplantation. *Lancet,* **344,** 151–5.

Freed, C.R., Greene, P.E., Breeze, R.E. *et al.* (2001). Transplantation of embryonic dopamine neurons for severe Parkinson's disease. *New England Journal of Medicine,* **344,** 710–9.

Gallardo, D., Arostegui, J.I., Balas, A. *et al.* (2001). Disparity for the minor histocompatibility antigen HA-1 is associated with an increased risk of acute graft-versus-host disease (GvHD) but it does not affect chronic GvHD incidence, disease-free survival or overall survival after allogeneic human leucocyte antigen-identical sibling donor transplantation. *British Journal of Haematology,* **114,** 931–6.

Ginsburg, D., Antin, J.H., Smith, B.R. *et al.* (1985). Origin of cell populations after bone marrow transplantation. Analysis using DNA sequence polymorphisms. *Journal of Clinical Investigation,* **75,** 596–603.

Giralt, S., Estey, E., Albitar, M. *et al.* (1997). Engraftment of allogeneic hematopoietic progenitor cells with purine analog-containing chemotherapy: harnessing graft-versus-leukemia without myeloablative therapy. *Blood,* **89,** 4531–6.

Griffin, J.D. (2001). Point mutations in the FLT3 gene in AML. *Blood,* **97,** 2193A–2193.

Grumet, F.C., Hiraki, D.D., Brown, B.W.M. *et al.* (2001). CD31 mismatching affects marrow transplantation outcome. *Biology of Blood and Marrow Transplantation,* **7,** 503–12.

Halushka, M.K., Fan, J.B., Bentley, K. *et al.* (1999). Patterns of single-nucleotide polymorphisms in candidate genes for blood-pressure homeostasis. *Nature Genetics,* **22,** 239–47.

Hochberg, E.P., Chillemi, A.C., Wu, C.J. *et al.* (2002). Quantitation of T-cell neogenesis in vivo after allogeneic bone marrow transplantation in adults. *Blood,* **98,** 1116–21.

Hochberg, E.P., Miklos, D.B., Neuberg, D. *et al.* (2003). A novel rapid single polymorphism (SNP) based method for assessment of hematopoietic chimerism after allogeneic stem cell transplantation. *Blood,* **101,** 363–9.

Hosoi, T., Yahara, S., Kunitomo, K. *et al.* (1977). Blood chimeric twins: an example of blood cell chimerism. *Vox Sanguinis,* **32,** 339–41.

http://www.atcc.org/Products/str.cfm

http://www.cstl.nist.gov/biotech/strbase/

http://ystr.charite.de/index_gr.html

Huss, R., Deeg, H.J., Gooley, T. *et al.* (1996). Effect of mixed chimerism on graft-versus-host disease, disease recurrence and survival after HLA-identical marrow transplantation for aplastic anemia or chronic myelogenous leukemia. *Bone Marrow Transplantion,* **18,** 767–76.

Immervoll, T., Loesgen, S., Dutsch, G. *et al.* (2001). Fine mapping and single nucleotide polymorphism association results of candidate genes for asthma and related phenotypes. *Human Mutation,* **18,** 327–36.

Jonsson, J.R., Hogan, P.G., Thomas, R. *et al.* (1997). Peripheral blood chimerism following human liver transplantation. *Hepatology,* **25,** 1233–6.

Kapelushnik, J., Or, R., Filon, D. *et al.* (1995). Analysis of beta-globin mutations shows stable mixed chimerism in patients with thalassemia after bone marrow transplantation. *Blood,* **86,** 3241–6.

Kernan, N.A., Flomenberg, N., Dupont, B., & O'Reilly, R.J. (1987). Graft rejection in recipients of T-cell-depleted HLA-nonidentical marrow transplants for leukemia. Identification of host-derived anti-donor allocytotoxic T lymphocytes. *Transplantation, 43,* 842–7.

Khouri, I.F., Keating, M., Korbling, M. *et al.* (1998). Transplant-lite: induction of graft-versus-malignancy using fludarabine-based nonablative chemotherapy and allogeneic blood progenitor-cell transplantation as treatment for lymphoid malignancies. *Journal of Clinical Oncology, 16,* 2817–24.

Knowlton, R.G., Brown, V.A., Braman, J.C. *et al.* (1986). Use of highly polymorphic DNA probes for genotypic analysis following bone marrow transplantation. *Blood, 68,* 378–85.

Korbling, M., Katz, R.L., Khanna, A. *et al.* (2002). Hepatocytes and epithelial cells of donor origin in recipients of peripheral-blood stem cells. *New England Journal of Medicine, 346,* 738–46.

Korver, K., de Lange, G.G., van den Bergh, R.L. *et al.* (1987). Lymphoid chimerism after allogeneic bone marrow transplantation. Y-chromatin staining of peripheral T and B lymphocytes and allotyping of serum immunoglobulins. *Transplantation, 44,* 643–50.

Lau, Y.L., Kwong, Y.L., Lee, A.C. *et al.* (1995). Mixed chimerism following bone marrow transplantation for severe combined immunodeficiency: a study by DNA fingerprinting and simultaneous immunophenotyping and fluorescence in situ hybridisation. *Bone Marrow Transplantation, 15,* 971–6.

Lum, L.G., Seigneuret, M.C., Orcutt-Thordarson, N. *et al.* (1985). The regulation of immunoglobulin synthesis after HLA-identical bone marrow transplantation: VI. Differential rates of maturation of distinct functional groups within lymphoid subpopulations in patients after human marrow grafting. *Blood, 65,* 1422–33.

Mackinnon, S., Barnett, L., Bourhis, J.H. *et al.* (1992). Myeloid and lymphoid chimerism after T-cell-depleted bone marrow transplantation: evaluation of conditioning regimens using the polymerase chain reaction to amplify human minisatellite regions of genomic DNA. *Blood, 80,* 3235–41.

Mackinnon, S., Papadopoulos, E.B., Carabasi, M.H. *et al.* (1995). Adoptive immunotherapy evaluating escalating doses of donor leukocytes for relapse of chronic myeloid leukemia after bone marrow transplantation: separation of graft-versus-leukemia responses from graft-versus-host disease. *Blood, 86,* 1261–8.

McSweeney, P.A., Niederwieser, D., Shizuru, J.A. *et al.* (2001). Hematopoietic cell transplantation in older patients with hematologic malignancies: replacing high-dose cytotoxic therapy with graft-versus-tumor effects. *Blood, 97,* 3390–400.

Mielcarek, M., Leisenring, W., Torok-Storb, B., & Storb, R. (2000). Graft-versus-host disease and donor-directed hemagglutinin titers after ABO-mismatched related and unrelated marrow allografts: evidence for a graft-versus-plasma cell effect. *Blood, 96,* 1150–6.

Mielcarek, M., Sandmaier, B.M., Maloney, D.G. *et al.* (2002). Nonmyeloablative hematopoietic cell transplantation: status quo and future perspectives. *Journal of Clinical Immunology, 22,* 70–4.

Morisaki, H., Morisaki, T., Nakahori, Y. *et al.* (1988). Genotypic analysis using a Y-chromosome-specific probe following bone marrow transplantation. *American Journal of Hematology, 27,* 30–3.

Najfeld, V., Burnett, W., Vlachos, A. *et al.* (1997). Interphase FISH analysis of sex-mismatched BMT utilizing dual color XY probes. *Bone Marrow Transplantation, 19,* 829–34.

Nuckols, J.D., Rasheed, B.K., McGlennen, R.C. *et al.* (2000). Evaluation of an automated technique for assessment of marrow engraftment after allogeneic bone marrow transplantation using a commercially available kit. *American Journal of Clinical Pathology, 113,* 135–40.

Oberkircher, R., Strout, M., Herzig, G. *et al.* (1995). Description of an efficient and highly informative method for the evaluation of hematopoietic chimerism following allogeneic bone marrow transplant. *Bone Marrow Transplantation, 16,* 695–702.

Oliver, D.H., Thompson, R.E., Griffin, C.A., & Eshleman, J.R. (2000). Use of single nucleotide polymorphisms (SNP) and real-time polymerase chain reaction for bone marrow engraftment analysis. *Journal of Molecular Diagnostics, 2,* 202–28.

Orsini, E., Alyea, E.P., Chillemi, A. *et al.* (2000). Conversion to full donor chimerism following donor lymphocyte infusion is associated with disease response in patients with multiple myeloma. *Biology of Blood and Marrow Transplantation, 6,* 375–86.

Palka, G., Stuppia, L., Di Bartolomeo, P. *et al.* (1996). FISH detection of mixed chimerism in 33 patients submitted to bone marrow transplantation. *Bone Marrow Transplantation, 17,* 231–6.

Petz, L.D., Yam, P., Wallace, R.B. *et al.* (1987). Mixed hematopoietic chimerism following bone marrow transplantation for hematologic malignancies. *Blood, 70,* 1331–7.

Pichert, G., Roy, D.C., Gonin, R. *et al.* (1995). Distinct patterns of minimal residual disease associated with graft-versus-host disease after allogeneic bone marrow transplantation for chronic myelogenous leukemia. *Journal of Clinical Oncology, 13,* 1704–13.

Pierce, R.A., Field, E.D., Mutis, T. *et al.* (2001). The HA-2 minor histocompatibility antigen is derived from a diallelic gene encoding a novel human class I myosin protein. *Journal of Immunology, 167,* 3223–30.

Quaini, F., Urbanek, K., Beltrami, A.P. *et al.* (2002). Chimerism of the transplanted heart. *New England Journal of Medicine, 346,* 5–15.

Ranade, K., Jorgenson, E., Sheu, W.H. (2002). A polymorphism in the beta1 adrenergic receptor is associated with resting heart rate. *American Journal of Human Genetics, 70,* 935–42.

Rondon, G., Giralt, S., Pereira, M. *et al.* (1997). Analysis of chimerism following allogeneic bone marrow transplantation by fluorescent-in-situ hybridization. *Leukemia & Lymphoma, 25,* 463–7.

Roth, M.S., Antin, J.H., Bingham, E.L., & Ginsburg, D. (1990). Use of polymerase chain reaction-detected sequence polymorphisms to document engraftment following allogeneic bone marrow transplantation. *Transplantation, 49,* 714–20.

Roux, E., Helg, C., Chapuis, B. *et al.* (1992). Evolution of mixed chimerism after allogeneic bone marrow transplantation as determined on granulocytes and mononuclear cells by the polymerase chain reaction. *Blood, 79,* 2775–83.

Roy, D.C., Tantravahi, R., Murray, C. *et al.* (1990). Natural history of mixed chimerism after bone marrow transplantation with CD6-depleted allogeneic marrow: a stable equilibrium. *Blood, 75,* 296–304.

Schaap, N., Schattenberg, A., Mensink, E. *et al.* (2002). Long-term follow-up of persisting mixed chimerism after partially T cell-depleted allogeneic stem cell transplantation. *Leukemia, 16,* 13–21.

Sparkes, R.S., Sparkes, M.C., & Gale, R.P. (1979). Immunoglobulin synthesis following allogeneic bone marrow transplantation in man. Conversion to donor allotype. *Transplantation, 27,* 212–3.

Spriewald, B.M., Wassmuth, R., Carl, H.D. *et al.* (1998). Microchimerism after liver transplantation: prevalence and methodological aspects of detection. *Transplantation,* **66,** 77–83.

Soiffer, R.J., Bosserman, L., Murray, C. *et al.* (1990). Reconstitution of T-cell function after CD6-depleted allogeneic bone marrow transplantation. *Blood,* **75,** 2076–84.

Spitzer, T.R., McAfee, S., Sackstein, R. *et al.* (2000). Intentional induction of mixed chimerism and achievement of antitumor responses after nonmyeloablative conditioning therapy and HLA-matched donor bone marrow transplantation for refractory hematologic malignancies. *Biology of Blood and Marrow Transplantation,* **6,** 309–20.

Sreenan, J.J., Pettay, J.D., Tbakhi, A. *et al.* (1997). The use of amplified variable number of tandem repeats (VNTR) in the detection of chimerism following bone marrow transplantation. A comparison with restriction fragment length polymorphism (RFLP) by Southern blotting. *American Journal of Clinical Pathology,* **107,** 292–8.

Sykes, M. & Spitzer, T.R. (2002). Non-myeloablative induction of mixed hematopoietic chimerism: application to transplantation tolerance and hematologic malignancies in experimental and clinical studies. *Cancer Treatment and Research,* **110,** 79–99

Sykes, M., Preffer, F., McAfee, S. *et al.* (1999). Mixed lympho-haemopoietic chimerism and graft-versus-lymphoma effects after non-myeloablative therapy and HLA-mismatched bone-marrow transplantation. *Lancet,* **353,** 1755–9.

Tait, B.D., Maddison, R., McCluskey, J. *et al.* (2001). Clinical relevance of the minor histocompatibility antigen HA-1 in allogeneic bone marrow transplantation between HLA identical siblings. *Transplantation Proceedings,* **33,** 1760–1.

Tseng, L.H., Lin, M.T., Martin, P.J. *et al.* (1998). Definition of the gene encoding the minor histocompatibility antigen HA-1 and typing for HA-1 from genomic DNA. *Tissue Antigens,* **52,** 305–11.

Ulrich, C.M., Yasui, Y., Storb, R. *et al.* (2001). Pharmacogenetics of methotrexate: toxicity among marrow transplantation patients varies with the methylenetetrahydrofolate reductase C677T polymorphism. *Blood,* **98,** 231–4.

van Dekken, H., Hagenbeek, A., & Bauman, J.G. (1989). Detection of host cells following sex-mismatched bone marrow transplantation by fluorescent in situ hybridization with a Y-chromosome specific probe. *Leukemia,* **3,** 724–8.

van Tol, M.J., Gerritsen, E.J., de Lange, G.G. *et al.* (1996). The origin of IgG production and homogeneous IgG components after allogeneic bone marrow transplantation. *Blood,* **87,** 818–26.

Viard, F., Merel, P., Bilhou-Nabera, C. *et al.* (1993). Mixed chimerism after sex-mismatched allogeneic BMT: evaluation of two molecular techniques. *Bone Marrow Transplantion,* **11,** 27–31.

Walters, M.C., Patience, M., Leisenring, W. *et al.* (2001). Stable mixed hematopoietic chimerism after bone marrow transplantation for sickle cell anemia. *Biology of Blood and Marrow Transplantion,* **7,** 665–73.

Wang, D.G., Fan, J.B., Siao, C.J. *et al.* (1998). Large-scale identification, mapping, and genotyping of single-nucleotide polymorphisms in the human genome. *Science,* **280,** 1077–82.

Weinberg, K., Blazar, B.R., Wagner, J.E. *et al.* (2001). Factors affecting thymic function after allogeneic hematopoietic stem cell transplantation. *Blood,* **97,** 1458–66.

Wessman, M., Ruutu, T., Volin, L., Knuutila, S. (1989). In situ hybridization using a Y-specific probe—a sensitive method for distinguishing residual male recipient cells from female donor cells in bone marrow transplantation. *Bone Marrow Transplantion,* **4,** 283–6.

Witherspoon, R.P., Lum, L.G., Storb, R. (1984). Immunologic reconstitution after human marrow grafting. *Seminars in Hematology,* **21,** 2–10.

Witherspoon, R.P., Schanfield, M.S., Storb, R. *et al.* (1978). Immunoglobulin production of donor origin after marrow transplantation for acute leukemia or aplastic anemia. *Transplantation,* **26,** 407–8.

Wu, C.J., Chillemi, A., Alyea, E.P. *et al.* (2000). Reconstitution of T-cell receptor repertoire diversity following T-cell depleted allogeneic bone marrow transplantation is related to hematopoietic chimerism. *Blood,* **95,** 352–9.

Yam, P.Y., Petz, L.D., Knowlton, R.G. *et al.* (1987). Use of DNA restriction fragment length polymorphisms to document marrow engraftment and mixed hematopoietic chimerism following bone marrow transplantation. *Transplantation,* **43,** 399–407.

Zuazu, J., Duran-Suarez, J.R., Julia, A. *et al.* (1988). Demonstration of chimerism after bone marrow transplantation by reticulocyte blood group typing. *Bone Marrow Transplantation,* **3,** 521–52.

31 Use of hematopoietic growth factors, interleukins, and interferons following autologous hematopoietic stem cell transplantation

DAVID S. RITCHIE AND ANDREW P. GRIGG

Royal Melbourne Hospital, Melbourne, Australia

Introduction

The major complications of myeloablative chemotherapy/chemoradiation are hematologic toxicity and organ damage. While peripheral blood progenitor cell (PBPC) transplantation leads to faster hematologic recovery than infusion of bone marrow (Schmitz *et al.,* 1996), there is still a period of pancytopenia after high-dose chemotherapy. Following autografting, myeloid and platelet recovery may take weeks, and recovery of lymphoid function takes years (Domenech *et al.,* 1995). The early posttransplant period is associated with red cell and platelet transfusion dependence, considerable morbidity, and a small but significant mortality from sepsis or hemorrhage. These complications also contribute to the considerable cost of treatment and prolonged supportive care.

In an attempt to reduce the cost, morbidity, and mortality of delayed hematopoietic reconstitution, a number of recombinant colony-stimulating factors (CSFs) have been widely evaluated, particularly after autologous bone marrow transplantation (BMT). The most widely used are the cytokines that stimulate granulocyte recovery, granulocyte CSF (G-CSF), and granulocyte-macrophage CSF (GM-CSF). An emerging issue concerns the role of myeloid cytokines after PBPC transplantation.

The role of early acting cytokines, such as interleukin-3 (IL-3) and flt-3-ligand (flt-3L), and lineage-specific cytokines, such as thrombopoietin (TPO) and erythropoietin (EPO) have also been studied. Preclinical studies have also examined the use of nonhematopoietic cytokines such as keratinocyte growth factor (Zeeh *et al.,* 1996,) and IL-11 (Du *et al.,* 1994) to attenuate the effects of chemotherapy and radiotherapy on the gastrointestinal mucosa. Cytokines such as interleukin-2 (IL-2) and interferon-α (IFN-α) have also been investigated as immunotherapy in an attempt to harness a putative graft-versus-tumor effect and thereby reduce the risk of disease recurrence.

This chapter reviews the use of growth factors and cytokines following autografting to accelerate hematopoietic recovery and to decrease the rate of disease relapse. The use of growth factors for the mobilization of hematopoietic stem and progenitor cells is dealt with in Chapter 24.

Use of colony-stimulating factors to accelerate count recovery

Granulocyte and granulocyte-macrophage colony-stimulating factors

Autologous bone marrow transplantation

As PBPC transplantation results in faster hematological recovery (and hence reduced costs) than autologous BMT (Schmitz *et al.,* 1996), the former is now the standard of therapy in autologous hematopoietic stem cell grafting. Autologous marrow is now utilized uncommonly in this context. However, a small proportion of patients undergoing autografting will not mobilize adequate numbers of PBPC. This problem seems in part determined by the intensity of prior treatment, the prior use of stem cell toxins such as melphalan, and the age of the patient. Other factors are also involved, since a small percentage of normal volunteers receiving G-CSF mobilize progenitors poorly (Grigg *et al.,* 1995). Some patients will, therefore, undergo autologous marrow harvest. The effect of myeloid CSFs given after marrow infusion on count recovery has been evaluated extensively in the past, but has not been the subject of extensive clinical study in recent years.

G-CSF G-CSF regulates the production, maturation, and function of cells of the neutrophil lineage. No major effects are observed on other hematopoietic lineages. Both glycosylated (lenograstim) and nonglycosylated (filgrastim) forms are commercially available, with minor differences in biological potency, attributable to the slightly greater half-life of the glycosylated form (Oh-eda *et al.,* 1990).

The first demonstration of the ability of G-CSF to accelerate neutrophil recovery after autologous BMT was shown by Sheridan and colleagues in 1989 (Fig. 31.1). The results of randomized studies comparing the use of G-CSF with placebo following autologous BMT are summarized in Table 31.1. These demonstrate that administration of G-CSF (lenograstim or filgrastim) at doses between 2 and 30 μg/kg/day, by subcutaneous or intravenous injection, results in a significantly shorter time to neutrophil recovery (Linch *et al.,* 1993; Gisselbrecht *et al.,* 1994;

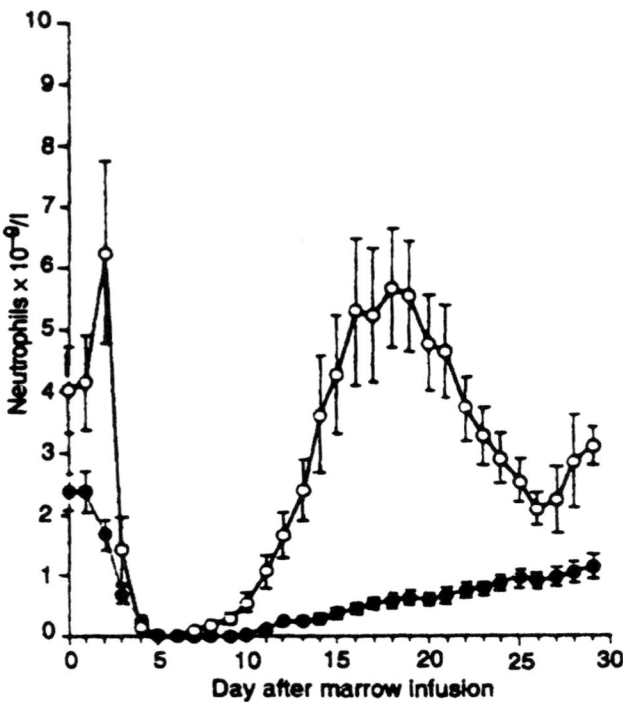

Fig. 31.1. Mean (SEM) total white cell count and neutrophil count following G-CSF=○, n=15) as compared to 18 historical controls=●. Reproduced, with permission, from Sheridan *et al.* (1989).

Significant reductions in febrile neutropenia, antibiotic usage, and duration of hospitalization were reported in one study (Klumpp *et al.,* 1995), but not in others (Stahel *et al.,* 1994; Schmitz *et al.,* 1995). The interpretation of duration of hospitalization as an endpoint in particular is problematic, since in some, but not all, institutions discharge is directly predicated on neutrophil counts in the absence of a clinical contraindication. Thus, clinical benefits from the use of G-CSF have been less consistently demonstrated and no study has yet reported a survival benefit from administration of G-CSF. The American Society of Clinical Oncology (ASCO) guidelines in 1996 recommended the use of CSFs following autologous bone marrow transplantation; this conclusion was not specifically commented upon further in the 2000 review (Ozer *et al.,* 2000).

The toxicity of G-CSF at doses used after transplantation (usually 5 µg/kg/day) is minor, with bone pain being the most common side-effect. This usually responds to non-narcotic analgesia. Less frequently observed are fever, weight gain, and splenomegaly with chronic administration. Intravenous administration of G-CSF may induce transient neutropenia, due to upregulation of neutrophil adhesion receptors and intravascular margination. Transient hypoxemia has been reported during neutrophil recovery in febrile patients receiving G-CSF, but the mechanism of this is not clear (White & Cebon, 1995). Of particular note, there is no published evidence to indicate whether G-CSF affects the likelihood of relapse following autografting for myeloid leukemias.

An early complication of both autologous BMT and PBPC transplantation is the engraftment syndrome, characterized by fever, skin rash, capillary leakage, and pulmonary infiltrates. The frequency of this complication in a retrospective series of 248 patients was almost 60% (Lee *et al.,* 1995). The onset of symptoms and signs coincides with neutrophil recovery (Cahill, Spitzer, & Mazumbder, 1996), occurring at 7 days postinfusion of stem cells and lasting a median of 11 days (Lee *et al.,* 1995). The administration of G-CSF appears to increase the likelihood of developing this syndrome. Steroid treatment results in rapid defervescence, shortens the duration of the ill-

Stahel *et al.,* 1994; Schmitz *et al.,* 1995). Randomized dose-finding studies suggest that 5 µg/kg/day represents an optimal dose (Linch *et al.,* 1993; Stahel *et al.,* 1997). No differences in efficacy or toxicity can be attributed to the route of administration. In the majority of studies G-CSF was commenced within 24 hours of marrow infusion. Studies have suggested that similar benefit may be obtained with delayed (starting day 6, 7, or 8 posttransplant) administration of G-CSF, with considerably reduced cost (Khwaja *et al.,* 1993; Vey *et al.,* 1994; Torres Gomez *et al.,* 1995; Faucher *et al.,* 1996).

Table 31.1. *Prospective controlled trials of G-CSF following autologous bone marrow transplantation*

Reference	Disease	Growth factor	Dose (µg/kg/day)	Number of patients	Days to ANC >0.5	Febrile days	Antibiotic days	Hospital days
Linch *et al.,* 1997	NHL/HD/MM/ALL/ solid tumors	G-CSF placebo	2–20	72 25	13–15 19[a]	4–7 6	17–20 23	21–25 36
Gisselbrecht *et al.,* 1994	NHL/HD/MM/ALL/ solid tumors	G-CSF placebo	5	127 118	14 20[a]	3 5	15 19[a]	25 29
Stahel *et al.,* 1994	NHL	G-CSF placebo	10/20	29	10	5		
Schmitz *et al.,* 1995	NHL/HD	G-CSF placebo	10/30	36 18	12/14 20[a]	NS	NS	NS

Abbreviations: ANC, absolute neutrophil count; NHL, non-Hodgkin's lymphoma; HD, Hodgkin's disease; ALL, acute lymphoblastic leukemia; MM, multiple myeloma; NS, no significant difference between G-CSF and placebo; no symbol means no significant difference.

[a] $P < .05$.

ness, and reduces the risk of fatal acute respiratory distress syndrome (ARDS) (Lee *et al.*, 1995).

GM-CSF GM-CSF promotes the survival, proliferation, and maturation of myeloid cells, and also enhances the function of mature neutrophils and monocytes. Glycosylated yeast-derived (sargramostim) and nonglycosylated *E. coli*-derived (molgramostim) forms are commercially available. Glycosylation appears to enhance the half-life of GM-CSF, and may reduce the incidence of side-effects, although no formal comparative studies have been undertaken.

The results of prospective controlled studies using GM-CSF following autologous BMT are summarized in Table 31.2. With the exception of one study (Advani *et al.*, 1992), these indicate that the use of GM-CSF following autologous BMT shortens the time to neutrophil recovery (Nemunaitis *et al.*, 1991; Gorin *et al.*, 1992; Khwaja *et al.*, 1992; Link *et al.*, 1992) (Fig. 31.2). However, only one study demonstrated reduced antibiotic use (Nemunaitis *et al.*, 1991), although several found that GM-CSF decreased the duration of hospitalization (Nemunaitis *et al.*, 1991; Gorin *et al.*, 1992; Gulati *et al.*, 1992). The use of GM-CSF following autologous BMT appears cost-effective (Gulati *et al.*, 1992). Only one study suggested an effect of GM-CSF on platelet recovery (Gulati *et al.*, 1992), and fewer red cell transfusions were reported in another study (Nemunaitis *et al.*, 1991). Long-term follow-up of patients treated with GM-CSF following autologous BMT has generally not demonstrated an increase in graft failure, secondary leukemia, or relapse rate (Rabinowe *et al.*, 1993), although a single historically controlled study comparing relapse rate and survival in children given autologous BMT for acute myeloid leukemia after condi-

tioning with busulfan and cyclophosphamide showed a significantly higher relapse rate and poorer overall survival compared with a group of children not given GM-CSF (Calderwood *et al.*, 1996). With the exception of this study, no effect on disease-free or overall survival due to the use of GM-CSF has been demonstrated.

Toxicities are reversible, and appear to be dependent on dose and route of administration. Most commonly observed are fever, nausea, fatigue, headaches, bone pain, myalgias and chills, and injection site reactions (Antman *et al.*, 1988). The assessment of febrile days as an endpoint in studies may be confounded by the high incidence of fever as a direct side-effect of GM-CSF. Less commonly reported toxicities are diarrhea, anorexia, arthralgias, rashes, flushing, capillary leak syndromes, and hypotension. For sargramostim, doses above 250 $\mu g/m^2/day$, and continuous intravenous infusion over 24 hours are more commonly associated with side effects than shorter infusions or subcutaneous administration. While doses as high as 60 $\mu g/kg/day$ of molgramostim have been given, 5 $\mu g/kg/day$ appears to represent an optimal dose. A "first-dose" effect has been described with molgramostim given intravenously, characterized by transient flushing, tachycardia, hypotension, musculoskeletal pain, dyspnea, rigors, nausea, and leg spasms (Lieschke *et al.*, 1989).

Priming prior to marrow harvest
The use of G-CSF prior to autologous BM harvest has been shown in a controlled study of 100 patients to result in higher numbers of CFU-GM in the harvest product, faster neutrophil and platelet recovery, and shorter hospitalization (Damiani *et al.*, 1999). It is not clear whether there is any benefit of primed mar-

Table 31.2. *Prospective controlled trials of GM-CSF following autologous bone marrow transplantation*

Reference	Disease	Growth factor	Dose	Number of patients	Days to ANC >0.5	Febrile days	Antibiotic days	Hospital days
Nemunaitis *et al.*, 1991	NHL/HD/ALL	GM-CSF	250 $\mu g/m^2$	65	19	NS	24	27
		placebo		63	26[a]		27[a]	33[a]
Link *et al.*, 1992	ALL/NHL	GM-CSF	250 $\mu g/m^2$	39	15	NA	NS	NS
		placebo		40	28[a]			
Advani *et al.*, 1992	NHL/HD	GM-CSF	10 $\mu g/kg/day$	14	19	NA	NA	NA
		placebo		16	19			
Gorin *et al.*, 1992	NHL	GM-CSF	250 $\mu g/m^2$	44	14	NS	NS	23
		placebo		47	21[a]			29[a]
Khwaja *et al.*, 1992	NHL	GM-CSF	250 $\mu g/m^2$	29	14	NS	11	24
		placebo		29	20[a]		10	25
Gulati *et al.*, 1992[b]	HD	GM-CSF	10 $\mu g/kg/day$	12	17	NS	NA	32
		placebo		12	27[a]			40[a]
Greenberg *et al.*, 1996[b]	Mixed	GM-CSF	10 $\mu g/kg/day$	343	19[a]	NS	NS	29[a]
		placebo			27			32

Abbreviations: NA, not available; NS, no significant difference between GM-CSF and placebo, no symbol means no significant differences; ANC, absolute neutrophil count; NHL, non-Hodgkin's lymphoma; HD, Hodgkin's disease; ALL, acute lymphoblastic leukemia.
[a] $P < .05$.
[b] Days to ANC > $1.0 \times 10^9/l$.

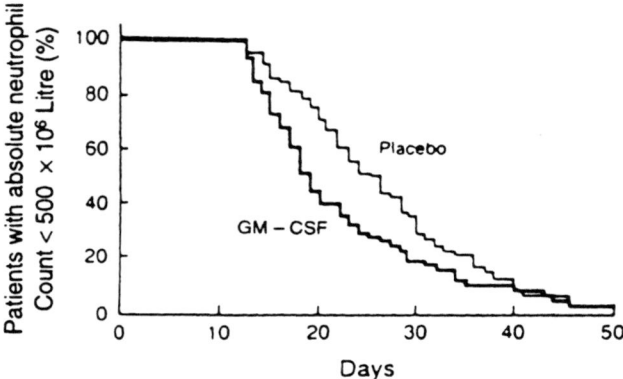

Fig. 31.2. Kaplan-Meier analysis of the time required for the absolute neutrophil count to reach or exceed 500 cells per cubic millimeter on two consecutive days in 65 patients who received rhGM-CSF and 63 patients who received placebo. There was significant difference ($P < .001$) in values between the two groups. Reproduced, with permission, from Nemunaitis *et al.* (1991).

row versus PBPCs in the autologous setting or of cytokine priming of marrow in patients who mobilise poor numbers of PBPCs.

Autologous peripheral blood progenitor cell transplantation

G-CSF G-CSF hastens neutrophil recovery by one to two days after PBPC transplantation (Table 31.3) and may abrogate the dose effect of stem cell numbers on rate of neutrophil recovery (Pierelli *et al.*, 1996a). Despite this, the clinical benefit as measured by reduction in the incidence of febrile days, antibiotic usage, and duration of hospitalization has been inconsistent and no survival benefit has been documented. There is no consistent evidence to show a cost saving with the use of G-CSF. Some studies have shown a delay in platelet

recovery with the use of G-CSF (Kawano *et al.*, 1998; Ojeda *et al.*, 1999) (Fig. 31.3).

The optimal dose and schedule remains unclear. One randomized study found no difference between 5, 10, and 16 µg/kg/day assessed by time to neutrophil engraftment, with a trend toward earlier platelet recovery for patients receiving 5 µg/kg/day (Bolwell *et al.*, 1997). The lower dose resulted in a halving of the cost for cytokine use (U.S. $2900 versus $6500 per patient). As described for patients undergoing autologous BMT, delaying G-CSF administration to day 5 or 6 following infusion of PBPC appears not to compromise time to neutrophil recovery or clinical outcome in some studies (Faucher *et al.*, 1996; Bolwell *et al.*, 1998; Hornedo *et al.*, 2002), but others have shown improved clinical outcome and cost savings when G-CSF is administered from day 1 (Colby *et al.*, 1998).

Based on these findings the routine use of G-CSF following autologous PBPC transplantation shows no clear clinical or financial benefit when the numbers of progenitor cells infused are adequate. Nevertheless, the 2000 ASCO guidelines recommend CSFs after PBPC infusion. Another approach is to use CSFs in selected cases only, such as after infusion of low CD34 numbers or in patients with delayed or inadequate neutrophil engraftment.

GM-CSF A similar picture emerges from studies using GM-CSF (Table 31.4). While two studies demonstrated more rapid neutrophil recovery (Advani *et al.*, 1992; Spitzer *et al.*, 1994), this was not confirmed in a small, single-center randomized study of GM-CSF 5 µg/kg/day compared to placebo after PBPC transplantation (Legros *et al.*, 1997). The difficulties inherent in using febrile days as a surrogate endpoint of clinical benefit in studies of GM-CSF are illustrated by the lower incidence of febrile days on the placebo arm (Legros *et al.*, 1997). Furthermore, the one study demonstrating a clinical benefit (reduction in duration of hospitalization) from the use

Table 31.3. *Trials of G-CSF following autologous peripheral blood progenitor cell transplantation*

Reference	Disease	Randomized	CSF	Dose (µg/kg/day)	Number of patients	Days to ANC>0.5	Febrile days	Antibiotic days	Hospital days
Klumpp *et al.*, 1995	NHL/HD/MM/ breast cancer	Yes	G-CSF placebo	5	10 10	11 17[a]	NS	NA	NA
Cortelazzo *et al.*, 1995	NHL	No	G-CSF placebo	5	20 20	10 12	NS	NS	NS
Brice *et al.*, 1996	NHL/HD	No	G-CSF placebo	5	43 34	11 16	NA	NA	NA
McQuaker *et al.*, 1997	NHL/HD/MM	Yes	G-CSF placebo	50 µg/m²/d	19 19	10 14[a]	NS	NS	13 16[a]
Ojeda *et al.*, 1999	NHL/HD/AML/ breast cancer	Yes	G-CSF placebo	5	30 32	10 12[a]	NS	NS	NA

Abbreviations: NA, not available; NS, no significant difference between treatment and placebo arms; ANC, absolute neutrophil count; NHL, non-Hodgkin's lymphoma; HD, Hodgkins's disease; ALL, acute lymphoblastic leukemia; MM, multiple myeloma; AML, acute myeloblastic leukemia.

[a] $P < .05$.

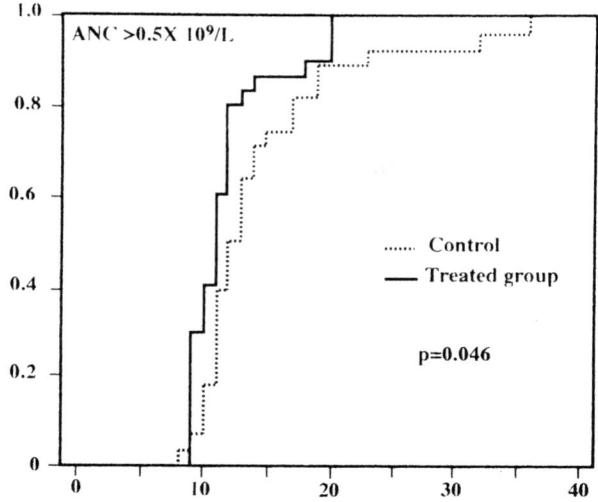

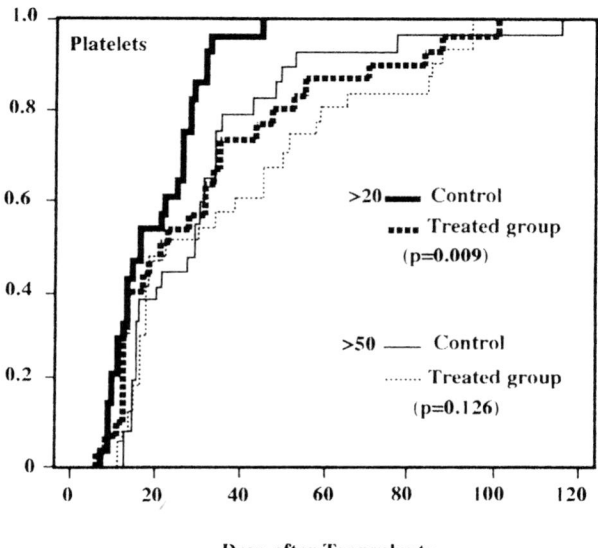

Days after Transplants

Fig. 31.3. Kaplan-Meier probability of achieving $0.5 \times 10^9/l$ of ANC (top graph, $P = .046$), and those of 20 or $50 \times 10^9/l$ of platelet counts independent of platelet transfusion (bottom graph, $P = .009$ for $20 \times 10^9/l$ or $P = .126$ for $50 \times 10^9/l$). Reproduced, with permission, from Kawano et al. (1998).

of GM-CSF after PBPC transplantation was confounded by the use of a combination of GM-CSF with G-CSF (Spitzer et al., 1994). One study showed no difference in hematologic recovery or clinical outcome of sequential G-CSF/GM-CSF versus G-CSF alone following autologous PBPC (Recchia et al., 2000).

Purged stem cell transplantation

Disease relapse following autografting may be due to tumor cells surviving conditioning treatment, reinfusion of tumor cells contaminating the graft, or, more likely, to a combination

of these possibilities. Tumor cells have been shown to contaminate marrow and PBPC inocula with a disturbing frequency (Negrin & Pesando, 1994). This is due in part to sensitive methods of detection, including reverse-transcriptase polymerase chain reaction analysis (Gribben et al., 1991). To address this issue, attempts have been made to purge contaminating malignant cells by a variety of methods. These include the ex vivo use of chemotherapy such as 4-hydroperoxycyclophosphamide (4HC), monoclonal antibodies directed to tumor-associated antigens in the presence of complement, or the use of agents such as interleukin-2 (see below) to enhance immunologic means of killing contaminating cells. These treatments probably result in prolongation of the time to hematopoietic recovery compared to unpurged autologous BMT, and therefore growth factor support may be required.

Several uncontrolled studies have examined the role of growth factors in this context. The administration of G-CSF after the infusion of marrow purged with 4HC to women with breast cancer accelerated neutrophil recovey, reduced the number of febrile days, and reduced the length of hospitalization (Kennedy et al., 1993a). Patients receiving mafosfamide-purged autologous BMT for lymphoid malignancies, who were treated with GM-CSF following autografting, had more rapid neutrophil recovery, although no effect was seen on platelet or erythrocyte recovery (Albin et al., 1994). G-CSF at approximately 10 μg/kg/day appeared to accelerate recovery compared to placebo- or GM-CSF-treated historical controls in patients receiving marrow purged using monoclonal antibody (Schriber et al., 1993).

Graft failure (and see Chapter 70)

Although uncommon, marrow graft failure after hematopoietic stem cell transplantation is associated with a high mortality. There appears to be benefit from the use of GM-CSF, with one study reporting improved long-term survival from early graft failure compared with a historical control group (40% versus 20%, respectively) (Nemunaitis et al., 1990) (Fig. 31.4). This study included allograft recipients. In a similar study of both allograft and autograft recipients, Weisdorf and colleagues (1995) also reported a survival advantage at 100 days in those experiencing graft failure who were treated with GM-CSF plus G-CSF versus those treated with G-CSF alone. This survival advantage occurred despite the absence of differences in neutrophil, red cell, or platelet recovery between the two groups.

Erythropoietin

Erythropoietin (EPO) expands the number of immature erythroid burst-forming units, in turn generating more mature colony-forming units and promoting their differentiation. Recombinant human EPO (rh-EPO) is useful in the anemia associated with renal failure, in which EPO levels are low. A number of studies have suggested that administration of rh-EPO reduces the requirement for red cell transfusion after allo-

Table 31.4. *Trials of GM-CSF following autologous peripheral blood progenitor cell transplantation*

Reference	Disease	Randomized	CSF	Dose (µg/kg/day)	Number of patients	Days to ANC>0.5	Febrile days	Antibiotic days	Hospital days
Avdani *et al.*, 1992	NHL/HD	Yes	GM-CSF	10	22	12	NA	NA	NA
			placebo		17	15			
Spitzer *et al.*, 1994	NHL/HD/solid tumors	Yes	GM-/G-CSF	2.5/7.5	18	10	NA	NA	19
			placebo		19	16[a]			21[a]
Legros *et al.*, 1997	Solid tumors	Yes	GM-CSF	5	25	12	6	NS	NS
			placebo		25	14	2[a]		

Abbreviations: NA, not available; NS, no significant difference between treatment and placebo arms; ANC, absolute neutrophil count; NHL, non-Hodgkin's lymphoma; HD, Hodgkins's disease.

geneic BMT (Klaesson *et al.*, 1994; Link *et al.*, 1994; Mitus *et al.*, 1994).

In contrast, a benefit for EPO has not been shown after auto-grafting (Locatelli *et al.*, 1994; Klaesson, 1999). In one study, EPO 200 IU/kg/day following autografting was well tolerated and produced a brisk reticulocytosis, but there was no reduction in red cell transfusion requirement (Ayash *et al.*, 1994). In another randomized study of 114 patients, there was no difference in reticulocyte generation or time to red cell transfusion independence (Link *et al.*, 1994). Other studies have demonstrated no evidence of a reduction in the number of red cell transfusions for patients receiving both EPO and G-CSF compared to patients receiving G-CSF alone (Chao *et al.*, 1994; Vanucchi *et al.*, 1996). Another study reported faster white cell, neutrophil, and platelet recovery in patients given a combination of G-CSF 5 mg/kg daily and erythropoietin 150 IU/kg daily after peripheral blood stem cell transplantation compared to a small group of historical control patients not given any cytokines posttransplant (Pierelli *et al.*, 1996b). Clearly, how-

ever, the accelerated leukocyte and neutrophil recovery could have been due to the G-CSF alone.

The reduction of transfusion requirements by EPO after allogeneic, but not autologous, transplantation may be due to several factors. Transfusion requirements after allogeneic transplantation are higher due to graft-versus-host disease (GVHD) and ABO incompatibility (Link *et al.*, 1994; Mehta *et al.*, 1996). In addition, red cell recovery appears to be slower after allogeneic than after autologous transplantation (Beguin, Oris, & Fillet, 1993). This may reflect different EPO responses to anemia: in one report, endogenous EPO responses to anemia were impaired in 15% of autologous compared with 72% of allogeneic transplant patients (Ireland *et al.*, 1990). Accordingly, the routine use of EPO following autografting cannot be recommended.

Interleukins

The failure of either G-CSF or GM-CSF to accelerate recovery of non-myeloid lineages has stimulated investigation of whether administration of cytokines acting at earlier steps in hematopoiesis may have effects on platelet and red cell reconstitution. Inconsistent evidence of benefit has been demonstrated with various interleukins, and their use in this context is associated with considerable toxicity. At present, the narrow therapeutic window of these compounds prohibits their use in routine clinical practice, but studies are in progress to improve efficacy with fewer side-effects.

Interleukin-1

Interleukins-1α and β (IL-1α and β) are pleiotropic cytokines with multiple effects in many organ systems. IL-1 acts as a costimulatory growth factor for hematopoietic stem cells. Phase I/II studies following autologous BMT suggested that IL-1β (0.01–0.05 µg/kg/day intravenously) may induce slightly earlier neutrophil recovery compared to historical controls, with no effect on platelet kinetics (Nemunaitis *et al.*, 1994). Side effects included fever and chills within 30 minutes of administration, and dose-limiting hypotension, and severe pain at the injection site (Elkordy *et al.*, 1997). IL-1α has also

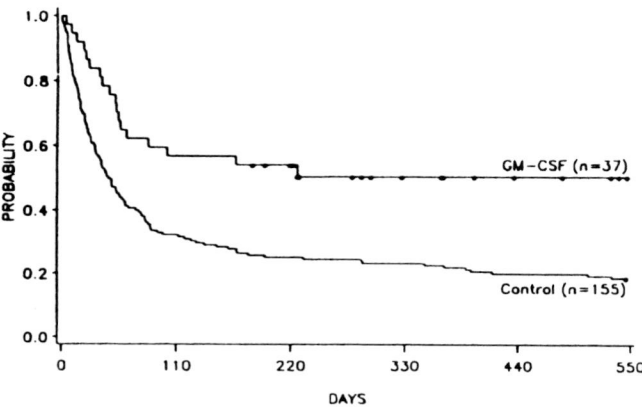

Fig. 31.4. Kaplan-Meier estimates of survival for 155 historical controls with graft failure and 37 marrow graft failure patients who received rhGM-CSF. Day 0 in the control patients was the day on which they met the definition of graft failure. Day 0 in the rhGM-CSF group was the day rhGM-CSF therapy was initited. Reproduced, with permission, from Nemunaitis *et al.* (1990).

been investigated, with similar toxicities in a phase I/II study (Weisdorf *et al.,* 1994). In this trial of 40 patients, neutrophil engraftment occurred significantly earlier and by day 14 the bone marrow of patients receiving IL-1α (0.1–10 μg/m2/day) were significantly enriched in committed myeloid progenitors. A trend to earlier platelet and red cell engraftment was noted, and patients receiving higher doses of IL-1α were discharged from the hospital earlier with a concomitant reduction in median hospital charges. These findings await confirmation in larger studies.

IL-1β has also been included in experimental protocols for the ex vivo expansion of CD34$^+$ hematopoietic progenitors (Mobest, Mertelsmann, & Henschler, 1998) and/or megakaryocytes (van den Oudenrijn *et al.,* 1999) from autologous stem cell collections, although these approaches have not yet been trialed in clinical practice.

Interleukin-3

Interleukin-3 (IL-3) is a multilineage growth factor that induces proliferation and differentiation of a broad spectrum of hematopoietic stem cells (Metcalf, 1989). As with IL-1, IL-3 has shown some utility in experimental protocols to expand hematopoietic progenitors (Drouet *et al.,* 2001). Phase I studies, however, have demonstrated a modest benefit in shortening the period of neutropenia from the use of recombinant human IL-3 (Nemunaitis *et al.,* 1993) and also enhanced platelet and reticulocyte recovery (Fibbe *et al.,* 1991). A randomized study of 198 patients with lymphoma showed no benefit from IL-3 in neutrophil or platelet recovery, the number of platelet transfusions, hemorrhagic complications, or major infections after autologous bone marrow transplantation (Brouwer *et al.,* 1999). Importantly, treatment could be completed in only 54% of the patients in the IL-3 group versus 75% in the placebo group ($P < .004$). Adverse events, including fever, myalgias, headaches, skeletal pain, nausea, and diarrhea were reported as reasons for premature discontinuation in the IL-3 group (23% for IL-3 versus 5% for placebo).

To enhance the previously observed modest effects of IL-3, the co-administration of a "late" acting cytokine such as GM-CSF or G-CSF has also been investigated. Subcutaneous IL-3 (2.5 or 5 μg/kg/day) was administered for either 5 or 10 days starting 4 hours post autologous BMT. Twenty-four hours after the last dose of IL-3, GM-CSF was administered as a 2-hour infusion until neutrophil recovery (Fay *et al.,* 1994). In this phase I/II study, neutrophil and platelet recovery were more rapid compared to historical controls receiving GM-CSF, G-CSF, or IL-3 alone. In addition, fewer red cell transfusions were required. These findings have been confirmed in a subsequent study combining IL-3 and G-CSF in patients undergoing autologous BMT for lymphoma (Lemoli *et al.,* 1996). While further study may better define the optimal usage of this cytokine, it currently has no role following autologous BMT.

PIXY321

A novel approach concerns the generation of a fusion protein called PIXY321, derived from both GM-CSF and IL-3. Animal studies indicate that binding to both the IL-3 and GM-CSF receptor components are preserved, without apparent additional toxicity (Williams *et al.,* 1991). Toxicities include mild to moderate fevers and injection site erythema, stomatitis, rash, headache, and edema. Data from a randomized double-blind study of 127 patients with lymphoma undergoing autologous transplantation comparing PIXY321 and GM-CSF found a statistically non-significant neutrophil recovery 2 days earlier in patients receiving PIXY321 (Vose *et al.,* 1997). No difference was seen in time to platelet independence. The therapeutic application of PIXY321 is potentially limited by the development of neutralizing antibodies (Miller *et al.,* 1999). Like a number of other agents which act on hematopoietic precursors, PIXY321 may have its greatest clinical utility in the ex vivo expansion of stem cells (Stiff *et al.,* 2000).

Interleukins 6 and 11

Interleukin-6 (IL-6) is a multifunctional cytokine with effects on T cells, myeloid differentiation, regulation of acute phase reactants, and megakaryopoiesis (Bruno & Hoffman, 1989). Studies have demonstrated an equivocal effect of IL-6 in the acceleration of neutrophil engraftment after autografting, and no effect on platelet recovery. The maximum tolerated dose after autologous BMT appears to be 1 mg/kg/day s.c. (Lazarus *et al.,* 1995). A small phase II study of IL-6 with G-CSF demonstrated no benefit over G-CSF alone (Devine *et al.,* 1994).

Interleukin-11 (IL-11) enhances the growth of IL-3-dependent megakaryopoiesis and stimulates production of acute phase proteins. A beneficial effect in reducing platelet transfusion requirements after conventional dose chemotherapy has been reported. Preclinical studies in mice indicate that IL-11 accelerated both neutrophil and platelet recovery posttransplant (Du *et al.,* 1993). However, in a subsequent prospective, randomized, controlled study in women receiving high-dose chemotherapy followed by autologous PBPC support, there was no demonstrable decrease in platelet transfusion requirements in the IL-11 arms (Vredenburgh *et al.,* 1998).

Thrombopoietin

The cloning of thrombopoietin (TPO), also known as megakaryocyte growth and differentiation factor (MGDF), represented a major breakthrough in understanding the later steps of megakaryopoiesis (Lok *et al.,* 1994). Thrombopoietin has been shown to stimulate megakaryocytopoiesis, as well as myelopoiesis and expansion of CD34$^+$ progenitor cells from single human CD34$^+$ Thy1$^+$ Lin$^-$ primitive progenitor cells (Young *et al.,* 1996). In preclinical and clinical studies, recombinant human TPO produced a dose-dependent increase in platelet counts in normal mice (Kabaya *et al.,* 1996; Ulich *et al.,* 1996) and humans, and enhancement of platelet recovery following chemotherapy (Basser *et al.,* 1996, 1997). Toxicities were minimal; of note, thrombotic events were equally uncommon in control and TPO-treated patients. Platelets were morphologically and functionally normal in the latter study. Serum TPO levels rise between days 0 and 10 after conditioning treatment prior to autologous PBPC transplantation, and gradually decline as platelet recovery occurs (Shimazaki *et al.,* 1997). In preclinical autograft models, TPO was highly effective in reducing the thrombocytopenia associated with PBPC transplantation in mice (Molineux *et al.,* 1996a, 1996b) and in clinical trials reduced the severity of thrombocytopenia induced by conventional dose cytotoxic chemotherapy.

Clinical application of TPO after high-dose chemotherapy, however, has shown limited success. In a phase I randomized, controlled study in women with breast cancer given PBSC autografts, there was no effect on the platelet count when TPO at doses from 2.5 to 10 µg/kg/day was given from the day of transplant until the platelet count reached $100 \times 10^9/l$ (Bolwell *et al.,* 2000). Similar results were observed following autologous BMT (Wolff, 2001). In a placebo-controlled study with dose escalation of pegylated recombinant human (PEG-rh) TPO up to 25 µg/kg/day in patients with delayed platelet recovery post autografting, results were similar for the placebo and TPO groups (Fields *et al.,* 2000). Of potential concern is the development of TPO-neutralizing antibodies, which may cross-react with endogenous TPO and cause severe refractory thrombocytopenia (Li *et al.,* 2001). At this time there appears to be no clear evidence to support the use of TPO in the post-autograft setting.

Use of cytokines to reduce nonhematopoietic toxicity

Mucositis is a common and distressing side effect of high-dose chemotherapy or chemoradiotherapy. Damaged mucosa also acts as a portal of entry for bacteria and other infectious agents. Dehydration can occur as a result of diarrhea from gastrointestinal inflammation and decreased oral intake of fluids. In many patients, mucositis is sufficiently severe to require intravenous alimentation, which is costly and associated with complications.

Keratinocyte growth factor (KGF) stimulates the growth of gut epithelial cells and enhances crypt survival, following exposure to chemoradiation (Finch *et al.,* 1989; Farrell *et al.,* 1998). Furthermore, KGF also promotes TGF-α production (Bajaj-Elliott *et al.,* 1998), which mediates mucosal healing (Egger *et al.,* 1997). A recombinant human product (rh-KGF) has been tested in preclinical studies, demonstrating a protective effect on gastrointestinal mucosa damaged by chemical injury, and improved survival of treated animals over controls (Housley *et al.,* 1994; Zeeh *et al.,* 1996). In a murine model of syngeneic bone marrow and PBPC transplantation, KGF promoted the survival of lethally irradiated mice, without impairment of hematopoietic engraftment (Lacey *et al.,* 1996). No effects on tumor cell proliferation in vitro or in vivo have been demonstrated in these studies. Phase II clinical studies in patients receiving autologous PBPC transplantation are in progress (Stiff, 2001).

Use of cytokines to prevent disease relapse

Immunologic antitumor effects play a key role in the curative capacity of allogeneic hematopoietic stem cell transplantation. Relapse rates are higher in patients with hematologic malignancy who receive autologous or syngeneic grafts compared to allografts, and attempts to minimize the sequelae of GVHD by T-cell depletion of marrow grafts from allogeneic donors have been associated with increased disease recurrence. A syndrome resembling GVHD has been described in 5% to 10% of patients receiving syngeneic or autologous BMT, which is clinically mild in character and predominantly affects the skin. In animal models cyclosporine (CSP) administered for brief periods induces GVHD after autologous BMT. This is thought to be due to inhibition by CSP of clonal deletion of autocytotoxic T lymphocytes in the thymus. A clinical study based on this observation suggested that 80% of patients treated with CSP following autografting developed GVHD. Preliminary data from this study suggest that the relapse rate may be reduced in these patients compared to historical controls, without deaths attributable to GVHD (Kennedy *et al.,* 1993b). Based on these observations, attempts have been made to generate an autologous GVHD effect with the use of cytokines, including IL-2 and interferon-γ (Higuchi *et al.,* 1991; Baumgarten *et al.,* 1994; Kennedy *et al.,* 1994; Lopez-Jimenez *et al.,* 1997).

Interleukin-2

Interleukin-2 promotes the generation and proliferation of natural killer (NK) cells in the peripheral blood and bone marrow both in vitro and in vivo (Charak *et al.,* 1992). When employed in preclinical studies in a syngeneic BMT setting, murine bone marrow cells activated by IL-2 demonstrate graft-versus-leukemia effects and anti-cytomegalovirus activity. These cells retain the ability to reconstitute the hematopoietic system in both normal and leukemic mice, without causing GVHD.

Interleukin-2 immunotherapy has been used after autologous stem cell transplantation for hematologic malignancies in an attempt to decrease disease relapse. The optimal dose, route, and timing of administration of IL-2 are still being determined. In one study comparing i.v. versus s.c. administration of IL-2, significantly less toxicity was seen in the s.c. group despite the induction of higher levels of CD56[+] cells (Lopez-Jimenez *et al.,* 1997). While earlier administration of IL-2 is desirable because of lower tumor burden, hepatic, renal, and pulmonary toxicities make administration of IL-2 soon after stem cell infusion difficult to tolerate and require dose attenuation (Weisdorf *et al.,* 1993). Toxicities seen in early studies include mild to moderate fever, nausea, diarrhea, and skin rash. Blaise and colleagues (1992) reported a high incidence of bacterial infections with intensive IL-2 immunotherapy after autologous BMT.

Late administration of subcutaneous IL-2 has also been investigated starting 2 to 3 months post-autograft. Interleukin-2 produced an approximately two-fold increase in circulating levels of CD56+ cells, markers of the NK cell and cytotoxic T-cell subset of lymphocytes (Lopez-Jimenez et al., 1997).

In a small study IL-2 appeared to induce histologic changes on skin biopsy consistent with GVHD (Massumoto et al., 1996). However, clinical benefit of this approach has not been established. A small randomized trial in patients with acute lymphoblastic leukemia treated with IL-2 following autografting failed to demonstrate a survival advantage (Attal et al., 1995). Similarly no clinical benefit was observed with IL-2 following autografting for breast cancer (Gravis et al., 2000), acute myeloid or acute lymphoid leukemia (Blaise et al., 2000), or a range of pediatric malignancies (Vlk et al., 2000).

Interferon-γ

The immunologic mechanisms underlying antitumor cell-mediated immunity depend on recognition of tumor-specific antigens in the context of MHC antigens on cells. The eradication of residual malignant cells by immunologic mechanisms after allografting (the graft-versus-leukemia effect related to GVHD) may involve similar mechanisms. Interferon-γ (IFN-γ) upregulates expression of MHC class I and class II antigens in a variety of normal and neoplastic tissues (Schwartz et al., 1985). This has led investigators to ask whether an autologous graft-versus-tumor effect may be augmented by the use of interferon-γ following autologous stem cell transplantation. In a phase I study of 36 patients with metastatic breast cancer, the combination of cyclosporine and interferon-γ (0.025 mg/kg/day s.c., days 7–28 posttransplant) resulted in clinical GVHD without delay in hematopoietic recovery (Kennedy et al., 1994, Vogelsang et al., 1999). The combination of IL-2 and interferon-γ to enhance immune responses by recruitment of NK and cytotoxic T cells has been studied following autologous stem cell transplantation in pediatric patients with high-risk acute leukemia (Baumgarten et al., 1994) and in adult patients with lymphoma, leukemia, and solid tumors (Vey et al., 1997). No benefit in relapse-free survival was seen, but significant increases in NK cells in the peripheral blood were observed. Larger clinical trials will be needed to demonstrate a benefit of interferon-γ following autologous transplantation.

Interferon-α

Cytokines have been used to maintain remission following autologous transplantation for non-Hodgkin's lymphoma (NHL), Hodgkin's disease (HD), CML, and multiple myeloma. Besides any direct effect of interferon-α on tumor cell proliferation, there is disputed evidence that immunoregulatory activity by T cells, NK cells, and lymphocyte-activated killer cells in response to interferon-α may play a role in maintenance of remission posttransplant (Uchida et al., 1984; Millar, Bell, & Powles, 1996).

The use of interferon-α following autologous transplantation has been associated with improved survival in patients with multiple myeloma (Cunningham et al., 1998; Bjorkstrand et al., 2001). The Cunningham study randomized 84 patients to receive interferon-α (3×10^6 units 3 times weekly) or no treatment postautograft. Median progression-free survival following stem cell transplantation was 27 months in the control group and 39 months in patients receiving interferon ($P <$ .025). Toxicities were mainly flu-like symptoms, malaise, and rashes. The study by Bjorkstrand et al. (2001) was a retrospective registry-based analysis, in which 473 patients with multiple myeloma receiving IFN maintenance treatment after autologous SCT were compared with 419 patients who did not receive IFN treatment. Patients who were evaluable for response and in complete or partial remission at 6 months posttransplant were eligible, after excluding patients with graft failure. Overall survival (OS) and progression-free survival (PFS) were significantly better in the IFN group. The difference was most strongly pronounced in the partial remission patients. The difference in median survival between the two groups was up to 2.5 years. No assessment of quality of life was performed.

Interferon-α has been used to try to prevent relapse following autografting for patients with relapsed NHL or HD. Published in abstract form, a randomized study of interferon-α2b versus no therapy demonstrated no difference in event-free or overall survival (Bosly et al., 2001). Another study combined IL-2 with interferon-α for patients with malignant lymphoma responding to autologous transplantation (Nagler et al., 1997). Treatment with both cytokines was commenced a median of 4 months posttransplant. Both disease-free and overall survival appeared better than historical controls, although again these results require confirmation in a randomized study.

Long term follow up of CML patients treated with autografting and interferon-α maintenance has shown a ten year survival of 55% with median survival not yet reached (Meloni et al., 2001). These data need to be confirmed in controlled trials comparing this approach with new agents such as imatinib (STI-571).

Conclusions

Such studies as have been done for PBPC transplantation do not provide convincing evidence of a clinical benefit with the routine use of myeloid CSFs post-infusion. There appears to be no current role for TPO or EPO following autografting. Cytokines such as KGF show significant promise in the attenuation of non-hematologic transplant-related toxicity. Much work remains to be done in order to determine the optimal use of immuno-potentiating cytokines to reduce the risk of relapse posttransplant.

References

Advani, R., Chao, N. J., Horning, S. J. et al. (1992). Granulocyte-macrophage colony-stimulating factor (GM-CSF) as an adjunct to autologous hematopoietic stem cell transplantation for lymphoma. *Annals of Internal Medicine*, **116**, 183–9.

Albin, N., Douay, L., Fouillard, L. *et al.* (1994). In vivo effects of GM-CSF and IL-3 on hematopoietic cell recovery in bone marrow and blood after autologous transplantation with mafosfamide-purged marrow in lymphoid malignancies. *Bone Marrow Transplantation*, **14**, 253–9.

Antman, K. S., Griffin, J. D., Elias, A. *et al.* (1988). The effect of recombinant human granulocyte-macrophage colony-stimulating factor (rhGM-CSF) on chemotherapy-induced myelosuppression. *New England Journal of Medicine*, **319**, 593–8.

Attal, M., Blaise, D., Marit, G. *et al.* (1995). Consolidation treatment of acute lymphoblastic leukemia: a prospective, randomized trial comparing allogeneic versus autologous bone marrow transplantation and testing the impact of recombinant interleukin-2 after autologous bone marrow transplantation. *Blood*, **86**, 1619–28.

Ayash, L. J., Elias, A., Hunt, M. *et al.* (1994). Recombinant human erythropoietin for the treatment of the anemia associated with autologous bone marrow transplantation. *British Journal of Haematology*, **87**, 153–61.

Bajaj-Elliott, M., Poulsom, R., Pender, S. L. *et al.* (1998). Interactions between stromal cell derived keratinocyte growth factor and epithelial transforming growth factor in immune-mediated crypt cell hyperplasia. *Journal of Clinical Investigation*, **102**, 1473.

Basser, R. L., Rasko, J.E.J., Clarke, K. *et al.* (1996). Thrombopoietic effects of pegylated recombinant human megakaryocyte growth and development factor (PEG-rhMGDF) in patients with advanced cancer. *Lancet*, **348**, 1279–81.

Basser, R. L., Rasko, J.E.J., Clarke, K. *et al.* (1997). Randomized, blinded, placebo-controlled phase I trial of pegylated recombinant human megakaryocyte growth and development factor with filgrastim after dose-intensive chemotherapy in patients with advanced cancer. *Blood*, **89**, 3118–28.

Baumgarten, E., Schmid, H., Pohl, U. *et al.* (1994). Low-dose natural interleukin-2 and recombinant interferon-gamma following autologous bone marrow grafts in pediatric patients with high-risk acute leukemia. *Leukemia*, **8**, 850–5.

Beguin, Y., Oris, R., & Fillet, G. (1993). Dynamics of erythropoietic recovery following bone marrow transplantation: role of marrow proliferative capacity and erythropoietin production in autologous versus allogeneic transplants. *Bone Marrow Transplantation*, **11**, 285–92.

Bjorkstrand, B., Svensson, H., Goldschmidt, H. *et al.* (2001). Alpha-interferon maintenance treatment is associated with improved survival after high-dose treatment and autologous stem cell transplantation in patients with multiple myeloma: a retrospective registry study from the European Group for Blood and Marrow Transplantation (EBMT). *Bone Marrow Transplantation*, **27**, 369–73.

Blaise, D., Stoppa, A. M., Viens, P. *et al.* (1992). Intensive immunotherapy with recombinant IL-2 after autologous bone marrow transplantation is associated with a high incidence of bacterial infections. *Bone Marrow Transplantation*, **10**, 193–5.

Blaise, D. Attal, M. Reiffers, J. *et al.* (2000). Randomized study of recombinant interleukin-2 after autologous bone marrow transplantation for acute leukemia in first complete remission. *European Cytokine Network*, **11**, 91–8.

Bolwell, B., Goormastic, M., Dannley, R. *et al.* (1997). G-CSF post-autologous progenitor cell transplantation: a randomized study of 5, 10, and 16 micrograms/kg/day. *Bone Marrow Transplantation*, **19**, 215–19.

Bolwell, B., Vredenburgh, J., Overmoyer, B. *et al.* (2000). Phase I study of pegylated recombinant human megakaryocyte growth and development factor (PEG-rHuMGDF) in breast cancer patients after autologous peripheral blood progenitor (PBPC) transplantation. *Bone Marrow Transplantation*, **26**, 141–5.

Bolwell, B. J., Pohlman, B., Andresen, S. *et al.* (1998). Delayed G-CSF after autologous progenitor cell transplantation: a prospective randomized trial. *Bone Marrow Transplantation*, **21**, 369–73.

Bosly, A., Lepage, E., Grigg, A. P. *et al.* (2001). Interferon α2b does not prolong response after intensive therapy and autologous stem cell transplantation for relapsing lymphoma. An international randomised study on 221 patients. American Society of Hematology 43rd Annual Meeting, Orlando; presentation #3579.

Brice, P., Marolleau, J. P., Pautier, P. *et al.* (1996). Hematologic recovery and survival of lymphoma patients after autologous stem-cell transplantation: comparison of bone marrow and peripheral blood progenitor cells. *Leukemia and Lymphoma*, **22**, 449–56.

Brouwer, R. E., Vellenga, E., Zwinderman, K. H. *et al.* (1999). Phase III efficacy study of interleukin-3 after autologous bone marrow transplantation in patients with malignant lymphoma. *British Journal of Haematology*, **106**, 730–6.

Bruno, E. & Hoffman, R. (1989). Effect of interleukin-6 on in vitro human megakaryocytopoiesis: its interactions with other cytokines. *Experimental Hematology*, **17**, 1038–42.

Cahill, R. A., Spitzer, T. R., & Mazumder, A. (1996). Marrow engraftment and clinical manifestations of capillary leak syndrome. *Bone Marrow Transplantation*, **18**, 177–84.

Calderwood, S., Doyle, J. J., Hitzler, J. K. *et al.* (1996). Administration of recombinant human granulocyte-macrophage colony-stimulating factor after autologous bone marrow transplantation in children with acute myelogenous leukemia; a note of caution. *Bone Marrow Transplantation*, **18**, 87–91.

Chao, N. J., Schriber, J. R., Long, G. D. *et al.* (1994). A randomized study of erythropoietin and granulocyte colony-stimulating factor (G-CSF) versus placebo and G-CSF for patients with Hodgkin's and non-Hodgkin's lymphoma undergoing autologous bone marrow transplantation. *Blood*, **83**, 2823–8.

Charak, B. S., Choudhary, G. D., Tefft, M., & Mazumder, A. (1992). Interleukin-2 in bone marrow transplantation: preclinical studies. *Bone Marrow Transplantation*, **10**, 103–11.

Colby, C., McAfee, S. L., Finkelstein, D. M., Spitzer, T. R. (1998). Early vs delayed administration of G-CSF following autologous peripheral blood stem cell transplantation. *Bone Marrow Transplantation*, **21**, 1005–10.

Cortelazzo, S., Viero, P., Bellavita, P. *et al.* (1995). Granulocyte colony-stimulating factor following peripheral-blood progenitor-cell transplant in non-Hodgkin's lymphoma. *Journal of Clinical Oncology*, **13**, 935–41.

Cunningham, D., Powles, R., Malpas, J. *et al.* (1998). A randomized trial of maintenance interferon following high-dose chemotherapy in multiple myeloma: long-term follow-up results. *British Journal of Haematology*, **102**, 495–502.

Devine, S. M., Winton, E. F., Holland, H. K. *et al.* (1994). Simultaneous administration of interleukin 6 (rhIL-6) and Neupogen (rhG-CSF) following autologous bone marrow transplantation (autologous BMT) in patients with poor-prognosis breast cancer. *Blood*, **84**, 343 (Abstract).

Damiani, D., Grimaz, S., Infanti, L. *et al.* (1999). Autologous bone marrow transplantation in non-Hodgkin's lymphoma patients: effect of a brief course of G-CSF on harvest and recovery. *Bone Marrow Transplantation,* **24,** 757–61.

Domenech, J., Linassier, C., Gihana, E. *et al.* (1995). Prolonged impairment of hematopoiesis after high-dose therapy followed by autologous bone marrow transplantation. *Blood,* **85,** 3320–7.

Drouet, M., Herodin, F., Norol, F. *et al.* (2001). Cell cycle activation of peripheral blood stem and progenitor cells expanded ex vivo with SCF, FLT-3 ligand, TPO and IL-3 results in accelerated granulocyte recovery in a baboon model of autologous transplantation but G0/G1 and S/G2/M graft cell content does not correlate with transplantability. *Stem Cells,* **19,** 436–42.

Du, X. X., Neben, T., Goldman, S., & Williams, D. A. (1993). Effects of recombinant human interleukin-11 on hematopoietic reconstitution in transplant mice: acceleration of recovery of peripheral blood neutrophils and platelets. *Blood,* **81,** 27–34.

Egger, B., Procaccino, F., Lakshmanan, J. *et al.* (1997). Mice lacking transforming growth factor alpha have an increased susceptibility to dextran sulfate-induced colitis. *Gastroenterology,* **113,** 825.

Elkordy, M., Crump, M., Vredenburgh, J. J. *et al.* (1997). A phase 1 trial of recombinant human interleukin-1β (OCT-43) following high-dose chemotherapy and autologous bone marrow transplantation. *Bone Marrow Transplantation,* **19,** 315–22.

Farrell, C. L., Bready, J. V., Rex, K. L. *et al.* (1998). Keratinocyte growth factor protects mice from chemotherapy and radiation-induced gastrointestinal injury and mortality. *Cancer Research,* **58,** 933–9.

Faucher, C., Le Corroller, A. G., Chabannon, C. *et al.* (1996). Administration of G-CSF can be delayed after transplantation of autologous G-CSF-primed blood stem cells: a randomized study. *Bone Marrow Transplantation,* **17,** 533–6.

Fay, J. W., Lazarus, H., Herzig, R. *et al.* (1994). Sequential administration of recombinant human interleukin 3 and granulocyte-macrophage colony-stimulating factor after autologous bone marrow transplantation for malignant lymphoma: a phase I/II multicenter study. *Blood,* **1,** 2151–7.

Fibbe, W. E., Raemakers, J., Verdonck, L. F. *et al.* (1991). Recombinant human interleukin 3 after bone marrow transplantation for malignant lymphoma: a phase I/II study. *Blood,* **78** (Suppl 1), 163a (Abstract).

Fields, K. K., Crump, M., Bence-Bruckler, I. *et al.* (2000). Use of PEG-rHuMGDF in platelet engraftment after autologous stem cell transplantation. *Bone Marrow Transplantation,* **26,** 1083–8.

Finch, P. W., Rubin, J. S., Miki, T. *et al.* (1989). Human KGF is FGF-related with properties of a paracrine effector of epithelial cell growth. *Science,* **245,** 752–5.

Gisselbrecht, C., Prentice, H. G., Bacigalupo, A. *et al.* (1994). Placebo-controlled phase III trial of lenograstim in bone-marrow transplantation. *Lancet,* **343,** 696–700.

Gorin, N. C., Coiffier, B., Hayat, M. *et al.* (1992). Recombinant human granulocyte-macrophage colony-stimulating factor after high dose chemotherapy and autologous bone marrow transplantation with unpurged and purged marrow in non-Hodgkin's lymphoma: a randomized double-blind placebo-controlled study. *Blood,* **80,** 1149–57.

Gravis, G., Viens, P., Vey, N. *et al.* (2000). Pilot study of immunotherapy with interleukin-2 after autologous stem cell transplantation in advanced breast cancers. *Anticancer Research,* **20,** 3987–91.

Greenberg, P., Advani, R., Keating, A. *et al.* (1996). GM-CSF accelerates neutrophil recovery after autologous hematopoietic stem cell transplantation. *Bone Marrow Transplantation,* **18,** 1057–64.

Gribben, J. G., Freedman, A. S., Woo, S. D. *et al.* (1991). All advanced stage non-Hodgkin's lymphomas with a polymerase chain reaction-amplification breakpoint of bcl-2 have residual cells containing the bcl-2 rearrangement at evaluation and after treatment. *Blood,* **78,** 3275–80.

Grigg, A. P., Roberts, A. W., Raunow, H. *et al.* (1995). Optimizing dose and scheduling of filgrastim (granulocyte-colony-stimulating factor) for mobilizing and collection of peripheral blood progenitor cells in normal volunteers. *Blood,* **86,** 4437–45.

Gulati, S. C. & Bennett, C. L. (1992). Granulocyte-macrophage colony-stimulating factor (GM-CSF) as adjunct therapy in relapsed Hodgkin disease. *Annals of Internal Medicine,* **116,** 177–82.

Higuchi, C. M., Thompson, J. A., Petersen, F. B. *et al.* (1991). Toxicity and immunomodulatory effects of interleukin-2 after autologous bone marrow transplantation for hematologic malignancies. *Blood,* **77,** 2561–8.

Hornedo, J., Sola, C., Solano, C. *et al.* (2002). The role of granulocyte colony-stimulating factor (G-CSF) in the posttransplant period. *Bone Marrow Transplantation,* **29,** 737–43.

Housley, R. M., Morris, C. F., Boyle, W. *et al.* (1994). Keratinocyte growth factor induces proliferation of hepatocytes and epithelial cells throughout the rat gastrointestinal tract. *Journal of Clinical Investigation,* **94,** 1764–77.

Ireland, R. M., Atkinson, K., Concannon, A. *et al.* (1990). Serum erythropoietin changes in autologous and allogeneic bone marrow transplant patients. *British Journal of Haematology,* **76,** 128–34.

Kabaya, K., Shibuya, K., Torii, Y. *et al.* (1996). Improvement of thrombocytopenia following bone marrow transplantation by pegylated recombinant human megakaryocyte growth and development factor in mice. *Bone Marrow Transplantation,* **18,** 1035–41.

Kawano, Y., Takaue, Y., Mimaya, J. *et al.* (1998). Marginal benefit/disadvantage of granulocyte colony-stimulating factor therapy after autologous blood stem cell transplantation in children: results of a prospective randomized trial. The Japanese Cooperative Study Group of PBSCT. *Blood,* **92,** 4040–6.

Kennedy, M. J., Davis, J., Passos-Coelho, J. *et al.* (1993a). Administration of human recombinant granulocyte colony-stimulating factor (filgrastim) accelerates granulocyte recovery following high-dose chemotherapy and autologous marrow transplantation with 4-hydroperoxycyclophosphamide-purged marrow in women with metastatic breast cancer. *Cancer Research,* **53,** 5424–8.

Kennedy, M. J., Vogelsang, G. B., Beveridge, R. A. *et al.* (1993b). Phase I trial of intravenous cyclosporine to induce graft-versus-host disease in women undergoing autologous bone marrow transplantation for breast cancer. *Journal of Clinical Oncology,* **11,** 478–84.

Kennedy, M. J., Vogelsang, G. B., Jones, R. J. *et al.* (1994). Phase I trial of interferon gamma to potentiate cyclosporine-induced graft-versus-host disease in women undergoing autologous bone marrow transplantation for breast cancer. *Journal of Clinical Oncology*, **12**, 249–57.

Khwaja, A., Linch, D. C., Goldstone, A. H. *et al.* (1992). Recombinant human granulocyte-macrophage colony stimulating factor after autologous bone marrow transplantation for malignant lymphoma: a British National Lymphoma Investigation double-blind placebo-controlled trial. *British Journal of Haematology*, **82**, 317–23.

Khwaja, A., Mills, W., Leveridge, K. *et al.* (1993). Efficacy of delayed granulocyte colony-stimulating factor after autologous BMT. *Bone Marrow Transplantation*, **11**, 479–82.

Klaesson, S. (1999). Clinical use of rHuEPO in bone marrow transplantation. *Medical Oncology*, **16**, 2–7.

Klaesson, S., Ringden, O., Ljungman, P. *et al.* (1994). Treatment with erythropoietin after allogeneic bone marrow transplantation: a randomized, double-blind study. *Transplantation Proceedings*, **26**, 1827–8.

Klumpp, T. R., Mangan, K. F., Goldberg, S. L. *et al.* (1995). Granulocyte colony-stimulating factor accelerates neutrophil engraftment following peripheral-blood stem-cell transplantation: a prospective, randomized trial. *Journal of Clinical Oncology*, **13**, 1323–7.

Lacey, D., Whitcomb, L., Farrell, C. *et al.* (1996). Keratinocyte growth factor promotes the survival of mice transplanted with syngeneic bone marrow or G-CSF-mobilized peripheral stem cells following lethal irradiation. *Blood*, **88**, 593a (Abstract).

Lazarus, H. M., Wintom, E. F., Williams, S. F. *et al.* (1995). Phase I multicenter trial of interleukin 6 therapy after autologous bone marrow transplantation in advanced breast cancer. *Bone Marrow Transplantation*, **15**, 935–42.

Lee, C.-K., Gingrich, R. D., Hohl, R. J., & Ajram, K. A. (1995). Engraftment syndrome in autologous bone marrow and peripheral stem cell transplantation. *Bone Marrow Transplantation*, **16**, 175–82.

Legros, M., Fleury, J., Bay, J. O. *et al.* (1997). rhGM-CSF versus placebo following rhGM-CSF-mobilized PBPC transplantation: a phase III double-blind randomized trial. *Bone Marrow Transplantation*, **19**, 209–13.

Lemoli, R. M., Rosti, G., Visani, G. *et al.* (1996). Concomitant and sequential administration of recombinant human granulocyte colony stimulating factor and recombinant interleukin-3 to accelerate hematopoietic recovery after bone marrow transplantation for malignant lymphoma. *Blood*, **14**, 3018–25.

Li, I., Yang, C., Xia, Y. *et al.* (2001). Thrombocytopenia caused by the development of antibodies to thrombopoietin. *Blood*, **98**, 3241–8.

Lieschke, G. J., Cebon, J., & Morstyn, G. (1989). Characterization of the clinical effects after the first dose of bacterially synthesized recombinant human granulocyte-macrophage colony-stimulating factor. *Blood*, **74**, 2634–43.

Linch, D. C., Milligan, D. W., Winfield, D. A. *et al.* (1997). G-CSF after peripheral blood stem cell transplantation in lymphoma patients significantly accelerated neutrophil recovery and shortened time in hospital: results of a randomized BNLI trial. *British Journal of Haematology*, **99**, 933–8.

Linch, D. C., Scarffe, H., Proctor, S. *et al.* (1993). Randomized vehicle-controlled dose-finding study of glycosylated recombinant human granulocyte colony-stimulating factor after bone marrow transplantation. *Bone Marrow Transplantation*, **11**, 307–11.

Link, H., Boogaerts, M. A., Carella, M. A. *et al.* (1992). A controlled trial of recombinant human granulocyte-macrophage colony-stimulating factor after total body irradiation, high-dose chemotherapy and autologous bone marrow transplantation for acute lymphoblastic leukemia or malignant lymphoma. *Blood*, **80**, 2188–95.

Link, H., Boogaerts, M. A., Fauser, A. A. *et al.* (1994). A controlled trial of recombinant human erythropoietin after bone marrow transplantation. *Blood*, **84**, 3327–35.

Locatelli, F., Zecca, M., Pedrazzoli, P. *et al.* (1994). Use of recombinant human erythropoietin after bone marrow transplantation in pediatric patients with acute leukemia: effect on erythroid repopulation in autologous versus allogeneic transplants. *Bone Marrow Transplantation*, **13**, 403–10.

Lok, S., Kaushansky, K., Holly, R. D. *et al.* (1994). Cloning and expression of murine thrombopoietin cDNA and stimulation of platelet production in vivo. *Nature*, **369**, 565–8.

Lopez-Jimenez, J., Perez-Oteyza, J., Munoz, A. *et al.* (1997). Subcutaneous versus intravenous low-dose IL-2 therapy after autologous transplantation: results of a prospective, non-randomized study. *Bone Marrow Transplantation*, **19**, 429–34.

Massumoto, C., Benyunes, M. C., Sale, G. *et al.* (1996). Close simulation of acute graft-versus-host disease by interleukin-2 administered after autologous bone marrow transplantation for hematologic malignancy. *Bone Marrow Transplantation*, **17**, 351–6.

McQuaker, I. G., Hunter, A. E., Pacey, S. *et al.* (1997). Low-dose filgrastim significantly enhances neutrophil recovery following autologous peripheral blood stem-cell transplantation in patients with lymphoproliferative disorders: evidence for clinical and economic benefit. *Journal of Clinical Oncology*, **15**, 451–7.

Mehta, J., Powles, R., Singhal, S. *et al.* (1996). Transfusion requirements after bone marrow transplantation from HLA-identical siblings: effects of donor-recipient ABO incompatibility. *Bone Marrow Transplantation*, **18**, 51–6.

Meloni, G., Capria, S., Vignetti, M. *et al.* (2001). Ten-year follow-up of a single center prospective trial of unmanipulated peripheral blood stem cell autograft and interferon-alpha in early phase chronic myeloyd leukemia. *Haematologica*, **86**, 596–601.

Metcalf, D. (1989). Hematopoietic growth factors 1. *Lancet*, **1**, 825–7.

Millar, B. C., Bell, J. B., & Powles, R. L. (1996). Lymphocyte recovery and clinical response in multiple myeloma patients receiving interferon alpha 2 beta after intensive therapy. *British Journal of Cancer*, **73**, 236–40.

Miller, L. L. Korn, E. L. Stevens, D. S. *et al.* (1999). Abrogation of the hematological and bilogical activities of the interleukin-3/granulocyte-macrophage colony-stimulating factor fusion protein PIXY321 by neutralizing anti-PIXY321 antibodies in cancer patients receiving high-dose carboplatin. *Blood*, **93**, 3250–8.

Mitus, A. J., Antin, J. H., Rutherford, C. J. *et al.* (1994). Use of recombinant human erythropoietin in allogeneic bone marrow transplant donor/recipient pairs. *Blood*, **83**, 1952–7.

Mobest, D., Mertelsmann, R., & Henschler, R. (1998). Serum-free ex vivo expansion of CD34(+) hematopoietic progenitor cells. *Biotechnology & Bioengineering*, **60**, 341–7.

Molineux, G., Hartley, C., McElroy, P. *et al.* (1996a). Megakaryocyte growth and development factor accelerates platelet recovery in peripheral blood progenitor cell transplant recipients. *Blood,* **88,** 366–76.

Molineux, G., Hartley, C. A., McElroy, P. *et al.* (1996b). Megakaryocyte growth and development factor stimulates enhanced platelet recovery in mice after bone marrow transplantation. *Blood,* **88,** 1509–14.

Nagler, A., Ackerstein, A., Or, R. *et al.* (1997). Immunotherapy with recombinant human interleukin-2 and recombinant interferon-alpha in lymphoma patients post autologous marrow or stem cell transplantation. *Blood,* **89,** 3951–9.

Negrin, R. S. & Pesando, J. (1994). Detection of tumor cells in purged bone marrow and peripheral-blood mononuclear cells by polymerase chain reaction amplification of bcl-2 translocations. *Journal of Clinical Oncology,* **12,** 1021–7.

Nemunaitis, J., Appelbaum, F. R., Lilleby, K. *et al.* (1994). Phase I study of recombinant interleukin-1 beta in patients undergoing autologous bone marrow transplant for acute myelogenous leukemia. *Blood,* **83,** 3473–9.

Nemunaitis, J., Appelbaum, F. R., Singer, J. W. *et al.* (1993). Phase I trial with recombinant human interleukin-3 in patients with lymphoma undergoing autologous bone marrow transplantation. *Blood,* **82,** 3273–8.

Nemunaitis, J., Rabinowe, S. N., Singer, J. W. *et al.* (1991). Recombinant granulocyte-macrophage colony-stimulating factor after autologous bone marrow transplantation for lymphoid cancer. *New England Journal of Medicine,* **324,** 1773–8.

Nemunaitis, J., Singer, J., Buckner, C. *et al.* (1990). Use of recombinant human granulocyte-macrophage colony-stimulating factor in graft failure after bone marrow transplantation. *Blood,* **76,** 245–53.

Oh-eda, M., Hasegawa, M., Hattori, K. *et al.* (1990). O-Linked sugar chain of human granulocyte colony stimulating factor protects it against polymerization and denaturation allowing it to retain its biological activity. *Journal of Biological Chemistry,* **265,** 11432–5.

Ojeda, E., Garcia-Bustos, J., Aguado, M. J. *et al.* (1999). Is filgrastim as useless after peripheral blood stem cell transplantation for adults as it could be for children? *Blood,* **93,** 3565–70.

Ozer, H., Armitage, J. O., Bennett, C. L. *et al.* (2000). 2000 update of recommendations for the use of hematopoietic colony-stimulating factors: evidence-based, clinical practice guidelines. American Society of Clinical Oncology Growth Factors Expert Panel. *Journal of Clinical Oncology,* **18,** 3558–85.

Pierelli, L., Menichella, G., Foddai, M. L. *et al.* (1996a). The administration of growth factors post-PBPC transplantation abrogates the dose-effect of CFU-GM on the rate of PMN recovery. *Bone Marrow Transplantation,* **17,** 1189–90.

Pierelli, L., Scambia, G., Menichella, A. *et al.* (1996b). The combination of erythropoietin and granulocyte colony-stimulating factor increases the rate of haemopoietic recovery with clinical recovery after peripheral blood progenitor cell transplantation. *British Journal of Haematology,* **92,** 287–94.

Rabinowe, S. N., Neuberg, D., Bierman, P. J. *et al.* (1993). Long-term follow-up of a phase III study of recombinant human granulocyte-macrophage colony-stimulating factor after autologous bone marrow transplantation for lymphoid malignancies. *Blood,* **81,** 1903–8.

Recchia, F., Accorsi, P., Bonfini, T. *et al.* (2000). Randomised trial of sequential administration of G-CSF and GM-CSF vs G-CSF alone following peripheral blood progenitor cell autograft in solid tumors. *Journal of Interferon and Cytokine Research,* **20,** 171–7.

Schmitz, N., Dreger, P., Zander, A. R. *et al.* (1995). Results of a randomized, controlled, multicenter study of recombinant human granulocyte colony-stimulating factor (filgrastim) in patients with Hodgkin's disease and non-Hodgkin's lymphoma undergoing autologous bone marrow transplantation. *Bone Marrow Transplantation,* **15,** 261–6.

Schmitz, N., Linch, D. C., Dreger, P. *et al.* (1996). Randomized trial of filgrastim-mobilized peripheral blood progenitor cell transplantation versus autologous bone-marrow transplantation in lymphoma patients. *Lancet,* **347,** 353–7.

Schriber, J. R., Negrin, R. S., Chao, N. J. *et al.* (1993). The efficacy of granulocyte colony-stimulating factor following autologous bone marrow transplantation for non-Hodgkin's lymphoma with monoclonal antibody purged bone marrow. *Leukemia,* **7,** 1491–5.

Schwartz, R., Momburg, F., Moldenhauer, G. *et al.* (1985). Induction of HLA class-II antigen expression on human carcinoma cell lines by IFN-gamma. *International Journal of Cancer,* **35,** 245–50.

Sheridan, W. P., Morstyn, G., Woolf, M. *et al.* (1989). Granulocyte colony-stimulating factor (G-CSF) and neutrophil recovery following high-dose chemotherapy and autologous bone marrow transplantation. *Lancet,* **2,** 891–5.

Shimazaki, C., Inaba, T., Uchiyama, H. *et al.* (1997). Serum thrombopoietin levels in patients undergoing autologous peripheral blood progenitor cell transplantation. *Bone Marrow Transplantation,* **19,** 771–5.

Spitzer, G., Adkins, D. R., Spencer, V. *et al.* (1994). Randomized study of growth factors post-peripheral-blood stem cell transplant: neutrophil recovery is associated with modest clinical benefit. *Journal of Clinical Oncology,* **12,** 661–70.

Stahel, R. A., Jost, L. M., Cerny, T. *et al.* (1994). Randomized study of recombinant human granulocyte colony-stimulating factor after high-dose chemotherapy and autologous bone marrow transplantation for high-risk lymphoid malignancies. *Journal of Clinical Oncology,* **12,** 1931–8.

Stahel, R. A., Jost, L. M., Honegger, H. *et al.* (1997). Randomized trial showing equivalent efficacy of filgrastim 5 μg/kg/d and 10 μg/kg/d following high-dose chemotherapy and autologous bone marrow transplantation for high-risk lymphomas. *Journal of Clinical Oncology,* **15,** 1730–5.

Stiff, P. (2001). Mucositis associated with stem cell transplantation: current status and innovative approaches to management. *Bone Marrow Transplantation,* **27,** S3–S11.

Stiff, P., Chen, B., Franklin, W. *et al.* (2000). Autologous transplantation of ex vivo expanded bone marrow cells grown from small aliquots after high-dose chemotherapy for breast cancer. *Blood,* **95,** 2169–74.

Torres Gomez, A., Jimenez, M. A., Alvarez, M. A. *et al.* (1995). Optimal timing of granulocyte colony-stimulating factor (G-CSF) administration after bone marrow transplantation. A prospective randomized study. *Annals of Hematology,* **71,** 65–70.

Uchida, A., Yanagawa, E., Kokoschka, E. M. *et al.* (1984). In vitro modulation of human natural killer cell activity by interferon: generation of adherent suppressor cells. *British Journal of Cancer,* **50,** 483–92.

Ulich, T. R., del Castillo, J., Senaldi, G. *et al.* (1996). Systemic hematologic effects of PEG-rHuMGDF-induced megakaryocyte hyperplasia in mice. *Blood,* **87,** 5006–15.

van den Oudenrijn, S., de Haas, M., Calafat, J. *et al.* (1999). A combination of megakaryocyte growth and development factor and interleukin-1 is sufficient to culture large numbers of megakaryocytic progenitors and megakaryocytes for transfusion purposes. *British Journal of Haematology,* **106,** 553–63.

Vanucchi, A. M., Bosi, A., Leri, A. *et al.* (1996). Combination therapy with G-CSF and erythropoietin after autologous bone marrow transplantation for lymphoid malignancies: a randomized trial. *Bone Marrow Transplantation,* **17,** 527–31.

Vey, N., Molnar, S., Faucher, C. *et al.* (1994). Delayed administration of granulocyte colony-stimulating factor after autologous bone marrow transplantation: effect on granulocyte recovery. *Bone Marrow Transplantation,* **14,** 779–82.

Vey, N., Viens, P., Fossat, C., *et al.* (1997). Clinical and biological effects of gamma interferon and the combination of gamma interferon and interleukin-2 after autologous bone marrow transplantation. *European Cytokine Network,* **8,** 389–94.

Vlk, V., Eckschlager, T., Kavan, P. *et al.* (2000). Clinical ineffectiveness of IL-2 and/or IFN alpha administration after autologous PBSC transplantation in pediatric oncological patients. *Pediatric Hematology & Oncology,* **17,** 31–44.

Vogelsang, G., Bitton, R., Piantadosi, S., *et al.* (1999). Immune modulation in autologous bone marrow transplantation: cyclosporine and gamma-interferon trial. *Bone Marrow Transplantation,* **24,** 637–40.

Vose, J. M., Anderson, J. E., Bierman, P. J. *et al.* (1997). Granulocyte-macrophage colony-stimulating factor/interleukin-3 fusion protein versus granulocyte-macrophage colony-stimulating factor after autologous bone marrow transplantation for non-Hodgkin's lymphoma: results of a randomized double-blind trial. *Journal of Clinical Oncology,* **15,** 1617–23.

Vredenburgh, J. J., Hussein, A., Fisher, D. *et al.* (1998). A randomized trial of recombinant human interleukin-11 following autologous bone marrow transplantation with peripheral blood progenitor cell support in patients with breast cancer. *Biology of Blood and Marrow Transplantation,* **4,** 134–41.

Weisdorf, D., Katsanis, E., Verfaillie, C. *et al.* (1994). Interleukin-1 alpha administered after autologous transplantation: a phase I/II clinical trial. *Blood,* **15,** 2044–9.

Weisdorf, D. J., Anderson, P. M., Blazar, B. R. *et al.* (1993). Interleukin-2 immediately after autologous bone marrow transplantation for acute lymphoblastic leukemia—a phase I study. *Transplantation,* **55,** 61–6.

Weisdorf, D. J., Verfaillie, C. M., Davies, S. M. *et al.* (1995). Hematopoietic growth factors for graft failure after bone marrow transplantation: a randomized trial of granulocyte-macrophage-colony-stimulating factor (GM-CSF) versus sequential GM-CSF plus granulocyte CSF. *Blood,* **85,** 3452–6.

White, K. & Cebon, J. (1995). Transient hypoxemia during neutrophil recovery in febrile patients. *Lancet,* **345,** 1022–4.

Williams, D. E., Park, L. S., & Broxmeyer, H. E. (1991). Hybrid cytokines as hematopoietic growth factors. *International Journal of Cell Cloning,* **9,** 542–7.

Wolff, S. N., Herzig, R.Lynch, J. *et al.* (2001). Recombinant human thrombopoietin (rhTPO) after autologous bone marrow transplantation: a phase I pharmacokinetic and pharmacodynamic study. *Bone Marrow Transplantation,* **27,** 261–8.

Young, J. C., Bruno, E., Luens, K. M. *et al.* (1996). Thrombopoietin stimulates megakaryococytopoiesis, myelopoiesis, and expansion of CD34+ progenitor cells from single CD34+Thy–1+ Lin-primitive progenitor cells. *Blood,* **88,** 1619–31.

Zeeh, J. M., Procaccino, F., Hoffmann, P. *et al.* (1996). Keratinocyte growth factor ameliorates mucosal injury in an experimental model of colitis in rats. *Gastroenterology,* **110,** 1077–83.

32 Use of hematopoietic growth factors following allogeneic hematopoietic stem cell transplantation

DAVID S. RITCHIE AND ANDREW GRIGG

Royal Melbourne Hospital, Melbourne, Australia.

Introduction

The three key components of mammalian hematopoiesis are hematopoietic stem cells (HSC), marrow stromal cells, and hematopoietic growth factors (HGFs). Mature blood cells derived from stem and progenitor cells represent the end stage of an orderly process of proliferation, differentiation, and maturation in the marrow and eventual export to the periphery. Cell production is of the order of 4×10^{11} cells per day in a normal adult human and is boosted considerably when demand is increased. To date at least 18 molecularly cloned proteins have been identified that have a stimulatory effect on human hematopoiesis (Chapter 3). Those shown to elevate the circulating neutrophil count, platelet count, or red cell mass are shown in Table 32.1. A number of proteins have also been identified that have an inhibitory effect on human hematopoiesis (Table 32.2). This complex, integrated cytokine network is the homeostatic mechanism for the production of effector blood cells. The identified glycosylated polypeptides with a demonstrated role in hematopoiesis are granulocyte-macrophage colony-stimulating factor (GM-CSF), granulocyte colony-stimulating factor (G-CSF), macrophage colony-stimulating factor (M-CSF), interleukin-3 (IL-3), and thrombopoietin (TPO), otherwise known as megakaryocyte growth and development factor (MGDF).

There is considerable overlap in the target cells of different hematopoietic growth factors (Fig. 32.1). Growth factors are produced by marrow stromal cells (particularly macrophages, endothelial cells, and fibroblasts), by activated T cells, and in the case of erythropoietin and thrombopoietin, by kidney parenchymal cells and liver cells (Shimada *et al.*, 1995; Sungaran, Markovic, & Chong, 1997), respectively (Fig. 32.2). Growth factors can be identified in almost all tissues in the body, perhaps related to their role in inducing functional maturation in differentiated cells. Local production is particularly important in the marrow where the discrete regulatory microenvironment determines the fate of primitive hematopoietic cells (Metcalf, 1988). It has also been suggested that hematopoietic stem cells may retain the ability to differentiate into a number of mature cell types (demonstrating plasticity) under the influence of a range of growth factors. This area of research remains one of intense activity and debate (reviewed by Orkin & Zon, 2002, and see Chapter 7), and although outside the scope of this chapter, represents a potentially revolutionary application of autologous and allogeneic hematopoietic stem cells in a therapeutic setting.

Table 32.1. *Effect of hematopoietic growth factors on circulating blood cells*

Cytokine	Elevated neutrophil count	Elevated platelet count	Increased red cell production
G-CSF	+	−	−
M-CSF	+	−	−
GM-CSF	+	−	−
IL-1	+	+	−
IL-3	+	+	−
IL-4	+	−	−
IL-5	+ (Eos)	−	−
IL-6	+	+	?
IL-7	−	+	−
IL-11	−	+	−
EPO	−	−	+
TPO	−	+	−
SCF	+	+	−

Abbreviations: CSF, colony-stimulating factor; G, granulocyte; M, macrophage; TPO, thrombopoietin; IL, interleukin; EPO, erythropoietin; LIF, leukemia inhibitory factor; SCF, stem cell factor; Eos, eosinophils

Table 32.2. *Proteins with inhibitory activity on human hematopoiesis*

Alpha-interferon (α-IFN)
Tumor necrosis factor (TNF)
Transforming growth factor-β (TGF-β)
Macrophage inflammatory protein (MIP)
Interleukin-2 (IL-2)

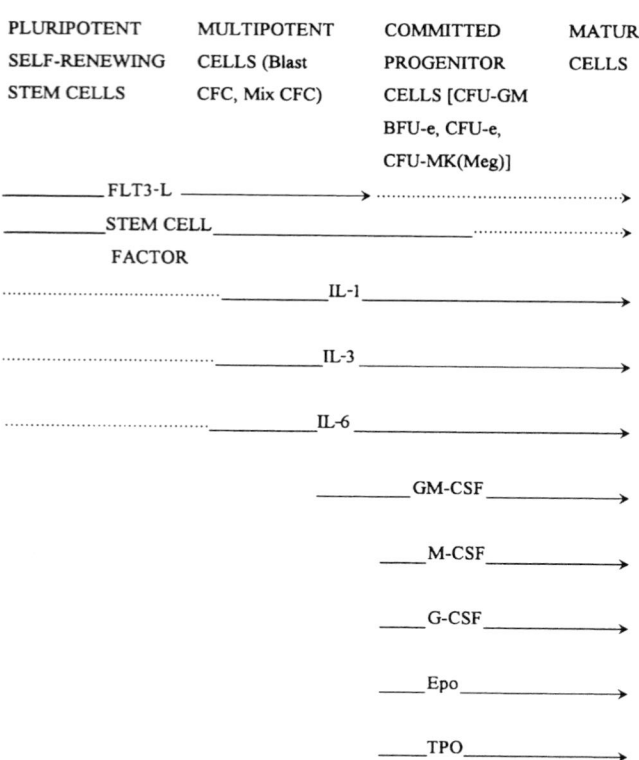

PLURIPOTENT	MULTIPOTENT	COMMITTED	MATURE
SELF-RENEWING	CELLS (Blast	PROGENITOR	CELLS
STEM CELLS	CFC, Mix CFC)	CELLS [CFU-GM	
		BFU-e, CFU-e,	
		CFU-MK(Meg)]	

Fig. 32.1. Target cells for hematopoietic growth factors acting alone. Adapted, with permission, from Testa and Dexter (1991).

The actual and potential uses of HGFs in HSC transplantation are shown in Table 32.3. To date most clinical activity has concentrated on accelerating hematopoietic recovery posttransplant by direct in vivo administration of HGFs. Prior to the introduction into the clinic of HGFs, there were concerns that recipient leukemic cells still viable after the pretransplant conditioning regimen would be stimulated by the administration of growth factors for which they carried cell surface receptors (for example, GM-CSF), thus leading to early recurrence of the leukemia posttransplant.

Animal models of acceleration of hematopoiesis posttransplant

In mice given T-replete allogeneic marrow and spleen HSC transplants, a number of different HGFs have been shown to accelerate recovery of neutrophils posttransplant (Atkinson *et al.*, 1991a). These include G-CSF, GM-CSF, IL-1, IL-3, IL-4, and IL-6. The effect of IL-6 on myeloid proliferation may be indirect, and induced by the upregulation of stem cell factor and flt-3-L (Peters *et al.*, 2001). In mice given T-depleted allogeneic transplants, several factors have been shown to improve survival including G-CSF, GM-CSF, and interleukin-1 (Blazar, Taylor, & Vallera, 1992). G-CSF has been shown to accelerate neutrophil recovery in dogs given total body irradiation and DLA-identical littermate marrow (Schuening *et al.*, 1990), and GM-CSF likewise after autologous marrow transplantation in primates (Nienhuis *et al.*, 1987). TPO has been shown to

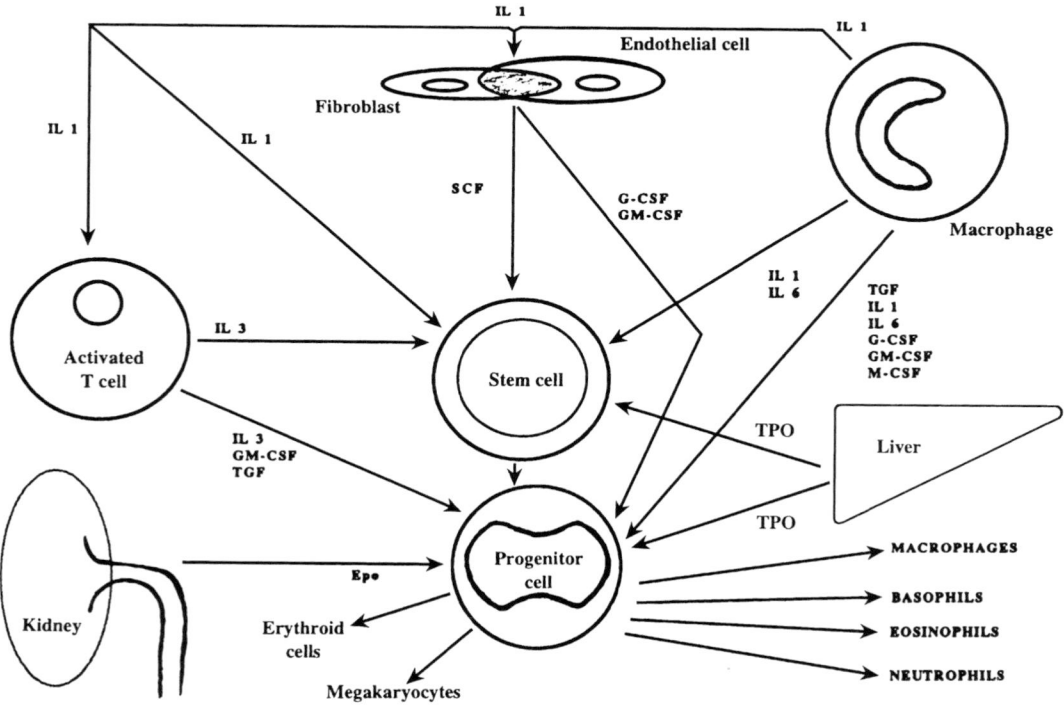

Fig. 32.2. The interaction of hematopoietic stem cells, marrow stromal cells, T cells, parenchymal cells (liver and kidney), and hematopoietic growth factors in human hematopoiesis. Adapted, with permission, from Testa and Dexter (1991).

Table 32.3. *Possible utilization of cytokines in hematopoietic stem cell transplantation*

1. Acceleration of hematopoiesis
   In vivo administration to recipient[a]
   In vivo mobilization of stem/progenitor cells for transplantation[b]
   Ex vivo expansion of stem/progenitor cells for transplantation[c]
2. Prevention/treatment of graft-versus-host disease (by cytokine or cytokine antagonists)[d]
3. Eradication of leukemic cells administration posttransplant[e]

[a] See Chapter 31 and this Chapter.
[b] See Chapter 24.
[c] See Chapter 110.
[d] See Chapter 71.
[e] See Chapters 31, 65 and this chapter.

enhance platelet recovery after murine bone marrow transplantation (Molineux *et al.,* 1996).

Use of HGFs to accelerate hematopoiesis after allogeneic HSC transplantation

The first CSF used to promote hematopoiesis after human allogeneic marrow transplantation was urinary CSF, a purified form of M-CSF (Masaoka *et al.,* 1988, 1990) (Table 32.4). M-CSF was administered from 1 day posttransplant to day 14 posttransplant. Lymphocytes, followed by monocytes and then neutrophils increased, and in a double-blind controlled study, the recovery of neutrophils was significantly faster than in the placebo arm (Masaoka *et al.,* 1990). M-CSF recipients in this study survived significantly better than placebo recipients due to a reduction in fatal GVHD, hemorrhage, and failure of engraftment. Furthermore, the leukemia relapse rate (including that in patients transplanted for leukemia with a monocytic component), was not increased by the administration of M-CSF. Side effects of M-CSF were slight and transient.

G-CSF (Table 32.5)

G-CSF induces more rapid neutrophil recovery and a greater reduction in the number of febrile days than M-CSF after allogeneic bone marrow transplantation. A typical hematological response seen with G-CSF following BMT is shown in Figure 32.3 (Masaoka *et al.,* 1989). The enhancement of neutrophil recovery, reduction in the number of febrile days, and/or reduction in duration of hospitalization has subsequently been reproduced in a number of studies where G-CSF has been used after sibling allogeneic BMT (Gisselbrecht *et al.,* 1994; Hiraoka *et al.,* 1994; Lickliter *et al.,* 1994; Schriber *et al.,* 1994; Martin-Algarra *et al.,* 1995). In at least one study, a significant cost saving (through reduction in antibiotic days and total days of admission and readmission to day 50) was obtained by the use

of G-CSF from day +1 (Lee *et al.,* 1998). No increase in GVHD or early mortality has been identified in the majority of studies to date of HLA-matched sibling bone marrow allografts. One small randomized study, however, revealed higher transplant-related mortality by day 100 (in part due severe hepatic veno-occlusive disease) in recipients of G-CSF from day zero as compared to those receiving G-CSF from day 6 (Lee *et al.,* 1999). No differences were observed between the two treatment schedules in the speed of neutrophil recovery.

In the unrelated marrow transplant setting, the use of G-CSF posttransplant also results in faster neutrophil recovery. However, no reduction in infective episodes or duration of hospitalization has been observed, in part due to higher rates of acute GVHD compared to patients receiving no growth factor therapy (Berger *et al.,* 1999). Rapid neutrophil recovery by day 16 has also been confirmed with the use of filgrastim from day 10 following HLA-matched unrelated donor transplants, with no difference between filgrastim started at day 0 or day 5 posttransplant (Hagglund *et al.,* 1998).

The impact of G-CSF following allogeneic peripheral blood progenitor cell transplantation is more complex, since G-CSF-mobilized allogeneic peripheral blood stem cell (PBSC) are clearly associated with faster rates of neutrophil and platelet recovery as compared to those with steady state marrow (Hagglund *et al.,* 1998; Schmitz *et al.,* 1998; Lickliter *et al.,* 2000). In addition to the faster rate of recovery with the use of PBSC, two controlled, randomized trials of filgrastim after HLA-identical related PBSC transplantation (both with methotrexate as part of the GVHD prophylaxis) have shown a significantly shorter time to achieve an absolute neutrophil count of $>0.5 \times 10^9/l$ in the filgrastim arm, but no difference in time to a platelet count of $20 \times 10^9/l$, red blood cell transfusion independence, the incidence of acute GVHD or 100 day mortality (Fig. 32.4) (Bishop *et al.,* 2000a; Przepiorka *et al.,* 2001). In the latter study the time to a neutrophil count of $0.5 \times 10^9/l$ was 12 days for the group receiving filgrastim versus 15 days for those receiving no growth factor posttransplant ($P = .002$). Despite the more rapid neutrophil recovery in patients treated with G-CSF, no significant cost saving has been demonstrated (Stinson *et al.,* 2000).

A cautionary note has been sounded regarding the impact of high numbers ($>8 \times 10^6$/kg) of mobilized allogeneic CD34[+] stem cells and the risk of inducing acute (Przepiorka *et al.,* 1999) or extensive chronic GVHD (Zaucha *et al.,* 2001).

The impact of G-CSF following non-myeloablative conditioning and allogeneic PBSC transplant has not been reported. Adverse side effects including hypoxia and anaphylaxis have, however, been reported following the administration of G-CSF to chronic phase CML patients undergoing allogeneic peripheral blood stem cell transplantation (Koury *et al.,* 2000).

The use of G-CSF-primed bone marrow has been studied in two separate randomized trials. Time to hematopoietic recovery, GVHD incidence, and survival were compared in patients transplanted with G-CSF mobilized PBSC compared to G-CSF stimulated bone marrow. No difference in time to neutrophil or platelet recovery was observed, although there was signifi-

Table 32.4.   *Summary of clinical studies of M-CSF or GM-CSF following allogeneic hematopoietic stem cell transplantation*

Reference	Study design	Number of patients	Randomized	Dose	Donor source	GVHD prophylaxis	Days to ANC >0.5	Febrile days	Antibiotic days	Hospital days	Cost saving
Masaoka et al., 1990	M-CSF	59	Yes	2×10^5 µg/kg/day	Related marrow	CSP	24*	NA	NA	NA	NA
	Placebo	60		–			27				
Powles et al., 1990	GM-CSF	20	Yes	8 µg/kg/day	Related marrow	CSP	18^{ns}	NA	16*	ND	NA
	Placebo	20		–			21		13		
Atkinson et al., 1991b	GM-CSF	10	No	250 µg/m²/day	Related marrow	CSP + MTX	17^{ns}	ND	NA	ND	NA
	Historical controls	16		–			19				
Nemunaitis et al., 1992	GM-CSF	40	No	250 µg/m²/day	Unrelated marrow	CSP + prednisone	21^{ns}	7*	NA	ND	NA
	Historical controls	78				CSP + MTX	21	4			
Hiraoka et al., 1994	GM-CSF	28	Yes	10 µg/kg/day	Related marrow	CSP ± MTX	17*	ND	ND	ND	NA
	Placebo	25					21				
Nemunaitis et al., 1995	GM-CSF	53	Yes	250 µg/m²/day	Related marrow	CSP + prednisolone	13*	ND	11^{ns}	25*	NA
	Placebo	56					17		14	26	

Abbreviations: ANC, absolute neutrophil count; CSP, cyclosporine; MTX, methotrexate; NA, not assessed; ND, no difference detected; ns, not statistically significant over controls;
* Statistically significant over controls ($P < .05$).

cantly more acute and chronic GVHD in those receiving PBSC, commensurate with the higher CD3+ cell dose (Serody et al., 2000; Morton et al., 2001).

GM-CSF (Table 32.4)

Several studies, including a placebo-controlled randomized double-blind trial, have shown the neutrophil count to recover to $0.5 \times 10^9/l$ 2 to 3 days earlier in recipients of GM-CSF after HLA-identical sibling transplants for hematologic malignancy (Powles et al., 1990). The lymphocyte count was also significantly higher in the GM-CSF group, and in one study the monocyte count was also significantly higher in recipients of GM-CSF. In the randomized placebo-controlled trial (Powles et al., 1990), there was no evidence for either an increased incidence of GVHD or leukemic relapse in the short term (Gupta et al., 1992), or at five year follow up (Singhal et al., 1997). In a historically controlled study in recipients of matched unrelated transplants, GM-CSF use was associated with a lesser number of febrile days and less septicemic episodes within the first 28 days (Nemunaitis et al., 1992). The use of GM-CSF was subsequently explored in a phase III trial by Nemunaitis and colleagues (1995), which confirmed that the time to myeloid engraftment was shortened, the incidence and severity of mucositis lessened, and the duration of hospitalization shorthened by GM-CSF without an increase in the incidence or severity of GVHD or the incidence of relapse. Overall survival was not different between the two groups. There is no clinical evidence that CSFs promote recurrence of leukemic clones either post-chemotherapy or posttransplantation, and the American Society of Clinical Oncology guidelines (2000) do not exclude patients with myeloid malignancies from those who are likely to benefit from CSF therapy (Ozer et al., 2000).

Although clearly effective in promoting neutrophil recovery after allogeneic BMT, the use of GM-CSF has been surpassed by G-CSF in clinical usage, in part due to the wider side effect profile of GM-CSF (Table 32.6).

Erythropoietin (EPO)

EPO acts primarily on committed erythroid progenitor cells to expand the number of immature erythroid burst-forming units (BFU-E). EPO induces an influx of BFU-E into the compartment of the more mature erythroid colony-forming units (CFU-E) and promotes their further differentiation. In addition, EPO prevents programmed death of CFU-E, enabling the cells to differentiate into erythrocytes. At least four randomized trials of recombinant human EPO (rh-EPO) after allogeneic BMT have been completed, and while all showed accelerated erythroid engraftment, only two showed a significant decrease in transfusion requirements for packed red blood cells (Link et al., 1994; Biggs et al., 1995). In one of the larger studies, 17 centers participated in a randomized double-blind, placebo-controlled trial (Link et al., 1994). The randomization was stratified according to major ABO-blood group incompatibility. A total of 106

patients received rh-EPO after allogeneic BMT and 109 patients received placebo. The dose was 150 IU/kg/day as a continuous intravenous infusion. Therapy started after bone marrow infusion and lasted until independence from red blood cell transfusions for 7 consecutive days with stable hemoglobin levels of >9 g/dl or until day 41 posttransplant. Reticulocyte counts were significantly higher with rh-EPO from day 21 to day 42 posttransplant. The median time to erythrocyte transfusion independence was 19 (range 16–21.6) days with EPO and 27 (range 22 to >42) days with placebo ($P < .003$). The mean (± 1 SD) numbers of red blood cell transfusions up to day 20 posttransplant were not different between the groups. However, from day 21 to day 41 the EPO-treated patients received 1.4 ± 2.5 transfusions while the control group received 2.7 ± 4.0 transfusions ($P = .004$). The investigators concluded that EPO significantly accelerated the reconstitution of erythropoiesis and reduced the number of packed cell transfusions after day 20 and found this effect to be strongest in patients with acute GVHD.

The development of late onset (beyond 50 days from transplant) anemia following allogeneic BMT is often associated with the development of GVHD. In a study of 9 such patients, EPO administration resulted in hemoglobin increases of 2 g/dl in 6. The remaining three patients, all of whom had severe GVHD, were unresponsive (Fujimori et al., 1998).

Thrombopoietin (TPO)

Clinical evaluation has involved two recombinant preparations. One consists of the full length, recombinant human molecule (rh-TPO); the other consists of the Mpl receptor-binding domain with the carbohydrate-rich carboxy terminus replaced by a polyethyeleneglycol moiety to improve in vivo stability (pegylated recombinant human megakaryocyte growth and development factor, PEG-rHuMGDF).

When administered subcutaneously (to non-transplant recipients) for a maximum of 10 days, PEG-rHuMGDF caused a dose-related increase in the platelet count, with no changes in white or red blood cell parameters (Basser et al., 1996). The platelet count began to rise from day 6 of treatment with maximum levels occurring between days 12 and 18. Similar results have been seen in studies with rh-TPO (Vadhan-Raj et al., 1997). With both molecules an increase in bone marrow megakaryocytes, with no changes in other cell lineages, was seen. Of concern is the potential risk of the development of neutralising antibodies following exposure to PEG-rhuMGDF. These antibodies may be associated with thrombocytopenia or, as in one case, marrow apalsia (Basser et al., 2002).

Studies of rh-TPO or PEG-rHuMGDF administered early after allografting have been reported. In a phase-I dose-escalating study of rh-TPO in 38 recipients of autologous or allogeneic HSC transplants who had persistent severe thrombocytopenia >35 days posttransplant, no significant adverse events (including no neutralizing TPO-specific antibodies) were seen. The study however showed no improvement in time to platelet

Table 32.5. *Summary of clinical studies of G-CSF following allogeneic hematopoietic stem cell transplantation*

Reference	Study design	Number of patients	Randomized	Dose	Donor source	GVHD prophylaxis	Days to ANC > 0.5	Febrile days	Antibiotic days	Hospital days	Cost saving
Schriber et al., 1994	G-CSF	50	No	5 µg/kg	Sibling/VUD marrow	CSP+prednisone+MTX	10*	13*	NA	NA	NA
	Historical controls	52				CSP+prednisone+MTX	16	19	NA	NA	NA
Gisselbrecht et al., 1994	G-CSF	163	Yes	5 µg/kg	Related marrow	NS	14*	3*	25*	NA	
	Placebo	152					20	5	29		
Lickliter et al., 1994	G-CSF	13	No	5 µg/kg	Related marrow	CSP+MTX	15*	ND	ND	NA	
	Historical controls			—	Related marrow		18.5	ND			
Martin-Algarra et al., 1995	G-CSF or GM-CSF	26	No	5–10 µg/kg/day (G) 250–500 µg/m²/day (GM)	Related marrow	CSP+MTX	17*	20*	33.5*	NA	
	Historical controls			—			NA				
Lee et al., 1998	Historical controls	38			Related marrow	T cell depletion	20	34	39		
	G-CSF	81	No	5 µg/kg			12*	NA	17*	Yes	
Lee et al., 1999	Matched controls	115		—	Related marrow	CD6 T cell depletion	20	NA	23	NA	
	G-CSF day 1	30	Yes	450 µg/day			16	NA	ND		
Berger et al., 1999	G-CSF day 6	30			Unrelated marrow	CSP+prednisone or CSP+MTX	16	ND	ND	NA	
	G-CSF	22	No	5 µg/kg/day			14*	ND	ND		
	Matched controls	25		—			16				
Hagglund et al., 1998	G-CSF day 0				Unrelated marrow	CPM+MTX	17	ND	ND	NA	
	G-CSF day 5	54	Yes	5 µg/kg/day			16	ND	ND		
	G-CSF day 10						16				
Bishop et al., 2000a	G-CSF	26	Yes	10 µg/kg/day	Related PBSC	CSP+MTX	11*	NA	NA	NA	
Przepiorka et al., 2001	Placebo	24			Related PBSC	Tacrolimus+prednisone or tacrolimus+MTX	15	ND	ND	No	
	G-CSF	21	Yes	10 µg/kg/day			12*	ND	ND		
Stinson et al., 2000	Placebo	21			Related PBSC	CSP+MTX	15	ND	ND	No	
	G-CSF	23	Yes	10 µg/kg/day			10.5*	ND	ND		
	Placebo	21					15				

Abbreviations: ANC, absolute neutrophil count; CSP, cyclosporine; MTX, methotrexate; PBSC, peripheral blood stem cells; NA, not assessed; ND, no difference detected; NS, not stated; VUD, volunteer unrelated donor.

* Statistically significant over controls (*P* < .05).

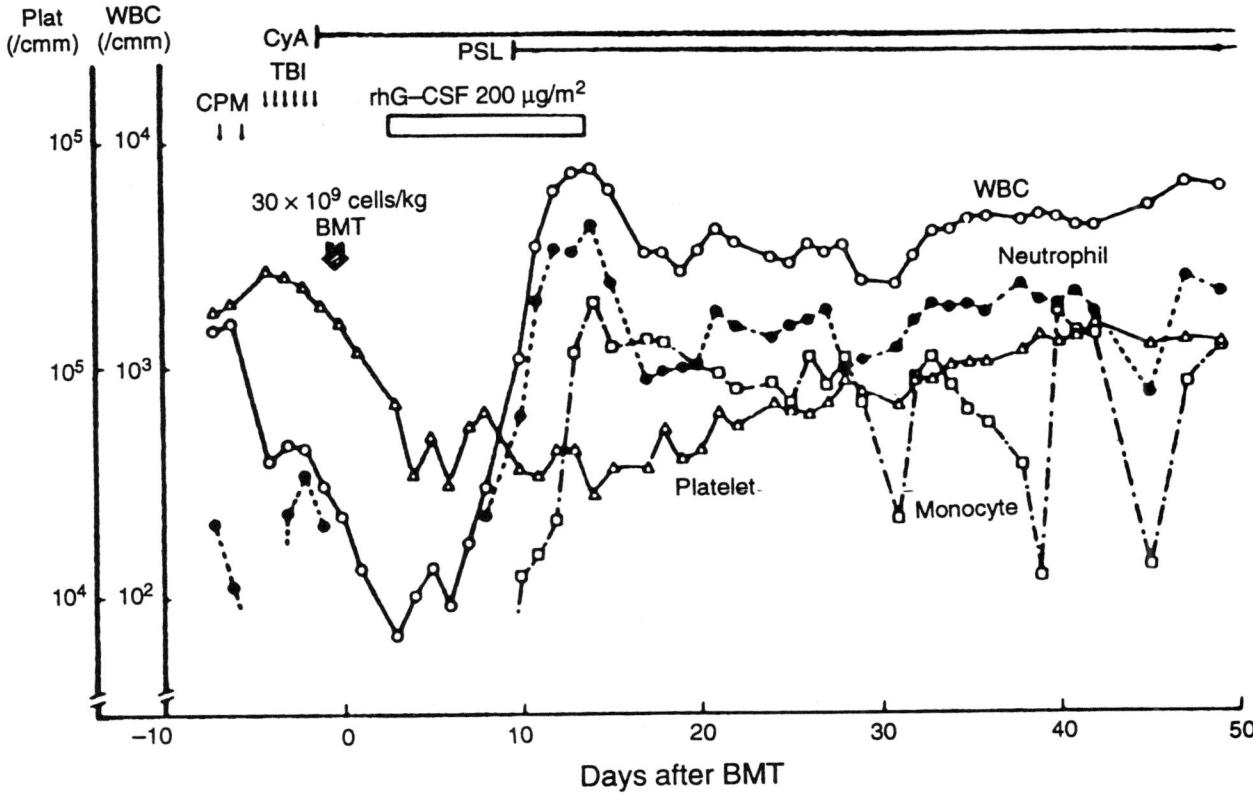

Fig. 32.3. Hematologic response of a typical patient treated with recombinant human G-CSF (24-year-old female with acute lymphoblastic leukemia). CyA, cyclosporine; PSL, prednisolone; CPM, cyclophosphamide; TBI, total body irradiation; BMT, bone marrow transplant. Reproduced, with permission, from Masaoka *et al.* (1989).

recovery (Nash *et al.*, 2000). Similar findings were made by Wolff *et al.* (2001).

Use of HGFs to enhance graft-versus-leukemia (GVL) effect (and see Chapter 65)

The success of donor lymphocyte infusions in the treatment of relapsed hematological malignancies following allogeneic stem cell transplantation has promoted the concept that the function of immunologically reactive cells contained within the initial graft or subsequent DLI may be enhanced by the use of cytokine therapy. In vitro and murine models have further advanced the understanding of the role of growth factors and other cytokines in stimulating NK and T lymphocytes to eradicate malignant cells.

Experiments demonstrated the anti-tumor effects of IL-2-stimulated allogeneic NK cells against a B cell leukemia line (Zeis *et al.*, 1994). A role has been established for IL-2 in the stimulation of anti-leukemic cytotoxic T lymphocytes (Leshem, Vourka-Karussis, & Slavin, 2000). Additional studies have shown a role for a range of cytokines in enhancing the GVL effect after allografting in murine models. These include IL-12 (Yang *et al.*, 1997; Yang & Sykes, 1999), IL-11 (Teshima *et al.*, 1999), and IL-7 (Alpdogan *et al.*, 2001). Phase I and II clinical studies have been reported which show that IL-2 may be delivered with

acceptable toxicity and with some suggestion of enhancement of an anti-leukemic effect (Soiffer *et al.*, 1994; Robinson *et al.*, 1996). A phase-II study suggested a benefit for interferon-α in the induction of GVL with DLI therapy following relapse of CML or AML after allogeneic BMT (Grigg *et al.*, 2001).

G-CSF has also demonstrated promise in its immunomodulatory effects after allografting. Animal models of allogeneic transplantation for leukemia have shown enhanced perforin-mediated GVL effects in mice transplanted with G-CSF-mobilized PBSC (Pan *et al.*, 1999). Additional enhancement of the GVL effect was observed when PBSC were mobilized with G-CSF and IL-3 compared to G-CSF mobilization alone (Hartung *et al.*, 1998). Others have suggested that the lower rates of GVHD observed in experimental models are due to alterations in donor dendritic cell function induced by G-CSF (Reddy *et al.*, 2000). In the clinic, filgrastim has been used as an alternative to DLI in the induction of GVL in patients with relapsed leukemia post BMT (Giralt *et al.*, 1993; Carral *et al.*, 1996; Bishop *et al.*, 2000b).

Use of HGFs to treat graft failure (and see Chapter 70)

Nemunaitis and colleagues (1990) reported the effect of recombinant human GM-CSF in 37 patients with marrow graft failure

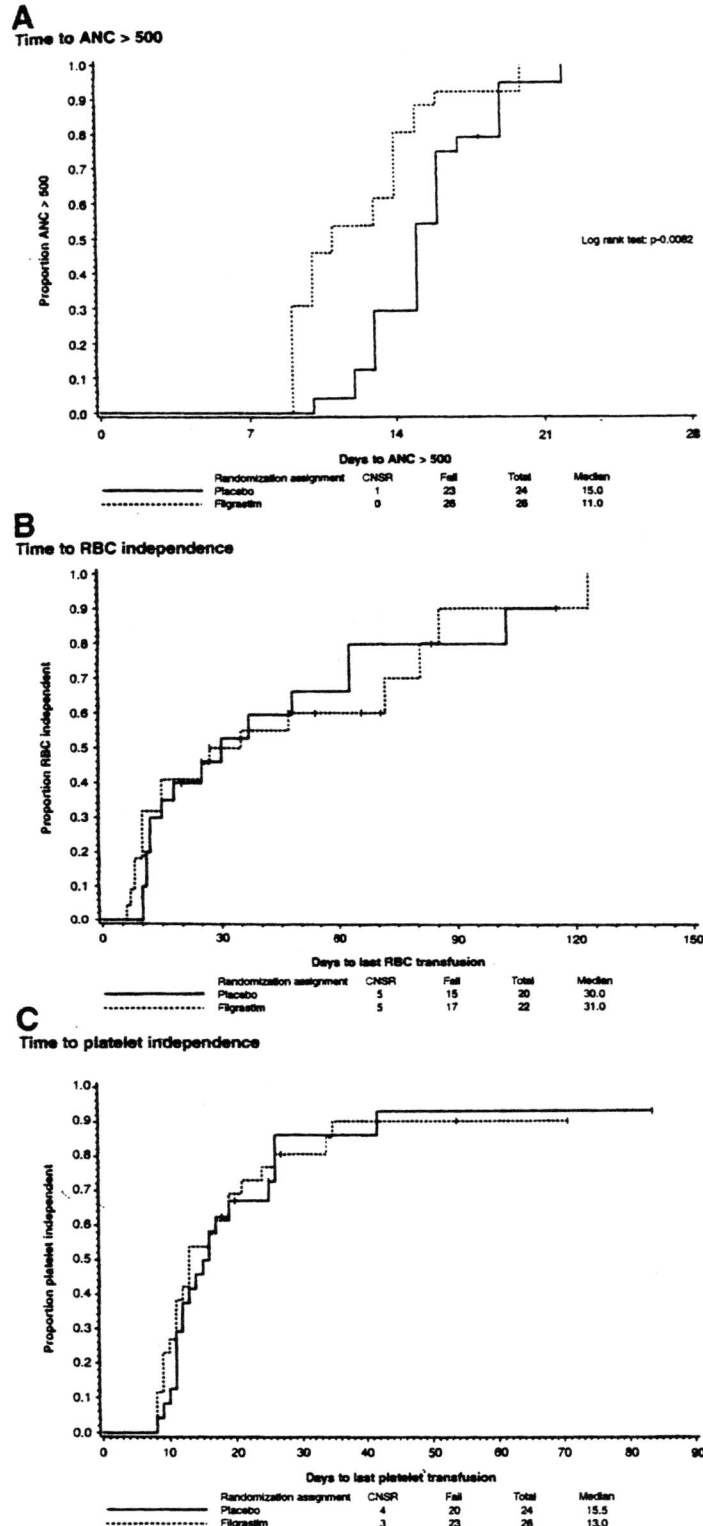

Fig. 32.4. Median times to hematopoietic recovery with G-CSF or placebo after allogeneic blood stem cell transplantation. Reproduced, with permission, from Bishop *et al.* (2000a).

Table 32.6. *Reported side effects of GM-CSF*

Headache
Fatigue
Confusion
Anorexia
Nausea/vomiting
Abnormal taste
ECG changes
Bone pain
Flu-like symptoms (fever, myalgia, chills)
Pericardial effusion[a]
Pleural effusion[a]
Capillary leak syndrome[a]
Hypotension[a]

[a] Indication to discontinue GM-CSF

after allogeneic ($n = 15$), autologous ($n = 21$), or syngeneic ($n = 1$) BMT. Twenty-one patients reached an absolute neutrophil count of 0.5×10^9/l (or greater) within 2 weeks of starting treatment, while 16 did not. At doses less than 500 μg/m² GM-CSF was well tolerated and did not exacerbate GVHD in allogeneic transplant recipients. No patient with myeloid leukemia relapsed while receiving treatment. The survival rate of those given GM-CSF was significantly better than that of a historical control group. The addition of G-CSF to GM-CSF in one randomized study did not enhance neutrophil recovery over GM-CSF alone in the treatment of graft failure (Weisdorf *et al.*, 1995). A single case report indicated the possible benefit of combined IL-3 and GM-CSF therapy for the treatment of graft failure (Vannucchi *et al.*, 1995).

Use of HGFs in the management of fungal infection after allogeneic HSC transplantation

The use of recombinant human M-CSF in the management of invasive fungal infection after allogeneic marrow transplantation has been reported (Nemunaitis *et al.*, 1991a). When given in combination with conventional antifungal therapy, 6 patients had resolution of their infection, 6 did not respond, and 12 were inevaluable. Transient dose-related thrombocytopenia was observed. Other isolated case reports have been published in which GM-CSF in combination with antifungal antibiotics have been used; however, the direct impact of GM-CSF on outcome in these situations is difficult to assess.

Conclusions

At this time the routine administration of HGFs after HSC transplantation is not of proven benefit. With the advent of allogeneic PBPC transplantation, which results in rapid hematopoietic reconstitution, there is little to suggest that the additional use of HGFs positively affects infection incidence, antibiotic usage, or duration of hospitalization after HLA-identical sib-ling transplantation. Attention is now being directed away from the role of HGFs to speed hematopoietic recovery and towards their role in enhancing patient survival via promoting GVL whilst limiting severe GVHD.

References

Alpdogan, O., Schmaltz, C., Muriglan, S. J. *et al* (2001). Administration of interleukin-7 after allogeneic bone marrow transplantation improves immune reconstitution without aggravating graft-versus-host disease. *Blood,* **98,** 2256–65.

Atkinson, K., Biggs, J. C., Downs, K. *et al.* (1991b). GM-CSF after allogeneic bone marrow transplantation: accelerated recovery of neutrophils, monocytes and lymphocytes. *Australia and New Zealand Journal of Medicine,* **21,** 686–92.

Atkinson, K., Matias, C., Guiffre, A. *et al.* (1991a). In vivo administration of G-CSF, GM-CSF, IL-1, IL-4 alone and in combination, after allogeneic murine hematopoietic stem cell transplantation. *Blood,* **77,** 1376–82.

Basser, R. L., O'Flaherty, E., Green, M. *et al.* (2002). Development of pancytopenia with neutralizing antibodies to thrombopoietin after multicycle chemotherapy supported by megakaryocyte growth and development factor. *Blood,* **99,** 2599–2602.

Basser, R. L., Rasko, J.E.J., Clarke. K. *et al.* (1996). Thrombopoietic effects of pegylated recombinant human megakaryocyte growth and development factor (PEG-rHuMGDF) in patients with advanced cancer. *Lancet,* **348,** 1279–81.

Berger, C., Bertz, H., Schmoor, C. *et al.* (1999). Influence of recombinant human granulocyte colony-stimulating factor (filgrastim) on hematopoietic recovery and outcome following allogeneic bone marrow transplantation (BMT) from volunteer unrelated donors. *Bone Marrow Transplantation,* **10,** 983–90.

Biggs, J. C., Atkinson, K. A., Booker, V. *et al.* (1995). Prospective randomised double-blind trial of the in vivo use of recombinant human erythropoietin in bone marrow transplantation from HLA-identical sibling donors. The Australian Bone Marrow Transplant Study Group. *Bone Marrow Transplantation,* **15,** 129–34.

Bishop, M. R., Tarantolo, S. R., Geller, R. B. *et al.* (2000a). A randomized, double-blind trial of filgrastim (granulocyte colony-stimulating factor) versus placebo following allogeneic blood stem cell transplantation. *Blood,* **96,** 80–5.

Bishop, M. R., Tarantolo, S. R., Pavletic, S. *et al.* (2000b). Filgrastim as an alternative to donor leukocyte infusion for relapse after allogeneic stem-cell transplantation. *Journal of Clinical Oncology,* **18,** 2269–72.

Blazar, B., Taylor, P., & Vallera, D. A. (1992). In vivo infusions of cytokines in murine recipients of T cell depleted bone marrow allografts. *Journal of Cellular Biochemistry,* **16a** (Suppl), 172.

Carral, A., Sanz, G. F., & Sanz, M. A. (1996). Filgrastim for the treatment of leukemia relapse after bone marrow transplantation. *Bone Marrow Transplantation,* **18,** 817–19.

Fanucchi, M., Glaspy, J., Crawford, J. *et al.* (1997). Effects of polyethylene glycol-conjugated recombinant human megakaryocyte growth and development factor on platelet counts for chemotherapy for lung cancer. *New England Journal of Medicine,* **336,** 404–9.

Fujimori, Y., Kanamaru, A., Saheki, K., *et al.* (1998). Recombinant human erythropoietin for late-onset anemia after allogeneic bone marrow transplantation. *International Journal of Hematology,* **67,** 131–6.

Giralt, S., Escudier, S., Kantarijan, H. *et al.* (1993). Preliminary results of treatment with filgastrim for relapse of leukemia and myelodysplasia after allogeneic bone marrow transplantation. *New England Journal of Medicine,* **329,** 757–61.

Gisselbrecht, C., Prentice, H. G., Bacigalupo, A. *et al.* (1994). Placebo-controlled phase III trial of lenograstim in bone marrow transplantation. *Lancet,* **343,** 696–700.

Grigg, A., Kannan, K., Schwarer, A. P. *et al.* (2001). Chemotherapy and granulocyte colony stimulating factor-mobilized blood cell infusion followed by interferon-alpha for relapsed malignancy after allogeneic bone marrow transplantation. *Internal Medicine Journal,* **31,** 15–22.

Gupta, P., Tiley, C., Powles, R. *et al.* (1992). No increase in relapse in patients with myeloid leukemias receiving rhGM-CSF after allogeneic bone marrow transplantation. *Bone Marrow Transplantation,* **9,** 491–3.

Hagglund, H., Ringden, O., Remberger, M. *et al.* (1998). Faster neutrophil and platelet engraftment, but no differences in acute GVHD or survival, using peripheral blood stem cells from related and unrelated donors, compared to bone marrow. *Bone Marrow Transplantation,* **22,** 131–6.

Hartung, G., Uharek, L., Zeis, M. *et al.* (1998). Superior antileukemic activity of murine peripheral blood progenitor cell (PBPC) grafts mobilized by G-CSF and stem cell factor (SCF) as compared to G-CSF alone. *Bone Marrow Transplantation,* **21** (Suppl 3), S16–20.

Hiraoka, A., Masaoko, T., Mizoguchi, H. *et al.* (1994). Recombinant human non-glycosylated granulocyte-macrophage colony-simulating factor in allogeneic bone marrow transplantation: double-blind placebo-controlled phase III clinical trial. *Japanese Journal of Clinical Oncology,* **24,** 205–11.

Koury, H., Adkins, D., Brown, R. *et al.* (2000). Adverse side-effects associated with G-CSF in patients with chronic myeloid leukemia undergoing allogeneic peripheral blood stem cell transplantation. *Bone Marrow Transplantation,* **25,** 1197–1201.

Lee, K. H., Lee, J. H., Choi, S. J. *et al.* (1999). Randomized comparison of two different schedules of granulocyte colony-stimulating factor administration after allogeneic bone marrow transplantation. *Bone Marrow Transplantation,* **24,** 591–9.

Lee, S. J., Weller, E., Alyea, E. P. *et al.* (1998). Efficacy and costs of granulocyte colony-stimulating factor in allogeneic T-cell depleted bone marrow transplantation. *Blood,* **92,** 2725–9.

Leshem, B., Vourka-Karussis, U., Slavin, S. (2000). Correlation between enhancement of graft-versus-leukemia effects following allogeneic bone marrow transplantation by rIL-2 and increased frequency of cytotoxic T-lymphocyte precursors in murine myeloid leukemia. *Cytokines and Cellular Molecular Therapy,* **6,** 141–7.

Lickliter, J. D., McGlave, P. B., DeFor, T. E. *et al.* (2000). Matched-pair analysis of peripheral blood stem cells compared to marrow for allogeneic transplantation. *Bone Marrow Transplantation,* **26,** 723–8.

Lickliter, J. D., Roberts, A. W., & Grigg, A. P. (1994). Phase II study of glycosylated recombinant human granulocyte colony-stimulating factor after HLA-identical sibling bone marrow transplantation. *Australian and New Zealand Journal of Medicine,* **24,** 541–6.

Link, H., Boogaerts, M. A., Fauser, A. A. *et al.* (1994). A controlled trial of recombinant human erythropoietin after bone marrow transplantation. *Blood,* **84,** 3327–35.

Martin-Algarra, S., Bishop, M. R., Tarantolo, S. *et al.* (1995). Hematopoietic growth factors after HLA-identical allogeneic bone marrow transplantation in patients treated with methotrexate-containing graft-vs-host disease prophylaxis. *Experimental Hematology,* **23,** 1503–8.

Masaoka, T., Motoyoshi, K., Takaku, F. *et al.* (1988). Administration of human colony-stimulating factor after bone marrow transplantation. *Bone Marrow Transplantation,* **3,** 121–8.

Masaoka, T., Shibata, H., Ohno, R. *et al.* (1990). Double blind trial of human urinary macrophage colony-stimulating factor for allogeneic and syngeneic bone marrow transplantation: effectiveness of treatment and two year follow up for relapse of leukemia. *British Journal of Haematology,* **76,** 501–5.

Masaoka, T., Takaku, F., Kato, S. *et al.* (1989). Recombinant human granulocyte colony-stimulating factor in allogeneic bone marrow transplantation. *Experimental Hematology,* **17,** 1047–50.

Metcalf, D. (1988). In *The Molecular Control of Blood Cells.* Cambridge, Massachusetts: Harvard University Press.

Molineux, G., Hartley, C. A., McElroy, P. *et al.* (1996). Megakaryocyte growth and development factor stimulates enhanced platelet recovery in mice after bone marrow transplantation. *Blood,* **88,** 1509–14.

Morton, J., Hutchins, C., & Durrant, S. (2001). Granulocyte-colony-stimulating factor (G-CSF)-primed allogeneic bone marrow: significantly less graft-versus-host disease and comparable engraftment to G–CSF-mobilized peripheral blood stem cells. *Blood,* **98,** 3186–91.

Nash, R. A., Kurzrock, R., DiPersio, J. *et al.* (2000). A phase I trial of recombinant human thrombopoietin in patients with delayed platelet recovery after hematopoietic stem cell transplantation. *Biology of Blood and Marrow Transplantation,* **6,** 25–34.

Nemunaitis, J., Anasetti, C., Storb, R. *et al.* (1992). Phase II trial of recombinant human granulocyte-macrophage colony-stimulating factor in patients undergoing allogeneic bone marrow transplantation from unrelated donors. *Blood,* **79,** 2572–7.

Nemunaitis, J., Meyers, J. D., Buckner, C. D. *et al.* (1991a). Phase 1 trial of recombinant human macrophage colony-stimulating factor in patients with invasive fungal infection. *Blood,* **78,** 907–13.

Nemunaitis, J., Rabino, W.E.S., Singer, J. W. *et al.* (1991b). Recombinant granulocyte-macrophage colony-stimulating factor after autologous bone marrow transplantation for lymphoid cancer. *New England Journal of Medicine,* **324,** 1773–8.

Nemunaitis, J., Rosenfeld, C. S., Ash, R. *et al.* (1995). Phase III randomized, double-blind placebo-controlled trial of rhGM-CSF following allogeneic bone marrow transplantation. *Bone Marrow Transplantation,* **15,** 949–54.

Nemunaitis, J., Singer, J. W., Buckner, C. D. *et al.* (1990). Use of recombinant human granulocyte-macrophage colony-stimulating factor in graft failure after bone marrow transplantation. *Blood,* **76,** 245–53.

Nienhuis, A. W., Donahue, R. E., Karlsson, S. *et al.* (1987). Recombinant human granulocyte-macrophage colony-stimulating factor (GM-CSF) shortens the period of neutropenia after autologous bone marrow transplantation in a primate model. *Journal of Clinical Investigation,* **80,** 537–77.

Orkin, S. H., Zon, L. I. (2002). Hematopoiesis and stem cells: plasticity versus developmental heterogeneity. *Nature Immunology,* **3,** 323–8.

Ozer, H., Armitage, J. O., Bennett, C. L. *et al.* (2000). 2000 update of recommendations for the use of hematopoietic colony-stimulating factors: evidence-based, clinical practice guidelines. *Journal of Clinical Oncology,* **18,** 3558–85.

Pan, L., Teshima, T., Hill, G. R. *et al.* (1999). Granulocyte colony-stimulating factor-mobilized allogeneic stem cell transplantation maintains graft-versus-leukemia effects through a perforin-dependent pathway while preventing graft-versus-host disease. *Blood,* **93,** 4071–8.

Peters, M., Solem, F., Goldschmidt, J., Schirmacher, P., Rose-John, S. (2001). Interleukin-6 and the soluble interleukin-6 receptor induce stem cell factor and Flt-3L expression in vivo and in vitro. *Experimental Hematology,* **29,** 146–55.

Powles, R., Smith, C., Milan, S. *et al.* (1990). Human recombinant GM-CSF in allogeneic bone marrow transplantation for leukemia: double blind, placebo-controlled trial. *Lancet,* **336,** 1417–20.

Przieporka, D., Smith, T. L., Folloder, J. *et al.* (2001). Controlled trial of filgrastim for acceleration of neutrophil recovery after allogeneic blood stem cell transplantation from human leukocyte antigen-matched related donors. *Blood,* **97,** 3405–10.

Reddy, V., Hill, G. R., Pan, L., *et al.* (2000). G-CSF modulates cytokine profile of dendritic cells and decreases acute graft-versus-host disease through effects on the donor rather than the recipient. *Transplantation,* **69,** 691–3.

Robinson, N., Sanders, J. E., Benyunes, M. C. *et al.* (1996). Phase I trial of interleukin-2 after unmodified HLA-matched sibling bone marrow transplantation for children with acute leukemia. *Blood,* **87,** 1249–54.

Serody, J. S., Sparks, S. D., Lin, Y. *et al.* (2000). Comparison of granulocyte colony-stimulating factor (G-CSF)–mobilized peripheral blood progenitor cells and G-CSF–stimulated bone marrow as a source of stem cells in HLA-matched sibling transplantation. *Biology of Blood and Marrow Transplantation,* **6,** 434–40.

Schmitz, N., Bacigalupo, A., Hasenclever, D. *et al.* (1998). Allogeneic bone marrow transplantation vs filgrastim-mobilised peripheral blood progenitor cell transplantation in patients with early leukaemia: first results of a randomised multicentre trial of the European Group for Blood and Marrow Transplantation. *Bone Marrow Transplantation,* **21,** 995–1003.

Schriber, J. R., Chao, N. J., Long, G. D. *et al.* (1994). Granulocyte colony-stimulating factor after allogeneic bone marrow transplantation. *Blood,* **84,** 680–4.

Schuening, F. G., Storb, R., Goehle, S. *et al.* (1990). Recombinant human granulocyte colony-stimulating factor accelerates hematopoietic recovery after DLA-identical littermate marrow transplants in dogs. *Blood,* **76,** 636–40.

Shimada, Y., Kato, T., Ogami, K. *et al.* (1995). Production of thrombopoietin (TPO) by rat hepatocytes and hepatoma cell lines. *Experimental Hematology,* **23,** 1388–96.

Singhal, S., Powles, R., Treleaven, J. *et al.* (1997). Long-term safety of GM-CSF (molgramostim) administration after allogeneic bone marrow transplantation for hematologic malignancies: five-year follow-up of a double-blind randomized placebo-controlled study. *Leukemia and Lymphoma,* **24,** 301–7.

Soiffer, R. J., Murray, C., Gonin, R., Ritz, J. (1994). Effect of low-dose interleukin-2 on disease relapse after T-cell-depleted allogeneic bone marrow transplantation. *Blood,* **84,** 964–71.

Stinson, T. J., Adams, J. R., Bishop, M. R. *et al.* (2000). Economic analysis of a phase III study of G-CSF vs placebo following allogeneic blood stem cell transplantation. *Bone Marrow Transplantation,* **26,** 663–6.

Sungaran, R., Markovic, B., & Chong, B. H. (1997). Localization and regulation of thrombopoietin mRNA-expression in human kidney, liver, bone marrow, and spleen using in situ hybridization. *Blood,* **89,** 101–7.

Teshima, T., Hill, G. R., Pan, L. *et al.* (1999). IL-11 separates graft-versus-leukemia effects from graft-versus-host disease after bone marrow transplantation. *Journal of Clinical Investigation,* **104,** 317–25.

Testa, N. G. & Dexter, T. M. (1991). *Interferons and Cytokines,* **17,** 43–5.

Vadhan-Raj, S., Murray, L. J., Bueso-Ramos, C. *et al.* (1997). Stimulation of megakaryocyte and platelet production of a single dose of recombinant human thrombopoietin in patients with cancer. *Annals of Internal Medicine,* **126,** 673–81.

Vannucchi, A. M., Bosi, A., Laszlo, D., *et al.* (1995). Treatment of a delayed graft failure after allogeneic bone marrow transplantation with IL-3 and GM-CSF. *Haematologica,* **80,** 341–3.

Weisdorf, D. J., Verfaillie, C. M., Davies, S. M. *et al.* (1995). Hematopoietic growth factors for graft failure after bone marrow transplantation: a randomized trial of granulocyte-macrophage colony-stimulating factor (GM-CSF) versus sequential GM-CSF plus granulocyte-CSF. *Blood,* **85,** 3452–6.

Wolff, S. N., Herzig, R., Lynch, J. *et al.* (2001). Recombinant human thrombopoietin (rhTPO) after autologous bone marrow transplantation: a phase I pharmakokinetic and pharmacodynamic study. *Bone Marrow Transplantation,* **27,** 261–8.

Yang, Y. G., Sergio, J. J., Pearson, D. A. *et al.* (1997). Interleukin-12 preserves the graft-versus-leukemia effect of allogeneic CD8 T cells while inhibiting CD4-dependent graft-versus-host disease in mice. *Blood,* **90,** 4651–60.

Yang, Y. G. & Sykes, M. (1999). The role of interleukin-12 in preserving the graft-versus-leukemia effect of allogeneic CD8 T cells independently of GVHD. *Leukemia and Lymphoma,* **33,** 409–20.

Zaucha, J. M., Gooley, T., Bensinger, W. I. *et al.* (2001). CD34 cell dose in granulocyte colony-stimulating factor-mobilized peripheral blood mononuclear cell grafts affects engraftment kinetics and development of extensive chronic graft-versus-host disease after human leukocyte antigen-identical sibling transplantation. *Blood*, **98**, 3221–7.

Zeis, M., Uharek, L., Glass, B. *et al.* (1994). Induction of graft-versus-leukemia (GVL) activity in murine leukemia models after IL-2 pretreatment of syngeneic and allogeneic bone marrow grafts. *Bone Marrow Transplantation,* **14,** 711–5.

33 Therapeutic drug monitoring in hematopoietic stem cell transplant recipients

HAI TRAN AND SUSAN TETT

MD Anderson Hospital, Houston, USA and The University of Queensland, Brisbane, Australia

Introduction

Therapeutic drug monitoring (TDM) is one approach which clinicians have utilized to follow an individual patient's therapy in order to maximize efficacy, while minimizing or reducing the risk of associated toxicities with the many agents that are used in the hematopoietic stem cell (HSC) transplant recipient.

Figure 33.1 demonstrates the theory upon which drug concentration targeting is based. A given effect is proposed to be more closely related to the drug concentration than it is to the dose of the drug. Many common agents that are prescribed by physicians do not require this close monitoring due to the extremely wide range of concentration between the limits of a therapeutic effect and unwanted adverse effects.

Some drugs have very poor correlations between dose and concentration, such that the same dose given to a number of individuals, or even to the same individual at different times, gives rise to vastly different concentrations. This is due to a variety of physiologic factors (gender, age, weight, body mass) and pathophysisologic factors (hepatic, renal or cardiac impairment, genetic polymorphism).

Variability in the relationship between dose and concentration is introduced because of intra- and interpatient differences in pharmacokinetic factors, such as clearance or bioavailability. Physiologic factors, such as age and weight, or pathophysiologic factors such as renal and hepatic disease can contribute to pharmacokinetic variability. Targeting a concentration, rather than administering standard doses, eliminates this source of variability, leading to a more predictable effect (Thomson & Whiting, 1992; Holford & Tett, 1997).

Specific drugs are monitored because they have narrow therapeutic ranges, such that concentrations at which toxic effects are more likely to occur are not much greater than those required for efficacy. Other reasons for monitoring concentrations include difficulty in clinical measurement of the endpoints of therapy (e.g., cardiac glycosides) or to ensure adequate prophylaxis because the endpoints are an absence of an event (for example, antiarrhythmic drugs, anticonvulsant drugs). Patients with rapidly changing clinical conditions, such as those with deteriorating renal or hepatic function, often require close monitoring of drug concentrations to ensure that the risk of toxicity is minimized. Specialists in dosage regimen design, based on pharmacokinetic principles, are available in the clinical pharmacology departments of most hospitals for consultation.

Table 33.1 provides a list of the drugs that are commonly monitored by concentration determination, together with the common therapeutic concentration ranges. These ranges are based on probabilities (of efficacy and toxicity) and are not comparable to the "normal ranges" used in biochemistry. They are not derived from the 95% confidence intervals around a "normal" value. It is important to adjust dose based on knowledge about an individual patient; for example, the phenytoin concentration targeted in a patient with low serum albumin will be lower than the usual therapeutic concentration range, because the unbound, active concentration is likely to be proportionately higher. It is important to remember that therapeutic concentration ranges are often not rigorously defined, provide only a guide to therapy, and the patients' clinical condition is always the prime consideration.

Assay methodologies

Several different assay methodologies are used for drug concentration determination, including immunoassay [fluorescence polarization immunoassay (FPIA), radioimmunoassay (RIA), enzyme multiplied immunoassay (EMIT)], high-performance liquid chromatography (HPLC), and gas chromatography (GC). These differ in specificity, sensitivity, and assay

DOSE ⇒ CONCENTRATION ⇒ EFFECT

Fig. 33.1. Relationship between dose of a drug, concentration, and effect. The arrows indicate connections between these, but also indicate sources of variability. One source of variability, inter- or intrasubject variability in the dose-concentration relationship, the pharmacokinetics of a drug, can be eliminated by designing drug dosage regimens to specifically target predefined drug concentrations.

Table 33.1. *Drugs that may be used in HSC transplant recipients that are often subject to concentration targeting strategies, showing the therapeutic ranges commonly used*[a]

Drug	Therapeutic concentration range	Comments
Amikacin	Trough less than 5 mg/l	For t.d.s. regimens
Carbamazepine	5–10 mg/l	
Clonazepam	10–70 μg/l	
Cyclosporine	See text	See text
Digoxin	0.5–2.0 μg/l	
5-fluorocytosine	35–70 mg/l	
Gentamicin	Trough less than 2 mg/l	For t.d.s. regimens
	AUC less than 101 mg·hr/l	For once daily dosing
Methotrexate	See text	
Netilmicin	Trough less than 2 mg/l	For t.d.s. regimens
	AUC less than 101 mg·hr/l	For once daily dosing
Phenobarbitone	15–40 mg/l	
Phenytoin	10–20 mg/l	
Tacrolimus (FK-506)	<20 μg/l	
Theophylline	10–20 mg/l (adult)	
Tobramycin	Trough less than 2 mg/l	For t.d.s. regimens
	AUC less than 101 mg·hr/l	For once daily dosing
Valproic acid	50–100 mg/l	
Vancomycin	Trough 5–10 mg/l	
	Peak 30–40 mg/l	

Abbreviation: AUC, area under curve.

[a] Other drugs that can be readily monitored include the antiarrhythmic drugs, such as amiodarone, disopyramide, flecainide, lignocaine, mexiletine, procainamide, and quinidine, and the antidepressant drugs, such as amitriptyline, nortriptyline, imipramine, doxepin, and lithium.

time. In general, immunoassays are quick, with a turnaround time, from delivery of an urgent sample to the laboratory to the final result, of about 1 hour. Chromatographic assays are generally slower, as the sample usually undergoes preliminary processing (for example, extraction of the drug into organic solvent, filtration, or protein precipitation) before quantitation. However, chromatographic assays are often more specific than immunoassays, separately quantitating parent drug and metabolites, and these are often required for sufficient sensitivity (Taylor *et al.*, 1996).

Dosage prediction

There are numerous nomograms, formulas, and computer programs available to assist with accurate dosage prediction. Some of these estimate dosage according to a patient's characteristics, such as weight, height, serum creatinine, etc., while others use drug concentration-time data to estimate the patient's own pharmacokinetic parameters, thus further individualizing dosing regimens. One of the most accurate methods of individualizing dos-

ing using the single concentration-time point generally available utilizes a computer program to obtain Bayesian estimates (based on Bayes' probability theory) of an individual's pharmacokinetics parameters (Thomson & Whiting, 1992). An individual's parameters are then used to predict future dosing requirements.

Commonly monitored drugs

Chemotherapeutic agents

Busulfan

Over the past 20 years, a growing body of work has been accumulating in the use of high-dose busulfan (HD-Bu) which was initiated by Santos and colleagues in 1983. Since then, high-dose busulfan has become an important component of many myeloablative regimens for patients undergoing hematopoietic stem cell (HSC) transplantation. However, the use of HD-Bu is not without inherent problems. Busulfan can cause significant hepatic toxicities, specifically veno-occlusive disease (VOD). In addition, busulfan disposition after oral administration is highly variable, so control of drug exposure is difficult. In children this problem is further complicated by their more rapid, age-dependent clearance of the drug (Growchow *et al.*, 1990; Regazzi *et al.*, 1992; Hassan *et al.*, 1996; Pawlowska *et al.*, 1997). Using oral busulfan doses equivalent to those administered to adults, on a mg/kg basis, resulted in lower busulfan area under the concentration-time curve (AUC), less regimen-related toxicity (RRT), and higher relapse rates in pediatric patients. It had been suggested that busulfan clearance rates in children are not significantly different from those of adults if the rates are normalized to body surface area (BSA). Thus, busulfan dosages based on BSA, rather than body weight, should lead to a busulfan exposure more approximate to that observed in adults. In later pediatric studies, when fixed doses of busulfan (600–640 mg/m²) were administered in combination with cyclophosphamide, the incidences of mucositis, VOD, and neurotoxicity approached those seen in the adult population (Vassal *et al.*, 1990, 1992, 1996; Yeager *et al.*, 1992; Hassan *et al.*, 1994).

Many investigators have described the relationships between clinical outcome and oral busulfan pharmacokinetics (Grochow *et al.*, 1990; Hassan *et al.*, 1991; Regazzi *et al.*, 1992; Yeager *et al.*, 1992; Embree *et al.*, 1993; Grochow, 1993; Vassal *et al.*, 1993; Hassan *et al.*, 1994; Schuler *et al.*, 1994; Shaw *et al.*, 1994; Slattery *et al.*, 1995; Chattergoon *et al.*, 1997; McCune *et al.*, 2002). In an adult population, Slattery *et al.* (1995) reported that busulfan concentration in plasma is an important determinant of graft survival as well as of regimen-related toxicity (including hepatic veno-oclusive disease), and that the variability of busulfan pharmacokinetics is marked and precludes the use of a fixed dose for all ages and indications. In one study in which patients received 16 to 30 mg/kg of busulfan followed by cyclophosphamide in preparation for autologous, syngeneic, or allogeneic grafts, only busulfan concentration remained a significant determinant of graft rejection. An average concentration of busulfan at steady state of at least 200

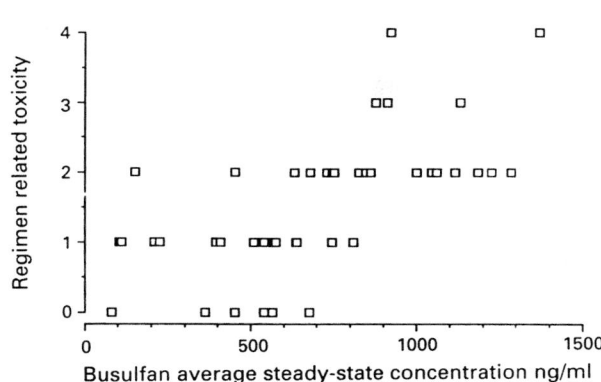

Fig. 33.2. Relationship between regimen-related toxicity score and busulfan average concentration at steady-state, $r_S = 0.717$; $P = .0001$. Reproduced, with permission, from Slattery et al. (1995).

ng/ml was needed to avoid rejection of an HLA-matched sibling graft, while 600 ng/ml was needed to avoid rejection of HLA-partially matched related, or HLA-matched unrelated, donor grafts. The toxicity of the cytoreductive regimen correlated with busulfan average concentration at steady state (Fig. 33.2), and busulfan clearance, when expressed in relation to body size, declined precipitously over the first decade of life (Fig. 33.3), confirming numerous previous observations that busulfan plasma levels are considerably lower in children in comparison to adults when administered at a fixed mg/kg dose.

Others have also reported the correlation between busulfan area under the curve and hepatic veno-occlusive disease (Dix et al., 1996; Vassal et al., 1996). Ljungman and colleagues (1995) reported a relationship between minimum busulfan concentration and posttransplant alopecia and subsequently (Ljungman et al., 1997) between busulfan concentration and transplant-related mortality (Fig. 33.4) and disease-free survival (Fig. 33.5). Slattery et al. (1997) described a relationship between

steady-state plasma busulfan concentration and relapse of chronic myeloid leukemia posttransplant (Fig. 33.6), as well as with posttransplant survival (Fig. 33.7). In a retrospective survey of patients allografted for treatment-related AML or myelodysplasia, the 5-year disease-free survival was higher, and the incidence of non-relapse mortality lower, in patients conditioned with a busulfan/cyclophosphamide regimen determined by targeted busulfan levels compared to that in patients prepared for transplant with a non-targeted busulfan/cyclophosphamide regimen or in patients given a cyclophosphamide/TBI regimen (Witherspoon et al., 2001).

In contrast to the above, Pawlowska et al. (1997) found no correlation with clinical outcome and busulfan plasma levels in a thalassemia transplant population. The reason for this disparity is unclear, although another study in thalassemic recipients did show an association between a high busulfan AUC and treatment-related mortality (Li et al., 1999). No correlation was found between busulfan pharmacokinetics and relapse risk in children transplanted for AML (Baker et al., 2000). In children given busulfan orally, a limited blood sampling technique (at 1, 1.5, 4, and 6 hours after an initial dose of 40 mg/m^2) has been recommended (Dupuis, Najdova, & Saunders, 2000).

Attempts to alter patient outcome by adjusting the dosages of oral busulfan dosages based on pharmacokinetic data of individual patients have met with various degrees of success (Dix et al., 1996; Tran et al., 2000). These studies included both adults and pediatric autologous and allogeneic transplant recipients who received various preparative regimens. The principle problems of excessive variability in the bioavailability and vomiting still remain with the administration of the high-dose busulfan as an oral formulation.

The bioavailability problem no longer remains an issue with availability of an FDA-approved intravenous formulation of busulfan (Busulfex) for use in adults undergoing high-dose busulfan therapy as part of the preparative regimen in combination with cyclophosphamide. Andersson et al. (2000) reported the results of a phase I study of this water-soluble formulation, which showed that this new formulation was safe and provided a consistent method by which to deliver high-dose busulfan. The authors recommended a dose of Busulfex of 0.8

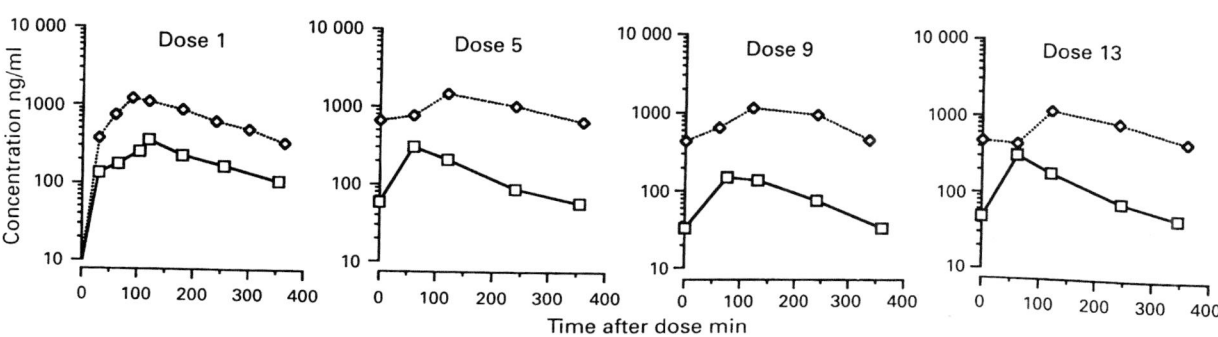

Fig. 33.3. Busulfan concentration-time curve for a child (UPN 6384; -□-) and an adult (UPN 5932; …◇…). Reproduced, with permission, from Slattery et al. (1995).

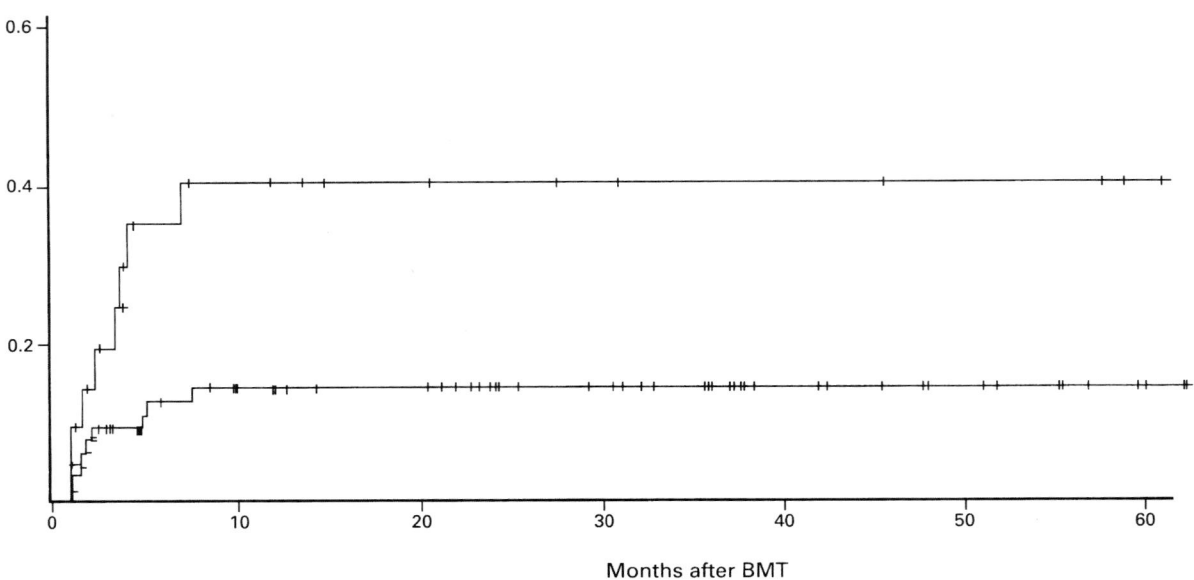

Fig. 33.4. Transplant-related mortality in allogeneic BMT patients in the highest quartile of busulfan concentrations (upper line) compared to patients with lower busulfan concentrations. Reproduced, with permission, from Ljungman *et al.* (1997).

mg/kg/dose to be administered over 2 hours (dose-equivalent to 1 mg/kg/dose of oral busulfan). This dose was estimated to reach a mean population area under the concentration-time curve (AUC) of 1100–1200 μM × min of single dose exposure. A completed phase II study from the same group using the BuCy2 (busulfan/cyclophosphamide) regimen with busulfan now administered intravenously at 0.8 mg/kg/dose every 6 hours for 16 doses demonstrated that the new regimen was well tolerated with excellent antitumor efficacy (Andersson *et al.*, 2002). Of the 61 adult patients, 86% of the individuals had an AUC between 800–1500 μM × min (Fig. 33.8). The intravenous preparation appears to reduce interpatient and interdose

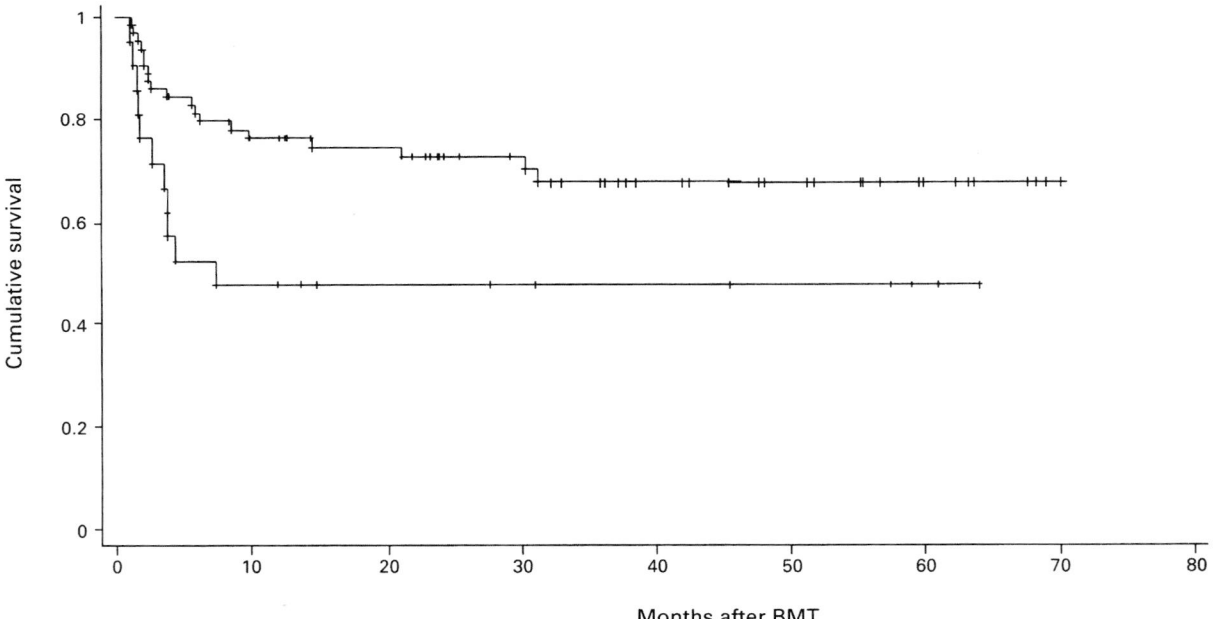

Fig. 33.5. Estimated disease-free survival in allogeneic BMT patients in the highest quartile of busulfan concentrations (lower line) compared to patients with lower busulfan concentrations. Reproduced, with permission, from Ljungman *et al.* (1997).

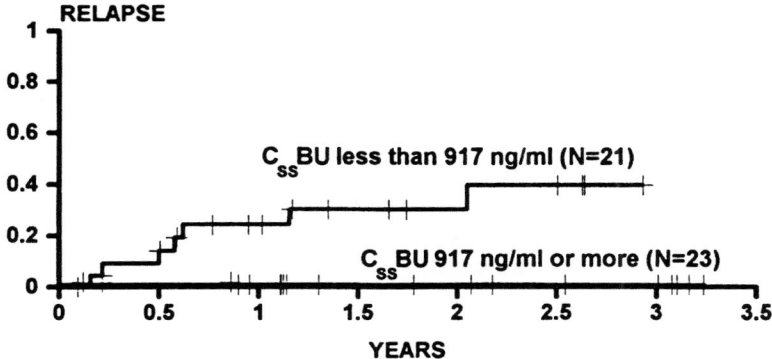

Fig. 33.6. The cumulative incidence of relapse for patients transplanted for CML in CP or AP categorized on the basis of busulfan steady-state concentrations (C_{SS}BU) greater than or less than the median (917 ng/ml) during conditioning. Patients were censored on the date of last cytogenetic examination. One patient who died on day 34 did not have any posttransplant cytogenetic examinations and was not evaluated for relapse. Tick marks denote patients at risk of relapse. The difference between the groups is statistically significant ($P = .0009$). Reproduced, with permission, from Slattery et al. (1997). Abbreviations: CP, chronic phase; AP, accelerated phase.

variability. Several questions still remain, such as optimal exposure (AUC or Css), administration schedule, and dosing for the pediatric population. In addition, a liposomal busulfan preparation has also been described and a significant linear correlation found between its dose and the area under the plasma concentration-time curve (Hassan et al., 2001, 2003).

Cyclophosphamide

Slattery and colleagues (1996) also studied the pharmacokinetics of cyclophosphamide and 4-hydroperoxycyclophosphamide (4HC) in patients being prepared for bone marrow transplantation with either busulfan/cyclophosphamide or cyclophosphamide/total body irradiation (TBI) to determine whether exposure to cyclophosphamide and its proximate toxic metabolite 4HC was modulated by other agents used in the preparative regimen. Patients receiving the busulfan/cyclophosphamide regimen also received phenytoin to minimize the risk of busulfan-related seizures. They found that prior administration of

busulfan (and/or phenytoin) significantly altered patient exposure to cyclophosphamide and 4HC: in busulfan/cyclophosphamide recipients, cyclophosphamide clearance was 112% greater, half-life 54% less, and the ratio of area under the plasma concentration-time curves of 4HC to cyclophosphamide 166% greater than in cyclophosphamide/TBI patients. McDonald and colleagues (2003) found the metabolism of cyclophosphamide to be highly variable, particularly for the metabolite o-carboxyethyl-phosphoramide mustard, whose area under the curve varied 16-fold. Exposure to this metabolite was related to development of VOD, non-relapse mortality, and survival after adjusting for age and irradiation dose.

Antibacterial and antifungal agents

Aminoglycoside antibiotics

Amikacin, gentamicin, netilmicin, and tobramycin are frequently used to treat aerobic, Gram-negative infections in

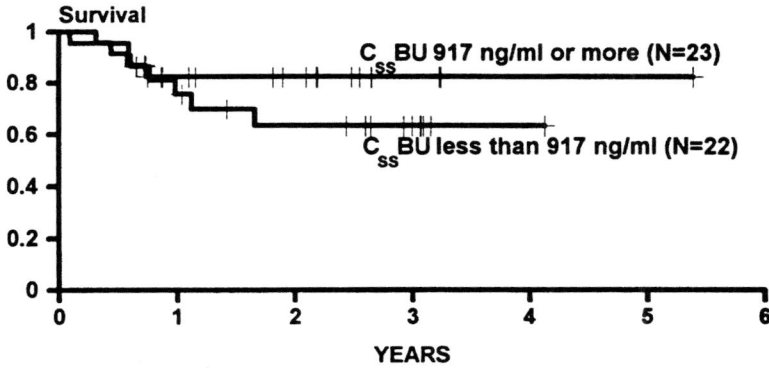

Fig. 33.7. Kaplan-Meier statistics on the survival of patients transplanted for CML in CP or AP categorized on the basis of busulfan steady-state concentrations (C_{SS}BU) greater than or less than the median (917 ng/ml) during conditioning. Patients were censored on the date of last contact. Tick marks denote survivors. The difference between the groups is not statistically significant ($P = .33$). Reproduced, with permission, from Slattery et al. (1997). Abbreviations: CP, chronic phase; AP, accelerated phase.

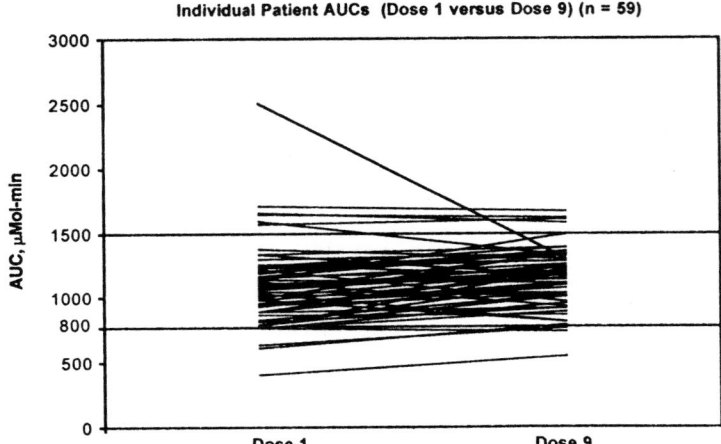

Fig. 33.8. Individual patient AUC values for dose 1 and dose 9 (59 patients). Interpatient results for the entire group ($n = 59$) for both dose 1 and dose 9 are represented vertically and show consistency and predictability across all patients. Results for each patient are represented horizontally where each line joins a single patient's dose 1 and dose 9 AUC value (intrapatient results). Reproduced, with permission, from Andersson et al. (2002).

immunosuppressed hematopoietic stem cell transplant recipients and are often commenced empirically in febrile, neutropenic patients. Specific immunoassays are readily available to assay these drugs. These antibiotics are principally eliminated by renal excretion. Clearance is decreased in patients with impaired renal function, and drug accumulation will occur. Several investigators observed alteration in the disposition of aminoglycoside clearance in patients with cancer (Hary et al., 1989; Higa et al., 1987; Zeitany et al., 1990). These alterations included increases in the mean clearance and volume of distribution of the aminoglycosides, which may lead to subtherapeutic concentration during treatment. Thus, dosage needs to be individualized according to estimated creatinine clearance and drug concentrations. Drug concentrations should be monitored closely, at least every 48 hours, to minimize the risk of toxicity. The principal concentration-related toxicities are ototoxicity, including auditory and vestibular dysfunction, and nephrotoxicity. Increased risk factors for developing these toxicities are well recognized to be related to prior exposure to aminoglycosides, cumulative dose, trough concentrations above 2 mg/l (amikacin trough concentrations above 5 mg/l), prolonged duration of therapy, concurrent administration of other potential nephrotoxic agents, impaired renal function, dehydration, advanced age, and underlying disease state.

Once-daily dosing of aminoglycosides has been advocated to maximize efficacy (the concentration-dependent bacterial kill) while minimizing toxicity (Begg, Barclay, & Duffull, 1995). Even though the half-life of aminoglycosides is short in most patients (around 2 to 4 hours), and concentrations fall below the minimum inhibitory concentration (MIC) for most organisms for a large part of such dosing intervals, a "postantibiotic" effect, whereby bacterial kill continues long after concentrations have fallen below the laboratory-determined MIC, has been described.

In such a regimen, high peak concentrations maximize the concentration-dependent bactericidal effect, ensuring bacterial kill, and trough concentrations are low, thus minimizing the risk of toxicity. Dosing can be totally individualized based on measured concentrations, with starting doses for a patient with normal renal function being in the range of 5 to 7 mg/kg (Begg, Barclay, & Duffull, 1995). A retrospective review of the use of once-daily gentamicin administration in thirty-three HSC transplant recipients was reported to show significant toxicities, including nephrotoxicity (3%) and ototoxicity (12%) (Warkentin et al., 1999). While the incidence of nephrotoxicity was within the reported range, the incidence of ototoxicity was higher than normally observed, and was attributed to the longer duration of therapy.

Vancomycin

Vancomycin is another antibiotic that is mainly eliminated by the kidneys. Patients with renal impairment are reported to be at risk of ototoxicity and nephrotoxicity if vancomycin dosage is not reduced and individualized based on creatinine clearance. It is not clear whether elevated peak or trough concentrations are associated with development of these toxicities. Histamine-like reactions, characterized by flushing, pruritic rash, and tachycardia, due to transiently high vancomycin concentrations, are generally avoided by administering the drug in a slow intravenous infusion, limited to 15 mg/minute. Samples for estimation of peak concentration are generally collected one-half to one hour after the end of the infusion. It is important if peak concentrations are to be monitored that the exact time of infusion and blood sampling are documented (Duffull, Chambers, & Begg, 1993). Trough concentrations are more often monitored, and any patient with a trough concentration reported above 5 to 10 mg/l should be investigated. Specific immunoassays are available for vancomycin quantitation. Similar to the aminoglycosides, alteration in the disposition of vancomycin in patients with hematologic malignancies has been described. Once again a mandate for dose individualization and close monitoring is required, to ensure the safe and effective administration of the optimal dose of vancomycin (and other antimicrobial agents).

Immune suppressive agents

Cyclosporine

Cyclosporine is used to prevent rejection and graft-versus-host disease (GVHD) in allogeneic HSC transplant recipients. The major concentration-related toxicity is nephrotoxicity, but a clear "cut-off" concentration for this adverse effect has not been determined. Many centers monitor this effect by close attention to serum creatinine concentrations, rather than an upper limit of cyclosporine concentration. Hepatoxicity, neurotoxicity and hypertension are also of concern.

Many different assays are used to monitor cyclosporine concentrations (Table 33.2). Some of these measure parent drug together with metabolites (for example, some of the immunoassays), while the HPLC assays, which are more expensive and time-consuming, generally separate parent drug from metabolites. Some of the metabolites of cyclosporine are reported to have immunosuppressive activity, so that any quoted therapeutic concentration range should clearly state whether any metabolites are included in this range. As cyclosporine binds to erythrocytes, lipoproteins, and other constituents of blood, whole blood concentrations are significantly higher than those measured in plasma or serum. Due to the temperature dependence of binding and difficulty of reproducibly separating plasma or serum from cells, most laboratories now measure whole blood concentrations. Different cyclosporine monitoring guidelines have been established (Shaw *et al.*, 1990; Holt *et al.*, 1994; Morris, Tett, & Ray, 1994). Commonly for allogeneic HSC transplant recipients, a minimum trough whole blood concentration of 200 µg/l (200 ng/ml) is aimed for in the immediate posttransplant period, with a tapering dose regimen (5% per week) often commenced 50 days posttransplant, although this may vary between institutions.

Neoral is a microemulsion formulation of cyclosporine which has improved bioavailability through increased intestinal absorption, with less variable pharmacokinetic parameters, at least in non-BMT patients. In one study, doubling the last i.v. dose of cyclosporine during the switch to oral administration of Neoral was found to give the best therapeutic range concentration of Neoral (Parquet *et al.*, 2000).

Tacrolimus (FK-506)

Tacrolimus (previously known as FK-506) has a similar mechanism of action to cyclosporine and is useful in allogeneic HSC transplantation (Przepiorka *et al.*, 1999). Pharmacokinetic studies have been conducted in this group of patients (Mekki, Piscitelli, & Fitzsimmons, 1993; Boswell *et al.*, 1998) (Fig. 33.9). In the latter study, all patients received i.v. tacrolimus initially and were subsequently switched to oral dosing. Patients received methotrexate by i.v. bolus on days 1, 3, 6, and 11 posttransplant. Patients were started on i.v. corticosteroids beginning on day 7 posttransplant. The noncompartmental pharmocokinetics of tacrolimus based on whole blood concentrations were determined following the i.v. and oral doses and were not different at steady-state compared to those following a single dose. The mean terminal elimination half-life of tacrolimus was 18.2 hours following i.v. administration; the total body clearance was 71 ml/hr/kg, and the volume of distribution was 1.67 l/kg. Coadministration of methylprednisolone or methotrexate did not significantly alter tacrolimus pharmacokinetics. The oral bioavailability was 31% to 49%. Trough blood concentrations [C_{min} at 0 hr (r = 0.92) and at 12 hr (r = 0.93)] indicated that either time point can be used for therapeutic drug monitoring in patient management. In solid organ transplant recipients, whole blood concentrations (measured by

Table 33.2. Cyclosporine assays

Assay	Target whole blood trough (12 hour) level (ng/ml)	Metabolites measured
Monoclonal radioimmunoassay	200–400	Yes
Monoclonal fluorescence polarization assay	200–400	Yes
Polyclonal immunoassay (TDX)	400–900	Yes
High-pressure liquid chromatography	150–250	No

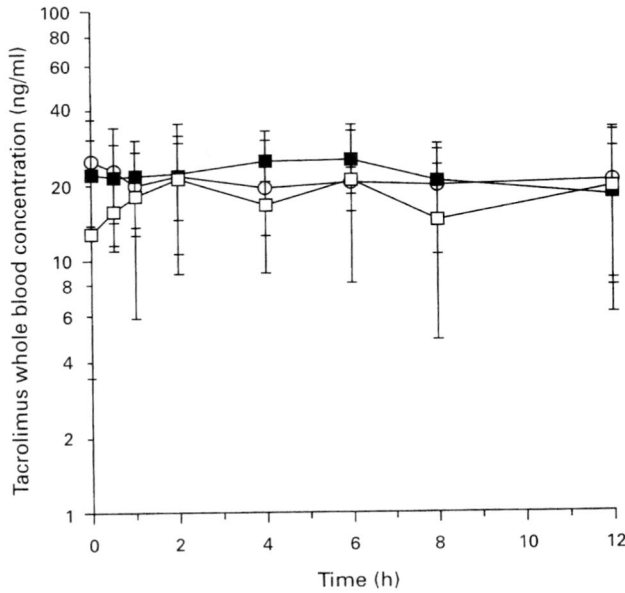

Fig. 33.9. Mean (S.D.) tacrolimus whole blood concentrations at steady state following continuous i.v. infusion of tacrolimus alone (○), tacrolimus plus methylprednisolone (■) or tacrolimus plus methotrexate (□). Reproduced, with permission, from Boswell *et al.* (1998).

immunoassay or the more sensitive and specific HPLC/electro-spray tandem mass spectometry) of 2 to 15 μg/l are targeted (Taylor *et al.,* 1996). For allogeneic HSC transplant recipients the trough whole blood concentration should be kept below 20 ng/ml (20 μg/l) (see Chapter 83). Children appear to have more rapid tacrolimus clearance than adults and may need to begin therapy earlier in order to obtain stable and optimal levels (Mehta *et al.,* 1999). Plasmapheresis does not appear to affect the blood concentration (Hale *et al.,* 2000).

Methotrexate

Methotrexate is often used in low doses posttransplant as a component of GVHD prophylaxis (usually with cyclosporine or tacrolimus) Renal excretion is the major route of elimination. Assays are available to ensure that concentrations are minimal before subsequent doses are administered, thus minimizing the risk to the nascent hematopoietic stem cells. For example, plasma concentrations of methotrexate are often measured, using an immunoassay, in samples collected 12 and 24 hours after the first methotrexate dose. If the concentration is below the limit of sensitivity of the assay (0.03 mmol/l), subsequent doses of methotrexate can be given. Careful monitoring needs to be performed if renal impairment or large extravascular fluid collections (e.g., pleural effusions, ascites) are present. A relatively well-defined range for bone marrow toxicity allows initiation of folinic acid rescue for high concentrations (Fig. 33.10 and see Chapter 83).

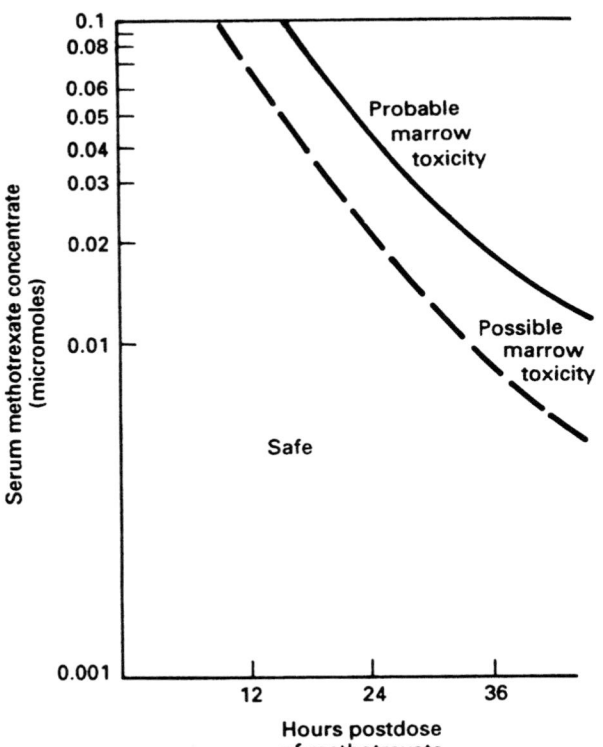

Fig. 33.10. Relationship between plasma methotrexate concentration (μmol) and bone marrow toxicity early posttransplantation. (Reproduced by kind permission of Dr. Archie Bleyer.)

Mycophenolate mofetil

Mycophenolic acid (MPA) is the active metabolite of mycophenolate mofetil (MMF) which has been used successfully as an immunosuppressant in solid organ transplantation in combination with cyclosporine and corticosteroids. After oral ingestion, MMF is rapidly converted to MPA in the liver. Mycophenolic acid is inactivated by glucuronidation and then excreted in the urine and bile. The elimination half-life is approximately 14 hours. Enterohepatic recirculation may occur with MPA, which may lead to enhanced exposure. Mycophenolic acid inhibits inosine monophosphate dehydrogenase, the principle enzyme responsible for the de novo synthesis of purines. Since T and B cell proliferation requires this pathway to synthesize GTP and dGTP, inhibition of purine synthesis leads to the inhibition of T and B cell proliferation (Mele & Halloran, 2000).

Several small series have utilized MMF in combination with cyclosporine (Jenke *et al.,* 2001), or cyclosporine and methotrexate (Basara *et al.,* 2000) for the prevention of GVHD. These studies showed that MMF in the combination regimen was well tolerated and effective in reducing the incidence of acute GVHD. Jenke *et al.* observed more grade II–III acute GVHD in patients with lower MPA trough concentrations. Additionally, the same group observed a much lower trough concentration of MPA when administered in equal dosing to patients after HSCT than seen in patients after solid organ transplantation or in healthy volunteers. MMF has also been combined with tacrolimus (Mookerjee *et al.,* 1999) as a salvage regimen for patients with refractory chronic GHVD, with satisfactory responses observed in this small retrospective analysis. Additional investigation is needed to determine if there is any correlation between MPA trough concentration and the development of acute GVHD, and to study the effects of the pretransplant conditioning regimen on the disposition of MMF.

Anticonvulsants

Hematopoietic stem cell transplant recipients may receive anticonvulsant therapy with drugs such as phenytoin, carbamazepine, or clonazepam (e.g., as prophylaxis for busulfan-induced seizures). Immunoassays are available for most of these drugs. Phenytoin is a difficult drug to dose because its kinetics are not linear in the therapeutic concentration range and there is wide interindividual variability in kinetic parameters. In practice, this means that doubling the dose is likely to more than double the concentration, and dosage adjustments of less than 100 mg/day can take certain patients from below the lower limit of the range to well above the concentrations where toxicity might be expected. If enzyme saturation occurs, steady state will never be reached, as more is entering the body than can be eliminated. Bayesian dosage prediction programs are particularly useful for drugs such as phenytoin (Garcia *et al.,* 1994). Similarly, carbamazepine is quite difficult to dose correctly. Carbamazepine induces its own metabolism, such that doses need to be gradually increased (to about twice the starting dose) over the first month to maintain the same concentration.

The future

There are many drugs for which it would be useful to use concentration targeting strategies in bone marrow and blood stem cell transplant recipients (for example, some of the other agents used against infections, such as fluconazole). On-going investigations into the utilization of a single, small test dose for intravenous busulfan days prior to receiving intravenous busulfan-based preparative regimen for HSCT may assist in dose individualization of this agent. Studies in the dosing schedule and monitoring strategy to maximize the immunosupresive effects of MMF will assist clinicians to best utilize this new agent in the prevention and treatment of GVHD. As assay methodology improves and more drugs are rigorously studied to determine the relationship between drug concentration, efficacy, and toxicity, therapeutic concentration monitoring is likely to become a more useful tool for clinicians. In all developmental work, the effect on the patient's outcome should be the major consideration.

References

Andersson, B. S., Kashyap, A., Gian, V. et al. (2002). Conditioning therapy with intravenous busulfan and cyclophosphamide (IV BuCy2) for hematologic maglignancies prior to allogeneic stem cell transplantation: a phase II study. Biology of Blood and Marrow Transplantation, 8, 145–54.

Andersson, B. S., Madden, T., Tran, H. T. et al. (2000). Acute safety and pharmacokinetics of intravenous busulfan when used with oral busulfan and cyclophosphamide as pretransplantation conditioning therapy: a phase I study. Biology of Blood and Marrow Transplantation, 6, 548–54.

Basara, N., Blau, W. I., Kiehl, M. G. et al. (2000). Mycophenolate mofetil for the prophylaxis of acute GVHD in HLA-mismatched bone marrow transplant patients. Clinical Transplanatation, 14, 121–126.

Baker, K. S., Bostrom, B., DeFor, T. et al. (2000). Busulfan pharmakokinetics do not predict relapse in acute myeloid leukemia. Bone Marrow Transplantation, 26, 607–14.

Begg, E. J., Barclay, M. L., & Duffull, S. B. (1995). A suggested approach to once-daily aminoglycoside dosing. British Journal of Clinical Pharmacology, 39, 605–9.

Boswell, G. W., Berkersky, I., Fay, J. et al. (1998). Tacrolimus pharmacokinetics in BMT patients. Bone Marrow Transplantation, 21, 23–8.

Chattergoon, D. S., Saunders, E. F., Klein, J. et al. (1997). An improved limited sampling method for individualised busulphan dosing in bone marrow transplantation in children. Bone Marrow Transplantation, 20, 347–54.

Dix, S. P., Wingard, J. R., Mullins, R. E. et al. (1996). Association of busulfan area under the curve with veno-occlusive disease following BMT. Bone Marrow Transplantation, 17, 225–30.

Duffull, S. B., Chambers, S. T., & Begg, E. J. (1993). How vancomycin is used in Australasia—a survey. Australian and New Zealand Journal of Medicine, 23, 662–6.

Dupuis, L. L., Najdova, M., & Saunders, E. F. (2000). Retrospective appraisal of busulfan dose adjustment in children. Bone Marrow Transplantation, 26, 1143–7.

Embree, L., Burns, R. B., Heggie, J. R. et al. (1993). Gas-chromatographic analysis of busulphan for therapeutic drug monitoring. Cancer Chemotherapy and Pharmacology, 32, 137–42.

Garcia, M. J., Gavira, R., Buelga, D. S. et al. (1994). Predictive performance of two phenytoin pharmacokinetic dosing programs from non-steady-state data. Therapeutic Drug Monitoring, 16, 380–7.

Grochow, L. B. (1993). Busulfan disposition: the role of therapeutic drug monitoring in bone marrow transplantation induction regimens. Seminars in Oncology, 20 (Suppl 4), 18–25.

Grochow, L. B., Krivit, W., Whitley, C. B., & Blazar, B. (1990). Busulfan disposition in children. Blood, 75, 1723–27.

Hale, G. A., Reece, D. E., Munn, R. K., Kniska, A. B., & Phillips, G. L. (2000). Blood tacrolimus concentrations in bone marrow transplant patients undergoing plasmapheresis. Bone Marrow Transplantation, 25, 449–51.

Hary, L., Andreak, M., Beraert, F. R. et al. (1989). Pharmacokinetics of amikacin in febrile neutropenic patients. Current Therapeutic Research, 46, 821–27.

Hassan, M., Fasth, A., Gerritsen, B. et al. (1996). Busulfan kinetics and limited sampling model in children with leukemia and inherited disorders. Bone Marrow Transplant, 18, 843–850.

Hassan, M., Ljungman, P., Bolme, P. et al. (1994). Busulfan bioavailability. Blood, 84, 2144–50.

Hassan, Z., Ljungman, P. Ringden, O. et al. (2001). Pharmacokinetics of liposomal busulphan in man. Bone Marrow Transplantation, 27, 479–85.

Hassan, M., Oberg, G., Bekassy, A. N. et al. (1991). Pharmacokinetics of high-dose busulphan in relation to age and chronopharmacology. Cancer Chemotherapy and Pharmacology, 28, 130–4.

Hassan, M., Nilsson, C., Gungor, T. et al. (2003). A phase II trial of liposomal busulphan as an intravenous myeloablative agent prior to stem cell transplantation: 500 mg/m^2 as an optimal total dose for conditioning. Bone Marrow Transplantation, 30, 833–41.

Higa, G. M., Murray, W. E. (1987). Alteration in aminoglycoside pharmacokinetics in patients with cancer. Clinical Pharmacy, 6, 963–66.

Holford, N.H.G. & Tett, S. (1997). Therapeutic drug monitoring: the strategy of target concentration intervention. In Avery's Drug Treatment, ed. T. Speight & N. Holford, pp. 225–229. Auckland, New Zealand: Adis International Limited.

Holt, D. W., Johnston, A., Roberts, N. B. et al. (1994). Methodological and clinical aspects of cyclosporine monitoring: report of the Association of Clinical Biochemists' Task Force. Annals of Clinical Biochemistry, 31, 420–46.

Jenke, A., Renner, U., Richte, M., et al. (2001). Pharmacokinetics of intravenous mycophenolate mofetil after allogeneic blood stem cell transplantation. Clinical Transplantation, 15, 176–84.

Li, C. K., Yuen, P.M.P., Wong, R. et al. (1999). Busulphan level and early mortality in thalassemia patients after BMT. Bone Marrow Transplantation, 23, 307–10.

Ljungman, P., Hassan, M., Békássy, A. N. et al. (1995). Busulfan concentration in relation to permanent alopecia in recipients of bone marrow transplants. Bone Marrow Transplantation, 15, 869–71.

Ljungman, P., Hassan, M., Békássy, A. N. et al. (1997). High busulfan concentrations are associated with increased transplant-related mortality in allogeneic bone marrow transplant patients. Bone Marrow Transplantation, 20, 909–13.

McCune, J. S., Gooley, T., Gibbs, J. P. et al. (2002). Busulfan concentration and graft rejection in pediatric patients undergoing hematopoietic stem cell transplantation. *Bone Marrow Transplantation,* **30,** 167–73.

McDonald, G. B., Slattery, J. T., Bouvier, M. E. et al. (2003). Cyclophosphamide metabolism, liver toxicity, and mortality following hematopoietic stem cell transplantation. *Blood,* **101,** 2043–8.

Mehta, P., Beltz, S., Kedar, A. et al. (1999). Increased clearance of tacrolimus in children: need for higher doses and earlier initiation prior to bone marrow transplantation. *Bone Marrow Transplantation,* **24,** 1323–7.

Mekki, Q. A., Piscitelli, D., & Fitzsimmons, W. E. (1993). Pharmacokinetics of tacrolimus in bone marrow transplant recipients. *Clinical Pharmacology and Therapeutics,* **55,** 149.

Mele, T. S. & Halloran, P. F. (2000). The use of mycophenolate mofetil in transplant recipients. *Immunopharmacology,* **47,** 215.

Mookerjee, B., Altomonte, V., & Volgelsang, G. (1999). Salvage therapy for refractory chronic graft versus-host disease with mycophenolate mofetil and tacrolimus. *Bone Marrow Transplanation,* **24,** 517–520.

Morris, R. G., Tett, S. E., & Ray, J. E. (1994). Cyclosporine-A monitoring in Australia: consensus recommendations. *Therapeutic Drug Monitoring,* **16,** 570–6.

Parquet, N., Reigneau, O., Humbert, H. et al. (2000). New oral formulation of cyclosporin A (Neoral) pharmacokinetics in allogeneic bone marrow transplant recipients. *Bone Marrow Transplantation,* **25,** 965–8.

Pawlowska, A. B., Blazar, B. R., Angelucci, E. et al. (1997). Relationship of plasma pharmacokinetics of high-dose oral busulfan to the outcome of allogeneic bone marrow transplantation in children with thalassemia. *Bone Marrow Transplantation,* **20,** 915–20.

Przepiorka, D., Devine, S. M., Fay, J. W., Uberti, J. P, & Wingard, J. R. (1999). Practical considerations in the use of tacrilomus for allogeneic marrow transplantation. *Bone Marrow Transplantation,* **24,** 1053–6.

Regazzi, M. B., Locatelli, F., Buggia, I. et al. (1992). Disposition of high-dose busulfan in pediatric patients undergoing bone marrow transplantation. *Clinical Pharmacology and Therapy,* **53,** 45–52.

Santos, G. W., Tutschka, P. J., Brookmeyer, R. et al. (1983). Marrow transplanation for acute nonlymphocytic leukemia after treatment with busulfan and cyclophosphamide. *New England Journal of Medicine,* **309,** 1347–1353.

Schuler, U., Schroer, S., Kühnle, A. et al. (1994). Busulphan pharmacokinetics in bone marrow transplant patients: is drug monitoring warranted? *Bone Marrow Transplantation,* **14,** 759–65.

Shaw, P. J., Scharping, C. E., Brian, R. J., & Earl, J. W. (1994). Busulfan pharmacokinetics using a single daily high-dose regimen in children with acute leukemia. *Blood,* **84,** 2357–62.

Shaw, L. M., Yatscoff, R. W., Bowers, L. D. et al. (1990). Canadian consensus meeting on cyclosporine monitoring: report of the consensus panel. *Clinical Chemistry,* **36,** 1841–6.

Slattery, J. T., Clift, R. A., Buckner, C. D. et al. (1997). Marrow transplantation for chronic myeloid leukemia: the influence of plasma busulfan levels on the outcome of transplantation. *Blood,* **89,** 3055–60.

Slattery, J. T., Kalhorn, T. F., McDonald, G. B. et al. (1996). Conditioning regimen-dependent disposition of cyclophosphamide and hydroxycyclophosphamide in human marrow transplantation patients. *Journal of Clinical Oncology,* **14,** 1484–94.

Slattery, J. T., Sanders, J. E., Buckner, C. D. et al. (1995). Graft-rejection and toxicity following bone marrow transplantation in relation to busulfan pharmacokinetics. *Bone Marrow Transplantation,* **16,** 31–42.

Taylor, P. J., Jones, A., Balderson, G. A. et al. (1996). Sensitive and specific quantitative analysis of tacrolimus (FK506) in blood by liquid chromatography–electrospray tandem mass spectrometry. *Clinical Chemistry,* **42,** 279–85.

Thomson, A. H. & Whiting, B. (1992). Bayesian parameter estimation and population pharmacokinetics. *Clinical Pharmacokinetics,* **22,** 447–67.

Tran, H. T., Madden, T., Petropoulos, D. et al. (2000). Individualizing high-dose oral busulfan: prospective dose adjustment in a pediatric population undergoing allogeneic stem cell transplantation for advanced hematologic malignancies. *Bone Marrow Transplantation,* **26,** 463–70.

Vassal, G., Deroussent, A., Challine, D. et al. (1992). Is 600mg/m^2 the appropriate dose of busulfan in children undergoing bone marrow transplantation? *Blood,* **79,** 2475–9.

Vassal, G., Deroussent, A., Hartmann, O. et al. (1990). Dose-dependent neurotoxicity of high-dose busulfan in children: a clinical pharmacological study. *Cancer Research,* **50,** 6203–6207.

Vassal, G., Fischer, A., Challine, D. et al. (1993). Busulphan disposition below the age of three: alteration in children with lysosomal storage disease. *Blood,* **82,** 1030–4.

Vassal, G., Koscielny, S., Challine, D. et al. (1996). Busulfan disposition and hepatic veno-occlusive disease in children undergoing bone marrow transplantation. *Cancer Chemotherapy and Pharmacology,* **37,** 247–53.

Warkentin, D., Ippoliti, C., Bruton, J. et al. (1999). Toxicity of single dose gentamicin in stem cell transplantation. *Bone Marrow Transplantation,* **24,** 57–61.

Witherspoon, R. P., Deeg, H. J., Storer, B. et al. (2001). Hematopoietic stem cell transplantation for treatment-related leukemia or myelodysplasia. *Journal of Clinical Oncology,* **19,** 2134–41.

Yeager, A. M., Wagner, J. E. Jr., Graham, M. L. et al. (1992). Optimisation of busulphan dosage in children undergoing bone marrow transplantation: a pharmacokinetic study of dose escalation. *Blood,* **80,** 2425–8.

Zeitany, R. G., Saghir, N. E., Santhosh-Kumar, C. R. et al. (1990). Increased aminoglycoside dosage requirements in hematologic malignancy. *Antimicrobial Agents and Chemotherapy,* **34,** 702–708.

PART III CLINICAL RESULTS I: AUTOLOGOUS HEMATOPOIETIC STEM CELL TRANSPLANTATION

34 Autologous hematopoietic stem cell transplantation for non-Hodgkin's lymphoma

PHILIP J. BIERMAN AND ARNOLD S. FREEDMAN

University of Nebraska Medical Center, Omaha and Dana-Farber Cancer Institute, Harvard University, Boston, USA

Introduction

According to data from the Surveillance, Epidemiology, and End Results (SEER) program of the National Cancer Institute there were predicted to be 53,900 new cases of non-Hodgkin's lymphoma (NHL) in the United States in 2002, and 24,400 people will die with this diagnosis. Approximately 4% of all new cancers in the United States are NHL. The incidence rate for NHL increased approximately 3–4% yearly over the last four decades, although there is evidence that there is now a plateau in this "epidemic" of lymphoma. The increase in NHL incidence is largely unexplained, but it is partially related to the aging population as well as to cases of NHL attributable to infection with the human immunodeficiency virus (HIV). In addition, some of the increase in incidence can be explained by improvements in our ability to diagnose lymphoma in cases that might have previously been called pseudolymphoma or atypical lymphoid hyperplasia, and cases that would have previously been classified as Hodgkin's disease. Improved imaging techniques and less invasive biopsy methods have also likely accounted for some of the increase in NHL incidence, although in aggregate these factors only account for a fraction of the increase and unknown environmental exposures have been proposed to account for the remainder.

A number of factors have been associated with the development of NHL, although studies have often shown conflicting results regarding causation. Some of the factors that have been reported to be associated with the development of NHL are shown in Table 34.1. Until recently, the most common lymphoma classification system in use in the United States was the Working Formulation, while the Kiel Classification was used more commonly in Europe. The Revised European-American Classification System (REAL) was developed by the International Lymphoma Study Group to incorporate additional tools such as immunophenotyping and cytogenetics, and to make the classification of lymphomas more clinically relevant. This classification is shown in Table 34.2 (Harris *et al.*, 1994). Table 34.3 shows the new World Health Organization (WHO) classification of lymphoid neoplasms, which is largely a modification of the REAL classification (Harris, 2001; Jaffe & Ralfkiaer, 2001). The immunophenotype of lymphoid neoplasms (Table 34.4) can be useful for diagnosis and prognosis and for identification of a monoclonal population of tumor cells in blood, marrow, or other tissue, particularly in situations of minimal residual disease. It may also be useful for the assessment of the efficacy of tumor-purging procedures on blood stem cell or bone marrow preparations. Cytogenetic abnormalities associated with lymphoid neoplasms are shown in Table 34.5.

The Ann Arbor staging system, originally developed for the staging of Hodgkin's disease, is routinely used for NHL patients

Table 34.1. *Possible causative factors in non-Hodgkin's lymphoma*

Occupational/environmental
  Pesticides
    Phenoxy herbicides
    Triazine herbicides
    Organophosphate insecticides
  Organic solvents
  Ultraviolet light
  Hair dyes
  Ionizing radiation
  Diet
Infectious agents
  Epstein-Barr virus
  HTLV-1
  HHV-8
  Hepatitis C virus
  Helicobacter pylori
Immunodeficiency
  Congenital
    Ataxia-telangiectasia
    Severe combined immunodeficiency
    Wiskott-Aldrich syndrome
    X-linked lymphoproliferative syndrome
  Acquired
    Autoimmune diseases
      Rheumatoid arthritis
      Sjögren syndrome
    Iatrogenic immunodeficiencies
      Organ transplantation
      Azathioprine, cyclosporine, or anti-CD3 treatment
  HIV infection/AIDS

Table 34.2. *A list of lymphoid neoplasms recognized by the International Lymphoma Study Group*

B-cell neoplasms
I. Precursor B-cell neoplasm: Precursor B-lymphoblastic leukemia/lymphoma
II. Peripheral B-cell neoplasms
  1. B-cell chronic lymphocytic leukemia/prolymphocytic leukemia/small lymphocytic lymphoma
  2. Lymphoplasmacytoid lymphoma/immunocytoma
  3. Mantle-cell lymphoma
  4. Follicle-center lymphoma, follicular
    Provisional cytologic grades: I (small cell), II (mixed small and large cell), III (large cell)
  5. Marginal-zone B-cell lymphoma
  6. Provisional entity: splenic marginal-zone lymphoma (+ villous lymphocytes)
  7. Hairy-cell leukemia
  8. Plasmacytoma/plasma-cell myeloma
  9. Diffuse large B-cell lymphoma Subtype: primary mediastinal (thymic) B-cell lymphoma
  10. Burkitt's lymphoma[a]
  11. Provisional entity: high-grade B-cell lymphoma, Burkitt-like

T-cell and putative NK-cell neoplasms
I. Precursor T-cell neoplasm: Precursor T-lymphoblastic lymphoma/leukemia
II. Peripheral T-cell and NK-cell neoplasms
  1. T-cell chronic lymphocytic leukemia/prolymphocytic leukemia
  2. Large granular-lymphocyte leukemia (LGL) T-cell type NK-cell type
  3. Mycosis fungoides/Sézary syndrome[b]
  4. Peripheral T-cell lymphomas, unspecified
    Provisional cytologic categories: medium-sized cell, mixed medium and large cell, large cell, lymphoepithelioid cell
    Provisional subtype: hepatosplenic γδ T-cell lymphoma
    Provisional subtype: subcutaneous panniculitic T-cell lymphoma
  5. Angioimmunoblastic T-cell lymphoma (AILD)
  6. Angiocentric lymphoma
  7. Intestinal T-cell lymphoma (+ enteropathy associated)
  8. Adult T-cell lymphoma/leukemia (ATL/L)
  9. Anaplastic large-cell lymphoma (ALCL), CD30+, T- and null-cell types
  10. Provisional entity: anaplastic large-cell lymphoma; Hodgkin's-like

Reproduced, with permission, from Harris *et al.* (1994).
[a]Denis Burkitt, British surgeon, 1911–1993.
[b]A. Sezary, French dermatologist, 1880–1956.

Table 34.3. *WHO histological classification of mature B-cell, T-cell, and NK-cell neoplasms*

B-cell neoplasms
Precursor B-cell neoplasm; Precursor B lymphoblastic leukemia/lymphoma

Mature B-cell neoplasms
  Chronic lymphocytic leukemia/small lymphocytic lymphoma
  B-cell prolymphocytic leukemia
  Lymphoplasmacytic lymphoma
  Splenic marginal zone lymphoma
  Hairy cell leukemia
  Plasma cell myeloma
  Monoclonal gammopathy of undetermined significance (MGUS)
  Solitary plasmacytoma of bone
  Extraosseous plasmacytoma
  Primary amyloidosis
  Heavy chain diseases
  Extranodal marginal zone B-cell lymphoma of mucosa-associated lymphoid tissue (MALT-lymphoma)
  Nodal marginal zone B-cell lymphoma
  Follicular lymphoma
  Mantle cell lymphoma
  Diffuse large B-cell lymphoma
  Mediastinal (thymic) large B-cell lymphoma
  Intravascular large B-cell lymphoma
  Primary effusion lymphoma
  Burkitt lymphoma/leukemia

B-cell proliferations of uncertain malignant-potential
  Lymphomatoid granulomatosis
  Post-transplant lymphoproliferative disorder, polymorphic

T-cell and NK-cell neoplasms
Leukemic/disseminated
  T-cell prolymphocytic leukemia
  T-cell large granular lymphocytic leukemia
  Aggressive NK cell leukemia
  Adult T-cell leukemia/lymphoma

Cutaneous
  Mycosis fungoides
  Sézary syndrome
  Primary cutaneous anaplastic large cell lymphoma
  Lymphomatoid papulosis

Other extranodal
  Extranodal NK/T cell lymphoma, nasal type
  Enteropathy-type T-cell lymphoma
  Hepatosplenic T-cell lymphoma
  Subcutaneous panniculitis-like T-cell lymphoma

Nodal
  Angioimmunoblastic T-cell lymphoma
  Peripheral T-cell lymphoma, unspecified
  Anaplastic large cell lymphoma

Neoplasm of uncertain lineage and stage of differentiation
  Blastic NK cell lymphoma

Adapted from Jaffe, Harris, Stein, & Vardiman (2001).

also (Carbone *et al.,* 1971). This and the Cotswald modifications are shown in Table 34.6. The stage of disease at presentation, however, is only one of a number of important prognostic predictors of response and disease-free survival developed initially for patients with aggressive NHL treated with CHOP (cyclophosphamide, doxorubicin, vincristine, prednisone)-type conventional dose chemotherapy. The outcome with such chemotherapy according to the risk groups defined by the International Prognostic Index (IPI) and age-adjusted International Prognostic Index are shown in Table 34.7 and in Figures 34.1 and 34.2.

Table 34.4. *Immune phenotype of lymphoid neoplasms*

	Tdt	CD19	CD20	CD22	CD79a	CD10	DR	SIg	cMU	CD34	CD13	CD33	SIgM	SIgD	cIg	CD5	CD23	CD43	CD11c	CD25
B-cell neoplasms																				
I. Precursor B cell neoplasm: Precursor B lymphoblastic leukemia/lymphoma	+	+	-/+	+	+	+/-	+	-	-/+	+/-	occ	occ								
II. Peripheral B cell neoplasms																				
B cell chronic lymphocytic leukemia/prolymphocytic leukemia/small lymphocytic lymphoma		+	+	weak	+	-							+	+/-	-/+	+ (not PLL)	+	+	+	-/+
Lymphoplasmacytoid lymphoma/immunocytoma		+	+	+	+	-	+	+	+				+	-	+	-	+/-	occ	occ	
Mantle cell lymphoma		+	+	+	+	-/+	+						+	+	-	+	-	+	-	
Follicle centre lymphoma, follicular		+	+	+	+	+/-	+	+					+/-	+/-	-/+	-	-/+	-	-	
Marginal zone B cell lymphoma Extranodal (MALT-type ± monocytoid B cells). Provisional subtype nodal ± monocytoid B cells)		+	+	+	+	-	+	+					+	-	-/+	-	-	-/+	+/-	
Hairy cell leukemia		+	+	+	+	-	+	+		-			+			-	-	+	+	+
Plasmacytoma/plasma cell myeloma		-	-	-	+/-	+/-	-/+	-							+	-	+/-	+/-		
Diffuse large B cell lymphoma Subtype: Primary mediastinal (thymic) B cell lymphoma		+	+	+	+	-/+	+	+/-						-/+	-/+	-/+				
Burkitt's lymphoma		+	+	+	+	+							+			-	-			
Provisional entity: High-grade B cell lymphoma, Burkitt-like		+	+	+	+	-	+/-	+/-								-	-			

	CD103	CD45	CD38	CD56	CD30	CD3	CD7	CD1a	CD4	CD8	CD16	CD57	CD2	TCRαβ	EMA	CD15	CDw75

I. B cell neoplasms
  Precursor B cell neoplasm: Precursor B lymphoblastic leukemia/lymphoma
II. Peripheral B cell neoplasms
  B cell chronic lymphocytic leukemia/prolymphocytic leukemia/small lymphocytic lymphoma
  Lymphoplasmacytoid lymphoma/immunocytoma
  Mantle cell lymphoma
  Follicle centre lymphoma, follicular

(continues)

Table 34.4. *(continued)*

	CD103	CD45	CD38	CD56	CD30	CD3	CD7	CD1a	CD4	CD8	CD16	CD57	CD2	TCRαβ	EMA	CD15	CDw75
Marginal zone B cell lymphoma Extranodal (MALT-type +/− monocytoid B cells). Provisional subtype nodal +/− monocytoid 0B cells)																	
Hairy cell leukemia	+																
Plasmacytoma/plasma cell myeloma		−/+	+	+/−											−/+		
Diffuse large B cell lymphoma Subtype: Primary mediastinal (thymic) B cell lymphoma																	
Burkitt's lymphoma																	
Provisional entity: High-grade B cell lymphoma, Burkitt-like																	

	Tdt	CD19	CD20	CD22	CD79a	CD10	DR	SIg	cMU	CD34	CD13	CD33	SIgM	SIgD	cIg	CD5	CD23	CD43	CD11c	CD25
T cell and putative NK cell neoplasms																				
I. Precursor T cell neoplasm; precursor T lymphoblastic lymphoma/leukemia	+	−	−	−	−											var				
II. Peripheral T cell and NK cell neoplasms																				
T cell chronic lymphocytic leukemia/ prolymphocytic leukemia																+				
Large granular lymphocyte leukemia (LGL), T cell type																−				−
NK cell type																−				−
Mycosis fungoides/ Sézary syndrome															+		+		occ	
Peripheral T cell lymphomas, unspecified Provisional subtype: hepatosplenic γδ T cell lymphoma		−	−	−												+/−				
Provisional subtype: subcutaneous panniculitic T cell lymphoma																				
Angioimmunoblastic T cell lymphoma (AILD)																+				
Angiocentric lymphoma																				
Intestinal T cell lymphoma (± enteropathy associated)																				
Adult T cell lymphoma/ leukemia (ATL/L)																+		+		+

Table (continued)

	CD103	CD45	CD38	CD56	CD30	CD3	CD7	CD1a	CD4	CD8	CD16	CD57	CD2	TCRαβ	EMA	CD15	CDw75
Anaplastic large cell lymphoma (ALCL), CD30⁺, T and null-cell types						−									var	−/+	+/−
Provisional entity: anaplastic large cell lymphoma, Hodgkin's like																	
Hodgkin's disease (HD)																	
Lymphocyte predominance		+	+		+											−	
Nodular sclerosis		+	−		−											−	
Mixed cellularity		−	−		−											−	
Lymphocyte depletion		−	−		−											−	
Provisional entity: lymphocyte-rich Classic HD		−			−											−	

	CD103	CD45	CD38	CD56	CD30	CD3	CD7	CD1a	CD4	CD8	CD16	CD57	CD2	TCRαβ	EMA	CD15	CDw75
T cell and putative NK cell neoplasms																	
I. Precursor T cell neoplasm; precursor T-lymphoblastic lymphoma/leukemia						+	+	+/−	+ or −	+ or −	+ or − or occ	occ	var	var			
II. Peripheral T cell and NK cell neoplasms																	
T cell chronic lymphocytic leukemia/prolymphocytic leukemia						+	+		+/−	−/+		+	+				
Large granular lymphocyte leukemia (LGL), T cell type			−			+	−		−	+	+	+/−	+	+			
NK cell type				+/−		−	−/+		−	+/−	+	+/−	+	−			
Mycosis fungoides/Sézary syndrome						+	−/+		+	−/+							
Peripheral T cell lymphomas, unspecified						+/−	−/+		+/−	−/+			+/−				
Provisional subtype: hepatosplenic γδ T cell lymphoma																	
Provisional subtype: subcutaneous panniculitic T cell lymphoma																	
Angioimmunoblastic T cell lymphoma (AILD)						+	+		+				+				
Angiocentric lymphoma																	
Intestinal T cell lymphoma (+/− enteropathy associated)	+					+	+		−	+/−							
Adult T cell lymphoma/leukemia (ATL/L)						+	+		+	−/+			+				
Anaplastic large cell lymphoma(ALCL), CD30⁺, T and null-cell types		−/+			+	−/+	var						var		+/−	−/+	
Provisional entity: anaplastic large cell lymphoma, Hodgkin's-like																	
Hodgkin's disease (HD)																	
Lymphocyte predominance		+			−/+										+/−	−	+
Nodular sclerosis		−			+										−	+/−	
Mixed cellularity		−			+										−	+/−	
Lymphocyte depletion		−			+										−	+/−	
Provisional entity: lymphocyte-rich Classic HD		−			+										−	+/−	

Abbreviations: S, surface; c, cytoplasmic; EMA, epithelial membrane antigen; var, variable; +, over 90% of cases positive; +/−, over 50% of cases positive; −/+, less than 50% of cases positive; −, less than 10% of cases positive.

Table 34.5. *Cytogenetic abnormalities in lymphoid neoplasms*

Neoplasm	Ig heavy chain rearrangement	Light chain rearrangement	T cell receptor rearrangement	Other
B cell neoplasms				
I. Precursor B cell neoplasm: Precursor B lymphoblastic leukemia/lymphoma	Usually	Maybe	Minority	Variable, including t(9;22), t(4;11), t(1;19), del(11), (q23), hyperdiploidy
II. Peripheral B cell neoplasms				
B cell chronic lymphocytic leukemia/ prolymphocytic leukemia/small lymphocytic lymphoma	Usually	Usually		Trisomy 12, 30%; abnormal 13q, 25%
Lymphoplasmacytoid lymphoma/ immunocytoma	Usually	Usually		
Mantle cell lymphoma				t(11;14)
Follicle center lymphoma, follicular				t(14;18)
Marginal zone B-cell lymphoma				Trisomy 3 reported
Extranodal (MALT type ± monocytoid B cells). Provisional subtype: nodal ± monocytoid B cells				t(11;18) (reported in extranodal cases)
Hairy cell leukemia	Yes	Yes		
Plasmacytoma/plasma cell myeloma	Yes	Yes		
Diffuse large B cell lymphoma				t(14;18), 30%; c-*myc* rearrangement in some
Subtype: primary mediastinal (thymic) B cell lymphoma	Yes	Yes		
Burkitt's lymphoma				t(8;14); t(2;8); t(8;22)
Provisional entity: high-grade B cell lymphoma, Burkitt-like				t(14;18), 30%; c-*myc* rearrangement in some
T cell and putative NK cell neoplasms				
I. Precursor T cell neoplasm: Precursor T lymphoblastic lymphoma/leukemia	Maybe		Variable	Variable, including inv(14), t(8;14), t(10;14), t(11;14)
II. Peripheral T cell and NK cell neoplasms T cell chronic lymphocytic leukemia/ prolymphocytic leukemia			Yes	inv(14), 75%; trisomy 8
Large granular lymphocyte leukemia (LGL), T cell type			Yes	
NK cell type			Germ line	
Mycosis fungoides/Sézary syndrome			Yes	
Peripheral T cell lymphomas, unspecified	Germ line		Yes	
Provisional subtype: hepatosplenic γδ T cell lymphoma				
Provisional subtype: subcutaneous panniculitic T cell lymphoma				
Angioimmunoblastic T cell lymphoma (AILD)	Yes (10%)		Yes (75%)	Trisomy 3; trisomy 5 may occur
Angiocentric lymphoma	Usually germ line		Usually germ line	
Intestinal T cell lymphoma (± enteropathy associated)			Yes (TCR-β)	
Adult T cell lymphoma/leukemia (ATL/L)			Yes	Clonally integrated HTLV-1 genomes (100%)
Anaplastic large cell lymphoma (ALCL), CD30+, T and null cell types			Yes (60%)	t(2;5)
Provisional entity: anaplastic large cell lymphoma, Hodgkin's-like				
Hodgkin's disease[a]				
Lymphocyte predominance	Germ line	Germ line	Germ line	
Nodular sclerosis	Usually germ line		Usually germ line	
Mixed cellularity	Usually germ line		Usually germ line	
Lymphocyte depletion	Usually germ line		Usually germ line	
Provisional entity: lymphocyte-rich classic HD	Usually germ line		Usually germ line	

[a]Thomas Hodgkin, English physician and pathologist, 1798–1866.

Table 34.6. *Ann Arbor Staging Classification and Cotswald modifications*

Stage I: Involvement of a single lymph node region or lymphoid structure.

Stage II: Involvement of two or more lymph node regions on the same side of the diaphragm.

Stage III: Involvement of lymph node regions or structures on both sides of the diaphragm.

Stage IV: Involvement of extranodal site(s) beyond the designated "E".

For All Stages:
    A. No symptoms
    B. Fever (>38°C), sweats, weight loss (>10% body weight over 6 months)

For Stages I to III:
    E. Involvement of a single, extranodal site contiguous or proximal to known nodal site.

Cotswald Modifications
Subscript *"X"* to be used if bulky disease is present.
The number of anatomic regions involved should be indicated by a subscript (e.g., II_3).
Stage III may be subdivided into:
    III1: with or without splenic, hilar, celiac, or portal nodes
    III2: with para-aortic, iliac, mesenteric nodes
Staging should be identified as clinical stage *(CS)* or pathologic stage *(PS)*. PS at a given site will be denoted by a subscript (i.e., M = bone marrow; H = liver; L = lung; O = bone; P = pleura; D = skin).
Unconfirmed/uncertain complete remission *(CR[u])* if persistent radiologic abnormalities of uncertain significance.

Rationale for transplantation

Modern chemotherapy regimens cure a substantial fraction of patients with aggressive histology NHL (Fisher *et al.*, 1993). In the United States, CHOP has until recently been the most widely used regimen for diffuse large B-cell lymphoma,

Table 34.7. *Factors independently prognostic of overall survival with conventional therapy*

Factor	Relative risk	*P* value
All patients (*n* = 1,385)		
Age (<60 vs. >60)	1.96	<0.001
Serum LDH (<1 × normal vs. >1 × normal)	1.85	<0.001
Performance status (0 or 1 vs. 2–4)	1.80	<0.001
Stage (I or II vs. III or IV)	1.47	<0.001
Extranodal involvement (≤1 site vs. >1 site)[a]	1.48	<0.001
Patients ≤60 years old (*n* = 685)		
Stage (I or II vs. III or IV)	2.17	<0.001
Serum LDH (≤1 × normal vs. >1 × normal)	1.95	<0.001
Performance status (0 or 1 vs. 2–4)	1.81	<0.001

[a] This was the only factor that did not retain independent prognostic significance in patients ≤60 years old (≤1 site vs. >1 site: relative risk, 1.20; *P* = 0.134).
Reproduced, with permission, from The International Non-Hodgkin's Lymphoma Prognostic Factors Project (1993).

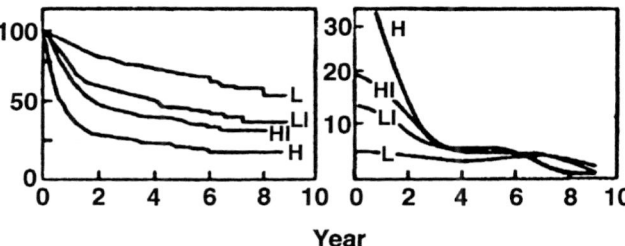

Fig. 34.1. Survival according to risk group defined by the International Prognostic Index. The left panel shows Kaplan-Meier survival curves for the four risk groups for whom complete data were available (*n* = 2,031); L, low risk; LI, low-intermediate risk; HI, high-intermediate risk; H, high risk. The right panel shows death rates during the study period. Reproduced, with permission, from Shipp *et al.* (1993).

although it is possible that other regimens are more effective (Tilly *et al.*, 2002). The addition of the anti-CD20 monoclonal antibody, rituximab, to CHOP has been shown to improve survival compared with CHOP alone, and this combination has now become accepted therapy for patients with newly diagnosed NHL (Coiffier *et al.*, 2002). Despite improvements in initial therapy, a significant proportion of patients will relapse or fail to attain a remission with front-line therapy, and the results of conventional chemotherapy salvage regimens in this population are poor (Ezzat *et al.*, 1994; Rodriguez *et al.*, 1995). Several chemotherapeutic agents exhibit steep dose-response curves against lymphoma, and are dose-limited primarily by hematopoietic toxicity (Frei & Canellos, 1980). This provides the rationale for the use of high-dose therapy followed by autologous hematopoietic stem cell transplantation (HSCT) for patients with relapsed and refractory NHL.

Reports dating back more than forty years document attempts at using stored autologous bone marrow to treat NHL patients with chemotherapy- or radiation-induced myelosuppression (McFarland, Granville, & Dameshek, 1959; Clifford, Clift, & Duff, 1961; Kurnick, 1962; Pegg, Humble, & Newton, 1962). However, techniques for bone marrow harvest and

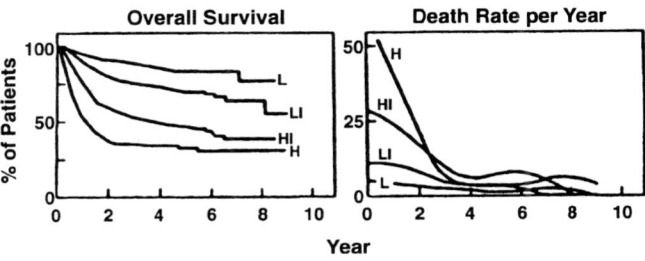

Fig. 34.2. Survival among the 1,274 younger patients (<60 years) according to risk group defined by the age-adjusted International Prognostic Index. The left panel shows the Kaplan-Meier curves for this age group, and the right panel the death rates during the study period; L, low risk; LI, low-intermediate risk; HI, high-intermediate risk; H, high risk. Reproduced, with permission, from Shipp *et al.* (1993).

cryopreservation had not been perfected, and it was difficult to demonstrate that the reinfused marrow actually accelerated hematopoietic recovery. In the late 1970s Appelbaum *et al.* (1978a, 1978b) demonstrated that reinfusion of cryopreserved autologous bone marrow did accelerate hematopoietic recovery following intensive chemotherapy and that some patients with resistant NHL were apparently cured by this approach.

The use of autologous HSCT transplantation for patients with relapsed and refractory NHL has increased rapidly. More than 3,600 autologous transplants for diffuse large cell lymphoma were recorded with the Autologous Blood and Marrow Transplant Registry (ABMTR) between 1994 and 1999, and approximately 1,700 autologous transplants for follicular lymphoma were recorded during the same time period (Horowitz, 2002). It is estimated that these represent approximately 50% of the actual number of transplants performed for NHL during this period, and NHL is the most common indication for autologous HSCT in North America. In 1999, 3,815 autologous HSC transplants for NHL were reported to the European Group for Blood and Marrow Transplantation (EBMT) (Gratwohl, Passweg, Baldomero, & Urbano-Ispizua, 1999). NHL was also the most common indication for autologous HSC transplantation in this survey.

Transplantation for NHL has become safer and less expensive (Bennett *et al.*, 1995), and can be performed in an outpatient setting (Meisenberg *et al.*, 1997; Rizzo *et al.*, 1999). These advances are the result of increased experience at individual institutions, better patient selection, and the introduction of technical improvements such as the use of hematopoietic growth factors and peripheral blood stem cells (Khan *et al.*, 1997).

Disease-specific pretransplant work-up

The pretransplant evaluation must be individualized and certain tests may not be appropriate for all transplant candidates. Nevertheless, pretransplant pulmonary function, renal function, cardiac function, and hepatic function have been demonstrated to be predictive of transplant-related mortality (Goldberg, Klumpp, Magdalinski, & Mangan, 1998). Guidelines for testing prior to HSC collection and initiation of high-dose therapy are shown in Table 34.8.

Preparative regimens

Some of the high-dose therapy regimens commonly used prior to autologous HSC transplantation for NHL are listed in Table 34.9. The wide variety of drug and radiation doses that have been used within individual high-dose therapy regimens should be noted.

Regimens are frequently divided into those that contain total body irradiation (TBI) and those containing only drugs. The use of TBI eliminates sparing of "sanctuary" sites, allows homogeneous dosing independent of blood supply, is not cross-resistant with chemotherapy, and has the potential for tailoring doses at specific sites or organs (Shank, 1998). Retrospective analyses

Table 34.8. *Selected tests useful prior to autologous hematopoietic stem cell transplantation for non-Hodgkin's lymphoma*

Expert hematopathologist review of diagnostic material
Verification of eligibility for transplant protocol(s)
Informed consent
Bone marrow aspiration and biopsy prior to marrow harvest
  (consider cytogenetics)
Pre-stem cell collection testing mandated by the Foundation for
  the Accreditation of Cell Therapy (FACT)
  Pregnancy testing when appropriate
  ABO and Rh typing
  Infectious disease tests (anti-HIV-1, anti-HIV-2, HIV-1-antigen,
  anti-HTLV,
  HBV sAg, anti-HBV, anti-HCV, anti-CMV, serologic test for
  syphilis)
CBC, chemistry screen, PT, PTT
Pulmonary function tests
Dental evaluation
Cardiac ejection fraction
Staging (CT scan, PET scan, etc.)

Abbreviations: HIV, human immunodeficiency virus; HTLV, human T-lymphotropic virus; sAg, surface antigen; HBV, hepatitis B virus; HCV, hepatitis C virus; CMV, cytomegalovirus; CBC, complete blood count; PT, prothrombin time; PTT, partial thromboplastin time; CT, computed tomography; PET, positron emission tomography.

have generally failed to find a significant survival advantage when TBI-containing regimens have been compared with drug-only regimens (Philip *et al.*, 1987; Petersen *et al.*, 1990; Weisdorf *et al.*, 1991; Schouten *et al.*, 1994; Bastion *et al.*, 1995; Bierman *et al.*, 1997; Stiff *et al.*, 1998; Aristei & Tabilio, 1999; Gutierrez-Delgado *et al.*, 2001; Stein *et al.*, 2001). However, investigators from Stanford University noted that

Table 34.9. *Commonly used high-dose therapy regimens for non-Hodgkin's lymphoma*

Regimen	Total dose administered
CBV	Cyclophosphamide, 4.8–7.2 g/m²
	Carmustine, 300–600 mg/m²
	Etoposide, 750–2,400 mg/m²
BEAC	Carmustine, 200–300 mg/m²
	Etoposide, 600–1,200 mg/m²
	Cytosine arabinoside, 800–1,200 mg/m²
	Cyclophosphamide, 140–180 mg/kg
BEAM	Carmustine, 300 mg/m²
	Etoposide, 400–800 mg/m²
	Cytosine arabinoside, 400–1,600/m²
	Melphalan, 140 mg/m²
CY-TBI	Cyclophosphamide, 120–200 mg/kg
	Total body irradiation, 800–1,320 cGy
VP-16, CY, TBI	Etoposide, 60 mg/kg
	Cyclophosphamide, 100–120 mg/kg
	Total body irradiation, 1,200–1,375 cGy

overall survival for NHL patients receiving autologous bone marrow transplants after cyclophosphamide, etoposide, and TBI was better than that of patients treated with cyclophosphamide, carmustine, and etoposide (Stockerl-Goldstein *et al.*, 1996). This difference was not observed in patients rescued with autologous peripheral blood stem cells. Other investigators have suggested that the addition of etoposide to combinations of cyclophosphamide and TBI improved results compared with historical controls (Gulati *et al.*, 1992; Stiff *et al.*, 1998).

Regimens containing TBI have been associated with increased toxicity, and posttransplant mortality in some series, particularly in patients who have received prior chest irradiation (Philip *et al.*, 1987; Petersen *et al.*, 1990; Goldberg *et al.*, 1998; Salar *et al.*, 2001). An increased incidence of interstitial pneumonitis in previously irradiated patients has also been noted in patients receiving drug-only regimens (Wheeler *et al.*, 1990). In addition, there is evidence that use of TBI may be an independent risk factor for the development of acute myeloid leukemia and myelodysplasia following autologous HSC transplantation for NHL, as well as Hodgkin's disease (Darrington *et al.*, 1994; Milligan *et al.*, 1999; Sureda *et al.*, 2001) (and see Chapter 86).

A retrospective EBMT analysis demonstrated that NHL patients transplanted with the CBV (cyclophosphamide, carmustine, etoposide) high-dose regimen had longer progression-free survival than those who received the BEAM (carmustine, etoposide, cytosine arabinoside, melphalan) regimen (Fielding *et al.*, 1994). In contrast, a Spanish registry analysis showed that the 8-year overall survival of patients who received BEAM or BEAC (carmustine, etoposide, cytosine arabinoside, cyclophosphamide) prior to autologous transplantation for diffuse large cell lymphoma was significantly longer than patients who received CBV (Salar *et al.*, 2001). Mills *et al.* (1995b) noted increased gastrointestinal toxicity without improvement in survival when the dose of etoposide in the BEAM regimen was increased from 800 mg/m^2/day to 2,400mg/m^2/day.

Dose escalation of carmustine in the CBV regimen has also been associated with increased toxicity. Wheeler *et al.* (1990) noted that interstitial pneumonitis was seen in 2 of 40 patients receiving 450 mg/m^2 carmustine, compared to 5 of 18 patients who received 600 mg/m^2 ($P = .02$). Weaver *et al.* (1993) noted that idiopathic pneumonitis was not observed in patients receiving 300 mg/m^2 carmustine, but was seen in 23% of patients who received 600 mg/m^2 ($P = .05$).

Other regimens incorporating carboplatin, hydroxyurea, and thiotepa have been used prior to autologous transplantation for NHL (Wilson *et al.*, 1992; Przepiorka *et al.*, 1995; Vaughan *et al.*, 1995), but have not been evaluated in phase III trials. Tandem transplants have also been tested at several institutions, although it is unclear whether this approach leads to better outcomes (Haioun *et al.*, 2001; Papadopoulos, Noguera-Irizarry, & Hesdorffer 2001).

Another approach that is being investigated involves the substitution of radiolabeled antibodies in place of TBI. It is felt that this approach may allow higher doses of radiation to be administered to tumor sites, while decreasing radiation doses to normal tissues (see Chapter 108). Phase I/II trials have demonstrated the feasibility of administering ^{131}I-labeled anti-CD20 antibodies followed by autologous HSC transplantation alone, or in combination with high-dose chemotherapy regimens for patients with relapsed and refractory NHL (Liu *et al.*, 1998; Press *et al.*, 2000; Gopal *et al.*, 2002). A retrospective analysis from Seattle demonstrated improved survival in B-cell NHL patients treated with radioimmunotherapy combined with cyclophosphamide and etoposide, when compared with historical controls who received cyclophosphamide, etoposide, and TBI (Fig. 34.3).

Peripheral blood stem cell transplantation

The use of peripheral blood as a source of stem cells for hematopoietic rescue has largely replaced bone marrow (Gratwohl *et al.*, 1999; Horowitz, 2002). Peripheral blood stem cells can be collected without general anesthesia and can sometimes be obtained with a single apheresis (Pettengell *et al.*, 1993; Negrin *et al.*, 1995). More important, peripheral blood stem cells can be collected from patients whose marrow cannot be harvested due to prior pelvic irradiation or malignant cell contamination.

In vitro techniques have demonstrated that malignant cells can be cultured more frequently from bone marrow harvests of NHL patients than from peripheral blood stem cell collections (Sharp *et al.*, 1995). Similarly, Gribben *et al.* (1994) used PCR techniques to demonstrate a higher frequency of tumor contamination in bone marrow as compared with peripheral blood. However, other investigators have demonstrated similar rates of contamination between blood and marrow (Hardingham *et al.*, 1993; McCann *et al.*, 1996; Léonard *et al.*, 1998).

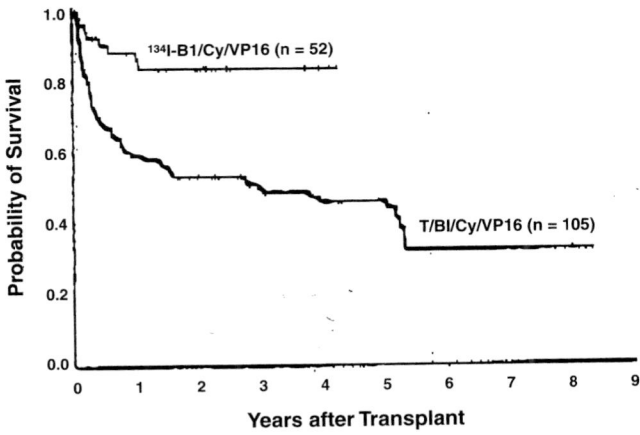

Fig. 34.3. Overall survival of 52 patients with relapsed B-cell lymphomas treated with ^{131}I-tositumomab, etoposide, cyclophosphamide, and autologous stem cell transplantation (thin line), and 105 patients treated with external-beam total body irradiation, etoposide, cyclophosphamide, and autologous stem cell transplantation (thick line). Reproduced, with permission, from Press *et al.* (2000).

Prospective trials have demonstrated more rapid hematopoietic reconstitution with mobilized peripheral blood stem cells compared to autologous bone marrow (Weisdorf *et al.*, 1993; Schmitz *et al.*, 1996; Vellenga *et al.*, 2001; Vose *et al.*, 2002). This has led to shorter hospitalizations (Weisdorf *et al.*, 1993; Ager *et al.*, 1995; Brice *et al.*, 1996; Smith *et al.*, 1997; Vellenga *et al.*, 2001), less blood product usage (Ager *et al.*, 1995; Schmitz *et al.*, 1996; Vellenga *et al.*, 2001), and lower costs (Ager *et al.*, 1995; Smith *et al.*, 1997; Vellenga *et al.*, 2001). Improved quality of life following transplantation with peripheral blood stem cells has also been demonstrated when compared with use of bone marrow (Vellenga *et al.*, 2001). Nevertheless, prospective comparisons (Weisdorf *et al.*, 1993; Schmitz *et al.*, 1996; Vellenga *et al.*, 2001; Vose *et al.*, 2002), retrospective comparisons (Rapoport *et al.*, 1993; Ager *et al.*, 1995; Brice *et al.*, 1996; Brunv *et al.*, 1996), and a case-matching study (Majolino *et al.*, 1997) have failed to find a significant difference in survival favoring the use of peripheral blood stem cells (Fig. 34.4). Retrospective analyses of autologous HSC transplantation in patients with low-grade NHL have also generally failed to show survival advantages for peripheral blood stem cell transplantation (Colombat *et al.*, 1994; Schouten *et al.*, 1994; Cervantes *et al.*, 1995; Bierman *et al.*, 1997). A retrospective analysis from Stanford University did show superior overall survival among NHL patients who received peripheral blood stem cell transplants when compared to those who received autologous marrow transplants (Stockerl-Goldstein *et al.*, 1996).

Most analyses have compared mobilized peripheral blood stem cells with bone marrow collected in the steady state. However, engraftment rates with bone marrow harvested after growth factor administration may be as rapid as those following mobilized peripheral blood stem cell transplantation (Janssen, Smilee, & Elfenbein, 1995; Damiani *et al.*, 1997; Weisdorf *et al.*, 1997).

Clinical results

Intermediate and high-grade lymphoma

Results of selected phase II trials of autologous HSC transplantation for intermediate and high-grade NHL are shown in Table 34.10. It is difficult to compare results because of differences in patient selection, supportive care, preparative regimens, and length of follow-up. In addition, the definition of important variables such as response rate and mortality are not standardized. However, these results demonstrate that long-term disease-free survival is possible following autologous HSC transplantation for NHL, and that transplants can be performed with low morbidity and mortality. In one report all 39 patients in complete remission at 5 years posttransplant were still in complete remission at 10 years posttransplant (Bolwell *et al.*, 2002).

Prognostic variables for outcome after high-dose therapy and autologous transplantation

Philip *et al.* (1984) noted that survival after autologous bone marrow transplantation (BMT) could be predicted by sensitivity to conventional salvage chemotherapy. This observation was validated in one of the first large series of autologous BMT for relapsed and refractory NHL (Philip *et al.*, 1987). Patients who failed to achieve an initial remission and then failed to respond to salvage therapy (primary refractory disease) had a poor prognosis, without any long-term survivors (Fig. 34.5). The remaining patients had achieved a remission with primary therapy, but had subsequently relapsed. The relapsed patients who were still responsive to conventional chemotherapy at the time of transplant (sensitive relapse) had an actuarial disease-free survival of 36% at 3 years, while resistant patients (resis-

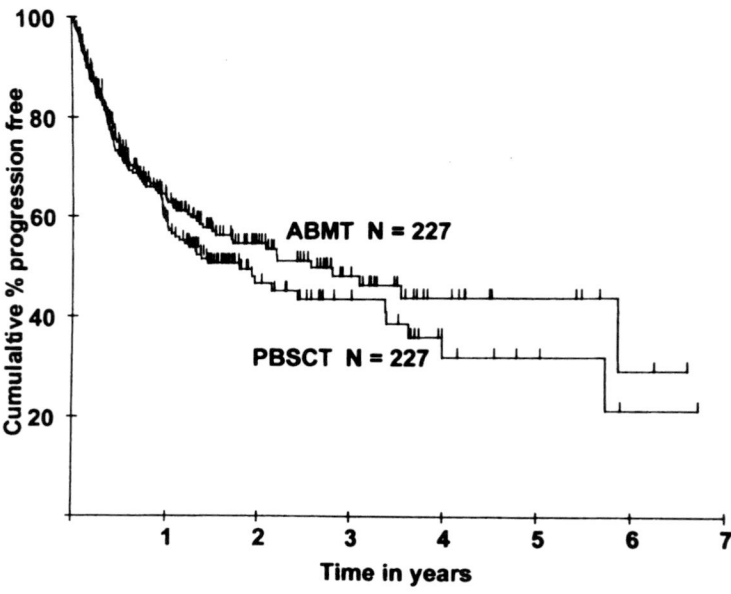

Fig. 34.4. Progression-free survival of matched non-Hodgkin's lymphoma patients who received autologous bone marrow transplantation or peripheral blood stem cell transplantation. Reproduced, with permission, from Majolino *et al.* (1997).

Table 34.10. *Autologous hematopoietic stem cell transplantation for intermediate and high-grade non-Hodgkin's lymphoma*

Reference	Number of Patients	Transplant Regimen	Early Purging	Death Rate	Outcome	Comments
Philip *et al.* (1987)	100	Various	No	21%	19% actuarial 3 yr DFS	
Colombat *et al.* (1990)	46	Various	Yes in 20	9%	60% actuarial 3 yr DFS	Included patients with low grade histology and in first CR
Petersen *et al.* (1990)	101	Various	Yes in 27	21%	11% actuarial 5 yr EFS	Included patients with low grade histology, Hodgkin's disease, and malignant histiocytosis
Phillips *et al.* (1990)	68	Cy + TBI	No	21%	11% actuarial PFS (median 4.6 yrs)	Included patient with malignant histiocytosis and one with mycosis fungoides
Weisdorf *et al.* (1991)	70	Cy + TBI, BCNU + Cy + CA	Yes in 54	13%	41% actuarial DFS for CRs (median 3 yrs)	Included patients with low grade histology and in first CR
Lazarus *et al.* (1992)	44	BEP	Yes in some	3%	24 (55%) CCR (12–57 mo)	Included patients with low grade histology
Gulati *et al.* (1992)	44	Cy+VP–16+TBI	Yes in 21	36%	57% DFS (median 42 mo)	Included patients with low grade histology
Vose *et al.* (1993)	158	Various	No	NS	29% actuarial 3 yr FFS	
Wheeler *et al.* (1993)	78	CBV	No	7%	43% actuarial 3 yr FFS	Included patients in first CR
Weaver *et al.* (1994)	53	Cy+VP–16+TBI	Yes in 33	17%	45% actuarial 2 yr EFS	Included patients with low grade histology, Hodgkin's disease, and in first CR
van Besien *et al.* (1995c)	48	BEAC	No	23%	30% actuarial 3 yr FFS	Included patients in first CR
Mills *et al.* (1995a)	107	BEAM	No	7%	35% actuarial 5 yr PFS	Included patients in first CR
Stockerl-Goldstein *et al.* (1996)	221	CBV, Cy+VP–16+TBI	Yes	10%	55% CCR (median 2.4 yrs)	Included patients with low grade histology and in first CR
Caballero *et al.* (1997)	112	BEAM	No	3%	71% actuarial 3 yr DFS (intermediate grade)	Included patients with low grade histology and in first CR
Rapaport *et al.* (1997)	136	BEAC in 117	No	4.4%	34% actuarial 5 yr EFS	Included patients with low grade histology
Stiff *et al.* (1998)	94	CBV, Cy+VP–16+TBI	Yes in 9	10.6%	33% actuarial 3 yr PFS	
Popat *et al.* (1998)	90	Various	No	NS	40% actuarial 4 yr DFS	

Abbreviations: Cy, cyclophosphamide; TBI, total body irradiation; BCNU, carmustine; CA, cytosine arabinoside; BEP, carmustine, etoposide, cisplatin; BEAC, carmustine, etoposide, cytosine arabinoside, cyclophosphamide; CBV, cyclophosphamide, carmustine, etoposide; BEAM, carmustine, etoposide, cytosine arabinoside, melphalan; TACC, 6-thioguanine, cytosine arabinoside, lomustine, cyclophosphamide; NS, not stated; DFS, disease-free survival; EFS, event-free survival; PFS, progression-free survival; CR, complete remission; FFS, failure-free survival; CCR, continuous complete remission.

tant relapse) had an actuarial 3-year disease-free survival of 14% (Fig. 34.5). The superior outcome following autologous HSC transplantation for patients with chemotherapy-sensitive disease has been verified in other reports (Colombat *et al.*, 1990; Weisdorf *et al.*, 1991; Lazarus *et al.*, 1992; Vose *et al.*, 1993; Wheeler *et al.*, 1993; Mills *et al.*, 1995a; van Besien *et al.*, 1995c; Ladenstein *et al.*, 1997; Stiff *et al.*, 1998), and may be the most important variable relating to transplant outcome.

Extensively pretreated patients are also more likely to have inferior outcomes following autologous HSC transplantation (Petersen *et al.*, 1990; Vose *et al.*, 1993; Weaver *et al.*, 1994; van Besien *et al.*, 1995c; Stockerl-Goldstein *et al.*, 1996). These results have been used to suggest that autologous HSC transplantation should be performed early in the course of disease, before chemotherapy resistance develops.

Other prognostic factors associated with adverse outcome include poor performance status (Petersen *et al.*, 1990; Phillips *et al.*, 1990; Cabellero *et al.*, 1997), bulky disease (Rapoport *et al.*, 1997; Stiff *et al.*, 1998) elevated lactic dehydrogenase (LDH) level (Vose *et al.*, 1993; van Besien *et al.*, 1995c; Popat

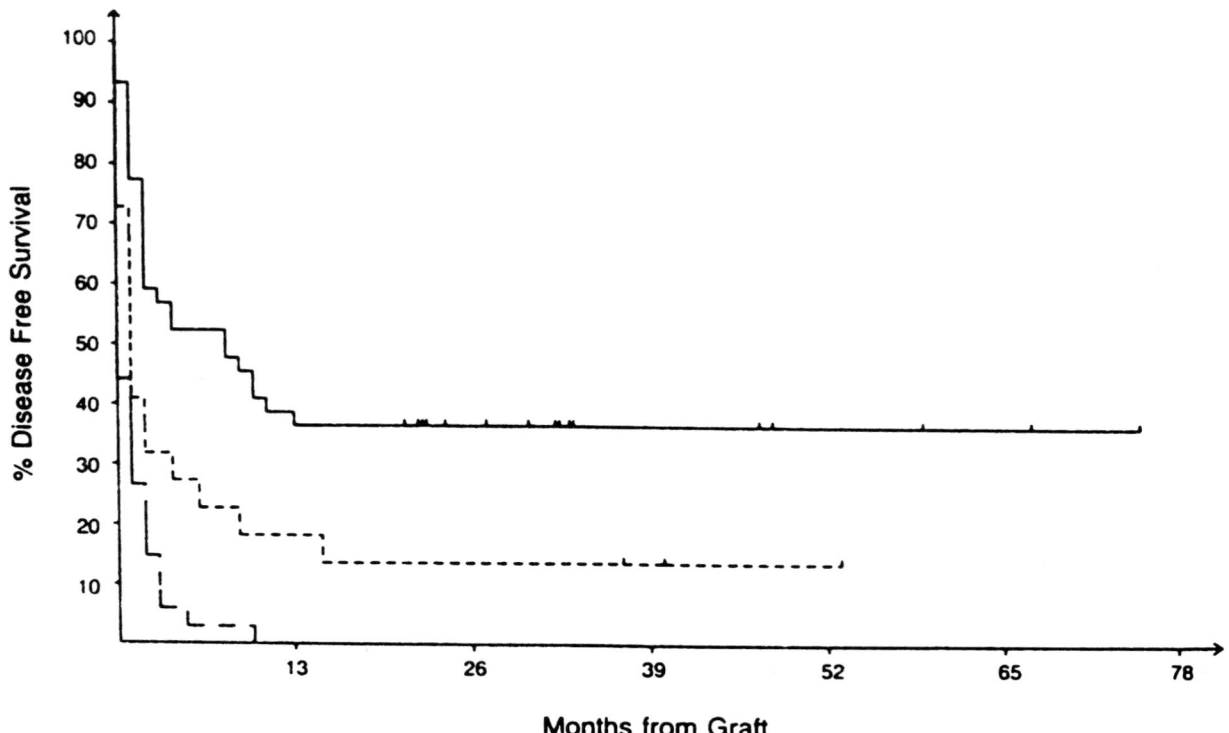

Fig. 34.5. Actuarial 3-year disease-free survival following autologous bone marrow transplantation for non-Hodgkin's lymphoma. The solid line indicates patients with sensitive relapses, the dashed line (—) patients with resistant relapse, and the broken line (– –) patients with no complete remission. Reproduced, with permission, from Philip *et al.* (1987).

et al., 1998), high-grade histology (Colombat *et al.*, 1990; Petersen *et al.*, 1990; Wheeler *et al.*, 1993; Weaver *et al.*, 1994; Caballero *et al.*, 1997), and obesity (Tarella *et al.*, 2000) (Table 34.11). In addition to its use for newly diagnosed patients, the IPI has also been shown to be useful in predicting outcome for patients undergoing autologous HSC transplantation for NHL in some series (Caballero *et al.*, 1997; Moskowitz *et al.*, 1999), although other analyses have not demonstrated a correlation between the IPI and response to autologous bone marrow transplantation (Blay *et al.*, 1998).

It should be noted that the significance of individual prognostic factors has not always been confirmed in various publications. Analyses are generally retrospective and may lack statistical power to detect differences among subgroups

Mediastinal large B-cell lymphoma, peripheral T-cell lymphoma, cutaneous T-cell lymphoma (mycosis fungoides), nasal NK/T cell lymphoma, and anaplastic large cell lymphoma

Mediastinal large B-cell lymphoma is a distinct entity recognized by the WHO classification (Jaffe *et al.*, 2001). A retrospective analysis by Popat *et al.* (1998) compared transplant results in patients with mediastinal large B-cell lymphoma with results of transplantation for diffuse large B-cell lymphoma. Patients with primary mediastinal disease had significantly bet-

ter disease-free survival and overall survival (Fig. 34.6). Another series of 35 patients from Dana-Farber Cancer Center showed a 5-year progression-free survival rate of 57% following autologous HSCT (Sehn *et al.*, 1998).

The outcome of primary chemotherapy for peripheral T-cell lymphoma is generally inferior to diffuse large B-cell lymphoma. There is less information on transplantation for T-cell lymphomas as compared with those having a B-cell phenotype, although most comparisons have failed to show significant differences in outcome when results of transplantation for B-cell and peripheral T-cell lymphomas have been compared (Vose *et al.*, 1990; Gordon *et al.*, 1992; Blystad *et al.*, 2001; Rodriguez *et al.*, 2001; Song *et al.*, 2002) (Fig. 34.7).

High response rates following autologous HSCT for advanced cutaneous T-cell lymphoma (mycosis fungoides) have also been reported, although remission durations have generally been limited (Bigler *et al.*, 1991; Olavarria *et al.*, 2001).

Encouraging results of autologous transplantation for relapsed nasal NK/T cell lymphoma have been reported (Liang *et al.*, 1997) (see below).

Results of autologous HSCT for anaplastic large cell lymphoma may be significantly better than results of transplanation for other aggressive histologic subtypes (Deconinck *et al.*, 2000).

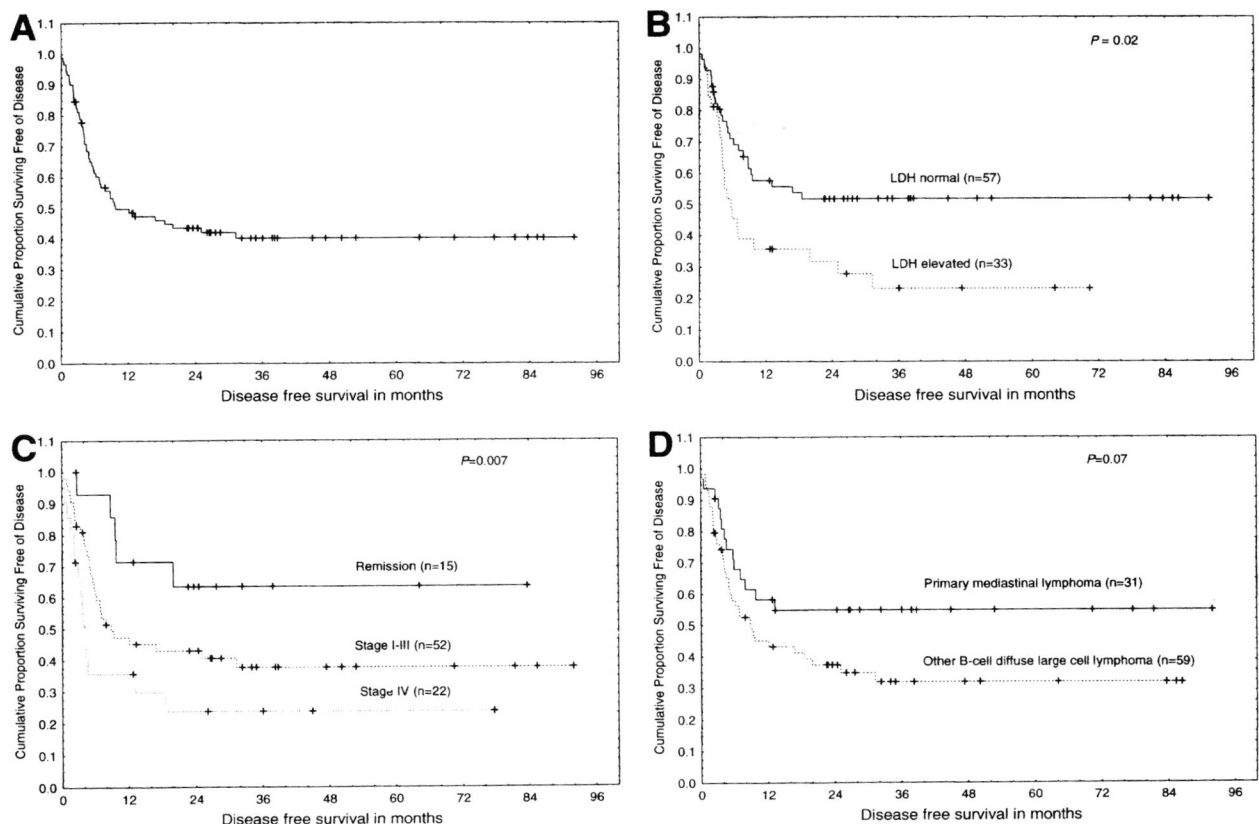

Fig. 34.6. Disease-free survival (A) for all patients and (B) by serum LDH at transplantation. (C) Disease-free survival by Ann Arbor stage at transplantation. Remission indicates patients without measurable disease. Stage I–III indicates patients with measurable nodal disease only. Stage IV indicates patients with measurable extranodal ≥ nodal disease at the time of transplantation. (D) Disease-free survival for primary mediastinal lymphoma and others. *P* values are those of univariate analyses. Reproduced, with permission, from Popat *et al.* (1998).

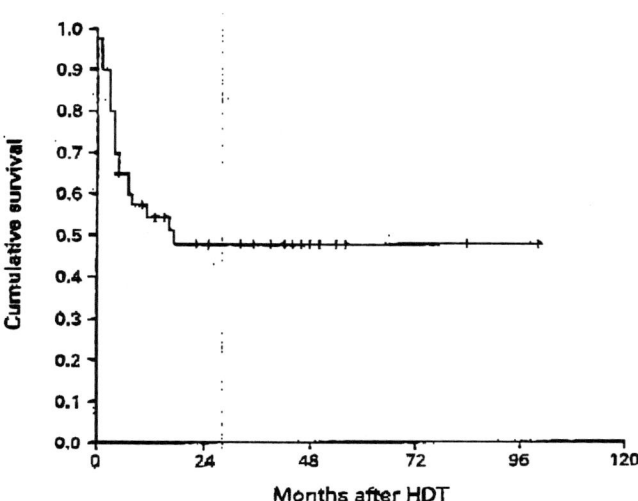

Fig. 34.7. Event-free survival of 40 patients with peripheral T-cell lymphoma following autologous hematopoietic stem cell transplantation. Reproduced, with permission, from Blystad *et al.* (2001).

Primary refractory disease

Early reports of autologous HSCT for aggressive NHL showed that results were extremely poor for patients with primary refractory disease (Philip *et al.*, 1987). However, there is no standard definition of primary refractoriness. In some series, this definition may encompass patients who progress on initial therapy, or fail to respond to initial therapy, even if they subsequently respond to second-line treatment and attain a remission prior to transplantation. Some series may include patients who attain a partial remission after primary therapy, while others may include only patients that are truly refractory to all treatments. More recent results have demonstrated that these various clinical situations are different and that some patients with primary refractory disease may have prolonged disease-free survival after autologous HSC transplantation. Interpretation of results is also complicated by the fact that persistent disease following primary therapy is not always pathologically confirmed and some patients categorized as having residual disease might actually have been in remission at the time of transplantation.

Investigators at Memorial Sloan-Kettering Cancer Center identified 85 NHL patients with aggressive histology who achieved at best a partial response with primary therapy (Kewalramani *et al.*, 2000). High-dose therapy followed by autologous HSCT was then performed for patients who subsequently responded to conventional salvage chemotherapy. The actuarial 3-year event-free survival was 44% for these patients. In addition, there were no differences in outcome between patients who had a partial remission with primary therapy, as compared with patients with true induction failure. Another series from the ABMTR analyzed results of autologous HSCT in 184 patients with aggressive NHL who had never achieved an initial complete remission (Vose *et al.*, 2001b). The 5-year progression-free survival was estimated at 31% (Fig. 34.8). The majority of patients received second-line conventional salvage chemotherapy prior to transplantation and results were significantly better in patients who were sensitive to this therapy. Similar results of autologous hematopoietic stem cell transplantation for primary refractory NHL have been reported in other series, particularly if patients are responsive to salvage chemotherapy (Prince *et al.*, 1996; Stiff *et al.*, 1998).

Transplantation versus conventional salvage chemotherapy

The results in Table 34.10 appear to be superior to those reported for conventional salvage chemotherapy. However, only a fraction of patients with relapsed and refractory NHL that are considered for transplantation may ultimately proceed to transplant, and the role of selection bias must be considered (Surbone, Armitage, & Gale, 1991), although retrospective and prospective data support the superiority of transplantation in certain situations.

A retrospective analysis identified 244 patients from the French Groupe d'Etude des Lymphomes de l'Adulte (GELA) who progressed after treatment with an identical chemotherapy regimen (Bosly *et al.*, 1992). Overall survival at 4 years was projected to be 14% among 200 patients who received conven-

tional salvage chemotherapy, as compared with 33% for transplanted patients (40 autologous BMT, 4 allogeneic; *P* < .001). A subsequent GELA analysis evaluated the outcome of patients who relapsed after randomization to the chemotherapy arm on their LNH87-2 trial (Haioun *et al.*, 2000). The 8-year overall survival rates of transplanted and non-transplanted patients were 36% and 8%, respectively. A similar trial evaluated pediatric NHL patients who relapsed following initial therapy (Philip *et al.*, 1993). Four out of 15 transplanted patients (14 autologous BMT, 1 allogeneic) were alive and in remission at 4 years, while there were no long-term survivors among the 12 patients who were not transplanted.

The most convincing evidence for the superiority of autologous HSC transplantation for relapsed NHL comes from the international PARMA trial (Philip *et al.*, 1995). Patients with relapsed intermediate- or high-grade NHL received two cycles of DHAP (dexamethasone, cytosine arabinoside, cisplatin) salvage chemotherapy. Patients with complete or partial responses were randomized to receive four additional cycles of DHAP or treatment with autologous BMT. Patients in each arm could also receive additional involved field radiation. Event-free survival at 5 years was estimated at 46% following autologous BMT and 12% for those who received conventional salvage chemotherapy (*P* = .001). Overall survival rates were 53% and 32%, respectively (Fig. 34.9). A follow-up analysis indicated that overall survival was only better for patients with IPI scores >0 at relapse, and that good-prognosis patients with scores of 0 had similar outcomes whether continued on DHAP salvage or if transplanted (Blay *et al.*, 1998).

Additional analyses have demonstrated that costs associated with autologous HSC transplantation for relapsed NHL compare favorably with other medical treatments (Messori *et al.*, 1997), and suggest that autologous HSC transplantation should be considered standard therapy for chemotherapy-sensitive patients with relapsed aggressive NHL.

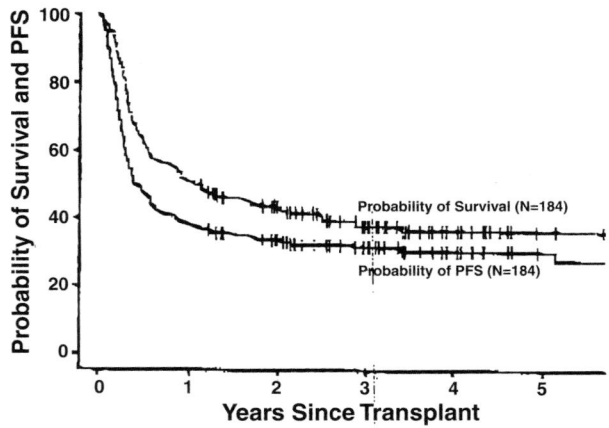

Fig. 34.8. Overall survival and progression-free survival in 184 patients who never achieved a complete remission prior to autologous hematopoietic stem cell transplantation. Reproduced, with permission, from Vose *et al.* (2001b).

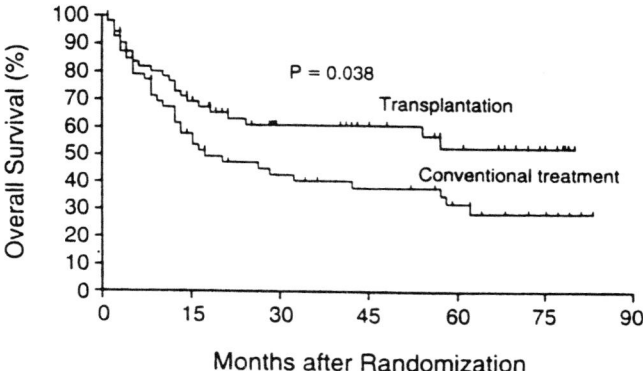

Fig. 34.9. Overall survival for patients with chemosensitive relapsed intermediate- or high-grade non-Hodgkin's lymphoma following autologous bone marrow transplantation or conventional salvage chemotherapy. Reproduced, with permission, from Philip *et al.* (1995).

Pretransplant therapy

The presence of bulky disease has been considered to be an adverse prognostic factor for patients undergoing autologous HSC transplantation for NHL (Philip *et al.*, 1987; Vose *et al.*, 1993; Mills *et al.*, 1995a; Caballero *et al.*, 1997; Stiff *et al.*, 1998). Rapoport *et al.* (1993) noted that actuarial 3-year event-free survival for patients transplanted with minimal disease (all sites ≥2 cm in diameter) was 48%, compared with 25% for patients with more extensive disease (*P* = .04).

Although the presence of bulky disease may simply be a manifestation of chemotherapy resistance, it is common practice to administer conventional salvage chemotherapy to reduce tumor burden before the transplant (Press *et al.*, 1991; Girouard *et al.*, 1997; Moskowitz *et al.*, 1999). There is relatively little information regarding the value of this approach, although this practice does provide important prognostic information about chemotherapy sensitivity. A prospective GELA trial indicated that aggressive debulking therapy prior to transplantation led to improved disease-free survival and overall survival (Bosly *et al.*, 1997). However, results of allogeneic BMT for acute myeloid leukemia (AML) are similar for patients transplanted in early first relapse or in second remission (Clift *et al.*, 1987). Similarly, the use of pretransplant chemotherapy may not improve the outcome for patients with Hodgkin's disease (HD) (Sweetenham *et al.*, 1996). Furthermore, the practice of administering debulking chemotherapy can result in significant toxicity and may exclude good candidates from receiving transplants (Phillips *et al.*, 1997).

In some series patients with untested relapse have been grouped with sensitive relapse patients (Petersen *et al.*, 1990; Phillips *et al.*, 1990). However, Mills *et al.* (1995a) noted that 3-year progression-free survival was 59% (estimated from survival curve) for patients transplanted in untested relapse. Weaver *et al.* (1994) noted that actuarial 2-year event-free survival was 59% for patients who received pretransplant cytoreduction compared with 38% for patients transplanted in untested relapse (*P* = .41).

Other investigators have used involved-field radiation to sites of bulky disease prior to transplantation (Phillips *et al.*, 1990; Gulati *et al.*, 1992; Lazarus *et al.*, 1992; Philip *et al.*, 1995; van Besien *et al.*, 1995b; Moskowitz *et al.*, 1999; Friedberg *et al.*, 2001). In these studies no clear benefit was demonstrated with this approach (Phillips *et al.*, 1990; Lazarus *et al.*, 1992), and it may be associated with significant morbidity including pulmonary toxicity and secondary myelodysplasia (Gulati *et al.*, 1992; Friedberg *et al.*, 2001). Nevertheless, the use of pretransplant radiotherapy may allow some patients to proceed to transplant who might otherwise have been considered ineligible. These patients may have outcomes that are similar to patients who did not receive radiation (Friedberg *et al.*, 2001). Occasionally, surgical debulking has been performed prior to transplantation (Rapoport *et al.*, 1993).

It is unlikely that a benefit from pretransplant cytoreduction can be conclusively demonstrated without a prospective trial. It may be reasonable to proceed directly to transplant for relapsed NHL patients with low tumor burden, although debulking ther-apy will likely be used for the majority of patients with significant tumor burden at relapse.

Low-grade lymphoma and Waldenstrom's macroglobulinemia[1]

Low-grade lymphoma

There is less experience with transplantation for low-grade NHL compared with aggressive histologic subtypes. The majority of patients treated have had follicular NHL, with a minority having other indolent histologies. Results from representative series are shown in Table 34.11. These series contain patients with a variety of prognostic factors treated in a heterogeneous manner (see Table 34.12). In addition, some series contained patients with follicular large cell histology (Bartlett *et al.*, 1994; Martin *et al.*, 1995), as well as other entities that may have a different clinical behavior. A study of 26 patients with follicular large cell lymphoma reported a 4 year overall survival and disease-free survival of 58% and 51%, respectively (Cao *et al.*, 2001).

Chemotherapy sensitivity prior to autologous HSC transplantation appears to be an important prognostic variable for patients with low-grade NHL (Freedman *et al.*, 1991; Colombat *et al.*, 1994; Schouten *et al.*, 1994; Cervantes *et al.*, 1995; Stein *et al.*, 1999). Heavily pretreated patients also do less well after autologous HSC transplantation (Rohatiner *et al.*, 1994; Bastion *et al.*, 1995; Bierman *et al.*, 1997). Patients with follicular small cleaved cell lymphoma and those with follicular mixed histology appear to have similar outcomes (Colombat *et al.*, 1994; Bierman *et al.*, 1997), although a large cell component may be associated with inferior survival (Bierman *et al.*, 1996). However, patients with follicular large cell histology may have superior survival when compared with patients having diffuse large cell histology (Vose *et al.*, 1998). Other negative prognostic factors which have been reported include male gender, involvement of greater than 8 sites, extranodal disease (exclusive of the marrow), and prior radiotherapy (Voso *et al.*, 2000a).

These results demonstrate that autologous HSC transplantation can be performed with low mortality for patients with low-grade histology, and that long-term disease-free survival is possible. However, the majority of these series and ABMTR data show a continuous pattern of treatment failure for most patient groups. It is unclear from these trials whether any patients are cured or whether survival is prolonged. Rohatiner *et al.* (1994) demonstrated that freedom from recurrence for follicular lymphoma patients receiving autologous BMT in second remission was significantly better than historical controls treated with conventional chemotherapy. However, no significant differences in overall survival were observed. With 8 year overall and disease-free survival rates of 66% and 42% respectively, Freedman and colleagues (1999) felt that myeloablative therapy and autologous BMT were likely to prolong survival in patients transplanted for relapsed follicular lymphoma. In a

---

[1]Jan Gösta Waldenstrom, Swedish physician, 1906–1996.

Table 34.11. *Autologous hematopoietic stem cell transplantation for low-grade non-Hodgkin's lymphoma*

Reference	Number of patients	Transplant regimen	Stem cell source	Purging	Early death rate	Outcome	Comments
Freedman *et al.* (1991)	51	Cy+TBI	Marrow	Yes	2%	47% 4 yr DFS	Included patients with small lymphocytic and diffuse inter-mediate histology
Fouillard *et al.* (1991)	10	TACC, BEAM	Marrow	Yes in 9	0%	80% CCR (15–43 mo)	Included patients in first CR
Colombat *et al.* (1994)	42	Various	Marrow, blood	Yes in 15	7%	58% 4 yr EFS	Included patients with follicular large-cell histology
Schouten *et al.* (1994)	92	Various	Marrow	Yes in 27	NS	52% 4 yr PFS	Included patients in first CR
Rohatiner *et al.* (1994)	64	Cy+TBI	Marrow	Yes	5%	35% (55%) CCR (1–8 yrs)	Included patients with follicular large cell histology
Cervantes *et al.* (1995)	34	Cy+TBI, BAC	Marrow, blood	Yes in 13	12%	18% 2 yr DFS	Included patients with small lymphocytic histology
Bastion *et al.* (1995)	60	Various	Blood	No	8%	53% 2 yr FFS	Included patients with follicular large cell histology
Haas *et al.* (1996b)	48	Cy+TBI, BEAM	Blood	No	4%	76% 2 yr DFS	Included patients in first CR
Bierman *et al.* (1997)	100	Various	Marrow, blood	No	8%	44% 4 yr FFS	

Abbreviations: Cy, cyclophosphamide; TBI, total body irradiation; TACC, 6-thioguanine, cytosine arabinoside, cyclophosphamide, lomustine; BEAM, carmustine, etoposide, cytosine arabinoside, melphalan; BAC, carmustine, cytosine arabinoside, cyclophosphamide; DFS, disease-free survival; CCR, continous complete remission; EFS, event-free survival; PFS, progression-free survival; FFS, failure-free survival; CR, complete remission

non-randomized study from the GELF group (Brice *et al.*, 2000) patients who underwent autologous SCT after first relapse had significantly longer freedom from progression (42% vs. 16%) and overall survival (58% vs. 38%) at 5 years than patients treated with conventional therapy. It remains unclear whether patients are cured by autologous HSC transplantation. In both retrospective analysis and prospective randomized trials it appears that remission duration is prolonged with high dose therapy and stem cell support (Lopez *et al.*, 1999; Horning *et al.*, 2001). Ninety-two patients with high-risk follicular lymphoma treated at diagnosis by intensive sequential high-dose therapy and autografting had a four year disease-free survival of 67% (Ladetto *et al.*, 2002). Posttransplant, 65% of molecularly evaluable patients achieved a clinical and molecular remission, and the projected DFS at 4 years for this subgroup was 85%. Prolonged follow-up is mandatory for patients transplanted for low-grade NHL. Late relapses up to 9 years following autologous HSC transplantation have been observed (Fouillard *et al.*, 1991; Colombat *et al.*, 1994; Bierman *et al.*, 1997). Relapse can occur as transformation of follicular lymphoma to diffuse large B cell lymphoma (Kojima *et al.*, 2000).

The absence of a definite plateau in disease-free survival following autologous HSC transplantation for low-grade lymphoma has led to attempts at transplantation in first remission. At Dana-Farber Cancer Institute, the actuarial 3-year disease-free survival and overall survival rates were 63% and 89%,

respectively, following autologous BMT in first complete remission or with minimal disease following CHOP chemotherapy (Freedman *et al.*, 1996). Although overall survival might be prolonged by early transplantation, it remains uncertain whether there is evidence of a plateau in disease-free survival (Fig 34.9). Horning and co-workers at Stanford have reported results of patients transplanted in first CR or PR. The estimated 10 year disease specific survival was 97% with overall survival of 86% (Horning *et al.*, 2001). Other reports of autologous HSC transplantation in first remission for low-grade lymphoma have also shown a continuous pattern of treatment failure without evidence of cure (Morel *et al.*, 1995; Haas *et al.*, 1996b). Remission duration is longer following autologous HSCT than after conventional therapy (Gonzalez-Barca *et al.*, 2000). Whether first remission transplant is superior to transplant for relapsed disease is unclear. The overall survival from diagnosis for patients transplanted in first remission is similar to that seen in patients transplanted in second or greater remission (Seyfarth *et al.*, 2001).

Waldenstrom's macroglobulinemia

Autologous peripheral blood stem cell transplantation for Waldenstrom's macroglobulinemia has been described (Desikan *et al.*, 1999; Yang *et al.*, 1999; Dreger *et al.*, 1999a). In the latter report both mobilization and engraftment may have been hindered by pretansplant fludaribine treatment. A marked improvement in, or normalization of, bone marrow infiltration and serum IgM levels was seen in some patients. A literature review described 24 patients with a median age of 51: 14 were transplanted with refractory or relapsed disease and 10 when their disease was chemosensitive. Twenty-three achieved remission and only 1 transplant-related death occurred. Fifteen were alive and well at the time of the report, two at 4.5 and 12 years posttransplant (Anagnostopoulos & Giralt, 2002).

The apparent inability of autologous HSC transplantation to cure low-grade lymphoma has led to increasing interest in allogeneic transplantation for these patients. van Besien et al. (1995a) reported that 8 of 10 patients who received an allogeneic BMT for low-grade NHL were alive and in remission between 1 and 5 years later. A subsequent report showed a 2-year disease-free survival estimated at 59% among 15 patients (van Besien et al., 1996c). International Bone Marrow Transplant Registry results showed an actuarial 3-year disease-free survival of 43% among 81 patients following HLA-matched BMT for low-grade NHL (van Besien et al., 1995a), although treatment-related mortality was 44%. Verdonck et al. (1997) retrospectively compared allogeneic and autologous BMT for recurrent and refractory low-grade lymphoma. The actuarial relapse rate was 0% following allogeneic transplantation, and 83% following autologous transplantation, leading to 2-year progression-free survival rates of 68% and 22%, respectively ($P = .049$). Forrest and colleagues (2002) reported on 24 patients with follicular lymphoma, none of whom were in complete remission at the time of transplant, and all of whom received myeloablative conditioning prior to an HLA-identical sibling graft in 23 or an HLA-matched unrelated graft in one. The transplant-related mortality was 21% and actuarial disease-free survival was 78% with a median follow-up of 28 months for the 19 patients alive at the time of the report. Non-myeloablative approaches are being intensively studied in indolent lymphomas. The M. D. Anderson group reported on 20 patients that the probability of remission was 84% at 2 years, with no relapses seen (Khouri et al., 2001) (see Chapters 22 and 57).

Despite lower relapse rates following allogeneic transplantation for low-grade lymphoma, use of this approach using myeloablative conditioning is limited by high procedure-related mortality as well as by donor availability. Nevertheless, the apparent lack of cure in most patient groups following autografting makes allogeneic transplantation worthy of additional study.

A literature review reported six patients with Waldenstrom's macroglobulinemia who had undergone allografting (Anagnostopoulos & Giralt, 2002). Their median age was 45 and all had been heavily pretreated because of refractory or relapsed disease. Four received myeloablative conditioning and two reduced intensity conditioning. Three were reported alive and well at 5+, 34+, and 112+ months posttransplant respectively.

Transformed lymphoma

Transformation of low-grade NHL to more aggressive histology is a frequent occurrence. Transformation has been associated with a poor prognosis in most reports, although good outcomes have sometimes been reported with conventional therapy (Yuen et al., 1995). In some series autologous HSC transplantation for transformed NHL has been associated with a worse prognosis than de novo aggressive histology NHL (Schouten et al., 1989, 1994; Bastion et al., 1995), while other investigators have failed to note inferior outcomes for patients transplanted after histologic transformation (Freedman et al., 1991; Wheeler et al., 1993; Bolwell et al., 2000; Williams et al., 2001).

Investigators from St. Bartholomew's Hospital noted that 14 of 27 patients who received autologous transplants for transformed lymphoma were alive and in remission at a median follow-up of 2.4 years (Foran et al., 1998). The actuarial 5-year disease-free survival rate was 46% in a series of transformed lymphoma patients following autologous HSC transplantation at Dana-Farber Cancer Institute (Friedberg et al., 1999a); the 4-year event-free survival was estimated to be 38% in a series from the Cleveland Clinic (Bolwell et al., 2000), and the 5-year progression-free survival rate was 36% in a series from Princess Margaret Hospital (Chen et al., 2001). The 5-year progression-free survival rate was estimated at 30% in an EBMT analysis of autologous HSC transplantation for transformed lymphoma (Williams et al., 2001). Prognostic factors reported to be associated with poorer outcome following autologous HSC transplantation for transformed lymphoma include elevated LDH and chemotherapy resistance (Williams et al., 2001), transformation more than 18 months from initial diagnosis of low-grade lymphoma (Friedberg et al., 1999a), and age greater than 60 years (Chen et al., 2001). Interpretation of results is hindered by differences in the definition of "transformed" among series, but these results suggest that transplantation should be considered for these patients, especially if they are sensitive to conventional salvage chemotherapy.

Mantle cell lymphoma

Mantle cell lymphoma is a distinct entity with a poor prognosis following treatment with conventional chemotherapy (Weisenburger & Armitage, 1996). Several series have investigated the role of autologous HSC transplantation for patients with relapsed and refractory mantle cell lymphoma (Haas et al., 1996a; Blay et al., 1998; Freedman et al., 1998; Kröger et al., 1998; Milpied et al., 1998; Decaudin et al., 2000; Vose et al., 2000; Sweetenham, 2001; Gopal et al., 2002). Although long-term disease-free survival may be observed, the majority of these series have failed to show evidence of a plateau in disease-free survival. These results have led to trials of transplantation in first remission for patients with mantle cell lymphoma.

Investigators from the Dana-Farber Cancer Institute failed to achieve polymerase chain reaction (PCR) negativity with immunologic purging in patients with mantle cell lymphoma (Andersen et al., 1997). No evidence of a disease-free survival plateau was demonstrated when patients with mantle cell lymphoma patients were treated with autologous HSCT in first remission (Freedman et al., 1998; Fig. 34.10). Other institutions have reported more optimistic results with disease-free survival rates of 70–80% at 2–4 years in small series (Dreger et al., 1999b; Geisler et al., 2000; Malone et al., 2001). Investigators

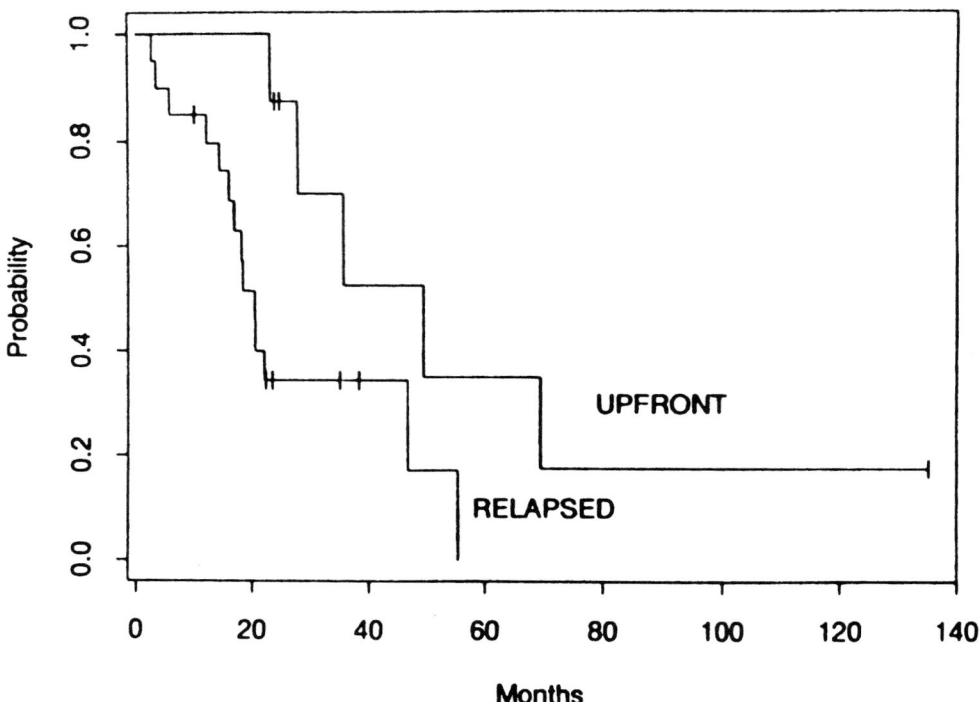

Fig. 34.10. Disease-free survival following autologous bone marrow transplantation for patients with mantle cell lymphoma in first remission following CHOP induction (upfront) or for relapsed patients treated in ≥ second remission (relapsed). Reproduced, with permission, from Freedman *et al.* (1998).

from M. D. Anderson Cancer Center reported a 72% 3-year event-free survival rate in 25 patients with previously untreated mantle cell lymphoma given 4 courses of Hyper-CVAD (cyclophosphamide, doxorubicin, vincristine, and dexamethasone, alternating with high-dose methotrexate and cytarabine) prior to HSC transplantation (autologous 21; allogeneic 4) (Khouri *et al.*, 1998). This result was significantly better than historical controls treated with CHOP-like regimens. The 5-year overall survival rate was estimated at 61% among mantle cell lymphoma patients transplanted in first remission in an EBMT analysis (Vandenberghe *et al.*, 2000). These results have been used to suggest that autologous transplantation in first remission may improve overall survival for mantle cell lymphoma patients, although definite plateaus in disease-free survival have not been observed. Results should also be interpreted with caution, since most series have only reported survival following transplantation for patients who achieved remission with initial therapy and were able to proceed to transplant. Definite survival advantages can only be shown if outcomes are reported using the entire denominator of patients identified at the time of diagnosis.

Case reports and small series of allogeneic transplantation for mantle cell lymphoma have also been reported (Corradini *et al.*, 1996; Sohn *et al.*, 1997; Adkins *et al.*, 1998; Khouri *et al.*, 1999; Vandenberghe *et al.*, 2000). At the University of Nebraska the 4-year event-free survival is 37% in 16 patients who received allogeneic transplants for mantle cell lymphoma (unpublished data). Evidence of a plateau in disease-free survival has been shown in some of these reports, and this approach may be considered for younger patients. However,

clear survival advantages over autologous HSC transplantation, and other approaches, have not been observed because of higher rates of transplant-related toxicity.

Primary nasal natural killer (NK/T) cell lymphoma

The prognosis for both nasal and non-nasal NK/T cell lymphoma is generally poor. Patients with advanced disease usually die despite intensive chemotherapy, with or without radiotherapy. Long-term disease-free survival has been described following autologous and allogeneic HSCT for patients with relapsed and refractory disease (Liang *et al.*, 1997; Nawa *et al.*, 1999; Takenaka *et al.*, 2001), although experience is limited.

Central nervous system disease

The prognosis for NHL patients with central nervous system (CNS) relapse is poor (van Besien, Forman, & Champlin, 1997a), and these patients have frequently been considered ineligible for transplantation. However, results from the EBMT demonstrated that 5-year progression-free survival was 42% for patients with prior CNS disease that had been eradicated prior to autologous HSC transplantation (Williams *et al.*, 1994). This outcome was in contrast to 9% progression-free survival for patients with active CNS disease at the time of transplant (*P* = .001). Patients with CNS disease at the time of diagnosis had significantly better survival than those with CNS relapse. Similar results have been noted by other investigators (van Besien *et al.*, 1996a; Alvarnas *et al.*, 2000). Some authors have suggested that the combination of pretransplant intrathecal chemotherapy and irradiation was most likely to eradicate CNS disease and result in prolonged survival (Williams *et al.*, 1994), while others have recommended different approaches (van Besien, Forman, & Champlin, 1997a; Alvarnas *et al.*, 2000). Prolonged follow-up is required for these patients because of concerns about delayed leukoencephalopathy.

Prolonged disease-free survival has also been described following high-dose therapy with HSC transplantation for patients with primary central nervous system lymphoma (Khalfallah *et al.*, 1996; Alvarnas *et al.*, 2000; Soussain *et al.*, 2001). The 3-year event-free survival was estimated at 53% following autologous transplantation in a series of 22 patients with relapsed and refractory primary central nervous system lymphoma (Soussain *et al.*, 2001). Long-term disease-free survival has also been described following allogeneic transplantation for relapsed primary central nervous system lymphoma (Varadi *et al.*, 1999).

HIV-associated lymphoma (and see Chapter 121)

The advent of highly active anti-retroviral therapy (HAART) has enabled the exploration of autologous HSC transplantation for HIV-associated lymphoma. At the City of Hope, nine patients with HIV-associated Hodgkin's disease or NHL received high-dose cyclophosphamide, carmustine, and etoposide followed by autologous G-CSF-mobilized peripheral blood stem cells. CD4+ T cell counts recovered to pretransplant levels and HIV viral load was controlled in those compliant with anti-retroviral therapy. Seven of the nine remained in remission at a median of 19 months posttransplant (Krishnan *et al.*, 2001).

Transplantation in the elderly

Decreasing procedure-related morbidity and mortality has allowed older patients to be considered for autologous HSC transplantation. The ABMTR demonstrated somewhat higher mortality and lower overall survival among NHL patients transplanted between the ages of 60 to 69, although these differences were not statistically significant (Lazarus, Horowitz, & Nugent, 1996). Investigators from Stanford University reported that 5-year event-free survival among patients transplanted for hematologic malignancy (49% NHL) was 46% for patients under age 50, compared to 34% for patients aged 51 to 65 ($P = .03$) (Kusnierz-Glaz *et al.*, 1997). Regimen-related mortality rates were 7.4% and 12.7%, respectively ($P = .07$). Miller *et al.* (1996) analyzed the influence of age in a cohort of patients (33% NHL) following autologous transplantation. Patients over age 50 had a significantly higher risk of transplant-related mortality and a slight decrease in event-free survival. A study from Mayo Clinic evaluated results of autologous HSC transplantation in NHL patients over age 65 (Inwards *et al.*, 2000). The median survival for these patients was 10.3 months, whereas the median had not been reached for younger patients ($P = .03$). The 4-year progression-free survival was estimated to be 24% among 53 NHL patients who received autologous transplants at Seattle (Gopal *et al.*, 2001). Treatment-related mortality was 22%.

Table 34.12. *Prognostic variables associated with autologous HSC transplantation for non-Hodgkin's lymphoma*

Chemotherapy sensitivity of NHL
Amount of prior therapy for NHL
Performance status at time of transplant (poor is bad)
Serum lactic acid dehydrogenase level (elevated is bad)
High-grade histology (high is bad)
Bulky disease

These results suggest that autografting can be performed relatively safely for patients at least into their seventh decade. Although results are somewhat poorer than younger patients, this population should not be excluded from potentially curative therapy on the basis of age alone.

Early transplantation

A variety of prognostic factors can identify NHL patients who are less likely to achieve remission, or more likely to relapse than others (Table 34.12) (Shipp, 1994). Several investigators have tested the hypothesis that use of autografting early in the course of disease might improve survival for patients who are unlikely to be cured with standard therapy. This approach requires the ability to identify poor-prognosis patients and the ability to perform autologous transplantation with low morbidity and mortality.

One of the first series of early autologous HSC transplantation for poor-prognosis NHL was reported by Gulati *et al.* (1988). Thirty-one patients with large cell NHL and poor prognostic features were treated with a conventional chemotherapy regimen. Fourteen patients in first complete or partial remission received high-dose therapy followed by an autologous transplant, and the remainder received additional conventional chemotherapy and had the option of subsequent transplant at relapse. Disease-free survival was significantly better for patients transplanted immediately after attaining remission.

Several other phase II trials of early autografting for patients with poor-prognosis aggressive NHL have been reported and selected results are displayed in Table 34.13. The ABMTR data for patients given autotransplants for intermediate-grade or immunoblastic NHL, are shown in Figure 34.11. The estimated 3-year overall survival was 68% among 362 patients transplanted in first remission (Horowitz, 2002).

These studies demonstrate that patients can be transplanted in first remission with little associated mortality. In addition, survival appears better than in conventionally treated patients. However, these patients may represent only a fraction of the total number of poor-prognosis patients who might have been considered for early transplant at the time of initial diagnosis. This denominator is rarely reported (Santini *et al.*, 1991; Jost *et al.*, 1995), but must be known to help evaluate the true impact of early transplantation, unless randomized trials are performed.

Several randomized trials have now been performed to evaluate the role of early autografting for patients with poor-prognosis NHL. The GELA LNH87-2 trial randomized 541 patients

Table 34.13. *Autologous hemopoietic stem cell transplantation in first remission for poor-prognosis non-Hodgkin's lymphoma*

Reference	Number of patients	Early death rate	Outcome	Comments
Gulati *et al.* (1988)	14	0%	11 (79%) CCR (31–71 mo)	6 patients in CR at transplant 8 patients in PR at transplant Disease-free survival significantly better than concurrent controls treated with chemotherapy alone
Milpied *et al.* (1989)	13	0%	70% 4 yr DFS	
Santini *et al.* (1991)	21	5%	66% DFS	40 patients initially entered on trial
Baro *et al.* (1991)	12	17%	8 (67%) CCR (8–52 mo)	Survival significantly better than historical controls treated with chemotherapy alone
Verdonck *et al.* (1992)	9	0%	6 (67%) CCR (12–113 mo)	
Freedman *et al.* (1993)	26	0%	85% 28 mo DFS	16 patients in CR at transplant 10 patients with minimal disease state at transplant
Jackson *et al.* (1994)	28	0%	83% 3 yr EFS	Outcome includes 2 patients who relapsed prior to transplant
Sweetenham *et al.* (1994)	102	4%	70% 5 yr PFS	
Sweetenham *et al.* (1996a)	70	3%	73% 3 yr PFS	All patients had diffuse small noncleaved cell histology
Jost *et al.* (1995)	17	0%	48% 3 yr EFS	26 patients initially entered on trial
Fanin *et al.* (1996)	16	0%	100% DFS	All patients had CD30 (Ki-1)+ anaplastic large cell lymphoma 12 patients in CR at transplant 4 patients in PR at transplant
Pettengell *et al.* (1996)	33	6%	61% 2 yr EFS	Survival significantly better than historical controls treated with chemotherapy alone
Vitolo *et al.* (1997)	39	6%	50% 32 mo FFS	Outcome includes all 50 patients entered on trial
Nademanee *et al.* (1997)	52	2%	82% 3 yr DFS	39 patients in CR at transplant 13 patients in PR at transplant
Schenkein *et al.* (1997)	32	6%	67% 18 mo RFS	

Abbreviations: CCR, continuous complete remission; DFS, disease-free survival; EFS, event-free survival; PFS, progression-free survival; RFS, relapse-free survival; CR, complete remission; PR, partial remission.

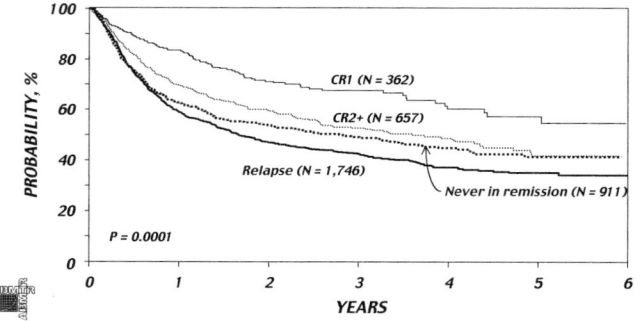

Fig. 34.11. Probability of survival after autotransplants for diffuse large cell lymphoma in patients reported to the ABMTR, 1994–1999. Three-year probabilities of survival were 68% ± 6% for 362 patients in first remission, 53% ± 5% for 657 in second remission, 42% ± 3% for 1,746 in relapse, and 49% ± 4% for 911 never achieving complete remission with conventional chemotherapy. Reproduced, with permission, from *ABMTR Newsletter, 9,* 4–11, 2002.

with aggressive NHL, who were in complete remission after the induction phase of the LNH84 regimen, to receive sequential chemotherapy or to receive high-dose chemotherapy followed by autologous BMT (Haioun *et al.,* 2000). Survival advantages were not associated with transplantation when the entire population of eligible patients was analyzed. However, a retrospective analysis was performed on 451 of 916 eligible patients in the high-intermediate and high-risk groups identified by the IPI (Shipp *et al.,* 1993). The 8-year disease-free survival among the 236 randomized poor-prognosis patients was 39% following sequential chemotherapy, as compared with 55% following autologous HSC transplantation (*P* = .02). Overall survival rates were 49% and 64%, respectively (*P* = .04; Fig. 34.12). In addition, the use of early transplantation in high-risk patients was associated with improvements in quality of life in this study (Mounier *et al.,* 2000). These results led to the subsequent GELA LNH93-3 trial for NHL patients with at least two adverse prognostic factors from the age-adjusted IPI (Gisselbrecht *et al.,* 2002). Patients were randomized to receive a novel shortened initial therapy with peripheral blood stem cell transplantation on day 60, or to treatment with standard ACVBP (doxorubicin, cyclophosphamide, vindesine, bleomycin, and prednisone, followed by methotrexate, etoposide, ifosfamide, and cytarabine). The 5-year event-free survival was

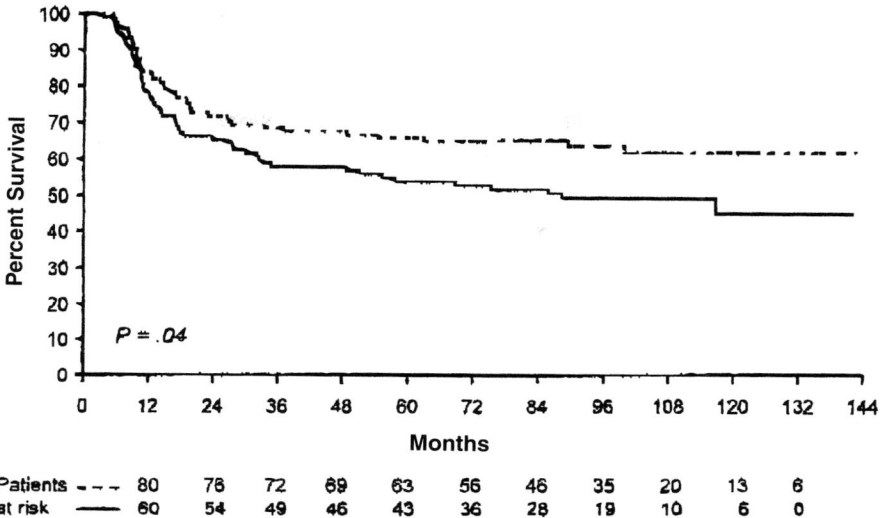

Fig. 34.12. Estimated overall survival for high/intermediate and high-risk patients following autologous BMT in first remission. Sequential chemotherapy (solid line). Autologous bone marrow transplantation (dashed line). Reproduced, with permission, from Haioun *et al.* (2000).

estimated at 39% for patients who received the novel regimen followed by autologous HSC transplantation, as compared with 51% for patients who received standard chemotherapy (*P* = .01). The overall survival rates were 46% and 60%, respectively (*P* = .007). The differing results of the two GELA trails suggest that early transplantation for poor-prognosis patients cannot be performed too soon before significant reduction of tumor burden is achieved with primary therapy.

Another trial comparing early autografting and conventional chemotherapy was reported by Gianni *et al.* (1997). Patients with untreated large cell lymphoma were randomized to receive MACOP-B (methotrexate, doxorubicin, cyclophosphamide, vincristine, prednisone, and bleomycin) or a high-dose sequential regimen consisting of debulking chemotherapy followed by high-dose chemotherapy and autologous HSC transplantation. Patients who failed either treatment could then be treated on the other arm. With a median follow-up of 55 months, event-free survival rates were 76% for patients who initially received high-dose sequential therapy, compared with 49% for patients who were first treated with MACOP-B (*P* = .004). At 7 years, overall survival rates were 81% and 55%, respectively (*P* = .09; Fig. 34.13). Use of similar high-dose sequential regimens for NHL have been successful at some institutions (Schenkein *et al.*, 1997), while this approach has been excessively toxic at other centers (Johnston *et al.*, 2000; Santini *et al.*, 2002).

Another prospective randomized trial compared conventional consolidation therapy with autologous HSCT for lymphoblastic lymphoma patients in first complete remission (Sweetenham *et al.*, 2001). The actuarial 3 year relapse-free survival rate was 24% for the conventionally treated arm as compared with 55% for the transplant arm (*P* = .065). Overall survival rates were 45% and 56% respectively (*P* = .71).

Several other randomized trials of early autologous HSC transplants have been performed for aggressive NHL with mixed results when compared with standard therapy (Santini *et al.*, 1998; Kaiser *et al.*, 1999; Milpied *et al.*, 1999; Intragumtornchai *et al.*, 2000; Kluin-Nelemans *et al.*, 2001; Kaiser *et al.*, 2002). These trials, as well as those previously mentioned, have differing trial designs. Some have randomized patients at diagnosis, while others have only randomized patients if they respond to initial conventional therapy. Some have included all patients, while others have only included poor-prognosis patients (defined in various ways). Finally, some trials have performed transplants after a full course of standard chemotherapy, while others have utilized abbreviated induction regimens. It appears that early transplantation is most likely to be beneficial for poor-prognosis patients who achieve maximal cytoreduction after a full course of conventional therapy.

Transplantation in first partial remission

Slow response to primary chemotherapy has been associated with poor outcome for patients with NHL (Haq *et al.*, 1994). A Dutch trial evaluated whether early transplantation would improve survival for patients who had only achieved partial remission after three cycles of CHOP chemotherapy (Verdonck *et al.*, 1995). Patients were randomized to receive five additional cycles of CHOP or to receive one additional cycle of CHOP followed by an autograft. No significant differences in event-free survival or overall survival were noted.

A similar Italian trial evaluated the role of early autologous transplantation for patients who were in partial remission after completing two-thirds of front-line chemotherapy (Martelli *et al.*, 1996). Patients were randomized to receive conventional DHAP chemotherapy or to treatment with autologous HSC transplantation. Progression-free survival at 55 months was estimated at 73% following transplant and 52% for those who

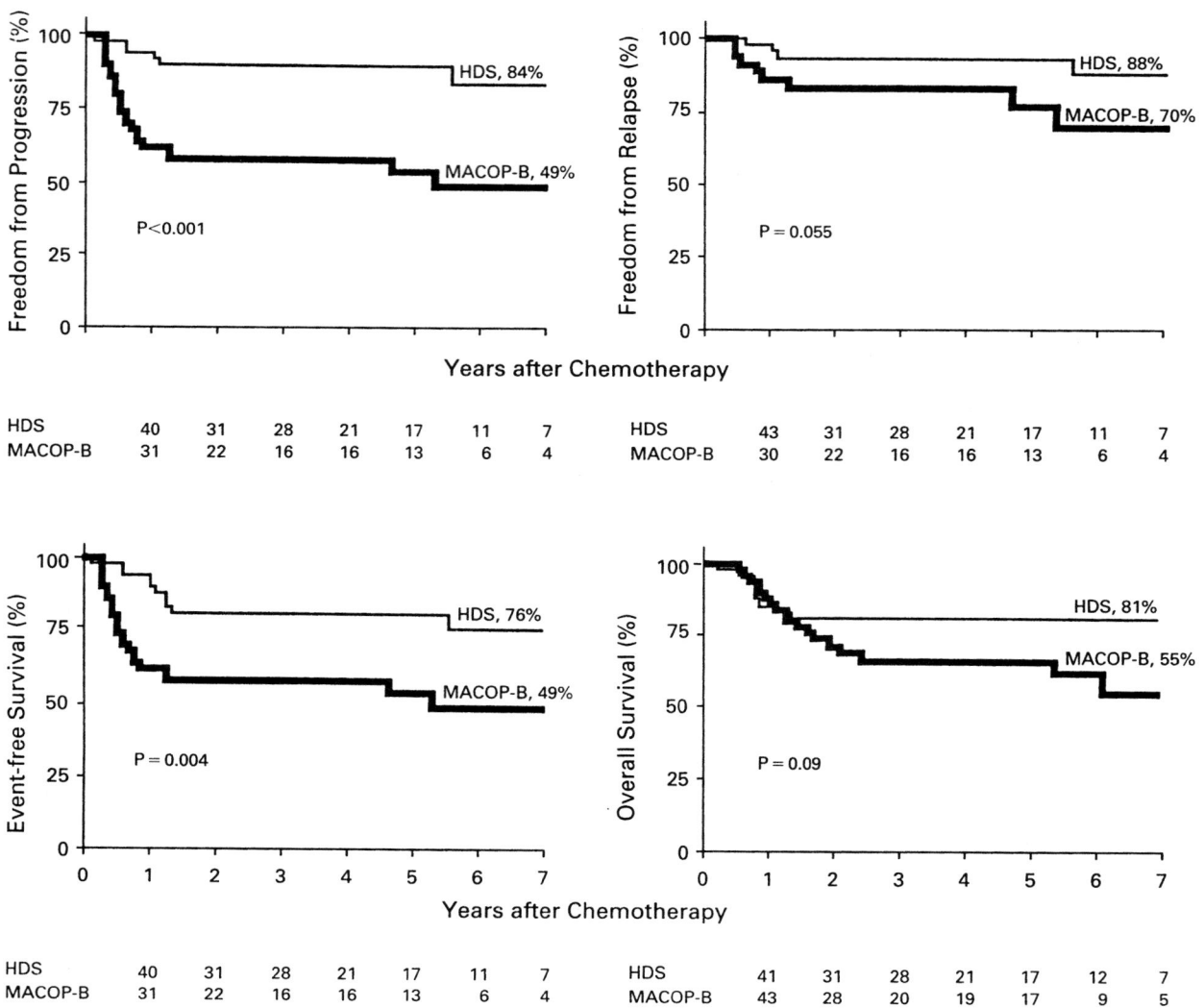

Fig. 34.13. Kaplan-Meier plots of freedom from disease progression, freedom from relapse, event-free survival, and overall survival for 48 patients initially assigned to high-dose sequential therapy (HDS) and 50 assigned to MACOP-B. The initial number of patients in complete remission and at risk for relapse was 46 for HDS and 35 for MACOP-B. The median follow-up was 55 months. The number of patients at risk is shown below each time point. Percentages at right are for each category of survival (free from disease progression, free from relapse, event-free, and overall) at 7 years. Reproduced, with permission, from Gianni *et al.* (1997).

received DHAP (*P* = .3). Overall survival rates were 73% and 59%, respectively (*P* = .4).

However, a retrospective analysis of patients achieving partial remission after the induction phase of the LNH87-2 regimen noted that 4-year overall survival was 63% for patients who received an autotransplant, compared to 46% for patients who received other salvage therapy (*P* = .03) (Haioun *et al.*, 1995). In addition, other trials suggest that patients who achieve a partial remission after primary chemotherapy may have good outcomes if they proceed directly to transplantation (Philip *et al.*, 1988; Verdonck *et al.*, 1992; Mills *et al.*, 1995a; Fouillard *et al.*, 1998).

These results suggest that patients transplanted for slow response assessed after partial completion of initial chemotherapy may not be directly comparable to patients transplanted in

first partial remission after a full course of initial therapy. Slow responders may not have achieved sufficient cytoreduction prior to transplant and might benefit by transplant after additional conventional therapy. Patients in first partial remission after completion of their initial treatment appear to be good transplant candidates if sufficient cytoreduction can be achieved.

Purging

Transplantation of autologous blood or marrow results in the possibility of reinfusing malignant cells. Various methods of removing (purging) tumor cells from autologous stem cells have been developed (Rizzoli & Carlo-Stella, 1995) (see Chapter 17). Few issues of HSC transplantation are as controversial as those dealing with purging. However, several lines of evidence suggest that the reinfusion of malignant cells may contribute to relapse and support the use of purging.

Gene marking studies have demonstrated that contaminated marrow can contribute to relapse in some patients with AML, chronic myeloid leukemia, and neuroblastoma (Hanania et al., 1995). Similar evidence for the origin of relapse is not available for NHL, however. Early disseminated relapse in some patients undergoing autologous BMT for NHL also suggests that infused cells might contribute to relapse (Vaughan et al., 1987; Rossetti, Deeg, & Hackman, 1995).

Sharp et al. (1996) used an in vitro culture system and Southern blot analysis to detect lymphoma cells in the marrow harvests of patients undergoing autologous BMT for NHL. The 5-year relapse-free survival rate was 57% for patients without detectable tumor, as compared to 17% for patients with marrow that contained tumor. The same group, however, subsequently found that lymphoma contamination of apheresis products had no apparent impact on event-free or overall survival (Demirkazik et al., 2001). Gribben et al. (1991) reported on 114 NHL patients who had bone marrow tumor cells detectable by PCR prior to purging. Following purging with monoclonal antibodies and complement, 57 patients had residual detectable tumor contamination, while 57 patients had no detectable tumor cells. At the time of median follow-up, 39% of patients transplanted with contaminated marrow had relapsed, as compared to 5% of patients without detectable lymphoma cells ($P < .00001$; Fig. 34.14). In addition, a retrospective French analysis showed a lower rate of relapse and improved event-free survival in NHL patients who received more aggressive purging (Fouillard et al., 1998).

Relapse also occurs, however, after syngeneic and allogeneic transplantation for NHL, and at least some relapses must result from failure to eradicate lymphoma with the preparative regimen. This is supported by the fact that most relapses occur at sites of prior disease (Phillips et al., 1990; Gribben et al., 1991). Furthermore, retrospective analyses, matched-pair analyses, and one prospective trial have failed to show a benefit from purging in NHL (Petersen et al., 1990; Weisdorf et al., 1991; Gulati et al., 1992; Schouten et al., 1994; Williams et al., 1996; Brunvand et al., 1996; Schouten et al., 2002).

Several groups are investigating the use of rituximab prior to autologous stem cell collection as a means of in vivo purging. Magni and colleagues (2000) used rituximab to effectively purge peripheral blood stem autografts in patients with CD20+ follicular or mantle cell lymphoma. CD34+ cells harvested from rituximab recipients were PCR-negative for tumor markers in 93% of cases, as compared to 40% of controls who did not receive rituximab. In addition, clinical and molecular remission was obtained in all 14 evaluable rituximab recipients, as compared to 70% of controls. Others have reported similar findings (Flinn et al., 2000; Voso et al., 2000b). Positive selection techniques as a means of purging have also been investigated (Gorin et al., 1995; McQuaker et al., 1997; Vose et al., 2001a), although an increased incidence of infectious complications has been reported with this approach (Crippa et al., 2002).

It is unlikely that the value of purging will be proven without a prospective randomized trial. Since purging makes intuitive sense and can be accomplished without apparent harm, many investigators will continue to use this approach in the absence of definitive studies proving benefit.

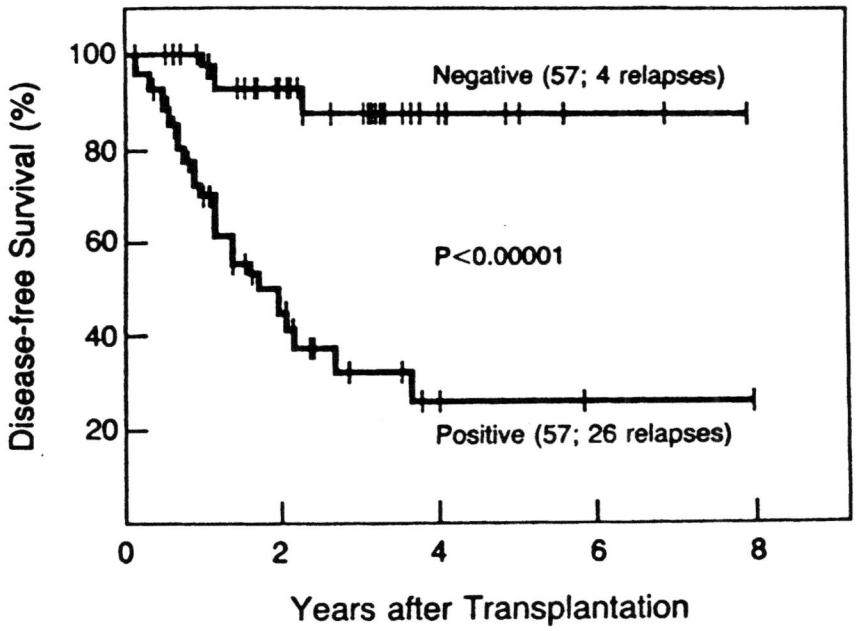

Fig. 34.14. Probability of disease-free survival after autologous bone marrow transplantation in 114 patients with B-cell non-Hodgkin's lymphoma. "Negative" denotes the patients in whom PCR did not detect residual lymphoma cells after purging, and "Positive" the patients in whom PCR did detect residual disease. Reproduced, with permission, from Gribben et al. (1991).

Late effects

Quality of life following HSC transplantation has been examined in several studies, although none have specifically addressed quality of life after autologous HSC transplantation for NHL (Wingard et al., 1991; Chao et al., 1992; Vose et al., 1992; Andrykowski et al., 1995). A multi-institutional study found that quality of life following BMT for NHL was similar to that of patients transplanted for leukemia and Hodgkin's disease (Andrykowski et al., 1995).

In general, recipients of autografts report significantly less functional impairment than allogeneic BMT recipients (Andrykowski et al., 1995). Most patients are able to return to a normal or nearly normal functional status, although significant numbers report problems with fatigue and sexual function. Chao et al. (1992) noted that mean quality of life was 8.9 (scale 1 to 10) at 1 year following autologous HSC transplantation for NHL.

Although infertility is very common following BMT for hematologic malignancies, successful pregnancies have been reported following autografting for NHL (Brice et al., 1994; Jackson et al., 1997). These results indicate the need for counseling regarding birth control for patients of childbearing age.

Several reports have documented an actuarial risk of 3% to 18% of developing cytogenetic abnormalities, AML, or myelodysplastic syndrome within 3 to 7 years following autologous transplantation for lymphoma (Darrington et al., 1994; Stone et al., 1994; Traweek et al., 1994; Bhatia et al., 1996; Krishnan et al., 2000; Micallef et al., 2000). Risk factors associated with the development of secondary leukemia have included older age (Darrington et al., 1994; Stone et al., 1994; Bhatia et al., 1996; Milligan et al., 1999; Micallef et al., 2000), use of TBI-containing regimens (Darrington et al., 1994; Milligan et al., 1999; Sureda et al., 2001) or any pretransplant radiotherapy (Stone et al., 1994; Krishnan et al., 2000; Friedberg et al., 2001), prior use of fludarabine (Micallef et al., 2000), etoposide priming for peripheral stem cell collections (Krishnan et al., 2000), and use of peripheral blood as opposed to marrow (Bhatia et al., 1996). The prognosis for patients who develop myelodysplastic syndromes is extremely poor, even if allogeneic transplantation is performed (Friedberg et al., 1999b) (see Chapter 86).

There is now increasing evidence that secondary AML and myelodysplastic syndromes are largely related to therapy administered prior to transplant, rather than to the high-dose therapy, itself. Abruzzese and colleagues (1999) used FISH to demonstrate in 9 of 12 cases that the cytogenetic abnormality present when MDS was diagnosed was also present in specimens taken before the high-dose transplant conditioning regimen was administered. Similar findings were noted by the group from St. Bartholomew's Hospital (Lillington et al., 2001).

Posttransplant therapy

Patients who achieve a complete remission after autologous transplantation for NHL are still at significant risk for relapse, and various posttransplant treatment strategies have been evalu-

ated. Rapoport et al. (1993; 1997) noted that posttransplant radiation therapy was associated with improved event-free survival following autografting for NHL. A retrospective French analysis noted similar results in the subgroup of patients transplanted in first remission (Fouillard et al., 1998). The use of posttransplant radiotherapy was associated with improved overall survival in an ABMTR analysis of transplantation for patients who had never achieved remission (Vose et al., 2001b). In contrast, an analysis from Dana-Farber Cancer Center found no significant differences in survival when patients who received posttransplant irradiation were compared with others (Friedberg et al., 2001). Some groups advocate posttransplant radiation for patients with persistently positive gallium scans following transplant (Wheeler et al., 1993). Interpretation of results is difficult in the absence of randomized trials, since patients who relapse early, those with poor performance status, or those with delayed engraftment may not be able to receive this treatment.

Several investigators have tested posttransplant immunotherapy. A prospective randomized trial of anti-B4-blocked ricin demonstrated no prolongation of survival following autologous BMT for NHL (Grossbard et al., 1998). Schenkein et al. (1994) demonstrated that posttransplant alpha-interferon led to improved overall survival in a nonrandomized trial for patients with lymphoma. The use of interleukin-2 has been investigated following autografting for NHL (Robinson et al., 1997). Israeli investigators reported improved disease-free survival and overall survival in patients treated with alpha-interferon and interleukin-2 following transplant, when compared with historical controls (Nagler et al., 1997). Additional trials of immunotherapy after autografting for NHL have been reported (Benyunes et al., 1995; Gryn et al., 1997). Rituximab has been used with some success to treat relapse after autologous transplantation (Tsai et al., 1999), and its potential to prevent relapse posttransplant is currently being explored.

Allogeneic HSC transplantation (and see Chapter 57)

Allogeneic HSCT for NHL is used less frequently than autologous transplantation (Gratwohl et al., 1999; Horowitz, 2002). Allogeneic transplantation eliminates the possibility of infusing malignant cells and may result in a graft-versus-lymphoma effect, similar to the graft-versus-leukemia effect associated with allogeneic transplantation for leukemia (Horowitz et al., 1990). However, allogeneic transplantation is limited by donor availability and increased morbidity and mortality.

In an early study, investigators from Seattle noted no significant differences in disease-free survival or relapse probability in lymphoma patients transplanted with autologous, allogeneic, or syngeneic marrow (Appelbaum et al., 1987). Investigators from Johns Hopkins Oncology Center and Wayne State University also compared autologous and allogeneic BMT in patients with lymphoma (Jones et al., 1991; Ratanatharathorn et al., 1994). Both studies noted significantly lower relapse rates among recipients of allogeneic transplants. However transplant-related

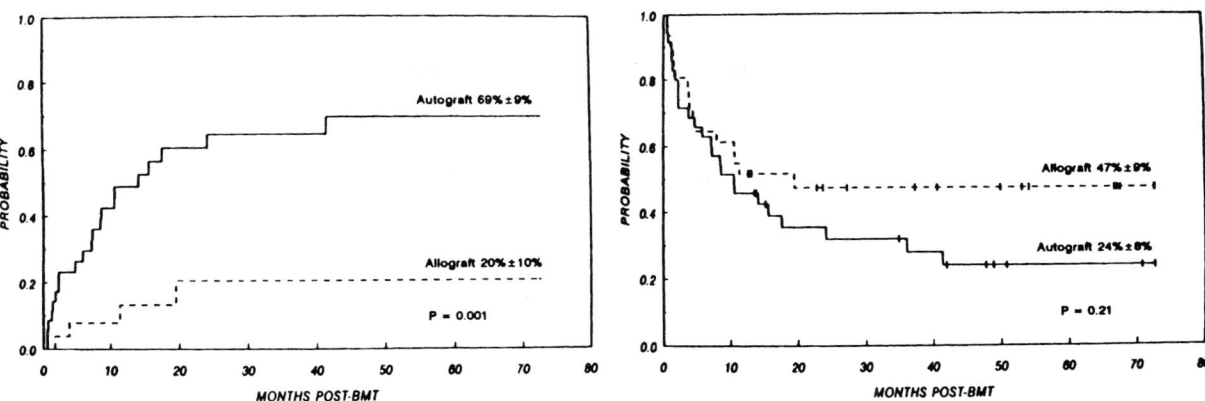

Fig. 34.15. Probability of disease progression (left panel) and progression-free survival (right panel) for non-Hodgkin's lymphoma patients following autologous or allogeneic bone marrow transplantation. Reproduced, with permission, from Ratanatharathorn *et al.*, 1994.

mortality was higher in allogeneic recipients (Fig. 34.15). A case-controlled analysis found no significant differences in progression-free survival between autologous and allogeneic BMT (Chopra *et al.*, 1992). Three-year probabilities of recurrence, survival, and disease-free survival in 113 patients reported to IBMTR with low-grade NHL given an HLA identical sibling transplant were 16%, 49%, and 49%, respectively (van Besien *et al.*, 1998; Fig. 34.16). Higher survival was associated with a pretransplant Karnofsky performance score of 90% or above, chemotherapy-sensitive disease, use of a TBI-containing conditioning regimen, and age <40 years.

A retrospective analysis of NHL transplants performed in Ontario noted that the 3-year actuarial probability of relapse

was 41% following autologous SCT as compared to 6% following allogeneic transplantation (*P* = .0006; Schimmer *et al.*, 2000). Nevertheless, overall survival rates were 62% and 71%, respectively. Another EBMT multivariate analysis noted that the relapse rate following allogeneic transplantation for intermediate/high grade NHL was significantly lower than the relapse rate following autologous transplanation (*P* = .0006), although autologous transplantation was associated with better overall survival (*P* = .0173) (Peniket *et al.*, 1997).

A retrospective registry study compared 128 patients with lymphoblastic lymphoma given an autotransplant with 76 given an HLA-identical sibling transplant (Levine *et al.*, 2003). Treatment-related mortality at 6 months was lower in the autograft recipients

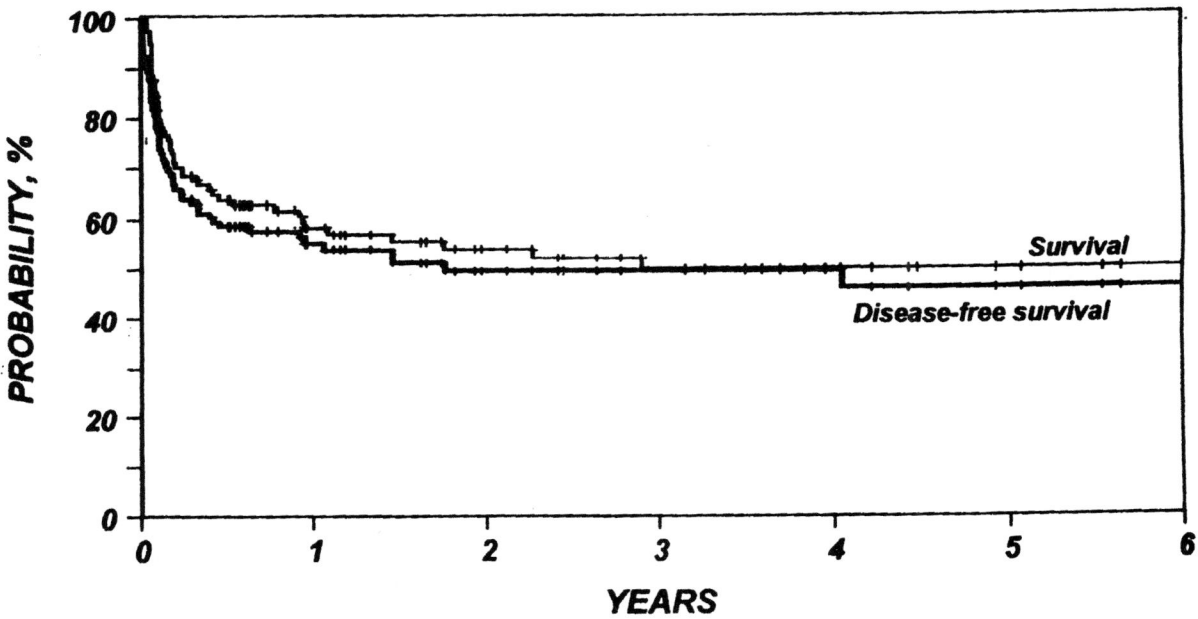

Fig. 34.16. Probability of survival and disease-free survival after HLA-identical donor bone marrow transplant for low-grade non-Hodgkin's lymphoma. Reproduced, with permission, from van Besien *et al.* (1998).

Table 34.14.   *Possible indications for allogeneic transplantation in patients with non-Hodgkin's lymphomas*

Younger age
High-grade histology
Low-grade histology
Mantle cell lymphoma
Other poor prognostic features for which a graft-versus-lymphoma effect might be useful

Table 34.15.   *Role for autologous hematopoietic stem cell transplantation in the management of non-Hodgkin's lymphomas*

Non-Hodgkin's lymphoma	Role of autologous transplantation
Chemosensitive, relapsed intermediate- or high-grade NHL	Treatment of choice
Aggressive NHL in first remission	Controversial. May be of value in IPI high-intermediate and high-risk patients (or those with other adverse prognostic characteristics) who have received a full course of initial therapy
Aggressive NHL in first partial remission	Probably beneficial
Aggressive NHL slow to respond to initial chemotherapy	Not beneficial if performed after partial course of initial chemotherapy. Possibly beneficial if sensitive to additional therapy.
Primary refractory aggressive NHL	Probably beneficial if sensitive to additional therapy
Low-grade lymphoma	Long-term disease-free suvival is possible. Ability to cure less clear-cut
Mantle cell lymphoma in first remission or in relapse	Controversial

(3% versus 18% respectively), while relapse rate was significantly higher in the autograft recipients at 1 and 5 years posttransplant (46% versus 32% and 56% versus 34%). There was no difference in disease-free or overall survival at 5 years.

These results provide evidence for the existence of a graft-versus-lymphoma effect, although lower relapse rates following allogeneic transplantation might be explained by the absence of tumor contamination. The existence of a graft-versus-lymphoma effect is also supported by findings of lower relapse rates in patients who develop chronic graft-versus-host disease (Chopra *et al.*, 1992; Ratanatharathorn *et al.*, 1994), by regression of NHL in patients who relapse after withdrawal of immunosuppression following allogeneic BMT (van Besien *et al.*, 1997b; Petersen *et al.*, 1989), and by reports of response to donor lymphocyte infusion (Mandigers *et al.*, 1998).

Despite a lower rate of relapse, virtually all comparisons have failed to show overall survival advantages with this approach because of higher transplant-related mortality. In most situations, autologous transplantation is probably the preferred approach, although there is increasing interest in allogeneic transplantation, especially for younger patients with low-grade histology (Table 34.14).

Most patients who might be considered for allogeneic transplantation lack an HLA-matched donor. An analysis from the National Marrow Donor Program analyzed results of matched unrelated allogeneic bone marrow transplantation in 158 NHL patients (Bierman *et al.*, 1999). The 2-year progression-free survival was estimated to be 30%. The actuarial day 100 mortality was 45%. Progression-free survival at 2 years was estimated to

be only 16% among adults who received matched unrelated allogeneic transplants in an EBMT analysis (Singer *et al.*, 1999).

The use of reduced intensity conditioning regimens is being studied in an attempt to decrease the mortality associated with allogeneic transplantation for NHL (Kottaridis *et al.*, 2000; Dey *et al.*, 2001; Khouri *et al.*, 2001; McSweeney *et al.*, 2001) (see Chapters 22 and 57). Despite enthusiasm for this approach, long-term follow-up is not available and comparisons with standard conditioning regimens have not been performed. In addition complications such as graft-versus-host disease occur. Nevertheless, this approach appears to result in relatively low rates of early posttransplant complications and may be appropriate for older patients or those who have relapsed after a prior autologous transplant. In the latter regard, Branson and colleagues (2002) reported on 38 patients with refractory, progressive or relapsed disease after a prior autograft. The conditioning regimen was Campath 1-H, fludarabine and melphalan. Actuarial 14-month overall survival was 53% and disease-free survival 50%. Transplant-related mortality was 79% at 100 days and 20% at 14 months.

Indications for autologous transplantation

Despite the widespread use of HSC transplantation for NHL, there is considerable uncertainty regarding the indications for this approach. Recommendations regarding indication for transplantation for NHL have been developed by two expert panels (Shipp *et al.*, 1999; Hahn *et al.*, 2001). Guidelines regarding use of HSC transplantation for NHL are shown in Table 34.15.

The current practice of HSC transplantation for NHL in Europe has been described (Urbano-Ispizua *et al.*, 2002) (and see also Chapter 124).

Future directions

High-dose therapy followed by autologous hematopoietic stem cell transplantation for NHL has become easier, safer, and less costly. It is hoped that ongoing trials, such as those combining radiolabeled antibodies with high-dose chemotherapy, will result in improved preparative regimens. Several trials are examining the role of transplantation in first remission. Other phase III trials are examining the role of posttransplant immunotherapy and several institutions are examining the use of maintenance rituximab. The role of allogeneic transplantation is becoming investigated and the use of low-intensity regimens is being actively studied. The role of transplantation will continue to evolve as improvements in primary therapy and non-transplant salvage treatments for NHL are developed.

References

Abruzzese, E., Radford, J. E., Miller, J. S. *et al.* (1999). Detection of abnormal pretransplant clones in progenitor cells of patients who developed myelodysplasia after autologous transplantation. *Blood,* **94,** 1814–9.

Adkins, D., Brown, R., Goodnough, L. T. *et al.* (1998). Treatment of resistant mantle cell lymphoma with allogeneic bone marrow transplantation. *Bone Marrow Transplantation,* **21,** 97–9.

Ager, S., Scott, M. A., Mahendra, P. *et al.* (1995). Peripheral blood stem cell transplantation after high-dose therapy in patients with malignant lymphoma: a retrospective comparison with autologous bone marrow transplantation. *Bone Marrow Transplantation,* **16,** 79–83.

Anagnostopoulos, A., & Giralt, S. (2002). Stem cell transplantation (SCT) for Waldenstrom's macroglobulinemia (WM). *Bone Marrow Transplantation,* **29,** 943–7.

Alvarnas, J. C., Negrin, R. S., Horning, S. J. *et al.* (2000). High-dose therapy with hematopoietic cell transplantation for patients with central nervous system involvement by non-Hodgkin's lymphoma. *Biology of Blood and Marrow Transplantation,* **6,** 352–8.

Andersen, N. S., Donovan, J. W., Borus, J. S. *et al.* (1997). Failure of immunologic purging in mantle cell lymphoma assessed by polymerase chain reaction detection of minimal residual disease. *Blood,* **90,** 4212–21.

Andrykowski, M. A., Greiner, C. B., Altmaier, E. M. *et al.* (1995). Quality of life following bone marrow transplantation: findings from a multicentre study. *British Journal of Cancer,* **71,** 1322–9.

Appelbaum, F. R., Deisseroth, A. B., Graw, R. G. *et al.* (1978a). Prolonged complete remission following high dose chemotherapy of Burkitt's lymphoma in relapse. *Cancer,* **41,** 1059–63.

Appelbaum, F. R., Herzig, G. P., Ziegler, J. L. *et al.* (1978b). Successful engraftment of cryopreserved autologous bone marrow in patient with malignant lymphoma. *Blood,* **52,** 85–95.

Appelbaum, F. R., Sullivan, K. M., Buckner, C. D. *et al.* (1987). Treatment of malignant lymphoma in 100 patients with chemotherapy, total body irradiation, and marrow transplantation. *Journal of Clinical Oncology,* **5,** 1340–7.

Aristei, C. & Tabilio, A. (1999). Total-body irradiation in the conditioning regimens for autologous stem cell transplantation. *The Oncologist,* **4,** 386–397.

Baro, J., Richard, C., Calavia, J. *et al.* (1991). Autologous bone marrow transplantation as consolidation therapy for non-Hodgkin's lymphoma patients with poor prognostic features. *Bone Marrow Transplantation,* **8,** 283–9.

Bartlett, N. L., Rizeq, M., Dorfman, R. F. *et al.* (1994). Follicular large-cell lymphoma: intermediate or low grade? *Journal of Clinical Oncology,* **12,** 1349–57.

Bastion, Y., Price, P., Haioun, C. *et al.* (1995). Intensive therapy with peripheral blood progenitor cell transplantation in 60 patients with poor-prognosis follicular lymphoma. *Blood,* **86,** 3257–62.

Bennett, C. L., Armitage, J. L., Armitage, G. O. *et al.* (1995). Costs of care and outcomes for high-dose therapy and autologous transplantation for lymphoid malignancies: results from the University of Nebraska 1987 through 1991. *Journal of Clinical Oncology,* **13,** 969–73.

Benyunes, M. C., Higuchi, C., York, A. *et al.* (1995). Immunotherapy with interleukin 2 with or without lymphokine-activated killer cells after autologous bone marrow transplantation for malignant lymphoma: a feasibility trial. *Bone Marrow Transplantation,* **16,** 283–8.

Bhatia, S., Ramsay, N., Steinbuch, M. *et al.* (1996). Malignant neoplasms following bone marrow transplantation. *Blood,* **87,** 3633–9.

Bierman, P., Molina, A., Nelson, G. *et al.* (1999). Matched unrelated donor (MUD) allogeneic bone marrow transplantation for non-Hodgkin's lymphoma (NHL): results from the National Marrow Donor Program (NMDP). *Proceedings of the American Society of Clinical Oncology,* **18,** 3a (Abstract).

Bierman, P., Vose, J., Anderson, J. *et al.* (1996). High-dose therapy with autologous hematopoietic rescue for follicular non-Hodgkin's lymphoma. *Proceedings of the American Society of Clinical Oncology,* **16,** 415 (Abstract).

Bierman, P. J., Vose, J. M., Anderson, J. R. *et al.* (1997). High-dose therapy with autologous hematopoietic rescue for follicular low-grade non-Hodgkin's lymphoma. *Journal of Clinical Oncology,* **15,** 445–50.

Bigler, R. D., Crilley, P., Micaily, B. *et al.* (1991). Autologous bone marrow transplantation for advanced stage mycosis fungoides. *Bone Marrow Transplantation,* **7,** 133–37.

Blay, J-Y., Sebban, C., Surbiguet, C. *et al.* (1998). High-dose chemotherapy with hematopoietic stem cell transplantation in patients with mantle cell or diffuse centrocytic non-Hodgkin's lymphomas: a single center experience on 18 patients. *Bone Marrow Transplantation,* **21,** 51–4.

Blystad, A. K., Enblad, G., Kvaløy, S. *et al.* (2001). High-dose therapy with autologous stem cell transplantation in patients with peripheral T cell lymphomas. *Bone Marrow Transplantation,* **27,** 711–6.

Bolwell, B., Kalaycio, M., Andresen, S. *et al.* (2000). Autologous peripheral blood progenitor cell transplantation for transformed diffuse large-cell lymphoma. *Clinical Lymphoma,* **1,** 226–31.

Bolwell, B., Kalaycio, M., Sobecks, R. *et al.* (2002). Autologous hematopoietic cell transplantation for non-Hodgkin's lymphoma: 100 month follow-up. *Bone Marrow Transplantation,* **29,** 673–9.

Bosly, A., Coiffier, B., Gisselbrecht, C. et al. (1992). Bone marrow transplantation prolongs survival after relapse in aggressive-lymphoma patients treated with the LNH-84 regimen. *Journal of Clinical Oncology*, **10**, 1615–23.

Bosly, A. Sonet, A., Salles, G. et al. (1997). Superiority of late over early intensification in relapsing/refractory aggressive non-Hodgkin's lymphoma: a randomized study from the GELA: LNH RP 93. *Blood,* **90** (Suppl 1), 594a (Abstract).

Branson, K., Chopra, R., Kottaridis, P. D. et al. (2002). Role of non-myeloablative allogeneic stem-cell transplantation after failure of autologous transplantation in patients with lymphoproliferative malignancies. *Journal of Clinical Oncology,* **20**, 4022–31.

Brice, P., Marolleau, J. P., Puatier, P. et al. (1996). Hematologic recovery and survival of lymphoma patients after autologous stem-cell transplantation: comparison of bone marrow and peripheral blood progenitor cells. *Leukemia and Lymphoma,* **22**, 449–56.

Brice, P., Pautier, P., Marolleau, J. P. et al. (1994). Pregnancy after autologous bone marrow transplantation for malignant lymphomas. *Nouvelle Revue Francaise Hématologie,* **36**, 387–8.

Brice, P., Simon, D., Bouabdallah, R. et al. (2000). High-dose therapy with autologous stem-cell transplantation (ASCT) after first progression prolonged survival of follicular lymphoma patients included in the prospective GELF 86 protocol. *Annals of Oncology,* **11**, 1585–90.

Brunvand, M. W., Bensinger, W. I., Soll, E. et al. (1996). High-dose fractionated total-body irradiation, etoposide and cyclophosphamide for treatment of malignant lymphoma: comparison of autologous bone marrow and peripheral blood stem cells. *Bone Marrow Transplantation,* **18**, 131–41.

Caballero, M. D., Rubio, V., Rifon, J. et al. (1997). BEAM chemotherapy followed by autologous stem cell support in lymphoma patients: analysis of efficacy, toxicity, and prognostic factors. *Bone Marrow Transplantation,* **20**, 451–8.

Cao, T. M., Horning, S., Negrin, R. S. et al. (2001). High-dose therapy and autologous hematopoietic-cell transplantation for follicular lymphoma beyond first remission: the Stanford University experience. *Biology of Blood and Marrow Transplantation,* **7**, 294–301.

Carbone, P. P., Kaplan, H. S., Musshoff, K. et al. (1971). Report of the committee on Hodgkin's disease staging classification. *Cancer Research,* **31**, 1860–1.

Cervantes, F., Shu, X. O., McGlave, P. B. et al. (1995). Autologous bone marrow transplantation for non-transformed low-grade non-Hodgkin's lymphoma. *Bone Marrow Transplantation,* **16**, 387–92.

Chao, N. J., Tierney, D. K., Bloom, J. R. et al. (1992). Dynamic assessment of quality of life after autologous bone marrow transplantation. *Blood,* **80**, 825–30.

Chen, C. I., Crump, M., Tsang, R. et al. (2001). Autotransplants for histologically transformed follicular non-Hodgkin's lymphoma. *British Journal of Haematology,* **113**, 202–8.

Chopra, R., Goldstone, A. H., Pearce, R. et al. (1992). Autologous versus allogeneic bone marrow transplantation for non-Hodgkin's lymphoma: a case-controlled analysis of the European Bone Marrow Transplant Group registry data. *Journal of Clinical Oncology,* **10**, 1690–5.

Clifford, P., Clift, R. A., & Duff, J. K. (1961). Nitrogen-mustard therapy combined with autologous marrow infusion. *Lancet,* **1**, 687–90.

Clift, R. A., Buckner, C. D., Thomas, E. D. et al. (1987). The treatment of acute non-lymphoblastic leukemia by allogeneic marrow transplantation. *Bone Marrow Transplantation,* **2**, 243–58.

Coiffier, B., Lepage, E., Briere, J. et al. (2002). CHOP chemotherapy plus rituximab compared with CHOP alone in elderly patients with diffuse large B cell lymphoma. *New England Journal of Medicine,* **346**, 235–42.

Colombat, P., Donadio, D., Fouillard, L. et al. (1994). Value of autologous bone marrow transplantation in follicular lymphoma: a France Autogreffe retrospective study of 42 patients. *Bone Marrow Transplantation,* **13**, 157–62.

Colombat, P., Gorin, N.-C., Lemonnier, M.-P. et al. (1990). The role of autologous bone marrow transplantation in 46 adult patients with non-Hodgkin's lymphomas. *Journal of Clinical Oncology,* **8**, 630–7.

Corradini, P., Ladetto, M., Astolfi, M. et al. (1996). Clinical and molecular remission after allogeneic blood cell transplantation in a patient with mantle-cell lymphoma. *British Journal of Haematology,* **94**, 376–8.

Crippa, F., Holmberg, L., Carter, R. A. et al. (2002). Infectious complications after autologous CD34-selected peripheral blood stem cell transplantation. *Biology of Blood and Marrow Transplantation,* **8**, 281–9, 2002.

Damiani, E., Fanin, R., Silvestri, F. et al. (1997). Randomized trial of autologous filgrastim-primed bone marrow transplantation versus filgrastim-mobilized peripheral blood stem cell transplantation in lymphoma patients. *Blood,* **90**, 36–42.

Darrington, D. L., Vose, J. M., Anderson, J. R. et al. (1994). Incidence and characterization of secondary myelodysplastic syndrome and acute myelogenous leukemia following high-dose chemoradiotherapy and autologous stem-cell transplantation for lymphoid malignancies. *Journal of Clinical Oncology,* **12**, 2527–34.

Decaudin, D., Brousse, N., Brice, P. et al. (2000). Efficacy of autologous stem cell transplantation in mantle cell lymphoma: a 3-year follow-up study. *Bone Marrow Transplantation,* **25**, 251–6.

Deconinck, E., Lamy, T., Foussard, C. et al. (2000). Autologous stem cell transplantation for anaplastic large-cell lymphomas: results of a prospective trial. *British Journal of Haematology,* **109**, 736–42.

Demirkazik, A., Kessinger, A., Armitage, J. O et al. (2001). Progenitor and lymphoma cell harvests: impact on survival following transplantation. *Bone Marrow Transplantation,* **28**, 207–12.

Desikan, R., Dhodapkar, M., Siegel, D. et al. (1999). High-dose therapy with autologous haemopoietic stem cell support for Waldenström's macroglobulinemia. *British Journal of Haematology,* **105**, 993–6.

Dey, B. R., McAfee, S., Sackstein, R. et al. (2001). Successful allogeneic stem cell transplantation with nonmyeloablative conditioning in patients with relapsed hematologic malignancy following autologous stem cell transplantation. *Biology of Blood and Marrow Transplantation,* **7**, 604–12.

Dreger, P., Glass, B., Kuse, R. et al. (1999a). Myeloablative radiochemotherapy followed by reinfusion of purged autologous stem cells for Waldenström's macroglobulinemia. *British Journal of Haematology,* **106**, 115–8.

Dreger, P., Martin, S., Kröger, N. et al. (1999b). The impact of early stem cell transplantation on the prognosis of mantle cell lymphoma. *Blood,* **94** (Suppl 1), 172a (Abstract).

Ezzat, A. A., Khalifa, F., Berry, J. *et al.* (1994). E-SHAP: an effective treatment in selected patients with relapsed non-Hodgkin's lymphoma. *Annals of Oncology*, **5**, 453–6.

Fanin, R., Silvestri, F., Geromin, A. *et al.* (1996). Primary systemic CD30 (Ki-1)-positive anaplastic large cell lymphoma of the adult: sequential intensive treatment with the F-MACHOP regimen (? radiotherapy) and autologous bone marrow transplantation. *Blood*, **87**, 1243–8.

Fielding, A. K., Philip, T., Carella, A. *et al.* (1994). Autologous bone marrow transplantation for lymphomas—a 15 year European Bone Marrow Transplant Registry (EBMT) experience of 3325 patients. *Blood*, **84** (Suppl 1), 536a (Abstract).

Fisher, R. I., Gaynor, E. R., Dahlberg, M. S. *et al.* (1993). Comparison of a standard regimen (CHOP) with three intensive chemotherapy regimens for advanced non-Hodgkin's lymphoma. *New England Journal of Medicine*, **328**, 1002–6.

Flinn, I. W., O'Donnell, P. V., Goodrich, A., *et al.* (2000). Immunotherapy with rituximab during peripheral blood stem cell transplantation for non-Hodgkin's lymphoma. *Biology of Blood and Marrow Transplantation*, **6**, 628–32.

Foran, J. M., Apostolidis, J., Papamichael, D. *et al.* (1998). High-dose therapy with autologous haematopoietic support in patients with transformed follicular lymphoma: a study of 27 patients from a single center. *Annals of Oncology*, **9**, 865–9.

Forrest, D. L., Thompson, K., Nevill, T. J., *et al.* (2002). Allogeneic hematopoietic stem cell transplantation for progressive follicular lymphoma. *Bone Marrow Transplantation*, **29**, 973–8.

Fouillard, L., Gorin, N. C., Laporte, J.Ph. *et al.* (1991). Feasibility of autologous bone marrow transplantation for early consolidation of follicular non-Hodgkin's lymphoma. *European Journal of Haematology*, **46**, 279–84.

Fouillard, L., Laporte, J. P., Labopin, M. *et al.* (1998). Autologous stem-cell transplantation for non-Hodgkin's lymphomas: the role of graft purging and radiotherapy posttransplantation—results of a retrospective analysis on 120 patients autografted in a single institution. *Journal of Clinical Oncology*, **16**, 2803–16.

Freedman, A. S., Gribben, J. G., Neuberg, D. *et al.* (1996). High-dose therapy and autologous bone marrow transplantation in patients with follicular lymphomas during first remission. *Blood*, **88**, 2780–6.

Freedman, A. S., Neuberg, D., Gribben, J. G. *et al.* (1998). High-dose chemoradiotherapy and anti-B-cell monoclonal antibody-purged autologous bone marrow transplantation in mantle-cell lymphoma: no evidence for long-term remission. *Journal of Clinical Oncology*, **16**, 13–18.

Freedman, A. S., Neuberg, D., Mauch, P. *et al.* (1999). Long-term follow-up of autologous bone marrow transplantation in patients with relapsed follicular lymphoma. *Blood*, **94**, 3325–33.

Freedman, A. S., Ritz, J., Neuberg, D. *et al.* (1991). Autologous bone marrow transplantation in 69 patients with a history of low-grade B-cell non-Hodgkin's lymphoma. *Blood*, **77**, 2524–9.

Freedman, A. S., Takvorian, T., Neuberg, D. *et al.* (1993). Autologous bone marrow transplantation in poor-prognosis intermediate-grade and high-grade B-cell non-Hodgkin's lymphoma in first remission: a pilot study. *Journal of Clinical Oncology*, **11**, 931–6.

Frei, E. & Canellos, G. P. (1980). Dose: a critical factor in cancer chemotherapy. *American Journal of Medicine*, **69**, 585–94.

Friedberg, J. W., Neuberg, D., Gribben, J. G. *et al.* (1999a). Autologous bome marrow transplantation after histologic transformation of indolent B cell malignancies. *Biology of Blood and Marrow Transplantatrion*, **5**, 262–8.

Friedberg, J. W., Neuberg, D., Monson, J., Jallow, H., Nadler, L. M., & Freedman, A. S. (2001). The impact of external beam radiation therapy prior to autologous bone marrow transplantation in patients with non-Hodgkin's lymphoma. *Biology of Blood and Marrow Transplantation*, **7**, 446–53.

Friedberg, J. W., Neuberg, D., Stone, R. M. *et al.* (1999b). Outcome in patients with myelodysplastic syndrome after autologous bone marrow transplantation for non-Hodgkin's lymphoma. *Journal of Clinical Oncology*, **17**, 3128–35.

Gianni, A. M., Bregni, M., Siena, S. *et al.* (1997). High-dose chemotherapy and autologous bone marrow transplantation compared with MACOP-B in aggressive B-cell lymphoma. *New England Journal of Medicine*, **336**, 1290–7.

Geisler, C. H., Elonen, E., Johnson, A. *et al.* (2000). Primary autologous stem cell transplantation in mantle cell lymphoma: Clinical and molecular response. *Blood*, **96** (Suppl 1), 794a (Abstract).

Girouard, C., Dufresne, J., Imrie, K. *et al.* (1997). Salvage chemotherapy with mini-BEAM for relapsed or refractory non-Hodgkin's lymphoma prior to autologous bone marrow transplantation. *Annals of Oncology*, **8**, 675–80.

Gisselbrecht, C., Lepage, E., Molina, M. *et al.* (2002). Shortened first-line high-dose chemotherapy for patients with poor-prognosis aggressive lymphoma. *Journal of Clinical Oncology*, **20**, 2472–9.

Goldberg, S. L., Klumpp, T. R., Magdalinski, A. J., & Mangan, K. F. (1998). Value of the pretransplant evaluation in predicting toxic day-100 mortality among blood stem-cell and bone marrow transplant recipients. *Journal of Clinical Oncology*, **16**, 3796–3802.

Gonzalez-Barca, E., Fernandez de Sevilla, A., Domingo- Claros, A. *et al.* (2000). Autologous stem cell transplantation (ASCT) with immunologically purged progenitor cells in patients with advanced stage follicular lymphoma after early partial or complete remission: toxicity, follow-up of minimal residual disease and survival. *Bone Marrow Transplantation*, **26**, 1051–6.

Gopal, A. K., Gooley, T. A., Golden, J. B. *et al.* (2001). Efficacy of high-dose therapy and autologous hematopoietic stem cell transplantation for non-Hodgkin's lymphoma in adults 60 years of age and older. *Bone Marrow Transplantation*, **27**, 593–9.

Gopal, A. K., Rajendran, G., Petersdorf, S. H. *et al.* (2002). High-dose chemo-radioimmunotherapy with autologous stem cell support for relapsed mantle cell lymphoma. *Blood*, **99**, 3158–3162.

Gordon, B. G., Warkentin, P. I., Weisenburger, D. D. *et al.* (1992). Bone marrow transplantation for peripheral T-cell lymphoma in children and adolescents. *Blood*, **80**, 2938–42.

Gorin, N-C., Lopez, M., Laporte, J-P. *et al.* (1995). Preparation and successful engraftment of purified CD34+ bone marrow progenitor cells in patients with non-Hodgkin's lymphoma. *Blood*, **85**, 1647–54.

Gratwohl, A., Passweg, J., Baldomero, H., & Urbano-Ispizua, A. (1999). Hematopoietic stem cell transplantation activity in Europe 1999. *Bone Marrow Transplantation*, **27**, 899–916.

Gribben, J. G., Freedman, A. S., Neuberg, D. *et al.* (1991). Immunologic purging of marrow assessed by PCR before autologous bone marrow transplantation for B-cell lymphoma. *New England Journal of Medicine*, **325**, 1525–33.

Gribben, J. G., Neuberg, D., Barber, M. *et al.* (1994). Detection of residual lymphoma cells by polymerase chain reaction in peripheral blood is significantly less predictive for relapse than detection in bone marrow. *Blood*, **83**, 3800–7.

Grossbard, M. L., Niedzwiecki, D., Nadler, L. M. *et al.* (1998). Anti-B4-blocked ricin (Anti-B4-bR) adjuvant therapy post-autologous bone marrow transplant (autologous BMT) (CALGB 9254): a phase III intergroup study. *Proceedings of the American Society of Clinical Oncology*, **17**, 3a (Abstract).

Gryn, J., Johnson, E., Goldman, N. *et al.* (1997). The treatment of relapsed or refractory intermediate grade non-Hodgkin's lymphoma with autologous bone marrow transplantation followed by cyclosporine and interferon. *Bone Marrow Transplantation*, **19**, 221–6.

Gulati, S., Yahalom, J., Acaba, L. *et al.* (1992). Treatment of patients with relapsed and resistant non-Hodgkin's lymphoma using total body irradiation, etoposide, and cyclophosphamide and autologous bone marrow transplantation. *Journal of Clinical Oncology*, **10**, 936–41.

Gulati, S. C., Shank, B., Black, P. *et al.* (1988). Autologous bone marrow transplantation for patients with poor-prognosis lymphoma. *Journal of Clinical Oncology*, **6**, 1303–13.

Gutierrez-Delgado, F., Maloney, D. G., Press, O. W. *et al.* (2001). Autologous stem cell transplantation for non-Hodgkin's lymphoma: comparison of radiation-based and chemotherapy-only preparative regimens. *Bone Marrow Transplantation*, **28**, 455–461.

Haas, R., Brittinger, G., Meusers, P. *et al.* (1996a). Myeloablative therapy with blood stem cell transplantation is effective in mantle cell lymphoma. *Leukemia*, **10**, 1975–9.

Haas, R., Moos, M., Möhle, R. *et al.* (1996b). High-dose therapy with peripheral blood progenitor cell transplantation in low-grade non-Hodgkin's lymphoma. *Bone Marrow Transplantation*, **17**, 149–55.

Haioun, C., Lepage, E., Gisselbrecht, C. *et al.* (1995). Autologous transplantation versus conventional salvage therapy in aggressive non-Hodgkin's lymphoma (NHL) partially responding to first line chemotherapy. A study of 96 patients enrolled in the LNH87–2 protocol. *Blood*, **86** (Suppl 1), 211a (Abstract).

Haioun, C., Lepage, E., Gisselbrecht, C. *et al.* (2000). Survival benefit of high-dose therapy in poor-risk aggressive non-Hodgkin's lymphoma: final analysis of the prospective LNH87–2 protocol—a Groupe D'Etude des Lymphomes de l'Adulte study. *Journal of Clinical Oncology*, **18**, 3025–30.

Haioun, C., Mounier, N., Quesnel, B. *et al.* (2001). Tandem auto-transplant as first-line consolidative treatment in poor-risk aggressive lymphoma: A pilot study of 36 patients. *Annals of Oncology*, **12**, 1749–55.

Hahn, T., Wolff, S. N., Czuczman, M. *et al.* (2001). The role of cytotoxic therapy with hematopoietic stem cell transplantation in the therapy of diffuse large cell B-cell non-Hodgkin's lymphoma: an evidence-based review. *Biology of Blood and Marrow Transplantation*, **7**, 308–31.

Hanania, E. G., Kavanagh, J., Hortobagyi, G. *et al.* (1995). Recent advances in the application of gene therapy to human disease. *American Journal of Medicine*, **99**, 537–52.

Haq, R., Sawka, C. A., Franssen, E. *et al.* (1994). Significance of a partial or slow response to front-line chemotherapy in the management of intermediate-grade or high-grade non-Hodgkin's lymphoma: a literature review. *Journal of Clinical Oncology*, **12**, 1074–84.

Hardingham, J. E., Kotasek, D., Sage, R. E. *et al.* (1993). Molecular detection of residual lymphoma cells in peripheral blood stem cell harvests and following autologous transplantation. *Bone Marrow Transplantation*, **11**, 15–20.

Harris, N. L. (2001). Mature B-cell neoplasms. In *Pathology and Genetics of Tumours of Haematopoietic and Lymphoid Tissues*, eds. E. Jaffe, N. Harris, H. Stein, and J. Vardiman, pp. 119–187. Lyon: IARC Press.

Harris, N. L., Jaffe, E. S., Stein, N. H. *et al.* (1994). A revised European-American Classification of Lymphoid Neoplasms: a proposal from the International Lymphoma Study Group. *Blood*, **84**, 1361–92.

Horning, S., Negrin, R. S., Hoppe, R. T. *et al.* (2001). High-dose therapy and autologous bone marrow transplantation for follicular lymphoma in first complete or partial remission: results of a phase II clinical trial. *Blood*, **97**, 404–9.

Horowitz, M. M. (2002). Report on state of the art in blood and marrow transplantation. IBMTR/ABMTR newsletter, **9**, 1–12.

Horowitz, M. M., Gale, R. P., Sondel, P. M. *et al.* (1990). Graft-versus-leukemia reactions after bone marrow transplantation. *Blood*, **75**, 555–62.

Intragumtornchai, T., Prayoonwiwat, W., Numbenjapon, T. *et al.* (2000). CHOP versus CHOP plus ESHAP and high-dose therapy with autologous peripheral blood progenitor cell transplantation for high-intermediate-risk and high-risk aggressive non-Hodgkin's lymphoma. *Clinical Lymphoma*, **1**, 219–25.

Inwards, D. J., Ansell, S. M., Gertz, M. A. *et al.* (2000). High dose therapy with stem cell transplant is effective for non-Hodgkin's lymphoma patients age 65 and over. *Proceedings of the American Society of Clinical Oncology*, **19**, 51a (Abstract).

Jackson, G. H., Lennard, A. L., Taylor, P.R.A. *et al.* (1994). Autologous bone marrow transplantation in poor-risk high-grade non-Hodgkin's lymphoma in first complete remission. *British Journal of Cancer*, **70**, 501–5.

Jackson, G. H., Wood, A., Taylor, P.R.A. *et al.* (1997). Early high dose chemotherapy intensification with autologous bone marrow transplantation in lymphoma associated with retention of fertility and normal pregnancies in females. *Leukemia and Lymphoma*, **28**, 127–32.

Jaff, E., Harris, N., Stein, H., & Vardiman, H. (2001). *Tumours of Haematopoietic and Lymphoid Tissue*. Lyon: IARC Press.

Jaffe, E. S. & Ralfkiaer, E. (2001). Mature T-cell and NK-cell neoplasms. In *Pathology and Genetics of Tumours of Haematopoietic and Lymphoid Tissues*, eds. E. Jaffe, N. Harris, H. Stein and J. Vardiman, pp. 189–235. Lyon: IARC Press

Janssen, W., Smilee, R., & Elfenbein, G. (1995). A prospective randomized trial comparing blood- and marrow-derived stem cells for hematopoietic replacement following high-dose chemotherapy. *Journal of Hematotherapy*, **4**, 139–40.

Johnston, L. J., Stockerl-Goldstein, K. E., Hu, W. W. *et al.* (2000). Toxicity of high-dose sequential chemotherapy and purged autologous hematopoietic cell transplantation precludes its use in refractory/recurrent non-Hodgkin's lymphoma. *Biology of Blood and Marrow Transplantation*, **6**, 555–62.

Jones, R. J., Ambinder, R. F., Piantadosi, S. *et al.* (1991). Evidence of a graft-versus-lymphoma effect associated with allogeneic bone marrow transplantation. *Blood*, **77**, 649–53.

Jost, L. M., Jacky, E., Dommann-Scherrer, C. *et al.* (1995). Short-term weekly chemotherapy followed by high-dose therapy with autologous bone marrow transplantation for lymphoblastic and Burkitt's lymphomas in adult patients. *Annals of Oncology*, **6**, 445–51.

Kaiser, U., Uebelacker, I., Birkmann, J., Havemann, K. *et al.* (1999). High dose therapy with autologous stem cell transplantation in aggressive NHL: Results of a randomized multicenter study. *Blood*, **94** (Suppl 1), 610a–11a (Abstract).

Kaiser, U., Uebelacker, I., Abel, U. *et al.* (2002)., Randomized study to evaluate the use of high-dose therapy as part of primary treatment for "aggressive lymphoma." *Journal of Clinical Oncology*, **20**, 4413–9.

Kewalramani, T., Zelenetz, A. D., Hedrick, E. E. *et al.* (2000). High-dose chemoradiotherapy and autologous stem cell transplantation for patients with primary refractory aggressive non-Hodgkin's lymphoma: an intention-to-treat analysis. *Blood*, **96**, 2399–404.

Khalfallah, S., Stamatoullas, A., Fruchart, C. *et al.* (1996). Durable remission of a relapsing primary central nervous system lymphoma after autologus bone marrow transplantation. *Bone Marrow Transplantation*, **18**, 1021–3.

Khan, A. M., Yamase, H., Tutschka, P. J., & Bilgrami, S. (1997). Autologous peripheral blood progenitor cell transplantation for non-Hodgkin's lymphoma with extensive bone marrow necrosis. *Bone Marrow Transplantation*, **19**, 1037–9.

Khouri, I. F., Lee, M.-S., Romaguera, J. *et al.* (1999). Allogeneic hematopoietic transplantation for mantle-cell lymphoma: molecular remissions and evidence of graft-versus-malignancy. *Annals of Oncology*, **10**, 1293–9.

Khouri, I. F., Romaguera, J., Kantarjian, H. *et al.* (1998). Hyper-CVAD and high-dose methotrexate/cytarabine followed by stem cell transplantation: an active regimen for aggressive mantle cell lymphoma. *Journal of Clinical Oncology*, **16**, 3803–9.

Khouri, I. F., Saliba, R. M., Giralt, S. A. *et al.* (2001). Nonablative allogeneic hematopoietic transplantation as adoptive immunotherapy for indolent lymphoma: low incidence of toxicity, acute graft-versus-host disease, and treatment-related mortality. *Blood*, **98**, 3595–9.

Kluin-Nelemans, H. C., Zagonel, V., Anastasopoulou, A. *et al.* (2001). Standard chemotherapy with or without high-dose chemotherapy for aggressive non-Hodgkin's lymphoma: Randomized phase III EORTC trial. *Journal of the National Cancer Institute*, **93**, 22–30.

Kojima, K., Mannami, T., Yoshino, T. *et al.* (2000). Histologic transformation of follicular lymphoma after allogeneic bone marrow transplantation. *Bone Marrow Transplantation*, **26**, 581–3.

Kottaridis, P. D., Milligan, D. W., Chopra, R. *et al.* (2000). In vivo CAMPATH-1H prevents graft-versus-host disease following non-myeloablative stem cell transplantation. *Blood*, **96**, 2419–25.

Krishnan, A., Bhatia, S., Slovak, M. L. *et al.* (2000). Predictors of therapy-related leukemia and myelodysplasia following autologous transplantation for lymphoma: an assessment of risk factors. *Blood*, **95**, 1588–93.

Krishnan, A., Molina, A., Zaia, J. *et al.* (2001). Autologous stem cell transplantation for HIV-associated lymphoma. *Blood*, **98**, 3857–9.

Kröger, N., Hoffknecht, M., Dreger, P. *et al.* (1998). Long-term disease-free survival of patients with advanced mantle-cell lymphoma following high-dose chemotherapy. *Bone Marrow Transplantation*, **21**, 55–7.

Kurnick, N. B. (1962). Autologous and isologous bone marrow storage and infusion in the treatment of myelo-suppression. *Transfusion*, **2**, 178–87.

Kusnierz-Glaz, C. R., Schlegel, P. G., Wong, R. M. *et al.* (1997). Influence of age on the outcome of 500 autologous bone marrow transplant procedures for hematologic malignancies. *Journal of Clinical Oncology*, **15**, 18–25.

Ladenstein, R., Pearce, R., Hartmann, O. *et al.* (1997). High-dose chemotherapy with autologous bone marrow rescue in children with poor-risk Burkitt's lymphoma: a report from the European Lymphoma Bone Marrow Transplantation Registry. *Blood*, **90**, 2921–30.

Ladetto, M., Corradini, P., Vallet, S. *et al.* (2002). High rate of clinical and molecular remissions in follicular lymphoma patients receiving high-dose sequential chemotherapy and autografting at diagnosis: a multicenter, prospective study by the Gruppo Italiano Trapilanto Midollo Osseo (GITMO). *Blood*, **100**, 1559–65.

Lazarus, H. M., Crilley, P., Ciobanu, N. *et al.* (1992). High-dose carmustine, etoposide, and cisplatin and autologous bone marrow transplantation for relapsed and refractory lymphoma. *Journal of Clinical Oncology*, **10**, 1682–9.

Lazarus, H. M., Horowitz, M. M., & Nugent, M. L. (1996). Outcome of autotransplants in older adults. *Proceedings of the American Society of Clinical Oncology*, **15**, 338 (Abstract).

Léonard, B. M., Hétu, F., Busque, L. B. *et al.* (1998). Lymphoma cell burden in progenitor cell grafts measured by competitive polymerase chain reaction: less than one log difference between bone marrow and peripheral blood sources. *Blood*, **91**, 331–9.

Levine, J. E., Harris, R. E., Loberiza, F. R. *et al.* (2003). A comparison of allogeneic and autologous bone marrow transplantation for lymphoblastic lymphoma. *Blood*, **101**, 2476–82.

Liang, R., Chen, F., Lee, C. K. *et al.* (1997). Autologous bone marrow transplantation for primary nasal T/NK cell lymphoma. *Bone Marrow Transplantation*, **19**, 91–3.

Lillington, D. M., Micallef, I. N., Carpenter, E., *et al.* (2001). Detection of chromosome abnormalities pre-high-dose treatment in patients developing therapy-related myelodysplasia and secondary acute myelogenous leukemia after treatment for non-Hodgkin's lymphoma. *Journal of Clinical Investigation*, **19**, 2472-81.

Liu, S. Y., Eary, J. F., Petersdorf, S. H. *et al.* (1998). Follow-up of relapsed B cell lymphoma patients treated with iodine-131-labelled anti-CD20 antibody and autologous stem cell rescue. *Journal of Clinical Oncology*, **16**, 3270–8.

Lopez, R., Martino, R., Sureda, A. *et al.* (1999). Autologous stem cell transplantation in advanced follicular lymphoma. A single center experience. *Haematological*, **84**, 350–5.

Magni, M., Di Nicola, M., Devizzi, L. *et al.* (2000). Successful in vivo purging of CD34-containing peripheral blood harvests in mantle cell and indolent lymphoma: evidence for a role of both chemotherapy and rituximab infusion. *Blood*, **96**, 864–9.

Majolino, I., Pearce, R., Taghipour, G. *et al.* (1997). Peripheral-blood stem-cell transplantation versus autologous bone marrow transplantation in Hodgkin's and non-Hodgkin's lymphomas: a new matched-pair analysis of the European Group for Blood and

Marrow Transplantation Registry Data. *Journal of Clinical Oncology*, **15**, 509–17.

Malone, J. M., Molina, A., Stockerl-Goldstein, K. *et al.* (2001). High dose therapy and autologous hematopoietic cell transplantation for mantle cell lymphoma: the Stanford/City of Hope experience. *Proceedings of the American Society of Clinical Oncology*, **20**, 13a (Abstract).

Mandigers, C. M., Raemaekers, J. M., Schattenberg, A. V. *et al.* (1998). Allogeneic bone marrow transplantation with T-cell depleted marrow grafts for patients with poor-risk relapsed low-grade non-Hodgkin's lymphoma. *British Journal of Haematology*, **100**, 198–206.

Martelli, M., Vignetti, M., Zinzani, P. L. *et al.* (1996). High-dose chemotherapy followed by autologous bone marrow transplantation versus dexamethasone, cisplatin, and cytarabine in aggressive non-Hodgkin's lymphoma with partial response to front-line chemotherapy: a prospective randomized Italian multicenter study. *Journal of Clinical Oncology*, **14**, 534–42.

Martin, A. R., Weisenburger, D. C., Chan, W. C. *et al.* (1995). Prognostic value of cellular proliferation and histologic grade in follicular lymphoma. *Blood*, **85**, 3671–8.

McCann, J. C., Kanteti, R., Shilepsky, B. *et al.* (1996). High degree of occult tumor contamination in bone marrow and peripheral blood stem cells of patients undergoing autologous transplantation for non-Hodgkin's lymphoma. *Biology of Blood and Marrow Transplantation*, **2**, 37–43.

McFarland, W., Granville, N. B., & Dameshek, W. (1959). Autologous bone marrow infusion as an adjunct in therapy of malignant disease. *Blood*, **14**, 503–21.

McQuaker, I. G., Haynes, A. P., Anderson, S. *et al.* (1997). Engraftment and molecular monitoring of CD34+ peripheral-blood stem-cell transplants for follicular lymphoma: a pilot study. *Journal of Clinical Oncology*, **15**, 2288–95.

McSweeney, P. A., Niederwieser, D., Shizuru, J. A. *et al.* (2001). Hematopoietic cell transplantation in older patients with hematologic malignancies: replacing high-dose cytotoxic therapy with graft-versus-tumor effects. *Blood*, **97**, 3390–400.

Micallef, I.N.M., Lillington, D. M., Apostolidis, J. *et al.* (2000). Therapy-related myelodysplasia and secondary acute myelogenous leukemia after high-dose therapy with autologous hematopoietic progenitor-cell support for lymphoid malignancies. *Journal of Clinical Oncology*, **18**, 947–55.

Meisenberg, B. R., Miller, W. E., McMillan, R. *et al.* (1997). Outpatient high-dose chemotherapy with autologous stem-cell rescue for hematologic and nonhematologic malignancies. *Journal of Clinical Oncology*, **15**, 11–17.

Messori, A., Bonistalli, L., Costantini, M. *et al.* (1997). Cost-effectiveness of autologous bone marrow transplantation in patients with relapsed non-Hodgkin's lymphoma. *Bone Marrow Transplantation*, **19**, 275–81.

Miller, C. B., Piantadosi, S., Vogelsang, G. B. *et al.* (1996). Impact of age on outcome of patients with cancer undergoing autologous bone marrow transplant. *Journal of Clinical Oncology*, **14**, 1327–32.

Milligan, D. W., Carmen Ruiz De Elvira, M., Kolb, H.-J. *et al.* (1999). Secondary leukaemia and myelodysplasia after autografting for lymphoma: results from the EBMT. *British Journal of Haematology*, **106**, 1020–1026.

Mills, W., Chopra, R., McMillan, A. *et al.* (1995a). BEAM chemotherapy and autologous bone marrow transplantation for patients with relapsed or refractory non-Hodgkin's lymphoma. *Journal of Clinical Oncology*, **13**, 588–95.

Mills, W., Strang, J., Goldstone, A. H. *et al.* (1995b). Dose intensification of etoposide in the BEAM autologous BMT protocol for malignant lymphoma. *Leukemia and Lymphoma*, **17**, 263–70.

Milpied, N., Deconninck, E., Colombat, Ph. *et al.* (1999). Frontline high-dose chemotherapy (HDC) with autologous stem cell transplantation compared to standard CHOP regimen: A randomized trial for adult patients with non IPI high-risk intermediate or high grade lymphomas (NHL). *Blood*, **94** (Suppl 1), 610a (Abstract).

Milpied, N., Gaillard, F., Moreau, P. *et al.* (1998). High-dose therapy with stem cell transplantation for mantle cell lymphoma: results and prognostic factors, a single centre experience. *Bone Marrow Transplantation*, **22**, 645–50.

Milpied, N., Ifrah, N., Kuentz, M. *et al.* (1989). Bone marrow transplantation for adult poor prognosis lymphoblastic lymphoma in first complete remission. *British Journal of Haematology*, **73**, 82–7.

Morel, P., Laporte, J. P., Noel, M. P. *et al.* (1995). Autologous bone marrow transplantation as consolidation therapy may prolong remission in newly diagnosed high-risk follicular lymphoma: a pilot study of 34 cases. *Leukemia*, **9**, 576–82.

Moskowitz, C. H., Nimer, S. D., Glassman, J. R. *et al.* (1999). The international prognostic index predicts for outcome following autologous stem cell transplantation in patients with relapsed and primary refractory intermediate-grade lymphoma. *Bone Marrow Transplantation*, **23**, 561–567.

Mounier, N., Haioun, C., Cole, B. F. *et al.* (2000). Quality of life-adjusted survival analysis of high-dose therapy with autologous bone marrow transplantation versus sequential chemotherapy for patients with aggressive lymphoma in first complete remission. *Blood*, **95**, 3687–92.

Nademanee, A., Molina, A., O'Donnell, M. R. *et al.* (1997). Results of high-dose therapy and autologous bone marrow/stem cell transplantation during remission in poor-risk intermediate- and high-grade lymphoma: International index high and high-intermediate risk group. *Blood*, **90**, 3844–52.

Nagler, A., Ackerstein, A., Or, R. *et al.* (1997). Immunotherapy with recombinant human interleukin-2 and recombinant interferon-α in lymphoma patients postautologous marrow or stem cell transplantation. *Blood*, **89**, 3951–9.

Nawa, Y., Takenaka., Shinagawa. *et al.* (1999). Successful treatment of advanced natural killer cell lymphoma with high-dose chemotherapy and syngeneic peripheral blood stem cell transplantation. *Bone Marrow Transplantation*, **23**, 1321–2.

Negrin, R. S., Kusnierz-Glaz, C. R., Still, B. J. *et al.* (1995). Transplantation of enriched and purged peripheral blood progenitor cells from a single apheresis product in patients with non-Hodgkin's lymphoma. *Blood*, **85**, 3334–41.

Olavarria, E., Child, F., Woolford, A. *et al.* (2001). T-cell depletion and autologous stem cell transplantation in the management of tumour stage mycosis fungoides with peripheral blood involvement. *British Journal of Haematology*, **114**, 624–31.

Papadopoulos, K. P., Noguera-Irizarry, W., & Hesdorffer, C. S. (2001). Tandem transplantation in lymphoma. *Bone Marrow Transplantation*, **28**, 529–35.

Pegg, D. E., Humble, J. G., & Newton, K. A. (1962). The clinical application of bone marrow grafting. *British Journal of Cancer,* **16,** 417–35.

Peniket, A. J., Ruiz de Elvira, M. C., Taghipour, G. *et al.* (1997). Allogeneic transplantation for lymphoma produces a lower relapse rate than autologous transplantation but survival is worse because of higher treatment related mortality—a report of 764 cases from the EBMT lymphoma registry. *Blood,* **90,** 255a (Abstract).

Petersen, F. B., Appelbaum, F. R., Bigelow, C. L. *et al.* (1989). High-dose cytosine arabinoside, total body irradiation and marrow transplantation for advanced malignant lymphoma. *Bone Marrow Transplantation,* **4,** 483–8.

Petersen, F. B., Appelbaum, F. R., Hill, R. *et al.* (1990). Autologous marrow transplantation for malignant lymphoma: a report of 101 cases from Seattle. *Journal of Clinical Oncology,* **8,** 638–47.

Pettengell, R., Morgenstern, G. R., Woll, P. J. *et al.* (1993). Peripheral blood progenitor cell transplantation in lymphoma and leukemia using a single apheresis. *Blood,* **82,** 3770–7.

Pettengell, R., Radford, J. A., Morgenstern, G. R. *et al.* (1996). Survival benefit from high-dose therapy with autologous blood progenitor-cell transplantation in poor-prognosis non-Hodgkin's lymphoma. *Journal of Clinical Oncology,* **14,** 586–92.

Philip, T., Armitage, J. O., Spitzer, G. *et al.* (1987). High-dose therapy and autologous bone marrow transplantation after failure of conventional chemotherapy in adults with intermediate-grade or high-grade non-Hodgkin's lymphoma. *New England Journal of Medicine,* **316,** 1493–8.

Philip, T., Biron, P., Maraninchi, D. *et al.* (1984). Role of massive chemotherapy and autologous bone-marrow transplantation in non-Hodgkin's malignant lymphoma. *Lancet,* **2,** 391.

Philip, T., Guglielmi, C., Hagenbeek, A. *et al.* (1995). Autologous bone marrow transplantation as compared with salvage chemotherapy in relapses of chemotherapy-sensitive non-Hodgkin's lymphoma. *New England Journal of Medicine,* **333,** 1540–5.

Philip, T., Hartmann, O., Biron, P. *et al.* (1988). High-dose therapy and autologous bone marrow transplantation in partial remission after first-line induction therapy for diffuse non-Hodgkin's lymphoma. *Journal of Clinical Oncology,* **6,** 1118–24.

Philip, T., Hartmann, O., Pinkerton, R. *et al.* (1993). Curability of relapsed childhood B-cell non-Hodgkin's lymphoma after intensive first line therapy: a report from the Société Francaise d'Oncologie Pédiatrique. *Blood,* **81,** 2003–6.

Phillips, G. L., Fay, J. W., Herzig, R. H. *et al.* (1990). The treatment of progressive non-Hodgkin's lymphoma with intensive chemoradiotherapy and autologous marrow transplantation. *Blood,* **75,** 831–8.

Phillips, G. L., Reece, D. E., Wolff, S. N. *et al.* (1997). The use of conventional salvage chemotherapy before dose-intensive cytotoxic therapy and autologous transplantation for aggressive-histology lymphoma: a case for re-evaluation. *Leukemia and Lymphoma,* **26,** 507–13.

Popat, U., Prezepiork, D., Champlin, R. *et al.* (1998). High-dose chemotherapy for relapsed and refractory diffuse large B-cell lymphoma: mediastinal localization predicts for a favorable outcome. *Journal of Clinical Oncology,* **16,** 63–9.

Press, O. W., Eary, J. F., Gooley, T. *et al.* (2000). A phase I/II trial of iodine-131-tositumomab (anti-CD20), etoposide, cyclophosphamide, and autologous stem cell transplantation for relapsed B-cell lymphomas. *Blood,* **96,** 2934–2942.

Press, O. W., Livingston, R., Mortimer, J. *et al.* (1991). Treatment of relapsed non-Hodgkin's lymphomas with dexamethasone, high-dose cytarabine, and cisplatin before marrow transplantation. *Journal of Clinical Oncology,* **9,** 423–31.

Prince, H. M., Crump, M., Imrie, K. *et al.* (1996). Intensive therapy and autotransplant for patients with an incomplete response to front-line therapy for lymphoma. *Annals of Oncology,* **7,** 1043–9.

Przepiorka, D., Nath, R., Ippoliti, C. *et al.* (1995). A phase I-II study of high-dose thiotepa, busulfan and cyclophosphamide as a preparative regimen for autologous transplantation for malignant lymphoma. *Leukemia and Lymphoma,* **17,** 427–33.

Rapoport, A. P., Lifton, R., Constine, L. S. *et al.* (1997). Autotransplantation for relapsed or refractory non-Hodgkin's lymphoma (NHL): long-term follow-up and analysis of prognostic factors. *Bone Marrow Transplantation,* **19,** 883–90.

Rapoport, A. P., Rowe, J. M., Kouides, P. A. *et al.* (1993). One hundred autotransplants for relapsed or refractory Hodgkin's disease and lymphoma: value of pretransplant disease status for predicting outcome. *Journal of Clinical Oncology,* **11,** 2351–61.

Ratanatharathorn, V., Uberti, J., Karanes, C. *et al.* (1994). Prospective comparative trial of autologous versus allogeneic bone marrow transplantation in patients with non-Hodgkin's lymphoma. *Blood,* **84,** 1050–5.

Rizzo, J. D., Vogelsang, G. B., Krumm, S. *et al.* (1999). Outpatient-based bone marrow transplantation for hematologic malignancies: Cost saving or cost shifting. *Journal of Clinical Oncology,* **17,** 2811–8.

Rizzoli, V. & Carlo-Stella, C. (1995). Stem cell purging: an intriguing dilemma. *Experimental Hematology,* **23,** 296–302.

Robinson, N., Benyunes, M. C., Thompson, J. A. *et al.* (1997). Interleukin-2 after autologous stem cell transplantation for hematologic malignancy: a phase I/II study. *Bone Marrow Transplantation,* **19,** 435–42.

Rodriguez, J., Munsell, M., Yazji, S. *et al.* (2001). Impact of high-dose chemotherapy on peripheral T-cell lymphomas. *Journal of Clinical Oncology,* **19,** 3766–70.

Rodriguez, M. A., Cabanillas, F. C., Velasquez, W. *et al.* (1995). Results of a salvage treatment program for relapsing lymphoma: MINE consolidated with ESHAP. *Journal of Clinical Oncology,* **13,** 1734–41.

Rohatiner, A.Z.S., Johnson, P.W.M., Price, C.G.A. *et al.* (1994). Myeloablative therapy with autologous bone marrow transplantation as consolidation therapy for recurrent follicular lymphoma. *Journal of Clinical Oncology,* **12,** 1177–84.

Rossetti, F., Deeg, H. J., & Hackman, R. C. (1995). Early pulmonary recurrence of non-Hodgkin's lymphoma after autologous marrow transplantation: evidence for reinfusion of lymphoma cells. *Bone Marrow Transplantation,* **15,** 429–32.

Salar, A., Sierra, J., Gandarillas, M. *et al.* (2001). Autologous stem cell transplantation for clinically aggressive non-Hodgkin's lymphoma: the role of the preparative regimen. *Bone Marrow Transplantation,* **27,** 405–12.

Santini, G., Congiu, A. M., Coser, P. *et al.* (1991). Autologous bone marrow transplantation for adult advanced stage lymphoblastic lymphoma in first CR. A study of the NHLCSG. *Leukemia,* **5** (Suppl 1), 42–5.

Santini, G., Olivieri, A., Majolino, I. *et al.* (2002). VACOP-B vs VACOP-B + high-dose sequential therapy (HDS) for aggressive non-Hodgkin's lymphoma (NHL). *Annals of Oncology,* **13** (Suppl 2), 75 (Abstract).

Santini, G., Salvagno, L., Leoni, P. *et al.* (1998). VACOP-B versus VACOP-B plus autologous bone marrow transplantation for advanced diffuse non-Hodgkin's lymphoma: Results of a prospective randomized trial by the non-Hodgkin's lymphoma cooperative study group. *Journal of Clinical Oncology,* **16,** 2796–802.

Schenkein, D. P., Dixon, P., Desforges, J. F. *et al.* (1994). Phase I/II study of cyclophosphamide, carboplatin, and etoposide and autologous hematopoietic stem-cell transplantation with post-transplant interferon alfa-2b for patients with lymphoma and Hodgkin's disease. *Journal of Clinical Oncology,* **12,** 2423–31.

Schenkein, D. P., Roitman, D., Miller, K. B. *et al.* (1997). A phase II multicenter trial of high-dose sequential chemotherapy and peripheral blood stem cell transplantation as initial therapy for patients with high-risk non-Hodgkin's lymphoma. *Biology of Blood and Marrow Transplantation,* **3,** 210–16.

Schimmer, A. D., Jamal, S., Messner, H. *et al.* (2000). Allogeneic or autologous bone marrow transplantation (BMT) for non-Hodgkin's lymphoma (NHL): results of a provincial strategy. *Bone Marrow Transplantation,* **26,** 859–64.

Schmitz, N., Linch, D. C., Dreger, P. *et al.* (1996). Randomized trial of filgrastim-mobilized peripheral blood progenitor cell transplantation versus autologous bone-marrow transplantation in lymphoma patients. *Lancet,* **347,** 353–7.

Schouten, H. C., Bierman, P. J., Vaughan, W. P. *et al.* (1989). Autologous bone marrow transplantation in follicular non-Hodgkin's lymphoma before and after histologic transformation. *Blood,* **74,** 2579–84.

Schouten, H. C., Colombat, Ph., Verdonck, L. F. *et al.* (1994). Autologous bone marrow transplantation for low-grade non-Hodgkin's lymphoma: the European Bone Marrow Transplant Group experience. *Annals of Oncology,* **5** (Suppl 2), S147–49.

Schouten, H. C., Qian, W., Sydes, M. R. *et al.* (2002). High dose therapy improves progression free survival in relapsed follicular non-Hodgkin's lymphoma (NHL). Results from the randomized European CUP trial. *Annals of Oncology,* **13** (Suppl 2), 26 (Abstract).

Sehn, L. H., Antin, J. H., Shulman, L. N. *et al.* (1998). Primary diffuse large B-cell lymphoma of the mediastinum: outcome following high-dose chemotherapy and autologous hematopoietic cell transplantation. *Blood,* **91,** 717–23.

Seyfarth, B., Kuse, R., Sonnen, R. *et al.* (2001). Autologous stem cell transplantation for follicular lymphoma: no benefit for early transplant? *Annals of Hematology,* **80,** 398–405.

Shank, B. (1998). Total body irradiation for marrow or stem-cell transplantation. *Cancer Investigation,* **16,** 397–404.

Sharp, J. G., Kessinger, A., Mann. S. *et al.* (1996). Outcome of high-dose therapy and autologous transplantation in non-Hodgkin's lymphoma based on the presence of tumor in the marrow or infused hematopoietic harvest. *Journal of Clinical Oncology,* **14,** 214–19.

Sharp, J. G., Mann, S., Murphy, B. *et al.* (1995). Culture methods for the detection of minimal tumor contamination of hematopoietic harvests: a review. *Journal of Hematotherapy,* **4,** 141–8.

Shipp, M. A. (1994). Prognostic factors in aggressive non-Hodgkin's lymphoma: who has "high-risk" disease? *Blood,* **83,** 1165–73.

Shipp, M. A., Abeloff, M. D., Antman, K. H. *et al.* (1999). International consensus conference on high-dose therapy with hematopoietic stem cell transplantation in aggressive non-Hodgkin's lymphomas: report of the jury. *Journal of Clinical Oncology,* **17,** 423–9.

Shipp, M. A., Harrington, D. P., Anderson, J. R. *et al.* (1993). A predictive model for aggressive non-Hodgkin's lymphoma. *New England Journal of Medicine,* **329,** 987–94.

Singer, C.R.J., Taghipour, G., Boogaerts, M. A. *et al.* (1999). Matched unrelated donor (MUD) bone marrow transplantation for adults and children with non-Hodgkin's lymphoma and Hodgkin's lymphoma: preliminary analysis of 56 cases reported to EBMT lymphoma registry. *Blood,* **94** (Suppl 1), 560a (Abstract).

Smith, T. J., Hillner, B. E., Schmitz, N. *et al.* (1997). Economic analysis of a randomized clinical trial to compare filgrastim-mobilized peripheral-blood progenitor-cell transplantation and autologous bone marrow transplantation in patients with Hodgkin's and non-Hodgkin's lymphoma. *Journal of Clinical Oncology,* **15,** 5–10.

Sohn, S. K., Bensinger, W., Holmberg, L. *et al.* (1997). High-dose chemotherapy with allogeneic or autologous stem cell transplantation for relapsed mantle cell lymphoma: the Seattle experience. *Proceedings of the American Society of Clinical Oncoloy,* **17,** 17a (Abstract).

Song, K. W., Mollee, P., Keating, A., & Crump, M. (2002). Autologous stem cell transplantation (ASCT) for relapsed/refractory T-cell lymphoma: similar outcome to diffuse large B cell lymphoma. *Annals of Oncology,* **13** (Suppl 2), 76 (Abstract).

Soussain, C., Suzan, F., Hoang-Xuan, F. *et al.* (2001). Results of intensive chemotherapy followed by hematopoietic rescue in 22 patients with refractory or recurrent primary CNS lymphoma or intraocular lymphoma. *Journal of Clinical Oncology,* **19,** 742–9.

Stein, R. S., Greer, J. P., Goodman, S. *et al.* (1999). High-dose therapy with autologous or allogeneic transplantation as salvage therapy for small cleaved cell lymphoma of follicular center cell origin. *Bone Marrow Transplantation,* **23,** 227–33.

Stein, R. S., Greer, J. P., Goodman, S. *et al.* (2001). Is total body irradiation a necessary component of preparative therapy for autologous transplantation in non-Hodgkin's lymphoma? *Leukemia and Lymphoma,* **41,** 97–103.

Stiff, P. J., Dahlberg, S., Forman, S. J. *et al.* (1998). Autologous bone marrow transplantation for patients with relapsed or refractory diffuse aggressive non-Hodgkin's lymphoma: value of augmented preparative regimens—a Southwest Oncology Group trial. *Journal of Clinical Oncology,* **16,** 48–55.

Stockerl-Goldstein, K. E., Horning, S. F., Negrin, R. S. *et al.* (1996). Influence of preparatory regimen and source of hematopoietic cells on outcome of autotransplantation for non-Hodgkin's lymphoma. *Biology of Blood and Marrow Transplantation,* **2,** 76–85.

Stone, R. M., Neuberg, D., Soiffer, R. *et al.* (1994). Myelodysplastic syndrome as a late complication following autologous bone marrow transplantation for non-Hodgkin's lymphoma. *Journal of Clinical Oncology,* **12,** 2535–42.

Surbone, A., Armitage, J. O., & Gale, R. P. (1991). Autotransplantations in lymphoma: better therapy or healthier patients? *Annals of Internal Medicine,* **114,** 1059–60.

Sureda, A., Arranz, R., Iriondo, A. et al. (2001). Autologous stem-cell transplantation for Hodgkin's disease: results and prognostic factors in 494 patients from the Grupo Español de Linfomas/ Transplante Autó logo de Médula Ósea Spanish Cooperative Group. Journal of Clinical Oncology, 19, 1395–1404.

Sweetenham, J. W. (2001). Stem cell transplantation for mantle cell lymphoma: should it ever be used outside clinical trials? Bone Marrow Transplantation, 28, 813–20.

Sweetenham, J. W., Pearce, R., Taghipour, G. et al. (1996a). Adult Burkitt's and Burkitt-like non-Hodgkin's lymphoma-outcome for patients treated with high-dose therapy and autologous stem-cell transplantation in first remission or at relapse: results from the European Group for Blood and Marrow Transplantation. Journal of Clinical Oncology, 14, 2465–72.

Sweetenham, J. W., Proctor, S. J., Blaise, D. et al. (1994). High-dose therapy and autologous bone marrow transplantation in first complete remission for adult patients with high-grade non-Hodgkin's lymphoma: the EBMT experience. Annals of Oncology, 5 (Suppl 2), S155–9.

Sweetenham, J. W., Santini, G., Qian, W. et al. (2001). High-dose therapy and autologous stem-cell transplantation versus conventional-dose consolidation/maintenance therapy as postremission therapy for adult patients with lymphoblastic lymphoma: results of a randomized trial of the European Group for Blood and Marrow Transplantation and the United Kingdom Lymphoma Group. Journal of Clinical Oncology, 19, 2927–36.

Sweetenham, J. W., Taghipour, G., Milligan, D. et al. (1996b). High dose therapy (HDT) and autologous stem cell transplantation (ASCT) for adults with Hodgkin's disease (HD) in first relapse after chemotherapy—conventional dose salvage therapy prior to ASCT has no effect on outcome: results from the EBMT. Blood, 6 (Suppl 1), 486a (Abstract).

Takenaka, K., Shinagawa, K., Maeda, Y. et al. (2001). High-dose chemotherapy with hematopoietic stem cell transplantation is effective for nasal and nasal-type CD56+ natural killer cell lymphomas. Leukemia and Lymphoma, 42, 1297–303.

Tarella, C., Caracciolo, D., Gavarotti, P. et al. (2000). Overweight as an adverse prognostic factor for non-Hodgkin's lymphoma patients receiving high-dose chemotherapy and autograft. Bone Marrow Transplantation, 26, 1185–91.

Tilly, H., Coiffier, B., Casasnovas, O. et al. (2002). Survival advantage of ACVBP regimen over standard CHOP in the treatment of advanced aggressive non-Hodgkin's lymphoma (NHL). The LNH 93–5 study. Annals of Oncology, 13 (Suppl 2), 28 (Abstract).

Traweek, S. T., Slovak, M. L., Nademanee, A. P. et al. (1994). Clonal karyotypic hematopoietic cell abnormalities occurring after autologous bone marrow transplantation for Hodgkin's disease and non-Hodgkin's lymphoma. Blood, 84, 957–63.

Tsai, D. E., Moore, H.C.F., Hardy, C. L. et al. (1999). Rituximab (anti-CD20 monoclonal antibody) therapy for progressive intermediate-grade non-Hodgkin's lymphoma after high-dose therapy and autologous peripheral stem cell transplantation. Bone Marrow Transplantation, 24, 521–6.

Urbano-Ispizua, A., Schmitz, N., de Witte, T. et al. (2002). Allogeneic and autologous transplantation for haematological diseases, solid tumors and immune disorders: definition and current practices in Europe. Bone Marrow Transplantation, 29, 639–46.

van Besien, K., Forman, A., & Champlin, R. (1997b). Central nervous system relapse of lymphoid malignancies in adults: the role of high-dose chemotherapy. Annals of Oncology, 8, 515–24.

van Besien, K., Przepiorka, D., Mehra, R. et al. (1996b). Impact of preexisting CNS involvement on the outcome of bone marrow transplantation in adult hematologic malignancies. Journal of Clinical Oncology, 14, 3036–42.

van Besien, K., Rowlings, P. A., Sobocinski, K. A. et al. (1995b). Allogeneic bone marrow transplantation for low grade lymphoma. Blood, 86 (Suppl 1), 209a (Abstract).

van Besien, K., Sobocinski, K. A., Rowlings, P. A. et al. (1998). Allogeneic bone marrow transplantation for low-grade lymphoma. Blood, 92, 1832–6.

van Besien, K., Tabocoff, J., Rodriguez, M. et al. (1995c). High-dose chemotherapy with BEAC regimen and autologous bone marrow transplantation for intermediate grade and immunoblastic lymphoma: durable complete remission, but a high rate of regimen-related toxicity. Bone Marrow Transplantation, 15, 549–55.

van Besien, K. W., de Lima, M., Giralt, S. A. et al. (1997a). Management of lymphoma recurrence after allogeneic transplantation; the relevance of graft-versus-lymphoma effect. Bone Marrow Transplantation, 19, 977–82.

van Besien, K. W., Khouri, I. F., Giralt, S. A. et al. (1995a). Allogeneic bone marrow transplantation for refractory and recurrent low-grade lymphoma: the case for aggressive management. Journal of Clinical Oncology, 13, 1096–102.

van Besien, K. W., Mehra, R. C., Giralt, S. A. et al. (1996a). Allogeneic bone marrow transplantation for poor-prognosis lymphoma: response, toxicity, and survival depend on disease histology. American Journal of Medicine, 100, 299–307.

Vandenberghe, E., Ruiz de Elvira, C., Isaacson, P. et al. (2000). Does transplantation improve outcome in mantle cell lymphoma (MCL)? Blood, 96 (Suppl 1), 482a (Abstract).

Varadi, G., Or, R., Kapelushnik, J. et al. (1999). Graft-versus-lymphoma effect after allogeneic peripheral blood stem cell transplantation for primary central nervous system lymphoma. Leukemia and lymphoma, 34, 185–90.

Vaughan, W. P., Kris, E., Vose, J. et al. (1995). Phase I/II study incorporating intravenous hydroxyurea into high-dose chemotherapy for patients with primary refractory or relapsed and refractory intermediate-grade and high-grade malignant lymphoma. Journal of Clinical Oncology, 13, 1089–95.

Vaughan, W. P., Weisenburger, D. C., Sanger, W. et al. (1987). Early leukemic recurrence of non-Hodgkin lymphoma after high-dose anti-neoplastic therapy with autologous marrow rescue. Bone Marrow Transplantation, 1, 373–8.

Vellenga, E., van Agthoven, M., Crookewit, A. J. et al. (2001). Autologous peripheral blood stem cell transplantation in patients with relapsed lymphoma results in accelerated haematopoietic reconstitution, improved quality of life and cost reduction compared with bone marrow transplantation: the Hovon 22 study. British Journal of Haematology, 114, 319–26.

Verdonck, L. F., Dekker, A. W., de Gast, G. C. et al. (1992). Autologous bone marrow transplantation for adult poor-risk lymphoblastic lymphoma in first remission. Journal of Clinical Oncology, 10, 644–6.

Verdonck, L. F., Dekker, A. W., Lokhorst, H. M. *et al.* (1997). Allogeneic versus autologous bone marrow transplantation for refractory and recurrent low-grade non-Hodgkin's lymphoma. *Blood,* **90,** 4201–5.

Verdonck, L. F., van Putten, W.L.J., Hagenbeek, A. *et al.* (1995). Comparison of CHOP chemotherapy with autologous bone marrow transplantation for slowly responding patients with aggressive non-Hodgkin's lymphoma. *New England Journal of Medicine,* **332,** 1045–51.

Vitolo, U., Cortellazzo, S., Liberati, A. M. *et al.* (1997). Intensified and high-dose chemotherapy with granulocyte colony-stimulating factor and autologous stem-cell transplantation support as first-line therapy in high-risk diffuse large-cell lymphoma. *Journal of Clinical Oncology,* **15,** 491–8.

Vose, J. M., Anderson, J. R., Kessinger, A. *et al.* (1993). High-dose chemotherapy and autologous hematopoietic stem-cell transplantation for aggressive non-Hodgkin's lymphoma. *Journal of Clinical Oncology,* **11,** 1846–51.

Vose, J. M., Bierman, P. J., Lynch, J. C. *et al.* (1998). Effect of follicularity on autologous transplantation for large-cell non-Hodgkin's lymphoma. *Journal of Clinical Oncology,* **16,** 844–9.

Vose, J. M., Bierman, P. J., Lynch, J. C. *et al.* (2001a). Transplantation of highly purified CD34$^+$Thy-1$^+$ hematopoietic stem cells in patients with recurrent indolent non-Hodgkin's lymphoma. *Biology of Blood and Marrow Transplantation,* **7,** 680–7.

Vose, J. M., Bierman, P. J., Weisenburger, D. D. *et al.* (2000). Autologous hematopoietic stem cell transplantation for mantle cell lymphoma. *Biology of Blood and Marrow Transplantation,* **6,** 640–5.

Vose, J. M., Kennedy, B. C., Bierman, P. J. *et al.* (1992). Long-term sequelae of autologous bone marrow or peripheral stem cell transplantation for lymphoid malignancies. *Cancer,* **69,** 784–9.

Vose, J. M., Peterson, C., Bierman, P. J. *et al.* (1990). Comparison of high-dose therapy and autologous bone marrow transplantation for T-cell and B-cell non-Hodgkin's lymphomas. *Blood,* **76,** 424–31.

Vose, J. M., Sharp, G., Chan, W. C. *et al.* (2002). Autologous transplantation for aggressive non-Hodgkin's lymphoma: Results of a randomized trial evaluating graft source and minimal residual disease. *Journal of Clinical Oncology,* **20,** 2344–2352.

Vose, J. M., Zhang, M-J., Rowlings, P. A. *et al.* (2001b). Autologous transplantation for diffuse aggressive non-Hodgkin's lymphoma in patients never achieving remission: a report from the Autologous Blood and Marrow Transplant Registry. *Journal of Clinical Oncology,* **19,** 406–13.

Voso, M. T., Martin, S., Hohaus, S. *et al.* (2000a). Prognostic factors for the clinical outcome of patients with follicular lymphoma following high-dose therapy and peripheral blood stem cell transplantation. *Bone Marrow Transplantation,* **25,** 957–64.

Voso, M. T., Pantel, G., Weis, M. *et al.* (2000b). In vivo depletion of B cells using a combination of high-dose cytosine arabinoside/mitoxantrone and rituximab for autografting in patients with non-Hodgkin's lymphoma. *British Journal of Haematology,* **109,** 729–35.

Weaver, C. H., Appelbaum, F. R., Petersen, F. B. *et al.* (1993). High-dose cyclophosphamide, carmustine, and etoposide followed by autologous bone marrow transplantation in patients with lymphoid malignancies who have received dose-limiting radiation therapy. *Journal of Clinical Oncology,* **11,** 1329–35.

Weaver, C. H., Petersen, F. B., Appelbaum, F. R. *et al.* (1994). High-dose fractionated total-body irradiation, etoposide, and cyclophosphamide followed by autologous stem-cell support in patients with malignant lymphoma. *Journal of Clinical Oncology,* **12,** 2559–66.

Weisdorf, D., Daniels, K., Miller, W. *et al.* (1993). Bone marrow vs. peripheral blood stem cells for autologous lymphoma transplantation: a prospective randomized trial. *Blood,* **82** (Suppl 1), 444a (Abstract).

Weisdorf, D. J., Haake, R., Miller, W. J. *et al.* (1991). Autologous bone marrow transplantation for progressive non-Hodgkin's lymphoma: clinical impact of immunophenotype and in vitro purging. *Bone Marrow Transplantation,* **8,** 135–42.

Weisdorf, D., Miller, J., Verfaillie, C. *et al.* (1997). Cytokine-primed bone marrow stem cells vs. peripheral blood stem cells for autologous transplantation: a randomized comparison of GM-CSF vs. G-CSF. *Biology of Blood and Marrow Transplantation,* **3,** 217–23.

Weisenburger, D. C. & Armitage, J. O. (1996). Mantle cell lymphoma—an entity comes of age. *Blood,* **87,** 4483–94.

Wheeler, C., Antin, J. H., Churchill, W. H. *et al.* (1990). Cyclophosphamide, carmustine, and etoposide with autologous bone marrow transplantation in refractory Hodgkin's disease and non-Hodgkin's lymphoma: a dose finding study. *Journal of Clinical Oncology,* **8,** 648–56.

Wheeler, C., Strawderman, M., Ayash, L. *et al.* (1993). Prognostic factors for treatment outcome in autotransplantation of intermediate-grade and high-grade non-Hodgkin's lymphoma with cyclophosphamide, carmustine, and etoposide. *Journal of Clinical Oncology,* **11,** 1085–91.

Williams, C. D., Goldstone, A. H., Pearce, R. *et al.* (1996). Purging of bone marrow in autologous bone marrow transplantation for non-Hodgkin's lymphoma: a case-matched comparison with unpurged cases by the European Blood and Marrow Transplant Lymphoma Registry. *Journal of Clinical Oncology,* **14,** 2454–64.

Williams, C. D., Harrison, C. N., Lister, T. A. *et al.* (2001). High-dose therapy and autologous stem cell support for chemosensitive transformed low-grade follicular non-Hodgkin's lymphoma: a case-matched study from the European Bone Marrow Transplant Registry. *Journal of Clinical Oncology,* **19,** 727–35.

Williams, C. D., Pearce, R., Taghipour, G. *et al.* (1994). Autologous bone marrow transplantation for patients with non-Hodgkin's lymphoma and CNS involvement: those transplanted with active CNS disease have a poor outcome—a report by the European Bone Marrow Transplant Lymphoma Registry. *Journal of Clinical Oncology,* **12,** 2415–22.

Wilson, W. H., Jain, V., Bryant, G. *et al.* (1992). Phase I and II study of high-dose ifosfamide, carboplatin, and etoposide with autologous bone marrow rescue in lymphomas and solid tumors. *Journal of Clinical Oncology,* **10,** 1712–22.

Wingard, J. R., Curbow, B., Baker, F. *et al.* (1991). Health, functional status, and employment of adult survivors of bone marrow transplantation. *Annals of Internal Medicine,* **114,** 113–18.

Yang, L., Wen, B. P., Li, H. M. *et al.* (1999). Autologous peripheral blood stem cell transplantation for Waldenström's macroglobulinemia. *Bone Marrow Transplantation,* **24,** 929–30.

Yuen, A. R., Kamel, O. W., Halpern, J., & Horning, S. J. (1995). Long-term survival after histologic transformation of low-grade follicular lymphoma. *Journal of Clinical Oncology,* **13,** 1726–33.

35 Autologous hematopoietic stem cell transplantation for Hodgkin's disease

IRIT AVIVI AND ANTHONY H. GOLDSTONE

University College London Hospitals, London, UK

Introduction

Hodgkin's disease[1] (HD) is a relatively uncommon malignancy with an incidence of 2.5 cases per 100,000 per annum, resulting in approximately 8,000 new cases each year in the United States. The age distribution is biphasic with age peaks at 25 to 30 years and over 60 years. The disease arises in lymph nodes and usually spreads to contiguous node groups. The current World Health Organization (WHO) classification divides patients into two main groups: classical HD and lymphocyte predominant HD (Table 35.1), based on the biological features of these two main subtypes (Pileri *et al.*, 2002). Staging of disease at presentation is determined using the Ann Arbor staging system (Table 35.2).

The natural history of HD is variable. It is usually chronically progressive if untreated and ultimately fatal. However, with current optimal conventional therapy (primarily chemotherapy (Table 35.3) with or without adjuvant radiotherapy), most patients can be cured (Table 35.4).

Different prognostic factors have been suggested (Table 35.5 and 35.6), aiming to identify patients with higher risk for relapsed/refractory disease, who may be considered for escalated first-line chemotherapy instead of conventional chemotherapy (Bartlett *et al.*, 1995; Hasenclever, Loeffler, & Diehl, 1996; Horning, Rosenberg, & Hoppe, 1996; Reuss *et al.*, 1996; Rüffer & Sieber, 1996) (Table 35.7).

Some of these new intensive protocols appear to be achieving better outcomes by exploring dose and time intensification or by combining chemotherapy and radiotherapy modalities. Indeed,

regimens such as the Stanford V and the German BEACOPP (bleomycin, etoposide, doxorubicin, cyclophosphamide, vincristine, procarbazine, prednisone) protocols show a freedom from disease progression (FFDP) of almost 90% (Bartlett *et al.*, 1995; Hasenclever, Loeffler, & Diehl, 1996; Horning, Rosenberg, & Hoppe, 1996; Reuss *et al.*, 1996; Rüffer & Sieber, 1996). However, follow-up is limited at the present time and long-term side effects including the incidence of secondary malignancies have to be followed further and quantitated. Nevertheless, even with these intensive first-line regimens, there are still patients who fail to respond or eventually relapse. It is

Table 35.1.   *WHO classification for Hodgkin's lymphoma*

Nodular lymphocyte predominance Hodgkin's lymphoma
Classical Hodgkin's lymphoma
    Hodgkin's lymphoma, nodular sclerosis (Grade 1 and 2)
    Classical Hodgkin's lymphoma, lymphocyte-rich
    Hodgkin's lymphoma, mixed cellularity
    Hodgkin's lymphoma, lymphocyte depletion

[1]Thomas Hodgkin, English physician and pathologist, 1798–1866.

Table 35.2.   *Ann Arbor Staging Classification and Cotswald modifications*

Stage I: Involvement of a single lymph node region or lymphoid structure.
Stage II: Involvement of two or more lymph node regions on the same side of the diaphragm.
Stage III: Involvement of lymph node regions or structures on both sides of the diaphragm.
Stage IV: Involvement of extranodal site(s) beyond the designated "E"

For All Stages:
  A. No symptoms
  B. Fever (>38° C), sweats, weight loss (>10% body weight over 6 months)

For Stages I to III:
  E: Involvement of a single, extranodal site contiguous or proximal to known nodal site.

Cotswald Modifications
Subscript "X" to be used if bulky disease is present.
The number of anatomic regions involved should be indicated by a subscript (e.g., II_3).
Stage III may be subdivided into:
    III1: with or without splenic, hilar, celiac, or portal nodes
    III2: with para-aortic, iliac, mesenteric nodes
Staging should be identified as clinical stage *(CS)* or pathologic stage *(PS)*. PS at a given site will be denoted by a subscript (i.e., M = bone marrow; H = liver; L = lung; O = bone; P = pleura; D = skin).
Unconfirmed/uncertain complete remission *(CR[u])* if persistent radiologic abnormalities of uncertain significance.

Table 35.3. *Conventional dose combination cytotoxic chemotherapy regimens commonly used in Hodgkin's disease*

Drug	Dose	Dosing schedule
MOPP regimen		
Mechlorathamine	6 mg/m^2 i.v.	Days 1 and 8
Vincristine	1.4 mg/m^2 i.v.	Days 1 and 8
Procarbazine	100 mg/m^2 po	Days 1–14
Prednisone	40 mg/m^2 po	Days 1–14
ABVD regimen		
Doxorubicin	25 mg/m^2 i.v.	Days 1 and 15
Bleomycin	10 U/m^2 i.v.	Days 1 and 15
Vinblastine	6 mg/m^2 i.v.	Days 1–15
Darabazine	375 mg/m^2 i.v.	Days 1–15
MOPP/ABV hybrid regimen		
Mustine	6 mg/m^2 i.v.	Day 1
Vincristine	1.4 mg/m^2 i.v. (max 2 mg)	Day 1
Procarbazine	100 mg/m^2 po	Days 1–7
Prednisone	40 mg/m^2 po	Days 1–14
Adriamycin	36 mg/m^2 i.v.	Day 8
Bleomycin	10 U/m^2 i.v.	Day 8
Vinblastine	6 mg/m^2 i.v.	Day 8
ChlorVPP regimen		
Chlorambucil	6 mg/m^2 po (not > 10 mg)	Daily × 14 days
Vinblastine	6 mg/m^2 i.v.	Days 1 and 8
Prednisone	40 mg/m^2 po	Daily × 14 days
Procarbazine	100 mg/m^2 po	Daily × 14 days

here that high-dose therapy (HDT) followed by autologous hematopoietic stem cell transplantation (HSCT) is felt to have the greatest potential impact. The dose-response effect that exists in HD makes high-dose therapy an attractive treatment for these patients. Reinfusion of autologous hematopoietic stem cells following the HDT allows the administration of therapy at an intensity that would otherwise be precluded by myelotoxicity.

Indications for autologous HSC transplantation

The main indication for autografting in HD remains relapsed disease (Baker *et al.*, 1999; Lazarus *et al.*, 2001; Sureda *et al.*,

Table 35.4. *Outcome with conventional therapy*

Stage		Treatment	10-year disease-free survival
IA	peripheral[a]	RT	>90%
I–IIA	supradiaphragmatic[a]	RT	85–90%
I–IIA	infradiaphragmatic	RT	85–90%
I–IIB	supradiaphragmatic[a]	RT	70–75%
I–IIB	infradiaphragmatic	RT + CT	~80%
I–II	bulky, mediastinal	RT + CT	~80%
IIIA[b]		CT	75–80%
IIIB–IV[b]			CT 55–65%

Abbreviations: RT, radiotherapy; CT, chemotherapy.
[a] With staging laparotomy. Spleen included in para-aortic field if no laparotomy done.
[b] Some patients might benefit from involved field radiation.

Table 35.5. *Prognostic factors for outcome with conventional therapy*

Factor	Better prognosis	Worse prognosis
Stage	Stage I–II	Stage III–IV
Histology	Lymphocyte predominant Nodular sclerosis	Mixed cellularity Lymphocyte depletion
Systemic symptoms	None	Fevers, night sweats, weight loss
Age	<40 years	>40 years
Sex	Female	Male

2001). An Autologous Blood and Marrow Transplant Registry (ABMTR) study of 414 patients in first relapse ($n = 295$) or in second complete remission ($n = 119$) showed a 3-year disease-free survival rate of 46% for those transplanted in first relapse and 64% for those transplanted in second complete remission ($P < .001$) (Fig. 35.1) (Lazarus *et al.*, 2001).

However, primary refractory disease may also be an indication (Sweetenham *et al.*, 1999; Lazarus *et al.*, 2001; Sureda *et al.*, 2001). HDT followed by HSCT in first complete remission (CR) had been considered for patients with HD who have a high probability of relapse (Carella *et al.*, 1991, 1996). However, an update of the European Bone Marrow Transplant EBMT/HD10 trial has failed to prove any advantage for upfront transplantation in this group of patients (Federico *et al.*, 2002). A summary of the current indications for HSCT in HD is presented in Table 35.8.

The current practice of HSC transplantation for Hodgkin's disease in Europe has been described (Urbano-Ispizua *et al.*, 2002) (and see Chapter 124, Breaking News…).

Relapsed or progressive Hodgkin's disease

Patients with relapsed or primary progressive Hodgkin's disease are usually treated with salvage (second-line) chemotherapy followed by HSCT. These salvage regimens (including ESHAP, IVE, mini-BEAM, MIME, DHAP, DICEP) (see Table 35.9) may obtain a response in up to 85%, including a 26%–62% CR rate, depending on whether patients are treated

Table 35.6. *Prognostic factors in Hodgkin's lymphoma*

Risk factor	P value	Relative risk[a]
Serum albumin <4 g/dl	<.001	1.49
Hemoglobin <10.5 g/dl	.006	1.35
Male (vs. female)	.001	1.35
Stage 4 disease	.011	1.26
Age >45 yr	.001	1.39
White blood cell count >15,000/mm^3	.001	1.41
Lymphocyte count <600/mm^3 or less than 8% of total white cell count	.002	1.38

[a] Relative risk for progression of disease in patients who presented with the risk factor, as compared with those without it.
Adapted from Hasenclever *et al.* (1998).

Table 35.7. *Escalated chemotherapy regimens for patients with high-risk Hodgkin's lymphoma*

| BEACOPP | Bleomycin, etoposide, doxorubicin, cyclophosphamide, vincristine, procarbazine, prednisone (Diehl *et al.*, 1998) |
| Stanford V | Bleomycin, etoposide, doxorubicin, vincristine, vinblastine, mechlorethamine, procarbazine, prednisone (Bartlett *et al.*, 1995) |

for first relapse, later relapse, or primary resistant disease (Longo, 1990; Chopra *et al.*, 1992; Martin *et al.*, 2001; Moskowitz *et al.*, 2001). Unfortunately, these post-salvage remissions are not durable in the majority of patients, particularly in those refractory to first-line therapy, or who relapse within a year of initial treatment, for which the cure rate is approximately 10%. Even those with an initial remission of 12 months or more have only a 25% to 35% chance of long-term disease-free survival (Longo *et al.*, 1992; Gause & Longo, 1996).

Compared with historical controls, autografting appears to confer a significant survival advantage in these groups of poor prognosis patients (Linch *et al.*, 1993; Yuen *et al.*, 1994) (Fig 35.2). Long-term freedom from progression (FFP) with high-dose therapy in patients with relapsed/refractory HD approaches 40–60% (Chopra *et al.*, 1993; [Fig. 35.3]; Reece *et al.*, 1994 [Fig 35.5]; Nademanee *et al.*, 1995 [Fig. 35.4]; Sweetenham *et al.*, 1997).

Pfreundschuh *et al.* (1994) have suggested that intensified salvage regimens, such as Dexa-BEAM (dexamethasone, carmustine, etoposide, cytosine arabinoside, melphalan) might improve survival in poor prognosis patients and are at least as good as high-dose therapy (Pfreundschuh *et al.*, 1994; Gause & Longo, 1996). However, a prospective randomized trial comparing Dexa-BEAM with Dexa-BEAM followed by BEAM and an autograft, showed a significantly increased freedom from treatment failure (FFTF) in patients treated with autograft (FFTF=55% versus 34 %, P = .019) (Schmitz

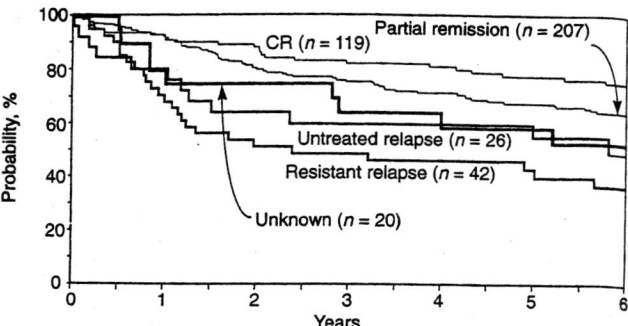

Fig. 35.1. Probability of survival after autotransplant for Hodgkin's disease in second complete remission or first relapse, according to sensitivity to salvage chemotherapy. Reproduced, with permission, from Lazarus *et al.* (2001).

Table 35.8. *Current indications for autologous stem cell transplantation in Hodgkin's lymphoma*

Accepted indications	1. Relapse after first-line therapy, especially if CR/PR obtained pretransplant using salvage therapy. 2. Failure to enter CR with standard first-line therapy (usually excluding patients who continue to progress on second-line therapy)
Controversial indication	Progressive disease on salvage chemotherapy
Not accepted indication	Transplantation of high-risk HD patients in CR1

et al., 2002). A previous prospective randomized trial comparing mini-BEAM (salvage therapy) with BEAM plus autograft for patients with early relapse/induction failure confirmed a significant advantage for BEAM plus autograft, with an event-free survival (EFS) of 53% in the autograft group compared with 10% in the mini-BEAM group (P = .025) (Linch *et al.*, 1993; Fig. 35.2). There was no significant difference in overall survival (OS), which might be explained by the fact that a relatively high number of patients in the mini-BEAM arm who relapsed were subsequently rescued with a BEAM/autograft.

A unique, though small subgroup of patients, mainly those who have lymphocyte predominance HD expressing CD20 antigen, may respond to rituximab (Keilholz *et al.*, 1999; Lush *et al.*, 2001). However, follow-up is still short and further studies are needed to confirm the superiority of this strategy versus HSCT for relapsed patients.

Contraindications for HSC transplantation

The main contraindication for HSCT in HD is disease progression on treatment. Patients with non-progressive (stable) chemorefractory disease may still be considered for HSCT,

Table 35.9. *Salvage chemotherapy regimens*

ESHAP	Etoposide, cisplatin, cytosine arabinoside, methylprednisolone (Watts *et al.*, 2000)
DHAP	Dexamethasone, cytosine arabinoside, cisplatin (Martelli *et al.*, 1996)
DVIP	Dexamethasone, etoposide, ifosfamide, cisplatin (Haim *et al.*, 1997)
DICEP	Dose-intensified cyclophosphamide, etoposide, cisplatin (Stewart *et al.*, 2000)
MINE	Ifosfamide, mitoxantrone, etoposide (Aydogdu *et al.*, 1997)
IVE	Ifosfamide, etoposide, epirubicin (Proctor *et al.*, 2002)
Mini-BEAM	Carmustine, etoposide, cytosine arabinoside, melphalan (Martin *et al.*, 2001)
ICE	Ifosfamide, carboplatin, etoposide (Moskowitz *et al.*, 2001)

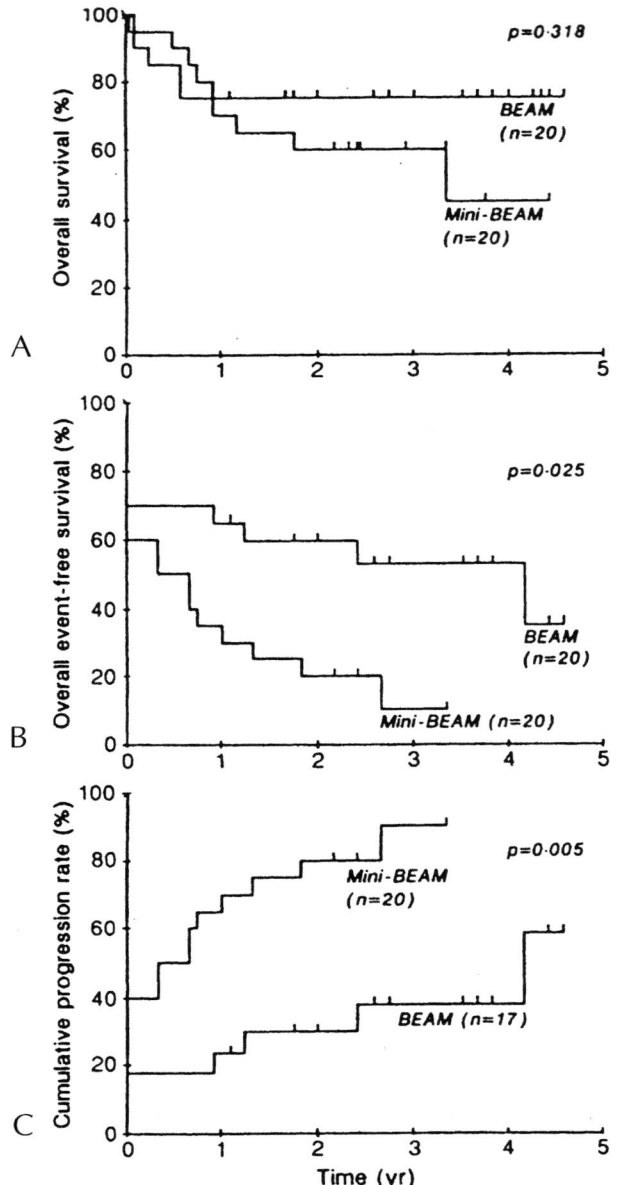

Fig. 35.2. Overall survival (**A**), event-free survival (**B**), and cumulative progression rate (**C**) in ABMT and mini-BEAM groups. Reproduced, with permission, from Linch *et al.* (1993).

Pretransplant work-up

Patient eligibility for transplantation should be carefully assessed by evaluation of disease response to pretransplant chemotherapy, as well as by the normal components of the work-up prior to HSCT (see Chapter 20). Most studies have used CT scans for evaluating response of Hodgkin's disease to chemotherapy prior to transplant. It is sometimes difficult to determine if the patient has residual disease or a fibrotic scar—in which case he/she will have achieved a CR instead of partial response (PR). In some cases, positron emission tomography (PET) scan can be helpful (Dittman *et al.*, 2001; Spaepen & Mortelmans, 2001). However, there will likely still be patients whose disease status pretransplantation is misinterpreted.

Conditioning regimens and sources of stem cells

The selection of an HDT regimen depends on the use of agents that are active against Hodgkin's disease, preferably including some to which the patient has not been previously exposed, while limiting the associated side effects. A number of regimens have been employed, the most frequently included agents being carmustine (BCNU), cyclophosphamide, and etoposide with (BEAM regimen) or without melphalan (CBV regimen), which generally meet these criteria (Table 35.10). Some groups have attempted escalation of individual agents in these regimens, but have reached a ceiling imposed by non-hematologic toxicities (Wheeler *et al.*, 1990; Weaver *et al.*, 1993; Snyder *et al.*, 1994; Mills *et al.*, 1995). Escalating the etoposide dose included in BEAM-HDT (600 mg/m^2 instead of 400 mg/m^2) has failed to improve outcome, but was associated with a significant increase in gastrointestinal toxicity (Mills *et al.*, 1995). Similarly, escalated BACE (carmustine, cytosine arabinoside, cyclophosphamide, and etoposide) appears to have increased pulmonary toxicity without improving transplant results (Snyder *et al.*, 1994).

The inclusion of total body irradiation (TBI) in the conditioning regimen exploits the inherent radiosensitivity of Hodgkin's disease, but carries the disadvantage of increased complications, particularly after previous exposure to irradiation. Additionally, TBI-based conditioning regimens produce more profound and lasting defects in immune response, which may be particularly relevant in Hodgkin's disease, in which patients are often immunocompromised prior to transplantation. Radiotherapy may be considered as an adjuvant therapy posttransplantation (see below).

Stem cell source

The stem cell source may be bone marrow or peripheral blood stem cells (PBSC), the latter being harvested after priming with cytotoxic agents, growth factors, or a combination of the two. The standard approach is now with PBSC, carrying the advantages that harvesting may be performed as

although outcome is relatively poor (Goldstone & McMillan, 1993). Poor performance status and age above 70 are often considered relative contraindications for transplantation. Bone marrow involvement by Hodgkin's disease at time of harvesting is not necessarily a contraindication for transplant, a surprising finding never fully explained (Chopra *et al.*, 1994). However, Nachbaur *et al.* (2001) reported a superior outcome in patients with bone marrow involvement at transplantation, who received an allograft compared to those who received an autograft.

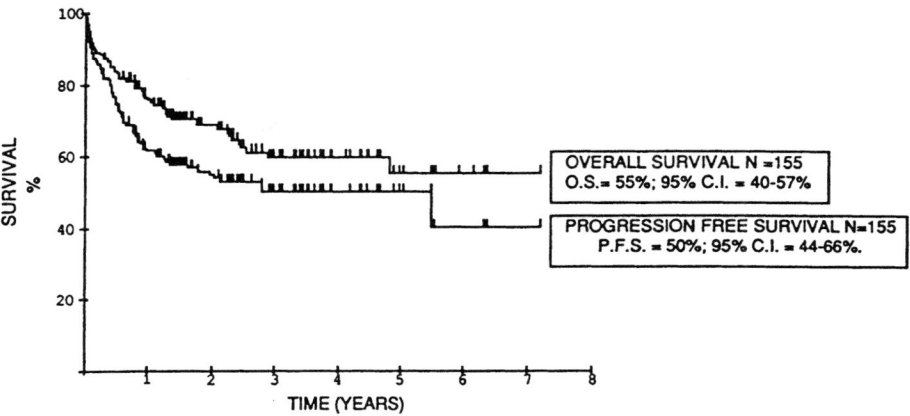

Fig. 35.3. Progression-free and overall survival for 155 patients treated with BEAM and ABMT. Reproduced, with permission, from Chopra *et al.* (1993). Eligibility criteria used: 1. No CR with MOPP and high-grade histology or erythrocyte sedimentation rate (ESR) >59 at diagnosis; 2. no CR with alternating regimens or hybrid regimen; 3. relapse within 1 year of alternating regimens or hybrid regimen; 4. failure after two or more chemotherapy regimens. Status at time of transplant:

	BEAM	Mini-BEAM
Never showing complete response	10	10
Responding relapse	2	2
Refractory relapse	2	0
Untested relapse	6	8

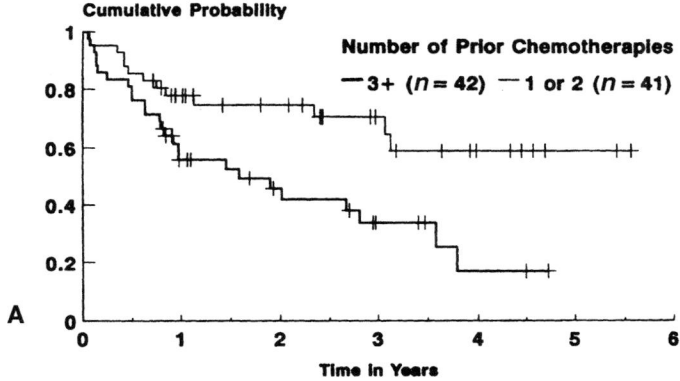

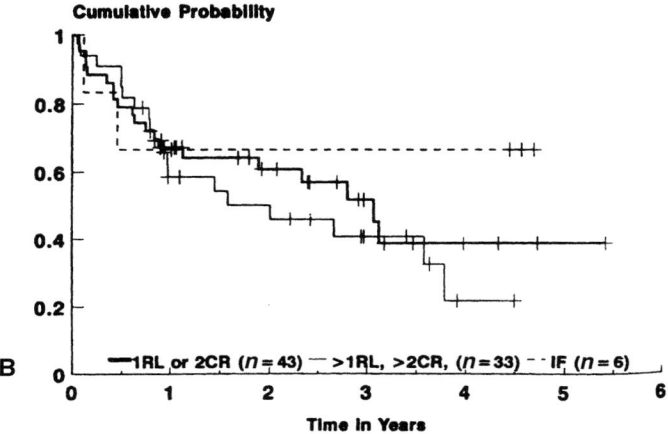

Fig. 35.4. **(A)** DFS curves comparing patients with ≤ 2 prior chemotherapy regimens and those with >2 chemotherapy regimens before ABMT (log-rank test, *P* = .006). **(B)** Probability of DFS by disease status at ABMT (log-rank test, *P* = .51). Reproduced, with permission, from Nademanee *et al.* (1995).

Table 35.10. *Conditioning protocols for autologous hematopoietic stem cell transplantation in Hodgkin's disease (total doses)*

	Cyclophosphamide	Etoposide	Carmustine	Melphalan	Cytosine arabinoside	Cisplatin	Total body irradiation	Total lymphoid irradiation
CBV	5.4–7.2 g/m² or 100 mg/kg	450–2,400 mg/m² or 60 mg/kg	300–800 mg/m² or 15 mg/kg					
CBV+P	7.2 g/m²	2.4 g/m²	500 mg/m²			150 mg/m²		
BEAM		800–1,600 mg/m²	300 mg/m²	140 mg/m²	1,600 mg/m²			
BEAC	140–150 mg/kg	800–1,500 mg/m²	300–700 mg/m²		800–1,500 mg/m²			
CV+TBI	100 mg/kg	60 mg/kg					12 Gy	
CV+TLI	120 mg/kg	750 mg/m²						20 Gy
C+TBI	120 mg/kg						12 Gy	
MBE		300 mg/m²	300–600 mg/m²	140 mg/m²				

Abbreviations: C, cyclophosphamide; B, carmustine (BCNU); V, etoposide (VP-16); P, cisplatin; A, cytosine arabinoside (Ara-C); M, melphalan; TBI, total body irradiation; TLI, total lymphoid irradiation.

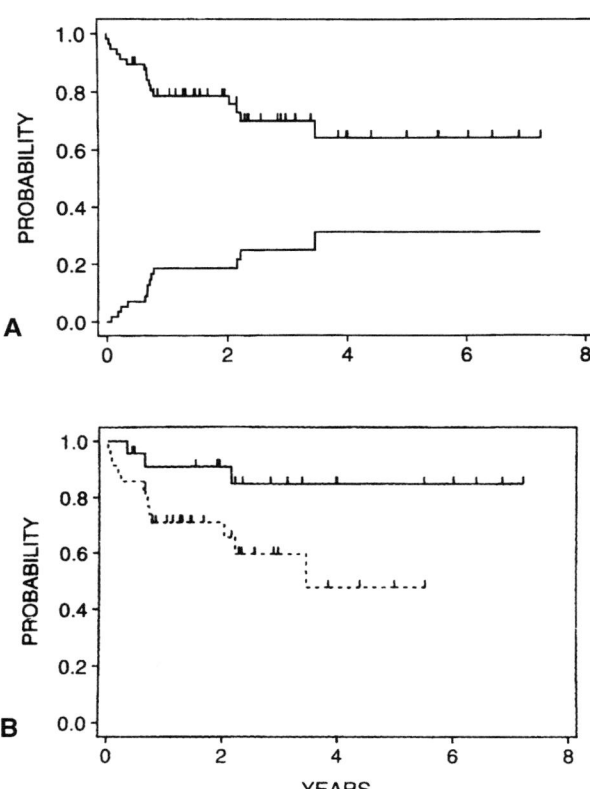

Fig. 35.5. (**A**) Actuarial progression-free survival (upper curve) and probability of disease progression (low curve) after intensive chemotherapy and autologous BMT in 58 patients treated at the time of first relapse. (**B**) Actuarial progression-free survival curves in patients with length of intial complete remission ≥1 year or more ($n = 23$) (solid line) or <1 year ($n = 35$) (dotted line). Reproduced, with permission, from Reece *et al.* (1994).

an outpatient procedure without the need for a general anesthetic, that harvesting may be performed in patients whose bone marrow is unattainable due to marrow fibrosis or previous pelvic irradiation (Körbling *et al.,* 1990), and, most importantly, that engraftment is more rapid following PBSC transplantation, leading to shorter hospital stays and an attendant reduction in treatment cost (Schmitz *et al.,* 1996; Smith *et al.,* 1997). Both retrospective (Perry *et al.,* 1999) and prospective (Schmitz *et al.,* 1996) studies failed to show any significant differences in transplant outcome between patients treated with granulocyte colony-stimulating factor mobilized PBSC versus bone marrow.

There are some reports suggesting a higher frequency (Andre *et al.,* 1998) or earlier development (Del Canizo *et al.,* 2000) of secondary malignancies in patients transplanted with PBSC compared with bone marrow stem cells. However, it is not clear if this is related to the chemotherapy used for stem cell mobilization, or mediated by the source of the stem cells. Further studies are needed to confirm those reports and clarify these issues.

Outcome of autologous HSC transplantation in Hodgkin's disease

Outcome of autologous HSC transplantation in patients with relapsed disease

It now seems clear that HDT followed by HSCT can improve outcome of patients with refractory/relapsed HD. The success rate of HDT for relapsed Hodgkin's disease varies between 40% and 60% in terms of long-term freedom from progression (Carella *et al.,* 1988; Chopra *et al.,* 1993; Reece *et al.,* 1994, 1995 [Fig. 35.6]; Nademanee *et al.,* 1995; Horning *et al.,* 1997; Sweetenham *et al.,* 1997, 1999). Clearly, this figure will vary according to selection criteria, and perhaps also according to

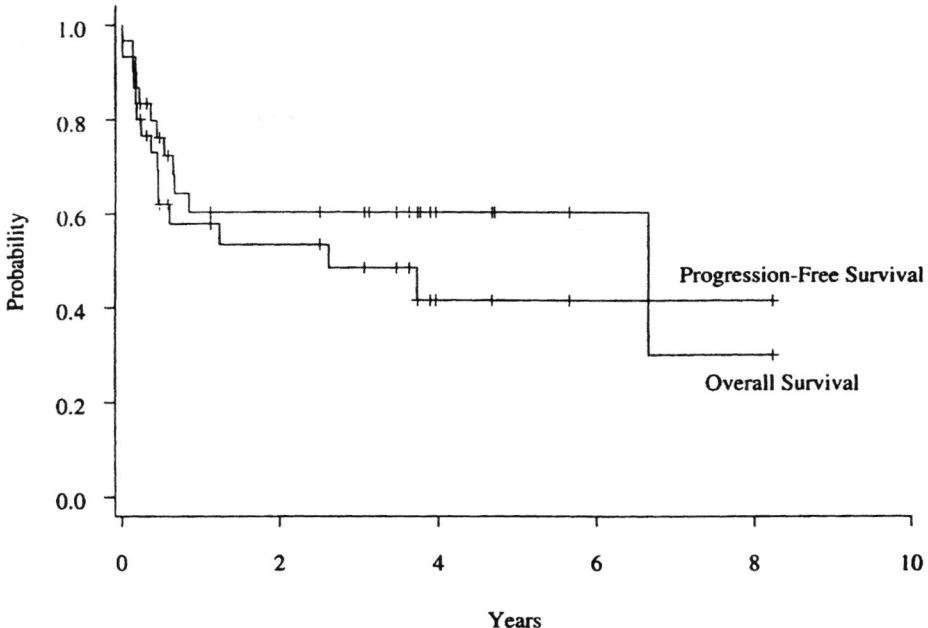

Fig. 35.6. Actuarial survival and PFS in 30 IF patients receiving CBV ± P and ASCT. IF, induction failure. Reproduced, with permission, from Reece *et al.* (1995).

the choice of high-dose regimen and local clinical practice. The outcome data for the larger series are shown in Table 35.11, and survival curves for four series (Chopra *et al.*, 1993; Reece *et al.*, 1994, 1995; Nademanee *et al.*, 1995) are shown in Figs. 35.3, 35.4, 35.5, and 35.6.

Outcome of autologous HSC transplantation in patients with refractory HD

Some patients with chemoresistant disease may benefit from HDT followed by an HSCT. A few studies have reported 3-year OS of 32–50% in patients transplanted with resistant disease (Lazarus *et al.*, 1999; Sureda *et al.*, 2001). Sureda analyzed the outcome of 494 HD patients who had undergone HSCT for relapsed/refractory HD disease or as consolidation in first CR. Two hundred and three patients (41%) were in CR, 216 had chemosensitive disease and 75 had resistant disease (49 primary refractory disease, 26 resistant relapse) at transplantation. Nine percent of the patients died in the first 100 days posttransplant. Five-year time to treatment failure (TTF) was 63.2% for patients transplanted in CR, 37.3% for patients with sensitive disease and 17.4% for patients transplanted with resistant disease. Five-year OS in these three groups was 70.4%, 41.4%, and 32.8% respectively.

Lazarus *et al.* (2001) reported a 3-year OS of 50% in patients who received an HSCT after failing to enter remission with induction chemotherapy. Poor performance status at transplantation and the presence of B symptoms at diagnosis were found to be the most significant prognostic factors affecting transplant outcome (Lazarus *et al.*, 1999).

The outcome of HD patients transplanted with refractory disease remains disappointing, but there are some patients that respond to transplant and might even be cured.

Outcome of autologous HSC transplantation in patients with primary induction failure

Attention has been given to patients who fail to remit with first-line conventional chemotherapy (primary induction failure) (Sweetenham *et al.*, 1999; Josting *et al.*, 2000; Lazarus *et al.*, 2001). Chopra *et al.* (1993) reported 5-year actuarial progression free survival of 33% in 46 patients with primary refractory HD treated with HDT followed by stem cell rescue.

The German Hodgkin's Lymphoma Study Group (GHSG) analyzed retrospectively the outcome of 206 patients with early progressive HD (70% progressed during first-line treatment, 30% progressed within the first 3 months after completing first-line therapy) (Josting *et al.*, 2000). Two hundred patients had been treated with salvage radiotherapy (*n* = 47) or salvage chemotherapy (*n* = 153). Seventy patients, including 62 who had responded to salvage therapy, were then treated with HSCT. Five-year OS and freedom from second failure rates for patients who had salvage therapy followed by HSCT were 43% and 31% respectively. Multivariate analysis revealed that low performance status, age >50 years, and failure to achieve temporary remission on first-line chemotherapy were significant adverse prognostic factors for OS. In the presence of the three risk factors, 5-year OS was 0% compared with 55% for a patient who had none of them. The relatively good results obtained with transplant were interpreted to be related mainly

Table 35.11. *Major studies of autologous HSC transplantation for Hodgkin's lymphoma*

Reference	Number of patients	Selection Criteria	Conditioning	Stem cell source	CR	OS	DFS	TRM
Carella *et al.*, 1988	50	Relapse/refractory	CBV	BM	48%		45%	4%
Jagannath *et al.*, 1989	61	Relapsed	CBV	BM	47%	46%	50%	7%
Reece *et al.*, 1991	56	Relapse/refractory	CBV	BM	80%	53%	47%	21%
Yahalom *et al.*, 1993	47	Relapse/refractory	CV+TLI	BM	74%		50%	17%
Chopra *et al.*, 1993	155	Relapse/refractory	BEAM	BM	28%	55%	50%	11%
Linch *et al.*, 1993[a]	40	Resistant/relapse (active disease)[a]	BEAM	BM		$P > .05$	53% vs. 10%[a] $P = .025$	2/20
Reece *et al.*, 1994	58	First relapse	CBV ± P	BM			64%	7%
Reece *et al.*, 1995	30	Refractory	CBV ± AP	BM/PB		60%	42%	18%
Nademanee *et al.*, 1995	85	Relapse/refractory	CBV or CV/TBI	BM/PB	76%	45%	39%	13%
Lumley *et al.*, 1996	42	Relapse/refractory	BEAM	BM/PB	61%	50%	65%	2%
Yuen *et al.*, 1997	60	Relapse/refractory	CBV or CV/TBI	BM/PB		54%	50%	10%
Lazarus *et al.*, 1999	122	Failure to achieve CR	CBV	BM/PB	50	50	38% (PFS)	12%
Lazarus *et al.*, 2001	414	First relapse/CR2	CBV (most pt)	BM/PB	56%-R[b]	58%-R[b] 75%-CR[c]	46%-R[b] 64%-CR[c]	7%
Sureda *et al.*, 2001	494	Relapse/refractory	CBV or BEAM or BEAC	BM/PB		54.5%	45%	9%
Schmitz *et al.*, 2002[d]	161[d]	Relapsed	BEAM	BM/PB		$P > .05$	55% vs.43%[d] $P = .019$	1/51

Abbreviations: BM, bone marrow; BM/PB, bone marrow/peripheral blood; CR, complete remission; OS, overall survival; DFS, disease-free survival; TRM, treatment-related mortality; PFS, progression-free survival; R, relapse. FFTF, freedom from treatment failure. Conditioning regimens, see Table 35.10.

[a] Patients with active resistant/relapsed disease were prospectively randomized to receive mini-BEAM salvage chemotherapy vs. BEAM followed by autologous BM.

[b] Data for patients transplanted with relapsed disease

[c] Data for patients transplanted in CR2

In most of these studies, patients received a second-line therapy for relapse/refractory disease pre-transplantation

[d] 161 patients were prospectively randomized to receive Dexa-BEAM (second-line therapy) versus Dexa-BEAM followed by BEAM and autograft. FFTF = 55% with autograft versus 34% with second line therapy. DFS = 53% versus 10% for autografted patients versus non-autgrafted patients.

to patient selection and not necessarily to HSCT itself (Josting *et al.*, 2000).

Andre *et al.* (1999) compared the outcome of primary refractory HD patients treated with salvage chemotherapy followed by HSCT ($n = 86$) with matched, conventionally treated (mechlorethamine, vincristine, procarbazine, and prednisone [MOPP]) patients ($n = 258$). Six-year OS (counted from diagnosis) for autografted patients was 38%, compared with 29% for conventionally treated patients ($P = .058$). Response to salvage therapy prior to transplantation was the only significant prognostic factor for survival (partial response had a relative risk of +2.8; progressive disease had a relative risk of 5.26, $P < .001$).

However, a different strategy for treating patients with primary induction failure has been suggested by ABMTR and EBMT studies, both supporting early transplantation, rather than a pretransplant salvage therapy followed by HSCT in HD patients refractory to induction chemotherapy (Sweetenham *et al.*, 1999; Lazarus *et al.*, 2001). In the ABMTR study, probabilities of progression-free survival and OS 3 years posttransplant were 38% and 50% respectively. There was no correlation

between disease sensitivity pretransplant (although this information was not available for all patients) and transplant outcome (Lazarus *et al.*, 2001). It is worth noting that in this particular study, patients were defined as having a primary induction failure if their CT scan showed progression rather than no response.

The EBMT group analyzed the outcome of 175 HD patients treated with HSCT after failing to respond to induction chemotherapy (Sweetenham *et al.*, 1999). Seventy-five patients were treated with salvage HSCT without further attempts to induce remission with conventional chemotherapy. The remaining 100 patients had an HSCT after failing to respond to second-line therapy. Thirty percent of all patients ($n = 175$) succeeded in achieving CR following transplant, 28% had a PR, 28% had no response or continued to progress, and 14% died of transplant-related complication. Actuarial 5 year OS and progression-free survival (PFS) were 36% and 32% respectively. Patients who had an HSCT without prior salvage therapy ($n = 75$) had a better PFS and OS compared with patients who had been transplanted after failing to respond to second-line treatment.

Both these studies suggest an advantage for early transplantation, rather than salvage chemotherapy followed by autografting, for primary refractory HD patients.

Thus it appears that patients failing to remit with induction chemotherapy might benefit from autologous transplantation. All studies reported to date, however, are retrospective and have not adequately separated patients failing induction therapy but responding to salvage (second-line) therapy from those failing both induction therapy and second-line therapy. Additionally, those with resistant relapse must be examined separately from those transplanted for untested relapse. Further analysis of each of these subgroups is needed in order to understand whom to transplant and whom to preclude.

Outcome of autologous HSC transplantation in first CR for patients with high-risk Hodgkin's disease

Consolidation therapy with HDT followed by HSCT has been investigated as a means to improve the outcome of HD patients with high risk of relapse (Carella et al., 1991, 1996; Moreau et al., 1998). Despite the encouraging results of a phase II trial (Carella et al., 1996), a phase III trial failed to show any advantage for upfront HSCT in high-risk HD patients (Federico et al., 2002). In this study, high-risk HD patients were randomized to HSCT versus 4 additional chemotherapy courses, after having achieved CR with 4 courses of induction chemotherapy. The 5-year failure-free survival was 85% in the transplant arm versus 83% in the chemotherapy arm ($P = .61$). No difference was found in terms of overall survival ($P = .76$) or relapse free survival ($P = .55$). The outcome was similar also in the subset of 93 patients in PR at time of randomization (Federico et al., 2002).

It seems that there is currently no place for upfront HSCT in high risk HD patients.

Prognostic factors for transplantation

Retrospective analyses of prognostic factors predicting outcome of HSCT in patients with HD (Table 35.12), have consistently shown that bulky/non-responsive disease at transplantation has a significant negative influence on posttransplant

Table 35.12. *Reported adverse prognostic factors for outcome after high-dose therapy for Hodgkin's disease*

Tumor bulk at time of transplant
More previous lines of therapy
Refractory disease
Short initial prior remissions
Poor performance status
B symptoms at relapse
Extranodal disease at relapse
Bone marrow involvement at time of transplant
High LDH at transplant
Female sex

disease-free survival (DFS) (Gribben et al., 1989; Jagannath et al., 1989; Chopra et al., 1993; Crump et al., 1993; Rapoport et al., 1993; Reece et al., 1995; O'Brien et al., 1996; Brice et al., 1997; Kusnierz-Glaz et al., 1997; Sureda et al., 2001). Baker et al. (1999) reported 5-year failure-free survival FFS of 9% in children and adolescents with resistant disease, compared with 35% for patients with sensitive relapse (Baker et al., 1999).

The apparent importance of tumor bulk has led many groups to attempt reduction of tumor mass as a prerequisite to undergoing HDT, rather than administering high-dose treatment in untested relapse (Brandwein et al., 1990, Rüffer & Sieber, 1996; Martin et al., 2001; Sureda et al., 2001). This approach does carry the theoretical risk of inducing drug resistance, but has the additional advantage of selecting out those with chemoresistant relapse that might fare poorly with HDT.

Other factors variously identified as poor prognostic factors include female sex (Chopra et al., 1993), a higher number of treatments pretransplantation (Chopra et al., 1993; Nademanee et al., 1995; O'Brien et al., 1996), initial remission of less than 12 months (Reece et al., 1994), poor performance status (Jagannath et al., 1989; Lazarus et al., 2001), B symptoms at relapse (Reece et al., 1994; Horning et al., 1997), extranodal disease at relapse (Reece et al., 1994; Nademanee et al., 1995; Horning et al., 1997), bone marrow disease at transplantation (Kessinger et al., 1991; Del Canizo et al., 2000), and high LDH at transplant (Lumley et al., 1996; Lazarus et al., 2001). Lynch et al. (2001) have suggested that the HD prognostic index (Hasenclever et al., 1998) used at diagnosis can also predict the outcome of autologous stem cell transplantation. Low serum albumin, low hemoglobin, lymphopenia, and advanced stage of disease at transplantation were found to be the most powerful prognostic factors, associated with reduced OS and EFS.

Evaluation of response to transplantation including early detection of disease relapse

Evaluation of patient's response to HSCT, as well as the assessment of new lesions posttransplant, remains complex. Some HD patients may retain abnormal appearances on CT scans (due to fibrotic scarring), although succeeding in achieving CR.

Positron emission tomography, based on radionuclide scanning, is currently being evaluated for this (Dittman et al., 2001; Spaepen & Mortelmans, 2001). This radionuclide scanning, 18-FDG-6 phosphate PET, is based on the fact that malignant tumors, including HD, rely largely on anerobic glycolysis (by amplification of the glucose transporter protein at the tumor cell surface as well as from increased activity of hexokinase). Therefore, a radiolabelled glucose (18-fluoro-deoxy-glucose; 18-FDG) injected into patients with active HD will be predominantly absorbed by the tumor cells. A localized increase of FDG uptake in the PET scan is considered as indicating active HD (Gallagher et al., 1978; Hoh et al., 1997; Jerusalem et al., 1999). A false positive PET scan can be caused by a co-existing infection/inflammation, increasing the glucose uptake (Dittmann et al., 2001; Spaepen & Mortelmans, 2001).

Dittman *et al.* have evaluated the ability of PET scanning, compared with CT scanning, to detect relapsed disease in HD patients. Seven of 8 patients with increased FDG uptake had histologically/clinically proven relapse; only 2 of 10 patients with a CT scan that was interpreted as showing relapse were eventually diagnosed with recurrent HD. The false negative rate was also higher with CT scanning: 6 of 16 compared with 1 of 8 with PET scan. The positive and negative predictive value of PET and CT scans were 87%, 94% and 20%, 62.5% respectively (Dittmann *et al.*, 2001). PET scanning has also been shown to be able to detect disease relapse earlier than CT scanning (Spaepen & Mortelmans, 2001). Thus PET scanning enables early detection of relapse, a better discrimination between active disease and scar tissue, and thus might prevent unnecessary treatment (Spaepen & Mortelmans., 2001).

A molecular method for detection of minimal residual HD has been introduced. Vockerodt *et al.* (1998) have studied the potential use of PCR to identify Reed[2]-Sternberg[3] cells with immunoglobulin (Ig) clonal gene rearrangement.

Adverse effects of autologous HSC transplantation

The high mortality rate (20–25%) initially reported with HSCT in HD was mainly related to the population of patients who were transplanted in the later stages of their disease. Pulmonary toxicity associated with prior mediastinal radiotherapy, TBI or chemotherapy (particularly carmustine and bleomycin) contributed (Pecego *et al.*, 1986; Goldstone & McMillan, 1993; Gause & Longo, 1996).

Mortality rates have decreased over the past decade, reflecting not only increasing experience in managing these patients, but also changing patient selection criteria. By performing HSCT at an earlier stage (first relapse or second remission), along with the introduction of less toxic high-dose chemotherapy regimes (CBV, BEAM) and an increasing usage of peripheral blood stem cells, instead of bone marrow stem cells, transplant-related mortality has been decreased to less then 5%.

Secondary malignancies

An increasingly important risk for HD patients undergoing autologous HSCT is the relatively high incidence of secondary myelodysplastic syndrome (MDS) and acute myeloid leukemia (AML) that occurs posttransplant, approaching 9%–18% at 5 to 7 years after the graft (Darrington *et al.*, 1994; Stone *et al.*, 1994; Yuen *et al.*, 1997; Andre *et al.*, 1998; Wheeler *et al.*, 2001 and see Chapter 86).

The pathogenesis of secondary MDS/AML in these patients treated prior to transplant with chemoradiotherapy is complex

and the contribution of each of these treatments to leukemia development is not fully elucidated. There have been reports of clonal abnormalities in the harvest or preharvest marrow, which may predict for subsequent myelodysplasia, and perhaps this should be considered a contraindication to autologous transplantation (Chao *et al.*, 1991). However, clonal cytogenetic changes have been shown to develop even after normal pretransplant karyotypic studies (Traweek *et al.*, 1994), while other patients displaying oligoclonality after transplantation have not progressed to myelodysplasia (Gale *et al.*, 1996).

Various studies have reported different risk factors for developing a secondary leukemia/MDS in autografted HD patients (Andre *et al.*, 1998; Krishnan *et al.*, 2000; Sureda *et al.*, 2001). Retrospective analysis of HD patients treated through the British National Lymphoma Investigation (BNLI) with (*n* = 595) or without HSCT (*n* = 4,576) revealed that the amount of prior therapy and treatment with MOPP or lomustine chemotherapy were the main risk factors for secondary MDS/AML. Sureda found age >40 at transplantation, pretransplant radiotherapy, and use of TBI in the conditioning regimen to be associated with an increased risk of developing secondary malignancy posttransplant. Sixteen out of 494 HD patients who had been transplanted developed a secondary malignancy (12 MDS/AML,1 ALL,1 NHL, 2 solid tumors), with a 5-year cumulative incidence of 4.3% (Sureda *et al.*, 2001). Krishnan analyzed the incidence of transplant-related MDS/AML in 218 HD patients who had been treated with HDT and HSCT rescue (Krishnan *et al.*, 2000). Eleven of 218 patients developed MDS/AML, characterized by 11q23/21q22 abnormalities, with an estimated cumulative probability of 8.1% ± 2.5% at six years posttransplant. Median time to develop secondary MDS/AML was 3.8 years from diagnosis and 0.9 years from transplant. Multivariate analyses showed priming with etoposide to be the only risk factor for secondary MDS/AML in this group of patients, where HD by itself was not found to be a risk factor for secondary AML/MDS (risk was compared to that observed in NHL patients, analysed in the same study).

There is no typical chromosomal change for transplant-related leukemia in HD patients. While some patients showed abnormalities in 11q23/21q22 (Krishnan *et al.*, 2000), partial/complete deletion of chromosome 7 (Andre *et al.*, 1998), translocations involving chromosome 8 [t(8:16) t(21:8)] (Park *et al.*, 2000), or other chromosomal changes, others may have no detectable chromosomal abnormalities (Park *et al.*, 2000).

An increased incidence of solid cancers has also been reported (Andre *et al.*, 1998). Ten out of 467 (2.1%) patients who had been transplanted developed secondary cancers (8 solid cancers, 2 NHL). Andre found age >40 years and the use of PBSC to be associated with increased risk of a secondary malignancy (Andre *et al.*, 1998). The risk of non-hematologic second malignancies is also increased after conventional treatment (Schnell *et al.*, 1996; Henry-Amar & Joly, 1996).

---

[2]Dorothy Reed, U.S. pathologist, 1874–1964.
[3]Carl Sternberg, Austrian pathologist, 1872–1935.

Other transplant-related complications

Other complications depend on the regimen used. Endocrine dysfunction and infertility are not uncommon (see Chapters 94 and 97).

Relapse posttransplant

At present, nearly half of those patients who undergo autologous HSCT for Hodgkin's disease will relapse posttransplant. Most relapses occur in the first 2 years after HDT (Vose et al., 1992; Varterasian et al., 1995). For these patients there is usually little in the way of curative therapy that can be offered. Nevertheless, palliative and semi-palliative regimens can successfully prolong the life of the patient for months or years following relapse (Longo, 1990; Bolwell et al., 1997). Patients with lymphocyte predominance HD (though a minority of HD patients) express CD20 antigen, and might therefore respond to anti-CD20 monoclonal antibodies as a salvage therapy for relapse post autograft (Lush, Jones, & Haynes, 2001).

Attempts at second autologous stem cell transplants as rescue have produced anecdotal successes (Avalos & Copelan, 1993; Lin et al., 2002), although morbidity and mortality are likely to be increased.

The efficacy of conventional allogeneic transplant in HD remains controversial and possible benefit has been countered by a very high non-relapse mortality rate (Jones et al., 1991; Anderson et al., 1993; Gajewski et al., 1996; Milpied et al., 1996).

In recent years, however, low or reduced intensity conditioning regimens prior to allogeneic stem cell transplantation have been developed, aiming to combine a graft-versus-tumor effect with less regimen-related toxicity (Kottaridis et al., 2000). The latter investigators have utilized this approach in 24 patients with advanced HD (17 patients had already failed an autograft). At transplant, 6 patients were in CR, 13 were in PR, and 6 had refractory disease. Patients received a low-intensity conditioning regimen consisting of Campath-1H, fludarabine, and melphalan. All patients achieved donor engraftment and 70% attained full myeloid and lymphoid chimerism. The incidence of treatment-related mortality (TRM), as well as the incidence and the severity of GVHD, were low.

Three out of the 6 patients transplanted with refractory disease progressed and died within 3 months posttransplantion. All five patients who relapsed posttransplant (19, 18, 17, 9, and 6 months posttransplant) were treated with donor lymphocyte infusions (DLI) with/without adjuvant chemotherapy. Four of these 5 patients achieved and maintained remission, but one died of grade IV graft-versus-host disease (GVHD), which developed after DLI. At a median follow-up of 23 months, the actuarial survival, progression-free survival, and actual progression free-survival following DLI ± chemotherapy were 72%, 45%, and 57% respectively.

The long-term effect of this kind of transplant and its curative potential is currently unknown. However, this treatment protocol is associated with a relatively low incidence of TRM and GVHD. Initial response to DLI supports the existence of graft-versus-Hodgkin's disease effect.

Approaches to improve outcome and future directions

Reduction of the morbidity and mortality of autologous HSC transplantation

Improving the outcome of autologous transplants in Hodgkin's disease rests in part on measures to reduce procedure-related complications and in part on ways to reduce posttransplant relapse. The use of hematopoietic growth factors, particularly granulocyte and granulocyte-macrophage colony-stimulating factors, has shortened the neutropenic period and, in some reports, the length of hospitalization posttransplantation (Devereux et al., 1989; Taylor et al., 1989; Gulati & Bennett, 1992). As growth factor technology evolves, other side effects such as thrombocytopenia and mucositis may also be reduced.

Reduction of relapse rate

Tumor cell purging

Controversy reigns over the question of whether posttransplant relapse is due to the reinfusion of malignant cells or to the inadequacy of the conditioning regimen in eliminating residual disease. There is no clear evidence that bone marrow purging can improve the outcome of HSCT in Hodgkin's (or any other) disease. Indeed, there is evidence of successful autotransplant in patients whose bone marrow has been involved with HD.

Pretransplant ex vivo purging performed in NHL patients had been demonstrated to reduce tumor cells by several logs. However, it risks loss and damage of stem and committed progenitor cells (Gribben et al., 1991). Elimination of lymphoid and accessory cells might also adversely affect immune reconstitution, including a physiological anti-tumor effect (Gribben et al., 1991). In vivo purging may be more effective then ex vivo purging in this regard.

Both ex vivo and in vivo purging can be carried out using monoclonal antibodies (Mabs) directed against antigens expressed by the tumor cells. The CD30 antigen expressed by the majority of HD cells could be a suitable target. Anti-CD30 Mabs, unconjugated or conjugated to immunotoxins (Falini et al., 1992; Matthey, Engert, & Barth, 2000) or radioisoptopes (Bierman et al., 1993) have been reported as having an in vitro and in vivo efficacy against Hodgkin's disease cells (Matthey, Engert, & Barth, 2000; Koon & Junghans, 2000).

Since most cases of HD express the CD25 antigen, anti-CD25 Mabs might also be useful. Anti-CD25 Mabs, unconjugated or conjugated to immunotoxins, have been shown to have activity against HD cells (Schnell et al., 1998). Rituximab, an anti-CD 20 Mab, has been anecdotally reported to be active in some HD patients characterized by high CD20 expression of their tumor cells (usually lymphocyte predominant HD) (Lush *et al.*, 2001).

Experience with all these antibodies remains limited and their use for pretransplant purging needs further investigation.

Posttransplant adjuvant therapy

Relapse after HSCT is mainly caused by residual lymphoma cells that survive the HDT. Therefore, posttransplant therapy with, for example, appropriate monoclonal antibodies might have a role in eradicating residual HD cells in order to reduce relapse rate and increase DFS and OS.

A number of such studies are on-going in patients receiving autologous transplants for non-Hodgkin's lymphoma, but none have been reported yet in patients with HD.

Posttransplant adjuvant radiotherapy   It remains true that most sites of disease relapse posttransplant represent original sites of disease involvement (Phillips *et al.*, 1989; Mundt *et al.*, 1995; Poen *et al.*, 1996). For this reason, the use of involved field radiotherapy to supplement HDT has been advocated, especially when radiation has not formed a substantial part of previous treatment. The involved field selected may be the site of previous bulk disease or the site of residual disease on posttransplant scanning. There is accumulating evidence that use of such radiotherapy does improve outcome (Mundt *et al.*, 1995; Pezner *et al.*, 1995; Hoppe, 1996; Poen *et al.*, 1996). The disadvantage is that toxicities may be increased by the additive effects of chemotherapy and radiotherapy, leading, for example, to pneumonitis or veno-occlusive disease (Poen *et al.*, 1996). This appears more likely to occur when radiotherapy is performed prior to transplant, especially within the preceding 3 months (Weaver *et al.*, 1993). It may be that delaying irradiation until after HDT is the safer option, although this can cause suppression of the still fragile marrow (Price *et al.*, 1994). One option is to delay radiotherapy until 3 months post-HDT, and then carefully monitor the blood counts, temporarily interrupting the radiation if necessary.

Posttransplant immunomodulation   Another theoretical way of reducing the relapse rate posttransplantation is by augmenting the immune response against residual malignant cells. Different cytokines, including interferon-alpha (Schenkein *et al.*, 1994) and interleukin-2 (Benyunes *et al.*, 1995) have been investigated. However, none of them have yet been shown to change transplant outcome significantly.

There are some reports supporting maintenance therapy with interferon-alfa 2b (IFN) in (non-transplanted) HD patients who achieve CR (Aviles *et al.*, 1998). A better DFS and OS have been reported in patients that were treated with INF-α compared with those who were randomized to no maintenance therapy ($P = .01$) (Aviles *et al.*, 1998). Posttransplant INF-α studied in 14 NHL/HD patients failed to reduce relapse rate, although it was reportedly associated with increased OS (Schenkein *et al.*, 1994).

Efforts to induce a graft-versus-tumor effect after autologous transplantation by using immunomodulatory drugs such as cyclosporine and INF-γ (the latter to upregulate MHC class II expression on cells) have been carried out (Vogelsang *et al.*, 1999).

Posttransplant therapy with different interleukins (IL-1, IL-2) have been suggested to augment the immune anti-tumor response (Katsanis *et al.*, 1994). Nagler *et al.* (1997) have reported an improved DFS in NHL/HD patients who received IL-2 following autografting, compared with historical controls. Prospective randomized trials are needed to confirm this.

Modifications of autologous HSC transplantation

Newer approaches continue to be investigated with the aim of reducing the relapse rate of Hodgkin's disease post-HDT. These include sequential double autograft protocols, which are potentially quite toxic strategies, with the series as yet being too small to yield valuable information (Ahmed *et al.*, 1991).

An alternative approach is the use of radiolabelled anti-CD30 Mabs given as part of the conditioning regimen protocol. Bierman *et al.* (1993) treated 14 patients with chemo-resistant/bulky HD with Yttrium 90-labelled anti-ferritin followed by HDT using the CBV regimen. Four patients were still alive 2 years posttransplantation, three of them in continued CR. However, effectiveness and toxicity of this treatment should be assessed in patients with less advanced disease and compared to results of conventional HSCT.

A different strategy based on autologous HSCT followed electively by reduced intensity conditioning and an allogeneic transplant has been suggested by Carella *et al.* (2000). Ten patients, all with progressive or advanced relapsed HD were treated with BEAM-HDT followed by an autograft, and then by an HLA-matched related allograft two months later. Treatment was well tolerated. Patients who did not achieve full chimerism following transplantation were treated with DLI. Three of 10 patients achieved CR post autograft, while 8 of 10 obtained CR following the allogeneic transplant, including 6 remaining in CR at 340 days posttransplantation. Follow-up is still short and the number of patients small, but this is an interesting approach.

Autologous or allogeneic transplantation?

There remains the question of whether allogeneic transplantation is ever preferable to HDT with autologous stem cell support. There are theoretical advantages of transplanting disease-free marrow (which is also free of dysplastic potential), and of inducing a graft-versus-lymphoma effect. There is currently some evidence that relapse rates are indeed lower after allogeneic transplantation for Hodgkin's disease, particularly in the presence of GVHD, suggesting that a graft-versus-lymphoma effect does exist (Jones *et al.*, 1991; Anderson *et al.*, 1993; Milpied *et al.*, 1996; Kottaridis & Mackinnon, 2001). Such advantages are offset by the increased morbidity and mortality of the allogeneic transplant; indeed, overall survival appears to be identical or even higher in autologous stem cell transplants (Jones *et al.*, 1991; Anderson *et al.*, 1993; Gajewski *et al.*, 1996; Milpied *et al.*, 1996).

There may be a subgroup of Hodgkin's disease patients for whom allogeneic transplantation might be preferable—young patients who relapse after autologous HSCT, who have an HLA-matched sibling and are in good performance status, and who are therefore at lower risk of transplant-related mortality.

The introduction of reduced intensity conditioning followed by an allograft deserves careful evaluation in appropriate categories of HD patients. Currently, however, any kind of allogeneic transplantation cannot really be considered a treatment of choice for HD patients in CR2 or first relapse, but might be offered as a part of a clinical trial to patients who relapse following an autograft.

Conclusions

Improvements in the outcome of first-line therapy for advanced Hodgkin's disease are likely to reduce the number of patients who may benefit from autologous stem cell transplantation. For the shrinking minority who fail to remit or who relapse after initial treatment, HDT with autologous stem cell support remains the most effective means of potential cure. Even so, this approach will fail in about half the patients, and as the procedure itself becomes safer, attention is being focused on ways to reduce the posttransplant relapse rate. The use of radiotherapy or immunotherapy to supplement high-dose chemotherapy may improve outcome. Similarly, clearer definition of patients who may do better with some kind of allogeneic transplant will aid in individually tailored treatment strategies. Autologous hematopoietic stem cell transplantation is undoubtedly an important contribution toward the goal of making Hodgkin's disease a curable disease. This goal will not be achieved without cost, in terms of the adverse consequences of therapy, and reducing the risks associated with intensive treatment remains one of the challenges of the future.

References

Ahmed, T., Feldman, E., Ciavearella, D. *et al.* (1991). Sequential autologous bone marrow transplantation for high risk Hodgkin's disease. *Proceedings of the American Society of Clinical Oncology,* **10,** 223 (Abstract).

Andre, M., Henry-Amar, M., Blaise, D. *et al.* (1998). Treatment-related deaths and second cancer risk after autologous stem-cell transplantation for Hodgkin's disease. *Blood,* **92,** 1933–40.

Andre, M., Henry-Amar, M., Pico, J. L. *et al.* (1999). Comparison of high-dose therapy and autologous stem-cell transplantation with conventional therapy for Hodgkin's disease induction failure: a case-control study. Societe Francaise de Greffe de Moelle. *Journal of Clinical Oncology,* **17,** 222–9.

Anderson, J. E., Litzow, M. R., Appelbaum, F. R. *et al.* (1993). Allogeneic, syngeneic and autologous marrow transplantation for Hodgkin's disease: the 21-year experience. *Journal of Clinical Oncology,* **11,** 2342–50.

Avalos, B. R. & Copelan, E. A. (1993). Second autologous bone marrow transplantation in Hodgkin's disease. *Bone Marrow Transplantation,* **12,** 665–7.

Aviles, A., Diaz-Maqueo, J. C., Talavera, A. *et al.* (1998). Maintenance therapy with interferon alfa 2b in Hodgkin's disease. *Leukemia and Lymphoma,* **30,** 651–6.

Aydogdu, I., Koc, H., Ilhan, O. *et al.* (1997). Administration of MINE protocol in untreated patients with intermediate and high grade non-Hodgkin's lymphoma. *Haematologia,* **28,** 207–13.

Baker, K. S., Gordon, B. G., Gross, T. G. *et al.* (1999). Autologous hematopoietic stem-cell transplantation for relapsed or refractory Hodgkin's disease in children and adolescents. *Journal of Clinical Oncology,* **17,** 825–31.

Bartlett, N. L., Rosenberg, S. A., Hoppe, R. T. *et al.* (1995). Brief chemotherapy, Stanford V and adjuvant radiotherapy for bulky or advanced stage Hodgkin's disease: a preliminary report. *Journal of Clinical Oncology,* **13,** 1080–8.

Benyunes, M. C., Higuchi, C., York, A. *et al.* (1995). Immunotherapy with interleukin 2 with or without lymphokine-activated killer cells after autologous bone marrow transplantation for malignant lymphoma: a feasibility trial. *Bone Marrow Transplantation,* **16,** 283–8.

Bierman, P. I., Vose, J. M., Leichner, P. K. *et al.* (1993). Yttrium 90-labelled antiferritin followed by high-dose chemotherapy and autologous bone marrow transplantation for poor-prognosis Hodgkin's disease. *Journal of Clinical Oncology,* **11,** 698–703.

Bolwell, B. J., Kalaycio, M., Goormastic, M. *et al.* (1997). Progressive disease after ABMT for Hodgkin's disease. *Bone Marrow Transplantation,* **20,** 761–5.

Brandwein, J. M., Callum, I., Sutcliffe, S. B. *et al.* (1990). Evaluation of cytoreductive therapy prior to high-dose treatment with autologous bone marrow transplantation in relapsed and refractory Hodgkin's disease. *Bone Marrow Transplantation,* **5,** 99–103.

Brice, P., Bouabdallah, R., Moreau, P. *et al.* (1997). Prognostic factors for survival after high-dose therapy and autologous stem cell transplantation for patients with relapsing Hodgkin's disease: analysis of 280 patients from the French registry. *Bone Marrow Transplantation,* **20,** 21–6.

Carella, A. M., Carlier, P., Congiu, A. *et al.* (1991). Autologous bone marrow transplantation as adjuvant treatment for high-risk Hodgkin's disease in first complete remission after MOPP/ABVD protocol. *Bone Marrow Transplantation,* **8,** 99–103.

Carella, A. M, Cavaliere, M., Lerma, E. *et al.* (2000). Autografting followed by nonmyeloablative immunosuppressive chemotherapy and allogeneic peripheral-blood hematopoietic stem-cell transplantation as treatment of resistant Hodgkin's disease and non-Hodgkin's lymphoma. *Journal of Clinical Oncology,* **18,** 3918–24.

Carella, A. M., Congiu, A. M., Gaozza, E. *et al.* (1988). High-dose chemotherapy with autologous bone marrow transplantation in 50 advanced resistant Hodgkin's disease patients: an Italian Study Group report. *Journal of Clinical Oncology,* **6,** 1411–6.

Carella, A. M., Prencipe, E., Pungolino, E. *et al.* (1996). Twelve years experience with high-dose therapy and autologous stem cell transplantation for high-risk Hodgkin's disease in first remission after MOPP/ABVD chemotherapy. *Leukemia and Lymphoma,* **21,** 63–70.

Chao, N. J., Nademanee, A. P., Long, G. D. *et al.* (1991). Importance of bone marrow cytogenetic evaluation before autologous bone marrow transplantation for Hodgkin's disease. *Journal of Clinical Oncology,* **9,** 1575–9.

Chopra, R., Linch, D. C., McMillan, A. K. *et al.* (1992). Mini-BEAM followed by BEAM and ABMT for very poor risk Hodgkin's disease. *British Journal of Haematology,* **81,** 197–202.

Chopra, R., McMillan, A. K., Linch, D. C. *et al.* (1993). The place of high-dose BEAM therapy and autologous bone marrow transplantation in poor risk Hodgkin's disease. A single center eight year study of 155 patients. *Blood,* **81,** 1137–45.

Chopra, R., Wotherspoon, A. C., Blair, S. *et al.* (1994). Detection and significance of bone marrow infiltration at the time of autologous bone marrow transplantation in Hodgkin's disease. *British Journal of Haematology,* **87,** 647–9.

Crump, M., Smith, A. M., Brandwein, J. *et al.* (1993). High-dose etoposide and melphalan, and autologous bone marrow transplantation for patients with advanced Hodgkin's disease: importance of disease status at transplant. *Journal of Clinical Oncology,* **11,** 704–11

Darrington, D. L, Vose, J. M., Anderson, J. R. *et al.* (1994). Incidence and characterization of secondary myelodysplastic syndrome and acute myelogenous leukemia following high-dose chemoradiotherapy and autologous stem-cell transplantation for lymphoid malignancies. *Journal of Clinical Oncology,* **12,** 2527–34.

Del Canizo, M. F., Amigo, M. F., Hernandez, J. M. *et al.* (2000). Incidence of myelodysplastic syndromes following autologous stem cell transplsantation. *Haematologica,* **85,** 403–409.

Deveraux, S., Linch, D. C., Gribben, I. G. *et al.* (1989). GM-CSF accelerates neutrophil recovery after autologous bone marrow transplantation for Hodgkin's disease. *Bone Marrow Transplantation,* **4,** 49–54.

Dittmann, H., Sokler, M., Kollmannsberger, C. *et al.* (2001). Comparison of 18FDG-PET with CT scans in the evaluation of patients with residual and recurrent Hodgkin's lymphoma. *Oncology Reports,* **8,** 1393–9.

Federico, M., Carella, A. M., Brice, P. *et al.* (2002). High dose therapy (HDT) and autologous stem cell transplantation (ASCT) versus conventional therapy for patients with advanced Hodgkin's disease (HD) responding to initial therapy. *Proceedings of the American Society of Clinical Oncology,* **21,** 263A.

Falini, B., Flenghi, L., Fedeli, L. *et al.* (1992). In vivo targeting of Hodgkin and Reed-Sternberg cells of Hodgkin's disease with monoclonal antibody Ber-H2 (CD30): immunohistological evidence. *British Journal of Haematology,* **82,** 38–45.

Gajewski, J. L., Phillips, G. L., Sobocinski, K. A. *et al.* (1996). Bone marrow transplants from HLA-identical siblings in advanced Hodgkin's disease. *Journal of Clinical Oncology,* **14,** 572–8.

Gale, R. E., Bunch, C., Moir, D. J. *et al.* (1996). Demonstration of developing myelodysplasia/acute myeloid leukemia in hematological normal patients after high-dose chemotherapy and autologous bone marrow transplantation using X-chromosome inactivation patterns. *British Journal of Haematology,* **93,** 53–8.

Gallagher, B. M., Fowler, J. S., Gutterson, N.I. *et al.* (1978). Metabolic trapping as a principle of oradiopharmaceutical design: some factors resposible for the biodistribution of [18F] 2-deoxy-2-fluoro-D-glucose. *Journal of Nuclear Medicine,* **19,** 1154–61.

Gause, B. L. & Longo, D. L. (1996). Treatment of relapsed Hodgkin's disease. *Bailliere's Clinical Haematology,* **9,** 559–72.

Goldstone, A. H. & McMillan, A. K. (1993). The place of high-dose therapy with haemopoietic stem cell transplantation in relapsed and refractory Hodgkin's disease (Review). *Annals of Oncology,* **4** (Suppl 1), 21–7.

Gribben, J. G., Linch, D. C., Singer, C.R.J. *et al.* (1989). Successful treatment of refractory Hodgkin's disease by high-dose combination chemotherapy and autologous bone marrow transplantation. *Blood,* **73,** 340–4.

Gribben, J. G., Freedman, A. S., Neuberg, D. *et al.* (1991). Immunologic purging of marrow assessed by PCR before autologous bone marrow transplantation for B-cell lymphoma. *New England Journal of Medicine,* **325,** 1525–33.

Gulati, S. C. & Bennett, C. L. (1992). Granulocyte-macrophage colony-stimulating factor as adjunct therapy in relapsed Hodgkin's disease. *Annals of Internal Medicine,* **116,** 177–82.

Haim, N., Ben-Shahar, M., Faraggi, D. *et al.* (1997). Dexamethasone, etoposide, ifosfamide, and cisplatin as second-line therapy in patients with aggressive non-Hodgkin's lymphoma. *Cancer,* **80,** 1989–96.

Hasenclever, D. & Diehl, V. (1998). A prognostic score for advanced Hodgkin's disease. *New England Journal of Medicine,* **339,** 1506–14.

Hasenclever, D., Loeefler, M., & Diehl, V. (1996). Rationale for dose escalation of first-line conventional chemotherapy in advanced Hodgkin's disease. *Annals of Oncology,* **7** (Suppl 4), S95–8.

Henry-Amar, M. & Joly, F. (1996). Late complications after Hodgkin's disease. *Annals of Oncology,* **7** (Suppl 4), S115–26.

Hoh, C. K., Glaspy, J., Rosen, P. *et al.* (1997). Whole-body FDG-PET imaging for staging of Hodgkin's disease and lymphoma. *Journal of Nuclear Medicine,* **38,** 343–8.

Hoppe, R. T. (1996). Hodgkin's disease—the role of radiation therapy in advanced disease. *Annals of Oncology,* **7** (Suppl 4), S99–103.

Horning, S. J., Chao, N. J., Negrin, R. S. *et al.* (1997). High-dose therapy and autologous hematopoietic progenitor cell transplantation for recurrent or refractory Hodgkin's disease: analysis of the Stanford University results and prognostic indices. *Blood,* **89,** 801–3.

Horning, S. J., Rosenberg, S. A., & Hoppe, R. T. (1996). Brief chemotherapy (Stanford V) and adjuvant radiotherapy for bulky or advanced Hodgkin's disease: an update. *Annals of Oncology,* **7** (Suppl 4), S105–8.

Jagannath, S., Armitage, J. O., Dicke, K. A. *et al.* (1989). Prognostic factors for response and survival after high-dose cyclophosphamide, carmustine and etoposide with autologous bone marrow transplantation for relapsed Hodgkin's disease. *Journal of Clinical Oncology,* **7,** 179–85.

Jerusalem, G., Beguin, Y., Fassotte, M. F. *et al.* (1999). Whole-body positron emission tomography using 18F-fluorodeoxyglucose for posttreatment evaluation in Hodgkin's disease and non-Hodgkin's lymphoma has higher diagnostic and prognostic value than classical computed tomography scan imaging. *Blood,* **94,** 429–33.

Jones, R. J., Ambinder, R. F., Piantodosi, S. *et al.* (1991). Evidence of a graft-versus-lymphoma effect associated with allogeneic bone marrow transplantation. *Blood,* **77,** 649–53.

Josting, A., Rueffer, U., Franklin, J. *et al.* (2000). Prognostic factors and treatment outcome in primary progressive Hodgkin lymphoma: a report from the German Hodgkin Lymphoma Study Group. *Blood,* **96,** 1280–6.

Katsanis, E., Weisdorf, D. J., Xu, Z. *et al.* (1994). Infusions of inter-leukin-1 alpha after autologous transplantation for Hodgkin's disease and non-Hodgkin's lymphoma induce effector cells with antilymphoma cytolytic activity. *Journal of Clinical Immunology,* **14,** 205–11.

Keilholz, U., Szelenyi, H., Siehl, J. *et al.* (1999). Rapid regression of chemotherapy refractory lymphocyte predominant Hodgkin's disease after administration of rituximab (anti-CD20 monoclonal antibody) and interleukin-2. *Leukemia and Lymphoma,* **35,** 641–2.

Kessinger, A., Bierman, P. J., Vose, J. M., & Armitage., J. O. (1991). High-dose cyclophosphamide, carmustine and etoposide fol-lowed by autologous peripheral stem cell transplantation for patients with relapsed Hodgkin's disease. *Blood,* **77,** 2322–5.

Koon, H. B. & Junghans, R. P. (2000). Anti-CD30 antibody-based therapy (Review). *Current Opinion in Oncology,* **12,** 588–93.

Körbling, M., Holle, R., Haas, R. *et al.* (1990). Autologous blood stem-cell transplantation in patients with advanced disease and prior radiation to the pelvic site. *Journal of Clinical Oncology,* **8,** 978–85.

Kottaridis, P. D., Milligan, D. W., Chopra, R. *et al.* (2000). In vivo CAMPATH-1H prevents graft-versus-host disease following non-myeloablative stem cell transplantation. *Blood,* **96,** 2419–25.

Krishnan, A., Bhatia, S., Slovak, M. L. *et al.* (2000). Predictors of therapy-related leukemia and myelodysplasia following autolo-gous transplantation for lymphoma: an assessment of risk factors. *Blood,* **95,** 1588–93.

Kusnierz-Glaz, C. R., Schlegel, P. G., Wong, R. M. *et al.* (1997). Influence of age on the outcome of 500 autologous bone marrow transplant procedures for hematological malignancies. *Journal of Clinical Oncology,* **15,** 18–25.

Lazarus, H. M., Rowlings, P. A., Zhang, M. J. *et al.* (1999). Autotransplants for Hodgkin's disease in patients never achieving remission: a report from the Autologous Blood and Marrow Transplant Registry. *Journal of Clinical Oncology,* **17,** 534–55.

Lazarus, H. M., Loberiza, F. R., Zhang, M.-J. *et al.* (2001). Autotransplants for Hodgkin's diseae in first relapse or second remission: a report from the Autologous Blood and Marrow Transplant Registry (ABMTR). *Bone Marrow Transplantation,* **27,** 387–96.

Lin, T. S., Avalos, B. R., Penza, S. L. *et al.* (2002). Second autolo-gous stem cell transplant for multiply relapsed Hodgkin's dis-ease. *Bone Marrow Transplantation,* **24,** 763–7.

Linch, D. C., Winfield, D., Goldstone, A. H. *et al.* (1993). Dose intensification with autologous bone-marrow transplantation in relapsed and resistant Hodgkin's disease: results of a BNLI ran-domized trial. *Lancet,* **341,** 1051–4.

Longo, D. L. (1990). The use of chemotherapy in the treatment of Hodgkin's disease. *Seminars in Oncology,* **17,** 716–35.

Longo, D. L., Duffey, P. L., Young, R. C. *et al.* (1992). Conventional-dose salvage combination chemotherapy in patients relapsing with Hodgkin's disease after combination chemotherapy: the low probability for cure. *Journal of Clinical Oncology,* **10,** 210–18.

Lumley, M. A., Milligan, D. W., Knechtle, C. J. *et al.* (1996). High lactate dehydrogenase level is associated with an adverse outlook in autografting for Hodgkin's disease. *Bone Marrow Transplantation,* **17,** 383–8.

Lush, R. J., Jones, S. G., Haynes, A. P. (2001). Advanced-stage, chemorefractory lymphocyte-predominant Hodgkin's disease: long-term follow-up of allografting and monoclonal antibody therapy. *British Journal of Haematology,* **114,** 734–5.

Lynch, J. C., Bierman, P. J., Bociek, G. *et al.* (2001). The Hodgkin's disease prognostic index predicts outcome of autologous stem cell transplantation (ASCT). *Proceedings of the American Society of Clinical Oncology,* (Abstract).

Martelli, M., Vignetti, M., Zinzani, P. L. *et al.* (1996). High-dose chemotherapy followed by autologous bone marrow transplanta-tion versus dexamethasone, cisplatin, and cytarabine in aggres-sive non-Hodgkin's lymphoma with partial response to front-line chemotherapy: a prospective randomized Italian multicenter study. *Journal of Clinical Oncology,* **14,** 534–42.

Martin, A., Fernandez-Jimenez, M. C., Cabellero, M. D. *et al.* (2001). Long-term follow-up in patients treated with mini-BEAM as salvage therapy for relapsed or refractory Hodgkin's disease. *British Journal of Haematology,* **113,** 161–71.

Matthey, B., Engert, A., & Barth, S. (2000). Recombinant immuno-toxins for the treatment of Hodgkin's disease (Review). *International Journal of Molecular Medicine,* **5,** 509–14.

Mills, W., Strang, J., Goldstone, A. H., & Linch, D. C. (1995). Dose intensification of etoposide in the BEAM ABMT protocol for malignant lymphoma. *Leukemia and Lymphoma,* **17,** 263–70.

Milpied, N., Fielding, A. K., Pearce, R. M. *et al.* (1996). Allogeneic bone marrow transplant is not better than autologous transplant for patients with relapsed Hodgkin's disease. European Group for Blood and Bone Marrow Transplantation. *Journal of Clinical Oncology,* **14,** 1291–6.

Moreau, P., Fleury, J., Brice, P. *et al.* (1998). Early intensive therapy with autologous stem cell transplantation in advanced Hodgkin's disease: retrospective analysis of 158 cases from the French reg-istry. *Bone Marrow Transplantation,* **21,** 787–93.

Moskowitz, C. H., Nimer, S. D., Zelenetz, A. D. *et al.* (2001). A 2-step comprehensive high-dose chemoradiotherapy second-line program for relapsed and refractory Hodgkin disease: analysis by intent to treat and development of a prognostic model. *Blood,* **97,** 616–23.

Mundt, A. J., Sibley, G., Williams, S. *et al.* (1995). Patterns of failure following high-dose chemotherapy and autologous bone marrow transplantation with involved field radiotherapy for relapsed/refractory Hodgkin's disease. *International Journal of Radiation Oncology, Biology, Physics,* **33,** 261–70.

Nachbaur, D., Oberaigner, W., Fritsch, E. *et al.* (2001). Allogeneic or autologous stem cell transplantation (SCT) for relapsed and refrac-tory Hodgkin's disease and non-Hodgkin's lymphoma: a single-centre experience. *European Journal of Haematology,* **66,** 43–9.

Nademanee, A., O'Donnell, M. R., Snyder, D. S. *et al.* (1995). High-dose chemotherapy with or without total body irradiation fol-lowed by autologous bone marrow and/or peripheral blood stem cell transplantation for patients with relapsed and refractory Hodgkin's disease: results in 85 patients with analysis of prog-nostic factors. *Blood,* **85,** 1381–90.

Nagler, A., Ackerstein, A., Or, R., Naparstek, E., & Slavin, S. (1997). Immunotherapy with recombinant human interleukin-2 and recombinant interferon-alpha in lymphoma patients postautolo-gous marrow or stem cell transplantation. *Blood,* **89,** 3951–9.

O'Brien, M. E., Milan, S., Cunningham, D. *et al.* (1996). High-dose chemotherapy and autologous bone marrow transplant in relapsed Hodgkin's disease—a pragmatic prognostic index. *British Journal of Cancer,* **73,** 1272–7.

Park, S., Brice, P., Noguerra, M. E. *et al.* (2000). Myelodysplasias and leukemias after autologous stem cell transplantation for lymphoid malignancies. *Bone Marrow Transplantation,* **26,** 321–6.

Pecego, R., Hill, R., Appelbaum, F. R. *et al.* (1986). Interstitial pneumonitis following autologous bone marrow transplantation. *Transplantation,* **42,** 515–17.

Perry, A. J., Peniket, A. J., Watts, M. J. *et al.* (1999). Peripheral blood stem cell versus autologous bone marrow transplantation for Hodgkin's disease: equivalent survival outcome in a single-centre matched-pair analysis. *British Journal of Haematology,* **105,** 280–7.

Pezner, R. D., Nademanee, A., Niland, J. C. *et al.* (1995). Involved field radiation therapy for Hodgkin's disease autologous bone marrow transplantation regimens. *Radiotherapy and Oncology,* **34,** 23–9.

Pfreundschuh, M. G., Ruefer, U., & Lathan, B. (1994). Dexa-BEAM in patients with Hodgkin's disease refractory to multidrug chemotherapy regimens: a trial of the German Hodgkin's Disease Study Group. *Journal of Clinical Oncology,* **12,** 580–6.

Pileri, S. A., Ascani, S., Leoncini, L. *et al.* (2002). Hodgkin's lymphoma: the pathologist's viewpoint (Review). *Journal of Clinical Pathology,* **55,** 162–76.

Poen, J. C., Hoppe, R. T., & Horning, S. J. (1996). High-dose therapy and autologous bone marrow transplantation for relapsed/refractory Hodgkin's disease: the impact of involved field radiotherapy on patterns of failure and survival. *International Journal of Radiation Oncology, Biology, Physics,* **36,** 3–12.

Price, A., Cunningham, D., Horwich, A. *et al.* (1994). Hematological toxicity of radiotherapy following high-dose chemotherapy and autologous bone marrow transplantation in patients with recurrent Hodgkin's disease. *European Journal of Cancer,* **30A,** 903–7.

Proctor, S. J., Taylor, P. R., Angus, B. *et al.* (2001). High-dose ifosfamide in combination with etoposide and epirubicin (IVE) in the treatment of relapsed/refractory Hodgkin's disease and non-Hodgkin's lymphoma: a report on toxicity and efficacy. *European Journal of Haematology,* **64** (Suppl), 28–32.

Rapoport, A. P., Rowe, J. M., Kouides, P. A. *et al.* (1993). One hundred autotransplants for relapsed or refractory Hodgkin's disease and lymphoma: value of pre-transplant disease status for predicting outcome. *Journal of Clinical Oncology,* **11,** 2351–61.

Reece, D. E., Barnett, M. J., Connors, J. M. *et al.* (1991). Intensive chemotherapy with cyclophosphamide, carmustine, and etoposide followed by autologous bone marrow transplantation. *Journal of Clinical Oncology,* **9,** 1871–9.

Reece, D. E., Barnett, M. J., Shephers, J. D. *et al.* (1995). High-dose cyclophosphamide, carmustine and etoposide with or without cisplatin and autologous transplantation for patients with Hodgkin's disease who fail to enter a complete remission after combination chemotherapy. *Blood,* **86,** 451–6.

Reece, D. E., Conners, J. M., Spinelli, J. J. *et al.* (1994). Intensive therapy with cyclophosphamide, carmustine, etoposide +/– cisplatin, and autologous bone marrow transplantation for Hodgkin's disease in first relapse alter combination chemotherapy. *Blood,* **83,** 1193–9.

Reuss, K., Engert, A., Tesch, H., & Diehl, V. (1996). Current clinical trials in Hodgkin's disease. *Annals of Oncology,* **7,** S109–13.

Rüffer, J. U. & Sieber, M. (1996). Report of the workshop on clinical trials. *Annals of Oncology,* **7,** S127–9.

Schenkein, D. P., Dixon, P., Desforges, J. F. *et al.* (1994). Phase I/II study of cyclophosphamide, carboplatin, and etoposide and autologous hematopoietic stem-cell transplantation with post-transplant interferon alfa-2b for patients with lymphoma and Hodgkin's disease. *Journal of Clinical Oncology,* **12,** 2423–31.

Schmitz, N., Linch, D. C., Dreger, P. *et al.* (1996). Randomized trial of filgrastim-mobilized peripheral blood progenitor cell transplantation versus autologous bone marrow transplantation in lymphoma patients. *Lancet,* **347,** 353–7.

Schmitz, N., Pfistner, B., Sextro, M. *et al.* (2002). Aggressive conventional chemotherapy compared with high-dose chemotherapy with autologous haemopoietic stem-cell transplantation for relapsed chemosensitive Hodgkin's disease: a randomised trial. *Lancet,* **359,** 2065–71.

Schnell, R., Barth, S., Diehl, V., & Engert, A. (1996). Future treatment strategies: fact or fiction? Bailliere's *Clinical Haematology,* **9,** 573–93.

Schnell, R., Vitetta, E., Schindler, J. *et al.* (1998). Clinical trials with an anti-CD25 ricin A-chain experimental and immunotoxin (RFT5-SMPT-dgA) in Hodgkin's lymphoma. *Leukemia and Lymphoma,* **30,** 525–37.

Smith, T. J., Hillner, B. E., Schmitz, N. *et al.* (1997). Economic analysis of a randomized clinical trial to compare filgrastim-mobilised peripheral-blood-progenitor-cell transplantation and autologous bone marrow transplantation in patients with Hodgkin's and non-Hodgkin's lymphoma. *Journal of Clinical Oncology,* **15,** 5–10.

Snyder, M. J., Johnson, D. B., Daly, M. B. *et al.* (1994). Carmustine, Ara C, cyclophosphamide and etoposide with autologous bone marrow transplantation in relapsed or refractory lymphoma: a dose-finding study. *Bone Marrow Transplantation,* **14,** 595–600.

Spaepen, K. & Mortelmans, L. (2001). Evaluation of treatment response in patients with lymphoma using [18F]FDG-PET: differences between non-Hodgkin's lymphoma and Hodgkin's disease (Review). *The Quarterly Journal of Nuclear Medicine,* **45,** 269–73.

Stewart, D. A., Guo, D., Gluck, S. *et al.* (2000). Double high-dose therapy for Hodgkin's disease with dose-intensive cyclophosphamide, etoposide, and cisplatin (DICEP) prior to high-dose melphalan and autologous stem cell transplantation. *Bone Marrow Transplantation,* **26,** 383–8.

Stone, R. M., Neuberg, D., Soiffer, R. *et al.* (1994). Myelodysplastic syndrome as a late complication following autologous bone marrow transplantation for non-Hodgkin's lymphoma. *Journal of Clinical Oncology,* **12,** 2535–42.

Sureda, A., Arranz, R., Iriondo, A. *et al.* (2001). Autologous stem cell transplantation for Hodgkin's disease: results and prognostic factors in 494 patients from the Group Español de Linfomas/ Transplante Autólogo de Médula Ósea Spanish Cooperative Group. *Journal of Clinical Oncology,* **19,** 1395–1404.

Sweetenham, J. W., Carella, A. M., Taghipour, G. *et al.* (1999). High-dose therapy and autologous stem-cell transplantation for adult patients with Hodgkin's disease who do not enter remission after induction chemotherapy: results in 175 patients reported to the European Group for Blood and Marrow Transplantation.

Lymphoma Working Party. *Journal of Clinical Oncology*, **17**, 3101–9.

Sweetenham, J. W., Taghipour, G., Milligan, D. *et al.* (1997). High-dose therapy and autologous stem cell rescue for patients with Hodgkin's disease in first relapse after chemotherapy: results from the EBMT. *Bone Marrow Transplantation*, **20**, 745–52.

Taylor, K. M., Jagannath, S., Spitzer, G. *et al.* (1989). Recombinant human granulocyte colony-stimulating factor hastens granulocyte recovery after high-dose chemotherapy and autologous bone marrow transplantation in Hodgkin's disease. *Journal of Clinical Oncology*, **7**, 1791–9.

Traweek, S. T., Slovak, M. L., Nademanee, A. P. *et al.* (1994). Clonal karyotypic abnormalities occurring after autologous bone marrow transplantation for Hodgkin's disease and non-Hodgkin's lymphoma. *Blood*, **84**, 957–63.

Urbano-Ispizua, A., Schmitz, N., de Witte, T. *et al.* (2002). Allogeneic and autologous transplantation for haematological diseases, solid tumors and immune disorders: definition and current practice in Europe. *Bone Marrow Transplantation*, **29**, 639–46.

Varterasian, M., Ratanatharathorn, V., Uberti, J. P. *et al.* (1995). Clinical course and outcome of patients with Hodgkin's disease who progress after autologous transplantation. *Leukemia and Lymphoma*, **29**, 59–65.

Vockerodt, M., Soares, M., Kanzler, H. *et al.* (1998). Detection of clonal Hodgkin and Reed-Sternberg cells with identical somatically mutated and rearranged VH genes in different biopsies in relapsed Hodgkin's disease. *Blood*, **92**, 2899–907.

Vogelsang, G., Bitton, R., Piantadosi, S. *et al.* (1999). Immune modulation in autologous bone marrow transplantation: cyclosporine and gamma-interferon trial. *Bone Marrow Transplantation*, **24**, 637–40.

Vose, J. M., Bierman, P., Anderson, J. R. *et al.* (1992). Progressive disease after high-dose therapy and autologous transplantation for lymphoid malignancy: clinical course and patient follow-up. *Blood*, **80**, 2142–8.

Watts, M. J., Ings, S. J., Leverett, D. *et al.* (2000). ESHAP and G-CSF is a superior blood stem cell mobilizing regimen compared to cyclophosphamide 1.5 g m(–2) and G-CSF for pre-treated lymphoma patients: a matched pairs analysis of 78 patients. *British Journal of Cancer*, **82**, 278–82.

Weaver, C. H., Appelbaum, F. R., Peterson, F. B. *et al.* (1993). High-dose cyclophosphamide, carmustine, and etoposide followed by autologous bone marrow transplantation in patients with lymphoid malignancies who have received dose-limiting radiation therapy. *Journal of Clinical Oncology*, **11**, 1329–35.

Wheeler, C., Antin, J. H., Churchill, W. H. *et al.* (1990). Cyclophosphamide, carmustine and etoposide with autologous bone marrow transplantation in refractory Hodgkin's disease and non-Hodgkin's lymphoma: a dose finding study. *Journal of Clinical Oncology*, **8**, 648–56.

Wheeler, C., Khurshid, A., Ibrahim, J. *et al.* (2001). Incidence of post transplant myelodysplasia/acute leukemia in non-Hodgkin's lymphoma patients compared with Hodgkin's disease patients undergoing autologous transplantation following cyclophosphamide, carmustine, and etoposide (CBV). *Leukemia and Lymphoma*, **40**, 499–509.

Yahalom, J., Gulati, S. C., Toia, M. *et al.* (1993). Accelerated hyperfractionated total-lymphoid irradiation, high-dose chemotherapy, and autologous bone marrow transplantation for refractory and relapsing patients with Hodgkin's disease. *Journal of Clinical Oncology*, **11**, 1062–70.

Yuen, A. R., Rosenberg, S. A., Hoppe, R. T. *et al.* (1997). Comparison between conventional salvage therapy and high-dose therapy with autografting for recurrent or refractory Hodgkin's disease. *Blood*, **89**, 814–22.

36 Autologous hematopoietic stem cell transplantation for acute myeloid leukemia

ALAN K. BURNETT

University of Wales College of Medicine and University Hospital of Wales, Cardiff, UK

Introduction

Acute myeloid leukemia (AML) has an incidence of 3 to 5 per 100,000 annually, increases in incidence with age, and accounts for approximately 85% of all adult acute leukemias. The FAB and WHO classifications are shown in Table 36.1.A and B respectively. A correlation of the FAB subtypes with special stains, immune phenotype, and associated cytogenetic abnormalities are shown in Tables 36.2 and 36.3. Prognostic factors for outcome with conventional therapy are shown in Table 36.4, of which the most important are karyotype (Grimwade *et al.,* 1998, 2001), de novo or secondary disease, and age. Approximately 70% of all patients achieve a complete remission with remission induction chemotherapy, although rates of 84% can consistently be achieved in patients under 60

Table 36.1.A *French-American British (FAB) classification of acute myeloid leukemia (AML)*

Subtype	Frequency	FAB type	Description
Acute myeloblastic leukemia without differentiation	2%	AML-M0	Undifferentiated blasts with no azurophilic granules, MPO = negative by electron microscopy; <3% MPO positivity by light microscopy, but significant amounts of CD33. May be CD7+ or Tdt+.
Acute myeloblastic leukemia without differentiation	19%	AML-M1	More than 30% blasts, with ≥3% MPO positivity, occasionally containing Auer rods or azurophilic granules and showing little maturation beyond the myeloblast stage. The blasts can be NASD-negative.
Acute myeloblastic leukemia with differentiation	24%	AML-M2	More than 30% myeloblasts (≥3% MPO-positive) with >10% maturing granulocytic elements (progranulocytes through granulocytes) and <20% monocytic cells. Auer rods are often present, and some blasts show NASD positivity. Some cases are associated with t(8;21).
Acute promyelocytic leukemia (APML or APL)	10%	AMO-M3	Strong MPO positivity often obscuring the nuclei, showing a predominance of abnormal promyelocytes with reniform or bilobed nuclei, with abnormally heavy granulation and occasional cells with bundles of Auer rods (faggot cells). A microgranular variant (M3r) lacks the heavy granulation usually associated with the disease, but maintains the other features, including cells with multiple Auer rods and strong MPO positivity. Both forms show NASD positivity and are associated with t(15;17).
Acute myelomonocytic leukemia (AMML)	30%	AML-M4	MPO-positive; resembles M2 except that 20% of the cells are promonocytes (NSE-positive). A distinct subtype, associated with inv(16), also has an increase in eosinophils with basophilic granules (M4EO).
Acute monocytic leukemia (AMoL) (M5a, monoblastic; M5b, promonocytic)	10%	AML-M5	Leukemic cells are either monoblasts (M5a) or promonocytes (M5b), with abundant cytoplasm and eccentric nuclei. Cytoplasm may contain many salmon-colored granules and shows diffuse staining with NSE. NASD staining may also be present, and MPO staining is usually rare (<3%).
Acute erythroleukemia	4%	AML-M6	As originally conceived by the FAB classification, consisted of M1, M2, or M4 blasts with dysplastic erythroid precursors, which were often PAS-positive.
Acute megakaryoblastic leukemia	1%	AML-M7	Blast morphology variable. Cytochemical stains usually negative, occasionally PAS-positive. Usually CD13 or CD33 positive. Some CD41a+. Electron-microscopic platelet peroxidase (PPO) reaction positivity is the most sensitive and specific test.

Abbreviations: MPO, myeloperoxidase; NASD, naphthol AS-D chloroacetate esterase; NSE, nonspecific esterase; PAS, periodic acid-Schiff. Adapted from Hirsch-Ginsberg *et al.* (1993).

Table 36.1.B *WHO histological classification of acute myeloid leukemias*

Acute myeloid leukemia with recurrent genetic abnormalities
Acute myeloid leukemia with t(8;21)(q22;q22); (AML1(CBFa)/ETO)
Acute myeloid leukemia with abnormal bone marrow eosinophils
    inv(16)(p12q22) or t(16;16)(p13;q22); (CBFb/MYH11)
Acute promyelocytic leukemia (AML with t(15;17)(q22;q12) (PML/RARa) and variants)
Acute myeloid leukemia with 11q23 (MLL) abnormalities
Acute myeloid leukemia with multilineage dysplasia
Acute myeloid leukemia and myelodysplastic syndromes, therapy-related
Acute myeloid leukemia not otherwise categorized
Acute myeloid leukemia minimally differentiated
Acute myeloid leukemia without maturation
Acute myeloid leukemia with maturation
Acute myelomonocytic leukemia
Acute monoblastic and monocytic leukemia
Acute erythroid leukemia
Acute megakaryoblastic leukemia
Acute basophilic leukemia
Acute panmyelosis with myelofibrosis
Myeloid sarcoma
Acute leukemia of ambiguous lineage
Undifferentiated acute leukemia
Bilineal acute leukemia
Biphenotypic acute leukemia

years (Hann *et al.,* 1997). Examples of such regimens are shown in Table 36.5. Disease-free survival with chemotherapy alone is approximately 40% to 45% for those less than 45 years of age and approximately 30% to 35% for those between 45 and 60 years (Mayer *et al.,* 1994; Hann *et al.,* 1997) (Fig. 36.1). The type of induction chemotherapy is independent of FAB

Table 36.2 *Correlation between morphology and cytochemical stains in the FAB classification of AML*

Subtype	Morphology	Cytochemical stains				
		Peroxidase	Sudan black	CAE	NBE	PAS
M0[a] Minimally differentiated AML	Large agranular blasts	−	−	−	−	−
M1 AML without maturation	Few if any azurophilic granules	+ −	+ −	−	−	−
M2 AML with differentiation	Blasts with promyelocytic granules; Auer rods may be present	++	++	++	−	−
M3 Promyelocytic	Hypergranular promyelocytes with multiple Auer rods	++++	++++	+++	−	+/−
M4 Myelomonocytic	Monocytoid-appearing cells in peripheral blood	++	++	++	++	−
M5 Monocytic	Immature monoblasts resemble monocytes	+ −	−	−	++++	+/−
M6 Erythroleukemia	>30% erythroblasts; megaloblastic erythroid precursors	−	−	−	−	+/− to ++++
M7[b] Megakaryocytic	Dry aspirate; biopsy shows fibrosis, dysplastic megakaryocytes	−	−	−	−	++

Abbreviations: CAE, chloroacetate esterase (specific), NBE, naphthylbuterate esterase (nonspecific); PAS, periodic acid-Schiff.
[a] AML-M0 requires monoclonal antibody testing to exclude B- and T-lineage markers and confirm expression of at least one myeloid antigen, CD13 or CD33.
[b] AML-M7 cells must be identified by platelet peroxidase reaction on electron microscopy or with platelet-specific monoclonal antibodies.

Table 36.3. *Correlation between FAB subtypes, special stains, immune phenotype, and cytogenetic abnormalities*

FAB type	Subtype	Immune phenotype														Cytogenetic abnormality
		MPO	SE	NSE	CD11	CD13	CD14	CD15	CD33	CD34	DR	Glyc.A	CD41	CD42	CD61	
M0	Myeloblastic without maturation	–	–	–		+			+							
M1	Myeloblastic without differentiation	±	±	–	–	±	–	–	±	±	±	–	–			+8; t(9;22); inv (3)
M2	Myeloblastic with differentiation	++	++	–	±	±	±	±	±	±	±	–	–			t(8;21); t(6;19)
M3	Promyelocytic	+++	+++	–	±	±	–	±	±	–	–	–	–			t(15;17)
M4	Myelomonocytic	++	++	++	+	+	+	+	+	±	±	–	–			+4; +8
M4EO	Myelomonocytic with eosinophilia in marrow	++			±	±	±	±	±	±	±	–	–			inv(16); t(16;16); del(16)
M5	Monocytic	±	–	+++	±	±	±	±	±	±	±	–	–			t(9;11); +8; 11q23 abnormalities; t(10;11)
M6	Erythroleukemia	–	–	–	–	–	–	±	±	–	±	±	–			Complex rearrangement del(5q); +8
M7	Megakaryoblastic	–	–	–	–	–	–	–	±	±	±	–	+	+	+	Complex rearrangement involving –5 or del(5q); +8

Abbreviations: MPO, myeloperoxidase; SE, specific esterase (naphthol ASD chloroacetate esterase); NSE, nonspecific esterase (naphthylbutyrate); Glyc. A, glycophorin A.

Table 36.4. *Prognostic factors for outcome in AML*

Better prognosis	Worse prognosis
De novo AML	AML secondary to myelodysplasia or prior therapy
	WHO performance score >2 (for induction therapy)
FAB type 2, 3, 4	FAB type 0, 1, 5, 6, 7
t(8:21), t(15;17), inv(16)	Complex abnormalities of chromosomes 5, 7, 3q–, t(10;11)
Younger age[a]	Older age (>60 years)
	High WBC at diagnosis (>100 × 10^9/l)
	FLT-3 mutation
CR with first course	Complete remission with >1 course

[a] Age is a continuous variable

classification except for acute promyelocytic leukemia (FAB M3), for which the addition of all-*trans* retinoic acid (ATRA) to chemotherapy markedly improves the outcome (Fig. 36.2) (Fenaux *et al.*, 1999; Burnett *et al.*, 1999; Tallman *et al.*, 1997). Following remission induction one or more consolidation courses of chemotherapy are normally given.

The major therapeutic problem facing younger patients (<60 years) with AML is the prevention of relapse in those who initially enter remission. Seventy-five to 85% of patients in this age group will respond to induction chemotherapy and achieve complete remission (CR), the majority with the first course of treatment. About half of those who fail succumb to problems related to failure of supportive care. While it will be difficult to improve further on induction treatment, there are several pieces of evidence that suggest that more intensive induction, while not necessarily increasing the proportion of cases entering CR,

Table 36.5. *Commonly used remission induction and consolidation chemotherapy regimens for AML*

Induction 5 + 2:
Cytosine arabinoside 100 mg/m²/d continuous infusion days 1–5
Daunorubicin 45 mg/m²/d days 1 and 2
Induction 7 + 3:
Cytosine arabinoside 100 mg/m²/d continuous infusion days 1–7
Daunorubicin 45 mg/m²/d days 1, 2, and 3
Induction HDAC:
Cytosine arabinoside 1–3 g/m² i.v. over 2–3 hours q 12 hours ×
   12 doses days 1–6
Induction IC:
Idarubicin 12 mg/m²/d i.v. days 1–3
Cytosine arabinoside 100 mg/m² continuous infusion days 1–7
Consolidation HDAC:
Cytosine arabinoside 1–3 g/m² i.v. over 2–3 hours q 12 hours ×
   12 doses days 1–6
or
Cytosine arabinoside 1–3 g/m² i.v. over 2–3 hours q 12 hours ×
   6 doses days 1, 3, and 5

Abbreviations: HDAC, high-dose cytosine arabinoside; IC, idarubicin and cytosine arabinoside.

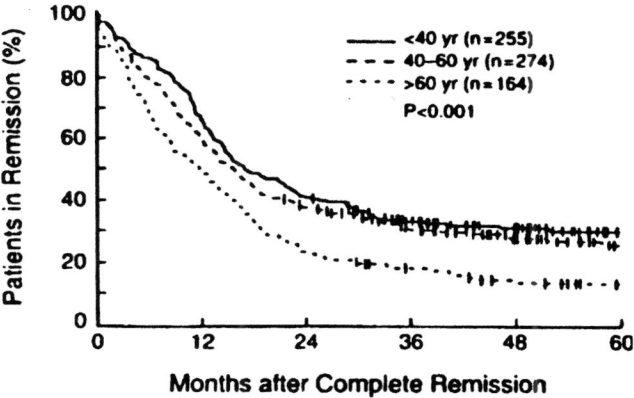

Fig. 36.1. Probability of disease-free survival for all patients with a complete response, according to age. The *P* value is for the differences among the three groups. The median follow-up was 52 months. Tick marks indicate surviving patients in continuous complete remission. Reproduced, with permission, from Mayer *et al.* (1994).

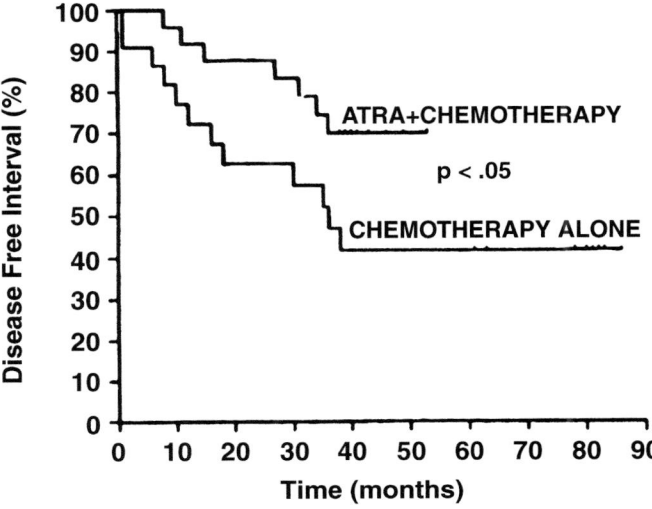

Fig. 36.2. Actuarial DFI in API patients treated with ATRA followed by chemotherapy and with chemotherapy alone. Reproduced, with permission, from Fenaux *et al.* (1994).

Table 36.6. *Summary of prospective randomized trials of autografting for AML in CR1*

Study	Age	Number randomized	Prior chemotherapy	Myeloablation	Purging	Median follow-up	Relapse rate (auto vs other)	Disease-free survival	Survival
BGMT 84	Adults }	112	1 consolidation	Melphalan × 2	No	–	– }	42% vs 25/5	NS
BGMT 87	Adults		1 consolidation	Busulfan + melphalan	No	–	–		
EORTC–GIMEMA	Adults	254	1 consolidation	Cy/TBI or BuCy	No	40 months	40% vs 57% (P = .05)	48% vs 30% (P = .05)	56% vs 46% (NS)
GOELAM	Adults	164	1 consolidation	BuCy	No	62 months	–	44% vs 40% (NS)	50% vs 54% (NS)
Intergroup	Adults	229	1 consolidation	BuCy	4HC	36 months	–	37% vs 35% (NS)	47% vs 54% (NS)
MRC	Adults and children	381	3 consolidation	Cy/TBI	No	66 months	37% vs 58% (P = .006)	54% vs 40%	57% vs 45%
POG	Children (21 years)	232	2 consolidation	BuCy	4HC	32 months	31% vs 58% (P = .001)	38% vs 36% (NS)	
AIEOP	Children (<1 5 years)	72	1 consolidation	BAVC	No	28 months	78% vs 70% (NS)	21% vs 27% (NS)	

Abbreviations: NS, not significant; Cy, cyclophosphamide, TBI, total body irradiation; Bu, busulfan; 4HC, 4-hydroperoxycyclophosphamide; BAVC, carmustine (BCNU), amsacrine, etoposide, cytosine arabinoside.

may achieve a better quality of remission and thereby prolong disease-free survival (Bishop *et al.*, 1996; Rees *et al.*, 1996). A number of strategies to maintain remission are available. Clearly allogeneic hematopoietic stem cell (HSC) transplantation must be considered and will be an option for those with an HLA-matched sibling donor (see Chapter 50), although when trials are carefully examined on a donor versus no donor basis, this preference may not be as clearcut as previously thought (Burnett *et al.*, 2002). Of those for whom a donor cannot be identified, intensive chemotherapy and/or autologous HSC transplantation are likely to be used.

Since the risk of relapse is highly variable, reflecting the biological, cytogenetic, and immunophenotypic heterogeneity of this disease (these diseases), the individual characteristics of the patient or their disease may influence the treatment choice. Contemporary chemotherapy protocols offer this age group of patients about a 45% chance of prolonged survival. Once a patient relapses, the prognosis is largely determined by the length of the first remission and the patient's age, both for the prospects of achieving a second remission and for survival from relapse. Some patients who fail first-line treatment can still be cured by an autograft for which stem cells were collected in first remission (Zittoun *et al.*, 1995). Approximately 20% of patients who fail first-line treatment can be cured, if autografted in second complete remission (CR2).

Factors that determine treatment choice

Once a patient enters complete remission a number of factors have been clearly identified that have value in predicting relapse. These factors are only now being incorporated into treatment planning, and few of the studies comparing the different treatment strategies so far completed have taken them into account when assessing the trial outcomes.

Age

The age of the patient has long been known to influence the response to initial chemotherapy and the duration of CR. The effect is evident over the total age span. Even in younger patients, age is a major factor in determining the duration of CR, with patients younger than 35 years having a survival of 50% whereas patients older than 45 years have a survival of around 30% (Hann *et al.*, 1997). While there are transplant centers that perform allogeneic transplants on patients up to 60 years old, many have an age threshold of around 50 years, beyond which the patient may be offered chemotherapy only or autologous HSC transplantation. In one historically controlled retrospective study, the 4-year leukemia-free survival for 111 patients aged 50 years or older (median 53, range 50–63) given an autologous bone marrow transplant (BMT) in CR1 was $34 \pm 5\%$ compared to $43 \pm 2\%$ for 786 patients transplanted between 16 and 49 years of age. This difference was due to increased transplant-related mortality (Cahn *et al.*, 1995). Further statistical analysis of existing trials may help to define if there is a useful age

threshold that can be identified that determines who should or should not receive an allogeneic transplant. In an analysis of data from the MRC 10 trial, there was no survival advantage for patients over 35 years (Burnett *et al.*, 2002).

Cytogenetics

The importance of cytogenetic abnormalities in relation to treatment response in AML has been recognized for a number of years (Yunis *et al.*, 1984; Keating *et al.*, 1988; Schiffer *et al.*, 1989; Burnett 1994; Dastugue *et al.*, 1995; Mrozek *et al.*, 1997). Several contemporary trials demonstrate broad agreement that t(8;21), inversion 16, and t(15;17) lesions confer a more favorable prognosis, and that abnormalities of chromosomes 3q–, 5, 7 or complex abnormalities represent an unfavorable group, which has a lower chance of entering remission, and if remission is achieved, a higher chance of subsequent relapse (Grimwade *et al.*, 1998; Slovak *et al.*, 2000). In 43 patients receiving an autologous BMT in first complete remission, leukemia-free survival was 100%, 33%, and 20%, respectively, for those with a favorable, intermediate, or unfavorable karyotype (Ferrant, Doyen, & Delannoy, 1995). These cytogenetic subgroups are known to similarly predict the relapse risk after allogeneic BMT (Gale *et al.*, 1995; Ferrant *et al.*, 1997). In the UK Medical Research Council (MRC) AML 10 trial, a careful analysis was unable to demonstrate any survival advantage in patients for whom an HLA-matched sibling donor was available compared with those with no donor for patients in the favorable or unfavorable group (Burnett *et al.*, 2002). In the former group this was accounted for by the fact that, although allogeneic BMT was able to reduce the relapse risk, the procedural mortality partially offset this benefit. A further confounding effect was that the survival of good risk patients who relapsed was about 30%, suggesting that all is not lost for such patients. These findings support the view that in this group of patients transplants should not be part of first-line treatment, an observation that is endorsed by taking into account the morbidity that the procedure brings to some surviving patients. In the poor risk group of patients even a transplant may not overcome the adverse biology of the disease.

One of the benefits of autologous HSC transplantation is its potentially wide availability. It is generally considered safe up to the age of 60 years and is available to those who do not have a sibling donor and are confirmed to be in remission.

Autologous hematopoietic stem cell transplantation

Several issues require consideration with respect to the use of autologous HSC transplantation. These relate to the optimization of the procedure itself and include issues relating to timing, characteristics of the autograft, the myeloablative protocol, and postgraft treatment. In addition, there are issues as to the efficacy of the treatment itself, and in what circumstances it may be most beneficial.

Optimization of the autograft

Several questions exist about how to optimize autologous HSC transplantation for AML. Included are questions such as, Is it beneficial to use an autograft early in first remission as consolidation or as intensification of consolidation? What is the best myeloablative treatment? Should the autograft be purged? What dose of cells is optimal? Are bone marrow stem cells or peripheral blood stem cells better? Does adding posttransplant treatment improve outcome and is it feasible?

The purist would argue that many of these issues should be answered by prospective randomized trials, but this will never be achieved because of the patient numbers required and the difficulties in ensuring the international collaboration to achieve this. Nonrandomized and/or registry experience has so far been the major influence in shaping opinion (Fig. 36.3 and 36.4). It is widely recognized that selection biases (Gray & Wheatley, 1991) will make such information indicative only, but perhaps useful in delineating which issues would be practical to address in a prospective manner. In this respect the Registry of the European Bone Marrow Transplant (EBMT) Group has been of value.

Is consolidation before the autograft valuable?

The interval between remission and autograft is a prognostic factor for the response to the autograft. This was concluded from the EBMT registry data (Gorin et al., 1990), but it is not found in all series. Such an effect is not surprising and it can be demonstrated from chemotherapy trials that the prognosis for patients improves with time as the relapse risk diminishes (Gray & Wheatley, 1991). Autografting within 6 months of remission being obtained resulted in a relapse risk of 46% compared with 33% for autografting beyond 6 months. Consolidation chemotherapy is very likely to be in part responsible for this effect. In the first place it may cytoreduce further disease remaining in the patient. Second, if the autograft is obtained

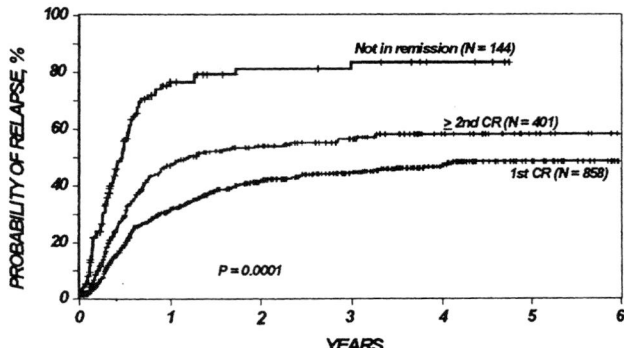

Fig. 36.4. Probability of relapse after autotransplants for acute myeloid leukemia, 1989–1995. Three-year probabilities of relapse were 44±4%, 56±6%, and 83±5%, respectively. Reproduced, with permission, from *ABMTR Newsletter,* 3, 10, 1996.

after consolidation, the chances of contamination of the autograft will be reduced, so-called in vivo purging. Two or more courses of consolidation prior to harvest and transplant was the most significant factor associated with decreased relapse risk in one study (Mehta et al., 1995). The use of high-dose cytosine arabinoside as consolidation therapy has been reported (Stein et al., 1996), but it is not clear whether there is a "best choice" consolidation treatment. On the other hand, there is common concern that the more exposure the marrow has to chemotherapy before harvest, the greater the possibility that hematopoietic reconstitution posttransplant will be compromised. The strategy of harvesting marrow or blood stem cells early in consolidation, applying more consolidation and then performing the autograft (thereby avoiding excessive exposure of the harvested cells to chemotherapy), has not been formally evaluated. All trials have deployed the autograft after some consolidation has been given, but may not have used extensive cytoreduction. This point will be discussed again when the results of prospective trials with different designs are noted.

Which myeloablative treatment?

A number of different schedules were given in the early days of autografting. Single- or double-dose melphalan, and single or double BACT-type treatment have fallen out of favor. There appears to be little to choose between cyclophosphamide/total body irradiation (Cy/TBI) or busulfan/cyclophosphamide (BuCy), with the latter the more favored of the two for second remission autografts. There is interest in the prospect of adding targeted therapy to the preparatory schedule using the immunoconjugate gemtuzumab ozogamicin (Mylotarg) (see Chapter 108).

What is the role of purging?

The field has enjoyed friendly rivalry between those who felt that optimizing in vitro purging was top priority and those who

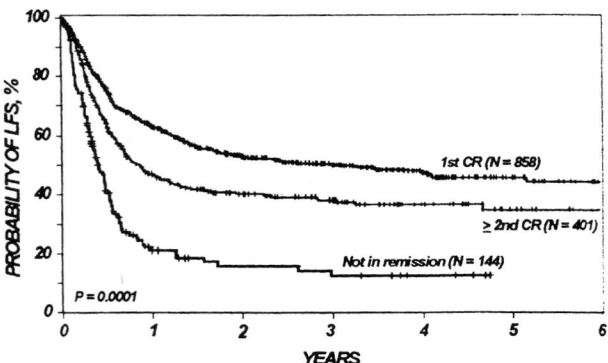

Fig. 36.3. Probability of leukemia-free survival after autotransplant for acute myeloid leukemia, 1989–1995. Three-year probabilities of LFS were 50±4%, 38±5%, and 12±7%, respectively. Reproduced, with permission, from *ABMTR Newsletter,* 3, 10, 1996.

did not. In fact, both sides believe in minimizing contamination of the autograft, because most in the nonpurging camp recognize the importance of prior consolidation chemotherapy as a means of "in vivo" purging.

The evidence in favor of in vitro purging is from two sources. The elegant gene marking studies of Brenner's group provide powerful evidence that in some cases of relapse after autologous BMT, the relapse derives in part from the autograft (Brenner *et al.*, 1993). Second, as mentioned previously, patients autografted early in first remission have a relapse risk of 46%. However, in patients autografted in a similar time frame, but with purged marrow, the relapse risk was 33% (Gorin *et al.*, 1991). This was not a prospective comparison but it has been taken as an important piece of evidence to support purging.

There have been a number of purging strategies adopted, some of which have provided anecdotal encouragement. Several monoclonal antibody-based techniques (Ball *et al.*, 1990, 1997) and an in vitro culture technique (Chang *et al.*, 1989) have reported survival of up to 80% in small series of patients. Whether these exceptional results are entirely, or at all, due to the procedure or to unconscious patient selection is not clear.

The most popular approach to purging to date has been in vitro incubation with 4-hydroperoxycyclophosphamide (4HC). This approach was pioneered by the Baltimore group (Sharkis, Santos, & Colvin, 1980), who had demonstrated dose-dependent efficacy in a myeloid leukemia model in the Brown-Norway rat. While the effect was clear, it should be pointed out that this leukemia was particularly sensitive to cyclophosphamide. The same group derived the appropriate dose (which did not unduly compromise marrow regenerative potential) and applied a standard dose in patients in second remission following myeloablation with busulfan/cyclophosphamide, with encouraging clinical results (Kaizer *et al.*, 1985; Yeager *et al.*, 1986). This gave the field considerable momentum. A subsequent study in similar patients in the UK produced identical results using the same myeloablative treatment, but did not use purged marrow (Chopra *et al.*, 1991).

Enthusiasm in Europe has been led by the Paris group at Hopital St Antoine, who devised the "adjusted purging" approach (Gorin *et al.*, 1986). The concept here is that a marrow sample taken from the patient is tested to find the concentration that kills 95% of granulocyte-macrophage colony-forming unit (CFU-GM) progenitor cells. This concentration is subsequently used on the full marrow harvest. The EBMT Registry data show that recipients of purged marrow following total body irradiation (TBI) have a reduced relapse risk (Gorin *et al.*, 1991). This effect is particularly noticeable in those patients at high risk of relapse; for example, those autografted early in remission, or those patients who originally took longer to enter CR (>40 days). No benefit could be demonstrated for patients who entered remission promptly (<40 days) or who received the transplant beyond 6 months. The EBMT Registry suggests that adjusted dose purging produces better results than

purging with a standard dose. The fact that the recipients of a higher purging dose in the adjusted dose cohort had a lower relapse risk has been presented as evidence of a dose-response effect.

Those who have not regarded in vitro purging as a priority issue—and it must be pointed out that the author is of this view—raise a number of points for debate.

The relapse risk in recipients of identical twin marrow (which represents the "perfect" autograft) is not dissimilar to that seen in recipients of unpurged autografts (Gale, Horowitz, & Ash, 1994), which can be extrapolated to suggest that the risk of relapse from the patient's endogenous tumor burden (rather than from the graft), in the absence of a graft-versus-leukemia effect, is around 40% to 50%. The demonstration, as mentioned above, that purging can make an impact on the relapse risk of patients autografted early when a syngeneic graft cannot do this means that it is not possible to explain the effect on the basis of tumor cell removal. An alternative explanation is required. It has been suggested that purged marrows are more immunologically reactive as autologous grafts than unmanipulated marrows (Mangoni *et al.*, 1991). Testing purging in a prospective manner may be feasible in high-risk cases (slower remitters and/or those who have the autograft early). These represent a minority of younger AML patients entering clinical trials; of practical concern, apart from patient recruitment, is the extent to which the purging technique can be standardized between centers and the fact that there is no robust method of measuring efficacy in vitro. There are also some doubts about the safety of purging, even if it is accepted that the relapse risk is reduced, since there have been some deaths and toxicity due to delayed hematopoietic engraftment in recipients of manipulated marrows.

How many cells are needed for optimal engraftment?

The answer to this question is not known. It does not seem that the total nucleated cell dose correlates well with the rate of hematologic recovery. Initially, a suggested minimum nucleated cell dose was 1×10^8/kg. In a single center study, a nucleated cell dose of $>2 \times 10^8$/kg improved disease-free survival by decreasing transplant-related mortality (Mehta *et al.*, 1995). In other autograft contexts, which may not involve myeloablative conditioning schedules, desirable CD34$^+$ cell doses of $\geq 2 \times 10^6$/kg have been suggested. Poor engraftment, especially of platelets, is well known after autografting AML. In one analysis of this problem the only correlate with protracted thrombocytopenia was the platelet count at the time of the harvest (Pendry, Alcorn, & Burnett, 1993). Growth in long-term culture has not been shown to predict engraftment, although it was highly predictive of those who would subsequently relapse (Burnett *et al.*, 1993). In the MRC AML 10 trial a range of cell doses were harvested, of which the median was 1.9×10^8/kg. There was a highly significant survival advantage for recipients above, as compared with below, this value (K. Wheatley, personal communication). The use of granulocyte colony-stimulating factor (G-CSF)-moblized peripheral blood stem cells used either as the sole source of reconstituting cells (Demirer *et al.*, 1996) or in combination with non-G-CSF-stimulated bone marrow (Demirer *et al.*, 1995) appears to enhance engraftment rates, with an absolute neutrophil count of $0.5 \times 10^9/l$ reached at a median of 12 and 13 days, respectively, in the two latter studies. A platelet count of $20 \times 10^9/l$ was obtained at a median of 15 and 14 days, respectively. Interestingly, peripheral blood stem cells (PBSCs) have also been mobilized (using chemotherapy and G-CSF) from patients with AML secondary to myelodysplasia or prior therapy, all of whom had abnormal karyotypes. Two patients in this series with secondary AML who were autografted had karyotypically normal marrow posttransplant (Carella *et al.*, 1996). The potential danger of giving an unnecessarily large dose is the increased danger of reinfusing occult leukemia. In the MRC 10 trial experience, at least, this did not seem to be a concern. Data from the European Organisation for Research and Treatment of Cancer (EORTC) however, suggests that, when large yields of PBSCs are obtained at leukapheresis, the risk of subsequent relapse is increased (de Witte *et al.*, 2001).

Source of the autologous graft

Most of the information available relates to bone marrow as the source of stem cells. In most autograft centers BMT has now been superseded by the use of PBSC autografts (Gondo *et al.*, 1997) (Fig. 36.5). This would appear at first sight to have particular attraction in AML in view of the faster hematopoietic recovery, especially of platelets, associated with PBSC transplantation. A retrospective comparison of the EBMT Registry data suggested that, although there was acceleration of neutrophil recovery, a benefit for platelet recovery was less clear. There was also a suggestion of a nonsignificant excess of relapses in the PBSC recipients (Reiffers *et al.*, 1997).

The Seattle group used PBSC transplantation as a supplement to autologous marrow in AML patients and were able to show a more rapid recovery of neutrophils and platelets compared with historical controls (Demirer *et al.*, 1995).

Not all cases of AML can be successfully mobilized. If PBSC mobilization is part of the treatment protocol, it is better that it take place after one of the early chemotherapy courses, since the yield drops with each successive chemotherapy course. In the current UK MRC AML 12 trial an "adequate" dose could be obtained after one leukapheresis in 70% to 80% of cases, but this dropped considerably after three courses, and some patients failed to mobilize at any stage (Goldstone *et al.*, 1997).

Persistence of cytogenetic abnormalities in harvested marrow is associated with a poor outcome posttransplant (Grimwade *et al.*, 1997) (Fig. 36.6).

Postautograft treatment

Relapse has always been, and remains, the principal reason for treatment failure. One approach to address this problem is to add further treatment after the autograft. This strategy, however, has been little used. In AML such an approach is unlikely to be practical because of the existing problems of slow engraftment. There have been some efforts to enhance the effects of autoreactive T cells reported to be in the circulation after autologous and allogeneic BMT, but not after chemotherapy (Reittie *et al.*, 1989). These cells have been shown to be capable of lysing autologous leukemic blast cells, thus providing evidence for an immune-based antileukemic effect in the autograft setting. While the use of conventional dose chemotherapy has little to offer for relapse post autograft, a second autograft or an allograft may offer an improved outcome (Ringden *et al.*, 2000).

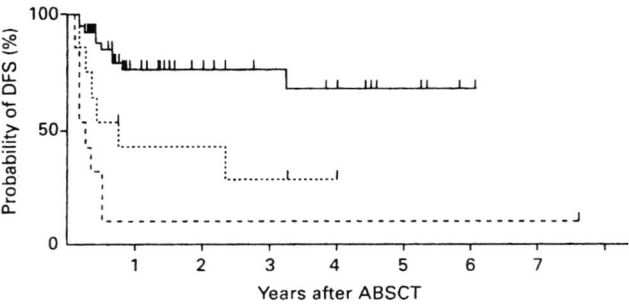

Fig. 36.5. Kaplan-Meier estimates of DFS for AML patients transplanted in first remission (—, $n = 42$), in second or third remission (..., $n = 9$), and in relapse (—, $n = 9$). The median follow-up time of AML patients transplanted in first remission was 17 months. First remission vs. second/third remission $P < .01$; first remission vs. relapse, $P < .01$. Reproduced, with permission, from Gondo *et al.* (1997).

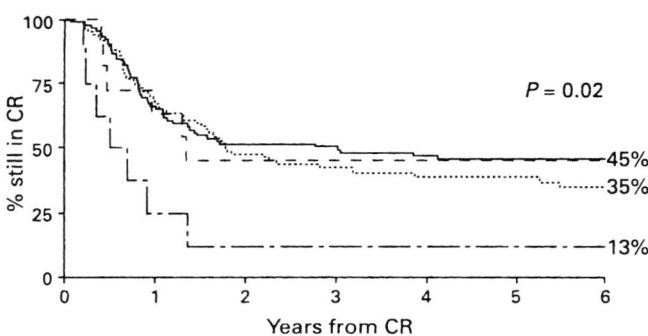

Fig. 36.6. Disease-free survival of patients entered into MRC AML 10 trial with successful karyotype analysis at diagnosis in whom cytogenetic assessment was performed at bone marrow harvest.—Cytogenetics abnormal at diagnosis, normal at harvest, $n = 89$; ..., cytogenetics normal at diagnosis and harvest, $n = 82$; - - -, cytogenetic abnormalities present at bone marrow harvest, not detected at diagnosis, $n = 11$; - — - persistence of same cytogenetic abnormality at diagnosis and harvest, $n = 8$. Reproduced, with permission, from Grimwade *et al.* (1997).

Monitoring for residual disease posttransplant (and see Chapters 105 and 106)

Some consistent conclusions are emerging from studies using reverse transcriptase-polymerase chain reaction (RT-PCR) monitoring of disease following chemotherapy (Yin & Tobal, 1999). Similar data are also available using aberrant immunophenotype monitoring (San Miguel *et al.*, 2001). Most of this body of information relates to patients with lesions associated with favorable karyotypes (Venditti *et al.*, 2000; Burnett *et al.*, 1999; Diverio *et al.*, 1998; Morschhauser *et al.*, 2000). Molecular monitoring is also valuable after allogeneic HSC transplantation because of the option of using donor lymphocyte infusions; however, there are few if any prospective studies in AML after autologous stem cell transplantation. Persistent molecular positivity following first-line induction and consolidation treatment (including the use of all-*trans* retinoic acid (ATRA)) is highly predictive of relapse. In that context autografting with RT-PCR negative stem cells has been effective (Meloni *et al.*, 1997). Molecular information may be useful in selected cases for predicting patients from risk categories not normally considered candidates for transplant, who would benefit from it. Using such methods to confirm the lack of marrow contamination is also logical. Currently, monitoring disease after autografting is worthwhile in order to develop an understanding of what to expect; however, the opportunities to intervene are limited other than in special cases such as acute promyelocytic leukemia for which ATRA or arsenic trioxide are available as non-toxic therapies.

Timing

It was established early that autografting patients who had relapsed and failed reinduction therapy had limited benefit (Dicke *et al.*, 1979). Some patients achieved a further CR, but this was invariably short-lived. As consolidation treatment for patients who relapsed and achieved a second remission, it promised to be more helpful, with about 30% of patients having durable remissions and several having "remission inversion" (i.e., longer second than first remissions; Yeager *et al.*, 1986; Rowley *et al.*, 1989). Such a result has been reported consistently from single center and registry studies, whether or not purged marrow was used (Chopra *et al.*, 1991). There is some evidence in this context that BuCy is superior to Cy/TBI. An exceptional experience was reported by the Rome Group using their carmustine, amsacrine, etoposide, and cytosine arabinoside (BAVC) protocol (Meloni *et al.*, 1990). This resulted in an approximately 50% survival, which interestingly enough was superior to their experience using the same regimen in CR1 patients. A follow-up report projected a 42% disease-free survival rate at 10 years posttransplant (Meloni *et al.*, 1996). There are some highly potent selection pressures operating on patients with AML in CR2. The prognosis for a patient who relapses from first-line treatment is heavily dependent on the patient's age and duration of first CR. Similarly, the time-cen-

soring effect that has been clearly recognized in CR1 is even more substantial in CR2. It is therefore very difficult to compare treatment modalities in CR2, but, for what it is worth, autografting at this point seems as good an option as any, possibly including allografting. This relatively useful effect in second CR creates the option of reserving an autograft as a salvage option by cryopreserving stem cells in CR1. While this appears to be logical, it is not known what proportion of patients who relapse will respond to reinduction treatment and survive unscathed in order to undergo an autograft in CR2. If this approach is planned, it would be important to be confident that patients "allowed" to relapse had a good chance of reaching the salvage treatment. This appears to be valid in patients with good risk cytogenetics.

An alternative approach is to use the autograft as the primary treatment of relapse, thereby avoiding the risk of losing patients. While it is entirely predictable that the relapse rate, and possibly procedural mortality, will be greater, this may be more than compensated for by more patients getting access to the treatment. The allogeneic transplant experience from Seattle makes this point (Clift *et al.*, 1992). Only one study has prospectively examined this approach (Petersen *et al.*, 1993). As they had previously described with allogeneic transplantation, the Seattle group compared the strategy of using an autograft harvested in CR1 to support myeloablation either as primary treatment of relapse or after the patient had been induced into CR2. Only 47 patients were randomized in the study. The actuarial probabilities of relapse-free survival at 2 years were 45% for those transplanted in relapse and 32% for those transplanted in CR2 (Fig. 36.7). These were not significantly different, suggesting that either approach is acceptable.

In summary, the key issues regarding the use of autologous HSC transplantation in the management of AML are (1) Is it better than chemotherapy alone? and (2) If so, when should it be deployed?

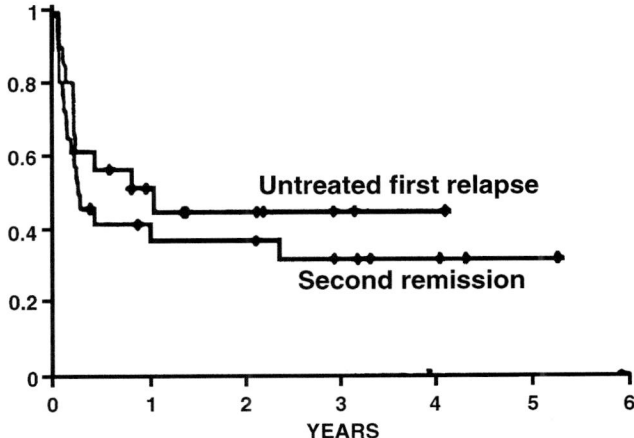

Fig. 36.7. Probability of relapse-free survival for patients with AML transplanted during untreated first relapse or second remission. Reproduced, with permission, from Petersen *et al.* (1993).

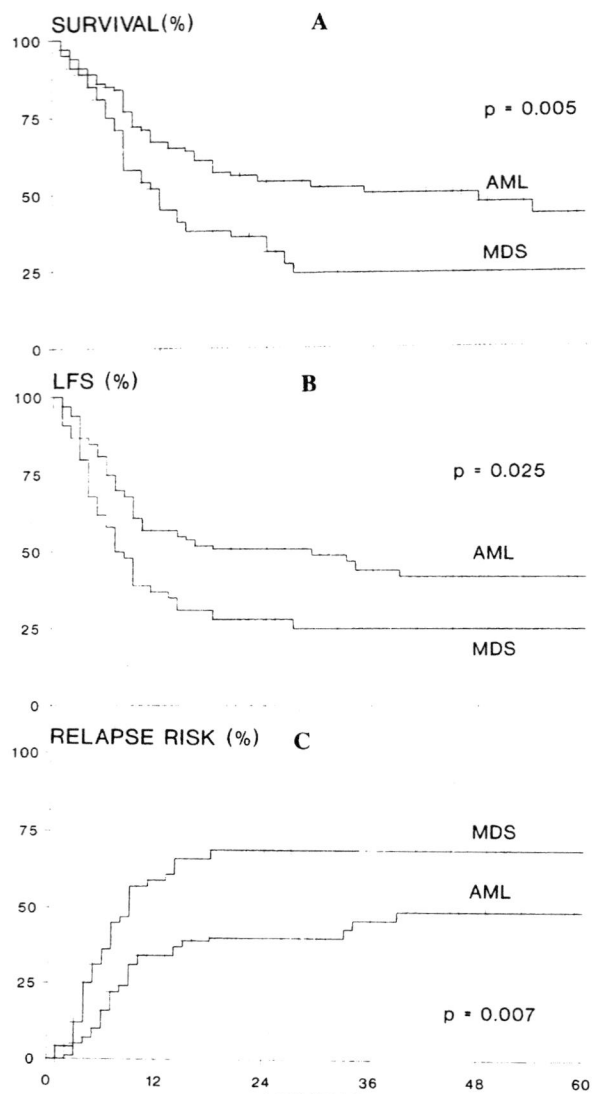

Fig. 36.8. (A) Actuarial survival, **(B)** leukemia-free survival (LFS), and **(C)** relapse risk of 55 patients transplanted in first CR for MDS, sAML, or therapy-related MDS/leukemia compared with 110 matched patients transplanted in first CR for de novo AML. MDS refers to myelodysplastic syndromes, secondary AML, and therapy-related MDS/AML; AML refers to de novo AML. Reproduced, with permission, from de Witte *et al.* (1997).

One interesting situation in which transplantation in CR1 would appear optimal is for myelodysplasia or secondary AML following myelodysplasia (de Witte *et al.,* 1997) (Fig. 36.8), although, not surprisingly, the outcome does not appear as good as for de novo AML transplanted in CR1.

Randomized trials of autologous transplantation in CR1

Of interest have been the results of the extensive efforts of most of the major AML trial groups to address the value of autograft-

ing in CR1. These studies fall into two categories: (1) those that compare chemotherapy to autograft, and (2) those that add the autograft as an extra course of treatment.

There have been additional differences between trials that may well have influenced outcome, for example, whether or not children were included, intensity and extent of prior chemotherapy, the myeloablative protocol used, the use of purging or not, and sample size (and therefore reliability of the result). Several of these studies are published in full or abstract form (Table 36.6).

The first study published was the French BGMT-84 trial (Reiffers *et al.,* 1989). This compared two courses of high-dose melphalan, each supported by ABMT, between which was a course of etoposide and cytosine arabinoside versus four courses of chemotherapy, one of which used high-dose cytosine arabinoside (3 g/m^2). No children were studied. Those receiving an autograft had a better outcome; however, the chemotherapy outcome was poorer than expected. A follow-up study, BGMT-87, randomized patients who had received consolidation courses, including high-dose cytosine arabinoside, to receive maintenance treatment for 2 years or an autograft after melphalan-busulfan conditioning. When these two studies were combined (Reiffers *et al.,* 1997), 54 patients were randomized to receive autotransplant and 58 chemotherapy. The survival was 42% and 25%, respectively, but the difference did not reach statistical significance. Clearly the sample sizes were too small.

The EORTC–GIMEMA trial

This large multicenter trial conducted in Europe recruited 941 patients, of whom 623 entered remission (Zittoun *et al.,* 1995). Those with an HLA-matched sibling were to receive an allogeneic BMT, while the remainder were available for randomization between an autograft following either Cy/TBI or BuCy ablation or a second course of intensive chemotherapy (Fig. 36.9). It should be noted that only one consolidation course was planned after the achievement of CR, which meant that most patients had two courses of chemotherapy before the autograft and three courses in all since two-thirds of patients entered CR after the first course. Of 408 patients eligible for randomization, 254 were randomized (60%). Of 128 randomized to autograft, 95 received it. The autograft resulted in a significant reduction in relapse with better disease-free survival. However, the overall survival at the time of reporting (median follow-up 3.3 years) (56% vs. 46%) was not significantly different, because it was possible to rescue some of the relapsed patients with an autograft. Of 58 patients who relapsed from the chemotherapy arm, 36 (62%) entered CR2, of whom 22 received an autograft (35%); in contrast only 11 of 29 (38%) who relapsed postautograft achieved a further CR, of whom 2 had a second autograft.

Even allowing for the absence of children in this study, the outcome from the chemotherapy arm is disappointing, so it could be argued that the chemotherapy used was insufficient to

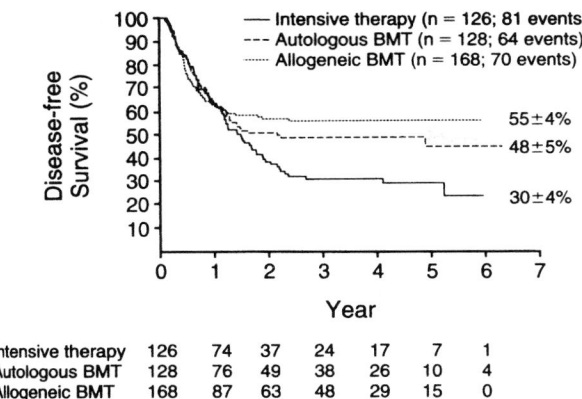

Fig. 36.9. Kaplan-Meier plots of disease-free survival, according to whether patients were assigned to autologous or allogeneic bone marrow transplantation (BMT) or a second course of intensive consolidation therapy. The number of patients at risk is shown below each time point. Plus-minus values are the projected disease-free survival rates (±SE) at 4 years. The events considered were relapse or death during a first complete remission. Reproduced, with permission, from Zittoun *et al.* (1995).

mount a serious challenge to the autograft. A common feature of trials of this design is that a substantial proportion of patients who are eligible do not get randomized, mostly due to reasons other than relapse. In addition, some patients do not receive the randomized treatment. In this respect the small number of courses before the autograft may explain the relatively better performance of the autografted arm in this trial compared with others, for example, the MRC or Intergroup trials.

The GOELAM Trial

The study conducted by the French GOELAM Group was initiated in 1987 (Harousseau *et al.,* 1997). It did not recruit children (<15 years) and compared autografting using unpurged marrow after BuCy conditioning with intensive chemotherapy. Most patients had only two previous courses of treatment. As with most of these trials, the proportion of eligible patients who were randomized—even though they had only two courses—was low at 32%. Excluding 88 patients who had an HLA-matched donor, 164 (58%) were randomized. Of the 86 assigned to auto-BMT, 75 (70%) received it. This trial had one of the lowest death rates in the autograft arm (6.5%). There was no difference in disease-free survival (DFS) or overall survival between the autograft arm and the intensive treatment arm. The design of this trial and that of EORTC–GIMEMA are similar. The observation of a difference in DFS in the EORTC trial, and not in the GOELAM trial, may well be due to less effective chemotherapy in the former study, in which the DFS in the chemotherapy arm was 30% compared with 40% in the latter.

The Intergroup trial

The major effort in the United States has been the collaborative Intergroup trial (Cassileth *et al.,* 1998). Eligible patients aged 16 to 55 were initially treated with idarubicin/cytosine arabinoside induction for 1 to 2 courses. Following a short consolidation course of the same drugs (2 + 5 days), patients were randomized either to auto-BMT using 4 HC-purged marrow after BuCy ablation, or to one course of high-dose cytosine arabinoside (HDAC) (3 g/m² b.i.d. for 6 days). Of 513 patients who entered CR, 120 were found to have an HLA-matched donor, 164 went off the protocol for a number of reasons (relapse, toxicity, refusal, other), and 229 were randomized to auto-BMT (*n* = 111) or HDAC (*n* = 118). However, only 67 of the 111 actually received the autograft. On an intention to treat analysis, the DFS and survival at 4 years for auto-BMT versus HDAC were 37% vs. 35% and 47% vs. 54% (not significant).

The UK MRC AML 10 trial

The largest study to date is that conducted by the UK MRC (Burnett *et al.,* 1998). Children were included and the question asked was, "Does an early or late autograft (i.e., in first or second remission) confer any advantage on patients who have already received four courses of intensive treatment?" The design meant that for most cases the patients received 1 to 2 more courses of treatment than those in the EORTC–GIMEMA or Intergroup trials. Again, only a relative minority of patients who could have been randomized were randomized (35%), but this still represents the largest number thus far reported (381). Only 126 of the 190 randomized to autograft received it. This was largely due to the fact that randomization took place at the end of 3 courses of chemotherapy, after which another treatment course was given. This fourth course was not without additional toxicity and explains why a number of patients did not receive the autograft. A notable feature of this trial was that the overall survival from diagnosis was fairly good (40% at 7 years), and the survival for the control (chemotherapy) arm was 45%. There can, therefore, be no caveats in this study of a weak control arm. Even so, the addition of an autograft on an intention-to-treat basis substantially reduced the relapse risk (37% vs. 58%) and improved DFS (54% vs. 40%). However, the antileukemic benefit of the autograft arm was decreased by two features. First, there were excess deaths in the autotransplant arm and, second, there was a suggestion of better survival after relapse in the chemotherapy arm (similar to that seen in the EORTC study). This latter difference was small but more obvious in patients with good risk disease. It has taken prolonged follow-up for the significant late survival benefit of the autograft arm to become apparent (57% vs. 45%).

The Pediatric Oncology Group trial

A large study in children (defined as <21 years) has been conducted by the Pediatric Oncology Group (POG) (Ravindranath *et al.,* 1996). Two hundred and thirty-two patients were randomized to auto-BMT (*n* = 115) or chemotherapy (*n* = 117), which comprised six courses of high-dose therapy. There was no significant difference between the autograft and chemotherapy arms for DFS (38% vs. 36%), in spite of the fact that the relapse risk was significantly reduced in the autograft arm (31% vs. 58%). The failure to convert the antileukemic benefit to superior survival was partly explained by a higher mortality rate in the autograft arm (15% vs. 27%).

The AIEOP Group trial

The Associazione Italiana Ematologica ed Oncologia Paediatrica (AIEOP) Cooperative Group conducted a prospective trial in children up to 15 years old. Of 127 who entered CR, 72 were randomized between auto-BMT using the BAVC protocol (Meloni et al., 1990), or 6 further courses of chemotherapy. The actuarial relapse rate on an intention to treat analysis was 78% versus 72% (auto-BMT vs. chemotherapy) and the DFS survival rates were 21% and 27%. It is notable that there were poorer outcomes in each of the randomized arms than would normally be expected in this good prognosis age group.

Two trials have compared the addition of an autograft in patients who are judged to have received adequate chemotherapy. The Dutch Trial (HOVON 4) compared the addition (or not) of an autograft (using BuCy) to 3 courses of intensive chemotherapy from diagnosis. One hundred seventeen patients have been randomized and the results are awaited. In an earlier study, patients were allocated to an allogeneic BMT if a donor was available, or to an autograft if not. The value of this study was that it prewarned us that a substantial number of patients expected to receive an autograft would not do so (Lowenberg et al., 1990). There were a variety of reasons for this, most a consequence of the toxicity of prior treatment rather than relapse.

The Children's Cancer Group trial

In this study of 652 children and adolescents (up to age 20), Woods et al. (2001) found actuarial 8-year survival in those receiving an HLA-identical related donor transplant (60%) to be significantly superior to those receiving autologous transplantation (48%) or aggressive high-dose cytarabine-based chemotherapy (53%) as intensive post-remission treatment. The actuarial probability of relapse was significantly lower in the allograft recipients. There have been criticisms of this large trial, and it should also be noted that the results of chemotherapy in children have continued to improve.

Are there patients who preferentially benefit from autologous HSC transplantation in CR1?

A major feature of most of the large trials reviewed here has been the difficulty in getting the majority of available patients randomized. In addition, some trials had significant failure to comply with the treatment allocated by randomization. This may compromise the generalization of the findings. However, in the MRC trial there was no significant difference in outcome

dependent on whether patients were randomized to, or elected to receive, treatment. Similarly, the proportion of good, standard, and poor risk patients was not different at the time of randomization when compared with the proportions at entry into CR. This in part gives reassurance that those randomized may be representative.

There may be important subgroups of patients who do not benefit from an autograft (or any form of transplant) as first-line treatment, either because the prognosis with chemotherapy is already favorable or because such patients, if they relapse, have a high prospect of successful salvage treatment (the delayed transplant option). This applies to children and those with good risk disease (i.e., a favorable karyotype [Nabhan, Mehta, & Tallman, 2001]). Finally, poor-risk patients may not benefit from autografting because the disease biology mitigates against the success of any form of therapy.

In children in particular the delayed effects of high-dose therapy such as intellectual development, growth, and fertility must also be taken into account.

Conclusions from trials

Although there are important differences between the major trials (for example, in design, the inclusion of children or not), some general observations can be made. In almost all risk groups and age groups those allocated to the autograft arm had a reduced relapse rate. This was achieved in spite of the fact that not all patients actually received the autograft. In general, compliance was higher in children. This benefit in some of the studies provided improved disease-free survival, but was partially counteracted by treatment-related mortality. Some of this mortality was associated with poor hematopoietic recovery, so there has been optimism that peripheral blood stem cell autografting would make a favorable impact on this. Randomized data from an unpublished EORTC trial indicated that, although there was an improved pattern on hematopoietic regeneration, this has not resulted in an improvement in overall survival.

The EORTC-GIMEMA trial demonstrated that a useful proportion of patients who have stem cells stored can be salvaged in second remission. Planning for this carries the risk that second remission may not be achieved. This is likely to be the case for high-risk patients (i.e., those who have adverse cytogenetics or who have failed to clear blast cells with the first course of induction chemotherapy). Standard-risk patients who relapse have a variable chance of achieving a CR and delay may be unproductive. Good-risk cytogenetic groups and children have a good chance of achieving a second remission, so storage and delay of the autograft is much more likely to be successful. This also includes the subgroup that can be molecularly assessed, so when to store and when to apply the autograft can be decided in the light of this more accurate assessment.

A message that could be taken from these trials is that more consolidation treatment is better. This raises the question of whether this could be achieved with additional chemotherapy. This issue has been addressed by the UK MRC AML12 trial in which a total of four courses were compared with five courses.

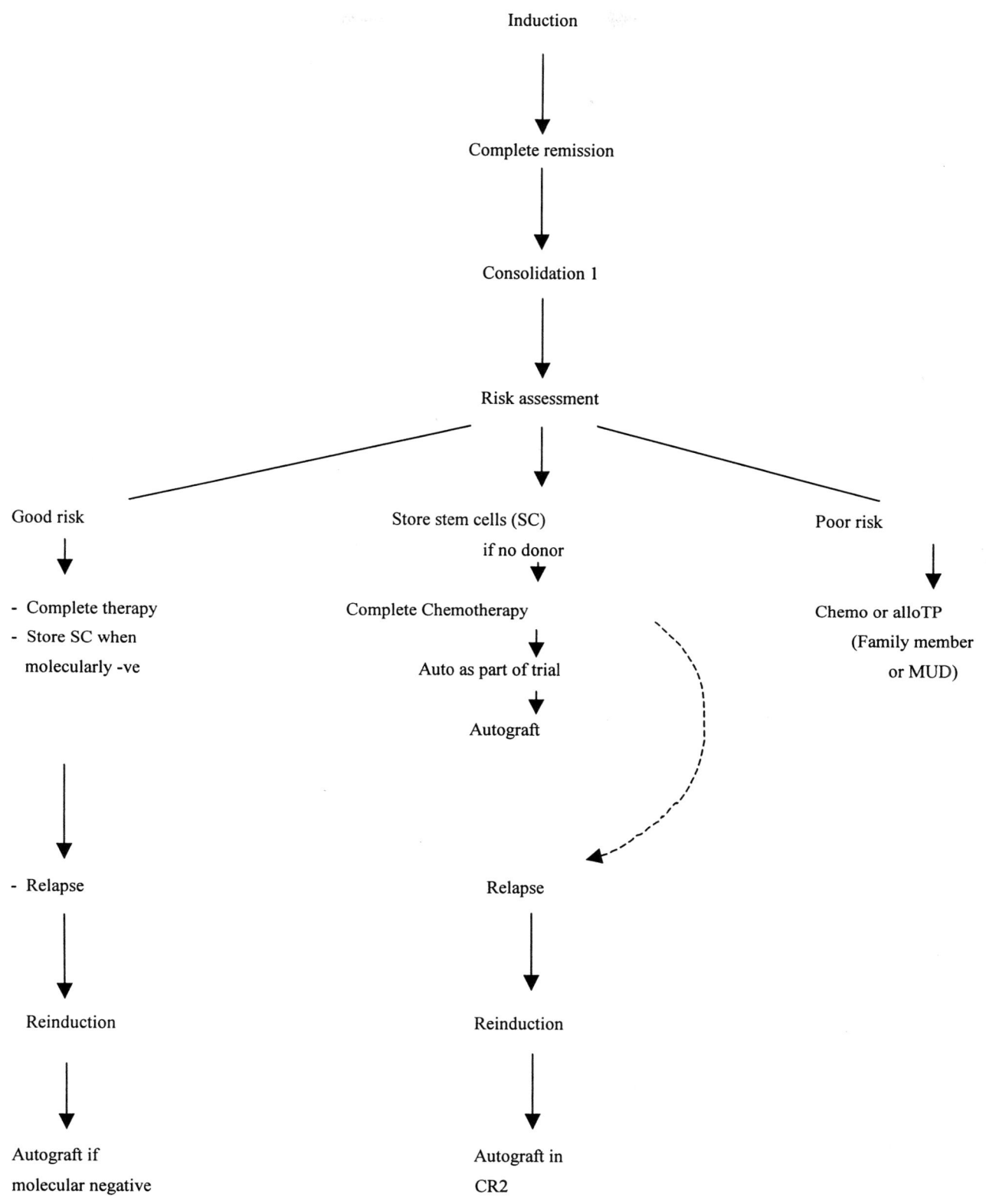

Fig. 36.10. A suggested algorithm for the treatment of AML.

Preliminary analysis suggests that there is no major difference in outcome (Wheatley *et al.*, 2002).

The current practice of HSC transplantation for AML in Europe has been described (Urbano-Ispizua *et al.*, 2002) (and see Chapter 124, Breaking News ...).

A suggested algorithm for the treatment of patients with AML is shown in Fig. 36.10.

The future

It is not likely that major new findings will emerge from other phase III trials. The Intergroup trial from the United States is smaller than the European studies and compliance has been at least as big a problem. More evidence should be collected if possible but lessons in trial design also have to be learned. There is a significant risk of treatment-related mortality following autografting, most noticeably in the POG and MRC trials. In the latter this was frequently associated with delayed engraftment. It needs to be determined if engraftment can be improved by using PBSC in addition to, or instead of, bone marrow, and whether improved engraftment can be achieved without increasing the relapse risk.

The anecdotal experience of autografting derived from single centers in uncontrolled studies has been validated prospectively, with approximately 45% to 55% of patients becoming long-term survivors. However, at least in the MRC and GOELAM experience, chemotherapy has improved such that 40% of patients survive. It has also been possible to salvage some patients who relapse, as best shown in the EORTC–GIMEMA study, but also to some extent in the MRC trial. Single-center experience suggests that transplant-related mortality can be as low as 6% to 8%. In some of the randomized trials it has been double that. The reasons for this discrepancy are not clear but it may be due to inadequate hematopoietic reconstitution.

Despite the fact that the MRC protocol resulted in a 40% survival from diagnosis, the substantial additional reduction in relapse risk from autografting (58% to 37%) is impressive, particularly when it is remembered that only two-thirds of those randomized received the autograft. This effect was apparent in each patient risk category. There are clearly other approaches available for good risk (favorable cytogenetics and children) cases. Careful overview analysis of all randomized data may be able to shed light on whether there is an age or risk subgroup in adults that particularly benefit. For example, in a preliminary analysis of mononuclear cell (MNC) dose harvested in the MRC AML 10 trial, there was a strong relationship to survival. Patients who had an above average number (1.9×10^8 MNC/kg) did well compared with those given a lower dose.

New prognostic factors may emerge which will be useful in predicting response. For example, FLT-3 mutations carry a higher risk of relapse and appear particularly useful in dividing the standard-risk group (Kottaridis *et al.*, 2001). However, there are few data yet available to provide guidelines as to whether those with mutations will benefit from transplantation.

References

Ball, E. D., Mills, L. E., Cornwell, III G. G. *et al.* (1990). Autologous bone marrow transplantation for acute myeloid leukaemia using monoclonal antibody purged bone marrow. *Blood*, **75**, 1199–1206.

Ball, E. D., Phelps, V., & Wilson, J. (1997). Autologous bone marrow transplantation for acute myeloid leukaemia in remission or first relapse using monoclonal antibody purged marrow. In *Autologous Marrow and Blood Transplantation VIII*, ed. K. A. Dicke & A. Keating, pp. 45–53. Charlottesville: Carden Jennings Ltd.

Bishop, J. F., Matthews, J. P., Young, G. A. *et al.* (1996). A randomized study of high-dose cytarabine in induction in acute myeloid leukemia. *Blood*, **87**, 1710–17.

Brenner, M. K., Rill, D. R., Moen, R. C. *et al.* (1993). Gene marking to trace origin of relapse after autologous bone marrow transplantation. *Lancet*, **341**, 85–6.

Burnett, A. K. (1994). Karyotypically defined risk groups in acute myeloid leukaemia. *Leukemia Research*, **18**, 889–90.

Burnett, A. K., Goldstone, A. H., Stevens, R. F. *et al.* (1998). Randomized comparison of addition of autologous bone marrow transplantation to intensive chemotherapy for acute myeloid leukaemia in first remission: results of MRC AML 10 trial. *Lancet*, **351**, 700–8.

Burnett, A. K., Graham, S., & Alcorn, M. (1993). Sustained growth in long term bone marrow culture of AML remission marrow predicts a high probability of remaining relapse free after auto BMT in first complete remission. *Experimental Hematology*, **21**, 1020.

Burnett, A. K., Grimwade, D., Solomon, E. *et al.* (1999). Presenting white cell count and kinetics of molecular remission predict prognosis acute promyelocytic leukaemia treated with all-*trans* retinoic acid: Result of the randomised MRC Trial. *Blood*, **93**, 4131–4143.

Burnett, A. K., Wheatley, K., Goldstone, A. H. *et al.* (2002). The value of allogeneic bone marrow transplant in patients with acute myeloid leukaemia at differing risk of relapse: results of the UK MRC AML10 Trial. *British Journal of Haematology*, **118**, 385–400.

Cahn, J. Y., Labopin, N., Mandelli, F. *et al.* (1995). Autologous bone marrow transplantation for first remission acute myeloblastic leukemia in patients older than 50 years: a retrospective analysis of the European Bone Marrow Transplant Group. *Blood*, **85**, 575–9.

Carella, A. M., Dejana, A., Lerma, E. *et al.* (1996). In vivo mobilization of karyotypically normal blood progenitor cells in high-risk MDS, secondary or therapy-related acute myelogenous leukaemia. *British Journal of Haematology*, **95**, 127–30.

Cassileth, P. A., Harrington, D. P., Appelbaum, F. R. *et al.* (1998). Chemotherapy compared with autologous or allogeneic bone marrow transplantation in the management of acute myeloid leukemia in first remission. *New England Journal of Medicine*, **339**, 1649–56.

Chang, J., Morgenstern, G., Coutinho, L. H. *et al.* (1989). The use of bone marrow cells grown in long-term culture for autologous bone marrow transplantation in acute myeloid leukaemia: an update. *Bone Marrow Transplantation*, **4**, 5.

Chopra, R., Goldstone, A. H., McMillan, A. K. *et al.* (1991). Successful treatment of acute myeloid leukemia using busulfan/cyclophosphamide as conditioning: the British autograft group experience. *Journal of Clinical Oncology*, **9**, 1840–7.

Clift, R. A., Buckner, C. D., Appelbaum, F. R. *et al.* (1992) Allogeneic marrow transplantation during untreated first relapse of acute myeloid leukaemia. *Journal of Clinical Oncology*, **10**, 1723–9.

Dastugue, N., Payen, C., Lafage-Pochitaloff, M. *et al.* (1995). Prognostic significance of karyotype in de novo adult acute myeloid leukemia. *Leukemia*, **9**, 1491–8.

Demirer, T., Buckner, C. D., Appelbaum, F. R. *et al.* (1995). Rapid engraftment after autologous transplantation utilizing marrow and recombinant granulocyte colony-stimulating factor-mobilized peripheral blood stem cells in patients with acute myelogenous leukemia. *Bone Marrow Transplantation*, **15**, 915–22.

Demirer, T., Petersen, F. B., Bensinger, W. I. *et al.* (1996). Autologous transplantation with peripheral blood stem cells collected after granulocyte colony-stimulating factor in patients with acute myelogenous leukemia. *Bone Marrow Transplantation*, **18**, 29–34.

de Witte, T., Keating, S., Suciu, S. *et al.* (2001). A randomized comparison of the value of autologous BMT versus autologous PSCT for patients with AML in first CR in the AML 10 trial of the EORTC LCG and GIMEMA. *Blood*, **98**, (Abstract).

de Witte, T., Van Biezen, A., Hermans, J. *et al.* (1997). Autologous bone marrow transplantation for patients with myelodysplastic syndrome (MDS) or acute myeloid leukemia following MDS. *Blood*, **90**, 3853–62.

Dicke, A., Spitzer, G., Peters, L. *et al.* (1979). Autologous bone marrow transplantation in relapsed adult acute leukaemia. *Lancet*, **1**, 514–17.

Diverio, D., Rossi, V., Avvisati, G. *et al.* (1998). Early detection of relapse by prospective RT-PCR analysis of the PML/RARα fusion gene in patients with acute promyelocytic leukemia enrolled in the GIMEMA-AIEOP mutlicenter "AIDA" trial. *Blood*, **92**, 784–789.

Fenaux, P., Chastang, C., Chevret, S. *et al.* (1999). A randomized comparison of all transretinoic acid (ATRA) followed by chemotherapy and ATRA plus chemotherapy and the role of maintenance therapy in newly diagnosed acute promyelocytic leukemia. *Blood*, **94**, 1192–1200.

Fenaux, P., Wattel, E., Archimbaud, E. *et al.* (1994). Prolonged follow-up confirms that all-trans retinoic acid followed by chemotherapy reduces the risk of relapse in newly diagnosed acute promyelocytic leukemia. *Blood*, **84**, 666–7.

Ferrant, A., Doyen, C., & Delannoy, A. (1995). Karyotype in acute myeloblastic leukemia; prognostic significance in a prospective study assessing bone marrow transplantation in first remission. *Bone Marrow Transplantation*, **15**, 685–90.

Ferrant, A., Labopin, M., Frassoni, F. *et al.* (1997). Karyotype in acute myeloblastic leukaemia: prognostic significance for bone marrow transplantation in first remission. A European Group for Blood and Marrow Transplantation Study. *Blood*, **90**, 2931–8.

Gale, R. P., Horowitz, M. M., & Ash, R. C. (1994). Identical twin bone marrow transplants for leukemia. *Annals of Internal Medicine*, **120**, 646–52.

Gale, R. P., Horowitz, M. M., Weiner, R. S. *et al.* (1995). Impact of cytogenetic abnormalities on outcome of bone marrow transplants in acute myelogenous leukaemia in first remission. *Bone Marrow Transplantation*, **16**, 203–8.

Goldstone, A. H., Perry, A. R., Robinson, L. G. *et al.* (1997). Stem cell transplants in acute myeloid leukaemia (AML). In *Acute Leukaemias VII: Experimental Approaches and Novel Therapies*, ed. W. Hiddeman *et al.*, pp. 906–10. Berlin: Springer-Verlag.

Gondo, H., Harada, M., Miyamoto, T. *et al.* (1997). Autologous peripheral blood stem cell transplantation for acute myelogenous leukemia. *Bone Marrow Transplantation*, **20**, 821–6.

Gorin, N. C., Aegerter, P., Auvert, B. *et al.* (1990). Auntologous bone marrow transplantation for acute myelocytic leukemia in first remission: a European survey of the role of marrow purging. *Blood*, **75**, 1606–14.

Gorin, N. C., Douay, L., Laporte, J. P. *et al.* (1986). Autologous bone marrow transplantation using marrow incubated with Asta Z 7557 in adult acute leukemia. *Blood*, **67**, 1367–76.

Gorin, N. C., Labopin, M., Meloni, G. *et al.* (1991). Autologous bone marrow transplantation for acute myeloid leukemia in Europe: further evidence of the role of marrow purging by mafosfamide. *Leukemia*, **5**, 896–904.

Gray, R., & Wheatley, K. (1991). How to avoid bias when comparing bone marrow transplantation with chemotherapy. *Bone Marrow Transplantation*, **7** (Suppl 3), 9–12.

Grimwade, D., Walker, H., Harrison, G. *et al.* (2001). The predictive value of hierarchical cytogenetic classification in older adults with acute myeloid leukemia (AML): analysis of 1065 patients entered into the United Kingdom Medical Research Council AML11 trial. *Blood*, **98**, 1312–20.

Grimwade, D., Walker, H., Oliver, F. *et al.* (1998). The importance of diagnostic cytogenetics on outcome of AML: analysis of 1,612 patients entered into the MRC AML 10 trial. *Blood*, **92**, 2322–33.

Grimwade, D., Walker, H., Oliver, F. *et al.* on behalf of the Medical Research Council Leukaemia Working Parties. (1997). What happens subsequently in AML when cytogenetic abnormalities persist at bone marrow harvest? Results of the 10th UK MRC AML trial. *Bone Marrow Transplantation*, **19**, 1117–23.

Hann, I. M., Stevens, R. F., Goldstone, A. H. *et al.* (1997). Randomized comparison of DAT versus ADE as induction chemotherapy in children and younger adults with acute myeloid leukemia. Results of the Medical Research Council's 10th AML Trial (MRC AML 10). *Blood*, **89**, 2311–18.

Harousseau, J. L., Cahn, J. Y., Pignon, B. *et al.* (1997). Comparisons of autologous bone marrow transplantation and intensive chemotherapy as post remission therapy in adult acute myeloid leukemia. *Blood*, **90**, 2978–86.

Hirsch-Ginsberg, C., Huh, Y. O., Kagan, K. *et al.* (1993). Advances in the diagnosis of acute leukemia. In *Management of Acute Leukemia*, ed. C. D. Bloomfield & G. P. Herzig, pp. 1–46. Philadelphia: Saunders.

Kaizer, H., Stuart, R. K., Brookmeyer, R. *et al.* (1985). Autologous bone marrow transplantation in acute leukemia: a phase I study of in vitro treatment of marrow with 4-hydroperoxycyclophosphamide to purge tumor cells. *Blood*, **6**, 1504–10.

Keating, M. J., Smith, T. L., Kantarjian, H. *et al.* (1988). Cytogenetic pattern in acute myelogenous leukemia: a major reproducible determinant of outcome. *Leukemia*, **2**, 403–12.

Kottaridis, P. D., Gale, R. E., Frew, M. E. *et al.* (2001). The presence of a FLT3 internal tandem duplication in patients with acute myeloid leukemia (AML) adds important prognostic information to cytogenetic risk group and response to the first cycle of chemotherapy: analysis of 854 patients from the United Kingdom Medical Research Council AML 10 and 12 Trials. *Blood*, **98**, 1752–1759.

Lowenberg, B., Verdonck, L. J., Dekker, A. W. *et al.* (1990). Autologous bone marrow transplantation in acute myeloid leukemia in first remission: results of a Dutch prospective study. *Journal of Clinical Oncology*, **8**, 287–94.

Mangoni, L., Carlo-Stella, C., Caffo, O. *et al.* (1991). Autologous bone marrow transplantation in acute non-lymphoid leukemia in first remission: effect of mafosfamide purging versus adjusted dose. In *Autologous Bone Marrow Transplantation, Proceedings of the Fifth International Symposium*, ed. K. A. Dicke, J. O. Armitage, & M. J. Dicke-Evinger, pp. 43–54. The University of Nebraska Medical Center, Nebraska.

Mayer, R. J., David, R. D., Schiffer, C. A. *et al.* (1994). Intensive post remission chemotherapy in adults with acute myeloid leukemia. *New England Journal of Medicine*, **331**, 896–903.

Mehta, J., Powles, R., Singhal, S. *et al.* (1995). Autologous bone marrow transplantation for acute myeloid leukemia in first remission: identification of modifiable prognostic factors. *Bone Marrow Transplantation*, **16**, 499–506.

Meloni, G., De Fabritiis, P., Petti, M. C. *et al.* (1990). BAVC regimen and autologous bone marrow transplantation in patients with acute myelogenous leukemia in second remission. *Blood*, **12**, 2282–5.

Meloni, G., Diverio, D., Vignetti, M. *et al.* (1997). Autologous bone marrow transplantation for acute promyelocytic leukemia in second remission: prognostic relevance of pretransplant minimal residual disease assessment by reverse-transcription polymerase chain reaction of the PML/RARα fusion gene. *Blood*, **90**, 1321–1325.

Meloni, G., Vignetti, M., Avvisati, G. *et al.* (1996). BAVC regimen and autograft for acute myelogenous leukemia in second complete remission. *Bone Marrow Transplantation*, **18**, 693–8.

Morschhauser, F., Cayuela, J. M., Martini, S. A. *et al.* (2000). Evaluation of minimal residual disease using reverse-transcription polymerase chain reaction in t(8;21) acute myeloid leukemia: A multicenter study of 51 patients. *Journal of Clinical Oncology*, **18**, 788–794.

Mrozek, K., Heinonen, K., De La Chapelle, A., & Bloomfield, C. D. (1997). Clinical significance of cytogenetics in acute myeloid leukemia. *Seminars in Oncology*, **24**, 17–31.

Nabhan, C., Mehta, J., & Tallman, M. S. (2001). The role of bone marrow transplantation in acute promyelocytic leukemia. *Bone Marrow Transplantation*, **28**, 219–26.

Pendry, K., Alcorn, M. J., & Burnett, A. K. (1993). Factors influencing hematological recovery in 53 patients with acute myeloid leukemia in first remission after autologous bone marrow transplantation. *British Journal of Haematology*, **83**, 45–52.

Petersen, F. B., Lynch, M.H.E., Clift, R. A. *et al.* (1993). Autologous marrow transplantation for patients with acute myeloid leukemia in untreated first relapse or in second complete remission. *Journal of Clinical Oncology*, **11**, 1353–60.

Ravindranath, Y., Yeager, A. M., Chang, M. N. *et al.* (1996). Autologous bone marrow transplantation versus intensive consolidation chemotherapy for acute myeloid leukemia in childhood. *New England Journal of Medicine*, **334**, 1428–34.

Rees, J.K.H., Gray, R. G., & Wheatley, K. (1996). Dose intensive in acute myeloid leukemia: greater effectiveness at lower cost. Principal report of the MRC's AML 9 Study. *British Journal of Haematology*, **94**, 89–98.

Reiffers, J., Gaspard, M. H., Maraninchi, D. *et al.* (1989). Comparison of allogeneic or autologous bone marrow transplantation and chemotherapy in patients with acute myeloid leukaemia in first remission: a prospective controlled trial. *British Journal of Haematology*, **72**, 57–63.

Reiffers, J., Stoppa, A. M., Attal, M. *et al.* (1997). Autologous stem cell transplantation for acute myelogenous leukaemia in adults. In *The BGMT experience in Autologous Marrow and Blood Transplantation VIII*, ed. K. A. Dicke & A. Keating, pp. 22–34. Charlottesville: Carden Jennings Ltd.

Reittie, J. E., Gottlieb, D., Heslop, H. E. *et al.* (1989). Endogenously generated activated killer cells circulate after autologous and allogeneic marrow transplantation but not after chemotherapy. *Blood*, **73**, 1351–8.

Ringden, O., Labopin, M., Gorin, N. C. *et al.* (2000). The dismal outcome in patients with acute leukemia who relapse after an autograft is improved if a second autograft or a matched allograft is performed. *Bone Marrow Transplantation*, **25**, 1053–8.

Rowley, S. D., Jones, R. J., Piantadosi, S. *et al.* (1989). Efficacy of ex vivo purging for autologous bone marrow transplantation in the treatment of acute nonlymphoblastic leukemia. *Blood*, **74**, 501–6.

San Miguel, J. F., Vidriales, M. B., Lopez-Berges, C. *et al.* (2001). Early immunophenotypical evaluation of minimal residual disease in acute myeloid leukemia identifies different patient risk-groups and may contribute to post-induction treatment stratification. *Blood*, **98**, 1746–1751.

Schiffer, C. A., Lee, E. J., Tomiyasu, T. *et al.* (1989). Prognostic impact of cytogenetic abnormalities in patients with de novo acute non-lymphocytic leukemia. *Blood*, **73**, 263–70.

Sharkis, S. J., Santos, G. W., & Colvin, O. M. (1980). Elimination of acute myelogenous leukemia cells from marrow and tumor suspensions in the rat with 4 hydroperoxycyclophosphamide. *Blood*, **55**, 521–3.

Slovak, M., Kopecky, K., Cassileth, P. A. *et al.* (2000). Karyotypic analysis predicts outcome of preremission and postremission therapy in adult acute myeloid leukemia: a Southwest Oncology Group/Eastern Cooperative Oncology Group Study. *Blood*, **96**, 4075–4083.

Stein, A. S., O'Donnell, M. R., Chai, A. *et al.* (1996). In vivo purging with high-dose cytarabine followed by high-dose chemoradiotherapy and reinfusion of unpurged bone marrow for adult acute myelogenous leukemia in first complete remission. *Journal of Clinical Oncology*, **14**, 2206–16.

Tallman, M. S., Anderson, J. W., Schiffer, C. A. *et al.* (1997). All-transretinoic acid in acute promyelocytic leukemia. *New England Journal of Medicine*, **337**, 1021–1028.

Urbano-Ispizua, A., Schmitz, N., de Witte, T. *et al.* (2002). Allogeneic and autologous transplantation for haematological diseases, solid tumors and immune disorders: definition and current practice in Europe. *Bone Marrow Transplantation*, **29**, 639–46.

Venditti, A., Buccisano, F., Del Poeta, C. *et al.* (2000). Level of minimal residual disease after consolidation therapy predicts outcome in acute myeloid leukemia. *Blood,* **96,** 3948–3952.

Wheatley, K., Burnett, A. K., & Gibson, B. (2002). Optimising consolidation therapy: Four versus five courses SCT versus chemotherapy—preliminary results of MRC AML12. *The Hematology Journal,* **3,** 159–160.

Woods, W. G., Neudorf, S., Gold, S. *et al.* (2001). A comparison of allogeneic bone marrow transplantation, autologous bone marrow transplantation, and aggressive chemotherapy in children with acute myeloid leukemia in remission: a report from the Children's Cancer Group. *Blood,* **97,** 56–62.

Yeager, A. M., Kaizer, H., Santos, G. W. *et al.* (1986). Autologous bone marrow transplantation in patients with acute non lymphoblastic leukemia using ex vivo marrow treatment with 4 hydroperoxycyclophosphamide. *New England Journal of Medicine,* **315,** 141–7.

Yin, A. L. & Tobal, K. (1999). Detection of minimal residual disease in acute myeloid leukaemia: methodologies, clinical and biological significance. *British Journal of Haematology,* **106,** 578–590.

Yunis, J. J., Brunning, R. D., Howe, R. B., & Lobell, M. (1984). High-resolution chromosomes as an independent prognostic indicator in adult acute non-lymphocytic leukemia. *New England Journal of Medicine,* **311,** 812–18.

Zittoun, R. A., Mandelli, F., Willemze, R. *et al.* (1995). Autologous or allogeneic bone marrow transplantation compared with intensive chemotherapy in acute myelogenous leukemia. *New England Journal of Medicine,* **332,** 217–23.

37 Autologous hematopoietic stem cell transplantation for acute lymphoblastic leukemia

DANIEL J. WEISDORF

University of Minnesota, Minneapolis, USA

Introduction

Acute lymphoblastic leukemia (ALL) is predominantly a disease of childhood with a peak incidence at age 5 to 6. In adults the incidence increases with age and is highest over age 60. ALL accounts for 15% to 20% of adult acute leukemias. The French-American-British (FAB) classification of ALL is based on morphology and cytochemical staining (Tables 37.1 and 37.2). Additional information on immune phenotype and associated cytogenetic abnormalities and clinical features is shown in Table 37.3. Prognostic factors for outcome with conventional therapy are shown in Table 37.4. Adult ALL is generally thought of as having a worse prognosis than childhood ALL (Table 37.5). The treatment of adult ALL is modeled on the successful therapy of childhood ALL, involving remission induction chemotherapy, various schedules of consolidation, prolonged maintenance therapy, and central nervous system (CNS) prophylaxis. A typical regimen for treatment of adult ALL is shown in Table 37.6 and typical results of conventional therapy in adults in Table 37.7 and Figure 37.1.

Dramatic improvements in the efficacy of multiagent cytotoxic chemotherapy for treatment of ALL have progressively increased the curable fraction of both children (Fig. 37.2) and adults (Copelan & McGuire, 1995; Hoelzer *et al.*, 1996; Kamps *et al.*, 1999; Gokbuget *et al.*, 2000; Thomas *et al.*, 2001). However, those with high-risk ALL in first remission and nearly all patients who relapse will predictably fail conventional approaches to treatment. Although allogeneic hematopoietic stem cell (HSC) transplantation from histocompatible sibling or unrelated donors can be curative, only a proportion (25%–40% in one study) of individuals will have a compatible donor available (Ringdén *et al.*, 1997).

Autologous transplantation utilizes the patient's own bone marrow or peripheral blood progenitor cells for hematopoietic reconstitution after intensive chemotherapy with or without total body irradiation (TBI) conditioning. Successful application of autologous HSC transplantation, however, requires the collection and cryopreservation of suitable numbers of hematopoietic progenitor cells to allow prompt hematologic and immunologic reconstitution. Additionally, measures to address potential contamination of the harvested stem cell inoculum with viable leukemic progenitor cells must be considered. These have included ex vivo bone marrow purging after harvest and before cryopreservation, using either leukemia-associated antigen-directed immunologic purging techniques or ex vivo chemotherapy of the harvested autologous stem cells. Additionally, successful leukemia control after autologous transplantation requires effective antileukemic pretransplant conditioning therapy and, in some recent approaches, posttransplant adjunct treatment to prevent leukemia relapse (Powles *et al.*, 2002). Clinical studies, to date, have variably addressed all these elements in the ongoing development of optimized autologous transplantation for ALL (Fiere *et al.*, 1993; Sebban *et al.*, 1994; Attal *et al.*, 1995; Powles *et al.*, 1995; Marco *et al.*, 2000; Balduzzi *et al.*, 2001; Houtenbos *et al.*, 2001; Martin & Linker, 2001; Gorin, 2002).

Patient selection

ALL comprises a heterogeneous group of leukemias that differ in clinical presentation, immunophenotype, cytogenetics, molecular genetics, and response to therapy. Features that have

Table 37.1. *FAB classification of acute lymphoblastic leukemia (ALL)*

ALL-L1: MPO-negative, with small cells predominating. Cells have a high N/C ratio (scant amount of cytoplasm), regular nuclear borders, and inconspicuous nucleoli. Tdt is usually positive.

ALL-L2: MPO-negative heterogeneous population, often with larger blasts. The cells have a low N/C ratio (moderate amount of cytoplasm), with irregular nuclear borders and prominent nucleoli. Tdt is usually positive.

ALL-L3: Burkitt type: MPO-negative, homogeneous population of large blasts. The cells have a moderate amount of deeply basophilic cytoplasm and prominent cytoplasmic vacuolation. The nuclei are regular, with one or more prominent nucleoli. The blasts are Tdt-negative and may be associated with t(2;8), t(8;14), or t(8;22) chromosomal abnormalities.

Abbreviation: MPO, myeloperoxidase; N/C, nuclear–cytoplasmic.

Table 37.2. *Detailed cytological features of the FAB subtypes of ALL*

Cytological features	L1	L2	L3
Cell size	Small cells predominate	Large, heterogeneous	Large, homogeneous
Nuclear chromatin	Homogeneous	Variable; heterogeneous	Finely stippled and homogeneous
Nuclear shape	Regular, occasional clefting or indentation	Irregular; clefting and indentation common	Regular—oval to round
Nucleoli	Not visible, or small and inconspicuous	One or more present, often large	Prominent; one or more vesicular
Amount of cytoplasm	Scanty	Variable; often moderately abundant	Moderately abundant
Basophilia of cytoplasm	Slight or moderate, rarely intense	Variable; deep in some	Very deep
Cytoplasmic vacuolation	Variable	Variable	Often prominent

been cited as high-risk and predictive of poor response to conventional therapy are shown in Table 37.4 (Ramsay & Kersey, 1990; Copelan & McGuire, 1995; Hagemeijer & Grosveld, 1996; Smith *et al.*, 1996), and the reasons why adults with ALL have a poorer outcome than children with ALL are shown in Table 37.5. Rapid developments in molecular genetic analysis of ALL may refine these clinical prognostic factors to better predict outcome and guide therapeutic decision-making. Outside of prospective controlled research studies, autologous HSC transplantation should be reserved only for patients whose clinical characteristics or response to therapy predict a poor outcome with conventional treatment alone.

Table 37.3. *Immune phenotype, cytogenetic abnormalities, and clinical features*

ALL subtype	CD2	CD5	CD10	CD19	Cμ	SIg	Cytogenetic abnormalities	Frequency Adults	Frequency Children	Clinical features
T ALL	+	+	−	−	−	−	inv(14); t(8;14); t(10;14); t(11;14); t(1;14); t(7;9); del(1); rearrangements 7q32–36; del(6q); del(11); t(7;10); t(10;14); t(14;14); t(4;11)	24%	13%	Often young males; mediastinal mass; increased incidence of hepatosplenomegaly, CNS disease and high WBC count
Early pre-B ALL (sometimes known as pro-B ALL, or pre pre-B ALL)	−	−	+	+	−	−	t(4;11)	11%	5%	Children often less than 1 year old; high WBC, count; increased incidence of hepatosplenomegaly, CNS disease, and high WBC count
Common ALL	−	−	+	+	−	−	Hyperdiploidy; t(9;22); t(1;19); t(9;11); t(5;14); del(9); del(6); +21; t(12;13)	52%	63%	Few significant differences
Pre-B ALL	−	−	±	+	+	−	t(17;19); t(9;22); t(4;11); t(1;19); t(5;14); t(9;11); t(8;14); t(14;18); t(11;19)	9%	16%	Few significant differences
B ALL	−	−	+	+	−	+	t(1;19); t(2;22); del(6q); del(11); t(9;22). Burkitt type: t(8;14); t(2;6)	3%	3%	Abdominal masses; CNS involvement; high incidence of renal involvement; low WBC count; male prevalence

Abbreviations: CNS, central nervous system; WBC, white blood cell.

Table 37.4. *Risk factors predictive of poor response to conventional therapy in ALL*

Beyond first complete remission
Higher white cell count at diagnosis
Delayed achievement of first remission
Extramedullary leukemia
Older patient age
Immunophenotype other than common (pre-B) ALL
Karyotype: Ph⁺; t(4;11); t(8;14); hypodiploidy
Molecular genotype:
    rearrangements or fusions in *MLL/HRX/ALL-1: AF4/FEL: BCR-ABL; E2A-PBX; IgH-MYC; TAL-1; TCR*

Abbreviations: ALL, acute lymphoblastic leukemia; Ph⁺, Philadelphia chromosome.

In first remission, transplantation should only be considered for children exhibiting leukemic characteristics definitively predictive of a poor outcome. These would include the Philadelphia chromosome [t(9;22)] or other structural chromosome anomalies such as t(4;11) or t(8;14). In addition, those failing to achieve first complete remission by 12 weeks of chemotherapy might be considered for transplantation.

Adults (older than 18 years) generally have poorer responses to chemotherapy and shorter duration of remission, thus suggesting the potential value of early intensive therapy including HSC transplantation (Barrett *et al.*, 1989; Copelan & McGuire, 1995). HSC transplantation can be considered as consolidation treat-

Table 37.5. *Features of adult ALL that contribute to poor prognosis compared with children*

Disease biology
1. Cytogenetics
    Increased incidence of poor prognostic changes, e.g., t(9;22), t(8;14)
2. Immunophenotype
    Increased incidence of expression of myeloid antigens; less frequent early pre B-immunophenotype
3. Drug metabolism
    Decreased formation of methotrexate polyglutamates; increased incidence of MDR-1 expression at relapse
4. Other
    Increased incidence of high leukocyte count at presentation
    Slow response to therapy
    Increased frequency of mediastinal masses
Treatment tolerance
1. Marrow
    Decreased tolerance predisposing to treatment delays, increased life-threatening infections
2. Extramedullary organs
    Increased toxicity—hepatic, cardiac
3. Poor tolerance of specific agents, e.g., high doses of L-asparaginase
4. Poorer compliance with intensive protocols

Reproduced with permission from Copelan & McGuire, 1995

Table 37.6. *An example of a conventional chemotherapy regime for adult acute lymphoblastic leukemia*

Drug	Dose	Route/Day
Induction		
Phase 1 (4 weeks)		
prednisone	60 mg/m²	po day 1–28
vincristine	1.5 mg/m² (max 2.0 mg)	i.v. day 1, 8, 15, 22
daunorubicin	25 mg/m²	i.v. day 1, 8, 15, 22
L-asparaginase	5000 U/m²	i.v. day 1–14
Phase 2 (4 weeks)		
cyclophosphamide	650 mg/m²	i.v. day 29, 43, 57
cytosine arabinoside	75 mg/m²	i.v. day 31–34, 38–41, 45–48, 52–55
6-mercaptopurine	60 mg/m²	po day 29–57
methotrexate	10 mg/m² (max 15 mg)	i.t. day 31, 38, 45, 52
First maintenance (8 weeks)		
6-mercaptopurine	60 mg/m²	po daily weeks 10–18
methotrexate	20 mg/m²	Po or i.v. weekly for weeks 10–18
Consolidation (begins week 20)		
Phase 1 (4 weeks)		
dexamethasone	10 mg/m²	po day 1–26
vincristine	1.5 mg/m² (max 2.0 mg)	i.v. day 1, 8, 15, 22
doxorubicin	25 mg/m²	i.v. day 1, 8, 15, 22
Phase 2 (2 weeks)		
cyclophosphamide	650 mg/m² (max 1000 mg)	i.v. day 29
cytosine arabinoside	75 mg/m²	i.v. day 31–34, 38–41
thioguanine	60 mg/m²	po day 29–42
Second maintenance (2 years)		
6-mercaptopurine	60 mg/m²	po daily 29–130
methotrexate	20 mg/m²	po or i.v. weekly for weeks 29–130

Note: CNS prophylaxis—if CR obtained in Phase 1, CNS prophylaxis starts during Phase 2. If CR not obtained by completion of Phase 2, prophylaxis begun when CR obtained. Prophylaxis consists of cranial radiation (2400 cGy) and i.t. methotrexate (10 mg/m²) once a week for 4 weeks.

Reproduced, with permission, from Hoelzer *et al.* (1988).

ment in first complete remission for adults with particular high-risk features including slow response to therapy (no remission within 4 weeks), elevated initial leukocyte count, structural chromosome anomalies, hypodiploidy, or extramedullary leukemia.

Patients of all ages suffering an isolated extramedullary or bone marrow relapse and achieving second remission are suitable candidates for transplantation (Messina *et al.*, 1998) (Fig. 37.3). Some studies have reported extended disease-free survival in second complete remission (CR2) for children relapsing after completion of first remission maintenance therapy (i.e., CR1 greater than 24 months). However, even in this most

Table 37.7. *Results with conventional therapy of ALL in adults*

Risk Factor	CR1 (%)	DFS (%)
Age <60 years	75	35
Age >60 years	40	0–20
t(9;22) or *bcr-abl* positive	50	0–10
T-lineage ALL	80	45–60
B-lineage ALL	70	40

favorable CR2 subgroup, most patients will again relapse after conventional treatment.

Disease-specific pretransplant work-up

Because the major reason for failure after autotransplantation is leukemia recurrence, the critical factor establishing patient suitability for autologous transplantation is confirmation of complete bone marrow and extramedullary remission. Bone marrow morphology as well as cytogenetic, flow cytometry, and molecular (PCR) assays, if they were informative at diagnosis, must be repeated and confirmed in remission prior to autotransplantation. Additionally, extended, multiparameter flow cytometry may identify a leukemia-associated phenotype (e.g., CD10+, CD19+ for pre-B ALL) characteristic of leukemia precursors. Identification of detectable minimal residual disease by cytogenetics, molecular profile, or immunophenotype must be considered a relative, and probably an absolute, contraindication to proceeding with autologous harvest and subsequent transplantation unless confirmed complete remission can be established after additional therapy.

In addition, examination of cerebrospinal fluid by routine cytology should be performed preharvest and, as indicated, pretransplant. While the specific outcomes of patients with minimal, asymptomatic pretransplant central nervous system (CNS) leukemia have not been reported, identification of occult, asymptomatic CNS disease may be an indication for additional intrathecal chemotherapy to establish CNS remission. Occult CNS leukemia prior to autotransplantation may also indicate the need to use TBI and/or supplemental cranial radiotherapy.

General multi-organ screening and documentation of suitable performance status, as well as evaluation for occult opportunistic infection are also important. These may be less critical prior to autotransplantation since the degree of immunocompromise and risk of opportunistic mycotic or viral infection posttransplant are substantially lower than after an allograft.

Purging

During morphologically confirmed complete remission, marrow blasts are not recognizable microscopically, but it is generally accepted that viable clonogenic leukemia progenitor cells might proliferate and result in relapse if reinfused along with the cryopreserved autologous HSCs (Uckun *et al.,* 1987; Yamada *et al.,* 1990). Most clinical experience to date has, therefore, utilized ex vivo purging to deplete or eliminate leukemic progenitors from the HSC inoculum. The varying methods utilized are shown in Table 37.8.

Purging techniques in ALL have used primarily immunologic methods directed toward leukemia-associated antigens expressed on the cell surface. Monoclonal antibodies against B-lineage antigens (CD9, CD10, CD19, CD20, CD22, CD24) or T-lineage antigens (CD5, CD7) have been used to opsonize cells and trigger the lytic capacity of exogenous complement.

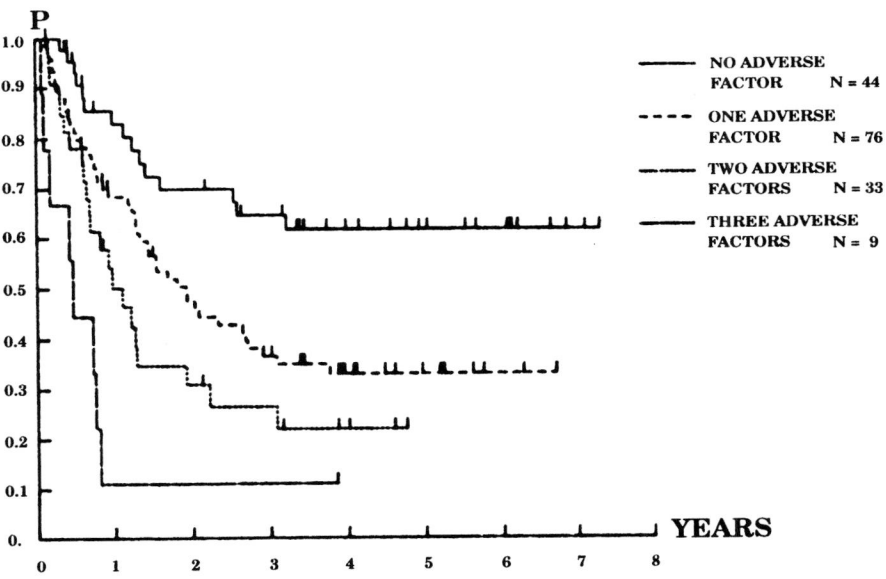

Fig. 37.1. Probability of continuous complete remission for patients having 0, 1, 2, or 3 adverse prognostic factors defined as: time to CR >4 weeks; age >35 years; WBC at diagnosis >30 × 10⁹/L; null (now pre pre-B) ALL. Reproduced, with permission, from Hoelzer *et al.* (1988).

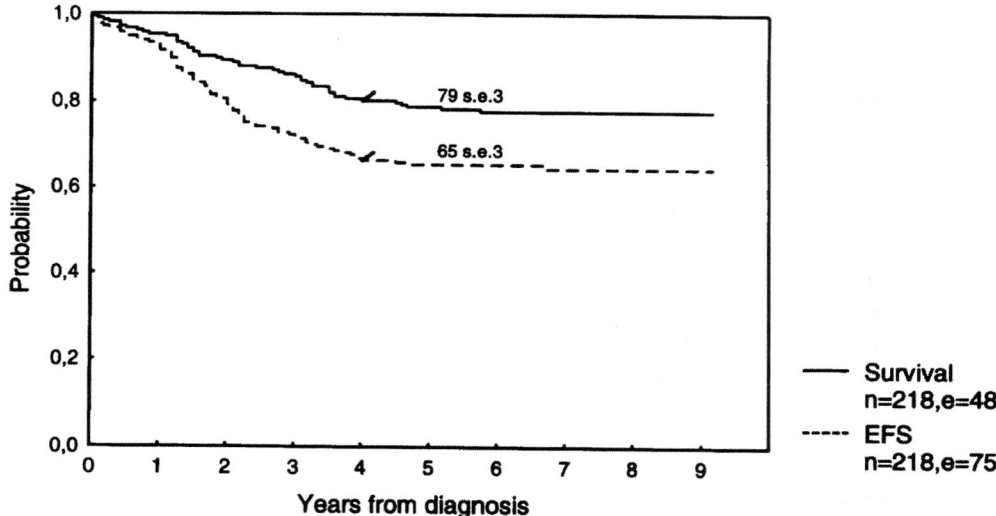

Fig. 37.2. Survival and EFS of 218 newly diagnosed ALL patients treated according to DCSLG protocol ALL-7. Reproduced, with permission, from Kamps *et al.* (1999).

Alternatively, such antibodies have been combined with chemical toxins (ricin, pokeweed antiviral protein) as chemical or recombinant immune conjugates. These immunotoxins use the specificity of the monoclonal antibody and are able to selectively poison cells expressing the leukemia-associated antigen while sparing hematopoietic progenitors (Uckun *et al.*, 1987, 1990; Roy *et al.*, 1990).

Ex vivo incubation of marrow with low-dose chemotherapy designed to exploit the therapeutic window between leukemic

cell sensitivity and hematopoietic progenitor sensitivity has also been used. Most frequently, 4-hydroperoxycyclophosphamide (4HC) has been used either alone or in combination with immunological purging techniques. Some reports have correlated the number of clonogenic leukemia progenitors present after purging with the clinical results of autologous transplantation (Simonsson *et al.*, 1989; Uckun *et al.*, 1990, 1992;

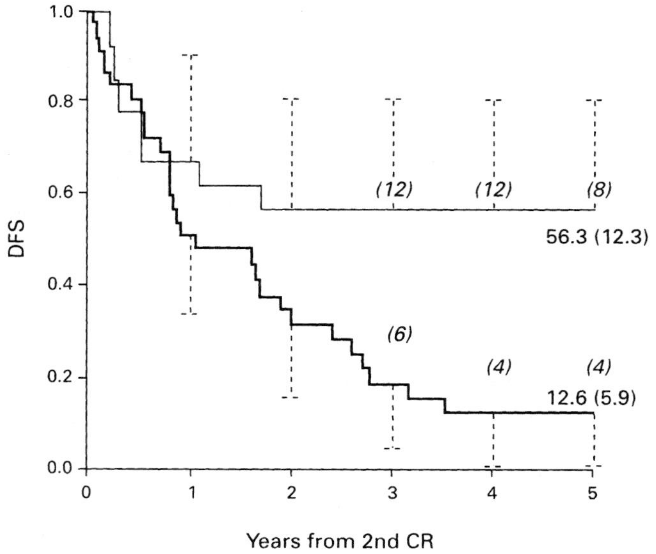

Table 37.8. *Purging techniques in ALL*

Immunological techniques
  Antileukemia monoclonal antibodies
    B lineage CD9, 10, 19, 20, 22, 24
    T lineage CD2, 3, 5, 7
  Targeted cell depletion
    Complement lysis
    Depletion with immunomagnetic beads
    Antibody conjugated to toxins (immunotoxins) (e.g., ricin or
      pokeweed antiviral protein)
    CD34 selection
Ex vivo chemotherapy
  4-hydroperoxycyclophosphamide (4HC)
  Vincristine
  Corticosteroids
Combined immunochemotherapy
  Antibody + complement + 4HC
  Immunotoxin + 4HC
Assessment of purging efficacy
  Clonogenic cell culture assay (CFU-L)
  FACS sorting (CD19+, surface immunoglobulin) followed by
    colony forming assay (LPC)
  Immunophenotype plus TdT immunostaining
  Polymerase chain reaction (PCR)

Abbreviations: ALL, acute lymphoblastic leukemia; CFU-L, colony forming unit-leukemia; FACS, fluorescence activated cell sorter; LPC, leukemia progenitor cell.

Fig. 37.3. Adjusted DFS curves comparing the outcome in the chemo (bottom curve) and ABMT groups (the number of patients at risk is reported on curves in parentheses). Pointwise 95% confidence intervals (CI) are indicated for the curve (only one side of the symmetric CI is plotted for simplicity). Reproduced, with permission, from Messina *et al.* (1998).

Campana & Pui, 1995). Such correlations have been interpreted as supporting the efficacy of ex vivo purging. Pretransplant or peritransplant administration of imatinib could be valuable for Ph+ ALL, though formal studies evaluating its utility in this setting have not been reported.

Pretransplant conditioning

Autologous transplantation usually produces less transplant-related morbidity and mortality than allogeneic transplantation. In most studies, similar pretransplant conditioning has been employed for autologous and allogeneic transplants (Kersey et al., 1987; Buckner et al., 1989; Blaise et al., 1990; Zintl et al., 1990; Cahn et al., 1991; Uderzo et al., 1991; Fiere et al., 1993; Sebban et al., 1994; Attal et al., 1995; Thiebaut et al., 2000; Mori et al., 2001; Al-Khasim et al., 2002; Soto et al., 2002). However, the additional safety of autologous transplantation might justify using more intensive and possibly more effective conditioning regimens. This approach has not yet been fully explored. Pretransplant conditioning has most often included TBI in single or multiple fractions delivered at varying dose rates, energies, and total doses. Fractionated TBI is often used and is reported to induce less acute toxicity than single-dose TBI. Techniques to protect vulnerable tissues (lung shielding) and intensify antileukemic radiation (chest wall boosting) have also been evaluated. Imaginative delivery techniques including radioimmune conjugates or radiochemicals that accumulate in the marrow cavity are being developed experimentally to more effectively deplete the body leukemia burden. Although high-dose cyclophosphamide (100–200 mg/kg) has been the standard chemotherapy agent used with TBI before transplantation, some reports have shown favorable results using cytosine arabinoside, etoposide, melphalan, or combination drug chemoradiotherapy (Table 37.9). No new regimen has shown results definitively superior to cyclophosphamide and TBI.

Minimal residual disease (and see Chapters 105 and 106)

After autologous HSC transplantation for ALL, the most frequent cause of treatment failure is leukemia relapse. As discussed above, this may be due to residual clonogenic leukemia reinfused within the purged HSCs, but more likely may represent residual resistant leukemia surviving in vivo despite intensive pretransplant conditioning. Detection of minimal residual disease (MRD) remaining at the time of clinical remission or following pretransplant conditioning has been difficult, although several techniques show promise in their ability to reliably determine the quality of residual leukemia (Simonsson et al., 1989; Uckun et al., 1990, 1992; Yamada et al., 1990; Campana & Pui, 1995).

At the University of Minnesota, fluorescence-activated cell sorter analysis in combination with in vitro culture has been used to quantify residual leukemia progenitor cells (LPC) within the marrow graft both before and after ex vivo purging. This assay has been used to test the efficacy of ex vivo purging, to determine the radiosensitivity of residual leukemia, and, most important perhaps, to define the quality of remission in patients undergoing transplantation. In two series of ALL patients undergoing autologous transplantation, residual leukemia before purging (representing the whole body leukemia burden before conditioning) was the most important factor predicting posttransplantation relapse. Patients with more than the median number of LPC (50 to 80 LPC/10^6 marrow mononuclear cells) had a greater than 90% chance of relapse within 1 year of autologous transplantation. Those with fewer LPC in their remission marrows had only a 60% chance of relapse and, accordingly, superior disease-free survival (Uckun et al., 1990, 1992). More precise determination of minimal residual disease in this fashion might allow tailoring of additional therapies (more intense conditioning, posttransplant maintenance chemotherapy or immunotherapy), for patients in demonstrably higher risk categories.

Molecular genetic determinations of rearranged fusion genes have been used as markers of MRD. Using the sensitive polymerase chain reaction (PCR), the rearranged leukemia-associated clonal gene products (e.g., IgH or *TCR* genes) or fusion proto-oncogenes (e.g., BCL-2, BCR-ABL, TAL-1, BCR-Abl) have been tested for their ability to quantify MRD during remission. PCR may also be applicable in evaluating residual clonal cells within a graft (purged or not). The utility of such highly sensitive assays requires additional study and clinical correlation (Campana & Pui, 1995).

Clinical results

More than 20 centers have reported results on autografts for patients with ALL and the results of the largest series are summarized in Table 37.9, and data from the Autologous Blood and Marrow Transplant Registry (ABMTR) in Figure 37.4. As shown, results are superior for patients undergoing transplantation earlier in their disease course (first complete remission). In all series reviewed, leukemia relapse is both frequent and early and is by far the most common cause of treatment failure. One study with 12-year follow-up described a disease-free and overall survival rate of 38% for adults transplanted in second or subsequent remission or in first remission with high-risk disease (Abdallah et al., 2001).

Peritransplant morbidity in most series is modest, and nonrelapse mortality averages 10% (range 5% to 22%). In 214 autograft recipients at the University of Minnesota and the Dana-Farber Cancer Institute, nonrelapse mortality was 15% and was similar in adults and children (Weisdorf et al., 1997). Transplant-related complications may be less frequent in patients transplanted during first or second complete remission, but this was not observed in all reports.

The heterogeneity between reported studies of autotransplantation in ALL makes direct comparisons difficult. Patient age, remission status at time of transplantation, and leukemia

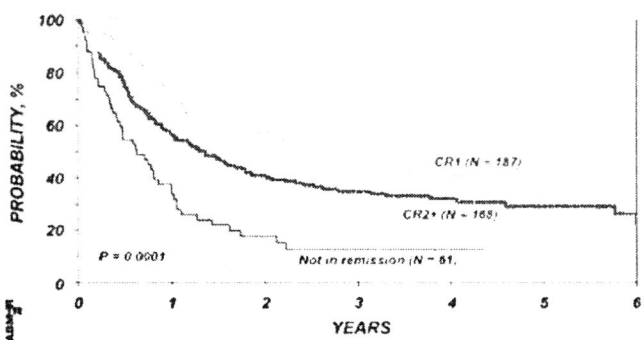

Fig. 37.4. Probability of survival after autotransplants for acute lymphoblastic leukemia, 1994–99. Three-year probabilities of survival were 44 ± 9%, 36 ± 9%, and 12 ± 9% in CR1, CR2+ or in relapse, respectively. Reproduced, with permission, from ABMTR Newsletter, **9**, 1.

characteristics including immunophenotype, white blood count at diagnosis, karyotype, and extramedullary leukemic involvement differ widely between centers and are often unreported. In addition, conditioning regimens and purging techniques are also heterogeneous (Table 37.9). Overall, leukemia relapse after autologous transplantation for ALL occurs in 45% to 90% of patients and yields 2-year disease-free survival ranging from an average of 35% to 45% during first complete remission and 15% to 40% during second or third complete remission. The conclusions drawn in nearly every report indicate the need for more effective antileukemic therapy and suggest the need for future studies of improved pretransplant conditioning, maintenance therapy, or posttransplant immunotherapy.

The innate chemotherapeutic sensitivity of the leukemia, reflected in the duration of first CR, may be the best clinical predictor of response, as favorable results have been seen in young recipients of CR2 autografts following a very long initial remission (Billett et al., 1993). This has not been corroborated in adults or other series (Soiffer et al., 1993).

A single-center report comparing disease-free survival after autologous or unrelated donor transplantation for patients with advanced acute leukemia (ALL or acute myeloid leukemia) found no significant difference between the two regardless of whether the transplant procedure was undertaken in remission (Fig. 37.5) or in relapse (Fig. 37.6) (Busca et al., 1994).

A similar study from the University of Minnesota and Dana-Farber Cancer Center found greater transplant-related mortality, less relapse, and superior disease-free survival in patients given unrelated transplants in CR2 (Weisdorf et al., 1997) (Figs. 37.7 and 37.8).

A large analysis has compared autologous transplants for ALL from ABMTR to unrelated donor (URD) transplants facilitated through the National Marrow Donor Program. This study found greater transplant-related mortality, lower relapse, and superior disease-free survival in patients receiving unrelated transplants, but only those with favorable fea-

tures suggesting lower risk disease (i.e., white blood cell count <50,000/μl; CR1 >1 year; Karnofsky ≥90%). In this lower risk group 3 year disease-free survival after autologous grafting was inferior in both children and adults (autologous ≤20 years 30%; >20 years; 32% vs. URD ≤20 years 53%; >20 years 48%). Patients with higher risk ALL had similar outcomes using autologous or unrelated grafts resulting in similar 3 year leukemia-free survival (1 risk factor autologous 41 ± 15% versus URD 42 ± 8%; 2+ risk factors autologous 20 ± 25% versus URD 25 ± 11%) (Weisdorf et al., 2002) (Fig 37.9).

Monitoring for residual disease posttransplant

Similar to the multiparameter assays used to determine minimal residual disease and/or confirm complete remission prior to autotransplantation, bone marrow cytogenetic, molecular and/or multiparameter flow cytometry studies may be used to identify occult minimal residual disease after chemotherapy or grafting (Mortuza et al., 2002; Sanchez et al., 2002). Importantly, however, outside of a research setting used to determine the clinical association or predictive value of MRD testing post-autotransplantation, routine screening for occult leukemia is only valuable if therapeutic interventions are available. Early identification of post-autograft MRD may be useful if alternative therapies such as imatinib for Ph+ ALL, immunoconjugate therapy (using immunotoxins or radioimmunotoxins) or investigational chemotherapy or immunotherapy (molecular or cellular vaccines) are available. Alternatively, if allogeneic stem cell transplantation using available donors is to be considered, early donor identification and consideration of early allografting for definitive or progressing MRD may be indicated and thus also justify serial assays for MRD post-autografting.

Adjunct antileukemia therapy after autologous HSC transplantation

The first reports of curative therapy for childhood ALL emphasized that extended duration of maintenance chemotherapy was critical for long-term disease control. However, the compromised marrow reserve of autograft recipients has impaired attempts to test maintenance therapy after transplantation. In one small controlled trial at the University of Minnesota, posttransplant maintenance therapy (after allogeneic and autologous transplantation) was both difficult to deliver and ineffective at preventing or delaying leukemia relapse (Weisdorf et al., 1987), although others have had a better experience (Tiley et al., 1993; Powles et al., 2002).

Current approaches to adjunct therapy have focused on nonspecific immunotherapy or immunotoxins directed at leukemia-associated antigens. Activation of cytotoxic T lymphocytes (CTL) or natural killer (NK) cells with recombinant interleukin 2 (IL-2) has received considerable interest. Interleukin-2 has been given in high doses, often in conjunc-

Table 37.9.   Results of autologous hematopoietic stem cell transplantation in ALL

Author	Remission status	n (total)	Conditioning	Purging	Disease-free survival	Time post-BMT	Relapse
Attal et al. (1995)	CR1	77	Cy TBI	Mafosfamide or immunobeads	26%	3 years	73%
Abdallah (2001)	CR1	14	TBI, variable		38%	4 years	47%[b]
	CR2+	18					
Balduzzi et al. (2001)	CR2	11	TBI, Cy, VP-16	Mab beads	89%	2 years	10%
Billett et al. (1993)	CR2+	51	Cy,CA, VM-26 TBI	Mab + C'	53%	3 years	42%
Blaise et al. (1990)	CR1	22	TBI + Cy or Melphalan	–	40%	3 years	52%
Buckner et al. (1989)	CR1	143	TBI + CY	Mab + C'	54%	2 years	36%
	CR2	23			17%		75%
Cahn et al. (1991)	CR1	6 (26)	TBI, CA	Mafosfamide or Mab + C'	28%	3.6 years	62%
	CR2	16	Melphalan				
	CR3+	4					
Carey et al. (1991)	CR1	15	Melphalan + TBI	–	48%	3 years	NR
Colleselli et al. (1994)	CR2	75	Variable	Mafosfamide or VCR + steroids	28%	5 years	59%[b]
Doney et al. (1993)	CR1	10	Cy TBI + other	Mab + C'	50%	2 years	30%
	CR2+	52			27%		69%
	Relapse	27			8%		
Fiere et al. (1993)	CR1	63[c] (95)	Cy TBI	Mab + C'	39%[c] (51%)	3 years	57%[b,c]
Gilmore et al. (1991)	CR1	27	CY + TBI ± CA	Mab + C'	32%	7 years	67%
Gonzales-Chambers et al. (1991)	CR1,2 Relapse	7 (10) 3	CY + TBI ±VCR + steriods	Mab + C' 4 HC	32% 3/10[b]	43 months	60%
Gorin et al. (1990)	CR1	233 (438) 205	Variable	Variable	41% 27%	>3 years	53% 70%
Gorin et al. (2002)	CR1 (adult)	366	Variable	Variable	36%	5 years	60%
	CR1 (children)	269			50%	5 years	
Houtenbos et al. (2001)	CR2+ (Peds)	19 (24)	TBI, Cy, VP-16, Ver	Ver, VCR, VP-16	42%	2 years	58%[b]
Laporte et al. (1994)	CR1	35	Cy, TBI	Mafosfamide	56%	8 years	37%
Marco et al. (2000)	CR1, 2 (infants)	18 (26)	Bu + Cy, variable	Mab, variable	56%	5 years	40%[b]
Meloni et al. (1990)	CR1	9 (30)	Bu + Cy	Mafosfamide	3/9[b]	–	5/9[b]
	CR2	16			6/16	–	9/16
	CR3	5			3/15	–	2/5
Parsons et al. (1996)	CR2+	57	Cy, VP-16, TBI	Immunomagnetic beads	47%	3 years	47%
Schmid et al. (1993)	CR2,3+	22	VP-16, fTBI		18%	4 years	80%
Schroeder et al. (1991)	CR2	17 (24)	Melphalan + TBI	Campath-1	12/24[a,b]	25 months	NR
	CR3	7					
Sebban et al. (1994)	CR1	40	Cy + TBI		31%	5 years	62%
Simonsson et al. (1989)	CR1	21 (54)	TBI + CY ± multidrug	Mab + C'	65%	> 2 years	6/21[b]
	CR2	29			31%		18/32
	CR3+	4					
Soiffer (1990)	CR1	2 (80)	Cy + fTBI ± CA	Mab + C'	34%	4 years	29/80[b]
	CR2	48					
	CR3+	30					
Spinolo et al. (1990)	CR1	26	CY, BCNU, VP-16	–	54%	4 years	10/26[b]

(Continues)

Table 37.9. (Continued)

Author	Remission status	n (total)	Conditioning	Purging	Disease-free survival	Time post-BMT	Relapse
Stoppa et al. (1990)	CR1 CR2, 3+	6 (12) 6	TBI ± Melphalan ± Cy	Immunomagnetic beads (CD10, CD19)	3/6[b] 3/6	1 year	3/6[b] 3/6
Thiebaut et al. (2000)	CR	95	Cy TBI	Mab + C'	34%[a]	10 years	
Uderzo et al. (1991)	CR1	12 (35)	Vincristine, Cy fTBI	Vincristine Mafosfamide + steroids	50%	2 years	47%
	CR2	13					
	CR3+	10					
Vey et al. (1994)	CR1	24	Cy TBI; Mel TBI	Mab + variable	27%	6 years	65%
Weisdorf et al. (1997)	CR1	51	fTBI + Cy or CA	Mab + C' or immunotoxin + 4HC	42%	3 years	53%
	CR2+	98			20%		76%
	CR3	40			19%		74%
Weisdorf (2002)	CR1	74	Variable	Variable (57%)	31%	5 years	49%
	CR2	121			27%		64%
Zintl et al. (1990)	CR1	6 (15)	TBI + Cy	–	43%	2.5 years	54%
	CR2,3	9					

Summary	Disease-free survival	Relapse
CR1	35–45%	45–60%
CR2	20–40%	50–75%
CR3+	15–30%	60–90%

Abbreviations: Mab, monoclonal antibody; NR, not reported; EBMTG, European Bone Marrow Transplant Group; f, fractionated; C', complement; Bu, busulfan; CA, cytosine arabinoside; CR, complete remission; Cy, cyclophosphamide; TBI, total body irradiation; ALL, acute lymphoblastic leukemia; BMT, bone marrow transplant; Ver, verapamil; VCR, vincristine.

[a] Survival, not disease free
[b] Not Kaplan-Meier projection
[c] 95 randomized to ABMT reported as intention to treat; (63 actually transplanted)

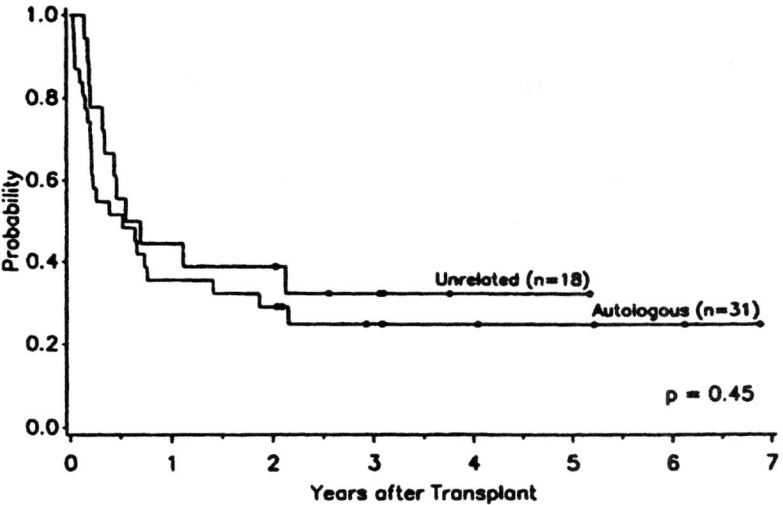

Fig. 37.5. Probability of disease-free survival in unrelated or autologous marrow recipients who were transplanted in remission (P = .45). Reproduced, with permission, from Busca *et al.* (1994).

tion with exogenously cultured lymphokine-activated killer (LAK) cells, and has demonstrated antineoplastic activity in various human tumors, including some lymphoid neoplasms. However, excessive toxicity associated with high-dose IL-2/LAK cell therapy has stimulated interest in more modest, and hopefully less toxic, applications of IL-2 after autologous transplantation. No reports have yet demonstrated clinically useful antineoplastic activity of IL-2 given after autologous transplantation, but immune activation (either CTL, NK, or LAK) has been observed. An earlier Minnesota trial of IL-2 given immediately postautologous transplantation for ALL resulted in enhancement of CTL activity against ALL target cells (Weisdorf *et al.*, 1993). In other studies, low-dose, long-duration IL-2 therapy induced potent NK/LAK activation in autologous bone marrow transplant recipients (Soiffer *et al.*, 1992). One randomized trial showed no benefit of postautograft IL-2 (Attal *et al.*, 1995). Ongoing studies will be required to test the clinical utility of immune effector mechanisms induced by IL-2 administration.

Monoclonal antibodies or immunotoxins (Uckun *et al.*, 1992; Roy *et al.*, 1990) have also been considered for in vivo use in the posttransplant setting. Because of their specificity in targeting leukemia-associated antigens and because they are not suppressive of marrow function, this approach is theoretically well suited to the eradication of MRD posttransplant.

These and other adjunct therapies may substitute for the missing graft-versus-leukemia effect, which accounts for some of the antileukemic potential of allogeneic transplantation

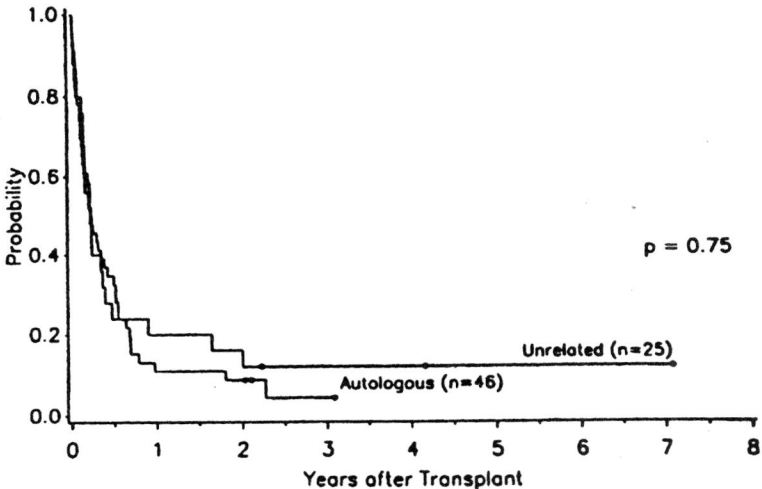

Fig. 37.6. Probability of disease-free survival in unrelated or autologous marrow recipients who were transplanted in relapse (P = .75). Reproduced, with permission, from Busca *et al.* (1994).

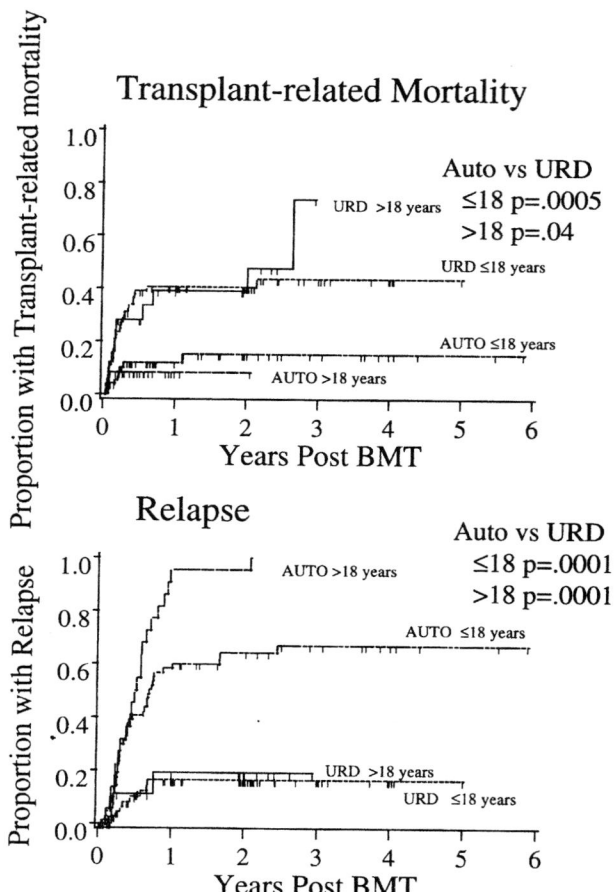

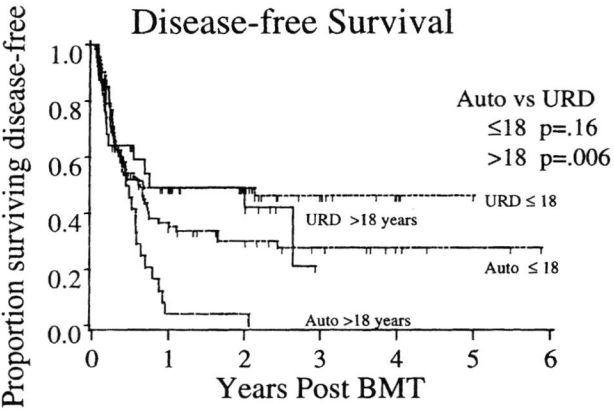

Fig. 37.7. TRM and relapse after autologous or URD BMT for ALL in CR2. Reproduced, with permission, from Weisdorf *et al.* (1997).

Fig. 37.8. DFS after transplantation for ALL in CR2. Shown are Kaplan-Meier projections of outcome for autologous and unrelated donor allogeneic marrow: recipients divided by age >18 years. *P* values shown represent log-rank tests of significance between autologous and age strata. Reproduced, with permission, from Weisdorf *et al.* (1997).

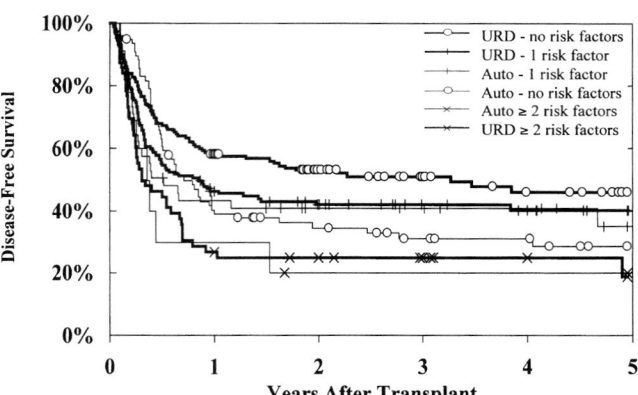

Fig. 37.9. DFS after either URD or autologous BMT using risk factors of short (<1 year) initial remission, WBC $\geq 50 \times 10^9/l$ and/or Karnofsky <90%. DFS for patients with 0, 1 or ≥ 2 risk factors were compared. Reproduced, with permission, from Weisdorf *et al.*, 2002.

(Weisdorf *et al.*, 1987). Future experimental and clinical studies have the potential to expand the applicability and effectiveness of autologous transplantation in ALL.

Indications and contraindications for autologous transplantation

Because of progressive improvements in chemotherapy management of ALL for both children and adults, autotransplant approaches must still be reserved for those expected to fail, or having failed, conventional chemotherapy. Autologous transplantation still requires improvement but may be indicated in atients with high-risk ALL in CR1 (Ph+, white blood cell count >50,000–100,000/μl, no CR after 30 days) or all patients in CR2 or CR3. Because allografts may be valuable in this setting, autograft candidates must lack an available sibling donor or be unsuited for unrelated bone marrow or peripheral blood transplants (Saarinen-Pihkala *et al.*, 2001; Woolfrey *et al.*, 2002). Autografts may also be indicated in older adults (>35 years) or younger adults (18–35) with no well-matched unrelated donor (allele-matched at HLA-A, -B, -C, and DRB1) available. Umbilical cord blood allografts may be considered, though formal data comparing their outcome to autografts has not been reported (Barker *et al.*, 2001; Rocha *et al.*, 2001).

The current practice of HSC transplantation for ALL in Europe has been described (Urbano-Ispizua *et al.*, 2002) (and see Chapter 124, Breaking News...).

Contraindications to autologous transplantation include no sustained bone marrow and extramedullary complete remission, especially as documented by cytogenetic, molecular, or immunophenotypic profile. Additional relative contraindications may include disease beyond CR3, even if in remission. Patients without a graft containing sufficient CD34 cells, or with a graft known to be contaminated with recognizable residual leukemia by either cytologic or more sensitive techniques, should not proceed to autotransplantation.

An algorithm for the treatment of patients with acute lymphoblastic leukemia

Interpreting these indications and contraindications for auto-transplantation suggest that conventional multi-drug induction and consolidation therapy are still the mainstays of management for all patients with ALL. Those with high-risk disease can be considered for allotransplantation in first remission and, if no allogeneic donor is available, autografts can be considered as well. In CR2 and CR3, sibling donor allografts are preferred, but unrelated donor marrow or peripheral blood or cord blood transplants can be considered. Autografts in CR2 or CR3, for patients with standard risk disease, are appropriate. Leukemia risk features, performance status, and clinical morbidity should guide the choice of unrelated donor allogeneic versus autologous transplantation.

References

Abdallah, A., Egerer, G., Goldschmidt, H. *et al.* (2001). Continuous complete remission in adult patients with acute lymphocytic leukaemia at a median observation of 12 years after autologous bone marrow transplantation. *British Journal of Haematology,* **112,** 1012–15.

ABMTR Newsletter (2002). **9,** 1.

Al-Kasim, F. A., Thornley, I., Rolland, M. *et al.* (2002). Single-centre experience with allogeneic bone marrow transplantation for acute lymphoblastic leukaemia in childhood: similar survival after matched-related and matched-unrelated donor transplants. *British Journal of Haematology,* **116,** 483–90.

Attal, M., Blaise, D., Marit, G. *et al.* (1995). Consolidation treatment of adult acute lymphoblastic leukemia: a prospective, randomized trial comparing allogeneic versus autologous bone marrow transplantation and testing the impact of recombinant interleukin-2 after autologous bone marrow transplantation. *Blood,* **86,** 1619–28.

Balduzzi, A., Gaipa, G., Bonanomi, S. *et al.* (2001). Purified autologous grafting in childhood acute lymphoblastic leukemia in second remission: evidence of long-term clinical and molecular remissions. *Leukemia,* **15,** 50–6.

Barker, J. N., Davies, S. M., DeFor, T. *et al.* (2001). Survival after transplantation of unrelated donor umbilical cord blood is comparable to that of human leukocyte antigen-matched unrelated donor bone marrow: results of a matched-pair analysis. *Blood,* **97,** 2957–61.

Barrett, A. J., Horowitz, M. M., Gale, R. *et al.* (1989). Marrow transplantation for acute lymphoblastic leukemia: factors affecting relapse and survival. *Blood,* **74,** 862–71.

Billett, A. L., Kornmehl, E., Tarbell, N. J. *et al.* (1993). Autologous bone marrow transplantation after a long first remission for children with recurrent acute lymphoblastic leukemia. *Blood,* **81,** 1651–7.

Blaise, D., Gaspard, M. H., Stopa, A. M. *et al.* (1990). Allogeneic or autologous bone marrow transplantation for acute lymphoblastic leukemia in first complete remission. *Bone Marrow Transplantation,* **5,** 7–12.

Buckner, C. D., Sanders, J. E., Hill, R. *et al.* (1989). Allogeneic versus autologous marrow transplantation for patients with acute lymphoblastic leukemia in first or second marrow remission. In *Autologous Bone Marrow Transplantation, Proceedings of the Fourth International Symposium,* ed. K. A. Dicke, G. Spitzer, S. Jagannath, & M. J. Evinger-Hodges, pp. 145–149, The University of Texas: M. D. Anderson Cancer Center.

Busca, A., Anasetti, C., Anderson, G. *et al.* (1994). Unrelated donor or autologous marrow transplantation for treatment of acute leukemia. *Blood,* **83,** 3077–84.

Cahn, J. Y., Bordingoni, P., Souillet, G. *et al.* (1991). The TAM regimen prior to allogeneic and autologous bone marrow transplantation for high-risk acute lymphoblastic leukemias: a cooperative study of 62 patients. *Bone Marrow Transplantation,* **7,** 1–4.

Campana, D. & Pui, C-H. (1995). Detection of minimal residual disease in acute leukemia: methodologic advances and clinical significance. *Blood,* **85,** 1416–34.

Carey, P. J., Proctor, S. J., Taylor, P. *et al.* (1991). Autologous bone marrow transplantation for high-grade lymphoid malignancy using melphalan/irradiation conditioning without marrow purging or cryopreservation. The Northern Regional Bone Marrow Transplant Group. *Blood,* **77,** 1593–8.

Colleselli, P., Rossetti, F., Messina, C. *et al.* (1994). Autologous bone marrow transplantation for childhood acute lymphoblastic leukemia in remission: first choice for isolated extramedullary relapse. *Bone Marrow Transplantation,* **14,** 821–5.

Copelan, E. A. & McGuire, E. A. (1995). The biology and treatment of acute lymphoblastic leukemia in adults. *Blood,* **85,** 1151–68.

Doney, K., Buckner, C. D., Fisher, L. *et al.* (1993). Autologous bone marrow transplantation for acute lymphoblastic leukemia. *Bone Marrow Transplantation,* **12,** 315–21.

Fiere, D., Lepage, E., Sebban, C. *et al.* (1993). Adult acute lymphoblastic leukemia: a multicentric randomized trial testing bone marrow transplantation as post remission therapy. *Journal of Clinical Oncology,* **11,** 1990–2001.

Gilmore, M.J.M.L., Hamon, M. D., Prentice, H. G. *et al.* (1991). Failure of purged autologous bone marrow transplantation in high-risk acute lymphoblastic leukemia in first complete remission. *Bone Marrow Transplantation,* **8,** 19–26.

Gokbuget, N., Hoelzer, D., Arnold, R. *et al.* (2000). Treatment of adult ALL according to protocols of the German Multicenter Study Group for Adult ALL (GMALL). *Hematology and Oncology Clinics of North America,* **14,** 1307–25.

Gonzales-Chambers, R., Przepiorka, D., Shadduck, R. K. *et al.* (1991). Autologous bone marrow transplantation with 4-hydroperoxycyclophosphamide-purged marrow for acute lymphoblastic leukemia. *Medical Pediatric Oncology,* **19,** 160–4.

Gorin, N. C. (2002). Autologous stem cell transplantation in acute lymphocytic leukemia. *Stem Cells,* **20,** 3–10.

Gorin, N. C., Aegerter, P., & Auvert, B. (1990). Autologous bone marrow transplantation for acute leukemia in remission: an analysis of 1322 cases. In *Haematology and Blood Transfusion, Vol. 33, Acute Leukemias II,* ed. T. Büchner, G. Schellong, W. Hiddemann, & J. Ritter, pp. 660–666. Berlin: Springer-Verlag.

Hagemeijer, A. & Grosveld, G. (1996). Molecular cytogenetics of leukemia. In *Leukemia, 6th Ed.,* ed. E. S. Henderson, T. A. Lister, & M. F. Greaves, p. 133. Philadelphia: WB Saunders.

Hoelzer, D., Ludwig, W. D., Thiel, E. *et al.* (1996). Improved outcome in adult B-cell acute lymphoblastic leukemia. *Blood,* **87,** 495–508.

Hoelzer, D., Thiel, E., Loeffler, H. *et al.* (1988). Prognostic factors in a multicenter study for acute lymphoblastic leukemia in adults. *Blood,* **71,** 123–31.

Houtenbos, I., Bracho, F., Davenport, V. *et al.* (2001). Autologous bone marrow transplantation for childhood acute lymphoblastic leukemia: a novel combined approach consisting of ex vivo marrow purging, modulation of multi-drug resistance, induction of autograft vs. leukemia effect, and post-transplant immuno- and chemotherapy (PTIC). *Bone Marrow Transplantation,* **27,** 145–53.

Kamps, W. A., Bokkerink, J.P.M., Hahlen, K. *et al.* (1999). Intensive treatment of children with acute lymphoblastic leukemia according to ALL-BFM-86 without cranial radiotherapy results of Dutch childhood leukemia study group protocol ALL-7 (1988–1991). *Blood,* **94,** 1226–36.

Kersey, J. H., Weisdorf, D., Nesbit, M. E. *et al.* (1987). Comparison of autologous and allogeneic bone marrow transplantation for treatment of high-risk refractory acute lymphoblastic leukemia. *New England Journal of Medicine,* **317,** 461–7.

Laporte, J.P.H., Douay, L., Lopez, M. *et al.* (1994). One hundred twenty-five adult patients with primary acute leukemia autografted with marrow purged by mafosfamide: a 10-year single institution experience. *Blood,* **84,** 3810–18.

Marco, F., Bureo, E., Ortega, J. J. *et al.* (2000). High survival rate in infant acute leukemia treated with early high-dose chemotherapy and stem-cell support. Grupo Español de Trasplante de Médula Ósea en Ninos. *Journal of Clinical Oncology,* **18,** 3256–61.

Martin, T. G. & Linker, C. A. (2001). Autologous stem cell transplantation for acute lymphocytic leukemia in adults. *Hematology and Oncology Clinics of North America,* **15,** 121–43.

Meloni, G., DeFabritiis, P., Mandelli, F. *et al.* (1990). Busulfan and cyclophosphamide as conditioning regimen for autologous bone marrow transplant in acute lymphoblastic leukemia. In *Autologous Bone Marrow Transplantation, Proceedings of the Fifth International Symposium, Vol. 5,* ed. K. A. Dicke, J. O. Armitage, & M. J. Dicke-Evinger, pp. 199–203. Omaha: The University of Nebraska.

Messina, C., Valsecchi, M. G., Arico, M. *et al.* (1998). Autologous bone marrow transplantation for treatment of isolated central nervous system relapse of childhood acute lymphoblastic leukemia. *Bone Marrow Transplantation,* **21,** 9–14.

Mori, T., Manabe, A., Tsuchida, M. *et al.* (2001). Allogeneic bone marrow transplantation in first remission rescues children with Philadelphia chromosome-positive acute lymphoblastic leukemia: Tokyo Children's Cancer Study Group (TCCSG) studies L89–12 and L92–13. *Medical and Pediatric Oncology,* **37,** 426–31.

Mortuza, F. Y., Papaioannou, M., Moreira, I. M. *et al.* (2002). Minimal residual disease tests provide an independent predictor of clinical outcome in adult acute lymphoblastic leukemia. *Journal of Clinical Oncology,* **20,** 1094–1104.

Parsons, S. K., Castellino, S. M., Lehmann, L. E. *et al.* (1996). Relapsed acute lymphoblastic leukemia: similar outcomes for autologous and allogeneic marrow transplantation in selected children. *Bone Marrow Transplantation,* **17,** 763–8.

Powles, R., Mehta, J., Singhal, S. *et al.* (1995). Autologous bone marrow or peripheral blood stem cell transplantation followed by maintenance chemotherapy for adult acute lymphoblastic

leukemia in first remission: 50 cases from a single center. *Bone Marrow Transplantation,* **16,** 241–7.

Powles, R., Sirohi, B., Treleaven, S. *et al.* (2002). The role of post-transplantation maintenance chemotherapy in improving the outcome of autotransplantation in adult acute lymphoblastic leukemia. *Blood,* **100,** 1641–7.

Ramsay, N.K.C. and Kersey, J. H. (1990). Indications for marrow transplantation in acute lymphoblastic leukemia. *Blood,* **75,** 815–18.

Ringdén, O., Labopin, M., Gluckman, E. *et al.* (1997). Donor search or autografting in patients with acute leukemia who lack an HLA-identical sibling? A matched pair analysis. *Bone Marrow Transplantation,* **19,** 963–8.

Rocha, V., Cornish, J., Sievers, E. L. *et al.* (2001). Comparison of outcomes of unrelated bone marrow and umbilical cord blood transplants in children with acute leukemia. *Blood,* **97,** 2962–71.

Roy, D. C., Ish, C., Blattler, W. *et al.* (1990). Anti-B4 blocked ricin: a new immunotoxin for purging of acute lymphoblastic leukemia cells prior to autologous bone marrow transplantation. *Proceedings of the Annual Meeting of the American Association for Cancer Research,* **31,** A1737 (Abstract).

Saarinen-Pihkala, U. M., Gustafsson, G., Ringden, O. *et al.* (2001). No disadvantage in outcome of using matched unrelated donors as compared with matched sibling donors for bone marrow transplantation in children with acute lymphoblastic leukemia in second remission. *Journal of Clinical Oncology,* **19,** 3406–14.

Sanchez, J., Serrano, J., Gomez, P. *et al.* (2002). Clinical value of immunological monitoring of minimal residual disease in acute lymphoblastic leukaemia after allogeneic transplantation. *British Journal of Haematology,* **116,** 686–94.

Schmid, H., Henze, G., Schwerdtfeger, R. *et al.* (1993). Fractionated total body irradiation and high-dose VP-16 with purged autologous bone marrow rescue for children with high-risk relapsed acute lymphoblastic leukemia. *Bone Marrow Transplantation,* **12,** 597–602.

Schroeder, H., Pinkerton, C. R., Powles, R. L. *et al.* (1991). High dose melphalan and total body irradiation with autologous marrow rescue in childhood acute lymphoblastic leukemia after relapse. *Bone Marrow Transplantation,* **7,** 11–15.

Sebban, C., Lepage, E., Vernant, J.-P. *et al.* (1994). Allogeneic bone marrow transplantation in adult acute lymphoblastic leukemia in first complete remission: a comparative study. *Journal of Clinical Oncology,* **12,** 2580–7.

Simonsson, B., Burnett, A. K., Prentice, H. G. *et al.* (1989). Autologous bone marrow transplantation with monoclonal antibody purged marrow for high-risk acute lymphoblastic leukemia. *Leukemia,* **3,** 631–6.

Smith, M., Arthur, D., Camitta, B. *et al.* (1996). Uniform approach to risk classification and treatment assignment for children with acute lymphoblastic leukemia. *Journal of Clinical Oncology,* **14,** 18–24.

Soiffer, R. J., Billett, A. L., Roy, D. C. *et al.* (1990). Autologous bone marrow transplantation for acute lymphoblastic leukemia in second or subsequent remission: ten years experience at Dana-Farber Cancer Institute. In *Autologous Bone Marrow Transplantation. Proceedings of the Fifth International Symposium,* ed. K. A. Dicke, J. O. Armitage, & M. J. Dicke-

Evinger, pp 167–176. Omaha: The University of Nebraska Medical Center.

Soiffer, R. J., Murray, C., Cochran, K. et al. (1992). Clinical and immunologic effects of prolonged infusion of low-dose recombinant interleukin-2 after autologous and T-cell-depleted allogeneic bone marrow transplantation. Blood, 79, 517–26.

Soiffer, R. J., Roy, D. C., Gonin, R. et al. (1993). Monoclonal antibody-purged autologous bone marrow transplantation in adults with acute lymphoblastic leukemia at high-risk of relapse. Bone Marrow Transplantation, 12, 243–51.

Soto, E. M., Piantadosi, S., Miller, C. B. et al. (2002). Long-term follow-up of intensive ara-C-based chemotherapy followed by bone marrow transplantation for adult acute lymphoblastic leukemia: Impact of induction Ara-C dose and post-remission therapy. Leukemia Research, 26, 461–71.

Spinolo, J. A., Dicke, K. A., Horwitz, L. J. et al. (1990). High dose chemotherapy and ABMT for adult acute lymphoblastic leukemia in remission. In Autologous Bone Marrow Transplantation, Proceedings of the Fifth International Symposium, Vol. 5, ed. K. A. Dicke, J. O. Armitage, & M. J. Dicke-Evinger, pp. 151–160. Omaha: The University of Nebraska.

Stoppa, A. M., Hirn, J., Blaise, D. et al. (1990). Autologous bone marrow transplantation for B cell malignancies after in vitro purging with floating immunobeads. Bone Marrow Transplantation, 6, 301–7.

Thiebaut, A., Vernant, J. P., Degos, L. et al. (2000). Adult acute lymphocytic leukemia study testing chemotherapy and autologous and allogeneic transplantation. A follow-up report of the French protocol LALA 87. Hematology and Oncology Clinics of North America, 14, 1353–66.

Thomas, X., Danaila, C., Le, Q. H. et al. (2001). Long-term follow-up of patients with newly diagnosed adult acute lymphoblastic leukemia: a single institution experience of 378 consecutive patients over a 21-year period. Leukemia, 15, 1811–22.

Tiley, C., Powles, R., Treleaven, J. et al. (1993). Feasibility and efficacy of maintenance chemotherapy following autologous bone marrow transplantation for first remission acute lymphoblastic leukaemia. Bone Marrow Transplantation, 12, 449–55.

Uckun, F. M., Gajl-Peczalska, K., Meyers, D. E. et al. (1987). Marrow purging in autologous bone marrow transplantation for T-lineage acute lymphoblastic leukemia: efficacy of ex vivo treatment with immunotoxins and 4-hydroperoxycyclophosphamide against fresh leukemic marrow progenitor cells. Blood, 69, 361–6.

Uckun, F. M., Kersey, J. H., Haake, R. et al. (1992). Autologous bone marrow transplantation (BMT) in high-risk remission B-lineage acute lymphoblastic leukemia using a cocktail of three monoclonal antibodies (BA-1/CD24, BA-2/CD9, BA-3/CD10) plus complement and 4-hydroperoxycyclo-phosphamide for ex vivo bone marrow purging. Blood, 79, 1094–104.

Uckun, F. M., Kersey, J. H., Vallera, D. A. et al. (1990). Autologous bone marrow transplantation in high-risk remission T-lineage acute lymphoblastic leukemia using immunotoxins plus 4-hydroperoxycyclophosphamide for marrow purging. Blood, 76, 1723–33.

Uderzo, C., Colleselli, P., Dini, G. et al. (1991). An Italian study comparing allogeneic and autologous BMT in childhood acute lymphoblastic leukemia using HD-vincristine, F-TBI and cyclophosphamide. Bone Marrow Transplantation, 7 (Suppl 3), 19–21.

Urbano-Ispizua, A., Schmitz, N., de Witte, T. et al. (2002). Allogeneic and autologous transplantation for haematological diseases, solid tumors and immune disorders: definition and current practice in Europe. Bone Marrow Transplantation, 29, 639–46.

Vey, N., Blaise, D., Stoppa, A. M. et al. (1994). Bone marrow transplantation in 63 adult patients with acute lymphoblastic leukemia in first complete remission. Blood, 14, 383–8.

Weisdorf, D., Nesbit, M. E., Ramsay, N.K.C. et al. (1987). Allogeneic bone marrow transplantation for acute lymphoblastic leukemia in remission: prolonged survival associated with acute graft-versus-host disease. Journal of Clinical Oncology, 5, 1348–55.

Weisdorf, D. J., Anderson, P., Blazar, B. et al. (1993). Interleukin-2 immediately after autologous marrow transplantation for acute lymphoblastic leukemia—a phase I study. Transplantation, 55, 61–6.

Weisdorf, D. J., Billett, A. L., Hannan, P. et al. (1997). Autologous versus unrelated donor allogeneic marrow transplantation for acute lymphoblastic leukemia. Blood, 90, 2962–8.

Weisdorf, D., Bishop, M., Dharan, B. et al. (2002). Autologous versus allogeneic unrelated donor transplantation for acute lymphoblastic leukemia: comparative toxicity and outcomes. Biology of Blood and Marrow Transplantation, 8, 213–20.

Woolfrey, A. E., Anasetti, C., Storer, B. et al. (2002). Factors associated with outcome after unrelated marrow transplantation for treatment of acute lymphoblastic leukemia in children. Blood, 99, 2002–8.

Yamada, M., Wasserman, R., Lange, B. et al. (1990). Minimal residual disease in childhood B-lineage lymphoblastic leukemia. Persistence of leukemic cells during the first 18 months of treatment. New England Journal of Medicine, 323, 448–55.

Zintl, F., Hermann, J., Fuchs, D. et al. (1990). Comparison of allogeneic and autologous bone marrow transplantation for treatment of acute lymphocytic leukemia in childhood. In Haematology and Blood Transfusion, Vol. 33, Acute Leukemias II, ed. T. Büchner, G. Schellong, W. Hiddemann, & J. Ritter, pp. 692–698. Berlin: Springer-Verlag.

38 Autologous hematopoietic stem cell transplantation for chronic myeloid leukemia

TARIQ I. MUGHAL AND JOHN M. GOLDMAN

Imperial College School of Medicine, London, UK

Introduction

Chronic myeloid leukemia (CML) is a clonal disorder of hematopoiesis in which the progeny of a leukemic stem cell acquires a consistent cytogenetic abnormality, the Philadelphia (Ph) chromosome. The Ph chromosome bears the *BCR-ABL* chimeric gene and the encoded BCR-ABL protein is now believed to be the principal cause of the chronic phase of CML as a consequence of its enhanced tyrosine kinase activity. The discovery that the kinase activity of the BCR-ABL protein could be inhibited in a highly specific manner by drugs such as imatinib mesylate provides the proof for this notion and should prove to be a significant landmark in the treatment of patients with CML (Goldman & Melo, 2001; Kantarjian *et al.*, 2002).

Currently allogeneic stem cell transplantation (allo-SCT) using HLA-matched donors is the only treatment that induces long-lasting hematological and cytogenetic remissions for patients with CML. However, the majority of patients with CML are not eligible for this treatment largely because of the lack of a suitable donor and the increased incidence of potentially lethal graft-versus-host disease (GVHD) in older recipi-ents. Conventionally such patients have been treated with interferon alpha (IFN-α), either alone or in combination with cytosine arabinoside and about 20% to 30% obtain some degree of reduction in the proportion of Ph-positive marrow metaphases (Table 38.1) and some of these patients become long-term survivors (Figure 38.1) (Baccarani *et al.*, 2002). Thus, it seems probable that IFN-α can prolong life in some cases, but does not indefinitely delay the inexorable transformation of chronic phase CML into the more advanced phases. Other treatment approaches such as autologous SCT (auto-SCT; autografting) therefore deserve consideration.

The transplant-related mortality (TRM) associated with autografting is less than 5% in most published series (Bhatia *et al.*, 1997; O'Brien & Goldman, 1997, 1998). Hematopoietic reconstitution is usually rapid and the 5-year overall survival rates following the procedure are in the order of 50 to 70%, although the majority of patients have persistent chronic phase disease. The concept gained popularity in the 1970s when it was established that stem cells collected and cryopreserved at the time of diagnosis could be used successfully at the time of transformation to re-establish a second chronic phase. It is also possible that the autograft procedure substantially reduces the number of leukemic stem cells and may confer a short-term proliferative advantage to the Ph-negative stem cells. In this chapter, we briefly review the possible place of this treatment for a patient with CML in chronic or advanced phase.

Clinical features and risk-stratification

The incidence of CML in North America and Europe is approximately 1.5 per 100,000 of population per annum and the disease represents approximately 15% of all adult leukemias. The median age of onset is 50 years. Characteristically CML is a biphasic or triphasic disease that is usually diagnosed in a stable or chronic phase. This initial chronic phase lasts typically 3 to 6 years but its duration may be shorter or occasionally very much longer. Other genetic events then occur that underlie disease progression to accelerated and blast phase (Table 38.2). About a third of such patients are diagnosed following a routine blood test and the remainder present with signs and symp-

Table 38.1. *Commonly used definitions of hematologic and cytogenetic responses*

Term	Definition
Complete hematologic remission	WBC <10 × 10⁹/l; platelets <400 × 10⁹/l; no splenomegaly
Partial hematologic remission	Counts improved, but not normal
Complete cytogenetic response	Absence of Philadelphia chromosome, with at least 20 metaphases studied
Major cytogenetic response	Suppression of Philadelphia chromosome to <35% of metaphases
Minor cytogenetic response	Philadelphia chromosome present in 35–95% of cells studied

Abbreviation: WBC, white blood cells.

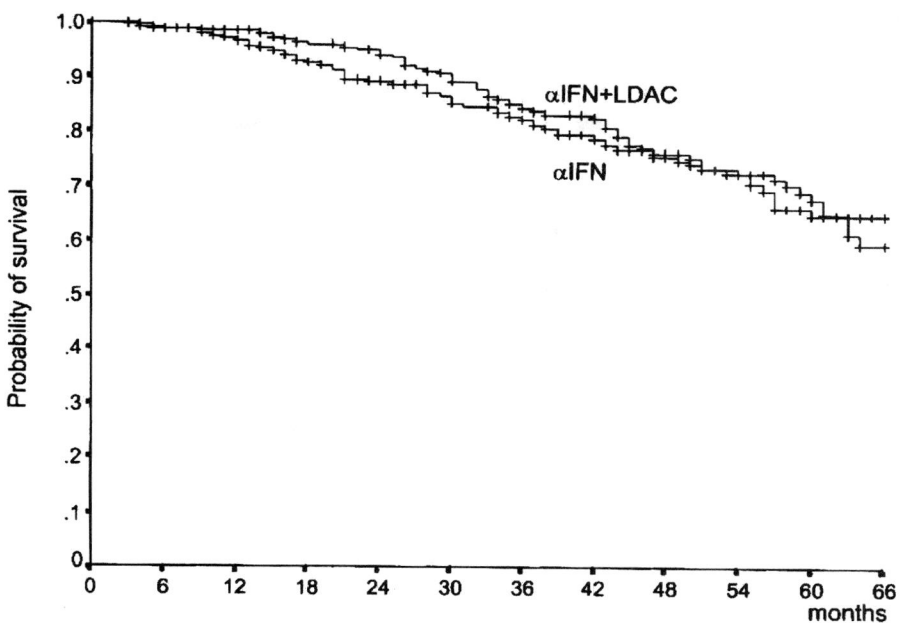

Fig. 38.1. Survival from randomization ($p = .77$, log rank test). The patients who received allo-BMT in first chronic phase were censored at the date of BMT. The number of cases at risk at 12, 24, 36, 48, and 60 months is 246, 217, 181, 111, and 53, respectively, in the IFN-α-plus-LDAC arm, and 225, 178, 151, 100, and 49, respectively, in the IFN-α arm. Reproduced, with permission, from Baccarani et al. (2002).

toms related to anemia and splenomegaly (Table 38.2). The most frequently used method to establish criteria definable at diagnosis that may help to predict survival for individual patients is the Sokal index (Sokal *et al.*, 1984) or the more recent Euro system (Table 38.4 and Figure 38.2) (Hasford *et al.*, 1998). Patients can be divided into various risk categories

based on Sokal's mathematical formula that takes into account the patient's age, blood blast cell percentage, spleen size and platelet count at diagnosis (Table 38.5, Figure 38.3); the Euro system is based on results of treating patients with IFN-α and includes assessment of basophil and eosinophil numbers. Other possible prognostic factors are the presence or absence of deletions in the derivative 9q+ chromosome and the rate of shortening of telomeres in the leukemia clone (Huntly *et al.*, 2001; Brummendorf *et al.*, 2000).

Molecular biology

About 90% of CML patients have a Ph chromosome in all cells of the myeloid series and in some B lymphocytes. This acquired cytogenetic abnormality is the result of a reciprocal

Table 38.2.   *The different phases of chronic myeloid leukemia*

Chronic phase
　Ability to reduce spleen size and restore and maintain 'normal'
　　blood count with appropriate therapy
Accelerated phase
　Presence of any one of the following:
　　Anemia (<8.0 g/dl)[a]
　　Leucocytosis (>100 × 10⁹/l)[a]
　　Thrombocytopenia (<100 × 10⁹/l)[a]
　　Thrombocytosis (>1000 × 10⁹/l)[a]
　　Splenomegaly[a]
　　>10% blasts in blood or marrow
　　>20% blasts plus promyelocytes in blood or marrow
　　>20% basophils plus eosinophils in blood
　　New cytogenetic changes (in addition to Ph)
Blastic phase
　More than 30% blasts plus promyelocytes in blood or marrow

Note: Classification of phase of disease must take account of the treatment the patient is receiving. Thus ([a]) indicates features that are indications of accelerated phase disease only if a patient is already receiving therapy that would be considered adequate for control of chronic phase disease.

Table 38.3.   *Clinical features of patients with CML*

Signs	n	%
Spleen palpable[a]	314	76
1–10 cm	153	37
>10 cm	161	39
Spleen not palpable	100	24
Purpura	66	16
Palpable liver	9	2
No signs	85	20

[a] in cms below the left costal margin

Table 38.4.   *Sokal index for predicting survival*

Prognostic Indices:
Good prognosis   < 0.8
Moderate prognosis   0.8–1.2
Poor prognosis   >1.2
Mathematical Expression:
  exp[0.0116(Age – 43.4) + 0.0345 (Spleen size – 7.51) + 0.188 ({Platelet count/700}^{2} – 0.563) + 0.0887 (percentage of blasts – 2.10)]

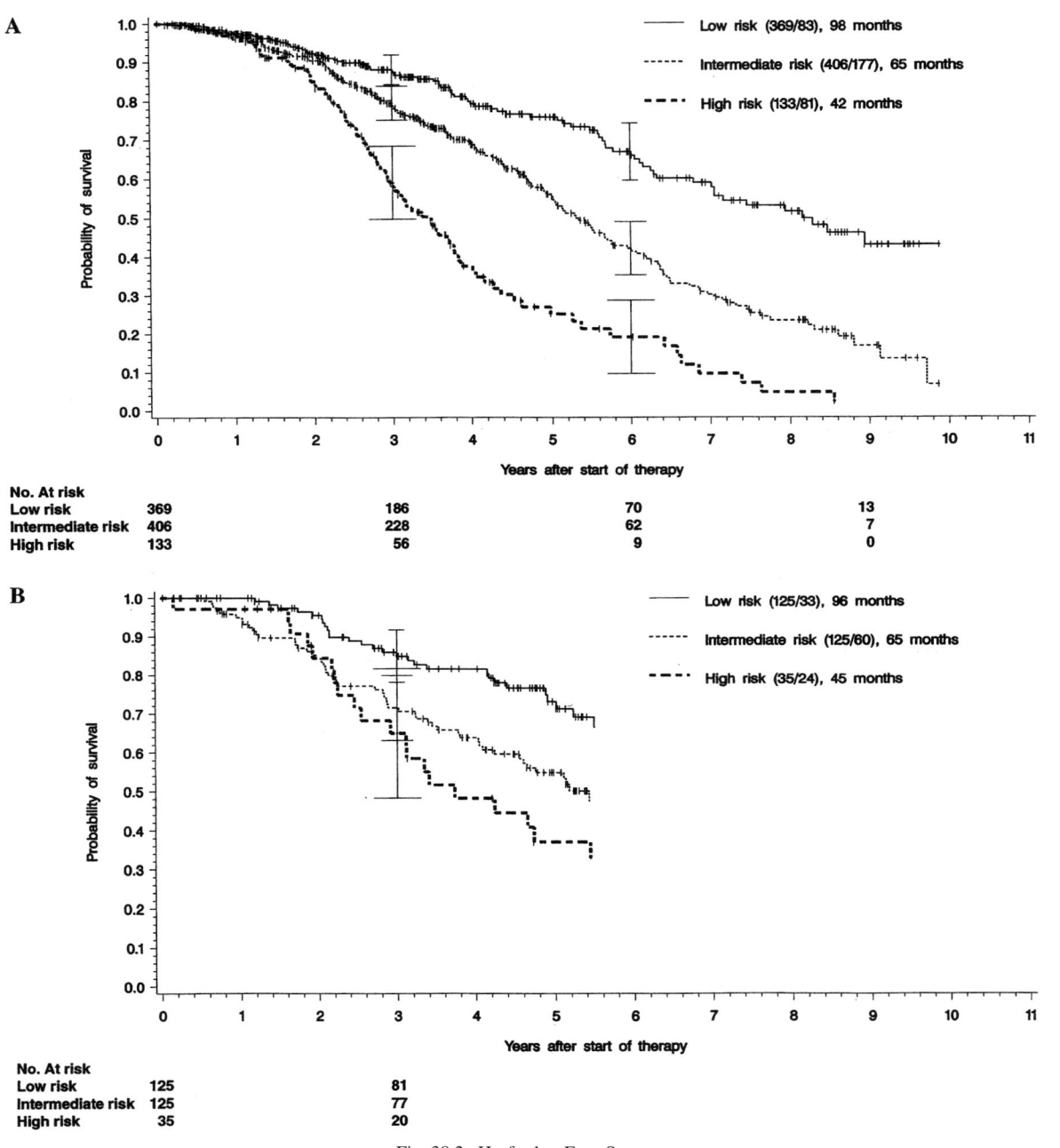

Fig. 38.2. Hasford or Euro Score

Table 38.5. *Prognostic factors for outcome with conventional chemotherapy of chronic myeloid leukemia*

An indication of likely outcome (with busulfan or hydroxyurea treatment) may be obtained at diagnosis. The following factors indicate a poor prognosis:
  Marked splenomegaly
  High circulating numbers of blast cells
  High platelet count ($>700 \times 10^9$/l)
  Blood or marrow basophilia (basophils plus eosinophils >15%)
  Ph negativity
  Older age
The impact of splenomegaly and circulating blast cells is illustrated in Figure 38.3.

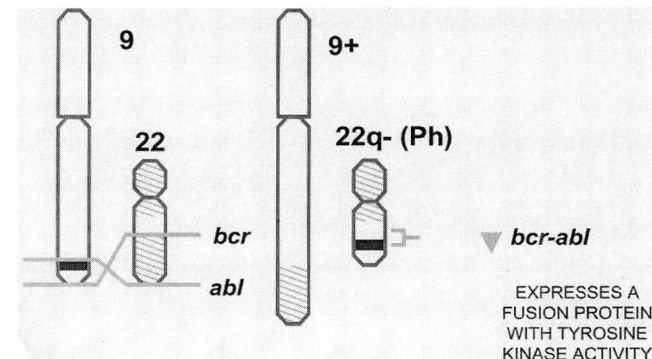

Fig. 38.4. Schematic representation of the Ph chromosome.

translocation of chromosomal material involving the long arm of one 9 chromosome and one 22 chromosome, referred to as t(9;22)(q34;q11) (Figure 38.4). The remaining 10% of patients with hematologically "acceptable" CML lack the Ph chromosome and are described as Ph-negative CML. About half of such patients have a cytogenetically occult *BCR-ABL* gene and are referred to as Ph-negative, BCR-ABL positive cases; the remainder are BCR-ABL negative and some of these have mutations in the *RAS* gene (Melo, 1996). The BCR-ABL oncoprotein (p210$^{BCR-ABL}$) has a much greater tyrosine kinase activity than its normal ABL counterpart and must play a central role in the pathogenesis of CML, though the precise mechanism remains enigmatic (Deininger *et al.*, 2000). It may act by constitutively activating mitogenic signaling, by reducing apoptosis, by impairing adhesion of CML cells to the stroma and extracellular matrix, or by proteasome-mediated degradation of ABL inhibitory proteins (Epstein, 1999).

At the cytokinetic level, the mechanism by which the BCR-ABL oncoprotein enhances proliferation and differentiation of myeloid progenitors is unclear. It is likely that normal myeloid progenitors cells are preferentially maintained in G_0 as a result of proliferation of leukemic cells, but conversely there are also quiescent Ph-positive progenitor cells which can under certain circumstances be induced to proliferate (Holyoake *et al.*, 1999; Graham *et al.*, 2002).

BCR-ABL junctional peptides can induce in vitro cytotoxic T lymphocyte (CTL) activity, and antigen-presenting cells loaded with BCR-ABL junctional 9-mers elicit specific class I-restricted CTL activity from autologous peripheral blood mononuclear cells (Bocchia *et al.*, 1996; Yotnda *et al.*, 1998). Clark and colleagues (2001) demonstrated HLA-restricted surface expression of the b3a2 peptide in CML patients, who were able to mount a CTL response against the junctional peptide. Furthermore, HLA-restricted, peptide-specific T cells were detected in the blood of patients with CML, and could be expanded in vitro, thus providing a sound basis of studies for immunization of CML patients against the BCR-ABL protein.

Rationale for autografting

The administration of high doses of cytotoxic drugs followed by autografting with a finite number of progenitor or stem cells may establish a major kinetic benefit if progression of CML is in any way related to the total number of leukemic stem cells in the patient's body. Thus, autografting perforce is likely to reduce this total number and perhaps thereby delay the occurrence of transformation. Conversely, one must not ignore the possibility that residual leukemic stem cells may be exposed to a mitogenic effect that acts to expedite transformation, but this risk may be small if the myeloablative therapy that precedes the autograft is effective.

Autografting may also have the capacity to restore durable Ph-negative hematopoiesis and thereby prolong survival (Hehlmann *et al.*, 2000). Various lines of evidence support the view that most or all newly diagnosed CML patients have residual Ph-negative stem cells in their marrow and these cells are probably normal. For example, the occasional patient "overtreated" with busulfan recovers predominantly Ph-negative hematopoiesis, which may

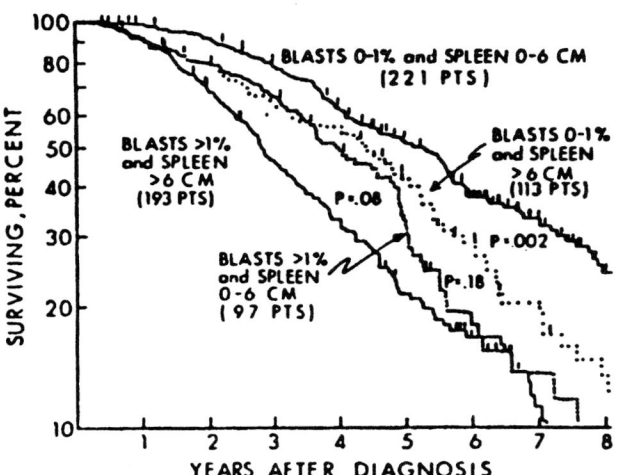

Fig. 38.3. Survival, according to spleen size and percentage of circulating blasts, among 624 patients diagnosed before 1978. Reproduced, with permission, from Sokal *et al.* (1984).

be durable. Ph-negative progenitor cells can be collected by leukapheresis after administration of high-dose chemotherapy (Carella et al., 1991), and some patients have achieved Ph-negative hematopoiesis after autografting with unmanipulated mononuclear cells, both in transformation and in chronic phase (Korbling et al., 1981; Haines et al., 1984; Brito-Babapulle et al., 1989). Moreover, it is sometimes possible to restore Ph-negative hematopoiesis in chronic phase CML by high-dose chemotherapy (Goto et al., 1982). IFN-α also induces partial or total Ph-negative hematopoiesis in 20% to 30% of patients (Talpaz et al., 1991). The most compelling argument for the persistence of Ph-negative stem cells at diagnosis is the observation that 65% of newly diagnosed patients treated with imatinib have achieved a complete cytogenetic response (Druker et al., 2002).

Autografting may restore IFN-α sensitivity and prolong survival in patients with IFN-α resistant CML (Boiron et al., 1999). Likewise it may be possible to restore responsiveness to imatinib in the cohort who acquires resistance to it, as appears to be the case in a number of patients, in particular those in the advanced phases. In some of the patients who fail to respond to imatinib or who lose a hematologic response, it may imply disease progression. An innovative strategy combining autografting with imatinib for such a cohort is being assessed and preliminary results appear encouraging.

When to autograft

Initial experience with autografting for CML was restricted to treatment of patients in transformation (Haines et al., 1984). In general, hematopoiesis characteristic of chronic phase was re-established but transformation recurred within a few months. The real benefit for the patient was therefore questionable. In recent years a number of groups have focused on the possibility of prolonging life by autografting while the patient is still in chronic phase. Because the value of this approach is still uncertain, it seems essential to discuss the procedure fully with a patient before proceeding and to ensure that the patient is fully aware of the rationale underlying the treatment and, perhaps, impose an arbitrary upper age limit of about 65 years. Until its value is established, the decision to undertake an autograft and the timing within the chronic phase must remain essentially arbitrary decisions. One might suggest that the autograft should be undertaken immediately or within 1 year of diagnosis. The autograft could then be repeated once or twice at perhaps 2-year intervals.

It is difficult to evaluate the clinical benefit of autografting in an individual patient but some criteria can be considered. One might speculate that durable induction of Ph-negative hematopoiesis might be associated with prolonged survival, but this is in no sense prima facie evidence that the link is causal; instead one might succeed in establishing Ph-negative hematopoiesis only in patients already destined for long survival. If, however, one could devise an autografting schedule that induced Ph-negative hematopoiesis in the majority of treated patients, and if this Ph-negativity were maintained for

months or years, it would be reasonable to predict that survival could be prolonged for at least some patients. Blood and marrow from Ph-negative patients should be studied for residual leukemia-specific (BCR/ABL) transcripts with the polymerase chain reaction (PCR) as discussed below.

For the present, perhaps, the best measure of benefit is the interval after autografting during which the patient has a normal leukocyte and/or platelet count, or the interval during which no further chemotherapy is required. Undoubtedly the eventual proof or disproof of the value of autografting must hinge on a study of survival in a prospective trial in which comparable patients are randomized to receive or not to receive treatment by autografting. Such studies were activated in the mid-1990s, but patient recruitment was poor after introduction of imatinib (Spencer, O'Brien, & Goldman, 1995).

Cytoreduction before autografting

For patients in transformation anti-leukemia or cytoreductive treatment before autografting was designed originally to eradicate the transformed clone, and therefore incorporated high-dose chemotherapy and "supralethal" irradiation. In contrast, for patients in chronic phase the objective is a substantial reduction in the numbers of Ph-positive stem cells and progenitor cells, but to aim for total eradication may be illogical since most methods of autografting will involve re-transfusing at least some leukemia cells (Deisseroth et al., 1994). Thus originally we at the Hammersmith Hospital used a combination of busulfan and cyclophosphamide at high dosage but our current protocol for cytoreduction before autografting involves only busulfan 4 mg/kg daily for 4 days (total 16 mg/kg) (O'Brien & Goldman, 1998; Olavarria et al., 2000).

What cells to use for reconstitution

There are various possible approaches to treating the patient or manipulating the peripheral blood or marrow inoculum after harvesting in order to favor reconstitution with Ph-negative hematopoiesis. In some cases preliminary clinical results have already been presented, while in others the principles are supported only by logic or laboratory studies.

Collecting Ph-negative stem cells

The Memorial Sloan-Kettering Cancer Center (New York) group showed in the late 1970s that about one-third of patients with newly diagnosed CML who were treated with high-dose chemotherapy, recovered partially negative hematopoiesis (Goto et al., 1982). The Baltimore group was the first to autograft a patient with Ph-negative stem cells collected from the peripheral blood after high-dose chemotherapy in chronic phase (Korbling et al., 1981). The same approach may be used for patients in transformation; the Genova group treated advanced phase patients with cytotoxic drugs (idarubicin, cytosine arabinoside, and etoposide), and subsequently autografted them with Ph-negative progenitors collected from their peripheral blood (Carella *et al.*, 1991). Long-term culture–initiating cells (LTC-IC) were found predominantly in Ph-negative, as opposed to Ph-positive or mixed, aphereses collected in this way (Podesta *et al.*, 1995). The same group has reported their experience with patients in chronic phase (Carella *et al.*, 1997). This approach resulted in a collection of Philadelphia-negative cells if the cells were harvested in early chronic phase in the early phase of recovery after chemotherapy-induced marrow aplasia in patients not extensively pretreated with IFN-α.

In the early 1980s it was speculated that similar results might be achieved by treating patients with IFN-α alone and autografting them with marrow collected during the subsequent phase of Ph-negativity. In practice, the marrow from patients who have responded to IFN-α is often hypocellular and may be difficult to aspirate. Nevertheless, this approach has been used with considerable success by the Uppsala group (Simonsson *et al.*, 1992). The administration of hematopoietic growth factors, especially G-CSF and GM-CSF, to patients with acute leukemia or lymphoma in remission may release into the circulation relatively large numbers of myeloid progenitor cells; it is likely that growth factors may have a similar effect in patients with CML, but to what extent this preferentially involves Ph-negative progenitor cells is not yet clear (Archimbaud *et al.*, 1997).

Choice of progenitor cells: blood or bone marrow?

There is currently no consensus as to whether peripheral blood or bone marrow would constitute a better source of stem cells (including Ph-negative stem cells) for autografting. Progenitor cells from the peripheral blood are easier to collect in large numbers and more convenient for the patient (Lowenthal *et al.*, 1975), but residual Ph-negative stem cells may be present in larger proportion in the marrow. Blood-derived progenitors may have reduced self-replicative capacity compared with marrow cells (Brito-Babapulle *et al.*, 1989), a feature which might or might not favor their use for autografting. Bone marrow cells are sometimes technically more difficult to collect and their use may be associated with an inferior survival compared to peripheral blood cells (Spencer *et al.*, 1998).

Manipulation of the autograft

Negative selection in vitro

It should in theory be possible to collect bone marrow from a CML patient, treat it in vitro with an agent that selectively suppresses Ph-positive myelopoiesis while leaving Ph-negative stem cells unaffected, and use the resulting cells for the autograft. Treating marrow in vitro with 4-hydroperoxycyclophosphamide favors survival of Ph-negative progenitor cells in culture, and such treated marrow cells can be used for autografting (Degliantoni *et al.*, 1985). The Minneapolis group has autografted a small series of patients with marrow incubated in vitro with gamma interferon (IFN-γ) (McGlave *et al.*, 1990). It

is not clear whether this in vitro treatment was or was not useful. The use of ribozymes and antisense oligodeoxynucleotides has been explored by some groups. Antisense oligomers directed against *BCR-ABL* and *MYB* sequences have been tested in the clinic and initial results were encouraging (de Fabritiis *et al.*, 1995, 1998). The use of agents that block the function of the ABL kinase, such as imatinib, appeared especially promising in this regard (Druker *et al.*, 1996; Deininger *et al.*, 1997), and a range of tyrphostins has been studied in some detail since (le Coutre *et al.*, 1999).

Another approach to in vitro manipulation has been developed in Vancouver as a result of the observation that Ph-positive progenitors survive less well than their Ph-negative counterparts in a modified Dexter-type long-term culture system (Coulombel *et al.*, 1983). Marrow was harvested from selected patients and incubated for 10 days in liquid culture (Barnett *et al.*, 1994).

Positive selection in vitro

CML progenitor cells express HLA-DR on their surface much more strongly than their normal counterparts. A number of groups have studied a primitive population of myeloid progenitor cells characterized as CD34+, HLA-DR−. The majority (Verfaillie *et al.*, 1992) of such cells are Ph-negative and therefore presumably residual normal cells. It might theoretically be possible to develop techniques that would permit collection of large numbers of CD34+, HLA-DR− (Verfaillie *et al.*, 1996). An alternative approach to positive selection of residual normal cells would exploit the known alterations in the adherence properties of CML cells. CML progenitor cells adhere poorly to a preformed marrow stromal layer grown in the presence of steroids in comparison with normal cells (Gordon *et al.*, 1987); conversely, their adherence to stromal layers grown in the absence of steroids is increased. CML cells also show increased binding to laminin and type IV collagen (Verfaillie *et al.*, 1991).

Positive selection in vivo

Much attention has focused on the notion that Ph-negative stem or progenitor cells may be collected from patients in chronic phase after initial treatment with IFN-α or cytotoxic drugs. The group in Uppsala treated patients first with IFN-α (Simonsson *et al.*, 1992); those who failed to achieve Ph-negativity received combinations of cytotoxic drugs. Once a patient achieved a Ph-negative marrow, marrow stem cells were harvested and used for a subsequent autograft. The majority of patients autografted in this manner recovered Ph-negative hematopoiesis, which has been durable in most cases. Of equal interest has been the program initiated in Genova (Carella *et al.*, 1991). Chronic phase patients who received chemotherapy with the combination idarubicin, cytosine arabinoside, and etoposide early after diagnosis could be subjected to leukapheresis in the recovery phase and mononuclear cells were predominantly or exclusively Ph-negative in most cases. Such cells were collected and cryopreserved and later used for autografting.

Clinical results of autografting

Autografting in advanced disease

A number of uncontrolled studies have been reported in which patients with CML in transformation were treated with high-dose chemotherapy or chemoradiotherapy and autografts of unmanipulated marrow or blood-derived stem cells (Butturini et al., 1990). Most patients engrafted. There were a few long-term survivors, but most patients relapsed within 3 to 6 months with evidence of the same transformed clone as had been present originally. This observation confirms the well-known aggressiveness of transformed CML and serves again to focus attention on possible benefits of autografting in chronic phase (Khouri et al., 1996). The Bordeaux group reported that patients autografted in transformation, who then receive a second autograft in "second chronic phase" and subsequent maintenance with IFN-α may survive longer than patients not so treated (Reiffers et al., 1994).

Autografting in chronic phase

The Hammersmith group reported preliminary results of autografting 21 patients with CML in chronic phase using chemotherapy or chemoradiotherapy and blood-derived stem cells (Mughal et al., 1993; Hoyle et al., 1994). At the time of these reports there were 12 survivors (median 82 months, range 9 to 105 months postautografting). Of special interest was the observation that one patient, autografted 2 months after diagnosis (Brito-Babapulle et al., 1989), is still 100% Ph-negative (but with low numbers of BCR-ABL transcripts in the blood) 11 years after autografting. A second patient was Ph-negative for 4 years, but showed slow re-emergence of the Ph-positive clone over the next 2 years. When busulfan alone was used as the conditioning regimen, the actuarial 3 year survival was 76% for patients in chronic phase as opposed to 30% for those trans-

planted with advanced phase disease (Olavarria et al., 2000). McGlave et al. (1994) collected clinical data from eight centers where a total of 142 patients had received autografts for CML; the 4-year probability of survival for the selected group of patients autografted in chronic phase was about 60%. Although patient age in this series affected clinical outcome, neither the source of stem cells (blood vs. marrow) nor the use of in vitro purging techniques influenced survival. The Vancouver group has reported the results of autografting in chronic phase with incubated marrow (see also above). Of 14 patients so treated, 3 failed to engraft, but one of these was successfully "rescued." There were 12 survivors; 10 were in hematologic remission and 9 of these in cytogenetic remission at intervals after autografting of 3 to 36 months (Barnett et al., 1994). Some of the remission patients had been treated with IFN-α.

Of the 31 patients autografted in Genova with stem cells collected after chemotherapy very early after diagnosis, 18 yielded Ph-negative leukapheresis collections (Carella et al., 1997). Eighteen patients underwent autograft procedures and 14 remained in complete or partial cytogenetic remission 3 to 28 months postautograft at the time of the report. This perhaps is the most interesting approach to autografting at present, and similar studies have been initiated in other centers.

The results of two retrospective, multicenter studies are shown in Figures 38.5 and 38.6.

For the reasons mentioned, it is extremely difficult to design a prospective study to answer the question: does autografting prolong survival compared with optimal alternative treatment? This said, the European Group for Blood and Marrow Transplantation designed a study in which patients are randomly allocated at diagnosis to receive either IFN-α (with or without cytosine arabinoside), or an autograft using either unmanipulated stem cells or stem cells collected after ifosfamide, carboplatin, and etoposide (ICE) mobilization. It would have taken 5 or more years before the results of this study

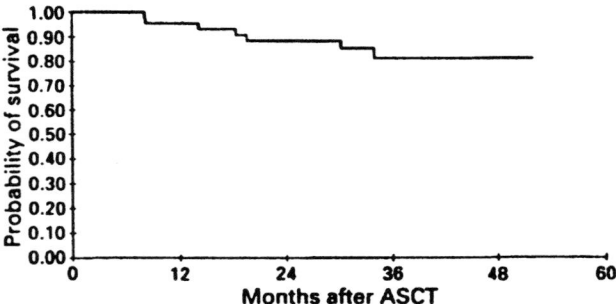

Fig. 38.5. Actuarial survival of the population of 44 patients transplanted during chronic phase and evaluable for response. Reproduced, with permission, from Reiffers et al. (1994).

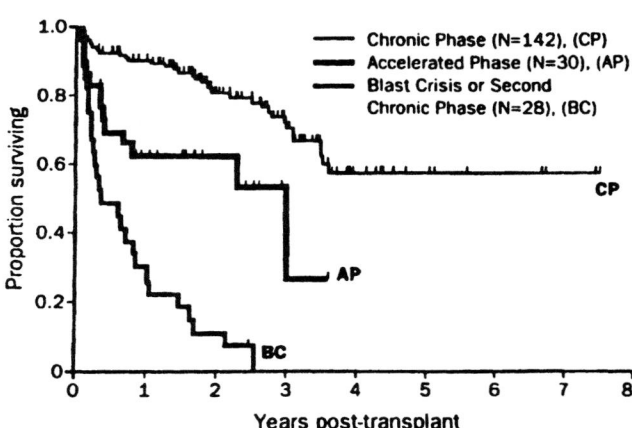

Fig. 38.6. Survival for patients receiving autologous transplants. Chronic phase (CP), accelerated phase (AP), blast crisis or second chronic phase (BC). Hatch marks represent surviving patients. Reproduced, with permission, from McGlave et al. (1994).

could be assessed, but the study will probably never be completed in the current imatinib era.

Monitoring for minimal residual disease postautograft

The principal aim of achieving exclusively Ph-negative hematopoiesis is obtained in only a minority of patients with CML by an autografting procedure, in contrast to allo-SCT (Mughal *et al.*, 2001). The degree of leukemic load reduction is, however, an important independent prognostic factor. Response is often expressed as a molecular response, defined in accordance to the methodology used as the proportion of the residual BCR-ABL transcripts. A cytogenetic response is defined as the proportion of residual Ph-positive metaphases and a hematological response is defined as the normalization of the peripheral blood counts and of the spleen size. Currently, quantitative real-time PCR is the preferred method for the determination of residual disease after autografting for patients with CML (Hochhaus, 2002)

An algorithm incorporating autografting

The issue of whether one should recommend an allogeneic SCT to any patient with CML in chronic phase and, if yes, to which patients, remains a challenge (Goldman & Druker 2001). One possible approach is to balance the perceived benefits and risks of a transplant against the likelihood of long-term survival with best available non-transplant therapy. Insofar as one cannot accurately predict the results of a given transplant and one does not currently know the long-term outcome for patients treated with imatinib or imatinib-containing combinations, one possibility would be to give all new patients a trial of treatment with imatinib and then to offer a transplant to those

who, after 6 or 9 months, are judged to have failed the trial, provided the estimated risk of transplant-related mortality was reasonably low, say less than 20%; other patients could be offered alternative non-transplant therapy. The best approach to managing the younger patient with a suitable transplant donor may be clearer in one or two years when we have gained more experience with the use of imatinib mesylate (Mughal & Goldman, 2001; Marin *et al.*, 2002). For patients who are not suitable for an allo-SCT and have had no cytogenetic response to imatinib, it is reasonable to consider alternative treatments, including autografting. It may also be reasonable to combine autografting with imatinib for patients who fail to respond to imatinib alone or who have severe toxicity from imatinib (Hsiao *et al.*, 2002). Such an algorithm is shown in Figure 38.7.

The current practice of HSC transplantation for CML in Europe has been described (Urbano-Ispizua *et al.*, 2002) (and see Chapter 124, Breaking News…).

Conclusions

Most, if not all, CML patients have substantial numbers of normal hematopoietic stem cells in their marrow at diagnosis. Methods are available today that can induce durable complete cytogenetic remission in a majority of patients. Further exploitation of the use of IFN-α, imatinib, and other cytokines, cytotoxic drugs, and autograft technology offers the possibility of inducing complete remission in all patients.

Though much has been achieved, many important issues in the biology and treatment of CML remain unresolved. To mention just a few, we know little of the mechanisms that cause the chromosomal rearrangement or underlie the proliferative advantage of the Ph-positive clone. We still need to identify the key signal transduction pathway or pathways perturbed by the BCR-ABL oncoprotein. We need a much better understanding

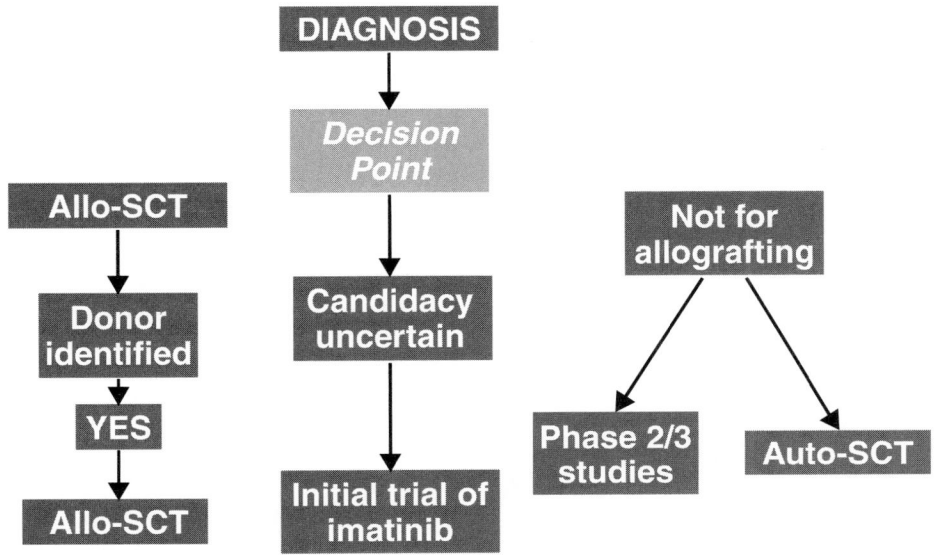

Fig. 38.7. An algorithm incorporating autografting for patients with CML in chronic phase.

of the molecular basis of disease progression. It would tremendously valuable if we could identify with certainty the target antigens for the graft-versus-leukemia effect. In therapeutic terms we need as rapidly as possible to define the true clinical potential of imatinib and to ascertain whether combining this agent with other kinase inhibitors, with other cytotoxic drugs, or with differentiating agents can improve its efficacy. We need to know whether imatinib, immunological (Cervantes et al., 1996), or genetic (Zhao et al., 1997) treatment can prolong survival or contribute to disease eradication following an autograft. We also need to establish if autografting has the potential to restore responsiveness to imatinib in the cohort who become resistant. It seems that at least some of these outstanding problems will be solved during the present decade.

References

Archimbaud, E., Michallet, M., Philip, I. et al. (1997). G-CSF (filgrastim) administered in addition to interferon-α to mobilize peripheral blood stem cells (PBSC) for autologous transplantation in chronic myeloid leukemia (CML). Data presented at the 26th Annual Meeting of the International Society for Experimental Hematology, Cannes, France.

Baccarani, M., Rosti, G., de Vivo, A. et al. (2002). A randomized study of interferon-α and low-dose arabinosyl cytosine in chronic myeloid leukemia. Blood, 99, 1527–1535.

Barnett, M. J., Eaves, C. J., Phillips, G. L. et al. (1994). Autografting with cultured marrow in chronic myeloid leukemia. Results of a pilot study. Blood, 84, 724–32.

Bhatia, R., Verfaillie, C. M., Miller, J. S., & Mcglave, P. B. (1997). Autologous transplantation therapy for chronic myelogenous leukemia. Blood, 89, 2623–34.

Bocchia, M., Korontsvit, T., Xu, Q. et al. (1996). Specific human cellular immunity to bcr-abl oncogene-derived peptides. Blood, 87, 3587–92.

Boiron, J. M., Cahn, J. Y., Meloni, G. et al. (1999). Chronic myeloid leukaemia in first chronic phase not responding to α-interferon: outcome and prognostic factors after autologous transplantation. Bone Marrow Transplantation, 24, 259–64.

Brito-Babapulle, F., Bowcock, S. J., Marcus, R. E. et al. (1989). Autografting for patients with chronic myeloid leukemia in chronic phase: peripheral blood stem cells may have a finite capacity for maintaining hematopoiesis. British Journal of Haematology, 73, 76–81.

Brummendorf, T. H., Holyoake, T. I., Rufer, N. et al. (2000). Prognostic implications of differences in telomore length between normal and malignant cells from patients with chronic myeloid leukemia measured by flow cytometry. Blood, 95, 1883–90.

Butturini, A., Keating, A., Goldman, J., & Gale, R. P. (1990). Autotransplants in chronic myelogenous leukemia: strategies and results. Lancet, 335, 1255–8.

Carella, A., Gaozza, E., Raffo, M. R. et al. (1991). Therapy of acute phase chronic myelogenous leukemia with intensive chemotherapy, blood cell autograft and cyclosporine A. Leukemia, 5, 517–21.

Carella, A. M, Cunningham, I., Lerma, E. et al. (1997). Mobilization and transplantation of Philadelphia-negative peripheral blood progenitor cells early in chronic myelogenous leukemia. Journal of Clinical Oncology, 15, 1575–82.

Cervantes, F., Pierson, B. A., McGlave, P. B. et al. (1996). Autologous activated natural killer cells suppress primitive chronic myelogenous leukemia progenitors in long-term culture. Blood, 87, 2476–85.

Clark, R. E., Dodi, I. A., Hill, S. C. et al. (2001). Direct evidence that leukemic cells present HLA-associated immunogenic peptides derived from the BCR-ABL b3a2 fusion protein. Blood, 98, 2887–93.

Coulombel, L., Kalousek, D. K., Eaves, C. J. et al. (1983). Long term marrow culture reveals chromosomally normal hematopoietic progenitor cells in patients with Philadelphia chromosome positive chronic myelogenous leukemia. New England Journal of Medicine, 309, 1493–9.

de Fabritiis, P., Amadori, S., Petti, M. C. et al. (1995). In vitro purging with bcr-abl antisense oligodeoxynucleotides does not prevent hematological reconstitution after autologous bone marrow transplantation. Leukemia, 9, 662–4.

de Fabritiis, P., Petti, M. C., Montefusco, E. et al. (1998). BCR-ABL antisense oligodeoxynucleotide in vitro purging and autologous bone marrow transplantation for patients with chronic myelogenous leukemia in advanced phase. Blood, 91, 3156–62.

Degliantoni, G., Mangoni, L., & Rizzoli, V. (1985). In vitro restoration of polyclonal hematopoiesis in chronic myelogenous leukemia after in vitro treatment with 4-hydroperoxycyclophosphamide. Blood, 65, 753–7.

Deininger, M. W., Goldman, J. M., & Melo, J. V. (2000). The molecular biology of chronic myeloid leukemia. Blood, 96, 3343–56

Deininger, M.W.N., Goldman, J. M., Lydon, N. B., & Melo, J. V. (1997). The tyrosine kinase inhibitor CGP57148B selectively inhibits the growth of BCR-ABL positive cells. Blood, 90, 3691.

Deisseroth, A. B., Zu, Z., Claxton, D. et al. (1994). Genetic marking shows that Ph+ cells present in the autologous transplants of chronic myelogenous leukemia (CML) contribute to relapse after autologous marrow. Blood, 83, 3068–76.

Druker, B. J., Tamura, S., Buchdunger, E. et al. (1996). Effects of a selective inhibitor of the ABL tyrosine kinase on the growth of bcr-abl positive cells. Nature Medicine, 2, 561–6.

Druker, B. J. (2002). Imatinib and chronic myeloid leukemia: validating the promise of molecularly targeted therapy. European Journal of Cancer, 38, Suppl 5, S70–6.

Epstein, F. H. (1999). The biology of chronic myeloid leukemia. New England Journal of Medicine, 341, 164–72.

Goldman, J. M. & Druker, B. (2001). Chronic myeloid leukemia: current treatment options. Blood, 98, 2039–42.

Goldman, J. M. & Melo, J. V. (2001). Targeting the BCR-ABL tyrosine kinase in chronic myeloid leukemia. New England Journal of Medicine, 344, 1084–86.

Gordon, M., Dowding, C. R., Riley, G. P. et al. (1987). Disordered regulation of primitive hematopoietic progenitor cells in chronic myeloid leukemia is associated with altered adhesive interactions with marrow stroma. Nature, 328, 342–4.

Goto, T., Nishikori, M., Arlin, Z. et al. (1982). Growth characteristics of leukemic and normal hematopoietic cells in Ph+ chronic myelogenous leukemia in vivo and in vitro and effects of intensive treatment with the L-15 protocol. Blood, 59, 793–808.

Graham, S. M., Jørgensen, H. G., Allan, E. *et al.* (2002). Primitive, quiescent, Philadelphia-positive stem cells from patients with chronic myeloid leukemia are insensitive to STI571 in vitro. *Blood,* **99,** 319–325.

Haines, M. E., Goldman, J. M., Worsley, A. M. *et al.* (1984). Chemotherapy and autografting for patients with chronic granulocytic leukemia in transformation: probable prolongation of life for some patients. *British Journal of Haematology,* **58,** 711–22.

Hasford, J., Pfirrmann, M., Hehlmann, R. *et al.* (1998). A new prognostic score for survival of patients with chronic myeloid leukaemia treated with interferon alfa. *Journal of the National Cancer Institute,* **90,** 850–8.

Hehlmann, R., Hochhaus, A., Berger, U. *et al.* (2000). Current trends in the management of chronic myelogenous leukemia. *Annals of Hematology,* **79,** 345–54.

Hochhaus, A. (2002). Lack of a molecular remission in patients with chronic myeloid leukemia following a complete cytogenetic remission with STI571. *Personal Communication.*

Holyoake, T., Jiang, X., Eaves, C., & Eaves, A. (1999). Isolation of a highly quiescent subpopulation of primitive leukemic cells in chronic myeloid leukemia. *Blood,* **94,** 2056–64.

Hoyle, C., Gray, R., Goldman, J. M. *et al.* (1994). Autografting for patients with CML in chronic phase—an update. *British Journal of Haematology,* **86,** 76.

Hsiao, L. T., Chung, H. M., Lin, J. T. *et al.* (2002). Stevens-Johnson syndrome after treatment with STI571: a case report. *British Journal of Haematology,* **117,** 620–22.

Huntly, B. I., Reid, A. G., Bench, A. J. *et al.* (2001). Deletions of the derivative chromosome 9 occur at the time of the Philadelphia translocation and provide a powerful and independent prognostic indicator in chronic myeloid leukemia. *Blood,* **98,** 1732–38.

Kantarjian, H., Sawyers, C., Hochhaus, A. *et al.* (2002). Hematologic and cytogenetic responses to imatinib mesylate in chronic myelogenous leukemia. *New England Journal of Medicine,* **346,** 645–52.

Khouri, I. F., Kantarjian, H. M., Talpaz, M. *et al.* (1996). Results with high-dose chemotherapy and unpurged autologous stem cell plantation in 73 patients with chronic myelogenous leukemia: the M. D. Anderson experience. *Bone Marrow Transplantation,* **17,** 775–9.

Korbling, M., Burke, P., Braine, H. *et al.* (1981). Successful engraftment of blood-derived normal hemopoietic stem cells in chronic myelogenous leukemia. *Experimental Hematology,* **9,** 684–90.

le Coutre, P., Mologni, L., Cleris, L. *et al.* (1999). In vivo eradication of human BCR/ABL positive leukemia cells with an ABL kinase inhibitor. *Journal of the National Cancer Institute,* **91,** 163.

Lowenthal, R. M., Buskard, N. A., Goldman, J. M. *et al.* (1975). Intensive leukapheresis as initial therapy of chronic granulocytic leukemia. *Blood,* **46,** 835.

Marin, D., Marktel, S., Bua, M. *et al.* (2002). The use of imatinib (STI571) in chronic myeloid leukemia: some practical considerations. *Haematologica,* **87,** 979–88.

McGlave, P. B., Arthur, D., Miller, W. J. *et al.* (1990). Autologous transplantation for CML using marrow treated ex vivo with recombinant interferon gamma. *Bone Marrow Transplantation,* **6,** 115–20.

McGlave, P. B., de Fabritiis, P., Deisseroth, A. *et al.* (1994). Autologous transplant therapy for chronic myelogenous

leukemia prolongs survival: results from eight transplant groups. *Lancet,* **343,** 1486–91.

Melo, J. V. (1996). The molecular biology of chronic myeloid leukaemia. *Leukemia,* **10,** 751–6.

Mughal, T. I., Hoyle, C., & Goldman, J. M. (1993). Autografting for patients with chronic myeloid leukemia—the Hammersmith experience. *Stem Cells,* **11,** 20–22.

Mughal, T. I. & Goldman, J. M. (2001). Chronic myeloid leukaemia: STI571 magnifies the therapeutic dilemma. *European Journal of Cancer,* **37,** 561–8.

Mughal, T. I., Yong, A., Szydlo, R. *et al.* (2001). The probability of long-term leukaemia free survival for patients in molecular remission 5 years after allogeneic stem cell transplantation for chronic myeloid leukaemia in chronic phase. *British Journal of Haematology,* **115,** 569–74.

O'Brien, S. G. & Goldman, J. M. (1997). Autografting for chronic myeloid leukemia. In *Blood Stem Cell Transplantation,* ed. J. Reiffers, J. M. Goldman, & J. O. Armitage, pp. 72–89. London: Martin Dunitz & Co.

O'Brien, S. G. & Goldman, J. M. (1998). "Busulfan alone" as cytoreduction before autografting for CML. *Blood,* **91,** 1091–2.

Olavarria, E., Kanfer, E., Szydlo, R. *et al.* (2000). High-dose busulphan alone as cytoreduction before allogeneic or autologous stem cell transplantation for chronic myeloid leukaemia: a single-centre experience. *British Journal of Haematology,* **108,** 769–77.

Podesta, M., Piaggio, G., Frassoni, F. *et al.* (1995). Very primitive hematopoietic (LTC-IC) are present in Philadelphia negative cytaphereses collected during early recovery after chemotherapy for chronic myeloid leukemia (CML). *Bone Marrow Transplantation,* **16,** 549–55.

Reiffers, J., Goldman, G., Meloni, G. *et al.* (1994). Autologous stem cell transplantation in chronic myelogenous leukemia: a retrospective analysis of the European group for bone marrow transplantation. *Bone Marrow Transplantation,* **14,** 407–10.

Simonsson, B., Oberg, G., Bjorkman, M. *et al.* (1992). Intensive treatment in order to minimize the Ph-positive clone in chronic myelogenic leukemia. *Leukemia and Lymphoma,* **7,** 55–7.

Sokal, J. E., Cox, E. V., Baccarani, M. *et al.* (1984). Prognostic discrimination in 'good-risk' chronic granulocytic leukemia. *Blood,* **63,** 789–99.

Spencer, A., Granter, N., Fagan, K. *et al.* (1998). Collection and analysis of peripheral blood mononuclear cells during haemopoietic recovery for PBSCT for CML: autografting as an in vivo purging manoeuvre? *Bone Marrow Transplantation,* **21,** 101–3.

Spencer, A., O'Brien, S. G., & Goldman, J. M. (1995). Chronic myeloid leukemia—options for therapy. *British Journal of Haematology,* **91,** 2–7.

Talpaz, M., Kantarjian, H., Kurzrock, R. *et al.* (1991). Interferon alpha induces sustained cytogenetic responses in chronic myelogenous leukemia. *Annals of Internal Medicine,* **114,** 532–8.

Urbano-Ispizua, A., Schmitz, N., de Witte, T. *et al.* (2002). Allogeneic and autologous transplantation for haematological diseases, solid tumors and immune disorders: definition and current practice in Europe. *Bone Marrow Transplantation,* **29,** 639–46.

Verfaillie, C. M., Bhatia, R., Miller, W. *et al.* (1996). BCR/ABL-negative primitive progenitors suitable for transplantation can be selected from the marrow of most early chronic phase, but not accelerated phase chronic myelogenous leukemia patients. *Blood,* **87,** 4770–9.

Verfaillie, C. M., McCarthy, J. B., Miller, W. J., & McGlave, P. B. (1991). Abnormal trafficking of malignant bone marrow progenitors in CML can be explained by their decreased adhesion to stroma and fibronectin but increased adhesion to the basement membrane components laminin and collagen and collagen type IV. *Blood,* **78** (Suppl 1), 172 (Abstract).

Verfaillie, C. M., Miller, W. J., Boylan, K., & McGlave, P. B. (1992). Selection of benign primitive hemopoietic progenitors in chronic

myelogenous leukemia on the basis of DR antigen expression. *Blood,* **79,** 1003–10.

Yotnda, P., Firat, P., Garcia-Pons, F. *et al.* (1998). Cytotoxic T cell response against the chimeric p210 BCR-ABL protein in patients with chronic myelogenous leukemia. *Journal of Clinical Investigation,* **101,** 2290–6.

Zhao, R.C.H., McIvor, R. S., Griffin, J. D., Verfaillie, C. M. (1997). Gene therapy for chronic myelogenous leukemia (CML): a retroviral vector that renders hematopoietic progenitors methotrexate-resistant and CML progenitors functionally normal and nontumorigenic in vivo. *Blood,* **90,** 4687–98.

39 Autologous hematopoietic stem cell transplantation for myelodysplasia

MICHEL DELFORGE AND MARC A. BOOGAERTS

University Hospital, Leuven, Belgium

Introduction

The myelodysplastic syndromes (MDS) are clonal disorders of an immature hematopoietic progenitor cell. MDS hematopoiesis is characterized by abnormal progenitor proliferation and differentiation, with frequently an increase in intramedullary apoptosis. These progenitor defects contribute to progressive bone marrow failure, cytopenia in the peripheral blood, and an increased risk for leukemic transformation. As a consequence, the natural evolution of MDS can vary from relatively indolent to highly aggressive. Information on the incidence, disease classification, prognostic factors, cytogenetic abnormalities and scoring systems is given in Chapter 54. The poor survival of patients with advanced myelodysplastic syndromes (refractory anemia with excessive blasts [RAEB], RAEB in transformation [RAEB-t]) and secondary AML (sAML) has stimulated the demand for improved therapeutic strategies, including intensified cytotoxic treatment with or without stem cell support. Until now, only the transplantation of allogeneic stem cells has proven to be a curative treatment, but at the expense of considerable transplant-related morbidity and mortality (de Witte, Zwaan, & Hermans, 1990; Boogaerts *et al.*, 1996; Boogaerts, 1998; Oosterveld & de Witte, 2000).

Therapeutic strategies in MDS have been inspired by either trying to convert the abnormal behavior of (pre-)malignant cells into normal behavior, or by destroying non-compliant elements at the expense of innocent bystanders. These approaches may now become complementary rather than conflicting with the advent of immunotherapy (non-myeloablative allogeneic transplants) and/or monoclonal antibodies (e.g. anti-CD33).

The elaboration of risk-adapted treatment algorithms has been much facilitated by the use of the International Prognostic Scoring System (IPSS), which uses marrow blast percentage, cytogenetic data, and number of cytopenias to delineate low-, intermediate (1 and 2)- and high-risk categories (Greenberg *et al.*, 1997). While not much controversy exists regarding treatment options for the older low-risk patient or the younger high-risk patient, the IPSS has intensified the discussion around optimal treatment for younger low- or intermediate-risk, and older (>5 years) intermediate- and high-risk patients.

Intensive cytotoxic treatment

AML-type chemotherapy can induce complete remission rates varying from 40% to 60%. Complete remission (CR) rates in MDS are lower than those in de novo AML patients, treated with similar or identical (mostly cytosine arabinoside-containing) regimens. Two reasons account for this: prolonged cytopenia, leading to higher early death rates, and increased drug resistance, mostly MDR P-glycoprotein-related. Factors predictive for reaching CR include younger age, RAEB or RAEB-t versus sAML, primary versus therapy-related MDS (t-MDS), the absence of cytogenetic abnormalities and the type of anthracyclines (e.g. mitoxantrone or idarubicin) used (Tricot & Boogaerts, 1986; de Witte *et al.*, 1995; Estey *et al.*, 1997). Based on a large retrospective analysis, results with chemotherapy treatment in children with MDS are disappointing compared to adults, presumably due to the inclusion of patients with other hematological diseases in the published trials (Novitzky & Prindull, 2000).

Maintaining remission after CR remains a major problem. The median duration of disease-free survival (DFS) rarely exceeds 12 months. For patients achieving remission, age seems to become less important as a predictor for overall survival (OS) and DFS. This may have much to do with initial performance status. Unfavorable cytogenetics are the major determinant for poor survival after intensive chemotherapy (de Witte *et al.*, 1996). MDS patients achieving either CR or partial remission (PR) after intensive chemotherapy may expect a >5 year survival of around 15%, and some of these will be cured (Wattel *et al.*, 1997). Long-term survivors are more likely to have suffered from RAEB-t at diagnosis, with normal or favorable cytogenetic findings. Earlier treatment in the course of the disease confers a better prognosis. This indicates that at least some patient categories—even some that only achieve PR—may benefit from intensive cytotoxic treatment.

At present it is unclear if newer induction regimens containing fludarabine (Parker *et al.*, 1997), topotecan (Beran *et al.*, 1999), or monoclonal antibodies (anti-CD33) (Estey *et al.*, 2002) give higher CR rates or if remission duration can be prolonged with newer drugs such as decitabine, azacytidine, or anti-CD33 monoclonal antibody. The use of myeloid growth factors such as G-CSF or GM-CSF may decrease the duration of granulocytopenia, but does not seem to increase survival.

Recommendations for allogeneic transplantation in MDS (and see Chapter 54)

Allogeneic hematopoietic stem cell transplantation (allo-SCT) can lead to long-term DFS and cure in a selected group of MDS patients. The high to very high non-relapse mortality remains disappointing. Moreover, most MDS patients lack a suitable HLA-identical sibling donor. The results of transplants using alternative, partially matched family donors and phenotypically matched unrelated donors, remain unsatisfactory and display a high transplant-related mortality (TRM) rate of about 50%. The probability of DFS is only 18% to 30%, depending largely on age and interval between diagnosis and transplant. Many investigators regard the high to very high allo-transplant mortality rates as unacceptable. However, for high- and intermediate 2-risk MDS patients who have a compatible sibling or unrelated donor by molecular HLA typing, allogeneic stem cell transplantation (bone marrow or peripheral blood) is the treatment of choice. The DFS after allogeneic transplantation for patients with MDS after chemo- or radiotherapy (t-MDS) is not different compared to that of patients with primary MDS (Boogaerts, 1998; Anderson, 2000; Deeg, 2000; Oosterveld & de Witte, 2000).

The best results with allo-SCT are obtained in younger patients, with low blast counts, transplanted early in the course of their disease. This subgroup was shown by IPSS analysis to have a median survival of more than 11 years without treatment. IPSS low- and intermediate 1-risk categories thus hardly form an indication for early transplant, unless complex unfavorable cytogenetics or a life threatening cytopenia is present. Unrelated donor transplants are, at present, not indicated in this category. In the Seattle series of unrelated donor transplants the actuarial non-relapse mortality at 2 years for RA patients (n = 20) was 46%. Similar figures were observed in our own series (Demuynck et al., 1996a). According to IPSS, these patients, if left untreated, can be predicted to have a 50% chance of survival beyond 11 years. Moreover, if the total Seattle data on 241 transplanted patients were subjected to IPSS score evaluation, slightly more than half of their patients (n = 145) belonged to intermediate 2- or high-risk categories before transplant and had a DFS of only 32% and 24% respectively. This included sibling transplant recipients. (Anderson et al., 1996; Anderson & Thomas, 1997; Appelbaum & Anderson, 1998; Anderson, 2000). As stated above, long-term DFS with chemotherapy alone in this category amounts to about 15%, with a 16% death rate from aplasia.

Therefore, definite recommendations regarding the early use of allogeneic transplants in MDS, outside well controlled and randomized studies, cannot be made. Attempts at reducing the risk of TRM are under way. Substitution of "supralethal" conditioning regimens by less toxic, tolerance-inducing regimens (the so-called "mini-transplant" approach), supplemented with delayed donor lymphocyte infusions (DLI) may improve outcome considerably. The availability of large numbers of allogeneic peripheral blood stem cells—partially or totally T-cell depleted, with or without add-backs—offers new opportunities for improved allogeneic transplant technology.

Autologous transplantation in MDS

Feasibility of autologous stem cell transplantation

As previously mentioned, the success of intensive chemotherapy in MDS is hampered by short remission durations and high relapse rates. Moreover, even in the most optimal setting, transplant-related mortality and morbidity after allogeneic transplantation remain high, and the number of MDS patients eligible for this procedure is low. Therefore, given its success in AML and lymphoma, treatment with high-dose chemotherapy followed by autologous hematopoietic stem cell transplantation (AHSCT) has also been explored in patients with MDS. However, since MDS is a clonal disease and marrow failure is one of the hallmarks of the pathogenesis of MDS, serious concerns have been raised about the feasibility of stem cell harvesting, about the clonal nature of the harvested progenitor cells, and about their in vivo repopulating capacity.

Hematological remissions in MDS: polyclonal or monoclonal?

The monoclonal nature of MDS hematopoiesis was demonstrated more than 20 years ago, (Prchal et al., 1978). During the following years, karyotyping, in situ hybridization, and X-chromosome inactivation (XCI) assays detecting polymorphisms in X-linked genes, have proven the monoclonality of erythro-, myelomono- and megakaryopoiesis in MDS (reviewed by Weimar et al., 1994). In contrast, clonal mutations are not detectable in T-lymphocytes, which is supported by the observation that transformation to acute lymphoblastic leukemia does not occur in MDS. Therefore, clonality experiments on mature MDS cells argue in favour of a clonal mutation in a committed myeloids progenitor cell. However, the scarcity of evidence for mature lymphocytes being derived from the MDS clone does not exclude the possibility that the primary transformation event can occur at a more immature progenitor level. Clonality data on highly purified committed and immature marrow progenitor cells do in fact suggest a heterogeneous pattern of progenitor involvement. Whereas some cytogenetic abnormalities such as trisomy 8 are found in more committed progenitor cells (Saitoh et al., 1998), immature progenitors seem to be more susceptible to other mutations such as del(5q) (Nilsson et al., 2000).

Despite the predominantly clonal involvement of MDS myelopoiesis at the time of diagnosis, some reports have suggested that residual non-clonal myeloid cells coexist with the malignant monoclonal ones. This has been demonstrated by FISH (Gerritsen et al., 1992; Kibbelaar et al., 1992), and has been confirmed by X-chromosome inactivation (XCI)-based experiments where allelic patterns in patients with early or advanced MDS have demonstrated the persistence of a minor fraction of non-clonally involved myeloid cells (Anan *et al.*, 1995; Delforge *et al.*, 1998). Earlier clonality studies with XCI (Ito *et al.*, 1994; Delforge *et al.*, 1998; Aivado *et al.*, 2000) and cytogenetics (de Witte *et al.*, 1995; Carella *et al.*, 1996) proved that by eradication of the monoclonal cells, intensive chemotherapy could stimulate the growth of this minor population of residual normal progenitor cells. Although these reports indicate that at least part of complete hematological remissions in MDS are polyclonal in origin, it still needs to be elucidated if polyclonal remissions are more durable than the monoclonal ones. The EORTC trial no. 06961 might give an answer to this important question. This multicenter trial was designed to compare an intensive chemotherapy consolidation course with autologous transplantation in high-risk MDS patients younger than 60 years not eligible for allogeneic transplantation. Patients were treated with a common remission-induction and consolidation course followed by stem cell harvesting. Subsequently, patients in remission were randomized to receive either an additional consolidation course with high-dose cytosine arabinoside, or an autologous transplantation with mobilized peripheral blood progenitor cells. Clonality patterns of mature myeloid cells and T lymphocytes were studied by conventional cytogenetics, FISH, and XCI at diagnosis, after the first consolidation course, in the stem cell harvest, and during follow-up. In 58% of 259 evaluable patients, remission induction with a combination of idarubicin, cytosine arabinoside, and etoposide resulted in a complete hematological remission. CR rates were 75%, 43%, and 46% respectively in the good, intermediate, and poor prognostic IPSS cytogenetic subgroups. In patients who reached CR, 73% achieved a cytogenetic remission and 27% of patients had persisting cytogenetic abnormalities in bone marrow and blood. Interim analysis after 2 years follow-up showed a significantly better DFS for patients in CR with a cytogenetic remission compared to patients with residual abnormal metaphases (44% vs. 15%; $P = 0.03$). In addition, the 2-year cumulative relapse incidence was 39% versus 85% in the 2 groups (de Witte *et al.*, 2001a). In female patients informative for polymorphisms in the human androgen receptor locus (HUMARA), 60% had polyclonal remissions in their myeloid cells when achieving a CR. Based on HUMARA results, the clinical outcome between clonal and polyclonal CR was not statistically different, but a longer observation period is needed to clarify if the XCI status at remission will have a prognostic impact (Van Dijk *et al.*, 2001). In summary, whereas the majority of remission marrows in primary AML are polyclonal, more than half of the MDS patients who achieve a CR after intensive chemotherapy have restoration of a polyclonal and cytogenetically normal hematopoiesis.

Can sufficient numbers of progenitors be mobilized in MDS?

Besides monoclonality, marrow failure is a typical feature of the pathogenesis of MDS. Although the majority of MDS patients have a hypercellular bone marrow, a significant percentage of these MDS marrow progenitors are doomed to become apoptotic and proliferate and differentiate abnormally. In other MDS patients autologous stem cell harvesting can be hampered by severe bone marrow hypocellularity, making an autologous hematopoietic stem cell transplant (HSCT) impossible (Demuynck *et al.*, 1996b; Wattel *et al.*, 1999). As with other hematological malignancies, mobilized peripheral blood progenitor cells (PBPC) have become a more attractive stem cell source for autografting in MDS (de Witte *et al.*, 2002). There are currently only a few reports on the feasibility of PBPC mobilization with either chemotherapy and G-CSF, or G-CSF alone, for MDS. Generally, a threshold of $1-2 \times 10^6$ $CD34^+$ cells/kg can be obtained in approximately half of the MDS patients after mobilization with cytosine arabinoside-containing regimens followed by G-CSF (Demuynck *et al.*, 1996b; Wattel *et al.*, 1999; de Witte, personal communication). In patients achieving a polyclonal CR, stem cell harvests have been found to be polyclonal (Delforge *et al.*, 1995) and cytogenetically normal (Carella *et al.*, 1996). Mobilization with G-CSF alone at 10 μg/kg/d for 5 days has also been reported in 16 patients with low-grade MDS. More than 2×10^6 $CD34^+$ cells/kg were harvested in 7 of 16 (44%) patients. In 4 out of 6 patients with an abnormal karyotype at diagnosis, the cytogenetic abnormality persisted in the majority of metaphases in the stem cell harvest. In the 2 other patients a significant amount of non-clonal cells was harvested (Mijovic *et al.*, 2001). These data, although limited, could argue in favour of PBPC harvesting after G-CSF in younger patients without leukemic blast cells, who lack a compatible related or unrelated donor. Although it seems logical that MDS patients with hypocellular marrows are "poor mobilizers," other disease characteristics that might predict a succesful harvest (e.g. clonal or polyclonal remission marrow) are yet to be identified.

What is the in vivo repopulating capacity of transplanted MDS progenitor cells?

In vitro experiments have proven that committed (Sawada *et al.*, 1995) and immature (Flores Figueroa *et al.*, 1999) marrow progenitors in MDS have a reduced proliferative capacity and shorter survival. However, although hematopoietic reconstitution after HSCT in MDS tends to be slower when compared with primary AML, transplant-related mortality was not found to be higher (de Witte *et al.*, 1997; Wattel *et al.*, 1999) This would suggest that the engraftment capabilities of stem cells derived from patients with MDS are usually sufficient to restore hematopoiesis to levels that prevent fatal infectious and hemorrhagic complications. Repopulation of hematopoiesis after autologous transplantation in MDS can be accelerated when PBPC are used instead of bone marrow (BM) (Demuynck *et al.*, 1996b; Carella *et al.*, 1996). Analysis of more than 30 MDS stem cell harvests collected at the University of Leuven failed to reveal a positive correlation between the number of $CD34^+$ cells and the number of CFU-GM, an in vitro surrogate marker for in vivo progenitor proliferation (Delforge and Boogaerts, unpublished results). Nevertheless, initial reports have shown more rapid, and sustained, hematopoietic recovery with PBPC compared to BM (Demuynck *et al.*, 1996b; Wattel *et al.*, 1999). Consistent with this rapid recovery, days of fever, need for parenteral antibiotics, empiric antifungal therapy, transfusions of red cells and platelets, and total duration of hospitalization are significantly decreased when compared with a historical matched autologous bone marrow transplantation (ABMT) group. Early relapse rates are not different from ABMT, while direct TRM is less prominent. Another argument in favor of the use of PBPC instead of BM comes from the observation that the use of PBPC as the source for autografting in MDS results in a

better outcome compared to bone marrow in patients younger than 55 years (de Witte *et al.*, 2002).

Clinical experience with autologous hematopoietic stem cell transplantation in MDS

The Chronic Leukemia Registry of the European Group for Blood and Marrow Transplantation (EBMT) contains data on almost 200 patients autografted for MDS or secondary leukemia. Data on 79 of those transplanted in first CR were published in 1997. The 2-year OS, DFS, and relapse rates were respectively 39%, 34%, and 64%. Patients younger than 40 years had a significantly better DFS (39%) than patients older than 40 (25%).

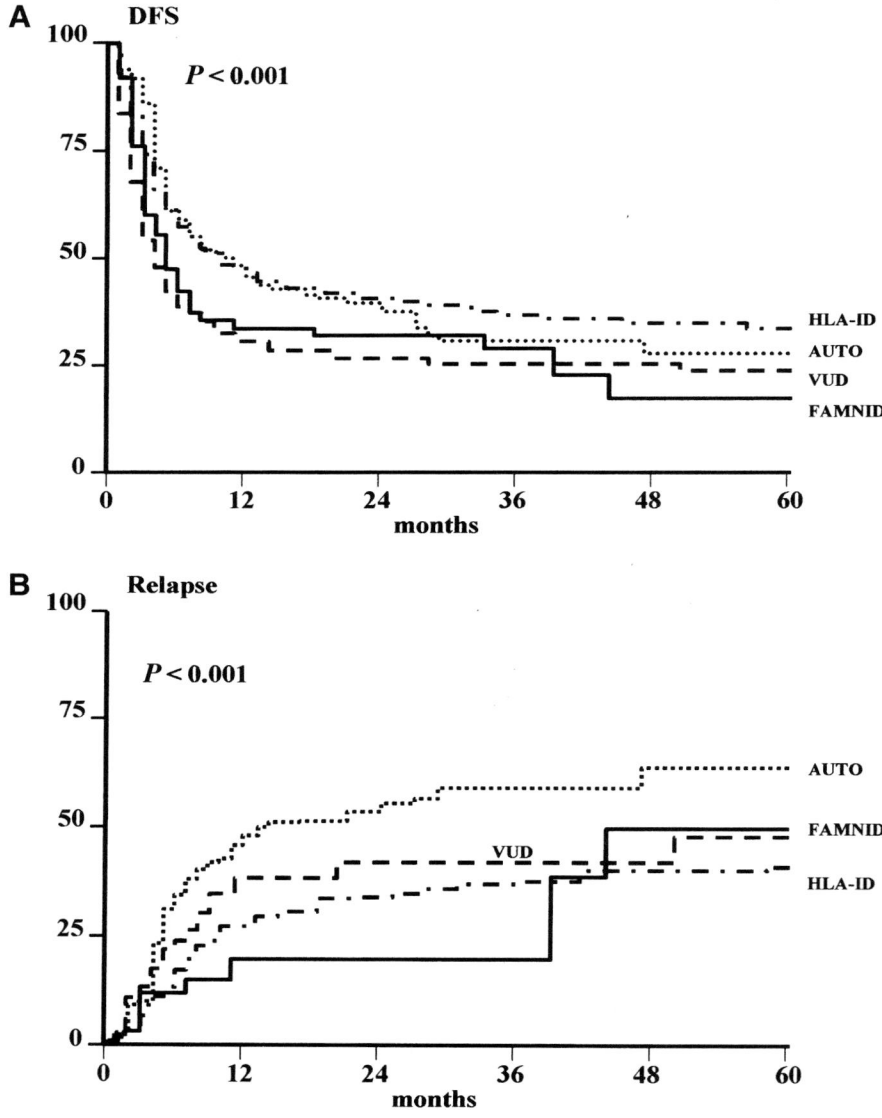

Fig. 39.1. **(A)** Disease-free survival (DFS) of MDS patients transplanted with stem cells derived from: histocompatible siblings (HLA-ID); genotypically matched non-identical relatives (FAMNID); volunteer unrelated donors (VUD); autologous stem cells (AUTO). Reproduced, with permission, from de Witte *et al.* (2000). **(B)** Risk of relapse of MDS patients transplanted with stem cells derived from: histocompatible siblings (HLA-ID); genotypically matched non-identical relatives (FAMNID); volunteer unrelated donors (VUD); autologous stem cells (AUTO). Reproduced, with permission, from de Witte *et al.* (2000).

The large majority of these patients were transplanted for a secondary leukemia or t-MDS, and only 19 underwent ABMT for primary RAEB or RAEB-T. The survival of the latter was slightly better (46%) than that of the whole group. The TRM was lower than 10% (de Witte et al., 1997). However, these data have to be interpreted with caution. Only patients in CR were included in this retrospective analysis, excluding those not recovering from, or resistant to, induction chemotherapy. Moreover, no data are available on the number of patients with MDS in whom no adequate marrow harvest could be performed (persistent hypoplasia, fibrosis, poor performance, etc.). In the same study, a cohort of 55 patients was compared with a matched control group of 110 patients with de novo AML. The MDS/sAML cohort showed a lower DFS (28%) when compared with de novo AML patients (51%), primarily due to a higher relapse rate.

Preliminary results on the influence of cytogenetic data on the outcome of autologous transplantation in MDS confirm previous data on intensive chemotherapy, i.e. actuarial 2-year survival of 52% in patients with good- or intermediate-risk, versus 28% in the poor risk group (de Witte et al., 1996).

The French MDS group has prospectively assessed the role of autologous stem cell transplantation as consolidation treatment in high-risk MDS patients after intensive chemotherapy. In this trial, patients aged 55 years or less, without an HLA-identical sibling donor and achieving CR, were scheduled to receive an unmanipulated HSCT preceded by a consolidation chemotherapy course. Twenty-four of the 39 patients (62%) received either an autologous BMT ($n = 16$) or an autologous PBPC transplant ($n = 8$) after conditioning with cyclophosphamide and busulfan. Hematological reconstitution tended to be faster after blood than marrow transplantation, although not significantly so. Median DFS after transplantation was 29 months (Wattel et al., 1999).

In another retrospective EBMT study (de Witte et al., 2001b), autologous HSCT and allo-SCT were compared as consolidation therapy after a similar remission-induction and consolidation course. Patients with a histocompatible sibling were candidates for allo-SCT and the remainder for autologous HSCT. In summary, 72% of patients with a donor were allografted in first CR, and 61% without a donor received HSCT. DFS at 4 years was 31% in the allo-SCT group, and 27% in the HSCT group. These early results of autologous HSCT, either with marrow or mobilized peripheral blood, indicate that survival may approach that of related allogeneic transplant recipients and even surpass those of unrelated transplants, because of low TRM. Support for this statement is found in an EBMT survey on 1378 transplants for MDS reported to the registry between 1983 and 1998 comparing autologous HSCT with allo-SCT using non-identical family members or unrelated donors (de Witte et al., 2000). The estimated DFS at 3 years was 25% for the 198 patients with volunteer unrelated donor transplants, 28% for 91 patients with alternative family donor transplants, and 33% for the 126 patients autografted in first CR (Figure 39.1A). The non-relapse mortality was 58% for patients with unrelated donors, 66% for patients with non-identical family donors, and 25% for autografted patients (Figure 39.1B). As expected, relapse rates were higher in the autologous HSCT group compared to allo-transplanted patients. Nevertheless, DFS after autologous HSCT is not inferior to allogeneic transplantation using non-identical family donors, and the intensity of the treatment is much lower. Similar observations were made in our own retrospective single center study in Leuven comparing autologous transplants ($n = 10$) with myeloablative sibling transplants ($n = 12$), matched unrelated transplants ($n = 10$), and non-myeloablative allogeneic transplants ($n = 9$). Kaplan-Meier estimated 2-year DFS was 49%, 40%, 47%, and 64% respectively (Boogaerts et al., 2002).

The current practice of HSC transplantation for myelodysplasia in Europe has been described (Urbano-Ispizua et al., 2002) (and see Chapter 124, Breaking News...).

Conclusions

Allogeneic stem cell transplantation, using either a compatible sibling or matched unrelated donor, has been advocated as the only possibility for cure in MDS. Data from the International Bone Marrow Transplant Registry, National Marrow Donor Program, and European Bone Marrrow Transplant/European Organisation for Research and Treatment of Cancer cooperative groups have consistently shown long-term DFS rates around 30% at the cost of a (sometimes excessive) high TRM. Only in younger patients with low-risk IPSS MDS subtypes with a short disease duration does DFS seem to outweigh TRM. This is only a small minority of the total MDS population. Therefore, in patients without a compatible donor, or in those in whom excessive TRM is feared, autologous HSCT can offer a valuable alternative. Although the procedure is still hampered by difficulties in stem cell harvesting in about half of the patients in complete remission, current studies have unequivocally proven the feasibility of autologous HSCT in MDS. Moreover, long-term DFS in the range of 30% can be expected without excessive TRM. Therefore, the outcome of autologous HSCT in MDS seems similar to that of allogeneic stem cell transplantation with donors other than HLA-identical siblings. Unfortunately, relapse rates above 50% are indicative of incomplete eradication of the malignant clone by current conditioning regimens, and/or contamination of the autografts with residual disease. The feasibility of harvesting cytogenetically, polyclonal progenitor cells in the majority of MDS patients in complete hematological remission should fuel further clinical trials. However, it still needs to be shown if this is associated with a better outcome due to lower relapse rates.

References

Aivado, M., Rong, A., Germing, U. et al. (2000). Long-term remission after intensive chemotherapy in advanced myelodysplastic syndromes is generally associated with restoration of polyclonal haemopoiesis. British Journal of Haematology, **110**, 884–86.

Anan, K., Ito, M., Misawa, M. et al. (1995). Clonal analysis of peripheral blood and haemopoietic colonies in patients with aplastic anaemia and refractory anaemia using the short tandem repeat on the human androgen-receptor (HUMARA) gene. *British Journal of Haematology*, **89**, 838–44.

Anderson, J., Anasetti, C., Appelbaum, F. *et al.* (1996). Unrelated donor bone marrow transplantation for myelodysplasia and MDS related acute myeloid leukemia. *British Journal of Haematology*, **93**, 59–67.

Anderson, J. E. (2000). Bone marrow transplantation for myelodysplasia. *Hematological Oncology*, **14**, 63–77.

Anderson, J. E. & Thomas, E. D. (1997). The Seattle experience with bone marrow transplantation for myelodysplasia. *Leukemia Research*, **51**, S21.

Appelbaum, F. & Anderson, J. (1998). Allogeneic bone marrow transplantation for myelodysplastic syndrome: outcomes analysis according to IPSS score. *Leukemia*, **12**, S1, S25–29.

Asano, H., Ohashi, H., Ichihara, M. *et al.* (1994). Evidence for non-clonal hematopoietic progenitor cell populations in bone marrow of patients with myelodysplastic syndromes. *Blood*, **84**, 588–94.

Beran, M., Estey, E., O'Brien, S. *et al.* (1999). Topotecan and cytarabine is an active combination regimen in myelodysplastic syndromes and chronic myelomonocytic leukemia. *Journal of Clinical Oncology*, **17**, 2819–30.

Boogaerts, M. (1998). Stem cell transplantation and intensified cytotoxic treatment for myelodysplasia. *Current Opinion in Hematology*, **5**, 465–71.

Boogaerts, M., Maertens, J., Delforge, M. *et al.* (2002). Comparison of different modalities of stem cell transplantation for myelodysplasia. *Hematology Journal*, **3** (Suppl 1) (Abstract 1062).

Boogaerts, M., Verhoef, G., & Demuynck, H. (1996). Treatment and prognostic factors in myelodysplastic syndromes. *Bailliere's Clinical Haematology*, **9**, 161–83.

Carella, A. M., Dejana, A., Lerma, E. *et al.* (1996). In vivo mobilisation of karyotypically normal peripheral blood progenitor cells in high-risk MDS, secondary or therapy-related acute myelogenous leukemia. *British Journal of Haematology*, **95**, 127–30.

Deeg, H. & Appelbaum, F. (2000). Hemopoietic stem cell transplantation for myelodysplastic syndrome. *Currrent Opinion in Oncology*, **12**, 116–20.

Delforge, M., Demuynck, H., Vandenberghe, P. *et al.* (1995). Polyclonal primitive hematopoietic progenitors can be detected in mobilized peripheral blood from patients with high-risk myelodysplastic syndromes. *Blood*, **86**, 3660–67.

Delforge, M., Demuynck, H., Verhoef, G. *et al.* (1998). Patients with high-risk myelodysplastic syndrome can have polyclonal or clonal haemopoiesis in complete haematological remission. *British Journal of Haematology*, **102**, 486–94.

Demuynck, H., Delforge, M., Verhoef, G. *et al.* (1996a). Feasibility of peripheral blood progenitor cell harvest and transplantation in patients with poor-risk myelodysplastic syndromes. *British Journal of Haematology*, **92**, 351–9.

Demuynck, H., Verhoef, G., Emonds, M. P. *et al.* (1996b). Treatment of patients with myelodysplastic syndromes with allogeneic bone marrow transplantation from genotypically HLA-identical siblings and alternative donors. *Bone Marrow Transplantation*, **17**, 745–51.

de Witte, T., Zwaan, F., & Hermans, J. (1990). Allogeneic bone marrow transplantation for secondary leukemia and myelodysplastic syndrome. A survey by the Leukemia Working Party of the EBMT. *British Journal of Haematology*, **74**, 151–5.

de Witte, T., Hagemeijer, A., Suciu, S. *et al.* (2001a). Cytogenetic risk group and cytogenetic response predict outcome of patients with poor-risk MDS and secondary AML treated with intensive chemotherapy and stem cell transplantation in a joint study (CRIANT) of the EORTC, EBMT, SAKK, HOVON and GIMEMA leukemia groups. *Blood*, **98**, Abstract 2595.

de Witte, T., Hermans, J., Vossen, J. *et al.* (2000). Haematopoietic stem cell transplantation for patients with myelodysplastic syndromes and secondary acute myeloid leukaemias: a report on behalf of the Chronic Leukemia Working Party of the European Group for Blood and Marrow Transplantation. *British Journal of Haematology*, **110**, 620–30.

de Witte, T., Suciu, S., Boogaerts, M. *et al.* (1996). The influence of cytogenetic abnormalities on treatment outcome after intensive antileukemic therapy for patients with high risk MDS and AML following MDS. A joint study of the EORTC, EBMT, SAKK, GIMEMA. *Blood*, **88**, Abstract 1806.

de Witte, T., Suciu, S., Peetermans, P., & Fenaux, P. (1995). Intensive chemotherapy for poor prognosis myelodysplasia and secondary acute myeloid leukemia following MDS of more than 6 months duration. A pilot study by the leukemia cooperative group of the EORTC. *Leukemia*, **9**, 1805–11.

de Witte, T., Suciu, S., Verhoef, G. *et al.* (2001b). Intensive chemotherapy followed by allogeneic or autologous stem cell transplantation for patients with myelodysplastic syndromes (MDSs) and acute myeloid leukemia following MDS. *Blood*, **98**, 2326–31.

de Witte, T., Van Biezen, A., Brand, R. *et al.* (2002). Peripheral stem cells are the preferred source of stem cells for autologous stem cell transplantation (HSCT) of young patients with high-risk MDS or AML following MDS. *The Hematology Journal*, **3** (Suppl 1) Abstract 0603.

de Witte, T., Van Biezen, A., Hermans, J. *et al.* (1997). Autologous bone marrow transplantation for patients with myelodysplastic syndromes or acute myeloid leukemia following MDS. *Blood*, **90**, 3853–57.

Estey, E., Thall, P., Beran, M. *et al.* (1997). Effect of diagnosis (refractory anemia with excess blasts, refractory anemia with excess blasts in transformation, or acute myeloid leukemia (AML) on outcome of AML-type chemotherapy. *Blood*, **90**, 2969–77.

Estey, E., Thall, P., Giles, F. *et al.* (2002). Gemtuzumab ozogamicin with or without interleukin 11 in patients 65 years of age or older with untreated acute myeloid leukemia and high-risk myelodysplastic syndrome: comparison with idarubicin plus continuous-infusion, high-dose cytosine arabinoside. *Blood*, **99**, 4343–9.

Flores Figueroa, E., Gutierrez Espindola, G., Guerrero Rivera, S., Pizzuto Chavez, J., & Mayani, H. (1999). Hematopoietic progenitor cells from patients with myelodysplastic syndromes: in vitro colony growth and long-term proliferation. *Leukemia Research*, **23**, 385–94.

Gerritsen, W., Donohue, J., Bauman, J. *et al.* (1992). Clonal analysis of myelodysplastic syndrome: monosomy 7 is expressed in the myeloid lineage, but not in the lymphoid lineage as detected by fluorescent in situ hybridization. *Blood*, **80**, 217–24.

Greenberg, P., Cox, C., Le Beau, M. *et al.* (1997). International scoring system for evaluating prognosis in myelodysplastic syndromes. *Blood,* **89,** 2079–88.

Heaney, M. L. & Golde, D. W. (1999). Myelodysplasia. *New England Journal Medicine,* **340,** 1649.

Ito, T., Ohashi, H., Ichikawa, A., Saito, H., & Hotta, T. (1994). Recovery of polyclonal hematopoiesis in patients with myelodysplastic syndromes following successful chemotherapy. *Leukemia,* **8,** 839–43.

Kibbelaar, R., Van Kamp, H., Dreef, E. *et al.* (1992). Combined immunophenotyping and DNA in situ hybridization to study lineage involvement in patients with myelodysplastic syndromes. *Blood,* **79,** 1823–8.

Mijovic, A., Delforge, M., Sekhavat, M., Czepulkowski, B., & Mufti, G. (2001). Do patients with low-grade myelodysplastic syndrome mobilise normal hemopoietic progenitors? *Leukemia Research,* **25** (Suppl 1) Abstract.

Nilsson, L., Astrand-Grundstrom, I., Arvidsson, I. *et al.* (2000). Isolation and characterization of hematopoietic progenitor/stem cells in 5q-deleted myelodysplatic syndromes: evidence for involvement at the hematopoietic stem cell level. *Blood,* **96,** 2012–21.

Novitzky, N. & Prindull, G. (2000). Myelodysplastic syndromes in children. A critical review of the clinical manifestations and management. *American Journal of Hematology,* **63,** 212–22.

Oosterveld, M. & de Witte, T. (2000). Intensive treatment strategies in patients with high-risk myelodysplastic syndrome and secondary acute leukemia. *Blood Reviews,* **14,** 182–9.

Parker, J., Pagliuca, A. *et al.* (1997). Fludarabine, cytarabine, G-CSF and idarubicin (FLAG-IDA) for the treatment of poor-risk myelodysplastic syndromes and acute myeloid leukemia. *British Journal of Haematology,* **99,** 939–44.

Prchal, J., Throckmorton, D., Carroll, A. *et al.* (1978). A common progenitor for human myeloid and lymphoid cells. *Nature,* **274,** 590–1.

Saitoh, K., Miura, I., Takahashi, N., & Miura, A. (1998). Fluorescence in situ hybridization of progenitor cells obtained by fluorescence-activated cell sorting for the detection of cells affected by chromosome abnormality trisomy 8 in patients with myelodysplastic syndromes. *Blood,* **92,** 2886–92.

Sawada, K., Sato, N., Notoya, A. *et al.* (1995). Proliferation and differentiation of myelodysplastic CD34+ cells: phenotypic subpopulations of marrow CD34+ cells. *Blood,* **85,** 194–202.

Tricot, G. & Boogaerts, M. (1986). The role of aggressive chemotherapy in the treatment of the myelodysplastic syndromes. *British Journal of Haematology,* **63,** 477–483.

Urbano-Ispizua, A., Schmitz, N., de Witte, T. *et al.* (2002). Allogeneic and autologous transplantation for haematological diseases, solid tumors and immune disorders: definition and current practice in Europe. *Bone Marrow Transplantation,* **29,** 639–46.

Van Dijk, J., Aivado, M., Delforge, M. *et al.* (2001). Analysis of clonality by Humara PCR in high risk MDS patients before and after intensive anti-leukemic treatment. *Blood,* **98,** Abstract 3519.

Wattel, E., De Botton, S., Lai, J., & Fenaux, P. (1997). Long-term follow-up of de novo myelodysplastic syndromes treated with intensive chemotherapy: incidence of long-term survivors and outcome of partial responders. *British Journal of Haematology,* **98,** 983–91.

Wattel, E., Solary, E., Leleu, X. *et al.* (1999). A prospective study of autologous bone marrow or peripheral blood stem cell transplantation after intensive chemotherapy in myelodysplastic syndromes. Groupe Français de myelodysplasies. Group Ouest-Est d'etude des leucemies aigues myeloides. *Leukemia,* **13,** 524–9.

Weimar, I., Bourhis, J., De Gast, G., & Gerritsen, W. (1994). Clonality in myelodysplastic syndromes. *Leukemia and Lymphoma,* **13,** 215–21.

40 Autologous hematopoietic stem cell transplantation for multiple myeloma and AL amyloidosis

BHAWNA SIROHI, NOOPUR RAJE, AND RAYMOND POWLES

Royal Marsden Hospital, Sutton, UK and Dana-Farber Cancer Center, Boston, USA

Introduction

Myeloma is one of the few hematologic malignancies in which autologous hematopoietic stem cell (HSC) transplantation is now accepted as front-line treatment in the majority of patients. For more than 30 years melphalan and prednisolone (Alexanian *et al.*, 1969), and other chemotherapy combinations such as ABCM, VCMP/VBAP, and MOCCA (Palva *et al.*, 1987; MacLennan *et al.*, 1992; Blade *et al.*, 1993; Salmon *et al.*, 1994), have been used and tumor responsiveness has been documented. This response is, however, restricted to 60% to 70% of the patients and median survival did not exceed 3 years. Thalidomide, used to treat myeloma based on its antiangiogenic activity and the increased angiogenesis observed in myeloma marrow, can achieve responses even in refractory, relapsed disease (Singhal *et al.*, 1999). Immunomodulatory drugs (ImiDs) derived from thalidomide, such as CC-5013, stimulate T-cell proliferation, as well as interleukin (IL)-2 and interferon-γ production and decrease production of cytokines mediating growth and survival of myeloma cells such as IL-6 and vascular endothelial factor. CC-5013 also decreases angiogenesis and stimulates anti-myeloma NK cell activity. It has clinical activity in relapsed and refractory myeloma (Richardson *et al.*, 2002). The use of dose-intensive chemotherapy has been challenging in patients with myeloma as the patients' median age is 65 years and almost 50% of patients have renal failure at some time point during the course of their disease. With the refinement of autologous transplantation, "operational cures" are now being described in patients with myeloma and we are beginning to see plateaus in a small group of patients who have been in continuous first complete remission (CR) for more than 10 years (Powles *et al.*, 2000a and b; Sirohi *et al.*, 2002).

The incidence of multiple myeloma is approximately 4 per 10,000 per annum. It accounted for 1.1% of estimated new cancer cases in the United States in 1996. The types of myeloma and their relative frequency are shown in Table 40.1. The minimal criteria for diagnosis of myeloma consist of more than 10% plasma cells in the bone marrow or a plasmacytoma and one of the following: (1) monoclonal (M)-protein in the serum usually more than 3 g/dl; (2) M-protein in the urine; or (3) lytic bone lesions, these findings being unrelated to carcinoma, lymphoma, connective tissue disorders, chronic infections, or other disorders associated with polyclonal hyperglobulinemia such as sarcoidosis or cirrhosis (Table 40.2).

The main conditions to consider in the differential diagnosis are monoclonal gammopathy of undetermined or unknown significance (MGUS), smoldering multiple myeloma, primary systemic amyloidosis (AL), lymphoma, and metastatic carcinoma. An M-protein value <3 g/dl, fewer than 10% bone marrow plasma cells, absence of lytic lesions, anemia, hypercalcemia, or renal insufficiency in an asymptomatic patient are characteristic of monoclonal gammopathy of undetermined

Table 40.1. *Frequency of different types of myeloma*

Myeloma	Relative frequency[a]
IgG	55%
IgA	20%
IgD	1%
Light chain	24%

[a] IgE and IgM myelomas are extremely rare.

Table 40.2. *Diagnostic criteria for myeloma*

1. Cytologic criteria
   (a) Marrow morphology: plasma cells and/or myeloma cells in excess of 10% when 1,000 or more cells have been counted.
   (b) Biopsy-proven plasmacytoma, either in bone or in soft tissues.
2. Clinical and laboratory criteria
   (a) Myeloma protein (M component) demonstrable by immunoelectrophoresis of plasma, usually <20 g/l.
   (b) Myeloma protein (M component) demonstrable by immunoelectrophoresis of urine, usually >1 g in 24 hours.
   (c) Radiologic evidence of osteolytic lesions: generalized osteoporosis qualifies as a criterion if the marrow contains in excess of 30% plasma or myeloma cells.
   (d) Myeloma cells in at least two peripheral blood smears.

Table 40.3. *Staging of myeloma (Salmon-Durie)*

Stage	Criteria
Stage I	All of the following: 1. Hemoglobin >10 g/dl 2. Serum calcium concentration normal 3. Normal bone structure (scale 0)[a] or solitary bone plasmacytoma only 4. Low paraprotein production rates 　(a) IgG value <5 g/dl 　(b) IgA value <3 g/dl 　(c) Urine light chain paraprotein on electrophoresis <4 g in 24 hours
Stage II	Neither stage I nor stage III
Stage III	One or more of the following: 1. Hemoglobin <8.5 g/dl 2. Serum calcium concentration elevated 3. Advanced lytic bone lesions (scale 3)[a] 4. High paraprotein production 　(a) IgG value >7 g/dl 　(b) IgA value >5 g/dl 　(c) Urine light chain paraprotein on electrophoresis >12 g in 24 hours

Subclassification: A, normal renal function; B, abnormal renal function.

[a] Scale for bone lesions: normal bones (0), osteoporosis (1), lytic bone lesions (2), extensive skeletal destruction and major fractures (3).

significance (MGUS) (see below). An M protein value <3 g/dl and more than 10% bone marrow plasma cells fulfill the diagnostic criteria for smoldering multiple myeloma in asymptomatic patients.

Differentiation from primary systemic amyloidosis is arbitrary because both are plasma cell proliferative disorders. In AL amyloidosis the proportion of bone marrow plasma cells is usually <20%, there are no osteolytic lesions, and the amount of Bence Jones protein in the urine is modest. A nephritic urinary protein pattern is common and the monoclonal light chain band is small and overshadowed by the albumin component.

Myeloma is usually staged using the Salmon-Durie staging system (Table 40.3). Details of the immune phenotype and cytogenetic abnormalities associated with myeloma are shown in Tables 34.4 and 34.5 in Chapter 34.

Serum protein electrophoresis shows a monoclonal spike in 90% of myeloma patients, and urine electrophoresis a globulin spike in 75% of patients. Immunoelectrophoresis is based on diffusion in an Ouchterlony plate of the M-protein against anti-isotope antibody to form a precipitant arc. Immunofixation uses electrophoresis to separate serum proteins and subsequent immunoprecipitation with monospecific antibodies to identify the heavy or light chain isotype.

Prognostic factors for outcome with conventional therapy are shown in Table 40.4. "Standard" chemotherapy treatment utilizes prednisone and melphalan or various combinations of agents, some examples of which are shown in Table 40.5. In a number of randomized trials superior survival has been shown

Table 40.4. *Prognostic factors for outcome with conventional therapy*

Factors reflecting the inherent proliferative capacity of the malignant clone
　Labeling index
　Serum thymidine kinase
Factors reflecting tumor bulk
　β_2 microglobulin (β_2m)
　Stage (see below)
Factors reflecting renal function
　Creatinine
　β_2m
Factors reflecting host-tumor interactions
　IL-6 and soluble IL-6 receptor

Durie-Salmon Stage	Median Survival
Stage I	>60 months
Stage II	36–48 months
Stage III	6–24 months

utilizing multidrug combinations compared to melphalan/prednisone (Table 40.6). Definitions of response to therapy have been revised and are given in Table 40.7 (Blade *et al.*, 1998), but generally outcome is poor with conventional dose chemotherapy (Fig. 40.1 to 40.3).

Table 40.5. *Some conventional dose chemotherapy drug regimens used in myeloma*

Regimen	Drug	Dose	Repeat cycle
MP	Melphalan	8 mg/m²/d po days 1–4	q 28 days
	Prednisone	40 mg/m²/d po days 1–7	
VAD	Vincristine	0.4–0.5 mg/d CI days 1–4	q 35 days
	Doxorubicin	10 mg/m²/d CI days 1–4	
	Dexamethasone	40 mg/d po days 1–4, 9–12, 17–20	
VBMCP	Vincristine	1.2 mg/m² i.v. day 1	q 35–42 days
	Carmustine	20 mg/m² i.v. day 1	
	Melphalan	8 mg/m²/d po days 1–4	
	Cyclophosphamide	400 mg/m² i.v. day 1	
	Prednisone	40 mg/m²/d po days 1–7	
EDAP	Etoposide	100 mg/m²/d CI days 1–4	q 35–42 days
	Dexamethasone	40 mg/m²/d po days 1–5	
	Cytosine arabinoside	1 g/m² i.v. day 5	
	Cisplatin	20–25 mg/m²/d CI days 1–4	

Abbreviation: CI, continuous infusion.

Table 40.6 *Outcome in randomized trials comparing melphalan and prednisone with multidrug combinations to treat newly diagnosed myeloma*

	Median survival (months)	
Reference	Melphalan and prednisone	Multidrug combination
Bergsagel *et al.* (1979)	28	31
Salmon *et al.* (1983)	23 $P < .01$	43
Pavlovsky *et al.* (1984)	39	41
Cooper *et al.* (1986)	34	29
Peest *et al.* (1988)	>40	40
Boccadoro *et al.* (1991)	37	32

Table 40.7. *EBMT, IBMT, and ABMT criteria for definition of response, relapse, and progression in patients with multiple myeloma treated by high-dose therapy and hematopoietic stem cell transplantation*

Complete response (CR) requires all the following:
1. Absence of the original monoclonal paraprotein in serum and urine by immunofixation, maintained for a minimum of 6 weeks. The presence of oligoclonal bands consistent with oligoclonal immune reconstruction does not exclude CR.
2. <5% plasma cells in a bone marrow aspirate and also on trephine bone biopsy, if biopsy is performed. If absence of monoclonal protein is sustained for 6 weeks it is not necessary to repeat the bone marrow, except in patients with non-secretory myeloma where the marrow examinations must be repeated after an interval of at least 6 weeks to confirm CR.
3. No increase in size or number of lytic bone lesions (development of a compression fracture does not exclude response).
4. Disappearance of soft tissue plasmacytomas.
   Patients in whom some, but not all the criteria for CR are fulfilled are classified as PR, providing the remaining criteria satisfy the requirements for PR. This includes patients in whom routine electrophoresis is negative, but in whom immunofixation has not been performed.

Partial response (PR) requires all of the following:
1. ≥50% reduction in the level of the serum monoclonal paraprotein, maintained for a minimum of 6 weeks.
2. Reduction in 24 hour urinary light chain excretion either by ≥90% or to <200 mg: maintained for a minimum of 6 weeks.
3. For patients with non-secretory myeloma only: ≥50% reduction in plasma cells in a bone marrow aspirate and on trephine biopsy, if biopsy is performed, maintained for a minimum of 6 weeks.
4. >50% reduction in the size of soft tissue plasmacytomas (by radiography or clinical examination).
5. No increase in the size or number of lytic bone lesions (development of a compression fracture does not exclude response).
   Patients in whom some, but not all, the criteria for PR are fulfilled are classified as MR, provided the remaining criteria satisfy the requirements for MR.

Minimal response (MR) requires all of the following:
1. 25–49% reduction in the level of the serum monoclonal paraprotein maintained for a minimum of 6 weeks.
2. 50–89% reduction in 24 hour urinary light chain excretion, which still exceeds 200 mg/24 h, maintained for a minimum of 6 weeks.

3. For patients with non-secretory myeloma only: 25–49% reduction in plasma cells in a bone marrow aspirate and on trephine biopsy, if biopsy is performed, maintained for a minimum of 6 weeks.
4. 25–49% reduction in the size of soft tissue plasmacytomas (by radiography or clinical examination).
5. No increase in the size or number of lytic bone lesions (development of a compression fracture does not exclude response).
   MR also includes patients in whom some of, but not all, the criteria for PR are fulfilled, provided the remaining criteria satisfy the requirement for MR.

No change (NC)
   Not meeting the criteria of either minimal response or progressive disease.

Plateau
   Stable values (within 25% above or below value at the time response is assessed) maintained for at least 3 months.

Time point for assessing response
1. Response to the transplant procedure will be assessed by comparison with results immediately prior to conditioning.
2. If transplant is part of a treatment program response to the whole treatment program will be assessed by comparison with the results at the start of the program.

Relapse from CR requires at least one of the following:
1. Reappearance of serum or urinary paraprotein on immunofixations or routine electrophoresis, confirmed by at least one further investigation and excluding oligoclonal immune reconstitution.
2. ≥5% plasma cells in a bone marrow aspirate or on trephine bone biopsy.
3. Development of new lytic bone lesions or soft tissue plasmacytomas or definite increase in the size of residual bone lesions (development of a compression fracture does not exclude continued response and may not indicate progression).
4. Development of hypercalcemia (corrected serum calcium >11.5 mg/dl or 2.8 mmol/l) not attributable to any other cause.

Progressive disease (for patients not in CR) requires one or more of the following:
1. >25% increase in the level of the serum monoclonal paraprotein, which must also be an absolute increase of at least 5 g/l and confirmed by at least one repeated investigation.
2. >25% increase in the 24 hour urinary light chain excretion, which must also be an absolute increase of at least 200 mg/24h and confirmed by at least one repeated investigation.
3. >25% increase in plasma cells in a bone marrow aspirate or on trephine biopsy, which must also be an absolute increase of at least 10%.
4. Definite increase in the size of the existing bone lesions or soft tissue plasmacytomas.
5. Development of new bone lesions or soft tissue plasmacytomas (development of a compression fracture does not exclude continued response and may not indicate progression).
6. Development of hypercalcemia (corrected serum calcium >11.5 mg/dl or 2.8 mmol/l) not attributable to any other cause.

Complete remission (CR) in myeloma was first documented in the early 1980s when McElwain and Powles (1983) treated eight patients with myeloma and one patient with plasma cell leukemia with escalating doses of melphalan (100–140 mg/m^2). All patients responded and three of five previously untreated patients achieved a biochemical and

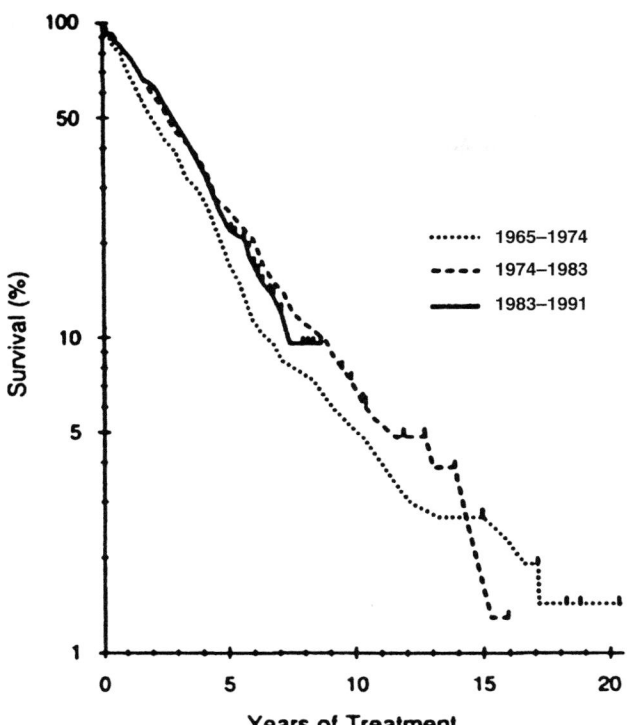

Fig. 40.1. Survival of 1,047 previously untreated patients with multiple myeloma. Consecutive patients were treated with a series of drug combinations during the periods indicated. A total of 357 patients were treated during the first period, 366 during the second, and 324 during the third. Patients still living after 5 years are denoted by tick marks. Reproduced, with permission, from Alexanian and Dimopoulos (1994).

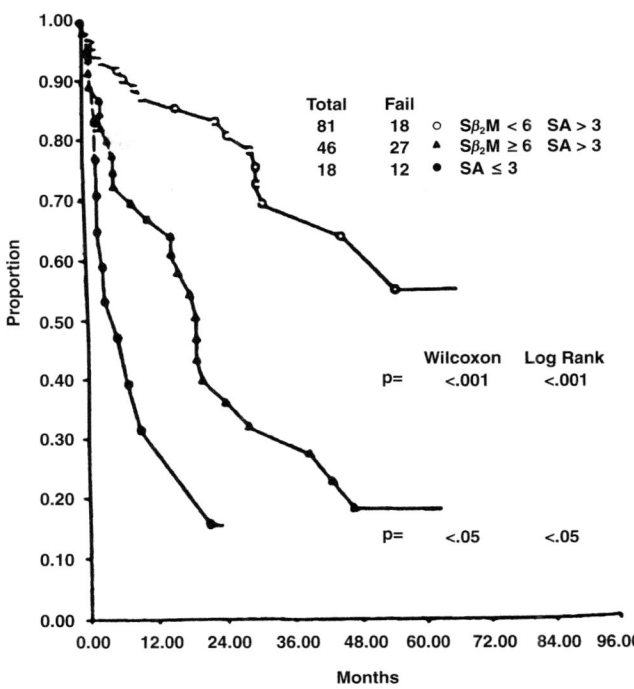

Fig. 40.2. Survival of myeloma patients staged on the basis of serum, β2 microglobulin (β2m), and serum albumin (SA). Kaplan-Meier actuarial survival curves are plotted for groups of patients with (1) β2m (<6 µg/ml) and high serum albumin (>3 g/dl) (open circles), (2) high β2m (<6 µg/ml) and high serum albumin (>3 g/dl) (triangles), and (3) low serum albumin (<3 g/dl) (filled circles). Reproduced, with permission, from Bataille *et al.* (1986).

bone marrow CR (i.e., disappearance of serum paraprotein and clearance of bone marrow plasma cells). Data using escalating doses of melphalan started accumulating and a dose-response effect was noted, even in patients who were resistant to conventional doses of melphalan. This dose-response effect of high-dose melphalan has led to its wide application in the treatment of myeloma in the transplant setting. The last decade has witnessed the use of high-dose chemotherapy or chemoradiotherapy and autologous hematopoietic stem cell (HSC) transplantation in a large proportion of patients with myeloma. Autologous transplantation is now considered to be the standard of care for newly diagnosed patients with myeloma. Experience in the allogeneic setting is somewhat limited due to the advanced median age of myeloma patients, and their innate susceptibility to infection, although occasionally myeloma occurs in patients younger than 30 years (Blade, Kyle, & Greipp, 1996): in one series of such patients the presenting findings and response to conventional therapy were similar to those in patients of all ages. Due to a high treatment-related mortality associated with allogeneic transplantation, reduced intensity conditioning regimens followed by allogeneic transplantation are currently being explored. Preliminary data in patients receiving a reduced intensity conditioning allotransplant preceded by an autologous transplant

appear encouraging (Badros *et al.*, 2001c; Maloney *et al.*, 2001; Kroger *et al.*, 2002). Syngeneic transplantation for myeloma has also been described (Bensinger *et al.*, 1996a) (Chapter 49).

Autologous hematopoietic stem cell transplantation

Current experience

Autologous HSC transplantation is an important therapeutic option in the treatment of patients with myeloma. Besides producing substantial remissions in a large proportion, it has contributed greatly to an improved quality of life, with most patients leading a normal lifestyle while the disease is controlled. The relative safety of the procedure (a transplant-related mortality of <5%) allows most specialist centers to autograft patients up to the age of 70 years or even older. Results of some selected series are shown in Table 40.8. The current practice of HSC transplantation for myeloma in Europe has been described (Urbano-Ispizua *et al.*, 2002) (and see also Chapter 124).

The initial encouraging results with high-dose melphalan (without stem cell support) (McElwain & Powles, 1983) led to a larger evaluation of this treatment strategy (Selby *et al.*, 1987,

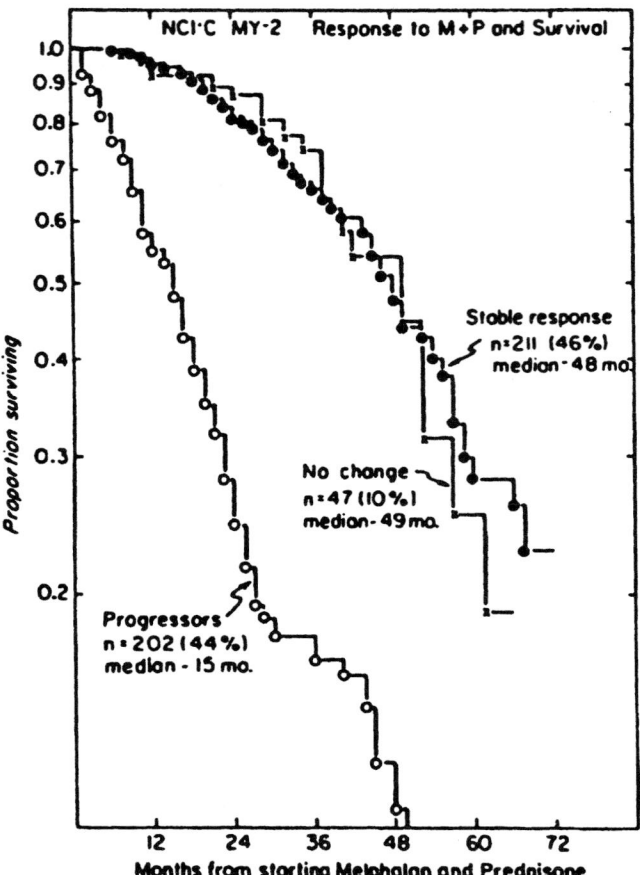

Fig. 40.3. Response and survival of myeloma patients treated with melphalan and prednisone. Patients were classified as responding, progressing, or unchanged. Reproduced, with permission, from Bergsagel (1979).

recover a white blood cell count of $1 \times 10^9/l$ was 28 days in patients who had not received previous treatment. The myelosuppression was associated with a significant infection risk and eight early deaths due to infection or bleeding occurred. Long-term follow-up of these 63 patients (Cunningham *et al.*, 1994a; Powles *et al.*, 2000a) showed an overall response rate of 82%, with 32% achieving a CR; 51 patients experienced disease progression 1–128 (median 19) months after high-dose therapy, and all but one of these eventually died of disease or consequences of further therapy at 2–176 (median 32) months. An improvement in quality of life was documented in the majority of the patients (pain grade 89%, performance status 92%). As of 2002, 3 patients are still alive: 2 in continuous CR (16 and 17 years after high-dose therapy) and 1 is in stable PR (progression after initial CR). The median overall survival (OS) of the whole group is 4 years (range, 2 days–16 years), and the median event-free survival (EFS) 16 months (range, 2 days–16 years). The actuarial 5-year and 10-year OS is 46% (95% confidence interval (CI), 34–58) and 19% (95% CI, 11–30) respectively. These data provide the longest available follow-up on patients treated with high-dose melphalan. While it is clear that the majority of patients relapse following therapy, the two long-term survivors raise the intriguing possibility that a small minority may not relapse. The availability of growth factors, effective maintenance therapy, and ability to harvest peripheral stem cells at diagnosis may make this approach worth exploring again.

The predictable hematologic toxicity and the initial high infection-related mortality led to investigation of the use of bone marrow as a source of hematopoietic stem cells following high-dose chemotherapy. Besides ameliorating hematologic toxicity, this approach led to further intensification of high-dose melphalan. The prerequisite for a bone marrow harvest, however, was a low level of marrow infiltration by disease prior to transplant. Therefore, a large proportion of patients were thought unable to benefit from autologous transplantation, because of a tumor-contaminated harvest. This resulted in the use of induction chemotherapy prior to the transplant procedure. The rationale for this approach was to reduce tumor burden and improve performance status prior to high-dose therapy. At approximately the same time as high-dose melphalan was introduced, Barlogie *et al.* (1984) introduced the concept of infusional chemotherapy for the treatment of myeloma. The

1988). In the follow-up study, the use of melphalan 140 mg/m² as a single intravenous injection was tested in 63 previously untreated myeloma patients and was associated with a high response rate. Seventy-eight percent of the patients responded, with 27% achieving a CR. In this study complete and partial remissions lasted a median duration of 19 months, but relapse occurred in almost all patients. High-dose melphalan resulted in a predictable period of myelosuppression. The median time to

Table 40.8 *Results of autologous transplantation for multiple myeloma*

Reference	Number of patients	TRM (%)	CR (%)	OS (median)	EFS (median)
Fermand *et al.* (1993)	63	11	20	59 mths	43 mths
Harousseau *et al.* (1995a)	133	3.7	37	46 mths	33 mths
Vesole *et al.* (1996)[a]	496	7	36	41 mths	26 mths
Attal *et al.* (1996)[a]	100	2	30	52% (5 yrs)	27 mths
Powles *et al.* (1997)[a]	195	4.9	53	54 mths	25 mths

Abbreviations: TRM, transplant-related mortality; CR, complete remission; OS, overall survival; EFS, event-free survival.

[a] Includes patients who were intended to receive an autograft but did not necessarily receive it.

rationale for this was to provide continuous exposure of the myeloma cells to chemotherapy in view of their slow growth fraction (Drewinka *et al.*, 1981). Barlogie used continuous infusions of vincristine and doxorubicin together with oral dexamethasone (VAD). We modified this regimen slightly and used methylprednisolone (VAMP) instead of dexamethasone (Forgeson *et al.*, 1988) and later on added cyclophosphamide (C-VAMP), which significantly increases CR rate compared to VAMP alone (Raje *et al.*, 1997b). Courses of infusional chemotherapy were given to patients to reduce tumor burden prior to transplant. Most patients required between 4 and 6 courses of this induction treatment. A combination of infusional chemotherapy and high-dose treatment have been crucial in the development of further intensive treatment requiring the use of hematopoietic stem cell support (Barlogie *et al.*, 1986; Selby *et al.*, 1988; Gore *et al.*, 1989; Powles *et al.*, 1997).

Autologous bone marrow transplantation

In 1986 Barlogie *et al.* treated seven patients with high-dose melphalan (HDM) followed by autologous bone marrow transplantation (ABMT) as supportive treatment. These initial reports of ABMT were primarily in patients who had relapsed or had resistant disease. Bone marrow had been harvested during prior remissions, and contained from 2% to 7% plasma cells. However, remissions were short and no patient given ABMT survived longer than 9 months. An attempt was subsequently made to induce more frequent and durable remissions by adding total body irradiation (TBI) (8.5 Gy in 5 fractions) to HDM 140 mg/m^2 (Barlogie *et al.*, 1987). Seven patients with advanced refractory disease were treated. Bone marrow had been collected either during previous remissions or after failure to respond to initial therapy, and contained from 6% to 30% plasma cells. There were two transplant-related deaths and the median remission duration was 15 months. The marked cytoreduction in patients with previous refractory disease proved that apparent drug resistance could be overcome by dose escalation. Data on HDM and TBI was further updated in 1990 (Jagannath *et al.*, 1990) with special reference to prognostic factors. Of 55 patients, 14 were in first remission and 20 in later remission. Twenty-one had resistant disease, of whom 7 were refractory to primary treatment and 14 had resistant relapse. Of the latter patients, none entered CR and there were 5 early deaths, with an overall median survival at 4 years of 82%. A high serum β_2 microglobulin level and non-IgG myeloma were identified as poor prognostic factors. Several studies have reported on the limited value of myeloablative treatment in late stages of the disease (Alexanian *et al.*, 1994; Demirer *et al.*, 1994; Bensinger *et al.*, 1996b). Ten to 25% of patients have died of transplant-related causes and median remission durations have not exceeded a year.

Purged autologous bone marrow transplantation

Although a high proportion of patients achieve remission with ABMT, relapse is inevitable. Most of these relapses are probably due to residual myeloma cells surviving the conditioning regimen. There is, however, the theoretical possibility of re-infusion of the malignant clone in the autologous bone marrow inoculum. To circumvent this problem, marrow purging using monoclonal antibodies (Mabs), either with complement (Anderson *et al.*, 1993) or as part of an immunotoxin involving momordin (Gobbi *et al.*, 1991), has been applied to myeloma patients undergoing ABMT. Reece *et al.* (1993) have used autologous marrow purged with 4-hydroperoxycyclophosphamide (4HC). Among the 14 patients transplanted, 2 died of hepatic veno-occlusive disease (VOD) and 1 from fungal infection. The remaining 11 patients achieved responses (6 CRs and 5 PRs) associated with a normal performance status. Seven patients have developed progressive myeloma at a median of 17 (range 5–30) months after BMT, while 4 patients remain free of progression at a median of 20 (range 6–42) months following transplant. Anderson *et al.* (1993) reported 26 patients given chemoradiotherapy followed by autologous marrow purged using in vitro lysis with Mabs and complement. With 24 months median follow-up, 16 of 26 patients are alive free from progression at 2+ to 55+ months posttransplant. Though these results appear promising, the procedure is expensive and has not gained popularity because newer alternative approaches are currently available.

Peripheral blood stem cell transplantation

An alternative approach to purged ABMT is the use of autologous peripheral blood stem cell transplants (PBSCT) on the theoretical basis that this source of stem cells will be less contaminated with tumor cells. One study used immunoglobulin heavy chain gene rearrangement and limiting dilution polymerase chain reaction to quantify myeloma cells in bone marrow and peripheral blood stem cell collections taken at a similar time from eight patients with myeloma (Henry *et al.*, 1996). Peripheral blood stem cells collections contained 1.7 to 23,700-fold fewer myeloma cells compared with bone marrow and would have resulted in re-infusion of 0.08- to 59,480-fold fewer myeloma cells based on total re-infused granulocyte-macrophage colony-forming units (CFU-GM), or 0.24- to 24,700-fold fewer myeloma cells based on total reinfused nucleated cells. The existence of circulating stem cells capable of producing sustained engraftment was demonstrated during the 1960s and 1970s in a variety of animal species (for review, see McCarthy & Goldman, 1984). PBSCT was an attractive option in myeloma patients due to the fact that patients with marrow infiltration, and those with prior radiotherapy to the spine and pelvis, could still be considered for this form of treatment.

The first report of PBSCT in myeloma came from Henon *et al.* in 1988. PBSC were collected in two patients during the recovery phase after HDM 140 mg/m^2. A total of 10×10^4 and 30×10^4 CFU-GM/kg, respectively, were obtained. No plasma cells were identified by cytology or immunofluorescence. Both patients were autografted after a further course of HDM and fractionated TBI, but the patient with the lower number of harvested PBSC also received bone marrow. The second received PBSC alone. Engraftment was prompt and he remained in CR 2 months after PBSCT. PBSCT has since been carried out in all phases of the disease and many studies have reported the combined results of ABMT and PBSCT.

Jagannath *et al.* (1992) attempted PBSC collections in 75 previously treated patients after the administration of high-dose cyclophosphamide (6 g/m^2) with or without granulocyte-macrophage colony-stimulating factor (GM-CSF). Sixty patients subsequently received high-dose treatment followed by rescue with both autologous bone marrow and PBSC; 38 patients received GM-CSF posttransplant. Among 72 patients undergoing apheresis, good mobilization was achieved when prior chemotherapy did not exceed 1 year and when GM-CSF was used after high-dose cyclophosphamide. These same variables also predicted rapid engraftment. The cumulative response rate for all 75 patients was 68% with 12-month event-free and overall survival projections of approximately 85%. The exact role of PBSCT could not, however, be ascertained from this study, because of the combined use of ABMT and PBSCT and the use of growth factors posttransplant.

A feasibility study followed by a phase II study of PBSCT after high-dose chemoradiotherapy was tested by Fermand *et al.* (1989, 1993). They treated 63 patients with high tumor mass multiple myeloma using high-dose chemotherapy comprising etoposide, carmustine, melphalan, and cyclophosphamide in the last 26 patients together with TBI, which was delivered in a single fraction of 10 Gy in 31 patients or in 6 fractions of 2Gy days −3 to −1 in 32 patients. Blood stem cell collection was performed at the time of diagnosis in 30 patients, while 33 had been previously treated. Mobilization included semi-intensive chemotherapy containing cyclophosphamide, doxorubicin, vincristine, and corticosteroids. This treatment resulted in a short period of cytopenia and PBSCs were collected at hematologic recovery by 3 to 5 leukapheresis procedures performed on consecutive days. Twenty-three patients received maintenance treatment with alpha-interferon (α-IFN) for a median of 6 months. Seven patients died from early toxicity. At 6 months post engraftment, 40 (71%) of the surviving patients had minimal residual disease and 11 (20%) were in apparent CR. During follow-up, 25 out of the 63 patients relapsed and 16 of these died. The median overall and event-free survival after transplantation were 59 and 43 months, respectively. The serum β$_2$ microglobulin (greater than or less than 2.8 mg/l) value at presentation and the length of previous therapy (greater than or less than 6 months of chemotherapy) were the only significant prognostic factors.

We have treated 222 myeloma patients (Singhal *et al.,* 2001) with high-dose melphalan 200 mg/m^2 followed by rescue with PBSCT. All patients received induction treatment with C-VAMP (infusional vincristine and doxorubicin plus weekly bolus cyclophosphamide and oral methylprednisolone). Our mobilization schedule included granulocyte colony-stimulating factor (G-CSF, filgrastim) alone followed by leukapheresis on 2 consecutive days. PBSC collection was performed on an outpa-

tient basis. All patients received maintenance treatment with α-IFN following transplant. This was based on results of our previous randomized trial comparing maintenance interferon treatment versus no treatment (Cunningham *et al.,* 1993; Powles *et al.,* 1995). Overall, 130 patients (59%) attained or remained in CR posttransplant; including 40% of NR, 53% of PR, and 97% of CR after C-VAMP ($P < .0001$). The overall (OS) and event-free (EFS) survival of patients with chemosensitive disease was somewhat better than those with primary refractory disease post C-VAMP. However, amongst the 130 CR patients, the 5-year OS was independent of response to C-VAMP (NR 79%, PR 74%, CR 60%; $P = .69$), as were relapse (NR 52%, PR 56%, CR 60%; $P = .86$) and EFS (NR 48%, PR 43%, CR 37%; $P = .81$). Similarly, among the 69 PR patients, the 5-year relapse, OS, and EFS were independent of response to C-VAMP. By Cox analysis, OS and EFS were higher in those with β2-microglobulin <2.5 mg/L, and lack of response to C-VAMP did not affect outcome significantly. We conclude that lack of response to induction therapy does not automatically predict poor long-term outcome in myeloma, since a substantial proportion of these patients attain CR after autografting and enjoy extended survival.

Thus, myeloma patients should not be disqualified from an autograft based upon lack of response to induction chemotherapy. With the increasing use of PBSCT in the autologous setting for myeloma, doubts as to its efficacy in comparison to ABMT started to develop, especially with the use of growth factors for mobilization and the possibility of the mobilization of the malignant clone in addition to the stem cells. We have previously shown in a group of 63 newly diagnosed myeloma patients that PBSC patients had a significantly faster engraftment (Raje *et al.,* 1997a). This resulted in a reduced need for platelet transfusions and intravenous antibiotics, and ultimately a significantly faster discharge from hospital in the PBSC population. Consequently, the cost of PBSC transplant was significantly lower than that of bone marrow transplant in a cost-minimization analysis. A French prospective randomized study (IFM 94 01) compared ABMT versus PBSCT (Attal & Harousseau, 2001). Of the 403 patients enrolled in the main study, 343 patients were randomized to receive ABMT ($n = 163$) or PBSCT ($n = 180$). The use of PBSC significantly shortened the period of neutropenia (0.5×10^9/l; 12 vs. 10 days; $P = .001$) and thrombocytopenia (50×10^9/l; 21 vs. 12 days; $P = .001$). No significant difference was observed with respect to response rate or EFS. A trend in favor of PBSC was observed for OS ($P = .07$). For the 180 patients randomized to receive PBSC, CD34 selection was allowed; 130 patients received an unselected graft and 50 a selected one—no significant difference in terms of engraftment, response rate, and survival were observed. PBSC should be the recommended source of stem cells for autotransplantation in patients with myeloma.

With the fast accumulating data on autologous transplantation in myeloma (Alegre *et al.,* 1998), Tricot *et al.* (1995b) have identified favorable variables for rapid engraftment in 225 patients of myeloma. All PBSCs were collected after high-dose cyclophosphamide and hematopoietic growth factor mobilization. A highly significant correlation was observed between the number of CD34$^+$ cells per kilogram infused and prompt recovery of both granulocytes (P = .0001) and platelets (P = .0001). Exposure to even 6 months or less of alkylating agents was associated with significantly delayed engraftment posttransplantation. The threshold dose of CD34$^+$ cells necessary for prompt engraftment was ≥2.0 × 10^6/kg for patients with less than 2 years of treatment prior to transplantation, whereas ≥5 × 10^6/kg CD34$^+$ cells were required to ensure rapid engraftment in patients exposed to longer durations of treatment.

Bearing in mind the problems with mobilization and engraftment and the long-term outcome of patients transplanted in late stages of the disease, a logical approach appeared to be to treat patients as early as possible with myeloablation followed by a transplant procedure of some sort. Data on ABMT in previously untreated patients have been reported (Gore *et al.*, 1989; Attal *et al.*, 1992; Cunningham *et al.*, 1994b). The French Registry (Harousseau *et al.*, 1995b) described 133 autologous stem cell transplants performed after first remission induction in myeloma. The source of stem cells was marrow (n = 81), blood (n = 51), or marrow plus blood (n = 1). Thirty-seven percent of patients entered CR and 46% achieved PR. There were 17 failures and 5 treatment-related deaths. With a median follow-up of 35 months, the median remission duration was 33 months, and the median time to treatment failure was 22 months. The median survival was 46 months overall, 54 months for the 103 responding patients and 30 months for the 30 non-responders (Figs. 40.4 and 40.5). A multivariate analysis revealed the quality of response after transplantation as the most important prognostic variable for outcome.

Our data (Powles *et al.*, 1997) on 195 previously untreated patients under the age of 70 years looked at outcome following autologous transplantation. All patients received induction chemotherapy and were intended to receive high-dose treatment. One hundred forty-one patients received high-dose treatment, with 112 patients receiving HDM plus an autograft (bone marrow or blood stem cells); 29 received modified high-dose treatment with melphalan alone (n = 23) or busulfan (n = 6). A total of 57 patients also received interferon maintenance following HDM and autografting. The CR rate in the whole group was 53%, while 74% of those receiving HDM and an autograft entered CR. Not all patients who were planned to receive HDM plus an autograft received it, because of increasing age or a raised serum creatinine level. Median overall survival from first treatment for the whole group and for the HDM/autograft group (from transplant) is 4.5 years and 6.6 years, respectively. The median overall survival of the patients in the HDM/autograft group receiving interferon has not been reached at 8 years. The median progression-free survival (PFS) for the whole group is 25 months (from first treatment), 27 months for the HDM/autograft group, and 44 months (from HDM) for patients on maintenance interferon.

The issue of the optimal timing of autologous transplantation (early vs. late) was answered by a randomized trial by the French group Myeloma Autogreffe (Fermand *et al.*, 1998),

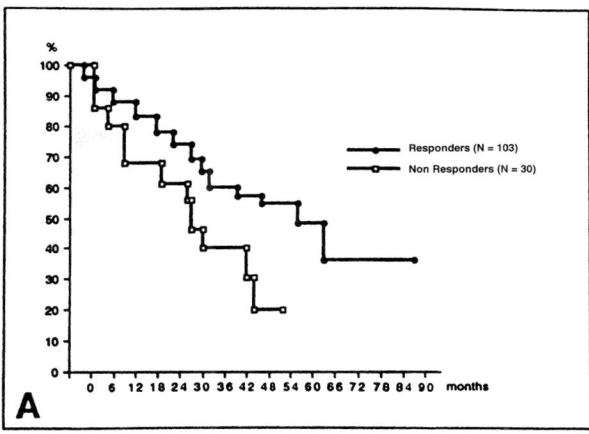

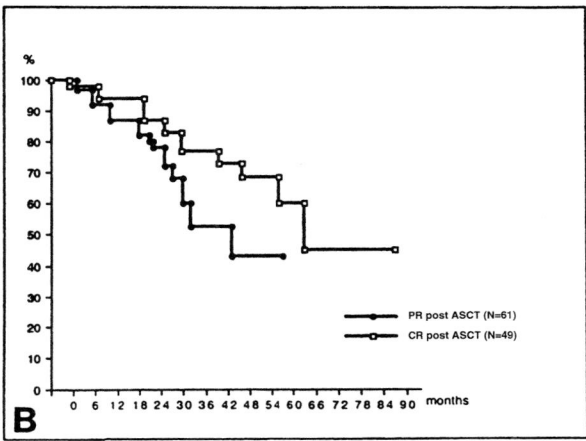

Fig. 40.4. **(A)** Impact of the response to previous chemotherapy (log-rank test, P = .06). **(B)** Impact of the quality of response achieved after ASCT (log-rank test, P = .04). Reproduced, with permission, from Harousseau *et al.* (1995b).

which compared the outcome of the disease in two groups of younger patients (<56 years); 91 received an autotransplant after a short induction (early transplant) and 94 received the transplant as rescue treatment either at relapse or for primary refractory disease (late transplant). The OS was identical in both groups with a median follow-up of 58 months (64.6 vs. 64 months); the early transplant group had a superior EFS. The period spent without chemotherapy was longer in the early transplant group. The potential advantages of early transplantation are better quality of life because of longer EFS, as well as a possible decrease in the development of drug resistance in the clonal population of plasma cells. Waiting for the disease to relapse in order to receive an autotransplant may have major disadvantages in the form of poor performance status, renal dysfunction, increasing age, and extensive skeletal morbidity at the time of relapse, as well as a higher risk of eventual myelodysplasia. We recommend early autotransplantation as consolidative treatment in patients with myeloma.

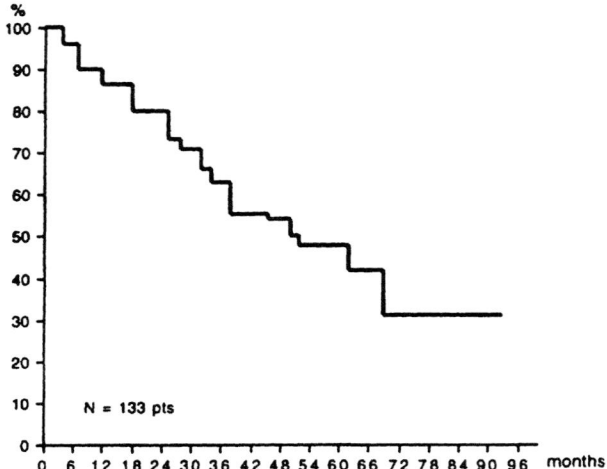

Fig. 40.5. Overall survival of the entire population. Reproduced, with permission, from Harousseau *et al.* (1995b).

In a series of 496 consecutive myeloma patients enrolled in clinical trials of tandem (double) transplants with PBSC support, Vesole *et al.* (1996) reported 95% patients completing the first autologous transplant with HDM, and 73% completing the second transplant with either HDM alone, or TBI plus HDM, or a combination of alkylating agents, depending on the response status prior to the second transplant. Thirty-one patients up to the age of 60 years received an allograft as the second transplant. The median interval from first to second transplant was 5 months. Treatment-related mortality during the first year after transplantation was 7%, and CR was obtained in 36% of the patients. The median durations of event-free survival and overall survival after transplant were 26 and 41 months, respectively (Fig. 40.6). Low serum β_2 microglobulin and C-reactive protein values were significant parameters associated with prolonged event-free and overall survival. Cytogenetic analysis revealed the

presence of 11q abnormalities, and/or complete or partial deletion of chromosome 13, as negative prognostic variables with respect to event-free and overall survival. Attainment of CR and application of two transplants within 6 months both significantly extended event-free and overall survival. Barlogie and colleagues (1999) in a single-center study have also reported on the use of tandem autologous transplantation in 231 patients with symptomatic myeloma. Remission induction was with non-cross-resistant induction chemotherapy (2 or 3 cycles of VAD; high-dose cyclophosphamide with GM-CSF was used for PBSC mobilization; conditioning was with etoposide-dexamethasone-cytarabine-cisplatin (EDAP)) followed by tandem transplantation (200 mg/m^2 melphalan $\times$ 2 or the second transplant with added TBI or cyclophosphamide in patients not attaining PR after first transplant), followed by maintenance interferon; 84% received the first transplant and 71% received the second transplant. An incremental response was seen with each stage of therapy, with final CR and PR rates of 41% and 42% for the whole group of 231 patients and 51% and 44% for those completing 2 transplants. The median OS and EFS were 5.7 and 3.6 years respectively, and the median CR duration close to 4 years.

An update by the same group on 1000 tandem autotransplants with prognostic factors has been published (Desikan *et al.*, 2000). All 1000 patients received melphalan (MEL) 200 mg/m^2 as the first high-dose therapy (HDT) cycle; 76% received a second HDT cycle (94% within 12 months). Major second HDT regimens were MEL 200 mg/m^2 in 39%, MEL 140 mg/m^2 + total body irradiation (850–1020 cGy) in 15%, MEL 200 mg/m^2 + cyclophosphamide 120 mg/kg in 8%, BEAM (carmustine 300 mg/m^2, etoposide 200 mg/m$^2 \times 4$ days, cytarabine 400 mg/m$^2 \times 4$ days, melphalan 140 mg/m^2) in 2%, and other regimens in the remainder; 10% received allotransplants. TRM was low (2.7% with first, 4.8% with second AHSCT-supported HDT); 44% achieved CR, which lasted a median of 2.4 years. Projected EFS and OS at 5 years were 25% (SE 2%) and 40% (SE 2%), respectively. Both EFS and OS were significantly longer in the absence of chromosome 13 abnormalities, with low pre-HDT β_2-microglobulin and C-reactive protein (CRP) levels, standard-dose chemotherapy (SDT) $\leq$ 12 months before HDT, chemosensitive disease, and, in contrast to CR, the absence of IgA isotype (Table 40.9). The 5-year CR rate was 52% among the 112 CR patients without chromosome 13 abnormalities and with β_2-microglobulin $\leq$ 2.5 mg/l, C-reactive protein $\leq$ 4 mg/l, and standard-dose chemotherapy $\leq$ 12 months. Of all 390 CR patients without chromosome 13 abnormalities, 35% enjoyed 5-year continuous CR. CR was more durable without chromosome 13 abnormalities (RR: 0.6, $P = .01$), standard-dose chemotherapy (SDT) $\leq$ 12months (RR: 0.6, $P < .0001$), CRP $\leq$ 4.0 mg/l (RR: 0.7, $P = .02$), and β_2-microglobulin $\leq$2.5 mg/l (RR: 0.8, $P = .03$).

These data show that myeloma with chromosome 13 abnormalities should be considered as a separate incurable disease entity even after tandem autotransplants. CR and a second HDT cycle applied within 6 months both extended EFS and OS significantly, justifying further pursuit of high-dose therapy.

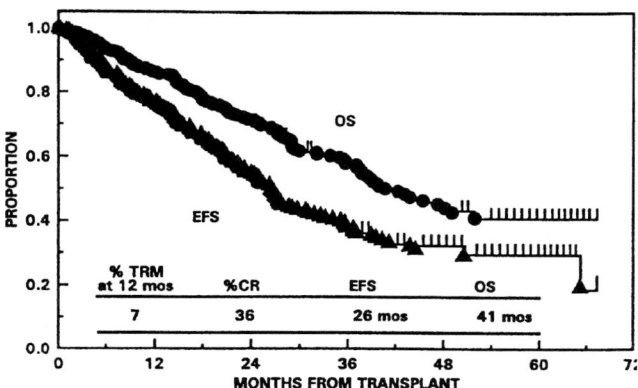

Fig. 40.6. EFS and OS from the first transplant ($n = 470$). TRM within 12 months of first transplant was 7%; 36% of patients achieved CR. Median durations of EFS and OS were 26 and 41 months, respectively. Reproduced, with permission, from Vesole *et al.* (1996).

Table 40.9. *Multivariate analysis of parameters predicting event-free survival and overall survival*

Event-free survival	RR	95% CI	P	Overall survival	RR	95% CI	P
No Δ13	0.5	0.4–0.5	< .0001	No Δ13	0.4	0.4–0.6	< .0001
β₂m ≤2.5 mg/l	0.7	0.6–0.8	< .0001	β₂m ≤2.5 mg/l	0.6	0.5–0.7	< .0001
≤12 months SDT	0.7	0.6–0.8	< .0001	≤12 months SDT	0.7	0.6–0.9	.0001
Sensitive to SDT	0.8	0.7–0.9	< .0001	CRP ≤4.0 mg/l	0.7	0.6–0.9	< .0002
Any 2nd HDT[a]	0.8	0.6–0.9	.0004	Sensitive to SDT	0.8	0.6–0.9	.0002
Non-IgA isotype	0.7	0.6–0.9	.002	(Days to 2nd HDT)[1a]	0.5	0.4–0.6	.001
Any CR[a]	0.8	0.6–0.9	.002	Any 2nd HDT[a]	0.04	0.01–0.1	< .0001
CRP ≤4.0 mg/l	0.8	0.7–0.9	.03	Non-IgA isotype	0.7	0.6–0.9	.002
(Days to 2nd HDT)⁻¹			.07	Any CR	0.8	0.7–1.0	.04

Abbreviations: Δ13, chromosome 13 abnormalities; β₂m, β₂-microglobulin; CR, complete remission; CRP, C-reactive protein; SDT, standard-dose therapy; HDT, high-dose therapy; RR, relative risk of experiencing event in favorable versus unfavorable categories; CI, confidence interval.
[a] Time-dependent covariate
Reproduced, with permission, from Desikan *et al.* (2000).

To see whether it is possible to predict long-term EFS in patients with myeloma following a tandem transplant, Tricot *et al.* (2002) identified a subset of 515 patients from the 1000 patients described above who had been transplanted at least 5 years prior to the date of analysis. They showed that factors associated with EFS of ≥ 5 years were absence of chromosome 11 and 13 abnormalities (odds ratio: 6.1), ≤ 12 months of preceding standard-dose therapy (SDT) (odds ratio: 2.6) and β₂-microglobulin ≤ 2.5mg/l at the time of first autotransplant (odds ratio: 1.7) (Fig. 40.7).

A non-randomized comparison of data submitted to the European Bone Marrow Transplant Registry demonstrated superior progression-free survival in patients undergoing tandem transplantation; the study detected no survival difference. Björkstrand and coworkers (1995) reported on 15 patients of whom 11 successfully underwent double autologous transplantation. Four of 5 patients in CR examined by PCR analysis of the clone-specific immunoglobulin gene rearrangement were PCR negative up to 33 months after transplant.

We at the Royal Marsden Hospital reported on 451 patients autotransplanted with 200 mg/m² melphalan with results comparable to tandem transplants (Sirohi *et al.,* 2002). The characteristics of these patients are shown in Table 40.10. Therapy was:

induction (VAMP/C-VAMP for untreated patients) to 1 cycle beyond maximum response → marrow or G-CSF-mobilized PBSC harvest → melphalan 200 mg/m² → interferon-α2b maintenance; 27 patients (6%) died of toxicity, all within 3 months; 266 patients (59%) remained in, or attained, CR. Overall response rate was 91%. The median (95% CI) times to relapse, EFS and OS of the whole group were 2.7 (2.2–3.2), 2.3 (2.0–2.6), and 5.7 (5.0–6.5) years, respectively (Figures 40.8 and 40.9). The 5-year probabilities of relapse, EFS and OS were 66%, 31%, and 57%, respectively. On multivariate analysis, patients with age < median 53 years (RR = 1.63), albumin >39 g/l (RR = 0.63), β₂-microglobulin ≤ 2.3 mg/l (RR = 1.47) had a significantly superior OS, while patients with age < 53 years (RR = 1.36), albumin >39 g/l (RR = 0.79), and in CR at the time of autotransplant (RR = 0.67) had a longer EFS. The only variable that predicted for a significantly longer relapse-free survival was being in CR at the time of autotransplant (RR = 0.69). The combination of albumin ≥ 40 g/L and β₂-microglobulin ≤ 2 mg/l identified 70 patients with a strikingly good outcome. The median time to relapse, EFS, and OS (Figure 40.10) of these and the other 381 patients was 3.3/2.6 years (*P* = .1), 3.3/2.2 years (*P* = .013), and >8.6/5.4 years (*P* < .0001), respectively. The 5-year

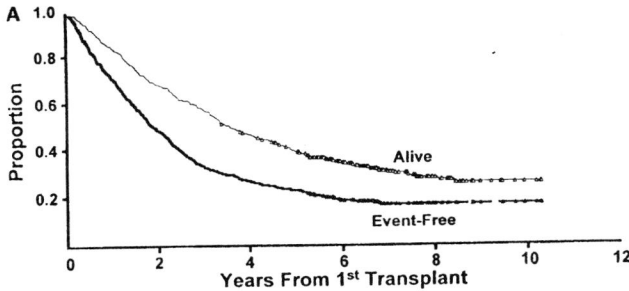

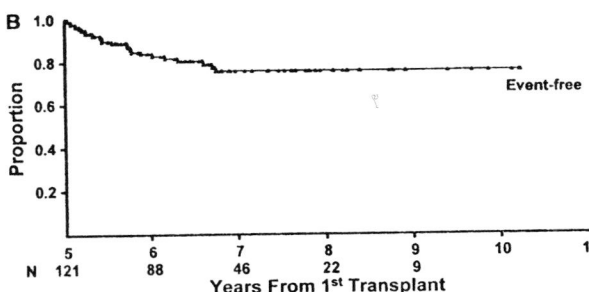

Fig. 40.7. (**A**) Event-free and overall survival of 515 myeloma patients receiving autotransplants and a follow-up period of at least 5 years. (**B**) Event-free survival of only those patients alive and without disease progression at 5 years (*n* = 121). Reproduced, with permission, from Tricot *et al.* (2002).

Table 40.10. *Patient characteristics at the time of autologous HSC transplantation*

Variable	Median value	Range	Proportion
Age (years)	53	31–75	
Calcium (mmol/l)	2.29	1.66–2.87	
Creatinine (μmol/l)	81	43–732	
β_2M (μg/ml)	2.3	0.1–54.6	
Albumin (g/l)	39	22–48	
Male			66%
Stage IIIA/IIIB			73%
BL >2			62%
PS: 1 to 4			27%
IgG/IgA			79%
CR at transplantation			17%
Source of cells: PBSC			67%

Abbreviations: β_2M, β_2-microglobulin; BL, bone lesion score; PS, performance score; CR, complete remission; PBSC, peripheral blood stem cells.
Data for 451 patients.
Reproduced, with permission, from Sirohi *et al.* (2002).

probabilities of relapse, EFS, and OS were 60/67%, 40/30%, and 71/55%, respectively. None of these 70 patients died after 9 years and the 10-year OS probability was 51%. The dramatically higher OS despite modestly higher EFS suggests that they continued to respond to salvage therapy after relapse.

High-dose melphalan 200mg/m^2 as part of a single autotransplant described here results in excellent outcome in myeloma, and should be regarded as standard of care. The results are comparable to tandem transplantation, raising questions about the latter as a routine therapy. Patients with poor prognostic factors or poor-risk disease seem to do poorly even with tandem transplants; hence this is a group of patients who should receive newer agents such as thalidomide or its analogs, proteasome inhibitor PS-341 or non-myeloablative allogeneic transplants as consolidative or maintenance therapy after a single autotransplant.

Tandem transplantation

The role of tandem or double autologous stem cell transplantation remains uncertain. The Intergroupe Francophone du Myelome (IFM) has addressed the issue in a randomized trial in patients less than 60 years. The latest analysis of this study, which enrolled 400 patients, was in favor of the double transplant in terms of CR rate (39 vs. 49%) and long-term survival, which became more evident with increasing follow-up, suggesting that probably it was the good-risk patients that benefitted most from the tandem transplant. The results of this study are shown in Figure 40.8. Three other groups are also trying to answer the same question (HOVON, Bologna, Myeloma Autogreffe), and the preliminary results do not show any added benefit for tandem autotransplantation; however, follow-up is short (Fermand *et al.*, 2001; Segeren *et al.*, 2001).

In conclusion, one or two autologous peripheral blood stem cell transplants with a conditioning regimen consisting of high-dose melphalan alone now seems to be the core treatment for younger myeloma patients. If the patients are correctly selected, transplant-related mortality is 1–3%, with CR rates between 30 and 50% and a median OS of over 5 years, which is 2–3 years longer than that achieved with conventional chemotherapy. Regarding the question of whether one or two transplants should be given as consolidative therapy, the single-center data from Little Rock and the Royal Marsden Hospital are similar. The French randomized trial IFM 94 has tried to answer this question and shown that there seems to be a significant advantage for the double transplant arm, but some other randomized studies that are not mature yet do not support this. Hence, it is still an open question.

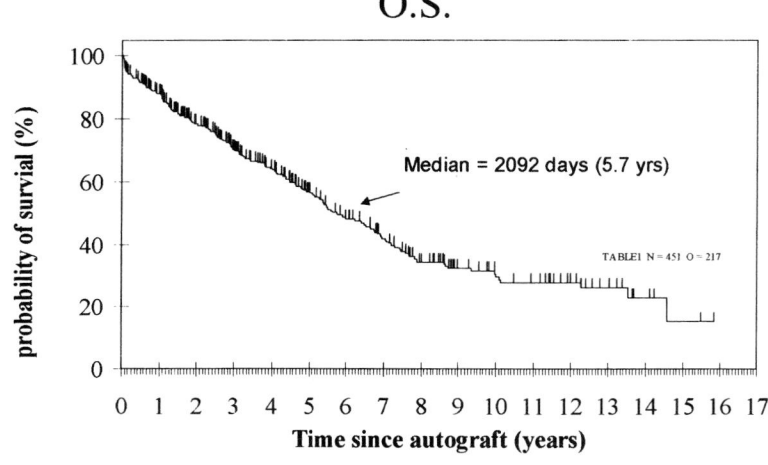

Fig. 40.8. Overall survival of 451 patients with myeloma given high-dose melphalan 200 mg/m^2 and an autologous HSC transplant.

E.F.S.

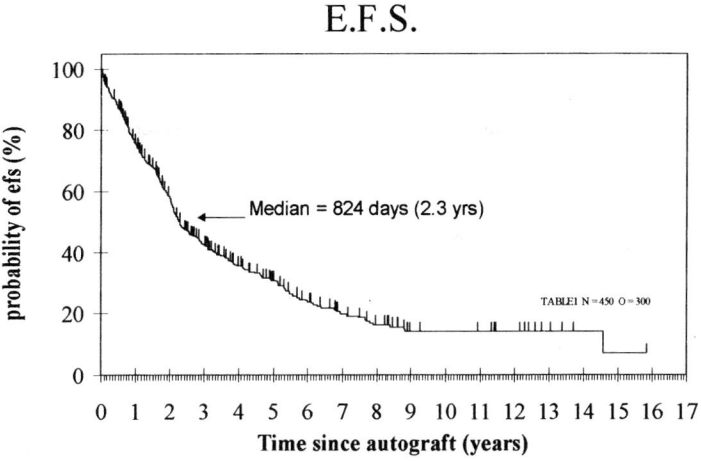

Fig. 40.9. Event-free survival of 451 patients with myeloma given high-dose melphalan 200 mg/m² and an autologous HSC transplant.

Singhal *et al.* (1995) at the Royal Marsden Hospital described the kinetics of paraprotein clearance after autografting for multiple myeloma (Figs. 40.11 and 40.12). Twenty-four of 33 patients eventually cleared their serum paraprotein at a median of 47 (range 5–783) days posttransplant. The probability of clearance was lower, and the time taken to clear paraprotein longer, in patients with a higher level (>19 g/dl) at the time of transplant. However, clearance occurred within 6 months in 23 of 24 patients who ultimately cleared their paraprotein. The administration of α2b-IFN posttransplant did not appear to influence the clearing of the paraprotein.

The above data suggested that an autologous transplant irrespective of the stem cell source was of benefit to patients early in the course of the disease. The studies, however, did not throw any light on the benefits of autografting over conventional chemotherapy for similar stage disease. Blade *et al.* (1996) have published data on 77 of 487 patients who could

have been candidates for early intensification therapy, but instead were treated with conventional chemotherapy. Their median age was 56 years. Thirty-six patients were initially treated with melphalan and prednisolone and 41 with VCMP/VBAP (vincristine, cyclophosphamide, melphalan, prednisone/vincristine, BCNU, doxorubicin, prednisone). The median response duration to initial chemotherapy was 22 months, and the actuarial probability of being in continued first response at 5 years was 14% after a median follow-up of 58 months; 59 patients have died, 1 was lost to follow-up, and 17 are alive, 69 to 119 months after initial chemotherapy. The median survival from initiation of treatment was 60 months and from the time when autotransplantation would have been considered, 52 months. Because of similarities in survival trends of these patients treated with conventional chemotherapy to those having received intensive treatment, it became crucial to compare these two treatment options in a prospective randomized trial

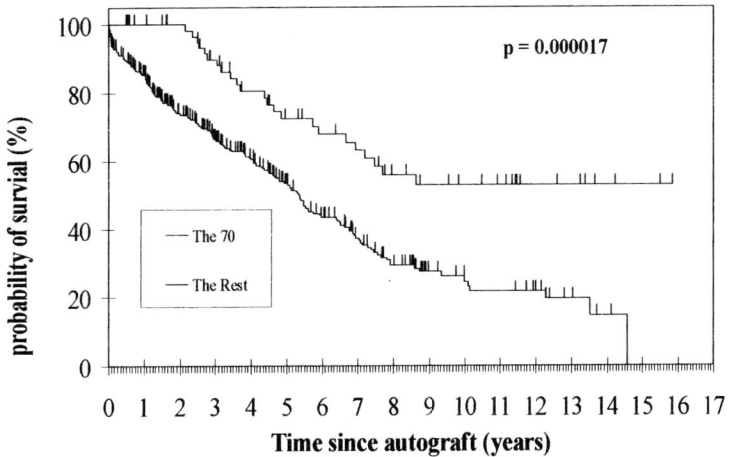

Fig. 40.10. Log rank comparison of overall survival of patients with myeloma (received high-dose melphalan 200 mg/m²) between those with albumin ≥ 40 g/l and β2-microglobulin ≤ 2 mg/l (*n* = 70) versus the rest.

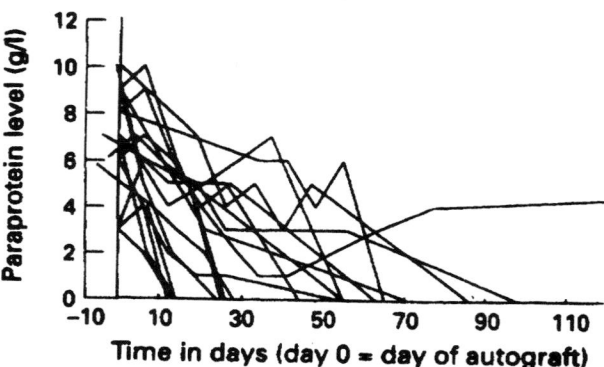

Fig. 40.11. Temporal profile of paraprotein levels after autografting in 15 patients with a paraprotein level of >10 g/l at the time of transplant. Plots for individual patients have been terminated when the paraprotein disappeared. One patient's paraprotein disappeared on day 783 (not shown). Reproduced, with permission, from Singhal *et al.* (1995).

and the Intergroupe Francais du Myeloma (Attal *et al.*, 1996) undertook this.

The results of this landmark trial are published and favored high-dose therapy over conventional treatment. Two hundred previously untreated patients under the age of 65 years who had myeloma were randomly assigned at the time of diagnosis to receive either conventional chemotherapy or high-dose therapy and ABMT. All analyses were on an intention to treat basis. The patients enrolled in the conventional-dose arm received a median of 18 cycles of VCMP and VBAP. Seventy-four patients enrolled in the high-dose arm underwent transplantation. The median time from diagnosis to transplantation was 5.5 months. This was usually after 4 to 6 alternating courses of VCMP and VBAP. High-dose treatment comprised HDM and TBI. Interferon was started in both groups, three times weekly, from cycle 9 in the conventional-dose group and upon hematologic recovery in the transplant group. The response rate among the patients who received high-dose treatment was 81%

(including CR in 22% and very good PR in 16%), whereas it was 57% (CR in 5% and very good PR in 9%) of the patients treated with conventional chemotherapy ($P < .001$). The probability of event-free survival at 5 years was 28% in the high-dose group and 10% in the conventional-dose group ($P = .01$) (Fig. 40.13). The overall estimated survival at 5 years was 52% and 12% in the high-dose and conventional-dose group, respectively ($P = .03$) (Fig. 40.14). Treatment-related mortality was similar in both groups. In a multivariate analysis of all 200 patients, event-free survival was significantly related to the level of serum β_2-microglobulin ($P < .001$) and the treatment assignment ($P = .01$). Overall survival was related to the level of β_2-microglobulin only ($P = .01$). An update of this study showed that in the conventional chemotherapy arm the 7-year EFS and OS were 8% and 25% respectively compared to 16% and 43% in the high-dose therapy arm ($P = .01$ and $P = .03$) respectively (Attal *et al.*, 2001). A study by the Southwest Oncology Group (Barlogie *et al.*, 1995) has also shown a similar advantage for the patients treated with intensive therapy up front, as has a study by the Nordic Myeloma Study Group using a population-based historical control group (Lenhoff *et al.*, 2000). The Medical Research Council Myeloma VII trial (Child, 1994) addresses the same issue. Patients under the age of 65 are eligible and it has compared the less intensive ABCM (adriamycin, BCNU, cyclophosphamide, melphalan) with infusional C-VAMP followed by high-dose therapy and either an ABMT or a PBSCT. All responding patients receive maintenance treatment with IFN. Preliminary data from this study show that there is a definite advantage to the high-dose therapy arm (Dr. Child, personal communication).

Disappointingly, a study by Corradini and colleagues (1999) showed only 7% of autograft recipients achieving a molecular remission posttransplant (as opposed to 50% of allograft recipients).

Autologous PBSCT has also been reported as treatment for plasma cell leukemia (Hovenga *et al.*, 1997).

Patients with renal dysfunction

Several reports have indicated that marked renal impairment is not necessarily a contraindication to transplantation (Ballester *et al.*, 1997; Rebibou *et al.*, 1997). The studies by Tricot *et al.* (1996) and Kergueris *et al.* (1994) showed that high-dose melphalan pharmacokinetics are not affected by renal function and therefore HDM 200 mg/m^2 could be an appropriate regimen. Accordingly, renal insufficiency should not constitute a criterion for exclusion from transplantation, and only patients with poor performance status should be excluded as potential candidates. We have shown that it is feasible and safe to administer HDM 140 mg/m^2 to patients with severe renal failure (serum creatinine >4 mg/dl). Two of the four patients who received HDM 140 mg/m^2, changed over from thrice weekly hemodialysis to twice weekly hemodialysis, an important factor for quality of life (Sirohi *et al.*, 2001), and two others who were dialysis-dependent pretransplant became dialysis-independent posttransplant

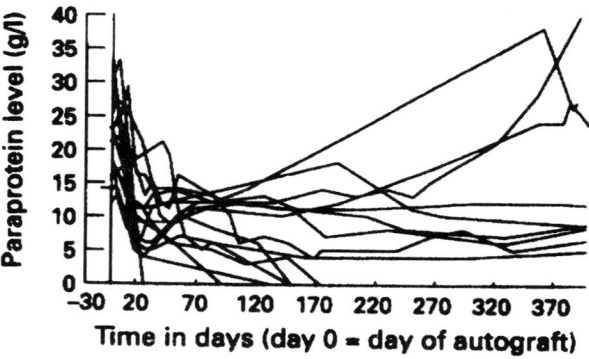

Fig. 40.12. Temporal profile of paraprotein levels after autografting in patients with a paraprotein level of ≥ 10g/l at the time of transplant. Plots for individual patients have been terminated when the paraprotein disappeared. Reproduced, with permission, from Singhal *et al.* (1995).

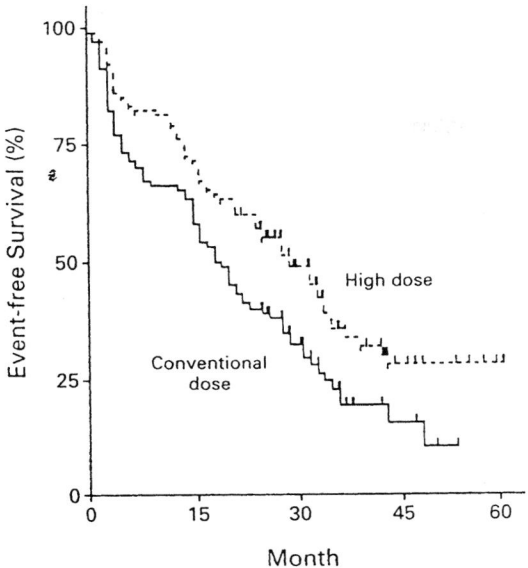

| Conventional dose | 58 (48–68) | 32 (23–42) | 15 (7–28) | 10 (3–27) |
| High dose | 71 (61–79) | 50 (39–55) | 28 (18–40) | 28 (18–40) |

Fig. 40.13. Event-free survival according to treatment group. The numbers shown below the time points are probabilities of event-free survival (the percentages of patients surviving event-free and 95% confidence interval). Reproduced, with permission, from Attal et al. (1996).

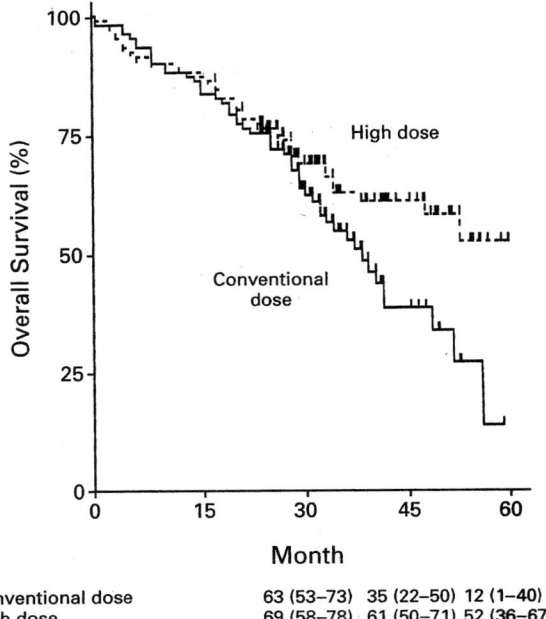

| Conventional dose | 63 (53–73) | 35 (22–50) | 12 (1–40) |
| High dose | 69 (58–78) | 61 (50–71) | 52 (36–67) |

Fig. 40.14. Overall survival according to treatment group. The numbers shown below the time points are probabilities of overall survival (the percentages of patients surviving) and 95 percent confidence intervals. Reproduced, with permission, from Attal et al. (1996).

(Tauro et al., 2002). Badros et al. (2001) have presented data on 81 patients with renal failure (creatinine >177 μmol/l) at the time of autotransplantation and shown that it is possible to mobilize stem cells in these patients without problems; 60 patients received melphalan 200 mg/m^2 (27 on dialysis), but, due to excessive toxicity, the dose was reduced to 140 mg/m^2 in the next 21 patients; 38% patients received a tandem transplant. The treatment-related mortality was 6% and 13% after first and second transplant. CR was attained in 38% of patients and 2 patients discontinued dialysis after the autotransplant. The 3-year OS and EFS were 55% and 48%, respectively. Sensitive disease prior to autotransplant, normal albumin level, and younger age were independent prognostic markers for better OS. In our experience, and that of the Arkansas group, lowering the dose of melphalan has an adverse impact on anti-tumor activity; all our patients who received melphalan 140 mg/m^2 have progressed, and, in the Arkansas experience, the EFS is significantly worse with melphalan 140 mg/m^2 ($P = .04$), suggesting that we still do not know the optimal dose of melphalan in patients with renal failure.

As the data stand, in patients with renal failure a modified dose of melphalan 140 mg/m^2 should be offered, and in patients with a low albumin the dose of melphalan should be lowered further to 70–100 mg/m^2. Studies should aim to further optimize the dose of melphalan.

Elderly patients

Age is no longer a prognostic variable in patients with myeloma (Siegel et al., 1999). The difficulty is in delivering intensive therapy in patients with myeloma. The upper age limit in various studies for delivery of high-dose therapy has been 65 years. We and others have shown that it is safe to deliver high-dose therapy in older patients. Prospective evaluation of high-dose chemotherapy in patients over the age of 70 years must also assess morbidity and quality of life issues as well as disease-related end-points.

We have shown in a matched-pair analysis (Sirohi et al., 2000) in 17 patients aged 65–74 (median 67) treated with high-dose therapy (usually melphalan 200 mg/m^2) that there are no differences in terms of tolerance, relapse rate, treatment-related mortality, and OS in comparison with 17 younger matched control patients. The Arkansas group has presented the outcome of 49 patients aged 65 years or older compared with that of 49 younger controls matched for critical prognostic factors (Badros et al., 2001b). The patients received high-dose melphalan therapy, and neither the ability to collect a sufficient number of peripheral blood stem cells nor the transplant-related mortality differed significantly between the two groups. Similarly, median durations of EFS and OS were comparable (2.8/1.5 and 4.8/3.3 years for younger and older patients, respectively). The Torino group also reported on the feasibility and the superiority of dose-intensive melphalan with stem cell support in elderly myeloma patients (Palumbo et al., 1999). These authors treated 71 patients between 55 and 75 years of age (median 64) with 2 or 3 cycles of melphalan 100 mg/m^2

and the clinical outcome of these patients was compared with that of 71 controls treated with standard-dose melphalan and prednisone (MP) and matched for age and β_2-microglobulin values. Melphalan 100 mg/m^2 was feasible (89% of the patients completed the program) and well-tolerated. No toxic deaths occurred. Melphalan 100 mg/m^2 was superior to MP in terms of CR rate (47 vs. 5%; $P \leq .01$), EFS (median 34 vs. 17.7 months; $P \leq .001$), and OS (56+ vs. 48 months; $P \leq .01$). A later study from the same group found a similar efficacy of melphalan 100 mg/m^2 and melphalan 200mg/m^2–based strategies (Palumbo et al., 2000).

Autologous HSC transplantation followed by elective reduced intensity conditioning and allografting

A new approach involves the use of a standard autograft for tumor debulking purposes followed by an elective allograft (using reduced intensity conditioning) and an allograft to exploit the graft-versus-myeloma effect (Maloney et al., 2001; Kröger et al., 2002). Kröger and colleagues (2002) treated 17 patients with advanced stage II/III myeloma with melphalan 200 mg/m^2 and an autologous transplant. After a median interval of 119 days, a reduced intensity conditioning regimen of fludarabine 180 mg/m^2, melphalan 100 mg/m^2, and ATC 10 mg/kg for 3 doses was administered prior to an allogeneic transplant from an HLA-matched related donor in 7 patients, an HLA-mismatched related donor in 2 patients, and an unrelated donor in 8 patients. Complete donor chimerism was detected after a median of 30 days. The 100-day mortality rate post allograft was 11%. The complete remission rate with negative immunofixation increased from 0% after induction or salvage chemotherapy to 18% after autologous transplantation to 73% after allografting. At a median follow-up of 13 months post allografting, the 2-year estimated event-free survival was 56% (see also Chapter 124).

Prognostic factors for outcome after high-dose therapy and autologous transplantation

The serum β_2-microglobulin level (<2.5 mg/l associated with better outcome) has been shown to be an important prognostic factor for outcome after high-dose therapy and autologous transplantation by a number of groups (see above), as have abnormalities (monosomy and/or deletions) of chromosome 13 (Tricot et al., 1995a; Facon et al., 2001). Rajkumar and colleagues (1999a) reported that overall and progression-free survival were better in patients with primary refractory myeloma than in those with relapsed disease. The same investigators found that low (<2.7 mg/l) serum β_2-microglobulin and low bone marrow plasma cell involvement (<40%) pretransplant predicted complete response posttransplant (Rajkumar et al., 1999b). Patients transplanted for Bence Jones myeloma had worse overall and event-free survival than those transplanted for IgG myeloma (Sirohi et al., 2001a). The various immunologic

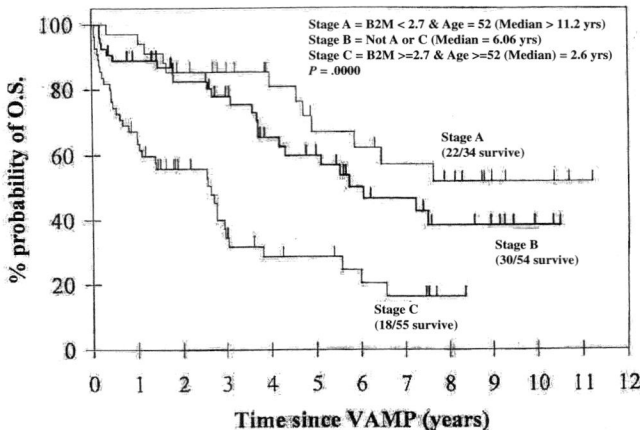

Fig. 40.15. Log rank comparison of overall survival of the three stages in IgG myelomas: stage A ($n = 34$), stage B ($n = 54$) and stage C ($n = 55$).

subtypes of myeloma have different predictors of outcome. We have examined IgG myeloma patients presenting to our unit between April 1985 and December 1997 ($n = 153$) to see if we can define a circumscribed disease entity with clear end points of disease remission and relapse (Sirohi et al., 2000b). Multivariate analysis of presentation variables in this group of patients showed that OS was significantly prolonged for patients with β_2-microglobulin (β_2M) <2.7 mg/l and age < median 52 years, while β_2M <2.7 mg/l and hemoglobin >8.5 g/dl predicted for longer EFS Based on the two dominant prognostic factors, patients could be stratified into three stages: stage A, those with favorable variables: β_2M <2.7 mg/l and age <52 years; stage B, those with one favorable variable; and stage C, those with only unfavorable variables. This system predicted highly significantly the patients with the best chance of obtaining CR and surviving longest ($P < .0001$, Figure 40.15). The 34 patients in the good risk group had a median OS not yet reached of >11.2 years (Table 40.11). Secretory myelomas may thus lend themselves to an accurate staging system predictive of specific end-points of disease response and relapse.

Additionally, age has been shown not to be a prognostic variable for outcome after autotransplantation (Siegel et al., 1999). Indeed, Palumbo and colleagues (1999) found dose-intensive therapy and stem cell support to be superior to standard treatment in older patients (median age 64) (Figure 40.16). Other factors shown in some series to favorably affect outcome posttransplant include less than 12 months therapy pretransplant, non-IgA isotype, plasma cell labelling index, plasmablastic morphology of plasma cells in the bone marrow, low soluble IL-6 receptor level, low plasma cell labelling index, absence of circulating plasma cells in PBSC harvests, and achievement of CR.

Conditioning regimens for autologous transplantation

Various different high-dose regimens have been used for autografting in myeloma, but by far the most commonly used proto-

Table 40.11. *Staging system for predicting overall survival based on presentation variables in patients with IgG myeloma*

	Number of patients ($n = 143$)[a] (%)	Patients receiving HDT (%)	Patients in CR (%)	Median CR length (years)	Number alive (%)
Stage A	34 (23.8)	30 (88)	24 (70.6)	2.9	22 (64.7)
Stage B	54 (37.8)	45 (83.3)	30 (55.5)	2.3	30 (55.5)
Stage C	55 (38.4)	34 (62)	20 (36.4)	2.1	18 (32.7)
P value		0.013[b]	0.012[c]	NS[c]	0.013[c]

Data for 153 patients.
[a] β_2M not available in 10 patients
[b] Chi-square with Yates correction
[c] Log rank comparison
Reproduced, with permission, from Sirohi *et al.* (1999).

cols have utilized melphalan alone at a dose of 200 mg/m^2 or melphalan at a dose of 140 mg/m^2 plus TBI. Schiller *et al.* (1994), as well as the Seattle group, have explored the use of busulfan/cyclophosphamide. Dimopoulos *et al.* (1993) used a new conditioning regimen, incorporating thiotepa (750mg/m^2), busulfan (10 mg/kg), and cyclophosphamide (120 mg/kg) followed by either an ABMT or PBSCT. Sixty-five percent of all patients responded to treatment. Thirteen percent of the patients died of regimen-related toxicity, but the response duration and survival outcomes were comparable to other studies. Adkins *et al.* (1994) investigated the feasibility of escalating doses of dacarbazine (DTIC) in combination with high-dose cyclophosphamide, carmustine, and etoposide (CBV) in patients with refractory myeloma and lymphoma in a phase I trial. Treatment-related mortality (TRM) was 18%, but the feasibility of combining high-doses of DTIC with CBV was demonstrated. Dose-limiting hypotension was transient and reversible when DTIC was administered at 3,900 mg/m^2 with CBV. We have used busulfan alone (Mansi *et al.*, 1992) at a dose of 16 mg/kg in a group of myeloma patients with renal impairment and short remission duration following HDM. The TRM was high (3 of 15), but 46% of the patients responded,

demonstrating the efficacy of busulfan in heavily pretreated patients and the safety of its administration in patients with renal impairment. However, we have also shown that patients receiving high-dose busulphan as well as those receiving high-dose melphalan at 140 mg/m^2 had a significantly worse progression-free ($P = .0003$) and overall ($P < .0001$) survival compared with those receiving melphalan 200 mg/m^2 (Powles *et al.*, 1997). The commonest conditioning regimens used for patients with myeloma have been high-dose melphalan 140 mg/m^2 with total-body irradiation and high-dose melphalan 200 mg/m^2. The French group (Moreau *et al.*, 2002) conducted a randomized study (IFM 9502 trial), which compared these two most widely used conditioning regimens in newly diagnosed symptomatic patients younger than 65 years old: 8 Gy total body irradiation plus 140 mg/m^2 melphalan ($n = 140$) versus 200 mg/m^2 melphalan ($n = 142$). Baseline characteristics and disease response to 4 cycles of the VAD regimen performed before randomization and autologous stem cell transplantation were identical in the two treatment arms. Patients receiving melphalan 200 mg/m^2 had a significantly faster hematologic recovery for both neutrophils and platelets, transfusion requirements were significantly lower, and the median

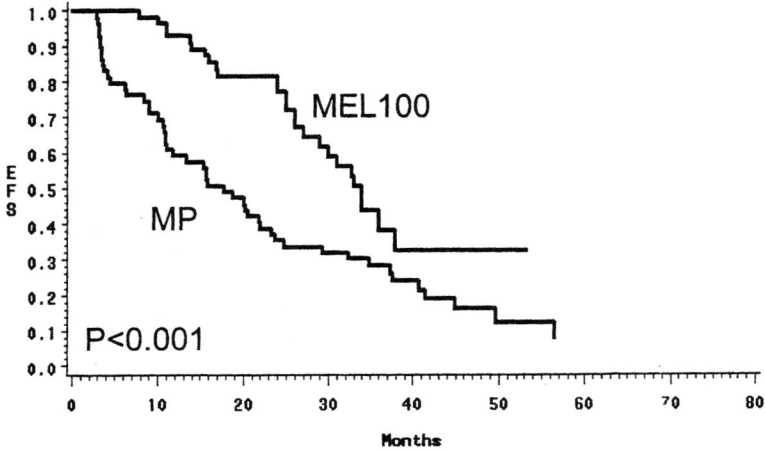

Fig. 40.16. Event-free survival of myeloma patients treated with MP or MEL 100. Reproduced, with permission, from Palumbo *et al.* (1999).

duration of hospitalization was significantly shorter. The median duration of EFS was similar in both arms (21 vs. 20.5 months, P = .6), but the 45-month survival was 65.8% in patients receiving melphalan 200 mg/m^2 versus 45.5% in those receiving melphalan plus TBI (P = .05). This difference was probably due to better salvage regimens after relapse in the melphalan 200 mg/m^2 arm.

Thus, 200 mg/m^2 melphalan significantly reduced transplant-related toxicity and was associated with a better OS than 140 mg/m^2 melphalan plus TBI and should be considered as the standard of care before autologous stem cell transplantation in patients with myeloma. Doses of melphalan as high as 220 mg/m^2 have been used with acceptable toxicity (Moreau *et al.*, 1999). The Spanish Registry has compared three conditioning regimens: melphalan 200 mg/m^2, melphalan 140 mg/m^2 plus TBI, and melphalan 140 mg/m^2 with busulfan 12 mg/kg. There were no differences in engraftment or transplant-related mortality and all three had a comparable antimyeloma effect with a trend in favor of busulfan-melphalan for better EFS (Lahuerta *et al.*, 2000)

From all these studies, it is clear that autologous transplantation in myeloma is currently the superior mode of treatment compared to conventional chemotherapy, and results are summarized in Table 40.8. This form of intensive treatment results in biochemical and hematologic CR in 30% to 50% of patients. Transplant-related mortality is around 5% in most series. The EFS and OS approximates 30 months and 4–5 years posttransplant, respectively. It is also apparent that patients who benefit most are those who are treated early in the course of the illness.

There is some evidence with emerging long-term follow-up data that there is a plateau in the survival curves. The question remains whether patients who have been in continuous first complete remission, living a normal quality of life, but probably with disease still present at a molecular level, for more than 10 years, are "operationally cured" (Powles *et al.*, 2000b; Sirohi *et al.*, 2001a). In this context, we tried to define a subset of patients in long-lasting CR for more than 10 years. Among 363 patients treated between January 1979 and December 1990, 14 (4%) were in first CR for more than 10 years. Comparison of this group with the remaining 349 patients showed that these patients were significantly younger (45 vs. 50 years, P = .01), but there was no difference in other pretreatment variables; 3 of 14 patients had received 140 mg/m^2 melphalan as primary therapy and the other 11 patients had received induction chemotherapy followed by an autograft. These patients had significantly higher CR rate with induction therapy as compared to others (63% vs. 12%, P < .0001) and this was also true for patients who received infusional VAMP/C-VAMP (70% vs. 9%, P < .0001). This supports our observation that early response to infusional chemotherapy is an independent predictor of better outcome for patients with myeloma. Two patients relapsed at 11 and 12 years (1 continues in stable PR and 1 died in second CR, suggesting that there is a possibility that these groups of patients will not die of myeloma but of other reasons, i.e., they are operationally cured

but living in harmony with their minimal residual disease). Among the operationally cured group, 79% had a normal Karnofsky performance status; 1 developed breast cancer, 1 had a cadaveric renal transplant and 1 developed Parkinson's disease. This suggests that operational cure may be possible in certain group of myeloma patients and this may be improved by obtaining early CR. The issue needs to be evaluated in randomized trials, but supports the concept of intensification of early treatment such as upfront high-dose therapy. To this end, we have tried to explore whether it is possible to harvest patients with myeloma at presentation, so that they can then be transplanted early.

As discussed above, primary treatment with melphalan 140 mg/m^2 without rescue resulted in high response rates in patients with myeloma with very long-term survival in some patients. Also, the early response to infusional chemotherapy is an independent prognostic factor for newly diagnosed patients with myeloma. It is on this background that a study to collect peripheral stem cells at diagnosis was performed to see if enough stem cells ($\geq 1 \times 10^6$ CD34$^+$ cells/kg) could be collected to perform an autograft as primary therapy in order to escalate the dose of melphalan to 200 mg/m^2 to produce rapid remission. Patients received 1 g/m^2/day of methylprednisolone (days 1–6) and 12–16 µg/kg/day G-CSF (days 3–6), and were apheresed (2 × blood volume) on days 6 and 7; 31 patients (21 M, 10 F; 34–67 years, 19 IgG, 7 IgA, 4 light chain, 1 nonsecretory) were harvested from October 1999 to January 2001. Of the 31 patients, 1 patient could not be harvested because of progressive renal failure requiring dialysis; 0.23–5.63 × 10^6 CD34$^+$ cells/kg (median 1.31) were harvested from the remaining 30. The yield was $\geq 1 \times 10^6$ CD34$^+$ cells/ kg in 22 patients (74%), the minimum required for autotransplantation. Thus, it is possible to harvest enough stem cells for 1 autograft at the time of diagnosis.

We have autotransplanted 3 patients at diagnosis using PBSC collected at diagnosis, whereby the patients receive melphalan 200 mg/m^2 and an autotransplant followed by 4 courses of C-VAMP for patients in CR or multiple courses of C-VAMP until maximum response in those not in CR, followed by IFN-α2b maintenance. Though polymerase chain reaction (PCR)-based techniques have shown that clonogenic myeloma cells are detectable in the peripheral blood of all patients, even those in CR, they have not been correlated with relapse after autografting. This approach would also be of benefit to the 20% of patients who do not respond to induction chemotherapy. This constitutes our first step towards using melphalan 200 mg/m^2 as primary therapy with a view to increasing the proportion of operationally cured patients.

Posttransplantation maintenance therapy

The role of maintenance therapy in multiple myeloma is controversial. Various agents have been evaluated. Those being considered as candidates for maintenance therapy include interferon-α2b, prednisone, thalidomide, the newer bisphosphonates, idiotype vaccination, and dendritic cell infusions. The use of IFN-α2b in the posttransplant setting has been tested by our group in a randomized trial (Cunningham *et al.,* 1998; Powles *et al.,* 1995). Interest in the use of interferon in myeloma was evoked after Mellstedt *et al.* (1979) demonstrated its efficacy as a single agent in previously untreated patients with myeloma. Following induction with conventional chemotherapy, two European studies (Mandelli *et al.,* 1990; Westin *et al.,* 1991) have demonstrated that interferon can prolong partial response, but a beneficial effect appears limited to patients who achieve an objective response to induction treatment. When Mandelli reported the results of the first trial of maintenance interferon, the greatest benefit was reported in patients with the lowest tumor burden at the start of maintenance therapy. Based on these results, we concluded that an ideal group of patients to test the role of maintenance therapy would be those with evidence of minimal residual disease. Since high-dose therapy resulted in very high CR rates and a majority of the patients have the lowest tumor burden so far seen, we tested this approach following ABMT. Eighty-four patients with myeloma were randomized to receive either IFN-α2b 3 mega units/m^2 s.c. three times weekly or no maintenance treatment, following induction chemotherapy and high-dose treatment. At a median follow-up of 52 months, the median progression-free survival was 27 months in the control arm and 46 months in the interferon-treated patients (*P* < .025). For the 65 patients who achieved a CR, there was a significant prolongation of remission (*P* = .02) for those on interferon treatment, and 33% of these patients remain in remission 6 years after high-dose treatment (updated data). Most studies to date have examined the effect of interferon maintenance following conventional treatment (Cooper *et al.,* 1993; Salmon *et al.,* 1994). Our study was the first to compare the use of interferon maintenance therapy following high-dose treatment. Attal *et al.* (1992) have reported, in a nonrandomized study, a 33-month PFS post-ABMT of 85% in CR patients. Their results, though encouraging, were in a small number of patients with a short follow-up. Data from the French registry (Harousseau *et al.,* 1995a), although unable to confirm our findings in a phase II nonrandomized trial, did demonstrate a favorable trend for CR patients on interferon maintenance following high-dose treatment. We have compared the tolerance for interferon after PBSCT versus ABMT (Powles *et al.,* 1996) and have demonstrated no difference. In a retrospective EBMT registry analysis of 892 patients, overall and progression-free survival were significantly better in the interferon group compared to the group which did not receive interferon posttransplant (78 vs. 47 months and 29 vs. 20 months, respectively) (Fig. 40.17) (Björkstrand *et al.,* 2001).

The meta-analysis conducted by Ludwig *et al.* (1998), which evaluated IFN maintenance therapy from 8 randomized trials comprising 929 patients, demonstrated benefit for IFN therapy in terms of prolongation of remission duration and survival. IFN maintenance treatment appeared to prolong the average relapse-free survival by 7 months and the average overall survival by 5

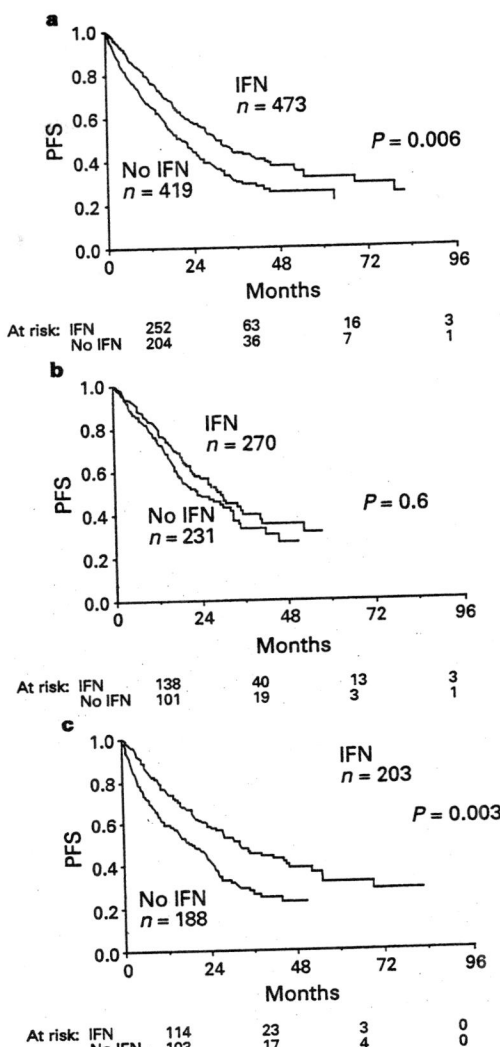

Fig. 40.17. Progression-free survival from the time point 6 months after transplantation. (**a**) All patients; (**b**) patients in partial remission after transplantation; (**c**) patients in complete remission after transplantation. The appearance of the curves is dependent on all prognostic factors analyzed, but the *P* values are statistically corrected to demonstrate the effect of IFN treatment alone. Reproduced, with permission, from Björkstrand *et al.* (2001).

months. Younger patients, those with a good performance status and those with a low tumor burden appear to benefit most from IFN maintenance. Another meta-analysis, by the Myeloma Trialists Collaborative group (2001), evaluated 24 randomized IFN trials (12 induction and 12 maintenance), which included 4,012 patients. Overall survival was better with IFN, the 3-year survival being 53% with IFN and 49% without IFN (*P* = .01). An effect of similar magnitude was observed in both induction and maintenance trials, with increases in median survival of about 2 and 7 months respectively. Progression-free survival was significantly better with IFN in both induction (*P* = .0003) and maintenance (*P* < .0001) trials. However, survival after recurrence was worse (*P* = .02) with IFN. The conclusion was that the benefits of IFN therapy must be weighed against its cost and its effect on the patient's quality of life.

Purging of the stem cell graft

Positive stem cell selection

The potential for re-infusion of the malignant clone is a concern in all autografting procedures for cancer patients. PBSCTs are currently being used preferentially instead of ABMT, because of the advantages of more rapid engraftment, less morbidity, lower cost, and the theoretical possibility of less tumor cell contamination in blood harvests. Several authors (Marriette *et al.*, 1994; Corradini *et al.*, 1995, 1999; Belch *et al.*, 1995) have, however, identified myeloma cells in PBSC harvests, as well as in the peripheral blood of these patients. Corradini *et al.* (1995, 1999) have demonstrated, by a PCR-based strategy using clone-specific sequences derived from the rearrangement of Ig heavy chain (IgH) genes, the presence of both pre- and postswitch B cells in both bone marrow and blood stem cell harvests. The complementarity-determining regions (CDR) of IgH genes were used to generate tumor-specific primers and probes. Their data suggested that blood-derived stem cell harvests may have a lower rate of contamination compared to bone marrow. Szczepek *et al.* (1997) showed that CD34+ cells in the blood of patients with myeloma expressed CD19 and mRNA for IgH, and had patient-specific IgH VDJ gene rearrangements. Other investigators have concluded that the CD34 antigen is not expressed on the malignant cells in myeloma (Vescio *et al.*, 1994). Contrarily, growth factors like G-CSF and GM-CSF used in most mobilization schedules for PBSC harvesting have been implicated in the mobilization of tumor cells (de la Rubia *et al.*, 1994). The fear of introducing tumor cells at the time of grafting has led to trials involving positive stem cell selection (see Chapters 17 and 27). Indeed, one study of unmanipulated PBSCT showed a correlation between the number of monoclonal plasma cells in the harvest and a shortened relapse-free survival posttransplant (Gertz *et al.*, 1997) (Fig. 40.18). Hematopoietic cells positively selected for CD34, an antigen expressed on early hematopoietic cells, can support hematopoietic recovery following myeloablative chemotherapy. Schiller *et al.* (1995) have reported a multi-institutional study of purified CD34-selected peripheral blood progenitor cell transplantation in 37 patients with advanced myeloma (Fig. 40.19). The positive selection for hematopoietic progenitor cells was carried out using the CEPRATE system (Cellpro, Bothell, WA), a continuous-flow-column-selection system that relied on the high affinity between avidin and biotin to select antibody-labeled hematopoietic progenitor cells. After CD34 selection, a greater than 2.7 to 4.5 log reduction in myeloma cell contamination was achieved in the harvests. Engraftment was prompt in patients treated with CD34-selected grafts and blood and platelet requirements were minimal. A dose of 2×10^6 CD34+ cells/kg was considered adequate for prompt and sustained engraftment. The 1-year PFS in this study was $67 \pm 19\%$. However, after a median follow-up of 33 months, the actuarial 3

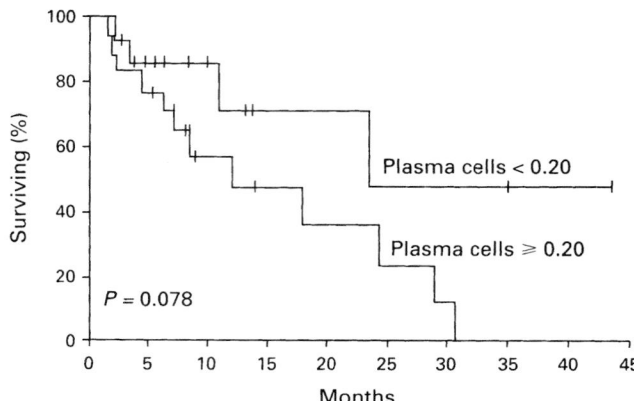

Fig. 40.18. Kaplan-Meier survival plot for overall survival stratified by number of circulating plasma cells ($P = .078$). Number of plasma cells expressed as $\times 10^6$/l. Reproduced, with permission, from Gertz *et al.* (1997).

year progression-free survival of 55 patients who underwent high-dose therapy and transplantation of CD34+ PBSCs was only $29 \pm 14\%$, suggesting that the majority of patients, as in other autografting studies, are destined to relapse (Schiller *et al.*, 1998; Stewart *et al.*, 2001).

A multi-center phase III, randomized trial compared the hematologic recovery and toxicity after autotransplantation with either CD34-selected PBSC or unselected PBSC (Vescio *et al.*, 1999). There was no significant difference in engraftment rate, although platelet engraftment was slightly delayed by 1–2 days in the CD34-selected arm without clinical sequelae. The incidence and type of infections were similar in both arms. There was no difference in the EFS and OS between the arms. With growing experience of CD34-selected transplantation, it has become evident that there is a delayed quantitative and functional recovery of T-cell subsets, associated with an

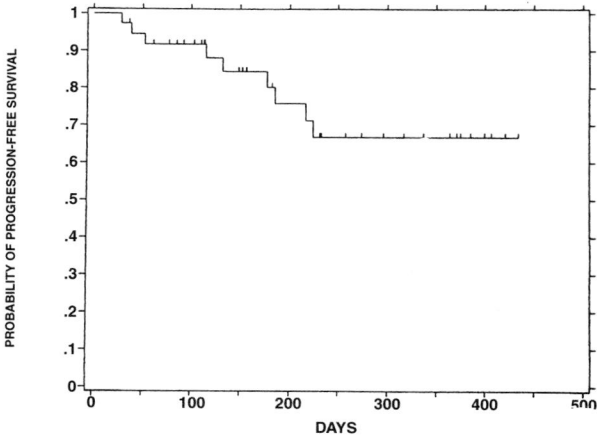

Fig. 40.19. Progression-free survival for MM patients undergoing CD34-selected peripheral blood progenitor cell transplantation for multiple myeloma. Reproduced, with permission, from Schiller *et al.* (1995).

increased risk of viral, fungal, and other opportunistic infections (Brugger *et al.*, 1996; Nachbaur *et al.*, 1997; Laurenti *et al.*, 1998; Gupta *et al.*, 1999). It is possible that CD34-selection could have an adverse effect on relapse risk by impairing immune reconstitution.

In an attempt to eradicate the PBSC product of contamination by tumor cells, Gazitt *et al.* (1995) purified CD34+ Lin⁻ Thy+ stem cells from mobilized PBSC harvests of 10 myeloma patients by sequentially using counterflow elutriation centrifugation, and flow cytometric sorting, using 5 parameter gating. Stem cell purification led to an overall stem cell enrichment of about 50-fold in all 10 patients. Quantitative PCR amplification of patient-specific complementarity-determining region III (CDRIII) DNA sequences showed depletion of clonal B cells by 2.7 to 7.3 logs, with the highest log reductions seen in samples initially containing the most tumor cells. A clinical trial using CD34+ Lin⁻ Thy1+ stem cells has been reported (Tricot *et al.*, 1998). Fluorescence-activated cell sorting (FACS)-sorted CD34+ Lin⁻ Thy1+ peripheral blood cells were substantially enriched for stem cell activity, yet contained virtually no clonal myeloma cells. A study was performed in patients with symptomatic myeloma, who had received <12 months of standard dose therapy (SDT), to evaluate the feasibility of large-scale purification of primitive hematopoietic stem cells and to study engraftment kinetics posttransplantation, as well as the degree of tumor cell contamination (based on PCR analysis for the patient-specific CDRIII). PBSC were mobilized with cyclophosphamide and GM-CSF. Of the 10 evaluable patients, nine met the required minimum criteria of ≥ 7.2 × 10⁵ CD34+ Thy1+ cells/kg to support tandem transplants. After 200 mg/m² melphalan, 8 patients engrafted successfully, although neutrophil and platelet recovery was substantially delayed when compared with unmanipulated PBSC grafts. The clinical impact of tumor-free grafts on the outcome of myeloma patients remains questionable at this time. It appears more likely that posttransplantation immune-based strategies will improve outcome in myeloma, since such interventions should affect both myeloma cells remaining in the patient posttransplant and myeloma cells reinfused with the graft.

Retroviral gene marking

CD34-enriched bone marrow and peripheral blood have been retrovirally marked by Dunbar *et al.* (1995). The main aims of their study were to investigate the efficiency of retroviral gene transfer to CD34-enriched hematopoietic cells, to compare the use of peripheral blood versus bone marrow cells as targets for retroviral gene transfer, to study the kinetics of reconstitution after autologous transplantation, and finally to determine if marked tumor cells were detected posttransplantation. Eleven patients with myeloma or breast cancer had cyclophosphamide and filgrastim-mobilized peripheral blood cells CD34-enriched and transduced with a retroviral-marking vector containing the neomycin resistance gene (Neo); CD34-enriched bone marrow cells were transduced with a second marking vector also containing a neomycin resistance gene. After high-dose conditioning therapy, both transduced cell populations were re-infused and patients were followed over time for the presence of the marker gene and any adverse effects related to the gene transfer procedure. All 10 evaluable patients had the marker gene detected at the time of engraftment, and 3 of 9 patients had persistence of the marker gene for greater than 18 months posttransplantation. The source of the marking was both the transduced peripheral blood graft and the bone marrow graft, with a suggestion of better long-term marking originating from the peripheral blood graft. There was no toxicity noted, and patients did not develop detectable replication-competent helper virus at any time posttransplant. The Neo signal was not detectable in residual CD38+ plasma cells isolated from two patients posttransplant.

Immune modulation

There are a number of possible approaches to immune modulation in conjunction with autologous transplantation (Jagannath & Dimopoulos, 1995). PBSC harvests can be incubated with interleukin (IL)-2. These harvests, once re-infused show prompt engraftment and contain cells that recognize and destroy tumor cells, including the autologous tumor cells in the harvest. Seven-day cultures of bone marrow with IL-2 have led to effective purging in diseases such as myeloma, CLL, and CML. A more specific approach will include patients with secretory myelomas, who will undergo plasmapheresis and have their idiotype protein isolated, conjugated to keyhole limpet hemocyanin (KLH), and used for in vivo and ex vivo immunization. The ability to generate ex vivo functional dendritic cells has made it possible to fuse them with patients' myeloma cells, thus producing a vaccine. Dendritic cells are also a crucial reagent to generate myeloma-specific cytotoxic T lymphocytes (CTLs) for reinfusion into the patient as adoptive immunotherapy (Ruffini & Kwak, 2001)

The minimal residual disease status achievable in most patients with high-dose therapy and the accelerated immune reconstitution after the use of PBSCT provides an optimal clinical setting to test such immunotherapy.

Relapse after autologous transplantation

With the increasing use of high-dose therapy and autografting, relapse following transplantation is becoming a common problem and poses a therapeutic dilemma for the clinician. Tricot *et al.* (1995c) studied 94 patients who relapsed following autologous transplantation. Salvage treatment consisted of either standard dose therapy (*n* = 53) or a second transplant procedure [autograft (31) or allograft (10)]. With a median follow-up of 11 months, the projected overall survival of all patients at 18 months was 59%. A multivariate analysis revealed presalvage serum β₂-microglobulin and late relapse after the preceding transplant (>12 months) as independent significant variables for overall survival. Transplantation performed as primary salvage therapy was associated with significantly prolonged sur-

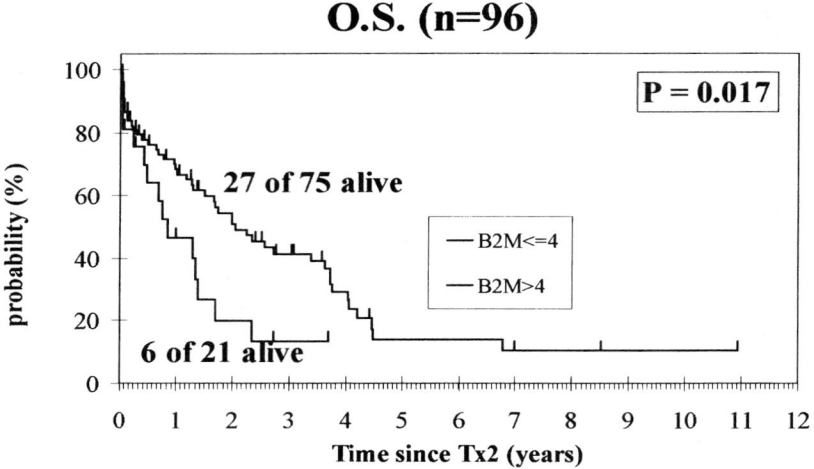

Fig. 40.20. Log rank comparison of patients with myeloma receiving a salvage autotransplant: influence of serum β₂-microglobulin at the time of salvage ASCT on overall survival (≥4 vs > 4 mg/l)

vival. These data confirm that a second transplant is feasible and may produce long-term survival in patients with good prognostic factors. Attal and colleagues (1996) in their randomized trial compared the effect of salvage treatment in both the previously treated conventional-dose group and the previously treated high-dose group. In the conventional-dose group 45 of 50 patients who relapsed received treatment, of whom 9 received high-dose therapy. With a median follow-up among the surviving patients of 11 months from the time of relapse, the probability of survival at 2 years after relapse was 25%. In the high-dose group, 46 patients relapsed and 41 received salvage treatment. Eight of these patients were given a second high-dose treatment. With a median follow-up among the surviving patients of 15 months from the time of relapse, the probability of further relapse was 35%, not significantly different from that in the conventional-dose group.

We have analyzed a group of 96 patients who relapsed after receiving a first autograft with 200 mg/m² (Sirohi *et al.*, 2001c). These patients (34–77 years, median 55) underwent a second autograft with melphalan 200 mg/m². The intervals between the first and second autograft, first autograft and relapse, and second/salvage autograft were 6 weeks to 11.8 years (median 3.2 years), 3 months to 8.8 years (median 2.1, years), and 1 week to 7.4 years (median 10 months), respectively. The treatment-related mortality with the salvage autograft was 9%; 32% patients attained CR, and the overall response rate was 76%. The actuarial 3-year probabilities of relapse, disease-free survival, and overall survival from salvage autograft were 84%, 13%, and 35%, respectively. Figure 40.20 shows that patients with β₂-microglobulin of more than 4 mg/l at the time of second autograft had a significantly poorer survival. Figure 40.21 shows the impact of being in CR with the first autograft on the probability of attaining a second CR. The results of the Cox analysis are shown in Table 40.12. From the time of first autograft, the actuarial survival of the group was 61% at 5 years and the median survival was 6.4 years. The latter is comparable to that reported with tandem autotransplantation, suggesting that salvage autotransplantation at relapse produces results that are equivalent to

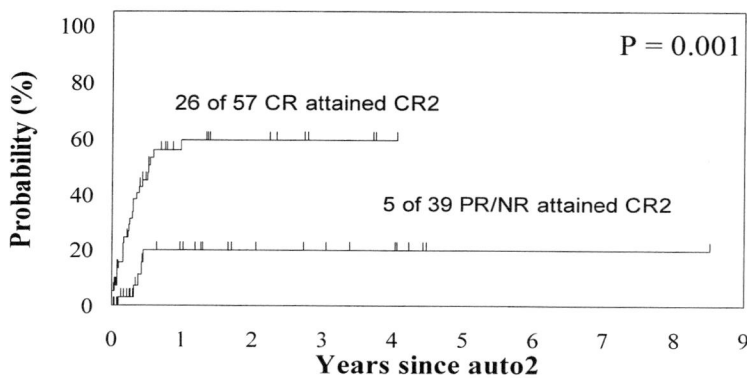

Fig. 40.21. Log rank comparison of patients with myeloma receiving a salvage autotransplant: influence of being in complete remission at the time of first ASCT on the probability of attaining second complete remission with the salvage ASCT.

Table 40.12. *Multivariate analysis of factors influencing outcome at the time of the second autologous HSC transplant*

Favorable covariate	RR	*P*
Interval between first auto and second autograft >2 years	0.25	.0004
Interval between first auto and second autograft >2 years	0.44	.007
β_2M ≤4 mg/l	2.43	.048
Creatinine <85 µmol/l	0.58	.036
β_2M ≤4 mg/l	3.26	.02
Creatinine <85 µmol/l	0.5	.02
In CR after first autograft	5.1	.0005
Chemosensitive disease at second autograft	2.2	.02
β_2M ≤4 mg/l	0.38	.048

Abbreviations: RR, relative risk; β_2M, β_2-microglobulin; CR, complete remission.

those seen with tandem autografts. Melphalan 200 mg/m² with an autograft is a reasonable treatment option in selected patients relapsing after one autograft. For patients with shorter interval between the first and second autograft, higher β_2-microglobulin values, higher creatinine values and lack of entering CR after the first autograft, salvage autotransplant along with newer agents should be the preferred option. A policy of autografting at relapse prevents a high proportion of patients receiving an unnecessary second autograft because they either would not need it (long-term survivors) or would not benefit from it due to refractory disease. Prospective, randomized trials are required to determine the optimum time for second autotransplantation.

Increasingly, the use of reduced intensity conditioning regimens followed by allogeneic transplantation (mini allografts) is being explored in this setting (Kottaridis *et al.*, 2000; Badros *et al.*, 2001c; Vesole, Simic, & Lazarus, 2001; Dey *et al.*, 2001) (see Chapters 22 and 55).

Because of the prominent vascularization of the bone marrow that occurs in myeloma, thalidomide (which has antiangiogenic properties) has been used to treat relapse occurring after high-dose chemotherapy (Singhal *et al.*, 1999). The dose used was 200 to 800 mg daily. Marked and durable responses were seen in some patients. An update of this study with 169 patients (Barlogie *et al.*, 2001) showed a 2-year survival of 60% in these patients. On multivariate analysis, EFS and OS were longer in the presence of normal cytogenetics, low plasma cell labeling index (PCLI), and a low β_2-microglobulin value (≤ 3 mg/l). The main side effects were sedation (25%), constipation (16%), sensory neuropathy (9%), and deep vein thrombosis (2%). Studies of thalidomide in combination with dexamethasone have also shown good results.

Monitoring for residual disease posttransplant

In a study by Martinelli and colleagues (2000), minimal residual disease in the bone marrow was monitored posttransplant using PCR technology to identify the rearranged variable region (VDJ) of the immunoglobulin heavy chain (IgH) using two primers designed from the patient-specific IgH CDRs II and III. Five of 30 evaluable patients who achieved a clinical complete remission posttransplant became PCR-negative (16%). One of these 5 patients subsequently relapsed, compared to 10 of 25 evaluable patients who never achieved a molecular complete remission (MCR) (Fig. 40.22). In the same report, 7 of 14 evaluable allograft recipients achieved MCR (50%). This was significantly higher than the incidence in the autograft recipients. In the study as a whole, relapse-free survival was longer in those achieving MCR (Fig. 40.23).

Monoclonal gammopathy of unknown significance

Monoclonal gammopathy of unknown significance (MGUS) is a term used to describe the presence of a paraprotein in serum in the absence of clinical or laboratory evidence of a malignant plasma cell dyscrasia. It was previously known as benign monoclonal gammopathy, but this was considered misleading since a significant proportion of cases eventually develop a plasma cell dyscrasia. Treatment depends on severity and includes various combinations of plasmapheresis, IVIG, corticosteroids, and cytotoxic agents. Autologous PBSC transplantation has been utilized in a patient whose illness was characterized by a severe peripheral neuropathy (Lee *et al.*, 2002).

Systemic AL amyloidosis

Systemic AL amyloidosis is a plasma cell dyscrasia that results from an excess production of Ig light chains, which form insoluble amyloid fibrillar deposits in the kidneys, heart, liver, and autonomic and peripheral nerves. Eighty-five percent of patients have evidence of a plasma cell dyscrasia with serum and/or urine monoclonal proteins and with low-level bone marrow plasmacytosis showing clonal dominance by either kappa or lambda light chain isotypes.

For patients with AL amyloidosis death usually occurs 1 to 2 years from diagnosis despite current standard treatment with oral melphalan and prednisone (Kyle *et al.*, 1997) (Fig. 40.24). An early report (Comenzo *et al.*, 1996) described five patients treated with dose-intensive melphalan and autologous blood stem cell support and followed for a period of 1 year. Patients were diagnosed with AL amyloidosis by tissue biopsy and categorized by performance status and organ involvement. Their plasma cell dyscrasias were evaluated with immunofixation electrophoresis of serum and urine specimens, quantitative serum Igs, and immunohistochemical staining of bone marrow biopsy specimens. After treatment with dose-intensive intravenous melphalan followed by infusion of autologous growth-factor-mobilized blood stem cells, clinical evaluations and plasma cell studies were repeated at 3 and 12 months. Three men and two women aged 38 to 53 years were treated. Median performance status (SWOG) was 2 (1 to 3), and clinical presentations included nephrotic syndrome (*n* = 1), symptomatic car-

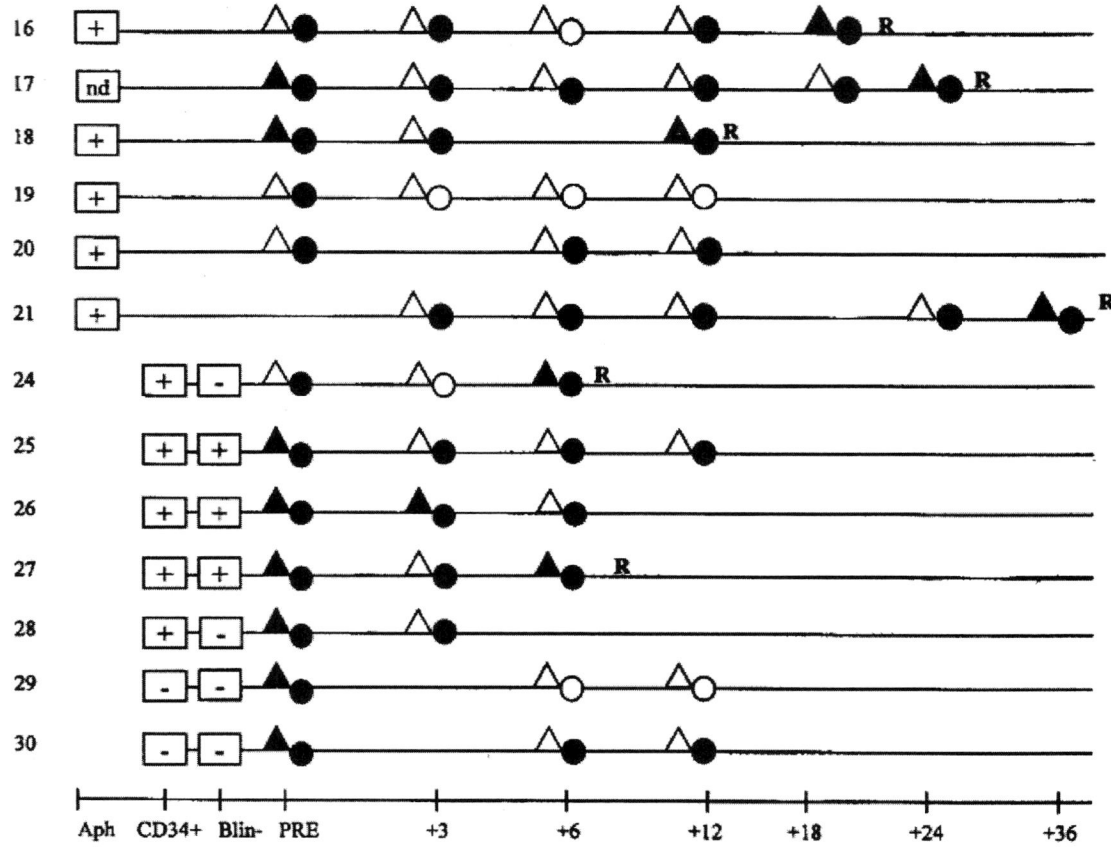

Fig. 40.22. Molecular monitoring of myeloma cells after single autograft procedures. Y-axis numbers represent patient numbers. nd, not determined; Aph, apheresis; PRE, pretransplant; R, relapse; (○), PCR-negative; (●), PCR-positive; (△), immunofixation-negative; (▲), immunofixation-positive. Reproduced, with permission, from Martinelli *et al.* (2000).

diomyopathy ($n = 1$), gastrointestinal involvement with polyneuropathy ($n = 2$), and hepatomegaly ($n = 1$). With a median follow-up of 13 months (12 to 17 months), all five patients were well and had shown stable or improved performance status and clinical remission of organ-related dysfunction, including a 50% reduction in daily proteinuria with no change in creatinine, reversal of symptoms of cardiomyopathy and reductions of posterior wall and septal thickening, reversal of polyneuropathy and gastric atony, and resolution of hepatomegaly by computed tomographic (CT) scan. In three of the five patients (60%) at 12 months after treatment, plasma cell dyscrasias could not be detected. Acquired factor X deficiency occurs in this disease, presumably due to adsorption of factor X to amyloid fibrils. Amelioration of this deficiency has been reported in those patients showing complete or partial hematologic responses (decrease in degree of plasma cell dyscrasia or monoclonal gammopathy) posttransplant (Choufani *et al.,* 2001).

A clinical remission has also been described after high-dose melphalan and autologous BMT in a patient with biopsy-proven cardiac involvement (Moreau *et al.,* 1996). Moreau and colleagues (1998) also reported that the major prognostic factor for both response and survival was the number of clinical manifestations at the time of transplant. Patients with 2 or more of the following features had a 4 year overall survival and event-free survival of 11% compared to 91% and 46% respectively in patients with fewer than 2 such features: creatinine clearance <30 ml/min, nephrotic syndrome with urinary protein excretion >3000 mg/24h, congestive heart failure, neuropathy, or hepatomegaly associated with alkaline phosphatase level >200 IU/l. Dember *et al.* (2001) reported an improvement in nephrotic syndrome posttransplant, but this was largely restricted to patients achieving eradication of their plasma cell dyscrasia.

A subsequent study by Comenzo *et al.* (1998) described outcome in relation to the predominant organ involved by amyloid (Fig. 40.25, Table 40.13). In general, the morbidity and mortality appear higher than for myeloma: the incidence of gastrointestinal toxicity is high, with a significant incidence of gastrointestinal hemorrhage (Kumar *et al.,* 2001). Cardiac complications, including arrthymias, are unexpectedly prevalent. Additionally, severe

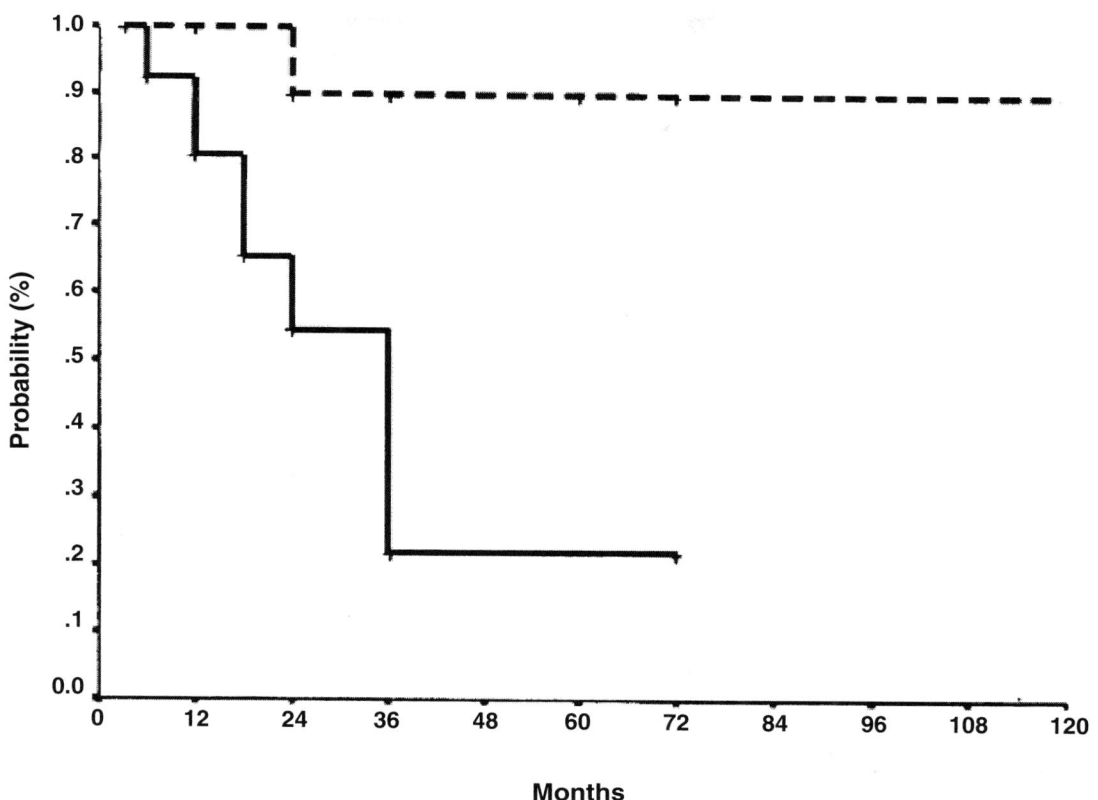

Fig. 40.23. Relapse-free survival according to PCR negativity. Solid line, persistently PCR-positive patients; dashed line, patients who became PCR-negative. Reproduced, with permission, from Martinelli *et al.* (2000).

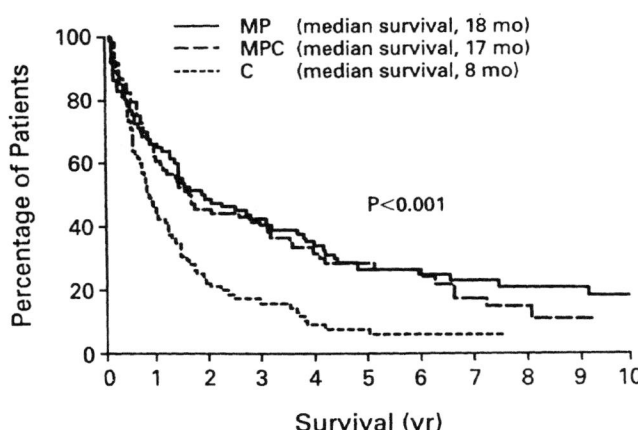

Fig. 40.24. Survival from the date of randomization among patients with primary systemic amyloidosis, according to treatment group. MP, melphalan and prednisone; MPC, melphalan, prednisone, and colchicine; C, colchicine. Reproduced, with permission, from Kyle *et al.* (1997).

episodes of fluid retention with progressive edema and bilateral pleural effusions have been reported (Gertz *et al.*, 2000).

A review of this approach to this disease in 205 patients noted the high peritransplant mortality (14% in this series), particularly in those with amyloid cardiomyopathy (Sancho-rawala *et al.*, 2001a and b). Their eligibility requirements included a left ventricular ejection fraction (LVEF) >40% and no evidence of symptomatic ventricular tachycardia, exertional syncope, or thrombo-embolic events from atrial dysfunction, oxygen saturation >95% on room air; and a baseline systolic blood pressure >90 mmHg. Pretransplant assessment of gastrointestinal function and mucosal integrity was also important with serial stool exams for occult blood, endoscopic evaluation if indicated, and a complete assessment of coagulation status. Patients with factor X deficiency were found to be at particularly high risk of bleeding complications during periods of thrombocytopenia. Additional unusual problems included difficulties with emergency intubation in patients with macroglossia, spontaneous splenic and esophageal rupture, and hypercoagulability in association with nephrotic syndrome. Neither age >65 years nor dialysis for end-stage renal disease were considered specific contraindications to transplantation. G-CSF alone was preferred over G-CSF and cyclophosphamide as the mobilization mechanism. The importance of a multidisciplinary team approach, with

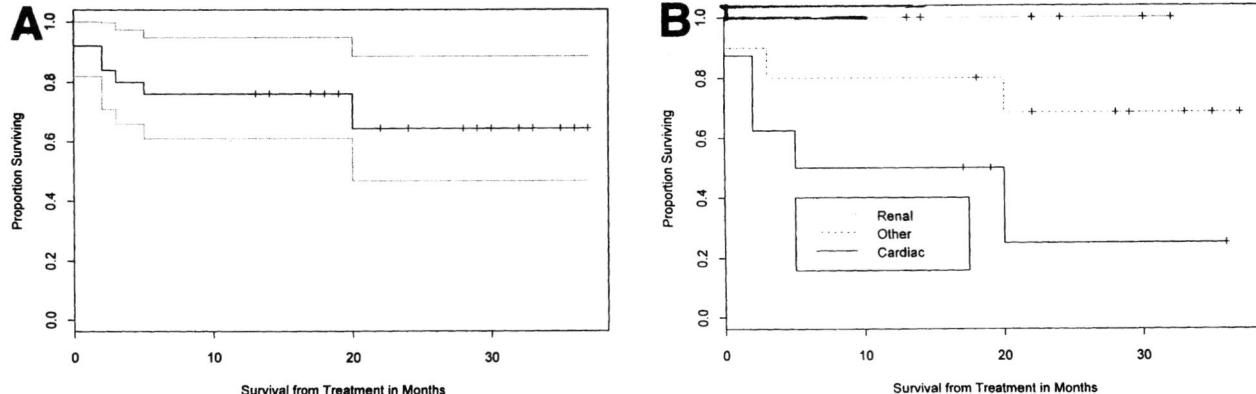

Fig. 40.25. Overall survival and survival by category of organ involvement. With median follow-up of 24 months (12 to 38), 17 of 25 patients (68%) survived, and the median survival has not yet been reached as depicted in (**A**), a Kaplan-Meier plot showing the 95% confidence interval (CI; proportional survival 0.65, 95% CI 0.48 to 0.88). (**B**) Survival by predominant organ involvement is shown. Total and mean times of follow-up for the three cohorts are 149 and 21.3 months (renal, $n = 7$), 225 and 22.5 months (other, $n = 10$), and 101 and 12.6 months (cardiac, $n = 8$). Patients without predominant cardiac involvement had better overall survival than cardiac patients (one-tailed Fisher's exact test, $P < .05$). Reproduced, with permission, from Comenzo et al. (1998).

involvement by subspecialists familiar with the manifestations and treatment of amyloid, was emphasized.

Suggested guidelines for the selection of patients for transplantation are shown in Table 40.14. A risk-adapted approach to melphalan dosing for the conditioning regimen has been proposed (Commenzo & Gertz, 2002) (see Breaking News chapter).

A favorable outcome has been reported after syngeneic transplantation for AL amyloidosis (van Buren et al., 1995) (Chapter 49), and objective response with disease regression

has been documented after allogeneic transplantation (Guillaume et al., 1997; Gillmore et al., 1998).

A prospective, randomized trail investigated the timing of stem cell transplantation in the treatment of AL amyloidosis (Sanchorawala et al., 2001b). Newly diagnosed patients were randomized to receive high-dose melphalan 140–200 mg/m² as initial therapy (early; $n = 52$) or following 2 cycles of oral standard-dose melphalan-prenisolone (delayed; $n = 48$); 100 patients were enrolled (median age 56 years); 65% of patients

Table 40.13 *Renal and hepatic responses*

		Proteinuria (<150 mg/d)		Alkaline phosphatase (<120 U/l)		Albumin (3.5–5.5 g/dl)		Creatinine (<1.5 mg/dl)	
		Pre	Post	Pre	Post	Pre	Post	Pre	Post
A	6	11,370	1,573	124	108	2.3	4.0	1.0	0.9
	7	12,800	11,400	104	77	2.2	2.5	1.0	4.1
	11	9,234	8,293	90	64	2.2	2.3	0.7	0.9
	13	9,653	7,320	135	111	2.1	3.1	0.8	0.9
	22	6,030	421	146	194	1.7	2.7	0.9	1.2
	23	16,390	21,625	59	61	1.2	1.7	0.9	7.1
	24	16,400	7,580	96	80	1.9	3.7	1.1	1.3
B	5	645	102	184	113	5.1	4.9	1.3	1.4
	8	16,300	4,218	490	520	3.4	4.8	1.6	1.3
	10	2,880	1,135	1,280	551	3.3	3.9	0.8	0.9
	12	3,548	1,595	413	199	3.3	5.7	0.8	0.7
	17	23,595	2,728	2,820	586	1.3	3.9	0.5	0.7
C	14	3,542	992	362	278	4.0	5.1	1.5	1.7
	18	2,420	4,189	1,488	160	2.7	3.3	0.9	1.3

All of these patients had amyloid-related renal involvement, and patients in groups B and C had both renal and hepatic involvement. The patients in group A had predominant renal involvement, those in B predominant hepatic, and in C predominant cardiac involvement. The columns give pre- and posttherapy values for laboratory tests obtained for each patient, the posttherapy value being from the most recent follow-up.
(Normal values)
Reproduced, with permission, from Comenzo et al. (1998).

Table 40.14. *Guidelines for selection of transplant patients*

Absolute contraindication
 Clinical congestive heart failure
 Total bilirubin >3.0 mg/dl
 Echocardiographic ejection fraction <55%
Relative contraindication
 Serum creatinine >2.0 mg/dl
 Interventricular septal thickness >15 mm
 Age >60 years
 More than two visceral organs involved

Reproduced, with permission, from Gertz *et al.* (2000).

in the early transplant group, and 48% in the delayed transplant group, had cardiac involvement. The OS of patients 1 year after randomization was significantly higher for the early transplant group (70%) than for the delayed group (58%; *P* = .04) when the distribution of cardiac patients was taken into account. For the subgroup of patients with cardiac involvement, median OS for the early transplant group was 19.6 months, significantly longer than for the delayed group (5.3 months; *P* = .02). Thus, new patients with AL amyloidosis eligible for high-dose therapy did not benefit from initial treatment with oral melphalan-prednisolone prior to high-dose therapy.

POEMS syndrome

The POEMS syndrome (polyneuropathy, organomegaly, endocrinopathy, serum monoclonal gammopathy, and skin changes) is a plasma cell dyscrasia that differs substantially from classic myeloma. It is often associated with disabling polyneuropathy in younger patients and current therapeutic approaches (local radiotherapy, prednisone, melphalan, plasmapheresis, intravenous immunoglobulin) are often inadequate and leave many patients wheelchair-bound. The disease occurs more frequently in Japan, where it is known as Crow-Fukase syndrome.[1]

A case report described a 41-year-old man prepared for autologous PBSC transplantation with the bone-seeking radio-pharmaceutical samarium-153 ethylene diamine tetramethylene phosphonate (^{153}Sm-EDTMP) followed by melphalan 200 mg/m^2 (Hogan *et al.*, 2001). Hepatomegaly resolved the week after transplant and neurologic function gradually improved until he could walk independently. At 23 months posttransplant neurologic function was stable, subclinical hypothyroidism had resolved, and serum and urine monoclonal protein was undetectable. A 58-year-old woman was conditioned with melphalan 200 mg/m^2 prior to autologous PBSC transplantation. She showed a dramatic and progressive improvement and was alive and well at 1 year posttransplant (Rovira *et al.*, 2001).

[1]R. S. Crowe, 20th Century British physician; Masaichi Fukase, 20th Century Japanese physician.

Jaccard *et al.* (2001) used autologous stem cell transplantation in 5 patients aged between 44 and 62 years, who were diagnosed with POEMS syndrome with multi-focal bone lesions or diffuse bone marrow plasma infiltration. All patients had distal bilateral sensory disturbance predominating in the lower limbs, associated with abolition of deep tendon reflexes. Two patients also presented with motor deficiency, including one who was bedridden because of tetraparesis. Electromyographic studies provided evidence for demyelinating lesions in all patients, either isolated (*n* = 2) or associated with axonal degeneration (*n* = 3). Other manifestations included POEMS-related nephropathy in 1 patient; organomegaly in 3 patients; impotence, diabetes mellitus, adrenal insufficiency and/or hypothyroidism in 4 patients; papilledema in 2 patients; hyperproteinorachia in 4 patients; and skin changes in 4 patients. HSC transplantation was performed about one month after stem cell collection in the 5 patients and 2 of them had a second transplant with total body irradiation 3 months later. No toxic death occurred during mobilization or transplantation. Posttransplant, monoclonal immunoglobulin was no longer detectable by immunofixation in the serum and urine of 4 patients. The last patient achieved a very good response with disappearance of abnormal bone marrow infiltration and with normal serum electrophoresis. In all cases, remission of plasma cell proliferation was associated with a marked improvement in performance and in neurological symptoms. Also, skin changes, edema (including papilledema) improved and organomegaly was no longer seen posttransplant in any case. With a median follow-up of 36 months from transplant, no patient has relapsed.

Conclusions

Data accumulated over the last decade suggest a convincing role for autografting in the management of myeloma, with suggestions of operational cures. Allogeneic transplantation offers the hope of attaining molecular CR and true cures, particularly since a graft-versus-myeloma effect has been demonstrated (Tricot *et al.*, 1996), but procedure-related mortality remains high and experience in this field remains limited. High-dose therapy and autografting has resulted in CR rates between 25% and 75%. Obviously, the meaning of CR depends on how one defines it and how closely one looks for evidence of residual disease. Most of the patients who achieve CR will show molecular evidence of disease. Most studies, whether in autografting or allografting, have identified the attainment of CR (based on hematologic and biochemical criteria) as a favorable prognostic indicator for survival, and therefore this should be the goal of future trials. Further dose-intensification and exploration of new high-dose combinations might improve our myeloablative strategies. Newer approaches such as IFN-α2b maintenance treatment, immune modulation with IL-2, gene therapy, dendritic cell vaccines, thalidomide and its analogs, PS-341, arsenic trioxide, vasoendothelial growth factor inhibitors, and monoclonal antibodies will be areas of future interest. Autografting, particularly with blood stem cells, has been crucial in decreasing the procedure-related mortality of high-dose therapy and therefore it is justifiable to offer this mode of treatment to all myeloma patients irrespective of age as front-line treatment, especially if they do not have an HLA-matched sibling donor. The dose of melphalan should be modified in patients with renal failure and the elderly, as described. Patients under the age of 55 years with a matched sibling donor should be considered for an allograft if they have associated poor prognostic indicators. Patients with an HLA-identical sibling donor and poor prognostic features should be considered for an allotransplant with non-myeloablative conditioning, with or without a prior debulking autograft. Table 40.15 presents on algorithm for the treatment of patients with myeloma. Treatment strategies today should aim at achieving maximum CR rate with minimal toxicity, in the hope that the higher response rates translate into better overall survival, and a higher proportion of operational cures in these patients. Whether up-front HDT with PBSC transplantation can contribute to improvement in this area remains to be determined.

Table 40.15. *An algorithm for the treatment of patients with myeloma*

New patients with good risk disease (low β_2M, normal albumin, no chromosome 11 or 13 abnormalities, low PCLI)
Infusional chemotherapy with VAD/VAMP/C-VAMP to maximum response + an additional course
↓
G-CSF mobilised peripheral blood stem cell harvest
↓
High-dose melphalan 200 mg/m^2
↓

Complete or partial remission Interferon-α2b maintenance	Non-responder Thalidomide IMiDs or PS-341 Non-myeloablative allotransplant ↓ Interferon maintenance

Patients with poor risk disease (high β_2M, low albumin, chromosome 11 and 13 abnormalities, high PCLI)
Infusional chemotherapy with VAD/VAMP/C-VAMP to maximum response + an additional course
↓
G-CSF mobilised peripheral blood stem cell harvest
↓
High-dose melphalan 200 mg/m^2
↓

Complete remission Interferon-α2b maintenance	Partial remission Nonmyeloablative allotransplant Thalidomide maintenance Immune-based strategies	Non-responder Thalidomide Non-myeloablative allotransplant IMiDs or PS-341

Abbreviations: β_2M, β_2-microglobulin; PCLI, plasma cell labeling index; VAD, vincristine, doxorubicin, dexamethasone; VAMP, vincristine, doxorubicin, methyl prednisolone; C-VAMP, cyclophosphamide, vincristine, doxorubicin, methyl prednisolone; G-CSF, granulocyte colony-stimulating factor.

References

Adkins, D. R., Salzman, D., Boldt, D. *et al.* (1994). Phase I trial of dacarbazine with cyclophosphamide, carmustine, etoposide, and autologous stem-cell transplantation in patients with lymphoma and multiple myeloma. *Journal of Clinical Oncology,* **12,** 1890–1901.

Alegre, A., Diaz-Mediavilla, J., San-Miguel, J. *et al.* (1998). Autologous peripheral blood stem cell transplantation for multiple myeloma: a report of 259 cases from the Spanish Registry. *Bone Marrow Transplantation,* **21,** 133–40.

Alexanian, R. & Dimopoulos, M. (1994). The treatment of multiple myeloma. *New England Journal of Medicine,* **330,** 484–9.

Alexanian, R., Dimopoulos, M., Smith, T. *et al.* (1994). Limited value of myeloablative therapy for late multiple myeloma. *Blood,* **83,** 512–16.

Alexanian, R., Haut, A., Khan, A. U. *et al.* (1969). Treatment for multiple myeloma: combination chemotherapy with different melphalan dose regimens. *Journal of the American Medical Association,* **208,** 1680–5.

Anderson, K. C., Anderson, J., Soiffer, R. *et al.* (1993). Monoclonal antibody-purged bone marrow transplantation therapy for multiple myeloma. *Blood,* **82,** 2568–76.

Attal, M. & Harousseau, J. L. (2001). Randomized trial experience of the Intergroupe Francophone du Myelome. *Seminars in Hematology,* **38,** 226–30.

Attal, M., Harousseau, J. L., Stoppa, A. M. *et al.* (1996). Prospective, randomized trial of autologous bone marrow transplantation and chemotherapy in multiple myeloma. *New England Journal of Medicine,* **355,** 91–7.

Attal, M., Huguet, F., Schlaifer, D. *et al.* (1992). Intensive combined therapy for previously untreated aggressive myeloma. *Blood,* **79,** 1130–6.

Badros, A., Barlogie, B., Morris, C. *et al.* (2001a). High response rate in refractory and high-risk multiple myeloma after allotransplantation using a nonmyeloablative conditioning regimen and donor lymphocyte infusions. *Blood,* **97,** 2574–9.

Badros, A., Barlogie, B., Siegel, E. *et al.* (2001b). Autologous stem cell transplantation in elderly multiple myeloma patients over the age of 70 years. *British Journal of Haematology,* **114,** 600–7.

Badros, A., Barlogie, B., Siegel, E. *et al.* (2001c). Results of autologous stem cell transplant in multiple myeloma patients with renal failure. *British Journal of Haematology,* **114,** 822–9.

Ballester, O. F., Tummala, R., Janssen, W. E. *et al.* (1997). High-dose chemotherapy and autologous peripheral blood stem cell transplantation in patients with multiple myeloma and renal insufficiency. *Bone Marrow Transplantation,* **20,** 653–6.

Barlogie, B., Alexanian, R., Dicke, K. A. *et al.* (1987). High-dose chemoradiotherapy and autologous bone marrow transplantation for resistant multiple myeloma. *Blood,* **70,** 869–72.

Barlogie, B., Crowley, J., Jagannath, S. *et al.* (1995). Superior outcome after early autotransplantation (AT) with "total therapy" (TT) compared to standard SWOG treatment (ST) for multiple myeloma (MM). *Blood,* **86** (Suppl 1), 207a (Abstract).

Barlogie, B., Hall, R., Zander, A. *et al.* (1986). High-dose melphalan with autologous bone marrow transplantation for multiple myeloma. *Blood,* **67,** 1298–301.

Barlogie, B., Jagannath, S., Desikan, K. R. *et al.* (1999). Total therapy with tandem transplants for newly diagnosed multiple myeloma. *Blood,* **93,** 55–65.

Barlogie, B., Jagannath, S., Vesole, D. H. *et al.* (1997). Superiority of tandem autologous transplantation over standard therapy over previously untreated multiple myeloma. *Blood,* **89,** 789–93.

Barlogie, B., Smith, L., & Alexanian, R. (1984). Effective treatment of advanced multiple myeloma refractory to alkylating agents. *New England Journal of Medicine,* **310,** 1353–6.

Barlogie, F., Desikan, R., Eddlemon, P. *et al.* (2001). Extended survival in advanced and refractory multiple myeloma after agent thalidomide: identification of prognostic factors in a phase 2 study of 169 patients. *Blood,* **98,** 492–4.

Bataille, R., Durie, B. G., Grenier, J., & Sany, J. (1986). Prognostic factors in staging multiple myeloma: a reappraisal. *Journal of Clinical Oncology,* **4,** 80–7.

Belch, A. R., Szczepek, A., Bergsagel, P. L. *et al.* (1995). Circulating CD34+ cells from peripheral blood in multiple myeloma include B cells with patient specific IGH CDR3 sequences and CD34mRNA as well as DNA hyperdiploidy and N-ras mutation. *Blood,* **86,** 276a (Abstract).

Bensinger, W. I., Demirer, T., Buckner, C. D. *et al.* (1996a). Syngeneic marrow transplantation in patients with multiple myeloma. *Bone Marrow Transplantation,* **18,** 527–31.

Bensinger, W. I., Rowley, S. D., Demirer, T. *et al.* (1996b). High-dose therapy followed by autologous hematopoietic stem-cell infusion for patients with multiple myeloma. *Journal of Clinical Oncology,* **14,** 1447–56.

Bergsagel, D. E. (1979). Treatment of plasma cell myeloma. *Annual Review of Medicine,* **30,** 431.

Bergsagel, D. E., Bailey, A. J., Langley, G. R. *et al.* (1979). The chemotherapy on plasma-cell myeloma and the incidence of acute leukemia. *New England Journal of Medicine,* **301,** 743–8.

Björkstand, B., Ljungman, P., Bird, J. M. *et al.* (1995). Double high-dose chemoradiotherapy with autologous stem cell transplantation can induce molecular remissions in multiple myeloma. *Bone Marrow Transplantation,* **15,** 367–71.

Björkstrand, B., Svennson, H., Goldschmidt, H. *et al.* (2001). Alpha-interferon maintenance is associated with improved survival after high-dose treatment and autologous stem cell transplantation in patients with multiple myeloma: a retrospective registry study from the European Group for Blood and Marrow Transplantation (EBMT). *Bone Marrow Transplantation,* **27,** 511–5.

Blade, J., Kyle, R. A., & Greipp, P. R. (1996). Multiple myeloma in patients younger than 30 years. Report of 10 cases and review of the literature. *Archives of Internal Medicine,* **156,** 1463–8.

Blade, J., Samson, D., Reece, D. *et al.* (1998). Criteria for evaluating disease response and progression in patients with multiple myeloma treated by high-dose therapy and haemopoietic stem cell transplantation. Myeloma Subcommittee of the EBMT. European Group for Blood and Marrow Transplant. *British Journal of Haematology,* **102,** 1115–23.

Blade, J., San Miguel, J. F., Alcala, A. *et al.* (1993). Alternating combination VCMP/VBAP chemotherapy versus melphalan/prednisolone in the treatment of multiple myeloma: a randomized multicentric study of 487 patients. *Journal of Clinical Oncology,* **11,** 1165–71.

Blade, J., San Miguel, J. F., Fontanillas, M. *et al.* (1996). Survival of multiple myeloma patients who are potential candidates for early high-dose therapy intensification/auto transplantation and who were conventionally treated. *Journal of Clinical Oncology,* **14,** 2167–73.

Boccadoro, M., Marmont, F., Tribalto, M. *et al.* (1991). Multiple myeloma: VMCP/VBAP alternating combination chemotherapy is not superior to melphalan and prednisone even in high-risk patients. *Journal of Clinical Oncology,* **9,** 444–8.

Brugger, S. A., Kahls, P., Keil, F. *et al.* (1996). Hematological and immunological reconstitution after high-dose radio- and/or chemotherapy with supportive infusion of unselected and CD34+ enriched peripheral stem cells. *Annals of Hematology,* **73** (Suppl 2), 165.

Child, J. A. (1994). Evolving strategies for the treatment of myelomatosis. *British Journal of Haematology,* **88,** 672–8.

Choufani, E. B., Sanchorawala, V., Ernst, T. *et al.* (2001). Acquired factor X deficiency in patients with amyloid light-chain amyloidosis: incidence, bleeding manifestations, and response to high-dose chemotherapy. *Blood,* **97,** 1885–7.

Comenzo, R. O., Vosburgh, E., Simms, R. W. *et al.* (1996). Dose-intensive melphalan with blood stem cell support for the treatment of AL amyloidosis: one year follow-up in 5 patients. *Blood,* **88,** 2801–6.

Comenzo, R. L., Vosburgh, E., & Falk, R. H. (1998). Dose-intensive melphalan with blood stem-cell support for the treatment of AL (amyloid light-chain) amyloidosis: survival and responses in 25 patients. *Blood,* **91,** 3662–70.

Comenzo, R. L., & Gertz, M. A. (2002). Autologous stem cell transplantation for primary systemic amyloidosis. *Blood,* **100,** 4276–82.

Cooper, M. R., Dear, K., McIntyre, O. R. *et al.* (1993). A randomized clinical trail comparing melphalan/prednisolone with or without interferon alfa 2b in newly diagnosed patients with multiple myeloma: a cancer and leukaemia group B Study. *Journal of Clinical Oncology,* **11,** 155–60.

Cooper, M. R., McIntyre, O. R., Propert, K. J. *et al.* (1986). Single, sequential and multiple alkylating agent therapy for multiple myeloma: a CALGB Study. *Journal of Clinical Oncology,* **4,** 1331–9.

Corradini, P., Voena, C., Astolfi, M. *et al.* (1995). High-dose sequential chemoradiotherapy in multiple myeloma: residual tumor cells are detectable in bone marrow and peripheral blood stem cell harvests and after autografting. *Blood,* **85,** 1596–602.

Corradini, P., Voena, C., Tarella, C. *et al.* (1999). Molecular and clinical remissions in multiple myeloma: role of autologous and allogeneic transplantation of hematopoietic cells. *Journal of Clinical Oncology,* **17,** 208–15.

Cunningham, D., Paz-Ares, L., Gore, M. E. *et al.* (1994a). High-dose melphalan for multiple myeloma: long term follow-up data. *Journal of Clinical Oncology,* **12,** 764–8.

Cunningham, D., Paz-Ares, L., Milan, S. *et al.* (1994b). High-dose melphalan and autologous bone marrow transplantation as consolidation in previously untreated myeloma. *Journal of Clinical Oncology,* **12,** 759–63.

Cunningham, D., Powles, R., Malpas, J. *et al.* (1993). A randomized trial of maintenance therapy with Intron-A following high-dose melphalan and ABMT in myeloma. *Proceedings of the American Society of Clinical Oncology,* **12,** 1232 (Abstract).

Cunningham, D., Powles, R., Malpas, J. *et al.* (1998). A randomised trial of maintenance interferon following high-dose chemotherapy in multiple myeloma: long-term follow-up results. *British Journal of Hematology,* **102**: 495–502.

de la Rubia, J., Bonanad, S., Palau, J. *et al.* (1994). Rapid progression of multiple myeloma following G-CSF mobilization. *Bone Marrow Transplantation,* **14,** 475–6.

Dember, L. M., Sanchorawala, V., Seldin, D. C. *et al.* (2001). Effect of dose-intensive intravenous melphalan and autologous blood stem cell transplantation on AL amyloidosis-associated renal disease. *Annals of Internal Medicine,* **134,** 746–53.

Demirer, T., Buckner, C., Lilleby, K. *et al.* (1994). Failure of a single cycle of high-dose cyclophosphamide followed by intensive myeloablative therapy and autologous stem cell transplantation to improve outcome in relapsed disease. *Cancer,* **74,** 715–21.

Desikan, R., Barlogie, B., Sawyer, J. *et al.* (2000). Results of high-dose therapy for 1000 patients with multiple myeloma: durable complete remissions and superior survival in the absence of chromosome 13 abnormalities. *Blood,* **95,** 4008–10.

Dey, B. R., McAfee, S., Sackstein, R. *et al.* (2001). Successful allogeneic stem cell transplantation with nonmyeloablative conditioning in patients with relapsed hematologic malignancy following autologous stem cell transplantation. *Biology of Blood and Marrow Transplantation,* **7,** 604–12.

Dimopoulos, M. A., Alexanian, R., Przepiorka, D. *et al.* (1993). Thiotepa, busulfan, and cyclophosphamide: a new preparative regimen for autologous marrow or blood stem cell transplantation in high-risk multiple myeloma. *Blood,* **82,** 2324–8.

Drewinka, B., Alexanian, R., Boyer, H. *et al.* (1981). The growth fraction of human myeloma cells. *Blood,* **57,** 333–8.

Dunbar, C. E., Cottler-Fox, M., O'Shaughnessy, J. A. *et al.* (1995). Retrovirally marked CD34-enriched peripheral blood and bone marrow cells contribute to long term engraftment after autologous transplantation. *Blood,* **85,** 3048–57.

Facon, T., Avet-Loiseau, H., Guillerm, G. *et al.* (2001). Chromosome 13 abnormalities identified by FISH analysis and serum β_2-microglobulin produce a powerful myeloma staging system for patients receiving high-dose therapy. *Blood,* **97,** 1566–71.

Fermand, J. P., Cherret, S., Ravaud, P. *et al.* (1993). High-dose chemoradiotherapy and autologous blood stem cell transplantation in multiple myeloma: results of a phase II trial involving 63 patients. *Blood,* **82,** 2005–9.

Fermand, J. P., Levy, Y., Gerota, J. *et al.* (1989). Treatment of aggressive multiple myeloma by high-dose chemotherapy and total body irradiation followed by blood stem cell autograft. *Blood,* **73,** 20.

Fermand, J. P., Marolleau, J. P., Albertini, C. *et al.* (2001). Single versus tandem high dose therapy (HDT) supported with autologous blood stem cell (ABSC) transplantation using unselected or CD34 enriched ABSC: preliminary results of a two by two designed randomized trial in 230 young patients with multiple myeloma (MM). *Blood,* **98,** 815a.

Fermand, J. P., Ravaud, P., Chevret, S. *et al.* (1998). High-dose therapy and autologous peripheral blood stem cell transplantation in multiple myeloma: up-front or rescue treatment? Results of a multicentre sequential randomised clinical trial. *Blood,* **92,** 3131–6.

Forgeson, G. V., Selby, P., Lakhani, S. *et al.* (1988). Infused vincristine and adriamycin with high-dose methyl prednisolone (VAMP) in advanced previously treated multiple myeloma patients. *British Journal of Cancer,* **58,** 469–73.

Gazitt, Y., Reading, C., Hoffman, R. *et al.* (1995). Purified CD34[+] Lin[−] Thy[+] stem cells do not contain clonal myeloma cells. *Blood,* **86,** 381–9.

Gertz, M. A., Lacy, M. Q., Gastineau, D. A. *et al.* (2000). Blood stem cell transplantation as therapy for systemic amyloidosis (AL). *Bone Marrow Transplantation,* **26,** 963–9.

Gertz, M. A., Witzig, T. E., Pineda, A. A. *et al.* (1997). Monoclonal plasma cells in the blood stem cell harvest from patients with multiple myeloma are associated with shortened relapse-free survival after transplantation. *Bone Marrow Transplantation,* **19,** 337–42.

Gillmore, J. D., Davies, J., Iqbal, A. *et al.* (1998). Allogeneic bone marrow transplantation for AL amyloidosis. *British Journal of Haematology,* **100,** 226–8.

Gobbi, M., Tazzari, P. L., Cavo, M. *et al.* (1991). Autologous bone marrow transplantation with immunotoxin purged for multiple myeloma, long term results in 14 patients with advanced disease. *Bone Marrow Transplantation,* **7** (Suppl 2), 30.

Gore, M. E., Selby, P. J., Viner, C. *et al.* (1989). Intensive treatment for multiple myeloma and criteria for complete remission. *Lancet,* **11,** 879–82.

Guillaume, J. D., Straetmans, N., Jadoul, M. *et al.* (1997). Allogeneic bone marrow transplantation for AL amyloidosis. *Bone Marrow Transplantation,* **20,** 907–8.

Gupta, D., Bybee, A., Cooke, F. *et al.* (1999). CD34[+]-selected peripheral blood progenitor cell transplantation in patients with multiple myeloma: tumour cell contamination and outcome. *British Journal of Haematology,* **104,** 166–77.

Harousseau, J. L., Attal, M., Divine, M. *et al.* (1995a). Comparison of autologous bone marrow transplantation and peripheral blood stem cell transplantation after first remission induction treatment in multiple myeloma. *Bone Marrow Transplantation,* **15,** 963–9.

Harousseau, J. L., Attal, M., Divine, M. *et al.* (1995b). Autologous stem cell transplantation after first remission induction treatment in multiple myeloma: a report of the French Registry on autologous transplantation in multiple myeloma. *Blood,* **85,** 3077–85.

Henon, P., Beck, G., Debecker, A. *et al.* (1988). Autograft using peripheral blood stem cells collected after high-dose melphalan in high risk multiple myeloma. *British Journal of Haematology,* **70,** 254–5.

Henry, J. M., Sykes, P. J., Brisco, M. J. *et al.* (1996). Comparison of myeloma cell contamination of bone marrow and peripheral blood stem cell harvests. *British Journal of Heamatology,* **92,** 614–19.

Hogan, W. J., Lacy, M. Q., Wiseman, G. A. *et al.* (2001). Successful treatment of POEMS syndrome with autologous hematopoietic progenitor cell transplantation. *Bone Marrow Transplantation,* **28,** 305–9.

Hovenga, S., de Wolf, J. T., Klip, H., & Vellenga, E. (1997). Consolidation therapy with autologous stem cell transplantation in plasma cell leukemia after VAD, high-dose cyclophosphamide and EDAP courses: a report of three cases and a review of the literature. *Bone Marrow Transplantation,* **20,** 901–4.

Jaccard, A., Royer, B., Bordesoulle, D. *et al.* (2001). High dose therapy and autologous blood stem cell transplantation in POEMS Syndrome. *Blood,* 98, 688a.

Jagannath, S., Barlogie, B., Dicke, K. *et al.* (1990). Autologous bone marrow transplantation in multiple myeloma: identification of prognostic factors. *Blood,* **76,** 1860–6.

Jagannath, S. & Dimopoulos. M. A. (1995). Workshop in multiple myeloma. *Bone Marrow Transplantation,* **15,** 240–6.

Jagannath, S., Vesole, D. H., Glenn, L. *et al.* (1992). Low-risk intensive therapy for multiple myeloma with combined autologous bone marrow and blood stem cell support. *Blood,* **80,** 1666–72.

Kergueris, M. F., Milpied, N., Moreau, N. *et al.* (1994). Pharmacokinetics of high-dose melphalan in adults: influence of renal function. *Anticancer Research,* **14,** 2379–82.

Kottaridis, P. D., Milligan, D. W., Chopra, R. *et al.* (2000). In vivo CAMPATH-1H prevents graft-versus-host disease following nonmyeloablative stem cell transplantation. *Blood,* **96,** 2419–25.

Kröger, N., Schwerdtfeger, R., Kiehl, M. *et al.* (2002). Autologous stem cell transplantation followed by a reduced-dose allograft induces high complete remission rate in multiple myeloma. *Blood,* **100,** 755-60.

Kumar, S., Dispenzieri, A., Lacy, M. Q., Litzow, M. R., & Gertz, M. A. (2001). High incidence of gastrointestinal tract bleeding after autologous stem cell transplant for primary systemic amyloidosis. *Bone Marrow Transplantation,* **28,** 381–5.

Kyle, R. A., Gentz, M. A., Greipp, P. R. *et al.* (1997). A trial of three regimens for primary amyloidosis: colchicine alone, melphalan and prednisone, and melphalan, prednisone, and colchicine. *New England Journal of Medicine,* **336,** 1202–7.

Lahuerta, J. J., Grande, C., Blade, J., Martinez-Lopez, J. *et al.* (2000). Myeloablative treatments for multiple myeloma: update of a comparative study of different regimens used in patients from the Spanish registry for transplantation in multiple myeloma. *British Journal of Haematology,* **109,** 138–47.

Laurenti, L., Sica, S., Salutari, P. *et al.* (1998). Assessment of hematological and immunological function during long-term follow-up after peripheral blood stem cell transplantation. *Hematologica,* **83,** 45–9.

Lee, Y. C., Came, N., Schwarer, A. & Day, B. (2002). Autologous peripheral blood stem cell transplantation for peripheral neuropathy secondary to monoclonal gammopathy of unknown significance. *Bone Marrow Transplantation,* **30,** 53–6.

Lenhoff, S., Hjorth, M., Holmberg, E. *et al.* (2000). Impact on survival of high-dose therapy with autologous stem cell support in patients younger than 60 years with newly-diagnosed multiple myeloma: a population-based study. *Blood,* **95,** 7–11.

Ludwig, H., Fritz, E., Zulian, G. B., Browman, G. P. *et al.* (1998). Should alpha-interferon be included as standard treatment in multiple myeloma? *European Journal of Cancer,* **34,** 12–24.

MacLennan, I.C.M., Chapman, C., Dunn, J., & Kelly, K. (1992). Combined chemotherapy with ABCM versus melphalan for treatment of myelomatosis. *Lancet,* **339,** 200–5.

Maloney, D. G., Sahebi, F., Stockerl-Goldstein, K. E. *et al.* (2001). Combining an allogeneic graft-versus-myeloma effect with high-dose autologous stem cell rescue in the treatment of multiple myeloma. *Blood,* **98,** 434–5a.

Mandelli, F., Avvisati, G., Amadori, S. *et al.* (1990). Maintenance treatment with recombinant alpha-2b interferon in patients with multiple myeloma responding to conventional induction chemotherapy. *New England Journal of Medicine,* **322,** 1430–34.

Mansi, J., da Costa, F., Viner, C. *et al.* (1992). High-dose busulfan in patients with myeloma. *Journal of Clinical Oncology,* **10,** 1569–73.

Mariette, X., Fermand, J. P., & Brouet, J. C. (1994). Myeloma cell contamination of peripheral blood stem cell grafts in patients with multiple myeloma treated by high-dose therapy. *Bone Marrow Transplantation,* **14,** 47–50.

Martinelli, G., Terragna, C., Zamagni, E. *et al.* (2000). Molecular remission after allogeneic or autologous transplantation of hematopoietic stem cells for multiple myeloma. *Journal of Clinical Oncology,* **18,** 2273–81.

McCarthy, D. M. & Goldman, J. M. (1984). Transfusion of circulating stem cells. *CRC Critical Reviews in Clinical Laboratory Science,* **20,** 1–24.

McElwain, T. J. & Powles, R. L. (1983). High-dose intravenous melphalan for plasma cell leukemia and myeloma. *Lancet,* **2,** 822–4.

Mellstedt, H., Ahre, A., Bjorkholm, M. *et al.* (1979). Interferon therapy in myelomatosis. *Lancet,* **1,** 245–7.

Moreau, P., Facon, T., Attal, M. *et al.* (2002). Comparison of 200 mg/m^2 melphalan and 8 Gy total body irradiation plus 140 mg/m^2 melphalan as conditioning regimens for peripheral blood stem cell transplantation in patients with newly diagnosed multiple myeloma: final analysis of the Intergroupe Francophone du Myélome 9502 randomized trial. *Blood,* **99,** 731–5.

Moreau, P., Leblond, V., Bourquelot, P. *et al.* (1998). Prognostic factors for survival and response after high-dose therapy and autologous stem cell transplantation in systemic AL amyloidosis: a report on 21 patients. *British Journal of Haematology,* **101,** 766–9.

Moreau, P., Milpied, N., de Faucal, P. *et al.* (1996). High-dose melphalan and autologous bone marrow transplantation for systemic AL amyloidosis with cardiac involvement. *Blood,* **87,** 3063–4 (Letter).

Moreau, P., Milpied, N., Mahe, B. *et al.* (1999). Melphalan 220 mg/m^2 followed by peripheral blood stem cell transplantation in 27 patients with advanced multiple myeloma. *Bone Marrow Transplantation,* **23,** 1003–6.

The Myeloma Trialists' Collaborative Group (MTCG). (2001). Interferon as therapy for multiple myeloma: an individual patient data overview of 24 randomised trials with over 4012 patients. *British Journal of Haematology,* **113,** 1020–34.

Nachbaur, D., Kropshofer, G., Feichtinger, H. *et al.* (1997). Cryptosporidiosis after CD34-selected autologous peripheral blood stem cell transplantation (PBSCT): treatment with paromycin, azithromycin and recombinant human interleukin-2. *Bone Marrow Transplantation,* **19,** 1261–63.

Palumbo, A., Triolo, S., Argentino, C. *et al.* (1999). Dose-intensive melphalan with stem cell support (MEL100) is superior to standard treatment in elderly myeloma patients. *Blood,* **94,** 1248–53.

Palumbo, A., Triolo, S., Bringhen, S. *et al.* (2000). In myeloma patients treated with melphalan 100 mg/m^2 or melphalan 200 mg/m^2 outcome is not significantly different. *Blood,* **96,** 419a.

Palva, I. P., Ahrenberg, P., Ala-Harja, K. *et al.* (1987). Treatment of multiple myeloma with an intensive 5-drug combination or intermittent melphalan and prednisolone; a randomized multicentre trial. *European Journal of Haematology,* **38,** 50–4.

Pavlovsky, S., Saslavsky, J., Tezanos Pinto, M. *et al.* (1984). A randomized trial of melphalan and prednisone versus melphalan, prednisone, cyclophosphamide, MeCCNU, and vincristine in untreated multiple myeloma. *Journal of Clinical Oncology*, **2**, 836–40.

Peest, D., Deicher, H., Coldeway, R. *et al.* (1988). Induction and maintenance therapy in multiple myeloma: a multcenter trial of MP versus VCMP. *European Journal of Cancer and Clinical Oncology*, **24**, 1061–7.

Powles, R., Raje, N., Horton, C. *et al.* (1996). Comparison of interferon tolerance after autologous bone marrow or peripheral blood stem cell transplants for myeloma patients who have responded to induction therapy. *Leukemia and Lymphoma*, **21**, 421–7.

Powles, R., Raje, N., Milan, S. *et al.* (1997). Outcome assessment of a population based group of 195 patients under 70 years of age offered intensive treatment. *Bone Marrow Transplantation*, **20**, 435–43.

Powles, R., Sirohi, B., Treleaven, J. *et al.* (2000a). 15 year follow-up of myeloma patients receiving 140 mg/m^2 melphalan without hematopoietic stem cell or growth factor support as initial therapy. *Blood*, **96**, 292b.

Powles, R., Sirohi, B., Treleaven, J. *et al.* (2000b) Continued first complete remission in multiple myeloma for over 10 years: a series of "operationally cured" patients. *Blood*, **96**, Abstract 2215.

Powles, R., Sirohi, B., Treleaven, J. *et al.* (2002). Collection of peripheral blood stem cells in newly-diagnosed myeloma patients without any prior cytoreductive therapy: the first step towards an "operational cure"? *Bone Marrow Transplantation*, **30**, 479–84.

Powles, R. L., Raje, N. S., Cunningham, D. *et al.* (1995). Maintenance therapy for remission in myeloma with Intron A following either an autologous bone marrow transplantation or peripheral stem cell rescue. *Stem Cells*, **13**, 114–17.

Raje, N., Powles, R., Horton, C. *et al.* (1997a). Comparison of marrow versus blood derived stem cells for autografting in previously untreated multiple myeloma. *British Journal of Cancer*, **75**, 1684–9.

Raje, N., Powles, R., Kulkarni, S. *et al.* (1997b). A comparison of vincristine and doxorubicin infusional chemotherapy with methylprednisolone (VAMP) with the addition of weekly cyclophosphamide (C-VAMP) as induction treatment followed by autografting in previously untreated myeloma. *British Journal of Haematology*, **97**, 153–60.

Raje, N. S., Powles, R. L., Horton, C.A.P. *et al.* (1995). Peripheral blood stem cell transplantation in multiple myeloma. *British Journal of Haematology*, **89** (Suppl 1), 84.

Rajkumar, S. V., Fonseca, R., Lacy, M. Q. *et al.* (1999a). Autologous stem cell transplantation for relapsed and primary refractory myeloma. *Bone Marrow Transplantation*, **23**, 1267–72.

Rajkumar, S. V., Fonseca, R., Lacy, M. Q. *et al.* (1999b). Beta2-microglobulin and bone marrow plasma cell involvement predict complete responders among patients undergoing blood cell transplantation for myeloma. *Bone Marrow Transplantation*, **23**, 1261–6.

Rebibou, J. M., Caillot, D., Casanova, R. O. *et al.* (1997). Peripheral blood stem cell transplantation in a multiple myeloma patient with end-stage renal failure. *Bone Marrow Transplantation*, **20**, 63–5.

Reece, D. E., Barnett, M. J., Connors, J. M. *et al.* (1993). Treatment of multiple myeloma with intensive chemotherapy followed by autologous BMT using marrow purged with 4-hydroperoxycyclophosphamide. *Bone Marrow Transplantation*, **11**, 139–46.

Reichardt, V. L., Okada, C., Liso, A. *et al.* (1999). Idiotype vaccination using dendritic cells after autologous peripheral blood stem cell transplantation for multiple myeloma—a feasibility study. *Blood*, **93**, 2411–9.

Richardson, P. G., Schlossman, R. L., Weller, E. *et al.* (2002). Immunomodulatory drug CC-5013 overcomes drug resistance and is well tolerated in patients with relapsed myeloma. *Blood*, **100**, 3063–7.

Rovira, M., Carreras, E., Blade, J. *et al.* (2001). Dramatic improvement of POEMS syndrome following autologous haematopoietic cell transplantation. *British Journal of Haematology*, **115**, 373–5.

Ruffini, A. & Kwak, L. W. (2001). Immunotherapy of multiple myeloma. *Seminars in Hematology*, **38**, 260–7.

Salmon, S. E., Crowley, J. J., Grogan, T. M. *et al.* (1994). Combination chemotherapy, glucocorticoids and interferon alfa in the treatment of multiple myeloma: a Southwest Oncology Group Study. *Journal of Clinical Oncology*, **12**, 2405–14.

Salmon, S. E., Haut, A., Bonnet, J. D. *et al.* (1983). Alternating combination chemotherapy and levamisole improves survival in multiple myeloma: a Southwest Oncology Group Study. *Journal of Clinical Oncology*, **1**, 453–61.

Sanchorawala, V., Wright, D. G., Seldin, D. C. *et al.* (2001a). An overview of the use of high-dose melphalan with autologous stem cell transplantation for the treatment of AL amyloidosis. *Bone Marrow Transplantation*, **28**, 637–42.

Sanchorawala, V., Wright, D. G., Seldin, D. C. *et al.* (2001b). High-dose intravenous melphalan and autologous stem cell transplantation as initial therapy or following two cycles of oral chemotherapy for the treatment of AL amyloidosis: results of a prospective randomized trial. *Blood*, **98**, 815a.

Schiller, G., Nimer, S., Vescio, R. *et al.* (1994). Phase I–II study of busulfan and cyclophosphamide conditioning for transplantation in advanced multiple myeloma. *Bone Marrow Transplantation*, **14**, 131–6.

Schiller, G., Vescio, R., Freytes, C. *et al.* (1995). Transplantation of CD34+ peripheral blood progenitor cells after high-dose chemotherapy for patients with advanced multiple myeloma. *Blood*, **86**, 390–7.

Schiller, G., Vescio, R., Freytes, C. *et al.* (1998). Autologous CD34-selected blood progenitor cell transplants for patients with advanced multiple myeloma. *Bone Marrow Transplantation*, **21**, 141–5.

Segeren, C. M., Sonneveld, P., Van der Holt, B. *et al.* (2001). Myeloablative treatment following intensified chemotherapy in untreated multiple myeloma: a prospective, randomized phase III study. *Blood*, **98**, 815a.

Selby, P., Zulian, G., Forgesson, G. *et al.* (1988). The development of high-dose melphalan and of autologous bone marrow transplantation in the treatment of multiple myeloma: Royal Marsden and St Bartholomew's Hospital studies. *Hematological Oncology*, **6**, 173–9.

Selby, P. J., McElwain, T. J., Nandi, A. C. *et al.* (1987). Multiple myeloma treated with high-dose intravenous melphalan. *British Journal of Haematology*, **66**, 52–5.

Siegel, D. S., Desikan, K. K., Mehta, J. *et al.* (1999). Age is not a prognostic variable with autotransplants for multiple myeloma. *Blood,* **93,** 51–4.

Singhal, S., Mehta, J., Desikan, R. *et al.* (1999). Antitumor activity of thalidomide in refractory multiple myeloma. *New England Journal of Medicine,* **341,** 1565–71.

Singhal, S., Powles, R., Milan, A. *et al.* (1995). Kinetics of paraprotein clearance after autografting for multiple myeloma. *Bone Marrow Transplantation,* **16,** 537–40.

Singhal, S., Powles, R., Sirohi, B. *et al.* (2001). J. Response to induction chemotherapy is not essential to obtain survival benefit from high-dose melphalan and autotransplantation in myeloma. *Blood,* **98,** 816a.

Sirohi, B., Kulkarni, S., Powles, R. (2001c). Some early phase II trials in previously untreated multiple myeloma: The Royal Marsden Experience. *Seminars in Hematology,* **38,** 209–18.

Sirohi, B., Powles, R., Kulkarni, S. *et al.* (2001a). Comparison of new patients with Bence-Jones, IgG and IgA myeloma receiving sequential therapy: the need to regard these immunologic subtypes as separate disease entities with specific prognostic criteria. *Bone Marrow Transplantation,* **28,** 29–37.

Sirohi, B., Powles, R., Mehta, J. *et al.* (1999). Complete remission rate and outcome after intensive treatment of 177 patients under 75 years of age with IgG myeloma defining a circumscribed disease entity with a new staging system. *British Journal of Haematology,* **107,** 656–66.

Sirohi, B., Powles, R., Mehta, J. *et al.* (2002). Single center results of 200 mg/m^2 melphalan (HDM200) and autograft (tx) in 451 myeloma patients: identifying patients with prolonged survival based upon albumin and β$_2$-microglobulin at transplant. *Proceedings of American Society of Clinical Oncology,* **21,** 269a.

Sirohi, B., Powles, R., Singhal, S. *et al.* (2001b). High-dose melphalan and second autografts for myeloma relapsing after one autograft: results equivalent to tandem autotransplantation. *Blood,* **98,** 402a.

Sirohi, B., Powles, R., Treleaven, J. *et al.* (2000a). High-dose melphalan and autotransplantation in myeloma patients with severe renal dysfunction (creatinine clearance ≤20 ml/min/m^2): high incidence of atrial fibrillation and treatment-related mortality. *Blood,* **96,** 1675a.

Sirohi, B., Powles, R., Treleaven, J. *et al.* (2000b). The role of autologous transplantation in patients with multiple myeloma aged 65 years and over. *Bone Marrow Transplantation,* **25,** 533–9.

Stewart, A. K., Vescio, R., Schiller, G. *et al.* (2001). Purging of autologous peripheral blood stem cells using CD34 selection does not improve overall or progression-free survival after high-dose chemotherapy for multiple myeloma: results of a multicenter randomized controlled trial. *Journal of Clinical Oncology,* **19,** 3771–9.

Szczepek, A. J., Bergsagel, P. L., Axelsson, L. *et al.* (1997). CD34+ cells in the blood of patients with multiple myeloma express CD19 in IgH mRNA and have patient-specific IgH VDJ gene rearrangements. *Blood,* **89,** 1824–33.

Tauro, S., Clark, F. J., Duncan, N. *et al.* (2002). Recovery of renal function after autologous stem cell transplantation in myeloma patients with end-stage renal failure. *Bone Marrow Transplantation,* **30,** 471–3.

Titzer, S., Christensen, O., Manske, O. *et al.* (2000). Vaccination of multiple myeloma patients with idiotype-pulsed dendritic cells: immunological and clinical aspects. *British Journal of Haematology,* **108,** 805–16.

Tricot, G., Alberts, D. S., Johnson, C. H. *et al.* (1996a). Safety of autotransplants with high-dose melphalan in renal failure: a pharmacokinetic and toxicity study. *Clinical Cancer Research,* **1,** 947.

Tricot, G., Barlogie, B., Jagannath, S. *et al.* (1995a). Poor prognosis in multiple myeloma is associated only with partial or complete deletions of chromosome 13 or abnormalities involving 11q and not with other karyotype abnormalities. *Blood,* **86,** 4250–6.

Tricot, G., Gazitt, Y., Leemhuis, T. *et al.* (1998). Collection, tumor contamination, and engraftment kinetics of highly purified hematopoietic progenitor cells to support high dose therapy in multiple myeloma. *Blood,* **91,** 4489–95.

Tricot, G., Jagannath, S., Vesole, D. *et al.* (1995b). Peripheral blood stem cell transplantation for multiple myeloma: identification of favorable variables for rapid engraftment in 225 patients. *Blood,* **85,** 588–96.

Tricot, G., Jagannath, S., Vesole, D. H. *et al.* (1995c). Relapse of multiple myeloma after autologous transplantation: survival after salvage therapy. *Bone Marrow Transplantation,* **16,** 7–11.

Tricot, G., Spencer, T., Sawyer, J. *et al.* (2002). Predicting long-term (≥ 5 years) event-free survival in multiple myeloma patients following planned tandem autotransplants. *British Journal of Haematology,* **116,** 211–17.

Tricot, G., Vesole, D. H., Jagannath, S. *et al.* (1996b). Graft-versus-myeloma effect: proof of principle. *Blood,* **87,** 1196–8.

Urbano-Ispizua, A., Schmitz, N., de Witte, T. *et al.* (2002). Allogeneic and autologous transplantation for haematological diseases, solid tumors and immune disorders: definition and current practice in Europe. *Bone Marrow Transplantation,* **29,** 639–46.

van Buren, M., Hene, R. J., Verdonck, L. F. *et al.* (1995). Clinical remission after syngeneic bone marrow transplantation in a patient with AL amyloidosis. *Annals of Internal Medicine,* **122,** 508–10.

Vescio, R. A., Hong, C. H., Cao, J. *et al.* (1994). The hematopoietic stem cell antigen, CD34, is not expressed on the malignant cells in multiple myeloma. *Blood,* **84,** 3283–90.

Vescio, R. A., Schiller, G., Stewart, A. K. *et al.* (1999). Multicenter phase III trial to evaluate CD34+ selected versus unselected autologous peripheral blood progenitor cell transplantation in mutiple myeloma. *Blood,* **93,** 1858–68.

Vesole, D. H., Crowley, J. J., Catchatourian, R. *et al.* (1999). High-dose melphalan with autotransplantation for refractory multiple myeloma: results of a Southwest Oncology Group phase II trial. *Journal of Clinical Oncology,* **17,** 2173–9.

Vesole, D. H., Simic, A., Lazarus, H. M. (2001). Controversy in multiple myeloma transplants: tandem autotransplants and mini-allografts. *Bone Marrow Transplantation,* **28,** 725–35.

Vesole, D. H., Tricot, G., Jagannath, S. *et al.* (1996). Autotransplants in multiple myeloma: what have we learned? *Blood,* **88,** 838–47.

Westin, J., Cortelezzi, A., Hjorth, M. *et al.* (1991). Interferon therapy during the plateau phase of multiple myeloma: an update of the Swedish study. *European Journal of Cancer,* **27,** 45–8.

41 Autologous hematopoietic stem cell transplantation for chronic lymphatic leukemia and prolymphocytic leukemia

JOHN G. GRIBBEN

Dana-Farber Cancer Institute, Harvard University, Boston, USA

Introduction

CLL: incidence, immune phenotype, cytogenetic abnormalities, outcome with conventional therapy

Chronic lymphatic leukemia (CLL) is the most common leukemia in the Western world and the incidence of this disease is increasing yearly. In 1998 almost 10,000 new cases were expected to be diagnosed in North America alone. The disease is generally considered to be a disease of the elderly, with a median age at presentation of greater than 65 years. However, 40% of patients with CLL are under age 60 and 12% are under age 50 and these patients almost invariably die of their disease or its complications. The immune phenotype of both CLL and prolymphocytic leukemia (PLL) is shown in Chapter 34. Most cases are of B-cell origin and T-cell CLL/PLL represents less than 5% of cases. Disease staging and prognostic factors are described below. Among the most important advances has been the identification of the importance of immunoglobulin gene rearrangement status and specific cytogenetic abnormalities as prognostic factors (Damle *et al.*, 1999; Hamblin *et al.*, 1999;

Dohner *et al.*, 2000). The cytogenetic abnormalities associated with each disease are shown in Chapter 34. Fludarabine has emerged as the treatment of choice in this disease (Keating *et al.*, 1993; O'Brien *et al.*, 1993; Rai *et al.*, 2000). Other chemotherapeutic agents are available (Table 41.1), and, like fludarabine, can induce complete and partial remissions in subsets of patients (Table 41.2) (Leporrier *et al.*, 2001). Additionally, the role of monoclonal antibodies directed at antigens present on the surface of B cells, such as CD20 and CD52, is being explored. Despite the high initial response rates (Osterborg *et al.*, 1997; Byrd *et al.*, 2001; O'Brien *et al.*, 2001), a number of ongoing clinical trials are assessing the addition of monoclonal antibody therapy to purine analogues, suggesting synergy of these agents when used in combination. Despite the high initial response rates reported with conventional chemotherapy, there are no data to date to suggest that these therapies are curative and patients invariably relapse and subsequently develop resistance to chemotherapy (Figs. 41.1 and 41.2). The definition of complete and partial remissions is shown in Table 41.3. At present the only potentially curative

Table 41.1 *Conventional dose chemotherapy used for chronic lymphatic leukemia*

Chlorambucil and prednisone
    Chlorambucil 0.1–0.4 mg/kg po day 1
    Prednisone 100 mg/d po for 2 days
    Repeat cycle every other week, increase chlorambucil by
        0.1 mg/kg increments every 2 weeks until control of disease
        or toxicity
Fludarabine
    Fludarabine 25–30 mg/m^2/d i.v. for 5 consecutive days
    Repeat cycle every 4 weeks × 4–6
2-CDA (2-chlorodeoxyadenosine)
    2-chlorodeoxyadenosine 0.09 mg/kg/day i.v. continuous
        infusion over 24 hours for 5–7 consecutive days
    Repeat every 4 weeks for 4–6 cycles
2-deoxycoformycin (pentostatin)
    Pentostatin 4 mg/m^2 i.v.
    Repeat weekly or every other week for 4–6 cycles

Table 41.2 *Response of chronic lymphatic leukemia to the purine analogues fludarabine and 2-chlorodeoxyadenosine (2-CDA)*

Agent	*n*	CR (%)	PR (%)	Reference
Previously untreated patients				
Fludarabine	36	36	8	Keating *et al.* (1993)
	95	30	19	O'Brien *et al.* (1993)
2-CDA	20	25	60	Saven *et al.* (1991)
Previously treated patients				
Fludarabine	169	12	14	O'Brien *et al.* (1993)
	637	4	27	Sorensen *et al.* (1997)
	20	20	35	Hiddemann *et al.* (1991)
2-CDA	90	4	40	Saven *et al.* (1993)
	18	39	28	Juliusson & Liliemark (1993)

Abbreviations: CR, complete remission; PR, partial remission.

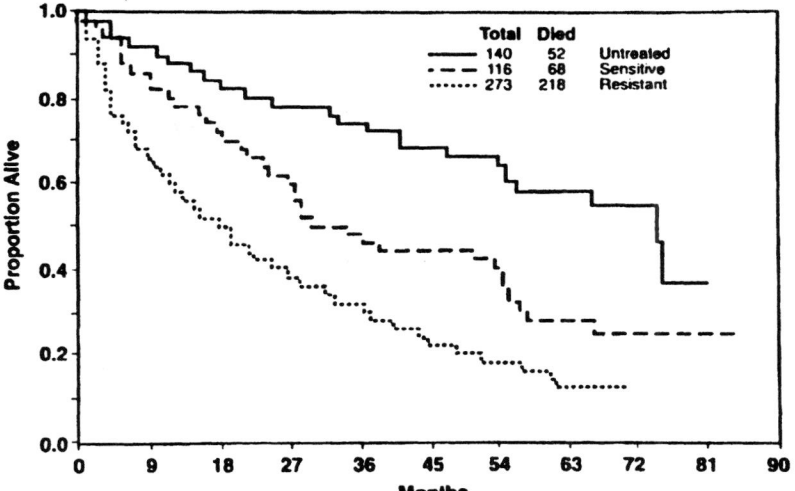

Fig. 41.1. Survival after fludarabine therapy according to pretreatment status. Reproduced, with permission, from Wright *et al.* (1994).

treatment for CLL is high-dose myeloablative hematopoietic stem cell (HSC) transplantation, although it remains to be concluded what the role of this treatment modality is in the management of this disease.

Prolymphocytic leukemia

PLL is a rare, aggressive lymphoid malignancy with distinct clinical, morphologic, and cytogenetic features. It is often resistant to conventional chemotherapy. As with CLL, the anti-CD52 monoclonal antibody CAMPATH-1H has shown significant, but temporary, therapeutic activity (Pawson *et al.*, 1997; Dearden *et al.*, 2001). Both autologous and allogeneic HSC transplantation have been reported for this disease (Collins *et al.*, 1998; Dearden *et al.*, 2001). In Dearden's study, 3 of 7 patients were alive in complete remission after

autologous transplantation at more than 5, 7, and 15 months posttransplant, respectively. The allograft outcomes are detailed below.

Problems with autologous HSC transplantation for CLL

HSC transplantation has become the treatment of choice for an increasing number of selected patients with hematologic and solid tumors. Despite the great increase in the use of HSC transplantation in the treatment of hematologic malignancies, historically few patients with CLL have been treated with this approach (Rozman & Montserrat, 1995) The reasons for this are shown in Table 41.4.

CLL is largely a disease of the elderly, with a median age at diagnosis of greater than 65 years. The majority of these

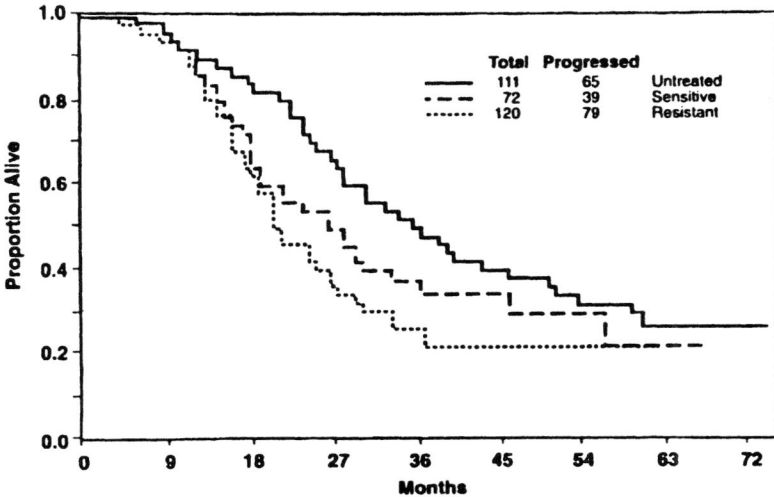

Fig. 41.2. Time to progression after fludarabine according to pretreatment status. Reproduced, with permission, from Wright *et al.* (1994).

Table 41.3 *Definition of complete and partial remission for chronic lymphatic leukemia*

Criteria	International Workshop[a] CR	NCI[b] CR	International Workshop PR	NCI PR
Lymphadenopathy/ organomegaly	None	None	Decrease in Binet stage	>50% decrease
Neutrophils	>1.5 × 10⁹/l	>1.5 × 10⁹/l		>1.5 × 10⁹/l or 50% increase
Platelets	>100 × 10⁹/l	>100 × 10⁹/l		>100 × 10⁹/l or >50% increase
Hemoglobin		>11 g/dl		>11 g/dl or >50% increase
Lymphocytes	<40 × 10⁹/l	<40 × 10⁹/l		>50% decrease
Bone marrow	Normal or local lymphoid infiltrate	<30% lymphocytes		

[a] International Workshop on CLL.
[b] National Cancer Institute Sponsored Working Group for CLL.

more elderly patients are not able to tolerate the toxicity associated with high-dose myeloablative treatment approaches. The disease has a very long natural history (Fig. 41.3) and under these circumstances there has been a hesitancy in subjecting patients to a treatment approach with a significant morbidity and potential mortality. The majority of patients do not have a suitable allogeneic donor and the use of autologous bone marrow (BM) or peripheral blood stem cells (PBSC) has been hampered by the extensive leukemic infiltration of the bone marrow, and peripheral blood involvement, that is invariable in this disease. Lastly, many of these patients have been very heavily pretreated, so that by the time of referral for HSC transplantation they have developed chemoresistant disease and have decreased stem cell reserve. There are, nonetheless, reasons why investigators have examined the role of myeloablative treatment regimens in the management of CLL, as shown in Table 41.5. There is, to date, no evidence that conventional therapy is curative in this disease. Although many patients are clearly not suitable (Catovsky & Murphy, 1995; Rozman & Montserrat, 1995; Rai *et al.*, 2000). However, the disease is characterized by chemosensitivity, at least in the earlier stages of the disease. This provides a rationale for attempting to overcome resistance to potentially curative therapy by the use of chemotherapy dose escalation. Although many patients are clearly not suitable candidates for such an approach, it is possible to identify patients with CLL who have a sufficiently poor prognosis to merit more experimental treatment approaches with curative intent. In addition, the use of purging techniques allows procurement of sources of autologous stem cells that are relatively free of tumor contamination.

Table 41.4 *Reasons why CLL is not suitable for autologous stem cell transplantation*

Majority of patients are elderly
Long natural history of disease
Bone marrow infiltration with leukemia
Patients often heavily pretreated

Identification of patients at high risk

Disease staging

The clinical course of CLL shows marked heterogeneity, with a median survival ranging from 2 to 20 years, depending on the stage at presentation. This range in clinical course has led clinicians to examine the clinical and biological factors that predict overall survival and disease progression. The most important factor determining prognosis is the stage of the disease at diagnosis (Fig. 41.4). Several staging systems have been proposed, two of which, the Rai and Binet staging systems (Rai *et al.*, 1975; Binet *et al.*, 1981) have become the most popular

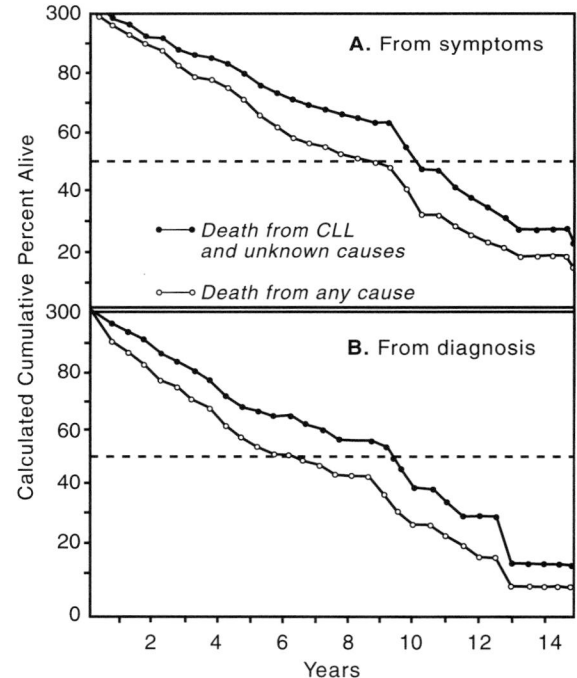

Fig. 41.3. Survival of 130 patients with chronic lymphocytic leukemia from onset of symptoms (**A**) or from time of diagnosis (**B**), based on deaths from all causes and deaths related to the leukemia. Reproduced, with permission, from Boggs (1966).

Table 41.5 *Reasons to use high-dose therapy in CLL*

Disease is incurable using standard therapy
Disease is chemoresponsive
Prognostic factors identify patients at high risk
Purging of leukemia cells is possible

because of their simplicity (Table 41.6). The Rai system describes five stages from stage 0 to stage IV. The Binet system uses three stages A, B, and C. The International Workshop on CLL recommended an integrated system incorporating the Binet criteria with the Rai criteria, defining three prognostic categories (Table 41.6): "low risk" with a median survival of greater than 100 months, "medium risk" with a median survival of 60 to 70 months, and "high risk" with a median survival of less than 36 months.

Prognostic factors

The staging systems do not provide sufficient information to determine the likelihood of disease progression in an individual patient. For this, other prognostic factors have to be examined and a number of additional prognostic factors, in addition to

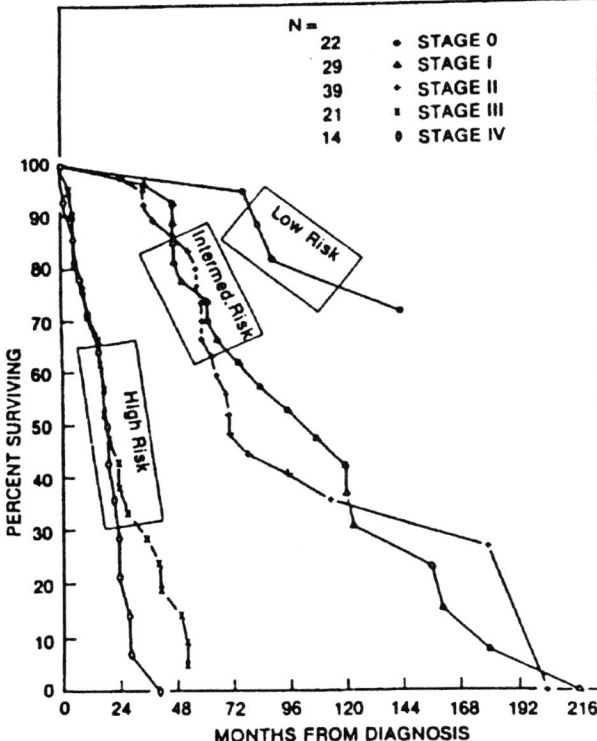

Fig. 41.4. Survival of patients with chronic lymphocytic leukemia staged according to the Rai system. Stages I and II are indistinguishable and are combined in the intermediate-risk group. Similarly, stages III and IV are combined in the high-risk group. Reproduced, with permission, from Rai and Han (1990).

Table 41.6 *Stage and prognosis in CLL*

a) International Workshop integrated system

Stage	Description	Median survival (years)
A	Lymphocytosis with clinical involvement of fewer than 3 lymph node groups; no anemia or thrombocytopenia	8–12+
	A (0) no enlarged node	
	A (I) nodes enlarged	
	A (II) hepatomegaly or splenomegaly	
B	More than three lymph node groups involved, no anemia or thrombocytopenia	5+
	B enlarged nodes	
	B (II) hepatomegaly or splenomegaly	
C	Anemia or thrombocytopenia regardless of number of lymph node groups involved	2.5
	C (III) anemia	
	C (IV) thrombocytopenia	

b) Rai classification (Rai *et al.*, 1975)

Stage	Survival (months)
Stage 0: Bone marrow (40%) and blood lymphocytosis (4×10^9/l); no enlarged nodes	>120
Stage I: Lymphocytosis with enlarged nodes	95
Stage II: Lymphocytosis with enlarged spleen or liver or both	72
Stage III: Lymphocytosis with anemia	30
Stage IV: Lymphocytosis with thrombocytopenia	30

c) Binet classification (Binet *et al.*, 1981)

Stage	Survival (months)
Stage A: Hb > 10 g/dl and platelets $\geq 100 \times 10^9$/l; fewer than 3 enlarged areas[a]	>120
Stage B: Hb > 10 g/dl and platelets >100 $\times 10^9$/l; 3 or more enlarged areas	61
Stage C: Hb <10 g/dl and/or platelets <100 $\times 10^9$/l; any number of enlarged areas	32

[a] The cervical, axillary, and inguinal areas (whether unilateral or bilateral) and the spleen and liver each count as one area; therefore the number of enlarged areas can take any value between 0 and 5.

clinical stage, have been shown to have an impact on survival (Table 41.7). Many factors have been examined including lymphocyte doubling time, pattern of bone marrow infiltration, lymphocyte and prolymphocyte count, surrogate markers in serum, immunoglobulin gene rearrangement status, and cytogenetic abnormalities. Patients with a lymphocyte doubling time of less than 12 months have a poor survival. Similarly, the pattern of bone marrow infiltration has been shown to have prognostic significance (Lipshutz *et al.*, 1980; Rozman *et al.*, 1984; Geisler *et al.*, 1986). Patients with a diffuse pattern of

Table 41.7. *Prognostic factors for outcome with conventional therapy for CLL*

Better outcome	Intermediate outcome	Worse outcome
Rai stage 0	Rai stage I–II	Rai stage III–IV
Binet stage A	Binet stage B	Binet stage C
(mean survival >10 yr)	(median survival 5–7 yr)	(median survival 1–2 yr)
Nondiffuse marrow involvement		Diffuse marrow involvement
Normal β₂-micro-globulin		Elevated β₂-micro-globulin
Absence of trisomy 12		Presence of trisomy 12 (30%)
Absence of p53 gene mutation		Presence of p53 gene mutation (15%)
CD11b, CD11c positive		CD11b, CD11a negative
Slower lymphocyte doubling time		Faster lymphocyte doubling time

bone marrow involvement have a worse outcome than patients with a nodular or interstitial pattern. Using these prognostic factors in addition to the absolute lymphocyte and prolympho-cyte count (Vallespi *et al.*, 1991) and cytogenetic abnormality (Juliusson *et al.*, 1990; Oscier, 1994; Dohner *et al.*, 2000), it is possible to identify patients who have a shortened median survival. Additionally, studies have assessed the prognostic significance of other biologic abnormalities. For example, serum beta-2-microglobulin and thymidine kinase values have been identified as independent prognostic parameters of disease (Hallek *et al.*, 1996, 1997). Of these factors, the lymphocyte doubling time, serum beta-2-microglobulin, immunoglobulin gene rearrangement status, and cytogenetic abnormalities may provide the most clinically useful information. It has been demonstrated that those patients with CLL who have unmu-tated immunoglobulin variable region genes have a poor prognosis compared to those whose immunoglobulin genes are mutated (Damle *et al.*, 1999; Hamblin *et al.*, 1999). This led to the suggestion that CLL might represent two different diseases, although this was not supported by gene microarray analysis studies (Klein *et al.*, 2001; Rosenwald *et al.*, 2001). Fluorescence in situ hybridization (FISH) has improved the detection of chromosomal abnormalities in patients with CLL and studies have eloquently assessed their prognostic implica-tions. In 325 patients chromosomal abnormalities were detected in 268 (82%). The most frequent changes were dele-tion in 13q (55%), deletion in 11q (18%), trisomy 12q (16%), and deletion in 17p (7%). The median survival time for patients with 17p deletion was 32 months, 11q deletion 79 months, 12q trisomy 114 months, normal karyotype 111 months, and 13q deletion as the sole abnormality 133 months. Patients in the 17p- and 11q-deletion groups had more advanced disease than those in the other three groups. Patients with 17p deletions had the shortest median treatment-free interval (9 months), and those with 13q deletions had the longest (92 months). Dohner

and his colleagues (2000) convincingly demonstrated that genomic aberrations in CLL are important independent predic-tors of disease progression and survival. These findings have clear implications for the design of risk-adapted treatment strategies. Several investigators have demonstrated clinical util-ity in assessing the lymphocyte doubling time (Montserrat *et al.*, 1986; Molica & Alberti 1987). Lastly, once patients become unresponsive to therapy, they have poor survival. In a study examining the role of fludarabine in patients who were refractory to alkylating agents, the median survival was approximately 1 year (Sorensen *et al.*, 1997).

Not all patients with CLL are elderly. Forty percent of patients with CLL are under age 60 and 12% are under age 50 at the time of initial presentation. Unlike more elderly patients who often die of other causes, these younger patients almost invariably die of their disease or its complications (Montserrat *et al.*, 1991). Since these younger patients are likely to die of their disease, younger patients with aggressive disease are candidates for more experimental treatment approaches, such as HSC transplantation (Rabinowe *et al.*, 1993; Khouri *et al.*, 1994; Khouri & Champlin 1996; Michallet *et al.*, 1996; Pavletic *et al.*, 2000; Doney *et al.*, 2002; Dreger & Montserrat, 2002). A significant concern about the use of high-dose therapy in CLL is the morbidity and mortal-ity associated with this approach. This is especially the case in treating patients who may have a prolonged natural history with-out aggressive treatment. For this reason, only patients deter-mined to have sufficiently adverse prognostic factors to severely limit their life expectancy should currently be eligible. Criteria that could be used for the selection of patients with CLL who are suitable for HSC transplantation are shown in Table 41.8. Since CLL is a disease in which the bone marrow and peripheral blood are infiltrated with tumor cells, even after conventional induction or salvage chemotherapy, patients who do not have an HLA-identical family member donor may be candidates for autolo-gous HSC transplantation if residual leukemic cells can be elimi-nated successfully from the bone marrow or peripheral blood.

Clinical studies of HSC transplantation in CLL

Disease-specific pretransplant work-up

In addition to the factors that determine end-organ function in patients prior to transplantation, the following features may have importance in outcome in patients with CLL and should be evaluated. The stage of disease at diagnosis, the time of

Table 41.8. *Selection of CLL patients suitable for HSC transplantation*

Stage C disease
Stage B disease with adverse prognostic factors
    Rapid doubling time
    Diffuse pattern of bone marrow infiltration
    Adverse cytogenetic abnormalities
    Elevated serum β₂-microglobulin level

commencing most recent therapy, and stage at transplant are all important factors. Response to previous therapy and documentation of best response to such therapy is also important to assess, not only in terms of disease status but also the impact of each therapy on eventual outcome. It is currently not clear whether the immune status of a patient impacts survival or morbidity after a transplant, although patients prone to recurrent infections prior to transplant might be expected to have increased infections in the early posttransplant period. In addition to using the available prognostic factors to assess whether patients should be candidates for transplant, it is important to assess the prognostic significance of these factors on outcome after HSC transplantation. The most important pretransplant work-up for patients with CLL is a risk-adjusted assessment of whether a particular patient has sufficient risk from his or her disease to merit this approach.

Autologous HSC transplantation

For patients with relapsed intermediate grade non-Hodgkin's lymphoma (NHL) autologous HSC transplantation has been offered as the treatment of choice rather than allogeneic HSC transplantation because of the reduced treatment-related mortality of autologous compared to allogeneic HSC transplantation. In this setting, autologous HSC transplantation has been shown to result in improved outcome compared to salvage therapy for patients with chemosensitive disease (Philip et al., 1987). In CLL, several studies for autologous HSC transplantation have been reported to date. In a pilot study from the Dana-Farber Cancer Institute 12 patients underwent autologous HSC transplantation (Rabinowe et al., 1993). These patients had been heavily pretreated and received an intensive conditioning regimen. Eligibility criteria for entry into this study included documented chemosensitivity at the time of HSC transplantation and patients had to achieve protocol-eligible minimal disease status before HSC transplantation. Complete remission after a median follow-up of 12 months was achieved in 6 out of nine patients.

Initial results of autologous HSC transplantation from the MD Anderson Cancer Center were less encouraging (Khouri et al., 1994). These patients were also heavily pretreated and underwent autologous HSC transplantation, not at a time of minimal tumor burden, but after subsequent relapse. Seven patients received stem cells purged by an immunomagnetic method; however, in five cases, residual clonal B cells were detectable. The outcome was poor. Three underwent a Richter's transformation, two died in complete remission and two relapsed. Only 2 achieved a complete remission and one a partial remission.

In a Finnish study, eight heavily pretreated patients received autologous HSC transplantation with partially purged CD34+ PBSC (Itala et al., 1997). Although four patients remained in complete remission, the median follow-up was very short at only 9 months.

In a study by Sutton and colleagues (1998), the outcome after autologous HSC transplantation was evaluated in heavily pretreated patients with advanced CLL. The majority of patients were not eligible for HSC transplantation because of inability to mobilize sufficient CD34+ cells, disease progression, or pretransplant therapy related deaths. Of eight patients, six achieved a complete remission with a median duration of 33 months. A high relapse rate after autologous HSC transplantation in CLL was observed by Pavletic and colleagues (1998). After a median follow-up of 41 months, 8 of 16 patients had relapsed and 6 had died (3 from progressive malignancy). Other groups observed better results. Dreger et al. (1998) investigated 18 patients with CLL including early stage patients. Transplantation was performed in 13 patients. Only 1 patient had relapsed at the time of publication. In this, and the following reports, polymerase chain reaction (PCR) analysis was used to follow MRD status. In a study by Esteve and colleagues (1998), five patients underwent autologous HSC transplantation. Four of these patients achieved a complete molecular remission. The median follow-up in this study was 13 months. In another study 10 patients undergoing autologous HSC transplantation were investigated and with a follow-up of 22 months, 5 patients remained in complete molecular remission (Schey et al., 1999).

Immunologic purging of autologous stem cells

One of the major obstacles to the use of autologous HSC transplantation after high-dose chemotherapy is that contaminating tumor cells will be infused back to the patient and could then contribute to subsequent relapse. To minimize this risk, most centers obtain autologous stem cells either when the patient is in complete remission or when there is no evidence of marrow infiltration by histologic examination. This is rarely possible in those patients with CLL who have a sufficiently poor prognosis to merit HSC transplantation. PBSC may provide a less contaminated source and most investigators now use exclusively PBSC except where patients fail to mobilize sufficient CD34+ stem cells. To enable the use of autologous HSC transplantation in patients with disease infiltrating the marrow or involving the blood, a variety of methods to purge malignant cells can be used. The aim of purging is to eliminate any contaminating malignant cells and leave intact the HSCs that are necessary for engraftment. The development of purging techniques has led to a number of studies of autologous HSC transplantation in patients with B-cell malignancies who had either a previous history of marrow infiltration or even overt marrow infiltration at the time of marrow harvest (Gribben et al., 1991; Gribben & Nadler, 1993; Gribben 1997, 1999). Numerous clinical studies have demonstrated that in vitro purging can deplete malignant cells without significantly impairing hematologic reconstitution in vivo.

The strategies used for immunologic purging of CLL are shown in Figure 41.5. Most studies performed have utilized immunologic maneuvers to remove malignant cells from autologous marrow by a process of negative selection. An alternative and attractive strategy is to select the HSC positively using monoclonal antibodies directed against the CD34 cell surface antigen. These studies have been hampered to date largely by

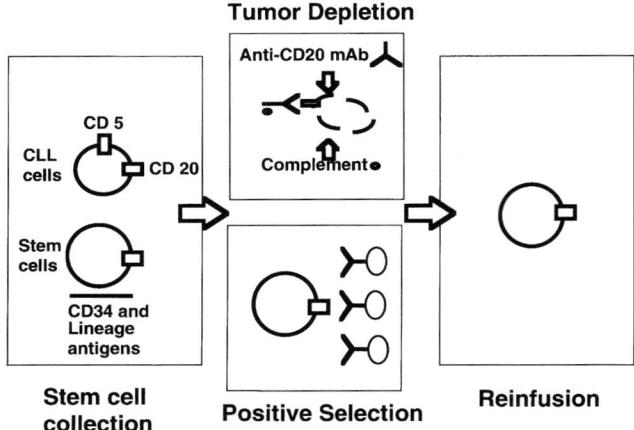

Fig. 41.5. Strategies for immunologic purging. Hematopoietic stem cells can be isolated that are free of leukemia cell contamination using either tumor depletion to eradicate tumor cells, or positive selection to select hematopoietic stem cells.

the relative inefficiency of the CD34 selection systems, several of which are now commercially available for clinical studies. Preclinical studies are now under way in many centers examining the potential role of positive selection of CD34 cells followed by negative depletion steps to remove residual contaminating tumor cells (Dreger *et al.*, 2000).

Although these immunologic purging techniques may be capable of eradicating minimal and overt disease from autologous HSCs, the evidence that such eradication of tumor cells results in improved disease-free or overall survival is circumspect at best. Techniques are also now available to assess whether such purging techniques have successfully eradicated leukemia cells from the autologous HSC using sensitive detection methodology, as described below. It is important to continue to assess whether successful eradication of detectable tumor from the source of autologous HSC results in improved outcome. While the rationale for removing tumor cells from hematopoietic cells might appear compelling, the clinical benefit of purging remains highly controversial. To date there have been no prospective, controlled clinical trials in CLL testing the efficacy of purging by comparison of infusion of purged versus unpurged autologous marrow or blood cells. In addition, the finding that the majority of patients who relapse after autologous transplantation do so at sites of prior disease has led to the widespread view that purging of autologous marrow could contribute little to subsequent outcome. Further studies will be required to determine definitively whether purging has a role to play in the management of patients with CLL.

Allogeneic HSC transplantation (and see Chapter 56)

Allogeneic HSC transplantation is associated with significant morbidity and mortality, both from regimen-related toxicity as well as from graft-versus-host disease (GVHD) and infection. In a report of Registry data, treatment-related mortality following allogeneic BMT was 46% in patients with CLL, the GVHD mortality being 20% (Michallet *et al.*, 1996). In this report, patients with Rai stage 0, I, and II disease were included. Clearly, this level of mortality is worrisome, especially in patients who may have survived for many years without therapy.

In contrast, studies from the M.D. Anderson Cancer Center have suggested that GVHD occurs at a lower frequency than anticipated in patients with CLL previously treated with fludarabine (Khouri *et al.*, 1994). These investigators assessed outcome after allogeneic BMT for patients with CLL that was refractory to, or had relapsed after, chemotherapy with fludarabine. One patient was transplanted from a one HLA-antigen mismatched unrelated donor. Three others received a one or two antigen-mismatched graft and 11 had HLA-identical sibling donors. The patients received cyclosporine or tacrolimus in addition to methotrexate or methylprednisolone for prophylaxis of GVHD. Fourteen patients engrafted; one patient had graft failure, but recovered after therapy with intravenous immunoglobulin. Thirteen (87%) achieved a complete remission posttransplant. At the time of reporting, nine patients (53%) remained alive and in complete remission with a median follow-up of 36 months. These data compared favorably to published reports in patients with other forms of leukemia, as well as with the results in patients with CLL who had received comparable prior therapy but without fludarabine exposure. Their data indicated that allogeneic hematopoietic transplantation can induce durable remission even in patients with CLL refractory to fludarabine. The authors suggested that prior exposure to fludarabine may decrease the incidence of severe acute GVHD, possibly through its immunosuppressive effects (Khouri *et al.*, 1997).

Results on 25 patients with CLL who had undergone allogeneic HSC at the Fred Hutchinson Cancer Center have been reported (Doney *et al.*, 2002). Twenty-one donors were HLA-matched siblings, one was an HLA-DR mismatched sibling, and three were syngeneic. Fourteen patients developed grades II–IV acute GVHD and 10 developed extensive chronic GVHD. Late clearance of CLL cells was associated with the development of chronic GVHD in one patient. Two patients had recurrent CLL. Nonrelapse mortality at day 100 was unacceptably high at 57% for the seven patients conditioned with BU/CY and 17% for the 18 patients conditioned with total body irradiation (TBI)-containing regimens. Actuarial survival at 5 years for the 25 patients was 32%. All patients who received BU/CY died within 3 years of transplant. For the 14 patients transplanted since 1992 and who received TBI, actuarial 5-year survival was 56%, suggesting that long-term disease-free survival might be achieved in this disease.

A small of number of cases of PLL have been treated by allogeneic HSC transplantation (Collins *et al.*, 1998; Dearden *et al.*, 2001). Of the four cases reported in the latter study, three were alive and in complete remission at the time of the report at more than 2, 11, and 24 months posttransplant, respectively. Two received myeloablative conditioning and a sibling transplant, one nonablative conditioning and a sibling transplant, and one nonablative conditioning and an unrelated donor transplant.

A major advantage of the use of allogeneic HSC transplantation is the potential for a graft-versus-leukemia (GVL) effect. This effect can potentially be exploited by infusion of donor lymphocytes following allografting. Evidence for the existence of GVL in CLL is scarce. However, a number of case reports in patients with CLL have suggested that a GVL effect is operative in this malignancy, either following infusion of donor lymphocytes (Rondon *et al.*, 1996), or after cessation of immunosuppressive therapy (deMagalhaes-Silverman *et al.*, 1997). In a patient with persistent lymphocytosis and lymphadenopathy after allogeneic transplantation, infusion of donor lymphocytes on day 87 posttransplant resulted in attainment of complete remission after development of chronic GVHD (Rondon *et al.*, 1996). A number of studies are under way addressing the issue of the number of lymphocytes required and the optimal timing of donor lymphocyte infusions after allogeneic HSC transplantation in this and other hematologic malignancies. In addition, preclinical studies are attempting to develop strategies to exploit maximal GVL without concomitant GVHD.

In studies at the Dana-Farber Cancer Institute, the incidence of severe GVHD is similar in patients with CLL compared to patients with other malignancies undergoing T-cell-depleted allogeneic BMT (see below).

Morbidity and mortality of HSC transplantation in CLL

Graft-versus-host disease

A significant concern in the use of HSC transplantation in CLL is the morbidity and mortality associated with this approach, including GVHD after allogeneic HSC transplantation. This is especially the case in treating patients who may have prolonged natural history without aggressive treatment. For this reason, only patients determined to have sufficiently adverse prognostic factors to severely limit their life expectancy should be eligible for this trial approach.

Infectious complications

The morbidity and mortality of patients undergoing autologous HSCT appears to be considerably lower than that for allogeneic HSCT. However, there does appear to be a higher incidence of opportunistic infections in patients undergoing autologous HSCT for CLL compared to other patient populations. Whether this is due to a greater degree of immune incompetence in patients with CLL, or is secondary to the immune suppressive effects of fludarabine and other therapy remains to be determined (Griffiths *et al.*, 1992; Robertson *et al.*, 1993; Zomas *et al.*, 1994). The use of prophylactic antimicrobial therapy appears to be indicated in CLL patients after HSC transplantation (Mehta *et al.*, 1997).

Comparison of autologous versus allogeneic HSC—studies of HSC transplantation at the Dana-Farber Cancer Institute

At the Dana-Farber Cancer Institute clinical trials assessing the role of HSC transplantation in CLL have been under way since 1989. The results of the pilot study have been published (Rabinowe *et al.*, 1993). Patients were eligible for this approach if they were 65 years of age or less and had poor prognosis disease assessed as stage C(III) or C(IV) disease (high risk), or stage B(II) disease with poor prognostic factors (intermediate risk) comprising a diffuse pattern of bone marrow involvement, a rapid lymphocyte doubling time (less than 1 year), a prolymphocyte count of >60/μl, or a complex karyotype with or without trisomy 12. Patients with stage IV small lymphocytic lymphoma were also eligible if they had anemia, thrombocytopenia, splenomegaly, or bulky adenopathy.

To be protocol-eligible and proceed to transplant, patients had to have chemosensitive disease and achieve a minimal disease state following induction or salvage therapy. In particular, after induction or salvage therapy patients had to achieve leukemic infiltration of 10% or less of the intertrabecular space. (Previously untreated patients most often require two or more regimens to achieve protocol-eligible minimal disease state.) In previously treated patients, only one-third of patients achieved protocol eligibility after a single regimen and up to 50% of such patients no longer had sufficiently chemoresponsive disease to ever achieve the eligibility criteria. Despite this extensive treatment very few patients achieved complete remission immediately prior to transplant. The majority of patients had persistent histologic evidence of marrow infiltration, more than one-third persistent lymphadenopathy, and 25% persistent splenomegaly (greater than 15 cm in craniocaudal diameter) requiring splenectomy before proceeding to BMT, since this was thought likely to contribute to improved outcome (Coad *et al.*, 1993).

The treatment plan is shown in Figure 41.6. Patients with an HLA-compatible sibling donor underwent allografting and those without a donor underwent autografting. The donor mar-

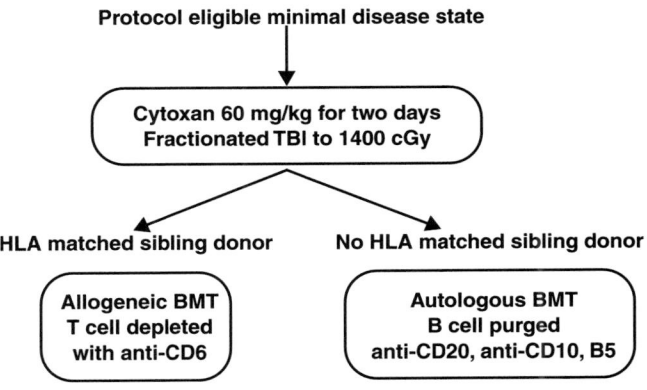

Fig. 41.6. HSC transplantation treatment plan for patients with high-risk CLL at Dana-Farber Cancer Institute.

row for allografting is T-cell depleted in vitro with anti-T12 monoclonal antibody (CD6) and complement (Rabinowe et al., 1993). Patients undergoing allogeneic BMT did not receive immunosuppressive therapy posttransplant unless they developed grade II or greater acute GVHD. Autologous bone marrow was purged using a cocktail of monoclonal antibodies (anti-CD20, anti-CD10, and B5) and complement (Rabinowe et al., 1993). The preparative regimen for both groups consisted of cyclophosphamide 60 mg/kg on each of two successive days (total dose 120 mg/kg) followed by fractionated TBI 200 cGy per fraction delivered over 3.5 days (total dose 1,400 cGy). Patients who did not achieve a protocol-eligible minimal disease state but who had an HLA-matched donor were still eligible for allogeneic HSC transplantation, but these patients were not included in the comparison with patients who had undergone autologous transplantation. Since 2001, allogeneic HSC transplantation has been offered following a reduced intensity conditioning regimen rather than an ablative TBI-containing regimen.

One hundred and eight-five patients attained protocol eligibility and have undergone BMT for CLL in this study. Thirty-four underwent allogeneic and 151 autologous BMT. At the time of transplant, only 2 patients had attained a complete remission while 183 patients still had histologic evidence of bone marrow infiltration.

Despite the heavy pretreatment required for patients to be able to undergo BMT, the median time to neutrophil engraftment (greater than 0.5×10^9/l granulocytes on two successive days) in patients undergoing auto-BMT was 18.5 (range 8–29) days, comparable to that seen in those undergoing allo-BMT, 16 (range 10–28) days. However, there was a delay in platelet engraftment in the patients undergoing auto-BMT; they took a median of 29 (range 16–78) days to reach a platelet count greater than 20×10^9/l compared to those undergoing allo-BMT, who took 20 (range 13–37) days. After auto-BMT six patients remained platelet transfusion-dependent for more than 8 weeks.

The treatment-related mortality in the immediate posttransplant period (less than 100 days) was low with three deaths, one following allo-BMT and two following auto-BMT. Six additional patients died of transplant-related causes more than 100 days after BMT. Four patients died of infectious complications associated with GVHD. One patient developed disseminated mucormycosis and died 8 months after auto-BMT. Five patients who relapsed have died of progressive disease. Projected overall survival (OS) is significantly better following auto-BMT than allo-BMT ($P = .001$). The finding of improved OS and disease-free survival (DFS) after auto-BMT compared to allo-BMT is surprising and appears largely related to mortality associated with GVHD.

Since patients undergoing HSC transplantation are treated with curative intent, stringent criteria must be used to assess response. Criteria for complete remission should include no evidence of disease on computed tomographic (CT) scanning, immunophenotyping of peripheral blood and bone marrow aspirates in addition to standard criteria as outlined by the National Cancer Institutes guidelines (Cheson et al., 1996). Of some concern in staging

these patients is the frequent finding on BM biopsy of nodular aggregates or clusters of lymphocytes comprising less than 5% of the intertrabecular space. The current practice at Dana-Farber Cancer Institute is to classify these patients as nodular complete remission. However, these minimal lymphoid aggregates may not represent disease since none of these patients had an increase in the CD19+/CD5+ or CD20+/CD5+ population on immunophenotyping of BM or blood and, in addition, in a number of cases PCR amplification of the IgH region failed to show evidence of the clonal population associated with the disease. The presence of such nodules in the marrow remains a consistent problem in assessing response on subsequent follow-up in these patients. For analysis of event-free survival (EFS) after BMT, patients in nodular complete remission are classified as remaining in CR until such time as clear evidence of relapse (as defined in the relapse criteria) are met.

Patients who underwent autologous BMT had improved EFS compared to those who underwent allogeneic BMT. The estimated EFS at 5 years after BMT is estimated to be 59% for patients undergoing autologous and 37% for patients undergoing allogeneic BMT. There was no significant difference in the time to relapse in the two patient groups ($P = .27$). The majority of patients who remain disease-free have no evidence of PCR-detectable minimal residual disease (Provan et al., 1996). In contrast, persistence of PCR detectable disease is invariably associated with subsequent relapse.

Minimal residual disease assessment in CLL

There are a number of techniques that can be used to increase the sensitivity of detection of minimal residual disease (MRD) in patients with CLL, including flow cytometric analysis, restriction fragment analysis with Southern blotting, and PCR analysis. The most sensitive of these techniques is PCR analysis, although multiparameter flow cytometric analysis is evolving as an alternative strategy to evaluate MRD in patients with CLL (Rawstron et al., 2001). Human lymphoid malignancies, including CLL, are characterized by proliferation of cells that have undergone transformation with subsequent clonal expansion. The underlying principle for the application of molecular biological techniques to the diagnosis and detection of these cancers is the detection of such clonal proliferation. In B cells, clonal immunoglobulin gene (Ig) diversity is generated by rearrangement of the germline sequences of the Ig heavy chain (IgH) region on chromosome 14. The most hypervariable region of the Ig molecule is the third complementarity-determining region (CDRIII). The CDRIII is generated early in B-cell development by the rearrangement of germline variable (V), diversity (D), and joining (J) region elements. The initial event joins the D segment with the J segment. The resulting D-J segment then joins one V region sequence producing a V-D-J complex. In a mechanism common to Ig and TCR gene assembly, the enzyme terminal deoxynucleotidyl transferase (TdT) inserts random nucleotides at both the V-D and D-J junctions. Further diversity is generated by random excision of nucleotides by exonucleases. Antibody diversity is further increased by subsequent somatic mutation of V, D, J, and N region nucleotides. The final V-N-D-N-J sequence that comprises the CDRIII region is unique to that cell. CLL cells usually rearrange either the Ig heavy chain or light chain genes or both, and their clonal progeny bear the identical antigen receptor rearrangement.

PCR amplification of the CDRIII region is possible due to the presence of highly conserved sequences within the V (Vcon) and J (Jcon) regions. Although the large number of V regions makes the design of single oligonucleotide primer pairs capable of amplifying all Ig rearrangements difficult, a combined approach with Vcon and primers specific to each family of V regions will amplify most rearrangements. The strategy used to PCR-amplify the CDRIII region is shown in Figure 41.7. The amplified rearrangements serve as clonal markers for detection of MRD when they are sequenced. Cloned allele-specific oligonucleotides (ASO) can be constructed and used as oligonucleotide probes for the subsequent detection of MRD or as primers for second round or nested PCR amplification (Jonsson *et al.*, 1990; Billadeau *et al.*, 1991).

At the time of initial presentation, DNA from patients with CLL can be PCR-amplified using consensus variable (VH) and joining (JH) region primers using CDRIII consensus region primers or a panel of V_H family-specific framework region 1 (FR1) primers, employing the strategy shown. The clonal product can then be directly sequenced and patient-specific probes constructed using N region nucleotide sequences. This strategy successfully amplifies and allows sequencing of the CDRIII to design patient ASO probes for the detection of MRD in almost 90% of patients with poor prognosis CLL who are referred for autologous or allogeneic HSC transplantation.

The clinical utility of PCR detection of MRD after HSC transplantation was previously suggested by studies from Dana-Farber Cancer Institute (Provan *et al.*, 1996). The aim of this study was to determine whether high-dose therapy was capable of eradicating PCR-detectable MRD in these patients, and to determine whether detection of MRD might act as a sur-

rogate endpoint for subsequent clinical disease relapse in patients with B-cell CLL undergoing HSC transplantation. PCR amplification was performed on patient samples at the time of, and following, autologous (21 patients) or allogeneic (10 patients) BMT, in whom serial bone marrow samples obtained after BMT were available for analysis. Persistence of MRD after BMT was found to be associated with increased probability of relapse. In all cases that have relapsed to date, the IgH CDRIII region was identical at the time of initial presentation and at relapse, suggesting that clonal evolution of the IgH locus is unusual in this disease. The finding that a significant number of patients remain disease-free and with no evidence of PCR-detectable MRD after BMT suggests that high-dose therapy may contribute to improved outcome in selected patients with CLL. The implication of these studies is that the eradication of detectable disease may lead to improved survival and this should be tested in future studies.

An algorithm for the treatment of patients with CLL

Based on our present understanding of this disease a case can be made for a risk-adjusted strategy in the management of this disease. Patients who present with good prognostic features should not be candidates for HSC transplantation based on their age at presentation but on their risk characteristics. In younger patients with poor-risk disease an attempt should be made to identify potential allogeneic HSC donors, since the lack of any potential allogeneic donor can have major implications for subsequent therapy. In those patients in whom no donor exists, approaches to manage the disease while leaving relatively intact the HSC population would seem indicated, since these are the patients in whom autologous HSC transplantation may have a role to play. Those patents who have an allogeneic donor can more safely receive more aggressive upfront chemotherapy regimens. The optimal timing of HSC transplantation is more difficult to determine and the role of HSC transplantation in first remission remains controversial. For those patients in whom autologous HSC transplantation

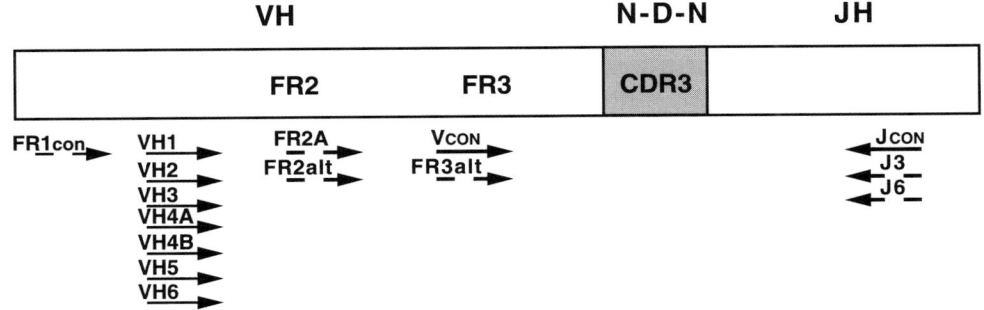

Fig. 41.7. Strategies to PCR amplify the CDRIII region in CLL. PCR can be performed using consensus framework region 1 (FR1 con) or family specific variable region primers (VH1-VH6). Alternatively, a number of FR2 or FR3 primers can be used. The 3′ primers are complementary to the joining (JH) region, which can be either a JH consensus primer (Jcon) or J family specific primers. The sequence of the CDRIII region can then be determined and an allele specific oligonucleotide (ASO) constructed for subsequent detection of minimal residual disease.

offers the most preferable option, the best outcome can be obtained in treating these patients while their disease remains chemosensitive. The more therapy required to achieve response, the more reasonable it is to offer high-dose therapy with autologous HSC transplantation early in the disease course. In those patients for whom an allogeneic donor exists, an allogeneic transplant can be offered in early relapse, since there is the opportunity to exploit a GVL effect in this disease.

The current practice of HSC transplantation for CLL in Europe has been described (Urbano-Ispizua et al., 2002) (and see Chapter 124, Breaking News...).

Conclusions

High-dose therapy and autologous HSC transplantation is feasible in younger patients with poor-risk CLL. Allogeneic HSC transplantation is associated with increased morbidity and mortality and should be restricted to patients with very poor prognosis. High-dose therapy is associated with a very high complete remission rate and results in long-term, event-free survival and eradication of PCR-detectable MRD in a cohort of these patients. Clearly, in terms of assessing the curability of CLL using HSC transplantation, current follow-up of the clinical trials is short. However, the median time to relapse after fludarabine therapy for previously untreated patients with advanced stage CLL patients is reported to be 12 to 26 months and is significantly shorter in previously treated patients (Keating et al., 1993; Gjedde & Hansen 1996; Johnson et al., 1996). It is therefore possible that autologous HSC transplantation will result in significant prolongation of overall and disease-free survival compared to conventional therapy.

Approaches to further improve DFS after HSC transplantation include immunologic approaches to attempt to eradicate MRD. Use of biological response modifiers have generally resulted in no improvement in outcome in CLL, but studies are under way examining the role of monoclonal antibody therapy or infusion of allogeneic donor lymphocytes (Rondon et al., 1996; Dyer et al., 1997; Osterborg et al., 1997). Future approaches to the management of this disease should take into account the balance between the increased morbidity and mortality of high-dose chemotherapy and HSC transplantation with the curative potential that this approach may offer. It seems likely that the use of non-myeloablative conditioning regimens will shortly become the standard method for preparing patients for allogeneic HSC transplantation in this and in other disease settings. This approach is likely to decrease at least the short-term morbidity and mortality associated with allogeneic HSC transplantation, which has been a limiting factor to the application of this modality to patients with CLL.

References

Billadeau, D., Blackstadt, M. et al. (1991). Analysis of B-lymphoid malignancies using allele-specific polymerase chain reaction: a technique for sequential quantitation of residual disease. Blood, 78(11), 3021–9.

Binet, J.L., Auquier, A. et al. (1981). A new prognostic classification of chronic lymphocytic leukemia derived from a multivariate survival analysis. Cancer, 48, 198–206.

Boggs, D.R. (1966). Factors influencing the duration of survival of patients with lymphocytic leukemia. American Journal of Medicine, 40, 243.

Byrd, J.C., Murphy, T. et al. (2001). Rituximab using a thrice weekly dosing schedule in B-cell chronic lymphocytic leukemia and small lymphocytic lymphoma demonstrates clinical activity and acceptable toxicity. Journal of Clinical Oncology, 19(8), 2153–64.

Catovsky, D. & Murphy, R.L. (1995). Key issues in the treatment of chronic lymphocytic leukemia. European Journal of Cancer, 31A, 2146–54.

Cheson, B.D., Bennett, J.M. et al. (1996). National Cancer Institute-sponsored Working Group guidelines for chronic lymphocytic leukemia: revised guidelines for diagnosis and treatment. Blood, 87, 4990–7.

Coad, J.E., Matutes, E. et al. (1993). Splenectomy in lymphoproliferative disorders: a report on 70 cases and review of the literature. Leukemia & Lymphoma, 10(4–5), 245–64.

Collins, R.H., Pineiro, L.A. et al. (1998). Treatment of T prolymphocytic leukemia with allogeneic bone marrow transplantation. Bone Marrow Transplantation, 21(6), 627–8.

Damle, R.N., Wasil, T. et al. (1999). Ig V gene mutation status and CD38 expression as novel prognostic indicators in chronic lymphocytic leukemia. Blood, 94(6), 1840–7.

Dearden, C.E., Matutes, E. et al. (2001). High remission rate in T-cell prolymphocytic leukemia with CAMPATH-1H. Blood, 98(6), 1721–6.

deMagalhaes-Silverman, M., Donnenberg, A. et al. (1997). Induction of graft-versus-leukemia effect in a patient with chronic lymphocytic leukemia. Bone Marrow Transplantation, 20, 175–7.

Dohner, H., Stilgenbauer, S. et al. (2000). Genomic aberrations and survival in chronic lymphocytic leukemia. New England Journal of Medicine, 343(26), 1910–6.

Doney, K.C., Chauncey, T. et al. (2002). Allogeneic related donor hematopoietic stem cell transplantation for treatment of chronic lymphocytic leukemia. Bone Marrow Transplantation, 29, 817–23.

Dreger, P. & Montserrat, E. (2002). Autologous and allogeneic stem cell transplantation for chronic lymphocytic leukemia. Leukemia, 16(6), 985–92.

Dreger, P., Viehmann, K. et al. (2000). A prospective study of positive/negative ex vivo B-cell depletion in patients with chronic lymphocytic leukemia. Experimental Hematology, 28(10), 1187–96.

Dreger, P., von Neuhoff, N. et al. (1998). Early stem cell transplantation for chronic lymphocytic leukaemia: a chance for cure?" British Journal of Cancer, 77(12), 2291–7.

Esteve, J., Villamor, N. et al. (1998). Hematopoietic stem cell transplantation in chronic lymphocytic leukemia: a report of 12 patients from a single institution [see comments]. Annals of Oncology, 19(2), 167–72.

Geisler, C., Ralfkiaer, E. et al. (1986). The bone marrow histological pattern has independent prognostic value in early stage chronic lymphocytic leukaemia. *British Journal of Haematology*, **62**, 47–54.

Gjedde, S.B. & Hansen, M.M. (1996). Salvage therapy with fludarabine in patients with progressive B-chronic lymphocytic leukemia. *Leukemia & Lymphoma*, **21**, 317–20.

Gribben, J.G. (1997). Bone marrow transplantation for low-grade B-cell malignancies. *Current Opinions in Oncology*, **9**(2), 117–21.

Gribben, J.G. (1999). Stem-cell transplantation for indolent lymphoma. *Seminars in Hematology*, **36**(4 Suppl 5), 18–25.

Gribben, J.G., Freedman, A.S. *et al.* (1991). Immunologic purging of marrow assessed by PCR before autologous bone marrow transplantation for B-cell lymphoma. *New England Journal of Medicine*, **325**(22), 1525–33.

Gribben, J.G. & Nadler, L.M. (1993). Purging of autologous bone marrow in the treatment of non-Hodgkin's lymphoma. *Important Advances in Oncology*, 139–56.

Griffiths, H., Lea, J. *et al.* (1992). Predictors of infection in chronic lymphocytic leukaemia. *Clinical and Experimental Immunology*, **89**, 347–7.

Hallek, M., Kuhn-Hallek, I. *et al.* (1997). Prognostic factors in chronic lymphocytic leukemia. *Leukemia*, **11**(2), S4–13.

Hallek, M., Wanders, L. *et al.* (1996). Serum beta(2)-microglobulin and serum thymidine kinase are independent. *Leukemia & Lymphoma*, **22**(5–6), 439–47.

Hamblin, T.J., Davis, Z. *et al.* (1999). Unmutated Ig V(H) genes are associated with a more aggressive form of chronic lymphocytic leukemia. *Blood*, **94**(6), 1848–54.

Hiddemann, W., Rottmann, R., Wormana, B. *et al.* (1991). Treatment of advanced chronic lymphocytic leukemia by fludarabine: results of a clinical phase-II study. *Annals in Hematology*, **63**, 1–4.

Itala, M., Pelliniemi, T.T. *et al.* (1997). Autologous blood cell transplantation in B-CLL: response to chemotherapy prior to mobilization predicts the stem cell yield. *Bone marrow Transplantation*, **19**(7), 647–51.

Johnson, S., Smith, A.G. *et al.* (1996). Multicenter prospective randomized trial of fludarabine versus cyclophosphamide, doxorubicin and prednisone (CAP) for treatment of advanced-stage chronic lymphocytic leukemia. *Lancet*, **347**, 1432–8.

Jonsson, O.G., Kitchens, R.L. *et al.* (1990). Detection of minimal residual disease in acute lymphoblastic leukemia using immunoglobulin hypervariable region specific oligonucleotide probes. *Blood*, **76**, 2072–9.

Juliusson, G. & Liliemark, J. (1993). High complete remission rate from 2-chioro-2'-deoxyadenosine in previously treated patients with B-cell chronic lymphocyte-leukemia: response predicted by rapid decrease of blood lymphocyte count. *Journal of Clinical Oncology*, **11**, 679–89.

Juliusson, G., Oscier, D.G. *et al.* (1990). Prognostic subgroups in B-cell chronic lymphocytic leukemia defined by specific chromosomal abnormalities. *New England Journal of Medicine*, **323**, 720–4.

Keating, M.J., O'Brien, S. *et al.* (1993). Long-term follow-up of patients with chronic lymphocytic leukemia treated with fludarabine as a single agent. *Blood*, **81**, 2878–84.

Khouri, I. & Champlin, R. (1996). Allogenic bone marrow transplantation in chronic lymphocytic leukemia. *Annals of Internal Medicine*, **125**(9), 780–7.

Khouri, I.F., Keating, M.J. *et al.* (1994). Autologous and allogeneic bone marrow transplantation for chronic lymphocytic leukemia: preliminary results. *Journal of Clinical Oncology*, **12**(4), 748–58.

Khouri, I.F., Przepiorka, D. *et al.* (1997). Allogeneic blood or marrow transplantation for chronic lymphocytic leukemia. *British Journal of Haematology*, **97**(2), 466–73.

Klein, U., Tu, Y. *et al.* (2001). Gene expression profiling of B cell chronic lymphocytic leukemia reveals a homogeneous phenotype related to memory B cells. *Journal of Experimental Medicine*, **194**(11), 1625–38.

Leporrier, M., Chevret, S., Cazin, B. *et al.* (2001). Randomized comparison of fludarabine, CAP, and ChOP in 938 previously untreated stage B and C chronic lymphocytic leukemia patients. *Blood*, **98**, 2319–25.

Lipshutz, M.D., Mir, R. *et al.* (1980). Bone marrow biopsy and clinical staging in chronic lymphocytic leukemia. *Cancer*, **46**, 1422–7.

Mehta, J., Powles, R. *et al.* (1997). Antimicrobial prophylaxis to prevent opportunistic infections in patients with chronic lymphocytic leukemia after allogeneic blood or marrow transplantation. *Leukemia & Lymphoma*, **26**, 83–8.

Michallet, M., Archimbaud, E. *et al.* (1996). HLA-identical sibling bone marrow transplantation in younger patients with chronic lymphocytic leukemia. European Group for blood and marrow transplantation and the International bone marrow transplant registry. *Annals of Internal Medicine*, **124**, 311–15.

Molica, S. & Alberti, A. (1987). Prognostic value of the lymphocyte doubling time in chronic lymphocytic leukemia. *Cancer*, **60**, 2712–17.

Montserrat, E., Gomis, F. *et al.* (1991). Presenting features and prognosis of chronic lymphocytic leukemia in younger adults. *Blood*, **78**, 1545–51.

Montserrat, E., Sanchez-Bisono, J. *et al.* (1986). Lymphocyte doubling time in chronic lymphocytic leukaemia: analysis of its prognostic significance. *British Journal of Haematology*, **62**, 567–75.

O'Brien, S., Kantarjian, H. *et al.* (1993). Results of fludarabine and prednisone therapy in 264 patients with chronic lymphocytic leukemia with multivariate analysis-derived prognostic model for response to treatment. *Blood*, **82**(6), 1695–700.

O'Brien, S.M., Kantarjian, H. *et al.* (2001). Rituximab dose-escalation trial in chronic lymphocytic leukemia. *Journal of Clinical Oncology*, **19**(8), 2165–70.

Oscier, D.G. (1994). Cytogenetic and molecular abnormalities in chronic lymphocytic leukemia. *Blood Reviews*, **8**, 88–97.

Osterborg, A., Dyer, M.J. *et al.* (1997). Phase II multicenter study of human CD52 antibody in previously treated. *Journal of Clinical Oncology*, **15**(4), 1567–74.

Pavletic, Z.S., Arrowsmith, E.R. *et al.* (2000). Outcome of allogeneic stem cell transplantation for B cell chronic lymphocytic leukemia. *Bone Marrow Transplantation*, **25**(7), 717–22.

Pavletic, Z.S., Bierman, P.J. *et al.* (1998). High incidence of relapse after autologous stem-cell transplantation for B-cell chronic lymphocytic leukemia or small lymphocytic lymphoma. *Annals of Oncology*, **19**(9), 1023–6.

Pawson, R., Dyer, M.J. *et al.* (1997). Treatment of T-cell prolymphocytic leukemia with human CD52 antibody. *Journal of Clinical Oncology*, **15**(7), 2667–72.

Philip, T., Armitage, J.O. *et al.* (1987). High-dose therapy and autologous bone marrow transplantation after failure of conventional chemotherapy in adults with intermediate-grade or high-grade non-Hodgkin's lymphoma. *New England Journal of Medicine,* **316,** 1493–8.

Provan, D., Bartlettpandite, L. *et al.* (1996). Eradication of polymerase chain reaction-detectable chronic lymphocytic leukemia. *Blood,* **88**(6), 2228–35.

Rabinowe, S.N., Soiffer, R.J. *et al.* (1993). Autologous and allogeneic bone marrow transplantation for poor prognosis patients with B-cell chronic lymphocytic leukemia. *Blood,* **82**(4), 1366–76.

Rai, K.R. & Han, T. (1990). Prognostic factors and clinical staging in chronic lymphocytic leukemia. *Haematology and Oncology Clinics of North America,* **4,** 447.

Rai, K.R., Peterson, B.L. *et al.* (2000). Fludarabine compared with chlorambucil as primary therapy for chronic lymphocytic leukemia. *New England Journal of Medicine,* **343**(24), 1750–7.

Rai, K.R., Sawitsky, A. *et al.* (1975). Clinical staging of chronic lymphocytic leukemia. *Blood,* **46,** 219–34.

Rawstron, A.C., Kennedy, B. *et al.* (2001). Quantitation of minimal disease levels in chronic lymphocytic leukemia using a sensitive flow cytometric assay improves the prediction of outcome and can be used to optimize therapy. *Blood,* **98**(1), 29–35.

Robertson, L.E., Huh, Y.O. *et al.* (1993). Response assessment in chronic lymphocytic leukemia after fludarabine plus prednisone: clinical, pathologic, immunophenotypic, and molecular analysis. *Blood,* **80,** 29–36.

Rondon, G., Giralt, S. *et al.* (1996). Graft-versus-leukemia effect after allogeneic bone marrow transplantation. *Bone Marrow Transplantation,* **18**(3), 669–72.

Rosenwald, A., Alizadeh, A.A. *et al.* (2001). Relation of gene expression phenotype to immunoglobulin mutation genotype in B cell chronic lymphocytic leukemia. *Journal of Experimental Medicine,* **194**(11), 1639–47.

Rozman, C. & Montserrat, E. (1995). Chronic lymphocytic leukemia. *New England Journal of Medicine,* **333,** 1052–7.

Rozman, C., Montserrat, E. *et al.* (1984). Bone marrow histologic pattern—the best single prognostic parameter in chronic lymphocytic leukemia: a multivariate survival analysis of 329 cases. *Blood,* **64,** 642–8.

Saven, A. & Piro, L.D. (1993). 2-Chlorodeoxy adenosine: a new nucleoside agent effective in the treatment of lymphoid malignancies. *Leukemia & Lymphoma,* **10**(Suppl), 43–9.

Schey, S., Ahsan, G. *et al.* (1999). Dose intensification and molecular responses in patients with chronic lymphocytic leukaemia: a phase II single centre study. *Bone Marrow Transplantation,* **24**(9), 989–93.

Sorensen, J.M., Vena, D.A. *et al.* (1997). Treatment of refractory chronic lymphocytic leukemia. *Journal of Clinical Oncology,* **15**(2), 458–65.

Sutton, L., Maloum, K. *et al.* (1998). Autologous hematopoietic stem cell transplantation as salvage treatment for advanced B cell chronic lymphocytic leukemia. *Leukemia,* **12**(11), 1699–707.

Urbano-Ispizua, A., Schmitz, N., de Witte, T. *et al.* (2002). Allogeneic and autologous transplantation for haematological diseases, solid tumors and immune disorders: definition and current practice in Europe. *Bone Marrow Transplantation,* **29,** 639–46.

Vallespi, T., Montserrat, E. *et al.* (1991). Chronic lymphocytic leukaemia: prognostic value of lymphocyte morphological subtypes. A multivariate survival analysis in 146 patients. *British Journal of Haematology,* **77,** 478–85.

Wright, S.J., Robertson, L.E., O'Brien, S. *et al.* (1994). The role of fludarabine in haematological malignancies. *Blood Reviews,* **8,** 125–34.

Zomas, A., Mehta, J. *et al.* (1994). Unusual infections following allogeneic bone marrow transplantation for chronic lymphocytic leukemia. *Bone Marrow Transplantation,* **14,** 799–803.

42 Autologous hematopoietic stem cell transplantation for breast cancer

AMY TIERSTEN AND KAREN ANTMAN

Columbia University College of Physicians and Surgeons, New York, USA

Introduction

United States cancer statistics document a decreasing mortality from breast cancer for the first time in the five decades for which such statistics are available. Nevertheless, breast cancer caused 40,000 deaths in 2002 and remains the major cause of death in 15- to 54-year-old American women (Anonymous, 2000; Jemal *et al.,* 2002).

Risk factors for the development of breast cancer include a positive family history of breast cancer particularly if more than one first-degree relative is affected, early menarche, late first pregnancy, and late menopause. The classification of invasive breast cancer (excluding inflammatory breast cancer) is shown in Table 42.1. Inflammatory breast cancer accounts for 1% to 4% of all breast cancers and is characterized by redness, warmth, and edema of the overlying skin. The underlying tissue is indurated, but a discrete mass is often not palpable. Noninvasive breast cancer (carcinoma in situ) may be ductal or lobular and is confined to the mammary ducts or lobules. The most common site for a primary tumor is in the upper outer quadrant of the breast (48%) and the most common sites of metastatic disease are lymph nodes (72%), lungs (59%), liver (58%), bone (44%), pleura (37%), skin (34%), and adrenal glands (31%).

Prognostic factors for outcome with conventional treatment are shown in Table 42.2. Of these, the most important is the number of axillary lymph nodes involved by tumor. The TNM staging for breast cancer is shown in Table 42.3. The serum concentration of carbohydrate antigen 15.3 (CA 15.3) is elevated in approximately 30% of patients with breast cancer. Its sensitivity is lowest in early disease. Fewer than 2% of healthy individuals have a CA15.3 concentration >30 U/ml. CA15.3 concentrations can also be elevated in cancers of the lung, colorectum, pancreas, ovary, and liver.

The key focus for conventional therapy is to obtain local and regional control of the tumor with surgery with or without radiotherapy and adjuvant cytotoxic chemotherapy. Commonly utilized regimens for such chemotherapy are shown in Table 42.4. Survival with such an approach is shown in Table 42.5.

High-risk primary breast cancer

While early detection has improved the outcome for early stage disease, survival at 10 years remains approximately 15% for those with 10 or more involved lymph nodes or large primary tumors. In addition, 10% of patients initially present with metastatic breast cancer. For those with metastatic disease the goal was, until recently, palliative and the median survival of 2 years had not changed appreciably in the last 50 years (Clark *et al.,* 1987; Mick *et al.,* 1989). Consequently, the development and evaluation of new treatment appropriately focuses not only on patients with metastatic disease, but also on patients who are at a particularly high risk of relapse.

Table 42.1. *Classification of invasive breast cancer (excluding inflammatory breast cancer).*

Type	Frequency	Characteristics	5-year survival
Ductal	78%	Stony hard on palpation: Gritty when cut; metastasizes to bone, lung, liver, & brain	59%
Lobular	9%	Ill-defined thickening on palpation; "Indian file" cells; predilection for metastasizing to meningeal and serosal surfaces	57%
Medullary	4%	Circumscribed; can be large; low-grade infiltrative properties	69%
Colloid or mucinous	3%	Can be bulky	76%
Comedo	5%		84%
Papillary	1%		89%

Table 42.2. *Prognostic factors for outcome with conventional therapy*

Number of axillary lymph nodes involved by tumor at time of initial surgery
Size of primary tumor (>5 cm)
Estrogen receptor status of tumor, progesterone receptor status of tumor
Overexpression of c-erb B-2 (Her-2/neu) oncogene
Grade of differentiation

The rationale for combination chemotherapy regimens for metastatic breast cancer is based on their superiority over single agents in decreasing the emergence of drug-resistant clones in the laboratory (Skipper *et al.*, 1964; Skipper, 1967, 1974a,b, 1983). The clinical objective is to maximize response while minimizing toxicity. Conventional dose chemotherapy regimens vary, with doxorubicin- and taxane-containing regimens producing higher response rates but at some cost of greater toxicity (Hayes & Henderson 1987; Reichman *et al.*, 1993; Gianni *et al.*, 1995; Trudeau *et al.*, 1996). While conventional dose chemotherapy regimens produce complete responses of up to

Table 42.3. *TNM staging system for cancer of the breast*

T	Tumor (indicates size or involvement)
TX	Primary tumor cannot be assessed
T0	No evidence of primary tumor
Tis	Carcinoma in situ; intraductal carcinoma, lobular carcinoma in situ, or Paget's disease of the nipple with no tumor
T1	Tumor <2 cm
T1a	Tumor <0.5 cm
T1b	Tumor <0.5 cm but not >1 cm
T1c	Tumor >1 cm but not >2 cm
T2	Tumor >2 cm but not >5 cm
T3	Tumor >5 cm
T4	Tumor of any size with direct extension to chest wall[a] or skin[b]
T4a	Extension to chest wall
T4b	Edema (including peau d'orange), ulceration of the skin of the breast, or satellite skin nodules confined to the same breast
T4c	Both of T4a and T4b
T4d	Inflammatory carcinoma
N	**Node (indicates regional lymph node involvement)**
NX	Regional lymph nodes cannot be assessed (e.g., previously removed)
N0	No regional lymph node metastases
N1	Metastases to movable ipsilateral axillary nodes
N2	Metastases to ipsilateral axillary nodes fixed to one another or to other structures
N3	Metastases to ipsilateral internal mammary lymph nodes
M	**Metastasis (indicates extent of metastasis)**
MX	Extent of metastasis cannot be determined
M0	No evidence of distant metastasis
M1	Distant metastases (including metastases to ipsilateral supraclavicular lymph nodes)
	Clinical stage
I	T1, N0, M0
IIA	T0, N1, M0
	T1, N1, M0
	T2, N0, M0
	T2, N0, M0
IIB	T2, N1, M0
	T3, N0, M0
IIIA	T0 or T1, N2, M0
	T2, N2, M0
	T3, N1 or N2, M0
IIIB	T4, any N, M0
	Any T, N3, M0
IV	Any T, any N, M1

[a] The chest wall includes the ribs, intercostal muscles, and serratus anterior muscle, but not the pectoral muscle.
[b] Dimpling of the skin, nipple retraction, or any other skin changes except those listed for T4b may occur in T1, T2, or T3 without affecting the classification.

Table 42.4. *Conventional-dose cytotoxic drug regimens commonly used in breast cancer*

Drug	Dose	Dosing schedule
FAC (Swenerton *et al.*, 1979)[a]		
Fluorouracil	500 mg/m^2 IVB	Days 1 and 8
Doxorubicin	50 mg/m^2 IVB	Day 1
Cyclophosphamide	500 mg/m^2 IVB	Day 1
CAF (Smalley *et al.*, 1977)[b]		
Cyclophosphamide	500 mg/m^2 IVB	Day 1
Doxorubicin	50 mg/m^2 IVB	Day 1
Fluorouracil	500 mg/m^2 IVB	Day 1
CMF (Tancini *et al.*, 1983)[c]		
Cyclophosphamide	100 mg/m^2	Days 1–14
Methotrexate	40 mg/ m^2 IVB	Days 1 and 8
Fluorouracil	600 mg/ m^2 IVB	Days 1 and 8

[a] Repeat the cycle every 21–28 days. Monitor WBC count, hematocrit, platelets, creatinine, bilirubin, AST, alkaline phosphatase, and total doxorubicin dose (maximum, 450 mg/m^2). Obtain a baseline cardiac ejection fraction before beginning doxorubicin treatment.
[b] Repeat the cycle every 21 days. The regimen is given for 24–30 weeks (9–10 doses), then discontinued. Monitor WBC count, hematocrit, platelets, creatinine, bilirubin, AST, alkaline phosphatase, and total doxorubicin dose (maximum, 450 mg/m^2). Obtain a baseline cardiac ejection fraction before beginning doxorubicin treatment.
[c] Repeat the cycles every 28 days. Monitor WBC count, hematocrit, platelets, creatinine, AST, and alkaline phosphatase.

40% in metastatic breast cancer (Gianni *et al.*, 1995), the median duration of response remains 6 to 12 months. Typically, successive chemotherapy regimens produce lower objective response rates of shorter duration. Hence, chemotherapy-induced complete remissions that persist beyond 5 years are rare, occurring in about 1.3% of patients in a large series from M.D. Anderson Hospital in Houston (Greenberg *et al.*, 1996).

Rationale for dose-intensive therapy in breast cancer

The initial development of bone marrow transplantation for leukemia (Thomas *et al.*, 1977), and its subsequent modification to support high-dose therapy for other malignancies, began

Table 42.5. *Survival after conventional treatment for breast cancer*

Prognostic factor	Nine-year disease-free survival (%)
Number of axillary nodes involved by tumor at diagnosis	
0	75
1–3	40
4–7	35
8–10	25
>10	22
Size of primary tumor at diagnosis	
<2 cm (T1)	70–80
2–5 cm (T2)	50–65
>5 cm (T3)	40–45

five decades ago. Once the techniques of autologous and allogeneic transplantation were optimized and accepted for leukemias, various groups initiated studies in lymphomas (Appelbaum & Thomas 1983; Armitage *et al.*, 1986). Promising pilot studies were followed by randomized trials in Hodgkin's and non-Hodgkin's disease with significantly improved disease-free survival and the emergence of significant differences in survival in intermediate and, later, low grade lymphomas (Hagenbeek *et al.*, 1991; Linch *et al.*, 1992; Philip *et al.*, 1992; Martelli *et al.*, 1996; Bosly *et al.*, 1997; Schouten *et al.*, 2000; Kluin-Nelemans *et al.*, 2001; Schouten *et al.*, 2002). Certainly the question of extension of the strategy to more common invariably fatal solid tumors such as metastatic breast cancer was a reasonable research question.

Curative therapy appears to be contingent on the delivery of the highest possible doses of chemotherapy in laboratory models of breast cancer (Frei & Canellos, 1980). In these models, cytotoxic chemotherapy dose correlates with cure, while cumulative dose correlates with longer survival for animals who are not cured (Skipper, 1990). An optimal strategy may be high doses of chemotherapy when cure is the objective but many repetitive smaller doses if palliation and longer survival are the goal. A combination of repetitive cycles of high-dose cytotoxic therapy, followed by appropriate hormonal and biologic agents based on the tumor's receptors, might optimally provide both the highest cure rate and the longest survival.

The concept of dose intensity (drug dose administered in mg/m^2 week) was emphasized for the purpose of quantifying dose response effects using breast cancer as a model (Hryniuk & Bush, 1984; Hryniuk & Levine, 1986; Hryniuk, 1987).

Table 42.6. *Randomized adjuvant studies of chemotherapy dose in breast cancer*

Group, reference, number of patients	Drug dose in mg/m^2			Number of cycles	Summation dose intensity (SDI)	Ratio of highest dose density arm compared to lowest	Outcome
	Cyclophosphamide	Doxorubicin	5FU				
CALGB (Wood *et al.*, 1994) 1,572 patients	300 400 600	30 40 60	300 400 600	4 6 4	1.0 2.0 2.0	2-fold increase in each of 3 drugs	Significantly improved DFS & survival for arm 2 & 3 over arm 1
CALGB (Henderson *et al.*, 1998) 3,170 patients	600 600 600	60 75 90	– – –	4 4 4	1.0 1.13 1.25	1.5-fold increase of 1 of 2 drugs	No significant differences
NSABP (Wolmark *et al.*, 1998) B-22: 2,305 patients	600 1,200 1,200	60 60 60	– – –	4 2 4	1.0 1.0 1.5	2-fold increase in 1 of 2 drugs	No significant differences
NSABP (Fisher *et al.*, 1999) B-25: 2,548 patients	1,200 2,400 2,400	60 60 60	– – –	4 2 4	1.0 1.0 1.5	2-fold increase of 1 of 2 drugs	No significant differences

Although the model does not adjust for many potentially relevant factors such as drug activity, synergy, cross-resistance, and pharmacokinetics, the authors conclude that chemotherapy regimens should be designed to maximize the overall dose administered over time (dose intensity).

Randomized studies of dose using conventional dose therapy

The first statistically robust positive study of higher doses of adjuvant chemotherapy was conducted by the CALGB (Table 42.6). Patients with node-positive breast cancer were randomized to one of three doses of CAF (Wood *et al.*, 1994). The high dose arm involved CAF at doses of 600, 60, and 600 mg/m^2 respectively, and the low dose arm 300, 30, and 300 mg/m^2. A 10% difference in the relapse-free curve developed by 2 years and has persisted through 10 years (i.e., an approximately 20% reduction in mortality). This study has been criticized in that the low dose is lower than the current standard dose, and may be below a threshold dose required for effect (i.e., within the "no treatment" range). The dose effect was seen most prominently in the 20% of patients whose tumors overexpressed Her2/neu. For tumors without Her2/neu overexpression, no dose effect was seen (Muss *et al.*, 1994).

However, two studies of cyclophosphamide conducted by the NSABP failed to show a dose effect for a doubling of the cyclophosphamide dose with the doxorubicin dose held constant, a 1.5-fold summation dose escalation (Wolmark *et al.*, 1998; Fisher et al; 1999). Finally, a two-by-two factorial study conducted by the CALGB failed to show a dose effect for a 25% and a 50% increase in doxorubicin dose (at most a 25% summation dose escalation) (Henderson *et al.*, 1998).

Thus for the first positive CALGB study, all three agents were increased twofold. In the second CALGB study, only the doxorubicin was increased 1.5 fold, a difference probably below the level of detection considering the dilutional effects of

the other one or two agents. At best, the dose intensity falls to 1.25 fold increase, an effect that would defy detection in a clinical trial. Because blood levels of most drugs vary about 2–3 fold, no significant differences even in serum levels emerge unless drug dosages are escalated substantially.

Thus while a threshold effect is one reasonable hypothesis, the lack of a significant escalation of the summation dose intensity (as low as 13% in the CALGB study of doxorubicin escalation) is also a reasonable and testable hypothesis.

Dose-intensive therapy with autologous stem cell support

Hematopoietic growth factors (Nemunaitis *et al.*, 1991) and autologous marrow or blood-derived stem cells (Gianni *et al.*, 1989; Siena *et al.*, 1989) limit the duration of the aplasia associated with very high-dose therapy and thus allowed the question of dose to be addressed relatively safely for the first time. The use of hematopoietic stem cells from peripheral blood produces more rapid hematologic recovery after high-dose chemotherapy, resulting in decreased morbidity and mortality.

Initial studies evaluated single agents, then combinations, in women with advanced refractory disease. While responses were observed supporting the importance of dose, responses were generally short and disease-free survival was rare.

Clinical trials of high-dose therapy for breast cancer preceded expeditiously and responsibly in an orderly progression of studies and publications to randomized evaluations. The first phase II studies of combination cytotoxic chemotherapy in untreated or responding patients with metastatic disease were published between 1988 and 1992 (Peters *et al.*, 1988; Williams *et al.*, 1989; Dunphy *et al.*, 1990; Jones *et al.*, 1990). Phase II studies in adjuvant patients appeared in 1993 (Peters *et al.*, 1993). The first randomized studies were published in 1995 and 2000 (Bezwoda *et al.*, 1995; Stadtmauer *et al.*, 2000).

The early emergence of a positive randomized trial in metastatic breast cancer from South Africa significantly hampered accrual onto randomized studies in the United States, where high-dose chemotherapy was also available off study. The use of high-dose chemotherapy on and off study for breast cancer increased rapidly in North America in the 1990s as supportive care technology became more readily available and mortality levels fell from about 22% in 1989 to 5% in 1995 (Antman *et al.*, 1997) and then fell sharply after four abstracts were presented at the May American Society of Clinical Oncology meeting in 1999. Of the four abstracts, three showed no significant advantage for high-dose therapy and the South African adjuvant study that did show significant differences was soon found to be fabricated. Nevertheless, accrual on several had been substantial or complete and after an additional 3 to 5 years additional larger studies have been presented and a few published.

Data from 19 randomized studies have been published, at least in abstract form (Table 42.7). Most investigators, patients, and insurers agree that the two discredited South African trials are uninterpretable at best, and thus they will not be included in this analysis and discussion, leaving 17 randomized studies.

Deaths from toxicity are variable depending on the high-dose regimens used, but are 0 to 2% in the majority of studies, particularly those using second- or third-generation regimens. Half of the studies randomized fewer than 300 patients and could not reliably exclude 15% differences, and thus are underpowered. Nevertheless, many of the studies have found statistically significant differences in time to relapse or disease-free survival. Follow-up in the adjuvant studies is still short—3 to 5 years. Significant differences in survival may or may not eventually emerge. Given the size of the studies, particularly those studies for metastatic disease for which the largest study is only 219 randomized patients, subset analysis is particularly hazardous. No firm conclusions can be drawn at all for patients transplanted in partial or complete response. Thus, the optimal regimen or schedule is unknown and these studies have a variety of different designs, schedules, and regimens.

Half of the studies randomized fewer than 300 patients and could not reliably exclude 15% differences, and thus are underpowered (Table 42.8). Examples of various sample sizes needed to reliably detect differences of a given size with 90% power and a *P* value of .05 are provided. In the setting of metastatic disease with perhaps 20% of patients in follow-up surviving on the standard therapy, the study would have to include almost 400 patients to reliably exclude a 15% difference (line shown in bold).

Autologous stem cell transplantation in patients with metastatic breast cancer

Untreated or responding metastatic breast cancer

Evidence exists both for and against restricting high-dose therapy only to patients who respond to conventional doses of chemotherapy. Presumed advantages include maximal tumor cytoreduction prior to a consolidative high-dose treatment as well as an in vivo assay of tumor sensitivity. If tumor cell contamination of the apheresis product is important, then several cycles of conventionally dosed chemotherapy prior to their collection may provide in vivo purging (Vredenburgh *et al.*, 1995). In contrast, conventional doses of chemotherapy could theoretically induce multidrug or specific resistance, or allow growth of moderately resistant clones. Most patients currently receive conventionally dosed induction therapy for purely practical reasons, such as disease control during evaluation, as well as planning for an available bed and obtaining insurance approval.

Breast cancer responding to standard-dose chemotherapy

Multiple high-dose regimens comprising a varied number and schedule of drugs have been used in patients responding to conventional dose chemotherapy. Autologous Transplant Registry data for North America on 2,134 patients with metastatic breast cancer revealed that 36% received CTCb (cyclophosphamide,

Table 42.7. *Seventeen randomized trials of high-dose therapy in breast cancer published to date*

Study	No. Randomized
Dutch	885
American Intergroup	783
Anglo-Celtic	605
Scandinavian	525
Milan HD sequential	382
French PEGASE 01	314
German Breast Cancer Study Group	302
NCI Canada	219
Philadelphia	184
French PEGASE 3	180
Duke CR crossover	98
Japan COG	97
German	92
Dutch pilot	81
M. D. Anderson Hospital	78
Duke bone mets crossover	69
French PEGASE 4	61

Table 42.8. *Sample sizes required for 90% power to detect various percentage differences (P = .05, two-sided)*

Control	Test	Difference	Total *n*
20	24	4	4,604
20	28	8	1,244
20	30	10	824
20	**35**	**15**	**396**
20	40	20	238
20	50	30	116

thiotepa, carboplatin) as the conditioning regimen (Antman *et al.*, 1997). In more than 42 single institution studies using a single high-dose cycle of therapy, complete response rates ranged from 18% to 72% and 10% to 20% of patients were disease-free at 5 years. Registry data corroborate these observations with an 18% estimated disease-free survival at 3 years (Antman *et al.*, 1997). Thirty-two percent of those in complete remission, 13% of those in partial remission, and 7% of those not responding to pretransplant conventional dose chemotherapy remained disease-free at 3 years.

Prognostic variables

Registry and institutional data have identified prognostic variables after high-dose chemotherapy. Complete response prior to (Antman *et al.*, 1997; Rowlings *et al.*, 1999), or following (Dasgupta *et al.*, 1994), high-dose chemotherapy (whether from previous chemotherapy, radiation, or surgical resection of residual disease) is the strongest predictor of long-term disease-free survival in virtually all studies. In registry data factors associated with significantly ($P < .05$) increased risk of treatment failure were: age greater than 45 years; Karnofsky performance score less than 90%; absence of hormone receptors; prior use of adjuvant chemotherapy; initial disease-free survival interval with adjuvant treatment <18 months; metastases in the liver or central nervous system (compared to soft tissue, bone, or lung); 3 or more sites of metastatic disease; and incomplete response (compared to a complete response) to standard dose chemotherapy. Receiving hormonal therapy post-transplant was associated with a reduced risk of treatment failure in women with hormone receptor positive tumors (Antman *et al.*, 1997; Rowlings *et al.*, 1999).

Multivariate analyses in institutional studies have identified liver metastases, prior adjuvant chemotherapy, a short disease-free interval after adjuvant chemotherapy, and in one series, presence of soft tissue disease as factors that correlate negatively with survival (Dunphy *et al.*, 1994; Doroshow *et al.*, 1995; Ayash *et al.*, 1998). Patients in a University of Colorado study with metastases confined to a single radiotherapy or operative field (stage IV with no evidence of disease) were a particularly favorable prognostic group, with 62% of patients progression-free at a median follow-up of 20 (range 4.6 to 34) months (Bearman *et al.*, 1994). The use of doxorubicin compared to non-doxorubicin containing high-dose chemotherapy regimens improved outcome (Somlo *et al.*, 1995). Her2/neu overexpression is a significant negative predictor of survival (Doroshow *et al.*, 1996; Palangie *et al.*, 1996).

Randomized trials in patients with metastatic breast cancer (Table 42.9)

The largest study published to date is from the National Cancer Institute of Canada (NCIC) (Crump *et al.*, 2001). Patients with no prior chemotherapy for metastatic breast cancer received induction anthracycline or taxane based therapy depending on

their prior adjuvant regimen. Of 386 patients entered, 223 patients responding after 4 cycles were stratified by site of disease, estrogen and progesterone receptor status, and response, and randomized to receive 2 to 4 additional cycles of standard chemotherapy (111 patients) or 1 to 2 cycles followed by high-dose therapy (112 patients) (cyclophosphamide 1.5 g/m^2, mitoxantrone 17.5 mg/m^2, carboplatin 450 mg/m^2 daily × 4). All estrogen receptor positive patients received hormone therapy and radiotherapy for solitary bone or soft tissue sites. The median age was 47. Forty-two percent had visceral disease. Prior to randomization, 12 percent were in complete response, 45% in partial response, and 43% had nonmeasurable disease. Of 112 randomized to high-dose therapy, 23 (21%) never received it. At 19 months median follow-up, no difference in survival was observed. However, disease-free survival (40% vs. 22%) significantly favored high-dose therapy.

In the Philadelphia Intergroup study, responders after 4 to 6 cycles of CAF or CMF chemotherapy were randomized to high-dose CTCb versus conventional dose chemotherapy continued until progression or for up to 24 cycles. This study randomized only 199 patients (36% of the 535 patients entered) (Stadtmauer *et al.*, 2000). An additional 18% of the randomized patients were deemed ineligible or did not receive their assigned treatment, leaving 164 eligible randomized patients who received their assigned treatment. Additional patients assigned to receive conventional dose therapy underwent high-dose therapy after they relapsed. The PR to CR rate of 7% is strikingly low. In an update with a median follow-up of 5.6 years, 27 patients were alive (16 after high-dose therapy, 11 with CMF). Survival at 5 years is 14% for high-dose therapy vs. 13% for CMF. In subset analysis, survival for patients under age 43 favored high-dose therapy; survival for those greater than 42 favored CMF ($P = .02$). Progression-free survival at 5 years is 4% for high-dose chemotherapy (HDC) and 3% for CMF. Subgroup analysis showed a trend towards longer time to tumor progression for hormone receptor positive patients with CMF ($P = .05$). Given the similar survival in the two arms and the less than 1% mortality rate for high-dose chemotherapy, many patients might prefer a short, intense treatment compared to up to 2 years of repetitive cycles of chemotherapy (Stadtmauer *et al.*, 2002).

In the South African trial 90 patients were randomized to two cycles of a high-dose anthracycline-based regimen vs. conventional dose therapy. Complete responders received tamoxifen therapy. Because of the demonstrated unreliability of the adjuvant trial by Bezwoda (Weiss *et al.*, 2000) this study is currently being audited. The complete response rate (4% vs. 51%), overall response rate (53% vs. 95%), disease-free survival (34 weeks vs. 80 weeks), and overall survival (45 weeks vs. 90 weeks) were reported to be superior in the high-dose arm (Bezwoda *et al.*, 1995; Bezwoda, 1998).

In the French PEGASE 3 trial, 308 women with metastatic breast cancer requiring first-line chemotherapy were entered and 180 responding to 4 cycles of 5FU 500 mg/m^2, cyclophosphamide 500 mg/m^2, and epirubicin 100 mg/m^2 were randomized to no additional therapy (91) vs. high-dose thiotepa 800 mg/m² and cyclophosphamide 6,000 mg/m². Of 89 randomized to intensification, 9 were not transplanted. One patient (1%) died of toxicity. Median age was 46 years and median follow-up was 48 months. The 1-year progression rate was 80% for conventional dose chemotherapy vs. 54% for high-dose therapy (P = .0005). The 1-year disease free survival was 19% vs. 46% respectively (P = .0001), also favoring the intensive arm. The 3 year OS was 30% for conventional vs. 38% for high-dose therapy (P = .7) (Biron et al., 2002).

In two Duke studies with a crossover design, 453 women with metastatic breast cancer were treated with conventional-dose AFM (doxorubicin, fluorouracil, and methotrexate). Of 120 women who attained a complete response, 98 were randomized to either immediate high-dose cyclophosphamide, BCNU and cisplatin (CBP) vs. CBP at the time of relapse. Sixty-nine women with only metastases to bone underwent a similar randomization with crossover to high-dose therapy for women randomized to conventional treatment at the time of relapse. Significant differences in disease-free survival favored high-dose therapy in both studies. In the bone metastases study, all patients randomized to conventional therapy relapsed and then underwent high-dose therapy (Madan et al., 2000). Although survival of the immediate bone marrow transplantation (BMT) group in the complete response study was initially reported to be shorter than for the group getting delayed BMT, with further follow-up this difference is no longer significant (Peters et al., 1996; Nieto et al., 2000). The first generation BCNU-based high-dose regimen used in this study resulted in a 9.7% mortality.

A German study randomized 92 women aged less than 60 with no prior treatment for metastatic breast cancer and stratified by menopausal status and hormone receptor status to 6 to 9 courses of doxorubicin 60 mg/m² and paclitaxel 200 mg/m² every 3 weeks (44 patients) or two high-dose cycles with blood stem cell support after cyclophosphamide 4.4 g/m², mitoxantrone 45 mg/m², and etoposide 2.5 g/m² repeated after 6 weeks (48 patients). Filgrastim-mobilized stem cells were collected before and after the first course of HDC. All of the 73% who had estrogen receptor positive tumors received tamoxifen. The median age was 50 years and the median number of metastatic sites was 2. Dominant disease was visceral in 86% and soft tissue in 14%. One treatment-related death (2%) occurred on the high-dose arm. Patients who relapsed after conventional dose therapy were crossed over to high-dose therapy. At a median follow-up of 14 months, the median progression free survival by intent to treat was 14.3 months versus 10.3 months favoring the high-dose therapy (P = .05), and survival was 28 months versus 25 months for high versus conventional dose therapy (P = .39) (Schmid et al., 2002).

In the small French PEGASE 4 trial 61 women with metastatic breast cancer or first relapse responding to 4 to 6 courses of conventional chemotherapy were randomized to high-dose mitoxantrone, cyclophosphamide, and melphalan versus continued conventional chemotherapy (Lotz et al., 1999). The populations were well balanced for prognostic factors except for pulmonary disease (15/32 in the intensive group vs. 4/29 in the standard group) and CNS metastasis (2 vs. none). Median event-free survivals were 20 versus 35.3 months in the standard and intensive groups (P = .05). The progression rates were 79% versus 51% at 3 years and 91% versus 91% at 5 years respectively. The median overall survivals were 20 and 43 months, with an overall survival rate of 18% versus 30% at 5 years (P = .12).

Summary of randomized metastatic trials: None of these available metastatic studies (Table 42.9) randomized more than 300 patients. The Canadian study, the two French PEGASE studies, and the two Duke crossover studies all have significant differences in disease-free survival. Because of the crossover design of the Duke trials, survival for conventional versus high-dose therapy cannot be compared. Based on the very few patients (approximately 907 excluding the South African study) randomized to date, no firm conclusions can be drawn

Table 42.9. *Nine randomized high-dose metastatic breast cancer studies: The South African metastatic study has been discredited (Weiss et al., 2000). Significant and borderline significant differences are shown in bold.*

	Number randomized	% Toxic deaths, median years			% 3-year EFS			% 3-year S		
		HDC	Control	Follow-up	HDC	Control	P value	HDC	Control	P value
NCI Canada	223	6.2	0	1.6	**40**	**22**	**.01**	60	59	.96
Philadelphia Intergroup	184	1.0	0	5.6	4	3	.31	14	13	.62
French PEGASE 3	180	1.1	0	4.0	**46**	**19**	**.0001**	38	30	.70
Duke CR crossover studies										
Complete responders only[b]	98	NA	NA	6.3	**25**	**10**	**<.01**	33	[a]38	.32
Bone mets only	69	9.7	NA	4.9	**17**	**0**	**<.01**	28	[b]22	NA
German	92	2.1	0	1.2	NA	NA	.05	NA	NA	.12
S. African (discredited)	90									
French PEGASE 4	61	0	0	4.4	**49**	**21**	**.05**	55	28	.12

Abbreviations: EFS, event-free survival; HDC, high-dose chemotherapy; NA, not available; NS, not significant.
[a] Patients who relapsed on the conventional dose arm then received high dose chemotherapy.
[b] Data at 6 years median follow-up.

for patients with metastases. Furthermore, analyses for the even smaller subsets of patients in either partial or complete response prior to transplant would be particularly hazardous.

Autologous stem cell transplantation in patients with stage II, III, or inflammatory breast cancer

Patients with 10 or more involved axillary lymph nodes or inflammatory breast cancer have a dismal prognosis, with less than 20% survival at 10 years despite combined modality conventional therapy, and thus high-dose therapy in high-risk primary disease was also studied. Autologous Blood and Marrow Transplant Registry (ABMTR) data estimated 63% to be without relapse at 3 years posttransplant for stage II and III disease and 42% for inflammatory breast cancer (Antman et al., 1997; Rowlings et al., 1999). Such Phase II data from ABMTR database and single institutions must be cautiously interpreted as patients for transplant are carefully selected and evaluated for metastases, resulting in stage migration.

Data from the ABMTR confirm that at least 1,240 patients with stage III or inflammatory breast cancer have been treated with at least 10 high-dose regimens. Patients with inflammatory breast cancer did significantly worse than their counterparts with high-risk stage II or stage III breast cancer (P < .0001) (Antman et al., 1997; Rowlings et al., 1999); however, there was no significant difference in disease-free survival or overall survival between stage II or III (noninflammatory) breast cancer. Results from individual centers for inflammatory breast cancer (Ayash et al., 1998; Cagnoni et al., 1998; Viens et al., 1998) have also been reported.

Randomized trials in high-risk stage II and III primary breast cancer (Table 42.10)

The Dutch Insurance Industry–funded trial with 885 randomized patients included most women eligible at the 10 participating centers (Rodenhuis et al., 2000). Patients received four cycles of 5-fluorouracil, epirubicin, cyclophosphamide (FEC) and then were randomized either to cyclophosphamide, thiotepa, carboplatin (CTCb), or an additional cycle of FEC, followed by surgery, radiation, and tamoxifen for 2 years. The toxic mortality was 1 of 443 patients on standard dose FEC and 4 of 442 on high-dose CTCb. At a median of 3 years follow-up, a trend (P = .057) in disease-free survival has emerged favoring high-dose therapy. In a planned analysis of the first 284 patients with a median follow-up of 6 years, disease-free and overall survival were significantly improved with high-dose CTCb. The Netherlands Cancer Institute phase 2 pilot, which had randomized 81 women with an involved apical axillary lymph node in a feasibility study of the same randomization design, had shown no differences in disease-free and overall survival with a median follow-up of 4 years, but could not exclude differences in survival of less than 30% (Rodenhuis et al., 1998). In fact, their 284-patient study described above had a survival difference of about 10%.

In the CALGB-Intergroup study patients received cyclophosphamide, adriamycin, and 5-fluorouracil (CAF) induction and were then randomized to high versus intermediate dose cyclophosphamide, BCNU, and cisplatin (CBP) (Peters et al., 1999). Although intermediate dose CBP is not a standard regimen, the design is a pure comparison between high and intermediate dose CBP. As in the Duke crossover studies above, this first-generation BCNU-based high-dose regimen resulted in a high (7.4%) mortality, which increased with patient age and varied significantly with the experience of the transplant center. Pulmonary and hepatic toxicity were also common. With a median of 3.6 years of follow-up, significantly fewer relapses have occurred in the high-dose arm although neither progression-free or overall survival were significantly improved. Because the study group was selected to have a tumor mortality of about 80% and survival is currently around 70% in both arms, significant differences may or may not emerge as larger numbers of relapses occur.

The Anglo-Celtic I study randomized 605 women with breast cancer involving 4 or more involved lymph nodes (median 9) following 4 cycles of doxorubicin 75 mg/m^2 to CMF versus a hematopoietic progenitor cell mobilization cycle of cyclophosphamide 4.0 g/m^2 supported by filgrastim, followed by cyclophosphamide 6.0 g/m^2 and thiotepa 800 mg/m^2. Five (1.7%) died of treatment-related toxicity on the high-dose arm. With a median of 4 years of follow-up, event-free survival rates at 5 years for high and conventional dose chemotherapy were 51% and 54%, respectively. Survivals were 63% versus 62% (Crown et al., 2002).

The Scandinavian trial compared conventional dose induction FEC followed either by one high-dose CTCb cycle versus six additional cycles of escalated doses of FEC tailored to individual tolerance (up to 1,800 of cyclophosphamide, 600 of 5-FU, and 120 of epirubicin per cycle). The planned and delivered cumulative doses for tailored therapy exceeded doses in the BMT arm (Bergh et al., 2000). Leukemia or myelodysplasia developed in 9 (3.6%) patients on the tailored dose arm, versus none on the marrow transplant arm. Topoisomerase-associated leukemias can occur early but alkylating agent-associated leukemias develop later than the current median follow-up of 3 years. Thus additional cases are likely. With a follow-up of just under 3 years, breast cancer relapsed in 81 patients on the tailored FEC group versus 113 in the CTCb group (P = .04). Sixty deaths occurred in the tailored FEC group and 82 in the CTCb group (P = .12).

The group in Milan randomized 382 women younger than 60 years with 4 or more positive nodes to 3 courses of epirubicin 120 mg/m^2, followed by 6 courses of CMF versus with high-dose sequential chemotherapy (one course of cyclophosphamide 7 g/m^2, followed by one course of methotrexate 8 g/m^2 with leucovorin rescue, by two courses of epirubicin 120 mg/m^2, and by one course of thiotepa 600 mg/m^2 plus melphalan 160–180 mg/m^2 with stem cell autografting) (Gianni & Bonadonna, 2001). Stratifications included the number of involved nodes (4–9 or >9). Patients received tamoxifen for 5 years regardless of receptor or menopausal status. One high-dose patient (0.5%) died of interstitial pneumonia. At a median follow-up of 52 months in an intent to treat analysis of the patients receiving conventional (197 patients) and high-dose sequential therapy (185 patients), the 5-year progression-free survivals were 62% and 65%, respectively, and overall survivals were 77% and 76%. A trend in favor of high-dose therapy was seen in the 112 patients younger than 36 years, and the 147 patients with 4–9 nodes (HR 0.66 and 0.69, respectively). Many patients are still receiving tamoxifen and thus a follow-up will continue.

The French PEGASE 01 randomized 314 women aged 60 or less with 7 or more positive axillary nodes to 5-FU 500 mg/m^2, epirubicin 100 mg/m^2, cyclophosphamide 500 mg/m^2 (FEC, 155 patients) with or without cyclophosphamide, 60 mg/kg per day for 2 days, mitoxantrone 45 mg/m^2 and melphalan 140 mg/m^2 (CMA, 159 patients) followed by radiation therapy and for patients with estrogen receptor positive diease, tamoxifen for 3 years. The median number of involved axillary nodes was 13. One CMA patient died of sepsis. At 3 years, disease-free survival was 55% versus 71% ($P = .002$) and overall survival was 84% versus 85% ($P = .33$), for conventional therapy versus high-dose treatment, respectively (Roche et al., 2001).

The German Breast Cancer Study Group randomized 307 breast cancer patients with 10 or more involved axillary lymph nodes who had received 4 cycles of EC epirubicin 90 mg/m^2, cyclophosphamide 600 mg/m^2, i.v. every 3 weeks to either high-dose chemotherapy (152 patients) of cyclophosphamide 1,500 mg/m^2, thiotepa 150 mg/m^2, and mitoxantrone 10 mg/m^2 on 4 consecutive days, respectively, with autologous hematopoietic stem cell support versus 3 cycles of a standard-dose CMF (155 patients, cyclophosphamide 500 mg/m^2, methotrexate mg/m^2, and 5-fluorouracil 600 mg/m^2, i.v. on day 1 and 8, respectively, every 4 weeks). Patients with tumors

with hormone receptors received 5 years of tamoxifen. Two patients died of toxicity. With a median follow-up of 3.7 years, event-free survival was 51% versus 41% favoring high-dose therapy ($P = .095$). Survival was 72% versus 67% (Zander et al., 2002).

The South African study was reported to compare conventional CAF versus two cycles of high-dose chemotherapy with no induction conventional dose therapy (Bezwoda 1999). In an independent audit, discrepancies in eligibility criteria and reported data were substantial. Control group patient records were not provided for review. The title of the protocol given to the audit team suggests that the control group was treated not with CAF but rather cyclophosphamide, mitoxantrone, and vincristine. Thus the data are best considered unreliable (Weiss et al., 2000).

The Japan Cooperative Oncology Group randomized 97 women aged 55 or less with 10 or more positive axillary nodes to cyclophosphamide 6 g/m^2 and thiotepa 600 mg/m^2 as consolidation after 6 courses of cyclophosphamide 500 mg/m^2, adriamycin 40 mg/m^2, and fluorouracil 500 mg/m^2 every 3 weeks followed by tamoxifen. The median number of involved axillary nodes was 16 (range 10–49). The standard treatment arm included 48 patients. Of the 49 patients randomized to high-dose therapy, 15 (31%) never actually received it. No treatment-related deaths occurred. After 4 years, an analysis based on intent to treat, relapse-free survival was 48% versus 60% ($P = .42$) and overall survival was 66% versus 67% ($P = .95$), for conventional therapy versus high-dose treatment, respectively (Tokuda et al., 2001).

The M. D. Anderson Cancer Center study randomized 78 patients to eight cycles of FAC with or without two cycles of high-dose cyclophosphamide, etoposide, and cisplatin. Three patients randomized to conventional dose therapy underwent transplant elsewhere; six randomized to transplant did not receive it. With a median 78-month follow-up, no advantage for

Table 42.10. *Ten randomized high-dose breast cancer adjuvant studies: The South African adjuvant study has been discredited (Weiss et al., 2000). Significant and borderline significant differences are shown in bold*

	Number randomized	% Toxic deaths, median years			% 3-year EFS			% 3-year S		
		HDC	Control	Follow-up	HDC	Control	P value	HDC	Control	P value
Dutch Phase 3	885	0.9	0.2	3.5	**72**	**65**	**.057**	NA	NA	.31
First 284 pt subset	284	NA	NA	7.0	77	**62**	**.009**	**89**	**79**	**.039**
CALGB Intergroup	783	7.4	0	3.6	71	64	NS	79	79	.29
Anglo-Celtic	605	1.7	0	4.0	51	54	NS	63	62	NS
Scandinavian	525	0.7	0	2.9	**72**	**63**	**.013**	83	77	.12
Milan HD sequential	382	0.5	0	4.3	65	62	NS	76	77	NS
French PEGASE 01	314	0.6	0	3.0	**71**	**55**	**.002**	85	84	.33
German	302	2.0	0	3.7	51	41	.095	72	67	NS
S. African (discredited)	154									
Japan COG	97	0	0	4.0	60	48	NS	67	66	NS
Dutch randomized Phase 2	81	0	0	4.1	70	65	.97	82	75	.84
M.D. Anderson Hospital	78	2.5	0	6.5	48	62	NS	58	77	NS

Abbreviations: EFS, event-free survival; HDC, high-dose chemotherapy; NA, not available; NS, not significant.

high-dose chemotherapy has emerged, but the study cannot exclude differences of less than 30% (Hortobagyi *et al.*, 2000).

Summary of randomized adjuvant trials: Seven of the 10 studies (Table 42.10) randomized more than 300 patients. The United States CALGB study has a significantly decreased relapse rate but also a substantial treatment-associated mortality. The Anglo-Celtic study shows not differences to date. Disease-free survival favors the higher dose tailored arm of the Scandinavian study, which compares one high-dose cycle versus six intermediate dose cycles.

In all studies except for the Anglo-Celtic and the M.D. Anderson hospital studies, the high-dose arm has a higher disease-free survival than the conventional dose arm. Given that the most optimistic data project about a 2% disease-free survival after the development of metastases (Greenberg *et al.*, 1996), and that the median time from relapse to death is about 2 years, event-free survival provides a preliminary indication of eventual survival data.

Special considerations in high-dose studies to date

Tumor involvement of a stem cell collection

A major issue is potential tumor involvement of a stem cell collection. As many as 40% of patients with metastatic breast cancer, and more than 55% of patients with bone involvement, also have detectable breast cancer in marrow using standard stains (Ingle *et al.*, 1978; Ellis *et al.*, 1989). More sensitive immunocytochemical and molecular techniques also reveal occult tumor in marrow in many otherwise normal appearing specimens (Ross *et al.*, 1993; Fields *et al.*, 1994; Ross *et al.*, 1994). The clinical significance of micrometastatic disease for patients with primary or metastatic breast cancer is unknown, using time to progression or survival as endpoints (Myers *et al.*, 1994; Seong *et al.*, 1994; Shpall *et al.*, 1995; Vredenburgh *et al.*, 1995, 1997).

Tumor cell recruitment and contamination of the blood-derived stem cell collection may occur in patients with clinically involved or apparently normal marrow (Douer *et al.*, 1993; Ross *et al.*, 1993a,b; Brugger *et al.*, 1994). Tumor cells can be detected in stem cell collections from blood significantly less frequently than from marrow; however, tumor cells from either source prove clonogenic in vitro. While gene marking studies have demonstrated relapse due at least in part to contamination of progenitor cell infusions in patients with leukemia or neuroblastoma (Rill *et al.*, 1994), definitive studies in breast cancer are still lacking. Due to uncertainties about the purity of the stem cell product, several institutions are presently studying purging techniques. Methods under investigation include chemotherapy (Passos-Coelho *et al.*, 1994), monoclonal antibody cocktails (Myklebust *et al.*, 1994), an antisense-based approach (Bergan *et al.*, 1996), as well as positive and negative selection methods (Shpall *et al.*, 1995). Insertion of suicide genes (Wu *et al.*, 1997), drug resistance genes, or genes that produce pro-drugs (Garcia-

Sanchez *et al.*, 1997), into the stem cell product are also in the initial testing phase.

Dose-intensive therapy with stem cell support harvested from an identical twin

The Autologous Blood and Marrow Transplant Registry (ABMTR) accrued 14 women at 13 centers with metastatic breast cancer for whom stem cells were collected from a healthy identical twin (Table 42.11). Their median age was 41 years (range 34–50). Tumors from 7 women expressed estrogen receptors. Of these, 3 received hormonal therapy pretransplant. Twelve were premenopausal at diagnosis.

All had received an anthracycline-based regimen; 9 also had received a taxane and 7 radiotherapy. Two women received one chemotherapy regimen pretransplant, 10 had two or three, 2 had four or five. At transplant, 4 women were in complete response, 5 had responded partially, 2 had stable disease, and 2 had progressive disease. One died of toxicity. Three-year survival was 63% and 3-year progression-free survival was 17%. Previous ABMTR reports have shown the 3-year survival and progression-free survival after autotransplants to be 31% and 13%, respectively. Thus progression-free survival for women transplanted with syngeneic grafts is not statistically better than for women receiving autologous grafts, supporting the premise that residual cancer in the patient is the major contributor to relapse (Rizzo *et al.*, 2003).

Autologous HSC transplantation for men with breast cancer

Few data exist for results of high-dose therapy for men with breast cancer, but they appear similar to those reported for women. Of 13 such men treated at 10 centers reported by the Autologous Blood and Marrow Transplant Registry (ABMTR), 6 had stage 2 cancer, four stage 3, and 3 had metastases (McCarthy *et al.*, 1999). All 12 tested tumors were estrogen receptor positive. The median age was 50 years. Of the 10 men receiving adjuvant high-dose therapy, three relapsed 3, 5, and 50 months and died at 16, 19, and 67 months posttransplant. The remaining 7 were disease-free with a median follow-up of 23 months (range 6–50 months). All three men treated for metastatic breast cancer had progressive or recurrent disease at 6, 7, and 16 months posttransplant.

Allogeneic HSC transplantation in breast cancer

The role of allogeneic stem cell transplant requires that immune cells recognize breast cancer HLA-class I bound peptide antigens. The group at Washington University in St. Louis has reported that at least in a mouse model, tumor-reactive, HLA-class I restricted cytotoxic T lymphocytes (CTL) can be produced by stimulating normal peripheral blood lymphocytes (PBL) against an HLA-class I matched breast cancer cell line (Nguyen *et al.*, 1999).

Table 42.11. *Three-year survival and three-year progression-free survival from the Autologous Blood and Marrow Transplant Registry (ABMTR) database*

	Survival	95% CI	Progression-free survival	95% CI
Syngeneic	63%	36–85%	17%	2–41%
Autologous	31%	28–34%	13%	10–16%

Clinical data in humans are limited. A case report by Eibl and colleagues in which the development of circulating minor histocompatibility antigen-specific CTLs recognizing breast carcinoma targets appeared to coincide with the clinical disappearance of liver metastases suggested a graft-versus-tumor effect (Eibl *et al.*, 1996). The group at M.D. Anderson conducted a trial in which 10 "poor-risk" (bone and liver metastases) women underwent HLA-identical sibling allo-peripheral blood stem cell transplants and standard graft-versus-host disease (GVHD) prophylaxis. The morbidity and mortality was greater than what would be expected with a conventional autotransplant with 2 toxic deaths. The response rate was 60% and the remission durations were short (median 238 days). Interestingly, in an attempt to forestall disease progression, 4 patients had their immunosuppression reduced and 1 received a donor lymphocyte infusion. Two patients had regression of liver lesions coincident with exacerbation of GVHD (Ueno *et al.*, 1998).

The group at Hadassah University Hospital, Jerusalem, attempted to produce a graft-versus-tumor effect in six patients with metastatic breast cancer (Or *et al.*, 1998). The patients first underwent high-dose chemotherapy and autologous stem cell transplantation and then as an outpatient received HLA-matched donor peripheral blood lymphocytes treated in vivo with human recombinant interleukin-2. If no GVHD developed, donor PBL were infused, again treated in vitro with rIL-2. Two patients developed grade I–II GVHD, one of whom was in complete response more than 34 months.

Five patients with metastatic breast cancer were treated at M.D. Anderson Hospital in Houston with mini-allogeneic transplantation using a conditioning regimen of fludarabine 30 mg/m^2 i.v. daily from day –6 to –2 and melphalan 70 mg/m^2 i.v. daily from day –3 to –2 and tacrolimus and mini-methotrexate GVHD prophylaxis. Tacrolimus was tapered for disease progression at 100 days after transplant. On day 30, all patients had 100% donor myeloid and lymphoid chimerism. One patient who presented with metastatic disease is in complete response. Three additional patients have had prolonged stable disease (Ueno *et al.*, 2002). In another study, two of 6 patients given a nonmyeloablative conditioning regimen of thiotepa, cyclophosphamide, and fludarabine prior to an HLA-identical sibling PBSC transplant showed a partial response after posttransplant donor lymophocyte infusions with or without interferon-γ (Bregnia *et al.*, 2002).

Graft-versus-tumor strategies are most likely to be effective in the setting of minimum residual disease. The means to better control onset and extent of GVHD would improve this approach.

Quality of life and cost effectiveness

Major advances in supportive care over the past 5 years have substantially reduced the time to engraftment, morbidity, and cost associated with transplant (Winer *et al.*, 1991). The net result is that dose-intense regimens can now be reasonably safely and efficiently tested in breast cancer.

Most patients resume a relatively normal lifestyle within 2 to 4 months after transplant in the absence of progressive disease. Most prospective evaluations correlate improved quality of life (QOL) with disease control (McQuellon *et al.*, 1996). It appears the same QOL issues (job situation, finances, appearance, insurability, intimate relationships) are also present in nontransplant patients (Hillner *et al.*, 1991; Hann *et al.*, 1997). Appropriate intervention strategies to improve QOL can be designed as the data become available.

If the complete remissions prove to be durable (15% disease-free beyond 5 years), the cost per year of life saved was estimated to be quite cost effective at $17,000 as compared to $45,000 per year of life saved for renal dialysis (Hillner *et al.*, 1992). In fact, many centers now administer high-dose chemotherapy in the outpatient setting, which may further contribute to decreased cost. Up to 1.6% patients have developed myelodysplasia and/or acute leukemia after high-dose chemotherapy for breast cancer (Laughlin *et al.*, 1998).

Current practice based on studies to date

Indications and contraindications for autologous transplantation for breast cancer

No audited large randomized trial has to date documented a significant survival advantage for high-dose therapy although a number of studies report significantly longer disease-free survival. Thus high-dose therapy for breast cancer is generally offered only in the context of a prospective clinical study. Eligibility criteria for studies generally include high-risk primary breast cancer or metastatic breast cancer responding to conventional dose therapy. High-dose therapy is generally hazardous for patients with renal or hepatic dysfunctions (which would result in unreliable metabolism or excretion of chemotherapy), or pulmonary or cardiac function inadequate to withstand possible additional drug toxicity. Pregnant or nursing mothers are excluded, as are those with active infections including hepatitis or HIV.

Disease-specific pretransplant work-up

The usual evaluation for high-dose chemotherapy include addressing safety, such as ensuring adequate renal and hepatic function for excretion and metabolism of the chemotherapy agents; HIV, HTLV, and hepatitis status; pulmonary and cardiac function; and head computed tomography (CT) for brain metastases. Many teams also evaluate marrow or peripheral blood involvement by tumor.

Monitoring for residual disease posttransplant

Criteria for relapse of breast cancer after high-dose therapy is that for after standard therapy. To date molecular markers for minimal residual disease remain unreliable. Appropriate follow-up for relapse (as opposed to residual toxicity) remains annual mammography and physician examination.

The future: new strategies in high-dose therapy for breast cancer

Single institution and ABMTR data reproducibly show that a complete response is the single most important prognostic factor associated with prolonged disease-free survival. Strategies used to attempt to increase the percentage of patients who achieve complete remission (CR), in the hope that a higher CR rate will translate into an increased proportion of patients with prolonged disease-free survival, include incorporation of new active drugs and the use of multiple high-dose cycles.

New drugs

Inclusion of newer cytotoxic agents (i.e., taxanes, navelbine) into established high-dose regimens is currently under way. Response rates vary from 17% to 100% with an extremely short follow-up period (Spitzer et al., 1994; Stemmer et al., 1994; Vukelja et al., 1994; Mayordomo et al., 1997; Rahman et al., 1997). Noncytotoxic approaches include the development of anti-angiogenesis agents (O'Reilly et al., 1997), inhibitors of signal transduction (Chou et al., 1997), and matrix metalloproteinases (Brown & Giavazzi, 1995). Newer chemotherapy drugs are being rapidly incorporated into established combination regimens. A tandem transplant regimen piloted by the group at Columbia University includes paclitaxel at doses up to 825 mg/m^2 as the first high-dose cycle in a regimen that builds on the tandem transplant regimen developed in Boston (Ayash et al., 1994, 1996).

Multicycle chemotherapy

Sequences of single-agent and combination chemotherapy regimens are currently under evaluation. An alternative approach to single high-dose regimens is the use of multicycle, escalated dose, but nonablative chemotherapy supported by blood stem cell infusions (Tepler et al., 1993; Basser et al., 1999).

Overall, multicycle chemotherapy produces complete response rates ranging from 0 to 93% depending on the regimen. Because many of the trials include patients with inevaluable bony disease, complete response rates are conservative and the best endpoints are freedom from progression and survival.

In the two randomized trials to date, the Scandinavian study suggested that six high-dose cycles may lead to significantly improved disease-free survival with a trend in survival (Bergh et al., 2000). However in an Italian study, sequential high-dose single agent and combinations did not lead to a benefit over conventional dose therapy (Gianni et al., 2001).

Immunologic strategies

Patients in complete response after high-dose therapy, but nevertheless at high risk of relapse (minimal residual disease) might benefit from various immunologic strategies (e.g., vaccines or induction of an autologous graft-versus-tumor effect). Patients with acute and chronic myeloid leukemia who develop even mild GVHD after allogeneic marrow transplantation have a reduced relapse rate (Wieden et al., 1979). Vaccines directed against a variety of epitopes (Gilewski et al., 1997), or growth factor receptors (Baselga & Mendelsohn, 1994), have been used.

Gene therapy

The human multidrug resistance (MDR) gene can be transduced into human marrow progenitor cells and these cells subsequently exhibit preferential resistance to paclitaxel chemotherapy (Ward et al., 1994). Thus, chemotherapy-resistant marrow populations could be selected. Preliminary results of Phase I trials in advanced cancers demonstrate that the MDR gene can be safely and efficiently transduced into stem cells and expression maintained for at least 4 months (Hesdorffer et al., 1998). Additional applications for gene therapy include the transduction of suicide genes into neoplastic cells (Talmadge et al., 1997).

Monoclonal antibodies after high-dose chemotherapy

Growth factors and their receptors play a regulatory role in cell proliferation and have been implicated in oncogenesis (Fan et al., 1993). In preclinical studies, Her-2/neu antibodies are capable of inhibiting tumor growth and greatly enhancing the effects of doxorubicin, paclitaxel, and cisplatin chemotherapy (Baselga et al., 1993, 1994). Future studies may include a combination of monoclonal antibodies and chemotherapy in the setting of minimal residual disease.

Summary

Of the 19 randomized studies reported to date, only 7 randomized more than 300 patients. Nevertheless, many studies document significant advantages in disease-free survival for the high-dose group. Whether an advantage in survival emerges is unknown. Additional follow-up of these randomized trials (see Chapter 124, Breaking News...), and the completion and presentation of the as yet unpublished randomized trials will provide a more reliable database on which to base treatment decisions in breast cancer. Certainly lessons from randomized high-dose trials for lymphoma should caution our early interpretation of the current breast cancer randomized trials. Good risk lymphoma patients and those with resistant disease do not appear to benefit from high-dose chemotherapy. Lymphoma studies required 4 to 7 years of follow-up for differences in survival to emerge; thus, any differences in a more indolent disease such as breast cancer may take longer. In one French lymphoma study conventional dose induction therapy significantly improved disease-free and overall survival. Maintenance therapy obscures differences. We may see these patterns in breast cancer as well.

Since the initial randomized trials were planned, the taxanes have been integrated into conventional dose therapy for metastatic disease and are being evaluated in the adjuvant setting. In the large randomized CALGB Intergroup study, adjuvant paclitaxel provided a 1% to 2% survival benefit that is significant if a Wilcoxon test is used but not a log rank (Henderson *et al.*, 1998). Two other studies show no survival differences thus far. In comparison, the 285 patient Dutch study has about a 15% disease-free survival advantage and a 10% survival advantage, with a cost in terms of mortality of 1%. Thus although the toxicity of high-dose therapy exceeds that of conventional dose paclitaxel, the potential survival difference may also be larger. Based on data showing a correlation of dose with response for taxanes in the laboratory (Hanauske *et al.*, 1992), higher doses of paclitaxel are now under study (Stemmer *et al.*, 1996; Vahdat *et al.*, 1998; Hudis *et al.*, 1999).

Some investigators postulate a threshold dose required for effectiveness, above which survival is not improved. Because blood levels of most drugs vary about 2- to 5-fold, significant differences in serum levels are difficult to detect unless drug dosages are escalated substantially. This observation provides an alternative hypothesis to explain the outcomes of the four available studies of modestly increased chemotherapy doses without stem cell support. In the three studies in which no differences in outcome were detected, the dose escalations were 1.13-fold in the CALGB (Henderson *et al.*, 1998) and to 1.5-fold in the two NSABP studies (Wolmark *et al.*, 1998; Fisher *et al.*, 1999), probably below the level of detection. In the positive CALGB study, the dose escalation was fully twofold. (Wood *et al.*, 1994). A 10% difference in the relapse-free survival developed by 2 years, which persisted through 10 years. The dose effect was most significant in the 20% of patients whose tumors overexpressed Her2/neu, suggesting that important therapeutic differences might be missed if biological subsets are ignored (Muss *et al.*, 1994). Although a threshold effect is one reasonable hypothesis to explain these data, the lack of a significant escalation in the summation dose intensity (as low as 13% in the CALGB doxorubicin escalation study) is also a reasonable and testable hypothesis.

Some have criticized the further development of high-dose therapies based on a higher priority for molecular targeted therapy. Although we all enthusiastically envision more effective, specific molecularly targeted treatments for breast cancer, few currently exist. First-generation monoclonal antibodies such as Herceptin are effective for a relatively small subset of breast cancer patients, and even for these women are not likely to be curative as single agents. Once more effective molecularly targeted therapies are developed, their evaluation would still generally take several years. Most new treatments do not replace standard therapy, but are added or integrated. Herceptin and other biologically based treatments can easily be incorporated into high-dose regimens, should they prove more effective than conventional dose therapy.

Ensuring the return of uncontaminated hematopoietic stem cells may prove necessary for improving outcome. Stem cell transplants selected to deplete contaminating breast cancer cells are already under way. Enormous technological developments related to hematopoietic stem cell support (including the recombinant hematopoietic growth factors) have already improved our methods of harvesting stem cells, and our understanding of the immune system, and provided tools to therapeutically modulate the immune response.

In addition to facilitating the evaluation of dose-intensive therapy, evolving technology has facilitated the development of cytokine therapy, recombinant vaccines, and gene therapy. Stem cell transplant technology already is used to deliver new biologically based therapies, and may be required for gene or immunotherapies. Sequential high-dose therapies, regimens incorporating new agents, and studies of cell therapies or vaccines using dendritic cells are currently under study.

References

Anonymous. (2000). Breast cancer statistics. *Journal of the National Cancer Institute,* **92,** 445.

Antman, K., Rowlings, P., Vaughn, W. *et al.* (1997). High dose chemotherapy with autologous hematopoietic stem cell support for breast cancer in North America. *Journal of Clinical Oncology,* **15,** 1870–9.

Appelbaum, F.R. & Thomas, E.D. (1983). Review of the use of marrow transplantation in the treatment of non-Hodgkin's lymphoma. *Journal of Clinical Oncology,* **1,** 440–7.

Armitage, J.O., Jagannath, S., Spitzer, G. *et al.* (1986). High dose therapy and autologous marrow rescue as salvage treatment for patients with large cell lymphoma. *European Journal of Cancer and Clinical Oncology,* **22,** 871–7.

Ayash, L., Elias, A., Ibrahim, J. *et al.* (1998). High dose multimodality therapy with autologous stem cell support for state IIIB breast carcinoma. *Journal of Clinical Oncology,* **16,** 1000–7.

Ayash, L., Elias, A., Schwartz, G. *et al.* (1996). Double dose-intense chemotherapy with autologous stem cell support for metastatic breast cancer: no improvement in progression-free survival by the sequence of high-dose melphalan followed by cyclophosphamide, thiotepa, and carboplatin. *Journal of Clinical Oncology,* **14,** 2984–92.

Ayash, L.J., Elias, A., Wheeler, C. *et al.* (1994). Double dose-intensive chemotherapy with autologous marrow and peripheral-blood progenitor-cell support for metastatic breast cancer: a feasibility study. *Journal of Clinical Oncology,* **12,** 37–44.

Baselga, J. & Mendelsohn, J. (1994). The epidermal growth factor receptor as a target for therapy in breast carcinoma. *Breast Cancer Research and Treatment,* **1,** 127–38.

Baselga, J., Norton, L., Masui, H. *et al.* (1993). Antitumor effects of doxorubicin in combination with anti-epidermal growth factor receptor monoclonal antibodies. *Journal of the National Cancer Institute,* **85,** 1327–33.

Basser, R.L., To, L.B., Collins, J.P. (1999). Multicycle high-dose chemotherapy and filgrastim-mobilized peripheral-blood progenitor cells in women with high-risk stage II or III breast cancer: five-year follow-up. *Journal of Clinical Oncology,* **17,** 82–92.

Bearman, S., Jones, R., Shpall, E. *et al.* (1994). High dose chemotherapy with autologous progenitor cell support for Stage 4 NED breast cancer. *Breast Cancer Research and Treatment,* **32,** 65 (Abstract 146).

Bergan, R., Hakim, F., Schwartz, G. *et al.* (1996). Electroporation of synthetic oligodeoxynucleotides: a novel technique for ex vivo bone marrow purging. *Blood,* **88,** 731–41.

Bergh, J., Wiklund, T., Erikstein, B. *et al.* (2000). Tailored fluorouracil, epirubicin, and cyclophosphamide compared with marrow-supported high-dose chemotherapy as adjuvant treatment for high- risk breast cancer: a randomised trial. Scandinavian Breast Group 9401 study. *Lancet,* **356,** 1384–91.

Bezwoda, W. (1998). Primary high dose chemotherapy for metastatic breast cancer: update and analysis of prognostic factors. *Proceedings of the American Society of Clinical Oncology,* **17,** 115a (Abstract 443).

Bezwoda, W., Seymour, L., & Dansey, R. (1995). High dose chemotherapy with hematopoietic rescue as primary treatment for metastatic breast cancer: A randomized trial. *Journal of Clinical Oncology,* **13,** 2483–9.

Bezwoda, W.R. (1999). Randomised, controlled trial of high dose chemotherapy versus standard dose chemotherapy for high risk, surgically treated, primary breast cancer. *Proceedings of the American Society of Clinical Oncology,* **18,** 2a.

Biron, P., Durand, M., Roche, H. *et al.* (2002). High dose thiotepa, cyclophosphamide and stem cell transplantation after 4 FEC 100 compared with 4 FEC alone allowed a better disease free survival but the same overall survival in first line chemotherapy for metastatic breast cancer. Results of the PEGASE 03 French Protocole. *Proceedings of the American Society of Clinical Oncology,* (Abstract 167).

Bosly, A., Sonet, A., Salles, G. *et al.* (1997). Superiority of late over early intensification in relapsing/refractory aggressive non-Hodgkin's lymphoma: A randomized study from the GELA: LNH RP 93. *Blood,* **90,** 594a.

Bregni, M., Dodero, A., Peccatori, J. *et al.* (2002). Nonmyeloablative conditioning followed by hematopoietic cell allografting and donor lymphocyte infusions for patients with metastatic renal and breast cancer. *Blood,* **99,** 4234–6.

Brown, P. & Giavazzi, R. (1995). Matrix metalloproteinase inhibition: a review of anti-tumour activity. *Annals of Oncology,* **6,** 967–74.

Brugger, W., Bross, K., Glatt, M. *et al.* (1994). Mobilization of tumor cells and hematopoietic progenitor cells into peripheral blood of patients with solid tumors. *Blood,* **83,** 636–40.

Cagnoni, P., Nieto, Y., Shpall, E. *et al.* (1998). High dose chemotherapy with autologous hematopoietic progenitor cell support as part of combined modality therapy in patients with inflammatory breast cancer. *Journal of Clinical Oncology,* **16,** 1661–8.

Chou, J., Moasser, M., Kohl, N. *et al.* (1997). The farnesyl transferase inhibitor induces G1 arrest in Ras-transformed human mammary epithelial cells in combination with epidermal growth factor receptor blockade. *Proceedings of the American Association of Cancer Research,* **38,** 63 (Abstract 426).

Clark, G., Sledge, G.W., Osborne, C.K., & McGuire, W.L. (1987). Survival from first recurrence: relative importance of prognostic factors in 1,015 breast cancer patients. *Journal of Clinical Oncology,* **5,** 55–61.

Crown, J.P., Lind, M., Gould, A. *et al.* (2002). High-dose chemotherapy with autograft support is not superior to cyclophosphamide methotrexate and 5-FU (CMF) following doxorubicin induction in patients with breast cancer and 4 or more involved axillary lymph nodes: the Anglo-Celtic I study. *Proceedings of the American Society of Clinical Oncology,* (Abstract 166).

Crump, M., Gluck, S., Stewart, D. *et al.* (2001). A randomized trial of high-dose chemotherapy (HDC) with autologous peripheral blood stem cell support (ASCT) compared to standard therapy in women with metastatic breast cancer: a National Cancer Institute of Canada (NCIC) Clinical Trials Group Study (Abstract 82).

Dasgupta, A., Rajagopal, C., Efird, J. *et al.* (1994). High dose cyclophosphamide/carboplatin and autologous bone marrow transplantation/peripheral blood stem cell transplantation for metastatic breast cancer: an analysis of prognostic factors. *Proceedings of the American Society of Hematology,* **85,** (Abstract 3757).

Doroshow, J., Simpson, J., Somlo, G. *et al.* (1996). Immunohistochemical and histopathologic factors predicting progression-free and overall survival following high-dose chemotherapy and stem cell rescue for responsive metastatic breast cancer. *Proceedings of the American Society of Clinical Oncology,* **15,** (Abstract 176).

Doroshow, J., Somlo, G., Ahn, C. *et al.* (1995). Prognostic factors predicting progression-free and overall survival in patients with responsive metastatic breast cancer treated with high-dose chemotherapy and bone marrow stem cell reinfusion. *Proceedings of the American Society of Clinical Oncology,* **14,** 319 (Abstract 942).

Douer, D., Chaiwun, B., Glaspy, J. *et al.* (1993). Analysis of peripheral blood progenitor cell harvests for occult breast cancer micrometastases using a sensitive immunohistochemical method. *Proceedings of the American Society of Clinical Oncology,* **12,** 62 (Abstract 51).

Dunphy, F., Spitzer, G., Fornoff, J.F. *et al.* (1994). Factors predicting long-term survival for metastatic breast cancer patients treated with high-dose chemotherapy and bone marrow support. *Cancer,* **73,** 2157–67.

Dunphy, F.R., Spitzer, G., Buzdar, A.U. *et al.* (1990). Treatment of estrogen receptor-negative or hormonally refractory breast cancer with double high-dose chemotherapy intensification and bone marrow support. *Journal of Clinical Oncology,* **8,** 1207–16.

Eibl, B., Schwaighofer, H., Nachbaur, D. *et al.* (1996). Evidence for a graft-versus-tumor effect in a patient treated with marrow ablative chemotherapy and allogeneic bone marrow transplantation for breast cancer. *Blood,* **88,** 1501–8.

Ellis, G., Ferguson, M., Yamanaka, E. *et al.* (1989). Monoclonal antibodies for detection of occult carcinoma cells in bone marrow of breast cancer patients. *Cancer,* **63,** 2509–14.

Fan, Z., Baselga, J., Masui, H., & Mendelsohn, J. (1993). Antitumor effect of anti-epidermal growth factor receptor monoclonal antibodies plus cis-diamminedichloroplatinum on well established A431 cell xenografts. *Cancer Research,* **53,** 4637–42.

Fields, K., Moscinski, L., Trudeau, W. *et al.* (1994). High incidence of bone marrow micrometastases using the polymerase chain reaction technique in patients with high risk Stage II and Stage III breast cancer following adjuvant therapy: clinical correlates. *Breast Cancer Research and Treatment,* **32** (Suppl), 63 (Abstract 139).

Fisher, B., Anderson, S., DeCillis, A. *et al.* (1999). Further evaluation of intensified and increased total dose of cyclophosphamide for the treatment of primary breast cancer: findings from National Surgical Adjuvant Breast and Bowel Project B-25. *Journal of Clinical Oncology,* **17,** 3374–88.

Frei III, E. & Canellos, G.P. (1980). Dose, a critical factor in cancer chemotherapy. *American Journal of Medicine,* **69,** 585–94.

Garcia-Sanchez, F., Pizzorno, G., Cooperberg, M. *et al.* (1997). Effective bone marrow purging using an adenovirus vector containing the prodrug activation unit cytosine deaminase. *Proceedings of the American Society of Clinical Oncology,* **16,** 91a (Abstract 320).

Gianni, A. & Bonadonna, G. (2001). Five-year results of the randomized clinical trial comparing standard versus high-dose myeloablative chemotherapy in the adjuvant treatment of breast cancer with > 3 positive nodes (LN+). *Proceedings of the American Society of Clinical Oncology,* (Abstract 80).

Gianni, A., Siena, S., Bregni, M. *et al.* (1995). 5-year results of high-dose sequential (HDS) adjuvant chemotherapy in breast cancer with > 10 positive nodes. *Proceedings of the American Society of Clinical Oncology,* **14,** 90 (Abstract 61).

Gianni, A.M., Bregni, M., Siena, S. *et al.* (1989). Rapid and complete hematapoietic reconstitution following combined transplantation of autologous blood and bone marrow cells. A changing role for high dose chemoradiotherapy. *Hematology and Oncology,* **7,** 139–48.

Gianni, L., Munzone, E., Capri, G. *et al.* (1995). Paclitaxel by 3-hour infusion in combination with bolus doxorubicin in women with untreated metastatic breast cancer: high antitumor efficacy and cardiac effects in a dose-finding and sequence-finding study. *Journal of Clinical Oncology,* **13,** 2688–99.

Gilewski, T., Adluri, R., Zhang, S. *et al.* (1997). MUC-1 keyhole limpet hemocyanin conjugate plus QS-21 vaccination of high risk breast cancer patients with no evidence of disease. *Proceedings of the American Society of Clinical Oncology,* **16,** 438a (Abstract 1569).

Greenberg, P., Hortobagyi, G., Smith, T. *et al.* (1996). Long-term follow-up of patients with complete remission following combination chemotherapy for metastatic breast cancer. *Journal of Clinical Oncology,* **14,** 2197–205.

Hagenbeek, A., Philip, T., Bron, D. *et al.* (1991). The Parma international randomized study in relapsed non Hodgkin lymphoma: 1st interim analysis of 128 patients (as 15 January 1991: 153 patients). *Bone Marrow Transplantation,* **7** (Suppl 2), 142.

Hanauske, A., Degen, D., Hilsenbeck, S. *et al.* (1992). Effects ot taxotere and taxol on invitro colony formation of freshly explanted human tumor cells. *Anti-Cancer Drugs,* **3,** 121–4.

Hann, D., Jacobsen, P., Martin, S. *et al.* (1997). Quality of life following bone marrow transplantation for breast cancer: a comparative study. *Bone Marrow Transplantation,* **19,** 257–64.

Hayes, D.F. & Henderson, I.C. (1987). CAF in metastatic breast cancer: standard therapy or another effective regimen? *Journal of Clinical Oncology,* **5,** 1497–9.

Henderson, I., Berry, D., Demetri, G. *et al.* (1998). Improved disease free and overall survival from the addition of sequential paclitaxel but not from the escalation of doxorubicin dose level in the adjuvant chemotherapy of patients with node positive primary breast cancer. *Proceedings of the American Society of Clinical Oncology,* **17,** 101a (Abstract 390a).

Hesdorffer, C., Awyello, J., Ward, M. *et al.* (1998). A Phase I trial of retroviral-mediated transfer of the human MDR-1 gene as marrow chemoprotection in patients undergoing high dose chemotherapy and autologous stem cell transplantation. *Journal of Clinical Oncology,* **16,** 165–72.

Hillner, B.E., Smith, T.J., & Desch, C.E. (1991). Estimating the cost-effectiveness of autologous bone marrow transplantation for metastatic breast cancer. *Proceedings of the American Society of Clinical Oncology,* **10,** 46 (Abstract 60).

Hillner, B.E., Smith, T.J., & Desch, C.E. (1992). Efficacy and cost-effectiveness of autologous bone marrow transplantation in metastatic breast cancer—estimates using decision analysis while awaiting clinical trial results. *Journal of the American Medical Association,* **267,** 2055–61.

Hortobagyi, G.N., Buzdar, A.U., Theriault, R.L. *et al.* (2000). Randomized trial of high-dose chemotherapy and blood cell autografts for high-risk primary breast carcinoma. *Journal of the National Cancer Institute,* **92,** 225–33.

Hryniuk, W. & Levine, M.N. (1986). Analysis of dose intensity for adjuvant chemotherapy trials in stage II breast cancer. *Journal of Clinical Oncology,* **4,** 1162–70.

Hryniuk, W.M. (1987). Average relative dose intensity and the impact on design of clinical trials. *Seminars in Oncology,* **14,** 65–74.

Hryniuk, W.M. & Bush, H. (1984). The importance of dose intensity in chemotherapy of metastatic breast cancer. *Journal of Clinical Oncology,* **2,** 1281–7.

Hudis, C., Seidman, A., Baselga, J. *et al.* (1999). Sequential dose-dense doxorubicin, paclitaxel, and cyclophosphamide for resectable high-risk breast cancer: feasibility and efficacy. *Journal of Clinical Oncology,* **17,** 93–100.

Ingle, J.N., Tormey, D.C., & Tan, K.H. (1978). The bone marrow examination in breast cancer: diagnostic considerations and clinical usefulness. *Cancer,* **41,** 670–4.

Jemal, A., Thomas, A., Murray, T., & Thun, M. (2002). Cancer statistics, 2002. *CA: A Cancer Journal for Physicians,* **52,** 23–47.

Jones, R.B., Shpall, E.J., Shogan, J. *et al.* (1990). The Duke AFM program. Intensive induction chemotherapy for metastatic breast cancer. *Cancer,* **66,** 431–6.

Kluin-Nelemans, H.C., Zagonel, V., Anastasopoulou, A. *et al.* (2001). Standard chemotherapy with or without high-dose chemotherapy for aggressive non-Hodgkin's lymphoma: randomized phase III EORTC study. *Journal of the National Cancer Institute,* **93,** 22–30.

Laughlin, M.J., McGaughey, D.S., Crews, J.R. *et al.* (1998). Secondary myelodysplasia and acute leukemia in breast cancer patients after autologous bone marrow transplant. *Journal of Clinical Oncology,* **16,** 1008–12.

Linch, D.C., Winfield, D., Goldstone, A.H. *et al.* (1992). A randomized trial of BEAM and ABMT versus mini-Beam in relapsed and resistant Hodgkin's disease. *Proceedings of the European Group for Bone Marrow Transplantation,* **18,** 203 (Abstract 403).

Lotz, J.P., Cure, H., Janvier, M. *et al.* (1999). High-dose chemotherapy with hematopoietic stem cells transplantation for metastatic breast cancer: results of the French protocol Pegase 04. *Proceedings of the American Society of Clinical Oncology,* **18,** 43a.

Madan, B., Broadwater, G., Rubin, P. *et al.* (2000). Improved survival with consolidation high-dose cyclophosphamide, cisplatin and carmustine compared with observation in women with metastic breast cancer and only bone metastases treated with induction Adriamycin, 5-fluorouracil and methotrexate: A phase III prospective radomized comparative trial. *Proceedings of the American Society of Clinical Oncology,* **19,** 48a.

Martelli, M., Vignetti, M., Zinzani, P.L. *et al.* (1996). High-dose chemotherapy followed by autologous bone marrow transplantation versus dexamethasone, cisplatin, and cytarabine in aggressive non-Hodgkin's lymphoma with partial response to front-line chemotherapy: a prospective randomized Italian multicenter study. *Journal of Clinical Oncology,* **14,** 534–42.

Mayordomo, J., Yubero, A., Cajal, R. *et al.* (1997). Phase I trial of high dose paclitaxel in combination with cyclophosphamide, thiotepa and carboplatin with autologous peripheral blood stem cell rescue. *Proceedings of the American Society of Clinical Oncology,* **16,** 102a (Abstract 358).

McCarthy, P., Hurd, D., Rowlings, P. *et al.* (1999). Autotransplants in men with breast cancer. ABMTR Breast Cancer Working Committee. Autologous Blood and Marrow Transplant Registry. *Bone Marrow Transplantation,* **24,** 365–8.

McNamee, D. (2000). High dose chemotherapy positive in breast cancer trial. *Lancet,* **355,** 1973.

McQuellon, R., Craven, B., Russell, G. *et al.* (1996). Quality of life in breast cancer patients before and after autologous bone marrow transplantation. *Bone Marrow Transplantation,* **18,** 579–84.

Mick, R., Begg, C.B., Antman, K. *et al.* (1989). Diverse prognosis in metastatic breast cancer: who should be offered alternative initial therapies? *Breast Cancer Research and Treatment,* **13,** 33–38.

Muss, H., Thor, A., Berry, D. *et al.* (1994). c-erbB-2 expression and response to adjuvant therapy in women with node-positive early breast cancer. *New England Journal of Medicine,* **330,** 1260–6.

Myers, S., Mick, R., & Williams, S. (1994). High-dose chemotherapy with autologous stem cell rescue in women with metastatic breast cancer with involved bone marrow: a role for peripheral blood progenitor transplant. *Bone Marrow Transplantation,* **13,** 449–54.

Myklebust, A., Godal, A., Juell, S. *et al.* (1994). Comparison of two antibody-based methods for elimination of breast cancer cells from human marrow. *Cancer Research,* **54,** 209–14.

Nemunaitis, J., Rabinowe, S.N., Singer, J.W. *et al.* (1991). Recombinant granulocyte-macrophage colony-stimulating factor after autologous bone marrow transplantation for lymphoid malignancy: Pooled results from three randomized double-blind, placebo controlled trials. *New England Journal of Medicine,* **324,** 1773–8.

Nguyen, T., Naziruddin, B., Dintzis, S. *et al.* (1999). Recognition of breast cancer-associated peptides by tumor-reactive, HLA-class I restricted allogeneic cytotoxic T lymphocytes. *International Journal of Cancer,* **81,** 607–15.

Nieto, Y., Nieto, Y., Champlin, R. *et al.* (2000). Status of high dose chemotherapy for breast cancer in the new mellennium. *Biology of Bone and Marrow Transplantation,* **6,** 476–95.

Or, R., Ackerstein, A., Nagler, A. *et al.* (1998). Allogeneic cell-mediated immunotherapy for breast cancer after autologous stem cell transplantation: a clinical pilot study. *Cytokines Cellular Molecular Therapy,* **4,** 1–6.

O'Reilly, M.S., Boehm, T., Shing, Y. *et al.* (1997). Endostatin: an endogenous inhibitor of angiogenesis and tumor growth. *Cell,* **88,** 277–85.

Palangie, T., Sastre, X., Scholl, S. *et al.* (1996). Her-2 overexpression and recurrence in inflammatory breast cancer treated with multiple-cycle high dose chemotherapy. *Breast Cancer Research and Treatment,* **41,** 227.

Passos-Coelho, J., Ross, A., Davis, J. *et al.* (1994). Bone marrow micrometastases in chemotherapy responsive advanced breast cancer: effect of ex vivo purging with 4-hydroperoxycyclophosphamide. *Cancer Research,* **54,** 2366–71.

Peters, W., Jones, R., Vredenburgh, J. *et al.* (1996). A large prospective randomized trial of high-dose combination alkylating agents (CPB) with autologous cellular support as consolidation for patients with metastatic breast cancer achieving complete remission after intensive doxorubicin-based induction therapy (AFM). *Proceedings of the American Society of Clinical Oncology,* **15,** 121 (Abstract 149).

Peters, W., Ross, M., Vredenburgh, J. *et al.* (1993). High-dose chemotherapy and autologous bone marrow support as consolidation after standard-dose adjuvant therapy for high risk primary breast cancer. *Journal of Clinical Oncology,* **11,** 1132–43.

Peters, W., Shpall, E., Jones, R. *et al.* (1988). High-dose combination alkylating agents with bone marrow support as initial treatment for metastatic breast cancer. *Journal of Clinical Oncology,* **6,** 1368–76.

Peters, W.P., Rosner, G., Vredenburgh, J. *et al.* (1999). A prospective, randomized comparison of two doses of combination alkyating agents as consolidation after CAF in high-risk primary breast cancer involving ten or more axillary lymph nodes: preliminary results of CALGB 9082/SWOG 9114/NCIC MA-13. *Proceedings of the American Society of Clinical Oncology,* **18,** 1a.

Philip, T., Guglielmi, C., Hagenbeek, A. *et al.* (1992). The Parma international randomized prospective study in relapsed non Hodgkin's lymphoma; second interim analysis of 172 patients. *Proceedings of the European Group for Bone Marrow Transplantation,* **18,** 203 (Abstract 402).

Rahman, Z., Frye, D., Champlin, R. *et al.* (1997). Phase I trial of multiple cycle escalating dose doxorubicin, paclitaxel and cyclophosphamide with peripheral blood progenitor cells and G-CSF support in patients with metastatic breast cancer. *Proceedings of the American Society of Clinical Oncology,* **16,** 92a (Abstract 326).

Reichman, B., Seidman, A., Crown, J. *et al.* (1993). Paclitaxel and recombinant human granulocyte colony-stimulating factor as initial chemotherapy for metastatic breast cancer. *Journal of Clinical Oncology,* **10,** 1943–51.

Rill, D., Santana, V., Roberts, W. *et al.* (1994). Direct demonstration that autologous bone marrow transplantation for solid tumors can return a multiplicity of tumorigenic cells. *Blood,* **84,** 380–3.

Rizzo, D., Williams, S., Wu J. T. *et al.* (2003). Syngeneic hematopoietic stem cell transplantation for women with metastatic breast cancer. *Bone Marrow Transplantation,* **32,** 151–5.

Roche, H., Pouillart, P., Meyer, N. *et al.* (2001). Adjuvant high dose chemotherapy (HDC) improves early outcomes for high risk

(N>7) breast cancer patients: the pegase 01 trial. *Proceedings of the American Society of Clinical Oncology*, **20**, 26a.

Rodenhuis, S., Bontenbal, M., Beex, E.L. *et al.* (2000). Randomized phase III study of high-dose chemotherapy with cyclophosphamide, thiotepa and carboplatin in operable breast cancer with 4 or more axillary lymph nodes. *Proceedings of the American Society of Clinical Oncology*, **19**, 74 (Abstract 286).

Rodenhuis, S., Richel, K.J., van der Wall, E. *et al.* (1998). Randomized trial of high-dose chemotherapy and hematopoietic progenitor cell support in operable breast cancer with extensive axillary lymph node involvement. *Lancet*, **352**, 515–21.

Ross, A., Cooper, B., Lazarus, H. *et al.* (1993a). Detection and viability of tumor cells in peripheral blood stem cell collections from breast cancer patients using immunocytochemical and clonogenic assay techniques. *Blood*, **82**, 2605–10.

Ross, A., Farmer, S., Moss, T. *et al.* (1994). Tumor contamination of peripheral blood stem cell collections from breast cancer patients: influence of clinical status at time of pheresis. *Breast Cancer Research and Treatment*, **32** (Suppl), 63 (Abstract 139).

Ross, A.A., Cooper, B.W., Lazarus, H.M. *et al.* (1993b). Incidence of tumor cell contamination in peripheral blood stem cell collections from breast cancer patients. *Proceedings of the American Society of Clinical Oncology*, **12**, 69 (Abstract 77).

Rowlings, P.A., Williams, S.F., Antman, K.H. *et al.* (1999). Factors correlated with progression-free survival after high-dose therapy and hematopoietic stem cell transplantation for metastatic breast cancer. *Journal of the American Medical Association*, **282**, 1335–43.

Schmid, P., Samonigg, H., Nitsch, T. *et al.* (2002). Randomized trial of up front tandem high-dose chemotherapy compared to standard chemotherapy with doxorubicin and paclitaxel in metastatic breast cancer. *Proceedings of the American Society of Clinical Oncology*, (Abstract 17).

Schouten, H.C., Kvaloy, S., Sydes, M. *et al.* (2000). The CUP trial: a randomized study analyzing the efficacy of high dose therapy and purging in low-grade non-Hodgkin's lymphoma (NHL). *Annals of Oncology*, **11** (Suppl 1), 91–4.

Schouten, H.C., Qian, W., Sydes, M.R. *et al.* (2002). High dose therapy improves outcome in relapsed follicular non-Hodgkin's lymphoma: results of a randomized clinical trial. *Proceedings of the American Society of Clinical Oncology*, (Abstract 1654).

Seong, D., Mehra, R., Andersson, B. *et al.* (1994). Autologous bone marrow infusion does not contribute to relapse following high dose tandem chemotherapy for recurrent or metastatic breast cancer. *Blood*, **84**(10), 210a (Abstract 827).

Shpall, E., Franklin, W., Jones, R. *et al.* (1995). Transplantation of CD34+ selected progenitor cells into breast cancer patients following high dose chemotherapy. *Proceedings of the American Society for Blood and Marrow Transplantation*, **1**, (Abstract 520).

Siena, S., Bregni, M., Brando, B. *et al.* (1989). Circulation of CD34-positive hematopoietic stem cells in the peripheral blood of high-dose cyclophosphamide treated patients: enhancement by intravenous recombinant human GM-CSF. *Blood*, **74**, 1905–14.

Skipper, H.E. (1967). Criteria associated with destruction of leukemia and solid tumor cells in animals. *Cancer Research*, **27**, 2636–45.

Skipper, H.E. (1974a). Combination therapy: some concepts and results. *Cancer Chemotherapy and Rep*, **4**, 137–45.

Skipper, H.E. (1974b). Thoughts on cancer chemotherapy and combination modality therapy (1974). *Journal of the American Medical Association*, **230**, 1033–5.

Skipper, H.E. (1983). Stepwise progress in the treatment of disseminated cancers. *Cancer*, **51**, 1773–6.

Skipper, H.E. (1990). Dose intensity versus total dose of chemotherapy: an experimental basis. In eds. V.T. DeVita, S. Hellman, & S.A. Rosenberg, pp. 43–64. *Important Advances in Oncology*, Philadelphia: Lippincott.

Skipper, H.E., Schabel, F.M., Jary, R., & Wilcox, W.S. (1964). Experimental evaluation of potential anticancer agents. XIII. On the criteria and kinetics associated with "curability" of experimental leukemia. *Cancer Chemotherapy Report*, **35**, 1–111.

Smalley, R.V., Carpenter, J., Bartolucci, A. *et al.* (1977). A comparison of cyclophosphamide, adriamycin, 5-fluorouracil (CAF) and cyclophosphamide, methotrexate, 5-fluorouracil, vincristine, prednisone (CMFVP) in patients with metastatic breast cancer: a Southeastern Cancer Study Group project. *Cancer*, **40**, 625–32.

Somlo, G., Doroshow, J., Foreman, S. *et al.* (1995). High dose chemotherapy and stem cell rescue for the treatment of primary high-risk breast cancer: prognostic indicators of overall survival and progression-free survival. *Proceedings of the American Society of Clinical Oncology*, **14**, 113 (Abstract 150).

Spitzer, G., Champlin, R., Seong, D. *et al.* (1994). Repetitive high-dose therapy (HDT) tolerance and outcome in stage IV breast cancer. *Seventh International Symposium on Autologous Bone Marrow Transplantation*, eds. K.A. Dicke & A. Keating, Arlington, TX.

Stadtmauer, E.A., O'Neill, A., Goldstein, L.J. *et al.* (2000). Conventional-dose chemotherapy compared with high-dose chemotherapy plus autologous hematopoietic stem-cell transplantation for metastatic breast cancer. Philadelphia Bone Marrow Transplant Group [see comments]. *New England Journal of Medicine*, **342**, 1069–76.

Stadtmauer, E.A., O'Neill, A., Goldstein, L.J. *et al.* (2002). Conventional-dose chemotherapy compared with high-dose chemotherapy (HDC) plus autologous stem-cell transplantation (SCT) for metastatic breast cancer: 5-year update of the 'Philadelphia Trial'. *Proceedings of the American Society of Clinical Oncology*, (Abstract 169).

Stemmer, S., Cagnoni, P., Shpall, E. *et al.* (1996). High dose paclitaxel, cyclophosphamide and cisplatin with autologous hematopoietic progenitor cell support: A phase I trial. *Journal of Clinical Oncology*, **14**, 1463–72.

Stemmer, S., Jones, R., Bearman, S. *et al.* (1994). Intensive taxol/cyclophosphamide/cisplatin with autologous hematopoietic cell support. *Proceedings of the American Society of Clinical Oncology*, **13**, 105 (Abstract 222).

Swenerton, K.D., Legha, S.S., Smith, T. *et al.* (1979). Prognostic factors in metastatic breast cancer treated with combination chemotherapy. *Cancer Research*, **39**, 1552–62.

Talmadge, J., Watanabe, T., Kuxzynski, C. *et al.* (1997). Purging properties of p53 adenovirus-mediated gene transfer into breast cancer cells using protocols which are nontoxic for human C34+ cells. *Proceedings of the American Association of Cancer Research*, **38**, 6 (Abstract 37).

Tancini, G., Bonadonna, G., Valagussa, P. *et al.* (1983). Adjuvant CMF in breast cancer: comparative 5-year results of 12 versus 6 cycles. *Journal of Clinical Oncology*, **1**, 2–10.

Tepler, I., Cannistra, S.A., Frei, E. *et al.* (1993). Use of peripheral-blood progenitor cells abrogates the myelotoxicity of repetitive outpatient high-dose carboplatin and cyclophosphamide chemotherapy. *Journal of Clinical Oncology*, **11**, 1583–91.

Thomas, E.D., Buckner, C.D., Banaji, M. *et al.* (1977). One hundred patients with acute leukemia treated by chemotherapy, total body irradiation and allogeneic marrow transplantation. *Blood,* **49**, 511–33.

Tokuda, Y., Tajima, T., Narabayashi, M. *et al.* (2001). "Randomized phase III study of high-dose chemotherapy (HDC) with autologous stem cell support as consolidation in high-risk postoperative breast cancer: Japan Clinical Oncology Group (JCOG9208). *Proceedings of the American Society of Clinical Oncology*, (Abstract 148).

Trudeau, M., Eisenhauer, E., Higgins, B.F. *et al.* (1996). Docetaxel in patients with metastatic breast cancer: a phase II study of the National Cancer Institute of Canada-Clinical Trials Group. *Journal of Clinical Oncology*, **14**, 422–8.

Ueno, N., Randon, G., Mirza, N. *et al.* (1998). Allogeneic peripheral blood progenitor cell transplantation for poor risk patients with metastatic breast cancer. *Journal of Clinical Oncology*, **16**, 986–93.

Ueno, N.T., Cheng, Y.C., Giralt, S.A. *et al.* (2002). Complete donor chimerism by fludarabine/melphalan in mini-allogeneic transplantation for metastatic renal cell carcinoma and breast cancer. *Proceedings of the American Society of Clinical Oncology*, (Abstract 1659).

Vahdat, L., Papadopoulos, K., Balmaceda, C. *et al.* (1998). Phase I trial of sequential high dose chemotherapy with escalating dose pacli-taxel, melphalan, and cyclophosphamide, thiotepa and carboplatin with peripheral blood progenitor support in women with responding metastatic breast cancer. *Clinical Cancer Research*, **4**, 1689–95.

Viens, P., Penault-Llorca, F., Jacquemier, J. *et al.* (1998). High dose chemotherapy and haematopoietic stem cell transplantation for inflammatory breast cancer: pathologic response and outcome. *Bone Marrow Transplantation*, **21**, 249–54.

Vredenburgh, J., Peters, W., Rosner, G. *et al.* (1995). Detection of tumor cells in the bone marrow of stage IV breast cancer patients receiving high-dose chemotherapy: the role of induction chemotherapy. *Bone Marrow Transplantation*, **16**, 815–21.

Vredenburgh, J., Tyer, C., Broadwater, G. *et al.* (1997). The inci-dence and significance of tumor cell contamination of the hematopoietic support from patients with breast cancer treated with high dose chemotherapy. *Proceedings of the American Society of Clinical Oncology*, **16**, 96a (Abstract 338).

Vukelja, S., Baker, W., Burrel, L. *et al.* (1994). High-dose taxol, cyclophosphamide, and cisplatin with stem cell support in treat-ment of metastatic breast cancer. *Autologous Bone Marrow Transplantation, Proceedings of the International Symposium*, eds. K.A. Dicke, J.O. Armitage, & M.J. Dicke-Evinger, Arlington, Texas, p. 74.

Ward, M., Richardson, C., Pioli, P. *et al.* (1994). Transfer and expression of the human multiple drug resistance gene in human CD34+ cells. *Blood,* **84**, 1408–14.

Weiss, R.B., Rifkin, R.M., Stewart, F.M. *et al.* (2000). High-dose chemotherapy for high-risk primary breast cancer: an on-site review of the Bezwoda study. *Lancet,* **355**, 999–1003.

Wieden, P., Sullivan, K., Fluornoy, N. *et al.* (1979). Antileukemic effect of graft-versus host disease in human recipients of allo-geneic-marrow autografts. *New England Journal of Medicine,* **300**, 1068–73.

Williams, S., Mick, R., Dresser, R. *et al.* (1989). High dose consoli-dation therapy with autologous stem cell rescue in stage IV breast cancer. *Journal of Clinical Oncology*, **7**, 1824–30.

Winer, E., Gold, D., Lees, J. *et al.* (1991). Evaluation of quality of life in patients with metastatic breast cancer undergoing high dose chemotherapy with autologous bone marrow support. *Proceedings of the American Society of Clinical Oncology*, **10**, 62 (Abstract 122).

Wolmark, N., Fisher, B., & Anderson, S. (1998). The effect of increasing dose intensity and cumulative dose of adjuvant cyclophosphamide in node positive breast cancer. *Breast Cancer Research and Treatment*, **46** (Suppl), 26.

Wood, W., Budman, D., Korzun, A. *et al.* (1994). Dose and dose inten-sity of adjuvant chemotherapy for stage II, node-positive breast carcinoma. *New England Journal of Medicine*, **330**, 1253–9.

Wu, A., Rabkin, S., Maruzas, R. *et al.* (1997). Bone marrow purging by attenuated multi-mutated herpes simplex virus-1. *Proceedings of the American Society of Clinical Oncology*, **16**, 91a (Abstract 319).

Zander, A.R., Krüger, W., Kröger, N. *et al.* (2002). High-dose chemotherapy with autologous hematopoietic stem-cell support vs. standard-dose chemotherapy in breast cancer patients with 10 or more positive lymph nodes: first results of a randomized trial. *Proceedings of the American Society of Clinical Oncology*, (Abstract 1658).

43 Autologous hematopoietic stem cell transplantation for germ cell tumors

BRANDON HAYES-LATTIN AND CRAIG R. NICHOLS

Oregon Health Sciences University, Portland, USA

Introduction

Malignant testicular tumors are the most common solid tumor among young men, with approximately 9,000 new cases diagnosed each year in the United States. Ninety-five percent of malignant testicular tumors are germ cell tumors (Bosl *et al.*, 1997). Germ cell tumors can also arise in extragonadal sites such as the retroperitoneum or mediastinum, often portending a poorer prognosis. Staging is based on pattern of spread and initial therapy is guided by the presenting stage (Table 43.1)

Table 43.1. *AJCC Staging system (Anonymous 1997b)*

A. TNM definitions

Primary tumor (T)

pTX	Cannot be assessed
pT0	No evidence of tumor
pTis	Intratubular neoplasia (carcinoma in situ)
pT1	Limited to testis and epididymis without lymphatic/vascular invasion
pT2	Limited to testis and epididymis with lymphatic/vascular invasion, or tumor extending through the tunica albuginea with involvement of the tunica vaginalis
pT3	Invades the spermatic cord with or without lymphatic/vascular invasion
pT4	Invades the scrotum with or without lymphatic/vascular invasion

Regional Lymph Nodes (N)

NX	Cannot be assessed
N0	No regional lymph node metastases
N1	Metastases in a single lymph node, 2 cm or less in greatest dimension
N2	Metastases in a single lymph node, more than 2 cm but not more than 5 cm in greatest dimension; or multiple lymph nodes, none more than 5 cm in greatest dimension
N3	Metastases in a lymph node, more than 5 cm in greatest dimension

Distant Metastasis (M)

MX	Cannot be assessed
M0	No distant metastasis
M1	Distant metastasis
	M1a: nonregional nodal or pulmonary metastasis
	M1b: distant metastasis other than nonregional nodes and lungs

Serum Markers (S)

SX	Not available or not performed
S0	Marker study levels within normal limits
S1	LDH <1.5 times the upper limit of normal AND HCG (mIU/ml) <5,000 AND AFP (mcg/ml) <1,000
S2	LDH 1.5–10 times the upper limit of normal OR HCG (mIU/ml) 5,000–50,000 OR AFP (mcg/ml) 1,000–10,000
S3	LDH >10 times the upper limit of normal OR HCG (mIU/ml) >50,000 OR AFP (mcg/ml) >10,000

B. Stage groupings

Stage 0		pTis, N0, M0, S0
Stage I		pT1–4, N0, M0, Sx
	Stage IA	pT1, N0, M0, S0
	Stage IB	pT2–3, N0, M0, S0
	Stage IS	Any pT, N0, M0, S1-3
Stage II		Any pT, N1-3, M0, Sx
	Stage IIA	Any pT, N1, M0, S0-1
	Stage IIB	Any pT, N2, M0, S0-1
	Stage IIC	Any pT, N3, M0, S0-1
Stage III		Any pT, any N, M1, Sx
	Stage IIIA	Any pT, any N, M1a, S0–1
	Stage IIIB	Any pT, N1–3, M0, S2
		Any pT, any N, M1a, S2
	Stage IIIC	Any pT, N1–3, M0, S3
		Any pT, any N, M1a, S3
		Any pT, any N, M1b, any S

(Anonymous 1997b). Standard therapies for early-stage germ cell tumors routinely cure greater than 95% of patients, and current research goals focus on limiting therapy while preserving high cure rates for these patients.

Before the advent of cisplatin-based chemotherapies, metastatic germ cell tumors were almost always fatal, but today the cure rate for metastatic disease reaches 70% to 80% (Tables 43.2 and 43.3). Unfortunately, 20% to 30% of patients with advanced disease require additional therapy after primary cisplatin-based treatments, including salvage surgery or chemotherapy.

In an effort to better care for and study patients with metastatic disease, many prognostic models based on the pattern of

683

Table 43.2. *Conventional primary therapy results*

Stage	Treatment	Disease-free survival
I	Radical orchiectomy and retroperitoneal lymph node dissection (RPLND)	95%
II, III	Radical orchiectomy plus bleomycin/etoposide/cisplatin (BEP) $\times$ 3–4 cycles plus RPLND for partial response plus BEP $\times$ 2 cycles for residual disease	80% (good risk) 60% (poor risk)

disease spread and serum tumor markers at disease presentation have been employed. (Samuels *et al.*, 1975; Peckham *et al.*, 1979; Bosl *et al.*, 1983; Anonymous, 1985; Birch *et al.*, 1986; Newlands *et al.*, 1986; Stoter *et al.*, 1987; Droz *et al.*, 1988; Aass *et al.*, 1991; Mead *et al.*, 1992). In 1995, a uniform system was developed based on 5,202 patients with nonseminomatous germ cell tumors and 660 patients with seminomas treated with cisplatin-containing regimens to guide decision-making and standardize patient enrollment in clinical trials (Table 43.4, Fig. 43.1) (Anonymous 1997a).

Conventional-dose salvage approaches to patients with poor risk, recurrent, or refractory germ cell tumors lead to remission in 30% to 60% of patients, but only 20% experience long-term survival, leading to investigation of alternate therapies including high-dose chemotherapy with autologous hematopoietic stem cell transplantation (Table 43.5). Herein, we will review the management of the small fraction of patients for whom initial treatments are incompletely effective, with emphasis on the role of high-dose chemotherapy.

Table 43.3. *Conventional-dose chemotherapy regimens*

Indication	Regimen
Primary treatment of disseminated disease (Stage II–III)	BEP (Williams *et al.*, 1987) Bleomycin 30 units intravenously (i.v.) on days 2, 9, and 16
	Etoposide 100 mg/m^2 day i.v. on days 1–5 Cisplatin 20 mg/m^2 day i.v. on days 1–5 Repeat cycle at 21 day intervals
Primary salvage treatment of relapsed disease	VelP(Loehrer *et al.*, 1988) Vinblastine 0.11 mg/kg/day i.v. on days 1–2 Ifosfamide 1.2 g/m^2/day i.v. on days 1–5 Cisplatin 20 mg/m^2/day i.v. on days 1–5 Repeat cycle at 21 day intervals
	VIP(Loehrer, *et al.*, 1988) Etoposide 75 mg/m^2/day i.v. on days 1–5 Ifosfamide 1.2 g/m^2/day i.v. on days 1–5 Cisplatin 20 mg/m^2/day i.v. on days 1–5 Repeat cycle at 21 day intervals

Conventional salvage therapies for germ cell tumors

A unique feature in the management of germ cell tumors is the ability to achieve long-term disease-free survival with secondary chemotherapies after initial treatment failures.

The current standard for comparison for all initial salvage therapies in germ cell tumors is the combination of vinblastine, ifosfamide, and cisplatin (VeIP). In one series, 135 patients with progressive disease after cisplatin and etoposide-based chemotherapy were treated with VeIP regardless of metastatic site or performance status. (Loehrer *et al.*, 1998). A 50% complete response rate after chemotherapy with or without surgical resection of residual disease was seen, with a long-term overall survival rate of 32% and disease-free survival rate of 24%. Importantly, none of the 32 patients with extragonadal nonseminomatous disease were continuously disease-free.

In addition to standard-dose chemotherapy, salvage surgery plays a significant role in the treatment of patients with recurrent germ cell tumors. Murphy *et al.* (1993) retrospectively reviewed all patients felt to have progressive chemorefractory yet resectable disease who underwent salvage surgery at Indiana University from 1977 to 1990. The majority underwent isolated retroperitoneal lymphadenectomy (69%). Thirty-eight of 48 patients (79%) were grossly disease-free after surgery and 29 (60%) obtained a serologic remission. Ten patients (21%) achieved event-free survival for 31 to 89 months. Six additional patients who relapsed after surgery achieved disease-free survival after additional surgery (4 patients) or high-dose chemotherapy and autologous transplant (2 patients). Notably, no patients with more than one site of metastatic disease, even when resectable, achieved long-term disease control. However, a definite potential for cure with salvage surgery was identified in selected patients with recurrent germ cell tumor.

High-dose chemotherapy for recurrent germ cell tumors

An active strategy to improve outcomes for patients with relapsed or refractory germ cell tumors is the use of high-dose chemotherapy with autologous hematopoietic stem cell rescue (Table 43.5). Initial attempts at dose-escalation with cisplatin (without stem cell support) increased toxicity without a survival advantage (Nichols *et al.*, 1991). However, several advances have led to substantial progress toward defining the role of high-dose therapy for germ cell tumors. Drugs such as carboplatin, etoposide, and alkylating agents such as thiotepa or the oxazaphosphorines (ifosfamide and cyclophosphamide) demonstrated antitumor activity, dose-responsiveness, and a wide dose range between dose-limiting myelotoxicity and dose-limiting extramedullary toxicities. Additional improvements in transplant procedures (peripheral blood rather than bone marrow stem cells), supportive care (hematopoietic growth factors and selective antibiotics), and patient selection have advanced the field.

The first investigations of high-dose chemotherapy with autologous hematopoietic stem cell transplantation for germ

Table 43.4. *International Germ Cell Consensus Classification prognostic staging system*

	Nonseminoma		Seminoma	
Good prognosis	Testis or retroperitoneal primary AND No nonpulmonary visceral metastases AND	56% of patients	Any primary site AND No nonpulmonary visceral metastases AND	90% of patients
	Good markers (AFP <1,000 ng/ml and HCG <5,000 IU/l and LDH <1.5 × upper limit of normal)	PFS 89% at 5 years OS 92% at 5 years	Normal AFP, any HCG, any LDH	PFS 82% at 5 years OS 86% at 5 years
Intermediate prognosis	Testis or retroperitoneal primary AND No nonpulmonary visceral metastases AND	28% of patients	Any primary site AND Nonpulmonary visceral metastases AND	10% of patients
	Intermediate markers (AFP 1,000–10,000 ng/ml or HCG 5,000–50,000 IU/l or LDH 1.5–10 × upper limit of normal)	PFS 75% at 5 years OS 80% at 5 years	Normal AFP, any HCG, any LDH	PFS 67% at 5 years OS 72% at 5 years
Poor prognosis	Mediastinal primary OR Nonpulmonary visceral metastases OR	16% of patients		
	Poor markers (AFP >10,000 ng/ml or HCG >50,000 IU/l or LDH >10 × upper limit of normal)	PFS 41% at 5 years OS 48% at 5 years		

Abbreviations: AFP, alpha-fetoprotein; HCG, human chorionic gonadotropin; LDH, lactic dehydrogenase.

cell tumors involved single agent etoposide or etoposide and cyclophosphamide (Blijham *et al.*, 1981; Mulder *et al.*, 1988; Wolff *et al.*, 1984). Although some patients were refractory to these agents in standard doses, 20% to 40% response rates and rare long-term cures were observed.

Most modern phase I/II trials of high-dose chemotherapy have included carboplatin and etoposide, sometimes with ifosfamide, cyclophosphamide, or thiotepa (Table 43.6). Several centers intended high-dose therapy to be repeated once after recovery (tandem transplants) to maximize potential benefit. Initial investigations focused on patients with either relapse after best standard salvage chemotherapies or cisplatin-refractory germ cell tumors who were felt unlikely to be cured by any available treatment. One of the first examples was the phase I/II study of two courses of high-dose carboplatin and etoposide in patients with germ cell tumors refractory to cisplatin (defined as progression on or within 4 weeks of the last cisplatin dose) or recurrent after primary cisplatin-based therapy and a salvage containing ifosfamide and cisplatin (Nichols *et al.*, 1989). The results were updated after the first 40 patients (Broun *et al.*, 1992). Over half of the patients had received 3 or more prior regimens and 70% were considered cisplatin-refractory. Therapy consisted of carboplatin 900 to 2,000 mg/m^2 and etoposide 1,200 mg/m^2. Ifosfamide was added to the regimen in 3 patients. Twenty-six of 40 (65%) received both courses of high-dose therapy. Overall, 7 of 40

(18%) died as a consequence of therapy, primarily due to infection. There were 12 patients (30%) who obtained a complete response and 14 (35%) who obtained a partial response, for an overall response rate of 65%. Six patients (15%) were long-term disease-free survivors, and a seventh patient died at 22 months free of germ cell tumor from a therapy-related acute myeloid leukemia. These results were confirmed in a phase II multi-institutional trial of similar patients receiving tandem high-dose carboplatin and etoposide, where 58% completed both transplants, a 13% treatment-related mortality was observed, 9 patients (24%) achieved a complete remission (2 after posttransplant surgical resections), and 5 patients (13%) were alive and free of disease with a minimum of 18 months follow-up (Nichols *et al.*, 1992).

Several features merit emphasis from this and similar early series. First, a portion of patients (perhaps 13% to 24%) with multiply recurrent germ cell tumors can achieve long-term disease-free survival with high-dose chemotherapy and hematopoietic stem cell transplantation. Second, nearly all relapses occur in the first 18 months posttransplant and disease status after high-dose therapy predicts long-term outcome. Third, in this series, the tandem approach was supported. In the phase I/II study, all of the long-term disease-free survivors received both transplants and 8 of 12 patients in partial remission after the first transplant achieved complete remission after the second transplant. The value of tandem cycles, however,

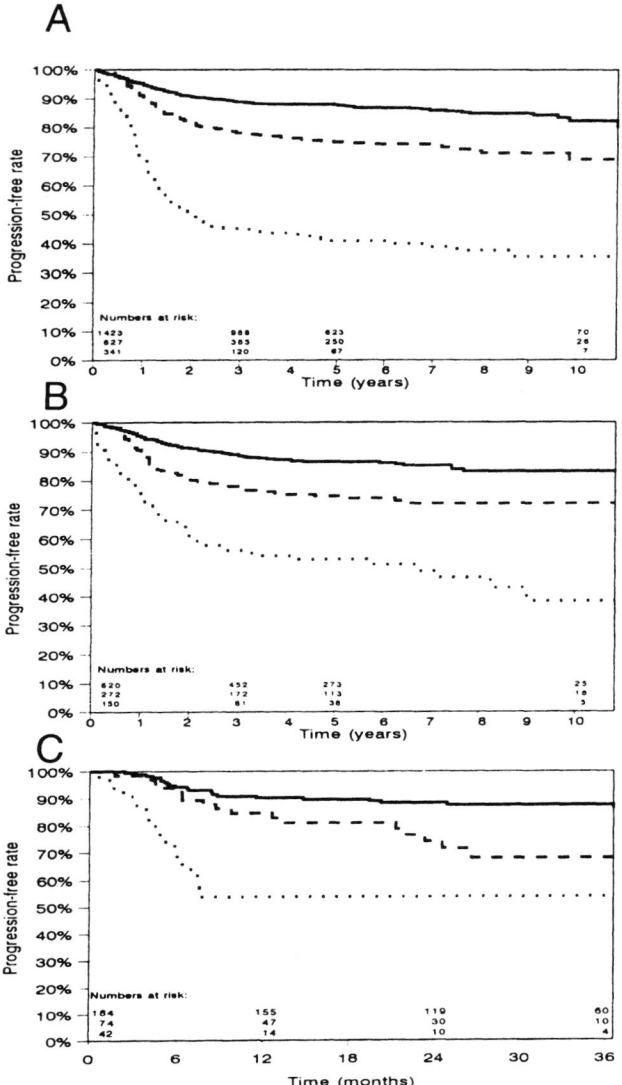

Fig. 43.1. (**A**) PFS rates in the "test" data set according to the IGCCC (—, good prognosis; - - -, intermediate prognosis; ..., poor prognosis). (**B**) PFS rates in the "validation" data set according to the IGCCC (—, good prognosis; - - -, intermediate prognosis; ..., poor prognosis). (**C**) PFS rates in the recent MRC/EORTC data set according to the IGCCC (—, good prognosis; - - -, intermediate prognosis; ..., poor prognosis). Reproduced, with permission from Group IGCCC (1997).

remains to be proven in a randomized trial. Fourth, surgical salvage remained an important treatment modality after transplant, leading to complete remissions and likely contributing to cures in several patients. Lastly, patients with primary mediastinal germ cell tumors failed to respond, with 0 of 8 patients in the phase I/II study and 0 of 11 patients in the phase II study achieving a complete remission. This is a population for whom conventional salvage therapies also have poor outcomes and such patients should be the focus of investigational approaches (Broun *et al.*, 1991; Saxman *et al.*, 1994).

Table 43.5. *Possible indications for high-dose chemotherapy in the management of germ cell tumors*

Salvage therapy for multiply relapsed or refractory germ cell tumor (GCT)	A small proportion of (otherwise incurable) patients will be cured.
Initial salvage for relapsed GCT	Single center studies suggest there may be a role. Currently being examined in European prospective randomized trial.
Primary treatment for poor-risk GCT	Role unclear. Currently being examined in North American prospective randomized trial.
Treatment for failure to achieve a complete remission	Suboptimal decline/plateau in serum tumor markers (see text). Persistent clinical disease (see text).

Subsequent trials of high-dose therapy began to enroll less heavily pretreated patients and incorporated the use of peripheral blood stem cells and growth factors, which all served to shorten the duration of cytopenia. These improvements led investigators to attempt further dose escalations or add additional agents such as ifosfamide or cyclophosphamide. One trial of dose escalation involved treating 33 patients with relapsed or refractory germ cell tumors with carboplatin, 1,650 to 2,100 mg/m^2 and etoposide 1,200 to 2,250 mg/m^2 for 2 tandem cycles (Broun *et al.*, 1995). The dose-limiting toxicities for this regimen were mucositis and peripheral neurotoxicity, and reversible transaminitis was common. Results were similar to earlier studies, with 20 of 33 patients (61%) completing both transplants, and a treatment-related mortality of 18%. Four of 29 evaluable patients (14%) achieved complete remission and 8 of 33 (24%) were long-term survivors.

The German Testicular Cancer Study Group added ifosfamide up to 10 g/m^2 to carboplatin 1,500 to 2,000 mg/m^2 and etoposide 1,200 to 2,400 mg/m^2 as a transplant regimen in 74 patients with relapsed or refractory germ cell tumors (Siegert *et al.*, 1994; Beyer *et al.*, 1997). Therapy was delivered regardless of response to 2 proceeding cycles of re-induction standard-dose cisplatin, etoposide, and ifosfamide. Treatment-related mortality was only 3%, but late toxicities included renal toxicity (21%), paresthesias (29%), and ototoxicity (18%). Approximately 50% of patients achieved a complete remission with this therapy, and 28 of 74 (38%) were alive from 3.2 to 5.6 years posttreatment.

In reviewing these trials, it is important to recognize the large variability in inclusion criteria, making comparisons of results difficult. A series from Margolin *et al.* (1996) with a long-term disease-free survival of 45% included 40% of patients treated during initial salvage (Fig. 43.2). Ayash *et al.* (2001) reported a 17% long-term disease-free survival but included only 10% of patients treated during initial salvage, and included 48% of patients with cisplatin-refractory disease including 34% who were absolutely refractory (having never achieved even stable disease on a cisplatin-containing regimen).

Table 43.6. *Selected phase I/II trials: relapsed/refractory disease*

Author	Patients	Therapy	Response	Survival	Comments
Mulder *et al.*, 1988	11 relapsed or refractory	Etoposide 2,500 mg/m^2, cyclophosphamide 7 g/m^2 ($n = 3$) Or Etoposide 2,500 mg/m^2, then: Etoposide 2,000 mg/m^2, cyclo-phosphamide 7 g/m^2 ($n = 8$)	RR 64% CR 18%	OS 18% at 66–72 weeks DFS 9% at 66 weeks TRM 0%	
Nichols *et al.*, 1989; Broun *et al.*, 1992	40 relapsed or refractory	Carboplatin 900–2,000 mg/m^2 etoposide 1,200 mg/m^2 (Ifosfamide added for 3 pts) (tandem)	RR 65% CR 30%	OS 15% at >24 months TRM 18%	10% initial salvage, 70% cisplatin-refractory 8 pts with mediastinal primary 26 pts received both transplants
Drroz *et al.*, 1991	17 relapsed or refractory	Salvage chemotherapy, then: Cisplatin 200 mg/m^2, etoposide 1,750 mg/m^2, cyclophospha-mide 6,400 mg/m^2	CR 50%	DFS 24% at 68–74 months TRM 6%	65% cisplatin-refractory
Nichols (ECOG) *et al.*, 1992	38 relapsed or refractory	Carboplatin 1,500 mg/m^2, etoposide 1,200 mg/m^2 (tandem)	RR 45% CR 24%	DFS 13% at >12 months TRM 13%	13% initial salvage, 50% cisplatin-refractory 11 pts with mediastinal primary 22 pts received both transplants
Motzer *et al.*, 1992	13 relapsed or refractory	Carboplatin 1,500 mg/m^2, etoposide 1,200 mg/m^2, cyclophosphamide 90–150 mg/kg (tandem)	CR 46%	DFS 23% at 8–24 months TRM 3%	62% cisplatin-refractory 13 pts received both transplants
Broun *et al.*, 1995	33 relapsed or refractory	Carboplatin 1,650–2,100 mg/m^2, etoposide 1,200–2,250 mg/m^2 (tandem)	RR 18/29 (64%) CR 4/29 (14%)	OS 8/33 (24%) at 10–30 mo, TRM 6/33 (18%) 4 pts with mediastinal primary	12% initial salvage, 21% cisplatin-refractory 20 pts received both transplants
Motzer, 1996	58 relapsed or refractory	Carboplatin 1,500 mg/m^2, etoposide 1,200 mg/m^2, cyclophosphamide 60–150 mg/kg (tandem)	CR 40%	OS 29% at 10–65 months DFS 21% at 16–65 months TRM 12%	17% initial salvage, 57% cisplatin-refractory (21% absolute) 7 pts with extragonadal primary 27 pts received both transplants
Margolin *et al.*, 1996	20 relapsed or refractory	1) Ifosfamide 6 g/m^2, carboplatin 1,200 mg/m^2, etoposide 60 mg/kg 2) Ifosfamide 9 g/m^2, carbo-platin 1,200 mg/m^2, etoposide 60 mg/kg (tandem)	RR 60%	DFS 45% at 23–70 months TRM 0%	40% initial salvage, 0% cisplatin-refractory 8 pts with extragonadal primary 18 pts received both transplants
Siegert *et al.*, 1994; Beyer *et al.*, 1997	74 relapsed or refractory	Salvage cisplatin, etoposide, and ifosfamide × 2, then: Carboplatin 1,500–2,000 mg/m^2, etoposide 1,200–2,400 mg/m^2, ifosfamide 0–10 g/m^2	CR 51% (at first report)	OS 38% at 3.2–5.6 years DFS 31% at 3.2–5.6 years TRM 3%	8% initial salvage, 32% cisplatin-refractory 17 pts with extragonadal primary (5 mediastinal)
Mandanas, 1998	21 relapsed or refractory	Various regimens (including cyclophosphamide and a platinum)	RR 79%	DFS 52% at 4–10 years TRM 7%	5% initial salvage, 43% cisplatin-refractory

(Continues)

Table 43.6.   *Continued*

Author	Patients	Therapy	Response	Survival	Comments
Ayash *et al.*, 2001	29 relapsed or refractory	Carboplatin 1,500–2,100 mg/m^2, etoposide 1,200–2,250 mg/m^2 (tandem)	RR 38% CR 10%	Median OS 14 months DFS 17% PFS 28% at 31–93 months TRM 10%	10% initial salvage, 48% cisplatin-refractory (34% absolute) All testis or retroperitoneal primary 15 pts received both transplants tandems
Rick, 2001	80 relapsed or refractory	Salvage paclitaxel, ifosfamide, and cisplatin (TIP) × 3, then: (*n* = 23) paclitaxel, ifosfamide mobilization, then: Carboplatin 1,500 mg/m^2, etoposide 2,400 mg/m^2, thiotepa 450–750 mg/m^2 (CET)	RR 69% to TIP RR 66% to CET	OS 33% at 22–46 months DFS 26% at 22–46 months TRM 3%	67% initial salvage, 11% absolute cisplatin-refractory 3 pts with mediastinal primary 62 pts received both transplants

Abbreviations: RR, response rate; CR, complete response rate; OS, overall survival; DFS, disease-free survival; PFS, progression-free survival; TRM, treatment-related mortality.

This heterogeneity led investigators to compile pooled data to identify prognostic variables for response and survival in male patients with relapsed or refractory germ cell tumors treated with high-dose chemotherapy (Beyer *et al.*, 1996). Three hundred and ten patients from four centers in the United States and Europe were retrospectively evaluated and data on 283 patients were complete. Overall, the treatment-related mortality was 8%. Fifty-five percent of patients achieved a favorable response (complete remission or partial remission with negative tumor markers), and 47% of those patients later relapsed. The actuarial overall survival rate was 51% at 1, 36% at 2, and 30% at 3 years, respectively. Multivariate analysis identified progressive disease before transplant, mediastinal nonseminomatous primary tumor, refractory or absolute refractory disease to conventional-dose cisplatin, and human chorionic gonadotropin (HCG) levels greater than 1,000 IU/l before transplant as independent adverse

prognostic factors. Importantly, response to first-line therapy did not predict outcomes. These variables were used to identify patients with good, intermediate, or poor prognoses with predicted failure-free survival rates at 2 years of 51%, 27%, and 5%, respectively (Table 43.7, Fig. 43.3).

In summary, the use of high-dose chemotherapy with autologous hematopoietic stem cell transplantation for the treatment of relapsed or refractory germ cell tumors can produce long-term survivors in roughly 15% to 40% of patients. The principal toxicities include nephrotoxicity, peripheral neurotoxicity, transaminitis, and gonadal toxicity. Treatment-related mortality rates range from 0 to 18%, with most recent series reporting 3% to 5%. Patients with primary mediastinal tumors do not benefit from salvage high-dose therapy. Treatment earlier in the course of relapsed or refractory disease appears to be associated with better outcomes.

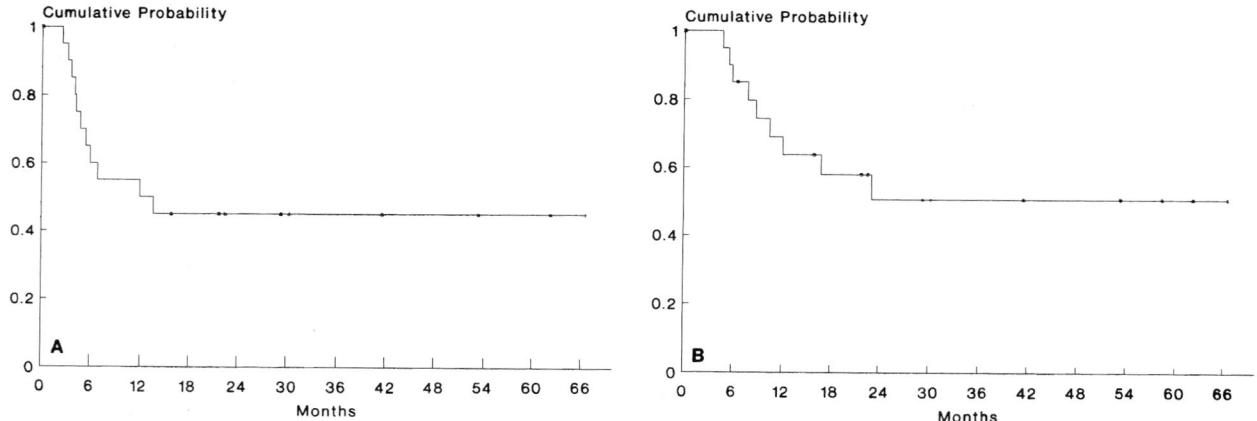

Fig. 43.2. (**A**) Disease-free survival of the 20 study patients, calculated from the time of completion of protocol therapy. (**B**) Overall survival of the 20 study patients, calculated from the time of completion of protocol therapy. Reproduced, with permission, from Margolin *et al.* (1996).

Table 43.7. *Beyer Prognostic Score for survival after high-dose salvage chemotherapy*

Factor	Score	Risk	2 yr FFS	2 yr OS
Progressive disease before transplant	1	Good (score 0)	51%	61%
Primary mediastinal tumor	1	Intermediate (score 1–2)	27%	34%
Cisplatin-refractory before transplant	1	Poor (score >2)	5%	8%
Absolute cisplatin-refractory before transplant	2			
HCG > 1,000 IU/l before transplant	2			

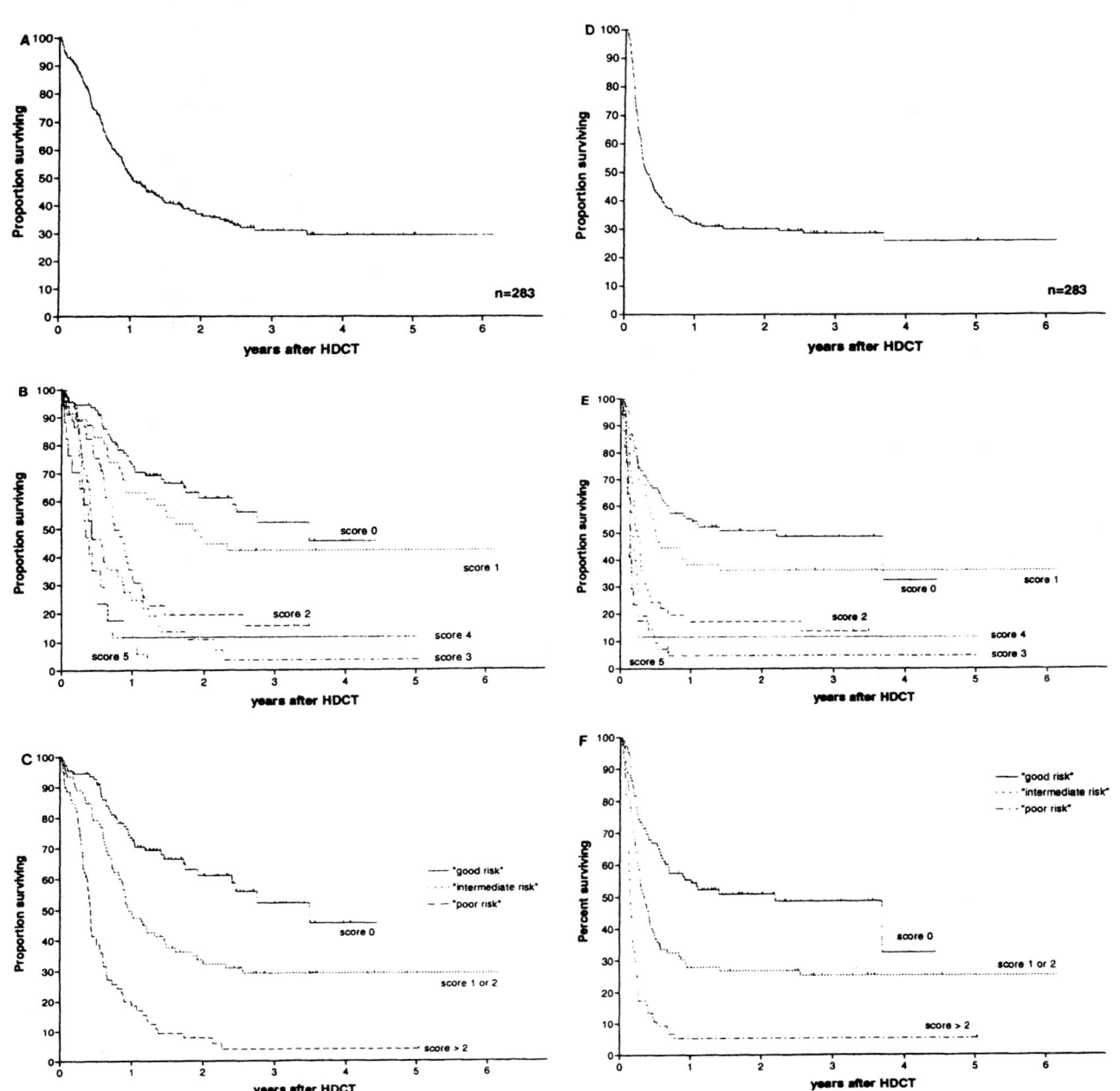

Fig. 43.3. Overall survival (left) and FFS (right) plotted according to (**A** and **D**) study population, (**B** and **E**) scores, and (**C** and **F**) prognostic categories. Reproduced, with permission, from Beyer *et al.* (1996).

Initial salvage and primary treatment with high-dose chemotherapy for germ cell tumors

The modest results of standard-dose salvage chemotherapies (24% long-term disease-free survival with VeIP discussed above) combined with improving rates of durable responses and decreasing morbidity and mortality associated with high-dose therapy have led to the investigation of high-dose therapy

for initial salvage of relapsed germ cell tumors (Table 43.8). The largest published experience is from Indiana University, where 65 patients with relapsed or persistent testicular cancer were given initial salvage treatment with 2 tandem courses of carboplatin 2,100 mg/m^2 and etoposide 2,250 mg/m^2 followed by autologous hematopoietic stem cell rescue (Bhatia *et al.*, 2000). All patients had primary testicular tumors. Fifty-six of the 65 patients (86%) received at least one cycle of standard-

Table 43.8. *Phase I/II trials: initial salvage/first-line therapy*

Author	Patients	Therapy	Response	Survival	Comments
Droz, 1992	28 poor risk (first-line)	2 cycles mPVeBV, then: Cisplatin 200 mg/m^2, etoposide 1,750 mg/m^2, cyclophosphamide 6,400 mg/m^2	CR 61%	DFS 43% at 7–72 months TRM 7%	9 pts with extragonadal primary 21 pts proceeded to transplant
Motzer *et al.*, 1992; Motzer, *et al.*, 1993	28 poor risk (first-line)	VAB-6 × 2 cycles, then: VAB-6 × 2 cycles (n = 5) OR Etoposide 1,200 mg/m^2, carboplatin 1,500 mg/m^2, (tandem) (n = 22)	RR 96% CR 56% VAB-6 alone: CR 60% Transplant: CR 55%	OS 57% at 2.5–47 months DFS 46% at 2.5–47 months TRM 4%	14 of 22 received both transplants
Barnett, 1993	21 poor risk or relapsed (first-line n = 6) (initial salvage n = 15)	(1) HIPE × 5–11 cycles, then: Ifosfamide 6 g/m^2, etoposide 3 g/m^2, carboplatin 1.2 g/m^2 OR (2) HIPE × 5 cycles, VIP × 1–2 cycles, then: Cyclophosphamide 7.2 g/m^2, etoposide 2.4 g/m^2, carboplatin 0.8 g/m^2		First-line: EFS 50% Salvage: EFS 73% EFS 67% at 6–78 months TRM 10%	Renal and mucosal toxicity prompted Regimen (2)
Broun, 1994	23 relapsed (initial salvage)	VeIP or VeBP × 2 cycles, then: Etoposide 1,200–2,250 mg/m^2, carboplatin 150–2,100 mg/m^2	Induction: RR 87% CR 35% Transplant: RR 83% CR 56%	Transplant: OS 50% at 10–36 months EFS 39% at 10–33 months TRM 4% (induction)	18 pts proceeded to transplant
Motzer *et al.*, 1997	30 poor risk (first-line)	VIP × 2 cycles, then: VIP × 2 more cycles (n = 16) OR Carboplatin 1,800 mg/m^2, etoposide 1,800 mg/m^2, cyclophosphamide 150 mg/kg (tandem) (n = 14)	Initial VIP: CR 57% VIP × 4: RR 81%, CR 63% Transplant: CR 50%	OS 67% at 15–47 months DFS 50% at 16–47 months TRM 0%	7 pts with mediastinal primary 9 of 14 received both transplants
Bokemeyer *et al.*, 1998	141 poor risk (first-line)	4 cycles in 8 escalating dose levels to maximum: Cisplatin 125–150 mg/m^2, etoposide 550–1,250 mg/m^2, ifosfamide 6–10 g/m^2		OS 78% at 2 years PFS 73% at 2 years Early death 8%	Transplant support used for dose levels 3–8 Analysis based on levels 1–5
Broun, 1997; Bhatia, *et al.*, 2000	65 relapsed (initial salvage)	Carboplatin 2,100 mg/m^2, etoposide 2,250 mg/m^2 (tandem)	RR 88% CR 43% Additional CR after chemo (n=1) or surgery (n=13)	Chemo: DFS 57% at 16–91 months DFS 62% TRM 0%	Excluded pts with extragonadal primary 86% received initial standard chemotherapy 26 pts received both transplants Gene therapy and maintenance oral etoposide used

Abbreviations: mPVeBV, modified cisplatin, vinblastine, bleomycin, etoposide; VAB-6, cisplatin, vinblastine, bleomycin, cyclophosphamide, dactinomycin; HIPE, high-intensity cisplatin-etoposide; VIP, etoposide, ifosfamide, cisplatin; VeIP, vinblastine, ifosfamide, cisplatin; VeBP, vinblastine, bleomycin, cisplatin; RR, response rate; CR, complete response rate; OS, overall survival; DFS, disease-free survival; EFS, event-free survival; PFS, progression-free survival; TRM, treatment-related mortality.

dose salvage chemotherapy (usually VeIP) prior to transplant. Ten of 65 (15%) received ex vivo cytokine-stimulated, mdr-1 transduced autologous CD34-positive stem cells and 26 of 65 (40%) received posttransplant maintenance oral etoposide. Using the Beyer prognostic score for outcomes with high-dose therapy (Table 43.7), 61% were good risk, 31% intermediate risk, and 8% poor risk. There were no treatment-related deaths. A complete remission was achieved in 28 patients (43%) with high-dose chemotherapy and in another 1 patient with additional VeIP after only one transplant and 13 patients (20%) with posttransplant surgical resections. With follow-up ranging 16 to 91 months, 37 patients (57%) were continuously disease-free and 40 (60%) remain disease-free after definitive therapy.

Reports of high-dose therapy and autologous HSC transplantation as salvage treatment for pure seminomas are scarce (Rick et al., 2002; Vuky et al., 2002), but one study of 13 patients described a 38% survival rate with a median follow-up of 4.5 years after a high-dose regimen of one cycle of carboplatin, and etoposide in combination with either ifosfamide or thiotepa in patients who had either failed cisplatin-based first-line treatments or cisplatin-based salvage treatments (Rick et al., 2002).

Another prognostic scoring system may be of use when interpreting the results of high-dose chemotherapy trials in patients who progress after platinum-based induction chemotherapy with or without surgery (Table 43.9) (Fossa et al., 1999). One hundred sixty-four patients were treated with "conventional" platinum-based chemotherapy. Multivariate analysis of prognostic factors demonstrated progression-free interval, response to induction treatment, and the level of serum HCG and AFP at relapse to be significant. A poor-prognosis group was identified in which none of 30 patients survived after 3 years. In contrast, the good-prognosis group consisted of 94 patients who had a 47% 5-year survival, including 38 patients with a progression-free interval of greater than 2 years who had a 61% 5-year survival. Validation with an independent data set gave 5-year survivals for good and poor-prognosis patients of 51% and 0%, respectively.

Incorporating high-dose chemotherapy as first-line for the treatment of patients with poor-risk germ cell tumors at presentation has also been investigated. One randomized trial of high-dose chemotherapy with autologous transplant support for the treatment of patients with poor-risk germ cell tumors failed to show a benefit (Chevreau et al., 1993). In this trial, patients deemed poor-risk were randomized either to receive 4 cycles of cisplatin 200 mg/m², vinblastine, etoposide, and bleomycin

(PVeVB) or to receive 2 cycles of PVeVB plus one cycle of high-dose therapy including cisplatin 200 mg/m² followed by autologous transplantation. This study has been criticized because the four-drug regimen is not considered a standard therapy, the dose-intensity and total cisplatin dose were lower in the "high-dose" arm, and a substantial number of patients randomized to the high-dose arm did not receive that therapy (Motzer et al., 1997; Bokemeyer et al., 1998).

One strategy for incorporating high-dose chemotherapy in the first-line therapy of patients with germ cell tumors has been to stratify poor-risk patients based on the observed decline in serum tumor markers with the first 2 cycles of standard chemotherapy (Toner et al., 1990). In two published phase II trials, patients whose serum markers were either rising or not falling according to their predicted serum half-life (prolonged half-life by >7 days for AFP and >3 days for HCG) were switched to treatment with high-dose chemotherapy. The first trial of 28 patients studied standard-dose cisplatin, vinblastine, bleomycin, cyclophosphamide, and dactinomycin (VAB-6) with or without 2 cycles of high-dose carboplatin 1,500 mg/m² and etoposide 1,200 mg/m² (Motzer et al., 1992, 1993). Twenty-two of 28 patients (79%) were treated with high-dose chemotherapy and transplant and the disease-free survival of 46% at 2.5 to 47 month follow-up compared favorably to earlier conventional dose trials in similar risk patients. These results led to the second trial with a similar design (Motzer et al., 1997). This trial changed the standard therapy to etoposide, ifosfamide, and cisplatin (VIP) and increased the high-dose therapy to carboplatin 1,800 mg/m², etoposide 1,800 mg/m², and cyclophosphamide 150 mg/kg. Thirty patients were enrolled in this trial, and 14 (47%) went on to high-dose therapy. There were no treatment-related deaths, and again a relatively favorable 50% long-term disease-free survival was noted.

An alternate strategy is being tested in a phase I trial of poor-risk nonseminomatous germ cell tumors in Germany (Bokemeyer et al., 1998). This trial is based on the front-line use of multiple high-dose cycles before drug resistance develops. Patients receive 4 consecutive cycles of cisplatin, etoposide, and ifosfamide (PEI) with granulocyte-macrophage colony-stimulating growth factor (GM-CSF) support in the initial 2 dose intensity levels, or granulocyte colony-stimulating factor (G-CSF) and peripheral blood stem cell support in dose levels 3 to 8. Data were reported on the first 141 patients treated at dose levels 1 through 5 (cisplatin 150 mg/m², etopo-

Table 43.9. *Fossa Prognostic Score for survival after standard-dose salvage chemotherapy*

Factors	Risk		
Progression-free interval < 2 years	Good (< 3 factors)	47% OS at 5 yr	Progression-free > 2 yr: OS 74% at 2 yr Progression-free <2 yr: OS 45% at 2 yr
Less than complete response to induction therapy AFP > 100 kU/l or HCG > 100 IU/l	Poor (3 factors)	0% OS at 3 yr	

side 1,250 mg/m^2, and ifosfamide 10 g/m^2). The treatment-related death rate was 8%. After a median follow-up of 2.6 years, the 2-year survival rate was 78% and the progression-free survival rate was 73%.

In the absence of randomized trial data, a multivariate and matched-pair analysis was performed on data from 3 large controlled clinical trials to compare first-line high-dose chemotherapy to standard-dose chemotherapy in males with advanced, poor-risk germ cell tumors (Bokemeyer et al., 1999c). Multivariate analysis of 423 patients demonstrated superiority of first-line high-dose therapy compared to standard-dose therapy for both progression-free survival (75% versus 62%, P = .002) and overall survival (81% versus 73%, P = .021) when adjusted for available prognostic factors. A matched-pair analysis of 147 patients from each therapy estimated a 2-year overall survival of 82% and progression-free survival of 72% among recipients of high-dose therapy versus 71% (P = .0184) and 59% (P = .0056), respectively, among recipients of standard-dose therapy.

Whether the results of these initial trials of high-dose chemotherapy in the setting of initial salvage or primary treatment of poor-risk disease represent a true therapeutic advance is now being tested in randomized clinical trials.

Ongoing studies and future directions

Two important randomized trials are investigating the role of high-dose therapy in the treatment of patients with germ cell tumors. In the United States, the issue of primary therapy for poor-risk disease is being addressed in an intergroup cooperative study by randomizing patients to receive either 4 cycles of bleomycin, etoposide, and cisplatin (BEP) or 2 cycles of BEP followed by 2 cycles of high-dose carboplatin, etoposide, and cyclophosphamide. In Europe, initial salvage therapy is being assessed by randomizing patients on first relapse to either 4 cycles of standard cisplatin, etoposide, and ifosfamide salvage or to 3 cycles of this standard salvage followed by high-dose carboplatin, etoposide, and cyclophosphamide. These trials are nearing the completion of accrual and analysis is imminent.

Newer compounds with single-agent response rates are being incorporated into trials including paclitaxel, gemcitabine, bendamustine, and oxaliplatin (Bokemeyer et al., 1999a, 1999b; Kollmannsberger et al. 2000). Unique dosing strategies such as multiple cycles or alternating agents may be incorporated in future high-dose algorithms. Adjunctive agents may reduce the toxicity of high-dose therapy such as amifostine or keratinocyte growth factor (Cronin et al., 2000). Concern has been raised over the generation of secondary hematologic malignancies, particularly with the use of high-dose etoposide. However, in one series, the incidence of secondary leukemia among 302 recipients of autologous stem cell transplant with cumulative doses of greater than 2 g/m^2 of etoposide was only 1.3% (Kollmannsberger et al., 1998). Advances in adjuvant or maintenance therapies with oral etoposide or immunmodulators such as interleukins have been considered (Cooper & Einborn, 1995).

Ultimately, advances in the molecular understanding of germ cell malignancies may lead to targeted therapies.

Conclusions

In the United States today, high-dose carboplatin and etoposide-based chemotherapy with autologous transplantation is accepted as a standard therapy for patients with germ cell tumors who have failed two prior standard-dose regimens as well as a component of salvage therapy for poor-risk patients. Study of the potential role of high-dose therapy for the treatment of initial relapse or for primary treatment of poor-risk disease has been slowed by the few number of patients and the relative success of standard-dose therapy. Randomized trials are under way to clarify these issues, and new treatment designs and agents are being pursued.

References

Aass, N. et al. (1991). Prognostic factors in unselected patients with nonseminomatous metastatic testicular cancer: a multicenter experience. Journal of Clinical Oncology, 9, 818–26.

Anonymous. (1985). Prognostic factors in advanced non-seminomatous germ-cell testicular tumours: results of a multicentre study. Report from the Medical Research Council Working Party on Testicular Tumours. Lancet, 1, 8–11.

Anonymous. (1997a). International Germ Cell Consensus Classification: a prognostic factor-based staging system for metastatic germ cell cancers. International Germ Cell Cancer Collaborative Group. Journal of Clinical Oncology, 15, 594–603.

Anonymous. (1997b). Testis. In American Joint Committee on Cancer: AJCC Cancer Staging Manual. 5th ed. pp. 225–30. Philadelphia, PA: Lippincott-Raven Publishers.

Ayash, L.J. et al. (2001). Double dose-intensive chemotherapy with autologous stem cell support for relapsed and refractory testicular cancer: the University of Michigan experience and literature review. Bone Marrow Transplantation, 27, 939–47.

Beyer, J. et al. (1996). High-dose chemotherapy as salvage treatment in germ cell tumors: a multivariate analysis of prognostic variables. Journal of Clinical Oncology, 14, 2638–45.

Beyer, J. et al. (1997). Long-term survival of patients with recurrent or refractory germ cell tumors after high dose chemotherapy. Cancer, 79, 161–8.

Bhatia, S. et al. (2000). High-dose chemotherapy as initial salvage chemotherapy in patients with relapsed testicular cancer. Journal of Clinical Oncology, 18, 3346–51.

Birch, R. et al. (1986). Prognostic factors for favorable outcome in disseminated germ cell tumors. Journal of Clinical Oncology, 4, 400–7.

Blijham, G. et al. (1981). The treatment of advanced testicular carcinoma with high dose chemotherapy and autologous marrow support. European Journal of Cancer, 17, 433–41.

Bokemeyer, C. et al. (1998). The use of dose-intensified chemotherapy in the treatment of metastatic nonseminomatous testicular germ cell tumors. German Testicular Cancer Study Group. Seminars in Oncology, 25, 24–32; discussion 45–8.

Bokemeyer, C. *et al.* (1999a). Gemcitabine in patients with relapsed or cisplatin-refractory testicular cancer. *Journal of Clinical Oncology*, **17**, 512–6.

Bokemeyer, C. *et al.* (1999b). Treatment of patients with cisplatin-refractory testicular germ-cell cancer. German Testicular Cancer Study Group (GTCSG). *International Journal of Cancer*, **83**, 848–51.

Bokemeyer, C. *et al.* (1999c). First-line high-dose chemotherapy compared with standard-dose PEB/VIP chemotherapy in patients with advanced germ cell tumors: a multivariate and matched-pair analysis. *Journal of Clinical Oncology*, **17**, 3450–6.

Bosl, G.J. *et al.* (1983). Multivariate analysis of prognostic variables in patients with metastatic testicular cancer. *Cancer Research*, **43**, 3403–7.

Bosl, G.J. & Motzer, R.J. (1997). Testicular germ-cell cancer. *New England Journal of Medicine*, **337**, 242–53.

Broun, E.R. *et al.* (1992). Long-term outcome of patients with relapsed and refractory germ cell tumors treated with high-dose chemotherapy and autologous bone marrow rescue. *Annals of Internal Medicine*, **117**, 124–8.

Broun, E.R. *et al.* (1995). Dose escalation study of high-dose carboplatin and etoposide with autologous bone marrow support in patients with recurrent and refractory germ cell tumors. *Bone Marrow Transplantation*, **16**, 353–8.

Broun, E.R., Nichols, C.R., Einhorn, L.H., & Tricot, G.J. (1991). Salvage therapy with high-dose chemotherapy and autologous bone marrow support in the treatment of primary nonseminomatous mediastinal germ cell tumors. *Cancer*, **68**, 1513–5.

Chevreau, C. *et al.* (1993). Early intensified chemotherapy with autologous bone marrow transplantation in first line treatment of poor risk non-seminomatous germ cell tumors. Preliminary results of a French randomized trial. *European Urology*, **23**, 213–7.

Cooper, M.A. & Einhorn, L.H. (1995). Maintenance chemotherapy with daily oral etoposide following salvage therapy in patients with germ cell tumors. *Journal of Clinical Oncology*, **13**, 1167–9.

Cronin, S. *et al.* (2000). Use of amifostine as a chemoprotectant during high-dose chemotherapy in autologous peripheral blood stem cell transplantation. *Bone Marrow Transplantation*, **26**, 1247–9.

Droz, J.P. *et al.* (1988). Prognostic factors in advanced nonseminomatous testicular cancer. A multivariate logistic regression analysis. *Cancer*, **62**, 564–8.

Fossa, S.D. *et al.* (1999). Prognostic factors in patients progressing after cisplatin-based chemotherapy for malignant non-seminomatous germ cell tumours. *British Journal of Cancer*, **80**, 1392–9.

Kollmannsberger, C. *et al.* (1998). Secondary leukemia following high cumulative doses of etoposide in patients treated for advanced germ cell tumors. *Journal of Clinical Oncology*, **16**, 3386–91.

Kollmannsberger, C. *et al.* (2000). Phase II study of bendamustine in patients with relapsed or cisplatin-refractory germ cell cancer. *Anticancer Drugs*, **11**, 535–9.

Loehrer, P.J., Sr. *et al.* (1988). Salvage therapy in recurrent germ cell cancer: ifosfamide and cisplatin plus either vinblastine or etoposide. *Annals of Internal Medicine*, **109**, 540–6.

Loehrer, P.J., Sr. *et al.* (1998). Vinblastine plus ifosfamide plus cisplatin as initial salvage therapy in recurrent germ cell tumor. *Journal of Clinical Oncology*, **16**, 2500–4.

Margolin, B.K. *et al.* (1996). Treatment of germ cell cancer with two cycles of high-dose ifosfamide, carboplatin, and etoposide with autologous stem-cell support. *Journal of Clinical Oncology*, **14**, 2631–7.

Mead, G.M. *et al.* (1992). The Second Medical Research Council study of prognostic factors in nonseminomatous germ cell tumors. Medical Research Council Testicular Tumour Working Party. *Journal of Clinical Oncology*, **10**, 85–94.

Mostofi, F.K., Sesterhenn, I.A., & Davis, C.J., Jr. (1988). Developments in histopathology of testicular germ cell tumors. *Seminars in Urology*, **6**, 171–88.

Motzer, R.J. *et al.* (1992). High-dose chemotherapy and autologous bone marrow rescue for patients with refractory germ cell tumors. Early intervention is better tolerated. *Cancer*, **69**, 550–6.

Motzer, R.J. *et al.* (1993). Phase II trial of high-dose carboplatin and etoposide with autologous bone marrow transplantation in first-line therapy for patients with poor-risk germ cell tumors. *Journal of the National Cancer Institute*, **85**, 1828–35.

Motzer, R.J. *et al.* (1997). High-dose carboplatin, etoposide and cyclophosphamide with autologous bone marrow transplantation in first-line therapy for patients with poor-risk germ cell tumors. *Journal of Clinical Oncology*, **15**, 2546–52.

Mulder, P.O. *et al.* (1988). Chemotherapy with maximally tolerable doses of VP 16-213 and cyclophosphamide followed by autologous bone marrow transplantation for the treatment of relapsed or refractory germ cell tumors. *European Journal of Cancer Clinical Oncology*, **24**, 675–9.

Murphy, B.R. *et al.* (1993). Surgical salvage of chemorefractory germ cell tumors. *Journal of Clinical Oncology*, **11**, 324–9.

Newlands, E.S. *et al.* (1986). Current optimum management of anaplastic germ cell tumours of the testis and other sites. *British Journal of Urology*, **58**, 307–14.

Nichols, C.R. *et al.* (1989). Dose-intensive chemotherapy in refractory germ cell cancer—a phase I/II trial of high-dose carboplatin and etoposide with autologous bone marrow transplantation. *Journal of Clinical Oncology*, **7**, 932–9.

Nichols, C.R. *et al.* (1991). Randomized study of cisplatin dose intensity in poor-risk germ cell tumors: a Southeastern Cancer Study Group and Southwest Oncology Group protocol. *Journal of Clinical Oncology*, **9**, 1163–72.

Nichols, C.R. *et al.* (1992). High-dose carboplatin and etoposide with autologous bone marrow transplantation in refractory germ cell cancer: an Eastern Cooperative Oncology Group protocol. *Journal of Clinical Oncology*, **10**, 558–63.

Peckham, M.J., McElwain, T.J., Barrett, A., & Hendry, W.F. (1979). Combined management of malignant teratoma of the testis. *Lancet*, **2**, 267–70.

Rick, O., Siegert, W., Schwella, N. *et al.* (2002). High-dose chemotherapy as salvage treatment for seminoma. *Bone Marrow Transplantation*, **30**, 157–60.

Samuels, M.L., Holoye, P.Y., & Johnson, D.E. (1975). Bleomycin combination chemotherapy in the management of testicular neoplasia. *Cancer*, **36**, 318–26.

Saxman, S.B., Nichols, C.R., & Einhorn, L.H. (1994). Salvage chemotherapy in patients with extragonadal nonseminomatous germ cell tumors: the Indiana University experience. *Journal of Clinical Oncology*, **12**, 1390–3.

Siegert, W. *et al.* (1994). High-dose treatment with carboplatin, etoposide, and ifosfamide followed by autologous stem-cell transplantation in relapsed or refractory germ cell cancer: a phase I/II study. The German Testicular Cancer Cooperative Study Group. *Journal of Clinical Oncology,* **12,** 1223–31.

Stoter, G. *et al.* (1987). Multivariate analysis of prognostic factors in patients with disseminated nonseminomatous testicular cancer: results from a European Organization for Research on Treatment of Cancer Multiinstitutional Phase III Study. *Cancer Research,* **47,** 2714–8.

Toner, G.C. *et al.* (1990). Serum tumor marker half-life during chemotherapy allows early prediction of complete response and survival in nonseminomatous germ cell tumors. *Cancer Research,* **50,** 5904–10.

Vuky, J., Tickoo, S. K., Sheinfeld, J. *et al.* (2002). Salvage chemotherapy for patients with advanced pure seminoma. *Journal of Clinical Oncology,* **20,** 297–301.

Williams, S.D. *et al.* (1987). Treatment of disseminated germ-cell tumors with cisplatin, bleomycin, and either vinblastine or etoposide. *New England Journal of Medicine,* **316,** 1435–40.

Wolff, S.N., Johnson, D.H., Hainsworth, J.D., & Greco, F.A. (1984). High-dose VP-16-213 monotherapy for refractory germinal malignancies: a phase II study. *Journal of Clinical Oncology,* **2,** 271–4.

44 Autologous hematopoietic stem cell transplantation for ovarian cancer

SAM MILLIKEN

St Vincent's Hospital, Sydney, Australia

Introduction

In the past several decades positive results using high-dose therapy with autologous blood or marrow stem cell transplantation for hematologic malignancies have invigorated interest for similar approaches in the management of solid tumors including ovarian carcinoma.

Ovarian cancer is a common malignancy affecting women predominantly over the age of 50 with a median age of 62 years (Neijt *et al.,* 1995). Reports of reduced toxicity of autologous hematopoietic stem cell (HSC) transplantation [with mortality figures approaching 1% for patients 65 years of age and less (Legros *et al.,* 1997; Stiff *et al.,* 1997)] indicate that the majority of such women would be suitable for consideration of a high-dose, intensive approach if proven effective. Premature death from this disease has a considerable social and economic impact on society. It is a common cancer in industrialized societies, ranking as the fifth most common cause of female death in the United States and the leading cause of death from gynecologic malignancy (Silverberg, Boring, & Squires, 1990). In the United States, 20,000 women develop the disease annually, and 12,500 die. Risk is increased in women with early menarche, late menopause, high dietary fats, and use of talc as a perineal dusting powder. There is also a genetic link in families with a high incidence of breast and ovarian cancers. Risk is decreased in women who have used oral contraceptives, had multiple pregnancies, and breast fed.

The large majority of ovarian cancers are epithelial carcinomas. Epithelial tumors of the ovary may be cystadenocarcinoma (42%), mucinous cystadenocarcinoma (12%), endometrial carcinoma (15%), undifferentiated carcinoma (17%), or clear cell carcinoma (6%). Epithelial carcinoma of the ovary arises from surface epithelial cells that cover the ovary, which then invaginate into the parenchyma of the ovary. The tumor may remain confined to the ovary for some time or spread by exfoliation into the peritoneal cavity or via lymphatics. Hematologic spread to parenchymal organs or bone may occur in more advanced stages. Disease staging requires surgery with removal of the primary tumor, multiple blind biopsies, peritoneal cytology, and a meticulous and thorough intraoperative search for disease throughout the pelvis and abdomen. Serologic markers of disease include carbohydrate antigen 125 (CA-125), CEA, and occasionally β-HCG. The serum concentration of CA-125 is greater than 35 U/ml in 80% of women with carcinoma of the ovary. Among patients with carcinoma that has disseminated beyond the ovary, 90% have serum concentrations greater than 35 U/ml; only 50% of patients whose disease is confined to the ovary are positive for CA-125.

More than 70% of women present with advanced disease (FIGO stage II or greater), requiring surgery and chemotherapy to achieve modest survival benefits. With aggressive surgical debulking and platinum-based chemotherapy, 20% to 30% of stage III patients (Neijt *et al.,* 1991; Ozols & Young, 1991; Alberts *et al.,* 1992; Runowicz, 1992; McGuire *et al.,* 1996) and only 5% of stage IV patients (Ozols, 1994; Berek & Hacker, 1985; Richardson *et al.,* 1985) will survive 5 years (Table 44.1). The addition of taxanes (e.g., paclitaxel, taxotere) to these protocols has only modestly improved these figures (McGuire *et al.,* 1996).

A number of factors have led investigators to examine the application of high-dose chemotherapy and autologous HSC transplantation for advanced (FIGO stages IIB to IV) ovarian cancer. These tumors are chemoresponsive with modest improvement in cure rates for patients given conventional dose therapies following surgical resection of advanced disease (Ozols, 1992). Early data supported a dose-response relationship for relapsed ovarian carcinoma (Levin & Hryniuk, 1987). Relapse is often limited to the abdominal cavity and strategies to debulk such disease with further surgery and/or radiotherapy may salvage some patients or provide improved remission from disease (Mychalczak & Fuks, 1992; Rubin, 1992). Involvement of marrow and peripheral blood stem cell products appears uncommon (McGuire, 1992; Ross *et al.,* 1995). Chemotherapy agents effective at conventional dosages such as melphalan, cyclophosphamide, carboplatin, and etoposide are suitable agents for dose-escalation protocols, as their major dose-limiting toxicity is marrow suppression (McGuire, 1992). These characteristics suggest that strategies to escalate effective chemotherapy dosages by as much as five- to tenfold beyond standard doses, may be beneficial.

Table 44.1. *Staging of ovarian cancer and survival with conventional therapy*

FIGO stage[a]	5-year survival
I Limited to ovaries	75–80%
IA One ovary involved, no ascites, capsule intact	
IB Both ovaries involved, no ascites, capsule intact	
IC IA or IB and tumor on surface of ovary or ruptured capsule or malignant cells in peritoneal wash or ascites present with malignant cells.	
II Pelvic extension	60–65%
IIA Pelvic wall extension	
IIB Extension to uterus or tubes	
IIC IIA or IIB and tumor on surface of ovary or ruptured capsule or malignant cells in peritoneal wash or ascites present with malignant cells	
III Peritoneal implants or positive retroperitoneal or inguinal nodes (liver capsule metastasis = stage III)	20–30%
IIIA Microscopic seeding of abdominal peritoneal surface	
IIIB Abdominal peritoneal implants not exceeding 2 cm	
IIIC Abdominal peritoneal implants exceeding 2 cm or positive retroperitoneal or inguinal nodes	
IV Distant metastasis (liver parenchymal metastasis = stage IV; pleural effusion must have malignant cells to be stage IV).	

[a] FIGO, International Federation of Gynecology and Obstetrics.

Table 44.2. *Possible indications for high-dose chemotherapy and autologous HSC transplantation in the management of ovarian cancer*

1. Consolidation therapy for advanced disease (FIGO stage II–IV) achieving minimal tumor burden at second-look surgery
Currently being examined in North American prospective randomized study (conventional dose platinum/paclitaxel versus high-dose platinum/mitoxantrone/cyclophosphamide), and in a French prospective randomized study (conventional dose carboplatin/cyclophosphamide versus high-dose carboplatin/cyclophosphamide).
2. Consolidation therapy for advanced disease with bulky tumor at second-look laparotomy
No evidence that high-dose chemotherapy/autotransplant prolongs survival. Role controversial.
3. Salvage therapy for relapsed disease
No evidence that high-dose chemotherapy/autotransplant prolongs survival. Role controversial.
4. Salvage therapy for disease refractory to conventional chemotherapy
No evidence that high-dose chemotherapy/autotransplant prolongs survival. Role controversial.
5. As part of initial therapy for advanced disease (e.g., sequential courses of high-dose chemotherapy each supported by autologous blood stem cell transplantation
Under investigation in single centers. Role unclear at present.

As indicated above, over 85% of ovarian cancers are of epithelial origin and these tumors have been the focus for studies of dose escalation. Rarer subtypes such as germ cell have been too infrequent to be a focus of such study. Even for epithelial tumors, small patient numbers and the lack of randomized studies have made assessment of the role of high-dose therapy difficult.

An editorial by Thigpen (1997) cogently summarized the issues concerning the role of high-dose therapy requiring stem cell support for ovarian cancer as follows: currently available studies are not randomized; existing studies include different high-dose regimens making comparison difficult; response rates are impressive; patient populations are highly selected; and finally, results are compared with those for standard therapies in less-selected patient populations.

The possible indications for high-dose chemotherapy and autologous HSC transplantation in the management of ovarian cancer are shown in Table 44.2.

Results of conventional dose therapy

Long-term results for conventional treatment have been extensively reported (see Table 44.1). Survival depends on initial stage, the success of initial debulking, and findings at second-look laparotomy. For women with no residual disease at a second-look laparotomy, 3-year survival is approximately 80%, while for those with less than 2 cm of disease 50%, and for those with more than 2 cm of disease it is 30%. In the last decade the overall 5-year survival rates for ovarian cancer have improved from 38% to 44% (Ozols & Vermoken, 1997). Combination therapy with cisplatin appeared to improve survival rates by more than 10% at 5 and 10 years. The addition of paclitaxel to cisplatin appears to have further improved results. McGuire *et al.* (1996) reported results of 410 women with FIGO stage III and IV ovarian cancer who were incompletely resected (residual disease >1 cm postsurgery), comparing cisplatin-cyclophosphamide to cisplatin-paclitaxel therapy. Both progression-free and overall survival were significantly better for the paclitaxel combination. Preliminary results of an international collaborative study comparing cisplatin/paclitaxel with cisplatin/cyclophosphamide (Piccart *et al.*, 1997) support the combination of paclitaxel and cisplatin as the best current standard protocol for comparing results to those of autologous HSC transplantation for advanced ovarian cancer. Despite these advances in conventional therapy, the majority of women with advanced ovarian cancer will succumb to their disease within 5 years.

Early retrospective results of conventional dose protocols suggested a dose-response relationship in ovarian cancer. An analysis by Levin and Hryniuk (1987) indicated such a relationship for advanced disease, particularly with the use of cisplatin. A later meta-analysis of randomized trials suggested increasing platinum dose-intensity, to 25 mg/m^2 week, resulted in better response rates and survival (Levin, Simon, & Hryniuk, 1993). However, a number of subsequent, prospective randomized studies have not confirmed this observation for dose intensities of approximately twofold, for which stem cell support is not required.

The Gynecological Oncology Group randomized 458 patients with advanced, bulk disease to either 8 cycles of cisplatin 50 mg/m^2 and cyclophosphamide 500 mg/m^2 or 4 cycles of the same agents at double dose both scheduled 3 weekly. Dose intensification did not demonstrate any benefit for either response or survival (McGuire et al., 1995). An Italian cooperative study (Colombo et al., 1993) of 306 patients with advanced disease randomized to either 6 cycles of cisplatin 75 mg/m^2 given every 3 weeks or 9 cycles of 50 mg/m^2 weekly showed no differences in pathologically staged response or survival. In these two studies, the total dose of cisplatin was the same with doubling of the dose-intensity. This suggests that the total dose of therapy may also be an important consideration.

Three randomized trials have increased the total dose of platinum as well as doubling dose-intensity. Conte et al. (1996) reported 145 patients with bulky, advanced disease randomized to either cisplatin 50 or 100 mg/m^2 plus cyclophosphamide 600 mg/m^2 and epirubicin 60 mg/m^2 given every 4 weeks to 6 cycles. No differences in response, including pathologic complete response, or survival were seen. Gore et al. (1996) reported 241 patients with advanced disease given single-agent carboplatin to an area under the curve (AUC) of either 6 or 12 every 4 weeks for 6 cycles with no differences in response or survival. Jakobsen et al. (1997) saw no difference in pathologic complete response or survival in 222 patients randomized to carboplatin of AUC either 4 or 8 for 6 cycles. In all three studies doubling dose-intensity with increased total therapy only increased toxicity.

Dittrich et al. (1996) examined increased dose-intensity of platinols by combining cisplatin and carboplatin. Patients were randomized to cisplatin 100 mg/m^2 with either carboplatin 300 mg/m^2 or cyclophosphamide 600 mg/m^2 every 4 weeks for 6 cycles in 253 patients with FIGO stage 1C to IV disease. Platinum dose-intensity was increased 1.6-fold with no improvement in response or survival and increased toxicity.

Two randomized studies have had positive results for this degree of dose-intensity. A study by the Scottish Cancer Group (Kaye et al., 1992) demonstrated a survival benefit for patients receiving 100 mg/m^2 cisplatin compared to half that dose. Both groups were also given cyclophosphamide 750 mg/m^2 to a maximum of six cycles. The improvement in overall survival was modest (28 versus 17 months), decreased with time, and came at the price of greater toxicity. Kaye (1997) has concluded the small benefit was not justified, particularly with most other randomized studies showing no such benefit. A smaller study of 50 patients (Ngan et al., 1989) of undetermined stage compared cisplatin 60 with 120 mg/m^2 given 4 times weekly and reported improved response rate and 3-year survival for the higher dose cohort. The size of this study and limited patient details, however, impair its value.

These studies imply a flattening of the dose-response relationship for advanced ovarian carcinoma at a threshold of twofold current standard chemotherapy dose levels. Autologous HSC transplantation allows dose escalation/intensification of between 5- and 10-fold and preliminary studies suggest improved response rates and a potential benefit for this approach. Most studies have employed autologous transplantation after conventional therapy. Improvements in mortality and morbidity risks for this approach allow consideration of multiple, sequential high-dose therapy. Preliminary data for such an approach are emerging (Lotz et al., 1996; Shea et al., 1997; Wandt et al., 1997). Randomized, prospective studies of appropriate statistical power are needed to address the role of high-dose therapy in ovarian cancer.

High-dose therapy

A number of different protocols have been employed for autologous HSC transplantation in ovarian cancer patients and no comparative data for efficacy are available. It is also difficult to compare toxicity of these different protocols as, over time, improvements in supportive care appear to have substantially reduced the risks of toxicity.

Most protocols employ agents known to be effective at conventional dose. In vitro studies have demonstrated benefits for dose-escalation of alkylating agents and mitoxantrone (Alberts et al., 1985; Beherns et al., 1987). Combinations of alkylating agents such as cisplatin and cyclophosphamide appear synergistic (Teicher et al., 1989; Lidor et al., 1991). Melphalan is a highly effective alkylating agent against ovarian cancer and suitable for high-dose therapy, with dose-escalations above 10-fold achievable when given as a single agent (Piver, 1984; Spitzer et al., 1984). However, it has been recognized for some time to induce second malignancies (Einhorn, 1978). Cyclophosphamide, another alkylating agent, is also highly effective against ovarian cancer, may be escalated 5- to 10-fold, and appears synergistic with the platinols, perhaps the most effective single agents for this tumor type (Lidor et al., 1991). Etoposide may be escalated above fivefold standard doses and appears an effective salvage therapy (Dunton, 1997). Anthracyclines, also effective for the treatment of ovarian cancer, are limited to dose-escalations of two- to threefold conventional dose because of nonhematologic (especially cardiac) toxicity. Of the platinols, dose escalation of cisplatin is also limited by nonhematologic toxicities (renal, neuropathic, and ototoxic), although dose escalations of twofold have been achieved with acceptable toxicity. Carboplatin may be escalated five- to sevenfold without nonhematologic toxicity (Shea et al., 1989; McGuire, 1992), and is likely as efficacious against ovarian cancer as cisplatin (Alberts, 1995). To date, the taxanes have not been widely employed in high-dose protocols. Experience of autologous transplantation for breast cancer suggests paclitaxel may be escalated to single doses above 800 mg/m^2 without unacceptable nonhematologic toxicity but recurrent dosing above 200 mg/m^2 results in unacceptable, progressive sensory peripheral neuropathy (Hortobyagi et al., 1997).

Levin and Hryniuk's (1987) study indicated that combination chemotherapy would be more effective in ovarian cancer and results of conventional therapy would support this paradigm. Consequently, most autotransplant studies have utilized combinations comprising cyclophosphamide and cisplatin, investigating the addition of other agents such as anthracyclines, etoposide, and taxanes.

Early studies used marrow stem cell support, but, with the emerging recognition of the ease of collection and improvement in engraftment kinetics of blood stem cells, these products have replaced marrow collections. A study by Ross *et al.* (1995) indicated an additional advantage for blood stem cell products as being less likely to contain contaminating ovarian cancer cells. Using a cytochemical technique they found 43% of marrow samples positive compared to 10% of peripheral blood stem cell collections.

Results of high-dose therapy

A number of early phase clinical studies have been undertaken investigating the role of autologous bone marrow transplantation (BMT) in advanced ovarian cancer. These studies have supplied valuable information on the feasibility of this approach, providing data on appropriate regimens, maximal tolerable dosages of various agents, and overall toxicity. None of these studies have been randomized against standard therapies and most have had too few patients, short durations of follow-up, and differed in patient characteristics with regard to burden of disease, chemosensitivity, and high-dose regimen to adequately assess results when compared to retrospective experience. These studies have been well reviewed by McGuire (1992) and Shpall *et al.* (1993). Few studies have had over 30 patients. The major reports have been for patients with advanced and chemoresistant disease. Generally, response rates have been higher than expected for conventional therapy, of the order of 55% to 75%, but response durations short, usually only 5 to 7 months (Mulder *et al.,* 1989; Shea *et al.,* 1989, 1990). However, a small cohort of patients (10% to 15%) appeared to remain disease free beyond 1 year.

Additional studies still contain small numbers of patients. Lotz *et al.* (1996) reported 37 patients with poor prognosis disease salvaged with tandem high-dose teniposide, ifosfamide, and carboplatin. Overall response was 56% with 5-year survival 14% and a median duration of survival of 18 months. Viens *et al.* (1990a, 1990b) reported 48 patients with advanced disease, initially treated with debulking surgery, then 4 to 12 cycles of conventional chemotherapy containing cisplatin. Of these, 44 had high-dose therapy, 31 with melphalan (140 to 240 mg/m^2), 12 with melphalan (140 mg/m^2) in combination with cyclophosphamide (120 mg/m^2), and 1 with a combination carboplatin, etoposide, and cyclophosphamide, followed by marrow transplantation. Fifteen patients with refractory disease did poorly: 4 were nonresponders and the remaining 11 had disease progression at a median of 3 months posttransplant. For 10 patients with residual disease greater than 2 cm, only 3

remained disease-free and 6 progressed at a median of 7 months. The remaining 23 patients with low tumor burden fared much better. Of these, 12 had disease less than 2 cm, 2 showed no evidence of progression with 9 progressing at a median of 14 months. For the 11 in complete remission, there were 5 relapses and 6 remained disease-free (4 for more than 20 months). The procedure-related death rate was 8% with 11 patients (25%) alive without disease at a median of 26 months. Stiff *et al.* (1995) reported 30 patients with relapsed/refractory disease given mitoxantrone (75 mg/m^2), carboplatin (1,500 mg/m^2), and cyclophosphamide (120 mg/m^2) followed by autologous marrow transplantation. Overall, 89% responded, with one treatment-related death due to fungal infection. Median survival was 29 months with 23% alive without evidence of disease at 3 years. Twenty of the patients were platinum-resistant and had poorer outcomes, with only 47% of this group achieving a complete response and having a median progression-free survival just greater than 5 months. For the remaining platinum-sensitive patients, 89% achieved a complete response and the median progression-free duration was just over 10 months.

Stiff *et al.* (1997) updated their experience with autologous BMT in 100 patients with persistent/relapsed ovarian cancer with a multivariate analysis to identify factors influencing survival. This was a poor prognostic group of patients with 66% demonstrating platinum resistance, 62% with high-grade tumors, 61% with bulky disease at time of transplant, and 70% having received two or more chemotherapy regimens prior to transplant. Of 87 patients assessable for response, there were 64% complete and 22% partial responses. Complete responses were longer for patients without bulky disease and whose tumors were considered platinum-responsive. However, survival figures were disappointing with median overall survival 13 months and median progression-free survival only 7 months (Fig. 44.1). Patients with platinum-sensitive disease and residual tumor <1 cm did best with a median progression-free survival of 18.6 months and a median overall survival of 29 months (Fig. 44.2). The authors identified absence of tumor bulk (disease >1 cm) and platinum sensitivity as the best indicators of improved progression-free survival and these two factors, as well as younger age (<48 years, the median age of the entire group), as predictors of improved overall survival. The toxicity of the high-dose protocols employed for transplant (mitoxantrone, carboplatin, and cyclophosphamide; or melphalan, mitoxantrone with or without paclitaxel; or thiotepa, cisplatin, and cyclophosphamide) (Table 44.3) was of concern with 10 patient deaths attributed to the procedure. The authors concluded that only patients with platinum-sensitive, nonbulky disease should be considered for autologous transplantation and proposed future studies should consider patients with minimal disease responsive to initial chemotherapy.

Shinozuka *et al.* (1997) have updated their experience of sequential high-dose cyclophosphamide, adriamycin, and cisplatin in 60 patients. This was a dose-escalation study and 6

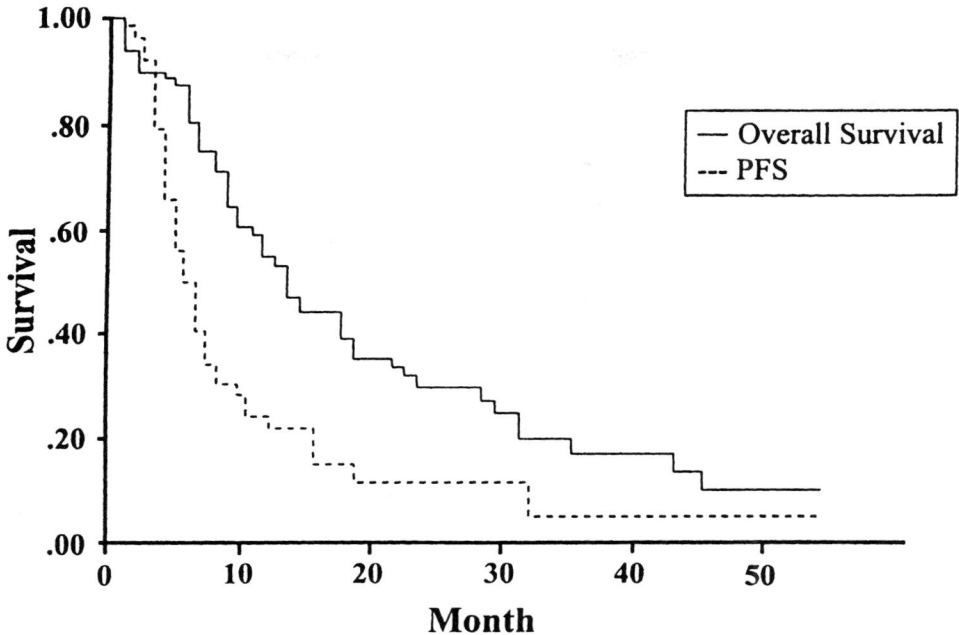

Fig. 44.1. Kaplan-Meier estimates of OS and PFS for all 100 patients. Reproduced, with permission, from Stiff *et al.* (1997).

patients received only one course. The majority were treated initially with conventional dose cyclophosphamide, adriamycin, and cisplatin with intraperitoneal and/or intrapleural cisplatin (46 patients). Seven patients had FIGO stage IC, 7 stage II, 25 stage III, 12 stage IV, and 9 recurrent/refractory dis-ease. Forty-two percent had a 5-year disease-free survival, with improved survivals in patients with stage IC to III disease rather than stage IV or refractory disease. For patients with less than 2 cm residual disease, 5-year disease-free survival was 25% and 14% for disease greater than 2 cm.

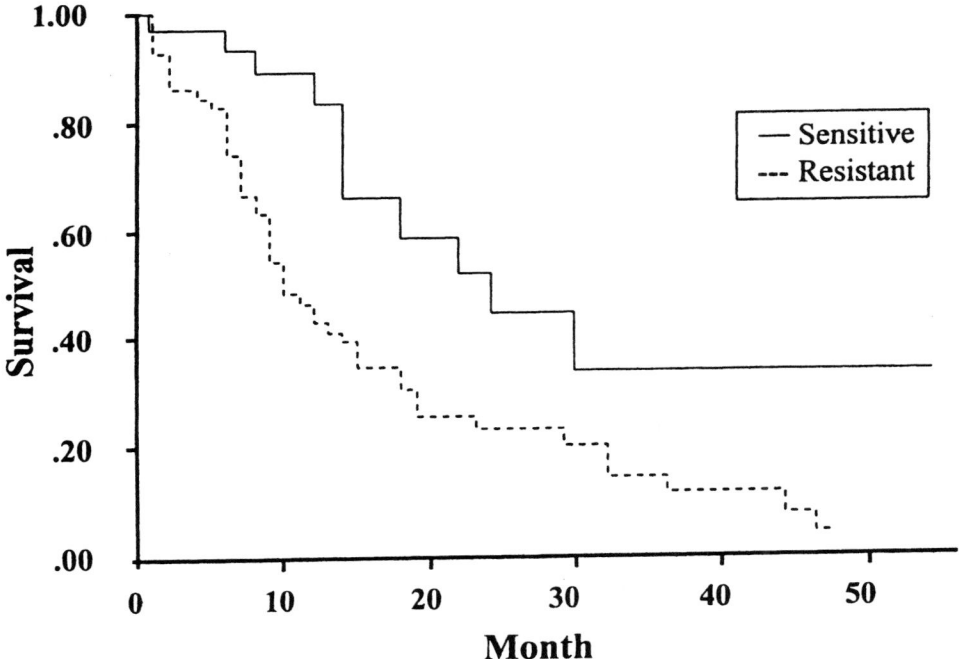

Fig. 44.2. Kaplan-Meier estimates of OS for the 66 platinum-resistant and 34 platinum-sensitive patients. Reproduced, with permission, from Stiff *et al.* (1997).

Table 44.3. *Pretransplant preparative regimens used in the study by Stiff et al., 1997*

1. Mitoxantrone	20–25 mg/m^2	Days 1, 3, 5
Carboplatin[a]	1,500 mg/m^2	Days 1–5
Cyclophosphamide	30–40 mg/kg	Days 1, 3, 5
±Cyclosporine	1.7–9.7 mg/m^2 bolus then 5.0–28.2 mg/m^2	Days 0–5
2. Melphalan	90 mg/m^2	Days 1, 2
Mitoxantrone	20–30 mg/m^2	Days 1, 2, 3
± Paclitaxel	250–350 mg/m^2	Days 1–4
3. Thiotepa	600 mg/m^2	Day 1
Cisplatin	55 mg/m^2	Days 2–4
Cyclophosphamide	1,875 mg/m^2	Days 2–4

[a] Changed to AUC dosing of 28 for last 9 patients.

Legros *et al.* (1997) have reported 53 patients with advanced ovarian cancer who underwent autologous BMT after initial debulking surgery, conventional doxorubicin, cyclophosphamide, and cisplatin chemotherapy, and second-look laparotomy. Complete remission was achieved in 31 patients who had poor prognostic factors and 22 patients had persistent disease after second-look surgery (18 <1 cm). The first 23 patients in the study were treated with high-dose melphalan, 140 mg/m^2 as a single dose, with autologous bone marrow as the source of stem cell rescue. Because of concern regarding risk of second malignancy with melphalan and emerging evidence of the improved efficacy of platinols, the remaining 30 patients received high-dose carboplatin (1,600 mg/m^2) and cyclophosphamide (6.4 g/m^2) administered over 4 days, followed by blood stem cell rescue. Peripheral stem cells were obtained by leukapheresis following etoposide (400 mg/m^2 over 2 days), cyclophosphamide (4 g/m^2 over 2 days), and G-CSF (5 μg/kg/day for 10 days). Minimum follow-up was 25 months with a mean of 85.5 months. The 5-year overall survival rate was 60% with a median of nearly 66 months. Disease-free survival at 5 years was 23.6% with a median of 30 months. Of 29 deaths, 26 were due to disease with 1 treatment-related death 25 days posttransplant and 2 other deaths possibly treatment-related, 1 due to cardiac failure at 6 months and 1 due to abnormal marrow function at 84 months posttransplant. Not surprisingly, survival was superior in the group of patients without persistent disease at transplant compared to the salvage group.

Overall, 5-year survivals were 71% (median 80 months) for the complete remission group versus 34% (median 39 months) for the salvage group; disease-free survival rates at 5 years were 27% (median 37 months) versus 19% (median 24 months), respectively, for the 2 groups (Fig. 44.3). Of the 39 patients who relapsed, the 5-year overall survival rate was 17% (median 19 months). For the entire group the median time without symptoms or treatment was 24 months posttransplant, implying good quality of life for these patients. There were no differences according to high-dose regimen utilized. These figures appear impressive compared to the results of conventional therapy, even for those patients who relapsed posttransplant.

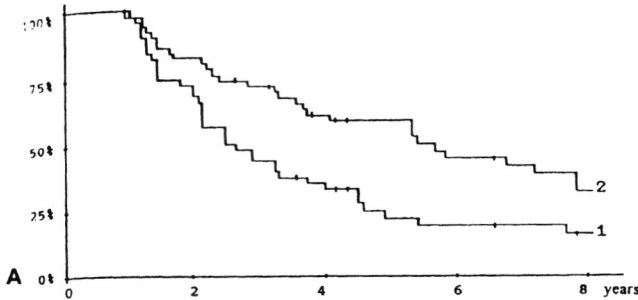

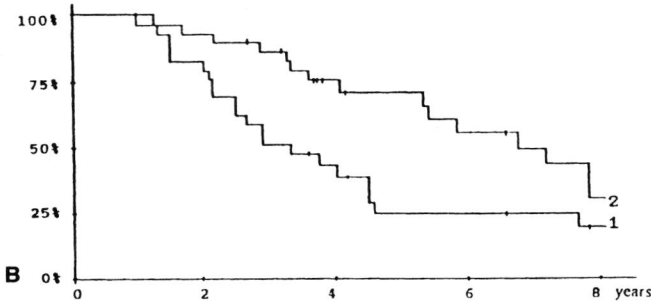

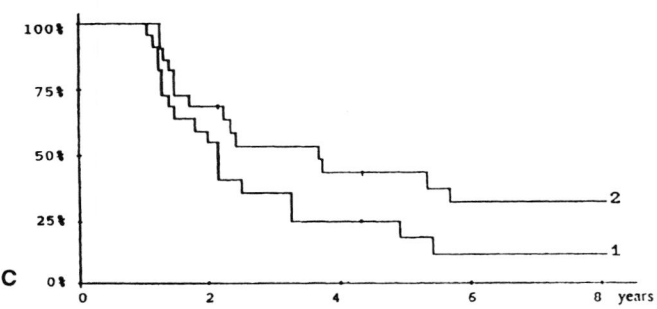

Fig. 44.3. **(A)** DFS (1) and overall survival (2) from diagnosis for the entire patient cohort (*N* = 53) (Kaplan-Meier method). Reproduced, with permission, from Legros *et al.* (1997). **(B)** DFS (1) and overall survival (2) from diagnosis for the consolidation group (group A, *n* = 31) (Kaplan-Meier method). Reproduced, with permission, from Legros *et al.* (1997). **(C)** DFS (1) and overall survival (2) from diagnosis for the salvage group (group B, *n* = 22) (Kaplan-Meier method). Reproduced, with permission, from Legros *et al.* (1997).

The North American Autologous Blood and Marrow Transplant Registry's Ovarian Cancer Working Committee has attempted to overcome some of the shortcomings of small study numbers by collecting data from a large number of centers, reporting on 390 women receiving autologous HSC transplantation for ovarian cancer between 1989 and 1996 (Horowitz *et al.*, 1997). Of 341 whose response was recorded prior to transplant, 37% achieved a complete response, 35% a partial response, 9% stable disease, and 19% progressive disease. Mortality by 30 days posttransplant was 7%. Two-year probability of survival was 37% overall, 51% for complete responders, 38% for partial responders, 29% for patients with stable disease, and 10% for patients with progressive disease prior to transplant. These data support earlier encouraging data for autologous BMT in this disease. The relatively high treatment-related mortality may reflect the inclusion of patients from early programs. Women with chemosensitive disease appear to derive the most benefit, supporting the findings of earlier, smaller studies. These data were subsequently updated to include 421 patients (Stiff *et al.*, 2000). Forty-one percent had platinum-resistant tumors and 38% had tumors at least 1 cm in diameter. Two-year progression-free survival was 12% and 2-year overall survival was 35%. Younger age, Karnofsky performance score of at least 90%, non-clear cell disease, remission at the time of transplant, and platinum sensitivity were associated with better outcomes. Progression-free and overall survival were 22% and 55%, respectively, for women with a high Karnovsky score and non-clear cell, platinum-sensitive tumors (Fig. 44.4).

These studies suggest that autologous HSC transplantation offers improved response rates for advanced disease, including relapsed or chemorefractory disease. These better responses do not appear to improve survival for patients with chemoresistant or bulk disease, and most investigators now suggest such patients are not suitable for autologous transplantation. Only patients with advanced disease achieving minimal tumor burden given autotransplantation early in their disease course might derive a survival benefit, and future trials should concentrate on these patient groups.

Future directions

Currently, two large prospective trials have begun to examine the role of autologous HSC transplantation as further therapy for patients with small-volume, minimal residual disease at second-look laparotomy following platinum and paclitaxel chemotherapy. In the United States an Intergroup phase III

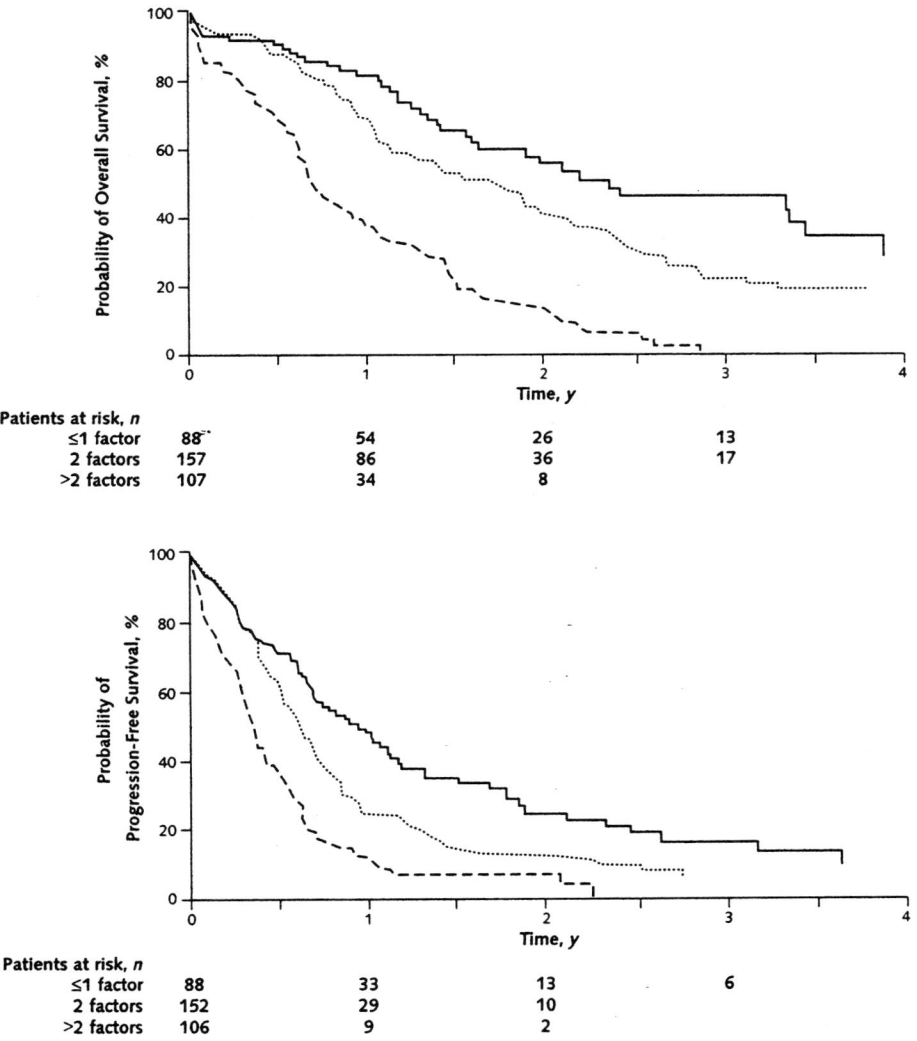

Fig. 44.4. Probabilities of survival (top) and progression-free survival (bottom) after autotransplantation according to number of adverse prognostic factors. Reproduced, with permission, from Stiff *et al.* (2000).

study commenced in late 1996 comparing continued conventional dose platinum/paclitaxel to high-dose combination carboplatin/mitoxantrone/cyclophosphamide. In France, the Groupe Investigation Nationale Etude Cancre Ovaie (GINECO) study is randomizing patients with minimal or no residual disease with demonstrable chemosensitivity to 3 cycles of conventional dose carboplatin/cyclophosphamide versus autotransplantation with high doses of the same agents.

Sequential high-dose therapy

The use of peripheral blood progenitor cells and hematopoietic growth factors allows consideration of a sequential high-dose strategy. The rationale of only using a single high-dose therapy is somewhat at odds with the standard paradigm of multiple courses of therapy to induce and consolidate complete remissions. One study demonstrated this approach to be feasible. Wandt *et al.* (1997) reported 21 patients with advanced disease in a sequential, dose-escalation study of 4 courses comprising high-dose cyclophosphamide, carboplatin, etoposide, melphalan, and conventional dose paclitaxel. Each course was supported with peripheral blood stem cells and G-CSF. All patients responded with 10 complete and 11 partial responses, no treatment-related deaths, and only two infectious episodes.

Intraperitoneal therapy

Intraperitoneal therapy may allow dose intensification and could be used as adjunct in patients with platinum-sensitive, minimal residual disease. One report suggested this approach may be superior to continued conventional therapy (Alberts *et al.*, 1996). In an Intergroup trial of 650 patients with small-volume residual disease, response rates were similar, but survival was improved for patients randomized to receive cisplatin 100 mg/m^2 intraperitoneally compared to the intravenous route, given every 3 weeks. Both groups also received cyclophosphamide 600 mg/m^2 intravenously every 3 weeks. Another preliminary report (Barakat *et al.*, 1997) suggested that 3 courses of intraperitoneal cisplatin and etoposide given as adjuvant therapy (following negative second-look laparotomy) improved disease-free survival.

Interleukin-2 (IL-2) has anticancer properties and early studies have shown favorable responses to this agent for chemoresistant disease when given intraperitoneally (Edwards *et al.*, 1995). Gamma-interferon appeared effective when given via intraperitoneal injection in a study by Pujade-Lauraine *et al.* (1996). Confirmation of these results would promote these strategies, perhaps in combination with other treatment modalities, as part of initial therapy or as adjunct treatment.

Topotecan

New chemotherapy agents may improve results of conventional or high-dose protocols. Topotecan, a topoisomerase I inhibitor and an analogue of campothecin, has demonstrated good activity as a second-line and salvage therapy for patients with ovarian cancer (Dunton, 1997). Its dose-limiting toxicity appears to be hematologic and noncumulative, making it a suitable agent for consideration in autologous HSC protocols.

Conclusions

While significant progress has been made in our understanding of the application of high-dose therapy and autologous transplantation for advanced ovarian cancer, the lack of randomized studies of sufficient power has prevented a definitive answer as to the role of this procedure. Fortunately, at least two such studies are in progress and should help to clarify the appropriate role of high-dose therapy and autografting in this disease. Some conclusions can be drawn regarding patients with chemorefractory disease, especially to platinum-containing regimens and with bulk disease following first-line therapy. While autotransplantation may improve responses for these patients, no significant survival benefits have been achieved. Consequently, autografting cannot be recommended for such patients and, if they wish to continue treatment, they should be considered for trials of other novel approaches.

It seems likely that, as therapeutic options for this disease increase, complex regimens of therapy, probably including autologous HSC transplantation will impact in a positive way on patient survival.

References

Alberts, D., Lui, P., Hannigan, E. *et al.* (1996). Intraperitoneal cisplatin plus intravenous cyclophosphamide versus intravenous cisplatin plus intravenous cyclophosphamide for stage III ovarian cancer. *New England Journal of Medicine,* **335,** 1950–5.

Alberts, D.S. (1995). Carboplatin versus cisplatin in ovarian cancer. *Seminars in Oncology,* **22** (Suppl 12), 88–90.

Alberts, D.S., Green S.G., Hannigan, E.V. *et al.* (1992). Improved therapeutic index of carboplatin plus cyclophosphamide versus cisplatin plus cyclophosphamide: final report of the Southwest Oncology Group of a phase III randomized trial in stage III and IV ovarian cancer. *Journal of Clinical Oncology,* **10,** 706–17.

Alberts, D.S., Young L., Mason, N. *et al.* (1985). In vitro evaluation of anticancer drugs against ovarian cancer at concentrations achievable by intraperitoneal administration. *Seminars in Oncology,* **12** (Suppl 4), 38–42.

Barakat, R., Almadrones, L., Venkatraman, E., & Spriggs, D. (1997). A phase II trial of intraperitoneal (IP) cisplatin (CDDP) and etoposide (VP-16) as consolidation therapy in patients with stage II–IV epithelial ovarian cancer (EOC) following negative surgical assessment. *Proceedings of the American Society of Clinical Oncology,* **16,** 354 (Abstract).

Beherns, B.C., Hamilton, T.C., Masuda, H. *et al.* (1987). Characterization of a cis-diamine dichloroplatinum (II)-resistant human ovarian cancer cell line and its use in evaluation of platinum analogs. *Cancer Research,* **47,** 414–18.

Berek, J.S. & Hacker, N.F. (1985). Staging and second-look operations in ovarian cancer. In *Ovarian Cancer*, ed. D.S. Alberts & E.A. Jorwitt, pp. 109–127. Boston: Martinus Nijkoff.

Colombo, N., Pitelli, M., Parma, G. *et al.* (1993). Cisplatin dose-intensity in advanced ovarian cancer: a randomized study of conventional dose versus dose-intense cisplatin monochemotherapy. *Proceedings of the American Society of Clinical Oncology*, **12**, 255 (Abstract).

Conte, P., Bruzzone, M., Carnino, F. *et al.* (1996). High-dose versus low-dose cisplatin in combination with cyclophosphamide and epidoxorubicin in suboptimal ovarian cancer: a randomized study of the Gruppo Oncologico Nord-Ovest. *Journal of Clinical Oncology*, **14**, 351–6.

Dittrich, C., Obermair, A., Kurz, C. *et al.* (1996). Prospective randomized trial of cisplatin/carboplatin versus conventional cisplatin/cyclophosphamide in epithelial ovarian cancer: first results of the impact of platinum dose-intensity on patient outcome. *Proceedings of the American Society of Clinical Oncology*, **15**, 279 (Abstract).

Dunton, C.J. (1997). New options for the treatment of advanced ovarian cancer. *Seminars in Oncology*, **24** (Suppl 5), 2–11.

Edwards, B.P., Lembersky, B.C., Kunschner, A.J. *et al.* (1995). Intraperitoneal interleukin-2 produces durable responses for refractory ovarian cancer. *Proceedings of the American Society of Clinical Oncology*, **14**, 333 (Abstract).

Einhorn, N. (1978). Acute leukemia after chemotherapy (melphalan). *Cancer*, **41**, 444–7.

Gore, M., Mainwaring, P., MacFarlane, V. *et al.* (1996). A randomized study of high versus standard dose carboplatin in patients with advanced epithelial ovarian cancer. *Proceedings of the American Society of Clinical Oncology*, **15**, 284 (Abstract).

Horowitz, M.M., Stiff, P.J., Veum-Stone, J., & Rowlings, P.A. (1997). Outcome of transplants for advanced ovarian cancer. *Proceedings of the American Society of Clinical Oncology*, **16**, 353 (Abstract).

Hortobyagi, G.N., Holmes, F.A., Ibrahim, N. *et al.* (1997). The University of Texas, M.D. Anderson Cancer Center experience with paclitaxel in breast cancer. *Seminars in Oncology*, **24** (Suppl 3), 30–3.

Jakobsen, A., Bertelsen, K., Andersen, J.E. *et al.* (1997). Dose-effect study of carboplatin in ovarian cancer: a Danish Ovarian Cancer Group Study. *Journal of Clinical Oncology*, **15**, 193–8.

Kaye, S., Paul, J., Cassidy, J. *et al.* (1996). Mature results of a randomized trial of two doses of cisplatin for the treatment of ovarian cancer. *Journal of Clinical Oncology*, **14**, 2113–19.

Kaye, S.B. (1997). The role of dose intensity in the treatment of ovarian cancer. *Proceedings of the 20th International Congress of Chemotherapy*, **122**, 4069 (Abstract).

Kaye, S.G., Lewis, C.R., Paul J. *et al.* (1992). Randomized study of two doses of cisplatin with cyclophosphamide in epithelial ovarian cancer. *Lancet*, **340**, 329–33.

Legros, M., Dauplat, J., Fleury, J. *et al.* (1997). High-dose chemotherapy with hematopoietic rescue in patients with stage III to IV ovarian cancer: long-term results. *Journal of Clinical Oncology*, **15**, 1302–8.

Levin, L. & Hryniuk, W. (1987). Dose-intensity analysis of chemotherapy regimens in ovarian carcinoma. *Journal of Clinical Oncology*, **5**, 756–67.

Levin, L., Simon, R., & Hryniuk, W. (1993). Importance of multiagent chemotherapy regimens in ovarian carcinoma: dose-intensity analysis. *Journal of the National Cancer Institute*, **85**, 1732–42.

Lidor, Y.J., Shpall, E.J., & Peters, W.P. (1991). Synergistic cytotoxicity of different alkylating agents for epithelial ovarian cancer. *International Journal of Cancer*, **49**, 704–10.

Lotz, J.P., Bouleuc, C., Andre, T. *et al.* (1996). Tandem high-dose chemotherapy with ifosfamide, carboplatin, and teniposide with autologous bone marrow transplantation for the treatment of poor prognosis common epithelial ovarian carcinoma. *Cancer*, **77**, 2550–9.

McGuire, W.P. (1992). Experimental chemotherapy. *Hematology/Oncology Clinics of North America*, **6**, 927–40.

McGuire, W.P., Hoskins, W.J., Brady, M.D. *et al.* (1995). Assessment of dose-intensive therapy in suboptimally debulked ovarian cancer: a Gynecologic Oncology Group study. *Journal of Clinical Oncology*, **13**, 1589–99.

McGuire, W.P., Hoskins, W.J., Brady, M.F. *et al.* (1996). Cyclophosphamide and cisplatin compared with paclitaxel and cisplatin in patients with stage III and stage IV ovarian cancer. *New England Journal of Medicine*, **334**, 1–6.

Mulder, P.O.M., Sleijfer, D.T., Willemse, P.H.B. *et al.* (1989). High-dose cyclophosphamide or melphalan with escalating doses of mitoxantrone and autologous bone marrow transplantation for refractory solid tumors. *Cancer Research*, **49**, 4654–8.

Mychalczak, B.R. & Fuks, Z. (1992). The current role of radiotherapy in the management of ovarian cancer. *Hematology/Oncology Clinics of North America*, **6**, 895–913.

Neijt, J.P., Allen, D.G., Colombo, N., and Vermorken, J.B. (1995). Carcinoma of the ovary. In *The Oxford Textbook of Oncology*, ed. M. Peckham, H.M. Pinedo, & U. Veronesi, pp. 1293–1308. Oxford, UK: Oxford University Press.

Neijt, J.P., ten Bokkel Huinink, W.W., van der Burg, M.E.L. *et al.* (1991). Long-term survival in ovarian cancer. Mature data from the Netherlands Joint Study Group for Ovarian Cancer. *European Journal of Cancer*, **27**, 1367–72.

Ngan, H., Choo, Y., Cheung, M. *et al.* (1989). A randomized study of high-dose versus low-dose cisplatin combined with cyclophosphamide in the treatment of advanced ovarian cancer. *Chemotherapy*, **35**, 221–7.

Ozols, R.F. (1992). Chemotherapy for advanced epithelial ovarian cancer. *Hematology/Oncology Clinics of North America*, **6**, 879–84.

Ozols, R.F. (1994). Treatment of ovarian cancer: current status. *Seminars in Oncology*, **21**, 1–9.

Ozols, R.F. & Vermoken, J.B. (1997). Chemotherapy of advanced ovarian cancer: current status and future directions. *Seminars in Oncology*, **24**, (Suppl), 1–9.

Ozols, R.F. & Young, R.C. (1991). Chemotherapy of ovarian cancer. *Seminars in Oncology*, **18**, 222–32.

Piccart, M.J., Bertelsen, K., Stuart, G. *et al.* (1997). Is cisplatin-paclitaxel (P-T) the standard in first-line treatment of advanced ovarian cancer (Ov Ca)? The EORTC-GCCG, NOCOVA, NCI-C and Scottish intergroup experience. *Proceedings of the American Society of Clinical Oncology*, **16**, 352 (Abstract).

Piver, M.S. (1984). Ovarian carcinoma. A decade of progress. *Cancer*, **54**, 2706–15.

Pujade-Lauraine, E., Guastalla, J.P., Colombo, N. *et al.* (1996). Intraperitoneal recombinant interferon gamma in ovarian cancer patients with residual disease at second-look laparotomy. *Journal of Clinical Oncology*, **14**, 343–50.

Richardson, G.S., Sculy, R.E., Nikrui, N. *et al.* (1985). Common epithelial cancer of the ovary. *New England Journal of Medicine*, **312**, 415–24.

Ross, A.A., Miller, G.W., Moss, T.J. *et al.* (1995). Immunocytochemical detection of tumor cells in bone marrow and peripheral blood stem cell collections from patients with ovarian cancer. *Bone Marrow Transplantation*, **15**, 929–33.

Rubin, S.C. (1992). Surgery for ovarian cancer. *Hematology/Oncology Clinics of North America*, **6**, 851–65.

Runowicz, C.D. (1992). Advances in the screening and treatment of ovarian cancer. *CA: A Cancer Journal for Clinicians*, **42**, 327–49.

Shea, T., Serody, J., Gabriel, D. *et al.* (1997). Phase I trial of two cycles of high-dose chemotherapy in patients (pts) with recurrent or refractory ovarian cancer. *Proceedings of the American Society of Clinical Oncology*, **16**, 377 (Abstract).

Shea, T.C., Flaherty, M., Elias, A. *et al.* (1989). A phase I clinical and pharmacokinetic study of carboplatin and autologous bone marrow support. *Journal of Clinical Oncology*, **7**, 651–61.

Shpall, E.J., Clark-Pearson, D., Soper, J.T. *et al.* (1990). High-dose alkylating agent chemotherapy with autologous bone marrow support in patients with stage III/IV epithelial ovarian cancer. *Gynecological Oncology*, **38**, 386–91.

Shpall, E.J., Stemmer, S.M., Bearman, S.I., and Jones, R.B. (1993). Role of auto transplantation in treatment of other solid tumors. *Hematology/Oncology Clinics of North America*, **7**, 663–86.

Shinozuka, T., Miyamoto, T., Muramatsu, T. *et al.* (1997). Long-term follow-up and prognostic analysis in epithelial ovarian cancer treated by high-dose cyclophosphamide, adriamycin and cisplatin (CAP) with autologous bone marrow transplantation (ABMT). *Proceedings of the American Society of Clinical Oncology*, **16**, 378 (Abstract).

Silverberg, E., Boring, C.S., and Squires, T.S. (1990). Cancer statistics 1990. *CA: A Cancer Journal for Clinicians*, **40**, 9–26.

Spitzer, G., Dicke, K., Zander, A.R. *et al.* (1984). High-dose chemotherapy with autologous bone marrow transplantation. *Cancer*, **54**, 1216–25.

Stiff, P., Bayer, R., Camarda, M. *et al.* (1995). A phase II trial of high-dose mitoxantrone, carboplatin, and cyclophosphamide with autologous bone marrow rescue for recurrent epithelial ovarian carcinoma: analysis of risk factors for clinical outcome. *Gynecological Oncology*, **57**, 278–85.

Stiff, P.J., Bayer, R., Kerger, C. *et al.* (1997). High-dose chemotherapy with autologous transplantation for persistent/relapsed ovarian cancer: a multivariate analysis of survival for 100 consecutively treated patients. *Journal of Clinical Oncology*, **15**, 1309–17.

Stiff, P.J., Veum-Stone, J., Lazarus, H.M. *et al.* (2000). High-dose chemotherapy and autologous stem-cell transplantation for ovarian cancer: an Autologous Blood and Marrow Transplant Registry Report. *Annals of Internal Medicine*, **133**, 504–15.

Teicher, B., Holden, S.A., Jones, S.M. *et al.* (1989). Influence of scheduling in two-day combinations of alkylating agents in vivo. *Cancer Chemotherapy and Pharmacology*, **25**, 161–6.

Thigpen, J.T. (1997). Dose-intensity in ovarian carcinoma: hold, enough? *Journal of Clinical Oncology*, **15**, 1291–93.

Viens, P., Maranchini, D., Legros, M. *et al.* (1990a). High-dose melphalan and autologous marrow rescue in advanced epithelial ovarian carcinomas: a retrospective analysis of 35 patients treated in France. *Bone Marrow Transplantation*, **5**, 227–33.

Viens, P., Stoppa, A.M., Legros, M. *et al.* (1990b). High-dose chemotherapy and autologous marrow rescue in poor prognosis ovarian carcinomas. In *Autologous Bone Marrow Transplantation: Proceedings of the Fifth International Symposium*, ed. K.A. Dicke, J.O. Armitage, and M.J. Dicke-Evinger, pp. 655–659. Omaha: University of Nebraska Medical Center.

Wandt, H., Birkmann, J., Schaefer-Echart, J. *et al.* (1997). Sequential cycles of high-dose chemotherapy supported by G-CSF (filgrastim) and peripheral blood progenitor cells (PBPC) in advanced ovarian cancer: a phase I/II dose escalation study for carboplatin. *Proceedings of the American Society of Clinical Oncology*, **16**, 92 (Abstract).

45 Autologous hematopoietic stem cell transplantation for small cell lung cancer

ANTHONY ELIAS

University of Colorado Cancer Institute and University of Colorado, Denver, USA

Introduction

Lung cancer is the leading cause of death from cancer in both men and women (Boring *et al.*, 1994), and is epidemic throughout the world due to increased tobacco consumption. It is the second most common malignancy in the United States, with more than 180,000 new cases per year, and is the first cause of cancer-related deaths with more than 160,000 deaths per year. Disappointingly, 5-year survival of lung cancer patients has improved only minimally during the past two decades. Of the two major histologic subtypes, small cell lung cancer usually is dose-responsive while it is unclear whether this effect holds true for the non-small-cell subtype (Lazarus & Elias, 1996).

Approximately 15% to 20% of all bronchogenic carcinomas are small cell lung cancer (SCLC). At diagnosis SCLC is staged as either limited disease or extensive disease. Limited disease is defined as disease that can be encompassed by a radiation port (i.e., hemithorax, ipsilateral mediastinal, and supraclavicular nodes). Some studies include malignant pleural effusion, contralateral supraclavicular, and ipsilateral and contralateral cervical nodes as limited stage. Extensive disease is defined as involvement of any organ/structure not included in the definition of limited stage. Excellent immediate palliation from combination chemotherapy is achieved. Many chemotherapeutic agents have major activity against SCLC. The most active of these are cisplatin (and carboplatin), etoposide (and teniposide), ifosfamide, cyclophosphamide, vincristine, and doxorubicin. Combination regimens constructed from the established agents achieve almost identical short- and long-term results. A reasonable consensus treatment approach consists of 4 to 6 cycles of etoposide and platinum with concurrent chest radiation therapy for the third of patients with limited stage disease (Johnson *et al.*, 1996) and combination chemotherapy alone for extensive stage disease. Only 20% to 40% of limited and 5% to 10% of extensive stage patients remain alive by 2 years (Osterlind *et al.*, 1986; Seifter & Ihde, 1988). About half of patients alive at 2 years remain alive at 5 years (Table 45.1). A number of new agents appear to have at least equivalent activity compared with these established drugs, particularly the topoisomerase I inhibitors (topotecan, irinotecan), as well as the taxanes (paclitaxel and taxotere) and gemcitabine. Trials to define the role of the new active agents as well as resistance modulators in first-line therapy are ongoing. The median age of 60 to 65 years, underlying smoking-related cardiovascular and pulmonary comorbidity, and an enhanced risk of secondary smoking-related malignancies contribute to an increased risk from the application of dose-intensive therapy in lung cancer patients.

Dose-intensive therapy—without cellular support

Preclinical in vitro and in vivo experiments indicate near log-linear dose-response relationships for many agents, particularly for the alkylating agents and radiation (Frei, 1972; Frei & Canellos, 1980; Teicher, 1992; Frei *et al.*, 1993). Cohen *et al.* (1977) were one of the first to demonstrate higher response rates, both complete and partial, and a modestly longer median survival time when administering higher, rather than lower, doses of cyclophosphamide, lomustine, and methotrexate.

The contribution of dose or dose intensity of chemotherapy to response and survival remains controversial. Klasa *et al.* (1991) analyzed numerous SCLC trials using the methodology of Hryniuk and Bush (1984) to determine whether dose intensity (expressed in drug dose administered per m² per week) of individual agents or regimens correlated with response or survival. Longer median survival in extensive disease patients receiving higher dose intensities of CAV (cyclophosphamide, doxorubicin, vincristine) and CAE (cyclophosphamide, doxorubicin, etoposide) but not EP (etoposide, cisplatin) was observed, but the effects and the dose ranges analyzed were

Table 45.1. *Outcome of standard treatment for small cell lung cancer*

Parameter	Limited stage	Extensive stage
Response rate	90%	60%
Complete response rate	40–60%	10–20%
Median survival	12–18 months	8 months
5-year survival	5–20%	<1%

small. This type of analysis makes the assumption that all drugs are therapeutically equivalent, and that cross-resistance (or synergy) between drugs, peak drug concentrations, or schedule and duration of drug exposure has no effect.

Seven randomized trials have evaluated dose intensity in SCLC, almost exclusively in the extensive stage setting (Cohen et al., 1977; Mehta & Vogl, 1982; Brower et al., 1983; Figueredo et al., 1985; Johnson et al., 1987; Arriagada et al., 1993; Ihde et al., 1994). The planned dose-intensity differences between the high and lower dose arms ranged between 1.2- and 2-fold, although the differences in actual delivered doses were less. Three of the seven randomized trials showed a modest survival advantage for the higher dose therapy. Two of these three trials compared less than standard dose therapy with full dose therapy. The trials without evident benefit generally compared full dose to a small incremental dose-intensity between one- and twofold full conventional dose. Currently established cytokines [e.g., granulocyte-macrophage colony-stimulating factor (GM-CSF) and granulocyte (G)-CSF] shorten chemotherapy-induced myelosuppression and consequent febrile neutropenia (Crawford et al., 1991). However, dose intensities can be increased by only 1.5- to 2-fold with cytokine use because of cumulative thrombocytopenia. Survival advantages have not been described. Thus, the effectiveness of various thrombopoietins or other cytokines to achieve increased dose-intensity remains to be demonstrated.

Arriagada et al. (1993) randomized patients to six cycles of conventional dose chemotherapy with a modestly intensified first cycle or not. It was surprising to observe a complete response and survival advantage for the patients receiving the intensified chemotherapy, since the relative difference in the two groups was so small. While this result could reflect chance, it is possible that dose intensity, particularly if given early in the course of treatment, may be more likely to impact on outcomes in the limited rather than the extensive stage setting. However, the same investigators did not observe an improvement in outcomes when giving an additional 25% increment in the cyclophosphamide dose for the first cycle in a follow-on randomized trial for 295 limited stage patients (LeChevalier et al., 2002). Both of these themes, early intensification and treatment of earlier stage disease, are important in considering new trial designs.

Multidrug cyclic weekly therapy was designed to intensify the number of drugs to which the cancer was exposed, with less compromise of dose given the differing toxicities of the weekly agents. Early phase II results were quite promising (Miles et al., 1991; Murray et al., 1994), although patient selection effects were evident. The randomized trials evaluating these regimens did not demonstrate a response or survival advantage (Furuse et al., 1996; Murray et al., 1997). Unfortunately in actual practice (Sculier et al., 1993; Souhami et al., 1994), the weekly schedules in the randomized trials had greater dose reductions and delays compared with every three weekly conventional therapy; thus, the actual delivered dose intensities were not very different. Not only did dose and schedule differ, but so did the regimens, leading to difficulties in interpretation.

In these studies, follow-up was too short to observe late disease-free survival differences.

Dose-intensive therapy—with cellular support

Data on patients with SCLC undergoing autologous hematopoietic stem cell (HSC) transplantation, on whom sufficient details were available, have been pooled to determine relapse-free and overall survival (Table 45.2). Required details included disease status (untreated; responding to first-line chemotherapy; relapsed; refractory) and extent of disease (limited or extensive stage).

For relapsed or refractory disease

Fourteen studies (with a median of 3, maximum patients 8) described outcome in 52 patients who had either relapsed or refractory disease (Spitzer et al., 1979, 1980; Douer et al., 1981; Harada et al., 1982; Phillips et al., 1983; Pico et al., 1983; Wolff et al., 1983; Rushing et al., 1984; Stahel et al., 1984; Pico et al., 1987; Eder et al., 1988; Postmus et al., 1988; Lazarus et al., 1990; Elias et al., 1995) (Table 45.2, group 1). Complete and partial remissions were observed in 19% and 37%, respectively. The median response durations and survivals were approximately 2 to 3 months. The overall regimen-related mortality rate was 13%. Combination chemotherapy regimens, especially those containing multiple alkylating agents were slightly more effective (response rate 58%, complete response 26%), but more toxic (18% vs. 6% deaths). The observed high complete response rate supported a dose-response relationship, but was insufficient to improve survival.

As initial treatment

Overall and complete response rates of 84% and 42% were achieved in 103 patients with SCLC (71% had limited disease)

Table 45.2. *High-dose intensification therapy and autologous bone marrow transplantation for small cell lung cancer*[a]

Patient group	Number	Complete remission rate (%)	Disease-free survival (%)	Treatment-related mortality (%)
1. Relapsed/refractory disease	52	19	0	13
2. Initial treatment	103	43	7	6
3. First PR/SD	189	42	8	11
4. First CR	110		33	3
Extensive disease	25		16	8
Limited disease	85		38	1

Abbreviations: PR, partial remission; SD, chemosensitive disease; CR, complete remission.

[a] Median follow-up 3 years with wide variability between studies.

receiving high-dose therapy as initial treatment (Johnson *et al.,* 1983; Littlewood *et al.,* 1985, 1986; Spitzer *et al.,* 1986; Souhami *et al.,* 1989; Nomura *et al.,* 1990; Lange *et al.,* 1991; Elias *et al.,* 1995) (Table 45.2, group 2). Disease-free, 2-year, and overall survivals were comparable to treatment with conventional multicycle regimens. Transplantation in the newly diagnosed SCLC setting may not be optimal because of the frequency of life-threatening complications from uncontrolled disease, and the potential for tumor cell contamination in non-purged autografts.

As consolidation treatment for patients responding to initial conventional chemotherapy

Approximately 300 patients responding to first-line chemotherapy received high-dose chemotherapy with autologous marrow support as intensification treatment (Farha *et al.,* 1983). Of those patients achieving a partial response only to induction therapy (n = 189), the conversion to complete response occurred in 42%, but without durable effect (Table 45.2, group 3). The best results (38% disease-free survival with a median follow-up >3 years at the time of publication) were reported in patients with limited disease in complete remission at the time of high-dose therapy. Those with extensive disease, but in complete remission at the time of high-dose therapy, had a disease-free survival of 16%, giving an overall disease-free survival of 33% for those given high-dose therapy when in complete remission (Table 45.2, group 4).

Much of the high-dose SCLC experience took place during the initial developmental phase of high-dose therapy for solid tumors. Thus, many of these high-dose trials employed either single chemotherapeutic agents (with or without low-dose agents in addition) (6 series; 2 with chest radiotherapy) (Banham *et al.,* 1982, 1983; Burnett *et al.,* 1983; Marangolo *et al.,* 1985; Smith *et al.,* 1985; Souhami *et al.,* 1989; Lange *et al.,* 1991; Jennis *et al.,* 1996), single alkylating agents (6 series; 4 with chest radiotherapy) (Klastersky *et al.,* 1982; Farha *et al.,* 1983; Cunningham *et al.,* 1985; Sculier *et al.,* 1985; Ihde *et al.,* 1986; Spitzer *et al.,* 1986; Lange *et al.,* 1991), or combination alkylating agents (10 series; 6 with chest radiotherapy) (Pico *et al.,* 1983; Stewart *et al.,* 1983; Cornbleet *et al.,* 1984; Stahel *et al.,* 1984; Humblet *et al.,* 1987; Wilson *et al.,* 1988; Nomura *et al.,* 1990; Elias *et al.,* 1993; Brugger *et al.,* 1995; Tomeczko *et al.,*

1996). Results are shown in Table 45.3, and suggest improved outcomes in those given combination alkylating agent chemotherapy and chest radiotherapy. Higher treatment-related morbidity and mortality occurred than is currently expected with the use of blood stem cell autografts.

Humblet *et al.* (1987) designed a randomized trial of five cycles of conventional therapy with prophylactic cranial irradiation followed by one further cycle of either high or conventional dose therapy using cyclophosphamide, etoposide, and carmustine. No chest radiotherapy was given. Of 101 SCLC patients entered, only 45 were eligible for randomization due to disease progression and morbidity of treatment. A clear dose-response was demonstrated. Conversion from partial to complete response occurred in 77% of evaluable patients after high-dose therapy, compared with none after conventional-dose treatment. Disease-free survival was significantly enhanced, and a trend toward improved survival was observed. However, an 18% treatment-related death rate in the transplant arm led the investigators to conclude that dose-intensive therapy should not be considered as standard therapy in SCLC. Moreover, since chest radiotherapy was not given in this trial, almost all patients who relapsed, recurred in the chest.

High rates of relapse in sites of prior tumor involvement (Sculier *et al.,* 1985; Souhami *et al.,* 1989), may be explained by greater tumor burden in the chest, the possible presence of drug-resistant clones or non-SCLC elements, poorer drug delivery, or intratumoral resistance factors such as hypoxia, or, in the case of autograft contamination by tumor cells, the possibility of homing and microenvironmental support for the tumor in local and regional sites. By 3-years posttransplant, chest relapse is expected in 90% of individuals following chemotherapy alone, and in 60% after conventional-dose radiotherapy. Thus, radiotherapy to sites of bulk disease is likely to represent an essential component in approaches to curative treatment.

Disease-specific pretransplant work-up

Eligibility for transplant studies generally includes patients who are physiologically under age 60 (i.e., patients with an ECOG performance score of 0–1 and limited comorbidity, those over age 60 accepted on a case by case basis). Routine restaging studies included head MRI, chest and upper abdominal computed tomography (CT) scans, bone scan, bilateral

Table 45.3. *High-dose intensification therapy and autologous bone marrow transplantation for small cell lung cancer*

High-dose regimen	Number of trials	Subset with chest RT	Number of patients	Disease-free survival (%)	Treatment-related mortality (%)
Single agent	6	2	93	10	4
Single alkylating agent	6	4	102	9	3
Combination alkylating agents	10	6	92	32	16
Without chest RT	4	–	41	17	24
With chest RT	6	6	76	39	7

Abbreviation: RT, radiotherapy.

marrow aspirates and biopsies and eligibility laboratory tests to confirm continued response to first-line conventional dose induction chemotherapy. Laboratory requirements included leukocytes ≥3,000/μl, platelets ≥100,000/μl, creatinine ≤ 1.5 × normal, creatinine clearance ≥ 60 cc/min, serum SGOT and bilirubin ≤ 1.5 × normal, forced vital capacity (FVC) and carbon monoxide diffusing capacity (DLCO) of ≥ 60% of predicted (corrected for hemoglobin), a left ventricular ejection fraction (LVEF) of ≥ 45%, and pathology review.

Monitoring for residual disease posttransplant

Because SCLC can progress so quickly, typical monitoring posttransplant includes chest radiographs every 2 months for 6 months, then every 3 months to 2 years, then every 6 months to 5 years, then yearly. CBC with differential and liver function tests are obtained on a similar schedule. CT scans of the chest and upper abdomen are obtained every 3 to 4 months to 2 years, and then repeated only if clinical suspicion is raised.

Newer reports with cellular support

Jennis et al. (1996) treated 10 extensive stage patients showing partial responses to conventional dose chemotherapy with high-dose cyclophosphamide in order to mobilize blood stem cells. Six were transplanted after high-dose methotrexate and etoposide chemotherapy. A near complete response was obtained in all; however, all relapsed a median of 4 months later. Of note, half had documented tumor contamination of their blood stem cells.

In a Polish trial, 6 limited and 20 extensive stage patients were treated with two cycles of high-dose cyclophosphamide and etoposide as induction therapy followed by the same drugs as pretransplant conditioning in 6, or with BCNU in 20. Seven of 18 converted from a partial to a complete response. Seven patients were already in complete response. Five patients remained progression-free 3 to 89 months later. Of the complete responders, 29% remained disease-free beyond 2 years from transplant (Tomeczko et al., 1996). Brugger et al. (1995) reported 18 limited stage patients who received two cycles of VIPE (vincristine, ifosfamide, cisplatin, etoposide) with mobilization of blood stem cells. Thirteen (72%) then received high-dose ICE (ifosfamide, carboplatin, etoposide) chemotherapy with epirubicin followed by an autologous transplant. At a median of 14 months follow-up, event-free survival was 69%. Nine patients remained progression-free. Several Japanese phase II trials were reported demonstrating feasibility in administration of high-dose therapy to the more elderly SCLC population. In Okayama, 11 patients received induction (cisplatin/irinotecan for the 5 extensive disease patients and cisplatin/etoposide/chest radiotherapy for the 6 limited disease patients) (Bessho et al., 1999). Eight were transplanted after high-dose ICE. All relapsed except 2 of the 4 LD patients.

At the Dana-Farber Cancer Institute and Beth Israel Hospital, over 50 patients with limited stage, and over 25 with extensive stage, SCLC have been treated with high-dose combination alkylating agents following a response to conventional dose induction therapy. Of the original cohort of 36 limited stage SCLC (all had N2 or N3 disease), 29 were in or near complete response prior to treatment with high-dose cyclophosphamide, carmustine, and cisplatin with bone marrow (plus peripheral blood stem cells in some) support, followed by chest and prophylactic cranial radiotherapy (Elias et al., 1993). With a minimum follow-up of 3 (range 3–10) years from completion of high-dose chemotherapy, the 5-year event-free survival is 53% (Fig. 45.1) (Elias et al., 1999). Similar results have been observed in a separate cohort of 24 limited stage patients in or near complete response receiving high-dose CBP supported with CD34-enriched peripheral blood progenitor cells (A.D. Elias, manuscript in preparation). Local regional relapse represented about 50% of all relapses.

These investigators also reported their experience with extensive stage lung and extrapulmonary small cell carcinoma

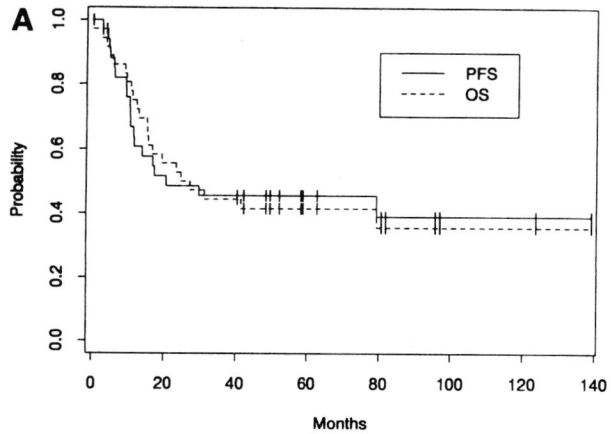

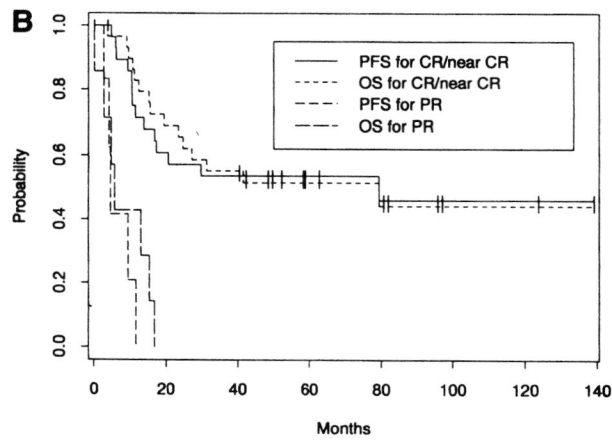

Fig. 45.1. Overall survival (OS; time from initiation of high-dose chemotherapy to death from any cause) and PFS [time from initiation of high-dose chemotherapy to first failure (progression of disease or death from any cause)] as determined by Kaplan-Meier method; | = follow-up time for patients. (A) All patients (n = 36); (B) patients in or near CR before intensification (n = 29) or in PR before intensification. Reproduced, with permission, from Elias et al. (1999).

(EPSC) (Elias *et al.*, 2002). Of 29 extensive disease SCLC, 24 had achieved complete or near complete response prior to high-dose CBP or ICE. Only two remained progression-free beyond 2 years. Of seven EPSC, three remain progression-free 8 to 72 months later. It was concluded that high-dose therapy did not provide any detectable benefit for extensive disease SCLC. The results for EPSC, however, were intriguing and in keeping with several other case reports in which two of five patients remain free from progression (Tetreault *et al.*, 1999; Buxhofer *et al.*, 2000).

The ABMTR analyzed 103 patients with SCLC from 22 centers whose data were submitted to the Registry (Rizzo *et al.*, 2002). The 100 day mortality was 11%. The 3-year progression-free and overall survival rates were 26% and 33% for all patients and 35% and 43% for limited stage patients. Poor prognosis was associated with age more than 50 years, extensive stage, and regimens other than CBP or ICE. These investigators also concluded that high-dose therapy held some promise for limited stage patients, but not for extensive stage patients.

Future directions

Intensification of involved field radiotherapy

As summarized by meta-analyses of randomized trials, chest radiotherapy provides a 25% improvement in local-regional control, and a 5% increase in long-term, progression-free survival for limited stage SCLC (Pignon *et al.*, 1992; Warde & Payne, 1992). With the commonly used 45 to 50 Gy thoracic radiotherapy approach, chest relapse remains unacceptably high (approximately 60% actuarial risk of local relapse by 3 years) (Bunn *et al.*, 1987; Kies *et al.*, 1987; Perry *et al.*, 1987), and may be underestimated due to the competing risk of systemic relapse (Arriagada *et al.*, 1992). Since chest-only relapse is observed in about 40% of patients, further enhancement of local-regional control may increase the proportion of long-term survivors. This concept has been supported by the survival benefit of chest radiotherapy after mastectomy for breast cancer. If systemic control is improved by high-dose chemotherapy, initial failure in local-regional sites may become more prevalent.

The dose intensity of chest radiotherapy has not been well studied. An ECOG/RTOG study (Turrisi *et al.*, 1994) reported a comparison of 45 Gy chest radiotherapy given either daily over 5 weeks or twice daily over 3 weeks concurrent with cisplatin and etoposide chemotherapy. Intensified chest radiotherapy reduced chest relapse from 61% to 48% at 2 to 3 years (*P* < .05). Further follow-up indicated that the daily radiotherapy regimen had a 75% local (with or without distant) failure rate whereas the twice daily radiotherapy regimen had a 42% overall local failure rate. There is now a survival advantage for the more intensive radiotherapy regimen. Choi *et al.* (personal communication) escalated the dose of radiotherapy in cohorts of 5 to 6 patients with limited stage SCLC. Thoracic radiotherapy was given concurrently with

cisplatin and etoposide either as daily 180 cGy fractions or as twice daily 150 cGy fractions. The maximal tolerated doses with respect to acute radiation esophagitis appeared to be 45 Gy for twice daily administration and 70 Gy when given once daily using a shrinking field technique. Five-year survival for the patients receiving high-dose radiotherapy in a daily fractionation schema was 36% (Choi *et al.*, 2002). Thus, marked intensification of radiotherapy dose appears possible and should be evaluated in a randomized setting.

The Cancer and Leukemia Group B and Southwest Oncology Group activated a phase II feasibility trial stemming from the above experience. Patients under age 60 with limited stage SCLC were treated with four cycles of cisplatin and etoposide and concurrent twice daily chest radiotherapy to 45 Gy (150 cGy fractions). Those patients achieving complete or near complete response received high-dose cyclophosphamide, cisplatin, and carmustine with autologous stem cell support. Upon recovery, prophylactic cranial irradiation was given. It was hoped that this would lead to a phase III trial. However, due in large part to the toxicity of the standard induction therapy, of 11 patients entered on trial, only 8 completed the induction therapy, and only 4 were able to receive high-dose therapy.

Intensification of induction therapy

Induction therapy reduces tumor burden, and allows selection of patients with chemosensitive tumors for subsequent intensification. Rapidly progressive systemic and local symptoms from SCLC can be controlled with marked improvement in performance status. Moreover, reduction of the degree of micrometastases in the marrow and/or blood may be obtained. Alternatively, it is possible that chemoresistant tumor cells might be induced by induction chemotherapy. Several strategies have been explored to intensify dose early in treatment. As previously discussed, the weekly multidrug regimens had greater planned dose intensity, but required sufficient dose reduction and delay due to unacceptable toxicity that the actual delivered dosing was not substantively enhanced (Sculier *et al.*, 1993; Souhami *et al.*, 1994). Similar findings were noted in cytokine-supported trials (Girling *et al.*, 1996).

As suggested by the Arriagada trial (Arriagada *et al.*, 1993), initial intensification of induction treatment may improve overall disease-free and overall survival. A logical extension of this concept would be to administer multicycle dose-intensive combination therapies supported by hematopoietic growth factors and blood progenitor cells infusion using either repeated cycles of the same regimen (Tepler *et al.*, 1993; Pettengell *et al.*, 1995; Perey *et al.*, 1996; Woll *et al.*, 1996) or a sequence of different agents (Gianni *et al.*, 1991; Crown *et al.*, 1992; Ayash *et al.*, 1994; Humblet *et al.*, 1996). Increasing experience with sequential cycles of stem cell supported therapy has been obtained in the treatment of good performance status SCLC patients. The doses delivered in individual cycles ranged from the conventional dosages (but given more frequently) to moderately intensified dosages (about two-thirds the doses of conventional pretransplant conditioning doses). Pettengell and colleagues (1995) have explored ways to achieve greater dose intensity with the ICE regimen. In a phase I trial, 25 patients received conventional dose ICE chemotherapy for six cycles. Autologous hematopoietic cell support was given on day 3 of chemotherapy. Cycle length was 3 weeks using cryopreserved pheresis products, or 2 weeks using either pheresis products or 750 cc of whole blood stored at 4°C. By repeating cycles when platelets had recovered above $30 \times 10^9/l$, the full planned dose intensity for each of the arms was achieved over the first three cycles, although only 56% completed all six cycles. Mortality was 12% and the complete response rate was 64%, but the median follow-up was only 10 months; thus, the longer term outcomes are unknown. The authors noted that the collection of whole blood without cryopreservation reduced the cost and complexity of treatment substantially. In a subsequent randomized phase II study, Woll et al. (1996) treated 50 "good prognosis" patients with ICE chemotherapy given either every 2 or 4 weeks. The median dose intensity delivered over the first three cycles was .99 (.33–1.02) versus 1.8 (.99–1.97) for the 4-week and 2-week cycles, respectively. More hematopoietic and infectious toxicity was encountered on the standard dose, 4-week arm.

Leyvraz et al. (1996) reported an EBMT experience with 69 patients (30 limited disease, 39 extensive disease). Mobilization was achieved with epirubicin and G-CSF followed by three monthly cycles of moderately intensive ICE chemotherapy. Radiation to the chest and head was recommended. An overall complete response was observed in 51%. Mortality was 9%, in part attributable to a learning curve. Median overall survival was 18 months for limited and 11 months for extensive disease. The delivered dose-intensity was 290% above the standard ICE regimen. These investigators are now conducting a randomized trial under the auspices of the EBMT.

Humblet et al. (1996) treated 37 limited stage patients with four intensive alternating cycles of ifosfamide with etoposide, and carboplatin with etoposide. Patients received 10 Gy thoracic radiotherapy in five fractions concurrently with each chemotherapy administration. The median follow-up was 15 months and the median overall survival was 25 months (van de Velde et al., 1999). Perhaps due to the fact that no prophylactic cranial irradiation was given, 12 of 25 relapses occurred in the brain. Mortality was 3%.

Minimal residual tumor and tumor involvement of the autograft

Tumor contamination of stem cells may be a source of relapse. As demonstrated by gene marking and other studies, residual tumor cells do contribute to relapse in certain hematologic malignancies and neuroblastoma (Gribben et al., 1991; Brenner et al., 1993; Brenner & Rill, 1994). It is less clear whether these cells are the sole cause for relapse or rather indicate that the patient has an increased endogenous chemotherapy-resistant tumor burden. Gene marking experiments in other solid tumors have not yet been informative (O'Shaughnessy et al., 1994).

In SCLC, the bone marrow is one of the most common metastatic sites. Of patients with untreated SCLC and histologically negative marrow biopsies at diagnosis, small trials have demonstrated that subclinical micrometastatic disease is detected in the marrow in 13% to 54% of limited, and in 44% to 77% of extensive stage SCLC by immunohistochemical techniques, with a sensitivity of detection of 1 in 104 cells (Stahel et al., 1985; Berendsen et al., 1988; Canon et al., 1988; Trillet et al., 1989; Beiske et al., 1992). Two small series suggested that two-thirds of patients with an excellent chemotherapy response had residual marrow contamination (Hay et al., 1988; Leonard et al., 1990). Leonard et al. (1990) suggested that residual marrow tumor predicted relapse. In patients with metastatic SCLC or breast cancer, peripheral blood cells mobilized with G-CSF during the first cycle of VIP chemotherapy had demonstrable circulating tumor cells, although their viability was not established (Brugger et al., 1994). Mobilization of tumor cells after the second cycle of chemotherapy was apparently not observed, supporting the contention that in vivo chemotherapy induction can "purge" the patient and the autologous stem cell source of tumor cells. In our own unpublished data, up to 85% of limited disease patients in or near complete response prior to high-dose therapy have detectable tumor cells in their marrow by keratin staining. Although CD34 selection can reduce the number of tumor cells infused, few autografts are rendered tumor-free using immunofluorescent detection methods (A.D. Elias, manuscript in preparation).

Numerous chemotherapeutic agents have major clinical activity against overt SCLC, although the uniformly dismal clinical outcomes suggest that systemic chemotherapy administration fails to eradicate a central core of tumor stem cells, presumably enriched for in vivo resistance mechanisms. Identification and characterization of these residual cancer cells may guide therapeutic strategies to specifically target these cells. Minimal residual tumor characterization could then be employed to determine additional treatment. Thus, the detection of heterogeneity and analysis of patterns of coexpression of various markers is the focus of our effort to detect rare cells. We are utilizing a confocal fluorescence microscope with automated computerized scanning with one set of fluorescent probes for detection and a second set with different fluorophores for biological characterization (Elias et al., 1996). Prospective trials to evaluate the clinical significance of marrow or peripheral blood tumor contamination and the impact of novel stem cell sources to support high-dose therapy are being initiated.

Indications and contraindications for autologous transplantation for small cell lung cancer

At this point, there is no indication that a single cycle of high-dose stem-cell supported therapy using the currently tested agents benefits patients with extensive disease, recurrent disease, or those in first partial response or worse. Whether such patients might benefit from multicycle intense therapy awaits further study. Selection of the limited stage patient for good physiology and lack of significant comorbid disease is paramount in avoiding the high mortality associated with many of the earlier studies.

An algorithm for the treatment of patients with small cell lung cancer

Those patients with limited stage disease and limited comorbidity, who present with a good performance status may be candidates for initial intensification and/or chemoradiotherapy induction followed by autologous HSC transplantation on a clinical trial. There is an additional cohort of patients, quite symptomatic at presentation, who have an excellent response to therapy and improve their performance status, who may then be candidates for later intensification strategies. Radiation therapy to the chest and brain appear to remain important components of an overall treatment strategy.

Conclusions

The two major strategies for administering high-dose therapy to patients with SCLC are the multicycle approach and the later, single intensification approach. Advantages for each approach are evident. The multicycle approach can achieve early dose intensity and maintain it for about 3 to 4 cycles. Its disadvantages include lower drug dosages than used pretransplant, high mortality rates, a general inability to deliver chest radiotherapy early (except in the Humblet trial, which used relatively low-dose thoracic radiation), and the collection of stem cells early in treatment when they are highly likely to be contaminated with tumor cells. On the other hand, the later single intensification approach can take advantage of initial therapy to control tumor-related symptoms with consequent improved performance status, a partial purge of tumor-contaminated stem cell sources, and the ability to give thoracic radiation early during intense induction therapy. Its major disadvantage is the later administration of the dose-intense cycle, although this drawback can be surmounted in part by intensification and shortening of induction chemoradiotherapy.

High-dose therapy kills more tumor cells. When toxicity is acceptable, it will result in prolonged progression-free survival. An additional group of patients may achieve minimal residual tumor burden (near-cure). If additional targets of residual tumor cells can be identified for novel treatment strategies and modalities, high-dose therapy may have increased value. The initial experience with the c-kit inhibitor STI571, however, will require more study (Johnson *et al.*, 2002). Most biological strategies, such as replacement of the retinoblastoma gene and/or p53 function, interference with autocrine or paracrine growth loops, or immunologic therapy (IL-2, IL-12, immunotoxins, tumor vaccines), will likely work best against minimal tumor burden. Multiple new agents with substantial SCLC

activity are now available for incorporation into high-dose treatment strategies including gemcitabine, irinotecan, and the taxanes.

References

Arriagada, R., Kramar, A., Le Chevalier, T., & De Cremoux, H. (1992). Competing events determining relapse-free survival in limited small-cell lung carcinoma. *Journal of Clinical Oncology*, **10**, 447–51.

Arriagada, R., Le Chevalier, T., Pignon, J-P. *et al.* (1993). Initial chemotherapeutic doses and survival in patients with limited small-cell lung cancer. *New England Journal of Medicine*, **329**, 1848–52.

Ayash, L., Elias, A., Wheeler, C. *et al.* (1994). Double dose-intensive chemotherapy with autologous marrow and peripheral blood progenitor cell support for metastatic breast cancer: a feasibility study. *Journal of Clinical Oncology*, **12**, 37–44.

Banham, S., Burnett, A., Stevenson, R. *et al.* (1982). Pilot study of combination chemotherapy with late dose intensification and autologous bone marrow rescue in small cell bronchogenic carcinoma. *British Journal of Cancer*, **42**, 486.

Banham, S., Loukop, M., Burnett, A. *et al.* (1983). Treatment of small cell carcinoma of the lung with late dosage intensification programmes containing cyclophosphamide and mesna. *Cancer Treatment Reviews*, **10** (Suppl A), 73–7.

Beiske, K., Myklebust, A.T., Aamdal, S. *et al.* (1992). Detection of bone marrow metastases in small cell lung cancer patients. *American Journal of Pathology*, **141**, 531–8.

Berendsen, H.H., De Leij, L., Postmus, P.E. *et al.* (1988). Detection of small cell lung cancer metastases in bone marrow aspirates using monoclonal antibody directed against neuroendocrine differentiation antigen. *Journal of Clinical Pathology*, **41**, 273–6.

Bessho, A., Ueoka, H., Kiura, K. *et al.* (1999). High-dose ifosfamide, carboplatin and etoposide with autologous peripheral blood progenitor cell transplantation for small-cell lung cancer. *Anticancer Research*, **19**, 693–8.

Boring, C.C., Squires, T.S., & Tong, T.T. (1994) Cancer Statistics, 1993. *CA: A Cancer Journal for Clinicians*, **44**, 19–51.

Brenner, M.K. & Rill, D.R. (1994). Gene marking to improve the outcome of autologous bone marrow transplantation. *Journal of Hematotherapy*, **3**, 33–6.

Brenner, M.K., Rill, D.R., Moen, R.C. *et al.* (1993). Gene-marking to trace origin of relapse after autologous bone-marrow transplantation. *Lancet*, **341**,(1), 85–6.

Brower, M., Ihde, D.C., Johnston-Early, A. *et al.* (1983). Treatment of extensive stage small cell bronchogenic carcinoma: effects of variation in intensity of induction chemotherapy. *American Journal of Medicine*, **75**, 993–1000.

Brugger, W., Bross, K.J., Glatt, M. *et al.* (1994). Mobilization of tumor cells and hematopoietic progenitor cells into peripheral blood of patients with solid tumors. *Blood*, **83**, 636–40.

Brugger, W., Frommhold, H., Pressler, K. *et al.* (1995). Use of high-dose etoposide/ifosfamide/carboplatin/epirubicin and peripheral blood progenitor cell transplantation in limited-disease small cell lung cancer. *Seminars in Oncology*, **22** (Suppl 2), 3–8.

Bunn, P.A., Lichter, A.S., Makuch, R.W. *et al.* (1987). Chemotherapy alone or chemotherapy with chest radiation therapy in limited stage small cell lung cancer. *Annals of Internal Medicine,* **106,** 655–62.

Burnett, A.K., Tansey, P., Hills, C. *et al.* (1983). Haematologic reconstitution following high-dose and supralethal chemoradiotherapy using stored non-cryopreserved autologous bone marrow. *British Journal of Haematology,* **54,** 309–16.

Buxhofer, V., Ruckser, R., Kier, P. *et al.* (2000). High dosage therapy with stem cell transplantation in neuroendocrine carcinoma. *Acta Medica Austriaca,* **27,** (Suppl 52), 37–9.

Canon, J.L., Humblet, Y., Lebacq-Verheyden, A.M. *et al.* (1988). Immunodetection of small cell lung cancer metastases in bone marrow using three monoclonal antibodies. *European Journal of Cancer and Clinical Oncology,* **24,** 147–50.

Choi, N.C., Herndon, J., Rosenman, J. *et al.* (2002). Long term survival data from CALGB 8837: radiation dose escalation and concurrent chemotherapy in limited stage small cell lung cancer (LD-SCLC): possible radiation dose-survival relationship. *Proceedings of the American Society of Clinical Oncology,* **21,** 298a (1190) (Abstract).

Cohen, M.H., Creaven, P.J., Fossieck, B.E. *et al.* (1977). Intensive chemotherapy of small cell bronchogenic carcinoma. *Cancer Treatment Reports,* **61,** 349–54.

Cornbleet, M., Gregor, A., Allen, S. *et al.* (1984). High-dose melphalan as consolidation therapy for good prognosis patients with small cell carcinoma of the bronchus (SCCB). *Proceedings of the American Society of Clinical Oncology,* **3,** 210 (Abstract).

Crawford, J., Ozer, H., Stoller, R. *et al.* (1991). Reduction by granulocyte colony-stimulating factor of fever and neutropenia induced by chemotherapy in patients with small-cell lung cancer. *New England Journal of Medicine,* **325,** 164–70.

Crown, J., Wasserheit, C., Hakes, T. *et al.* (1992). Rapid delivery of multiple high-dose chemotherapy courses with granulocyte colony-stimulating factor and peripheral blood-derived hematopoietic progenitor cells. *Journal of the National Cancer Institute,* **84,** 1935–6.

Cunningham, D., Banham, S.W., Hutcheon, A.H. *et al.* (1985). High-dose cyclophosphamide and VP-16 as late dosage intensification therapy for small cell carcinoma of lung. *Cancer Chemotherapy and Pharmacology,* **15,** 303–6.

Douer, D., Champlin, R.E., Ho, W.G. *et al.* (1981). High-dose combined-modality therapy and autologous bone marrow transplantation in resistant cancer. *American Journal of Medicine,* **71,** 973–6.

Eder, J.P., Antman, K., Shea, T.C. *et al.* (1988). Cyclophosphamide and thiotepa with autologous bone marrow transplantation in patients with solid tumors. *Journal of the National Cancer Institute,* **80,** 1221–6.

Elias, A. D. *et al.* (2002). Manuscript submitted for publication.

Elias, A., Li, Y., Wheeler, C. *et al.* (1996). CD34-selected peripheral blood progenitor cell (PBPC) support in high-dose therapy of small cell lung cancer (SCLC): use of a novel detection method for minimal residual tumor (MRT). *Proceedings of the American Association of Clinical Oncology,* **15,** 341 (Abstract).

Elias, A., Ibrahim, J., Skarin, A.T. *et al.* (1999). Dose-intensive therapy for limited-stage small-cell lung cancer: long-term outcome. *Journal of Clinical Oncology,* **17,** 1175–84.

Elias, A.D., Ayash, L., Frei, E. III *et al.* (1993). Intensive combined modality therapy for limited stage small cell lung cancer. *Journal of the National Cancer Institute,* **85,** 559–66.

Elias, A.D., Ayash, L.J., Wheeler, C. *et al.* (1995). A phase I study of high-dose ifosfamide, carboplatin, and etoposide with autologous hematopoietic stem cell support. *Bone Marrow Transplantation,* **15,** 373–9.

Farha, P., Spitzer, G., Valdivieso, M. *et al.* (1983). High-dose chemotherapy and autologous bone marrow transplantation for the treatment of small cell lung carcinoma. *Cancer,* **52,** 1351–5.

Figueredo, A.T., Hryniuk, W.M., Strautmanis, I. *et al.* (1985). Co-trimoxazole prophylaxis during high-dose chemotherapy of small-cell lung cancer. *Journal of Clinical Oncology,* **3,** 54–64.

Frei, E., III (1972). Combination cancer chemotherapy: Presidential address. *Cancer Research,* **32,** 2593–607.

Frei, E. III & Antman, K.H. (1993). Combination chemotherapy, dose, and schedule: section XV, principles of chemotherapy. In *Cancer Medicine,* ed. J.F. Holland, E. Frei, III, R.C. Bast, Jr. *et al.,* pp. 631–9. Philadelphia: Lea & Febiger.

Frei, E. III & Canellos, G.P. (1980). Dose, a critical factor in cancer chemotherapy. *American Journal of Medicine,* **69,** 585–94.

Furuse, K., Kubota, K., Nishiwaki, Y. *et al.* (1996). Phase III study of dose intensive weekly chemotherapy with recombinant human granulocyte-colony stimulating factor (G-CSF) versus standard chemotherapy in extensive stage small cell lung cancer (SCLC). *Proceedings of the American Society of Clinical Oncology,* **15,** 375 (Abstract).

Gianni, A.M., Siena, S., Bregni, M. *et al.* (1991). Prolonged disease-free survival after high-dose sequential chemo-radiotherapy and hemopoietic autologous transplantation in poor prognosis Hodgkin's disease. *Annals of Oncology,* **2,** 645–53.

Girling, D.J., Thatcher, N., Clark, P.I., & Stephens, R.J. (1996). Increasing the dose intensity of chemotherapy by means of granulocyte-colony stimulating factor (G-CSF) support in the treatment of small cell lung cancer (SCLC). *European Journal of Cancer,* **32,** 1263 (Letter).

Gribben, J.G., Freedman, A.S., Neuberg, D. *et al.* (1991). Immunologic purging of marrow assessed by PCR before autologous bone marrow transplantation for B-cell lymphoma. *New England Journal of Medicine,* **325,** 1525–33.

Harada, M., Yoshida, T., Funada, H. *et al.* (1982). Combined-modality therapy and autologous bone marrow transplantation in the treatment of advanced non-Hodgkin's lymphoma and solid tumors: the Kanawaza experience. *Transplantation Proceedings,* **14,** 733–7.

Hay, F.G., Ford, A., & Leonard, R.C.F. (1988). Clinical applications of immunocytochemistry in the monitoring of the bone marrow in small cell lung cancer (SCLC). *International Journal of Cancer,* **2,** Suppl 8–10.

Hryniuk, W. & Bush, H. (1984). The importance of dose intensity in chemotherapy of metastatic breast cancer. *Journal of Clinical Oncology,* **2,** 1281–8.

Humblet, Y., Bosquee, L., Weynants, P., & Symann, M. (1996). High-dose chemo-radiotherapy cycles for LD small cell lung cancer patients using G-CSF and blood stem cells. *Bone Marrow Transplantation,* **18** (Suppl 1), S36–9.

Humblet, Y., Symann, M., Bosly, A. *et al.* (1987). Late intensification chemotherapy with autologous bone marrow transplantation in selected small-cell carcinoma of the lung: a randomized study. *Journal of Clinical Oncology,* **5,** 1864–73.

Ihde, D.C., Diesseroth, A.B., Lichter, A.S. *et al.* (1986). Late intensive combined modality therapy followed by autologous bone marrow infusion in extensive stage small-cell lung cancer. *Journal of Clinical Oncology,* **4,** 1443–54.

Ihde, D.C., Mulshine, J.L., Kramer, B.S. *et al.* (1994). Prospective randomized comparison of high-dose and standard-dose etoposide and cisplatin chemotherapy in patients with extensive-stage small-cell lung cancer. *Journal of Clinical Oncology,* **12,** 2022–34.

Jennis, A., Levitan, N., Pecora, A.L. *et al.* (1996). Sequential high-dose chemotherapy (HDC) with filgrastim/peripheral stem cell support (PSCS) in extensive stage small cell lung cancer (SCLC). *Proceedings of the American Society of Clinical Oncology,* **15,** 349 (Abstract).

Johnson, B.E., Fisher, B., Fisher, T. *et al.* (2002). Phase II study of STI571 (Gleevec) for patients with small cell lung cancer. *Proceedings of the American Society of Clinical Oncology,* **21,** 293a (1171) (Abstract).

Johnson, D.H., Einhorn, L.H., Birch, R. *et al.* (1987). A randomized comparison of high-dose versus conventional dose cyclophosphamide, doxorubicin, and vincristine for extensive stage small cell lung cancer: a phase III trial of the Southeastern Cancer Study Group. *Journal of Clinical Oncology,* **5,** 1731–8.

Johnson, D.H., Hande, K.R., Hainsworth, J.D., & Greco, F.A. (1983). High-dose etoposide as single-agent chemotherapy for small cell carcinoma of the lung. *Cancer Treatment Reports,* **67,** 957–8.

Johnson, D.H., Kim, K., Sause, W. *et al.* (1996). Cisplatin and etoposide plus thoracic radiotherapy administered once or twice daily in limited stage small cell lung cancer: final report of Intergroup trial 0096. *Proceedings of the American Society of Clinical Oncology,* **15,** 374 (Abstract).

Kies, M.S., Mira, J.G., Crowley, J.J. *et al.* (1987). Multimodal therapy for limited small-cell lung cancer: a randomized study of induction combination chemotherapy with or without thoracic radiation in complete responders; and with wide-field versus reduced-field radiation in partial responders: a Southwest Oncology Group study. *Journal of Clinical Oncology,* **5,** 592–600.

Klasa, R.J., Murray, N., & Coldman, A.J. (1991). Dose-intensity meta-analysis of chemotherapy regimens in small-cell carcinoma of the lung. *Journal of Clinical Oncology,* **9,** 499–508.

Klastersky, J., Nicaise, C., Longeval, E. *et al.* (1982). Cisplatin, adriamycin and etoposide (CAV) for remission induction of small-cell bronchogenic carcinoma: evaluation of efficacy and toxicity and pilot study of a "late intensification" with autologous bone marrow rescue. *Cancer,* **50,** 652–8.

Lange, A., Kolodziej, J., Tomeczko, J. *et al.* (1991). Aggressive chemotherapy with autologous bone marrow transplantation in small cell lung carcinoma. *Archives of Immunology and Experimental Therapeutics,* **39,** 431–9.

Lazarus, H.M. & Elias, A.D. (1996). Autologous bone marrow and peripheral blood progenitor cell transplants in small cell lung cancer. *Bone Marrow Transplantation,* **17,** 1–3.

Lazarus, H.M., Spitzer, T.R., & Creger, R.T. (1990). Phase I trial of high-dose etoposide, high-dose cisplatin, and reinfusion of autologous bone marrow for lung cancer. *American Journal of Clinical Oncology,* **13,** 107–12.

LeChevalier, T., Alain, R., Jean Pierre, P. *et al.* (2002). Is there an optimal dose for frontline chemotherapy (CT) in limited small cell lung cancer (SCLC)? Results of a randomized trial in 295 patients from the French Cancer Centers Group. *Proceedings of the American Society of Clinical Oncology,* **21,** 294a (1172) (abstract).

Leonard, R.C.F., Duncan, L.W., & Hay, F.G. (1990). Immunocytological detection of residual marrow disease at clinical remission predicts metastatic relapse in small cell lung cancer. *Cancer Research,* **50,** 6545–8.

Leyvraz, S., Perey, L., Rosti, G. *et al.* (1999). Multiple courses of high-dose ifosfamide, carboplatin, and etoposide with peripheral-blood progenitor cells and filgrastim for small-cell lung cancer: a feasibility study by the European Group for Blood and Marrow Transplantation. *Journal of Clinical Oncology,* **17,** 3531–9.

Littlewood, T.J., Bentley, D.P., & Smith, A.P. (1986). High-dose etoposide with autologous bone marrow transplantation as initial treatment of small cell lung cancer—negative report. *European Journal of Respiratory Diseases,* **68,** 370–4.

Littlewood, T.J., Spragg, B.P., & Bentley, D.P. (1985). When is autologous bone marrow transplantation safe after high-dose treatment with etoposide. *Clinical and Laboratory Hematology,* **7,** 213–18.

Marangolo, M., Rosti, G., Ravaioli, A. *et al.* (1985). Small cell carcinoma of the lung (SCCL): high-dose (HD) VP-16 and autologous bone marrow transplantation (ABMT) as intensification therapy: preliminary results. *International Journal of Cell Cloning,* **3,** 277.

Mehta, C. & Vogl, S.E. (1982). High-dose cyclophosphamide in the induction therapy of small cell lung cancer: minor improvements in rate of remission and survival. *Proceedings of the American Association of Cancer Research,* **23,** 155 (Abstract).

Miles, D.W., Earl, H.M., Souhami, R.L. *et al.* (1991). Intensive weekly chemotherapy for good-prognosis patients with small-cell lung cancer. *Journal of Clinical Oncology,* **9,** 280–5.

Murray, N., Gelmon, K., Shah, A. *et al.* (1994). Potential for long-term survival in extensive stage small-cell lung cancer (ESCLC) with CODE chemotherapy and radiotherapy. *Lung Cancer,* **11** (Suppl 1), 99.

Murray, N., Livingston, R., Shepherd, F. *et al.* (1997). A randomized study of CODE plus thoracic irradiation versus alternating CAV/EP for extensive stage small cell lung cancer (ESCLC). *Proceedings of the American Society of Clinical Oncology,* **16,** 456 (Abstract).

Nomura, F., Shimokata, K., Saito, H. *et al.* (1990). High-dose chemotherapy with autologous bone marrow transplantation for limited small cell lung cancer. *Japanese Journal of Clinical Oncology,* **20,** 94–8.

O'Shaughnessy, J.A., Cowan, K.H., Cottler-Fox, M. *et al.* (1994). Autologous transplantation of retrovirally-marked CD34-positive bone marrow and peripheral blood cells in patients with multiple myeloma or breast cancer. *Proceedings of the American Association of Clinical Oncology,* **13,** 296 (Abstract).

Osterlind, K., Hansen, H.H., Hansen, M. *et al.* (1986). Long-term disease-free survival in small-cell carcinoma of the lung: a study of clinical determinants. *Journal of Clinical Oncology,* **4,** 1307–13.

Perey, L., Rosti, G., Lange, A. *et al.* (1996). Sequential high-dose ICE chemotherapy with circulating progenitor cells (CPC) in small cell lung cancer: an EBMT study. *Bone Marrow Transplantation,* **18** (Suppl 1), S40–3.

Perry, M.C., Eaton, W.L., Propert, K.J. *et al.* (1987). Chemotherapy with or without radiation therapy in limited small-cell carcinoma of the lung. *New England Journal of Medicine,* **316**, 912–18.

Pettengell, R., Woll, P.J., Thatcher, N. *et al.* (1995). Multicyclic, dose-intensive chemotherapy supported by sequential reinfusion of hematopoietic progenitors in whole blood. *Journal of Clinical Oncology,* **13**, 148–56.

Phillips, G.L., Fay, J.W., Herzig, G.P. *et al.* (1983). Nitrosourea (BCNU), NSC #4366650 and cryopreserved autologous marrow transplantation for refractory cancer: a phase I-II study. *Cancer,* **52**, 1792–802.

Pico, J.L., Beaujean, F., Debre, M. *et al.* (1983). High-dose chemotherapy (HDC) with autologous bone marrow transplantation (ABMT) in small cell carcinoma of the lung (SCCL) in relapse. *Proceedings of the American Society of Clinical Oncology,* **2**, 206 (Abstract).

Pico, J.L., Baume, D., Ostronoff, M. *et al.* (1987). Chimiotherapie à hautes doses suivie d'autogreffe de moelle osseuse dans le traitement du cancre bronchique a petites cellules. *Bulletin of Cancer,* **74**, 587–95.

Pignon, J.P., Arriagada, R., Ihde, D.C. *et al.* (1992). A meta-analysis of thoracic radiotherapy for small-cell lung cancer. *New England Journal of Medicine,* **327**, 1618–24.

Postmus, P.E., Mulder, N.H., & Elema, J.D. (1988). Graft versus host disease after transfusions of non-irradiated blood cells in patients having received autologous bone marrow. *European Journal of Cancer,* **24**, 889–94.

Rizzo, J.D., Elias, A.D., Stiff, P.J. *et al.* (2002). Autologous stem cell transplantation for small cell lung cancer. *Biology of Blood and Marrow Transplantation,* **8**, 273–80.

Rushing, D.A., Baldauf, M.C., Gehlsen, J.A. *et al.* (1984). High-dose BCNU and autologous bone marrow reinfusion in the treatment of refractory or relapsed small cell carcinoma of the lung (SCCL). *Proceedings of the American Society of Clinical Oncology,* **3**, 217 (Abstract).

Sculier, J.P., Klastersky, J., Stryckmans, P. *et al.* (1985). Late intensification in small-cell lung cancer: a phase I study of high-doses of cyclophosphamide and etoposide with autologous bone marrow transplantation. *Journal of Clinical Oncology,* **3**, 184–91.

Sculier, J.P., Paesmans, M., Bureau, G. *et al.* (1993). Multiple drug weekly chemotherapy versus standard combination regimen in small cell lung cancer: a phase III randomized study conducted by the European Lung Cancer Working Party. *Journal of Clinical Oncology,* **11**, 1858–65.

Seifter, E.J. & Ihde, D.C. (1988). Therapy of small cell lung cancer: a perspective on two decades of clinical research. *Seminars in Oncology,* **15**, 278–99.

Smith, I.E., Evans, B.D., Harland, S.J. *et al.* (1985). High-dose cyclophosphamide with autologous bone marrow rescue after conventional chemotherapy in the treatment of small cell lung carcinoma. *Cancer Chemotherapy and Pharmacology,* **14**, 120–4.

Souhami, R.L., Hajichristou, H.T., Miles, D.W. *et al.* (1989). Intensive chemotherapy with autologous bone marrow transplantation for small cell lung cancer. *Cancer Chemotherapy and Pharmacology,* **24**, 321–5.

Souhami, R.L., Rudd, R., Ruiz de Elvira, M.C. *et al.* (1994). Randomized trial comparing weekly versus 3-week chemotherapy in small cell lung cancer: a Cancer Research Campaign trial. *Journal of Clinical Oncology,* **12**, 1806–13.

Spitzer, G., Dicke, K.A., Latam, J. *et al.* (1980). High-dose combination chemotherapy with autologous bone marrow transplantation in adult solid tumors. *Cancer,* **45**, 3075–85.

Spitzer, G., Dicke, K.A., Verma, D.S. *et al.* (1979). High-dose BCNU therapy with autologous bone marrow infusion: preliminary observations. *Cancer Treatment Reports,* **63**, 1257–64.

Spitzer, G., Farha, P., Valdivieso, M. *et al.* (1986). High-dose intensification therapy with autologous bone marrow support for limited small-cell bronchogenic carcinoma. *Journal of Clinical Oncology,* **4**, 4–13.

Stahel, R.A., Mabry, M., Skarin, A.T. *et al.* (1985). Detection of bone marrow metastasis in small-cell lung cancer by monoclonal antibody. *Journal of Clinical Oncology,* **3**, 455–61.

Stahel, R.A., Takvorian, R.W., Skarin, A.T., & Canellos, G.P. (1984). Autologous bone marrow transplantation following high-dose chemotherapy with cyclophosphamide, BCNU, and VP-16 in small cell carcinoma of the lung and a review of current literature. *European Journal of Cancer and Clinical Oncology,* **20**, 1233–8.

Stewart, P., Buckner, C.D., Thomas, E.D. *et al.* (1983). Intensive chemoradiotherapy with autologous marrow transplantation for small cell carcinoma of the lung. *Cancer Treatment Reviews,* **67**, 1055–9.

Teicher, B.A. (1992). Preclinical models for high-dose therapy. In *High-Dose Cancer Therapy: Pharmacology, Hematopoietins, Stem cells,* ed. J.O. Armitage & K.H. Antman, pp. 14–2. Baltimore: Williams & Wilkins.

Tepler, I., Cannistra, S.A., Frei, E. III *et al.* (1993). Use of peripheral blood progenitor cells abrogates the myelotoxicity of repetitive outpatient high-dose carboplatin and cyclophosphamide chemotherapy. *Journal of Clinical Oncology,* **11**, 1583–91.

Tetreault, S.A., Kossman, C., & Mason, J. (1999). Syngeneic bone marrow transplantation for small cell carcinoma of the esophagus. *Bone Marrow Transplantation,* **24**, 813–4.

Tomeczko, J., Pacuszko, T., Napora, P., & Lange, A. (1996). Treatment intensification which includes high-dose induction improves survival of lung carcinoma patients treated by high-dose chemotherapy with hematopoietic progenitor cell rescue but does not prevent high rate of relapses. *Bone Marrow Transplantation,* **18**, (Suppl 1), S44–7.

Trillet, V., Revel, D., Combaret, V. *et al.* (1989). Bone marrow metastases in small cell lung cancer: detection with magnetic resonance imaging and monoclonal antibodies. *British Journal of Cancer,* **60**, 83–8.

Turrisi, A.T., Kim, K., Johnson, D.H. *et al.* (1994). Daily (qd) v twice-daily (bid) thoracic irradiation (TI) with concurrent cisplatin-etoposide (PE) for limited small cell lung cancer (LSCLC): preliminary results on 352 randomized eligible patients. *Lung Cancer,* **11** (Suppl 1), 172.

van de Velde, H., Bosquee, L., Weynants, P. *et al.* (1999). Moderate dose-escalation of combination chemotherapy with concomitant thoracic radiotherapy in limited-disease small-cell lung cancer: prolonged intrathoracic tumor control and high central nervous system relapse rate. *Annals of Oncology,* **10,** 1051–7.

Warde, P. & Payne, D. (1992). Does thoracic irradiation improve survival and local control in limited-stage small-cell carcinoma of the lung? A meta-analysis. *Journal of Clinical Oncology,* **10,** 890–5.

Wilson, C., Pickering, D., Stewart, S. *et al.* (1988). High-dose chemotherapy with autologous bone marrow rescue in small cell lung cancer. *In Vivo,* **2,** 331–4.

Wolff, S.W., Fer, M.F., McKay, C.M. *et al.* (1983). High-dose VP-16-213 and autologous bone marrow transplantation for refractory malignancies: a phase I study. *Journal of Clinical Oncology,* **1,** 701–5.

Woll, P.J., Lee, S.M., Lomax, L. *et al.* (1996). Randomized phase II study of standard versus dose-intensive ICE chemotherapy with reinfusion of hemopoietic progenitors in whole blood in small cell lung cancer (SCLC). *Proceedings of the American Society of Clinical Oncology,* **15,** 333 (Abstract).

46 Autologous hematopoietic stem cell transplantation after high-dose chemotherapy for primary malignant tumors of the central nervous system

SRIDHARAN GURURANGAN, SHARON GARDNER, AND JONATHAN FINLAY

Duke University Medical Center, Durham, USA and the Stephen D. Hassenfeld Cancer Center and New York University Cancer Institute, New York, USA

Introduction

Primary central nervous system (CNS) tumors are the second most common malignancies in children, with a frequency of 13 per 100,000 children per year (Duffner *et al.,* 1986; Rickert, 1998; Bleyer, 1999). The incidence of CNS tumors in adults is 6.5 per 100,000 population at 35 years and increases to 70 by 70 years of age (Annegers *et al.,* 1981). Decades of clinical investigation based on promising leads provided by well-conducted preclinical studies have failed to improve outcome for most patients with brain tumors and survival has generally lagged behind what has been achieved in childhood lymphoblastic leukemia and other solid tumors. Factors frequently cited as responsible for this therapeutic failure include the blood-tumor barrier (Stewart, 1994; Groothuis, 2000) and drug resistance (both inherent and acquired) (Scotto *et al.,* 2001). Overcoming such barriers to treatment has been the focus of recent research in developing more innovative therapies for patients with malignant CNS tumors. High-dose chemotherapy (HDC) with stem cell rescue is one such strategy that has been increasingly used in the last several years with the aim of overcoming the blood-tumor barrier and drug resistance both in patients with newly diagnosed and recurrent malignant brain tumors. This chapter will attempt to elucidate the underlying rationale of this strategy and the pharmacologic principles, efficacy, and toxicity of the various chemotherapeutic regimens used in HDC of malignant brain tumors.

Pharmacologic rationale for high-dose chemotherapy and choice of chemotherapeutic agents

HDC for brain tumors is based on the premise that there is a steep dose-response relationship for many chemotherapeutic agents, particularly alkylating drugs (Rosenblum *et al.,* 1977; Frei *et al.,* 1988, 1989). In preclinical in vitro and in vivo studies of human tumor cells including the MCF-7 breast cancer cell lines, the dose-response curve, analyzed over multiple logs of tumor stem cell depletion, revealed that the reduction in stem cell viability was linear for alkylating agents like nitrosoureas (BCNU or CCNU), thiotepa, cisplatin, 4-hydroxypercyclophosphamide,

melphalan, and busulfan (Frei *et al.,* 1989) (Figure 46.1). In contrast, nonalkylating drugs like methotrexate and vinca alkaloids demonstrated a response curve that was curvilinear, implying initial tumor cell kill followed by a lack of response related to innate drug resistance (Frei *et al.,* 1989). This characteristic of alkylators is critical for maintaining multiple logs of cell kill and consequent depletion of tumor stem cells to achieve cure. While drug resistance is a potential problem, tumor models using non-CNS tumor cell lines have shown that extensive and prolonged selection pressure results in minimal drug resistance when alkylating agents are employed in escalating doses (Frei *et al.,* 1985). Hence, for example, a 20-fold increase in dose, as can be attained in the setting of HDC, can theoretically produce total stem cell kill within a tumor cell population (Frei *et al.,* 1985, 1989). Since the number of

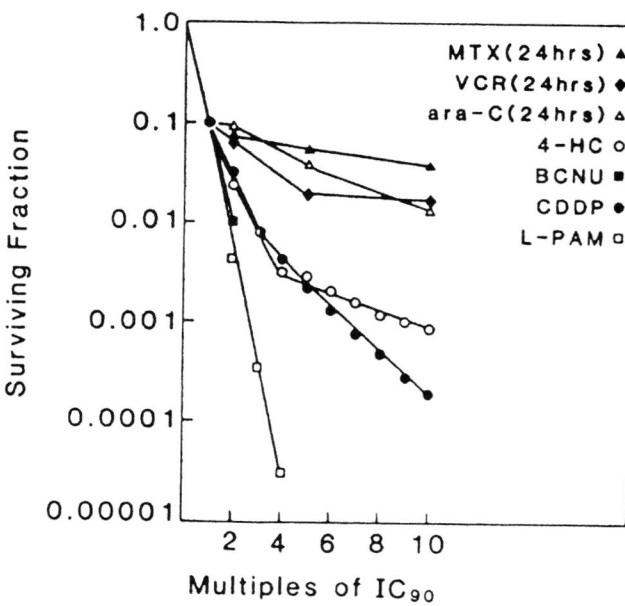

Fig. 46.1. Survival of the MCF-7 human breast carcinoma parent cell line exposed to several alkylating agents (4-HC, BCNU, CDDP, and L-PAM) for 1 hour or nonalkylating agents (MTX, VCR, and ara-C) for 24 hours. The results are expressed as multiples of the IC_{90} for each drug. Reproduced, with permission, from Frei *et al.* (1988).

resistant tumor cells is directly proportional to the size of the tumor, it is preferable to treat patients with the least tumor burden (minimal residual disease). This can be achieved with the use of surgery, and four to six cycles of conventional chemotherapy (which would also provide preliminary evidence that the tumor is chemosensitive), and/or radiotherapy. While the use of single alkylating agents in myeloablative therapy has produced objective responses in brain tumors, heterogeneity of malignant cells within the same tumor dictates that sustained clinical responses are hard to maintain by the use of monotherapy (Frei *et al.*, 1998). Instead, the use of two- or three-drug combinations, by virtue of lack of cross-resistance and the presence of synergism (Schabel *et al.*, 1978; Teicher *et al.*, 1990), will theoretically enable eradication of all stem cells within a tumor and enhance cure rates. The use of topoisomerase inhibitors like etoposide in combination with alkylating agents in high-dose chemotherapy regimens is an attractive approach and has been shown to be synergistic in preclinical studies involving brain tumor xenografts (Lilley *et al.*, 1990; Janss *et al.*, 1998; Castellino *et al.*, 2000). Pourquier *et al.* (2001) have shown that alkylation of DNA at the O^6 position of guanidine results in increased topoisomerase I cleavage and decreased religation of DNA, an effect that can potentially be enhanced in the presence of topoisomerase inhibitors. Drugs like etoposide and topotecan also exhibit significant penetration into the CNS and have been utilized in high doses both as a single agent and in multidrug combinations (Leff *et al.*, 1988; Long *et al.*, 1989; Kushner *et al.*, 2001). However, it is important to select these agents carefully when using combination chemotherapy. Additive toxicity might offset any therapeutic advantage obtained from increase in cell kill due to the combination.

A thorough understanding of the clinical pharmocokinetics of drugs used in high doses is crucial in order to use them effectively and safely in patients with brain tumors. Increased doses of a drug can easily saturate elimination pathways and result in nonlinear and unpredictable pharmacokinetics (Huitema *et al.*, 2000). In addition, schedule of administration may be important when multiple agents are used in HDC. For example, the area under the concentration time curve (AUC) of cyclophosphamide and its metabolite 4-hydroperoxycyclophosphamide is schedule dependent when given in combination with thiotepa, with increased AUC of the former and decreased AUC of the latter when thiotepa is given before cyclophosphamide. This is due to inhibition of hepatic cytochrome P-450 (CYP) enzymes by thiotepa and the consequent decreased metabolism of cyclophosphamide (Huitema *et al.*, 2000). Similarly, medications that are used during HDC like phenytoin, phenobarbital, and ondansetron can induce CYP enzymes and have a profound influence on the metabolism of drugs like cyclophosphamide (Huitema *et al.*, 2000). Additional factors that need to be considered when choosing drugs for HDC in patients with brain tumors include organ function status, the possible disrupted blood-brain barrier in the vicinity of brain tumors (Long, 1970; Stewart, 1994; Groothuis, 2000), lipid solubility, molecular size, degree of ionization, and protein binding of chemotherapeutic agents (Wolff, 1995). Table 46.1 summarizes the various HDC regimens used in patients with malignant brain tumors.

Table 46.1. *Myeloablative chemotherapy regimens used in patients with malignant CNS tumors*

Myeloablative regimen	Drug doses	Reference
Single agents		
Carmustine (BCNU)	600–1,400 mg/m^2 over 3 to 4 days	Phillips *et al.* (1986); Abrey *et al.* (1996); Johnson *et al.* (1987); Biron *et al.* (1991)
Aziridinylbenzoquinone	125–150 mg/m^2 over 5 days	Abrams *et al.* (1985)
Etoposide	1,800–2,400 mg/m^2 over 3 days	Long *et al.* (1989); Left *et al.* (1988); Giannone *et al.* (1987)
Thiotepa	600–900 mg/m^2 over 3 days	Ascensao *et al.* (1989); Ahmed *et al.* (1990)
Multidrug regimens		
Thiotepa and etoposide	Thiotepa 900 mg/m^2 and etoposide 750 mg/m^2 over 3 days	Finlay *et al.* (1996)
Carboplatin, thiotepa, and etoposide	Carboplatin 1,500 mg/m^2, thiotepa 900 mg/m^2, and etoposide 750 mg/m^2 over 3 days	Finlay (1993)
Thiotepa, etoposide, and BCNU	Thiotepa 600 mg/m^2, etoposide 750 mg/m^2, and BCNU 600 mg/m^2 over 3 days	Finlay *et al.* (1990); Abrey *et al.* (1998)
Cyclophosphamide and melphalan	Cyclophosphamide 6 g/m^2 over 4 days and melphalan 75–150 mg/m^2 over 3 days	Mahoney *et al.* (1996); Graham *et al.* (1997)
Melphalan and bulsulfan	Melphalan 140–180 mg/m^2 single dose and busulfan 600 mg/m^2 over 4 days	Graham *et al.* (1997)
Cyclophosphamide and thiotepa	Cyclophosphamide 3–6 g/m^2 over 3 to 4 days and thiotepa 600–900 mg/m^2 over 3 days	Heideman *et al.* (1993); Kedar *et al.* (1994)
Cyclophosphamide, cisplatin, and vincristine	Cyclophosphamide 4 g/m^2, cisplatin 75 mg/m^2, and vincristine 1.5 mg/m^2 over 3 days	Strother *et al.* (2001)
Topotecan, thiotepa, and carboplatin	Topotecan 10 mg/m^2 over 4 days, thiotepa 900 mg/m^2 over 3 days, and carboplatin 1,500 mg/m^2 over 3 days	Kushner *et al.* (2001)

Disease-specific pretransplant work-up

Selection of patients with recurrent malignant brain tumors for HDC requires meticulous planning and attention to detail since the procedure carries a definite risk for permanent organ damage and possibly even death from serious organ dysfunction. Most patients with recurrent brain tumors who are candidates for HDC have already been exposed to chemotherapy and irradiation and have suffered some organ damage as a consequence of these interventions. Comorbid conditions including hypertension, diabetes mellitus, or cardiac, pulmonary, or hepatic diseases can further contribute to organ dysfunction. Hence, the importance of assessing organ function before embarking on this intensive procedure cannot be overemphasized.

Since the success of HDC in solid tumors is best achieved in the setting of minimal residual disease, it is imperative that the physician establishes the extent of disease prior to considering this treatment and exclude patients with bulky local disease and those with metastatic spread that cannot be reduced to minimal status. Extent of disease in patients with brain tumors is readily assessed with contrast-enhanced magnetic resonance imaging of the brain and spine and cerebrospinal fluid cytology for malignant cells, preferably within 14 days of HDC. Due to the risk of tumor spread to the bone and bone marrow in a small proportion of patients with primitive neuroectodermal tumor (PNET) of the brain, a technetium (Tc^{99m}) radiolabeled bone scan and a bone marrow aspirate and biopsy (preferably from four sites) are required in such patients to ensure the absence of

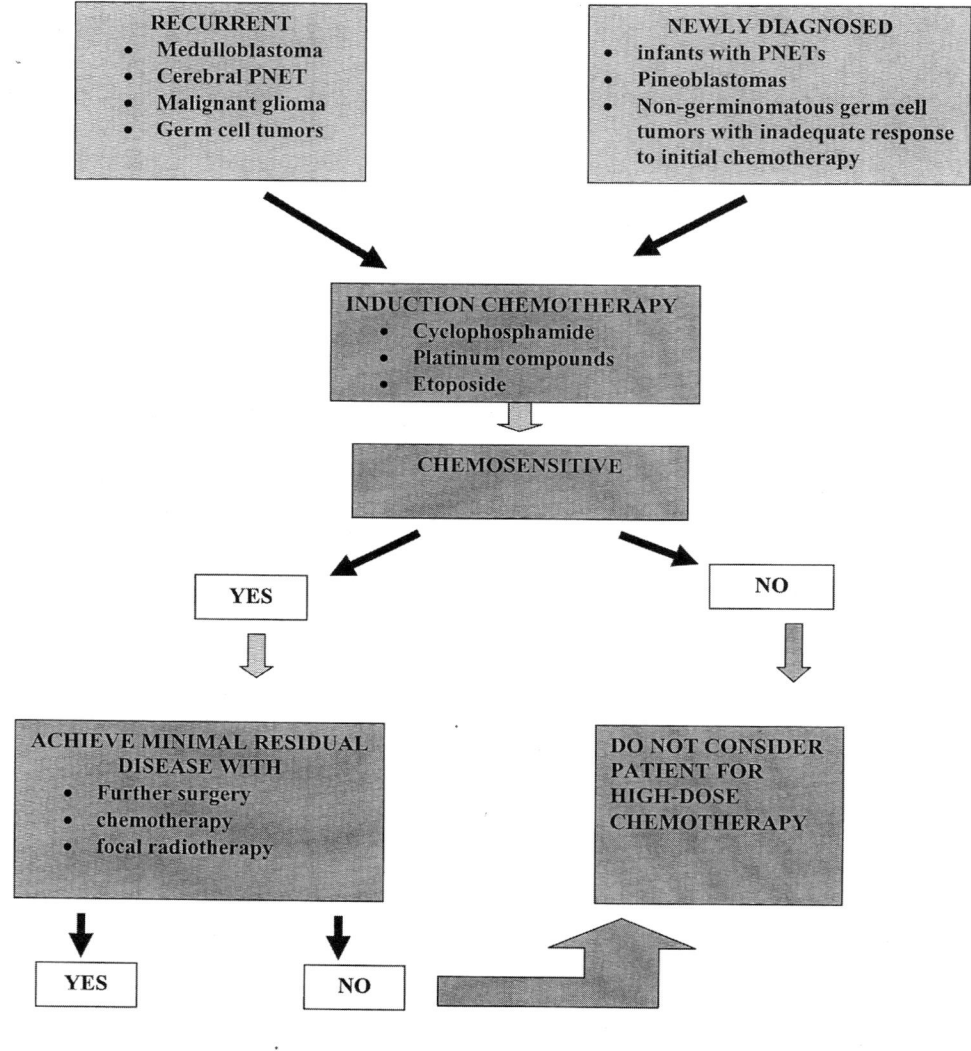

Fig. 46.2. An algorithm for high-dose chemotherapy with stem cell rescue in patients with malignant brain tumors.

tumor in these areas prior to bone marrow harvest and to avoid collection of tumor-contaminated marrow cells.

A peripheral blood CD34 count obtained 3 days following granulocyte colony-stimulating factor (G-CSF) administration can be a useful predictor of hematopoietic stem cell yield following peripheral blood stem cell harvest and marrow recovery following HDC, particularly in patients who have received intensive chemo/radiotherapy previously (Duggan et al., 2000; Heuft et al., 2001; Peng et al., 2001; Stewart et al., 2001). A recommended pretransplant work-up is summarized in Table 46.2.

Clinical studies of high-dose chemotherapy in malignant brain tumors

Malignant glial tumors

Supratentorial anaplastic astrocytoma and glioblastoma multiforme

Anaplastic astrocytoma (AA) and glioblastoma multiforme (GBM) in the supratentorial region are rare in children and constitute approximately 6% of all pediatric brain tumors (Duffner et al., 1986; Bleyer, 1999; Rickert et al., 2001). In adults, however, these tumors account for over 40% of all CNS malignancies (Duncan et al., 1992).

The outcome for these tumors in adults is dismal with conventional therapy, which includes surgery, chemotherapy, and local irradiation, with median survivals of less than 12 months (Duncan et al., 1992). The addition of BCNU both during radiotherapy and every 8 weeks for a year thereafter did not improve survival (Nelson et al., 1993). A meta-analysis of all randomized clinical trials in high-grade gliomas has found a marginal benefit (about 6% improvement in 1-year survival from 40% to 46%) for patients who receive radiotherapy and chemotherapy (Stewart, 2002). An improved outcome was

Table 46.2. *Recommended diagnostic workup for patients with brain tumors considered for high-dose chemotherapy*

Complete blood count with differential
Peripheral blood CD34 count following SC G-CSF for 3 days
Electrolytes, BUN, creatinine
Serum bilirubin, SGOT, SGPT, serum alkaline phosphatase, GGT
GFR as estimated by $TC^{99}DTPA$ clearance or 24-hour urine
   creatinine clearance
Chest X-ray, pulmonary function tests including DLCO
12-lead electrocardiogram and MUGA scan
MRI of the brain and spine
CSF cytology for malignant cells
Bone marrow aspirate and biopsy

Abbreviations: SC, subcutaneous; G-CSF, granulocyte colony-stimulating factor; BUN, blood urea nitrogen; SGOT, serum glutamate oxalacetate transaminase; SGPT, serum glutamate pyruvate; GGT, gamma glutamyl transaminase; GFR, glomerular filtration rate; DLCO, diffusion capacity of carbon monoxide; MUGA, multigated equilibrium TC^{99m} radionuclide cineangiography; CSF, cerebrospinal fluid.

noted in pediatric patients with non-midline tumors who underwent radical surgical resection, adjuvant chemotherapy, and local irradiation (Sposto et al., 1989; Marchese & Chang, 1990; Finlay et al., 1995). However, the overall prognosis for these tumors with conventional chemotherapy remains poor.

HDC with autologous stem cell rescue has been evaluated in AA and GBM since the 1980s due to their poor response to conventional therapies (Table 46.3). The early studies in adults used single-agent therapy with BCNU (Phillips et al., 1986; Johnson et al., 1987; Biron et al., 1991). These studies included patients with newly diagnosed or recurrent tumors. The dose of BCNU ranged from 600 to 1,400 mg/m² over 3 to 4 days. Local irradiation was given either preceding or following myeloablative therapy. While impressive durable remissions were observed in one report (Johnson et al., 1987), other studies have reported median survivals of less than 12 months (Phillips et al., 1986; Biron et al., 1991). Also, prohibitive pulmonary hepatic, and CNS toxicities were observed. In a large series of 98 patients reported by Biron et al., BCNU was given at a dose of 800 mg/m² over 3 days followed by radiotherapy 6 weeks later. The toxic death rate was approximately 6% and serious pulmonary toxicity was encountered in 20 patients.

Other single agents used include aziridinylbenzoquinone (125–150 mg/m² over 5 days) (Abrams et al., 1985), etoposide (125–150 mg/m² over 3 days) (Giannone et al., 1987; Leff et al., 1988; Long et al., 1989), and thiotepa (600–900 mg/m² over 3 days) (Ascensao et al., 1989; Ahmed et al., 1990; Abrey et al., 1999). Responses to these agents have been variable and have not been sustained in most cases.

Myeloablation using combination chemotherapy has also been used in adult patients with malignant glial tumors. Abrey et al. (1999) have reported on 26 adults with malignant glioma treated with myeloablative chemotherapy consisting of a thiotepa- and etoposide-based regimen with the addition of BCNU or carboplatin, followed by autologous stem cell transplantation. Of these 26 patients, 9 underwent high-dose chemotherapy at diagnosis and the rest following recurrence. In the group of patients with newly diagnosed disease, 6 of the 9 patients had residual bulky disease at the time of HDC. Two patients with glioblastoma were reportedly alive and progression-free 68+ and 74+ months. In the group with recurrent gliomas only 1 of the 17 patients was alive at 86 months. The 2-year event-free survival (EFS) was 33% for the former, and 26% for the latter group. Toxic mortality for all patients in the study was 12% for patients treated at recurrence versus 33% for those treated at diagnosis.

In summary, the results of myeloablative therapy and autologous stem cell transplantation in adults with AA or GBM, while interesting, are not convincingly superior to those obtained with conventional therapy. High-dose chemotherapy with two or three agents appears to be slightly better than monotherapy.

Pediatric studies of myeloablative therapy with autologous stem cell transplantation for AA and GBM have for the most part used multidrug regimens, with either two- or three-drug combinations: thiotepa and etoposide , thiotepa-etoposide-carboplatin (Finlay *et al.,* 1990), thiotepa-etoposide-BCNU (Finlay, 1993), cyclophosphamide and melphalan (Mahoney *et al.,* 1996; Graham *et al.,* 1997), cyclophosphamide with thiotepa (Heideman *et al.,* 1993; Kedar *et al.,* 1994), and busulfan plus thiotepa (Kalifa *et al.,* 1992) (Table 46.3).

In 1990, Finlay *et al.* reported on nine patients with histologically confirmed malignant astrocytoma (seven with recurrent disease) who were treated with thiotepa 600–900 mg/m^2 over 3 days and etoposide 1,500 mg/m^2 over 3 days (five patients) or thiotepa and etoposide in the same doses in combination with BCNU 600 mg/m^2 over 3 days (four patients). An objective response rate of 60% was achieved with durable remissions in two patients. This result led the Children's Cancer Group (CCG) to explore myeloablative chemotherapy and autologous transplantation for recurrent brain tumors in children and young adults. High-dose thiotepa 900 mg/m^2 over 3 days and etoposide 750 mg/m^2 over 3 days were employed in 45 patients, 18 of whom had malignant gliomas (Finlay *et al.,* 1996). Most of the patients in this study had received radiotherapy (involved field or craniospinal) prior to myeloablative chemotherapy. Four of 18 patients with malignant gliomas demonstrated objective responses to HDC. Five of 18 patients are long-term survivors (39+ to 59+ months) (Fig. 46.3). Durable remission was dependent on the extent of surgical resection prior to myeloablative chemotherapy with patients who underwent radical resection having a significantly better outcome. Seven of 45 patients (16%) died of treatment-related causes, mainly hepatic veno-occlusive disease, bacterial sepsis, or multiorgan failure.

In a subsequent study, 43 patients (39 with AA or GBM) with a median age of 13 years were treated at Memorial Sloan-Kettering Cancer Center with thiotepa-etoposide, thiotepa-etoposide-BCNU, or thiotepa-carboplatin-etoposide combinations (Finlay, 1993). Eight patients with GBM or AA (20%) are alive and disease-free between 12+ and 52+ months posttransplant. However, an unacceptable treatment-related mortality rate of 27% was reported with the thiotepa-etoposide-BCNU combination. In another Children's Cancer Group (CCG-9922) study, Grovas and colleagues (1999) treated 11 patients with GBM using thiotepa (900 mg/m^2 over 3 days), etoposide (750 mg/m^2 over 3 days), and BCNU (600 mg/m^2 over 3 days) followed by involved field external beam irradiation; three patients are alive disease-free 399 to 811 days from study entry. However, five patients suffered grade III or IV pulmonary or neurologic toxicities. Selected adult and pediatric studies of myeloablative therapy and autologous stem cell transplantation in patients with AA and GBM are listed in Table 46.3.

The role of HDC in patients with supratentorial AA or GBM appears promising, at least in pediatric patients, with impressive event-free survivals in a disease that is normally almost uniformly fatal. The presence of bulky tumor at the time of transplant could partly explain the dismal outcome in some studies (Heideman *et al.,* 1993; Mahoney *et al.,* 1996). Minimal residual disease achieved either by surgery, chemotherapy, or irradiation prior to high-dose chemotherapy appears to improve survival. Local involved field radiotherapy may augment cure rates, although we have observed three long-term survivors in four children less than 3 years of age with recurrent GBM or AA who were treated with myeloablative therapy without local irradiation (Gururangan *et al.,* 1998). Given the heterogeneity of tumor cells found in these tumors, a multidrug regimen should theoretically enhance cell kill. BCNU-containing regimens shall be avoided due to prohibitive pulmonary and neurologic toxicity.

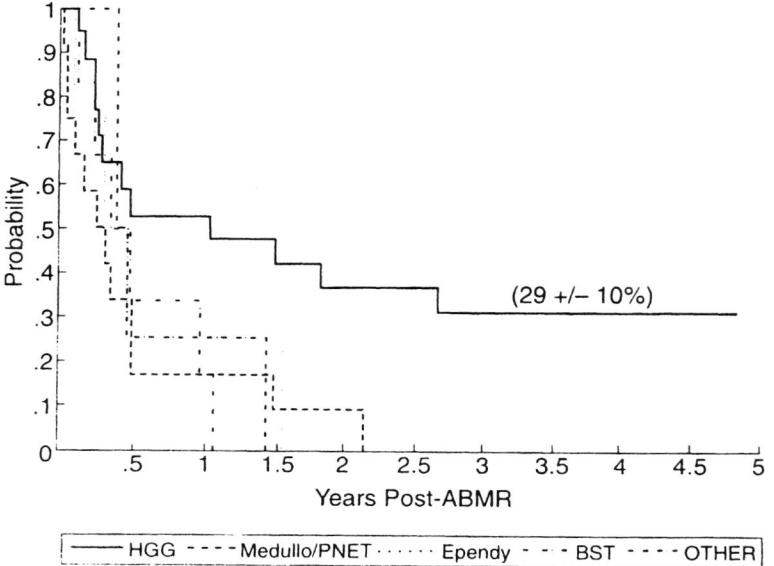

Fig. 46.3. OS according to pathologic diagnosis. BST, brain stem tumor; Medullo, medulloblastoma; Ependy, ependymoma; HGG, high-grade glioma. Reproduced, with permission, from Finlay *et al.* (1996).

Table 46.3. *High-dose chemotherapy and autologous stem cell rescue in patients with supratentorial malignant glial tumors*

Study	Number of patients	Myeloablative regimen	Response to chemotherapy	Radiotherapy following hematopoietic recovery	Median survival	Number alive without disease
Phillips *et al.* (1986)	27[a]	BCNU	NA	Local	3 months	4
	18[b]				18 months	
Biron *et al.* (1991)	98	BCNU	NA	Local	11 months	None
Finlay *et al.* (1990)	18	T, E	4 (PR + CR)	None	13 months	5
Finlay *et al.* (1993)	43	T, E *or* T, E, BCNU *or* T, E, C	NA	None	NA	8
Mahoney *et al.* (1996)	3	CY, PAM	None	None	4 months	None
Graham *et al.* (1997)	6	CY, PAM *or* Bu, PAM *or* C, E	NA	None	NA	1
Heideman *et al.*[c] (1993)	13	CY, T	4 (PR + CR)	Local	9 months	1
Kedar *et al.* (1994)	3	CY, T	1 (PR)	Local	NA	1
Fernandez-Hidalgo *et al.* (1996)	34	BCNU, CDDP	NA	Local	15.5 months	8

Abbreviations: BCNU, carmustine; T, thiotepa; E, etoposide; C, carboplatin; CY, cyclophosphamide; PAM, melphalan; Bu, busulfan; CDDP, cisplatin; NA, not available; CR, complete response; PR, partial response.
[a] Patients with progressive disease.
[b] New patients treated adjuvantly with myeloablative therapy.
[c] Two patients with brain stem and spinal cord tumors, respectively.

Diffuse pontine gliomas

Brain stem tumors comprise approximately 10% to 20% of posterior fossa tumors in children (Duffner *et al.*, 1986; Bleyer, 1999; Rickert *et al.*, 2001). Approximately 85% of these are of the diffuse variety involving the pons and are histologically either AA or GBM (Packer *et al.*, 1994c). Diffuse pontine gliomas are extremely lethal with only a handful of patients surviving beyond 2 years from diagnosis (Freeman *et al.*, 1996). Conventional therapy for these tumors has traditionally been radiotherapy in doses of 54 to 60 Gy (unfractionated) or 72 to 78 Gy (fractionated) with 3-year progression-free survival rates of less than 15% (Freeman *et al.*, 1993; Packer *et al.*, 1993, 1994a, 1994c). With poor outcome from conventional treatment, investigators, noting the impressive responses to HDC in supratentorial AA and GBM, have attempted to employ such a strategy in patients with diffuse pontine gliomas with disappointing results.

Dunkel and colleagues (1998b) treated 16 patients (10 recurrent, 6 newly diagnosed) with diffuse pontine tumors using thiotepa (900 mg/m^2 over 3 days), etoposide (750 mg/m^2 over 3 days) (6 patients), thiotepa, etoposide, and BCNU (600 mg/m^2 over 3 days) (8 patients), and thiotepa, etoposide, and carboplatin (1 patient) (1.5 g/m^2 over 3 days). Newly diagnosed patients received 72 to 78 Gy approximately 6 weeks following myeloablative therapy. Event-free survival for all patients lasted only 0.1 to 19 months from treatment (median duration of survival of 4 and 7 months for patients with recurrent and newly diagnosed disease, respectively). Results of other studies of HDC with autologous stem cell transplantation in brain stem tumors have been equally dismal (Finlay *et al.*, 1990; Kalifa *et al.*, 1992; Kedar *et al.*, 1994; Bouffet *et al.*,

2000). Based on these results, we do not recommend myeloablative chemotherapy and autologous transplantation in patients with this tumor.

Anaplastic oligodendroglioma

Anaplastic oligodendroglioma is an uncommon tumor that occurs mostly in adults (median age at diagnosis is 40 to 50 years) (Peterson & Cairncross, 1996). Only 6% of oligodendrogliomas occur in children (Duffner *et al.*, 1986). These tumors are invariably located in the cerebral hemispheres. Conventional treatment includes wide surgical resection and focal radiotherapy. Anaplastic oligodendrogliomas are also chemosensitive tumors and respond well to procarbazine, CCNU, and vincristine (PCV) combination chemotherapy (Cairncross, 1994).

High-dose chemotherapy in patients with anaplastic oligodendroglioma has mainly been used at the time of recurrence. A report by Cairncross *et al.* described the use of high-dose thiotepa (900 mg/m2 over three days) in adult patients with recurrent anaplastic oligodendroglioma (Cairncross *et al.*, 2000). Twenty patients underwent this procedure following induction chemotherapy with an intensive procarbazine based regimen. Only four patients were reported alive at a median of 42 months (range, 22 to 77 months) from induction chemotherapy. There was a toxic mortality rate of 20% in this study. The authors concluded that the procedure was of marginal benefit in this group of patients with an unacceptable toxicity. Further high-dose chemotherapy trials are therefore not being pursued in patients with recurrent anaplastic oligodendrogliomas (Doolittle *et al.*, 2001). However, this strategy is being tested in newly diagnosed adults who are found to be chemosensitive to induction therapy with PCV. This study is ongoing and has currently accrued 69 patients with 37 of them having undergone the entire regimen of PCV induction and high-dose thiotepa thus far (Doolittle *et al.*, 2001; Abrey *et al.*, 2001). The median progression-free survival for these patients is 69 months with acceptable toxicity (Abrey *et al.*, 2001).

Malignant embryonal tumors

Medulloblastoma

Medulloblastoma, a neoplasm of primitive neuroectodermal origin (PNET), is typically a posterior fossa tumor of childhood and constitutes about 20% of all pediatric CNS tumors (Duffner *et al.*, 1986; Bleyer, 1999). Infants (age less than 3 years), patients with unresectable tumor or gross residual disease postsurgery, and those with metastases (within and beyond the CNS) constitute a high-risk group requiring more intensive treatment (Evans *et al.*, 1990; Packer *et al.*, 1999a). Conventional therapy for patients with low-risk medulloblastoma is surgical resection followed by craniospinal irradiation (24 to 36 Gy) and a focal boost to the primary site (54 to 56 Gy) with a 5-year event-free survival rate of approximately 60% (Merchant *et al.*, 1996, 1999; Thomas *et al.*, 2000). The addition of chemotherapy (vincristine, procarbazine, with or without cisplatin) appears to benefit patients with high-risk features and might help to decrease the dose of neuraxis irradiation in patients with average risk disease (Evans *et al.*, 1990; Packer *et al.*, 1994b, 1999a, 1999b; Zeltzer *et al.*, 1999). Patients with recurrent tumors fare very poorly despite conventional retrieval therapy with few or no long-term survivors reported (Belza *et al.*, 1991; Torres *et al.*, 1994). There have been many reports of the use of high-dose chemotherapy as a retrieval strategy in such patients (Table 46.4). In a study by the French Society of Pediatric Oncology (SFOP), Dupois-Girod *et al.* (1996) treated 20 patients less than 3 years of age (median age 23 months) with myeloablative chemotherapy using busulfan and thiotepa (Table 46.4). Seven of these patients had metastatic disease. Patients with disease localized to the primary site received radiotherapy confined to the posterior fossa following recovery from chemotherapy. An objective response to chemotherapy was observed in 12 of 16 evaluable patients (75%). The median progression-free interval was 31 months posttransplant and the 2-year event-free survival (EFS) rate 50%. Ten of 13 patients with local recurrence were alive and disease-free compared to only one of seven patients with metastatic disease. Only one treatment-related death was reported. Gururangan *et al.* (1998) have similarly reported impressive disease control in three of five young children who progressed following initial chemotherapy and subsequently received HDC with a carboplatin-thiotepa-etoposide regimen. However, these children also received reduced dose craniospinal irradiation with a focal boost following recovery from HDC. In another study from the Duke University Medical Center, Graham *et al.* (1997) treated 18 patients with recurrent medulloblastoma using a myeloablative regimen consisting of cyclophosphamide and melphalan (Table 46.4). Sixteen of these patients had received radiotherapy as part of this initial treatment for relapse. Four patients remained disease-free at a median of 10 months (range, 8 to 20 months) from transplant. This study also demonstrated significantly better EFS for patients with localized disease at the time of recurrence. Toxicity in this study was mild and reversible. Similarly, Mahoney *et al.* (1996) treated eight patients with cyclophosphamide (750 to 1,500 mg/m² over 4 days) and melphalan (180 mg/m² over 3 days). There were four objective responses. Two patients died of toxicity. Two patients with localized disease at the time of HDC were reported to be alive and disease-free 24+ and 25+ months from transplant. In another study reported from the Memorial Sloan Kettering Cancer Center, Dunkel *et al.* (1998a) treated 23 patients with recurrent medulloblastoma (median age 13 years, range 2 to 44 years) with a myeloablative regimen consisting of carboplatin, thiotepa, and etoposide. There were three toxic deaths (two of multiorgan failure , one of aspergillus infection). Seven patients, all with localized recurrence, survived progression-free at a median of 35 months posttransplant (3-year EFS of 30%). It must be noted that in this series, 21 patients had also received conventional salvage therapy following relapse (surgical resection 7

Table 46.4. *High-dose chemotherapy and autologous stem cell transplantation in patients with medulloblastoma*

Study	Number of patients	Myeloablative regimen	Response to chemotherapy	Radiotherapy following hematopoietic recovery	Median disease-free interval	Number alive without disease
Dupuis-Girod *et al.* (1991)	20	Bu, T	12 (CR + PR)	Local ± CNS	31 months	11
Finlay *et al.* (1996)	9	T, E	1 (PR)	None	None	None
Dunkel *et al.* (1998a)	23	C, T, E	NA	Local ± CNS	54 months	7
Mahoney *et al.* (1996)	8	CY, PAM	4 (CR + PR)	None	NA	2
Graham *et al.* (1997)	19	CY, PAM or Bu, PAM or C, E	NA	None[a]	10 months	4
Abrey *et al.* (1999)	9	C, T, E or T only	NA	None	33 months	None

Abbreviations: T, thiotepa; E, etoposide; C, carboplatin; CY, cyclophosphamide; PAM, melphalan; Bu, busulfan; NA, not available; CR, complete response; PR, partial response; CNS, central nervous system.
[a] 16 patients received radiotherapy as part of initial treatment of relapse.

patients, chemotherapy 17 patients, and radiotherapy 11 patients) (Fig. 46.4).

Following these impressive results using HDC in patients with recurrent tumors, we implemented this strategy in young children less than 6 years of age with newly diagnosed primary malignant brain tumors with the primary intent of avoiding radiotherapy in this group of children at high-risk of neurocognitive deficits from this treatment. The reasoning behind this strategy is that in selected patients, dose intensification can potentially eradicate residual tumor cells in the primary site and other areas of the neuraxis and help avoid radiotherapy. In a report of this study called the "Head-Start I" program from the Memorial Sloan-Kettering Cancer Center by Mason *et al.* (1998a), 11 young children with newly diagnosed medulloblastoma were treated with induction chemotherapy using vincristine, cyclophosphamide, cisplatin, and etoposide followed by HDC using carboplatin, thiotepa, and etoposide in patients whose tumors were responsive or stable to induction chemotherapy. Radiotherapy was avoided unless patients suffered progression either following induction or high-dose chemotherapy or had stable unresectable tumor following recovery from myeloablative therapy. The EFS for these patients was 44% at 2 years from stem cell rescue (Fig. 46.5) and has subsequently remained stable at 5 years following the procedure (Mason *et al.*, 1998a; Finlay, 2001). Gross total tumor resection afforded a longer median EFS and 5-year EFS. Age at diagnosis and use of irradiation postconsolidation did not impact on survival (Finlay, 2001). The results of this study compare favorably to a 2-year EFS of 34% reported by Duffner *et al.* (1993) in infants with medulloblastomas treated with prolonged conventional chemotherapy and delayed irradiation. The current "Head Start II" study was modified to include high-dose methotrexate (8 g/m^2 on day four) in the induction

regimen for patients with medulloblastoma/PNET, ependymomas with neuraxis dissemination, and atypical teratoid/rabdoid tumors. The addition of methotrexate has been particularly useful in patients with metastatic medulloblastoma with 10 of 12 patients demonstrating a complete response to the induction regimen (Finlay, 2001). In another multi-institutional study, Strother *et al.* (2001) administered four cycles of high-dose cyclophosphamide together with cisplatin and vincristine at conventional doses followed by stem cell rescue to 53 children with newly diagnosed medulloblastoma or supratentorial PNETs. All patients received surgical resection and craniospinal irradiation with a focal boost to the primary site prior to HDC. Children with metastatic disease also received topotecan in a 6-week phase II window prior to radiotherapy. The 2-year PFS for patients with average and high-risk disease are 94% and 74%, respectively. While further follow-up is clearly required to assess the durability of these results, it clearly shows the importance of dose intensity of cyclophosphamide in the treatment of PNETs (all chemotherapy delivered over a 4-month period) and such therapy is possible with the help of stem cell rescue even in the context of prior craniospinal irradiation.

The use of high-dose chemotherapy as a retrieval strategy in adults with recurrent medulloblastoma has not shown promising results as it has in children. In a single-institution study, Abrey *et al.* (1999) treated 11 adults with recurrent medulloblastoma who received myeloablative chemotherapy with either carboplatin- or thiotepa-based regimens. Two patients died of toxicity in this study. Seven of the remaining nine patients have suffered recurrent disease posttransplant. It is possible that most patients had a high disease burden at the time of transplant since almost 75% of the treated patients had metastatic disease at the time of high-dose chemotherapy. This might explain higher rates of progressive disease in this study.

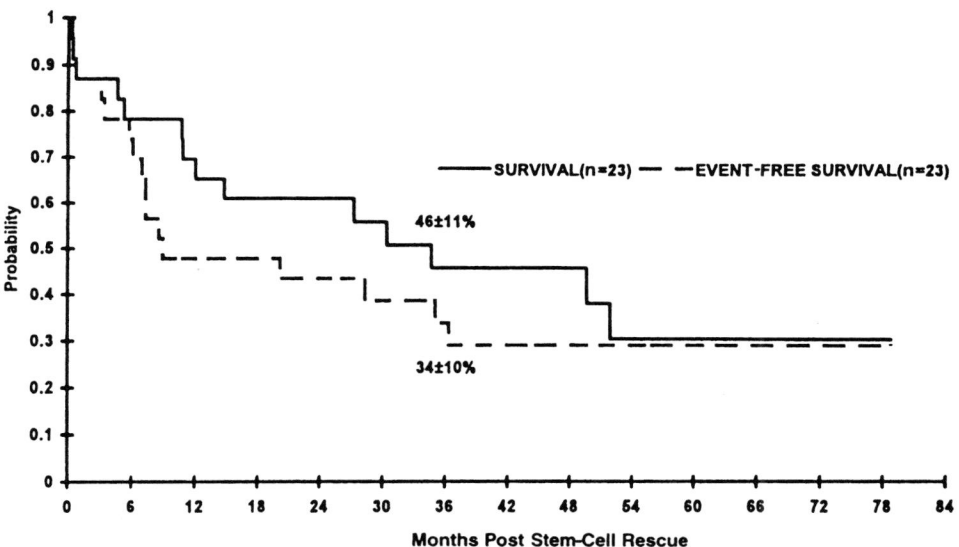

Fig. 46.4. Kaplan-Meier plots of survival and EFS after high-dose chemotherapy and ASCR in children with recurrent medulloblastoma. Reproduced, with permission, from Dunkel *et al.* (1998a).

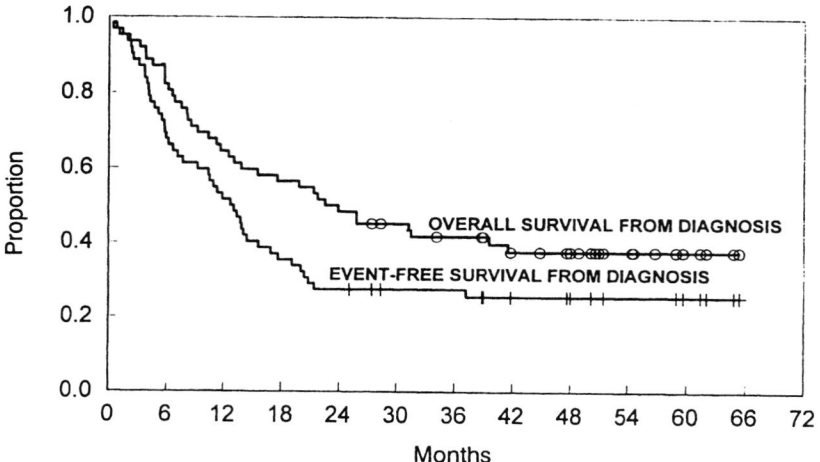

Fig. 46.5. OS and EFS from diagnosis in 62 children with primary brain tumors. (O and +) Censored times. Reproduced, with permission, from Mason *et al.* (1998a).

The above studies indicate that HDC with stem cell rescue appears to be a promising modality of retrieval treatment in a selected group of children with medulloblastoma who suffer recurrence that is restricted to the primary site. While the SFOP study indicates that neuraxis irradiation can be avoided safely in a selected group of young patients with localized recurrence, larger studies are needed to confirm these results. The HDC strategy is also useful in young children with newly diagnosed medulloblastoma and could help avoid irradiation altogether or reduce the dose of radiotherapy to the neuraxis.

Supratentorial primitive neuroectodermal tumor

Supratentorial PNETs may be separated into cerebral PNETs and pineoblastomas.

Cerebral PNETs account for 2.5% of childhood brain tumors (Cohen *et al.*, 1995). In a report by the Children's Cancer Group (CCG-921), the 3-year progression-free survival of 44 evaluable patients over 18 months of age with cerebral PNET treated by surgery, chemotherapy, and radiotherapy was 45% (Cohen *et al.*, 1995). Localized disease and age over 3 years were good prognostic factors. Survival for infants (children less than 3 years of age) was poor with an OS at 5 years of 25% to 27% in studies reported by the Pediatric Oncology and Children's Cancer Groups (Duffner *et al.*, 1993; Cohen *et al.*, 1995; Duffner *et al.*, 1999b). The outcome of patients with recurrent tumor is dismal.

The use of HDC with stem cell rescue has mainly been reported in patients with recurrent cerebral PNETs (Kalifa *et al.*, 1992; Mahoney *et al.*, 1996; Graham *et al.*, 1997; Johnson *et al.*, 1997). Johnson *et al.* (1997) treated 16 patients with recurrent supratentorial PNETs (including cerebral and pineal) with either thiotepa/etoposide (four patients) or thiotepa/etoposide/carboplatin regimens (12 patients). Twelve patients died of progressive disease. Four patients, all with minimal residual disease at the time of treatment, have survived disease-free at a median interval of 31 months posttransplant. Three of these

patients also received involved field radiotherapy following hematopoietic recovery (Johnson *et al.*, 1997; Gururangan *et al.*, 1998). Graham *et al.* (1997) treated three patients with recurrent cerebral PNET with high-dose chemotherapy using a carboplatin-thiotepa regimen and reported two disease-free survivors at 33+ and 35+ months.

The use of a high-dose chemotherapy strategy in young children with newly diagnosed supratentorial PNETs (including cerebral PNET and pineoblastomas) has been reported by Mason *et al.* (1998a) with a reported 2-year EFS of 43%. Similarly, excellent results have been reported by Strother *et al.* (2001) in children with newly diagnosed supratentorial PNETs treated with craniospinal irradiation with a focal boost followed by high-dose cyclophosphamide along with cisplatin and vincristine.

Pineoblastoma is a PNET of the pineal region, comprises 3% to 11% of CNS tumors that occur in children, and is much less common in adults (Jakacki *et al.*, 1995). Conventional therapy includes surgical resection when possible, chemotherapy, and radiotherapy (local plus craniospinal). In the CCG-921 study conducted between 1986 and 1992, a 3-year EFS of 61% ± 13% was observed (Jakacki *et al.*, 1995). However, survival for infants with pineoblastoma is dismal with no survivors reported with conventional chemotherapy and delayed irradiation (Duffner *et al.*, 1993; Cohen *et al.*, 1995; Duffner *et al.*, 1999a).

Patients with pineoblastomas have been treated with HDC both at diagnosis and recurrence. Mason *et al.* (1998a) treated 14 children with supratentorial PNET (including pineoblastoma) at diagnosis with a high-dose carboplatin, thiotepa, and etoposide regimen and achieved a 4-year EFS of 43%. A study from Duke University Medical Center reported in abstract form, included 11 patients with pineoblastoma treated with either high-dose busulfan-melphalan or cyclophosphamide-melphalan regimens. Eight of these patients received craniospinal irradiation and a focal boost to the pineal region following recovery from high-dose chemotherapy. Nine of 11 patients are alive with no evidence of disease at a median of 37 months from diagnosis (range, 13–96), including 3 infants with pineoblastoma following bilateral retinoblastoma who did not receive any radiotherapy and two patients with metastatic disease (McLaughlin *et al.*, 2001).

The outcome for patients with recurrent pineoblastoma treated with HDC regimens has been uniformly disappointing (Graham *et al.*, 1997; Johnson *et al.*, 1997; Gururangan *et al.*, 1998).

High-dose chemotherapy with stem cell rescue in patients with cerebral PNETs and pineoblastomas appears promising; however, achieving minimal residual disease prior to high-dose chemotherapy, and timing this treatment prior to recurrence, particularly in patients with pineoblastomas, will improve the chance of durable disease-free remissions.

Retinoblastoma

Retinoblastoma is a tumor of the embryonic neural retina or rarely the pineal gland that occurs exclusively in children. About 95% of tumors occur prior to 5 years of age (Donaldson *et al.*, 1997; Young *et al.*, 1999). About 300 new cases are diagnosed each year in the United States. Children can have unilateral (hereditary or sporadic, about 75% of cases) or bilateral (always heritable, 25% of cases) tumors (Donaldson *et al.*, 1997). Histologically, retinoblastomas are malignant neuroblastic tumors that arise from the nucleated layers of the retina. Children with retinoblastoma are usually treated with a combination of enucleation of the involved eye or cryotherapy with external beam radiotherapy in some patients with residual disease involving the optic nerve or orbital tissues. Conventional chemotherapy including carboplatin, cyclophosphamide, vincristine, doxorubicin, and etoposide is used in patients with certain unfavorable features (Donaldson *et al.*, 1997). Survival can be over 90% for children with unilateral disease. However, patients with bilateral retinoblastoma have an inferior survival due to the high incidence of second malignancies in these patients (Donaldson *et al.*, 1997). Patients with high-risk features include those with involvement of the optic nerves beyond the lamina cribrosa, orbits, and systemic disease and prognosis for these patients is extremely poor.

HDC plus stem cell rescue has been tried in patients with high-risk retinoblastoma. In a report from the SFOP, 25 of 34 patients with high-risk retinoblastoma received high-dose carboplatin, etoposide, and cyclophosphamide followed by stem cell rescue (Namouni *et al.*, 1997). Six of these patients had newly diagnosed localized disease and received this HDC regimen as consolidation treatment following enucleation and adjuvant chemotherapy due to involvement of the optic nerve. The remaining 19 patients had recurrent or advanced stage retinoblastoma and received the HDC regimen following confirmation of chemosensitivity of the tumor with conventional chemotherapy. Thirteen patients also received radiotherapy to the orbit and/or neuraxis following recovery from HDC. Response to HDC was evaluable in eight patients and included a complete response in two patients and stable disease in six

patients. Seventeen of 25 patients are alive and disease-free at a median of 10 months (range, 5 to 26) from HDC. Relapses occurred in eight patients following HDC and were predominantly within the CNS. Eleven of 15 patients with orbital or systemic metastases without CNS disease are alive and disease-free compared with only one of four patients with CNS involvement at the time of HDC. Toxicity was predominantly mucositis and eighth cranial nerve damage. In a study from the Memorial Sloan-Kettering Cancer Center, four patients with systemic metastasis from retinoblastoma but without CNS disease were treated with a high-dose carboplatin plus thiotepa or a carboplatin, thiotepa, and etoposide regimen (Dunkel *et al.*, 2000). In addition, all four patients received adjuvant focal radiotherapy to sites of bulky involvement. All four patients are alive and disease-free 46 to 80+ months from therapy. Clearly, it appears that this strategy is effective in patients with localized or systemic relapse. However, patients with overt CNS involvement fare poorly despite intensification of therapy.

Ependymomas

Ependymomas comprise 5% to 10% of pediatric brain tumors and occur predominantly in children and young adults (Duffner *et al.*, 1986; Robertson *et al.*, 1998). There is considerable debate regarding the histologic grade and appropriate treatment of this malignancy. This tumor rarely presents with neuraxis spread but has a propensity to recur locally (Goldwein *et al.*, 1990; Robertson *et al.*, 1998). Conventional treatment includes surgical resection and radiotherapy with 5-year EFS of 39% to 50% (Evans *et al.*, 1996; Robertson *et al.*, 1998). The role of adjuvant chemotherapy in this malignancy has been questioned. Children with recurrent ependymomas have a poor prognosis (Goldwein *et al.*, 1990).

HDC has been employed for both newly diagnosed and recurrent ependymomas with variable outcomes (Grill *et al.*, 1996; Graham *et al.*, 1997; Mason *et al.*, 1998b). Mason *et al.* (1998b) treated 10 children less than 6 years of age with newly diagnosed ependymoma with HDC using carboplatin, thiotepa, and etoposide, following surgery and induction chemotherapy. The 2-year PFS and OS following HDC were 56% and 67%, respectively. However, survival following HDC in patients with recurrent tumors has been disappointing (Grill *et al.*, 1996; Graham *et al.*, 1997; Grill & Kalifa, 1998). While HDC could potentially be explored in patients with ependymomas in the setting of newly diagnosed disease, it is our impression that the role of myeloablative therapy and autologous transplantation for those with recurrent tumors remains questionable until more effective chemotherapeutic agents are identified.

Germ cell tumors

Primary germ cell tumors of the CNS are very rare and comprise 2% of all intracranial malignancies below 20 years of age (Balmaceda *et al.*, 1996). CNS germ cell tumors are of two broad categories: germinomas and nongerminomatous germ cell tumors (NGGCT). The latter include endodermal sinus tumor, embryonal carcinoma, choriocarcinoma, and teratoma. These tumors favor midline structures with about 80% of tumors occurring in the pineal or suprasellar region. About 15% of patients present with dissemination within the CNS. Conventional treatment for patients with germinomas, an extremely radiosensitive tumor, is surgery with periventricular field irradiation and a focal boost to the primary site. Patients with NGGCT have poor survival with radiotherapy alone and require intensive adjuvant chemotherapy (carboplatin/cisplatin, bleomycin, etoposide). Event-free survival for CNS germinoma has been reported at 85% to 92% at 5 years and 27% to 67% at 4 years for NGGCT (Balmaceda et al., 1996; Matsutani et al., 1997). Survival is dismal for patients with recurrent germ cell tumors and those with newly diagnosed NGGCT that demonstrate an inadequate response to chemotherapy. Such patients have benefited from HDC with stem cell rescue. Modak et al. (1997) have treated nine patients with recurrent CNS germ cell tumors (four germinomas, five NGGCT) with thiotepa-based myeloablative regimens and autologous transplantation; three patients with germinomas survived disease-free while all five patients with NGGCT died of progressive disease. Graham et al. (1997) treated two patients with recurrent mixed germinomas with conventional chemotherapy and radiotherapy followed by HDC. Both patients were alive and disease-free 30+ and 21+ months following treatment. Mahoney et al. (1996) treated two patients with recurrent germinoma with a high-dose cyclophosphamide-melphalan regimen and achieved CR in both patients. One patient was alive and disease-free at 32+ months. We recommend HDC either for patients with recurrent germ cell tumors or those with newly diagnosed NGGCT that are slow to respond (as evidenced by marker or radiologic studies) to conventional therapy.

Toxicity associated with high-dose chemotherapy in malignant brain tumors

The potential for treatment-related toxicity is an important consideration when evaluating a patient with a malignant brain tumor for HDC. Toxicities associated with the chemotherapeutic agents used in myeloablative chemotherapy of brain tumor patients are listed in Table 46.5.

Pancytopenia

Severe pancytopenia is universal with HDC. Additionally, patients who receive spinal irradiation have delayed marrow recovery when given marrow derived from the posterior iliac crests (Faulkner et al., 1996). In our own practice, we usually obtain marrow from the anterior iliac crests or use peripheral blood stem cells from patients who have had craniospinal irradiation.

Neurotoxicity

The alkylating agents used in myeloablative chemotherapy are very lipophilic and enter brain tissue readily. Thus, neurotoxicity is frequently seen in patients treated with these agents, particularly at high doses, and can occur from the time of administration

Table 46.5. *Toxicities associated with myeloablative chemotherapy in patients with malignant CNS tumors*

Severe pancytopenia
SIADH
Neurotoxicity
    Somnolence
    Seizures
    Coma
    Sensorineural deafness
    Optic neuropathy and retinopathy
Nausea and poor appetite
Hepatic veno-occlusive disease
Mucositis
Dermatitis
Multiorgan failure syndrome
Renal dysfunction
Pneumonitis and pulmonary fibrosis

Abbreviation: SIADH, syndrome of inappropriate anti-diuretic hormone secretion.

of these agents until approximately 3 months posttransplant (Leff et al., 1988; Kramer et al., 1997). Factors that contribute to this toxicity include concurrent administration of high volume fluids, sedatives, and narcotics, as well as electrolyte and metabolic imbalances. Neurotoxicity usually manifests as hallucinations, encephalopathy, seizures, or coma (Leff et al., 1988; Kramer et al., 1997; Vassal et al., 1990;). It should be remembered that intracranial hemorrhage due to thrombocytopenia and/or tumor progression can also cause acute neurologic dysfunction in patients who have undergone myeloablative chemotherapy.

White matter changes in the brain have been noted by neuroimaging studies within 6 months posttransplant in patients who received high-dose regimens containing carmustine, carboplatin, and cyclophosphamide (Brown et al., 1998). Ototoxicity in the form of high-frequency hearing loss seems to occur frequently among patients who receive high-dose carboplatin. Prior exposure to cisplatin, cranial irradiation, and aminoglycoside antibiotics are risk factors for such hearing loss (Freilich et al., 1996). We do not routinely administer aminoglycoside antibiotics during febrile neutropenic episodes following myeloablative chemotherapy in patients with brain tumors for fear of aggravating the auditory nerve damage from inadvertent high serum concentrations of this antibiotic. Optic neuropathy has been observed in patients receiving conditioning regimens containing cisplatin or carmustine within 1 to 4 months of treatment and is associated with swollen optic discs followed by pallor and can be associated with blurring or loss of vision. Retinal changes consisting of cotton wool spots, hemorrhages, and macular exudates have also been observed in these patients (Khawly et al., 1996; Johnson et al., 1999).

Mucositis and dermatitis

Oropharyngeal mucositis and diarrhea are common following myeloablative chemotherapy with two- or three-drug regimens. Oropharyngeal mucositis can be severe enough to cause upper

Table 46.6. *Possible indications for high-dose chemotherapy and autologous HSC transplantation in the management of malignant tumors of the central nervous system*

Tumor	Use of HDC / autotransplant
Supratentorial anaplastic astrocytoma	Promising results in children
Supratentorial GBM	Not convincingly superior to results of conventional therapy in adults
Diffuse pontine glioma	Not currently recommended
Anaplastic oligodendroglioma	Not currently recommended for patients with recurrent tumors
Medulloblastoma	Promising as salvage therapy for selected patients with a localized recurrence after primary treatment. Potential benefit as upfront treatment in infants with the possibility of avoiding radiotherapy.
Cerebral PNET	May be of value in a minority of patients with recurrent disease after primary treatment. Potential benefit as upfront treatment in infants with the possibility of avoiding radiotherapy.
Pineoblastoma	Promising as upfront therapy in newly diagnosed patients. Not recommended at recurrence.
Ependymoma	Of questionable value at recurrence
Germ cell tumors	Recommended for newly diagnosed NGGCTs that show a slow response to conventional treatment
Retinoblastoma	Recommended for high-risk patients without CNS disease

Abbreviations: HDC, high-dose chemotherapy; GBM, glioblastoma multiforme; PNET, primitive neuroectodermal tumor; NGGCT, non-germinomatous germ cell tumor; CNS, central nervous system.

airway obstruction and we have occasionally had to resort to endotracheal intubation to maintain airway patency. These patients also require parenteral nutrition and pain control with narcotic analgesics. Skin involvement in the form of erythema, blistering, desquamation, and dark pigmentation is a characteristic feature of regimens containing thiotepa.

Multiorgan failure syndrome

Multiorgan failure syndrome (MOFS) is characterized by fluid retention, weight gain, capillary leak, hepatic dysfunction, renal insufficiency, pulmonary edema, and respiratory failure in the immediate transplant period (George *et al.*, 1994). We have reported 11 treatment-related deaths in which MOFS was the sole ($n = 6$) or a contributory factor ($n = 5$) in 67 patients with malignant brain tumors who were treated with thiotepa-etoposide regimens with or without BCNU or carboplatin (George *et al.*, 1994). All patients who died solely of MOFS had received carboplatin-containing regimens. Six of 16 patients who received carboplatin by dosing based on body surface area died of MOFS compared with only of 1 of 33 patients dosed using Calvert's formula (Calvert *et al.*, 1989; Newell *et al.*, 1993). Thus, dosing carboplatin based on this formula can avoid undue toxicity from this agent.

Other toxicities that have been noted in patients treated with high-dose chemotherapy include hepatic veno-occlusive disease, pneumonia leading to pulmonary fibrosis, and renal dysfunction including hemolytic-uremic syndrome (Seiden *et al.*, 1992; van der Lelie *et al.*, 1995; Merouani *et al.*, 1996).

Monitoring for residual disease posttransplant

Patients with malignant brain tumors who recover from HDC require close follow-up to monitor for residual or progressive disease following treatment. We routinely perform neuroimag-ing of the brain and spine every 3 months for the first year, every 4 months in the second year, and every 6 months for 3 to 5 years thereafter.

Conclusions

High-dose chemotherapy with autologous hematopoietic stem cell support is a promising treatment approach for children with malignant CNS tumors. It has brought a glimmer of hope for patients with certain malignant CNS tumors that carry a poor prognosis with conventional therapy. To date, the HDC strategy has not had the same degree of success in adults, mainly due to the higher treatment-related mortality associated with the nitrosourea-containing HDC regimens used in this patient population. Possible indications for this approach are listed in Table 46.6 and a treatment algorithm is given in Fig. 46.2.

Future strategies for high-dose chemotherapy should aim at minimizing toxicity without compromising therapeutic benefit. Further investigation of newer chemotherapeutic agents in different combinations and doses needs to be carried out in patients with tumors refractory to existing drug regimens. Approaches to facilitate dose escalation without causing hematopoietic toxicity are being refined in animal models. Introduction of retroviral constructs that carry drug resistance genes into hematopoietic stem cells may protect them from chemotherapy damage (Wang *et al.*, 1996). Engraftment of such resistant stem cells following high-dose chemotherapy may more readily allow further treatment in patients who relapse following high-dose therapy.

References

Abrams, R.A., Casper, J., Kun, L. *et al.* (1985). In *Autologous Bone Marrow Transplantation: Proceedings of the First International*

Symposium, ed. K.A. Dicke, G. Spitzer, A.R. Zander, & N.C. Gorin, pp. 227–30. Houston: The University of Texas, MD Anderson Hospital and Tumor Institute.

Abrey, L.E., Paleologos, N., Rosenfeld, S. *et al.* (2001). Intensive PCV chemotherapy followed by high dose thiotepa with autologous stem cell rescue (ASCR) for patients with newly diagnosed anaplastic oligodendroglioma. *Neuro-oncology,* **3,** 354 (Abstract).

Abrey, L.E., Rosenblum, M., Malkin, M. *et al.* (1996). High dose chemotherapy with autologous stem cell rescue in adults with malignant brain tumors. *Proceedings of the Society of Neuro-Oncology.* (Abstract).

Abrey, L.E., Rosenblum, M.K., Papadopoulos, E. *et al.* (1999). High dose chemotherapy with autologous stem cell rescue in adults with malignant primary brain tumors. *Journal of Neurooncology,* **44,** 147–53.

Ahmed, T., Feldman, E., Helson, L. *et al.* (1990). Phase I-2 trial of high dose thiotepa (HDT) with autologous bone marrow transplantation (ABMT) and localized radiotherapy (RT) for patients (pts) with astrocytoma grade III-IV. *Proceedings of the American Society for Clinical Oncology,* **21,** A1023.

Annegers, J.F., Schoenberg, B.S., Okazaki, H. *et al.* (1981). Epidemiologic study of primary intracranial neoplasms. *Archives of Neurology,* **38,** 217–9.

Ascensao, J., Ahmed, T., Feldman, E. *et al.* (1989). High-dose thiotepa with autologous bone marrow transplantation and localized radiotherapy for patients with astrocytoma grade II–IV: a promising approach. *Proceedings of American Society for Clinical Oncology,* **8,** A353.

Balmaceda, C., Heller, G., Rosenblum, M. *et al.* (1996). Chemotherapy without irradiation: a novel approach for newly diagnosed CNS germ cell tumors: results of an international cooperative trial. *Journal of Clinical Oncology,* **14,** 1–8.

Belza, M.G., Donaldson, S.S., Steinberg, G.K. *et al.* (1991). Medulloblastoma: freedom from relapse longer than 8 years—a therapeutic cure? *Journal of Neurosurgery,* **75,** 572–82.

Biron, P., Vial, C., Chauvin, F. *et al.* (1991). In *Autologous Bone Marrow Transplantation: Proceedings of the Fifth International Symposium,* ed. K.A. Dicke, J.O. Armitage & M.J. Dicke-Evinger. Omaha: The University of Nebraska Medical Center.

Bleyer, W.A. (1999). Epidemiologic impact of children with brain tumors. *Child's Nervous System,* **15,** 758–63.

Bouffet, E., Raquin, M., Doz, F. *et al.* (2000). Radiotherapy followed by high dose busulfan and thiotepa: a prospective assessment of high dose chemotherapy in children with diffuse pontine gliomas. *Cancer,* **88,** 685–92.

Brown, M.S., Stemmer, S.M., Simon, J.H. *et al.* (1998). White matter disease induced by high-dose chemotherapy: longitudinal study with MR imaging and proton spectroscopy. *American Journal of Neuroradiology,* **19,** 217–21.

Cairncross, G., Swinnen, L., Bayer, R. *et al.* (2000). Myeloablative chemotherapy for recurrent aggressive oligodendroglioma. *Neurooncology,* **2,** 114–9.

Cairncross, J.G. (1994). Aggressive oligodendroglioma: a chemosensitive tumor. *Recent Results in Cancer Research,* **135,** 127–33.

Calvert, A.H., Newell, D.R., Gumbrell, L.A. *et al.* (1989). Carboplatin dosage: prospective evaluation of a simple formula based on renal function. *Journal of Clinical Oncology,* **7,** 1748–56.

Castellino, R.C., Elion, G.B., Keir, S.T. *et al.* (2000). Schedule-dependent activity of irinotecan plus BCNU against malignant glioma xenografts. *Cancer Chemotherapy and Pharmacology,* **45,** 345–9.

Cohen, B.H., Zeltzer, P.M., Boyett, J.M. *et al.* (1995). Prognostic factors and treatment results for supratentorial primitive neuroectodermal tumors in children using radiation and chemotherapy: a Childrens Cancer Group randomized trial. *Journal of Clinical Oncology,* **13,** 1687–96.

Donaldson, S.S., Egbert, P.R., Newsham, I. *et al.* (1997). In *Principles and Practice of Pediatric Oncology,* ed. P.A. Pizzo & D.G. Poplack, pp. 699–715. Philadelphia: Lippincott-Raven.

Doolittle, N.D., Anderson, C.P., Bleyer, W.A. *et al.* (2001). Importance of dose intensity in neuro-oncology clinical trials: summary report of the Sixth Annual Meeting of the Blood-Brain Barrier Disruption Consortium. *Neuro-oncology,* **3,** 46–54.

Duffner, P.K., Cohen, M.E., Myers, M.H. *et al.* (1986). Survival of children with brain tumors: SEER Program, 1973–1980. *Neurology,* **36,** 597–601.

Duffner, P.K., Horowitz, M.E., Krischer, J.P. *et al.* (1999a). The treatment of malignant brain tumors in infants and very young children: an update of the Pediatric Oncology Group experience. *Neuro-oncology,* **1,** 152–61.

Duffner, P.K., Horowitz, M.E., Krischer, J.P. *et al.* (1999b). The treatment of malignant brain tumors in infants and very young children: an update of the Pediatric Oncology Group experience. *Neuro-oncology,* **1,** 152–61.

Duffner, P.K., Horowitz, M.E., Krischer, J.P. *et al.* (1993). Postoperative chemotherapy and delayed radiation in children less than three years of age with malignant brain tumors. *New England Journal of Medicine,* **328,** 1725–31.

Duggan, P.R., Guo, D., Luider, J. *et al.* (2000). Predictive factors for long-term engraftment of autologous blood stem cells. *Bone Marrow Transplantation,* **26,** 1299–304.

Duncan, G.G., Goodman, G.B., Ludgate, C.M. *et al.* (1992). The treatment of adult supratentorial high grade astrocytomas. *Journal of Neurooncology,* **13,** 63–72.

Dunkel, I.J., Aledo, A., Kernan, N.A. *et al.* (2000). Successful treatment of metastatic retinoblastoma. *Cancer,* **89,** 2117–21.

Dunkel, I.J., Boyett, J.M., Yates, A. *et al.* (1998a). High-dose carboplatin, thiotepa, and etoposide with autologous stem-cell rescue for patients with recurrent medulloblastoma. Children's Cancer Group. *Journal of Clinical Oncology,* **16,** 222–8.

Dunkel, I.J., Garvin, J.H., Jr., Goldman, S. *et al.* (1998b). High dose chemotherapy with autologous bone marrow rescue for children with diffuse pontine brain stem tumors. Children's Cancer Group. *Journal of Neurooncology,* **37,** 67–73.

Dupuis-Girod, S., Hartmann, O., Benhamou, E. *et al.* (1996). Will high dose chemotherapy followed by autologous bone marrow transplantation supplant cranio-spinal irradiation in young children treated for medulloblastoma? *Journal of Neurooncology,* **27,** 87–98.

Evans, A.E., Anderson, J.R., Lefkowitz-Boudreaux, I.B. *et al.* (1996). Adjuvant chemotherapy of childhood posterior fossa ependymoma: cranio-spinal irradiation with or without adjuvant CCNU, vincristine, and prednisone: a Children's Cancer Group study. *Medical and Pediatric Oncology,* **27,** 8–14.

Evans, A.E., Jenkin, R.D., Sposto, R. *et al.* (1990). The treatment of medulloblastoma. Results of a prospective randomized trial of radiation therapy with and without CCNU, vincristine, and prednisone. *Journal of Neurosurgery*, **72**, 572–82.

Faulkner, L.B., Lindsley, K.L., Kher, U. *et al.* (1996). High-dose chemotherapy with autologous marrow rescue for malignant brain tumors: analysis of the impact of prior chemotherapy and cranio-spinal irradiation on hematopoietic recovery. *Bone Marrow Transplantation*, **17**, 389–94.

Fernandez-Hidalgo, O.A., Vanaciocha, V., Vicitcz, J.M. *et al.* (1996). High-dose BCNU and autologous progenitor cell transplantation given with intra-arterial cisplatinum and simultaneous radiotherapy in the treatment of high-grade gliomas: benefit for selected patients. *Bone Marrow Transplantation*, **18**, 143–9.

Finlay, J. (1993). High-dose chemotherapy with autologous marrow rescue (HDCx + ABMR) improves survival of patients with recurrent malignant glioma (MG) compared with conventional or no chemotherapy. *Journal of Neurooncology*, **15** (Abstract).

Finlay, J.L. (2001). Chemotherapy only strategy for young children with newly diagnosed malignant brain tumors: a ten year review of the "Head Start" regimens. *Neuro-oncology*, **3**, 371 (Abstract).

Finlay, J.L., August, C., Packer, R. *et al.* (1990). High-dose multi-agent chemotherapy followed by bone marrow 'rescue' for malignant astrocytomas of childhood and adolescence. *Journal of Neurooncology*, **9**, 239–48.

Finlay, J.L., Boyett, J.M., Yates, A.J. *et al.* (1995). Randomized phase III trial in childhood high-grade astrocytoma comparing vincristine, lomustine, and prednisone with the eight-drugs- in-1-day regimen. Childrens Cancer Group. *Journal of Clinical Oncology*, **13**, 112–23.

Finlay, J.L., Goldman, S., Wong, M.C. *et al.* (1996). Pilot study of high-dose thiotepa and etoposide with autologous bone marrow rescue in children and young adults with recurrent CNS tumors. The Children's Cancer Group. *Journal of Clinical Oncology*, **14**, 2495–503.

Freeman, C.R., Bourgouin, P.M., Sanford, R.A. *et al.* (1996). Long term survivors of childhood brain stem gliomas treated with hyperfractionated radiotherapy. Clinical characteristics and treatment related toxicities. The Pediatric Oncology Group. *Cancer*, **77**, 555–62.

Freeman, C.R., Krischer, J.P., Sanford, R.A. *et al.* (1993). Final results of a study of escalating doses of hyperfractionated radiotherapy in brain stem tumors in children: a Pediatric Oncology Group study. *International Journal of Radiation Oncology, Biology, and Physics*, **27**, 197–206.

Frei, E., 3rd, Antman, K., Teicher, B. *et al.* (1989). Bone marrow autotransplantation for solid tumors—prospects. *Journal of Clinical Oncology*, **7**, 515–26.

Frei, F., 3rd Cucchi, C.A., Rosowsky, A. *et al.* (1985). Alkylating agent resistance: in vitro studies with human cell lines. *Proceedings of the National Academy of Science USA*, **82**, 2158–62.

Frei, E., 3rd, Elias, A., Wheeler, C. *et al.* (1998). The relationship between high-dose treatment and combination chemotherapy: the concept of summation dose intensity. *Clinical Cancer Research*, **4**, 2027–37.

Frei, E., 3rd, Teicher, B.A., Holden, S.A. *et al.* (1988). Preclinical studies and clinical correlation of the effect of alkylating dose. *Cancer Research*, **48**, 6417–23.

Freilich, R.J., Kraus, D.H., Budnick, A.S. *et al.* (1996). Hearing loss in children with brain tumors treated with cisplatin and carboplatin-based high-dose chemotherapy with autologous bone marrow rescue. *Medical and Pediatric Oncology*, **26**, 95–100.

George, D., Ginsberg, J., & Weingast, R. (1994). Multi-organ failure syndrome in patients undergoing myeloablative chemotherapy and autologous bone marrow rescue for malignant brain tumors. *Experimental Hematology*, **22**, 379.

Giannone, L. & Wolff, S.N. (1987). Phase II treatment of central nervous system gliomas with high-dose etoposide and autologous bone marrow transplantation. *Cancer Treatment Reports*, **71**, 759–61.

Goldwein, J.W., Glauser, T.A., Packer, R.J. *et al.* (1990). Recurrent intracranial ependymomas in children. Survival, patterns of failure, and prognostic factors. *Cancer*, **66**, 557–63.

Graham, M.L., Herndon, J.E., 2nd, Casey, J.R. *et al.* (1997). High-dose chemotherapy with autologous stem-cell rescue in patients with recurrent and high-risk pediatric brain tumors. *Journal of Clinical Oncology*, **15**, 1814–23.

Grill, J. & Kalifa, C. (1998). High dose chemotherapy for childhood ependymona. *Journal of Neurooncology*, **40**, 97.

Grill, J., Kalifa, C., Doz, F. *et al.* (1996). A high-dose busulfan-thiotepa combination followed by autologous bone marrow transplantation in childhood recurrent ependymoma. A phase-II study. *Pediatric Neurosurgery*, **25**, 7–12.

Groothuis, D.R. (2000). The blood-brain and blood-tumor barriers: a review of strategies for increasing drug delivery. *Neuro-oncology*, **2**, 45–59.

Grovas, A.C., Boyett, J.M., Lindsley, K. *et al.* (1999). Regimen-related toxicity of myeloablative chemotherapy with BCNU, thiotepa, and etoposide followed by autologous stem cell rescue for children with newly diagnosed glioblastoma multiforme: report from the Children's Cancer Group. *Medical and Pediatric Oncology*, **33**, 83–7.

Gururangan, S., Dunkel, I.J., Goldman, S. *et al.* (1998). Myeloablative chemotherapy with autologous bone marrow rescue in young children with recurrent malignant brain tumors. *Journal of Clinical Oncology*, **16**, 2486–93.

Heideman, R.L., Douglass, E.C., Krance, R.A. *et al.* (1993). High-dose chemotherapy and autologous bone marrow rescue followed by interstitial and external-beam radiotherapy in newly diagnosed pediatric malignant gliomas. *Journal of Clinical Oncology*, **11**, 1458–65.

Heuft, H.G., Dubiel, M., Rick, O. *et al.* (2001). Inverse relationship between patient peripheral blood CD34+ cell counts and collection efficiency for CD34+ cells in two automated leukapheresis systems. *Transfusion*, **41**, 1008–13.

Huitema, A.D., Smits, K.D., Mathot, R.A. *et al.* (2000). The clinical pharmacology of alkylating agents in high-dose chemotherapy. *Anticancer Drugs*, **11**, 515–33.

Jakacki, R.I., Zeltzer, P.M., Boyett, J.M. *et al.* (1995). Survival and prognostic factors following radiation and/or chemotherapy for primitive neuroectodermal tumors of the pineal region in infants and children: a report of the Childrens Cancer Group. *Journal of Clinical Oncology*, **13**, 1377–83.

Janss, A.J., Cnaan, A., Zhao, H. *et al.* (1998). Synergistic cytotoxicity of topoisomerase I inhibitors with alkylating agents and etoposide in human brain tumor cell lines. *Anticancer Drugs,* **9,** 641–52.

Johnson, D.B., Thompson, J.M., Corwin, J.A. *et al.* (1987). Prolongation of survival for high-grade malignant gliomas with adjuvant high-dose BCNU and autologous bone marrow transplantation. *Journal of Clinical Oncology,* **5,** 783–9.

Johnson, D.W., Cagnoni, P.J., Schossau, T.M. *et al.* (1999). Optic disc and retinal microvasculopathy after high-dose chemotherapy and autologous hematopoietic progenitor cell support. *Bone Marrow Transplantation,* **24,** 785–92.

Johnson, J.H., Boyett, J., Yates, A. *et al.* (1997). Recurrent supratentorial primitive neuroectodermal tumors treated with intensive chemotherapy and autologous bone marrow rescue. *Journal of Neurooncology,* **33,** 288.

Kalifa, C., Hartmann, O., Demeocq, F. *et al.* (1992). High-dose busulfan and thiotepa with autologous bone marrow transplantation in childhood malignant brain tumors: a phase II study. *Bone Marrow Transplantation,* **9,** 227–33.

Kedar, A., Maria, B.L., Graham-Pole, J. *et al.* (1994). High-dose chemotherapy with marrow reinfusion and hyperfractionated irradiation for children with high-risk brain tumors. *Medical and Pediatric Oncology,* **23,** 428–36.

Khawly, J.A., Rubin, P., Petros, W. *et al.* (1996). Retinopathy and optic neuropathy in bone marrow transplantation for breast cancer. *Ophthalmology,* **103,** 87–95.

Kramer, E.D., Packer, R.J., Ginsberg, J. *et al.* (1997). Acute neurologic dysfunction associated with high-dose chemotherapy and autologous bone marrow rescue for primary malignant brain tumors. *Pediatric Neurosurgery,* **27,** 230–7.

Kushner, B.H., Cheung, N.K., Kramer, K. *et al.* (2001). Topotecan combined with myeloablative doses of thiotepa and carboplatin for neuroblastoma, brain tumors, and other poor-risk solid tumors in children and young adults. *Bone Marrow Transplantation,* **28,** 551–6.

Leff, R.S., Thompson, J.M., Daly, M.B. *et al.* (1988). Acute neurologic dysfunction after high-dose etoposide therapy for malignant glioma. *Cancer,* **62,** 32–5.

Lilley, E.R., Rosenberg, M.C., Elion, G.B. *et al.* (1990). Synergistic interactions between cyclophosphamide or melphalan and VP-16 in a human rhabdomyosarcoma xenograft. *Cancer Research,* **50,** 284–7.

Long, D.M. (1970). Capillary ultrastructure and the blood-brain barrier in human malignant brain tumors. *Journal of Neurosurgery,* **32,** 127–44.

Long, J., Leff, R.S., Daly, M.B. *et al.* (1989). Phase II trial of high-dose etoposide and autologous bone marrow transplantation for treatment of progressive glioma. *Proceedings of the American Society of Clinical Oncology,* **8,** 92.

Mahoney, D.H., Jr., Strother, D., Camitta, B. *et al.* (1996). High-dose melphalan and cyclophosphamide with autologous bone marrow rescue for recurrent/progressive malignant brain tumors in children: a pilot pediatric oncology group study. *Journal of Clinical Oncology,* **14,** 382–8.

Marchese, M.J. & Chang, C.H. (1990). Malignant astrocytic gliomas in children. *Cancer,* **65,** 2771–8.

Mason, W.P., Grovas, A., Halpern, S. *et al.* (1998a). Intensive chemotherapy and bone marrow rescue for young children with

newly diagnosed malignant brain tumors. *Journal of Clinical Oncology,* **16,** 210-21.

Mason, W.P., Goldman, S., Yates, A.J. *et al.* (1998b). Survival following intensive chemotherapy with bone marrow reconstitution for children with recurrent intracranial ependymoma—a report of the Children's Cancer Group. *Journal of Neurooncology,* **37,** 135–43.

Matsutani, M., Sano, K., Takakura, K. *et al.* (1997). Primary intracranial germ cell tumors: A clinical analysis of 153 histologically verified cases. *Journal of Neurosurgery,* **86,** 446–55.

McLaughlin, C.A., Gururangan, S., Halperin, E.C. *et al.* (2001). High dose chemotherapy with stem cell rescue for patients with newly diagnosed pineoblastoma—The Duke experience. *Neurooncol-ogy,* **3,** 372 (Abstract).

Merchant, T.E., Happersett, L., Finlay, J.L. *et al.* (1999). Preliminary results of conformal radiation therapy for medulloblastoma. *Neuro-oncology,* **1,** 177–87.

Merchant, T.E., Wang, M.H., Haida, T. *et al.* (1996). Medulloblastoma: long-term results for patients treated with definitive radiation therapy during the computed tomography era. *International Journal of Radiation Oncology, Biology, and Physics,* **36,** 29–35.

Merouani, A., Shpall, E.J., Jones, R.B. *et al.* (1996). Renal function in high dose chemotherapy and autologous hematopoietic cell support treatment for breast cancer. *Kidney International,* **50,** 1026–31.

Modak, S., Gardner, S., Dunkel, I.J. *et al.* (1997). In *Childhood Cancer into the 21st century: An international conference to mark the 20th anniversary of the UKCCSG,* London, United Kingdom.

Namouni, F., Doz, F., Tanguy, M.L. *et al.* (1997). High-dose chemotherapy with carboplatin, etoposide and cyclophosphamide followed by a haematopoietic stem cell rescue in patients with high-risk retinoblastoma: a SFOP and SFGM study. *European Journal of Cancer,* **33,** 2368–75.

Nelson, D.F., Curran, W.J., Jr., Scott, C. *et al.* (1993). Hyperfractionated radiation therapy and bis-chlorethyl nitrosourea in the treatment of malignant glioma—possible advantage observed at 72.0 Gy in 1.2 Gy B.I.D. fractions: report of the Radiation Therapy Oncology Group Protocol 8302. *International Journal of Radiation Oncology, Biology, and Physics,* **25,** 193–207.

Newell, D.R., Pearson, A.D., Balmanno, K. *et al.* (1993). Carboplatin pharmacokinetics in children: the development of a pediatric dosing formula. The United Kingdom Children's Cancer Study Group. *Journal of Clinical Oncology,* **11,** 2314–23.

Packer, R.J., Boyett, J.M., Zimmerman, R.A. *et al.* (1994a). Outcome of children with brain stem gliomas after treatment with 7800 cGy of hyperfractionated radiotherapy. A Childrens Cancer Group Phase I/II Trial. *Cancer,* **74,** 1827–34.

Packer, R.J., Boyett, J.M., Zimmerman, R.A. *et al.* (1993). Hyperfractionated radiation therapy (72 Gy) for children with brain stem gliomas. A Childrens Cancer Group Phase I/II Trial. *Cancer,* **72,** 1414–21.

Packer, R.J., Cogen, P., Vezina, G. *et al.* (1999a). Medulloblastoma: clinical and biologic aspects. *Neuro-oncology,* **1,** 232–50.

Packer, R.J., Goldwein, J., Nicholson, H.S. *et al.* (1999b). Treatment of children with medulloblastomas with reduced-dose craniospinal radiation therapy and adjuvant chemotherapy: A

Children's Cancer Group Study. *Journal of Clinical Oncology,* **17,** 2127–36.

Packer, R.J., Sutton, L.N., Elterman, R. *et al.* (1994b). Outcome for children with medulloblastoma treated with radiation and cisplatin, CCNU, and vincristine chemotherapy. *Journal of Neurosurgery,* **81,** 690–8.

Packer, R.J. & Vezina, G. (1994c). Pediatric glial neoplasms including brain-stem gliomas. *Seminars in Oncology,* **21,** 260–72.

Peng, L., Yang, J., Yang, H. *et al.* (2001). Determination of peripheral blood stem cells by the Sysmex SE-9500. *Clinical and Laboratory Haematology,* **23,** 231–6.

Peterson, K. & Cairncross, J.G. (1996). Oligodendroglioma. *Cancer Investigation,* **14,** 243–51.

Phillips, G.L., Wolff, S.N., Fay, J.W. *et al.* (1986). Intensive 1,3-bis (2-chloroethyl)-1-nitrosourea (BCNU) monochemotherapy and autologous marrow transplantation for malignant glioma. *Journal of Clinical Oncology,* **4,** 639–45.

Pourquier, P., Waltman, J.L., Urasaki, Y. *et al.* (2001). Topoisomerase I-mediated cytotoxicity of N-methyl-N′-nitro-N-nitrosoguanidine: trapping of topoisomerase I by the O6-methylguanine. *Cancer Research,* **61,** 53–8.

Rickert, C.H. (1998). Epidemiological features of brain tumors in the first 3 years of life. *Child's Nervous System,* **14,** 547–50.

Rickert, C.H. & Paulus, W. (2001). Epidemiology of central nervous system tumors in childhood and adolescence based on the new WHO classification. *Child's Nervous System,* **17,** 503–11.

Robertson, P.L., Zeltzer, P.M., Boyett, J.M. *et al.* (1998). Survival and prognostic factors following radiation therapy and chemotherapy for ependymomas in children: a report of the Children's Cancer Group. *Journal of Neurosurgery,* **88,** 695–703.

Rosenblum, M.K., Knebel, K.D., Vasquez, D.A. *et al.* (1977). Brain-tumor therapy. Quantitative analysis using a model system. *Journal of Neurosurgery,* **46,** 145–54.

Schabel, F.M., Jr., Trader, M.W., Laster, W.R., Jr. *et al.* (1978). Patterns of resistance and therapeutic synergism among alkylating agents. *Antibiotics and Chemotherapy,* **23,** 200–15.

Scotto, K.W. & Bertino, J.R. (2001). In *The Molecular Basis of Cancer,* ed. J. Mendelsohn, P.M. Howley, M.A. Israel & L.A. Liotta, pp. 387–400. Philadelphia: W.B. Saunders Company.

Seiden, M.V., Elias, A., Ayash, L. *et al.* (1992). Pulmonary toxicity associated with high dose chemotherapy in the treatment of solid tumors with autologous marrow transplant: an analysis of four chemotherapy regimens. *Bone Marrow Transplantation,* **10,** 57–63.

Sposto, R., Ertel, I.J., Jenkin, R.D. *et al.* (1989). The effectiveness of chemotherapy for treatment of high grade astrocytoma in children: results of a randomized trial. A report from the Children's Cancer Study Group. *Journal of Neurooncology,* **7,** 165–77.

Stewart, D.A., Guo, D., Luider, J. *et al.* (2001). The CD3– 16+ 56+ NK cell count independently predicts autologous blood stem cell mobilization. *Bone Marrow Transplantation,* **27,** 1237–43.

Stewart, D.J. (1994). A critique of the role of the blood-brain barrier in the chemotherapy of human brain tumors. *Journal of Neurooncology,* **20,** 121–39.

Stewart, L.A. (2002). Chemotherapy in adult high-grade glioma: a systematic review and meta-analysis of individual patient data from 12 randomised trials. *Lancet,* **359,** 1011–8.

Strother, D., Ashley, D., Kellie, S.J. *et al.* (2001). Feasibility of four consecutive high-dose chemotherapy cycles with stem-cell rescue for patients with newly diagnosed medulloblastoma or supratentorial primitive neuroectodermal tumor after craniospinal radiotherapy: results of a collaborative study. *Journal of Clinical Oncology,* **19,** 2696–704.

Teicher, B.A., Holden, S.A., Eder, J.P. *et al.* (1990). Preclinical studies relating to the use of thiotepa in the high-dose setting alone and in combination. *Seminars in Oncology,* **17,** 18–32.

Thomas, P.R., Deutsch, M., Kepner, J.L. *et al.* (2000). Low-stage medulloblastoma: final analysis of trial comparing standard-dose with reduced-dose neuraxis irradiation. *Journal of Clinical Oncology,* **18,** 3004–11.

Torres, C.F., Rebsamen, S., Silber, J.H. *et al.* (1994). Surveillance scanning of children with medulloblastoma. *New England Journal of Medicine,* **330,** 892–5.

van der Lelie, H., Baars, J.W., Rodenhuis, S. *et al.* (1995). Hemolytic uremic syndrome after high dose chemotherapy with autologous stem cell support. *Cancer,* **76,** 2338–42.

Vassal, G., Deroussent, A., Hartmann, O. *et al.* (1990). Dose-dependent neurotoxicity of high-dose busulfan in children: a clinical and pharmacological study. *Cancer Research,* **50,** 6203–7.

Wang, G., Weiss, C., Sheng, P. *et al.* (1996). Retrovirus-mediated transfer of the human O6-methylguanine-DNA methyltransferase gene into a murine hematopoietic stem cell line and resistance to the toxic effects of certain alkylating agents. *Biochemical Pharmacology,* **51,** 1221–8.

Wolff, S.N. (1995). In *High-Dose Cancer Therapy. Pharmacology, Hematopoietins, Stem Cells,* ed. J.O. Armitage & K. Antman, pp. 879–88. Baltimore: Williams & Wilkins.

Young, J.L., Smith, M.A., Roffers, S.D. *et al.* (1999). In *Cancer incidence and survival among children and adolescents: United States SEER Program 1975–1995, National Cancer Institute, SEER Program,* ed. S.M. Ries, J.G. Gurney, M. Linet *et al.,* pp. 73–78. NIH Pub No. 99-4649, Bethesda, MD.

Zeltzer, P.M., Boyett, J.M., Finlay, J.L. *et al.* (1999). Metastasis stage, adjuvant treatment, and residual tumor are prognostic factors for medulloblastoma in children: conclusions from the Children's Cancer Group 921 randomized phase III study. *Journal of Clinical Oncology,* **17,** 832–45.

47 Autologous hematopoietic stem cell transplantation for neuroblastoma

MATTHIAS SCHELL, CHRISTOPHE BERGERON, AND THIERRY PHILIP

Centre Léon Bérard, Lyon, France

Introduction

Neuroblastoma is a malignancy of neural crest cells which usually give rise to the sympathetic nervous system. It is the most common extracranial solid tumor of childhood. Its annual incidence is approximately 9 per million children with only approximately 650 new cases diagnosed yearly in the United States (Parkin *et al.*, 1988; Hayes & Smith, 1989; Bernstein *et al.*, 1992). Neuroblastoma is a tumor of infants and young children (5 years and less in 90% of all cases). It may arise at any site in the sympathetic nervous system, while an abdominal primary is most common.

At diagnosis the tumor may be limited to a single organ, locally or regionally invasive, or widely disseminated. Bone, bone marrow, liver, and skin are among the most common metastatic sites. The two major clinical staging systems (International Neuroblastoma Staging System (INSS) and the Evans/Children's Cancer Study Group Staging systems) are shown in Table 47.1. Most localized tumors have an excellent prognosis when treated by surgical resection, with or sometimes without chemotherapy (Kushner *et al.*, 1996). Infants less than 1 year have stage-independent better prognosis than children. Some of these tumors may even show spontaneous regression (localized or stage IVs) (Evans *et al.*, 1971; Evans, D'Angio, & Koop, 1984; Matthay *et al.*, 1989, Rubie *et al.*, 1997; Castleberry 1997; Cotterill *et al.*, 2000). In contrast, approximately 60% of children with neuroblastoma present with metastatic disease at diagnosis with poor outcome even after intensive treatment protocols. The clinical diversity is related to several biological and molecular characteristics including DNA content, amplified expression of N-*myc* oncogene, and expression of TRK neurotrophin receptors (Seeger *et al.*, 1991; Look *et al.*, 1991; Nakagawara *et al.*, 1993; Kamani, 1996; Rubie *et al.*, 1997). Other variables correlated with poor survival include elevated serum ferritin, lactate dehydrogenase and neuron-specific enolase levels, lack of CD44 expression, and unfavorable histologic features at diagnosis (Evans *et al.*, 1987; Kamani, 1996; Combaret *et al.*, 1996; Lau, 2002) (Table 47.2). Taken together, three different types of neuroblastoma were identified by Brodeur (1994) (Table 47.3). In this chapter we will focus on high-risk neuroblastoma patients with poor outcome such as patients with disseminated stage IV disease and/or N-*myc* amplified neuroblastoma, who may benefit from high-dose therapy followed by hematopoietic stem cell (HSC) transplantation. Over the past 10 to 15 years there has been a steady improvement in outcome for these high-risk patients with 5-year projected survival increasing from 10% to approximately 30% (DeBernardi *et al.*, 1992; Matthay *et al.*, 1995; Kamani, 1996; Kamani *et al.*, 1996; Stram *et al.*, 1996; Ladenstein *et al.*, 1998; Matthay *et al.*, 1999) (Figs. 47.1 to 47.5). It is unclear to what extent this is due to improved induction therapy, high-dose therapy with bone marrow or blood stem cell transplantation, posttransplant treatment with retinoic acid, and/or selection of patients.

Disease specific work-up before high-dose therapy for high-risk neuroblastoma

High-dose therapy forms part of a strategy that starts with induction chemotherapy. A large number of studies indicate that remission status prior to myeloablative therapy is important for outcome of high-risk neuroblastoma patients. Therefore, much effort has been made to design new, non–cross-resistant agents and effective induction regimens.

Since 1985 platinum compounds, epipodophyllotoxins, and ifosfamide have been added to the regular induction chemotherapeutic agents (vincristine, doxorubicin, cyclophosphamide) and shown to improve response rates. In an early-randomized phase II study, McWilliams *et al.* (1995) compared the activity of teniposide (100 mg/m^2) and cisplatin (90 mg/m^2) to the standard induction of the 1980s, cyclophosphamide (1,000 mg/m^2) and doxorubicin (35 mg/m^2). They found a trend toward higher complete and partial remission for the cisplatin regimen but no significant difference for event-free survival. Notable response rates were further noted in a phase II study for carboplatin and etoposide (Frappaz *et al.*, 1992). A phase II study showed excellent and almost identical response rates of approximately 70% for ifosfamide, carboplatin, and iproplatin, but an inferior response rate with epirubicin (Castleberry *et al.*, 1994). These and other studies led to the use of multidrug induction

Table 47.1. *The International Neuroblastoma Staging System and the Evans/CCSG Staging System*

The International Neuroblastoma Staging System

Stage   *Definition*

1   Localized tumor with complete gross excision, with or without microscopic residual disease; representative ipsilateral lymph nodes negative for tumor microscopically (nodes attached to and removed with the primary tumor may be positive).

2A   Localized tumor with incomplete gross excision; representative ipsilateral nonadherent lymph nodes negative for tumor microscopically.

2B   Localized tumor with or without complete gross excision, with ipsilateral nonadherent lymph nodes positive for tumor. Enlarged contralateral lymph nodes must be negative microscopically.

3   Unresectable unilateral tumor infiltrating across the midline[a] with or without regional lymph node involvement; or localized unilateral tumor with contralateral regional lymph node involvement; or midline tumor with bilateral extension by infiltration (unresectable) or by lymph node involvement.

4   Any primary tumor with dissemination to distant lymph nodes, bone, bone marrow, liver, skin, and/or other organs (except as defined for stage 4S).

4S   Localized primary tumor (as defined for stage 1, 2A, or 2B), with dissemination limited to skin, liver, and/or bone marrow (limited to infants <1 year of age).

The Evans/CCSG Staging System

Stage I   Tumor confined to the organ or structure of origin.

Stage II   Tumor extending in continuity beyond the organ or structure of origin but not crossing the midline. Regional lymph nodes on the homolateral side may be involved.

Stage III   Tumors extending in continuity beyond the midline. Regional lymph nodes bilaterally may be involved.

Stage IV   Remote disease involving bone, parenchymatous organs, soft tissues, distant lymph node groups, or marrow.

Stage IV-S   Patients who would otherwise be stage I or II but who have remote disease confined to one or more of the following sites: liver, skin, or marrow (without evidence of bone metastases).

[a] The midline is defined as the vertebral column. Tumors originating on one side and crossing the midline must infiltrate to or beyond the opposite side of the vertebral column. Marrow involvement in stage 4S should be minimal, i.e. <10% of total nucleated cells identified as malignant on bone marrow biopsy or on marrow aspirate. More extensive marrow involvement would be considered to be stage 4. The MIBG scan (if performed) should be negative in the marrow.

Abbreviation: MIBG, I-metaiodobenzylguanidine.

regimens. The most relevant published studies are shown in Table 47.4.

The most commonly used drugs were etoposide/teniposide, cisplatin/carboplatin, cyclophosphamide (ifosfamide), doxorubicin, and vincristine. Doses per course or 21 days varied widely between studies: the range for cyclophosphamide varied from 0.6 g/m^2 (Shafford *et al.*, 1984; De Bernardi *et al.*, 1992b;

Table 47.2. *Outcome according to risk group*

Low risk (survival > 80–100% with surgery alone)
   All stage I[a]
   Stage II
     without amplification of N-*myc*
   Stage IV-S
     without amplification of N-*myc*

Intermediate risk (survival > 80% with surgery, conventional chemotherapy, ± local irradiation)
   Stage III
     without amplification of N-*myc*
     without elevated serum ferritin or neuron-specific enolase
     with no or few occult tumor cells in marrow by immunocytology
     with favorable histopathology (Shimada)
   Stage IV (diagnosed <1 year of age)
     without amplification of N-*myc*
     without elevated serum ferritin or neuron-specific enolase
     with no or few occult tumor cells in marrow by immunocytology
     with hyperdiploid DNA content
     with favorable histopathology

High risk (survival <10–15% with conventional chemotherapy, surgery, ± local irradiation)
   Stage IV (diagnosed at 1 year of age or older)
   Any clinical stage or age
     with N-*myc* amplification

[a] Evans/CCSG staging system.

Donfrancesco *et al.*, 1995) to approximately 4 g/m^2 (Kushner *et al.*, 1987, 1990, 1994). Doxorubicin and etoposide doses ranged from 30 (Kushner *et al.*, 1987; Stram *et al.*, 1996) to 75 mg/m^2 (Kushner *et al.*, 1994) and from 300 (Donfrancesco *et al.*, 1995) to 600 mg/m^2 (Kushner *et al.*, 1994), respectively.

As suggested by Cheung & Heller (1991), it seems that dose intensification may increase response rate. Doubling the dose of cyclophosphamide more than doubled the response rate in the N4 regimen (Kushner *et al.*, 1987). Later, induction regimens using high-dose cisplatin (CDDP) had high rates of complete

Table 47.3. *Types of neuroblastoma*

Feature	Type 1	Type 2	Type 3
MYCN	1 copy	1 copy	Amplified
DNA ploidy	Hyperdploid/ near triploid	Near diploid/ near tetraploid	Near diploid/ near tetraploid
1p LOH	Absent	± Present	Usually present
14q LOH	Absent ?	± Present	Usually present
TRK-A expression	High	Variable	Low or absent
Age	Usually < 1 yr	Any age	Usually 1–5 years
Stage	Usually I, II, IV-S	Usually III, IV	Usually III, IV
3-yr survival	95%	20–25%	< 5%

Reproduced, with permission from Brodeur (1994).

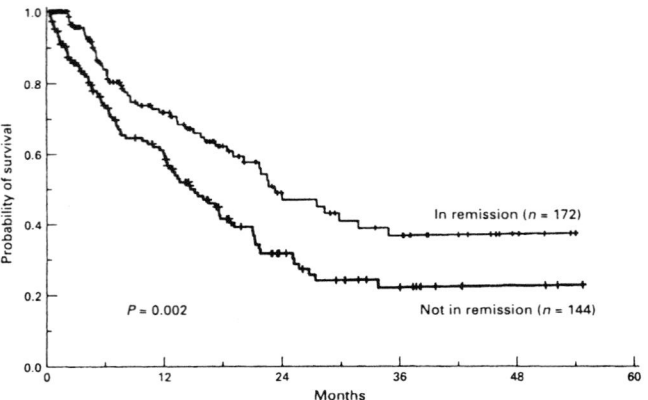

Fig. 47.1. Probability of survival after autologous bone marrow transplantation for 316 patients for whom complete data were reported to the Autologous Blood and Marrow Transplant Registry, as of January 1995. Reproduced, with permission, from Kamani (1996).

response, although comparable results were also documented in the N4 regimen that lacked cisplatin, or with the OPEC and PE/CADO regimens with standard cisplatin doses. In regimens containing high doses of cisplatin, the drug was given in alternate courses. Therefore, the dose intensity was unremarkable (Pinkerton *et al.*, 2000). The impressive response rates with N5 and N6 regimens could not be reproduced elsewhere with larger number of patients (Valteau-Couanet *et al.*, 2000b). The interpretation and comparison of most results is limited with regard to the small number of patients studied. The differences in definition of stage IV (more or less extensive bone marrow investigation, MIBG scanning), as well as different ways of assessing response, make it difficult to draw firm conclusions about any individual drug or regimen (Pinkerton *et al.*, 2000).

High-dose therapy versus conventional chemotherapy

Until recently the prognosis of high-risk patients following conventional therapeutic approaches remained substantially

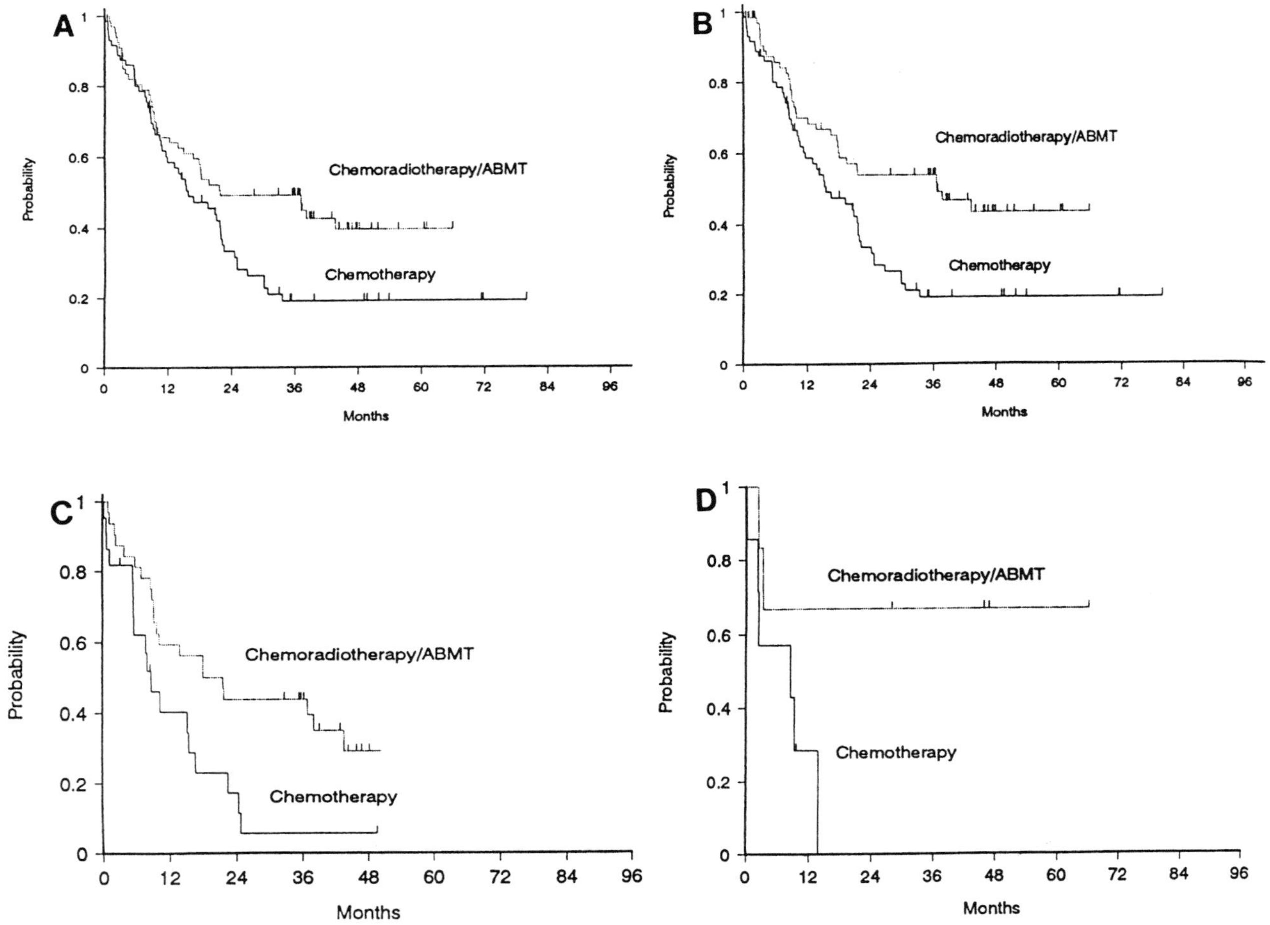

Fig. 47.2. Event-free survival (EFS) for stage IV neuroblastoma, chemoradiotherapy/ABMT vs continued chemotherapy. (**A**) All patients (P = .020); (**B**) all patients, censoring therapy-related deaths (P = .004); (**C**) patients with partial response to induction chemotherapy (P = .011); (**D**) patients with amplified N-*myc* (P = .066). Reproduced, with permission, from Stram *et al.* (1996).

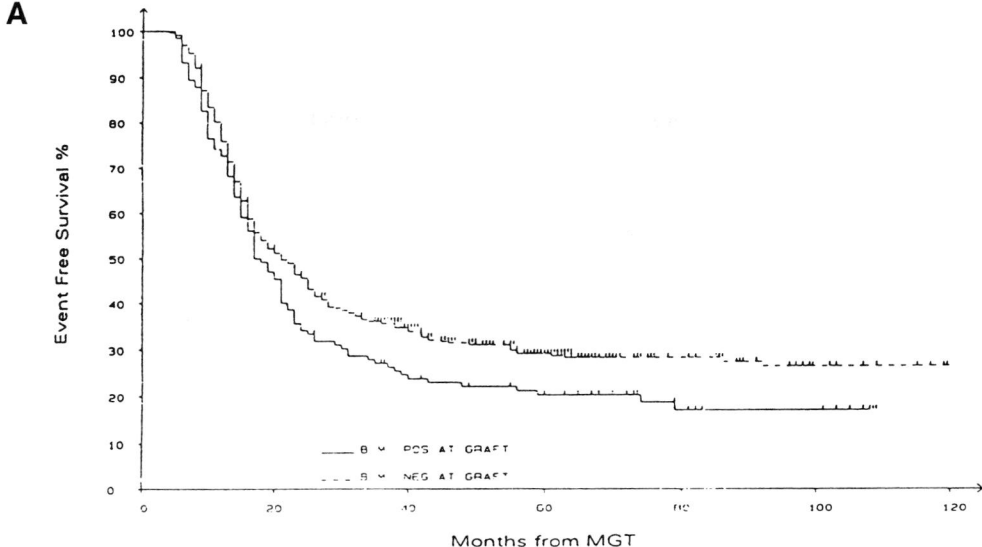

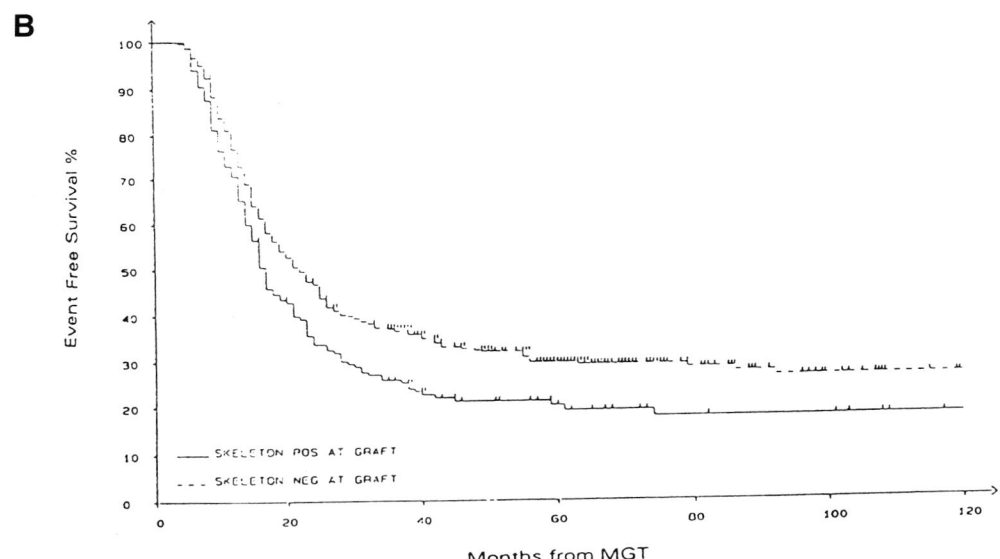

Fig. 47.3. (A) Event-free survival (EFS) according to bone marrow response status before MGT. Bone marrow involvement before MGT: 5-year EFS rate for bone-marrow-positive patients (132 patients) is 20%, and for bone-marrow-negative patients (399 patients), 29% (*P* = .03). (B) Event-free survival according to skeletal response status before MGT. Skeletal disease before MGT as defined by 99Tc and/or mIBG scan: 5-year EFS rate for skeleton-positive patients (170 patients) is 20%, and for skeleton-negative patients (369 patients), 30% (*P* = .004). Reproduced, with permission, from Ladenstein *et al.* (1998). *Abbreviation:* MGT, megatherapy.

unchanged from the observation made by Ariel and Pack (1960) almost 40 years ago: "A review of 275 cases of adrenal neuroblastoma collected from the literature painted a very gloomy picture indicating that in most of these children the disease ran a rapidly fatal course."

The demonstration that hematopoiesis could be restored by autologous HSC infusion opened the way for the use of much higher doses of chemotherapy with autologous bone marrow support for treatment of solid tumors. In 1982, Pritchard *et al.*

published a prospective study showing a response of the primary tumor in 6 out of 11 patients following a high-dose melphalan regimen with autologous bone marrow support. Subsequently, when 25 newly diagnosed patients were treated by high-dose melphalan and nonpurged marrow rescue, after a significant tumor response to induction therapy, the median duration of survival doubled from 8.5 to 16 months when compared retrospectively to previous studies. Ten patients survived disease-free 21 to 50 months after diagnosis (Shafford *et al.*,

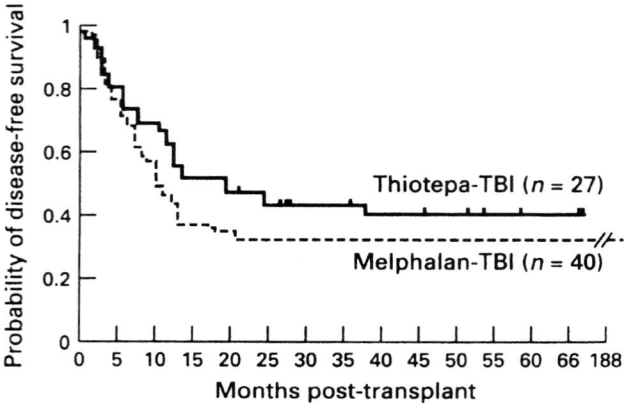

Fig. 47.4. Kaplan-Meier life table analysis of the probability of disease-free survival after bone marrow transplantation for 27 patients treated with VP-16, thiotepa, and TBI (—). The tick marks represent individual patients continuing at risk. DFS analysis for patients treated with melphalan/TBI containing regimens is also shown (----). Reproduced, with permission, from Kamani *et al.* (1996).

1984). Many other subsequent single arm studies suggested the improvement in outcome following high-dose therapy compared to historical series with conventional chemotherapy (Matthay *et al.,* 1993; Philip *et al.,* 1987; Seeger *et al.,* 1991).

Comparable survival rates, however, have also been reported with conventional chemotherapeutic approaches. In a study by Green and colleagues (1986), 35 of 44 children with disseminated neuroblastoma obtained a good partial response (PR) or complete response (CR) following treatment with cyclophosphamide, cisplatin, doxorubicin, and teniposide, with subsequent surgery for residual disease. Maintenance therapy with the same

drugs was given for a total of 8 months. Eight patients (24%) survived, 6 disease-free, with a follow-up of 36 to 58 months. In a subsequent study in which these same four drugs were given in a more intensive fashion, all 28 patients obtained a significant or complete response and 10 (42%) remained disease-free at a median of 17 (range, 9–34) months from diagnosis.

The first randomized study comparing high-dose chemotherapy versus no further therapy was performed by the European Neuroblastoma Study Group. This study showed a significant advantage in progression-free survival for patients with stage IV disease over 1 year of age at diagnosis given high-dose melphalan with unpurged bone marrow infusion (Pinkerton *et al.,* 1987). The overall progression-free survival time was 23 months in the high-dose chemotherapy group ($n = 32$) compared to 6 months in the chemotherapy alone group ($n = 33$; $P < .02$). However, applicability of these results is limited since the number of randomized patients was small (65 out of 130 patients) and bias may have been introduced by a high proportion of nonrandomized patients. With a follow-up between 3.5 and 6 years 8 of 24 patients treated by myeloablative therapy and 5 of 26 treated by chemotherapy alone remained disease progression-free (Pinkerton, 1991). This mirrored the results of a previous study using the same chemotherapeutic agents and high-dose preparative regimen, where the event-free survival of 35% at 2.5 years dropped to 18% at 5-year follow-up (Pritchard *et al.,* 1989). Thus, although high-dose therapy improved the rate and duration of remission, it did not appear to improve the overall cure rate.

Published cooperative group studies also raise the question of whether high-dose therapy offers any advantage over conventional therapy in the long term. Fifty-four out of 103 patients treated by the "NB 85" protocol from the Italian Association of Pediatric Hematology and Oncology (AIEOP)

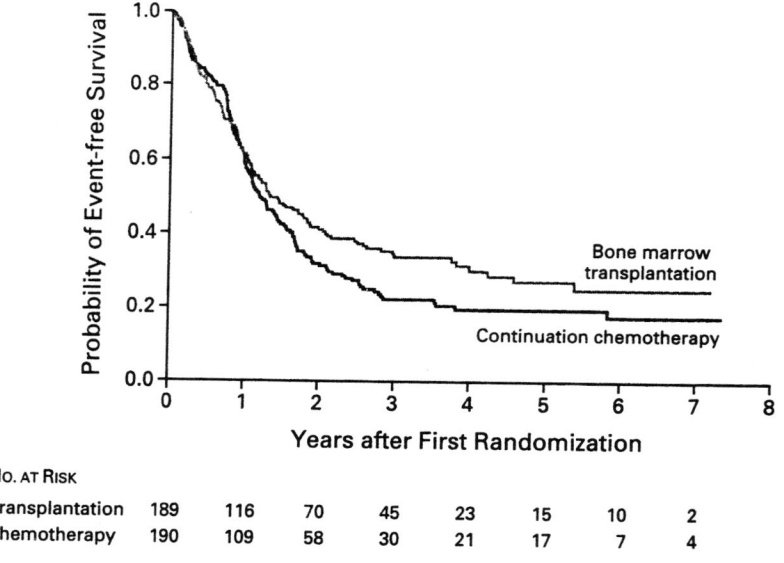

No. at Risk							
Transplantation	189	116	70	45	23	15	10	2
Chemotherapy	190	109	58	30	21	17	7	4

Fig. 47.5. Probability of event-free survival among patients assigned in a randomized fashion to megatherapy or continuation chemotherapy. Reproduced, with permission, from Matthay *et al.* (1999).

Table 47.4. *Induction regimens and their results*

Reference	Protocol	Chemotherapy regimen	Number of patients	Time of response assessment (months)	Method of response assessment				CR (%)
					Bone	MIBG	Trephines	Aspirates	
Shafford et al. (1984)	OPEC(D)	VCR, Cyclo, CDDP, Tenipo (Doxo)	42	6–12	Tc	–	2	2	74
Bernard et al. (1987)	PE/Cado	CDDP, Tenipo/Cyclo, Doxo, VCR	35	6	Tc	–	6	4	68
Kushner et al. (1987)	N4	Doxo, Cyclo, 5-FU, VCR, Ara-C, Hydroxyurea	33	5	Tc	–	"Multiple"		70
Kushner et al. (1990)	N5	Doxo, Cyclo, VCR/CDDP, Etopo	14	6	Tc	+/–	2	4	90
Kushner et al. (1994)	N6	Doxo, Cyclo, VCR/CDDP, Etopo	24	5	Tc	+	2	4	96
Stram et al. (1996)	CCG321-P2	Cyclo, CDDP, Tenipo, Doxo	157	8	Tc	–	"Multiple"		57
DeBernardi et al. (1992)	NB82	Peptichi/CDDP, Tenipo	75	3	Tc	–	?	yes	57
DeBernardi et al. (1992)	NB 85	Peptichi/Cyclo, VCR, CDDP / Doxo, Tenipo	106	3	Tc	–	?	yes	76
Pinkerton et al. (1990)	ENSG3	Ifos, VCR, Doxo / CDDP, Etopo	36	3	Tc	+	2	2	47
Coze et al. (1997)	SFOP NB87	Cyclo, Doxo, VCR/CDDP, Etopo	164	3	–	+	2	2	66
		Doxo, Cyclo	70	4	Tc	–	?	yes	27
McWilliams et al. (1995)	POG 81	Randomized CDDP Tenipo	64	4	Tc	–	?	yes	34
Castel et al. (1995)	SNSG	Cyclo, Doxo/CDDP, Tenipo	58	4	Tc	+	?	yes	47
Donfrances et al. (1995)	DCECaT	Desferoxamine, Cyclo, Etopo, TP, Carbo	43	3	Tc	+	4	?	50

Abbreviations: Ara-C, cytosine arabinoside; Carbo, carboplatin; CDDP, cisplatin; Cyclo, cyclophosphamide; Doxo, doxorubicin; Etopo, etoposide; Ifos, ifosfamide; Peptichi, peptichimio; Tenipo, teniposide; TP, thiotepa; VCR, vincristine; 5-FU, fluorouracil.

achieved CR or very good PR after induction therapy. In a nonrandomized fashion, 32 out of these 54 patients were then treated with vincristine, melphalan, and total body irradiation (TBI) followed by nonpurged autologous marrow rescue, while 22 of 54 patients continued conventional chemotherapy with drugs used in the induction regimen. The outcome was similar in both groups, with 23% in the high-dose chemotherapy group and 33% in the chemotherapy group being progression-free (projected) at 5 years ($P = .6$) (Lanino et al., 1991). The latest relapse occurred 5 years following diagnosis in a transplanted patient. The median survival in both groups was 33 months, and in this study myeloablative therapy did not appear to offer an advantage over conventional chemotherapy.

A retrospective Pediatric Oncology Group study that compared conventional chemotherapy and high-dose therapy reported on 116 patients who achieved greater than 50% tumor reduction after surgery and five courses of chemotherapy with cisplatin, cyclophosphamide, an epipodophyllotoxin, and adriamycin (Shuster et al., 1991). Forty-nine patients were then entered in a study involving localized radiation therapy to sites of bulk disease, followed by melphalan 180 mg/m², TBI 1,200 cGy, and rescue with immunomagnetically purged marrow. Sixty-seven patients continued on the original conventional therapy protocol with three to five additional courses of chemotherapy with the same agents and were treated with further surgery when appropriate. With a follow-up of 43 to 70 months, the projected 4-year survival rate of all patients achieving a complete or partial response was 30%. There was no significant difference in overall survival between patients treated by high-dose therapy or conventional chemotherapy.

The Study Group of Japan completed a nonrandomized study of 161 newly diagnosed patients with advanced neuroblastoma (stage III and stage IV, Children's Cancer Group and International Staging Criteria). All patients received identical courses of induction chemotherapy with aggressive surgical debulking. Patients were then treated with conventional chemotherapy or high-dose therapy. The 5-year event-free survival rate after high-dose therapy and maintenance chemotherapy was 50% ($n = 31$) and 38.8% ($n = 79$), respectively. Comparing only patients in CR undergoing high-dose therapy ($n = 27$) to those treated with maintenance chemotherapy ($n = 55$), the 5-year EFS rate was not statistically different (64.6% versus 56.6% respectively) (Ohnuma et al., 1995).

The Children's Cancer Group studied 141 nonrandomized patients following similar induction chemotherapeutic protocols who were in CR or PR at the time of scheduled autologous BMT. Sixty-seven patients received an immunomagnetically purged rescue. Seventy-four patients were treated with continued maintenance chemotherapy. The high-dose therapy/autologous transplant group showed a significant improved event-free survival at 4 years when compared to the chemotherapy group (40% and 19%, respectively, $P = .02$) (Stram et al., 1996). The advantage for autologous BMT was greatest for certain very high-risk subgroups including those >2 years of age at diagnosis, those with bone or bone marrow metastases, those with N-

myc amplification, and those with partial rather then complete response to induction chemotherapy.

The first randomized, controlled collaborative group study was completed to try to determine whether high-dose therapy followed by bone marrow rescue is more effective than intensive chemotherapy alone in the treatment of high-risk neuroblastoma. For the Children's Cancer Group, Matthay and colleagues (1999) reported a study of 539 eligible children with high-risk features (including Evan's stage IV, stage IV infants with N-myc oncogene amplification, localized neuroblastoma with N-myc oncogene amplification, serum ferritin >142 nmol, and unfavorable histology features). All patients received the same initial chemotherapy regimen (5 cycles of cisplatin 60 mg/m², doxorubicin 30 mg/m², etoposide 200 mg/m², and cyclophosphamide 2,000 mg/m²). Three hundred seventy-nine patients without disease progression were then randomly assigned to receive myeloablative chemotherapy (CEM/TBI and infusion of purged autologous bone marrow; $n = 189$) or 3 cycles of conventional chemotherapy (cisplatin/etoposide/adriamycin/ifosfamide; $n = 190$). One hundred eighteen patients were nonrandomly assigned to continuation chemotherapy and 42 patients never underwent randomization because of progression, withdrawal, or treatment deviation. The mean 3-year EFS for the whole population ($n = 539$), the randomized patients ($n = 379$), and the nonrandomly treated patients ($n = 118$) was 30 ± 2%, 28 ± 3%, and 33 ± 4%, respectively. The 3-year EFS from time of randomization was 34 ± 4% among patients assigned to transplantation, a significantly higher value than the rate of 22 ± 4% among those assigned to continuation chemotherapy ($P = .034$). Subsequently, the benefit of myeloablative therapy was evident in each subgroup analysis and it was most pronounced among patients who were older than 2 years at diagnosis ($P = .01$) and those with N-MYC amplification ($P = .03$) (Fig. 47.5).

Role of multiple high-dose therapies

Attempts to intensify therapy further using double transplants have been reported. In two pilot studies from the LCME group, 25 patients in first partial remission and 8 patients who had relapsed but obtained another partial (6 patients) or complete response (2 patients), were treated with a double round of intensive cytotoxic therapy and purged autologous BMT. The preparatory regimen prior to the first transplant included BCNU, teniposide, and cisplatin or carboplatin. The preparatory regimen prior to the second transplant included vincristine, TBI, and melphalan. The overall survival for 25 patients undergoing double transplantation in first PR was 34% at 5 years. For the 8 patients who underwent double transplantation after relapse, the overall survival was 25% at 2 years. In this group of extremely poor-risk neuroblastoma patients (newly diagnosed patients in PR or relapsed patients), double high-dose therapy showed an overall survival of 32% at 5 years (Philip et al., 1993). A rapid-sequence tandem transplant as a first-line treatment for children with high-risk neuroblastoma after induction therapy was published by Grupp et al. (2000). The first high-dose chemotherapy regimen comprised carboplatin, etoposide, and cyclophosphamide, followed by a second regimen of melphalan and TBI within 6 weeks. This treatment approach was shown to be feasible and treatment-related mortality (7%) was similar to that of single transplant studies. The 3-year EFS in this study was 59%. Further dose escalation by a triple-tandem high-dose therapy was shown to be feasible in a study of Kletzel et al. (2002). Twenty-six high-risk patients were treated by an induction regimen including cisplatin, etoposide, cyclophosphamide, and doxorubicin, followed by surgery and three cycles of cyclophosphamide for PBSC collection. High-dose chemotherapy with two cycles of carboplatin and etoposide followed by a third cycle including thiotepa and cyclophosphamide was utilized. Of the patients enrolled in this study, 21 patients underwent one, 19 underwent two, and 17 patients completed all three high-dose chemotherapy regimens. With a median follow-up of 38 months from diagnosis, the estimated 3-year EFS for the 26 patients was 57%.

Further follow-up, as well as randomized comparison between single and multiple high-dose therapies are needed to evaluate the impact on long-term EFS.

Indications for high-dose therapy in neuroblastoma

With the publication of the study of the Children's Cancer Group (Matthay et al., 1999) there is strong evidence that high-dose therapy is indicated in children with stage IV neuroblastoma.

However, a few studies have documented that high-dose chemotherapy appears to be most effective in children with high-risk neuroblastoma who have obtained a significant response (either CR or a good PR) to initial therapy after diagnosis: a report from the Italian bone marrow transplant registry (Garaventa et al., 1996) described outcome for 135 children undergoing myeloablative therapy between 1984 and 1993 for disseminated neuroblastoma, of whom 117 received unpurged autologous bone marrow. Of the 135 children, 57 were in first CR at the time of transplant, 11 in second or subsequent CR, 42 in first PR, and 25 had more advanced disease. The disease-free survival was 26% for the whole group, 34.6% for those grafted in first CR, and 23.6%, 36.4%, and 8% for patients grafted, respectively, in first PR, in subsequent CR, or with advanced disease.

The LMCE group using a preparative regimen of melphalan and TBI with immunomagnetically purged marrow, demonstrated that the probability of disease-free survival at 4 years was 25% for patients grafted after obtaining greater than a 90% response to induction chemotherapy compared to only 16% for patients obtaining a PR (Philip et al., 1991a). Subsequently, a significantly higher progression-free survival at 7 years was also observed in 27 CR–very good PR patients when compared to 68 patients with a less good response to induction therapy (52% versus 19%) (Frappaz et al., 2000). This trend of a poorer prognosis being associated with lesser response to initial chemotherapy was also observed in a study of 81 patients treated with high-dose therapy and TBI followed by immunomagnetically purged marrow rescue. With a median follow-up of approximately 18 months, disease-free survival was 57% for patients with a CR or very good partial response (VGPR), compared to 37% for patients transplanted following a lesser response. Subsequently, a retrospective study of the European Group for Bone Marrow Transplantation indicated that patients with persisting bone marrow involvement and/or skeletal lesions before high-dose therapy, defined by technetium and/or MIBG scans, have worse outcome (Ladenstein et al., 1998). Thus, obtaining significant response to induction chemotherapy seems necessary prior to high-dose therapy. Representative high-dose therapy regimens currently being used are summarized in Table 47.5 and published results in Table 47.6.

Early studies indicated that high-dose therapy is less efficacious at relapse than as first-line treatment. The Pediatric Oncology Group published results with an actuarial 2-year event-free survival of 32% to 43% when patients were treated by high-dose therapy respectively in CR or following a first PR, but only 5% in patients treated during a second PR (Graham Pole et al., 1991a). For the Children's Cancer Group, Seeger et al. (1991) published an estimated survival of 53% at 4.5 years for patients transplanted before progressive disease occurred compared to 7% at 2.5 years for those transplanted after disease progression.

There are some data, however, that raise the question of whether there may be a select group of stage IV neuroblastoma patients who should have high-dose therapy postponed until relapse occurs (Ladenstein et al., 1993). This retrospective study involved 48 patients who had achieved a CR with initial therapy and then relapsed. Thirty patients had initially received conventional chemotherapy before relapse and an additional 18 patients obtained their first CR with conventional chemotherapy followed by myeloablative therapy. Following chemotherapy for relapse, 14 of 30 patients in the conventional chemotherapy group, and 2 of 18 in the group with prior myeloablative therapy, obtained a second CR. The overall survival rate at 2 years was 27% for those who were initially treated with conventional chemotherapy compared to no long-term survivors in those receiving high-dose therapy as part of their

Table 47.5. *Preparative regimens used prior to autotransplantation for neuroblastoma*

Chemotherapy only	Chemotherapy and TBI
Melphan	Melphalan/TBI
Melphalan/etoposide	Melphalan/vincristine/TBI
Melphalan/BCNU/teniposide	Melphalan/teniposide/doxorubicin/cisplatin/TBI
Busulfan/cyclophosphamide	Melphalan/BCNU/teniposide/carboplatin/vincristine/TBI
Busulfan/melphalan	Thiotepa/etoposide/TBI
Carboplatin/etoposide/melphalan	Carboplatin/etoposide/melphalan/TBI

Table 47.6. *Current results of autologous HSC transplantation for neuroblastoma*

Group Institution	Patient number	Purge	Conditioning regimen	TBI	DFS 2-year	DFS 4-5 year
EBMTG	1,070	Y/N	Multiple	Y/N	49[a]	33[a]
CCG	189	Y	CEM-TBI	Y	34 (3 yrs)	28
POG	94	Y	Multiple	Y	40	32
CHOP/MCH	67	Y	Multiple	Y	38	32
LMCE	87	Y/N	Multiple	Y/N	54+	30[b]

[a] Survival rates shown are overall survival rates.
[b] Survival rates shown are progression-free survival rates.

initial treatment. Subsequently, in a study at the Children's Hospital of Philadelphia, 41 patients with high-risk neuroblastoma were treated by high-dose therapy followed by either a purged autologous marrow rescue (70%) or an allogeneic transplant (30%). Twenty-six patients were treated by high-dose therapy at relapse and 15 as part of their initial therapy. The disease-free survival at 24 months in patients undergoing high-dose therapy was 27% when performed at relapse and 25% when included in first-line treatment, a difference that was not statistically significant (Ikeda *et al.*, 1992).

In addition to stage IV children, some other subgroups of patients may also be considered as high-risk neuroblastoma and justify high-dose therapy: a few studies identified a small subgroup of patients (10%) with localized neuroblastoma with unfavorable outcome. Among 316 consecutive patients with localized neuroblastoma, the SFOP group found N-*myc* amplification to be the most powerful unfavorable predictive indicator with EFS rates of 32% compared to 90% in nonamplified tumors (Rubie *et al.*, 1997). In a Children's Cancer Group study of 228 Evans stage III patients, the only independent factors were age and N-*myc* amplification (Matthay *et al.*, 1998). In both studies more intensive treatment for these patients was advocated. However, these observations are at variance with the study of Cohn *et al.* (1995). In their retrospective study, N-*myc* was not necessarily associated with an adverse outcome (*n* = 6), but unresectable primary tumors were not included in this study. As the small number of patients does not permit a randomized study in a reasonable time frame, more and more investigators include these groups of patients into treatment protocols for high-risk neuroblastoma (Sibley *et al.*, 1995; Matthay *et al.*, 1999; Grupp *et al.*, 2000; Castel *et al.*, 2001; Cheung *et al.*, 2001c).

Infants less than 1 year of age at diagnosis with localized or stage IV-S neuroblastoma have an excellent prognosis even in the presence of unfavorable biologic markers with event-free survival at 4 years >90% (Strother *et al.*, 1995; Matthay *et al.*, 1998). Also, stage IV neuroblastoma in this age group has a much better prognosis than in older children with 50% to 75% EFS (Paul *et al.*, 1991; De Bernardi *et al.*, 1992; Strother *et al.*, 1995). However, a study of 134 infants with stage IV neuroblastoma, treated by four-drug induction chemotherapy including cisplatin, cyclophosphamide, doxorubicin, and etoposide, delin-

eated a subgroup of infants with worse prognosis. The 3-year EFS of infants with N-*myc* amplified stage IV disease was 10% compared to 93% in nonamplified patients (Schmidt *et al.*, 2000). Subsequently, infants with bone metastases were shown to have worse outcome in a multivariate analysis of 51 infants with a 5-year EFS of 27.2% compared to 90% for infants without bone lesions (*P* < .0001; Minard *et al.*, 2000).

In a study including 12 infants with poor prognosis neuroblastoma, a combination of busulfan and melphalan conditioning followed by stem cell transplantation resulted in a 5-year event-free survival rate of 64%: transplant was performed after metastatic relapse for 5 patients, because of persistent bone metastases in 1 patient and as first-line consolidation in six patients whose tumor exhibited N-*myc* amplification (Valteau-Couanet *et al.*, 2000a). High-dose therapy should therefore be discussed for infants with high-risk neuroblastoma.

An algorithm for the treatment of patients with neuroblastoma is shown in Figures 47.6 and 47.7.

Peripheral blood as a source of stem cells for autotransplantation

Autologous peripheral blood stem cells (PBSC) provide an alternative source to marrow for patients undergoing myeloablative chemotherapy (Henn, 1990). PBSCs can be obtained without the use of anesthesia and without the discomfort involved in multiple bone marrow aspirations, and can be obtained from infants weighing less than 10 kg without difficulty. In one study, three infants weighing 6.9 to 9.4 kg had autologous PBSCs mobilized following high-dose chemotherapy with G-CSF. A median of 4 (range 4–7) procedures were needed to collect at least 4×10^8/kg nucleated cells. All three children were then successfully transplanted with myeloid engraftment occurring in 8 (range 7–9) days and independence from packed cell and platelet transfusions in 15 (range 10–20) days and 25 (range 14–29) days, respectively after PBSC reinfusion (Nussbaumer *et al.*, 1996). Investigators from the University of Minnesota reported the use of autologous PBSCs in nine patients with neuroblastoma, all of whom had evidence of marrow involvement at the time of apheresis. All patients engrafted. Tumor cell contamination may also prove to be a problem using PBSC, however, as circulating neuroblastoma

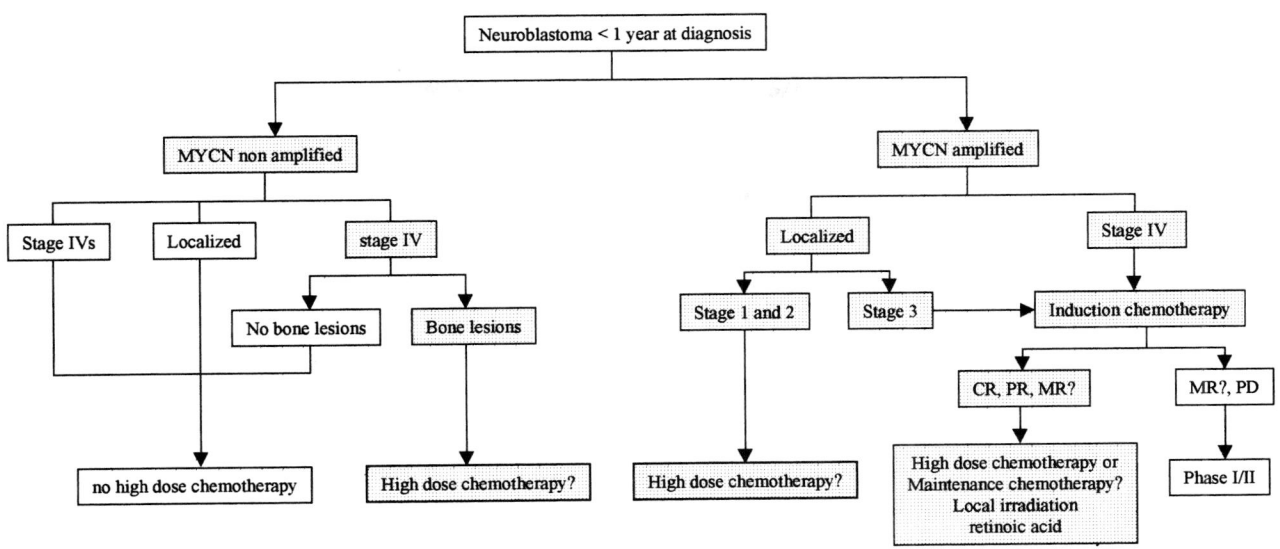

Fig. 47.6. An algorithm for treatment of infants less than 1 year of age at diagnosis.

cells were demonstrated in three of the nine patients (Di Caro *et al.*, 1994). Because tumor cell contamination is a potential contributing cause of relapse after myeloablative therapy and autologous reconstitution, Moss and colleagues (1994) examined the potential risk of re-infusing circulating neuroblastoma cells. They performed immunocytologic and tumor cell clonogenic assays on 74 blood samples from 56 children with advanced stage neuroblastoma. Thirty patients had concurrent bone marrow evaluations. Twenty percent of the PBSC specimens had circulating neoplastic cells demonstrated immunocytologically. Thirteen patients had identifiable clonogenic tumor colonies. Interestingly, 3 of 53 samples (6%) negative by immunocytology had tumor cells demonstrated by the clonogenic assay.

In a study of 466 stage IV patients, immunocytologically identified neuroblastoma cells were compared in bone marrow and blood. At the time of bone marrow collection, persisting neuroblastoma cells were identified in the bone marrow in 19% of patients and in the blood in 5% (Seeger *et al.*, 2000). In another study, blood and bone marrow disease were evaluated by immunocytochemistry at diagnosis and during induction chemotherapy in 57 patients. Cytoreduction was found to be much faster in blood compared to bone marrow. Circulating tumor cells were more likely found in patients with bone metastases (Faulkner *et al.*, 2000). The persistence of tumor cells in a small number of patients emphasizes the importance of testing peripheral blood stem collections for tumor. One report utilizing CD34 selection of PBSCs by the CliniMACS device described detectable neuroblastoma cells in 17 patients before selection and in 4 after selection (Handgretinger et al., 2002). Large clinical studies of ex vivo purging of PBSCs are needed.

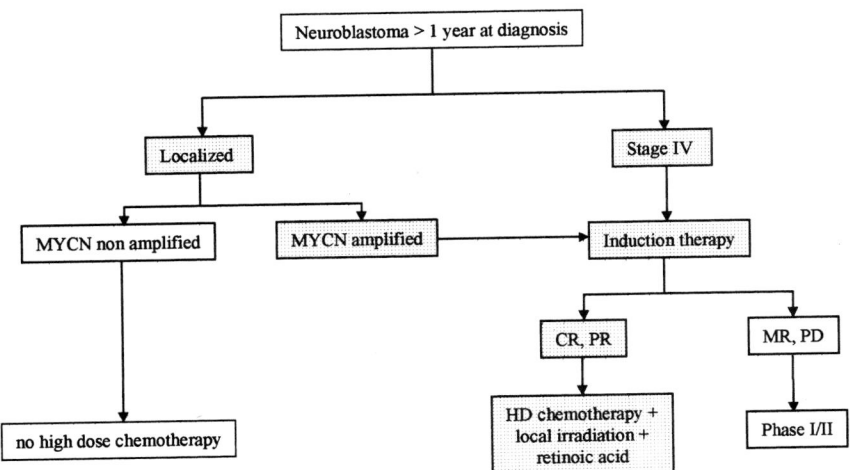

Fig. 47.7. An algorithm for treatment of children older than 1 year at diagnosis.

The role of marrow purging

Purging of marrow in patients with previous marrow involvement should reduce or eliminate the risk of the infused marrow being contaminated with viable neuroblastoma cells and thus perhaps improve the outcome of autologous HSC transplantation. This was clearly demonstrated by Brenner et al. (1994). In a study including 8 neuroblastoma patients in clinical and cytological remission, the residual cancer cells in harvested bone marrow were marked with a neomycin resistance gene using a retroviral vector. In all 3 neuroblastoma patients who relapsed, the recurrent cells contained the neomycin resistance marker identified by polymerase chain reaction. Therefore, residual cancer cells in harvested marrow were shown to contribute to relapse.

Between 30% and 50% of patients with stage IV neuroblastoma have metastatic disease detectable in the marrow harvested prior to autotransplantation (Combaret, Favrot, & Kremens, 1989b; Seeger et al., 1991). Current methods of purging marrow, particularly immunomagnetic techniques, appear to be effective in eradicating residual neuroblastoma cells from contaminated marrow and do not appear to significantly damage hematopoietic stem cells (Combaret et al., 1989a; Seeger et al., 1991). Purging techniques that have been studied or proposed are summarized in Table 47.7. Of all the different physical methods for purging marrow, the immunomagnetic separation technique involving marrow sedimentation, filtration, and depletion with magnetic microspheres coated with a cocktail of antineuroblastoma monoclonal antibodies (e.g., 390, 459, HSAN 1.2, BA-1) has been most commonly used in clinical trials. This method offers the advantages of simplicity, reproducibility, and lack of toxicity and permits a 3–4 log malignant cell depletion (Kemshead et al., 1986; Combaret et al., 1989a; Rogers et al., 1998; Reynolds et al., 1994b).

Because there is a significant loss of mononuclear cells with immunomagnetic purging (average mononuclear cell recovery 35%), there has been concern about slow or failed engraftment observed in some studies utilizing marrow purged with monoclonal antibodies or pharmacologic agents such as mafosfamide (Beaujean et al., 1987; Favrot et al., 1988). In studies utilizing unpurged marrow, the median time to achieve an absolute neutrophil count of $0.5 \times 10^9/1$ and a platelet count of over $50 \times 10^9/1$ has been approximately 2 and 4 weeks, respectively (Hartmann et al., 1986; Dini et al., 1991; Pinkerton,

Table 47.7.   *Purging techniques*

Method	Approximate log depletion of neuroblastoma cells
Density sedimentation	0.5–1
Velocity sedimentation	0.5–1
Mafosfamide	3
Monoclonal antibodies/complement	2–4
Magnetic immunobeads	2–4

1991). The corresponding recovery times in studies utilizing either immunomagnetic or pharmacologic purged marrow have been approximately 4 and 7 weeks (Hartmann et al., 1987; Philip et al., 1987; Pinkerton et al., 1987; Kushner et al., 1990; Seeger et al., 1991).

The largest study examining the rate of hematopoietic recovery involved 123 patients who received immunomagnetically purged marrow following a preparative regimen of melphalan and TBI. The rate of hematopoietic recovery depended mainly on pre-existing factors including the amount of prior chemotherapy, the interval from the most recent chemotherapy, the time of harvest, and only marginally on the manipulation of the marrow after harvest (Graham Pole et al., 1991b).

The results in most studies using unpurged marrow, however, have not been substantially different from studies using purged marrow. In a French study, 23 patients with stage IV neuroblastoma involving the marrow received "in vivo bone marrow purging" during induction chemotherapy prior to intensive therapy and unpurged marrow support. Posttransplant serial bone marrows were examined using immunofluorescence with the anti-GD2 monoclonal antibody 3A7. Four-year disease-free survival for 5 patients with "perfect in vivo purging" was 100%; for 8 patients with "eventually perfect in vivo purging" (with continued chemotherapy) it was 67%; and for 5 patients with "unsuccessful in vivo purging" it was 0. The authors concluded that autografting with immunofluorescent-antibody-negative unpurged marrow gave a disease-free survival rate comparable to that of studies using ex vivo purging (Philip et al., 1991a, 1991b). A further study of Saarinen and colleagues (1996) described a correlation between the success of in vivo purging and outcome posttransplant (Fig. 47.8). In the absence of randomized trials, the clinical benefit of ex vivo purging remains to be demonstrated.

Autologous versus allogeneic HSC transplantation

There have been few reports of the use of allogeneic HSCT in the treatment of neuroblastoma. One retrospective review comparing 350 patients treated by autotransplantation with 124 patients receiving allogeneic transplants found no difference in recurrence or survival, but an increased toxicity in the allogeneic transplant group (Graham-Pole et al., 1989, 1991a). The heterogeneity of the patients' clinical conditions, cytotoxic therapy, and transplant protocols used in these studies from several centers over many years limits any definitive conclusions being made from this analysis. Increased early mortality has been observed in other studies of allogeneic marrow transplantation (Seeger et al., 1988). In the CCG-321 series of studies, 56 patients who did not progress following induction chemotherapy were then treated by marrow transplantation. The myeloablative preparatory regimen included etoposide, melphalan, cisplatinum, and TBI. Twenty patients underwent HLA-identical allogeneic BMT and 36 patients received purged autologous marrow transplantation. Both groups had similar CR and PR rates of 52% and 55%, respectively, at the

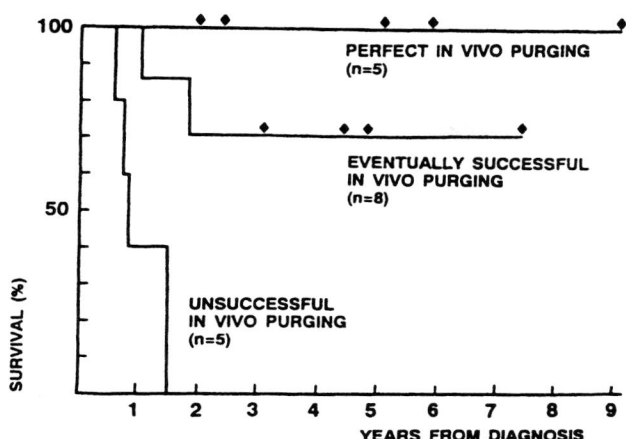

Fig. 47.8. Kaplan-Meier plot of survival of children with poor-risk neuroblastoma and initial bone marrow involvement, divided into three groups by the success in in vivo purging. Two children with toxic deaths after ABMT, both with eventually successful purging, were censored at the time of death. Of the children with unsuccessful in vivo purging and resistant disease, only one underwent autografting (double transplant with PBSCs). All current survivors, marked on the curves, are disease-free. Statistical significance of differences: all three groups, $P < .001$; perfect versus eventually successful, $P < .1$ (log rank test). Confidence intervals: see Results section. Reproduced, with permission, from Saarinen *et al.* (1996).

time of myeloablative therapy. Four of 20 patients treated by allogeneic BMT and 3 of 36 patients treated by autologous BMT suffered therapy-related deaths ($P = .21$). The relapse rate was 69% in the allogeneic and 46% in the autologous group. The estimated disease-free survival at 4 years was lower for the allogeneic group compared to the autologous group (25% versus 49%, $P = .051$) (Matthay *et al.*, 1994, 1995). The European Group for Bone Marrow Transplantation performed a case control study of allogeneic versus autologous bone marrow transplantation for advanced or poorly responding patients with neuroblastoma in first remission. Seventeen allogeneic and 34 autologous BMT patients were matched for a number of prognostic factors including age, sex, prior treatment duration, pretransplant response status, and bone marrow involvement pretransplant. Progression-free survival at 2 years posttransplant was 35% and 41%, respectively (not significantly different) (Philip *et al.*, 1997).

In another study, 6 of 12 patients receiving allogeneic transplants following a VAMP-TBI preparative regimen died within 1 month of transplant from renal failure, hepatic veno-occlusive disease, or disseminated bacterial or fungal infection (Seeger *et al.*, 1988). This high early mortality was thought due to added toxicity from methotrexate given for the prevention of graft-versus-host disease in patients with impaired renal function secondary to previous chemotherapy with platinum compounds and/or nephrotoxic antibiotics. Such severe toxicity has not been observed in other studies comparing autotransplantation and allogeneic transplantation following a preparative regimen of cyclophosphamide and TBI. With only a small number

of patients entered on another study, the projected 2-year disease-free survival was 67% for 8 patients receiving allogeneic and 41% for 17 patients receiving autologous transplantation (Dinndorf *et al.*, 1991).

As neuroblastoma is a disease of young children, the number of siblings, and therefore the chance of an HLA-matched sibling donor is often low. Additionally, the absence of benefit for allogeneic compared to autologous transplantation may be related to the absence of HLA class I expression on neuroblastoma cells. A graft-versus-tumor effect may not exist in this disease.

Posttransplant treatment

Several different therapies given after high-dose cytotoxic therapy and stem cell support are currently being investigated. When neuroblastoma cell lines are exposed to *trans*-retinoic acid or *cis*-retinoic acid in vitro, they exhibit decreased proliferation, decreased expression of the N-*myc* oncogene, and morphologic differentiation (Sidell *et al.*, 1983; Thiele *et al.*, 1985; Reynolds *et al.*, 1991, 1994a). Furthermore, growth arrest and differentiation in response to *cis*-retinoic acid has been observed in neuroblastoma cell lines from tumors at the time of progression after chemotherapy and radiation (Thiele *et al.*, 1985; Reynolds *et al.*, 1991). A phase I trial following autologous BMT has been completed by the Children's Cancer Group showing a maximal tolerated dosage of 160 mg/m^2/day (Villablanca *et al.*, 1995). In a study of Matthay *et al.* (1999), such treatment was associated with a significantly better 3-year EFS (46% versus 29%; $P = .027$) among the 130 patients who were randomized to receive 13-*cis*-retinoic acid compared to patients assigned to receive no further therapy (Fig. 47.9). In contrast, no advantage in EFS was shown in children receiving retinoic acid at a dosage of 0.75 mg/kg/day following high-dose chemotherapy in a double-blind randomized, placebo-controlled study (Kohler *et al.*, 2000). However, the dose of 13-*cis*-retinoic acid in this study was low and administered chronically, whereas Matthay and colleagues used the high-dose pulsed schedule as published by Villablanca *et al.* (1995).

IL-2 has also been shown to induce the regression of established cancers in animal models and in some patients with metastatic renal cell carcinoma and melanoma. During the first 4 months after autologous BMT, immunologic studies have demonstrated a T-cell deficiency with an excess of natural killer (NK) cells. IL-2 stimulates T-cell reconstitution and LAK activity in NK cells. Furthermore, neuroblastoma cell lines have been demonstrated to be sensitive to NK cell lysis (Main *et al.*, 1991). Valteau-Couanet *et al.* (1995) performed a phase I–II study of IL-2 following autologous BMT in 12 patients with relapsed neuroblastoma, and four are alive in CR 36 to 54 months posttransplant. Of the seven patients evaluable for response to IL-2, two achieved CR, two PR, and three exhibited persistent disease. Another phase I/II trial utilized low-dose recombinant human IL-2 following high-dose chemotherapy and autologous transplantation in 17 consecutive patients with

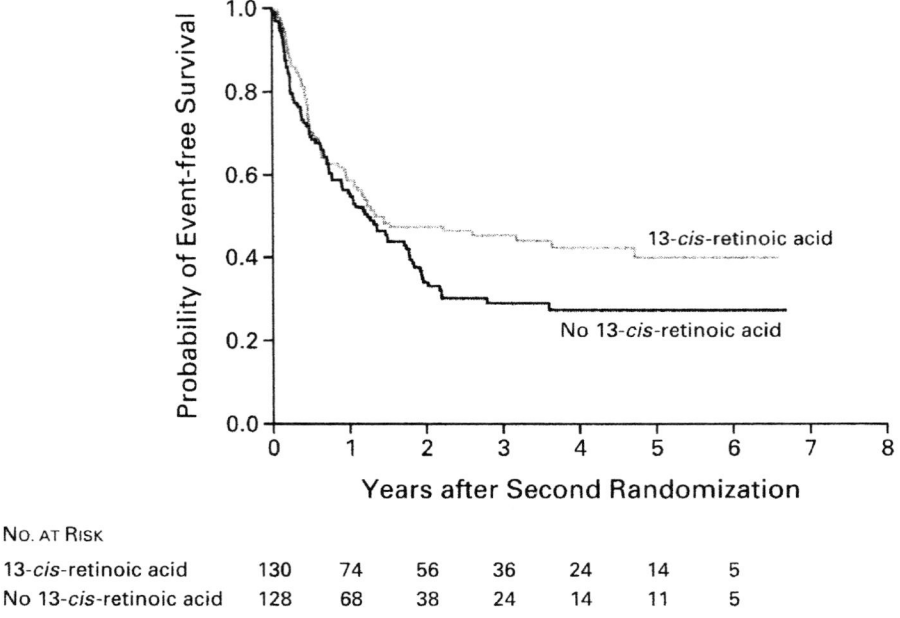

Fig. 47.9. Probability of event-free survival among patients following megatherapy assigned in a randomized fashion to receive 13-*cis*-retinoic acid (*n* = 130) compared to patients assigned to receive no further therapy. Reproduced, with permission, from Matthay *et al.* (1999).

stage IV or relapsed neuroblastoma. Twelve patients are alive and well with a 2-year EFS of 67% (Pession *et al.*, 1998).

Numerous monoclonal antibodies (Mab) have been generated against tumor-associated antigens. This technology holds promise for tumor-targeted cancer therapy. Cheung *et al.* (1987) reported in vivo clinical efficacy of a murine anti-disialoganglioside (anti-GD-2) Mab 3F8 in some patients with neuroblastoma and melanoma. The antigen disialoganglioside GD-2 is suited for targeting therapy because of its high density on human neuroblastoma cells ($5-10 \times 10^6$ molecules/cell) and its persistence on the cell surface upon binding to antibodies. The antibody 3F8 is a murine IgG$_3$ suitable for immunotherapy because it mediates efficient tumor cell kill by human complement and by human lymphocytes, neutrophils, and activated monocytes and macrophages in vitro. A phase II trial of 3F8 monoclonal antibody involving 16 patients with relapsed or chemotherapy-resistant stage IV neuroblastoma documented one PR and one minor response. Response rates further defined by responses at specific sites of diseases revealed two of seven patients with bone lesions and three of eight with marrow involvement demonstrating tumor shrinkage at those sites (Cheung *et al.*, 1994; Uttenreuther-Fischer *et al.*, 1995). In a phase I study, 22 patients were treated with a chimeric human/murine anti-GD2 antibody (ch14.18). Of 19 evaluable patients 14 were in first, and 5 in second, remission. The maximal tolerated dose was 40 mg/m2/day for 4 days with significant, but manageable toxicity (pain, fever, urticaria, hypotension, neurotoxicity). Despite previous high-dose chemotherapy, five patients developed an antichimeric antibody response. However, this phenomenon was not noted until after the second

course of ch14.18. The authors suggested that in subsequent trials two or three courses could be given with little risk from the development of a human antichimeric antibody response (Ozkaynak *et al.*, 2000). In a phase II study including 27 patients assessable for anti-GD2 antibody (ch14.18) response, Yu *et al.* (1997) observed 1 CR, 3 PR, 2 stable diseases, and 1 mixed response. Complete and partial response of marrow disease was observed in 4 of 18 and 1 of 18 patients, respectively. Out of 21 patients with bone involvement, there were 1 CR and 2 PR. Two of 16 patients with large tumor masses showed size reduction of 63% and 70%.

Causes of failure

Relapse or refractory disease remains the major cause of failure following intensive cytotoxic therapy and hematopoietic stem cell support. Relapse occurs in approximately 45% to 65% of patients, 1 to 7 years following high-dose therapy. However, 5-year survivors after high-dose therapy do have an 80% chance of becoming long-term survivors (Graham Pole *et al.*, 1991a; Philip *et al.*, 1997). Patients who have received nonpurged marrow have been reported to have developed metastatic disease in a pattern suggestive of tumor embolization, for example, lung or brain metastases (Graeve *et al.*, 1988; Gaze *et al.*, 1995; Bouffet *et al.*, 1997). Generally the pattern of recurrence in both purged or unpurged marrow transplant recipients has been similar, occurring at the site of the primary tumor, residual gross disease, or bone and bone marrow, suggesting that inability to eradicate tumor with cytotoxic therapy is a major cause of relapse (Matthay *et al.*, 1991; Seeger *et al.*, 1991). In a

Children's Cancer Group study of 99 patients, 49% of 84 evaluable patients relapsed. Twenty-two of these patients relapsed in their primary site, 8 in the primary site alone and 14 in both the primary site and with distant metastases. Nineteen patients relapsed outside the primary site. Incomplete resection of the primary tumor during initial therapy appeared to be a significant risk factor for relapse in the primary site (Matthay et al., 1993).

In a study from the University of Chicago, 26 patients were treated with autologous or allogeneic marrow transplantation for newly diagnosed or recurrent high-risk neuroblastoma. Fifty percent (13 of 26) of the patients received an involved field boost of 8 to 24 Gy to primary and/or metastatic sites prior to BMT. Three of the 10 evaluable "boost" patients relapsed, 1 in new sites and 2 in both new and previous sites of disease, whereas 7 of 10 "no boost" patients relapsed, 4 in primary sites, 1 in a new site, and 2 in both new and old sites, with a trend toward improved 5-year progression-free survival in patients receiving a boost (68% vs 33%, $P = .23$) (Sibley et al., 1995).

As indicated above, the contamination of the stem cell inoculum by tumor cells is also a potential cause of relapse, as demonstrated by gene marking studies in which neuroblastoma cells contaminating hematopoietic grafts were demonstrated to contribute to recurrent disease (Brenner et al., 1993).

More intensive cytotoxic preparative regimens prior to autologous marrow infusion have been associated with fatal toxicity observed in between 3% and 24% of patients, depending on the preparative regimen, rate of engraftment, and clinical condition of the patient at the time of transplant (August et al., 1984; Philip et al., 1987; Dini et al., 1991a, 1991b; Philip et al., 1991a, 1991b; Seeger et al., 1991). Most toxic deaths are due to infection, frequently due to disseminated aspergillus or Candida albicans infections, bacterial infection, idiopathic or cytomegalovirus interstitial pneumonitis, or encephalitis. The risk of fatal infections increases with duration of aplasia. Therefore BMT has a higher risk compared to PBSC transplantation. Multiorgan failure (presumably due to drug toxicity), hemolytic-uremic syndrome, gastrointestinal hemorrhage, and hepatic veno-occlusive disease have also been described; this last complication occurred in 6 of 62 patients in one study (Philip et al., 1991b).

Preparative regimens prior to stem cell infusion need to be developed with an awareness of the increased risk for delayed complications in this patient population. Young children are particularly susceptible to late effects of intensive therapy, especially growth retardation and endocrine defects associated with TBI (Sanders, 1990).

Monitoring for residual disease posttransplant

The inability to eradicate tumor with cytotoxic therapy is a major cause of relapse (Matthay et al., 1991; Seeger et al., 1991; Seeger et al., 2000). When disease is microscopic, standard methods with conventional sampling of bone marrow have limited sensitivity compared to immunocytology (Moss et al., 1991). Molecular detection of tumor markers has been described for neuroblastoma. As catecholamines are produced by approximately 98% of neuroblastomas, the first enzyme in the catecholamine synthesis pathway, tyrosine hydroxylase, was proposed as an mRNA target for neuroblastoma cell detection by reverse transcriptase polymerase chain reaction (RT-PCR). Tyrosine hydroxylase mRNA in peripheral blood from clinically disease-free children off treatment ($n = 112$) was shown to identify those patients who were destined to relapse ($P = .0014$; Burchill et al., 2001). The expression of genes named GAGE and MAGE in combination with immunocytology and tyrosine hydroxylase mRNA were shown to be useful for the detection of minimal residual disease (Cheung et al., 2001a). GAGE positivity in bone marrow 24 months following diagnosis was also shown to be associated with poorer outcome ($P < .001$; Cheung et al., 2000a). The same authors developed a model for quantitative tumor cell detection. Real time quantitative PCR of GD2 synthetase levels correlated well with the number of GD2 positive cells, and the transcript level correlated closely with the clinical status in patients. Positivity for GD2 synthetase mRNA 24 months after diagnosis was strongly associated with an adverse clinical outcome in 44 patients ($P < .005$; Cheung & Cheung, 2001b).

For N-myc amplified patients, the study of Combaret et al. (2002) showed that 25–600-fold higher levels of N-myc DNA sequences are present in peripheral blood of patients with N-myc amplified neuroblastomas when compared to neuroblastoma patients without N-myc amplification or controls. In 8 N-myc amplified patients available for follow-up, this study showed that tumor response was consistently associated with a significant decrease in serum N-myc levels. Therefore, the authors suggested that circulating N-myc may be used as a prognostic marker in localized or metastatic neuroblastomas with N-myc amplification. In one patient the authors observed a significant increase of N-myc serum levels 2 months before clinical diagnosis of relapse, suggesting that N-myc DNA in the serum may be an early marker of relapse.

Monitoring of all such parameters should be investigated to define treatment strategies such as indications for high-dose therapy.

Conclusions

The observation that more aggressive multimodality therapy can produce a higher percentage of remissions and longer duration of response in children with advanced neuroblastoma has led to studies of further intensification of cytotoxic therapy enabled by support with autologous hematopoietic stem cells. The results of studies using intensive cytotoxic therapy and hematopoietic stem cell support have demonstrated an improvement in short-term disease-free survival over historical experience, particularly in those children who have obtained significant tumor response from conventional induction therapy prior to harvesting and high-dose therapy with PBSCT or BMT. These observations have been confirmed in a randomized study. Subsequently, the same study also demonstrated the benefit of maintenance therapy for residual disease with retinoic acid (Matthay *et al.*, 1999).

Current issues relate to increasing the response rates to induction therapy, improving the efficacy of purging and determining the most effective and practical purging method, and further exploring additional therapeutic strategies after autologous stem cell infusion such as humoral immunotherapy (Ozkaynak *et al.*, 2000). Later it will be important to determine whether these therapeutic approaches improve the cure rate in children with advanced disease.

References

Ariel, I.M. & Pack, G.T. (1960). *Cancer and Allied Diseases of Infancy and Childhood*, p. 377. Boston: Little, Brown & Company.

August, C.S., Serota, F.T., Koch, P.A. *et al.* (1984). Treatment of advanced neuroblastoma with supralethal chemotherapy, radiation, and allogeneic or autologous marrow reconstitution. *Journal of Clinical Oncology*, **2**, 609–16.

Beaujean, F., Hartrnann, O., Pico, J.L. *et al.* (1987). Incubation of autologous bone marrow graft with Asta-Z (7557): comparative studies of hematologic reconstitution after purged or not purged bone marrow transplantation. *Pediatric Hematology and Oncology*, **4**, 105–15.

Bernard, J.L., Philip, T., Zucker, J.M. *et al.* (1987). Sequential cisplatin/ VM26 and vincristine/ cyclophosphamide/ doxorubicin in metastatic neuroblastoma: an effective alternating non cross resistant regimen. *Journal of Clinical Oncology*, **5**, 1952–9.

Bernstein, M.L., Leclerc, J.M., Bunin, G. *et al.* (1992). A population-based study of neuroblastoma incidence, survival, and mortality in North America. *Journal of Clinical Oncology*, **10**, 323–9.

Bouffet, E., Doumi, N., Thiesse, P. *et al.* (1997). Brain metastases in children with solid tumors. *Cancer*, **79**, 403–10.

Brenner, M.K., Rill, D.R., Moen, R.C. *et al.* (1993). Gene-marking to trace origin of relapse after autologous bone marrow transplantation. *Lancet*, **341**, 85–6.

Brenner, M.K., Rill, D.R., Moen, R.C. *et al.* (1994). Gene-marking and autologous bone marrow transplantation. *Annals of the New York Academy of Science*, **716**, 204–14.

Brodeur, G.M. (1994). Molecular pathology of human neuroblastoma. *Seminars in Diagnostic Pathology*, **11**, 118–25.

Burchill, S.A., Lewis, I.J., Abrams, K.R. *et al.* (2001). Circulating neuroblastoma cells detected by reverse transcriptase polymerase chain reaction for tyrosine hydroxylase mRNA are an independent poor prognostic indicator in stage IV neuroblastoma in children over 1 year. *Journal of Clinical Oncology*, **19**, 1795–801.

Castel, V., Canete, A., Navarro, S. *et al.* (2001). Outcome of high-risk neuroblastoma using a dose intensity approach: improvement in initial but not in long-term results. *Medical and Pediatric Oncology*, **37**, 537–2.

Castel, V., Garcia-Miguel, P., Melero, C. *et al.* (1995). The treatment of advanced neuroblastorna. Results of the Spanish Neuroblastoma Study Group (SNSG) studies. *European Journal of Cancer*, **31A**, 642–5.

Castleberry, R.P. (1997). Paediatric update. Neuroblastoma. *European Journal of Cancer*, **33**, 1430–8.

Castleberry, R.P., Cantor, A.B., & Green, A.A. (1994). Phase II investigational window using carboplatin, iproplatin, ifosfamide and epirubicin in children with disseminated neuroblastoma: a pediatric oncology group study. *Journal of Clinical Oncology*, **12**, 1616–20.

Cheung, I.Y. & Cheung, N.V. (2001a). Detection of microscopic disease: comparing histology, immunocytology, and RT-PCR of tyrosine hydroxylase, GAGE, and MAGE. *Medical and Pediatric Oncology*, **36**, 210–2.

Cheung, I.Y. & Cheung, N.V. (2001b). Quantitation of marrow disease in neuroblastoma by real-time reverse transcription-PCR. *Clinical Cancer Research*, **7**, 1698–705.

Cheung, I.Y., Chi, S.N., & Cheung, N.V. (2000a). Prognostic significance of GAGE detection in bone marrows on survival of patients with metastatic neuroblastoma. *Medical and Pediatric Oncology*, **35**, 632–4.

Cheung, N.V. & Heller, G. (1991). Chemotherapy dose intensity correlates strongly with response, median survival, and median progression-free survival in metastatic neuroblastoma. *Journal of Clinical Oncology*, **9**, 1050–8.

Cheung, N.V., Guo, H., & Cheung, I.Y. (2000b). Correlation of anti-idiotype network with survival following anti-GD2 monoclonal antibody 3F8 therapy of stage IV neuroblastoma. *Medical and Pediatric Oncology*, **35**, 635–7.

Cheung, N.V., Kushner, B.H., LaQuaglia, M. *et al.* (2001c). N7: a novel multi-modality therapy of high-risk neuroblastoma (NB) in children diagnosed over 1 year of age. *Medical and Pediatric Oncology*, **36**, 227–30.

Cheung, N.V., Kushner, B.H., Yeh, S.J. *et al.* (1994). 3F8 monoclonal antibody treatment of patients with stage IV neuroblastoma: a phase II study. *Advances in Neuroblastoma Research*, **4**, pp. 319–29. New York: Alan R. Liss, Inc.

Cheung, N.V., Lazarus, H., Miraldi, F.D. *et al.* (1987). Ganglioside GD2 specific monoclonal antibody 3F8: a phase I study in patients with neuroblastoma and malignant melanoma. *Journal of Clinical Oncology*, **5**, 1430–40.

Cohn, S.L., Look, A.T., Joshi,V.V. *et al.* (1995). Lack of correlation of N-myc gene amplification with prognosis in localized neuroblastoma: a pediatric Oncology Group study. *Cancer Research*, **55**, 721–6.

Combaret, V., Audoynaud, C., Iacono, I. *et al.* (2002). Circulating N-MYC DNA as tumor specific marker and indicator of tumor progression in neuroblastoma patients. *Cancer Research*, **62**, 346–8.

Combaret, V., Favrot, M.C., Chauvin, F. *et al.* (1989a). Immunomagnetic depletion of malignant cells from autologous bone marrow graft: from experimental models to clinical trials. *Journal of Immunogenetics*, **16**, 125–36.

Combaret, V., Favrot, M.C., & Kremens, B. (1989b). Immunological detection of neuroblastoma cells in bone marrow harvested for autologous transplantation. *British Journal of Cancer*, **59**, 844–7.

Combaret, V., Gross, N., Lasset, C. *et al.* (1996). Clinical relevance of CD44 cell-surface expression and N-myc gene amplification in a multicentric analysis of 121 pediatric neuroblastomas. *Journal of Clinical Oncology*, **14**, 25–34.

Cotterill, S.J., Pearson, A.D.J., Pritchard, J. *et al.* (2000). Clinical prognostic factors in 1277 patients with neuroblastoma: results of The European Neuroblastoma Study Group Survey 1982–92. *European Journal of Cancer*, **36**, 901–8.

Coze, C., Hartmann, O., Frappaz, D. *et al.* (1997). NB87 induction protocol for stage 4 neuroblastoma in children over 1 year of age: a report from the French Society of Pediatric Oncology. *Journal of Clinical Oncology,* **15,** 3433–40.

DeBernardi, B., Carli, M., Casale, F. *et al.* (1992a). Standard dose and high-dose peptichimio and cisplatin in children with disseminated poor risk neuroblastoma: two studies by the Italian Cooperative Group for Neuroblastoma. *Journal of Clinical Oncology,* **10,** 1870–8.

DeBernardi , B., Pianca, C., Boni, L. *et al.* (1992b). Disseminated neuroblastoma (stage IV and IV-S) in the first year of life. Outcome related to age and stage. Italian Cooperative Group on neuroblastoma. *Cancer,* **70,** 1625–33.

Di Caro, A., Bostrum, B., Moss, T.J. *et al.* (1994). Autologous peripheral blood cell transplantation in the treatment of advanced neuroblastoma. *American Journal of Pediatric Hematology/ Oncology,* **16,** 200–6.

Dini, G., Lanino, E., Garaventa, A. *et al.* (1991). Unpurged autologous bone marrow transplantation for neuroblastoma: the AIEOP-BMT group experience. *Bone Marrow Transplantation,* **7** (Suppl 3), 109–11.

Dinndorf, P., Johnson, L., Gaynon, P. *et al.* (1991). Outcome of autologous (auto)-versus-allogeneic (allo) bone marrow transplantation (BMT) in 25 children with neuroblastoma (NB) and unfavorable prognostic features (UPF). *Journal of Cellular Biochemistry,* **16A** (Suppl), 201 (Abstract).

Donfrancesco, A., DeBernardi, B., Carli, M. *et al.* (1995). Deferoxamine followed by cyclophosphamide, etoposide, carboplatin, thiotepa induction regimen in advanced neuroblastoma/ preliminary results. *European Journal of Cancer,* **31A,** 612–5.

Evans, A.E., D'Angio, G.J., & Koop, C.E. (1984). The role of multimodal therapy in patients with local and regional neuroblastoma. *Journal of Pediatric Surgery,* **19,** 77–80.

Evans, A.E., D'Angio, G.J., & Propert, K. (1987). Prognostic factors in neuroblastoma. *Cancer,* **59,** 1853–9.

Evans, A.E., D'Angio, G.J., & Randolph, J. (1971). A proposed staging for children with neuroblastoma. *Cancer,* **27,** 374–8.

Faulkner, L.B., Garaventa, A., Paoli, A. *et al.* (2000). In vivo cytoreduction studies and cell sorting-enhanced tumor-cell detection in high-risk neuroblastoma patients: implications for leukapheresis strategies. *Journal of Clinical Oncology,* **18,** 3829–36.

Favrot, M.C., Philip, T., Combaret, V. *et al.* (1988). Very long delay to engraftment after ABMT in neuroblastoma patients and effect of CD8 monoclonal antibody in vivo therapy. In *Advances in Neuroblastoma Research,* Vol. **2,** ed. A.E. Evans, G. D'Angio, A. Knudson, & R.C. Seeger, p. 225. New York: Alan R. Liss, Inc.

Frappaz, D., Michon, J., & Hartmann, O. (1992). Etoposide and carboplatin in neuroblastoma: a French Society of Pediatric Oncology phase II study. *Journal of Clinical Oncology,* **10,** 1592–601.

Frappaz, D., Michon, J., Coze, C. *et al.* (2000). LMCE3 treatment strategy: results in 99 consecutively diagnosed stage IV neuroblastomas in children older than 1 year at diagnosis. *Journal of Clinical Oncology,* **18,** 468–76.

Garaventa, A., Rondelli, R., Lanino, E. *et al.* (1996). Myeloablative therapy and bone marrow rescue in advanced neuroblastoma. Report from the Italian Bone Marrow Registry. *Bone Marrow Transplantation,* **18,** 125–30.

Gaze, M.N., Wheldon, T.E., O'Donoghue, J.A. *et al.* (1995). Multi-modality megatherapy with (131 J) meta-iodobenzylguanidine, high-dose melphalan and total body irradiation with bone marrow rescue: feasibility study of a new strategy for advanced neuroblastoma. *European Journal of Cancer,* **31 A,** 252–6.

Graeve, J.L., De Alarcon, P.A., Sato, Y. *et al.* (1988). Miliary pulmonary neuroblastoma. A risk of autologous bone marrow transplantation. *Cancer,* **56,** 2125–7.

Graham Pole, J., August, C., Ramsay, N. *et al.* (1989). Is there an advantage to allogeneic over autologous marrow transplantation in patients with metastatic neuroblastoma? *Experimental Hematology,* **17,** 586 (Abstract).

Graham Pole, J., Casper, J., Elfenbein, G. *et al.* (1991a). High-dose chemo-radiotherapy supported by marrow infusions for advanced neuroblastoma: a Pediatric Oncology Group study. *Journal of Clinical Oncology,* **9,** 152–8.

Graham Pole, J., Gee, A., Emerson, S. *et al.* (1991b). Myeloablative chemoradiotherapy and autologous bone marrow infusions for treatment of neuroblastoma: factors influencing engraftment. *Blood,* **78,** 1607–14.

Green, A., Hayes, F.A., & Rao, B. (1986). Disease control and toxicity of aggressive 4 drug therapy for children with disseminated neuroblastoma (DNb). *Proceedings of the American Society of Clinical Oncology,* **5,** 210 (Abstract).

Grupp, S.A., Stern, J.W., Bunin, N. *et al.* (2000). Tandem high-dose therapy in rapid sequence for children with high-risk neuroblastoma. *Journal of Clinical Oncology,* **18,** 2567–75.

Haase, G.M., O'Leary, M.C., Ramsay, N.K.C. *et al.* (1991). Aggressive surgery combined with intensive chemotherapy improves survival in poor-risk neuroblastoma. *Journal of Pediatric Surgery,* **26,** 1119–23.

Handgretinger, R., Lang, P., Ihm, K. *et al.* (2002). Isolation and transplantation of highly purified autologous peripheral CD34+ progenitor cells: purging efficacy, hematopoietic reconstitution and long-term outcome in children with high-risk neuroblastoma. *Bone Marrow Transplantation,* **29,** 731–6.

Hartmann, O., Benhamou, E., Beaujean, F. *et al.* (1987). Repeated high-dose chemotherapy followed by purged autologous bone marrow transplantation as consolidation therapy in metastatic neuroblastoma. *Journal of Clinical Oncology,* **5,** 1205–11.

Hartmann, O., Kalifa, C., Benhamon, E. *et al.* (1986). Treatment of advanced neuroblastoma with high-dose melphalan and autologous bone marrow transplantation. *Cancer Chemotherapy and Pharmacology,* **16,** 165–9.

Hayes, F.A., Green, A.A., Casper, J. *et al.* (1981). Clinical evaluation of sequentially scheduled cisplatin and VM26 in neuroblastoma: response and toxicity. *Cancer,* **48,** 1715–8.

Hayes, F.A. & Smith, E.I. (1989). Neuroblastoma. In *Principles and Practice of Pediatric Oncology,* ed. P.A. Pizzo & D.G. Poplack, p. 607. Philadelphia: J.B. Lippincott.

Henn, P.R. (1990). Consideration underlying the use of autologous blood stem cell transplantation and malignancies. *Haematologica,* **75,** 497.

Ikeda, H., August, C.S., Goldwein, J.W. *et al.* (1992). Sites of relapse in patients with neuroblastoma following bone marrow transplantation in relation to preparatory "debulking" treatments. *Journal of Pediatric Surgery,* **27,** 1438–41.

Kamani, N.R. (1996). Autotransplants for neuroblastoma. *Bone Marrow Transplantation, 17,* 301–4.

Kamani, N.R., August, C.S., Bunin, N. *et al.* (1996). A study of thiotepa, etoposide and fractionated total body irradiation as a preparative regimen prior to bone marrow transplantation for poor prognosis patients with neuroblastoma. *Bone Marrow Transplantation, 17,* 911–6.

Kemshead, J.T., Heath, L., Gibson, F.M. *et al.* (1986). Magnetic microspheres and monoclonal antibodies for the depletion of neuroblastoma cells from bone marrow: experiences, improvements and observations. *British Journal of Cancer, 54,* 771–8.

Kletzel, M., Katzenstein, H.M., Haut, P.R. *et al.* (2002). Treatment of high-risk neuroblastoma with triple tandem high-dose therapy and stem-cell rescue: results of the Chicago Pilot II Study. *Journal of Clinical Oncology, 9,* 2284–92.

Kohler, J.A., Imeson, J., & Ellershaw, C. (2000). A randomized trial of 13-Cis retinoic acid in children with advanced neuroblastoma after high-dose therapy. *British Journal of Cancer, 83,* 1124–7.

Kushner, B.H. & Helson, L. (1987). Co-ordinated use of sequentially escalated cyclophosphamide and cell cycle specific chemotherapy (N4SE protocol) for advanced neuroblastoma: experience with 100 patients. *Journal of Clinical Oncology, 5,* 1746–51.

Kushner, B.H., Cheung, N.V., LaQuaglia, M.P. *et al.* (1996). Survival from locally invasive or widespread neuroblastoma without cytotoxic therapy. *Journal of Clinical Oncology, 14,* 373–81.

Kushner, B.H., Gulati, S.C., O'Reilly, R.J. *et al.* (1990). Autografting with bone marrow exposed to multiple courses of very high-dose cyclophosphamide in vivo and to 4-hydroxypercyclophosphamide in vitro. *Medical and Pediatric Oncology, 18,* 454–8.

Kushner, B.H., O'Reilly, R.J., LaQauglia, M. *et al.* (1990). Dose-intensive use of cyclophosphamide in ablation of neuroblastoma. *Cancer, 66,* 1095–100.

Kushner, B.H., LaQuaglia, M.P., Bonilla, M.A. *et al.* (1994). Highly effective induction therapy for stage 4 neuroblastoma in children over 1 year of age. *Journal of Clinical Oncology, 12,* 2607–13.

Ladenstein, R., Lasset, C., Hartmann, O. *et al.* (1993). Impact of megatherapy on survival after relapse from stage IV neuroblastoma in patients over one year of age at diagnosis: report from the European Group for Bone Marrow Transplantation. *Journal of Clinical Oncology, 11,* 2330–41.

Ladenstein, R., Lasset, C., Hartmann, O. *et al.* (1994). Comparison of auto versus allografting as consolidation of primary treatments in advanced neuroblastoma over one year of age at diagnosis: report from the European Group for Bone Marrow Transplantation. *Bone Marrow Transplantation, 14,* 37–46.

Ladenstein, R., Philip, T., Lasset, C. *et al.* (1998). Multivariate analysis of risk factors in stage 4 neuroblastoma patients over the age of one year treated with megatherapy and stem-cell transplantation: a report from the European Bone Marrow Transplant Solid Tumor Registry. *Journal of Clinical Oncology, 16,* 953–65.

Lanino, E., Boni, L., Corciulo, P. *et al.* (1991). Did BMT change the clinical course of neuroblastoma? *Bone Marrow Transplantation, 7* (Suppl 3), 114–7.

Lau, L. (2002). Neuroblastoma: a single institution's experience with 128 children and an evaluation of clinical and biological prognostic factors. *Pediatric Hematology and Oncology, 19,* 79–89.

Look, A.T., Hayes, F.A., Shuster, J.J. *et al.* (1991). Clinical relevance of tumor cell ploidy and N-myc gene amplification in childhood neuroblastoma: a Pediatric Oncology Group study. *Journal of Clinical Oncology, 9,* 581–91.

Main, E.K., Lampson, L.A., Hart, M.K. *et al.* (1991). Human neuroblastoma cell lines are susceptible to lysis by natural killer cells but not by cytotoxic T lymphocytes. *Journal of Immunology, 135,* 242–6.

Matthay, K.K., Atkinson, J., Reynolds, C.P. *et al.* (1991). Pattern of relapse after autologous bone marrow transplant for neuroblastoma. *Proceedings of the American Society of Clinical Oncology, 10,* 312 (Abstract).

Matthay, K.K., Atkinson, J.B., Stram, D.O. *et al.* (1993). Pattern of relapse after autologous purged bone marrow transplantation for neuroblastoma. A Children's Cancer Group Pilot Study. *Journal of Clinical Oncology, 11,* 2226–33.

Matthay, K.K., O'Leary, M.C., Ramsay, N.K. *et al.* (1995). Role of myeloablative therapy in improved outcome for high-risk neuroblastoma: review of recent Children's Cancer Group Results. *European Journal of Cancer, 31A,* 572–5.

Matthay, K.K., Perez, C., Seeger, R.C. *et al.* (1998). Successful treatment of stage III neuroblastoma based on prospective biologic staging: a Children's Cancer Group study. *Journal of Clinical Oncology, 16,* 1256–64.

Matthay, K.K., Sather, H.N., Seeger, R.C. *et al.* (1989). Excellent outcome for stage II neuroblastoma is independent of residual disease and radiation therapy. *Journal of Clinical Oncology, 7,* 236–44.

Matthay, K.K., Seeger, R.C., Reynolds, C.P. *et al.* (1994). Allogeneic versus autologous purged bone marrow transplantation for neuroblastoma: a report from the Children's Cancer Group. *Journal of Clinical Oncology, 12,* 2382–9.

Matthay, K.K., Villablanca, J.G., Seeger, R.C. *et al.* (1999). Treatment of high-risk neuroblastoma with intensive chemotherapy, radiotherapy, autologous bone marrow transplantation, and 13-cis-retinoic acid. *New England Journal of Medicine, 341,* 1165–73.

McWilliams, N.B., Hayes, F.A., Green, A.A. *et al.* (1995). Cyclophosphamide/doxorubicin vs cisplatin/teniposide in the treatment of children older than 12 months of age with disseminated neuroblastoina: a Pediatric Oncology Group randomised phase 2 study. *Medical and Pediatric Oncology, 24,* 176–80.

Minard, V., Hartmann, O., Peyroulet, M.C. *et al.* (2000). Adverse outcome of infants with metastatic neuroblastoma, N-MYC amplification and/or bone lesions: results of the French society of pediatric oncology. *British Journal of Cancer, 83,* 973–9.

Moss, T.J., Cairo, M., Santana, V.M. *et al.* (1994). Clonogenicity of circulating neuroblastoma cells: implications regarding peripheral blood stem cell transplantation. *Blood, 83,* 3085–9.

Moss, T.J., Reynolds, C.P., Sather, H.N. *et al.* (1991). Prognostic value of immunocytologic detection of bone marrow metastases in neuroblastoma. *New England Journal of Medicine, 324,* 219–26.

Nakagawara, A., Arima Nakagawara, M., Scavarda, N.J. *et al.* (1993). Association between high levels of expression of the TRK gene and favorable outcome in human neuroblastoma. *New England Journal of Medicine, 328,* 847–54.

Ninane, J., Pritchard, J., & Malpas, J.S. (1981). Chemotherapy of advanced neuroblastoma: dees adriamycin help? *Archives of Diseases of Childhood, 56,* 544–8.

Nitschke, R., Cangir, A., Crist, W. *et al.* (1982). Intensive chemotherapy for metastatic neuroblastoma: a Southwest Oncology Group study. *Medical and Pediatric Oncology, 8*, 281–8.

Nussbaumer, W., Schonitzer, D., Trieb, T. *et al.* (1996). Peripheral blood stem cell (PBSC) collection in extremely low birth weight infants. *Bone Marrow Transplantation, 18*, 15–7.

Ohnuma, N., Takahashi, H., Kaneko, M. *et al.* (1995). Treatment combined with bone marrow transplantation for advanced neuroblastoma: an analysis of patients who were pretreated intensively with the protocol of the Study Group of Japan. *Medical and Pediatric Oncology, 24*, 181–7.

Ozkaynak, M.F., Sondel, P.M., Krailo, M.D. *et al.* (2000). Phase I study of chimeric human/murine anti-ganglioside GD2 monoclonal antibody (ch14.18) with granulocyte-macrophage colony-stimulating factor in children with neuroblastoma immediately after hematopoietic stem-cell transplantation: a Children's Cancer Group Study. *Journal of Clinical Oncology, 18*, 4077–85.

Parkin, D.M., Stiller, C.A., Drapper, G.J. *et al.* (1988). The international incidence of childhood cancer. *International Journal of Cancer, 42*, 511–20.

Paul, S.R., Tarbell, N.J., Korf, B. *et al.* (1991). Stage IV neuroblastoma in infants. Long term survival. *Cancer, 67*, 1493–7.

Pession, A., Prete, A., Locatelli, F. *et al.* (1998). Immunotherapy with low-dose recombinant interleukin 2 after high-dose chemotherapy and autologous stem cell transplantation in neuroblastoma. *British Journal of Cancer, 78*, 528–33.

Philip, T., Benard, J.L., Zucker, J.M. *et al.* (1987). High-dose chemoradiotherapy with bone marrow transplantation as consolidation treatment in neuroblastoma. An unselected group of stage IV patients over 1 year of age. *Journal of Clinical Oncology, 5*, 266–71.

Philip, T., Ladenstein, R., Lasset, C. *et al.* (1997). 1070 myeloablative megatherapy procedures followed by stem-cell rescue for neuroblastoma: 17 years of European experience and conclusions. *European Journal of Cancer, 33*, 2130–5.

Philip, T., Ladenstein, R., Zucker, J.M. *et al.* (1993). Double megatherapy and autologous bone marrow transplantation for advanced neuroblastoma: the LMCE2 Study. *British Journal of Cancer, 67*, 119–27.

Philip, T., Zucker, J.M., Bemard, J.L. *et al.* (1991a). Improved survival at 2 and 5 years in the LMCEI unselected group of 72 children with stage IV neuroblastoma older than one year of age at diagnosis: is cure possible in a small subgroup? *Journal of Clinical Oncology, 9*, 1037–44.

Philip, T., Zucker, J.M., Bemard, J.L. *et al.* (1991b). The LMCE1 unselected group of stage IV neuroblastoma revisited with a median follow-up of 59 months after BMT. In *Advances in Neuroblastoma Research*, Vol. 3, ed. A.E. Evans, G. D'Angio, A. Knudson, & R.C. Seeger, pp. 517–25. New York: Wiley-Liss, Inc.

Pinkerton, C.R. (1991). ENSG 1 - randomized study of high-dose melphalan in neuroblastoma. *Bone Marrow Transplantation, 7* (Suppl 3), 112–13.

Pinkerton, C.R., Blanc Vincent, M.P., Bergeron, C. *et al.* (2000). Induction chemotherapy in metastatic neuroblastoma—does dose influence response? A critical review of published data standards, options and recommendations (SOR) project of the National Federation of French Cancer Centers (FNCLCC). *European Journal of Cancer, 36*, 1808–15.

Pinkerton, C.R., Philip, T., Biron, P. *et al.* (1987). High-dose melphalan, vincristine, and total-body irradiation with autologous bone marrow transplantation in children with relapsed neuroblastoma: a phase II study. *Medical and Pediatric Oncology, 15*, 236–40.

Pinkerton, C.R., Zucker, J.M., Hartmann, O. *et al.* (1990). Short duration, high-dose, alternating chemotherapy in metastatic neuroblastoma. (ENSG 3C induction regimen). *British Journal of Cancer, 62*, 319–23.

Pritchard, J., Kiely, E., Rogers, D.W. *et al.* (1989). Long term survival after advanced neuroblastoma. *New England Journal of Medicine, 617*, 1026–7.

Pritchard, J., McElwain, T.J., & Graham Pole, J. (1982). High-dose melphalan with autologous marrow for treatment of advanced neuroblastoma. *British Journal of Cancer, 45*, 86–94.

Reynolds, C.P., Kane, D.J., Einhorn, P.A. *et al.* (1991). Responsive neuroblastoma to retinoic acid in vitro and in vivo. *Progress in Clinical and Biologic Research, 366*, 203–11.

Reynolds, C.P., Schindler, P., Jones, D. *et al.* (1994a). Comparison of 13 cis-retinoic acid to trans-retinoic acid using human neuroblastoma cell lines. In *Advances in Neuroblastoma Research*, Vol. 4, pp. 237–44. New York: Wiley-Liss, Inc.

Reynolds, C.P., Seeger, R.C., Vo, D.D. *et al.* (1994b). Model system for removing neuroblastoma cells from bone marrow using monoclonal antibodies and magnetic immunobeads. *Cancer Research, 46*, 5882–6.

Rogers, D.W., Treleaven, J.G., Kemshead, J.T. *et al.* (1989). Monoclonal antibodies for detection of bone marrow invasion by neuroblastoma. *Journal of Clinical Pathology, 42*, 422–6.

Rosen, E.M., Cassady, J.R., Franz, C.N. *et al.* (1984). Neuroblastoma: the Joint Center for Radiation Therapy/Dana-Farber Cancer Institute/Children's Hospital experience. *Journal of Clinical Oncology, 2*, 719–32.

Rubie, H., Hartmann, O., Michon, J. *et al.* (1997). N-Myc gene amplification is a major prognostic factor in localized neuroblastoma: results of the French NBL 90 study. *Journal of Clinical Oncology, 15*, 1171–82.

Saarinen, U.M., Wikström, S., Mäkipemaa, A. *et al.* (1996). In vivo purging of bone marrow in children with poor-risk neuroblastoma for marrow correction and autologous bone marrow transplantation. *Journal of Clinical Oncology, 14*, 2791–802.

Sanders, J.E. (1990). Later effects following marrow transplantation. In *Bone Marrow Transplantation in Children*, ed. F.L. Johnson & C. Pochedly, p. 471. New York: Raven Press.

Schmidt, M.L., Lukens, J.N., Seeger, R.C. *et al.* (2000). Biologic factors determine prognosis in infants with stage IV neuroblastoma: a prospective Children's Cancer Group study. *Journal of Clinical Oncology, 18*, 1260–8.

Seeger, R.C., Moss, T.J., Feig, S.A. *et al.* (1988). Bone marrow transplantation for poor prognosis neuroblastoma. In *Advances in Neuroblastoma Research*, Vol. 2, ed. A.E. Evans, G.D. Angio, A. Knudson, & R.C. Seeger, pp. 203–13. New York: Alan R. Liss, Inc.

Seeger, R.C., Reynolds, C.P., Gallego, R. *et al.* (2000). Quantitative tumor cell content of bone marrow and blood as a predictor of outcome in stage IV neuroblastoma: a Children's Cancer Group study. *Journal of Clinical Oncology, 18*, 4067–76.

Seeger, R.C., Villablanca, J.G., Matthay, K.K. *et al.* (1991). Intensive chemoradiotherapy and autologous bone marrow transplantation for poor prognosis neuroblastoma. In *Advances in Neuroblastoma Research,* Vol. 3, ed. A.E. Evans, G. D'Angio, A. Knudson, & R.C. Seeger, p. 527. New York: Wiley-Liss, Inc.

Shafford, E.A., Rogers, D.W., & Pritchard, J. (1984). Advanced neuroblastoma: improved response rate using a multiagent regimen (OPEC) including cisplatinum and VM-26. *Journal of Clinical Oncology, 2,* 742–7.

Shuster, J.L., Cantor, A.B., McWilliams, N. *et al.* (1991). The prognostic significance of autologous bone marrow transplantation in advanced neuroblastoma. *Journal of Clinical Oncology, 9,* 1045–9.

Sibley, G.S., Mundt, A.J., Goldman, S. *et al.* (1995). Patterns of failure following total body radiation and bone marrow transplantation with or without a radiotherapy boost for advanced neuroblastoma. *International Journal of Radiation Oncology, Biology and Physics, 32,* 1127–35.

Sidell, N., Altrnan, A., Haussier, M.R. *et al.* (1983). Effect of retinoic acid on the growth and phenotypic expression of several human neuroblastoma cell lines. *Experimental Cell Research, 148,* 21–30.

Stram, D.O., Matthay, K.K., O'Leary, M. *et al.* (1996). Consolidation chemoradiotherapy and autologous bone marrow transplantation versus continued chemotherapy for metastatic neuroblastoma: a report of two concurrent Children's Cancer Group studies. *Journal of Clinical Oncology, 14,* 2417–26.

Strother, D., Shuster, J.J., McWilliams, N. *et al.* (1995). Results of pediatric oncology group protocol 8104 for infants with stage D and DS neuroblastoma. *Journal of Pediatric Hematology and Oncology, 17,* 254–9.

Thiele, C.J., Reynolds, C.P., & Israel, M.A. (1985). Decreased expression of N-myc precedes retinoic acid induced morphologic differentiation of human neuroblastoma. *Nature, 313,* 404–6.

Uttenreuther-Fischer, M.M., Huang, C.S., Reisfield, R.A. *et al.* (1995). Pharmacokinetics of anti-ganglioside GD2 niab 14G2a in a phase I trial in pediatric cancer patients. *Cancer Immunology Immunotherapy, 41,* 229–36.

Valteau-Couanet, D., Benhamou, E., Vassal, G. *et al.* (2000a). Consolidation with a busulfan-containing regimen followed by stem cell transplantation in infants with poor prognosis stage 4 neuroblastoma. *Bone Marrow Transplantation, 25,* 937–42.

Valteau-Couanet, D., Michon, J., & Parel, Y. (2000b). Preliminary results of stage 4 neuroblastoma (NB) NB 97 protocol. *Medical and Pediatric Oncology, 35,* 759 (Abstract).

Valteau-Couanet, D., Rubie, H., Meresse, V. *et al.* (1995). Phase I–II study of interleukin 2 after high-dose chemotherapy and autologous bone marrow transplantation for poorly responding neuroblastoma. *Bone Marrow Transplantation, 16,* 515–20.

Villablanca, J., Khan, A.A., Avramis, V.L. *et al.* (1995). Phase I trial of 13-cis-retinoic acid in children with neuroblastoma following bone marrow transplantation. *Journal of Clinical Oncology, 13,* 894–901.

Yu, A.L., Batova, A., Alvarado, C. *et al.* (1997). Usefulness of chimeric anti-GD2 (ch14.18) and GM CSF for refractory neuroblastoma: a POG phase II study. *Proceedings of the American Society of Clinical Oncology, 16,* 513a (Abstract).

48 Autologous hematopoietic stem cell transplantation for poor-risk sarcomas and nephroblastoma

MITCHELL S. CAIRO, IFEYINWA OSUNKWO, VIRGINIA DAVENPORT, LAUREN HARRISON, AND KAREN H. ANTMAN

Herbert Irving Comprehensive Cancer Center, Columbia University College of Physicians and Surgeons, New York, USA

Introduction

Soft tissue sarcomas comprise approximately 7.4% of all malignancies in children and adolescents (0–20 years) but only 1% of malignancies in adults (≥21 years) (Landis *et al.*, 1998; Ries *et al.*, 1999). Rhabdomyosarcoma (RMS) represents the majority of childhood and adolescent soft tissue sarcomas. Nonmetastatic embryonal histology (embryonal rhabdomyosarcoma, ERMS) tumors arising in favorable primary sites are associated with a 5-yr event-free survival (EFS) and overall survival (OS) of approximately 85% and 95%, respectively (Crist *et al.*, 1995, 2001). However, children and adolescents with newly diagnosed stage IV (metastatic) disease and recurrent or progressive disease with RMS have a dismal outcome (<20% 5-yr OS) with conventional therapy (Koscielniak *et al.*, 1992; Crist *et al.*, 1995; Pappo *et al.*, 1999). Similarly, adults with newly diagnosed metastatic (stage IV) disease and recurrent/progressive soft tissue sarcomas have a dismal outcome with adjuvant conventional therapy (≤10% 5-yr OS) (chemotherapy, radiotherapy, surgery) (Sarcoma Meta Analysis, 1997; Keohan & Taub, 1997).

Ewing's sarcoma (ES) and primitive neuroectodermal tumors (PNET) represent another large group of sarcomas that belong to the Ewing's sarcoma family of tumors (ESFT). Similar to RMS, children, adolescents, and adults with both newly diagnosed stage IV (metastatic) disease and recurrent/progressive disease have a poor prognosis with conventional therapy (chemotherapy, radiation therapy, and surgery) (5–25% 5-yr OS) (Bacci *et al.*, 1989; Kinsella *et al.*, 1991; Antman, 1992; Keohan & Taub, 1997; Cotterill *et al.*, 2000; Kushner & Meyers; 2001). In this chapter we review the treatment and prognosis for patients with poor-risk sarcomas with both stage IV disease at diagnosis and recurrent/progressive disease treated with and without myeloablative therapy and autologous-hematopoietic stem cell transplantation (HSCT).

Ewing's sarcoma[1]: description and outcome without autologous HSCT

Description and demographics

ES consists of a family of tumors (ESFT) distinguished by small round blue cells of endothelial origin that may arise

[1] James Ewing, American pathologist, 1866-1943.

either in bone (skeletal Ewing's) or soft tissue (extraosseous Ewing's). ESFT also includes the primitive PNETs, which exhibit varying degrees of neuroepithelial differentiation (Horowitz *et al.*, 1997). Approximately 2.7 per million children in the United States present each year with skeletal Ewing's sarcoma (excluding PNET and soft tissue ES) (Gurney *et al.*, 1996). In a review by Horowitz *et al.* (1997) over a 10-year period of over 1,500 patients with ESFT, 87% of patients had skeletal ES, 8% had extraosseous ES, and 5% had PNET. The peak age at presentation usually occurs within the first two decades of life (Antman, 1992). ES is unusual in patients of non-Caucasian ethnic background and rarely occurs as a secondary malignancy (Fraumeni & Glass, 1970).

The diagnosis of ES is usually made by a combination of morphology, immunohistochemistry, and cytogenetics. ESFTs are usually MIC-2 (CD99) positive with varying degrees of expression of neural markers including NSE, Leu 7, and synaptophysin. ESFTs also commonly stain positive for vimentin and for 013/HBA71 in a characteristic nonspeckled pattern (Fellinger *et al.*, 1991; Delattre *et al.*, 1994; Weidner & Tjoe, 1994). ES may be negative for S-100, neuron specific antigen (NSA), desmin, actin, and leukocyte common antigen (LCA).

Over 90% of ES patients exhibit a chromosome 22 translocation, that is a t(11;22)(q24;q12) or a variant, leading to a variety of gene fusion products between the ES gene and ETS-related oncogenes, especially the FL-1 or ERG gene (Delattre *et al.*, 1992). Presence of this marker is virtually diagnostic of ESFT. This gene fusion product is readily detectable by reverse-transcriptase polymerase chain reaction (RT-PCR) and has been used in some studies as a means of detecting early relapse (Zoubek *et al.*, 1996; Kushner *et al.*, 1999). Prognostically, some investigators have linked improved relapse-free survival to the presence of the EWS-FL1 gene fusion transcript rather than to the presence of other genetic rearrangements (Nesbit *et al.*, 1990).

ES is staged as either localized or metastatic disease with metastatic disease occurring mostly in lung, bone, and/or marrow. Presence of metastatic disease at diagnosis is perhaps the most significant predictor of a poor outcome in patients with ESFT (Cotterill *et al.*, 2000). Patients with metastasis to the lungs may have a slightly improved outlook compared to those with dissemination to the bone or marrow or disease involving multiple sites. The Children's Oncology Group/Pediatric Oncology Group (COG/POG) Intergroup study (1988–92) reported less than 20% survival rates for patients with metastatic disease at diagnosis, with approximately one-third of metastases occurring in the lungs, a third in bone or marrow, and a third involving more than one site (Miser *et al.*, 1988; Kushner & Meyers, 2001) (Table 48.1).

The most common site of primary disease for ES is the pelvis and for PNET is the central axis, and each of these primary sites confers a poor prognosis [25% 2-yr disease-free survival (DFS); Nesbit *et al.*, 1990; Evans *et al.*, 1991]. Rib lesions and distal extremity primaries are associated with improved outcomes. Other adverse prognostic factors include:

1. large tumor size/volume;
2. extraosseous extension in bone primaries;
3. filigree or dark cell histology pattern;
4. persistence of macro or micro nodules on surgical biopsies after induction chemotherapy;
5. presence of any neural differentiation;
6. elevated LDH/ESR;
7. and/or age less than 10 years or greater than 20 at diagnosis

(Oberlin *et al.*, 1985; Hayes *et al.*, 1989; Cangir *et al.*, 1990; Nesbit *et al.*, 1990; Dunst *et al.*, 1991; Evans *et al.*, 1991; Picci *et al.*, 1993; McClean *et al.*, 1999; Bacci *et al.*, 2000).

Treatment and prognosis for newly diagnosed metastatic Ewing's sarcoma without autologous HSCT

ESFTs are notably very radiosensitive but extremely prone to hematogenous spread and therefore require multimodal therapy (chemotherapy, radiotherapy, and surgery) to prevent relapse (Rosen *et al.*, 1981). A review of all the major Ewing's sarcoma clinical trials for nonmetastatic disease have demonstrated that most regimens were composed of a VACD backbone (vincristine, actinomycin, cyclophosphamide, and doxorubicin), with non-pelvic primaries portending the best prognosis. Using this approach, investigators from Memorial Sloan-Kettering Cancer Center reported a 79% 2-yr DFS with a VACD (vincristine, actinomycin, cyclophosphamide, doxorubicin)/bleomycin/ BCNU regimen (Rosen *et al.*, 1981), and Bacci *et al.* (1989) reported a 54% 9-yr DFS using VACD therapy for patients with nonmetastatic ES.

The outcome following treatment of metastatic disease, however, has remained disappointing, despite the addition of local radiation to sites of metastatic disease (less than 4 bone lesions, lung, etc.) and removal of 1 to 3 lung metastases (Lanza *et al.*, 1987). Results from the German Cooperative Ewing's Sarcoma studies (CESS81&86, EICESS92) suggested a survival advantage for higher doses of lung radiation therapy (RT) for patients with lung metastasis (1 of 6 that received no RT, 4 of 10 who received 12–16 Gy, and 5 of 6 who received 18–21 Gy survived) (Dunst *et al.*, 1993). Five-year OS among patients with ES metastatic to lung only was 36% (Paulussen *et al.*, 1998), but only 27% for those with bone and/or bone mar-

row involvement, and a disappointing 14% for disseminated disease involving multiple sites (Table 48.1).

In two consecutive studies without autologous HSCT conducted by the National Cancer Institute (NCI), EFS was 7% and 13%, respectively, for metastatic (stage IV) ES (Table 48.1). Patients with metastatic disease to the lung who underwent thoracotomy (*n* = 19) achieved an overall 5-year DFS of only 15% (Kinsella *et al.*, 1991; Wexler *et al.*, 1996). The Intergroup Ewing's Sarcoma Study-II (IESS-II) demonstrated no statistically significant improvement in outcome over IESS-I for patients with metastatic disease (5-year OS of 30% vs. 28%, respectively) (Table 48.1) (Cangir *et al.*, 1990). The third Intergroup Ewing's Sarcoma trial, conducted by CCG/POG, reported less than 20% OS utilizing the regimen of alternating VACD with ifosfamide/etoposide (IE) (Miser *et al.*, 1996). St Jude's Children's Research Hospital reported a 54% 3-year EFS for 18 patients utilizing the VACD regimen with BCNU (EW179 study) (Hayes *et al.*, 1987) and a 27% 3-year EFS utilizing VACD with IE (Marina *et al.*, 1999). Other investigators have also reported EFS of 7% to 30% using variations of the VACD regimen (Wessalowski *et al.*, 1988; Michon *et al.*, 1993; Koscielniak *et al.*, 1996; Craft *et al.*, 1998; Paulussen *et al.*, 1998) (Table 48.1).

Treatment and prognosis for progressive/relapsed Ewing's sarcoma without autologous HSCT

Survival is generally poor after relapse with ESFT and is directly proportional to length of time from diagnosis to relapse/progression. Recurrent ES occurring less than 2 years from diagnosis produces an OS of less than 5% at 10 years (Cotterill *et al.*, 2000). McLean *et al.* (1999) reported on the long-term follow-up of 82 patients treated with ESFT at the Dana Farber Cancer Institute. After 5 additional years, of the 31 long-term survivors, 5 had relapsed and another 5 developed a secondary malignancy. Relapse rates for patients with metastatic disease at diagnosis are even higher. In one study, there were no disease-free survivors with PNET after first relapse, while patients with relapsed ES had a 12% DFS at 4 years (Bacci *et al.*, 1989). Thus, in patients with newly diagnosed metastatic or stage IV ES or patients with recurrent ES, the available data suggest that survival is less than 25% and that alternative treatment strategies should be investigated and compared to current conventional therapy (chemotherapy, surgery, and radiotherapy) (Table 48.2).

Autologous HSCT for Ewing's sarcoma and PNET

We retrospectively reviewed 12 publications (1989–2001) reporting the outcome in children, adolescents, and young adults with either metastatic disease (stage IV) at diagnosis or relapsed or progressive ES or PNET, who received high-dose consolidation therapy (chemotherapy ± TBI) with autologous HSCT. We have summarized these experiences according to

Table 48.1. *Outcome of poor-risk stage IV newly diagnosed Ewing's sarcoma/PNET treated without autologous HSCT*

Autor (year)	Study	No. of patients/ age (yrs)	Stage	Regimen, dose per course	Outcome
Kinsella et al. (1991)	NCI (1968–80)	N = 27 3–45	IV	Vinc 0.025–0.04 mg/kg; Cy 40 mg/kg or Vinc 0.025–0.04 mg/kg; Cy 40 mg/kg; Dact 0.1–0.15 mg/kg or Vinc 0.025–0.04 mg/kg; Cy 40 mg/kg; Dox 75 mg/m²	<7% 5-yr DFS
Wexler et al. (1996)	NCI (1986–92)	N = 23 7–24	IV	Vinc 2 mg/m²; Dox 70–90 mg/m²; Cy 1.2–1.5 g/m²; Ifos 300–500 mg/m²; Etop 300–500 mg/m²	13% 5-yr EFS
Cangir et al. (1990)	IESS-MD I (1975–77)	N = 39 N/A	IV	Vinc 1.5 mg/m²; Dact 0.075 mg/m²; Cy 500 mg/m²; Dox 60 mg/m² + RT	30% 5-yr OS
Cangir et al. (1990)	IESS-MD II (1980–83)	N = 48 N/A	IV	Vinc 1.5 mg/m²; Dact 2 mg/m²; Cy 500 mg/m²; Dox 75 mg/m² + 5-FU 300 mg/m² + RT	28% 5-yr OS
Miser et al. (1996)	CCG-POG (1988–92)	N = 121 N/A	IV	Vinc 1.5 mg/m², Dact 1.25 mg/m²; Cy 1.2–4.2 g/m²; Dox 75 mg/m² ± Ifos 9–12 g/m²; Etop 500 mg/m² + RT	<20% OS
Hayes et al. (1987)	St Jude's (1978–85)	N = 18 7–18	IV	Vinc 1.5 mg/m²; Dact 1.5 mg/m²; Cy 1.05 g/m²; Dox 35 mg/m² ± BCNU 50 mg/m² + RT	50% 4-yr PFS
Marina et al. (1999)	St Jude's (1992–96)	N = 18 4–24	IV	Vinc 1.5 mg/m²; Dact 1.5 mg/m²; Cy 2–7.5 g/m²; Dox 60–225 mg/m²; Ifos 10 g/m²; Etop 450 mg/m² + high dose Ifos 10 g/m²; Etop 750 mg/m²	27% EFS
Craft et al. (1997)	ET-1 (1978–85)	N = 22 1–33	IV	Vinc 2 mg/m²; Dact 1.4 mg/m²; Dox 50 mg/m²; Cy 400–1,000 mg/m² + RT	9% 4-yr OS
Craft et al. (1998)	ET-2 (1987–93)	N = 42 1–27	IV	Vinc 2 mg/m²; Dact 1.5 mg/m²; Dox 60 mg/m²; Ifos 6–9 g/m² ± Cy 300 mg/m²/week (during RT) + RT	23% 5-yr OS
Verrill et al. (1997)	Royal Marsden (1980–95)	N = 17 14–51	IV	Vinc 1.4 mg/m²; Dact 1.4 mg/m²; Dox 60 mg/m²; Ifos 6–9 g/m² ± Cy + RT or Vinc 1.4 mg/m²; Dact 1.4 mg/m²; Dox 60 mg/m²; Cy 1.2 g/m² + RT	7% 5-yr EFS
Michon et al. (1993)	EW-88 (1988–90)	N = 25 4–41	IV	Vinc 1.5 mg/m²; Dact 1.5 mg/m²; Dox 35 mg/m²; Cy 1.05 g/m² ± BCNU 50 mg/m² + RT	12% 3-yr OS
Wessalowski et al. (1988)	CESS (1981–87)	N = 48 N/A	IV	Vinc 1.5 mg/m²; Dact 1.5 mg/m²; Dox 60 mg/m²; Cy 1.2 g/m² or Vinc 1.5 mg/m²; Dact 1.5 mg/m²; Ifos 6 g/m² + RT	18% 7-yr DFS
Koscielniak et al. (1996)	CESS (1981–90)	N = 16 0–21	IV	Vinc 1.5 mg/m²; Dact 1.5 mg/m²; Dox 30 mg/m²; Cy 1.2 g/m² or Vinc 1.5 mg/m²; Dact 1.5 mg/m²; Ifos 6 g/m² + RT	13% 2-yr OS
Paulussen et al. (1998a)	CESS EICESS 92 (1997)	N = 114 2–45	IV	Vinc 1.5 mg/m²; Dact 1.5 mg/m²; Dox 60 mg/m²; Cy 1.2 g/m² or Vinc 1.5 mg/m²; Dact 1.5 mg/m²; Ifos 6–9 g/m² ± Etop 450 mg/m² + RT	36% 5-yr OS
Paulussen et al. (1998b)	EICESS 92 (1990–1995)	N = 171 1–44	IV	Vinc 1.5 mg/m²; Dact 1.5 mg/m²; Dox 30 mg/m², or Vinc 1.5 mg/m²; Dact 1.5 mg/m²; Ifos 6–9 g/m² ± Etop 450 mg/m² + RT ? WLRT	27% 4-yr EFS

Abbreviations: NCI, National Cancer Institute; IESS, Intergroup Ewing's Sarcoma Study; CCG, Children's Cancer Group; POG, Pediatric Oncology Group; ET, Ewing's Tumor; EW, Ewing's Sarcoma Study; CESS, Cooperative Ewing Sarcoma Studies; EICESS, European Intergroup Cooperative Ewing Sarcoma Studies; N/A, not available; Vinc, vincristine; Cy, cyclophosphamide; Dact, actinomycin D; Dox, doxorubicin; Ifos, ifosfamide; Etop, etoposide; RT, radiotherapy; 5FU, 5-fluorouracil; BCNU, 3-bis (2-chloroethyl)-1-nitrosurea; WLRT, whole lung radiotherapy; DFS, disease-free survival; EFS, event-free survival; OS, overall survival.

Table 48.2. *Outcome of poor-risk patients with relapsed/progressive rhabdomyosarcoma/Ewing's sarcoma treated without autologous HSCT*

Author	No. of patients/ age (yrs)	Diagnosis	Regimen, dose per course	Outcomes: Alive/Dead
Nitschke *et al.* (1998)	$N = 141$ 1–23	RMS ($n = 22$) ES ($n = 29$)	Topo 10 g/m^2 + G-CSF	N/A
Klingebiel *et al.* (1998)	$N = 44$ N/A	ERMS ($n = 17$) ARMS ($n = 13$) PNET ($n = 6$)	Carbo 600 mg/m^2; Etop 600 mg/m^2 + Ifos 8 g/m^2 + RT/Surgery/RHT	ERMS 9-A, 8-D ARMS 3-A, 10-D PNET 0-A, 6-D
Kushner *et al.* (2000)	$N = 25$ 2–33	RMS ($n = 3$) ES ($n = 5$)	Cy 4.2 g/m^2; Topo 6 mg/m^2	EWS N/A RMS N/A
Saylors *et al.* (2001)	$N = 83$ 1–21	RMS ($n = 15$) ES ($n = 17$) Other STS ($n = 2$)	Cy 1.25 g/m^2; Topo 3.75 mg/m^2 + G-CSF	RMS 2-A, 2-D, 11-N/A EWS 3-A, 1-D, 13-N/A
van Hoff *et al.* (1995)	$N = 10$ 1–22	RMS/STS ($n = 4$) ES ($n = 2$)	Ifos 4.5 g/m^2; Cisp 60 mg/m^2; Etop 300 mg/m^2	RMS 1-A, 3-N/A EWS-N/A
Magrath *et al.* (1986)	$N = 75$ 0–64	RMS ($n = 9$) ES ($n = 20$)	Ifos 9 g/m^2	N/A
Kung *et al.* (1995/1995)	$N = 241$ 0–30	RMS/STS ($n = 70$) ESS ($n = 62$)	Ifos 4.5 g/m^2; Carbo 300–635 mg/m^2; Etop 300 mg/m^2 Ifos 6 g/m^2; Etop 300 mg/m^2	N/A
Miser *et al.* (1987)	$N = 77$ N/A	RMS ($n = 13$) ES/PNET ($n = 25$)	Etop 500 mg/m^2; Ifos 9 g/m^2	N/A
Grabois *et al.* (1994)	$N = 9$ <16	RMS ($n = 5$)	Carbo 200 mg/m^2; Etop 500 mg/m^2	N/A
Carpenter *et al.* (1997)	$N = 38$ 1–20	RMS ($n = 9$) ES ($n = 4$)	Vinc 0.05 mg/kg × 2; Etop 75 mg/kg; Cy 90–165 mg/kg	RMS 1-A, 8-D EWS 1-A, 3-D
Raney (1987)	$N = 16$ 0–16	RMS ($n = 9$)	Cisp 75–100 mg/m^2; Etop 300–750 mg/m^2	0-A, 16-D
Castello *et al.* (1990)	$N = 23$ 0–16	RMS ($n = 2$) ES ($n = 3$)	Carbo 1 g/m^2; Etop 300 mg/m^2	N/A
Pappo *et al.* (1999)	$N = 605$ 0–20	ARMS = 273 ERMS-313 BRMS-19	As per institution	ARMS: St. 1–60-A, 10-D St. 2–4-A, 249-D ERMS: St. 1–44-A, 40-D; St. 2-3–325-A, 98-D;St.4–11-A, 83-D BRMS: 10-A, 6-D
Blaney *et al.* (1998)	$N = 85$ 1–21	RMS ($n = 15$) ES/PNET ($n = 26$)	Topo 1–1.3 mg/m^2	N/A

Abbreviations: N/A, not available; RMS, rhabdomyosarcoma; ES, Ewing's sarcoma; ERMS, embryonal rhabdomyosarcoma; ARMS, alveolar rhabdomyosarcoma; STS, soft tissue sarcoma; PNET, primitive neuroectodermal tumor; BRMS, botyroid rhabdomyosarcoma; Topo, topotecan; Carbo, carboplatin; Etop, etoposide; Ifos, ifosfamide; RT, radiotherapy; RHT, regional hyperthermia; Cy, cyclophosphamide; G-CSF, granulocyte colony-stimulating factor; Cisp, cisplatin; A, alive; D, dead.

their disease status at diagnosis in two tables (Table 48.3— newly diagnosed stage IV, and Table 48.4—relapsed disease). We have briefly summarized the OS and EFS for all patients, and (when available) reported the ES and PNET survival.

Treatment and prognosis for poor-risk patients with newly diagnosed metastatic (stage IV) ES/PNET following autologous HSCT

Perentesis *et al.* (1999) reported on 5 patients with ES from a total of 24 patients with metastatic solid tumors (Wilms', rhabdomyosarcoma, neuroblastoma) who underwent myeloablative therapy and autologous HSCT. Two preparative regimens were used: etoposide 1.8 g/m^2, thiotepa 900 mg/m^2, and cyclophosphamide 1.2 g/m^2; or busulfan 12 mg/kg, melphalan 100 mg/m^2, and thiotepa 500 mg/m^2. The DFS for the entire group (24 patients) at 2 and 4 years was 39% and 34%, respectively. Of the 5 patients with ES, two patients with stage IV ES at diagnosis who were transplanted in CR were alive and disease-free, and one patient transplanted in PR had stable disease at a median of 29 months post–autologous HSCT. The other two ES patients died, one of relapse and one of veno-occlusive disease (VOD) (Table 48.3).

Emminger *et al.* (1991) reported on 5 patients with ES and PNET from a total of 20 patients with solid tumors (neuroblastoma and rhabdomyosarcoma) who received myeloablative

Table 48.3. *Outcome of poor-risk patients with newly diagnosed stage IV Ewing's sarcoma/PNET treated with autologous HSCT*

Author	No. of patients/ age (yrs)	Histology	Stage	Primary sites	Metastasis at diagnosis	Status at autologous HSCT	Conditioning regimen/dose	Outcome
Perentesis et al. (1999)	N = 5 9–17	ES	IV	Forearm Ilium Pelvic Femur	Lung, BM, bone	1 CR1 1 CR2 3 PR1	Etop 1.8 g/m², Thio 900 mg/m², Cy 1.2 g/m² Bu 12 mg/kg, Mel 100 mg/m², Thio 500 mg/m²	3 – A (2 CR, 1 SD) 2 – D (1 Rel, 1 VOD)
Emminger et al. (1991)	N = 5 1.8–23	ES/PNET	IV	N/A	Bone, BM	2 CR1 3 CR2	12 Gy FTBI, Mel 120–240 mg/m², ± Etop 60 mg/kg, ± Carbo 4.5 g/m²	4 – A (2 CR, 2 Rel) 1 – D
Ozkaynak et al. (1998)	N = 5 2–21	ES/PNET	IV	N/A	Bone and/or BM	5 CR1	Mel 200 mg/m², Carbo 1.2 g/m², Etop 800 mg/m², ± Cy 3 g/m²	5 – A (4 CR, 1 PD)
Bader et al. (1989)	N = 19 4–35	ES/PNET	IV	N/A	BM, bone, lung	N/A	TBI 8 Gy, Vinc 2 mg/m², Dox 70 mg/m², Cy 2.4 g/m²	N/A
Kushner et al. (2001)	N = 11 8–39	ES/PNET	IV	Pelvis/femur Spine Chest	BM, lung, bone	11 CR/VGPR	TBI 15 Gy, Mel 180 mg/m² OR Thio 900 mg/m², Carbo 1.5 g/m²	10 – D (7 PD, 3 toxic) 1 – A (CR)
Burdach et al. (1993)	N = 7 6–31	ES	IV	Multifocal, bone	Lung, BM	5 CR1 2 PR	Mel 120–180 mg/m², TBI 12 Gy, ± Etop 60 mg/kg–1.2 g/m², ± Carbo 600–800 mg/m²	3 – A 4 – D
Atra et al.[a] (1997)	N = 18 2.75–30	ES	IV (11 pts)	Femur Pelvis Humerus Scapula Skull	Lung, BM	12 CR1 4 CR2 1 PR 1 PD	Bu 16 mg/kg, Mel 140–160 mg/m²	14 – A 4 – D (Rel)
Meyers et al. (2001)	N = 22 1–22	ES	IV	N/A	Bone, BM	22 CR/VGPR	TBI 12 Gy, Mel 120 mg/m², Etop 750 g/m²	N/A
Diaz et al.[a] (1999)	N = 15 2–21	ES/PNET	IV	N/A	N/A	11 CR1 2 CR2 2 PR	Bu 16 mg/kg, Mel 140 mg/m²	64% 4-yr EFS
Horowitz et al.[a] (1993)	N = 44 2–38	ES/PNET	N/A	N/A	Bone, BM, lung, node	44 CR	TBI 8 Gy, Vinc 2 mg/m², Dox 60 mg/m², Cy 2.4 g/m²	10% 6-yr EFS

Abbreviations: ES, Ewing's sarcoma; PNET, primitive neuroectodermal tumor; N/A, not available; BM, bone marrow; CR, complete response; PR, partial response; VGPR, very good partial response; PD, progressive disease; Etop, etoposide; Thio, thiotepa; Cy, cyclophosphamide; Bu, busulfan; Mel, Melphalan; FTBI, fractionated total body irradiation; Carbo, carboplatin; Vinc, vincristine; Dox, doxorubicin; A, alive; D, dead; Rel, relapse; SD, stable disease; VOD, veno-occlusive disease; EFS, event-free survival.
[a] Report did not separate out newly diagnosed and relapsed patients.

Table 48.4. *Outcome of poor-risk patients with relapsed Ewing's sarcoma/PNET treated with autologous HSCT*

Author	No. of patients/ age (yrs)	Histology	Status at HSCT	Conditioning regimen/dose	Outcome
Perentesis *et al.* (1999)	*N* = 4 Age 5–28	ES	1 CR2 1 CR3 1 PR2 1 PR4	Etop 1.8 g/m^2, Thio 900 mg/m^2, Cy 1.2 g/m^2; OR Bu 12 mg/kg, Mel 100 mg/m^2, Thio 500 mg/m^2	1 – A – CR 3 – D – Rel
Emminger *et al.* (1991)	*N* = 4 Age 1.8–23	ES/PNET	3 CR2 1 PR2	12 Gy FTBI, Mel 180 mg/m^2, 12 Gy FTBI, Mel 240 mg/m^2 12 Gy FTBI, Mel 120 mg/m^2, Etop 60 mg/kg	3 – Rel 1 – CR
Ozkaynak *et al.* (1998)	*N* = 9 Age 2–21	ES/PNET	CR/VGPR	Mel 200 mg/m^2, Carbo 1.2 g/m^2, Etop 800 mg/m^2; OR Mel 200 mg/m^2, Cy 3 g/m^2, Carbo 1.2 g/m^2, Etop 800 mg/m^2	5 – A (2 PD, 3 CR) 4 – D (2 toxic, 2 PD)
Bader *et al.* (1989)	*N* = 27 Age 4–35	ES/PNET	N/A	8 Gy TBI, vinc 2 mg/m^2, Dox 70 mg/m^2, Cy 2.4 g/m^2	N/A
Chan *et al.*[a] (1997)	*N* = 6 Age 1–17	ES	3 PR1 1 CR2 1 PR2 1 PD	Thio 450–750 mg/m^2, Mel 180 mg/m^2	N/A
Burdach *et al.* (1993)	*N* = 9 Age 6–31	ES	3 CR2 1 CR1 3 PR2 1 CR3 1 PR3	Mel 120–180 mg/m^2, TBI 12 Gy, +/– Etop 40–60 mg/kg to 1.2 g/m^2, +/– Carbo 600–800 mg/m^2	4 – A – CR 5 – D – PD
Stewart *et al.*[a] (1996)	*N* = 4 Age 16–30	ES/PNET	N/A	Mel 140–200 mg/m^2, +/– TBI 5 Gy	N/A

Abbreviations: ES, Ewing's sarcoma; PNET, primitive neuroectodermal tumor; CR, complete response; PR, partial response; VGPR, very good partial response; N/A, not available; Etop, etoposide; Thio, thiotepa; Cy, cyclophosphamide; Bu, busulfan; FTBI, fractionated total body irradiation; Mel, melphalan; Carbo, carboplatin; Vinc, vincristine; Dox, doxorubicin; A, alive; D, dead; Rel, Relapse; PD, progressive disease.
[a] Report did not separate out newly diagnosed and relapsed patients.

therapy and autologous HSCT. The preparative regimen included fractionated TBI, melphalan 120–240 mg/m^2, ± etoposide 60 mg/kg, ± carboplatin 4.5 g/m^2. Both patients with ES are alive, one of whom is disease-free at 29 months. Two of the three patients with PNET were alive, and one was disease-free at 9 months (Table 48.3).

We have reported on 5 children with ES and PNET from a total of 27 children with various solid tumors, 7 in first complete remission/very good partial remission (CR/VGPR) who underwent myeloablation and autologous HSCT (Ozkaynak *et al.*, 1998). The preparative regimen included melphalan 200 mg/m^2, carboplatin 1.2 g/m^2, etoposide 800 mg/m^2, ± cyclophosphamide 3 g/m^2. All 5 patients with ES/PNET were alive, 4 in continuous CR, and one with progressive disease. Patients with ES/PNET transplanted in first CR had a 66% 3-year EFS (Table 48.3).

Bader *et al.* (1989) reported on the NCI experience in 19 patients with ES and PNET from a total of 75 patients who underwent induction chemotherapy. Those who obtained a CR then received chemoradiotherapy and autologous HSCT. The preparative regimen included TBI 8 Gy, vincristine 2 mg/m^2, cyclophosphamide 2.4 g/m^2, and doxorubicin 70 mg/m^2. The 7-years EFS for all patients with PNET and ES was 34% and 28%, respectively (Table 48.3).

Kushner *et al.* (2001) reported the results of 11 patients with newly diagnosed metastatic (bone/bone marrow) ES/PNET who obtained a CR/VGPR following induction chemoradiotherapy and subsequently received myeloablative therapy and autologous HSCT. Only one patient is alive in CR. There were 8 patients treated with a preparative regimen of TBI 15 Gy, melphalan 180 mg/m^2 or thiotepa 900 mg/m^2 and carboplatin 1.5 g/m^2. Among the 8 patients, 4 relapsed, 3 died of toxicity, and 1 was in CR at 7 years (Table 48.3).

Burdach *et al.* (1993) reported on 7 patients with ES from a total of 17 patients with newly diagnosed stage IV or relapsed ES who underwent myeloablation and autologous HSCT. The preparative regimen consisted of TBI 12 Gy, melphalan 120–180 mg/m^2, ± etoposide 60 mg/kg to 1.2 g/m^2, ± carboplatin 600–800 mg/m^2. Three of 7 patients transplanted survived event-free (Table 48.3).

Atra *et al.* (1997) reported on 11 patients with stage IV ES from a total of 18 patients that underwent myeloablation and autologous HSCT. The preparative regimen included busulfan 16 mg/kg and melphalan 140–160 mg/m^2. Six of the 11 patients survived with a median follow-up of 2 years (Table 48.3).

Meyers *et al.* (2001) reported on 22 patients with stage IV ES undergoing myeloablative therapy and autologous HSCT. The preparative regimen consisted of TBI 12 Gy, melphalan

120 mg/m^2, and etoposide 750 g/m^2. The 2-year EFS was only 24%, with the majority of patients relapsing and/or dying of progressive disease (Table 48.3).

Diaz et al. (1999) reported on 15 patients with ES and PNET from a total of 30 patients with high-risk solid tumors (neuroblastoma and rhabdomyosarcoma) who underwent myeloablative therapy and autologous HSCT. The preparative regimen included busulfan 16 mg/kg and melphalan 120 mg/m^2. Patients were not separated into newly diagnosed and relapsed. The 4-year EFS was 64% in patients with ES/PNET. Overall, 20 patients were alive, 19 in CR, 1 in relapse, and 10 died (Table 48.3).

Horowitz et al. (1993) reported on 44 patients with high-risk ES and PNET who went on to achieve a CR and underwent consolidation therapy with TBI/chemotherapy and autologous HSCT from a total of 91 patients with solid tumors (rhabdomyosarcoma). The study did not separate out newly diagnosed metastatic patients and those in relapse. For the 44 patients with ES, the 6-year EFS and OS were 10% and 14%, respectively. A total of 31 patients with metastatic disease went on to consolidation therapy, and the EFS and OS for that subgroup were 19% and 29%, respectively. The EFS and OS rate for 34 patients with localized disease who underwent autologous HSCT was somewhat better at 41% and 46%, respectively (Table 48.3).

Treatment and prognosis of poor-risk patients with relapsed/progressive ES/PNET following autologous HSCT

Perentesis et al. (1999) reported on 4 patients with relapsed/progressive ES from a total of 24 patients with relapsed/progressive solid tumors (Wilms', rhabdomyosarcoma, neuroblastoma) following myeloablative therapy and autologous HSCT. Only one patient with ES was alive in CR (Table 48.4).

Emminger et al. (1991) reported on 4 patients with relapsed/progressive ES and PNET from a total of 20 patients with solid tumors (neuroblastoma and rhabdomyosarcoma). All four patients were alive. Two patients with ES relapsed, one patient with PNET is in CR, and one patient with PNET relapsed (Table 48.4).

We reported on 9 children with relapsed/progressive ES and PNET from a total of 27 children with various solid tumors (medulloblastoma, rhabdomyosarcoma) following myeloablation and autologous HSCT (Ozkaynak et al., 1998). At the time of our previous report, 5 patients were alive, 3 in CR and 2 in PD (Table 48.4).

Bader et al. (1989) reported on the NCI experience in 27 patients with relapsed/progressive ES and PNET from a total of 75 patients following myeloablation and autologous HSCT. The outcome results in the specific subgroup with the relapsed/progressive disease, however, are unavailable (Table 48.4).

Chan et al. (1997) reported on 6 patients with relapsed/progressive ES from a total of 21 patients with solid tumors (neuroblastoma and osteosarcoma) following myeloablative therapy and autologous HSCT. The report did not differentiate between patients diagnosed with metastatic disease and those who relapsed. The conditioning regimen included thiotepa 450–750 mg/m^2 and melphalan 180 mg/m^2. At a median of 7 months, one patient with ES was alive and in CR (Table 48.4).

Burdach et al. (1993) reported on 9 patients with ES from a total of 17 patients with newly diagnosed stage IV or relapsed ES who underwent myeloablation and autologous HSCT. Four of the original nine patients with relapsed/progressive disease with ES/PNET were alive and in CR (Table 48.4).

Lastly, Stewart et al. (1996) reported on four adult patients with relapsed/progressive ES/PNET following high-dose therapy with melphalan and TBI and autologous HSCT. Three of 4 patients had less than a 5-month progression-free survival, and one was a long-term survivor (Table 48.4).

In summary, we have reviewed the results of over 147 patients with newly diagnosed stage IV ES/PNET who were treated in first CR/VGPR with various combinations of myeloablative chemoradiotherapy and autologous HSCT. The ages ranged between 1 and 39 years and the outcomes varied, but averaged around 40% to 50% of patients alive and in continuing complete remission (CCR).

This approach may be slightly better than conventional nontransplant approaches for newly diagnosed patients with stage IV ES/PNET (surgery, chemotherapy, local/metastatic radiation) (Table 48.1) (estimated average 25% 3-year EFS) (Table 48.3 vs. Table 48.1, respectively).

We have also reviewed the results of 63 patients with relapsed ES/PNET, ages 1.8 to 35 years, who received a variety of myeloablative chemoradiotherapy regimens. The outcome results were variable but 25% to 40% of patients achieved either CR or had stable disease (SD). In comparison, 5-year survival after a conventional nontransplant (chemotherapy, radiation, surgery) approach was approximately 10% to 25% (Table 48.4 vs. Table 48.2, respectively).

Prospective randomized trials in both newly diagnosed stage IV patients and in patients with relapsed/progressive ES/PNET disease will be required to determine if myeloablation and autologous HSCT offers any advantage over conventional dose therapy.

Rhabdomyosarcoma: description and outcome without autologous HSCT

Description and demographics

RMS is a malignant tumor of immature mesenchymal cells committed to some skeletal muscle differentiation (Horn & Enterline, 1958). RMS is the most common soft tissue sarcoma of childhood and adolescence, with an incidence of 4.6 cases per million children (Wexler & Helman, 1997). RMS is classified into two major histological subtypes (embryonal and alveolar) depending on the degree of mesenchymal differentiation. Significant prognostic factors include histological type, age at presentation, and location of primary tumor (Lawrence et al., 1987; Crist et al., 1990).

Embryonal RMSs (ERMS) comprise about 50% of RMS cases and affect mostly children 0–15 (median 4) years of age. ERMS occurs most commonly in the head and neck region, followed by the genitourinary tract and retroperitoneum (bladder, prostate, and vagina), and orbit. ERMS commonly demonstrate a loss of heterozygosity on chromosome 11. The ERMS botyroid variant and the spindle cell variant make up an additional 10% of RMS and exhibit more favorable clinical outcomes (Wexler & Helman, 1997; Snyder et al., 1998). The remaining RMS consist mainly of the alveolar (ARMS) subtype (approximately 30%) (Newton et al., 1995; Wexler & Helman, 1997; Snyder et al., 1998). ARMS is associated with a characteristic chromosome 13 translocation and near tetraploidy (Crist et al., 1990). Seventy percent of ARMS have the t(2:13)(q35;q14) translocation (PAX3-FKHR), while t(1;13)(p36;q14) (PAX7-FKHR) comprises 10% to 15% of cases (Whang Peng et al., 1986; Pappo et al., 1993). ARMS is more common in older patients (ages 10–25 years), and has a predilection for extremities and paratesticular region. Trunk (central) primaries confer a poor prognosis (Neifeld et al., 1979; Crist et al., 1995). Pleomorphic RMS (PRMS) is a rare subtype (5% to 7%) that occurs almost exclusively in adults over 45 years old.

The 35% to 44% of RMS that occur in the head and neck area confer a less favorable outcome due to the risk of involvement of parameningeal structures and intracranial extension.

Treatment and prognosis of poor-risk patients with newly diagnosed metastatic rhabdomyosarcoma treated without autologous HSCT

Multimodal therapies such as surgical resection, chemotherapy, and radiation have improved survival in patients with non-metastatic RMS from 20% to 30% in the 1960s to over 70% today (Crist et al., 1995; Pappo et al., 1995). The 5-year OS is 82% for patients with completely resected and localized RMS. However, for patients with metastatic disease at diagnosis, the prognosis is dismal—an estimated 5-year survival of only 20% to 25% (Neifeld et al., 1979; Maurer et al., 1988, 1993; Crist et al., 1995; Pappo et al., 1995).

Despite multiagent intensified therapeutic regimens developed by the Intergroup Rhabdomyosarcoma Study group (IRS) and other groups for treatment of RMS, cure rates have not improved significantly over the past 20 years for patients with metastases or disease at unfavorable sites or with unfavorable histology. In the IRS-I-III study, the 5-year OS for patients with stage IV disease ranged between 20% and 30%, with multiple sites of disease in bone and/or bone marrow sites having the worst prognosis (Maurer et al., 1988, 1993; Crist et al., 1995) (Table 48.5). In the IRS-IV study, an up-front treatment window approach achieved only minimal improvement in outcome for patients with metastatic disease. OS was 33% to 34% at 5 years using ifosfamide in combination with doxorubicin or etoposide and 46% at 2 years using ifosfamide with topotecan (Breitfeld et al., 2001; Pappo et al., 2001; Sandler et al., 2001) (Table 48.5).

The German CWS-81 study reported only an 11% 5-year DFS, while the European Malignant Mesenchymal Tumor (MMT)-89 study reported a 25% 3-year OS for patients with stage IV disease (Koscielniak et al., 1992; Frascella et al., 1996) (Table 48.5). In a review by Koscielniak et al. (1991) of four major European Trials for metastatic RMS (SIOP, MMT-75, CWS 81 and CWS 86), overall survival was approximately 18%. Ferrari et al. (2002) reviewed the results of 16 patients treated with multimodal therapy by the Italian German Cooperative Group (IGCG). The overall survival at 5 years was only 22% (Table 48.5).

Treatment and prognosis of poor-risk patients with progressive relapsed rhabdomyosarcoma treated without autologous HSCT

Approximately 30% of patients relapse after primary therapy for RMS. About 50% to 95% of these relapsed patients die of progressive disease (Rousseau et al., 1994; Crist et al., 1995; Klingbiel et al., 1998). Based on the available data from IRSG studies I–IV, tumor histology, type, and intensity of initial therapy (chemotherapy, surgery, and/or radiation) independently predicted survival after first relapse (Pappo et al., 1999). Embryonal and botyroid histiotypes had a survival advantage over alveolar or undifferentiated subtypes (5-year OS of 64% for botyroid, 26% for embryonal, and 5% for alveolar/undifferentiated RMS, respectively) (Table 48.2).

Local versus metastatic recurrence and longer time to relapse predict longer survival for patients with alveolar RMS, while IRSG clinical stage/group at initial diagnosis was identified as a predictor of outcome for recurrent embryonal RMS (20% 5-year OS for groups I/II vs. 12% for group IV embryonal RMS) (Pappo et al., 1999). Recurrent orbital RMS previously treated with only vincristine and actinomycin D (VA) had an encouraging 86% 5-year OS. Overall, the results of IRS-IV demonstrated only a 16% survival at 5 years for patients who progress or relapse with RMS (Table 48.2).

The German CESS/CWS REZ 91 trial using a carboplatin/etoposide-based regimen demonstrated a 41% 5-yr EFS for ERMS and 25% for ARMS after recurrence (Klingbiel et al., 1998), while the Malignant Mesenchymal Tumor Study (MMT 84) reported an OS of 0% for metastatic disease, 41% for local recurrence of previously nonmetastatic RMS, and over 80% OS for relapsed orbital RMS (Rousseau et al., 1994).

These results have identified a favorable risk group with improved survival postrecurrence for patients with embryonal histology, local or regional relapse, particularly at favorable sites, and an early stage/group disease at initial diagnosis (Bader et al., 1989). Patients who relapse with unfavorable characteristics including alveolar or undifferentiated histology, group II–IV disease at initial diagnosis, metastases (Flamant et al., 1998) and surgically unresectable disease (Klingbiel et al., 1998) have a poor outcome. In Table 48.2 we have reviewed some of the larger reports of retrieval regimens for relapsed soft tissue sarcomas, including RMS and EFST using combination chemotherapy without autologous HSCT. Overall survival

Table 48.5. *Outcome of poor-risk stage IV newly diagnosed rhabdomyosarcoma treated without autologous HSCT*

Author	Study	No. of patients/ age (yrs)	Stage	Regimen, dose per course	Outcome
Maurer *et al.* (1988)	IRS I	N/A 0–21	IV	Vinc 2 mg/m^2; Dact 0.075 mg/m^2; Cy 2.5 mg/m^2/d × 1–2 yrs or 50 mg/kg; ± Dox 60 mg/m^2 + RT	20% 5-yr OS
Maurer *et al.* (1993)	IRS II	N = 172 0–21	IV	Vinc 2 mg/m^2; Dact 0.075 mg/kg; Cy 2.5 mg/kg/d × 2 yrs or 20–30 mg/kg ± Dox 60 mg/m^2 + RT	27% 5-yr OS
Crist *et al.* (1995)	IRS III	N = 150 0–21	IV	Vinc 2 mg/m^2; Dact 0.075 mg–3.6 mg/m^2; Cy 30 mg/kg ± Dox 60 m/m^2 (± DTIC 1 g/m^2); ± Cisp 90 mg/m^2;± Etop 300 mg/m^2 + RT	32% 5-yr OS
Sandler *et al.* (2001)	IRS IV pilot	N = 152 0–21	IV	Vinc 5 mg/m^2; Dact 1.2 mg/m^2; Cy 1.2 g/m^2 + Ifos 9 g/m^2; Dox 60 mg/m^2 + RT	34% 5-yr OS
Breitfeld *et al.* (2001)	IRS IV up front window	N = 128 0–21	IV	Vinc 1.5 mg/m^2; Dact 0.075 mg/kg; Cy 2.2 g/m ± Ifos 9 g/m^2; Etop 500 mg/m^2 or Vinc 1.5 mg/m^2; Mel 30 mg/m^2 + RT	19–33% 5-yr OS
Pappo *et al.* (1999)	IRS IV up front window	N = 48 0–21	IV	Vinc 1.5 mg/m^2; Dact 1.5 mg/m^2; Cy 1.25–2.2 g/m^2 + Topo 3.75–12 mg/m^2 + RT	46% 2-yr OS
Koscielniak *et al.* (1992)	CWS 81	N/A 0–91	IV	Vinc 1.5 mg/m^2; Dox 60 mg/m^2; Cy 1.2 g/m^2 + Ifos 6 g/m^2 + RT	11% 5-yr DFS
Koscielniak *et al.* (1992)	SIOP MMT75 CWS 81 & 86	N = 146 1–18	IV	N/A	18% OS
Frascella *et al.* (1996)	MMT 89	N = 56 0–18	IV	Vinc 1.5 mg/m^2; Dact 1.5 mg/m^2; Ifos 9 g/m^2; Carbo, 500 mg/m^2; Epi 150 mg/m^2; Etop 600 mg/m^2 ± RT	25% 3-yr OS
Ferrari *et al.* (2002)	IGCG	N = 16 0–21	IV*	Vinc 1.5 mg/m^2; Dact 1.5 mg/m^2; Dox 60 mg/m^2; Cy 1.2 mg/m^2; Vinc 1.5 mg/m^2; Dact 1.5 mg/m^2; Dox 80 mg/m^2; Ifos 6 g/m^2; Vinc 1.5 mg/m^2; Dact 1.5 mg/m^2; Epi 150 mg/m^2; Ifos 9 g/m^2; Etop 600 mg/m^2; Carbo 500 mg/m^2 + RT	22% 5-yr OS

Abbreviations: IRS, Intergroup Rhabdomyosarcoma; CWS, German Cooperative Soft Tissue Sarcoma Study; SIOP, Societe Francaise d'Oncologie Pediatrique; MMT, Malignant Mesenchymal Tumor; IGCG, Italian German Cooperative Group comprising ICG, RMS-79,88, & 96; CWS 81, 86, 91 & 96 and MMT 4; N/A, not available; *, paratesticular disease only; Vinc, vincristine; Dact, actinomycin D; Cy, Cyclophosphamide; Dox, doxorubicin; RT, radiotherapy; DTIC, dacarbazine; Cisp, cisplatin; Etop, etoposide; Ifos, ifosfamide; Mel, melphalan; Topo, topotecan; Carbo, carboplatin; Epi, epirubicin; OS, overall survival; DFS, disease-free survival.

remains dismal despite reports of initial tumor response. Drugs that have shown efficacy in retrieval protocols for RMS/ES include topotecan, etoposide, carboplatin, and ifosfamide; however, long-term remissions remain elusive.

This subgroup of refractory/relapsed patients should be considered for innovative experimental therapeutic investigations such as high-dose therapy with newer agents active against RMS followed by autologous HSCT.

Autologous hematopoietic stem cell transplantation for rhabdomyosarcoma

High-dose chemoradiotherapy followed by autologous HSCT has been investigated over the past decade in an effort to eliminate micrometastatic residual disease in high-risk (stage IV) patients with RMS in first complete remission after conven-

tional chemotherapy, or in patients with relapsed or progressive disease in second CR or second PR (Carli *et al.*, 1999). The rationale in part for the use of high-dose chemoradiotherapy and autologous HSCT includes:

1. sensitivity of rhabdomyosarcoma cells in vitro and in xenograft models to high-dose alkylating agents;
2. steep dose-response curves of alkylating agents in conditioning regimens for autologous transplants and little cross-reactivity with agents generally used for upfront therapy to overcome drug resistance;
3. dose-limiting myelosuppression, which can be ameliorated with autologous stem cell transplantation (Weigel *et al.*, 2001).

We have reviewed nine publications reporting the outcome of children, adolescents, and young adults with primary metastatic stage IV RMS, and six publications on relapsed

RMS, treated with high-dose chemotherapy and autologous HSCT. Demographics, histology, conditioning regimen, and outcome are summarized in Table 48.6 (newly diagnosed stage IV) and Table 48.7 (relapsed/progressive disease).

Treatment and prognosis for poor-risk patients with newly diagnosed metastatic (stage IV) rhabdomyosarcoma following autologous HSCT

Pinkerton *et al.* (1991) reported on 43 children and young adults newly diagnosed with RMS. Thirty-six of the 43 patients, 12 of whom had stage IV disease, received vincristine, actinomycin, cyclophosphamide (VAC) induction, high-dose melphalan (140–220 mg/m^2) consolidation followed by autologous HSCT. In the 12 stage IV patients, 8 relapsed, 3 were alive, and 9 died. The 3- and 5-year progression-free and overall survival in the stage IV patients were 20% and 25%, respectively (Table 48.6).

Dumontet *et al.* (1992) reported on 22 children and young adults with locally advanced or metastatic soft tissue sarcomas (hemangiopericytoma, fibrohistiocytomas, leiomyosarcoma, undifferentiated sarcoma, esthesioneuroblastoma, and 11 RMS) who received high-dose chemotherapy and autologous HSCT. High-dose chemotherapy regimens consisted of either melphalan 140 mg/m^2, ± vincristine 3 mg/m^2, ± carboplatin 1.7 g/m^2, ± fractionated total body irradiation or etoposide 1 g/m^2, ifosfamide 12 g/m^2, cisplatin 200 mg/m^2 or busulfan 600 mg/m^2 and cyclophosphamide 4 g/m^2. Four of the 11 patients with RMS had metastatic disease (stage IV). The overall survival rates for the entire group of patients for 2 and 5 years was 40% and 32%, respectively. Two out of the 11 RMS patients were disease-free at a median of 15 months, and the 2-year OS for the RMS group of patients was 40% (Table 48.6).

Horowitz *et al.* (1993) reported on the results of 25 children and young adults newly diagnosed with high-risk RMS receiving TBI/chemotherapy followed by autologous HSCT. Nineteen patients achieved a CR from induction chemotherapy and went on to consolidation with 2 days of TBI (8 Gy), vincristine 2 mg/m^2, doxorubicin 70 mg/m^2, and cyclophosphamide 2.4 g/m^2 and autologous HSCT. Seven patients were alive and 18 were dead. The 6-year EFS and OS for the total patients with RMS was 24% and 28%, respectively (Table 48.6).

Koscielniak *et al.* (1997) reported on the results of 36 children and young adults with metastatic or recurrent RMS treated with high-dose chemotherapy and hematopoietic rescue. Twenty-seven patients had primary metastatic disease (stage IV) at diagnosis. Patients received melphalan 120–180 mg/m^2, ± etoposide 40–60 mg/kg, ± carboplatin 1.2 g/m^2, ± fractionated total body irradiation (12 Gy), ± BCNU, ± cyclophosphamide, ± busulfan, and ± total lymphoid irradiation. Of the total 36 patients, 27 obtained CR1, 2 CR2 and 1 VGPR prior to transplant. Five of the 27 (18.5%) stage IV RMS patients had no evidence of disease (NED) at 57 months. (Table 48.6).

Boulad *et al.* (1998) reported on a prospective study to improve the response and survival rates of children and adolescents with high-risk RMS, extraosseous ES, and undifferenti-

ated sarcoma utilizing a short multiagent induction, hyperfractionated radiotherapy, and consolidation with melphalan 90 mg/m^2 and etoposide 1.5 g/m^2 followed by autologous HSCT for those patients attaining CR or GPR. Twenty-one patients were enrolled, including 14 stage IV patients (12 RMS and 2 ES). Nine of the 14 stage IV patients obtained CR or VGPR and went on autologous HSCT. Relapse occurred in 5 of 9 patients with stage IV disease. The 2-year overall and progression-free survival for the 14 stage IV patients was 50% (Table 48.6).

Malogolowkin *et al.* (1999) reported on the survival of children with metastatic (stage IV) RMS treated with intensive therapy and autologous HSCT. Twenty-three of the 36 patients reported had stage IV RMS. At the time of this report, 4 patients were receiving induction therapy, 1 was lost to follow-up, and 4 had developed progressive disease (PD). Nine patients obtained CR and 5 PR and received a conditioning regimen of carboplatin 1.2 g/m^2, etoposide 480 mg/m^2, and melphalan 210 mg/m^2 followed by autologous HSCT (14 patients). Six patients were alive with NED, 6 had PD, and 2 died. The one- and two-year EFS was 61 ± 11% and 44% ± 12%, respectively (Table 48.6).

Carli *et al.* (1999) reported on a prospective nonrandomized study of children and adolescents comparing high-dose melphalan (200 mg/m^2) and autologous HSCT versus conventional chemotherapy. Fifty-two stage IV RMS patients with metastatic disease obtained CR after induction and proceeded to conditioning and autologous HSCT. Twenty-three patients were alive and 29 were dead at 36 months. The 3-year EFS and OS for these patients was 30% and 40%, respectively, compared to 19% and 28%, respectively, for patients who received conventional chemotherapy consolidation (Table 48.6).

Walterhouse *et al.* (1999) reported on 4 newly diagnosed stage IV metastatic RMS patients who achieved CR after induction and subsequently received high-dose chemotherapy and autologous HSCT. The preparative regimen consisted of thiotepa 900 mg/m^2, carboplatin 6 g/m^2, and cyclophosphamide 1.2 g/m^2. One patient was alive with NED at 53 months, and 3 were dead at 10 to 19 months posttransplant (Table 48.6).

Lastly, Diaz *et al.* (1999) reported on the role of high-dose busulfan and melphalan as conditioning for autologous HSCT in children and adolescents with high-risk solid tumors There were 5 patients with RMS in the total of 30 patients enrolled on this prospective study either at the time of diagnosis or relapse. Patients were not separated out in this report by newly diagnosed or relapsed/progressive status. One patient was in CR1, 2 in CR2, and 2 in PR at the time of autologous HSCT and received busulfan 16 mg/kg and melphalan 140 mg/m^2 followed by autologous HSCT. The 4-year EFS for the entire group was 55% (Table 48.6).

Treatment and prognosis for poor-risk patients with relapsed rhabdomyosarcoma following autologous HSCT

Koscielniak *et al.* (1997) reported on the results of 9 children and young adults with recurrent RMS treated with high-dose

Table 48.6.   *Outcome of poor-risk patients with newly diagnosed stage IV rhabdomyosarcoma treated with autologous HSCT*

Author	No. of patients/ age (yrs)	Histology	Stage	Metastasis at diagnosis	Status at HSCT	Conditioning regimen/dose	Outcome: Alive/Dead	Survival
Pinkerton et al. (1991)	N = 12 0.8–21	Alveolar Embryonal Undiff Botryoid	IV	Lung, bone, BM	NA	Mel 140–220 mg/m²	A-3 D-9	25% 5-yr OS
Dumontet et al. (1992)	N = 4 4–23	N/A	IV	N/A	N/A	Mel 140 mg/m² + Vinc 3 mg/m² + Carbo 1.7 g/m² ± FTBI OR Etop 1 g/m² + Ifos 12 g/m² + Cisp 200 mg/m² OR Bu 600 mg/m² + Cy 4 g/m²	NA	NA
Horowitz et al. (1993)	N = 19 2–38	Alveolar Embryonal	NA	N/A	19 CR	TBI 8 Gy, Vinc 2 mg/m², Dox 70 mg/m², Cy 2.4 g/m²	NA	NA
Koscielniak et al. (1996)	N = 27 0–22	Alveolar Embryonal Undiff	IV	N/A	N/A	Mel 120–180 mg/m², ± Etop 40–60 mg/kg, ± Carbo 1.2 g/m², ± FTBI 12 Gy, ± BCNU, ± Cy, ± Bu, ± TBI	A-5 D-22	NA
Boulad et al. (1998)	N = 7 1.1–23	Alveolar Embryonal	IV	N/A	N/A	Mel 90 mg/m²/BID, Etop 1.5 g/m²/d	NA	NA
Malogolowkin et al. (1999)	N = 14	N/A	IV	N/A	9 CR 5 PR	Carbo 1.2 g/m², Etop 480 mg/m², Mel 210 mg/m²	A-6 D-8	61% 1-yr EFS
Carli et al. (1999)	NA N = 52 0.25–18	Alevolar Embryonal	IV	Bone, BM, lung	52 CR	Mel 200 mg/m²	A-23 D-29	44% 2-yr EFS 30% 3-yr EFS 40% 3-yr OS
Walterhouse et al. (1999)	N = 4 3–17	Alevolar Embryonal Undiff	IV	Lungs, BM, liver, bone	4 CR	Thio 900 mg/m², Carbo 6 g/m², Cy 1.2 g/m²	A-1 D-3	NA
Diaz et al.[a] (1999)	N = 5 2–21	N/A	IV	N/A	1 CR1 2 CR 2 2 PR	Bu 16 mg/kg, Mel 140 mg/m²	NA	NA

Abbreviations: NA, not available; BM, bone marrow; CR, complete response; PR, partial response; Mel, melphalan; Vinc, vincristine; Carbo, carboplatin; FTBI, fractionated total body irradiation; Etop, etoposide; Ifos, ifosfamide; Cisp, cisplatinum; Bu, Busulfan; Cy, cytoxan; TBI, total body irradiation; Dox, doxorubicin; carbo, carboplatin; Thio, thiotepa; A, alive; D, dead; OS, overall survival; EFS, event-free survival.
[a] Report did not separate newly diagnosed and relapsed patients.

Table 48.7. *Outcome of poor-risk patients with relapsed rhabdomyosarcoma treated with autologous HSCT*

Author	No. of Patients/ age (yrs)	Histology	Status at HSCT	Conditioning regimen/dose	Outcome: Alive/Dead
Koscielniak *et al.* (1996)	$N = 9$ 0–22	Alveolar Embryonal Undiff	5 CR2 4 VGPR	Mel 120–180 mg/m^2, ± Etop 40–60 mg/kg, ± Carbo 1.2 g/m^2, ± FTBI 12 Gy, ± BCNU, ± Cy, ± Bu, ± TLI	A-5 D-4
Ozkaynak *et al.* (1998)	$N = 2$ 2–21	NA	1 VGPR 1-CR	Mel 200 mg/m^2, Carbo 1.2 g/m^2, Etop 800 mg/m^2, ± Cy 750 mg/m^2	A-0 D-2
Hara *et al.* (1998)	$N = 2$ 1–19	Embryonal	2 CR D-0	Thio 600–1,000 mg/m^2, Mel 150–300 mg/m^2, Bu 8–10 mg/kg	A-2
Lucidarme *et al.* (1998)	$N = 8$ 2–17	N/A	2 PR 6 PD	Thio 900 mg/m^2	A-1 D-7
Parentesis *et al.* (1999)	$N = 2$ 10–12	Alveolar Embryonal	1 CR2 1 PR3	Etop 1.8 g/m^2, Thio 900 mg/m^2, Cy 1.2 g/m^2 OR Bu 12 mg/kg, Mel 100 mg/m^2, Thio 500 mg/m^2	A-0 D-2

Abbreviations: N/A, not available; CR, complete response; VGPR, very good partial response; PR, partial response; PD, progressive disease; Mel, melphalan; Etop, etoposide; Carbo, carboplatin; FTBI, fractionated total body irradiation; BCNU, 3-bis (2-chloroethyl)-1-nitrosurea; Cy, cytoxan; Bu, busulfan; TBI, total body irradiation; Thio, thiotepa; A, alive; D, dead.

chemotherapy and autologous HSCT. Patients received melphalan 120–180 mg/m^2, ± etoposide 40–60 mg/kg, ± carboplatin 1.2 g/m^2, ± fractionated total body irradiation (12 Gy), ± BCNU, ± cyclophosphamide, ± busulfan, and ± total lymphoid irradiation. Four of the 9 (44%) relapsed patients had NED at 57 months (Table 48.7).

We reported on the results of a double-alkylator and non-TBI conditioning regimen followed by autologous HSCT in patients with a variety of solid tumors (Ozkaynak *et al.,* 1998). Twenty-seven children and adolescents were treated in first remission or at relapse. There were 2 RMS patients, 1 in CR and 1 in VGPR after consolidation. The conditioning regimen utilized melphalan 200 mg/m^2, carboplatin 1.2 g/m^2, etoposide 800 mg/m^2, and ± cyclophosphamide 3 g/m^2. One patient developed PD at 8 months and died and one patient died of toxicity (Table 48.7).

Hara *et al.* (1998) reported on the results of 28 children and adolescents with poor prognosis solid tumors receiving two tandem conditioning regimens of thiotepa 600–1000 mg/m^2, busulfan 8–10 mg/kg, and ± melphalan 150–300 mg/m^2 followed by autologous HSCT. These patients had either advanced, chemoresistant and/or relapsed disease. There were 2 RMS patients, 1 in first relapse and one in third relapse, both in CR at time of transplant. Both patients were alive at 21 and 32 months, respectively, with no evidence of disease (Table 48.7).

Lucidarme *et al.* (1998) reported on a phase II study of thiotepa 900 mg/m^2 and autologous HSCT in children with various solid tumors. There were 8 RMS patients, 6 in first relapse, 1 in second, and 1 in third relapse. At the time of autologous HSCT, 2 patients had achieved PR and 6 had PD. One patient was alive in CR and 7 died (Table 48.7).

Perentesis *et al.* (1999) reported on autologous HSCT for 24 children and young adults with various relapsed or metastatic solid tumors (Wilms', Ewing's sarcoma, neuroblastoma, osteosarcoma, yolk sac, and RMS). There were 2 RMS patients

in CR2 and PR3, respectively, at the time of transplantation. The conditioning regimen consisted of etoposide 1.8 g/m^2, thiotepa 900 mg/m^2, cyclophosphamide 1.2 g/m^2 or busulfan 12 mg/kg, melphalan 100 mg/m^2 and thiotepa 500 mg/m^2. Both patients died of progressive disease after transplant (Table 48.7).

We have reviewed 13 publications on children, adolescents, and young adults either with newly diagnosed and/or relapsed/progressive rhabdomyosarcoma treated with various combinations of myeloablative chemoradiotherapy and autologous HSCT. We have reviewed the results of over 130 patients (8 months to 38 years) with newly diagnosed stage IV RMS, treated in first CR/PR. The overall disease-free survival ranged from 20% to 45%. The use of myeloablative therapy and autologous HSCT may be associated with improved outcome compared to the conventional therapy (surgery, chemotherapy, radiation) in patients with newly diagnosed stage IV RMS or the results could have occurred because of selection bias (Table 48.6 vs. Table 48.5, respectively).

Of 23 patients with relapsed/progressive RMS aged 0 to 22 years receiving various myeloablative chemoradiotherapy regimens and autologous HSCT, 8 patients were alive and in CR (35%). Although these data appear favorable compared to the <10% survival achieved with conventional therapy at 5 years after relapse, the numbers are small and the prognostic factors vary between studies (Table 48.7 vs. Table 48.2).

Only prospective randomized trials in both newly diagnosed stage IV RMS and in relapsed/progressive RMS can determine if high-dose therapy and autologous HSCT is superior to conventional dose therapy.

Autologous HSCT for osteogenic sarcoma

There are few reports of autologous transplantation in osteogenic sarcoma. In an Italian sarcoma group study, 32 patients with high-grade osteosarcoma in metastatic relapse received high-dose carboplatin and etoposide with stem cell support. A second course was planned 4 to 6 weeks after the first. Surgery was allowed before or after chemotherapy. One died of toxicity (3%). Twenty-five patients achieved complete remission, six were alive with disease progression. At the time of publication, 14 patients were alive at a median of 23 months (4 in first CR, 3 in second CR, and 1 in fourth CR). Six were alive with disease; 18 (56%) died (17 of disease and 1 of toxicity). The 3-year overall survival rate was 20% and the 3-year disease-free survival rate was 12% (Fagioli et al., 2002).

In a smaller adjuvant study, 6 patients with osteosarcoma received 25 mg/kg cyclophosphamide i.v. every other day for 5 doses. Three remained alive with no evidence of disease at 2.5, 3, and 5 years following diagnosis (Shepp et al., 1978). One patient, transplanted in Australia after 200 mg/m^2 of melphalan, had stable pulmonary metastases but complete resolution of scalp lesions (Mauger, 1982) (Table 48.8).

Autologous HSCT in adults with soft tissue sarcoma

Most studies of high-dose therapy in adults with sarcomas include ifosfamide, carboplatin, and etoposide. In a Dana-Farber Cancer Institute (DFCI) study of escalating doses of ifosfamide, dose-limiting renal toxicity was observed at 20 g/m^2 and thus 18 g/m^2 was the recommended maximum tolerated dose. Twenty patients with sarcoma were evaluated, of whom 1 responded completely and 6 partially, for an overall response rate of 35% (Elias et al., 1990). In the subsequent phase I study of ifosfamide at 12 g/m^2 and escalating doses of carboplatin (400 to 1,600 mg/m^2), both given by continuous infusion over 4 days with mesna and autologous marrow support, renal toxicity precluded further dose escalation. Of 8 patients with advanced refractory sarcoma, 4 responded partially or completely (Elias et al., 1991).

In the next phase I study, high-dose ifosfamide, carboplatin, and etoposide were given as consolidation to patients with sarcomas responding to conventional dose therapy. The maximum tolerated doses were 16 g/m^2 ifosfamide, 1.8 g/m^2 carboplatin, and 1.2 g/m^2 etoposide; renal toxicity again precluded further dose escalation. Twenty sarcoma patients were entered, of whom 16 were evaluable for response. Two responded completely and one partially for an overall response rate of 19% (Elias et al., 1995).

Fields et al. (1995) also reported a study of escalating doses of ifosfamide 6 to 24 g/m^2, carboplatin 1.2 to 2.1 g/m^2, and etoposide 1.8 to 3 g/m^2 (ICE) divided over 6 days with mesna and stem cell support. The MTD of the ICE regimen in this study was considerably higher than the MTD in the DFCI study—20.1 g/m^2 of ifosfamide, 1.8 g/m^2 of carboplatin, and 3.0 g/m^2 of etoposide. Dose-limiting toxicities included CNS toxicity and renal failure. Severe but reversible mucositis and enteritis occurred at the MTD in 78% and 33% of patients, respectively. Regimen-related deaths occurred in 8% of patients treated at all dose levels and 4% treated at the MTD. Four patients with sarcoma were treated; one had a partial response. Renal toxicity of high-dose ifosfamide, carboplatin, and etoposide was dose-related and reversible in the majority of patients. Serum bicarbonate, potassium, and magnesium levels fell despite massive replacement (Agaliotis et al., 1997).

Dumontet et al. (1992) treated 22 patients with locally advanced or metastatic soft tissue sarcoma with various high-dose chemotherapy regimens followed by marrow support. Six patients (4 CRs and 2 PRs) were treated as front-line therapy, 8 in second or subsequent CR, 1 in first and 4 in second or subsequent PR, 13 after chemosensitive relapse, and 3 with primary refractory disease. One patient died of infection. The median overall and disease-free survival rates were 19 and 15 months, respectively. The actuarial survival rates at 2 and 5 years were 40% and 32%, respectively. Eight patients remained free of disease.

Between 1988 and 1994, 30 patients with locally advanced, unresectable soft tissue sarcoma who were responding to a standard chemotherapy regimen received ifosfamide (12 g/m^2), etoposide (800 mg/m^2), and cisplatin (200 mg/m^2) (VIC). Nineteen patients (63%) experienced some renal toxicity. Eight patients were in complete remission before high-dose therapy. Of the 22 patients with partial or minor responses to conventional chemotherapy, 4 (18%) achieved CR, 3 (13%) PR, 12 (54%) stable disease, and 3 (14%) progressed by day 60. After a median follow-up of 94 months, overall and progression-free survival rates at 5 years were 23% and 21%, respectively. Of patients in complete response at the time of high-dose therapy, 75% survived 5 years compared with 5% of other patients (P = .001) (Blay et al., 2000) (Table 48.9).

Table 48.8. *Outcome of poor-risk patients with osteosarcoma treated with autologous HSCT*

Author	Study/Group	No. of patients	Stage	Regimen	Outcome: Alive/Dead	Survival
Fagioli et al. (2002)	Italian Sarcoma Group	32	Metastatic/relapse	Carboplatin/etoposide	A-14 D-18	20% 3-yr OS 12% 3-yr DFS
Shepp et al. (1978)		6	Metastatic	Cyclophosphamide	A-3 D-3	NA
Mauger (1982)		1	Metastatic/relapse	Melphalan	A-1	NA

Abbreviation: NA, not available.

Table 48.9. *Outcome of adult patients with poor-risk soft tissue sarcomas treated with autologous HSCT*

Author	Study/Group	No. of patients	Regimen	Response	Survival
Elias *et al.* (1990)	DFCI	20	Ifosfamide	CR-1 PR-6	NA
Elias *et al.* (1991)	DFCI	8	Ifosfamide, carboplatin	ORR-4	NA
Elias *et al.* (1995)	DFCI	16	Ifos 16 g/m^2, Carbo 1.8 g/m^2, Etop 1.2 g/m^2	ORR-3	NA
Fields *et al.* (1995)	Florida	4	Ifos 6–24 g/m^2, Carbo 1.2–2.1 g/m^2, Etop 1.8–3 g/m^2	PR-1	NA
Dumontet *et al.* (1992)	Centre Leon Berard	22	Varied regimens	NA	32% 5-yr OS
Blay *et al.* (2000)	Centre Leon Berard	30	Ifos 12 g/m^2, Cis 200 mg/m^2, Etop 800 mg/m^2	NA	23% 5-yr OS

Abbreviations: DFCI, Dana Farber Cancer Institute; Ifos, ifosfamide; Carbo, carboplatin; Etop, etoposide; Cis, cisplatin; CR, complete response; PR, partial response; ORR, overall response rate; NA, not available; OS, overall survival.

Table 48.10. *Future strategies to enhance stem cell transplantation for poor-risk sarcomas*

Strategy	Reference
Incorporation of chemoprotective agents (amifostine, etc.)	Capizzi (1999)
Circumvention of drug resistance (verapamil, etc.)	Houtenbos *et al.* (2001)
Investigation of new cytotoxic agents (camptothecins, etc.)	Pappo *et al.* (2001)
	Pappo *et al.* (2002)
Ex vivo purging of autologous stem cells (immunomagnetic separation, etc.)	Ghavimi *et al.* (1981)
	Merino *et al.* (2001)
	Moss *et al.* (1994)
	Rill *et al.* (1994)
Dendritic cell based immunotherapy (peptide pulsing, etc.)	Geiger *et al.* (2000)
Immunoregulatory cytokines post stem cell transplantation (IL-2, etc.)	Sosman *et al.* (2001)
Identification of new target genes (CD99)	Liu *et al.* (2000)
	Scotlandi *et al.* (2000)
Tumor vaccination therapy (Pax7-FKHR, etc.)	Mackall *et al.* (1998)
	Mackall *et al.* (2000)
Reduced-intensity allogeneic stem cell transplantation (fludarabine/cyclophosphamide, etc.)	Childs *et al.* (2000)

Autologous hematopoietic stem cell transplantation for nephroblastoma (Wilms' tumor[1])

The prognosis for childhood Wilms' tumor, even those patients with metastatic disease at diagnosis and/or those with recurrent disease, is excellent with conventional chemotherapy with or without local radiotherapy. However, there is a subset of patients that may benefit from high-dose chemotherapy and autologous HSCT. Patients expected to have less than a 20% chance of survival include those with unfavorable histology, relapse within 6 months of diagnosis, failure of 3-drug chemotherapy, involvement of sites of recurrence other than lung and abdomen, or abnormal recurrence after abdominal radiation therapy (Chen and Civin, 1999).

The European Bone Marrow Transplantation Solid Tumor Registry has reported the results of 25 patients with Wilms' tumor who received myeloablative therapy and HSCT from 1984-1991. Seventeen patients were in CR and 8 had measur-

able disease. Seven different high-dose regimens were administered. Of the 17 patients grafted in CR, 8 were alive and event-free, but only one of 8 patients grafted with measurable disease was alive and disease-free (Garaventa *et al.*, 1994). The Societe Francaise d'Oncologie Pediatrique (SFOP) conducted a phase II trial of myeloablative therapy with melphalan, etoposide and carboplatin and autologous HSCT in 29 patients with Wilms' tumor (15-2nd CR, 3-2nd PR, 3-3rd CR, 5-3rd PR, 1-5th PR, and 2 with stage IV anaplastic histology at diagnosis). Fourteen patients (50%) remained alive and disease-free 3 years post-transplant (Pein *et al.*, 1998) These results suggest that in patients with poor prognosis Wilms' tumor, myeloablative therapy and autologous HSCT may provide long-term disease-free survival. Future randomized and prospective studies are needed to more specifically address the role of this therapy in this subgroup of patients.

Future directions

The results of myeloablative therapy and autologous HSCT in poor-risk patients with stage IV and/or recurrent/progressive

[1]Max Wilms, German surgeon, 1867-1918.

RMS and ES are sufficiently interesting to justify well-controlled prospective randomized multicenter trials to definitively determine clinical benefit, if any. Potential reasons for disease progression and death despite myeloablative therapy and autologous HSCT include the number of tumor cells at the time of high-dose therapy, virtually guaranteeing the presence of tumor cells with intrinsic and acquired multidrug resistance. If a dose effect was proven in randomized trials, reasonable research strategies to eliminate residual disease after high-dose therapy would include induction of graft-versus-tumor effect or the use of other specific targeted therapy (e.g., therapy directed against the fusion proteins produced by the characteristic translocations in Ewing's sarcoma or alveolar RMS or downstream targets).

New therapeutic stem and immune cell strategies to potentially improve the outcome in patients with poor-risk rhabdomyosarcoma and Ewing's sarcoma are summarized in Table 48.10. Carefully designed translational and clinical trials will be required to determine if any of these stem cell transplant strategies, alone or in combination, will enhance long-term survival in this poor-risk group of patients.

References

Agaliotis, D.P., Ballester, O.F., Mattox, T. et al. (1997). Nephrotoxicity of high-dose ifosfamide/carboplatin/etoposide in adults undergoing autologous stem cell transplantation. American Journal of the Medical Sciences, 314, 292–8.

Antman, K.H. (1992). Chemotherapy of advanced sarcomas of bone and soft tissue. Seminars in Oncology, 19(6 Suppl 12), 13–20.

Atra, A., Whelan, J.S., Calvagna, V. et al. (1997). High-dose busulphan/melphalan with autologous stem cell rescue in Ewing's sarcoma. Bone Marrow Transplantation, 20, 843–6.

Bacci, G., Ferrari, S., Bertoni, F. et al. (2000). Neoadjuvant chemotherapy for peripheral malignant neuroectodermal tumor of bone: recent experience at the Istituto Rizzoli. Journal of Clinical Oncology, 18, 885–92.

Bacci, G., Toni, A., Avella, M. et al. (1989). Long-term results in 144 localized Ewing's sarcoma patients treated with combined therapy. Cancer, 63, 1477–86.

Bader, J.L., Horowitz, M.E., Dewan, R. et al. (1989). Intensive combined modality therapy of small round cell and undifferentiated sarcomas in children and young adults: local control and patterns of failure. Radiotherapy and Oncology, 16, 189–201.

Blaney, S.M., Needle, M.N., Gillespie, A. et al. (1998). Phase II trial of topotecan administered as 72-hour continuous infusion in children with refractory solid tumors: a collaborative Pediatric Branch, National Cancer Institute, and Children's Cancer Group Study. Clinical Cancer Research, 4, 357–60.

Blay, J.Y., Bouhour, D., Ray-Coquard, I. et al. (2000). High-dose chemotherapy with autologous hematopoietic stem-cell transplantation for advanced soft tissue sarcoma in adults. Journal of Clinical Oncology, 18, 3643–50.

Boulad, F., Kernan, N.A., LaQuaglia, M.P. et al. (1998). High-dose induction chemoradiotherapy followed by autologous bone marrow transplantation as consolidation therapy in rhabdomyosarcoma, extraosseous Ewing's sarcoma, and undifferentiated sarcoma. Journal of Clinical Oncology, 16, 1697–706.

Breitfeld, P.P., Lyden, E., Raney, R.B. et al. (2001). Ifosfamide and etoposide are superior to vincristine and melphalan for pediatric metastatic rhabdomyosarcoma when administered with irradiation and combination chemotherapy: a report from the Intergroup Rhabdomyosarcoma Study Group. Journal of Pediatric Hematology and Oncology, 23, 225–33.

Burdach, S., Jurgens, H., Peters, C. et al. (1993). Myeloablative radiochemotherapy and hematopoietic stem-cell rescue in poor-prognosis Ewing's sarcoma. Journal of Clinical Oncology, 11, 1482–8.

Cangir, A., Vietti, T.J., Gehan, E.A. et al. (1990). Ewing's sarcoma metastatic at diagnosis. Results and comparisons of two intergroup Ewing's sarcoma studies. Cancer, 66, 887–93.

Capizzi, R.L. (1999). Clinical status and optimal use of amifostine. Oncology (Huntingt), 13, 47–59; discussion 63, 67.

Carli, M., Colombatti, R., Oberlin, O. et al. (1999). High-dose melphalan with autologous stem-cell rescue in metastatic rhabdomyosarcoma. Journal of Clinical Oncology, 17: 2796–803.

Carpenter, P.A., White, L., McCowage, G.B. et al. (1997). A dose-intensive, cyclophosphamide-based regimen for the treatment of recurrent/progressive or advanced solid tumors of childhood: a report from the Australia and New Zealand Children's Cancer Study Group. Cancer, 80, 489–96.

Castello, M.A., Clerico, A., Jenkner, A., & Dominici, C. (1990). A pilot study of high-dose carboplatin and pulsed etoposide in the treatment of childhood solid tumors. Pediatric Hematology and Oncology, 7, 129–35.

Chan, K.W., Petropoulos, D., Choroszy, M. et al. (1997). High-dose sequential chemotherapy and autologous stem cell reinfusion in advanced pediatric solid tumors. Bone Marrow Transplantation, 20, 1039–43.

Chen, A.R. and C.I. Civin (1999). Hematopoietic cell transplantation for pediatric solid tumors. Hematopoietic Cell Transplantation, E.D. Thomas, K.G. Blume and S.J. Forman. Malden, MA: Blackwell Science, Inc: 1092–1104.

Childs, R., Chernoff, A., Contentin, N. et al. (2000). Regression of metastatic renal-cell carcinoma after nonmyeloablative allogeneic peripheral-blood stem-cell transplantation. New England Journal of Medicine, 343, 750–8.

Cotterill, S.J., Ahrens, S., Paulussen, M. et al. (2000). Prognostic factors in Ewing's tumor of bone: analysis of 975 patients from the European Intergroup Cooperative Ewing's Sarcoma Study Group. Journal of Clinical Oncology, 18, 3108–14.

Craft, A., Cotterill, S., Malcolm, A. et al. (1998). Ifosfamide-containing chemotherapy in Ewing's sarcoma. The Second United Kingdom Children's Cancer Study Group and the Medical Research Council Ewing's Tumor Study. Journal of Clinical Oncology, 16, 3628–33.

Craft, A.W., Cotterill, S.J., Bullimore, J.A., & Pearson, D. (1997). Long-term results from the first UKCCSG Ewing's Tumour Study (ET-1). United Kingdom Children's Cancer Study Group (UKCCSG) and the Medical Research Council Bone Sarcoma Working Party. European Journal of Cancer, 33, 1061–9.

Crist, W., Gehan, E.A., Ragab, A.H. et al. (1995). The Third Intergroup Rhabdomyosarcoma Study. Journal of Clinical Oncology, 13, 610–30.

Crist, W.M., Anderson, J.R., Meza, J.L. et al. (2001). Intergroup rhabdomyosarcoma study-IV: results for patients with non-metastatic disease. Journal of Clinical Oncology, 19, 3091–102.

Crist, W.M., Garnsey, L., Beltangady, M.S. et al. (1990). Prognosis in children with rhabdomyosarcoma: a report of the intergroup rhabdomyosarcoma studies I and II. Intergroup Rhabdomyosarcoma Committee. Journal of Clinical Oncology, 8, 443–52.

Delattre, O., Zucman, J., Melot, T. et al. (1994). The Ewing family of tumors—a subgroup of small-round-cell tumors defined by specific chimeric transcripts. New England Journal of Medicine, 331, 294–9.

Delattre, O., Zucman, J., Plougastel, B. et al. (1992). Gene fusion with an ETS DNA-binding domain caused by chromosome translocation in human tumours. Nature, 359, 162–5.

Diaz, M.A., Vicent, M.G., & Madero, L. (1999). High-dose busulfan/melphalan as conditioning for autologous PBPC transplantation in pediatric patients with solid tumors. Bone Marrow Transplantation, 24, 1157–9.

Dumontet, C., Biron, P., Bouffet, E. et al. (1992). High-dose chemotherapy with ABMT in soft tissue sarcomas: a report of 22 cases. Bone Marrow Transplantation, 10, 405–8.

Dunst, J., Paulussen, M., & Jurgens, H. (1993). Lung irradiation for Ewing's sarcoma with pulmonary metastases at diagnosis: results of the CESS-studies. Strahlentherapie Onkologic, 169, 621–3.

Dunst, J., Sauer, R., Burgers, J.M. et al. (1991). Radiation therapy as local treatment in Ewing's sarcoma. Results of the Cooperative Ewing's Sarcoma Studies CESS 81 and CESS 86. Cancer, 67, 2818–25.

Elias, A.D., Ayash, L.J., Eder, J.P. et al. (1991). A phase I study of high-dose ifosfamide and escalating doses of carboplatin with autologous bone marrow support. Journal of Clinical Oncology, 9, 320–7.

Elias, A.D., Ayash, L.J., Wheeler, C. et al. (1995). Phase I study of high-dose ifosfamide, carboplatin and etoposide with autologous hematopoietic stem cell support. Bone Marrow Transplantation, 15, 373–9.

Elias, A.D., Eder, J.P., Shea, T. et al. (1990). High-dose ifosfamide with mesna uroprotection: a phase I study. Journal of Clinical Oncology, 8, 170–8.

Emminger, W., Emminger-Schmidmeier, W., Peters, C. et al. (1991). Is treatment intensification by adding etoposide and carboplatin to fractionated total body irradiation and melphalan acceptable in children with solid tumors with respect to toxicity? Bone Marrow Transplantation, 8, 119–23.

Evans, R.G., Nesbit, M.E., Gehan, E.A. et al. (1991). Multimodal therapy for the management of localized Ewing's sarcoma of pelvic and sacral bones: a report from the second intergroup study. Journal of Clinical Oncology, 9, 1173–80.

Fagioli, F., Aglietta, M., Tienghi, A. et al. (2002). High-dose chemotherapy in the treatment of relapsed osteosarcoma: an Italian sarcoma group study. Journal of Clinical Oncology, 20, 2150–6.

Fellinger, E.J., Garin-Chesa, P., Triche, T.J. et al. (1991). Immunohistochemical analysis of Ewing's sarcoma cell surface antigen p30/32MIC2. American Journal of Pathology, 139, 317–25.

Ferrari, A., Bisogno, G., Casanova, M. et al. (2002). Paratesticular rhabdomyosarcoma: report from the Italian and German Cooperative Group. Journal of Clinical Oncology, 20, 449–55.

Fields, K.K., Elfenbein, G.J., Lazarus, H.M. et al. (1995). Maximum-tolerated doses of ifosfamide, carboplatin, and etoposide given over 6 days followed by autologous stem-cell rescue: toxicity profile. Journal of Clinical Oncology, 13, 323–32.

Flamant, F., Rodary, C., Rey, A. et al. (1998). Treatment of non-metastatic rhabdomyosarcomas in childhood and adolescence. Results of the second study of the International Society of Paediatric Oncology: MMT84. European Journal of Cancer, 34, 1050–62.

Frascella, E., Pritchard-Jones, K., Modak, S. et al. (1996). Response of previously untreated metastatic rhabdomyosarcoma to combination chemotherapy with carboplatin, epirubicin and vincristine. European Journal of Cancer, 32A, 821–5.

Fraumeni, J.F., Jr. & Glass, A.G. (1970). Rarity of Ewing's sarcoma among U.S. Negro children. Lancet, 1, 366–7.

Garaventa, A.O., Hartmann, J.L., Bernard, J.M. et al. (1994). Autologous bone marrow transplantation for pediatric Wilm's tumor: the experience of the European Bone Marrow Transplantation Solid Tumor Registry. Medical and Pediatric Oncology, 22, 11–14.

Geiger, J., Hutchinson, R., Hohenkirk, L. et al. (2000). Treatment of solid tumours in children with tumour-lysate-pulsed dendritic cells. Lancet, 356, 1163–5.

Ghavimi, F., Exelby, P.R., Jereb, B. et al. (1981). Multidisciplinary treatment of advanced stages of embryonal rhabdomyosarcoma in children. National Cancer Institute Monograph, (56), 103–9.

Grabois, M., Frappaz, D., Bouffet, E. et al. (1994). High-dose VP16 cisplatinum in soft tissue sarcoma of children. Cancer Chemotherapy and Pharmacology, 33, 355–7.

Gurney, J.G., Davis, S., Severson, R.K. et al. (1996). Trends in cancer incidence among children in the U.S. Cancer, 78, 532–41.

Hara, J., Osugi, Y., Ohta, H. et al. (1998). Double-conditioning regimens consisting of thiotepa, melphalan and busulfan with stem cell rescue for the treatment of pediatric solid tumors. Bone Marrow Transplantation, 22, 7–12.

Hayes, F.A., Thompson, E.I., Meyer, W.H. et al. (1989). Therapy for localized Ewing's sarcoma of bone. Journal of Clinical Oncology, 7, 208–13.

Hayes, F.A., Thompson, E.I., Parvey, L. et al. (1987). Metastatic Ewing's sarcoma: remission induction and survival. Journal of Clinical Oncology, 5, 1199–204.

Horn, R.C.J. & Enterline, H.T. (1958). Rhabdomyosarcoma: a clinicopathological study and classification of 39 cases. Cancer, 11, 181–99.

Horowitz, M.E., Kinsella, T.J., Wexler, L.H. et al. (1993). Total-body irradiation and autologous bone marrow transplant in the treatment of high-risk Ewing's sarcoma and rhabdomyosarcoma. Journal of Clinical Oncology, 11, 1911–18.

Horowitz, M.E., Malawer, M.M., Woo, S.Y., & Hicks, M.J. (1997). Ewing's sarcoma family of tumors: Ewing's sarcoma of bone and soft tissue and the peripheral primitive neuroectodermal tumors. In Principles and Practice of Pediatric Oncology, 3rd ed, ed. P.A. Pizzo & D.G. Poplack, pp. 831–64. Philadelphia: Lippincott-Raven.

Houtenbos, I., Bracho, F., Davenport, V. et al. (2001). Autologous bone marrow transplantation for childhood acute lymphoblastic leukemia: a novel combined approach consisting of ex vivo marrow purging, modulation of multi-drug resistance, induction of autograft vs leukemia effect, and post-transplant immuno- and chemotherapy (PTIC). *Bone Marrow Transplantation*, **27**, 145–53.

Keohan, M.L. & Taub, R.N. (1997). Chemotherapy for advanced sarcoma: therapeutic decisions and modalities. *Seminars in Oncology*, **24**, 572–9.

Kinsella, T.J., Miser, J.S., Waller, B. *et al.* (1991). Long-term follow-up of Ewing's sarcoma of bone treated with combined modality therapy. *International Journal of Radiation Oncology, Biology, and Physics*, **20**, 389–95.

Klingebiel, T., Pertl, U., Hess, C.F. *et al.* (1998). Treatment of children with relapsed soft tissue sarcoma: report of the German CESS/CWS REZ 91 trial. *Medical and Pediatric Oncology*, **30**, 269–75.

Koscielniak, E., Harms, D., Jurgens, H. *et al.* (1996). Malignant peripheral neuroectodermal tumors (MPNT) and extraosseous Ewing sarcoma (EES) in childhood and adolescence: results of the German Cooperative Soft Tissue Sarcoma Studies CWS-81 + 86. *Medical and Pediatric Oncology*, **21**, 265.

Koscielniak, E., Jurgens, H., Winkler, K. *et al.* (1992). Treatment of soft tissue sarcoma in childhood and adolescence. A report of the German Cooperative Soft Tissue Sarcoma Study. *Cancer*, **70**, 2557–67.

Koscielniak, E., Klingebiel, T.H., Peters, C. *et al.* (1997). Do patients with metastatic and recurrent rhabdomyosarcoma benefit from high-dose therapy with hematopoietic rescue? Report of the German/Austrian Pediatric Bone Marrow Transplantation Group. *Bone Marrow Transplantation*, **19**, 227–31.

Koscielniak, E., Treuner, J., Jurgens, H. *et al.* (1991). Treatment of soft tissue sarcomas in childhood and adolescence: results of the CWS-81 multicenter therapy study. *Klinische Padiatrie*, **203**, 211–9.

Kung, F.H., Harris, M.B., & Krischer, J.P. (1999). Ifosfamide/carboplatin/etoposide (ICE), an effective salvaging therapy for recurrent malignant non-Hodgkin lymphoma of childhood: a Pediatric Oncology Group phase II study. *Medical and Pediatric Oncology*, **32**, 225–6.

Kung, F.H., Pratt, C.B., Vega, R.A. *et al.* (1993). Ifosfamide/etoposide combination in the treatment of recurrent malignant solid tumors of childhood. A Pediatric Oncology Group Phase II study. *Cancer*, **71**, 1898–903.

Kushner, B.H., Kramer, K., Meyers, P.A. *et al.* (2000). Pilot study of topotecan and high-dose cyclophosphamide for resistant pediatric solid tumors. *Medical and Pediatric Oncology*, **35**, 468–74.

Kushner, B.H., LaQuaglia, M.P., Cheung, N.K. *et al.* (1999). Clinically critical impact of molecular genetic studies in pediatric solid tumors. *Medical and Pediatric Oncology*, **33**, 530–35.

Kushner, B.H. & Meyers, P.A. (2001). How effective is dose-intensive/myeloablative therapy against Ewing's sarcoma/primitive neuroectodermal tumor metastatic to bone or bone marrow? The Memorial Sloan-Kettering experience and a literature review. *Journal of Clinical Oncology*, **19**, 870–80.

Landis, S.H., Murray, T., Bolden, S., & Wingo, P.A. (1998). Cancer statistics, 1998. *CA Cancer Journal for Clinicians*, **48**, 6–29.

Lanza, L.A., Miser, J.S., Pass, H.I., & Roth, J.A. (1987). The role of resection in the treatment of pulmonary metastases from Ewing's sarcoma. *Journal of Thoracic and Cardiovascular Surgery*, **94**, 181–7.

Lawrence, W., Jr., Gehan, E.A., Hays, D.M. *et al.* (1987). Prognostic significance of staging factors of the UICC staging system in childhood rhabdomyosarcoma: a report from the Intergroup Rhabdomyosarcoma Study (IRS-II). *Journal of Clinical Oncology*, **5**, 46–54.

Liu, X.F., Helman, L.J., Yeung, C. *et al.* (2000). XAGE-1, a new gene that is frequently expressed in Ewing's sarcoma. *Cancer Research*, **60**, 4752–5.

Lucidarme, N., Valteau-Couanet, D., Oberlin, O. *et al.* (1998). Phase II study of high-dose thiotepa and hematopoietic stem cell transplantation in children with solid tumors. *Bone Marrow Transplantation*, **22**, 535–40.

Mackall, C.L., Goletz, T.J., Berzofsky, J.A., & Helman, L.J. (1998). *Toward New Approaches: Targeting Tumor Specific Molecular Alterations with Immune-Based Therapy*. Georgetown, MD: Medical Intelligence Unit Landes Publishers.

Mackall, C.L., Stein, D., Fleisher, T.A. *et al.* (2000). Prolonged CD4 depletion after sequential autologous peripheral blood progenitor cell infusions in children and young adults. *Blood*, **96**, 754–62.

Magrath, I., Sandlund, J., Raynor, A. *et al.* (1986). A phase II study of ifosfamide in the treatment of recurrent sarcomas in young people. *Cancer Chemotherapy and Pharmacology*, **18**(Suppl 2), S25–28.

Malagolowkin, M., Sposto, R., Grovas, L. *et al.* (1999). Lack of improvement in survival of children with metastatic rhabdomyosarcoma (RMS) treated with intensive therapy followed by stem cell transplant (SCT) for control of minimal residual disease. *Proceedings of the American Society of Clinical Oncology*, **18**, 551, #2143 (Abstract).

Marina, N.M., Pappo, A.S., Parham, D.M. *et al.* (1999). Chemotherapy dose-intensification for pediatric patients with Ewing's family of tumors and desmoplastic small round-cell tumors: a feasibility study at St. Jude Children's Research Hospital. *Journal of Clinical Oncology*, **17**, 180–90.

Mauger, D.C. (1982). Complete regression of osteogenic sarcoma scalp metastases following one pulse of high-dose melphalan combined with a bone marrow autograft: case report. *New Zealand Medical Journal*, **95**, 455–6.

Maurer, H.M., Beltangady, M., Gehan, E.A. *et al.* (1988). The Intergroup Rhabdomyosarcoma Study-I. A final report. *Cancer*, **61**, 209–20.

Maurer, H.M., Gehan, E.A., Beltangady, M. *et al.* (1993). The Intergroup Rhabdomyosarcoma Study-II. *Cancer*, **71**, 1904–22.

McLean, T.W., Hertel, C., Young, M.L. *et al.* (1999). Late events in pediatric patients with Ewing sarcoma/primitive neuroectodermal tumor of bone: the Dana-Farber Cancer Institute/Children's Hospital experience. *Journal of Pediatric Hematology and Oncology*, **21**, 486–93.

Merino, M.E., Navid, F., Christensen, B.L. *et al.* (2001). Immunomagnetic purging of Ewing's sarcoma from blood and bone marrow: quantitation by real-time polymerase chain reaction. *Journal of Clinical Oncology*, **19**, 3649–59.

Meyers, P.A., Krailo, M.D., Ladanyi, M. *et al.* (2001). High-dose melphalan, etoposide, total-body irradiation, and autologous stem-cell reconstitution as consolidation therapy for high-risk Ewing's sarcoma does not improve prognosis. *Journal of Clinical Oncology*, **19**, 2812–20.

Michon, J., Oberlin, O., Demeocq, F. et al. (1993). Poor results in metastatic Ewing's sarcomas (ES) treated according to the scheme of the Saint Jude 19781985 study. A study of the French Society of Pediatric Oncology. *Medical and Pediatric Oncology*, **21**, 572 (Abstract).

Miser, J.S., Kinsella, T.J., Triche, T.J. et al. (1987). Ifosfamide with mesna uroprotection and etoposide: an effective regimen in the treatment of recurrent sarcomas and other tumors of children and young adults. *Journal of Clinical Oncology*, **5**, 1191–8.

Miser, J.S., Kinsella, T.J., Triche, T.J. et al. (1988). Preliminary results of treatment of Ewing's sarcoma of bone in children and young adults: six months of intensive combined modality therapy without maintenance. *Journal of Clinical Oncology*, **6**, 484–90.

Miser, J.S., Krailo, M.D., Meyers, P.A. et al. (1996). Metastatic Ewing's sarcoma (ES) and primitive neuroectodermal tumor (PNET) of bone: failure of new regimens to improve outcome. *Proceedings of the American Society of Clinical Oncology*, **15**, 1472.

Moss, T.J., Cairo, M., Santana, V.M. et al. (1994). Clonogenicity of circulating neuroblastoma cells: implications regarding peripheral blood stem cell transplantation. *Blood*, **83**, 3085–9.

Neifeld, J.P., Maurer, H.M., Godwin, D. et al. (1979). Prognostic variables in pediatric rhabdomyosarcoma before and after multimodal therapy. *Journal of Pediatric Surgery*, **14**, 699–703.

Nesbit, M.E., Jr., Gehan, E.A., Burgert, Jr., E.O. et al. (1990). Multimodal therapy for the management of primary, nonmetastatic Ewing's sarcoma of bone: a long-term follow-up of the First Intergroup study. *Journal of Clinical Oncology*, **8**, 1664–74.

Newton, W.A., Jr., Gehan, E.A., Webber, B.L. et al. (1995). Classification of rhabdomyosarcomas and related sarcomas. Pathologic aspects and proposal for a new classification—an Intergroup Rhabdomyosarcoma Study. *Cancer*, **76**, 1073–85.

Nitschke, R., Parkhurst, J., Sullivan, J. et al. (1998). Topotecan in pediatric patients with recurrent and progressive solid tumors: a Pediatric Oncology Group phase II study. *Journal of Pediatric Hematology and Oncology*, **20**, 315–18.

Oberlin, O., Patte, C., Demeocq, F. et al. (1985). The response to initial chemotherapy as a prognostic factor in localized Ewing's sarcoma. *European Journal of Cancer and Clinical Oncology*, **21**, 463–7.

Ozkaynak, M.F., Matthay, K., Cairo, M. et al. (1998). Double-alkylator non-total-body irradiation regimen with autologous hematopoietic stem-cell transplantation in pediatric solid tumors. *Journal of Clinical Oncology*, **16**, 937–44.

Pappo, A.S., Anderson, J.R., Crist, W.M. et al. (1999). Survival after relapse in children and adolescents with rhabdomyosarcoma: A report from the Intergroup Rhabdomyosarcoma Study Group. *Journal of Clinical Oncology*, **17**, 3487–93.

Pappo, A.S., Crist, W.M., Kuttesch, J. et al. (1993). Tumor-cell DNA content predicts outcome in children and adolescents with clinical group III embryonal rhabdomyosarcoma. The Intergroup Rhabdomyosarcoma Study Committee of the Children's Cancer Group and the Pediatric Oncology Group. *Journal of Clinical Oncology*, **11**, 1901–5.

Pappo, A.S., Lyden, E., Breitfeld, P.P. et al. (2002). Irinotecan (CPT-11) is active against pediatric rhabdomyosarcoma (RMS): a phase II window trial from the Soft Tissue Sarcoma Committee (STS) of the Children's Oncology Group (COG). *Proceedings of the American Society of Clinical Oncology*, **21**, 393a (Abstract).

Pappo, A.S., Lyden, E., Breneman, J. et al. (2001). Up-front window trial of topotecan in previously untreated children and adolescents with metastatic rhabdomyosarcoma: an intergroup rhabdomyosarcoma study. *Journal of Clinical Oncology*, **19**, 213–19.

Pappo, A.S., Shapiro, D.N., Crist, W.M., & Maurer, H.M. (1995). Biology and therapy of pediatric rhabdomyosarcoma. *Journal of Clinical Oncology*, **13**, 2123–39.

Paulussen, M., Ahrens, S., Burdach, S. et al. (1998a). Primary metastatic (stage IV) Ewing tumor: survival analysis of 171 patients from the EICESS studies. European Intergroup Cooperative Ewing Sarcoma Studies. *Annals of Oncology*, **9**, 275–81.

Paulussen, M., Ahrens, S., Craft, A.W. et al. (1998b). Ewing's tumors with primary lung metastases: survival analysis of 114 (European Intergroup) Cooperative Ewing's Sarcoma Studies patients. *Journal of Clinical Oncology*, **16**, 3044–52.

Pein, F.J., Michon, D., Valteau-Couanet, E. et al. (1998). High-dose melphalan, etoposide, and carboplatin followed by autologous stem cell rescue in pediatric high-risk recurrent Wilm's tumor: a French Society of Pediatric Oncology study. *Journal of Clinical Oncology*, **16**, 3295-3301.

Perentesis, J., Katsanis, E., DeFor, T. et al. (1999). Autologous stem cell transplantation for high-risk pediatric solid tumors. *Bone Marrow Transplantation*, **24**, 609–15.

Picci, P., Rougraff, B.T., Bacci, G. et al. (1993). Prognostic significance of histopathologic response to chemotherapy in nonmetastatic Ewing's sarcoma of the extremities. *Journal of Clinical Oncology*, **11**, 1763–9.

Pinkerton, C.R., Groot-Loonen, J., Barrett, A. et al. (1991). Rapid VAC high-dose melphalan regimen, a novel chemotherapy approach in childhood soft tissue sarcomas. *British Journal of Cancer*, **64**, 381–5.

Raney, R.B., Jr. (1987). Inefficacy of cisplatin and etoposide as salvage therapy for children with recurrent or unresponsive soft tissue sarcoma. *Cancer Treatment Report*, **71**, 407–8.

Ries, L.A.G., Smith, M.A., Gurney, J.G. et al. (1999). *Cancer Incidence and Survival Among Children and Adolescents: United States SEER Program 1975–1995*. Bethedsa, MD: National Cancer Institute, SEER Program.

Rill, D.R., Santana, V.M., Roberts, W.M. et al. (1994). Direct demonstration that autologous bone marrow transplantation for solid tumors can return a multiplicity of tumorigenic cells. *Blood*, **84**, 380–3.

Rosen, G., Caparros, B., Nirenberg, A. et al. (1981). Ewing's sarcoma: ten-year experience with adjuvant chemotherapy. *Cancer*, **47**, 2204–13.

Rousseau, P., Flamant, F., Quintana, E. et al. (1994). Primary chemotherapy in rhabdomyosarcomas and other malignant mesenchymal tumors of the orbit: results of the International Society of Pediatric Oncology MMT 84 Study. *Journal of Clinical Oncology*, **12**, 516–21.

Sandler, E., Lyden, E., Ruymann, F. et al. (2001). Efficacy of ifosfamide and doxorubicin given as a phase II "window" in children with newly diagnosed metastatic rhabdomyosarcoma: a report from the Intergroup Rhabdomyosarcoma Study Group. *Medical and Pediatric Oncology*, **37**, 442–8.

Sarcoma Meta-Analysis Collaboration. (1997). Adjuvant chemotherapy for localised resectable soft-tissue sarcoma of adults: meta-analysis of individual data. *Lancet, 360,* 1647–54.

Saylors, R.L., 3rd, Stine, K.C., Sullivan, J. *et al.* (2001). Cyclophosphamide plus topotecan in children with recurrent or refractory solid tumors: a Pediatric Oncology Group phase II study. *Journal of Clinical Oncology, 19,* 3463–9.

Scotlandi, K., Baldini, N., Cerisano, V. *et al.* (2000). CD99 engagement: an effective therapeutic strategy for Ewing tumors. *Cancer Research, 60,* 5134–42.

Shepp, M., Necheles, T.F., Banks, H.H. *et al.* (1978). Adjuvant treatment of osteogenic sarcoma with high-dose cyclophosphamide. *Cancer Treatment Report, 62,* 295–6.

Snyder III, H.M., D'Angio, G.J., Evans, A.E., & Raney, R.B. (1998). Pediatric oncology. In *Campbell's Urology,* 7th ed., eds. P.C. Walsh, E.D. Vaughan Jr., & A.J. Wein, pp. 2240–5. St. Louis, WB Saunders Company.

Sosman, J.A., Stiff, P., Moss, S.M. *et al.* (2001). Pilot trial of interleukin-2 with granulocyte colony-stimulating factor for the mobilization of progenitor cells in advanced breast cancer patients undergoing high-dose chemotherapy: expansion of immune effectors within the stem-cell graft and post-stem-cell infusion. *Journal of Clinical Oncology, 19,* 634–44.

Stewart, D.A., Gyonyor, E., Paterson, A.H. *et al.* (1996). High-dose melphalan +/– total body irradiation and autologous hematopoietic stem cell rescue for adult patients with Ewing's sarcoma or peripheral neuroectodermal tumor. *Bone Marrow Transplantation, 18,* 315–18.

van Hoff, J., Grier, H.E., Douglass, E.C., & Green, D.M. (1995). Etoposide, ifosfamide, and cisplatin therapy for refractory childhood solid tumors. Response and toxicity. *Cancer, 75(,* 2966–70.

Verrill, M.W., Judson, I.R., Harmer, C.L. *et al.* (1997). Ewing's sarcoma and primitive neuroectodermal tumor in adults: are they different from Ewing's sarcoma and primitive neuroectodermal tumor in children? *Journal of Clinical Oncology, 15,* 2611–21.

Walterhouse, D.O., Hoover, M.L., Marymont, M.A., & Kletzel, M. (1999). High-dose chemotherapy followed by peripheral blood stem cell rescue for metastatic rhabdomyosarcoma: the experience at Chicago Children's Memorial Hospital. *Medical and Pediatric Oncology, 32,* 88–92.

Weidner, N. & Tjoe, J. (1994). Immunohistochemical profile of monoclonal antibody O13: antibody that recognizes glycoprotein p30/32MIC2 and is useful in diagnosing Ewing's sarcoma and peripheral neuroepithelioma. *American Journal of Surgical pathology, 18,* 486–94.

Weigel, B.J., Breitfeld, P.P., Hawkins, D. *et al.* (2001). Role of high-dose chemotherapy with hematopoietic stem cell rescue in the treatment of metastatic or recurrent rhabdomyosarcoma. *Journal of Pediatric Hematology and Oncology, 23,* 272–6.

Wessalowski, R., Jurgens, H., Bodenstein, H. *et al.* (1988). Results of treatment of primary metastatic Ewing sarcoma. A retrospective analysis of 48 patients. *Klinische Padiatrie, 200,* 253–60.

Wexler, L.H., DeLaney, T.F., Tsokos, M. *et al.* (1996). Ifosfamide and etoposide plus vincristine, doxorubicin, and cyclophosphamide for newly diagnosed Ewing's sarcoma family of tumors. *Cancer, 78,* 901–11.

Wexler, L.H. & Helman, L.J. (1997). Rhabdomyosarcoma and the undifferentiated sarcomas. In *Principles and Practice of Pediatric Oncology,* eds. P.A. Pizzo & D.G. Poplack, pp. 799–829. Philadelphia: Lippincott-Raven.

Whang-Peng, J., Triche, T.J., Knutsen, T. *et al.* (1986). Cytogenetic characterization of selected small round cell tumors of childhood. *Cancer Genetics and Cytogenetics, 21,* 185–208.

Zoubek, A., Dockhorn-Dworniczak, B., Delattre, O. *et al.* (1996). Does expression of different EWS chimeric transcripts define clinically distinct risk groups of Ewing tumor patients? *Journal of Clinical Oncology, 14,* 1245–51.

PART IV   CLINICAL RESULTS II: IDENTICAL TWIN HEMATOPOIETIC STEM CELL TRANSPLANTATION

49 Identical twin hematopoietic stem cell transplantation

ANNA BUTTURINI, MARY M. HOROWITZ, AND ROBERT PETER GALE

Childrens' Hospital, Los Angeles, USA; International Bone Marrow Transplant and Autologous Blood and Marrow Transplant Registries, Milwaukee, USA; and Center for Advanced Studies in Leukemia, Los Angeles, USA

Introduction

Blood or bone marrow transplants are commonly used to treat leukemia and other bone marrow disorders. Most transplants are autotransplants or are from HLA-identical related or unrelated persons otherwise genetically disparate from the recipient. However, 1% to 5% of transplants are between genetically identical twins (Gluckman *et al.*, 1989; Bortin, Horowitz, & Rimm, 1992; Gratwohl & Hermans, 1994). Analyzing results of these transplants is important in understanding the biology of leukemia and aplastic anemia and how transplants work in these diseases (Fefer *et al.*, 1974, 1977, 1979, 1981, 1982; Goldman *et al.*, 1981; Kolb *et al.*, 1989; Gale *et al.*, 1994). For example, comparing outcomes of identical-twin versus allo- and autotransplants can help distinguish graft-versus-leukemia (GVL) from graft-versus-host disease (GVHD) and determine whether cancer cells in an autograft contribute to relapse risk.

In this chapter we review results of identical-twin transplants reported in the literature and data from the International Bone Marrow Transplant (IBMTR) and Autologous Blood and Marrow Transplant Registries (ABMTR; Bortin, Horowitz, & Rimm, 1992; Gale *et al.*, 1994; Barrett *et al.*, 2000). Most twin transplants used bone marrow; blood cells were used in some reports (Weaver *et al.*, 1993) with similar outcomes.

Leukemia

Acute lymphoblastic leukemia

IBMTR analyses contain data on 24 persons with acute lymphoblastic leukemia (ALL) receiving identical-twin transplants in first remission (Gale *et al.*, 1994). The 3-year relapse probability was 36% (95% confidence interval, 20%–32%); 3-year leukemia-free survival (LFS) was 57% (37%–57%; Fig. 49.1). Results of identical-twin transplants in more advanced ALL were worse: relapse risk was greater than 50% in persons transplanted in second remission and greater than 60% in persons with more advanced leukemia.

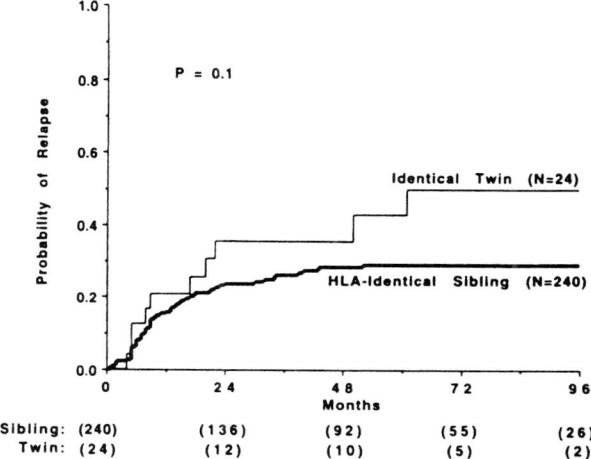

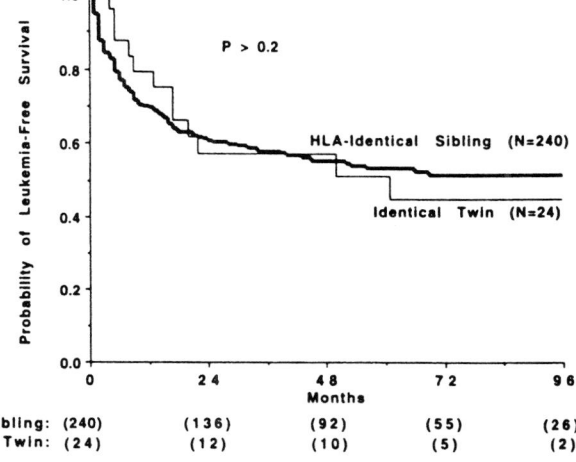

Fig. 49.1. Outcome of transplants for acute lymphoblastic leukemia. Actuarial probability of relapse (top) and leukemia-free survival (bottom) after identical-twin and HLA-identical sibling transplants for acute lymphoblastic leukemia in first remission. Numbers in parentheses are numbers at risk (alive in continuous complete remission) at indicated intervals. Reproduced, with permission, from Gale *et al.* (1994).

Acute myeloid leukemia

IBMTR analyses contain data on 45 persons with acute myeloid leukemia (AML) receiving identical-twin transplants in first remission (Gale *et al.,* 1994). The 3-year relapse probability was 52% (37%–67%); 3-year LFS was 42% (27%–57%; Fig. 49.2). Results of identical-twin transplants in more advanced leukemia are worse: relapse risk was greater than 80%.

Chronic myeloid leukemia

IBMTR analyses contain data on 34 persons with chronic myeloid leukemia (CML) receiving identical-twin transplants in chronic phase (Gale *et al.,* 1994). The 3-year relapse probability was 40% (23%–53%); 3-year LFS was 59% (42%–76%; Fig. 49.3). Results of identical-twin transplants

in more advanced leukemia are worse: relapse risk was greater than 80%.

Nonrelapse outcomes

Overall treatment-related mortality is low after identical-twin transplants: 5-year risk in an IBMTR study was 6%, significantly less than after allotransplants (Barrett *at al.,* 2000). Variables associated with treatment-related mortality after identical-twin transplants are graft dose and disease stage. Because there is no genetic disparity between identical twins, transplants between them should not be accompanied by graft-rejection and GVHD. This is so in most instances. However, about 10% of recipients of identical-twin transplants have clinical features consistent with acute GVHD (Rappeport *et al.,* 1979; Hinterberger *et al.,* 1997; Barrett *et al.,* 2000). Whether these persons really have acute

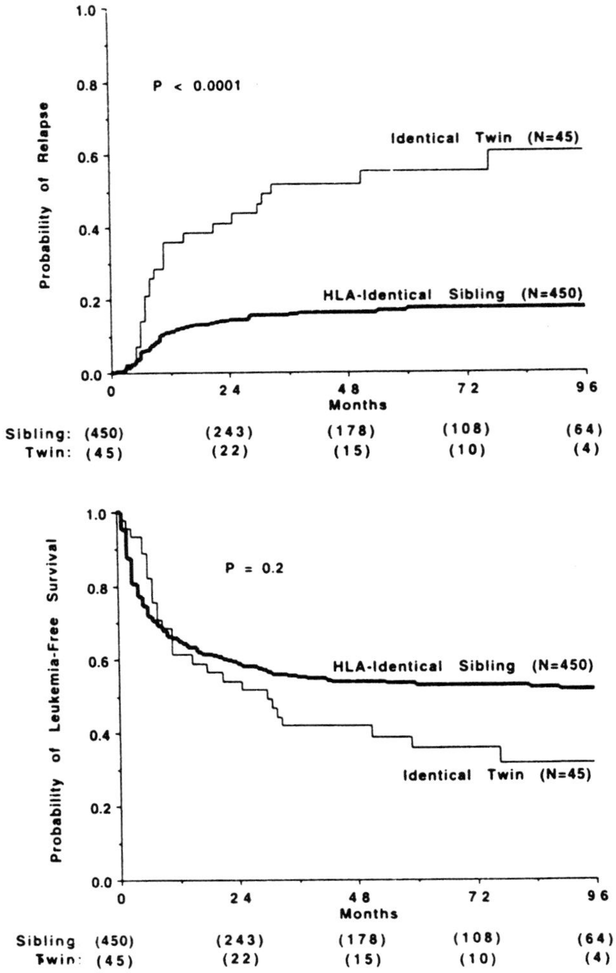

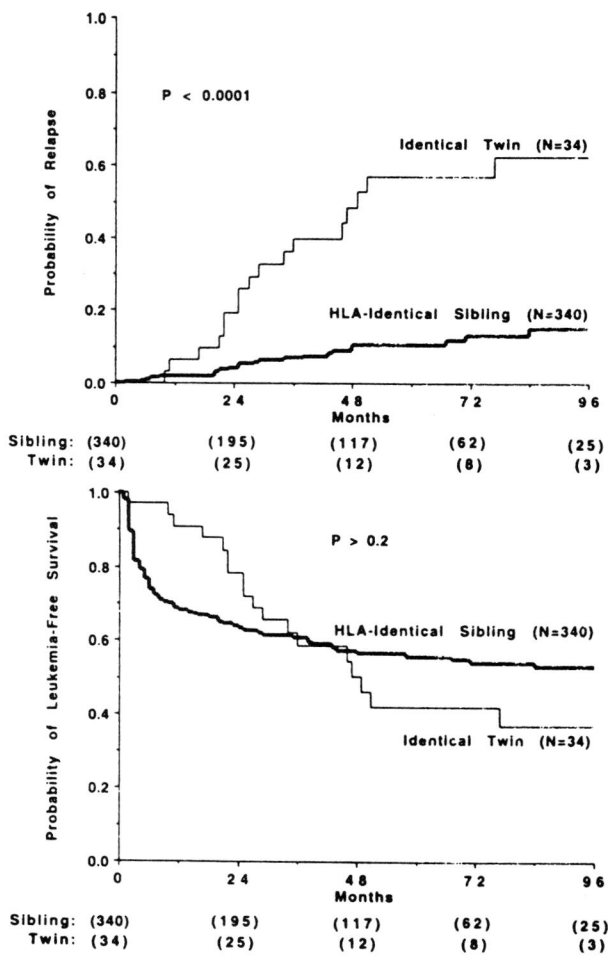

Fig. 49.2. Outcome of transplants for acute myelogenous leukemia. Actuarial probability of relapse (top) and leukemia-free survival (bottom) after identical-twin and HLA-identical sibling transplants for acute myelogenous leukemia in first remission. Numbers in parentheses are numbers at risk (alive in continuous complete remission) at indicated intervals. Reproduced, with permission, from Gale *et al.* (1994).

Fig. 49.3. Outcome of transplants for chronic myelogenous leukemia. Actuarial probability of relapse (top) and leukemia-free survival (bottom) after identical-twin and HLA-identical sibling transplants for chronic myelogenous leukemia in chronic phase. Numbers in parentheses are numbers at risk (alive in continuous complete remission) at indicated intervals. Reproduced, with permission, from Gale *et al.* (1994).

GVHD is uncertain; we have previously emphasized the considerable difficulty in accurate diagnosis (Atkinson *et al.*, 1988) and questioned the precision of this diagnosis in identical twins (Sallerfors & Gale, 1987). Chronic GVHD is rarely reported as are graft rejection and interstitial pneumonia.

Relapse

Considerable data in animals and humans suggest immune-mediated antileukemia effects operate in the setting of genetic disparity (Okunewick & Meredith, 1981; Truitt, Gale, & Bortin, 1987; Butturini, Bortin, & Gale, 1987; Butturini & Gale, 1992). We and others have shown potent antileukemia effects correlated with GVHD after conventional and T-cell-depleted transplants (Weiden *et al.*, 1979, 1981; Weisdorf *et al.*, 1987; Sullivan *et al.*, 1989; Horowitz *et al.*, 1990; Marmont *et al.*, 1991). Antileukemia mechanisms other than GVHD collectively termed GVL, also operate in the context of genetic disparity between donor and recipient. These effects are shown predominantly in AML and CML but less in ALL, and appear predominantly mediated by T cells.

Because of these considerations, it is not surprising that identical-twin relapse risk is higher than HLA-identical sibling relapse risk in AML in first remission and CML in chronic phase (Butturini, Bortin, & Gale, 1987; Horowitz *et al.*, 1990; Butturini & Gale, 1992). This increase persists after adjusting for relapse-correlated variables like immune phenotype, FAB type, WBC at diagnosis, and absence of GVHD. In contrast, relapse risk is not higher after identical-twin transplants for ALL in first remission (Butturini, Bortin, & Gale, 1987; Horowitz *et al.*, 1990; Marmont *et al.*, 1991). This may be because of the limited statistical power of the analysis in ALL or lack of GVL in ALL.

There are few data suggesting an impact of conditioning regimen on relapse risk relapse after identical-twin transplants. One study in CML suggested fewer relapses when dimethylmyeleran was used for conditioning (Fefer *et al.*, 1982). An IBMTR study reported fewer relapses in subjects receiving total-body irradiation (TBI) and cyclophosphamide versus those receiving busulfan and cyclophosphamide (Barrett *et al.*, 2000).

Although identical-twin transplants are associated with more relapses (except ALL), leukemia-free survival is similar to recipients of HLA-identical sibling transplants because of less treatment-related mortality.

Other cancers

Multiple myeloma

About 50 identical-twin transplants are reported in subjects with multiple myeloma (Osserman *et al.*, 1982; Fefer *et al.*, 1986; Bensinger *et al.*, 1996; Gahrton *et al.*, 1999). Remission (variably defined) is reported in about one-half. A few have had very long remissions including some with persisting monoclonal immunoglobulin production (Trullemans *et al.*, 2000).

A European Bone Marrow Transplant Registry (EBMTR) study compared results of identical-twin transplants with allo- and autotransplant (Gahrton *et al.*, 1999) (Figs. 49.4 and 49.5). Myeloma relapse was similar after identical-twin and allotransplants but higher after autotransplants, suggesting that myeloma cells in the graft may contribute to relapse. Treatment-related mortality was less with identical-twin and auto- compared to allotransplants. Identical-twin transplants had the best progression-free survival.

Polycythemia rubra vera

A patient with spent-phase polycythemia rubra vera with massive splenomegaly received TBI and busulfan followed by a syngeneic PBSC graft, but failed to engraft (Richard *et al.*, 2002). At day 40 posttransplant he underwent splenectomy followed by a marrow boost from his donor. He engrafted with subsequent resolution of marrow fibrosis.

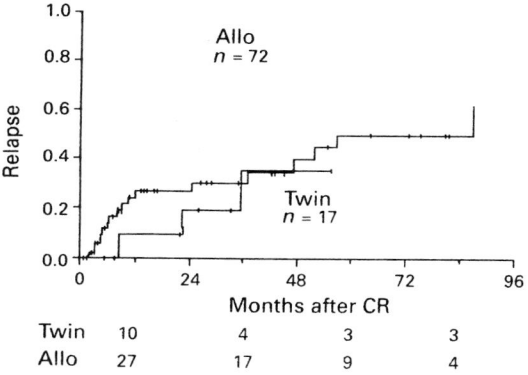

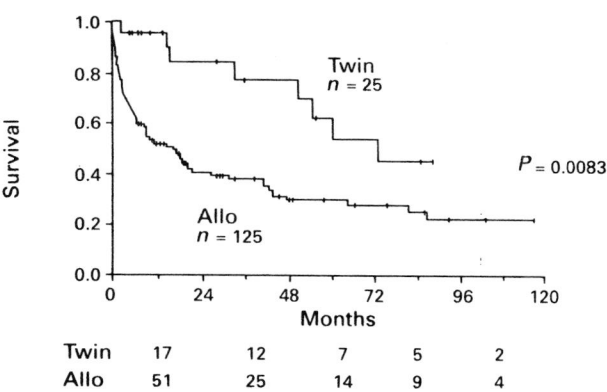

Fig. 49.4. Outcome of transplants for multiple myeloma. Actuarial probability of relapse (top) and survival (bottom) after identical-twin and HLA-identical sibling transplants for multiple myeloma. Numbers in parentheses are numbers at risk (alive in remission) at indicated intervals. Reproduced, with permission, from Gahrton *et al.* (1999).

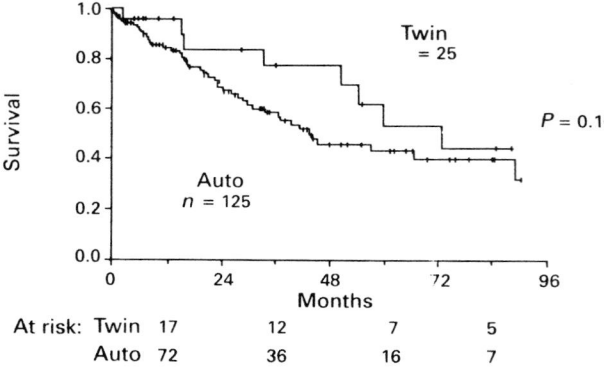

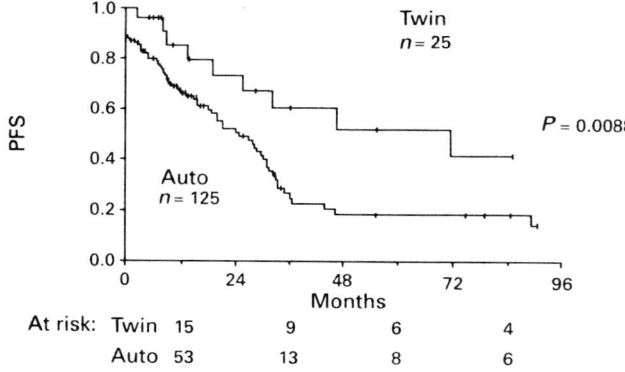

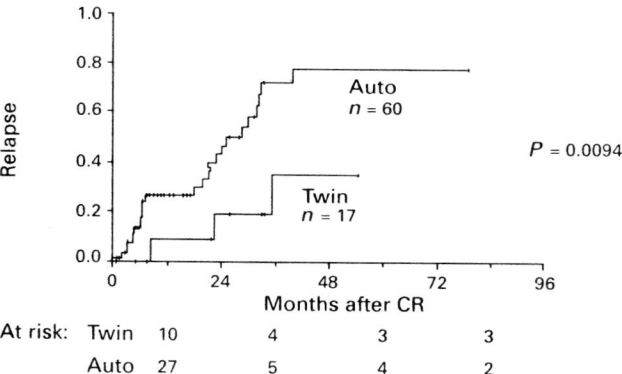

Fig. 49.5. (Top) Overall survival in twin transplantation (median 73 months; CI 53–∞) compared to autologous transplantation (median 44 months; CI 31–89). The difference was not significant (P = .10). (Middle) Progression-free survival in twin transplantation (median 72 months; CI 26–∞) compared to autologous transplantation (median 25 months; CI 18–31). The difference was statistically significant (P = .009). (Bottom) Relapse risk in twin transplantation (36% at 48 months) compared to autologous transplantation (78% at 48 months). The difference was statistically significant. (P = .009). Reproduced, with permission, from Gahrton et al. (1999).

Myelodysplastic syndrome

Five persons with myelodysplastic syndrome received identical-twin transplants (Stuart & Mangan, 1986; Deeg et al.,

2000). Three were alive and disease-free more than 2 years posttransplant.

Non-Hodgkin's lymphoma

The IBMTR and European Group for Blood and Marrow Transplantation reported data from 89 subjects with non-Hodgkin's lymphoma (NHL) receiving identical-twin transplants (Bierman et al., submitted). There was substantial diversity in histology, disease stage, and prior therapy. In 30 subjects with low-grade histology, 5-year relapse-risk and progression-free survival at 5 years were 9% (2%–25%) and 73% (51% to 86%), respectively. In 31 subjects with intermediate-grade histology corresponding results were 29% (15%–45%) and 42% (17%–65%). In 38 subjects with high-grade histology corresponding results were 32% (15%–49%) and 46% (28%–62%). These data were compared to similar subjects receiving allo- and autotransplants. Identical-twin and allotransplant recipients had similar relapse rates, suggesting no graft-versus-lymphoma effect. There were more relapses after autotransplants than identical-twin transplants, suggesting lymphoma cells in the graft may contribute to relapse.

Nawa and colleagues (1999) described a case of syngeneic transplantation for CD56+, CD2+, CD3− nasopharyngeal non-Hodgkin's lymphoma that resulted in an ongoing complete remission at 30 months posttransplant. Prior conventional chemotherapy had produced only a partial response.

Breast cancer

IBMTR analyzed the outcome of 14 women with metastatic breast cancer receiving high-dose chemotherapy followed by an identical-twin transplant (Williams et al., submitted). Treatment-related mortality was 7% (2% to 26%), 3-year progression-free survival was 17% (2% to 41%), and 3-year survival was 63% (36% to 84%). There was no comparison to allo- or autotransplants so it is not possible to determine if there is an immune-mediated anticancer effect.

Other diseases

Aplastic anemia

An IBMTR study reported data on 40 subjects receiving identical-twin transplants (Hinterberger et al., 1997) (Fig. 49.6). Twenty-three patients received their first bone marrow transplant without conditioning and 17 received conditioning. Six received posttransplant immune suppression. Seven of 23 unconditioned subjects had sustained complete bone marrow recovery. One more subject recovered after a second transplant, also without conditioning. The other 15 subjects received two to five more transplants with conditioning; 13 recovered bone marrow function; 2 died. Twelve of 17 conditioned subjects had sustained bone marrow recovery (1 after a second transplant also with conditioning); 5 died. The 10-year survival of

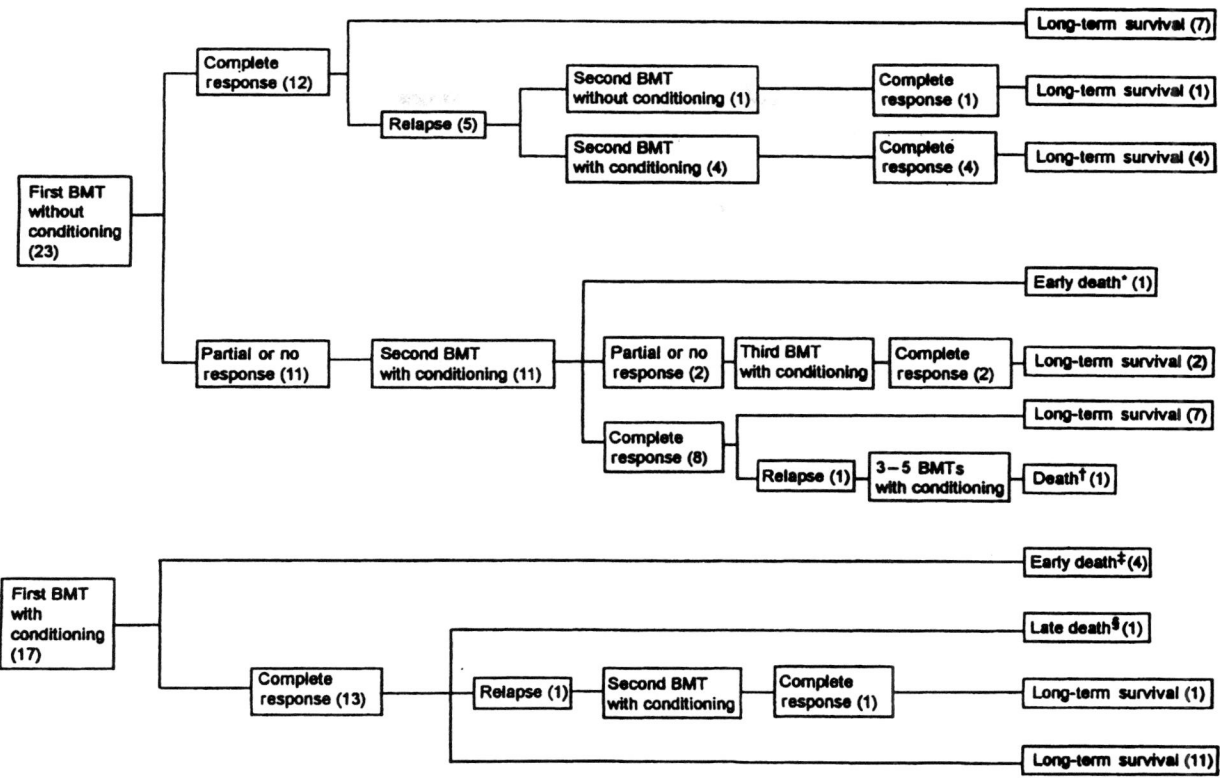

Fig. 49.6. Outcome of transplanting bone marrow from genetically identical twins into 40 patients with aplastic anemia. *Patient died of fungal pneumonia 3.5 months after first transplantation; †Patient died of septicemia 3.5 years after first transplantation; ‡Patients died of fungal pneumonia (1 patient), the acute respiratory distress syndrome (1 patient), and diffuse alveolar hemorrhage (2 patients) 7, 12, 16, and 20 days after first transplantation, respectively. §Patient died of interstitial pneumonia, pneumothorax, and GVHD 5 months after first transplantation. Values in parentheses are numbers of patients. BMT, bone marrow transplantation. Reproduced, with permission, from Hinterberger *et al.* (1997).

the 40 subjects was 78% (59% to 92%). Conditioning increased the likelihood of rapid bone marrow recovery but did not improve survival.

Paroxysmal nocturnal hemoglobinuria (PNH)

There are several reports of identical-twin transplants for PNH (Fefer *et al.,* 1976; Hershko *et al.,* 1979; Saso *et al.,* 1999). Most subjects were cured (variably defined; Kawahara *et al.,* 1992). In some instance conditioning appeared needed to eradicate the PNH clone (Endo *et al.,* 1996).

Rheumatoid arthritis

A subject with rheumatoid arthritis received an identical-twin transplant after conditioning followed by clinical improvement (McColl *et al.,* 1999).

Idiopathic thrombocytopenic purpura

A 19-year-old man with chronic idiopathic thrombocytopenic purpura, refractory to corticosteroids, IVIG, splenectomy, RhoGAM, cyclophosphamide, vincristine, cyclosporine, and rituxan, had resolution of the disease after a syngeneic periph-

eral blood stem cell transplant preceded by conditioning with TBI 5.5 Gy and cyclophosphamide 150 mg/kg (Zaydan *et al.,* 2002). He required four platelet transfusions posttransplant and his platelet count rose to $98 \times 10^9/l$ by day 50, $148 \times 10^9/l$ by day 55, and $374 \times 10^9/l$ at 6 months posttransplant.

Conclusions

Data from identical-twin transplants show that immune-mediated anticancer effects operate after some, but not all, allotransplants. Effects are detectable in AML and CML but not ALL, multiple myeloma, or lymphoma. Other cancers are not yet been studied but this effect also seems to operate in kidney cancer. It is also uncertain whether this effect is distinct from GVHD (reviewed in Horowitz *et al.,* 1990; Butturini & Gale, 1992). Data from identical-twin transplants also suggest that cancer cells in the graft contribute to relapse risk as in multiple myeloma and lymphoma.

Results of identical-twin transplants can help determine the best donor when there is a choice between an identical-twin and an HLA-identical sibling. Despite a higher relapse risk after identical-twin transplants, leukemia-free survival is comparable to HLA-identical sibling transplants because of less treatment-related mortality. Consequently, use of either type of donor is reasonable, although early mortality is higher with HLA-identical sibling transplants. Because of increased concordance for ALL in identical twins less than 5 years old (Boice, 1988), using an HLA-identical sibling donor is reasonable in this setting.

References

Atkinson, K., Horowitz, M.M., Biggs, J.C. *et al.* (1988). The clinical diagnosis of acute graft-versus-host disease: a diversity of views amongst marrow transplant centers. *Bone Marrow Transplantation,* **3,** 5–10.

Barrett, A.J., Ringden, O., Zhang, M-J. *et al.* (2000). Effect of nucleated marrow cell dose on relapse and survival in identical twin bone marrow transplants for leukemia. *Blood,* **95,** 3323–7.

Bensinger, W.I., Demirer, T., Buckner, C.D. *et al.* (1996). Syngeneic marrow transplantation in patients with multiple myeloma. *Bone Marrow Transplantation,* **18,** 527–31.

Bierman, P.J., Sweetenham, J.W., & Loberiza, F.R. Identical-twin blood and bone marrow transplants for non-Hodgkin lymphoma. Submitted.

Boice, J.D. (1988). Carcinogenesis—a synopsis of human experience with external exposure in medicine. *Health Physics,* **55,** 621–30.

Bortin, M.M., Barrett, A.J., & Horowitz, M.M. (1992). Progress in allogeneic bone marrow transplantation for acute lymphoblastic leukemia in the 1980's: a report from the IBMTR. *Leukemia,* **6** (Suppl 2), 196–7.

Bortin, M.M., Horowitz, M.M., & Rimm, A.A. for The International Bone Marrow Transplant Registry. (1992). Increasing utilization of allogeneic bone marrow transplantation. Results of the 1988–1990 survey. *Annals of Internal Medicine,* **116,** 505–12.

Butturini, A., Bortin, M.M., & Gale, R.P. (1987). Graft-versus-leukemia following bone marrow transplantation. *Bone Marrow Transplantation,* **2,** 233–42.

Butturini, A. & Gale, R.P. (1992). Graft-versus-leukemia. *Immunology Research,* **11,** 24–33.

Deeg, H.J., Shulman, H.M., Anderson, J.E. *et al.* (2000). Allogeneic and syngeneic marrow transplantation for myelodysplastic syndrome in patients 55 to 66 years of age. *Blood,* **95,** 1188–94.

Endo, M., Beatty, P.G., Vreeke, T.M. *et al.* (1996). Syngeneic bone marrow transplantation without conditioning in a patient with paroxysmal nocturnal hemoglobinuria : in vivo evidence that the mutant stem cells have a survival advantage. *Blood,* **88,** 742–50.

Fefer, A., Buckner, C.D., Thomas, E.D. *et al.* (1977). Cure of hematologic neoplasia with transplantation of marrow from identical twins. *New England Journal of Medicine,* **297,** 146–8.

Fefer, A., Cheever, M.A., & Greenberg, P.D. (1986). Identical twin (syngeneic) marrow transplantation for hematologic cancers. *Journal of the National Cancer Institute,* **76,** 1269–73.

Fefer, A., Cheever, M.A., Greenberg, P.D. *et al.* (1982). Treatment of chronic granulocytic leukemia with chemoradiotherapy and transplantation of marrow from identical twins. *New England Journal of Medicine,* **306,** 63–8.

Fefer, A., Cheever, M.A., Thomas, E.D. *et al.* (1979). Disappearance of Ph1-positive cells in four patients with chronic granulocytic leukemia after chemotherapy, irradiation and marrow transplan-

tation from an identical twin. *New England Journal of Medicine,* **300,** 333–7.

Fefer, A., Cheever, M.A., Thomas, E.D. *et al.* (1981). Bone marrow transplantation for refractory acute leukemia in 34 patients with identical twins. *Blood,* **57,** 421–30.

Fefer, A., Einstein, A.B., Thomas, E.D. *et al.* (1974). Bone marrow transplantation for hematologic neoplasia in 16 patients with identical twins. *New England Journal of Medicine,* **290,** 1389–93.

Fefer, A., Freeman, H., Strob, R. *et al.* (1976). Paroxysmal nocturnal hemoglobinuria and marrow failure treated by infusion of marrow from an identical twin. *Annals of Internal Medicine,* **84,** 692–5.

Gahrton, G., Svensson, H., Bjorkstrand, B. *et al.* (1999). Syngeneic transplantation in multiple myeloma—a case-matched comparison with autologous and allogeneic transplantation. *Bone Marrow Transplantation,* **24,** 741–5.

Gale, R.P., Horowitz, M.M., Ash, R.C. *et al.* (1994). Identical-twin bone marrow transplants for leukemia. *Annals of Internal Medicine,* **120,** 646–52.

Gluckman, E., Esperou, H., Devergie, A. *et al.* (1989). Pediatric bone marrow transplantation for leukemia and aplastic anemia. Report of 222 cases transplanted in a single center. *Nouvelle Revue Francaise d Hematologie,* **31,** 111–4.

Goldman, J.M., Johnson, S.A., Catovsky, D. *et al.* (1981). Identical twin marrow transplantation for patients with leukemia and lymphoma. *Transplantation,* **31,** 140–1.

Gratwohl, A. & Hermans, J. (1994). Bone marrow transplantation activity in Europe 1992: report from the European Group for Bone Marrow Transplantation (EBMT). *Bone Marrow Transplantation,* **13,** 5–10.

Hershko, C., Gale, R.P., Ho, W.G., & Cline, M.J. (1979). Cure of aplastic anemia in paroxysmal nocturnal hemoglobinuria by marrow transfusion from an identical twin: failure of peripheral leucocyte transfusion to correct marrow aplasia. *Lancet,* **1,** 945–7.

Hinterberger, W., Rowlings, P.A., Hinterberger-Fischer, M. *et al.* (1997). Results of transplanting bone marrow from genetically identical twins into patients with aplastic anemia. *Annals of Internal Medicine,* **126,** 116–22.

Horowitz, M.M., Gale, R.P., Sondel, P.M. *et al.* (1990). Graft-versus-leukemia reactions after bone marrow transplantations. *Blood,* **75,** 555–62.

Kawahara, K., Witherspoon, R.P., & Storb, R. (1992). Marrow transplantation of paroxysmal nocturnal hemoglobinuria. *American Journal of Hematology,* **39,** 283–8.

Kolb, H.J., Bender-Gotze, C., Haas, R.J. *et al.* (1989). Bone marrow transplantation for the treatment of leukaemia—results of the Munich Cooperative Group. *Folia Haematologica,* **116,** 397–402.

Marmont, A.M., Horowitz, M.M., Gale, R.P. *et al.* (1991). T-cell depletion of HLA-identical transplants in leukemia. *Blood,* **78,** 2120–30.

McColl, G., Kohsaka, H., Szer, J., & Wicks, I. (1999). High-dose chemotherapy and syngeneic hemopoietic stem-cell transplantation for severe, seronegative rheumatoid arthritis. *Annals of Internal Medicine,* **131,** 507–9.

Nawa, Y., Takenaka, K., Shinagawa, K. *et al.* (1999). Successful treatment of advanced natural killer cell lymphoma with high-dose chemotherapy and syngeneic peripheral blood stem cell transplantation. *Bone Marrow Transplantation,* **23,** 1321–2.

Okunewick, J.P. & Meredith, R.F. (eds). (1981). *Graft-versus-Leukemia in Man and Animal Models*. Boca Raton, FL: CRC Press, Inc.

Osserman, E.D., Di Re, L.B., Di Re, J. *et al.* (1982). Identical twin marrow transplantation in patients with multiple myeloma. *Acta Haematologica*, **68**, 215–23.

Rappeport, J., Mihm, M., Reinherz, E. *et al.* (1979). Acute graft-versus-host disease in recipients of bone-marrow transplants from identical twin donors. *Lancet*, **2**, 717–20.

Richard, S., Isola, L., Scigliano, E, *et al.* (2002). Syngeneic stem cell transplant for spent-phase polycythaemia vera: eradication of myelofibrosis and restoration of normal haematopoiesis. *British Journal of Haematology*, **117**, 245-6.

Rizzo, J.D., Williams, S., Wu, J.T. *et al.* (2003). Syngeneic hematopoietic stem cell transplantation for women with metastatic breast cancer. *Bone Marrow Transplantation*, **32**, 151-5.

Sallerfors, B. & Gale, R.P. (1987). A critical analysis of acute graft-versus-host disease in twins. In *Progress in Bone Marrow Transplantation*, ed. R.P. Gale & R.E. Champlin, pp. 281–93. New York: Alan R. Liss.

Saso, R., Marsh, J., Cevreska, L. *et al.* (1999). Bone marrow transplants for paroxysmal nocturnal haemoglobinuria. *British Journal of Haematology*, **104**, 392–6.

Stuart, R.K. & Mangan, K.F. (1986). Hematologic and cytogenetic remission of 5q-refractory anemia after syngeneic bone marrow transplantation. *American Journal of Medicine*, **80**, 503–7.

Sullivan, K.M., Weiden, P.L., Storb, R. *et al.* (1989). Influence of acute and chronic graft-versus-host disease on relapse and survival after bone marrow transplantation from HLA-identical siblings as treatment of acute and chronic leukemia. *Blood*, **73**, 1720–8.

Truitt, R.L., Gale, R.P., & Bortin, M.M. (eds.) (1987). *Cellular Immunotherapy of Cancer*, pp. 371–90. New York: Alan R. Liss.

Trullemans, F., Schots, R., Storme, G., & Van Camp, B. (2000). Late and localized extramedullary relapse of a light chain kappa myeloma after syngeneic bone marrow transplantation. *Bone Marrow Transplantation*, **25**, 115–7.

Weaver, C.H., Buckner, C.D., Longin, K. *et al.* (1993). Syngeneic transplantation with peripheral blood mononuclear cells collected after the administration of recombinant human granulocyte colony-stimulating factor. *Blood*, **82**, 1981–4.

Weiden, P.L., Flournoy, N., Thomas, E.D. *et al.* (1979). Antileukemic effect of graft-versus-host disease in human recipients of allogeneic marrow grafts. *New England Journal of Medicine*, **300**, 1068–73.

Weiden, P.L., Sullivan, K.M., Flournoy, N. *et al.* (1981). Antileukemic effect of chronic graft-versus-host disease: contribution to improved survival after allogeneic marrow transplantation. *New England Journal of Medicine*, **304**, 1529–33.

Weisdorf, D.J., Nesbit, M.E., Ramsay, N.K.C. *et al.* (1987). Allogeneic bone marrow transplantation for acute lymphoblastic leukemia in remission: prolonged survival associated with acute graft-versus-host disease. *Journal of Clinical Oncology*, **5**, 1348–55.

Zaydan, M.A., Turner, C., & Miller, A.M. (2002). Resolution of chronic idiopathic thrombocytopenic purpura following syngeneic peripheral blood progenitor transplant. *Bone Marrow Transplantation*, **29**, 87–9.

PART V   CLINICAL RESULTS III: ALLOGENEIC HEMATOPOIETIC STEM CELL TRANSPLANTATION

50 Allogeneic hematopoietic stem cell transplantation for acute myeloid leukemia

ANDREA BACIGALUPO, V. GALBUSERA, AND FRANCESCO FRASSONI

Ospedale San Martino, Genova, Italy

Introduction

Allogeneic hematopoietic stem cell transplantation (HSCT) is one of the treatment options for patients with acute myeloid leukemia (AML): the donor can be an HLA-identical sibling, a family member mismatched donor, or an unrelated individual selected from the international registries.

Risk factors, such as cytogenetic abnormalities, have a significant influence on the outcome of AML patients, including after transplantation, and should be factored into the therapeutic decision-making process (Ferrant *et al.,* 1997) (Table 50.1). Information on disease incidence, classification, immune phenotype, cytogenetic abnormalities, prognostic factors, outcome with conventional therapy, disease-specific pretransplant workup, and monitoring for residual disease posttransplant is given in Chapter 36.

Results of HLA-identical sibling transplantation

AML in first remission

Thomas and co-workers (1979) first reported their experience with HLA-identical sibling bone marrow transplantation (BMT) in 19 AML patients in first complete remission. At the time of their report, only 1 patient had died of leukemic relapse, 6 patients had died of infection and/or graft-versus-host disease (GVHD), and 12 patients were alive in remission 473 to 1,102 (median 680) days posttransplant. The Kaplan-Meier estimate of survival was 62%. When these results were subsequently updated (Thomas, 1983), 2 of these latter 12 patients had died, 1 of pneumothorax and 1 of leukemic relapse, so that the estimated chance of surviving without recurrent disease at 5 years was approximately 50%.

Twenty years after this first report, the results of HLA-identical sibling HSCT for AML in first remission have been confirmed in large number of patients: transplants performed during 1987–2001 registered with the European Group for Blood and Marrow Transplantation (EBMT) show a 5-year survival of 63% for 623 children and 55% for 3,255 adults (Fig. 50.1) (EBMT web site, ebmt.org). One large prospective randomized study compared HLA-identical sibling BMT in first remission with autologous transplantation and with chemotherapy (Zittoun *et al.,* 1995). The projected disease-free survival (DFS) rates at 4-years posttransplant were 55%, 48%, and 30% respectively, for allogeneic, autologous transplants, and chemotherapy (Fig. 50.2).

Results have improved with time: an IBMTR analysis indicates that DFS for first remission transplants has risen from 45% in 1983 to 59% in 1996 (ABMTR Newsletter, 1996). An EBMT analysis showed a similar improvement in DFS from 45% between 1979 and 1987 to 57% in the period 1987 to 1991 (Frassoni *et al.,* 1996). Single-center studies have reported 5-year survival in excess of 75% for adults with first remission AML (Zikos *et al.,* 1998).

Conditioning regimens

In most reports, the combination of cyclophosphamide (CY) (60 mg/kg/day for 2 days) and single dose or fractionated total body irradiation (TBI) (8 Gy to 12.5 Gy) was used as the preparative regimen. The Baltimore group introduced a combi-

Table 50.1. *HLA-identical sibling transplantation for AML in first complete remission: impact of cytogenetic abnormality on outcome posttransplant*

Type of chromosome abnormality	n	Probability of leukemia-free survival (%)	Probability of relapse (%)
None	424	55	20
Good prognosis[a]	123	56	22
Intermediate prognosis[b]	117	50	22
Poor prognosis[c]	44	24	56

[a] Good prognosis for outcome (with conventional chemotherapy): t(8;21); t(15;17); inv(16): del(16).

[b] Intermediate prognosis for outcome (with conventional chemotherapy): +8; +21; t(6;9); other translocation or numerical or structural abnormality.

[c] Poor prognosis for outcome (with conventional chemotherapy): t(9;22); −5; −7; del(11).

Adapted, with permission, from Gale *et al.* (1995).

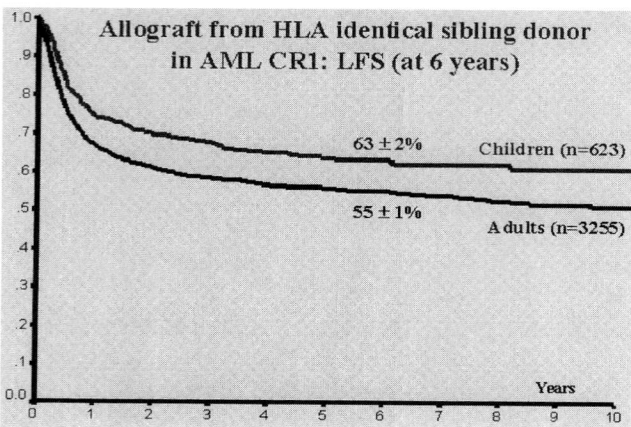

Fig. 50.1. Actuarial leukemia-free survival of adults and children with AML in first remission undergoing an allogeneic transplant from an HLA-identical sibling.

nation of busulfan (4 mg/kg/day for 4 days) and CY (50 mg/kg/day for 4 days), and obtained survival results that did not differ significantly from those reported with the CY-TBI regimen (Santos *et al.*, 1983). To decrease the toxic effects of this latter regimen, the dose of CY was subsequently decreased to 60 mg/kg/day for 2 days (Tutschka *et al.*, 1987), but in one prospective randomized study, this new regimen appeared to be less effective than the standard CY-TBI regimen (Blaise *et al.*, 1992). The comparison of the two regimens CY-TBI and BU-CY has been the object of several large randomized studies (Clift *et al.*, 1994; Ringden *et al.*, 1994; Devergie *et al.*, 1995; Blaise *et al.*, 2001). Sociè and co-workers (2001) have pub-

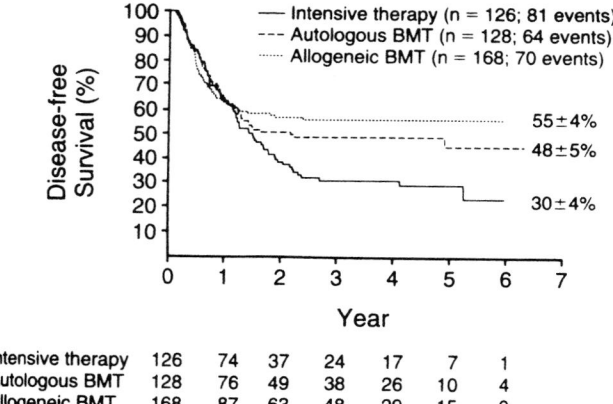

Fig. 50.2. Kaplan-Meier plots of disease-free survival, according to whether patients were assigned to autologous or allogeneic bone marrow transplantation (BMT) or a second course of intensive consolidation therapy. The number of patients at risk is shown below each time point. Plus–minus values are the projected disease-free survival rates (±SE) at 4 years. The events considered were relapse or death during a first complete remission. Reproduced. With permission, from Zittoun *et al.* (1995).

lished a meta-analysis of these four studies showing superior disease-free survival with CY-TBI compared to BU-CY. Other TBI regimens include fractionated or hyperfractionated TBI (Brochstein *et al.*, 1987). There is only one prospective randomized trial, performed in Seattle, comparing two different doses of radiation, 12 Gy (2 Gy/day × 6 days) versus 15.75 Gy (2.25 × 7 days). It showed that the use of a higher dose of irradiation reduced the risk of relapse ($P = .06$), but increased transplant-related mortality ($P = .04$) and did not modify the final outcome (Clift *et al.*, 1990). Other attempts to improve the efficacy of the conditioning regimen have been proposed. They involve the use of drugs known for their antileukemic efficacy (for example, high-dose cytosine arabinoside, melphalan, or etoposide). The efficacy of these new conditioning regimens has been tested in children or young adult patients with AML beyond first remission (see below), as well as in first remission (Snyder *et al.*, 1993). At the present time there is no evidence that these regimens are superior to the combination of CY and TBI as initially described by Thomas, at least for patients with AML in first remission.

Early complications

There is evidence that outcome for children transplanted for AML in first remission has improved, largely due to a decrease in treatment-related mortality (TRM) to less than 10% (Michel *et al.*, 1996). A significant reduction of TRM has been achieved also in adults (Wahlin *et al.*, 2002). Reduced TRM is the result of combined immunosuppressive therapy posttransplant (Deeg *et al.*, 1997), better supportive care including preemptive treatment of cytomegalovirus disease (Reusser *et al.*, 2002), and new antibacterial and antifungal agents (Walsh *et al.*, 2002). GVHD is the major direct or indirect cause of non-relapse mortality after allogeneic transplantation, and several programs have been developed to prevent this complication: depletion of donor T cells from the stem cell harvest (Marmont *et al.*, 1991) (ex vivo T-cell depletion), aggressive immunosuppression pretransplant, also referred to as in vivo T-cell depletion (Hows *et al.*, 1993), and combined immunosuppressive therapy posttransplant (Deeg *et al.*, 1997). Combined therapy (cyclosporine and methotrexate) significantly decreased the incidence of moderate to severe acute GVHD (grades II–IV) and improved survival in a series of 92 patients with AML in first remission or chronic myeloid leukemia (Storb *et al.*, 1986). Similar results have been reproduced by Zikos *et al.* (1998) (Fig. 50.3).

Graft-versus-leukemia (GVL) effect

Ex vivo T-cell depletion is one way to prevent GVHD: in a retrospective analysis of 719 AML patients in first remission reported to the IBMTR, the use of T-cell depletion was followed by a reduction in the risk of severe acute GVHD, but did not improve survival. Actuarial leukemia-free survival at 2 years was 57% for 560 patients without T-cell depletion versus 45% for 159 patients undergoing T-cell depletion (Marmont *et al.*, 1991). The difference was statistically significant ($P < .02$), and was due to a twofold increase in the risk of relapse (relative

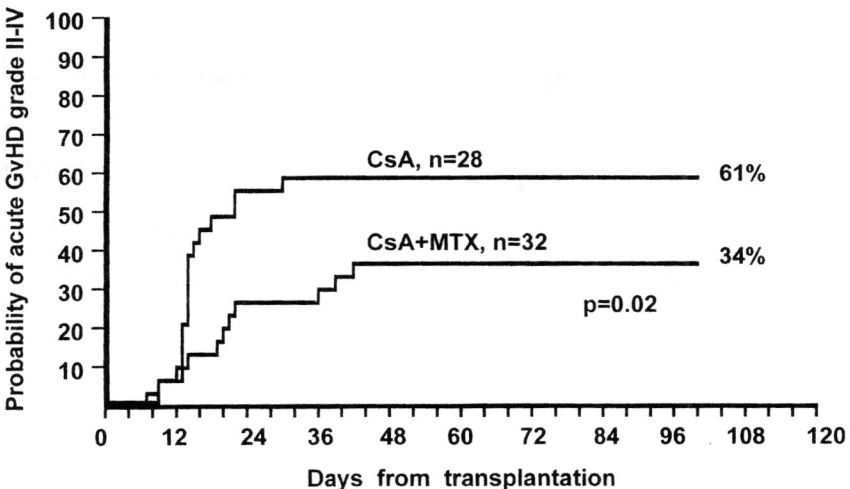

Fig. 50.3. Actuarial probability of developing a GVHD grade II–IV, showing a significant difference between the two groups: CSA + MTX, 34% versus CSA alone, 61% (*P* = .02). Reproduced, with permission, from Zikos *et al.* (1998).

risk = 1.94) for patients undergoing T-cell depletion. These results are in agreement with those reported by Bacigalupo *et al.* (1991) and Fagioli *et al.* (1994), who showed that patients with acute leukemia in first remission given "high-dose" cyclosporine (5 mg/kg/day) as GVHD prophylaxis had a higher incidence of recurrent leukemia (43%) than patients given lower doses of cyclosporine (1 mg/kg/day) (9%). A long-term follow-up of that study, with minimum observation exceeding 10 years, confirmed the impact of early posttransplant immunosuppression on long-term control of leukemia relapse (Bacigalupo *et al.*, 2001) (Fig. 50.4). Therefore, a potent GVL effect is seen in AML patients undergoing allogeneic HSCT and correlates with GVHD and its prophylaxis (Horowitz *et al.*, 1990).

Late complications

Chronic GVHD is the major late complication of allogeneic BMT, and has a significant impact on quality of life (Chiodi *et al.*, 2000) and mortality (Lee *et al.*, 2002). The 3-year risk of nonrelapse mortality is 28% for limited and 48% for extensive chronic GVHD (Lee *et al.*, 2002). Chronic GVHD is increased in patients receiving alternative donor grafts, both unrelated (UD) and family member mismatched, when compared to transplants from HLA-identical siblings (Storb *et al.*, 1983; Marks *et al.*, 1993; Weisdorf *et al.*, 2002). In severe cases patients may develop extensive scleroderma, crippling contractures, and severe infections with mortality up to 80% (Shulman *et al.*, 1980; Storb *et al.*, 1983; Deeg *et al.*, 1988). Treatment of chronic GVHD unfortunately has made little

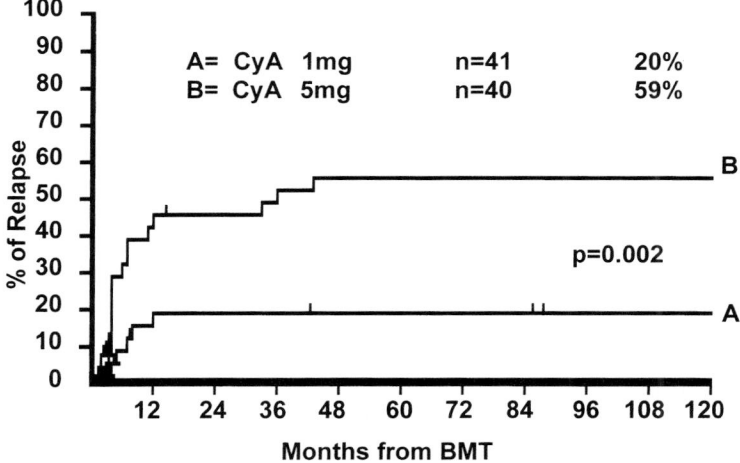

Fig. 50.4. Risk of relapse for patients with acute leukemia randomized to receive cyclosporine 1 mg/kg/day versus cyclosporine 5 mg/kg/day. This is the update of a study published in 1991 (Bacigalupo *et al.*, 2001). The minimum follow-up for these patients is 10 years, and the difference highly significant. The two groups differ in the dose of cyclosporine and in cyclosporine serum levels between day +1 and day +10.

progress over the past 3 decades, with average mortality remaining stable at 24% (Goerrner *et al.*, 2002), and intensified immunosuppression does not seem to improve survival (Koc *et al.*, 2002). Chronic GVHD, however, has an important GVL effect, so that one may want to use different strategies according to risk factors for relapse in AML: patients at high risk can receive marrow from unrelated donors, or from peripheral blood, with intensified conditioning regimens, all procedures associated with a high incidence of chronic GVHD (Clift *et al.*, 1990; Champlin *et al.*, 2000; Przepiorka *et al.*, 2001; Weisdorf *et al.*, 2002). The opposite may be true for patients in first remission with no adverse risk factors.

Center effect

The issue of a possible center effect has been debated, although little evidence is available in the literature. We have conducted within the EBMT a large study on AML first remission patients to test whether we could identify a center effect (Frassoni *et al.*, 2000).The analysis was restricted to centers performing at least 30 transplants for AML in first remission between 1987 and 1995. The overall leukemia-free survival at 3 years was 57%, and ranged from 75% to 39%, due to a difference in transplant-related mortality (from 5% to over 50%). The conclusion of the study was that the outcome of BMT for AML in first remission is influenced by the center in which the procedure is performed, suggesting significant variations in transplant practice around Europe. This confirms the need to document transplant activity and define minimum requirements and standards of practice (Urbano-Ispizua *et al.*, 2002). It also calls for careful analysis of different transplant procedures in order to identify optimal treatment protocols.

An interesting study by the EORTC/GIMEMA group showed a significant center effect in treatment strategy, such that more patients were transplanted if they had received induction chemotherapy in a transplant center. However, there was no overall effect on survival (Keating *et al.*, 1999).

Postremission chemotherapy

A retrospective IBMTR survey found that the intensity of postremission chemotherapy had no impact on leukemia-free survival, relapse incidence, or incidence of treatment-related mortality, when they compared patients with AML in first CR who had received no consolidation therapy with those who received standard-dose cytosine arabinoside and with those who received high-dose cytosine consolidation therapy prior to grafting (Tallman *et al.*, 2000).

AML beyond first remission

The outcome of allografts for AML beyond first remission is poorer when compared to first remission patients, due to both an increase in the transplant-related mortality and in the risk of relapse. An analysis of the EBMT data showed an actuarial survival at 6 years of 62% for patients in first CR (*n* = 3,419), of 45% for patients in second remission (*n* = 659), and of 23% for patients

beyond second remission or in relapse (*n* = 717) (Fig. 50.5). The cause of poorer outcome in patients with advanced AML was a high risk of transplant-related mortality and of relapse. The IBMTR data showed an actuarial risk of relapse of 25%, 45%, and 67% for AML transplanted in first, second, and subsequent remission/relapse (ABMTR Newsletter, 1996), with leukemia-free survival rates of 47%, 35%, and 25% respectively. The Seattle group found that a substantial proportion of patients with AML in untreated first relapse could be salvaged by allogeneic BMT (Clift *et al.*, 1991). For a subgroup of 29 patients transplanted using CY and fractionated TBI 15.75 Gy, with cyclosporine and methotrexate as GVHD prophylaxis, the risk of relapse was 26% and the estimated chance of surviving without disease at 3 years was 38%.

A retrospective study comparing HLA-identical sibling transplants with chemotherapy for AML in second remission found significantly longer leukemia-free survival in those transplanted aged 30 or less and whose first remissions lasted 1 year or longer (41% vs 17%) and in those transplanted aged over 30 with first remissions of 1 year or less. Other patients had comparable survival with each treatment approach (Gale *et al.*, 1996b).

Using a regimen of high-dose etoposide, cyclophosphamide, and TBI, the 44-month actuarial probabilities of disease-free survival, persistent or recurrent leukemia, and transplant-related mortality in 40 patients given a family-member allograft for untreated first relapse of AML were 29%, 44%, and 47%, respectively (Brown *et al.*, 1995). Disease-free survival was improved and the risk of persistent leukemia reduced among patients with grade II acute GVHD. The relapse rate was 58% and 5-year disease-free survival only 7% in 14 AML patients with 11q23 abnormalities allografted in relapse or with primary refractory disease (Appelbaum *et al.*, 2000).

Primary induction failure

In 21 leukemic patients who failed to achieve remission after induction chemotherapy (two courses of conventional dose

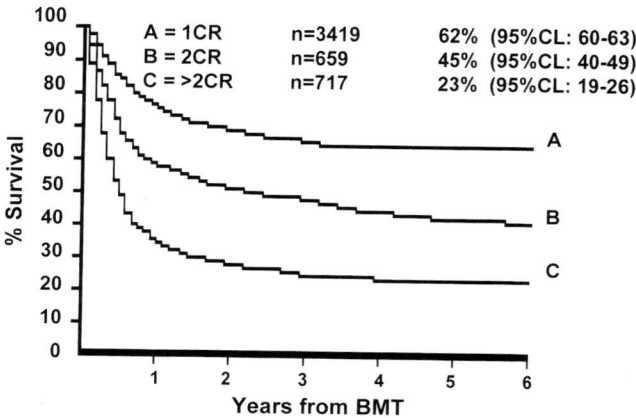

Fig. 50.5. The effect of disease phase on actuarial survival of AML patients allografted 1990–2000 from HLA-identical siblings: first remission 62%, 2nd remission 45%, beyond second remission 23%. Analysis 2002, EBMT Acute Leukemia Working Party 2002.

cytosine arabinoside and anthracycline), Forman *et al.* (1991) reported that complete remission was achieved in 90% after allogeneic BMT, and the actuarial risk of relapse-free survival after 5 years was estimated to be 43%. An IBMTR multicenter study (Biggs *et al.*, 1992) reported a 3-year leukemia-free survival rate of 21% for 88 patients with AML refractory to remission induction chemotherapy.

Another study showed 15% long-term survival in primary refractory patients with AML (Singhal *et al.*, 2002). The 2002 EBMT analysis (unpublished) shows an 18% survival at 6 years for 407 patients with AML classified as primary refractory (Fig. 50.6). Therefore patients failing induction chemotherapy should be considered for an allogeneic transplant as soon as possible. Patients who received an allograft as primary treatment (most with dysplasia) (*n* = 43) had a 30% survival at 6 years (Figure 50.6). Although this is a small patient population, it is interesting to note that allografting as first-line therapy is feasible.

Acute promyelocytic leukemia (APL) (FAB M3)

AML cases with features of APL, including the hypergranular (FAB AML-M3) or microgranular (FAB AML-M3v) morphology variants, usually have an associated t(15;17)(q21;q11) chromosomal abnormality. The t(15;17) results in the fusion of the PML gene on chromosome 15q with the RARα on chromosome 17q. Preliminary studies of the use of reverse-transcriptase polymerase chain reaction (RT-PCR) for minimal residual disease monitoring suggested that APL was one form of acute leukemia in which the combination of *trans* retinoic acid (ATRA) and chemotherapy led to complete elimination of the leukemic clone. Additionally, arsenic trioxide appears to be an effective agent for this disease (Shen *et al.*, 1997; Soignet *et al.*, 2001).

Achievement of PCR negativity for the PML/RARα transcript is predictive of continuous complete remission: a review by Diverio and colleagues (1994) showed that 5 of 86 patients in first molecular remission relapsed as compared to 27 of 36 who were in remission but had persistent PCR positivity.

A patient with APL in first remission and an HLA-identical sibling, should be quantitatively monitored for PML/RARα transcripts and considered for an allograft only if RT-PCR positivity persists or recurs. Equally, autologous HSCT could be employed, particularly if cells negative for PML-RARα are available (Nabhan *et al.*, 2001) (Figs. 50.7 and 50.8).

Acute erythroleukemia (FAB M6)

A retrospective EBMT survey reported the outcome on 106 adult patients given an autograft, and 104 given an HLA-identical allograft, for acute erythroleukemia in first complete remission (Fouillard *et al.*, 2002). The median follow-up was 24 months for the autograft recipients and 44 months for the allograft recipients. For the autograft recipients the 5-year leukemia-free survival rate, the relapse incidence, and the transplant-related mortality rate was $26 \pm 5\%$, $70 \pm 6\%$, and $13 \pm 9\%$, respectively. In contrast, the results for the allograft recipients were $57 \pm 5\%$, $21 \pm 5\%$, and $27 \pm 5\%$, respectively, indicating that an HLA-matched allograft can improve the otherwise poor prognosis of this disease.

Acute megakaryoblastic leukemia (FAB M7)

Acute megakaryoblastic leukemia (AML M7, acute myelosclerosis) is a severe form of AML with medullary overgrowth of reticular fibers, marrow infiltration by sheets and clusters of large and small dysplastic mononuclear megakaryoblasts, and terminal megakaryoblastemia with severe pancytopenia. The clinical course rarely exceeds 1 year and is more often fatal within a matter of months. It may arise secondarily as a variant of CML in blast transformation. It represents 8% to 10% of AML cases in adults and 3% in children. While initial therapy

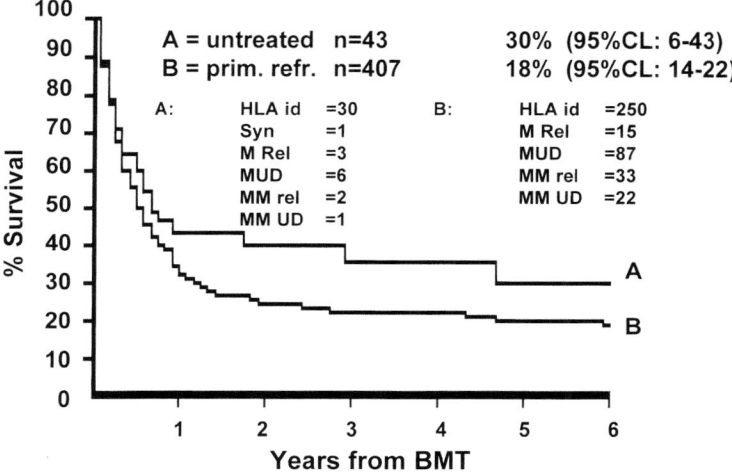

Fig. 50.6. Primary induction failure: actuarial survival of AML patients allografted 1990–2000 after failing induction chemotherapy: 18% survival at 6 years, with transplants being performed from HLA-identical siblings, but also alternative donors. Survival of patients allografted as first-line therapy is also shown (30% survival at 6 years). Analysis 2002, EBMT Acute Leukemia Working Party 2002.

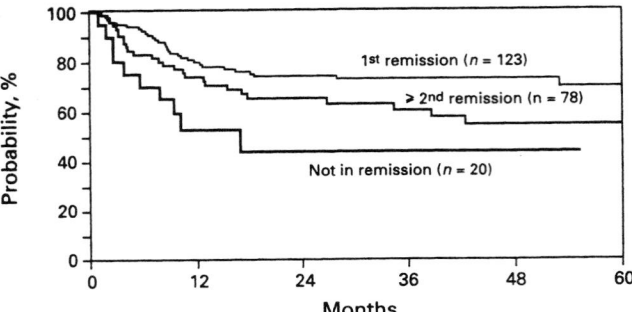

Fig. 50.7. Leukemia-free survival of patients in CR1 and CR2 undergoing autologous hematopoietic stem cell transplantation for APL 1990–1999 (data from IBMTR). Reproduced, with permission, from Nabhan *et al.* (2001).

utilizes AML remission induction chemotherapy, allogeneic marrow transplantation has been reported in a small number of cases with or without preceding chemotherapy (Mehta *et al.*, 1983; Bullorsky *et al.*, 1990; de Oliveira *et al.*, 1992). As in chronic idiopathic myelofibrosis, the marrow fibrosis resolves with successful allografting (Masauzi *et al.*, 1994). Engraftment can be rapid.

A literature review of seven cases treated with allogeneic BMT described a 12- and 24-month survival of 86% without relapses (Ruiz-Arguelles *et al.*, 1992). This was in marked contrast to 57 patients in the same report treated either by combination chemotherapy or low-dose cytosine arabinoside in which the 12-month survival rates were 37% and 26%, respectively, and 24-month survival rates were 12% and 11%. The relapse rates were 68% and 94%, respectively. It was concluded that eligible patients with a histocompatible donor should be offered allogeneic transplantation.

Treatment of relapse

Relapse of AML after an allograft can be treated with chemotherapy, donor lymphocyte infusions (DLI), and/or a

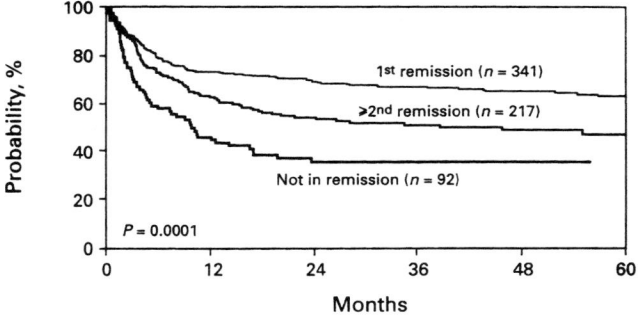

Fig. 50.8. Leukemia-free survival of patients in CR1 and CR2 undergoing matched sibling allogeneic hematopoietic stem cell transplantation for APL 1990–1999 (data from IBMTR). Reproduced, with permission, from Nabhan *et al.* (2001).

second allograft. Induction chemotherapy is usually the first choice and is aimed at reducing the proportion of leukemic cells in the marrow; it is of interest that once remission is achieved, this is sustained by residual normal donor stem cells. DLI should be used to consolidate remission and not to treat relapse; some patients may become long-term remitters after DLI given in remission.

A second allograft is a potentially curative approach. In an EBMT survey, 170 patients with acute leukemia relapsing postallograft, received a second allogeneic transplant. Of these 26% were alive at 5 years (Bosi *et al.*, 2001), although transplant-related mortality was 46% and relapse 59%; favorable prognostic factors were a late relapse (>292 days after the first transplant), complete remission, and TBI conditioning for second transplant. In patients who received a second allograft when the relapse occurred beyond 292 days from first transplant, the long-term survival was 50% (Bosi *et al.*, 2001). Therefore, this treatment modality should be kept in mind when a patient with AML experiences a relapse posttransplant.

Donors other than HLA-identical siblings

Results of HLA-mismatched family member transplantation

Patients with AML who lack an HLA-identical sibling are eligible for an HSCT from an alternative donor; this may be an unrelated or a family member mismatched donor. The latter has the great advantage of not requiring a time-consuming and expensive donor search through the international registries because almost everybody has a mismatched donor in the family. In patients with AML refractory to remission induction chemotherapy, a 3-year actuarial disease-free survival rate of 19% has been reported, similar to the outcome with HLA-identical sibling grafts (Chiang *et al.*, 2001).

The Perugia group has developed a program for 1-haplotype-mismatched family transplants: donor peripheral blood stem cells (PBSC) are mobilized with G-CSF, collected with several leukaphereses, and purified using a CD34+ positive selection approach (Aversa *et al.*, 1998). The aim is to give a "megadose" of CD34+ cells stringently depleted (4 logs) of T cells, which will engraft following intensive cytoreductive chemo/radiotherapy (TBI, thiotepa, fludarabine, ATG). Some patients with AML, although in advanced phase of the disease, have become long-term survivors, possibly due to natural killer (NK) cell-mediated eradication of the leukemic clone (Ruggeri *et al.*, 2002). This is not seen in ALL patients, whose blasts are not killed by NK cells (see Chapters 16 and 66). The same group has provided evidence that only recipients who lack the inhibitory NK receptor (KIR) for donor NK cells will experience a low risk of relapse, contrary to AML patients with a KIR match with their donor, who have the expected 70% relapse rate (Ruggeri *et al.*, 2002). The possibility of using cells to eradicate a leukemia that is otherwise incurable is exciting. The induction of BCR-ABL negativity in NOD-SCID mice engrafted with a human myeloid blast crisis of chronic myeloid leukemia, using NK cells only, is provocative, although in keeping with this hypothesis (Ruggeri *et al.*, 2002).

Results of unrelated donor transplantation

Despite significant improvement over the past decade, survival of patients undergoing an unrelated graft is somewhat lower compared to that of recipients of HLA-identical sibling transplants. The EBMT database currently contains 13,041 patients with AML, of whom 5,187 were autografted and 7,807 allografted (EBMT web site, ebmt.org). The proportion of unrelated donor transplants for AML increased from less than 400/year in 1997 to over 600/year in 2000. Survival at 5 years for patients grafted in first remission is shown in Fig. 50.9. In the pediatric population, survival for HLA-identical siblings (*n* = 388) was 66% compared with 43% for patients grafted from an unrelated donor (*n* = 334). In adults the figures were 58% (*n* = 2,306) for HLA-identical sibling transplants and 47% for unrelated transplants (*n* = 109). In children allografted in second remission, survival was 51% for siblings (*n* = 59) versus 47% unrelated donors (*n* = 62). In adults the figures in second remission were 47% for siblings (*n* = 420) and 37% for unrelated donors (*n* = 109). The Fred Hutchinson Cancer Research Center has reported 161 patients with primary AML conditioned with cyclophosphamide and TBI prior to an unmanipulated unrelated donor BMT followed by cyclosporine/methotrexate (Sierra *et al.*, 2000) (Fig. 50.10). With a median follow-up of 2.9 years, the leukemia-free survival was 50% ± 12% for those transplanted during first complete remission, 28 ± 8% during second remission, 7 ± 3% for those transplanted in relapse, and 19 ± 10% for those with primary induction failure. The cumulative incidences of relapses was 19%, 23%, 44%, and 63%, respectively. Favorable prognostic factors were transplantation during remission, a marrow cell dose above 3.5 × 10^8/kg, and CMV seronegative status.

Results of identical twin transplantation (and see Chapter 49)

We have analyzed 5,224 AML patients who received a bone marrow transplant while in first remission from an HLA-identical sibling (*n* = 4,876), an identical twin (*n* = 84), or an unrelated HLA-matched donor (*n* = 264) between 1980 and 2000. The actuarial survival at 6 years was 62% for the syngeneic grafts, 62% for the HLA-identical siblings, and 46% for the unrelated grafts (Fig. 50.11). Causes of death were different in the three groups: relapse was 61%, 35%, and 21% for syngeneic, HLA-identical, and unrelated transplants, respectively, whereas TRM was 33%, 33%, and 21%. Thus, in the unrelated setting the low relapse compensates for the high TRM, and in the syngeneic setting it is the opposite: little TRM, but a higher proportion of patients experiencing leukemia relapse (Fig. 50.12). This emphasizes the importance of both high-dose chemoradiotherapy conditioning and of the GVL effect: that they both contribute to cure AML is clear in the unrelated setting. It is also true that over 60% of AML patients receiving high-dose chemoradiotherapy and syngeneic stem cells (with no GVL effect by definition) are cured of their disease.

Stem cell source

Bone marrow or peripheral blood

Mobilized peripheral blood (PB) transplants are being increasingly used in the allogeneic setting, and are now often preferred to conventional bone marrow (BM) transplants. Comparison of the two stem cell sources has been performed in retrospective and prospective trials but adequate follow-up is available only for HLA-identical sibling transplants (Schmitz *et al.*, 1998; Vigorito *et al.*, 1998; Champlin *et al.*, 2000; Powles *et al.*, 2000; Bensinger *et al.*, 2001; Flowers *et al.*, 2002) (and see Chapter 11). The results of retrospective and prospective studies can be summarized as follows. Hematologic and immune

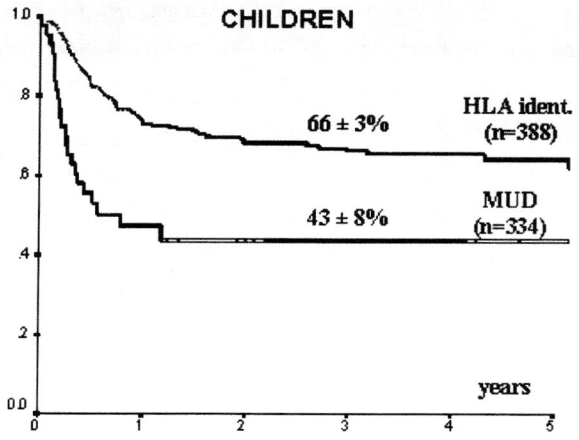

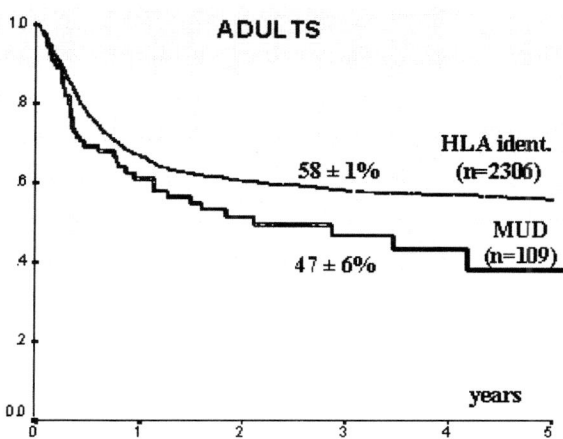

Fig. 50.9. The effect of donor type on actuarial survival of AML patients allografted 1990–2000 in first CR: HLA-identical siblings, 66% in children and 58% in adults. Unrelated transplants, 43% in children and 47% for adults. Analysis 2002, EBMT Acute Leukemia Working Party 2002.

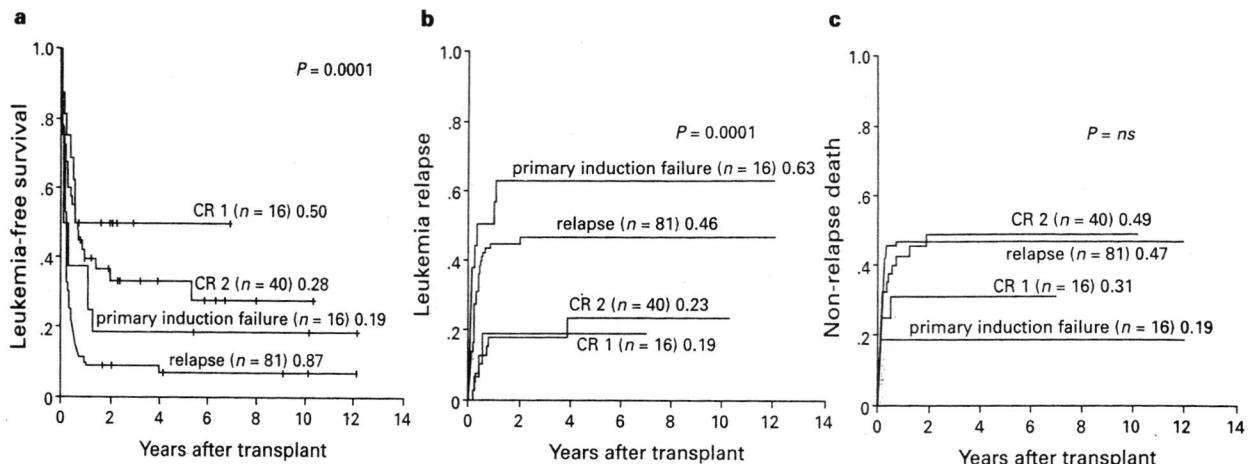

Fig. 50.10. Outcome of unrelated BMT for AML according to disease status (*n* = 161); leukemia-free survival (**a**), leukemia recurrence (**b**), and cumulative incidence of nonrelapse death. Reproduced, with permission, from Sierra *et al.* (2000).

recovery is faster after PB grafts, but the quality of graft function is comparable. The incidence and severity of acute graft-versus-host disease is similar, whereas that of chronic GVHD is increased in recipients of PB transplants. Transplant-related mortality is similar in the two groups, whereas disease recurrence is lower after PB grafts. The general feeling is that PB grafts are indicated for patients with advanced disease, whereas for early phase patients the two sources may give comparable results.

As with all innovative medical procedures, the use of peripheral blood cells should be considered with caution. For example, one randomized trial showed no significant difference in chronic GVHD (Bensinger *et al.*, 2001), but this was no longer true after additional follow-up of one year (Flowers *et al.*, 2002). Because chronic GVHD is a serious complication, a long-term follow-up of PB transplant recipients will need to

look at quality of life and time to discontinuation of immuno-suppressive therapy.

Results of cord blood transplantation

Cord blood (CB) is a relatively new source of stem cells that has been explored over the past decade. Three publications have set the stage for CB transplants from HLA-identical siblings (Rocha *et al.*, 2000), from unrelated donors in children (Rocha *et al.*, 2001), and for adults grafted with unrelated CB (Laughlin *et al.*, 2001). Common to the results of these three studies is the low risk of acute and chronic GVHD for patients receiving CB transplants: in the HLA-identical IBMTR/EUROCORD study, the risk of acute GVHD was 0.41 compared to bone marrow (*P* = .001), and was 0.35 for chronic GVHD (*P* = .02). In order to compare the outcome of unrelated grafts, 541 children with

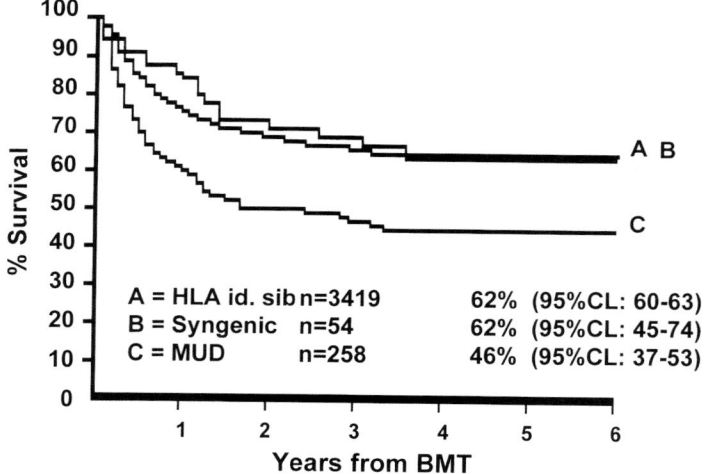

Fig. 50.11. Syngeneic transplants for AML allografted 1990–2000 in first remission. The actuarial survival is 62%. It is 62% also for HLA-identical sibling transplants and 46% for unrelated grafts. Analysis 2002, EBMT Acute Leukemia Working Party 2002.

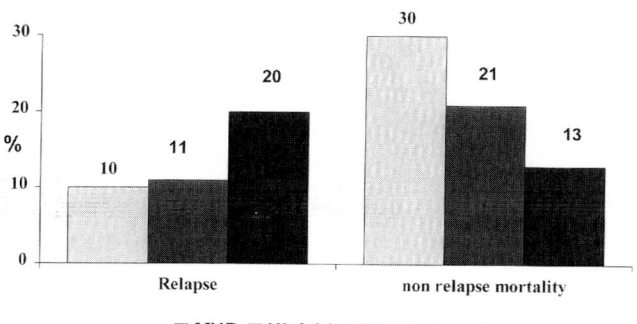

Fig. 50.12. Syngeneic transplants for AML allografted 1990–2000 in first remission. Causes of death differ between syngeneic and allogeneic transplants. Leukemia relapse predominates in the syngeneic transplants, whereas nonrelapse mortality is higher in the unrelated donor grafts As seen in Fig. 50.11 the final outcome depends on the sum of failure causes. Analysis 2002, EBMT Acute Leukemia Working Party 2002.

acute leukemia were stratified according to whether they received stem cells from CB ($n = 99$), T-cell-depleted bone marrow ($n = 180$), or T-cell-replete bone marrow ($n = 262$) (Rocha *et al.*, 2001). Nonadjusted estimates of 2-year survival were 35% for CB, 41% for T-cell-depleted marrow, and 49% for T-cell-replete marrow recipients. The conclusion was that unrelated CB transplantation is a reasonable option for children with acute leukemia. In adults the issue is complicated by the cell dose effect, since it is more difficult to achieve a high CB cell dose; nevertheless, an analysis of 68 adults showed that 28% were alive with a median follow-up of 22 months (Laughlin *et al.*, 2001).

Results using reduced intensity conditioning regimens

Allogeneic HSC transplants following reduced intensity regimens have been investigated over the past 5 years in an attempt to reduce transplant-related toxicity and mortality. Due to the independent work from Houston, Seattle, and Jerusalem (Giralt *et al.*, 1997; Slavin *et al.*, 1998; Storb *et al.*, 1999), it has become clear that the use of small doses of fludarabine or TBI in combination with each other or other agents can allow permanent engraftment of donor hematopoietic stem cells. This approach allows the exploration of the GVL effect without the toxicity of myeloablative therapy and warrants further study in patients with leukemia who are ineligible for conventional transplantation, either because of age or concurrent medical conditions.

Investigators at the M.D. Anderson Hospital performed a pilot trial to determine whether purine analogue-containing non-myeloablative chemotherapy could be sufficiently immunosuppressive to enable engraftment of allogeneic hematopoietic progenitor cells in patients with acute leukemia or myelodysplasia (MDS) considered ineligible for myeloabla-

tive therapy either because of age or medical condition (Giralt *et al.*, 2001).

Fifteen patients were treated [13 with acute myeloid leukemia (AML), 2 with MDS]. The median age was 59 (range 27–71) years; 12 patients were either refractory to therapy or beyond first relapse of AML. Eight patients were given fludarabine 30 mg/m² daily for 4 days with idarubicin 12 mg/m² for 3 days and cytosine arabinoside 2 g/m² daily for 4 days ($n = 7$) or melphalan 140 mg/m² ($n = 1$); 7 patients were given 2-chlorodeoxyadenosine 12 mg/m² daily for 5 days and cytosine arabinoside 1 g/m² daily for 5 days. Thirteen patients received HLA-compatible allogeneic PBSC and 1 received bone marrow after the chemotherapy. One treatment-related death occurred in a patient who developed multiorgan failure before receiving stem cells. GVHD prophylaxis consisted of cyclosporine and methylprednisolone.

Thirteen patients achieved a neutrophil count of greater than $0.5 \times 10^9/l$ at a median of 10 (range 8–17) days postinfusion. Ten patients achieved platelet counts of $20 \times 10^9/l$ a median of 13 (range 7–78) days postinfusion. Eight patients achieved complete remission (bone marrow blasts <5% with neutrophil recovery and platelet transfusion independence); 6 of these 8 patients had greater than 90% donor cells using either RFLP or conventional cytogenetic analyses; 1 patient showed autologous reconstitution and 1 patient could not have chimerism analysis performed. At 2 to 3 months posttransplant 4 patients remained in remission, with 3 having greater than 80% donor cells by RFLP or cytogenetic techniques. One patient remains alive and disease-free with 100% donor cells as documented by RFLP and cytogenetic testing. It was concluded from this experience that purine analogue-containing non-myeloablative regimens allow engraftment of HLA-compatible hematopoietic progenitor cells, and that this approach could allow exploration of the GVL effect without the toxicity of myeloablative therapy in patients with leukemia ineligible for conventional myeloablative regimens either because of age or concurrent medical conditions (Giralt *et al.*, 1997).

Slavin and colleagues (1998) have also described their initial experience with non-myeloablative conditioning in 26 patients, 10 of whom had acute leukemia. They found that a regimen comprising fludarabine, anti-T-lymphocyte globulin, and low-dose busulfan (8 mg/kg) was extremely well tolerated, with no severe procedure-related toxicity. Granulocyte colony-stimulating factor (G-CSF)-mobilized blood stem cell transplantation with standard dose of cyclosporine as the sole anti-GVHD prophylaxis resulted in stable partial ($n = 9$) or complete ($n = 17$) chimerism. In 9 patients the absolute neutrophil count (ANC) did not decrease to below $0.1 \times 10^9/l$ whereas 2 patients never experienced ANC less than $0.5 \times 10^9/l$. ANC $0.5 \times 10^9/l$ or greater was accomplished within 10 to 32 (median 15) days. Platelet counts did not decrease to below $20 \times 10^9/l$ in 4 patients requiring no platelet support at all; overall platelet counts greater than $20 \times 10^9/l$ were achieved within 0 to 35 (median 12) days. Fourteen patients experienced no GVHD at all; severe GVHD (grades 3 and 4) was the single major complication and

the cause of death in 4 patients, occurring after early discontinuation of cyclosporine. Relapse was reversed by allogeneic cell
therapy in 2 of 3 cases, with no residual host DNA detected by
cytogenetic analysis and PCR. To date, with an observation
period extending over 1 year (median 8 months), 22 of 26
patients (85%) treated by allogeneic non-myeloablative stem
cell transplantation are alive, and 21 (81%) are disease-free. The
actuarial probability of disease-free survival at 14 months is
77.5% (95% confidence interval 53% to 90%) (Fig. 50.13).

A study using fludarabine and busulfan included 17 patients
with AML, as well as 20 with MDS. The 1 year TRM and progression-free survival rates were 5% and 66%, respectively
(Martino et al., 2002). The 1 year incidence of disease progression was 13% and 58% in those with and without acute GVHD
grade II-IV or chronic GVHD, suggesting a significant role for a
GVL effect in minimizing relapse after this regimen.

Other regimens using reduced doses of thiotepa or melphalan have also been proposed (Raiola et al., 2000; Chakraverty
et al., 2002). Several meetings have summarized the preliminary results. An EBMT workshop focused on transplant-related
mortality and GVHD (Bacigalupo, 2002). Retrospective and
prospective studies from the EBMT, national groups, and single institutions included over 900 patients: the incidence of
acute GVHD grade III–IV was 12% (1%–17%), extensive
chronic GVHD 42% (25%–51%), and TRM 20% (14%–38%).
Conditioning regimens could be classified into 4 major groups
based on (1) total body irradiation (TBI) 200 cGy, (2) busulfan
8 mg/kg, (3) thiotepa 10 mg/kg, and (4) melphalan 140 mg/m^2.
Most of these regimens were administered in association with
fludarabine in different doses and used mobilized peripheral
blood as the source of stem cells. The incidence of TRM was
similar if not identical for all four regimens, whereas the risk of
acute GVHD and chronic GVHD varied according to whether
T-cell antibodies (such as CAMPATH) were used in the conditioning regimen (Bacigalupo, 2002).

Reduced intensity conditioning, followed by an allograft,
has been used successfully to treat patients with AML at high
risk of not entering remission after conventional induction
chemotherapy (Platzbecker et al., 2001).

Comparison of allogeneic transplantation with chemotherapy or autologous transplantation

The issue of allogeneic transplantation versus autologous transplantation or even versus intensive consolidation chemotherapy
for patients with AML in first remission has been debated for at
least 2 decades

In a large registry study, 901 patients given an HLA-identical
sibling transplant for AML in first remission were compared to
198 patients given chemotherapy (Gale et al., 1996a). Five-year
leukemia-free survival, TRM, and relapse for the two groups
were 46% versus 35% (P = .01), 43% versus 7% (P < .0001),
and 24% versus 63% (P < .0001), respectively. Five-year probability of survival was similar (48% versus 42%, P = .24). The
results of these different strategies are overlapping, and their
interpretation is further complicated by biases in patient selection, and, most importantly, by censoring of patients who
relapse before undergoing transplantation or consolidation
chemotherapy. Another study of 652 children and adolescents
(up to age 20), found actuarial 8-year survival in those receiving
an HLA-identical related donor transplant to be significantly
superior (60%) to those receiving autologous transplantation
(48%) or aggressive high-dose cytarabine-based chemotherapy
as intensive postremission treatment (53%) (Woods et al., 2001)
(Fig. 50.14). The actuarial probability of relapse was significantly lower in the allograft recipients.

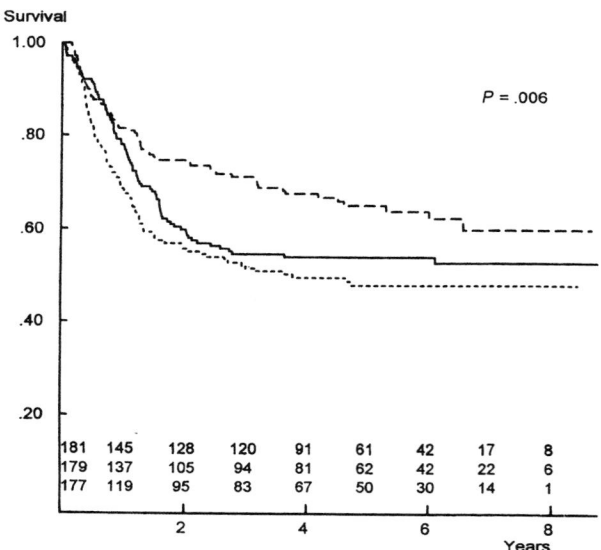

Fig. 50.14. Actuarial survival from AML remission, comparing the three
postremission regimens from CCG-2891. Numbers are patients at risk at
yearly intervals; rows are in the same order as curves. P value is for homogeneity. Dashed line indicates allogeneic BMT; solid line, intensive non-
marrow-ablative chemotherapy; dotted line, autologous BMT. Reproduced,
with permission, from Woods et al. (2001).

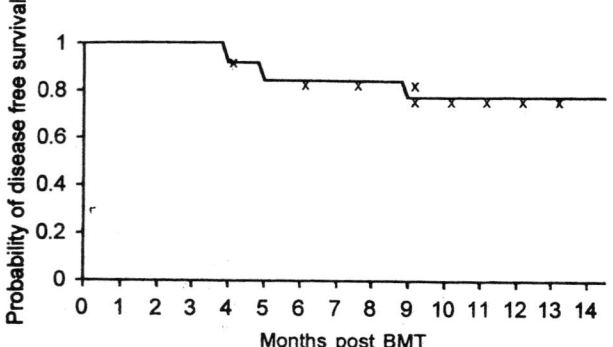

Fig. 50.13. Kaplan-Meier actuarial disease-free survival at 14 months of
the entire group of 26 patients treated with allogeneic non-myeloablative
stem cell transplantation. Reproduced, with permission, from Slavin et al.
(1998).

Table 50.2. *The impact of treatment strategy (chemotherapy, autologous transplants, allogeneic transplants) in patients with AML in first CR, stratified for risk category*

		Chemotherapy	Autologous transplant	Allogeneic transplant
Good	No. pts	411	49	50
	Relapse	40%	23%	8%
	Survival	70%	77%	72%
Standard	No. pts	750	127	135
	Relapse	59%	34%	19%
	Survival	45%	57%	66%
Poor	No. pts	204	23	16
	Relapse	83%	73%	38%
	Survival	19%	29%	38%

Reproduced, with permission, from Wheatly *et al.* (1999).

Censoring of patients who are excluded before they receive the planned treatment is difficult, but can be achieved by analyzing the results according to the "intention to treat" as well as by the treatment patients actually receive (Suciu, 1991). In order to avoid bias due to patient selection, comparisons must be made in prospective studies.

In the BGMT 87 study (Reiffers *et al.*, 1996), which prospectively compared HLA-identical sibling transplantation in first remission (*n* = 36) with either autologous stem cell transplantation or chemotherapy (*n* = 60), the 3-year disease-free survival was 66% for the former and 43% for the latter (*P* < .05), with a lower relapse rate in the allografted patients.

Two large multicenter prospective trials have been published: one by the GIMEMA/EORTC group (Zittoun *et al.*, 1995) (Fig. 50.3), and one from the UK involving close to 1,000 patients each (Table 50.2). In the study by Zittoun, allogeneic transplants results proved borderline better than those of autologous transplants, and significantly better than those with chemotherapy (Fig. 50.3).

In the UK trial, risk groups were identified: good risk patients had favorable cytogenetic abnormalities [t(15;17),

t(8,21) and inv(16)], and had achieved remission after one course of chemotherapy. High-risk were patients with unfavorable cytogenetic findings (monosomy 5 or 7, abnormalities of the long arm of chromosome 3, or complex karyotype), or had required two courses of chemotherapy to enter remission. Intermediate risk patients were all the others. The numbers were 421 for good risk, 765 for intermediate, and 305 for poor risk patients (Wheatly *et al.*, 1999). Best results were obtained in good-risk patients with all 3 treatment options (chemo, auto, allograft), and worst outcome in high-risk patients (Table 50.2; Figs. 50.15 and 50.16). The allotransplant patients were the ones with lowest relapse rate and best survival in all three categories; in the intermediate group (which was the largest) the survival advantage was significant—66% for allografts, 57% for autografts, and 45% for chemotherapy. We believe this study exemplifies well the heterogeneity of patients with AML, and the need to take into account cytogenetic data as well as remission induction data. It also suggests that when a matched donor is available, an allogeneic transplant is probably the best choice, in all risk categories, but especially in the intermediate and high-risk group (Wheatly *et al.*, 1999).

Other markers of outcome may be identified and could be used to further refine decision making in AML patients; the FLT3 length mutation (FLT3-LM) is one example (Schnittger *et al.*, 2002).

When choosing the treatment strategy not only survival data should be taken into account but also quality of life assessment; overall, patients treated with an allograft have a slightly poorer quality of life, due to chronic GVHD, as compared to those given autologous grafts or chemotherapy (Zittoun *et al.*, 1997). Thus, improved survival rate in allografts must be balanced against reduced quality of life.

Indications and contraindications for allogeneic transplantation

An allogeneic transplant is indicated if a suitable donor is available, and when the patient is clinically fit. The age limit has

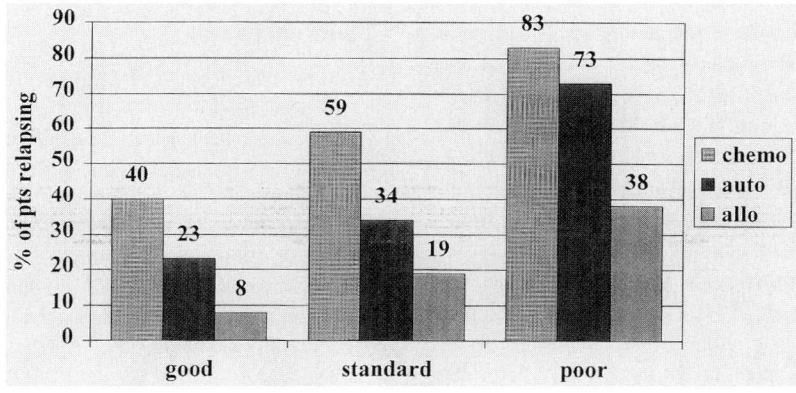

Fig. 50.15. The impact of treatment strategy (chemotherapy, autologous transplants, allogeneic transplants) in patients with AML in first CR, stratified for risk category. Reproduced, with permission, from Wheatly *et al* 1999).

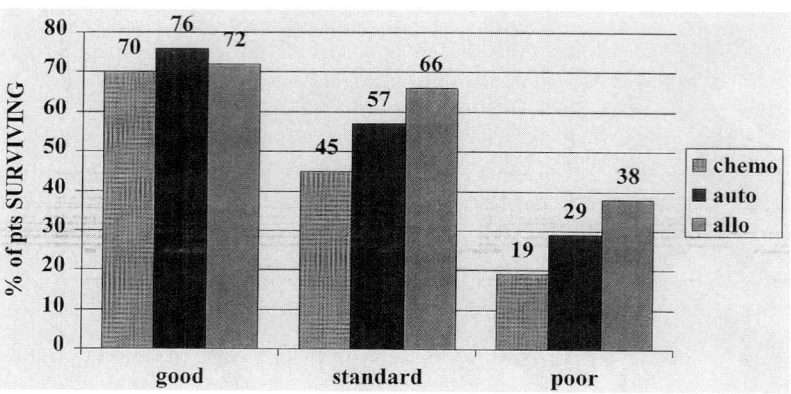

Fig. 50.16. The impact of treatment strategy (chemotherapy, autologous transplants, allogeneic transplants) in patients with AML in first CR, stratified for risk category. Reproduced, with permission, from Wheatly *et al.* (1999).

been increasing; it was 40 to 45 years in the 1980s and it is now up to 65 to 70. The median age was 20 in 1985, 35 in 1995, and is now 45 years (unpublished data). Twenty years ago it was contraindicated to allograft a 60-year-old patient with AML in first remission. Today, with reduced intensity conditioning regimens, this is feasible and may enhance the control of the underlying disease. An "indication" paper from the EBMT defines transplant procedures in four different categories (Urbano-Ispizua *et al.*, 2002): standard, clinical research protocol, developmental, not recommended. The category standard (S) refers to transplants with well-defined results that compare favorably (or are superior) to results of nontransplant treatment approaches.

The category clinical protocol (CP) refers to transplants the value of which is not fully defined, and are performed in the context of a clinical protocol. Developmental (D) are transplants with little or no national or international experience. The category also covers fundamentally new approaches to the management of a disease that in a different status or phase may already be classified under (S) or (CP) above. Finally, the category not recommended (NR) covers procedures contemplated for a disease in a phase or status in which patients are not conventionally treated by hematopoietic HSCT. Clearly, there will be some overlap between NR and D. NR also includes early disease stages when results of conventional treatment do not justify the additional risk of TRM, or when the disease is so advanced that the chance of success is so small that the risk of the harvest procedure for the normal donor is difficult to justify. NR may not apply to specific situations where there exists a syngeneic donor.

For patients with AML, transplants from HLA-identical siblings are standard in all phases of disease. Unrelated transplants are clinical protocol for patients in remission and "not recommended" applies to those with AML-M3 in molecular remission or in those with AML in refractory relapse. Additionally, some European groups discourage allografts for patients in first remission with other cytogenetically favorable subtypes, such as t(8;21) and inv(16) (Urbano Ispizua *et al.*, 2002) (see Chapter 124).

Conclusions

HLA-identical sibling HSCT is an effective treatment for AML patients. It remains the only curative treatment for patients with primary induction failure, and the best treatment for many of those who achieve a first remission following induction chemotherapy and for those who later relapse.

The use of a reduced intensity conditioning regimen has raised the age limit to 70 and possibly above. Despite increasing age, TRM is being gradually and constantly reduced. The large file of bone marrow donors worldwide (BMDWW) provides a donor for the majority of patients activating an unrelated donor search. Extended family HLA typing may identify partially mismatched family donors for many patients. The use of one full haplotype mismatched donor is a new promising venue of investigation, which may help us understand NK mediated-leukemic cell kill.

New stem cell sources have been explored, and now peripheral blood is widely used and cord blood has proven valuable, especially in the pediatric population. Documentation and quality control remain important challenges for the next decade, and will hopefully further improve the outcome of those undergoing an allogeneic HSCT.

References

ABMTR Newsletter. (1996). IBMTR/ABMTR Statistical Center, Milwaukee, **3**, 10–11.

Appelbaum, F.R., Bryant, E., & Garrido, S.M. (2000). Allogeneic stem cell transplantation for relapsed and refractory acute myeloid leukemia patients with 11q23 abnormalities. *Leukemia Research*, **24**, 481–6.

Aversa, F., Tabilio, A., Velardi, A. *et al.* (1998). Treatment of high-risk acute leukemia with T-cell-depleted stem cells from related donors with one fully mismatched HLA haplotype. *New England Journal of Medicine*, **339**, 1238–9.

Bacigalupo, A. (2002). Second EBMT workshop on reduced intensity conditioning regimen. *Bone Marrow Transplantation*, **29**, 191–5.

Bacigalupo, A., Lamparelli, T., Gualandi, F. et al. (2001). Increased risk of leukemia relapse with high-dose cyclosporine A after allogeneic marrow transplantation for acute leukemia: a 10 year follow-up of a randomized study. *Blood,* **98,** 3174–5.

Bacigalupo, A., Van Lint, M.T., Occhini, D. et al. (1991). Increased risk of leukemia relapse with high-dose cyclosporine A after allogeneic marrow transplantation for acute leukemia. *Blood,* **77,** 1423–8.

Bensinger, W.I., Martin, P.J., Storer, B. et al. (2001). Transplantation of bone marrow as compared with peripheral-blood cells from HLA-identical relatives in patients with hematologic cancers. *New England Journal of Medicine,* **344,** 175–81.

Biggs, J.C., Horowitz, M., Gale, R.P. et al. (1992). Bone marrow transplants may cure patients with acute leukemia never achieving remission with chemotherapy. *Blood,* **80,** 1090–3.

Blaise, D., Maraninchi, D., Archimbaud, E. et al. (1992). Allogeneic bone marrow transplantation for acute myelogenous leukemia in first remission. Busulfan-cytoxan versus cytoxan-total body irradiation as preparative regimens. A report from the Groupe d'Etudes de la Greffe de Moelle Osseuse. *Blood,* **79,** 2578–82.

Blaise, D., Maranchini, D., Michallet, M. et al. (2001). Long-term follow-up of a randomized trial comparing the combination of cyclophosphamide with total body irradiation or busulfan as conditioning regimen for patients receiving HLA-identical marrow grafts for acute myeloblastic leukemia in first complete remission. *Blood,* **97,** 3669–71.

Bleakley, M., Lau, L., Shaw, P.J., & Kaufman, A. (2002). Bone marrow transplantation for paediatric AML in first remission: a systematic review and meta-analysis. *Bone Marrow Transplantation,* **29,** 843–52.

Bosi, A., Laszlo, D., Labopin, M. et al. (2001). Acute Leukemia Working Party of the European Blood and Marrow Transplant Group. *Journal of Clinical Oncology,* **19,** 3675–84.

Brochstein, J.A., Kernan, N.A., Groshen, S. et al. (1987). Allogeneic bone marrow transplantation after hyperfractionated total body irradiation and cyclophosphamide in children with acute leukemia. *New England Journal of Medicine,* **317,** 1618–24.

Brown, R.A., Wolff, S.N., Fay, J.W. et al. (1995). High-dose etoposide, cyclophosphamide, and total body irradiation with allogeneic bone marrow transplantation for patients with acute myeloid leukemia in untreated first relapse: a study by the North American Marrow Transplant Group. *Blood,* **85,** 1391–5.

Bullorsky, E.O., Shanley, C.M., Stemmelin, G. et al. (1990). Acute megakaryoblastic leukemia with massive myelofibrosis: complete remission and reversal of marrow fibrosis with allogeneic bone marrow transplantation as the only treatment. *Bone Marrow Transplantation,* **6,** 449–52.

Chakraverty, R., Peggs, K., Chopra, R. et al. (2002). Limiting transplantation-related mortality following unrelated donor stem cell transplantation by using a nonmyeloablative conditioning regimen. *Blood,* **99,** 1071–8.

Champlin, R.E., Schmitz, N., Horowitz, M.M. et al.. (2000). Blood stem cells compared with bone marrow as a source of hematopoietic cells for allogeneic transplantation. IBMTR Histocompatibility and Stem Cell Sources Working Committee and the European Group for Blood and Marrow Transplantation (EBMT). *Blood,* **95,** 3702–9.

Chiang, K.Y., Van Rhee, F., Godder, K. et al. (2001). Allogeneic bone marrow transplantation from partially mismatched related donors as therapy for primary induction failure acute myeloid leukemia. *Bone Marrow Transplantation,* **27,** 507–10.

Chiodi, S., Spinelli, S., Ravera, G. et al. (2000). Quality of life in 244 recipients of allogeneic bone marrow transplantation. *British Journal of Haematology,* **110,** 614–9.

Clift, R.A., Buckner, C.D., Appelbaum, F.R. et al. (1990). Allogeneic marrow transplantation in patients with acute myeloid leukemia in first remission: a randomized trial of two irradiation regimens. *Blood,* **76,** 1867–71.

Clift, R.A., Buckner, C.D., Thomas, E.D. et al. (1994). Marrow transplantation for chronic myeloid leukemia: a randomized study comparing cyclophosphamide and total body irradiation with busulfan and cyclophosphamide. *Blood,* **84,** 2036–43.

Clift, R.A., Peterson, F.B., Buckner, C.D. et al. (1991). The timing of transplantation for acute myeloid leukemia. *Experimental Hematology,* **19,** 574 (Abstract).

Deeg, H.J., Leinsenring, W., Storb, R. et al. (1988). Long-term outcome after marrow transplantation for severe aplastic anemia. *Blood,* **91,** 3637–45.

Deeg, H.J., Lin, D., Leisenring, W. et al. (1997). Cyclosporine or cyclosporine plus methylprednisone for prophylaxis of graft-versus-host disease: a prospective randomized trial. *Blood,* **89,** 3880.

de Oliveira, J.S., Sale, G.E., Bryant, E.M. et al. (1992). Acute megakaryoblastic leukemia in children: treatment with bone marrow transplantation. *Bone Marrow Transplantation,* **10,** 399–403.

Devergie, A., Blaise, D., Attal, M. et al. (1995). Allogeneic bone marrow transplantation for chronic myeloid leukemia in first chronic phase: a randomized trial of busulfan-cytoxan versus cytoxan-total body irradiation as preparative regimen: a report from the French Society of Bone Marrow Graft (SFGM). *Blood,* **85,** 2263–8.

Diverio, D., Pandolfi, P.P., Rossi, V. et al. (1994). Monitoring of treatment outcome in acute promyelocytic leukemia by RT-PCR. *Leukemia,* **8,** 1105–7.

Fagioli, F., Bacigalupo, A., Frassoni, F. et al. (1994). Allogeneic bone marrow transplantation for acute myeloid leukemia in first complete remission: the effect of FAB classification and GVHD prophylaxis. *Bone Marrow Transplantation,* **13,** 247–52.

Ferrant, A., Labopin, M., Frassoni, F. et al. (1997). Karyotype in acute myeloblastic leukemia: prognostic significance for bone marrow transplantation in first remission: a European Group for Blood and Marrow Transplantation Study. *Blood,* **90,** 2931–8.

Flowers, M.E.D., Parker, P.M., Johnston, L.J. et al. (2002). Comparison of chronic graft-versus-host disease after transplantation of peripheral blood stem cells versus bone marrow in allogeneic recipients: long-term follow-up of a randomized trial. *Blood,* **100,** 415–9.

Forman, S.J., Schmidt, G.M., Nademanee, A.P. et al. (1991). Allogeneic bone marrow transplantation as therapy for primary induction failure for patients with acute leukemia. *Journal of Clinical Oncology,* **9,** 1570–4.

Fouillard, L., Labopin, M., Gorin, N-C. et al. (2002). Hematopoietic stem cell transplantation for de novo erythroleukemia: a study of the European Group for Blood and Marrow Transplantation (EBMT). *Blood,* **100,** 3135–40.

Frassoni, F., Labopin, M., Gluckman, F. et al. (1996). Results of allogeneic bone marrow transplantation for acute leukemia have improved in Europe with time: a report from the Acute Leukemia

Working Party of the European Group for Bone Marrow Transplantation (EBMT). *Bone Marrow Transplantation,* **17,** 13–8.

Frassoni, F., Labopin, M., Powles, R. *et al.* for the Acute Leukemia Working Party of the European Group for Blood and Marrow Transplantation (2000). Effect of center on outcome of bone-marrow transplantation for acute leukaemia. *Lancet,* **355,** 1393–8.

Gale, R.P., Buchner, T., Zhang, M.J. *et al.* (1996a). HLA-identical sibling bone marrow transplants versus chemotherapy for acute myelogenous leukemia in first remission. *Leukemia,* **10,** 1687–91.

Gale, R.P., Horowitz, M.M., Rees, J.K. *et al.* (1996b). Chemotherapy versus transplants for acute myelogenous leukemia in second remission. *Leukemia,* **10,** 13–9.

Gale, R.P., Horowitz, M.M., Weiner, R.S. *et al.* (1995). Impact of cytogenetic abnormalities on outcome of bone marrow transplants in acute myelogenous leukemia in first remission. *Bone Marrow Transplantation,* **16,** 203–8.

Giralt, S., Thall, P.F., Khouri, I. *et al.* (2001). Melphalan and purine analog-containing preparative regimens: reduced-intensity conditioning for patients with hematologic malignancies undergoing allogeneic progenitor cell transplantation. *Blood,* **97,** 631–7.

Goerner, M., Gooley, T., Flowers, M.E. *et al.* (2002). Morbidity and mortality of chronic GVHD after hematopoietic stem cell transplantation from HLA-identical siblings for patients with aplastic or refractory anemias. *Biology of Blood and Marrow Transplantation,* **8,** 47–56.

Horowitz, M.M., Gale, R.P., Sondel, P.M. *et al.* (1990). Graft-versus-leukemia reactions after bone marrow transplantation. *Blood,* **75,** 555–62.

Hows, J., Bradley, B., Gore, S. *et al.* (1993). Prospective evaluation of unrelated donor bone marrow transplantation. *Bone Marrow Transplantation,* **12,** 371–80.

Keating, S., de Witte, T., Suciu, S. *et al.* (1999). Centre effect on treatment outcome for patients with untreated acute myelogenous leukaemia? An analysis of the AML8A Study of the Leukemia Cooperative Group of the EORTC and GIMEMA. European Organization for Research and Treatment of Cancer (EORTC) Leukemia Cooperative Group and the Gruppo Italiano Malattie Ematologiche Maligne dell'Adulto (GIMEMA). *European Journal of Cancer,* **35,** 1440–7.

Koc, S., Leisenring, W., Flowers, M.E. *et al.* (2002). Therapy for chronic graft-versus-host disease: a randomized trial comparing cyclosporine plus prednisone versus prednisone alone. *Blood,* **100,** 48–51.

Laughlin, M.J., Barker, J., Bambach, B. *et al.* (2001). Hematopoietic engraftment and survival in adult recipients of umbilical-cord blood from unrelated donors. *New England Journal of Medicine,* **344,** 1860–1.

Lee, S.J., Vogelsang, G., Gilman, A. *et al.* (2002). A survey of diagnosis, management and grading of chronic GVHD. *Biology of Blood and Marrow Transplantation,* **8,** 32–9.

Marks, D.I., Cullis, J.O., Ward, K.N. *et al.* (1993). Allogeneic bone marrow transplantation for chronic myeloid leukemia using siblings and volunteer unrelated donors. A comparison in complications in the first 2 years. *Annals of Internal Medicine,* **119,** 204–14.

Marmont, A.M., Horowitz, M.M., Gale, R.P. *et al.* (1991). T cell depletion of HLA-identical transplants in leukemia. *Blood,* **78,** 2120–30.

Martino, R., Caballero, M.D., Perez Simon, J.A. *et al.* (2002). Evidence for a graft-versus-leukemia effect after allogeneic peripheral blood stem cell transplantation with reduced-intensity conditioning in acute myelogenous leukemia and myelodysplastic syndromes. *Blood,* **100,** 2243–5.

Masauzi, N., Tanaka, J., Ohizumi, H. *et al.* (1994). Reversal of myelofibrosis is an important pretransplant factor for bone marrow grafting—a successful case of allogeneic bone marrow transplantation for an acute megakaryoblastic leukemia. *Rinsho Ketsueki,* **35,** 148–53.

Mehta, A.B., Baugham, A.S.J., Catoversusky, D. *et al.* (1983). Reversal of marrow fibrosis in acute megakaryoblastic leukemia after remission-induction and consolidation chemotherapy followed by bone marrow transplantation. *British Journal of Haematology,* **53,** 445–9.

Michel, G., Leverger, G., Leblanc, T. *et al.* (1996). Allogeneic bone marrow transplantation for children with acute myeloid leukemia in first complete remission: a prospective study from the French Society of Pediatric Hematology and Immunology (SHIP). *Bone Marrow Transplantation,* **18,** 455–63.

Nabhan, C., Mehta, J., & Tallman, M.S. (2001). The role of bone marrow transplantation in acute promyelocytic leukemia. *Bone Marrow Transplantation,* **28,** 219–26.

Platzbecker, U., Thiede, C., Freiberg-Richter, J. *et al.* (2001). Early allogeneic blood stem cell transplantation after modified conditioning therapy during marrow aplasia: stable remission in high-risk acute myeloid leukemia. *Bone Marrow Transplantation,* **27,** 543–6.

Powles, R., Mehta, J., Kulkami, S. *et al.* (2000). Allogeneic blood and bone-marrow stem-cell transplantation in haematological malignant diseases: a randomised trial. *Lancet,* **355,** 1231–7.

Przepiorka, D., Anderlini, P., Saliba, R. *et al.* (2001). Chronic graft-versus-host disease after allogeneic blood stem cell transplantation. *Blood,* **98,** 1695–700.

Raiola, A.M., Van Lint, M.T., Lamparelli, T. *et al.* (2000). Reduced intensity thiothepa-cyclophosphamide conditioning for allogenic hematopoietic stem cell transplants (HSCT) in patients up to 60 years of age. *British Journal of Haematology,* **109,** 716–21.

Reiffers, J., Stoppa, A.M., Attal, M. *et al.* (1996). Allogeneic versus autologous stem cell transplantation versus chemotherapy in patients with acute myeloid leukemia in first remission: the BGMT 87 study. *Leukemia,* **10,** 1874–82.

Reusser, P., Einsele, H., Lee, J. *et al.* for the infectious disease working party of the European Group for Blood and Marrow Transplantation. (2002). Randomized multicenter trial of foscarnet versus ganciclovir for preemptive therapy of cytomegalovirus infection after allogenic stem cell transplantation. *Blood,* **99,** 1159–64.

Ringden, O., Ruutu, T., Remberger, M. *et al.* (1994). A randomized trial comparing busulfan with total body irradiation as conditioning in allogeneic marrow transplant recipients with leukemia—a report from the Nordic Bone Marrow Transplantation Group. *Blood,* **83,** 2723–30.

Rocha, V., Cornish, J., Sievers, E.L. *et al.* (2001). Comparison of outcomes of unrelated bone marrow and umbilical cord blood transplants in children with acute leukemia. *Blood,* 97, 2962–71.

Rocha, V., Wagner, J.E., Jr, Sobocinski, K.A. *et al.* (2000). Graft-versus-host disease in children who have received a cord-blood or bone marrow transplant from an HLA-identical sibling. Eurocord and International Bone Marrow Transplant Registry Working Committee on Alternative Donor and Stem Cell Sources. *New England Journal of Medicine,* 342, 1846–54.

Ruggeri, L., Capanni, M., Urbani, E. *et al.* (2002). Effectiveness of donor natural killer cell alloreactivity in mismatched hematopoietic transplant. *Science,* 29, 2097–100.

Ruiz-Arguelles, G.J., Lobato-Mendizabal, E., San-Miguel, J.F. *et al.* (1992). Long-term treatment results for acute megakaryoblastic leukaemia: a multicentre study. *British Journal of Haematology,* 82, 671–5.

Santos, G.W., Tutschka, P.J., Brookmeyer, R. *et al.* (1983). Marrow transplantation for acute nonlymphocytic leukemia after treatment with busulfan and cyclophosphamide. *New England Journal of Medicine,* 309, 1347–53.

Schmitz, N., Bacigalupo, A., Hasenclever, D. *et al.* (1998). Allogeneic bone marrow transplantation versus filgrastim-mobilised peripheral blood progenitor cell transplantation in patients with early leukemia: first results of a randomised multicentre trial of the European Group for Blood and Marrow Transplantation. *Bone Marrow Transplantation,* 21, 995–1003.

Schnittger, S., Schoch, C., Dugas, M. *et al.* (2002). Analysis of FLT3 length mutation in 1003 patients with acute myeloid leukemia: correlation to cytogenetics, FAB subtype, and prognosis in the AMLCG study and usefulness as a marker for the detection of minimal residual disease. *Blood,* 100, 59–66.

Shen, Z-X., Chen, G-Q., Ni, J-H. *et al.* (1997). Use of arsenic trioxide (As203) in the treatment of acute promyelocytic leukemia (APL): II. Clinical efficacy and pharmacokinetics in relapsed patients. *Blood,* 89, 3354–60.

Shulman, H.M., Sullivan, K.M., Weiden, P.L. *et al.* (1980). Chronic graft-versus-host syndrome in man: a long-term clinicopathologic study of 20 Seattle patients. *American Journal of Medicine,* 69, 204–17.

Sierra, J., Storer, B., Hansen, J.A. *et al.* (2000). Unrelated donor marrow transplantation for acute myeloid leukemia: an update of the Seattle experience. *Bone Marrow Transplantation,* 26, 397–404.

Singhal, S., Powles, R., Henslee-Downey, P.J. *et al.* (2002). Allogeneic transplantation from HLA-matched sibling or partially HLA-mismatched related donors for primary refractory acute leukemia. *Bone Marrow Transplantation,* 29, 291–5.

Slavin, S., Nagler, A., Naparstek, E. *et al.* (1998). Nonmyeloablative stem cell transplantation and cell therapy as an alternative to conventional bone marrow transplantation with lethal cytoreduction for the treatment of malignant and nonmalignant hematologic diseases. *Blood,* 91, 756–63.

Snyder, D.S., Chao, N.J., Amylon, M.D. *et al.* (1993). Fractionated total body irradiation and high-dose etoposide as a preparatory regimen for bone marrow transplantation for 99 patients with acute leukemia in first complete remission. *Blood,* 82, 2920–8.

Sociè, G., Reginald, A., Clift, D. *et al.* (2001). Busulfan plus cyclophosphamide compared with total-body irradiation plus cyclophosphamide before marrow transplantation for myeloid leukemia: long-term follow-up of 4 randomized studies. *Blood,* 98, 3569–74.

Soignet, S.L., Frankel, S.R., Douer, D. *et al.* (2001). United States multicenter study of arsenic trioxide in relapsed acute promyelocytic leukemia. *Journal of Clinical Oncology,* 19, 3852–60.

Storb, R., Prentice, R.L., Sullivan, K.M. *et al.* (1983). Predictive factors in chronic graft-versus-host disease in patients with aplastic anemia treated by marrow transplantation from HLA-identical siblings. *Annals of Internal Medicine,* 98, 461–6.

Storb, R., Deeg, H.J., Whitehead, J. *et al.* (1986). Methotrexate and cyclosporine compared with cyclosporine alone for prophylaxis of acute graft-versus-host disease after marrow transplantation for leukemia. *New England Journal of Medicine,* 314, 729–35.

Storb, R., Yu, C., Sanmeier, B.M. *et al.* (1999). Mixed hematopoietic chimerism after marrow allografts. Transplantation in the ambulatory care setting. *Annals of the New York Academy of Sciences,* 872, 372–5.

Suciu, S. (1991). The value of BMT in AML patients in first remission. A statistician's viewpoint. *Annals of Haematology,* 62, 41–4.

Tallman, M.S., Rowlings, P.A., Milone, G. *et al.* (2000). Effect of post-remission chemotherapy before human leukocyte antigen-identical sibling transplantation for acute myelogenous leukemia in first complete remission. *Blood,* 96, 1254–8.

Thomas, E.D. (1983). Marrow transplant for acute nonlymphoblastic leukemia in first remission: a follow-up. *New England Journal of Medicine,* 308, 1539–40.

Thomas, E.D., Buckner, C.D., Clift, R.A. *et al.* (1979). Marrow transplantation for acute nonlymphoblastic leukemia in first remission. *New England Journal of Medicine,* 301, 597–9.

Tutschka, P.J., Copeland, E.A., & Klein, J.P. (1987). Bone marrow transplantation for leukemia following a new busulphan and cyclophosphamide regimen. *Blood,* 70, 1382.

Urbano-Ispizua, A., Schmitz, N., de Witte, T. *et al.* for the European Group for Blood and Marrow Transplantation (2002). Allogeneic and autologous transplantation for haematological diseases, solid tumours and immune disorders: definitions and current practice in Europe in 2001. *Bone Marrow Transplantation,* 29, 639–46.

Vigorito, A.C., Azevedo, W.M., Marques, J.F.C. *et al.* (1998). A randomised, prospective comparison of allogeneic bone marrow and peripheral blood progenitor cell transplantation in the treatment of haematological malignancies. *Bone Marrow Transplantation,* 22, 1145–51.

Wahlin, A., Markervarn, B., Golovleva, I., & Nilsson, M. (2002). Improved outcome in adult acute myeloid leukemia is almost entirely restricted to young patients and associated with stem cell transplantation. *European Journal of Haematology,* 68(1), 54–65.

Walsh, T.J., Pappas, P., Winston, D.J. *et al.* for the National Institute of Allergy and Infectious Diseases Mycoses Study Group. (2002). Voriconazole compared with liposomal amphotericin B for empirical antifungal therapy in patients with neutropenia and persistent fever. *New England Journal of Medicine,* 346, 225–34.

Weisdorf, D.J., Anasetti, C., Antin, J.H. *et al.* (2002). Allogeneic bone marrow transplantation for chronic myelogenous leukemia: comparative analysis of unrelated versus matched sibling donor transplantation. *Blood,* 99, 1971–7.

Wheatley, K., Burnett, A.K., Goldstone, A.H. *et al.* (1999). A simple, robust, validated and highly predictive index for the determination of risk-directed therapy in acute myeloid leukaemia derived from the MRC AML 10 trial. United Kingdom Medical Research Council's Adult and Childhood Leukaemia Working Parties. *British Journal of Haematology,* **107,** 69–79.

Woods, W.G., Neudorf, S., Gold, S. *et al.* (2001). A comparison of allogeneic bone marrow transplantation, autologous bone marrow transplantation, and aggressive chemotherapy in children with acute myeloid leukemia in remission: a report from the Children's Cancer Group. *Blood,* **97,** 56–62.

Zikos, P., Van Lint, M.T., Frassoni, G. *et al.* (1998). Low transplant-related mortality in allogeneic bone marrow transplantation for acute myeloid leukemia: a randomized study of low-dose cyclosporine versus low-dose cyclosporin and low-dose methotrexate. *Blood,* **91,** 3503–8.

Zittoun, R., Suciu, S., Watson, M. *et al.* (1997). Quality of life in patients with acute myelogenous leukemia in prolonged first complete remission after bone marrow transplantation (allogeneic or autologous) or chemotherapy: cross-sectional study of the EORTC-GIMEMA AML 8A trial. *Bone Marrow Transplantation,* **20,** 307–15.

Zittoun, R.A., Mandelli, F., Willemze, R. *et al.* for the European Organization for Research and Treatment of Cancer (EORTC) and the Gruppo Italiano Malattie Ematologiche Maligne Dell' Adulto (GIMEMA) Leukemia Cooperative Groups. (1995). Autologous or allogeneic bone marrow transplantation compared with intensive chemotherapy in acute myelogenous leukemia. *New England Journal of Medicine,* **332,** 217–23.

51 Allogeneic stem cell transplantation for acute lymphoblastic leukemia[1]

JOSEPH H. ANTIN

Dana-Farber Cancer Institute and Brigham and Women's Hospital, Harvard University, Boston, USA

Introduction

The use of hematopoietic stem cell (HSC) transplantation in acute lymphoblastic leukemia (ALL) is limited by the excellent long-term disease-free survivals routinely achieved in this disease, especially in children. Current multidrug chemotherapy regimens induce sustained remissions in 70% to 90% of children with standard risk features (Clavell *et al.*, 1986; Steinherz *et al.*, 1986; Chessells *et al.*, 1995; Kersey, 1998; Pui & Evans, 1998). Even children with high-risk features are doing well with disease-free survival rates of 60% to 84% (Chessells *et al.*, 1995; Silverman *et al.*, 2001). Long-term outcome in adults is less favorable, but in good risk patients (BCR/ABL negative or T-cell disease) survival rates of 30% to 50% may be observed (Henze *et al.*, 1991; Boucheix *et al.*, 1994; Pui & Evans 1998; Czuczman *et al.*, 1999). Traditionally, allogeneic HSC transplantation is reserved for those patients who fail to enter remission or who relapse. However, well-established high-risk groups of patients with ALL in first remission, such as those who have a BCR/ABL gene rearrangement, a high white blood cell count (WBC) at diagnosis, the L3 FAB morphologic type (Burkitt's-like), certain other cytogenetic abnormalities including t(4;11) and t(1;19), −7, +8, the MLL gene rearrangement, hypodiploidy, failure to respond to corticosteroids, or failure to achieve complete remission rapidly, do poorly with conventional therapy and are candidates for stem cell transplantation in first remission (Wetzler *et al.*, 1999). As described below, large-scale trials are now suggesting that transplantation is a valid alternative for a broader group of patients in first remission. Clearly, to the degree that transplant-related toxicity can be diminished, this is a more attractive alternative.

The current practice of HSC transplantation for ALL in Europe has been described (Urbano-Ispizua *et al.*, 2002) (and see Chapter 124).

Information on disease incidence, classification, immune phenotype, cytogenetic abnormalities, prognostic factors, outcome with conventional therapy, disease-specific pretransplant work-up, and monitoring for residual disease posttransplant, are given in Chapter 37.

Results with HLA-identical sibling transplantation

Over 10,000 bone marrow transplants from HLA-identical siblings have been performed in people with ALL (Rowlings *et*

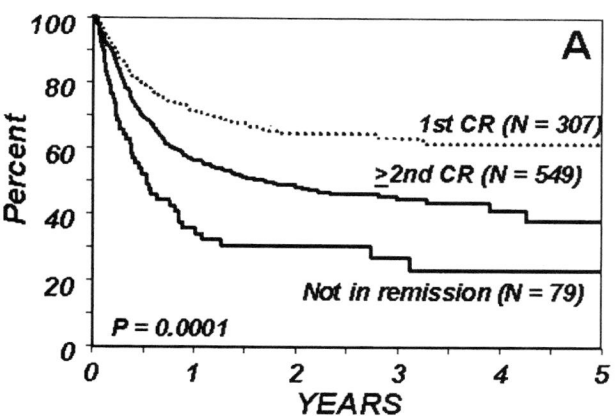

Fig. 51.1. Probability of leukemia-free survival after histocompatible family-member transplantation for ALL in patients less than 20 years of age (excluding Ph+ disease), 1996–2000. Patients registered with IBMTR. (Courtesy of IBMTR/ABMTR Statistical Center; these data have not yet been reviewed by the IBMTR/ABMTR Advisory Committee.)

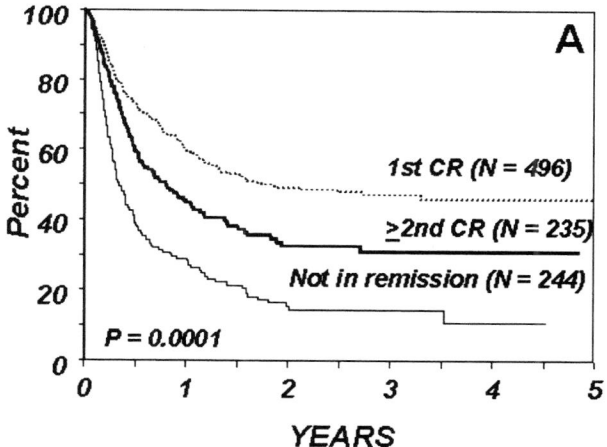

Fig. 51.2. Probability of leukemia-free survival after histocompatible family-member transplantation for ALL in patients 20 years of age or older (excluding Ph+ disease), 1996–2000. Patients registered with IBMTR. (Courtesy of IBMTR/ABMTR Statistical Center; these data have not yet been reviewed by the IBMTR/ABMTR Advisory Committee.)

[1]Anna Butturini, Robert Gale, and Mary M. Horowitz contributed significantly to this chapter in the Second Edition.

al., 1996). Outcome correlates with age and leukemia stage, and while these variables are confounded, both are important. Older patients are more likely to have high-risk disease, as well as more treatment-related mortality (Figs. 51.1 and 51.2). Other variables correlated with transplant outcome in first remission include WBC at diagnosis, cytogenetic abnormalities, and time to obtain remission (Weisdorf *et al.,* 1994). These variables are similar to those correlated with results of conventional chemotherapy and relate predominantly to relapse risk. The duration of first remission is a major correlate of outcome in those transplanted after relapse. In contrast to the substantial impact of subject- and disease-related variables on transplant outcome, transplant-related variables such as conditioning regimen, T-cell depletion, and graft-versus-host disease (GVHD) prophylaxis, have a lesser impact on leukemia-free survival.

ALL in first remission

Studies of marrow transplantation in first remission have been carried out in patients considered to be at high risk of relapse. Actuarial disease-free survival rates of 42% to 89% and actuarial relapse rates of 0% to 31% have been reported (Zwaan *et al.,* 1984; Blume *et al.,* 1987; Brochstein *et al.,* 1987; Forman *et al.,* 1987; Herzig *et al.,* 1987; Vernant *et al.,* 1988; Chao *et al.,* 1991; Biggs *et al.,* 1992; Chao *et al.,* 1995; Zhang *et al.,* 1995; Saarinen *et al.,* 1996; Deconinck *et al.,* 1997; Uderzo *et al.,* 1997; Oh *et al.,* 1998; Snyder *et al.,* 1999; Snyder, 2000; Wheeler *et al.,* 2000; Cornelissen *et al.,* 2001; Martin & Gajewski, 2001; Rowe *et al.,* 2001). Some of these studies are summarized in Table 51.1 and IBMTR data are shown in Figures 51.1 and 51.2.

Three prospective randomized trials have been performed for adult patients at high risk for relapse comparing marrow grafts to chemotherapy in these patients. Patients in all three studies were assigned allogeneic transplantation based on the availability of an HLA-identical sibling. Patients without a donor were randomized to receive chemotherapy alone versus chemotherapy plus an autologous transplant. In the LALA87 study (France) the 5-year survival rates were no different between the cohorts for patients with standard risk ALL. When only patients with high-risk ALL were considered (Ph chromosome, null or undifferentiated ALL, or either age greater than 35 years or WBC count $>30 \times 10^9$ cells/l or time to achieve complete remission >4 weeks), overall survival (OS) and disease-free-survival (DFS) were better for the allogeneic group compared with the control group (5-year OS, 44% versus 20%, $P = .03$; 5-year DFS, 39% versus 14%, $P = .01$ (Sebban *et al.,* 1994). A similar study performed as a collaboration between the Medical Research Council (MRC) in the United Kingdom and the Eastern Cooperative Oncology Group (ECOG) showed an advantage to allogeneic transplantation in both standard risk [5-year event-free survival (EFS) 66% versus 44%] and Ph-negative high-risk groups (5-year EFS 44% versus 26%) (Rowe *et al.,* 2001). In the third study (also French), patients received an allogeneic or autologous transplant. Recipients of autologous marrow were randomized to receive or not receive infusions of interleukin-2 (IL-2). The three-year DFS probability was significantly higher for recipients of HLA-identical sibling allogeneic transplants: 68% versus 26% with no benefit seen in the group that received IL-2 (Attal *et al.,* 1995) (Fig. 51.3). Taken together, these studies demonstrate that there is a role for allogeneic transplantation in patients with adult ALL in first remission, especially those patients with high-risk features; however, the MRC/ECOG study also suggests that improvements in transplantation may make it the preferred therapy for all adults with ALL.

No similar prospective trials have been reported for children with ALL. Several comparative or cohort studies have been reported. In a Scandinavian analysis of stem cell transplantation (SCT) in very high risk children, DFS at 10 years was 73%

Table 51.1. *Stem cell transplantation from a histocompatible family member for the treatment of acute lymphoblastic leukemia in first remission*

Study	Risk category	Treatment	No.	Actuarial DFS (%)	Relapse Rate (%)
EGBMT (Zwaan *et al.,* 1984)	Varied	Varied	57	~60	6
MSKCC (Brochstein *et al.,* 1987)		HFTBI/Cy	31	64	13
GEGMO (Vernant *et al.,* 1988)	Adults	Varied	27	59	14
IBMTR (Horowitz *et al.,* 1991)	Adult	Varied	251	44	
IBMTR (Barrett *et al.,* 1992)	Ph	Varied	33	38	
Chao (Chao *et al.,* 1991)	High risk		53	61	10
Italy (Uderzo *et al.,* 1997)	High risk	Varied—mainly Cy/TBI	30	58.5	31.5
France (Deconinck *et al.,* 1997)	High risk	TBI, high-dose Ara-c, melphalan	42	40	31
United Kingdom (Wheeler *et al.,* 2000)	High risk	Cy/TBI	76	45	31
Scandanavia (Saarinen *et al.,* 1996)	High risk	Varied—mainly Cy/TBI	22	73	9

Abbreviations: Ara-c, cytosine arabinoside; Cy, cyclophosphamide; DFS, disease-free survival; IBMTR, International Bone Marrow Transplant Registry; EGBMT, European Group for Bone Marrow Transplantation; GEGMO, Groupe d'Etudes de la Greffe de Moelle Osseuse; MSKCC, Memoial Sloan-Kettering Cancer Center; TBI, total body irradiation (F, fractionated; HF, hyperfractionated; SF, single fraction).

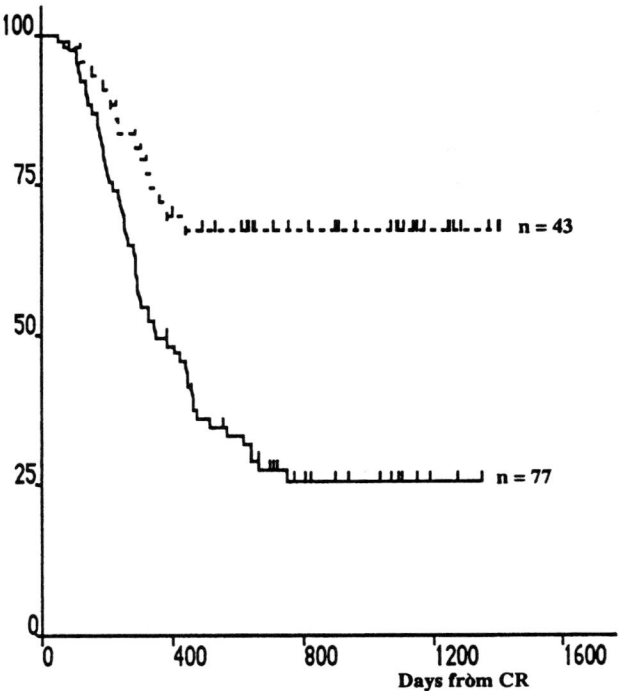

Fig. 51.3. DFS was significantly superior ($P < .001$) for patients with an HLA-identical sibling (——) than for patients without an HLA-identical sibling (—). Reproduced, with permission, from Attal *et al.* (1995).

in children receiving allogeneic transplants in first remission and 50% in the matched controls ($P = .02$). The improved prognosis of the group was due to a much lower relapse rate (9% versus 41%) (Saarinen *et al.,* 1996). A similar Italian study compared the outcome of children with high-risk ALL in first complete remission treated with chemotherapy or with allogeneic bone marrow transplantation. A cohort of nontransplanted patients was matched on prognostic factors and duration of first remission in an effort to control the selection and time-to-transplant biases. At a median follow-up of 4 years, the DFS was 58.5% in the transplanted group and 47.7% in the conventional therapy group, and the estimated cumulative incidence of relapse at 1.5 years was 31.5% versus 29.2%. Interestingly, the risk of relapse after transplantation was constant, but without transplantation it continued to increase to 48.2% at 4 years (Uderzo *et al.,* 1997). This study suggests that the higher risk of early failure in the group is outweighed by the lower risk of relapse after 1 year. Finally, an analysis by the MRC examined 3,676 patients (aged 1 to 15 years) entered into trials UKALL X and XI from 1985 to 1997. Of these patients, 473 patients (13%) were classified as very high risk and were eligible for transplantation from a matched histocompatible sibling donor, and only 76 patients were transplanted. The 10-year EFS adjusted for the time to transplantation, diagnostic WBC count, Ph chromosome status, and ploidy was better for the transplanted patients (45.3% versus 39.3%). The transplan-

tation group had fewer relapses (31%) compared to relapses in the chemotherapy group (55%); however, the transplantation group had more remission deaths (18%) compared to the chemotherapy group (3%). The authors concluded that transplantation did not significantly improve survival in this cohort (Wheeler *et al.,* 2000). Infants but not older children with MLL gene rearrangements have a poor prognosis, but there is improving outcome data using chemotherapy for these infants and no good data to show that allogeneic transplant improves EFS for this high-risk group.

ALL beyond first remission

SCT is the preferred therapy for advanced ALL (Fig. 51.1 and 51.2). Most transplants in children and about 50% of transplants in adults for ALL are performed in second or subsequent remission. Although recent intensive regimens have improved remission duration in patients who have relapsed, most centers have poor long-term survival of patients who are no longer in first remission. The timing of treatment is important. There is still controversy about its role for children in late marrow relapse (Chessells *et al.,* 1986; Pinkel, 1989; Harrison *et al.,* 2000). There have been few prospective studies comparing chemotherapy to marrow transplantation following initial relapse, and the results are at odds (Johnson *et al.,* 1981; Henze *et al.,* 1991; Barrett *et al.,* 1994; Chessells *et al.,* 1994; Boulad *et al.,* 1999). Children with a particularly long first remission may have favorable results for allogeneic transplantation in third remission. The Berlin-Frankfurt-Munster Relapse Study showed excellent long-term EFS with chemotherapy if there were no circulating blasts (Buhrer *et al.,* 1996); however, it requires 2 years of continued therapy. The presence of blasts in the blood in this study was a poor prognostic finding and the data suggest that marrow grafting might be a good alternative. A Nordic retrospective analysis recommended transplantation for children who had relapsed on therapy or within 6 months of stopping primary therapy but could find no advantage in transplanting children with later relapses (Schroeder *et al.,* 1999). However, other single center and multicenter retrospective studies indicate that children with ALL in second remission fare significantly better if they receive an allogeneic transplant as compared to chemotherapy alone. For recipients of HLA identical transplants, the 5-year DFS ranged from 30% to 56%, while EFS for patients with chemotherapy alone ranged from 17% to 38% (Fig. 51.1). The observation appeared to be true for children with poor risk features at initial presentation or whose initial remission lasted less than 18 or 24 months, as well as for those patients whose first remissions were longer than 24 months (Barrett *et al.,* 1994) (Fig. 51.4). The results observed for pediatric patients with ALL in remission transplanted with an unrelated donor are encouraging, but the long-term effects of the increased incidences of acute or chronic GVHD are unknown (Bordigoni *et al.,* 1998; Boulad *et al.,* 1999). The site of relapse is also important since at least one study indicated that chemotherapy plus central nervous system (CNS)-directed therapy resulted in an EFS greater than 80% for late isolated CNS relapse (Ritchey *et al.*, 1999). On the other hand, transplantation for isolated CNS disease results in good outcomes in children as well (Bordigoni *et al.*, 1998).

Results of marrow transplantation reflect heterogeneity in conditioning regimens, risk groups, and time of relapse. DFS rates of 22% to 62% have been reported, with relapse rates of 13% to 62% (Buckner & Clift, 1984; Brochstein *et al.*, 1987; Herzig *et al.*, 1987; Sanders *et al.*, 1987; Weisdorf *et al.*, 1987; Coccia *et al.*, 1988; Barrett *et al.*, 1989). The lowest relapse rates appear to be seen after hyperfractionated total body irradiation with or without etoposide in the conditioning regimen (Table 51.2). TBI and cyclophosphamide are thought to be a superior conditioning regimen to busulfan and cyclophosphamide for HLA-identical transplantation in children with ALL (Davies *et al.*, 2000).

Survival rates of patients treated in relapse parallel the results observed in relapsed AML or CML in blast crisis— 10% to 15% (Badger *et al.*, 1982; Buckner & Clift 1984; Thomas *et al.*, 1999). HLA-identical sibling transplants in children and adults with advanced ALL result in about 20% 5-year leukemia-free survival, an outcome clearly better than that from chemotherapy. Similar results have been reported in adults never achieving remission with induction chemotherapy (Forman *et al.*, 1991; Biggs *et al.*, 1992). In patients with very high risk disease leukemia relapse is the major cause of treatment failure; actuarial relapse risk is about 60%. Children with isolated CNS relapse appear to do particularly well and better than children with marrow involvement (Bordigoni *et al.*, 1998).

Based on these data HLA-identical sibling transplants are recommended for adults and most children in second or subsequent remission. Possible exceptions are in children with very late relapses and perhaps isolated CNS relapse. When the MRC/ECOG trial is more mature, we may need to reconsider recommendations regarding adults with standard risk disease in first remission. In children relapsing after a first remission, it seems worthwhile to give chemotherapy to try to achieve a second remission before the transplant. This may not be necessary in adults who can be transplanted in relapse without additional chemotherapy.

Prognostic factors

If transplantation is undertaken in first remission, non–T-cell phenotype, leukocyte count at diagnosis of 50,000 cells/µl or higher, male donor to female recipient, and GVHD may be associated with a reduction in leukemia-free survival, while use of corticosteroids appears to increase leukemia-free survival (Barrett *et al.*, 1989). It has been difficult to identify prognostic factors that predict relapse after marrow transplantation in second or subsequent remission (Sanders *et al.*, 1987), although the Westminster group found standard prognostic factors in ALL to apply to marrow transplantation (Barrett *et al.*, 1986). An analysis by the IBMTR identified age 16 years or older, relapse while on therapy, GVHD prophylaxis without methotrexate, and absence of GVHD as factors

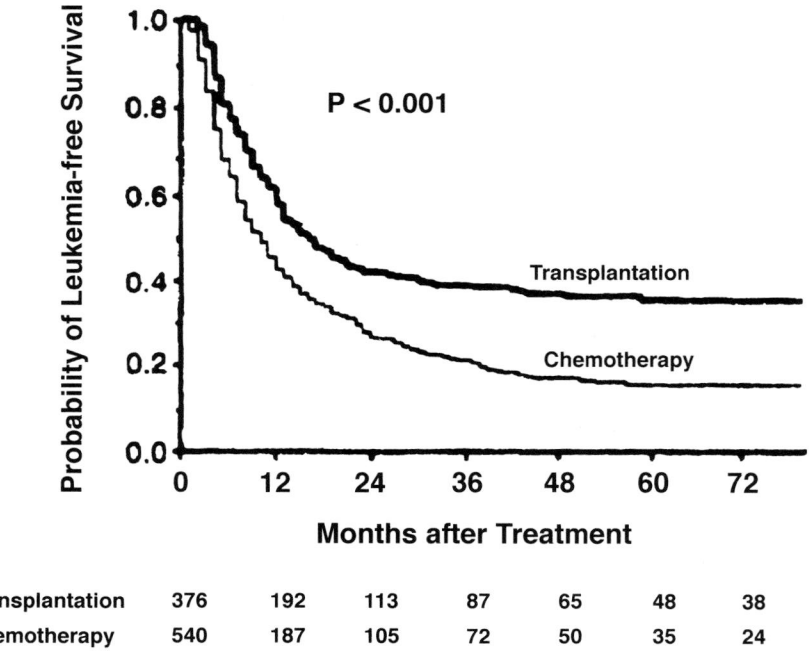

Transplantation	376	192	113	87	65	48	38
Chemotherapy	540	187	105	72	50	35	24

Fig. 51.4. Actuarial probability of leukemia-free survival in unmatched cohorts of children receiving chemotherapy or undergoing transplantation. The numbers below the figure indicate the numbers of children at risk. Reproduced, with permission, from Barrett *et al.* (1994).

Table 51.2. *Family member stem cell transplantation for the treatment of acute lymphoblastic leukemia beyond first remission*

Study	Donor	Remission status	Treatment	No.	Actuarial DFS (%)	Relapse (%)
MSKCC (Brochstein *et al.*, 1987)	Family member	Second, third, or relapse	HFTBI/Cy	12	42	25
				16	23	64
EGBMT (Zwann *et al.*, 1984)	Family member	Second, third, or more	Varied	96	~40	34
				39	~12	73
Seattle (Sanders *et al.*, 1987)	Family member	Second	Cy/SFTBI or Cy/FTBI	57	40	42
IBMTR (Barrett *et al.*, 1994)	Family member	Second	Varied	391	40	45
GITMO (Uderzo *et al.*, 1995)	Family member	Second	Varied	57	41	—
Minnesota/DFCI (Weisdorf *et al.*, 1997)	Unrelated donor	Second, third, fourth, relapse	Varied, primarily Cy/FTBI	106	42	17
				79	23	47
				14	31	73
				83	16	60
Scandinavia (Saarinen-Pihkala *et al.*, 2001)	Family member	Second	Varied	37	39	76
	Unrelated			28	54	40

Abbreviations: Cy, cyclophosphamide; DFCI, Dana-Farber Cancer Institute; IBMTR, International Bone Marrow Transplant Registry; EGBMT, European Group for Bone Marrow Transplantation; GITMO, Gruppo Italiano Trapianti di Midolio Osseo; MSKCC, Memorial Sloan-Kettering Cancer Center; TBI, total body fradiation (F, fractionated; HF, hyperfractionated; SF, single fraction).

that predict for a poor outcome (Barrett *et al.*, 1989). Difficulty in comparing studies may arise in part from the high relapse rates observed in these patients and the heterogeneity of chemotherapy regimens as well as transplantation-conditioning regimens.

Patients with the Ph chromosome are at particularly high risk for relapse with conventional treatment.

Thirty to 40% of ALL patients have the BCR/ABL gene rearrangement (p190, 77%; p210, 20%; simultaneous p190/p210, 3%). BCR/ABL positivity is often associated with the high-risk features of older age, and higher white blood cell counts (Gleissner *et al.*, 2002). Several studies have analyzed results of transplants in persons with the t(9;22) translocation

(Forman *et al.*, 1987; Horowitz *et al.*, 1991; Barrett *et al.*, 1992; Chao *et al.*, 1995; Stockschlader *et al.*, 1995; Dunlop *et al.*, 1996; Sierra *et al.*, 1997; Snyder *et al.*, 1999; Arico *et al.*, 2000; Snyder, 2000) (Figs. 51.5 and 51.6). These data generally indicate a 30% to 50% 3-year leukemia-free survival, similar to other smaller series. A large international collaboration between MRC and ECOG examined the outcome of 203 Ph+ patients. Stable complete remission was achieved in 167 and these patients received matched family member (*n* = 49), unrelated donor (*n* = 23), autologous (*n* = 7), or chemotherapy alone (*n* = 88). Interestingly the trial started in 1993 and there was initially a high rate of death in remission in the allogeneic groups (matched related donor = 37% and unrelated donor =

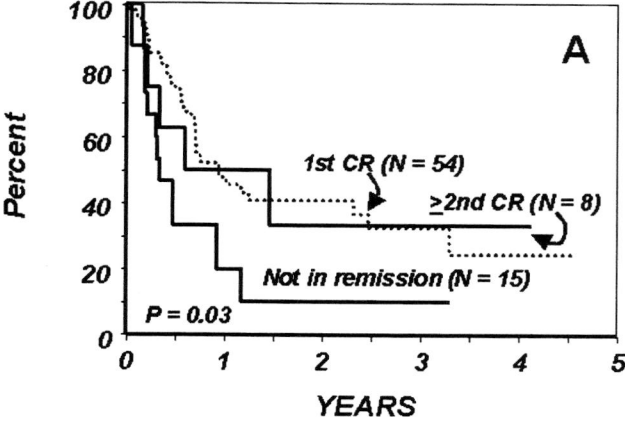

Fig. 51.5. Probability of leukemia-free survival after histocompatible family-member transplantation for Ph+ ALL, 1996–2000. Patients registered with IBMTR. (Courtesy of IBMTR/ABMTR Statistical Center; these data have not yet been reviewed by the IBMTR/ABMTR Advisory Committee.)

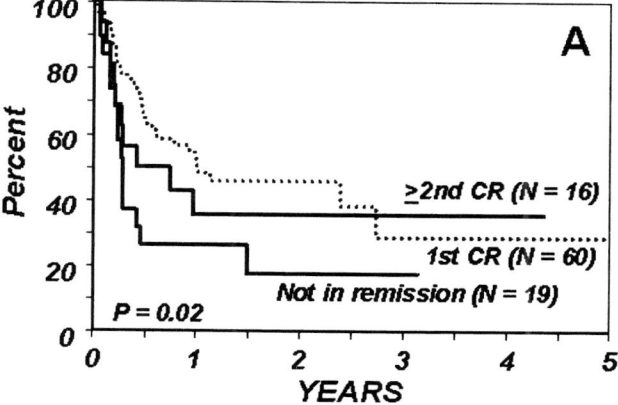

Fig. 51.6. Probability of leukemia-free survival after unrelated donor transplantation for Ph+ ALL, 1996–2000. Patients registered with IBMTR. (Courtesy of IBMTR/ABMTR Statistical Center; these data have not yet been reviewed by the IBMTR/ABMTR Advisory Committee.)

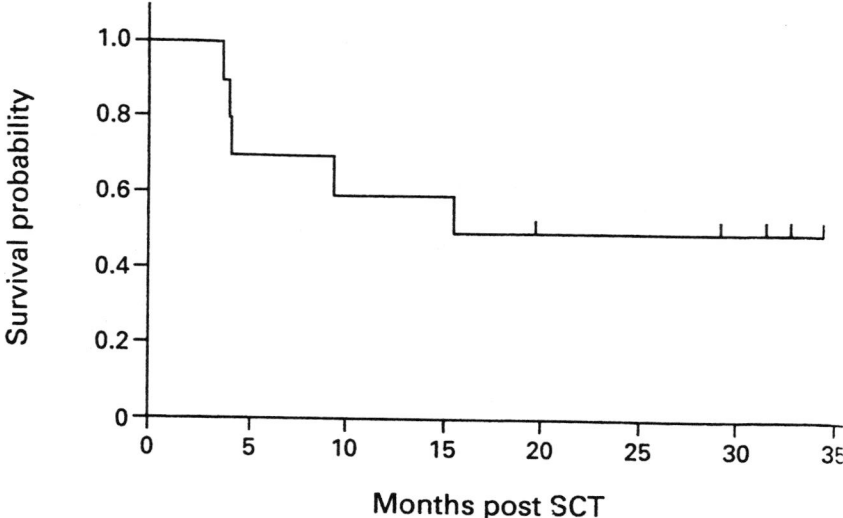

Fig. 51.7. Kaplan-Meier plot of leukemia-free survival following allogeneic stem cell transplantation for adult T-cell leukemia/lymphoma. Reproduced, with permission, from Utsunomiya *et al.* (2001).

43%) but the rate appeared to diminish with time (27% in 1997 to 2000). The actuarial relapse risk for patients receiving allogeneic transplants (either matched family member or unrelated donor) was 29% at 5 years compared with 81% (95% CI = 66–95%) in the 66 patients receiving autologous transplants or chemotherapy who were in remission at the median time to transplant (*P* < .001). At 5 years their event-free (38%) and overall survivals (43%) were higher after allogeneic transplantation than in the autologous/chemotherapy group (EFS=17%, OS=19%) (Goldstone *et al.*, 2001).

Since the outcome of patients receiving conventional chemotherapy for this ALL variant is so poor, the results of allogeneic transplantation are encouraging. Specific inhibition of the BCR-ABL tyrosine kinase with imitinab mesylate (Gleevec®) results in a high remission rate in patients with Ph+ ALL (Druker *et al.*, 2001). However, the remissions are short-lived. It will be critical to determine whether therapy with imitinab mesylate either as pretransplant induction therapy or posttransplant maintenance therapy improves the relapse rate.

HTLV-1-associated adult ALL

HTLV-1-associated adult T-cell leukemia/lymphoma (ATLL) is a highly aggressive malignancy with a median survival of 6 months or less. A small number of patients, described primarily as case reports and small series, have undergone transplantation for this disease. Some have apparently had eradication of the malignancy as well as evidence of viral infection (Borg *et al.*, 1996; Kawa *et al.*, 1998; Kanda *et al.*, 1999; Leclercq *et al.*, 1999; Obama *et al.*, 1999; Tajima *et al.*, 2000; Kishi *et al.*, 2001; Utsunomiya *et al.*, 2001; Ogata *et al.*, 2002) (Fig. 51.7).

Results with donors other than histocompatible family members

Clearly, most people who need transplantation do not have family member donors, so alternative sources of stem cells are an important resource. Typically, stem cells can be obtained from a histocompatible unrelated donor or a mismatched family member. Limited data are available on mismatched unrelated donor transplants. One limitation in projecting probable outcome from unrelated donor transplantation data is the recognition that many patients who were thought to be histocompatible based on serologic typing were in fact mismatched by high-resolution molecular typing. Thus, it is reasonable to extrapolate that results of unrelated donor transplantation are substantially better than some of the early studies suggest. Primary concerns in alternative donor transplantation are (1) risk of graft rejection, (2) risk of acute and chronic GVHD, (3) risk of Epstein-Barr virus lymphoproliferative disorders, and (4) slow immunologic recovery. The expected counterpoint to these risks is a more potent graft-versus-leukemia (GVL) response resulting in a lower relapse rate.

HLA-mismatched transplantation is more problematic, and the success is in large measure dependent on the age of the recipient (younger do better) and stem cell source (cord blood is better). An IBMTR analysis compared the outcomes of marrow transplants for leukemia from HLA-identical siblings, haploidentical HLA-mismatched relatives, and HLA-matched and mismatched unrelated donors. The diseases analyzed were not limited to ALL, but data are likely to be generalizable. A total of 2,055 recipients of allogeneic bone marrow transplants performed between 1985 and 1991 were evaluated. Donors were HLA-identical siblings (*n* = 1,224); haploidentical relatives mismatched for one (*n* = 238) or two (*n* = 102) HLA-A,

-B, or -DR antigens; or unrelated donors who were HLA-matched (*n* = 383) or mismatched for one HLA-A, -B, or -DR antigen (*n* = 108) by serologic methods. Transplant-related mortality was significantly higher after alternative donor transplants than after HLA-identical sibling transplants. Among patients with early leukemia the 3 year transplant-related mortality was 21 ± 2% after matched sibling transplants and greater than 50% after alternative donor transplants. For patients with advanced leukemia, differences in treatment failure were less striking—probably because the matched family member transplants were relatively less effective (Szydlo *et al.*, 1997).

Results of unrelated donor transplantation

A study from Seattle examined 88 consecutive children and adolescents with ALL. Transplants were from histocompatible (*n* = 56) or partly matched (*n* = 32) unrelated donors during first complete remission (*n* = 10), second remission (*n* = 34), third remission (*n* = 10), or relapse (*n* = 34). Three-year rates of leukemia-free survival according to stage of disease were 70%, 46%, 20%, and 9%, respectively (*P* < .0001) and 3-year cumulative relapse rates were 10%, 33%, 20%, and 50%, respectively. Grades III and IV acute GVHD was observed in 43% of recipients of HLA-matched transplants and in 59% of recipients of partly matched transplants (*P* = .1). Extensive chronic GVHD occurred in 32% and 38%, respectively (*P* = .23). Outcomes were worse with advanced disease (*P* < .0001), age 10 years or older (*P* = .002), and short duration of first remission (*P* = .007) (Woolfrey *et al.*, 2002) (Fig. 51.8). These results are comparable to studies reported from the United Kingdom where EFS was approximately 50% after unrelated donor transplantation and 45% in family member transplantation (Oakhill *et al.*, 1996; Lawson *et al.*, 2000). A Nordic multi-

center study of a similar cohort in second remission received allogeneic transplants from 1990 to 1997. Of the allografts, 37 were from HLA-matched siblings and 28 were from unrelated donors. Interestingly, the recipients of unrelated donor stem cells seemed to do better—5-year EFS of 39% versus 54%, due to a lower relapse rate (76% versus 40%), although these differences did not achieve statistical significance. The trend in improved outcome occurred despite more GVHD in the unrelated donor group [grade II to IV acute GVHD was 38% versus 64% (*P* < .05) and chronic GVHD was 26% versus 57% (*P* < .05)] (Saarinen-Pihkala *et al.*, 2001).

In an NMDP study of 363 children with ALL in second remission who underwent an unrelated donor transplant between 1988 and 2000, leukemia-free survival was 36% at 5 years and was improved in patients less than 15 years of age or receiving HLA-matched grafts (Bunin *et al.*, 2002). Transplant-related mortality was 42%. The 5 year estimate for relapse was 33%, with first remission of at least 6 months associated with a lower risk.

If the recipient is an adult, results are similar in unrelated and family member transplantation (Goldstone *et al.*, 2001). A retrospective analysis of 127 patents with high-risk ALL was undertaken by the National Marrow Donor Program (Cornelissen *et al.*, 2001) (Fig. 51.9). High risk was defined by the presence of the translocations t(9;22) (*n* = 97), t(4;11) (*n* = 25), or t(1;19) (*n* = 5). Sixty-four patients underwent transplantation in first remission, 16 in second or third remission, and 47 patients were in relapse or primary induction failure. Multivariable analysis showed that first remission, shorter interval from diagnosis to transplantation, DRB1 match, negative cytomegalovirus (CMV) serology (patient and donor), and presence of the Ph chromosome were independently associated with better disease-free survival. Transplantation in remission and, surprisingly, presence of t(9;22) were associated with lower risk of relapse. While transplant-related mortality was high, the low relapse rate

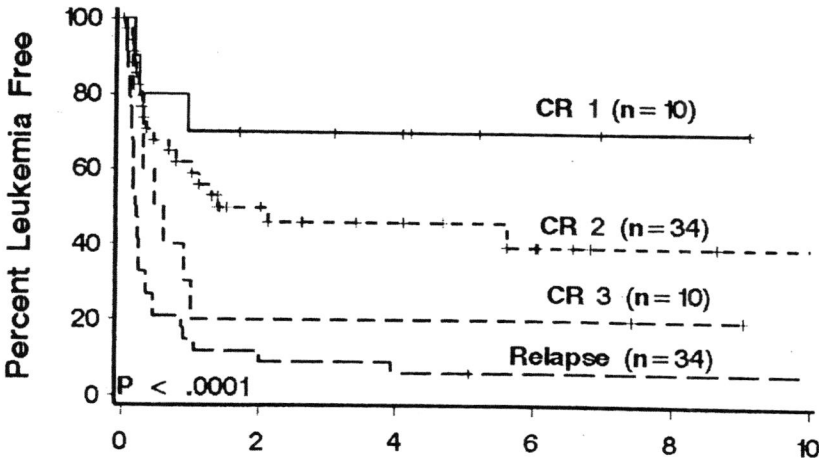

Fig. 51.8. Kaplan-Meier estimates of LFS in 88 patients with ALL according to phase of disease at transplantation. Phase of disease was defined by the number of medullary relapses. Significance was determined by log rank test. Censored patients are indicated by hatch marks. Reproduced, with permission, from Woolfrey *et al.* (2002).

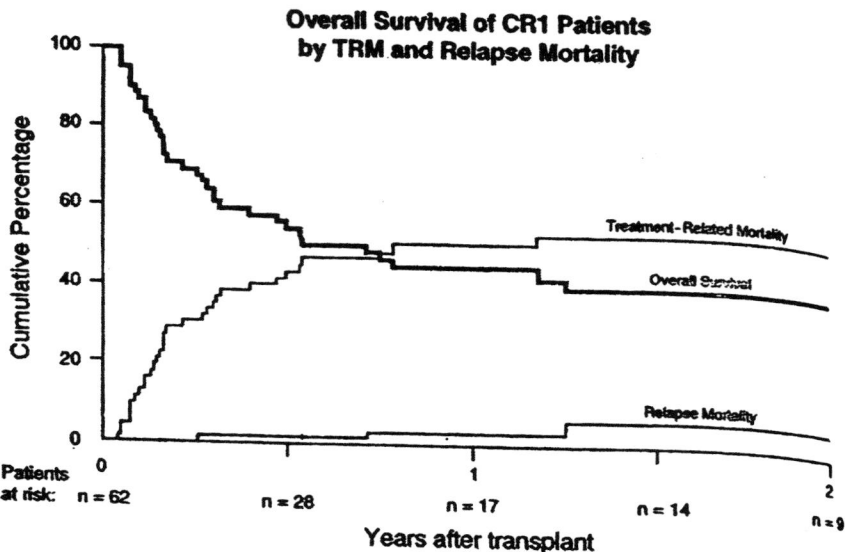

Fig. 51.9. Overall survival in CR1, as determined by competing risk factors, relapse mortality, and treatment-related mortality. Reproduced, with permission, from Cornelissen *et al.* (2001).

resulted in a 37 ± 13% disease-free survival for patients in first remission.

Data from the IBMTR summarizing outcomes in unrelated donor transplantation are shown in Figures 51.10 and 51.11.

Two patients with Down's syndrome complicated by acute leukemia have had successful unrelated donor marrow transplants (Pawlowska *et al.*, 1996). One child was transplanted in third remission of ALL and at the time of the report had been disease-free for 8 months. The second child was disease-free 15 months after transplantation for AML.

Results of cord blood transplantation

When unrelated donor umbilical cord blood is used as the source of stem cells, results are similar. A comparison with bone marrow transplants in 541 children with acute leukemia transplanted with umbilical cord blood (n = 99), T-cell-depleted bone marrow transplants (n = 180), or unmanipulated marrow (n = 262) were analyzed in a retrospective multicenter study. The donor was HLA mismatched in 92% of cord blood, in 18% of unmanipulated BMT, and in 43% of T-cell-depleted BMT (P < .001). Cord blood recipients had slower hematopoietic recovery, higher transplant-related mortality, but less acute

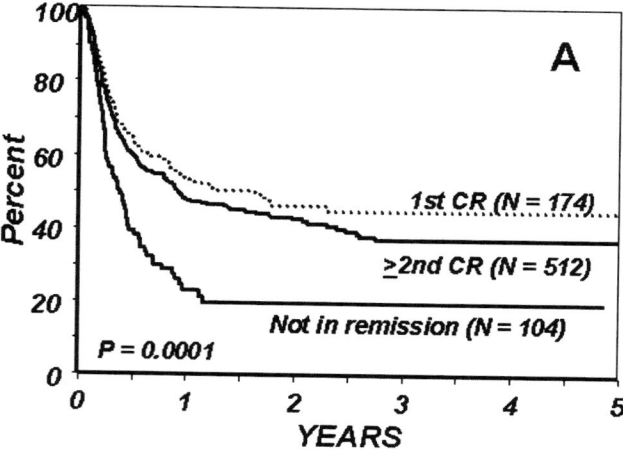

Fig. 51.10. Probability of leukemia-free survival after unrelated donor transplantation for ALL in patients less than 20 years of age (excluding Ph+ disease), 1996–2000. Patients registered with IBMTR. (Courtesy of IBMTR/ABMTR Statistical Center; these data have not yet been reviewed by the IBMTR/ABMTR Advisory Committee.)

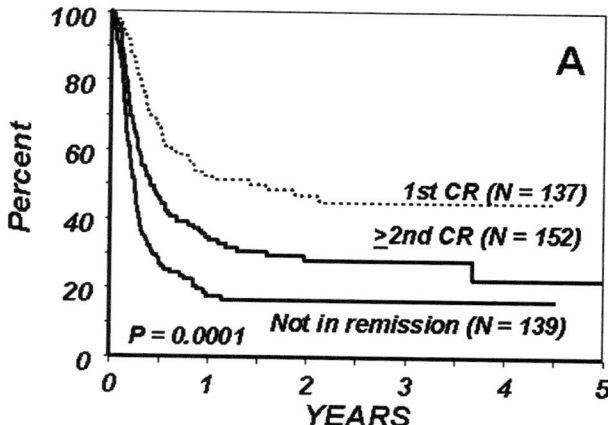

Fig. 51.11. Probability of leukemia-free survival after unrelated donor transplantation for ALL in patients 20 years of age or older (excluding Ph+ disease), 1996–2000. Patients registered with IBMTR. (Courtesy of IBMTR/ABMTR Statistical Center; these data have not yet been reviewed by the IBMTR/ABMTR Advisory Committee.)

and chronic GVHD than unmanipulated marrow recipients. After day 100 the three groups achieved similar results in terms of relapse (Rocha *et al.*, 2001).

Results of HLA-mismatched family member transplantation (and see Chapter 66)

Efforts to improve the outcome in patients receiving highly mismatched transplants have been promising, but require confirmation. Aversa and colleagues (1998) treated 43 patients with total body irradiation, thiotepa, fludarabine, and antithymocyte globulin conditioning followed by infusion of either filgrastim-mobilized peripheral blood stem cells (PBSC) alone or PBSC and bone marrow in 28 cases. Bone marrow from the donor was depleted of T lymphocytes by processing with soybean agglutinin and E-rosetting. T-cell depletion of peripheral-blood mononuclear cells was achieved by E-rosetting followed by positive selection of CD34+ cells. Interestingly, 11 of the 23 patients with ALL relapsed, compared with 2 of the 20 patients with acute myeloid leukemia (AML), suggesting that the GVL response was not robust in patients with ALL. Transplant-related mortality was 40%. After a median follow-up of 18 months (range, 8 to 30), 12 of the 43 patients were alive and free of disease. Most of the nonrelapse deaths were due to opportunistic infections (Aversa *et al.*, 1998). Another approach to mismatched transplantation consisted of partial T-cell depletion combined with posttransplant immunosuppression in a high-risk group of 43 patients with ALL and 24 with AML. More than half of the donors were disparate at two or three HLA antigens. Estimated probability of engraftment was 96% and was not affected by donor-antigen mismatch. Grades II to IV acute GVHD was observed in 24% and DFS was 26% at 3 years [45% when donors were younger than 30 years ($P < .001$)] (Godder *et al.*, 2000).

In a report of 39 children given CD34-positively selected histoincompatible PBSC, of whom the majority with malignant disease had ALL (Handgretinger *et al.*, 2001), the mean number of purified CD34+ cells infused was 20.7×10^6/kg, and the mean number of CD3+ T cells was 15.5×10^3/kg. The first seven patients received short-term (<4 weeks) GVHD prophylaxis with cyclosporine, whereas in all the following 32 patients, no GVHD prophylaxis was used. Rapid engraftment was seen in 36 patients with a median time to reach a neutrophil count of greater than 0.5×10^9/l of 11 days. Three patients failed to engraft, and two of those who did engraft subsequently rejected their graft. After reconditioning with methylprednisolone and OKT3 monoclonal antibody followed by re-infusion of purified CD34+ cells from the same donor, 4 of these 5 subsequently engrafted. In 38 evaluable patients, 5 experienced grade I acute GVHD after the stem cell infusion and 1 grade II. Twenty-one patients were given donor T cells posttransplant at CD3+ doses of 2.5×10^4/kg to 1×10^5/kg on between 1 and 4 occasions, either because of high relapse risk or because they showed evidence of transient autologous recovery. After donor lymphocyte

infusion, acute GVHD grade I occurred in 2 patients, grade II in 3, and grade IV in one. T-cell reconstitution was more rapid if the number of infused CD34+ cells was greater than 20×10^6/kg. Of the 39 patients, 15 were alive and well at the time of the report, 13 died from relapse, and 10 from transplant-related mortality. Viral infection was the cause of death in 5 and fungal infection in 2 (Fig. 51.12).

Results with reduced intensity conditioning regimens

Despite uncertainty over the potency of GVL in the control of ALL, many groups are studying ways to eradicate the disease by depending on the GVL effect. These trials typically use conditioning regimens that are substantially less intense than the commonly used regimens of cyclophosphamide and total body irradiation. Thus, it is unlikely that the conditioning regimen per se eradicates the leukemia. As yet, there are no studies that either specifically target ALL or have enough patients with ALL to make any inferences about the efficacy of reduced intensity transplantation for this disease.

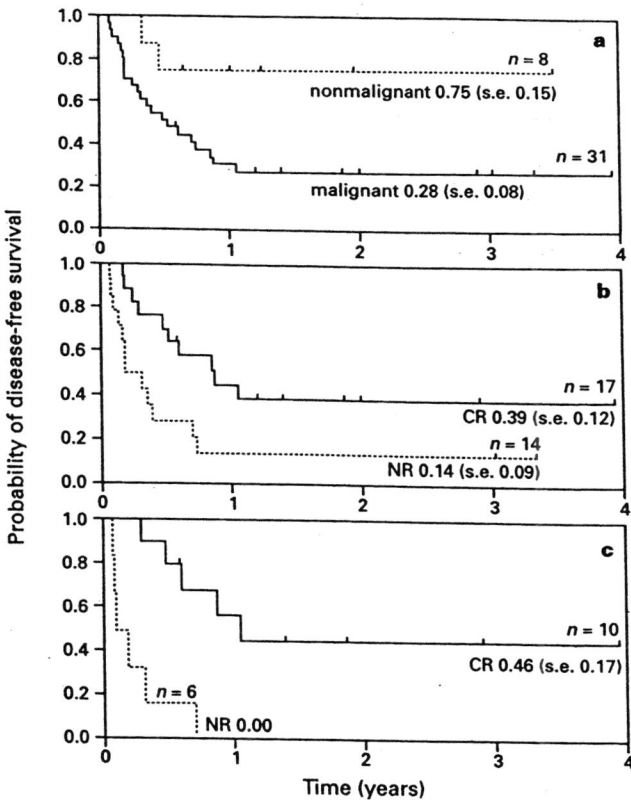

Fig. 51.12. Disease-free survival of patients after haploidentical transplantation with malignant and nonmalignant diseases ····· (a), malignant diseases in remission and not in remission (b), and in patients with ALL in remission or not in remission (c) at the time of transplant. Reproduced, with permission, from Handgretinger *et al.* (2001).

Comparison of allogeneic transplantation with chemotherapy and autologous transplantation

Limitations to the use of autologous HSC transplantation include concerns about infusing viable, clonogenic leukemic cells, a limited ability to detect minimal residual disease, and absence of a GVL response. It is expected that the results of autologous transplantation will be somewhat worse than the results of syngeneic transplantation. Therefore, the relapse rate after syngeneic transplantation probably reflects the asymptote that can be achieved with autologous transplantation. We know that patients relapse after allogeneic or syngeneic transplants, indicating that conditioning regimens are not completely effective in eradicating residual leukemia.

In considering the results of autologous transplantation in ALL, the duration of the preceding remission is a critical variable. Patients with long chemotherapy-induced remissions tend to have long remissions after autologous transplantation. Therefore, the benefit of autologous transplantation may be exaggerated unless the follow-up is at least as long as the chemotherapy-induced remissions. Moreover, the interval between achievement of remission and autologous transplantation is important, since patients who can sustain long remissions before autologous transplantation have more favorable prognoses. The administration of chemotherapy before autologous transplantation is likely to favor the transplant, because it both reduces the number of harvested leukemic cells as well as the number of residual leukemic cells in the body. However, it tends to select for patients with better prognosis, since the early relapsers are not considered for transplantation. Finally, patients with ALL who experienced relapses while on maintenance or consolidation therapy had a shorter survival compared with patients who relapsed after completing treatments in some series (Billett *et al.*, 1993) but not in others (Kersey *et al.*, 1987). Patients with Ph⁺ ALL are also unlikely to do well

with autologous transplantation. Nevertheless, a DFS rate of 50% to 70% at 2 to 4 years can be achieved in ALL in first remission (Boucheix *et al.*, 1994; Attal *et al.*, 1995). Transplants performed in second or subsequent remission have been reported to produce long-term survival rates of up to 50% (Billett *et al.*, 1993; Lawson *et al.*, 2000; Vaidya *et al.*, 2000). Several groups have demonstrated that in patients with high-risk ALL, allogeneic and purged autologous transplantations have similar outcomes. As noted in previous studies, the relapse rate was lower in the allogeneic patients with GVHD, but the toxicity related to the procedure was greater, and the overall DFS rates were not statistically different (Boucheix *et al.*, 1994; Attal *et al.*, 1995; Parsons *et al.*, 1996; Weisdorf *et al.*, 1997; Lawson *et al.*, 2000). Long-term quality of life and function seem to be well preserved after autologous transplantation (Singhal *et al.*, 1999).

Relapse

Methotrexate used for GVHD prophylaxis may have antileukemic activity (Barrett *et al.*, 1989), but attempts to exploit antimetabolites as maintenance therapy have been unsuccessful (Weisdorf *et al.*, 1987). Intrathecal methotrexate to prevent CNS relapse is effective but associated with a severe and devastating incidence of leukoencephalopathy in patients who received prior CNS therapy (Thompson *et al.*, 1986). Occasional patients who relapse after marrow grafting for ALL can achieve a complete remission with standard antileukemia therapy, although they relapse eventually (Bostrom *et al.*, 1987). Imitinab mesylate is likely to be more effective for Ph⁺ ALL, although the data are too immature to assess the durability of response.

Graft-versus-leukemia is a critical component of the antileukemia effect of allogeneic transplantation. Large retrospective studies indicate substantially reduced leukemic relapse rates in patients with GVHD, particularly chronic GVHD, although the effect is less prominent in ALL than that observed in myeloid diseases (Weiden *et al.*, 1981; Kersey *et al.*, 1987; Weisdorf *et al.*, 1987; Sullivan *et al.*, 1989). It appears to operate equally in B- and T-cell lineage ALL (Passweg *et al.*, 1998) (Fig. 51.13). One study of posttransplant immune modulation using alpha-interferon (given to prevent CMV infection) reported fewer relapses (Meyers *et al.*, 1987); this was not confirmed in subsequent analyses. Unrelated donor transplantation typically has been reported to be associated with very low relapse rates; however, it was hard to detect a prominent GVL effect in haploidentical transplantation. Unfortunately, while donor leukocyte infusions can be a highly effective method of inducing remission in CML, the results observed for treatment of posttransplant relapse of ALL are disappointing with only anecdotal responses reported (Kolb *et al.*, 1995; Porter *et al.*, 1999, 2000). Furthermore, despite promising early data, it does not appear that the large number of T cells intrinsic to peripheral blood stem cell grafts confer an improved GVL effect when compared with marrow grafts (Ringden *et al.*, 2001). It is likely that the stage of the dis-

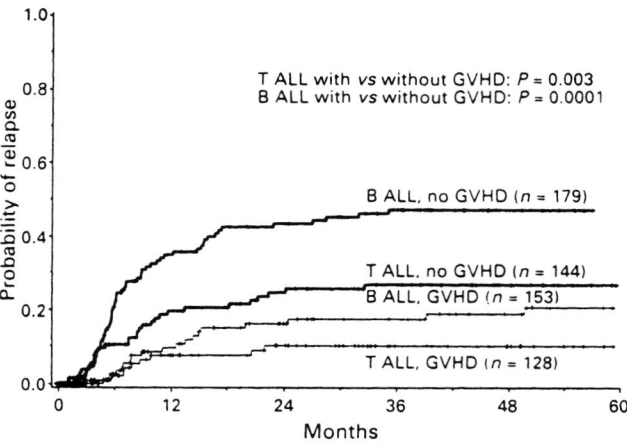

Fig. 51.13. Unadjusted (for other prognostic variables) probabilities of relapse in recipients of HLA-identical sibling bone marrow transplants for ALL in first complete remission with and without GVHD by ALL phenotype. Reproduced, with permission, from Passweg *et al.* (1998).

ease at the onset of the GVL effect, the ability of the lymphoblasts to present antigen or co-stimulate effectively, and the proliferative rate of the blasts are important variables that may influence the sensitivity to a GVL effect. Thus, GVL is observed less reliably after transplantation or immunotherapy for ALL for reasons that are presently obscure.

Decreasing relapse

There are two strategies to decrease relapse after transplants: (1) more effective antileukemia drugs and/or radiation; and (2) more effective immune-mediated antileukemic mechanisms. Conditioning regimens using hyperfractionated total body irradiation (Brochstein *et al.,* 1987), high-dose cytosine arabinoside (Coccia *et al.,* 1988), etoposide (Giralt *et al.,* 1994; Carpenter *et al.,* 1996), and/or busulfan (von Bueltzingsloewen *et al.,* 1995) report fewer relapses than typical pretransplant therapy. However, none are convincingly superior in careful comparisons or randomized trials (Blume *et al.,* 1993; Giralt *et al.,* 1994; Demirer *et al.,* 1995), and some are markedly toxic (Deconinck *et al.,* 1997). Radiolabeled monoclonal antibodies (Matthews *et al.,* 1995) have been added to conditioning regimens. There are too few data to comment whether relapse risk is decreased. Attempts to decrease relapse by increased immune-mediated antileukemia effects such as the prophylactic use of donor leukocyte infusions are entering clinical trials.

Conclusions

HLA-identical sibling transplants in first remission are probably comparable to, or better than, chemotherapy in children with high or very high risk features and in adults less than 30 years old (especially those with high-risk features). Otherwise, transplants are typically reserved to treat relapse after chemotherapy, those patients never achieving remission with chemotherapy, and children and adults with advanced leukemia. The dynamics of transplantation and conventional therapies suggest that as the effectiveness of therapy continues to improve, more patients are being cured. Early evidence from large-scale trials is starting to demonstrate an overall benefit from transplantation in adults with standard risk disease in first complete remission. Our challenge has previously been to determine who should receive a transplant and when. Our challenge now is to be sure that clinical investigation remains a priority, so we can determine the most efficient and effective means of curing this disease.

References

Arico, M., Valsecchi, M.G., Camitta, B. *et al.* (2000). Outcome of treatment in children with Philadelphia chromosome-positive acute lymphoblastic leukemia. *New England Journal of Medicine,* **342,** 998–1006.

Attal, M., Blaise, D., Marit, G. *et al.* (1995). Consolidation treatment of adult acute lymphoblastic leukemia: a prospective, randomized trial comparing allogeneic versus autologous bone marrow

transplantation and testing the impact of recombinant interleukin-2 after autologous bone marrow transplantation. BGMT Group. *Blood,* **86,** 1619–28.

Aversa, F., Tabilio, A., Velardi, A. *et al.* (1998). Treatment of high-risk acute leukemia with T-cell-depleted stem cells from related donors with one fully mismatched HLA haplotype. *New England Journal of Medicine,* **339,** 1186–93.

Badger, C., Buckner, C.D., Thomas, E.D. *et al.* (1982). Allogeneic marrow transplantation for acute leukemia in relapse. *Leukemia Research,* **6,** 383–7.

Barrett, A.J., Horowitz, M.M., Ash, R.C. *et al.* (1992). Bone marrow transplantation for Philadelphia chromosome-positive acute lymphoblastic leukemia. *Blood,* **79,** 3067–70.

Barrett, A.J., Horowitz, M.M., Gale, R.P. *et al.* (1989). Marrow transplantation for acute lymphoblastic leukemia: factors affecting relapse and survival. *Blood,* **74,** 862–71.

Barrett, A.J., Horowitz, M.M., Pollock, B.H. *et al.* (1994). Bone marrow transplants from HLA-identical siblings as compared with chemotherapy for children with acute lymphoblastic leukemia in a second remission. *New England Journal of Medicine,* **331,** 1253–8.

Barrett, A.J., Joshi, R., Kendra, J.R. *et al.* (1986). Prediction and prevention of relapse of acute lymphoblastic leukaemia after bone marrow transplantation. *British Journal of Haematology,* **64,** 179–86.

Biggs, J.C., Horowitz, M.M., Gale, R.P. *et al.* (1992). Bone marrow transplants may cure patients with acute leukemia never achieving remission with chemotherapy. *Blood,* **80,** 1090–3.

Billett, A.L., Kornmehl, E., Tarbell, N.J. *et al.* (1993). Autologous bone marrow transplantation after a long first remission for children with recurrent acute lymphoblastic leukemia. *Blood,* **81,** 1651–7.

Blume, K.G., Forman, S.J., Snyder, D.S. *et al.* (1987). Allogeneic bone marrow transplantation for acute lymphoblastic leukemia during first complete remission. *Transplantation,* **43,** 389–92.

Blume, K.G., Kopecky, K.J., Henslee-Downey, J.P. *et al.* (1993). A prospective randomized comparison of total body irradiation-etoposide versus busulfan-cyclophosphamide as preparatory regimens for bone marrow transplantation in patients with leukemia who were not in first remission: a Southwest Oncology Group study. *Blood,* **81,** 2187–93.

Bordigoni, P., Esperou, H., Souillet, G. *et al.* (1998). Total body irradiation-high-dose cytosine arabinoside and melphalan followed by allogeneic bone marrow transplantation from HLA-identical siblings in the treatment of children with acute lymphoblastic leukaemia after relapse while receiving chemotherapy: a Societe Francaise de Greffe de Moelle study. *British Journal of Haematology,* **102,** 656–65.

Borg, A., Yin, J.A., Johnson, P.R. *et al.* (1996). Successful treatment of HTLV-1-associated acute adult T-cell leukaemia lymphoma by allogeneic bone marrow transplantation. *British Journal of Haematology,* **94,** 713–5.

Bostrom, B., Woods, W.G., Nesbit, M.E. *et al.* (1987). Successful reinduction of patients with acute lymphoblastic leukemia who relapse following bone marrow transplantation. *Journal of Clinical Oncology,* **5,** 376–81.

Boucheix, C., David, B., Sebban, C. *et al.* (1994). Immunophenotype of adult acute lymphoblastic leukemia, clinical parameters, and outcome: an analysis of a prospective trial including 562 tested patients (LALA87). French Group on Therapy for Adult Acute Lymphoblastic Leukemia. *Blood,* **84,** 1603–12.

Boulad, F., Steinherz, P., Reyes, B. *et al.* (1999). Allogeneic bone marrow transplantation versus chemotherapy for the treatment of childhood acute lymphoblastic leukemia in second remission: a single-institution study. *Journal of Clinical Oncology,* **17,** 197–207.

Brochstein, J.A., Kernan, N.A., Groshen, S. *et al.* (1987). Allogeneic bone marrow transplantation after hyperfractionated total-body irradiation and cyclophosphamide in children with acute leukemia. *New England Journal of Medicine,* **317,** 1618–24.

Buckner, C.D. & Clift, R.A. (1984). Marrow transplantation for acute lymphoblastic leukemia. *Seminars in Hematology,* **21,** 43–7.

Buhrer, C., Hartmann, R., Fengler, R. *et al.* (1996). Peripheral blast counts at diagnosis of late isolated bone marrow relapse of childhood acute lymphoblastic leukemia predict response to salvage chemotherapy and outcome. Berlin-Frankfurt-Munster Relapse Study Group. *Journal of Clinical Oncology,* **14,** 2812–7.

Bunin, N., Carston, M., Wall, D. *et al.* (2002). Unrelated marrow transplantation for children with acute lymphoblastic leukemia in second remission. *Blood,* **99,** 3151–7.

Carpenter, P.A., Marshall, G.M., Giri, N. *et al.* (1996). Allogeneic bone marrow transplantation for children with acute lymphoblastic leukemia conditioned with busulfan, cyclophosphamide and melphalan. *Bone Marrow Transplantation,* **18,** 489–94.

Chao, N.J., Blume, K.G., Forman, S.J., & Snyder, D.S. (1995). Long-term follow-up of allogeneic bone marrow recipients for Philadelphia chromosome-positive acute lymphoblastic leukemia. *Blood,* **85,** 3353–4.

Chao, N.J., Forman, S.J., Schmidt, G.M. *et al.* (1991). Allogeneic bone marrow transplantation for high-risk acute lymphoblastic leukemia during first complete remission. *Blood,* **78,** 1923–7.

Chessells, J.M., Bailey, C., & Richards, S.M. (1995). Intensification of treatment and survival in all children with lymphoblastic leukaemia: results of UK Medical Research Council trial UKALL X. Medical Research Council Working Party on Childhood Leukaemia. *Lancet,* **345,** 143–8.

Chessells, J.M., Leiper, A.D., & Richards, S.M. (1994). A second course of treatment for childhood acute lymphoblastic leukaemia: long-term follow-up is needed to assess results. *British Journal of Haematology,* **86,** 48–54.

Chessells, J.M., Rogers, D.W., Leiper, A.D. *et al.* (1986). Bone-marrow transplantation has a limited role in prolonging second marrow remission in childhood lymphoblastic leukaemia. *Lancet,* **1,** 1239–41.

Clavell, L.A., Gelber, R.D., Cohen, H.J. *et al.* (1986). Four-agent induction and intensive asparaginase therapy for treatment of childhood acute lymphoblastic leukemia. *New England Journal of Medicine,* **315,** 657–63.

Coccia, P.F., Strandjord, S.E., Warkentin, P.I. *et al.* (1988). High-dose cytosine arabinoside and fractionated total-body irradiation: an improved preparative regimen for bone marrow transplantation of children with acute lymphoblastic leukemia in remission. *Blood,* **71,** 888–93.

Cornelissen, J.J., Carston, M., Kollman, C. *et al.* (2001). Unrelated marrow transplantation for adult patients with poor-risk acute lymphoblastic leukemia: strong graft-versus-leukemia effect and risk factors determining outcome. *Blood,* **97,** 1572–7.

Czuczman, M.S., Dodge, R.K., Stewart, C.C. *et al.* (1999). Value of immunophenotype in intensively treated adult acute lymphoblastic leukemia: cancer and leukemia Group B study 8364. *Blood,* **93,** 3931–9.

Davies, S.M., Ramsay, N.K., Klein, J.P. *et al.* (2000). Comparison of preparative regimens in transplants for children with acute lymphoblastic leukemia. *Journal of Clinical Oncology,* **18,** 340–7.

Deconinck, E., Cahn, J.Y., Milpied, N. *et al.* (1997). Allogeneic bone marrow transplantation for high-risk acute lymphoblastic leukemia in first remission: long-term results for 42 patients conditioned with an intensified regimen (TBI, high-dose Ara-C and melphalan). *Bone Marrow Transplantation,* **20,** 731–5.

Demirer, T., Weaver, C.H., Buckner, C.D. *et al.* (1995). High-dose cyclophosphamide, carmustine, and etoposide followed by allogeneic bone marrow transplantation in patients with lymphoid malignancies who had received prior dose-limiting radiation therapy. *Journal of Clinical Oncology,* **13,** 596–602.

Druker, B.J., Sawyers, C.L., Kantarjian, H. *et al.* (2001). Activity of a specific inhibitor of the BCR-ABL tyrosine kinase in the blast crisis of chronic myeloid leukemia and acute lymphoblastic leukemia with the Philadelphia chromosome. *New England Journal of Medicine,* **344,** 1038–42.

Dunlop, L.C., Powles, R., Singhal, S. *et al.* (1996). Bone marrow transplantation for Philadelphia chromosome-positive acute lymphoblastic leukemia. *Bone Marrow Transplantation,* **17,** 365–9.

Forman, S.J., O'Donnell, M.R., Nademanee, A.P. *et al.* (1987). Bone marrow transplantation for patients with Philadelphia chromosome-positive acute lymphoblastic leukemia. *Blood,* **70,** 587–8.

Forman, S.J., Schmidt, G.M., Nademanee, A.P. *et al.* (1991). Allogeneic bone marrow transplantation as therapy for primary induction failure for patients with acute leukemia. *Journal of Clinical Oncology,* **9,** 1570–4.

Giralt, S.A., LeMaistre, C.F., Vriesendorp, H.M. *et al.* (1994). Etoposide, cyclophosphamide, total-body irradiation, and allogeneic bone marrow transplantation for hematologic malignancies. *Journal of Clinical Oncology,* **12,** 1923–30.

Gleissner, B., Gokbuget, N., Bartram, C.R. *et al.* (2002). Leading prognostic relevance of the BCR-ABL translocation in adult acute B-lineage lymphoblastic leukemia: a prospective study of the German Multicenter Trial Group and confirmed polymerase chain reaction analysis. *Blood,* **99,** 1536–43.

Godder, K.T., Hazlett, L.J., Abhyankar, S.H. *et al.* (2000). Partially mismatched related-donor bone marrow transplantation for pediatric patients with acute leukemia: younger donors and absence of peripheral blasts improve outcome. *Journal of Clinical Oncology,* **18,** 1856–66.

Goldstone, A.H., Prentice, H.G., Durrant, J. *et al.* (2001). Allogeneic transplant (related or unrelated donor) is the preferred treatment for adult Philadelphia chromosome positive (Ph+) acute lymphoblastic leukaemia (ALL). Results from the International ALL Trial (MRC UKALLXII/ECOG E2993). *Blood,* **98** (Suppl 1), 856a.

Handgretinger, R., Klingbiel, T., Lang, P. *et al.* (2001). Megadose transplantation of purified peripheral blood CD34+ progenitor cells from HLA-mismatched parental donors in children. *Bone Marrow Transplantation,* **27,** 777–83.

Harrison, G., Richards, S., Lawson, S. *et al.* (2000). Comparison of allogeneic transplant versus chemotherapy for relapsed childhood acute lymphoblastic leukaemia in the MRC UKALL R1 trial. MRC Childhood Leukaemia Working Party. *Annals of Oncology,* **11,** 999–1006.

Henze, G., Fengler, R., Hartmann, R. *et al.* (1991). Six-year experience with a comprehensive approach to the treatment of recurrent childhood acute lymphoblastic leukemia (ALL-REZ BFM 85). A relapse study of the BFM group. *Blood,* **78,** 1166–72.

Herzig, R.H., Bortin, M.M., Barrett, A.J. *et al.* (1987). Bone-marrow transplantation in high-risk acute lymphoblastic leukaemia in first and second remission. *Lancet,* **i,** 786–9.

Horowitz, M.M., Messerer, D., Hoelzer, D. *et al.* (1991). Chemotherapy compared with bone marrow transplantation for adults with acute lymphoblastic leukemia in first remission. *Annals of Internal Medicine,* **115,** 13–8.

Johnson, F.L., Thomas, E.D., Clark, B.S. *et al.* (1981). A comparison of marrow transplantation with chemotherapy for children with acute lymphoblastic leukemia in second and subsequent remission. *New England Journal of Medicine,* **305,** 846–51.

Kanda, Y., Taketazu, F., Chiba, S. *et al.* (1999). Persistent infection with human T lymphotropic virus type 1 after allogeneic bone marrow transplantation from a seronegative donor. *Bone Marrow Transplantation,* **24,** 349.

Kawa, K., Nishiuchi, R., Okamura, T., & Igarashi, H. (1998). Eradication of human T-lymphotropic virus type 1 by allogeneic bone-marrow transplantation. *Lancet,* **352,** 1034–5.

Kersey, J.H. (1998). Fifty years of studies of the biology and therapy of childhood leukemia. *Blood,* **92,** 1838.

Kersey, J.H., Weisdorf, D., Nesbit, M.E. *et al.* (1987). Comparison of autologous and allogeneic bone Marrow transplantation for treatment of high-risk refractory acute lymphoblastic leukemia. *New England Journal of Medicine,* **317,** 461–7.

Kishi, Y., Kami, M., Oki, Y. *et al.* (2001). Successful bone marrow transplantation for adult T-cell leukemia from a donor with oligoclonal proliferation of T-cells infected with human T-cell lymphotropic virus. *Leukemia and Lymphoma,* **42,** 819–22.

Kolb, H.J., Schattenberg, A., Goldman, J.M. *et al.* (1995). Graft-versus-leukemia effect of donor lymphocyte transfusions in marrow grafted patients. *Blood,* **86,** 2041–50.

Lawson, S.E., Harrison, G., Richards, S. *et al.* (2000). The UK experience in treating relapsed childhood acute lymphoblastic leukaemia: a report on the medical research council UKALLR1 study. *British Journal of Haematology,* **108,** 531–43.

Leclercq, I., Mortreux, F., Morschhauser, F. *et al.* (1999). Semiquantitative analysis of residual disease in patients treated for adult T-cell leukaemia/lymphoma (ATLL). *British Journal of Haematology,* **105,** 743–51.

Martin, T.G. & Gajewski, J.L. (2001). Allogeneic stem cell transplantation for acute lymphocytic leukemia in adults. *Hematology/Oncology Clinics of North America,* **15,** 97–120.

Matthews, D.C., Appelbaum, F.R., Eary, J.F. *et al.* (1995). Development of a marrow transplant regimen for acute leukemia using targeted hematopoietic irradiation delivered by 131I-labeled anti-CD45 antibody, combined with cyclophosphamide and total body irradiation. *Blood,* **85,** 1122–31.

Meyers, J.D., Flournoy, N., Sanders, J.E. *et al.* (1987). Prophylactic use of human leukocyte interferon after allogeneic marrow transplantation. *Annals of Internal Medicine,* **107,** 809–16.

Oakhill, A., Pamphilon, D.H., Potter, M.N. *et al.* (1996). Unrelated donor bone marrow transplantation for children with relapsed acute lymphoblastic leukaemia in second complete remission. *British Journal of Haematology,* **94,** 574–8.

Obama, K., Tara, M., Sao, H. *et al.* (1999). Allogenic bone marrow transplantation as a treatment for adult T-cell leukemia. *International Journal of Hematology,* **69,** 203–5.

Oh, H., Gale, R.P., Zhang, M.J. *et al.* (1998). Chemotherapy vs HLA-identical sibling bone marrow transplants for adults with acute lymphoblastic leukemia in first remission. *Bone Marrow Transplantation,* **22,** 253–7.

Ogata, M., Ogata, Y., Imamura, T. *et al.* (2002). Successful bone marrow transplantation from an unrelated donor in a patient with adult T cell leukemia. *Bone Marrow Transplantation,* **30,** 699–701.

Parsons, S.K., Castellino, S.M., Lehmann, L.E. *et al.* (1996). Relapsed acute lymphoblastic leukemia: similar outcomes for autologous and allogeneic marrow transplantation in selected children. *Bone Marrow Transplantation,* **17,** 763–8.

Passweg, J.R., Tiberghien, P., Cahn, J.Y. *et al.* (1998). Graft-versus-leukemia effects in T lineage and B lineage acute lymphoblastic leukemia. *Bone Marrow Transplantation,* **21,** 153–8.

Pawlowska, A.B., Davies, S.M., Orchard, P.J. *et al.* (1996). Unrelated donor Bone Marrow transplantation for acute leukemia in patients with Down's syndrome. *Bone Marrow Transplantation,* **18,** 453–5.

Pinkel, D. (1989). Allogeneic bone marrow transplantation in children with acute leukemia: a practice whose time has gone. *Leukemia,* **3,** 242–4.

Porter, D.L., Collins, R.H., Jr., Hardy, C. *et al.* (2000). Treatment of relapsed leukemia after unrelated donor marrow transplantation with unrelated donor leukocyte infusions. *Blood,* **95,** 1214–21.

Porter, D.L., Collins, R.H., Jr., Shpilberg, O. *et al.* (1999). Long-term follow-up of patients who achieved complete remission after donor leukocyte infusions. *Biology of Blood and Marrow Transplantation,* **5,** 253–61.

Pui, C.H. & Evans, W.E. (1998). Acute lymphoblastic leukemia. *New England Journal of Medicine,* **339,** 605–15.

Ringden, O., Labopin, M., Bacigalupo, A. *et al.* (2001). Transplantation of peripheral blood stem cells as compared with bone marrow from HLA Identical siblings in patients with acute myeloid leukemia and acute lymphoblastic leukemia. *Blood,* **99** (Suppl 1), 482a.

Ritchey, A.K., Pollock, B.H., Lauer, S.J. *et al.* (1999). Improved survival of children with isolated CNS relapse of acute lymphoblastic leukemia: a pediatric oncology group study. *Journal of Clinical Oncology,* **17,** 3745–52.

Rocha, V., Cornish, J., Sievers, E.L. *et al.* (2001). Comparison of outcomes of unrelated bone marrow and umbilical cord blood transplants in children with acute leukemia. *Blood,* **97,** 2962–71.

Rowe, J.M., Richards, S.M., Burnett, A.K. *et al.* (2001). Favorable results of allogeneic bone marrow transplantation (BMT) for adults with Philadelphia (Ph)-chromosome-negative acute lymphoblastic leukemia (ALL) in first complete remission (CR): results from the international ALL trial (MRC UKALL XII/ECOG E2993). *Blood,* **98** (Suppl 1), 481a.

Rowlings, P.A., Passweg, J.R., Armitage, J.O. *et al.* (1996). Current status of allogeneic and autologous blood and marrow transplantation. Report from the IBMTR and ABMTR-North America. In *Yearbook of Cell and Tissue Transplantation,* eds. R.P. Lanza & W.L. Chick, pp. 19–34. Dordrecht, The Netherlands: Kluwer Academic Publishers.

Saarinen, U.M., Mellander, L., Nysom, K. *et al.* (1996). Allogeneic bone marrow transplantation in first remission for children with very high-risk acute lymphoblastic leukemia: a retrospective case-control study in the Nordic countries. Nordic Society for Pediatric Hematology and Oncology (NOPHO). *Bone Marrow Transplantation,* **17,** 357–63.

Saarinen-Pihkala, U.M., Gustafsson, G., Ringden, O. *et al.* (2001). No disadvantage in outcome of using matched unrelated donors as compared with matched sibling donors for Bone Marrow transplantation in children with acute lymphoblastic leukemia in second remission. *Journal of Clinical Oncology,* **19,** 3406–14.

Sanders, J.E., Thomas, E.D., Buckner, C.D., & Doney, K. (1987). Marrow transplantation for children with acute lymphoblastic leukemia in second remission. *Blood,* **70,** 324–6.

Schroeder, H., Gustafsson, G., Saarinen-Pihkala, U.M. *et al.* (1999). Allogeneic Bone Marrow transplantation in second remission of childhood acute lymphoblastic leukemia: a population-based case control study from the Nordic countries. *Bone Marrow Transplantation,* **23,** 555–60.

Sebban, C., Lepage, E., Vernant, J.P. *et al.* (1994). Allogeneic bone marrow transplantation in adult acute lymphoblastic leukemia in first complete remission: a comparative study. French Group of Therapy of Adult Acute Lymphoblastic Leukemia. *Journal of Clinical Oncology,* **12,** 2580–7.

Sierra, J., Radich, J., Hansen, J.A. *et al.* (1997). Marrow transplants from unrelated donors for treatment of Philadelphia chromosome-positive acute lymphoblastic leukemia. *Blood,* **90,** 1410–4.

Silverman, L.B., Gelber, R.D., Dalton, V.K. *et al.* (2001). Improved outcome for children with acute lymphoblastic leukemia: results of Dana-Farber Consortium Protocol 91-01. *Blood,* **97,** 1211–8.

Singhal, S., Powles, R., Treleaven, J. *et al.* (1999). Long-term outcome of adult acute leukemia patients who are alive and well 2 years after autologous blood or marrow transplantation. *Bone Marrow Transplantation,* **23,** 875–9.

Snyder, D.S. (2000). Allogeneic stem cell transplantation for Philadelphia chromosome-positive acute lymphoblastic leukemia. *Biology of Blood and Marrow Transplantation,* **6,** 597–603.

Snyder, D.S., Nademanee, A.P., O'Donnell, M.R. *et al.* (1999). Long-term follow-up of 23 patients with Philadelphia chromosome-positive acute lymphoblastic leukemia treated with allogeneic bone marrow transplant in first complete remission. *Leukemia,* **13,** 2053–8.

Steinherz, P.G., Gaynon, P., Miller, D.R. *et al.* (1986). Improved disease-free survival of children with acute lymphoblastic leukemia at high risk for early relapse with the New York regimen—a new intensive therapy protocol: a report from the Children's Cancer Study Group. *Journal of Clinical Oncology,* **4,** 744–52.

Stockschlader, M., Hegewisch-Becker, S., Kruger, W. *et al.* (1995). Bone marrow transplantation for Philadelphia-chromosome-positive acute lymphoblastic leukemia. *Bone Marrow Transplantation,* **16,** 663–7.

Sullivan, K.M., Storb, R., Buckner, C.D. *et al.* (1989). Graft-versus-host disease as adoptive immunotherapy in patients with advanced hematologic neoplasms. *New England Journal of Medicine,* **320,** 828–34.

Szydlo, R., Goldman, J.M., Klein, J.P. *et al.* (1997). Results of allogeneic bone marrow transplants for leukemia using donors other than HLA-identical siblings. *Journal of Clinical Oncology,* **15,** 1767–77.

Tajima, K., Amakawa, R., Uehira, K. *et al.* (2000). Adult T-cell leukemia successfully treated with allogeneic bone marrow transplantation. *International Journal of Hematology,* **71,** 290–3.

Thomas, D.A., Kantarjian, H., Smith, T.L. *et al.* (1999). Primary refractory and relapsed adult acute lymphoblastic leukemia: characteristics, treatment results, and prognosis with salvage therapy. *Cancer,* **86,** 1216–30.

Thompson, C.B., Sanders, J.E., Flournoy, N. *et al.* (1986). The risks of central nervous system relapse and leukoencephalopathy in patients receiving marrow transplants for acute leukemia. *Blood,* **67,** 195–9.

Uderzo, C., Valsecchi, M.G., Bacigalupo, A. *et al.* (1995). Treatment of childhood acute lymphoblastic leukemia in second remission with allogeneic bone marrow transplantation and chemotherapy: ten-year experience of the Italian Bone Marrow Transplantation Group and the Italian Pediatric Hematology Oncology Association. *Journal of Clinical Oncology,* **13,** 352–8.

Uderzo, C., Valsecchi, M.G., Balduzzi, A. *et al.* (1997). Allogeneic bone marrow transplantation versus chemotherapy in high-risk childhood acute lymphoblastic leukaemia in first remission. Associazione Italiana di Ematologia ed Oncologia Pediatrica (AIEOP) and the Gruppo Italiano Trapianto di Midollo Osseo (GITMO). *British Journal of Haematology,* **96,** 387–94.

Urbano-Ispizua, A., Schmitz, N., de Witte, T. *et al.* (2002). Allogeneic and autologous transplantation for haematological diseases, solid tumors and immune disorders: definition and current practice in Europe. *Bone Marrow Transplantation,* **29,** 639–46.

Utsunomiya, A., Miyazaki, Y., Takatsuka, Y. *et al.* (2001). Improved outcome of adult T cell leukemia/lymphoma with allogeneic hematopoietic stem cell transplantation. *Bone Marrow Transplantation,* **27,** 15–20.

Vaidya, S.J., Atra, A., Bahl, S. *et al.* (2000). Autologous bone marrow transplantation for childhood acute lymphoblastic leukaemia in second remission—long-term follow-up. *Bone Marrow Transplantation,* **25,** 599–603.

Vernant, J.P., Marit, G., Maraninchi, D. *et al.* (1988). Allogeneic bone marrow transplantation in adults with acute lymphoblastic leukemia in first complete remission. *Journal of Clinical Oncology,* **6,** 227–31.

von Bueltzingsloewen, A., Esperou-Bourdeau, H., Souillet, G. *et al.* (1995). Allogeneic bone marrow transplantation following a busulfan-based conditioning regimen in young children with acute lymphoblastic leukemia: a Cooperative Study of the

Societe Francaise de Greffe de Moelle. *Bone Marrow Transplantation,* **16,** 521–7.

Weiden, P.L., Sullivan, K.M., Flournoy, N. *et al.* (1981). Antileukemic effect of chronic graft-versus-host disease: contribution to improved survival after allogeneic marrow transplantation. *New England Journal of Medicine,* **304,** 1529–33.

Weisdorf, D.J., Billett, A.L., Hannan, P. *et al.* (1997). Autologous versus unrelated donor allogeneic marrow transplantation for acute lymphoblastic leukemia. *Blood,* **90,** 2962–8.

Weisdorf, D.J., Nesbit, M.E., Ramsay, N.K. *et al.* (1987). Allogeneic bone marrow transplantation for acute lymphoblastic leukemia in remission: prolonged survival associated with acute graft-versus-host disease. *Journal of Clinical Oncology,* **5,** 1348–55.

Weisdorf, D.J., Woods, W.G., & Nesbit, M.E.J. (1994). Allogeneic bone marrow transplantation for acute lymphoblastic leukaemia: risk factors and clinical outcome. *British Journal of Haematology,* **86,** 62–9.

Wetzler, M., Dodge, R.K., Mrozek, K. *et al.* (1999). Prospective karyotype analysis in adult acute lymphoblastic leukemia: the Cancer and Leukemia Group B experience. *Blood,* **93,** 3983–93.

Wheeler, K.A., Richards, S.M., Bailey, C.C. *et al.* (2000). bone marrow transplantation versus chemotherapy in the treatment of very high-risk childhood acute lymphoblastic leukemia in first remission: results from Medical Research Council UKALL X and XI. *Blood,* **96,** 2412–8.

Woolfrey, A.E., Anasetti, C., Storer, B. *et al.* (2002). Factors associated with outcome after unrelated marrow transplantation for treatment of acute lymphoblastic leukemia in children. *Blood,* **99,** 2002–8.

Zhang, M.J., Hoelzer, D., Horowitz, M.M. *et al.* (1995). Long-term follow-up of adults with acute lymphoblastic leukemia in first remission treated with chemotherapy or bone marrow transplantation. The Acute Lymphoblastic Leukemia Working Committee. *Annals of Internal Medicine,* **123,** 428–31.

Zwaan, F.E., Hermans, J., Barrett, A.J., & Speck, B. (1984). Bone marrow transplantation for acute lymphoblastic leukaemia: a survey of the European Group for Bone Marrow Transplantation (E.G.B.M.T.). *British Journal of Haematology,* **58,** 33–42.

52 Allogeneic hematopoietic stem cell transplantation for chronic myeloid leukemia

DAVID G. SAVAGE AND JOHN M. GOLDMAN

*Columbia University College of Physicians and Surgeons, New York City, USA, and
Imperial College School of Medicine, London, UK*

Introduction

Treatment decisions for a patient with newly diagnosed chronic myeloid leukemia (CML) have become increasingly complex, but only allogeneic hematopoietic stem cell (HSC) transplantation has been shown to be curative (Goldman *et al.*, 1986, 1988; Thomas *et al.*, 1986; van Rhee *et al.*, 1997; Gale *et al.*, 1998) (Figs. 52.1 to 52.3). Chemotherapy with busulfan or hydroxyurea results in median survivals of about 5 years, but hydroxyurea has fewer side effects and is easier to administer. Interferon-alpha (IFN-α) appears to prolong survival compared with hydroxyurea (Talpaz *et al.*, 1991; Italian Cooperative Study Group on CML, 1993; CML Trialists Collaborative Study, 1997), but probably does not cure any patients; complete cytogenetic responders (only 10%–20% of all those treated)

remain positive for BCR-ABL (break point cluster region-Abelson) transcripts using the reverse transcriptase polymerase chain reaction (RT-PCR) (Hochhaus *et al.*, 1996) and do eventually relapse (Talpaz *et al.*, 1991). A specific inhibitor of the tyrosine kinase activity encoded by the BCR-ABL oncogene, known as imatinib mesylate (STI 571), has shown promising ability to induce hematologic and cytogenetic remissions, but follow-up is currently short (see Chapter 38). High-dose therapy with infusion of autologous progenitor cells may prolong survival but does not cure patients. Its role is also discussed in Chapter 38.

Information on disease incidence, classification, immune phenotype, cytogenetic abnormalities, prognostic factors, outcome with conventional therapy, disease-specific pretransplant

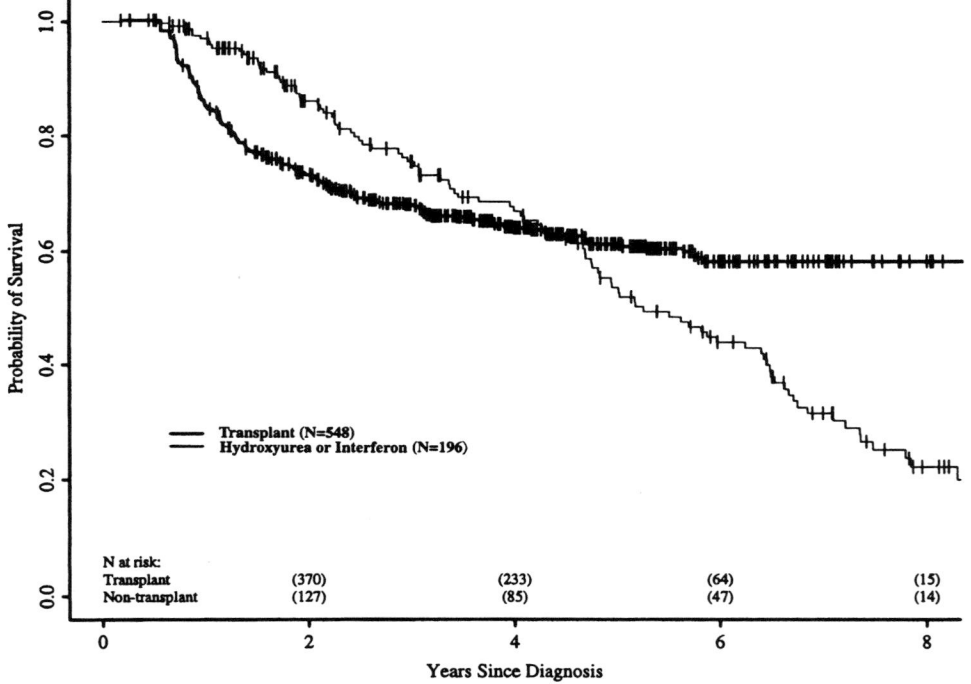

Fig. 52.1. Adjusted probabilities (from Cox regression model) of survival after diagnosis of CML in persons receiving HLA-identical sibling bone marrow transplants or nontransplant therapy with hydroxyurea or interferon. Reproduced, with permission, from Gale *et al.* (1998).

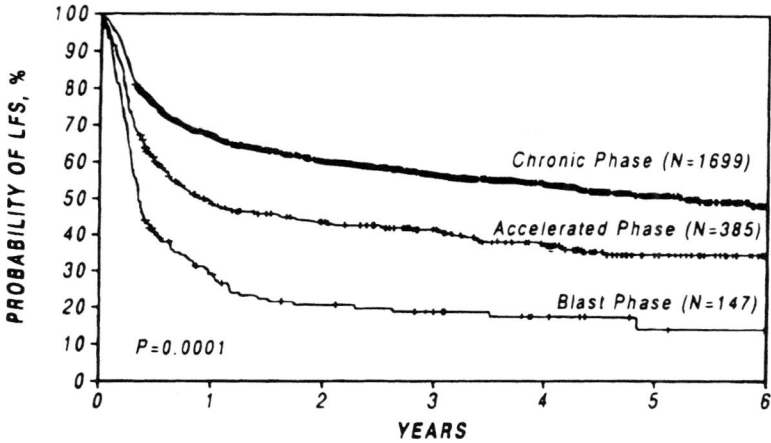

Fig. 52.2. Actuarial probability of LFS after HLA-identical sibling bone marrow transplantation for CML according to phase of disease at time of transplant. Reproduced, with permission, from Horowitz *et al.* (1996).

work-up, and monitoring for residual disease posttransplant are given in Chapter 38.

Whom to transplant?

The results of allogeneic HSC transplantation using HLA-identical sibling donor marrow seem to be improving. Transplant-related complications are fewer in this decade than in the 1980s, and cytomegalovirus (CMV) infections can be managed effectively, at least in recipients of HLA-identical sibling transplants. The observation that HLA-identical sibling transplants can in many cases cure patients with CML led naturally to consideration of allogeneic transplantation for those lacking sibling donors. The use of alternative donors (i.e., partially matched family members or unrelated volunteers) has been studied extensively during the past 10 years. The clinical results, although generally less good than those of sibling

donor transplants, are encouraging (Laporte *et al.*, 1996; Szydlo *et al.*, 1997; Hansen *et al.*, 1998), and in some reports show outcomes comparable to those achieved with sibling donors (Lamparelli *et al.*, 1997) (Fig. 52.4).

The upper age limit for allogeneic HSC transplantation for CML patients remains a matter of some debate because of the well-recognized increased risk of severe graft-versus-host disease (GVHD) and other complications with increasing age. For patients with HLA-identical sibling donors, it is probably reasonable to offer transplantation up to the age of 60 years provided they are medically fit; for those with alternative donors, a somewhat lower upper age may be advisable. The use of non-myeloablative conditioning regimens (see Chapter 22) for older, or medically infirm, patients may be a useful development. Guidelines for the treatment of patients with CML, based on specific risk factors are provided in Table 52.1.

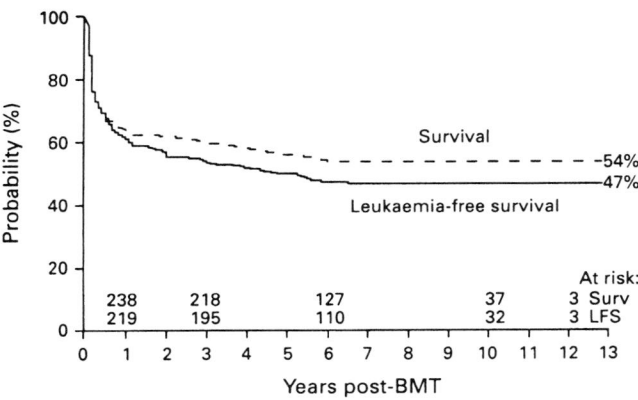

Fig. 52.3. Probability of survival and LFS after HLA-identical sibling BMT for CML in first chronic phase. Reproduced, with permission, from van Rhee *et al.* (1997).

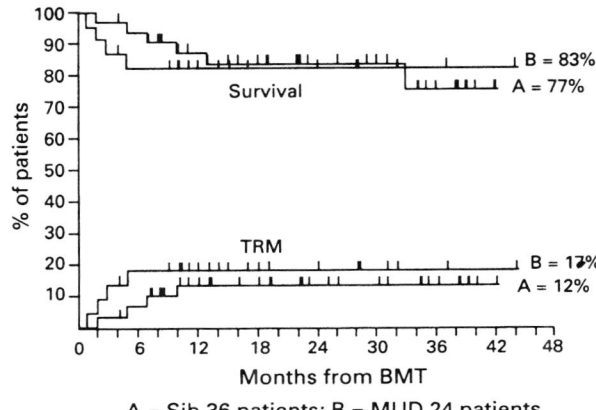

Fig. 52.4. Actuarial survival and transplant-related mortality. Reproduced, with permission, from Lamparelli *et al.* (1997).

When to transplant?

There is general agreement that results achieved with patients transplanted in chronic phase are superior to those obtained in patients with more advanced disease. Furthermore, the results of allogeneic transplantation in chronic phase are significantly better in younger patients and if the transplant occurs within 1 year of diagnosis (Thomas *et al.,* 1986; Goldman *et al.,* 1993; Clift & Storb, 1996; Hansen *et al.,* 1998) (Figs. 52.5 and 52.6). The use of busulfan prior to transplant is associated with an increased risk of transplant-related mortality (Goldman *et al.,* 1993). It is worth noting that for patients prepared for transplant with busulfan/cyclophosphamide, the improved survival for transplants performed in chronic phase within 1 year of diagnosis only occurred in the group given prior maintenance therapy with hydroxyurea rather than with busulfan (Biggs *et al.,* 1992). Prolonged (6–12 months) use of IFN-α prior to allo-BMT (using related or unrelated donors) may also be associated with inferior survival (Beelen *et al.,* 1995; Morton *et al.,* 1998) (Fig. 52.7), although there are conflicting reports on this (Giralt *et al.,* 1993; Hehlmann *et al.,* 1999; Lee *et al.,* 2001). An International Bone Marrow Transplant Registry (IBMTR) study of 873 patients found that a short course (median 2 months) of IFN-α pretransplant did not adversely affect survival after a subsequent HLA-identical sibling BMT for chronic phase CML (Giralt *et al.,* 2000) . In contrast, Hehlmann's study found that, while duration of IFN-α therapy pretransplant did not influence outcome, the interval between cessation of treatment and BMT did: use of IFN within 90 days of transplant was associated with a worse outcome. In a second retrospective IBMTR study, IFN-α therapy did not influence

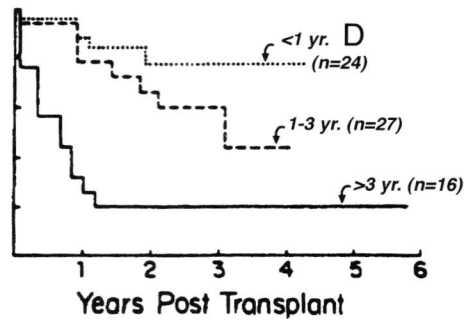

Fig. 52.5. The effect of the interval from diagnosis to transplant on survival. The dotted line shows less than 1 year; the broken line, 1–3 years; the solid line, greater than 3 years. Reproduced, with permission, from Thomas *et al.* (1986).

outcome in 489 patients who received allografts from unrelated donors (Lee *et al.,* 2001). Preliminary EBMT data suggest that treatment with imatinib mesylate does not have a deleterious effect on subsequent allogeneic transplantation (Deininger *et al.,* 2001), but this will require further observation.

An analysis from the IBMTR suggested a 30% long-term disease-free survival for patients transplanted in accelerated phase (Horowitz *et al.,* 1996) (Fig. 52.2). The Ohio group reported remarkable results in a small group of patients with accelerated phase disease (55% 3-year disease-free survival) who received busulfan and cyclophosphamide conditioning (Copelan *et al.,* 1989), but these results have not been confirmed. The Seattle group has also reported encouraging results in some subsets of patients transplanted in acceleration (Figs. 52.8 to 52.11). The prognostic impact of the different IBMTR criteria for acceleration varies considerably, but it is clear that increased numbers of blast cells and cytogenetic evolution are associated with a poor outcome. The long-term results of allogeneic transplantation in overt blastic phase are poorer still (Fig. 52.2). Hematologic relapse posttransplant is (predictably) more common for advanced phase disease, but so are GVHD (Savage *et al.,* 1997) and pneumonitis, the reasons for which are unknown.

Conditioning regimens and source of hematopoietic stem cells

Pretransplant conditioning should cause sufficient immune suppression to permit engraftment, but it may not be necessary that the conditioning alone eradicates the last malignant stem cell. Thus, cytoreduction by the conditioning regimen must be important, but cure probably depends also on a graft-versus-leukemia (GVL) effect.

Cyclophosphamide (2×60 mg/kg) and fractionated total body irradiation (TBI; 1,200 cGy) is a standard conditioning regimen. Cyclophosphamide and TBI have been combined with high-dose etoposide, resulting in an event-free survival at 5-years posttransplant of 64% for patients transplanted in first

Table 52.1. *Proposed risk classification for allogeneic stem cell transplantation (SCT)*

Risk factors	Results at 5 years		
	Percent of Patients with risk factors	Leukemia-free survival (%)	Transplant-related mortality (%)
0	2	60	20
1	18	60	23
2	28	47	31
3	28	37	46
4	15	35	51
5	7	19	71
6–7	2	16	73

Risk factors are donor type (0 for HLA-identical sibling donor, 1 for a matched unrelated donor); disease stage (0 for first chronic phase, 1 for accelerated phase, and 2 for blast crisis or higher chronic phase); age of recipient (0 for <20 years, 1 for 20–40 years, and 2 for >40 years); sex combination (0 for all, except 1 for male recipient/female donor); and time from diagnosis to stem cell transplantation (0 for <12 months, 1 for >12 months) Adapted from Gratwohl *et al.* (1998).

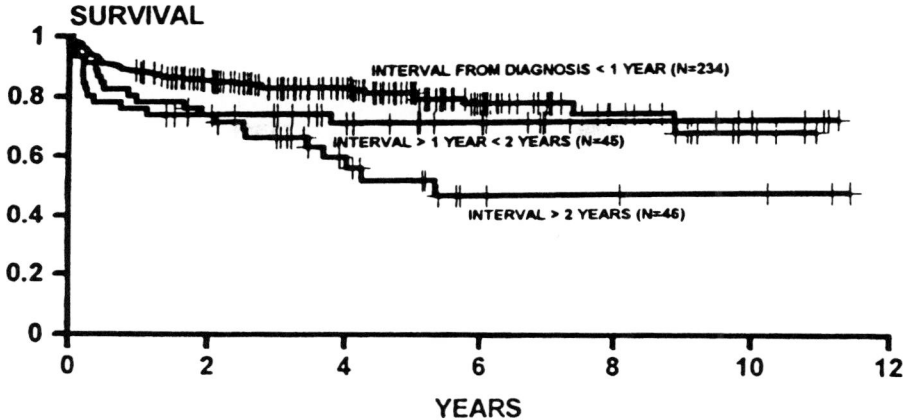

Fig. 52.6. Overall survival for patients with CML in chronic phase receiving transplants from HLA-identical related donors in Seattle according to interval from diagnosis to transplant. Reproduced, with permission, from Clift & Storb (1996).

chronic phase (Snyder *et al.*, 1994). Higher doses of TBI achieve better long-term disease control, but cause more pulmonary toxicity (Clift *et al.*, 1991). The combination of busulfan (16 mg/kg) and cyclophosphamide (120 mg/kg) appears to achieve similar results (Biggs *et al.*, 1992; Clift *et al.*, 1994; Devergie *et al.*, 1995; Clift *et al.*, 1999). This combination causes a later neutrophil nadir and may occasionally cause permanent hair thinning. It should probably not be used if there has been substantial prior exposure to busulfan. Relapse rates appear low but currently there is no evidence that busulfan/

cyclophosphamide is superior to cyclophosphamide/TBI for chronic phase disease (Fig. 52.12). Adjusting the busulfan dose according to the drug's plasma concentration appears to reduce toxicity (Radich *et al.*, 2001b).

Conventionally, allogeneic transplants have employed bone marrow as the source of HSC. The demonstration that pluripotential stem cells can be mobilized into the peripheral blood of normal persons by administration of filgastrim (G-CSF) led to interest in the possibility that blood might be a better source of stem cells than marrow. Current studies show that engraftment

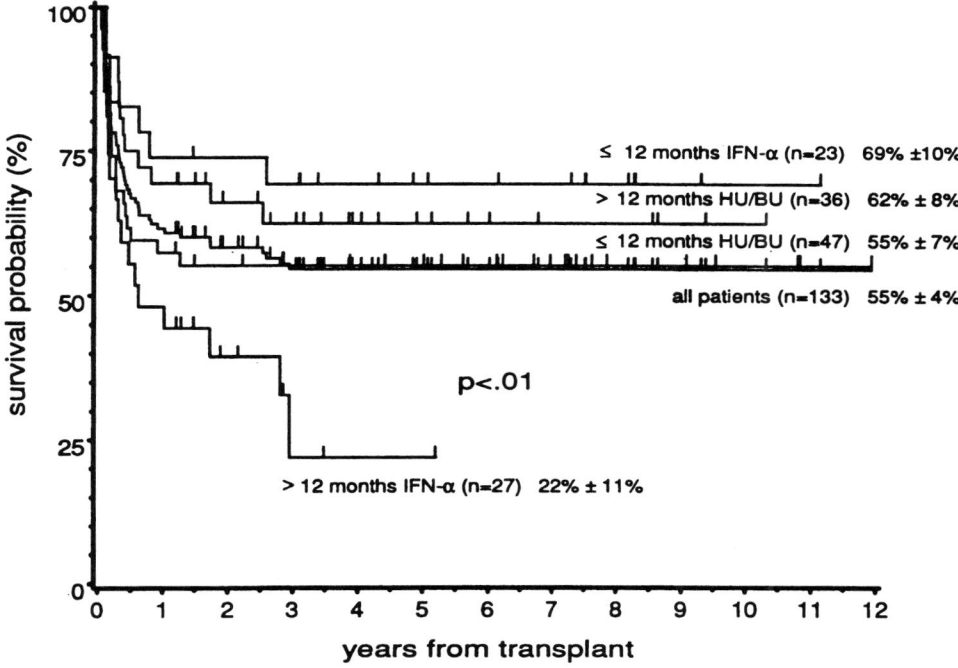

Fig. 52.7. Product-limit estimates of survival categorized according to type and duration of pretransplant therapy. The indicated significance was derived from testing differences in the survival distribution functions between patients with more than 12 months of pretransplant IFN-α administration and all other patients by the log-rank test. Reproduced, with permission, from Beelen *et al.* (1995).

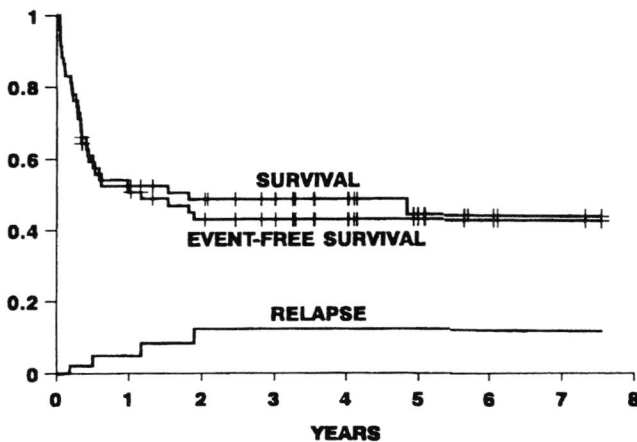

Fig. 52.8. The Kaplan-Meier probabilities of survival, event-free survival, and relapse for 58 patients receiving transplants from HLA-identical siblings during the accelerated phase of CML. Reproduced, with permission, from Clift *et al.* (1994).

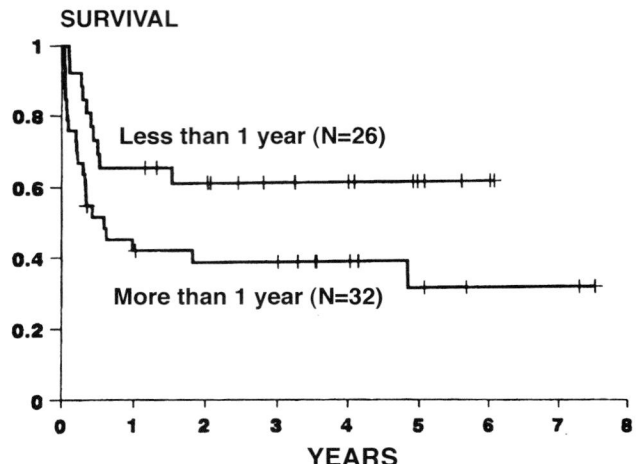

Fig. 52.10. The Kaplan-Meier probabilities of survival for 58 patients receiving transplants during the accelerated phase of CML. Twenty-six patients receiving transplants less than 1 year after diagnosis had a significantly better survival than those receiving transplants after a delay of more than 1 year (*P* = .03). Reproduced, with permission, from Clift *et al.* (1994).

is more rapid after transfusion of peripheral blood stem cells, but the incidence of chronic GVHD may be increased (Storek *et al.*, 1997; Bensinger *et al.*, 2001; Brunet *et al.*, 2001; Schmitz *et al.*, 2001). The increased risk of chronic GVHD correlates with the CD34 count in the blood stem cell allograft (Zaucha *et al.*, 2001). Allogeneic blood stem cell transplantation appears to reduce transplant-related mortality (TRM) in patients transplanted for advanced phase CML, but may increase TRM for those in early stage disease (Schmitz *et al.*,

2001). It remains unclear whether the risk of relapse differs significantly following transplantation of allogeneic blood cells rather than marrow cells (Elmaagacli *et al.*, 1999; Körbling & Anderlini, 2001). Allogeneic transplantation has also been performed using filgastrim-primed bone marrow; engraftment appears to be comparable to that achieved with filgastrim-mobilized blood stem cells, but with less GVHD (Morton *et al.*, 2001). Stem cells present in the umbilical cord of neonates have also been used with success to transplant a few patients with CML (Bogdanic *et al.*, 1993).

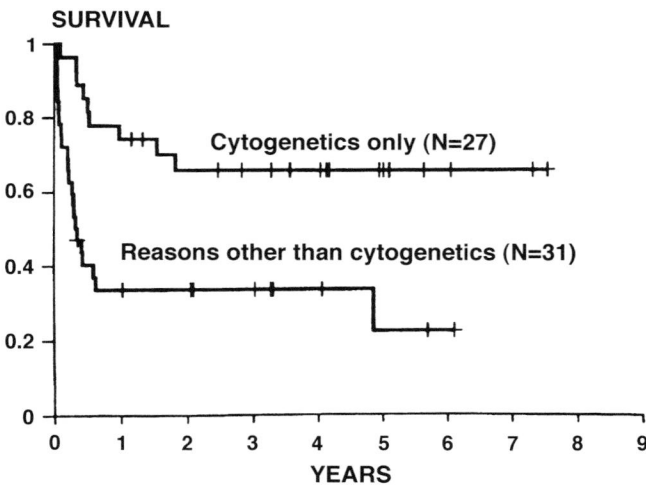

Fig. 52.9. The Kaplan-Meier probabilities of survival for 58 patients receiving transplants during the accelerated phase of CML. Twenty-seven patients were categorized as accelerated phase solely because of cytogenetic abnormalities additional to a single Ph chromosome. These patients had significantly better survival than did those categorized as accelerated phase for other reasons (*P* < .001). Reproduced, with permission, from Clift *et al.* (1994).

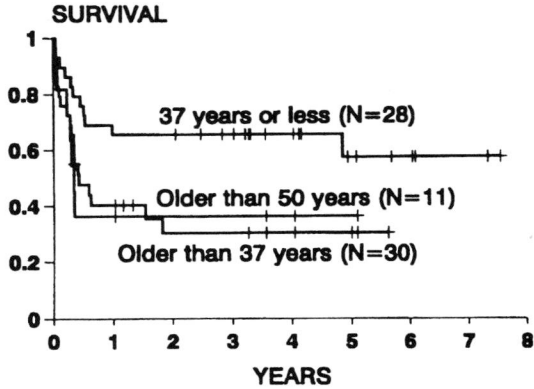

Fig. 52.11. The Kaplan-Meier probabilities of survival for 58 patients receiving transplants during the accelerated phase of CML. Twenty-eight patients aged 37 years or less had a significantly better survival than those who were older than 37 years (*P* = .01). Also displayed is the survival curve for the 11 patients older than 50 years. Reproduced, with permission, from Clift *et al.* (1994).

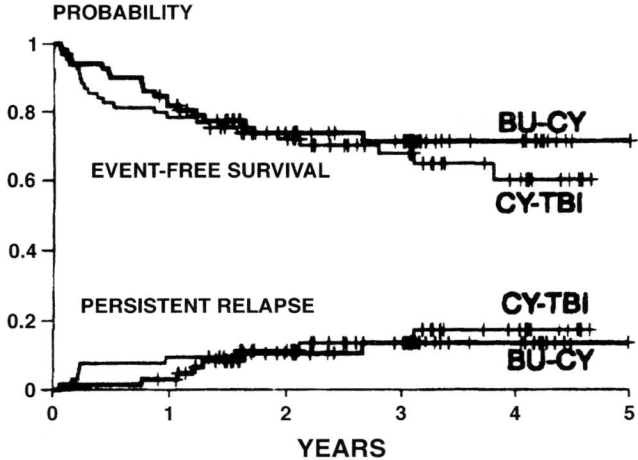

Fig. 52.12. The probabilities of event-free survival and of developing persistent cytogenetic relapse for patients transplanted after the Cy-TBI or Bu-Cy regimens are shown. Reproduced, with permission, from Clift *et al.* (1994a).

Graft-versus-host disease prophylaxis

The best approach to prophylaxis of GVHD remains controversial. The standard method involves administration of "short-course" methotrexate (MTX) on four occasions posttransplant in association with cyclosporine (CSP) given for a period of approximately 6 months. Experience in Seattle has shown that the CSP/MTX combination reduces the incidence of severe acute GVHD to about 30%. This reduction in GVHD may be associated with less GVL effect. For Seattle patients conditioned with cyclophosphamide and 1,200 cGy of TBI and given CSP/MTX prophylaxis, the actuarial relapse rate at 4 years was 25%. Relapse could be prevented by increasing the dose of radiotherapy to 1,575 cGy (Clift *et al.*, 1991) although, as indicated above, increased pulmonary toxicity was seen.

The relapse rate at the Hammersmith Hospital (with 1,200 cGy in 6 doses in 3 days) is low using CSP/MTX, but 54% of our patients have grade II to IV acute GVHD. Our method of giving radiotherapy differs from that used in Seattle and the amount of MTX is lower. The majority of Hammersmith patients with GVHD have grade II disease and respond readily to corticosteroids (Marks *et al.*, 1992). Disease-free survival in the CSP/MTX group may be better than in the patient group given CSP alone, but the difference is not statistically significant.

The removal of T cells from donor marrow substantially reduces the incidence of acute and chronic GVHD, but also increases the risk of relapse (Goldman *et al.*, 1988). Thus, ex vivo T-cell depletion (TCD) with the CD52 monoclonal antibody Campath-1 results in an actuarial relapse rate after transplantation in chronic phase of 60% to 70%. Other methods of TCD, including use of other antibodies and E rosette formation/soybean lectin agglutination, also reduce the incidence of GVHD but increase to varying degrees the incidence of relapse. Prophylactic donor lymphocyte infusions after T-cell depleted (including CD34-selected) allografts may prevent hematologic relapse posttransplant (Elmaagacli *et al.*, 2003).

Management of the spleen

The presence of an enlarged spleen influences survival adversely after bone marrow transplantation. Splenic irradiation appears to provide some survival benefit in patients transplanted early in chronic phase, but not in patients with features of advanced phase disease or those receiving T-cell depleted transplants (Gratwohl *et al.*, 1999; Jabro *et al.*, 1999). There is no consensus as to whether pretransplant splenectomy alters disease-free survival, but the presence of a palpably enlarged spleen does appear to be associated with delayed engraftment or failure to engraft (Helenglass *et al.*, 1990), and this can be corrected by splenectomy (Richard *et al.*, 1996). In one retrospective study of 358 patients receiving HLA-identical marrow grafts for CML, 68 (19%) had undergone splenectomy pretransplant. The overall risk of leukemic relapse was significantly increased in splenectomized patients (56% vs. 32% for controls, $P = .001$) and for control patients with splenomegaly ($P < .001$). In this study splenectomy and splenomegaly remained significant and independent hazards for relapse. In this patient population pretransplant splenectomy had no impact on the incidence of late infectious complications posttransplant or on the incidence or severity of acute or chronic GVHD (Kalhs *et al.*, 1995).

Results of HLA-identical sibling transplantation

The best overall picture of the clinical results of allogeneic bone marrow transplantation for CML is provided by the data collated by the IBMTR (Horowitz, Rowlings, & Passweg, 1996) (Fig. 52.2). Among 2,231 recipients of HLA-identical sibling transplants performed worldwide between 1987 and 1994 and reported to the IBMTR, the actuarial probability of leukemia-free survival (LFS) at 3 years (95% ± confidence intervals) was 57% ± 3%, 41% ± 5%, and 18% ± 7% for patients transplanted in first chronic phase, accelerated phase, and blastic phase, respectively. Corresponding figures for probability of relapse were 13% ± 2%, 26% ± 6%, and 58% ± 11%. For 331 patients allografted in chronic phase with marrow from an unrelated donor the probability of LFS at 3 years was 38% ± 6%. The Seattle group published excellent results for allografting in chronic phase using marrow stem cells from HLA-matched unrelated donors (Hansen *et al.*, 1998). The actuarial survival at 5 years for 196 patients was 57%. For the best subset, those under 50 years of age who received transplants from HLA-matched donors within 1 year of diagnosis, the actuarial survival at 5 years was 74%. These results are little different from what would be expected with HLA-identical sibling donor transplants, and do not by themselves help the clinician advise a given patient whether or not to proceed to allogeneic transplantation. An attempt has therefore been made to develop a "risk score" for individual patients that takes account of the patient's age, disease phase, duration of disease, HLA match with the prospective donor, and patient-donor gender relationship (Gratwohl *et al.*, 1998; Passweg *et al.*, 2001) (Table 52.1). The probability of transplant-related mortality is significantly related to the pretransplant risk score. For example, a given patient with newly diagnosed disease in chronic phase who has an HLA-identical brother may score 0, while an older patient with CML diag-

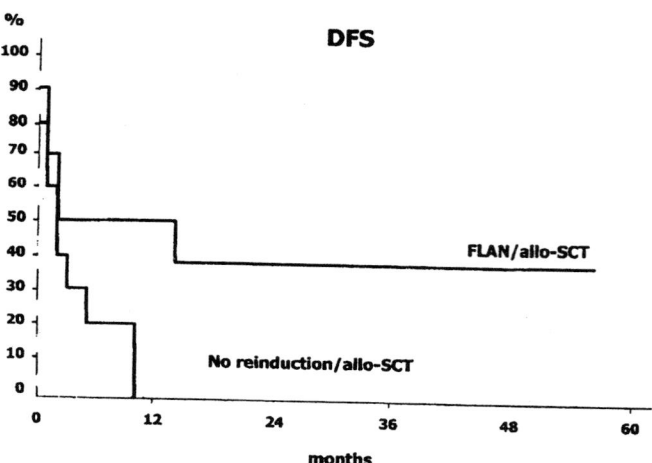

Fig. 52.13. Disease-free survival (FLAN/allo-SCT vs. no reinduction/allo-SCT). Reproduced, with permission, from Visani et al. (2000).

nosed some years earlier and now in transformation, who only has an unrelated donor, would score 6.

The pretransplant cytogenetic status has also been shown to predict posttransplant outcome. Konstantinidou and colleagues (2000) analyzed 418 patients in first or second chronic phase or in accelerated phase and divided them into five categories: those with just the Philadelphia (Ph) chromosome, those who were Ph-negative but BCR-ABL positive, those with a variant Ph chromosome, those with a Ph chromosome and at least one of trisomy 8, +Ph or chromosome 17 abnormalities, and those with abnormalities in addition to the Ph chromosome. Ph-negative patients had a better LFS and none relapsed. Moreover, those with +8, a second Ph, or i(17q) did not show a worse outcome compared to those with no additional abnormalities. Przepiorka and Thomas (1988) found a higher risk of relapse in patients transplanted in accelerated phase with a variant Ph as well as those with a +8 or second Ph.

As indicated above, outcome of transplantation in blastic phase is poor, although it has been suggested that it can be considerably improved by inducing a second chronic phase prior to transplant. Visani and colleagues (2000) used fludarabine, cytosine arabinoside, and mitoxantrone for this purpose. The mean duration of survival posttransplant was 22.7 months with remission induction therapy versus 6.4 months without such treatment (Fig. 52.13).

A possible scheme for planning treatment for patients with CML is shown in Figure 52.14. It is based on the notion that immediate allogeneic transplantation should not be offered to older patients and those lacking an HLA-identical sibling donor who respond well to IFN-α or imatinib mesylate. However, this notion can be challenged.

Results of transplantation using family member donors other than HLA-identical siblings

Family members who are not genetically HLA-identical with the patient have occasionally served as donors with acceptable

results (Hows et al., 1986; Anasetti et al., 1990; Ash et al., 1991; Bishop et al., 1996; Schipper et al., 1996; Speiser et al., 1997). These donors are usually classified as "phenotypically" HLA-identical because they share with the recipient the 6 major HLA-A, -B, and -DR antigens. If the "matched" donor is a child or parent, he/she must be genetically identical for one HLA haplotype and phenotypically identical for the other. Family members mismatched for one or two HLA antigens have also served as donors. The European Group for Blood and Marrow Transplantation (EBMT) has published the results of haploidentical family member transplants in 103 patients with CML (Speiser et al., 1997). The 2-year probability of survival was 47% for patients transplanted in first chronic phase and 25% for those receiving allografts in advanced phase. Outcome also correlated strongly with degree of HLA mismatch.

Results of unrelated donor transplantation

The therapeutic approach to patients with CML who lack an HLA-identical family member donor, but who have an HLA-identical unrelated donor, has become increasingly difficult. On the one hand, the availability of nontransplant strategies that can effectively achieve cytogenetic remission, such as imatinib mesylate and IFN-α, offers the possibility of long-term disease control without allografting. On the other hand, the increasing size and number of volunteer donor registries, as well as improvements in tissue typing and supportive care, have improved the outcomes of unrelated donor transplantation.

McGlave and colleagues (1993, 2000) have described unrelated donor marrow transplantation in 1,423 patients with CML using donors provided by the National Marrow Donor Program (NMDP) between 1988 and 1996. The median age of the recipients was 35 (range 1.9–59) years. At the time of transplant, 65% of patients were in first chronic phase, 7% in second or subsequent chronic phase, 21% in accelerated phase, and 7% in blastic phase. Eighty-one percent of donor-recipient pairs were serologically matched for HLA-A, -B, and -DR; in the remainder there was nonidentity at one HLA locus. The conditioning regimen consisted of high-dose chemotherapy and TBI in 86% of patients and high-dose chemotherapy alone in 14%. Twenty-three percent of patients received a T-cell depleted graft. Ten percent of patients failed to engraft, and an additional 7% experienced late graft failure. The incidence of grade III–IV acute GVHD was 33% and that of extensive chronic GVHD 60%. Only 6% of patients transplanted in chronic phase suffered hematological relapse at 3 years. There was no association between T-cell depletion and rejection or loss of the graft; however, T-cell depletion was associated with significantly less GVHD and more relapse. Superior disease-free survival was associated with the following: transplant in chronic phase, transplant in the first year following diagnosis, young patients, recipient CMV seronegativity, and the occurrence of little or no GVHD. Disease-free survival was 63% in a subset of 157 patients less than 35 years of age, still in chronic phase, and who received transplants from HLA-matched donors.

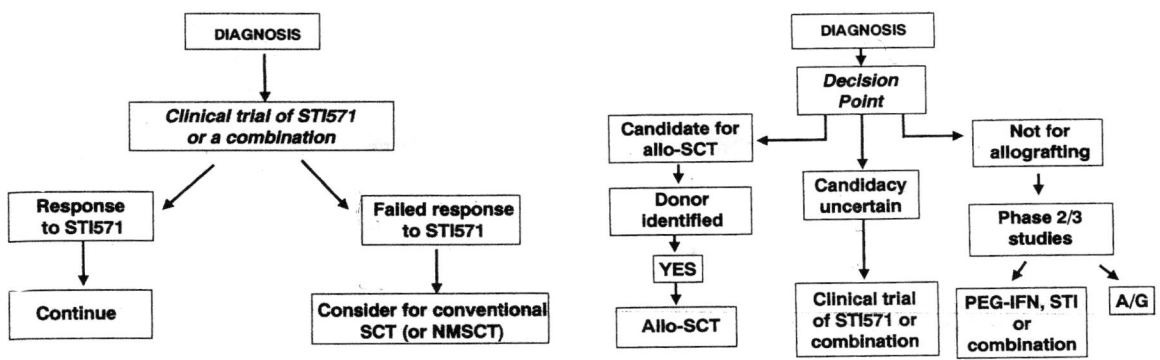

Fig. 52.14. Algorithm setting out a possible approach to management for a patient with newly diagnosed CML. (SCT, stem cell transplantation; STI571, imatinib mesylate; A/G, autograft). Reproduced, with permission, from Goldman & Druker (2001).

Cullis and colleagues (1993) compared ex vivo and in vivo T-cell depletion for patients receiving matched unrelated donor transplants for CML in chronic phase. Forty-eight patients with chronic phase CML received transplants from an unrelated donor with whom they were serologically identical at HLA-A, -B, and -DR loci. Of the 48, 19 received marrow depleted of T cells ex vivo by incubation with Campath monoclonal antibodies, while 29 patients received unmanipulated marrow and cyclosporine/methotrexate prophylaxis for GVHD; in addition, 28 of these 29 received intravenous antilymphocyte therapy from day +1 to day +5 posttransplant. Overall, actuarial survival at 3 years posttransplant was 50% and LFS 38%. Three patients had hematologic relapse. There was no difference in overall survival between the ex vivo T-cell-depleted recipients and those receiving in vivo T-cell depletion, although primary graft-failure ($n = 4$) occurred only in those depleted ex vivo, and grade II–IV acute GVHD occurred more frequently in those depleted in vivo (61% vs. 29%).

In an EBMT summary of data from eight European countries (Dini et al., 1996), 44 children with CML aged less than 17 years underwent unrelated donor transplantation. Twenty-four of 33 evaluable patients were matched while 7 were mismatched at 1 HLA locus. Engraftment occurred in 32 of the 33 with an absolute neutrophil count of 0.5×10^9/l being reached at a median of 21 days posttransplant. Additionally, 2 children developed secondary graft failure. Nine children never recovered a platelet count in excess of 50×10^9/l. Fourteen of the 33 evaluable children developed grade II–IV acute GVHD and 7 developed chronic GVHD, which was limited in 4 cases and extensive in 3. Relapse occurred in 3 of the 44 children included in this study at a median of 14 months posttransplant and with an incidence of 14%. The TRM rate was 38% and event-free survival was 50%. In a series of 88 children given unrelated donor transplants for hematologic malignancy in Seattle, 16 had CML of whom the actuarial disease-free survival and relapse rates were 75% and 0% (Balduzzi et al., 1995). These children received cyclophosphamide and TBI followed by T-replete marrow and cyclosporine/methotrexate as posttransplant GVHD prophylaxis.

The Seattle group (Hansen et al., 1998) has reported their experience with unrelated donor transplants performed between May 1985 and December 1994 for 196 patients with Ph-positive CML in chronic phase. The median follow-up was 5 years (range, 1.2–10.1). Graft failure occurred in 5% of patients who could be evaluated. Acute GVHD of grade III or IV severity was observed in 35% of patients who received HLA-matched transplants, and grade II–IV severity in 77%. It was 89% among those with a minor mismatch of HLA-A or B, and 95% among those with a minor mismatch of HLA-DRB1. The cumulative incidence estimate of clinically extensive chronic GVHD was 67% among patients surviving without relapse for at least 80 days, and the estimated cumulative incidence of relapse at 5 years was 10%. The Kaplan-Meier estimate of survival at 5 years was 57%. Survival was adversely affected by an interval from diagnosis to transplantation of 1 year or more, and HLA-DR $\geq$ 1 mismatch, a high body-weight index, and an age of more than 50 years. Survival was improved by the prophylactic use of fluconazole and ganciclovir. The Kaplan-Meier estimate of survival at 5 years was 74% (95% confidence interval, 62%–86%) for patients who were 50 years of age or younger who received a transplant from an HLA-matched donor within 1 year of diagnosis (Figs. 52.15 and 52.16).

A retrospective registry analysis compared the outcome of 2,464 unrelated donor transplants (63% HLA-A, -B and DRB1 matched) with that of 450 HLA-identical sibling transplants (Weisdorf et al., 2002). The unrelated donor transplants were performed later after diagnosis than the sibling transplants, and were associated with a significantly higher risk of graft failure and GVHD. Survival and disease-free survival was significantly poorer after unrelated transplantation (Fig. 52.17), although for those in chronic phase transplanted within 1 year of diagnosis, 5-year disease-free survival was similar, or only slightly inferior, to that of matched sibling transplantation (Fig. 52.18).

Identification of an optimal donor is crucial to the success of unrelated donor transplantation. The NMDP have confirmed the Seattle experience that molecular matching at DRB1 reduces GVHD and improves survival in patients transplanted in chronic phase (Petersdorf et al., 2001). Additional factors associated with more favorable outcomes include relatively young donor age and a lack of multiparity in female donors (Kollman *et al.*, 2001).

Results of cord blood transplantation

UCB transplantation is not feasible for most patients with CML because of the constraints of patient size and cell dose (Bogdanic *et al.*, 1993; Abecasis *et al.*, 1996; Fernández *et al.*, 1996; Kurtzberg *et al.*, 1996; Laporte *et al.*, 1996; Sanz *et al.*, 2001). A single institution study of 9 adult patients transplanted for CML reported a median time to reach a neutrophil count of greater than $0.5 \times 10^6/l$ of 22 (range 19–52) days in 7 evaluable patients (Sanz *et al.*, 2001). The median number of nucleated cells infused was 1.7 (range 1.2–4.9) $\times 10^7/kg$. Four of 6 patients transplanted in chronic phase were alive in complete molecular remission at 18 to 42 months posttransplant, while 3 of 3 transplanted with advanced disease died of transplant-related complications 0.3 to 5 months posttransplant.

Results with reduced intensity conditioning regimens

Another alternative to conventional bone marrow transplantation is allogeneic transplantation after non-myeloablative or low-dose conditioning. This procedure is predicated on the concept of partial ablation of the host marrow and immune system, in order to establish tolerance to the newly engrafting, immunologically competent donor-derived cells. The GVL effect is thereby preserved, and the milder conditioning regimen is less toxic. Greater numbers of patients are thus eligible for potentially curative treatment.

Numerous different regimens have been explored (Slavin *et al.*, 1998; Bacigalupo *et al.*, 2000; Craddock *et al.*, 2000; Bornhäuser *et al.*, 2001; Giralt *et al.*, 2001; McSweeney *et al.*, 2001; Michallet *et al.*, 2001). For example, Raiola and col-

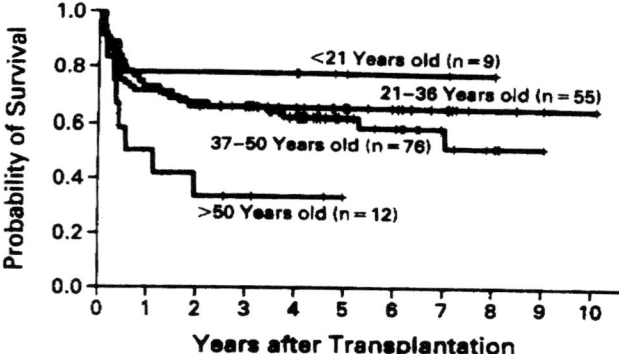

Fig. 52.15. Probability of survival in 152 patients with CML in chronic phase who received a transplant matched for HLA-A, B, and DRB1 from an unrelated donor, according to age. Tick marks represent patients alive at the last follow-up. Reproduced, with permission, from Hansen *et al.* (1998).

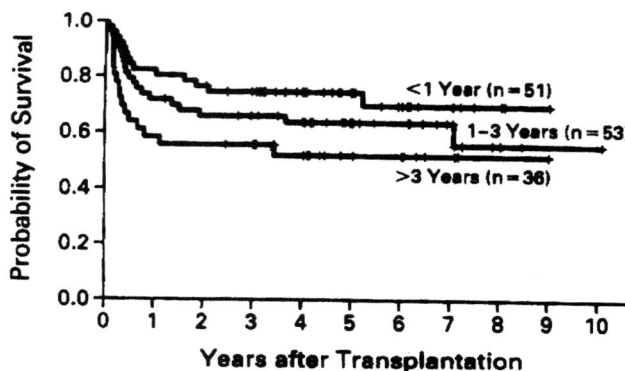

Fig. 52.16. Probability of survival in 140 patients with CML in chronic phase who were ≤ 50 years old and received a transplant matched for HLA-A, B, and DRB1 from an unrelated donor, according to the time from diagnosis to transplantation. Tick marks represent patients alive at the last follow-up. Reproduced, with permission, from Hansen *et al.* (1998).

leagues (2000) treated 33 patients, 15 of whom had CML, with thiotepa 10 mg/kg and cyclophosphamide 100 mg/kg prior to a T-replete HLA-identical sibling allograft. The median age was 53 (range 43–60) years. Full donor chimerism was detected in 79% of patients by day 100. The actuarial probability of survival at 3 years posttransplant was 72% (Fig. 52.19).

Khoury and colleagues (2001) showed that low-dose TBI (550 cGy), together with cyclophosphamide 60 mg/kg for 2 days, was associated with a low incidence of acute toxicity and a low nonrelapse mortality rate in a relatively older cohort of patients (median age 47 years) given a T-replete, HLA-identical sibling peripheral blood stem cell transplant. The day 100 mortality was 10% and actuarial 2-year survival was 83%.

Or *et al.* (2003) used fludarabine, busulfan and ATG in 24 patients in first chronic phase, with cyclosporine and methotrexate as GVHD prophylaxis. At a median follow-up of 42 months, 21 patients remained alive and disease-free. The five year actuarial probability of disease-free survival was 85% ± 8%.

In preliminary form, the EBMT have summarized results of nonablative allogeneic transplantation in 46 patients with CML, 23 of whom were in advanced phase at the time of transplant (Goldman, 2001). Ten patients received allografts from unrelated donors. All patients engrafted and only 6 developed severe GVHD. Of 39 evaluable patients, donor chimerism exceeded 95% in 32. At 1 year of follow-up, TRM was 35% and survival was 65%.

High BCR/ABL transcript levels have been reported early after non-myeloablative conditioning, although a complete molecular remission subsequently occurred in most patients (Uzunel *et al.*, 2003).

Comparison of allogeneic transplantation with chemotherapy and autologous transplantation

A prospective, randomized study comparing chemotherapy to allogeneic transplantation has not been performed in CML.

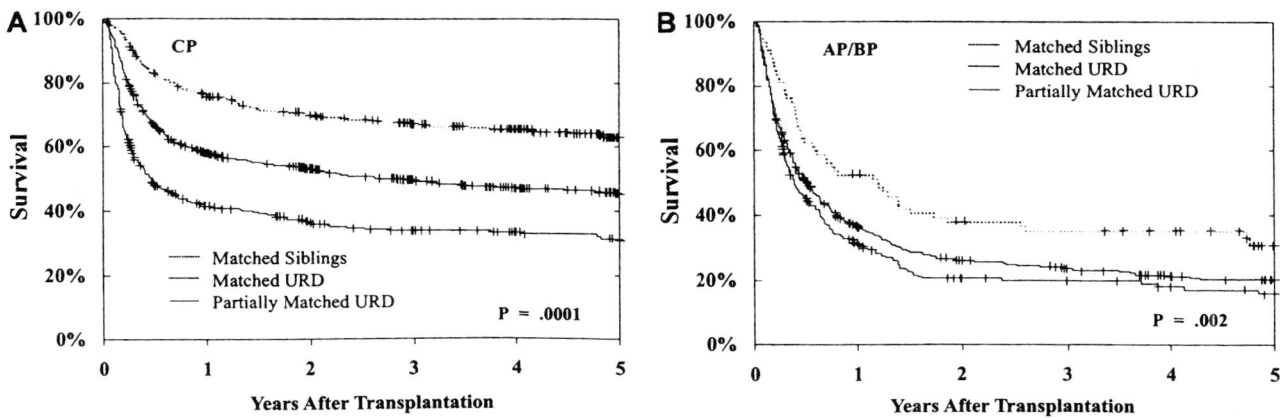

Fig. 52.17. Survival following bone marrow transplantation during chronic phase (CP) ([**A**] P = .001) and beyond CP ([**B**] P = .002). Reproduced, with permission, from Weisdorf *et al.* (2002).

Nevertheless, Gale and colleagues (1998) retrospectively compared outcomes in 548 patients in the IBMTR series who had undergone HLA-matched sibling transplantation to 121 patients treated with hydroxyurea and 75 patients receiving IFN-α by the German CML Study Group. For the first 18 months after diagnosis, mortality was higher in the transplant group than in the nontransplant group. During the 18 to 56 month period, however, mortality was equivalent, and after 56 months, the transplant group fared far better (Fig. 52.1). Survival advantage for transplants was greater and occurred earlier in patients with poor risk features than those with good risk features. Seven-year survival probabilities were 58% for the transplant group and 32% for the patients treated with hydroxyurea or IFN-α. This study thus confirmed a long-term survival advantage for HLA-identical sibling transplants over hydroxyurea or IFN-α in CML.

Although imatinib mesylate appears to be exceptionally potent in the treatment of CML, it is not known whether this agent is curative (Goldman & Druker, 2001; Savage & Antman, 2002). Thus, in young patients in chronic phase with an HLA-identical sibling, allogeneic transplantation remains the primary treatment. In older patients and those lacking an HLA-identical sibling, a trial of imatinib is reasonable first-line therapy (Fig. 52.14).

Autologous transplantation is safer than allogeneic transplantation and may provide some benefit in disease control and survival, but does not offer the possibility of cure (Savage & Goldman, 1999). Autografting should be considered for a patient in chronic phase who is not eligible for allografting and who prefers to be treated by a method that can still be considered "investigational." It is reasonable to offer autologous HSC transplantation soon after diagnosis, or after an initial trial of imatinib or IFN-α has failed to induce cytogenetic conversion in the bone marrow.

Indications and contraindications for allogeneic transplantation

Curative therapy should be the goal in all patients less than 60 years of age (Fig. 52.14). If an HLA-identical sibling is avail-

able, allogeneic transplantation should generally be performed as early as feasible for younger patients. For those 40 years of age or older, one might postpone the transplant to allow a trial of imatinib mesylate or IFN-α. If the patient has a cytogenetic response, allo-HSC transplantation could be postponed until there is evidence of resistance. If blastic phase is present, an attempt should be made to induce a second chronic phase with intensive chemotherapy (Visani *et al.*, 2000) or, possibly, imatinib. Patients over the age of 60 years and those with comorbid conditions preventing conventional allografting might be offered transplantation with reduced intensity conditioning if an HLA-identical sibling is available. Some debatable points include the upper age limit for allogeneic transplantation, the age at which an initial trial of imatinib or IFN-α is appropriate, and the duration of drug therapy if a cytogenetic response is not achieved within 6 months.

If a patient has no HLA-identical sibling, an initial trial of imatinib or IFN-α would seem reasonable. If a durable cytogenetic response is obtained, drug therapy should probably be continued indefinitely. For patients who cannot tolerate imatinib or IFN-α or who fail to achieve Ph negativity, consideration should be given to a different strategy such as autologous transplantation. If an appropriate alternative donor has been identified in the interim, allografting should be considered. Major points that are still a matter of debate include the duration of therapy with IFN-α, whether to proceed to allografting rather than autografting, and what degree of HLA mismatch is acceptable.

The current practice of HSC transplantation for CML in Europe has been described (Urbano-Ispizua *et al.*, 2002) (and see Chapter 124).

Minimal residual disease and cure

The evidence that CML is cured by allografting is based on survival curves (Goldman *et al.*, 1986, 1988; Thomas *et al.*, 1986; Hansen *et al.*, 1998) and the results of PCR studies. Of 154 patients with chronic phase CML transplanted at the Hammersmith Hospital through June 1995, more than half are

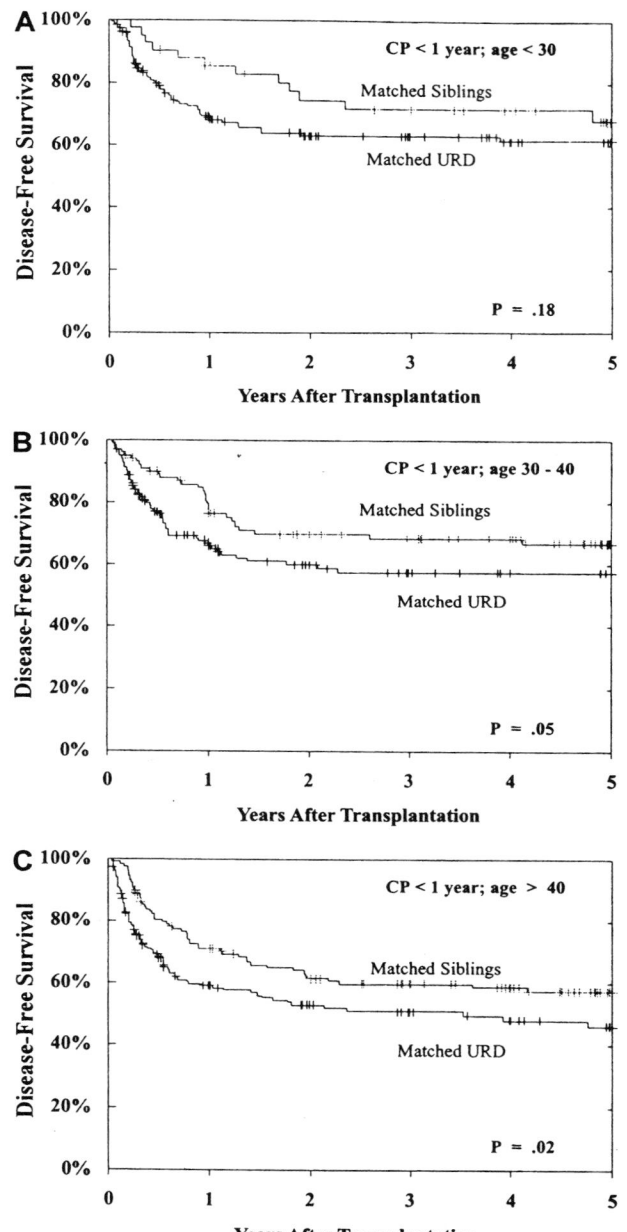

Fig. 52.18. DFS following BMT during chronic phase (CP) within 1 year from diagnosis: effect of patient age. Reproduced, with permission, from Weisdorf *et al.* (2002).

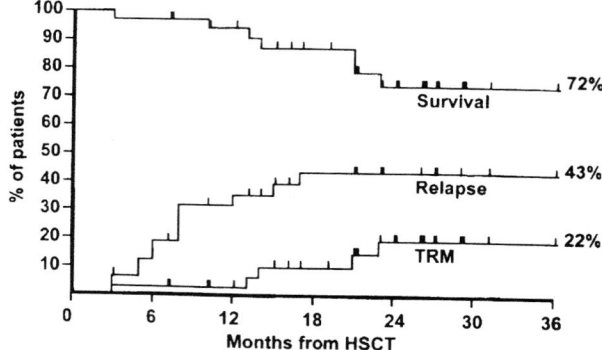

Fig. 52.19. Actuarial proportion of patients surviving (survival 72%), together with the probability of relapsing (relapse 43%) and the risk of transplant-related mortality (TRM 22%). Reproduced, with permission, from Raiola *et al.*, 2000.

level of BCR-ABL transcripts then steadily increases (molecular relapse). Thereafter, Ph-positive metaphases appear in the marrow (cytogenetic relapse). When their level reaches 100%, the patient develops a leukocytosis and other features typical of hematologic relapse.

These observations provide the rationale for the routine use of RT-PCR to monitor the presence of BCR-ABL transcript numbers in patients in complete cytogenetic remission post-transplant (Hughes *et al.*, 1989; Negrin & Blume, 1991; Roth *et al.*, 1991; Cross *et al.*, 1993; Radich *et al.*, 1995; Chomel *et al.*, 2000) (Fig. 52.20). With this technique, RNA is extracted from the buffy coat of peripheral blood or bone marrow and reverse transcribed into cDNA. Using oligonucleotide primers, a defined junctional region of cDNA is then amplified by a two-step PCR, electrophoresed, and probed for the BCR-ABL gene rearrangement. The use of a "competing" molecule of known concentration that co-amplifies with material from the patient permits quantification of BCR-ABL transcripts (Cross, 1997). The Taqman-based "real-time" PCR method has now largely replaced the competitor PCR technique to quantitate BCR-ABL RNA transcripts (Branford *et al.*, 1999), but it is unclear which of these methods is most sensitive.

In a study of 138 patients allografted for CML, Olavarria *et al.* (2001) used quantitative PCR at 3 to 5 months posttransplant to classify the recipients as either being negative for BCR-ABL transcripts, or being positive at a low level (<100 transcripts/100 μg RNA and/or a BCR-ABL/ABL ratio of < 0.02%), or being positive at a high level. The 3-year cumulative incidence of relapse in these three groups was 16.7%, 42.9%, and 86.4%, respectively (*P* = .001). This relationship was apparent regardless of whether the transplants were T-cell-depleted or not, and regardless of whether a sibling or an unrelated donor was used. Radich and colleagues (2001a) examined the significance of BCR/ABL positivity in 379 patients at 18 months or later post-transplant. Ninety (24%) had at least one positive test, and 13 (14%) relapsed, compared to 3 relapses (1%) in the 289 BCR/ABL-negative patients. The median time from BCR/ABL

now 5 to 15 years post-BMT (Savage *et al.*, 1997). However, 1 patient relapsed 14 years after transplant (Yong & Goldman, 1999). An EBMT study reported a small number of relapses more than 5-years posttransplant (van Rhee *et al.*, 1994).

Patients who relapse usually do so in an orderly manner, which may recapitulate the natural history of the original disease. Thus, typically a patient who has been negative on RT-PCR study of peripheral blood, and whose marrow has also been Ph-negative for some while, becomes PCR-positive. The detection to relapse was 916 (range 251–2,654) days. Using quantitative PCR the median BCR/ABL level at relapse was 40,443 copies/μg of RNA compared to a median value of 24 copies/μg in BCR/ABL-positive patients who did not relapse. Patients continuously negative for BCR-ABL by RT-PCR for 5 years posttansplant had a probability of relapse of 2.6%, while those with one (or more) low-level result in the same time period had 54% probability (Fig. 52.21) (Mughal et al., 2001).

Patients who satisfy the criteria for molecular relapse are probably best treated with donor lymphocyte transfusions at a relatively early stage (see below), but IFN-α or imatinib can be considered if donor lymphocytes are not available. It should be noted, however, that typical and atypical BCR-ABL fusion genes can be detected in the leukocytes of normal individuals at very low levels and could theoretically cause confusion in a patient being monitored after allogeneic HSC transplantation (Bose et al., 1998). While quantitative RT-PCR can be used to estimate the risk of relapse, fluorescence in situ hybridization (FISH) for BCR-ABL can be used to evaluate residual disease (Chomel et al., 2000). Hypermetaphase FISH (combining FISH with long-term colcemid exposure) detects low levels of Ph-positive cells undetectable by standard G-band cytogenetic analysis, thus enabling earlier therapeutic intervention (Seong et al., 2000).

Graft-versus-leukemia effect

There is now considerable evidence that a GVL effect plays a major role in the cure of CML after allografting. The increased risk of relapse seen in patients without GVHD (Enright et al., 1996; Gratwohl et al., 2002), in recipients of T-cell-depleted marrow (Hessner et al., 1996), and in syngeneic transplants all lend support to this concept. The observation that patients who relapse may re-enter complete remission after transfusion of donor-derived lymphoid cells is further evidence for a GVL effect (Kolb et al., 1990; Cullis et al., 1992a; Kolb et al., 1995). Much effort

has been devoted to defining the antigen target for this GVL effect and to the production of cytotoxic T lymphocytes that recognize leukemia cells (Falkenberg et al., 1999). Possible targets include putative leukemia-specific antigens, such as BCR-ABL peptides, lineage-specific oligopeptides, and minor histocompatibility antigens (Barrett & Malkovska, 1996; Clark et al., 2001).

Relapse after allogeneic transplantation

Relapse continues to be a problem after allogeneic bone marrow transplantation for chronic phase CML, occurring in 8% to 20% of patients given unmanipulated donor marrow (Thomas et al., 1986; Horowitz et al., 1996). The corresponding figure for advanced phase disease is 40% to 60%. The first indication of relapse may be a rising percentage of Ph-positive metaphases in an unduly cellular marrow. Peripheral blood counts remain normal for some time, but eventually a leukocytosis develops with basophilia, eosinophilia, and increasing spleen size. In a retrospective registry series of 500 patients who relapsed postallograft, the actuarial 5-year survival from relapse was 34% (Guglielmi et al., 2000). Survival after relapse was significantly related to five factors: time from diagnosis to transplant (>2 years worse), disease phase at transplant (beyond first chronic phase worse), disease phase at relapse (acceleration or blast phase worse), time from transplant to relapse (>1 year worse), and donor type (unrelated donor worse). The effects of these individual adverse risk factors were cumulative.

Additionally, nonleukemic autologous reconstitution can occur posttransplant, usually manifests initially as mixed chimerism, and is usually followed by relapse, although relapse-free survival may be prolonged (Brunstein et al., 2000).

Molecular and cytogenetic relapses

Molecular relapse can be defined as the finding of persistently high BCR-ABL transcript numbers or a rising number of tran-

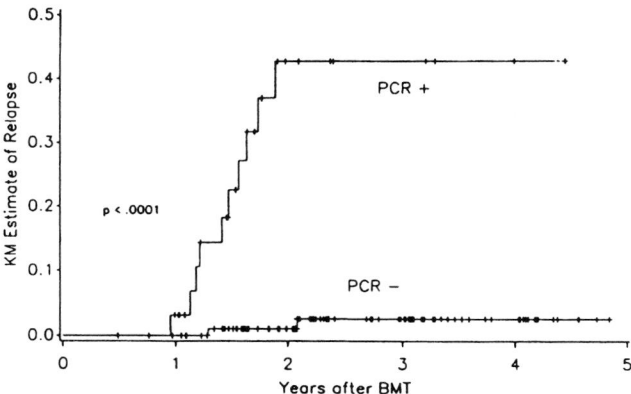

Fig. 52.20. The Kaplan-Meier estimates of relapse for patients testing PCR-positive (N = 38) at 6 to 12 months compared with patients who were PCR-negative (N = 112) for BCR-ABL mRNA. Tick marks represent patients alive and still at risk of relapse. Reproduced, with permission, from Radich et al. (1995).

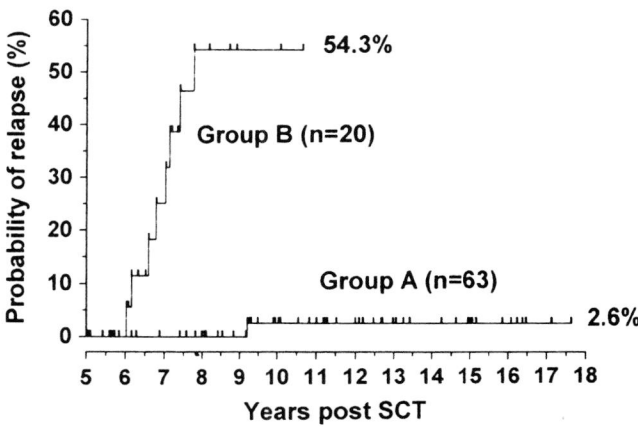

Fig. 52.21. Cumulative incidence estimation of the probability of relapse for patients surviving in remission more than 5 years post-SCT. Reproduced, with permission, from Mughal et al. (2001).

scripts more than 9 months after transplant (van Rhee *et al.*, 1994). A small percentage of patients in the first year after BMT are transiently found to have some Ph-positive metaphases in their bone marrow (Arthur *et al.*, 1988). These Ph-positive cells commonly disappear and many of these patients are long-term survivors. The pattern tends to be different in the cytogenetic relapse that precedes hematologic relapse. At about 12 to 36 months posttransplant there is a progressive increase in the percentage of Ph-positive cells, usually in the absence of symptoms. Patients with rising numbers of BCR-ABL transcripts in blood or Ph-positive metaphases in bone marrow are candidates for treatment by donor lymphocyte infusion (DLI) (van Rhee *et al.*, 1994). Relapse of BCR-ABL positive disease as BCR-ABL negative disease has been described (at 1.5- and 5-years posttransplant) (Au *et al.*, 2001).

Hematologic relapse

Most relapses occur in the first 3 years after transplant, but some occur many years later. The patient usually enters the same phase of CML as before transplantation, but some patients allografted in chronic phase relapse directly into blastic phase (Cullis *et al.*, 1992b). It is possible that a preceding relapse to chronic phase may have escaped detection. Alternatively, transformed cells present at the time of transplant may have persisted posttransplant. Third, it is possible that leukemic stem cells survive allografting in many patients and that these cells retain the capacity to transform.

Donor cell relapse

Relapse in cells of donor origin is a well-documented, but rare, event (Marmont *et al.*, 1984; Smith *et al.*, 1985); its mechanism is unexplained. It is most easily proven in sex-mismatched transplants where cells with the sex chromosomes of the donor are shown to contain the Philadelphia chromosome. Residual leukemic cells of host origin or the marrow microenvironment might in some way affect normal donor cells and render them leukemic.

Donor lymphocyte infusions (and see Chapter 65)

In some cases established relapse evolves slowly and may require no treatment for some time (Hughes *et al.*, 1989); in others, only small doses of hydroxyurea are required. Relapse may be reversed following abrupt discontinuation of CSP or other immune suppression (Collins *et al.*, 1992). Preliminary observations suggest that imatinib mesylate is highly active against posttransplant leukemic relapse (Chambon-Pautas *et al.*, 2001; Kantarjian *et al.*, 2001; Rodriguez *et al.*, 2001; Soiffer *et al.*, 2001; Ullman *et al.*, 2001), but long-term safety and efficacy have not been established. Relapse may respond to treatment with IFN-α alone (Arcese *et al.*, 1993; Higano, Raskind, & Singer, 1992), or to the combination of IFN-α and infusion of lymphocytes from the original marrow donor (Kolb *et al.*,

1990). However, IFN-α is unlikely to cure patients who relapse, and DLI without IFN-α is probably the best initial treatment.

The conventional approach to DLI has been to collect as many lymphoid cells as possible by leukapheresis of the original transplant donor. Without further manipulation these cells are then transfused into the patient in relapse. Most patients do not receive prophylaxis for GVHD. The response rate for those patients relapsed into chronic phase is approximately 70%, and most patients are restored to molecular remission (Drobyski *et al.*, 1992), which may prove to be permanent (Kolb *et al.*, 1995; Dazzi *et al.*, 2000b, Klein *et al.*, 2000).

Nevertheless, DLI can be complicated by acute GVHD, which has on occasion proved fatal, and also by marrow hypoplasia (probably as a manifestation of GVHD), which can be corrected by transfusion of additional donor-derived stem cells. The latter complication may be prevented by implementation of DLI therapy before the onset of hematologic relapse (van Rhee *et al.*, 1994). To reduce the incidence of GVHD, the Sloan-Kettering group (New York) introduced the concept of escalating dose DLI starting with a low dose of donor CD3+ cells and then giving further doses at increased levels at 3-month intervals according to response (Mackinnon *et al.*, 1995). With this approach, efficacy against leukemia is retained and the risk of GVHD seems to be reduced substantially (Dazzi *et al.*, 2000a). To achieve the same goal, investigators at M.D. Anderson have reported promising results with selective CD8 depletion of DLI (Shimoni *et al.*, 2001).

Imatinib mesylate

Preliminary observations suggest that imatinib mesylate is highly active against posttransplant leukemic relapse (Chambon-Pautas *et al.*, 2001; Rodriguez *et al.*, 2001; Ullman *et al.*, 2001; Kantarjian *et al.*, 2001; Soiffer *et al.*, 2001; Olivarria *et al.*, 2002), but long-term safety and eficacy have not been established. The MD Anderson group reported on 28 patients given 400-1000 mg/day for relapse occurring a median of 9 (range 1-137) months posttransplant. Thirteen patients had undergone salvage DLI. Complete hematologic responses occurred in 100% of those in chronic phase, 83% for accelerated phase, and 43% for blast phase. Cytogenetic response rates were 63% for chronic or acccelerated phase and 43% for blast phase. The 1 year estimated survival was 74%. Recurrence of GVHD occurred in 5 patients. Severe granulocytopenia occurred in 43% and thrombocytopenia in 27% (Kantarjian *et al.*, 2002). Imatinib has been shown to induce a complete hematologic response and complete restoration of donor-type hematopoiesis in a patient who did not benefit from DLI (Olivarria *et al.*, 2002).

Future developments

Although TCD is not currently used in the majority of transplant centers, the procedure might return to favor if the cells responsible for GVHD could be eliminated while leaving intact those responsible for facilitating engraftment and mediating GVL effects. Conversely, the increased risk of relapse could be offset by T-cell "add-back" on a routine basis or at the earliest signs of relapse (Drobyski *et al.*, 1999; Sehn *et al.*, 1999; Ho & Soiffer, 2001). Elucidation of the mechanism of action of GVL will hopefully lead to immunotherapeutic approaches to management of CML that do not involve intensive conditioning regimens. In this regard the introduction of mini-allografting, by which the intensity of the conditioning is reduced and reliance is placed on the capacity of donor-derived lymphoid cells to eradicate leukemia (Giralt *et al.*, 1997; Slavin *et al.*, 1998), is of great interest. The role of imatinib before transplant and in the treatment of posttransplant relapse (Olivarria et al., 2002) is an object of intensive investigation. The results of allogeneic transplantation of CML in blastic transformation are currently unsatisfactory and highlight the need to perform allografting early in the course of the disease or not at all, unless a second chronic phase can be induced prior to transplant.

References

Abecasis, M.M., Machado, A.M., Boavida, G. *et al.* (1996). Haploidentical cord blood transplantation contaminated with maternal T cells in a patient with advanced leukaemia. *Bone Marrow Transplantation, 17,* 891–5.

Anasetti, C., Beatty, P.G., Storb, R. *et al.* (1990). Effect of HLA incompatibility on graft-versus-host disease, relapse, and survival after marrow transplantation for patients with leukemia or lymphoma. *Human Immunology, 29,* 79–91.

Arcese, W., Gratwohl, A., Niederwieser, D. *et al.* (1993). Outcome for patients who relapse after allogeneic bone marrow transplantation for chronic myeloid leukemia. *Blood, 82,* 3211–9.

Arthur, C.K., Apperley, J.F., Guo, A.P. *et al.* (1988). Cytogenetic events after bone marrow transplantation for chronic myeloid leukemia in chronic phase. *Blood, 80,* 1179–86.

Ash, R.C., Horowitz, M.M., Gale, R.P. *et al.* (1991). Bone marrow transplantation from related donors other than HLA-identical siblings: effect of T-cell depletion. *Bone Marrow Transplantation, 7,* 443–52.

Au, W.Y., Lie, A.K.W., Ma, S.K. *et al.* (2001). Philadelphia (Ph) chromosome-positive chronic myeloid leukaemia relapsing as Ph-negative leukaemia after allogeneic bone marrow transplantation. *British Journal of Haematology, 114,* 365–8.

Balduzzi, A., Gooley, T., Anasetti, C. *et al.* (1995). Unrelated donor marrow transplantation in children. *Blood, 86,* 3247–56.

Barrett, A.J. & Malkovska, V. (1996). Graft-versus-leukemia: understanding and using the alloimmune response to treat haematological malignancies. *British Journal of Haematology, 93,* 754–61.

Beelen, D.W., Graefen, U., Elmaagacli, A.H. *et al.* (1995). Prolonged administration of interferon-α in patients with chronic-phase Philadelphia chromosome-positive chronic myelogenous leukemia before allogeneic bone marrow transplantation may adversely affect transplant outcome. *Blood, 85,* 2981–90.

Bensinger, W., Martin, P.J., Storer, B. *et al.* (2001). Transplantation of bone marrow as compared with peripheral blood cells from HLA-identical relatives in patients with hematologic cancers. *New England Journal of Medicine, 344,* 175–81.

Biggs, J.C., Szer, J., Crilley, P. *et al.* (1992). Treatment of chronic myeloid leukemia with allogeneic bone marrow transplantation after preparation with BuCy2. *Blood, 80,* 1352–7.

Bishop, M.R., Henslee-Downey, P.J., Anderson, J.R. *et al.* (1996). Long-term survival in advanced chronic myelogenous leukemia following bone marrow transplantation from haploidentical related donors. *Bone Marrow Transplantation, 18,* 747–53.

Bogdanic, V., Nemet, D., Kastelan, A. *et al.* (1993). Umbilical cord blood transplantation in a patient with Philadelphia chromosome positive chronic myeloid leukemia. *Transplantation, 56,* 477–8.

Bornhäuser, M., Kiehl, M., Siegert, W. *et al.* (2001). Dose-reduced conditioning for allografting in 44 patients with chronic myeloid leukaemia: a retrospective analysis. *British Journal of Haematology, 115,* 1129–4.

Bose, S., Deininger, M., Gora-Tybor, J. *et al.* (1998). The presence of typical and atypical BCR-ABL fusion genes in leukocytes of normal individuals: biologic significance and implications for the assessment of minimal residual disease. *Blood, 92,* 3362–7.

Branford, S., Hughes, T.P., & Rudzki, Z. (1999). Monitoring chronic myeloid leukaemia therapy by real-time quantitative PCR in blood is a reliable alternative to bone marrow cytogenetics. *British Journal of Haematology, 107,* 587–99.

Brunet, S., de Soria, V.G.G., Sanz, G. *et al.* (2001). Allogeneic bone marrow stem cell transplantation (allo-BMT) vs peripheral blood (allo-PBT) in chronic myeloid leukemia (CML): the Spanish experience. *Blood* (Abstract 1717).

Brunstein, C.G., Hirsch, B.A., Miller, J.S. *et al.* (2000). Non-leukemic autologous reconstitution after allogeneic bone marrow transplantation for Ph-positive chronic myelogenous leukemia: extended remission preceding eventual relapse. *Bone Marrow Transplantation, 26,* 1173–7.

Chambon-Pautas, C., Cony-Makhoul, C., Giraudier, S. *et al.* (2001). Glivec (STI571) treatment for chronic myelogenous leukemia in relapse after allogeneic stem cell transplantation: a report of the French experience (on behalf of SFGM and FILMC). *Blood* (Abstract 587).

Childs, R., Epperson, E., Bahceci, E. *et al.* (1999). Molecular remission of chronic myeloid leukaemia following a non-myeloablative allogeneic peripheral blood stem cell transplant: in vivo and in vitro evidence for a graft-versus-leukaemia effect. *British Journal of Haematology, 107,* 396–400.

Chomel, J-C., Brizard, F., Veinstein, A. *et al.* (2000). Persistence of BCR-ABL genomic rearrangement in chronic myeloid leukemia patients in complete and sustained remission after interferon-α therapy or allogeneic bone marrow transplantation. *Blood, 95,* 404–9.

Clark, R.E., Anthony-Dodi, L.A., Hill, S.C. *et al.* (2001). Direct evidence that leukemic cells present HLA-associated immunogenic peptides derived from the BCR-ABL b3a2 fusion protein. *Blood, 98,* 2887–93.

Clift, R., Radich, J., Appelbaum, F.R. *et al.* (1999). Long-term follow-up of a randomized study comparing cyclophosphamide and total body irradiation with busulfan and cyclophosphamide for patients receiving allogeneic marrow transplants during chronic phase of chronic myeloid leukemia. *Blood, 94,* 3960–2.

Clift, R.A., Buckner, C.D., Appelbaum, F.R. *et al.* (1991). Allogeneic marrow transplantation in patients with chronic myeloid leukemia in the chronic phase: a randomized trial of two irradiation regimens. *Blood,* **77,** 1660–5.

Clift, R.A., Buckner, C.D., Thomas, E.D. *et al.* (1994a). Marrow transplantation for chronic myeloid leukemia: a randomized study comparing cyclophosphamide and total body irradiation with busulfan and cyclophosphamide. *Blood,* **84,** 2036–43.

Clift, R.A., Buckner, C.D., Thomas, E.D., *et al.* (1994b). Marrow transplantation for patients in accelerated phase of chronic myeloid leukemia. *Blood,* **84,** 4368–73.

Clift, R.A. & Storb, R. (1996). Marrow transplantation for CML: the Seattle experience. *Bone Marrow Transplantation,* **17** (Suppl 3), S1–S3.

CML Trialists Collaborative Group. (1997). Interferon alfa versus chemotherapy for chronic myeloid leukemia: a meta-analysis of seven randomized trials. *Journal of the National Cancer Institute,* **89,** 1616–20.

Collins, R.H., Rogers, Z.R., Bennett, M. *et al.* (1992). Hematologic relapse of chronic myelogenous leukemia following allogeneic bone marrow transplantation: apparent graft-versus-leukemia effect following abrupt discontinuation of immunosuppression. *Bone Marrow Transplantation,* **10,** 391–5.

Copelan, E.A., Grever, M.R., Kapoor, N., & Tutschka, P.J. (1989). Marrow transplantation following busulphan and cyclophosphamide for chronic myeloid leukemia in accelerated or blastic phase. *British Journal of Haematology,* **71,** 487–91.

Craddock, C., Bardy, P., Kreiter, S. *et al.* (2000). Engraftment of T-cell-depleted allogeneic haematopoietic stem cells using a reduced intensity conditioning regimen. *British Journal of Haematology,* **111,** 797–800.

Cross, N.C., Hughes, T.P., Feng, L. *et al.* (1993). Minimal residual disease after allogeneic bone marrow transplantation for chronic myeloid leukemia in first chronic phase: correlation with acute graft-versus-host disease and relapse. *British Journal of Haematology,* **84,** 67–74.

Cross, N.C.P. (1997). Minimal residual disease. *Bailliere's Clinical Haematology,* **10,** 389–403.

Cullis, J.O., Jiang, Y.Z., Schwarer, A.P. *et al.* (1992a). Donor leukocyte infusions for chronic myeloid leukemia after allogeneic bone marrow transplantation. *Blood,* **79,** 1379–81.

Cullis, J.O., Marks, D.I., Schwarer, A.P. *et al.* (1992b). Relapse into blast crisis following bone marrow transplantation for chronic phase chronic myeloid leukemia: a report of five cases. *British Journal of Haematology,* **81,** 378–81.

Cullis, J.O., Szydlo, R.M., Cross, N.C. *et al.* (1993). Matched unrelated donor bone marrow transplantation for chronic myeloid leukemia in chronic phase: comparison of ex vivo and in vivo T cell depletion. *Bone Marrow Transplantation,* **11** (Suppl 1), 107–11.

Dazzi, F., Szydlo, R.M., Craddock, C. *et al.* (2000a). Comparison of single-dose and escalating-dose regimens of donor lymphocyte infusion for relapse after allografting for chronic myeloid leukemia. *Blood,* **95,** 67–71.

Dazzi, F., Szydlo, R.M., Cross, N.C.P. *et al.* (2000b). Durability of responses following donor lymphocyte infusions for patients who relapse after allogeneic stem cell transplantation for chronic myeloid leukemia. *Blood,* **96,** 2712–6.

Deininger, M.W.N., Schleuning, M., Olavarria, E. *et al.* (2001). Glivec prior to allografting is safe and not associated with increased transplant-related toxicity. *Blood* (Abstract 5146).

Devergie, A., Blaise, D., Attal, M. *et al.* (1995). Allogeneic bone marrow transplantation for chronic myeloid leukemia in first chronic phase: a randomised trial of busulfan-cytoxan versus cytoxan-total body irradiation as preparative regimen: a report from the French Society of Bone Marrow Graft (SFGM). *Blood,* **85,** 2263–8.

Dini, G., Rondelli, R., Miano, M. *et al.* (1996). Unrelated donor bone marrow transplantation for Philadelphia chromosome-positive chronic myelogenous leukemia in children: experience of 8 European countries. *Bone Marrow Transplantation,* **18** (Suppl 2), 80–5.

Drobyski, W.R., Roth, M.S., Thibodeau, S.N. *et al.* (1992). Molecular remission occurring after donor leukocyte infusions for the treatment of relapsed chronic myelogenous leukemia after allogeneic bone marrow transplantation. *Bone Marrow Transplantation,* **10,** 301–4.

Drobyski, W.R., Hessner, M.J., Klein, J.P. *et al.* (1999). T-cell depletion plus salvage immunotherapy with donor leukocyte infusions as a strategy to treat chronic-phase chronic myelogenous leukemia patients undergoing HLA-identical sibling marrow transplantation. *Blood,* **94,** 434–41.

Elmaagacli, A.H., Beelen, D.W., Opalka, B. *et al.* (1999). The risk of residual molecular and cytogenetic disease in patients with Philadelphia-chromosome positive first chronic phase chronic myelogenous leukemia is reduced after transplantation of allogeneic peripheral blood stem cells compared with bone marrow. *Blood,* **94,** 384–9.

Elmaagacli, A.H., Beelen, D.W., & Schaefer, U.W. (1997). A retrospective single centre study of the outcome of five different therapy approaches in 48 patients with relapse of chronic myelogenous leukemia after allogeneic bone marrow transplantation. *Bone Marrow Transplantation,* **20,** 1045–55.

Elmaagacli, A.H., Peceny, R., Steckel, N. *et al.* (2003). Outcome of transplantation of highly purified blood CD34+ cells with T-cell add-back compared with unmanipulated bone marrow or peripheral blood stem cells from HLA-identical sibling donors in patients with first chronic phase chronic myeloid leukemia. *Blood,* **101,** 446–53.

Enright, H., Davies, S.M., DeFor, T. *et al.* (1996). Relapse after non-T-cell-depleted allogeneic bone marrow transplantation for chronic myelogenous leukemia: early transplantation, use of an unrelated donor, and chronic graft-versus-host disease are protective. *Blood,* **88,** 714–20.

Falkenburg, J.H.F., Wafelman, A.R., Joosten, P. *et al.* (1999). Complete remission of accelerated phase chronic myeloid leukemia by treatment with leukemia-reactive cytotoxic T lymphocytes. *Blood,* **94,** 1201–8.

Fernández, M.N., Regidor, C., Diez, J.L. *et al.* (1996). HLA haploidentical cord blood cell transplant in a 15-year-old, 50 kg weight patient: successful treatment for chronic myeloid leukemia after myeloid blastic transformation. *Bone Marrow Transplantation,* **17,** 1175–8.

Gale, R.P., Hehlmann, R., Zhang, M-J. *et al.* (1998). Survival with bone marrow transplantation versus hydroxyurea or interferon for chronic myelogenous leukemia. *Blood,* **91,** 1810–19.

Giralt, S.A., Kantarjian, H.M., Talpaz, M. *et al.* (1993). Effect of prior interferon alfa therapy on the outcome of allogeneic bone marrow transplantation for chronic myelogenous leukemia. *Journal of Clinical Oncology,* **11,** 1055–61.

Giralt, S., Estey, E., Albtar, M. *et al.* (1997). Engraftment of allogeneic hematopoietic progenitor cells with purine analog-containing chemotherapy: harnessing graft-versus-leukemia without myeloablative therapy. *Blood,* **89,** 4531–7.

Giralt, S., Szydlo, R., Goldman, J.M. *et al.* (2000). Effect of short-term interferon therapy on the outcome of subsequent HLA-identical sibling bone marrow transplantation for chronic myelogenous leukemia: an analysis from the International Bone Marrow Transplant Registry. *Blood,* **95,** 410–5.

Giralt, S., Thall, P.F., Khouri, I. *et al.* (2001). Melphalan and purine analog-containing preparative regimens: reduced-intensity conditioning for patients with hematologic malignancies undergoing progenitor cell transplantation. *Blood,* **97,** 631–7.

Goldman, J.M. (2001). Implications of imatinib mesylate for hematopoietic stem cell transplantation. *Seminars in Hematology,* 38 (Suppl 8), 28–34.

Goldman, J.M., Apperley, J.F., Jones, L. *et al.* (1986). Bone marrow transplantation for patients with chronic myeloid leukemia. *New England Journal of Medicine,* **314,** 202–7.

Goldman, J.M., Gale, R.P., Horowitz, M.M. *et al.* (1988). Bone marrow transplantation for chronic myelogenous leukemia in chronic phase: increased risk of relapse associated with T cell depletion. *Annals of Internal Medicine,* **108,** 806–14.

Goldman, J.M., Szydlo, R., Horowitz, M.M. *et al.* (1993). Choice of pre-transplant treatment and timing of transplants for chronic myelogenous leukemia in chronic phase. *Blood,* **82,** 2235–8.

Goldman, J.M. & Druker, B.J. (2001). Chronic myeloid leukemia: current treatment options. *Blood,* **98,** 2039–42.

Gratwohl, A., Hermans, J., Goldman, J.M. *et al.* (1998). Risk assessment for patients with chronic myeloid leukemia before allogeneic blood or marrow transplantation. *Lancet,* **352,** 1087–92.

Gratwohl, A., van Biezen, A., Hermans, J. *et al.* (1999). Role of splenic irradiation in patients with chronic myeloid leukemia undergoing allogeneic bone marrow transplantation. *Biology of Blood and Marrow Transplantation,* **6,** 211–2.

Gratwohl, A., Brand, R., Apperley, J. *et al.* (2002). Graft-versus-host disease and outcome in HLA-identical sibling transplantations for chronic myeloid leukemia. *Blood,* **100,** 3877–86.

Guglielmi, C., Arcese, W., Hermans, J. *et al.* (2000). Risk assessment in patients with Ph+ chronic myelogenous leukemia at first relapse after allogeneic stem cell transplant: an EBMT retrospective analysis. *Blood,* **95,** 3328–34.

Hansen, J.A., Gooley, T.A., Martin, P.J. *et al.* (1998). Bone marrow transplantation from unrelated donors for patients with chronic myeloid leukemia. *New England Journal of Medicine,* **338,** 962–8.

Hehlmann, R., Hochaus, A., Kolb, H-J. *et al.* (1999). Interferon-α before allogeneic bone marrow transplantation in chronic myelogenous leukemia does not affect outcome adversely, provided it is discontinued at least 90 days before the procedure. *Blood,* **94,** 3668–77.

Helenglass, G., Treleaven, J., Parikh, P. *et al.* (1990). Delayed engraftment associated with splenomegaly in patients undergoing bone marrow transplantation for chronic myeloid leukemia. *Bone Marrow Transplantation,* **5,** 247–51.

Hessner, M.J., Endean, D.J., Casper, J.T. *et al.* (1996). Use of unrelated marrow grafts compensates for reduced graft-versus-leukemia reactivity after T-cell-depleted allogeneic marrow transplantation for chronic myelogenous leukemia. *Blood,* **86,** 3987–96.

Higano, C.S., Raskind, Y.H., & Singer, J.W. (1992). Use of α interferon for the treatment of relapse of chronic myelogenous leukemia in chronic phase after allogeneic bone marrow transplantation. *Blood,* **80,** 1437–42.

Ho, V.T. & Soiffer, R.J. (2001). The history and future of T-cell depletion as graft-versus host disease prophylaxis for allogeneic hematopoietic stem cell transplantation. *Blood,* **98,** 3192–205.

Hochhaus, A., Lin, F., Reiter, A. *et al.* (1996). Quantification of residual disease in chronic myelogenous leukemia on interferon-α therapy by competitive polymerase chain reaction. *Blood,* **87,** 1549–55.

Horowitz, M.M., Rowlings, P.A., & Passweg, J.R. (1996). Allogeneic bone marrow transplantation for CML: a report from the International Bone Marrow Transplant Registry. *Bone Marrow Transplantation,* **17** (Suppl 3), S5–6.

Hows, J.M., Yin, J.L., Marsh, J. *et al.* (1986). Histocompatible unrelated volunteer donors compared with HLA nonidentical family donors in marrow transplantation for aplastic anemia and leukemia. *Blood,* **68,** 1322–8.

Hughes, T.P., Economou, K., Mackinnon, S. *et al.* (1989). Slow evolution of chronic myeloid leukemia relapsing after BMT with T-cell depleted donor marrow. *British Journal of Haematology,* **73,** 462–7.

Italian Cooperative Study Group on Chronic Myeloid Leukemia. (1993). Interferon alfa-2a as compared with conventional chemotherapy for the treatment of chronic myeloid leukemia. *New England Journal of Medicine,* **330,** 820–5.

Jabro, G., Koc, Y., Boyle, T. *et al.* (1999). Role of splenic irradiation in patients with chronic myeloid leukemia undergoing allogeneic bone marrow transplantation. *Biology of Blood and Marrow Transplantation,* **5,** 173–9.

Kalhs, P., Schwarzinger, I., Anderson, G. *et al.* (1995). A retrospective analysis of the long-term effect of splenectomy on late infections, graft-versus-host disease, relapse, and survival after allogeneic marrow transplantation for chronic myeloid leukemia. *Blood,* **86,** 2028–32.

Kantarjian, H., Melo, J.V., Tura, S. *et al.* (2000). Chronic myelogenous leukemia: disease biology and current and future therapeutic strategies. In *Hematology 2000,* ed., G.P. Schechter, N. Berliner, & M.J. Telen, pp. 90–109. American Society of Hematology.

Kantarjian, H., O'Brien, S., Cortes, J. *et al.* (2001). Results of imatinib mesylate (STI571) therapy in patients with chronic myelogenous leukemia in relapse after allogeneic stem cell transplantation. *Blood* (Abstract 575).

Kantarjian, H.M., O'Brien, S., Cortes, J.E. *et al.* (2002). Imatinib mesylate therapy for relapse after allogeneic stem cell transplantation for chronic myelogenous leukemia. *Blood,* **100,** 1590–5.

Khoury, H., Adkins, D., Brown, R. *et al.* (2001). Low incidence of transplantation-related acute complications in patients with chronic myeloid leukemia undergoing allogeneic stem cell transplantation with a low-dose (550 cGy) total body irradiation conditioning regimen. *Biology of Blood and Marrow Transplantation,* **7,** 352–8.

Klein, J.P., Keiding, N., Shu, Y. *et al.* (2000). Summary curves for patients transplanted for chronic myeloid leukaemia salvaged by a donor lymphocyte infusion: the current leukaemia-free survival curve. *British Journal of Haematology,* **109,** 148–52.

Kolb, H.J., Mittermuller, J., Clemm, C. *et al.* (1990). Donor leukocyte transfusions for treatment of recurrent chronic myelogenous leukemia in marrow transplant patients. *Blood,* **76,** 2462–5.

Kolb, H.J., Schattenberg, A., Goldman, J.M. *et al.* (1995). Graft-versus-leukemia effect of donor lymphocyte transfusion in marrow grafted patients. *Blood,* **86,** 2041–50.

Kollman, C., Howe, W.S., Anasetti, C. *et al.* (2001). Donor characteristics as risk factors in recipients after transplantation of bone marrow from unrelated donors: the effect of donor age. *Blood,* **98,** 2043–51.

Konstantinidou, P., Szydlo, R.M., Chase, A., & Goldman, J.M. (2000). Cytogenetic status pre-transplant as a predictor of outcome post bone marrow transplantation for chronic myelogenous leukaemia. *Bone Marrow Transplantation, 25,* 143–6.

Körbling, M. & Anderlini, P. (2001). Peripheral blood stem cell versus bone marrow allotransplantation: does the source of hematopoietic stem cells matter? *Blood,* **98,** 2900–8.

Kurtzberg, J., Laughlin, M., Graham, M.L. *et al.* (1996). Placental blood as a source of hematopoietic stem cells for transplantation into unrelated recipients. *New England Journal of Medicine,* **335,** 157–66.

Lamparelli, T., Van Lint, M.T., Gualandi, F. *et al.* (1997). Bone marrow transplantation for chronic myeloid leukemia (CML) from unrelated and sibling donors: single center experience. *Bone Marrow Transplantation, 20,* 1057–62.

Laporte, J.P., Gorin, N.C., Rubinstein, P. *et al.* (1996). Cord-blood transplantation from an unrelated donor in an adult with chronic myelogenous leukemia. *New England Journal of Medicine,* **335,** 167–70.

Lee, S.J., Klein, J.P., Anasetti, C. *et al.* (2001). The effect of pretransplant interferon therapy on outcome of unrelated donor hematopoietic stem cell transplantation for patients with chronic myelogenous leukemia in first chronic phase. *Blood,* **98,** 3205–11.

Mackinnon, S., Papadopoulos, E.P., Carabasi, M.H. *et al.* (1995). Adoptive immunotherapy evaluating escalating doses of donor leukocytes for relapse of chronic myeloid leukemia following bone marrow transplantation: separation of graft-versus-leukemia responses from graft-versus-host disease. *Blood,* **86,** 1261–7.

Marks, D.I., Hughes, T.P., Szydlo, R. *et al.* (1992). HLA-identical sibling donor bone marrow transplantation for chronic myeloid leukemia in first chronic phase: influence of GVHD prophylaxis on outcome. *British Journal of Haematology, 81,* 383–90.

Marmont, A., Frassoni, F., Bacigalupo, A. *et al.* (1984). Recurrence of Ph-positive leukemia after marrow transplantation for chronic granulocytic leukemia. *New England Journal of Medicine,* **310,** 903–6.

McGlave, P.B., Bartsch, G., Anasetti, C. *et al.* (1993). Unrelated donor marrow transplantation therapy for chronic myelogenous leukemia: initial experience of the National Marrow Donor Program. *Blood,* **81,** 543–50.

McGlave, P.B., Shu, X.O., Wen, W. *et al.* (2000). Unrelated donor marrow transplantation for chronic myelogenous leukemia: 9 years' experience of the National Marrow Donor Program. *Blood,* **95,** 2219–25.

McSweeney, P.A., Niederweiser, D., Shizuru, J.A. *et al.* (2001). Hematopoietic cell transplantation in older patients with hematologic malignancies: replacing high-dose cytotoxic therapy with graft-versus-tumor effects. *Blood,* **97,** 3390–400.

Michallet, M., Bilger, K., Garban, F. *et al.* (2001). Allogeneic hematopoietic stem-cell transplantation after non-myeloablative preparative regimens: impact of pretransplantation and posttransplantation factors on outcome. *Journal of Clinical Oncology,* **19,** 3340–9.

Morton, A.J., Gooley, T., Hansen, J.A. *et al.* (1998). Association between pretransplant interferon-alpha and outcome after unrelated donor marrow transplantation for chronic myelogenous leukemia in chronic phase. *Blood,* **92,** 394–401.

Morton, J., Hutchins, C., & Durrant, S. (2001). Granulocyte-colony-stimulating factor (G-CSF)-primed allogeneic bone marrow: significantly less graft-versus-host disease and comparable engraftment to G-CSF-mobilized peripheral blood stem cells. *Blood,* **98,** 3186–91.

Mughal, T., I., Yong, A., Szydlo, R. *et al.* (2001). Molecular studies in patients with chronic myeloid leukaemia in remission 5 years after allogeneic stem cell transplant define the risk of subsequent relapse. *British Journal of Haematology, 115,* 569–74.

Negrin, R.S. & Blume, K.G. (1991). The use of the polymerase chain reaction for the detection of minimal residual disease. *Blood,* **78,** 255–8.

Olavarria, E., Kanfer, E., Szydlo, R. *et al.* (2001). Early detection of BCR-ABL transcripts by quantitative reverse transcriptase-polymerase chain reaction predicts outcome after allogeneic stem cell transplantation for chronic myeloid leukemia. *Blood,* **97,** 1560–5.

Olavarria, E., Craddock, C., Dazzi, F. *et al.* (2002). Imatinib mesylate (ST1571) in the treatment of relapse of chronic myeloid leukemia after allogneic stem cell transplantation. *Blood,* **99,** 3861–2.

Passweg, J., Walker, I., Sobocinski, K. *et al.* (2001). Validation of the EBMT risk score for recipients of allogeneic hematopoietic stem cell transplants for chronic myeloid leukemia (CML). *Blood* (Abstract 1470).

Przepiorka, D. & Thomas, E.D. (1988). Prognostic significance of cytogenetic abnormalities in patients with chronic myelogenous leukemia. *Bone Marrow Transplantation, 3,* 113–9.

Radich, J.P., Gehly, G., Gooley, T. *et al.* (1995). Polymerase chain reaction detection of the BCR-ABL fusion transcript after allogeneic transplantation for chronic myeloid leukemia: results and implications in 346 patients. *Blood,* **85,** 2632–8.

Radich, J.P., Gooley, T., Bryant, E. *et al.* (2001a). The significance of bcr-abl molecular detection in chronic myeloid leukemia patients "late," 18 months or more after transplantation. *Blood,* **98,** 1701–7.

Radich, J.P., Gooley, T., Clift, R. *et al.* (2001b). Allogeneic-related transplantation for chronic phase chronic myeloid leukemia (CML) using a targeted busulfan and Cytoxan preparative regimen. *Blood* (Abstract 3239).

Raiola, A.M., Van Lint, M.T., Lamparelli, T. *et al.* (2000). Reduced intensity thiotepa-cyclophosphamide conditioning for allogeneic haematopoietic stem cell transplants (HSCT) in patients up to 60 years of age. *British Journal of Haematology, 109,* 716–21.

Richard, C., Romon, I., Perez-Encinas, M. *et al.* (1996). Splenectomy for poor graft function after bone marrow transplantation in patients with chronic myeloid leukemia. *Leukemia, 10,* 1615–8.

Rodriguez, R., Snyder, D., Nademanee, A. *et al.* (2001). Gleevec for relapsed CML after allogeneic transplant may overcome need for donor leukocyte infusions or interferon. *Blood* (Abstract 1684).

Roth, M.S., Antin, J.H., Ash, R. *et al.* (1991). Prognostic significance of Philadelphia chromosome-positive cells detected by the polymerase chain reaction after allogeneic bone marrow transplant for chronic myelogenous leukemia. *Blood*, 79, 276–82.

Sanz, G.F., Saavedra, S., Jimenez, C. *et al.* (2001). Unrelated donor cord blood transplantation in adults with chronic myelogenous leukemia: results in nine patients from a single institution. *Bone Marrow Transplantation, 27*, 693–701.

Savage, D.G. & Antman, K.H. (2002). Imatinib mesylate: a new oral targeted therapy. *New England Journal of Medicine, 28*, 683–96.

Savage, D.G. & Goldman, J.M. (1999). Chronic myelogenous leukemia. In *High Dose Therapy: Pharmacology, Hematopoietins, Stem Cells,* 3rd eds. J.O. Armitage & K.H. Antman, pp. 705–731. Baltimore: Williams & Wilkins.

Savage, D.G., Szydlo, R.M., Chase, A. *et al.* (1997). Bone marrow transplantation for chronic myeloid leukemia: the effects of differing criteria for defining chronic phase on probabilities of survival and relapse. *British Journal of Haematology, 99*, 30–5.

Schipper, R.F., DíAmaro, J., & Oudshoorn, M. (1996). The probability of finding a suitable related donor for bone marrow transplantation in extended families. *Blood, 87*, 800–4.

Schmitz, N., Champlin, R.E., Loberiza, F.R. Jr. *et al.* (2001). Long-term follow-up of allogeneic blood stem cell and bone marrow transplantation: a collaborative study of EBMT and IBMTR. *Blood* (Abstract 3099).

Sehn, L.H., Alyea, E.P., Weller, E. *et al.* (1999). Comparative outcomes of T-cell-depleted and non-T-cell-depleted allogeneic bone marrow transplantation for chronic myelogenous leukemia: impact of donor lymphocyte infusion. *Journal of Clinical Oncology, 17*, 561–8.

Seong, C-M., Giralt, S., Kantarjian, H. *et al.* (2000). Early detection of relapse by hypermetaphase fluorescence in situ hybridization after allogeneic bone marrow transplantation for chronic myeloid leukemia. *Journal of Clinical Oncology, 18*, 1831–6.

Shimoni, A., Gajewski, J., Donato, M. *et al.* (2001). Long-term follow-up of recipients of CD8-depleted donor lymphocyte infusions for the treatment of chronic myelogenous leukemia relapsing after allogeneic progenitor cell transplantation. *Biology of Blood and Marrow Transplantation, 7*, 568–75.

Slavin, S., Nagler, A., Naparstek, E. *et al.* (1998). Nonmyeloablative stem cell transplantation and cell therapy as an alternative to conventional bone marrow transplantation with lethal cytoreduction for the treatment of malignant and nonmalignant hematologic diseases. *Blood, 91*, 756–63.

Smith, J.L., Heerema, N.A., Provisor, A.J. *et al.* (1985). Leukaemic transformation of engrafted bone marrow cells. *British Journal of Haematology, 60*, 415–22.

Snyder, D.S., Negrin, R.S., O'Donnell, M.R. *et al.* (1994). Fractionated total body irradiation and high-dose etoposide as a preparatory regimen for bone marrow transplantation in 94 patients with chronic myelogenous leukemia in chronic phase. *Blood, 84*, 1672–9.

Soiffer, R.J., Galinsky, I., DeAngelo, D. *et al.* (2001). Imatinib mesylate (Gleevec) for disease relapse following allogeneic bone marrow transplantation. *Blood* (Abstract 1682).

Speiser, D.E., Hermans, J., van Biezen, A. *et al.* (1997). Haploidentical family member transplants for patients with chronic myeloid leukaemia: a report of the Chronic Leukaemia Working Party of the European Group for Blood and Marrow Transplantation (EBMT). *Bone Marrow Transplantation, 19*, 1197–203.

Storek, J., Gooley, T., Siadak, M. *et al.* (1997). Allogeneic peripheral blood stem cell transplantation may be associated with a high risk of chronic graft-versus-host disease. *Blood, 90*, 4705–9.

Szydlo, R., Goldman, J.M., Klein, J.P. *et al.* (1997). Results of allogeneic bone marrow transplants using donors other than HLA-identical siblings. *Journal of Clinical Oncology, 15*, 1767–77.

Talpaz, M., Kantarjian, H., Kurzrock, R. *et al.* (1991). Interferon-alpha produces sustained cytogenetic responses in chronic myelogenous leukemia. *Annals of Internal Medicine, 114*, 532–8.

Thomas, E.D., Clift, R.A., Fefer, A. *et al.* (1986). Marrow transplantation for the treatment of chronic myelogenous leukemia. *Annals of Internal Medicine, 105*, 155–63.

Ullmann, A.J., Beck, J., Kolbe, K. *et al.* (2001). Clinical and laboratory evaluation of patients treated with STI-571 (Gleevec) after allogeneic and syngeneic stem cell transplantation with relapsed Philadelphia chromosome-positive leukemia. *Blood* (Abstract 1685).

Urbano-Ispizua, A., Schmitz, N., de Witte, T. *et al.* (2002). Allogenic and autologous transplantation for haematological diseases, solid tumors and immune disorders: definition and current practice in Europe. *Bone Marrow Transplantation, 29*, 639–46.

Uzunel, M., Mattsson, J., Bruce, M. *et al.* (2003). Kinetics of minimal residual disease and chimerism in patients with chronic myeloid leukemia after nonmyeloablative conditioning and allogeneic stem cell transplantation. *Blood, 101*, 469-72.

van Rhee, F., Feng, L., Cullis, J.O. *et al.* (1994). Relapse of chronic myeloid leukemia after allogeneic bone marrow transplant: the case for giving donor leukocyte transfusions before the onset of hematologic relapse. *Blood, 83*, 3377–83.

van Rhee, F., Szydlo, R.M., Hermans, J. *et al.* (1997). Long-term results after allogeneic bone marrow transplantation for chronic myelogenous leukemia in chronic phase: a report from the Chronic Leukemia Working Party of the European Group for Blood and Marrow Transplantation. *Bone Marrow Transplantation, 20*, 553–60.

Visani, G., Rosti, G., Bandini, G. *et al.* (2000). Second chronic phase before transplantation is crucial for improving survival of blastic phase chronic myeloid leukemia. *British Journal of Haematology, 109*, 722–8.

Weisdorf, D.J., Anasetti, C., Antin, J.H. *et al.* (2002). Allogeneic bone marrow transplantation for chronic myelogenous leukemia: comparative analysis of unrelated versus matched sibling donor transplantation. *Blood, 99*, 1971–7.

Yong, A. & Goldman, J.M. (1999). Relapse of chronic myeloid leukaemia 14 years after allogeneic bone marrow transplantation. *Bone Marrow Transplantation, 23*, 827–28.

Zaucha, J.M., Gooley, T., Bensinger, W.I. *et al.* (2001). CD34 cell dose in granulocyte colony-stimulating factor-mobilized peripheral blood mononuclear cell grafts affects engraftment kinetics and development of extensive chronic graft-versus-host disease after human leukocyte antigen-identical sibling transplantation. *Blood, 98*, 3221–7.

53 Allogeneic hematopoietic stem cell transplantation for juvenile myelomonocytic leukemia, chronic neutrophil leukemia, hypereosinophilic syndrome, and chronic myeloproliferative disorders other than chronic myeloid leukemia

JANE APPERLEY

Imperial College School of Medicine, London, UK

Introduction

This chapter deals with allogeneic hematopoietic stem cell (HSC) transplantation for juvenile myelomonocytic leukemia (JMML), chronic neutrophil leukemia (CNL), hypereosinophilic syndrome (HES), and the three chronic myeloproliferative disorders other than chronic myeloid leukemia (CML)—agnogenic myeloid metaplasia (chronic myelofibrosis) (AMM), polycythemia rubra vera (PRV), and essential thrombocythemia (ET). Bone marrow fibrosis is a cytokine-mediated reaction that can accompany any of these latter three chronic myeloproliferative disorders and their diagnosis requires the absence of the chromosomal translocation t(9;22)(q34;q11) and dyserythropoiesis. Substantial bone marrow fibrosis can be associated with both CML and myelodysplasia. Other laboratory features that distinguish these three chronic myeloproliferative syndromes from CML are shown in Table 53.1.

PRV is defined by an increased red cell mass, and ET by clonal thrombocytosis not otherwise classifiable as PRV, CML, agno-genic myeloid metaplasia, or myelodysplasia. Disease progression to a clinical picture identical to agnogenic myeloid metaplasia occurs in approximately 9% of patients with PRV (post-polycythemic myelofibrosis) and in less than 2% of those with essential thrombocythemia (post-thrombocythemic myelofibrosis). Patients with these later stages of PRV and ET are managed in a fashion similar to that for agnogenic myeloid metaplasia. The term myelofibrosis with myeloid metaplasia encompasses agnogenic myeloid metaplasia and these later stages of PRV and ET.

Agnogenic myeloid metaplasia (idiopathic or chronic myelofibrosis) must be distinguished from acute or "malignant" myelofibrosis—now classified as acute megakaryoblastic leukemia (FAB M7); the latter disease is dealt with in Chapter 50.

Agnogenic myeloid metaplasia (chronic idiopathic myelofibrosis)

Agnogenic myeloid metaplasia (idiopathic myelofibrosis) is a chronic myeloproliferative disorder characterized by marrow

Table 53.1. *Laboratory features that distinguish the chronic myeloproliferative syndromes*

Laboratory parameter	Agnogenic myeloid metaplasia (chronic idiopathic myelofibrosis)	PRV	ET	CML
Hemoglobin	Usually decreased	Increased	Normal or decreased	Usually decreased
White blood count × 10⁹/l	Usually less than 30	Usually less than 25	Usually less than 25	Usually more than 50
Differential white blood cell count	Occasional immature cells	Moderate neutrophilia	Normal or moderate neutrophilia	Myelocytes and earlier stage at diagnosis
Basophilia >1%	Usually	Sometimes	Sometimes	Usually
Red cell morphology	Teardrop poikilocytes	Normal to hypochromic, microcytic	Normal to hypochromic, microcytic	Normal
Nucleated red cells in blood	Yes	Seldom	Seldom	Yes
Platelet count	Normal, increased, or decreased	Normal or increased	Markedly elevated	Normal or increased
Leukocyte alkaline phosphatase	Usually increased	Usually increased	Normal	Low
Bone marrow	Fibrotic	Hypercellular, decreased iron stores	Hypercellular, increased megakaryocytes	Myeloid hyperplasia

Abbreviations: PRV, polycythemia rubra vera; ET, essential thrombocythemia; CML, chronic myeloid leukemia.

fibrosis, splenomegaly due to extramedullary hematopoiesis, leukoerythroblastic blood changes, and tear-drop deformities of red blood cells. The marrow fibrosis and extramedullary hematopoiesis are early concurrent but independent processes instigated by clonal proliferation of defective pluripotent hematopoietic stem cells. Blood cell abnormalities are secondary to the hematopoietic dysplasia. The incidence is approximately one-third that of CML; it is diagnosed most frequently in the seventh decade, but it can occur at a younger age and has been described in children (Sekhar *et al.,* 1996), including one set of identical twins. The fibrosis can resolve with successful therapy. The incidence of cytogenetic abnormalities is higher than was originally recognized. In a retrospective study of 112 patients, an abnormal karyotype was identified in 55% at some stage in their disease. Forty-nine percent of patients had identifiable cytogenetic changes at diagnosis (Tefferi *et al.,* 2001). Several recurrent chromosomal abnormalities are overrepresented, notably 13q–; 20q–; +8; and abnormalities of chromosomes 1, 7, and 9, which constitute more than 80% of the changes. 13q–, 20q–, and +8 are usually seen as single events whereas abnormalities of chromosomes 1, 5, 7, and 9 co-exist with other changes. This suggests that these latter abnormalities represent secondary events reflecting genomic instability while the former changes may be earlier events with pathological relevance.

Work in mice has shown that overexpression of thrombopoietin (TPO) (using retroviral-mediated gene transfer into bone marrow cells) results in the development of myelofibrosis and osteosclerosis, most likely produced by platelet-derived cytokines (Yan *et al.,* 1995); indeed, subsequent work showed that serum contained a two- to five-fold increase in the amount of transforming growth factor-beta-1 and platelet-derived growth factor (Yan *et al.,* 1996). In these mice, platelet levels increased four- to eight-fold above baseline levels and remained elevated. Interestingly, hematopoietic stem cell (HSC) transplantation resulted in return of megakaryocyte and platelet numbers to normal and complete resolution of the myelofibrosis and osteosclerosis. This work was later confirmed and extended by Villeval *et al.* (1997) to produce a murine model with many of the features of the human disease.

The median survival from diagnosis is approximately 5 years. Factors associated with long survival include lack of symptoms, absence of circulating blasts, hemoglobin levels above 10 g/dl, platelet counts above $100 \times 10^9/l$, and absence of splenomegaly. Poor prognostic indicators include older age, the presence of severe ineffective hematopoiesis, excessive hemolysis, a reduced red cell mass, massive splenomegaly, and portal hypertension, resulting in an average survival of only 1 to 2 years. Evaluation of prognosis is particularly important if allogeneic HSC transplantation is an option, since this is the only currently available curative treatment. Cytotoxic chemotherapy with busulfan or 6-thioguanine can reduce spleen size and control thrombocytosis but has little effect on anemia. Hydroxyurea can be useful for controlling compensatory hepatic hematopoiesis following splenectomy. About 50% of

patients respond to a combination of androgen (e.g., oxymetholone 200 mg daily or testosterone enanthate 400 mg i.m. weekly) and glucocorticosteroid therapy. Imatinib mesylate (Gleevec, STI571) is ineffective in the management of AMM (Tefferi *et al.,* 2002). Splenectomy may be considered for painful or massive splenomegaly, refractory life-threatening thrombocytopenia, portal hypertension with bleeding varices, or uncontrollable hemolytic or dilutional anemia sufficient to cause cardiopulmonary symptoms. Operative mortality under these conditions is considerable.

Until recently the total published experience of allogeneic transplantation for AMM was restricted to fewer than 20 cases. Four patients with "chronic myelofibrosis" (equivalent to agnogenic myeloid metaplasia) were included in a report of 47 patients transplanted for a variety of diseases with the common histological feature of bone marrow fibrosis (Rajantie *et al.,* 1986). Fifteen patients with "severe" fibrosis (grades 3 or 4 according to Bauermeister, 1971) were compared to a group of 32 patients with "mild" fibrosis (grades 1 or 2) and to a control group of 28 patients without fibrosis. Remarkably, reversal of fibrosis was observed in 12 of the 15 patients with severe fibrosis, confirming previously reported experience in acute myelosclerosis (Smith *et al.,* 1981; Wolf *et al.,* 1982). Unfortunately 50% of these responders experienced recurrent fibrosis at the time of either graft rejection ($n = 3$) or leukemic relapse ($n = 3$). Survival was similar in all three groups. However, the group with severe fibrosis experienced delays in neutrophil and platelet engraftment and prolonged blood product dependence compared to the other two groups. This effect appeared independent of other risk factors such as marrow cell dose, type of GVHD prophylaxis, and the degree of HLA compatibility (although the numbers of patients receiving HLA non-identical marrow or T-cell depleted products were very small in this series). Thus, very early in the history of transplantation for myelofibrotic conditions, the presence of fibrosis was thought to be associated with an increased risk of delayed or failed engraftment. The mechanism by which fibrosis might impair engraftment was unknown. The authors speculated that a marrow obliterated by dense fibrosis might be unable to provide an adequate micro-environment for hematopoietic reconstitution. An alternative hypothesis was that failure to ablate the malignant process itself impaired engraftment.

There followed a number of case reports or small series (Cahn *et al.,* 1987; Dokal *et al.,* 1989; Ifrah *et al.,* 1989; Creemers *et al.,* 1992; Iwata *et al.,* 1992; Schmitz *et al.,* 1992; Bandini *et al.,* 1994; Jouet *et al.,* 1994; Sutton *et al.,* 1994; Singhal *et al.,* 1995; Rossbach *et al.,* 1996) until a more definitive analysis of 55 patients (including most of those previously reported in the case studies) from an international collaborative group in 1999 (Guardiola *et al.,* 1999). A recurrent theme throughout these case reports was the issue of delayed or failed engraftment, sometimes with autologous recovery. The patients were hetereogeneous with respect to prior therapy, pretransplant splenectomy, conditioning regimens, GVHD prophylaxis (including T-cell depletion), and donor identity. A later retrospective study from the Seattle group cast doubt on the association between myelofibrosis and delayed neutrophil engraftment (Soll *et al.*, 1995). Two hundred and three patients whose pretransplant marrow examinations showed varying degrees of fibrosis (including 33 with severe fibrosis) were compared with matched controls. There was no significant difference in the time to neutrophil engraftment between the two groups, although platelet recovery and the time to blood product independence were slower in the former group.

Schmitz *et al.* (1992) described an interesting case in which the patient remained pancytopenic for 10 months posttransplant until he underwent splenectomy which was followed by a prompt recovery of donor hematopoiesis. Histology of the spleen confirmed extensive sequestration of blood cells. Cytogenetic analyses of metaphases from cells derived from the spleen detected residual clonal malignant cells. Consideration of pretransplant splenectomy was recommended for all patients for whom allografting was proposed, both to remove a potential sanctuary site of disease and to avoid hypersplenism.

Routine splenectomy prior to transplantation remains a controversial issue. A review of 223 patients who were splenectomized for AMM reported a surgery-related mortality of 9% and a morbidity of 31%. Approximately 50% of patients derive a benefit in excess of 12 months from splenectomy (Tefferi, 2000; Benbassat, 2000). The Seattle group reviewed 26 patients who had received allogeneic transplants for AMM; 11 patients had been splenectomized prior to transplant and the remaining 15 all had palpable splenomegaly at the time of allografting. Hematopoietic recovery was more rapid in splenectomized patients but the incidence of relapse and the overall survival were similar in both groups (Li *et al.*, 2001). The two groups were not identical with respect to other potential risk factors such as age, duration of disease prior to transplant, and donor identity, but the authors concluded that routine splenectomy could not be justified. Splenectomy can be reserved for those patients with massive splenomegaly or with other features associated with poor engraftment such as severe fibrosis.

Guardiola *et al.* (1999) initially summarized the outcome of 55 patients allografted for AMM and later updated the analysis to include a further 11 patients. The majority were transplanted from HLA-identical donors (*n* = 49). With a median follow-up of 36 months (range 6–223) the one year transplant-related mortality was 27%. Actuarial overall and event-free survivals at 5 years were 47% and 39% respectively for the entire group and 54% and 48% for patients receiving T-replete transplant products from HLA-identical sibling donors (Fig. 53.1). The incidence of grade III–IV acute GVHD was 33% with 16 of 45 patients experiencing extensive chronic GVHD. With respect to engraftment, a Hb >100 g/l at time of transplant, pretransplant splenectomy, the absence of osteomyelosclerosis, and a high number of infused nucleated cells were significantly associated with more rapid neutrophil recovery. Pretransplant splenectomy did not affect the risk of acute or chronic GVHD, which were associated with pretransplant osteomyelosclerosis and the use of total

body irradiation in the conditioning regimen. In the multivariate analysis of pretransplant variables affecting survival, increasing age, hemoglobin <100 g/l, and the presence of osteomyelosclerosis were adverse risk factors. Patients under the age of 45 years had a 5 year overall survival of 62% compared to 14% for those over 45 at the time of transplant.

Complete resolution of fibrosis was observed in 22 patients and occurred between 21 days and 23 months posttransplant. Three patients had persistent disease and 10 evaluable patients experienced disease recurrence at a median of 12 (range 4–67) months after grafting. Older age at transplant, presence of a cytogenetic abnormality, and the absence of grade II–IV GVHD were all associated with disease persistence or relapse, the risk of which reached 28% at 5 years. As with CML, recurrence of the original disease can be associated with prolonged survival with 8 patients alive at 1–108 months after detection of recurrent disease. The management of disease recurrence could include withdrawal of immunosuppression, donor lymphocyte infusions, or second transplant. The efficacy of donor lymphocytes, suggested by the association of GVHD with a reduced risk of relapse, has been confirmed. Two case reports have described the successful re-induction of remission with regression of fibrosis using donor lymphocyte infusions (Cervantes *et al.*, 2000; Byrne *et al.*, 2000).

The study of Guardiola *et al.*, confirmed the value of allografting in AMM, and the results appear superior to those obtained using conventional, non-aggressive therapy where the 5 year survival is approximately 40% (Dupriez *et al.*, 1996). Optimal timing of transplant, as in CML, is more problematic. The prognostic scores of Dupriez *et al.* (1996) and Cervantes *et al.* (1998) identify groups of patients with short median survivals. Dupriez and her colleagues used two adverse prognostic factors, namely Hb <100 g/l and white cell count <4 or >30 × 10^9/l to separate patients into three groups. Patients with low (0 factor), intermediate (1 factor), and high (2 factors) scores had median survivals of 93, 26, and 13 months, respectively. Cervantes *et al.* used three variables—Hb <100 g/l, presence of constitutional symptoms, and >1% circulating blasts to identify 2 groups. The low-risk group with up to one adverse factor had a median survival of 176 months and the high-risk group (2 or 3 factors) had more aggressive disease with a median survival of 33 months. Irrespective of the scoring system used, it would seem appropriate to offer early transplant to patients not in either low-risk group. For low-risk patients the decision for early transplant is more controversial, as these patients can have an excellent outcome from both conservative therapy and transplantation (Figure 53.1C). A compromise solution might be to recommend transplant at the appearance of one or more of the adverse features. Older patients also present a management dilemma. In the study of Guardiola *et al.*, patients over the age of 45 years fared particularly poorly. Deeg and Appelbaum (2001) reported a rather different outcome. At the Fred Hutchinson Cancer Research Center, 23 patients over the age of 44 years received allogeneic transplants for AMM. The three- and five-year overall survivals for these individuals were 63% and 50%, respectively.

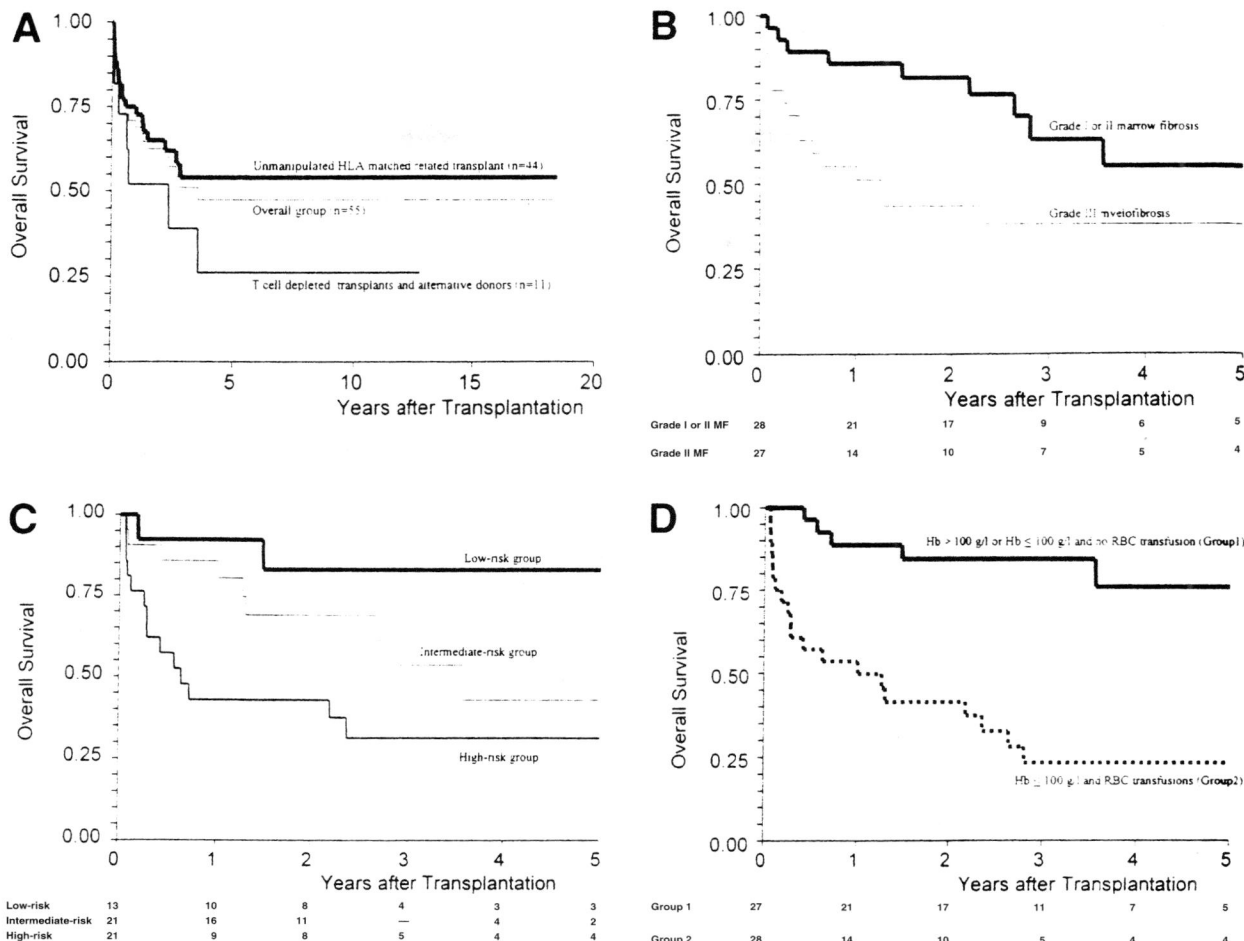

Fig. 53.1. **(A)** Actuarial probability of survival in 55 patients who received an allogeneic SCT for AMM. The 5-year probability of survival was 47% for the overall group, 54% for patients receiving an unmanipulated HLA-matched related transplant, and 26% for those receiving a T cell depleted graft or a graft coming from an alternative donor ($P = .18$). **(B)** Outcome according to the severity of myelofibrosis prior to transplant. The 5-year probability of survival was 55% if there was grade I or II marrow fibrosis, and 38% if there was grade III marrow fibrosis (osteomyelosclerosis) ($P = .027$). **(C)** Outcome according to the score proposed by Dupriez et al. (1996) before transplant. The 5-year probability of survival was 83% for the patients in the low-risk group, 43% for the patients in the intermediate-risk group, and 31% for the patients in the high-risk group ($P = .018$). **(D)** Outcome according to the hemoglobin level at transplant and the requirement of red blood cell transfusions before transplant. The 5-year probability of survival was 76% for patients with hemoglobin > 10 g/dl or with hemoglobin < 10 g/dl and no red blood cell transfusion before transplant, and 23% for patients with hemoglobin < 10 g/dl receiving pretransplant red blood cell transfusions ($P < .0001$). Reproduced, with permission, from Guardiola et al. (1999).

Awareness of the existence of a "graft-versus-myelofibrosis" effect suggests that reduced intensity conditioning regimens may provide improved outcome with respect to transplant-related mortality without necessarily jeopardizing disease ablation. Devine and colleagues (2002) reported 4 patients aged between 48 and 58 years, and Hessling et al. (2002) three between 44 and 58 years, who received reduced intensity conditioning prior to HLA-identical sibling or unrelated donor transplant. All patients engrafted and at a median follow-up of 13 (range 11–19) months were in hematological remission with regression of splenomegaly and bone marrow fibrosis and with full donor hematopoietic chimerism. The long-term efficacy with respect to disease control is less clear given that grade I fibrosis was still detectable in all patients at one year and 2

patients still had palpable splenomegaly. Donor lymphocyte infusions had not been administered at the time of the report, presumably in part due to the development of chronic GVHD in 3 of the 4 patients.

Autologous transplantation is an interesting and novel therapy for AMM. Anderson and colleagues (2001) reported a pilot study of the feasibility and efficacy of peripheral blood stem cell mobilization and subsequent transplantation: 26 of 27 patients aged 45–75 years of age were successfully mobilized (defined as >4.8 × 10^6 CD34+ cells/kg). The presence of increased numbers of clonogenic cells in the peripheral blood of patients with AMM has long been recognized (Wang et al., 1983; Hibbin et al., 1984; Craig et al., 1991); 21 patients have since received autografts following myeloablation with busulfan alone. Three patients experienced failure of neutrophil engraftment and one further patient received additional cells on day 26 because of life-threatening infection. Eight patients had prolonged thrombocytopenia and two of these also required further stem cells. Six of the 8 patients had undergone stem cell mobilization after chemotherapy. The median follow-up was 390 (range 70–1,623) days and the actuarial survival was 61% at 2 years (Figure 53.2). With respect to efficacy, 15 of the 21 patients showed evidence of clinical improvement particularly in the degree of cytopenia. Seven of 10 patients with pretransplant splenomegaly achieved a reduction in spleen size following the autograft. In 6 patients there was evidence of some reduction in the degree of fibrosis, although in those with osteomyelosclerosis there was no change in the marrow appearances after transplant. The mechanism of response is uncertain. The authors proposed a number of explanations including a reduction in fibrosis allowing improved intramedullary hematopoiesis, a reduction in splenic sequestration consequent on decreased spleen size, providing nonclonal stem cells with a proliferative advantage and the effect of overall debulking of the disease. Autologous transplantation is perceived as a potentially useful but largely palliative procedure that might offer an attractive treatment option for those unsuitable for allogeneic transplantation.

Polycythemia rubra vera

Polycythemia rubra vera (PRV) is an insidious clonal myeloproliferative disorder of pluripotential HSCs characterized by excessive erythropoiesis accompanied by low serum erythropoietin (EPO) levels. Two populations of erythroid progenitors have been identified in the marrow of patients with PRV (Bilgrami & Greenberg, 1995). One population responds normally to EPO and the other, the malignant clone, is exquisitely sensitive to EPO. The latter phenomenon is regarded as the most readily accepted explanation for the pathophysiology of this disease. The annual incidence is intermediate between that of CML and AMM and the mean age at onset is 60 with a range

of 15 to 85 years. Two phases of polycythemia are recognized; first the initial proliferative phase associated with an increased red cell mass and later a "spent," or post-polycythemic, phase in which cytopenias are associated with bone marrow fibrosis, extramedullary hematopoiesis, and hypersplenism. Clinical evolution occurs gradually over many years. Patients usually present with symptoms related to an increase in blood volume or viscosity. Thrombohemorrhagic complications, which usually correlate with the hematocrit level, are the most important because of their frequency and severity. Preventing such complications represents one of the most important therapeutic goals. Criteria for the diagnosis of PRV are shown in Table 53.2. Patients may also develop acute leukemia, which is increased in incidence if myelosuppressive therapy is used, compared to the use of phlebotomy alone.

Initial treatment is with phlebotomy to obtain a hematocrit of 45% or less. Phlebotomy is associated with the same survival as with the use of the radioisotope ^{32}P. Survival with each is superior to that with the alkylating agent chlorambucil, which produces excessive mortality from secondary malignancy. Hydroxyurea appears less leukemogenic than alkylating agents or ^{32}P, although some reports have questioned this. Interferon-α shows promise and may become a standard form of therapy in the future (for review see Bilgrami & Greenberg, 1995). The use of ^{32}P in the treatment of PRV has been reviewed by Parmentier and Gardet (1994). The efficacy and tolerability of interferon-α was evaluated in 17 patients (Taylor et al., 1996). Complete disease control was achieved after 1 to 12 months in nine patients with partial control in another five cases. Three patients failed to respond. Pruritus significantly improved in

Table 53.2. *WHO criteria for polycythemia rubra vera*

Category A
A1 Elevated red cell mass > 25% above mean normal predicted value, or Hb > 18.5 g/dl in men, >16.5 g/dl in women
A2 No cause of secondary erythrocytosis including
    Absence of familial erythrocytosis
    No elevation of EPO due to
    • Hypoxia (pO_2<92%)
    • High oxygen affinity hemoglobin
    • Truncated EPO receptor
    • Inappropriate EPO production by tumor
A3 Splenomegaly
A4 Clonal genetic abnormality other than the Ph chromosome or BCR/ABL fusion gene in marrow cells
A5 Endogenous erythroid colony formation in vitro

Category B
B1 Thrombocytosis >400 × 10^9/l
B2 White blood cell count >12 × 10^9/l
B3 Bone marrow biopsy showing panmyelosis with prominent erythroid and megakaryocytic proliferation
B4 Low serum erythropoietin levels
Diagnose PRV when A1 + A2 and any other category A are present, or when A1 + A2 and any two category B are present.

Abbreviations: Hb, hemoglobin; EPO, erythropoietin; PRV, polycythemia rubra vera.

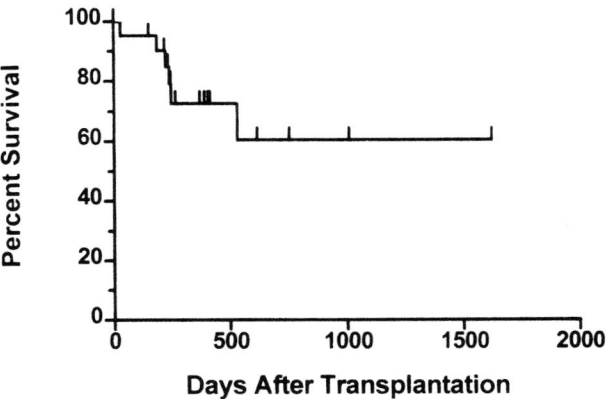

Fig. 53.2. Actuarial survival from day 0 for 21 patients who underwent transplantation. Tick marks represent surviving patients. Reproduced, with permission, from Anderson et al. (2001).

83% of cases. Six patients, however, were unable to tolerate interferon because of weight loss, myalgia, and mental changes. Interferon therapy significantly improved venesection requirements, platelet counts, pruritus scores, and the degree of splenomegaly. In the same study, analysis of pooled published data (100 evaluable patients) revealed an overall complete remission rate of 60%, a partial remission rate of 27%, and a failure rate of 13%.

The first report of a successful allogeneic transplant for fibrosis complicating spent PRV was described by de Revel et al. in 1995. This 35-year-old woman was prepared for a T-replete marrow graft with cyclophosphamide and total body irradiation. Hematologic recovery was rapid with an absolute neutrophil count of $0.5 \times 10^9/l$ by day 16 and a platelet count > $50 \times 10^9/l$ by day 35. Six months posttransplant, bone marrow histology was normal with disappearance of the fibrosis and a repeat ^{111}In study demonstrated normalization of medullary activity. The red cell volume studied by ^{51}Cr was not increased. These data were thought consistent with complete remission of both the myelofibrosis and the polycythemia vera. Since this case study there have been a number of further reports of transplantation for either spent phase polycythaemia or after progression to myelodysplasia and/or acute leukemia. Richard et al. (2002) described a 57-year-old man who received a transplant from his syngeneic twin twenty-five years after the original diagnosis. The conditioning regimen included total body irradiation and busulfan. Primary graft failure occurred and the patient was splenectomized and received further marrow-derived stem cells without additional conditioning therapy. This was followed by a prompt rise in peripheral counts and regression of fibrosis over the first year posttransplant. Unfortunately, recurrence of bone marrow hypercellularity, chromosomal abnormalities, and endogenous erythropoiesis were observed at day 446.

A small series of 10 patients allografted for polycythaemia have been described by the Seattle group together with 9 patients with an original diagnosis of essential thrombocythemia (Jurado et al., 2001). Ten patients received cells from HLA-identical sibling donors and the remainder from unrelated volunteers (n = 8) or a partially mismatched family member (n = 1). Three of the patients with polycythemia were in the spent phase and 7 others had transformed to myelodysplasia and/or acute leukemia. Eighteen of the 19 patients engrafted and once again, engraftment appeared to be more rapid in splenectomized patients. Twelve patients survived at a median follow-up of 41 (range 5–116) months including 5 of the 10 patients transplanted for polycythemia. The outcome was better for patients transplanted in the spent phase of either disease with 9 of 10 patients surviving compared to 3 of the 9 cases transplanted after transformation.

Allogeneic transplantation has also been performed for a small number of cases before the development of fibrosis and/or leukemic progression. One of these was a 14-year-old female who received an HLA-identical sibling transplant 34 months from diagnosis after preparation with busulfan 16 mg/kg and cyclophosphamide 200 mg/kg. The total dose of nucleated marrow cells was $3.9 \times 10^8/kg$. At the time of report, the patient was well 15 months posttransplant with a normal blood count, no splenomegaly, and no longer met the diagnostic criteria for polycythemia vera (Stobart & Rogers, 1994).

Interestingly, the presence of a graft-versus-tumor effect induced by donor lymphocyte infusions has been reported in a case of PRV with myelofibrosis who relapsed posttransplant: a complete response was obtained (Kolb et al., 1995).

Essential thrombocythemia

Essential thrombocythemia (ET) is the least common of the myeloproliferative disorders and is characterized primarily by the expansion of the megakaryocyte lineage. Diagnostic laboratory findings are shown in Table 53.3. The average age at diagnosis is in the 50s, although occasionally younger patients are seen. Many cases are diagnosed by the finding of a raised platelet count on investigation for other reasons. The most common presenting symptoms involve thromboembolic events, both of the microcirculation and of large vessels. Splenomegaly is detected in approximately 50% of patients and hepatomegaly in 20%. The platelet count is usually > $600 \times 10^9/l$ accompanied by hyperplasia of marrow megakaryocytes. Liver function is abnormal. Patients with ET have an almost normal life expectancy if thrombohemorrhagic complications are prevented or controlled.

The Philadelphia chromosome and the BCR-ABL rearrangement are absent in ET and this allows differentiation from cases of CML characterized primarily by an increased platelet count (Crisan et al., 1996). One review favored treatment of asymptomatic patients who have cardiovascular risk factors, but not of asymptomatic women who are pregnant or of childbearing age

Table 53.3. *WHO diagnostic criteria for essential thrombocythemia*

Positive criteria
Sustained platelet count > $600 \times 10^9/l$
Bone marrow biopsy specimen showing proliferation mainly of the megakaryocytic lineage with increased numbers of enlarged mature megakaryocytes
Criteria of exclusion
No evidence of polycythemia (see Table 53.2)
No evidence of CML
   No Philadelphia chromosome and no BCR/ABL fusion gene
No evidence of agnogenic myeloid metaplasia (chronic idiopathic myelofibrosis)
   Collagen fibrosis absent
   Reticulin fibrosis minimal or absent
No evidence of myelodysplastic syndrome
   No del 5q, t(3;3)(q21;q26), inv(3)(q21q26)
   No significant granulocyte dysplasia; few if any micromegakaryocytes
No evidence that the thrombocytosis is reactive due to
   Underlying inflammation or infection
   Underlying neoplasm
   Prior splenectomy

(Tefferi & Hoagland, 1994). Treatment may also be warranted in younger patients: in a study of patients with ET younger than 40, 12 of 36 had thrombohemorrhagic symptoms at diagnosis and 13 of 36 during follow-up. Four of the 36 patients experienced major complications, but leukemic transformation did not occur and none of the patients had died at the time of the report. Thus, young age does not appear to be a favorable prognostic factor for this disease.

New therapies have been reported: anagrelide, a drug that appears to inhibit megakaryocyte maturation and platelet release, has been shown to be effective in reducing platelet counts for prolonged periods of time in patients with ET (Silverstein et al., 1988; Chintagumpala, Kennedy, & Steuber, 1995; Storen & Tefferi, 2001). Interferon-α has also been utilized (Sacchi, 1995). The latter study summarized several reports in patients with ET who had shown a reduction in abnormal proliferation of megakaryocytes and splenomegaly, together with an improvement in hematologic parameters and clinical symptomatology. Long-term control can be obtained with a well-tolerated, low dose of interferon-α.

Nine patients transplanted for ET were reported in the analysis from Seattle of PRV and ET (Jurado et al., 2001) (see above under PRV); 7 were in the spent phase of the disease and 2 had experienced progression to more aggressive disease. Seven of the patients were alive at the time of the report. Five of the 7 were in complete hematological remission, although one had residual fibrosis and a further patient was being treated with interferon-α for a rising platelet count together with mixed donor chimerism.

Allogeneic HSC transplantation is a reasonable option for younger patients, and for those at risk of thrombohemorrhagic complications, who have an HLA-identical donor available and in whom other non-transplant therapies have failed.

Juvenile myelomonocytic leukemia

Juvenile myelomonocytic leukemia (JMML) is a rare disease of childhood defined by hyperleukocytosis with the presence of immature myeloid cells, monocytosis, hypercellularity of the bone marrow with a blast cell count <30%, and absence of the Philadelphia chromosome. Other features include the presence of fetal hemoglobin in excess of 10% and progressive thrombocytopenia. The incidence of JMML is approximately 1.3 per million children aged 0–14 years. Although it is a highly unusual cause of childhood leukemia, accounting for 2–3% of new presentations, JMML forms 20–30% of the myelodysplastic and myeloproliferative syndromes of childhood. Many patients are less than 2 years of age at diagnosis and 95% are less than age 4. Approximately 10% of cases occur in children affected by neurofibromatosis type 1.

JMML has variably been referred to as juvenile granulocytic leukemia, infantile monosomy 7, chronic and subacute myelomonocytic leukemia, and juvenile chronic myelogenous leukemia (JCML). However, an international consensus panel comprised of the JMML Working Group and the European Working Group of Myelodysplastic Syndromes in Childhood (EWOG-MDS) agreed upon the term JMML in 1994, and in addition agreed on clinical and laboratory criteria for diagnosis (Table 53.4) (Niemeyer et al., 1998). This nomenclature has helped distinguish JMML from Ph-positive chronic myeloid leukemia which can also occur in children, but some confusion continues to exist with respect to the adult disease, chronic myelomonocytic leukemia (CMML). The two conditions are similar but some important differences exist such as the absence of an elevated fetal hemoglobin level and the tendency to more complex cytogenetic abnormalities in CMML.

Patients present with malaise, bleeding, fever, and on examination pallor, hepatosplenomegaly, lymphadenopathy, and an eczematous facial rash are common. The white count is often over 100×10^9/l at presentation. A clonal chromosomal abnormality is found in 40% of patients at diagnosis. One study reported that patients with JCML have activating point mutations in Ras genes, while others show loss of the NF1 (neurofibromatosis type 1) gene, encoding a Ras GTPase-activating protein, resulting in hypersensitivity to granulocyte-macrophage colony-stimulating factor (GM-CSF) (Largaespada et al., 1996). The disease is usually extremely aggressive and resistant to conventional chemotherapy such as those normally utilized for CML or for acute myeloid leukemia. Most patients die within one year of diagnosis. Some may respond initially to chemotherapy but inevitably relapse and progress. Rare long-term survivors have been described. In general three therapeutic strategies have been used, either alone or successively.

- Single agent chemotherapy, e.g, 6-mercaptopurine, cytosine arabinoside, inteferon-α 13-cis retinoic acid. Transient responses have been recorded.
- Intensive remission induction chemotherapy protocols
- Allogeneic hematopoietic stem cell (HSC) transplantation from HLA-identical siblings or alternative donors, with or without prior chemotherapy.

There is little doubt that allogeneic stem cell transplantation is currently the only curative therapy for this disease. The first

Table 53.4. *Diagnostic criteria of juvenile myelomonocytic leukemia*

Peripheral blood monocytosis $>1 \times 10^9$/l
Blasts (including promyelocytes) are <20% of the white blood cells in the blood and of the nucleated bone marrow cells
No Philadelphia chromosome and no BCR/ABL fusion gene
Plus two or more of the following
    Fetal hemoglobin increased for age
    Immature granulocytes in the peripheral blood
    White cell count $>10 \times 10^9$/l
    Clonal chromosomal abnormality (e.g., monosomy 7)
    GM-CSF hypersensitivity of myeloid progenitors in vitro

Abbreviation: GM-CSF, granulocyte-macrophage colony-stimulating factor. Reproduced, with permission, from Niemeyer et al. (1998).

successful transplant for this condition was reported by Sanders *et al.* in 1979. Since then sizable numbers of transplants have been reported from both single institutions and collaborative groups. Matthes-Martin *et al.* (2000) reported not only their own experience of 11 children with JMML, but also summarized the outcome of 65 patients reported by single institutions (Sanders *et al.*, 1988; Urban *et al.*, 1990; Bunin *et. al.*, 1992; Rassam *et al.*, 1993; Donadieu *et al.*, 1994; Chown *et al.*, 1996; Locatelli *et al.*, 1996; MacMillan *et al.*, 1998; Orchard *et al.*, 1998). These patients were heterogeneous with respect to a number of important features, namely pretransplant therapy, degree of HLA compatibility, GVHD prophylaxis (including T-cell depletion), and conditioning regimens. Because of the fatal nature of the disease and the young age of the patients, partially matched family members are the most frequently used donors.

The overall transplant-related mortality was 21%, but was higher in recipients of alternative donor cells (unrelated and family mismatched donors) at 32% than in recipients of HLA-identical sibling marrow at 7%. Fourteen of the 65 patients were transplanted without any prior chemotherapy and 29 had received infusional combination chemotherapy. There was no significant difference in the transplant-related mortality between the treatment groups. An evaluation of the incidence of GVHD was complicated by the range of donors and the methods of prophylaxis employed. However, GVHD was a very uncommon cause of death. Twenty-four of 51 evaluable patients (47%) experienced disease relapse. Pretransplant chemotherapy, transplant within 6 months of diagnosis, and the use of total body irradiation did not protect against relapse. Rather surprisingly, the occurrence of GVHD also did not affect the incidence of relapse although any graft-versus-leukemia effect may have been obscured by the use of T-cell depletion; 11 of the 24 relapsed patients received additional therapy. In 6, immunosuppressive therapy was withdrawn with 2 children subsequently achieving complete remission. Donor lymphocyte infusions were successful in restoring remission in one of 2 patients. A second transplant was attempted in 7 children and effective in 3. A later report (Ohta *et al.*, 2000) described the successful use of interferon-α in restoring remission in a child who relapsed 9 months after stem cell transplantation.

Locatelli and colleagues (1997) reported data from the EBMT registry on 43 children. Twenty-five received transplants from an HLA-identical or one antigen disparate family member, 4 a more disparate family member transplant, and 14 from an HLA-matched unrelated donor. Total body irradiation and chemotherapy were used in 22 patients, whereas busulfan with other cytotoxic drugs was used in the remaining patients. Six of 43 patients failed to engraft, 5 of whom received a transplant from an alternative donor. Transplant-related mortality was 9% in those given HLA-identical or one-antigen disparate family member transplants and 46% in those given more mismatched family member transplant or a matched unrelated transplant. The probability of relapse for the entire group was 58% and the 5-year event-free survival was 31% (38% in those

given an HLA-identical sibling or a one antigen disparate family member transplant). In the latter group, patients who received busulfan had a better event-free survival compared to those given total body irradiation (62% vs. 11%). The suggestion that busulfan-containing conditioning regimens may result in a lower incidence of relapse compared to the use of total body irradiation was not substantiated by a retrospective review of Matthes-Martin *et al.* (2000). This documented an increased incidence of relapse in children conditioned with total body irradiation (61%) compared to chemotherapy-only regimens (21%). However the incidence of disease recurrence in patients given both total body irradiation and busulfan was 53%. Such retrospective studies are difficult to interpret when the reasons for choosing one or other conditioning regimens are not provided.

The efficacy of HSC transplantation for JMML was confirmed in an EWOG-MDS study (Hasle *et al.*, 1996), which described the outcome of 43 children treated with one of the three strategies. Fifteen children received no or low dose single agent therapy only. Six of the 15 were alive at the time of the report with two reaching 28 and 110 months from diagnosis. None of the 12 children treated with intensive chemotherapy survived. 16 patients were allografted, 8 after prior intensive chemotherapy. There were 8 survivors including 6 of the 8 who had not received prior therapy.

Smith *et al.* (2002) described 46 children who received marrow from unrelated donors facilitated by the National Marrow Donor Program (NMDP). Fory-three children engrafted. The incidence of acute (grades II–IV) and chronic GVHD was 73% and 40% respectively. At a median follow-up of 2 years, the probabilities of survival and disease-free survival were 42% and 24% respectively. Relapse remained the most important cause of treatment failure, being 58% at 2 years. Multivariate analysis showed that the presence of chronic GVHD was associated with a reduced risk of relapse and improved survival and event-free survival. Survival was inferior in patients with acute GVHD. Outcome was not affected by age, gender, disease bulk, fetal hemoglobin levels, or white cell count at diagnosis.

Interestingly, Grainger *et al.* (2002) described the successful outcome of autografting for an infant with JMML. A search for an unrelated donor was unsuccessful and the patient was progressing on 6-mercaptopurine. The disease was characterized by a t(1;5) chromosomal abnormality. Long-term marrow cultures were initiated in the laboratory and showed a gradual loss of clonal cells. These findings prompted the group to perform the autograft with cells cultured in vitro prior to infusion. The patient engrafted and initial bone marrow cytogenetics showed no evidence of the malignant clone. However, by 2 years post autograft the translocation was present in the majority of bone marrow derived cells. The child remained stable with a mildly increased white cell count with eosinophilia for a further 5 years. At 7 years posttransplant the malignant clone began to decline, becoming undetectable 9 years after the original autograft. This remarkable case may simply reflect the heterogeneity of the underlying disease or may suggest that the process of autografting gave a proliferative advantage to the normal stem cells.

Clearly, allogeneic transplantation is curative in this disease and is the treatment of choice, particularly for those with an HLA-identical or one-antigen disparate family member donor. However, results remain poor and there is considerable scope for improvement. Late complications may be a particular problem for survivors of transplant. Sanders *et al.* (1988) reported cataract development, learning difficulties, delayed puberty, and short stature in six long-term survivors.

Chronic neutrophil leukemia

Chronic neutrophil leukemia is a rare myeloproliferative disorder predominantly reported in elderly patients. In 20% of reported cases there was a co-existing second malignancy, most commonly multiple myeloma (Tursz *et al.*, 1974). In such cases clonal abnormalities have not been identified in the neutrophils and it remains possible that the neutrophilia is secondary to stimulation by cytokines produced by the malignant plasma cells. The disease is also sometimes known as neutrophilic chronic myeloid leukemia and generally runs a much more benign course than typical CML. The large majority of the circulating myeloid cells consist of mature granulocytes, the total white blood cell count is usually lower, anemia less severe, splenomegaly less prominent, and blastic transformation occurs much later. Three patients with chronic neutrophil leukemia were described who had the Philadelphia chromosome but a rare type of BCR-ABL rearrangement. The breakpoint on chromosome 22 was located between exon c3 and exon c4 of the BCR gene (i.e., distal to the M-BCR of typical CML) and gave rise to a 230 kd fusion protein (Pane *et al.*, 1996).

There is one report of a 15-year-old girl and a 25 year old male with chronic neutrophil leukemia, both of whom were treated successfully by allogeneic marrow transplantation (Hasle *et al.*, 1996). Clonal cytogenetic abnormalities were detected in both patients pretransplant. One showed trisomy 21 evolving into tetrasomy 21. The second showed a unique aberration during blast crisis: t(2;2)(q32;p24). Thus, allografting also appears to represent a potentially curative treatment for this rare disorder and should be seriously considered in appropriate patients.

Hypereosinophilic syndrome and chronic eosinophil leukemia

Chronic eosinophil leukemia (CEL) is characterized by the clonal proliferation of eosinophilic precursors resulting in peripheral eosinophilia. Damage to body organs can occur as a result of both leukemic infiltration and cytokine release from the malignant eosinophils. The diagnosis of CEL rests not only on the presence of eosinophilia ($>1.5 \times 10^9$/l) in the absence of the Philadelphia chromosome, but also on an increased number of blast cells in the blood or bone marrow and evidence of clon-

ality of the eosinophils. The latter evidence is absent in the majority of cases, which are then classified as idiopathic hypereosinophilic syndrome (HES), i.e., persistent eosinophilia for which no underlying cause can be found. The diagnosis of HES is frequently one of exclusion (Table 53.6). HES usually presents between the ages of 20 and 50 years and is almost 10-fold more common in men. The clinical manifestations are heterogeneous, perhaps reflecting the etiology of the syndrome, but also the organ damage induced by excessive numbers of eosinophils, and include fatigue, myalgia, fever, rash, cardiac disease, thromboembolic phenomena, peripheral neuropathy, encephalopathy, and gastrointestinal disturbance (Weller & Bubley, 1994).

No single or specific cytogenetic event has been identified in CEL or HES. One particular cytogenetic abnormality that may be associated with CEL is t(8;13)(p11;q12) and other 8p11 translocations which involve dysregulation of the *FGFR1* gene

Table 53.5   *WHO Criteria for chronic eosinophil leukemia and hypereosinophilic syndrome*

Required: persistent eosinophilia $>1.5 \times 10^9$/l in blood, increased numbers of bone marrow eosinophils and myeloblasts <20% in blood or marrow
Exclude all causes of reactive eosinophilia secondary to
• Allergy
• Parasitic disease
• Infectious disease
• Pulmonary disease (hypersensity pneumonitis, Loeffler's syndrome, etc).
• Collagen vascular disease
Exclude all neoplastic disorders with secondary, reactive eosinophilia
• T-cell lymphomas
• Hodgkin's disease
• Acute lymphoblastic leukemia
• Mastocytosis
Exclude other neoplastic disorders in which eosinophils are part of the neoplastic clone
• Chronic myeloid leukemia (Ph chromosome positive or BCR/ABL fusion gene positive)
• Acute myeloid leukemia, including those with inv(16), t(16;16)(p13;q22)
• Other myeloproliferative disorders, e.g., ET, PRV, AMM
• Myelodysplastic syndromes
Exclude T-cell population with aberrant phenotype and abnormal cytokine production
If there is no demonstrable disease that could cause the eosinophilia, no abnormal T-cell population and no evidence of a clonal myeloid disorder, diagnose HES.
If all of the requirements including the above conditions 1–4 have been met and if the myeloid cells demonstrate a clonal chromosomal abnormality, or are shown to be clonal by other means, or if blast cells are present in the peripheral blood (>2%) or are increased in the bone marrow (>5% but <19% of nucleated bone marrow cells) diagnose CEL.

Abbreviation: ET, essential thrombocythemia; PRV, polycythemic rubra vera; AMM, agnogenic myeloid metaplasia; HES, hypereosinophilic syndrome; CEL, chronic eosinophil leukemia.

normally located at 8p11 (Xiao *et al.*, 1998; Demiroglu *et al.*, 2001). The chronic myeloproliferative disorder characterised by the t(5;12) is associated with peripheral eosinophilia. This may represent a distinct disease entity and has some clinical features resembling chronic myelomonocytic leukemia (CMML) with peripheral blood monocytosis and evidence of myelodysplasia. The important molecular feature appears to be the involvement of the platelet-derived growth factor receptor-β (PDGFR-β) on chromosome 5q33. Steer and Cross (2002) reviewed the clinical features of myeloproliferative disorders with translocations of 5q31–35. The literature includes 34 patients with the classical t(5;12)(q31–33:p13), though in some cases involvement of PDGFR-β) was not definitely demonstrated. Most patients presented with myeloproliferative disorders variously designated MPD (myeloproliferative disorder), CMML, or Ph-negative CML. The great majority of patients were male with peripheral blood eosinophilia, monocytosis, and splenomegaly. Details of disease progression and overall outcome were incomplete, but a number of patients progressed to blastic transformation and the 2-year survival for the 18 evaluable patients was only 55%. An additional 20 patients were reported with reciprocal translocations involving 5q31–35 but not 12p13. The phenotype in this group was more diverse but certain similarities persist. Male predominance was less pronounced, the median age of onset was younger and the 2-year survival was 76%. However, all 11 evaluable patients had peripheral blood eosinophilia. There are anecdotal reports of good outcome in response to interferon-α, but a report of rapid and complete responses using imatinib mesylate may indicate that this tyrosine kinase inhibitor of PDGFR-β is now the treatment of choice (Apperley *et al.*, 2002). Rather surprisingly, imatinib mesylate also appears to have efficacy in cases of HES without any cytogenetic abnormality or obvious activation of any of its targets (Gleich *et al.*, 2002). If this initial report can be confirmed in further cases, imatinib mesylate may become first-line therapy for the more diverse syndrome.

A number of case reports have described the use of allogeneic HSC transplantation for HES. Sadoun and colleagues (1997) reported a 33 year old man with atypical HES who achieved complete remission with resolution of organ damage after an HLA-identical sibling transplant. Unfortunately his disease recurred 40 months after transplant. They also reviewed the three other cases in the literature at that time (Archimbaud *et al.*, 1988; Fukushima *et al.*, 1995; Sigmund & Flessa, 1995). All 3 patients were transplanted from HLA-identical sibling donors and only one had severe organ damage at the time of transplant. This individual died at day 83 of CMV pneumonitis, but the other two patients were alive in complete remission at 1 and 5 years postgraft. Vazquez (2000) described a successful HLA-identical sibling transplant using peripheral blood-derived stem cells in a 38-year-old woman with HES and extensive myelofibrosis. Allografting has a role in younger patients before the onset of severe organ damage and for whom chemotherapy is unlikely to be beneficial.

References

Anderson, J. E., Tefferi, A., Craig, F. *et al.* (2001). Myeloablation and autologous peripheral blood stem cell rescue results in hematologic and clinical responses in patients with myeloid metaplasia with myelofibrosis. *Blood*, **98**, 586–93.

Apperley, J. F., Gardembas, M., Melo, J. V. *et al.* (2002). Chronic myeloproliferative diseases involving rearrangements of the platelet derived growth factor beta receptor (PDGFRB) showing rapid responses to the tyrosine kinase inhibitor STI571. *New England Journal of Medicine*, **347**, 481–7.

Archimbaud, E., Guyotat, D., Guillaume, C. *et al.* (1988). Hypereosinophilic syndrome with multiple organ dysfunction treated by allogeneic bone marrow transplantation. *American Journal of Hematology*, **27**, 302–3.

Bandini, G., Ljungman, P., Arcese, G. *et al.* (1994). Allogeneic bone marrow transplantation for primary myelofibrosis. *Bone Marrow Transplantation*, **13**, 105a.

Bauermeister, D. E. (1971). Quantitation of bone marrow reticulin: a normal range. *American Journal of Clinical Pathology*, **56**, 24–31.

Benbassat, J. (2000). Myelofibrosis with myeloid metaplasia. *New England Journal of Medicine*, **343**, 659 (Letter).

Bilgrami, S. & Greenberg, B. R. (1995). Polycythemia rubra vera. *Seminars in Oncology*, **22**, 307–26.

Bunin, N. J., Casper, J. T., Lawton, C. *et al.* (1992). Allogeneic marrow transplantation using T-cell depletion for patients with juvenile chronic myelogenous leukemia without HLA-identical siblings. *Bone Marrow Transplantation*, **9**, 119–22.

Byrne, J. L., Beshti, H., Clark, D. *et al.* (2000). Induction of remission after donor leukocyte infusion for the treatment of relapsed chronic idiopathic myelofibrosis following allogeneic transplantation: evidence for a "graft vs. myelofibrosis" effect. *British Journal of Haematology*, **108**, 430–3.

Cahn, J. Y., Plouvier, E., Flesch, M., Carbillet, J. P., & Herve, P. (1987). T cell-depleted allogeneic bone marrow transplantation in case of childhood idiopathic myelofibrosis. *Bone Marrow Transplantation*, **2**, 209–11.

Cervantes, F., Barosi, G., Demory, J. L. *et al.* (1998). Myelofibrosis with myeloid metaplasia in young individuals: disease characteristics, prognostic factors and identification of risk groups. *British Journal of Haematology*, **102**, 684–90.

Cervantes, F., Rovira, M., Urbano-Ispizua, A. *et al.* (2000). Complete remission of idiopathic myelofibrosis following donor lymphocyte infusion after failure of allogeneic transplantation: demonstration of a graft-versus-myelofibrosis effect. *Bone Marrow Transplantation*, **26**, 697–9.

Chintagumpala, M. N., Kennedy, L. L., & Steuber, C. P. (1995). Treatment of essential thrombocythemia with anagrelide. *Journal of Pediatrics*, **127**, 495–8.

Chown, S. R., Potter, M. N., Cornish, J. *et al.* (1996). Matched or mismatched unrelated donor bone marrow transplantation for juvenile chronic myeloid leukemia. *British Journal of Haematology*, **93**, 674–6.

Craig, J. I. O., Anthony, R. S., & Parker, A. C. (1991). Circulating progenitor cells in myelofibrosis: the effect of recombinant alpha 2b interferon in vivo and in vitro. *British Journal of Haematology*, **78**, 155–60.

Creemers, G. J., Löwenberg, R., & Hagenbeek, A. (1992). Allogeneic bone marrow transplantation for primary myelofibrosis. *British Journal of Haematology,* **82,** 772–3.

Crisan, D., Mattson, J. C., O'Malley, B. A. *et al.* (1996). *bcr* gene rearrangement analysis in myeloproliferative disorders other than chronic myelogenous leukemia. *Cancer Detection and Prevention,* **20,** 263–9.

Deeg, H. J. Appelbaum, F. R. (2001). Stem cell transplantation for myelofibrosis. *New England Journal of Medicine,* **344,** 775 (Letter).

Demiroglu, A., Steer, E. J., Heath, C. *et al.* (2001). The t(8;22) in chronic myeloid leukemia fuses BCR to FGFR1: transforming activity and specific inhibition of FGFR1 fusion proteins. *Blood,* **98,** 3778–83.

de Revel, T., Girandier, S., Nedellec, G. *et al.* (1995). Allogeneic bone marrow transplantation for postpolycythemic myeloid metaplasia with myelofibrosis: a case report. *Bone Marrow Transplantation,* **16,** 187–9.

Devine, S. M., Hoffman, R., Verma, A. *et al.* (2002). Allogeneic blood cell transplantation following reduced-intensity conditioning is effective therapy for older patients with myelofibrosis with myeloid metaplasia. *Blood,* **99,** 2255–8.

Dokal, I., Jones, L., Deenmamode, M. *et al.* (1989). Allogeneic bone marrow transplantation for primary myelofibrosis. *British Journal of Haematology,* **71,** 158–9.

Donadieu, J., Stephan, J. L., Blanche, S. *et al.* (1994). Treatment of juvenile chronic myelomonocytic leukemia by allogeneic bone marrow transplantation. *Bone Marrow Transplantation,* **13,** 777–82.

Dupriez, B., Morel, P., Demory, J. L. *et al.* (1996). Prognostic factors in agnogenic myeloid metaplasia: a report of 195 cases with a new scoring system. *Blood,* **88,** 1013–8.

Fukushima, T., Kuriyama, K., Itom H. *et al.* (1995). Successful bone marrow transplantation for idiopathic hypereosinophilic syndrome. *British Journal of Haematology,* **90,** 213–5.

Gleich, G. J., Leiferman, K. M., Pardanani, A., Tefferi, A., & Butterfield, J. H. (2002). Treatment of hypereosiniphilic syndrome with imatinib mesilate. *Lancet,* **359,** 1577–8.

Grainger, J. D., Will, A. M., & Stevens, R. F. (2002). Cultured autografting for juvenile myelomonocytic leukaemia. *British Journal of Haematology,* **117,** 477–9.

Guardiola, P., Anderson, J. E., Bandini, G. *et al.* (1999). Allogeneic stem cell transplantation for agnogenic myeloid metaplasia. *Blood,* **93,** 2831–8.

Hasle, H., Olesen, G., Kerndrup, G. *et al.* (1996). Chronic neutrophil leukemia in adolescence and young adulthood. *British Journal of Haematology,* **94,** 628–30.

Hessling, J., Kröger, N., Werner, M. *et al.* (2002). Dose-reduced conditioning regimen followed by allogeneic stem cell transplantation in patients with myelofibrosis with myeloid metaplasia. *British Journal of Haematology,* **119,** 769–72.

Hibbin, J. A., Njoku, O. S., Matutes, E., Lewis, S. M., & Goldman, J. M. (1984). Myeloid progenitor cells in the circulation of patients with myelofibrosis and other myeloproliferative disorders. *British Journal of Haematology,* **57,** 495–503.

Ifrah, N., Gardembas-Pain, M., Hunault, M. *et al.* (1989). Allogeneic bone marrow transplantation for primary myelofibrosis. *British Journal of Haematology,* **73,** 575–6.

Iwata, N., Inoue, N., Tamura, A. *et al.* (1992). Primary myelofibrosis successfully treated with allogeneic bone marrow transplantation. *Japanese Journal of Clinical Hematology,* **33,** 1703–7.

Jouet, J. P., Noel, M. P., Facon, T. *et al.* (1994). BMT in a case of primary myelofibrosis. *Bone Marrow Transplantation,* **13** (Suppl 1), 42a.

Jurado, M., Deeg, H. J., Gooley, T. *et al.* (2001). Haemopoietic stem cell transplantation for advanced polycythemia vera or essential thrombocythaemia. *British Journal of Haematology,* **112,** 392–6.

Kolb, H. J., Schattenberg, A., Goldman, J. M. *et al.* (1995). Graft-versus-leukemia effective donor lymphocyte transfusions in marrow grafted patients. *Blood,* **86,** 2041–50.

Largaespada, D. A., Brannan, C. I., Jenkins, N. A., & Copeland, N. G. (1996). NF1 deficiency causes Ras-mediated granulocyte/macrophage colony stimulating factor hypersensitivity and chronic myeloid leukemia. *Nature Genetics,* **12,** 137–43.

Li, Z., Gooley, T., Appelbaum, F. R., & Deeg, H. J. (2001). Splenectomy and hemopoietic stem cell transplantation for myelofibrosis. *Blood,* **97,** 2180–1.

Locatelli, F., Niemeyer, C., Angelucci, E. *et al.* (1997). Allogeneic bone marrow transplantation for chronic myelomonocytic leukemia in childhood: a report from the European Working Group on Myelodysplastic Syndrome in Childhood. *Journal of Clinical Oncology,* **15,** 566–73.

Locatelli, F., Pession, A., & Comoli, P. (1996). Role of allogeneic bone marrow transplantation from an HLA-identical sibling or a matched-unrelated donor in the treatment of children with juvenile chronic myeloid leukaemia. *British Journal of Haematology,* **92,** 49–54.\

MacMillan, M. L., Davies, S. M., Orchard, P. J., Ramsay, N. K. C., & Wagner, J. E. (1998). Haemopoietic cell transplantation with juvenile myelomonocytic leukaemia. *British Journal of Haematology,* **103,** 552–8.

Matthes-Martin, S., Mann, G., Peters, C. *et al.* (2000). Allogeneic bone marrow transplantation for juvenile myelomonocytic leukaemia: a single centre experience and review of the literature. *Bone Marrow Transplantation,* **26,** 377–82.

Niemeyer, C. M., Fenu, S., Hasle, H. *et al.* (1998). Response: differentiating juvenile myelomonocytic leukemia from infectious disease. *Blood,* **91,** 365–66.

Ohta, H., Kawai, M., Sawada, A. *et al.* (2000). Juvenile myelomonocytic leukemia relapsing after allogeneic bone marrow transplantation successfully treated with interferon-alpha. *Bone Marrow Transplantation,* **26,** 681–3.

Orchard, P. J., Miller, J. S., McGlennan, R., Davies, S. M., Ramsay, N. K. C. (1998). Graft versus leukaemia is sufficient to induce remission in juvenile myelomonocytic leukaemia. *Bone Marrow Transplantation,* **22,** 201–3.

Pane, F., Frigeri, F., Sindona, M. *et al.* (1996). Neutrophilic chronic myeloid leukemia: a distinct disease with a specific molecular marker (BCR/ABL with C3/A2 junction). *Blood,* **88,** 2410–14.

Parmentier, C. & Gardet, T. (1994). The use of 32 phosphorus (^{32}P) in the treatment of polycythemia vera. *Nouvelle Revue Francaise Hematologie,* **36,** 189–92.

Rajantie, J., Sale, G. E., Deeg, H. J. *et al.* (1986). Adverse effect of severe marrow fibrosis on hematologic recovery after chemoradiotherapy and allogeneic bone marrow transplantation. *Blood,* **67,** 1693–7.

Rassam, S. M. B., Katz, F., Chessells, J. M., & Morgan, G. (1993). Successful allogeneic bone marrow transplantation in juvenile CML: conditioning or graft versus leukaemia effect? *Bone Marrow Transplantation,* **11,** 1247–50.

Richard, S., Isola, L., Scigliano, E. *et al.* (2002). Syngeneic stem cell transplantation for spent phase polycythaemia vera: eradication of myelofibrosis and restoration of normal haematopoiesis. *British Journal of Haematology,* **117,** 245–6.

Rossbach, H. C., Grana, N. H., Chamizo, W. *et al.* (1996). Successful allogeneic bone marrow transplantation for agnogenic myeloid metaplasia in a 3-year-old boy. *Journal of Pediatric Hematology and Oncology,* **18,** 213–15.

Sacchi, S. (1995). The role of alpha-interferon in essential thrombocythaemia, polycythemia vera and myelofibrosis with myeloid metaplasia (MMM): a concise update. *Leukemia and Lymphoma,* **19,** 13–20.

Sadoun, A., Lacotte, L., & Delwail, V. (1997). Allogeneic bone marrow transplantation for hypereosinophilic syndrome with advanced myelofibrosis. *Bone Marrow Transplantation,* **19,** 741–3.

Sanders, J. E., Buckner, C. D., Stewart, P., & Thomas, E. D. (1979). Successful treatment of juvenile chronic granulocytic leukemia with marrow transplantation. *Pediatrics,* **63,** 44–6.

Sanders, J. E., Buckner, C. D., Thomas, E. D. *et al.* (1988). Allogeneic marrow transplantation for children with juvenile chronic myelogenous leukemia. *Blood,* **71,** 1144–6.

Schmitz, N., Suttorp, M., Schlegelberger, B. *et al.* (1992). The role of the spleen after bone marrow transplantation of primary myelofibrosis. *British Journal of Haematology,* **81,** 616–18.

Sekhar, M., Prentice, H. G., Popat, U. *et al.* (1996). Idiopathic myelofibrosis in children. *British Journal of Haematology,* **93,** 394–7.

Sigmund, D. A. & Flessa, H. C. (1995). Hypereosinophilic syndrome: successful allogeneic bone marrow transplantation. *Bone Marrow Transplantation,* **15,** 647–8.

Silverstein, M. N., Petitt, R. M., Solberg, L. A, Jr. *et al.* (1988). Anagrelide: a new drug for treating thrombocytosis. *New England Journal of Medicine,* **318,** 1292–4.

Singhal, S., Powles, R., Treleaven, J. *et al.* (1995). Allogeneic bone marrow transplantation for primary myelofibrosis. *Bone Marrow Transplantation,* **16,** 743–6.

Smith, F. O., King, R., Nelson, G. *et al.* (2002). Unrelated donor bone marrow transplantation for children with juvenile myelomonocytic leukaemia. *British Journal of Haematology,* **116,** 716–24.

Smith, J. W., Shulman, H. M., Thomas, E. D., Fefer, A., & Buckner, C. D. (1981). Bone marrow transplantation for acute myelosclerosis. *Cancer,* **48,** 2198–203.

Soll, E., Massumoto, C., Clift, R. A. *et al.* (1995). Relevance of marrow fibrosis in bone marrow transplantation: a retrospective analysis of engraftment. *Blood,* **86,** 4667–73.

Steer, E. J. & Cross, N. C. P. (2002). Myeloproliferative disorders with translocations of chromosome 5q31–35: role of the platelet derived growth factor receptor. *Acta Haematologica,* **107,** 113–22.

Stobart, K. & Rogers, P. C. J. (1994). Allogeneic bone marrow transplantation for an adolescent with polycythemia vera. *Bone Marrow Transplantation,* **13,** 337–9.

Storen, E. C., & Tefferi, A. (2001). Long-term use of anagrelide in young patients with essential thrombocythemia. *Blood,* **97,** 863–6.

Sutton, L., Soussain, C., Travade, P., Binet, J. L., & Leblond, V. (1994). Unusual rise of peripheral blood erythroblats preceding peutrophil recovery after allogeneic BMT for primitive myelofibrosis with myeloid metaplasia. *Bone Marrow Transplantation,* **13** (Suppl 1), 40a.

Taylor, P. C., Dolan, G., Ng, J. P. *et al.* (1996). Efficacy of recombinant interferon-alpha (rIFN-alpha) in polycythemia vera: a study of 17 patients and an analysis of published data. *British Journal of Haematology,* **92,** 55–9.

Tefferi, A. (2000). Myelofibrosis with myeloid metaplasia. *New England Journal of Medicine,* **342,** 1255–65.

Tefferi, A. & Hoagland, H. C. (1994). Issues in the diagnosis and management of essential thrombocythemia. *Mayo Clinic Proceedings,* **69,** 651–5.

Tefferi, A., Mesa, R. A., Gray, L. A. *et al.* (2002). Phase 2 trial of imatinib mesylate in myelofibrosis with myeloid metaplasia. *Blood,* **99,** 3854–6.

Tefferi, A., Mesa, R. A., Schroeder, G. *et al.* (2001). Cytogenetic findings and their clinical relevance in myelofibrosis with myeloid metaplasia. *British Journal of Haematology,* **113,** 763–71.

Tursz, T., Flandrin, G., Brouet, J. C., & Seligmann, M. (1974). Coexistence of myeloma and a granulocytic leukaemia in the absence of any treatment: a study of four cases. *Nouvelle Revue Francaise Hematologie,* **14,** 693–704.

Urban, C., Schwinger, I., Slavc, I. *et al.* (1990). Busulfan/cyclophosphamide plus bone marrow transplantation is not sufficient to eradicate the malignant clone in juvenile chronic myelogenous leukemia. *Bone Marrow Transplantation,* **5,** 353–6.

Vazquez, L., Cabellero, D., Del Canizo, C. *et al.* (2000). Allogeneic peripheral blood cell transplantation for hypereosinophilic syndrome with myelofibrosis. *Bone Marrow Transplantation,* **25,** 217–8.

Villeval, J. L., Cohen-Solal, K., Tulliez, M. *et al.* (1997). High thrombopoietin production by hematopoietic cells induces a fatal myeloproliferative syndrome in mice. *Blood,* **90,** 4369–83.

Wang, J. C., Cheung, C. P., Ahned, F., Steier, W., & Tobin, M. S. (1983). Circulating granulocyte and macrophage progenitor cells in primary and secondary myelofibrosis. *British Journal of Haematology,* **54,** 301–7.

Weller, P. F. & Bubley, G. J. (1994). The idiopathic hypereosiniphilic syndrome. *Blood,* **83,** 2759–79.

Wolf, J. L., Spruce, W. E., Bearman, R. M. *et al.* (1982). Reversal of acute (malignant) myelosclerosis by allogeneic bone marrow transplantation. *Blood,* **59,** 191–3.

Xiao, S., Nalabolu, S. R., Aster, J. C. *et al.* (1998). FGFR1 is fused with a novel zinc-finger gene ZNF198 in the t(8;13) leukaemia/lymphoma syndrome. *Nature Genetics,* **18,** 84–87.

Yan, X. Q., Lacey, D., Fletcher, F. *et al.* (1995). Chronic exposure to retroviral vector encoded MGDF (mpl-ligand) induces lineage-specific growth and differentiation of megakaryocytes in mice. *Blood,* **86,** 4025–33.

Yan, X. Q., Lacey, D., Hill, D. *et al.* (1996). A model of myelofibrosis and osteosclerosis in mice induced by over-expressing thrombopoietin (mpl-ligand): reversal of disease by bone marrow transplantation. *Blood,* **88,** 402–9.

54 Allogeneic hematopoietic stem cell transplantation for myelodysplastic syndrome

THEO DE WITTE

University Hospital, Nijmegen, The Netherlands

Introduction

The myelodysplastic syndrome (MDS) consists of a group of clonal hematopoietic disorders characterized by ineffective hematopoiesis, refractory cytopenias, and a tendency to progress to acute myeloid leukemia (AML). MDS has been classified pathologically into five groups defined by the French-American-British (FAB) group (Bennett *et al.*, 1982) (Table 54.1): refractory anemia (RA), RA with ringed sideroblasts (RAS), RA with excess blasts (RAEB), RAEB in transformation (RAEBt), and chronic myelomonocytic leukemia (CMML). Additional categories that do not fit strictly into one of these FAB categories include MDS with myelofibrosis, hypoplastic MDS, refractory cytopenias with trilineage dysplasia, and therapy-related MDS (Kouides & Bennett, 1996; Rosati *et al.*, 1996). More recently the International Prognostic Scoring System (IPSS) (Greenberg *et al.*, 1997) (Table 54.1) has used a risk-based classification system to facilitate clinical decision-making. The score has a strong correlation with predicted median survival and use of the classification has achieved international acceptance. However, the IPSS excluded patients who have been treated with intensive antileukemic therapy. The IPSS might be less useful for predicting outcome after intensive chemotherapy and/or stem cell transplantation.

The incidence of MDS is increasing in younger patients due to better survival following irradiation or chemotherapy for primary malignancies. Overall, however, the median age at diagnosis is 65 years. Survival and risk of leukemic transformation in those given conventional therapy is shown in Table 54.2. A clonal chromosomal abnormality is seen in 40% to 60% of patients and the principal karyotypic changes in MDS are shown in Table 54.3. The characteristics of myleodysplasia (and AML) secondary to prior cytotoxic chemotherapy are shown in Table 54.4. Prognostic factors for outcome using both the Bournemouth scoring system (Mufti *et al.*, 1985) and the International Scoring System (Greenberg *et al.*, 1997) are shown in Table 54.5. Survival of patients with MDS categorized using the Bournemouth scoring system are shown in Figure 54.1; a comparison of survival between primary de novo MDS and chemotherapy-related MDS is shown in Figure 54.2.

Conventional treatment

The generally accepted policy of treatment for MDS of most patients is supportive therapy (Kantarjian *et al.*, 1986), mainly in view of the high average age of patients with MDS. The prognosis of MDS is variable, but most patients die of life-threatening cytopenias or evolution of the disease to acute leukemia. Younger patients have been treated with combination cytotoxic chemotherapy. Young patients with the morphologic picture of RAEBt (who have not been treated previously with cytotoxic therapy) may achieve prolonged, disease-free survival with this approach, but overall median remission duration appears to be shorter compared to de novo AML treated with chemotherapy only (de Witte *et al.*, 1990a, 1995). Low-dose cytosine arabinoside and vitamin A and D analogs have been assessed in several feasibility studies, but all approaches failed to induce a substantial percentage of complete remission. Improvement of leukocyte counts after administration of recombinant granulocyte-macrophage colony-stimulating factor (GM-CSF) and interleukin-3 (IL-3) have been observed, but responses have been incomplete and of short duration.

The median survival of patients with RAEB, RAEBt, or AML evolving from MDS is less than 12 months despite any treatment given (Bennett *et al.*, 1982). Patients with a Bournemouth score A (which excludes profound cytopenias) (Mufti *et al.*, 1985), patients without cytogenetic abnormalities, and patients with a normal growth pattern and normal in vitro differentiation in the CFU-GM assay have a median survival of more than 18 months. These categories of patients constitute a minority of patients with MDS. For this reason allogeneic hematopoietic stem cell (HSC) transplantation is the treatment of choice in the majority of young patients with histocompatible siblings.

Results of HLA-identical sibling transplantation

The first reported cases were transplanted more than 15 years ago (Marmont & Tura, 1986). Larger series of patients have been reported from Seattle (Appelbaum *et al.*, 1984, 1990; Anderson *et al.*, 1993) (Figs. 54.3 and 54.4) and City of Hope Hospital (O'Donnell *et al.*, 1987, 1995) (Figs. 54.5 to 54.7).

Table 54.1.   *The FAB and IPSS classification schemes for myelodysplasia*

FAB Classification System	IPSS Risk-Based Classification System

FAB Classification System

Refractory Anemia (RA): Cytopenia of one PB lineage; normo- or hypercellular marrow with dysplasias; <1% PB blasts and <5% BM blasts.

Refractory Anemia with Ringed Sideroblasts (RAS): Cytopenia, dysplasia and the same % blast involvement in BM and PB as RA. Ringed sideroblasts account for >15% of nucleated cells in marrow.

Refractory Anemia with Excess Blasts (RAEB): Cytopenia of two or more PB lineages; dysplasia involving all 3 lineages; <5% PB blasts and 5–20% BM blasts.

Refractory Anemia with Excess Blasts in Transformation (RAEBt): Hematologic features identical to RAEB. >5% blasts in PB or 21–30% blasts in BM or the presence of Auer rods in the blasts.

Chronic Myelomonoeytic Leukemia (CMML): Monocytosis in PB (>1 × 10^9 per liter); >5% blasts in PB and up to 20% BM blasts.

IPSS Risk-Based Classification System

Overall IPSS Risk Score Based On:

Marrow Blast Percentage

Blast%	IPSS Score
<5	0
5–10	0.5
11–20	1.5
21–30	2.0

Cytogenetic Features[a]

Karyotype	IPSS Score
Good prognosis (−Y, 5q−,20−)	0
Intermediate prognosis	0.5
Poor prognosis (abn. 7; complex)	1.0

Cytopenias[b]

Cytopenia	IPSS Score
None or 1 type	0
2 or 3 types	0.5

Overall IPSS Score and Survival

Overall Score	Median Survival
Low(0)	5.7 Yrs.
Intermediate	
1 (0.5 or 1.0)	3.5 Yrs
2 (1.5 or 2.0)	1.2 Yrs
High (≥2.5)	0.4 Yrs.

Abbreviations: FAB, French-American-British; IPSS, International Prognostic Scoring System; PB, peripheral blood; BM, bone marrow.
[a] IPSS Cytogenetic Classification: Good prognosis: −Y only, normal, del(5q) only, del(20q) only; Intermediate prognosis: +8, Single miscellaneous abnormality, double abnormalities: Poor prognosis: (i.e., ≥ 3 abnormalities), any chromosome 7 abnormality.
[b] IPSS Types of Cytopenia: Hemoglobin <10 g/dl; absolute neutrophil count <1500/mm³; platelet count <100,000/mm³.

Additionally, eight children with MDS at the Dana-Farber Cancer Institute (Guinan *et al.,* 1989) and 6 infants (less than 2 years of age) at the Fred Hutchinson Cancer Research Center (Woolfrey *et al.,* 1998) received an allogeneic transplant. Successful transplants have also been described in patients older than 55 (Deeg *et al.,* 2000). Bone marrow transplant (BMT) registries have collected data on many hundreds of

patients transplanted for myelodysplasia and the first analysis from the European registry (EBMT) was reported in 1990 (de Witte *et al.,* 1990b) (Fig. 54.8) and has been updated subsequently (de Witte *et al.,* 2000). Published reports of allogeneic bone marrow transplantation for MDS (series of at least 20 patients) are shown in Table 54.6.

The results of treatment with allogeneic BMT vary considerably depending on the stage of disease at the time of transplantation and other prognostic factors such as the presence of

Table 54.2.   *Survival and risk of leukemic transformation for patients with myelodysplasia treated conventionally*

FAB subtype (%)	Median survival (months) (range)	Leukemic transformation (%) (range)
RA (25)	37 (19–64)	11 (0–20)
RAS (18)	49 (21–76)	5 (0–15)
RAEB (28)	9 (7–15)	23 (11–50)
RAEBt (12)	6 (5–12)	48 (11–75)
CMML (17)	22 (8–60)	20 (3–55)
All patients		19

Reproduced, with permission, from Sanz & Sanz (1992).

Table 54.3.   *Principal karyotypic changes in myelodysplasia*

Subtype	5q−	−5	−7	+8	del/t(11q)
RA	70	<5	5	15	<15
RAS	30	<5	<5	25	20
RAEB/RAEBt	30	10	30	10	10
CMML	<5	<5	20	20	<5

Note: Data expressed as percentage of abnormal karyotypes in each group.

Reproduced, with permission, from Heim & Mitelman (1987).

Table 54.4. *Characteristics of myelodysplasia (MDS) and acute myeloid leukemia (AML) secondary to prior chemotherapy*

In addition to de novo presentation, MDS and AML can occur secondary to prior cytotoxic chemotherapy, in which case there is a poorer prognosis than with de novo disease.
Secondary MDS/AML has been found to be associated with use of the following agents:

1. Alkylating agents (e.g., MOPP, especially if radiotherapy also used): MDS with abnormalities of chromosome 5 or 7
2. Epipodophyllotoxins: AML with short latency (1–3 years); M4 or MS FAB subtype; 11q23 abnormalities
3. Anthracyclines: AML with properties similar to those of epipodophyllotoxin-induced AML
4. Anthracycline/cyclophosphamide: increased risk with high-dosage regimens using these agents; AML with properties similar to those of anthracycline-induced AML

Compared with de novo AML, secondary AML (or treatment-related AML)

1. Is less likely to enter CR1 with conventional chemotherapy
2. Is more likely to show prolonged cytopenia during remission induction

Abbreviation: MOPP, mechlorethamine, vincristine, procarbazine, prednisone.

Table 54.5. *Prognostic factors for outcome of myelodysplasia treated conventionally*

(1) Bournemouth scoring system (Mufti *et al.*, 1985)

Risk factor	Points
Hb <10 g/dl	1
Neutrophils <2.5 × 10^9/l	1
Platelets <100 × 10^9/l	1
Marrow blasts ≥5%	1

(2) International Scoring System (Greenberg *et al.*, 1997)

Risk group	Score[a]	Median survival (years) All patients	Median survival (years) ≤60 years	Time to 25% risk of AML evolution (years) All patients	Time to 25% risk of AML evolution (years) ≤60 years
Low	0	5.7	11.8	9A	>9.4
Intermediate-1	0.5–1.0	3.5	5.2	3.3	6.9
Intermediate-2	1.5–2.0	1.2	1.8	1.1	0.7
High	≥2.5	0.44	0.3	0.2	0.2

[a] Total score is based on sum of individual scores for marrow blast percentage, karyotype, and peripheral cytopenias. For marrow blast percentage, a score of 0 is given for blasts <5%; 0.5 for 5%–10%; 1.5 for 11%–20%; and 2.0 for 21%–30%. For karyotype, a score of 0 is given for normal, –Y, del(5q), or del(20q); 1.0 for ≥3 abnormalities or chromosome 7 anomalies; and 0.5 for other abnormalities. For peripheral cytopenias, a score of 0 is given for none or a single cytopenia and 0.5 for two or three cytopenias.

cytogenetic abnormalities, age, the percentage of blasts in the bone marrow at time of transplantation (Guinan *et al.*, 1989; de Witte *et al.*, 1990b; de Witte & Gratwohl, 1993; Anderson *et al.*, 1996b; Demuynck *et al.*, 1996b; Sutton *et al.*, 1996), and marrow fibrosis (O'Donnell *et al.*, 1995). The French Registry Study (Sutton *et al.*, 1996) reported on 71 consecutive patients with de novo MDS and found a better outcome among young patients, patients in an early stage of the FAB classification or with a low percentage of marrow blasts before transplantation, patients who did not undergo cytoreductive chemotherapy before transplantation, and those conditioned with total body irradiation (TBI) and cyclophosphamide. In contrast, Anderson *et al.* (1996b) found no difference in a historical comparison between cyclophosphamide and TBI versus busulfan and

cyclophosphamide. In their study variables independently associated with improved survival included younger age, shorter disease duration, a lower neutrophil count pretransplant, and a low hematocrit pretransplant. In another study Anderson and colleagues (1996c) explored a preparative regimen of busulfan, cyclophosphamide, and TBI for patients with advanced disease

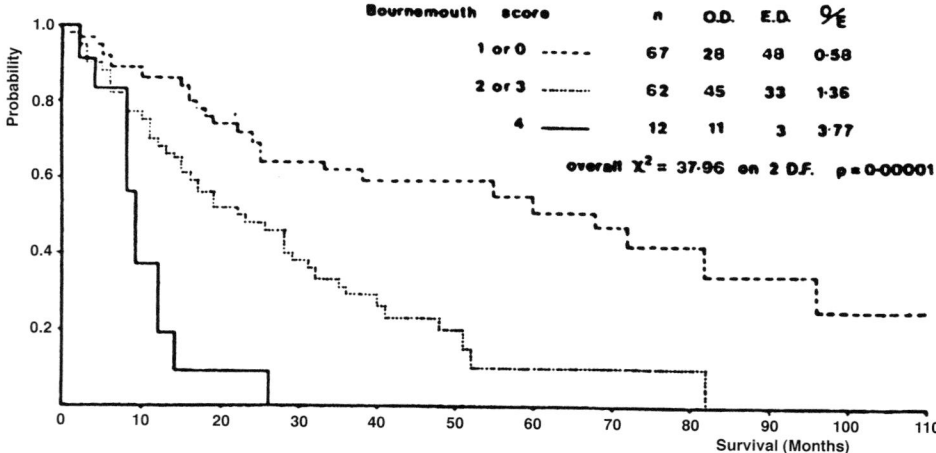

Fig. 54.1. Survival of patients with myelodysplastic syndrome categorized using the Bournemouth scoring system. Adapted from Mufti *et al.* (1985).

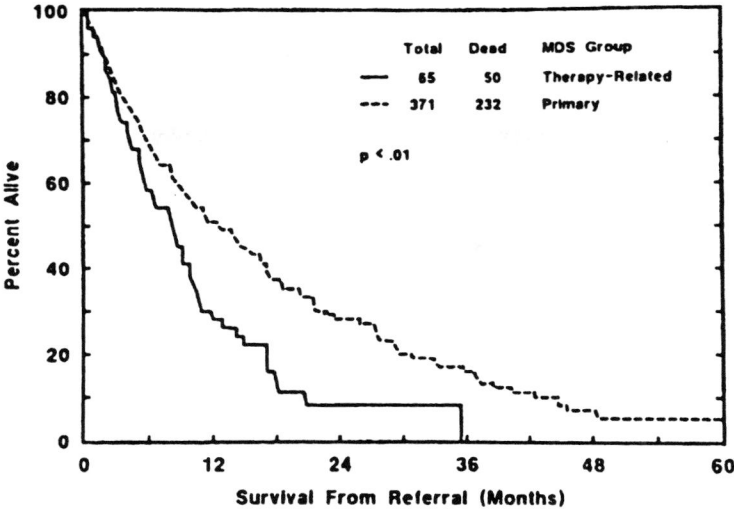

Fig. 54.2. Survival of patients at M. D. Anderson Cancer Center, Houston. Comparison of survival with primary MDS and treatment-related MDS. Reproduced, with permission, from Kantarjian, Estey, & Keating, (1993).

and found that they tolerated this intensified combination poorly (Figure 54.9).

A retrospective comparison of HLA-identical sibling PBSC transplantation versus marrow transplantation found a lower two-year transplant mortality rate in the PBSC recipients and improved 2 year event-free survival rate in all groups except those with refractory anemia or high-risk cytogenetics (Guadiola et al., 2002).

Refractory anemia with or without ringed sideroblasts

Refractory anemia (RA) or RA with ringed sideroblasts (RAS) without profound neutropenia or thrombocytopenia is characterized by a low risk of transformation and a median survival usually exceeding 30 months (Mufti et al., 1985). The remaining patients with MDS have median survival times of less than

18 months and they are generally considered good candidates for allogeneic HSC transplantation. Relapses are rare when a patient has been transplanted for RA(S), provided that the pre-transplant conditioning includes a bone marrow–ablative regimen, such as TBI and high-dose cyclophosphamide. Disease-free survival usually exceeds 50% after allogeneic transplantation (Appelbaum et al., 1990; de Witte et al., 1990b, 2000; Mattijssen et al., 1997; Runde et al., 1998;) (Figs. 54.10 and 54.11). Patients with the clinical picture of severe aplastic anemia (SAA) including a hypocellular marrow and severe pancytopenia, but with specific cytogenetic changes associated with MDS (such as monosomy 7) should also receive a bone marrow–ablative regimen. Three patients, prepared for transplantation with cyclophosphamide alone, showed either a persisting, or rapidly re-emerging, abnormal clone (Appelbaum et al., 1984). In the study by Runde and colleagues (1998),

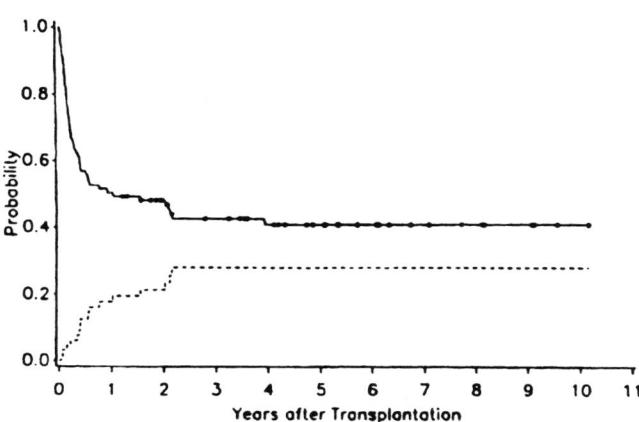

Fig. 54.3. Probability of DFS (solid line) and relapse (dashed line) for all 93 patients transplanted for MDS. Points represent patients alive in continuous complete remission. Reproduced, with permission, from Anderson et al. (1993).

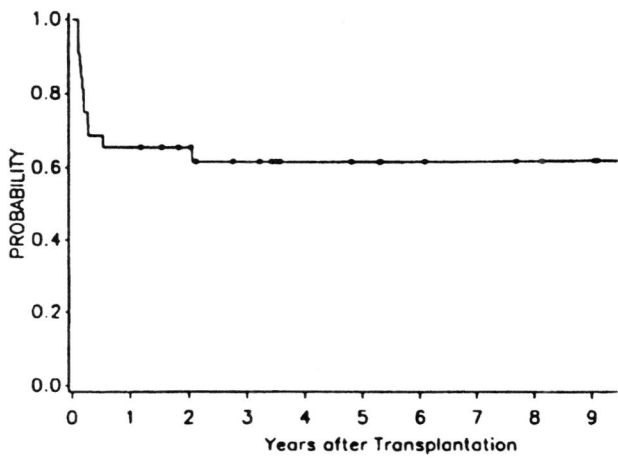

Fig. 54.4. Probability of DFS for 32 patients younger than 40 and without excess blasts. Points represent patients alive in continuous complete remission. Reproduced, with permission, from Anderson et al. (1993).

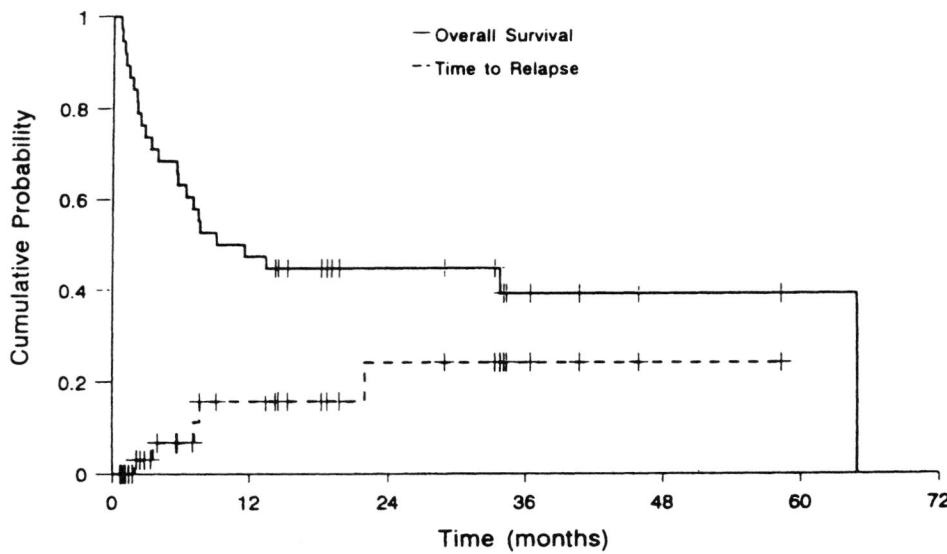

Fig. 54.5. Kaplan-Meier survival estimates and estimate of relapse for 38 MDS patients who received allogeneic BMT using BU/CY as conditioning regimen. Tick marks represent censored data points. Reproduced, with permission, from O'Donnell *et al.* (1995).

improved outcome posttransplant was associated with younger age (Fig. 54.12), shorter disease duration (Fig. 54.13), and absence of excess blasts in multivariate analysis. In the Seattle analysis disease duration was found to have a significant effect on transplanted-related complications, but not on disease-free survival in multivariate analysis (Appelbaum *et al.*, 1990). For this reason if an HLA-identical sibling donor is available, one should aim at early transplantation before sensitization due to transfusion of blood products has occurred, and before the development of iron overload and opportunistic infections.

However, postponement of the transplant may be justified in patients with a relatively good prognosis. These patients are

characterized by an absence of profound and life-threatening cytopenias and an absence of transfusion requirement.

RAEB and RAEBt

Twenty patients were transplanted for RAEB or RAEBt at the City of Hope Hospital (O'Donnell *et al.*, 1987). An increase in marrow blasts of >10% appeared to have a negative impact on disease-free survival, since three out of four relapses were in this group. Only 2 of 10 patients with this characteristic survived, compared to 6 of 10 patients who had less than 10% marrow blasts at the time of BMT. The EBMT analysis showed

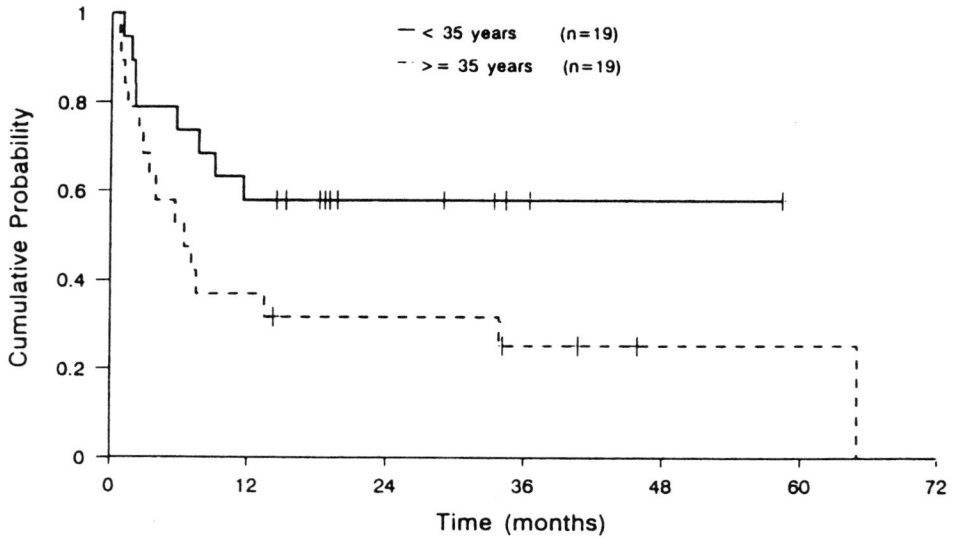

Fig. 54.6. Kaplan-Meier survival estimate for patients who received allogeneic BMT for MDS stratified by age ($P = .07$, log-rank test). Tick marks represent censored data points. Reproduced, with permission, from O'Donnell *et al.* (1995).

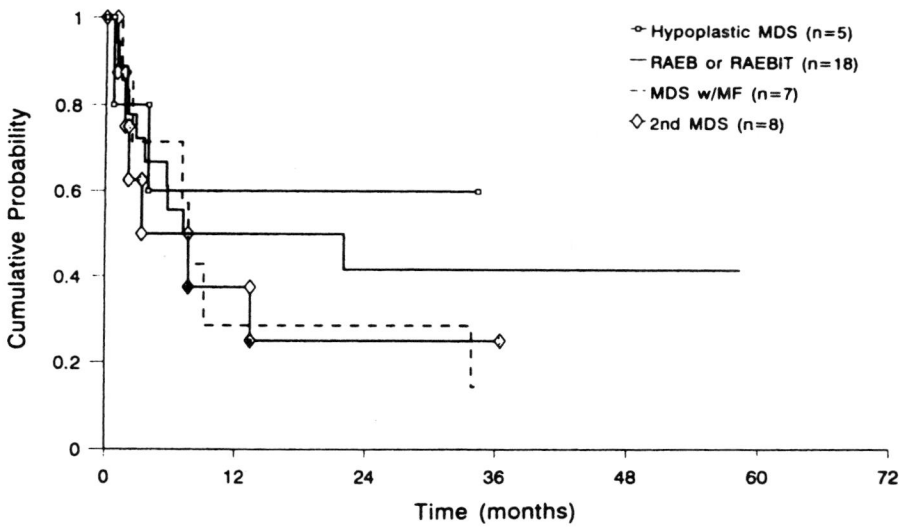

Fig. 54.7. Relapse-free survival probability stratified by histology (*P* = .64, log-rank test). Reproduced, with permission, from O'Donnell *et al.* (1995).

an actuarial disease-free survival (DFS) of 74% when the transplant was performed for a patient with RAEB and 50% for RAEBt (de Witte *et al.*, 1990b). A later reanalysis of the EBMT data showed a 3-year DFS of 32% for 18 patients transplanted for RAEB, and 27% of 11 patients transplanted for RAEBt. Late relapses occurred, especially in patients with RAEB, showing a relapse pattern similar to that of late phase chronic myeloid leukemia (CML) after allogeneic BMT. The actuarial relapse rate at 3 years posttransplant was more than 50% in this group (de Witte & Gratwohl, 1993). One of the analyses from

Seattle (Appelbaum *et al.*, 1990) showed a similar cumulative relapse risk of 45% in 30 patients transplanted with RAEB or RAEBt. Half of the relapses occurred more than 1 year after transplantation. It was hypothesized that more intensive conditioning regimens are needed to eradicate the disease in this category of patients (Appelbaum *et al.*, 1990).

An IBMTR study of 452 recipients included 136 patients with RAEB and 136 with RAEBt (Sierra *et al.*, 2002). The proportion of blast cells in the marrow before transplantation was the most important parameter predicting disease-free survival.

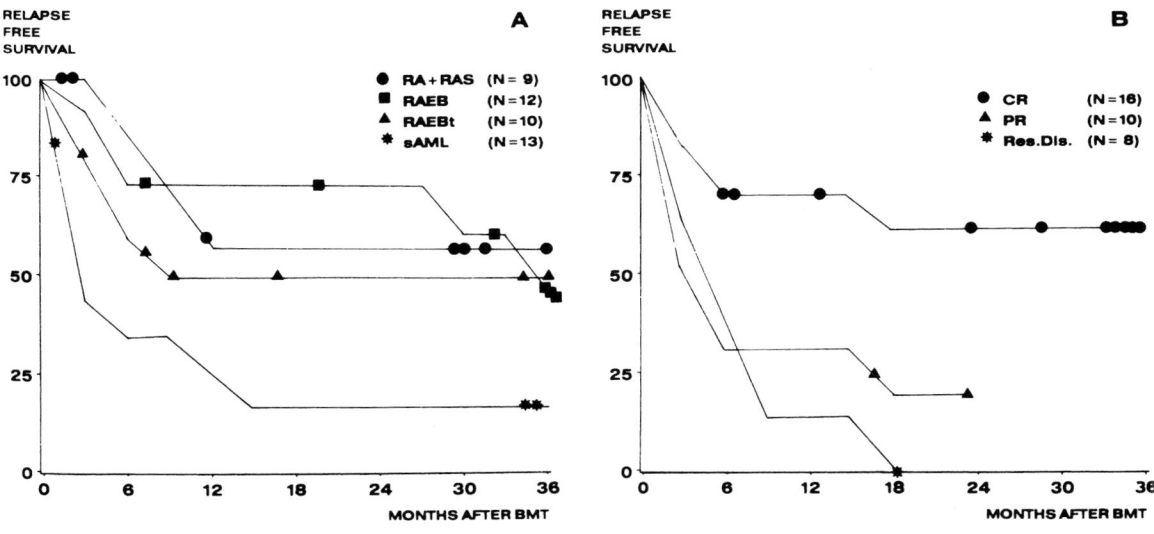

Fig. 54.8. Probability of relapse-free survival, according to the diagnosis and to stage of disease. (**A**) No prior intensive chemotherapy: RA + RAS (●), refractory anemia + RA with ring sideroblasts; RAEB (■), refractory anemia with excess of blasts; RAEBt (▲), RAEB in transformation; sAML (*), secondary acute myelogenous leukemia. (**B**) Prior intensive chemotherapy: CR (●), complete remission; PR (▲), partial responder; Res. Dis. (*), advanced disease. Symbols indicate surviving patients without evidence of leukemia or MDS, except for the symbol of advanced disease (*), which indicated the end of the curve; patients surviving beyond 33 months after BMT are indicated by symbols between 33 and 36 months post-BMT. Reproduced, with permission, from de Witte *et al.* (1990b).

Table 54.6.   *Published reports of allogeneic bone marrow transplantation (BMT) for myelodysplasia series comprising more than 20 patients*

Author, year	No. of patients Median age Median disease duration	Morphology at BMT, no. of patients	Preparative regimen, no. of patients	Donor, no. of patients	Median follow-up	Actuarial DFS (actual no. of patients)	Actuarial relapse (actual no. of patients)	Actuarial NRM (actual no. of patients)
Anderson *et al.*, 1993	93 30 yrs 10 mos	RA, 40 RAEB, 31 RAEBt, 14 CMML, 2 Other, 6	CY-TBI, 88 BU-CY, 5	HLA-id sib, 64 Syngeneic, 3 Other family, 20 Unrelated, 6	4 yrs	41%	28% (*n* = 17)	43% (*n* = 36)
de Witte *et al.*, 1990b	78 32 yrs 7 mos	RA, 9 RAEB, 16 RAEBt, 20 sAML, 32 CMML, 1	Chemotherapy +TBI, 69 –TBI, 9	HLA-id sib, 74 Syngeneic, 3 Other family, 1	2.3 yrs	Not stated (*n* = 35)	Not stated (*n* = 18)	Not stated (*n* = 25)
Sutton *et al.*, 1996	71 37 yrs 201 days	RA, 11 RAEB, 21 RAEBt, 21 sAML, 11 CR7	CY-TBI, 26 BU-CY, 17 Other, 28	HLA-id sib, 70 Syngeneic, 1	6 yrs	32%	48% (*n* = 24)	39% (*n* = 24)
Locatelli *et al.*, 1997	43 2 yrs 7 mos	CMML, 43	Chemotherapy +TBI, 22 –TBI, 21	Related, 29 Unrelated, 14	11 mos	31%	58% (*n* = 22)	20% (*n* = 7)
O'Donnell *et al.*, 1995	38 35 yrs 7 mos	Blasts <10%, 20 Blasts ≥10%, 18	BU-CY, 38	HLA-id sib, 38	Approx 2 yrs	38%	24% (*n* = 5)	Not stated (*n* = 19)
Anderson *et al.*, 1996c	31 41 yrs 5 mos	RAEB, 15 RAEBt, 8 CMML, 8	BU-CY-TBI, 31	HLA-id sib, 22 Other family, 3 Unrelated, 6	1.7 yrs	23%	28% (*n* = 6)	68% (*n* = 17)
Anderson *et al.*, 1996b	30 29 yrs 8 mos	RA, 30	BU-CY, 30	HLA-id sib, 16 Other family, 1 Unrelated, 13	2.1 yrs	63%	0% (*n* = 0)	37% (*n* = 11)

Ratanatharathorn et al., 1993	27	33 yrs 5.6 mos	RA, 9 RAEB, 8 RAEBt, 3 sAML, 6 Other, 1	BU-CY, 1 BU-AraC-CY, 24 BU-TLI, 2	HLA-id sib, 18 Other family, 6 Unrelated, 3	1.7 yrs	56%	Not stated (n = 1)	Not stated (n = 9)
Demuynck et al., 1996	24	30 yrs 5 mos	RA, 4 RAEB, 4 RAEBt, 9 CMML, 1 sAML, 6	CY-TBI ± chemotherapy, 24	HLA-id sib, 16 Other family, 5 Unrelated, 3	3.3 yrs	35%	25% (n = 6)	50% (n = 11)
Nevill et al., 1992	23	35 yrs 3 mos	RA, 2 RAEB, 2 RAEBt, 13 CMML, 1 Other, 5	BU-CY, 23 Other family, 1	HLA-id sib, 22	2.3 yrs	35%	Not stated (n = 5)	Not stated (n = 10)
Longmore et al., 1990	23	23 yrs 3 mos	RA, 6 RAEB, 6 RAEBt, 5 sAML, 6	Chemotherapy +TBI, 19 −TBI, 4	HLA-id sib, 21 Syngeneic, 1 Other family, 1	3.1 yrs	Not stated (n = 10)	Not stated (n = 4)	Not stated (n = 9)

Abbreviations: RA, refractory anemia; RAEB, RA with excess blasts; RAEBt, RAEB in transformation; sAML, secondary AML; CMML, chronic myelomonocytic leukemia; CY, cyclophosphamide; TBI, total body irradiation; BU, busulfan; AraC, cytosine arabinoside; TLI, total lymphoid irradiation; HLA-id sib, human leukocyte antigen identical sibling; DFS, disease-free survival; NRM, nonrelapse mortality; CR, complete remission.

Reproduced, with permission, from Gilliland *et al.* (1997).

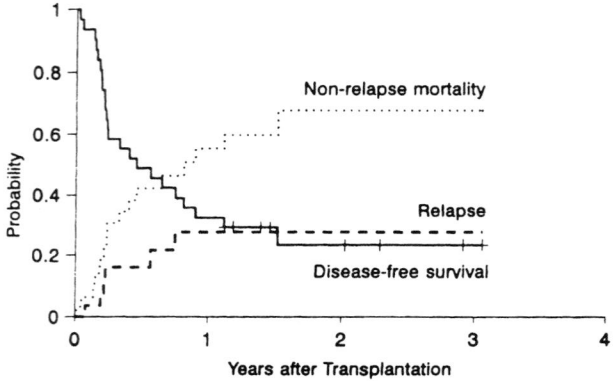

Fig. 54.9. DFS (—), relapse (- - - -), and nonrelapse mortality (......) following allogeneic marrow transplantation in 31 patients with advanced-
morphology MDS treated with BU/TBI. Tick marks represent patients alive
in continuous complete remission. Reproduced, with permission, from
Anderson *et al.* (1996b).

Secondary AML

Both therapy-related AML and AML evolved from a preceding phase of myelodysplasia can be considered secondary
AML (sAML). Many transplant centers will only consider
allogeneic transplantation after remission induction therapy.
The EBMT Leukemia Working Party conducted a survey
among member transplant centers. Ten of 14 responding centers preferred to perform allogeneic BMT after an attempt to
induce remission. The results of allogeneic BMT for patients
with overt sAML were worse compared to results of patients
transplanted for RAEB or RAEBt, with prolonged DFS of
around 20%. Some patients with sAML, with a hypocellular
marrow and unlikely to respond favorably to intensive
chemotherapy, have achieved prolonged disease-free interval
after allogeneic BMT without chemotherapy prior to the conditioning regimen (Marmont & Tura, 1986; Anderson *et al.*,
1997) (Fig. 54.14).

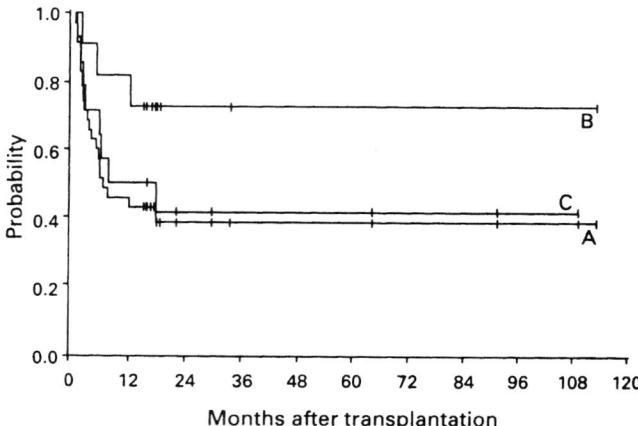

Fig. 54.11. Probability of DFS following BMT for patients with MDS. (A)
Total group (*n* = 35); (B) subgroup of patients with RA transplanted with
marrow from HLA-identical and MLC-negative siblings (*n* = 11); (C) sub-
group of patients with RAEB, RAEBt, CMML, or sAML, transplanted in
CR with marrow from HLA-identical and MLC-negative siblings (*n* = 14).
Log rank *P*, B vs C = 0.2. Bars represent patients alive in continuous CR.
Reproduced, with permission, from Mattijssen *et al.* (1997).

Therapy-related MDS or AML

Therapy-related MDS and AML occurring after chemotherapy
and/or radiotherapy are characterized by cytogenetic abnormalities most commonly associated with primary myelodysplasia
[abnormalities involving chromosome 5, 7, or 11, and complex
abnormalities (Rubin *et al.*, 1991)]. In 30% to 55% of patients
with therapy-related MDS evolution to AML occurs at a median
of 3 to 5 months, and median survival is usually short (12 to 30
weeks) (Kantarjian *et al.*, 1986). The clinical outcome after
chemotherapy is usually poor with only an occasional patient
surviving 1 year (Vaughan, Karp, & Burke, 1983). The actuarial
DFS of 11 patients transplanted for therapy-related MDS/AML
was 27% compared to a DFS of 56% of 12 patients transplanted

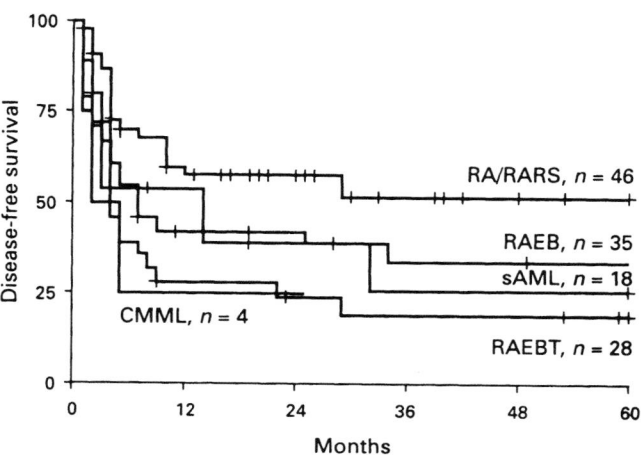

Fig. 54.10. Probability of DFS according to FAB diagnosis at the time of
transplant. Reproduced, with permission, from Runde *et al.* (1998).

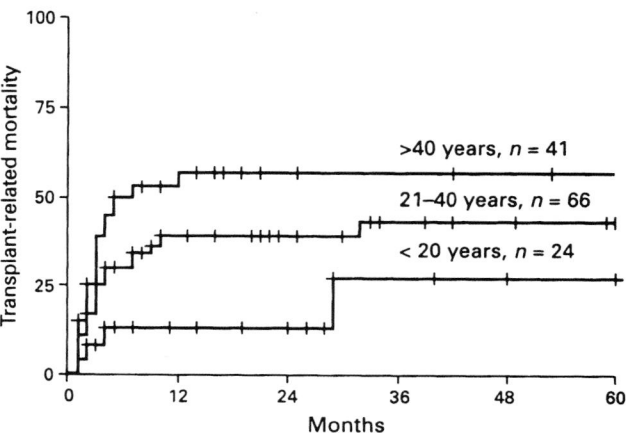

Fig. 54.12. Probability of transplant-related mortality according to age.
Reproduced, with permission, from Runde *et al.* (1998).

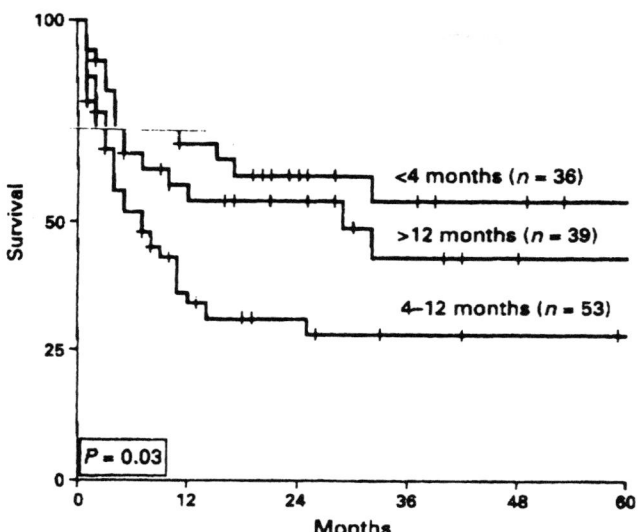

Fig. 54.13. Probability of survival according to interval between diagnosis and bone marrow transplantation. Reproduced, with permission, from Runde *et al.* (1998).

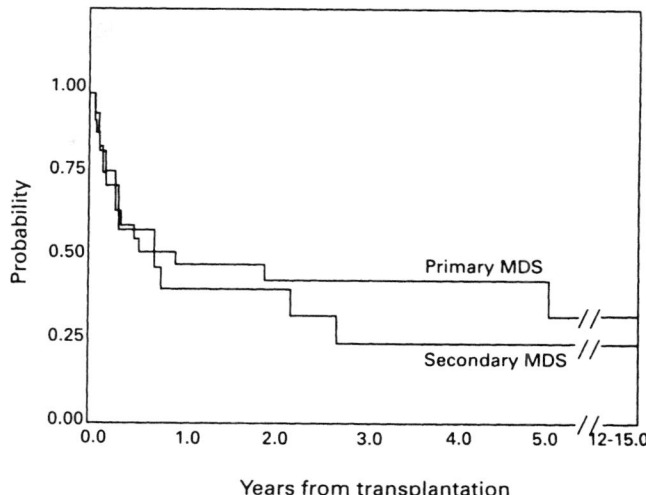

Fig. 54.15. Allogeneic BMT for myelodysplasia: all patients. Actuarial DFS of patients with primary MDS compared with secondary MDS. Reproduced, with permission, from Ballen *et al.* (1997).

for primary MDS. These two groups were not completely comparable, however, since the number of patients with overt AML was five in the therapy-related group compared to none in the control group (Longmore *et al.*, 1990). Similar outcome results were reported in a study by Ballen *et al.* (1997) (Fig. 54.15). All seven patients transplanted for AML secondary to treatment for Hodgkin's disease died of multiorgan failure (four patients) or leukemia (Sargur *et al.*, 1987). In another study, four patients with AML secondary to treatment for Hodgkin's disease were transplanted in first complete remission. Two patients were alive

and disease-free at the time of the report (Geller *et al.*, 1988). Only 4 of 21 children who developed secondary AML after treatment for ALL or NHL (and all of whom had received epipodophyllotoxin-containing regimens) became long-term disease-free survivors (Hale *et al.*, 1999). One of the analyses of the EBMT data (de Witte & Gratwohl, 1993) compared transplant results of 28 patients with therapy-related RAEBt or AML with the results of 53 patients with de novo RAEBt or AML evolved from MDS. The overall DFS was identical, but the relapse rate was slightly higher in the therapy-related group.In a retrospective survey of patients allografted for treatment-related

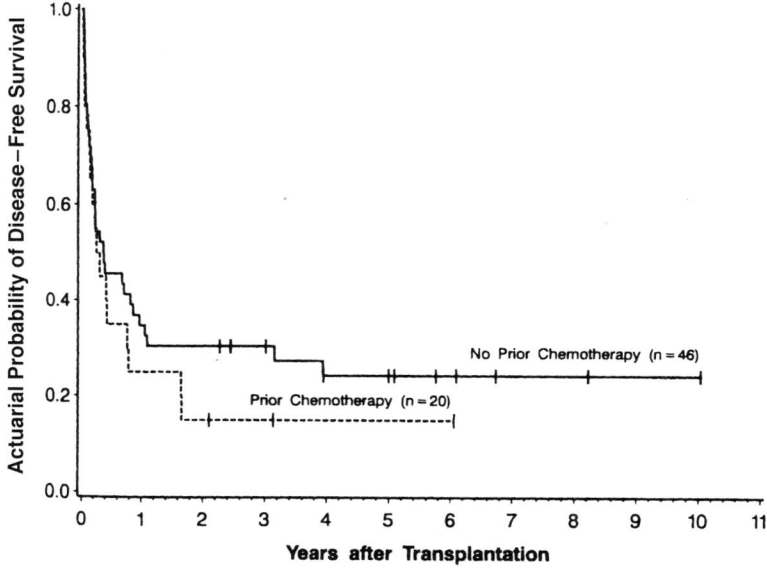

Fig. 54.14. Actuarial probability curves of DFS for patients with secondary AML who received induction chemotherapy before transplantation and were in first or second CR or first untreated relapse at time of transplantation (*n* = 20) compared to patients with secondary AML who received no induction chemotherapy before transplantation (*n* = 46). Tick marks represent patients alive in continuous CR. Reproduced, with permission, from Anderson *et al.* (1997).

AML or myelodysplasia, the 5 year disease-free survival was higher, and the incidence of non-relapse mortality lower, in patients conditioned with a busulfan/cyclophosphamide regimen determined by targeted busulfan levels compared to that in patients prepared for transplant with a non-targeted busulfan/cyclophosphamide regimen or in patients given a cyclophosphamide/TBI regimen (Witherspoon *et al.,* 2001). Other variables changed during this study, including the use of prophylactic fluconazole and prophylactic ganciclovir.

Chronic myelomonocytic leukemia

The modified Bournemouth score for CMML identified patients with a good prognosis and a clinical course similar to refractory anemia as well as those with a more aggressive course. Marrow infiltration with more than 5% monoblasts, a neutrophil count of more than $16 \times 10^9/l$, and/or a monocyte count of more than 2.6 $\times 10^9/l$ was associated with a poor prognosis. These patients are good candidates for allogeneic transplantation. The City of Hope Hospital report contained data on two patients with CMML. One patient was alive almost 3 years after BMT, whereas the other died of transplant-related complications (O'Donnell *et al.,* 1987). The European data for allogeneic transplantation for CMML in children showed a 38% event-free survival rate. Patients prepared with a busulfan-containing regimen did better than those receiving a TBI-containing regimen (Locatelli *et al.,* 1997) (Fig. 54.16). An EBMT study of 50 adults with CMML reported a treatment-related mortality rate of 52%, a 5-year estimated relapse rate of 49%, and a 5-year estimated disease-free survival rate of only 18% (Kroger *et al.,* 2002). A series from Seattle described a 3-year event-free survival rate for 21 patients of 39% and an actuarial relapse rate of 25% (Zang *et al.,* 2000).

Results of HLA-mismatched family member transplantation

Transplantation with family donors, other than HLA-identical siblings, is an option for patients without HLA-identical siblings. Updated analyses of the EBMT evaluated transplantation with genotypically nonidentical family member donors and compared the results to those obtained with unrelated donors and autologous stem cell transplantation (de Witte *et al.,* 2000, 2001b) (Figs 54.17 and 54.18). Overall three-year survival was 35% for the 79 patients transplanted using genotypically nonidentical donors; DFS was 31%, relapse risk 16%, and the treatment-related mortality (TRM) 62%. Patients transplanted using phenotypically identical family donors had a significantly superior survival and a lower TRM than patients transplanted with mismatched family donors. Age had no influence on the outcome of transplantation. The DFS of patients transplanted in early stage of the disease was 42% compared to 28% in patients transplanted with more advanced disease (*P* = .03).

The results of transplantation with mismatched family donors were comparable to those obtained with unrelated donor transplantation. This suggests that nonidentical family

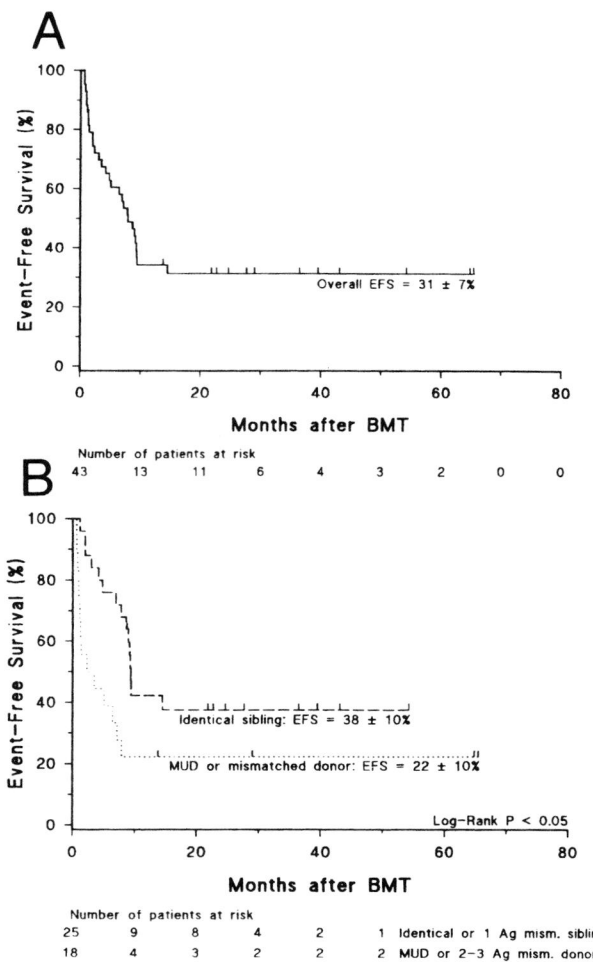

Fig. 54.16. Overall probability of EFS (**A**) for the entire cohort of patients and (**B**) for children transplanted using an HLA-identical sibling/1-antigen-disparate relative or a MUD/2 to 3-antigen-disparate relative. Reproduced, with permission, from Locatelli *et al.* (1997).

donors may be considered if a fully matched unrelated donor is not available. The TRM of patients transplanted with nonidentical family donors is significantly higher than the TRM of patients transplanted with autologous stem cells. The disease-free survival of autologous HSCT is not inferior to allogeneic transplantation using nonidentical family donors, and the intensity of the treatment is much lower. The choice of autotransplant or alternative donor transplantation must be influenced by the age of the patient and the risk of relapse.

Results of unrelated donor transplantation

The development of efficient, world-wide registries of HLA-typed volunteer unrelated donors (VUD) has made allogeneic HSCT with fully or partially matched unrelated donors a realistic possibility. Three analyses reported an 18 to 38 percent disease-free survival (Kernan *et al.,* 1993; Anderson *et al.,* 1996c; Arnold *et al.,* 1998). Non-relapse mortality was higher com-

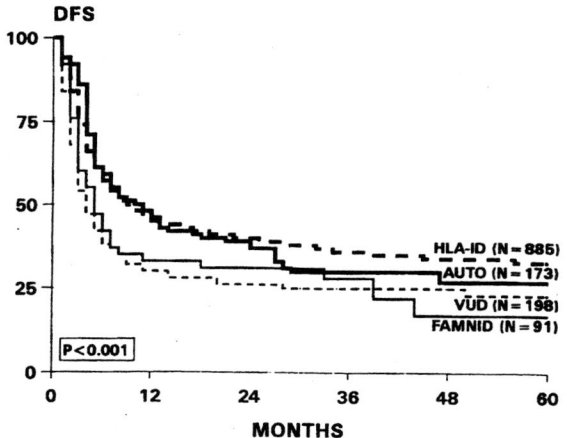

Fig. 54.17. Disease-free survival (DFS) of patients with myelodysplastic syndromes transplanted with stem cells from: histocompatible siblings (HLA-ID); genotypically non-identical relatives (FAMNID); volunteer unrelated donors (VUD); autologous stem cells (AUTO). Reproduced, with permission, from de Witte *et al.* (2000).

pared to that of HLA-identical related recipients. Increasing age was significantly associated with increased risk of death from non-relapse causes (Anderson *et al.*, 1996c; Arnold *et al.*, 1998). Fifty-two patients with MDS or MDS-related AML treated with unrelated donor marrow transplantation had a median age of 33 (range 1–53) years. Thirty-three of the 52 patients received chemotherapy and TBI as pretransplant conditioning, while 19 received busulfan and cyclophosphamide (Anderson *et al.*, 1996c). The donors were phenotypically identical at the HLA-A, -B, and -DRB1 loci in 34 cases, and mismatched for 1 HLA locus in 17 cases, and 2 loci in 1 case. T-replete marrow was administered and methotrexate with cyclosporine or tacrolimus (FK-506) was used as posttransplant

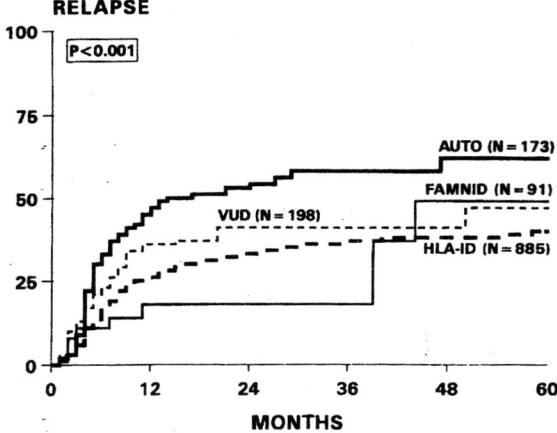

Fig. 54.18. Relapse risk of patients with myelodysplastic syndromes transplanted with stem cells from: histocompatible siblings (HLA-ID); genotypically non-identical relatives (FAMNID); volunteer unrelated donors (VUD); autologous stem cells (AUTO). Reproduced, with permission, from de Witte *et al.* (2000).

prophylaxis for graft-versus-host disease (GVHD). The 2-year disease-free survival and relapse rates were 38% and 28%, respectively, and the transplant-related mortality was 48%. Patients with MDS in transformation or with AML had a significantly higher risk of relapse than patients with less advanced disease. Increased nonrelapse mortality was significantly associated with higher recipient age, longer disease duration pretransplant, a lower neutrophil count on admission, and, unexpectedly, being seronegative for CMV. The report concluded that the outcome with transplantation using unrelated donors was similar to reported results using related donors and that, while cure was possible with this treatment, future studies should focus on reducing treatment-related toxicity. A subsequent Seattle study utilizing oral busulfan, with plasma concentrations targeted at 800-900 ng/ml, in combination with cyclophosphamide as conditioning reported a 56% probability of 3-year relapse-free survival for recipients of HLA-identical sibling transplants compared to 59% for recipients of HLA-identical unrelated grafts (Deeg *et al.*, 2002). The 3-year DFS probabilities for RA/RAS, RAEB, and RAEB-T/AML were 65%, 32%, and 18%, respectively. The 3-year DFS probabilities for IPPS risk low, intermediate-1, intermediate-2, and high were 80%, 64%, 40%, and 29%, respectively.

In an EBMT Registry study that included 198 patients transplanted from an unrelated donor, the estimated 3-year disease-free survival rate was 25% (Fig. 54.8) (de Witte *et al.*, 2000). The transplant-related mortality rate was 58% and the relapse risk 41% (Fig. 54.18). An NMDP registry study of 510 patients reported an incidence of graft rejection rate of 3%, a late graft failure rate of 8%, a grade II–IV acute GVHD rate of 47% and a two year cumulative incidence of treatment-related mortality of 54% (Castro-Malaspino *et al.*, 2002). The probability of disease-free survival at 2 years was 29%.

Results of cord blood transplantation

Seven adult patients with MDS-associated secondary AML were conditioned with total body irradiation 12 Gy, cytosine arabinoside 3 g/m^2 every 12 hours for a total dose of 12 g/m^2 and cyclophosphamide 60 mg/kg/day for two days prior to an unrelated cord blood transplant (Ooi *et al.*, 2001). Four of the grafts differed with the recipient at one, and three at two, HLA alleles. The number of nucleated cells infused ranged from 2.09 to 4.06 × 10^7/kg. Cyclosporine and methotrexate were used for GVHD prophylaxis. All patients engrafted; grade II–III acute GVHD occurred in two and extensive chronic GVHD in one. Two patients died of relapse at 3 and 10 months posttransplant respectively. The others were alive at 7+ to 31+ months posttransplant at the time of the report.

Results with reduced intensity conditioning regimens

The principle idea of reduced intensity conditioning regimen is to minimize the toxicity associated with myeloablative regimens and to allow the graft-versus-MDS effect of the infused donor lymphocytes to eradicate disease. Reduced intensity conditioning regimens have been explored because of the high treatment-related mortality after conventional marrow-ablative conditioning regimens, but results for MDS patients have been reported in abstract form only and the follow-up of these reported patients was limited. A fludarabine-based regimen was tested in 12 patients with MDS. Complete donor chimerism was observed in all 12 patients. The 2-year estimated DFS was 19% with failure due to relapse (4 patients) and toxicity (4 patients) (Kroger *et al.*, 2001). Parker and colleagues (2002) reported on 23 patients prepared for either a sibling or an unrelated donor allograft with fludarabine, busulfan, and Campath 1-H. Two-year actuarial disease-free survival was 39%, which was similar to that of a comparator group given myeloablative conditioning. A study using fludarabine and busulfan included 20 patients with MDS, as well as 17 with AML. The 1-year TRM and progression-free survival rates were 5% and 66%, respectively (Martino *et al.*, 2002). The 1-year incidence of disease progression was 13% and 58% in those with and without acute GVHD grade II-IV or chronic GVHD, suggesting a significant role for a GVL effect in minimizing relapse after this regimen. Investigational studies on reduced intensity regimens are warranted, especially in MDS patients older than 50 years and in patients with poor performance status.

Effect of cytogenetic abnormalities on treatment outcome

In an earlier Seattle analysis, cytogenetic abnormalities were significantly associated with better DFS compared to that of patients without a cytogenetic abnormality, largely due to a significantly increased incidence of transplant-related mortality in patients without cytogenetic abnormalities (Appelbaum *et al.*, 1990). A larger cohort of patients with longer follow-up in a more recent analysis from Seattle showed that cytogenetic abnormalities were no longer significantly associated with an improved outcome (Anderson *et al.*, 1993). The group with noncomplex abnormalities (monosomy 7, trisomy 8, or 5q–) had a significantly lower chance of relapse than did those with more complex abnormalities or those with no abnormalities (Appelbaum *et al.*, 1990). The EBMT analysis (de Witte & Gratwohl, 1993) showed an identical overall DFS when survival of patients with and without chromosomal abnormalities was compared. However, the relapse rate was significantly higher in the subgroup with cytogenetic abnormalities: 45% versus 8% in the group without cytogenetic abnormalities ($P = .03$). A French registry study showed a higher relapse rate for patients with complex cytogenetic abnormalities, resulting in low (14%) event-free survival (Sutton *et al.*, 1996). A retrospective study of 60 adult patients from Vancouver found that cytogenetic abnormalities were the only parameter predictive of event-free survival in multivariate analysis (Nevill *et al.*, 1998). The cytogenetic abnormalities were categorized according to the International MDS Workshop system (Greenberg *et al.*, 1997).

Influence of marrow cellularity on treatment outcome

Marrow cellularity may influence the transplant results in various ways. A hypercellular marrow may indicate a high tumor load and may be associated with a high relapse risk posttransplant. A hypocellular marrow and myelofibrosis may result in slow engraftment or graft failure. DFS was 38% at 1 year postgrafting in two comparable groups subdivided according to marrow cellularity, but no plateau was reached in the normo/hypercellular group due to continuous relapses occurring beyond 12 months from transplant. This resulted in a DFS of 26% in this group at 3 years posttransplant (de Witte & Gratwohl, 1993). Twelve patients with hypoplastic MDS had an outcome similar to the overall MDS population in the Seattle analysis. However, among six patients with grade 3 or 4 myelofibrosis, none survived (Appelbaum *et al.*, 1990). Patients with extensive marrow fibrosis appear to be at a higher risk for regimen-related mortality compared with those with little or no fibrosis (O'Donnell *et al.*, 1995).

Myelodysplastic syndrome treated with remission-induction chemotherapy prior to transplant

Patients with the morphologic picture of RAEB or RAEBt (Fenaux *et al.*, 1991a), patients of young age (de Witte *et al.*, 1990a), or patients treated within 3 months of diagnosis (Fenaux *et al.*, 1991a) respond favorably to cytotoxic chemotherapy, with remission rates approaching those of de novo AML. Remission duration of these patients, however, is usually short (de Witte *et al.*, 1990a, 1995), especially in those with cytogenetic abnormalities (Fenaux *et al.*, 1991b). These results suggest that these patients should be offered allogeneic transplantation as consolidation therapy in complete or partial remission after cytotoxic chemotherapy. The 2-year DFS was 60% for 16 patients transplanted in chemotherapy-induced complete remission (de Witte *et al.*, 1990b). Patients with a partial response after chemotherapy responded less well and showed a 2-year DFS of 18%, while none of those who either relapsed or were resistant to chemotherapy survived beyond 2 years from BMT.

Comparison with chemotherapy and autologous transplantation

Autologous stem cell transplantation (ASCT) may be a treatment option for MDS or secondary AML (sAML) patients without an HLA-identical sibling donor (de Witte *et al.*, 1997). A primary requisite for ASCT is complete remission with sufficient numbers of normal stem cells available for harvesting. Chemotherapy is capable of inducing cytogenetically normal complete remissions in the majority of MDS and sAML patients (de Witte *et al.*, 1995) and long-term polyclonal remissions in some patients (Aivado *et al.*, 2000). The peripheral stem cell harvests of patients with MDS are usually polyclonal, when assessed by PCR techniques based on X-chromosome inactivation patterns (Delforge *et al.*, 1995). Preliminary data indicate that hematopoietic reconstitution after transplantation with mobilized peripheral stem cells is much faster compared to reconstitution after autologous bone marrow transplantation (Demuynck *et al.*, 1996a).

An analysis of 79 patients from the Chronic Leukemia Working Party (CLWP) of the EBMT showed a 2-year DFS of 34% (de Witte *et al.*, 1997) after ASCT. This was statistically significantly inferior to the DFS achieved for an age-matched group of patients transplanted in first remission for de novo AML (de Witte *et al.*, 1997).

A prospective French study evaluated autologous stem cell transplantation in myelodysplastic syndromes (Wattel *et al.*, 1999). A complete remission was attained in 51% of patients (42 of 83). In 39 of these patients, 24 had either a transplant with autologous bone marrow cells (16 patients) or autologous peripheral stem cells (8 patients). Hematological reconstitution occurred in all autografted patients. However, this study did not demonstrate faster hemopoietic recovery for peripheral blood stem cells compared to bone marrow cells. The median DFS of the autografted patients was 29 months from transplantation.

A recently completed study from the EORTC Leukemia Study Group compared the results of intensive antileukemic therapy with the form of transplantation depending on the presence of a donor (de Witte *et al.*, 2001a). Twenty-eight of 39 patients (72%) with a donor, who were in remission after consolidation therapy, were allografted in CR1, and 36 of 59 patients (61%) without a donor received autologous stem cell transplantation in CR1. The 4-year DFS rates in the group of patients with or without a donor were 31% and 27%. The 4-year survival rates from CR were 36% and 33%, respectively. These results show the feasibility of ASCT in CR1 in a large prospective study. This is a reasonable treatment approach for those patients who lack a histocompatible sibling donor.

Indications and contraindications for allogeneic transplantation

Elderly patients, patients with significant comorbidity and MDS patients with a good prognosis should not receive intensive antileukemic therapy. For the remaining patients an allogeneic stem cell transplantation should be performed as soon as the diagnosis of MDS has been established if an HLA-identical sibling donor is available. In general, the treating physician should try to induce a complete remission with intensive chemotherapy if the percentage of marrow blasts exceeds 10%. The value of this approach will be explored in a planned prospective study in Europe. The intensity of the conditioning regimen is a matter of debate. The treatment-related mortality of 40% and higher after conventional conditioning justifies exploration of reduced intensity conditioning regimens, especially in patients older than 50 years and in patients with poor performance status.

If an HLA-identical donor is not available, transplantation with a phenotypically identical family donor (sibling, parent,

cousin) gives similar results to transplantation with histocompatible sibling donors. Second, transplantation from a nonidentical family member gives results not inferior to those obtained with matched unrelated donors. This implies that nonidentical family donors may be considered if a matched unrelated donor is not available. Third, if an sAML patient without a matched sibling is in first complete remission one may choose autologous stem cell transplantation. The disease-free survival is not inferior, and the intensity of the treatment is much lower. The decision may be influenced by the estimation of the relapse risk after autologous stem cell transplantation, which may be higher in some patients. For instance, patients in morphological remission with persistent cytogenetic abnormalities are considered at high risk for relapse after autologous stem cell transplantation. Therefore, the preferred treatment for these patients may be an allogeneic transplantation with a mismatched family member or an unrelated donor.

References

Aivado, M., Rong, A., Germing, U. *et al.* (2000). Long-term remission after intensive chemotherapy in advanced myelodysplastic syndromes is generally associated with restoration of polyclonal haemopoiesis. *British Journal of Haematology*, **110**, 884–6.

Anderson, E., Gooley, T. A., Schoch, G. *et al.* (1997). Stem cell transplantation for secondary acute myeloid leukemia: evaluation of transplantation as initial therapy or following induction chemotherapy. *Blood*, **89**, 2578–85.

Anderson, J. E., Anasetti, C., Appelbaum, F. R. *et al.* (1996c). Unrelated donor marrow transplantation for myelodysplasia (MDS) and MDS-related acute myeloid leukemia. *British Journal of Haematology*, **93**, 59–67.

Anderson, J. E., Appelbaum, F. R., Fisher, L. D. *et al.* (1993). Allogeneic bone marrow transplantation for 93 patients with myelodysplastic syndromes. *Blood*, **82**, 677–81.

Anderson, J. E., Appelbaum, F. R., Schoch, G. *et al.* (1996a). Allogeneic marrow transplantation for refractory anemia: a comparison of two preparative regimens and analysis of prognostic factors. *Blood*, **87**, 51–8.

Anderson, J. E., Appelbaum, F. R., Schoch, G. *et al.* (1996b). Allogeneic marrow transplantation for myelodysplastic syndrome with advanced disease morphology: a phase II study of busulfan, cyclophosphamide, and total-body irradiation and analysis of prognostic factors. *Journal of Clinical Oncology*, **14**, 220–6.

Appelbaum, F. R., Barrall, J., Storb, R. *et al.* (1990). Bone marrow transplantation for patients with myelodysplasia. *Annals of Internal Medicine*, **112**, 590–7.

Appelbaum, F. R., Storb, R., Ramberg, R. E. *et al.* (1984). Allogeneic transplantation in the treatment of preleukemia. *Annals of Medicine*, **100**, 689–93.

Arnold, R., de Witte, T., van Biezen, A. *et al.* (1998). Unrelated bone marrow transplantation in patients with myelodysplastic syndromes and secondary acute myeloid leukemia: an EBMT survey. *Bone Marrow Transplantion*, **21**, 1213–6.

Ballen, K.K., Gilliland, D. G., Guinan, E. C. *et al.* (1997). Bone marrow transplantation for therapy-related myelodysplasia: comparison with primary myelodysplasia. *Bone Marrow Transplantation,* **20,** 737–43.

Bennett, J.M., Catovsky, D., Daniel, M.D. *et al.* (1982). Proposals for the classification of the myelodysplastic syndromes. *British Journal of Haematology,* **51,** 189–99.

Castro-Malaspino, H., Harris, R. E., Gajewski, J. *et al.* (2002). Unrelated donor marrow transplantation for myelodysplastic syndromes: outcome analysis in 510 transplants facilitated by the National Marrow Donor Program. *Blood,* **99,** 1943–51.

Deeg, H.J., Shulman, H. M., Anderson, J. E. *et al.* (2000). Allogeneic and syngeneic marrow transplantation for myelodysplastic syndrome in patients 55 to 66 years of age. *Blood,* **95,** 1188–94.

Deeg, H.J., Storer B., Slattery, J.T. *et al.* (2002). Conditioning with targeted busulfan and cyclophosphamide for hemopoietic stem cell transplantation from related and unrelated donors in patients with myelodysplastic syndrome. *Blood,* **100,** 1201–7.

Delforge, M., Demuynck, H., Vandenberghe, P. *et al.* (1995). Polyclonal primitive hematopoietic progenitors can be detected in mobilized peripheral blood from patients with high-risk myelodysplastic syndromes. *Blood,* **86,** 3660–7.

Demuynck, H., Delforge, G., Verhoef, P. *et al.* (1996a). Feasibility of peripheral blood progenitor cell harvest and transplantation in patients with poor-risk myelodysplastic syndromes. *British Journal of Haematology,* **92,** 351–9.

Demuynck, H., Vernoet, G. E. G., Zachee, P. *et al.* (1996b). Treatment of patients with myelodysplastic syndromes with allogeneic bone marrow transplantation from genotypically HLA-identical siblings and alternative donors. *Bone Marrow Transplantation,* **17,** 745–51.

de Witte, T. & Gratwohl, A. (1993). Bone marrow transplantation for myelodysplastic syndromes and secondary leukaemias. *British Journal of Haematology,* **84,** 361–4.

de Witte, T., Hermans, J., Vossen, J. *et al.* (2000). Haematopoietic stem cell transplantation for patients with myelodysplastic syndromes and secondary acute myeloid leukemias: a report on behalf of the Chronic Leukemia Working Party of the European Group for Blood and Marrow Transplantation. *British Journal of Haematology,* **110,** 620–30.

de Witte, T., Muus, P., De Pauw, B., & Haanen, C. (1990a). Intensive antileukemic treatment of patients younger than 65 years with myelodysplastic syndromes and secondary acute myelogenous leukemia. *Cancer,* **66,** 831–7.

de Witte, T., Pikkemaat, T., Hermans, J. *et al.* (2001a). Genotypically nonidentical related donors for transplantation of patients with myelodysplastic syndromes: comparison with unrelated donor transplantation and autologous stem cell transplantation. *Leukemia,* **15,** 1878–84.

de Witte, T., Suciu, S., Peetermans, M. *et al.* (1995). Intensive chemotherapy for poor prognosis myelodysplasia (MDS) and secondary acute myelogenous leukemia following MDS of more than 6 months duration. A pilot study by the Leukemia Cooperative Group of the European Organization for Research and Treatment in Cancer. (EORT-LCG). *Leukemia,* **9,** 1805–10.

de Witte, T., Suciu, S., Verhoef, G. *et al.* (2001b). Intensive chemotherapy followed by allogeneic or autologous stem cell transplantation for patients with myelodysplastic syndromes (MDSs) and acute myeloid leukemia following MDS. *Blood,* **98,** 2326–31.

de Witte, T., van Biezen, A., Hermans, J. *et al.* (1997). Autologous bone marrow transplantation for patients with myelodysplastic syndrome (MDS) or acute myeloid leukemia following MDS. *Blood,* **90,** 3853–7.

de Witte, T., Zwaan, F., Hermans, J. *et al.* (1990b). Allogeneic bone marrow transplantation for secondary leukemia and myelodysplastic syndrome: a survey by the Leukaemia Working Party of the European Bone Marrow Transplantation Group (EBMTG). *British Journal of Haematology,* **74,** 151–7.

Fenaux, P., Laï, J. L., Quiquandon, I. *et al.* (1991b). Therapy-related myelodysplastic syndrome and leukemia with no "unfavourable" cytogenetic findings have a good response to intensive chemotherapy: a report on 15 cases. *Leukemia and Lymphoma,* **5,** 117–25.

Fenaux, P., Morel, P., Rose, C. *et al.* (1991a). Prognostic factors in adult de novo myelodysplastic syndromes treated by intensive chemotherapy. *British Journal of Haematology,* **77,** 497–501.

Geller, R. B., Vogelsang, G. B., Wingard, J. R. *et al.* (1988). Successful marrow transplantation for acute myelocytic leukemia following therapy for Hodgkin's disease. *Journal of Clinical Oncology,* **6,** 1558–61.

Gilliland, D. G., Silverstein, M. N., Anderson, J. E. *et al.* (1997). Myeloproliferative disorders and myelodysplastic syndromes. In *Hematology 1997,* ed. J. R. McArthur, G. P. Schechter, O. S. Platt, & J. L. Bajus, pp. 167–76, Washington, D.C: American Society of Hematology.

Greenberg, P., Cox, C., LeBeau, M. M. *et al.* (1997). International scoring system for evaluating prognosis in myelodysplastic syndromes. *Blood,* **89,** 2079–88.

Guardiola, P., Runde, V., Bacigalupo, A. *et al.* (2002). Retrospective comparison of bone marrow and granulocyte colony-stimulating factor-mobilized peripheral blood progenitor cells for allogeneic stem cell transplantation using HLA identical sibling donors in myelodysplastic syndromes. *Blood,* **99,** 4370–8.

Guinan, E. C., Tarbell, N. J., Tantravahi, R. *et al.* (1989). Bone marrow transplantation for children with myelodysplastic syndromes. *Blood,* **73,** 919–22.

Hale, G. A., Heslop, H. E., Bowman, L. C. *et al.* (1999). Bone marrow transplantation for therapy-induced acute myeloid leukemia in children with previous lymphoid malignancies. *Bone Marrow Transplantation,* **24,** 735–9.

Heim, S. & Mitelman, F. (1987). In *Cancer Cytogenetics.* New York: Alan R. Liss.

Kantarjian, H. M., Estey, E. H., & Keating, K. J. (1993). Treatment of therapy-related leukemia and myelodysplastic syndrome. In *Management of Acute Leukemia,* ed. C. D. Bloomfield & G. P. Herzig, pp. 81–107. Philadelphia: Saunders.

Kantarjian, H. M., Keating, M. J., Walters, R. S. *et al.* (1986). Therapy-related leukemia and myelodysplastic syndrome: clinical, cytogenetic, and prognostic features. *Journal of Clinical Oncology,* **4,** 1748–57.

Kernan, N. A., Bartsch, G., Ash, R. C. *et al.* (1993). Analysis of 462 transplantations from unrelated donors facilitated by the National Marrow Donor Program. *New England Journal of Medicine,* **328,** 593–602.

Kouides, P. A. & Bennett, J. M. (1996). Morphology and classification of the myelodysplastic syndromes and their pathologic variants. *Seminars in Hematology,* **33,** 95–110.

Kroger, N., Schetelig, J., Zabelina, T. *et al.* (2001). A fludarabine based dose-reduced condtioning regimen followed by allogeneic stem cell transplantation from related or unrelated donors in patients with myelodysplastic syndrome. *Bone Marrow Transplantation,* **28,** 643–7.

Kroger, N., Zabelina, T., Guardiola, P. *et al.* (2002). Allogeneic stem cell transplantation of adult chronic myelomonocytic leukaemia. A report on behalf of the Chronic Leukemia Working Party of the European Group for Blood and Marrow Transplantation (EBMT). *British Journal of Haematology,* **118,** 76–78.

Locatelli, F., Niemeyer, C., Angelucci, E. *et al.* and the European Working Group on Myelodysplastic Syndrome in Childhood. (1997). Allogeneic bone marrow transplantation for chronic myelomonocytic leukemia in childhood: a report from the European Working Group on Myelodysplastic Syndrome in Childhood. *Journal of Clinical Oncology,* **15,** 566–73.

Longmore, G., Guinan, E. C., Weinstein, H. J. *et al.* (1990). Bone marrow transplantation for myelodysplasia and secondary acute non-lymphoblastic leukemia. *Journal of Clinical Oncology,* **8,** 1707–14.

Marmont, A. M. & Tura, S. (1986). Bone marrow transplantation for secondary leukemia. Report of two cases. *Bone Marrow Transplantation,* **1** (Suppl 1), 191–2.

Martino, R., Caballero, M.D., Perez Simon, J.A. *et al.* (2002). Evidence for a graft-versus-leukemia effect ater allogeneic peripheral blood stem cell transplantation with reduced-intensity conditioning in acute myelogenous leukemia and myelodysplastic syndromes. *Blood,* **100,** 2243–5.

Mattijssen, V., Schattenberg, A., Schaap, N. *et al.* (1997). Outcome of allogeneic bone marrow transplantation with lymphocyte-depleted marrow grafts in adult patients with myelodysplastic syndromes. *Bone Marrow Transplantation,* **19,** 791–4.

Mufti, G. J., Stevens, J. R., Oscier, D. G. *et al.* (1985). Myelodysplastic syndromes: a scoring system with prognostic significance. *British Journal of Haematology,* **59,** 425–33.

Nevill, T. J., Fung, H. C., Shepherd, J. D. *et al.* (1998). Cytogenetic abnormalities in primary myelodysplastic syndrome are highly predictive of outcome after allogeneic bone marrow transplantation. *Blood,* **92,** 1910–7.

Nevill, T. J., Shepherd, J. D., Reece, D. E. *et al.* (1992). Treatment of myelodysplastic syndrome with busulfan-cyclophosphamide conditioning followed by allogeneic BMT. *Bone Marrow Transplantation,* **10,** 445–50.

O'Donnell, M. R., Long, G. D., Parker, P. M. *et al.* (1995). Busulfan/cyclosphosphamide as conditioning regimen for allogeneic bone marrow transplantation for myelodysplasia. *Journal of Clinical Oncology,* **13,** 2973–9.

O'Donnell, M. R., Nademanee, A. P., Snyder, D. S. *et al.* (1987). Bone marrow transplantation for myelodysplastic and myeloproliferative syndromes. *Journal of Clinical Oncology,* **5,** 1822–6.

Ooi, J., Iseki, T., Nagayama, H. *et al.* (2001). Unrelated cord blood transplantation for adult patients with myelodysplastic syndrome–related secondary acute myeloid leukemia. *British Journal of Haematology,* **114,** 834–6.

Parker, J.A., Safi, T., Pagliuca, A. *et al.* (2002). Allogeneic stem cell transplantation in the myelodysplastic syndromes: interim results of outcome following reduced-intensity conditioning compared with standard preparative regimens. *British Journal of Haematology,* **119,** 144–54.

Ratanatharathorn, V., Karanes, C., Uberti, J. *et al.* (1993). Busulfan-based regimens and allogeneic bone marrow transplantation in patients with myelodysplastic syndromes. *Blood,* **81,** 2194–9.

Rosati, S., Anastasi, J., & Vardiman, J. (1996). Recurring diagnostic problems in the pathology of the myelodysplastic syndromes. *Seminars in Hematology,* **33,** 111–26.

Rubin, C. M., Arthur, D. C., Woods, W. G. *et al.* (1991). Therapy-related myelodysplastic syndrome and acute myeloid leukemia in children: correlation between chromosomal abnormalities and prior chemotherapy. *Blood,* **78,** 2982–8.

Runde, V., de Witte, T., Arnold, R. *et al.* (1998). Bone marrow transplantation from HLA-identical siblings as first-line treatment in patients with myelodysplastic syndromes: early transplantation is associated with improved outcome. *Bone Marrow Transplantation,* **21,** 255–61.

Sanz, G. F. & Sanz, M. A. (1992). Prognostic factors in myelodysplastic syndromes. *Leukemia Research,* **16,** 77.

Sargur, M., Buckner, C. D., Appelbaum, F. R. *et al.* (1987). Marrow transplantation for acute nonlymphocytic leukemia following therapy for Hodgkin's disease. *Journal of Clinical Oncology,* **5,** 731–4.

Sierra, J., Perez, W.S., Rozman, C. et al. (2002). Bone marrow transplantation from HLA-identified siblings as treatment for myelodysplasia. *Blood,* **100,** 1997–2000.

Sutton, L., Chastang, C., Ribaud, P. *et al.* (1996). Factors influencing outcome in de novo myelodysplastic syndromes treated by allogeneic bone marrow transplantation: a long-term study of 71 patients. *Blood,* **88,** 358–65.

Vaughan, W. P., Karp, J. E., & Burke, P. J. (1983). Effective chemotherapy of acute myelocytic leukemia occurring after alkylating agent or radiation therapy for prior malignancy. *Journal of Clinical Oncology,* **1,** 204–7.

Wattel, E., Solary, E., Leleu, X. *et al.* (1999). A prospective study of autologous bone marrow or peripheral blood stem cell transplantation after intensive chemotherapy in myelodysplastic syndromes. *Leukemia,* **13,** 524–9.

Witherspoon, R. P., Deeg, H. J., Storer, B. *et al.* (2001). Hematopoietic stem cell transplantation for treatment-related leukemia or myelodysplasia. *Journal of Clinical Oncology,* **19,** 2134–41.

Woolfrey, A. E., Gooley, T. A., Sievers, E. L. *et al.* (1998). Bone marrow transplantation for children less than 2 years of age with acute myelogenous leukemia or myelodysplastic syndrome. *Blood,* **92,** 3546–56.

Zang, D. Y., Deeg, H. J., Gooley, T. *et al.* (2000). Treatment of chronic myelomonocytic leukaemia by allogeneic marrow transplantation. *British Journal of Haematology,* **110,** 217–22.

55 Allogeneic hematopoietic stem cell transplantation for myeloma and AL amyloidosis

GÖSTA GAHRTON

Karolinska Institute and Huddinge University Hospital, Stockholm, Sweden

Introduction

Multiple myeloma is an invariably fatal neoplastic disorder with a median survival of about 36 months with conventional chemotherapy treatment (Alexanian *et al.*, 1969). Using either low-dose continuous melphalan or intermittent melphalan and prednisolone therapy, about 50% of patients respond with a decrease in monoclonal immunoglobulin secretion and a reduction in the number of plasma cells in the bone marrow. However, complete remissions, defined as disappearance of monoclonal immunoglobulin from the serum, or of light chains from the urine and no detectable myeloma cells in the bone marrow, are rare using such treatment. There are considerable data regarding prognostic factors for response to conventional dose chemotherapy (Bataille *et al.*, 1986) (Table 55.1). The most important are age, Salmon-Durie stage (Table 55.2), serum β_2 microglobulin levels, and plasma cell labeling index.

In the early 1980s attempts were made to induce complete remission by high-dose melphalan therapy. This, indeed, increased the fraction of patients entering complete remission (CR) (McElwain & Powles, 1983; Selby *et al.*, 1987). Further studies showed that there was a dose-response relationship.

Thus, the remission rate could be increased if the melphalan dose was increased from 70 to 100 to 140 mg/m². Also, increased frequency of remission was associated with a progressive extension of relapse-free and overall survival duration (Barlogie *et al.*, 1988). At higher dosages, or if high-dose melphalan treatment was combined with total body irradiation (TBI), even higher frequencies of remission could be obtained, but rescue with autologous bone marrow transplantation (ABMT) was required (Barlogie *et al.*, 1987; Selby *et al.*, 1987). High-dose chemoradiotherapy followed by autologous hematopoietic stem cell (HSC) transplantation is an interesting approach for the treatment of patients with multiple myeloma

Table 55.1. *Prognostic factors in multiple myeloma*

Patient related
  Age
  Performance status
Disease-related
  Salmon-Durie stage
  Bone marrow plasmacytosis
  Extent of lytic bone lesions
  Labeling index
  DNA content and RNA content by flow cytometry
  β_2-microglobulin
  Albumin
  Hemoglobin
  Serum calcium
  Serum creatinine
  Lactic dehydrogenase
  Chemotherapy response

Table 55.2. *Staging of multiple myeloma*

Stage	Criteria

I.	All of the following:
	1. Hemoglobin value >10 g/dl
	2. Serum calcium value normal
	3. Normal bone structure (scale 0)[a] or solitary bone plasmacytoma only
	4. Low paraprotein production rates
	  a. IgG value <5 g/dl
	  b. IgA value <3 g/dl
	  c. Urine light chain paraprotein on electrophoresis <4 g/24 hours

II.	Neither stage I nor stage III

III.	One or more of the following:
	1. Hemoglobin value <8.5 g/dl
	2. Serum calcium value raised
	3. Advanced lytic bone lesions (scale 3)[a]
	4. High paraprotein production
	  a. IgG value >7 g/dl
	  b. IgA value >5 g/dl
	  c. Urine light chain paraprotein (Bence Jones protein[b]) on electrophoresis >12 g/24 hours

[a] Scale of bone lesions: normal bones (0); osteoporosis (1); lytic bone lesions (2); extensive skeletal destruction and major fractures (3).
Subclassification: A = normal renal function; B = abnormal renal function.
[b] Henry Bence Jones, British physician, 1814–1907.

(Barlogie & Gahrton, 1991). However, the lesson from the use of such treatment in patients with leukemia is that, in comparison to treatment with allogeneic bone marrow transplantation (BMT), the relapse rate is relatively high. One reason for this may be that the autologous graft contains neoplastic cells. Another, and perhaps more likely explanation, is that the allogeneic graft may induce a graft-versus-tumor effect (Weiden et al., 1981; Horowitz et al., 1990), which is lacking following autologous transplantation.

The first two myeloma patients who received allogeneic bone marrow transplants survived 6 and 36 months, respectively (Ozer et al., 1984). Promising results in the use of allogeneic marrow transplantation for treatment of multiple myeloma were published independently by the Huddinge Group (Gahrton et al., 1986) and the Bologna group (Tura et al., 1986). One of the first three patients who received a bone marrow graft at Huddinge Hospital, and who had disease that was resistant to conventional prednisolone/melphalan therapy, entered a CR that lasted 4 years. Such results triggered further attempts to treat multiple myeloma with allogeneic marrow transplantation (Gahrton et al., 1987; Buckner et al., 1989). The European Group for Blood and Marrow Transplantation (EBMT) opened a registry for myeloma transplants in 1983 and started to publish the results in 1987 (Gahrton et al., 1987). Since then more than 1,800 patients with multiple myeloma have received allogeneic grafts from HLA-matched sibling donors at more than 200 European transplant centers (Gahrton et al., 2001).

Information on disease incidence, classification, immune phenotype, cytogenetic abnormalities, prognostic factors, outcome with conventional therapy, disease-specific pretransplant work-up, monitoring for residual disease posttransplant, and a treatment algorithm are given in Chapter 40.

Results of HLA-identical sibling transplantation

The results of HSC transplantation for myeloma are very dependent on the condition of the patient before transplantation. Thus, patients who are in stage I at diagnosis irrespective of the stage before allografting, patients who already are in CR before transplantation or patients who have received only one type of treatment prior to transplantation appear to have a higher chance of entering CR following transplantation. In the EBMT study (Gahrton et al., 1991, 1995) 56% of patients who received only one type of pretransplant treatment entered a CR posttransplant, but only 35% of those who had received three or more types of treatment did so. Similarly, of the patients who were in CR before transplantation, 83% were also in remission following engraftment while only 24% of the patients who had progressive disease pretransplant entered a CR posttransplant. Immunoglobulin isotype and serum β_2 microglobulin level at diagnosis also have an impact.

The time from transplant to CR varies considerably. Most patients will enter CR within the first 3 months, but in other patients monoclonal immunoglobulin may persist in the serum or light chains in the urine for several months or even years. Likewise, myeloma cells may persist for several months in the marrow. Then, without further treatment (except for graft-versus-host prophylaxis), patients who engraft may eventually enter a CR. This seems to indicate that the graft itself has a graft-versus-myeloma effect similar to the previously demonstrated graft-versus-leukemia effect (Weiden et al., 1981; Horowitz et al., 1990).

Bone lesions

Radiologic bone lesions are usually not significantly affected by HSC transplantation. In only 7 out of 58 evaluable patients in the EBMT study (Gahrton et al., 1991) did the severity of the lesions decrease (i.e., major lytic lesions changed to minor lesions in three patients and minor lesions disappeared in four patients). It is not known whether the lesions harbor viable myeloma cells. In those patients who later relapse, it seems likely that they do; however, in those patients who stay in remission for many years, they may not. Biopsy results have not been reported in long-term survivors following HSC transplantation.

Survival and disease-free survival

The overall 4-year survival in patients with multiple myeloma given HLA-identical sibling allografts was 32% in a previous EBMT study (Gahrton et al., 1995). In an update in 1998 (Gahrton et al., 1998), 35 patients were still alive more than 4 years following transplantation, and 17 of these patients were still in CR. The outcome seemed to be dependent on the same factors important for obtaining a complete response. Thus, in the EBMT study the best results were obtained in patients who were in stage I (Fig. 55.1), in CR, or had received only one type of treatment before BMT (Fig. 55.2). In these patients, the 4-year survival was between 42% and 52%. For those who were in stage III, had progressive disease, or had received two or more types of treatment, the 4-year survival was between 20% and 30%. Similarly, in a report on 26 patients, 21 of whom had chemosensitive disease, Reece et al. (1995) reported a progression-free survival rate of 52% in chemoresponsive patients versus 0% in chemoresistant patients with a median follow-up of 14 months.

The most important posttransplant factor for long-term survival was obtaining CR (Fig. 55.3). Patients that engrafted and obtained CR had a median survival of approximately 4 years following transplantation.

A significant improvement in outcome due to less transplant-related mortality has been documented for transplants performed between 1994 and 1998 versus those performed during 1983–1993. The transplant-related mortality was reduced from 30% to 21% at 6 months (Fig. 55.4) and the overall 4-year survival improved from 32 months to 50 months (Fig. 55.5). The improvement was apparently related to fewer deaths from bacterial and fungal infections, and from interstitial pneumonitis,

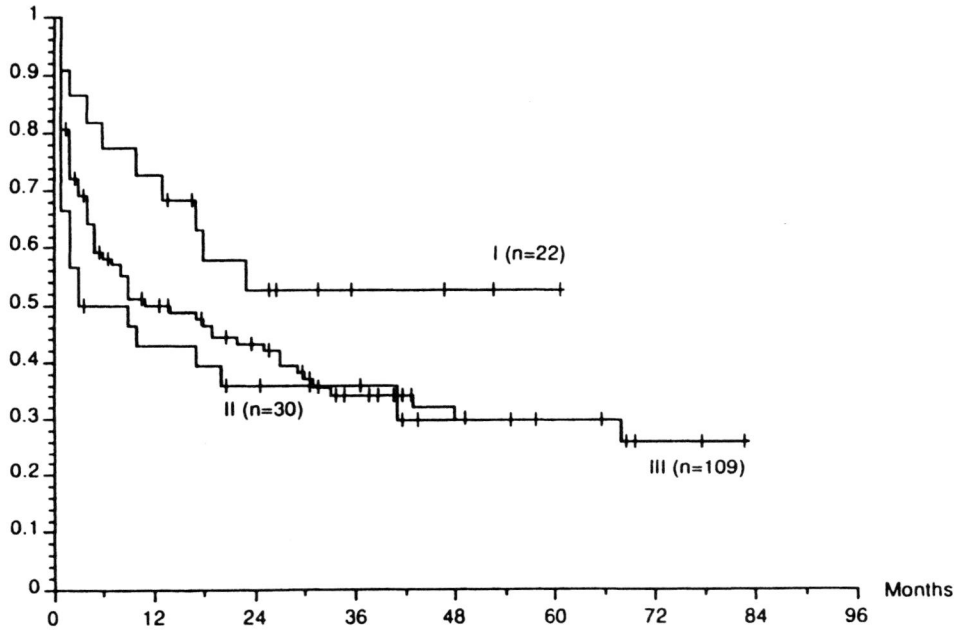

Fig. 55.1. Actuarial survival after BMT according to stage of disease at diagnosis. Kaplan-Meier curves show significantly better survival among patients with stage I disease at diagnosis than among those with stages II and III (*P* = .05). Reproduced, with permission, from Gahrton *et al.* (1995).

in turn a result of earlier transplantation, less prior chemotherapy and to the use of more effective new antiviral and antifungal drugs (Gahrton *et al.*, 2001).

Alyea and colleagues (2001) described a two year progression-free survival rate of 42% in 24 recipients of CD6 T-cell-depleted, HLA-identical sibling bone marrow transplants, 14 of

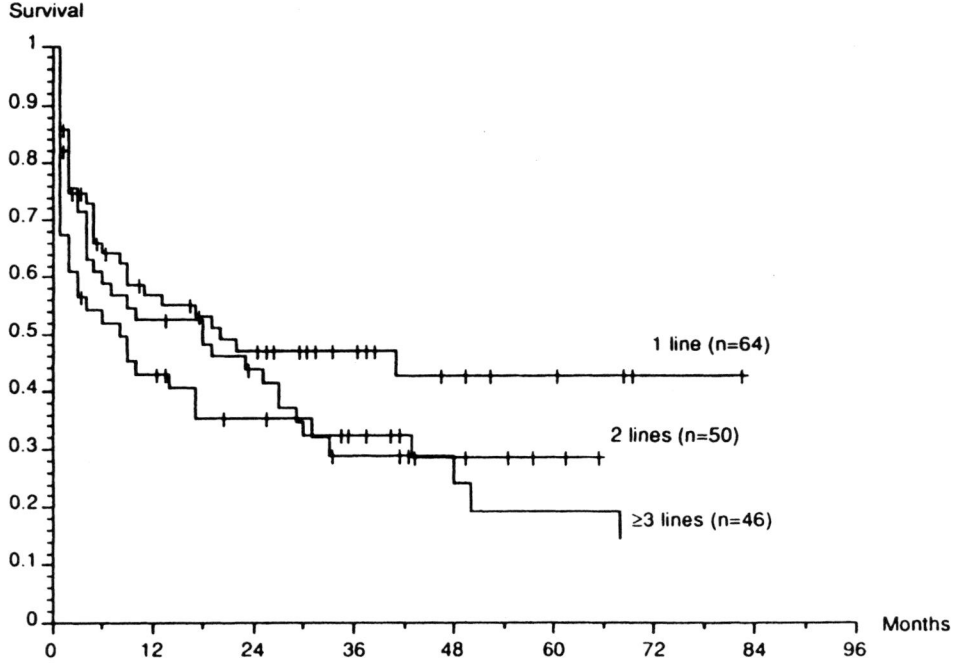

Fig. 55.2. Actuarial survival after BMT according to number of lines of treatment regimens used pretransplantation. Kaplan-Meier curves show significantly better survival among patients who received only one line of treatment versus those who received three lines of treatment (*P* = .02). There was also a tendency for better survival among patients who received only one line of treatment versus those who received two lines of treatment (not significant). Reproduced, with permission, from Gahrton *et al.* (1995).

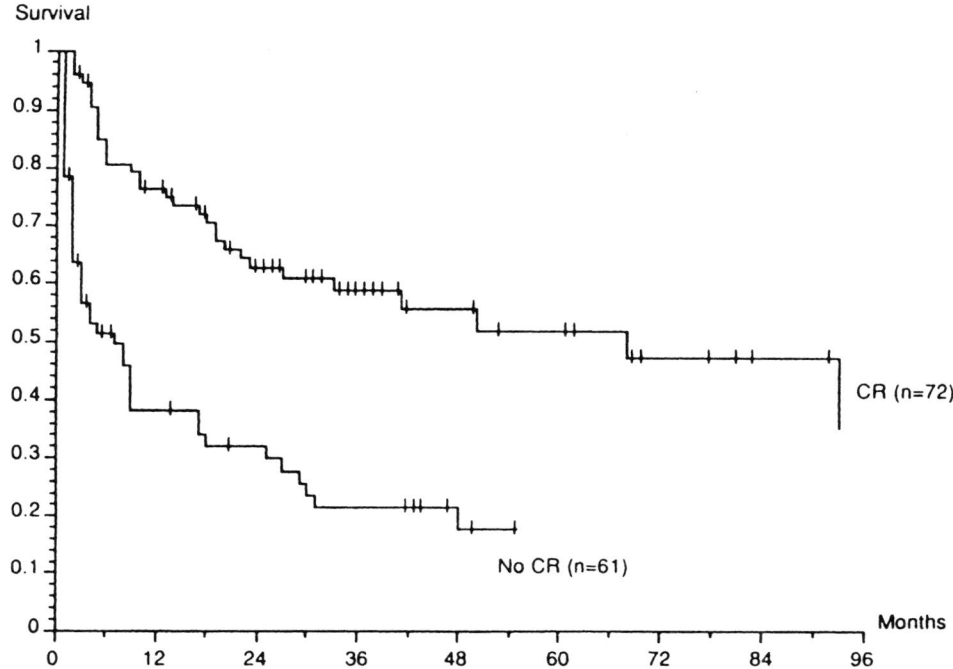

Fig. 55.3. Actuarial survival after BMT according to whether patients were in complete remission (CR) after engraftment. Kaplan-Meier curves show significantly better survival among patients who entered CR after engraftment than among those who did not ($P = .001$). Reproduced, with permission, from Gahrton *et al.* (1995).

whom subsequently received a donor lymphocyte infusion at 6–9 months posttransplant to elicit a graft-versus-myeloma effect.

Age and survival

Multiple myeloma is a disorder of the elderly. In Sweden, the incidence of multiple myeloma is 545 patients yearly, but only 7% are under 55 years of age, a common age limit for allogeneic HSC transplantation. Thus, the fraction of multiple myeloma patients that can benefit from allogeneic transplanta-

tion is limited. In the EBMT registry data there was a tendency for better survival in patients below 35 years of age, but no significant difference between patients 35 to 45 as compared to those between 45 and 55. However, patients more than 55 years of age seemed to have a poor prognosis.

Conditioning regimens and survival

As for other neoplastic disorders, a number of conditioning regimens have been used to prepare patients with multiple

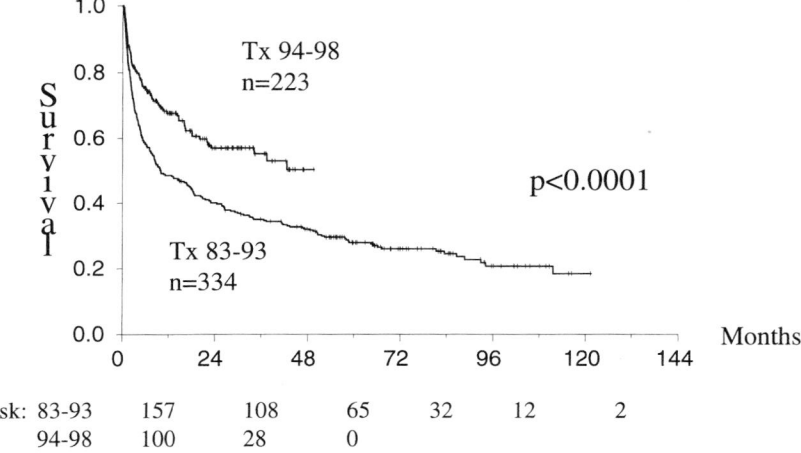

Fig. 55.4. Actuarial survival after BMT according to the time of transplantation. Kaplan-Meier curves show a significantly better survival among patients who received the transplant (Tx) 1994–98 than among those who received the transplant 1983–93. Reproduced, with permission, from Gahrton *et al.* (2001).

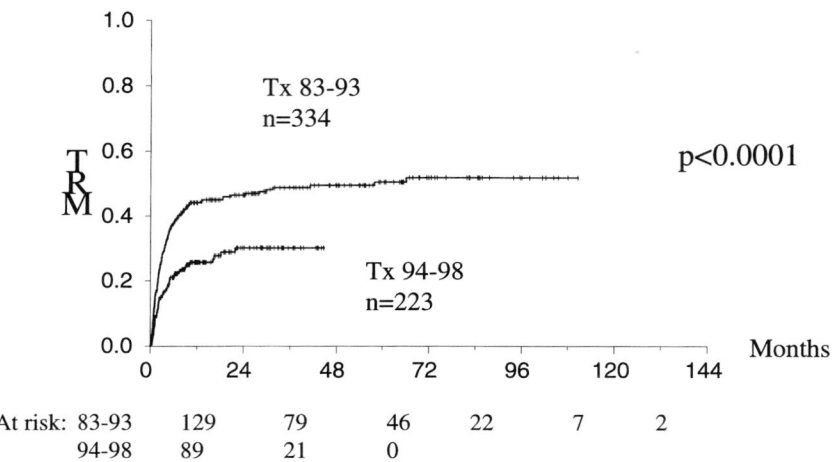

Fig. 55.5. Transplant-related mortality (TRM) according to the time of BMT. Kaplan-Meier curves show significantly less transplant-related mortality among patients who received the transplant 1994–98 than those who received the transplant 1983–93. Reproduced, with permission, from Gahrton *et al.* (2001).

myeloma for transplant. The most common regimen has been a combination of cyclophosphamide and TBI. Although there was no clear difference in survival between this regimen and other regimens (for example, those using melphalan and TBI, or melphalan and cyclophosphamide, or TBI and several cytotoxic drugs), the EBMT database shows that such differences exist. Transplant-related mortality appears to be high with most regimens; however, a report using TBI fractionated in 6 doses for a total of 12 Gy combined with a relatively low dose of melphalan (110 mg/m^2) (Russell *et al.,* 1997) indicated that this kind of regimen may be less toxic than those used previously combining TBI and cyclophosphamide. Other studies have claimed advantages with busulfan and cyclophosphamide (Buckner *et al.,* 1989; Bensinger *et al.,* 1992). In a subsequent study (Bensinger *et al.,* 1996), 57 patients with myeloma were prepared for allografting with busulfan and cyclophosphamide and 23 had this combined with modified TBI (7.5–10.5 Gy). The type of pretransplant conditioning regimen was not a factor in outcome endpoints. In this study adverse factors for outcome included transplantation beyond 1 year from diagnosis, a serum β_2 microglobulin level of >2.5 mg/l at the time of transplant, females transplanted from male donors, patients who had received greater than eight cycles of chemotherapy pretransplant, and those who were in a Salmon-Durie stage 3 at the time of transplant (Table 55.3). Overall actuarial probability of progression-free survival was 24% ± 17% at 4.5 years, but was 50 ± 21 for those in whom CR was obtained (Figs. 55.6 and 55.7).

Complications and causes of death

The complications and causes of death following allogeneic transplantation in patients with multiple myeloma are in general the same as those in patients who undergo allogeneic transplantation for other hematologic malignancies. In earlier EBMT studies (Gahrton *et al.,* 1991 and 1995), 40% of patients died within 6 months of transplantation. The most common

causes of death were interstitial pneumonitis, acute graft-versus-host disease (GVHD), bacterial and fungal infections, and hemorrhage. GVHD does not appear to be more severe in patients transplanted for multiple myeloma than in those transplanted for other diseases. Those patients who had acute GVHD grade III or IV had poor survival. Interestingly, those with grade I acute GVHD had the best long-term survival, in concordance with observations in leukemia and again suggestive of a graft-versus-myeloma effect. The causes of death were mainly the same in the latest follow-up; however, the frequency of death due to bacterial and fungal infections as well as to interstitial pneumonitis was lower (Gahrton *et al.,* 2001).

Results of HLA-mismatched family member, unrelated, donor, and cord blood transplantation

Only a few transplants have been performed with family members other than siblings or unrelated donors. Cord blood donors do not yet appear to have been used for myeloma. Results using non-sibling donors have so far been poor. Bensinger *et al.* (1996) reported a 64% treatment-related mortality in 14 patients who received conventional conditioning followed by a transplant from an unrelated or mismatched related donor. However, the use of nonmyeloablative regimens appears to improve results (see below).

Results with reduced intensity conditioning regimens

Investigators at the M.D. Anderson Hospital have begun to explore a combination of melphalan 140 mg/m^2 in combination with fludarabine 30 mg/m^2 daily for 4 days. In 10 patients treated to date, 9 have engrafted (including 3 receiving bone marrow from unrelated donors). One patient died early from multiorgan failure, and 3 have died from complications associated with GVHD. Six patients remain alive, 2 in complete remission

Table 55.3. *Factors affecting posttransplant outcome*

Variables	Death <100 days			Survival			Relapse or progression			Relapse/progression-free survival		
	Univariate	Multivariate	Relative risk	Univariate	Multivariate	Relative risk	Univariate	Multivariate	Relative Risk	Univariate	Multivariate	Relative risk
Age >40	0.527			0.409			0.848			0.551		
Sex D/R	0.449			0.249			0.014	0.026	3.5 (1.1–11.5)	0.490		
No. cycles chemo	0.196			0.180			0.010	0.010	4.3 (1.2–15.9)	0.052		
No. chemo regimens	0.838			0.865			0.102			0.741		
Plasma cells >10%	0.466			0.221			0.919			0.571		
Previous XRT	0.127			0.541			0.934			0.423		
Stage 3	0.051			0.951			0.794			0.021	0.021	1.9 (1.1–3.2)
β_2-Microglobulin	0.859			0.009	0.009	2.0 (1.1–3.7)	0.091			0.934		
Chemosensitive	0.318			0.373			0.511			0.349		
Time Dx to Tx	0.006	0.005	2.5 (1.3–4.9)	0.019	0.033	1.8 (1.0–3.1)	0.729			0.038		
Regimen (TBI)	0.985			0.568			0.635			0.435		
Donor type	0.922			0.930			0.563			0.891		

Reproduced, with permission, from Bensinger *et al.* (1996).

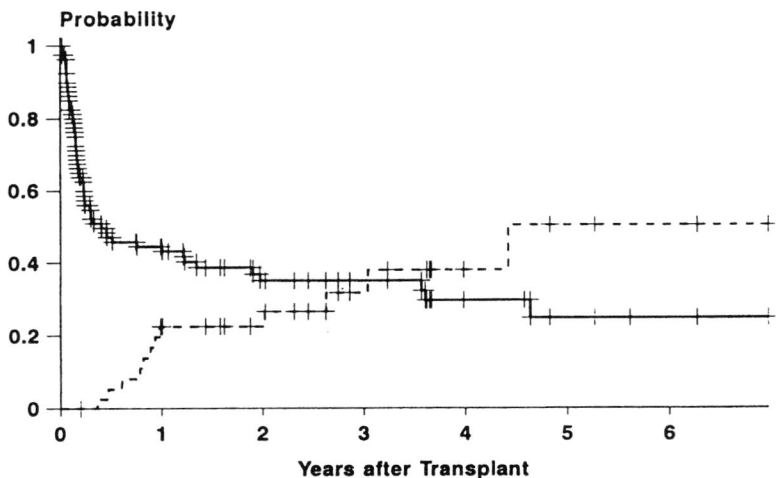

Fig. 55.6. The probabilities of survival and relapse or disease progression for all 80 patients undergoing allogeneic transplant for multiple myeloma. Survival: ——— ; relapse or progression: - - - - . Reproduced, with permission, from Bensinger *et al.* (1996).

between 30 and 180 days posttransplant. Three of the other 4 patients received CD8-depleted donor lymphocyte infusions because of persistent disease and require further evaluation. Thus, this strategy appears feasible, but further study is required before concluding that this approach could potentially improve the outcome of allogeneic transplantation in multiple myeloma.

Badros and colleagues (2001) prepared 16 poor-risk patients, all of whom had received at least one prior autograft, with melphalan 100 mg/m^2 prior to infusion of an HLA-identical ($n =$ 14) or non-identical ($n = 2$) sibling peripheral blood stem cell transplant. Ten had refractory relapse, 4 sensitive relapse, and 2 were in near complete remission. Donor lymphocyte infusions were given posttransplant to 14 patients with no clinical evidence of GVHD, either to obtain full donor chimerism ($n = 4$) or to eradicate residual disease ($n = 10$). Fifteen patients

showed myeloid engraftment and 12 were full donor chimeras at day 21 posttransplant. Acute GVHD occurred in ten, and chronic GVHD in seven. At a median follow-up of 1 year, five patients achieved and sustained a complete remission (CR), 3 a near CR, and 4 a partial remission. Remarkable graft-versus myeloma responses were seen in chemotherapy-refractory patients, although 3 patients died of GVHD-related complications. However, in another study, two patients who relapsed with extramedullary disease after autologous transplantation also relapsed soon after reduced conditioning with the busulfan, fludarabine, ATG regimen, and an HLA-identical sibling transplant (Ornstein *et al.*, 2002).

An EBMT survey of non-myeloablative transplants collected results of 54 patients. All patients had received previous therapy. One was in complete remission at the time of transplant,

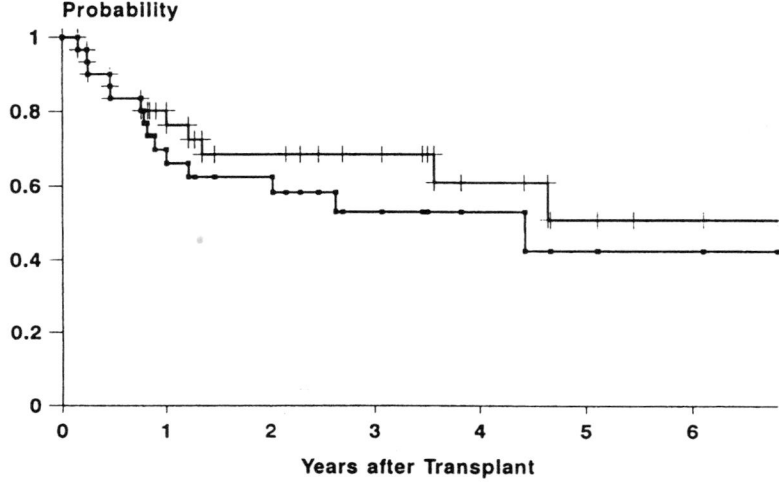

Fig. 55.7. The probabilities of survival and relapse-free survival for the 29 patients who achieved CR following allogeneic transplant. Survival: ——— ; relapse-free survival: •–•–• . Reproduced, with permission, from Bensinger *et al.* (1996).

29 in partial remission, and 18 were refractory. All patients engrafted. Following the transplant, 24 were in complete remission and 6 refractory patients had responded. The transplant-related mortality for good risk patients (CR and PR before transplant) was only 13%, but was 63% for poor risk patients (refractory or relapse). The one year survival for good risk patients was 83%, but 25% for poor risk ones. Kröger and colleagues (2002a) used fludarabine 150/m^2 melphalan 100-140 mg/m^2, and rabbit ATG 10 mg/kg for 3 days as conditioning prior to an unrelated transplant for 21 patients with stage II/III myeloma, all of whom had received a prior autologous graft (in 9 as part of an autologous/allogneic tandom procedure). Forty per cent achieved a complete, and 50% a partial, response, with a nonrelapse mortality rate at 100 days of 10% and of 26% at 1 year. The estimated 2-year overall and progression-free survival rates were 74% and 53%, respectively.

Use of 200 cGY total body irradiation with or without fludarabine 30 mg/m^2 for three days by the Seattle group seems promising (McSweeney et al., 2001; Bensinger et al., 2001). The best results were obtained if the non-myeloablative allogeneic transplant was performed 2–4 months after an autologous transplant. The response rate in 32 previously treated patients (43% refractory or in relapse after autologous transplantation) was 84% and 53% entered a complete hematologic remission. With a median follow-up time of 423 days after the autologous transplantation and 328 days after the non-myelablative allogeneic transplant, the overall survival was 81%.

Comparison of allogeneic transplantation with chemotherapy and autologous transplantation

Allogeneic transplantation has not been compared to conventional chemotherapy in prospective or retrospective studies. However, a case-matched study of patients in the EBMT registry was performed to compare allogeneic and autologous transplantation (Björkstrand et al., 1996). The comparison comprised 378 patients, 189 for each transplant modality. Matching was made for the most important prognostic factors for allogeneic transplantation, that is, the gender (females do better than males) and the number of pretransplant treatment lines (one line is better than several lines). Most other parameters were similar. However, differences were seen in the median age (autologous 49 years, allogeneic 43 years), and in the follow-up time, which was shorter for autologous transplant recipients. The study showed a significantly better overall survival for autologous transplantation due to a higher transplant-related mortality for allogeneic transplantation. However, the survival curves merged at about 4 years posttransplant and long-term survival appeared similar, because the relapse rate was lower after allogeneic transplantation than after autologous transplantation (Fig. 55.8). Prognostic factors analyzed for their potential impact on survival and progression-free survival are shown in Table 55.4. However the difference in outcome was only seen in males (Fig. 55.9). Since results of allogeneic transplants have improved considerably during the time after

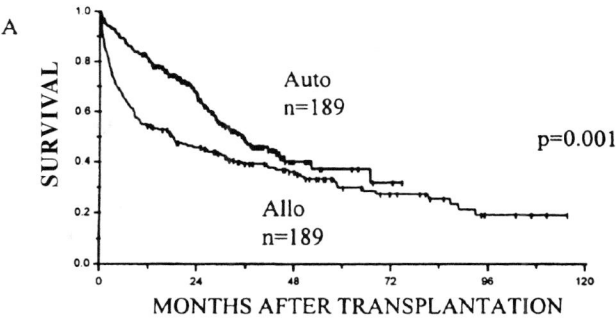

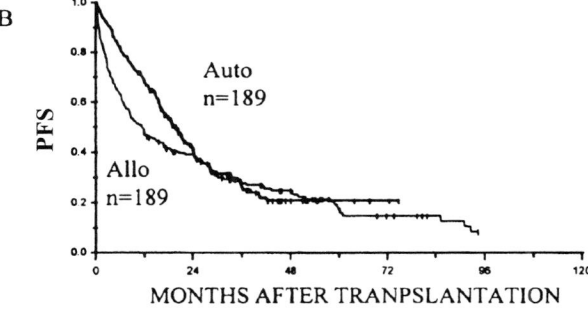

Fig. 55.8. Probability of (A) overall survival (OS) and (B) PFS for all patients. The curve with the thicker line indicates the autologous stem cell transplantation (ASCT) group. A P value cannot be given in (B) because the curves cross and therefore the log-rank test cannot be applied. Reproduced, with permission, from Björkstrand et al. (1996).

this investigation, while results of autologous ones have not, a comparison of more recent transplants may be more favorable for allogeneic transplantation (Gahrton et al., 2001). Also, a further reduction in transplant-related mortality following non-myeloablative allogeneic transplantation is likely. Additionally, complete molecular remissions are rare following autologous transplantation, while about half of those who enter a hematologic complete remission following allogeneic transplantation also obtain a molecular remission (Corradini et al., 1999; Cavo et al., 2000) (Fig. 55.10). Thus the prospect for cure appears better with allogenic transplantation than with autologous transplantation.

The graft-versus-myeloma effect

In the study by Björkstrand et al. (1996) described above, the relapse rate was lower after allogeneic transplantation than after autologous transplantation, again suggesting a graft-versus-myeloma effect in the allogeneic setting (Mehta & Singhal, 1998; Libura et al., 1999; Le Blanc et al., 2001). In another study of 56 patients with myeloma prepared with the same conditioning regimen of TBI, busulfan and cyclophosphamide, there was a trend to improved progression-free and overall survival (60% versus 30% and 60% versus 42% respectively) for the allograft recipients (Reynolds et al., 2001). This was not a randomized study, however; the choice of graft was determined

Table 55.4.   *Prognostic factors analyzed for their potential impact on survival and progression-free survival (PFS) from the time of transplantation in the comparison between allo-BMT and autologous stem cell transplantation*

Group analyzed (no. allo/no. auto)	Median survival (confidence interval) in months			Median PFS (confidence interval) in months		
	Allo	Auto	*P* value	Allo	Auto	*P* value
All patients (189/189)	18 (9–30)	34 (28–44)	.001	11 (8–16)	20 (16–23)	†
Male (112/112)	9 (6–18)	31 (26–45)	.0003	7 (5–12)	19 (15–22)	†
Female (77/77)	31 (18–58)	36 (25–∞)	†	20 (9–29)	20 (14–33)	†
1 line of chemotherapy (76/76)	31 (11–86)	41 (31–∞)	†	16 (7–35)	24 (20–33)	†
≥2 lines of chemotherapy (113/113)	14 (7–26)	29 (24–43)	.0002	8 (6–12)	16 (13–20)	†
Age <46 yr (131/58)	18 (8–31)	33 (24–45)	†	11 (7–17)	21 (16–24)	†
Age ≥46 yr (58/131)	17 (6–41)	35 (28–66)	.04	9 (5–26)	18 (15–24)	.2
Responsive to chemotherapy (143/143)	17 (8–31)	37 (29–66)	.0002	10 (7–18)	23 (18–26)	†
CR at transplant (27/21)	18 (5–86)	31 (22–∞)	.3	15 (5–28)	20 (17–∞)	†
PR at transplant (117/122)	17 (8–33)	37 (29–∞)	.0008	9 (7–20)	24 (18–28)	†
Responsive/1 line of chemo (62/69)	31 (10–86)	41 (31–∞)	†	16 (6–48)	24 (20–40)	†
Unresponsive to chemotherapy (44/43)	18 (6–41)	20 (9–29)	†	11 (5–18)	9 (5–14)	†
IgG subtype (97/110)	8 (6–21)	32 (28–52)	.0005	7 (5–11)	21 (17–24)	.002
Non-IgG subtype (92/79)	18 (5–49)	33 (19–∞)	.2	12 (5–28)	21 (6–24)	.8
Stage I (28/24)	65 (17–∞)	67 (29–∞)	.5	26 (12–50)	33 (18–∞)	†
Stage II (39/38)	10 (3–41)	NR (37–∞)	.003	9 (3–15)	33 (16–∞)	.004
Stage III (122/126)	17 (7–31)	28 (24–33)	†	9 (6–19)	17 (14–21)	†
β₂m <4 mg/l (37/53)	58 (16–81)	66 (44–∞)	.03	28 (11–36)	28 (18–40)	.3
β₂m ≥4 mg/l (25/27)	5 (3–18)	22 (13–43)	.03	5 (3–16)	14 (7–20)	.2
CR posttransplant (90/75)	65 (33–88)	35 (25–52)	†	36 (18–58)	22 (17–33)	†

† The curves crossed; therefore, the significance analysis (stratified log-rank test) cannot be applied and no *P* value can be given. Reproduced, with permission, from Björkstrand *et al.* (1996).

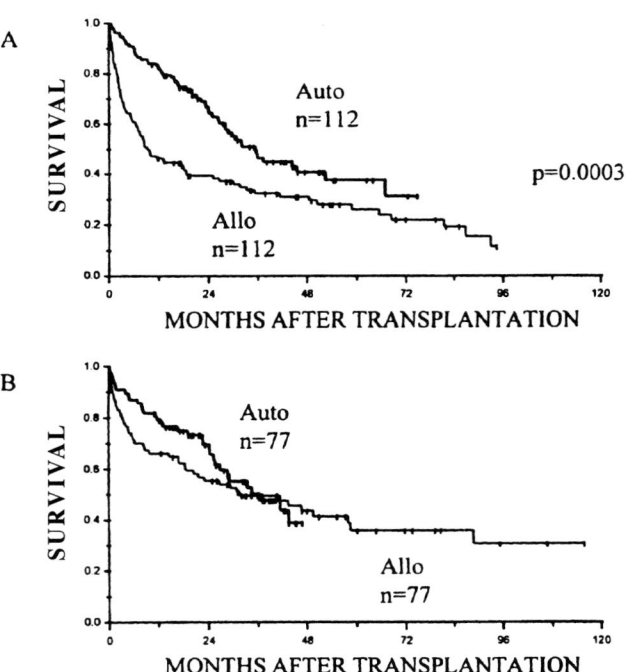

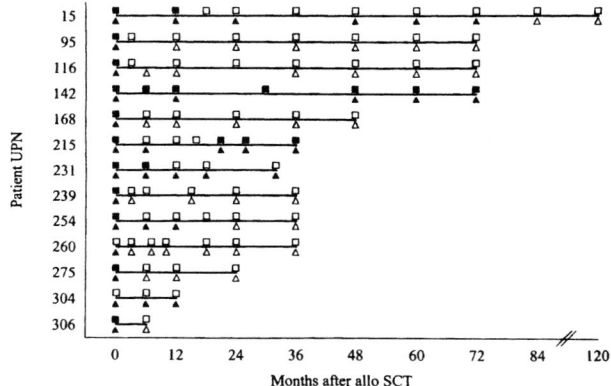

by patient preference. An association between achieving complete remission and the presence of chronic GVHD was noted in the study by Le Blanc *et al.* (2001).

The evidence for a graft-versus-myeloma effect have been further strengthened by findings that donor lymphocyte transfusions (DLI) can induce remissions following relapse after allogeneic transplantation (Aschan *et al.*, 1996; Tricot *et al.*, 1996; Verdonck *et al.*, 1996). In a series by Lokhorst and col-

Fig. 55.9. Probability of overall survival (OS) for (**A**) male and (**B**) female patients. The curve with the thicker line indicates the autologous stem cell transplantation (ASCT) group. A *P* value cannot be given in (**B**) because the curves cross and therefore the log rank test cannot be applied. Reproduced, with permission, from Björkstrand *et al.* (1996).

Fig. 55.10. Results of PCR analysis for MRD detection on serial bone marrow samples taken before and after allo SCT. The figure represents positive (■) and negative (□) results of immunofixation analysis and positive (▲) and negative (△) results of the PCR-based assay. Reproduced, with permission, from Cavo *et al.* (2000).

leagues (2000), 14 of 27 relapsed patients responded to DLI, including 6 who attained a complete remission. Salama *et al.* (2000) reviewed data in 25 patients treated at 15 centers: complete remissions occurred in 2 of 22 patients receiving DLI alone, and in a further 3 who received DLI after chemotherapy. Nine patients received additional DLI due to the absence of a complete response, and two complete and three partial responses were seen. Alyea and co-workers (1998) infused a CD8-depleted DLI (consisting predominantly of CD4$^+$ T cells): 5 of 6 relapsed myeloma patients responded. Byrne and colleagues (1998) have administered interferon-α after allogeneic transplantation for myeloma in an attempt to minimize the risk of relapse, possibly by augmenting a GVM effect.

Autologous HSC transplantation followed by elective reduced intensity conditioning and allografting

A new approach involves the use of a standard autograft for tumor debulking purposes followed by an elective allograft (using reduced intensity conditioning) and an allograft to exploit the graft-versus-myeloma effect (Maloney *et al.*, 2001; Kröger *et al.*, 2002b). Kröger and colleagues (2002b) treated 17 patients with advanced stage II/III myeloma with melphalan 200 mg/m^2 and an autologous transplant. After a median interval of 119 days, a reduced intensity conditioning regimen of fludarabine 180 mg/m^2, melphalan 100 mg/m^2, and ATG 10 mg/kg for 3 doses was administered prior to an allogeneic transplant from an HLA-matched related donor in 7 patients, an HLA-mismatched related donor in 2 patients, and an unrelated donor in 8 patients. Complete donor chimerism was detected after a median of 30 days. The 100 day mortality rate post allograft was 11%. The complete remission rate with negative immunofixation increased from 0% after induction or salvage chemotherapy to 18% after autologous transplantation to 73% after allografting. At a median follow-up of 13 months post allografting, the 2-year estimated event-free survival was 56% (see also Chapter 124).

Indications and contraindications for allogeneic transplantation

Myeloablative conditioning followed by allogeneic transplantation remains associated with significant transplant-related mortality. However, the prospects for cure are probably better than with any other presently available treatment. Therefore, carefully selected patients with stage IIIA disease are candidates. The best candidates appear to be females of younger age who have not been heavily pretreated and who have an HLA-identical female sibling donor available. The current practice of HSC transplantation for myeloma in Europe has been described (Urano-Ispizua *et al.*, 2002) (and see Chapter 124).

The place of non-myelablative conditioning followed by allotransplantation has yet to be determined. However, the low initial transplant-related mortality indicates that this may be the treatment of choice, possibly after an autologous transplant (for tumor debulking), and with the option of later donor lymphocyte transfusions. Patients treated with non-myeloablative transplantation should be entered into trial protocols. A prospective trial comparing non-myelablative transplantation following autologous transplantation to autologous transplantation alone is currently running under the supervision of the Myeloma Subcommittee of the EBMT.

Monitoring minimal residual disease posttransplant

Minimal residual disease in the bone marrow can be monitored posttransplant using PCR technology to identify the rearranged variable region (VDJ) of the immunoglobulin heavy chain (IgH) using primers designed from the patient-specific IgH complementarity-determining regions (CDRs) II and III. In a study by Martinelli and colleagues (2000), 7 of 14 evaluable allograft recipients achieved a molecular complete remission (MCR) posttransplant (50%). This was significantly higher than the incidence in autograft recipients in the same study (16%). Relapse-free survival was longer in those achieving MCR. In a different study, 9 of 12 patients who attained complete remission remained persistently PCR-negative for a median of 36 months posttransplant (Cavo *et al.*, 2000) (Fig. 55.10).

Allogeneic HSC transplantation for AL amyloidosis

Several cases of allogeneic transplantation has been reported for AL amyloidosis, with improvement posttransplant (Guillaume *et al.*, 1997; Gillmore *et al.*, 1998). More commonly autologous transplantation has been performed (see Chapter 40).

Prospects for the future

Allogeneic transplantation is an option for younger patients with multiple myeloma. However, the report that overall survival is superior with autologous transplantation, due to a higher transplant-related mortality with allogeneic transplantation (Björkstrand *et al.*, 1996), indicates that caution is necessary in selection of patients for allogeneic transplantation. Although transplant-related mortality has been reduced, and survival improved significantly during the latest 5–7 years, transplant-related mortality needs to be further reduced before early transplantation can be recommended for most patients.

Protocols are now being designed that attempt to reduce transplant-related mortality by lowering the intensity of the conditioning regimens (non-myeloablative transplantation). Such approaches may be hampered by an increased relapse rate. Therefore, attempts will be made to use donor lymphocyte transfusions in poorly responding, nonresponding, or relapsing patients. GVHD might be reduced by the use of selected cell populations such as CD34$^+$ peripheral blood stem cells.

Besides the use of donor lymphocyte infusions to treat relapse posttransplant thalidomide has demonstrated activity in patients with relapsed or refractory myeloma, and its use has been described in patients relapsing after allogeneic HSC transplantation (Biagi *et al.*, 2001).

With these approaches it may be possible to reduce transplant-related mortality without increasing the relapse rate. It may also be possible to increase the number of transplants by using unrelated HLA-matched volunteer donors.

Conclusions

Allogeneic HSC transplantation is a potentially curative method for treating patients with multiple myeloma. Treatment-related mortality is still high and autologous transplantation may therefore be preferential for most patients at the present time. Allogeneic transplantation may still be an option for younger patients with early poor prognostic parameters for other treatment modalities, for those with optimal donors (identical siblings with the same sex) and for patients that are nonresponsive, have received more than one line of treatment, or have relapsed following autologous transplantation. If measures now being used to decrease transplant-related mortality (non-myeloablative conditioning) are successful, the lower relapse rate with allogeneic transplantation compared to autologous transplantation will likely increase the indications for allogeneic transplantation.

References

Alexanian, R., Haut, A., Khan, A. *et al.* (1969). Treatment for multiple myeloma: combination chemotherapy with different melphalan dose regimens. *Journal of the American Medical Association,* **208,** 1680–5.

Alyea, A. P., Soiffer, R. J., Cunning, C. *et al.* (1998). Toxicity and efficacy of defined doses of CD4+ donor lymphocytes for treatment of relapse after allogeneic bone marrow transplantation. *Blood,* **91,** 3671–88.

Alyea, E., Weller, E., Schlossman, R. *et al.* (2001). T-cell-depleted allogeneic bone marrow transplantation followed by donor lymphocyte infusion in patients with multiple myeloma: induction of graft-versus-myeloma effect. *Blood,* **98,** 934–9.

Aschan, J., Lönqvist, B., Ringdén, O. *et al.* (1996). Graft-versus-myeloma effect. *Lancet,* **348,** 346.

Badros, A., Barlogie, B., Morris, C. *et al.* (2001). High response rate in refractory and high-risk multiple myeloma after allotransplantation using a nonmyeloablative conditioning regimen and donor lymphocyte infusions. *Blood,* **97,** 2574–9.

Barlogie, B. & Gahrton, G. (1991). Bone marrow transplantation in multiple myeloma. *Bone Marrow Transplantation,* **7,** 71–9.

Barlogie, B., Alexanian, R., Dicke, K. *et al.* (1987). High-dose chemoradiotherapy and autologous bone marrow transplantation for resistant multiple myeloma. *Blood,* **70,** 869–72.

Barlogie, B., Alexanian, R., Smallwood, L. *et al.* (1988). Prognostic factors with high-dose melphalan for refractory multiple myeloma. *Blood,* **72,** 2015–9.

Bataille, R., Durie, B. G. M., Genier, J., & Sany, J. (1986). Prognostic factors and staging in multiple myeloma: a reappraisal. *Journal of Clinical Oncology,* **3,** 80–7.

Bensinger, W. I., Buckner, C. D., Anasetti, C. *et al.* (1996). Allogeneic transplantation for multiple myeloma: an analysis of risk factors on outcome. *Blood,* **88,** 2787–93.

Bensinger, W. I., Buckner, C. D., Clift, R. A. *et al.* (1992). Phase I study of busulfan and cyclophosphamide in preparation for allogeneic marrow transplant for patients with multiple myeloma. *Journal of Clinical Oncology,* **10,** 1492–7.

Bensinger, W. I., Maloney, D., Storb, R. (2001). Allogeneic hematopoietic cell transplantation for multiple myeloma. *Seminars in Hematology,* **38,** 243–9

Biagi, J. J., Mileshkin, L., Grigg, A. P., Westerman, D. W. & Prince, H. M. (2001). Efficacy of thalidomide therapy, for extramedullary relapse of myeloma following allogeneic transplantation. *Bone Marrow Transplantation,* **28,** 1145–50.

Björkstrand, B., Ljungman, P., Svensson, H. *et al.* (1996). Allogeneic bone marrow transplantation versus autologous stem cell transplantation in multiple myeloma—a retrospective case-matched study from the European Group for Blood and Marrow Transplantation. *Blood,* **88,** 4711–8.

Buckner, C. D., Fefer, A., Bensinger, W. I. *et al.* (1989). Marrow transplantation for malignant plasma cell disorders: summary of the Seattle experience. *European Journal of Haematology,* **51** (Suppl), 86–90.

Byrne, J. L., Carter, G. I., Bienz, N. *et al.* (1998). Adjuvant α-interferon improves complete remission rates following allogeneic transplantation for multiple myeloma. *Bone Marrow Transplantation,* **22,** 639–43.

Cavo, M., Terragna, C., Martinelli, G. *et al.* (2000). Molecular monitoring of minimal residual disease in patients in long-term complete remission after allogeneic stem cell transplantation for multiple myeloma. *Blood,* **96,** 355–7.

Corradini, P., Voena, C., Tarella, C. *et al.* (1999). Molecular and clinical remissions in multiple myeloma: role of autologous and allogeneic transplantation of hematopoietic cells. *Journal of Clinical Oncology,* **17,** 208–215.

Gahrton, G., Ringdén, O., Lönnqvist, B. *et al.* (1986). Bone marrow transplantation in three patients with multiple myeloma. *Acta Medica Scandinavica,* **219,** 523–7.

Gahrton, G., Tura, S., Flesch, M. *et al.* (1987). Bone marrow transplantation in multiple myeloma. Report from the European Cooperative Group for Bone Marrow Transplantation. *Blood,* **69,** 1262–4.

Gahrton, G., Tura, S., Ljungman, P. *et al.* (1991). Allogeneic bone marrow transplantation in multiple myeloma. *New England Journal of Medicine,* **325,** 1267–73.

Gahrton, G., Tura, S., Ljungman, P. *et al.* (1995). Prognostic factors in allogeneic bone marrow transplantation for multiple myeloma. *Journal of Clinical Oncology,* **13,** 1312–22.

Gahrton, G., Tura, S., Svensson, H. *et al.* (1998). Allogeneic bone marrow transplantation in multiple myeloma. *Bone Marrow Transplantation,* **21** (Suppl 1), S204.

Gahrton, G., Svensson, H., Cavo, M. *et al.* (2001). Progress in allogeneic bone marrow and peripheral blood stem cell transplantation for multiple myeloma: a comparison between transplants performed 1983–93 and 1994–98 at European Group for Blood and Marrow Transplantation Centers. *British Journal of Haematology,* **113,** 209–16.

Gillmore, J. D., Davies, J., Iqbal, A. *et al.* (1998). Allogeneic bone marrow transplantation for systemic AL amyloidosis. *British Journal of Haematology,* **100,** 226–8.

Guillaume, B., Straetmans, N., Jadoul, M. *et al.* (1997). Allogeneic bone marrow transplantation for AL amyloidosis. *Bone Marrow Transplantation,* **20,** 907–8.

Horowitz, M. M., Gale, R. P., Sondel, P. M. *et al.* (1990). Graft-versus-leukemia reactions after bone marrow transplantation. *Blood,* **75,** 555–72.

Kröger, N., Sayer, H.G., Schwertfeger, R. *et al.* (2002a). Unrelated stem cell transplantation in multiple myeloma after a reduced-intensity conditioning with pretransplantation antithymocyte globulin is highly effective with low transplantation-related mortality. *Blood,* **100,** 3919–24.

Kröger, N., Schwerdtfeger, R., Kiehl, M. *et al.* (2002b). Autologous stem cell transplantation followed by a reduced-dose allograft induces high complete remission rate in multiple myeloma. *Blood,* **100,** 755–60.

Le Blanc, R., Montminy-Metivier, S., Belanger, R. *et al.* (2001). Allogeneic transplantation for multiple myeloma: further evidence for a GVHD-associated graft-versus-myeloma effect. *Bone Marrow Transplantation,* **28,** 841–8.

Libura, J., Hoffmann, T., Passweg, J. R. *et al.* (1999). Graft-versus-myeloma after withdrawal of immunosuppression following allogeneic peripheral stem cell transplantation. *Bone Marrow Transplantation,* **24,** 925–7.

Lokhorst, H. M., Schattenberg, A., Cornelissen, J. J. (2000). Donor lymphocyte infusions for relapsed multiple myeloma after allogeneic stem-cell transplantation: predictive factors for response and long-term outcome. *Journal of Clinical Oncology,* **18,** 3031–7.

Maloney, D.G., Sahebi, F., Stockerl-Goldstein, K.E. *et al.* (2001). Combining an allogeneic graft-vs-myeloma effect with high-dose autologous stem cell rescue in the treatment of multiple myeloma. *Blood,* **98,** 434–5a (abstract).

Martinelli, G., Terragna, C., Zamagni, E. *et al.* (2000). Molecular remission after allogeneic or autologous transplantation of hematopoietic stem cells for multiple myeloma. *Journal of Clinical Oncology,* **18,** 2273–81.

McElwain, T. J. & Powles, R. L. (1983). High-dose intravenous melphalan for plasma cell leukaemia and myeloma. *Lancet,* **1,** 822–4.

McSweeney, P. A., Niederwieser, D., Shizuru, J. A. *et al.* (2001). Hematopoietic cell transplantation in older patients with hemato-logic malignancies: replacing high-dose therapy with graft-versus-tumor effects. *Blood,* **97,** 3390–400.

Mehta, J. & Singhal, S. (1998). Review. Graft-versus-myeloma. *Bone Marrow Transplantation,* **22,** 835–43.

Ornstein, D. L., Ririe, D. W., Shaughnessy, P. J., Neuhauser, T. & Bee, C. (2002). Nonmyeloablative allogeneic peripheral blood stem cell transplantation for extramedullary plasmacytomas progressing after autologous transplantation. *Bone Marrow Transplantation,* **29,** 71–4.

Ozer, H., Han, T., Nussbaum-Blumenson, A. *et al.* (1984). Allogeneic BMT and idiotypic monitoring in multiple myeloma. AACR *Abstracts,* **84,** 161.

Reece, D. E., Shepherd, J. D., Klingemann, H.-G. *et al.* (1995). Treatment of myeloma using intensive therapy and allogeneic bone marrow transplantation. *Bone Marrow Transplantation,* **15,** 117–23.

Reynolds, C., Ratanatharathorn, V., Adams, P. *et al.* (2001). Allogeneic stem cell transplantation reduces disease progression compared to autologous transplantation in patients with multiple myeloma. *Bone Marrow Transplantation,* **27,** 801–7.

Russell, N. H., Miflin, G., Stainer, C. *et al.* (1997). Allogeneic bone marrow transplant for multiple myeloma. *Blood,* **89,** 2610–7.

Salama, M., Nevill, T., Marcellus, D. *et al.* (2000). Donor leukocyte infusions for multiple myeloma. *Bone Marrow Transplantation,* **26,** 1179–84.

Selby, P., McElwain, T. J., Nandi, A. C. *et al.* (1987). Multiple myeloma treated with high-dose intravenous melphalan. *British Journal of Haematology,* **66,** 55–62.

Tricot, G., Vesole, D. H., Jagannath, S. *et al.* (1996). Graft-versus-myeloma effect: proof of principle. *Blood,* **8,** 1196–8.

Tura, S., Cavo, M., Baccarani, M. *et al.* (1986). Bone marrow transplantation in multiple myeloma. *Scandinavian Journal of Haematology,* **36,** 176–9.

Urbano-Ispizua, A., Schmitz, N., de Witte, T. *et al.* (2002). Allogeneic and autologous transplantation for haematological diseases, solid tumors and immune disorders: definition and current practice in Europe. *Bone Marrow Transplantation,* **29,** 639–46.

Verdonck, L. F., Lokhorst, H. M., Dekker, A. W. *et al.* (1996). Graft-versus-myeloma effect in two cases. *Lancet,* **347,** 800–1.

Weiden, P. L., Sullivan, K. M., Flournoy, N. *et al.* (1981). Antileukemic effect of chronic graft-versus-host disease: contribution to improved survival after allogeneic marrow transplantation. *New England Journal of Medicine,* **304,** 1529–33.

56 Allogeneic hematopoietic stem cell transplantation for chronic lymphatic leukemia and prolymphocytic leukemia

GIUSEPPE BANDINI AND SANTE TURA

Institute of Haematology and Clinical Oncology "L. A. Seragnoli," St. Orsola Hospital, University of Bologna, Italy

Introduction

Conventional treatment of chronic lymphatic leukemia (CLL) has aimed at prolonging survival and improving quality of life (see Chapter 41). Since hematopoietic stem cell (HSC) transplantation can cure a wide range of hematologic neoplasms, it is logical to explore this in CLL, for which no other curative treatments exist. At the present time, approximately 130 CLL patients worldwide have been reported, in peer-reviewed journals, to have undergone high-dose chemoradiotherapy and hematopoietic stem cell (HSC) transplantation, mostly from HLA-identical siblings (Michallet *et al.*, 1991, 1996; Bandini *et al.*, 1991a; Rabinowe *et al.*, 1993; Khouri *et al.*, 1994, 1997; Pavletic *et al.*, 2000; Toze *et al.*, 2000; Esteve *et al.*, 2001). Considering that CLL is the most common form of leukemia in the West, and that nearly 100,000 allogeneic HSC transplants have been performed for acute and chronic leukemias, it is clear that the place of HSC transplantation in the management of CLL remains to be defined. In the first part of this chapter we examine the rationale for allografting in CLL, and in the second we summarize the results of allotransplants performed to date. Autologous HSC transplantation for CLL is described in Chapter 41.

Information on disease incidence, classification, immune phenotype, cytogenetic abnormalities, prognostic factors, outcome with conventional therapy, disease-specific pretransplant work-up, and monitoring for residual disease posttransplant are given in Chapter 41, as is information on prolymphocytic leukemia.

Age of patients

The median age of onset of CLL is 60 years, currently beyond the commonly used upper age limit for HLA-identical sibling transplantation of 55 years. However, about 10% of patients with CLL are less than 50 years old at diagnosis. The prognosis of these younger patients is in general much better than that of the general population with CLL; in fact, their median survival was 9 years in one series, was not reached at 5 years in a second study (Bandini *et al.*, 1991a), and was 12.3 years in a survey by the Spanish Cooperative Group for CLL (Montserrat *et*

al., 1991). Increasing age is known to adversely affect the results of transplantation. Thus, one of the management dilemmas facing the physicians of such patients is clear: the passage of time may be an advantage for younger patient who are diagnosed now, because new, effective drugs might be developed. However, it may also be disadvantageous to them because the risk of transplant-related mortality increases with increasing age. Enthusiasm for the use of so-called "non-ablative transplants" (Khouri *et al.*, 1998) might be particularly relevant to CLL patients, because many of them are too old or too sick for conventional transplants: if successful, there is a potential multi-fold expansion of these procedures to a large number of patients. A few such cases have been reported and are discussed later in the chapter.

Prognostic factors

The clinical course of CLL is so variable that a search for prognostic factors has been thorough. There are two well-known staging systems, the Rai classification (Rai *et al.*, 1975) and the Binet classification (Binet *et al.*, 1981), which both identify patients at low, intermediate, and high risk (Table 56.1). These staging systems can be supplemented with additional data such as lymphocyte count at diagnosis, cytogenetic findings, pattern of marrow infiltration, and lymphocyte doubling time, so that patients at one extreme can be identified with a survival similar to that of an age- and sex-matched control population and those at the other extreme with a median survival of less than 2 years (see Bandini *et al.*, 1991a; Rozman & Montserrat, 1995). The decision to undertake allogeneic HSC transplantation and its timing should be made with regard to these prognostic factors. They have been shown to be valid for younger patients (Montserrat *et al.*, 1991). Those with the worst risk should be candidates for an early transplant.

Conventional therapy of chronic lymphatic leukemia

A number of antimitotic agents (alone or in combination) are active in CLL, including chlorambucil, cyclophosphamide, vin-

Table 56.1. *Staging systems for chronic lymphatic leukemia*

Rai classification[a]	Binet classification[b]
Stage 0: bone marrow (40%) and blood lymphocytosis (4×10^9/l); no enlarged nodes	Stage A Hb > 10 g/dl and platelets $\geq 100 \times 10^9$/l. Less than 3 enlarged areas [c]
Stage I: lymphocytosis with enlarged nodes	Stage B Hb >10 g/dl and platelets $\geq100 \times 10^9$/l. Three or more enlarged areas
Stage II: lymphocytosis with enlarged spleen or liver or both	Stage C Hb <10 g/dl and platelets $<100 \times 10^9$/l. Any number of enlarged areas
Stage III: lymphocytosis with anemia	
Stage IV: lymphocytosis with thrombocytopenia	

[a] From Rai *et al.* (1975).

[b] From Binet *et al.* (1981).

[c] Each of cervical, axillary, inguinal area (whether unilateral or bilateral), spleen and liver count as one area; therefore the number of enlarged areas can take any value between 0 and 5.

cristine, corticosteroids, melphalan, busulfan, and anthracycline antibiotics. Additionally, CLL lymphocytes are very radiosensitive. Radiation therapy is effective and has been employed in several ways, including total body irradiation (TBI), total nodal irradiation, extracorporeal blood radiation, and low-dose splenic irradiation (for review see Gale & Foon, 1985). These data suggest that a conditioning regimen incorporating irradiation should be used pretransplant. A dose-response effect, an ideal prerequisite for the application of HSC transplantation, has not been shown in the majority of more intensive regimens, such as those employing moderately high doses of cyclophosphamide, vincristine, cytosine arabinoside, and anthracyclines (for review see Bandini & Michallet, 1992). There is, however, one prospective, randomized study comparing CHOP (cyclophosphamide, doxorubicin, vincristine, prednisone) with COP (cyclophosphamide, vincristine, prednisone) in advanced CLL, which demonstrated superiority for the doxorubicin-containing regimen (French Cooperative Group on CLL, 1989). Finally, a new class of drug, purine analogues—fludarabine monophosphate (Keating *et al.*, 1989) and 2-chlorodeoxyadenosine (Piro *et al.*, 1988)—have shown promising results and are likely to play a significant role in the treatment of CLL. In particular, fludarabine has been shown to be the most effective single agent in CLL, both in previously treated and untreated patients (Keating *et al.*, 1996). This drug, now widely employed, may well become, alone or in combination, the standard treatment of CLL in the future.

Evaluation of response to treatment

After conventional treatment a complete response is broadly defined as the normalization of the blood and bone marrow, resolution of organomegaly, and absence of symptoms. However, these criteria do not apply if the aim of treatment is the elimination of the neoplastic clone. More stringent criteria of complete remission include the normalization of T and B cell numbers and the kappa/lambda light chain ratio, and the presence of very low numbers of cells phenotypically characteristic of B CLL (for example CD5+ CD20+) by dual marker analysis. Finally, direct evidence for the eradication of CLL can be provided by the absence of markers of the neoplastic clone; immunoglobulin gene rearrangement studies can detect low numbers of CLL cells (1% to 2%) if the pattern of rearrangement of the individual patient is known (Rechavi *et al.*, 1989). By use of molecular biological techniques, such as polymerase chain reaction amplification of the rearranged immunoglobulin heavy chain locus (IgH), it is possible to detect residual tumor at a much lower threshold level (Billadeau *et al.*, 1991; Provan *et al.*, 1996). Conventional cytogenetic analysis is of less practical value, because of the very low mitotic yield commonly observed in CLL cells.

Results of HLA-identical sibling transplantation

Chronic lymphatic leukemia

There are now a few reports from single institutions involving small numbers of patients (Rabinowe *et al.*, 1993; Khouri *et al.*, 1994, 1997; Pavletic *et al.*, 2000; Toze *at al.*, 2000; Esteve at al., 2001; Doney *et al.*, 2002) and a single relatively large, multicenter study (Michallet *et al.*, 1996). This analysis, from the International Bone Marrow Transplant Registry and the European Group for Blood and Marrow Transplantation, described 54 patients who underwent HLA-identical sibling bone marrow transplantation (BMT). Detailed information is given in Table 56.2 and a summary in Table 56.3. Thirty-nine patients were male and 15 female, with a median age of 41 (range 21–57) years; 10 had been splenectomized. The median interval from diagnosis to transplant was 37 (range 5–130) months. The disease stage was reported at time of BMT in 52 patients. The immunologic phenotype was known in 47 patients: they all had B-CLL. Over half of the cases had advanced disease: 22 were Rai stage IV and 7 stage III, while 22 were stage I–II and three stage 0. Of 49 patients in whom prior chemotherapy data were available, 45 had received multiple courses of chemotherapy before transplant—in 26 cases including the COP or CHOP regimens—while 4 patients were untreated prior to transplant. Two patients had received local irradiation and three total lymphoid irradiation. None was in complete remission at the time of BMT: 7 patients were considered to have responsive, 19 stable, and 28 progressive disease. Conditioning before BMT consisted of cyclophosphamide in all 54 patients; however, 19 received one or more additional agents: etoposide, 13; cytosine arabinoside, 5; chlorambucil, 1; melphalan, 1; and daunorubicin, 1. TBI was administered in 51 patients, at doses varying between 8 and 14 Gy, usually in multiple fractions (48 of 51 patients). Three patients received a

Table 56.2. *Characteristics and transplant outcomes for 54 patients receiving HLA-identical sibling transplants for chronic lymphocytic leukemia*

Patient	Age (yr)	Sex	Rai stage at diagnosis	Rai stage at transplantation	Splenectomy	Interval from diagnosis to transplant (mo)	Grade of acute GVHD	Extent of chronic GVHD	Disease status	Primary cause of death (if any)
1	32	Male	4	0	N	7	1	0	HR	
2	29	Female	2	0	Y	15	2	0	HR	
3	48	Female	0	0	N	23	1	0	HR	
4	38	Male	1	1	N	10	1	Limited	HR	
5	4	Male	NA	1	N	24	4	NE	HR	Acute GVHD
6	48	Female	1	1	N	36	1	0	HR	
7	33	Male	1	1	N	39	0	0	HR	
8	37	Male	2	1	Y	40	3	Limited	HR	
9	48	Male	1	1	N	41	2	Extensive	Relapse	Chronic GVHD
10	34	Female	1	1	N	43	1	0	HR	
11	40	Male	1	1	N	51	4	NE	HR	Acute GVHD
12	51	Male	2	1	N	77	1	0	HR	
13	38	Male	1	1	Y	88	1	Limited	HR	
14	49	Male	2	2	N	6	4	NE	HR	Acute GVHD
15	37	Male	2	2	N	6	0	0	Relapse	Unknown
16	40	Male	2	2	N	10	NE	NE	HR	VOD
17	45	Male	1	2	N	14	NE	NE	HR	VOD
18	45	Male	1	2	N	22	0	Extensive	HR	Chronic GVHD
19	44	Female	NA	2	N	24	1	Limited	HR	
20	42	Male	2	2	N	25	3	Extensive	HR	IPN
21	51	Male	4	2	N	29	3	Limited	HR	
22	44	Male	NA	2	N	36	0	Extensive	HR	Chronic GVHD
23	32	Male	2	2	N	96	4	Limited	HR	
24	44	Female	3	3	N	5	1	0	HR	
25	45	Male	NA	3	N	12	1	Extensive	HR	Chronic GVHD
26	44	Male	3	3	N	20	1	Limited	HR	
27	37	Male	2	3	N	48	1	0	HR	
28	30	Male	3	3	Y	62	2	NE	HR	Bacterial infection
29	36	Male	1	3	N	96	1	NE	HR	IPN
30	45	Male	3	3	Y	106	1	Limited	HR	
31	43	Female	4	4	Y	14	0	0	HR	
32	43	Male	4	4	N	16	2	0	HR	Bacterial infection
33	44	Male	2	4	N	23	3	Extensive	HR	Chronic GVHD
34	37	Male	2	4	N	24	1	Limited	HR	
35	39	Male	2	4	N	26	4	NE	FIR	Acute GVHD
36	48	Female	1	4	N	26	3	NE	HR	Acute GVHD
37	36	Male	4	4	N	28	1	0	Relapse	CLL
38	23	Male	4	4	N	36	1	0	HR	
39	39	Male	2	4	N	39	0	0	HR	
40	32	Male	4	4	Y	41	2	NE	HR	Graft failure
41	49	Male	2	4	N	41	0	NE	HR	Graft failure
42	47	Female	1	4	N	46	0	0	HR	
43	48	Male	1	4	N	48	NE	NE	HR	Graft failure
44	41	Female	2	4	N	50	3	Limited	HR	Acute GVHD
45	49	Male	NA	4	N	51	NE	NE	HR	VOD
46	36	Female	2	4	N	60	NE	NE	HR	Viral infection
47	35	Male	1	4	N	63	0	0	HR	
48	36	Female	2	4	Y	68	1	0	Relapse	CLL
49	39	Female	2	4	Y	73	NE	NE	HR	Graft failure
50	36	Female	1	4	N	77	2	0	Relapse	CLL
51	45	Male	2	4	Y	91	1	NE	HR	Hemorrhage
52	58	Male	1	4	N	130	0	NE	HR	VOD
53	21	Male	NA	NA	N	36	NE	NE	HR	Fungal infection
54	41	Female	NA	NA	N	48	1	Limited	HR	

Abbreviations: CLL, chronic lymphatic leukemia; GVHD, graft-versus-host disease; HR, hematologic remission; IPN, interstitial pneumonitis; N, no; NA, not available; NE, not evaluable; VOD, veno-occlusive disease of the liver; Y, yes.

Reproduced, with permission, from Michallet *et al.* (1996)

Table 56.3. *Outcome after HLA-identical sibling bone marrow transplantation for 54 patients with CLL*

Number of patients	Median age (yr)	Median interval from diagnosis to transplant (mo)	Rai stage at BMT	Conditioning regimen	CLL status posttransplant	Survival
54	41 (21–57)	37 (5–130)	0, 3 I, 10 II, 10 III, 7 IV, 22 NA, 2	TBI+CY, 32 TBI+CY+other, 19 BU/CY, 3	Hematologic remission, 38 Relapse, 5	Alive, 24 Dead, 30 Transplant-related, 25 Relapse, 5

Abbreviations: CLL, chronic lymphatic leukemia; TBI, total body irradiation; CY, cyclophosphamide; BU, busulfan; NA, not available. Reproduced, with permission, from Michallet *et al.* (1996).

combination of busulfan and cyclophosphamide, without irradiation. GVHD prophylaxis was varied and included cyclosporine in 8 patients, cyclosporine and methotrexate in 35, T-cell depletion in 8, and methotrexate in 2.

The posttransplant outcome is summarized in Table 56.2. Stable engraftment occurred in 45 of 49 evaluable patients. Engraftment of neutrophils and platelets occurred within the usual time frame. Of the 45 who engrafted, 2 had a late (7 and 12 months) autologous reconstitution: both had received a T-cell-depleted graft. The disappearance of splenomegaly/hepatomegaly and lymph node enlargement usually occurred between the first and third week, while blood lymphocytosis decreased slowly, generally between the third and fourth week. However, normalization of the lymphocyte count took a long time (several months) in some patients, as we and others have observed after syngeneic (Bandini *et al.*, 1991b), or allogeneic (Jarque *et al.*, 1993) transplantation. Acute GVHD was absent in 10 patients, was grade I in 20, grade II in 6, grade III in 6, and grade IV in 5. Of 35 patients at risk, 17 developed chronic GVHD: it was extensive in 6 and limited in 11. Thirty-eight

patients achieved hematologic remission; five relapsed at 4, 7, 11, 48, and 58 months, respectively. Three of the five relapses occurred in recipients of T-cell-depleted transplants and two in recipients of unmanipulated transplants. In four patients studies of the immunoglobulin JH region rearrangement were performed before and after BMT on peripheral blood lymphocytes; the rearrangements demonstrated pretransplant were no longer present. Thirty patients died after BMT: the cause of death was relapsed CLL in 5 cases and treatment-related in 25: failure of engraftment, 4; acute GVHD, 6; chronic GVHD, 4; cerebral hemorrhage, 1; infection, 4; hepatic veno-occlusive disease, 4; and interstitial pneumonitis, 2. Twenty-four patients were alive at the time of the report, of whom 23 were in hematologic remission, at a median of 27 (range 5–80) months posttransplant. Three-year survival probability was 46% (CI, 32%–60%). Actuarial survival is shown in Fig. 56.1. There was no statistical difference in survival for patients transplanted in stages 0–III (stage 0: 100%; stage I: 68%, CI, 38%–98%; stage II: 30%, CI, 2%–58%; stage III: 57%, CI, 21%–93%). Patients with stage IV disease had a 34% (CI, 12%–56%) probability of 3-year survival. Three-year probability of survival was 86% (CI, 62%–100%) in patients with responsive disease; 61% (CI, 38%–84%) in those with stable disease, and 23% (CI, 2%–44%) in those with progressive disease.

A report from the Fred Hutchinson Cancer Research Center of 25 patients transplanted between 1980 and 1999 indicated a 5 year actuarial survival of 32%; all 7 patients conditioned with busulfan/cyclophosphamide died within 3 years of transplant, while 14 patients transplanted since 1992 and who received a TBI-containing conditioning had an actuarial 5 year survival of 56% (Doney *et al.*, 2002).

Rodriguez and colleagues (2000) reported on 8 patients with Richter's syndrome[1] (CLL transformed to an aggressive lymphoma, usually diffuse large cell lymphoma). At the time of transplant all had been heavily pretreated, 2 had failed to respond to autologous transplantation, 5 had refractory disease, 5 had B symptoms, and 7 had stage III or IV disease. At the time of the report, 3 were alive and in remission at 14, 47, and

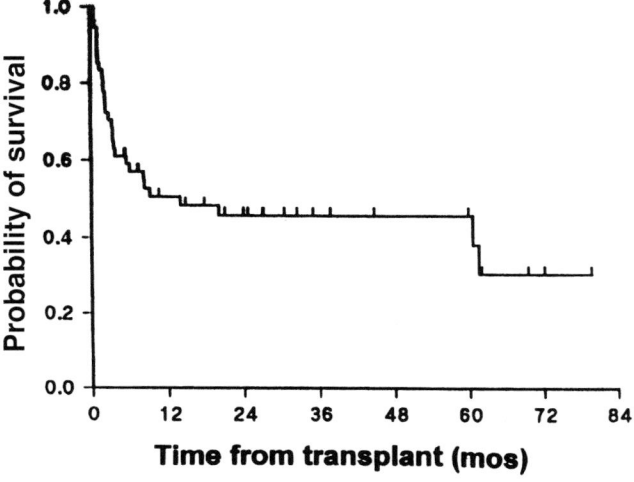

Fig. 56.1. Actuarial probability of survival after HLA-identical sibling bone marrow transplantation for chronic lymphatic leukemia. Reproduced, with permission, from Michallet *et al.* (1996).

[1] Maurice Richter, U.S. pathologist, born 1897.

67 months posttransplant respectively. Two of these three had received non-myeloablative regimens.

Prolymphocytic leukemia (PLL)

A small of number of cases of prolymphocytic leukemia have been treated by allogeneic HSC transplantation (Collins *et al.,* 1998; Dearden *et al.,* 2001). Of the four cases reported in the latter study, three were alive and in complete remission at the time of the report at >2, >11, and >24 months posttransplant respectively. Two received myeloablative conditioning and a sibling transplant, one non-ablative conditioning and a sibling transplant, and one non-ablative conditioning and an unrelated donor transplant. Another case of unrelated transplantation was reported by Toze *et al.* (2000), in a larger series of CLL transplants. The patient, a 46-year-old male achieved complete remission after transplant but died of progressive multifocal leukoencephalopathy after 13 months. A patient with refractory PLL who received a non-ablative regimen has been reported (Garderet *et al.,* 2001). The patient relapsed at day 84 and died of progressive disease at five months, despite DLI and chemotherapy.

Results of HLA-mismatched family member transplantation

Three cases of 1 or 2 HLA antigen family member mismatched grafts have been reported in a larger series of CLL transplants (Khouri *et al.,* 1997). All had refractory disease, received myeloablative TBI/cyclophophsamide based regimens and cyclosporine/methotrexate (CSP/MTX) or tacrolimus/methotrexate for GVHD prophylaxis. Two patients were alive (one after a second transplant), with no evidence of disease at the time of writing, while the third died of GVHD and infections after DLI.

Another patient with refractory disease received marrow from a DRB1-mismatched sibling after a 200 cGy TBI non-ablative regimen (Kreiter *et al.,* 2001). He died of GVHD on day +112, with no evidence of disease by immunophenotypic analysis.

Results of unrelated donor transplantation

Few cases have been reported. One patient, with progressive disease, received a partially mismatched unrelated transplant, which was T-depleted; the posttransplant course was uneventful and he was alive, in remission, at 10 months (Mehta *et al.,* 1996b) (Fig. 56.2). One patient with refractory disease (Khouri *et al.,* 1997) received a conventional transplant and was alive in remission, with limited chronic GVHD at the time of writing. A third patient (Toze *et al.,* 2000) was reported alive without evidence of disease at two years after a T-cell depleted transplant.

Results of cord blood transplantation

No transplants for CLL or PLL with cord blood as the source of stem cells have been described so far.

Results with reduced intensity conditioning regimens

At the M.D. Anderson Hospital nine patients with CLL or NHL have been treated, of whom eight were older than age 50. Two regimens have been explored in patients with CLL and lymphoma and are summarized in Table 56.4 (and see Chapters 22 and 57).

All patients had failed to respond to, or had recurring disease after, primary chemotherapy. Five patients had CLL in relapse after a prior fludarabine response and four patients had trans-

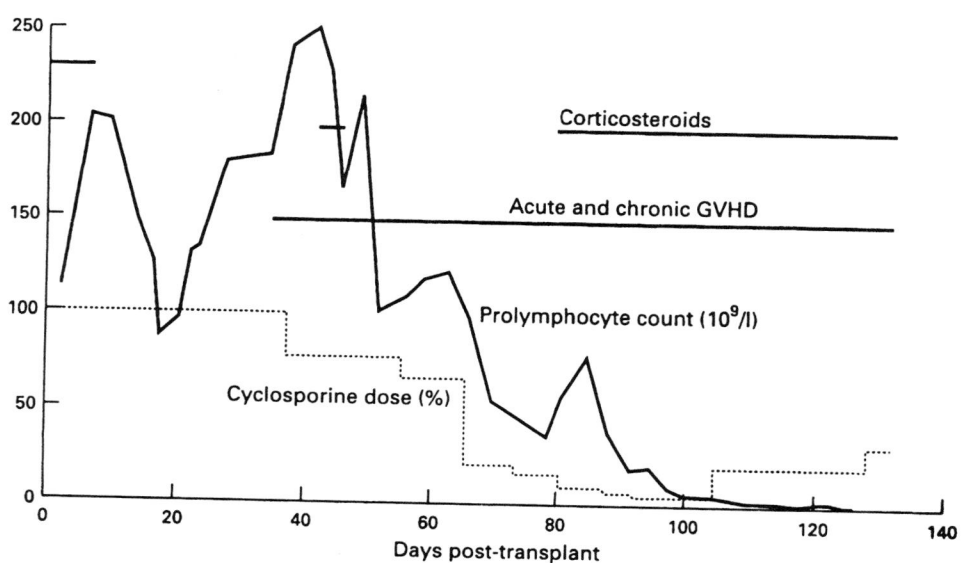

Fig. 56.2. Temporal relationship between cyclosporine dose, GVHD, steroid therapy, and leukocyte count after allogeneic bone marrow transplantation in a patient with PLL. Reproduced, with permission, from Mehta *et al.* (1996a).

Table 56.4. *Preparative regimens for "mini-transplants" in lymphoid malignancies*

Chronic lymphatic leukemia

Days	−5	−4	−3	−2	−1	0
	F	F	F			
	30 mg/m²	30 mg/m²	30 mg/m²			Allo SCT
	C	C	C			
	300 mg/m²	300 mg/m²	300 mg/m²			

Lymphoma

Days	−6	−5	−4	−3	−2	−1	0
	P	P	P	P			
	25 mg/m²	25 mg/m²	25 mg/m²	25 mg/m²			Allo SCT
			F	F			
			30 mg/m²	30 mg/m²			
			C	C			
			500 mg/m²	500 mg/m²			

Abbreviations: F, fludarabine; C, cyclophosphamide; P, cisplatin; SCT, stem cell transplant.

formed lymphoma. All patients had active disease at the time of transplant; three had a performance status of 3 (SWOG criteria), one had elevated liver function tests, and all had received extensive prior therapy. Despite these features, no patient had a nonhematologic toxicity of greater than grade 2 with the preparative regimens used.

These chemotherapy regimens are known to be non-myeloablative and mixed chimerism was anticipated. Six of the nine patients had evidence of engraftment documented by marrow RFLP testing. The percentage of donor cells in the marrow ranged from 50% to 100% at 1 month posttransplant. One had 75% donor cells in his marrow at 6 weeks posttransplant, and converted to 100% donor cells following a donor lymphocyte infusion.

Of the patients who engrafted, one never had an absolute neutrophil count (ANC) of less than $1.0 \times 10^9/l$; and one had an ANC of less than $0.5 \times 10^9/l$ for only 2 days. Neither of these patients required platelet transfusions. Four patients received donor lymphocyte infusions between 55 and 100 days posttransplant to augment the graft-versus-tumor effect. One achieved an initial partial remission and converted to complete response 9 months after the donor lymphocyte infusion. Of the engrafted patients, four achieved complete remission and two had decreased tumor burden. The patients failing to engraft recovered endogenous hematopoiesis promptly and had no serious adverse effects. Increasing the intensity of the preparative regimen might increase the rate of engraftment. The minimal toxicity and mild cytopenia suggest that this procedure could be administered on an outpatient basis.

Seven patients with CLL, part of a larger group with various hematological malignancies, were treated with 200 cGy TBI and CSP/mycophenolate mofetil as GVHD prophylaxis (McSweeney et al., 2001). Donors were HLA-identical siblings; the stem cell source was mobilized peripheral blood. Four patients had refractory disease. All engrafted, but extensive chronic GVHD occurred in 6 of 7. Two died, one of pneumonia and one of disease. Of the 5 alive, with a follow-up ranging between 10 and 17 months, 2 were in molecular remission, 1 in clinical remission, and 2 had evidence of disease; 4 had extensive chronic GVHD. In two patients DLIs were necessary for disease progression or relapse. Another patient received a similar TBI regimen, with the addition of fludarabine from days −4 to −2 (Nieto et al., 2001). Because of early, explosive tumor growth posttransplant, he was treated with rituximab and high-dose chemotherapy. A rapid response was achieved, demonstrating that posttransplant chemotherapy did not compromise donor cell engraftment or establishment of stable donor chimerism.

Comparison with chemotherapy and autologous transplantation

A formal statistical comparison is not yet possible, since CLL patients subjected to allogeneic transplantation represent a highly selected group. Additionally, there are no results of trials comparing chemotherapy to autologous transplantation, although some studies are in progress. We can, however, make some qualitative observations about the type of response achieved with these different forms of therapy. Intensive chemotherapy or, the monoclonal antibody Campath 1, can induce high remission rates at the clinical level and, to a lesser degree, at the molecular level. However, these responses, although remarkably sustained, eventually are lost in the majority of patients (Dearden et al., 2001; Rawstron et al., 2001). In the autologous transplantation setting, the possibility of achieving molecular remission is well documented and its likelihood is strictly related to the sensitivity of the technique. Employing the exquisitively sensitive assay of the rearrangement pattern of the CDR III region of the heavy chain immunoglobulin (IgH) gene, Esteve et al. (2001) found a 64% negativity rate for minimal residual disease (MRD) in 14 cases of autologous transplantation. However, with prolonged follow-up, two of the nine patients had a clinical relapse and four became MRD-positive. In contrast, of 8 allotransplant recipients who achieved a clinical complete remission, all became MRD-negative (in two patients requiring up to 22 months), and none subsequently demonstrated MRD or clinical relapse. Similarly, a study at the Huddinge Hospital, showed that after allogeneic transplantation patients slowly became MRD-negative, and did not relapse (Mattson *et al.*, 2000). These data suggest that the type of response achieved after allogeneic transplantation is durable, may result in true "cure" in some cases and is related to the allogeneic effect of the graft, be it coincident or not with GVHD. This is in contrast to what is seen after chemotherapy or after autologous transplantation, when the disease eventually always recurs, although some of the remissions may be quite long.

Another study on the clinical usefulness of molecular methods to assess residual disease after high-dose therapy described three patients with CLL who were persistently polymerase chain reaction (PCR)-negative for 4 years after HLA-identical sibling BMT (Provan *et al.*, 1996). A similar outcome was described in a single patient by Sardoun *et al.* (1994) (see also Chapter 41 on autologous HSC transplantation for CLL).

Indications and contraindications for allogeneic transplantation

The existing data indicate that the choice of allogeneic transplantation should be based on disease risk on the one hand, and the transplant risk on the other. In patients with high-risk CLL, allogeneic transplantation should be considered as first-line treatment if the transplant-related mortality risk is not high— for example, younger patients with no co-existing infections or other co-morbidities, those with younger donors and perfect HLA matching. In the remaining cases, allogeneic transplantation should be employed as a second or third line therapy. Since there are several reports of response, even in cases of advanced disease, the deferral of transplantation may not be detrimental and the increased risk of transplant-related mortality may thus be justified by the disease status. Clearly, an accurate assessment of disease risk and transplant risk is not always easy to determine in everyday clinical practice. Nonetheless, it should be the approach used to guide the physician in the therapeutic strategy for each individual patient.

The current practice of HSC transplantation for CLL in Europe has been described (Urbano-Ispizua *et al.*, 2002) (see also Chapter 124).

Conclusions

The number of patients so far reported is too small to allow in-depth statistical analysis. However, from the analysis of the largest reported group of CLL patients treated by HLA-identical sibling BMT (Michallet *et al.*, 1996), a few observations can be made. Firstly, allogeneic BMT can be successfully performed in CLL, resulting in long-term leukemia-free survival in patients with either early or advanced disease; the main causes of death were transplant-related and occurred early after BMT, a finding similar to that observed by us in multiple myeloma (Tura *et al.*, 1990) or after transplants for Hodgkin's disease (Gajewski *et*

al., 1996). A similar, although slightly less high transplant-related mortality was reported by Pavletic *et al.* (2000); of 23 patients, 8 died of a transplant-related cause and only one of disease. These data somewhat contrast with the low mortality reported in some small studies from single institutions. At the Dana-Farber Cancer Institute, eight patients with CLL were allotransplanted in complete remission, having responded to fludarabine: seven of them were alive with a follow-up period ranging from 6 to 18 months (Rabinowe *et al.*, 1993). Of six patients who received HLA-identical sibling transplants at the Vancouver Hospital, two died, one of infection and one of relapse (Toze *et al.*, 2000). Of 12 patients transplanted at Hospital Clinic in Barcelona, 3 died of transplant-related causes and one of disease relapse. Ten patients were allotransplanted at the M.D. Anderson Cancer Center, after unsuccessful treatment with fludarabine; seven had advanced disease. Nine were alive 2 to 36 months posttransplant (Khouri *et al.*, 1994). Two updates, however, reported a higher mortality rate in a larger number of patients (Khouri, 1996; Khouri *et al.*, 1997): of 15 patients with advanced disease, 7 died after transplant, only one case being due to disease progression and five being transplant-related. It is matter of speculation whether the prior use of fludarabine, patient selection, or other factors contributed to the low incidence of acute GVHD and overall transplant-related mortality in the earlier reports. However, these data are generally encouraging and it can be expected that transplant-related morbidity and mortality will in the future be reduced in CLL patients, similarly to that observed in other malignancies, especially the acute leukemias, during the past decade (Frassoni *et al.*, 1996).

A second point of note is that overall survival was best in patients with Rai stages 0 to III, and in those with stable or responsive disease. Such findings are analogous to results in most hematologic malignancies. Patients with more advanced CLL, and more prior therapy, are more likely to have a poorer performance status at transplant than those with less advanced disease. A report from the Royal Marsden Hospital has underlined the occurrence of unusual opportunistic infections in six CLL or PLL patients following allogeneic HSC transplantation (Zomas *et al.*, 1994; Mehta *et al.*, 1997). Thus, it is likely to be advantageous to transplant earlier in the course of the disease, soon after achieving a stable decrease of the leukemic mass. It is of interest in this respect that the three patients transplanted in Rai stage 0 became long-term survivors. The incidence of severe acute GVHD was high, with 10 patients having grade III–IV disease; this finding could perhaps have been expected in view of the median age of the patient population (Gale *et al.*, 1987).

Interestingly, there are at least five reports suggesting that a graft-versus-leukemia effect is operative in this malignancy and in the related PLL (Rondon *et al.*, 1996; Mehta *et al.*, 1996a; de Magalhaes-Silverman *et al.*, 1997; Khouri *et al.*, 1998; Dreger *et al.*, 2000). In these reports, disease remission occurred after withdrawal of immunosuppression, infusion of donor lymphocytes, or the onset of GVHD. Also the delayed clearance of CLL, taking up to one year or longer in a few patients, (Jarque *et al.*, 1993; Mattson *et al.*, 2000; Esteve *et al.*, 2001) has been explained by the modulation of the graft-versus-tumor effect on residual leukemic cells.

We think that further studies of the use of allogeneic HSC transplantation in selected patients with CLL are justified and should be encouraged, with the aim of better defining the indications and timing of transplant, while taking into account the availability of the newer chemotherapy agents. Such studies should help establish the precise role of allotransplantation in the management of CLL.

References

Bandini, G., Michallet, M., Rosti, G., & Tura, S. (1991a). Bone marrow transplantation for chronic lymphocytic leukemia. *Bone Marrow Transplantation,* **7,** 101–3.

Bandini, G., Miggiano, C., Calori, E. *et al.* (1991b). Slow kinetics of disappearance of peripheral blood lymphocytes after syngeneic bone marrow transplantation for chronic lymphocytic leukemia. Presented at the 17th meeting of the EBMT, Cortina d'Ampezzo, January 27–31, 1991 (abstract 389).

Bandini, G. & Michallet, M. (1992). High-dose therapy and allogeneic bone marrow transplantation in chronic lymphocytic leukemia. In *High-dose Cancer Therapy: Pharmacology, Hematopoietins, Stem Cells,* ed. J. O. Armitage & K. Antman, pp. 626–37. Baltimore: Williams & Wilkins.

Billadeau, D., Blackstadt, M., Greipp, P. *et al.* (1991). Analysis of B-lymphoid malignancies using allele specific polymerase chain reaction: a technique for sequential quantitation of residual disease. *Blood,* **78,** 3021–19.

Binet, J., Auquir, A., Dighiero, G. *et al.* (1981). A new prognostic classification of chronic lymphocytic leukemia derived from multivariate survival analysis. *Cancer,* **48,** 198–206.

Collins, R. H., Pineiro, L. A., Agura, E. D., & Fay, J. W. (1998). Treatment of T prolymphocytic leukemia with allogeneic bone marrow transplantation. *Bone Marrow Transplantation,* **21,** 627–8.

Dearden, C. E., Matutes, E., Cazin, B. *et al.* (2001). High remission rate in T-cell prolymphocytic leukemia with CAMPATH-1H. *Blood,* **98,** 1721–6.

Dreger, P., Glass, B., Seygarth, B. *et al.* (2000). Reduced-intensity allogeneic stem cell transplantation as salvage treatment for patients with indolent lymphoma or CLL after failure of autologous SCT. *Bone Marrow Transplantation,* **26,** 131–6.

de Magalhaes-Silverman, M., Donnenberg, A., Hammert, L. *et al.* (1997). Induction of graft-versus-leukemia effect in a patient with chronic lymphocytic leukemia. *Bone Marrow Transplantation,* **20,** 175–77.

Doney, K. C., Chauncey, T., & Appelbaum, F. R. for the Seattle Bone Marrow Transplant Team (2002). Allogeneic related donor hematopoietic stem cell transplantation for treatment of chronic lymphocytic leukemia. *Bone Marrow Transplantation,* **29,** 817–23.

Esteve, J., Villamor, N., Colomer, D. *et al.* (2001). Stem cell transplantation for chronic lymphocytic leukemia: different outcomes after autologous and allogeneic transplantation and correlation with minimal residual disease status. *Leukemia,* **15,** 445–451.

Frassoni, F., Labopin, M., Gluckman, E. *et al.* (1996). Results of allogeneic transplantation for acute leukemia have improved in Europe with time: a report of the Acute Leukemia Working party of the European Group for Blood and Marrow Transplantation (EBMT). *Bone Marrow Transplantation,* **17,** 13–18.

French Cooperative Group on Chronic Lymphocytic Leukaemia (CLL) (1989). Long-term results of the CHOP regimen in stage C chronic lymphocytic leukaemia. *British Journal of Haematology,* **73,** 334–40.

Gajewski, J. L., Phillips, G. L., Sobocinski, K. A. *et al.* (1996). Bone marrow transplants from HLA-identical siblings in advanced Hodgkin's disease. *Journal of Clinical Oncology,* **14,** 572–8.

Gale, R. P. & Foon, K. A. (1985). Chronic lymphocytic leukemia. Recent advances in biology and treatment. *Annals of Internal Medicine,* **103,** 101–20.

Gale, R., Bortin, M. M., Van Bekkum, D. W. *et al.* (1987). Risk factors for acute graft-versus-host disease. *British Journal of Haematology,* **67,** 397–406.

Garderet, L., Bittencourt, H., Kaliski, A. *et al.* (2001). Treatment of T-prolymphocytic leukemia with nonmyeloablative allogeneic stem cell transplantation. *European Journal of Haematology,* **66,** 137–9.

Jarque, I., Palan, J., Sanz, F. G. *et al.* (1993). Delayed complete response after allogeneic bone marrow transplantation in chronic lymphocytic leukemia. *Blood,* **82,** 1036–8 (letter).

Keating, M. J., Kantarjian, H., Talpaz, M. *et al.* (1989). Fludarabine: a new agent with major activity against chronic lymphocytic leukemia. *Blood,* **74,** 19–25.

Keating, M. J., O'Brien, S., McLaughlin, P. *et al.* (1996). Clinical experience with fludarabine in hemato-oncology. *Hematology and Cell Therapy,* **38** (Suppl 2), 83–91.

Khouri, I. (1996). Allogeneic bone marrow transplantation in chronic lymphocytic leukemia. *Annals of Internal Medicine,* **125,** 780 (Letter).

Khouri, I. F., Keating, M., Korbling, M. *et al.* (1998). Transplant-lite: induction of graft-versus-malignancy using fludarabine-based nonablative chemotherapy and allogeneic blood progenitor-cell transplantation as treatment for lymphoid malignancies. *Journal of Clinical Oncology,* **16,** 2817–24.

Khouri, I. F., Keating, M. J., Vriesendorp, H. M. *et al.* (1994). Autologous and allogeneic bone marrow transplantation for chronic lymphocytic leukemia: preliminary results. *Journal of Clinical Oncology,* **12,** 748–58.

Khouri, I. F., Przepiorka, D., van Besien, K. *et al.* (1997). Allogeneic blood or marrow transplantation for chronic lymphocytic leukemia: timing of transplantation and potential effect of fludarabine on acute graft-versus-host disease. *British Journal of Haematology,* **97,** 466–73.

Kreiter, S., Winkelmann, N., Schneider, P. M. *et al.* (2001). Failure of sustained engraftment after non-myeloablative conditioning with low-dose TBI and T-cell reduced allogeneic peripheral stem cell transplantation. *Bone Marrow Transplantation,* **28,** 157–161.

Mattson, J., Uzunel, M., Remberger, M. *et al.* (2000). Minimal residual disease is common after allogeneic stem cell transplantation in patients with B-cell chronic lymphocytic leukemia and may be controlled by graft-versus-host disease. *Leukemia,* **14,** 247–254.

McSweeney, P., Niederwieser, D., Shizuru, J. A. *et al.* (2001). Hemopoietic cell transplantation in older patients with hematologic malignancies: replacing high-dose cytotoxic therapy with graft-versus-tumor effects. *Blood,* **97,** 3390–3400.

Mehta, J., Powles, R., Singhal, S. *et al.* (1996a). Clinical and hematologic response of chronic lymphocytic and prolymphocytic leukemia persisting after allogeneic bone marrow transplantation with the onset of acute graft-versus-host disease: possible role of graft-versus-leukemia. *Bone Marrow Transplantation,* **17,** 371–5.

Mehta, J., Powles, R., Singhal, S. *et al.* (1996b). T cell-depleted allogeneic bone marrow transplantation from a partially HLA-mismatched unrelated donor for progressive chronic lymphocytic leukemia and fluadarabine-induced bone marrow failure. *Bone Marrow Transplantation,* **17,** 881–83.

Mehta, J., Powles, R. L., Singhal, S. *et al.* (1997). Antimicrobial prophylaxis to prevent opportunistic infections in patients with chronic lymphocytic leukemia after allogeneic blood or marrow transplantation. *Leukemia and Lymphoma,* **26,** 83–88.

Michallet, M., Archimbaud, E., Bandini, G. *et al.* (1996). HLA-identical sibling bone marrow transplantation in younger patients with chronic lymphocytic leukemia. *Annals of Internal Medicine,* **124,** 311–15.

Michallet, M., Corront, B., Hollard, D. *et al.* (1991). Allogeneic bone marrow transplantation in chronic lymphocytic leukemia: 17 cases. Report from the EBMTG. *Bone Marrow Transplantation,* **7,** 275–9.

Montserrat, E., Gomis, F., Vallespi, T. *et al.* (1991). Presenting features and prognosis of chronic lymphocytic leukemia in younger adults. *Blood,* **78,** 1545–51.

Nieto, Y., Bearman, S. I., Sphall, E. J. *et al.* (2001). Intensive chemotherapy for progressive chronic lymphocytic leukemia administered early after a non myeloablative allograft. *Bone Marrow Transplantation,* **28,** 1083–86.

Pavletic, Z. S., Arrowsmith, E. R., Bierman, P. J. *et al.* (2000). Outcome of allogeneic stem cell transplantation for B cell chronic lymphocytic leukemia. *Bone Marrow Transplantation,* **25,** 717–22.

Piro, L. D., Carrera, C. J., Beutler, E., & Carson, D. A. (1988). 2-Chlorodeoxyadenosine: an effective new agent for the treatment of chronic lymphocytic leukemia. *Blood,* **72,** 1069–73.

Provan, D., Bartlett-Pandite, L., Zwicky, C. *et al.* (1996). Eradication of polymerase chain reaction-detectable chronic lymphocytic leukemia cells is associated with improved outcome after bone marrow transplantation. *Blood,* **88,** 2228–35.

Rabinowe, S. N., Soiffer, R. J., Gribben, J. G. *et al.* (1993). Autologous and allogeneic bone marrow transplantation for poor prognosis patients with B-cell chronic lymphocytic leukemia. *Blood,* **82,** 1366–76.

Rai, K. R., Sawitsky, A., Cronkite, E. P. *et al.* (1975). Clinical staging of chronic lymphocytic leukemia. *Blood,* **46,** 219–34.

Rawstron, A. C., Kennedy, B., Evans, P. A. S. *et al.* (2001). Quantitation of minimal disease levels in chronic lymphocytic leukemia using a sensitive flow cytometric assay improves the prediction of outcome and can be used to optimize therapy. *Blood,* **98,** 29–35.

Rechavi, G., Mandel, M., Katzir, N. *et al.* (1989). Immunoglobulin heavy chain gene rearrangements in chronic lymphocytic leukaemia: correlation with clinical stage. *British Journal of Haematology,* **72,** 524–9.

Rodrigez, J., Keating, M. J., O'Brien, S. *et al.* (2000). Allogeneic haematopoietic transplantation for Richter's syndrome. *British Journal of Haematology,* **110,** 897–9.

Rondon, G., Giralt, S., Huh, Y. *et al.* (1996). Graft-versus-leukemia effect after allogeneic bone marrow transplantation for chronic lymphocytic leukemia. *Bone Marrow Transplantation,* **18,** 669–72.

Rozman, C. & Montserrat, E. (1995). Chronic lymphocytic leukemia. *New England Journal of Medicine,* **333,** 1052–7.

Sardoun, A., Patri, S., Delwail, V. *et al.* (1994). Molecular remission after allogeneic bone marrow transplantation for chronic lymphocytic leukemia. *Bone Marrow Transplantation,* **13,** 217–19.

Toze, C. L., Sheperd, J. D., Connors, J. M. *et al.* (2000). Allogeneic bone marrow transplantation for low-grade lymphoma and chronic lymphocytic leukemia. *Bone Marrow Transplantation,* **25,** 605–12.

Tura, S., Cavo, M., Gobbi, M. *et al.* (1990). High-dose chemoradiotherapy and allogeneic bone marrow transplantation in multiple myeloma. *European Journal of Haematology,* **43** (Suppl 51), 191–5.

Urbano-Ispizua, A., Schmitz, N., de Witte, T. *et al.* (2002). Allogeneic and autologous transplantation for haematological diseases, solid tumors and immune disorders: definition and current practice in Europe. *Bone Marrow Transplantation,* **29,** 639–46.

Zomas, A., Mehta, J., Powles, R. *et al.* (1994). Unusual infections following allogeneic bone marrow transplantation for chronic lymphocytic leukemia. *Bone Marrow Transplantation,* **14,** 799–803.

57 Allogeneic hematopoietic stem cell transplantation for the non-Hodgkin's and Hodgkin's lymphomas

GREGORY HALE, DONNA E. REECE, AND GORDON L. PHILLIPS

St. Jude Children's Research Hospital, Memphis, Princess Margaret Hospital, Toronto, Canada, and University of Rochester, Rochester, USA

Introduction

Allogeneic hematopoietic stem cell (HSC) transplantation has been used less frequently in the treatment of non-Hodgkin's lymphoma (NHL) and Hodgkin's lymphoma than has autologous transplantation; the latter is a well-accepted component of the overall treatment schema in selected patients with these diagnoses (Reece & Phillips, 1994; Salzman, Briggs, & Vaughan, 1997; Mink & Armitage, 2001). Specifically, data from the International and Autologous Blood and Marrow Transplant Registries (IBMTR/ABMTR) for 1999 indicated a ratio of 3.3:1 of autologous to allogeneic transplants for NHL, and an even higher ratio for Hodgkin's lymphoma (M. Horowitz, personal communication, 2002). The requirements for a closer degree of histocompatibility between donor and recipient and a younger age limit reduce the relative number of allografts. That said, there are unique advantages to the use of allogeneic transplants; obviously, there are disadvantages as well. To further consider this issue, an encyclopedic review of the published literature will not be attempted; rather, registry data (including that of the IBMTR/ABMTR and the European Group for Blood and Marrow Transplantation [EBMT]) will be emphasized, with other selected published sources used to highlight current patterns of usage, frequent problems, and specific considerations regarding transplantation for the lymphomas. Moreover, since an emerging literature (Linch *et al.*, 1993; Philip *et al.*, 1995; Haioun *et al.*, 1997, 2000) suggests the superiority of autologous stem cell transplants to conventional therapy in some circumstances, the comparison of allografts to autotransplants will be emphasized, and a tentative listing of recommendations for the preferential use of allogeneic stem cell transplantation proposed.

Overview

Non-Hodgkin's lymphoma

The NHLs are a diverse set of hematologic malignancies; they are, in the main, of uncertain etiology and have differing histologies, immune phenotypes, molecular and cytogenetic abnormalities, clinical courses, and responses to conventional therapy (Norton, 1996) (and see Chapter 35). For reasons only partially explained, these diseases continue to increase in frequency, affecting 56,200 Americans per year and were anticipated to claim the lives of roughly 26,000 Americans in 2001 (Greenlee *et al.*, 2001). Although a new classification schema of NHL—The Revised European-American Classification of Lymphoid Neoplasms—is evolving (Pittaluga *et al.*, 1996) (Chapter 34), it is not yet widely utilized in the published literature (De Wolf-Peeters & Pittaluga, 1996). The Working Formulation (Non-Hodgkin's Lymphoma Classification Project, 1982) that subclassifies NHL into three grades has been used for most reported cases to date. The low-grade NHLs are usually widely disseminated (often including the marrow) B-cell diseases with frequently indolent courses that occur in older individuals, although exceptions are not rare. These diseases are responsive to, but minimally curable with, conventional chemotherapy; a small proportion may be cured with loco-regional radiotherapy. The intermediate-grade NHLs (for this discussion, immunoblastic lymphoma is included) are disseminated slightly less frequently, and also involve the marrow less often. Unlike the majority of low-grade NHL cases, most intermediate-grade cases are rapidly fatal unless successfully treated with combination chemotherapy. The high-grade NHLs more often occur in younger patients, resemble to various degrees acute lymphoblastic leukemia (ALL), and are treated accordingly; as with intermediate-grade NHL, cures are also observed in patients who achieve a durable initial remission with conventional chemotherapy.

The incidence of low- and intermediate-grade NHL is roughly equal; approximately 10% of patients have high-grade NHL (Skarin & Dorfman, 1997). Many NHL patients are aged more than 60 years, a fact relevant to all forms of stem cell transplantation, but especially allogeneic stem cell transplantation.

One problem with the Working Formulation classification is the difficulty in classifying some of the more recently defined entities such as mucosa-associated lymphoid tissue (MALT) and mantle cell lymphoma. Less-than-definitive information exists regarding both autologous, and especially allogeneic, stem cell transplants for many specific lymphomatous entities, providing less than optimal assistance to the clinician trying to delineate the precise role of these modalities for these diseases.

Additional information on disease incidence, classification, immune phenotype, cytogenetic abnormalities, prognostic factors, outcome with conventional therapy, disease-specific pretransplant work-up, and monitoring for residual disease posttransplant are given in Chapter 34.

Hodgkin's lymphoma

Hodgkin's lymphoma[1] is a malignancy of unknown etiology. The incidence appears to be stable, afflicting roughly 7,500 Americans per year, with 1,200 expected to die from the disease in 2001 (Greenlee *et al.*, 2001). Histologically, the tumor mass is comprised mainly of reactive cells; the derivation of the characteristic Hodgkin/Reed[2]-Sternberg[3] cell has been uncertain, although some studies indicate a B-cell origin in at least some cases (Marafioti *et al.*, 1997; Stein & Hummel, 1999). These characteristic cells occur with differing frequencies in the recognized histologic subtypes (i.e., nodular sclerosis, mixed cellularity, lymphocyte predominance, and lymphocyte depletion). Both localized and disseminated presentations are common. Details of classification and staging are given in Chapter 35. Optimal use of radiotherapy and conventional chemotherapy cures approximately 75% of Hodgkin's lymphoma patients (Longo, Banks, & Hoppe, 1994; Fung & Nadamanee, 2002); however, only a minority of those who fail optimal primary chemotherapy are curable by conventional salvage treatment (Longo *et al.*, 1992).

Allogeneic stem cell transplantation

Dose-intensive cytotoxic therapy with allogeneic stem cell transplantation is an attractive therapeutic modality for those diseases with a steep dose-response effect to cytotoxic agents (Frei & Canellos, 1980), and in which an immune therapeutic effect analogous to the graft-versus-leukemia phenomenon (Horowitz *et al.*, 1990) is present. These features apply to the lymphomas. Furthermore, in allogeneic hematopoietic stem cell (HSC) transplantation, the stem cells have not been exposed to cytotoxic therapy.

A detailed discussion of various conditioning regimens used for allografting will not be undertaken herein, for several reasons: (1) the general principles of such are outlined elsewhere in this volume; (2) there are few data indicating special requirements for lymphoma—save for the avoidance of total body irradiation (TBI) in patients previously given thoracic irradiation (Friedberg *et al.*, 2001); (3) a wide variety of regimens are utilized, but few comparative data are available. That said, it is at least possible that there are differences in sensitivity to conditioning regimens for different types of lymphoma.

[1]Thomas Hodgkin, English physician and pathologist, 1798–1866.
[2]Dorothy Reed, U.S. pathologist, 1874–1964.
[3]Carl Sternberg, Austrian pathologist, 1872–1935.

The graft-versus-lymphoma effect, however, will be discussed in detail; its utilization is critical to the ongoing, and certainly the expanded, use of allografts for malignant lymphoproliferative diseases.

Results of HLA-identical sibling transplantation

Non-Hodgkin's lymphoma

Table 57.1 shows selected features of patients reported to the IBMTR regarding details of patient characteristics, therapeutic modalities utilized, and results. Figure 57.1 shows an overall survival curve for a larger group of less-fully analyzed patients.

As noted above, many fewer patients have been allografted then autografted. Given the heterogeneity of clinical and treatment-related features, this finding limits confidence in statements regarding potential prognostic parameters. Secondly, a relative disproportionate number of patients with high-grade NHL have been transplanted, considering that they comprise a minority of NHL patients; the explanation for this is likely the younger median patient age and similarities to ALL, a disease in which allografting is, in some situations, a standard of care. Of note, outcome data in lymphoma patients are similar to those of other hematologic malignancies when corrected for disease status (Passweg *et al.*, 1995). If similar considerations exist as in autotransplantation (Bolwell, Goormastic, & Andresen, 1997), longer follow-up is required to fully assess the possibility of cure, especially for those allografted for low-grade NHL.

Low-grade NHL

Several groups have reported on allogeneic transplantation for these diseases, mostly follicular center cell lymphoma. Workers at the M.D. Anderson Cancer Center reported the results of such therapy in 15 low-grade NHL patients (van Besien *et al.*, 1995, 1996a) (Fig. 57.2). Overall survival and relapse-free survival were higher, and relapse rates were lower, than in other allografted NHL patients; interestingly, even patients with refractory low-grade NHL had surprisingly favorable outcomes. Verdonck *et al.* (1997) reported similar findings in 28 low-grade NHL patients, of whom 10 were allografted. Relapse rates were 0% for the allografts versus 83% for the autografts, resulting in an improved 3-year progression-free survival of 68% versus 22% (Fig. 57.3). These findings suggested to these authors that allogeneic transplants might be preferred to autografts in low-grade NHL. Similar results have been reported after allografts depleted of T cells by antibody and complement treatment (Juckett *et al.*, 1998) (Fig. 57.4). Cull and colleagues (2000) used the in vivo administration of Campath-1G from day −5 to day −1 before transplant, in association with the carmustine, etoposide, cytosine arabinoside, and melphalan (BEAM) regimen, to treat patients with lymphoma or CLL. Eleven of 12 patients engrafted and only one developed acute GVHD. Toxicity appeared similar to that experienced when using BEAM for autologous transplantation.

The IBMTR experience in low-grade lymphoma, partially summarized in Table 57.1, has been reviewed (van Besien *et*

Table 57.1. *Summary of allogeneic transplants for NHL reported to the IBMTR*

Parameter	Grade of NHL[a]		
	Low	Intermediate	High
Number analyzed	113	225	205
Age in years: median (range)	38 (15–61)	39 (2–57)	26 (<1–55)
Male sex (%)	58	64	70
Disease status at transplant: CR/relapse/PIF (%)	2/37/53	37/21/42	16/60/24
TBI-containing conditioning regimen (%)	82	57	66
Bone marrow as source of stem cells (%)	100	86	96
T-cell depletion as GVHD prophylaxis (%)	22	5	4
3-year overall survival (%)	49	29	38

Abbreviations: CR, complete remission; PIF, primary induction failure; TBI, total body irradiation; GVHD, graft-versus-host disease.

[a] Working Formulation Classification.

al., 1998). This retrospective study consisted of 113 patients, including 52 with follicular small cleaved cell and 41 with follicular mixed cell histology. As expected in an allograft series, the median age at transplant (38 years) was below the usual median age of such patients. At the time of transplant, 68% had marrow involvement. Most patients were heavily pretreated (median number of prior chemotherapy cycles was two); 29% had Karnofsky scores less than 80%, and 37% had refractory disease. All donors were HLA-matched siblings. Treatment modalities regarding conditioning, graft manipulation, and various supporting techniques were variable. Results were encouraging, with the 3-year probability of survival, disease-free survival, relapse, and nonrelapse mortality being 49% (95% confidence interval, [CI], 39%–60%), 49% (95% CI, 39%–59%), 16% (95% CI, 9%–27%), and 40% (95% CI, 30%–50%), respectively. Not surprisingly, improved survival was associated with patient age less than 40 years, better pretransplant performance status, chemosensitive disease, and the use of TBI in the conditioning regimen. Other investigators have demonstrated that allogeneic stem cell transplantation in patients with

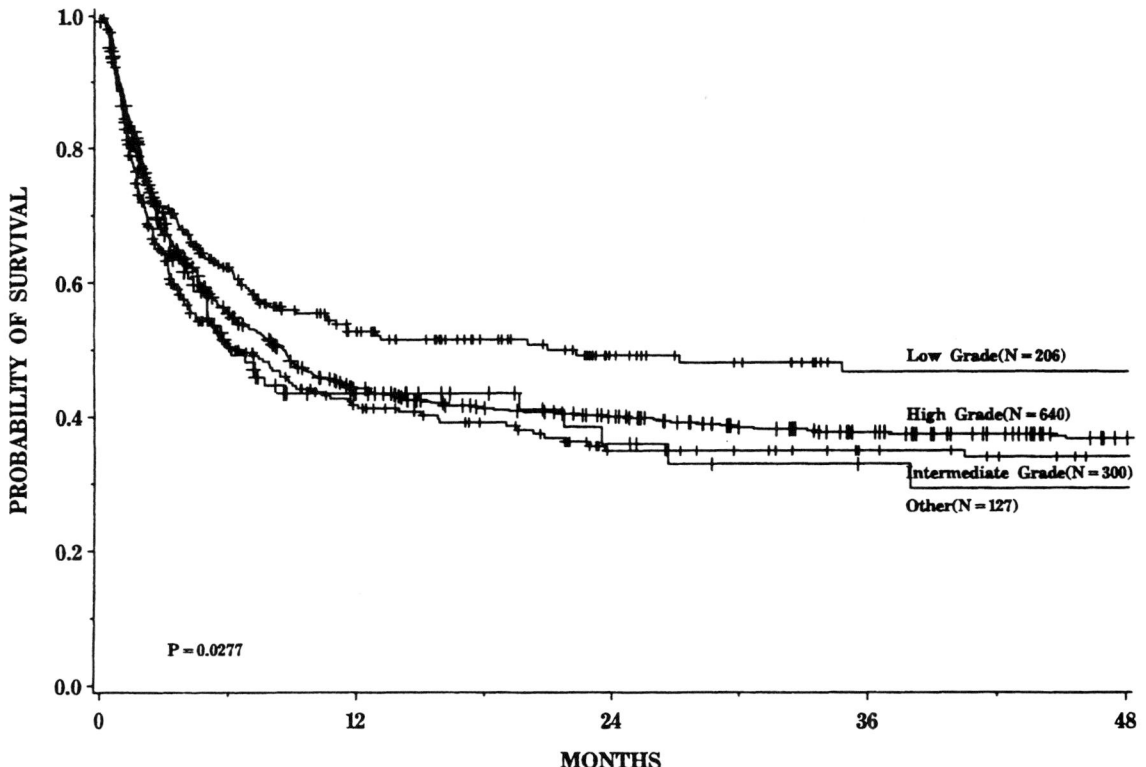

Fig. 57.1. Survival after HLA-identical sibling BMT for NHL (IBMTR data).

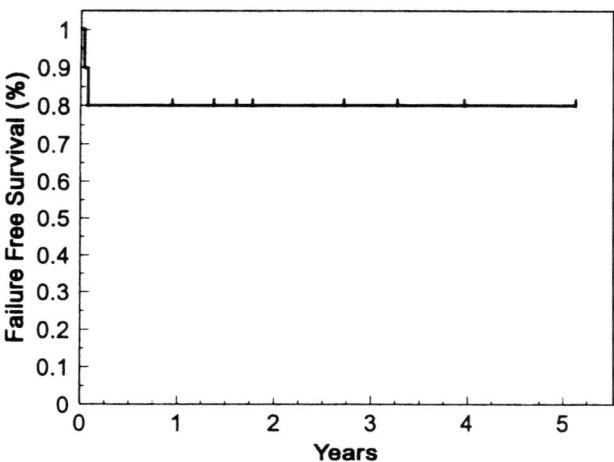

Fig. 57.2. Survival and failure-free survival curves. The curves are identical. Reproduced, with permission, from van Besien *et al.* (1995).

recurrent or refractory disease may result in long-term disease-free survival (Toze *et al.,* 2000).

Again, these data taken together are neither definitive nor mature—considering the natural history of these diseases (Gribben, 1997). Nonetheless, they add to the impression that allografts, at least those using HLA-matched related donors, should be considered for younger, low-grade NHL patients who are not in an initial, conventional chemotherapy-induced remission (Toze *et al.,* 2000)—probably in those with more clinically aggressive disease. Whether patients in a complete or very good partial remission, but with an anticipated poor prognosis, should be considered as well is a reasonable question, but such is not currently the standard of care.

Aggressive lymphoma

French investigators have published their experience with allogeneic bone marrow transplantation in 73 patients for treatment of aggressive NHL from 1984 to 1994 (Dhedin *et al.,* 1999). Patients with low grade, Burkitt's, and lymphoblastic lym-

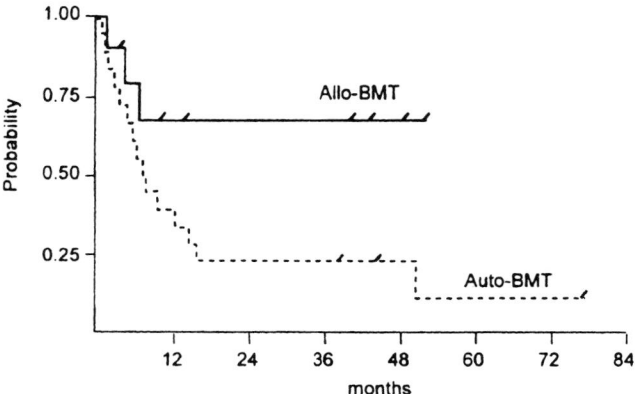

Fig. 57.3. Estimated PFS after autologous versus allogeneic BMT (log rank test, *P* = .049). Tick marks depict patients alive. Reproduced, with permission, from Verdonck *et al.* (1997).

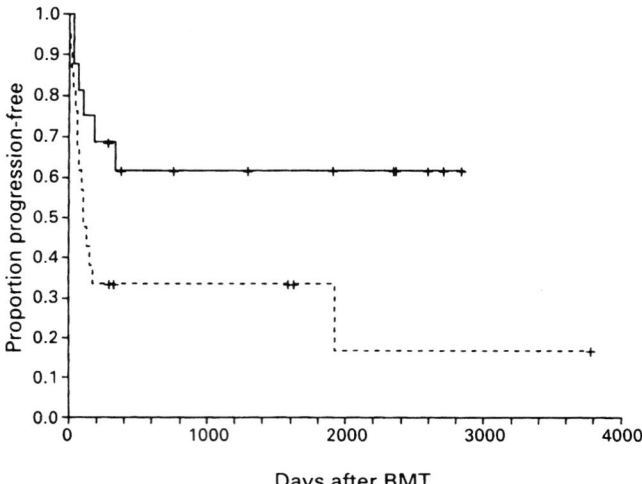

Fig. 57.4. Proportion surviving progression-free by histology: (—) aggressive (*n* = 21), or (—) indolent (*n* = 16). Reproduced, with permission, from Juckett *et al.* (1998).

phoma were excluded. The majority of patients (*n* = 39) had diffuse large cell lymphoma; 13 had anaplastic large cell lymphoma. The overall and disease-free survival rates at 5 years were 41% and 40%, respectively. In this series, 32 patients died of regimen-related toxicity. The probability of relapse was 30% at 5 years, with only one recurrence beyond 15 months posttransplant. The authors found that patients in remission at transplantation, and those receiving fewer than 3 treatment regimens prior to transplantation, had improved outcomes. However, acute and chronic GVHD did not influence relapse rates.

Lymphoblastic lymphoma

Lymphoblastic lymphoma is at the opposite end of the clinical spectrum from low-grade lymphomas, resembling ALL (Zinzani *et al.,* 1996) in biology, presentation, and outcome. Accordingly, one may consider the indications for allogeneic transplants in these patients to be similar to those for ALL in age-matched groups. The clearest indications for allografts in ALL require the identification of adverse prognostic factors despite an initial, chemotherapy-induced complete remission, or, alternatively, the absence of remission (Weisdorf, 1997).

A case-controlled, matched-pair analysis performed by the EBMT (Chopra *et al.,* 1992) noted a 50% reduction in relapse rate (i.e., 24% vs. 48%) using allogeneic versus autologous transplants for lymphoblastic lymphoma—more reduction than in the entire NHL group as a whole (23% vs. 38%). However, a higher rate of nonrelapse mortality occurred in the allograft group (i.e., 24% vs. 10%), and decreased the progression-free survival to statistically insignificant levels between the two groups.

A retrospective IBMTR study compared 128 patients with lymphoblastic lymphoma given an autotransplant with 76 given an HLA-identical sibling transplant (Levine *et al.*, 2003). Treatment-related mortality at 6 months was lower in the autograft recipients (3% versus 18% respectively), while relapse rate was significantly higher in the autograft recipients at 1 and 5 years posttransplant

(46% versus 32% and 56% versus 34%). There was no difference in disease-free or overall survival at 5 years.

Adult T cell leukemia/lymphoma

Utsunomiya *et al.* (2001) reported their experience with allogeneic transplantation in 10 patients with adult T-cell leukemia/lymphoma. Six patients developed acute GVHD; 2 did not develop GVHD and developed disease recurrence. Four patients remained alive in remission a median of 17.5 months after transplantation.

Mantle cell lymphoma

This lymphoma has specific clinicopathologic features and a poor prognosis with conventional therapy. Several reports of specifically defined autotransplant series have appeared (Stewart *et al.*, 1995; Dreger *et al.*, 1997; Ketterer *et al.*, 1997; Freedman *et al.*, 1998) A 4-year disease-free survival rate of 31% was reported in the study by Freedman, but there was no evidence for a plateau in the survival curve, despite the use of tumor-purged grafts.

Allogeneic transplants have also been reported (Corradini *et al.*, 1996; Khouri *et al.*, 1998a; Adkins *et al.*, 1998; Khouri *et al.*, 1999; Kroger *et al.*, 2000; Martinez *et al.*, 2000). In the study by Khouri, both disease-free and overall survival at 3 years were significantly higher in the allogeneic recipients compared to the autologous recipients. Although not definitive, the failure to detect evidence of disease by sensitive molecular methods at 1 year after transplant in the single patient reported by Corradini suggests the possibility of cure. Additionally, in the report by Martinez, two patients who had relapsed at 13 and 24 months after an autograft, were alive and disease-free 24 months after an allograft. In the case report by Kroger (2000), the patient remained in remission 8 years following transplantation. Taken together, these data indicate the potential utility of an allograft in mantle cell NHL early after initial therapy.

Chronic lymphatic leukemia (see Chapter 56)

Chronic lymphatic leukemia (CLL) is closely related to certain NHL, such as diffuse small cell type. In any event, few would disagree that the conventional therapy for CLL is wanting— despite the introduction of newer purine analogs (Bergmann, 1997) and the availability of alemtuzumab (Campath-1H). Consequently, interest in both autologous and allogeneic transplantation in this disease is increasing (Dreger & Schmitz, 1997; Cull *et al.*, 2000).

In 1996, a series of 54 CLL patients who had received allografts was reported by the EBMT and the IBMTR (Michallet *et al.*, 1996). Only CLL patients less than 60 years of age with HLA-matched donors were described; the median age was 41 (range 21–58) years and the median interval from diagnosis to transplant was 37 (range 5–130) months. Most, but not all, had advanced stage disease. Routine transplant techniques using HLA-matched sibling donors were utilized.

Remission was achieved in 70% of patients, and 44% remained alive at a median follow-up of slightly beyond 2 years. Actuarial 3-year probability of survival was 46%. As expected, patients with the most advanced CLL had poorer outcomes. Interestingly, only five patients died of CLL, while 46% died of complications. Again, these data suggest careful consideration of allografts in CLL patients who are beyond early stage disease (see Chapter 56).

Rodriguez and colleagues (2000) described 8 patients with Richter's syndrome[4] (CLL transformed to an aggressive lymphoma, usually diffuse large cell lymphoma). At the time of transplant all had been heavily pretreated, 2 had failed to respond to autologous transplantation, 5 had refractory disease, 5 had B symptoms, and 7 had stage III or IV disease. At the time of the report, 3 were alive and in remission at 14, 47, and 67 months after transplant, respectively. Two of these three had received non-myeloablative regimens. Five patients died of non-relapse mortality. This study suggests that allogeneic transplantation using a less toxic conditioning regimen may improve outcome in this patient population.

Large granular lymphocyte (CD56+, natural killer cell) leukemia/lymphoma

NK cell leukemia/lymphoma is an aggressive, rare disorder originating from the clonal proliferation of CD3−, CD56+ large granular lymphocytes. This disorder is typically rapidly fatal despite therapy. Allogeneic bone marrow transplantation from an HLA-matched sibling donor has been used successfully to treat a child with this disorder (Ohnuma *et al.*, 1997). The patient, who developed acute GVHD, remained in remission 12 months after transplantation.

Waldenström's macroglobulinemia[5]

Two cases of HLA-identical sibling transplantation for Waldenstrom's macroglobulinemia have been reported (Martino *et al.*, 1999). The patients, aged 34 and 39 respectively, were alive 3 and 9 years posttransplant at the time of the report. One had a normal IgM level; the other had a monoclonal serum IgM kappa level of 2.25 g/l. The patient with no evidence of disease posttransplant had previously relapsed after an autologous graft, suggesting the likelihood of a graft-versus-lymphoma effect. In addition, a non-myeloablative regimen has been used to treat a 62 year-old man (Ueda *et al.*, 2001). The M.D. Anderson Cancer Center has reported 3 patients with refractory disease who underwent allogeneic transplantation (Anagnostopoulos *et al.*, 2001). Only one had a partial response, temporally associated with GVHD.

Mycosis fungoides/Sézary syndrome[6]

There are at least two case reports of successful allogeneic transplants for advanced mycosis fungoides (Molina *et al.*, 1999; Burt *et al.*, 2000). In the former report, the patient remained in remission 36 months after transplantation from an unrelated donor, the longest durable remission experienced by the patient. In the case reported by Burt, a putative graft-ver-

---

[4] Maurice Richter, U.S. pathologist, born 1897.

[5] Jan Waldenström, Swedish physician, 1906–1998.

[6] Albert Sézary, French dermatologist, 1880–1956.

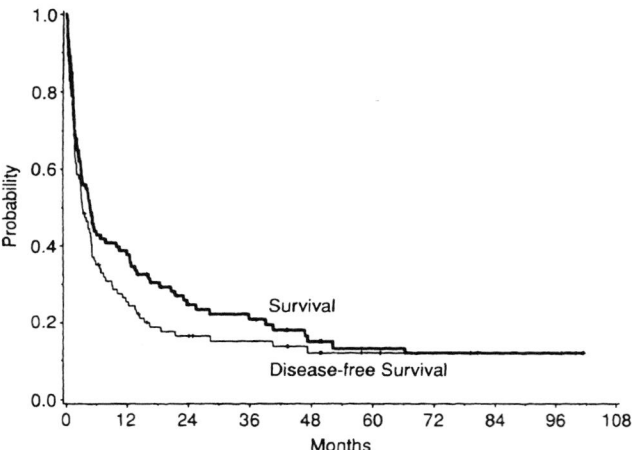

Fig. 57.5. Probability of survival and disease-free survival after HLA-identical sibling bone marrow transplantation for Hodgkin's disease. Reproduced, with permission, from Gajewski *et al.* (1996).

sus-tumor effect was seen with resolution of recurrent tumor posttransplant when immune suppression was withdrawn.

Hodgkin's lymphoma

Just as the role of autologous transplantation is now relatively clear (Reece, 2002; Reece & Phillips, 1994), the role of allogeneic transplantation for Hodgkin's lymphoma is also becoming more apparent, primarily due to two analyses. First, the EBMT described 49 patients with Hodgkin's lymphoma who underwent allogeneic transplantation from related donors; 45 with sufficient data were compared to 45 who had autotransplants using a matched-pair analysis. The 4-year actuarial probabilities of survival, progression-free survival, relapse, and nonrelapse mortality were 25%, 15%, 61%, and 48%, respectively, for allogeneic grafts, compared to 37%, 24%, 61%, and 27% for autologous grafts. While patients with grade II–IV acute graft-versus-host disease (GVHD) had lower recurrence rates, they

also had a lower survival rate (Milpied *et al.*, 1996). These authors concluded that allogeneic transplants "cannot be recommended" in most circumstances for Hodgkin's lymphoma. Gajewski and colleagues (1996) analyzed results of 100 consecutive allotransplants for Hodgkin's patients reported to the IBMTR between 1982 and 1992. Patients were, in general, heavily pretreated and in poor condition. For example, 50% had performance status scores less than 90% and fewer than 80% were in remission at transplant. The 3-year probabilities of survival, progression-free survival, and relapse were 21%, 15%, and 65%, respectively (Figs. 57.5 and 57.6). These authors concluded that allogeneic transplantation has a "limited role" in such patients.

A study of 157 patients with Hodgkin's lymphoma suggested a clinical graft-versus-lymphoma effect in the patients undergoing allogeneic transplantation (Akpek *et al.*, 2001). In this series, 53 patients underwent allogeneic transplantation, while 104 underwent autologous transplantation. There was a trend toward lower relapse rates after allogeneic transplantation for patients with chemosensitive disease (34% vs. 51%, *P* = .17). For patients undergoing autologous transplantation, there was a continuing risk of relapse or therapy-related myelodysplastic syndrome/acute myeloid leukemia (MDS/AML) at 12 years after transplant; there were no cases of relapse or therapy-related AML/MDS beyond 3 years after allogeneic transplantation.

Clearly, these data are not encouraging for the routine use of allogeneic stem cell transplantation in Hodgkin's lymphoma, and given the current technologies available for the therapy of such patients, it is difficult to disagree with these authors: as currently practiced, allogeneic transplants have little impact on Hodgkin's lymphoma. That said, some patients with Hodgkin's lymphoma who require transplantation for prolonged survival simply cannot be autografted, and it is these patients in whom an allograft should be considered. Examples include patients with severely hypoplastic (and/or dysplastic), or tumor-involved, or fibrotic marrows, and those patients who have relapsed after an autograft. In addition, non-myeloablative regimens may allow a graft-versus-lymphoma effect to be exploited with less regimen-related toxicity.

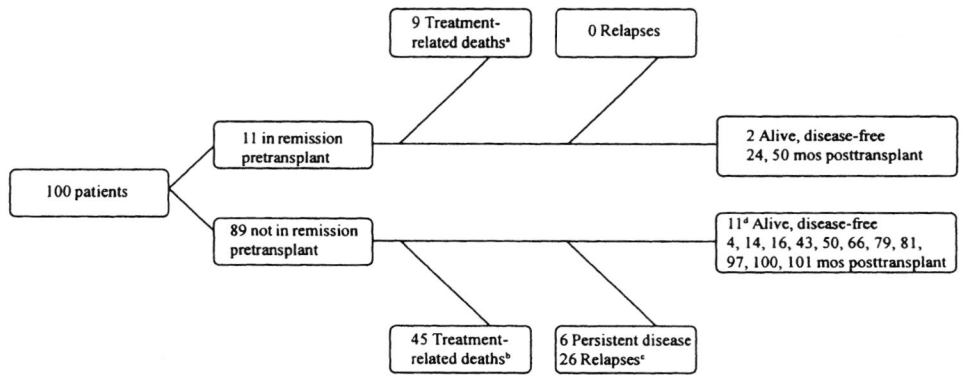

Fig. 57.6. Outcome of 100 HLA-identical sibling transplants for Hodgkin's disease. [a]Causes of death: 1 graft failure, 5 pulmonary, 3 other; [b]Causes of death: 1 graft failure, 37 pulmonary toxicity or infection, 2 nonpulmonary infections, 5 other; [c]3 alive with Hodgkin's disease 19, 22, and 37 months posttransplant; [d]1 additional patient alive 28 months posttransplant—disease status unknown. Reproduced, with permission, from Gajewski *et al.* (1996).

Results of HLA-mismatched family member and unrelated donor transplantation

The vast majority of published experience in allografting for the lymphomas deals with HLA-identical sibling donors. In these series, there are occasionally a small number of alternate donors included. There are only a few published reports—mainly case reports—describing the use of alternate donors, primarily using reduced intensity conditioning. Transplantation from an unrelated donor has been used successfully to treat a 16 year old with nodal gamma/delta lymphoma (Aoyama *et al.*, 2001). This patient remained in remission 35 months after transplantation. However, published experience with larger numbers of patients undergoing alternate donor transplantation is limited. The National Marrow Donor Program (NMDP) has described its experience with 158 patients with NHL (Bierman *et al.*, 1999). Progression-free survival at 2 years was 30%, and was significantly higher for patients with chemosensitive disease at transplant compared to those with resistance disease (40% vs. 24%, *P* = .07). The EBMT registry has reported a similar series that also included patients with Hodgkin's lymphoma (Singer *et al.*, 1999). Progression-free survival was higher in patients less than 16 years of age than for older patients (51% vs. 16%).

Results of cord blood transplantation

Published reports of cord blood transplantation for the lymphomas is limited. The first report of cord blood transplantation was in a child with refractory mediastinal T-cell lymphoma who received a graft from an HLA-identical sibling (Brichard *et al.*, 1995). The patient developed grade II acute GVHD and remained in remission one year after transplantation. Subsequently, Weinthal and colleagues (2000) reported an unrelated donor cord blood transplant for a child with disseminated recurrent Burkitt's lymphoma. He experienced grade II acute GVHD and was in remission 24 months after transplantation. Investigators at Duke University have used non-myeloablative regimens followed by infusion of unrelated donor cord blood grafts matched at 4 of 6 HLA loci to treat 2 adults with NHL (Rizzieri *et al.*, 2001). One patient with mantle cell lymphoma was in second remission and the other patient had large cell NHL, which had failed autologous transplantation. Both patients engrafted and remained in remission at 6 months and 12 months following transplantation.

Results using reduced intensity conditioning

Reduced intensity conditioning regimens have been used to treat patients with Waldenström's macroglobulinemia and CLL, and have been used in alternate donor and cord blood transplantation. Additional discussion is provided in those specific sections of this chapter. Khouri and colleagues (1998a; 2001), Grigg *et al.* (1999), and Nagler *et al.* (2000) have described the use of reduced intensity or non-myeloablative conditioning regimens in patients with lymphoid malignancies. In the series by Khouri *et al.* (2001), twenty patients with indolent (18 follicu-

lar, 2 small lymphocytic) lymphoma were conditioned with fludarabine and cyclophosphamide with (9 patients) or without rituxan pre- and posttransplant on days –6, +1, +8 and +15 prior to a T-replete PBSC transplant. Tacrolimus and methotrexate were administered as immune suppression posttransplant. The median age was 51 years and the median follow-up 21 months. The two-year disease-free survival was 84% (Figure 57.7). All patients achieved engraftment of donor cells, and the cumulative incidence of acute GVHD grades II–IV was 20%. All patients achieved complete remission, including a molecular remission for *bcl-2* gene rearrangement in six patients.

Nagler and colleagues (2000) treated 19 NHL and 4 Hodgkin's lymphoma patients with a fludarabine-based regimen. While all patients engrafted, 4 patients developed grade III–IV acute GVHD, and died from this complication. The probability of disease-free survival at 37 months was 40%, and the probability of relapse was 26%. These studies suggest a graft-versus-lymphoma effect is operative in these diseases; however, GVHD remained a significant cause of morbidity and mortality.

Similar results have been confirmed in other reports (Bertz *et al.*, 2002; Corradini *et al.*, 2002). In the former report, 25 patients with refractory lymphomas who received conventional conditioning regimens had inferior survival at one year compared with those who received non-myeloablative regimens (67% vs. 23%), largely due to lower nonrelapse mortality rates in the group treated with nonmyeloablative conditioning regimens (54% vs. 17%). In the study by Corradini, 45 patients with hematologic malignancies who were unable to undergo conventional transplantation received a fludarabine-based non-myeloablative regimen. All patients engrafted, and regimen-related mortality was quite low at 13%. At a median of 385 days following transplantation, 25 patients (55%) were alive in remission. This study demonstrated that non-myeloablative regimens can permit durable engraftment with low regimen-related toxicity, while still inducing remissions in high-risk patients.

An EBMT Registry series of 188 patients, 48% of whom had received a prior autologous transplant, described an overall

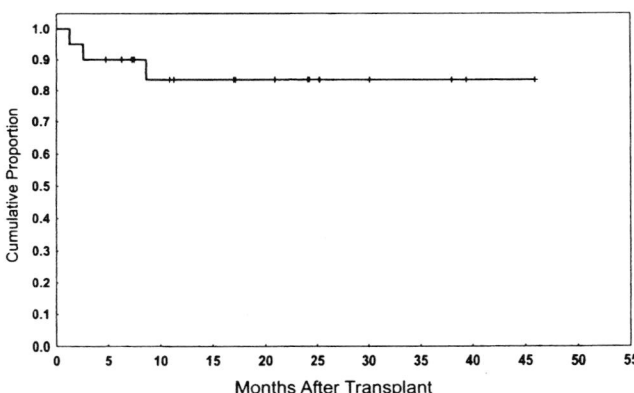

Fig. 57.7. Overall survival and event-free survival of the study population. The actuarial probability of being alive and in remission at 2 years was 84%. Reproduced, with permission, from Khouri *et al.* (2001).

progression-free survival rate of 46%, but the rate was significantly better than this in patients with low-grade NHL, Hodgkin's disease and in those with chemosensitive disease (Robinson *et al.*, 2002). Patients with high-grade lymphoma, mantle cell lymphoma and those with chemoresistant lymphoma had a poor outcome.

Sykes and colleagues (1999) have demonstrated that a non-myeloablative conditioning regimen utilizing cyclophosphamide, ATG, and thymic irradiation can induce mixed chimerism in adults with refractory lymphoma receiving grafts from HLA-mismatched related donors. Furthermore, all patients developed grade II–III acute GVHD and a striking antilymphoma response was seen in three patients; one of the 5 patients died prior to engraftment. In a separate study, the same group has described the use of donor lymphocyte infusion beginning 5 to 6 weeks after transplantation for conversion to full donor hematopoiesis and to optimize a GVL effect in 21 patients with refractory malignancies who received grafts from phenotypically or genotypically HLA-matched donors (Spitzer *et al.*, 2000) (Fig. 57.8). Five of 10 patients who received donor lymphocyte infusions attained a remission compared with only 3 of 11 patients who did not receive this intervention. This study demonstrated that following a non-myeloablative regimen, the early administration of donor lymphocyte infusions was able to induce complete donor chimerism and a remarkable antitumor response in patients with refractory malignancies.

At M.D. Anderson Cancer Center, six patients with advanced Hodgkin's lymphoma who had failed autologous transplantation were treated with a fludarabine-based non-myeloablative regimen. Three of the 4 patients with responses also developed GVHD. However, only one of six was alive without disease at greater than 9 months after transplant (Anderlini *et al.*, 2000).

Carella and associates (2000) have reported their experience with a planned tandem autologous/allogeneic transplant approach in 15 patients with resistant Hodgkin's (*n* = 10) and non-Hodgkin's (*n* = 5) lymphomas. After recovering from an initial autologous transplant, these patients received a cyclophosphamide/fludarabine non-myeloablative regimen followed by infusion of HLA-identical donor peripheral blood stem cells. Eleven patients achieved a complete remission after the combined therapy. Grade II–IV acute GVHD was observed in 7 patients and two developed chronic GVHD. At the time of publication, 10 patients were alive and 5 were in remission. Five patients had died: one of progressive disease, one of chronic GVHD, one of infection, and two of progressive disease and chronic GVHD. These response rates suggest that after debulking with autologous transplantation, allogeneic transplantation allows a graft-versus-lymphoma effect to be more effective in patients with previously advanced disease.

Advantages of allogeneic transplantation

Allogeneic stem cells have certain advantages over autologous stem cells, most obviously related to their normalcy—a feature that permits rapid and reliable hematologic reconstitution, reduction in disease- or treatment-related stem cell abnormalities (i.e., hypoplasia or treatment-related myelodysplasia/acute myeloid leukemia), and occult or overt lymphomatous contamination. Additionally, as mentioned above, an immunotherapeutic (i.e., graft-versus-lymphoma) effect is presumably operative.

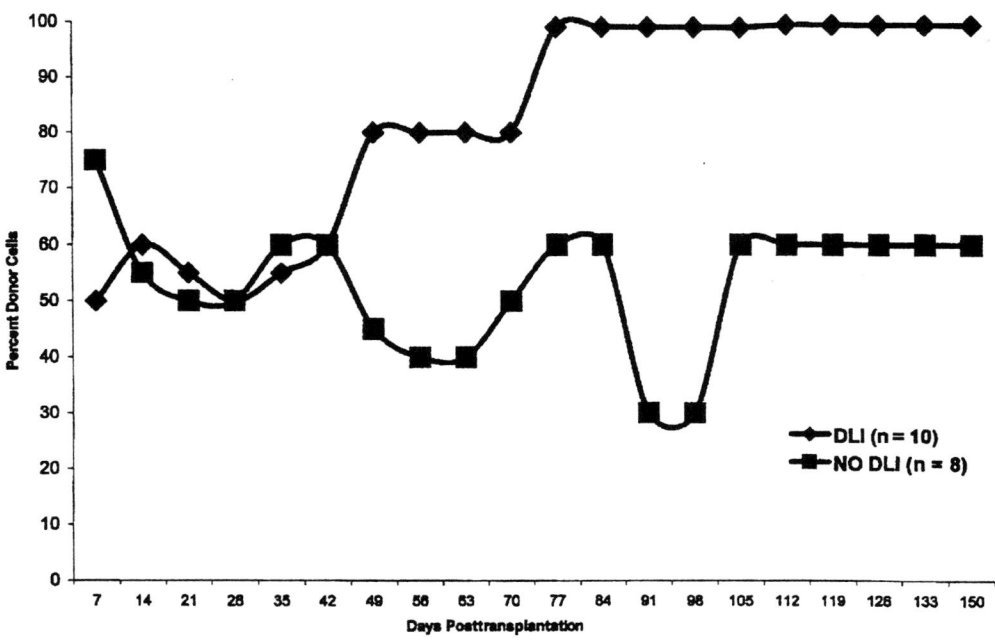

Fig. 57.8. The median percentage of donor cells found in peripheral white cells over time in 10 recipients of an HLA-matched donor BMT who received DLI on day 35 and between days 56 and 64 posttransplant, and 8 patients who did not receive DLI posttransplant because of the presence or suspicion of GVHD. Patterns of chimerism were determined by microsatellite analysis and are shown as estimates of the percentage of donor DNA present. Reproduced, with permission, from Spitzer *et al.* (2000).

Table 57.2. *Allogeneic stem cell transplants for malignant lymphoma*

Advantages	Disadvantages
Normalcy of stem cells	Greater need for age restriction
Reliably prompt hematopoietic reconstitution	Insufficient number of suitable donors
Reduction of secondary myelodysplasia/AML	Need for immunosuppression
No tumor cell contamination	Greater treatment-related mortality
Graft-versus-lymphoma effect	Second malignancies

Abbreviation: AML, acute myeloid leukemia.

Both of these features, as well as prominent disadvantages, are summarized in Table 57.2.

Normal stem cells

Although most have rapid hematologic recovery, some patients with lymphoma undergoing autologous stem cell transplantation have delayed recovery, presumably due to the effects of prior chemotherapy or radiotherapy (Mauch *et al.,* 1995). Of course, this variable is avoided with the use of normal allogeneic donors. On the other hand, some allogeneic stem cell transplants are also associated with engraftment problems. These may be due to several different etiologies, but are mainly seen with the use of histoincompatible donors, T-cell depleted grafts, and certain myelosuppressive treatments posttransplant (such as methotrexate to reduce the incidence and severity of GVHD and ganciclovir for cytomegalovirus prevention or treatment).

Nevertheless, an unknown, but probably substantial number of NHL patients cannot be (or at least are not) autotransplanted due to extensive HSC damage from prior chemotherapy and/or radiotherapy utilized in conventional dose. In fact, some patients are unable to have adequate numbers of stem cells collected due to marrow damage from disease or prior therapy (Stiff, 1999). If the patient is otherwise suitable, an allograft is an obvious approach.

In addition, the use of allogeneic stem cells may minimize the development of treatment-related MDS/AML (see Chapter 86). This complication, initially observed in the absence of dose-intensive chemotherapy/radiotherapy and stem cell transplants (Henry-Amar & Joly, 1996), is likely potentiated in the auto-transplant population, perhaps by allowing prolonged survival of heavily pretreated patients (Darrington *et al.,* 1994; Miller *et al.,* 1994; Traweek *et al.,* 1996; Pedersen-Bjergaard *et al.,* 2000). The contribution of prior stem cell damage to the development of MDS/AML after autologous transplantation has been evaluated by one group (Abruzzese *et al.,* 1999). These investigators studied a cohort of patients with posttransplant MDS characterized by chromosomal aberrations for which an appropriate probe (FISH, fluorescent in situ hybridization) was available. They examined either archived bone marrow slides or pretransplant stem cell collections for the presence of the cytogenetic abnormality, which was identified in 9 of 10 cases.

Therefore, prior cytotoxic therapy plays an important role in the development of this complication. Conversely, additional damage to surviving stem cells by the transplant conditioning regimen is suggested by the finding that TBI-containing conditioning regimens may predispose to the development of MDS/AML (Darrington *et al.,* 1994). If damaged endogenous stem cells are ablated, these malignancies should be less frequent with allografting. This indeed appears to be the case, although allogeneic transplantation is associated with an increased incidence of other secondary hematologic (Witherspoon *et al.,* 1989) or solid cancers, at least some of which may be related to GVHD (Curtis *et al.,* 1997) (see Chapter 87).

Absence of tumor cell contamination

Another positive feature of allogeneic transplantation is the assured absence of contamination with lymphoma in the stem cell product. Conversely, it must be admitted that, in autotransplants for NHL and Hodgkin's lymphoma, a role for contamination, reinoculation, and ultimately relapse is assumed, rather than proven (Gribben, 1997). Clearly, the high recurrence rates, even with syngeneic transplantation, (Appelbaum *et al.,* 1987; Santos *et al.,* 1987) implicate the inadequacy of current conditioning regimens to deplete the patient of lymphoma cells as the chief cause of relapse after any type of stem cell transplantation. Nonetheless, a tumor-free graft can only be viewed as an advantage—it is only the degree of advantage that is arguable.

Graft-versus-lymphoma effect

The issue of defining—and then optimizing—a graft-versus-lymphoma effect is critically important in broadening the use of allografting for the lymphomas.

The difficulty in defining a graft-versus-tumor effect in human cancer has led to the use of a variety of indirect parameters, including (1) relapse rates after syngeneic versus allogeneic transplants; (2) relapse rates in patients with and without clinically apparent GVHD; and (3) relapse rates after T-cell-depleted (TCD) versus T-replete transplants (Horowitz *et al.,* 1990). The comparison of relapse rates after autografts versus allografts is potentially compromised due to the possible contribution to relapse of co-transplantation of malignant cells. Unfortunately, many series suggesting the presence of a graft-versus-lymphoma effect minimize this variable, although almost all report decreased recurrence rates after allografts versus autografts.

The extent of clinical data regarding a graft-versus-tumor effect is less extensive and less clear in the lymphomas than in the leukemias (Horowitz *et al.,* 1990). Selected studies are summarized in Table 57.3. Appelbaum *et al.* (1987) noted reduced relapse rates after allogeneic versus syngeneic (vs. autologous) stem cell transplantation for both Hodgkin's lymphoma and NHL. Although this decrease was not statistically significant, this may have been due, in part, to relatively low patient numbers (e.g., 13 syngeneic transplants). Jones *et al.* (1991) reported a statistically significant difference in relapse rates in patients with both Hodgkin's and non-Hodgkin's lymphomas;

Table 57.3. *Comparative clinical studies evaluating a graft-versus-lymphoma effect*

Reference	Comparison	Antitumor effects
Appelbaum *et al.* (1987)	Allogeneic vs syngeneic transplants (NHL and Hodgkin's)	Reduced relapse rate, but not statistically significant
Jones *et al.* (1991)	None formalized (NHL and Hodgkin's)	Acute GVHD in 5 of 9 and chronic GVHD in 3 of 9 durable CR patients transplanted in sensitive relapse
Chopra *et al.* (1992)	Chronic GVHD vs none (NHL)	Relapse/progression rate 0 vs 35%
Gajewski *et al.* (1996)	Acute vs chronic GVHD vs none (Hodgkin's)	Reduced relapse rate, but not statistically significantly, in GVHD patients
Ratanatharathon *et al.* (1994)	Acute vs chronic GVHD vs none	Nonstatistically significant reduction in chronic GVHD
Collins *et al.* (1997)	Donor leukocyte infusions for NHL	No CR in 6 patients
van Besien *et al.* (1997a)	Cessation of immunosuppression; donor leukocyte infusions for NHL	2 of 9 CR with cessation, one durable; 0 of 3 with DLI

Abbreviations: NHL, non-Hodgkin's lymphoma; GVHD, graft-versus-host disease; DLI, donor leukocyte infusions; CR, complete remission.

however, this comparison also involved autografts (treated ex vivo with 4-hydroxycyclophosphamide) and allografts, but there was no comparison of data regarding relapse rates in patients who developed clinical GVHD compared to those who did not.

Chopra and co-workers (1992) used EBMT data to compare autologous and allogeneic transplants, and also found an insignificantly different result in relapse rates in allogeneic recipients (23% at 31 months) versus autologous recipients (38% at 46 months). More directly, a significantly reduced relapse rate (i.e., 0% vs. 35%) was observed in allogeneic recipients developing chronic GVHD compared to those who did not. A nonsignificant increase in progression-free survival was noted in the former patients. A review of IBMTR data on 100 patients with Hodgkin's lymphoma who underwent allografting from HLA-identical siblings revealed lower, but not significantly different, relapse rates in those patients who

developed acute or chronic GVHD (Gajewski *et al.*, 1996). Ratanatharathorn *et al.* (1994) compared autologous and allogeneic patients prospectively, and found lower recurrence rates not only in allograft compared to autograft recipients, but also in allograft patients with, compared to those without, GVHD (Figs. 57.9 and 57.10). Again, however, the differences were not significant, possibly due to small sample size.

Investigators in Utrecht reported their experience in patients with low grade NHL in a non-randomized study of autologous and allogeneic transplantation from HLA-identical sibling donors (Verdonck, 1999). While all 18 autologous recipients had chemosensitive disease, only 8 of 14 allogeneic patients did. In addition, 14 of 15 allograft recipients had marrow involvement at transplant. At 3 years posttransplant, the probabilities of relapse, overall survival, and event-free survival were 0%, 70%, and 70% for allogeneic recipients compared with 78%, 33%, and 22% for

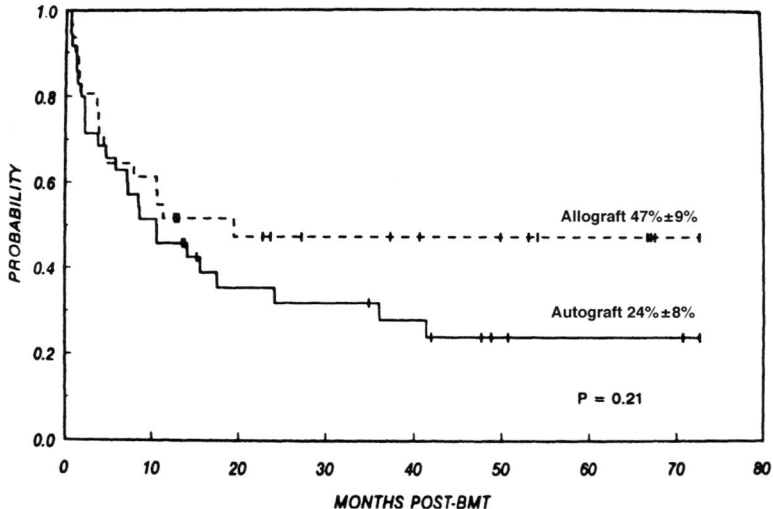

Fig. 57.9. The probability of PFS of 31 allograft recipients (----) and 35 autograft recipients (—) is shown. Reproduced, with permission, from Ratanatharathorn *et al.* (1994).

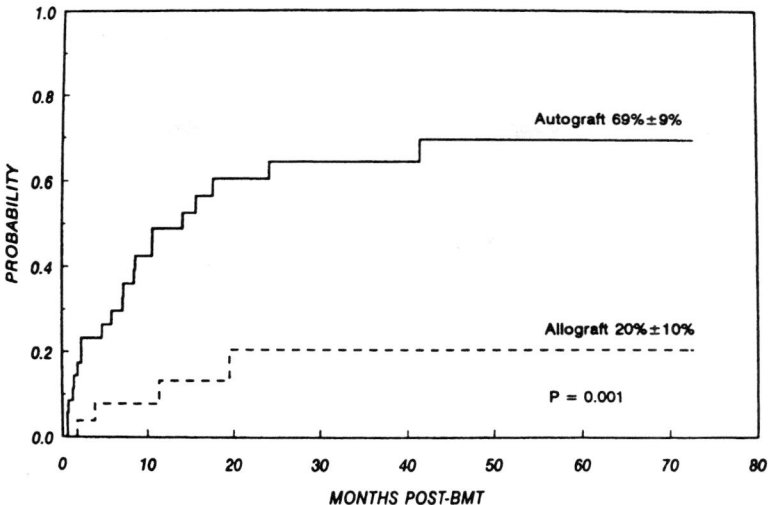

Fig. 57.10. The probability of disease progression of 31 allograft recipients (----) and 35 autograft recipients (—) is shown. Reproduced, with permission, from Ratanatharathorn *et al.* (1994).

autologous patients. This observation suggests a graft-versus-lymphoma effect in patients with low-grade NHL.

Little information regarding T-cell depletion of hematopoietic grafts has been reported for patients with NHL or Hodgkin's lymphoma. Soiffer and colleagues (1998) reported on 22 patients with recurrent or refractory NHL who received T-cell depleted grafts from closely matched relatives. The disease-free survival at a median follow-up of 30 months was 54%. Only one patient died in remission and GVHD was infrequent. Similar findings have been observed by other investigators (Juckett *et al.*, 1998; Mandigers *et al.*, 1998).

In order to harness a graft-versus-lymphoma effect, investigators omitted GVHD prophylaxis in 12 patients receiving unmanipulated peripheral blood stem cells from HLA-identical sibling donors (Fassas *et al.*, 2000). All patients developed grade III–IV acute GVHD, and 7 of 9 evaluable patients developed chronic GHVD. Of the 7 with NHL, 2 were alive without disease at 14 and 24 months posttransplant. Nachbauer *et al.* (2001) published their results with 24 autologous and 14 allogeneic stem cell transplants as treatment for recurrent or relapsed lymphoma. The probabilities of overall survival, disease-free survival, treatment-related mortality, and relapse were 57%, 51%, 29%, and 30% for autografted patients compared with 43%, 43%, 29%, and 38% for allograft recipients. In patients with elevated LDH and bone marrow involvement, allogeneic transplantation resulted in a superior survival, suggesting a graft-versus-lymphoma effect.

While the response of some diseases, most notably CML, relapsed after allogeneic transplantation to donor leukocyte infusions (DLI) has been striking (Kolb & Holler, 1997), fewer data have been reported in this regard for NHL and Hodgkin's lymphoma. Collins *et al.* (1997), in a review of 140 patients treated with allografts, reported no responses in six NHL patients, although only two developed GVHD. More encouraging results, albeit in a small number of patients, were reported by the M.D.

Anderson group (van Besien *et al.*, 1997a); of nine NHL patients who relapsed after allografts, four responded, all to withdrawal of immunosuppression, with one durable remission in a lymphoblastic lymphoma patient. Donor leukocyte infusion produced a minor response in one of three so treated. An interesting, if anecdotal, report by Salutari *et al.* (1996) noted extramedullary relapse after the use of prophylactic DLI (obtained after priming with granulocyte colony-stimulating factor) following allogeneic bone marrow transplantation for two NHL patients with refractory disease. Donor lymphocyte infusions have been used successfully in a patient with mantle cell lymphoma to convert a partial response to a complete response (Sohn *et al.*, 2000).

More data are clearly required, but it appears that a graft-versus-lymphoma effect does occur, although it is not as potent as in CML. This raises the question of how such an effect can be exploited to the benefit of patients.

Unfortunately, these antilymphoma effects have not usually translated into improved survival rates due to an increased incidence of death due to graft-versus-host disease. Therefore, it is unlikely that the full potential of the graft-versus-lymphoma will be reached with current techniques. More sophisticated techniques are forthcoming, however. For example, novel methods of T-cell depletion of grafts from alternate donors may reduce the incidence and severity of GVHD (Handgretinger *et al.*, 2000). In addition, the transduction of donor lymphocytes with the herpes simplex virus thymidine kinase (HSV-Tk) suicide gene and the subsequent control of GVHD by administration of ganciclovir is likely a useful step in this direction (Bonini *et al.*, 1997) (see Chapter 117). Additionally a potent graft-versus-lymphoma effect would be of potential benefit to autotransplant recipients. Such an attempt has been made using various cytokines felt important in the pathogenesis of GVHD—mainly, but not exclusively, interleukin-2 (Massumoto *et al.*, 1996) and/or alpha-interferon (Nagler *et al.*, 1997; Nakao *et al.*, 1997).

Disadvantages of allogeneic transplantation

The main disadvantages of allogeneic HSC transplantation for NHL and Hodgkin's lymphoma include (1) age limitation (more so than for autologous transplants); (2) unavailability of suitable HLA-matched donors in many cases; (3) the need for posttransplant immune suppression; (4) the complications of allogenicity—rejection, GVHD, and delayed immune reconstitution; and (5) late effects, mainly, but not exclusively, secondary malignancies.

The issue of patient age is critically important in any discussion regarding allogeneic stem cell transplantation. This issue was analyzed by the Rochester group (Rapoport et al., 1995) in patients undergoing autologous or allogeneic transplants. Somewhat surprisingly, patients older than 40 years had better outcomes, although some of this effect was felt (undoubtedly correctly) to be due to patient selection. Over the years, the age limit for allografting has been increased toward 60 years for recipients with histocompatible donors, and this may be extended in the future with the used of reduced intensity conditioning regimens. However, the age limit is likely to remain lower for less well-matched pairs.

Several other points should be made regarding age. First, age is also important as a physiologic variable; for instance, some patients at age 50 are in poorer condition than some at 60 years, and this point should be considered in addition to chronologic age. Second, the processes of GVHD and, more broadly, nonrelapse mortality, are complex ones that depend on factors other than histocompatibility alone, including the toxicity of current conditioning regimens for normal tissues (Ferrara et al., 1996). Accordingly, regimens that produce less toxicity, notably but not exclusively, non-myeloablative regimens (Giralt et al., 1997), may allow greater utilization of allogeneic transplants in older patients than currently deemed acceptable. Nonetheless, with presently available techniques, only selected patients older than 50 years of age should be allografted, even with HLA-matched donors; patients older than 60 years should be considered only in exceptional circumstances. Newer techniques will allow this ceiling to be raised, as the management of such patients remains inadequate (O'Reilly et al., 1997).

Comparison of allogeneic transplantation with autologous transplantation

Several points must be emphasized in regard to the "choice" between allogeneic and autologous stem cells for transplantation. First, a choice is not always present. For instance, the features of certain marrow abnormalities (dense tumor infiltration, severe hypocellularity, extensive fibrosis) preclude autologous stem cell procurement; conversely, many patients are too old and/or lack a suitably histocompatible donor for an allograft. Given the inherent limitation on numbers of allografts due to these age and histocompatibility considerations, it is unreasonable to expect a randomized clinical trial of allogeneic versus autologous stem cell transplants for lymphoma therapy.

Nonetheless, some sort of comparison is required for situations in which either source is available. The EBMT has published two matched-pair analyses. The first, for NHL (Chopra et al., 1992), compared 101 patients in each group. While relapse rates were lower in allogeneic recipients (although statistically significant only in lymphoblastic lymphoma patients), nonrelapse mortality was lower in the autologous recipients (11% vs. 25%); these factors resulted in a similar progression-free survival (49% vs. 46%). Subsequently, this group reported a similar analysis of Hodgkin's lymphoma (Milpied et al., 1996) with 45 patients in each group. Although similar relapse rates were identified, the higher nonrelapse mortality in the allogeneic group (48% vs. 27%) resulted in little difference in progression-free survival (Figure 57.11).

Thus, these analyses mirror others in the literature in which the frequent reduction in the relapse rate with allografting is counterbalanced by death due to "allogenicity-related" problems—usually GVHD. A marked change in the balance of this equation, with less nonrelapse mortality in allogeneic recipients, and no change in relapse rates in the autologous situation, would have major consequences.

As well as age, disease status is also important. Perhaps the clearest example of a situation in which an allograft is recommended is an NHL patient with "chemoresistant" disease who not only has a suitable donor but is also in relatively good clinical condition. Beyond that, it is unclear whether the "balance" of increased nonrelapse mortality versus relapse mortality is favorable for any other situation. The features discussed above are summarized in Table 57.4.

Definitive information is not yet available to make a decision regarding allo versus auto in most patients who are eligible for either. For the present, an individual approach is advocated.

Indications and contraindications for allogeneic transplantation

In general, autologous hematopoietic stem cell transplantation is the standard salvage therapy for patients with high-risk lym-

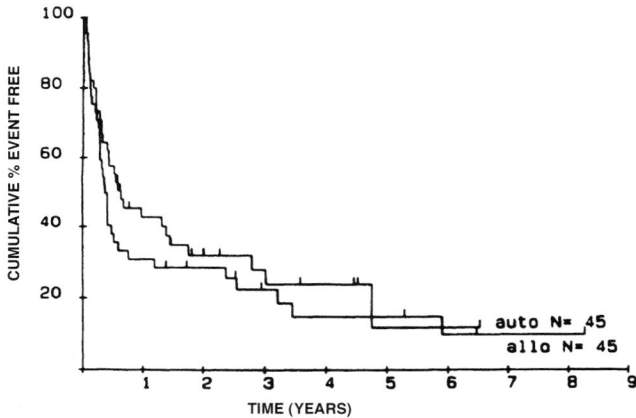

Fig. 57.11. Probability of PFS: ABMT versus allo BMT. Reproduced, with permission, from Milpied et al. (1996).

Table 57.4. *Indications for preferential allogeneic transplantation*[a]

Non-Hodgkin's lymphoma
    Primary refractory or "resistant relapse" disease status
    Low-grade histology[b]
    Lymphoblastic histology[b]
    Severe stem cell compromise (or dysplasia) due to prior therapy
    Dense marrow infiltration with tumor, or fibrosis
    Second transplants after failure of an initial autograft[b]
Hodgkin's disease
    None routinely
    Severe stem cell compromise (or dysplasia) due to prior therapy
    Dense marrow infiltration with tumor or fibrosis
    Second transplants after failure of an initial autograft (probable)[b]

[a] In patients generally suitable for an allograft.
[b] Especially in "refractory" patients.

phoma. However, there are several scenarios in which allogeneic hematopoietic stem cell transplantation should be considered based on published data. In patients with NHL and Hodgkin's lymphoma, prior cytotoxic therapy, marrow disease, or marrow fibrosis often make stem cell procurement difficult or impossible. In addition, many of the patients have received intensive therapy that includes autologous hematopoietic stem cell transplantation, and are unlikely to benefit from further dose escalation of cytotoxic therapy. In these circumstances, an allogeneic transplant should be considered, even earlier in patients with refractory disease. In addition, the cure rates of some subtypes of NHL (lymphoblastic lymphoma, low grade lymphoma, and mantle cell lymphoma) using autologous transplantation are poor. In these cases, allogeneic transplantation offers an immunologic graft-versus-lymphoma effect in addition to the use of cytotoxic therapy.

The current practice of HSC transplantation for Hodgkin's disease and NHL in Europe has been described (Urbano-Ispizua *et al.* 2002) (and see Chapter 124, Breaking News…).

Timing

The optimal timing for an autologous stem cell transplant is only becoming clear after decades of clinical research (Armitage, 1992; Philip *et al.*, 1995; Reece, 1995). Because of less experience, the optimal timing of an allograft remains uncertain.

A very effective method of decreasing the relapse rate is to transplant patients earlier in the disease course. However, it is unclear exactly which NHL patients should be transplanted in first remission, although selected patients with poor prognostic signs for continuous remission are the most appropriate group to study (International Non-Hodgkin's Lymphoma Prognostic Factors Project, 1993). However, patients in an initial remission are often those in whom one is most reluctant to risk the substantial toxicity currently intrinsic to allografting. Another consideration is the possibility of improved outcome using conventional primary therapy; this is more obvious for selected categories of high-grade NHL, especially in children (Shad & Magrath, 1997), as opposed to adults with intermediate grade NHL (Fisher *et al.*, 1993) or Hodgkin's lymphoma (Canellos,

1996). A number of series have included patients given allografts in first remission; while many series have included patients in first remission, some have comprised these patients exclusively (Nademanee *et al.*, 1987; Milpied *et al.*, 1989; Troussard *et al.*, 1990; de Witte *et al.*, 1994). No prospective comparative studies, however, have been reported.

Accordingly, patients with NHL and Hodgkin's lymphoma should be transplanted at a time when conventional therapy is unlikely to be curative, but before the features of end-stage disease are present. In general, this may be considered to be at the first sign of treatment failure—or in the presence of prognostic signs that portend eventual failure—with conventional multiagent cytotoxic chemotherapy.

Some disease status categories can be regarded as preferential indications for allografting. In particular, NHL patients with "refractory disease" status (failure to achieve at least a partial remission or very early recurrence after effective primary or salvage conventional-dose chemotherapy) have poor results with autografting and should be allografted if a suitable donor is available and if adequate clinical performance persists (Mendoza *et al.*, 1995) (Fig. 57.12). In this situation, the increased nonrelapse mortality may be justified by a potentially beneficial graft-versus-lymphoma. Similar statements cannot be as clearly rendered for Hodgkin's lymphoma (Reece & Phillips, 1994; Milpied *et al.*, 1996).

Specific considerations of lymphomas with regard to HSC transplantation

Bulky tumor masses

This is a common issue, and bulky lymphomatous masses increase the relapse risk. The usual approach to this problem is the use of localized radiation therapy, and experience in autotransplantation indicates that substantial (if somewhat reduced) antilymphoma doses of radiation may usually be given safely to nonmediastinal structures, even with the use of TBI in the

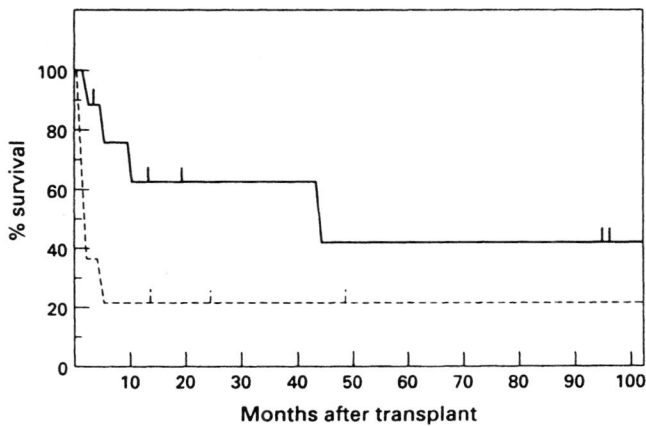

Fig. 57.12. Probability of survival based on disease status for patients with Hodgkin's disease and NHL who underwent allogeneic BMT from HLA-identical sibling donors: those with chemotherapy-sensitive disease (—) versus those with refractory disease (----). Reproduced, with permission, from Mendoza *et al.* (1995).

conditioning regimen (Mundt *et al.*, 1995; Abrams *et al.*, 1997). This strategy should be considered for allograft recipients as well.

High-dose thoracic radiation prior to stem cell transplantation poses problems, however, as it increases the risk of interstitial pneumonitis posttransplant several fold (Pecego *et al.*, 1986). It may be possible to decrease the risk by giving the radiotherapy to areas of bulky disease after, rather than before, the transplant. This approach also allows the potential use of smaller radiation ports if the conditioning has been effective.

Conditioning regimens that do not include TBI are, in theory, less problematic with respect to interstitial pneumonitis, and several have been utilized, including busulfan and cyclophosphamide (Van der Jagt *et al.*, 1991) and cyclophosphamide, carmustine (BCNU), and etoposide (Demirer *et al.*, 1995). In the former study, 37 patients (including 22 allogeneic recipients) who had received limiting doses of prior chest radiotherapy that precluded the routine use of TBI received busulfan/cyclophosphamide. Only two patients developed pneumonitis; however, 32% died of other toxicities and only 19% remained alive and well at the time of the report. The rate of interstitial pneumonia was below that observed with cyclophosphamide and TBI (32%), and a modest event-free survival advantage was noted when compared to historical controls.

In the latter study, also performed at the Fred Hutchinson Center, 56 patients (26 with NHL, 17 with Hodgkin's lymphoma, and 13 with ALL), who had received prior dose-limiting radiotherapy were treated with cyclophosphamide 7.2 g/m^2, carmustine 300 to 600 mg/m^2, and etoposide 2,400 mg/m^2 prior to allografting. The probabilities of nonrelapse mortality, relapse, and event-free survival at 2 years were 62%, 59%, and 17%, respectively. In particular, the carmustine dose of 600 mg/m^2 was thought to be excessively toxic, although the lower dose was also toxic. This regimen may be inferior to busulfan and cyclophosphamide for this situation.

The use of non-myeloablative conditioning regimens has been explored, with emphasis placed on various manipulations, especially donor leukocyte transfusions, to maximize a graft-versus-lymphoma effect (Giralt *et al.*, 1997) (see Chapter 22). This innovative approach deserves more evaluation; at present it should be used only in patients in whom a high nonrelapse mortality is anticipated—perhaps especially those with significant co-morbid problems and those who have relapsed following autotransplantation.

Central nervous system lymphoma

Two series detailing central nervous system (CNS) lymphoma have been reported (Williams *et al.*, 1994; van Besien *et al.*, 1996b). Both studies noted that the presence of CNS disease before transplant did not adversely affect outcome. In contrast, patients with CNS involvement at the time of autotransplantation have a poor prognosis, although a small number survive in complete remission. These data indicate the need for CNS remission induction before transplant; it is likely that similar considerations apply to allografting.

The possibility of using a graft-versus-lymphoma effect to provide additional control of CNS lymphoma is more speculative. No firm data exist, but if substantiated in the future, this would be a clear indication for allografting. There is a case report of a patient with primary CNS lymphoma who had resolution of the CNS disease following allogeneic transplantation from an HLA-identical sibling (Varadi *et al.*, 1999). A similar report for patients with posttransplant lymphoproliferative disease involving the CNS indicated responsiveness to donor lymphocytes (Emanuel *et al.*, 1997).

Disease recurrence after autologous transplantation

With the large number of autotransplants performed, plus the attendant high relapse rates, it is inevitable that some autografted patients will be considered for second transplants. The possibility of increasing tumor resistance to traditional cytotoxic therapy, as well as the marginal status of the autotransplanted stem cell pool, make allogeneic grafts attractive for at least some of these patients (Moreau *et al.*, 1996). However, outcomes for patients with NHL undergoing allogeneic transplantation following autotransplantation are poor with standard transplant techniques (Radich *et al.*, 2000; Hale *et al.*, 2001).

Experience remains limited. The EBMT analyzed 34 patients with either Hodgkin's lymphoma or NHL who had second transplants; only three had allografts. Some patients clearly benefited and may have been cured; these included patients with intermediate/high-grade NHL and Hodgkin's lymphoma, but not low-grade NHL or chemotherapy-resistant patients. All three allografted patients died of disease recurrence (Vandenberghe *et al.*, 1997).

The M.D. Anderson group (de Lima *et al.*, 1997) described 12 patients who relapsed following autografting; subsequent allografts were used for 8. Disease status varied from resistant relapse ($n = 3$) to responsive relapse ($n = 2$) to complete remission ($n = 2$). They were treated with standard (if heterogeneous) regimens. At the time of the report 3 were in remission at 7, 22, and 25 months, while 4 died of treatment-related toxicity and 1 from relapse.

While one might be tempted to postulate a unique role for allografting in this case, it is important to note that 2 of the 4 patients who underwent second autografting were also free of disease at 12 and 30 months. Unlike most of the allograft recipients, all had chemosensitive disease. Although this finding supports the use of second transplants in highly selected patients, it does not clearly delineate the role of allogeneic transplantation. Nonetheless, individual patients who relapse after autografts may be considered for allografts, especially, although not exclusively, if they are younger (i.e., less than 50 years) and have well-matched donors, little residual nonhematologic toxicity from the prior autograft, relatively little tumor bulk, and a long interval from transplant to relapse.

While clearly applicable in some patients, it is difficult to consider subsequent allografts as a planned approach, and either an autograft or an allograft should be approached as the definitive procedure initially.

Disease recurrence after allogeneic transplantation

In general, patients should be offered a therapeutic spectrum from supportive care to local radiation or chemotherapy to donor leukocyte transfusions or second transplants, as appropriate, with the usual notation that increased toxicity should be anticipated. Slavin et al. (1996) reported an experience in patients with leukemia relapsed after allogeneic transplantation in whom IL-2 primed "activated cell therapy" was given; results were anecdotal but encouraging. Obviously, a highly individualized approach is required. Patients with recurrent disease after allogeneic transplantation may be candidates for maneuvers such as donor lymphocyte infusions or non-myeloablative transplantation to employ a graft-versus-lymphoma effect.

Posttransplant lymphoproliferative disorder (see also Chapter 88)

The posttransplant lymphoproliferative disorder (PTLD) is a recognized complication of allografting that is more frequent with greater degrees of immunosuppression, especially involving the use of T-cell depletion. In the solid organ transplant setting, PTLD is usually of host origin and polyclonal; in HSC transplants, they are usually of donor origin and monoclonal. In both situations, PTLD appears to be related to Epstein-Barr virus (EBV) infection or reactivation, resulting in a B-cell hyperproliferation in the absence of effective T-cell control (Swinnen, 1997).

Previous attempts at prophylaxis and treatment have included cessation of immunosuppression, conventional anti-lymphoma chemotherapy, and, in some cases, antiviral drugs and biologics; none were very successful. Investigators have also utilized therapeutic DLI at relatively low doses (i.e., 10^5 CD3$^+$ cells/kg) as well as donor-derived cytotoxic lymphocytes given prophylactically to patients at high risk of developing PTLD, with encouraging results (Heslop & Rooney, 1997). The former is now arguably a standard of care, the latter a promising developmental approach. Also, the use of anti-CD20 monoclonal antibody (rituximab) with or without donor leukocyte infusions has been efficacious (Cook et al., 1999; McGuirk et al., 1999; Faye et al., 1998).

HIV-related lymphoma (and see Chapter 121)

Aggressive NHL, usually B cell in origin, occurs as a frequent complication in some patients with human immunodeficiency virus (HIV) infection. Due to a variety of factors, related to host problems, outcome with conventional therapy is very poor (Straus, 1997).

The IBMTR has information on 8 patients who underwent allogeneic transplantation (M. Horowitz, personal communica-

tion, 2002). All had a diagnosis of NHL, and seven of the eight recipients have died, only one from progressive disease. These limited data suggest that standard allogeneic transplant regimens may be too toxic for this patient group. Anecdotal reports for allogeneic (Holland et al., 1989), autologous (Gabarre et al., 1996) and syngeneic (Campbell et al., 1999) transplantation have been published. While tumor regression was noted in all patients, complications can be formidable. Investigators at the National Institutes of Health have demonstrated that non-myeloablative allogeneic stem cell transplantation is feasible in patients with refractory malignancies and concomitant HIV infection (Kang et al., 2002). Two patients, one with therapy-related AML and another with refractory Hodgkin's lymphoma, attained remissions following this treatment. While the patient with Hodgkin's lymphoma eventually developed recurrent disease, the patient with AML was in remission 24 months following transplantation. The use of such therapy awaits a greater ability to control HIV infection, and patients should not, at present, be transplanted outside of a clinical trial.

Conclusions

An unresolved area in stem cell transplantation for lymphoma is whether to offer allogeneic or autologous transplantation to a patient eligible for either. A prognostic assessment based on the patient's risk of GVHD-related mortality and the perceived need for a graft-versus-lymphoma effect should be balanced in individual cases. Some published reports indicate that some patients with lymphomas may be cured with allogeneic hematopoietic stem cell transplantation, even if heavily pretreated.

It is likely that allogeneic stem cell transplantation is under-utilized at present, although it is unlikely that it will ever be applied to the majority of patients with Hodgkin's lymphoma or NHL. This statement may not hold true if the current, relatively strict requirements for histocompatibility matching are abrogated, and/or if a potent graft-versus-lymphoma effect can be safely and reliably produced by allografting. This latter point bears emphasis, as the harnessing of this effect (i.e., markedly reduced relapse rate without increased toxicity) would greatly increase the use of allografts. Moreover, a trend in the direction of a favored use of allografts may occur without such measures, if continued progress in reducing relapse or, to a lesser extent, the incidence of therapy-related MDS/AML after autologous transplantation, is not forthcoming.

References

Abbruzzese, E., Radford, J. E., Miller, J. S. et al. (1999). Detection of abnormal pretransplant clones in progenitor cells of patients who developed myelodysplasia after autologous transplantation. Blood, 94, 1814–1819.

Abrams, R. A., Liu, P. J., Ambinder, R. F. et al. (1997). Hodgkin and non-Hodgkin lymphoma: local radiation therapy after bone marrow transplantation. Radiology, 203, 865–70.

Adkins, D., Brown, R., Goodnough, L. T. *et al.* (1998). Treatment of resistant mantle cell lymphoma with allogeneic bone marrow transplantation. *Bone Marrow Transplantation, 21,* 97–9.

Akpek, G., Ambinder, R. F., Piantadosi, S. *et al.* (2001). Long-term results of blood and marrow transplantation for Hodgkin's lymphoma. *Journal of Clinical Oncology, 19,* 4314–21.

Anagnostopoulos, A., Dimopoulos, M. A., Aleman, A. *et al.* (2001). High-dose chemotherapy followed by stem cell transplantation in patients with resistant Waldenström's macroglobulinemia. *Bone Marrow Transplantation, 27,* 1027–1029.

Anderlini, P., Giralt, S., Andersson, B. *et al.* (2000). Allogeneic stem cell transplantation with fludarabine-based, less intensive conditioning regimens as adoptive immunotherapy in advanced Hodgkin's disease. *Bone Marrow Transplantation, 26,* 615–20.

Aoyoma, L. K. Y., Yamane, T., Hino, M. *et al.* (2001). Nodal gamma/delta T cell lymphoma in complete remission following allogeneic bone marrow transplantation from an HLA-matched unrelated donor. *Acta Haematologica, 105,* 49–52.

Appelbaum, F. R., Sullivan, K. M., Buckner, C. D. *et al.* (1987). Treatment of malignant lymphoma in 100 patients with chemotherapy, total body irradiation, and stem cell transplantation. *Journal of Clinical Oncology, 5,* 1340–7.

Armitage, J. O. (1992). Autologous bone marrow transplantation for patients with aggressive non-Hodgkin's lymphoma. *Bone Marrow Transplantation, 10* (Suppl 1), 62–3.

Bergmann, L. (1997). Present status of purine analogs in the therapy of chronic lymphocytic leukemia. *Leukemia, 11* (Suppl 2), S29–34.

Bertz, H., Illerhaus, G., Veelken, H., Finke, J. (2002). Allogeneic heamatopoietic stem-cell transplantation for patients with relapsed or refractory lymphomas: comparison of high-dose conventional conditioning versus fludarabine-based reduced-intensity regimens. *Annals of Oncology, 13,* 135–9.

Bierman, P., Molina, A., Nelson, G. *et al.* (1999). Matched unrelated donor (MUD) allogeneic bone marrow transplantation for non-Hodgkin's lymphoma (NHL): results from the National Marrow Donor Program (NMDP). *Proceedings of the American Society of Clinical Oncology, 18,* 3.

Bolwell, B., Goormastic, M., & Andresen, S. (1997). Durability of remisssion after ABMT for NHL: the importance of the 2-year evaluation point. *Bone Marrow Transplantation, 19,* 443–8.

Bonini, C., Ferrari, G., Verzeletti, S. *et al.* (1997). HSV-TK gene transfer into donor lymphocytes for control of allogeneic graft-versus-leukemia. *Science, 276,* 1719–24.

Brichard, B., Vermylen, C., Ninane, J. *et al.* (1995). Transplantation of umbilical cord blood in a refractory lymphoma. *Pediatric Hematology Oncology, 12,* 79–81.

Burt, R. K., Guitart, J., Traynor, A. *et al.* (2000). Allogeneic hematopoietic stem cell transplantation for advanced mycosis fungoides: evidence of a graft-versus-tumor effect. *Bone Marrow Transplantation, 25,* 111–3.

Campbell, P., Iland, H., Gibson, J., & Joshua, D. (1999). Syngeneic stem cell transplantation for HIV-related lymphoma. *British Journal of Haematology, 105,* 795–8.

Canellos, G. P. (1996). Current strategies for early Hodgkin's disease. *Annals of Oncology, 7* (Suppl 4), 91–3.

Carella, A. M., Cavaliere, M., Lerma, E. *et al.* (2000). Autografting followed by nonmyeloablative immunosuppressive chemother-

apy and allogeneic peripheral-blood hematopoietic stem-cell transplantation as treatment of resistant Hodgkin's disease and non-Hodgkin's lymphoma. *Journal of Clinical Oncology, 18,* 3918–24.

Chopra, R., Goldstone, A. H., Pearce, R. *et al.* (1992). Autologous versus allogeneic bone marrow transplantation for non-Hodgkin's lymphoma: a case-controlled analysis of the European Bone Marrow Transplant Group Registry data. *Journal of Clinical Oncology, 10,* 1690–5.

Collins, R. H. Jr., Shpilberg, O., Drobyski, W. R. *et al.* (1997). Donor leukocyte infusions in 140 patients with relapsed malignancy after allogeneic bone marrow transplantation. *Journal of Clinical Oncology, 15,* 433–44.

Cook, R. C., Connors, J. M., Gascoyne, R. D. *et al.* (1999). Treatment of post-transplant lymphoproliferative diseas with rituximaab monoclonal antibody after lung transplantation. *Lancet, 354,* 1698–1699.

Corradini, P., Ladetto, M., Astolfi, M. *et al.* (1996). Clinical and molecular remission after allogeneic blood cell transplantation in a patient with mantle-cell lymphoma. *British Journal of Haematology, 94,* 376–8.

Corradini, P., Tarella, C., Olivieri, A. *et al.* (2002). Reduced-intensity conditioning followed by allografting of hematopoietic cells can produce clinical and molecular remissions in patients with poor-risk hematologic malignancies. *Blood, 99,* 75–82.

Cull, G. M., Haynes, A. P., Byrne, J. L. *et al.* (2000). Preliminary experience of allogeneic stem cell transplantation for lymphoproliferative disorders using BEAM-CAMPATH conditioning: an effective regimen with low procedure-related toxicity. *British Journal of Haematology, 108,* 754–60.

Curtis, R. E., Rowlings, P. A., Deeg, H. J. *et al.* (1997). Solid cancers after bone marrow transplantation. *New England Journal of Medicine, 336,* 897–904.

Darrington, D. L., Vose, J. M., Anderson, J. R. *et al.* (1994). Incidence and characterization of secondary myelodysplastic syndrome and acute myelogenous leukemia following high-dose chemoradiotherapy and autologous stem-cell transplantation for lymphoid malignancies. *Journal of Clinical Oncology, 12,* 2527–34.

de Lima, M., van Besien, K. W., Giralt, S. A. *et al.* (1997). Bone marrow transplantation after failure of autologous transplant for non-Hodgkin's lymphoma. *Bone Marrow Transplantation, 19,* 121–7.

Demirer, T., Weaver, C. H., Buckner, C. D. *et al.* (1995). High-dose cyclophosphamide, carmustine, and etoposide followed by allogeneic bone marrow transplantation in patients with lymphoid malignancies who had received prior dose-limiting radiation therapy. *Journal of Clinical Oncology, 13,* 596–602.

de Witte, T., Awwad, B., Boezeman, J. *et al.* (1994). Role of allogeneic bone marrow transplantation in adolescent or adult patients with acute lymphoblastic leukaemia or lymphoblastic lymphoma in first remission. *Bone Marrow Transplantation, 14,* 767–74.

De Wolf-Peeters, C. & Pittaluga, S. (1996). Further considerations on the Revised European-American Lymphoma classification. *Current Opinions in Oncology, 8,* 366–70.

Dhedin, N., Giraudier, S., Gaulard, P. *et al.* (1999). Allogeneic bone marrow transplantation in aggressive non-Hodgkin's lymphoma (excluding Burkitt and lymphoblastic lymphoma) a series of 73 patients from the SFGM database. *British Journal of Haematology,* **107,** 154–161.

Dreger, P. & Schmitz, N. (1997). The role of stem cell transplantation in the treatment of chronic lymphocytic leukemia. *Leukemia,* **11** (Suppl 2), S42–5.

Dreger, P., Von Neuhoff, N., Kuse, R. *et al.* (1997). Sequential high-dose therapy and autologous stem cell transplantation for treatment of mantle cell lymphoma. *Annals of Oncology,* **8,** 1997.

Emanuel, D. J., Lucas, K. G., Mallory, G. B. *et al.* (1997). Treatment of post-transplant lymphoproliferative disease in the central nervous system of a lung transplant recipient using allogeneic leukocytes. *Transplantation,* **63,** 1691–1694.

Eyrich, M., Lang, P., Lal, S. *et al.* (2001). A prospective analysis of the pattern of immune reconstitution in a paediatric cohort following transplantation of positively selected human leucocyte antigen-disparate haematopoietic stem cells from parental donors. *British Journal of Haematology,* **114,** 422–32.

Fassas, A. B., Rapoport, A. P., Cottler-Fox *et al.* (2000). Encouraging preliminary results in 12 patients with high-risk haematological malignancies by omitting graft-versus-host disease prophylaxis after allogeneic transplantation. *British Journal of Haematology,* **111,** 662–667.

Faye, A., Van Den Abeele, T., Peuchjmaur, M. *et al.* (1998). Anti-CD20 monoclonal antibody for post-transplant lymphoproliferative disorders. *Lancet,* **352,** 1285.

Ferrara, J. L., Cooke, K. R., Pan, L., & Krenger, W. (1996). The immunopathophysiology of acute graft-versus-host-disease. *Stem Cells,* **14,** 473–89.

Fisher, R. I., Gaynor, E. R., Dahlberg, S. *et al.* (1993). Comparison of a standard regimen (CHOP) with three intensive chemotherapy regimens for advanced non-Hodgkin's lymphoma. *New England Journal of Medicine,* **328,** 1002–6.

Freedman, A. S., Neuberg, D., Gribben, J. G. *et al.* (1998). High-dose chemo-radiotherapy and anti-B-cell monoclonal antibody-purged autologous bone marrow transplantation in mantle-cell lymphoma: no evidence for long-term remission. *Journal of Clinical Oncology,* **16,** 13–8.

Frei, E. & Canellos, G. P. (1980). Dose: a critical factor in cancer chemotherapy. *American Journal of Medicine,* **69,** 585–94.

Friedberg, J. W., Neuberg, D., Monson, E. *et al.* (2001). The impact of external beam radiation therapy prior to autologous bone marrow transplantation in patients with non-Hodgkin's lymphoma. *Biology of Blood and Marrow Transplantation,* **7,** 446–453.

Fung, H. C. & Nademanee, A. P. (2002). Approach to Hodgkin's lymphoma in the new millennium. *Hematology Oncology,* **20,** 1–15.

Gabarre, J., Leblond, V., Sutton, L. *et al.* (1996). Autologous bone marrow transplantation in relapsed HIV-related non-Hodgkin's lymphoma. *Bone Marrow Transplantation,* **18,** 1195–7.

Gajewski, J. L., Phillips, G. L., Sobocinski, K. A. *et al.* (1996). Bone marrow transplants from HLA-identical siblings in advanced Hodgkin's disease. *Journal of Clinical Oncology,* **14,** 572–8.

Giralt, S., Estey, E., Albitar, M. *et al.* (1997). Engraftment of allogeneic hematopoietic progenitor cells with purine analog-containing chemotherapy: harnessing graft-versus-leukemia without myeloablative therapy. *Blood,* **89,** 4531–6.

Greenlee, R., Hill-Harmon, M., Murray, T. *et al.* (2001). Cancer Statistics, 2001. *CA, A Cancer Journal for Clinicians,* **51,** 15–36.

Gribben, J. G. (1997). Bone marrow transplantation for low-grade B-cell malignancies. *Current Opinions in Oncology,* **9,** 117–21.

Grigg, A., Bardy, P., Byron, K. *et al.* (1999). Fludarabine-based non-myeloablative chemotherapy followed by infusion of HLA-identical stem cells for relapsed leukaemia and lymphoma. *Bone Marrow Transplantation,* **23,** 107–10.

Haioun, C., Lepage, E., Gisselbrecht, C. *et al.* (1997). Benefit of autologous bone marrow transplantation over sequential chemotherapy in poor-risk aggressive non-Hodgkin's lymphoma: updated results of the prospective study LNH87–2. Groupe d'Etude des Lymphomes de l' Adulte. *Journal of Clinical Oncology,* **15,** 1131–7.

Haioun, C., Lepage, E., Gisselbrecht, C. *et al.* (2000). Survival benefit of high-dose therapy in poor-risk aggressive non-Hodgkin's lymphoma: final analysis of the prospective LNH87-2 protocol— a Group d'Etude des Lymphomes de l'Adulte study. *Journal of Clinical Oncology,* **18,** 3025–30.

Hale, G., Tong, X., Benaim, E. *et al.* (2001). Allogeneic bone marrow transplantation in children failing prior autologous bone marrow transplantation. *Bone Marrow Transplantation,* **27,** 155–162.

Handgretinger, R., Klingebiel, T., Land, P. *et al.* (2001). Megadose transplantation of purified peripheral blood CD34(+) progenitor cells from HLA-mismatched parental donors in children. *Bone Marrow Transplantation,* **27,** 777–783.

Henry-Amar, M. & Joly, F. (1996). Late complications after Hodgkin's disease. *Annals of Oncology,* **7** (Suppl 4), 11–26.

Heslop, H. E. & Rooney, C. M. (1997). Adoptive cellular immunotherapy for EBV lymphoproliferative disease. *Immunological Reviews,* **157,** 217–22.

Holland, H. K., Saral, R., Rossi, J. J. *et al.* (1989). Allogeneic bone marrow transplantation, zidovudine, and human immunodeficiency virus type 1 (HIV-1) infection. Studies in a patient with non-Hodgkin's lymphoma. *Annals of Internal Medicine,* **111,** 973–81.

Horowitz, M. M., Gale, R. P., Sondel, P. M. *et al.* (1990). Graft-versus-leukemia reactions after bone marrow transplantation. *Blood,* **75,** 555–62.

International Non-Hodgkin's Lymphoma Prognostic Factors Project. (1993). A predictive model for aggressive non-Hodgkin's lymphoma. *New England Journal of Medicine,* **329,** 987–94.

Jones, R. J., Ambinder, R. F., Piantadosi, S., & Santos, G. W. (1991). Evidence of a graft-versus-lymphoma effect associated with allogeneic bone stem cell transplantation. *Blood,* **77,** 649–53.

Juckett, M., Rowlings, P., Hessner, M. *et al.* (1998). T cell-depleted allogeneic bone marrow transplantation for high-risk non-Hodgkin's lymphoma: clinical and molecular follow-up. *Bone Marrow Transplantation,* **21,** 893–9.

Kang, E. M., de Witte, M., Malech, H. *et al.* (2002). Nonmyeloablative conditioning followed by transplantation of genetically modified HLA-matched peripheral blood progenitor cells for hematologic malignancies in patients with acquired immunodeficiency syndrome. *Blood,* **99,** 698–701.

Ketterer, N., Salles, G., Espinouse, D. *et al.* (1997). Intensive therapy with peripheral stem cell transplantation in 16 patients with mantle cell lymphoma. *Annals of Oncology,* **8,** 701–4.

Khouri, I. F., Keating, M., Korbling, M. *et al.* (1998a). Transplant-lite: induction of graft-versus-malignancy using fludarabine-based nonablative chemotherapy and allogeneic blood progenitor cell transplantation as treatment for lymphoid malignancies. *Journal of Clinical Oncology*, **16**, 2817–24.

Khouri, I. F., Lee, M. S., Romaguera, J. *et al.* (1999). Allogeneic hematopoietic transplantation for mantle-cell lymphoma: molecular remissions and evidence of graft-versus-malignancy. *Annals of Oncology*, **10**, 1293–9.

Khouri, I. F., Romaguera, J., Kantarjian, H. *et al.* (1998b). Hyper-CVAD and high-dose methotrexate/cytarabine followed by stem cell transplantation: an active regimen for aggressive mantle cell lymphoma. *Journal of Clinical Oncology*, **16**, 3803–9.

Khouri, I. F., Saliba, R. M., Giralt, S. A. *et al.* (2001). Nonablative allogeneic hematopoietic transplantation as adoptive immunotherapy for indolent lymphoma: low incidence of toxicity, acute graft-versus-host disease and transplant-related mortality. *Blood*, **98**, 3595–9.

Kolb, H. J. & Holler, E. (1997). Adoptive immunotherapy with donor lymphocyte transfusions. *Current Opinions in Oncology*, **9**, 139–45.

Kroger, N., Hoffknecht, M., Kruger, W. *et al.* (2000). Allogeneic bone marrow transplantation for refractory mantle cell lymphoma. *Annals of Hematology*, **79**, 578–580.

Levine, J. E., Harris, R. E., Loberiza, F. R. *et al.* (2003). A comparison of allogeneic and autologous bone marrow transplantation for lymphoblastic lymphoma. *Blood*, **101**, 2476–82.

Linch, D. C., Winfield, D., Goldstone, A. H. *et al.* (1993). Dose intensification with autologous bone-marrow transplantation in relapsed and resistant Hodgkin's disease: results of a BNLI randomised trial. *Lancet*, **341**, 1051–4.

Longo, D. L., Duffey, P. L., Young, R. C. *et al.* (1992). Conventional-dose salvage combination chemotherapy in patients relapsing with Hodgkin's disease after combination chemotherapy: the low probability for cure. *Journal of Clinical Oncology*, **10**, 210–18.

Longo, D. L., Banks, P. M., & Hoppe, R. T. (1994). Hodgkin's disease. Revista, De Investigation Clinica, Suppl, 73–83.

Mandigers, C.M.P.W., Raemaekers, J.M.M., Schattenberg, A.V.M.B. *et al.* (1998). Allogeneic bone marrow transplantation with T-cell–depleted marrow grafts for patients with poor-risk relapsed low-grade non-Hodgkin's lymphoma. *British Journal of Haematology*, **100**, 198–206.

Marafioti, T., Hummel, M., Anagnostopoulos, I. *et al.* (1997). Origin of nodular lymphocyte-predominant Hodgkin's disease from a clonal expansion of highly mutated germinal-center B cells. *New England Journal of Medicine*, **337**, 453–8.

Martinez, C., Carreras, E., Rovira, M. *et al.* (2000). Patients with mantle-cell lymphoma relapsing after autologous stem cell transplantation may be rescued by allogeneic transplantation. *Bone Marrow Transplantation*, **26**, 677–9.

Martino, R., Shah, A., Romero, P. *et al.* (1999). Allogeneic bone marrow transplantation for advanced Waldenström's macroglobulinemia. *Bone Marrow Transplantation*, **23**, 747–9.

Massumoto, C., Benyunes, M. C., Sale, G. *et al.* (1996). Close simulation of acute graft-versus-host disease by interleukin-2 administered after autologous bone marrow transplantation for hematologic malignancy. *Bone Marrow Transplantation*, **17**, 351–6.

Mauch, P., Constine, L., Greenberger, J. *et al.* (1995). Hematopoietic stem cell compartment: acute and late effects of radiation therapy and chemotherapy. *International Journal of Radiation Oncology, Biology, Physics*, **31**, 1319–39.

McGuirk, J. P., Seropian, S., Howe, G. *et al.* (1999). Use of rituximab and irradiated donor-derived lymphocytes to control Epstein-Barr virus–associated lymphoproliferation in patients undergoing related haplo-identical stem cell transplantation. *Bone Marrow Transplantation*, **24**, 1253–1258.

Mendoza, E., Territo, M., Schiller, G. *et al.* (1995). Allogeneic bone marrow transplantation for Hodgkin's and non-Hodgkin's lymphoma. *Bone Marrow Transplantation*, **15**, 299–303.

Michallet, M., Archimbaud, E., Bandini, G. *et al.* (1996). HLA-identical sibling bone marrow transplantation in younger patients with chronic lymphocytic leukemia. European Group for Blood and Marrow Transplantation and the International Bone Marrow Transplant Registry. *Annals of Internal Medicine*, **124**, 311–15.

Miller, J. S., Arthur, D. C., Litz, C. E. *et al.* (1994). Myelodysplastic syndrome after autologous bone marrow transplantation: an additional late complication of curative cancer therapy. *Blood*, **83**, 3780–6.

Milpied, N., Fielding, A. K., Pearce, R. M. *et al.* (1996). Allogeneic bone marrow transplant is not better than autologous transplant for patients with relapsed Hodgkin's disease. European Group for Blood and Bone Marrow Transplantation. *Journal of Clinical Oncology*, **14**, 1291–6.

Milpied, N., Ifrah, N., Kuentz, M. *et al.* (1989). Bone marrow transplantation for adult poor prognosis lymphoblastic lymphoma in first complete remission. *British Journal of Haematology*, **73**, 82–7.

Mink, S. A. & Armitage, J. O. (2001). High-dose therapy in lymphomas: a review of the current status of allogeneic and autologous stem cell transplantation in Hodgkin's disease and non-Hodgkin's lymphoma. *The Oncologist*, **6**, 247–56.

Molina, A., Nademanee, A., Arber, D., & Forman, S. J. (1999). Remission of refractory Sézary syndrome after bone marrow transplantation from a matched unrelated donor. *Biology of Blood and Marrow Transplantation*, **5**, 400–4.

Moreau, P., Mechinaud, F., Mahe, B. *et al.* (1996). Successful allogeneic bone marrow transplantation for early relapse after autologous bone marrow transplantation in two cases of aggressive high-grade non-Hodgkin's lymphoma. *Bone Marrow Transplantation*, **18**, 665–7.

Mundt, A. J., Sibley, G., Williams, S. *et al.* (1995). Patterns of failure following high-dose chemotherapy and autologous bone marrow transplantation with involved field radiotherapy for relapsed/refractory Hodgkin's disease. *International Journal of Radiation Oncology, Biology, Physics*, **33**, 261–70.

Nachbauer, D., Oberaigner, W., Fritsch, E. *et al.* (2001). Allogeneic or autologous stem cell transplantation (SCT) for relapsed and refractory Hodgkin's disease and non-Hodgkin's lymphoma: a single-centre experience. *European Journal of Haematology*, **66**, 43–49.

Nademanee, A. P., Forman, S. J., Schmidt, G. M. *et al.* (1987). Allogeneic bone marrow transplantation for high risk non-Hodgkin's lymphoma during first complete remission. *Blut*, **55**, 11–18.

Nagler, A., Ackerstein, A., Or, R. *et al.* (1997). Immunotherapy with recombinant human interleukin-2 and recombinant interferon-alpha in lymphoma patients postautologous marrow or stem cell transplantation. *Blood,* **89,** 3951–9.

Nagler, A., Slavin, S., Varadi, G. *et al.* (2000). Allogeneic peripheral blood stem cell transplantation using a fludarabine-based low intensity conditioning regimen for malignant lymphoma. *Bone Marrow Transplantation,* **25,** 1021–8.

Nakao, S., Miura, Y., Zeng, W. *et al.* (1997). Induction of autocytotoxic T cells with cyclosporine and interferon-gamma for patients with non-Hodgkin's lymphoma after transplantation of peripheral blood stem cells. *Journal of Allergy and Clinical Immunology,* **100,** S65–9.

Non-Hodgkin's Lymphoma Pathologic Classification Project. (1982). National Cancer Institute sponsored study of classifications of non-Hodgkin's lymphomas: summary and description of a working formulation for clinical usage. *Cancer,* **49,** 2112–35.

Norton, A. J. (1996). Classification of non-Hodgkin's lymphomas. *Baillieres Clinical Haematology,* **9,** 641–52.

Ohnuma, K., Toyoda, Y., Nishihira, H. *et al.* (1997). Aggressive natural killer (NK) cell lymphoma: report of a pediatric case and review of the literature. *Leukemia and Lymphoma,* **25,** 387–92.

O'Reilly, S. E., Connors, J. M., Macpherson, N. *et al.* (1997). Malignant lymphomas in the elderly. *Clinical Geriatric Medicine,* **13,** 251–63.

Park, S., Brice, P., Noguerra, M. E. *et al.* (2000). Myelodysplasias and leukemias after autologous stem cell transplantation for lymphoid malignancies. *Bone Marrow Transplantation,* **26,** 321–326.

Passweg, J. R., Rowlings, P. A., Armitage, J. O. *et al.* (1995). Report from the International Bone Marrow Transplant Registry and Autologous Blood and Marrow Transplant Registry—North America. *Clinical Transplantation,* 117–27.

Pecego, R., Hill, R., Appelbaum, F. R. *et al.* (1986). Interstitial pneumonitis following autologous bone marrow transplantation. *Transplantation,* **42,** 515–17.

Pedersen-Bjergaard, J., Andersen, M. K., & Christiansen, D. H. (2000). Therapy-related acute myeloid luekemia and myelodysplasia after high-dose chemotherapy and autologous stem cell transplantation. *Blood,* **95,** 3273–79.

Philip, T., Guglielmi, C., Hagenbeek, A. *et al.* (1995). Autologous bone marrow transplantation as compared with salvage chemotherapy in relapses of chemotherapy-sensitive non-Hodgkin's lymphoma. *New England Journal of Medicine,* **333,** 1540–5.

Pittaluga, S., Bijnens, L., Teodorovic, I. *et al.* (1996). Clinical analysis of 670 cases in two trials of the European Organization for the Research and Treatment of Cancer Lymphoma Cooperative Group subtyped according to the Revised European-American Classification of Lymphoid Neoplasms: a comparison with the Working Formulation. *Blood,* **87,** 4358–67.

Radich, J., Gooley, T., Sanders, J. *et al.* (2000). Second allogeneic transplantation after failure of first autologous transplantation. *Biology of Blood and Marrow Transplantation,* **6,** 272–279.

Rapoport, A. P., DiPersio, J. F., Martin, B. A. *et al.* (1995). Patients > or = age 40 years undergoing autologous or allogeneic BMT have regimen-related mortality rates and event-free survivals comparable to patients < age 40 years. *Bone Marrow Transplantation,* **15,** 523–30.

Ratanatharathorn, V., Uberti, J., Karanes, C. *et al.* (1994). Prospective comparative trial of autologous versus allogeneic bone marrow transplantation in patients with non-Hodgkin's lymphoma. *Blood,* **84,** 1050–5.

Reece, D. (1995). Should high-risk patients with Hodgkin's disease be singled out for heavier therapeutic regimens while low risk patients are spared such therapies? *Leukemia and Lymphoma,* **15** (Suppl 1), 19–21.

Reece, D. E. (2002). Hematopoietic stem cell transplantation in Hodgkin disease. *Current Opinions in Oncology,* **14,** 165–170.

Reece, D. E. & Phillips, G. L. (1994). Intensive therapy and autotransplantation in Hodgkin's disease. *Stem Cells,* **12,** 477–93.

Rizzieri, D. A., Long, G. D., Vrendenburgh, J. J. *et al.* (2001). Successful allogeneic engraftment of mismatched unrelated cord blood following a nonmyeloablative preparative regimen. *Blood,* **98,** 3486–3488.

Robinson, S. P., Goldstone, A. H., Mackinnon, S. *et al.* (2002), Chemoresistant or aggressive lymphoma predicts for a poor outcome following reduced-intensity allogeneic progenitor cell transplantation: an analysis from the Lymphoma Working Party of the European Group for Blood and Marrow Transplantation. *Blood,* **100,** 4310–6.

Rodrigez, J., Keating, M. J., O'Brien, S. *et al.* (2000). Allogeneic haematopoietic transplantation for Richter's syndrome. *British Journal of Haematology,* **110,** 897–9.

Salutari, P., Sica, S., Micciulli, G. *et al.* (1996). Extramedullary relapse after allogeneic bone marrow transplantation plus buffycoat in two high risk patients. *Haematologica,* **81,** 182–5.

Salzman, D. E., Briggs, A. D., & Vaughan, W. P. (1997). Bone marrow transplantation for non-Hodgkin's lymphoma: a review. *American Journal of Medical Science,* **313,** 228–35.

Santos, G. W., Saral, R., Burns, W. H. *et al.* (1987). Allogeneic, syngeneic and autologous marrow transplantation in the acute leukemias and lymphomas—Baltimore experience. *Acta Haematologica,* **78** (Suppl 1), 175–80.

Shad, A. & Magrath, I. (1997). Non-Hodgkin's lymphoma. *Pediatric Clinics of North America,* **44,** 863–90.

Singer, C. R., Taghipour, G., Boogaerts, M. A. *et al.* (1999). Matched unrelated donor (MUD) bone marrow transplantation for adults and children with non-Hodgkin's lymphoma and Hodgkin's lymophoma: Preliminary analysis of 56 cases reported to EBMT lymphoma registry. *Blood,* **94** (Suppl 1), 560a.

Skarin, A. T. & Dorfman, D. M. (1997). Non-Hodgkin's lymphomas: current classification and management. *CA, A Cancer Journal for Clinicians,* **47,** 351–72.

Slavin, S., Naparstek, E., Nagler, A. *et al.* (1996). Allogeneic cell therapy with donor peripheral blood cells and recombinant human interleukin-2 to treat leukemia relapse after allogeneic bone marrow transplantation. *Blood,* **87,** 2195–204.

Sohn, S. K., Baek, J. H., Kim, D. H. *et al.* (2000). Successful allogeneic stem-cell transplantation with prophylactic stepwise G-CSF primed-DLIs for relapse after autologous transplantation in mantle cell lymphoma: a case report and literature review on the evidence of GVL effects in MCL. *American Journal of Hematology,* **65,** 75–80.

Soiffer, R. J., Freedman, A. S., Neuberg, D. *et al.* (1998). CD6+ T cell-depleted allogeneic bone marrow transplantation for non-Hodgkin's lymphoma. *Bone Marrow Transplantation,* **21,** 1177–1181.

Spitzer, T. R., McAfee, S., Sackstein, R. *et al.* (2000). Intentional induction of mixed chimerism and achievement of antitumor responses after nonmyeloablative conditioning therapy and HLA-matched donor bone marrow transplantation for refractory hematologic malignancies. *Biology of Blood and Marrow Transplantation,* **6,** 309–20.

Stein, H. & Hummel, M. (1999). Cellular origin and clonality of classic Hodgkin's lymphoma: Immunophenotypic and molecular studies. *Seminars in Hematology,* **36,** 233–241.

Stewart, D. A., Vose, J. M., Weisenburger, D. D. *et al.* (1995). The role of high-dose therapy and autologous hematopoietic stem cell transplantation for mantle cell lymphoma. *Annals of Oncology,* **6,** 263–6.

Stiff, P. Management strategies for the hard-to-mobilize patient. (1999). *Bone Marrow Transplantation,* **23** (Suppl 2), S29-S33.

Straus, D. J. (1997). HIV-associated lymphomas. *Current Opinions in Oncology,* **9,** 450–4.

Swinnen, L. J. (1997). Treatment of organ transplant-related lymphoma. *Hematology/Oncology Clinics of North America,* **11,** 963–73.

Sykes, M., Preffer, F., McAfee, S. *et al.* (1999). Mixed lymphohematopoietic chimerism and graft-versus-lymphoma effects after non-myeloablative therapy and HLA-mismatched donor bone marrow transplantation. *Lancet,* **353,** 1755–9.

Toze, C. L., Shepherd, J. D., Connors, J. M. *et al.* (2000). Allogeneic bone marrow transplantation for low-grade lymphoma and chronic lymphocytic leukemia. *Bone Marrow Transplantation,* **25,** 605–12.

Traweek, S. T., Slovak, M. L., Nademanee, A. P. *et al.* (1996). Myelodysplasia and acute myeloid leukemia occurring after autologous bone marrow transplantation for lymphoma. *Leukemia and Lymphoma,* **20,** 365–72.

Troussard, X., Leblond, V., Kuentz, M. *et al.* (1990). Allogeneic bone marrow transplantation in adults with Burkitt's lymphoma or acute lymphoblastic leukemia in first complete remission. *Journal of Clinical Oncology,* **8,** 809–12.

Ueda, T., Hatanaka, K., Kosugi, S. *et al.* (2001). Successful non-myeloablative allogeneic peripheral blood stem cell transplantation (PBSCT) for Waldenstrom's macroglobulinemia with severe pancytopenia. *Bone Marrow Transplantation,* **28,** 609–11.

Urbano-Ispizua, A., Schmitz, N., de Witte, T. *et al.* (2002). Allogeneic and autologous transplantation for haematological diseases, solid tumors and immune disorders: definition and current practice in Europe. *Bone Marrow Transplantation,* **29,** 639–46.

Utsunomiya, A., Miyazaki, Y., Takatsuka, Y. *et al.* (2001). Improved outcome of adult T cell leukemia/lymphoma with allogeneic hematopoietic stem cell transplantation. *Bone Marrow Transplantation,* **27,** 15–20.

van Besien, K., Sobocinski, K. A., Rowlings, P. A. *et al.* (1998). Allogeneic bone marrow transplantation for low-grade lymphoma. *Blood,* **92,** 1832–6.

van Besien, K. W., de Lima, M., Giralt, S. A. *et al.* (1997a). Management of lymphoma recurrence after allogeneic transplantation: the relevance of graft-versus-lymphoma effect. *Bone Marrow Transplantation,* **19,** 977–82.

van Besien, K. W., Forman, A., & Champlin, R. (1997b). Central nervous system relapse of lymphoid malignancies in adults: the role of high-dose chemotherapy. *Annals of Oncology,* **8,** 515–24.

van Besien, K. W., Khouri, I. F., Giralt, S. A. *et al.* (1995). Allogeneic bone marrow transplantation for refractory and recurrent low-grade lymphoma: the case for aggressive management. *Journal of Clinical Oncology,* **13,** 1096–102.

van Besien, K. W., Mehra, R. C., Giralt, S. A. *et al.* (1996a). Allogeneic bone marrow transplantation for poor-prognosis lymphoma: response, toxicity and survival depend on disease histology. *American Journal of Medicine,* **100,** 299–307.

van Besien, K. W., Przepiorka, D., Mehra, R. *et al.* (1996b). Impact of preexisting CNS involvement on the outcome of bone marrow transplantation in adult hematologic malignancies. *Journal of Clinical Oncology,* **14,** 3036–42.

Van der Jagt, R. H., Appelbaum, F. R., Petersen, F. B. *et al.* (1991). Busulfan and cyclophosphamide as a preparative regimen for bone marrow transplantation in patients with prior chest radiotherapy. *Bone Marrow Transplantation,* **8,** 211–15.

Vandenberghe, E., Pearce, R., Taghipour, G. *et al.* (1997). Role of a second transplant in the management of poor-prognosis lymphomas: a report from the European Blood and Bone Marrow Registry. *Journal of Clinical Oncology,* **15,** 1595–600.

Varadi, G., Or, R., Kapelushnik, J. *et al.* (1999). Graft-versus-lymphoma effect after allogeneic peripheral blood stem cell transplantation for primary central nervous system lymphoma. *Leukemia and Lymphoma,* **34,** 185–190.

Verdonck, L. F. (1999). Allogeneic versus autologous bone marrow transplantation for refractory and recurrent low-grade non-Hodgkin's lymphoma: updated results of the Utrecht experience. *Leukemia and Lymphoma,* **34,** 129–136.

Verdonck, L. F., Dekker, A. W., Lokhorst, H. M. *et al.* (1997). Allogeneic versus autologous bone marrow transplantation for refractory and recurrent low-grade non-Hodgkin's lymphoma. *Blood,* **90,** 4201–5.

Weinthal, J. A., Goldman, S. C., Lenarsky, C. (2000). Successful treatment of relapsed Burkitt's lymphoma using unrelated cord blood transplantation as consolidation therapy. *Bone Marrow Transplantation,* **25,** 1311–3.

Weisdorf, D. J. (1997). Bone marrow transplantation for acute lymphocytic leukemia (ALL). *Leukemia,* **11** (Suppl 4), S20–2.

Williams, C. D., Pearce, R., Taghipour, G. *et al.* (1994). Autologous bone marrow transplantation for patients with non-Hodgkin's lymphoma and CNS involvement: those transplanted with active CNS disease have a poor outcome—a report by the European Bone Marrow Transplant Lymphoma Registry. *Journal of Clinical Oncology,* **12,** 2415–22.

Witherspoon, R. P., Fisher, L. D., Schoch, G. *et al.* (1989). Secondary cancers after bone marrow transplantation for leukemia or aplastic anemia. *New England Journal of Medicine,* **321,** 784–9.

Zinzani, P. L., Bendandi, M., Visani, G. *et al.* (1996). Adult lymphoblastic lymphoma: clinical features and prognostic factors in 53 patients. *Leukemia and Lymphoma,* **23,** 577–82.

58 Allogeneic hematopoietic stem cell transplantation for severe aplastic anemia

GEORGE GEORGES AND RAINER STORB

Fred Hutchinson Cancer Research Center and the University of Washington, Seattle, USA

Introduction

Severe aplastic anemia, characterized by pancytopenia and a hypocellular marrow (Table 58.1), is generally an acquired disease that has been associated with hepatitis, chemicals, drugs, and rarely, pregnancy, although in most patients, no etiologic factor for the disease can be identified (Table 58.2). Although both hepatitis A virus (HAV) and hepatitis B virus (HBV) have been associated with severe aplastic anemia in a small number of patients, most cases of hepatitis-associated severe aplastic anemia are related to non-A, non-B, non-C (and non-D, non-E, and non- G) viral hepatitis (Safadi *et al.*, 2001). Successful bone marrow transplantation for hepatitis-associated severe aplastic anemia has been reported following successful orthotopic liver transplantation (Kawahara *et al.*, 1991).

The acquired failure of hematopoiesis has heterogeneous pathophysiologic mechanisms including a lack of, or defect in, hematopoietic stem cells, an immunologically mediated destruction of hematopoiesis, or an abnormal marrow stromal microenvironment. In its severe form, aplastic anemia has a mortality of 80% to 90% despite supportive care, with most patients dying within 6 months of diagnosis. Criteria for severe aplastic anemia include the presence of at least two of the following three peripheral blood findings:

(1) a neutrophil count of less than $0.5 \times 10^9/l$;
(2) a platelet count of less than $20 \times 10^9/l$; and
(3) a corrected reticulocyte count of less than 1%.

The bone marrow must be hypocellular, with lymphoid cells being predominant without morphologic evidence of myeloid or megakaryocytic dyspoiesis. In addition, it is essential to obtain cytogenetic studies to rule out evidence of clonal genetic abnormalities consistent with myelodysplasia, and it is helpful to screen for the presence of glycosylphosphatidyl-inositol anchored proteins to exclude paroxysmal nocturnal hemoglobinuria.

An appreciation of the pathophysiologic mechanisms of the disease has led to treatment strategies that include immunosuppressive therapy and allogeneic hematopoietic stem cell (HSC) transplantation. The observation that acquired aplastic anemia can be corrected in some patients by infusion of syngeneic

Table 58.1. *Diagnosis of severe aplastic anemia*

Parameter	Severe aplastic anemia[a]	Very severe aplastic anemia
Blood		
Neutrophils	$<0.5 \times 10^9/l$	$<0.2 \times 10^9/l$
Platelets	$<20 \times 10^9/l$	
Reticulocytes	<1% (corrected)	
Marrow	Severe hypocellularity	
	or	
	Moderate hypocellularity with hematopoietic cells <30% of residual cells	

[a] Any two of the three blood parameters or either marrow criteria.

Table 58.2. *Etiology of aplastic anemia*

Acquired	Congenital
1. Direct toxicity to stem cells Iatrogenic causes Radiation Chemotherapy Benzene Intermediate metabolites of some common drugs[b]	Fanconi anemia (Chapter 59) Schwachman-Diamond syndrome (Chapter 64) Dyskeratosis congenita (Chapter 64)
2. Immune-mediated causes Iatrogenic causes Transfusion-associated graft-versus-host disease Eosinophilic fasciitis Hepatitis-associated disease[a] Pregnancy Intermediate metabolites of some common drugs[b] Idiopathic aplastic anemia	

[a] Usually non-A, non-B, non-C, non-G hepatitis.

[b] Drugs associated with acquired aplastic anemia include nonsteroidal anti-inflammatory agents, antithyroid agents, anticonvulsants, chloramphenicol, gold, D-penicillamine, sulfonamides, phenothothiazines, quinacrine, allopurinol.

marrow led, in the early 1970s, to the exploration of allogeneic HLA-identical sibling marrow transplants following immunosuppressive conditioning regimens for the treatment of this disease. Improved patient survival as a result of better transplant conditioning regimens and supportive care has led to the widespread acceptance of HLA-identical sibling HSC transplantation as the treatment of choice for patients with severe aplastic anemia. However, not all patients have HLA-identical siblings. Treatment outcomes with HLA-matched unrelated donor HSC transplantation have also improved significantly over the past two decades, making this an important treatment option for many patients. This chapter will review the results of immunosuppressive therapy, HLA-identical sibling HSC transplantation, and outcomes with alternative donor HSC transplantation including HLA-matched unrelated donors.

Outcome with immunosuppressive therapy

A treatment alternative to allogeneic HSC transplantation has been immunosuppression without marrow transplant, usually involving antithymocyte globulin (ATG) and cyclosporine. The long-term outcome in patients treated with immunosuppressive therapy alone or immunosuppressive therapy plus hematopoietic growth factors, however, remains generally inferior to that of HLA-identical sibling transplantation (Fig. 58.1; Fig. 58.2) (Doney et al., 1997; Fouladi et al., 2000; Kojima et al., 2000; Paquette et al., 1995), although some studies have shown good results with immunosuppressive therapy (Bacigalupo et al., 2000b; Frickhofen et al., 1991). Furthermore, late clonal complications including myelodysplasia and paroxysmal nocturnal hemoglobinuria developed in up to 42% by 11 to 15 years after immune suppressive treatment versus 0% in those treated by

allogeneic transplantation (Tichelli et al., 1994; Frickhofen et al., 2003). Increased age of onset of severe aplastic anemia does not appear to affect the risk for developing clonal disorders (Tichelli et al., 1999). The risk of late clonal complications and the requirement for chronic immunosuppressive therapy for the majority of patients have led many clinicians to consider immunosuppressive therapy only as front-line treatment for older patients or those without a suitable HSC donor.

More intensive immunosuppressive therapy with high-dose cyclophosphamide alone has been studied, but substantial toxicity observed in a randomized trial significantly diminished enthusiasm for this approach. Cyclophosphamide at a dose of 45 mg/kg/day for 4 consecutive days with or without cyclosporine, but without a subsequent transplant was initially reported to induce complete remissions in severe aplastic anemia (Brodsky, Sensenbrenner, & Jones, 1996). A complete response was achieved in 7 of 10 patients. Six remained alive in continuous complete remission with a median follow up of 10.8 (range 7.3–17.8) years and none had relapsed or developed a clonal disease. A study of 19 patients treated with cyclophosphamide 50 mg/kg/day for 4 consecutive days without cyclosporine but with G-CSF support reported an 84% probability of 2-year survival and a 65% probability of complete remission at 4 years (Brodsky et al., 2001). Recovery of neutrophil counts was delayed and the median time to independence from transfusion of red blood cells and platelets was 11 months. However, a randomized trial conducted at the National Institutes of Health (NIH) that compared high-dose cyclophosphamide with ATG (both treatment groups included cyclosporine) was terminated early due to excessive infectious mortality in the cyclophosphamide treatment arm (Tisdale et al., 2000). In the NIH study, cyclophosphamide induced pro-

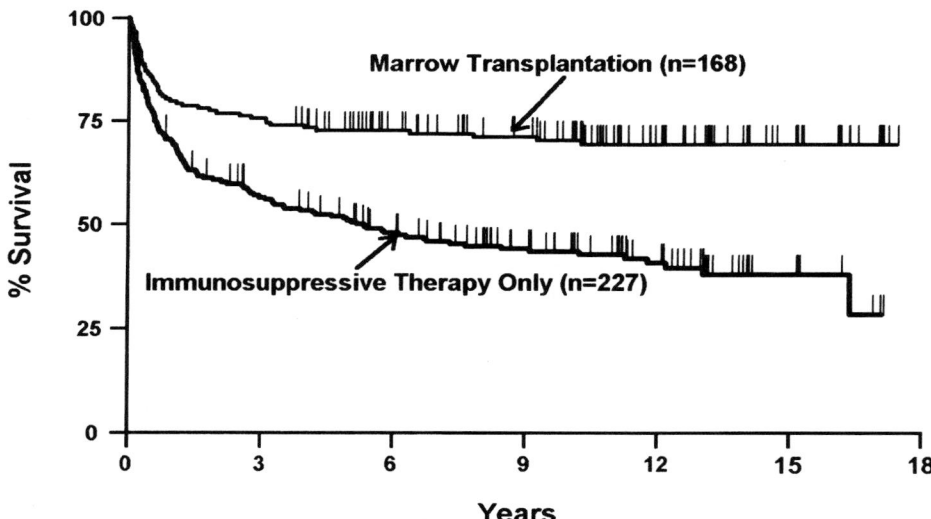

Fig. 58.1. Survival after therapy for acquired aplastic anemia for all patients treated in Seattle between January 1978 and December 1991. Bone marrow transplantation included cyclophosphamide conditioning (no TBI given). In addition, 78 patients received donor buffy coat cells after bone marrow infusion and, starting in June 1988, 21 patients received antithymocyte globulin (ATG). GVHD prophylaxis included: methotrexate (MTX) only (78 patients), MTX and cyclosporine (CSA) (42 patients), CSA only (8 patients), MTX + CSA + prednisone (3 patients). Immunosuppressive therapy included ATG only (162 patients), ATG plus mismatched bone marrow (50 patients), and GM-CSF plus ATG (13 patients). Modified from Doney et al. (1997).

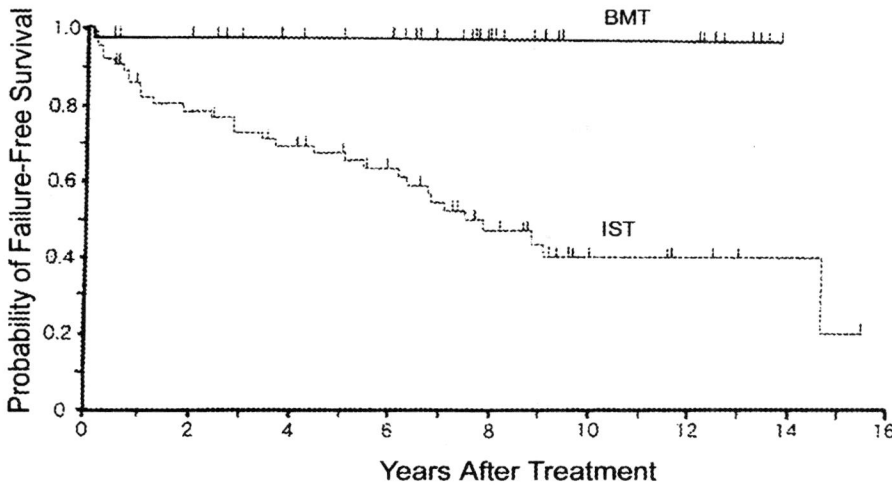

Fig. 58.2. Failure-free survival of children with aplastic anemia initially treated with bone marrow transplantation (BMT) or immunosuppressive therapy (IST) in the Japanese Marrow Donor Program registry. Failure-free survival was measured from the time of start of treatment to the time of last follow-up or death for patients who underwent BMT, and last follow-up, death or BMT for patients who received IST. Reproduced, with permission, from Kojima *et al.* (2000).

longed pancytopenia, particularly in patients with a pretreatment absolute neutrophil count of greater than $0.5 \times 10^9/l$, which contributed to the increased risk of infectious deaths. The authors concluded that high-dose cyclophosphamide without allogeneic HSC transplantation was a dangerous choice for treatment of aplastic anemia. In a subsequent report of late complications, relapse of disease and clonal evolution of cytogenetic abnormalities occurred in both ATG and cyclophosphamide treatment groups (Tisdale *et al.*, 2002). Given these results, high dose cyclophosphamide alone, without subsequent HSC transplant, is unlikely to become a widely used alternative regimen for the treatment of severe aplastic anemia. Also of interest was a report of a successful autologous transplant for severe aplastic anemia, using G-CSF mobilized blood leukocytes harvested upon immunosuppression-induced hematopoietic recovery (Koza *et al.*, 1998).

Disease-specific pretransplant work-up

Although the criteria for severe aplastic anemia are well established, the diagnosis of severe aplastic anemia may be difficult to establish since marrow hypocellularity without karyotypic abnormalities or morphologic dysplasia may occur in other hematological diseases. In children and young adults, Fanconi anemia should be ruled out by tests for chromosomal susceptibility to chemical cross-linking agents. Other constitutional syndromes such as dyskeratosis congenita or ataxia-pancytopenia can be diagnosed with pedigree-associated physical stigmata or neurologic signs, respectively. Marrow cytogenetic analysis is essential to evaluate aplastic anemia and to distinguish it from the hypocellular form of myelodysplastic syndrome (MDS). Normal marrow cytogenetics are the hallmark of aplastic anemia. However, chromosome testing may be unsuccessful due to

low numbers of cells. In this case, repeat sampling of marrow is indicated. Furthermore, some patients with hypocellular MDS may have normal cytogenetic studies. In this situation, careful evaluation of marrow morphology is necessary to attempt to distinguish these diseases. Although MDS can be cured with allogeneic HSC transplantation, the conditioning regimen for MDS is in general more intensive and includes alkylating agents such as busulfan (see Chapter 54), so the distinction between severe aplastic anemia and hypoplastic MDS is important therapeutically as well. Cytogenetic abnormalities such as monosomy 7 and trisomy 8 have been reported to occur in patients with severe aplastic anemia following immunosuppressive treatment (Kojima *et al.*, 2002b; Maciejewski *et al.*, 2002). Clonal evolution is in general associated with poor prognosis, particularly complex cytogenetic abnormalities.

There has been the recognition of considerable clinical overlap between severe aplastic anemia, MDS and paroxysmal nocturnal hemoglobinuria (PNH). T-cell mediated suppression of hematopoiesis may be a pathogenetic mechanism in all three of these marrow failure syndromes. In one report, 32% of patients with newly diagnosed severe aplastic anemia had PNH clones in the peripheral blood with greater than 1% glycosylphosphatidyl-anchored protein (GPI-AP)-deficient granulocytes (Maciejewski *et al.*, 2001). However, conversion to pure hemolytic PNH was infrequent over the relatively short follow-up time. T-cell large granular lymphocytic leukemia (also known as lymphoproliferative disease of granular T-lymphocytes) is a clonal disorder of cytotoxic T lymphocytes that can present as aplastic anemia (Go *et al.*, 2000; Karadimitris *et al.*, 2001). Large granular lymphocytes have a distinctive phenotype and have a clonal T cell receptor rearrangement. Younger patients with large granular lymphocytic leukemia presenting with severe aplastic anemia and good performance status can be excellent candidates for allogeneic HSC transplantation.

Transfusion support should be provided for patients with severe aplastic anemia, but should be given per specific clinical thresholds to decrease the risk of allosensitization. For example, in asymptomatic patents it is appropriate to transfuse with platelets if the platelet count is less than $10 \times 10^9/l$ and to transfuse with red blood cells for hemoglobin of less than 8 gm/dl if the HSC transplant is not imminent. As discussed in the subsequent section, to decrease the risk of sensitization to minor histocompatibility antigens of the HSC donor, only blood products that are both irradiated and leukodepleted should be used. To reduce the overall transfusion support needed prior to transplantation, HLA-typing of the patient and family members should be performed as promptly and efficiently as possible.

Results of HLA-identical sibling transplantation

From early on, three major problems were recognized that limited the success of allogeneic HSC transplantation in this disease: graft rejection, and acute and chronic graft-versus-host disease (GVHD). In addition, organ toxicity from more intensive immunosuppressive preparative regimens limited the effectiveness of HSC transplantation. The impact of these problems on the outcome of transplantation has changed significantly over the past three decades. As a result of the introduction of an optimal conditioning regimen, effective GVHD prophylaxis, and improved supportive care, the impact of graft rejection, as well as acute and chronic graft versus host disease has been significantly reduced. The following section reviews these changes and updates the results of HLA-matched sibling marrow grafting for aplastic anemia.

Graft rejection

Before allogeneic marrow transplantation, recipients are given intensive immunosuppressive therapy to prevent graft rejection. Immunosuppression has included agents such as cyclophosphamide, given alone or in combination with total body irradiation (TBI) or limited field irradiation such as total lymphoid irradiation (TLI) or thoracoabdominal irradiation (TAI). More recently, the combination of cyclophosphamide plus ATG has been shown to be very successful in preventing rejection. In the 1970s, graft rejection was the major cause of failure of marrow transplants following cyclophosphamide conditioning with a rejection rate of 34% and survival on the order of 45% (Storb *et al.*, 1984). With the conditioning regimen of cyclophosphamide (50 mg/kg/day for 4 days) given concurrently with ATG (30 mg/kg/day for 3 days) used for all patients in Seattle since June 1988, the incidence of graft rejection is now 4% (Storb *et al.*, 2001). Combined with other improvements in management of patients transplanted for severe aplastic anemia, the use of an optimal conditioning regimen has dramatically increased patient survival.

The need for intensive immunosuppressive conditioning was emphasized by studies in dogs that showed that previous blood

product transfusions increase the risk of graft rejection despite otherwise adequate immunosuppression, presumably by sensitizing recipients to minor transplantation antigens on donor cells. Avoiding transfusions before transplantation has decreased the problem of rejection and improved survival (Fig. 58.3) (Doney *et al.*, 1997). Factors predicting rejection among multiply transfused patients conditioned with cyclophosphamide were a low marrow cell dose ($<3 \times 10^8$ nucleated marrow cells/kg recipient body weight) and positive in vitro assays of cell-mediated immunity of recipient against donor cells, consistent with the concept of transfusion-induced sensitization (Storb *et al.*, 1984).

Two forms of graft rejection may occur. Patients may experience either primary rejection with no sign of hematologic function of the graft or, more commonly, late rejection following initial recovery of hematopoiesis. Late graft rejection may be seen weeks to years after the transplant. One reported case occurred at 10 years after transplantation (Eapen *et al.*, 2000). The outcome is poor for patients with primary graft rejection, although occasional patients have been successfully retransplanted. Patients with late graft rejection can frequently be rescued by a second transplant from the same or alternative donors. Second transplant regimens include those that employ cyclophosphamide combined with TBI. In Seattle, a combination of cyclophosphamide and ATG, followed by combined methotrexate and cyclosporine immunosuppression, resulted in successful engraftment in 66% of patients and 83% long-term survival (Stucki *et al.*, 1998). In addition, investigational agents such as an anti-CD3 monoclonal antibody (BC3) plus high-dose corticosteroids have been successfully used for conditioning prior to second transplant (Bjerke *et al.*, 1995).

Over the past three decades, several centers have reported on various approaches to reduce the risk of graft rejection. The following paragraphs will summarize the major historical developments in this area. In addition, Table 58.3 summarizes the transplant outcomes of some the major center trials for severe aplastic anemia over time. One approach that decreased rejection was to maximize the number of donor marrow cells infused. In a randomized comparative trial initiated in 1976, multiply transfused patients conditioned by cyclophosphamide were given, in addition, unirradiated donor lymphocyte infusions or buffy coat cells after the marrow graft. A decrease in graft rejection was seen, and there was no increase in acute GVHD; however, there was an increased incidence of chronic GVHD. This complication required prolonged immunosuppressive therapy and associated chronic GVHD mortality was 27%. In the Seattle study, long-term survival was improved compared to patients not given donor lymphocyte infusions (62% vs. 46%) (Storb *et al.*, 1992). This finding was not confirmed in a retrospective analysis by the International Bone Marrow Transplantation Registry (IBMTR) (Gluckman *et al.*, 1992), possibly because most patients were conditioned for transplant with more intense immunosuppression containing not only cyclophosphamide but also TBI or limited field irradiation.

Other transplant teams have shown that increasing the intensity of pretransplant immunosuppression by combining

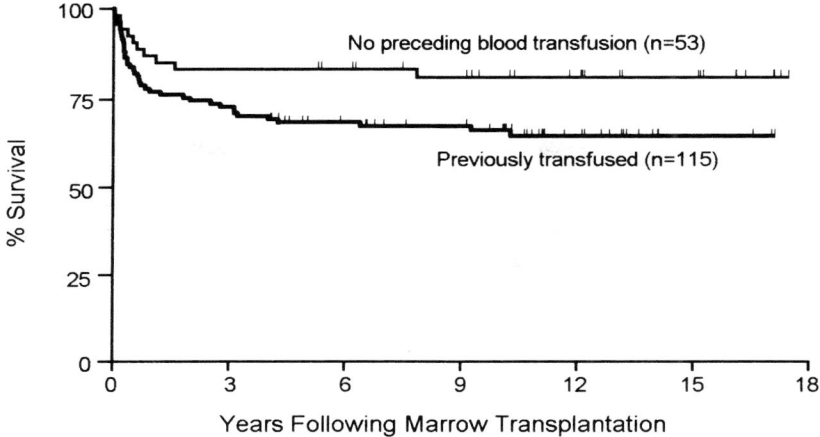

Fig. 58.3. Effect of transfusion status on survival. Patients were defined as untransfused if the first blood product was given within 72 hours of the start of the cyclophosphamide conditioning regimen. Patients were transplanted between 1978 and 1991 and included cyclophosphamide-based conditioning as described in the legend for Fig. 58.1. The transfused group of patients had an increased incidence of graft rejection, presumably due to sensitization to the donor's non-HLA antigens resulting from prior blood transfusions. Modified from Doney *et al.* (1997).

cyclophosphamide with TBI or with limited field irradiation resulted in a decreased risk of graft rejection. However, relatively high-dose limited field irradiation, in the range of 600 to 750 cGy, was necessary to prevent graft rejection. In addition, the toxicity associated with TBI or limited field irradiation was significant and contributed to increased transplant-related mortality. In subsequent long-term follow-up, patients who received irradiation were at an increased risk for secondary malignancies (Deeg *et al.*, 1996; Socié *et al.*, 1993).

In the 1980s, the Seattle team noted that the year of transplant emerged as an independent risk factor for predicting rejection (Fig. 58.4). Results of a randomized, prospective trial suggested that reduction in rejection rates was not due to the introduction of cyclosporine in lieu of methotrexate for GVHD prevention. Instead, an important factor shown to decrease the risk of rejection in aplastic patients was minimizing the recipients' exposure to potentially immunogeneic blood products before transplantation. The incidence of rejection was significantly reduced in previously untransfused patients compared to that in patients receiving preceding blood and platelet transfusions (Storb *et al.*, 1992). Avoidance of all transfusion products before transplant can be difficult. The use of leukocyte-depleted red blood cells and platelet transfusions decreased the risk of sensitization to donor antigens in experimental animals (Storb *et al.*, 1979). In addition, gamma irradiation of blood effectively minimized recipient sensitization to donor minor histocompatibility antigens in animal studies (Bean *et al.*, 1994, 1996). Thus, with the use of either leukocyte depletion or gamma irradiation (both before transplant), it is possible to provide blood product support for patients with severe aplastic anemia without increasing the risk of increasing rejection.

Important progress in reducing the incidence of rejection has been made with improved immunosuppressive conditioning therapy. Because of the proven efficacy of the cyclophos-

phamide/ATG regimen in conditioning patients for second transplants after failure of the first, the Seattle team began using this regimen for first marrow grafts in July 1988 (Storb *et al.*, 1994). This regimen omits buffy coat cell transfusions, thereby reducing the risk of chronic GVHD. Combining ATG with cyclophosphamide did not increase the acute toxicities of the conditioning regimen but provided increased immunosuppression as indicated by the low incidence of graft rejection (4%), even though most patients had been multiply transfused prior to transplantation. Updated results from a multicenter study of cyclophosphamide and ATG for patients with severe aplastic anemia confirmed that graft rejection had become a minor problem (Storb *et al.*, 2001) (Fig 58.5A). Of the 94 consecutive patients enrolled, 87 had received multiple transfusions and 38 had failed immunosuppressive therapy. The ages of the patients ranged from 2 to 59 years. After transplantation, 89 patients received a methotrexate and cyclosporine regimen for GVHD prophylaxis, a drug combination found to be superior to either drug alone in two randomized prospective trials (Storb *et al.*, 1986b, 1990). There was a 4% incidence of graft rejection between 2 and 7 months after transplantation. Of the four patients with graft rejection, three were alive following successful second HSC transplantation. With a median follow-up of 6.0 years (range, 0.5–11.6 years), the overall survival rate was 88% (Fig 58.6). This survival was significantly better than the 72% survival rate of a cohort of historical patients conditioned with cyclophosphamide alone, of whom 62% had received marrow grafts and added buffy coat cell infusions (Storb *et al.*, 2001).

Some transplant centers have continued to use cyclophosphamide without ATG as the conditioning regimen for younger patients receiving HLA-identical sibling HSC transplants. Results from a multicenter trial sponsored by the Gruppo Italiano Trapianti di Midollo Osseo (GITMO) and the

Table 58.3. *Results of HLA-identical marrow grafts in the 1980s and 1990s*

Investigators	Year of report	Year of transplant	Number of patients	Age in years (median)	Trans-fused	Conditioning regimen	GVHD prevention	Rejection (%)	GVHD (%) Acute	GVHD (%) Chronic	Long-term survival (%)	Follow-up (median)
UCLA (Feig et al., 1983)	1983	1977–1981	46	2–44 (19)	+	CY+3 Gy TBI	MTX	2	70	–	63	9 mo–4.5 yrs (2 yrs)
Boston (Smith et al., 1985)	1985	1977–1984	40	2–35 (17)	+	PAPAPA+Cy	MTX	10	53	>35	61	<10 mo–11 yrs (5 yrs)
Seattle (Sanders et al., 1986)	1986	1971–1981	81	2–17 (13)	+	CY	MTX	18	30	30	71	10–20 yrs
Seattle (Anasetti et al., 1986)	1986	1972–1984	50	3–32 (17)	–	CY	MTX	10	23	37	82	1–12 yrs (7 yrs)
Minneapolis (McGlave et al., 1987)	1987	1977–1986	58	2–45 (18)	+	CY+7.5 Gy TLI	MTX/ATG+Pred	5	38	12–54	70	<6 mo–8 yrs
EBMT (Bacigalupo et al., 1988)	1988	1981–1988	218	1–50	+	CY±TLI, TAI, or TBI	MTX or CSA	–	–	–	63	<1–6 yrs
Seattle (Anasetti et al., 1988)	1988	1976–1981	42	1–49 (20)	+	CY	MTX	14	36	60	67	7–11 yrs
London (Hows et al., 1989)	1989	1979–1985	49	3–47 (22)	+	CY	CSA	17	50	37	69	1.8–7.8 yrs (5.8 yrs)
IBMTR (Champlin et al., 1989)	1989	1978–1986	625	–	+	CY / CY+TLI or TAI / CY+TBI	MTX or CSA	20 / 9 / 5	–	–	–	–
UCLA (Champlin et al., 1990)	1990	1984–1988	29	0.7–41 (19)	+	CY+3 Gy TLI	MTX/CSA	23	22	–	78	7 mo–5 yrs (2 yrs)
EBMT (Locasciulli et al., 1990)	1990	1970–1988	171	1–15	+	CY±TLI, TAI, or TBI	MTX or CSA	–	–	–	63	1 mo–15 yrs (4.5 yrs)
Seattle (Storb et al., 1991)	1991	1981–1988	26	1–18 (10)	+	CY	MTX/CSA	26	12	27	92	2–10 yrs (5.7 yrs)
Paris (Gluckman et al., 1991)	1991	1980–1989	107	5–46 (19)	+	CY+6 Gy TAI	MTX, CSA, or MTX/CSA	3	32	55	62	1–10 yrs (3.7 yrs)
IBMTR (Gluckman et al., 1992)	1992	1980–1987	595	1–<40	+	CY±TLI, TAI, or TBI	MTX, CSA, or MTX/CSA	10	40	45	63	>2–>7 yrs
Seattle (Storb et al., 1992)	1992	1988–1991	29	2–46 (24)	+	CY/ATG	MTX/CSA	3	15	30	93	6 mo–3½ yrs (2 yrs)
Baltimore (May et al., 1993)	1993	1984–1991	24	4–53 (21)	+	CY	CSA	29	4.5	0	79	0.8–8 yrs (approx. 5 yrs)
Memorial Sloan-Kettering (Castro-Malaspina et al., 1994)	1994	1983–1990	23	2.5–32 (13)	+	CY+6 Gy TLI	CSA, MTX, or CSA/MTX	13	31	17	65	3–10 yrs (5.6 yrs)
Hamburg (Horstmann et al., 1995)	1995	1990–1993	9	7–30 (25)	+	CY+ATG	MTX/CSA	0	0	0	88	1.2–4.4 yrs (2.5 yrs)
Philadelphia (Bunin et al., 1996)	1996	1989–1993	11	1.5 mo–5 yrs (3)	+	CY+ATG	CSA	0	36	9	100	0.5 mo–4.2 yrs (2.1 yrs)
Mie, Japan (Azuma et al., 1997)	1997	1993–1996	10	1.5–14 (8)	+	CY+ATG	MTX/CSA	0	0	10	100	7 mo–3.5 yrs (2 yrs)
IBMTR (Passweg et al., 1997)	1997	1976–1980	186	2–56 (19)	+	CY (48%), CY+TBI (27%), CY+TLI or TAI (15%)	Multiple agents including: MTX±other (83%), CSA±other (12%)	20	39	37	48	6 yrs
		1981–1987	648	1–57 (20)	+	CY (46%), CY+TBI (12%), CY+TLI or TAI (39%)	MTX±other (33%), CSA±Other (46%), MTX+CSA (15%)	11	37	47	61	6 yrs
		1988–1992	471	1–51 (20)	+	CY (46%), CY+TLI or TAI (36%), CY+ATG (9%)	CSA±other (27%), MTX+CSA (67%)	16	19	32	66	5 yrs
Seattle (Storb et al., 1997a)	1997	1988–1993	39	2–52 (24.5)	+	CY+ATG	MTX/CSA	5	15	8	92	3.6–8.2 yrs (5.2 yrs)
Seattle/Stanford/City of Hope (Storb et al., 2001)[a]	2001	1988–1999	94	2–59 (26)	+	CY+ATG	MTX+CSA	4	29	32	88	0.5–11.6 yrs (6.0 yrs)
GITMO/EBMT (Locatelli et al., 2000)	2000	1991–1998	71	4–46 (19)	+	CY	CSA vs. MTX+CSA	8	33	35	86[b]	0.6–7.8 yrs (4.0 yrs)
IBMTR (Horowitz, 2000)	2000	1991–1997	874	1–20	+	–	–	–	–	–	75±3	0.2–5.0 yrs
			696	20–40				–	–	–	68±4	
			129	>40				–	–	–	35±18	
EBMT (Bacigalupo et al., 2000a)[c]	2000	1974–1990	583	1–50 (18)	+	–	–	–	–	–	54	0.2–5.0 yrs
		1991–1996						–	–	–	77	

Abbreviations: CY = cyclophosphamide; TBI = total body irradiation; PAPAPA = alternating days of procarbazine and antithymocyte globulin; TLI = total lymphoid irradiation; ATG = antithymocyte globulin; MTX = methotrexate; CSA = cyclosporine; Pred = prednisone; MTX±Other = methotrexate alone or with a second agent (not CSA).

[a] Includes 39 patients previously reported (Storb et al., 1997a).

[b] 5-year Kaplan-Meier survival estimate for CSA patients 78%, for MTX+CSA patients 94% (Locatelli et al., 2000).

[c] Additional interactive Cox survival model analysis for transplant outcome based on EBMTR data of neutrophil count, age and year of transplant is available at the following website: www.ebmt.org/4Registry/registry5.html.

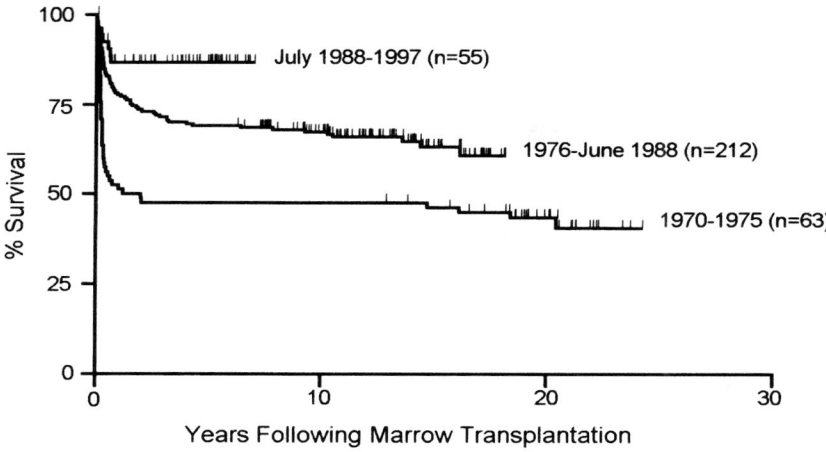

Fig. 58.4. Survival after HLA-identical marrow grafts following conditioning with cyclophosphamide in Seattle over three different time periods. All patients transplanted since July 1988 were conditioned with cyclophosphamide and ATG and received methotrexate and cyclosporine for GVHD prophylaxis. Tick marks indicate surviving patients as of last follow-up. Seventeen patients died at 2.5 to 20.4 years after transplant: 13 of these had chronic GVHD and had developed septicemia ($n = 3$), pulmonary failure ($n = 5$), oropharyngeal squamous cell carcinoma ($n = 3$), or HIV infection ($n = 2$).

European Group for Blood and Marrow Transplantation (EBMT) that compared cyclosporine alone versus methotrexate/cyclosporine for GVHD prophylaxis in 71 patients with severe aplastic anemia showed an overall incidence of graft rejection of 8% (Locatelli *et al.,* 2000). Several factors may explain why the GITMO/EBMT results with cyclophosphamide alone were superior to the historic data from the Seattle group in the 1980s. Since the 1980s there has been increased awareness in the medical community of the benefit of leukodepleted, irradiated blood products for patients with severe aplastic anemia. Although not specifically addressed in the GITMO/EBMT study, the widespread use of irradiated and leukodepleted blood products for transfusion support prior to transplantation for patients with aplastic anemia may have contributed to the lower incidence of graft rejection. The GITMO/EBMT study included predominantly younger patients transfused with a median of 6 units of blood products, many of whom were not treated with a trial of immunosuppression prior to proceeding to allogeneic HSC transplant. In contrast, the multicenter Seattle regimen trial of cyclophosphamide and ATG included older, heavily transfused patients whose prior treatment with immunosuppressive therapy had failed. These factors suggest that transfusion of leukodepleted, irradiated blood products along with prompt referral for transplantation of patients with HLA-identical sibling donors may decrease the necessity for ATG in the conditioning regimen, especially for younger patients.

Recently there has been great interest in the use of granulocyte colony-stimulating factor (G-CSF) mobilized peripheral blood stem cells (G-PBSCs) as the source of HSC for allogeneic transplantation. G-PBSCs contain an increased number of CD34[+] stem cells and an approximately 10-fold increased number of T-cells compared to marrow (Korbling & Anderlini, 2001). Infusion of G-PBSC could potentially decrease the risk of graft rejection in patients with severe aplastic anemia. Data from EBMT indicate that approximately 20% of HLA-identical sibling transplants for severe aplastic anemia in the years 1998–1999 used G-PBSC as the stem cell source (EBMT Registry, 2001). However, many transplant centers have refrained from the use of G-PBSC from HLA-identical siblings for patients with severe aplastic anemia because of concerns of the significantly increased long-term risk of chronic GVHD (Flowers *et al.,* 2002).

Finally, improved postgrafting immunosuppression with the combination of cyclosporine/methotrexate compared with either methotrexate or cyclosporine alone for GVHD prophylaxis may have also decreased the rejection rate by suppressing the host-versus-graft reactions, as shown in animal studies (Storb *et al.,* 1997b). Postgrafting immunosuppression will be discussed in greater detail in the next section.

Acute graft-versus-host disease

Patients transplanted for severe aplastic anemia who develop acute GVHD have worse survival than those without. Important risk factors for the development of acute GVHD include increased patient age and prior pregnancy of the female marrow donor. In order to reduce the risk of GVHD, virtually all allograft recipients are given posttransplant immunosuppression. Methotrexate was the first effective widely used agent. Approximately 40% of patients so treated developed acute GVHD grades II–IV. Laminar airflow isolation was of some benefit in preventing acute GVHD in methotrexate-treated patients (Storb *et al.,* 1983a). When compared to methotrexate, cyclosporine alone failed to change the incidence of acute GVHD. The combination of methotrexate and cyclosporine significantly reduced the risk of acute GVHD compared to either

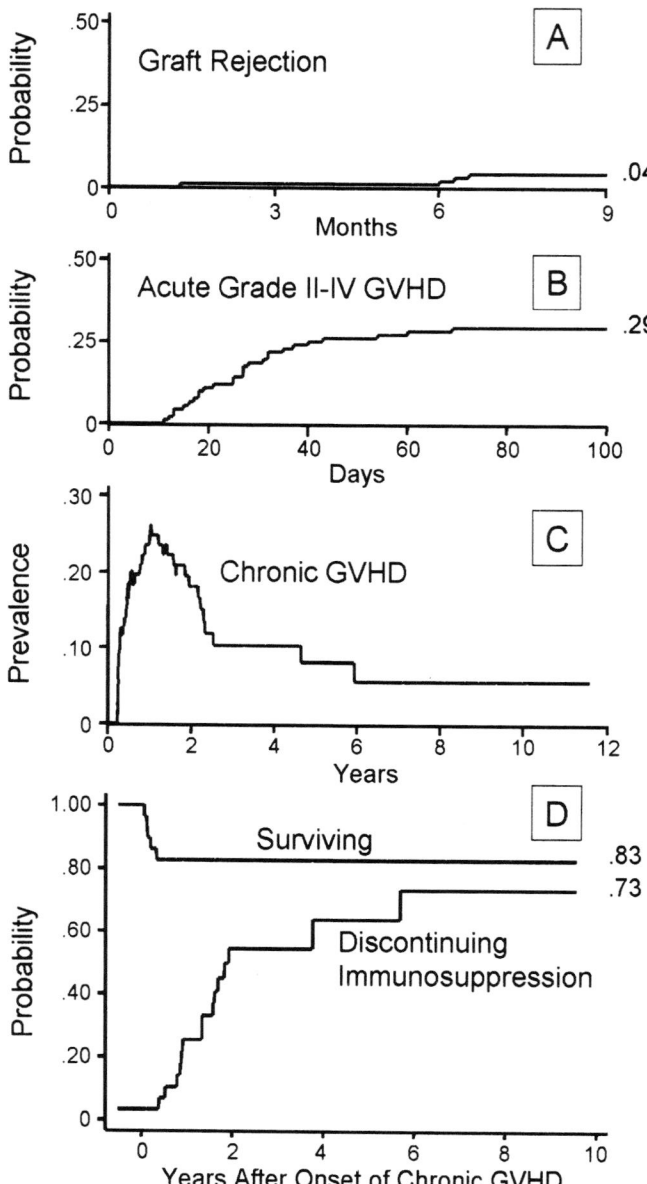

Fig. 58.5. Cumulative incidences of graft rejection (**A**) and acute grade II to IV graft-versus-host disease (GVHD) (**B**) in patients with aplastic anemia given HLA-identical marrow grafts following cyclophosphamide and antithymocyte globulin and GVHD prophylaxis with methotrexate and cyclosporine. (**C**) Prevalence of chronic GVHD. (**D**) Probability of surviving among the 29 patients with chronic GVHD and probability of discontinuing immunosuppression given for chronic GVHD. Reproduced, with permission, from Storb *et al.* (2001).

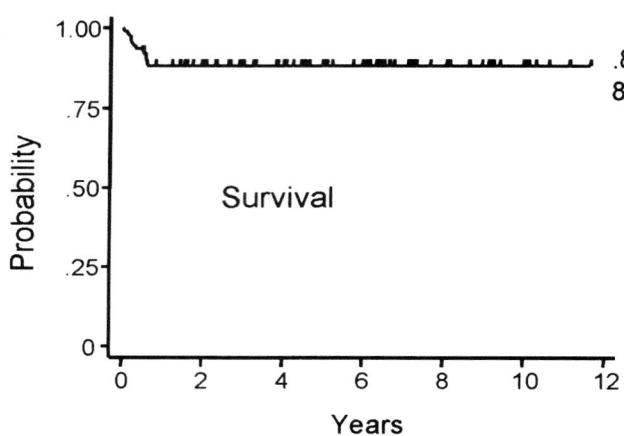

Fig. 58.6. Kaplan-Meier curve of survival among the 94 patients with aplastic anemia who underwent HLA-identical sibling bone marrow transplants. The age range was 2 to 59 years. In this multi-center study, the conditioning regimen was cyclophosphamide/antithymocyte globulin and GVHD prophylaxis was methotrexate/cyclosporine. The event-free survival rate was 88%. Reproduced, with permission, from Storb *et al.* (2001).

the combination of cyclosporine and methotrexate resulted in superior 5-year estimated survival compared to the use of cyclosporine alone for patients transplanted with an HLA-identical sibling marrow graft for severe aplastic anemia. The benefit in survival, however, could not be ascribed to a reduction in the incidence of acute or chronic GVHD (Locatelli *et al.*, 2000) (Fig. 58.7).

The updated results of the multicenter study of cyclophosphamide/ATG conditioning, HLA-identical marrow followed by combined methotrexate/cyclosporine immunosuppression in 94 consecutive patients showed that the cumulative incidence of grades II to IV acute GVHD was 29% (Storb *et al.*, 2001) (Fig. 58.5B). The GVHD observed was grade II (21%), grade III (7%) and grade IV (1%). Despite the increased patient age compared to the GITMO/EBMT study, the overall incidence of acute GVHD was lower in the multicenter cyclophosphamide and ATG study. ATG can be detected in the serum of treated patients days to weeks after infusion. The use of ATG in the conditioning regimen may have helped to decrease the incidence of acute GVHD compared to conditioning regimens without ATG. However, in an earlier cohort of severe aplastic anemia patients conditioned with cyclophosphamide alone, only 23% of patients developed acute GVHD (Storb *et al.*, 1986a). The possible beneficial effect of ATG in decreasing the incidence and severity of GVHD may be particularly relevant for older patients.

A combination of cyclosporine and prednisone has also been used for preventing acute GVHD, but is not as successful as methotrexate plus cyclosporine. In a randomized controlled study comparing cyclosporine as a single agent with the combination of prednisone and cyclosporine for prophylaxis of GVHD, the combination regimen had only limited efficacy in acute GVHD prevention, and an increased incidence of chronic GVHD was seen (Deeg *et al.*, 1997, 2000). Triple therapy with

methotrexate alone or cyclosporine alone, and no grade IV acute GVHD was observed (Storb *et al.*, 1986a, 1986b). The reduction in acute GVHD resulted in improved survival (Storb *et al.*, 1991). Administration of optimal doses of both methotrexate and cyclosporine is important to prevent acute GVHD (Nash *et al.*, 1992). In the GITMO/EBMT multicenter randomized study,

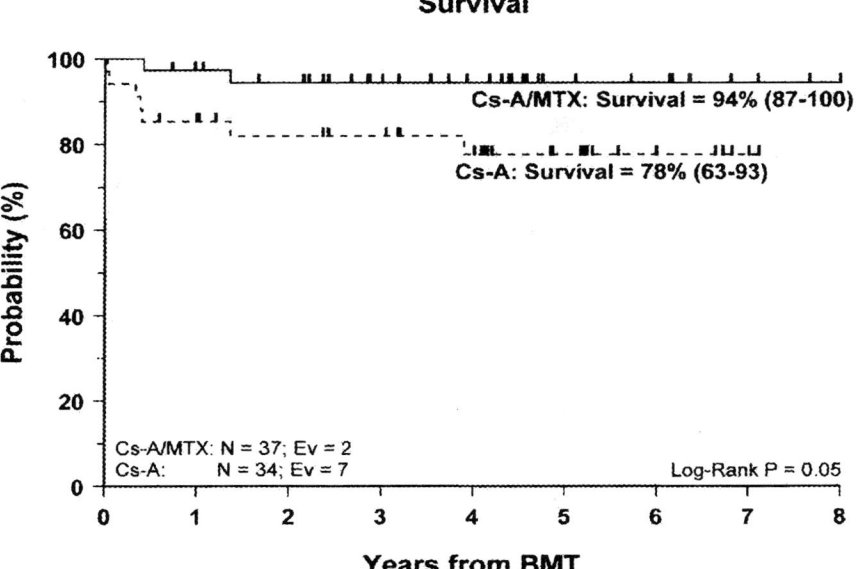

Fig. 58.7. Probability of survival following HLA-identical bone marrow transplantation for aplastic anemia in the multicenter GITMO/EBMT study. Conditioning was with cyclophosphamide only. Patients were prospectively randomized to receive post-grafting immunosuppression consisting of cyclosporine (CSA, dotted line) versus CSA and methotrexate (CSA/MTX, solid line). The cumulative probabilities of survival for the CSA group (n = 34) and the CSA/MTX group (n = 37) are shown. EV, number of events occurring in each arm of randomization. Reproduced, with permission, from Locatelli *et al.* (2000).

methotrexate, cyclosporine, and prednisone did not result in an improved outcome compared to double therapy with cyclosporine and methotrexate in Seattle (Storb *et al.,* 1990). Similarly, a City of Hope/Stanford study indicated that long-term outcome with the three-drug regimen was not statistically different from the two-drug regimen of cyclosporine and methotrexate (Chao *et al.,* 2000).

T-cell depletion of bone marrow cells is a strategy that has been shown to decrease the incidence of acute GVHD. However, an IBMTR study showed that T-cell–depleted transplants for severe aplastic anemia were associated with a high risk of graft failure (Champlin *et al.,* 1989). A subsequent IBMTR report of a retrospective, nonrandomized study indicated that survival of patients receiving T-cell–depleted transplants conditioned with irradiation-based regimens was comparable to patients receiving non-T-cell–depleted transplants with posttransplant methotrexate and cyclosporine. The number of patients receiving T-cell–depleted transplants was small (n = 43), and the inclusion of irradiation as part of the conditioning regimen makes it difficult to draw any conclusions about the effects of T-cell depletion on outcome. Eleven of 39 evaluable patients receiving T-cell–depleted transplants had graft failure, but some were successfully rescued with a second transplant; 5-year survival was 76% (Passweg *et al.,* 1997).

Chronic graft-versus-host disease

Chronic GVHD has persisted as a problem in a minority of patients transplanted for severe aplastic anemia ever since the first report in 1976 from Seattle of patients with this condition (Storb *et al.,* 1976). Risk factors for chronic GVHD include preceding acute GVHD, increasing patient age, use of supplemental buffy coat cell infusions, and possibly the use of radiation-based conditioning regimens (Storb *et al.,* 1983b). Chronic GVHD is associated with significant morbidity and requires prolonged immunosuppressive therapy. Prednisone, cyclosporine, azathioprine, and thalidomide have been given either alone or in combination for the treatment of chronic GVHD since 1976 (Sullivan *et al.,* 1991), and newer agents such as tacrolimus (FK-506) and mycophenolate mofetil (MMF) have shown promise as effective immunosuppressive agents (Furlong *et al.,* 1997; Nash *et al.,* 1997, 2000). Up to 27% of patients with chronic GVHD may die, frequently from Gram-positive infections. This finding emphasizes the need to prevent chronic GVHD. Many cases of chronic GVHD are diagnosed either at the time of cyclosporine taper or shortly after complete discontinuation of the drug, typically at 6 months after transplant (Sullivan *et al.,* 1986). Patients at highest risk of developing chronic GVHD, such as those with preceding acute GVHD or older patients, may benefit from a prolonged course of cyclosporine treatment at therapeutic levels for a longer period of time after transplant.

Since the introduction of the cyclophosphamide and ATG conditioning regimen for HLA-matched sibling marrow grafts and, thereby, the discontinuation of added buffy coat cell infusions, the prevalence of chronic GVHD has significantly decreased. Chronic GVHD was not only less frequent but also appeared to be more responsive to therapy in patients condi-

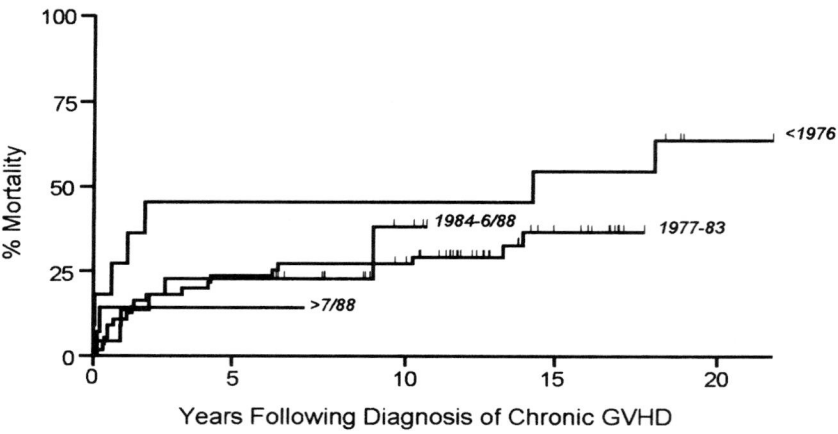

Fig. 58.8. Mortality after diagnosis of chronic GVHD following HLA-identical marrow grafts conditioned with cyclophosphamide in Seattle over four different time periods. Tick marks indicate surviving patients at the time of most recent follow-up.

tioned with cyclophosphamide and ATG and given marrow alone compared to historical control patients treated with cyclophosphamide and marrow plus buffy coat. In the multicenter study, following cyclophosphamide/ATG, unmanipulated marrow, and postgrafting methotrexate/cyclosporine immunosuppression, the cumulative incidence of chronic GVHD observed was 32% (Fig. 58.5C). In most patients chronic GVHD responded to therapy with complete responses. Of the patients with chronic GVHD, 83% survived. At a median of 2.6 (range, 1.5–10) years after transplantation, 8% of patients still required immunosuppressive therapy for chronic GVHD (Storb et al., 2001) (Fig 58.5D).

The overall incidence of chronic GVHD in the GITMO/ EBMT trial with cyclophosphamide conditioning and postgrafting immunosuppression with either cyclosporine alone or methotrexate and cyclosporine was 35%. Patients treated with cyclosporine or methotrexate combined with cyclosporine had a 30% and 44% incidence of chronic GVHD, respectively. This difference in incidence of chronic GVHD was not significant. The majority of patients with chronic GVHD had limited disease of the skin; the overall incidence of extensive chronic GVHD was 9% (Locatelli et al., 2000). Most of the patients in the GITMO/EBMT study were children, who have a lower incidence of chronic GVHD compared with adults.

Taken together, the cyclophosphamide and ATG regimen followed by HLA-identical marrow transplantation with methotrexate and cyclosporine immunosuppression provides the lowest risk of development of graft rejection, acute GVHD, and chronic GVHD compared to other preparative regimens. With prompt diagnosis of chronic GVHD combined with aggressive initiation of immunosuppressive treatment with a combination of cyclosporine and prednisone, the duration of time needed for inducing remission of chronic GVHD appears to have decreased and the overall response to treatment has improved (Goerner et al., 2002) (Fig 58.8). Because of the increased risk of chronic GVHD associated with G-PBSC, bone marrow with a target cell

dose of at least 3.0×10^8 nucleated cells per kilogram body weight remains the preferred source of stem cells. Future progress in improving the outcome of allogeneic HSC transplantation for severe aplastic anemia will depend on reducing the incidence of, and developing better treatment for, chronic GVHD.

Survival

In the 1970s, a long-term survival probability of 40% to 45% was standard for patients undergoing HLA-identical sibling marrow transplantation for severe aplastic anemia. Over the past 30 years, survival rates have markedly improved (Table 58.3 and Fig. 58.4). Improvement has been primarily due to reductions in the incidence of graft rejection and acute and chronic GVHD. Earlier results from Seattle showed that patients conditioned with cyclophosphamide and given methotrexate alone for GVHD prophylaxis had an overall survival of 67% for multiply transfused patients at 11 to 17 years posttransplant, 82% for untransfused patients observed for 8 to 17 years, and 71% for pediatric patients observed for 15 to 25 years. Pediatric patients conditioned with cyclophosphamide followed by methotrexate and cyclosporine for GVHD prophylaxis had a survival probability of 90% with the observation period ranging from 5 to 15 years. More recent results showed survival for both pediatric and adult patients conditioned with cyclophosphamide plus ATG followed by methotrexate and cyclosporine for GVHD prophylaxis to be 92%, with an observation period of 3 to 8 years.

Since the initial reports by the Seattle team (Storb et al., 1992, 1994, 2001), other centers have reported on the success of the cyclophosphamide/ATG conditioning regimen (Azuma et al., 1997; Bunin et al., 1996; Horstmann et al., 1995) (Table 58.3). The multicenter study of cyclophosphamide/ATG strongly supports the superiority of this regimen over other transplant regimens, particularly for patients over age 20 who have received blood product transfusion support.

The randomized GITMO/EBMT trial comparing cyclosporine alone versus combined methotrexate/cyclosporine for patients conditioned with cyclophosphamide alone showed an estimated 5-year 94% survival in the methotrexate/cyclosporine group and 78% for those in the cyclosporine alone group (Locatelli *et al.*, 2000) (Fig 58.7). This difference in survival was significant. Thus, this Italian study confirmed the initial Seattle results demonstrating the superiority of combined methotrexate/cyclosporine postgrafting immunosuppression.

Analysis of transplant registry data has been helpful for identifying important trends over time. A retrospective multicenter, multiregimen IBMTR study (Passweg *et al.*, 1997) reported that 5-year survival after HLA-identical sibling transplants had increased from 48% in 1976 to 1980 to 66% in 1988 to 1992. Due to the introduction of methotrexate plus cyclosporine for GVHD prophylaxis, the risk of GVHD decreased. Improved long-term survival was due to decreased mortality in the first 3 months posttransplant. The incidence of reported graft failure did not change significantly, ranging from 20% in 1976–1980 to 16% in 1988–1992; only 9% of reported transplants in 1988–1992 included cyclophosphamide/ATG conditioning.

IBMTR data for 1,699 patients receiving HLA-identical sibling transplants for severe aplastic anemia between 1991 and 1997 showed a 5-year probability of survival (95% confidence intervals) of 75% ± 3% for 874 patients ≤ 20 years of age, 68% ± 4% for 696 who were 21 to 39 years, and 35% ± 18% for 129 who were 40 years or older (Horowitz, 2000). These results are reflected in the updated IBMTR data (Fig. 58.9). Survival was

highest in untransfused patients transplanted early in the course of their disease and who were without active infection at the time of transplant. Only a minority of patients recorded in the registry received cyclophosphamide/ATG conditioning and cyclosporine/methotrexate postgrafting immunosuppression. It is likely that the registry data are inferior to the Seattle data because relatively few of the transplant centers have adopted the cyclophosphamide/ATG conditioning and cyclosporine/ methotrexate postgrafting immunosuppression.

EBMT data for 1799 patients receiving HLA-identical sibling transplant between 1971 and 1998 confirmed the IBMTR results. The year of the transplant and the age of the patient predicted outcome after HSC transplantation. There has been a striking improvement in 5-year survival rates comparing patients transplanted before or after 1990. In the years 1990–1998 actuarial survival was 77% for patients aged 16 years or less, 68% for those 17 to 40, and 54% for patients greater than 40 years of age (Fig. 58.9). Cyclophosphamide alone as conditioning, and cyclosporine with or without methotrexate for GVHD prophylaxis, were given to 551 patients and their survival rate was 69%. Based on the EBMT registry data, anti-lymphocyte globulin (ALG) was added to the conditioning regimen in 28 patients and their survival was 87% (Bacigalupo *et al.*, 2000a).

Immune suppressive therapy versus allogeneic hematopoietic stem cell transplantation

The current results of excellent long-term survival of patients transplanted with an HLA-identical sibling marrow graft have

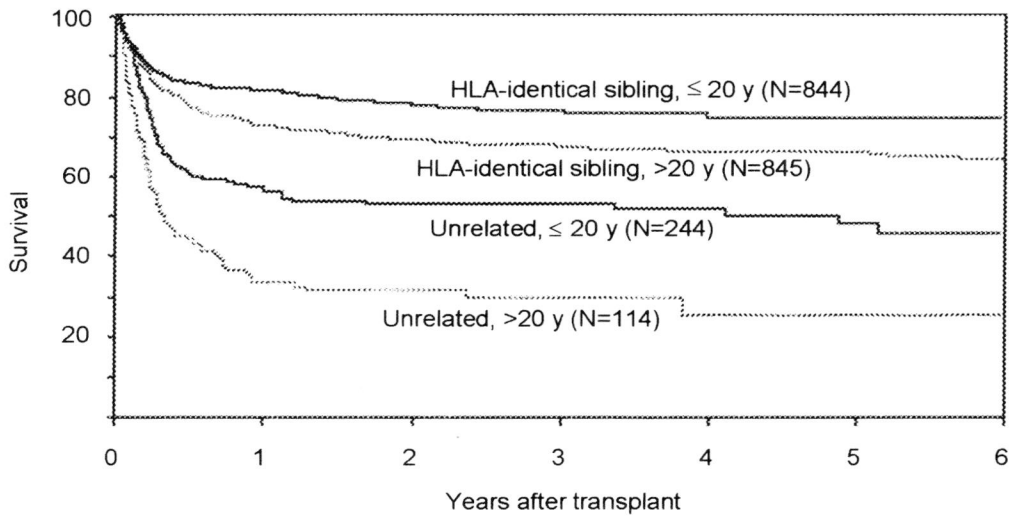

Fig. 58.9. International Bone Marrow Transplant Registry (IBMTR) data indicating the probability of survival after allogeneic bone marrow transplantation for severe aplastic anemia by donor type and age for patients treated between 1994–1999. Allogeneic transplantation is the treatment of choice for young patients with aplastic anemia who have HLA-identical siblings. Three-year probabilities of survival after 1,689 HLA-identical sibling transplants were 76 ± 3% for 844 patients ≤ 20 years of age and 67 ± 3 % for 845 older patients. Results were less favorable in 358 recipients of unrelated donor transplants: 53 ± 6 % in 244 patients ≤ 20 years of age and 32 ± 10 % in 114 older patients. Adapted, with permission, from the IBMTR website. http://instruct.mcw.edu/IBMTR/ BWebServer/summarysldset/SummarySet2002_files/v3_document.htm

led most physicians to the conclusion that allogeneic hematopoietic stem cell transplantation is the first-line, definitive therapy for patients with severe aplastic anemia under age 40. These recommendations are supported by results of two randomized studies, although the Japanese study looked at children only (Doney *et al.,* 1997; Kojima *et al.,* 2000). While there has been significant improvement in outcome following immunosuppressive therapy with the combination of ATG and cyclosporine, the long-term risk of development of MDS and acute leukemia, as well the high risk of relapse of aplastic anemia, significantly limit enthusiasm for this treatment for younger patients who have HLA-identical siblings. Furthermore, over the past decade, improvement in supportive care has led to the increased survival of older patients undergoing allogeneic HSC transplantation. For this reason the number of older patients with hematologic malignancies transplanted with allogeneic HSC grafts has progressively increased. Similarly, for patients with severe aplastic anemia above age 40, a strong case can be made for definitive therapy with HLA-identical sibling marrow transplantation. In practice, however, most patients over age 40 are referred for allogeneic HSC transplant only after failure of immunosuppressive therapy.

In contrast, a retrospective analysis of survival outcome was based on initial treatment offered to patients with severe aplastic anemia reported to the European Bone Marrow Transplant (EBMT) registry from 1974 to 1996 (Bacigalupo *et al.,* 2000a). On multivariate analysis, outcome was primarily affected by neutrophil counts at the time of treatment and patient age. Patients up to age 20 had consistently superior 5-year survival with BMT. Adults between the ages of 20 to 40 with neutrophil counts below $300 \times 10^9/l$ had better 5-year survival with BMT. For patients with neutrophil counts greater than $300 \times 10^9/l$, the predicted 5-year survival appeared comparable to BMT or slightly superior with immunosuppressive therapy. For patients older than 40 years, immunosuppressive therapy offered a better survival advantage than BMT at 5 years of follow-up. However, this recommendation carries the caveat that the majority of patients reported to the registry database did not receive what is now considered the optimal transplant regimen, cyclophosphamide and ATG conditioning, followed by HLA-identical BMT and combined postgrafting methotrexate and cyclosporine. As suggested by the Seattle studies, it is likely that older patients over age 40 have long-term survival benefit from allogeneic HSC transplantation if treated with the optimal transplant regimen.

Summary of HLA-identical sibling hematopoietic stem cell transplantation

In summary, the survival of patients transplanted for aplastic anemia with HLA-identical siblings has improved over the past three decades. These improvements are in part due to a decrease in the incidence of rejection as a result of more intensified conditioning regimens, as well as from changes in transfusion practice before transplant. Improvement is also due, in part, to a decline in the incidence of, and mortality from, acute GVHD with the introduction of combined methotrexate and cyclosporine immunosuppression after transplantation. The transplant registry data confirm the improvement in the outcome of patients transplanted for severe aplastic anemia over the past three decades. Of all the transplant regimens studied, the one that consistently results in the most favorable long-term survival is the combination of cyclophosphamide and ATG conditioning, HLA-identical unmanipulated bone marrow, and methotrexate with cyclosporine postgrafting immunosuppression. Despite the favorable results, the transplant registry data suggest that many transplant centers have yet to adopt this regimen for their patients with aplastic anemia. More uniform adoption of this regimen would likely result in further improvement in outcome for patients undergoing allogeneic transplantation. Consideration could be made for withholding ATG or ALG from the conditioning regimen for children who proceed immediately to transplant and who have been only minimally transfused with irradiated and leukodepleted blood products. However, the inclusion of ATG in the preparative regimen is not typically associated with excessive toxicity and appears to reduce the risk of graft rejection and, possibly, GVHD. The registry data reflect the fact that many physicians are hesitant to recommend allogeneic transplantation for patients over age 40. However the efficacy of the cyclophosphamide and ATG conditioning, combined with methotrexate and cyclosporine postgrafting immunosuppression suggests that marrow transplantation for older patients should be strongly considered especially if there is poor response to first-line immunosuppressive therapy or if there is relapse of disease.

Delayed effects of transplantation

Growth and development

A survey of patients transplanted in Seattle for aplastic anemia following high-dose cyclophosphamide (200 mg/kg) found there were no thyroid function abnormalities, in contrast to children receiving cyclophosphamide/TBI for hematologic malignancies (Sanders *et al.,* 1991). Similarly, children transplanted following cyclophosphamide have normal growth velocity and growth hormone levels, while decreased growth was seen among those given cyclophosphamide/TBI. Some patients with chronic GVHD had decreased growth velocity during the time of disease activity. However, once chronic GVHD was controlled and treatment discontinued, their growth rates returned to normal and catch-up growth occurred.

A subsequent Seattle survey (Deeg *et al.,* 1998) defined the cumulative incidence of delayed complications dependent, at least in part, on the occurrence of acute and chronic GVHD, including cataracts, lung disease, bone and joint disease, secondary malignancy, and depression (Fig. 58.10).

Fertility

Findings similar to those on growth and development have been reported with regard to gonadal function during and after

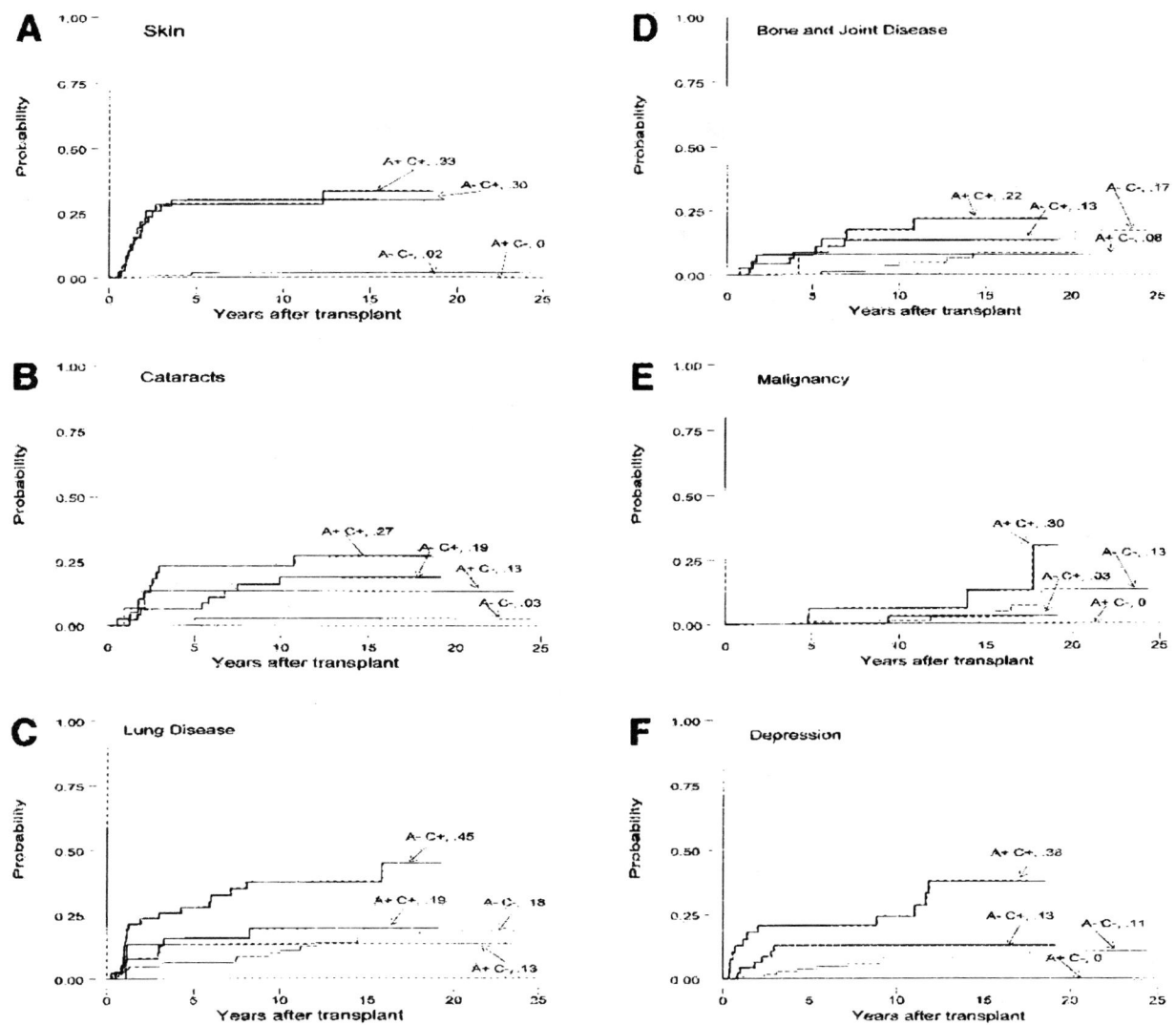

Fig. 58.10. Cumulative incidence of delayed complications dependent on acute and chronic GVHD. (A) Skin disease; (B) cataracts; (C) lung disease; (D) bone and joint disease; (E) posttransplant malignancy; (F) depression. For any patient, only the first event was considered. While only 2-year survivors were included in the analysis, the onset of a given complication could have been before the 2-year mark. A, acute GVHD; C, chronic GVHD; "+", present; "–", absent. Reproduced, with permission, from Deeg *et al.* (1998).

puberty, although there is evidence that cyclophosphamide may result in amenorrhea in women older than 40 years at the time of transplant (Sanders & the Seattle Marrow Transplant Team, 1991). Long-term follow-up among children prepubertal at transplant and receiving cyclophosphamide showed that all had normal development of secondary sexual characteristics. In the Seattle experience, 95 children have been born to patients conditioned with cyclophosphamide, a figure that is disproportionately higher than that seen in patients conditioned with cyclophosphamide/TBI (Sanders *et al.,* 1996). Thus, among 212 transplanted aplastic anemia patients followed for up to 20 years, the probability that a female patient would become pregnant was 47% and the probability that a male patient had fathered a child was 50%.

Secondary cancer

Previous observations from Seattle in a canine marrow transplant model indicated that secondary malignant tumors were significantly increased with radiation-based treatment compared to chemotherapy-based regimens. A collaborative analysis from Paris and Seattle of long-term follow-up of 621 aplastic anemia patients (Deeg *et al.,* 1996) showed that there was a 14% probability (Kaplan-Meier estimate) of developing any type of secondary malignancy by 20 years after transplantation. Of the 193 patients who received irradiation in the conditioning regimen, 7 developed solid tumors. Only 6 of 428 patients conditioned without irradiation developed malignancies. By multivariate analysis, there was a 3.9-fold increased risk of development of solid tumors in those who received irradiation (total body or thoraco-abdominal) compared to those who received cyclophosphamide as conditioning regimen. The hazard of developing a solid tumor increased progressively with time posttransplant with peaks at 8 and 17 years after transplant. In view of the good survival seen following conditioning with cyclophosphamide, irradiation-based regimens should be avoided in HLA-identical marrow transplant recipients because of the associated risk of late cancer.

Chronic GVHD is a risk factor for the development of sold tumors after transplant, with a 30% probability at 20 years for patients with both acute and chronic GVHD (Fig. 58.10E) (Deeg et al., 1998). Carcinomas of the oropharyngeal mucosa developed in patients with chronic GVHD. The severity of chronic GVHD and duration of immunosuppressive therapy appear to be risk factors for secondary malignancy. These findings emphasize the importance of avoiding infusion of buffy coat or PBSC to minimize the risk of chronic GVHD in patients with severe aplastic anemia.

Results of HLA-mismatched family member transplantation

Wagner and colleagues reported on the Seattle experience of bone marrow transplantation from HLA non-identical relatives for patients with severe aplastic anemia. Nine patients, conditioned with cyclophosphamide 200 mg/kg and who received marrow from HLA-phenotypically identical relatives, were all alive and disease-free 3 to 18 years after transplantation with the exception of one patient who died from an accident. Thus, transplants from phenotypically HLA-identical family members can be carried out with the same regimen and with comparable results as for HLA-genotypically identical siblings.

Thirty-one patients received marrow from HLA-mismatched relatives who differed by one or more HLA loci. Fifteen of these patients received cyclophosphamide, 50 mg/kg for 4 doses, without TBI and none survived; deaths mostly resulted from primary graft rejection. Because of this, the conditioning regimen was intensified to include 12 Gy TBI and cyclophosphamide, 60 mg/kg for 2 doses. Sixteen patients who had previously failed to respond to immunosuppressive therapy were treated and 8 remained alive without disease between 1.5 and 11.3 years after transplant (Wagner et al., 1996).

Similar results using HLA-haploidentical family donors were reported by the Taipei transplant group. Six patients were conditioned with cyclophosphamide 200 mg/kg and 8 Gy TBI prior to marrow grafting and were given methotrexate and cyclosporine postgrafting immunosuppression. Two deaths occurred during treatment for acute GVHD and four patients survived long-term (Tzeng et al., 1996).

These results show that transplants from related donors mismatched for one or more HLA loci require more intensive conditioning than cyclophosphamide alone to achieve sustained engraftment after transplantation for aplastic anemia. Due to the poorer outcome of HLA-mismatched transplants, this approach should be reserved for patients who have failed immunosuppressive treatment and do not have HLA-matched unrelated donors.

Results of unrelated donor transplantation

Patients with aplastic anemia who do not have suitably HLA-matched related donors receive immunosuppressive therapy as the first-line treatment of choice. They are considered candidates for unrelated donor HSC transplantation only if they fail to respond to immunosuppressive treatment. Historically, rates of transplant-related morbidity and mortality have been high. In a National Marrow Donor Program (NMDP) retrospective analysis of 141 patients transplanted between 1988 and 1995, the overall survival at a median of 36 months after transplant was 36% (Deeg et al., 1999). Eighty-six percent received radiation-containing conditioning regimens; 74% received HLA-matched marrow, while 26% received marrow mismatched for at least one HLA-A, -B or -DR antigen; 32% received T-cell–depleted marrow and all but 13% received cyclosporine-containing regimens to prevent GVHD. Eighty-nine percent achieved sustained engraftment, and 52% of those evaluable developed grades II–IV acute GVHD.

In a pilot study of 5 patients who received unrelated donor transplants following cyclophosphamide/ATG conditioning, as used for recipients of HLA-identical donor marrow, three patients experienced graft failure and only 1 patient survived long-term (Deeg et al., 1994). Other groups reported that high-dose irradiation regimens, although effective in achieving engraftment, resulted in an increased incidence of fatal organ toxicity without increasing the probability of survival.

A collaborative multicenter prospective NMDP-sponsored study was undertaken to define the minimum effective dose of TBI sufficient to achieve engraftment for patients with aplastic anemia transplanted with unrelated donor marrow. The starting dose of TBI was 6 Gy given after 3 doses of 30 mg/kg/day ATG combined with 4 consecutive infusions of 50 mg/kg/day cyclophosphamide. The TBI dose was to be escalated in increments of 2 Gy if graft failure occurred in the absence of prohibitive toxicity, and de-escalated for toxicity in the absence of graft failure.

A total of 50 patients were enrolled: 38 patients received HLA-A-, B-, and DR-phenotypically matched marrow transplants and 12 patients received marrow from donors who differed by 1 HLA-antigen. Patient ages ranged from 1.3 to 46.5 (median, 14.4) years. The time intervals from diagnosis to transplantation were 2.8 to 264 (median, 14.5) months. All patients had received multiple transfusions and a median of four courses of immunosuppressive treatments. All 20 patients treated with 6 or 4 Gy TBI, cyclophosphamide/ATG, and HLA-matched marrow engrafted, and survival was 50%. Of the 13 patients receiving 2 Gy TBI and HLA-matched marrow grafts, 1 rejected and 8 were alive. Severe pulmonary toxicity occurred in 8 of 30 patients conditioned with 6 or 4 Gy TBI and in 2 of 13 patients conditioned with 2 Gy TBI (Deeg et al., 2001).

Patients who underwent transplantation within 1 year of diagnosis had a 73% probability of survival, while patients who delayed transplantation beyond 3 years after initial diagnosis had a 39% survival (Fig. 58.11). In addition, patients who were less than 20 years old at the time of transplantation had a 67% survival compared with 43% for patients greater than 20 years old. The incidence of acute GVHD was 61%, with 3 deaths attributable to GVHD and infection. Chronic GVHD requiring therapy developed in 37% of evaluable patients.

A phase II study with a conditioning regimen of 2 Gy TBI, cyclophosphamide/ATG is currently underway. Preliminary results confirm that that this dose of TBI is sufficient to sustain engraftment of both HLA-matched unrelated donor marrow and 1 HLA-antigen mismatched unrelated donor marrow without excessive organ toxicity (H.J. Deeg, oral communication, June 2002).

Before the ongoing multicenter study with unmanipulated marrow, the role of T-cell depletion of unrelated donor marrow was examined. However, as discussed above with matched sibling marrow transplantation, the intensity of the conditioning regimen was substantially increased to prevent graft rejection. In a single center study of children and young adults, twenty-eight previously transfused patients received T-cell–depleted, unrelated donor marrow grafts. The conditioning regimen consisted of cytosine arabinoside, cyclophosphamide, and TBI. Marrow was T-cell depleted with the anti-CD3 antibody T10B9 and complement, and patients received posttransplant cyclosporine. Nine recipients were HLA-matched with their donors, while 19 were not. Overall, 54% of patients were alive, transfusion-independent, and well with a median follow-up of 2.75 years. Three patients failed to engraft and died, and three patients who developed grades III–IV acute GVHD also died. The overall incidence of ☁ grade II acute GVHD was 28%.

The authors concluded that in children with severe aplastic anemia who failed immune suppression and who lacked family member donors, unrelated donor transplantation offered a reasonable hope of long-term survival (Margolis et al., 1996). The use of CD34+ megadose PBSC transplants that were effectively T-cell depleted using immunomagnetic separation technology (CliniMACS device) resulted in prompt hematopoietic recovery in 3 patients (Schwinger et al., 2000).

Other transplant regimens for aplastic anemia have been reported using HLA-matched unrelated donor marrow. The Nagoya transplant group reported on results of 15 children conditioned with cyclophosphamide/ATG and 5 Gy TBI (Kojima et al., 2001). All patients survived and were alive at a median follow-up of 51 months. Transplant teams in London and Bristol reported that the combination of Campath-1G, cyclophosphamide, and 3 Gy TBI followed by unrelated donor BMT in 8 young children resulted in engraftment and uniform survival (Vassiliou et al., 2001). The higher doses of TBI were well tolerated in children, but as discussed previously, lower TBI doses are preferable in order to decrease the risk of organ toxicities and the risk of secondary malignancies.

The results of 154 aplastic anemia patients transplanted from unrelated donors identified through the Japan Marrow Donor Program (JMDP) have been reported (Kojima et al., 2002a). With DNA-based methods of typing, 79 patients were matched at HLA-A, -B, and -DRB1 loci, while 22 were HLA-DRB1 mismatched, 29 were mismatched at either HLA-A or -B, and 12 were mismatched at 2 or more loci. None of the grafts were T-cell depleted. The median age of the patients was 17 years. The conditioning regimens used were varied and predominantly included TBI or limited field irradiation and cyclophosphamide with or without ATG. The majority of patients (73%) received the combination of methotrexate/cyclosporine for GVHD pro-

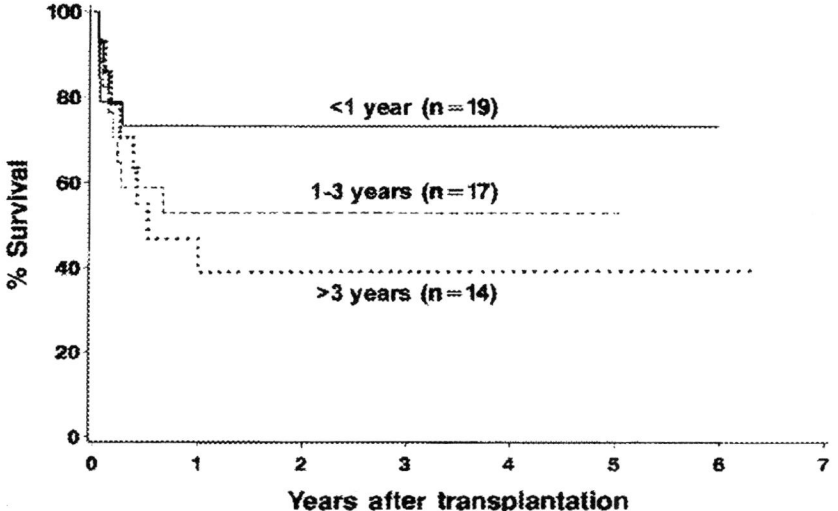

Fig. 58.11. Survival by pretransplantation disease duration for patients with aplastic anemia who underwent HLA-matched unrelated donor transplantation. The survival rate was 73% with a pretransplantation disease duration of <1 year(—), 53 % for 1 to 3 years (- - - -), and 39% for > 3 years (.... .) (P = .32). Reproduced, with permission, from Deeg et al. (2001).

phylaxis. The overall incidence of graft rejection was 11%. The incidence of grade II–III acute GVHD was 49%, and the incidence of chronic GVHD was 30%. The median follow-up after transplant was 29 months and the overall probability of survival at 5 years was 56%. Patients treated with the conditioning regimen that included TBI/cyclophosphamide/ATG had the highest probability of 5-year survival (75%). Most of the 56 patients conditioned with TBI/cyclophosphamide/ATG received 10 Gy TBI and the incidence of graft rejection was low (2%). However, the toxicity associated with this intensive regimen was substantial. Consistent with the NMDP multicenter study described above, a subset of 10 patients received TBI doses of 2 to 5 Gy, cyclophosphamide, and ATG; 9 of the 10 were surviving. Other unfavorable risk factors for survival included transplantation more than 3 years after diagnosis, patient age greater than 20 years, transplantation following a conditioning regimen without ATG, and transplantation from an HLA class I mismatched donor. The adverse effect of HLA-mismatching was restricted to class I HLA alleles since patients with 6 of 6 antigen matched donors had a 59.5% 5-year survival and those with HLA-DRB1 mismatched donors had 71% survival, while HLA-A and HLA-B mismatched recipients had 46% and 32% survival, respectively. These findings were consistent with the previous JMDP study of unrelated donor transplant recipients, which showed that mismatching of class I HLA alleles was a strong risk factor for increased incidence of GVHD and poor survival, while mismatching for HLA class II alleles did not affect survival. In contrast, the NMDP study involving North American unrelated donor recipients showed that mismatching of HLA-DRB1 was the most crucial risk factor for survival.

The IBMTR data showed that among 288 patients transplanted with unrelated donor marrow between 1991 and 1997, the 5-year survival probabilities were $53 \pm 6\%$ for those ≤ 20 years of age and $32 \pm 10\%$ for older patients (Fig. 58.9) (Horowitz, 2000). There were multiple sub-optimal preparative regimens used, and the results are inferior to the new regimen identified by Deeg et al. for unrelated donor BMT. Most unrelated donor transplants were performed late in the course of disease after failure to respond to one or more courses of immune suppression. In the future, it is anticipated that the widespread adoption of improved molecular techniques for HLA-typing will result in better outcomes for recipients of HLA-matched unrelated donor transplants.

In summary, the NMDP-sponsored study reported by Deeg et al. showed improved outcome of patients transplanted less than 1 year after diagnosis and identified a conditioning regimen of 2 Gy TBI/cyclophosphamide/ATG that achieved reliable engraftment with significantly decreased organ toxicity. These results combined with advances in molecular HLA-typing suggest that patients who have fully HLA-matched unrelated donors for both class I and class II antigens, including HLA-C, by high resolution DNA-based typing, may have superior long-term outcome with BMT over immunosuppressive therapy. If a high resolution HLA-matched donor can be identified, then unrelated donor BMT should be considered early in the course of treatment of

patients with acquired severe aplastic anemia. Due to the time interval involved in the donor search, unrelated donor BMT is unlikely to be used as first line therapy for acquired aplastic anemia. However, patients could proceed to unrelated donor BMT within 3 to 5 months if response to immunosuppressive therapy was unsatisfactory. As with the HLA-identical sibling setting, transfusion with leukodepleted, irradiated blood products pre-transplant is critical to decrease the risk of graft rejection. Younger patients (≤ 35 years of age) with 1 HLA antigen minor mismatched donors could also proceed to bone marrow transplantation if treatment with one or possibly more optimal immunosuppressive therapy regimens had failed.

Results of cord blood transplantation

Very limited data are available for patients with severe aplastic anemia transplanted with cord blood cells. Cord blood appears to have a reduced risk of development of GVHD, but is associated with delayed engraftment or graft rejection. Retrospective studies of cord blood recipients with primarily hematological malignancies suggest that children have better outcomes than adults (Rubinstein et al., 1998). In addition, in adults total nucleated cell doses of $\geq 1.87 \times 10^7$/kg and CD34$^+$ cell doses $\geq 1.7 \times 10^5$/kg are important for improved survival and sustained engraftment (Wagner et al., 2002). Among 562 recipients of cord blood, the 19 patients with severe aplastic anemia had the highest occurrence of events after transplant (death, autologous reconstitution, or receipt of a second transplant) (Rubinstein et al., 1998). In that report, of the 19 patients with severe aplastic anemia, only 2 had event-free survival at 270 days after transplant. The currently limited data on cord blood transplantation for severe aplastic anemia are not very encouraging. However, children with severe aplastic anemia who lack HLA-matched siblings or unrelated donors and who have failed more than two courses of immunosuppressive therapy, may be considered candidates for unrelated cord blood transplantation if no other suitable alternative donor is identified.

Future directions

Experimental animal studies have demonstrated an important role of postgrafting immunosuppression, not only for preventing GVHD, but also for suppressing host-versus-graft reactions, and thereby improving the rate of engraftment. In a canine model of hematopoietic stem cell transplantation, the combination of methotrexate and cyclosporine was found to be superior to cyclosporine alone in enhancing engraftment, and the best results were seen with a combination of a new immunosuppressive agent, mycophenolate mofetil, and cyclosporine (Storb et al., 1997b). Thus, enhanced postgrafting immunosuppression may allow reduction in the intensity and toxicity of conditioning programs in future years.

Beyond the question of whether the addition of ATG to the conditioning regimen is necessary for patients previously transfused with irradiated and leukodepleted blood products, future progress in allogeneic HSC transplantation will involve the use of less toxic immunosuppressive agents and more effective prevention and treatment of chronic GVHD. For conditioning regimens, potential alternatives to the combination of high dose cyclophosphamide and ATG include such agents as fludarabine, monoclonal antibodies to the T cell receptor, and second signal blockers such as cytotoxic T-lymphocyte associated antigen-4 immunoglobulin (CTLA4Ig) or monoclonal antibody to CD40 ligand.

Conclusions

Survival of patients with aplastic anemia treated by marrow grafts during the early 1970s was adversely influenced by graft rejection, acute GVHD, and chronic GVHD. The problem of graft rejection has gradually declined. This success is due to the more judicious use of transfusions before transplant, the removal of white blood cells from transfusion products, and improvements in the immunosuppressive qualities of the conditioning regimens. As shown by experimental studies in animals, it is likely that the risk of sensitization to minor transplantation antigens may be further reduced by irradiation of blood products. The incidence and severity of acute GVHD have declined with the introduction of the combined cyclosporine/methotrexate prophylaxis regimen. With these changes, survival of patients transplanted in the late 1980s and 1990s has been significantly improved over that of those grafted in the 1970s. Although chronic GVHD continues to be a cause of morbidity and even mortality, avoidance of buffy coat infusion and the use of the cyclophosphamide and ATG regimen combined with methotrexate and prolonged cyclosporine have decreased the prevalence and severity of chronic GVHD. As more patients become long-term survivors, delayed effects from the initial conditioning regimen and postgrafting immune suppression must be considered. Irradiation-based regimens are not advisable in HLA-identical sibling recipients because of growth retardation in children, sterility, and the higher risk of developing secondary malignancies.

The outcome of unrelated donor HSC transplantation has also improved significantly with the rational identification of a preparative regimen with less toxicity combined with the development of high-resolution DNA-based HLA-typing to identify optimally matched unrelated marrow donors. Patients with fully HLA-matched unrelated donors should be considered candidates for transplantation before exposure to repeat courses of immunosuppression. This will require immediate initiation of unrelated donor searches.

The current practice of HSC transplantation for severe aplastic anemia in Europe has been described (Urbano-Ispizua et al., 2002) (and see Chapter 124, Breaking News...).

Future progress in HSC transplantation for aplastic anemia will be directed toward further decreasing the acute toxicity and decreasing the delayed effects of the conditioning regimens. This must be achieved while maintaining highly reliable rates of sustained engraftment and prevention of both acute and chronic GVHD.

References

Anasetti, C., Doney, K. C., Storb, R. et al. (1986). Marrow transplantation for severe aplastic anemia: long-term outcome in fifty "untransfused" patients. Annals of Internal Medicine, 104, 461–466.

Anasetti, C., Storb, R., Longton, G. et al. (1988). Donor buffy coat cell infusion after marrow transplantation for aplastic anemia. Blood, 72, 1099–1100 (Letter).

Azuma, E., Kojima, S., Kato, K. (1997). Conditioning with cyclophosphamide/antithymocyte globulin for allogeneic bone marrow transplantation from HLA-matched siblings in children with severe aplastic anemia. Bone Marrow Transplantation, 19, 1085–1087.

Bacigalupo, A., Hows, J., Gluckman, E. et al. for the EBMT Working Party on Severe Aplastic Anaemia (1988). Bone marrow transplantation (BMT) versus immunosuppression for the treatment of severe aplastic anaemia (SAA): a report of the EBMT SAA Working Party. British Journal of Haematology, 70, 177–182.

Bacigalupo, A., Brand, R., Oneto, R. et al. (2000a). Treatment of acquired severe aplastic anemia: bone marrow transplantation compared with immunosuppressive therapy—The European Group for Blood and Marrow Transplantation experience (Review). Seminars in Hematology, 37, 69–80.

Bacigalupo, A., Bruno, B., Saracco, P. et al. (2000b). Antilymphocyte globulin, cyclosporine, prednisolone, and granulocyte colony-stimulating factor for severe aplastic anemia: an update of the GITMO/EBMT study on 100 patients. European Group for Blood and Marrow Transplantation (EBMT) Working Party on Severe Aplastic Anemia and the Gruppo Italiano Trapianti di Midolio Osseo (GITMO). Blood, 95, 1931–1934.

Bean, M. A., Graham, T., Appelbaum, F. R. et al. (1994). Gamma-irradiation of pretransplant blood transfusions from unrelated donors prevents sensitization to minor histocompatibility antigens on dog leukocyte antigen-identical canine marrow grafts. Transplantation, 57, 423–426.

Bean, M. A., Graham, T., Appelbaum, F. R. et al. (1996). Gamma radiation of blood products prevents rejection of subsequent DLA-identical marrow grafts: Tolerance vs. abrogation of sensitization to non-DLA antigens. Transplantation, 61, 334–335.

Bjerke, J. W., Lorenz, J., Martin, P. J. et al. (1995). Treatment of graft failure with anti-CD3 antibody BC3, glucocorticoids and infusion of donor hematopoietic cells. Blood, 86, 107a (Abstract).

Brodsky, R. A., Sensenbrenner, L. L., & Jones, R. J. (1996). Complete remission in severe aplastic anemia after high-dose cyclophosphamide without bone marrow transplantation. Blood, 87, 491–494.

Brodsky, R. A., Sensenbrenner, L. L., Smith, B. D. et al. (2001). Durable treatment-free remission after high-dose cyclophosphamide therapy for previously untreated severe aplastic anemia. Annals of Internal Medicine, 135, 477–483.

Bunin, N., Leahey, A., Kamani, N., & August, C. (1996). Bone marrow transplantation in pediatric patients with severe aplastic anemia: cyclophosphamide and anti-thymocyte globulin conditioning followed by recombinant human granulocyte-macrophage colony stimulating factor. Journal of Pediatric Hematology/Oncology, 18, 68–71.

Castro-Malaspina, H., Childs, B., Laver, J. et al. (1994). Hyperfractionated total lymphoid irradiation and cyclophosphamide for preparation of previously transfused patients under-going HLA-identical marrow transplantation for severe aplastic anemia. *International Journal of Radiation Oncology, Biology, Physics,* **29,** 847–854.

Champlin, R. E., Horowitz, M. M., van Bekkum, D. W. *et al.* (1989). Graft failure following bone marrow transplantation for severe aplastic anemia: risk factors and treatment results. *Blood,* **73,** 606–613.

Champlin, R. E., Ho, W. G., Nimer, S. D. *et al.* (1990). Bone marrow transplantation for severe aplastic anemia. Effect of a preparative regimen of cyclophosphamide-low-dose total-lymphoid irradiation and posttransplant cyclosporine-methotrexate therapy. *Transplantation,* **49,** 720–724.

Chao, N. J., Snyder, D. S., Jain, M. *et al.* (2000). Equivalence of 2 effective graft-versus-host disease prophylaxis regimens: results of a prospective double-blind randomized trial. *Biology of Blood and Marrow Transplantation,* **6,** 254–261.

Deeg, H. J., Amylon, M. D., Harris, R. E. *et al.* (2001). Marrow transplants from unrelated donors for patients with aplastic anemia: minimum effective dose of total body irradiation. *Biology of Blood and Marrow Transplantation,* **7,** 208–215.

Deeg, H. J., Anasetti, C., Petersdorf, E. *et al.* (1994). Cyclophosphamide plus ATG conditioning is insufficient for sustained hematopoietic reconstitution in patients with severe aplastic anemia transplanted with marrow from HLA-A, B, DRB matched unrelated donors. *Blood,* **83,** 3417–3418 (Letter).

Deeg, H. J., Flowers, M.E.D., Leisenring, W. *et al.* (2000). Cyclosporine (CSP) or CSP plus methylprednisolone for graft-versus-host disease prophylaxis in patients with high-risk lymphohemopoietic malignancies: long-term follow-up of a randomized trial. *Blood,* **96,** 1194–1195 (Letter).

Deeg, H. J., Leisenring, W., Storb, R. *et al.* (1998). Long-term outcome after marrow transplantation for severe aplastic anemia. *Blood,* **91,** 3637–3645.

Deeg, H. J., Lin, D., Leisenring, W. *et al.* (1997). Cyclosporine or cyclosporine plus methylprednisolone for prophylaxis of graft-versus-host disease: a prospective, randomized trial. *Blood,* **89,** 3880–3887.

Deeg, H. J., Seidel, K., Casper, J. *et al.* (1999). Marrow transplantation from unrelated donors for patients with severe aplastic anemia who have failed immunosuppressive therapy. *Biology of Blood and Marrow Transplantation,* **5,** 243–252.

Deeg, H. J., Socié, G., Schoch, G. *et al.* (1996). Malignancies after marrow transplantation for aplastic anemia and Fanconi anemia: a joint Seattle and Paris analysis of results in 700 patients. *Blood,* **87,** 386–392.

Doney, K., Leisenring, W., Storb, R., & Appelbaum, F. R., for the Seattle Bone Marrow Transplant Team (1997). Primary treatment of acquired aplastic anemia: outcomes with bone marrow transplantation and immunosuppressive therapy. *Annals of Internal Medicine,* **126,** 107–115.

Eapen, M., Ramsay, N. K., Mertens, A. C. *et al.* (2000). Late outcomes after bone marrow transplant for aplastic anaemia. *British Journal of Haematology,* **111,** 754–760.

Feig, S. A., Champlin, R., Arenson, E. *et al.* (1983). Improved survival following bone marrow transplantation for aplastic anaemia. *British Journal of Haematology,* **54,** 509–517.

Flowers, M. E. D., Parker, P. M., Johnston, L. J. *et al.* (2002). Comparison of chronic graft-versus-host disease after transplantation of peripheral blood stem cells versus bone marrow in allogeneic recipients: long-term follow up of a randomized trial. *Blood,* **100,** 415–419.

Fouladi, M., Herman, R., Rolland-Grinton, M. *et al.* (2000). Improved survival in severe acquired aplastic anemia of childhood. *Bone Marrow Transplantation,* **26,** 1149–1156.

Frickhofen, N., Kaltwasser, J. P., Schrezenmeier, H. *et al.* (1991). Treatment of aplastic anemia with antilymphocyte globulin and methylprednisolone with or without cyclosporine. *New England Journal of Medicine,* **324,** 1297–1304.

Frickhofen, N., Heimpel, H., Kaltwasser, J. P. & Schrezenmeier, H. (2003). Antithymocyte globulin with or without cyclosporin A: 11 year follow-up of a randomized trial comparing treatments of aplastic anemia. *Blood,* **1001,** 1236–42.

Furlong, T., Storb, R., Anasetti, C. *et al.* (1997). Conversion to FK506 for cyclosporine (CSP)-resistant acute GVHD or CSP-associated toxicity. *Blood.* **90** (Supp. 1), 104a, (Abstract).

Gluckman, E., Horowitz, M. M., Champlin, R. E. *et al.* (1992). Bone marrow transplantation for severe aplastic anemia: influence of conditioning and graft-versus-host disease prophylaxis regimens on outcome. *Blood,* **79,** 269–275.

Gluckman, E., Socié, G., Devergie, A. *et al.* (1991). Bone marrow transplantation in 107 patients with severe aplastic anemia using cyclophosphamide and thoraco-abdominal irradiation for conditioning: long-term follow-up. *Blood,* **78,** 2451–2455.

Go, R. S., Tefferi, A., Li, C. Y., Lust, J. A., & Phyliky, R. L. (2000). Lymphoproliferative disease of granular T lymphocytes presenting as aplastic anemia. *Blood,* **96,** 3644–3646.

Goerner, M., Gooley, T., Flowers, M.E.D. *et al.* (2002). Morbidity and mortality of chronic GVHD after hematopoietic stem cell transplantation from HLA-identical siblings for patients with aplastic or refractory anemias. *Biology of Blood and Marrow Transplantation,* **8,** 47–56.

Horowitz, M. M. (2000). Current status of allogeneic bone marrow transplantation in acquired aplastic anemia (Review). *Seminars in Hematology,* **37,** 30–42.

Horstmann, M., Stockschlaeder, M., Kabisch, H., & Zander, A. (1995). Cyclophosphamide/antithymocyte globulin conditioning of patients with severe aplastic anemia transplanted with bone marrow from HLA-identical related donors. *Blood,* **85,** 1404–1405 (Letter).

Hows, J. M., Marsh, J. C., Yin, J. L. *et al.* (1989). Bone marrow transplantation for severe aplastic anaemia using cyclosporin: long-term follow-up. *Bone Marrow Transplantation,* **4,** 11–16.

Karadimitris, A., Li, K., Notaro, R. *et al.* (2001). Association of clonal T-cell large granular lymphocyte disease and paroxysmal nocturnal haemoglobinuria (PNH): further evidence for a pathogenetic link between T cells, aplastic anaemia and PNH. *British Journal of Haematology,* **115,** 1010–1014.

Kawahara, K., Storb, R., Sanders, J., & Petersen, F. B. (1991). Successful allogeneic bone marrow transplantation in a 6.5- year-old male for severe aplastic anemia complicating orthotopic liver transplantation for fulminant non-A-non-B hepatitis. *Blood,* **78,** 1140–1143.

Kojima, S., Horibe, K., Inaba, J. *et al.* (2000). Long-term outcome of acquired aplastic anaemia in children: comparison between immunosuppressive therapy and bone marrow transplantation. *British Journal of Haematology*, **111**, 321–328.

Kojima, S., Inaba, J., Yoshimi, A. *et al.* (2001). Unrelated donor marrow transplantation in children with severe aplastic anaemia using cyclophosphamide, anti-thymocyte globulin and total body irradiation. *British Journal of Haematology*, **114**, 706–711.

Kojima, S., Matsuyama, T., Kato, S. *et al.* (2002a). Outcome of 154 patients with severe aplastic anemia who received transplants from unrelated donors: the Japan Marrow Donor Program. *Blood*, **100**, 799–803.

Kojima, S., Ohara, A., Tsuchida, M. *et al.* (2002b). Risk factors for evolution of acquired aplastic anemia into myelodysplastic syndrome and acute myeloid leukemia after immunosuppressive therapy in children. *Blood*, **100**, 786–790.

Korbling, M. & Anderlini, P. (2001). Peripheral blood stem cell versus bone marrow allotransplantation: does the source of hematopoietic stem cells matter? *Blood*, **98**, 2900–2908.

Koza, V., Jindra, P., Svojgrova, M., & Cetkovsky, P. (1998). Successful autologous transplantation in a patient with severe aplastic anemia (SAA). *Bone Marrow Transplantation*, **21**, 957–959.

Locasciulli, A., van't Veer, L., Bacigalupo, A. *et al.* (1990). Treatment with marrow transplantation or immunosuppression of childhood acquired severe aplastic anemia: a report from the EBMT SAA Working Party. *Bone Marrow Transplantation*, **6**, 211–217.

Locatelli, F., Bruno, B., Zecca, M. *et al.* (2000). Cyclosporin A and short-term methotrexate versus cyclosporin A as graft versus host disease prophylaxis in patients with severe aplastic anemia given allogeneic bone marrow transplantation from an HLA-identical sibling: results of a GITMO/EBMT randomized trial. *Blood*, **96**, 1690–1697.

Maciejewski, J. P., Rivera, C., Kook, H., Dunn, D., & Young, N. S. (2001). Relationship between bone marrow failure syndromes and the presence of glycophosphatidyl inositol-anchored protein-deficient clones. *British Journal of Haematology*, **115**, 1015–1022.

Maciejewski, J. P., Risitano, A., Sloand, E. M., Nunez, O., & Young, N. S. (2002). Distinct clinical outcomes for cytogenetic abnormalities evolving from aplastic anemia. *Blood*, **99**, 3129–3135.

Margolis, D., Camitta, B., Pietryga, D. *et al.* (1996). Unrelated donor bone marrow transplantation to treat severe aplastic anaemia in children and young adults. *British Journal of Haematology*, **94**, 65–72.

May, W. S., Sensenbrenner, L. L., Burns, W. H. *et al.* (1993). BMT for severe aplastic anemia using cyclosporine. *Bone Marrow Transplantation*, **11**, 459–464.

McGlave, P. B., Haake, R., Miller, W. *et al.* (1987). Therapy of severe aplastic anemia in young adults and children with allogeneic bone marrow transplantation. *Blood*, **70**, 1325–1330.

Nash, R. A., Pepe, M. S., Storb, R. *et al.* (1992). Acute graft-versus-host disease: analysis of risk factors after allogeneic marrow transplantation and prophylaxis with cyclosporine and methotrexate. *Blood*, **80**, 1838–1845.

Nash, R. A., Furlong, T., Storb, R. *et al.* (1997). Mycophenolate mofetil (MMF) as salvage treatment for graft-versus-host-disease (GVHD) after allogeneic hematopoietic stem cell transplantation (HSCT): safety analysis. *Blood*, **90** (Suppl 1), 105a, (Abstract).

Nash, R. A., Antin, J. H., Karanes, C. *et al.* (2000). Phase 3 study comparing methotrexate and tacrolimus with methotrexate and cyclosporine for prophylaxis of acute graft-versus-host disease after marrow transplantation from unrelated donors. *Blood*, **96**, 2062–2068.

Paquette, R. L., Tebyani, N., Frane, M. *et al.* (1995). Long-term outcome of aplastic anemia in adults treated with antithymocyte globulin: comparison with bone marrow transplantation. *Blood*, **85**, 283–290.

Passweg, J. R., Socié, G., Hinterberger, W. *et al.* (1997). Bone marrow transplant for severe aplastic anemia: has outcome improved? *Blood*, **90**, 858–864.

Rubinstein, P., Carrier, C., Scaradavou, A. *et al.* (1998). Outcomes among 562 recipients of placental-blood transplants from unrelated donors. *New England Journal of Medicine*, **339**, 1565–1577.

Sanders, J. E., Whitehead, J., Storb, R. *et al.* (1986). Bone marrow transplantation experience for children with aplastic anemia. *Pediatrics*, **77**, 179–186.

Sanders, J. E. & the Seattle Marrow Transplant Team (1991). The impact of marrow transplant preparative regimens on subsequent growth and development. *Seminars in Hematology*, **28**, 244–249.

Sanders, J. E., Hawley, J., Levy, W. *et al.* (1996). Pregnancies following high-dose cyclophosphamide with or without high-dose busulfan or total-body irradiation and bone marrow transplantation. *Blood*, **87**, 3045–3052.

Schwinger, W., Urban, C., Lackner, H. *et al.* (2000). Unrelated peripheral blood stem cell transplantation with 'megadoses' of purified CD34+ cells in three children with refractory severe aplastic anemia. *Bone Marrow Transplantation*, **25**, 513–517.

Smith, B. R., Guinan, E. C., Parkman, R. *et al.* (1985). Efficacy of a cyclophosphamide-procarbazine-antithymocyte serum regimen for prevention of graft rejection following bone marrow transplantation for transfused patients with aplastic anemia. *Transplantation*, **39**, 671–673.

Socié, G., Henry-Amar, M., Bacigalupo, A. *et al.* for the European Bone Marrow Transplantation-Severe Aplastic Anaemia Working Party (1993). Malignant tumors occurring after treatment of aplastic anemia. *New England Journal of Medicine*, **329**, 1152–1157.

Storb, R., Blume, K. G., O'Donnell, M. R. *et al.* (2001). Cyclophosphamide and antithymocyte globulin to condition patients with aplastic anemia for allogeneic marrow transplantations: the experience in four centers. *Biology of Blood and Marrow Transplantation*, **7**, 39–44.

Storb, R., Deeg, H. J., Farewell, V. *et al.* (1986a). Marrow transplantation for severe aplastic anemia: methotrexate alone compared with a combination of methotrexate and cyclosporine for prevention of acute graft-versus-host disease. *Blood*, **68**, 119–125.

Storb, R., Deeg, H. J., Weiden, P. L. *et al.* (1979). Marrow graft rejection in DLA-identical canine littermates: antigens involved are expressed on leukocytes and skin epithelial cells but probably not on platelets and red blood cells. *Transplantation Proceedings*, **11**, 504–506.

Storb, R., Deeg, H. J., Whitehead, J. *et al.* (1986b). Methotrexate and cyclosporine compared with cyclosporine alone for prophylaxis of acute graft versus host disease after marrow transplantation for leukemia. *New England Journal of Medicine*, **314**, 729–735.

Storb, R., Etzioni, R., Anasetti, C. *et al.* (1994). Cyclophosphamide combined with antithymocyte globulin in preparation for allogeneic marrow transplants in patients with aplastic anemia. *Blood,* **84,** 941–949.

Storb, R., Leisenring, W., Anasetti, C. *et al.* (1997a). Long-term follow-up of allogeneic marrow transplants in patients with aplastic anemia conditioned by cyclophosphamide combined with antithymocyte globulin. *Blood,* **89,** 3890–3891 (Letter).

Storb, R., Longton, G., Anasetti, C. *et al.* (1992). Changing trends in marrow transplantation for aplastic anemia (Review). *Bone Marrow Transplantation,* **10,** 45–52.

Storb, R., Pepe, M., Anasetti, C. *et al.* (1990). What role for prednisone in prevention of acute graft-versus-host disease in patients undergoing marrow transplants? *Blood,* **76,** 1037–1045.

Storb, R., Prentice, R. L., Buckner, C. D. *et al.* (1983a). Graft-versus-host disease and survival in patients with aplastic anemia treated by marrow grafts from HLA-identical siblings. Beneficial effect of a protective environment. *New England Journal of Medicine,* **308,** 302–307.

Storb, R., Prentice, R. L., Sullivan, K. M. *et al.* (1983b). Predictive factors in chronic graft-versus-host disease in patients with aplastic anemia treated by marrow transplantation from HLA-identical siblings. *Annals of Internal Medicine,* **98,** 461–466.

Storb, R., Sanders, J. E., Pepe, M. *et al.* (1991). Graft-versus-host disease prophylaxis with methotrexate/cyclosporine in children with severe aplastic anemia treated with cyclophosphamide and HLA-identical marrow grafts. *Blood,* **78,** 1144–1145 (Letter).

Storb, R., Thomas, E. D., Buckner, C. D. *et al.* (1984). Marrow transplantation for aplastic anemia. *Seminars in Hematology,* **21,** 27–35.

Storb, R., Thomas, E. D., Buckner, C. D. *et al.* (1976). Allogeneic marrow grafting for treatment of aplastic anemia: a follow-up on long-term survivors. *Blood,* **48,** 485–490.

Storb, R., Yu, C., Wagner, J. L. *et al.* (1997b). Stable mixed hematopoietic chimerism in DLA-identical littermate dogs given sublethal total body irradiation before and pharmacological immunosuppression after marrow transplantation. *Blood,* **89,** 3048–3054.

Stucki, A., Leisenring, W., Sandmaier, B. M. *et al.* (1998). Decreased rejection and improved survival of first and second marrow transplants for severe aplastic anemia (a 26-year retrospective analysis). *Blood,* **92,** 2742–2749.

Sullivan, K. M. (1986). Acute and chronic graft-versus-host disease in man (Review). *International Journal of Cell Cloning,* **4** (Suppl 1), 42–93.

Sullivan, K. M., Agura, E., Anasetti, C. *et al.* (1991). Chronic graft-versus-host disease and other late complications of bone marrow transplantation. *Seminars in Hematology,* **28,** 250–259.

Tichelli, A., Gratwohl, A., Nissen, C., & Speck, B. (1994). Late clonal complications in severe aplastic anemia. *Leukemia and Lymphoma,* **12,** 167–175.

Tichelli, A., Socie, G., Henry-Amar, M. *et al.* (1999). Effectiveness of immunosuppressive therapy in older patients with aplastic anemia. European Group for Blood and Marrow Transplantation Severe Aplastic Anaemia Working Party. *Annals of Internal Medicine,* **130,** 193–201.

Tisdale, J. F., Dunn, D. E., Geller, N. *et al.* (2000). High-dose cyclophosphamide in severe aplastic anaemia: a randomised trial. *Lancet,* **356,** 1554–1559.

Tisdale, J. F., Maciejewski, J. P., Nuñez, O., Rosenfeld. S. J., & Young, N. S. (2002). Late complications following treatment for severe aplastic anemia (SAA) with high-dose cyclophosphamide (Cy): follow up of a randomized trial. *Blood,* **100,** 4668–4670.

Tzeng, C. H., Chen, P. M., Fan, S. *et al.* (1996). CY/TBI-800 as a pretransplant regimen for allogeneic bone marrow transplantation for severe aplastic anemia using HLA-haploidentical family donors. *Bone Marrow Transplantation,* **18,** 273–277.

Urbano-Ispizua, A., Schmitz, N., de Witte, T. *et al.* (2002). Allogeneic and autologous transplantation for haematological diseases, solid tumors and immune disorders: definition and current practice in Europe. *Bone Marrow Transplantation,* **29,** 639–46.

Vassiliou, G. S., Webb, D. K., Pamphilon, D., Knapper, S., & Veys, P. A. (2001). Improved outcome of alternative donor bone marrow transplantation in children with severe aplastic anaemia using a conditioning regimen containing low-dose total body irradiation, cyclophosphamide and Campath. *British Journal of Haematology,* **114,** 701–705.

Wagner, J. E., Barker, J. N., Defor, T. E. *et. al.* (2002). Transplantation of unrealated donor umbilical cord blood in 102 patients with malignant and nonmalignant diseases: influence of CD34 cell dose and HLA disparity on treatment-related mortality and survival. *Blood,* **100,** 1611–1618.

Wagner, J. L., Deeg, H. J., Seidel, K. *et al.* (1996). Bone marrow transplantation for severe aplastic anemia from genotypically HLA-nonidentical relatives: An update of the Seattle experience. *Transplantation,* **61,** 54–61.

59 Allogeneic hematopoietic stem cell transplantation for Fanconi anemia

ELIANE GLUCKMAN AND PHILIPPE GUARDIOLA

Hôpital Saint Louis, Paris, France

Introduction

Fanconi[1] anemia (FA) is a rare autosomal disease that affects 1 in 100,000 people and is associated with birth defects, progressive aplastic anemia, and cancer susceptibility (Auerbach, Rogato, & Schroeder-Kurth, 1989). FA cells show a high level of chromosomal breakage, both spontaneously or induced by cross-linking agents such as mitomycin C (MMC), nitrogen mustard, diepoxybutane (DEB), or photo-activated psoralens (Auerbach & Wolman, 1976; Berger, Bernheim, & Gluckman, 1980). Based on the correction of the characteristic hypersensitivity of FA cells to DNA cross-linking agents such as MMC and DEB, eight different complementation groups have been identified in somatic cell hybrids (Joenje et al., 2001): FA-A, FA-B, FA-C, FA-D1, FA-D2, FA-E, FA-F, and FA-G. The genes for FA complementation group A (FANCA), group C (FANCC), group D2 (FANCD2), group E (FANCE), group F (FANCF), and group G (FANCG) have been identified. Molecular cloning has localized FANCA on chromosome 16q24.3, FANCE on 9q22.3, FANCF on 11p13-p15, and FANCG on 9p13. Retroviral vectors containing cDNA for FA-A, FA-C, and FA-G, the most frequent complementation groups in Europe and North America, allow rapid identification of the defective gene by complementation of primary T cells (Hanenberg et al., 2002). The six known FA proteins interact in a common pathway. Five of the FA proteins (A, C, E, F, G) assemble in a multi-subunit nuclear complex. In response to DNA damage or during S phase of the cell cycle, this complex activates the monoubiquitination of the downstream D2 protein, thereby targeting D2 to BRCA1-containing nuclear foci. Biallelic mutation of an upstream FA gene disrupts the monoubiquitination of FANCD2 resulting in loss of FANCD2 foci and hypersensitivity to MMC. Studies suggest genetic interactions among the breast cancer susceptibility genes, BRCA1 and BRCA2, and the FA genes (Howlett et al., 2002). FANCD2 protein is vital for cellular resistance to DNA cross-linking. It has also been shown to be involved in a second, independent function, and the arrest of DNA synthesis after ionizing radiation (Grompe, 2002). Ubiquitination of FANCD2 has been used as a test for diagnosis of FA.

FA is a heterogeneous disorder with both genetic and phenotypic variability (Gillio et al., 1997). Bone marrow failure is the most frequent hematological abnormality, occurring typically around 5 years of age, but it can appear later. Clonal abnormalities, including a high frequency of monosomy 7 and duplications involving chromosome 11, may occur, indicating transformation to myelodysplastic syndrome or acute myeloid leukemia (Auerbach & Allen, 1991; Butturini et al., 1994). Without an attempt at curative treatment survival is poor, with death occurring during the second decade from aplastic anemia, leukemia, or cancer.

Bone marrow studies including clonogenic assays and long-term marrow cultures have shown a decrease in the hematopoietic stem cell (HSC) pool without a gross microenvironmental defect (Stark et al., 1993b). Although the molecular expression of the *c-kit* proto-oncogene and kit ligand in long-term marrow culture cells are normal (Stark et al., 1993a), there is evidence of a subtle microenvironment defect, consisting of dysregulation of cytokines such as interleukin-6 (IL-6), tumor necrosis factor (TNF), and granulocyte-macrophage colony-stimulating factor (GM-CSF), which may contribute to marrow failure (Rosselli et al., 1994). Inactivation of the FANCC gene augments gamma interferon-induced apoptotic responses in hematopoietic cells (Rathbun et al., 1997). The FA genes inhibit growth of hematopoietic progenitor cells (Segal et al., 1994). Treatment with androgens, corticosteroids, or hematopoietic growth factors can produce transient improvement, but not cure of, Fanconi anemia (Guinan et al., 1994). An association of complementation group and mutation type with clinical outcome has been shown, explaining the heterogeneity of the disease and the differences in transplant results (Faivre et al., 2000). FA-G patients had more severe cytopenia and higher leukemia incidence. Somatic abnormalities were less prevalent in FA-C, but were more common in the rare groups FA-D, FA-E, and FA-F. In FA-A, patients homozygous for null mutations had an earlier onset of anemia and a higher incidence of leukemia than those with mutations producing an altered pro-

[1] Guido Fanconi, Swiss pediatrician, 1892–1979.

tein. In FA-C, there was a later age of onset of aplastic anemia and fewer somatic abnormalities in patients with the 322delG mutation, but there were more somatic abnormalities in patients with IVS4+4A→T. This study indicates that FA patients with mutations in the FANCG gene and patients homozygous for null mutations in FANCA are high-risk groups with a poor hematological outcome and should be considered as candidates for frequent monitoring and early therapeutic intervention.

Disease-specific pretransplant work-up

FA being a heterogeneous disease, clinical diagnosis is not always sufficient to assess the correct diagnosis in children or young adults with aplastic anemia. Other constitutional aplastic anemia may have similar congenital abnormalities and FA patients may have no abnormalities. The most frequent abnormalities in FA are low birth weight, growth retardation, café-au-lait spots, thumb abnormalities, and urinary tract and kidney malposition with or without renal failure.

Diagnosis is suspected with:

- Blood counts: pancytopenia with macrocytic anemia
- Raised alfa fetoprotein and hemoglobin F

Diagnosis is confirmed with:

- Peripheral blood lymphocyte cytogenetic analysis with clastogenic agents—nitrogen mustard, DEB, or MMC showing increased chromosome breaks with tri- and quadri-radial figures
- Study of the cell cycle showing a G2/M arrest increased by incubation with clastogenic agents

Other tests

- Bone marrow cytogenetic abnormalities for diagnosis of leukemia or myelodysplastic syndrome including monosomy 7, 5, 8 and abnormalities of chromosomes 1 and 11

New tests

- Ubiquitination of FANCD2: specific and sensitive, allows the detection of mosaicism
- Phenotypic correction with retroviral vectors

Results of HLA-identical sibling transplantation

Hematopoietic stem cell (HSC) transplantation is the only treatment that definitively restores normal hematopoiesis. Cyclophosphamide (CY), which is used for the pretransplant condition of patients with idiopathic aplastic anemia at a total dose of 200 mg/kg, has been shown to be too toxic for FA patients, leading to a high transplant-related mortality rate (Gluckman et al., 1980). Radiosensitivity studies, both in vitro and in vivo, have shown delayed development of skin lesions, an increased degree of skin damage, and an absence of repair after fractionated irradiation (Dutreix & Gluckman, 1983). Therefore we modified the conditioning regimen for bone marrow transplantation in 1980 to include CY 20 mg/kg given i.v.

over 4 days and 5 Gy thoraco abdominal irradiation (TAI), followed by cyclosporine alone for prevention of graft-versus-host disease (GVHD) (Gluckman, Devergle, & Dutreix, 1983; Gluckman, 1989). A total of 50 patients with FA received transplants from an HLA-identical sibling donor between October 1981 and April 1996 with a median follow-up of 57 months (Socié et al., 1998). Bone marrow was given to 46 patients and cord blood to 4 patients. The median age at transplant was 11 (range 4–26) years. All patients received CY at a total dose of 20 mg/kg, except four patients with myelodysplastic changes in the marrow who received 40 mg/kg. All received 5 Gy TAI and cyclosporine. The 5-year actuarial disease-free survival was 74.4% ± 6% at 54 months (Fig. 59.1). In univariate analysis, a small number of transfusions pretransplant and the absence of acute or chronic GVHD were associated with improved survival. In the Cox's model analysis, the number of transfusions before transplant was the only factor associated with survival (relative risk [RR] 7.08, 2.47–20.2; P = .0003). Patients without chronic GVHD had 100% survival. Early complications included hemorrhagic cystitis in four patients, interstitial pneumonitis in four, and hepatic veno-occlusive disease in one. Graft rejection was observed in three patients. Acute GVHD grade ≥II was observed in 26 patients with 10 patients having grade III–IV. Chronic GVHD was absent in 19 cases, limited in 18, and extensive in 2. The actuarial survival of 159 patients collected by the European Blood and Marrow Transplant (EBMT) Group was 68% (unpublished data). Most of them had received the low-dose cyclosporine and irradiation protocol.

Reports from the International Bone Marrow Transplant Registry (IBMTR) (Gluckman et al., 1995), and from individual centers, had confirmed that conditioning regimens including low-dose CY give a better survival than regimens using greater than 100 mg/kg (Hows et al., 1989; Kohli-Kumar et al., 1994). The IBMTR study analyzed the results of allogeneic bone marrow transplantation (BMT) in 151 patients transplanted from an HLA-identical sibling and in 48 patients transplanted with an alternative related or unrelated donor. FA was

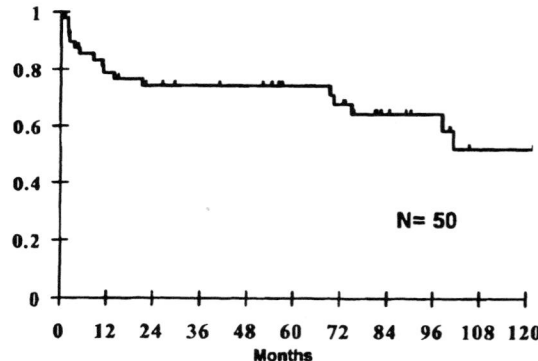

Fig. 59.1. Results of HLA-identical sibling bone marrow transplantation for Fanconi anemia performed at Hôpital Saint Louis, Paris. Cyclophosphamide and thoracoabdominal irradiation were used for pretransplant conditioning. Tick marks indicate patients alive.

documented by cytogenetic analysis in all cases. Two-year probability of survival was 66% after HLA-identical sibling transplants and 29% after alternative donor transplants. Younger patient age, higher pretransplant platelet counts, use of antithymocyte globulin (ATG) pretransplant, use of low-dose CY plus limited field irradiation, and cyclosporine for graft-versus-host disease prophylaxis were associated with improved survival. These results show that early transplant improves the prognosis and confirms again that decreasing the dose of CY reduces regimen-related toxicity without increasing the risk of graft rejection. However, some centers have reported that doses of CY in the order of 100 to 140 mg/kg, with or without ATG, and without irradiation, gave long-term survival of about 50% to 80% (Flowers *et al.*, 1992; Zanis-Neto *et al.*, 1995). In the series by Zanis-Neto and colleagues (1995), 24 patients were described, 22 of whom received a transplant from an HLA-identical sibling and two from a 1 or 2 HLA-antigen mismatched relative. The CY dose was 200 mg/kg in 10 patients and 140 mg/kg in 12, none of whom received total body irradiation (TBI). At the time of the report, 14 of the 24 patients were alive with normal hematopoietic function, including 8 of the 10 patients with an HLA-identical sibling donor conditioned with CY 140 mg/kg (Fig. 59.2). The Seattle group used reduced doses of CY without radiation in the conditioning regimen (Flowers *et al.*, 1996). Nine patients received an HLA-identical sibling transplant, in whom the total CY dose was 140 mg/kg in 2 and 120 mg/kg in 7. GVHD prophylaxis was with cyclosporine and methotrexate in 8 and with cyclosporine alone in 1. Four patients had sustained engraftment and two developed grade II or greater acute GVHD. CY toxicity included grade II or greater mucositis in all evaluable patients and hemorrhagic cystitis in two patients. With a median follow-up of 285 (range 56–528) days the actuarial survival estimate was 89%. These were small series and the overall toxicity was reported as high, but these results raise the possibility that the sensitivity to alky-

lating agents might vary according to the specific genetic defect that is reflected in vivo by the heterogeneity of phenotypic expression and in vitro by the variability in the number of chromosomal breaks. Some genetic defects might be more severe than others and cases of spontaneous mosaicism have been observed (Lo Ten Foe *et al.*, 1997).

A retrospective registry review of 27 Italian patients reported a survival rate at 36 months of 81.5% (Dufour *et al.*, 2001). In this series, the use of a high-dose cyclophosphamide conditioning regimen and the presence of genital malformations were significantly associated with an increased incidence of acute GVHD grade II–IV. The use of busulfan 8 mg/kg and CY 40 mg/kg has been reported (Maschan *et al.*, 1997), as has a combination of fludarabine, ATG, and CY (Kapelushnik *et al.*, 1997). Severe esophagitis occurring both early and late after allogeneic transplantation (and not associated with GVHD) has been described in patients transplanted for Fanconi anemia despite the use of a reduced intensity conditioning regimen (Yakoub-Agha *et al.*, 2000), possibly due to increased sensitivity of the mucosal cells to cytotoxic agents. Several patients had severe stenosis of the esophagus, but none developed secondary cancer there. The observation of secondary tumors posttransplant is of major concern. The probability of developing such tumors is very high in this population because of the additive effect of several risk factors, including the pretransplant conditioning regimen with or without irradiation, environmental exposure, and the chromosome instability characteristic of the disease.

Our results have been updated on 112 patients transplanted from 1976 to 2002. The major long-term risk is head and neck squamous cell carcinoma (SCC), which appeared at a median time of 8.8 years (median 5–22) with a cumulative incidence of 40%. Ten patients developed SCC (4 of the tongue and 5 of the oropharynx). The median age at transplant was 10 years (range 4.5–19). All were transplanted with bone marrow (8 HLA-identical siblings and 2 unrelated donors). All except 1 had received total lymphoid irradiation. All had previous chronic GVHD (8 limited and 2 extensive). Multivariate analysis of risk factors associated with SCC were acute GVHD (RR 7.7 (2–2,926), P = .0193), and age (RR 1.3 (0.97–1.32), P = .076). The prognosis of the SCC was very poor: most patients relapsed after surgery and did not respond or did not tolerate irradiation or chemotherapy. Two patients relapsed with leukemia at 10 and 5 years posttransplant. One patient died of post hepatitis B liver carcinoma. Hypothyroidism was observed in 4 patients and cataracts in 4; 2 patients had growth hormone deficiency and were treated; 6 boys had a normal puberty and 1 girl had spontaneous normal menstruation. One patient had vaginal stenosis that required surgery; 3 had esophageal stenosis, 1 femoral head osteonecrosis, 1 bronchiolitis, and 1 hemolytic-uremic syndrome. Chimerism studies showed that all engrafted patients had hematopoiesis of donor origin with no residual host cells. This confirms that the decrease in the intensity of the pretransplant conditioning was sufficient to induce long-term tolerance and complete donor reconstitution (Socié *et al.*, 1993). The good results of HLA-identical sibling

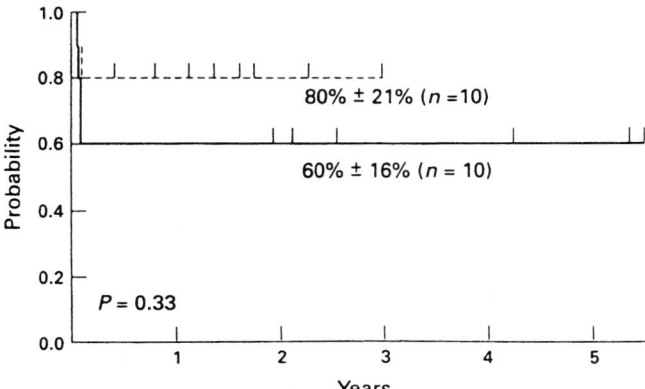

Fig. 59.2. Kaplan-Meier estimates (±S.E.) of event-free survival for 20 patients who received HLA-identical sibling bone marrow. (- - - -) Ten patients conditioned with CY at 140 mg/kg; (——) 10 patients who received 200 mg/kg CY. Numbers on the curves reflect the event-free survival rates at the time. Reproduced, with permission, from Zanis-Neto *et al.* (1995).

marrow transplantation raise several questions regarding the optimal timing of BMT and the best conditioning regimen. Concerning the former, there is a general agreement that HLA-identical sibling transplantation should be performed as first-line therapy, without first using androgens or corticosteroids, which have considerable side effects. When blood counts fulfill the criteria of severe aplastic anemia (Hb <8 g/100 ml, neutrophils <0.5 × 10⁹/l, or platelets <20 × 10⁹/l), transfusions are necessary and, therefore, this seems a suitable time to perform BMT. During the waiting period, it is important to regularly perform bone marrow aspiration and cytogenetic analysis for detection of clonal abnormalities or of leukemic transformation. Results show that transplants performed late (after a long period of aplasia or during leukemic transformation) give poor results, although survivors are reported (Philpott et al., 1994).

The question of the best conditioning regimen is more difficult to answer for several reasons. First, the number of patients is too small for prospective, randomized, multicenter studies. Second, there is not, at the present time, any in vitro test for predicting the sensitivity of a given patient to the conditioning regimen. There is no information about the sensitivity of cell subsets to alkylating agents. The chemosensitivity of leukemic cells seems to be increased since some remissions have been obtained after low-dose chemotherapy or after conditioning with low-dose CY without any attempt to induce remission; however, such cases are rare and most patients treated for acute leukemia do not tolerate standard dose chemotherapy (and have a very poor prognosis). It is possible that genetic diagnosis, which will be performed in the future, will delineate criteria for disease severity (Gillio et al., 1997, Faivre et al., 2000).

Third, it will be difficult to show further marked improvement, when most survival curves show more than 75% long-term survival. Finally, the absence of irradiation in the conditioning regimen did not abolish the risk of secondary tumors, which are likely also related to the specific genetic defect present and to the environment, as shown by different phenotypic expression of the disease in homozygous twins (Lo Ten Foe et al., 1997) (see Table 59.1).

Table 59.1. *A proposed protocol for HLA-matched related bone marrow transplantation in Fanconi anemia*

Objective	
Absence of irradiation (in order to minimize risk of secondary tumor)	
Conditioning	
Busulfan	1.5 mg/kg/day on days −8, −7, −6, −5. (Total dose 6 mg/kg)
Cyclophosphamide	10 mg/kg/day on days −5, −4, −3, −2. (Total dose 40 mg/kg)
Prevention of GVHD	
Cyclosporine	3 mg/kg starting on day −1 for at least 6 months
Methotrexate	5 mg/m² on days +1, +3, +6

The best recommendation at this time is to avoid irradiation because of the risk of cancer, to prefer non-myeloablative regimens using, for example, low dose fludarabine, cyclophosphamide, and antithymocyte globulin. GVHD is particularly severe in FA patients because of the tissue DNA repair defect, and must also be prevented because lichen planus lesions can give rise to squamous cell carcinoma. The association of cyclosporine and mycophenolate mofetil is currently being tested.

Results of HLA-mismatched family member transplantation

In FA, the results of HLA-mismatched family member transplants or transplants performed with HLA-identical unrelated donors have been disappointing (Davies et al., 1996; Zwaan et al., 1998; Macmillan et al., 2000). In our series of 18 patients transplanted with a standard protocol, only 2 are surviving. The causes of death have been multiorgan failure (6 patients), acute GVHD (5 patients), rejection (2 patients), and interstitial pneumonitis (2 patients). Of 41 patients with alternative donors reported to the IBMTR, actuarial 2-year survival was 29%; the probability of graft rejection was 24%, the probability of grade II–IV acute GVHD was 51%, of chronic GVHD 46%, and of interstitial pneumonitis 25%. The number of patients was too small for an analysis of risk factors (Gluckman et al., 1995). Boulad and colleagues (2000) reported successful outcomes after non-myeloablative conditioning in 2 patients with Fanconi anemia given HLA-DRB1-disparate family member PBSC grafts that were T-cell depleted by CD34 selection followed by E-rosetting.

Results of unrelated donor transplantation

Seven patients with Fanconi anemia received unrelated donor transplants at the University of Minnesota (Davies et al., 1996). Two of the patients had marrow failure with normal chromosomes and no dysplasia prior to transplant while the remaining five had clonal chromosomal abnormalities. One patient had RAEB-t and two had early AML. The conditioning regimen was cyclophosphamide 40 mg/kg and TBI 4 to 4.5 Gy. Marrow was infused T replete and posttransplant prophylaxis for GVHD used a methotrexate-based regimen. Two patients died before day 28 without evidence of engraftment, one of veno-occlusive disease and one of fungal infection. Four of the remaining five patients achieved sustained engraftment after the first infusion, while one patient had secondary graft failure and required a second marrow infusion to achieve engraftment. Three of five evaluable patients had grade I–II acute GVHD and two had grade IV, which was fatal in both cases. Two of three evaluable survivors had chronic GVHD controlled with immune suppression. At the time of the report three patients survived 9 months to 3 years posttransplant. Two of these had early leukemia and one severe aplasia at the time of transplant. This regimen utilized a higher dose of cyclophosphamide (40 mg/kg) than has been widely used for patients with Fanconi anemia receiving a radiation-containing conditioning regimen with cyclophosphamide (20 mg/kg). Thus, although this report demonstrated that Fanconi anemia patients could be successfully engrafted with unrelated donor marrow with a likelihood of cure, significant problems with GVHD and engraftment remained and improvement in these areas is required. The European Blood and Marrow Transplantation work party on aplastic anemia has analyzed the outcome of alternative donors transplants in FA (Guardiola *et al.*, 2000). Sixty-seven patients were transplanted; the median age at transplant was 10 (range 3–31) years. The median time from diagnosis to transplant was 37 months, and five patients were transplanted before 1985. The donor was an HLA-matched unrelated donor, defined by serology for HLA class 1 antigens and low-resolution DRB1 typing in 40 cases. In 11 cases there was at least 1 HLA antigen difference between donor and recipient. In 16 cases the donor was an HLA-mismatched family donor. Fifty-eight patients received bone marrow and 9 cord blood cells. Six patients received CD34 selected bone marrow, and six T-cell-depleted bone marrow (negative selection). Forty-eight patients received ATG or a monoclonal anti-T-cell antibody as part of the conditioning regimen or for prevention of GVHD. Thirty patients received TAI and 22 TBI (various doses). Cyclosporine was used alone in 11 cases and with methotrexate in 15 cases. The median number of nucleated cells infused was 2.9×10^8/kg.

The median 2-year survival was 28% ± 8% (Fig. 59.3). Engraftment was complete in 46 cases, while 18 patients had primary graft failure, excluding 3 patients who died before day 21. Twelve patients had secondary graft failure. Thirteen patients received a second transplant with two patients alive at 35 and 32 months. Acute GVHD grade II–IV was observed in 65% with grade III–IV in 45.7%. Chronic GVHD was observed in 8 of 28 evaluable cases. Causes of death included infection, hemorrhage, acute GVHD, chronic GVHD, veno-occlusive disease, and multiorgan failure.

Factors associated with survival were analyzed in Cox's model (Table 59.2). Factors associated with improved survival

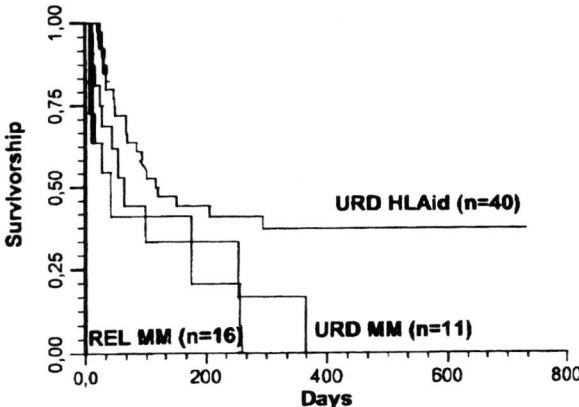

Fig. 59.3. Survival after alternative donor transplantation for Fanconi anemia (EBMT data). URD HLA id, unrelated HLA-identical donor; URD MM, unrelated HLA-mismatched donor; REL MM, HLA-mismatched related donor.

Table 59.2. *Analysis of risk of transplantation*

Factor	Univariate analysis *P*	Multivariate analysis *P*	Relative risk
Time from diagnosis to transplant	.052		
Source of stem cells: marrow/cord blood	.015	.018	1.62
Irradiation in conditioning regimen: TBI/No TBI or TAI	.009	.007	3.15
T-cell depletion: Yes/No	.007	.02	6.59
HLA match between donor and recipient: match/mismatch	.006		

Abbreviations: TBI, total body irradiation, TAI, thoracoabdominal irradiation.

in multivariate analysis were the use of bone marrow rather than cord blood cells, irradiation in the conditioning regimen, and T-cell depletion. Younger age also improved survival (RR 1.06, *P* = .009). Better engraftment occurred with male donors (*P* = .09) and the use of an HLA-matched donor compared to a mismatched donor (*P* = .004). GVHD was more common in female recipients (*P* = .03). Younger age (*P* = .02) and use of T-cell depletion (*P* = .027) were associated with less GVHD.

In our center, we have used a modified conditioning regimen with a higher dose of CY (total dose 40 mg/kg), 4.5 Gy TBI, and ATG (6 doses) from day 6 followed by CD34 selected unrelated bone marrow cells. This has improved our results with four of six patients alive with good engraftment and absence of GVHD. One patient rejected the transplant and 1 died of aspergillosis associated with acute GVHD. This improvement may be due also to better selection of patients and improved HLA matching using high-resolution techniques. More patients and longer follow-up are necessary to evaluate this approach. This small series and the results of the EBMT study indicate that T-cell depletion is worth considering in future prospective protocols.

T-cell depletion can be performed either by positive selection of CD34$^+$ cells (on columns or with magnetic beads), or by negative selection of T cells using elutriation or complement-mediated lysis. T-cell depletion is likely to increase the frequency of rejection. Since increasing the intensity of the conditioning regimen will certainly increase the risk of toxicity, agents not yet tested such as busulfan or thiothepa should be explored. Additionally, increasing the number of stem cells infused by adding G-CSF–mobilized peripheral blood CD34$^+$ cells to the donor marrow cells may be tried. Adding back lymphocytes after the transplant may also improve engraftment and immunity in patients without GVHD.

Results of cord blood transplantation

The first successful HLA-identical cord blood transplant was performed in a patient with FA (Gluckman *et al.*, 1997). The donor was known, before birth, to be HLA-identical to the patient and not affected by FA. His cord blood was collected at birth, cryopreserved, and subsequently transplanted to his brother who had severe aplastic anemia due to FA. The patient was conditioned with low-dose CY and TAI, and received cyclosporine posttransplant for prevention of GVHD. This patient had complete hematological and immunological reconstitution with complete donor chimerism. At current follow-up of more than 7 years, he is doing well and is apparently cured of his disease. Since this first successful transplant, the number of cord blood transplants has increased worldwide to more than 2,000 (adults and children), with various hematological diseases reported. Simultaneously, cord blood banks have been initiated, mostly in the United States and in Europe, for unrelated HLA-matched or mismatched cord blood transplants. Several patients with FA have been transplanted successfully with partially matched unrelated cord blood transplants, including one conditioned with fludarabine and low-dose TBI (200 cGy) (de Medeiros *et al.*, 2001). It seems that one of the advantages of using cord blood instead of bone marrow is a reduction in the severity of GVHD due to the relative immaturity of neonatal T cells.

Posttransplant monitoring

Patients with FA require particular attention because of their sensitivity to toxic agents, development of various organ dysfunctions due to congenital malformations and increased risk of developing malignancies.

This should include at least yearly endocrinological and growth follow-up, bone marrow cytogenetics and oral examination.

Patients with oral lichen planus lesions should be biopsied regularly and the lesions removed.

Gene therapy

Autologous transplantation seems of very limited value in FA; the few CD34+ isolated from G-CSF–mobilized peripheral blood cells (Croop *et al.*, 2001) do not grow in long-term culture and are unlikely to produce short- or a long-term engraftment. Collection of cord blood at birth or of peripheral blood CD34+ stem cells can be performed at an early phase of the disease for gene transfer (Liu, Buchwald, Walsh, & Young, 1994). The localization of new genes and the demonstration in vitro that transfected cells have a selective growth advantage over FA cells has increased interest in the design of gene therapy protocols in FA. Several questions remain unsolved, including the integration of the gene in primitive HSCs, the level of integration necessary for correction of the disease, the long-term expression of the transfected gene, the selective growth advantage of transfected cells, and the function of the proteins of the FA genes. New retrovirus and lentivirus vectors should make this therapeutic option available in the future, taking advantage of the selective growth of transduced cells.

Alternatively, prenatal diagnosis and early recognition of the disease, as well as detection of the heterozygous state, may likely lead to a diminished incidence of the disease.

Conclusions

FA is a hereditary disorder characterized by chromosomal breaks increased by cross-linking agents. HSC transplantation is the treatment of choice when an HLA-identical sibling donor is identified. Results have improved since it was realized that in vitro sensitivity to alkylating agents explained the in vivo toxicity of high-dose CY used for conditioning. The reduction of the dose of CY to 20 mg/kg with 5 Gy TAI or TLI produces a 75% long-term survivorship. Most patients are completely cured of the bone marrow disease, but there is concern about the increased frequency of secondary tumors (head and neck squamous cell carcinomas). Results of HLA-matched family member transplants or unrelated HLA-matched transplants need improvement. New approaches are being explored including cord blood transplantation and gene therapy.

References

Auerbach, A. D. & Allen, R. G. (1991). Leukemia and preleukemia in Fanconi anemia patients. *Cancer Genetics and Cytogenetics,* **51,** 1–12.

Auerbach, A. D. & Wolman, S. R. (1976). Susceptibility of Fanconi anemia fibroblasts to chromosome damage by carcinogens. *Nature,* **261,** 494–6.

Auerbach, A. D., Rogatko, A., & Schroeder-Kurth, T. M. (1989). International Fanconi anemia registry: relation of clinical symptoms to diepoxybutane sensitivity. *Blood,* **73,** 391–6.

Berger, R., Bernheim, A., & Gluckman, E. (1980). In vitro effect of cyclophosphamide metabolites on chromosomes of Fanconi anemia patients. *British Journal of Haematology,* **45,** 565–8.

Boulad, F., Gillio, A., Small, T. N. *et al.* (2000). Stem cell transplantation for the treatment of Fanconi anaemia using a fludarabine-based regimen and T-cell-depleted related HLA-mismatched peripheral blood stem cell grafts. *British Journal of Haematology,* **111,** 1153–7.

Butturini, A., Gale, R. P., Verlander, P. C. *et al.* (1994). Hematological abnormalities in Fanconi anemia: an international Fanconi anemia registry study. *Blood,* **84,** 1650–5.

Croop, J. M., Cooper, R., Fernandez, C. *et al.* (2001). Mobilization and collection of peripheral blood CD34+ cells from patients with Fanconi anemia. *Blood,* **98,** 2917–21.

Davies, S. M., Khan, S., Wagner, J. E. *et al.* (1996). Unrelated donor bone marrow transplantation for Fanconi anemia. *Bone Marrow Transplantation,* **17,** 43–7.

de Medeiros, C. R., Silva, L. M., & Pasquini, R. (2001). Unrelated cord blood transplantation in a Fanconi anemia patient using fludarabine-based conditioning. *Bone Marrow Transplantation,* **28,** 110–11 (Letter).

Dufour, C., Rondelli, R., Locatelli, F. *et al.* (2001). Stem cell transplantation from HLA-matched donor for Fanconi's anemia: a retrospective review of the multicentric Italian experience on behalf of Assocciazone Italiana di Ematologia ed Oncologia Pediatrica

(AIEOP)–Gruppo Italiano Trapianto di Midollo Osseo (GITMO). *British Journal of Haematology*, **112**, 796–805.

Dutreix, J. & Gluckman, E. (1983). Skin test of radiosensitivity. Application to Fanconi anemia. *Journal of European Radiotherapy*, **4**, 3–8.

Faivre, L., Guardiola, P., Lewis, C. *et al.* (2000). Association of complementation group and mutation type with clinical outcome in Fanconi anemia. *Blood*, **96**, 4064–9.

Fanconi Anemia/Breast Cancer Consortium. (1996). Positional cloning of the Fanconi anemia group A gene. *Nature Genetics*, **14**, 324–8.

Flowers, M. E., Zanis, J., Pasquini, R. *et al.* (1996). Marrow transplantation for Fanconi anaemia following conditioning with reduced doses of cyclophosphamide without radiation. *British Journal of Haematology*, **92**, 699–706.

Flowers, M.E.D., Doney, K. C., Storb, R. *et al.* (1992). Marrow transplantation for Fanconi anemia with or without leukemic transformation: an update of the Seattle experience. *Bone Marrow Transplantation*, **9**, 167–73.

Gillio, A. P., Verlander, P. C., Batish, S. D. *et al.* (1997). Phenotypic consequences of mutations in the Fanconi anemia FAC gene: an international Fanconi anemia registry study. *Blood*, **90**, 105–10.

Gluckman, E. (1989). Bone marrow transplantation for Fanconi anemia. *Baillère's Clinical Haematology*, **2**, 153–82.

Gluckman, E., Auerbach, A. D., Horowitz, M. M. *et al.* (1995). Bone marrow transplantation in Fanconi anemia from the International Bone Marrow Transplant Registry. *Blood*, **86**, 2856–62.

Gluckman, E., Devergle, A., & Dutreix, J. (1983). Radiosensitivity in Fanconi anemia: application to the conditioning for bone marrow transplantation. *British Journal of Haematology*, **54**, 431–40.

Gluckman, E., Devergie, A., Schaison, G. *et al.* (1980). Bone marrow transplantation in Fanconi anemia. *British Journal of Haematology*, **45**, 557–64.

Gluckman, E., Rocha, V., Boyer-Chammard, A. *et al.*, for EURO-CORD Transplant Group and European Blood and Marrow Transplant Group (EBMT) (1997). Clinical outcome in recipients of cord blood transplants from related and unrelated donors. *New England Journal of Medicine*, **337**, 373–81.

Grompe, D. (2002). FANCD2: A branch-point in DNA damage response? *Nature Medicine*, **8**, 555–6.

Guardiola, Ph., Pasquini, R. Dokal, I. *et al.* (2000). Outcome of 69 allogeneic stem cell transplants for Fanconi anemia using HLA-matched unrelated donors: a study of the European Group for Blood and Marrow Transplantation. *Blood*, **95**, 422–9.

Guinan, E. C., Lopez, K. D., Huhn, R. D. *et al.* (1994). Evaluation of granulocyte-macrophage colony-stimulating factor for treatment of cytopenia in children with Fanconi anemia. *Journal of Pediatrics*, **124**, 144–50.

Hanenberg, H., Batish, S. D., Pollok, K. E. *et al.* (2002). Phenotypic correction of primary Fanconi anemia T cells with retroviral vectors as a diagnosis tool. *Experimental Hematology*, **30**, 410–20.

Howlett, N. G., Taniguchi, T., Olson, S. *et al.* (2002). Biallelic inactivation of BRCA2 in Fanconi anemia. Science express, www.science express.org.

Hows, J. M., Chapple, M., Marsch, J.C.W. *et al.* (1989). Bone marrow transplantation for Fanconi anemia: the Hammersmith experience 1977–1989. *Bone Marrow Transplantation*, **4**, 629–34.

Joenje, H., Lo Ten Foe, J.R.L., Oostra, A. B. *et al.* (1995). Classification of Fanconi anemia patients by complementation analysis: evidence for a fifth genetic subtype. *Blood*, **86**, 2156–60.

Kapelushnik, J., Or, R., Slavin, S., & Nagler, A. (1997). A fludarabine-based protocol for bone marrow transplantation in Fanconi's anemia. *Bone Marrow Transplantation*, **20**, 1109–10.

Kohli-Kumar, M., Morris, C., Delaat, C. *et al.* (1994). Bone marrow transplantation in Fanconi anemia using matched sibling donors. *Blood*, **84**, 2050–4.

Liu, J. M., Buchwald, M., Walsh, C. E., & Young, N. S. (1994). Fanconi anemia and novel strategies for therapy. *Blood*, **84**, 3995–4007.

Lo Ten Foe, J. R., Kwee, M. L., Rooimans, M. A. *et al.* (1997). Somatic mosaicism in Fanconi anemia: molecular basis and clinical significance. *European Journal of Human Genetics*, **5**, 137–48.

Lo Ten Foe, J. R., Rooimans, M. A., Bosnoyan-Collins, L. *et al.* (1996). Expression cloning of a cDNA for the major Fanconi anemia gene FAA. *Nature Genetics*, **14**, 320–3.

Macmillan, M. L., Auerbach, A. D., Dacie, S. M. *et al.* (2000). Haematopoietic cell transplantation in patients with Fanconi anaemia using alternate donors: results of a total body irradiation dose escalation trial. *British Journal of Haematology*, **109**, 121–9.

Maschan, A. A., Kryzanovskii, O. I., Yourlova, M. I. *et al.* (1997). Intermediate-dose busulfan and cyclophosphamide as a conditioning regimen for bone marrow transplantation in a case of Fanconi anemia in myelodysplastic transformation. *Bone Marrow Transplantation*, **19**, 385–7.

Philpott, N. J., Marsh, J.C.W., Kumaran, T. O. *et al.* (1994). Successful bone marrow transplant for Fanconi anemia in transformation. *Bone Marrow Transplantation*, **14**, 151–3.

Rathbun, R. K., Faulkner, G. R., Ostroski, M. H. *et al.* (1997). Inactivation of the Fanconi anemia group C gene augments interferon-γ induced apoptotic responses in hematopoietic cells. *Blood*, **90**, 974–85.

Rosselli, F., Sanceau, J., Gluckman, E. *et al.* (1994). Abnormal lymphokine production a novel feature of the genetic disease Fanconi anemia: II. In-vitro and in-vivo spontaneous overproduction of tumor necrosis factor alfa. *Blood*, **83**, 1216–25.

Segal, G. M., Magenis, R. E., Brown, M. *et al.* (1994). Repression of Fanconi anemia gene (FACC) expression inhibits growth of hematopoietic progenitor cells. *Journal of Clinical Investigation*, **94**, 846–52.

Socié, G., Devergie, A., Girinski, T. *et al.* (1998). Transplantation for Fanconi's anemia: long-term follow-up of fifty patients transplanted from a sibling donor after low-dose cyclophosphamide and thoraco-abdominal irradiation for conditioning. *British Journal of Haematology*, **103**, 249–55.

Socié, G., Gluckman, E., Raynal, B. *et al.* (1993). Bone marrow transplantation for Fanconi anemia using low dose cyclophosphamide/thoraco abdominal irradiation as conditioning regimen: chimerism study by the polymerase chain reaction. *Blood*, **82**, 2249–56.

Socié, G., Henry-Amar, M., Cosset, J. M. *et al.* (1991). Increased incidence of solid malignant tumors after bone marrow transplantation for severe aplastic anemia. *Blood*, **78**, 277–9.

Stark, R., André, C., Thierry, D. *et al.* (1993a). The expression of cytokine and cytokine receptor genes in long-term bone marrow culture in congenital and acquired bone marrow hypoplasias. *British Journal of Haematology,* **83,** 560–6.

Stark, R., Thierry, D., Richard, P., & Gluckman, E. (1993b). Long-term bone marrow culture in Fanconi anemia. *British Journal of Haematology,* **83,** 554–9.

Yakoub-Agha, I., Damaj, G., Guarderet, L. *et al.* (2000). Severe oesophagitis after allogeneic bone marrow transplantation for Fanconi's anemia. *Bone Marrow Transplantation,* **26,** 215–8.

Zanis-Neto, J., Ribeiro, R. C., Meideros, C. *et al.* (1995). Bone marrow transplantation for patients with Fanconi anemia: a study of 24 cases from a single institution. *Bone Marrow Transplantation,* **15,** 293–8.

Zwaan, C. M., Van Weel-Sipman, M. H., Fibbe, W. E. *et al.* (1998). Unrelated donor bone marrow transplantation in Fanconi anemia: the Leiden experience. *Bone Marrow Transplantation,* **21,** 447–53.

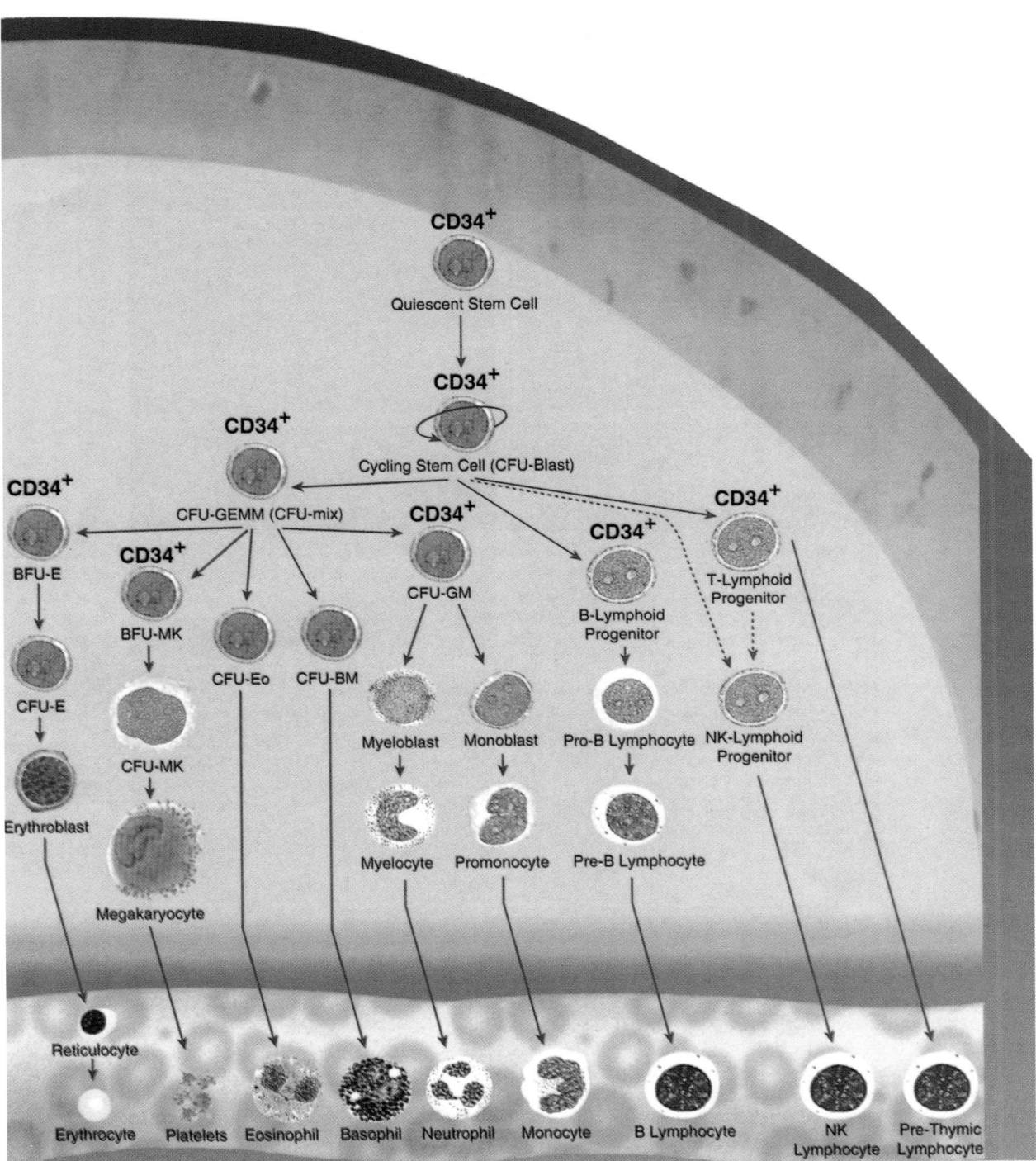

Color Plate 27.4. CD34 antigen expression on normal tissues. Abbreviations: BFU-E, burst forming unit-erythroid; BFU-MK, BFU-megakaryocyte; CFU-BM, colony forming unit-basophil/mast cell; CFU-E, CFU-erythroid; CFU-Eo, CFU-eosinophil; CFU-GEMM, CFU-granulocyte/erythroid/macrophage/megakaryocyte; CFU-GM, CFU-granulocyte/macrophage; CFU-MK, CFU-megakaryocyte; →, actual relationship; --→, potential relationship.

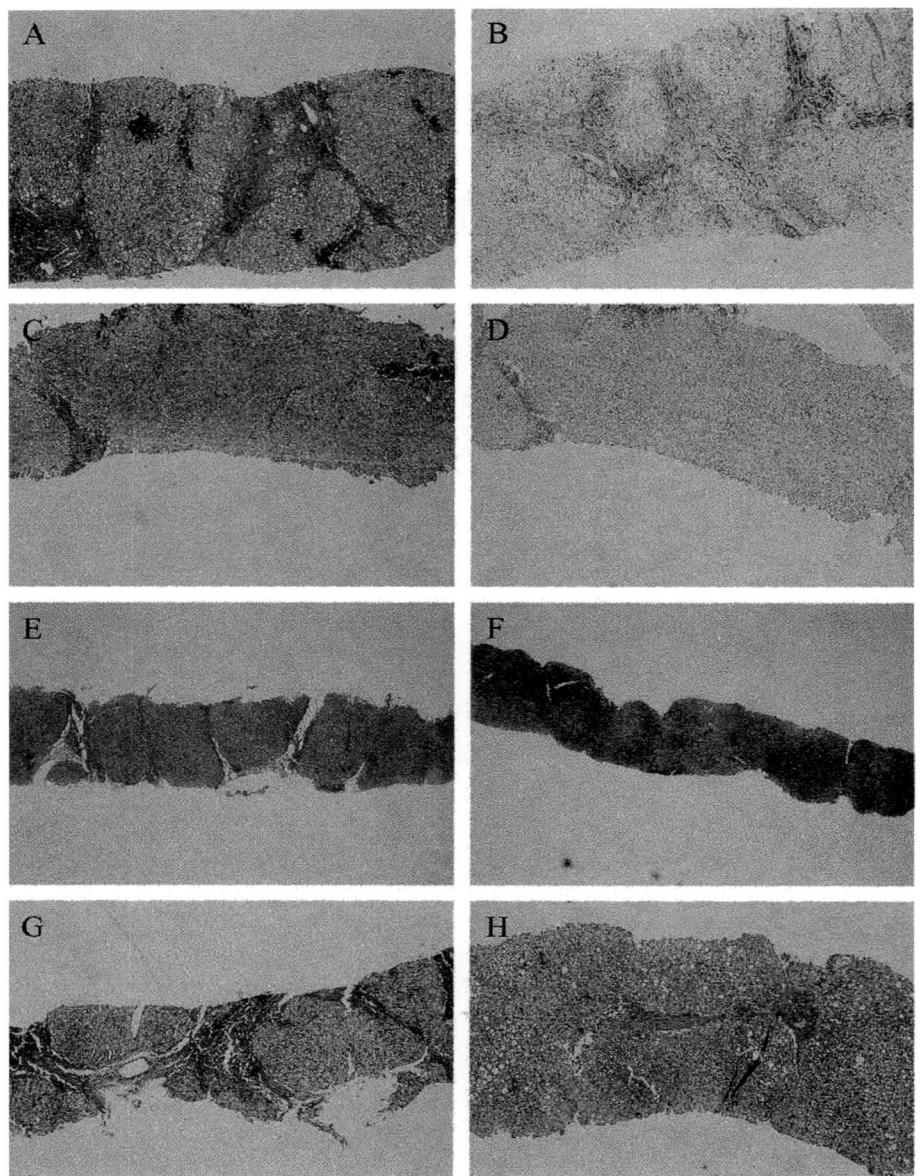

Color Plate 60.13. Percutaneous liver biopsy specimens. **A.** Patient 1. Specimen obtained at diagnosis of cirrhosis (4 years after marrow transplantation) shows cirrhosis with active hepatitis. (Masson trichrome stain; original magnification, ×60.) **B.** Patient 1. Specimen obtained at diagnosis shows severe iron overload (hepatic iron concentration, 22.94 mg/g of liver, dry weight). (Perls Prussian blue reaction; original magnification, ×60.) **C.** Patient 1. Specimen obtained 10 years after transplantation shows regression of cirrhosis and marked improvement of hepatitis. (Masson trichrome stain; original magnification, ×60.) **D.** Patient 1. Specimen obtained 10 years after transplantation shows absence of iron overload (hepatic iron concentration, 0.94 mg/g of liver, dry weight). (Perls Prussian blue reaction; original magnification, ×60.) **E.** Patient 2. Specimen obtained at diagnosis (4 years after transplantation) shows cirrhosis. (Masson trichrome stain; original magnification, ×25.) **F.** Patient 2. Specimen obtained 10 year after transplantation shows regression of cirrhosis. (Masson trichrome stain; original magnification, ×25.) **G.** Patient 6. Specimen obtained at diagnosis (before transplantation) shows definite cirrhosis. (Masson trichrome stain; original magnification, ×60.) **H.** Patient 6. Specimen obtained 5 years and 4 months after transplantation shows stage 2 fibrosis. (Masson trichrome stain; original magnification, × 60.) Reproduced, with permission, from Muretto *et al.* (2002).

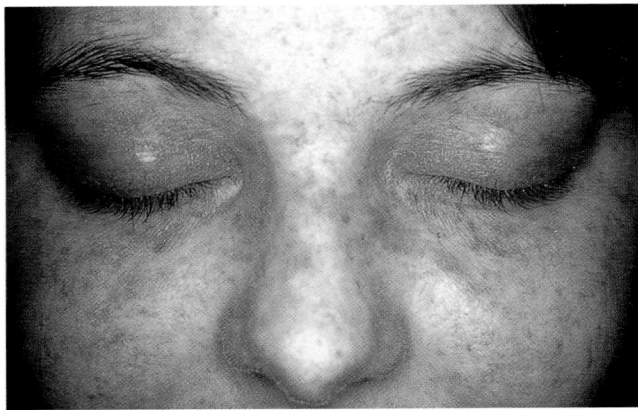

Color Plate 96.1. Macular rash of acute GVHD concentrated on eyelids simulating dermatomyositis.

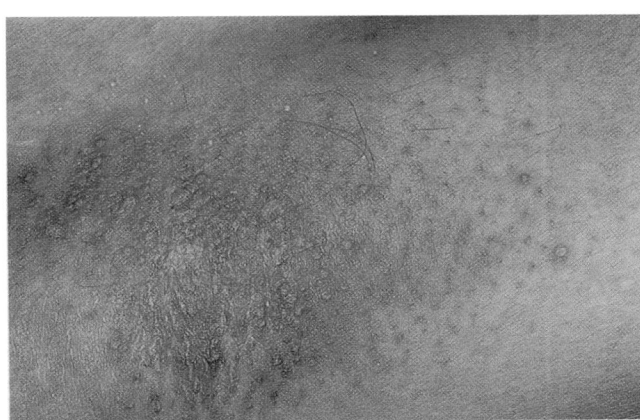

Color Plate 96.4. Lichenoid rash seen with early chronic GVHD in the skin.

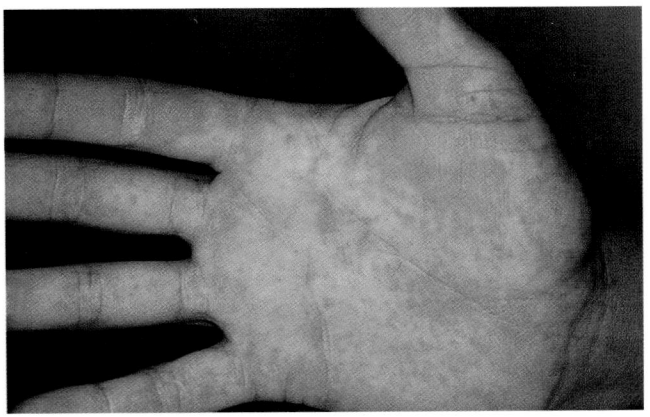

Color Plate 96.2. Acute GVHD involving palms characterized by patchy tender erythema.

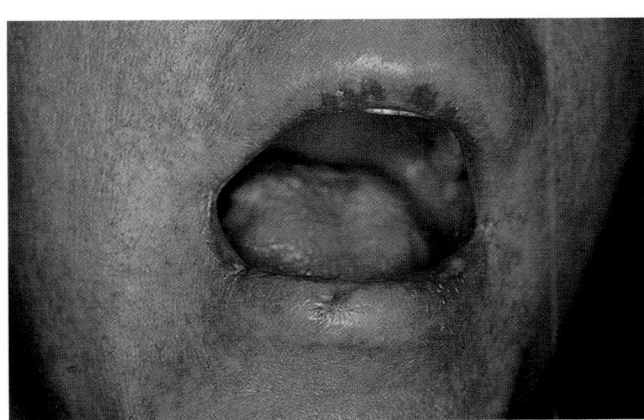

Color Plate 96.5. Mucous membrane erosions and white patches seen with chronic GVHD.

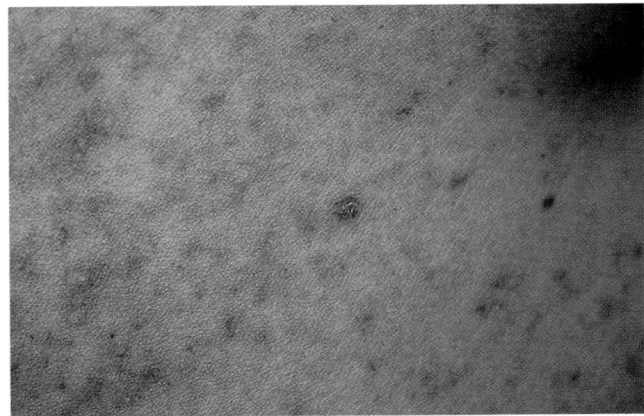

Color Plate 96.3. Acute GVHD of the skin with micropapular element reflecting appendageal involvement.

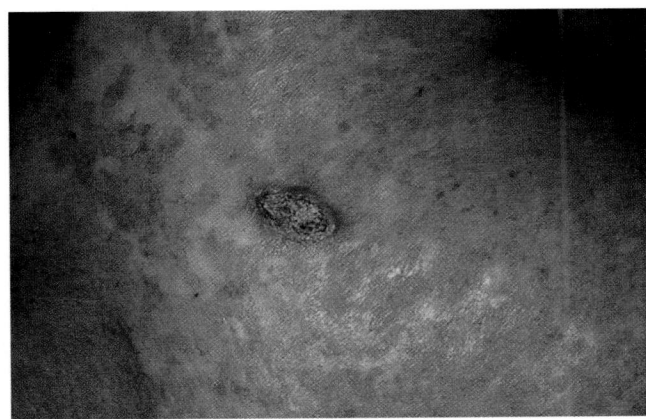

Color Plate 96.6. Advanced cutaneous chronic GVHD demonstrating sclerosis, patchy pigmentation, and focal ulceration.

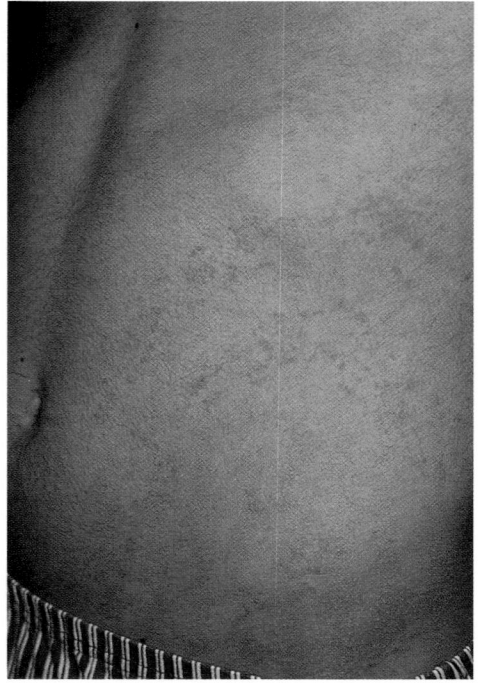

Color Plate 96.7. V-shaped lichenoid pattern seen in unilateral chronic GVHD along Blaschko's lines on back.

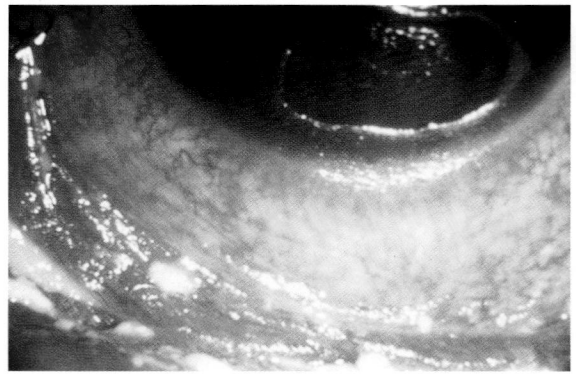

Color Plate 98.1. Stage IV ocular GVHD showing intense conjunctival injection, edema, and exudation associated with intense keratopathy and epithelial loss.

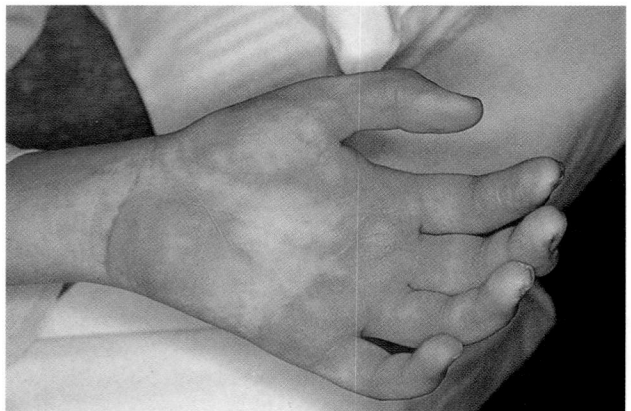

Color Plate 96.8. Well-demarcated dusky acral erythema with early blister formation induced by chemotherapy.

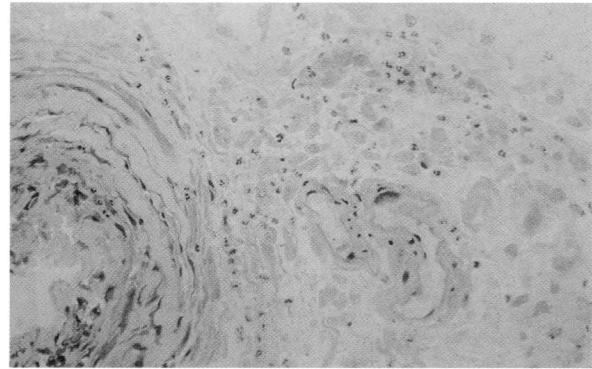

Color Plate 98.2. Conjunctival biopsy in acute GVHD showing perivascular inflammation.

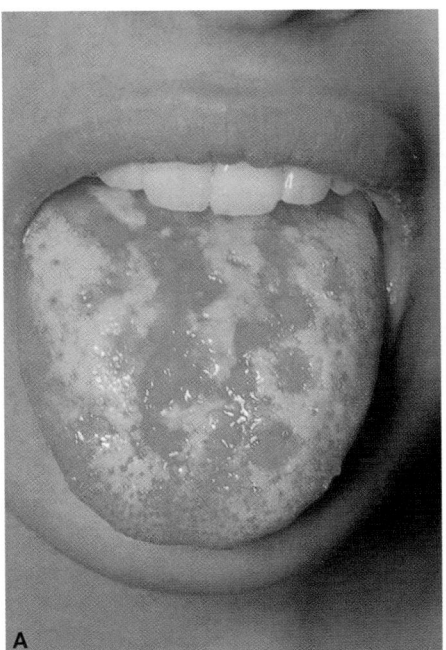

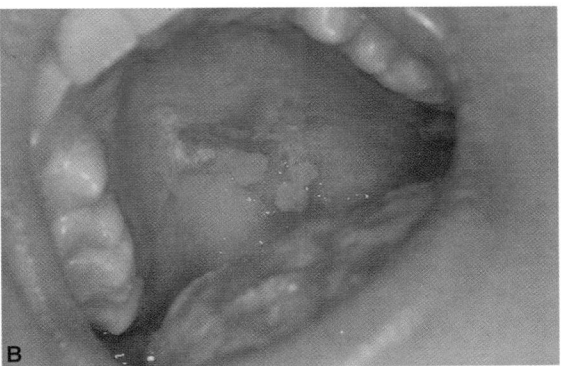

Color Plate 99.1. **(A)** Oral herpetic gingivostomatitis in a 19-year-old female bone marrow transplant recipient. Multiple aphthous ulcerations are present on the dorsum of the tongue. **(B)** Similar herpetiform aphthous ulceration is present on the hard palate. Herpes simplex virus was identified on immunofluorescence of the lesions.

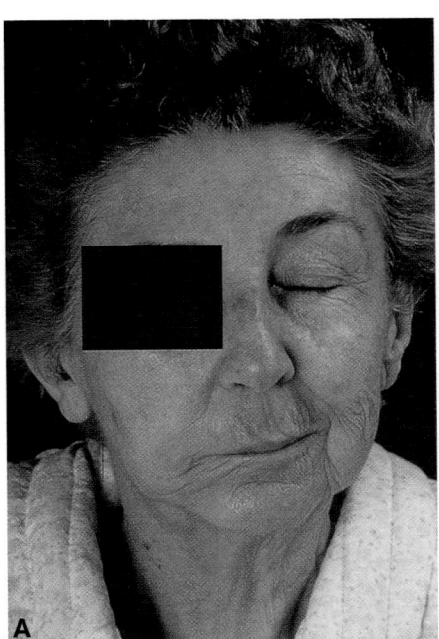

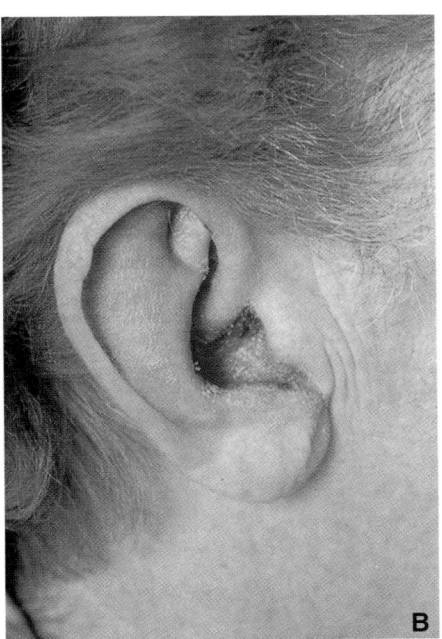

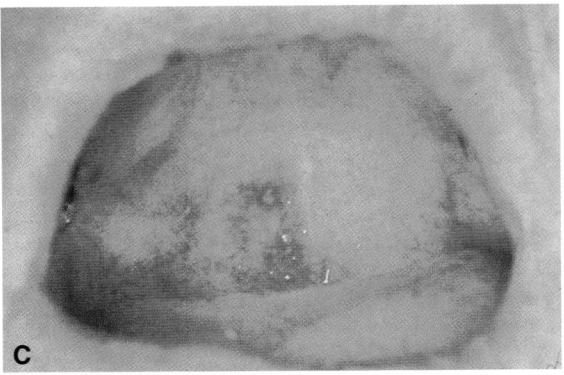

Color Plate 99.4. **(A)** A 65-year-old female immunocompromised after bone marrow transplantation with herpes zoster oticus. She presented with a right lower facial nerve palsy. **(B)** Vesicles with crusting were noted in the conchal bowl of the right ear. **(C)** Right palatal vesicles were also noted. She was successfully treated with systemic acyclovir.

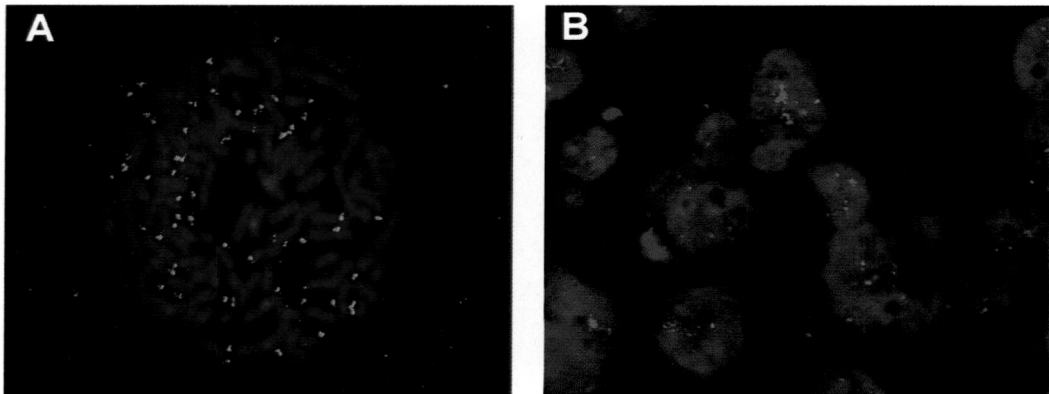

Color Plate 103.1. **(A)** *NYMC* amplification in neuroblastoma. Amplified *NMYC* gene sequences are visible in the form of multiple double minute (dmin) chromosomes in this mitotic neuroblastoma cell. *NMYC* amplification correlates with both advanced disease stage and rapid tumor growth. **(B)** *HER2/NEU* amplification detected by dual-color FISH in a paraffin-embedded breast cancer specimen. Four-micron tissue sections were hybridized using a cosmid probe for *HER2/NEU* [spectrum orange (red) signal] and a chromosome 17 centromere control reference probe (spectrum green signal). Clusters of red signals in the presence of 2 to 4 chromosome 17 centromeric signals [indicating diploid (G1) or tetraploid (G2) cells] indicate amplified *HER2/NEU* gene sequences. *HER2/NEU* amplification is observed in ~25% of breast cancers and has been associated with high-grade disease and short disease-free survival.

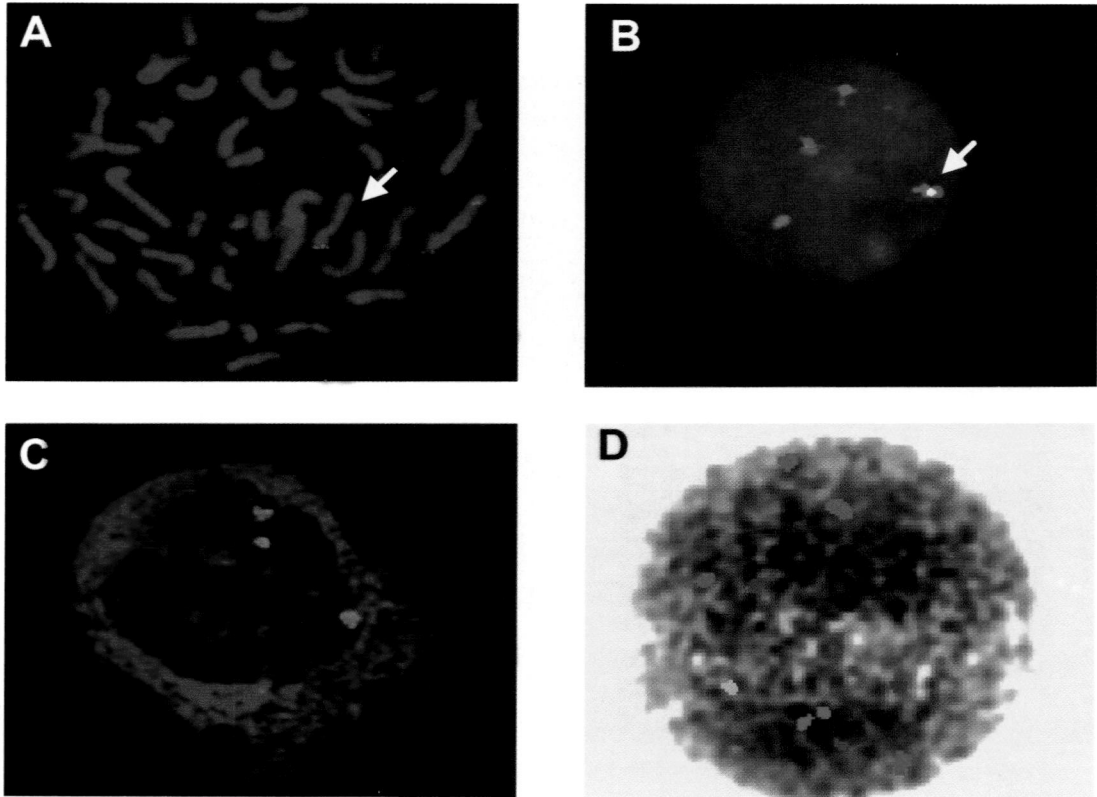

Color Plate 103.2. Various fluorescence in situ hybridization (FISH) techniques. **(A)** Dual color FISH exhibiting a deletion of the long arm of one chromosome 5 (arrow), specifically band 5q31 (spectrum green), in a patient with AML. The spectrum orange chromosome 5 p arm probe identifies the two chromosomes 5 in this metaphase cell. The normal chromosome 5 is seen on the far right. **(B)** Triple-color/triple-probe FISH detecting the Philadelphia chromosome rearrangement. The normal chromosome 22 is represented by the green signal. The red/aqua fusion represents the normal 9. The red/green fusion is the derivative 22 chromosome (arrow) and the lone aqua signal is the derivative 9 chromosome. Samples without the sole aqua signal would identify deletions in the derivative 9 chromosome. **(C)** *F*luorescence *I*mmunophenotyping and *I*nterphase *C*ytogenetics as a *T*ool for *I*nvestigation *o*f *N*eoplasms (FICTION) detection in acute myelogenous leukemia. Trisomy 8 (three blue-green signals) is detected in a CD15 negative cell (right) and a CD15 positive cell (left). FICTION characterizes karyotypically aberrant cells with immunophenotype to allow cell lineage analysis of single cells. **(D)** Spectral FISH cell with MDS/AML probe panel. This cell shows two 5p15 signals (red) with loss of EGR1 (5q31) (one yellow signal). The patient has two copies of chromosome 7 indicated by two centromeric 7 signals (aqua) and two CULT 1 signals (blue). The patient also has four copies of chromosome 8 indicated by four magenta signals that hybridize to the centromeric region of chromosome 8.

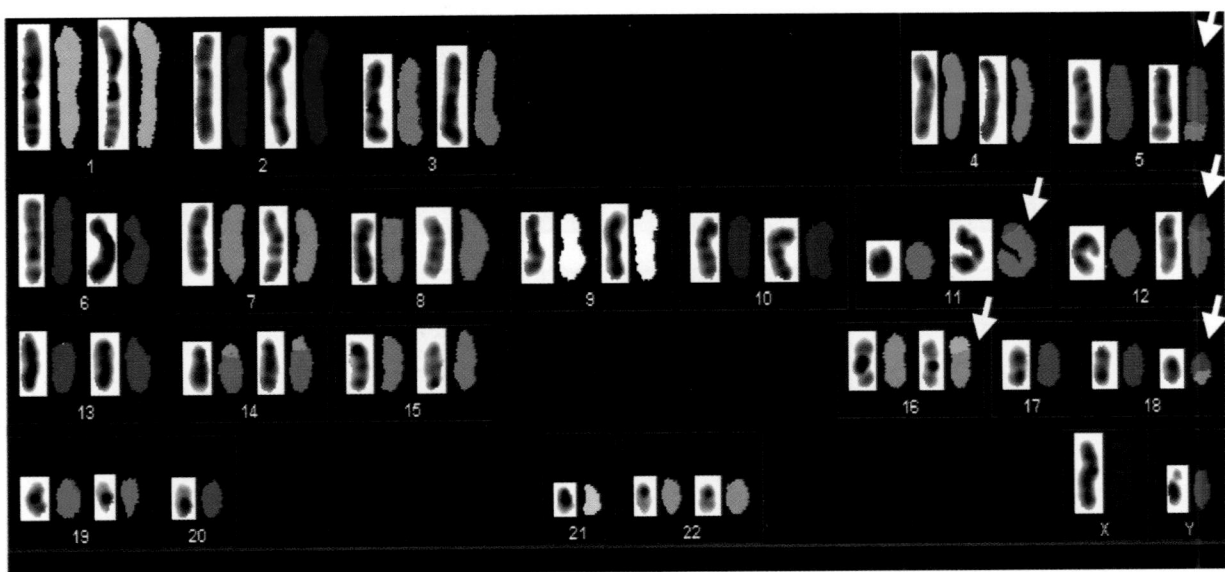

Color Plate 103.3. Example of spectral (24-color) karyotyping of chromosomes prepared from a AML bone marrow sample. The DAPI-banded image (left) and spectrally classified chromosomes (right) are shown. Abnormalities of chromosomes 1, 5, 11, 12, 16, 17, 18, 20, and 21 are identified by their classification colors.

Normal bone marrow

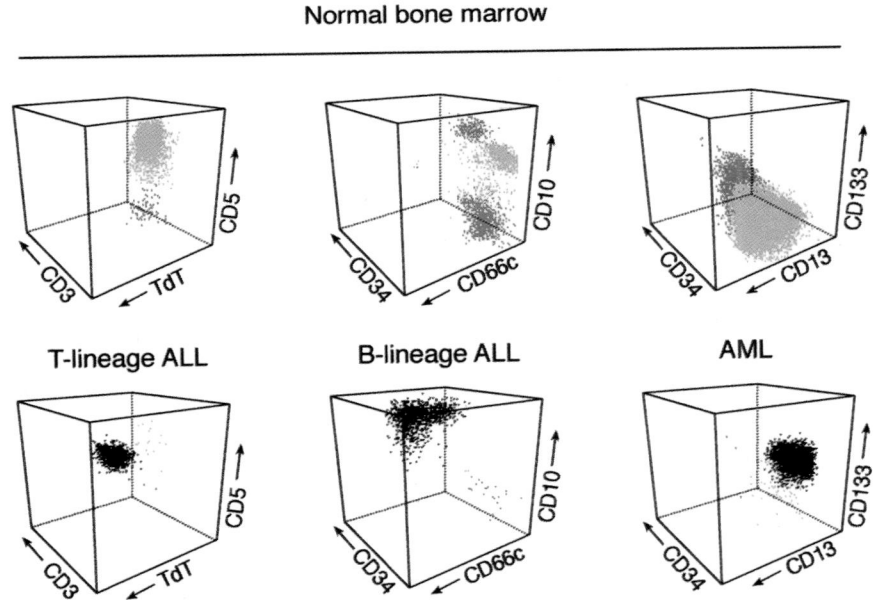

Color Plate 106.1. Immunophenotyic differences between normal and leukemic cells demonstrated by 4-color flow cytometry. Three-dimensional dot plots illustrate expression of the indicated markers on bone marrow cells obtained from healthy individuals (top row) and on bone marrow cells obtained from patients with leukemia at diagnosis (bottom row). The analysis was selectively performed on cells with lymphoblast morphology and lacking expression of HLA-DR, CD19, and CD33 (left panels), cells with lymphoblast morphology and expressing CD19 (center panels), and cells with myeloblast morphology and CD33 expression (right panels).

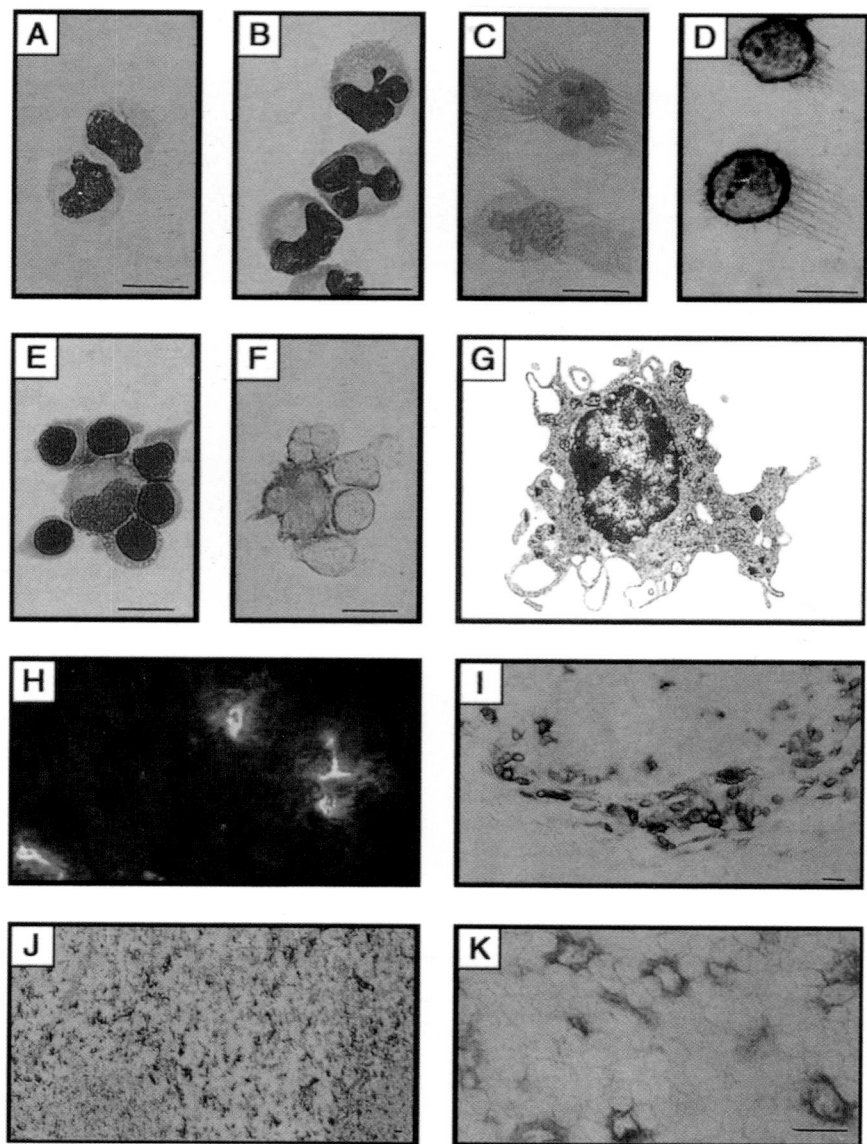

Color Plate 112.1. The morphology of human DC. (**A**) Fresh "lineage negative" blood DC, isolated without a period of tissue culture, using immunoselection (May-Grünwald-Giemsa [MGG], original magnification [OM] × 1,433). (**B**) CMRF-44 sorted, Nycodenz gradient purified cultured blood DC (MGG, OM × 1,433). (**C**) Tonsil low-density cultured DC stained with anti-HLA-DR. The veils and dendritic processes are more obvious in these preparations (OM × 1,433). (**D**) Mo-derived DC preparation stained with CMRF-44 using an immunoenzyme (brown, peroxidase-DAB) technique (in preparation) (OM × 1,433). (**E and F**) Fresh "lineage negative" blood DC clustered with CD4⁺ purified autologous T lymphocytes in the presence of staphylococcal enterotoxin A (SEA) and MGG stained. The DC is stained in another cluster (**F**) for the co-stimulator molecule CD86 using an immunoenzyme (alkaline phosphatase-fast blue) technique (OM × 1,197). (**G**) EM appearances of a CMRF-44-positive cultured blood DC. Note the mitochondria endosomes and lysosomal vacuoles (OM × 17,000). (**H**) DC in the interstitial tissues of rat heart identified by anti-MHC class II staining (immunofluorescence) (OM × 479). (**I**) Dermal CMRF-44⁺ DC (red, peroxidase-AEC) and T lymphocytes (blue, alkaline phosphatase-fast blue) within a section of normal skin adjacent to a hair follicle (OM × 479). (**J**) Lymph node interfollicular (T lymphocyte) area containing CMRF-44⁺ IDC (brown, peroxidase-DAB) compared with CD14 Mo and CD20 B lymphocytes (blue, alkaline phosphatase-fast blue) (OM × 143). (**K**) Lymph node interfollicular region with CMRF-44⁺ IDC (blue, alkaline phosphatase-fast blue) showing nuclear labeling for the transcription factor Rel B (brown, peroxidase-DAB) (OM × 1,197). Bar, 10 μm. Reproduced, with permission, from Hart (1997).

60 Allogeneic hematopoietic stem cell transplantation for thalassemia

GUIDO LUCARELLI AND EMANUELE ANGELUCCI

Ospedale di Pesaro, Pesaro, Italy

Introduction

Homozygous β-thalassemia (Cooley's anemia[1]) is a worldwide, inherited disease characterized by absent or defective globin β chain synthesis (Table 60.1). The defect in β chain synthesis causes imbalance in chain production and accumulation of free chains in red blood cells or red blood cell precursors, leading to intramedullary destruction (Schrier *et al.*, 1997), apoptosis (Yuan *et al.*, 1993), ineffective erythropoiesis, and hemolytic anemia.

The development of regular transfusion regimens and of chelation treatment with deferoxamine given subcutaneously for 8 to 12 hours every day by continuous infusion (Giardini, 1997; Olivieri & Brittenham, 1997) has led to the transformation of this disease from a fatal disease of infancy to a chronic disease with prolonged survival (Brittenham *et al.*, 1994; Olivieri *et al.*, 1994; Lucarelli, Clift, & Angelucci, 1995) (Figs. 60.1 and 60.2).

Allogeneic bone marrow transplantation has proved to be a radical form of cure in those patients with an HLA-identical donor (Lucarelli *et al.*, 1984, 1987, 1990, 1993b; Thomas, Buckner, & Sanders, 1982).

Homozygous α-thalassemia patients have hemoglobin Bart's disease and hydrops fetalis syndrome, which usually leads to stillbirth or neonatal death. With improvements in neonatal care, a few babies have survived after birth, and there is at least one report of a successful HLA-identical sibling transplant (Chik *et al.*, 1998) and one of a successful 1 HLA antigen-mismatched cord blood transplant (Zhou *et al.*, 2001).

The rest of this chapter will deal with allogeneic transplantation for homozygous β-thalassemia.

Results of HLA-identical sibling transplantation

Clinical transplant experience at Pesaro

Clinical outcome

From December 17, 1981, through December 31, 2001, 886 patients with homozygous β-thalassemia received marrow

transplants from HLA-identical related donors at Pesaro and the results are shown in Figure 60.3.

In our early experience the best results were obtained in younger patients (Lucarelli *et al.*, 1984, 1985, 1987). Of the first six patients over the age of 16 years, four died of graft-versus-host disease–related causes within the first 100 days, one died of infection on day 235, and one had recurrence of thalassemia on day 48 and died of consequent cardiac damage more than 6 years after transplantation (Lucarelli *et al.*, 1984).

In view of this experience, early studies concentrated on patients under the age of 17 years. Results in young patients were very encouraging, and in 1990 we reported our experience through August 1988 in treating 222 consecutive patients under the age of 16 years (Lucarelli *et al.*, 1990). All these patients received HLA-identical marrow, in 10 cases from parents and in the other cases from siblings, after conditioning with regimens containing cyclophosphamide 200 mg/kg.

Analysis of the influence of pretransplant characteristics on the outcome of transplantation was conducted in 116 patients

Table 60.1. *The β-thalassemia syndromes*

Syndrome	Main characteristics	Clinical features
Thalassemia major	Severe anemia Life-limiting iron overload from transfusions	Hb <7 g/dl Marked splenomegaly Skeletal changes Jaundice
Thalassemia intermedia	Less severe anemia Chronic transfusion not required Usually survive to adult life	Hb 7–10 g/dl Moderate splenomegaly Mild or no skeletal changes
Thalassemia minor	Asymptomatic Abnormal red cell morphology Little or no anemia	Hb > 10 g/dl Mild or no splenomegaly
Thalassemia minima	Undetectable except by inference from family studies	No abnormal clinical features

[1] Thomas Cooley, U.S. pediatrician, 1871–1945.

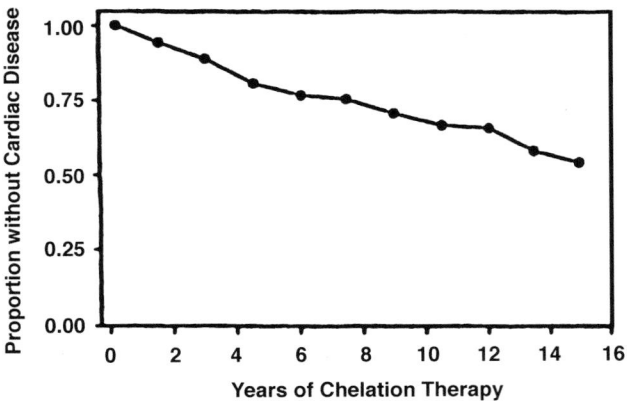

Fig. 60.1. Survival without cardiac disease during chelation therapy in 97 patients with thalassemia major. Reproduced, with permission, from Olivieri *et al.* (1994).

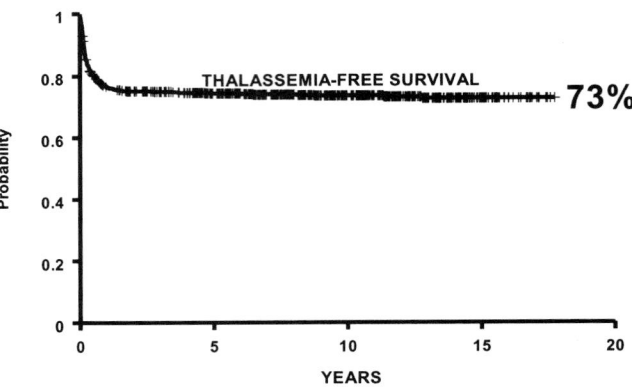

Fig. 60.3. The Kaplan-Meier probability of thalassemia-free survival for all 886 patients with thalassemia aged 1 through 35 years who received HLA-identical family member transplants from December 17, 1981, through December 31, 2001.

who were all treated with exactly the same regimen. It was demonstrated that hepatomegaly and portal fibrosis were associated with a significantly reduced probability of survival. In multivariate analysis a history of poor compliance with the chelation regimen could not be distinguished from hepatomegaly as a predictor of survival and rejection-free survival. The influence of pretransplant characteristics on the outcome of transplantation was re-examined in late 1989 (Lucarelli *et al.*, 1991), by which time 161 patients under the age of 17 had been treated with the same regimen. The quality of chelation was characterized as regular when desferoxamine therapy was initiated not later than 18 months after the first transfusion and administered subcutaneously for 8 to 10 hours continuously for at least 5 days each week. The chelation variable was defined as

irregular for any deviation from this requirement. The degree of hepatomegaly (greater, or not greater, than 2 cm), the presence or absence of portal fibrosis in the pretransplant liver biopsy (Angelucci *et al.*, 1995), and the quality of chelation given before transplant, were identified as variables permitting the categorization of patients into three risk classes. Class 1 patients had none of these adverse risk factors, class 2 patients had one or two adverse risk factors, and class 3 had all three. This analysis confirmed the prognostic significance for transplant outcome of risk class, particularly the strong influence of the quality of chelation therapy (Table 60.2). A thalassemia-specific pretransplant work-up protocol is shown in Table 60.3.

The results of bone marrow transplantation from HLA-identical family member donors obtained in 543 patients aged less than 17 years, of whom 124 were in class 1, 297 in class 2, and 122 in class 3, are shown in Figures 60.4 and 60.5. Patients in class 1 and in class 2 received busulfan 14 mg/kg (Pawlowska *et al.*, 1997) and cyclophosphamide 200 mg/kg as the preparative regimen, while those included in class 3 or in the group of

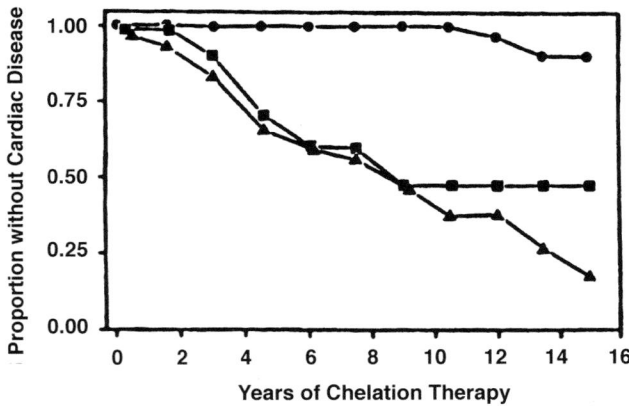

Fig. 60.2. Survival without cardiac disease, according to the proportion of serum ferritin measurements greater than 2,500 ng/ml. The circles show cardiac-disease-free survival among patients in whom fewer than 33% of ferritin measurements exceeded 2,500 ng/ml. Squares show survival among patients in whom 33% to 67% of ferritin measurements exceeded 2,500 ng/ml. Triangles show survival among patients in whom more than 67% of ferritin measurements exceeded 2,500 ng/ml. Reproduced, with permission, from Olivieri *et al.* (1994).

Table 60.2.   *Assessment of pretransplant risk category*

Risk factors
  Hepatomegaly
  Portal fibrosis in pretransplant liver biopsy
  Inadequate quality of pretransplant chelation therapy
Assessment of chelation therapy
  Adequate if desferoxamine was initiated within 18 months of
    first transfusion and was administered subcutaneously for
    8–10 hours, continuously, 5 or more days per week
  Inadequate if there was any deviation from that protocol
Assessment of risk category
  Class 1: no risk factors
  Class 2: 1–2 risk factors
  Class 3: all 3 risk factors

Table 60.3. *Thalassemia-specific pretransplant work-up*

1. Hb electrophoretogram (EPG)
   Hb A_2 and Hb F quantitation
2. Family studies, especially on marrow donor, as in item 1
3. Serum ferritin and iron-binding capacity
4. Ejection fraction
5. Pulmonary function testing
6. Fasting blood sugar
7. Liver biopsy to assess for hepatic siderosis, chronic active hepatitis, chronic persistent hepatitis, and portal fibrosis (except in children <3 years of age without hepatomegaly)
8. Assessment of growth and development and pubertal assessment using Tanner growth charts (Tanner & Whitehouse, 1976)

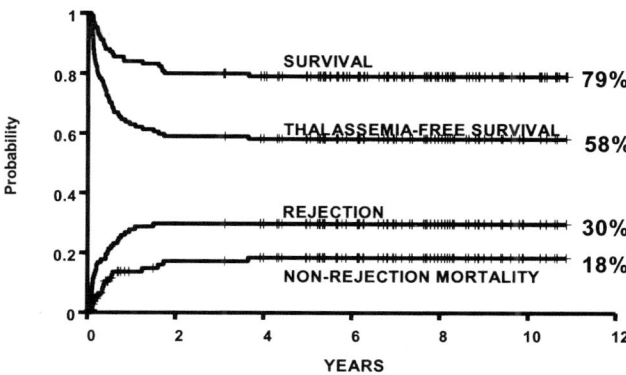

Fig. 60.5. The Kaplan-Meier probabilities of survival, event-free survival, rejection, and nonrejection mortality for the 122 class 3 patients aged less than 17 years.

adults received protocols with the dose of cyclophosphamide reduced to 120 or to 160 mg/kg (Lucarelli *et al.*, 1996, 1999). As described above, early experience with transplantation for patients older than 16 years was disastrous. Most adult patients presenting for transplantation have disease characteristics that place them in class 3, and because of the improved results in treating young class 3 patients using protocols with lower doses of cyclophosphamide, transplantation studies were resumed for patients older than 16 years. One hundred nine patients aged from 17 through 35 years have been transplanted from HLA-identical and mixed lymphocyte culture-nonreactive sibling donors using 200 mg/kg cyclophosphamide for 19 who were in class 2 and either 120 mg/kg or 160 mg/kg for 89 who were in class 3. Figure 60.6 describes the probabilities of survival, event-free survival, rejection, and nonrejection mortality of all the 109 adult patients transplanted after March 1989. In contrast to the results in younger class 3 patients receiving regimens with lower cyclophosphamide dosages, the cumulative incidence of rejection for adult patients was only 4%. The reason for this difference is unknown, but it is noteworthy that the adult patients had a history of more red cell transfusions than the class 3 patients less than 17 years old, and it has been demonstrated that for patients with thalassemia, the likelihood of rejection is inversely related to the transfusion burden (Lucarelli *et al.*, 1996) (Fig. 60.7).

To increase the engraftment rate without increasing the treatment-related mortality, a new conditioning regimen has been used for class 3 children as of April 1997. This regimen comprises 45 days of hydroxyurea 30 mg/kg/day, azathioprine 3 mg/kg/day, hypertransfusion and intensive chelation followed by fludarabine 20 mg/m²/day for 5 days, busulfan 14 mg/kg and cyclophosphamide 160 mg/kg. Preliminary results obtained with this regimen are shown in Figure 60.8.

The occurrence of sudden cardiac tamponade has been described as a complication affecting approximately 2% of thalassemic patients undergoing allogeneic marrow transplantation. In the first six cases that occurred at Pesaro, the diagnosis was only made postmortem. In the next two cases immediate echocardiography revealed the diagnosis and emergency pericardiocentesis led to complete resolution. In one patient the development of pericardial effusion was preceded by an episode of junctional tachycardia. Six patients developed cardiac tamponade after they accumulated 250 to 300 ml of fluid in the pericardium (Angelucci *et al.*, 1992). We have also reported a patient given an allograft for thalassemia after surgical correction of congenital transposition of the great arteries. Thirty-two months posttransplant her hematologic parameters

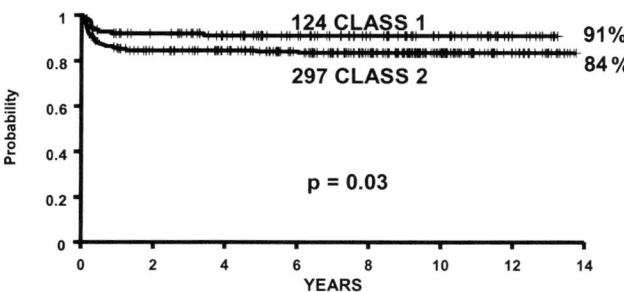

Fig. 60.4. The Kaplan-Meier probabilities of thalassemia-free survival 124 class 1 and 297 class 2 patients aged less than 17 years.

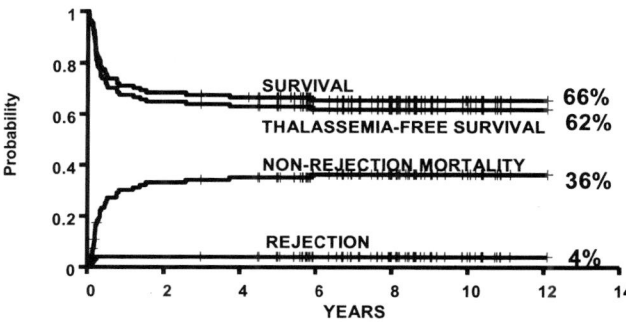

Fig. 60.6. The Kaplan-Meier probabilities of survival, event-free survival, rejection, and nonrejection mortality for the 109 patients older than 16 years.

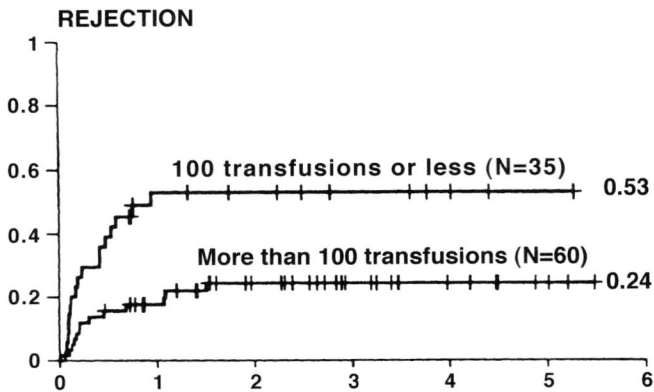

Fig. 60.7. Kaplan-Meier probabilities of rejection for 95 patients aged <17 years transplanted from HLA-identical related donors for treatment of class 3 homozygous β-thalassemia with conditioning regimens containing <200 mg/kg Cy. Patients are categorized on the basis of number of red blood cell transfusions received before transplantation. Reproduced, with permission, from Lucarelli et al. (1996).

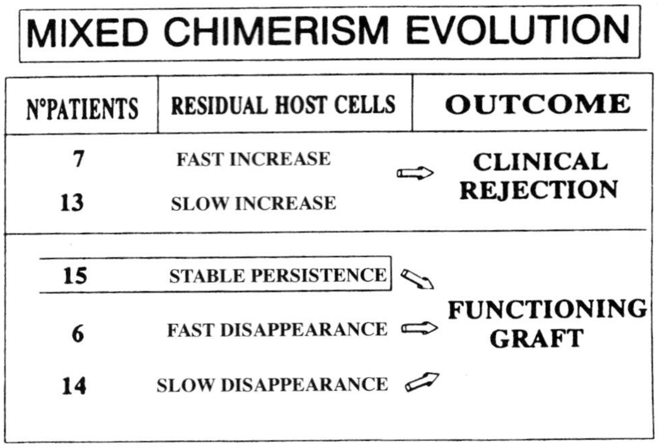

were normal and she had a substantial improvement in cardiac function (Baronciani et al., 1996).

Chimerism

The evolution and cellular distribution of persistent mixed chimerism was studied in 55 patients transplanted for thalassemia. Rejection occurred in 20 patients, the host component disappeared in 20, and mixed chimerism without transfusion requirements persisted for 1 to 7 years in the remaining 15 (Andreani, Manna, & Lucarelli, 1996) (Fig. 60.9). In three patients with stable mixed chimerism for 4, 5, and 7 years, respectively, host hematopoiesis fluctuated between 25% and 75%. Despite this, donor β-globin chain synthesis maintained hemoglobin levels between 10 and 13.5 g/dl without transfusion. In these three patients polymerase chain reaction (PCR) analysis of variable number tandem repeats and use of fluorescent in situ

MIXED CHIMERISM EVOLUTION

N°PATIENTS	RESIDUAL HOST CELLS	OUTCOME
7	FAST INCREASE	CLINICAL REJECTION
13	SLOW INCREASE	
15	STABLE PERSISTENCE	FUNCTIONING GRAFT
6	FAST DISAPPEARANCE	
14	SLOW DISAPPEARANCE	

Fig. 60.9. Mixed chimerism evolution in 55 thalassemic transplanted patients and clinical outcome. Reproduced, with permission, from Andreani et al. (1996).

hybridization revealed the coexistence of donor and host cells in different peripheral blood cell subpopulations and precursors including CD2+, CD4+, CD8+, CD19+, granulocytes, glycophorin- A+, erythrocyte burst-forming-units (BFU-E), and granulocyte macrophage colony-forming-units (CFU-GM) (Figs. 60.10 and 60.11). Thus rejection and disease recurrence occurred in approximately one-third of patients with mixed chimerism, but high levels of host type hematopoiesis can be present in patients not requiring transfusion (Andreani et al., 2000). Kapelushnik and colleagues (1996) have described a second transplant using peripheral blood stem cells to displace host cells in a patient displaying stable mixed chimerism with only 5% donor-derived cells for about 5 years after first transplant. The patient received nonmyeloablative conditioning for the second transplant with blood stem cells. Another study found that the risk of graft rejection was high when >15% host hematopoiesis was present at 3 months posttransplant—4 of 6 such patients rejected their graft. Conversely, none of 29 patients with <15% host hematopoiesis at 3 months rejected (Amrolia et al., 2001).

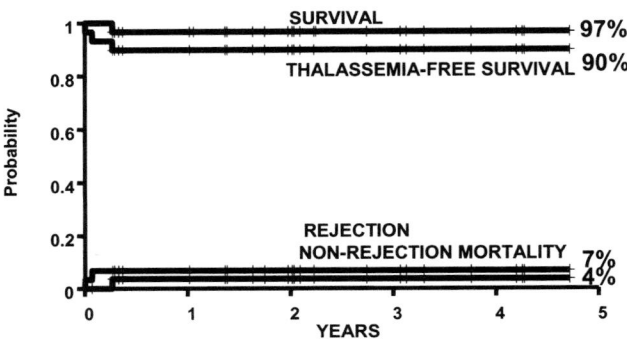

Fig. 60.8. The Kaplan-Meier probabilities of survival, event-free survival, rejection, and nonrejection mortality for the 29 class 3 patients aged less than 17 years treated after April 1997 with the new conditioning regimen (see text).

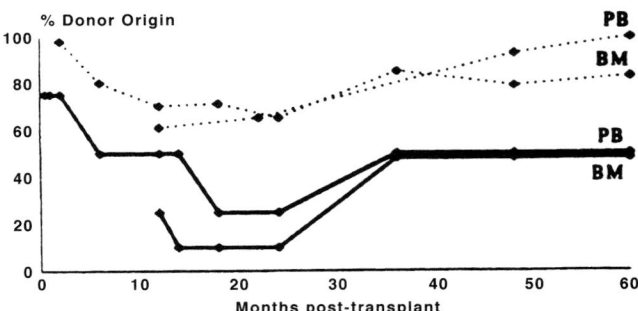

Fig. 60.10. Long-term stable mixed chimerism evaluated by VNTR-RFLP (—) in the peripheral blood (PB) and in the bone marrow (BM) of case UPN 572. High levels of adult β-globin chain synthesis as determined by HPLC (- - - -). Physiologic levels of peripheral Hb were observed for the whole posttransplant period studied. Reproduced, with permission, from Andreani et al. (1996).

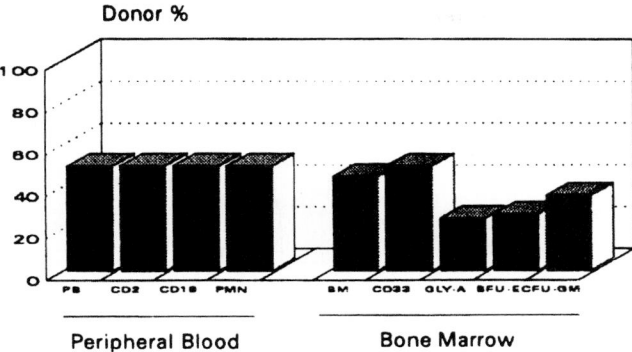

Fig. 60.11. Donor/recipient origin of different PB and BM cell subpopulations in patient UPN 572 at 4 years posttransplant. Reproduced, with permission, from Andreani *et al.* (1996).

Treatment of graft failure

In Pesaro, 32 patients received a second HLA-identical related marrow transplant for graft failure (Gaziev *et al.*, 1999). Most patients received BuCy or CY in association with TLI and/or ALG. Fifty-two percent had sustained engraftment after the second transplant. Transplant-related mortality was 28%. We recommend cryopreservation of autologous marrow before a second transplant, since the graft failure rate was 32.3%.

Transplantation has provided what is probably a permanent cure for the marrow defect in nearly all these patients, but prolonged follow-up is necessary to determine the long-term outcome. It is reasonable to hope that removal of the continuing cause for the extramedullary organ damage will modify disease progression and permit healing of the damaged organs.

Experience at other transplant centers

Many reports describe the experience of other groups in transplanting patients for the treatment of thalassemia (Table 60.4). These data clearly show that results obtained in Pesaro have been widely reproduced. Additionally, peripheral blood stem cells have been utilized successfully (Yesilipek *et al.*, 2001).

Results of HLA-mismatched family member transplantation

At Pesaro, 29 patients received a marrow transplant from a family member donor other than an HLA-identical sibling. Six of the 29 received a transplant from an HLA phenotypically identical donor and the rest a 1 (15 patients), or 2 (five patients), or 3 (2 patients) antigen-disparate graft (Gaziev *et al.*, 2000). The probability of graft failure or rejection was 55%, and was uninfluenced by the degree of HLA disparity. The probability of overall and disease-free survival was 65%

Table 60.4. *Reported transplants for thalassemia*

Center	Patient number	Survival (%)	Disease-free survival (%)
Pescara (Di Bartolomeo *et al.*, 1997)	102	91	87
Cagliari (Argiolu *et al.*, 1997)	37	88	88
United States (Clift & Johnson, 1997)	68	87	69
United Kingdom (Roberts *et al.*, 1997)	50	90	76
Tehran (Ghavamzadeh *et al.*, 1997)	60	83	73
Vellore (Dennison *et al.*, 1997)	50	76	68
Malaysia (Lin *et al.*, 1997)	28	86	75
Hong Kong (Li *et al.*, 1997)	25	86	83
Bangkok (Issaragrisil *et al.*, 1997)	21	76	53

and 21%, respectively. The transplant-related mortality was 34%. Alternative family member donor transplants should be restricted to patients with poor life expectancy because of inability to receive adequate conventional treatment or because of alloimunization to minor blood antigens.

Results of unrelated donor transplantation

The first trial of unrelated donor marrow transplantation for thalassemia was reported by La Nasa and colleagues (2002). Thirty-two consecutive patients were transplanted in five Italian centers. Four were class 1 patients, 11 class 2, and 17 class 3. Of the 32 donor/recipient pairs, 24 were identical for HLA-A, -B, -C, -DRB1, -DRB3, -DRB4, -DRB5, -DQA1, and -DQB1 loci; 7 pairs were identical for 2 extended haplotypes and 15 pairs shared one extended haplotype. Acute GVHD grade II–IV developed in 11 patients (41%) and chronic GVHD in 6 (25%) out of 24 patients at risk. After a median follow up of 30 (range 7–109) months, 22 patients (69%) were alive and thalassemia-free, 6 patients (19%) had died, and 4 (12%) had recurrence of thalassemia. Of the 6 patients who died, 5 belonged to class 3 and 1 to class 2. Of the 22 patients with a donor identical for at least one extended haplotype, 19 survived the transplant and 17 were thalassemia-free. Of the 10 patients who did not share any extended haplotype with the donor, 7 survived the transplant and 5 were thalassemia-free.

It was concluded that marrow transplantation from well-selected unrelated donors may offer results comparable to those with HLA-identical sibling transplantation. It should be noted that the prognostic significance of the risk classes was confirmed in the MUD transplant setting.

Results of cord blood transplantation

Forty-four patients (median age 5 years, range 1–20) underwent allogeneic related cord blood transplantation—33 with thalassemia and 11 with sickle cell disease (SCD) (Locatelli *et al.*, 2003). Thirty children were given cyclosporine (CSP) alone as GVHD prophylaxis, 10 received CSP and methotrexate (MTX) and 4 received other combinations of immunosuppressive drugs. The median number of nucleated cells infused was 4.0×10^7/kg (range 1.2-10). No patient died and 36 of the 44 remain disease-free, with a median follow-up of 24 (range 4–76) months. Graft failure occurred in one patient with SCD and in 7 patients with thalassemia; all of them had recurrence of the hemoglobinopathy. Acute grade II GVHD occurred in four patients; only 2 patients of 36 at risk developed limited chronic GVHD. The 2-year probability of event-free survival was 79% and 90% for patients with thalassemia and sickle cell disease, respectively. Use of MTX for GVHD prophylaxis was associated with a greater risk of treatment failure. The authors concluded that related cord blood transplantation for hemoglobinopathies offers a probability of success comparable to that following bone marrow transplantation; optimization of transplant strategies could further improve the results.

So far no report has been published on the use of unrelated cord blood transplantation in thalassemia.

Results with reduced intensity conditioning regimens

Hongeng and colleagues (2002) described a 10 year old girl with class 3 thalassemia who was conditioned for transplant using busulfan 8 mg/kg over 2 days, fludarbine 35 mg/m^2 daily for 5 days, Fressenius ALG 5 mg/kg daily for 5 days and a single fraction of TLI 500cGy prior to an HLA-identical sibling PBSC transplant. GVHD prophylaxis was cyclosporine and mycophenolate mofetil. She showed full donor chimerism at day 23 posttransplant and experienced no GVHD. One year posttransplant she was alive and well and had a Hb level of 12 g/dl.

The ex-thalassemic patient after bone marrow transplantation

The treatment of patients with thalassemia is not always complete once successful marrow transplants have been performed. Health and a normal life expectancy can only be achieved after resolution of the organ damage acquired during the years with thalassemia and its treatment (primarily iron overload and hepatitis C virus infection). Iron overload and hepatitis C virus infection are independent and mutually reinforcing risk factors for liver fibrosis progression and development of cirrhosis (Angelucci *et al.*, 2002). Patients not infected by hepatitis C virus and with low levels of iron overload at the time of the transplant usually do not require additional treatment after transplant (Lucarelli *et al.*, 1993a; Muretto *et al.*, 1994). Patients heavily overloaded with iron at the time of the transplant maintain such levels after the transplant. Because of the limited excretion of iron, phlebotomy

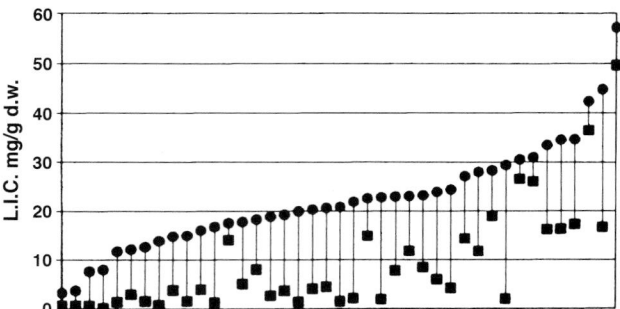

Fig. 60.12. Liver iron concentration (LIC) expressed as mg/g dry weight before the start of phlebotomy program (●) and at last follow-up (■) of all 41 patients treated. Data have been ordered on the basis of pretreatment liver iron concentration. Reproduced, with permission, from Angelucci *et al.* (1997).

appeared to be appropriate to remove iron overload from the ex-thalassemic after transplantation (Angelucci *et al.*, 1997). Phlebotomy has been able to normalize body iron stores in these patients and is the treatment of choice (Fig. 60.12). In those ex-thalassemic patients with high iron levels who cannot be treated with phlebotomy because of young age or difficult venous access, daily subcutaneous administration of desferoxamine has reduced the iron pool (Giardini *et al.*, 1993).

Reduction or normalization of the iron pool results in marked improvement in serum levels of liver enzymes and in liver histopathology in the majority of ex-thalassemic patients after bone marrow transplantation (Angelucci *et al.*, 1997). In some patients reversion of advanced liver damage has been observed (Muretto *et al.*, 2002) (Fig. 60.13).

For patients transplanted in childhood, those whose age at transplant was <7 years had a less impaired growth rate than those transplanted at >7 years of age (De Simone *et al.*, 2001) (and see Chapter 84).

The role of transplantation in the treatment of thalassemia.

The results of transplantation from HLA-identical family members are clear. Class 1 patients have a very high probability of cure with very low early and late morbidity and mortality rates. There is no reason to deny these patients the advantages of a life free from daily tedious, expensive, and uncomfortable therapy. We still do not know the likelihood that a patient receiving conventional therapy will deteriorate into a worse risk category, but the fact is that every day transplant centers are confronted with patients in risk classes 2 and 3 who represent failures of conventional treatment. Delay of transplantation until the patient is in a risk category beyond class 1 substantially reduces the probability of transplant success and jeopardizes the reversibility of liver and cardiac damage. We therefore believe that all patients with β-thalassemia who have a genotypically HLA-identical donor should be transplanted as soon as possible.

Approximately 60% of thalassemic children do not have HLA-identical family members. The use of family member

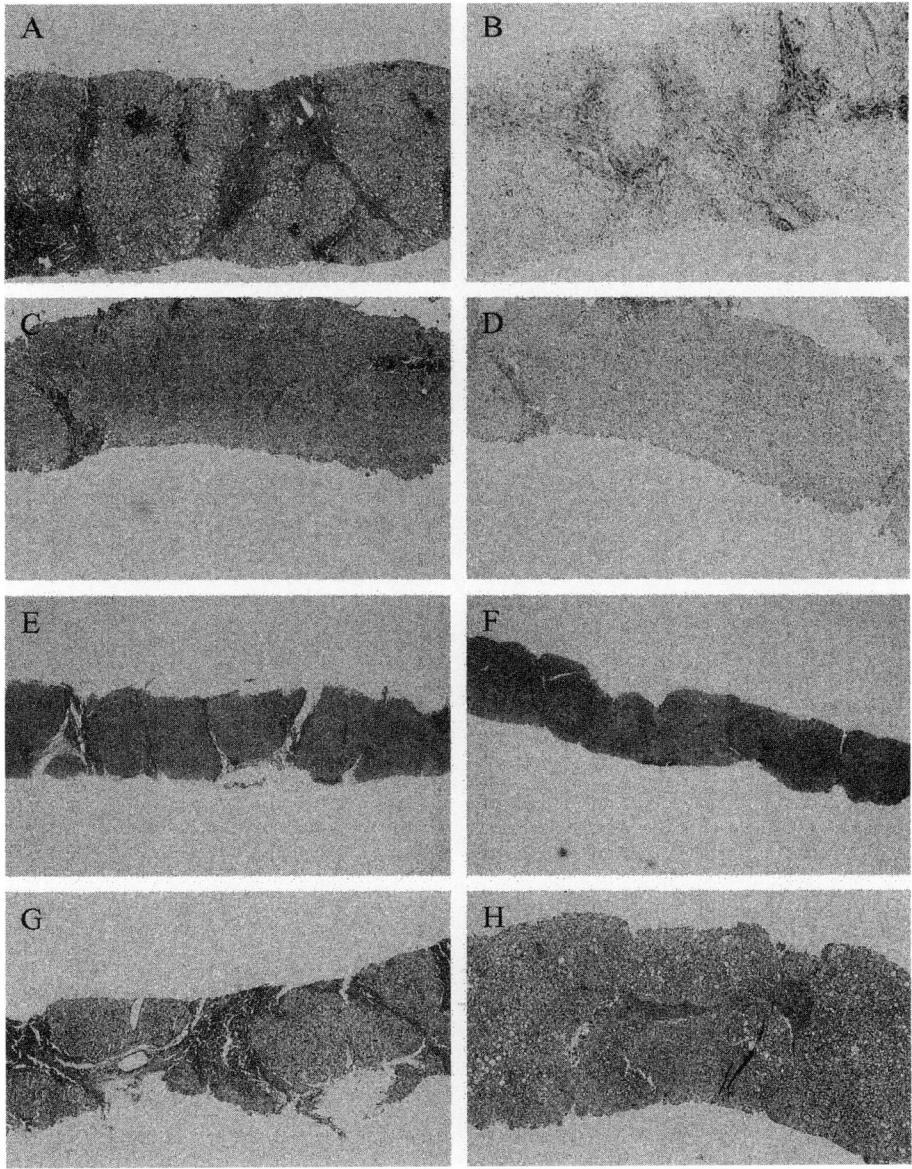

Fig. 60.13. Percutaneous liver biopsy specimens. **A.** Patient 1. Specimen obtained at diagnosis of cirrhosis (4 years after marrow transplantation) shows cirrhosis with active hepatitis. (Masson trichrome stain; original magnification, ×60.) **B.** Patient 1. Specimen obtained at diagnosis shows severe iron overload (hepatic iron concentration, 22.94 mg/g of liver, dry weight). (Perls Prussian blue reaction; original magnification, ×60.) **C.** Patient 1. Specimen obtained 10 years after transplantation shows regression of cirrhosis and marked improvement of hepatitis. (Masson trichrome stain; original magnification, ×60.) **D.** Patient 1. Specimen obtained 10 years after transplantation shows absence of iron overload (hepatic iron concentration, 0.94 mg/g of liver, dry weight). (Perls Prussian blue reaction; original magnification, ×60.) **E.** Patient 2. Specimen obtained at diagnosis (4 years after transplantation) shows cirrhosis. (Masson trichrome stain; original magnification, ×25.) **F.** Patient 2. Specimen obtained 10 year after transplantation shows regression of cirrhosis. (Masson trichrome stain; original magnification, ×25.) **G.** Patient 6. Specimen obtained at diagnosis (before transplantation) shows definite cirrhosis. (Masson trichrome stain; original magnification, ×60.) **H.** Patient 6. Specimen obtained 5 years and 4 months after transplantation shows stage 2 fibrosis. (Masson trichrome stain; original magnification, × 60.) Reproduced, with permission, from Muretto *et al.* (2002). For color reproduction, see Color Plate 60.13.

donors genotypically identical for one HLA haplotype with minimal mismatching on the other haplotype has not been very rewarding, Clearly, more studies of partially HLA-matched transplants are needed, but they are not at present an attractive option in the early management of patients who can obtain and tolerate conventional therapy. The first large multicenter trial experience in the use of unrelated donors has been published (La Nasa *et al.*, 2002) and showed that results comparable to those after HLA-identical sibling transplantation can be obtained if the transplant is performed at an early stage of the disease (class 1 and 2) and a high degree of histocompatibility between patient and donor exists.

References

Amrolia, P. J., Vulliamy, T., Vassiliou, G. *et al.* (2001). Analysis of chimaerism in thalassaemic children undergoing stem cell transplantation. *British Journal of Haematology,* **114,** 219–25.

Andreani, M., Manna, M., & Lucarelli, G. (1996). Persistence of mixed chimerism in patients transplanted for the treatment of thalassemia. *Blood,* **87,** 3494–9.

Andreani, M., Nesci, S., Lucarelli, G. *et al.* (2000). Long-term survival of ex-thalassemic patients with persistent mixed chimerism after bone marrow transplantation. *Bone Marrow Transplantation,* **25,** 401–4.

Angelucci, E., Baronciani, D., Lucarelli, G. *et al.* (1995). Needle liver biopsy in thalassemia: analyses of diagnostic accuracy and safety in 1,184 consecutive biopsies. *British Journal of Haematology,* **89,** 757–61.

Angelucci, E., Mariotti, E., Lucarelli, G. *et al.* (1992). Sudden cardiac tamponade after chemotherapy for marrow tranplantation in thalassemia. *Lancet,* **339,** 287–9.

Angelucci, E., Muretto, P., Lucarelli, G. *et al.* (1997). Phlebotomy to reduce iron overload in patients cured of thalassemia by bone marrow transplantation. *Blood,* **90,** 994–8

Angelucci, E., Muretto, P., Nicolucci, A. *et al.* (2002). Effects of iron overload and HCV positivity in determining progression of liver fibrosis in thalassemia following bone marrow transplantation. *Blood,* **100,** 17–21.

Argiolu, F., Sanna, M. A., Cossu, F. *et al.* (1997). Bone marrow transplant in thalassemia. The experience of Cagliari. *Bone Marrow Transplantation,* **19,** 65–7.

Baronciani, D., Angelucci, E., Agostinelli, F. *et al.* (1996). Bone marrow transplantation in a thalassemia patient with congenital heart disease. *Bone Marrow Transplantation,* **17,** 119–20.

Brittenham, G. M., Griffith, P. M., Nienhuis, A. W. *et al.* (1994). Efficacy of desferoxamine in preventing complications of iron overload in patients with thalassemia major. *New England Journal of Medicine,* **331,** 567–73.

Chik, K. W., Shing, M. M., Li, C. K. *et al.* (1998). Treatment of hemoglobin Bart's hydrops with bone marrow transplantation. *Journal of Pediatrics,* **132,** 1039–42.

Clift, R. A. & Johnson, F. L. (1997). Marrow transplants for thalassemia. The USA experience. *Bone Marrow Transplantation,* **19,** 57–9.

Dennison, D., Srivastava, A., & Chandy, M. (1997). Bone marrow transplantation for thalassemia in India. *Bone Marrow Transplantation,* **19,** 70.

De Simone, M., Verrotti, A., Iughetti, L. *et al.* (2001). Final height of thalassemic patients who underwent bone marrow transplantation during childhood. *Bone Marrow Transplantation,* **28,** 201–5.

Di Bartolomeo, P., Di Girolamo, G., Olioso, P. *et al.* (1997). The Pescara experience of allogeneic bone marrow transplantation in thalassemia. *Bone Marrow Transplantation,* **19,** 48–53.

Gaziev, D., Galimberti, M., Lucarelli, G. *et al.* (2000). Bone marrow transplantation from alternative donors for thalassemia: HLA-phenotypically identical relative and HLA-nonidentical sibling or parent transplants. *Bone Marrow Transplantation,* **25,** 815–21.

Gaziev, D., Polchi, P., Lucarelli, G. *et al.* (1999). Second marrow transplants for graft failure in patients with thalassemia. *Bone Marrow Transplantation,* **24,** 1299–1306.

Ghavamzadeh, A., Bahar, B., Djahani, M. *et al.* (1997). Bone marrow transplantation of thalassemia, the experience in Tehran (Iran). *Bone Marrow Transplantation,* **19,** 71–3.

Giardini, C. (1997). Treatment of β-thalassemia. *Current Opinion in Hematology,* **4,** 79–87.

Giardini, C., La Nasa, G., Contu, L. *et al.* (1993). Desferoxamine induces clearance of iron deposits after bone marrow transplantation for thalassemia: case report. *Bone Marrow Transplantation,* **12,** 108–10.

Hongeng, S., Chuansumrit, A., Hathirat, P. *et al.* (2002). Full chimerism in nonmyeloablative stem cell transplantation in a thalassemia major patient (class 3 Lucarelli). *Bone Marrow Transplantation,* **30,** 409–10.

Issaragrisil, S., Suvatte, V., Visuthisakchai, S. *et al.* (1997). Bone marrow and cord blood stem cell transplantation for thalassemia in Thailand. *Bone Marrow Transplantation,* **19,** 54–6.

Kapelushnik, J., Naparstek, E., Nagler, A. *et al.* (1996). Second transplantation using allogeneic peripheral blood stem cells in beta-thalassemia major patient featuring stable mixed chimaerism. *British Journal of Haematology,* **94,** 257–7.

La Nasa, G., Giardini, C., Argiolu, F. *et al.* (2002). Unrelated donor bone marrow transplantation in thalassemia: the effect of extended haplotypes. *Blood,* **99,** 4350–6.

Li, C. K., Yuen, P.M.P., Shing, M. K. *et al.* (1997). Stem cell transplant for thalassemia patients in Hong Kong. *Bone Marrow Transplantation,* **19,** 62–4.

Lin, H. P., Chan, L. L., Lam, S. K. *et al.* (1997). Bone marrow transplantation for thalassemia. The experience from Malaysia. *Bone Marrow Transplantation,* **19,** 74–7.

Locatelli, F., Rocha, V., Reed, W. *et al.* (2003). Related umbilical cord blood transplant in patients with thalassemia and sickle cell disease. *Blood,* **101,** 2137–43.

Lucarelli, G., Angelucci, E., Giardini, C. *et al.* (1993a). Fate of iron stores in thalassemia after bone marrow transplantation. *Lancet,* **342,** 1388–91.

Lucarelli, G., Clift, R., & Angelucci, E. (1995). Desferoxamine in thalassemia major. *New England Journal of Medicine,* **332,** 271.

Lucarelli, G., Clift, R. A., Galimberti, M. *et al.* (1996). Marrow transplantation for patients with thalassemia. Results in class 3 patients. *Blood,* **87,** 2082–8.

Lucarelli, G., Clift, R. A., Galimberti, M. *et al.* (1999). Bone marrow transplantation in adult thalassemic patients. *Blood,* **93,** 1164–7.

Lucarelli, G., Galimberti, M., Polchi, P. *et al.* (1987). Marrow transplantation in patients with advanced thalassemia. *New England Journal of Medicine,* **316,** 1050–5.

Lucarelli, G., Galimberti, M., Polchi, P. *et al.* (1990). Bone marrow transplantation in patients with thalassemia. *New England Journal of Medicine,* **322,** 417–21.

Lucarelli, G., Galimberti, M., Polchi, P. *et al.* (1991). Bone marrow transplantation in thalassemia. *Hematology/Oncology Clinics of North America,* **5,** 549–56.

Lucarelli, G., Galimberti, M., Polchi, P. *et al.* (1993b). Marrow transplantation in patients with thalassemia responsive to iron chelation therapy. *New England Journal of Medicine,* **329,** 840–4.

Lucarelli, G., Polchi, P., Galimberti, M. *et al.* (1985). Marrow transplantation for thalassemia following busulphan and cyclophosphamide. *Lancet,* **1,** 1355–7.

Lucarelli, G., Polchi, P., Izzi, T. *et al.* (1984). Allogeneic marrow transplantation for thalassemia. *Experimental Hematology,* **12,** 676–81.

Muretto, P., Angelucci, E., & Lucarelli, G. (2002). Reversibility of cirrhosis in patients cured of thalassemia by bone marrow transplantation. *Annals of Internal Medicine,* **136,** 667–72.

Muretto, P., Del Fiasco, S., Angelucci, E., & Lucarelli, G. (1994). Bone marrow transplantation in thalassemia: modification of hepatic iron overload and related pathologies after long-term engrafting. *Liver,* **14,** 14–24.

Olivieri, N. F. & Brittenham, G. M. (1997). Iron-chelation therapy and the treatment of thalassemia. *Blood,* **89,** 739–61.

Olivieri, N. F., Nathan, D. G., MacMillan, J. H. *et al.* (1994). Survival in medically treated patients with homozygous β-thalassemia. *New England Journal of Medicine,* **331,** 574–8.

Pawlowska, A. B., Blazar, B. R., Angelucci, E. *et al.* (1997). Relationship of plasma pharmacokinetics of high-dose oral busulfan to the outcome of allogeneic bone marrow transplantation in children with thalassemia. *Bone Marrow Transplantation,* **20,** 915–20.

Roberts, I.A.G., Darbyshire, P. J., & Will, A. M. (1997). BMT for children with β-thalassemia major in the UK. *Bone Marrow Transplantation,* **19,** 60–1.

Schrier, S., Ma, L., Angelucci, E., & Lucarelli, G. (1997). Advances in understanding of the abnormal cell biology in the thalassemias. *Bone Marrow Transplantation,* **19,** 1–3.

Tanner, J. M. & Whitehouse, R. H. (1976). Clinical longitudinal standards for height, weight, height velocity, weight velocity, and stages of puberty. *Archives of Disease of Childhood,* **51,** 170–9.

Thomas, E. D., Buckner, C. D., & Sanders, J. E. (1982). Marrow transplantation for thalassemia. *Lancet,* **2,** 227–9.

Yesilipek, M. A., Hazar, V., Küpesiz, A. *et al.* (2001). Peripheral blood stem cell transplantation in children with beta-thalassemia. *Bone Marrow Transplantation,* **28,** 1037–40.

Yuan, J., Angelucci, E., Lucarelli, G. *et al.* (1993). Accelerated programmed cell death (apoptosis) in erythroid precursors of patients with severe beta-thalassemia (Cooley's anemia). *Blood,* **82,** 374–7.

Zhou, X., Ha, S. Y., Chan, C.G.F. *et al.* (2001). Successful mismatched sibling cord blood transplant in Hb Bart's disease. *Bone Marrow Transplantation,* **28,** 105–7.

61 Allogeneic hematopoietic stem cell transplantation for sickle cell disease

F. LEONARD JOHNSON

Oregon Health and Science University, Portland, USA

Introduction

Sickle cell anemia, inherited in an autosomal codominant manner, results from the substitution of valine for glutamic acid in the sixth position of the β globin chain. This single amino acid substitution is associated with intracellular polymerization of sickle cell hemoglobin and abnormal interactions of sickle red cells with the vascular endothelium, leading to the clinical manifestations of hemolytic anemia, vascular occlusion causing pain, organ dysfunction and failure, and increased susceptibility to infection. Approximately 30 million individuals worldwide have the sickle cell trait including 8% of African-Americans (Lubin & Vichinsky, 1991).

Developments in newborn screening, comprehensive health maintenance to prevent complications, particularly prophylactic penicillin and pneumococcal vaccination, together with improvements in supportive care for specific complications, including pain management and transfusion and antibiotic therapy, have lengthened the lifespan and improved the quality of life for many affected patients, some of whom have now lived into their seventh decade. The mortality in the first decade of life has been reduced from 15% to 1%, and over 90% of children with sickle cell disease treated in medical centers with optimal comprehensive care are expected to live into their third decade (Vichinsky, 1991). In a study of life expectancy and risk factors for early death among over 3,000 patients with sickle cell disease, the median age at death for patients with sickle cell anemia was 42 years for males and 48 years for females (Platt *et al.*, 1994). The predicted survival to 50 years of age in one study of 381 sickle cell patients was 60% (Smith, 1991).

As children with sickle cell anemia survive longer, however, significant morbidity and early mortality (from vaso-occlusive crises and progressive central nervous system, renal, and pulmonary damage) are now frequent in early adult life. In a study of vaso-occlusive episodes in adult patients, two-thirds had moderately severe to severe disease (Lubin & Vichinsky, 1991). Similarly, data from several studies, including the U.S. Cooperative Study of Sickle Cell Disease, have documented that, while 40% of children do not have a vaso-occlusive crisis, between 5% and 18% suffer severe disease or evidence of organ failure, accounting for the majority of hospital visits.

Although drugs that induce fetal hemoglobin synthesis, such as hydroxyurea, have shown promise in some studies, the only curative therapy currently available for sickle cell anemia is allogeneic hematopoietic stem cell (HSC) transplantation (Steinberg, 1999). The dilemma is that HSC transplantation itself is associated with a substantial risk of morbidity and mortality, and is currently available only to a minority of patients (those who have a satisfactorily matched source of donor HSC).

Experience with allogeneic stem cell transplantation in sickle cell disease

In 1982, Thomas and colleagues demonstrated that bone marrow transplantation could be successfully used to treat human hemoglobinopathies when they reported the transplant of a child with thalassemia (Thomas *et al.*, 1982). This report followed studies in experimental animal models showing that bone marrow transplantation could cure inherited anemias, such as hereditary spherocytosis and hemolytic anemia due to pyruvate kinase deficiency (Weiden *et al.*, 1967).

The possibility of treating selected patients with sickle cell anemia by bone marrow transplantation was first demonstrated in an 8-year-old girl who was suffering from both acute myeloid leukemia and sickle cell anemia. Following bone marrow transplantation, the hemoglobin S level was reduced to that of the bone marrow donor, who had sickle cell trait (Fig. 61.1). The patient's course following transplant was complicated by moderately severe, but transient, acute and chronic graft-versus-host disease (GVHD) predominantly involving her skin and gastrointestinal tract, and hypogonadism. This patient is now 20 years from transplantation, in excellent general health and with no evidence of recurrence of her sickle cell anemia or leukemia (Johnson *et al.*, 1984).

Over 150 patients worldwide have subsequently been treated for sickle cell anemia by allogeneic bone marrow transplantation using HLA-matched sibling donors (the vast majority) or HLA-matched sibling umbilical cord blood as the source of HSC (Bernaudin, 1999; Brichard *et al.*, 1996; Johnson, 1996; Vermylen *et al.*, 1998; Walters *et al.*, 2000, 2001).

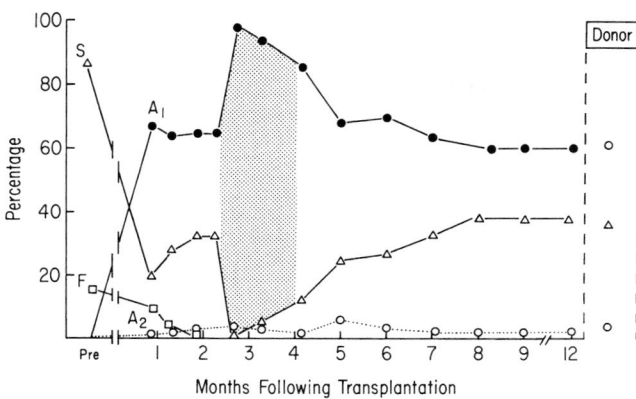

Fig. 61.1. Hemoglobin electrophoretic pattern before and after marrow transplantation for sickle cell anemia. Shaded area indicates a period of red cell transfusions during acute GVHD. Reprinted, with permission, from Johnson *et al.* (1984).

The criteria for selection for treatment by HSC transplantation has usually been younger patients with severe disease due to recurrent vaso-occlusive crises (the most common indication in European studies), stroke (the most common indications in North American studies), or recurrent infections. In a worldwide compilation of the results of marrow transplantation in 147 children with sickle cell disease treated by matched allogeneic HSC transplantation, the commonest indications for transplantation were veno-occlusive crises (66%), acute chest syndrome (31%—some overlap with patients with veno-occlusive crises), and a stroke or prior CNS event (29%) (Fixler *et al.*, 2001).

The most commonly used preparative regimen has been busulfan 3.5 to 4 mg/kg/day for 4 days and cyclophosphamide 50 mg/kg/day for 4 days, with or without antithymocyte globulin (ATG) or thoraco-abdominal irradiation. Complete engraftment has been achieved in over 75% of patients following such a preparative regimen (Walters, 1999). The most common GVHD prophylactic regimens have included cyclosporine with or without methotrexate, methotrexate alone, or corticosteroids added to either of these regimens.

Studies from the United States and Europe demonstrate survival and event-free survival of 92% to 94% and 75% to 84%, respectively (Walters, 1999). In the largest survey published to date involving 147 patients, the overall survival was 93% and the event-free survival was 82%. Graft failure occurred in 13 patients (9%), acute GVHD in 47 patients (32%), and chronic GVHD in 15 patients (10%) (Fixler *et al.*, 2001). In a study of 127 patients transplanted in centers in the United States and Europe, with a follow-up of 42 months (range 0.2–132 months), the overall survival and disease-free survival rates were 91% and 77%, respectively. The rejection rate was 13% and the incidence of acute and chronic GVHD was 26% and 13%, respectively. Six of the 11 patients who died posttransplant had severe chronic GVHD (Walters, 1999).

The most recent update on a trial involving 24 centers in the United States and Europe provides data on longer-term follow-up of children treated for sickle cell disease by matched sibling allogeneic marrow transplantation. Fifty children (median age 9.4 years, range 3.3–14.0 years) were so treated between 1991 and 1999 (Walters *et al.*, 2000). The criteria for selection for treatment by marrow transplantation included younger patients with severe sickle cell disease but without significant end organ dysfunction. With a median follow-up of 4.7 years (range 3.2–7.9 years), 47 of the 50 patients survive with the overall 6-year Kaplan-Meier probability of survival and event-free survival being 94% and 84%, respectively (Fig. 61.2) (Walters *et al.*, 2000). Graft failure and recurrence of the sickle cell disease occurred in 5 patients, 4 patients had stable mixed chimerism, and 38 patients had full donor chimerism. Three patients died, 1 due to an intracranial hemorrhage, and 2 from complications of chronic GVHD. All but one patient with full donor cell engraftment had Karnofsky or Lansky Play Performance scores of 100% and no engrafted patient suffered recurrence of vaso-occlusive crises. A further update of this experience confirmed the significant therapeutic effect of mixed chimerism (Walters *et al.*, 2001). Of 59 patients, 55 survived, 50 of them disease-free. Of the latter 50, 13 developed stable mixed chimerism: in 5 patients the level of donor chimerism measured more than 6 months posttransplant varied between 11% and 74%. Their Hb levels ranged from 11.2 to 14.2 g/dl. Three of these patients, whose donors had a normal Hb genotype, had Hb S fractions of 7%, 0%, and 0%, corresponding to donor chimerism levels of 11%, 67%, and 74%, respectively. The other two, whose donors had sickle trait, had Hb S fractions of 36% and 37%, corresponding to donor chimerism levels of 25% and 60%, respectively. Clearly, the use of non-myeloablative condition-

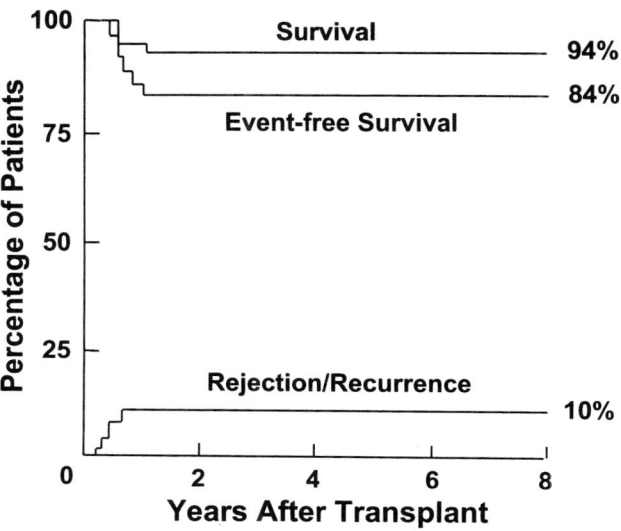

Fig. 61.2. Kaplan-Meier estimates of survival and event-free survival after bone marrow transplantation in 50 children with sickle cell disease. Modified and reprinted, with permission, from Walters *et al.* (2000).

ing regimens, to produce mixed chimerism with a lower risk of regimen-related toxicity may be of value in this regard (Kean *et al.*, 2002), although better control of GVHD is also necessary (Slavin *et al.*, 1998; van Besien *et al.*, 2000).

Twenty-six patients in this study had been followed for at least 2 years after transplantation and were evaluated for late effects. Three of these patients had developed grade I–III acute GVHD and two had chronic GVHD. Twenty-two patients had stable engraftment of donor cells, and four patients suffered graft rejection with return of their sickle cell disease.

Nineteen of the 26 patients had central nervous system (CNS) abnormalities related to sickle cell disease. After transplantation 10 patients with a prior history of stroke had stable or improved cerebral magnetic resonance imaging (MRI) and none had suffered a subsequent stroke. Similarly, none of 4 patients with an evidence of silent cerebral infarction had a stroke posttransplantation. Two of 3 patients had stable cerebral MRI scans and another who developed new MRI lesions 1 month after transplantation, subsequently had stable studies.

Pulmonary function studies were stable in 22 of 24 evaluable patients and worse in 2 patients. Seven of 8 patients transplanted because of recurrent acute chest syndrome demonstrated stable pulmonary function after transplantation and none had suffered another episode of the acute chest syndrome. One patient who died of obliterative bronchiolitis continued to suffer from obstructive pulmonary disease after transplantation.

Studies of linear growth also showed improvement in most patients after transplantation, although a decreased rate of growth velocity has been associated with chronic GVHD. All children tested had normal thyroid function after transplantation. Busulfan-containing conditioning regimens were associated with subsequent abnormal ovarian function in 5 of 7 evaluable females 13 years of age or older. None of 4 males tested had elevated gonadotropin levels. In a Belgian series, 5 of 6 prepubertal girls had primary amenorrhea and 4 of 6 boys with normal development demonstrated decreased testosterone and elevated FSH levels (Vermylen *et al.*, 1998).

Thus, although the majority of children treated by HSC transplantation appeared to be cured of sickle cell disease, significant morbidity due to transplant-related complications remains a challenge.

Recognition of these complications and therapeutic intervention have, however, led to decreased morbidity and mortality following transplantation. For example, initial studies indicated that patients with sickle cell anemia exhibited an increased risk of neurologic complications after marrow transplantation, particularly those with a history of prior stroke who appeared to have an increased risk of intracerebral bleeding. In a report of 21 patients treated by HLA-matched sibling marrow transplantation for sickle cell anemia, 7 developed neurologic complications at a median of 1 month (range 5–243 days) after transplantation (Walters *et al.*, 1995). All patients were prepared with busulfan and cyclophosphamide, with or without ATG and received cyclosporine, with or without methotrexate or prednisone, for GVHD prevention. Seizures were the most common

complication, occurring in 6 patients and completely resolving in all but 1 patient. Hypertension was present in 4 of these patients, in contrast to being detected in only one of the patients who did not suffer a seizure. Three patients suffered an intracranial hemorrhage posttransplant that proved fatal in two of these patients. In the 8 patients with a history of stroke prior to transplant, 4 developed a neurologic complication posttransplant compared with 3 of 13 patients who did not have a history of stroke. Of most concern was the observation that among the patients who had suffered a stroke prior to transplant, the incidence of posttransplant intracranial hemorrhage was 38% (3 of 8) versus zero for the 13 patients without such a history. Of the 7 patients who suffered a neurologic event after transplantation, 3 were thrombocytopenic and 3 relatively polycythemic at the time of the neurologic complication.

This experience was observed by other investigators who described an increased risk of seizures in this setting. Five of 12 patients in one study had a history of stroke before transplant. Three of these 5 patients suffered seizures after transplant, compared with only 1 of the 7 children who did not have a pretransplant neurologic event (Ferster *et al.*, 1995). In a survey of North American transplant centers, 16 of 22 evaluable patients had a prior history of a cerebrovascular accident, and 7 of these 16 patients developed a neurologic complication following transplantation, including 2 patients who died of intracerebral hemorrhage. None of the 6 patients who had not suffered a stroke pretransplant developed a neurologic complication posttransplant. Again, the use of cyclosporine to prevent GVHD, thrombocytopenia, and hypertension was associated with these neurologic complications (Johnson, 1996).

These experiences led to modification of the transplant regimen in 1993 including phenytoin prophylaxis with busulfan-containing preparative regimens and while the patient was receiving cyclosporine, strict control of hypertension, prompt repletion of magnesium deficiency, maintenance of hemoglobin levels between 9 and 11 g/dl, and platelet counts greater than 50,000/mm³. In the multicenter trial noted above, no patient has suffered an intracranial hemorrhage while these measures were used to prevent CNS complications (Walters *et al.*, 2000).

Controversies

Despite these promising results, the use of stem cell transplantation to treat sickle cell disease continues to be characterized by controversy including the iatrogenic risks of the treatment, the indications for, and timing of, transplantation, and acceptance of the therapy by affected patients and their families.

Iatrogenic risks

Table 61.1 summarizes the potential risks and benefits to be considered in the treatment of sickle cell disease by either supportive care or transplantation. In reviewing the results of the international cooperative transplant trial cited, Platt and Guinan

Table 61.1. *Risks and benefits of treatment of sickle cell disease by supportive care or HSC transplantation*

	Supportive care	HSC transplant
Benefits	Not immediately life-threatening	>75% chance of cure
Risks	Transfusion-related	Transplant-related
	Iron overload	Graft failure
	Infection	Acute GVHD
	CMV	Chronic GVHD
	Hepatitis	Infection
	HIV	Late effects
	Alloimmunization	
	Chronic organ damage	

Abbreviations: CMV, cytomegalovirus; HIV, human immuno-deficiency virus; GVHD, graft-versus-host disease; HSC, hematopoietic stem cell.

(1996) noted that of the 22 children with sickle cell disease treated by HLA-matched sibling transplantation, 15 (68%) were cured, but were at risk for infertility, chemotherapy-induced malignancy, or other late complications, and that the overall mortality rate following transplant approximated 10%. This is compared with a death rate of 1% among children with sickle cell disease in the first decade of life. The potential iatrogenic complications of transplantation are more readily accepted when the treatment is proposed for an immediately life-threatening disease, such as severe aplastic anemia. Sickle cell disease, however, is of uncertain prognosis in the individual patient and not immediately life-threatening.

One way to reduce posttransplant morbidity and mortality is to perform the procedure early in life, ideally in infancy. The incidence of severe GVHD appears to be age-related, and transplantation earlier in the patient's course avoids therapeutic failure due to already established complications of the disease or its conventional therapy. In the Belgian experience a significantly higher incidence of complications such as graft failure and recurrent sickle cell disease was observed in older patients following transplantation (Vermylen *et al.*, 1998). Some centers have proposed transplanting children as young as possible at the first sign of any complication. The suggestion has also been made that clinical trials comparing matched allogeneic HSC transplantation and other available therapies in infants with sickle cell disease should now be conducted before any complications have occurred (Piomelli, 1991). Although perhaps of objective scientific merit, these suggestions still appear premature, given that as many as one-half of infants with sickle cell anemia may never face a life-threatening event, and because it is currently impossible to predict the course of sickle cell anemia in an individual patient.

These risk-benefit issues related to treating sickle cell anemia by marrow transplantation were considered in a mock "trial" in London over a decade ago. The motion that "bone marrow transplantation should forthwith be offered to all children in the U.K. with sickle cell anemia who have HLA-compatible siblings" resulted in no unanimous verdict from a jury of seven individuals, each of whom had an interest in sickle cell anemia but no special expertise in marrow transplantation or the disease itself. They heard evidence from hematologists experienced in the treatment of sickle cell anemia who disagreed on the role of marrow transplantation. The majority verdict was against the motion as stated, but the jury did not feel qualified to suggest a suitable amendment to the motion (Roberts & Davies, 1993). This interesting exercise exemplifies the dilemma that still remains true today.

Indications and timing

Studies to identify those at risk who may benefit from early intervention with treatment by HSC transplantation, however, are becoming increasingly important as neurologic, renal, and pulmonary complications become more frequent causes of severe morbidity and premature death in young adults with sickle cell disease. Several genetic, clinical, and laboratory factors have been proposed to be of prognostic value, although most still need to be confirmed as larger cohort studies have produced conflicting results (Table 61.2). For example, identification of the β gene status and the β^s gene-cluster haplotype were thought to have predictive value. Sickle cell patients who inherit β-thalassemia were thought to suffer fewer complications with a lower mortality. Patients with the Sen (Senegalese) β gene cluster haplotype were thought to have less severe disease than patients who were homozygous for the CAR (Central African Republic) β globin gene haplotype. It was estimated that a newborn with a CAR chromosome who has the normal

Table 61.2. *Genetic, clinical, and laboratory features with potential prognostic significance in sickle cell anemia*

Prognostic feature	Prognosis		
	Better	Intermediate	Worse
β^s-GCH	Senegal	Benin	Central African Republic[a]
α gene	α thalassemia-2[a]		Frequent pain crises
Clinical	↑HbF[a]		Acute chest syndrome[a]
			Dactylitis in first year
			Renal failure
			Seizures
			↓HbF[a]
			Hemoglobin <7 g/dl
			WBC > 15,000/mm^3
			Silent cerebral ischemia

Abbreviations: GCH, gene-cluster haplotype.
[a] Not confirmed in Cooperative Study of Sickle Cell Disease (Miller *et al.*, 2000).

complement of genes would have an 80% risk of major organ damage by age 40 (Powars, 1991).

Laboratory findings thought to be indicative of more severe disease included decreased levels of fetal hemoglobin (HbF) and a baseline white cell count above 15,000/mm^3. A high level of fetal hemoglobin appeared to predict improved survival, and was considered a reliable forecaster of adult life expectancy, with patients having a fetal hemoglobin level above the 75th percentile showing statistically improved survival (Platt et al., 1994). In this study early mortality was highest among patients with symptomatic disease, with the occurrence of the acute chest syndrome, renal failure, and seizures being associated with an increased risk of early death (Platt et al., 1994). Other studies have also suggested that patients over the age of 20 with more frequent painful crises have higher mortality rates. Silent cerebral ischemia discovered on MRI scans results in impaired cognitive functioning, and recurrent episodes of the acute chest syndrome appeared to predispose to pulmonary failure in the second and third decades of life (Platt et al., 1991; Powars, 1991; Vichinsky, 1991).

However, an analysis from the Cooperative Study of Sickle Cell Disease of a cohort of 392 infants followed from infancy to age 10 years did not confirm many of these findings. For example, the percentage of steady-state fetal hemoglobin, the presence of α thalassemia trait, the β globin gene haplotype, and frequent episodes of the acute chest syndrome did not predict the future severity of disease (Miller et al., 2000). Three clinical features were found associated with more severe disease—dactylitis before age 1, a steady-state hemoglobin level of less than 7 g/dl, and leukocytosis in the absence of infection (>13,000/mm^3).

Of particular interest from this analysis is that leukocytosis in the absence of infection is confirmed as a prognostic factor, but the HbF level is not. This raises the question of the mechanism of action of cytotoxic drugs, such as hydroxyurea, in preventing crises. Historically it has been thought that such drugs are effective because they raise the HbF level, but perhaps such agents may be effective primarily because they decrease the number of circulating leukocytes.

The investigators concluded from this analysis that a group of patients could be identified as being at "high risk" for severe disease and in whom more intensive therapies such as HSC transplantation might be warranted. They constructed a model defining a group of children with early dactylitis, lower hemoglobin levels, and leukocytosis in the absence of infection whose probability of severe disease was 36%, twice the rate of severe disease in the general sickle cell disease population. This group, however, consisted of only 3% of the entire cohort studied.

Thus, accurate combinations of genetic, clinic, and laboratory predictive factors still remain to be defined to allow the certain identification of patients for whom the benefit of transplantation outweighs the risks. This is particularly important because, in the cited study of mortality and sickle cell disease, one in three patients who died during an acute sickle cell crisis did not have organ failure (Platt et al., 1994).

At the present time, then, it is difficult to justify allogeneic HSC transplantation in an infant before the particular clinical pattern of his or her illness becomes obvious. In addition, further blunting the overall impact of stem cell transplantation in curing sickle cell anemia is the apparent difficulty of finding a suitably HLA-matched family member donor. In a review of the medical records of 143 patients with sickle cell anemia under the age of 16 years, probability calculations indicated that an HLA-matched sibling would only be available as a donor for 18% of afflicted patients (Mentzer et al., 1994).

The role of HSC transplantation in children with evidence of CNS vasculopathy, either overt or covert, is particularly controversial. Studies involving large numbers of children and adolescents with sickle cell disease have demonstrated up to an 11% incidence of clinical stroke in the first 18 years of life (Steen et al., 2001). In addition, the Cooperative Study of Sickle Cell Disease showed 17% of patients with hemoglobin SS had silent infarcts (CNS ischemic changes in a patient with no clinical history of stroke) detected by cerebral MRI. These findings correlated with impaired neuropsychological performance, which worsened in older patients even in the absence of new MRI lesions (Walters et al., 1999; Steen et al., 2001). Magnetic resonance angiography (MRA) has expanded these findings, one study suggesting that about one-third of young sickle cell patients have vasculopathy involving the major arteries of the brain. About 36% of sickle cell patients under age 5 have abnormalities of the basilar artery and abnormally enlarged arteries can be present in children under 1 year of age (Steen et al., 2001). These findings indicate that vasculopathy may be one of the earliest indicators of significant neurologic disease and are consistent with previous clinical experience cited that existing vasculopathy predisposes patients who have had a stroke pretransplant to neurologic complications posttransplant.

Evidence suggests that allogeneic marrow transplantation may prevent infarctive strokes, reversing the progression of CNS vasculopathy associated with sickle cell disease by reversing stenotic lesions, enabling the diameter of the CNS vasculature to increase and reducing cranial blood flow velocity. Twenty-four patients with sickle cell disease aged 7 years or older were studied with baseline and follow-up MRA. Four patients who received an allogeneic bone marrow transplant were compared to 7 patients who received other therapy, and to 13 untreated patients. There was a 10% increase in the measured diameter of vessels following any treatment. The patients treated by allogeneic bone marrow transplantation exhibited a 12% increase in the lumen of 22 vessels and those treated with chronic transfusion or hydroxyurea exhibited an 8% increase in 42 vessels. In two transplanted patients with severe stenosis the artery normalized after transplantation. The blood flow rate was also reduced in patients treated by transplantation. In 13 untreated patients there was a trend for the size of the arterial lumen to decrease, consistent with disease progression (Steen et al., 2001).

In accordance with the observation by Steen and colleagues, other investigators have also demonstrated that chronic transfusion therapy can reverse CNS vasculopathy. Forty-seven (37%) of 127 patients evaluated in a study by Pegelow and colleagues had evidence of silent infarcts. Transfusion therapy lowered the risk for the development of new silent infarcts or stroke for children having both abnormal transcranial Doppler (TCD) ultrasonography velocity and MRI-detected silent infarcts (Pegelow *et al.*, 2001).

So what is the best treatment for a child with evidence of CNS vasculopathy who has a stroke identified by TCD, has a suitable source of HSCs for transplantation, but no other indications for treatment by transplantation—allogeneic HSC transplantation or chronic transfusion therapy? An interesting exercise addressed this question constructing Markov models with intent to treat, representing the clinical course after marrow transplantation and prophylactic red blood cell transfusions (Nietert *et al.*, 2000). This analysis indicated that for those patients whose only indication for transplantation is abnormal cerebral blood flow neither treatment has a substantial advantage, and that marrow transplantation is not the best strategy. From their decision analysis the outlook would be best for those patients who were treated by prophylactic red blood cell transfusions and chelation. In addition, it has been estimated that 40% of patients identified as having high stroke risk by TCD will never suffer a stroke (Cohen, 1998).

Thus, although no episodes of intracranial hemorrhages have been observed in the large multicenter trial since instituting the CNS preventative measures described above, further follow-up is still necessary to determine if HSC transplantation is superior to prophylactic red blood cell transfusion therapy and chelation in preventing intracranial hemorrhage in the long term (Walters *et al.*, 2000).

Stroke or silent cerebral ischemia remain controversial indications for HSC transplantation, but is there a time when the vasculopathy is so severe that transplantation is not indicated? In the Cooperative Group transplant study there appeared to be posttransplant stabilization of cerebrovascular disease in most patients, but progression of large vessel pathology occurred after transplantation in one child transplanted after suffering a stroke. This patient had multiple stenotic cerebral vessels and moyamoya disease demonstrated on MRI scanning pretransplant. Six months following the transplant the patient suffered a seizure and neurologic imaging revealed progression of large vessel pathology despite significant improvement in cortical perfusion on an MRI perfusion scan (Kalinyak *et al.*, 1995). In addition, reports on MRA findings posttransplant have been conflicting. Although patients have been reported to have qualitative improvements in the appearance of the cerebral vasculature, other patients with significant moyamoya vessel formation prior to transplant have shown deterioration on follow-up studies (Steen *et al.*, 2001).

These observations raise the question of whether transplantation is indicated in patients with extensive neuropathology associated with sickle cell disease, particularly moyamoya disease. Although the underlying sickle cell anemia may be cured, pretransplant damage to the cerebral vasculature in this setting is probably not reversible, or may even be worsened by the transplant procedure (Kalinyak *et al.*, 1995).

Acceptance of the therapy

Results of parent-patient questionnaires in two U.S. centers have indicated that parents want the opportunity to decide if transplantation is an option (Vickinsky, 1991). In the International Cooperative transplant study, only 10% of patients who met the eligibility criteria in this analysis for HSC transplantation declined to proceed with HLA typing, and among those with a suitable donor, only 16% refused transplantation (Sullivan *et al.*, 1996). These data conflict with a previously published survey to determine whether parents would accept significant iatrogenic risks of transplantation for the chance of cure of their child's sickle cell disease, where only a small minority consented to transplantation. Almost one in four parents would not accept any risk and only 13% would accept a 15% mortality risk and an additional 15% risk of GVHD (Kodish *et al.*, 1991). Surprisingly, the parents' decisions were not related to the severity of their child's illness.

In contrast, in a similar questionnaire study of adult patients (median age 36 years, range 19–60 years) a substantial proportion were interested in curative treatment at the expense of significant risk. Sixty-three of 100 patients were willing to accept some short-term risk of mortality in exchange for cure (van Besien *et al.*, 2001). Fifteen patients were willing to accept more than a 35% mortality risk. Twenty-eight patients were unwilling to accept any risk of death within 30 days for the chance of a cure. Of interest, the proportion of patients for whom transplant would be recommended varied greatly among the health care providers—from less than 10% to 60%, and there was an absolute lack of agreement between the provider's recommendation and the patient's decision. These investigators concluded that adults with sickle cell disease should be given the option of considering transplantation and reiterated the conclusion from the earlier pediatric study by Kodish and colleagues that "patients may not think about risks and benefits the way doctors do."

The study also confirms other data indicating a wide disparity in the concept of who is or who is not qualified for transplant. In a survey of 22 centers the proportion of patients who qualified for transplant protocols ranged from 0.9% to 36% in different centers, indicating radically different attitudes among physicians regarding indications for transplantation in children (van Besien *et al.*, 2001).

Future directions

Non-myeloablative conditioning regimens

Studies are now being undertaken, in both malignant and nonmalignant disorders, to develop non-myeloablative, and consequently less toxic, conditioning regimens aimed at enabling sufficient engraftment of donor cells to eliminate the underlying disease. This approach can establish durable mixed chimerism and utilizes posttransplant immunosuppression to control host-versus-graft and graft-versus-host reactions (Slavin *et al.,* 1998; van Besien *et al.,* 2000). Non-myeloablative matched sibling allogeneic marrow transplantation has been reported in the treatment of at least three children with sickle cell disease. In an 8-year-old girl with symptomatic sickle cell disease, including history of a stroke, veno-occlusive crises, and the acute chest syndrome, the conditioning regimen consisted of busulfan 2 mg/kg every 12 hours for 2 days, fludarabine 35 mg/m^2 i.v. daily for 5 days, ATG, and 500 cGy total lymphoid irradiation (TLI). GVHD prophylaxis consisted of cyclosporine and mycophenolate mofetil (MMF). The patient achieved full chimerism by day 60 and remained disease-free without complications 14 months after transplantation (Krishnamurti *et al.,* 2001). Two other children with symptomatic sickle cell disease were reported to have benefited at 6 months follow-up after treatment with a non-myeloablative TBI-fludarabine regimen, matched sibling marrow transplantation, and GVHD prophylaxis with tacrolimus and MMF (Iannone *et al.,* 2001). Two multiply transfused adult patients with end-stage sickle cell disease demonstrated durable engraftment following a fludarabine/melphalan/ATG-based non-myeloablative conditioning regimen followed by a matched sibling marrow transplant, but both died of complications related to severe GVHD (van Besien *et al.,* 2000).

Armado and Schiller (2000) described a clinical trial using a purine analogue-based non-myeloablative chemotherapy conditioning regimen followed by related allogeneic peripheral blood stem cell transplantation as an approach for the treatment of severe sickle cell disease in young adults. The ability to develop less toxic preparative regimens and rely on posttransplant immunological manipulation is illustrated in a report of a child with sickle cell disease whose matched sibling allograft was complicated by decreasing mixed chimerism. Following donor lymphocyte infusions, the patient developed grade II acute GVHD which responded well to corticosteroids and cyclosporine. Complete donor chimerism was established 2 months after a second infusion and the patient remained disease free with a follow-up of 2 years (Baron *et al.,* 2000).

Use of alternative donors

Based on experience in transplantation for a variety of malignant and nonmalignant disorders, the use of alternate sources of HSC, including umbilical cord blood (UCB) cells and matched unrelated marrow or peripheral blood cells, would increase the number of patients suffering from sickle cell disease who might benefit from HSC transplantation. A successful transplant in sickle cell disease using HLA-matched sibling UCB cells has been reported (Brichard *et al.,* 1996), but the overall impact of this approach in sickle cell disease remains to be determined. UCB transplantation is associated with a higher risk of rejection and some risk of GVHD.

Improvements in the results of HLA-matched unrelated HSC transplants have resulted in studies showing equivalent outcomes after transplantation in children and young adults with acute lymphoblastic leukemia and chronic myeloid leukemia in chronic phase treated by matched sibling or matched unrelated donor marrow transplantation (Hongeng *et al.,* 1997; Hansen *et al.,* 1998). This raises the possibility of using a matched unrelated donor in transplants for a variety of genetic disorders.

Conclusions

The results from studies to date indicate that HSC transplantation is effective in stabilizing or reversing the complications of severe sickle cell disease, including pre-existing neurologic damage, respiratory function in patients with a prior history of acute chest syndrome, and splenic recovery in patients with pretransplant splenic dysfunction (Abboud *et al.,* 1994; Walters *et al.,* 1996). However, the impact of HSC transplantation in the treatment of sickle cell disease still remains limited until problems related to the toxicity and immunologic complications of transplantation are solved, and better prognostic factors are identified and confirmed.

Table 61.3. *Suggested criteria for eligibility for stem cell transplantation in patients with sickle cell anemia[a]*

Indications
HLA-identical donor
One or more of the following:
　Stroke or central nervous system event lasting longer than 24 hours
　Acute chest syndrome with recurrent hospitalizations or previous exchange transfusions
　Recurrent vaso-occlusive pain (≥2 episodes per year for several years) or recurrent priapism
　Impaired neuropsychological function and abnormal cerebral MRI scan
　Stage I or II sickle lung disease
　Sickle nephropathy (moderate or severe proteinuria or a glomerular filtration rate 30% to 50% of the predicted normal value)
　Bilateral proliferative retinopathy and significant visual impairment in at least one eye
　Osteonecrosis involving multiple joints
　Red cell alloimmunization (≥2 antibodies) during long-term transfusion therapy
Exclusion criteria
One or more of the following:
　Karnofsky or Lansky functional performance score <70
　Acute hepatitis or evidence of moderate to severe portal fibrosis or cirrhosis on biopsy
　Severe renal impairment (glomerular filtration rate <30% of the predicted normal value)
　Severe residual functional neurologic impairment (other than hemiplegia alone)
　Stage III or IV sickle lung disease
　Demonstrated lack of compliance with medical care
　Seropositivity for the human immunodeficiency virus

[a] Modified from Walters *et al.* (1996).

In addition, while stem cell transplantation is restricted to patients with donors matched at the major histocompatibility complex, only a minority of patients with sickle cell anemia can be so treated. Expansion of relevant donor registries, decreased toxicity enabled by effective non-myeloablative transplant protocols, improvements in outcome of HLA-mismatched transplantation, and the ready availability of alternative sources of allogeneic stem cells, such as cord blood banks, may eventually increase the number of patients for whom HSC transplantation is an appropriate therapy.

The outcome for reported patients suggests that stem cell transplantation should be considered as a therapeutic option in selected younger patients suffering significant morbidity from sickle cell anemia as defined in the Cooperative Group transplant trial (Table 61.3). In settings where optimum supportive care is not available, it appears ethical to broaden these indications. A major aim of ongoing studies of large populations of sickle cell patients is to identify genetic and clinical features that will help to predict those patients who are likely to suffer significant morbidity from sickle cell disease and who will benefit most from allogeneic stem cell transplantation early in the course of their disease.

References

Abboud, M.R., Jackson, S.M., Barredo, J. *et al.* (1994). Bone marrow transplantation for sickle cell anemia. *American Journal of Pediatric Hematology/Oncology,* **16,** 86–9.

Armado, R.G. & Schiller, G.F. (2000). Nonmyeloablative approaches to the treatment of sickle hemoglobinopathies. *Seminars in Oncology,* **27,** 82–9.

Baron, F., Dresse, M.F., & Beguan, Y. (2000). Donor lymphocyte infusion to eradicate recurrent host hematopoiesis after allogeneic BMT for sickle cell disease. *Transfusion,* **40,** 1071–3.

Bernaudin, E. (1999). Resultats et indications actuelles de l'allogreffe de moelle dans drepanocytose. *Pathologie et Biologie,* **47,** 59–64.

Brichard, B., Vermylen, C., Ninane, J., & Cornu, G. (1996). Persistence of fetal hemoglobin production after successful transplantation of cord blood stem cells in a patient with sickle cell anemia. *Journal of Pediatrics,* **128,** 241–3.

Cohen, A.R. (1998). Sickle disease—new treatments and questions. *New England Journal of Medicine,* **339,** 42–4.

Ferster, A., Christopher, C., Dan, B. *et al.* (1995). Neurologic complications after bone marrow transplantation for sickle cell anemia. *Blood,* **86,** 408–9.

Fixler, J., Vichinsky, E., & Walters, M. (2001). Stem cell transplantation for sickle cell disease: can we reduce the toxicity? *Pediatric Pathology and Molecular Medicine,* **20,** 73–86.

Hansen, J.A., Gooley, T.A., Martin, P.J. *et al.* (1998). Bone marrow transplants from unrelated donors for patients with chronic myeloid leukemia. *New England Journal of Medicine,* **338,** 962–8.

Hongeng, S., Krance, R.A., Bowman, L.C. *et al.* (1997). Outcomes of transplantation with matched-sibling and unrelated-donor bone marrow in children with leukemia. *Lancet,* **350,** 767–71.

Iannone, R., Chen, A.R., Goodman, S.N. *et al.* (2001). Treatment of sickle cell anemia in two patients using non-myeloablative bone marrow transplantation. *Blood,* **98,** 490a (Abstract).

Johnson, F.L. (1996). Bone marrow transplantation for sickle cell anemia—the North American experience. Sixth Biennial Symposium on Blood Cell and Bone Marrow Transplants, Keystone, Colorado, January 1996.

Johnson, F.L., Look, A.T., Gockerman, J. *et al.* (1984). Bone marrow transplantation in a patient with sickle cell anemia. *New England Journal of Medicine,* **311,** 780–3.

Kalinyak, K.A., Morris, C., Ball, W.S. *et al.* (1995). Bone marrow transplantation for a young child with sickle cell anemia. *American Journal of Hematology,* **48,** 256–61.

Kean, L.S., Durham, M.M., Adams, A.B. *et al.* (2002). A cure for murine sickle cell disease through stable mixed chimerism and tolerance induction after nonmyeloablative conditioning and major histocompatibility complex-mismatched bone marrow transplantation. *Blood,* **99,** 1840–9.

Kodish, E., Lantos, J., Stocking, C. *et al.* (1991). Bone marrow transplantation for sickle cell disease. A study of parents' decisions. *New England Journal of Medicine,* **325,** 1349–53.

Krishnamurti, L., Bilazer, B.R. Wagner, J.E. (2001). Bone marrow transplantation without myeloablation for sickle cell disease. *New England Journal of Medicine,* **344,** 68.

Lubin, B. & Vichinsky, E.P. (1991). Sickle cell disease. In *Hematology, Basic Principles and Practice,* ed. R. Hoffman, E.J. Berg, Jr., S.J. Shattil, *et al.,* pp. 450–71. New York: Churchill Livingstone.

Mentzer, W.C., Heller, S., Pearle, P.R. *et al.* (1994). Availability of related donors for bone marrow transplantation in sickle cell anemia. *American Journal of Pediatric Hematology/ Oncology,* **16,** 27–9.

Miller, S.T., Sleeper, L.A., Pegelow, C.H. *et al.* (2000). Prediction of adverse outcomes in children with sickle cell disease. *New England Journal of Medicine,* **342,** 83–9.

Nietert, P.J., Abboud, M.R., Silverstein, M.D., & Jackson, S.M. (2000). Bone marrow transplantation versus periodic blood transfusion in sickle cell patients at high risk of ischemic stroke: a decision analysis. *Blood,* **95,** 3057–64.

Pegelow, C.H., Wang, W., Granger, S. *et al.* (2001). Silent infarcts in children with sickle cell anemia and abnormal cerebral artery velocity. *Archives of Neurology,* **58,** 2017–21.

Piomelli, S. (1991). Sickle cell disease in the 1990's: the need for active and preventive intervention. *Seminars in Hematology,* **28,** 227–32.

Platt, O., Brambilla, D., Rosse, W.F. *et al.* (1994). Mortality in sickle cell disease. Life expectancy and risk factors for early death. *New England Journal of Medicine,* **330,** 1639–44.

Platt, O. & Guinin, E.C. (1996). Bone marrow transplantation in sickle cell anemia—the dilemma of choice. *New England Journal of Medicine,* **335,** 426–7.

Platt, O.S., Thorington, B.C., Brambilla, D.T. *et al.* (1991). Pain in sickle cell disease: rates and risk factors. *New England Journal of Medicine,* **325,** 11–6.

Powars, D.R. (1991). Sickle cell anemia: β^s-gene-cluster haplotypes as prognostic indicators of vital organ failure. *Seminars in Hematology,* **28,** 202–8.

Roberts, I.A.G. & Davies, S.C. (1993). Sickle cell disease: the transplant issue. *Bone Marrow Transplantation,* **11,** 253–4.

Slavin, S., Nagler, A., Naparstek, E. *et al.* (1998). Nonmyeloablative stem cell transplantation and cell therapy cytoreduction for the treatment of malignant and nonmalignant hematologic diseases. *Blood,* **91,** 756–63.

Smith, J.A. (1991). What do we know about the clinical course of sickle cell disease? *Seminars in Hematology,* **28,** 299–312.

Steen, R.G., Helton, K.J., Horowitz, E.N. *et al.* (2001). Improved cerebrovascular patency following therapy in patients with sickle cell disease: Initial results in four patients who received HLA-identical hematopoietic stem cell allografts. *Annals of Neurology,* **49,** 222–9.

Steinberg, M.H. (1999). Management of sickle cell disease. *New England Journal of Medicine,* **340,** 1021–30.

Sullivan, K.M., Walters, M.C., & Ohene-Frempong, K. (1996). Bone marrow transplantation for sickle cell disease—reply. *New England Journal of Medicine,* **335,** 1845–6.

Thomas, E.D., Buckner, C.D., Sanders, J.E. *et al.* (1982). Marrow transplantation for thalassemia. *Lancet,* **2,** 227–9.

van Besien, K., Bartholomew, A., Stock, W. *et al.* (2000). Fludarabine-based conditioning for allogeneic transplantation in adults with sickle cell disease. *Bone Marrow Transplantation,* **26,** 445–9.

van Besien, K., Koshy, M., Anderson-Shaw, L. *et al.* (2001). Allogeneic stem cell transplantation for sickle cell disease. A study of patients' decisions. *Bone Marrow Transplantation,* **28,** 545–9.

Vermylen, C., Cornu, G., Ferster, A. *et al.* (1998). Haematopoietic stem cell transplantation for sickle cell anemia: the first 50 patients transplanted in Belgium. *Bone Marrow Transplantation,* **22,** 1–6.

Vichinsky, E.P. (1991). Comprehensive care in sickle cell disease: its impact on morbidity and mortality. *Seminars in Hematology,* **28,** 220–6.

Walters, M.C. (1999). Bone marrow transplantation for sickle cell disease: where do we go from here? *Journal of Pediatric Hematology Oncology,* **21,** 467–74.

Walters, M.C., Patience, M., Leisenring, W. *et al.* (1996). Bone marrow transplantation for sickle cell disease. *New England Journal of Medicine,* **335,** 369–76.

Walters, M.C., Patience, W., Leisenring, W. *et al.* (2001). Stable mixed hematopoietic chimerism after bone marrow transplantation for sickle cell disease. *Biology of Blood and Marrow Transplantation,* **7,** 665–73.

Walters, M.C., Storb, R., Patience, M. *et al.* (2000). Impact of bone marrow transplantation for symptomatic sickle cell disease: an interim report. *Blood,* **95,** 1918–24.

Walters, M.C., Sullivan, K.M., Bernaudin, R. *et al.* (1995). Neurologic complications after allogeneic marrow transplantation for sickle cell anemia. *Blood,* **85,** 879–84.

Weiden, P.L., Storb, R., Graham, T.C. *et al.* (1967). Severe hereditary hemolytic anaemia in dogs treated by marrow transplantation. *British Journal of Haematology,* **33,** 357–9.

62 Allogeneic hematopoietic stem cell transplantation for congenital immune deficiencies

ALAIN FISCHER

Hôpital Necker-Enfants Malades, Paris, France

Introduction

Most primary immune deficiencies represent intrinsic defects of lymphocytic and/or phagocytic cell lineages. Therefore, replacement of genetically impaired hematopoietic stem cells (HSC) by normal HSC is a logical therapeutic approach. The first reports of successful bone marrow transplantation (BMT) for primary immune deficiencies were published in 1968: Gatti *et al.* (1968) described correction of severe combined immune deficiency (SCID) and Bach *et al.* (1968) partial correction of Wiskott-Aldrich syndrome (WAS). Since that time, it is estimated that over 3,000 patients with primary immune deficiency have undergone allogeneic HSC transplantation. About 28 different inherited immune deficiencies have been cured by transplantation (Table 62.1), including the different forms of SCID, other T-cell immune deficiencies, WAS, various phagocytic cell diseases, and more recently hyper IgM and XL proliferative syndromes. BMT has also been used as a source of mature T cells to correct, at least for some time, the severe T-cell lymphocytopenia observed in DiGeorge syndrome.[1] Based on a better understanding of major histocompatibility complex (MHC) molecular biology and the identification of T-cell-associated antigens, alternatives to transplantation from HLA-genetically identical donors have been proposed, including the use of related, partially HLA-matched donors as well as HLA-matched unrelated donors. Results of T-cell-depleted haploidentical family member transplantation will be discussed as will transplantation using unrelated donors, and the use of fetal liver cells as a source of HSC.

Fetal liver cell transplantation

In the 1970s, the use of HLA-mismatched fetal liver cells as a source of HSC to cure SCID patients without an HLA-identical donor was proposed. This was based on the knowledge that MHC disparate HSC could engraft and then generate T lymphocytes, which differentiated in the host thymus to become tolerant to the recipient's tissues. In a low proportion of cases (11%),

fetal liver transplantation was successful, leading to T- (and sometimes B-) cell differentiation without causing GVHD, provided that the fetal liver originated from a fetus not older than 12 weeks (O'Reilly *et al.*, 1989b). Some patients are alive and well with normal immune function 20 years after this procedure. However, the procedure often failed, and it required a very long time (1 to 2 years) before patients could safely leave the protected environment. In long-term surviving patients, interesting observations were made with regard to chimerism and tolerance. In a context where T cells were of donor origin, while B cells and monocytes were of host, and natural killer (NK) cells either of donor or host origin (Bacchetta *et al.*, 1993, 1995), it was found that donor antihost-reactive CD4+ and CD8+ T-cell clones could be derived, although no GVHD occurred. This dis-

Table 62.1. *Immune deficiencies that have been cured by hematopoietic stem cell transplantation*

Severe combined immune deficiencies
  Alymphocytosis (SCID without T cells or B cells)
  Absence of T lymphocytes (autosomal recessive and X-linked inheritance) (SCID with B cells)
  Adenosine deaminase deficiency
  Reticular dysgenesis
T-cell deficiencies
  Omenn's syndrome
  Defective T-cell activation (combined immunodeficiencies)
  ZAP (zeta-associated protein) 70 deficiency
  Purine nucleoside phosphorylase deficiency
  Major histocompatibility complex Class II deficiency
  Immune deficiency with cartilage – hair hypoplasia
Hyper IgM syndrome (HIGM-CD40L deficiency)
X-linked proliferative syndrome (XLP, Purtilo's syndrome)
Wiskott-Aldrich syndrome
Phagocytic cell diseases
  Agranulocytosis
  Leukocyte adhesion deficiency
  Chronic granulomatous disease
  Chediak-Higashi syndrome
  Familial hemophagocytic lymphohistiocytosis
  Immune deficiency with partial albinism (Griscelli's disease)
fas deficiency (lymphoproliferative syndrome with autoimmunity)

---

[1] Angelo DiGeorge, U.S. pediatrician, born 1921.

crepancy is likely accounted for by the high level of immuno-suppressive interleukin (IL)-10 production by antihost T cells, as well as by host non-T cells (Bacchetta *et al.,* 1994) These T cells produced low levels of IL-2. These surprising findings indicate that tolerance in this setting is mainly the consequence of a peripheral control mechanism.

Results of HLA-identical sibling transplantation for SCID

The severe combined immune deficiencies represent a group of diseases characterized by an inherited defect in T-, with or without B-, cell differentiation, resulting in the absence of mature T, with or without B, cells. The overall frequency is estimated at 1 in 75,000 live births. The three main SCID syndromes (Table 62.2) are SCID without T cells or B cells (alymphocytosis), in which T and B lymphocytes are absent while NK cells are present (as in the murine SCID model); SCID with B-cell-selective blockade of T-cell and NK-cell differentiation, which can be inherited either as an autosomal recessive, or more frequently, as an X-linked recessive disorder; and adenosine deaminase (ADA) deficiency. A fourth, even rarer type, is reticular dysgenesis characterized by both defective myelopoiesis and lymphopoiesis. The molecular basis of several SCID syndromes has been unraveled including the IL-2 receptor common gamma chain deficiency in X-linked SCID, JAK3 (kinase) deficiency in autosomal recessive B+ SCID, recombinase activating gene (Rag) 1/2 deficiencies, and Artemis deficiency in autosomal recessive B– SCID and IL-7 receptor-α deficiency. About 4% of patients with SCID have a defect of purine nucleoside phosphorylase (PNP). In the absence of HSC transplantation, SCID syndromes are fatal, usually within the first year of life.

Gatti *et al.* (1968) first reported the successful correction of SCID by allogeneic BMT. Since then at least 200 children with SCID have received an HLA-identical marrow transplant. Results have gradually improved due to earlier diagnosis, prevention of life-threatening complications such as transfusion-induced graft-versus-host disease (GVHD), and the availability of more effective antibiotics. In Europe, the cure rate has exceeded 90% since 1983 (Fischer *et al.,* 1990).

The most remarkable features of HLA-identical sibling marrow transplantation for SCID are the lack of an absolute requirement for conditioning (although most, if not all, patients transplanted for PNP deficiency have received a myeloablative conditioning regimen) (Classen *et al.,* 2001), the rarity of acute and chronic GVHD, and the rapid development of T- and B-cell function posttransplant. In most cases, only lymphocytes of donor origin develop. All myeloid and erythroid precursors remain of recipient origin, although an occasional exception to this has been described (Rubocki *et al.,* 2001). In pure T-cell deficiency SCID, donor-derived T lymphocytes coexist effectively with host-derived B lymphocytes (Fischer *et al.,* 1986; O'Reilly *et al.,* 1989a, 1990; Friedrich *et al.,* 1993; Buckley *et al.,* 1993; Buckley, 1995). It is unknown whether engraftment of stem cells occurs in the marrow with selective lineage differentiation, or whether stem cells differentiate in the thymus, or whether only mature donor T cells expand (as observed after transfer of mature T cells in athymic nude mice). The latter hypothesis may account for the rapid (within a few weeks) development of full immune function and the success of marrow transplantation as a cure of DiGeorge syndrome (Goldsobel *et al.,* 1987). The low incidence of GVHD may be related to the absence of a marrow-ablative regimen pretransplant, thus possibly sparing natural suppressor cells. In some patients, a partial B-cell immune deficiency persists including impaired production of IgA and sometimes of IgG_2 and IgG_4. It is not presently clear whether in these cases B-cell immune deficiency results from intrinsic host B-cell deficiency (as observed in X-linked SCID in which B cells are unresponsive to IL-2 and IL-15 but responsive in part to IL-4 and to IL-13), or whether another mechanism causes residual B-cell immune deficiency. A minority (<10%) of SCID patients who undergo HLA-identical sibling BMT are supplemented with intravenous immunoglobulin in the long term.

Results of HLA-mismatched family member transplantation for SCID

Only approximately 20% to 30% of SCID patients (as other potential HSC transplant recipients) have an HLA-identical sibling. HLA-phenotypically identical transplantation from

Table 62.2. *The main SCID syndromes*

Name	Other names	Inheritance pattern	Cellular defect	Molecular defect
SCID without B or T cells	Alymphocytosis, classical SCID, Swiss SCID	Autosomal recessive	No T cells, no B cells (NK cells present)	Defect in RAG 1, 2 genes
SCID with B cells		X-linked recessive	No T cells (B cells present)	Defect in IL-2 receptor gamma chain (common gamma chain)
		or		
		Autosomal recessive	No T cells (B cells present)	JAK 3 (kinase) deficiency
ADA-deficient SCID			No T cells, no B cells	Lack of ADA gene

Abbreviations: SCID, severe combined immune deficiency; ADA, adenosine deaminase; RAG, recombinase activating genes; JAK, Janus kinase.

related donors has also been used successfully, although the success rate is significantly lower compared to that of HLA genotypically identical transplants [65% ($n = 23$) vs. 85% ($n = 60$), $P < .05$] in Europe. As soon as T-cell depletion methods became available, HLA-partially compatible marrow transplantation was proposed as an alternative to fetal liver transplantation. It was expected, from animal models, that T-cell-depleted marrow transplantation would give rise to normal lymphoid differentiation in the absence of GVHD. Reisner et al. (1983) successfully used a physical method (a combination of soybean agglutination and sheep erythrocyte rosetting) to remove mature T cells from the marrow. Results were reproduced in other centers using other T-cell depletion methods, including anti-T-cell antibodies or sheep erythrocyte rosetting alone. From the literature, it appears that at least 600 patients with SCID syndromes have received a T-cell-depleted marrow from a related donor, usually a parent. About 60% are alive with development of immune function. Some single centers reported success rates above 70% (Buckley et al., 1986, 1993; O'Reilly et al., 1990; Friedrich et al., 1993; Stephan et al., 1993; Buckley, 1995; Buckley et al., 1999 [Fig. 62.1]; De Santes, Lai, & Cowan, 1996; Dickinson et al., 1997). Overall 2-year survival in Europe is now 60% to 80% (Antoine et al., submitted). CD34+ cell selection has resulted in a reduced rate of GVHD, likely accounting for the improvement in survival over time. It has been shown that SCID patients transplanted under the age of 3 months have a likelihood of survival above 95% given the low risk of GVHD combined with the absence of infections (Buckley et al., 2000; Kane et al., 2001). It is also associated with superior thymic output and slightly faster kinetics of T-cell development (Myers et al., 2002) (Figs. 62.2 and 62.3).

Nevertheless, a number of failures are related to the time lapse required to get significant T-cell immunity, 3 to 6 months in most cases, sometimes more (Buckley et al., 1999; Haddad et al., 1999). The absence of a myeloablative conditioning regimen usually leads to an absence of myeloid engraftment and

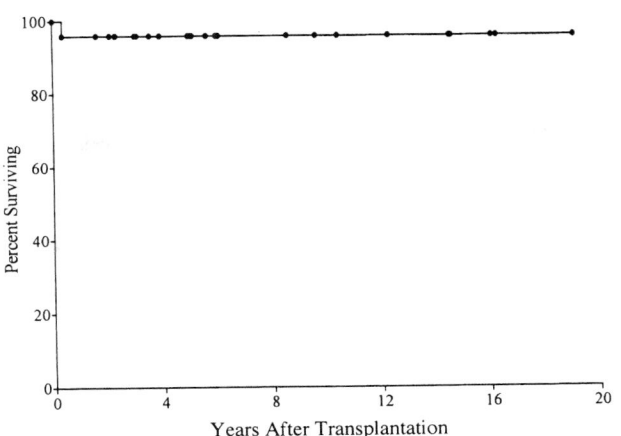

Fig. 62.2. Kaplan-Meier survival curve for 21 patients with SCID who received stem cell transplants in the first 28 days of life. One patient died at 4 months of age from CMV encephalitis. Reproduced, with permission, from Myers et al. (2002).

lack of donor B cells is found in 70% to 75% of cases, a persisting B-cell immunodeficiency requiring IVIG administration (Buckley et al., 1999; Haddad et al., 1999). Bertrand and colleagues (2002) reported on 10 patients with the reticular dysgenesis form of SCID given haploidentical transplants between 1979 and 1999: five received myeloablative conditioning with busulfan (16 mg/kg) and cyclophosphamide and 3 were alive and well with myeloid and T and B cell reconstitution. Transplantation without, or with other, conditioning in the other 5 cases led to absent or incomplete engraftment and none survived.

Patel et al. have shown that, with time, T-cell output from the thymus declines in patients transplanted for SCID. As shown by quantification of T cells containing T-cell receptor excision circles—a marker of recent thymic emigration—such cells are no longer detected beyond 14 years after hap-

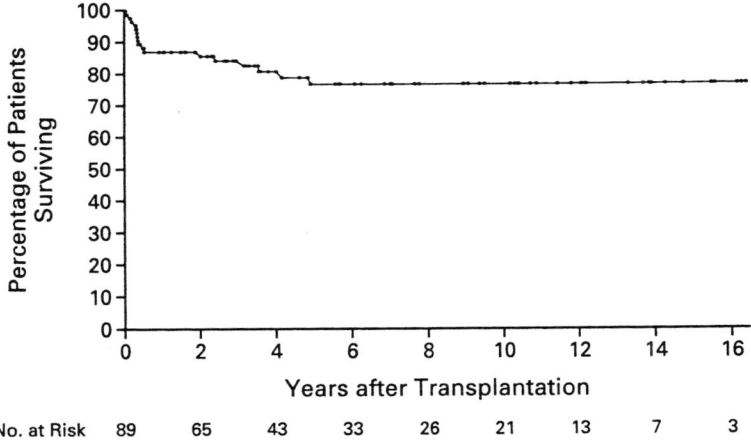

Fig. 62.1. Kaplan-Meier survival curve for 89 patients with severe combined immunodeficiency who received stem cell transplants. Eighty-one percent of the patients were alive at the most recent evaluation; only 12 received transplants from related identical donors. Reproduced, with permission, from Buckley et al. (1999).

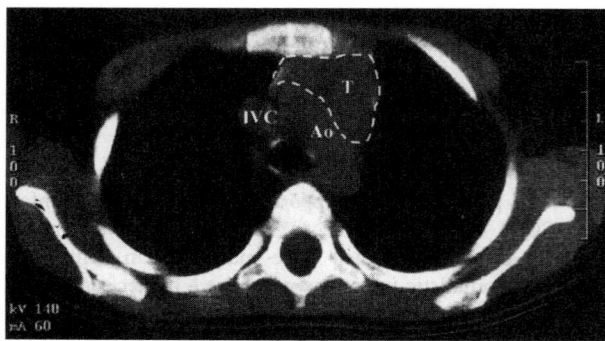

Fig. 62.3. Computed tomography scan of the anterior mediastinum of a Jak3-deficient SCID patient 4 years after transplantation. Thymic tissue is indicated by the dashed lines. It is in the normal position and measures 3.8 cm in its greatest transverse dimension, which is normal for age. Ao indicates aortic arch; IVC, inferior vena cava; T, thymus. Reproduced, with permission, from Myers *et al.* (2002).

loidentical BMT (Patel *et al.,* 2000). It is not known whether this is a consequence of premature thymus involution or loss of donor progenitors.

Ege and colleagues (2001) reported marked hepatosplenomegaly due to polyclonal CD8+ cell infiltration occurring 9 years after haploidentical paternal marrow transplantation for SCID was carried out in an infant at 1 month of age. This was reversed by a subsequent marrow transplant from a younger HLA-identical sibling.

Disseminated Bacille Calmette-Guérin[2] (BCG) infection due to prior BCG vaccination can complicate allogeneic HSC transplantation in SCID patients, but can be managed successfully (Minigishi *et al.,* 1985; Heyderman *et al.,* 1991; Ikinciogullari *et al.,* 2002).

Results of unrelated donor transplantation for SCID

Successes have been obtained using HLA-matched unrelated donors (Ash *et al.,* 1990; Filipovich *et al.,* 1992; Kernan *et al.,* 1993; Hallett *et al.,* 1999; Dalal *et al.,* 2000; Ortin *et al.,* 2000). Kernan *et al.* (1993) noted a success rate for patients with inborn errors of 50% and Filipovich *et al.* (1992) reported successful unrelated donor BMT in six of eight SCID recipients.

Some success using HLA-partially incompatible unrelated donor marrow has also been reported, especially when the degree of incompatibility was restricted to one HLA antigen and provided that the marrow was T-cell depleted (Ash *et al.,* 1990). Nevertheless, results do not look altogether superior to those of haploidentical SCT. Given the fact that SCID treatment is an emergency, search for an unrelated donor is usually therefore not justified.

[2]Léon Calmette, French bacteriologist, 1863–1933.
Camille Guerin, French veterinarian, 1872–1961.

Results of cord blood transplantation for SCID

Occasional reports have indicated that unrelated cord blood transplantation can effectively correct the immunodeficiency observed in SCID (Rocha *et al.,* 2000).

Prognostic factors

Analyses have been performed to delineate prognostic factors for the success of these transplants. It appeared that neither the syndrome nor the T-cell-depletion method used had any influence on outcome. Major factors were age at the time of transplant or the presence of a lung infection prior to transplant (the two variables are not independent), use of a protective environment, and, since 1986, use of a conditioning regimen (Table 62.3). A European survey showed that the outcome of T-cell-depleted, HLA-nonidentical BMT in B− SCID was poorer than that in B+ SCID. This was in part related to a lower rate of engraftment, possibly caused by the ability of patient NK cells to reject donor marrow (Bertrand *et al.,* 1999; Haddad *et al.,* 1999).

Results of HLA-nonidentical T-cell-depleted transplants for SCID syndromes in Europe differ significantly from those of HLA-identical transplants ($P <.01$). It has been recognized that a combination of favorable factors (protective environment, optimal donor, and use of a conditioning regimen) gives a 76% survival rate compared to 42% for all other patients.

Graft failure and GVHD

Several factors have been proposed to account for the surprisingly high graft failure rate of HLA-nonidentical, T-cell-depleted marrow transplants in SCID patients. In the murine SCID model, it has been demonstrated that NK cells con-

Table 62.3. *Factors influencing the outcome of HLA-nonidentical, T-cell-depleted BMT for severe combined immune deficiencies*

Factor	Relative risk[a]	*P*
Lung infection before BMT	9.3	.002
Absence of protective environment	11.1	.001
Female donor to male recipient	3.4	.065
Since 1986		
Absence of conditioning regimen	3.3	.02

	Cumulative 2-year survival (%)	
Lung infection before BMT	With	31
	Without	78
Protective environment	With	64
	Without	29
Female donor/male recipient		45
Other combinations		61
Conditioning regimen	With	71 (since 1986)
	Without	40

[a] Cox multivariate regression analysis.
Adapted from Fischer *et al.* (1990).

tributed to failure of marrow engraftment. This could be prevented by 4 Gy total body irradiation. NK cells may also prevent engraftment in SCID patients (Peter *et al.,* 1983; O'Reilly *et al.,* 1990; Haddad *et al.,* 1999). Other mechanism(s) could be also involved. Engraftment of maternal T cells is frequent (30% to 50%) in SCID patients. They contribute to graft rejection (Haddad *et al.,* 1999). It has therefore been suggested that the mother be the marrow donor if a conditioning regimen cannot be used pretransplant. Maternal T cells, however, are frequently oligoclonal (Scottini *et al.,* 1995) and likely have poor capacity to induce graft rejection, in the same way that they seldom induce GVHD in SCID recipients.

Provided that T-cell depletion of the marrow inoculum is sufficiently profound (producing an infusion of less than 1×10^5 T cells/kg), the risk of severe GVHD is limited. Recipients of marrow treated by soybean agglutination and sheep erythrocyte rosetting developed GVHD infrequently.

Use of a pretransplant conditioning regimen

In the absence of a conditioning regimen, failure of engraftment occurred in 50% of patients, while the use of busulfan (8 mg/kg) and cyclophosphamide (20 mg/kg) led to a 95% engraftment rate. It also appears that a myeloablative conditioning regimen promotes the rate of development of B-cell immune function, and that T- and B-cell function both recover more frequently. The latter observation seems to be correlated with the pattern of chimerism. In the absence of a conditioning regimen, engraftment of donor B (and myeloid) cell lineages occurs in 30% or less, while it is present in 75% of conditioned patients (Brady *et al.,* 1996). Moreover, donor B-cell chimerism is strongly associated with the development of B-cell function (antibody production), although host B cells have been shown to be functional in some cases (Van Leeuwen *et al.,* 1994; Haddad *et al.,* 1999). It seems that in order to prevent the high risk of graft rejection, myeloablative therapy is preferable for non HLA-identical HSC transplantation per-

formed for NK+ SCID. A high-dose conditioning regimen, however, may be detrimental in profoundly immune deficient patients. Thus, busulfan 16 mg/kg and cyclophosphamide is associated with significantly poorer survival compared to busulfan 8 mg/kg and cyclophosphamide (54.5% vs. 69.5% 2-year cumulative survival rate, $P < .05$). Some SCID patients infected at the time of transplant, however, cannot tolerate any conditioning regimen prior to transplant.

An interesting development in this regard is the use of nonmyeloablative regimens to achieve at least stable mixed chimerism posttransplant (see Chapter 22 and below).

Recovery of immune function

Infants with SCID given family member BMT develop T cells of donor origin that are functionally normal (Buckley *et al.,* 1986, 1999; Haddad *et al.,* 1999). It has been shown that the stem cell progenitors mature in the vestigial recipient thymus by measuring T-cell antigen receptor episomes in the recipient blood before and after transplant. [During intrathymic differentiation, progenitor cells undergo rearrangement of T-cell antigen receptor genes to become T cells, leading to the formation of extrachromosomal DNA circles, or episomes. These are also known as T-cell receptor recombination excision circles (TREC).] Patel and colleagues (2000) found TRECs in the blood within 3 to 6 weeks of transplantation (Fig. 62.4). The kinetics of development of T- and B-lymphocyte function are slower in recipients of T-depleted, HLA-incompatible marrow than in recipients of HLA-identical marrow (Buckley *et al.,* 1986; Roberts *et al.,* 1989; Wijnaendts *et al.,* 1989; O'Reilly *et al.,* 1990; Dror *et al.,* 1993). Indeed, we found that full T- and B-lymphocyte-mediated responses were present at day 186 in recipients of HLA-identical transplants, but at day 505 in recipients of HLA-nonidentical transplants (Wijnaendts *et al.,* 1989).

Factors associated with slower development of T-cell function are nonutilization of a conditioning regimen and development of GVHD. A European retrospective survey of 116 patients showed

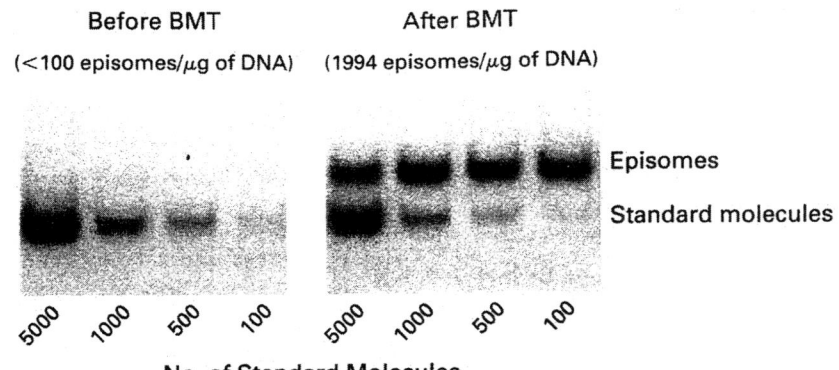

Before BMT

(<100 episomes/μg of DNA)

After BMT

(1994 episomes/μg of DNA)

Episomes

Standard molecules

5000   1000   500   100   5000   1000   500   100

No. of Standard Molecules

Fig. 62.4. Appearance of T-cell antigen-receptor episomes after bone marrow transplantation (BMT) in an infant with immunodeficiency. DNA was purified from the peripheral-blood mononuclear cells of Patient 2 before transplantation and 238 days after transplantation and assayed for the presence of T-cell antigen-receptor episomes by quantitative, competitive polymerase chain reaction (PCR). The autoradiographs show episomes and standard molecules amplified by PCR. The number of standard molecules in each reaction is indicated. Reproduced, with permission, from Patel *et al.* (2000).

that in addition to GVHD, B– SCID was an adverse factor for the development of T-cell function (Haddad *et al.*, 1998). B-cell function fails to develop in approximately 40% of transplanted patients. This appears strongly correlated with an absence of donor B cells and thus with lack of a conditioning regimen. The reason for the poor cooperation between donor T cells and host B cells (in T–, B+ SCID patients) is unclear. An intrinsic B-cell defect may contribute to this poor function, although in some cases host B cells have been shown to produce antibodies following HLA-identical and nonidentical transplantation (Fischer *et al.*, 1986; O'Reilly *et al.*, 1989a; Van Leeuwen *et al.*, 1994; Haddad *et al.*, 1999). Ineffective T-cell stimulation (because of donor-derived MHC Class II restriction) can be excluded because (1) donor and recipient always share at least one HLA haplotype and (2) engrafted Class II MHC responsive ("helper") T cells can recognize antigen in the context of host Class II HLA antigens as previously determined in murine models of BMT (Lo & Sprent, 1986). Van Leeuwen *et al.* (1994), however, found in a survey of the Leiden experience that, in nine long-term survivors of haploidentical BMT for SCID, IgG antibody responses were detectable whether donor B cells were present or not. Three patients had only IgA deficiency.

It has been found that patients with selective engraftment of donor T cells exhibit T-cell "autoreactivity" specific for donor MHC Class II molecules (De Villartay *et al.*, 1986). These results might be accounted for by the absence of donor-derived MHC Class II expressing cells of the monocyte lineage in host thymus, resulting in a lack of negative selection. The latter cells have been previously shown to be required for negative selection of autoreactive T cells. As in fetal liver transplant recipients, it was demonstrated in HLA-haploidentical, T-cell-depleted marrow recipients, that antihost T-cell clones could be derived. Lack of in vivo reactivity appeared to be associated with inability to produce high levels of cytokines including IL-2, IL-4, IL-5, IL-10, gamma-interferon, and granulocyte colony-stimulating factor (G-CSF) (Bacchetta *et al.*, 1994).

HSC transplantation for other immune deficiencies

In 1968, Bach and colleagues were successful in achieving HLA-identical lymphoid engraftment in a patient with WAS. Since then, allogeneic BMT has been found effective in at least 16 distinct non-SCID immune deficiencies (Tables 62.1 and 62.4).

The conditioning regimen

A major difference compared to SCID patients is the usual requirement of a conditioning regimen to achieve engraftment (Parkman *et al.*, 1978; O'Reilly *et al.*, 1989a). A few exceptions have been noted, particularly in the treatment of profound T-cell immune deficiency such as Omenn's syndrome. Initially, total body irradiation (TBI) was used to prepare immune deficiency patients for transplant. It was later recognized that TBI could be safely replaced by busulfan at dosages (16 to 20 mg/kg) that did not produce comparable adverse late effects. It was also found that such doses were sufficient for young patients (below the age of 2 to 4 years), despite the reduced bioavailability of busulfan in this age group (Blazar *et al.*, 1985). There is now a general consensus on the use of busulfan 16 to 20 mg/kg together with cyclophosphamide 200 mg/kg as a conditioning regimen for patients with non-SCID immune deficiency treated by HLA-identical sibling transplantation (Blazar *et al.*, 1985). One should note, however, that studies have reported high variability in busulfan disposition among young children (by a factor of 6) (Vassal *et al.*, 1993). These findings favor individual dose adjustment of busulfan. This regimen may, however, be insufficient in young patients with phagocytic cell disorders (see below). Other myeloablative drugs such as thiotepa could be utilized.

Table 62.4. *Survival in non-SCID congenital immune deficiency syndromes*

	Proportion (%) surviving to adulthood		
Syndrome	No transplant	HLA-identical transplant	HLA-nonidentical transplant
T-cell immune deficiencies			
Omenn's syndrome	0	80	50
Purine nucleoside phosphorylase deficiency	0	50	
MHC Class II deficiency	0	50	35
Others	0	60	50
Wiskott-Aldrich syndrome	50	>90	40
X-linked hyper IgM syndrome	20	>90	
XLP (X-linked proliferation) syndrome	25	>90	
Phagocytic cell disorders			
Agranulocytosis	90–100	>90 (see text)	–
Leukocyte adhesion deficiency			
Severe phenotype	0	>70	75
Moderate phenotype	50		
Chronic granulomatous disease	80–90	70–90 (see text)	–
Chediak-Higashi syndrome	5	90	20–50
Familial hemophagocytic lymphohistiocytosis	0	70	

Table 62.5. *Donor chimerism levels desirable for functional correction of genetic disorders*

Percentage donor cells[a]	Diseases	Comments
3–10	Sickle cell anemia	RBC graft required
	Chronic granulomatous disease	PMN graft required
	Leukocyte adhesion deficiency	PMN, lymphoid graft required
>10	Severe combined immunodeficiency	Usually T cells[b]
	Wiskott-Aldrich syndrome	Platelet graft required
	CD40 ligand deficiency	
	Hemophagocytic lymphohistiocytosis	NK-cell, CTL graft required
100	Autoimmune lymphoproliferative syndrome	
	Fanconi's anemia	

Abbreviations: RBC, red blood cells; PMN, polymorphonucleocytes; NK, natural killer; CTL, cytotoxic T lymphocyte.
[a] Peripheral blood nucleated cells.
[b] Many patients require lifetime intravenous immunoglobulin G because of lack of B-cell engraftment.
Reproduced, with permission, from Antin *et al.* (2001).

Results with reduced intensity conditioning regimens

Preliminary results in patients with congenital immune deficiencies are encouraging: eight patients who all had severe organ dysfunction pretransplant were conditioned with fludarabine, melphalan, and anti-thymocyte globulin prior to a T-replete, HLA-matched unrelated (six) or sibling (two) donor BMT (Amrolia *et al.*, 2000). All eight patients engrafted with predominantly donor hematopoiesis. One died of disease recurrence and three showed stable mixed chimerism. At a median of 1-year posttransplant, all patients showed good recovery of CD3[+] T cells and six of seven evaluable had normal phytohemagglutinin stimulation indices. Two patients who had CD40 ligand deficiency showed significant expression posttransplant and one patient with adenosine deaminase deficiency showed improved deoxy adenosine triphosphate metabolites. (See also the section on phagocytic disorders below.)

It should be noted that varying degrees of donor chimerism after non-myeloablative or reduced intensity conditioning regimens may be sufficient for functional correction of genetic disorders (Table 62.5).

Wiskott-Aldrich syndrome[3]

Wiskott-Aldrich syndrom (WAS) is an X-linked recessive disorder characterized by the triad of thrombocytopenia, eczema and immune deficiency, with a proclivity towards the development of lymphoid malignant disease. The responsible gene is the WASP gene (Wiskott-Aldrich syndrome protein). The protein appears to play a role in transducing signals related to cell growth. In addition, it specifically associates with the activated form of Cdc-42, suggesting its involvement in regulating cytoskeletal architecture through actin polymerization.

After the partial correction obtained in WAS in 1968, full correction of WAS was achieved in 1978 following the use of an appropriate conditioning regimen (Parkman *et al.*, 1978). HLA-identical marrow transplantation has been found efficient in 90% of patients who had an HLA-identical sibling (Brochstein *et al.*, 1991; Mullen *et al.*, 1993; Oszahin *et al.*, 1996) (Table 62.4). All aspects of WAS are corrected by marrow transplantation, including the eczema, autoimmunity, and the risk of lymphomas. This indicates that these disease complications are related to the immune deficiency. Similarly, thrombocytopenia and bleeding tendency disappear after transplantation. HLA-identical HSC transplantation is recommended for patients with WAS and should be performed as early as possible. A report from the IBMTR and the NMDP described outcome after 170 allografts (Filipovich *et al.*, 2001), 55 of which were from HLA-identical siblings, 48 from other relatives, and 67 from unrelated donors. The 5-year probability of survival was 87% for those receiving HLA-identical sibling transplants, 52% for those receiving other related donor grafts, and 71% for those receiving transplants from unrelated donors (Fig. 62.5). Conversion to full donor

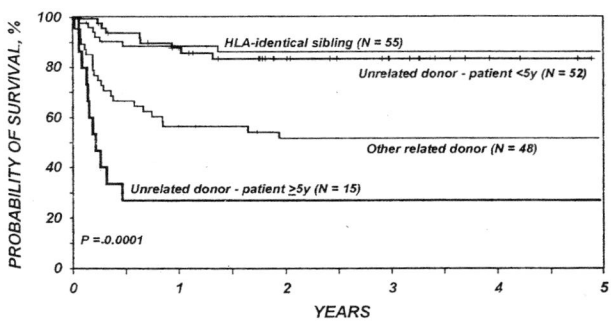

Fig. 62.5. Probabilities of survival for 170 patients receiving bone marrow transplants for Wiscott-Aldrich syndrome by donor type and age. There was not a significant difference in the risk of mortality after HLA-matched sibling transplants and after unrelated donor transplants in children younger than 5 years. Significantly worse survival was associated with use of related donors other than HLA-identical siblings, regardless of recipient age, and with use of unrelated donors over 5 years of age. Reproduced, with permission, from Filipovich *et al.* (2001).

[3] Alfred Wiskott, German pediatrician, 1898–1978; Robert Aldrich, U.S. pediatrician, born 1917.

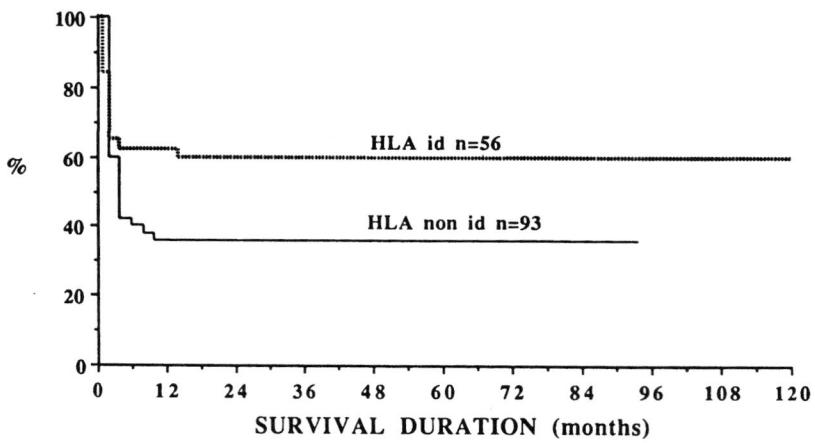

Fig. 62.6. Event-free survival of patients with immunodeficiencies except SCID who underwent either HLA genetically identical (HLA id) or nonidentical (HLA non id) BMT; log-rank test: statistics, 6.974; dof = 1; $P <.0083$. Reproduced, with permission, from Fischer *et al.* (1994).

No. of Patients Alive and Well (March 1, 1992)											
Months	12	24	36	48	60	72	84	96	108	120	132	144
HLA id	37	32	28	23	221	16	13	9	6	4	2	1
HLA non id	37	22	20	17	14	9	3	1				

chimerism may take time. Chimeric status can be assessed using flow cytometry for intracellular expression of the WAS protein (Yamaguchi *et al.*, 2002).

T-cell immune deficiencies

Extension of allogeneic transplantation to T-cell immune deficiencies has not been as successful, although cure of a number of them has been achieved.

Overall, HLA-identical BMT for various T-cell immune deficiency syndromes, including Omenn's syndrome[4] (Gomez *et al.*, 1995; Loechelt *et al.*, 1995), MHC Class II deficiency (Klein *et al.*, 1995), ZAP 70 deficiency, purine nucleoside phosphorylase deficiency (Broome *et al.*, 1996; Carpenter *et al.*, 1996), and others (Berthet *et al.*, 1994, 1996), cures approximately half the patients (a figure significantly inferior to that obtained for other immune deficiencies) (Table 62.4 and Fig. 62.6).

It appears that failure is often related to viral infection or organ failure. These complications are directly related to the pretransplant clinical status. Since the immune deficiencies are less pronounced than in SCID, they are compatible with life for several years, although infections caused by intracellular microorganisms develop and are exacerbated following marrow-ablative and immune suppressive conditioning. Early diagnosis of these immune deficiencies should be treated by allogeneic transplantation as early as possible, in order to offer maximal likelihood of cure. Indeed, in a European survey, including all non-SCID immune deficiency diseases, transplants performed before the age of 2 give a 79% success rate versus 48% over 4 years of age (Fischer *et al.*, 1994) (Table 62.6).

Hyper IgM syndrome (CD40 ligand deficiency)

X-linked hyper IgM syndrome is caused by mutations of the CD40 ligand gene (Notarangelo *et al.*, 1992). The CD40 ligand is expressed on activated T cells and other hematopoietic cells and its co-ligand, CD40, is expressed on monocytes, macrophages, B cells, dendritic cells and endothelial cells. CD40 ligand-CD40 interaction on B cell membranes transduces an essential signal for Ig class-switching and for differentiation of B cell memory in response to T cell-dependent antigens. This syndrome is severe because it predisposes to opportunistic infections that are often fatal during childhood. Serious pyogenic infections caused by encapsulated bacteria occur, as do infections with intracellular pathogens such as Pneumocystis carinil and Cryptosporidium parvum. The latter predisposes to sclerosing cholangitis with progression to cirrhosis and liver failure. Prompt prophylactic treatment with IVIG and antibiotics is portant. Allogeneic HSC transplantation is the sole curative treatment (Thomas *et al.*, 1995a; Duplantier *et al.*, 1997; Scholl *et al.*, 1998; Kawai *et al.*, 1999; Kato *et al.*, 1999; Leone *et al.*, 2002), and has been performed in conjunction with hepatic transplantation (Hadzic *et al.*, 2000).

X-linked proliferation syndrome (XLP, Purtilo's syndrome)[5]

XLP is invariably fatal (Sullivan & Woda, 1989). It is caused by poor control of Epstein-Barr virus (EBV) infection, although the disease mechanism is still unknown; bone marrow or cord blood cell transplantation can cure the disease and is therefore indicated, provided an HLA-matched donor is available (Vowels *et al.*, 1993; Williams *et al.*, 1993; Pracher *et al.*, 1994; Gross *et al.*, 1996).

---

[4] Gilbert Omenn, U.S. internist, born 1941.

[5] David T. Purtilo, 20th-century U.S. physician.

Table 62.6. *Survival according to date of transplantation and age at time of transplant*

	HLA identical			HLA phenotypically matched (related and unrelated) PMRD (1 HLA ag)			PMRD (≥2 HLA ag)		
	n	Percentage alive[a]		n	Percentage alive[a]		n	Percentage alive[a]	
Date of BMT									
<10/85	29	52		7	14.3		20	15	
≥10/85	27	81.5	P < .01	15	60	P = .05	51	47	P < .0001
Age at BMT (yr)									
<2	19	79		15	60		44	43	
>2<4	14	79	P < .0001	2	50		19	31.5	
>4	23	48		5	0		8	25	

Abbreviation: PMRD, partially matched related donor.
[a] One-year survival with functional graft.
Reproduced, with permission, from Fischer *et al.* (1994).

Phagocytic cell disorders

Some inherited phagocytic cell disorders remain lethal, either because of the severity of infections in the absence of alternative therapy, or because of the onset of specific complications such as the "acute phase" of the Chediak-Higashi syndrome.[6]

Leukocyte adhesion deficiency (LAD) is a rare disease characterized by defective expression of the beta-2 integrin subunit shared by the leukocyte adhesion proteins. Its complete absence leads to the severe phenotype of LAD, which predisposes to severe bacterial infections, often causing death within the first years of life. HLA-identical sibling transplantation is the treatment of choice. Aggressive pretransplant conditioning including the use of etoposide or TBI may be required for appropriate marrow ablation (Fischer *et al.*, 1986; Thomas *et al.*, 1995b). Results of sibling cord blood (Stary *et al.*, 1996) (Table 62.4) and unrelated donor (Mancias *et al.*, 1999; Farinha *et al.*, 2002) transplantation have been satisfactory (Fig. 62.7).

Chediak-Higashi syndrome, familial hemophagocytic lymphohistiocytosis and Griscelli's syndrome

Similarly, HLA-identical sibling transplantation can cure the hematologic manifestations of the Chediak-Higashi syndrome (Filipovich *et al.*, 1992; Haddad *et al.*, 1995), of familial hemophagocytic lymphohistiocytosis (Blanche *et al.*, 1991), and of immune deficiency with partial albinism (Griscelli's disease) (Schneider *et al.*, 1990; Klein *et al.*, 1994; Tezcan *et al.*, 1999; Schuster *et al.*, 2001). It should be noted that only patients with Griscelli's syndrome[7] who have mutations of

the RAB27A gene suffer from immunodeficiency and hemophagocytic lymphohistiocytosis, not those with mutations of the myosin Va gene. Transplantation prevents relapse of lymphohistiocytic activity. It is worth noting that mixed chimerism is sufficient to achieve disease control (Trigg & Schugar, 2001). This indicates that an abnormal regulatory process, rather than a malignant process, underlies these conditions. Use of TBI is not necessary; a combination of etoposide, busulfan, and cyclophosphamide appears both a safe and efficient conditioning regimen for these diseases. HLA-compatible unrelated BMT has also been used successfully to cure Griscelli's syndrome: the myeloablative conditioning regimen consisted of busulfan, thiotepa and fludarabine (Arico *et al.*, 2002).

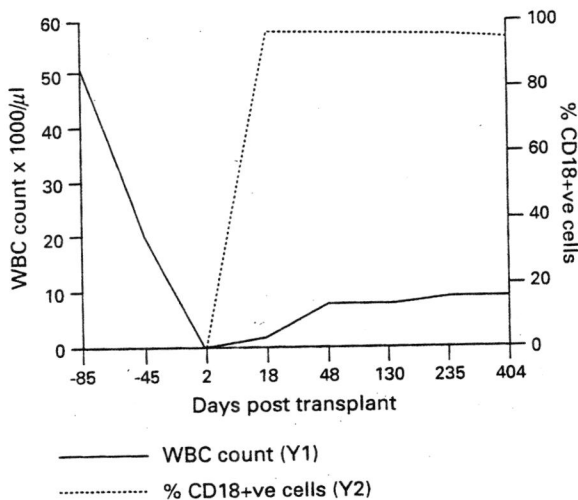

Fig. 62.7. Recovery of CD18 expression on patient leukocytes following bone marrow transplantation (dotted line) correlated with patient white blood cell count. Reproduced, with permission, from Mancias *et al.* (1999).

---

[6] Moises Chediak, Cuban physician, born 1903. Ototaka Higashi, Japanese physician.
[7] Claude Griscelli, French physician, born 1936.

Table 62.7. *Frequency of BMT complications (%) and event-free survival (%) according to date of transplantation*

	HLA identical BMT[a]			HLA nonidentical BMT[b]		
	<10/85	≥10/85		<10/85	≥10/85	
No. of patients	34	37		22	56	
Graft failure	13%	3%		52%	25%	P < .001
Acute GVHD ≥ grade II	37%	24%		27%	44%	
IP	30%	12%		47%	27%	
Bacterial and fungal infections	32%	14%		36%	27%	
BLPD	0	0		25%	17%	
Alive	45%	77%	P < .0001	18%	47.5%	P < .0001

Abbreviation: IP, interstitial pneumonitis; BLPD, B cell lymphoproliferative disease.

[a] Includes HLA genetically identical siblings, HLA identical related, and matched unrelated donors.

[b] Includes related 1, 2, or 3 HLA-ag-mismatched donors.

Congenital agranulocytosis (Kostmann syndrome) and chronic granulomatous disease

Although allogeneic transplantation has been demonstrated to cure congenital agranulocytosis (Kostmann syndrome)[8] and chronic granulomatous disease (CGD) (Ho *et al.*, 1996; review of the literature in Leung *et al.*, 1999), alternative therapies currently offer good quality, long-term survival (G-CSF in agranulocytosis, and cotrimoxazole with or without gamma-interferon in CGD). Thus, HSC transplantation should not usually be recommended for these conditions. Allogeneic transplantation should be considered in those patients with Kostmann syndrome refractory to G-CSF. Zeidler and colleagues (2000) described 11 patients, 8 of whom received grafts from HLA-identical siblings. All 8 survived. Some CGD patients still develop life-threatening fungal infections and/or granulomas. It has therefore been advocated that transplantation from an HLA-identical sibling donor could be proposed in this setting. Seger (2001) has shown that 16 of 19 transplants performed in CGD patients were successful, including 16 of 16 without risk factors or pulmonary compromise. This has been confirmed in a larger series: those transplanted with no overt infection or inflammation did better than those transplanted with active inflammation or inflammatory sequelae or with therapy-refractory infection (Seger *et al.*, 2002).

Additionally, the use of non-myeloablative conditioning (with cyclophosphamide, fludarabine, and ATG) followed by a T-cell-depleted, HLA-identical sibling PBSC transplant has been described in 5 children and 5 adults with CGD (Horwitz *et al.*, 2001). After a median follow-up of 17 months, the proportion of donor neutrophils in the circulation in 8 of the 10 patients ranged from 33% to 100%. Graft failure occurred in 2 patients; 3 patients died—of graft failure, pneumococcal pneumonia, and GVHD. Pre-existing granulomatous lesions resolved in the patients in whom transplantation was successful.

Complete interferon-γ receptor 1 deficiency

Complete interferon-γ receptor 1 (IFNγ R1) deficiency is an autosomal recessive inherited disorder with a very poor prognosis due

[8] Rolf Kostmann, Swedish pediatrician, born 1909.

to severe infections caused, in particular, by mycobacteria and other intracellular microorgansims. Mutations of the gene (on chromosome 6) can lead to lack of expression or function of IFNγ R1. In macrophages this results in failure to become activated on exposure to IFN-γ, leading to lack of tumor necrosis factor α production and a profound deficiency in intracellular killing of pathogens. An 8 year-old child with recurrent mycobacterial infections and hepatic cirrhosis was successfully treated by HLA-identical sibling BMT (Reuter *et al.*, 2002). Conditioning was with cyclophosphamide, ATG and TBI 12 Gy. Mixed chimerism was present posttransplant for which donor lymphocyte infusions were administered. Monocyte IFN-γ R1 expression revealed two populations, one with normal, and one with absent, expression.

The long-term (10-year) outcome of HLA-identical BMT for most immune deficiency syndromes appears reasonably satisfactory. Correction of the underlying deficiency is sustained, despite frequent mixed chimerism in the absence of TBI usage. Sequelae are generally limited to consequences of the primary disease. Chronic GVHD is of limited frequency in these young patients (Fischer *et al.*, 1986).

Over the past decade, increasing numbers of allogeneic transplants have been performed for immune deficiency syndromes. Younger age at the time of transplant is associated with excellent outcome (79% below 2 years of age vs. 48% over 4 years of age) (Fischer *et al.*, 1994), and progress has been made in recent years, particularly in infection prevention (intravenous immunoglobulin, antiviral drugs) and in GVHD prophylaxis (combination of "short" methotrexate and cyclosporine). In Europe, the success rate for BMT performed from October 1985 through March 1991 was 77% versus 47.5% before October 1985 (Tables 62.7 and 62.8).

BMT has also been shown to correct the autoimmune syndromes associated with fas deficiency (ALPS syndrome) (Benkerrou *et al.*, 1997) and IPEX syndrome (Baud *et al.*, 2001).

Results of HLA-mismatched family member, unrelated donor, and cord blood transplantation

Following the improving results in HLA-nonidentical BMT for the treatment of SCID syndromes, a similar approach was

Table 62.8. *Causes of death expressed as frequency among all patients (%)*

	HLA identical BMT		HLA nonidentical BMT	
	<10/85	>10/85	<10/85	>10/85
No. of patients	34	37	22	56
Died	55%	23%	72%	47.5%
IP	15%	3%	32%	10%
CMV IP	9%	3%	14%	0
Bacterial and fungal infections	12%	3%	9%	3.5%
Other viral infections	6%	6%	5%	5%
Toxic deaths	6%	3%	0	7%
GVHD	9%	6%	5%	5%
BLPD	0	0	14%	8.5%
Disease progression	3%	3%	14%	8.5%

Reproduced, with permission, from Fischer *et al.* (1994).

taken for the treatment of the other lethal immune deficiencies. Unfortunately, results were disappointing because of a high incidence of graft rejection (up to 75%) (Fischer 1991; Fischer *et al.*, 1986, 1991) and of infectious complications. More recently, successes have been obtained using HLA-matched unrelated donors (Ash *et al.*, 1990; Filipovich *et al.*, 1992; Kernan *et al.*, 1993; Mancias, Infante, & Kermani, 1999; Dalal *et al.*, 2000). An example in a patient with leukocyte adhesion deficiency is shown in Fig. 62.7. In a report of HLA-matched unrelated donor bone marrow transplantation, Kernan *et al.* (1993) noted a success rate for patients with inborn errors of 50%. Filipovich *et al.* (1992) reported successful unrelated donor BMT in 6 of 8 SCID recipients, 2 of 2 patients with WAS, and 2 of 2 patients with Chediak-Higashi syndrome. These promising results appear confirmed recently.

Some success using HLA-partially incompatible unrelated donor marrow has also been reported, especially when the degree of incompatibility was restricted to one HLA antigen and provided that the marrow was T-cell depleted (Ash *et al.*, 1990; Schwinger *et al.*, 2000). Delay in the recovery of T- and B-cell function (6 to 40 months) causes significant infectious complications that remain a major concern in recipients of T-cell-depleted, HLA-nonidentical transplants. For example, 16 of 71 patients who underwent 2 or 3 HLA-incompatible, T-depleted transplants for primary immune deficiencies (excluding SCID) developed EBV-induced B-lymphoproliferative syndromes, and 10 died. This complication is particularly frequent in Wiskott-Aldrich patients who undergo HLA-nonidentical BMT. In a European survey, 39% of such patients (compared with 12% of patients with T-cell deficiencies, and 3% of those with SCID) developed a lymphoproliferative disorder (EBMT Registry, unpublished data). This may have been caused by poor T-cell control of EBV replication.

Rumelhart *et al.* (1990) have described success in 3 of 4 WAS patients, while Brochstein *et al.* (1991) reported only 1 in 6 suc-

cessful. These contrasting results stress the need for careful evaluation of HLA-haploidentical family member HSC transplantation in patients who lack both an HLA-genetically identical and an HLA-matched unrelated donor. Indications depend on the patient's clinical status as well as the prognosis defined by the type of immune deficiency, age (results are poorer above 2 years of age), and degree of HLA incompatibility. For instance, Mullen *et al.* (1993) stressed that splenectomized WAS patients could survive at least until adulthood. Nevertheless, WAS patients who develop refractory thrombocytopenia and/or severe autoimmune manifestations could be considered for HLA-haploidentical family member transplantation. Similarly, patients with functional T-cell immune deficiencies (including HLA Class II deficiency) have a poor prognosis (median survival 5 to 8 years) in the absence of HLA-identical sibling transplantation (Klein *et al.*, 1995). Chronic granulomatous disease has been treated successfully by unrelated donor BMT (Hobbs *et al.*, 1992; Watanabe *et al.*, 2001), as has Kostmann syndrome (Toyoda *et al.*, 2001). Apart from LAD (see above), the indications for HLA-haploidentical family member transplantation in patients with phagocytic cell disorders remains investigational, given the high risk of failure. It is possible that acute phase Chediak-Higashi syndrome or familial hemophagocytic lymphohistiocytosis could be reasonable indications.

Transplantation of a very high number of stem cells is an attractive approach to try to circumvent graft failure. Aversa *et al.* (1994) have provided promising results in adults with hematologic malignancies and this appoach was successful in a child with WAS given a CD34-selected PBSC transplant from an unrelated donor mismatched at 1 HLA-C locus (Schwinger *et al.*, 2000). The dose of CD34+ cells infused was 24.5×10^6/kg.

Results with reduced intensity conditioning regimens

A 29-year-old man, who received a non-myeloablative conditioning regimen of CAMPATH 1-H, fludarabine, and cyclophosphamide prior to an unrelated donor bone marrow transplant for WAS (because of severe infections and vasculitis), achieved partial engraftment and immune restoration and was well at 1-year posttransplant (Longhurst *et al.*, 2002).

Anti-LFA-1 antibody pretreatment for graft rejection

In the mid-1980s, we were surprised by the consecutive success of three HLA-nonidentical bone marrow transplants for patients with the severe phenotype of LAD (Le Deist *et al.*, 1989). This has since been confirmed in seven of nine patients with the severe phenotype of LAD, who received an HLA-nonidentical BMT: engraftment occurred in all and seven are alive with partial or full correction of the LAD. This is in sharp contrast to the engraftment rate of marrow transplanted under the same conditions to other immune deficiency patients (excluding SCID), in whom the engraftment rate was 26% (Fischer *et al.*, 1991).

It was therefore postulated that the defective expression of the LFA-1 molecule on host effector cells of graft rejection (cytotoxic T cells and NK cells) impaired cell contact with donor marrow cells and thereby permitted engraftment. This led to the use of in vivo infusion of a monoclonal anti-LFA-1 (CD11a) antibody to inhibit LFA-1/ligand interactions.

In a multicenter trial, we showed that a 10-day course of 0.2 mg/kg/ of antibody/day reduced the graft failure rate from 74% to 28% following transplantation of T-cell-depleted marrow in patients with immune deficiencies and osteoporosis (Van Dijken et al., 1990; Fischer et al., 1991). No late rejection occurred. Acute GVHD was observed in 35.5% of cases, and chronic GVHD in 12.9%. The survival rate with a functioning graft was 47% in 42 patients (median follow-up 50 months), instead of 20% in similar patients who did not receive the anti-LFA-1 antibody. Updating of these data shows a 74% engraftment rate with 45% long-term survival in 38 immune deficient patients who were treated with anti-LFA-1 antibody, while engraftment occurred in only 37.5%, and survival in 20.8%, of 24 patients similarly treated except for anti-LFA-1 antibody administration (Fischer et al., 1991). Addition of in vivo injection of an anti-CD2 antibody might further improve engraftment (Jabado et al., 1996).

Other experimental strategies

Other strategies aimed at selectively inhibiting graft rejection have been developed experimentally and could be of potential clinical benefit: anti-CD4 and anti-CD8 antibody infusions promote engraftment of H2-incompatible marrow in mice (Cobbold et al., 1986).

Another major residual problem is the prolonged immune deficiency that follows T-cell-depleted stem cell transplantation. This 3- to 12-month period is characterized by a profound T-cell lymphocytopenia, which is responsible for lethal complications including EBV-induced B-lymphocyte proliferative disorder. The latter can, in some instances, be effectively treated by infusion of EBV-specific cytotoxic T cells from the donor (Heslop et al., 1994) (see Chapter 88).

An ultimate goal is to shorten the period during which T cells are virtually absent. Manipulation with cytokines (IL-7; Bolotin et al., 1997) or infusion of low doses of donor T cells transduced with a suicide gene or depleted of alloreactivity toward the host (Cavazzana-Calvo et al., 1994) represent possible solutions.

Alternative therapies

Alternative treatments (to allogeneic postnatal stem cell transplantation) have been devised for some congenital immune deficiencies over the past decade. For instance, congenital agranulocytosis is effectively treated by daily subcutaneous injections of G-CSF. The prognosis of CGD has been profoundly modified by the prophylactic use of antibiotics (cotrimoxazole) and possibly of gamma-interferon (The International CGD Cooperative Study Group, 1991).

ADA-negative SCID can now be treated by a weekly intramuscular injection of bovine ADA covalently coupled to the carbohydrate polyethyleneglycol (PEG), which stabilizes ADA and diminishes its immunogenicity (Hershfield et al., 1987). More than 40 patients have currently been treated worldwide. In most, a significant improvement occurred that allowed normal or close-to-normal lifestyle.

It is possible that gene transfer into mature T cells of, for example, adenine deaminase (Blaese et al., 1995) or into stem cells may be of benefit to immune deficient patients. ADA SCID, in which a selective advantage may be conferred on transduced cells, represents a good candidate disease. Recently, it has been shown that ex vivo gene transfer of γc gene into marrow cells from patients with X-linked SCID can result in sustained (3 years up to now) correction of the immunodeficiency (Cavazzana-Calvo et al., 2000), although a T cell leukemia or leukemia-like disease has developed in 2 of 10 patients (see Chapter 116).

In utero transplantation

Most primary immune deficiencies can now be diagnosed during pregnancy. If the family does not wish to terminate the pregnancy, stem cell transplantation in utero is an option as shown by the success of HLA-haploidentical CD34-selected transplantation into two SCID fetuses (Flake et al., 1996; Wengler et al., 1996) (Chapter 111). Cord blood gene transfer might also be envisaged, as attempted at birth in three ADA-deficient patients (Kohn et al., 1995).

References

Amrolia, P., Gasspar, H.B., Hassan, A. et al. (2000). Nonmyelablative stem cell transplantation for congenital immunodeficiencies. Blood, 96, 1239–46.

Antin, J.H., Childs, R., Filipovich, A.H. et al. (2001). Establishment of complete and mixed donor chimerism after allogeneic lymphohematopoietic transplantation: recommendations from a workshop at the 2001 Tandem Meetings. Biology of Blood and Marrow Transplantation, 7, 473–85.

Arico, M., Zecca M., Santoro, N. et al. (2002). Successful treatment of Griscelli syndrome with unrelated donor allogeneic hematopoietic stem cell transplantation. Bone Marrow Transplantation, 29, 995–8.

Ash, R.C., Casper, J.T., Chitambar, C.R. et al. (1990). Successful allogeneic transplantation of T cell depleted bone marrow from closely HLA-matched unrelated donors. New England Journal of Medicine, 322, 485–95.

Aversa, F., Tabilio, A., Terenzi, A. et al. (1994). Successful engraftment of T cell depleted haploidentical "three-loci" incompatible transplants in leukemia patients by addition of recombinant human granulocyte colony-stimulating factor-mobilized peripheral blood progenitor cells to bone marrow inoculum. Blood, 84, 3948–56.

Bacchetta, R., Bigler, M., Touraine, J.L. et al. (1994). High levels of interleukin 10 production in vivo are associated with tolerance in SCID patients transplanted with HLA mismatched hematopoietic stem cells. Journal of Experimental Medicine, 179, 493–502.

Bacchetta, R., Parkman, R., McMahon, M. et al. (1995). Dysfunctional cytokine production by host-reactive T cell clones isolated from a chimeric SCID patient transplanted with haploidentical bone marrow. *Blood*, **85**, 1944–53.

Bacchetta, R., Vanderkerckhove, B.A.E., Touraine, J.L. *et al.* (1993). Chimerism and tolerance to host and donor in SCID transplanted with fetal liver stem cells. *Journal of Clinical Investigation*, **91**, 1067–78.

Bach, F.H., Albertini, R.J., Anderson, J.L. *et al.* (1968). Bone marrow transplantation in a patient with the Wiskott-Aldrich syndrome. *Lancet*, **2**, 1364–6.

Baud, O., Goulet, O., Canioni, D. *et al.* (2001). Treatment of the immune dysregulation, polyendocrinopathy, enteropathy, X-linked syndrome (IPEX) by allogeneic bone marrow transplantation. *New England Journal of Medicine*, **344**, 1758–62.

Benkerrou, M., Le Deist, F., de Villartay, J.P. *et al.* (1997). Correction of Fas (CD95) deficiency by haploidentical bone marrow transplantation. *European Journal of Immunology*, **27**, 2043–7.

Berthet, F., Le Deist, F., Duliege, A.M. *et al.* (1994). Clinical consequences and treatment of primary immune deficiency syndromes characterized by functional T and B lymphocyte anomalies (combined immune deficiency). *Pediatrics*, **93**, 265–70.

Berthet, F., Siegrist, C.A., Ozsahin, H. *et al.* (1996). Bone marrow transplantation in cartilage hair hypoplasia: correction of the immuodeficiency but not of the chondrodysplasia. *European Journal of Pediatrics*, **155**, 286–90.

Bertrand, Y., Landais, P., Friedrich, W. *et al.* (1999). Influence of severe combined immunodeficiency phenotype on the outcome of HLA non-identical, T-cell-depleted bone marrow transplantation: a retrospective European survey from the European group for bone marrow transplantation and the European society for immunodeficiency. *Journal of Pediatric*, **134**, 740–8.

Bertrand, Y., Muller, S. M., Casanova, J. L. *et al.* (2002). Reticular dysgenesis: HLA non-identical bone marrow transplantation in a series of 10 patients. *Bone Marrow Transplantation*, **29**, 729–62.

Blaese, R.M., Culver, K.W., Miller, A.D. *et al.* (1995). T lymphocyte-directed gene therapy for ADA-SID; initial trial results after 4 years. *Science*, **270**, 475–80.

Blanche, S., Caniclia, M., Girault, D., Le Deist, F. *et al.* (1991). Treatment of hemophagocytic lymphohistiocytosis by chemotherapy and allogeneic bone marrow transplantation. *Blood*, **78**, 51–5.

Blazar, D.R., Ramsay, M.K.C, Kersey, J.H. *et al.* (1985). Pretransplant conditioning with busulfan and cyclophosphamide for non malignant diseases. *Transplantation*, **39**, 597–603.

Bolotin, E., Nolta, J., Smith, S. *et al.* (1997). Effective immune reconstitution in mice after co-transplantation of bone marrow and marrow stroma transduced with the IL 7 gene: gene therapy for post-BMT deficiency. *Journal of Allergy and Clinical Immunology*, **99S**, 100.

Brady, K.A., Cowan, M.J., & Leavitt, A.D. (1996). Circulating red cells usually remain of host origin after bone marrow transplantation for severe combined immunodeficiency. *Transfusion*, **36**, 314–7.

Brochstein, J., Gilio, A.P., Ruggiero, M. *et al.* (1991). Marrow transplantation from HLA-identical or haploidentical donors for correction of Wiskott-Aldrich. *Journal of Pediatrics*, **119**, 907–12.

Broome, C.B., Graham, M.L., Saulsbury, F.T. *et al.* (1996). Correction of purine nucleoside phosphorylase deficiency by transplantation of allogeneic bone marrow from a sibling. *Journal of Pediatrics*, **128**, 373–6.

Buckley, R.H. (1995). Bone marrow transplantation in primary immune deficiency. In *Clinical Immunology: Principles and Practice*, ed. R.R. Rich, pp. 1813–30. St. Louis: C.V. Mosby.

Buckley, R.H., Schiff, S.E., Sampson, H.A. *et al.* (1986). Development of immunity in human severe primary T cell deficiency following haploidentical bone marrow stem cell transplantation. *Journal of Immunology*, **136**, 2398–407.

Buckley, R.H., Schiff, S.E., Schiff, R.I. *et al.* (1993). Haploidentical bone marrow stem cell transplantation in human severe combined immune deficiency. *Seminars in Hematology*, **30**, 92–104.

Buckley, R.H., Schiff, S.E., Schiff, R.I. *et al.* (1999). Hematopoietic stem cell transplantation for the treatment of severe combined immunodeficiency. *New England Journal of Medicine*, **340**, 508–16.

Carpenter, P.A., Siegler, J.B., & Vowels, M.R. (1996). Late diagnosis and correction of purine nucleoside phosphorylase deficiency with allogenic bone marrow transplantation. *Bone Marrow Transplantation*, **17**, 121–4.

Cavazzana-Calvo, M., Hacein-Bey, S., de Saint Basile, G. *et al.* (2000). Gene therapy of human severe combined immunodeficiency (SCID)-X1 disease [see comments]. *Science*, **288**, 669–72.

Cavazzana-Calvo, M., Stephan, J.L., Sarnacki, S. *et al.* (1994). Attenuation of graft-versus-host disease and graft rejection by ex vivo immunotoxin elimination of alloreactive T cells in an H-2 haplotype disparate mouse combination. *Blood*, **83**, 288–98.

Classen, C.F., Schulz, A.S., Sigl-Kraetzig, M. *et al.* (2001). Successful HLA-identical bone marrow transplantation in a patient with PNP deficiency using busulfan and fludarabine for conditioning. *Bone Marrow Transplantation*, **28**, 93–6.

Cobbold, S.P., Martin, G., Qin, Z. *et al.* (1986). Monoclonal antibodies to promote marrow engraftment and tissue graft tolerance. *Nature*, **323**, 164–6.

Dalal, I., Reid, B., Doyle, J. *et al.* (2000). Matched unrelated bone marrow transplantation for combined immunodeficiency. *Bone Marrow Transplantation*, **25**, 613–21.

De Santes, K.B., Lai, S.S., & Cowan, M.J. (1996). Haploidentical bone marrow transplants for two patients with reticular dysgenesis. *Bone Marrow Transplantation*, **17**, 1171–3.

De Villartay, J.P., Griscelli, C., & Fisher, R.A. (1986). Self tolerance to host and donor following HLA-mismatched BMT. *European Journal of Immunology*, **16**, 117–22.

Dickinson, A.M., Reid, M.M., Abinum, A. *et al.* (1997). In vitro T cell depletion using Campath 1M for mismatched BMT for severe combined immunodeficiency (SCID). *Bone Marrow Transplantation*, **19**, 323–9.

Dror, Y., Gallagher, R., Wara, D.W. *et al.* (1993). Immune reconstitution in severe combined immune deficiency disease after lectin-treated, T cell depleted haplocompatible bone marrow transplantation. *Blood*, **81**, 2021–30.

Duplantier, J.E., Nelson, R.P. Jr., Ochs, H.D. *et al.* (1997). Successful bone marrow transplantation (BMT) for X-linked Hyper IgM (XHIM) syndrome. *Journal of Allergy and Clinical Immunology*, **99S**, 102.

Ege, M., Manfras, B.J., Barbi, G. *et al.* (2001). Eradication of a dysfunctional HLA-haploidentical T cell system by a second HLA-identical BMT. *Bone Marrow Transplantation*, **28**, 993–5.

Farinha, N. J., Duval, M., Wagner, E. *et al.* (2002). Unrelated bone marrow transplantation for leukocyte adhesion deficiency. *Bone Marrow Transplantation, 30,* 979–81.

Filipovich, A.H., Shapiro, R.S., Ramsay, N.K.C. *et al.* (1992). Unrelated donor bone marrow transplantation for correction of lethal congenital immunedeficiencies. *Blood, 80,* 270–6.

Filipovich, A.H., Stone, J.V., Tomany, S.C. *et al.* (2001). Impact of donor type on outcome of bone marrow transplantation for Wiskott-Aldrich syndrome: collaborative study of the International Bone Marrow Transplant Registry and the National Marrow Donor Registry. *Blood, 97,* 1598–603.

Fischer, A. (1991). Anti-LFA-1 antibody as immunosuppressive reagent in transplantation. *Clinical Immunology, 50,* 89–97.

Fischer, A., Friedrich, W., Fasth, A. *et al.* (1991). Reduction of graft failure by monoclonal antibody (anti-LFA-1 CD11a) after HLA-non identical bone marrow transplantation in children with immunodeficiencies, osteoporosis and Fanconi's anemia. *Blood, 77,* 249–56.

Fischer, A., Griscelli, C., Friedrich, W. *et al.* (1986). Bone marrow transplantation for immunodeficiencies and osteoporosis. A European survey, 1968–1985 *Lancet, 2,* 1079–82.

Fischer, A., Landais, P., Friedrich, W. *et al.* (1990). European experience of bone marrow transplantation for SCID. *Lancet, 2,* 850–4.

Fischer, A., Landais, P., Friedrich, W. *et al.* (1994). Bone marrow transplantation (BMT) in Europe for primary immunedeficiencies other than severe combined immunodeficiency: a report from the European group for BMT and the European group for immunodeficiency. *Blood, 83,* 1149–54.

Flake, A.W., Roncarolo, M.G., Puck, J.M. *et al.* (1996). Treatment of X-linked severe combined immunodeficiency by in utero transplantation of paternal bone marrow. *New England Journal of Medicine, 335,* 1806–10.

Friedrich, W., Knoblock, C., Greher, J. *et al.* (1993). Bone marrow transplantation in severe combined immunodeficiency: potential and current limitations. *Immunodeficiency, 4,* 315–22.

Gatti, R.A., Meuwissen, H.J., Allen, H.D. *et al.* (1968). Immunological reconstitution of sex-linked lymphogenic immunological deficiency. *Lancet, 2,* 1366–9.

Goldsobel, A.B., Haas, A., & Stiehm, E.R. (1987). Bone marrow transplantation in Di George syndrome. *Journal of Pediatrics, 11,* 40–4.

Gomez, L., Le Deist, F., Blanche, S. *et al.* (1995). Treatment of Omenn's syndrome by BMT. *Journal of Pediatrics, 127,* 76–81.

Gross, T.G., Filipovich, A.H., Conley, M.E. *et al.* (1996). Cure of X-linked lymphoproliferative disease (XLP) with allogeneic hematopoietic stem cell transplantation (HSCT): report from the XLP registry. *Bone Marrow Transplantation, 17,* 741–4.

Haddad, E., Landais, P., Friedrich, W. *et al.* (1998). Long-term immune reconstitution and outcome after HLA-nonidentical T-cell-depleted bone marrow transplantation for severe combined immunodeficiency: a European retrospective study of 116 patients. *Blood, 91,* 3646–53.

Haddad, E., Le Deist, F., Aucouturier, P. *et al.* (1999). Long-term chimerism and B-cell function after bone marrow transplantation in patients with severe combined immunodeficiency with B cells: a single-center study of 22 patients *Blood, 94,* 2923–30.

Haddad, E., Le Deist, F., Blanche, S. *et al.* (1995). Treatment of Chediak-Higashi syndrome by allogeneic bone marrow transplantation: report of 10 cases. *Blood, 85,* 3328–33.

Haddad, E., Paczesny, S., Leblond, V. *et al.* (2001). Treatment of B-lymphoproliferative disorder with a monoclonal anti-interleukin-6 antibody in twelve patients : a multicenter phase I-II clinical trial. *Blood, 97,* 1590–7.

Hadzic, N. Pagliuca, A., Rela, M. *et al.* (2000). Correction of hyperIgM syndrome after liver and bone marrow transplantation. *New England Journal of Medicine, 342,* 320–3.

Hallett, R.J., Gaspar, B., Duley, J.A. *et al.* (1999). Allogeneic bone marrow transplantation corrects the immunodeficiency in PNP deficiency but does not reverse the neurological abnormalities. *Cellular and Molecular Biology Letter, 4,* 374.

Hershfield, M.S., Buckley, R.H., Greenberg, M.L. *et al.* (1987). Treatment of adenosine deaminase deficiency with PEG modified ADA. *New England Journal of Medicine, 316,* 589–96.

Heslop, H.E., Brenner, M.K., & Rooney, C.M. (1994). Donor T cells to treat EBV-associated lymphoma. *New England Journal of Medicine, 331,* 679–80.

Heyderman, R. S., Morgan, G., Levinsky, R. J. *et al.* (1991). Successful bone marrow transplantation and treatment of BCG infection in two patients with severe combined immunodeficiency. *European Journal of Pedaitrics, 150,* 477–80.

Ho, C.M., Vowels, M.R., Lockwood, L., & Ziegler, J.B. (1996). Successful bone marrow transplantation in a child with X-linked chronic granulomatous disease. *Bone Marrow Transplantation, 18,* 213–15.

Hobbs, J.R., Monteil, M., McCluskey, D.R. *et al.* (1992). Chronic granulomatous disease 100% corrected by displacement bone marrow transplantation from a volunteer unrelated donor. *European Journal of Pediatrics, 151,* 806–10.

Horwitz, M.E., Barrett, A.J., Brown, M.R. *et al.* (2001). Treatment of chronic granulomatous disease with nonmyeloablative conditioning and a T-cell-depleted hematopoietic allograft. *New England Journal of Medicine, 344,* 881–8.

Ikinciogullari, A., Dogu, F., Ciftci, E. *et al.* (2002). An intensive approach to the treatment of disseminated BCG infection in a SCID patient. *Bone Marrow Transplantation, 30,* 45–7.

Jabado, N., Le Deist, F., Cant, A. *et al.* (1996). Bone marrow transplantation from genetically HLA-non identical donors in children with fatal inherited disorders excluding severe combined immunodeficiencies: use of two monoclonal antibodies to prevent graft rejection. *Pediatrics, 98,* 420–8.

Kane, L., Gennery, A.R., Crooks, B.N. *et al.* (2001). Neonatal bone marrow transplantation for severe combined immunodeficiency. *Archives of Disease of Childhood, Fetal Neonatal Ed., 85,* F110–3.

Kato, T., Tsuge, I., Inaba, J. *et al.* (1999). Successful bone marrow transplantation in a child with X-linked hyper-IgM syndrome. *Bone Marrow Transplantation, 23,* 1081–3.

Kawai, S., Sasahara, Y., Minigishi, M. *et al.* (1999). Immunological reconstitution by allogeneic bone marrow transplantation in a child with the X-linked hyper-IgM syndrome. *European Journal of Pediatrics, 158,* 394–7.

Kernan, N.A., Bartsch, G., Ash, R.C. *et al.* (1993). Analysis of 462 transplantations from unrelated donors facilitated by the National

Marrow Donor Program. *New England Journal of Medicine,* **328,** 593–602.

Klein, C., Cavazzana-Calvo, M., Le Deist, F. *et al.* (1995). Bone marrow transplantation in major histocompatibility complex class II deficiency: a single center study of 19 patients. *Blood,* **85,** 580–7.

Klein, C., Philippe, N., Le Deist, F. *et al.* (1994). Partial albinism with immunodeficiency (Griscelli syndrome). *Journal of Pediatrics,* **125,** 886–95.

Kohn, D.B., Weinberg, K.I., Nolta, J.A. *et al.* (1995). Engraftment of gene modified umbilical cord blood cells in neonates with adenosine deaminase deficiency. *Nature Medicine,* **1,** 1017–23.

Le Deist, F., Blanche, S., Keable, H. *et al.* (1989). Successful HLA-non-identical bone marrow transplantation in three patients with leukocyte adhesion deficiency. *Blood,* **74,** 512–19.

Leone, V., Tommasini, A., Andolina, M. *et al.* (2002). Elective bone marrow transplantation in a child with X-linked hyper-IgM syndrome presenting with acute respiratory distress syndrome. *Bone Marrow Transplantation,* **30,** 49–52.

Leung, T.F., Chik, K.W., Li, C.K. *et al.* (1999). Bone marrow transplantation, for chronic granulomatous disease: long-term follow-up and review of literature. *Bone Marrow Transplantation,* **24,** 567–70.

Lo, D. & Sprent, J. (1986). Identity of cells that imprint H-2 restricted T cell specificity in the thymus. *Nature,* **319,** 672–5.

Loechelt, B.J., Shapiro, R.S., Jyonouchi, H. *et al.* (1995). Mismatched bone marrow transplantation for Omenn syndrome: a variant of severe combined immune deficiency. *Bone Marrow Transplantation,* **16,** 381–5.

Longhurst, H.J., Taussig, D., Haque, T. *et al.* (2002). Non-myeloablative bone marrow transplantation in an adult with Wiscott-Aldrich syndrome. *British Journal of Haematology,* **116,** 497–9.

Mancias, C., Infante, A.J., & Kermani, N.R. (1999). Matched unrelated donor bone marrow transplantation in leukocyte adhesion deficiency. *Bone Marrow Transplantation,* **244,** 1261–3.

Minigishi, M., Tsuchiya, S., Imaizumi, M. *et al.* (1985). Successful transplantation of soy bean agglutinin-fractionated, histoincompatible, maternal marrow in a patient with a severe combined immunodeficiency and BCG infection. *European Journal of Pediatrics,* **143,** 291–4.

Mullen, C.A., Anderson, K.D., & Blaese, R.M. (1993). Splenectomy and/or bone marrow transplantation in the management of the Wiskott-Aldrich syndrome: long-term follow-up of 62 cases. *Blood,* **82,** 2961–6.

Myers, L.A., Patel, D.D., Puck, J.M. *et al.* (2002). Hematopoietic stem cell transplantation for severe combined immunodeficiency in the neonatal period leads to superior thymic output and improved survival *Blood,* **99,** 872–8.

Notarangelo, L.N., Duse, M., & Ugazio, A.G. (1992). Immune deficiency with hyper IgM (HIM). *Immunodeficiency Reviews,* **3,** 101–21.

O'Reilly, R.J., Brochstein, J., Dinsmore, R. *et al.* (1989a). Marrow transplantation for congenital disorders. *Seminars in Hematology,* **21,** 188–225.

O'Reilly, R.J., Keever, C.A., Small, T.N. *et al.* (1990). The use of HLA-non identical T cell depleted marrow transplants for correction of SCID. *Immunodeficiency Reviews,* **1,** 273–98.

O'Reilly, R.J., Pollock, M.S., Kapoor, N. *et al.* (1989b). Fetal liver transplantation in man and animals. In *Recent Advances in Bone Marrow Transplantation,* ed. R.P. Gale, pp. 789–830. New York: Alan R. Liss.

Ortin, M., Rhymes, H., Weightman, H., & Darbyshire, P.J. (2000). Unrelated donor bone marrow transplantation in the treatment of purine nucleoside phosphorylase deficiency. *Bone Marrow Transplantation,* **25** (Suppl 1), 112.

Ozsahin, H., Le Deist, F., Benkerrou, M. *et al.* (1996). Bone marrow transplantation in 26 patients with Wiskott-Aldrich syndrome from a single center. *Journal of Pediatric Surgery,* **129,** 238–44.

Parkman, R., Rappeport, J., Geha, R. *et al.* (1978). Complete correction of the Wiskott-Aldrich syndrome by allogenic bone marrow transplantation. *New England Journal of Medicine,* **208,** 921–7.

Patel, D.D., Gooding, M.E., Parrott, R.A. *et al.* (2000). Thymic function after hematopoietic stem cell transplantation for the treatment of severe combined immunodeficiency. *New England Journal of Medicine,* **342,** 1325–32.

Peter, H.H., Friedrich, W., Dopfer, R. *et al.* (1983). NK cell function in severe combined immunodeficiency (SCID): evidence of a common T and NK cell defect in some but not all SCID patients. *Journal of Immunology,* **131,** 2332–9.

Pracher, E., Panzer-Grümayer, E.R., Zoubek, A. *et al.* (1994). Successful bone marrow transplantation in a boy with X-linked lymphoproliferative syndrome and acute severe infectious mononucleosis. *Bone Marrow Transplantation,* **13,** 655–8.

Reisner, Y., Kapoor, N., Kirkpatrick, D. *et al.* (1983). Transplantation for SCID with HLA-A, B, D/DR incompatible marrow fractionated by soy bean agglutinin and sheep red blood cells. *Blood,* **61,** 341–8.

Reuter, U., Roessler, J., Thiede, C. *et al.* (2002). Correction of complete interferon-gamma receptor 1 deficiency by bone marrow transplantation. *Blood,* **100,** 4234–5.

Roberts, J.L., Volkman, D.J., & Buckley, R.H. (1989). Modified MHC restriction of donor origin T cells in humans with SCID transplanted with haploidentical bone marrow stem cells. *Journal of Immunology,* **143,** 1575–9.

Rocha, V., Wagner, Jr., J.E., Sobocinski, K.A. *et al.* (2000). Graft-versus-host disease in children who have received a cord-blood or bone marrow transplant from an HLA-identical sibling. Eurocord and International Bone Marrow Transplant Registry Working Committee on Alternative Donor and Stem Cell Sources. *New England Journal of Medicine,* **342,** 1846–54.

Rubocki, R.J., Parsa, J.R., Hershfield, M.S. *et al.* (2001). Full hematopoietic engraftment after allogeneic bone marrow transplantation without cytoreduction in a child with severe combined immunodeficiency. *Blood,* **97,** 809–11.

Rumelhart, S.L., Trigg, M.E., Horowitz, S.D. *et al.* (1990). Monoclonal antibody T cell depleted haploidentical bone marrow transplantation for Wiskott-Aldrich syndrome. *Blood,* **75,** 1031–5.

Schneider, L.C., Berman, R.S., Shea, C.R. *et al.* (1990). Bone marrow transplantation (BMT) for the syndrome of pigmentary dilution and lymphohistiocytosis (Griscelli's syndrome). *Journal of Clinical Immunology,* **10,** 146–53.

Scholl, P. R., O'Gorman, M. R. G., Pachman, L. M., *et al.* (1998). Correction of neutropenia and hypogammaglobulinemia in X-linked hyper-IgM syndrome by allogeneic bone marrow transplantation. *Bone Marrow Transplantation,* **22,** 1215–8.

Schuster, F., Stachel, D.K., Schmid, I. *et al.* (2001). Griscelli syndrome: report of the first peripheral blood stem cell transplant and the role of mutations of the RAB27A gene as an indication for BMT. *Bone Marrow Transplantation,* **28,** 409–12.

Schwinger, W., Urban, Ch., Lackner, H. *et al.* (2000). Unrelated partially matched peripheral blood stem cell transplantation with highly purified CD34+ cells in a child with Wiskott-Aldrich syndrome. *Bone Marrow Transplantation,* **26,** 235–7.

Scottini, A., Quirbs-Roldan, E., Notarangelo, L.D. *et al.* (1995). Engrafted maternal T cells in a SCID patient express T cell receptor variable segments characterized by a restricted V-D junctional diversity. *Blood,* **85,** 2105.

Seger, R.A. (2001). Bone marrow transplantation (BMT) for chronic granulomatous disease. *Bone Marrow Transplantation,* **27** (Suppl 1), S34 (Abstract).

Seger, R. A., Gungor, T., Belohradsky, B. H. *et al.* (2002). Treatment of chronic granulomatous disease with myeloablative conditioning and an unmodified hemopoietic allograft: a survey of the European experience, 1985–2000. *Blood,* **100,** 4344–50.

Stary, J., Bartunkova, J., Kobylka, P. *et al.* (1996). Successful HLA-identical sibling cord blood transplantation in a 6 year old boy with leukocyte adhesion deficiency syndrome. *Bone Marrow Transplantation,* **18,** 249–52.

Stephan, J.L., Vlekova, V., Le Deist, F. *et al.* (1993). Severe combined immunodeficiency: a retrospective single-center study of clinical presentation and outcome in 117 cases. *Journal of Pediatrics,* **123,** 564–72.

Sullivan, J.L. & Woda, B.A. (1989). X-linked lymphoproliferative syndrome. *Immunodeficiency Reviews,* **1,** 325–47.

Tezcan, I., Sanal, O., Ersoy, F. *et al.* (1999). Successful bone marrow transplantation in a case of Griscelli disease which presented in accelerated phase with neurological involvement. *Bone Marrow Transplantation,* **24,** 931–3.

The International Chronic Granulomatous Disease Cooperative Study Group. (1991). A controlled trial of interferon gamma to prevent infection in chronic granulomatous disease. *New England Journal of Medicine,* **324,** 509–6.

Thomas, C., de Saint Basile, G., Le Diest, F. *et al.* (1995a). Brief report: correction of X-linked hyper-IgM syndrome by allogeneic bone marrow transplantation. *New England Journal of Medicine,* **333,** 426–9.

Thomas, C., Le Deist, F., Cavazzana-Calvo, M. *et al.* (1995b). Results of allogeneic bone marrow transplantation in patients with leukocyte adhesion deficiency. *Blood,* **86,** 1629–35.

Toyoda, H., Azuma, E., Hori, H. *et al.* (2001). Successful unrelated BMT in a patient with Kostmann syndrome complicated by pre-transplant pulmonary 'bacterial' abscesses. *Bone Marrow Transplantation,* **28,** 413–5.

Trigg, M.E. & Schugar, R. (2001). Chediak-Higashi syndrome: hematopoietic chimerism corrects genetic defect. *Bone Marrow Transplantation,* **27,** 1211–3.

Van Dijken, P.J., Ghayur, T., Mauch, P. *et al.* (1990). Evidence that anti-LFA-1 in vivo improves engraftment and survival after allogeneic bone marrow transplantation. *Transplantation,* **49,** 882–6.

Van Leeuwen, J.E.M., Van Tol, M.J.D., Joosten, A.M. *et al.* (1994). Relationship between patterns of engraftment in peripheral blood and immune reconstitution after allogeneic BMT for SCID. *Blood,* **84,** 3936–47.

Vassal, G., Fischer, A., Challien, D. *et al.* (1993). Busulfan disposition below the age of three: alteration in children with lysosomal storage disease. *Blood,* **82,** 1030–4.

Vowels, M.R., Lam-Po-Tang, R., Berdoukas, V. *et al.* (1993). Correction of X-linked lymphoproliferative disease by transplantation of cord-blood stem cells. *New England Journal of Medicine,* **329,** 1623–5.

Watanabe, C., Yajima, S., Taguchi, T. *et al.* (2001). Successful unrelated bone marrow transplantation for a patient with chronic granulomatous disease and associated resistant pneumonitis and Aspergillus osteomyelitis. *Bone Marrow Transplantation,* **28,** 83–7.

Wengler, G.S., Lanfranchi, A., Frusca, T. *et al.* (1996). In utero transplantation of parental CD34 haematopoietic progenitor cells in a patient with X-linked severe combined immune deficiency (SCIDX1). *Lancet,* **348,** 1484–7.

Wijnaendts, L., Le Deist, F., Griscelli, C. *et al.* (1989). Development of immunologic functions after BMT in 33 patients with SCID. *Blood,* **74,** 2212–19.

Williams, L.L., Rooney, C.M., Conley, M.E. *et al.* (1993). Correction of Duncan's syndrome by allogeneic bone marrow transplantation. *Lancet,* **342,** 587–8.

Yamaguchi, K., Ariga, T., Yamada, M. *et al.* (2002). Mixed chimera status of 12 patients with Wiskott-Aldrich syndrome (WAS) after hematopoietic stem cell transplantation: evaluation by flow cytometric analysis of intracellular WAS protein expression. *Blood,* **100,** 1208–14.

Zeidler, C., Welte, K., Barak, Y. *et al.* (2000). Stem cell transplantation in patients with severe congenital neutropenia without evidence of leukemic transformation. *Blood,* **95,** 1195–8.

63 Allogeneic hematopoietic stem cell transplantation for metabolic disease

AMI SHAH, NEENA KAPOOR, GAY CROOKS, DONALD B. KOHN, KENNETH I. WEINBERG, AND ROBERTSON PARKMAN

Children's Hospital Los Angeles and University of Southern California School of Medicine, Los Angeles, USA

Introduction

The use of allogeneic hematopoietic stem cell transplantation (HSCT) to treat metabolic diseases (Table 63.1) is an area of continuing controversy. Metabolic diseases include the lysosomal storage disorders (LSDs), a group of at least 41 distinct genetic disorders, each resulting from a deficiency of a particular lysosomal protein, or, in a few cases, from nonlysosomal proteins involved in lysosomal biogenesis (Meikle *et al.*, 1999). In all the LSDs, accumulation of normally degraded substrate occurs within lysosomes. The LSDs can be grouped into broad categories that include the mucopolysaccaridoses, lipidoses, glycogenoses, and oligosaccaridoses. Common features of many LSDs include bone abnormalities, organomegaly, central nervous system (CNS) dysfunction, and coarse hair and facies.

Allogeneic HSCT has been used to treat metabolic diseases including Hurler syndrome, osteopetrosis, Gaucher disease, and adrenoleukodystrophy for over 20 years (Parkman, 1986; Krivit *et al.*, 1989; Parkman & Crooks, 1996; Krivit, Peters, & Shapiro, 1999). However, questions still exist as to which diseases and what patients are appropriate candidates for HSCT. Central to the evaluation of patients as potential candidates for transplantation to correct metabolic diseases is (1) whether the clinical symptomatology of their disease is restricted to lymphohematopoietically derived cells and (2) whether significant end organ damage has occurred prior to transplantation. The engraftment of enzymatically normal donor HSC will result in all lymphohematopoietic cells expressing donor level of enzyme. However, successful HSCT engraftment will not result in the production of enzyme by recipient nonlymphohematopoietic cells. In some diseases, however, enzyme produced by the donor-derived cells can be transported into the nonlymphohematopoietic recipient cells resulting in increased intracellular levels of the normal enzyme. Moreover, the differentiation of normal donor HSC into tissue-specific cells such as Kupfer cells, pulmonary or peritoneal macrophages, and microglia cells can result in the local production of the defective enzyme (Krivit *et al.*, 1995).

Clinical results

Osteopetrosis

Osteopetrosis is a clinical syndrome characterized by abnormal osteoclastic activity, defective resorption of bone, and bone sclerosis. Four main genetic types have been described: an autosomal recessive infantile "malignant" form, a milder autosomal recessive form, an autosomal dominant form, and a form due to deficiency of carbonic anhydrase II. The infantile form is charac-

Table 63.1. *Inheritance pattern and defect in some congenital metabolic diseases*

Disease	Inheritance pattern	Defect
Osteopetrosis	Autosomal recessive	Defective osteoclast activity
Osteogenesis imperfecta	Autosomal recessive	Defective type 1 collagen
Gaucher disease	Autosomal recessive	Defective β-glucocerebrosidase
Hurler syndrome	Autosomal recessive	Abnormal α-iduronidase
Hunter syndrome	X-linked recessive	Deficiency of iduronate sulfatase
Maroteaux-Lamy syndrome	Autosomal recessive	Deficiency arylsulfatase B
Sanfilippo A and B disease	Autosomal recessive	Four different enzymatic defects described
Metachromatic leukodystrophy	Autosomal	Deficiency of arylsulfatase A
Adrenoleukodystrophy	Peroxisomal X-linked	Abnormal lignoceroyl CoA ligase
Fucosidosis	Autosomal recessive	Deficiency of α-L-fucosidase
Farber disease	Autosomal recessive	Deficiency of ceramidase

terized by the rapid onset of severe symptoms including fractures, pancytopenia, blindness, deafness, and hydrocephalus. The milder autosomal recessive variant has a later age of onset with short stature, macrocephaly, mandibular osteomyelitis, dental abnormalities, and mild anemia. The autosomal dominant form is usually diagnosed coincidentally in the young adult with multiple fractures, bone pain, or cranial nerve palsy. The form due to carbonic anhydrase deficiency is characterized by pathologic fractures, renal tubular acidosis, and cerebral calcifications.

Although osteopetrotic mice had been cured by HSCT, when the initial patients with osteoperosis were transplanted, it was not known what the effects of successful donor lymphohematopoietic engraftment would be on their disease (Walker, 1975; Lajeunesse et al., 1996). Successful donor lymphohematopoietic engraftment following pretransplant preparation with busulfan and cyclophosphamide (to eliminate the recipient hematopoietic and lymphoid stem cells) resulted in clinical improvement (Coccia et al., 1980). Circulating mononuclear cells of donor ori-

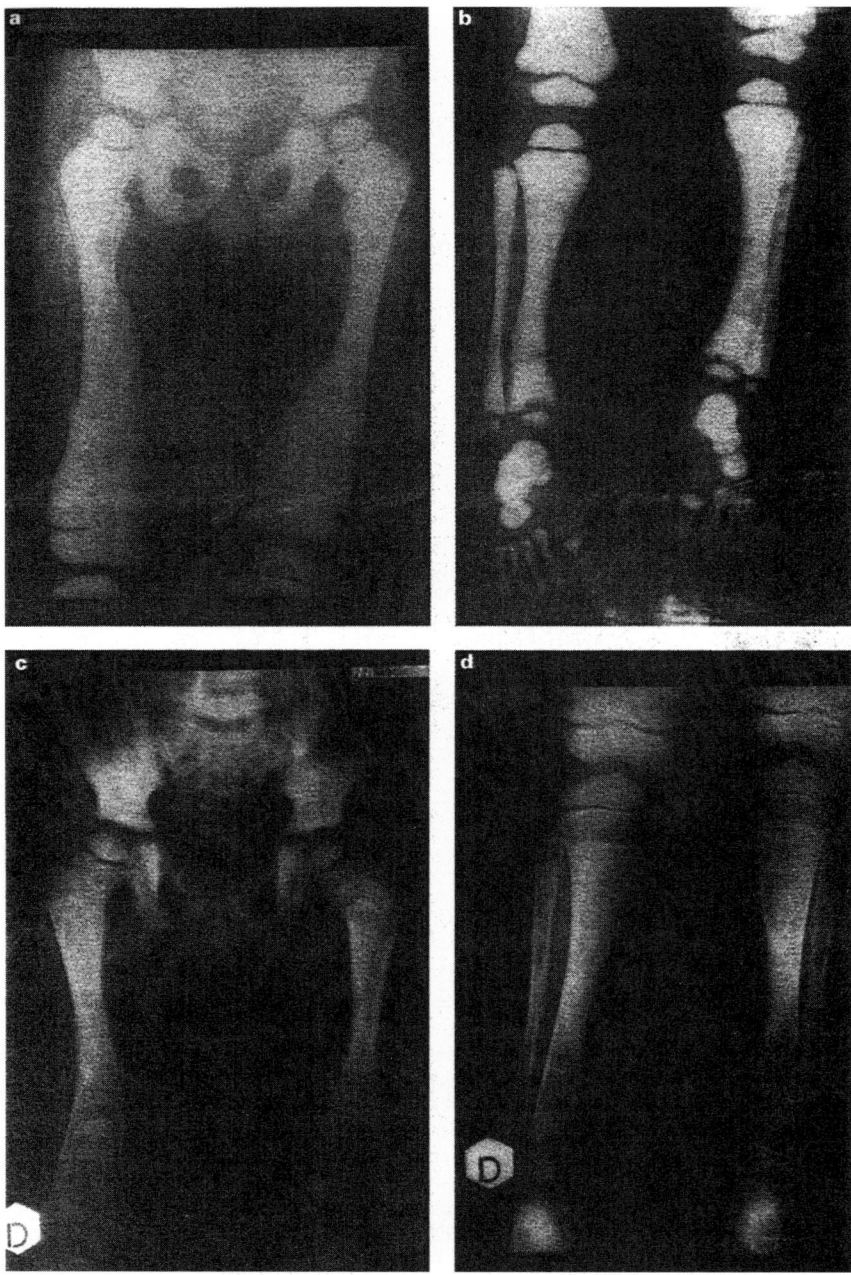

Fig. 63.1. Longitudinal radiographs of the pelvis and lower limbs before (**a, b**) and 48 months after (**c, d**) BMT (case 2). (**a**) Marked osteosclerosis with widened metaphyses (onion skin phenomenom). (**b**) Periosteal bone appositions consistent with previous pathological fractures. (**c, d**) A marked remodeling and consequent reduction of deformation is evident, as well as a dramatic decrease in bone radiodensity. Reproduced, with permission from Dini et al. (2000).

gin were detected by 3 to 4 weeks following transplantation. However, an increase in the diameter of the marrow cavity was not noted until 4 to 6 months following transplantation, at which time there was a decrease in extramedullary hematopoiesis with a secondary decrease in hepatosplenomegaly and an increase in urinary calcium excretion. Bone marrow biopsies following the normalization of hematopoiesis demonstrated that the patient's osteoclasts were of donor origin. Therefore, the primary defect in osteopetrosis is due to defective osteoclast activity and the cure of patients with osteopetrosis by HSCT confirms that osteoclasts are of hematopoietic origin.

Long-term follow-up of children transplanted for mild osteopetrosis have demonstrated extensive bone resorption with marked augmentation of osteoclasts, but no improvement in visual acuity, despite complete remodeling of skeletal abnormalities (Fig. 63.1) (Dini et al., 2000). Progressive visual impairment resulting in blindness has been reported in some patients despite complete donor lymphohematopoietic engraftment. Thus, progression of the neurological complications of osteopetrosis can occur following successful donor HSC engraftment (Kapelushnik et al., 2001). Therefore, patients have to be counseled about the possibility of neurological progression following HSCT.

Carbonic anhydrase II is present in renal tubules, brain, and osteoclasts and is critical in acid-base balance and bone remodeling. Two children with osteopetrosis due to carbonic anhydrase II deficiency received histocompatible HSCT (McMahon et al., 2001). Following successful engraftment the children demonstrated radiologic and histologic resolution of their osteopetrosis with stabilization of hearing and vision. However, the children remain developmentally delayed and continued to have renal tubular acidosis.

The major clinical question associated with the transplantation of patients with osteopetrosis is their clinical condition prior to transplantation. Patients with osteopetrosis develop blindness and deafness secondary to damage to their second and eighth cranial nerves by bony overgrowth. Successful donor HSC engraftment and normalization of hematopoietic function after deafness and blindness has developed will not result any improvement in neurological function. Magnetic resonance imaging (MRI) analysis of the optic foramens and electrophysiological assessment of auditory function is, therefore, a necessary part of the pretransplant workup of patients with osteopetrosis. Since no significant donor-derived osteoclast function can be detected until 4 to 6 months following transplantation, ongoing damage to the second and eighth cranial nerves may continue following transplant (Kapelushnik et al., 2001). Therefore, the clinical question is not "What is the patient's neurological function at the time of transplant?" but is "What will be the patient's neurological status 4 to 6 months following transplantation?"

If a histocompatible donor is available, donor bone marrow engraftment can be routinely achieved following pretransplant preparation with busulfan and cyclophosphamide. The use of T-cell-depleted haploidentical parental bone marrow has achieved a 50% engraftment rate (Fischer et al., 1986). Thus, patients with osteopetrosis can be successfully engrafted with parental bone marrow but have an increased incidence of graft-versus-host disease (GVHD).

Osteogenesis imperfecta

Osteogenesis imperfecta (OI) or "brittle bone disease" is a genetic disorder due to defects in type I collagen, the major structural protein of the extracellular matrix of bone. Patients with OI have multiple fractures, progressive deformities of their limbs, and retarded bone growth resulting in short stature. No curative therapy for OI exists. Biphosphonates may have therapeutic potential (Glorieux et al., 1998). Three children with OI were transplanted with HLA-identical bone marrow after myeloablative conditioning (Horwitz et al., 1999, 2001). Osteoblasts of donor origin were documented in all three recipients. The patients had a median of 7.5 cm increase in body length in the 6 months following transplantation compared to 1.25 cm for age-matched control children. The patients gained 21 to 65.3 g in body bone mineral content (45% to 77% of their baseline values) by 3 months following HSCT. However, their increase in linear growth was not sustained. The lack of sustained improvement suggests that donor-derived osteoblastic precursors rather than mesenchymal stem cells (MSC) were the origin of the donor-derived osteoblasts. As compared to osteoclasts, which are derived from HSC present in the bone marrow, osteoblasts are derived from MSC present in the bone marrow.

Gaucher disease[1]

Gaucher disease is due to defective glucocerebrosidase, which results in the lack of degradation of glucocerebroside. The use of HSCT in Gaucher disease has been modified by the commercial availability of glucocerebrosidase. Although effective, the enzyme therapy costs between $250–500,000 per year depending on the patient's size. Allogeneic HSCT has been used to treat two forms of Gaucher disease: Type I, in which the symptomatology is restricted to non-CNS tissues, and Type III, in which the later onset of neurological symptoms occurs. At present Type II Gaucher disease, in which there is the early onset of neurological symptoms, is not a candidate disease for HSCT. The first patient transplanted for Gaucher disease had Type I disease (Rappeport & Gins, 1984). He was prepared for transplantation with busulfan to eliminate his abnormal HSC and cyclophosphamide to eliminate his normal lymphoid cells and immune system. Although the correction of Gaucher disease is based on the successful engraftment of enzymatically normal HSC, engraftment of donor lymphoid stem cells is required to prevent the immunologically mediated rejection of the donor HSC. Following transplantation enzymatically normal peripheral blood leukocytes were detected by 1 month following transplantation, but bone marrow analysis showed the continued persistence of Gaucher cells. Repeated

[1] Philippe Gaucher, French physician, 1854–1918.

bone marrow examinations demonstrated that the percentage of Gaucher cells in the bone marrow began to decrease 6 months following HSCT with the appearance of normal hematopoietic cells. The persistence in the bone marrow of Gaucher cells following transplantation demonstrated that the in vivo survival of tissue macrophages is longer than that of circulating monocytes and that the tissue macrophages have a half-life of 4 to 6 months. Therefore, the replacement of abnormal recipient tissue macrophages by normal donor derived cells does not occur until 4 to 6 months following transplantation. Once the abnormal recipient tissue macrophages die, they can be replaced by enzymatically normal donor macrophages. Following successful HSCT, there is a reduction in the patient's hepatosplenomegaly and a normalization of bone marrow hematopoiesis. The initial patient transplanted for Gaucher disease had esophageal varices prior to transplantation. The successful engraftment of donor lymphohematopoietic cells did not reverse the pre-existing end organ damage, demonstrating that HSCT should be performed before significant end organ damage occurs.

Allogeneic HSCT has also been performed in patients with Type III Gaucher disease (Svennerhold et al., 1984) with some patients initially being diagnosed as having Type I disease. Molecular analysis permits a more precise definition of patients' disease than was possible using only enzymatic assays. Oculomotor ataxia is one of the early neurological signs of Type III Gaucher disease. Patients transplanted for Type III Gaucher disease have been followed for 13 to 15 years following transplantation (Ringden et al., 1988). Some Type III patients have had no increase in their neurological symptomatology or decrease in their intelligence, suggesting that HSCT prevented further CNS deterioration. The lack of further CNS deterioration suggests that enzymatically normal cells derived from HSC are present within CNS, most likely microglia cells, and is consistent with murine experiments in which donor-derived microglial cells were identified within the CNS (Krall et al., 1994). Further patient follow-up is necessary before definitive statements about the effect of HSCT on the neurological function of patients with Type III Gaucher disease can be made.

Successful engraftment of histocompatible bone marrow can be routinely achieved in patients with Gaucher disease following pretransplant preparation with busulfan and cyclophosphamide. Some centers advocate splenectomy prior to transplant to decrease the sequestration of HSC in the enlarged spleen (Hobbs et al., 1987). HSCT for Gaucher disease has also been performed with matched unrelated donors with successful donor lymphohematopoietic engraftment. However, the intravenous administration of modified human glucocerebroside has resulted in clinical improvement for most patients reducing the clinical indications for unrelated HSCT (Barton et al., 1991; Erikson et al., 1995).

Mucopolysaccharidoses

The group of metabolic diseases for which HSCT has had the greatest use is the mucopolysaccharidoses (Hobbs et al., 1981;

Parkman, 1986; Krivit & Shapiro, 1991). Most transplants have been performed for Hurler syndrome, followed by Maroteaux-Lamy syndrome, Hunter syndrome, and Sanfilippo A and B diseases. Successful HSCT will result in disease stabilization in mucopolysaccharidosis patients in contrast to the cure of disease that is the object of HSCT in patients with severe aplastic anemia, severe combined immune deficiency, leukemia, and genetic diseases of HSC such as the hemoglobinopathies. Successful donor HSC engraftment modifies the natural history of the disease in patients with Hurler syndrome and Maroteaux-Lamy syndrome whereas donor engraftment has had little impact on the natural history of patients with Hunter syndrome and Sanfilippo A and B diseases. It is recommended that the determination of the donor lysosomal enzyme level be a part of the pre-HSCT workup (de Gasperi et al., 2000).

Hurler syndrome[2]

Patients with Hurler syndrome are characterized by abnormal α-iduronidase. Although Hurler syndrome was initially felt to be a single disease, molecular heterogeneity has demonstrated that multiple genotypes exist as in Gaucher disease. A genotype/phenotype association has not been established yet. Therefore, accurate statements about the effects of allogeneic HSCT on an individual patient's disease are difficult.

If a histocompatible family member donor or HLA-matched unrelated donor is available, successful donor lymphohematopoietic engraftment can be achieved in most patients with Hurler syndrome following pretransplant preparation with busulfan and cyclophosphamide (Parkman, 1986; Krivit et al., 1989). Following successful donor engraftment, circulating donor lymphohematopoietic cells expressing donor levels of enzyme (either homozygote or heterozygote) can be detected 1 month following HSCT. Successful donor engraftment results in decreased corneal clouding and a reduction in hepatosplenomegaly. Central to the clinical use of HSCT to treat Hurler syndrome is the effect of donor HSC engraftment on the CNS function of affected patients. Murine experiments have demonstrated that microglial cells are of donor hematopoietic origin after successful HSCT (Krall et al., 1994). The effect of HSCT on the intellectual function of patients with Hurler syndrome is compounded by the genetic heterogeneity of patients, which may result in variations in the tempo of CNS deterioration. Longitudinal neuropsychological evaluation of donor engrafted patients suggests that patients transplanted before the age of 18 to 24 months have stabilization of their intellectual function that starts 6 months following transplantation (Hugh-Jones, 1986; Peters et al., 1998) (Fig. 63.2). Patients transplanted later than 24 to 30 months of age or with markedly reduced developmental quotations (DQ) prior to transplantation, derive little clinical benefit from transplantation with continued CNS deterioration. As in the cases of Gaucher disease and osteopetrosis, the turnover of recipient tissue macrophages within the CNS (microglial cells) takes 4 to 6 months.

---

[2] Gertrude Hurler, Austrian pediatrician, 1889–1963.

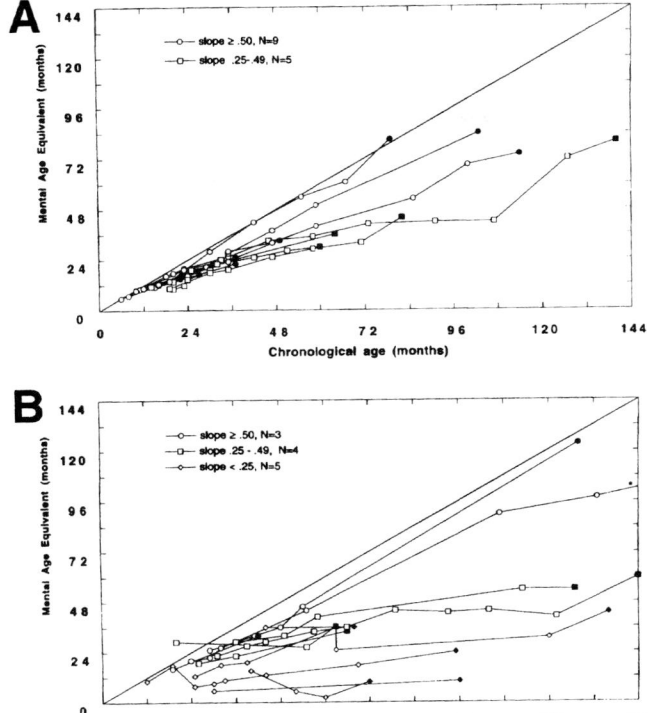

Fig. 63.2. **(A)** Mental age-equivalent scores of MPSIH (Hurler syndrome) patients receiving related-donor BMT before 24 months of age (normal, —; slope ≥.50, ○; slope .25 to .49, □; solid symbol denotes most recent neuropsychological evaluation). **(B)** Mental age-equivalent scores of MPSIH patients receiving related-donor BMT after 24 months of age (normal, —; slope ≥.50, ○; slope .25 to .49, □; slope <.25, ◇; solid symbol denotes most recent neuropsychological evaluation). *Latest neuropsychological evaluation at 159 months of age and a mental age-equivalent score of 108 months. Reproduced, with permission, from Peters *et al.* (1998).

Therefore, ongoing CNS damage will continue following HSCT. It is only when enzymatically normal, donor-derived cells are present within the CNS that further CNS deterioration is prevented. Thus, the clinical question is not what is the intellectual function of a patient at the time of transplantation, but what the intellectual function will be when enzymatically normal donor cells gain access to the CNS. Animal experiments have demonstrated that donor-derived blood monocytes can be detected within the areas of CNS degeneration early after transplantation; however, the presence of neurological degeneration means that significant end organ damage has already occurred. Therefore, HSCT for Hurler disease should be performed as early as possible, preferably before any CNS damage occurs. The diagnosis of Hurler disease is adequate justification for HSCT if an appropriate donor is available. If transplantation is delayed until signs of CNS deterioration occur, the CNS function of the patient may have declined to unacceptable levels before donor-derived microglial cells are present within the CNS in adequate numbers to provide clinical benefit. Second

transplantation can be of benefit if graft failure (as high as 27% in some series) occurs (Grewal *et al.*, 2002). The estimated 4-year survival after second transplant in this series of 11 patients with Hurler syndrome was 50%.

The outcome of unrelated donor HSCT in patients with Hurler syndrome has been reported (Peters *et al.*, 1996). The patients were transplanted at a median age of 1.7 years (range 0.9–3.2). Twenty-five of the 40 patients initially engrafted, and half were alive at 2 years. Eleven of the 15 patients, who rejected their initial graft, were successfully engrafted after a second unrelated HSCT. Neither T-cell depletion of the marrow nor irradiation influenced the likelihood of initial engraftment suggesting that HSC engraftment is compromised in patients with Hurler syndrome. Children who had a baseline mental development index of 70 or greater and engrafted, were more likely to achieve a favorable long-term outcome with improved cognitive function.

In addition to the use of both matched related and unrelated donor HSCT, some centers have transplanted patients with four and five antigen matched family donors following partial T-cell depletion. The use of unmatched family member donors has resulted in successful engraftment with acceptable degrees of acute and chronic GVHD (Henslee-Downey *et al.*, 1990; Fleming *et al.*, 1998; Peters *et al.*, 1998) (Fig. 63.3).

Maroteaux-Lamy syndrome[3]

Maroteaux-Lamy syndrome is an autosomal recessive disease due to a deficiency of the enzyme, arylsulfatase B, resulting in accumulation of glycoaminoglycans. Affected individuals exhibit coarse skin and facial features, hepatosplenomegaly, corneal cloudiness, upper airway narrowing, chronic middle ear effusion, valvular heart disease, and cardiomyopathy. Patients with severe disease die in early adult life from cardiopulmonary complications. Maroteaux-Lamy syndrome is unique among the mucopolysaccharidoses in that no significant CNS deterioration occurs.

Successful donor HSC engraftment results in the presence of enzymatically normal donor cells in the patient's peripheral circulation and a reduction in hepatosplenomegaly (Krivit *et al.*, 1984; Krivit, 1992b). The resolution of the patient's hepatosplenomegaly is due to the fact that circulating enzyme derived from the donor cells can be transported into recipient nonlymphohematopoietic cells, thus gaining access to the accumulated mucopolysaccharide. Co-culture experiments using normal and patient fibroblasts have demonstrated that donor-derived enzyme is actively transported into defective patient fibroblasts. Although some improvement in the facial features has been reported, the patients' orthopedic abnormalities do not show any improvement (Herskhovitz *et al.*, 1999). In the first report of an HLA-identical sibling cord blood transplant for this disease, the coarseness of the skin and facial features again improved, suppurative middle ear effusions did not recur, hepatosplenomegaly resolved, and height increased by 5 cm in

[3] Pierre Maroteaux, French geneticist, born 1926. Maurice Lamy, French physician, 1895–1975.

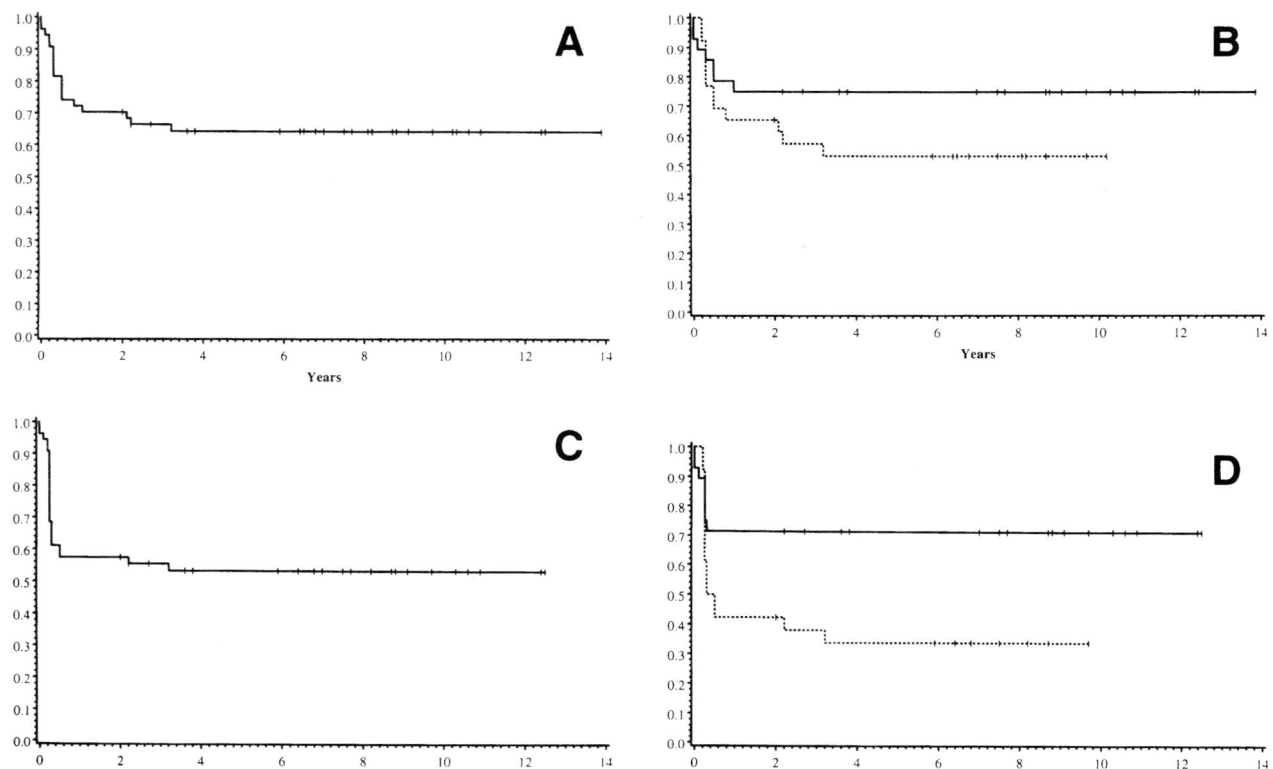

Fig. 63.3. (A) Overall actuarial probability of survival (—) of 54 MPSIH patients treated with related-donor BMT. (B) Overall actuarial probability of survival of MPSIH patients treated with GIS (—) or HIR (—) donor BMT. (C) Overall actuarial probability of survival (—) of MPSIH patients with donor cell engraftment following related-donor BMT. (D) Overall actuarial probability of survival of MPSIH patients with donor cell engraftment following GIS (—) or HIR (—) donor BMT. Abbreviations: MPSIH, Hurler syndrome; GIS, genotypically identical sibling; HIR, haploidentical related. Reproduced, with permission, from Peters et al. (1998).

10 months (Lee et al., 2000). The persistence of skeletal abnormalities in patients with Maroteaux-Lamy syndrome indicates that the donor-derived enzyme is not able to gain access to the mucopolysaccharide accumulations in chondrocytes. Patients with Maroteaux-Lamy syndrome have continuing skeletal deformities that result in a lack of growth particularly of their pelvic girdle. The unequal skeletal growth requires secondary orthopedic procedures in some patients.

Hunter syndrome[4]
While clinical experience has demonstrated clinical stabilization following donor HSC engraftment in young patients with Hurler syndrome, results in patients transplanted for Hunter syndrome have been less successful, with a lack of clinical stabilization and continued deterioration of neurocognitive function (Bergstrom et al., 1994; McKinnis et al., 1996). The lack of benefit following transplantation for Hunter syndrome is due to the fact that circulating donor-derived enzyme is not effectively transported into recipient cells. Therefore, most centers no longer consider patients with Hunter syndrome as candidates for HSCT.

Sanfilippo A and B Disease[5]
Although successful donor HSC engraftment has been achieved in patients with both Sanfilippo A and B diseases, clinical improvement or stabilization of CNS function has not been achieved. Therefore, most centers no longer believe that HSCT for Sanfilippo A and B disease is indicated.

Metachromatic leukodystrophy
Metachromatic leukodystrophy (MLD) is due to a deficiency in the lysosomal enzyme, arylsulfatase A. Deterioration of CNS function is due to the accumulation of galactosyl sulfatide in the white matter of the brain. Successful donor engraftment in patients with MLD has resulted in stabilization of the patient's intellectual function; however, progression of the patient's neurologic abnormalities, particularly of the peripheral nerves has occurred (Bayever et al., 1985; Krivit et al., 1990). An animal model for MLD exists in the Twitcher mouse. Successful engraftment in the mouse model shows the presence of donor-derived enzyme earlier in the CNS than in peripheral nerves (Yeager et al., 1984). The more rapid appearance of donor-derived enzyme within the CNS may explain the observation in

[4] Charles Hunter, Canadian physician, 1872–1955.

[5] Sylvester Sanfilippo, 20th-century U.S. physician.

patients that successful donor engraftment results in the stabilization of CNS function, but the progression of peripheral nerve abnormalities. As in the cases of other CNS metabolic diseases, transplantation will not reverse pre-existing abnormalities, and, therefore, patients should be transplanted prior to the development of CNS abnormalities, which will continue to progress for 4 to 6 months following transplantation. The patient's disease status and diagnosis are central to the likelihood of disease stabilization. Patients with moderate neurological abnormalities and the late infantile or juvenile forms of MLD have had continued disease progression. These results emphasize the importance of transplanting only presymptomatic children with infantile or early juvenile MLD (Malm *et al.,* 1996). Other reports have described prevention or stabilization, or slowing down of the progress of the disease. The series by Malm and colleagues emphasizes the importance of current recommendations to consider allografting for MLD only in the presymptomatic child with infantile MLD or early in the course of juvenile MLD. Donor origin lymphocytes have been described in the cerebrospinal fluid of patients with MLD postallografting (Yazaki *et al.,* 1995). Patients with a diagnosis of MLD should be transplanted as soon as possible if an appropriate donor is available since the clinical deterioration that occurs in MLD patients is predictable.

Adrenoleukodystrophy

Whereas the early transplantation of patients with MLD is unequivocally advocated, the timing of transplantation for adrenoleukodystrophy (ALD) is a topic of controversy. ALD is due to abnormalities in lignoceroyl CoA ligase, which is involved in the peroxisomal oxidation of very long chain fatty acids. The abnormalities result in either adrenal insufficiency or CNS deterioration. The clinical spectrum of ALD is diverse with infantile, juvenile, and adult onset forms (Moser *et al.,* 1987). Within families the time of onset and the clinical spectrum varies. Therefore, it is not possible to predict with certainty the age of onset or symptomatology even within kindreds. The initial transplants in patients with established ALD resulted in the accelerated deterioration of the patients' clinical status and their death shortly following transplantation despite donor HSC engraftment (Moser *et al.,* 1984). Patients are now transplanted at the first signs of radiological and/or clinical deterioration. Successful donor engraftment has resulted in the improvement/stabilization of neuropsychological function or MRI appearance in some patients (Aubourg *et al.,* 1990; Krivit *et al.,* 1992c). Long-term (5–10 years) follow-up of 12 children transplanted with ALD demonstrated the complete reversal of MRI abnormalities in 2 patients and improvement in 1 patient (Shapiro *et al.,* 2000). Eight patients, who showed an initial period of demyelination, stabilized and remained unchanged thereafter. Motor function remained normal or improved in 10 patients. Verbal intelligence remained within the normal range in 11 patients. Performance (nonverbal) abilities were improved or stabilized in 7 patients while a decline in performance abilities followed by stabilization occurred in 5 patients. Plasma

very-long chain fatty acid concentrations decreased by 55% and remained slightly above the upper limits of normal. Non-HSCT therapy with a low-fat diet and erucic acid (Lorenzo's oil) has not been shown to have significant clinical benefit.

The clinical problem associated with HSC transplantation for ALD patients is, "What is the appropriate time for transplantation if the patients have a variable time of onset of their disease?" At present no clear consensus about the appropriate timing for transplantation exists. Most centers follow patients with ALD closely to detect early signs of electrophysiologic or radiologic abnormalities and transplant patients at the first sign of disease progression. Like other CNS storage diseases, patients with ALD will have continued disease progression for 4 to 6 months following HSCT. Therefore, transplantation of ALD patients with significant pre-existing symptomatology is unlikely to produce clinical benefit.

Fucosidosis

Fucosidosis is an autosomal recessive lysosomal disorder caused by deficiency of α-L-fucosidase, resulting in accumulation of glycolipids and oligosaccharides, preferentially in the CNS. Patients with fucosidosis have progressive mental and motor deterioration, growth retardation, coarse facies, seizures, and hepatosplenomegaly. In a canine model of fucosidosis, HSCT has resulted in the delay or prevention of clinical disease. Although family member HSCT has not been performed in patients, unrelated HSCT has (Vellodi *et al.,* 1995; Miano *et al.,* 2001). In two patients, stabilization or a delay in disease progression was reported when patients were transplanted before significant clinical symptomatology was present (Miano *et al.,* 2001). A progressive rise in α-fucosidase levels in lymphocytes, plasma, and cerebrospinal fluid was documented. In the first report the transplant was performed on an 8-month-old boy. Although he was asymptomatic and his development normal at the time of transplant, abnormalities were found on an MRI scan pretransplant. Posttransplant the presence of donor levels of α-fucosidase were documented at 18 months posttransplant. There was evidence of mild neurodevelopmental delay but in contrast his elder sibling had shown far greater developmental delay at the same age. Improvement was also seen in a case with 4-year follow-up, although initially the patient deteriorated clinically. A progressive rise in α-fucosidase levels in lymphocytes, plasma, and cerebrospinal fluid was documented.

Farber disease[6]

Infantile ceramidase deficiency is an uncommon, progressive, autosomal recessive lysosomal storage disease characterized by multiple ceramidase-containing nodules (lipogranulomata) in the subcutaneous tissue and digestive tract and psychomotor retardation. Management is generally limited to supportive care, and few affected children have survived beyond 5 years.

[6] Sydney Farber, U.S. pediatrician, 1903–1973.

Although successful HSC engraftment has resulted in the resolution of the lipogranulomata, CNS deterioration continued in two patients (Souillet *et al.*, 1989; Yeager *et al.*, 2000). In the first patient, who had neurological involvement before transplant, the lipogranulomata regressed, but he died with progressive neurological involvement 6 months posttransplant. In the second patient, a 9.5-month-old female received a BMT from her HLA-identical sister, who was heterozygous for the condition, after conditioning with busulfan and cyclophosphamide. Ceramidase activity in peripheral blood leukocytes increased from 6% pretransplant to 44% 6 weeks posttransplant. By 2 months posttransplant, the lipogranulomata, pain on joint movement, and hoarseness had resolved. However, despite modest gains in cognitive and language development, hypotonia and delayed motor skills persisted. Gradual loss of circulating donor cells with autologous hematopoietic recovery occurred, and the patient died at 28 months posttransplant. The authors concluded that allografting may not prevent neurological deterioration even if performed in minimally symptomatic patients.

Diseases for which donor lymphohematopoietic engraftment has not resulted in clinical improvement

Allogeneic HSCT has been used to treat other metabolic disorders including Pompe disease[7] and Lesch-Nyhan syndrome[8] (Nyhan *et al.*, 1986; Watson *et al.*, 1986). In these diseases no clinical improvement or disease stabilization was associated with successful donor lymphohematopoietic engraftment. Patients with Pompe disease (Type IIA glycogen storage disease) have been transplanted following preparation with busulfan and cyclophosphamide. Successful donor engraftment was documented by the presence of enzymatically normal cells in the peripheral blood. Sequential evaluations of liver and muscle showed no increase in enzyme levels or any decrease in glycogen deposition. Patients, who were successfully engrafted, died as a result of their clinical symptomatology. In vitro co-culture experiments have failed to indicate that exogenous enzyme can be transported into patient cells. Thus, successful donor lymphohematopoietic engraftment in patients with Pompe disease does not result in the transport of the donor-derived enzyme into the affected tissues.

Lesch-Nyhan syndrome is due to the deficiency of the enzyme hypoxanthine-guanine phosphoribosyltransferase (HGPRT). Patients with Lesch-Nyhan syndrome have abnormalities of hypoxanthine metabolism, abnormal behavior, and self-mutilation. Successful lymphohematopoietic engraftment did not result in the modification of patient's abnormal behavior although some decrease in CNS hypoxanthine levels did occur.

Other diseases for which HSCT has been performed without consistent clinical improvement include Morquio syndrome[9], Niemann-Pick disease[10], Krabbe disease[11], Wolman disease[12] (Lenarsky *et al.*, 1990), and Alexander disease[13] (Staba *et al.*, 1997). A lack of disease progression was seen in one patient

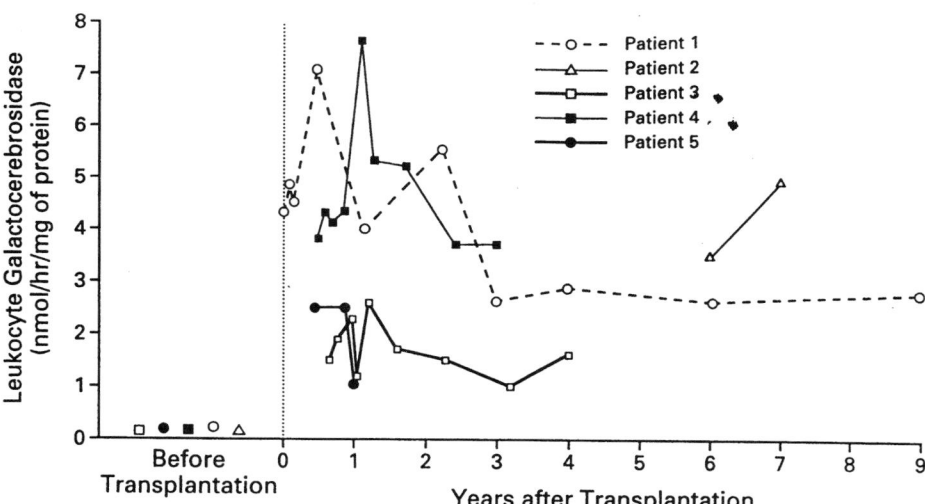

Fig. 63.4. Leukocyte galactocerebrosidase activity in five patients with globoid-cell leukodystrophy before and after hematopoietic stem-cell transplantation. The dotted lines indicate the time of transplantation. Reproduced, with permission, from Krivit *et al.* (1998).

[9] Louis Morquio, Uraguayan physician, 1867–1935.

[10] William Niemann, U.S. pediatrician, born 1926. Ludwig Pick, German physician, 1868–1935.

[11] Knud Krabbe, Danish neurologist, 1885–1961.

[12] Moshe Wolman, 20th-century Israeli neuropathologist, born 1914.

[13] William C. Alexander, New Zealand pathologist.

[7] J.C. Pompe, 20th-century Dutch physician.

[8] Michael Lesch, U.S. pediatrician, born 1939. Albert Nyhan, German physician, 1880–1921.

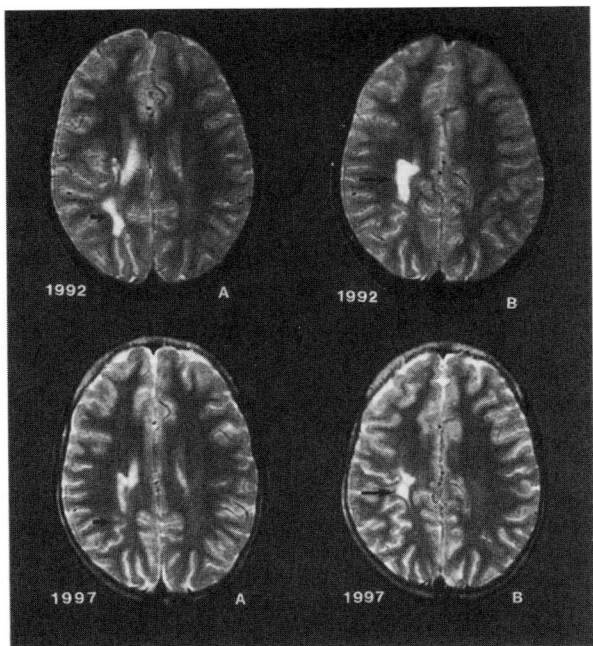

Fig. 63.5. Magnetic resonance imaging evidence of improvement after transplantation in globoid cell leukodystrophy. Reproduced, with permission, from Krivit *et al.* (1998).

Table 63.2. *Current recommendations of the Storage Disease Study Group for allogeneic HSC transplantation*

Disease	Recommendation
Gaucher Type 1	No
Type 2	No
Type 3	Yes
Hurler syndrome	Yes
Maroteaux-Lamy syndrome	Yes
Hunter syndrome	No
Sanfilipo A and B disease	No
Metachromatic leukodystrophy	
Late infantile	No if symptomatic
	Yes if presymptomatic
Juvenile, adolescent, adult	Yes
Adrenoleukodystrophy	Yes if early in course
	No if significant motor syndromes
Globoid cell leukodystrophy	
Infantile (Krabbe's disease)	No, unless diagnosed within a few weeks of birth
Juvenile and adult	Yes

with Niemann-Pick disease type C after HSCT (Hsu *et al.*, 1999). While an initial report of HSCT for Wolman disease showed no benefit, HSCT has been successful (Krivit *et al.*, 1992, 2000).

Krabbe disease is the infantile form of globoid cell leukodystrophy (GLD) and is characterized by rapid neurologic deterioration in infancy with intractable seizures and decerebration. HSCT for Krabbe disease is unlikely to produce clinical benefit unless it is performed within a few weeks of birth. The few patients that have been transplanted for the juvenile and adult forms of GLD have shown clinical benefit (Krivit *et al.*, 1998) (Figs. 63.4 and 63.5). This disease is usually much milder and more slowly progressive than the infantile form and associated initially with ataxia tremor and amnesia.

Conclusions

Histocompatible HSCT can result in reproducible donor lymphoid and hematopoietic engraftment in patients with metabolic diseases following pretransplant preparation with cyclophosphamide and busulfan. The likelihood of clinical success with histocompatible HSCT is related to the patients' age and clinical status at the time of transplant, especially in diseases with CNS involvement. The National Institutes of Health have funded a consortium known as the Storage Disease Collaborative Study Group in order to obtain information on the efficacy of allogeneic HSC transplantation in these rare diseases. The current recommendations of the consortium regarding transplantation are shown in Table 63.2.

Cell-based gene therapy using autologous cells transfected with a vector encoding the gene for normal enzyme may well be feasible in the future for at least some of these diseases (Baxter *et al.*, 2002).

References

Aubourg, P., Blanche, S., Jambaque, I. *et al.* (1990). Reversal of early neurologic and neuroradiologic manifestations of X-linked adrenoleukodystrophy by bone marrow transplantation. *New England Journal of Medicine*, **322**, 1860–6.

Barton, N.W., Brady, R.O., Dambrosia, J.M. *et al.* (1991). Replacement therapy for inherited enzyme deficiency-macrophage-targeted glucocerebrosidase for Gaucher's disease. *New England Journal of Medicine*, **324**, 1464–70.

Baxter, M.A., Wynn, R.F., Deakin, J.A. *et al.* (2002). Retrovirally mediated correction of bone marrow-derived mesenchymal stem cells from patients with mucopolysaccaridosis type I. *Blood*, **99**, 1857–9.

Bayever, E., Philippart, M., Nuwer, M. *et al.* (1985). Bone marrow transplantation for metachromatic leukodystrophy. *Lancet*, **1**, 471–3.

Bergstrom, S.K., Quinn, J.J., Greenstein, R., & Ascensao, J. (1994). Long-term follow up of a patient transplanted for Hunter's disease type IIB: a case report and literature review. *Bone Marrow Transplantation*, **14**, 653–8.

Chan, K.W., Wong, L.T.K., Applegarth, D., & Davidson. A.G.F. (1994). Bone marrow transplantation in Gaucher's disease: effect of mixed chimeric state. *Bone Marrow Transplantation*, **14**, 327–30.

Coccia, P.F., Krivit, W., Cervenka, J. *et al.* (1980). Successful bone marrow transplantation for infantile malignant osteopetrosis. *New England Journal of Medicine*, **302**, 701–8.

de Gasperi, R., Raghaven, S.S., Gama Sosa, M.A. *et al.* (2000). Measurements from normal umbilical cord blood of four lysosomal enzymatic activities: α-L-iduronidase (Hurler), galatocerebrosidase (globoid cell leukodystrophy), arylsulfatase A (metachromatic leukodystrophy), arylsulfatase B (Maroteaux-Lamy). *Bone Marrow Transplantation, 25,* 541–4.

Dini, G., Foris, R., Garaventa, A. *et al.* (2000). Long-term follow-up of two children with a variant of mild autosomal recessive osteopetrosis undergoing bone marrow transplantation. *Bone Marrow Transplantation, 26,* 219–24.

Erikson, A., Astrom, M., & Mansson, J.E. (1995). Enzyme infusion therapy of the Norrbottnian (type 3) Gaucher disease. *Neuropediatrics, 26,* 203–7.

Fischer, A., Friedrich, W., Levinsky, R. *et al.* (1986). Bone marrow transplantation for immunodeficiencies and osteopetrosis. *Lancet, 2,* 1080–3.

Fleming, D.R., Henslee-Downey, P.J., Ciocci, G. *et al.* (1998). The use of partially HLA-matched donors for allogeneic transplantation in patients with mucopolysaccharidosis-I. *Pediatric Transplantation, 2,* 299–304.

Glorieux, F.H., Bishop, N.J., Plotkin, H. *et al.* (1998). Cyclic administration of pamidronate in children with severe osteogenesis imperfecta. *New England Journal of Medicine, 339,* 947–52.

Grewal, S.S., Krivit, W., Defor, T.E. *et al.* (2002). Outcome of second hematopoietic cell transplantation in Hurler syndrome. *Bone Marrow Transplantation, 29,* 491–6.

Henslee-Downey, P.J., Pettogrew, A.L., Schmitt, F. *et al.* (1990). The use of alternative donors for marrow transplantation in the correction of Hurler's syndrome. *Blood, 76,* 544a (Abstract).

Herskhovitz, E., Young, E., Rainer, J. *et al.* (1999). Bone marrow transplantation for Maroteaux Lamy syndrome (MPS VI). *Journal of Inherited Metabolic Disease, 22,* 50–62.

Hobbs, J.R., Hugh-Jones, K., Barrett, A.J. *et al.* (1981). Reversal of clinical features of Hurler's disease and biochemical improvement after treatment by bone marrow transplantation. *Lancet, 2,* 709–12.

Hobbs, J.R., Hugh-Jones, K., Shaw, P.J. *et al.* (1987). Beneficial effect of pre-transplant splenectomy on displacement bone marrow transplantation for Gaucher's syndrome. *Lancet, 1,* 1111–5.

Horwitz, E.M., Prockop, D.J., Fitzpatrick, L.A. *et al.* (1999). Transplantability and therapeutic effects of bone marrow-derived mesenchymal cells in children with osteogenesis imperfecta. *Nature Medicine, 5,* 309–13.

Horwitz, E.M., Prockop, D.J., Gordon, P.L. *et al.* (2001). Clinical responses to bone marrow transplantation in children with severe osteogenesis imperfecta. *Blood, 97,* 1227–31.

Hsu, Y-S., Hwu, W-L., Huang, S-F. *et al.* (1999). Niemann-Pick disease type C (a cellular cholesterol lipidosis) treated by bone marrow transplantation. *Bone Marrow Transplantation, 24,* 103–7.

Hugh-Jones, K. (1986). Psychomotor development of children with mucopolysaccharidosis Type 1-H following bone marrow transplantation. In *Bone Marrow Transplantation for Treatment of Lysosomal Storage Disease,* ed. W. Krivit & N.W. Paul, pp. 25–29. New York: Alan R. Liss.

Kapelushnik, J., Shalev, C., Yaniv, I. *et al.* (2001). Osteopetrosis: a single center experience of stem cell transplantation and prenatal diagnosis. *Bone Marrow Transplantation, 27,* 129–32.

Kooma, H., Nose, M., Niida, S., & Yamasaki, A. (1991). Essential role of macrophage colony-stimulating factor in the osteoclast differentiation supported by stromal cells. *Journal of Experimental Medicine, 173,* 1291–4.

Krall, W.J., Challita, P.M., Perlmutter, L. *et al.* (1994). Cells expressing human glucocerebrosidase from a retroviral vector repopulate tissue macrophages and the CNS microglia after bone marrow transplantation. *Blood, 83,* 2737–48.

Krivit, W. (1992b). Maroteaux-Lamy syndrome (mucopolysaccharidosis type VI) treatment by allogeneic BMT in 6 patients and potential for autotransplantation bone marrow gene insertion. *International Pediatrics, 7,* 47–52.

Krivit, W., Freese, D., Chan, K.W., & Kulkarni, R. (1992a). Wolman's disease: review of treatment with bone marrow transplantation and considerations for the future. *Bone Marrow Transplantation, 10,* 97–101.

Krivit, W., Peters, C., Dusenbery, K. *et al.* (2000). Wolman disease successfully treated by bone marrow transplantation. *Bone Marrow Transplantation, 26,* 567–70.

Krivit, W., Pierpont, M.E., Ayaz, K. *et al.* (1984). Bone marrow transplantation in the Maroteaux, Lamy syndrome (mucopolysaccharidosis type VI). *New England Journal of Medicine, 3ll,* 1606–11.

Krivit, W. & Shapiro, E.G. (1991). BMT for storage diseases. In *Treatment of Genetic Diseases,* ed. R.J. Desnick, pp. 203–21. New York: Churchill-Livingstone.

Krivit, W., Shapiro, E., Kennedy, E. *et al.* (1990). Treatment of late infantile metachromatic leukodystrophy by bone marrow transplantation. *New England Journal of Medicine, 322,* 28–32.

Krivit, W., Shapiro, E.G., Lockmann, L.A. *et al.* (1992c). Recommendations for treatment of childhood cerebral form of adrenoleukodystrophy. In *COGENT II, correction of GEN diseases by transplantation,* ed. J.R. Hobbo & P.G. Riches, pp. 38–49. Westminster Medical School.

Krivit, W., Shapiro, E.G., Peters, C. *et al.* (1998). Hematopoietic stem cell transplantation in globoid-cell leukodystrophy. *New England Journal of Medicine, 338,* 1119–26.

Krivit, W., Sung, J.H., Shapiro, E.G. *et al.* (1995). Microglia: the effector cell for reconstitution of the central nervous system following bone marrow transplantation for lysosomal and peroxisomal storage disease. *Cell Transplantation, 4,* 385–92.

Krivit, W., Whitley, C.B., Chang, P-N. *et al.* (1989). Lysosomal storage disease treated by bone marrow transplantation. A report from the University of Minnesota Variety Club Children's Hospital. In *Bone Marrow Transplantation: Current Controversies,* ed. R.P. Gale & R.E. Champlin, pp. 367–78. New York: Alan R. Liss.

Lanjeunesse, D., Busque, L., Menard, P. *et al.* (1996). Demonstration of an osteoblast defect in two cases of human malignant osteopetrosis. Correction of the phenotype after bone marrow transplant. *Journal of Clinical Investigation, 98,* 1835–42.

Lee, V., Li, C.K., Shing, M.M.K. *et al.* (2000). Umbilical cord blood transplantation for Maroteaux-Lamy syndrome (mucopolysaccharidosis type VI). *Bone Marrow Transplantation, 26,* 455–8.

Lenarsky, C., Kohn, D.B., Weinberg, K.I., & Parkman, R. (1990). Bone marrow transplantation for genetic diseases. *Hematology/Oncology Clinic of North America, 4,* 589–602.

Malm, G., Ringden, O., Winiarsky, J. *et al.* (1996). Clinical outcome in four children with metachromatic leukodystrophy treated by bone marrow transplantation. *Bone Marrow Transplantation,* **17,** 1003–8.

McKinnis, E.J., Sulzbacher, S., Ruthledge, J.E. *et al.* (1996). Bone marrow transplantation in Hunter syndrome. *Journal of Pediatrics,* **129,** 145–8.

McMahon, C., Will, A., Hu, P. *et al.* (2001). Bone marrow transplantation corrects osteopetrosis in the carbonic anhydrase II deficiency syndrome. *Blood, 97,* 1947–50.

Meikle, P., Hopwood, J.J., Clague, A.E., & Carey, W.F. (1999). Prevalence of lysosomal storage disorders. *Journal of the American Medical Association,* **281,** 249–54.

Miano, M., Lanino, E., Gatti, R. *et al.* (2001). Four-year follow-up of a case of fucosidosis treated with unrelated donor bone marrow transplantation. *Bone Marrow Transplantation, 27,* 747–51.

Moser, H.W., Naisu, S., Kusar, A.J., & Roenbaum, A.E. (1987). The adrenoleukodystrophies. *Critical Reviews in Neurobiology,,* **3,** 29–88.

Moser, H.W., Tutschka, P.J., Brown, F.R., III *et al.* (1984). Bone marrow transplant in adrenoleukodystrophy. *Neurology, 34,* 1410–7.

Nyhan, W.L., Page, T., Truber, A.B. *et al.* (1986). Bone marrow transplantation in Lesch-Nyhan disease. In *Bone Marrow Transplantation for Treatment of Lysosomal Storage Disorders,* ed. W. Krivit & N.W. Paul, pp. 41–53, New York: Alan R. Liss.

Parkman, R. (1986). The application of bone marrow transplantation for the treatment of genetic diseases. *Science, 232,* 1373–8.

Parkman, R. & Crooks, G. (1996). Bone marrow transplantation for metabolic diseases. *Immunology & Allergy Clinics of North America,* **16,** 429–38.

Peters, C., Balthazor, M., Shapiro, E.G. *et al.* (1996). Outcome of unrelated donor bone marrow transplantation in 40 children with Hurler syndrome. *Blood,* **87,** 4894–902.

Peters, C., Shapiro, E.G., Anderson, J. *et al.* (1998). Hurler syndrome: 11. Outcome of HLA-genotypically identical sibling and HLA- haploidentical related donor bone marrow transplantation in fifty-four children. *Blood,* **91,** 2601–8.

Rappeport, J.M. & Gins, E.I. (1984). Bone marrow transplantation in severe Gaucher's disease. *New England Journal of Medicine,* **311,** 84–8.

Ringden, O., Groth, C.G., Erikson, A. *et al.* (1988). Long-term follow-up of the first successful bone marrow transplantation in Gaucher's disease. *Transplantation, 46,* 66–70.

Ringden, O., Roth, C.G., Erickson, A. *et al.* (1995). Ten years' experience of bone marrow transplantation for Gaucher disease. *Transplantation,* **59,** 864–70.

Shapiro, E., Krivit, W., Lockman, L. *et al.* (2000). Long-term effect of bone-marrow transplantation for childhood-onset cerebral X-linked adrenoleukodystrophy. *Lancet,* **356,** 713–8.

Souillet, G., Gouiband, P., Fensom, A.H. *et al.* (1989). Outcome of displacement bone marrow transplantation in Farber's disease: a report of a case. In *Correction of Certain Genetic Disease by Transplantation,* ed. J.R. Hobbs, pp. 137–41. London: COGENT.

Staba, M.-J., Goldman, S., Johnson, F.L., & Huttenlocher, P.R. (1997). Allogeneic bone marrow transplantation for Alexander's disease. *Bone Marrow Transplantation,* **20,** 247–9.

Svennerhold, L., Mansson, J.E. *et al.* (1984). Bone marrow transplantation in the Norrbottnian form of Gaucher disease. In *Molecular Basis of Lysosomal Storage Disorders,* ed. J.A. Barranger & R.O. Brandy, pp. 441–59. New York: Academic Press.

Vellodi, A., Cragg, H., Winchester, B. *et al.* (1995). Allogeneic bone marrow transplantation for fucosidosis. *Bone Marrow Transplantation,* **15,** 153–8.

Walker, D.G. (1975). Bone resorption restored in osteopetrotic mice by transplants of normal bone marrow and spleen cells. *Science,* **190,** 784–5.

Watson, J.G., Gardner-Medwin, D., Goldfinch, M.E. *et al.* (1986). Bone marrow transplantation for glycogen storage disease type II (Pompe's disease). *New England Journal of Medicine,* **314,** 385.

Yazaki, M., Ohno, T., Matsubayashi, T. *et al.* (1995). Detection of donor lymphocytes in the cerebrospinal fluid of a patient with metachromatic leukodystrophy following bone marrow transplantation. *Bone Marrow Transplantation,* **15,** 137–9.

Yeager, A.M., Armfield Uhas, K., Coles, C.D. *et al.* (2000). Bone marrow transplantation for infantile ceramidase deficiency. *Bone Marrow Transplantation,* **26,** 357–63.

Yeager, A.M., Bernnan, S., Tiffany, C. *et al.* (1984). Prolonged survival and remyelination after hematopoietic cell transplantation in the Twitcher mouse. *Science,* **225,** 1052–4.

64 Allogeneic hematopoietic stem cell transplantation for rare diseases

KERRY ATKINSON

Osiris Therapeutics Inc., Baltimore, and Weil Medical College, New York Presbyterian Hospital, New York, USA

Introduction

Increasingly, there are reports of rare or very rare diseases treated by allogeneic hematopoietic stem cell (HSC) transplantation. This chapter describes the reports of allografting for the following diseases: paroxysmal nocturnal hemoglobinuria, Diamond-Blackfan syndrome, Shwachman-Diamond syndrome, dyskeratosis congenita, Glanzmann's thrombasthenia, congenital amegakaryocytic thrombocytopenia, idiopathic CD4+ T lymphocytopenia, congenital red blood cell pyruvate kinase deficiency, congenital dysenthropoietic anemia type II, hereditary sideroblastic anemia, pure red cell aplasia, autoimmune hemolytic anemia, Evan's syndrome, congenital erythropoietic porphyria, hypereosinophilic syndrome, Langerhans cell histiocytosis, hemophagocytic lymphohistiocytosis, large granular lymphocyte proliferation, osteogenesis imperfecta, and chronic EBV infection with lymphoproliferation.

Paroxysmal nocturnal hemoglobinuria

Paroxysmal nocturnal hemoglobinuria (PNH) is a rare acquired clonal hematologic disorder characterized by an increased risk of thrombosis and intravascular hemolysis, reflecting exceptional sensitivity of red blood cells to complement-mediated lysis. PNH is caused by a somatic mutation of the phosphatidylinosotol glycan protein A (PIG-A) gene (Takeda *et al.*, 1993). The PIG-A protein is essential for formation of the glycocyl phosphatidylinosotol anchor by which many surface proteins attach to the cell membrane (Yeh & Rosse, 1994). Clinical features include hemoglobinuria, often occurring during sleep, thrombosis; bone marrow failure; and susceptibility to infections (Dacie, 1967; Oni, Osunkoya, & Luzzatto, 1970; Rotoli & Luzzatto, 1989; Rosse, 1989; Josten *et al.*, 1991; Rosse, 1993; Bessler *et al.*, 1994; Rosse & Ware, 1995). PNH is associated with bone marrow failure syndromes including aplastic anemia, myelodysplasia, and leukemia. There is a close relationship between PNH and bone marrow failure, particularly aplastic anemia. About one-third of patients with PNH die of marrow failure, and in some patients with aplastic anemia a small clone of PNH cells may arise, producing significant hemolysis and

identified only by test of increased erythrocyte susceptibility to complement-mediated lysis (Ham[1] and sugar-water tests).

There is both laboratory and clinical evidence that PNH cells have a survival advantage over normal stem cells. When injected into SCID mice, PNH hematopoiesis persisted for more than 10 months and did not always need human cytokines, in contrast to hematopoiesis from control grafts obtained from healthy volunteers (Iwamoto *et al.*, 1996). Substantiating this, a 10-year-old girl with PNH who received an infusion of syngeneic bone marrow without preparative marrow ablation or immune suppression improved clinically posttransplant and showed an increase in the percentage of peripheral blood cells with normal expression of GPI-anchored proteins. However, molecular analysis suggested engraftment of a relatively small number of donor stem cells and persistence of an abnormal stem cell clone with mutant PIG-A (Endo *et al.*, 1996). During 17 months of observation, the percentage of cells with normal GPI-anchored protein expression gradually decreased and intravascular hemolysis progressively increased. At 16 months posttransplant, the patient again became symptomatic.

Another study showed that peripheral blood mobilization from patients with PNH contained both normal CD34+ CD38− hematopoietic cells exhibiting normal expression of the GPI-anchored decay accelerating factor (DAF) and CD59, as well as CD34+ CD38− cells that did not express these surface proteins (Prince *et al.*, 1995).

The clinical course of PNH is usually chronic. A study from the Hammersmith Hospital, London, followed 80 consecutive patients with PNH between 1940 and 1970 (Hillman *et al.*, 1995). These patients were treated with supportive measures only, including oral anticoagulant therapy after established thromboses, and transfusion. The median age of the patients at diagnosis was 42 years (range 16–75), and the median survival after diagnosis was 10 years with 28% of patients surviving for 25 years. Sixty of the 80 patients died; 28 of the 48 for whom the cause of death was known died of either venous thrombosis or hemorrhage. Thirty-nine percent had one or more episodes of venous thrombosis dur-

---

[1] Thomas Hale Ham, U.S. physician, born 1905.

ing their illness. Of the 35 patients who survived for 10 years or more, 12 had a spontaneous clinical recovery and no PNH-affected cells were found among the erythrocytes or neutrophils of patients in prolonged remission, although a few PNH-affected lymphocytes were detectable in three of the four patients tested. The fact that spontaneous long-term remission can occur indicates the care that must be taken when considering therapy, albeit curative, such as allogeneic HSC transplantation. This study concluded that platelet transfusion should be given as appropriate and that long-term anticoagulation therapy should be considered for all patients. A similar study followed 21 patients diagnosed with PNH between 1970 and 1991 at La Fey University Hospital in Spain (Tudela et al., 1993). In this study hemolysis was monitored by reticulocyte count, unconjugated bilirubin and LDH levels, haptoglobin levels, and hemosiderinuria. The median age was 38 (range 18–72) years. The most common presenting symptoms were weakness, dark urine, jaundice, and purpura. All patients had anemia, 28% presenting with aplastic anemia. The complications most frequently seen included thrombosis (documented in 7, clinically suspected in 6), infection (6), and hemorrhage (6). One patient developed aplastic anemia after 16 years and another had acute myeloid leukemia (AML). Only 5 patients required no transfusions. Actuarial survival at 10 years was 68%. These authors also recommended that anticoagulant therapy be utilized unless severe thrombocytopenia was present.

PNH may be cured by either syngeneic (Fefer et al., 1976; Hershko et al., 1979) or allogeneic (Szer et al., 1984) transplantation. An algorithm for therapeutic decision making is shown in Figure 64.1. It should be noted that infusion of syngeneic HSC

may result in sustained engraftment without prior conditioning sometimes (Saso et al., 1999), but not always (Endo et al., 1996).

There are a number of reports of allogeneic transplantation (Szer et al., 1984; Antin et al., 1985; Kolb et al., 1989; Kawahara, Witherspoon, & Storb, 1992; Saso et al., 1999; Bemba et al., 2000; Woodard et al., 2001). The largest of these series is that by Saso et al. reported from the International Bone Marrow Transplant Registry. Forty-one patients received marrow transplants between 1978 and 1992 at 25 centers. Two of the transplants were from identical twins, 34 from HLA-identical siblings, and 5 from alternate donors. Thirty-seven of these patients had been transfused pretransplant with a median of 43 units and 3 of 29 tested patients were refractory to platelet transfusions. Conditioning was with cyclophosphamide alone in 3, combined with total body irradiation in 9, limited field irradiation in 7, or busulfan in 21. One of the identical twin transplant recipients received no conditioning and 4 patients received T-cell-depleted grafts. Two patients showed no engraftment and 8 engrafted with subsequent graft failure. Acute graft-versus-host disease (GVHD) grade II or greater developed in 41% and chronic GVHD in 37%. Five patients received a second transplant because of graft failure, and all 5 died of nonengraftment, GVHD or infection. The overall 2-year probability of survival (95% confidence interval) was 47% (27%–62%) (Fig. 64.2). Patients with sustained engraftment had better 2-year survival than those without sustained engraftment (65% vs. 10%, P = .004) (Fig. 64.3). Two patients received identical twin transplants; one without conditioning prior to first transplant showed graft failure; the second transplant preceded by cyclophos-

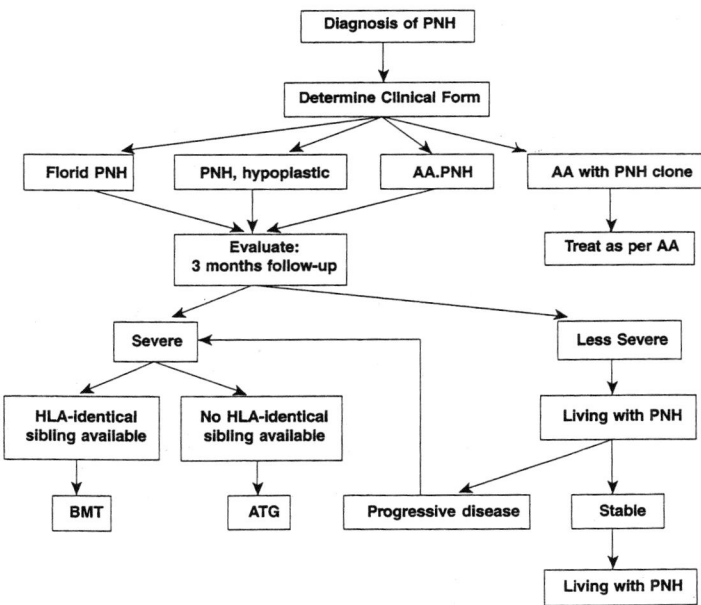

Fig. 64.1. An algorithm for therapeutic decision making in paroxysmal nocturnal hemoglobinuria. This algorithm is based on the consideration that patients with this condition vary considerably (a) in terms of clinical severity, and (b) in terms of the contributions of the PNH clone and of bone marrow failure (BMF) respectively to determining the overall clinical picture. Some patients have been cured by bone marrow transplantation (BMT); at the other end of the spectrum, some of the patients who for a long time have been 'living with PNH'—by choice or otherwise—have eventually experienced spontaneous recovery. Adapted from Tremml et al. (1998).

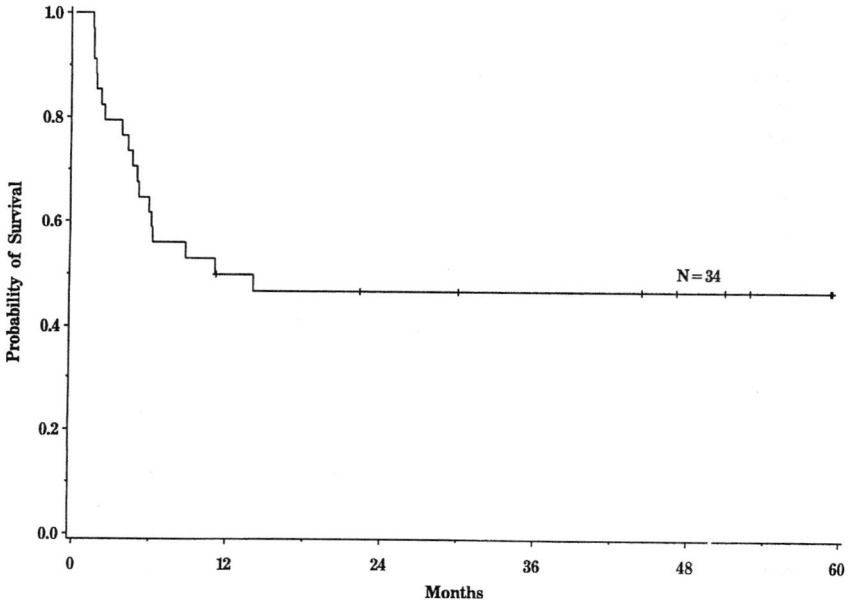

Fig. 64.2. Survival after 34 HLA-identical sibling bone marrow transplants for paroxysmal nocturnal hemoglobinuria. Reproduced, with permission, from Saso *et al.* (1999).

phamide and total body irradiation resulted in complete recovery for more than 12 years. The second patient conditioned with cyclophosphamide and busulfan was alive at the time of the report in complete remission for more than 8 years.

Of the five patients receiving alternate donor transplants, four received HLA-matched unrelated donor transplants after conditioning with cyclophosphamide and busulfan. Three of these

died of graft failure or interstitial pneumonia and one was alive 4 years posttransplant (and see Chapter 49). The single patient transplanted with bone marrow from an HLA-haplotype mismatched parental donor, after conditioning with cyclophosphamide and busulfan, died of graft failure. Interestingly, only one patient was thought to have hepatic veno-occlusive disease posttransplant. There was no excessive incidence of thrombosis.

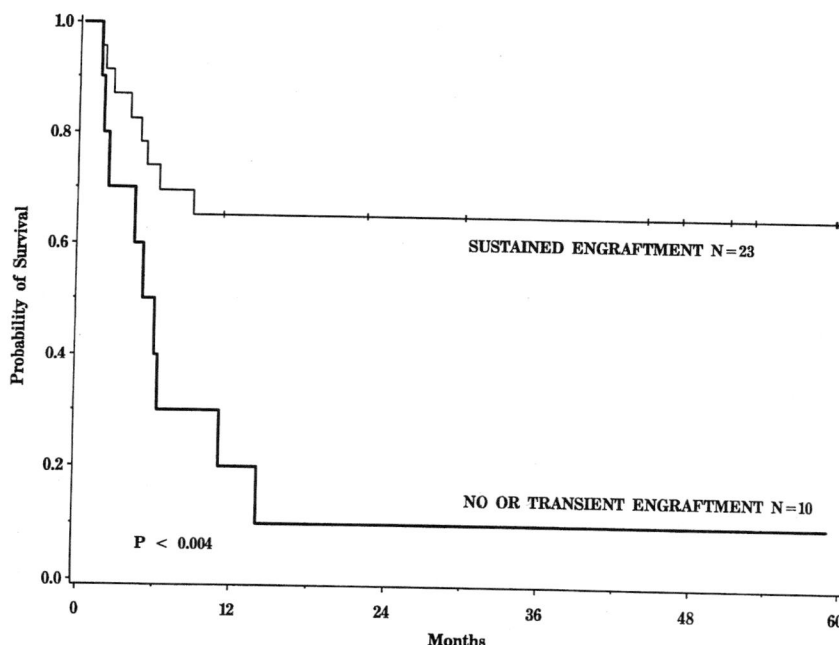

Fig. 64.3. Survival after 34 HLA-identical sibling bone marrow transplants for paroxysmal nocturnal hemoglobinuria in patients with and without sustained engraftment. Reproduced, with permission, from Saso *et al.* (1999).

As with other diseases, the use of cyclophosphamide and busulfan as conditioning prior to an alternate donor transplant may be inadequate to ensure consistent sustained engraftment. Thrombosis of the hepatic veins (Budd-Chiari syndrome)[2] is known to occur in PNH (Wyatt, Mowat, & Layton, 1995). This syndrome can resolve following bone marrow transplantation for PNH, as reported in a child who underwent a syngeneic transplant (Graham et al., 1996).

Diamond-Blackfan syndrome[3]

Diamond-Blackfan syndrome (previously known as congenital hypoplastic anemia) is a rare, inherited autosomal recessive disorder characterized by macrocytic anemia and a normal or slightly reduced white blood cell count. Congenital physical anomalies are present in 10% to 20% of cases and include exocrine insufficiency, skeletal abnormalities, and short stature. Typically, the disease is diagnosed within the first year of life, although some cases are first recognized in children aged 5 to 10 years, and infrequently later. The cause and pathogenesis are unknown. Most patients have selective deficiency of erythroid progenitor cells in a normocellular marrow. There are some data to suggest an intrinsic defect in erythroid precursors, partly or completely refractory to erythropoietin.

Although most patients respond to corticosteroids, more than 20% are, or become, steroid-refractory. There are no convincing data that other immune suppressive agents are effective and neither is treatment with recombinant human erythropoietin. Those patients unresponsive to corticosteroids receive many packed cell transfusions.

There are a number of reports of marrow transplantation for children with this disease. One small series of four patients, all of whom were resistant to corticosteroid treatment and red blood cell transfusion-dependent, received marrow grafts from HLA-identical sibling donors. Conditioning was with cyclophosphamide and busulfan. Three of four patients had sustained and complete marrow engraftment. The other showed early signs of hematopoietic recovery but died on day 35 of pulmonary toxicity. The three surviving patients were well at the time of the report with normal hematopoiesis at 3, 7.4, and 10.6 years posttransplant (Greinix, Storb, & Sanders, 1993). In a report from the International Bone Marrow Transplant Registry (Mugishima et al., 1995), 10 children received a marrow transplant from an HLA-identical sibling (n = 8), a maternal (n = 1), or an unrelated (n = 1) donor. Of the eight recipients of HLA-identical sibling transplants, six were alive 5 to 87 months posttransplant with no evidence of disease and with Karnofsky performance scores of 90% to 100%. The two recipients of alternate donor transplants died less than 2 weeks posttransplant. The actuarial 2-year probability of survival for the eight

sibling transplants was 72 (37%–92%) (95% confidence intervals). A French registry report described 13 patients (Willig et al., 1999). In a review of the literature the projected actuarial survival for allogeneic transplantation in 33 patients who received an HLA-identical sibling transplant was 66% (Alter, 1998). The Diamond-Blackfan Anemia Registry described 8 patients who underwent transplantation from an HLA-identical sibling donor and 12 from an alternate donor (Vlachos et al., 2001). The median age at transplant for all patients was 6 years 2 months. All the HLA-identical sibling recipients received a non-irradiation-containing regimen, whereas the majority of the alternate donor transplants were performed using total body irradiation. Survival for the HLA-matched sibling recipients was 87.5 ± 11.7% and for the alternate donor recipients 14.1 ± 12.1% (P < .015) (Fig. 64.4).

Okcu and colleagues (1998) emphasized that these patients frequently have underlying organ dysfunction and are prone to multiple severe complications after transplantation. Interestingly, a single case report described *Listeria monocytogenes* septicemia complicating allogeneic marrow transplantation for Diamond-Blackfan syndrome (Lee et al., 1995). Listeria infection is uncommon after marrow transplantation, but hemosiderosis appears to be a risk factor for it. The child was treated successfully with intravenous ampicillin.

Shwachman[4]-Diamond[5] syndrome

Shwachman-Diamond syndrome is a rare autosomal recessive disorder that usually manifests in infancy and is characterized

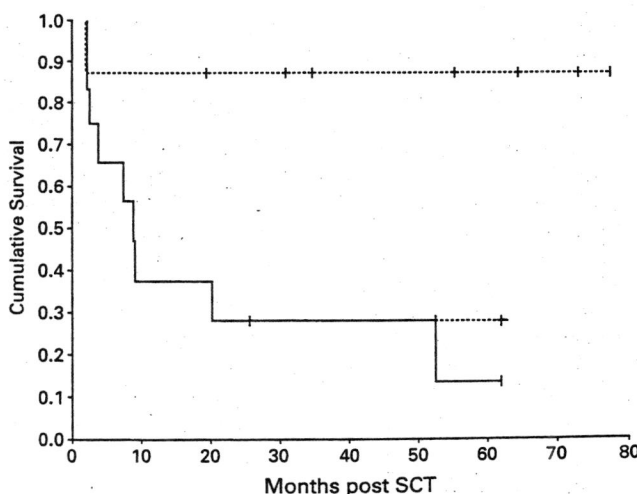

Fig. 64.4. Kaplan-Meier analysis of survival in Diamond-Blackfan syndrome patients undergoing HLA-matched sibling (...) versus alternate donor stem cell transplant. Alternate donor stem cell transplants are presented without (—) and with (...) the death from osteogenic sarcoma. Reproduced, with permission from Vlachos et al. (2001).

---

[2] George Budd, English Physician, 1808–1882. Hans Chiari, German pathologist, 1857–1916.

[3] Louis Diamond, U.S. physician, born 1902. Kenneth Blackfan, U.S. physician, 1883–1941.

[4] Harry Shwachman, 20th-century U.S. pediatrician.

[5] Louis Diamond, U.S. physician, born 1902.

by exocrine pancreatic insufficiency, metaphyseal dysostosis, and bone marrow dysfunction. The spectrum of hematologic manifestations seen includes intermittent neutropenia, impaired neutrophil chemotaxis, anemia, elevated levels of fetal hemoglobin, thrombocytopenia, and a predilection for development of aplastic anemia, myelodysplasia, or leukemia. The pathogenesis has not been fully elucidated. There are reports of a number of patients who have undergone allogeneic transplantation (reviewed in Fleitz et al., 2002), several of whom received marrow from an HLA-identical unrelated donor (Smith et al., 1995; Cesaro et al., 2001). Smith's patient was a 5-year-old boy who received cyclophosphamide 60 mg/kg × 2 and total body irradiation 12 Gy in 6 fractions prior to a T-replete HLA-identical unrelated donor marrow transplant. Immune suppression was cyclosporine and methotrexate. He showed temporary engraftment but eventually died of bone marrow failure 1 year posttransplant. A few years prior to transplant the patient had developed a clonal cytogenetic abnormality involving chromosome 7, and prior to transplant had transformed into acute monoblastic leukemia. Another patient who was transplanted because of progression to AML was prepared with busulfan 16 mg/kg and cyclophosphamide 120 mg/kg prior to a T-replete transplant and immunosuppressed with cyclosporine and methotrexate. Hematologic recovery was delayed but the patient was discharged at day 28 in complete remission with RFLP analysis showing complete donor engraftment. The patient's leukemia recurred 9 months posttransplant, and death occurred from cytomegalovirus (CMV) infection and multiorgan failure. Cesaro's patient, who was also a 5-year-old boy, was alive and well 32 months after an HLA-identical unrelated transplant (Cesaro et al., 2001). Conditioning was with busulfan, cyclophosphamide, thiotepa, and ATG. Hematopoietic reconstitution was complete and the other characteristics (pancreatic insufficiency and short stature) were stable.

Subclinical hepatic steatosis has been reported in up to 30% of patients with Schwachman-Diamond syndrome. A case in which non-alcoholic steatohepatitis developed, leading to rapidly progressive liver failure, has been described in an allograft recipient (Ritchie et al. 2002).

Allogeneic bone marrow transplantation (BMT) appears a potentially curative option for this rare disease, although the interaction of the transplant procedure with the pancreatic insufficiency still has to be ascertained (Arseniev, Diedrich, & Link, 1996).

Dsykeratosis congenital and Hoyeraal–Hreidarsson syndrome

Dyskeratosis congenita is a rare congenital cause of aplastic anemia and appears to be a disease of defective telomere maintenance. Affected tissues are those that require constant renewal. The syndrome is characterized clinically by hyperpigmentation, dystrophic nails, mucosal leukoplakia, and pancytopenia. It may be X-linked or inherited autosomally. The Fred Hutchinson Cancer Research Center reported the outcome of

allogeneic transplantation in eight patients, six of whom received HLA-identical sibling grafts and two of whom received transplants from HLA-matched unrelated donors. The recipients of HLA-identical sibling transplants were conditioned with cyclophosphamide 140 to 200 mg/kg, with or without antithymocyte globulin. Those who received unrelated donor marrow were conditioned with cyclophosphamide 120 mg/kg and total body irradiation 12 Gy. Three patients survived greater than 2 weeks posttransplant and all had evidence of engraftment. These three who survived at least 1 year posttransplant had normal hematologic function. Three patients died with respiratory failure and pulmonary fibrosis at 70 days, 8 years, and 20 years posttransplant. Three patients died during the neutropenic period of invasive fungal infections and one died at day 44 posttransplant of acute GVHD. One patient remained alive 463 days posttransplant at the time of the report (Langston et al., 1996). This patient subsequently underwent surgical resection of a Dukes' stage C rectal carcinoma diagnosed at 14 months posttransplant.

Hoyeraal–Hreidarsson syndrome (HHS) is severe multisystem disorder affecting male infants and characterized by growth retardation of prenatal onset, cerebellar hypoplasia, microcephaly, marrow failure and immune deficiency. Demonstration of mutations in the DKC1 gene have shown it to be a severe variant of X-linked dyskeratosis congenital. Cossu and colleagues (2002) described a 9-month-old infant with HHS who had T[+] B[−]NK[−] severe combined immune deficiency and marrow failure, who has given an HLA-identical sibling marrow graft after non-myeloablative conditioning. At 1 year posttransplant, the blood count was normal and immune reconstitution adequate. However, tongue leukoplakia remained and nail dystrophy developed at 9 months posttransplant.

Thus allogeneic transplantation appears able to treat the pancytopenia associated with dyskeratosis congenita but does not reverse other systemic manifestations of the syndrome.

Glanzmann's thrombasthenia[6]

Glanzmann's thrombasthenia is a rare, inherited bleeding disorder due to defective platelet function that occurs because of a decrease or absence of the functional platelet membrane glycoprotein (GP) complex, GPIIb/IIIa (alpha[IIb] beta[III]). This glycoprotein complex is a calcium-dependent heterodimer that combines fibrinogen, fibronectin, von Willebrand factor,[7] and vitronectin when platelets are activated. The complex plays a critical role in platelet aggregation and adhesion, as well as in the trafficking of fibrinogen into megakaryocytes and platelets. Glanzmann's thrombasthenia is characterized by a prolonged bleeding time with normal platelet count and morphology. The platelets do not aggregate in response to ADP and other agonists. A number of mutations for the genes encoding GPIIb and

---

[6] Eduard Glanzmann, Swiss clinician, 1887–1959.
[7] Erik A. von Willebrand, Finnish physician, 1870–1939.

GPIIIa have been described (Peretz *et al.*, 1995). The disease is broadly classifiable according to the amount of GPIIb/IIIa complex associated with the platelets as follows: type 1, 0.5% of normal; type 2, 6% to 20% of normal; and variant disease, 50% to 100% of normal. The disease is thought to fit a pattern of autosomal recessive inheritance.

The most common clinical features of the disease are purpura, epistasis, and gingival hemorrhage, with menorrhagia in the majority of female patients and severe intrapartum and postpartum hemorrhage. Gastrointestinal bleeding, intracranial hemorrhage, and hemarthrosis are also reported. Bleeding is rarely spontaneous. With careful management, mortality is low but morbidity is high.

Management has traditionally been supportive; bleeding may be controlled by local measures including topical thrombin and nasal packing, and systemic antifibrinolytic drugs. Platelet transfusions are often necessary for an acute situation and prophylactically prior to surgery, but carry the risk of alloimmunization.

There are several reported cases of treatment of Glanzmann's thrombasthenia by allogeneic marrow transplantation. One 4-year-old boy with a history of severe bleeding and multiple platelet and red cell transfusions was successfully transplanted from his HLA-identical brother resulting in complete correction of the disease. A 2-year-old girl with a history of frequent hospitalization was also successfully transplanted from her HLA-identical sibling (Johnson *et al.*, 1994). Engraftment was monitored by analysis of the platelet GPIIb/IIIa complex (Fig. 64.5) and complete donor engraftment was seen at day 25 posttransplant. At the time of writing, she had been clinically stable for 19 months posttransplant. One recipient, transplanted at age 2, remains alive and well 16 years later (Belluci *et al.*, 2000).

Congenital amegakaryocytic thrombocytopenia and acquired amegakaryocytic thrombocytopenia

Congenital amegakaryocytic thrombocytopenia is an uncommon cause of thrombocytopenia in childhood characterized by a marked reduction in bone marrow megakaryocytes. It usually presents with isolated thrombocytopenia but often progresses to marrow failure. The defective thrombopoiesis is not well understood nor is the etiology of the progressive marrow failure. It is not associated with skeletal abnormalities [as in the thrombocytopenia/absent radii syndrome (TAR syndrome) which is characterized by spontaneous improvement after the first year of life and a good response to platelet transfusion]. Congenital amegakaryocytic thrombocytopenia, in contrast, has a poor prognosis. There are X-linked and autosomal patterns of inheritance. Average survival of affected children without anomalies is approximately 6 years. In one study, 12 of 21 children developed aplastic anemia at a median age of 3.5 years.

There is no standard treatment. Temporary or partial therapeutic responses to corticosteroids and androgens have been reported, but these approaches are often ineffective.

One study of in vivo administration of interleukin-3 (IL-3) resulted in improved platelet counts in two of five patients with

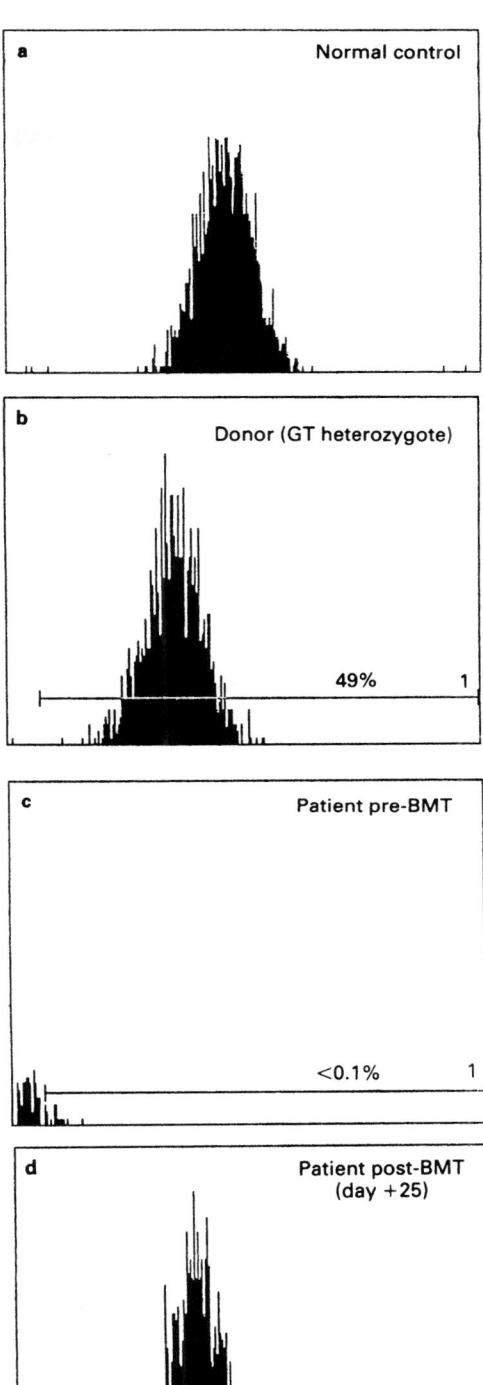

Fig. 64.5. Flow cytometric analysis of platelet GPIIb-IIIa. Platelets from a normal subject (**a**), the heterozygous donor (**b**), the patient pretransplant (**c**) and (**d**) posttransplant (day 25) were analyzed for GPIIb-IIIa expression, by whole blood flow cytometry. The relative fluorescence intensity is shown on the x-axis against cell count. Values represent the mean fluorescence intensity per platelet as a percentage of the control platelets. Reproduced, with permission, from Johnson *et al.* (1994).

decreased bleeding and transfusion requirement in the remaining three (Guinan *et al.*, 1993). In this report, in vitro studies demonstrated assayable numbers of CFU-MK colonies from bone marrows of all patients who responded in vitro to the addition of IL-3, GM-CSF, or a combination of both. GM-CSF was ineffective in vivo.

Henter and colleagues (1995) described two patients treated by allogeneic bone marrow transplantation. These children had failed to respond to steroids and intravenous immunoglobulin. The first child received an HLA-identical sibling marrow at 42 months of age, after conditioning with cyclophosphamide 50 mg/kg for 4 days, busulfan 1 mg/kg 4 times daily for 2 days, and antithymocyte globulin for 5 days. The marrow was infused T replete and posttransplant immune suppression utilized cyclosporine and methotrexate. The child engrafted satisfactorily and at the time of reporting was well at 2.5 years posttransplant.

The second child received an HLA-A and -B matched unrelated donor marrow at 22 months of age. Genomic typing showed that the donor had an HLA-DR 52c split while the recipient had an HLA-DR 52a. The child was prepared with antithymocyte globulin, cyclophosphamide 50 mg/kg for 3 days, and a single dose of total body irradiation 7.5 Gy. This patient also engrafted satisfactorily and at the time of report was well 12 months posttransplant.

MacMillan and colleagues (1998) described two children treated by an unrelated donor marrow and an unrelated cord blood transplant, respectively, who both rejected their initial grafts, but who both subsequently engrafted after further donor stem cell infusion. A 13-month-old girl engrafted rapidly and durably after conditioning with cyclophosphamide 200 mg/kg and ATG followed by G-CSF mobilized PBSC from her HLA-identical sibling (Yesilipek *et al.*, 2000). Lackner and colleagues (2000) described eight patients. All six receiving family member transplants were well with stable platelet counts 3 to 27 months posttransplant. Two patients given HLA-matched unrelated donor transplants died.

Allogeneic transplantation appears to represent a feasible treatment option for children with congenital amegakaryocytic thrombocytopenia. A case of acquired amegakaryocytic thrombocytopenia, which was unresponsive to IVIG, prednisone, splenectomy , danazol, cyclophosphamide, and vincristine, has been reported in which normal thromopoiesis was restored by HLA-identical sibling transplantation (Lional *et al.*, 1999).

Idiopathic CD4+ T lymphocytopenia

CD4+ T lymphocytopenia, in the absence of human immunodeficiency virus (HIV) infection, is a heterogeneous disorder of unknown cause. The Centers for Disease Control and Prevention define idiopathic CD4+ T lymphocytopenia as follows: CD4+ cells below 300 per cubic millimeter or a CD4+ count of less than 20% of total T cells on two occasions, while testing negative for HIV infection. The opportunistic infections described in these patients are very similar to those described in acquired immunodeficiency syndrome (AIDS) and include candidiasis, cryptococcosis, visceral leishmaniasis, *Pneumocystis carinii* infection, and disseminated tuberculosis. Additionally, immune thrombocytopenia and Kaposi's sarcoma have been reported in these patients. The pathogenesis of the disease is unknown. No curative therapy has been reported.

There is one case report of a successful allogeneic transplant carried out for this disease (Petersen *et al.*, 1996). The patient was a 22-year-old male who presented with a *Rhodococcus equi* infection. He subsequently developed severe aplastic anemia that warranted allogeneic marrow transplantation. This was uneventful and 2 years posttransplant he had normal blood counts, a normal CD4+ count, and no evidence of recurrent infection of any sort.

Again, allogeneic HSC transplantation appears a potentially curative therapy for this rare disease.

Congenital red blood cell pyruvate kinase deficiency

Pyruvate kinase (PK) deficiency is the most common hereditary red blood cell enzymopathy of the glycolytic pathway. The clinical manifestations are heterogeneous, ranging from fetal anemia, neonatal jaundice, or severe chronic hemolytic anemia to a fully compensated hemolytic anemia. Conventional treatment is primarily supportive and includes blood transfusion and splenectomy. BMT has been used to cure the disease in mice and dogs. A successful HLA-identical sibling transplant has been reported in a 5-year-old boy (Tanphaichitr *et al.*, 2000). Busulfan and cyclophosphamide were used as conditioning prior to a T-replete BMT, and cyclosporine/short methotrexate were given as GVHD prophylaxis. The posttransplant course was uneventful with 100% donor chimerism being obtained. He was placed on iron chelation therapy posttransplant. Two years after BMT both donor and recipient had PK activities at 110% of normal control, compared to a value of 20% in the recipient pretransplant.

Congenital dyserythropoietic anemia type I

The congenital dyserythropoietic anemias (CDAs) are rare inherited disorders affecting the normal differentiation-proliferation pathway of the erythroid lineage. They comprise a group of heterogeneous diseases characterized by ineffective erythropoiesis as the predominant mechanism of anemia and distinct morphologic abnormalities of the majority of erythroblasts in the marrow. The CDAs have been classified into 3 types based on morphologic and serologic findings. CDA type I can manifest during the neonatal period or at any age thereafter up to middle age. The severity of anemia is variable. Patients may also have jaundice, hepatosplenomegaly and dysmorphic features such as syndactyly, absence of phalanges and dysplastic nails. Interferon-α has been shown to have efficacy (Lavabre-Bertrand *et al.*, 1995).

Three children with transfusion-dependent CDA type I were conditioned with cyclophosphamide 50 mg/kg/day for 4 days, busulfan 4 mg/kg/day for 4 days and ATG 30 mg/kg for 4 doses prior to unmanipulated HLA-identical sibling BMT (Ayas *et al.*, 2002). Ages at transplant were 1.8, 10 and 4.4 years. Cyclosporine or cyclosporine and methotrexate were used for GVHD prophylaxis. All three patients engrafted and were alive and transfusion-independent at the time of reporting, 5, 2.5 and 2 years posttransplant respectively.

Congenital dyserythropoietic anemia type II

Congenital dyserythropoietic anemia type II (CDA-II) is the most frequent cause of congenital dyserythropoiesis. It is an autosomal recessive disorder characterized by normocytic anemia, jaundice, and hepatosplenomegaly. Bi- and multinucleated (10–40%) erythroblasts with karyorrhexis are detectable in the bone marrow. Electron microscopy of these cells shows the presence of a so-called double membrane, that is, peripheral cisternae running parallel to and beneath the plasma membrane. Clinical manifestations in the vast majority of patients are very mild. Gallbladder disease and secondary hemochromatosis are frequent late complications.

Iolascon and colleagues (2001) described a child with CDA-II who also had β-thalassemia trait, and who was transfusion-dependent with poor compliance with chelation therapy. At the time of transplant his serum ferritin was 3,500 ng/ml. Busulfan, thiotepa, and fludarabine were used for conditioning prior to a T-replete, HLA-identical sibling bone marrow transplant. Three years posttransplant the patient was well with normal Hb levels, and undergoing regular phlebotomy with a serum ferritin of 1,180 ng/ml. Another successfully transplanted case has been reported (Milledge *et al.*, 2002) (see Familial Mediterranean fever below).

Hereditary sideroblastic anemia

The sideroblastic anemias are a heterogeneous group of disorders that can be hereditary or acquired. The acquired sideroblastic anemias include the myelodysplastic syndromes, reflecting a clonal preleukemic disorder. Hereditary sideroblastic anemia (HAS) is usually transmitted as an X-linked trait, although unusual forms of autosomal recessive disease have been documented. HAS can respond, or be refractory, to pyridoxine. Management is directed toward maintenance of the hematocrit with transfusion and removal of excess iron load with desferrioxamine. Pyridoxine 50–200 mg/day is often given, but only one-third of patients respond.

Gonzalez and colleagues (2000) described a patient with hemoglobin levels of 5 to 7 g/dl, who was pyridoxine-refractory and who received an HLA-identical sibling peripheral blood stem cell transplant at age 19. The blood contained only donor cells at day 21 posttransplant, although the marrow showed mixed chimerism until day 221 posttransplant. When the hemoglobin was normal, a phlebotomy program reduced serum ferritin levels. Three years posttransplant, the patient's ECOG score was 0 and his hemoglobin 15 g/dl.

Pure red cell aplasia

Muller and colleagues (1999) described a 16-year-old female with pure red cell aplasia that was successfully treated with HLA-identical sibling BMT. Cyclophosphamide and ATG were used for conditioning. The patient showed mixed chimerism at 6 months posttransplant, but full autologous recovery at 12 months. The disease, however, continued in complete remission at the time of the report.

Autoimmune hemolytic anemia (AIHA)

A 12-year-old boy with AIHA and thalassemia failed to respond to thoraco-abdominal irradiation, cyclophosphamide, and Campath-1G conditioning followed by a T-cell-depleted autologous transplant, but the AIHA resolved entirely after a matched unrelated bone marrow transplant following conditioning with busulfan, thiotepa, and fludarabine (De Stefano *et al.*, 1999).

Evans syndrome[8]

Evans syndrome is a rare disorder characterized by combined autoimmune thrombocytopenia (ITP) and AIHA. Standard treatment consists of transfusions, corticosteroids, splenectomy, IVIG, anabolic steroids, vincristine, alkylating agents, or cyclosporine. Two cases treated by allografting have been described. Raetz *et al.* (1999) reported on a 4-year-old boy prepared for transplant with cyclophosphamide and total body irradiation prior to an allogeneic cord blood transplant. The disease went into complete remission, but the patient died of liver failure at 289 days posttransplant. Oyama and colleagues (2001) described a 28-year-old male with refractory disease in whom an HLA-identical sibling bone marrow transplant supplemented with PBSC resulted in complete clinical and serologic remission at 30 months posttransplant. Cyclophosphamide and ATG were used as conditioning. The PBSC graft (but not the marrow) was CD34-selected. Cyclosporine and corticosteroids were used as immune suppression posttransplant. The patient had major pretransplant morbidities including ICU transfer and respiratory support for renal and respiratory failure and pretansplant infections that included cryptococcal fungemia, persistent CMV viremia, and positive blood cultures for *Mycobacterium avium*. Posttransplant complications included TTP, grade IV acute GVHD, extensive chronic GVHD, and posttransplant infections that included *Nocardia* in blood cultures and CMV retinitis. The patient demonstrated 100% donor chimerism, became negative for antibodies to platelets and red cells, and transfusion-independent.

---

[8] Robert Evans, U.S. physician, 1912–1974.

Congenital erythropoietic porphyria (Günther's disease)[9]

Congenital erythropoietic porphyria is an inborn defect of heme biosynthesis, resulting from a deficiency of the enzyme uroporphyrinogen III synthase, the fourth enzyme of the heme biosynthesis pathway (Bottomley & Muller-Eberhard, 1988). It is a rare autosomal recessive disease, with less than 200 cases reported in 1986. The clinical features include extreme photosensitivity and skin fragility, leading to severe scarring, especially of the face and hands, hemolytic anemia, hirsutism, and stunted growth (Moore *et al.*, 1990).

The enzyme deficiency expresses itself mainly in bone marrow erythroblasts; it results in overproduction of porphyrins, especially uroporphyrin I and coproporphyrin I, which accumulate in bone marrow erythroblasts and erythrocytes, causing hemolytic anemia. The porphyrins released are excreted in the urine (colored red) and stool, and accumulate in the skin, causing severe oxidative damage in cells exposed to sunlight and extreme sensitivity to trauma. The porphyrins also deposit in bones, fingernails, and teeth, resulting in red-brown discoloration.

The major prognostic factor seems to be the age at which severe clinical symptoms first occur. If the dermatologic changes leading to early scarring occur in the first decade of life, prognosis is poor. Since the encoding DNA is known (Tsai, Bishop, & Desnick, 1988), gene therapy may be appropriate treatment for this disease in the future. However, at the present time, only allogeneic HSC transplantation offers curative potential.

The first report of treatment of this disease with BMT was in 1991 (Kauffmann *et al.*, 1991). Unfortunately the child died 11 months posttransplant from CMV infection. Uroporphyrinogen III synthase (UROIIIS) activity was normal 7 months posttransplant and her skin fragility had greatly improved.

In 1996, two additional case reports were published. Zix-Kieffer and colleagues (1996) reported a 3-year-old girl transplanted from her HLA-identical brother with umbilical cord blood cells. Ten months posttransplant she had no abnormal skin fragility or photosensitivity, no hemolytic anemia, and regression of the discoloration of teeth, fingernails, and skin. This was associated with the complete normalization of UROIIIS activity in the erythrocytes, demonstrating that allografting is curative for this disease. Thomas and colleagues (1996) reported a 2-year-old girl given an HLA-identical bone marrow transplant from her heterozygous sister. A second transplant was necessary to obtain full donor chimerism. Correction of the UROIIIS deficiency was obtained and the patient's clinical condition improved dramatically. At the time of the report, she was well 1 year posttransplant.

Lagarde and colleagues (1998) reported a 2-year-old girl clinically well 21 months after a second sibling transplant that

was likewise required to obtain sustained donor engraftment. Shaw *et al.* (2001) reported a 23-month-old boy alive and disease-free 15 months after an HLA-identical sibling transplant. Conditioning was with busulfan and cyclophosphamide.

Familial Mediterranean fever

Familial Mediterranean fever (FMF) is autosomal recessive disorder characterized by short episodic bouts of fever, inflammatory sinusitis causing arthritis, abdominal pain, pleurisy and pericarditis, and an erysipelas-like rash. The responsible gene, MEFV, encodes a 791-amino acid protein known as pyrin or marenostrin, which is predominantly expressed on granulocytes and synovium. Its function remains to be established, but it may be an interferon γ-mediated regulator of the acute inflammatory response. Colchicine has proved effective in minimizing acute episodes and in preventing the long-term complications of amyloiosis. Milledge and colleagues (2002) reported a 4 year-old child who had both congenital dyserythropoietic anemia (CDA) and FMF. The indication for transplant was the CDA. However, 2 years postransplant she appeared cured of both the CDA and the FMF. Conditioning was with busulfan, cyclophosphamide and ATG prior to an unmantableipulated HLA-identical sibling marrow graft. GVHD prophylaxis consisted of cyclosporine. The FMF symptoms resolved rapidly during conditioning regimen, and her previously persistent left elbow effusion and splenomegaly disappeared.

Idiopathic hypereosinophilic syndrome (and see Chapter 53)

The idiopathic hypereosinophilic syndrome (HES) is a leukoproliferative disorder, or a number of disorders, marked by a sustained overproduction of eosinophils (Weller & Bubley, 1994). A distinct feature of the syndrome, in addition to the eosinophilia, is its marked predilection to damage specific organs, including the heart. There are no specific tests diagnostic of HES. Rather, the syndrome is defined by the combination of unexplained, prolonged eosinophilia and evidence of organ involvement. Diagnostic criteria for HES have been established:

1. The patient must have sustained blood eosinophilia $\geq 1.5 \times 10^9/l$ present for ≥ 6 months.
2. Other apparent causes of eosinophilia must be absent, including parasitic infections and allergic diseases.
3. The patient must have signs and symptoms of organ involvement.

HES tends to occur between the ages of 20 and 50, although a few cases have been reported in children. Clinically, it has varied manifestations. The presenting manifestations may be caused by sudden cardiac or neurologic complications, but tend to be more insidious and evolve slowly.

The organ systems involved in three series of HES are shown in Table 64.1.

---

[9] Hans Günther, German physician, 1884–1956.

Table 64.1. *Frequency of organ involvement in the hypereosinophilic syndrome from three different series*

Organ system	Series (no. of patients)			
	American (50)	French (40)	English (15)	Overall (105)
Hematologic	100	100	100	100
Cardiovascular	50	58	73	58
Cutaneous	56	50	73	56
Neurologic	64	35	73	54
Pulmonary	40	63	40	49
Splenic	46	33	60	43
Hepatic	32	28	–	30
Ocular	18	15	60	23
Gastrointestinal	14	23	53	23

Values are percentages.
Reviewed by, and reproduced with permission from, Weller and Bubley (1994).

Table 64.2. *Therapies for the hypereosinophilic syndrome (HES)*

Therapy	Indications
None	If no evidence of organ involvement, i.e., those with eosinophilia but without defining features of HES
Corticosteroids	First-line agent for those with organ involvement; if effective in suppressing blood eosinophilia, dose may be tapered or changed to every other day; response to corticosteroids associated with a better prognosis
Hydroxyurea	Used in those with organ involvement and eosinophilia unresponsive to corticosteroids; anemia and/or thrombocytopenia common with chronic therapy
Vincristine	Especially useful for acute reductions when total eosinophil counts are excessive (=50,000 to 75,000/µl); can be administered episodically to control HES often with amelioration of thrombocytopenia
Alkylating agents	Chlorambucil and others; may be administered in 4-day pulse doses repeated as dictated by magnitude of blood eosinophilia
Other	α-interferon; cyclosporine
Cardiac surgery	Indicated for serious mitral regurgitation with bioprosthetic mitral valve replacement; less commonly, thrombectomy or endomyocardectomy

Reproduced, with permission, from Weller and Bubley (1994).

The defining hematologic abnormality is sustained eosinophilia. Often leukocyte counts are $<25 \times 10^9/l$ with between 30% and 70% eosinophils, but occasionally extremely high leukocyte counts ($>90 \times 10^9/l$) develop and are associated with a poor prognosis. A full description of the clinical involvement in other organ systems is given in the review by Weller and Bubley (1994).

The distinction between HES syndromes and a truly malignant eosinophilic leukemia can be difficult to make in patients who present with acute HES. Acute eosinophilic leukemia can be distinguished from HES when there is a marked increase in the number of immature eosinophils from the blood and/or marrow, with more than 10% blast forms in the marrow, infiltration of tissues with immature cells of predominantly eosinophilic type, and a clinical course similar to that of other acute leukemias, including pronounced anemia, thrombocytopenia, and susceptibility to infection. The cardiac and neurologic complications seen in HES can develop in acute eosinophilic leukemia as in other eosinophilic diseases, so these are not distinguishing clinical features. Eosinophilic leukemia is often associated with chromosomal abnormalities described in other acute myeloid leukemias, including trisomy 1, t(8:21), and 10p+11q– translocations. Additionally, eosinophilic leukemia has been described as a variant of the AML M4 phenotype of acute myelomonocytic leukemia, including the characteristic chromosome 16 abnormalities.

The differential diagnosis of HES involves the disparate diseases associated with eosinophilia. Eosinophilic syndromes limited to specific organ involvement such as eosinophilic pneumonia or eosinophilic gastroenteritis characteristically do not extend beyond their own target organs.

Therapies used for HES are shown in Table 64.2. Usually the goal is chronic maintenance therapy rather than aggressive therapy aiming to induce a remission of disease. The disease may subside in severity with time. More aggressive therapy may be indicated but it must be tailored to the needs and responsiveness of the individual patient.

There are a small number of case reports of the use of allogeneic BMT for HES. The first resulted in complete hematologic recovery but the patient died 3 months posttransplant of CMV infection (Archimbaud *et al.*, 1988). Two subsequent cases reported long-term survivors, one at 30 months posttransplant and one at 5 years posttransplant (Sigmund & Flessa, 1995; Esteva-Lorenzo *et al.*, 1996). The first patient, a 32-year-old man, presented with pulmonary dysfunction, thrombocytopenia, lymphadenopathy, and hepatosplenomegaly and his disease was progressive on prednisone and hydroxyurea therapy. Thirty months posttransplant, he was asymptomatic with no evidence of eosinophilia. The second patient, a 23-year-old woman, who had progressive and nearly fatal HES with neurologic and cardiac involvement, received an HLA-matched T-cell-depleted sibling bone marrow transplant after conditioning with cyclophosphamide 60 mg/kg on 2 consecutive days followed by fractionated total body irradiation 12 Gy. The cardiac and neurologic abnormalities resolved posttransplant as did the hepatosplenomegaly, and the abnormal blood count and marrow. Other studies have reported comparable outcomes (Fukushima *et al.*, 1995; Sadoun *et al.*, 1997; Vazquez *et al.*, 2000).

Allogeneic transplantation appears to represent a potentially curative therapeutic modality for some patients with this syndrome.

Langerhans[10] cell histiocytosis and hemophagocytic lymphohistiocytosis

The term *histiocyte* embraces cells of both monocyte/macrophage series and the Langerhans cell/dendritic cell series. Both macrophages and Langerhans/dendritic cells arise from CD34+ bone marrow stem cells, probably under the influence of GM-CSF, IL-3, and TNF-α. Macrophages develop from the progenitor cell designated colony-forming unit granulocyte-macrophage (CFU-GM). These progenitor cells give rise to promonocytes that mature in the marrow to monocytes, which then circulate briefly in the blood before entering the tissues. The Langerhans cell also develops from a blood cell that originates from the bone marrow. Its maturation commences in the epidermis but may not be completed before these migrate into the lymphatics of the dermis and then to the lymph nodes. There, in T-cell-rich regions, they complete the process of maturation into dendritic cells. Langerhans cells contain distinctive granules called Birbeck granules not found in macrophages or other cell types.

Functionally, monocytes and macrophages are "professional phagocytes" that defend the body against microorganisms and rid it of unwanted organic and inorganic particles by phagocytosis. Langerhans and dendritic cells in contrast are poor phagocytes but are highly evolved for the efficient presentation of new antigens to CD4+ T cells in the initiation of the class II cellular immune response. They present antigen in conjunction with their rich array of surface MHC class II and CD1a antigens. Among the antigenic, structural, and functional markers that are helpful in identifying macrophage and Langerhans cells in disease states are CD1a and 1c, CD15, CD30, CD45, CD68, acid phosphatase, and lysozyme. This subject has been reviewed by Cline (1994).

The categorization of diseases that arise from histiocytes is confusing. A classification proposed by the Histiocyte Society in 1987 is shown in Table 64.3. Cline (1994) proposed a different classification (Table 64.4).

In addition to some of the macrophage storage disorders (see Chapter 63), two disorders from this long list have been reported as curable with allogeneic BMT: Langerhans cell histiocytosis (LCH) and hemophagocytic lymphohistiocytosis.

Langerhans cell histiocytosis

The published literature reveals only a few cases of LCH treated by allogeneic transplantation and two by autologous BMT. It appears that the disease is curative at least by allografting. Conter and colleagues (1996) described a 4-year-old child whose disseminated refractory LCH was not controlled by front-line monotherapy with etoposide nor subsequently by combination chemotherapy or with corticosteroids and cyclosporine. Because of the high risk of fatal progressive disease, he underwent an HLA-identical sibling transplant and

Table 64.3. *Classification of histiocytosis syndromes in children*[a]

Class I	Langerhans cell histiocytosis
Class II	Histiocytosis of mononuclear phagocytes other than Langerhans cells
	Hemophagocytic lymphohistiocytosis (familial and reactive)
	Sinus histiocytosis with massive lymphadenopathy (Rosai-Dorfman disease)[11]
	Juvenile xanthogranuloma
	Reticulohistiocytoma
Class III	Malignant histiocytic disorders
	Acute monocytic leukemia (FAB M5)
	Malignant histiocytosis
	True histiocytic lymphoma

[a] Adopted by the Histiocyte Society in 1987.

engrafted satisfactorily. At the time of the report, he was in excellent condition, disease-free 25 months posttransplant. Frost and Wiersma (1996) described a 4-month-old infant with a seborrheic-appearing rash, respiratory collapse, and spontaneous pneumothorax at presentation. He progressed despite aggressive multiagent chemotherapy and therefore underwent allogeneic marrow transplantation at age 16 months. He had a satisfactory posttransplant outcome with complete donor chimerism.

Hemophagocytic lymphohistiocytosis

This disease is categorized clinically by fever, hepatosplenomegaly, and cytopenia. The histopathologic findings consist of a nonmalignant accumulation of lymphocytes and macrophages in the reticuloendothelial organs (Fig. 64.6). The familial (primary) form of the disease is inherited as an autosomal recessive. A secondary form consequent to infection or malignancy (lymphoma) also occurs. The natural course is usually rapidly fatal with median survival after onset being 2 to 3 months. Chemotherapy, including the epipodophyllotoxin derivatives etoposide and teniposide, combined with corticosteroids have markedly prolonged the survival of affected children, but have not resulted in cure (Hirst *et al.*, 1994).

In contrast, allogeneic transplantation has been associated with cure in a number of reports first described by Fischer *et al.* (1986), with a subsequent follow-up from the same center in 1991 (Blanche *et al.*, 1991).

In later studies, Bolme and colleagues (1995) described transplantation of 6 children aged 9 months to 10 years, 2 of whom received sibling marrow, 2 parental marrow, and 2 unrelated donor marrow. Conditioning consisted of etoposide, busulfan, and cyclophosphamide with the addition of ATG in 2 cases and OKT3 in 1 case. Marrow was given T replete and methotrexate

---

[10] Paul Langerhaus, German pathologist, 1847–1888.

[11] Juan Rosai, Argentine-U.S. pathologist; Ronald Dorfman, U.S. pathologist.

Table 64.4. *Histiocytic diseases*

Disease	Cell	Characteristic pathologic features	Clinical course	Etiology/pathogenesis (references)
Reactive macrophage histiocytoses				
M-I. Storage diseases				
A. Gaucher's disease[b]	MP	Intracellular storage material in macrophages	Chronic; ± organ infiltration and dysfunction	Enzyme deficiencies
B. Niemann-Pick disease[c]				
C. Sphingomyelinase deficiency, etc.				
M-II. Benign proliferative macrophage diseases				
Xanthoma disseminata Multicentric reticulohistiocytosis; juvenile xanthogranuloma		Macrophages with foamy cytoplasm and usually without particle phagocytosis	Nodules in skin ± joints ± viscera. Self-limited; sometimes recurrent	Unknown
M-III. Nonmalignant hemophagocytic macrophage diseases				
A. Fulminant hemophagocytic syndrome	MP	Macrophages phagocytizing blood cells	Benign to aggressive disease in children. Often fatal	A. Reactive: viruses, bacteria, drugs, SLE
B. Sinus histiocytosis with massive lymphadenopathy (*Rosai-Dorfman disease*)[h]	MP	Lymphocytophagocytosis	Benign to fatal; lymphadenopathy, ± visceral disease	B. Familial of unknown cause. Usually unknown; rare association with Herpes virus 6 or EBV
Malignant diseases of macrophages				
M-IV. Acute monocytic leukemia	Monoblast	Proliferation of primitive hematopoietic cells in BM	Aggressive; usually fatal	Unknown, malignant
M-V. Chronic myelomonocytic leukemia	Monoblast	Proliferation of primitive hematopoietic cells in BM	Aggressive; usually fatal	Unknown, malignant
M-VI. Malignant 5q35 histiocytosis	MP	Proliferating MPs without cellular phagocytosis	Cytopenias; infiltration of soft tissues and bone	Probably malignant with 5q35 translocation and cell lines
Reactive Langerhans cell histiocytosis				
L-1. Benign Langerhans cell histiocytosis				
A. Eosinophilic granuloma (*Hand[a]-Schüller-Christian disease*)[d]	LHC	Infiltration with Langerhans cells with characteristic Birbeck granules[g]	Variable; benign to aggressive. Involves bone ± lungs, pituitary, and rarely viscera	Usually unknown
B. Relapsing Langerhans cell histiocytosis	LHC	Infiltration with LHCs	Variable; benign to aggressive; rarely fatal. Relapsing	Unknown
C. Self-healing histiocytosis	LHC	Infiltration with LHCs	Skin involvement. Benign	Unknown
Presumptively malignant Langerhans cell histiocytoses				
L-II. Progressive Langerhans cell[a] histiocytosis (*Letterer-Siwe disease*)[e]	LHC	Infiltration with LHCs	Fatal, Infiltration of skin, marrow, and viscera	Possibly malignant, but monoclonality not proven; some progress to AMoL
L-III. Langerhans cell lymphoma[f]	LHC	Infiltration with LHCs with Birbeck granules[g]	Aggressive lymphoma	Probably malignant; only 2 cases reported
L-IV. Dendritic cell lymphoma	DC	Node replacement by cells with complex interdigitating processes	Generally limited to lymph nodes	Probably malignant; some have aneuploidy; 13 cases reported

Abbreviations: MP, macrophage; LHC, Langerhans cell; DC, dendritic cell; SLE, systemic lupus erythematosus; AMoL, acute monocytic leukemia.

Historical designation of disease is given in italics.

[a] Histiocytosis X was a term coined to encompass eosinophilic granuloma of bone, Hand-Schüller-Christian disease, and Letterer-Siwe disease.

[b] Philippe Gaucher, French physician, 1854–1918.

[c] William Niemann, U.S. pediatrician, born 1926. Ludwig Pick, German physician, 1868–1935.

[d] Alfred Hand, U.S. pediatrician, 1868–1949. Arthur Schüller, Austrian neurologist, born 1874. Henry Christian, U.S. internist, 1876–1951.

[e] Erich Letterer, German pathologist, born 1895. Sture Siwe, Swedish pediatrician, 1897–1966.

[f] Paul Langerhans, German anatomist, 1847–1888.

[g] Michael Birbeck, 20th-century British cancer researcher.

[h] Juan Rosai, Argentine-U.S. pathologist; Ronald Dorfman, U.S. pathologist.

Reproduced, with permission, from Cline (1994).

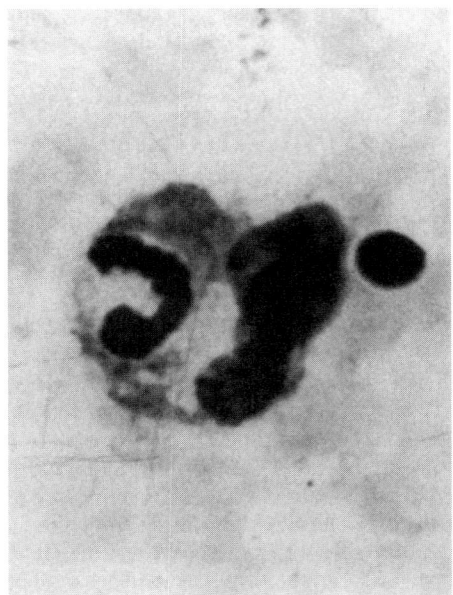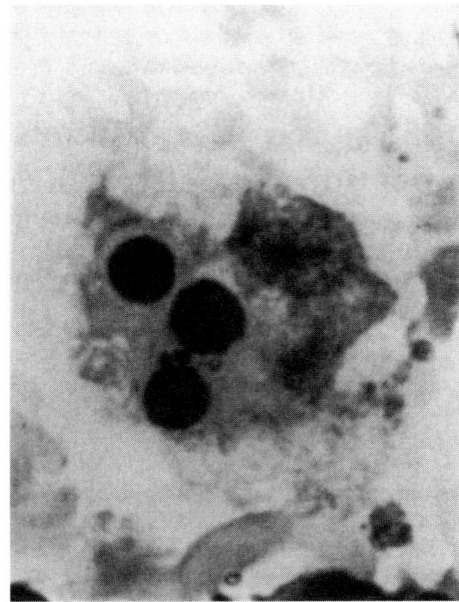

Fig. 64.6. Histiocytes in the bone marrow showing phagocytosis of neutrophils or erythroblasts. Reproduced, with permission, from Adachi *et al.* (1997).

and cyclosporine were used in 5, while cyclosporine and methylprednisolone were used in the sixth. Four of the 6 children were reported alive and well 2 years and 3 months to 3 years and 1 month posttransplant. The two children receiving unrelated marrow died. A French study also described 6 children transplanted with marrow from an HLA-identical sibling donor in five cases and from an HLA-nonidentical related donor (1 HLA-mismatch) in the sixth (Landman-Parker *et al.*, 1993). The conditioning regimen included etoposide 900 mg/m², busulfan 16 mg/kg, cyclophosphamide 200 mg/kg, and cytosine arabinoside in 1 case (2 g/m²). Four patients were alive at the time of the report of treatment more than 3 years posttransplant. The other two had a recurrence of the disease 1 year posttransplant. The four long-term survivors showed mixed chimerism, with recipient cells dominant in three. Other series successfully utilizing HLA-nonidentical related donors (Jabado *et al.*, 1997) or unrelated donors (Baker *et al.*, 1997) (Figs. 64.7 and 64.8) have been published. In another report, all 8 patients given HLA-identical unrelated donor bone marrow transplants were alive without disease at a median follow-up of 24.5 months (Dürken *et al.*, 1999). The conditioning regimen was busulfan 16 to 20 mg/kg, etoposide 30 to 60 mg/kg, cyclophosphamide 120 mg/kg, and ATG. Three of the patients showed slight to moderate developmental delay.

Successful haploidentical (maternal) peripheral blood stem cell transplantation, performed 2 months after receiving a living related liver transplant from the same donor, has been described (Matthes-Martin *et al.*, 2000). Conditioning comprised busulfan 16 mg/kg, cyclophosphamide 200 mg/kg, thiotepa 10 mg/kg, and ATG. However, posttransplant DLI was necessary to obtain complete donor T-cell chimerism.

A successful outcome was reported after a 1 HLA antigen-mismatched unrelated cord blood transplant in a patient with an EBV-associated form of the disease (Minegishi *et al.*, 2001). An international collaboration organized by the Histiocyte Society enrolled 113 patients with both the familial and secondary forms of the disease on a treatment protocol that included allogeneic transplantation (Henter *et al.*, 2002). Sixty-one children were transplanted—including 15 from a matched related donor, 25 from a matched unrelated donor, 4 from a mismatched unrelated donor, 14 from a haploidentical family member donor and 5 from cord blood. The 3 year probability of survival posttransplant was 62%.

Autologous HSC transplantation has also been used with success (Ohga *et al.*, 1997).

Large granular lymphocyte proliferation

Large granular lymphocyte (LGL) proliferation is characterized by expansion of cytotoxic lymphocytes with abundant cytoplasm containing multiple azurophilic granules (Chan *et al.*, 1986; Scott & Richards, 1992; Loughran, 1993). The disease usually presents in late middle age and is associated with neutropenia and autoimmune disorders (especially rheumatoid arthritis). The clinical course is benign in most patients but treatment is warranted should progressive disease with recurrent infections and organ infiltration occur. However, cytotoxic drugs, splenectomy, corticosteroids, and cyclosporine have all been of limited value.

Gentile *et al.* (1994) reported a more aggressive variant of LGL leukemia characterized by expression of CD3⁺ and CD56⁺. Clinical features of this disease were subsequently summarized (Kojima, Komeno, & Shinagawa, 1995) (Table 64.5). Most cases of T-cell LGL are T-cell receptor α/β^+, but a minority are T-cell receptor γ/δ^+.

Besides T-cell chronic lymphatic leukemia and prolymphocytic leukemia, there are several other T-cell lymphopro-

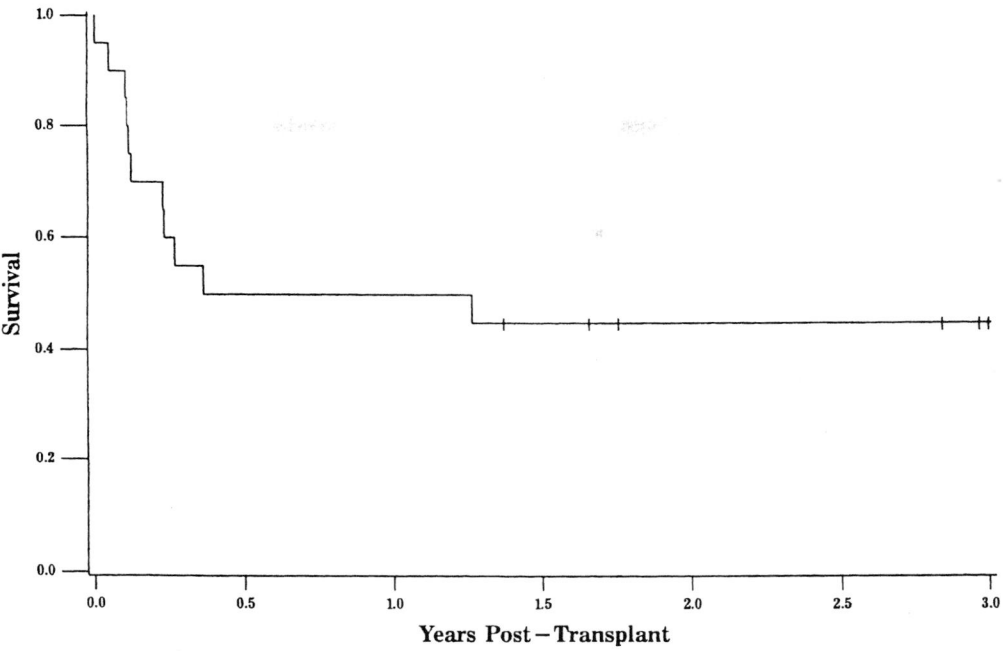

Fig. 64.7. The probability of survival for all patients was 45% at 3 years of follow-up (95% CL, 0.23, 0.67). Tick marks represent surviving patients censored as of the date of analysis, with a single tick mark at 3 years representing 4 patients who survive more than 3 years. Reproduced, with permission, from Baker *et al.* (1997)

liferative disorders that should be distinguished from LGL leukemia; one is S-100⁺ T-cell lymphoproliferative disease characterized by marked splenomegaly lymphadenopathy and a poor prognosis (Zarate-Osorno, 1994). In this disease T cells express the alpha/beta T-cell receptor with CD3, CD8, and the natural killer (NK)-associated markers CD16 and CD56.

Another T-cell malignancy expressing the CD56 antigen is γ/δ T-cell lymphoma, which presents with marked hepatosplenomegaly and only moderate peripheral blood involvement.

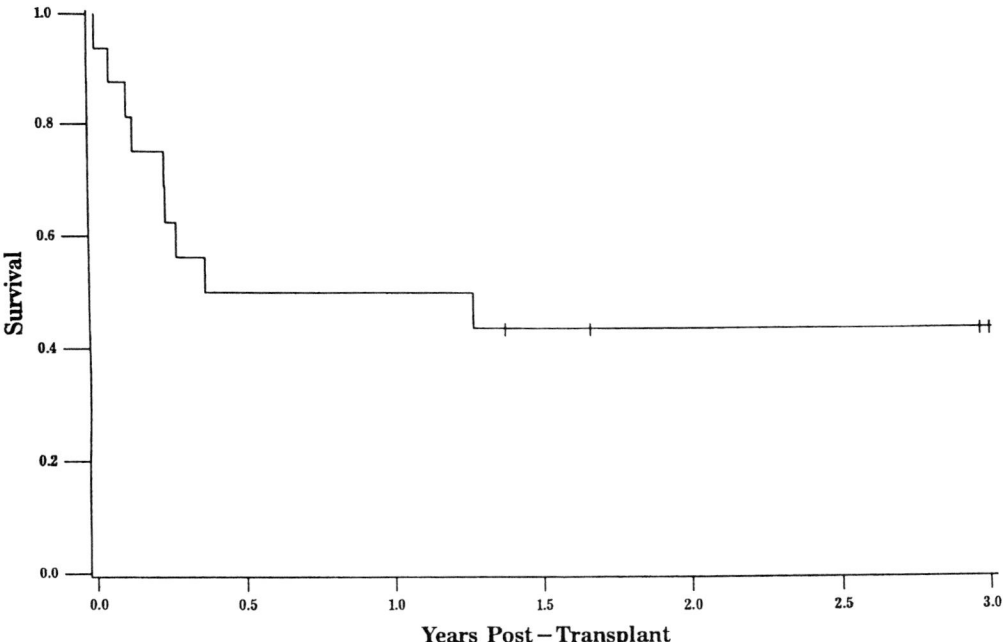

Fig. 64.8. The probability of survival for patients undergoing unrelated donor transplant was 44% at 3 years of follow-up (95% CL, 0.19, 0.68). Tick marks represent surviving patients censored as of the date of analysis, with a single tick mark at 3 years representing 4 patients who survive more than 3 years. Reproduced, with permission, from Baker *et al.* (1997).

Table 64.5. *Clinical features of CD3+, CD56+ LGL leukemia*

Patient	Age/sex	WBC count (/μl)	CD3	4	8	16	56	57	TCR β rearrangement	L/N	H/S	B symptoms	RA	Prognosis (months)	Reference
1	14/F	14,800	+	−	+	−	+	−	+	+	+	+	−	19	Gentile *et al.*, 1994
2	52/M	29,900	+	−	+	+	+	−	+	+	+	+	−	5	Gentile *et al.*, 1994
3	41/M	19,000	+	−	+	+	+		+	+	+	+	−	8	Gentile *et al.*, 1994
4	69/M	21,000	+	−	+	−	+	+	+	−	−			72+	Oshimi, 1988
5	88/F		+	−	−	+	+		+	−	−			9	Woessner *et al.*, 1994
6	68/M		+	+	−	−	+		+	−	−	−		18+	Woessner *et al.*, 1994
7	71/F	14,200	+	+	−	−	+		+	−	−	−	−	4+	Kojima *et al.*, 1995

Abbreviations: L/N, lymphadenopathy; H/S, hepatosplenomegaly; RA, rheumatoid arthritis.
Reproduced, with permission, from Kojima *et al.* (1995).

Patients are frequently anemic, leukopenic, and thrombocytopenic. Prognosis is generally poor. γ/δ T cells are usually double-negative for CD4 and CD8, although a subset of γ/δ T-cell lymphomas are CD8+. In addition to CD2 and CD3 these lymphoma cells express CD16 and CD56 (Gaulard *et al.*, 1990).

At least two cases of allogeneic bone marrow transplantation for LGL leukemia have been reported (Seebach, Speich, & Gmür, 1995; Teshima *et al.*, 1996). In the study reported by Seebach and colleagues, the patient was a 23-year-old woman first observed in 1983 when she suffered from infectious mononucleosis. During the following years, lymphocytosis, splenomegaly, and neutropenia developed. She suffered from recurrent infections. Immunophenotyping showed the peripheral blood mononuclear cells to have an increased population (85%) of CD3+/TCR γ/δ+, CD4−, CD8−, CD16−, CD56−, CD57+ with the typical morphology of large granular lymphocytes. Southern blot analysis of the T-cell receptor beta gene showed an exclusively germline fragment, whereas the TCR gamma and delta genes were clonally rearranged. Splenectomy was performed but did not affect the neutrophil count. The blood lymphocytosis increased and hepatomegaly developed rapidly. There was no response to hematopoietic growth factors. She was given a course of conventional chemotherapy (VACOP-B) prior to transplant conditioning with cyclophosphamide 60 mg/kg on 2 consecutive days and fractionated total body irradiation 12 Gy given in 6 fractions over 6 days. She received marrow from her HLA-identical brother. At the time of report she was in excellent health 29 months posttransplant with no clinical or histologic signs of disease.

Osteogenesis imperfecta (and see Chapter 63)

Osteogenesis imperfecta is a genetic disorder in which osteoblasts produce defective type I collagen, leading to osteopenia, multiple fractures, severe bony deformities, and considerably shortened stature. In principle, transplantation of mesenchymal progenitor cells could attenuate or correct such a disorder. This was shown to be the case by allografts performed for three children with the disease (Horwitz *et al.*, 1999). Three months after osteoblast engraftment (1.5% to 2% of donor cells), trabecular bone showed new dense bone formation. All three patients had increases in total body bone mineral content. These changes were associated with increases in growth velocity and reduced frequencies of bone fracture.

Chronic EBV[12] infection with lymphoproliferation

A boy with chronic active EBV infection, who developed bilateral exophthalmos due to infiltration by EBV-infected NK cells, achieved complete remission after allogeneic BMT (Okamura *et al.*, 2000).

References

Adachi, S., Kubota, M., Akiyama, Y. *et al.* (1997). Successful bone marrow transplantation from an HLA-identical unrelated donor in a patient with hemaphagocytic lymphohistiocytosis. *Bone Marrow Transplantation*, **19**, 183–5.

Alter, B.P. (1998). Bone marrow transplant in Diamond-Blackfan anemia. *Bone Marrow Transplantation*, **21**, 965 (Letter).

Antin, J.H., Ginsburg, D., Smith, B.R. *et al.* (1985). Bone marrow transplantation for paroxysmal nocturnal hemoglobinuria: eradication of the PNH clone and documentation of complete lympho hematopoietic engraftment. *Blood*, **66**, 1247–50.

Archimbaud, E., Guyotat, D., Guillaume, C. *et al.* (1988). Hypereosinophilic syndrome with multiple organ dysfunction treated by allogeneic bone marrow transplantation. *American Journal of Hematology*, **27**, 302–3.

Arseniev, F.L., Diedrich, H., & Link, H. (1996). Allogeneic bone marrow transplantation in a patient with Shwachman-Diamond syndrome. *Annals of Hematology*, **72**, 83–4.

Ayas, M., Al-Jefri, A., Baothman, A. *et al.* (2002). Transfusion-dependent congenital dyserythropoietic anemia type I successfully treated with allogeneic stem cell transplantation. *Bone Marrow Transplantation*, **29**, 618–2.

---

[12] Michael Epstein, British virologist, born 1921; Yvonne Barr, British scientist, born 1932.

Baker, K.S., DeLaat, C.A., Streinbuch, M. *et al.* (1997). Successful correction of hemophagocytic lymphohistiocytosis with related or unrelated bone marrow transplantation. *Blood*, **89**, 3857–63.

Bellucci, S., Damaj, G., Boval, B. *et al.* (2000). Bone marrow transplantation in severe Glanzmann's thrombasthenia with antiplatelet immunization. *Bone Marrow Transplantation*, **25**, 327–30.

Bemba, M., Guardiola, P., Garderet, L. *et al.* (2000). Bone marrow transplantation for paroxysmal nocturnal haemoglobinuria. *British Journal of Haematology*, **105**, 366–8.

Bessler, M., Mason, P., Shillmen, P., & Luzzatto, L. (1994). Somatic mutations and cellular selection in paroxysmal nocturnal haemoglobinuria. *Lancet*, **343**, 951–3.

Blanche, S., Caniglia, M., Girault, D. *et al.* (1991). Treatment of hemophagocytic lymphohistiocytosis with chemotherapy and bone marrow transplantation: a single center study of 22 cases. *Blood*, **78**, 51–4.

Bottomley, S.S. & Muller-Eberhard, U. (1988). Pathophysiology of heme synthesis. *Seminars in Hematology*, **25**, 282–302.

Bolme, P., Henter, J.I., Winiarski, J. *et al.* (1995). Allogeneic bone marrow transplantation for hemophagocytic lymphohistiocytosis in Sweden. *Bone Marrow Transplantation*, **15**, 331–5.

Cesaro, S., Guariso, G., Calore, E. *et al.* (2001). Successful unrelated bone marrow transplantation for Shwachman-Diamond syndrome. *Bone Marrow Transplantation*, **27**, 97–9.

Chan, W.C., Link, S., Mawle, A. *et al.* (1986). Heterogeneity of large granular lymphocyte proliferation: delineation of 2 major subtypes. *Blood*, **68**, 1142–53.

Cline, M.J. (1994). Histiocytes and histiocytosis. *Blood*, **84**, 2840–53.

Conter, V., Reciputo, A., Arrigo, C. *et al.* (1996). Bone marrow transplantation for refractory Langerhans cell histiocytosis. *Haematologica*, **81**, 468–71.

Cossu, F., Vulliamy, T. J., Marrone, A., Badiali, M. & Cao, A. (2002). A novel DKC1 mutation, severe combined immunodeficiency T+ B− NK− SCID) and bone marrow transplantation in an infant with Hoyeraal-Hreidarsson syndrome. *British Journal of Haematology*, **119**, 765–8.

Dacie, J.V. (1967). The nature of paroxysmal nocturnal hemoglobinuria. In *The Hemolytic Anemias: Congenital and Acquired*, Part IV, p. 1219. London: J & A Churchill.

De Stefano, P., Zecca, M., Giorgiani, G. *et al.* (1999). Resolution of immune hemolytic anemia with allogeneic bone marrow transplantation after unsuccessful autograft. *British Journal of Haematology*, **106**, 1063–4.

Dürken, M., Horstmann, M., Bieling, P. *et al.* (1999). Improved outcome in haemophagocytic lymphohistiocytosis after bone marrow transplantation from related and unrelated donors: a single centre experience of 12 patients. *British Journal of Haematology*, **106**, 1052–8.

Endo, M., Beatty, P.G., Vreeke, T.M. *et al.* (1996). Syngeneic bone marrow transplantation without conditioning in a patient with paroxysmal nocturnal hemoglobinuria: in vivo evidence that the mutant stem cells have a survival advantage. *Blood*, **88**, 742–50.

Esteva-Lorenzo, F.J., Meehan, K.R., Spitzer, T.R., & Mazumder, A. (1996). Allogeneic bone marrow transplantation in a patient with hypereosinophilic syndrome. *American Journal of Hematology*, **51**, 164–5.

Fefer, A., Freeman, H., Storb, R. *et al.* (1976). Paroxysmal nocturnal hemoglobinuria and marrow failure treated by infusion of marrow from an identical twin. *Annals of Internal Medicine*, **84**, 692–5.

Fischer, A., Cerf-Bensussan, N., Blanche, S. *et al.* (1986). Allogeneic bone marrow transplantation for erythrophagocytic lymphohistiocytosis. *Journal of Pediatrics*, **108**, 267–70.

Fleitz, J., Rumelhart, S., Goldman, F. *et al.* (2002). Successful allogeneic hematopoietic stem cell transplantation (HSCT) for Shwachman-Diamond syndrome. *Bone Marrow Transplantation*, **29**, 75–9.

Frost, J.D. & Wiersma, S.R. (1996). Progressive Langerhans cell histiocytosis in an infant with Klinefelter syndrome successfully treated with allogeneic bone marrow transplantation. *Journal of Pediatric Hematology/Oncology*, **18**, 396–400.

Fukushima, T., Kuriyama, K., Ito, H. *et al.* (1995). Successful bone marrow transplantation for idiopathic hypereosinophilic syndrome. *British Journal of Haematology*, **90**, 213–15.

Gaulard, P., Bourquelot, P., Kanavaros, P. *et al.* (1990). Expression of the alpha/beta and gamma/delta T-cell receptors in 57 cases of peripheral T-cell lymphomas: identification of a subset of γ/δ T-cell lymphomas. *American Journal of Pathology*, **137**, 617–28.

Gentile, T.C., Uner, A.H., Hutchison, R.E. *et al.* (1994). CD3+, CD56+ aggressive variant of aggressive variant of large granular lymphocyte leukemia. *Blood*, **84**, 2315–21.

Gonzalez, M.I., Caballero, D., Vazquez, L. *et al.* (2000). Allogeneic peripheral stem cell transplantation in a case of hereditary sideroblastic anaemia. *British Journal of Haematology*, **108**, 658–60.

Graham, M.L., Rosse, W.F., Halperin, E.C. *et al.* (1996). Resolution of Budd-Chiari syndrome following bone marrow transplantation for paroxysmal nocturnal hemoglobinuria. *British Journal of Haematology*, **92**, 707–10.

Greinix, H.T., Storb, R., & Sanders, J.E. (1993). Long-term survival and cure after marrow transplantation for congenital hypoplastic anemia (Diamond-Blackfan syndrome). *British Journal of Haematology*, **84**, 515–20.

Guinan, E.C., Lee, Y., Lopez, K.E.D. *et al.* (1993). Effects of interleukin-3 and granulocyte-macrophage colony-stimulating factor on thrombopoiesis in congenital amegakaryocytic thrombocytopenia. *Blood*, **81**, 1691–8.

Henter, J.-I., Winiarski, J., Ljungman, P. *et al.* (1995). Bone marrow transplantation in 2 children with congenital amegakaryocytic thrombocytopenia. *Bone Marrow Transplantation*, **15**, 799–801.

Henter, J-L., Samuelsson-Horn, A., Arico, M. *et al.* (2002). Treatment of hemophagocytic lymphohistiocytosis with HLH-94 immunochemotherapy and bone marrow transplantation. *Blood*, **100**, 2367–73.

Hershko, C., Gale, R.P., Ho, W.G. *et al.* (1979). Cure of aplastic anaemia in paroxysmal nocturnal haemoglobinuria by marrow transfusion from identical twin: failure of peripheral leukocyte transfusion to correct marrow aplasia. *Lancet*, **1**, 945–7.

Hillman, P., Lewis, S.M., Bessler, M. *et al.* (1995). Natural history of paroxysmal nocturnal hemoglobinuria. *New England Journal of Medicine*, **333**, 1253–8.

Hirst, W.J., Layton, D.M., Singh, S. *et al.* (1994). Hemophagocytic lymphohistiocytosis: experience at 2 UK centres. *British Journal of Haematology*, **88**, 731–9.

Horwitz, E.M., Prockop, D.J., Fitzpatrick, L.A. *et al.* (1999). Transplantability and therapeutic effects of bone marrow-derived mesenchymal cells in children with osteogenesis imperfecta. *Nature Medicine,* **5,** 309–13.

Iolascon, A., Sabato, V., de Mattia, D., & Locatelli, F. (2001). Bone marrow transplantation in a case of severe, type II congenital dyserythropoietic anaemia (CDA II). *Bone Marrow Transplantation,* **27,** 213–5.

Iwamoto, M., Kawaguchi, T., Horikawa, K. *et al.* (1996). Preferential hematopoiesis by paroxysmal nocturnal hemoglobinuria clone engrafted in SCID mice. *Blood,* **87,** 4944–8.

Jabado, N., de Graeff-Meeder, E.R., Cavazzana-Calvo, M. *et al.* (1997). Treatment of familial hemophagocytic lymphohistiocytosis with bone marrow transplantation from HLA genetically nonidentical donors. *Blood,* **90,** 4743–8.

Johnson, A., Goodall, A.H., Downie, C.J.C. *et al.* (1994). Bone marrow transplantation for Glanzmann's thrombasthenia. *Bone Marrow Transplantation,* **14,** 147–50.

Josten, K.M., Tooze, J.A., Borthwick-Clarke *et al.* (1991). Acquired aplastic anemia and paroxysmal nocturnal hemoglobinuria: studies on clonality. *Blood,* **78,** 3162–7.

Kauffmann, L., Evans, D.I.K., Stevens, R.F., & Weinkove, C. (1991). Bone marrow transplantation for congenital erythropoietic porphyria. *Lancet,* **337,** 1510–1.

Kawahara, K., Witherspoon, R.P., & Storb, R. (1992). Marrow transplantation for paroxysmal nocturnal hemoglobinuria. *American Journal of Hematology,* **39,** 283–8.

Kojima, H., Komeno, T., & Shinagawa, A. (1995). CD3$^+$, CD56$^+$ large granular lymphocyte leukemia. *Blood,* **85,** 3762–71.

Kolb, H.J., Holler, E., Bender-Gotze, C. *et al.* (1989). Myeloablative conditioning for marrow transplantation in myelodysplastic syndromes and paroxysmal nocturnal haemoglobinuria. *Bone Marrow Transplantation,* **4,** 29–34.

Lackner, A., Basu, O., Bierings, M. *et al.* (2000). Haematopoietic stem cell transplantation for amegakaryocytic thrombocytopenia. *British Journal of Haematology,* **109,** 773–5.

Lagarde, C., Hamel-Teillac, D., DeProst, Y. *et al.* (1998). Allogeneic bone marrow transplantation in congenital erythropoietic porphyria. *Annals of Dermatology and Venereology,* **125,** 114–7.

Landman-Parker, J., Le Deist, F., Blase, A. *et al.* (1993). Partial engraftment of donor bone marrow cells associated with long-term remission of haemophagocytic lymphohistiocytosis. *British Journal of Haematology,* **85,** 37–41.

Langston, A.A., Sanders, J.E., Deeg, H.J. *et al.* (1996). Allogeneic marrow transplantation for aplastic anaemia associated with dsykeratosis congenita. *British Journal of Haematology,* **92,** 758–65.

Lavabre-Bertrand, T., Blanc, P., Navarro, R. *et al.* (1995). Alpha-interferon therapy for congenital dyserythropoiesis type I. *British Journal of Haematology,* **89,** 929–32.

Lee, A.C., Ha, S.Y., Yuen, K.Y., & Lau, Y.L. (1995). Listeria septicemia complicating bone marrow transplantation for Diamond-Blackfan syndrome. *Pediatric Hematology/Oncology,* **12,** 295–9.

Lional, S., Bilodeau, P.A., Langston, A.A. *et al.* (1999). Acquired amegakaryocytic thrombocytopenia treated with allogeneic BMT: case report and review of the literature. *Bone Marrow Transplantation,* **24,** 1337–41.

Loughran, T.P. (1993). Clonal diseases of large granular lymphocytes. *Blood,* **82,** 1–14.

MacMillan, M.L., Davies, S.M., Wagner, J.E., & Ramsay, N.K.C. (1998). Engraftment of unrelated donor stem cells in children with familial amegakaryocytic thrombocytopenia. *Bone Marrow Transplantation,* **21,** 735–7.

Matthes-Martin, S., Peters, C., Königsrainer, A. *et al.* (2000). Successful stem cell transplantation following orthotopic liver transplantation from the same haploidentical family donor in a girl with hemophagocytic lymphohistiocytosis. *Blood,* **96,** 3997–9.

Milledge, J., Shaw, P. J., Mansour, A. *et al.* (2002). Allogeneic bone marrow transplantation: cure for familial Mediterranean fever. *Blood,* **100,** 774–7.

Minegishi, M., Ohashi, Y., Kumaki, S. *et al.* (2001). Successful umbilical cord blood transplantation from an unrelated donor for a patient with Epstein-Barr virus-associated hemophagocytic lymphohistiocytosis. *Bone Marrow Transplantation,* **27,** 883–6.

Moore, M.R., McColl, K.E.L., Fitzsimons, E.J. *et al.* (1990). The porphyrias. *Blood Reviews,* **4,** 84–96.

Mugishima, H., Gale, R.P., Rowlings, P.A. *et al.* (1995). Bone marrow transplantation for Diamond-Blackfan anemia. *Bone Marrow Transplantation,* **15,** 55–8.

Muller, B.U., Tichelli, A., Passweg, J.R. *et al.* (2001). Successful treatment of refractory acquired pure red cell aplasia (PRCA) by allogeneic bone marrow transplantation. *Bone Marrow Transplantation,* **23,** 1205–7.

Ohga, S., Nomura, A., Kai, T. *et al.* (1997). Prolonged resolution of hemophagocytic lymphohistiocytosis following myeloablative chemotherapy and subsequent autologous peripheral blood stem cell transplantation. *Bone Marrow Transplantation,* **19,** 633–5.

Okamura, T., Arai, H., Hatsukawa, Y. *et al.* (2000). Blood stem-cell transplantation for chronic active Epstein-Barr virus with lymphoproliferation. *Lancet,* **356,** 223–4 (Letter).

Okcu, F., Roberts, W.M., & Chan, K.W. (1998). Bone marrow transplantation in Shwachman-Diamond syndrome: report of two cases and review of the literature. *Bone Marrow Transplantation,* **21,** 849–51.

Oni, S.B., Osunkoya, B.O., & Luzzatto, L. (1970). Paroxysmal nocturnal hemoglobinuria: evidence for monoclonal origin of abnormal red cells. *Blood,* **36,** 145–52.

Oshimi, K. (1988). Granular lymphocyte proliferative disorder: report of 12 cases and review of literature. *Leukemia,* **12,** 617.

Oyama, Y., Papadopoulos, E.B., Miranda, M. *et al.* (2001). Allogeneic stem cell transplantation for Evan's syndrome. *Bone Marrow Transplantation,* **28,** 903–5.

Peretz, H., Rosenberg, N., Usher, S. *et al.* (1995). Glanzmann's thrombasthenia associated with deletion-insertion and alternative splicing in the glycoprotein IIb gene. *Blood,* **85,** 414–20.

Petersen, E.J., Rozenberg-Arska, M., Dekker, A.W. *et al.* (1996). Allogeneic bone marrow transplantation can restore CD4$^+$ T-lymphocyte count and immune function in idiopathic CD4$^+$ T-lymphocytopenia. *Bone Marrow Transplantation,* **18,** 813–5.

Prince, G.M., Nguyen, M., Lazarus, H.M. *et al.* (1995). Peripheral blood harvest of unaffected CD34$^+$ CD38$^-$ hematopoietic precursors in paroxysmal nocturnal hemoglobinuria. *Blood,* **86,** 3381–6.

Raetz, E., Beatty, P.G., & Adams, R.H. (1997). Treatment of severe Evans syndrome with an allogeneic cord blood transplant. *Bone Marrow Transplantation*, **20**, 427–9.

Ritchie, D. S., Angus, P. W., Bhathal, P. S. & Grigg, A. P. (2002). Liver failure complicating non-alcoholic steatohepatitis following allogeneic bone marrow transplantation for Schwachman-Diamond syndrome. *Bone Marrow Transplantation*, **29**, 931–3.

Rosse, W.F. (1989). Paroxysmal nocturnal haemoglobinuria: the biochemical defects and the clinical syndrome. *Blood Reviews*, **3**, 192–200.

Rosse, W.F. (1993). Evolution of clinical understanding: paroxysmal nocturnal hemoglobinuria as a paradigm. *American Journal of Hematology*, **42**, 122–6.

Rosse, W.F. & Ware, R.E. (1995). The molecular basis of paroxysmal nocturnal hemoglobinuria. *Blood*, **86**, 3277–86.

Rotoli, B. & Luzzatto, L. (1989). Paroxysmal nocturnal hemoglobinuria. *Bailliere's Clinical Haematology*, **2**, 113.

Sadoun, A., Lacotte, L., Delwail, V. *et al.* (1997). Allogeneic bone marrow transplantation for hypereosinophilic syndrome with advanced myelofibrosis. *Bone Marrow Transplantation*, **19**, 741–3.

Saso, R., Marsh, J., Cevreska, L. *et al.* (1999). Bone marrow transplants for paroxysmal nocturnal haemoglobinuria. *British Journal of Haematology*, **104**, 392–6.

Scott, C.S. & Richards, S.J. (1992). Classification of large granular lymphocyte (LGL) and NK-associated (NKa) disorders. *Blood Reviews*, **6**, 220–33.

Seebach, J., Speich, R., & Gmür, J. (1995). Allogeneic bone marrow transplantation for CD3⁺/TCR γ/δ^+ large granular lymphocyte proliferation. *Blood*, **85**, 853.

Shaw, P.H., Mancini, A.J., McConnell, J.P. *et al.* (2001). Treatment of congenital erythropoietic porphyria in children by allogeneic stem cell transplantation: a case report and review of the literature. *Bone Marrow Transplantation*, **27**, 101–5.

Sigmund, D.A. & Flessa, H.C. (1995). Hypereosinophilic syndrome: successful allogeneic bone marrow transplantation. *Bone Marrow Transplantation*, **15**, 647–8.

Smith, O.P., Chan, M.Y., Evans, J., & Veys, P. (1995). Shwachman-Diamond syndrome and matched unrelated donor BMT. *Bone Marrow Transplantation*, **16**, 717–8.

Szer, J., Deeg, H.J., Witherspoon, R.P. *et al.* (1984). Long-term survival after marrow transplantation for paroxysmal nocturnal hemoglobinuria with aplastic anemia. *Annals of Internal Medicine*, **1**, 193–5.

Takeda, J., Myata, T., Kawagoe, K. *et al.* (1993). Deficiency of the GPI anchor caused by a somatic mutation of the PIG-A gene in paroxysmal nocturnal hemoglobinuria. *Cell*, **73**, 703–11.

Tanphaichitr, V.S., Suvatte, V., Issaragrisil, S. *et al.* (2000). Successful bone marrow transplantation in a child with red blood cell pyruvate kinase deficiency. *Bone Marrow Transplantation*, **26**, 689–90.

Teshima, T., Gmiyaji, R., Fukuda, M., & Ohshima, K. (1996). Bone marrow transplantation for Epstein-Barr-virus-associated natural killer cell-large granular lymphocyte leukemia. *Lancet*, **347**, 1124.

Thomas, C., Ged, C., Nordmann, Y. *et al.* (1996). Correction of congenital erythropoietic porphyria by bone marrow transplantation. *Journal of Pediatrics*, **129**, 453–6.

Tremml, G., Karadimitris, A., & Luzzatto, L. (1998). Paroxysmal nocturnal hemoglobinuria: learning about PNH cells from patients and from mice. *Haematology*, **1**, 12–20.

Tsai, S.F., Bishop, D.F., & Desnick, R.J. (1988). Human uroporphyrinogen III synthase: molecular cloning, nucleotide sequence, and expression of a full length cDNA. *Proceedings of the National Academy of Science, USA*, **85**, 7049–53.

Tudela, M., Jarque, I., Perez-Sirvent, M.L. *et al.* (1993). Clinical profile and course of paroxysmal nocturnal hemoglobinuria. *Sangre*, **38**, 301–7.

Vazquez, L., Caballero, D., Del Canizo, C. *et al.* (2000). Allogeneic peripheral blood cell transplantation for hypereosinophilic syndrome with myelofibrosis. *Bone Marrow Transplantation*, **25**, 217–8.

Vlachos, A., Federman, N., Reyes-Haley, C. *et al.* (2001). Hematopoietic stem cell transplantation for Diamond-Blackfan anemia: a report from the Diamond-Blackfan Registry. *Bone Marrow Transplantation*, **27**, 381–6.

Weller, P.F. & Bubley, G.J. (1994). The idiopathic hypereosinophilic syndrome. *Blood*, **83**, 2759–79.

Willig, T.N., Niemeyer, C., Leblanc, T. *et al.* (1999). Identification of new prognosis factors from the clinical and epidemiologic analysis of a registry of 229 Diamond-Blackfan anemia patients. *Pediatric Research*, **46**, 553–61.

Woessner, S., Feliu, E., Vilamor, N. *et al.* (1994). Granular lymphocyte proliferative disorders: a multicenter study of 20 cases. *Annals of Hematology*, **68**, 285.

Woodard, P., Wang, W., Pitts, N. *et al.* (2001). Successful unrelated donor bone marrow transplantation for paroxysmal nocturnal hemoglobinuria. *Bone Marrow Transplantation*, **27**, 589–92.

Wyatt, H.A., Mowat, A.P., & Layton, M. (1995). Paroxysmal nocturnal haemoglobinuria and Budd-Chiari syndrome. *Archives of Diseases of Children*, **72**, 241–2.

Yeh, E.T. & Rosse, W.F. (1994). Paroxysmal nocturnal hemoglobinuria and the glycocyl phosphatidylinosotol anchor. *Journal of Clinical Investigation*, **93**, 2305–10.

Yesilipek, M.A., Hazar, V., Kupesiz, A., & Yegin, O. (2000). Peripheral stem cell transplantation in a child with amegakaryocytic thrombocytopenia. *Bone Marrow Transplantation*, **26**, 571–2.

Zarate-Osorno, A., Raffeld, M., Berman, E.L. *et al.* (1994). S-100 positive T-cell lymphoproliferative disorder: a case report and review of the literature. *American Journal of Clinical Pathology*, **102**, 478–82.

Zix-Kieffer, I., Langer, B., Eyer, D. *et al.* (1996). Successful cord blood stem cell transplantation for congenital erythropoietic porphyria (Gunther's disease). *Bone Marrow Transplantation*, **18**, 217–20.

65 Adoptive cellular immunotherapy for treatment or prevention of relapse of hematologic malignancy posttransplant

HANS-JOCHEM KOLB AND STEVEN MACKINNON

Klinikum Grosshadern, Ludwig Maximilians Universität, Munich, Germany, and University College Hospital, London, UK

Introduction

Allogeneic hematopoietic stem cell (HSC) transplantation has induced remissions of hematopoietic malignancies in patients with otherwise refractory disease (Thomas *et al.*, 1975, 1977). In many of these patients remissions persisted without further maintenance treatment for several decades, and some patients may be cured. However, relapse of the primary malignancy remains the most frequent cause of treatment failure in patients transplanted in both early and more advanced stages of disease (Sullivan *et al.*, 1989). The 3-year probability of relapse after allogeneic transplantation in early stage leukemia [i.e., first complete remission of acute leukemia and chronic phase of chronic myeloid leukemia (CML)] is in the range of 10% and 30% (Horowitz *et al.*, 1990). After transplantation in more advanced stages, the 3-year probability of relapse is between 20% and 70% (Barrett *et al.*, 1989; Sullivan *et al.*, 1989; Gale *et al.*, 1995; Horowitz, 1995). In patients surviving more than 3 years after transplantation for acute leukemia the risk of relapse decreases considerably, whereas for patients transplanted for CML in chronic phase the relapse risk remains significant (Horowitz, 1995). The relapse risk may be lower in patients with HLA-matched, unrelated donors, and it is higher in patients given a syngeneic transplant and after autografting. However, continued remissions have been observed even in a considerable proportion of patients with syngeneic donors: effective conditioning, as well as the absence of postgrafting immunosuppression, may contribute to such favorable results. In general, risk factors predicting a poor response to chemotherapy also apply to hematopoietic transplantation. For example, the presence of cytogenetic abnormalities with an adverse impact on the remission rate and probability of relapse after chemotherapy also predict a higher probability of relapse after transplantation (Barrett *et al.*, 1989; Goldman *et al.*, 1988; Zander *et al.*, 1988; Sullivan *et al.*, 1989; Horowitz *et al.*, 1990; Gale *et al.*, 1995).

Nature of, and risk factors for, relapse

Single patients with evidence for recurrent leukemia in donor cells have been reported (Fialkow *et al.*, 1971; Thomas *et al.*, 1972; Goh & Klemperer, 1977; Elfenbein *et al.*, 1978; Newburger *et al.*, 1981; Marmont *et al.*, 1984; Barrett *et al.*, 1985), indicating the persistence of a leukemogenic hazard. However, the great majority of leukemic relapses occur in the patient's own cells. In these patients the leukemic clone has not been eliminated by transplantation, and the relapse results from regrowth of the original clone.

Leukemia recurs from a minority of leukemic cells endowed with extensive proliferative and self-renewal capacity surviving high-dose chemotherapy and radiotherapy (Lapidot *et al.*, 1994). Several studies have compared the combination of cyclophosphamide (CY) and total body irradiation (TBI) with that of busulfan and CY as pretransplant conditioning (Blaise *et al.*, 1992; Buckner *et al.*, 1992; Ringden *et al.*, 1994) and have been unable to demonstrate unequivocal superiority of one regimen. The use of etoposide in combination with TBI has been promising in patients with advanced disease (Blume *et al.*, 1993). Most other preparatory regimens have failed to improve the disease-free survival of leukemic patients after allogeneic transplantation. In prospective studies from Seattle, higher TBI doses have been associated with less relapse, but more transplant-related toxicity, and no improvement in overall survival. In a retrospective comparison of various radiation regimens, no difference was found in patients given unmanipulated bone marrow; however, differences were observed in patients given T-cell-depleted marrow grafts (Marmont *et al.*, 1991). After T-cell depletion the relapse rate was higher in patients given lower doses of TBI or fractionated TBI. Therefore, the role of T cells in the graft may be more powerful than variations in the conditioning regimen.

Allogeneic HSC transplantation as a form of immunotherapy was first perceived by the Harwell group of scientists (Barnes & Loutit, 1957). Its potential for the treatment of leukemia was investigated by Mathé and colleagues (Mathé *et al.*, 1965). Only after the principles for successful transplantation with regard to the selection of histocompatible donors, effective preparatory regimens, and prophylaxis of acute graft-versus-host disease (GVHD) were defined, could the effect of acute and chronic GVHD on leukemia-free survival be evaluated (Weiden *et al.*, 1981). Chronic GVHD in particular has a beneficial effect on the relapse rate after transplantation. In patients with advanced disease both acute and chronic GVHD were found beneficial for relapse-free survival (Sullivan et al., 1989). Likewise, patients transplanted in early stage leukemia had an increased risk of relapse if GVHD was absent (Horowitz et al., 1990). Immunogenetically identical transplants from monozygotic twin donors resulted in an increased risk of relapse (Fefer et al., 1987; Gale et al., 1994), and recipients of marrow from unrelated HLA-identical donors have a lower probability of relapse of leukemia than that of recipients of HLA-identical family member transplants (Kernan et al., 1993; McGlave et al., 1993). However, the degree of immunogenetic disparity between donor and recipient may not solely determine the susceptibility to leukemic relapse; rather modification of the allogeneic immune reaction may influence the course of leukemia (Odom et al., 1978; Higano et al., 1990).

The graft-versus-leukemia (GVL) effect is closely associated with the graft-versus-host reaction, but it may be separable in certain instances. One example is the probability of relapse in CML patients given T-cell-depleted marrow grafts: patients who develop GVHD despite T-cell depletion still have an increased risk of relapse (Horowitz et al., 1990). T cells may exert a GVL effect without inducing (clinically apparent) GVHD.

Types of relapse

Leukemia relapse may be systemic, in many instances heralded by a drop in blood counts and sometimes by an improvement in GVHD. As a rule, progression is rapid, but it may be smoldering in some patients. Extramedullary relapses are not rare after allogeneic marrow transplantation: about 13% of patients with acute myeloid leukemia (AML) and 24% of patients with acute lymphoblastic leukemia (ALL) initially present with an isolated extramedullary relapse (Mortimer et al., 1989; Doney et al., 1991). Isolated extramedullary relapses tend to occur later than systemic relapses (Mortimer et al., 1989), often in the testes or central nervous system (CNS). The CNS and testes are sanctuary sites for chemotherapy and may be sanctuary sites for the immune system also (Odom et al., 1978). Most extramedullary relapses are followed by a systemic relapse.

In CML, cells carrying the Philadelphia (Ph) chromosome may persist or recur after allogeneic marrow transplantation. Small numbers of Ph-positive cells may disappear without therapeutic intervention in many patients (Thomas et al., 1986; Goldman et al., 1986). Larger and increasing proportions of Ph-positive cells may indicate persistence of the disease or cytogenetic relapse (Lin et al., 1996). Cytogenetic relapses progress to hematologic relapses unless they are treated and constitute an indication for giving donor lymphocyte infusion (DLI) (van Rhee et al., 1994).

A positive reverse transcriptase polymerase chain reaction (RT-PCR) for BCR/ABL transcripts in CML patients after transplantation does not necessarily indicate recurrence of the disease, since long-lived cells such as T cells may persist without a risk of relapse. An increasing signal in quantitative RT-PCR may predict a relapse of CML (Lin et al., 1996).

Hematologic relapse is characterized by the recurrence of the clinical disease with reappearance of immature cells and basophils in the blood, leukocytosis, and thrombocytosis unexplained by other causes such as infection or inflammatory responses. Relapse of leukemia with blast cells in the blood and marrow and clinical signs of transformation is common after transplantation for accelerated or blastic phase of CML.

Cellular adoptive immunotherapy

Experimental background

The chimeric state of the patient with leukemic relapse provides specific conditions for adoptive immunotherapy using lymphocytes and other immunocompetent cells of the stem cell donor. Persistent donor chimerism after discontinuation of immunosuppressive therapy indicates a state of tolerance. In DLA-identical canine chimeras graft-versus-host tolerance could not be abrogated by the transfusion of lymphocytes from the donor (Weiden et al., 1976). Transplantation of T-cell-depleted bone marrow can induce mixed chimerism in DLA-identical dogs without further immunosuppression after transplantation (Kolb et al., 1997a). In these chimeras, transfusion of donor lymphocytes did not produce GVHD if delayed for at least 2 months after transplantation. Nevertheless, mixed donor-host chimerism was converted to complete donor chimerism after transfusion of donor lymphocytes (Kolb et al., 1997a). Conversion of lymphoid chimerism occurred early (less than 50 days posttransplant). Conversion of myeloid chimerism could take several months. In these dogs 2 to 4×10^8/kg mononuclear blood cells could be transfused without risk of GVHD. In mice such delayed transfusion was able to cure leukemia without producing GVHD (Johnson et al., 1993).

In dogs immunity could be adoptively transferred by the transfusion of lymphocytes from immunized donors. For example, tetanus antibodies developed in animals transfused with cells from immunized donors and antibody levels persisted for several years after booster immunizations. Transfusions of donor lymphocytes also improved the antibody response of chimeras to neo-antigens such as diphtheria toxin (Kolb et al., 1997a).

Consistent with the results of the animal experiments, transfusion of donor lymphocytes at a dose of 2 to 4×10^8/kg induced complete remissions in patients with CML recurrent postallografting (Kolb et al., 1990). The first patients were treated for hematologic relapse. After the failure of treatment with interferon-α to induce cytogenetic remissions, donor lymphocytes were transfused. Complete cytogenetic remissions and negativity for BCR/ABL in RT-PCR developed several weeks to months after the lymphocyte transfusions. Side effects included mild GVHD in one patient (which responded to immunosuppressive treatment) and opsomyoclonic changes indicative of vasculitis (responsive to corticosteroids) in a second patient. Side effects were not observed in the third patient

(Kolb *et al.*, 1990). These patients remained in remission 13 and 14 years after lymphocyte transfusion. A patient with recurrent AML was treated with donor lymphocytes after failure of chemotherapy to induce remission. She developed moderately severe GVHD and a complete remission of the AML. Thirty-two months after the lymphocyte transfusion the patient died of a systemic relapse preceded by meningeal leukemia.

Response to donor lymphocyte transfusions— clinical data

Chronic myeloid leukemia

These preliminary results were confirmed in large studies performed by centers in Europe (Kolb *et al.*, 1995) and North America (Collins *et al.*, 1997; Porter *et al.*, 1999). Results obtained from EBMT centers demonstrated a response rate of 72% for patients with recurrent CML in hematologic relapse and 88% for patients in cytogenetic relapse (Table 65.1). Responses were complete clinical, cytogenetic, and, in most patients, molecular remissions, with the absence of BCR/ABL transcripts in an RT-PCR. Results were poor in patients with CML who relapsed into accelerated or blastic phase: only 22% of patients responded. In many patients the leukemia did not respond immediately (leukocytosis and thrombocytosis may even increase before a response occurs). Disappearance of Ph-positive metaphases and negativity for the BCR/ABL transcript may require several weeks or even months (Baurmann *et al.*, 1988; van Rhee & Goldman, 1996). The median time to PCR-negativity observed in one study was 4.5 months, with responses as late as 12 months.

In patients treated for cytogenetic or hematologic relapse the responses appear quite durable and the probability of survival at 5 years is 79% and 55%, respectively (Fig. 65.1). Dazzi and colleagues (2000) demonstrated that the probability of survival was much higher in those who entered molecular remission after DLI (Fig. 65.2). In the study reported by Collins *et al.* (1997), the actuarial probability of remaining in complete remission at 2 years was 89.6%. Second relapses have occurred, but remissions could be induced in many instances by repeated lymphocyte transfusions. In multivariate analysis, relapse in accelerated or blastic phase was unfavorable for a complete response. Patients with a monozygotic twin donor did not respond. The impact of chronic GVHD after allogeneic HSC transplantation on the response to donor lymphocytes is not clear; it was unfavorable in the European study and favorable in the North American study. Similar results to those obtained in these larger studies have been documented when CD4+ DLI have been utilized (by depletion of CD8+ cells) (Alyea *et al.*, 1998) (Table 65.2 and Fig. 65.3).

The value of BCR-ABL PCR in predicting relapse post-bone marrow transplantation (BMT) is controversial. However, there are data to suggest that qualitative PCR is predictive of relapse following T-cell-depleted BMT and that quantitative PCR is predictive following T-replete BMT (Cross *et al.*, 1993; Mackinnon *et al.*, 1996). A complete remission is even more likely if the DLI is administered when there is only evidence of molecular relapse (Dazzi *et al.*, 2000) (Table 65.3).

Table 65.1. *Graft-versus leukemia effect of donor lymphocyte transfusions: EBMT study follow-up (October 1997)*

Diagnosis	No. of patients studied	No. of patients evaluable[a]	Complete remission
CML			
Cytogenetic relapse (CP)	46	40	35 (88%)
Hematologic relapse (CP)	104	100	72 (72%)
Accelerated or blastic phase	33	27	6 (22%)
Polycythemia rubra vera/MPS	2	1	1
AML	64	42	12 (29%)
MDS	12	9	3 (33%)
ALL	43	22	1 (5%)
MM	18	11	4 (36%)

Abbreviations: EBMT, European Bone Marrow Transplant Registry; CML, chronic myeloid leukemia; CP, chronic phase; MPS, myeloproliferative syndrome; AML, acute myeloid leukemia; MDS, myelodysplasia; ALL, acute lymphoblastic leukemia; MM, multiple myeloma; NHL, non-Hodgkin's lymphoma.
[a] Patients in remission after chemotherapy and patients surviving less than 30 days after donor lymphocyte transfusions were excluded from analysis. 14 patients with recurrent CML were excluded because of unknown relapse phase; 7 patients with other diagnoses were also excluded: 2 NHL, 1 juvenile CML, and 4 unknown.

Number of cells transfused In the EBMT study (Kolb *et al.*, 1995) the role of the number of cells and concomitant treatment with interferon-α was studied retrospectively. There was no difference in response rate, nor in severity of GVHD, with cell numbers below and above the median of 3.0×10^8/kg mononuclear cells transfused. However, several groups have initially transfused very low numbers (1×10^5/kg) and subsequently increased the number, if neither a response nor GVHD was observed (Mackinnon *et al.*, 1995a and b) (Table 65.4). Responses were observed with the transfusion of 1×10^7/kg T cells. Many centers have started to transfuse escalating numbers of donor lymphocytes in patients with molecular or cytogenetic evidence of CML after transplantation, with favorable results (Bacigalupo *et al.*, 1997; Dazzi *et al.*, 2000) (Figs. 65.4 and 65.5). In a survey on 298 patients treated in EBMT centers a low initial dose of 2×10^7 mononuclear cells/kg or less had prognostic relevance for better survival and less treatment-related mortality than higher initial doses (Guglielmi *et al.*, 2002). In patients with unrelated or mismatched related (Pati *et al.*, 1995) donors, and in patients with alloimmune donors, the risk of GVHD is increased. In these patients a lower number of cells may be preferable. Similarly, very-low-dose donor lymphocyte infusions have been used successfully in a CML patient with extensive chronic GVHD (Rahman *et al.*, 1998).

Interferon-α and imatinib Interferon-α has been used in the treatment of recurrent CML without DLI. Its mechanism of action includes a direct antiproliferative effect on CML cells (Arcese *et al.*, 1990, 1993; Higano *et al.*, 1992) possibly by re-

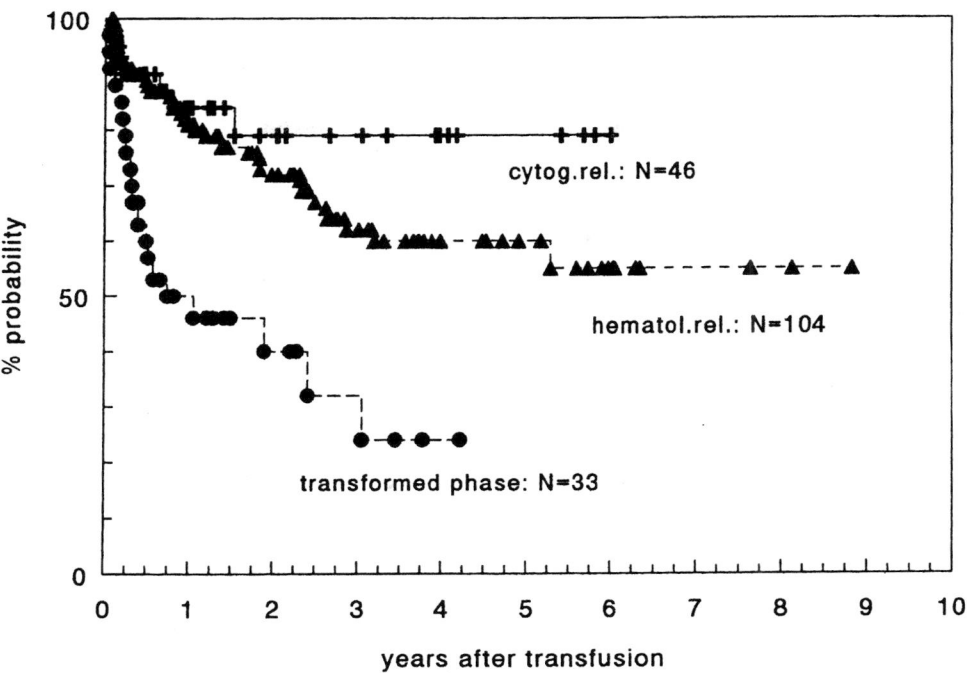

Fig. 65.1. Actuarial probability of survival of patients treated with transfusion of lymphocytes from the original marrow donor for recurrent chronic myeloid leukemia after allogeneic marrow transplantation. Data were collected from cooperative centers of the EBMT (evaluated October 1997).

establishing close contact with the supporting stroma (Dowding *et al.,* 1991), an immunomodulatory effect by up-regulating the expression of cell surface molecules, such as HLA-antigens, and the activation of immune effector cells (Baron *et al.,* 1991). Various schedules of interferon-α have been used. Doses ranged from 1 to 5×10^6 U/m² daily to 5×10^6 U/m² twice per week. Hematologic remissions were achieved in about 50%, and cytogenetic remissions in about 30%, of patients with relapse after allografting into the chronic phase of CML. In patients with cytogenetic relapse, complete cytogenetic remissions were achieved in up to 30%. In a retrospective analysis involving

multiple centers, interferon-α delayed progression of cytogenetic to hematologic relapse, but did not improve cytogenetic responses compared to untreated patients. It improved survival of patients with hematologic relapse in advanced phase (Arcese *et al.,* 1993). Observations in single centers are consistent with long-lasting remissions in some patients with cytogenetic relapses treated with interferon-α The role of interferon-α in the control of cytogenetic remission can be evaluated only by a prospective randomized trial. However, this would expose the patient to the risk of progression to clinical disease. The use of interferon-α in the treatment of relapse of AML and ALL is less well documented (Palva *et al.,* 1991), but may be supportive of immunotherapeutic approaches (Kolb *et al.,* 1995).

Interferon-α has been used in many patients as the primary method for treatment of CML relapse prior to the transfusion of donor lymphocytes, although some studies have electively combined the two approaches (Porter *et al.,* 1994). In the retrospective analysis interferon-α did not improve the response to donor lymphocyte transfusions (Kolb *et al.,* 1995). Again, this question cannot be answered adequately by such an analysis, since many patients were only treated with donor lymphocytes after interferon-α had failed. In some patients a response to donor lymphocytes was observed only after interferon-α had been added, while others only responded to the combination of donor lymphocytes with interferon-α and interleukin-2 (Lönnqvist *et al.,* 1996; Slavin *et al.,* 1996). Imatinib, at a dose of 400 to 600 mg per day, has been shown to re-induce hematological and cytogenetic remissions in patients with recurrent

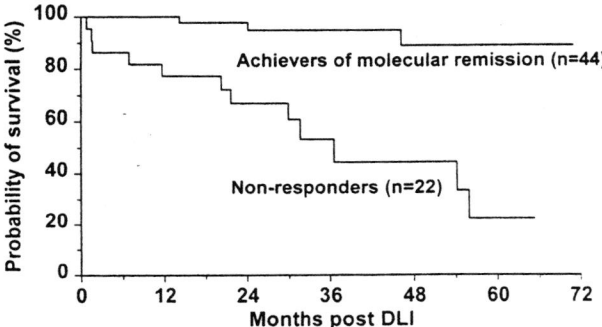

Fig. 65.2. Probability of survival for 44 patients who achieved molecular remission compared with survival for 22 patients who failed to achieve molecular remission dated from initiation of DLI. Reproduced, with permission, from Dazzi *et al.* (2000).

Table 65.2. *Characteristics of infused cells after ex-vivo CD8 depletion*

Dose level	N	Median no. of pheresis sessions/patient	CD3	CD4	CD8	CD56	CD20
1	28	1	3.5 (2.1–3.0)	3.0 (2.1–3.7)	<0.01 (0–0.2)	0.3 (0–0.9)	0.4 (0.1–0.7)
2	5	2	11.3 (8.1–13.1)	9.4 (7.9–10.3)	<0.01 (0–0.1)	1.0 (0.4–1.9)	0.9 (0.2–2.4)
3	7	2	13.2 (10.4–18.8)	13.2 (10.9–16.8)	<0.01 (0–0.1)	2.3 (1.4–6.4)	1.6 (0.7–2.7)

Values are the number of cells infused per patient $\times$ 10^7 cells/kg given as median (range in parentheses).
Reproduced, with permission, from Alyea *et al.* (1998).

CML following allogeneic transplantation (Soiffer *et al.,* 2001; Chambon-Pautas *et al.,* 2001). As follow-up is currently limited, it is unknown what the incidence of molecular remission will be or whether these responses will be durable.

Withdrawal of immune suppression

Single patients have been treated with DLI together with immunosuppressive treatment for prophylaxis of GVHD. Persistent remissions were not achieved in these patients. In contrast, successes have been reported by discontinuation of immunosuppressive therapy in some patients without DLI (Odom *et al.,* 1978; Higano *et al.,* 1990; Collins *et al.,* 1992). Discontinuation of the immunosuppressive therapy triggers development of GVHD in some patients, with an associated decline in leukemic cells. Without the development of GVHD the response may be only transient (personal observation). Abrupt discontinuation of cyclosporine may be indicated as a first step prior to DLI in patients who relapse posttransplant and who do not have severe GVHD.

Chimerism

The role of chimerism is crucial to the success of DLI. In CML most polymorphonuclear cells are part of the leukemia and are usually of host origin, while mononuclear cells may be of donor origin (Kolb *et al.,* 1990). As a rule T cells are not part of the leukemic clone, and T cells of host origin may be eliminated by donor lymphocytes together with the leukemia (Mackinnon *et al.,* 1995a). The presence of donor type hematopoiesis (Schattenberg *et al.,* 1996), in particular donor T cells (Schattenberg *et al.,* 1997) is of importance for the success of DLI. Presumably this reflects presence or absence of tolerance toward donor tissue.

Graft-versus-host disease

About 55% of patients treated by DLI for recurrent CML develop GVHD. It is mild (grade I) in 16%, moderately severe (grade II) in 25%, and severe (grade III and IV) in 14%. Response of CML to DLI correlates with the severity of GVHD (χ^2: P <.0001), but even 48% of patients without any sign of GVHD responded to the treatment (Kolb *et al.,* 1995).

GVHD after DLI differs in some respects from that seen after marrow transplantation, since inflammatory reactions exacerbated by the conditioning treatment are absent. Skin rashes are less pronounced and diarrhea may be absent. Liver abnormalities are frequent, and microangiopathic changes resembling thrombotic thrombocytic purpura (TTP) or hemolytic-uremic syndrome (HUS) may predominate. Presentation resembling acute hepatitis has been described (Akpek *et al.,* 2002).

Several attempts at preventing GVHD without losing the GVL effect have been explored. One report focused on the transfusion of small doses of cells, increasing the dose in a stepwise fashion until the disease responded or GVHD devel-

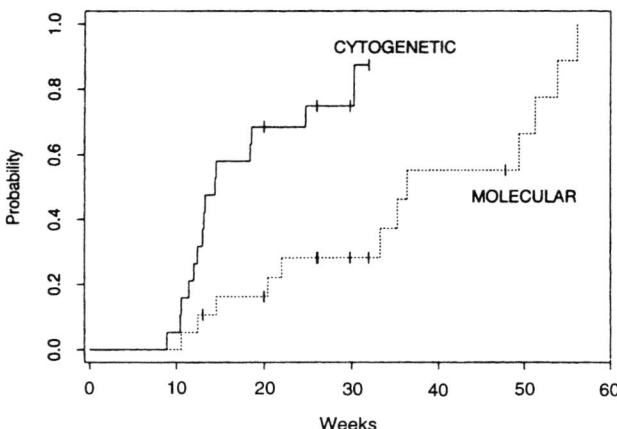

Fig. 65.3. Time to cytogenetic and molecular response. Reproduced, with permission, from Alyea *et al.* (1998).

Table 65.3. *Relationship between response to DLI, disease phase, and interval SCT relapse*

Relapse type	Interval SCT relapse	
	<9 months	>9 months
Molecular ($n = 8$)[a]	5/5 (100%)[b]	3/3 (100%)
Cytogenetic ($n = 19$)	3/5 (60%)	14/14 (100%)
Hematologic		
CP ($n = 30$)	5/11 (45%)	12/19 (73%)
AP ($n = 9$)	0/4 (0%)	2/5 (40%)

Abbreviations: DLI, donor lymphocyte infusion; SCT, stem cell transplantation; CP, chronic phase; AP, advanced phase.
[a] Total number of patients at each disease stage at DLI.
[b] Number of responder/number of patients (percentage).
Reproduced, with permission, from Dazzi *et al.* (2000).

Table 65.4. *Relationship between T-cell dose, leukemia remissions, and GVHD*

T-cell dose/kg	No. of patients treated with this cell dose	GVL effect	GVHD
1×10^5	10	0	0
5×10^5	10	0	0
1×10^6	9	0	0
5×10^6	8	0	0
1×10^7	21	8	1
5×10^7	14	4	3
$\geq 1 \times 10^8$	17	7	5

Reproduced, with permission, from MacKinnon *et al.* (1995a).

oped (Mackinnon *et al.,* 1995b). In some patients there appears to be a therapeutic window where a GVL reaction without GVHD occurs. Unfortunately, the GVL reaction may require several weeks or even months to effect elimination of the leukemic clone (van Rhee *et al.,* 1996). Discontinuing the cell dose increase may therefore be arbitrary unless GVHD occurs. Another approach used depletion of CD8+ T cells from the lymphocyte inoculum (Giralt *et al.,* 1995; Alyea *et al.,* 1998).

CD4+ T cells may exert a GVL effect without producing GVHD (Alyea *et al.,* 1996). A small randomized trial comparing prophylactic CD8-depleted DLI with unselected DLI after a T-cell-depleted marrow allograft described an incidence of acute GVHD of 67% in the unselected arm versus zero in the CD8-depleted arm, without an adverse effect on relapse or conversion to donor chimerism (Soiffer *et al.,* 2002). Regardless of the approach, patients treated with donor lymphocytes should be followed closely for the development of GVHD and treated as clinically indicated.

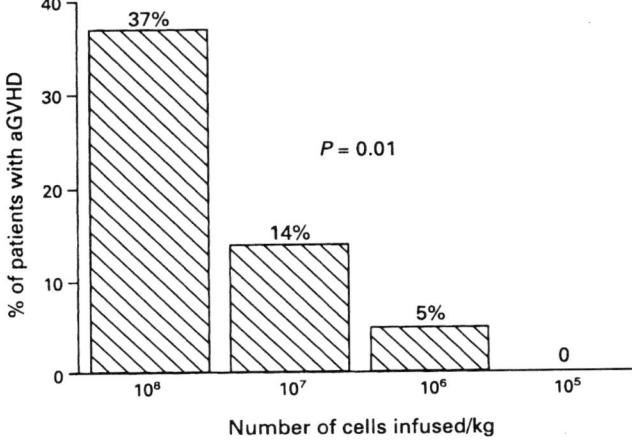

Fig. 65.4. Incidence of acute graft-versus-host disease (GVHD) grade II or more: it was recorded in 37% of infusions containing 1×10^8 cells/kg, 14% of the infusions with 2×10^7/kg cells, 5% with 2×10^6/kg cells, and none with 2×10^5/kg cells. The difference is statistically significant (*P* = .01). Reproduced, with permission, from Bacigalupo *et al.* (1997).

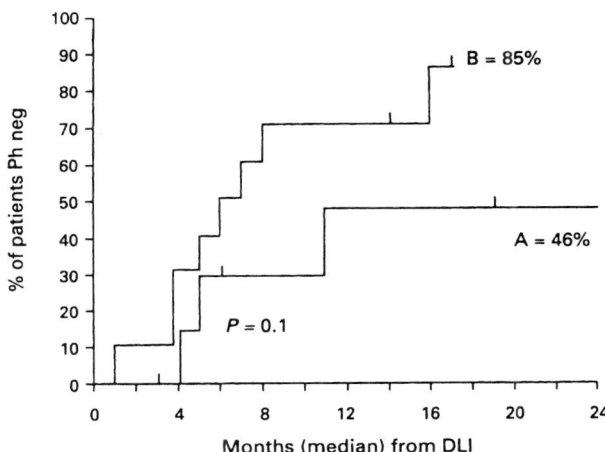

Fig. 65.5. Actuarial probability of becoming Ph-negative in eight patients receiving single high-dose DLI (group A) (46%) and in 10 patients receiving escalating doses of DLI (group B) (85%) (*P* = .1). Reproduced, with permission, from Bacigalupo *et al.* (1997).

Myelosuppression

A drop in blood counts resulting in white blood cell counts (WBC) less than 1.0×10^9/l, platelets less than 20×10^9/l, and reticulocytes less than 0.2% was observed in 40% of patients with hematologic relapse of chronic phase (CML). It was rare in patients with cytogenetic relapse only. In most cases, transfusion of donor stem cells (either marrow or blood) led to the recovery of hematopoiesis. In some patients with severe chronic GVHD, hematopoiesis did not recover despite infusion of stem cells. The mechanism of myelosuppression after DLI is probably similar to that associated with transfusion-induced GVHD (Anderson & Weinstein, 1990). It is thought that transfused T cells recognize hematopoietic cells of the recipient and eliminate them. It does not seem to occur when the hematopoietic cell is predominantly of donor origin (Keil *et al.,* 1997).

Prevention of myelosuppression secondary to DLI has been attempted by transfusing peripheral blood stem cells with the lymphocytes (Flowers *et al.,* 2000). Myelosuppression may best be prevented by earlier transfusion of donor lymphocytes before the malignant CML cells dominate hematopoiesis.

Diseases other than CML

Responses have been observed in a minority of patients with AML and myelodysplastic syndrome (MDS), and more rarely in patients with ALL (Table 65.1; Porter *et al.,* 1996; Levine *et al.,* 2002). The number of patients treated for recurrent or persistent myeloma is small, but responses occur (Tricot *et al.,* 1996; Verdonck *et al.,* 1996; Lokhorst *et al.,* 1997; Salama *et al.,* 2000). (Fig. 65.6), although generally a T-cell dose of 100 million/kg is required, in contrast to CML in chronic phase for which a dose of 10 million/kg is usually sufficient (Verdonck *et al.,* 1998). In one case DLI was given after the donor had been immunized with an immunogenic preparation of the recipient's monoclonal protein (Cabrera *et al.,* 2000). Analysis of the T-

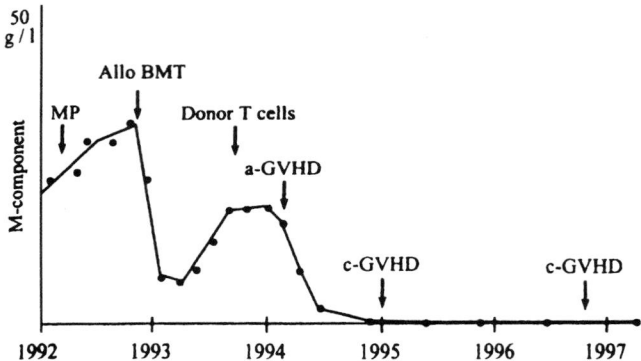

Fig. 65.6. Durable GVM effect as shown by response of serum M-protein to infusion of donor T cells in a patient with relapsed myeloma after allogeneic BMT. MP, melphalan and prednisone chemotherapy. Reproduced, with permission, from Lokhorst *et al.* (1997).

cell-receptor repertoire by PCR amplification of 24 Vβ gene subfamilies and analysis of CDR3 regions for each TCR Vβ gene subfamily revealed the appearance of clonal T-cell populations after DLI in each of three myeloma patients responding to DLI (Orsini *et al.*, 2000). The appearance of some clones coincided with an ongoing graft-versus-myeloma (GVM) response, while the appearance of others coincided with the development of GVHD. Other studies have shown increased restriction of the T-cell repertoire after DLI (Verfluerth *et al.*, 2000). A few patients with recurrent polycythemia vera or myeloproliferative syndrome have also responded to this form of adoptive immunotherapy and there are case reports of responses in patients allografted for chronic idiopathic myelofibrosis (Byrne *et al.*, 2000; Cervantes *et al.*, 2000).

A graft-versus-tumor effect has been described in patients receiving allografts for breast cancer (Eibl *et al.*, 1996; Ueno *et al.*, 1998), ovarian cancer (Bay *et al.*, 2000), renal cell carcinoma (Childs *et al.*, 1999, 2000) and non-small-cell lung cancer (Moscardo *et al.*, 2000) (see Chapters 42 and 120).

Additionally, in recipients of ABO-mismatched allografts, a more rapid disappearance of isohemagglutinins was noted after HLA-matched related transplants than after HLA-matched unrelated transplants and in those with GVHD compared to those without GVHD, suggesting a graft-versus-normal plasma cell effect (Mielcarek *et al.*, 2000) (Fig. 65.7).

Responses have not been as durable in patients with recurrent acute leukemia, but some patients with recurrent AML have survived more than 2 years (Fig. 65.8). The time to achieve complete remission appears shorter in AML compared to CML (Fig. 65.9). In patients with acute leukemia treatment frequently included chemotherapy. Four groups of patients could be defined: patients treated by DLI alone, patients treated by chemotherapy and DLI at the same time, patients treated with DLI in remission after chemotherapy, and patients treated with lymphocyte transfusions after chemotherapy had failed (Tables 65.5 and 65.6). Recurrent AML did respond to DLI without prior chemotherapy or after chemotherapy had failed (Table 65.5).

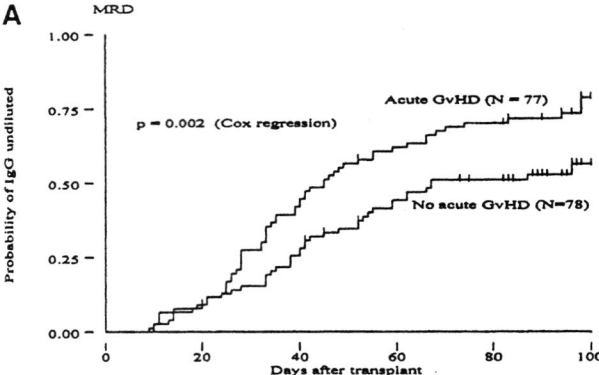

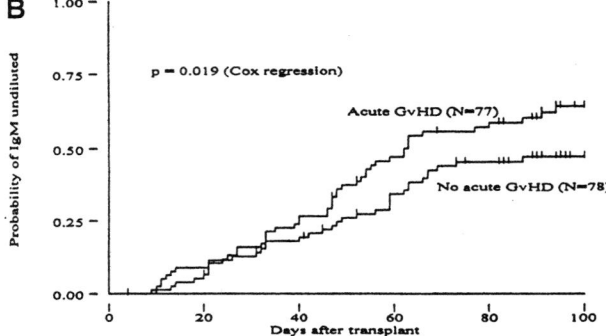

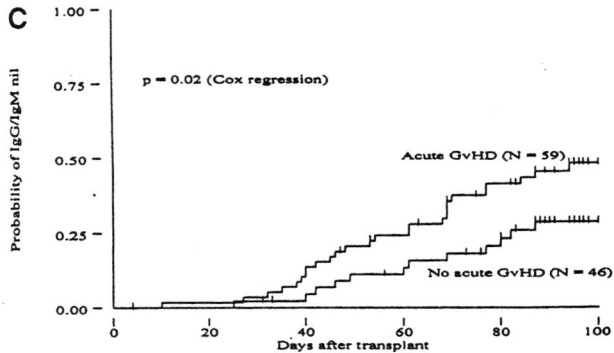

Fig. 65.7. Cumulative incidence curves showing probability of reaching different hemagglutinin titer endpoints during 100 days after transplant in recipients of marrow from HLA-matched related donors (MRD) in patients with or without acute GVHD. (**A**, "IgG-undiluted"), days after transplant when IgG-hemagglutinins were only detectable in undiluted serum; (**B**, "IgM-undiluted"), days after transplant when IgM-hemagglutinins were only detectable in undiluted serum; (**C**, "IgG/IgM-nil"), days after transplant when IgG plus IgM-hemagglutinins were undetectable. Reproduced, with permission, from Mielcarek *et al.* (2000).

Only two patients with relapses of ALL responded to lymphocyte transfusions without prior chemotherapy (Table 65.6).

In a North American registry study of 44 patients with recurrent ALL posttransplant, 2 of 15 patients received no chemotherapy pre-DLI and obtained a complete remission lasting >764 and 1,112 days, respectively (Collins *et al.*, 2000). Four patients received DLI as consolidation of remission induced by chemotherapy or withdrawal of immune sup-

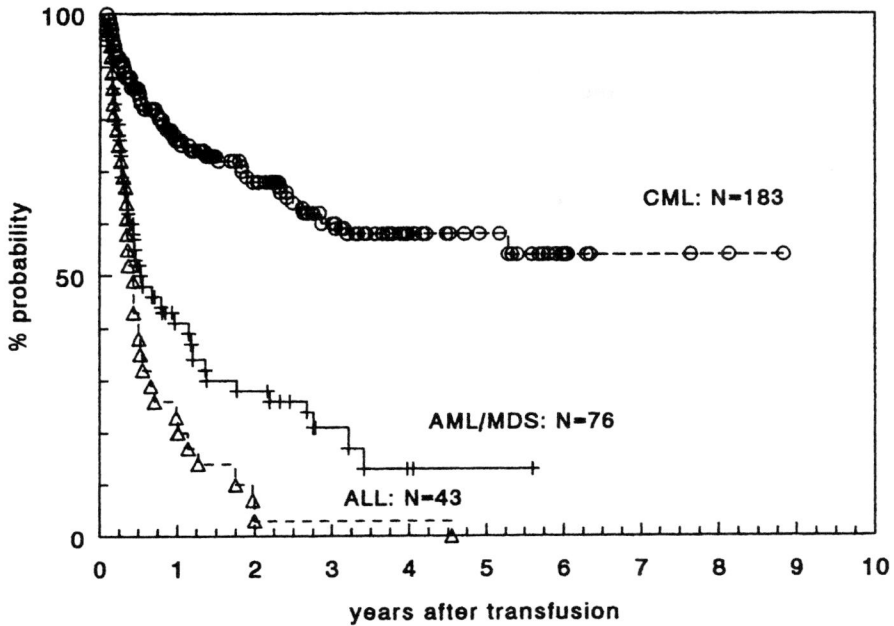

Fig. 65.8. Actuarial probability of survival of patients treated with transfusion of lymphocytes from the original marrow donor for recurrent chronic myeloid leukemia, acute myeloid leukemia, or acute lymphoblastic leukemia after allogeneic marrow transplantation. Data were collected from cooperative centers of the EBMT (evaluated October 1997).

pression: their remissions lasted 65 to >672 days. Twenty-five patients received DLI during the nadir after chemotherapy: 5 had remissions lasting 42 to 193 days. The actuarial survival rate of the whole group at 3 years was 13% (Fig. 65.10).

Chemotherapy and radiotherapy prior to donor lymphocyte transfusions

The pace of the disease recurrence may mandate the treatment regimen used (Barrett *et al.*, 1985). Most patients with acute

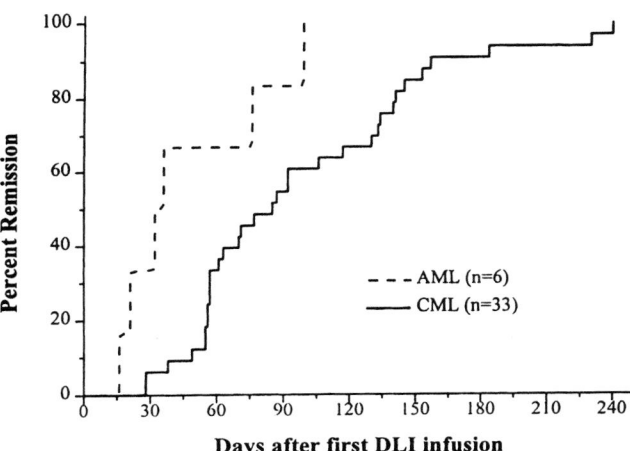

Fig. 65.9. Time to complete remission in AML and CML patients treated with DLI. Reproduced, with permission, from Collins *et al.* (1997).

Table 65.5. *Graft-versus-leukemia effect of donor lymphocyte transfusions: EBMT study follow-up (October 1997). Results in acute myeloid leukemia*

Treatment	No. of patients studied	No. of patients evaluable	Complete remission	Remission duration (days)
No chemo–DLT	32	26	5	301, 436, 1007+, 1014+, 2,045+
Chemo + DLT	9	6	2	96, 237
Chemo–CR–DLT	10	8	8	59, 68, 159+, 312+, 324, 791+, 849+, 897+, 1015+, 1245
Chemo–No CR–DLT	9	7	3	800, 977, 1018+

Abbreviations: EBMT, European Bone Marrow Transplant Registry; CR, complete remission; chemo, conventional dose cytotoxic chemotherapy; DLT, donor lymphocyte transfusion. + indicates remission at the time reported; the treatment groups received either DLT only, or chemotherapy and DLT at the same time, or chemotherapy with DLT given after achieving complete remission (CR), or DLT after failure of CR induction by chemotherapy. Patients were evaluable if they were in CR or had survived at least 30 days after DLT.

Table 65.6. *Graft-versus-leukemia effect of donor lymphocyte transfusions: EBMT study follow-up (October 1997). Results in acute lymphoblastic leukemia*

Treatment	No. of patients studied	No. of patients evaluable	Complete remission	Remission duration (days)
No chemo–DLT	12	10	1	417+
Chemo + DLT	10	8	1	442
Chemo–CR–DLT	14	14	12	21, 32, 47+, 71, 122+, 158+, 164, 185+, 200, 255, 370+, 539
Chemo–No CR–DLT	6	4	0	

Abbreviations: EBMT, European Bone Marrow Transplant Registry; CR, complete remission; chemo, conventional dose chemotherapy; DLT, donor lymphocyte transfusion.
+ indicates remission at the time reported; the treatment groups received either DLT only, or chemotherapy and DLT at the same time, or chemotherapy with DLT given after achieving complete remission (CR), or DLT after failure of CR induction by chemotherapy. Patients were evaluable if they were in CR or had survived at least 30 days after DLT.

leukemia or transformed CML recurring after marrow transplantation need cytotoxic chemotherapy. In a retrospective analysis of 76 patients with ALL and 41 patients with AML, remissions were induced by conventional chemotherapy in approximately 40% of treated patients (Frassoni *et al.*, 1988). The median survival of responders was 8 months for AML and 14 months for ALL, and only four patients remained in remission longer than 2 years. Even without transfusion of donor cells, hematopoietic recovery was derived exclusively from the graft.

In patients with slow tempo disease and smoldering forms of AML, low-dose cytosine arabinoside may be the treatment of

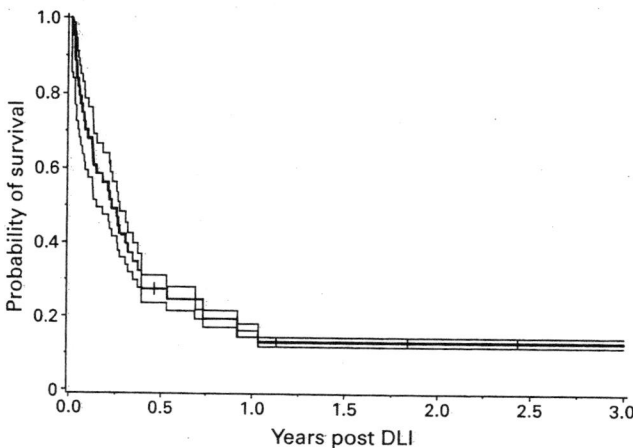

Fig. 65.10. Actuarial survival with 95% confidence intervals in 44 ALL patients treated with DLI. Reproduced, with permission, from Collins *et al.* (2000).

choice (Mittermüeller *et al.*, 1986, 1990; Trenschel *et al.*, 1997). Stable phase disease may be achieved for prolonged periods of time, and chemotherapy may be combined with adoptive immunotherapy.

Radiotherapy is the treatment of choice for isolated extramedullary relapses. These can involve any site in the body (Bekassy *et al.*, 1996) and may occur at either single or multiple sites. Radiation treatment is indicated in patients with large tumor masses prior to the transfusion of donor lymphocytes. Leukemic recurrences in the CNS or testes should be treated with radiation to the involved site and systemic chemotherapy (Charak *et al.*, 1983; Bowman *et al.*, 1984) prior to adoptive immunotherapy.

Ballen and colleagues (2002) used TBI 100 cGy followed by allogeneic lymphocyte infusion in patients with refractory cancer. Non-mobilized apheresed peripheral blood cells from family member donors or unrelated cord blood cells were used. Nine of 11 patients with hematologic malignancy demonstrated donor chimerism ranging from 5% to 100%, and 4 demonstrated sustained disease remission.

Hematopoietic growth factors and other cytokines

In a single case report, host-origin granulocytes appeared at the time of recurrence of AML posttransplant, indicating differentiation of leukemic blast cells (Mittermüeller *et al.*, 1986). Treatment with granulocyte colony-stimulating factor (G-CSF) induced complete remissions for a prolonged period of time in three of seven patients with leukemic relapse (Giralt *et al.*, 1993). Differentiation of the patient's blast cells was not observed, but hematologic recovery with donor cells occurred. Follow-up reports on this form of treatment have been less enthusiastic (Giralt & Champlin, 1994). G-CSF has been found to polarize T cells from Th1 toward Th2 type cytokine production and to reduce the severity of GVHD in mice (Pan *et al.*, 1995). Granulocyte-macrophage colony-stimulating factor (GM-CSF) stimulates proliferation and differentiation of myelopoiesis (Metcalf, 1979). Its immunomodulatory properties have also been of interest (Widmer-Pack *et al.*, 1987). GM-CSF has not been studied systematically for the treatment of relapse; experience in single patients has not been promising (unpublished data).

The use of interferon-α in the treatment of AML and ALL is less well documented than in CML (Palva *et al.*, 1991), but it may support immunotherapeutic approaches (Kolb *et al.*, 1995). Interleukin-2 (IL-2) has been used more commonly in the treatment of acute leukemia (Lotzova *et al.*, 1987; Verdonck *et al.*, 1991; Soiffer *et al.*, 1992; Charak *et al.*, 1993; Slavin *et al.*, 1996). It enhances antileukemic activity of natural killer (NK) cells and cytotoxic T cells (Charak *et al.*, 1992). In most studies, it has been used for the prevention of leukemic relapse (Blaise *et al.*, 1990; Fefer *et al.*, 1995). Activity of IL-2 as a single agent has been reported in a few patients only (Foa *et al.*, 1991; Verdonck *et al.*, 1991; Giralt *et al.*, 1994). Its efficacy may be greater in conjunction with adoptive immunotherapy (Lönnqvist *et al.*, 1996; Slavin *et al.*, 1996). Larger studies for the treatment of leukemic relapse after allogeneic transplantation are required before its utility can be defined.

Peripheral blood stem cells and marrow infusion after chemotherapy

In many patients with acute leukemia and transformed CML the pace of the disease is so rapid that a GVL reaction cannot evolve in time to be therapeutically useful. In such patients chemotherapy is required to control leukemic proliferation. It should not be immunosuppressive or myeloablative, because hematopoietic recovery of donor type is desired. Chemotherapy-induced remissions may allow time for a GVL reaction to develop.

Another potential defect of acute leukemia and transformed CML is inadequate presentation of antigen and co-stimulatory molecules. Only a small percentage of AML cells express the co-stimulatory molecule B7.1 (CD80). Dendritic cells of donor origin could present antigen from leukemic blast cells and activate donor T cells (Huang et al., 1994). Large numbers of dendritic cells may be produced by the exposure of stem cells to IL-4, GM-CSF (Romani et al., 1994), and Flt-3 ligand (Siena et al., 1995). Preliminary results of the transfusion of peripheral blood cells containing mobilized stem cells and treatment with GM-CSF are promising (Kolb et al., 1997b). Treatment with GM-CSF may be sufficient for the production of dendritic cells from stem cells in vivo. The combination of T cells and antigen-presenting cells may be preferable to lymphocytes for the treatment of acute leukemia and CML in transformation.

Reduced intensity conditioning regimens and allogeneic HSC transplantation

This approach to minimizing regimen-related toxicity and relying on a donor T cell-mediated graft-versus-leukemia effect to effect cure is being increasingly explored. Donor lymphocyte infusions posttransplant, either to promote conversion to full donor chimerism or to prevent or treat relapse of the underlying malignancy, has been an integral component of the approach in some protocols (Marks et al., 2002) (see Chapter 22).

Cause of death

Three hundred forty-three patients were reported in the EBMT study, and 166 patients died. In 9 patients the cause of death was not evaluated and 13 patients died early after treatment. One hundred seventeen patients died of leukemia and 27 patients died of causes other than leukemia. Major complications of lymphocyte transfusions were GVHD, myelosuppression, and infections.

Mechanism of the GVL reaction

The mechanism of the GVL reaction is unknown; T cells and NK cells may contribute to the effect (Jiang et al., 1993). Obviously an alloimmune reaction is involved, since syngeneic

DLI failed to induce remissions (Bunjes et al., 1996), and the response was excellent in patients with matched unrelated donors. GVL effects were also observed in patients with HLA-mismatched donors. Since the patient was HLA-identical with the donor in most cases, minor histocompatibility antigens might be involved in the reaction. However, the GVL reaction may be separable from a GVH reaction, because about 40% of patients without any clinical signs of GVHD, and 76% of patients with mild GVHD, demonstrate a GVL reaction. A GVL reaction directed against potential leukemia-specific antigens may exist. Cytotoxic T cells have been produced against the BCR-ABL fusion peptide (Bocchia et al., 1996; Mannering et al., 1996), but their potential clinical role has not yet been elucidated.

The spectrum of activity of the transfusion-induced GVL reaction is consistent with a role for dendritic cells produced by the leukemia. In CML, and sometimes in AML, differentiation toward mature dendritic cells can occur. These cells are well able to stimulate and sustain a reaction against the leukemia. It can be speculated that lymphoblastic leukemia and lymphomas cannot generate dendritic cells as part of the malignant clone. The role of CD4[+] T cells is supported by their demonstrated reactivity against HLA class II restricted developmental antigens shared by leukemic cells and hematopoietic progenitor cells (Mutis et al., 1997).

The future—prophylactic donor lymphocyte therapy

The possibility of treating leukemia relapse with lymphocytes from the marrow donor offers several new treatment choices in allogeneic HSC transplantation. First, induction of tolerance by depletion of T cells from the donor graft may be re-introduced into the treatment plan with less acute GVHD and associated complications.

Table 65.7. *Generation of 3 leukemia-reactive CTL lines*

	CTL line		
	1	2	3
No. of positive wells harvested	309	389	525
No. of T cells harvested	0.2×10^9	1.3×10^9	1.7×10^9
Phenotype of CTL line			
CD3	97%	97%	99%
CD4	92%	82%	86%
CD8	9%	18%	14%
TCR$\alpha\beta$	97%	96%	99%
TCR$\gamma\delta$	<1%	2%	<1%
Lysis[a] of CML-MNC	30	24	18
Lysis[a] of PHA-blast patient	0	0	0
Lysis[a] of BM stromal cells patient	8	NT	10
Lysis[a] of PHA-blast donor	3	0	1

Abbreviation: NT, not tested.
[a] Percentage specific lysis in a ^{51}Cr-release assay at a 10:1 effector: target ratio.
Reproduced, with permission, from Falkenburg et al. (1999).

Second, donor lymphocytes may be transfused prophylactically in patients at high risk for relapse earlier after transplantation before leukemic relapse occurs (Naparstek *et al.,* 1995;
Lee *et al.,* 1999; de Lima *et al.,* 2001). Experimental and clinical studies indicate that the longer the interval between transplant and T-cell add-back, the less is the risk of GVHD
(Johnson *et al.,* 1993; Johnson & Truitt, 1995; Lee *et al.,* 1999;
Naparstek *et al.,* 1995). A trial of 44 HLA-matched sibling
transplants for hematologic malignancies (Barrett *et al.,* 1998)
demonstrated that large T-cell doses of up to 5×10^7 CD3+
cells/kg could be added back safely 45 days after a T-cell-
depleted transplant in conjunction with cyclosporine prophylaxis. Doses of 1×10^7 CD3+ cells given earlier posttransplant

(for example, at day 30) can cause severe GVHD (de Lima *et
al.,* 2001). Another way to minimize the risk of GVHD is to
purge the DLI of alloreactive T cells. An initial attempt at this
(by purging the infusions of CD8+ cells) resulted in increased
numbers of CD20+ B cells, a more rapid improvement in TCR
V beta repertoire, and increased numbers of TRECs in CD3+ T
cells, as well as conversion to complete donor hematopoiesis
(Bellucci *et al.,* 2002).

Third, donor lymphocytes may be immunized ex vivo by co-
cultivation with dendritic cells presenting a leukemia-specific
antigen (Bocchia *et al.,* 1996; Mannering *et al.,* 1996; Osman
et al., 1999; Pawelec *et al.,* 1997). Another possibility is immunization against minor histocompatibility antigens (mHags)

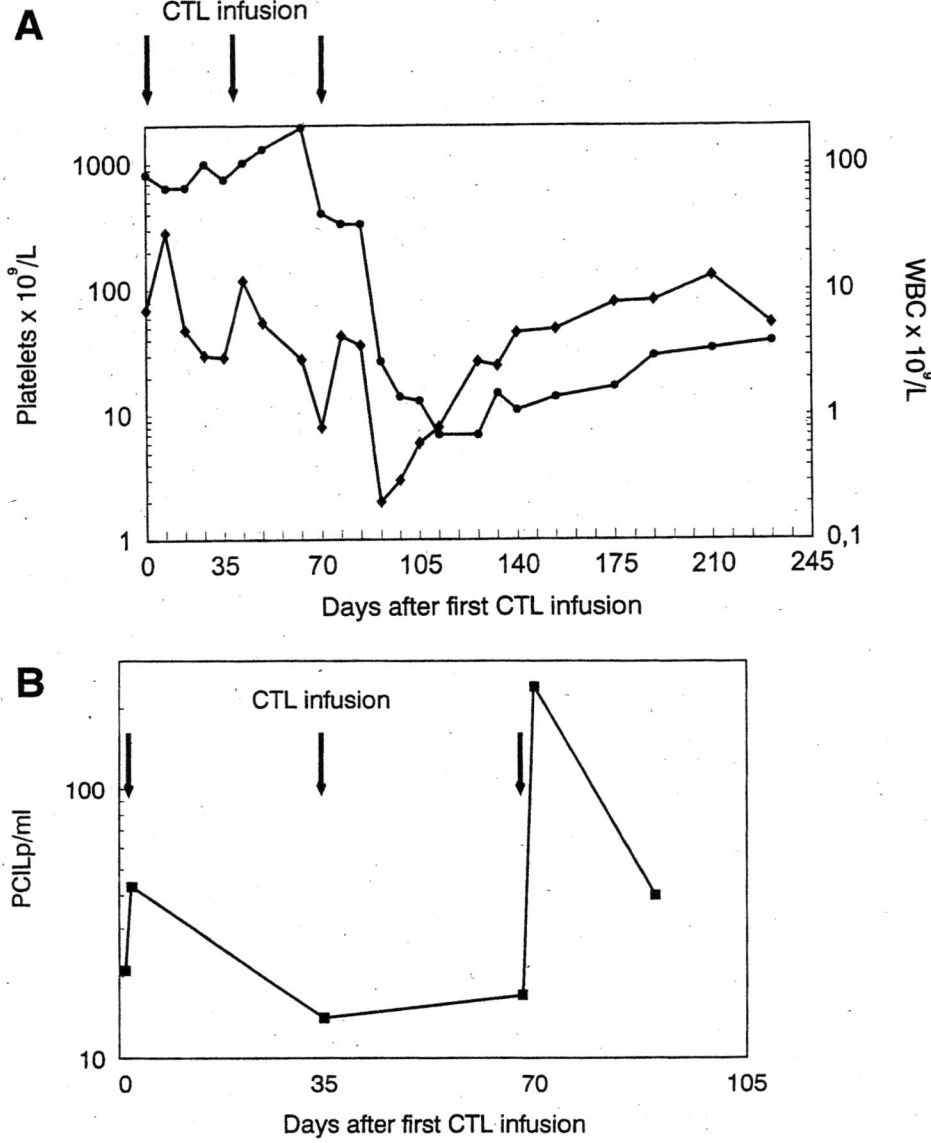

Fig. 65.11. Platelets, white blood cells (WBC), and PCIL_p before and after treatment with leukemia-reactive CTL lines 1, 2, and 3. **(A)** Between days 80 and
90, 10 to 20 days after the infusion of CTL line 3, a rapid decrease of (●) platelets and (◆) WBC was observed, followed by a gradual recovery. **(B)** A strong
increase in PCIL_p frequencies in PBL from the patient was observed between days 70 and 90. Reproduced, with permission, from Falkenburg *et al.* (1999).

preferentially expressed on host hematopoietic cells (Voogt *et al.*, 1988). Indeed, Falkenburg and colleagues (1999) have shown that donor CTL lines generated in vitro by a modification of limiting dilution technology can lyse leukemia cells from the patient and inhibit the growth of leukemic progenitor cells. These CTL did not react with lymphocytes from donor or recipient and did not affect donor hematopoietic progenitor cells. Infusion of a total dose of 3.2×10^9 CTL resulted in complete eradication of the accelerated phase of CML (Table 65.7, Fig. 65.11). The antigen specificity of these CTL is unknown, but it is possible that the majority were directed against mHags with at least a partially restricted tissue distribution. Lineage-specific antigens, such as proteinase-3, have been shown to be targets for leukemia-specific CTL (Molldrem *et al.*, 1997), as has the Wilm's tumor gene-encoded transcription factor WT1 (Gao *et al.*, 2000; Ohminami *et al.*, 2000). In a murine model of haploidentical transplantation, selection of leukemia-reactive Vβ+ T cells provided significant GVL responses with concomitant minimization of GVHD (Patterson & Korngold, 2001). Finally, immunized T cells can be transfected with a suicide gene that allows their selective and elective eradication as soon as they attack normal organs in the patient (Bonini *et al.*, 1997). T cells may be used in this setting for the treatment of viral diseases as well as relapse (Rooney *et al.*, 1995), and their use is being explored as primary therapy in patients with malignancy who have not undergone a prior allogeneic transplant (Porter *et al.*, 1999). These new developments give hope for patients with otherwise refractory disease.

References

Akpek, G., Boitnott, J. K., Lee, L. A. *et al.* (2002). Hepatic variant or graft-versus-host disease after donor lymphocyte infusion. *Blood*, **100**, 3903–7.

Alyea, E.P., Canning, C., Collins, H. *et al.* (1996). Efficacy and toxicity of CD4 positive donor T-lymphocyte transfusion for treatment of relapsed chronic myelogenous leukemia (CML) after allogeneic BMT. *Blood*, **88** (Suppl 1), 682a (Abstract).

Alyea, E.P., Soiffer, R.J., Canning, C. *et al.* (1998). Toxicity and efficacy of defined doses of CD4+ donor lymphocytes for treatment of relapse after allogeneic bone marrow transplant. *Blood*, **91**, 3671–80.

Anderson, K.C. & Weinstein, H.J. (1990). Transfusion-associated graft-versus-host disease. *New England Journal of Medicine*, **323**, 315.

Arcese, W., Goldman, J.M., Darcangelo, E. *et al.* (1993). Outcome for patients who relapse after allogeneic bone marrow transplantation for chronic myeloid leukemia. *Blood*, **82**, 3211–19.

Arcese, W., Mauro, F.R., Alimena, G. *et al.* (1990). Interferon therapy for Ph1-positive CML patients relapsing after T cell depleted allogeneic bone marrow transplantation. *Bone Marrow Transplantation*, **5**, 309–15.

Bacigalupo, A., Soracco, M., & Vassallo, F. (1997). Donor lymphocyte infusions (DLI) in patients with chronic myeloid leukemia following allogeneic bone marrow transplantation. *Bone Marrow Transplantation*, **19**, 927–32.

Ballen, K. K., Becker, P. S., Emmons, R.V.B. *et al.* (2002). Low-dose total body irradiation followed by allogeneic lymphocyte infusion may induce remission in patients with refractory hematologic malignancy. *Blood*, 442–50.

Barnes, D.H.W. & Loutit, J.F. (1957). Treatment of murine leukemia with X-rays and homologous bone marrow. *British Journal of Haematology*, **3**, 241–52.

Baron, S., Tyring, S.K., Fleischmann, W.R. *et al.* (1991). The interferons—mechanism of action and clinical applications. *Journal of the American Medical Association*, **266**, 1375–83.

Barrett, A.J., Horowitz, M.M., Gale, R.P. *et al.* (1989). Bone marrow transplantation for acute lymphoblastic leukemia: factors influencing relapse and survival. *Blood*, **74**, 862–71.

Barrett, A.J., Joshi, R., & Tew, C. (1985). How should acute lymphoblastic leukemia relapsing after bone marrow transplantation be treated? *Lancet*, **1**, 1188–91.

Barrett, A.J., Horowitz, M.M., Gale, R.P. *et al.* (1992). Bone marrow transplantation for Philadelphia-chromosome positive acute lymphoblastic leukemia. *Blood*, **79**, 3067–70.

Barrett, A.J., Mavroudis, D., Tisdale, J. *et al.* (1998). T-cell depleted bone marrow transplantation followed by delayed T-cell add-back to prevent severe acute GVHD. *Bone Marrow Transplantation*, **21**, 543–51.

Baurmann, H., Nagel, S., Binder, T. *et al.* (1998). Kinetics of graft-versus-leukemia response after donor leukocyte infusions for relapsed chronic myeloid leukemia after allogeneic bone marrow transplantation. *Blood*, **92**, 3582–90.

Bay, J.O., Choufi, C., Pomel, C. *et al.* (2000). Potential allogeneic graft-versus-tumor effect in a patient with ovarian cancer. *Bone Marrow Transplantation*, **25**, 681–2.

Bekassy, A.N., Hermans, J., Gorin, N.C. *et al.* (1996). Granulocytic sarcoma after allogeneic bone marrow transplantation: a retrospective European multicenter survey. *Bone Marrow Transplantation*, **17**, 801–8.

Bellucci, R., Alyea, E. P., Weller, E. *et al.* (2002). Immunologic effects of prophylactic donor lymphocyte infusion after allogeneic marrow transplantation for multiple myeloma. *Blood*, **99**, 4610–7.

Blaise, D., Maraninchi, D., Archimbaud, E. *et al.* (1992). Allogeneic bone marrow transplantation for acute myeloid leukemia in first remission: a randomized trial of busulfan-cytoxan versus cytoxan-total body irradiation as preparative regimen: a report of the Group d'Etudes de la Greffe de Moelle Osseuse. *Blood*, **79**, 2578–82.

Blaise, D., Olive, D., Stoppa, A. *et al.* (1990). Hematologic and immunologic effects of the systemic administration of recombinant interleukin-2 after autologous bone marrow transplantation for hematological malignancies. *Blood*, **76**, 1092–7.

Blume, K.G., Kopecky, K.J., Henslee-Downey, P.J. *et al.* (1993). A prospective comparison of total body irradiation-etoposide versus busulfan-cyclophosphamide as preparatory regimens for bone marrow transplantation in patients with leukemia who were not in first remission: a Southwest Oncology Group Study. *Blood*, **81**, 2187–93.

Bocchia, M., Korontsvit, T., Xu, Q. *et al.* (1996). Specific human cellular immunity to BCR-ABL oncogene-derived peptides. *Blood*, **87**, 3587–92.

Bonini, C., Ferrari, G., Verzelletti, S. *et al.* (1997). HSV-TK gene transfer into donor lymphocytes for control of allogeneic graft-versus leukemia. *Science,* **276,** 1719–24.

Bowman, W.P., Aur, R.J., Hustu, H.O. *et al.* (1984). Isolated testicular relapse in acute lymphocytic leukemia of childhood: categories and influence on survival. *Journal of Clinical Oncology,* **2,** 924–9.

Buckner, C.D., Clift, R.A., Appelbaum, F. *et al.* (1992). A randomized study comparing two transplant regimens for CML in chronic phase. *Blood,* **80,** 72a (Abstract).

Bunjes, D., Hertenstein, B., Wiesneth, M. *et al.* (1996). Donor lymphocyte transfusions and low-dose interleukin-2 in 2 patients with relapsed CML after syngeneic BMT. *Bone Marrow Transplantation,* **17,** (Suppl 1), S9.

Byrne, J.L., Beshti, H., Clark, D. *et al.* (2000). Induction of remission after donor leukocyte infusion for the treatment of relapsed chronic idiopathic myelofibrosis following allogeneic transplantation: evidence for a "graft vs. myelofibrosis" effect. *British Journal of Haematology,* **108,** 430–3.

Cabrera, R., Diaz-Espada, F.R., Barrios, Y. *et al.* (2000). Infusion of lymphocytes obtained from a donor immunized with the paraprotein idiotype as a treatment in a relapsed myeloma. *Bone Marrow Transplantation,* **25,** 1105–8.

Cervantes, F., Rovira, M., Urbano-Ispizua, A. *et al.* (2000). Complete remission of idiopathic myelofibrosis following donor lymphocyte infusion after failure of allogeneic transplantation: demonstration of a graft-versus-myelofibrosis effect. *Bone Marrow Transplantation,* **26,** 697–9.

Chak, L., Sapozink, M., & Cox, R. (1983). Extramedullary lesions in non-lymphocytic leukemia: results of radiation therapy. *International Journal of Radiation Oncology, Biology, Physics,* **9,** 1173–6.

Chambon-Pautas, C., Cony-Makhoul, P., Giraudier, S. *et al.* (2001). Glivec (STI571) treatment for chronic myelogenous leukemia (CML) in relapse after allogeneic stem cell transplantation (SCT): a report on the French experience. *Blood,* **98,** (Abstract).

Charak, B.S., Brynes, R.K., Chogyoji, M. *et al.* (1993). Graft versus leukemia effect after transplantation with interleukin-2-activated bone marrow. Correlation with eradication of residual disease. *Transplantation,* **56,** 31–7.

Charak, B.S., Choudary, G., Tefft, M. *et al.* (1992). Interleukin-2 in bone marrow transplantation: preclinical studies. *Bone Marrow Transplantation,* **10,** 103–11.

Childs, R., Chernoff, A., Contentin, A. *et al.* (2000). Regression of metastatic renal-cell carcinoma after nonmyeloablative allogeneic peripheral blood stem cell transplantation. *New England Journal of Medicine,* **343,** 750–8.

Childs, R.W., Clave, E., Tisdale, J. *et al.* (1999). Successful treatment of metastatic renal cell carcinoma with a nonmyeloablative allogeneic peripheral blood progenitor-cell transplant: evidence for a graft-versus-tumor effect. *Journal of Clinical Oncology,* **17,** 2044–9.

Collins, R.H., Goldstein, S., Giralt, S. *et al.* (2000). Donor leukocyte infusions in acute lymphocytic leukemia. *Bone Marrow Transplantation,* **26,** 511–6.

Collins, R.H., Shpilberg, O., Drobyski, W.R. *et al.* (1997). Donor leukocyte infusions in 140 patients with relapsed malignancy after allogeneic bone marrow transplantation. *Journal of Clinical Oncology,* **15,** 433–44.

Collins, R.H.J., Rogers, Z.R., Bennett, M. *et al.* (1992). Hematologic relapse of chronic myelogenous leukemia following allogeneic bone marrow transplantation: apparent graft-versus-leukemia effect following abrupt discontinuation of immunosuppression. *Bone Marrow Transplantation,* **10,** 391–5.

Cross, N.C.P., Feng, L., Chase, A. *et al.* (1993). Competitive polymerase chain reaction to estimate the number of BCR-ABL transcripts in chronic myeloid leukemia patients after bone marrow transplantation. *Blood,* **82,** 1929–36.

Dazzi, F., Szydlo, R.M., Craddock, C. *et al.* (2000a). Comparison of single-dose and escalating-dose regimens of donor lymphocyte infusion for relapse after allografting for chronic myeloid leukemia. *Blood,* **95,** 67–71.

Dazzi, F., Szydlo, R.M., Cross, N.C.P. *et al.* (2000b). Durability of responses following donor lymphocyte infusions for patients who relapse after allogeneic stem cell transplantation for chronic myeloid leukemia. *Blood,* **96,** 2712–6.

de Lima, M., Bonamino, M., Vasconcelos, Z. *et al.* (2001). Prophylactic donor lymphocyte infusions after moderately ablative chemotherapy and stem cell transplantation for hematological malignancies: high remission rate among poor prognosis patients at the expense of graft-versus-host disease. *Bone Marrow Transplantation,* **27,** 73–8.

Doney, K., Fisher, L., Appelbaum, F. *et al.* (1991). Treatment of adult acute lymphoblastic leukemia with allogeneic bone marrow transplantation. Multivariate analysis of factors affecting acute graft-versus-host disease, relapse and relapse-free survival. *Bone Marrow Transplantation,* **7,** 453–9.

Dowding, C., Guo, A.P., Osterholz, J. *et al.* (1991). Interferon-alpha overrides the deficient adhesion of chronic myeloid leukemia primitive progenitor cells to bone marrow stromal cells. *Blood,* **78,** 499–505.

Eibl, B., Schweighofer, H., Nachbaur, D. *et al.* (1996). Evidence for a graft-versus-tumor effect in a patient treated with marrow ablative chemotherapy and allogeneic bone marrow transplantation for breast cancer. *Blood,* 1501–8.

Elfenbein, G.J., Brogaonkar, D.S., Bias, W.B. *et al.* (1978). Cytogenetic evidence for recurrence of acute myelogeneous leukemia after allogeneic bone marrow transplantation in donor hematopoietic cells. *Blood,* **52,** 627–36.

Falkenburg, J.H.F., Wafelman, A.R., Joosten, P. *et al.* (1999). Complete remission of accelerated phase chronic myeloid leukemia by treatment with leukemia-reactive cytotoxic T lymphocytes. *Blood,* **94,** 1201–8.

Fefer, A., Benyunes, M.C., York, A. *et al.* (1995). Use of interleukin-2 after bone marrow transplantation. *Bone Marrow Transplantation,* **15** (Suppl 1), S162–6.

Fefer, A., Sullivan, K.M., Weiden, P.L. *et al.* (1987). Graft-versus-leukemia effect in man: the relapse rate of acute leukemia is lower after allogeneic than after syngeneic marrow transplantation. *Progress in Clinical and Biological Research,* **244,** 401–8.

Fialkow, P.J., Thomas, E.D., Bryant, J.I. *et al.* (1971). Leukemic transformation of engrafted human marrow cells in vivo. *Lancet,* **1,** 251–5.

Flowers, M.E.D., Leisenring, W., Beach, K. *et al.* (2000). Granulocyte colony-stimulating factor given to donors before apheresis does not prevent aplasia in patients treated with donor leukocyte infusion for recurrent chronic myeloid leukemia after bone marrow transplantation. *Biology of Blood and Marrow Transplantation*, **6**, 321–6.

Foa, R., Meloni, G., Tosti, S. *et al.* (1991). Treatment of acute myelogenous leukaemia patients with recombinant interleukin-2: a pilot study. *British Journal of Haematology*, **77**, 491–6.

Frassoni, F., Barrett, A.J., Granena, A. *et al.* (1988). Relapse after allogeneic bone marrow transplantation for acute leukaemia: a survey by the E.B.M.T. of 117 cases. *British Journal of Haematology*, **70**, 317–20.

Gale, R.P., Butturini, A., & Horowitz, M.M. (1995). HLA-identical sibling bone marrow transplants for acute lymphoblastic leukemia. *Bone Marrow Transplantation*, **15** (Suppl 1), S199–S202.

Gale, R.P., Horowitz, M.M., Ash, R. *et al.* (1994). Identical twin bone marrow transplantation for leukemia. *Annals of Internal Medicine*, **120**, 646–52.

Gale, R.P., Horowitz, M.M., Weiner, R.S. *et al.* (1995). Impact of cytogenetic abnormalities on outcome of bone marrow transplantation in acute myelogenous leukemia in first remission. *Bone Marrow Transplantation*, **16**, 203–8.

Gao, L., Bellantuono, I., Elsasser, A. *et al.* (2000). Selective elimination of leukemic CD34+ progenitor cells by cytotoxic T lymphocytes specific for WT1. *Blood*, **95**, 2198–203.

Giralt, S., Escudier, S., Kantarijan, H. *et al.* (1993). Preliminary results of treatment with filgastrim for relapse of leukemia and myelodysplasia after allogeneic bone marrow transplantation. *New England Journal of Medicine*, **329**, 757–61.

Giralt, S., Hester, J., Huh, Y. *et al.* (1995). CD8-depleted donor lymphocyte infusion as treatment for relapsed chronic myelogenous leukemia after allogeneic bone marrow transplantation. *Blood*, **86**, 4337–43.

Giralt, S.A. & Champlin, R.E. (1994). Leukemia relapse after allogeneic bone marrow transplantation: a review. *Blood*, **84**, 3603–12.

Goh, K. & Klemperer, M.R. (1977). In vivo leukemia transformation: cytogenetic evidence of in vivo leukemic transformation of engrafted marrow cells. *American Journal of Hematology*, **2**, 283–90.

Goldman, J.M., Apperley, J., Jones, L. *et al.* (1986). Bone marrow transplantation for patients with chronic myeloid leukemia. *New England Journal of Medicine*, **314**, 202–7.

Goldman, J.M., Gale, R.P., Horowitz, M.M. *et al.* (1988). Bone marrow transplantation for chronic myelogenous leukemia in chronic phase: increased risk of relapse associated with T cell depletion. *Annals of Internal Medicine*, **108**, 806–14.

Guglielmi, C. *et al.* (2002). Donor lymphocyte infusion for relapsed chronic myelogenous leukemia: prognostic relevance of the initial cell dose. *Blood*, **100**, 397–405.

Higano, C.S., Brixey, M., Bryant, E.M. *et al.* (1990). Durable complete remission of acute nonlymphocytic leukemia associated with discontinuation of immunosuppression following relapse after allogeneic bone marrow transplantation: a case report of a probable graft-versus-leukemia effect. *Transplantation*, **50**, 175–7.

Higano, C.S., Raskind, W.H., & Singer, J.W. (1992). Use of alpha interferon for the treatment of relapse of chronic myelogenous leukemia in chronic phase after allogeneic marrow transplantation. *Blood*, **80**, 1437–42.

Horowitz, M.M. (1995). New IBMTR/ABMTR slides summarize current use and outcome of allogeneic and autologous transplants. *IBMTR Newsletter*, **2**, 2–8.

Horowitz, M.M., Gale, R.P., Sondel, P.M. *et al.* (1990). Graft-versus-leukemia reactions after bone marrow transplantation. *Blood*, **75**, 555–62.

Huang, A.Y.C., Golumbek, P., Ahmadzadeh, M. *et al.* (1994). Role of bone marrow-derived cells presenting MHC class I-restricted tumor antigens. *Science*, **264**, 961–5.

Jiang, Y.Z., Cullis, J.O., Kanfer, E.J. *et al.* (1993). T cell and NK cell mediated graft-versus-leukaemia reactivity following donor buffy coat transfusion to treat relapse after marrow transplantation for chronic myeloid leukemia. *Bone Marrow Transplantation*, **11**, 133–8.

Johnson, B.D., Drobyski, W.R., & Truitt, R.L. (1993). Delayed infusion of normal donor cells after MHC-matched bone marrow transplantation provides an antileukemia reaction without graft-versus-host disease. *Bone Marrow Transplantation*, **11**, 329–36.

Johnson, B.D. & Truitt, R.L. (1995). Delayed infusion of immuno-competent donor cells after bone marrow transplantation breaks graft-host tolerance and allows for persistent antileukemic reactivity without severe graft-versus-host disease. *Blood*, **85**, 3302–12.

Keil, F., Haas, O.A., Fritsch, G. *et al.* (1997). Donor leukocyte infusion for leukemic relapse after allogeneic marrow transplantation: lack of residual donor hematopoiesis predicts aplasia. *Blood*, **89**, 3113–7.

Kernan, N.A., Bartsch, G., Ash, R.C. *et al.* (1993). Analysis of 462 transplantation from unrelated donors facilitated by the National Marrow Donor Program. *New England Journal of Medicine*, **328**, 593–602.

Kolb, H.J., Mittermueller, J., Clemm, C. *et al.* (1990). Donor leukocyte transfusions for treatment of recurrent chronic myelogenous leukemia in marrow transplant patients. *Blood*, **76**, 2462–5.

Kolb, H.J., Schattenberg, A., Goldman, J.M. *et al.* (1995). Graft-versus-leukemia effect of donor lymphocyte transfusions in marrow grafted patients. *Blood*, **86**, 2041–50.

Kolb, H.J., Günther, W., Schumm, M. *et al.* (1997a). Adoptive immunotherapy in canine chimeras. *Transplantation*, **63**, 1–7.

Kolb, H.J., Menzel, H., Holler, E. *et al.* (1997b). Donor cell transfusion for the treatment of recurrent leukemia after allogeneic bone marrow transplantation. *Blood*, **90**, 546a (Abstract).

Lapidot, T., Sirard, C., Vormoor, J. *et al.* (1994). A cell initiating human acute myeloid leukaemia after transplantation into SCID mice. *Nature*, **367**, 645–8.

Lee, C.-K., Gingrich, R.D., deMagalhaes-Silverman, M. *et al.* (1999). Prophylactic reinfusion of T cells for T cell-depleted allogeneic bone marrow transplantation. *Biology of Blood and Marrow Transplantation*, **5**, 15–27.

Levine, J.E., Braun, T., Penza, S.L. *et al.* (2002). Prospective trial of chemotherapy and donor leukocyte infusions for relapse of advanced myeloid malignancies after allogeneic stem-cell transplantation. *Journal of Clinical Oncology*, **20**, 405–12.

Lin, F., van Rhee, F., Goldman, J.M. *et al.* (1996). Kinetics of increasing BCR-ABL transcript numbers in chronic myeloid leukemia patients who relapse after bone marrow transplantation. *Blood*, **87**, 4473–8.

Lokhorst, H.M., Schattenberg, A., Cornelissen, J.J. *et al.* (1997). Donor leukocyte infusions are effective in relapsed multiple myeloma after allogeneic bone marrow transplantation. *Blood*, **90**, 4206–11.

Lönnqvist, B., Brune, M., & Ljungman, P. (1996). Lymphoblastoid human interferon and low dose IL-2 combined with donor lymphocyte infusion as therapy of a third relapse of CML—a case report. *Bone Marrow Transplantation*, **18**, 241–2.

Lotzova, E., Savary, C.A., & Herberman, R.B. (1987). Induction of NK cell activity against fresh human leukemia in culture with interleukin-2. *Journal of Immunology*, **138**, 2718–27.

Mackinnon, S., Barnett, L., & Heller, G. (1996). Polymerase chain reaction is highly predictive of relapse in patients following T cell-depleted allogeneic bone marrow transplantation for chronic myeloid leukemia. *Bone Marrow Transplantation*, **17**, 643–7.

Mackinnon, S., Papadopoulos, E.B., Carbasi, M.H. *et al.* (1995a). Adoptive immunotherapy using donor leukocytes following bone marrow transplantation for chronic myeloid leukemia: is T cell dose important in determining biological response? *Bone Marrow Transplantation*, **15**, 591–4.

Mackinnon, S., Papadopoulos, E.B., Carabasi, M.H. *et al.* (1995b). Adoptive immunotherapy evaluating escalating doses of donor leukocytes for relapse of chronic myeloid leukemia after bone marrow transplantation: separation of graft-versus-leukemia responses from graft-versus-host disease. *Blood*, **86**, 1261–8.

Mannering, S.I., McKenzie, J.L., & Hart, D.N. (1996). Generation of T-lymphocyte clones specific for the BCR-ABL fusion peptide presented by dendritic cells and other antigen presenting cells. *Bone Marrow Transplantation*, **17** (Suppl 1), S59.

Marks, D.I., Lush, R., Cavenagh, J. *et al.* (2002). The toxicity and efficacy of donor lymphocyte infusions given after reduced-intensity conditioning allogeneic stem cell transplantation. *Blood*, **100**, 3108–14.

Marmont, A.M., Frassoni, F., Bacigalupo, A. *et al.* (1984). Recurrence of Philadelphia-positive leukemia in donor cells after marrow transplantation for chronic granulocytic leukemia. *New England Journal of Medicine*, **310**, 903–6.

Marmont, A.M., Horowitz, M.M., Gale, R.P. *et al.* (1991). T cell depletion of HLA-identical transplants in leukemia. *Blood*, **78**, 2120–30.

Mathé, G., Amiel, J.L., Schwarzenberg, L. *et al.* (1965). Adoptive immunotherapy of acute leukemia: experimental and clinical results. *Cancer Research*, **25**, 1525–30.

McGlave, P., Bartsch, G., Anasetti, C. *et al.* (1993). Unrelated donor marrow transplantation therapy for chronic myelogenous leukemia: initial experience of the National Marrow Donor Program. *Blood*, **81**, 543–50.

Metcalf, D. (1979). Clonal analysis of the action of GM-CSF on the proliferation and differentiation of myelomonocytic leukemic cells. *International Journal of Cancer*, **24**, 616–23.

Mielcarek, M., Leisenring, W., Torok-Storb, B., & Storb, R. (2000). Graft-versus-host disease and donor-directed hemagglutinin titers after ABO-mismatched related and unrelated marrow allografts: evidence for a graft-versus-plasma cell effect. *Blood*, **96**, 1150–6.

Mittermüller, J., Kolb, H.J., Clemm, C. *et al.* (1990). Chimerism and treatment of recurrent leukemia after marrow transplantation. *Cancer Research and Clinical Oncology*, **116**, 577.

Mittermüeller, J., Kolb, H.J., Gerhartz, H.H. *et al.* (1986). In vivo differentiation of leukemic blasts and effect of low dose ara-c in a marrow grafted patient with leukemic relapse. *British Journal of Haematology*, **62**, 757–62.

Molldrem, J.J., Clave, E., Jiang, Y.Z. *et al.* (1997). Cytotoxic T-lymphocytes specific for a nonpolymorphic proteinase-3 peptide preferentially inhibit chronic myeloid leukemia colony-forming units. *Blood*, **90**, 2529–34.

Mortimer, J., Blinder, M.A., Schulman, S. *et al.* (1989). Relapse of acute leukemia after marrow transplantation: natural history and results of subsequent therapy. *Journal of Clinical Oncology*, **7**, 50–7.

Moscardo, F., Martinez, J.A., Sanz, G.F. *et al.* (2000). Graft-versus-tumour effect in non-small-cell lung cancer after allogeneic peripheral blood stem cell transplantation. *British Journal of Haematology*, **111**, 708–10.

Mutis, T., Schrama, E., van Luxemburg, Heijs, S.A. *et al.* (1997). HLA class II restricted T cell reactivity to a developmentally regulated antigen shared by leukemic cells and CD34+ early progenitor cells. *Blood*, **90**, 1083–90.

Naparstek, E., Or, R., Nagler, A. *et al.* (1995). T cell depleted allogeneic bone marrow transplantation for acute leukaemia using Campath-1 antibodies and posttransplant administration of donor's peripheral blood lymphocytes for prevention of relapse. *British Journal of Haematology*, **89**, 506–15.

Newburger, P.E., Latt, S.A., Pesando, J.M. *et al.* (1981). Leukemia relapse in donor cells after allogeneic bone marrow transplantation. *New England Journal of Medicine*, **304**, 712–14.

Odom, L., Githers, J., Morse, H. *et al.* (1978). Remission of relapsed leukemia during a graft-versus-host reaction. A graft-versus-leukemia reaction in man? *Lancet*, **2**, 537–40.

Ohminami, H., Yasukawa, M., Fujita, S. *et al.* (2000). HLA class I-restricted lysis of leukemia cells by a CD8(+) cytotoxic T-lymphocyte clone specific for WT1 peptide. *Blood*, **95**, 286–93.

Orsini, E., Alyea, E.P., Schlossman, R. *et al.* (2000). Changes in T cell receptor repertoire associated with graft-versus-tumor effect and graft-versus-host disease in patients with relapsed multiple myeloma after donor lymphocyte infusion. *Bone Marrow Transplantation*, **25**, 623–32.

Osman, Y., Takahshi, M., Zheng, Z. *et al.* (1999). Generation of bcr-abl specific cytotoxic T-lymphocytes by using dendritic cells pulsed with bcr-abl (b3a2) peptide: its applicability for donor leucocyte transfusions in marrow-grafted CML patients. *Leukemia*, **13**, 166–74.

Palva, I.P., Almqvist, A., Elonen, E. *et al.* (1991). Value of maintenance therapy with chemotherapy or interferon during remission of acute myeloid leukemia. *European Journal of Haematology*, **47**, 229–33.

Pan, L., Delmonte, J., Jalonen, C.K. *et al.* (1995). Pretreatment of donor mice with granulocyte colony-stimulating factor polarizes donor T-lymphocytes toward type-2 cytokine production and reduces severity of experimental graft-versus-host disease. *Blood*, **86**, 4422–9.

Pati, A.R., Godder, K., Lamb, L. *et al.* (1995). Immuno therapy with donor leukocyte infusions for patients with acute myeloid leukemia following partially mismatched related donor bone marrow transplantation. *Bone Marrow Transplantation*, **15**, 979–81.

Patterson, A.E. & Korngold, R. (2001). Infusion of select leukemia-reactive TCR Vβ+ T cells provides graft-versus-leukemia responses with minimization of graft-versus-host disease following murine hematopoietic stem cell transplantation. *Biology of Blood and Marrow Transplantation*, **7**, 187–96.

Pawelec, G., Max, H., Halder, T. *et al.* (1996). BCR/ABL leukemia oncogene fusion peptides selectively bind to certain HLA-DR alleles and can be recognized by T cells found at low frequency in the repertoire of normal donors. *Blood*, **88**, 2118–24.

Porter, D.L., Collins, R.H., Shpilberg, O. *et al.* (1999). Long-term follow-up of patients who achieved complete remission after donor leukocyte infusions. *Biology of Blood and Marrow Transplantation*, **5**, 253–61.

Porter, D.L., Connors, J.M., Van Deerlin, V.M.D. *et al.* (1999). Graft-versus-tumor induction with donor leukocyte infusions as primary therapy for patients with malignancies. *Journal of Clinical Oncology*, **17**, 1234–43.

Porter, D.L., Roth, M.S., Lee, S.J. *et al.* (1996). Adoptive immunotherapy with donor mononuclear cell infusions to treat relapse of acute leukemia or myelodysplasia after allogeneic bone marrow transplantation. *Bone Marrow Transplantation*, **18**, 975–80.

Porter, D.L., Roth, M.S., McGarigle, C. *et al.* (1994). Induction of graft-versus-host disease as immuno therapy for relapsed chronic myeloid leukemia. *New England Journal of Medicine*, **330**, 100–6.

Rahman, S.L., Mahendra, P., Nachva, E. *et al.* (1998). Achievement of complete cytogenetic remission after two very low-dose donor leucocyte infusions in a patient with extensive cGVHD relapsing in accelerated phase post allogeneic BMT for CML. *Bone Marrow Transplantation*, **21**, 955–6.

Ringden, O., Ruutu, T., Nikoskelainen, J. *et al.* (1994). A randomized trial comparing busulfan with total body irradiation as conditioning in allogeneic bone marrow transplant recipients with leukemia: a report from the Nordic Bone Marrow Transplantation Group. *Blood*, **83**, 2723–30.

Romani, N., Gruner, S., Brang, D. *et al.* (1994). Proliferating dendritic cell progenitors in human blood. *Journal of Experimental Medicine*, **180**, 83–93.

Rooney, C.M., Smith, C.A., Ng, C.Y.C. *et al.* (1995). Use of gene-modified virus-specific T lymphocytes to control Epstein-Barr-virus-related lymphoproliferation. *Lancet*, **345**, 9–13.

Salama, M., Nevill, T., Marcellus, D. *et al.* (2000). Donor leukocyte infusions for multiple myeloma. *Bone Marrow Transplantation*, **26**, 1179–84.

Schattenberg, A., van de Wiel-van Kemenade, E., Schaap, N. *et al.* (1996). Chimerism and outcome of the infusion of lymphocytes as a treatment for relapse after T cell depleted BMT. *Bone Marrow Transplantation*, **17**, (Suppl 1), S9.

Schattenberg, A., van de Wiel-van Kemenade, E., Schaap, N. *et al.* (1997). Chimerism status of T-lymphocytes at the time of relapse predicts outcome of donor lymphocyte transfusions for treatment of relapse after allogeneic BMT. *Bone Marrow Transplantation*, **19**, S68.

Siena, S., Di Nicola, M., Bregni, M. *et al.* (1995). Massive ex vivo generation of functional dendritic cells from mobilized CD34+ blood progenitors for anticancer therapy. *Experimental Hematology*, **23**, 1463–7.

Slavin, S., Naparstek, E., Nagler, A. *et al.* (1996). Allogeneic cell therapy with donor peripheral blood cells and recombinant human interleukin-2 to treat leukemia relapse after allogeneic bone marrow transplantation. *Blood*, **87**, 2195–204.

Soiffer, R., Galinsky, I., DeAngelo, D. *et al.* (2001). Imatinib mesylate (Gleevec) for disease relapse following allogeneic bone marrow transplantation. *Blood*, **98**, (Abstract).

Soiffer, R., Murray, C., Cochran, K. *et al.* (1992). Clinical and immunological effects of prolonged infusions of low dose recombinant interleukin-2 after autologous and T cell depleted allogeneic bone marrow transplantation. *Blood*, **79**, 517–26.

Soiffer, R.J., Alyea, E.P., Hochberg, E. *et al.* (2002). Randomized trial of CD8+ T-cell depletion in the prevention of graft-versus-host disease associated with donor lymphocyte infusion. *Biology of Blood and Marrow Transplantation*, **8**, 625–32.

Sullivan, K.M., Weiden, P.L., Storb, R. *et al.* (1989). Influence of acute and chronic graft-versus-host disease on relapse and survival after bone marrow transplantation from HLA-identical siblings as treatment of acute and chronic leukemia. *Blood*, **73**, 1720–8.

Thomas, E.D., Bryant, J.I., Buckner, C.D. *et al.* (1972). Leukemic transformation of engrafted human marrow cells in vivo. *Lancet*, **1**, 1310–3.

Thomas, E.D., Buckner, C.D., Banaji, M. *et al.* (1977). One hundred patients with acute leukemia treated by chemotherapy, total body irradiation and allogeneic marrow transplantation. *Blood*, **49**, 511–33.

Thomas, E.D., Clift, R.A., Fefer, A. *et al.* (1986). Marrow transplantation for the treatment of chronic myelogenous leukemia. *Annals of Internal Medicine*, **104**, 155–63.

Thomas, E.D., Storb, R., Clift, R.A. *et al.* (1975). Bone marrow transplantation. *New England Journal of Medicine*, **292**, 832–43.

Trenschel, R., Bernier, M., & Stryckmans, P. (1997). Case report. Complete remission following donor PBSC after low-dose cytarabine chemotherapy for early relapse of acute myelogenous leukemia after allogeneic stem cell transplantation. *Bone Marrow Transplantation*, **19**, 381–3.

Tricot, G., Vesole, D.H., Jagannath, S. *et al.* (1996). Graft-versus-myeloma effect: proof of principle. *Blood*, **87**, 1196–8.

Ueno, N.T., Rondon, G., Mirza, N.Q. *et al.* (1998). Allogeneic peripheral-blood progenitor-cell transplantation for poor-risk patients with metastatic breast cancer. *Journal of Clinical Oncology*, **16**, 986–93.

van Rhee, F. & Goldman, J.M. (1996). Donor lymphocyte therapy in bone marrow transplantation. In *Cell Therapy—Stem Cell Transplantation, Gene Therapy, and Cellular Immunotherapy*, ed. G. Morstyn & W. Sheridan, pp. 550–67. Cambridge: Cambridge University Press.

van Rhee, F., Lin, F., Cullis, J.O. *et al.* (1994). Relapse of chronic myeloid leukemia after allogeneic bone marrow transplantation: the case for giving donor leukocyte transfusions before the onset of hematologic relapse. *Blood*, **83**, 3377–83.

Verdonck, L.F., Lokhorst, H.M., Dekker, A.W. *et al.* (1996). Graft-versus-myeloma effect in two cases. *Lancet*, **347**, 800–1.

Verdonck, L.F., Petersen, E.J., Lokhorst, H.M. *et al.* (1998). Donor leukocyte infusions for recurrent hematologic malignancies after allogeneic bone marrow transplantation: impact of infused and residual donor T cells. *Bone Marrow Transplantation, 22,* 1057–63.

Verdonck, L.F., van Heugten, H.G., Giltay, J. *et al.* (1991). Amplification of the graft-versus-leukemia effect in man by interleukin-2. *Transplantation, 51,* 1120–4.

Verfluerth, S., Peggs, K., Vyas, P. *et al.* (2000). Longitudinal monitoring of immune reconstitution by CDR3 size spectratyping after T-cell-depleted allogeneic bone marrow transplant and the effect of donor lymphocyte infusions on T-cell repertoire. *Blood, 95,* 3990–5.

Voogt, P.J., Goulmy, E., Veenhof, W.F.J. *et al.* (1988). Cellularly defined minor histocompatibility antigens are differentially expressed on human hematopoietic progenitor cells. *Journal of Experimental Medicine, 168,* 2337–4.

Weiden, P.L., Storb, R., Tsoi, M.S. *et al.* (1976). Infusion of donor lymphocytes into stable canine radiation chimeras: implications for mechanism of transplantation tolerance. *Journal of Immunology, 116,* 1212–9.

Weiden, P.L., Sullivan, K.M., Flournoy, N. *et al.* (1981). Antileukemic effect of chronic graft-versus-host disease. Contribution to improved survival after allogeneic marrow transplantation. *New England Journal of Medicine, 304,* 1529–31.

Widmer-Pack, M.D., Olivier, W., Valinski, J. *et al.* (1987). Granulocyte-macrophage colony stimulating factor is essential for the viability and function of cultured murine epidermal Langerhans cells. *Journal of Experimental Medicine, 166,* 1494–8.

Zander, A., Keating, M., Dicke, K. *et al.* (1988). A comparison of marrow transplantation with chemotherapy for adults with acute leukemia of poor prognosis in first complete remission. *Journal of Clinical Oncology, 6,* 1548–57.

PART VI   FAMILY MEMBER MISMATCHED HEMATOPOIETIC STEM CELL TRANSPLANTATION

66 HLA-mismatched family member hematopoietic stem cell transplantation[1]

MASSIMO F. MARTELLI, FRANCO AVERSA, ANDREA VELARDI, AND YAIR REISNER

University of Perugia, Italy, and Weizmann Institute of Science, Rehovot, Israel

Introduction

Over the past 30 years hematopoietic stem cell (HSC) transplantation from human leukocyte antigen (HLA)-matched siblings has become treatment of choice for many hematologic diseases (Beatty, 1997a) with the only allogeneic barriers being "minor" histocompatibility antigens (Beatty, 1997b). With modern techniques for immunosuppression, such transplants usually result in rapid engraftment, a relatively low risk of fatal graft-versus-host disease (GVHD), and successful development of immune tolerance and immune reconstitution. However, any given sibling pair has only a 25% chance of inheriting the same HLA haplotypes from their parents and as there are, on average, fewer than three siblings per family in most developed countries and one is the patient, under 40% of patients will have such a match.

Consequently, worldwide volunteer donor registries have been established for HLA-matched, unrelated transplants. Even though this network includes over 8 million HLA-typed volunteers, the chance of finding a matched unrelated donor depends on the HLA diversity and varies with race, ranging from up to 90% in Caucasians to under 30% for ethnic minorities. Other limitations are the lapse in time from registering to identifying a donor, which may lead to disease progression in patients who urgently need a transplant (e.g., those with acute leukemia). Age is a further drawback as morbidity and mortality rise with age and paradoxically, so is closer matching, based on DNA techniques, since it reduces the odds of finding a suitably matched donor (Hansen *et al.*, 1997).

For all these reasons HSC transplantation for a matched sibling or unrelated donor is not feasible for over half of the patients requiring a transplant and so attention has focused on other sources of stem cells. Umbilical cord blood offers the advantages of easy procurement, absence of risks to donors, reduced risk of transmitting infections, and immediate availability of cryopreserved samples. However, engraftment is a major concern when the harvested cord blood contains under 3

$\times 10^7$ mononuclear cells/kg and the thawed graft CD34+ cell dose less than 2×10^5/kg. Risk factors include age over 15 and increased HLA disparity (Kurtzberg *et al.*, 2000; Gluckman *et al.*, 2001; Rocha *et al.*, 2001).

A viable alternative is a relative other than an HLA-matched sibling. These potential donors have one identical HLA haplotype and variable mismatches for zero, one, two, or three HLA-A, -B, and -DR loci of the unshared haplotype (Anasetti, 1999). In a German population the probability of finding a sibling mismatched at one HLA-A, -B, or -DR locus was 3.1%, which rose to 10.4% in the larger pool of one locus mismatched relatives (Ottinger *et al.*, 1994). When one of the patient's haplotypes is relatively common, an extended family search for a one locus mismatched relative may be justified (Fig. 66.1). On the other hand, almost all patients have at least one HLA-haploidentical mismatched family member, (parent, child, or sibling), who is immediately available as a donor. Unfortunately, in full haplotype mismatched transplants, the high frequency of alloreactive donor T cells in unmanipulated grafts that recognize major histocompatibility (MHC) antigens, is associated with an extremely high incidence of severe, acute GVHD (Anasetti *et al.*, 1990). Although extensive T-cell depletion prevents GVHD (Reisner *et al.*, 1981; Prentice *et al.*, 1984; O'Reilly *et al.*, 1986; Hale *et al.*, 1988; Marmont *et al.*, 1991) the rejection rates rise steeply (Gale & Reisner, 1986; Patterson *et al.*, 1986; Martin *et al.*, 1988) because the balance between competing host and donor T cells shifts in favor of the unopposed host-versus-graft reaction.

T-cell allorecognition, natural killer (NK) cell alloreactivity, a biological phenomenon that is unique to mismatched transplants, needs to be borne in mind (Ruggeri *et al.*, 2002). NK cells are regulated by inhibitory receptors for MHC class I molecules (Moretta & Moretta, 1997; Lanier, 1998). Some of these receptors, known as KIRs, are specific for epitopes shared by certain class I alleles and each KIR is expressed by a subset of NK cells. Therefore, in the NK repertoire, some NK cells recognize, and are blocked by, specific class I alleles (Fig. 66.2). These NK cells trigger alloreactions when the mismatched target cells do not express the specific class I alleles which block them. In the context of full haplotype-mis-

[1] Patrick Beatty and P. Jean Henslee-Downey contributed significantly to this chapter in the First and Second Editions of this book.

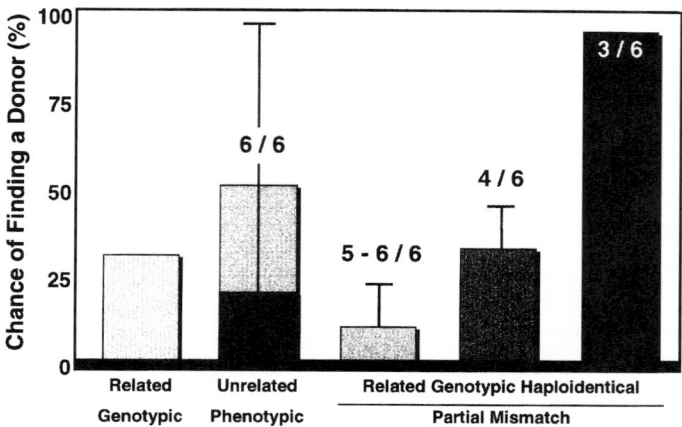

Fig. 66.1. Availability of different types of donor.

matched transplants, host and/or donor NK cells may be responsible for three situations:

1. A potential for graft-versus-host reactions, when donor NK cells do not recognize the host MHC and are, consequently, activated to lyse the recipient cells
2. A potential for host-versus-graft reactions, when the donor fails to express the recipient's KIR epitopes
3. No NK cell alloreactions, when the donor and recipient mismatched alleles express the same KIR epitopes.

This chapter describes results of haploidentical transplants from donors who are mismatched at one or more loci and concentrates on recent advances that have ensured the safe use of a related donor mismatched at two or three HLA-A, -B, or -DR loci.

Clinical results

Outcomes in several clinical trials indicate that complications of HSC transplantation from HLA-mismatched relatives depend on the degree of HLA disparity. A series of reports from Seattle described patients who, after conditioning with cyclophosphamide (CY) and total body irradiation (TBI), received unmanipulated bone marrow and either methotrexate alone or a combination of methotrexate and cyclosporine for GVHD prophylaxis (Beatty *et al.*, 1985, 1987; Anasetti *et al.*,

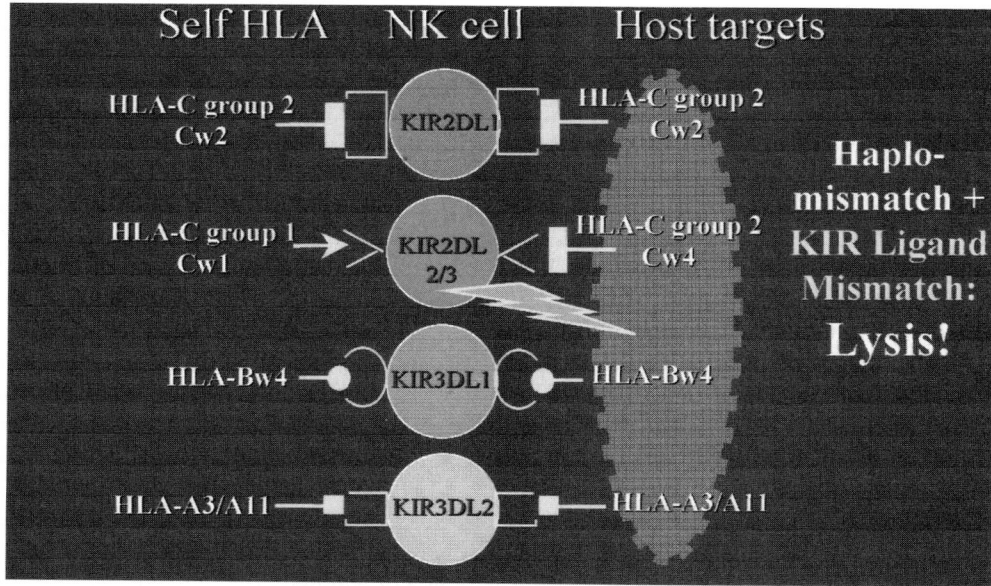

Fig. 66.2. NK cell lysis is negatively regulated by receptors for MHC class I. Some receptors (KIRs) are specific for determinants shared by certain class I alleles. Each KIR is expressed by a subset of NK cells (NK cell repertoire). NK cell bearing KIR2DL2/3 is blocked only by HLA-C group 1 alleles (Cw1,3,7,8,9), NK cell bearing KIR2DL1 is blocked only by HLA-C group 2 alleles (Cw2,4,5,6), NK cell bearing KIR3DL1 is blocked only by B alleles sharing the Bw4 supertypic specificity.

1989, 1990). Overall graft rejection increased to 12.3% versus the 2% in matched transplants and correlated with the degree of mismatch, with a 9% incidence of graft rejection in recipients of one HLA locus transplant and a 21% incidence in those incompatible for two loci (Anasetti *et al.*, 1989). Furthermore, circulating antidonor lymphocytotoxic antibodies were a major risk factor for graft rejection (RR = 2.3, P = .004). The risk of graft failure may be disease-related as data suggest patients with chronic myeloid leukemia (CML) have a higher risk of rejection than those with acute leukemia, who are generally more immunosuppressed at transplant after being treated with repeated cycles of chemotherapy (Anasetti, 1999).

The incidence and severity of acute GVHD also rose with increasing HLA disparity, from phenotypic match through three-locus mismatch (Fig. 66.3), reaching at least 80% with an earlier onset than in matched transplants (median time 14 days) (Beatty *et al.*, 1985; Cunningham *et al.*, 1997). Posttransplant immunosuppression with the cyclosporine-metrotrexate combination significantly reduced the risk of grade III–IV acute GVHD from 53% to 28% in one locus incompatible recipients and from 63% to 47% in two loci incompatible transplant recipients. Unfortunately recipients of HLA locus D disparity did not respond to this approach (Anasetti, 1999). The probability of clinically extensive chronic GVHD was higher (49% versus 33%) and the onset was earlier (159 versus 201 days posttransplant) (Sullivan *et al.*, 1991) than in transplants from HLA-identical siblings. Although the duration of chronic GVHD in recipients of partially HLA mismatched transplants has not been reported, its impact on the quality of life should not be underestimated.

The probability of relapse was expected to be lower in mismatched transplants because of the high incidence of GVHD which is linked with the graft-versus-leukemia (GVL) effect (Weiden *et al.*, 1979; Horowitz *et al.*, 1990). The Seattle report (Anasetti *et al.*, 1989) of a significant reduction was not, however, confirmed by a later International Bone Marrow Transplant Registry (IBMTR) study on 238 patients who received one locus incompatible transplants (Sierra *et al.*, 1997).

Besides HLA disparity, factors influencing survival after mismatched transplants are age, underlying disease, and remission status at transplant. In the Seattle series the probability of survival for patients receiving one-locus incompatible grafts as therapy for acute myeloid leukemia (AML) in first remission, acute lymphoblastic leukemia (ALL) in first and second remission or CML in the chronic phase overlapped with outcomes in recipients of transplants from HLA-identical siblings (Anasetti *et al.*, 1990; Szydlo *et al.*, 1997) (Fig. 66.4), independently of whether the posttransplant immunosuppression with either methotrexate alone or combined cyclosporine. Similar results were reported in recipients of 1 HLA antigen mismatched family member transplants by Przepiorka and colleagues (1999) using tacrolimus and "mini"-dose methotrexate (5 mg/m^2 i.v. on days 1, 3, 6, and 11) as posttransplant immune suppression. A large IBMTR study on over 1,000 patients, which included 340 transplants from HLA-mismatched relatives, adopted different definitions of donor-recipient histocompatibility and showed leukemia-free survival was poorer in the 238 recipients of one locus mismatched transplants than in the 1,224 recipients of transplants from identical siblings (33% versus 66%, P < .001) (Szydlo *et al.*, 1997) (Fig. 66.5). Transplant-related mortality (TRM) was higher (53% versus 21%, P < .001) but the relapse rates were similar. Of the 340 patients, 102 received a T-cell-replete graft from 2-loci mismatched relatives. The

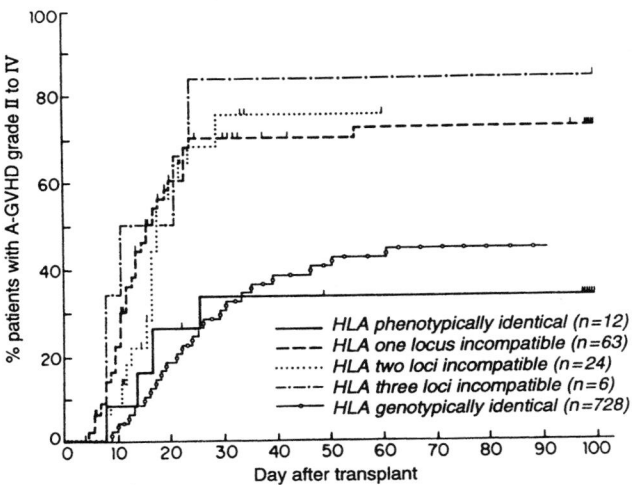

Fig. 66.3. Risk of acute graft-versus-host disease (GVHD) in relation to the number of disparate loci. The curves represent the cumulative probability of severe disease (grade II or higher) as a function of time after transplantation. Early tick marks indicate patients whose data were censored from further analysis at death. Tick marks at 100 days indicate patients who were alive without severe GVHD. Patients with graft rejection are included; some received second grafts and subsequently had acute GVHD. Reprinted, with permission, from Beatty *et al.* (1985).

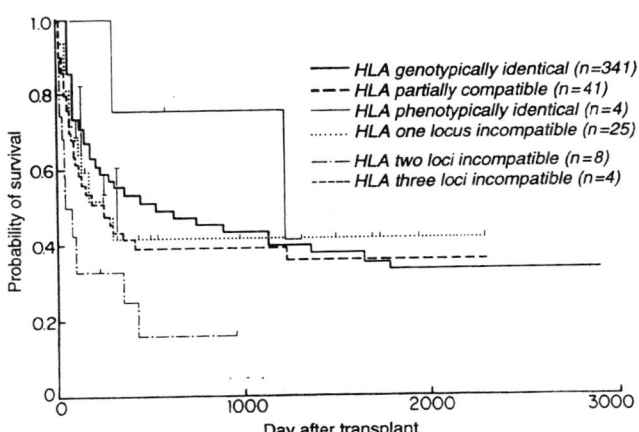

Fig. 66.4. Probability of survival in patients with acute leukemia undergoing transplantation during remission. Tick marks indicate patients who were alive at the time of analysis. Tick marks were omitted from control curves for clarity. The bars at 100 and 300 days represent 2 S.E. Reprinted, with permission, from Beatty *et al.* (1985).

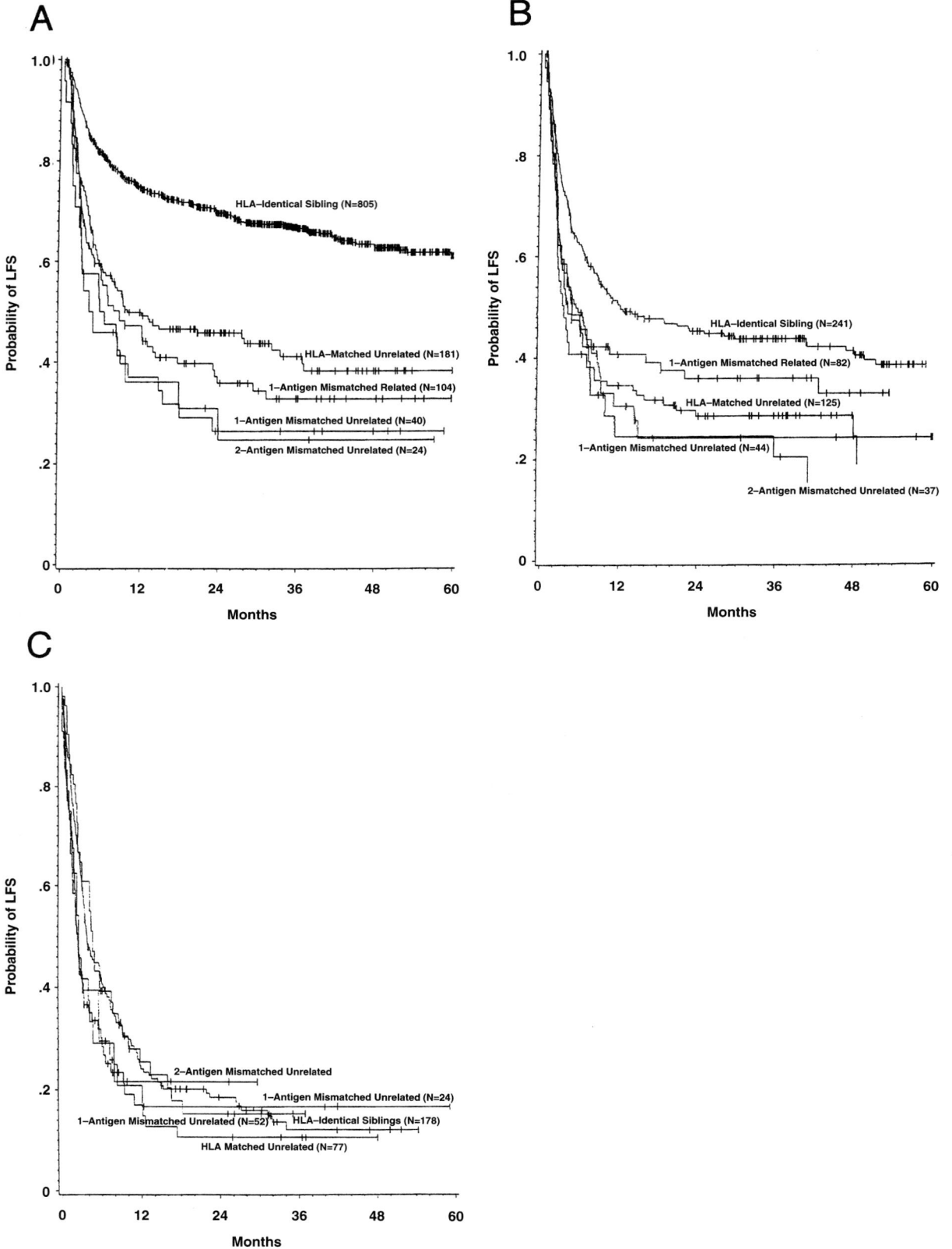

Fig. 66.5. Probability of leukemia-free survival after bone marrow transplants for early (**A**), intermediate (**B**), and advanced (**C**) leukemia by donor type. Reproduced, with permission, from Szydlo *et al.* (1997).

rejection rate was 16%, severe grade III–IV GVHD occurred in 36%, chronic GVHD in 60%, and leukemia-free survival at 3 years ranged from 20% to 25% according to disease status at transplant. Survival of patients receiving T-cell-replete grafts from two or three locus incompatible donors was undoubtedly much worse in all reports, mainly because of graft rejection and the extremely high incidence of severe GVHD (Ash *et al.*, 1991; Beatty, 1992).

In an update of the Seattle experience of bone marrow transplantation (BMT) from HLA non-genotypically identical relatives for patients with severe aplastic anemia, Wagner and colleagues (1996) reported on nine patients conditioned with cyclophosphamide 50 mg/kg for 4 doses who received marrow from HLA-phenotypically identical relatives who were all alive and disease-free 3 to 18 years posttransplant with the exception of one who died accidentally. Thirty-one patients received marrow from HLA-mismatched relatives who differed by one or more HLA loci. Fifteen of these patients received cyclophosphamide 50 mg/kg for 4 doses without TBI and none survived. Because of this, TBI 12 Gy was subsequently added to cyclophosphamide 60 mg/kg for 2 doses: of 16 patients thus treated (after failure to respond to immunosuppressive therapy), 8 remained alive at the time of the report without disease between 1.5 and 11.3 years posttransplant. Clearly transplants from related donors mismatched for one or more HLA loci required more intensive conditioning than cyclophosphamide alone to achieve sustained engraftment after transplantation for aplastic anemia.

In the early 1980s extensive (3 log) ex vivo T-cell depletion of the graft using soybean agglutination and E-rosetting was successfully pioneered by Reisner and O'Reilly (Reisner *et al.*, 1983) who showed it completely prevented acute and chronic GVHD even when using haploidentical parental bone marrow differing at the three major HLA loci in patients with severe combined immune deficiency (SCID). More than 300 full haplotype mismatched transplants have since been performed worldwide with a high rate of partial or complete immune reconstitution, confirming that GVHD is prevented in SCID patients by 3 log T-cell depletion (Fischer *et al.*, 1990; Buckley *et al.*, 1999).

Given these encouraging results it was reasonable to presume the same principle would apply in leukemia patients. Unfortunately, full haplotype mismatched, extensively T-cell-depleted BMT was associated with a high incidence of graft failure (O'Reilly *et al.*, 1985; Kernan *et al.*, 1987). The earliest trials used standard cyclophosphamide and fractionated TBI as conditioning for transplant and there was 60% to 100% graft failure, no matter whether lectin, an immunotoxin, CT2, or Campath (reviewed in Cunningham *et al.*, 1997) was used for T-cell depletion. Rejection in T-cell-depleted mismatched transplants is due mainly to residual host lymphocytes that exhibit donor-specific cytotoxic activity directed against donor MHC alleles (Reisner *et al.*, 1986). This resistance rarely occurs in the T-cell-replete transplant because the donor T cells in the graft contribute to suppression of the residual recipient immune system. Animal models of T-cell-depleted transplanta-

tion showed that the recipient immune system surviving after lethal TBI can be suppressed by increasing the dose of TBI (Schwartz *et al.*, 1987), or by combining the standard dose of TBI with selective anti-T-cell measures, with low non-hematological toxicity (Cobbold *et al.*, 1986; Lapidot *et al.*, 1988, 1990). Engraftment is also enhanced when myeloablative drugs (dimethyl-myleran, busulfan, or thiotepa) are combined with TBI (Lapidot *et al.*, 1989; Terenzi *et al.*, 1990). However enhancing immunosuppression and myeloablation by adding antithymocyte globulin and thiotepa to a standard conditioning protocol based on hyperfractionated TBI and cyclophosphamide in leukemia patients still did not ensure engraftment of conventional doses of full haplotype mismatched T-cell-depleted bone marrow cells (Aversa *et al.*, 1994, 2001b).

In an attempt to facilitate engraftment without excessive GVHD, Henslee-Downey and co-workers (1989, 1996) exploited the principle of sequential immunomodulation in the recipient of haploidentical transplants by combining partial ex vivo T-cell depletion of the donor bone marrow with T10B9 monoclonal antibody and posttransplant in vivo T-cell lysis with an immunotoxin H65-RTA. In 1997 they tested other T-lymphocyte targeted products (Henslee-Downey *et al.*, 1997). In a analysis of 72 consecutive patients, antithymocyte globulin was used for in vivo T depletion. Although most patients received 2 or 3 antigen mismatched grafts, the probability of engraftment was 88% at 32 days and the incidence of grade II–IV acute GVHD was 16%. Disease status at the time of transplant (early/remission versus late/relapse) was the only variable affecting long-term outcome. The probability of 2-year survival was significantly higher in low-risk versus high-risk patients (55% versus 27%, respectively, *P* = .048) (Fig. 66.6).

OKT3, an anti-CD3 monoclonal antibody, has also been tested for T-cell depletion of haploidentical marrow grafts. The engraftment rate improved significantly to 97%; there was no change in the incidence of acute GVHD, with a 0.24 estimated probability of grade II–IV. In this analysis of 67 pediatric

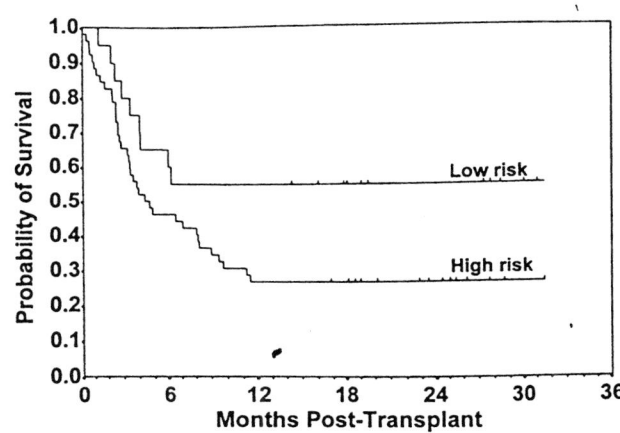

Fig. 66.6. Probability of survival for patients with low-risk and high-risk disease status. Estimated survival at 2 years was 0.55 and 0.27, respectively (*P* = .048). Reproduced, with permission, from Henslee-Downey *et al.* (1997).

patients (median age 8.3 years), the overall estimated probability of survival at 3 years was 0.26, which improved when the donor was under 30 years of age and when the blood blast count of the patients was low (Godder *et al.*, 2000) (Fig. 66.7). In patients with AML refractory to remission induction chemotherapy, a 3-year actuarial disease-free survival rate of 19% has been reported—similar to the outcome with HLA-identical sibling grafts (Chiang *et al.*, 2001).

Soiffer and co-workers (1997) transplanted 27 adult patients, 10 of whom were two loci mismatched. Grafts were T-cell depleted with an anti-CD6 monoclonal antibody, T12, and no posttransplant immunosuppression was given. Conditioning included total lymphoid irradiation, fractionated TBI, and standard-dose cyclophosphamide. Twenty-four of the 27 patients successfully engrafted; 40% developed grade II–IV acute GVHD. The estimated overall survival for HLA-mismatched patients was 56% at 2 years, and was independent of HLA disparity. Event-free survival significantly correlated with the timing of transplant, being 69% at 2 years for early disease status, and 20% for more advanced disease.

An alternative approach to partial T-cell depletion for the prevention of GVHD involves the co-incubation of recipient and donor cells with an antibody that blocks the co-stimulatory pathway, resulting in specific anergy to mismatched HLA. Guinan *et al.* (1999) tolerized alloreactive T cells in the graft by stimulating the donor bone marrow cells against host cells in the presence of CTLA-4. Primary engraftment was achieved in 9 of the 12 children, but 3 developed acute GVHD despite posttransplant immunosuppressive therapy.

Megadose stem cell transplantation

In a radically different approach to full haplotype mismatched transplants for advanced stage leukemia Aversa *et al.* (1994)

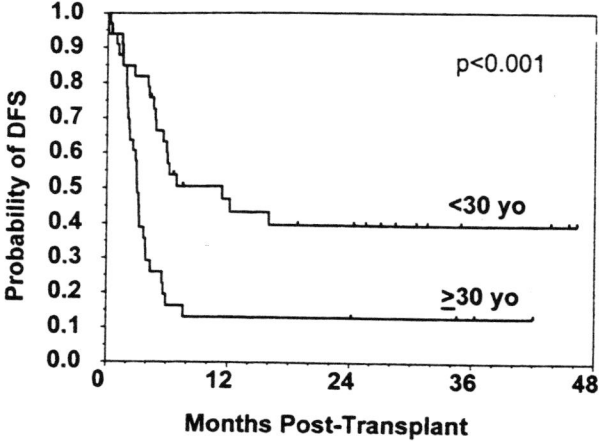

Fig. 66.7. Estimated probability of DFS by donor age. Patients who received grafts from donors who were younger than 30 years had an improved DFS (0.45) compared with those who received grafts from older donors (0.13). Abbreviation: yo, years old. Reproduced, with permission, from Godder *et al.* (2000).

employed only extensive ex vivo T-cell depletion to prevent GVHD and, at the same time, overcame the barrier to engraftment by adopting the escalated stem cell dose concept, the so-called megadose approach, that had been successfully pioneered in animal models in the late 1980s (Bachar-Lustig *et al.*, 1995; Lapidot *et al.*, 1989). To increase the overall number of CD34[+] cells infused by an order of magnitude, bone marrow was supplemented with granulocyte colony-stimulating factor (G-CSF)- mobilized peripheral blood progenitor cells (PBPC). Both sources were depleted of T cells by soybean agglutination and E-rosetting. Transplant recipients were conditioned with a highly immunosuppressive and myeloablative regimen that included TBI in a single fraction at a fast dose rate, cyclophosphamide, ATG, and thiotepa. Eighty percent of the 36 adult patients achieved primary, sustained engraftment and, although no posttransplant immunosuppressive therapy was administered, the incidence of GVHD was significantly lower than in T-cell-replete mismatched transplants.

Over the years modifications to this approach have led to remarkable progress. Fludarabine was substituted for cyclophosphamide in the conditioning regimen (Fig. 66.8) to minimize nonhematological toxicity (Aversa *et al.*, 1998). At the same time, with the aim of eliminating GVHD, the number of CD3[+] cells in the graft was reduced to a mean of 2×10^4/kg recipient weight (i.e., one log less than in the original study). Initially PBPCs were depleted of T lymphocytes by E-rosetting and positive selection of CD34[+] cells using the Ceprate technique (CellPro, Bothell, Washington, USA) but, since January 1999, the Clinimacs device (Miltenyi Biotech, Bergisch, Gladbach, Germany) has been used to purify CD34[+] cells in a one-step procedure (Table 66.9). Posttransplant G-CSF administration to the recipients was stopped because experimental data suggested it induced immunosuppression (Pan *et al.*, 1995; Sloand *et al.*, 2000).

This strategy has been tested in 93 high-risk acute leukemia patients since October 1995 (Table 66.10). Primary sustained engraftment was achieved in 87 (93%). Five successfully engrafted after second transplants. Hematopoietic recovery was extremely rapid. Neutrophil counts reached 1×10^9/l and platelet counts 25×10^9/l at a median of 12 days (range 8–19) and 18 days (range 12–84), respectively. Analysis of DNA polymorphism documented full donor-type chimerism in both the peripheral blood and the bone marrow of all evaluable patients. Only three patients developed acute GVHD grade II–IV, which progressed to chronic GVHD in one.

In a pediatric series by Handgretinger and colleagues, 39 children (median age 8.6 years) with high-risk acute leukemia received approximately 20×10^6/kg CD34[+] cells after a chemotherapy-alone based conditioning regimen (Fig. 66.9). Twenty-five achieved primary engraftment and the other 4 successfully engrafted after second transplants from the same donors (Handgretinger *et al.*, 1999, 2001) Once again, GVHD was prevented by an ex vivo T-cell depletion alone (CD34[+] selection with the Clinimacs system), with the graft containing a number of T lymphocytes ($\leq 1 \times 10^4$/kg) similar to the thresh-

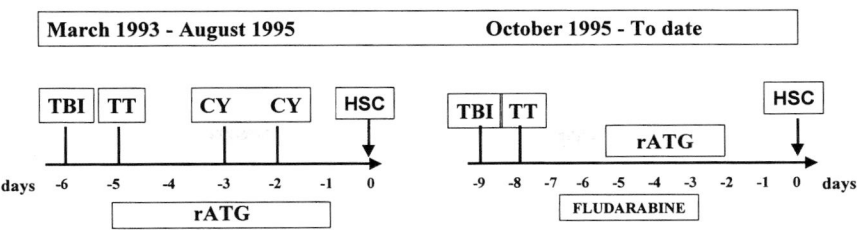

Fig. 66.8. The Perugia conditioning regimens in the periods March 1993–August 1995 and October 1995–to date. TBI, total body irradiation; TT, thiotepa; CY, cyclophosphamide; ATG, rabbit antithymocyte globulin; HSC, hematopoietic stem cells.

old dose that prevents GVHD in SCID patients receiving mismatched transplants. Another factor that may have contributed to T-cell depletion in vivo, thereby reducing the incidence of GVHD, was the OKT3 administered in the conditioning regimen and posttransplant. The same principle applies to the Perugia trial as the ATG administered during conditioning persisted in plasma for several days. Whether TBI is part of the conditioning or not does not seem to influence the engraftment rate when a stem cell megadose is given.

Using the same technique, Muller and colleagues (1999) determined that a residual T-cell content of less than 5×10^4/kg in the mobilized blood stem cell graft was adequate for the prevention of GVHD.

In another pediatric study Kato *et al.* (2000) transplanted 135 patients, 107 of whom were two loci mismatched. CD34+ cells were isolated with the Isolex device and the mean CD34+ cell dose for those receiving bone marrow was 3.2×10^6/kg, 5.5 $\times 10^6$/kg for those receiving PBSC, and 4.9×10^6/kg for those receiving both. These CD34+ counts were well below the dose employed in the studies reported above. Furthermore, the mean CD3+ T cell doses of 6.0, 9.4, and 12.1×10^4/kg, respectively were much higher than reported elsewhere. The majority of patients received posttransplant immunosuppressive therapy to prevent GVHD. Graft failure was reported in 13% of patients with neoplastic diseases and in 40% for patients with nonhematologic malignancies. The incidence of GVHD was 10% when ATG was included in the conditioning and 27% when it was not. The disease-free survival rate in standard and high-risk patients was 39% and 5%, respectively.

A feasible hypothesis to explain how the CD34+ cell megadose overcomes the barrier of residual donor specific host cytotoxic T lymphocyte precursors (CTL-p) after an immuno-myeloablative conditioning is that CD34+ cells exert "veto"

activity, that is, they neutralize CTL-p directed against their antigens (Rachamin *et al.*, 1998). Preliminary data suggest that the veto activity of human CD34+ cells, like other veto cells, is mediated by apoptosis (Gur *et al.*, 2002).

Besides the conditioning regimen and the stem cell megadose, donor NK cell alloreactivity facilitates engraftment in some donor-recipient pairs (Ruggeri *et al.*, 2002). In recipients of NK alloreactive donor HSCs (see above), the reconstituting NK cell repertoire contains a high frequency of donor NK cell clones that are alloreactive toward the recipient and are constantly activated to lyse the recipient's lympho-hematopoietic cells, without causing GVHD. All these patients achieve primary sustained engraftment, confirming donor alloreactive NK cells help ablate the host immune system in vivo. The few rejections were all in patients whose donors were unable to mount NK cell alloreactions against the host.

Biological evidence in support of these clinical observations comes from studies in animal models (Ruggeri *et al.*, 2002). Even after mild host immune suppression in mice the infusion of donor-versus-recipient alloreactive NK cells efficiently ablated the host immune and myeloid cells and engraftment was achieved even though transplantation was across major MHC barriers.

Eradication of leukemia in allogeneic hematopoietic transplantation is achieved by means of two mechanisms: the antileukemic effect of a high-intensity radio- and/or chemotherapy based conditioning regimen, and the ability of the immune cells in the graft to recognize and eliminate the leukemia cells that survive the conditioning regimen (T-cell alloreaction-mediated GVL effect) (Horowitz *et al.*, 1990; Marmont *et al.*, 1991). The removal of donor T cells from the graft, which is essential to the success of mismatched transplants, raises the question of whether this type of transplant exerts a GVL effect. In vitro leukemia killing assays demon-

Table 66.9. *Graft processing and graft composition*

Years	1993–95	1995–97	1999–2002
Patients	(n = 36)	(n = 44)	(n = 49)
Methods	SBA, E-rosette	E-rosette + CD34 selection (Ceprate SC)	CD34 selection (CliniMACS)
CD34+ × 10^6/kg	10.8	10.5	12
CD3+ × 10^4/kg	22.4	2.0	1.0

Table 66.10. *Immunoselected CD34⁺ cell haploidentical transplants (October 1995–February 2002)*

Demographics		Results	
No. of Patients	93	Graft composition:	
Age in Years:		CD34$^+$ ($\times 10^6$/kg)	12.0
Median	26	CD3$^+$ ($\times 10^4$/kg)	1.5
Range	4–62		
Diagnosis:		Engraftment:	
AML	53	Primary	87 (93%)
ALL	40	Overall	92 (99%)
Status at transplant:		Days to:	
CR I	16	ANC >1 $\times 10^9$/l	12
CR ≥ II	35	PLT > 25 $\times 10^9$/l	18
Relapse	42		
CD 34 selection:		Acute GVHD ≥ II	3/84
Ceprate	44	Chronic GVHD	1/61
Clinimacs	49		

strated 100% of acute myeloid leukemias (AML) and chronic myeloid leukemias are lysed by alloreactive NK clones. Most common acute lymphoblastic leukemias (ALL) are not susceptible to this in vitro lysis (Ruggeri *et al.,* 1999). In clinical practice, transplants with KIR epitope mismatches in the GVH direction are associated with almost complete control of AML relapse but, as predicted by the in vitro resistance to alloreactive NK cells, the relapse rate in ALL does not differ whether NK alloreactivity is present or not. Thus these observations show that donor-versus-recipient NK cell alloreactivity contributes to the eradication of minimal residual disease in AML patients.

Posttransplant immune reconstitution remains a major clinical issue (Figs. 66.10 and 66.11). The high incidence of infection-related deaths in mismatched transplants is linked to the delay in immune reconstitution and to the fact that most patients had a long history of disease, had been heavily pretreated, and/or were in relapse at time of transplant (Aversa *et al.,* 1998; 2001b; Kato *et al.,* 2000; Handgretinger *et al.,* 2001). Similar high infection-related mortality rates have been reported in patients at the same stage of disease who received unmanipulated or T-cell-depleted matched unrelated transplants (Small *et al.,* 1999).

Several mechanisms are responsible for the posttransplant immune deficiency. In adults, with thymic function in decline, early immune recovery stems from expansion of the mature T cells in the graft, and several months later, from de novo production of naïve T cells (Dumont-Girard *et al.,* 1998; Heitger *et al.,* 2000). In mismatched transplants the number of T lymphocytes in the graft has to be particularly low in order to prevent GVHD and their peripheral expansion is antagonized by ATG or similar drugs in the conditioning regimen. Furthermore, the highly intensive conditioning regimen itself induces tissue damage that prevents T-cell homing to peripheral lymphoid tissues, where generation and maintenance of T-cell memory take place

(Sallusto *et al.,* 1999). The impact of G-CSF in transplant recipients must not be underestimated because G-CSF blocks IL-12 production in antigen-presenting cells (APCs) and decreases pathogen-specific T-cell responses in donor cells in vitro and in vivo (Volpi *et al.,* 2001). In fact, since its posttransplant administration was suspended in the Perugia series, the engraftment rate remained unchanged, and IL-12 production by APCs was restored to normal much sooner, with CD4$^+$ cell numbers and function markedly improving. The better immune reconstitution in all likelihood contributed to the 15% TRM in 17 AML patients who were transplanted in remission and who did not receive G-CSF as compared to the 58% TRM in 15 patients who were transplanted in CR but who were included in the G-CSF program. In the former group the TRM rate approaches that reported for HLA-identical sibling transplants (Martelli & Aversa, 2002).

Other approaches to hasten immune reconstitution can be envisaged. One is the adoptive transfer of nonalloreactive T cells generated by purging IL-2 receptor (CD25)-positive, mixed lymphocyte response (MLR)-reactive T cells (Cavazzana-Calvo *et al.,* 1994). Another involves the infusion of lymphocytes co-cultured with irradiated cells from the recipients in the presence of CTLA4-Ig—an agent that inhibits B7/CD28-mediated costimulation (Gribben *et al.,* 1996; Greenwald *et al.,* 2001). Attempts are currently being made to transfer donor T lymphocytes specifically directed against pathogens (CMV, aspergillus) safely across the HLA barrier (Perruccio *et al.,* 2001). Thymic output of naive T cells could be enhanced by administering keratinocyte growth factor (KGF) to protect thymic stroma from radiation injury (Housley *et al.,* 1994)) or IL-7 to promote T-cell differentiation (Fry & Mackall., 2001).

One major factor has undoubtedly confounded interpretation of the outcome in full haplotype mismatched transplants: most recipients had advanced stage disease at transplant. In the 65

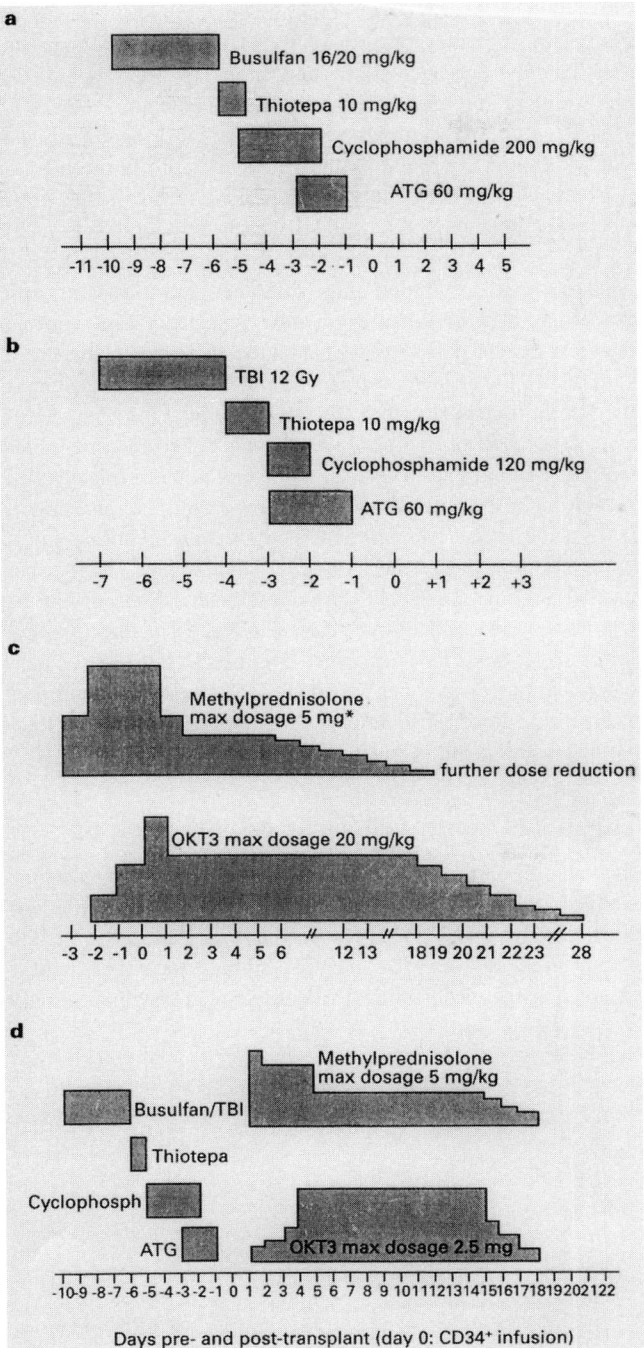

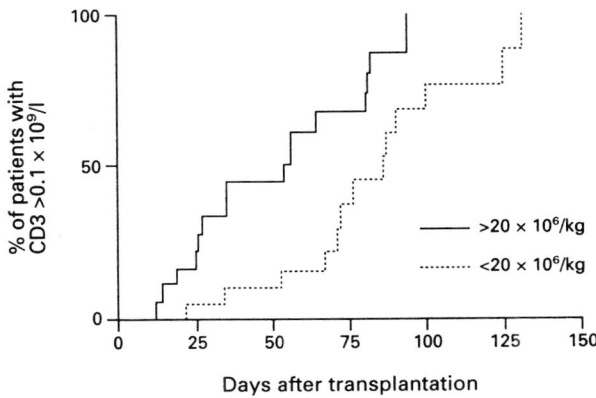

Fig. 66.10. Time to reach $>0.1 \times 10^9/l$ CD3$^+$ T lymphocytes in patients who were transplanted with $>20 \times 10^6$/kg purified CD34$^+$ progenitor cells. A significantly faster reconstitution of CD3$^+$ T lymphocytes ($P = .0065$) was seen in patients who were transplanted with $>20 \times 10^6$/kg CD34$^+$ cells. Reproduced, with permission, from Handgretinger *et al.* (2001).

patients with AML, who were transplanted in Perugia after March 1993, only 6 were under 18 years of age and 47 were in advanced stage disease at transplant (Aversa *et al.*, 2001a,b; 2002). Despite these poor prognostic factors, TRM was 44%, which overlaps with the cumulative 43% nonleukemic mortality in AML patients reported by Sierra *et al.* (2000) in the 26 children and 135 adults who received T-replete transplants from unrelated matched donors in Seattle.

Survival correlates with disease status at transplant in mismatched transplants as in matched unrelated transplants. Patients with AML who received a full haplotype mismatched transplant had, respectively, a 0.42 and 0.20 probability of EFS at 9 years (Fig. 66.12) when transplanted in hematological

Fig. 66.9. The myeloablative regimens based on chemotherapy (**a**) or on total body irradiation (TBI) (**b**), the reconditioning regimen for patients with nonengraftment or rejection (**c**), and the combination of the myeloablative regimen with the immunological rejection prophylaxis using the anti-CD3 monoclonal antibody OKT3 in combination with steroids (**d**) are shown. The doses of busulfan in regimen a were 16 mg/kg for children >3 years of age and 20 mg/kg <3 years of age (ATG = antithymocyte globulin). The doses in regimen d were: busulfan 16/20 mg/kg, thiotepa 10 mg/kg, cyclophosphamide 200 mg/kg or TBI 12 Gy, thiotepa 10 mg/kg, cyclophosphamide 120 mg/kg, and ATG 60 mg/kg. * Maximum dosage 5 mg, regardless of body weight. Reproduced, with permission, from Handgretinger *et al.* (2001).

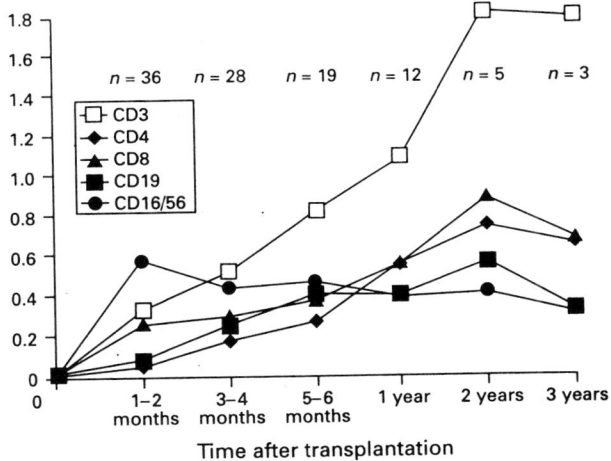

Fig. 66.11. Long-term reconstitution of CD3$^+$ T lymphocytes, CD4$^+$ helper cells, CD8$^+$ cytotoxic/suppressor cells, CD19$^+$ B lymphocytes, and CD56$^+$ natural killer (NK) cells in all evaluable patients. The mean absolute cell count for all evaluable patients is shown. Reproduced, with permission, from Handgretinger *et al.* (2001).

remission (CRI = 7; CRII = 25) or in relapse (No = 33). The Seattle report showed only 7% of the 81 patients in relapse, 19% of the 16 who never achieved remission, 28% for the 40 transplanted in second CR, and 50% of the 16 in first CR survived leukemia-free at 5 years. Age also influences outcome with only 14% of the adults surviving leukemia-free as compared to 32% of patients under 18 years of age. Similar data were reported by the National Marrow Donor Program (NMDP) in 756 AML patients transplanted from matched unrelated donors (Margolis *et al.,* 1999; Stockerl-Goldstein & Blume, 1999). In our experience EFS correlated with the age of patients (25% and 35% in adults and children, respectively) and stage of disease, with the difference being even more marked in patients in advanced stages of the disease at transplant (7% EFS for adults and 23% for children). In patients with AML receiving a full haplotype-mismatched transplant, besides the advanced disease status at transplant, the lack of donor-versus-recipient NK cell alloreactivity was a very significant risk factor for the clinical outcome with its hazard ratio of 6.1 (95% CI 2.6–14.9). Patients who received transplants from donors who were able to mount NK alloreactions had an EFS of 60% at 8 years versus the 5% of those without such donors (Ruggeri *et al.,* 2002).

In ALL disease status at transplant is the most significant risk factor influencing survival. In the series of 37 children who received a full haplotype mismatched transplant in Tübingen, the 21 in remission at transplant had a 0.39 probability of EFS as compared to the 0.13 for those not in remission at transplant (Handgretinger *et al.,* 2001) (Fig. 66.13). Almost all the 63 adult patients with ALL who were transplanted in Perugia, were at very high risk for leukemia relapse and nonleukemic death because many were in chemoresistant relapse at transplant. Their 9-year probability of EFS was 0.21 for the 31 patients in hematological remission (CRI = 10; CRII = 20) (Aversa *et al.,*

2001a,b) (Fig 66.12). The poor outcome, 5% for the 33 in relapse, is similar to the probability of leukemia-free survival after matched unrelated transplants in 321 patients with ALL who were not in remission at transplant (Appelbaum, 1997).

A different approach involves the selection of haploidentical family donors based on the presence of feto-maternal microchimerism. Feto-maternal microchimerism is the presence of fetal hematopoietic cells in the materal bood and maternal hematopoietic cells in the fetal circulation. This may be a mechanism of the immunologic tolerance that exists between mother and offspring. Van Rood and colleagues (2002) showed that recipients of non-T cell-depleted maternal transplants had a signifcantly lower incidence of chronic GVHD than recipients of paternal transplants; they also demonstrated a lower rate of acute GVHD in sibling transplants mismatched for non-inherited maternal antigens (NIMAs) compared to those mismatched for non-inherited paternal antigens. These observations support the hypothesis that recipients may be tolerant to haploidentical related donors expressing NIMAs (mother or NIMA-mismatched siblings), and that the microchimeric mother may be hyporesponsive to inherited paternal antigens in the offspring Shimazaki *et al.* (2003) performed five non-T cell-depleted haploidentical family member transplants based on this hypothesis. At the time of the report, three patients were alive at 105+, 390+ and 467+ days posttransplant respectively.

Patient and family histocompatibility work-up

Once an appropriate patient has been identified, all first-degree relatives (i.e., siblings, parents, and children) should be typed for HLA-A, -B, and -DR. This approach has three rationales: first, to attempt to identify an HLA-identical sibling; second, if there is not an HLA-identical sibling, to identify a relative who is closely

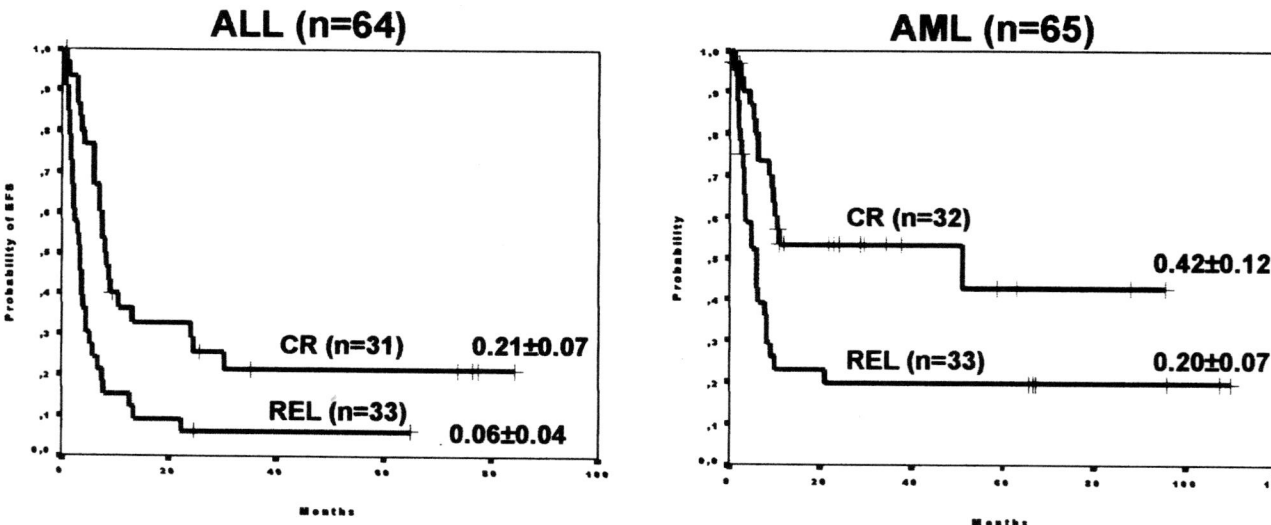

Fig. 66.12. Probability of event free survival (EFS) after haploidentical transplant in patients with acute lymphoblastic leukemia (ALL) or acute myeloid leukemia (AML) according to disease status at transplant. Upper curves refer to patients in any complete remission (CR) at transplant and lower curves to patients transplanted in relapse (REL).

enough matched to consider as a donor; and third, to identify the HLA haplotypes in the family in order to consider the feasibility of an extended family search for a donor. Table 66.11 illustrates a typical family study. In this example the patient and sib3 have inherited the same two HLA haplotypes from their parents, and hence are HLA-genotypically matched. Now assume that sib3 did not exist. Sib1 shares only one haplotype (A1-B8-DR3) with the patient and is mismatched for two antigens with respect to the nonshared haplotype. Both have A2, but they differ for B39 versus B27 and DR7 versus DR1. This would therefore be a two-antigen mismatch, and thus a candidate for an innovative approach, as described above. Sib2 is even more poorly matched, sharing neither haplotype with the patient.

Next, the presence or absence of first-degree relatives who might be appropriate donors should be determined. The mother is matched for HLA-A, but differs for both HLA-B and HLA-DR. The father differs for HLA-B and HLA-DR and hence is mismatched for at least two antigens. It is also noted that he is homozygous for HLA-A, and is therefore matched for HLA-A with respect to graft rejection (that is, the patient would see no HLA-A locus antigens on the father's cells that he/she does not have on his/her own cells). However, he/she differs for HLA-A with respect to GVHD (that is, the father would recognize HLA-A1 as foreign on the patient's cells). Therefore, the father is two locus mismatched with respect to rejection, and three locus mismatched with respect to GVHD. Finally, turning to the patient's children, we see no closer matches. As child 1 is homozygous for HLA-A, -B, and -DR, he/she and the patient are matched with respect to graft rejection, but are mismatched for three antigens with respect to GVHD. Close analysis of the haplotypes of the children and the patient's spouse reveal that there was a chance of

a fully matched child: the patient and spouse both carry the HLA-A1, -B8, -DR3 haplotype. If child1 had inherited the A2-B39-DR7 haplotype instead of the A1-B8-DR3 haplotype from the father, he/she would have been a match. He/she would have been genotypically matched by inheritance for A2-B39-DR7 from the father (the patient) and phenotypically matched for the A1-B8-DR3 haplotype, by chance carried by both patient and wife.

Although a matched or one-locus mismatched donor was not found within the patient's first-degree relatives, and assuming the patient was not a good candidate for a higher degree mismatched graft, a reasonable strategy presents itself. The patient has one very common haplotype (A1-B8-DR3) and one relatively uncommon haplotype (A2-B39-DR7) (see Table 66.12). The next step would be to "track" the A2-B39-DR7 haplotype through the extended family in the hope of finding an individual who also inherited the A2-B39-DR7 haplotype, and fortuitously also has inherited another A1-B8-DR3 haplotype. For each relative that has the 2,39,7 haplotype, there would be a 5.11% probability of that relative also by chance having the 1,8,3 haplotype, and hence would be a "zero-locus" mismatch with the patient. Thus, the patient's paternal uncles and aunts, then cousins should be evaluated. As long as the A2-B39-DR7

Table 66.11. *Family study of HLA haplotype segregation*

	Mother	Father	
HLA-A:	1 2	2 2	
HLA-B:	8 44	39 27	
HLA-DR:	3 2	7 1	

Patient	Sib1	Sib2	Sib3
1 2	1 2	2 2	1 2
8 39	8 27	44 27	8 39
3 7	3 1	2 1	3 7

Wife
1 3
8 35
3 1

Child1	Child2	Child3
1 1	3 2	3 1
8 8	35 39	35 8
3 3	1 7	1 3

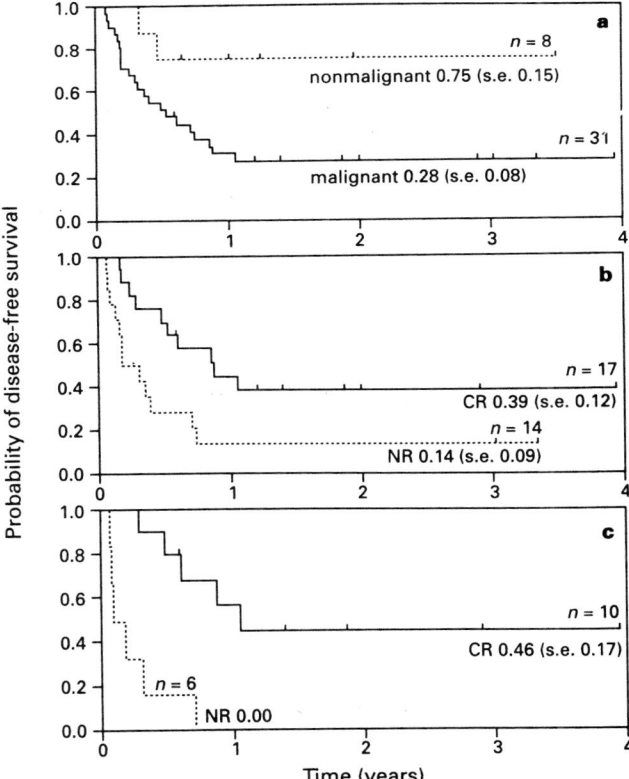

Fig. 66.13. Disease-free survival of patients after haploidentical transplantation with malignant and non-malignant diseases (**a**), malignant diseases in remission and not in remission (**b**), and in patients with ALL in remission or not in remission (**c**), at the time of transplant. Reproduced, with permission, from Handgretinger *et al.* (2001).

Table 66.12. *Common HLA haplotypes by race*

Caucasian		African-American		Asian-American		Hispanic		Native-American	
1,8,3[a]	5.11[b]	19,42,3	1.96	19,17,3	2.09	19,12,7	2.16	1,8,3	4.70
3,7,2	2.61	1,8,3	1.24	9,5,2	2.09	2,35,8	1.79	3,7,2	2.64
2,12,4	2.19	19,17,6	1.13	11,15,5	1.90	1,8,3	1.66	2,12,4	2.02
2,7,2	1.78	19,53,8	.96	19,12,6	1.56	2,35,4	1.35	2,7,2	1.87
19,12,7	1.67	28,17,5	.90	19,12,7	1.56	3,7,2	1.19	19,12,7	1.73
2,15,4	1.33	2,12,6	.81	2,46,9	1.49	19,14,1	1.13	2,15,4	1.51
1,17,7	1.15	2,12,5	.76	19,17,6	1.35	9,16,6	1.02	2,40,6	1.15
3,35,1	1.06	3,7,2	.76	19,13,7	1.27	28,16,4	1.02	1,17,7	1.01
2,40,6	.99	19,17,2	.72	9,40,4	1.21	2,16,4	1.00	19,40,4	.91
2,8,3	.78	2,12,4	.71	9,7,1	1.11	2,5,6	.94	3,35,1	.78
9,7,2	.77	19,35,6	.71	9,35,5	1.08	2,5,4	.93	9,5,4	.77
19,40,4	.76	19,7,5	.65	11,15,4	1.01	2,40,4	.86	19,5,4	.73
9,12,7	.74	19,12,7	.63	2,15,5	1.01	9,40,4	.84	2,12,5	.72
19,13,7	.71	10,12,2	.63	2,40,5	1.00	19,18,3	.84	2,40,4	.72
2,17,7	.71	19,53,6	.63	2,40,9	.91	9,35,5	.83	2,35,4	.67
9,35,5	.68	19,7,2	.60	9,40,2	.91	9,35,4	.82	2,15,6	.66
2,12,7	.64	2,7,2	.59	9,22,4	.90	2,12,4	.77	2,8,3	.65
2,12,5	.64	9,7,5	.56	9,40,5	.90	2,7,2	.69	2,17,7	.62
10,16,4	.61	19,53,5	.56	1,17,7	.88	2,15,4	.66	9,7,2	.61
19,14,1	.61	19,42,8	.55	2,16,2	.86	9,12,7	.64	19,35,4	.60

[a] "1,8,3" means the HLA-A1, B8, DR3 haplotype.

[b] Percent frequency of this haplotype in this race: 5.11% in this example.

haplotype can be demonstrated in a particular family branch, the search should continue in that branch. Common HLA haplotypes, sorted by race, which would make this strategy feasible, are listed in Table 66.12. A comprehensive listing of haplotype frequencies for patients of different races has been calculated (Beatty *et al.*, 1995; Milforde *et al.*, 1997), and a listing of such can be found on the World Wide Web site of the American Society for Histocompatibility and Immunogenetics (http://www.swmed.edu/home_pages/ASHI/ashi.htm). Computer programs are available to help in calculations (Kaufman, 1995; Schipper, D'Amaro, & Oudshoorn, 1996).

The average likelihood of finding a partially HLA-matched related donor is shown in Table 66.13. Tabulated by race are the probabilities of finding a "zero" locus mismatched donor (geno-

Table 66.13. *Average probability of a partial HLA-A,-B,-DR match assumes one HLA haplotype is matched by inheritance*

	Zero[a]	A[b]	B	DR	One[c]	A&B	A&DR	B&DR	Two[d]
Cauc	.68%	2.1%	2.5%	2.0%	5.3%	13.2%	8.0%	16.7%	31.2%
Afr	.31%	1.3%	2.4%	1.6%	4.8%	13.3%	8.2%	17.6%	34.1%
Asian	.52%	1.7%	2.9%	2.1%	5.7%	13.2%	8.6%	18.9%	34.3%
Hisp	.42%	1.6%	2.5%	1.7%	4.9%	13.3%	7.8%	17.4%	33.1%
Nat	.66%	1.9%	2.6%	2.0%	5.3%	13.1%	7.9%	17.3%	32.4%

Abbreviations: Cauc, Caucasian; Afr, African-American; Asian, Asian-American; His, Hispanic; Nat, Native-American.

[a] Given one shared haplotype, shown is the average probability of by chance being matched for HLA-A,-B,-DR with respect to the nonshared haplotypes.

[b] Probability of being mismatched only at this HLA locus: rest of loci on nonshared haplotype being matched.

[c] Probability of one- or zero-HLA mismatch.

[d] Probability of zero-, one-, or two-locus mismatch.

Table 66.14. *Probabilities of partial HLA-A,-B,-DR match based on a specific nonshared patient haplotype (assume one shared haplotype)*

	Zero	A	B	DR	One	A&B	A&DR	B&DR	Two
1,8,3	5.1%[a]	7.1%[b]	5.4%	6.7%	9.1%[c]	11%	9.4%	15.3%	21.5%
3,7,2	2.6%	6.7%	3.6%	4.6%	9.6%	15.4%	12.2%	13.5%	28.9%
2,12,4	2.2%	3.6%	6.2%	5.4%	1.8%	16.9%	14.2%	28.8%	46.9%
2,7,2	1.8%	6.7%	4.3%	3.2%	10.6%	15.4%	12.2%	28.8%	44.0%
19,12,7	1.7%	3.9%	3.3%	3.3%	7.2%	13.4%	14.2%	13.9%	32.7%
2,15,4	1.3%	2.4%	6.2%	3.0%	8.9%	16.9%	6.6%	28.8%	42.1%

[a] The probability of the related, one-haplotype matched, potential donor by chance also having the HLA-A1, -B8, -DR3 haplotype.

[b] The probability of the potential donor having HLA-B8, -DR3, and an A locus antigen other than A1.

[c] The probability of a zero or one antigen mismatch with respect to the HLA-A1, -B8, -DR3 haplotype.

typically matched by inheritance for one haplotype, fortuitously matched for all three antigens with respect to the nonshared haplotypes), a one-locus mismatch (subdivided by the probabilities for mismatch at a given locus), or a two-locus mismatch. The calculations assume one possible donor available: having additional haploidentical donors improves the odds. Returning to our example, again the chance of a zero-locus mismatch for the 1,8,3 haplotype is 5.11% (if the family is Caucasian). Table 66.13 takes the analysis of Table 66.12 one step forward. Examples are presented that show the chance of finding a partially matched related donor depends on the specific nonshared patient haplotype. If either a zero or one locus mismatch is considered acceptable, there is a 9.1% chance per candidate of finding such a donor.

All of these calculations are based on serologically defined HLA antigens. Each antigen can be subdivided into DNA-typing-defined alleles, as shown in Table 66.14 for HLA-DR1. Thus, these calculations should be considered best-case scenarios, and patients and candidate donors need to be HLA typed to the highest resolution possible.

Donor selection also requires cross-match testing to see if the recipient has been sensitized to the antigens of the donor through pregnancy or blood transfusions because sensitization to donor alloantigens may increase the risk of graft rejection (Anasetti, 1999). Standard procedures for cross-matching the patient's serum with donor lymphocytes use T cells as target cells to identify HLA Class I antibodies and B-cell cross-matching to identify HLA Class II antibodies.

Finally, in 2–3-loci mismatched transplants, given the role of alloreactive NK cells in preventing graft rejection, GVHD, and

acute myeloid leukemia relapse, donor-versus-recipient NK alloreactivity, which can be predicted by standard HLA-typing, should be a mandatory criteria when selecting the donor from among mismatched family members.

Conclusions

Nowadays allogeneic transplantation can be offered to virtually all patients. Until recently, even with a one-locus mismatch, there was a substantial risk of alloreactivity complications and going beyond it was potentially dangerous. Major breakthroughs came with the clinical application of a megadose of stem cells after extensive T-cell depletion. Currently transplantation from an HLA-mismatched family member is a viable option for patients with acute leukemia at high risk of relapse (Fig. 66.8) who urgently need a transplant and who do not have a well-matched unrelated donor.

In leukemia patients undergoing full-haplotype mismatched transplants, results in terms of TRM and EFS compare favorably with what is reported in patients at the same stage of disease receiving transplants from matched unrelated donors. Thus, mismatched transplantation should be offered, not as a last resort, but in the early stages of the disease to high-risk acute leukemia patients without a matched donor.

Interestingly, in AML patients transplanted from donors able to mount NK alloreactions, the extremely high probability of EFS is similar to what is reported in patients transplanted in

Table 66.15. *DNA-defined DRB1 allele frequencies within the DR1 antigen group, by race*

	Caucasian	African-American	Asian/Pacific	Hispanic	Native-American
0101	73%	38%	88%	50%	77%
0102	14%	56%	8%	41%	13%
0103	12%	5%	3%	8%	10%
0104	<0.01%	0%	0%	0%	0%

Table 66.16. *Full haplotype-mismatched HSC Transplantation: current indications[a]*

Acute myeloid leukemia	Acute lymphoid leukemia
High-risk CRI	High-risk CRI
CR ≥ II	High-risk CRII
Primary induction failure	
Relapse	

[a] For patients with AML in relapse haploidentical transplant is recommended only if the leukemia burden is low, if performance status is good, and if the donor is potentially NK alloreactive in the graft-versus-host direction.

first CR from HLA-identical siblings. NK cell alloreactivity may prove to be a powerful tool for enhancing the efficacy and safety of allogeneic hematopoietic transplantation. Furthermore, the tolerizing activity of facilitating cells such as expanded CD34+ cells or nonalloreactive cytotoxic T lymphocytes (CTLs) might be exploited in conditioning regimens to replace current myeloablative agents and minimize conditioning-related morbidity and mortality (Reich-Zeliger *et al.*, 2000; Bachar-Lustig *et al.*, 2001).

Future developments in these fields might extend the full-haplotype mismatched transplant to several categories of patients (e.g., the elderly) who cannot withstand highly intensive conditioning, patients with contraindications to intensive radio- and/or chemotherapy, and patients with nonmalignant hematological disorders in whom the current TRM rates are unacceptable.

References

Anasetti, C. (1999). Hematopoietic cell transplantation from HLA partially matched related donors. In *Hematopoietic Cell Transplantation*, 2nd ed., ed. E.D. Thomas, K.G. Blume, & S.J. Forman, pp. 904–14, New York: Blackwell Science Inc.

Anasetti, C., Amos, D., Beatty, P.G. *et al.* (1989). Effect of HLA compatibility on engraftment of bone marrow transplants in patients with leukemia or lymphoma. *New England Journal of Medicine*, **320**, 197–204.

Anasetti, C., Beatty, P.G., Storb, R. *et al.* (1990). Effect of HLA incompatibility on graft-versus-host disease, relapse, and survival after marrow transplantation for patients with leukemia or lymphoma. *Human Immunology*, **29**, 79–91.

Appelbaum, F.R. (1997). Allogeneic hematopoietic stem cell transplantation for acute leukemia. *Seminars in Oncology*, **24**, 114–23.

Ash, R.C., Horowitz, M.M., Gale, R.P. *et al.* (1991). Bone marrow transplantation from related donors other than HLA-identical siblings: effect of T cell depletion. *Bone Marrow Transplantation*, **7**, 443–52.

Aversa, F., Tabilio, A., Terenzi, A. *et al.* (1994). Successful engraftment of T-cell-depleted hapoidentical "three-loci" incompatible transplants in leukemia patients by addition of recombinant human granulocyte colony-stimulating factor-mobilized peripheral blood progenitor cells to bone marrow inoculum. *Blood*, **84**, 3948–55.

Aversa, F., Tabilio, A., Velardi, A. *et al.* (1998). Treatment of high risk acute leukemia with T-cell-depleted stem cells from related donors with one fully mismatched HLA haplotype. *New England Journal of Medicine*, **339**, 1186–93.

Aversa, F., Terenzi, A., Ballanti, S. *et al.* (2002). Full-haplotype mismatched HSCT is a valid option for high-risk acute myeloid leukemia (AML) patients. *Bone Marrow Transplantation*, **29**, (Suppl 2), O328 (Abstract).

Aversa, F., Terenzi, A., Carotti, A. *et al.* (2001a). Stem cell transplantation from full-haplotype mismatched donors in leukemia. *Haematologica*, **86**, (Suppl 10), CS016 (Abstract).

Aversa, F., Velardi, A., Tabilio, A. *et al.* (2001b). Haploidentical stem cell transplantation in leukemia. *Blood Reviews*, **15**, 111–9.

Bachar-Lustig, E., Rachamim, N., Li, H.W. *et al.* (1995). Megadose of T cell-depleted bone marrow overcomes MHC barriers in sublethally irradiated mice. *Nature Medicine*, **1**, 1268–73.

Bachar-Lustig, E., Reich-Zeliger, S., Gur, H. *et al.* (2001). Bone marrow transplantation across major genetic barriers: the role of magadose stem cells and nonalloreactive donor anti-third party CTLS. *Transplantation Proceedings*, **33**, 2099–100.

Beatty, P.G. (1992). Results of allogeneic bone marrow transplantation with unrelated or mismatched donors. *Seminars in Oncology*, **19**, 13–9.

Beatty, P.G. (1997a). Clinical and managed care issues in blood and marrow transplantation for hematologic diseases. *Experimental Hematology*, **25**, 1195–208.

Beatty, P.G. (1997b). Workshop on the importance of minor histocompatibility antigens. *Experimental Hematology*, **25**, 548–58.

Beatty, P.G., Clift, R.A., Mickelson, E.M. *et al.* (1985). Marrow transplantation from related donors other than HLA-identical siblings. *New England Journal of Medicine*, **313**, 765–71.

Beatty, P.G., Di Bartolomeo, P., Storb, R. *et al.* (1987). Treatment of aplastic anemia with marrow grafts from related donors other than HLA genotypically-matched siblings. *Clinical Transplantation*, **1**, 117–24.

Beatty, P.G., Mori, M., & Milford, E. (1995). Impact of racial genetic polymorphism on the probability of finding an HLA-matched donor. *Transplantation*, **60**, 778–83.

Buckley, R.H., Schiff, S.E., Schiff, R.I. *et al.* (1999). Hematopoietic stem-cell transplantation for the treatment of severe combined immunodeficiency. *New England Journal of Medicine*, **340**, 508–16.

Cavazzana-Calvo, M., Stephan, J.L., Sarnacki, S. *et al.* (1994). Attenuation of graft-versus-host disease and graft rejection by ex vivo immunotoxin elimination of alloreactive T cells in an H-2 haplotype disparate mouse combination. *Blood*, **83**, 288–98.

Chiang, K.Y., Van Rhee, F., Godder, K. *et al.* (2001). Allogeneic bone marrow transplantation from partially mismatched related donors as therapy for primary induction failure acute myeloid leukemia. *Bone Marrow Transplantation*, **27**, 507–10.

Cobbold, S.P., Martin, G., Quin, S. *et al.* (1986). Monoclonal antibodies to promote marrow engraftment and tissue graft tolerance. *Nature*, **323**, 164–6.

Cunningham, I., Aversa, F., & Martelli, M.F. (1997). Making successful haplotype-mismatched transplants possible. *Forum*, **7.2**, 203–11.

Dumont-Girard, F., Roux, E., van Lier, R.A. *et al.* (1998). Reconstitution of the T-cell compartment after bone marrow transplantation: restoration of the repertoire by thymic emigrants. *Blood*, **92**, 4464–71.

Fischer, A., Landais, P., Friedrich, W. *et al.* (1990). European experience of bone-marrow transplantation for severe combined immunodeficiency. *Lancet*, **336**, 850–4.

Fry, T.J. & Mackall, C.L. (2001). Interleukin-7: master regulator of peripheral T-cell homeostasis? *Trends in Immunology*, **22**, 564–71.

Gale, R.P. & Reisner, Y. (1986). Graft rejection and graft-versus-host disease: mirror images. *Lancet*, **1**, 1468–70.

Gluckman, E., Rocha, V., & Chevret, S. (2001). Results of unrelated umbilical cord blood hematopoietic stem cell transplantation. *Reviews in Clinical and Experimental Hematology*, **5**(2), 87–99.

Godder, K.T., Hazlett, L.J., Abhyankar, S.H. *et al.* (2000). Partially mismatched related donor bone marrow transplantation for pediatric patients with acute leukemia: younger donors and absence of peripheral blasts improve outcome. *Journal of Clinical Oncology,* **18**, 1856–66.

Greenwald, R.J., Boussiotis, V.A., Lorsbach, R.B. *et al.* (2001). CTLA-4 regulates induction of anergy in vivo. *Immunity,* **14**, 145–55.

Gribben, J.G., Guinan, E.C., Boussiotis, V.A. *et al.* (1996). Complete blockade of B7 family-mediated costimulation is necessary to induce human alloantigen-specific anergy: a method to ameliorate graft-versus-host disease and extend the donor pool. *Blood,* **87**, 4887–93.

Guinan, E.C., Boussiotis, V.A., Neuberg, D. *et al.* (1999). Transplantation of anergic histoincompatible bone marrow allografts. *New England Journal of Medicine,* **340**, 1704–14.

Gur, H., Krauthgamer, R., Berrebi, A. *et al.* (2002). Tolerance induction by megadose hematopoietic progenitor cells: expansion of veto cells by short-term culture of purified human CD34+ cells. *Blood,* **99**, 4174–81.

Hale, G., Cobbold, S., & Waldmann, H. (1988). T cell depletion with Campath-1 in allogeneic bone marrow transplantation. *Transplantation,* **45**, 753–9.

Handgretinger, R., Klingebiel, T., Lang, P. *et al.* (2001). Megadose transplantation of purified peripheral blood CD34(+) progenitor cells from HLA-mismatched parental donors in children. *Bone Marrow Transplantation,* **27**(8), 777–83.

Handgretinger, R., Schumm, M., Lang, P. *et al.* (1999). Transplantation of megadose of purified haploidentical stem cells. *Annals of the New York Academy of Sciences,* **872**, 351–61.

Hansen, J.A., Petersdorf, E., Martin, P.J., & Anasetti, C. (1997). Hematopoietic stem cell transplants from unrelated donors. *Immunology Review,* **157**, 141–51.

Heitger, A., Greinix, H., Mannhalter, C. *et al.* (2000). Requirement of residual thymus to restore normal T-cell subsets after human allogeneic bone marrow transplantation. *Transplantation,* **69**, 2366–73.

Henslee-Downey, P.J., Abhyankar, S.H., Parrish, R.S. *et al.* (1997). Use of partially mismatched related donors extends access to allogeneic marrow transplant. *Blood,* **89**, 3864–72.

Henslee-Downey, P.J., Byers, V.S., Jennings, C.D. *et al.* (1989). A new approach to the prevention of graft-versus-host disease using Xomazyme-H65 following histo-incompatible partially T-depleted marrow grafts. *Transplantation Proceedings,* **21**, 3004–7.

Henslee-Downey, P.J., Parrish, R.S., Macdonald, J.S. *et al.* (1996). Combined ex vivo and in vivo T-lymphocyte depletion for the control of graft-versus-host disease following haplo-identical marrow transplant. *Transplantation,* **61**, 738–45.

Horowitz, M.M., Gale, R.P., Sondel, P.M. *et al.* (1990). Graft-versus-leukemia reactions after bone marrow transplantation. *Blood,* **75**, 555–62.

Housley, R.M., Morris, C.F., Boyle, W. *et al.* (1994). Keratinocyte growth factor induces proliferation of hepatocytes and epithelial cells throughout the rat gastrointestinal tract. *Journal of Clinical Investigation,* **94**, 1764–77.

Kato, S., Yabe, H., Yasui, M. *et al.* (2000). Allogeneic hematopoietic transplantation of CD34+ selected cells from an HLA haplo-identical related donor. A long-term follow-up of 135 patients and a comparison of stem cell source between the bone marrow and the peripheral blood. *Bone Marrow Transplantation,* **26**, 1281–90.

Kaufman, R. (1995). HLA prediction model for extended family matches. *Bone Marrow Transplantation,* **15**, 279–82.

Kernan, N.A., Flomemberg, N., Dupont, B. *et al.* (1987). Graft rejection in recipients of T cell depleted HLA-nonidentical marrow transplants for leukemia: identification of host derived anti-donor allocytotoxic T lymphocytes. *Transplantation,* **43**, 482–7.

Kurtzberg, J., Martin, P., Chao, N. *et al.* (2000). Unrelated placental blood in marrow transplantation. *Stem Cells,* **18**, 153–4.

Lanier, L.L. (1998). NK cell receptors. *Annual Review of Immunology,* **16**, 359–93.

Lapidot, T., Lubin, I., Terenzi, A. *et al.* (1990). Enhancement of bone marrow allografts from nude mice into mismatched recipients by T cells void of graft-versus-host activity. *Proceedings of the National Academy of Science USA,* **87**, 4595–9.

Lapidot, T., Singer, T.S., Salomon, O. *et al.* (1988). Booster irradiation to the spleen following total body irradiation: a new immunosuppressive approach for allogeneic bone marrow transplantation. *Journal of Immunology,* **141**, 2619–24.

Lapidot, T., Terenzi, A., Singer, T.S. *et al.* (1989). Enhancement by dimethyl myleran of donor type chimerism in murine recipients of bone marrow allografts. *Blood,* **73**, 2025–32.

Margolis, D.A. & Casper, J.T. (1999). Allogeneic transplantation for acute myeloid leukemia in children. In *Hematopoietic Cell Transplantation,* 2nd Ed., ed. E.D. Thomas, K.G. Blume, & S.J. Forman, pp. 835–48. New York: Blackwell Science Inc.

Marmont, A.M., Horowitz, M.M., Gale, R.P. *et al.* (1991). T-cell depletion of HLA-identical transplants in leukemia. *Blood,* **78**, 2120–30.

Martelli, M.F. & Aversa, F. (2002). Full haplotype mismatched hematopoietic stem cell transplants. *Hematologia,* **5**, 73–6.

Martin, P.J., Hansen, J.A., Torok-Storb, B. *et al.* (1988). Graft failure in patients receiving T cell depleted HLA-identical allogeneic marrow transplants. *Bone Marrow Transplantation,* **3**, 445–56.

Milford, E.L., Mori, M., Graves, M. *et al.* (1997). HLA gene and haplotype frequencies in the North American population. *Transplantation,* **64**, 1017–27.

Moretta, A. & Moretta, L. (1997). HLA class I specific inhibitory receptors. *Current Opinion in Immunology,* **9**, 694–701.

Muller, S.M., Schulz, A.S., Reiss, U.M. *et al.* (1999). Definition of a critical T cell dose threshold for prevention of GVHD after HLA non-identical PBPC transplantation in children. *Bone Marrow Transplantation,* **24**, 575–81.

O'Reilly, R.J., Collins, N.H., Brochstein, J. *et al.* (1986). Soybean lectin agglutination and E-rosette depletion for removal of T-cells from HLA-identical marrow grafts: results in 60 consecutive patients transplanted for hematological malignancy. In *Minimal Residual Disease in Acute Leukemia 1986,* ed. A. Hagenbeek & B. Löwenberg, pp 337–44. Amsterdam: Martinus Nijhoff.

O'Reilly, R.J., Collins, N.H., Kernan, N. *et al.* (1985). Transplantation of marrow-depleted of T cells by soybean lectin agglutination and E-rosette depletion: major histocompatibility complex-related graft resistance in leukemia transplant recipients. *Transplantation Proceedings,* **17**, 455–9.

Ottinger, H., Grosse-Wilde, M., Schmitz, A., & Grosse-Wilde, H. (1994). Immunogenetic marrow donor search for 1012 patients: A retrospective analysis of strategies, outcome and costs. *Bone Marrow Transplantation,* **14** (Suppl 4), S34–8.

Pan, L., Delmonte, J. Jr, Jalonen, C.K., & Ferrara, J.L. (1995). Pretreatment of donor mice with granulocyte colony-stimulating factor polarizes donor T lymphocytes toward type-2 cytokine production and reduces severity of experimental graft-versus-host disease. *Blood,* **86,** 4422–9.

Patterson, J., Prentice, H.G., Brenner, M.K. *et al.* (1986). Graft rejection following HLA matched T-lymphocyte depleted bone marrow transplantation. *British Journal of Haematology,* **63,** 221–30.

Perruccio, K., Tosti, A., Posati, S. *et al.* (2001). Transfer of functional immune responses to aspergillus and CMV after haploidentical hematopoetic transplantation. *Bone Marrow Transplantation,* **27**(1), OS102 (Abstract).

Prentice, H.G., Janossy, G., Price-Jones, L. *et al.* (1984). Depletion of T lymphocytes in donor marrow prevents significant graft-versus-host disease in matched allogeneic leukemic marrow transplant recipients. *Lancet,* **1,** 472–5.

Przepiorka, D., Khouri, I., Ippoliti, C. *et al.* (1999). Tacrolimus and minidose methotrexate for prevention of acute graft-versus-host disease after HLA-mismatched marrow or blood stem cell transplantation. *Bone Marrow Transplantation,* **24,** 763–8.

Rachamin, N., Gan, J., Segall, R. *et al.* (1998). Tolerance induction by "megadose" hematopoietic transplants: donor-type human CD34 stem cells induce potent specific reduction of host anti-donor cytotoxic T lymphocyte precursors in mixed lymphocyte culture. *Transplantation,* **65,** 1386–93.

Reich-Zeliger, S., Zhao, Y., Krauthgamer, R. *et al.* (2000). Anti-third party CD8+ CTLs as potent veto cells: coexpression of CD8 and FasL is a prerequisite. *Immunity,* **13,** 507–15.

Reisner, Y., Ben-Bassat, I., Douer, D. *et al.* (1986). Demonstration of clonable alloreactive host T cells in a primate model for bone marrow transplantation. *Proceedings of the National Academy of Science USA,* **83,** 4012–5.

Reisner, Y., Kapoor, N., Kirkpatrick, D. *et al.* (1981). Transplantation for acute leukaemia with HLA-A and B nonidentical parental marrow cells fractionated with soybean agglutinin and sheep red blood cells. *Lancet,* **2,** 327–31.

Reisner, Y., Kapoor, N., Kirkpatrick, D. *et al.* (1983). Transplantation for severe combined immunodeficiency with HLA-A, B, D, DR incompatible parental marrow cells fractionated by soybean agglutinin and sheep red cells. *Blood,* **61,** 341–8.

Rocha, V., Cornish, J., Sievers, E.L. *et al.* (2001). Comparison of outcomes of unrelated bone marrow and umbilical cord blood transplants in children with acute leukemia. *Blood,* **97,** 2962–71.

Ruggeri, L., Capanni, M., Casucci, M. *et al.* (1999). Role of natural killer cell alloreactivity in HLA-mismatched hematopoietic stem cell transplantation. *Blood,* **94,** 333–9.

Ruggeri, L., Capanni, M., Urbani, E. *et al.* (2002). Effectiveness of donor natural killer cell alloreactivity in mismatched hematopoietic transplants. *Science,* **295,** 2097–100.

Sallusto, F., Lenig, D., Forster, R. *et al.* (1999). Two subsets of memory T lymphocytes with distinct homing potentials and effector functions. *Nature,* **401,** 708–12.

Shimazaki, C., Ochiai, N., Uchida, R. *et al.* (2003). Non-T-cell-depleted HLA-haploidentical stem cell transplantation in advanced hematologic malignancies based on the feto-maternal microchimerism. *Blood,* **101,** 3334–6.

Schipper, R.F., D'Amaro, J., & Oudshoorn, M. (1996). The probability of finding a suitable related donor for bone marrow transplantation in extended families. *Blood,* **87,** 800–4.

Schwartz, E., Lapidot, T., Gozes, D. *et al.* (1987). Abrogation of bone marrow allograft resistance in mice by increased total body irradiation correlates with eradication of host clonable T-cells and alloreactive cytotoxic precursors. *Journal of Immunology,* **138,** 460–5.

Sierra, J., Storer, B., Hansen, J.A. *et al.* (1997). Transplantation of marrow cells from unrelated donors for treatment of high risk acute leukemia: the effect of leukemia burden, donor HLA-matching and marrow cell dose. *Blood,* **89,** 4226–35.

Sierra, J., Storer, B., Hansen, J.A. *et al.* (2000). Unrelated donor marrow transplantation for acute myeloid leukemia: an update of the Seattle experience. *Bone Marrow Transplantation,* **26,** 397–404.

Sloand, E.M., Kim, S., Maciejewski, J.P. *et al.* (2000). Pharmacologic doses of granulocyte colony-stimulating factor affect cytokine production by lymphocytes in vitro and in vivo. *Blood,* **95,** 2269–74.

Small, T.N., Papadopoulos, E.B., Boulad, F. *et al.* (1999). Comparison of immune reconstitution after unrelated and related T-cell-depleted bone marrow transplantation: effect of patient age and donor leukocyte infusions. *Blood,* **93,** 467–80.

Soiffer, R.J., Mauch, P., Fairclough, D. *et al.* (1997). CD6+ T cell depleted allogeneic bone marrow transplantation from genotypically HLA non-identical related donors. *Biology of Blood & Marrow Transplantation,* **3,** 11–7.

Stockerl-Goldstein, K.E. & Blume, K.G. (1999). Allogeneic hematopoietic cell transplantation for adult patients with acute myeloid leukemia. In *Hematopoietic Cell Transplantation,* 2nd Ed., ed. E.D. Thomas, K.G. Blume, & S.J. Forman, pp. 823–34. New York: Blackwell Science.

Sullivan, K.M., Agura, E., Anasetti, C. *et al.* (1991). Chronic graft-versus-host disease and other late complications of bone marrow transplantation. *Seminars in Hematology,* **28,** 250–9.

Szydlo, R., Goldman, J.M., Klein, J.P. *et al.* (1997). Results of allogeneic bone marrow transplants for leukemia using donors other than HLA-identical siblings. *Journal of Clinical Oncology,* **15,** 1767–77.

Terenzi, A., Lubin, I., Lapidot, T. *et al.* (1990). Enhancement of T-cell-depleted bone marrow allografts in mice by thiotepa. *Transplantation,* **50,** 717–20.

van Rood, J. J., Loberiza, F. R., Zhang, M. J. *et al.* (2002). Effect of tolerance to noninherited maternal antigens on the occurrence of graft-versus-host disease after bone marrow transplantation from a parent or an HLA-haploidentical sibling. *Blood,* **96,** 1572–7.

Volpi, I., Perruccio, K., Tosti, A. *et al.* (2001). Post-grafting granulocyte colony-stimulating factor administration impairs functional immune recovery in recipients of HLA haplotype-mismatched hematopoietic transplants. *Blood,* **97,** 2514–21.

Wagner, J.L., Deeg, H.J., Seidel, K. *et al.* (1996). Bone marrow transplantation for severe aplastic anemia from genotypically HLA-nonidentical relatives. An update of the Seattle experience. *Transplantation,* **61,** 54–61.

Weiden, P.L., Flournoy, N., Thomas, E.D. *et al.* (1979). Antileukemic effect of graft-versus-host disease in human recipients of allogeneic-marrow grafts. *New England Journal of Medicine,* **300,** 1068–73.

PART VII UNRELATED DONOR HEMATOPOIETIC STEM CELL TRANSPLANTATION

67 Unrelated donor hematopoietic stem cell transplantation

CLAUDIO ANASETTI

Fred Hutchinson Cancer Research Center, Seattle, USA, and University of Washington, Seattle, USA

Introduction

The discovery that human leukocyte antigens (HLA) constitute the major histocompatibility complex (MHC) in humans led to successful transplantation of marrow stem cells from HLA-identical sibling donors. Transplants from partially HLA-incompatible relatives have been attempted for patients without a matched donor, but they are associated with an increased risk of graft rejection, graft-versus-host disease (GVHD), and lower survival that are correlated with the degree of genetic disparity. Progress in understanding the mechanisms for transplantation tolerance will continue to improve clinical results and lead to a predictable decrease in the requirement for HLA matching between donor and recipient. To date, however, the best option for curing patients .with congenital or acquired hematological disorders who are candidates for allogeneic transplantation is the use of hematopoietic stem cells (HSC) from HLA-compatible siblings or unrelated donors. The hurdle for a wider application and success of transplants from HLA-compatible unrelated donors resides in the great polymorphism of HLA genes. The discovery of HLA alleles, the development of precise and effective tissue typing techniques, and the assembly of large volunteer registries worldwide (currently approximately eight million HLA-typed individuals) have made feasible the transplantation of HSC from unrelated donors for the majority of patients.

Clinical results

Early reports

The first case of an HLA-compatible unrelated marrow transplant for severe aplastic anemia was reported in 1973 (Speck *et al.*, 1973) and that for hematologic malignancy in 1980 (Hansen *et al.*, 1980). These and other initial observations inspired the conception and assembly of large registries of HLA-typed volunteer marrow donors. The first national registry was the Anthony Nolan Research Center in London. The largest registry currently is the National Marrow Donor Program (NMDP) in the United States (Fig. 67.1). Nowadays, the probability of finding at least one HLA-A, B, and DR matched donor in the NMDP is greater than 85% for Caucasian patients and slightly less for non-Caucasian patients (Fig. 67.2). Updates can be found in the NMDP web site (www.marrow.org).

Transplant results from the NMDP

In 1993, Kernan and colleagues reported for the first time on the clinical results of unrelated donor transplants facilitated by the NMDP. This report detailed transplants for 459 patients with malignant ($n = 387$) or nonmalignant disorders ($n = 72$). The marrow transplants were performed in 29 centers and the transplant protocols varied considerably. The median age of the patients was 25.5 (range 0.3–54.5) years, while the median age of the donors was 37.9 (range 19–56) years. Donor compatibility testing in those early years almost exclusively relied on typing for antibody-defined antigens. Three hundred and four patients received marrow from HLA-A, B, DR compatible donors, and the remainder received marrow that differed by one HLA-A, B, or DR antigen. Ninety-three percent of patients engrafted, with an absolute neutrophil count of 0.5×10^9 per liter or greater at a median of 21 (range 6–121) days after transplant. Engraftment correlated significantly with the degree of HLA disparity. Acute GVHD grades II–IV occurred in 67% of patients and chronic GVHD in 51%. Increasing patient age correlated significantly with the occurrence of both acute and chronic GVHD.

The actuarial probability of disease-free survival at 1.5 years was 36% ± 0.4% (95% confidence intervals) for good prognosis patients transplanted for acute leukemia in first or second complete remission ($n = 58$), or chronic myeloid leukemia (CML) in first chronic phase ($n = 115$). This was significantly better than disease-free survival for patients with advanced leukemia or more advanced CML (20% ± 13%) (Fig. 67.3). Additional factors affecting disease-free survival included patient age, degree of HLA disparity, recipient's cytomegalovirus (CMV) serologic status, and the time between diagnosis and transplant. Disease-free survival for patients with aplastic anemia ($n = 29$) or myelodysplasia ($n = 32$) was poor at 16% ± 7% and 6% ± 6%, respectively. For 39 patients transplanted for an inherited disorder ($n = 39$), the survival rate was 64%. The primary cause of death for 302 patients included infection ($n = 60$), interstitial pneumonitis ($n = 52$), GVHD ($n = 45$), graft

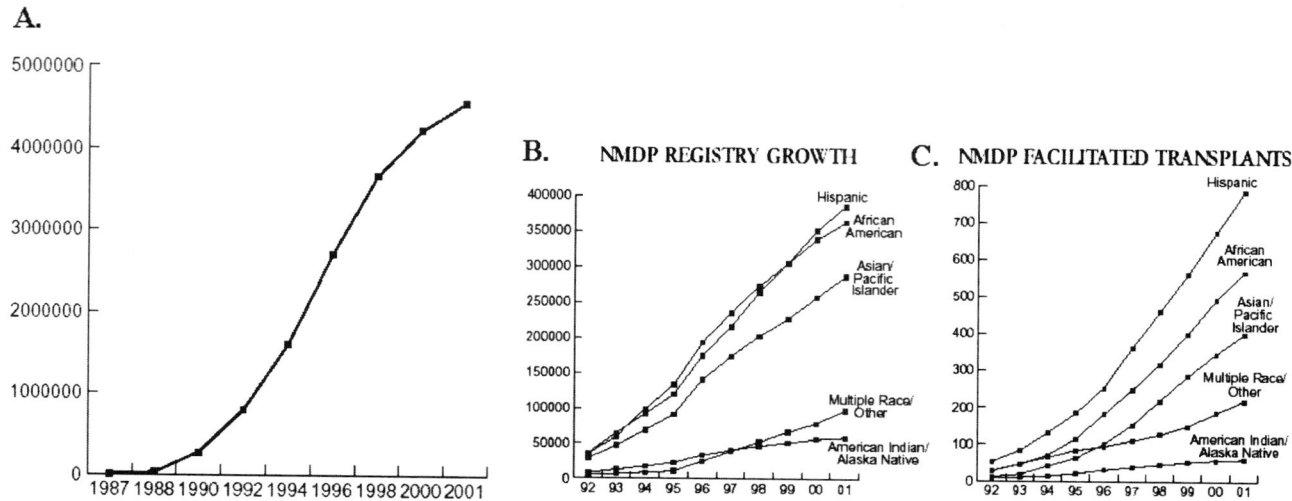

Fig. 67.1. **(A)** National Marrow Donor Program (NMDP) total registry growth. As of June 30, 2002, the number of potential volunteer donors was 4,713,296 and the number of unrelated stem cell transplants facilitated by the NMDP was 14,519. **(B)** NMDP Registry growth for non-Caucasian U.S. minorities. **(C)** As of June 30, 2002, the NMDP has facilitated 2,194 unrelated stem cell transplants for minority patients. Reproduced, with permission, by the NMDP (www.marrow.org).

failure ($n = 33$), relapse ($n = 36$), regimen-related toxicity ($n = 25$), hemorrhage ($n =$, secondary lymphoma ($n = 3$), and miscellaneous ($n = 29$). This large series reported from many transplant centers in the United States thus indicated that unrelated donor transplantation was feasible, but considerably more difficult than expected with the use of HLA-matched donors.

Milwaukee experience

Ash and colleagues (1990) reported a single-center study of T-cell-depleted marrow transplants from unrelated donors. Fifty-five patients, 47 of whom had malignancy, received transplants from unrelated donors that were compatible for 6 of 6 HLA-A, B, and DR loci and mixed leukocyte reaction (MLR) nonreactive ($n = 11$), or incompatible for 1 HLA locus ($n = 34$), or 2 HLA loci ($n = 10$). Pretransplant conditioning consisted of

high-dose cytosine arabinoside, cyclophosphamide, fractionated total body irradiation (TBI) 14 Gy, and methylprednisolone. Some patients with malignant disorders received oral busulfan before transplant in addition. Donor marrow was depleted of T cells with anti-T-cell receptor antibody T10B9 and complement. Cyclosporine (CSP) was administered after transplant. Engraftment occurred in 50 of 53 evaluable patients and acute GVHD grades II–IV in 46% (95% confidence intervals 27%–66%). The incidence was higher in those receiving mismatched than in those receiving matched transplants. The incidence of chronic GVHD and nonrelapse mortality was also higher in the latter patients. Disease-free survival for acute leukemia in first remission or CML in chronic phase was 48% (95% confidence limits 24%–73%), and was 32% for those with advanced leukemia (18%–51%). For the 8 patients with

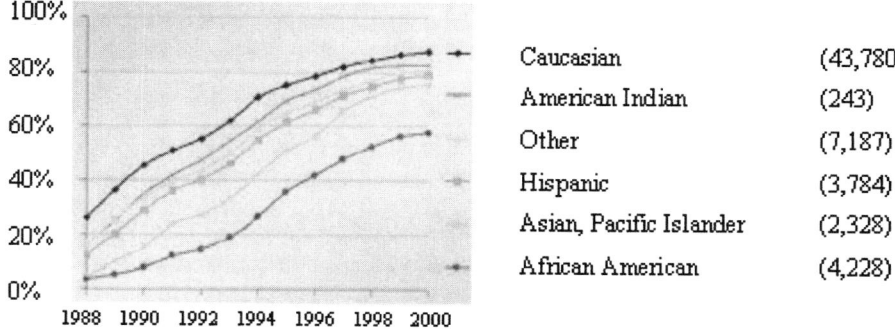

Fig. 67.2. Percentage of initial searches identifying at least one HLA-A, -B, and -DR compatible match in the NMDP registry, according to patient ethnic group. The numbers in parentheses represent the number of searches. Reproduced, with permission, by the NMDP (www.marrow.org).

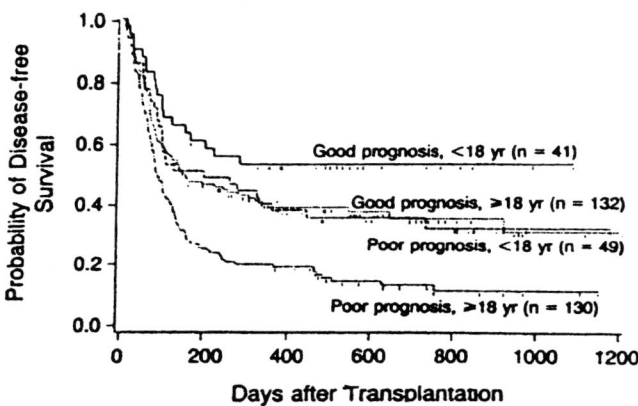

Fig. 67.3. Probability of disease-free survival according to prognostic factors for leukemia and age. Reproduced, with permission, from Kernan *et al.* (1993).

non-neoplastic disease, actuarial survival was 63%. Thirty-one of the 55 patients were dead at the time of the report, with interstitial pneumonitis being the most common single cause of death, followed in frequency by infection with aspergillus and pseudomonas. Two patients developed fatal B-cell lymphoproliferative disorders. Five patients died of recurrent disease. The actuarial probability of relapse for those transplanted for good risk neoplasia was 8% (1.5%–35%) and for those transplanted with advanced neoplasia was 16% (6%–34%). These results suggested that depletion of T cells from donor marrow could decrease the risk of acute GVHD, but it remained uncertain whether it could improve patient survival.

Morbidity and mortality compared to HLA-identical sibling transplants

International Bone Marrow Transplant Registry (IBMTR) data. A study of unrelated transplants in 37 centers reported to the IBMTR compared patients given HLA-A, B, and DR compatible unrelated transplants with those given transplants from siblings with an identical HLA genotype (Ash *et al.*, 1991). The incidence of acute GVHD grades II–IV was 32% and 53% in the sibling and unrelated donor cohorts, respectively (*P* < .0001) and 120-day mortality was 26% and 47%, respectively (*P* < .001). These data indicated that unrelated donor transplantation was considerably more difficult than HLA-identical sibling transplantation. Transplant complications were the same as those seen after HLA-identical sibling transplantation, but were more common and more severe.

IMUST study. The results of this cooperative group study on patients transplanted in 47 centers in Europe and North America (Howes *et al.*, 1993) showed a similar trend to those reported by Ash and colleagues (1991). The IMUST study also compared the results of unrelated donor transplantation to a matched cohort of HLA-identical sibling transplant recipients. The incidence of acute GVHD grades II–IV was 32% and 43%, and 100-day mortality was 22% and 47%. Thus, again unrelated donor transplant recipients had more acute GVHD and

worse survival than the control sibling group. Good prognostic factors for patient survival included being transplanted in a large center and being Caucasian.

Other single center experience. Single center studies also compared outcome for recipients of unrelated and sibling marrow allografts (Beatty *et al.*, 1991; Atkinson *et al.*, 1993; Bearman *et al.*, 1994). These studies comprised patients receiving HLA-A, B, and DR matched donor marrow. Recipients were prepared for transplant with cyclophosphamide and TBI; marrow was T-replete, and they received CSP/methotrexate (MTX) as GVHD prophylaxis. In the Sydney study, the unrelated recipients had a higher incidence of acute GVHD, which occurred earlier and was of greater severity compared to that in recipients of sibling allografts (Atkinson *et al.*, 1993). They also had a longer duration of posttransplant neutropenia [24 days to reach an absolute neutrophil count of $0.5 \times 10^9/l$ vs. 19.5 days (*P* = .07)], longer duration of first hospitalization, and a higher frequency of infection in the first 100 days posttransplant (*P* = .0004). Patient survival was similar in the two groups.

The preliminary Seattle experience with unrelated donor transplantation comprised 52 patients who received unrelated donor transplants and were compared for disease and disease stage with an age-matched cohort of 104 patients receiving HLA genotypically identical sibling transplants (Beatty *et al.*, 1991; Bearman *et al.*, 1994). There was no difference in engraftment rate or graft failure rate. However, acute GVHD grades II–IV occurred in 36% of the sibling transplants and 79% of the unrelated donor transplants (*P* < .001) (Fig. 67.4). Recipients of unrelated donor transplants had grade III–IV regimen-related toxicity of 31% compared to 21% after matched sibling transplantation (*P* = .1). The median duration of first hospitalization was 33 days for recipients of sibling marrow and 36 days for recipients of unrelated donor marrow (*P* = .02). In the Seattle study, the percentage of patients requiring readmission to the hospital and the actuarial probability of requiring either hemodialysis or mechanical ventilation were not statistically different between the two groups. There was similarity in disease-free survival, cause of death before day 100 (primarily pneumonia with or without acute GVHD), and cause of death after day 100 (relapse) in both groups. Thus, the increased severity of acute GVHD with unrelated donor grafts was also observed in this study. However, in contrast to the preceding reports, these small series of patients from single centers found similar disease-free survival between patients receiving unrelated and those receiving matched sibling transplants.

More recent results

A large IBMTR study of 2,055 recipients of allogeneic marrow transplants demonstrated significantly better leukemia-free survival in HLA-identical sibling recipients compared to HLA-compatible unrelated transplant recipients, particularly in those transplanted for early leukemia (Szydlo *et al.*, 1997) (Fig. 67.5). Even for transplants performed in recent years

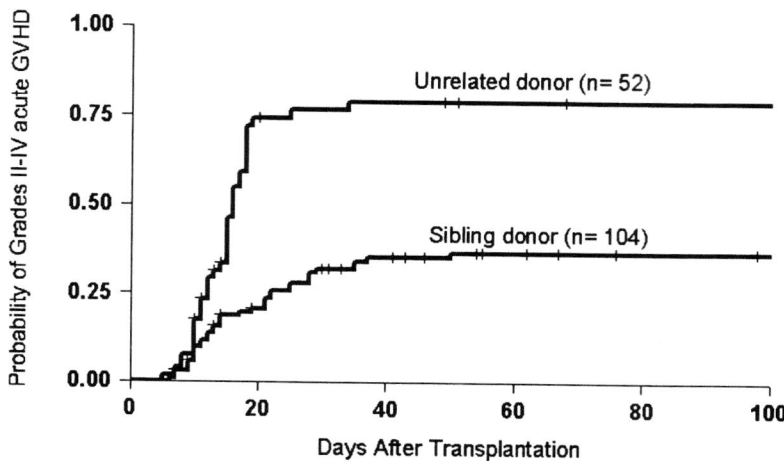

Fig. 67.4. Cumulative incidence of acute GVHD grades II to IV in recipients of marrow grafts from HLA-compatible unrelated or sibling donors. Reproduced, with permission, from Beatty *et al.* (1991).

(1994–2000), IBMTR data continue to show increased risk associated with the use of unrelated donors compared to HLA-identical sibling donors in patients otherwise comparable for age, diagnosis, and stage: the estimates for 100-day, 1-year, and 5-year mortality differ by up to 15% for the two types of donors (www.ibmtr.org). The fundamental reason for the increased morbidity and mortality associated with the use of unrelated donors must reside with the high degree of genetic disparity between donors and recipients that has remained undetected until recently by the unsophisticated tissue typing techniques employed for donor selection (Nademanee *et al.*, 1995; Petersdorf *et al.*, 1995; Petersdorf *et al.*, 1996; Petersdorf *et al.*, 1997; Hansen *et al.*, 1998; Petersdorf *et al.*, 1998; Sasazuki *et al.*, 1998; Petersdorf *et al.*, 2001b; Petersdorf *et al.*, 2001c; Flomenberg *et al.*, 2001; Morishima *et al.*, 2002). This issue will be discussed extensively below.

There are additional factors that may have produced a negative effect on the outcome of unrelated donor transplants. Because of the perceived increased risks associated with an unrelated donor graft, physicians have a tendency to reserve this procedure for patients with higher disease risk or a more advanced disease stage. For example, most transplant physicians would consider appropriate a sibling graft for acute myeloid leukemia (AML) patients with standard-risk cytogenetics, while they would only consider an unrelated donor graft for AML patients with high-risk cytogenetics (Burnett, 2001). An additional difference in risk between sibling and unrelated donor transplants may be associated with the choice of transplant protocol. Transplant physicians tend to enroll unrelated recipients on to transplant protocols with more intense conditioning regimens and postgrafting immunosuppression, with the hope of offsetting the increased risks of graft rejection and GVHD, but perhaps with the consequence of increasing the risks for organ toxicity and opportunistic infection.

Patients with CML in chronic phase represent the most homogeneous group of patients that can be utilized to assess the effects of donor type on outcome of allogeneic cell transplantation (McGlave *et al.*, 2000). Survival in this group of patients is better with younger patient age and short time interval from diagnosis to transplant. In order to minimize differences in the characteristics between study populations, Weisdorf and colleagues (2002) compared results of sibling and unrelated transplants for patients with CML transplanted in chronic phase within 1 year from diagnosis. The 5-year disease-free survival was inferior with unrelated transplantation by 7% to 11% in various age groups (Fig. 67.6).

Some single center studies have reported especially good results of unrelated transplants for CML. In a study from Seattle (Hansen *et al.*, 1998), survival was 74% at 5 years in patients up to 50 years of age with CML in chronic phase transplanted within the first year of diagnosis (Fig. 67.7). Survival improved over time with the use of more closely matched donors, preemptive therapy for CMV, and prophylaxis for *Candida albicans* (Goodrich *et al.*, 1991; Slavin *et al.*, 1995; Hansen *et al.*, 1998; Petersdorf *et al.*, 1998). The Italian Bone Marrow Transplant Group has also reported improved outcome over time (Dini *et al.*, 2001). The 1-year transplant-related mortality was 68% in patients grafted between 1979 and 1992 and 44% for patients grafted after 1993 ($P < .001$).

Influence of tissue typing on transplant outcome

In order to review the clinical results demonstrating the profound implications of improved tissue typing techniques and the more refined donor selection criteria that are in use nowadays, it is helpful to briefly review essential elements of histocompatibility (see also Chapter 8).

Essential elements of histocompatibility. Function and polymorphism of HLA. The HLA complex includes at least 12 genetic loci on the short arm of human chromosome 6. Each HLA locus is highly polymorphic because it can be occupied by multiple alternative forms of an HLA gene—designated HLA alleles. HLA alleles encode class I HLA-A, -B, and -C

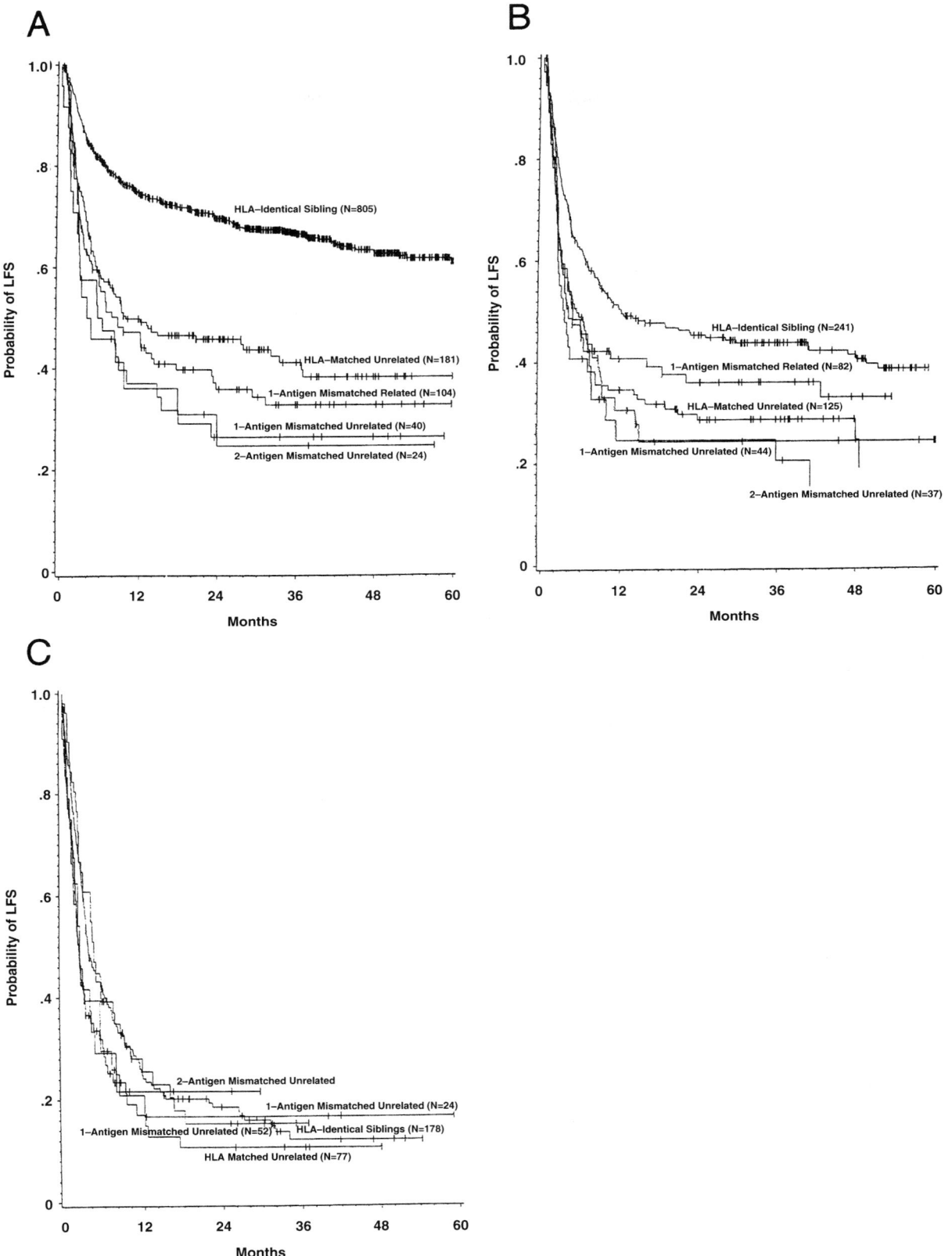

Fig. 67.5. Probability of leukemia-free survival after bone marrow transplants for early (**A**), intermediate (**B**), and advanced (**C**) leukemia by donor type. Reproduced, with permission, from Szydlo *et al.* (1997).

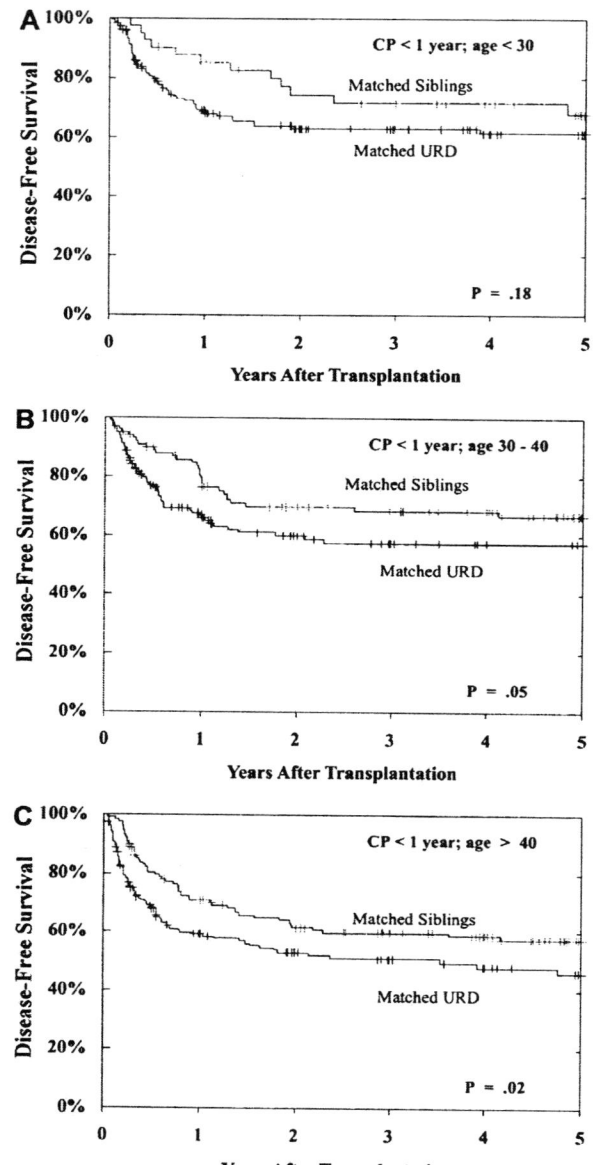

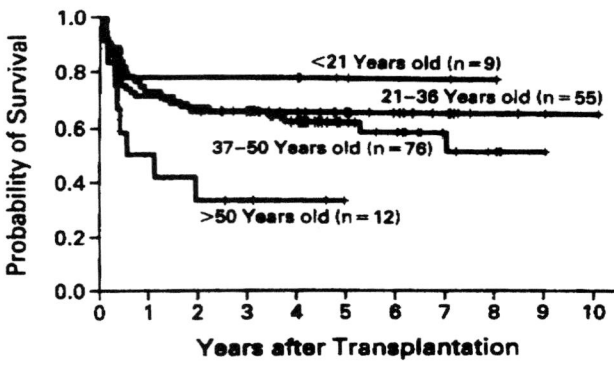

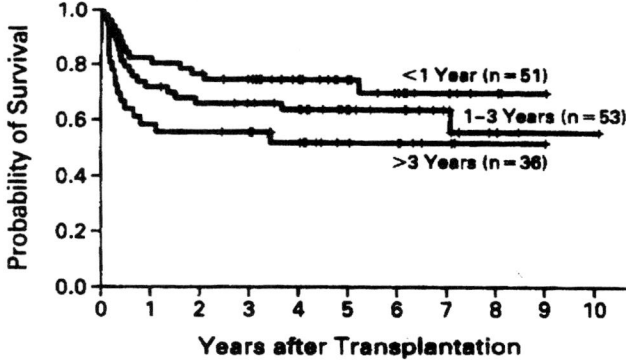

Fig. 67.7. (**A, top**) Probability of survival in 152 patients with chronic myeloid leukemia in chronic phase who received a transplant matched for HLA-A, -B, and -DRB1 from an unrelated donor in Seattle, according to age. (**B, bottom**) Probability of survival in 140 patients with chronic myeloid leukemia in chronic phase who were ≤ 50 years old and received a transplant matched for HLA-A, -B, and -DRB1 from an unrelated donor, according to the time from diagnosis to transplantation. Tick marks represent patients alive at the last follow-up. Reproduced, with permission, from Hansen *et al.* (1998).

Fig. 67.6. Probability of survival after bone marrow transplants for chronic myeloid leukemia (CML) in chronic phase within 1 year from diagnosis (**A**), 1–3 years (**B**), or more than 3 years (**C**) by donor type. Reproduced, with permission, from Weisdorf *et al.* (2002).

molecules, and class II HLA-DR, -DQ, and -DP molecules. Class I molecules are single chain glycoproteins expressed on the surface of all nucleated cells in the body in association with β_2-microglobulin and antigenic peptides. Class II molecules are expressed as α and β heterodimeric glycoproteins complexed with antigenic peptides on the surface of antigen-presenting cells such as dendritic cells, monocytes, and B cells, as well as on activated T cells. The function of HLA molecules is to bind antigenic peptides and activate adaptive immune responses in a specific manner. In order to accommodate the need for the binding of ever-changing environmental and microbial antigens, HLA molecules have evolved through gene duplication, gene conversion, recombination, and point mutation to acquire an enormous degree of polymorphism that is evident across different ethnic groups.

T-cell recognition. Disparity for minor histocompatibility antigens. Class I HLA molecules present cytosolic antigenic peptides and activate cytotoxic CD8+ T cells, while class II HLA molecules usually present processed extracellular antigenic peptides and activate helper CD4+ T cells. Both classes of HLA molecules lead to T-cell activation through the binding of specific T-cell antigen receptors. Immune responses are usually coordinated through the recognition of class II restricted peptides by CD4+ T cells that provide help through cytokine production and activation of antigen-presenting cells, and the induction of effector cytotoxic responses in CD8+ T cells, which recognize peptides in the context of class I. The best example of transplantation responses that require coordinated recognition of class I and class II-restricted peptides is rejection of skin transplants incompatible for HY-associated antigens. In this case, neither clonal responses directed to class I-restricted peptides nor those directed to class II-restricted peptides can result in skin graft rejection, while a coordinated response to both sets of peptides by CD4+ and CD8+ T cells leads to graft loss. In the case of HLA-identical sibling transplants, both rejection and acute GVHD occur, presumably as a result of incompatibility for polymorphic proteins that are presented as processed peptides that function as minor (non-HLA) histocompatibility antigens.

Disparity for HLA. Each HLA molecule binds a unique repertoire of antigenic peptides, which differs from the repertoire presented by other HLA molecules. In the case of an HLA-incompatible transplant, donor and recipient differ not only for one or more HLA molecules, but also for the thousands of antigenic peptides that each mismatched HLA molecule can bind and present to foreign T cells (direct recognition). It is also possible that mismatched HLA molecules are degraded and presented as peptides to responding T cells by self HLA (indirect recognition). Preclinical testing of human cells has predicted that the indirect recognition accounts for only 1% of the whole immune response to HLA incompatible molecules (Liu *et al.*, 1993). Studies in mice have confirmed the concept that acute GVHD mediated by CD8+ T cells depends on direct recognition of incompatible HLA molecules on host antigen-presenting cells (Shlomchik *et al.*, 1999). Since T cells can recognize the HLA sequence of amino acids that bind either antigenic peptides or T-cell receptors, disparity for an HLA allele with a single amino acid substitution could contribute to rejection or GVHD. Therefore, selection of HLA-compatible unrelated donors requires extremely sensitive typing techniques that must be able to distinguish between HLA alleles incompatible for a single amino acid polymorphism.

NK-cell recognition. Class I HLA molecules expressed on hematopoietic or lymphoid cells but not other cells also bind and activate specific receptors on natural killer (NK) cells. Target recognition and killing by NK cells are immediate and do not require immunity. The recognition process, however, is complex and only partially understood. On the one hand, recognition of allogeneic targets by one class of NK receptors can induce effector cell activation and immediate killing. On the other hand, a second class of NK receptors, the killing inhibitory receptors, bind HLA class I molecules on potential target cells and block NK effector function allowing NK cells to tolerate normal autologous cells, while destroying virally infected, mutated, or allogeneic cells. Therefore, NK cells only kill targets that do not express self-HLA molecules. NK-cell recognition is responsible for the rejection of MHC class I incompatible hematopoietic grafts in rodents, and the same process has been suggested to occur in humans (Ruggeri *et al.*, 2002). NK cells can kill leukemia cells but, since they only kill hematopoietic or lymphoid cells, NK cells do not cause tissue damage resulting in GVHD. Class I HLA mismatch for KIR-recognized allotypes appears to provide no certain benefit on the outcome of marrow transplantation from unrelated donors (Davies *et al.*, 2002).

Antibody recognition. HLA class I and II molecules also function as antigens by eliciting antibody responses by B cells. Anti-HLA antibodies can mediate hyperacute rejection of allogeneic stem cell transplants (Anasetti *et al.*, 1989; Ottinger *et al.*, 2002). Antibodies, however, do not distinguish all unique HLA molecules and, in fact, the development of genetic typing has demonstrated that very few antibody-defined antigens represent unique alleles. For example, HLA-A2 is defined as an individual antigen by specific antibodies, but DNA sequencing has identified at least 53 alleles, termed HLA-A*0201 through A*0258, that can be expressed as glycoprotein on the cell surface. Each allele has a unique DNA sequence, but all expressed glycoproteins cross-react with the same anti-HLA-A2 antibody. Thus, only selected combinations of HLA alleles, for example HLA-A*0101 and A*0201, function as antigens and can be distinguished by antibodies, in this case specific for HLA-A1 and A2, respectively.

HLA gene typing. Precise genetic methods have been developed to determine the allelic polymorphism of HLA genes, and the diversity found by DNA typing studies has greatly exceeded expectations (Tiercy *et al.*, 1991; Hurley, 1997; Scott *et al.*, 1998; Prasad *et al.*, 1999a, 1999b; Hurley *et al.*, 2000a, 2002). Most methods employ the polymerase chain reaction (PCR) to amplify genomic DNA. The primers utilized for the PCR can be specific for an entire locus, a group of alleles, or a specific allele. Typing is currently performed using one of the three most common technologies: sequence-specific primer amplification of genomic DNA (SSP), sequence-specific oligonucleotide probe hybridization of PCR-amplified DNA (SSOPH), or direct automated fluorescent sequencing. The level of resolution achieved depends on the individual test employed and the genetic probes utilized. Low or intermediate resolution typing discriminates between groups of HLA alleles that were formally recognized by serological typing, as for example, HLA-A*01XX versus HLA-A*02XX. High-resolution typing can distinguish between individual alleles that represent unique specificities, as for example, HLA-A*0101 versus HLA-A*0102. While SSP and SSOPH typing can generate commonly low or intermediate level resolution typing results, if a sufficient number of primers or probes are employed respectively in the two assays, high resolution typing can be achieved as well. More commonly, direct sequencing has been used for high-resolution DNA typing. Most tissue typing laboratories have implemented at least one DNA typing technology and algorithms have been developed for equating serologically defined specificities with DNA-defined alleles (Schreuder *et al.*, 2001). The complete and updated list of HLA alleles and their sequences is made available by the HLA informatics group web site (www.anthonynolan.com/HIG). The tables with HLA equivalents and a questionnaire for submission of serologic reaction patterns for poorly identified allelic products are also available on the World Marrow Donor Association web page (www.worldmarrow.org). Scott and colleagues (1998) used DNA-based typing methods for HLA-A and B on a cohort of 100 potential bone marrow donor/recipient pairs. They found that serological typing for HLA class I was limited in its ability to identify incompatibilities in unrelated pairs and that such incompatibilities were associated with a high frequency of alloreactive cytotoxic T-lymphocyte precursor cells. In another study, following DNA typing, only 52.9% of the originally 6/6 HLA- A, B, and DR matched unrelated donors remained 6/6, while 38.5%, 7.5%, and 1.1% were found to be 5/6, 4/6, and 3/6 matches, respectively (Prasad *et al.*, 1999b). Fleischhauer (1990) and Keever *et al.* (1994) proposed that mismatch for HLA-B*4402 vs. B*4403 can lead to rejection and GVHD after an otherwise HLA-matched unrelated donor graft. Thus, high-resolution DNA typing can uncover HLA disparities that are functional and not appreciated by old serological typing techniques.

Functional compatibility assays. Before DNA-based typing was developed, some laboratories used the MLR assay to assess compatibility between two individuals. Results of the mixed lymphocyte reaction (MLR) assay have a poor predictive value for acute GVHD after transplantation, which is better predicted by genotyping of HLA-DRB1, DQB1, and DPB1 alleles (Mickelson *et al.*, 1996). More sensitive assays have been developed to quantify the frequency of host-reactive helper T-lymphocyte and cytotoxic T-lymphocyte precursors in limiting dilution. Some investigators have proposed that both types of assays can detect mismatches for HLA and minor histocompatibility antigens and predict GVHD (Kaminski *et al.*, 1989). In other studies, however, these assays have not predicted for acute GVHD after transplantation (El Kassar *et al.*, 2001). At this time, there is no established role for functional assays in assessing donor and recipient pairs for HLA disparity and selecting donors (Oudshoorn *et al.*, 2002).

Minor histocompatibility antigens. Functional assays have been developed to define relevant minor histocompatibility antigens using antigen-specific, HLA-restricted clones, and experiments using HA-1-specific clones have established proof of principle that minor histocompatibility antigen mismatch between donor and recipient predicts for acute GVHD (Goulmy *et al.*, 1996). HA-1-reactive T cells expand after transplantation (Mutis *et al.*, 1999). The association between HA-1 mismatch and GVHD was confirmed in one study using HA-1 typing by SSOPH (Tseng *et al.*, 1999), although the study power to detect such an association was questioned in a follow-up report by the same laboratory (Lin *et al.*, 2001). It is likely that in the future routine typing of HLA and relevant minor histocompatibility antigens will be performed in prospective donor-recipient pairs using genetic rather than functional techniques, because the former provides superior standardization, reproducibility, and efficiency.

Immune regulation genes. Recent studies suggest that cytokine gene sequence polymorphisms may affect GVHD by regulating cytokine expression or function. Studies in small series HLA-identical sibling transplants have provided initial evidence that polymorphisms in interleukin (IL)-6, IL-10, tumor necrosis factor-α and interferon-γ genes (Middelton *et al.*, 1998; Cavet *et al.*, 2001; Cullup *et al.*, 2001; Socie *et al.*, 2001) may be associated with increased risk of GVHD. These studies will have obvious implications in the selection of unrelated donors.

Interpretation of results from clinical histocompatibility studies

Most published studies on the association between donor HLA mismatching and transplant outcome have one or more methodological limitations. In order to be interpretable, such epidemiological studies must evaluate typing data on all polymorphic HLA loci in both patient and donor, the typing techniques utilized must be sensitive enough to appreciate single amino acid substitutions in each HLA polymorphic domain, the analysis must be controlled for patient-, donor-, and treatment-associated variables, and there must be enough statistical power to detect relatively small differences in outcome. Using these criteria, the reader would find that few useful papers have been published so far, and such papers have included so few events that they have a very limited power to detect potentially important associations between HLA disparity and transplant outcome. Discussion will be limited to six papers (Petersdorf *et al.*, 1997; Petersdorf *et al.*, 1998; Sasazuki *et al.*, 1998; Petersdorf *et al.*, 2001b; Petersdorf *et al.*, 2001c; Morishima *et al.*, 2002) and one abstract (Flomenberg *et al.*, 2001), reporting studies that have evaluated donor and recipient typing for at least HLA-A, -B, -C, -DRB1, and -DQB1, have utilized DNA sequencing or equivalently sensitive typing techniques, and have utilized multivariable analyses controlling for variables extraneous to HLA. Questions addressed will be whether sufficient evidence was provided to demonstrate that a certain HLA locus is functional in unrelated donor transplantation, whether it is advisable that such a locus must be matched at the allele (DNA sequence) level in future transplants, and what type of outcome (i.e., rejection or GVHD) is affected by mismatch at that locus.

HLA-A, -B, and -C matching. Survival. Results of 1,874 unrelated donor marrow transplants facilitated by the NMDP were recently reported in abstract form (Flomenberg *et al.*, 2001). Treatment regimens were selected by the transplant center. DNA samples from patient and donor were typed at the sequence level for HLA-A, -B, -C, -DRB1, -DQB1, -DQA, -DPB1, and -DPA genes. The study revealed three major findings:

1. Mismatch for HLA-A, -B, -C, and -DRB1 loci is associated with worse survival compared to full match, while mismatch for -DQB1, -DQA, -DPB1, and -DPA is not significant (Table 67.1). Based on these data, it is advisable that future donors are matched not only at HLA-A, -B, and -DRB1 but also at HLA-C. Matching for HLA-DQ and -DP remains of unproven effect on survival.
2. Mismatching for one HLA-A, -B, or -DRB1 DNA sequence disparity (allele mismatch, i.e., A*0101 vs. A*0102, that is not recognized by anti-HLA antibodies) is associated with decreased survival compared to a full match. However, mismatching for one HLA-A, -B, and -DR disparity that is recognized by antibodies (antigen mismatch, i.e., A1 vs. A2) is associated with even worse survival. A Japanese study of 1,298 patients also found that high-resolution DNA typing of HLA-A and/or HLA-B allele mismatch reduced overall

Table 67.1. *Mismatch for HLA-A, -B, -C, and -DRBl alleles contribute to GVHD and death (n = 1,874)*

HLA locus mismatched	Typing resolution RR (95% CI)	Grade III/IV GVHD RR (95% CI)	P value	Death	P value
A	Low	1.52 (1.18–1.96)	.001	1.44 (1.20–1.73)	<.0001
A	High	1.33 (1.02–1.73)	.04	1.26 (1.02–1.55)	.03
B	Low	1.40 (1.07–1.83)	.01	1.51 (1.23–1.85)	<.0001
B	High	1.18 (.94–1.47)	.15	1.09 (.92–1.30)	.32
C	High	1.17 (.98–1.39)	.09	1.18 (1.03–1.34)	.02
DRB1	Low	1.43 (.90–2.29)	.13	1.51 (1.05–2.16)	.02
DRB1	High	1.26 (1.00–1.58)	.05	1.23 (1.04–1.47)	.02
DQ	High	1.02 (.83–1.25)	.86	.96 (.83–1.12)	.62
DP	High	1.19 (.99–1.43)	.06	1.06 (.88–1.26)	.55

Reproduced, with permission, from Flomenberg *et al.* (2001).

survival in both standard-risk and high-risk leukemia cases (Morishima *et al.*, 2002). Thus, high-resolution DNA typing at the DNA sequence level for HLA-A, -B, and -C is useful in selecting for more closely matched and safer donors. However, if a fully matched donor is not available, mismatch for an allele is preferable to mismatch for an antigen.

3. Mismatch for multiple alleles at HLA-A, -B, -C, and -DRB1 compounds the risk of mortality (Petersdorf *et al.*, 1998; Flomenberg *et al.*, 2001; Morishima *et al.*, 2002). The implications of such a finding are obvious.

In a separate study, Ferrara and colleagues (2001) have proposed that the position of amino acid disparity within the class I molecule may also have relevance to transplant outcome. The amino acid in position 116 forms the floor of the HLA molecule, and binds the C-terminal common motif of antigenic peptides thereby contributing to the selection of the peptide repertoire. Disparity for position 116 was associated with GVHD and mortality after unrelated donor transplants.

GVHD. The NMDP and the Japanese studies found that disparities for HLA-A, -B, -C, or -DRB1 alleles were independent risk factors for acute GVHD (Flomenberg *et al.*, 2001; Morishima *et al.*, 2002). HLA-A or -B allele mismatch was a significant risk factor for the occurrence of chronic GVHD (Morishima *et al.*, 2002).

Graft failure. The risk of graft failure is increased with donor disparity for HLA-A, -B, or -C (Peterdorf *et al.*, 1997, 2001b; Morishima *et al.*, 2002) and with patient homozygosity at the mismatched locus (Petersdorf *et al.*, 2001b), but not with mismatch for class II loci. When donors and recipients differ for a single HLA class I, the risk of graft failure varies according to whether the incompatibility is for an HLA antigen or an HLA allele. In the study by Petersdorf and colleagues (2001b) in patients transplanted from an unrelated donor, there were no episodes of rejection with a mismatch for a single allele (*n* = 47), compared to 14% rejection with a mismatch for a single antigen (*n* = 51) and 22% rejection if there was mismatch for multiple alleles (*n* = 9) (Table 67.2). These data on graft failure demonstrate that mismatch for an antigen has worse clinical consequences than mismatch for an allele, presumably because the former is associated with disparity for a greater number of amino acid residues in the HLA molecule. Furthermore, the effect of mismatching for multiple alleles is cumulative. These concepts are consistent with the survival data from a single center and national registry studies (Petersdorf *et al.*, 1998; Flomenberg *et al.*, 2001; Morishima *et al.*, 2002).

HLA-DRB1 matching. GVHD and mortality. Using HLA SSOPH for typing HLA-DRB1 and DQB1 in 50 donor-recipient pairs who were serologically matched for an HLA-A, B, and DR, Tiercy and colleagues (1991) found that 56% of the

Table 67.2. *Proportion of heterozygous unrelated donor marrow recipients with graft failure*

Matching category	Proportion with graft failure (%)	Odds ratio (95% CI)	P value
Matched	2/280 (0.7)	1.0	–
One class I mismatch			
HLA-A, -B, or -C allele	0/47	0 (∞–31.9)	1.0
HLA-A, -B, or -C antigen	7/51 (14)	21.8 (4.0–221.2)	<.001
Multiple class I mismatches			
Alleles	2/9 (22)	37.4 (2.4–585.9)	.005
Alleles and antigens	11/67 (16)	26.9 (5.7–256.5)	<.001

Reproduced, with permission, from Petersdorf *et al.* (2001c).

pairs were mismatched at either DRB1 or DQB1 loci. Petersdorf and colleagues (1995) analyzed 364 patients and their HLA-A, B, DR serologically matched donors to determine whether molecular typing of DRB1 alleles could allow more accurate donor-recipient matching and thereby improve clinical outcome after unrelated donor transplantation. The DRB1 alleles were typed by SSOPH. Of the 364 pairs, 305 were matched and 59 were mismatched for DRB1. The conditional probability of moderate to severe acute GVHD was 48% for the matched and 70% for the DRB1 mismatched recipients (Fig. 67.8). DRB1 matching was also associated with decreased transplant-related mortality rate and improved survival. This was the first study to demonstrate that DNA typing techniques have the power to identify functional HLA mismatches associated with poor transplant outcomes, and led the way to the transplant community adopting DNA-based typing as the gold standard for the selection of hematopoietic cell donors. The association between DRB1 mismatching with GVHD and mortality was later confirmed by studies from the European Bone Marrow Transplant Group (Devergie et al., 1997) and the NMDP (Petersdorf et al., 2001a). The limitation of these initial studies on the role of DRB1 on transplant outcome derives from the lack of consideration given to undetected mismatches for HLA-A, B, and C allele sequences. Despite matching for HLA-A, B, and DR antigens, HLA-DRB1 disparity predicts for additional mismatching for one or more HLA-A, B, and C alleles (Prasad et al., 1999b). Therefore, it is conceivable that all the three studies overestimated the risks associated with an isolated DRB1 allele mismatch, because of the confounding role of additional mismatching for HLA-A, B, or C.

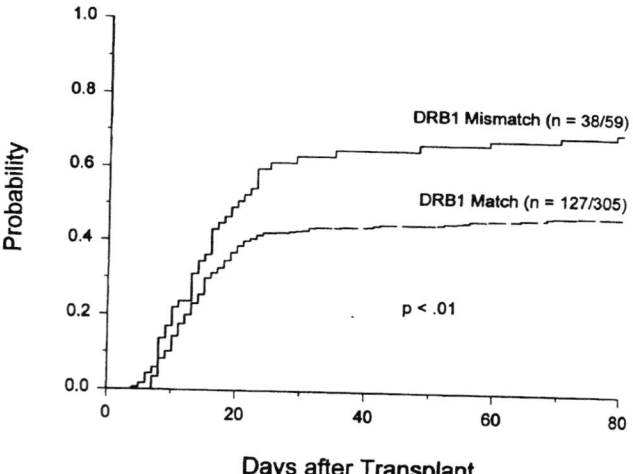

Fig. 67.8. Conditional probability of grades III–IV acute GVHD in DRB1-matched (*n* = 305) and mismatched (*n* = 59) groups. The probability of developing acute GVHD by day 80 after transplantation was .48 for DRB1-matched patients and 7.0 for mismatched patients. Data in parentheses denote the number of patients who developed grades III–IV GVHD. Reproduced, with permission, from Petersdorf et al. (1995).

A subsequent study from Petersdorf et al. (1998) used DNA sequencing to identify the HLA-A, B, and C alleles in 300 patients and their unrelated donors and SSOPH to type DRB1 and DQB1. The risk of acute GVHD was highest with DRB1 mismatch alone or in combination with DQB1. Mortality, however, was not significantly increased by a single DRB1 disparity, but it was increased by double or multiple disparities at DRB1 or DQB1 in combination with HLA-A, B, or C. The Japanese studies by Sasazuki et al. (1998) and Morishima et al. (2002) also failed to identify a significant association of single DRB1 allele mismatch with mortality. In contrast, a weak association between DRB1 allele mismatching and increased mortality was found in the larger NMDP study (Flomenberg et al., 2001) (Table 67.1). Thus, data suggest that DRB1 allele mismatching does not contribute to graft failure, but it contributes to acute GVHD and patient mortality, at least in the U.S. population that is predominantly Caucasian, even when donor and recipient are matched for HLA-A, B, and C alleles.

HLA-DQ and DP matching. HLA-DQ and DP incompatibilities contribute to T-cell reactivity in mixed lymphocyte culture, indicating that they are implicated in immune responses and that may act as transplantation antigens. In marrow transplantation performed between siblings, HLA-DP mismatches are extremely rare, but in unrelated donor-recipient pairs otherwise matched at HLA-A, B, C, DRB1, and DQB1, the proportion of HLA-DP mismatches is 80% to 85% (Petersdorf et al., 2001c). For this reason, it would not be practical to exclude unrelated donors solely on the basis of HLA-DP incompatibility. In the Seattle analyses, mismatches for DQB1 (Petersdorf et al., 1996) or DPB1 (Petersdorf et al., 2001c) were associated with an increased risk of acute GVHD. One report suggests that mismatching for DPB1 may increase mortality after transplantation (Varney et al., 1999). A French study found two HLA-DP incompatibilities to be associated with increased acute GVHD risk and poorer survival (Loiseau et al., 2002). The associations between DQ or DP incompatibility and GVHD or mortality after transplantation were not confirmed by the NMDP (Flomenberg et al., 2001) or by the Japanese studies (Sasazuki et al., 1998; Morishima et al., 2002). It is obvious, however, that given the multiple comparisons, the statistical power to detect significant differences was low in each study, and multivariable analyses of larger series of transplants are needed before mismatch for any HLA locus can be discounted as biologically irrelevant.

MHC haplotype matching. Tay and colleagues (1995) developed a simple and rapid method based on the amplification and electrophoretic analysis of duplicated polymorphic MHC sequences that distinguished between allelic blocks in the beta region (including HLA-B and C) and in the delta region (including HLA-DR and DQ). They proposed that unrelated recipients matched for the beta and delta blocks had survival comparable to that achieved with HLA-identical sibling transplant recipients, and better than if matched only for class I HLA by serology and for class II HLA by molecular technology. A thorough analysis of functional genes in the beta and the delta blocks will be of paramount importance for exploiting this technique.

Remaining challenges in defining acceptable histocompatibility criteria

Modern HLA typing using DNA technology can distinguish subtle polymorphisms previously undistinguishable by classical serological typing techniques. It is possible, however, that demanding donor matching at the DNA sequence level for all alleles at the HLA-A, B, C, and DRB1 loci will constitute an unnecessary stringency, and in some cases will prevent patient access to transplantation. The allowable limits of genetic disparity will likely differ according to the patient's underlying disease and stage. While patients with low-risk disease and fair life expectancy in the absence of transplant would want to avoid even the minimal risk associated with a mismatched donor, patients with high-risk disease in advanced stage will likely have to tolerate the risk associated with the use of a donor mismatched for a single antigen or multiple alleles, rather than face the greater risks of the underlying disease without transplantation (Ottinger *et al.*, 2001). Therefore, the definition of an acceptable mismatch will require analyses of a large number of patients with homogeneous disease risk and an identical treatment protocol.

Technical considerations

Donor search

Indications for an unrelated donor search

The diseases that can be considered for treatment by unrelated donor HSC transplantation are the same as those considered for family member donor transplantation, although some physicians would have reservations about proceeding to unrelated donor transplantation at the present time as early as they would proceed to HLA-identical sibling transplantation. The clinical indications for unrelated donor transplantation currently accepted by the NMDP are shown in Table 67.3. The most common indications are acute myeloid leukemia, acute lymphoblastic leukemia, chronic myeloid leukemia, myelodysplas-

Table 67.3. *Diseases treatable by hematopoietic stem cell transplantation*

Malignant disorders of the hematopoietic system
Leukemias
    Acute lymphoblastic leukemia (ALL)
    Acute myeloid leukemia (AML)
    Acute biphenotypic leukemia
    Acute undifferentiated leukemia
    Chronic myeloid leukemia (CML)
    Chronic lymphatic leukemia (CLL)
    Prolymphocytic leukemia
    Juvenile chronic myeloid leukemia
Myelodysplastic syndromes
    Refractory anemia
    Refractory anemia with ringed sideroblasts
    Refractory anemia with excess blasts
    Refractory anemia with excess blasts in transformation

Lymphomas
    Hodgkin's lymphoma
    Non-Hodgkin's lymphoma
Plasma cell disorders
    Multiple myeloma
    Plasma cell leukemia
    Waldenström's macroglobulinemia
Myeloproliferative disorders
    Acute myelofibrosis
    Chronic myelomonocytic leukemia (CMML)
    Essential thrombocythemia
    Myelofibrosis with agnogenic myeloid metaplasia
    Polycythemia vera
Histiocytic disorders
    Histiocytosis X
    Hemophagocytosis
Other malignancies
    Breast cancer
    Renal cell carcinoma
Nonmalignant disorders
Inherited erythrocyte abnormalities
    Beta thalassemia major
    Sickle cell disease
Inherited immune system disorders
    Ataxia-telangiectasia
    Severe combined immunodeficiency disorder
    Kostmann syndrome
    Leukocyte adhesion deficiency
    Chediak-Higashi syndrome
    Omenn syndrome
    Wiskott-Aldrich syndrome
    X-linked lymphoproliferative disorder
Inherited disorders of metabolism
    Adrenoleukodystrophy
    Sly syndrome, beta-glucuronidase deficiency
    Gaucher's disease
    Hunter syndrome
    Hurler syndrome
    Krabbe's disease
    Maroteaux-Lamy syndrome
    Metachromatic leukodystrophy
    Neiman-Pick disease
    Other mucopolysacharidoses
    Osteopetrosis
    Sanfilippo syndrome
    Wolman's disease
Inherited platelet abnormalities
    Amegakaryocytosis
    Congenital thrombocytopenia
Aplastic marrow disorders
    Severe aplastic anemia
    Pure red cell aplasia
    Fanconi anemia
    Paroxysmal nocturnal hemoglobinuria

tic syndrome, and severe aplastic anemia. The timing of transplantation varies depending on disease diagnosis and stage, prior results of transplantation, and available nontransplant therapies for the condition considered. Indications and results of unrelated donor transplantation are presented in detail in the chapters on allogeneic HSC transplantation for each disease.

Acute leukemia (and see Chapters 50 and 51). Marrow transplants from unrelated donors are usually performed in acute leukemia patients with primary induction failure or after first relapse. Transplant physicians prefer unrelated to autologous transplants for patients with high-risk features, including short duration of first remission (Busca *et al.,* 1994). There is active debate but little data about the indication for unrelated transplants for patients with AML with high-risk features in first remission, including high-risk cytogenetics and more than one cycle of chemotherapy to induce a first complete remission (Burnett, 2001). There is more enthusiasm and initial pilot data in unrelated transplants for patients with high-risk acute lymphoblastic leukemia (ALL) with t(4;11) or t(9;22) translocations, where 40% of patients (*n* = 64) survive disease-free at 2 years (Cornelissen *et al.,* 2001). Larger phase II studies of unrelated donor transplantation in patients with high-risk AML or ALL in first CR are warranted.

Chronic myeloid leukemia (and see Chapter 52). Unrelated donor transplantation within the first year provides better quality-adjusted survival than interferon-α in patients up to the age of 40 with newly diagnosed CML (Lee *et al.,* 1997). The benefits of transplantation decrease with a lower Sokal score, older patient age (Lee *et al.,* 1998). and the inexperience of the treatment center (Dresse *et al.,* 1999). A trial with single or combination therapy including interferon-α, cytarabine, and imatinib mesylate (Drucker *et al.,* 2001) should be considered as first-line therapy for all CML patients beyond 50 years of age, or patients above 40 with low-risk CML. Transplantation should be considered for patients up to the age of 40 with a matched sibling or unrelated donor, or older patients that fail to achieve complete cytogenetic response to nontransplant therapies (Appelbaum, 2001; Drucker *et al.,* 2001a and b).

Marrow failure, and myelodysplastic and myeloproliferative syndromes (and see Chapters 53, 54, and 58). Unrelated donor transplantation may represent the sole treatment modality for patients with life-threatening marrow failure, aplastic anemia unresponsive to immunosuppressive therapy, and high-risk myelodysplastic and myeloproliferative syndromes. Results are better in patients with aplastic anemia or refractory anemia, compared to those with advanced myelodysplasia and myeloproliferative syndromes, and patients with a short interval from diagnosis to transplant (Deeg *et al.,* 1999; Castro-Malaspina *et al.,* 2002). Results in patients with treatment-related myelodysplasia and AML have improved over time and with the use of less intense conditioning regimens (Witherspoon *et al.,* 2001).

Probability of finding a matched donor

Because of the enormous polymorphism of HLA genes, the probability of matching two random individuals for both alleles at HLA-A, -B, -C, -DR, -DQ, and -DP loci is extremely low. The success of matching, however, is higher than expected because of nonrandom association between certain alleles at one HLA locus and alleles at other loci, a phenomenon designated linkage disequilibrium. The DP locus represents an exception to this rule, because there is high frequency of DNA recombination between DQ and DP. HLA types are associated with the ethnic

group of an individual. The probability of matching a patient with a donor from a pool of unrelated volunteers depends on the HLA diversity of the patient ethnic group, the ethnic relationship of the patient to the donor pool, and the number of donors in the pool. Global efforts have led to the development of registries enlisting HLA-typed volunteer donors initially in the United Kingdom and the United States and later in the rest of Western and Eastern Europe, Australia, Asia, and the Americas. More than 8 million HLA-typed volunteer donors, including cord-blood cells, from over 51 registries in 37 countries appear in the Bone Marrow Donors Worldwide (BMDW) file available on the Internet from the Europdonor Foundation at the University of Leiden in the Netherlands (www.bmdw.org). An in-depth description of how to utilize the worldwide donor registry network is given in Chapter 23. HLA data for each potential volunteer donor varies for the number of typed genes and the level of resolution. Approximately 60% of the global donor pool has only been typed for HLA-A and -B antigens by low-resolution DNA or serological typing; the remaining 40% has also been typed for HLA-DR. Very few donors have been typed by high-resolution DNA for HLA-A, -B, and -DRB1 allele sequences and almost none for HLA-C and -DQ. More than 95% of the transplants are from donors who are already typed for at least HLA-A, -B, and -DR. The World Marrow Donor Association has published recommended guidelines for the histocompatibility testing of unrelated donors (Hurley *et al.,* 1999). These include the required use of DNA-based testing for HLA-DR and the recommended use of DNA-based testing for HLA-A and -B. Further, if serology is used for HLA-A and -B, then a DNA-based method must be used to define antigens in the population tested that are frequently missed and/or misassigned. As a minimum, all serologic splits should be resolved at a low level DNA-based resolution. It is likely that based on data from Flomenberg and colleagues (2001), consideration will be given by the WMDA for including in the recommendation upfront donor typing for HLA-C.

The probability of finding at least one HLA-A, -B, and -DR low-resolution match in the NMDP has grown as a function of the logarithm of the registry size from 15% in 1987 to greater than 80% in 2001 (Fig. 67.2). The probability of finding a match for HLA-A, -B, -C, -DR, and -DQ at the allele sequence level is postulated to be substantially less, 38% in one report from Europe (Tiercy *et al.,* 2000). For many patients it will not be feasible to find a complete match. Such likelihood varies greatly from one individual to another, however, and depends on how common or how rare that individual's combinations of HLA types are in the registry (Beatty *et al.,* 1988). For patients from minority ethnic groups, the chances of finding matched unrelated donors are lower than those for Caucasians (Beatty & Kollman, 1995). This issue is related not only to the smaller representation of minorities in the registries but also to their degree of HLA polymorphism (Freytes & Beatty, 1996). For example, the number of Hispanic and African-American volunteer donors is similar (Fig. 67.2a); however, the probability of finding at least an HLA-A, -B, -DR match is higher for Hispanics (Fig. 67.2b). For those patients with common HLA types, a well-matched donor will always be found;

for those with very rare HLA types there is a lower chance of finding a donor. This may change as the global donor pool enlarges, and as the matching requirements for donor-recipient pairs become less stringent with the development of new treatment modalities that may offset the risk of complications currently inherent in the use of mismatched donors.

Non-HLA criteria for donor selection. In a series of 6,978 transplants facilitated by the NMDP between 1987 and 1999, evaluation of donor characteristics as risk factors revealed age to be the only donor parameter besides HLA matching that was significantly associated with overall and disease-free survival (Kollman *et al.,* 2000). Five-year overall survival rates for recipients were 33%, 29%, and 25% with donors aged 18 to 30 years, 31 to 45 years, and greater than 45 years, respectively ($P = .0002$). A similar effect was noted among HLA-mismatched recipients. Additionally, the cumulative incidence of grade III to IV acute GVHD was 30%, 34%, and 34%, respectively ($P = .005$), and that of chronic GVHD at 2 years posttransplant was 44%, 48%, and 49% ($P = .02$). The use of male or nulliparous female donors was associated with lower risk of chronic GVHD compared to the use of multiparous female donors. The use of heavier donors was associated with higher yield of nucleated marrow cells (the role of a higher marrow cell dose on transplant outcome is discussed below). Donor and recipient combinations of gender, CMV serology, red cell ABO type, and race did not affect survival.

Non-HLA barriers to unrelated donor stem cell transplantation

A prospective survey involving 544 searches of the NMDP was conducted to identify reasons why many patients who have apparent HLA-compatible donors do not proceed to transplant (Kollman *et al.,* 2001). In 1 year, 41% of the patients received a transplant, 6% had their search continued, 9% had no survey follow-up, and 46% had their search terminated. Most commonly, a decision was made against transplant (21%) with preference given to other forms of treatment or no treatment. Death and worsening of the patient's medical condition in the face of a lengthy search process were common (17%) barriers to transplantation, while lack of finances was cited as the most important reason 3% of the time.

Speed of donor search

The time interval from the initiation of the search to transplant is a median of 4 months. In a study conducted through 1995 at the University of Minnesota, an unrelated donor search was initiated for 58 patients with ALL. A donor was identified for 22 patients (37% of searches) and 15 of the 22 patients underwent an unrelated transplant. The median time from patient referral to donor identification was 10 weeks. Nineteen percent of referred patients died prior to transplant despite all efforts to expedite the transplant (Davies, Ramsey, & Weisdorf, 1996). Thus, searching for an unrelated donor is a time-consuming process, although exceptions can occur, as indicated by a remarkable case in which an unrelated donor transplant was performed within 7 days of the need for it being identified (Oudshoorn *et al.,* 1996). In this case

report, a 27-year-old patient with acute myeloid leukemia was treated with an unrelated marrow transplant within 7 days of the accidental loss of his autologous marrow inoculum. Factors that allowed this very rapid identification and utilization of an unrelated donor included the recipient having a common HLA phenotype, the assistance of an experienced donor registry, a large donor file with fully HLA-A, -B, -DR typed donors, and good communication between the registry and the HLA laboratory in the hospital where the patient was located. With the use of molecular HLA typing technology and with the establishment of repositories containing donor DNA, it may no longer be necessary to call in specific donors for complete typing, resulting in further shortening of the donor search. There are, however, required steps including donor and recipient work-up and waiting lists at the transplant center that will likely prevent decreasing the time interval from initiation of the search to transplant below 2 to 3 months.

Alternative sources of allogeneic hematopoietic stem cells

For patients without an HLA-identical sibling donor, alternative sources of stem cells are partially HLA-matched relatives, matched unrelated volunteers, or unrelated cord blood. The impact of donor type on the outcome of marrow transplantation was investigated in children with Wiskott-Aldrich syndrome by the IBMTR and the NMDP (Filipovich *et al.,* 2001). Fifty-five transplants were from HLA-identical sibling donors, 48 from other relatives, and 67 from unrelated donors. The 5-year probability of survival differed by donor type: 87% (95% CI, 74–93%) with HLA-identical sibling donors, 71% (95% CI, 58–80%) with unrelated donors, and 52% (95% CI, 37–65%) with other related donors. Boys receiving an unrelated donor transplant before age 5 had survivals similar to those receiving HLA-identical sibling transplants.

A single center study in Milwaukee compared transplantation outcomes in patients with hematologic malignancies who received marrow grafts from either HLA-matched unrelated, one antigen mismatched unrelated, or highly mismatched family donors (Drobyski *et al.,* 2002). Between 1993 and 2000, 139 patients underwent transplantation from unrelated donors (81 matched and 58 mismatched) and 48 patients received marrow grafts from family donors that were mismatched at 2, 3, or 4 HLA-A, -B, -DR, and -DQ loci. All patients received a standardized conditioning regimen and a GVHD prophylaxis schedule with the exception of recipients of haploidentical marrow grafts, who received antithymocyte globulin (ATG) after bone marrow transplantation as additional immunosuppression. There was no statistically significant difference in the rate of engraftment, nor in the cumulative incidences of acute and chronic GVHD between any of the three groups. Transplant-related mortality was significantly higher in recipients of mismatched unrelated grafts (45%, $P = .01$) and haploidentical grafts (42%, $P = .001$) compared with recipients of matched unrelated marrow grafts (23%). This resulted in a significantly higher probability of overall survival for matched unrelated recipients (58%) versus either mismatched unrelated (34%, $P = .01$) or haploidentical (21%, $P = .002$) recipients. This study supports the contention that patients lacking a HLA matched family donor be offered a matched unrelated donor if available. With the limitations imposed by the low degree of HLa typing resolution employed, this single center data and IBMTR data (Fig. 67.5), there is no apparent advantage to using a one antigen mismatched unrelated donor versus a more HLA-disparate family donor.

A retrospective study by Eurocord compared unrelated cord blood or marrow transplants for children with leukemia (Rocha et al., 2001). Despite a higher degree of HLA incompatibility, cord blood was associated with less acute and chronic GVHD than was marrow. Relapse was similar after cord blood or marrow transplantation. Cord blood led to higher mortality during the first 100 days due to failed or delayed engraftment. This study supports the contention that transplantation of partially matched cord blood is effective treatment for children without a suitably matched unrelated marrow donor.

Transplant protocols

Conditioning regimens and engraftment

The standard regimen for conditioning patients before T-replete marrow grafts from unrelated donors consists of cyclophosphamide 60 mg/kg/day on 2 consecutive days and fractionated TBI 1,200 to 1,575 cGy given in 6 to 12 fractions over 3 to 7 days. Despite lower relapse rates, randomized trials in sibling transplants failed to show improved survival with 1,575 cGy compared to 1,200 cGy, because of increased nonrelapse mortality (Clift et al., 1994, 1998). Most transplant centers nowadays use 1,200 cGy TBI plus standard dose cyclophosphamide. Such a regimen before unrelated transplants appears very well tolerated in patients up to the age of 40 years, but is too toxic for those beyond 50 years (Hansen et al., 1998), begging the question as to whether older patients will fare better with a regimen that does not employ TBI. Topolsky and colleagues (1996) utilized busulfan 16 mg/kg and cyclophosphamide 50 mg/kg for 3 days. Patients also received cyclosporine (CSP)/methotrexate (MTX) for GVHD prophylaxis. All 25 patients engrafted and there were no cases of secondary graft failure. Ninety-four percent of patients engrafted in a series by Bertz and colleagues (1997) and there were no cases of secondary graft failure. Deeg and colleagues (2002) reported on a regimen of busulfan, with doses targeted to a blood level concentration at steady state of 800 to 900 nanograms per milliliter, plus standard dose cyclophosphamide in patients with myelodysplastic syndrome up to the age of 66 years. Graft failure occurred in 2 of 64 unrelated recipients and survival was similar after unrelated or sibling donor transplants.

Several centers have begun to investigate whether less intense conditioning regimens can decrease toxicity and improve survival, especially in older patients after marrow transplantation from HLA-compatible unrelated donors. No rejection of T-replete marrow occurred in 16 patients with hematologic malignancies conditioned with fludarabine 30 mg/m^2/day for 6 days, busulfan 4 mg/kg/day for 2 days plus anti-T lymphocyte globulin (ATG) 10 mg/kg/day for 4 days (Nagler et al., 2001). The minimal effective TBI dose sufficient to achieve engraftment in patients with aplastic anemia was 200 cGy when used in combination with cyclophosphamide 50 mg/kg/day for 4 days and ATG 30 mg/kg for 3 days (Deeg et al., 1994, 2001). A regimen consisting of the humanized anti-CD52 antibody CAMPATH-1H, 20 mg/day on days –8 to –4, fludarabine, 30 mg/m^2 on days –7 to –3, and melphalan, 140 mg/m^2 on day –2 led to engraftment in 42 of 44 patients with hematologic malignancies (Chakraverty et al., 2002). In this study, GVHD prophylaxis was with CSP alone. Three patients developed grade III to IV acute GVHD. The probability of nonrelapse mortality at day 100 was 15%, the overall and progression-free survivals at 1 year were 75% (95% CI, 63%–88%) and 62% (95% CI, 46%–77%), respectively (Fig. 67.9). These results indicate that certain low-intensity conditioning regimens without high-dose TBI can ensure stable engraftment of unrelated donor marrow grafts.

In an NMDP analysis of 5,246 recipients of unrelated donor transplants, the incidence of primary graft failure in patients surviving at least 28 days was 4% (Davies et al., 2000). Multivariate analysis showed that engraftment was associated with matching for HLA-A, HLA-B, and HLA-DRB1, higher cell dose, younger recipient, male recipient, and recipient from a non–African-American ethnic group. Secondary graft failure occurred in 10% of patients achieving initial engraftment, and was associated with poor survival. In multivariate analysis, factors associated with secondary graft failure were lower cell dose, older donor, DRB1 mismatch, recipient seropositivity for CMV, African-American ethnic group, Hispanic ethnic group, and initial engraftment after day 28. Quality of engraftment is an important predictor of survival after unrelated donor marrow transplantation.

Cell dose effect

The number of cells in the stem cell inoculum seems to be increasingly recognized as an important factor influencing a number of outcomes in addition to engraftment rate. In a study of 174 patients with acute leukemia receiving T-replete marrow from unrelated donors (median age 20, range 0.5–54 years), transplantation of a marrow nucleated cell dose above the median value of 3.65×10^8/kg was associated with faster neutrophil and platelet engraftment (Figs. 67.10A and B) and a decreased incidence of severe GVHD (Fig. 67.10C). In patients transplanted in remission, the use of a marrow cell dose above the median translated into less nonleukemic death (Figs. 67.10D and E) and better leukemia-free survival (Fig. 67.10F); transplant in remission with a high dose of marrow cells was associated with the best outcome in both children and adults (Sierra et al., 1997, 2000). A possible explanation for this finding is that a higher cell dose leads to a decreased incidence of early posttransplant infection, which itself may amplify GVHD.

A similar finding was reported in children receiving unrelated donor transplants for CML where event-free survival was 65% for those receiving $>3.5 \times 10^8$ mononuclear cells per kilogram compared to 49.7% for all patients overall (Dini et al., 1996). Similar findings have also been reported in children receiving unrelated donor transplants for Hurler syndrome (Peters et al., 1996): 62% of patients alive at 1 year who had

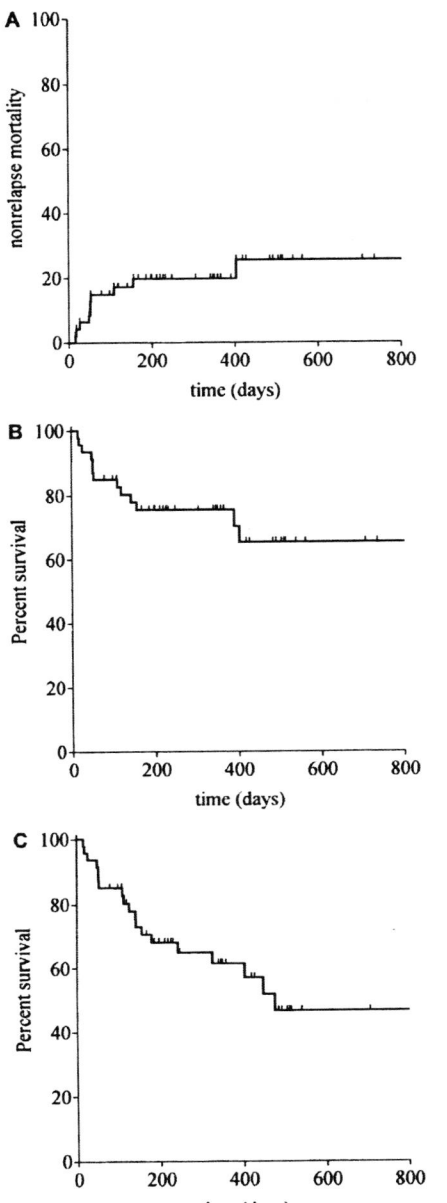

Fig. 67.9. Survival probabilities according to Kaplan-Meier curves for patients conditioned with fludarabine, melphalan, and Campath-1H and transplanted with unrelated donor marrow. (A) Nonrelapse mortality. (B) Overall survival. (C) Progression-free survival. Reproduced, with permission, from Chakraverty et al. (2002).

received a bone marrow cell dose >3.5 × 10^8/kg were estimated to be alive at 3 years in contrast to 24% receiving less than this dose. Similar findings have been described in recipients of T-replete HLA-matched sibling transplants for severe aplastic anemia, in recipients of umbilical cord blood transplants, and, in terms of CD34$^+$ cell number, in recipients of both HLA-identical family member transplants and haploidentical family member transplants (see also Chapter 13).

So far, there has been no improvement in survival with T-cell-depleted compared to T-cell-replete marrow transplants in unrelated donor transplantation (Wagner et al., 1998; Champlin et al., 2000). One of the possibilities that may explain the lack of improved survival despite the decreased incidence of GVHD, is that the ex vivo marrow manipulation has led to the loss of stem cells. Data have shown that in T-cell-depleted transplants, the CD34$^+$ cell dose in the graft is correlated with better outcome (Mavroudis et al., 1996). The concept that a higher stem cell dose can improve outcome relates also to the use of T-cell-depleted stem cell transplants (Aversa et al., 1998).

Peripheral blood stem cells

Studies of peripheral blood stem cell (PBSC) transplants should be considered for patients with acute leukemia with the goal of enhancing the stem cell dose and improving survival. In matched-cohorts studies by Ringden et al. (1999) and Remberger et al. (2001), PBSCs achieved faster neutrophil and platelet engraftment compared to marrow transplantation, but there was no difference in acute GVHD, relapse, treatment-related mortality, or survival. Elmaagacli and colleagues (2002) proposed that in patients with CML in chronic phase, PBSCs were associated with decreased relapse and improved survival compared with bone marrow from HLA-compatible unrelated donors.

T-cell depletion

Removal of CD4$^+$ cells, with retention of a defined number of CD8$^+$ cells, from HLA-mismatched unrelated marrow did not appreciably decrease the risk of grade III–IV acute GVHD (Martin et al., 1999). Depletion of CD8$^+$ cells was associated with an increased risk of rejection with either HLA-DRB1 or with HLA-A or B disparity between donor and recipient. Using CD6$^+$ cell depletion of the marrow as the sole form of GVHD prophylaxis, Soiffer and colleagues (2001) reported an incidence of grade II–IV acute GVHD of 42% in 48 patients conditioned with cyclophosphamide, TBI, and total lymphoid irradiation (TLI). All patients engrafted, the 100-day mortality was 19%, and estimated 2-year survival was 44% for the entire group and 58% for those less than 50 years. CD34 selection of unrelated donor PBSC has been used with some success in children with ALL given myeloablative conditioning and no posttransplant pharmacologic immune suppression (Lang et al., 2003).

To compare strategies for T-cell depletion and to compare T-cell-depleted with non-T-cell-depleted transplants, Champlin and colleagues (2000) studied 870 patients with leukemia who received T-cell-depleted transplants from unrelated or HLA-mismatched related donors from 1982 to 1994. Outcomes were compared with those of 998 non-T-cell-depleted transplants. Five categories of T-cell-depletion techniques were considered: narrow-specificity antibodies (i.e. specific for T-cell subsets), broad-specificity antibodies, Campath antibodies, elutriation, and lectins. Recipients of transplants T-cell depleted by narrow-specificity antibodies had higher leukemia-free survival than recipients of transplants T-cell depleted by other tech-

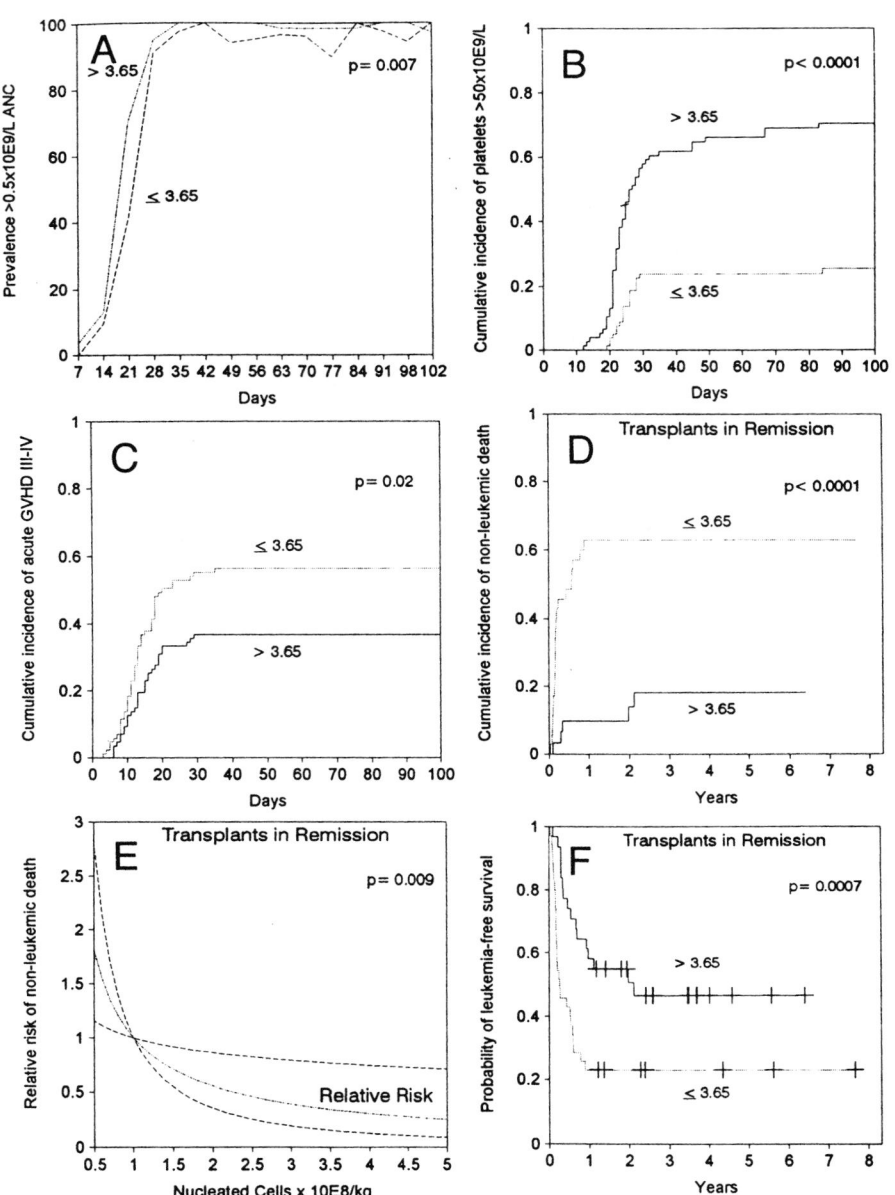

Fig. 67.10. Effect of marrow cell dose (nucleated cells × 10^8/kg of recipient body weight) on (**A**) prevalence of neutrophil count above 0.5×10^9/l; (**B**) cumulative incidence of achieving a self-sustained platelet count greater than 50×10^9/l; (**C**) cumulative incidence of grade III–IV acute GVHD; (**D**) cumulative incidence of nonleukemic death after transplant in remission; (**E**) estimated relative risk (RR) of nonleukemic death in transplants in remission showing a linear decrease in the RR by increasing marrow cell dose (the dashed lines indicate limit 95% CI); (**F**) leukemia-free survival after transplant in remission. Reproduced, with permission, from Sierra *et al.* (1997).

niques. The 5-year leukemia-free survival was 31% after T-replete transplants, 29% (*P* = ns) after transplants T-cell depleted by narrow-specificity antibodies, and 16% (*P* < .0001) after transplants T-cell depleted by other techniques. Thus, GVHD prophylaxis by marrow T-cell depletion by either type of techniques did not translate in improved survival.

Pharmacological prophylaxis and therapy for GVHD

One study compared CSP and MTX versus CSP, MTX and methylprednisolone (MP) in sequential cohorts of patients

(Leelasiri *et al.*, 1995). Twenty-nine patients with malignant hematologic disease were treated between May 1990 and November 1993. All donors were matched serologically for HLA-A, -B, and -DR. Sixteen patients received CSP/MTX and 13 received CSP/MTX/MP. CSP was given at a dose of 1.5 mg/kg i.v. every 12 hours beginning from day −1 and MTX at a dose of 10 mg/m^2 on days 1, 3, and 6 with folinic acid on days +2, +4, and +7. MP was administered at a dose of 0.25 mg/kg i.v. every 12 hours beginning at day +7 and increased to 0.5 mg/kg on day +14. Beginning on day +35 MP and CSP were tapered by 5% per week. GVHD occurred in 77% of the CSP/MTX group and in 50% of the CSP/MTX/MP group ($P > .1$). The conclusion from this study was that CSP/MTX remained suboptimal GVHD prophylaxis and that no benefit was derived by the addition of prednisone.

In a prospective, randomized multicenter trial, the combination of tacrolimus and MTX was significantly superior in preventing acute GVHD grades II–IV compared to CSP and MTX in recipients of T-replete, HLA-identical bone marrow transplants from unrelated donors (56% vs. 74%) (Nash et al., 2000). The former combination also allowed a reduced use of corticosteroids in the management of GVHD. Toxicity was not increased. Chronic GVHD, relapse, and survival were similar, indicating that tacrolimus can decrease morbidity early after transplantation without causing undue adverse events.

Several investigators have begun to employ pretransplant treatment with anti-T-cell antibodies to exploit their long half-life and prevent GVHD. Using Fresenius ATG at a dose of 60 to 90 mg/kg pretransplant, Finke and colleagues (2000) reported an incidence of acute GVHd grades II–IV of 15% and no graft rejection in 55 adult recipients of unrelated bone marrow transplants. Bacigalupo and colleagues (2001) enrolled 109 unrelated transplant recipients into two randomized trials to test the use of SangStat's rabbit ATG (Thymoglobuline) at 7.5 or 15 mg/kg before transplant against no ATG. Thymoglobuline at 15 mg/kg before transplant significantly reduced the risk for grade III–IV acute GVHD and chronic GVHD, increased the risk of infection, and survival was unchanged.

Not only is the incidence and severity of acute GVHD higher after HLA-matched unrelated compared to sibling donor transplants, but response to therapy for acute GVHD is more often unsatisfactory. In one study of 42 patients with moderate to severe acute GVHD, initial therapy consisted of prednisone 60 mg/m^2 orally daily for 7 days, followed by ATG 15 mg/kg i.v. twice daily for 8 to 10 doses if there was no adequate response to prednisone. Ten of 14 patients improved after prednisone, while only 4 of 21 who failed to respond to prednisone responded to ATG. Of the total 42 patients treated, only 9 achieved a complete and continuing response by day 100 (Roy et al., 1992). Neither age, diagnosis, recipient/donor gender status, histocompatibility matching, nor GVHD prophylaxis regimen was associated with more frequent responses.

CMV infection

CMV-positive patient serology confers a high risk for early disease and death, and CMV reactivation is very common after unrelated donor transplantation. Ganciclovir administered for prophylactic or preemptive therapy has decreased the incidence of CMV disease and mortality after unrelated donor marrow grafts (Hansen et al., 1998). The use of Campath-1H in the conditioning regimen appears to be associated with a low incidence of GVHD, but a high incidence of CMV infections and prolonged immune paresis. Chakrabarti and colleagues (2002) examined the pattern and outcome of CMV infections in 101 patients whose conditioning regimen contained in vivo

Campath-1H. The probability of CMV infection was 85% with onset at a median of 27 days after transplantation. The probability of recurrent CMV infection was more common in unrelated compared to sibling donor transplant recipients. All 3 patients who developed CMV disease died of this complication. In one study, prophylactic ganciclovir was not as effective in HLA-compatible unrelated marrow transplant recipients as in less heavily immune suppressed HLA-identical sibling transplant recipients (Atkinson et al., 1995). The actuarial incidence of CMV disease was 10% in 74 recipients of HLA-identical family member transplant recipients given prophylactic ganciclovir, but 33% in 14 recipients of HLA-identical unrelated donor transplants ($P = .006$).

Late infections

In a study of patients receiving either a related donor transplant ($n = 151$) or an unrelated donor transplant ($n = 98$) between 1989 and 1991, 367 late infectious events developed in 162 patients between day 50 posttransplant and 2 years posttransplant (Ochs et al., 1995). The incidence of late infection was greater in unrelated versus related recipients (84.7% vs. 68.2%, respectively, $P = .009$). In multivariate analysis, advanced GVHD was significantly associated with late infections. However, the effect of GVHD was apparent only in recipients of related donor transplants. Unrelated marrow transplant recipients, with or without GVHD, had more late infections when compared with related donor recipients without GVHD. Late posttransplant infections were the dominant independent factor associated with an increased nonrelapse mortality in the unrelated donor recipients. This prolonged period of increased infectious risk in unrelated donor recipients suggests the need for aggressive surveillance and therapy of late infections, perhaps including prolonged antibiotic prophylaxis in such recipients. Other studies have noted that late infections are common in patients with minimal GVHD, suggesting that immune deficiency is prolonged (Williamson et al., 1999).

Donor lymphocyte infusion for treatment of relapsed malignancy

A pilot multicenter study tested the efficacy of donor lymphocyte infusion, containing predominantly T cells, to treat 58 patients with a variety of malignancies that had relapsed after unrelated donor transplantation (Porter et al., 2000). Lymphocyte therapy was associated with a complete response rate of 42% (95% CI, 20–64%), a 37% incidence of acute GVHD grades II–IV, and a 31% incidence of chronic GVHD.

Recommendations from the World Marrow Donor Association on the practice of unrelated donor transplantation

The following recommendations (from "Donor selection" through "Second donation of marrow or blood cells for the same patient") are those of the World Marrow Donor Association, and are reproduced by permission from J.M. Goldman, *Blood*, **84**, 2833–9, 1994.

Donor selection

The donor and recipient should remain anonymous to each other and to each other's families and maintenance of donor confidentiality is of paramount importance. In most cases, such confidentiality should be maintained for life, although some centers accept the principle that donor and recipient may meet 6 months or more after a successful transplant, provided that both individuals have independently expressed a desire to do so. The donor should be counseled on three separate occasions: (1) when recruited to the Registry; (2) when selected for further testing; and (3) when definitely selected as a donor.

Counseling should aim to cover the following topics: (1) emphasis on anonymity for donor and patient; (2) requirement for further blood samples before donation; (3) requirement for virologic testing, especially human immunodeficiency virus (HIV) and HBsAg; (4) risks of anesthesia and harvest procedure; (5) loss of time from normal activities; (6) location of harvest procedure, that is, proximity to donor's home; (7) requirement for collection of autologous blood unit; (8) possibility of need for allogeneic blood unit and associated risks; (9) donor's right to withdraw and consequences for the patient if this right is exercised after the transplant protocol has started; (10) patient's need for transplantation and chance of success expressed in general terms; (11) possibility of second donation for the same patient (the fact that the donor is under no obligation to donate on a second occasion needs to be stressed); and (12) details of compensation for loss of income and details of insurance coverage affected.

Health. The donor should be examined by a physician not involved with the transplant procedure who should assess the patient's risk for undergoing general anesthesia. The following are absolute reasons for exclusion from donation: HIV seropositivity; human T-cell lymphotropic virus type 1 (HTLV-1) seropositivity; and pregnancy.

Infectious disease markers. Infectious disease markers should be assessed at three stages in relation to the actual donation. Requirements are essentially the same as for a sibling transplant. These three stages are (1) at time of donor recruitment—as for blood donation (e.g. hepatitis B, hepatitis C, HIV, CMV); (2) before selection decision—as for blood donation; (3) within 30 days before harvest—as for blood donation. Infectious-disease markers for consideration are the following: syphilis; hepatitis B surface antigen; HIV antigen; and antibodies to HIV, hepatitis B core antigen, hepatitis C, HTLV-1, herpes simplex virus, CMV, varicella-zoster virus, and Epstein-Barr virus (EBV).

Marrow collection, processing, labeling, and transportation (and see Table 67.4)

Marrow collection. Location of harvest procedure. The marrow collection should be performed at an accredited marrow collection center, ideally near the donor's normal residence.

Communications. Donor and recipient weight should be communicated to the harvest center in advance of the medical examination. A senior member of the harvest team should communicate with the recipient transplant center if the donor is dis-

Table 67.4. *Recommendations for collection, processing, labeling, and transportation of marrow*

1. Marrow should be collected in a minimum of 2 sealed plastic bags
2. ACD should be the only anticoagulant to be used in a ratio of 1 part to 8 parts marrow
3. Marrow bags should be labeled with:
   Donor number
   ABO and Rh type
   Harvest center—time and date of collection
   Transplant center—time and date of infusion (planned)
   Patient name
   Hospital
4. Marrow bags should be wrapped in surgical towel or water absorbent paper towel
5. Freezer packs should be wrapped in bubble plastic. These are then placed in a rigid container with insulating properties. They line the side and base of container. Freezer pack to be changed regularly to maintain desired temperature
6. Marrow bags should be vertically stacked or so arranged to be equally chilled
7. Marrow bags should be chilled to between 4° and 6°C and monitored by a standardized alcohol thermometer. Temperature to be checked several times during flight. Thermometers are best placed in between wrapped marrow bags (ensure broken thermometers will in no way pierce marrow bags)
8. Container should be labeled with "Human Bone Marrow For Transplantation. DO NOT X-RAY"
9. Peripheral blood samples to be collected:
   EDTA 5 ml
   Clot 10 ml
   Heparinized 30 ml
Should be labeled with:
   Donor number
   Harvest center and date of collection
Tubes should be placed in a plastic specimen bag wrapped with bubble plastic
Tubes should not be irradiated
It is suggested that a pair of examination gloves be included in the transport container for the security guard to examine marrow bags if required

proportionately small or there are other factors that might influence the success of the marrow collection.

Anesthesia. General anesthesia is recommended, but spinal or epidural anesthesia is acceptable if the donor and medical team agree. The duration of the general anesthetic should not exceed 2 hours.

Site of aspiration and collection. Marrow should be aspirated from the posterior and (if required) anterior iliac crests. The sternum should be avoided if possible, but may be used if the donor has agreed in advance. Marrow will ideally be collected using a closed system.

Cell counts. The harvest center must provide cell counts for each bag of marrow and the total number of cells collected. The target should be to collect no less than 2.0×10^8 cells/kg patient weight nucleated cells (uncorrected numbers).

Volume. The harvest team should aim to aspirate a total volume of 1,000 to 1,200 ml. In exceptional circumstances, this figure may be increased to 1,500 ml at the specific request of the harvest center. It should on no account be less than 500 ml (unless the recipient is a child). The volume of marrow harvested should be written on the bag (using the conversion factor 1 ml = 1.06 g).

Anticoagulant. For the donor, several centers use heparin (preservative-free) given intravenously with the premedication (100 U/kg, max 5,000 U). This approach may be used at a given transplant center, but it must be agreed to by the donor. The marrow should be anticoagulated with ACD-A (1 in 8) or equivalent unless heparin is requested by the transplant center. If the harvest center routinely uses heparin, they may use heparin for a volunteer donor harvest provided that the marrow transit time is not expected to exceed 12 hours. Whatever anticoagulant is used, it is the responsibility of the harvest center to ensure that their general policy is known and that each bag of marrow is labeled appropriately.

Autologous blood transfusion. The harvest center should aim to collect one or more units of autologous blood for transfusion to the donor during or after the harvest procedure. Every effort should be made to avoid the use of allogeneic blood; if its use is essential, it should be irradiated (>20 Gy).

Marrow processing. Filtration. Marrow should be filtered in accordance with the harvest center's routine practice, unless otherwise stipulated. The collection should employ a closed system incorporating the filter.

Labeling. The marrow should be labeled clearly with the donor's unique reference number (but not the name) and the unique reference number (but not the name) of the intended recipient, together with the name and address of the recipient transplant center, plus the donor ABO and Rhesus group. The nature of the anticoagulant used should be stated clearly.

Further marrow manipulation. Any further manipulation of the marrow will ordinarily be performed at the transplant center.

Transportation of marrow (and see Table 67.5). Courier. The designated courier should be a nurse, medical laboratory technician, doctor, or other person of comparable training or comparable level of responsibility. He/she should not be related to donor or patient and must have no other obligations until after the marrow is delivered.

Travel arrangements. The courier must keep the marrow in hand or in sight at all times. He/she must be prepared to communicate with the transplant center if any change occurs in travel arrangements and he/she must be prepared to improvise new travel arrangements if necessary. He/she should carry at least one major credit card. If necessary, airline agents should be informed of the urgency of the marrow delivery.

Travel documents. The courier should carry documents confirming the nature of the material, its destination, and the fact that it is HIV negative.

Irradiation. The marrow should not be subjected to irradiation in any airport security system. (However, note a report by Petzer *et al.* [2002] questioning the adverse impact of such radiological examination.)

Temperature. The marrow should be carried at room temperature (unless otherwise requested by the transplant center) in a

Table 67.5. *Guidelines for marrow couriers*

When marrow is collected at a hospital that is not the requesting transplant center, every effort must be made to ensure that the marrow arrives at the transplant site within 36 hours of collection

While the transport of marrow seems straightforward, there are problems that may arise. The courier is expected to take his/her responsibility seriously and use sound judgment in solving problems

Courier responsibilities are to ensure that:
- Marrow is transported in a rigid container, at 4°C (unless requested otherwise by the transplant center)
- Marrow is NEVER subjected to the airport X-ray screening devices. Any security check must be done by hand under direct supervision of the courier
- Alcohol is not consumed by the courier while transporting the marrow
- No drugs are allowed
- Immediate, alternate flights are obtained in case of delays
- All changes in original plans are communicated immediately to the donor and transplant centers involved
- Marrow is delivered directly to the designated person and no one else

When deciding who the courier will be, the following criteria must be assessed:
- The courier must know and understand the significance of the marrow he/she carries and have the maturity to take the task seriously
- The courier must be an experienced traveler
- The courier must have a major credit card

specially designed rigid container duly labeled. Transportation of 4°C may be optimal for long distances (i.e., greater than 12 hours ex vivo). The marrow cells must on no account be cooled below 4°C; neither dry ice nor liquid nitrogen should be used.

Marrow cryopreservation. The transplant center should specify the optimal amount and the minimum amount of marrow they require. The collected marrow should be transfused to the patient when it is received at the transplant center. Clinicians at the transplant center should not request additional marrow from the donor with the intention of cryopreserving a portion thereof.

If it is known that a given donor will not be available at the time when the marrow transplant is scheduled, it may in certain circumstances be permissible for harvested marrow to be cryopreserved at the harvest center or at the transplant center. This can only be undertaken with the approval of the donor and the medical director of the donor center. It should on no account be undertaken if there is any appreciable possibility that the transplant may not actually take place.

The feasibility and efficacy of cryopreserved unrelated donor marrow has been demonstrated (Stockschläder *et al.,* 1996). Ten patients received cryopreserved unrelated bone marrow between 1992 and 1995. All 9 evaluable patients engrafted. The time to reach an absolute neutrophil count of $>0.2 \times 10^9$/l and or $>0.5 \times 10^9$/l was 21.4×9.1 days and 22.6 ± 9.2 days, respectively. The incidence of acute GVHD $\geq$ grade II was 75% and that of chronic GVHD 20%.

Use of peripheral blood stem cells

Peripheral blood stem cells in place of, or in addition to marrow. Under certain circumstances there may be advantages in using PBSCs instead of bone marrow for allogeneic transplantation. Currently, the indications include inability or unwillingness for a donor to donate marrow or the treatment of marrow engraftment failure. However, this is a new and rapidly developing area and as such, the use of allogeneic PBSC transplants may (or may not) replace use of marrow stem cells for many purposes. The use of hematopoietic growth factors, including granulocyte-colony stimulating factor (G-CSF) and granulocyte-macrophage colony-stimulating factor, to mobilize blood stem cells for allogeneic use must be approved by the Research Ethics Committee and/or Institutional Review Board at the donor or transplant center.

A number of reports have demonstrated the feasibility and potential efficacy of G-CSF mobilized unselected PBSCs and CD34-enriched blood stem cells from unrelated donors (Stockschläder *et al.*, 1995; Hagglund *et al.*, 1998; Schwinger *et al.*, 2000[1]; Blau *et al.*, 2001).

Donor screening. The same criteria for donor selection and screening procedures should apply for donors being considered for allogeneic PBSC transplantation as for marrow transplantation. In addition, the prospective blood stem cell donor must have adequate venous access. Informed consent should take account of all aspects of the procedure including the administration of G-CSF and the leukapheresis procedure.

Stem cell harvesting. Leukaphereses should be performed in an appropriate setting according to institutional and blood bank center guidelines concerning the use of blood cell separators. Leukapheresis should be performed with a mechanical blood cell separator using peripheral venous access with the objective of processing a 9- to 12–1 lot of whole blood. Central venous access should be avoided. The necessary number of stem cells can probably be collected with one or two leukapheresis procedures in the majority of donors. It would be appropriate to confine allogeneic blood stem cell harvesting to units with an existing autologous stem cell harvesting program.

Informed consent and donor confidentiality

Donor consent. The donor should indicate general willingness to donate when he/she joins the panel. The donor should sign an approved form after the final selection has been made. This form should be approved by the local Institutional Review Board or Ethics Committee. The donor may at the same time be asked to consent to the use of marrow or blood cells for research purposes.

Donor confidentiality. Maintenance of donor confidentiality is of paramount importance. In most cases such confidentiality should be maintained for life. Some centers accept the principle that donor and recipient may meet 6 months or more after a successful transplant provided both individuals have independently expressed a desire to do so.

Second donation of marrow or blood cells for the same patient

A donor who has donated marrow in the past may on occasion be requested to repeat the donation for the same patient as a consequence of graft failure or relapse. The donation may take one of three forms: marrow stem cells, PBSCs, or PB mononuclear cells (PBMCs). The use of PBSCs is covered in part in the section above.

Second donation of marrow cells. The donor should be warned in advance of the original donation that there is a small possibility that he/she may be asked to donate again for the same patient. He/she should be asked soon after the first donation if he/she would be prepared to donate again. The donor should be informed as to the timing of possible second transplants. He/she should be asked to notify the donor center of any extended travel or change of address. Staff at the transplant center should consider collecting remission or chronic phase stem cells from the blood or marrow to permit an autologous rescue, but this may be unnecessary if the risk of graft failure is thought to be low. If the need for a second transplant for marrow (or blood) stem cells arises, the transplant center should contact its national hub and request that the need for a second transplant be transmitted rapidly to the national hub (or donor center) in the country of residence of the donor. The donor must on no account be contacted directly.

A senior staff member from the transplant center will prepare the case for a second donation in writing and submit it to the medical director of the hub. The document should include, as a minimum, details of (1) the patient's diagnosis; (2) the first transplant; (3) the patient's current clinical status; (4) the reasons for requesting a second donation; and (5) the clinician's estimate of the clinical outcome. On receipt of the request, the hub medical director will circulate the details to members of a review panel. This panel will operate under the direction of the medical director of the national hub and include representatives of the donor center and National Registry. The members of the panel will decide if the donor can be approached. The decision will take into account the clinical state of the patient, the likelihood that a second transplant will be successful, the condition of the donor, and other factors.

The review panel will endeavor to give its judgment within 48 hours of receiving the request. It will not normally reconsider the same request within a 7-day period. If the request is approved, the donor center is responsible for approaching the donor for a second marrow (or PB leukocyte) donation. Before the consent, the donor must be given a general explanation of the indications for, and results of, second marrow transplantation (or PBMC) donation, the procedure for the second marrow (or PBMC) donation, and the associated risks.

The donor must be given ample time to make his/her decision and must be free to ask all questions that he/she desires.

---

[1] The authors updated information that was not included in the original WMDA article.

The donor must feel free to decline. There must be no undue pressure on the prospective donor.

Second donation comprising peripheral blood leukocytes. A transplant center may request that the original marrow donor be asked to donate leukocytes rather than marrow cells for a second transplant procedure as treatment for graft failure. Moreover, leukocytes or (perhaps better) mononuclear cells from the PB of the original transplant donor have demonstrated activity in reversing relapse in patients previously allografted for leukemia, and thus, a marrow donor may on occasion be asked to undergo leukapheresis for leukocyte donation for either of these reasons. This request may be made months or years after the original marrow donation. The request for leukocyte donation should be handled in a manner strictly analogous to the request for a second marrow donation (see Second donation of marrow cells). The transplant center may request that the prospective leukocyte donor agrees to donate marrow on a future occasion if required. This request should then be discussed with the donor, who should not in any way be pressured to agree.

If the donor agrees to donate leukocytes, he/she should not be asked to travel to the transplant center. Leukocytes should be collected by means of a mechanical flow blood cell separator at a suitable center as near as possible to the donor's place of residence. The numbers of leukocytes to be collected should be specified by a senior clinician at the transplant center. Between two and five sessions should be performed within 5 to 9 days. Buffy coat should contain 2 to 4×10^8/kg nucleated cells unless otherwise stipulated by a senior clinician as described above.

If the second donation is to comprise only one unit of blood, as may be indicated for the management of EBV-related lymphoma developing in a patient after allografting, the donor center medical director may approve the request on his/her initiative without involvement of the review committee.

Conclusions

Transplants of HSCs from unrelated donors have become feasible for patients with a variety of disorders. The probability of finding a suitable donor has increased with the expansion of a registry network of approximately eight million HLA-typed donors worldwide. The selection of compatible donors has become more effective, because of the discovery of new HLA alleles and the development of precise and efficient HLA typing methods using DNA technology. Improved methods for transplantation may provide the opportunity to further decrease treatment-related toxicity and improve survival.

References

Anasetti, C., Amos, D., Beatty, P.G. *et al.* (1989). Effect of HLA compatibility on engraftment of bone marrow transplants in patients with leukemia or lymphoma. *New England Journal of Medicine*, **320**, 197–204.

Appelbaum, F.R. (2001). Perspectives on the future of chronic myeloid leukemia treatment. *Seminars in Hematology*, **38**, 35–42.

Ash, R.C., Casper, J.T., Christopher, R.C. *et al.* (1990). Successful allogeneic transplantation of T-cell depleted bone marrow from closely HLA-matched unrelated donors. *New England Journal of Medicine*, **322**, 485–94.

Ash, R.C., Horowitz, M.M., Gale, R.P. *et al.* (1991). Bone marrow transplantation from related donors other than HLA-identical siblings: effect of T cell depletion. *Bone Marrow Transplantation*, **7**, 443–52.

Atkinson, K., Arthur, C., Bradstock, K. *et al.* (1995). Prophylactic ganciclovir is more effective in HLA-identical family member marrow transplant recipients than in more heavily immune-suppressed HLA-identical unrelated donor marrow transplant recipients. *Bone Marrow Transplantation*, **16**, 401–5.

Atkinson, K., Dodds, A.J., Concannon, A.J. *et al.* (1993). Unrelated volunteer bone marrow transplantation: initial experience at St. Vincent's Hospital, Sydney. *Australian and New Zealand Journal of Medicine*, **23**, 450–7.

Aversa, F., Tabilio, A., Velardi, A. *et al.* (1998). Treatment of high-risk acute leukemia with T-cell-depleted stem cells from related donors with one fully mismatched HLA haplotype. *New England Journal of Medicine*, **339**, 1186–93.

Bacigalupo, A., Lamparelli, T., Bruzzi, P. *et al.* (2001). Antithymocyte globulin for graft-versus-host disease prophylaxis in transplants from unrelated donors: 2 randomized studies from Gruppo Italiano Trapianti Midollo Osseo (GITMO). *Blood*, **98**, 2942–7.

Bearman, S.I., Mori, M., Beatty, P.G. *et al.* (1994). Comparison of morbidity and mortality after marrow transplantation from HLA-genotypically identical siblings and HLA-phenotypically identical unrelated donors. *Bone Marrow Transplantation*, **13**, 31–5.

Beatty, P.G., Dahlberg, S., Mickelson, E.M. *et al.* (1988). Probability of finding HLA-matched unrelated marrow donors. *Transplantation*, **45**, 714–18.

Beatty, P.G., Hansen, J.A., Longton, G.M. *et al.* (1991). Marrow transplantation from HLA-matched unrelated donors for treatment of hematologic malignancies. *Transplantation*, **51**, 443–7.

Beatty, P.G. & Kollman, C. (1995). Unrelated donor marrow transplants: the experience of the National Marrow Donor Program. *Clinical Transplantation*, 271–7.

Bertz, H., Potthoff, K., Mertelsmann, R., & Finke, J. (1997). Busulfan/cyclophosphamide in volunteer unrelated donor (VUD) BMT: excellent feasibility and low incidence of treatment-related toxicity. *Bone Marrow Transplantation*, **19**, 1169–73.

Blau, I.W., Basara, N., Lentini, G. *et al.* (2001). Feasibility and safety of peripheral blood stem cell transplantation from unrelated donors: results of a single-center study. *Bone Marrow Transplantation*, **27**, 27–33.

Burnett, A.K. (2001). Treatment of acute myeloid leukaemia in younger patients. *Bailliere's Best Practice in Clinical Haematology*, **14**, 95–118.

Busca, A., Anasetti, C., Anderson, G. *et al.* (1994). Unrelated donor or autologous marrow transplantation for treatment with acute leukemia. *Blood*, **83**, 3077–84.

Castro-Malaspina, H., Harris, R.E., Gajewski, J. *et al.* (2002). Unrelated donor marrow transplantation for myelodysplastic syndromes: outcome analysis in 510 transplants facilitated by the National Marrow Donor Program. *Blood*, **99**, 1943–51.

Cavet, J., Dickinson, A.M., Norden, J. *et al.* (2001). Interferon-gamma and interleukin-6 gene polymorphisms associate with graft-versus-host disease in HLA-matched sibling bone marrow transplantation. *Blood*, **98**, 1594–600.

Chakrabarti, S., Mackinnon, S., Chopra, R. *et al.* (2002). High incidence of cytomegalovirus infection after nonmyeloablative stem cell transplantation: potential role of Campath-1H in delaying immune reconstitution. *Blood*, **99**, 4357–63.

Chakraverty, R., Peggs, K., Chopra, R. *et al.* (2002). Limiting transplantation-related mortality following unrelated donor stem cell transplantation by using a nonmyeloablative conditioning regimen. *Blood*, **99**, 1071–8.

Champlin, R.E., Passweg, J.R., Zhang, M.J. *et al.* (2000). T-cell depletion of bone marrow transplants for leukemia from donors other than HLA-identical siblings: advantage of T-cell antibodies with narrow specificities. *Blood*, **95**, 3996–4003.

Clift, R.A., Buckner, C.D., Appelbaum, F.R. *et al.* (1998). Long-term follow-up of a randomized trial of two irradiation regimens for patients receiving allogeneic marrow transplants during first remission of acute myeloid leukemia. *Blood*, **92**, 1455–6.

Clift, R.A., Buckner, C.D., Thomas, E.D. *et al.* (1994). Marrow transplantation for chronic myeloid leukemia: a randomized study comparing cyclophosphamide and total body irradiation with busulfan and cyclophosphamide. *Blood*, **84**, 2036–43.

Cornelissen, J.J., Carston, M., Kollman, C. *et al.* (2001). Unrelated marrow transplantation for adult patients with poor-risk acute lymphoblastic leukemia: strong graft-versus-leukemia effect and risk factors determining outcome. *Blood*, **97**, 1572–7.

Cullup, H., Dickinson, A.M., Jackson, G.H. *et al.* (2001). Donor interleukin 1 receptor antagonist genotype associated with acute graft-versus-host disease in human leucocyte antigen-matched sibling allogeneic transplants. *British Journal of Haematology*, **113**, 807–13.

Davies, S.M., Kollman, C., Anasetti, C. *et al.* (2000). Engraftment and survival after unrelated donor bone marrow transplantation: a report from the National Marrow Donor Program. *Blood*, **96**, 4096–102.

Davies, S.M., Ramsey, N.K.C., & Weisdorf, D.J. (1996). Feasibility and timing of unrelated donor identification for patients with ALL. *Bone Marrow Transplantation*, **17**, 737–40.

Davies, S.M., Ruggeri, L., DeFor, T. *et al.* (2002). Evaluation of KIR ligand incompatibility in mismatched unrelated donor hematopoietic transplants. *Blood*, **100**, 3825–7.

Davies, S.M., Shu, X.O., Blazar, B.R. *et al.* (1995). Unrelated donor bone marrow transplantation: influence of HLA A and b incompatibility on outcome. *Blood*, **86**, 1636–42.

Deeg, H.J., Amylon, M.D., Harris, R.E. *et al.* (2001). Marrow transplants from unrelated donors for patients with aplastic anemia: minimum effective dose of total body irradiation. *Biology of Blood and Marrow Transplantation*, **7**, 208–15.

Deeg, H.J., Anasetti, C., Petersdorf, E. *et al.* (1994). Cyclophosphamide plus ATG conditioning is insufficient for sustained hematopoietic reconstitution in patients with severe aplastic anemia transplanted with marrow from HLA-A, B, DR matched unrelated donors. *Blood*, **83**, 3417–21.

Deeg, H.J., Seidel, K., Casper, J. *et al.* (1999). Marrow transplantation from unrelated donors for patients with severe aplastic anemia who have failed immunosuppressive therapy. *Biology of Blood and Marrow Transplantation*, **5**, 243–52.

Deeg, H.J., Storer, B., Slattery, J.T. *et al.* (2002). Conditioning with targeted busulfan and cyclophosphamide for hemopoietic stem cell transplantation from related and unrelated donors in patients with myelodysplastic syndrome. *Blood*, **100**, 1201–7.

Devergie, A., Apperley, J.F., Labopin, M. *et al.* (1997). European results of matched unrelated donor bone marrow transplantation for chronic myeloid leukemia. Impact of HLA class II matching. *Bone Marrow Transplantation*, **20**, 11-N19.

Dini, G., Cancedda, R., Locatelli, F. *et al.* (2001). Unrelated donor marrow transplantation: an update of the experience of the Italian Bone Marrow Group (GITMO). *Haematologica*, **86**, 451–6.

Dini, G., Rondelli, R., Miano, M. *et al.* (1996). Unrelated-donor bone marrow transplantation for Philadelphia chromosome-positive chronic myelogenous leukemia in children: experience of eight European Countries. The EBMT Paediatric Diseases Working Party. *Bone Marrow Transplantation*, **18** (Suppl. 2) 80–5.

Dresse, M.F., Boogaerts, M., Vermylen, C. *et al.* (1999). The Belgian experience in unrelated donor bone marrow transplantation: identification of center experience as an important prognostic factor. *Haematologica*, **84**, 637–42.

Drobyski, W.R., Klein, J., Flomenberg, N. *et al.* (2002). Superior survival associated with transplantation of matched unrelated versus one-antigen-mismatched unrelated or highly human leukocyte antigen-disparate haploidentical family donor marrow grafts for the treatment of hematologic malignancies: establishing a treatment algorithm for recipients of alternative donor grafts. *Blood*, **99**, 806–14.

Drucker, B.J., Sawyers, C.J., Capdeville, R. *et al.* (2001b) Chronic mlyelogenous leukemia. *Hematology*, 87–112.

Drucker, B.J., Talpaz, M., Resta, D.J. *et al.* (2001a). Efficacy and safety of a specific inhibitor of the bcr-abl tyrosine kinase in chronic myeloid leukemia. *New England Journal of Medicine*, **344**, 1031–7.

El Kassar, N., Legouvello, S., Joseph, C.M. *et al.* (2001). High resolution HLA class I and II typing and CTL$_p$ frequency in unrelated donor transplantation: a single-institution retrospective study of 69 BMTs. *Bone Marrow Transplantation*, **27**, 35–43.

Elmaagacli, A.H., Basoglu, S., Peceny, R. *et al.* (2002). Improved disease-free-survival after transplantation of peripheral blood stem cells as compared with bone marrow from HLA-identical unrelated donors in patients with first chronic phase chronic myeloid leukemia. *Blood*, **99**, 1130–5.

Ferrara, G.B., Bacigalupo, A., Lamparelli, T. *et al.* (2001). Bone marrow transplantation from unrelated donors: the impact of mismatches with substitutions at position 116 of the human leukocyte antigen class I heavy chain. *Blood*, **98**, 3150–5.

Filipovich, A.H., Stone, J.V., Tomany, S.C. *et al.* (2001). Impact of donor type on outcome of bone marrow transplantation for Wiskott-Aldrich syndrome: collaborative study of the International Bone Marrow Transplant Registry and the National Marrow Donor Program. *Blood*, **97**, 1598–603.

Finke, J., Bertz, H., Schmoor, C. *et al.* (2000). Allogeneic bone marrow transplantation from unrelated donors using in vivo anti-T-cell globulin. *British Journal of Haematolpgy*, **11**, 303–13.

Fleischhauer, K., Kernan, N.A., O'Reilly, R.J. et al. (1990). Bone marrow-allograft rejection by T lymphocytes recognizing a single amino acid difference in HLA-B44. New England Journal of Medicine, 323, 1818–22.

Flomenberg, N., Baxter-Lowe, L.A., Confer, D. et al. (2001). Impact of HLA-class I and class II high resolution matching on outcomes of unrelated donor BMT. Blood, 98, 813 (Abstract).

Freytes, C.O. & Beatty, P.G. (1996). Representation of Hispanics in the National Marrow Donor Program. Bone Marrow Transplantation, 17, 323–7.

Goldman, J.M. for the WMDA Executive Committee (1994). A special report: bone marrow transplants using volunteer donors—recommendations and requirements for a standardized practice throughout the world—1994 update. Blood, 84, 2833–9.

Goodrich, J.M., Mori, M., Gleaves, C.A. et al. (1991). Early treatment with ganciclovir to prevent cytomegalovirus disease after allogeneic bone marrow transplantation. New England Journal of Medicine, 325, 1601–7.

Goulmy, E., Schipper, R., Pool, J. et al. (1996). Mismatches of minor histocompatibility antigens between HLA-identical donors and recipients and the development of graft-versus-host disease after bone marrow transplantation. New England Journal of Medicine, 334, 281–5.

Hagglund, H., Ringden, O., Remberger, M. et al. (1998). Faster neutrophil and platelet engraftment, but no differences in acute GVHD or survival, using peripheral blood stem cells from related and unrelated donors, compared to bone marrow. Bone Marrow Transplantation, 22, 131–6.

Hansen, J.A., Clift, R.A., Thomas, E.D. et al. (1980). Transplantation of marrow from an unrelated donor to a patient with acute leukemia. New England Journal of Medicine, 303, 565–7.

Hansen, J.A., Gooley, T.A., Martin, P.J. et al. (1998). Bone marrow transplantation from unrelated donors for patients with chronic myeloid leukemia. New England Journal of Medicine, 338, 962–8.

Hows, J., Bradley, B.A., Gore, S. et al. (1993). Prospective evaluation of unrelated donor bone marrow transplantation. The International Marrow Unrelated Search and Transplant (IMUST) Study. Bone Marrow Transplantation, 12, 371–80.

Hurley, C.K. (1997). Acquisition and use of DNA-based HLA typing data in bone marrow registries. Tissue Antigens, 49, 323–8.

Hurley, C.K., Baxter-Lowe, L.A., Begovich, A.B. et al. (2002). The extent of HLA class II allele level disparity in unrelated bone marrow transplantation: analysis of 1259 National Marrow Donor Program donor-recipient pairs. Bone Marrow Transplantation, 25, 385–93.

Hurley, C.K., Maiers, M., Ng, J. et al. (2000). Large-scale DNA-based typing of HLA-A and HLA-B at low resolution is highly accurate specific and reliable. Tissue Antigens, 55, 352–8.

Hurley, C.K., Wade, J.A., Oudshoom, M. et al. (1999). Histocompatibility testing guidelines for hematopoietic stem cell transplantation using voluteer donors: report from The World Marrow Donor Association. Bone Marrow Transplantation, 24, 119–21.

Kaminski, E., Hows, J., Man, S. et al. (1989). Prediction of graft-versus-host disease by frequency analysis of cytotoxic T cells after unrelated donor bone marrow transplantation. Transplantation, 48, 608–13.

Keever, C.A., Leong, N., Cunningham, I. et al. (1994). HLA-B44-directed cytotoxic T cells associated with acute graft-versus-host disease following unrelated bone marrow transplantation. Bone Marrow Transplantation, 14, 137–45.

Kernan, N.A., Kartsch, G., Ash, R.C. et al. (1993). Analysis of 462 transplantation from unrelated donors facilitated by the National Marrow Donor Program. New England Journal of Medicine, 328, 593–602.

Kollman, C., Howe, C.W.S., Anasetti, C. et al. (2000). Donor characteristics as risk factors in recipients after transplantation of bone marrow from unrelated donors: the effect of donor age. Blood, 98, 2043–51.

Kollman, C., Weis, T., Switzer, G.E. et al. (2001). Non-HLA barriers to unrelated donor stem cell transplantation. Bone Marrow Transplantation, 27, 581–7.

Lang, P., Handgretinger, R., Niethammer, D. et al. (2003). Transplantation of highly purified CD34+ progenitor cells from unrelated donors in pediatric leukemia. Blood, 101, 1630–6.

Lee, S.J., Anasetti, C., Horowitz, M.M., & Antin, J.H. (1998). Initial therapy for chronic myelogenous leukemia: playing the odds. Journal of Clinical Oncology, 16, 2897–903.

Lee, S.J., Kuntz, K.M., Horowitz, M.M. et al. (1997). Unrelated donor bone marrow transplantation for chronic myelogenous leukemia: a decision analysis. Annals of Internal Medicine, 127, 1080–8.

Leelasiri, A., Greer, J.P., Stein, R.S. et al. (1995). Graft-versus-host disease prophylaxis for matched unrelated bone marrow transplantation: comparison between cyclosporine-methotrexate and cyclosporine-methotrexate-methylprednisolone. Bone Marrow Transplantation, 15, 401–5.

Lin, M.T., Gooley, T., Hansen, J.A. et al. (2001). Absence of statistically significant correlation between disparity for the minor histocompatibility antigen-HA-1 and outcome after allogeneic hematopoietic cell transplantation. Blood, 15, 3172–3.

Liu, Z., Sun, Y.K., Xi, Y.P. et al. (1993). Contribution of direct and indirect recognition pathways to T-cell alloreactivity. Journal of Experimental Medicine, 177, 1643-N50.

Loiseau, P., Esperou, H., Busson, M. et al. (2002). DPBI disparities contribute to severe GVHD and reduced patient survival after unrelated donor bone marrow transplantation. Bone Marrow Transplantation, 30, 497–502.

Martin, P.J., Rowley, S.D., Anasetti, C. et al. (1999). A phase I-II clinical trial to evaluate removal of CD4 cells and partial depletion of CD8 cells from donor marrow for HLA-mismatched unrelated recipients. Blood, 94, 2192–9.

Mavroudis, D., Read, E., Cottier-Fox, M. et al. (1996). CD34+ cell dose predicts survival, posttransplant morbidity, and rate of hematologic recovery after allogeneic marrow transplants for hematologic malignancies. Blood, 88, 3223–9.

McGlave, P.B., Shu, X.O., Wen, W. et al. (2000). Unrelated donor marrow transplantation for chronic myelogenous leukemia: 9 years' experience of the National Marrow Donor Program. Blood, 95, 2219–25.

Mickelson, E.M., Longton, G., Anasetti, C. et al. (1996). Evaluation of the mixed lymphocyte culture (MLC) assay as a method for selecting unrelated donors for marrow transplantation. Tissue Antigens, 47, 27–36.

Middelton, P., Taylor, P., Jackson, G. *et al.* (1998). Cytokine genes polymorphisms associated with severe acute GVHD in HLA-identical sibling transplants. *Blood*, **92**, 3943–8.

Moreau, P. & Cesbron, A. (1994). HLA-DP and allogeneic bone marrow transplantation. *Bone Marrow Transplantation*, **13**, 675–81.

Morishima, Y., Sasazuki, T., Inoko, H. *et al.* (2002). The clinical significance of human leukocyte antigen (HLA) allele compatibility in patients receiving a marrow transplant from serologically HLA-A, HLA-B, and HLA-DR matched unrelated donors. *Blood*, **99**, 4200–6.

Mutis, T., Gillespie, G., Schrama, E. *et al.* (1999). Tetrameric HLA class I-minor histocompatibility antigen peptide complexes demonstrate minor histocompatibility antigen-specific cytotoxic T lymphocytes in patients with graft-versus-host disease. *Nature Medicine*, **5**, 839–42.

Nademanee, A., Schmidt, G.M., Parker, P. *et al.* (1995). The outcome of matched unrelated donor bone marrow transplantation in patients with hematologic malignancies using molecular typing for donor selection and graft-versus-host disease prophylaxis regimen of cyclosporine, methotrexate, and prednisone. *Blood*, **86**, 1228–34.

Nagler, A., Aker, M., Or, R. *et al.* (2001). Low-intensity conditioning is sufficient to ensure engraftment in matched unrelated bone marrow transplantation. *Experimental Hematology*, **29**, 362–70.

Nash, R.A., Antin, J.H., Karanes, C. *et al.* (2000). Phase 3 study comparing methotrexate and tacrolimus with methotrexate and cyclosporine for prophylaxis of acute graft-versus-host disease after marrow transplantation from unrelated donors. *Blood*, **96**, 2062–8.

Ochs, L., Shu, X.O., Miller, J. *et al.* (1995). Late infections after allogeneic bone marrow transplantations: comparison of incidence in related and unrelated donor transplant recipients. *Blood*, **86**, 3979–86.

Ottinger, H.D., Muller, C.R., Goldmann, S.F. *et al.* (2001). Second German consensus on immunogenetic donor search for allotransplantation of hematopoietic stem cells. *Annals of Hematology*, **80**, 706–14.

Ottinger, H.D., Rebmann, V., Pfeiffer, K.A. *et al.* (2002). Positive serum crossmatch as predictor for graft failure in HLA-mismatched allogeneic blood stem cell transplantation. *Transplantation*, **73**, 1280–5.

Oudshoorn, M., Doxiadis, I.I., van den Berg-Loonen, P.M. *et al.* (2002). Functional versus structural matching: can the CTL$_p$ test be replaced by HLA allele typing? *Human Immunology*, **63**, 176–84.

Oudshoorn, M., Falkenburg, J.H.F., Ebeling, L.J. *et al.* (1996). Unrelated bone marrow transplantation as a rescue procedure following inadvertent loss of an autologous bone marrow graft. *Bone Marrow Transplantation*, **18**, 461–3.

Peters, C., Balthazor, M., Shapiro, E.G. *et al.* (1996). Outcome of unrelated donor bone marrow transplantation in 40 children with Hurler syndrome. *Blood*, **87**, 4894–902.

Petersdorf, E.W., Gooley, T.A., Anasetti, C. *et al.* (1998). Optimizing outcome after unrelated marrow transplantation by comprehensive matching of HLA class I and class II alleles in the donor and recipient. *Blood*, **92**, 3515–20.

Petersdorf, E.W., Gooley, T., Malkki, M. *et al.* (2001a). The biological significance of HLA-DP variation in haematopoietic cell transplantation. *British Journal of Haematology*, **112**, 988–94.

Petersdorf, E.W., Hansen, J.A., Martin, P.J. *et al.* (2001b). Major-histocompatibility-complex class I alleles and antigens in hematopoietic-cell transplantation. *New England Journal of Medicine*, **345**, 1794–800.

Petersdorf, E.W., Kollman, C., Hurley, C.K. *et al.* (2001c). Effect of HLA class II gene disparity on clinical outcome in unrelated donor hematopoietic cell transplantation for chronic myeloid leukemia: the US National Marrow Donor Program Experience. *Blood*, **98**, 2922–9.

Petersdorf, E.W., Longton, G.M., Anasetti, C. *et al.* (1995). The significance of HLA-DRB1 matching on clinical outcome after HLA-A, -B B,-D DR, -identical unrelated donor marrow transplantation. *Blood*, **86**, 1606–13.

Petersdorf, E.W., Longton, G.M., Anasetti, C. *et al.* (1996). Definition of HLA-DQ as a transplantation antigen. *Proceedings of the National Academy of Sciences U.S.A.*, **93**, 15358–63.

Petersdorf, E.W., Longton, G.M., Anasetti, C. *et al.* (1997). Association of HLA-C disparity with graft failure after marrow transplantation from unrelated donors. *Blood*, **89**, 1818–23.

Petzer, A. L., Speth, H-G., Hoflehner, E. *et al.* (2002). Breaking the rules? X-ray examination of hematopoietic stem cell grafts at international ariports. *Blood*, **99**, 4632–3.

Porter, D.L., Collins, R.H. Jr, Hardy, C. *et al.* (2000). Treatment of relapsed leukemia after unrelated donor marrow transplantation with unrelated donor leukocyte infusions. *Blood*, **95**, 1214–21.

Prasad, V.K., Heller, G., Kernan, N.A. *et al.* (1999a). The probability of HLA-C matching between patient and unrelated donor at the molecular level: estimations based on the linkage disequilibrium between DNA typed HLA-B and HLA-C alleles. *Transplantation*, **68**, 1044–50.

Prasad, V.K., Kernan, N.A., Heller, G. *et al.* (1999b). DNA typing for HLA-A and HLA-B identifies disparities between patients and unrelated donors matched by HLA-A and HLA-B serology and HLA-DRB1 . *Blood*, **93**, 399–409.

Remberger, M., Ringden, O., Blau, I-W. *et al.* (2001). No difference in graft-versus-host disease, relapse, and survival comparing peripheral stem cells to bone marrow using unrelated donors. *Blood*, **98**, 1739–45.

Ringden, O., Remberger, M., Runde, V. *et al.* (1999). Peripheral blood stem cell transplantation from unrelated donors: a comparison with marrow transplantation. *Blood*, **94**, 455–64.

Rocha, V., Cornish, J., Sievers, E.L. *et al.* (2001). Comparison of outcomes of unrelated bone marrow and umbilical cord blood transplants in children with acute leukemia. *Blood*, **97**, 2962–71.

Roy, J., McGlave, P.B., Filipovich, A.H. *et al.* (1992). Acute graft-versus-host disease following unrelated donor marrow transplantation: failure of conventional therapy. *Bone Marrow Transplantation*, **10**, 77–82.

Ruggeri, L., Capanni, M., Urbani, E. *et al.* (2002). Effectiveness of donor natural killer cell alloreactivity in mismatched hematopoietic transplants. *Science*, **295**, 2097–100.

Sasazuki, T., Juji, T., Morishima, Y. *et al.* (1998). Effect of matching of class I alleles on clinical outcome after transplantation of hematopoietic stem cells from an unrelated donor. *New England Journal of Medicine,* **339,** 1177–85.

Schreuder, G.M., Hurley, C.K., Marsh, S.G. *et al.* (2001). The HLA Dictionary 2001: a summary of HLA-A, -B, -C, -DRB1/3/4/5, -DQB1 alleles and their association with serologically defined HLA-A, -B, -C, -DR and -DQ antigens. *Tissue Antigens,* **58,** 109–40.

Schwinger, W., Urban, Ch., Lackner, H. *et al.* (2000). Unrelated peripheral blood stem cell transplantation with "megadoses" of purified CD34+ cells in three children with refractory severe aplastic anemia. *Bone Marrow Transplantation,* **25,** 513–7.

Scott, I., O'Shea, J., Bunce, M. *et al.* (1998). Molecular typing shows a high level of HLA class I incompatibility in serologically well matched donor/recipient pairs: implications for unrelated bone marrow donor selection. *Blood,* **92,** 4864–71.

Shlomchik, W.D., Couzens, M.S., Tang, C.B. *et al.* (1999). Prevention of graft versus host disease by inactivation of host antigen-presenting cells. *Science,* **285,** 412–5.

Sierra, J., Storer, B., Hansen, J.A. *et al.* (1997). Transplantation of marrow cells from unrelated donors for treatment of high-risk acute leukemia: the effect of leukemic burden, donor HLA-matching, and marrow cell dose. *Blood,* **89,** 4226–35.

Sierra, J., Storer, B., Hansen, J.A. *et al.* (2000). Unrelated donor marrow transplantation for acute myeloid leukemia: an update of the Seattle experience: *Bone Marrow Transplantation,* **26,** 397–404.

Slavin, M.A., Osborne, B., Adams, R. *et al.* (1995). Efficacy and safety of fluconazole prophylaxis for fungal infections after marrow transplantation—a prospective, randomized, double-blind study. *Journal of Infectious Diseases,* **71,** 1545–52.

Socie, G., Loiseau, P., Tamouza, R. *et al.* (2001). Both genetic and clinical factors predict the development of graft-versus-host disease after allogeneic hematopoietic stem cell transplantation. *Transplantation,* **72,** 699–706.

Soiffer, R.J., Weller, E., Alyea, E.P. *et al.* (2001). CD6+ donor marrow T-cell depletion as the sole form of graft-versus-host disease prophylaxis in patients undergoing allogeneic bone marrow transplant from unrelated donors. *Journal of Clinical Oncology,* **19,** 1152–9.

Speck, B., Swann, F.E., van Rood, J.J. *et al.* (1973). Allogeneic bone marrow transplantation in a patient with aplastic anemia using a phenotypically HLA-identical unrelated donor. *Transplantation,* **16,** 24.

Stockschläder, M., Loliger, C., Kruger, W. *et al.* (1995). Transplantation of allogeneic rh G-CSF mobilized peripheral CD34+ cells from an HLA-identical unrelated donor. *Bone Marrow Transplantation,* **16,** 719–22.

Szydlo, R., Goldman, J.M., Klein, J.P. *et al.* (1997). Results of allogeneic bone marrow transplants for leukemia using donors other than HLA-identical siblings. *Journal of Clinical Oncology,* **15,** 1767–77.

Tay, G.K., Witt, C.S., Christiansen, F.T. *et al.* (1995). Matching for MHC haplotypes results in improved survival following unrelated bone marrow transplantation. *Bone Marrow Transplantation,* **15,** 381–5.

Tiercy, J-M., Bujan-Lose, M., Chapuis, B. *et al.* (2000). Bone marrow transplantation with unrelated donors: what is the probability of identifying an HLA-A/B/Cw/DRB1/B3/B5/DQB1-matched donor? *Bone Marrow Transplantation,* **26,** 437–41.

Tiercy, J-M., Morel, C., Freidel, A.C. *et al.* (1991). Selection of unrelated donors for bone marrow transplantation is improved by HLa class II genotyping with oligonucleotide hybridization. *Proceedings of the National Academy of Science USA,* **88,** 7121–5.

Topolsky, D., Crilley, P., Styler, M.G. *et al.*(1996). Unrelated donor bone marrow transplantation without T-cell depletion using a chemotherapy only conditioning regimen. Low incidence of failed engraftment and severe acute GVHD. *Bone Marrow Transplantation,* **17,** 549–54.

Tseng, L.H., Lin, M.T., Hansen, J.A. *et al.* (1999). Correlation between disparity for the minor histocompatibility antigen HA-1 and the development of acute graft-versus-host disease after allogeneic marrow transplantation. *Blood,* **15,** 2911–4.

Varney, M.D., Lester, S., McCluskey, J. *et al.* (1999). Matching for HLA DPA1 and DPB1 alleles in unrelated bone marrow transplantation. *Human Immunology,* **60,** 532–8.

Wagner, J.E., King, R., Kollman, K. *et al.* (1998). Unrelated donor bone marrow transplantation in 5075 patients with malignant and nonmalignant disorders: impact of marrow T-cell depletion. *Blood,* **92,** 686a (Abstract).

Weisdorf, D.J., Anasetti, C., Antin, J.H. *et al.* (2002). Allogeneic bone marrow transplantation for chronic myelogenous leukemia: comparative analysis of unrelated versus matched sibling donor transplantation. *Blood,* **99,** 1971–7.

Williamson, E.C.M., Millar, M.R., Steward, C.G. *et al.* (1999). Infections in adults undergoing unrelated donor bone marrow transplantation. *British Journal of Haematology,* **104,** 560–8.

Witherspoon, R.P., Deeg, H.J., Storer, B. *et al.* (2001). Hetnatopoietic stem-cell transplantation for treatment-related leukemia or myelodysplasia. *Journal of Clinical Oncology,* **19,** 2134–41.

PART VIII UMBILICAL CORD BLOOD TRANSPLANTATION

68 Umbilical cord blood transplantation

ELIANE GLUCKMAN AND VANDERSON ROCHA

Eurocord Registry and Hospital Saint Louis, Paris, France

Introduction

One of the most important advances in the field of allogeneic hematopoietic stem cell (HSC) transplantation has been the use of new sources of HSCs extending the indications for allogeneic transplants to patients lacking a human leukocyte antigen (HLA)-identical sibling donor. The principal limitations of allogeneic HSC transplantation are the absence of suitable HLA-matched donors and the complication of graft-versus-host disease (GVHD), which are more severe with increasing HLA disparity between donor and recipient. In the absence of an HLA-identical sibling donor, mismatched related or matched unrelated donors are sought. Clinical results have been improving, thanks to progress in molecular HLA typing, but the specificity of HLA high-resolution molecular typing decreases the probability of finding an HLA-identical donor for HLA-A, -B - C, -DR, -DQ, and -DP (Speiser *et al.*, 1996; Hansen *et al.*, 1998; Petersdorf *et al.*, 1998; Sasazuki *et al.*, 1998; Davies *et al.*, 2000). The relative contribution of major and minor histocompatibility polymorphisms to the relatively high frequency of transplant-related complications such as GVHD, rejection (host-versus-graft, HVG), immune deficiency, and leukemic relapse (graft-versus-leukemia, GVL) is unknown. Despite the increasing number of bone marrow donor registries that contain more than 8 million bone marrow donors worldwide, some patients cannot be transplanted because of the lack of a suitable donor. In these cases, alternative approaches are investigated. T-cell depletion has been used to decrease GVHD in matched or partially matched unrelated donor transplants (Oakhill *et al.*, 1996; Hongeng *et al.*, 1997; Hensley-Downey *et al.*, 1997, 1999; Szydlo *et al.*, 1997; Martin *et al.*, 1999; Green *et al.*, 1999; Woolfrey *et al.*, 2002). High-dose irradiation and chemotherapy with a mega dose of T-depleted peripheral blood CD34+ cells has been used in related haploidentical donor transplants. T-cell depletion of the graft has given interesting results, decreasing the probability of GVHD but the disadvantages are the increased risks of rejection, relapse, and delayed immune reconstitution (Aversa *et al.*, 1994, 1998; Ruggeri *et al.*, 2002).

Since the first successful allogeneic umbilical cord blood transplant (UCBT) performed in 1988 to treat a child with Fanconi anemia (Gluckman *et al.*, 1989), the development of cord blood banks and transplants has been increasing steadily. This first success opened the way to an entire new field in the domain of allogeneic HSC transplant with the demonstration that an umbilical cord blood unit could be collected at birth without any harm to the newborn infant, that umbilical cord blood HSCs could be cryopreserved, thawed, and transplanted in a myeloablated host and permanently engraft, and that a single umbilical cord blood contained enough HSCs to reconstitute the host's lympho-hematopoietic system. Table 68.1 describes the advantages and disadvantages of using unrelated cord blood cells for transplantation. Diseases treated to date by cord blood transplantation are shown in Table 68.2.

Umbilical cord blood banks (CBB) have been established for related or unrelated umbilical cord blood transplantation with more than 100,000 units available worldwide and more than 2,500 UCBT performed to date in children, and increasingly in adults, with malignant and nonmalignant diseases. Figure 68.1 describes the number of cord blood transplants reported to Eurocord. Table 68.3 describes the diagnosis and age of the patients.

Table 68.1. *Potential advantages and disadvantages of unrelated donor umbilical cord blood transplants*

Advantages	Disadvantages
For the recipient	Delay of engraftment
Decreased time of donor search	Delay of immunological
Low transmission of infectious	reconstitution
disease	Absence of donor infectious
Reduced risk of GVHD	immunization might
No risk of donor refusal	increase the risk of infection
	Decreased GVL
For the donor	
Absence of risk to the donor	
and the mother	
Absence of psychological	
problems for the donor	

Table 68.2. *Diseases treated by cord blood transplantation*

Malignant diseases
   Acute lymphocytic leukemia
   Acute myelocytic leukemia
   Chronic myelogeneous leukemia
   Juvenile chronic myelogeneous leukemia
   Myelodysplastic syndrome
   Neuroblastoma
Nonmalignant diseases
   Adrenoleukodystrophy
   Amegakaryocytic thrombocytopenia
   Blackfan-Diamond syndrome
   Dyskeratosis congenita
   Fanconi's anemia
   Globoid cell leukodystrophy
   Gunther's disease
   Hunter syndrome
   Hurler syndrome
   Idiopathic aplastic anemia
   Kostmann syndrome
   Lesch-Nyhan syndrome
   Osteopetrosis
   Severe combined immune deficiency
   Thalassemia
   X-linked lymphoproliferative syndrome

Reproduced, with permission, from Ballen *et al.* (2001b).

Compared to adult cells cord blood cells have distinct biological advantages. The HSCs in cord blood have a growth proliferation advantage, and immune cells are less reactive, decreasing the risk of severe allogeneic reactions. Compared to adult cells, umbilical cord blood HSCs grow larger colonies, have different growth factor requirements, are able to expand upon long-term culture in vitro, are able to engraft SCID mice in the absence of additional human growth factors, and have longer telomeres (Noort & Falkenburg, 2000). These properties should compen-

sate for the relatively low number of cells contained in a single umbilical cord blood unit and, through rapid expansion, reconstitute myeloablated recipients. A study investigating potential maternal and neonatal predictors of the hematopoietic potential of cord blood found that babies of longer gestational age had higher cell counts, but lower CD34+ cell counts and more colony-forming units–granulocyte-macrophage (CFU-GM) (Ballen *et al.*, 2001b). Bigger babies had higher cell counts, more CD34+ cell counts, and CFU-GM. Specifically, each 500 g increase in birth weight contributed to a 28% increase in CD34+ cell counts, each week of gestation contributed to a 9% decrease in CD34+ cell counts, and each previous birth contributed to a 17% decrease in CD34+ cell counts (all $P < .05$).

Wong and colleagues (2001) compared cell yields on cord blood taken either before or after delivery of the placenta and found higher numbers of nucleated cells and of CFUs in those collected before delivery. In pregnancies affected by pre-eclampsia, volume, nucleated cell count, and CD34+ cell count in the collected cord blood were all significantly lower compared to those of control subjects (Surbek *et al.*, 2001). These numbers are important since a clear correlation has been documented between the total number of nucleated cells infused and the speed of neutrophil and platelet engraftment as well as with the probability of long-term survival posttransplant (Kurtzberg *et al.*, 1996; Gluckman *et al.*, 1997; Rubinstein *et al.*, 1998).

The immaturity of the immune system at birth confers decreased lymphocyte alloreactivity and, as a consequence, reduces the incidence and severity of GVHD (De la Selle *et al.*, 1996, 1998; Madrigal *et al.*, 1997). Cord blood lymphocytes are naive and immature, are enriched in double negative CD3+ cells, and produce less cytokines; cord blood cells express mRNA transcripts for interferon (INF)-γ, interleukin (IL)-4, and IL-10 but very little IL-2, have a fully constituted polyclonal T cell repertoire (Garderet *et al.*, 1998), and could be protected from apoptosis because of low levels of CD95. Most of these functions are

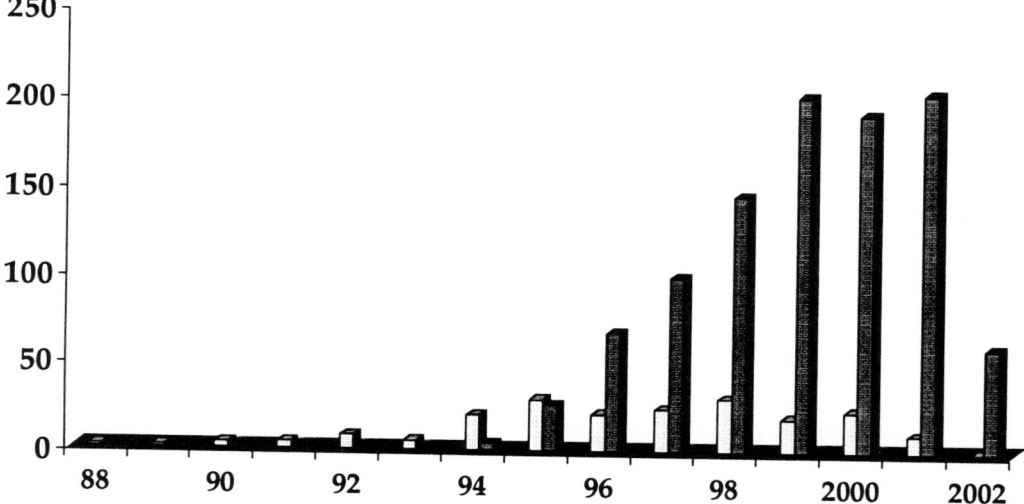

Fig. 68.1. Number of related cord blood transplants (white) (total *n* = 197) and unrelated cord blood transplants (total *n* = 1,002) reported to Eurocord.* Data still pending (June 2002).

Table 68.3. *Distribution of patients receiving UCBT according to type of donor, diagnosis, and age and reported to Eurocord*

Diagnosis	Related cord blood transplants (*n* = 197)		Unrelated cord blood transplants (*n* = 1,002)	
	Children *n* = 189 (<15 years)	Adults *n* = 8 (>15 years)	Children *n* = 667 (<15 years)	Adults *n* = 335 (>15 years)
Acute leukemias	70	1	382	194
MDS	8	–	50	26
CML	7	3	24	67
Lymphomas	2	–	14	27
Other malignancies	6	–	27	8
BMFs	30	1	59	11
Hemoglobinopathies	50	3	1	–
Immunodeficiencies	9	–	69	2
Metabolic diseases	8	–	42	–

Abbreviations: MDS, myelodysplastic syndrome; CML, chronic myeloid leukemia; BMFs, bone marrow failure syndromes.

inducible through in vitro or in vivo activation; as a consequence, early natural killer (NK) and T-cell cytotoxicity is impaired, but secondary activation can occur (Gardiner *et al.*, 1998). Therefore, one can speculate that despite the reduction of GVHD, an antileukemic effect (GVL) may still be observed. Since acute GVHD is an early event after allogeneic HSC transplantation and is in part triggered by cytokine release, it is reasonable to postulate that UCBT might induce less frequent and less severe acute and chronic GVHD than adult HSC transplants, which contain a higher number of mature T cells. This property in turn could lead to less stringent criteria for HLA donor-recipient matching.

Cord blood banking

Increasing success of reported UCBT resulted in the establishment of cord blood banks (Rubinstein *et al.*, 1993, 1995). Their number has been increasing, with more than 100,000 units collected and available for unrelated donor HSC transplant searches. The main practical advantages of using umbilical cord blood as an alternative source of HSCs are (1) the relative ease of procurement, (2) the absence of risks to donors, (3) the reduced risk of transmitting infection due to the low incidence of infection at birth, and (4) the prompt availability of cryopreserved samples to transplant centers. These advantages were first recognized in UCBT using related donors. Subsequently, large unrelated umbilical cord blood banks established criteria for standardization of umbilical cord blood collection, banking, processing, and cryopreservation for the treatment of various hematological malignant and nonmalignant diseases. Other advantages of UCBT are (5) the large donor pool, (6) the increased speed of search (Barker *et al.*, 2002) as the units are readily available, having been previously tested and cryopreserved, and (7) the low incidence of GVHD due to the immune immaturity of the newborn's immune cells.

Compared to unrelated bone marrow transplants where complete HLA identity for class I and class II antigens are normally required, most UCBTs have been performed with donors having 1, 2, or 3 HLA antigen mismatches with the recipient. It was realized that it was important to set minimum standards and reach international agreement on aspects essential for the safety of the donor and the mother and for providing the best possible chance of finding a suitable donor for the recipient. For this purpose, Netcord was founded in 1998; it currently includes large umbilical cord blood banks in the United States, Europe, Japan, and Australia. Netcord has developed a detailed set of standards for umbilical cord blood banking. These include national and international regulatory aspects [see Foundation for Accreditation of Cellular Therapy (FACT) standards www.unmc.edu]. Furthermore, a joint allocation system employing Internet technology is currently used to facilitate rapid allocation of umbilical cord blood units according to histocompatibility matching and number of nucleated cells. Table 68.4 lists inventories from Bone Marrow Donor Worldwide (BMDW) (www.bmdw.org) and Netcord (www.netcord.org). This list is not exhaustive and underestimates the total of cord blood units available worldwide. Considerations that should be taken into account when establishing a cord blood bank are listed in Table 68.5.

On average 100 ml of blood can be collected from the human umbilical cord taken while the placenta is in situ and from the placenta after expulsion. The procedure for cord blood collection is relatively standard: the cord is doubly clamped at the fetal end after birth; the umbilical vein and the placental veins are needled and blood collected into anticoagulant. The cells can then be either frozen unprocessed in 10% DMSO at a cooling rate of 1°C per minute and stored in liquid nitrogen at −180°C, or stored at 4°C for up 3 days without significant loss of viability. Occasionally the cell yield is suboptimal and some specimens have been infected. Methods for standardizing, and

Table 68.4. *Number of cord blood units registered with Bone Marrow Donor Worldwide (http://www.bmdw.org) and Netcord (http://www.netcord.org) as of July 2002*

Registry	Code	Number units
Argentina	ARCB	70
Australia	AUCB	6,447
Belgium	BCB	2,364
Bologna, Italy	BOCB	176
China (Sinocord)	CNCB	5,224
Czech Republic	CSCB	714
Düsseldorf	DUCB	4,802
Finland	FICB	1,389
France	FCB	3,134
Germany	DCB	2,394
Leuven	LVCB	2,774
Milan (Grace)	MICB	6,521
Netherlands	NLCB	944
Spain	ECB	5,728
Tokyo		1,849
UCBB		6,650
Jerusalem		549
London		4,327
New York		11,236
USA ARCCBP	WOCB	5,433
USA-CRIR	U3CB	2,122
USA-Michigan	GRCB	741
USA-NMDP	UICB	16,279
USA-Paramus	PMCB	1,390
USA-Stemcyte	ACBB	8,555
Number of banks	25	101,812

Abbreviations: NMDP, National Marrow Donor Program; CRIR, Caitlin Raymond International Registry; UCBB, Colorado University Cord Blood Bank; ARCCBP, American Red Cross Cord Blood Program; Grace, Italian Cord Blood Network.

partially automating, cord blood banking have been published (Reboredo *et al.*, 2000).

Table 68.5. *Considerations in establishing a cord blood bank*

Specific issues	Unresolved issues
Donor recruitment	Adequate cell dose
Consent	Speed of engraftment
Donor suitability	Histocompatibility requirement
Collection	Expansion potential
Stem cell selection or red cell depletion	Optimum processing procedures
	Duration of storage
Preservation	Autologous use potential
Histocompatibility testing	Role of maternal cells in cord blood
Genetic diseases testing	Role of genetic testing for disease
Transplant specimens	Approaches for testing opportunistic diseases
Transportation	
Thawing and transfusion	
Confidentiality	

Reproduced, with permission, from Ballen *et al.* (2001a).

Results of cord blood transplantation from Eurocord Registry

Eurocord is an international registry operating on behalf of the European Blood and Marrow Transplant (EBMT) group. Participation is open to European and non-European centers conducting UCBT. More than 172 transplant centers from 34 countries are currently reporting their data. Eurocord registry works in close collaboration with Netcord banks. Centers carrying out transplants with umbilical cord blood units from Netcord banks are invited to report their cases to Eurocord registry. From 1988 to June 2002, 1,199 UCBT have been reported to the Eurocord Registry. The donor was related in 197 cases and unrelated in 1,002 cases. Most of the patients were children ($n = 856$) but the number of adults is increasing ($n = 343$). Umbilical related and unrelated cord blood units were provided by the following Netcord umbilical cord blood banks: New York, USA 166; Düsseldorf, Germany 153; Milan, Italy 213; Barcelona, Spain 96; Tokyo, Japan 71; University of Colorado, USA 63; London, UK 41; Saint Louis, USA 52; Sydney, Australia 22; France 65; Belgium 17; Holland 3; and non-Netcord banks provided by the EBMT.

Results in children transplanted with related donor umbilical cord blood

Studies reported in the literature using family member cord blood transplants are shown in Table 68.6.

A comprehensive banking program of sibling donor cord blood has been described (Reed *et al.*, 2003). Families were eligible if they were caring for a child with a disorder treatable by HSC transplantation and expecting the birth of a full sibling. Five hundred and six cords were banked and 17 of them used subsequently for transplantation.

Results in patients with acute leukemia

In Eurocord the number of UCBT performed with a family donor has been relatively stable during the past 10 years in comparison with unrelated UCBT (Fig. 68.1). Outcomes of 40 related UCBT for children with acute leukemia (AL) have been published (Gluckman *et al.*, 1997; Locatelli *et al.*, 1999; Gluckman, 2000). We have updated the data and analyzed 62 children receiving a related UCBT for AL. Forty-four children had acute lymphoblastic leukemia (ALL) and 18 acute myeloid leukemia (AML). Most ALL cases were pre-B or B-cell origin ($n = 40$) and 4 were of T-cell origin. French-American-British (FAB) classification for AML was M0 ($n = 4$), M1 ($n = 4$), M2 ($n = 2$), M4 ($n = 1$), M5 ($n = 2$), and M7 ($n = 4$). The donor was HLA-identical in 45 cases or was mismatched for 1 ($n = 2$), 2 ($n = 6$), or 3 ($n = 9$) HLA antigens. The conditioning regimen varied according to age and diagnosis; however, 58% received an irradiation-containing regimen. Most often GVHD prevention consisted of cyclosporine (CSP) alone ($n = 35$) or CSP + methotrexate (MTX) ($n = 18$). The median follow-up was 56

Table 68.6. *Studies of cord blood transplantation from related (sibling) donors*

	International Cord Blood Transplantation Registry	Eurocord Registry
Number of patients	62	102
Median age, yr (range)	(0.5–16)	5 (0.2–20)
Median body weight, kg (range)	–	19 (5–50)
Diseases, *n*	–	Malignancies (61)
	–	Nonmalignancies (41)
Number of HLA mismatches, *n*	0 (51)	0 (80)
	1–3 (11)	1 (5)
		2 (6)
		3 (10)
		4 (10)
Overall survival at 1 yr	–	64%
Survival by HLA status	61% at 2 yr (0–1 HLA disparity)	73% at 1 yr (0 HLA disparity)
		50% at 1 yr (1–4 HLA disparity)
		(*p* = .006)
Survival at 1 year by disease	–	55% (malignancies)
		67% (bone marrow failure syndrome)
		100% (hemoglobinopathies)
		71% at 1 yr (inborn errors)
Incidence of GVHD	6/62 (grades 0–1)	24% (grade >II)
	3/62 (grades II–IV)	7% (grades II–IV)
	3/62 (chronic)	3 of 43 patients at risk (chronic)
Neutrophil engraftment, days (median)[a]	9–46 (22)	8–49 (28)
Platelet engraftment, days (median)[b]	15–117 (51)	4–180 (48)

[a] Neutrophil recovery defined as time to achieve an absolute neutrophil count $>5 \times 10^8/l$.
[b] Platelet count $>5 \times 10^{10}/l$ untransfused for 7 days.
Reproduced, with permission, from Ballen *et al.* (2001a).

months, median age 5 (range 1.7–13) years, and the median number of nucleated cells infused was $3 \times 10^7/kg$. Outcomes for children with ALL and AML as of April 2001 are listed in Table 68.7. These results are quite similar to those reported with bone marrow transplantation.

Results in patients with hemoglobinopathies

We studied 44 patients who received a related cord blood transplant for either thalassemia (*n* = 33) or sickle cell disease (SCD) (*n* = 11) (F. Locatelli, 2002, submitted). Median age was

Table 68.7. *Outcomes of children with acute leukemia transplanted with a related cord blood transplant*

Parameter[a]	ALL (*n* = 44)	AML (*n* = 18)	Total (= 62)
Neutrophil recovery at day 60	87%	94%	89%
Platelet recovery at day 180	92%	72%	88%
Acute GVHD at day 100	28%	35%	30%
Chronic GVHD at 2 years	4%	8%	6%
Relapse at 2 years	48%	40%	43%
Survival at 2 years	46%	50%	47%
Event-free survival at 2 years	36%	39%	37%

Abbreviations: ALL, acute lymphoblastic leukemia; AML, acute myeloid leukemia.
[a] Kaplan Meier estimates.

5 (range 1–20) years. Conditioning varied among centers and most patients received cyclosporine alone for prevention of GVHD. The median number of nucleated cells infused was 4.0 $\times 10^7/kg$ (range 1.2–10).

No patients died and 36 of the 44 children remain disease-free, with a median follow-up of 24 (range 3–76) months. Only one patient with SCD did not have sustained donor engraftment as compared to 7 out of the 33 patients with thalassemia. Three of these 8 patients had sustained donor engraftment after BMT from the same donor. Four patients experienced grade II acute GVHD, and only 2 of the 36 patients at risk developed limited chronic GVHD. The 2-year probability of event-free survival is 79% and 90% for patients with thalassemia and SCD, respectively. Use of MTX for GVHD prophylaxis was associated with a greater risk of treatment failure.

Related UCBT for hemoglobinopathies offers a probability of success comparable to that offered by BMT and is associated with lower risk of both treatment-related mortality (TRM) and chronic GVHD. This result can be further improved in optimizing the transplant procedure.

Results in patients with other nonmalignant diseases

Twenty-seven patients were transplanted for bone marrow failure syndromes (Fanconi anemia 12, idiopathic severe aplastic anemia 8, Blackfan-Diamond anemia 3, dyskeratosis congenita

2, amegakaryocytosis 1, and Kostmann's syndrome 1). Overall survival was 79%, engraftment 93%, acute GVHD 27%, chronic GVHD 8%, and transplant-related mortality 21%. Fifteen patients received a related UCBT for a metabolic storage disease (*n* = 8) or immunodeficiency (*n* = 7). Transplant-related mortality was 20% and survival 80%.

Comparison of related cord blood and bone marrow transplantation

In the group of patients receiving a related UCBT, we have shown that results were comparable to HLA-identical sibling transplantation using bone marrow as a source of HSCs (Rocha *et al.*, 2000). We utilized data from Eurocord and the International Bone Marrow Transplant Registry (IBMTR). We studied 113 children receiving an HLA-identical related UCBT and 2,052 children receiving an HLA-identical sibling BMT between 1990 and 1997.

Recipients of UCBT were younger (median 5 vs. 8 years, *P* < .001), weighed less (median 17 vs. 26 kg, *P* < .001), more frequently had major ABO incompatibility with their donor (25% vs. 15%, *P* < .001), and less frequently received MTX for GVHD prophylaxis (28% vs. 65%, *P* < .001) than BMT recipients. Interval from diagnosis to transplant was shorter for BMT recipients (median 10 vs. 25 months, *P* < .001). The median number of nucleated umbilical cord blood cells infused was 0.47 × 10^8/kg compared with 3.5 × 10^8/kg nucleated bone marrow cells (*P* < .001). Multivariate analysis demonstrated lower risks of grade II–IV acute GVHD [relative risk (RR) 0.40, 95% confidence interval (CI) 0.24–0.70; *P* = .001] and chronic GVHD (RR 0.35, 95% CI 0.14–0.85; *P* = .02) in UCBT recipients (Fig. 68.2, Panels A and B). Neutrophil recovery was significantly delayed after UCBT (RR 0.40, 95% CI 0.32–0.51; *P* < .001) (Fig 68.2, Panel C), as was platelet recovery in the first month after transplant (RR 0.20, 95% CI 0.13–0.29; *P* < .001). Survival was similar in both groups (RR 1.15, 95% CI 0.81–1.65; *P* = .43) (Fig. 68.2, Panel D). Platelet recovery from an earlier analysis (Gluckman *et al.*, 1997) is shown in Fig. 68.3.

This study demonstrated that recipients of HLA-identical sibling UCBT have less acute and chronic GVHD than recipients of HLA-identical sibling BMT. Survival was similar with cord blood and bone marrow transplantation (BMT), suggesting that umbilical cord blood is an acceptable source of HSCs for transplantation and justifying the collection of cord blood from siblings of a patient who might be cured by an allogeneic HSC transplant.

Results in children transplanted with unrelated donor umbilical cord blood

There are several reports of unrelated UCBT in children including those by Kurtzberg *et al.*, 1996; Wagner *et al.*, 1996; Gluckman *et al.*, 1997; Cairo & Wagner, 1997; and Rubinstein *et al.*, 1998. Studies reported in the literature using unrelated cord blood transplants are shown in Table 68.8.

In Eurocord, we analyzed 277 children; the diagnosis was ALL in 97 cases, AML in 47 cases, myelodysplastic syndrome (MDS) in 23 cases, chronic myeloid leukemia (CML) in 14 cases, non-Hodgkin's lymphoma (NHL) in 4 cases, and other malignancies in 5 cases. For nonmalignant diseases, the diagnosis was aplastic anemia in 29 cases and inborn errors of metabolism in 58 cases. Fifteen patients with acute leukemia had previously received an autologous transplant and 7 an allogeneic transplant. Most of the donors (87%) had 1 to 4 HLA mismatches and 31 were matched by serology and low-resolution DRB1 typing. The medium follow-up was 21 (range 1–64) months, the median age was 5 (0.3–15) years, the median weight was 18 (2.5–83) kg, and the median number of nucleated cells infused was 4.4 × 10^7/kg (0.6–36).

The 1-year survival was 48% ± 6%. It was 46% for malignant diseases, 32% for aplastic anemia, and 63% for inborn errors. The probability of day 60 granulocyte engraftment was 82% with a median time to reach more than 500/μl granulocytes of 29 days (range 10–60). The rate of engraftment was reduced in aplastic anemia where it was only 50%. The incidence of acute GVHD ≥II was 38%.

We performed a more detailed study in children with acute leukemia (Locatelli *et al.*, 1999). Children given an unrelated UCBT during 1st or 2nd complete remission were considered as belonging to the good risk group, whereas those transplanted in more advanced stage of the disease were assigned to the poor risk group. A Kaplan-Meier estimate for neutrophil recovery at day 60 was 79% ± 6%. In multivariate analysis, the most important factor influencing neutrophil engraftment was a nucleated cell dose infused greater than 3.7 × 10^7/kg (*P* = .05, RR 1.85, 95% CI 0.98–3.4). The incidence of grade II–IV GVHD was 37% ± 6%. A Kaplan-Meier estimate of 2-year event-free survival (EFS) was 30% ± 7%. In multivariate analysis, the most important factor influencing EFS was disease status at the time of transplantation: good-risk patients had a 2-year EFS of 49% ± 7% as compared to 8% ± 5% in patients with more advanced disease (*P* = .0003, RR 0.40, 95% CI 0.24–0.65). This was a consequence of both an increased 1-year transplant-related mortality rate and a higher 2-year relapse rate in the poor-risk group (65% ± 9% and 77% ± 14%, respectively), as compared to good risk patients (34% ± 6% and 31% ± 9%, respectively). Notably, there were no major differences in most outcomes between related and unrelated UCBT. These data confirm that allogeneic UCBT from an unrelated donor is a feasible procedure able to cure a significant proportion of children with acute leukemia, especially if transplanted in a favorable phase of disease.

More recently, we analyzed the results of unrelated UCBT in 195 children with ALL from 1994 to 2001 (unpublished data). At diagnosis, the median white blood cell count (WBC) was 35 × 10^9/l; cytogenetic analysis was normal in 34%, abnormal in 45%, and not available in 21% of patients. At transplant, the median age was 7 years (range 0.4–16) and median weight 25 kg (5–83). One hundred patients had a good prognostic status at transplant (CR1, *n* = 35 or CR2, *n* = 85), and 75 children

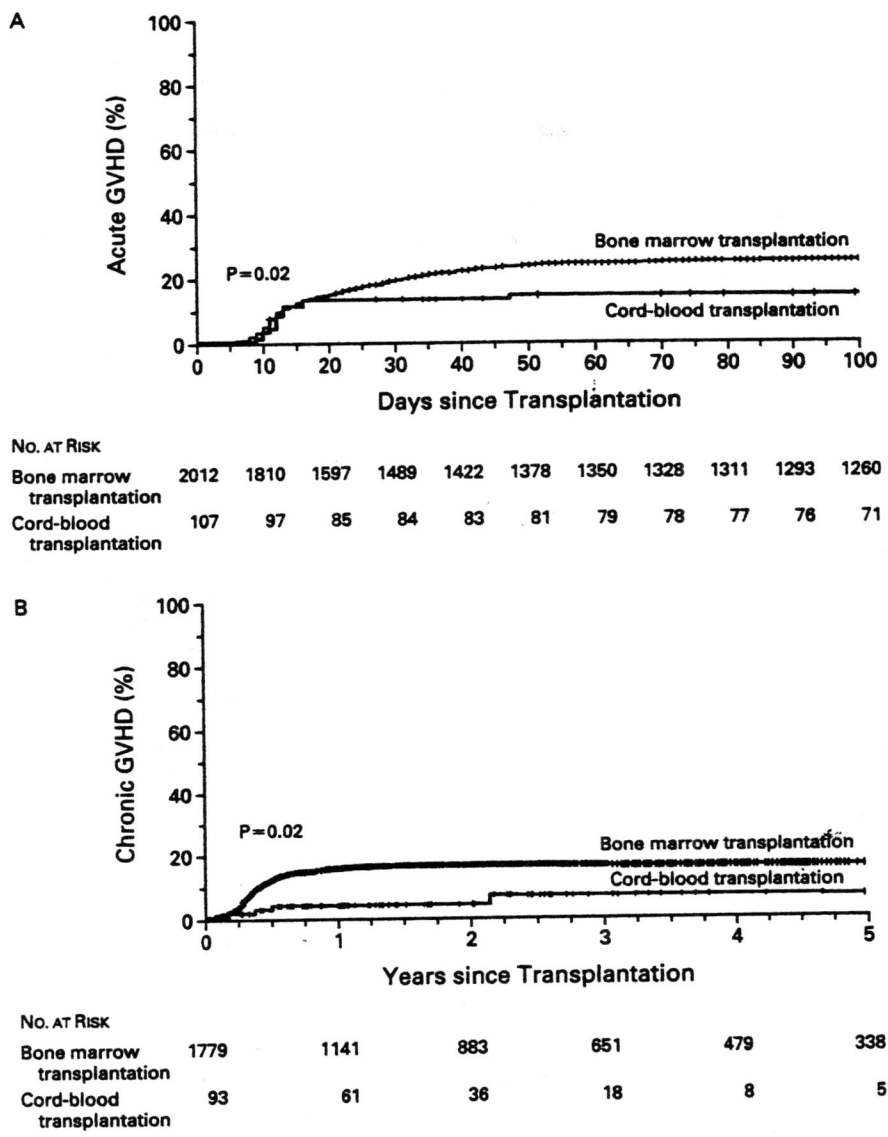

Fig. 68.2. Outcomes among recipients of a cord-blood transplant from an HLA-identical sibling and recipients of a bone marrow transplant from an HLA-identical sibling. The tick marks on the curve represent censored data. Panel **A** shows the cumulative incidence of grade II, III, and IV acute graft-versus-host disease (GVHD). Panel **B** shows the cumulative incidence of chronic GVHD. Panel **C** shows the cumulative incidence of neutrophil recovery to more than 500 cells per cubic millimeter. Panel **D** shows the Kaplan-Meier estimate of survival according to the underlying disease. Reproduced, with permission, from Rocha *et al.* (2000). *(Figure continues)*

were transplanted in more advanced phase of their disease. Sixteen patients had previously received either an autologous or an allogeneic BMT for high-risk leukemia or relapse. The median follow-up time was 31 months (0.6–78). Conditioning varied according to disease status, recipient age, and center protocols. Acute GVHD prophylaxis consisted of CSP alone in 17 patients, in combination with MTX in 39 patients and with prednisone in 129 patients. The median number of nucleated cells (NC) infused was 3.8×10^7/kg (0.6–21.3) and median number of CD34+ cells infused was 1.7×10^5/kg (0.03–39).

The donor was HLA-matched in 21 patients and mismatched in the others (5/6 matching, $n = 80$; 4/6, $n = 78$, and 3 or 2/6, $n = 8$). The probability of neutrophil recovery at day 60 was 84% and the median time to 500 neutrophils/µl was 29 days (95% CI 21–50). Patients receiving more than 3.7×10^7/kg NC had a 95% probability of neutrophil recovery compared to 81% in patients receiving less than 3.7×10^7/kg NC ($P < .001$). Multivariate analysis of neutrophil recovery showed that the number of nucleated cells infused ($P = .0007$) and remission status at transplant ($P = .03$) were both factors predicting

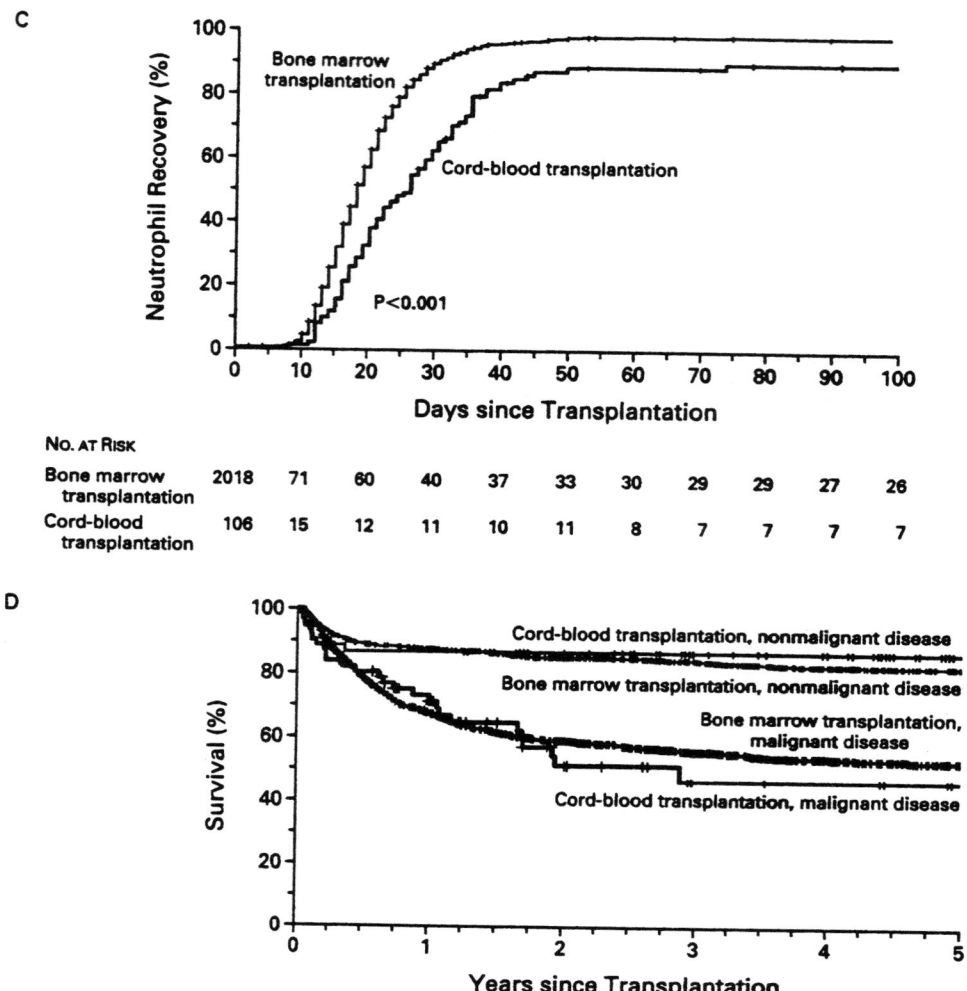

Fig. 68.2. *(Figure continued.)*

recovery. Platelet recovery at day 180 was 86% and was also influenced by the number of cells infused. Estimated probability of acute GVHD (≥ grade II) was 38%. Twenty-four patients had acute GVHD grade II, 19 grade III, and 17 grade IV. Chronic GVHD was observed in 11 of 89 patients at risk. Estimated 2-year EFS was 33%. It was 40% for patients transplanted in CR1, 34% for CR2, and 29% for more advanced phase (P = .41). Strikingly, the relapse rate was 43% in CR1, 35% in CR2, and 32% in advanced phase (P = .69). Cytogenetic abnormalities at diagnosis increased the risk of relapse. Relapse rate at 2 years was 47% in patients with cytogenetic abnormalities and 29% in patients with normal or unknown karyotypes (P = .02). There was a trend toward increased risk of relapse in T-ALL (P = .09), in patients receiving MTX for GVHD prophylaxis (P = .06) and in patients without acute GVHD (RR 0.48, 95% CI 0.20–1.18; P = .09). Relapse on therapy before transplant was an important factor with an increasing relapse rate in the group of patients transplanted in CR2 or beyond (P = .02). In multivariate analysis,

the most important factor influencing relapse was cytogenetic abnormalities at diagnosis, use of MTX for GVHD prophylaxis, and absence of acute GVHD.

Unrelated cord blood transplants compared to unrelated bone marrow transplants in children with acute leukemia

A comparison of results of unrelated UCBT to unrelated BMT has been published in 2 studies with similar results (Rocha *et al.*, 2001; Barker *et al.*, 2001a).

In our study, we compared the outcomes of 99 children with AL receiving an unrelated cord blood transplant (UD-UCBT) to those of 442 children receiving either a nonmanipulated unrelated BMT (UBMT) (n = 262) or a T-depleted unrelated BMT (T-UBMT) (n = 180). Comparisons were performed after adjustment for patient, disease, and transplant variables. The major difference between the three groups was the higher number of HLA mismatches (defined by serology for class I and

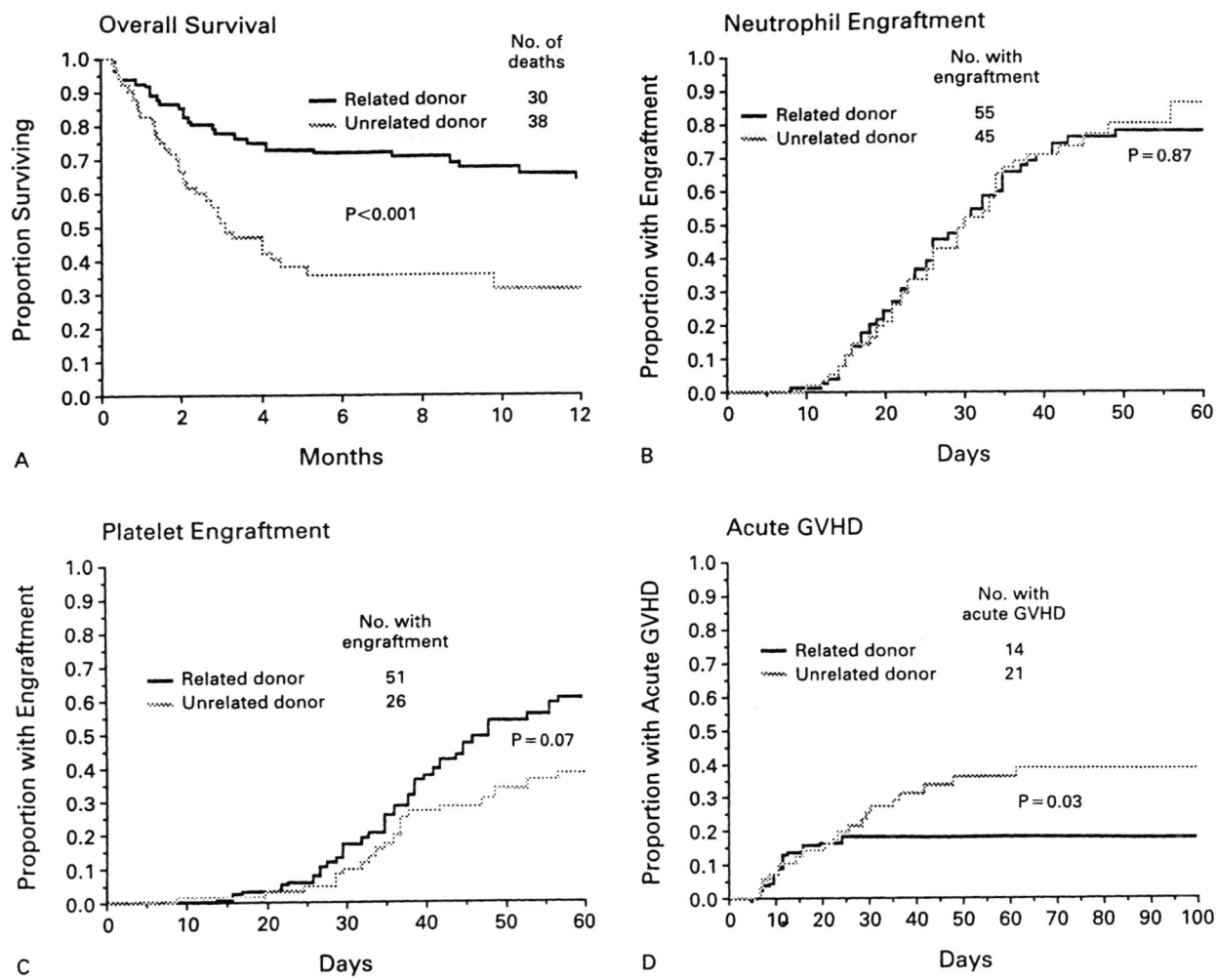

Fig. 68.3. Kaplan-Meier estimates of the probability of survival (Panel **A**), engraftment of neutrophils (Panel **B**), and platelets (Panel **C**) at day 60, and acute graft-versus-host disease (GVHD) (Panel **D**), according to whether the cord blood transplant originated from a related or an unrelated donor. Seventy-eight patients received cord blood from related donors, and 65 patients received cord blood from unrelated donors. Neutrophil engraftment was defined by an absolute neutrophil count of at least 500 per cubic millimeter, platelet engraftment by a count of at least 20,000 per cubic millimeter, and acute GVHD by disease of grade II or higher. Reproduced, with permission, from Gluckman *et al.* (1997).

molecular typing for DRB1) in the UD-UCBT group. The donor was HLA-mismatched with the recipient in 92% of UD-UCBT, in 18% of UBMT, and in 43% of T-UBMT ($P < .001$). Other significant differences were observed in pretransplant disease characteristics, preparative regimens, GVHD prophylaxis, and number of cells infused. Nonadjusted estimates of 2-year survival and EFS rates were 49% and 43%, respectively, in the UBMT group, 41% and 37% in the T-UBMT group, and 35% and 31% in the UD-UCBT group. After adjustment, differences in outcomes appeared in the first 100 days posttransplant. Compared to UBMT, UD-UCBT recipients had delayed hematopoietic recovery (HR 0.37; 95% CI 0.27–0.52; $P < .001$), increased 100-day transplant-related mortality (HR 2.13; 95% CI 1.20–3.76; $P < .01$), and decreased acute GVHD (HR 0.50; 95% CI 0.34–0.73; $P < .001$). T-UBMT recipients had

decreased acute GVHD (HR 0.25; 95% CI 0.17–0.36; $P < .0001$) and increased risk of relapse (HR 1.96; 95% CI 1.11–3.45; $P = .02$). After day 100 posttransplant, the three groups achieved similar results in terms of relapse. Chronic GVHD was decreased after T-UBMT (HR 0.21; 95% CI 0.11–0.37; $P < .0001$) and UD-UCBT (HR 0.24; 95% CI 0.01–0.66; $P .002$), and overall mortality was higher in T-UBMT recipients (HR 1.39; 95% CI 0.97–1.99; $P < .07$).

These data confirm that allogeneic UCBT from an unrelated HLA mismatched cord blood donor is a feasible procedure able to cure a significant proportion of children with acute leukemia. It is a reasonable option for children with AL lacking an acceptably matched unrelated marrow donor.

In conclusion, we recommend simultaneously searching bone marrow donor registries and cord blood banks. The final choice

Table 68.8.   *Studies of cord blood transplantation from unrelated donors*

	New York Blood Center	Eurocord Registry	Eurocord Registry	University of Minnesota/ Duke University[a]
Number of patients	562	158[b]	42[c]	257
Age, yr (n)	<2 (114) 2–5 (127) 6–11 (137) 12–17 (82) ≥18 (102)	Children: 0.2–14 (102) Adults: (44)	15–50 (median, 26)	0.2–58 (median, 8.1)
Body weight, kg (n)	<10 (77) 10–19 (148) 20–39 (152) 40–59 (91) ≥60 (94)	5–46 (102)	35–90 (median, 56)	3.9–102.8 (median, 24.5)
Diseases (n)	Leukemia or lymphoma (378) Genetic disease (137) Acquired disease (47)	Leukemia or lymphoma (72 children) Bone marrow failure syndrome (12 children) Inborn errors (18 children) Malignancies (42 adults)	Acute leukemia (16) Chronic myeloid leukemia (21) Non-Hodgkin's lymphoma (2) Myelodysplastic syndromes (3)	Malignancies (164) Nonmalignancies (93)
Number of HLA mismatches (n)	0 (40) 1 (218) 2 (261) 3 (37) 4 (3)	Children: 0 (14) 1 (64) 2 (23) 3 (1) Adults: 0 (6) 1 (17) 2 (14) 3 (5)	0 (2) 1 (8) 2 (21) 3 (10) 4 (1)	0 (18) 1 (91) 2 (124) 3 (15) Unresolved (9)
Platelets engraftment (median time)	85% at 180 days (90 days)	–	–	51% (6 mo)
Neutrophil engraftment (median time)	81% at 42 days (28 days)	74% for children	76 ± 12 at 60 days	87% (25 days)
Incidence of GVHD (grade)	23% acute (III–IV) 25% chronic	38% acute (≥II)	18 acute (≥II) 3 chronic	30% acute (≥II) 12% acute (III–IV) 7% chronic
Survival rate (disease)		Children: 37% (overall) 35% (malignancies) 10% (bone marrow failure syndrome) 70% (inborn errors) Adults: 16% (overall)	17% ± 6% (overall)	41% at 3 years

[a] Data presented at CME symposium.
[b] Patients analyzed were divided into 2 groups: children (*n* = 102) and adults (*n* = 44).
[c] Separate analysis of 42 adults patients with malignancies.
Reproduced, with permission, from Ballen *et al.* (2001a).

of the stem cell source must take into account the degree of HLA identity, the availability of the donor, the urgency of the transplant, and, of course, the cell dose in the cord blood unit.

Unrelated cord blood for adults with malignancies

The potential role of UD-UCBT in adults remains unclear. At present, information on the results of UCBT in adults comes only from heterogeneous registry series of patients with different diseases. This deficit is due mainly to grave concerns about the possibility of graft failure following UD-UCBT in adults.

At present, only two series of UD-UCBT in adults have been published (Laughlin *et al.*, 2001; Sanz *et al.*, 2001) as well as several abstracts (Goldberg *et al.*, 2000; Iseki *et al.*, 2001; Rocha *et al.*, 2000). Characteristics of the patients and outcomes are summarized in Table 68.9.

We analyzed 108 adult patients transplanted with an unrelated UCBT (Rocha *et al.*, 2001; unpublished data). Median age was 26 years (range 15–53), median weight was 60 kg (35–110), and median follow-up time was 20 months (6–60). Fifty-five patients had AL, 37 CML, 4 non-Hodgkin's lymphoma, and 12 MDS. Forty-seven patients were transplanted in

Table 68.9. *Summary of characteristics and outcome of unrelated cord blood transplants in adults*

	Laughlin	Sanz	Goldberg	Iseki	Rocha
No. of patients	68	22	19	30	108
Age (yr)	31 (18–58)	29 (18–46)	48 (20–59)	38	26 (15–53)
Weight (kg)	69 (41–116)	70 (41–85)	69 (52–126)	52	60 (35–110)
Malignancies	56	22	19	30	108
HLA (%)				NA	
6/6	2 (3)	1 (5)	4 (21)		6 (6)
5/6	18 (26)	13 (59)	8 (42)		38 (35)
4/6	37 (54)	8 (36)	7 (37)		51 (47)
3/6	11 (16)	0	0		13 (12)
NC infused $\times 10^7$/kg	1.6 (0.6–4)	1.7 (1–5)	1.8 (0.4–5.3)	2.39	1.7 (0.2–6)
Day ANC >500	27 (13–59)	22 (13–52)	28	22	32 (13–57)
Day PLTS >20	58 (35–142)	69 (49–153)	56	38	129 (26–176)
EFS	26% at 40 mo	53% at 12 mo	21% at 12 mo	76% at 36 mo	21% at 12 mo

good-risk status (1st and 2nd complete remission and chronic phase). Twenty (19%) patients had previously received an autologous HSC transplant. GVHD prophylaxis consisted mainly of CSP plus prednisone ($n = 77$). Conditioning regimen varied according to disease and center. Six patients received an HLA-identical unit (HLA-A, -B serology and -DRB1 allelic typing) and 102 an HLA-mismatched unit with 1 HLA difference (38 cases), 2 HLA differences (51 cases), or 3 HLA differences (13 cases). The median number of nucleated cells infused was 1.7×10^7/kg (0.2–6). Neutrophil recovery at day 60 occurred in 81% and platelet recovery at day 180 in 65%. Twenty-four patients died early between day 4 and 57, and 15 did not engraft. The median time for neutrophil recovery ≥ 500/mm^3 was 32 days (13–57) and for platelets $\geq 20,000$/mm^3 was 129 days (26–176). NC $\geq 1.7 \times 10^7$/kg was an important factor influencing neutrophil and platelet recovery ($P = .01$). Acute GVHD ($\geq$ grade II) was observed in 44 patients (grade II 16, grade III 12. and grade IV 15). The occurrence of grade III–IV GVHD was not influenced by the number of HLA disparities ($P = .12$). Chronic GVHD was observed in 15 of 58 patients at risk. Kaplan-Meier estimate for TRM at day 100 was 54%. In a univariate analysis the following factors increased 100-day TRM: poor-risk disease status at CBT ($P = .016$); $<1.7 \times 10^7$ NC/kg ($P = .03$), and UCBT performed before January 1998 ($P = .01$). Patients transplanted before this time received cord blood units containing fewer numbers of cells ($P = .03$) and with more HLA disparities ($P = .001$) compared to patients transplanted after. In a multivariate analysis, the risk of death at day 100 was influenced by the status of the disease at transplant (RR 1.85; $P = .03$), NC $\geq 1.7 \times 10^7$/kg (RR 1.2; $P = .04$), and transplant performed before January 1998 (RR 1.90; $P = .02$). One-year survival was 27% and EFS was 21%. In patients with AL, EFS was 23%. Favorable factors for survival were NC $\geq 1 \times 10^7$ /kg ($P = .014$) and good-risk status at transplant ($P = .007$). Ten out of 11 patients receiving less than 1×10^7 NC/kg died. Probability of survival at 1 year was 33% for patients receiving more than $\geq 2 \times 10^7$ NC/kg. Seventy-

four patients died: 7 (9%) of relapse, 30 (41%) of nonengraftment and infections, 17 of toxicity (23%), 13 (18%) of GVHD, and 7 of other causes.

These results suggest that UD-UCBT is an optional source of stem cells in adult patients with malignancies lacking a matched unrelated bone marrow donor. However, the choice of units containing large number of cells and good disease status at transplant might improve results.

Factors associated with outcome of unrelated cord blood transplantation: guidelines for donor choice

With the increasing number of unrelated cord blood transplants, it becomes possible to analyze factors associated with early outcomes. Previous studies have shown that most of the complications appear during the first 6 months and that in long-term follow-up the rate of death due to infections, chronic GVHD, and relapse is relatively low. We therefore analyzed 690 patients who received an unrelated cord blood transplant (unpublished results). There were 487 children (71%) and 203 adults (29%). Most patients had hematological malignances (80%), including 69% with acute leukemia; 13% had immune deficiencies or metabolic diseases, and 7% bone marrow failure syndromes. The median number of nucleated cells infused was 3.5×10^7/kg. Most were HLA mismatched (by serology for HLA-A and -B and -DRB1 molecular typing) with 1 (43%), 2 (40%), or 3–4 (6%) HLA incompatibilities. Forty-four percent had 1 or 2 HLA class I mismatches, 18% 1 or 2 HLA class II mismatches, and 27% both class I and class II mismatches. The cumulative incidence of neutrophil engraftment was 72% at 60 days; the cumulative incidence of platelet recovery at 6 months was 50%. In a multivariate analysis, factors associated with hematological recovery were:

1. Number of nucleated cells collected (more than 4.6×10^7/kg did better) (Fig. 68.4)
2. Diagnosis (patients with aplastic anemia had more rejection)

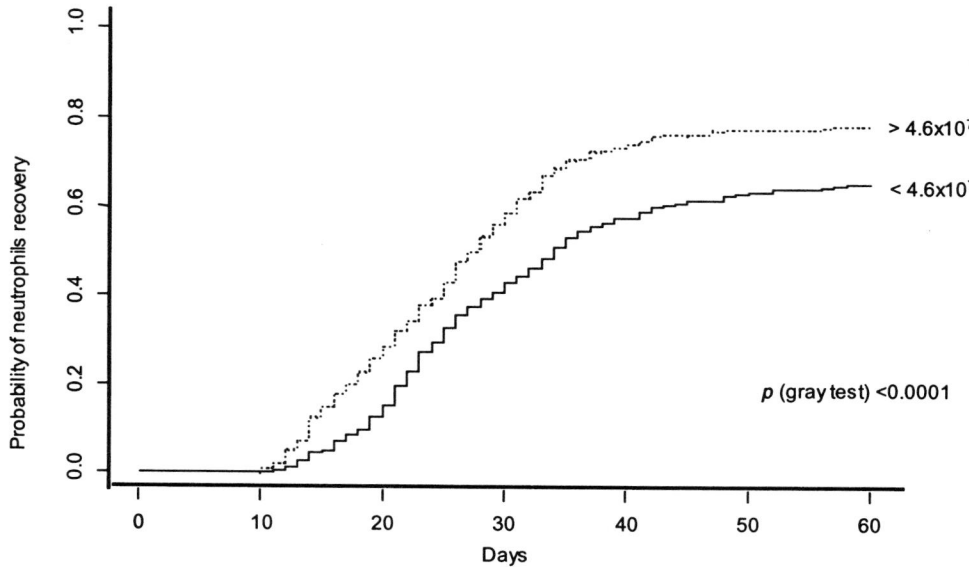

Fig. 68.4. Cumulative incidence of neutrophil recovery after unrelated cord blood transplantation according to number of cord blood cells before freezing.

3. HLA matching (there was a correlation between the number of HLA mismatches and engraftment) (Fig. 68.5); HLA mismatches for class I had better engraftment than mismatches for class II and for both class I and class II
4. ABO matching (compatibility associated with better engraftment)

The cumulative incidence of acute GVHD grade ≥II was 35%. There was no correlation between the number and type of HLA mismatches and the occurrence of GVHD (Fig. 68.6).

The cumulative incidence of day 100 TRM was 34%. In a multivariate analysis of factors associated with TRM, HLA mismatching, diagnosis of aplastic anemia, and number of nucleated cells collected were statistically significant prognostic factors.

Overall probability of survival was 46% for children and 26% for adults. Figure 68.7 shows 2-year survival according to diagnosis. Multivariate analysis of factors associated with decreased 2-year survival were:

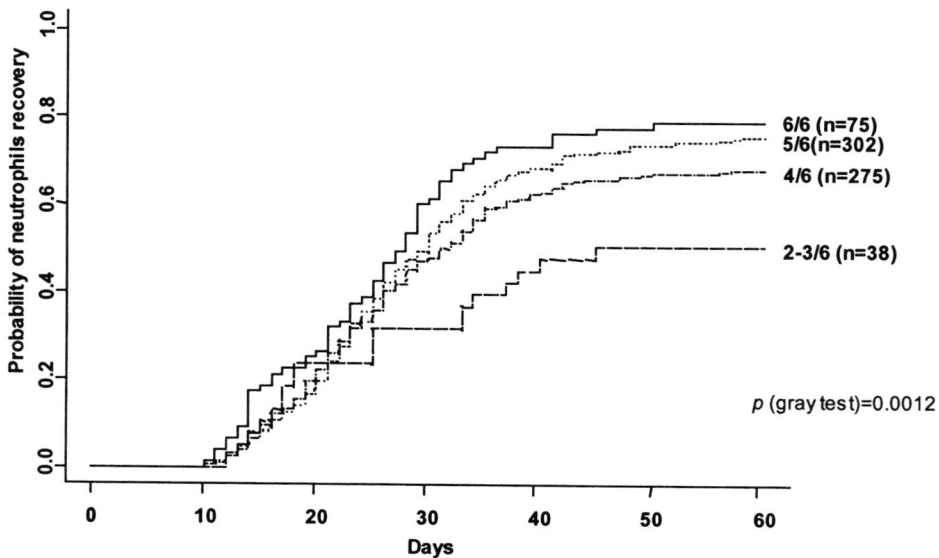

Fig. 68.5. Cumulative incidence of neutrophil recovery after unrelated cord blood transplantation according to number of HLA disparities between donor and recipient.

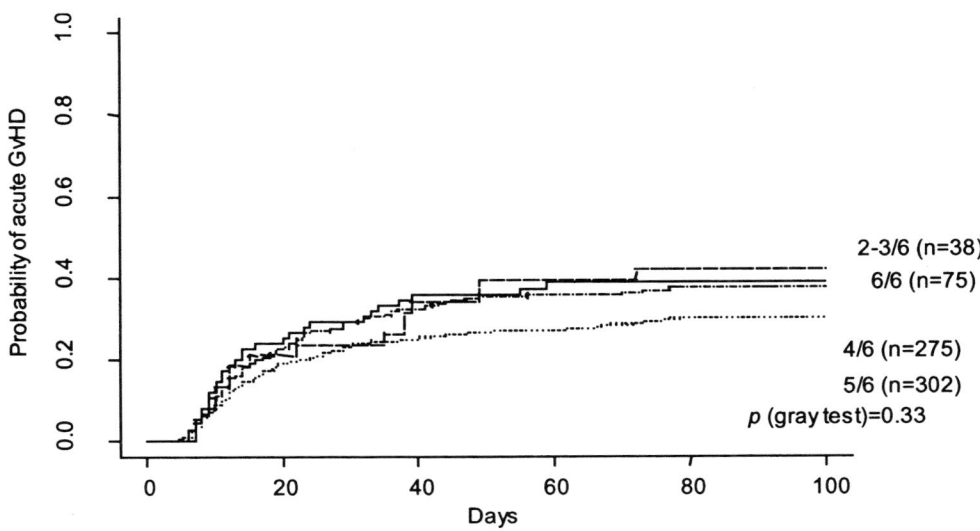

Fig. 68.6. Cumulative incidence of acute GVHD (II–IV) according to the number of HLA disparities between donor and recipient.

1. Age>15 years
2. Positive CMV serology
3. Cord blood transplants performed after 1998
4. Cell dose infused ($<3.7 \times 10^7$/kg)

The number and class of HLA mismatching had no influence on survival (Fig. 68.8). TRM in adults was 72% before 1998 and 44% after this period, indicating that better selection of patients and donors and better expertise of transplant centers

markedly improved results of unrelated HLA-mismatched cord blood transplants.

In some (Wagner *et al.*, 2002), but not all (Thompson *et al.*, 2000; Laughlin *et al.*, 2001), CD34+ cell content of the UCVB had a positive impact on engraftment and survival. In the study by Wagner and colleagues (2002), patients receiving a graft containing 1.7×10^6 CD34+ cells/kg, did better than those receiving grafts with $<1.7 \times 10^6$ CD34+ cells/kg.

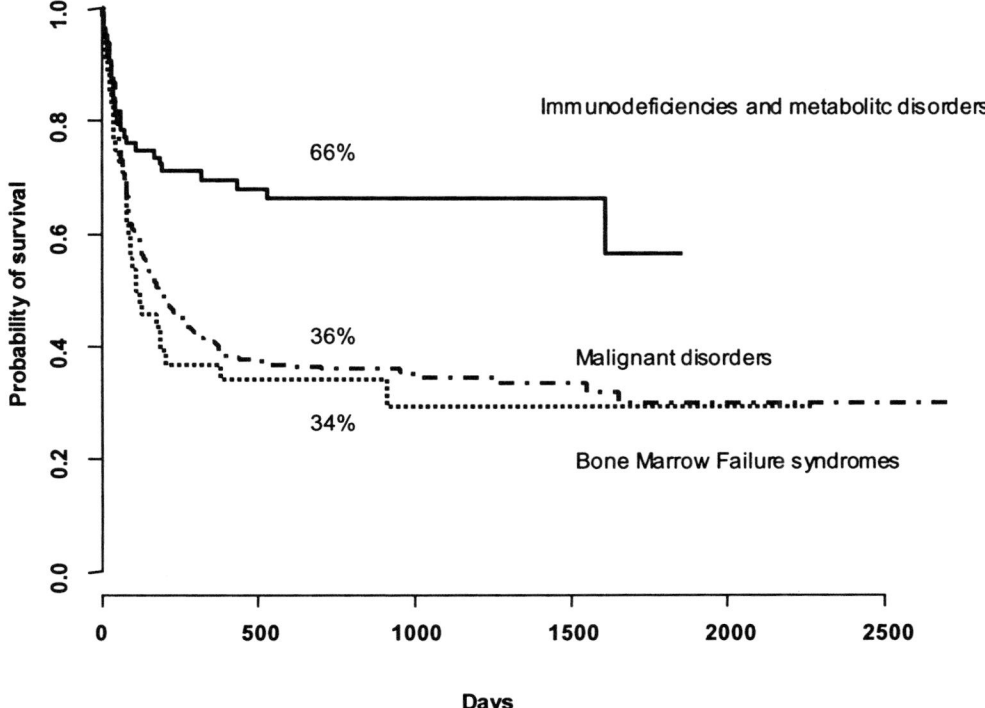

Fig. 68.7. Kaplan-Meier estimate of survival after cord blood transplantation according to diagnosis (% estimates at 2 years).

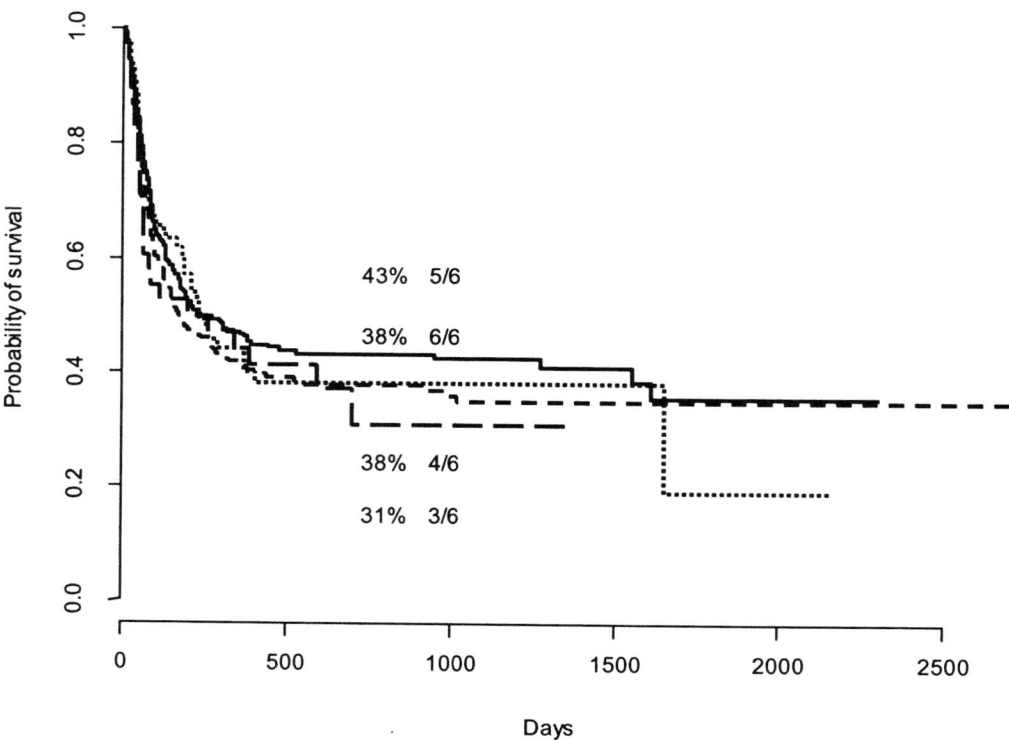

Fig. 68.8. Kaplan-Meier estimate of survival after cord blood transplantation according to number of HLA disparities (% estimates at 2 years).

Immune reconstitution after cord blood transplantation

There is some concern regarding the ability of cord blood cells to adequately reconstitute host immune responses because of the cumulative effect of the low number and immaturity of lymphocytes infused and the HLA mismatching between donor and recipient. Results published so far show that there is a delay of immunological reconstitution responsible for severe infections, but that in the long term immune reconstitution is reasonable.

In a study from Eurocord (Niehues *et al.,* 2001) of 63 children given either a related or an unrelated cord blood transplant, the median time to lymphocyte reconstitution was 3 months for NK cells, 6 months for B cells, and 8 months for CD8+ cells,

while it was 11.7 months for CD3+ and CD4+ lymphocytes. In multivariate analysis, factors favoring T-cell recovery were related donor (*P* = .002), higher nucleated cell infused/kg (*P* = .005), and recipient CMV seropositivity (*P* = .04). Presence of GVHD delayed T-cell recovery (*P* = .04). These results are not different from those after allogeneic BMT. Further, T-cell reconstitution has been evaluated using phenotyping, analysis of the αβ T-cell receptor (TCR) diversity, and assessment of ex vivo thymic function by measuring TCR rearrangement excision circles (TRECs) (Talvensaari *et al.,* 2002). Ten patients who underwent cord blood transplantation for high-risk hematological disorders were compared to a group of 19 age- and GVHD-matched patients who underwent transplantation with non-T-

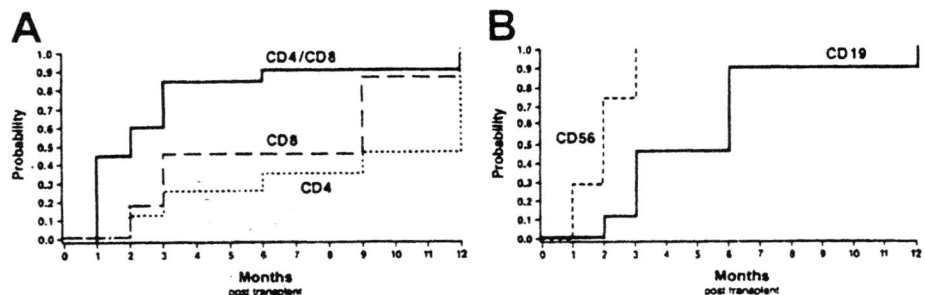

Fig. 68.9. Kaplan-Meier estimates of numerical immune reconstitution. (**A**) Cumulative probability of time to achieve an age-appropriate normal cell count for CD3+/CD4+ cells (dotted line), CD3+/CD8+ cells (dashed line), and CD4+-CD8+ ratio (solid line). Median time for CD4 and CD8 cell recovery was 12 and 9 months, respectively. (**B**) Cumulative probability of time to achieve an age-appropriate normal cell count for CD19+ cells (solid line) and NK (CD56+) cells (dashed line). Median time for CD19 and NK cell recovery was 6 and 2 months, respectively. Reproduced, with permission, from Thomson *et al.* (2000).

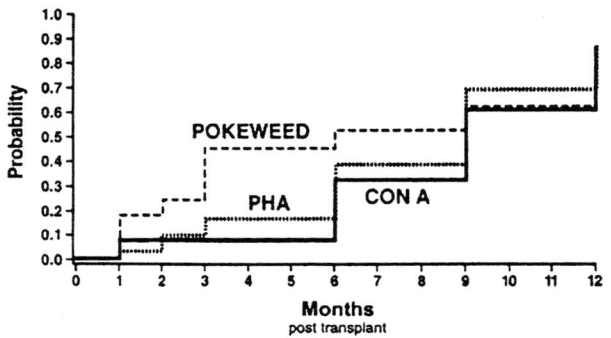

Fig. 68.10. Kaplan-Meier estimates of functional immune reconstitution. Cumulative probability of time to achieve an age-appropriate normal mitogen response to PHA (dotted line), Con A (solid line), and PWM (dashed line). Median time to recovery of normal mitogen responses was 6 to 9 months posttransplantation. Reproduced, with permission, from Thomson *et al.* (2000).

depleted bone marrow from an HLA-identical sibling donor. TREC values correlated with the relative number of naïve T cells and with TCR repertoire polyclonality. During the first year after transplantation, TCR repertoires were highly abnormal and TREC values low in both groups. Notably, 2 years after transplantation, TREC values and TCR diversity were higher in cord blood recipients than in bone marrow recipients. These data indicate an efficient thymic regeneration pathway from cord blood lymphoid progenitors despite the low number of cells infused compared to bone marrow, suggesting complete immune recovery after cord blood transplantation.

Another study of immunological reconstitution after unrelated cord blood transplantation found a delay in peripheral blood CD8[+] cell recovery compared to that reported for other HSC sources (9 months compared to 1–3 months; Fig. 68.9) (Thomson *et al.,* 2000). In contrast, recovery of other parameters, including mitogen responsiveness, was comparable (Fig. 68.10).

Discussion and conclusions

These registry-based analyses confirm other reported results and support the concept of establishing cryopreserved cord blood banks for clinical use. Several questions have been answered; others remain to be investigated.

Engraftment has been, and remains, the major concern, as all studies showed that neutrophil and platelet recoveries were delayed, while long-term engraftment was similar after UCBT compared to BMT. This result was expected as it has been shown that the number of cells infused predicted the outcome of UCBT. We have shown that a cord blood nucleated cell dose above 3.7×10^7/kg improved the speed and probability of engraftment. Recent results confirm our previous recommendation that units should be selected on the basis of the number of nucleated cells collected (above 3×10^7/kg recipient body weight before thawing). The cause for delayed recovery after UCBT might be due to the low number of cells infused, or to

other factors such as the immaturity of stem cells which might need more cell divisions before differentiation to marrow progenitors, to the lack of subpopulations facilitating engraftment, or to a homing defect. Whether current approaches being explored to speed hematopoietic recovery after cord blood transplantation, such as ex vivo expansion, will result in accelerated reconstitution and consequently decreased TRM is unknown. It is interesting to note that the number of cells infused is 1 log less than that in a standard allogeneic bone marrow harvest and 10 times less than a standard peripheral blood stem cell inoculum.

We have also shown that other factors interfere with engraftment such as diagnosis, HLA differences between donor and recipient, and major ABO incompatibility. Patients with severe aplastic anemia had a lower incidence of engraftment than patients with leukemia or inborn errors. This may be explained by pretransplant transfusion immunization and the reduced intensity of the conditioning regimens used for transplantation of aplastic anemia patients. We have shown that HLA incompatibilities are important for engraftment and early TRM, but not for GVHD and long-term survival.

In order to improve the speed of engraftment, several approaches can be investigated including the use of hematopoietic growth factors such as G-CSF, stem cell factor, or thrombopoietin (TPO). At this stage, the usefulness of these factors has not been demonstrated and they deserve further investigation. Other approaches include the co-infusion of mesenchymal stem cells, the co-infusion of related HLA-mismatched PBSC (Fernandez *et al.,* 2001), and ex vivo expansion of cord blood progenitors to improve short-term engraftment (Kögler *et al.,* 1999; Pecora *et al.,* 2000). This latter area of investigation seems particularly interesting, as in vitro studies have shown that expansion of cord blood was increased compared to bone marrow cells. Another avenue of research is the possibility of using several cord blood units in order to increase the stem cell yield (Barker *et al.,* 2001b). In the small number of multicord transplants reported, all have shown that only one unit engrafted while the other was rejected. From a practical point of view, these findings form the basis for recommending that umbilical cord blood banks collect as many cells as possible and improve the processing and volume reduction technique, in order to maximize the nucleated cell count of the stored units.

One of the first concerns raised by the use of umbilical cord blood for allogeneic transplant was the possibility of inadvertent transplantation of cells of maternal origin. We (Petit *et al.,* 1997), and other authors, have shown that, indeed, maternal cells were always present in cord blood but that their number was insufficient to induce GVHD. Their presence can be detected in cord blood by high-resolution molecular typing. As in previously published UCBT series, we observed GVHD, but it was usually not severe; the incidence of chronic GVHD was low; this is quite remarkable after HLA-mismatched transplants without T-cell depletion. The incidence of acute and chronic GVHD was lower after related HLA-identical UCBT than BMT. In unrelated transplants for acute leukemia in children, the difference was even more striking as the incidence of acute GVHD ≥II was lower after HLA-mismatched UCBT than after unmanipulated unrelated BMT. The incidence of chronic GVHD was the same after both UCBT and T-cell-depleted unrelated BMT, and was significantly lower than after unmanipulated unrelated BMT. This diminution of the incidence and severity of both acute and chronic GVHD was also found in adults transplanted with an HLA-mismatched unrelated cord blood donor. This study shows that the decreased incidence of acute and chronic GVHD after UCBT is observed in the presence of major class I and class II HLA differences. This observation lends support to the hypothesis that umbilical cord blood differs from bone marrow in its alloreactive potential. No studies have directly compared graft composition of umbilical cord blood and bone marrow transplants for lymphoid numbers and proportion of different subsets of T, B, and NK cells, but each of these cell types are expected to be lower in absolute numbers in UCB due to the low total cell dose of cord blood grafts. The hypothesis that reduced GVHD results from fewer T cells infused is plausible, since T-cell depletion of bone marrow transplants leads to lower GVHD risk. However, the number of T cells infused with UCBT is on the order of 8×10^6/kg and it is known that GVHD can be induced by as few as 1×10^5 CD3$^+$ cells/kg after HLA-identical sibling BMT, and even fewer (1×10^4/kg) in HLA-mismatched transplants. Since acute GVHD results from activation, clonal expansion, and proliferation of donor-derived T lymphocytes that recognize alloantigen presented by either host or donor antigen-presenting cells, the lower GVHD risk after UCBT might be due to impairment of these functions in umbilical cord blood cells. Therefore, looking for complete HLA identity does not seem to be an absolute prerequisite for a successful UCBT, as we did not find any correlation between the number of HLA mismatches and the outcome of UCBT. The role of HLA has been difficult to evaluate and discrepant results have emerged from different analyses. The methods of HLA typing have changed over time and new polymorphisms have been described, including minor histocompatibility antigens and cytokine polymorphisms. Among other confounding factors, the age of donor and recipient, CMV serology of the recipient, sex of the donor, and prior pregnancies of female donors must be included in multivariate analyses. This complexity emphasizes the need for large multi-institutional studies with registry data.

As the interaction between a lower risk of GVHD and a higher risk of leukemic relapse is well known, we expected a higher incidence of relapse in UCBT compared to unmanipulated BMT. However, we did not find any difference between the adjusted risk of relapse after unmanipulated BMT and after UCBT. The incidence of early relapse was higher after T-cell-depleted BMT. If confirmed with more patients and longer follow-up, this observation could indicate that NK or other cells present in cord blood have an antileukemic potential, despite the immaturity of the immune system at birth.

In conclusion, recommendations for the use of cord blood cells can be given. The best results are obtained when patients are transplanted at an early stage of the disease, indicating that a cord blood search should be performed as soon as possible in patients with acute leukemia or very severe aplastic anemia. The first criterion of choice in selecting a cord blood unit should be the number of cells collected, the second ABO compatibility, and the third HLA compatibility. A combination of class I and class II mismatches, or more than 2 HLA mismatches, should be avoided unless there is no other possible donor and the number of cells is greater than 2×10^7/kg.

References

Aversa, F., Tabilio, A., Terenzi, A. et al. (1994). Successful engraftment of T-cell depleted haploidentical three loci incompatible transplants in leukemia patients by addition of recombinant human granulocyte colony stimulating factor mobilized peripheral blood progenitor cells to bone marrow inoculum. *Blood*, **84**, 3948–55.

Aversa, F., Tabilio, A., Velardi, A. et al. (1998). Treatment of high risk acute leukemia with T cell depleted stem cells from related donors with one fully mismatched HLA haplotype. *New England Journal of Medicine*, **339**, 1186–93.

Ballen, K., Broxmeyer, H.E., McCullough, J. et al. (2001a). Current status of cord blood banking and transplantation in the United States and Europe. *Biology of Blood and Marrow Transplantation*, **7**, 635–45.

Ballen, K.K., Wilson, M., Wuu, J. et al. (2001b). Bigger is better: maternal and neonatal predictors of hematopoietic potential of umbilical cord blood units. *Bone Marrow Transplantation*, **27**, 7–14.

Barker, J.N., Davies, S.M., DeFor, T. et al. (2001a). Survival after transplantation of unrelated donor umbilical cord blood is comparable to that of human leukocyte antigen-matched unrelated donor bone marrow: results of a matched pair analysis. *Blood*, **97**, 2957–61.

Barker, J. N., Krepski, T. P., DeFor, T. E. et al. (2002). Searching for unrelated donor hematopoietic stem cells: availability and speed of umbilical cord versus bone marrow. *Biology of Blood and Marrow Transplantation*, **8**, 257–60.

Barker, J.N., Weisdorf, D.J., & Wagner, J.E. (2001b). Creation of a double chimera after transplantation of umbilical-cord blood from two partially matched unrelated donors. *New England Journal of Medicine*, **344**, 1870–1.

Cairo, M.S. & Wagner, J.E. (1997). Placental and/or umbilical cord blood an alternative source of haemopoietic stem cells for transplantation. *Blood*, **90**, 4665–78.

Chalmers, I.M.H., Janossy, G., Contreras, M. et al. (1998). Intracellular cytokine profile of cord and adult blood lymphocytes. *Blood*, **92**, 11–18.

Davies, S.M., Kollman, C., Anasetti, C. et al. (2000). Engraftment and survival after unrelated donor bone marrow transplantation: a report from the National Bone Marrow Donor Program. *Blood*, **96**, 4096–102.

De La Selle, V., Gluckman, E., Bruley-Rosset, M. (1996). Newborn blood can engraft adult mice without inducing graft versus host disease across non H-2 antigens. *Blood*, **87**, 3977–83.

De La Selle, V., Gluckman, E., Bruley-Rosset, M. (1998). Graft versus host disease and graft versus leukemia effect in mice grafted with newborn blood. *Blood,* **92,** 3968–75.

Fernandez, M.N., Regidor, C., Cabrera, R. *et al.* (2001). Cord blood transplants: early recovery of neutrophils from co-transplanted sibling haploidentical progenitor cells and lack of engaftment of cultured cord blood cells, as ascertained by analysis of DNA polymorphisms. *Bone Marrow Transplantation,* **28,** 355–63.

Garderet, L., Dulphy, N., Douay, C. *et al.* (1998). The umbilical cord blood αβ T cell repertoire: characteristics of a polyclonal and naive but completely formed repertoire. *Blood,* **91,** 340–6.

Gardiner, C.M., Meara, A.O., & Reen, D.J. (1998). Differential cytotoxicity of cord blood and bone marrow-derived natural killer cells. *Blood,* **91,** 207–13.

Gluckman, E. (2000). Current status of umbilical cord blood hematopoietic stem cell transplantation. *Experimental Hematology,* **28,** 1197–205.

Gluckman, E. (2001). Hematopoietic stem-cell transplants using umbilical cord blood. *New England Journal of Medicine,* **344,** 1860–1.

Gluckman, E., Broxmeyer, H.E., Auerbach, A.D. *et al.* (1989). Hematopoietic reconstitution in a patient with Fanconi's anemia by means of umbilical cord blood from an HLA-identical sibling. *New England Journal of Medicine,* **321,** 1174–8.

Gluckman, E., Rocha, V., Boyer Chammard, A. *et al.* (1997). Outcome of cord blood transplantation from related and unrelated donors. *New England Journal of Medicine,* **337,** 373–81.

Goldberg, S.L., Chedid, S., Jennis, A.A. *et al.* (2000). Unrelated cord blood transplantation in adults: a single institution experience. *Blood,* **96** (Suppl 1), 208a.

Green, A., Clarke, E., Hunt, L. *et al.* (1999). Children with acute lymphoblastic leukemia who receive T-cell depleted HLA mismatched marrow allografts from unrelated donors have an increased incidence of primary graft failure but a similar overall transplant outcome. *Blood,* **94,** 2236–46.

Hansen, J.A., Gooley, T.A., Martin, P.J. *et al.* (1998). Bone marrow transplants from unrelated donors for patients with chronic myeloid leukemia. *New England Journal of Medicine,* **338,** 962–8.

Henslee-Downey, P.J., Abhyankar, S.H., Parrish, R.S. *et al.* (1997). Use of partially mismatched related donors extends access to allogeneic marrow transplant. *Blood,* **89,** 3864–72.

Henslee-Donney, P.J., Gluckman, E. (1999). Allogeneic transplantation from donors other than HLA-identical siblings. *Hematology/ Oncology Clinics of North America,* **13,** 1017–39.

Hongeng, S., Krance, R.A., Bowman, L.C. *et al.* (1997). Outcomes of transplantation with matched-sibling and unrelated donor bone marrow in children with leukemia. *Lancet,* **350,** 767–71.

Iseki, T., Ooi, J., Tomonari, A. *et al.* (2001). Unrelated cord blood transplantation in adult patients with hematological malignancy: a single institution experience. *Blood,* **98** (Suppl 1), 665a.

Kögler, G., Nürberger, W., Fisher, J. *et al.* (1999). Simultaneous cord blood transplantation of ex vivo cells expanded together with non-expanded cells for high risk leukemia. *Bone Marrow Transplantation,* **24,** 397–403.

Kurtzberg, J., Laughlin, M., Graham, L. *et al.* (1996). Placental blood as a source of hematopoietic stem cells for transplantation

into unrelated recipients. *New England Journal of Medicine,* **335,** 157–66.

Laughlin, M.J., Barker, J., Bambach, B. *et al.* (2001). Hematopoietic engraftment and survival in adult recipients of unrelated donor umbilical cord blood. *New England Journal of Medicine,* **344,** 1815–22.

Locatelli, F., Rocha, V., Chastang, C. *et al.* (1999). Factors associated with outcome after cord blood transplantation in children with acute leukemia. *Blood,* **93,** 3662–71.

Madrigal, J.A., Cohen, S.B.A., Gluckman, E., Charron, D.J. (1997). Does cord blood transplantation result in lower graft versus host disease? It takes more than two to tango. *Human Immunology,* **56,** 1–5.

Martin, P.J., Rowley, S.D., Anasetti, C. *et al.* (1999). A phase I–II clinical trial to evaluate removal of CD4 cells and partial depletion of CD8 cells from donor marrow for HLA-mismatched unrelated recipients. *Blood,* **94,** 2192–9.

Niehues, T., Rocha, V., Filipovich, A.H. *et al.* (2001). Factors affecting lymphocyte subset reconstitution after either related or unrelated cord blood transplantation in children—a Eurocord analysis. *British Journal of Haematology,* **114,** 42–8.

Noort, W.A. & Falkenburg, J.H.F. (2000). Hematopoietic content of cord blood. In *Cord Blood Characteristics. Role in Stem Cell Transplantation,* ed. S.B.A. Cohen, E. Gluckman, A. Madrigal, & P. Rubinstein, pp. 13–37. London: Martin Dunitz.

Oakhill, A., Pamphilon, D.H., Potter, M.N. *et al.* (1996). Unrelated donor bone marrow transplantation for children with relapsed acute lymphoblastic leukaemia in second complete remission. *British Journal of Haematology,* **94,** 574–8.

Pecora, A.L., Stiff, P., Jennis, A. *et al.* (2000). Prompt and durable engraftment in two older adult patients with high risk chronic myelogenous leukemia (CML) using ex vivo expanded and unmanipulated umbilical cord blood. *Bone Marrow Transplantation,* **25,** 797–9.

Petersdorf, E.W., Gooley, T.A., Anasetti, C. *et al.* (1998). Optimizing outcome after unrelated marrow transplantation by comprehensive matching of HLA class I and II alleles in the donor and the recipient. *Blood,* **92,** 3515–20.

Petit, T., Dommergues, M., Socié, G. *et al.* (1997). Detection of maternal cells in human fetal blood during the third trimester of pregnancy using allele specific PCR amplification. *British Journal of Haematology,* **98,** 767–71.

Reboredo, N.M., Diaz, A., Castro, A., & Villaescusa, R.G. (2000). Collection, processing and cryopreservation of umbilical cord blood for unrelated transplantation. *Bone Marrow Transplantation,* **26,** 1263–70.

Reed, W., Smith, R., Dekovic, F. *et al.* (2003). Comprehensive banking of sibling donor cord blood for children with malignant and nonmalignant disease. *Blood,* **101,** 351–7.

Rocha, V., Arcese, W., Sanz, G. *et al.* (2000). Prognostic factors of outcome after unrelated cord blood transplant in adults with hematologic malignancies. *Blood,* **96** (Suppl 1), 587a.

Rocha, V., Cornish, J., Sievers, E. *et al.* (2001). Comparison of outcomes of unrelated bone marrow and umbilical cord blood transplants in children with acute leukemia. *Blood,* **97,** 2962–71.

Rocha, V., Wagner, J.E., Sobocinski, K. *et al.* (2000b). Comparison of graft-versus-host disease in children transplanted with HLA-identical sibling umbilical cord blood versus HLA-identical sibling bone marrow transplant. *New England Journal of Medicine,* **342,** 1846–54.

Rubinstein, P., Carrier, C., Scaradavou, A. *et al.* (1998). Outcomes among 562 recipients of placental blood transplants from unrelated donor. *New England Journal of Medicine,* **339,** 1565–77.

Rubinstein, P., Dobrila, L., Rosenfield, R.E. *et al.* (1995). Processing and cryopreservation of placental/umbilical cord blood for unrelated bone marrow reconstitution. *Proceedings of the National Academy of Sciences USA,* **92,** 10119–22.

Rubinstein, P., Rosenfield, R.D., Adamson, J.W. *et al.* (1993). Stored placental blood for unrelated bone marrow reconstitution. *Blood,* **81,** 1679–90.

Ruggeri, L., Capanni, M., Urbani, E. *et al.* (2002). Effectiveness of donor natural killer cell alloreactivity in mismatched hematopoietic transplants. *Science,* **295,** 2097–100.

Sanz, G.F., Saavedra, S., Planelles, D. *et al.* (2001). Standardized, unrelated donor cord blood transplantation in adults with hematological malignancies. *Blood,* **98,** 2332–8.

Sasazuki, T., Juji, T., Morishima, Y. *et al.* (1998). Effect of matching of class I HLA alleles on clinical outcome after transplantation of hematopoietic stem cells from an unrelated donor. *New England Journal of Medicine,* **339,** 1177–85.

Speiser, D.E., Tiercy, J.M., Rufer, N. *et al.* (1996). High resolution HLA matching associated with decreased mortality after unrelated bone marrow transplantation. *Blood,* **10,** 4455–62.

Szydlo, R., Goldman, J.M., Klein, J.P. *et al.* (1997). Results of allogeneic bone marrow transplants for leukemia using donors other than HLA-identical siblings. *Journal of Clinical Oncology,* **15,** 1767–77.

Talvensaari, K., Clave, E., Douay, C. *et al.* (2002). A broad T-cell repertoire diversity and an efficient thymic function indicate a favorable long-term immune reconstitution after cord blood stem cell transplantation. *Blood,* **99,** 1458–64.

Thomson, B.G., Robertson, K., Gowan, D. *et al.* (2000). Analysis of engraftment, graft-versus-host disease, and immune recovery following unrelated donor cord blood transplantation. *Blood,* **96,** 2703–11.

Wagner, J. E., Barker, J. N., DeFor, T. E. *et al.* (2002). Transplantation of unrelated donor umbilical cord blood in 102 patients with maligant and non-malignant diseases: influence of CD34 cell dose and HLA disparity on treatment-related mortality and survival. *Blood,* **100,** 1611–8.

Wagner, J.E., Rosenthal, J., Sweetman, R. *et al.* (1996). Successful transplantation of HLA matched and HLA mismatched umbilical cord blood from unrelated donors: analysis of engraftment and acute graft versus host disease. *Blood,* **88,** 795–802.

Woolfrey, A.E., Anasetti, C., Storer, B. *et al.* (2002). Factors associated with outcome after unrelated marrow transplantation for treatment of acute lymphoblastic leukemia in children. *Blood,* **99,** 2002–8.

PART IX   MAJOR TRANSPLANT-RELATED COMPLICATIONS

69   ABO incompatibility and blood product support

ANTHONY J. DODDS

St Vincent's Hospital and University of New South Wales, Sydney, Australia

Introduction

The problems of blood product support in patients undergoing bone marrow or blood stem cell transplantation [hematopoietic stem cell (HSC) transplantation] will be considered in two sections. The first is devoted to the unique complications arising when there is ABO incompatibility between the donor and recipient. Red blood cell antigens are not histocompatibility antigens and the possibility of red cell antigen-disparate, but HLA-matched, allogeneic transplantation results from the location of the pertinent genes on different chromosomes (Table 69.1). The second section describes the general principles of blood product support related to both allogeneic and autologous HSC transplantation. With the increasing use of allogeneic blood stem cell transplantation, a number of case reports of severe acute hemolytic reaction have been described (Toren *et al.*, 1996; Oziel-Taieb *et al.*, 1997), and guidelines for its prevention suggested (Lapierre *et al.*, 2000).

ABO incompatible HSC transplantation

Incompatibility of blood group antigens between donor and recipient is not a barrier to HSC transplantation. Red cell antigen disparity between recipient and donor does not result in an increased incidence of graft rejection or graft-versus-host disease. There are, however, potentially serious complications

(Table 69.2), that, if anticipated, can often be avoided. These are primarily hemolysis and delay of donor erythropoiesis. The first successful major ABO mismatched transplant was reported in 1978 (Buckner *et al.*, 1978). Allogeneic transplantation involves the (at least temporary) coexistence of recipient and donor immunologic and hematopoietic systems. Hence, the effects of an ABO mismatched transplant may persist for weeks to months posttransplant.

Alloimmune hemolysis is the most common complication. The likelihood of severe hemolysis is dependent on:

1. The amount and type of red cells (and red cell progenitors) infused
2. The quantity and nature of the specific red cell antibody present

The volume of red cells and plasma in an unmanipulated HSC marrow inoculum approximates that of whole blood. In blood stem cell collections these "contaminants" tend to be much less, due to the efficacy of apheresis protocols. However, in either case there may be sufficient red cells infused into the appropriate recipient to cause severe hemolysis, with a risk of renal failure and disseminated intravascular coagulation (DIC). Many of the features of alloimmune hemolysis posttransplant are typical of severe hemolysis from any cause. One exception is the lack of a compensatory reticulocytosis (Table 69.3).

Table 69.1.   *Genetics of HLA and red cell antigens*

Antigen	Chromosome
HLA	6
ABO	9
Rh	1
Kell (K)	7
Kidd (Jk)	18
Duffy (Fy)	1
Lewis (Le)	19
MNS	4

Shown are the chromosome locations of various antigens.
Reproduced, with permission, from Rowley (2001).

Table 69.2.   *Classification of alloimmune hemolytic anemia after allogeneic HSC transplantation*

1. Major ABO incompatibility
     Immediate or delayed hemolysis
     Delayed red cell engraftment
     Delayed neutrophil, lymphocyte, platelet engraftment
     Pure red cell aplasia
2. Minor ABO incompatibility
     Immediate or delayed hemolysis
3. Mixed ABO mismatch
     Combined features of major and minor ABO incompatibility
4. Mismatches of Rhesus or other antigen systems (MNSs, Kell, Kidd)
5. Mismatch of more than one antigen system

Table 69.3. *Clinical and laboratory features of alloimmune
hemolysis after allogeneic HSC transplantation*

Clinical features
   Immediate: Fever, back pain, dark urine, dyspnea
   Delayed: Unexpected drop in hemoglobin within 21 days
   Secondary signs of hemolysis
Laboratory features
   Positive direct Coomb's test[ab]
   Isoagglutinin directed against recipient red cells in patient's
      serum and/or red cell eluate
   Mixed field agglutination
   No compensatory reticulocytosis

[a] False negative if complete consumption of allosensitized cells.
[b] Robin Coombs, English veterinarian and immunologist, born 1921.

Severe hemolysis must be differentiated from DIC or the hemolytic-uremic/thrombotic thrombocytopenic purpura syndrome, which may occur in the posttransplant setting. The ABO mismatch can be major, minor, or mixed. The division has both clinical and laboratory implications.

Major ABO mismatch

A major ABO mismatch is defined as the expression of ABO antigens on donor red cells, which are not present on recipient red cells. The presence of isoagglutinins in the recipient plasma specific for those antigens will result in severe hemolysis when the stem cell inoculum is infused. Transplant candidates may sometimes lack these antibodies due to immune suppression, probably from prior chemotherapy (Buckner *et al.,* 1978). All major ABO-mismatched donor marrow stem cells should be depleted of red cells, irrespective of the recipient's isoagglutinin titer. This may not be necessary with blood stem cell collections that have already been depleted by the apheresis procedure. Major ABO mismatches occur in 10% to 15% of HLA-matched donor recipient pairs (Bensinger *et al.,* 1987). There is no significant effect on the incidence of graft rejection, graft-versus-host disease (GVHD), or overall survival (Buckner *et al.,* 1978; Bensinger *et al.,* 1987). Immediate hemolysis is due to the interaction between donor red cells and pre-existing isoagglutinins in the recipient plasma. Delayed hemolysis (which is clinically significant in only 10% of recipients) is less likely to be prevented by prophylaxis. It may begin as early as 3 days posttransplant (Sniecinski *et al.,* 1988). Early delayed hemolysis is thought to be due to the tissue pool of donor-specific IgG being released into the circulation, or to synthesis of IgG from host lymphocytes or plasma cells that survive the conditioning regimen (Bensinger *et al.,* 1982). The latter is likely if high titers of IgM antibody directed against donor antigens are present in recipient plasma. Delayed hemolysis persisting beyond 100 days posttransplant indicates hemolysis of engrafted erythroid progenitor cells. Delayed hemolytic reactions may be increased in patients receiving cyclosporine-based

GVHD prophylaxis regimens and patients with high pretransplant isoagglutinin titers (Sniecinski *et al.,* 1988). In recipients of ABO-mismatched allografts, a more rapid disappearance of isohemagglutinins was noted after HLA-matched related transplants than after HLA-matched unrelated transplants (Fig. 69.1) and in those with GVHD compared to those without GVHD (Fig. 69.2), suggesting a graft-versus-normal plasma cell effect (Mielcarek *et al.,* 2000).

The management of alloimmune hemolysis in the ABO-incompatible transplant is predominantly prophylactic. Table 69.4 details the various methods of prophylaxis. In general, the methods are better at preventing immediate hemolytic reactions

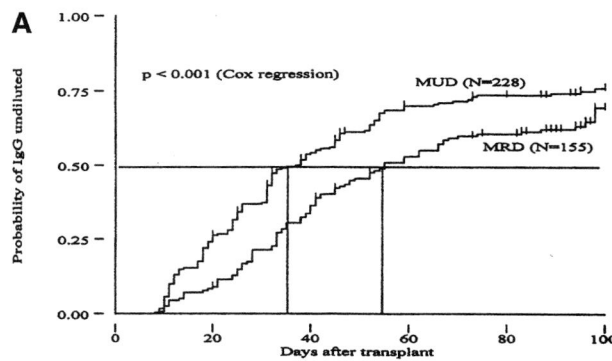

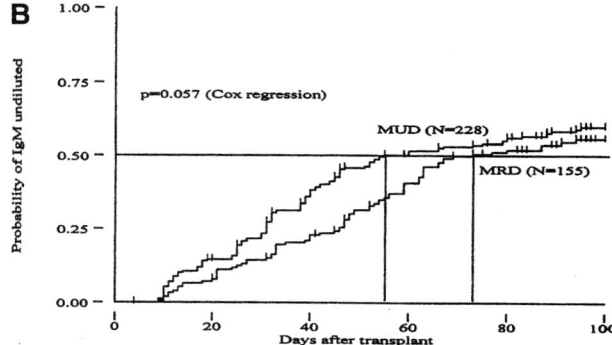

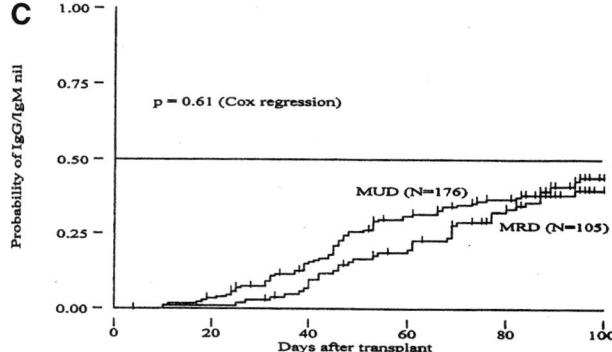

Fig. 69.1. Cumulative incidence curves showing probability of reaching different hemagglutinin titer endpoints during 100 days after transplant in recipients of marrow from HLA-matched related (MRD) or HLA-matched unrelated donors (MUD). Reproduced, with permission, from Mielcarek *et al.* (2000).

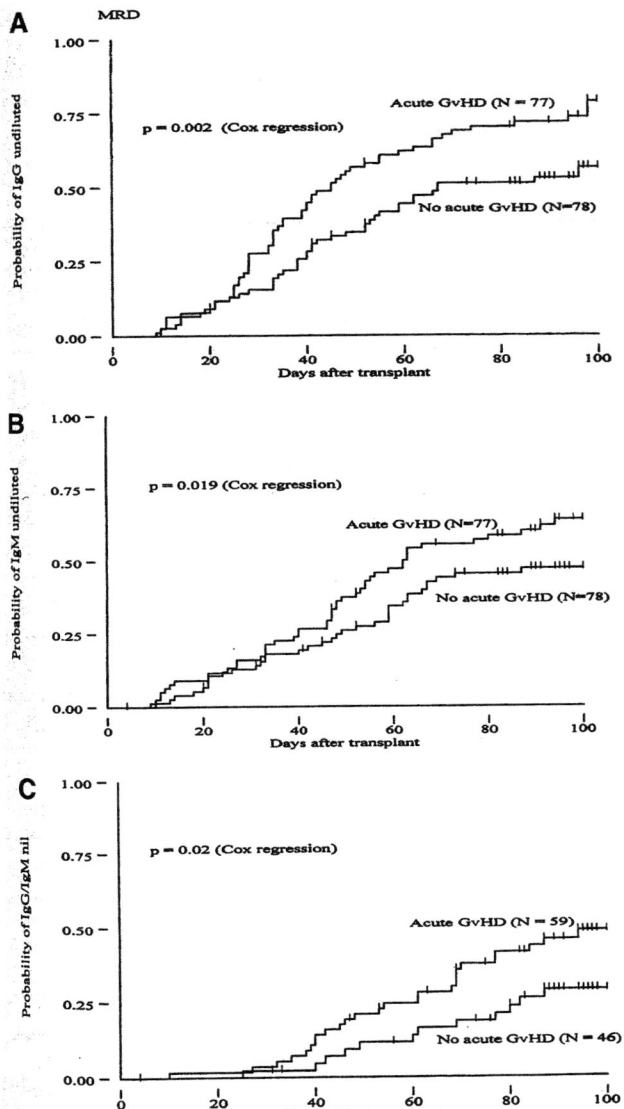

Fig. 69.2. Cumulative incidence curves showing probability of reaching different hemagglutinin titer endpoints during 100 days after transplant in recipients of marrow from HLA-matched related donors (MRD) in patients with or without acute GVHD. Reproduced, with permission, from Mielcarek *et al.* (2000).

Table 69.4. *Prophylaxis of alloimmune hemolysis in ABO major incompatible hematopoietic transplantation*

1. Remove red cells from stem cell inoculum (for example, by density gradient centrifugation, automated cell separation, or gravity sedimentation). This step is not required for blood stem cell collection(s) unless significant red cell contamination is present (hematocrit >10%).
2. Reduce titer of isoagglutinin in recipient plasma (for example, by plasma exchange, plasma immunoabsorption)
3. Infuse small volumes of donor red cells during the immediate pretransplant period—seldom practiced now (see text)

Stem cells collected from peripheral blood generally have less red cell contamination so red cell depletion is not required.

The second component of prophylaxis is reduction of the isoagglutinin titer in the recipient plasma. Plasma exchange has the added benefit of neutralization of residual isoagglutinin by A or B substance in the replacement plasma. Usually one to two plasma exchanges (depending on the titer of antibody) are necessary within the 24-hour period before marrow infusion. A common problem is rebound of isoagglutinin in the early post-transplant period. A third component of prophylaxis involving infusion of donor red cells in the pretransplant period is not commonly practiced now, due to the reported risk of hemolysis. However, it has been safely used in some patients (Buckner *et al.*, 1978; Bensinger *et al.*, 1987). The protocol practiced in our own unit is detailed in Table 69.5. Posttransplant, the patient is transfused with irradiated group O blood products until engraftment occurs. If donor platelets are given they should be collected red-cell–poor. An algorithm for the management of major ABO incompatibility between recipient and donor used at the Fred Hutchinson Cancer Research Center is shown in Figure 69.3a.

The treatment of an established hemolytic reaction consists of transfusions of compatible group O red cells (Buckner *et al.*, 1978), plasma exchange in severe cases, and possibly corticosteroids (Sniecinski *et al.*, 1988).

Delayed erythroid engraftment also occurs in this setting (Bensinger *et al.*, 1982; Marmont *et al.*, 1983; Sniecinski *et al.*, 1988; Gmur *et al.*, 1990; Bar *et al.*, 1995; Benjamin *et al.*, 1998), and may persist for over 100 days posttransplant. Risk factors are high titers of pretransplant isoagglutinins and possibly the use of cyclosporine, although this has been disputed. In a study of 258 T-cell-depleted allografts, 8 of 30 patients (27%) with major ABO incompatibility had no detectable donor erythrocytes 2 months after transplant (Bar *et al.*, 1995). Indeed donor erythroid reconstitution was significantly delayed up to 3 months posttransplant in the major ABO incompatible group, who required significantly more packed red cell transfusions than those without ABO incompatibility or with a minor incompatibility. Delayed neutrophil, platelet, and lymphocyte engraftment has also been reported (Bensinger *et al.*, 1982). The use of non-myeloablative conditioning regimens appears to enhance the delay of donor erythropoiesis: initial detection

than delayed reactions. No method is completely effective, and there are no clear data as to which is best. Depletion of red cells from the donor marrow inoculum should be performed in all major mismatches. An automated cell separator produces a closed processing system and a more objective and reproducible separation than the alternative methods of gravity sedimentation or density gradient centrifugation (Hows *et al.*, 1986). The aim is to reduce the red cell count to less than 10% of that in the unmanipulated marrow, while retaining 75% of the original mononuclear cell content (including stem cells). The loss of stem cells is the major disadvantage of this method.

Table 69.5. *Protocol for ABO incompatible HSC transplantation (St. Vincent's Hospital, Sydney)*

Major (A, B, or AB donor and O recipient)
  Pretransplant
     Deplete marrow inoculum of red cells on COBE 2991 cell separator. Goal is at least a 90% depletion. Blood stem cell inoculum does not need depletion unless hematocrit >10%.
     If isoagglutinin detected in recipient plasma against donor red cells, plasma exchange recipient. Give fresh frozen plasma after last exchange. Repeat isoagglutinin titers. Goal is hemolysin titer of O, agglutinin titer of 1 or 1/2.
  Transplant
     Intravenous hydration with 1 liter of normal saline during marrow infusion, with furosemide to maintain diuresis
     Graduated infusion of stem cells at 20 to 80 ml/hour
     Observe for signs of transfusion reaction
  Posttransplant
     Transfuse with irradiated recipient group blood products until engraftment occurs. If donor platelets cannot be avoided, then collect platelets red-cell–poor
Minor (O donor and A, B, or AB recipient or A_1 donor and A_2 recipient)
  Pretransplant
     If isoagglutinin detected in donor plasma directed against recipient red cells, deplete marrow inoculum of plasma on COBE 2991 cell separator. This step is not required for blood stem cell collection(s) where concentration has occurred during apheresis.
  Transplant
     Infusion as per ABO matched transplant. Observe for signs of transfusion reaction
  Posttransplant
     Transfuse with irradiated group O red cells and recipient group platelets. If donor platelets cannot be avoided, then collect plasma–poor
Mixed (A donor to B recipient, B donor to A recipient)
     Treat as major and/or minor mismatch as appropriate
     Deplete marrow inoculum of red cells or COBE 2991 cell separator
     Perform isoagglutinin titer in donor plasma against recipient red cells (major mismatch) and in recipient plasma against donor red cells (minor mismatch)
     If present in recipient plasma, then plasma exchange recipient
     If present in donor plasma, then deplete marrow inoculum of plasma

of donor-origin red cells was later after nonablative conditioning compared to that after ablative conditioning and the decline of anti-donor isohemagglutinins was slower (Fig. 69.4) (Bolan et al., 2001b). Pure red cell aplasia occurred in 29% of the patients in this study receiving nonablative conditioning versus none of 12 given an ablative regimen, and only resolved after the withdrawal of cyclosporine.

Pure red cell aplasia (Marmont et al., 1983) may present as primary failure of erythroid engraftment or late failure following a temporary period of erythroid engraftment. The latter may be due to the interaction of ABO antigens on donor-derived red cell progenitors with host-derived isoagglutinin. Treatment has been successful with plasma exchange (more

effective for IgM than for IgG antibodies), erythropoietin—primarily for those patients whose isoagglutinin levels have fallen to undetectable levels (Ohashi et al., 1994; Santamaria et al., 1997), and antithymocyte globulin (Labar et al., 1992). Spontaneous recovery has also been reported. In the study by Bar et al. (1995), six patients with blood group O developed pure red cell aplasia, which resolved in five without therapeutic intervention. In the six patients anti-A antibody titers were persistently high for the first 3 months posttransplant. This was in contrast to two patients with timely recovery of erythropoiesis, in whom anti-A and anti-B antibody titers showed a steady decrease posttransplant. Another case resolved when prophylactic immune suppression was withdrawn and chronic GVHD developed (Yamaguchi et al., 2002), possibly indicative of a graft-versus-plasma cell effect (Mielcarek et al., 2000).

The drop in isoagglutinin titers usually occurs over 6 to 8 weeks after transplantation (Rowley et al., 2000). Lee and colleagues (2000) have also reported that patients with anti-A isoagglutinins developed pure red cell aplasia more frequently than patients with anti-B (Fig. 69.5). Donor red blood cell engraftment was dependent on the disappearance of the anti-donor isoagglutinins (Fig. 69.6).

Minor ABO mismatch

A minor ABO mismatch is defined as the presence of recipient red cell ABO antigens, which are not present on donor red cells. Incompatible isoagglutinins may also be present in donor plasma. It occurs in 10% to 15% of HLA-matched donor-recipient pairs. Immediate hemolysis is rarely life threatening, with the underlying mechanism thought to be due to the interaction of recipient red cells and isoagglutinin infused in donor plasma. Delayed hemolytic reactions are more common with the reported incidence varying from 14% to 78% (Hows et al., 1986; Klumpp, 1991), and can be severe (Greeno et al., 1996), or even fatal (Oziel-Taieb et al., 1997; Bolan et al., 2001a) (Fig. 69.7). Pretransplant isoagglutinin titers are not predictive of the incidence or severity. The onset is usually within 7 to 21 days of HSC infusion. If occurring early, the synthesis of isoagglutinin by lymphocytes and plasma cells infused in the stem cell inoculum is probably the mechanism (Hows et al., 1986). If occurring later, then engrafted lymphoid stem cells may have synthesized the isoagglutinins. It has been suggested that posttransplant immunosuppressive regimens containing methotrexate reduce the risk of delayed hemolysis mediated by viable transferred lymphocytes (Gajewski et al., 1992). This may explain the suggestion that the risk of hemolysis is higher after transplantation of T-cell-depleted marrow administered without the posttransplant use of antimetabolite agents (Hazelhurst et al., 1986), such as methotrexate or mycophenolate mofetil, which suppress lymphocyte proliferation.

Prophylaxis consists of depleting the stem cell inoculum of plasma if isoagglutinins are detected in the donor plasma. In blood stem cell collections this is accomplished by the apheresis. Posttransplant, group O red cells and recipient group

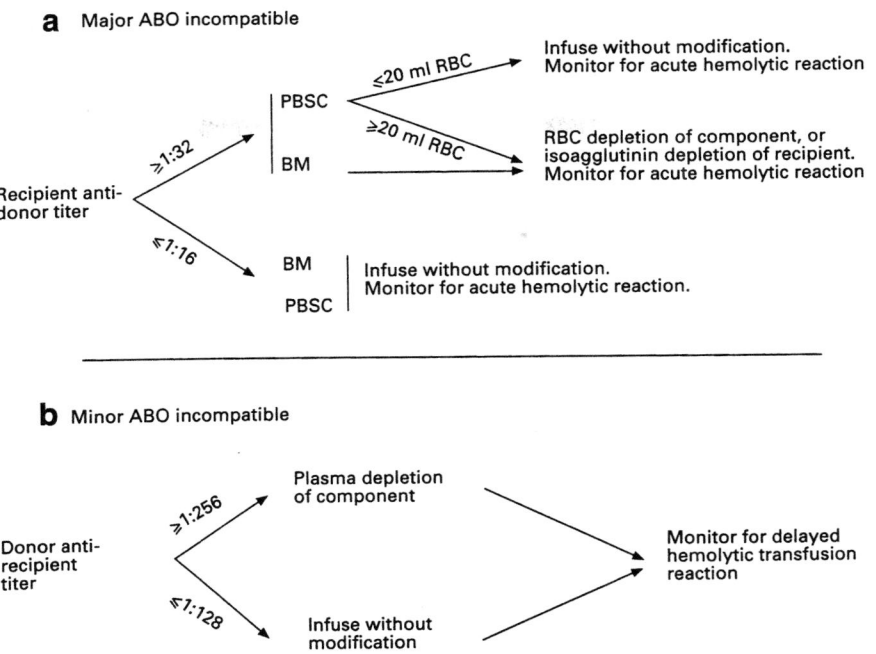

Fig. 69.3. Shown are suggested algorithms for the management of major red cell-incompatible transplants (**a**) and minor red cell-incompatible transplants (**b**). These algorithms are based on the experience of the author and are not tested in prospective studies of transplantation immunohematology. Reproduced, with permission, from Rowley (2001).

platelets are transfused. If donor platelets cannot be avoided, then they should be collected plasma-poor. In the event of established hemolysis, plasma exchange is the treatment of choice (Hows *et al.*, 1986).

There is mounting evidence of an increased risk of immune hemolysis when peripheral blood stem cells (PBSC), as opposed to bone marrow, grafts are used (Toren *et al.*, 1996; Bornhauser *et al.*, 1997; Laurencet *et al.*, 1997; Oziel-Taieb *et al.*, 1997; Salmon *et al.*, 1999; Bolan *et al.*, 2001a; Lapierre *et al.*, 2001). This may be due to the increased numbers of lymphoid cells present in the PBSC inoculum and capable of producing isohemagglutinins against recipient red cell antigens. This propensity may be enhanced by the use of non-myeloablative regimens (Bolan *et al.*, 2001a) (see above), possibly due to the utilization of cyclosporine alone as GVHD prophylaxis after such procedures (Hows *et al.*, 1986; Gajewski *et al.*, 1992). Vigilant monitoring during the first 2 weeks posttransplant (to include daily LDH estimation, daily direct antiglobulin test, and twice daily blood counts on days 5–12) should be practiced.

Mixed ABO mismatch

Patients receiving mixed ABO mismatched transplant (A to B or B to A) are at risk of complications relating to both major and minor ABO mismatches. Hence, prophylactic measures removing both red cells and plasma from the donor stem cells should be used to prevent immediate hemolysis.

It should be emphasized that a severe hemolytic reaction on the day of HSC infusion can be the disastrous initiation of a chain of events leading to acute renal failure, withholding of GVHD prophylactic medications such as cyclosporine and methotrexate, with subsequent high risk of severe GVHD and secondary infection.

Non-ABO antigen systems

Mismatches within other antigen systems also occur. There are reports of production of alloantibodies against Kidd and MNSs antigens and components of the Rhesus (Rh) system (anti-D, anti-C, anti-E, anti-G) (Hows *et al.*, 1986). Mismatches involving the Rh system do not appear to impair engraftment, affect overall survival, or increase the risk of GVHD. A positive direct Coomb's test may develop and rarely severe hemolysis has been reported with a major Rh mismatch. The probability of developing significant hemolysis following minor Rh mismatches is 10% to 15% (Hows *et al.*, 1986). Prophylactic Rh-negative blood products have been advocated. Interestingly, red cells continue to express recipient type Lewis antigens posttransplant, as these antigens are passively absorbed from the plasma. Young and colleagues (2001) described two cases of severe alloimmune hemolysis due to the formation of an anti-Jk^a antibody, in one of whom the duration of hemolysis was shortened by performing red blood cell exchange at the first sign of intravascular hemolysis. In contrast to cases of hemolysis due to ABO/Rh mismatches, cases of hemolysis due to non-ABO/Rh mismatches frequently involve donors and recipients with no prior evidence of alloantibodies, making it impossible to predict those patients at risk. The resulting hemolysis can be

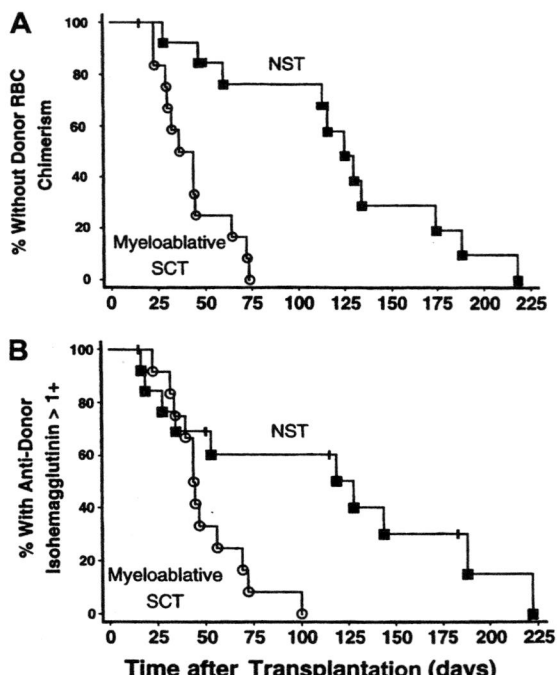

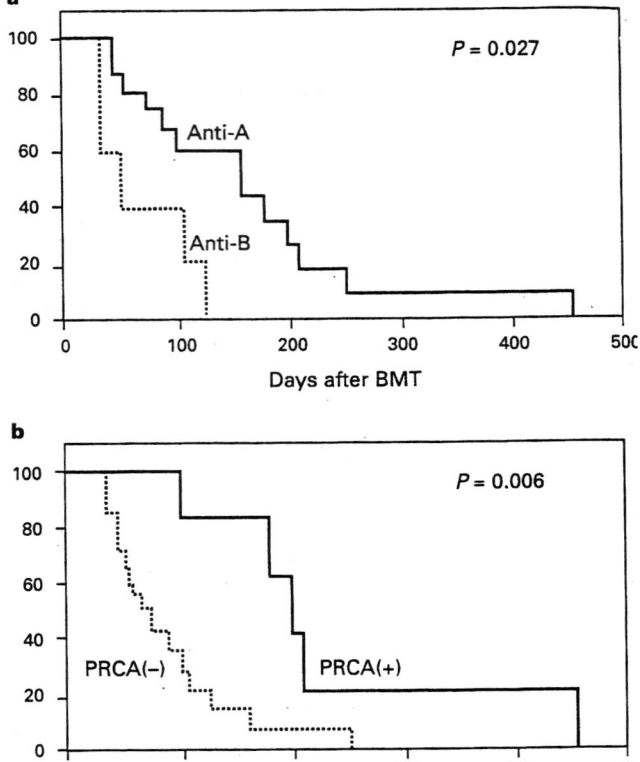

Fig. 69.4. The onset of donor red blood cell (RBC) chimerism and decline in antidonor isohemagglutinin levels after NST compared with myeloablative stem cell transplantation (SCT). The onset of donor RBC chimerism and decline of host antidonor isohemagglutinins to clinically insignificant levels were markedly delayed following major ABO-incompatible NST compared with myeloablative SCT. NST data are represented by solid squares; myeloablative SCT data, by open circles. (A) Kaplan-Meier plot of the percentage of patients without detectable donor RBC chimerism as a function of days after transplantation. The time until detection of donor RBC chimerism was significantly prolonged following NST versus myeloablative SCT; $P <$ .001. (B) Kaplan-Meier plot showing the percentage of patients with persistent host antidonor isohemagglutinins greater than 1+ in strength. Isohemagglutinins decreased significantly faster after myeloablative SCT than after NST; $P =$ .012. Reproduced, with permission, from Bolan et al. (2001b). Abbreviation: NST, non-myeloablative stem cell transplant.

Fig. 69.5. Time to disappearance of isoagglutinins against donor red blood cells (RBC). Median days were prolonged in patients with anti-A isoagglutinins (a) or in patients who developed pure red cell aplasia (PRCA) (b). Reproduced, with permission, from Lee et al. (2000).

severe (Hows et al., 1986; Myser et al., 1986; Robertson et al., 1987; Chen et al., 1997; Leo et al., 2000), thus emphasizing the importance of close immunohematologic monitoring of patients undergoing HSC transplantation.

Transfusion support

In the HSC transplant setting transfusion support is required for a finite time during the period of pancytopenia. This period is usually 4 to 12 weeks, but may occasionally be longer. In particular, delayed platelet engraftment is not uncommon (approximately 30%) after autologous bone marrow transplantation (BMT). The quantity of packed cell and platelet transfusions given to autologous and allogeneic HSC transplant recipients on our own unit during the first 3 months posttransplant is shown in Table 69.6. In a report from the Royal Marsden Hospital the median (range) number of red cells transfused in

the first, second, and third months after HLA-identical sibling transplantation for 477 patients with hematologic malignancies was 4 (0–32), 1 (0–39), and 0 (0–22), respectively. The number of random donor platelet concentrates infused was 32.5 (0–196), 0 (0–225), and 0 (0–135). ABO incompatibility, a conditioning regimen other than cyclophosphamide/total body irradiation (TBI), and age over 18 years increased red cell requirement significantly in the first month (Mehta et al., 1996). Platelet requirements in the second month posttransplant and red cell requirements in the second and third months posttransplant were increased significantly by the occurrence of acute GVHD, a diagnosis other than acute leukemia, and a conditioning regimen other than cyclophosphamide/TBI. Platelet requirements in the third month posttransplant were influenced only by acute GVHD. A summary of guidelines for blood product transfusion in the HSC transplant recipient is shown in Table 69.7 and Table 69.8, and the potential complications of blood product transfusion are listed in Table 69.9. The transmission rates of infectious diseases by blood product transfusion are shown in Table 69.10.

Optimal management pretransplant is to utilize leukocyte-poor red cells and single donor platelet concentrates from unre-

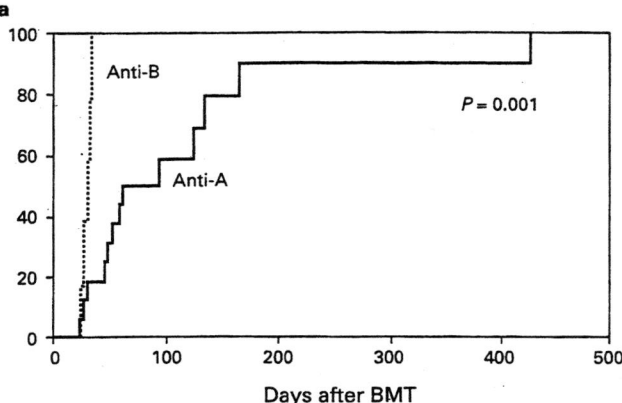

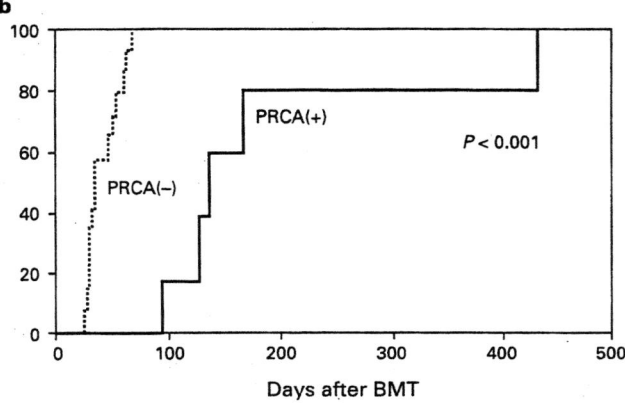

Fig. 69.6. Time to initial appearance of donor red blood cells (RBC). Median days were prolonged in patients with anti-A isoagglutinins (a) or in patients who developed pure red cell aplasia (PRCA) (b). Reproduced, with permission, from Lee *et al.* (2000).

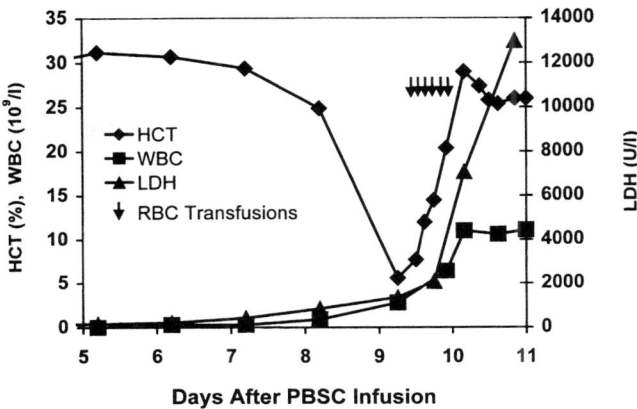

Fig. 69.7. Course of severe hemolysis in patient 1. On days 8 and 9 posttransplant, fever, hemodynamic instability, and renal insufficiency occurred, the hematocrit dropped precipitously, and the LDH doubled. Although the hematocrit responded to transfusions with group O red cells, cardiopulmonary arrest occurred, renal failure ensued, neurological function did not recover, and the patient died on day 16. Serological testing revealed that donor-type anti-A isohemagglutinins were the cause of the massive haemolysis. Reproduced, with permission, from Bolan *et al.* (2001a).

lated donors. Donations from family members should be avoided to minimize the risk of allosensitization to donor-specific histocompatibility antigens with subsequent risk of graft rejection. Posttransplant cellular blood products should be leukocyte-depleted and irradiated (15–25 Gy); irradiation is used to inactivate viable T cells in the transfusion product in order to prevent transfusion-induced GVHD. The major reason for leukocyte depletion is reduction of HLA alloimmunization, resulting in less platelet refractoriness. Other advantages are a reduction in cytomegalovirus (CMV) transmission and nonhemolytic febrile reactions. It has been estimated that depletion of lymphocytes to levels less than 5×10^6 will prevent primary HLA alloimmunization. The lymphocyte content of normal red cell concentrates is 1 to 2×10^9, of random donor platelet concentrates 4×10^7, and of single donor platelet concentrates 3×10^8 (Leitman, 1985).

CMV transmission from seropositive blood donors is thought to occur in approximately 20% of seronegative immune-suppressed recipients. Allogeneic HSC transplant recipients are particularly at risk, with CMV infections being a major cause of morbidity and mortality (Chapters 74 and 78). As there are seven subtypes of CMV, CMV-negative blood products should ideally be given to all recipients. This is impractical, however, due to unavailability. In our unit, CMV-negative blood products are only given to CMV-negative recipients (regardless of CMV status of the donor). Prophylactic or pre-emptive ganciclovir and CMV immunoglobulin are other therapeutic options. Cellular blood products should be leukocyte-depleted, as leukocytes are presumed to be the source of latent CMV infections. Nonhemolytic febrile reactions complicate 0.5% to 3% of transfusions and are predominantly due to leukoagglutinins present in the recipient's serum. Removing 85% to 90% of leukocytes will significantly reduce this incidence.

Various methods are available for leukocyte depletion. Cell washing by centrifugation separates blood components according to density. Variable results (70% to 95% leukocytes removed) and 15% red cell loss are major disadvantages. Frozen/thawed cells will also be depleted of approximately 95% leukocytes, but the method is too expensive for routine use. Bedside filtration is the method of choice. Leukocyte absorption filters are very efficient, removing up to 99.9% of leukocytes with minimal red cell loss, and are cost effective (Chambers, 1989). Microaggregate filters (pore size 20–40 nm) only deplete approximately 94% leukocytes, so do not prevent HLA alloimmunization, CMV transmission, or nonhemolytic febrile reactions.

In the United States in 1999, the infection risk from red blood cell transfusion for hepatitis B, hepatitis C, and HIV was 1/138,700 units, 1/233,000 units, and 1/1,326,300 units, respectively With the introduction of nucleic acid testing, the incidence of hepatitis C and HIV is projected to drop to 1/543,000 units and 1/1,930,000 units, respectively (American Red Cross data).

Table 69.6.   *Blood products received by recipients during the first 3 months after HSC transplantation*

Type of transplant (number of patients)	Average number of red cell units	Average number of multidonor platelet units (number of occasions)	Average number of single donor platelet units
Autologous BMT (10)	5	50 (7)	1
Allogeneic HLA-matched related BMT (10)	7	65 (10)	3
Allogeneic HLA-matched unrelated BMT (10)	28	97 (20)	7
Allogeneic HLA-matched related blood stem cell transplant (16)	8	38 (7)	1

Abbreviations: HSC, hematopoietic stem cell; BMT, bone marrow transplant.

Posttransfusion GVHD develops when immune competent allogeneic lymphocytes are transfused into a severely immunocompromised host. The high mortality rate (approximately 90%) makes prophylaxis essential. Gamma irradiation (15–25 Gy) is presently the most efficient way to do this, as it prevents proliferation of lymphocytes (Leitman, 1985).

Red cell transfusion

ABO compatible red cell concentrates from random community donors are used in the HSC transplant setting. Patients usually need red cell support for 6 to 12 weeks posttransplantation, primarily within the first 4 weeks. This may be prolonged if delayed engraftment, bleeding, or hemolysis develop. Although reconstitution of normal antimicrobial immunity is delayed for up to 12 months posttransplant, a study at our institution confirmed the early appearance of some red cell antibodies, 12 days to 11 months after allogeneic BMT (Ting *et al.,* 1987).

Platelet transfusion

Ten percent to 30% of individuals undergoing myeloablative therapy followed by an infusion of bone marrow or blood stem cells experience clinically significant bleeding and approximately 5% die due to thrombocytopenia-associated hemor-

Table 69.7.   *Guidelines for blood product transfusion in HSC transplant recipients*

1. All cellular blood products should be checked for the donor's CMV serologic status. If the patient is CMV-negative, only CMV-negative blood products should be given.
2. All cellular blood products should be irradiated with 15–25 Gy (1,500–2,500 rads) to inactivate lymphocytes, in order to prevent transfusion GVHD.
3. All packed red cells and platelet transfusions should be filtered using leukocyte filters to minimize the risk of allosensitization and CMV transfer.
4. *There are different filters for administration of red cells and platelets:* Marrow and granulocyte infusions must not be put through a leukocyte filter.
5. Acellular blood products such as fresh frozen plasma, albumin, or SPPS do not require leukocyte filtration.

rhage (Klumpp *et al.,* 1996). Prophylactic platelet concentrates are indicated to maintain a platelet count greater than $20 \times 10^9/l$ in an otherwise uncomplicated patient, although this "trigger point" has been debated (Gil-Fernandez *et al.,* 1996). These authors performed a retrospective analysis comparing major hemorrhages during hospitalization in 190 patients undergoing BMT during two different periods. In 87 patients transplanted from 1990 to 1991, the $20 \times 10^9/l$ level was used for prophylactic platelet transfusion. In 103 other patients transplanted from 1993 to 1994, the authors adopted a more stringent prophylactic policy: less than $10 \times 10^9/l$ for stable patients and less than $20 \times 10^9/l$ when higher platelet consumption factors were present. In the stringent group, 12 patients presented with 13 major hemorrhages and 4 died of hemorrhage. In the classical group 12 presented with 14 major hemorrhages and 3 died of hemorrhage. Platelet consumption factors were present in 12 of 13 hemorrhages in the stringent group and 12 of 14 in the classical group. By contrast, stable patients presented fewer hemor-

Table 69.8.   *Transfusion support for recipients of ABO-incompatible HSC components*

	Recipient	Donor	Red blood cell and granulocyte components	Platelet and plasma components
ABO major	0	A	0	A, AB
	0	B	0	B, AB
	0	AB	0	AB
	A	AB	A, O	AB
	B	AB	B, O	AB
ABO minor	A	O	O	A, AB
	B	O	O	B, AB
	AB	O	O	AB
	AB	A	A, O	AB
	AB	B	B, O	AB
ABO major and minor	A	B	O	AB
	B	A	O	AB

Red cell components should be packed or washed to reduce plasma volume, or components from donors with low isoagglutinin titers. Shown are the first choice for platelet support; platelets from other blood groups can also be infused but should similarly be concentrated to reduce plasma volume.
Reproduced, with permission, from Rowley (2001).

Table 69.9. *Potential complications of blood product transfusion*

Hemolytic transfusion reactions (1 in 12,000 transfusions)
Transmission of infectious disease (see Table 69.10)
Bacterial contamination of blood components (rare)
Alloimmunization of the recipient
Graft-versus-host disease (rare)
Febrile reactions (1 in 200 transfusions)
Allergic reactions (1 in 100–300 transfusions)
Circulatory overload
Iron overload (occurs after ~120 units of blood)
Clinically significant depletion of coagulation proteins and
  platelets can be a complication of massive transfusion
Microaggregates consisting of fibrin, white cells, and platelets
  can develop during storage of blood
Metabolic complications can occur when very large amounts of
  blood are transfused:
  Hypothermia
  Citrate toxicity
  Acidosis
  Alterations in potassium (hypokalemia or hyperkalemia)

rhages (2 of 14 and 1 of 13, respectively). The median number of platelets administered during the first 100 days posttransplant was 73 (3–943) in the classical group and 54 (0–647) in the stringent group ($P < .01$) The authors concluded that their policy of stringent prophylactic platelet transfusions was safe and reduced the overall use of this blood product.

The bleeding patient, and patients undergoing procedures such as central venous line insertions, gut biopsies, lumbar punctures, or surgery should have prophylactic platelet concentrates administered to obtain a platelet count of 50 to 100 × 10^9/l at the time of the procedure.

Pooled random donor platelet concentrates are usually adequate. Single donor concentrates collected by apheresis may have advantages by reducing the risk of alloimmunization and transmission of infection, but cost and inconvenience prohibit their routine use in most centers. Platelet donors undergo the same screening procedure as red cell donors. Their platelet count must be greater than 150×10^9/l, otherwise the collection may be unprofitable. The effect of ABO incompatible platelet transfusions is variable, with

Table 69.10. *Transmission rates of infectious diseases by blood product transfusion*

Disease	Transmission rate (United States)
Hepatitis A	Rare
Hepatitis B	1 per 200,000 units
Hepatitis C	1 per 3,000–5,000 units
HIV-1	1 per 225,000 units
HTLV-1/2	1 per 50,000 units
CMV	?
Syphilis	Rare
Malaria	Rare
Chagas' disease	Rare

reports ranging from no increment up to a 20% to 30% reduction in platelet survival.

Platelet refractoriness is a major clinical problem. Thirty percent to 70% of chronic multitransfused patients become refractory due to alloimmunization. Nonimmune platelet consumption is also important, with a study demonstrating DIC, amphotericin B administration, and splenomegaly as major causes. Other causes include bleeding, fever, and antibiotics (Bishop *et al.*, 1988). Platelet alloantibodies, particularly anti-HLA antibodies, are the most common cause of platelet refractoriness. The median time from first transfusion to detection of alloantibody is 4 weeks. This may be earlier if the recipient has been immunized previously by blood transfusion or pregnancy. Anti-HLA antibodies may disappear after discontinuation of transfusion, after switching to HLA-matched platelet transfusions, or even occasionally spontaneously. Hence, repeated anti-HLA antibody testing is important in patients receiving prolonged platelet support. Platelet-specific antibodies are present in 20% to 25% of cases showing anti-HLA antibodies. Only 30% of anti-HLA antibodies are associated with platelet refractoriness, in comparison to almost 100% of platelet-specific antibodies. Autoantibodies are detected in 50% of patients undergoing allogeneic or autologous BMT, but are usually transient and uncommonly cause platelet refractoriness.

Klumpp and colleagues (1996) studied factors associated with responses to platelet transfusion after HSC transplantation in 526 consecutive platelet transfusions. Poor responses to platelet transfusions (defined as increment of <7.5 × 10^9/l) occurred frequently with 310 of the 484 evaluable transfusions (64%) resulting in a postinfusion corrected count of less than this. Factors associated with a poor response to platelet transfusion by multivariate analysis included the following: presence of serum lymphocytotoxic antibodies, male sex, body surface area greater than 1.7 m², transfusion of red blood cells on the day of platelet transfusion, concurrent administration of corticosteroids, major ABO mismatch between the recipient and the platelet product, and in women a history of one or more pregnancies prior to transplant. Factors that showed little correlation with response to platelet transfusion included the age of the infused platelet product, concurrent fever, recent administration of intravenous immunoglobulin, and the absolute neutrophil count at the time of the infusion.

The TRAP study showed that leukocyte filtration or ultraviolet B irradiation of platelet concentrates were the most effective ways of reducing alloimmunization (TRAP Study Group, 1997). The cost effectiveness of leukocyte depletion is still debated (Heddle & Blajchman, 1995). Once platelet refractoriness develops and nonimmune causes are excluded, single donor concentrates from the bone marrow or blood stem cell donor should be tried. Other platelet donors and recipients should be matched for HLA-A and -B antigens. HLA-C matching has no additional benefit and matching for HLA class II antigens is not necessary. If the patient remains refractory, then the presence of platelet-specific alloantibodies should be tested for. However, there is no evidence that other treatments such as plasma exchange, high-dose immunoglobulin, or high-dose corticosteroids are effective.

Granulocyte transfusion

Granulocyte transfusions are now used much less frequently than previously because of hazards to the recipient, particularly noncardiogenic pulmonary edema due to sequestration of granulocytes in the lung, transmission of infection (particularly of CMV), and alloimmunization. The indications remain controversial. They may be of benefit in the severely neutropenic patient with a documented life-threatening infection unresponsive to 48 hours of appropriate antibiotics. Granulocyte colony-stimulating factor (G-CSF) stimulated granulocyte collection may offer some additional benefit but this is unproven.

Immunoglobulin

The National Institutes of Health (United States) supports the use of intravenous immunoglobulin for the prevention of local and disseminated infection in BMT patients. A dose of 400 to 500 mg/kg/week of intravenous immunoglobulin is often used. A large randomized prospective clinical trial also showed a reduction in risk of GVHD and interstitial pneumonitis in the immunoglobulin recipients (Sullivan et al., 1990; Lancet editorial, 1990). The best established role for prophylactic immunoglobulin in allogeneic transplantation is for minimization of GVHD risk (Guglielmo, Wong-Beringer, & Linker, 1994). As therapy it is useful in the management of hypogammaglobulinemic patients with chronic GVHD prone to repeated bacterial infections, and in the treatment of CMV pneumonitis in combination with ganciclovir.

The Jehovah's Witness patient

Occasionally patients present for HSC transplantation who cannot accept blood transfusion because of their religious beliefs. There has been a report of a patient surviving an autologous transplant in this situation (Ballen et al., 2000). Measures that may improve survival include the use of recombinant human erythropoietin, iron, antifibrinolytics, cytokines, and artificial blood substitutes if available. Pretransplant donation and storage of autologous red cells and platelets could also be employed if acceptable to the patient.

References

Ballen, K.K., Ford, P.A., Waitkus, H. et al. (2000). Successful autologous bone marrow transplant without the use of blood product support. Bone Marrow Transplantation, 26, 27–229.

Bar, B.M., Van Dijk, B.A., Schattenberg, A. et al. (1995). Erythrocyte repopulation after major ABO incompatible transplantation with lymphocyte-depleted bone marrow. Bone Marrow Transplantation, 16, 793–9.

Benjamin, R.J., Connors, J.M., McGurk, S. et al. (1998). Prolonged erythroid aplasia after major ABO-mismatched transplantation for chronic myelogenous leukemia. Biology of Blood and Marrow Transplantation, 4, 151–6.

Bensinger, W.I., Buckner, C.D., Clift, R.A. et al. (1987). Comparison of techniques for dealing with major ABO incompatible marrow transplants. Transplantation Proceedings, 19, 4605–8.

Bensinger, W.I., Buckner, C.D., Thomas, E.D., & Clift, R.A. (1982). ABO-incompatible marrow transplants. Transplantation, 33, 427–9.

Bishop, J.F., McGrath, K., Wolf, M.M. et al. (1988). Clinical features influencing the efficacy of pooled platelet transfusions. Blood, 71, 383–7.

Bolan, C.D., Childs, R.W., Procter, J.L. et al. (2001a). Massive immune hemolysis after allogeneic peripheral blood stem cell transplantation with minor ABO compatibility. British Journal of Haematology, 112, 787–95.

Bolan, C.D., Leitman, S.F., Griffith, L.M. et al. (2001b). Delayed donor red cell chimerism and pure red cell aplasia following major ABO-incompatible nonmyeloablative hematopoietic stem cell transplantation. Blood, 98, 1687–94.

Bornhauser, M., Ordemann, R., Paaz, U. et al. (1997). Rapid engraftment after ABO-incompatible peripheral blood progenitor cell transplantation complicated by severe hemolysis. Bone Marrow Transplantation, 19, 295–7.

Buckner, C.D., Clift, R.A., Sanders, J.G. et al. (1978). ABO-incompatible marrow transplants. Transplantation, 26, 233–8.

Chambers, L.A. (1989). Characteristics and clinical application of blood filters. Transfusion Science, 10, 207–18.

Chen, F.E., Owen, I., Savage, D. et al. (1997). Late onset haemolysis and red cell autoimmunization after allogeneic bone marrow transplant. Bone Marrow Transplantation, 19, 491–5.

Editorial. (1990). Consensus on IVIG. Lancet, 336, 470–2.

Gajewski, J.L., Petz, L.D., Calhoun, L. et al. (1992). Hemolysis of transfused group O red blood cells in minor ABO-incompatible unrelated-donor bone marrow transplants in patients receiving cyclosporine without posttransplant methotrexate. Blood, 79, 3076–85.

Gil-Fernandez, J.J., Alegre, A., Fernandez-Villalta, M.J. et al. (1996). Clinical results of a stringent policy on prophylactic platelet transfusion: non randomized comparative analysis in 190 bone marrow transplant patients from a single institution. Bone Marrow Transplantation, 18, 931–5.

Gmur, J.P., Burger, J., Schaffner, A. et al. (1990). Pure red cell aplasia of long duration complicating major ABO-incompatible bone marrow transplantation. Blood, 75, 290–5.

Greeno, E.W., Perry, E.H., Ilstrup, S.J., & Weisdorf, D.J. (1996). Exchange transfusion the hard way: massive hemolysis following transplantation of bone marrow with minor ABO incompatibility. Transfusion, 36, 71–4.

Guglielmo, B.J., Wong-Beringer, A., & Linker, C.A. (1994). Immune globulin therapy in allogeneic bone marrow transplant: a critical review. Bone Marrow Transplantation, 13, 499–510.

Hazelhurst, G.R., Brenner, M.K., Wimperis, J.Z. et al. (1986). Hemolysis after T-cell depleted bone marrow transplantation involving minor ABO incompatibility. *Scandanavian Journal of Haematology*, **37**, 1–3.

Heddle, N.M. & Blajchman, M.A. (1995). The leukodepletion of cellular blood products in the prevention of HLA-alloimmunization and refractoriness to allogeneic platelet transfusions. *Blood*, **85**, 603–6

Hows, J., Beddow, K., Gordon-Smith, E. *et al.* (1986). Donor-derived red blood cell antibodies and immune hemolysis after allogeneic bone marrow transplantation. *Blood*, **67**, 177–81.

Klumpp, T.R. (1991). Immunohematologic complications of bone marrow transplantation. *Bone Marrow Transplantation*, **8**, 159–70.

Klumpp, T.R., Herman, J.H., Innis, D. *et al.* (1996). Factors associated with response to platelet transfusion following hematopoietic stem cell transplantation. *Bone Marrow Transplantation*, **17**, 1035–41.

Labar, B., Bogdanic, V., Memet, D. *et al.* (1992). Antilymphocyte globulin for treatment of pure red cell aplasia after major ABO incompatible marrow transplant. *Bone Marrow Transplantation*, **10**, 471–2.

Lapierre, V., Kuentz, M., Tiberghien, P, for the Societe Francaise de Greffe de Moelle. (2000). Allogeneic peripheral blood hematopoietic stem cell transplantation: guidelines for red blood cell immuno-hematological assessment and transfusion practice. *Bone Marrow Transplantation*, **25**, 507–12.

Lapierre, V., Oubouzar, N., Auperin, A. *et al.* (2001). Influence of the hematopoietic stem cell source on early immunohematologic reconstitution after allogeneic transplantation. *Blood*, **97**, 2580–6.

Laurencet, F.M., Samii, K., Bressoud, A. *et al.* (1997). Masive delayed hemolysis following peripheral blood stem cell transplantation with minor ABO incompatibility. *Hematological Cell Therapy*, **39**, 159–62.

Lee, J.-H., Lee, K.-H., Kim, S. *et al.* (2000). Anti-A isoagglutinin as a risk factor for the development of pure red cell aplasia after major ABO-incompatible allogeneic bone marrow transplantation. *Bone Marrow Transplantation*, **25**, 179–84.

Leitman, S.F. (1985). Post-transfusion graft-versus-host disease. In *Special Considerations in Transfusing the Immunocompromised Patient*, ed. D.M. Smith & A.J. Silvergleid, pp. 15–37. Arlington, VA: American Association of Blood Banks.

Leitman, S.F. (1989). Use of blood cell irradiation in the prevention of post-transfusion graft-versus-host disease. *Transfusion Science*, **10**, 219–32.

Leo, A., Mytillineros, J., Voso, M.T. *et al.* (2000). Passenger lymphocyte syndrome with severe hemolytic anemia due to an anti-Jka after allogeneic PBPC transplantation. *Transplantation*, **40**, 632–6.

Marmont, A.M., Frassoni, F., Van Lint, M.T. *et al.* (1983). Isohemagglutinin-induced pure red cell aplasia following major ABO incompatible marrow transplant for severe aplastic anemia. Resolution after plasma exchange. *Experimental Hematology*, **11** (Suppl 13), 51–3.

Mehta, J., Powles, R., Singhal, S. *et al.* (1996). Transfusion requirements after bone marrow transplantation from HLA-identical siblings: effects of donor-recipient ABO incompatibility. *Bone Marrow Transplantation*, **18**, 151–6.

Mielcarek, M., Leisenring, W., Torok-Storb, B., & Storb, R. (2000). Graft-versus-host disease and donor-directed hemagglutinin titers after ABO-mismatched related and unrelated marrow allografts: evidence for a graft-versus-plasma cell effect. *Blood*, **96**, 1150–6.

Myser, T., Steedman, M., Hunt, K. *et al.* (1986). A bone marrow transplant with an acquired anti Le (a): a case study. *Human Immunology*, **17**, 102–6.

Ohashi, K., Akiyama, H., Takamoto, S. *et al.* (1994). Treatment of pure red cell aplasia after major ABO-incompatible bone marrow transplantation resistant to erythropoietin. *Bone Marrow Transplantation*, **13**, 335–6.

Oziel-Taieb, S., Faucher-Barbey, C., Chabannon, C. *et al.* (1997). Early and fatal immune haemolysis after so-called 'minor' ABO-incompatible peripheral blood stem cell allotransplantation. *Bone Marrow Transplantation*, **19**, 1155–6.

Robertson, V., Hill, M., Bryant, J. *et al.* (1987). Anti-Jk^b identified in Jk^b positive recipient following T cell depleted bone marrow transplant. *Transfusion*, **27**, 525 (Abstract).

Rowley, S.D. (2001). Hematopoietic stem cell transplantation between red cell incompatible donor-recipient pairs. *Bone Marrow Transplantation*, **28**, 315–21.

Rowley, S.D., Liang, P.S., & Ulz, L. (2000). Transplantation of ABO-incompatible bone marrow and peripheral blood stem cell components. *Bone Marrow Transplantation*, **26**, 749–57.

Salmon, J.P., Michaux, S., Hemanne, J.P. *et al.* (1999). Delayed massive immune hemolysis mediated by minor ABO incompatibility after allogeneic peripheral blood progenitor cell transplantation. *Transfusion*, **39**, 824–7.

Santamaría, A., Sureda, A., Martino, R. *et al.* (1997). Successful treatment of pure red cell aplasia after major ABO-incompatible T cell-depleted bone marrow transplantation with erythropoietin. *Bone Marrow Transplantation*, **20**, 1105–7.

Sniecinski, I.J., Oien, L., Petz, L.D., & Blume, K.G. (1988). Immunohematologic consequences of major ABO mismatched bone marrow transplantation. *Transplantation*, **45**, 530–4.

Sullivan, K.M., Kopecky, K.J., Jocum, J. *et al.* (1990). Immunomodulatory and antimicrobial efficacy of intravenous immunoglobulin in bone marrow transplantation. *New England Journal of Medicine*, **314**, 1006–10.

Ting, A., Pun, A., Dodds, A.J. *et al.* (1987). Red cell alloantibodies produced after bone marrow transplantation. *Transfusion*, **27**, 145–7.

Toren, A. Dacosta, Y., Manny, N. *et al.* (1996). Passenger B-lymphocyte-induced severe hemolytic disease after allogeneic peripheral blood stem cell transplantation (letter). *Blood*, **87**, 843–4.

TRAP Study Group. (1997). Leukocyte reduction and ultraviolet B irradiation of platelets to prevent alloimmunization and refractoriness to platelet transfusions. *New England Journal of Medicine*, **337**, 1861–9.

Yamaguchi, M., Sakai, K., Murata, R., Ueda, M. (2002). Treatment of pure red cell aplasia after major ABO-incompatible peripheral blood stem cell transplantation by induction of chronic graft-versus-host disease. *Bone Marrow Transplantation*, **30**, 539–41.

Young, P.P., Goodnough, L.T., Westervelt, P., & DiPersio, J.F. (2001). Immune hemolysis involving non-ABO/RhD alloantibodies following hematopoietic stem cell transplantation. *Bone Marrow Transplantation*, **27**, 1305–10.

70 Failure of sustained engraftment: clinical manifestations and treatment

GEORGE GEORGES AND RAINER STORB

Fred Hutchinson Cancer Research Center and the University of Washington, Seattle, USA

Introduction

Hematopoietic stem cell transplantation (HSCT) has been used therapeutically in at least three clinical settings. In patients with malignant diseases, transplants have served to rescue patients from the typically irreversible hematopoietic damage caused by myeloablative chemoradiation conditioning regimens and to exert a graft-versus-cancer (leukemia) effect. In patients with genetic diseases (e.g., sickle cell disease), grafts have been used as a replacement for the diseased marrow, thereby correcting disease manifestations. In patients with aplastic anemia, the stem cell graft restores the missing marrow function. Stem cells are transplanted by simple intravenous infusion. They circulate through the bloodstream and then home to the marrow. There they replicate and differentiate in response to genetically defined signals, which results in the reconstitution of hematopoiesis. In most stem cell transplant recipients, these signals for hematopoietic reconstitution are executed without major obstacles, thereby promptly accomplishing the aim of the transplant. In a significant minority of patients, however, the grafted stem cells may fail to produce hematopoietic reconstitution and graft failure may ensue, an event whose clinical manifestation is life-threatening pancytopenia. When graft failure occurs following a truly nonmyeloablative conditioning regimen, autologous reconstitution typically occurs without life-threatening pancytopenia.

The causes of graft failure vary. Some causes are uniquely linked to the source of stem cells used (i.e., autologous or allogeneic donors), while others may affect both autologous and allogeneic transplants. Unique to the autologous setting are adverse effects of preceding chemotherapy or irradiation on the quality of the transplanted cells. Unique to the allogeneic setting is the immunologic barrier of the host-versus-graft (HVG) reaction, which increases in direct relation to increasing degree of histoincompatibility between donors and recipients, and which can be further magnified by recipient sensitization to transplantation antigens via preceding transfusions. T-cell depletion has also been an important cause for failure of allogeneic grafts. In addition, transplantation of a low number of donor CD34+ stem cells is an important risk factor for graft failure. Causes of graft failure that may be seen in both autologous and allogeneic transplant settings are adverse effects on marrow function from drugs administered after transplant or from certain viral infections. In some patients, damage to the marrow stroma may contribute to graft failure, while in yet others, graft failure may herald relapse of the underlying disease for which the transplant had been carried out.

The treatment of graft failure includes (1) discontinuation of marrow suppressive drugs; (2) administration of hematopoietic growth factors; and (3) second transplantation of donor stem cells or buffy coat either with or without a second conditioning regimen or, alternatively, infusion of previously collected cryopreserved autologous peripheral blood stem cells (PBSC). The appropriate treatment depends on the etiology of graft failure and the time after transplant when failure of engraftment becomes evident.

This chapter will define graft failure, analyze the causes of graft failure, and discuss the treatment strategies that have been developed to deal with the major consequence of graft failure, life-threatening pancytopenia. As the mortality related to graft failure remains high, the best strategy for effectively dealing with graft failure is to attempt to optimize transplant-associated procedures that can decrease the patient's risk of developing graft failure.

Definition and diagnosis of graft failure

Primary and secondary graft failure

The general term *graft failure* is used to indicate inadequate hematopoietic function after marrow transplantation. It implies that a minimally acceptable level of function for the erythroid, myelomonocytic, megakaryocytic, and lymphoid lineages has not been reached at a time interval after transplant where such function would be expected. The time after transplant at which failure of engraftment develops distinguishes two clinical types of graft failure (Fig. 70.1). Primary graft failure indicates no evidence of transplanted marrow function after myeloablation, with no recovery of granulocyte counts. Secondary graft failure is the development of inadequate marrow function after initial

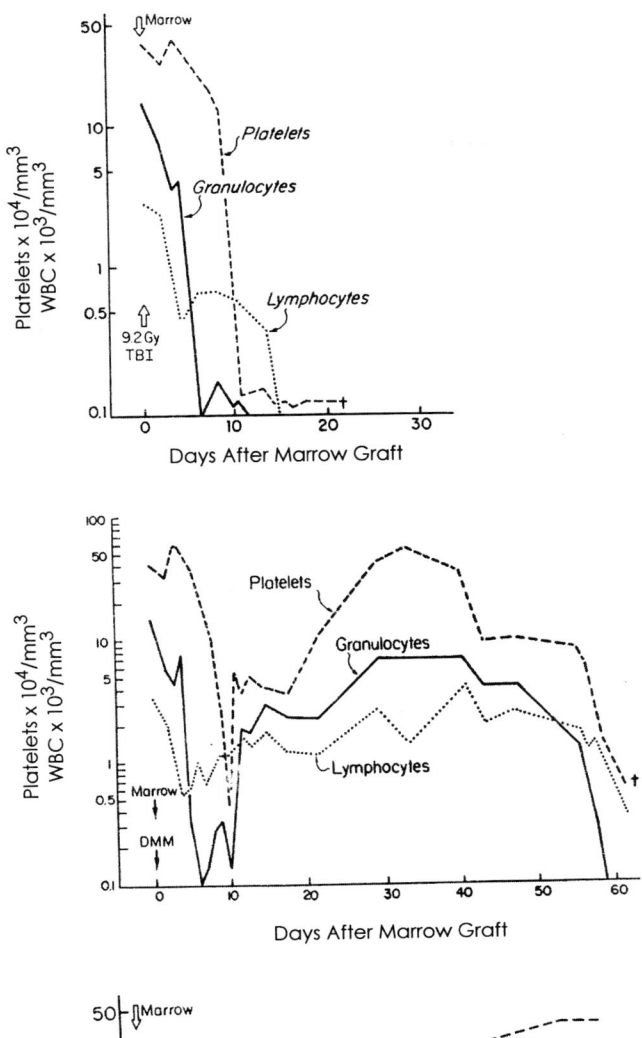

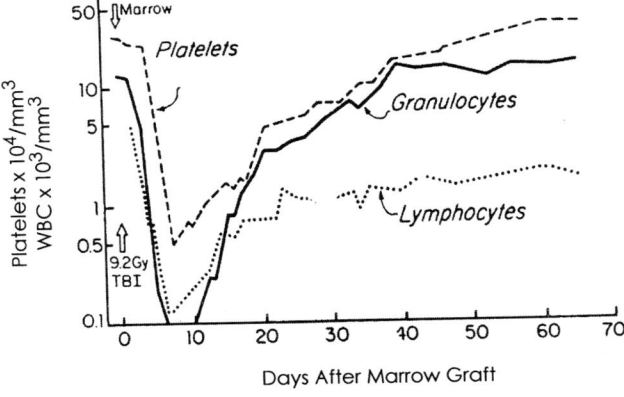

Fig. 70.1. **(A)** Primary graft failure. Peripheral blood count changes in a dog given 9.2 Gy TBI and marrow from an unrelated DLA-nonidentical donor. **(B)** Secondary graft failure. Peripheral blood count changes in a dog given 10 mg dimethylbusulfan/kg i.v. followed by marrow and buffy coat infusion from a DLA-identical littermate. Without postgrafting immunosuppression, 8 of 16 dogs failed to sustain engraftment. **(C)** Successful engraftment of DLA-identical littermate marrow following 9.2 Gy TBI. Adapted from Storb & Deeg (1986).

engraftment has already been achieved. An interval as long as 8 years between the initial transplant and development of secondary graft failure has been described (Dufour *et al.,* 1999). The cause of primary graft failure is not necessarily different from the cause of secondary graft failure; for example, recipient sensitization to donor antigens via previous transfusion of unirradiated blood products can result in either primary or secondary graft failure. Both primary and secondary graft failure can be manifestations of either graft rejection or poor graft function.

The diagnosis of primary graft failure is first suspected in patients who remain pancytopenic for a prolonged period of time following infusion of stem cells. Similarly, the diagnosis of secondary graft failure is suspected in patients who, after initial engraftment, experience recurrent pancytopenia. Once the diagnosis of graft failure is suspected, marrow cellularity is assessed by bone marrow biopsy, aspirate, or both. Graft failure is confirmed by findings of an empty marrow or low cellularity without evidence of myeloid, erythroid, or megakaryocytic precursors at a point in time after transplant at which patients are expected to show evidence of hematopoietic recovery.

Graft rejection

Graft rejection is defined as an immunologically mediated failure of donor hematopoiesis, and it results in the complete destruction of the donor cells. Graft rejection is seen only in the allogeneic HSCT setting and is due to immune reaction against major or minor histocompatibility differences between recipient and donor. Rejection of the graft is characterized by the emergence of immunocompetent host T lymphocytes and a simultaneous loss of all donor cells. Also, there may be a concurrent emergence of host hematopoiesis with either normal or malignant precursor cells. Increased donor-recipient human leukocyte antigen (HLA)-disparity, recipient sensitization to donor antigens by prior blood transfusions, and T-cell depletion of donor marrow can all be causes of graft rejection. In addition, inadequate postgrafting immunosuppression following a reduced-intensity conditioning regimen may predispose to graft rejection.

Poor graft function

Graft failure can also manifest itself as poor or inadequate graft function without evidence of immunologically mediated rejection. Poor graft function can occur within any hematopoietic lineage or may affect all hematopoietic lineages. The most important lineage for early patient survival following transplant is myeloid-derived neutrophil (or granulocyte) recovery, which provides a first-line defense against bacterial infections. In general, if there is failure of neutrophil recovery, there is inadequate function of other hematopoietic lineages. Inadequate megakaryocytic engraftment results in prolonged platelet transfusion–dependence with associated complications of donor platelet allosensitization and an increased risk of serious bleeding episodes. Other important causes of prolonged platelet transfusion dependence include the presence of high-risk chronic graft-versus-host disease (GVHD) (Sullivan *et al.,* 1988). Inadequate lymphoid engraftment is generally described as delayed immune reconstitution, which contributes to infectious mortality from viral and fungal pathogens and is most commonly associated with donor graft T-cell depletion procedures.

Poor erythroid engraftment results in prolonged red blood cell transfusion dependence. An example of this is seen in the setting of major ABO-mismatch (with the presence of hemagglutinins in the recipient against erythrocyte antigens of the donor, e.g., a donor with A and a recipient with type O blood groups). However, although persistence of anti-donor isohemagglutinins is associated with significantly increased red blood cell transfusion requirements compared with ABO-matched patients, the presence of host anti-donor isohemagglutinins is not associated with overall poor myeloid graft function as the following study illustrates. Of 383 major or major/minor ABO-mismatched unrelated and related HSCT allografts, recipients of HLA-matched unrelated donor grafts had a more rapid median time to reach undetectable anti-donor IgG and IgM titers, 46 days compared with 61 days in related recipients. Patients with acute GVHD had a significantly more rapid clearance of hemagglutinins compared to those without GVHD. However, when compared with concurrent recipients of ABO-compatible marrow, neutrophil, and platelet engraftment, incidence of acute GVHD and survival were not influenced by ABO-mismatching (Mielcarek *et al.,* 2000). An occasional patient may require 1 to 2 years for isohemagglutinin resolution (Gmur *et al.,* 1990). Until isohemagglutinin titers disappear, patients typically require support with frequent blood transfusions.

The absolute neutrophil count (ANC) has been used as a convenient indicator of graft function because neutrophils are the first to appear in the peripheral blood following engraftment, and they have a short lifespan. Primary graft failure is generally defined as failure to achieve an ANC of $>0.2 \times 10^9/l$ by day +21 (or at the latest, day +28) after transplantation of unmodified marrow or PBSC. The time period during which engraftment is expected to occur depends on the source of HSC. Neutrophils can appear in the peripheral blood as early as 8 days after transplantation, and following allogeneic marrow infusion, most patients reach 1.0×10^9 neutrophils/l by day +24 (Storb *et al.,* 1986). In general, recipients of both autologous or allogeneic cytokine-mobilized PBSC achieve engraftment 1 week earlier than those of unmodified marrow. On the other hand, delayed engraftment of T-cell-depleted marrow or cryopreserved cord blood beyond day +21 is frequently observed, and failure to achieve an ANC $>0.2 \times 10^9/l$ by the third week does not necessarily imply irreversible graft failure.

Mortality from graft failure

Since the diagnosis of primary graft failure is usually established between days 21 and 28 after transplant, and prolonged

neutropenia is associated with progressively increasing risk of fatal infection, early diagnosis of graft failure is essential to reduce that risk. In an attempt to identify patients at risk for developing primary graft failure, the group at the Royal Marsden Hospital, London, reported on predictors of graft failure or death in a retrospective analysis of over 700 first-marrow allograft recipients. The majority of patients did not receive day +11 methotrexate. In multivariate analysis, a leukocyte count of $<0.2 \times 10^9/l$ on day 16 was the most powerful predictor of subsequent graft failure or death (Mehta *et al.,* 1997a). In a retrospective analysis of 2,276 patients after marrow transplantation in Seattle, the risk of death before day 100 in patients with an ANC $<0.1 \times 10^9/l$ on any given day was compared with those alive on the same day with an ANC $>0.1 \times 10^9/l$ (Offner *et al.,* 1996). There was no increased risk of death in patients with an ANC $<0.1 \times 10^9/l$ on day +14, but by day +20 and after, there was an increased relative risk of death in allogeneic recipients who were neutropenic.

The mortality from graft failure is high due to infectious complications that develop from prolonged neutropenia. In the 1970s and early 1980s, primary graft failure had a mortality of 80% to 95%. Subsequently, the mortality decreased to 40% to 50% due to better treatment options and earlier intervention with identification of risk factors for primary graft failure. Secondary graft failure, depending on its cause, may have a lower mortality rate. Approximately half of all patients with secondary graft failure show subsequent recovery of neutrophil counts to levels $>0.5 \times 10^9/l$. Because of the transient initial recovery from preparative regimen-induced pancytopenia and mucositis, patients have improved tolerance of therapeutic interventions for secondary graft failure. In a report of second allogeneic HSCT for mostly secondary graft failure in 82 patients with acute leukemia, chronic myeloid leukemia (CML), and aplastic anemia, the overall survival after second HSCT was 30% with 53% transplant-related mortality (Fig. 70.2) (Guardiola *et al.,* 2000). However, results for 12 patients with aplastic anemia that experienced rejection of their HLA-identical sibling graft and underwent a second marrow transplant in Seattle showed a 10-year survival of 83%. The use of combined methotrexate and cyclosporine postgrafting immunosuppression was a significant factor accounting for the increase in survival after the second transplant (Stucki *et al.,* 1998). The high mortality of both primary and secondary graft failure points to the need to focus interventions aimed at prevention of this serious complication.

Distinction between graft rejection and other forms of graft failure

Graft failure in the autologous setting is either due to poor quality of transplanted stem cells or caused by drugs or viral infections after transplantation. Distinguishing between these causes may be difficult, and the distinction is often based on circumstantial evidence. In the allogeneic setting it is important to separate graft rejection from other causes of graft fail-

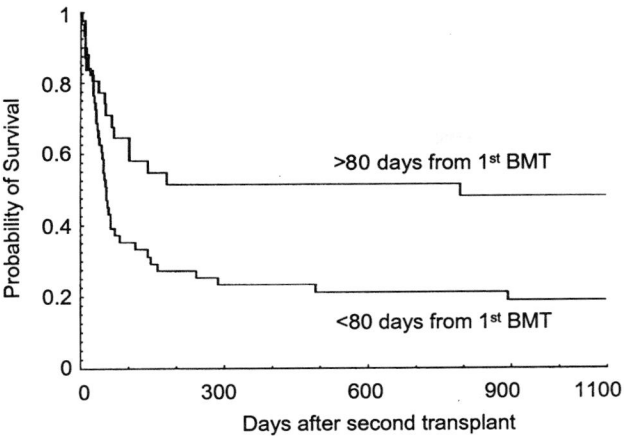

Fig. 70.2. Survival of patients treated with second allogeneic transplant for primary or early secondary graft failure. The graph shows the impact of the time interval from the first transplant to the second transplant on survival outcome. Patients with an intertransplant time interval of at least 80 days had a 3-year estimated survival of 47% (*n* = 31) compared with 19% survival for those who had a shorter intertransplant time interval (*n* = 51) (*P* = .01), univariate analysis. Reproduced, with permission, from Guardiola *et al.* (2000).

ure, given the different treatment options for these conditions. Blood genetic marker studies are indispensable for making this distinction. Genetic markers permit determination of whether marrow cells, peripheral blood neutrophils, and T lymphocytes are of donor or host origin. In this way, informative genetic markers can be used to determine hematopoietic chimerism status.

In the past, marker studies were limited to cytogenetics in the case of sex mismatched donor-recipient pairs or to determination of red blood cell groups and enzyme polymorphisms. Not infrequently, host cells could not be distinguished from donor cells, either because no marker existed, no analyzable metaphase spreads were obtained, or a given patient had received recent blood transfusions. DNA technologies have now evolved that enable clinicians to distinguish host from donor cells in all cases of allogeneic transplants (see Chapter 30).

Peripheral blood and marrow samples are obtained for DNA marker studies. Assessment of graft rejection involves flow cytometric isolation of T cells from peripheral blood or in vitro phytohemagglutinin stimulation to enhance T-lymphocyte proliferation. Once T cells are obtained, a polymerase chain reaction (PCR)-based technique to assess DNA polymorphism in minisatellite nucleotide repeat regions (also referred to as variable number of tandem repeats—VNTR) between donor and recipient, can be used to identify chimerism status. Percent donor chimerism is accurately quantified using either the storage phosphor imaging technique or the fluorescent-based short tandem repeat (STR). Additionally, real-time quantitative TaqMan assays have been developed that offer even more sensitive quantitative assessment of mixed chimerism (Alizadeh *et*

al., 2002). In a laboratory that performs this assay routinely, accurate and reproducible results of chimerism status can be expected with a 4- to 5-day turnaround. In general, quantitative PCR determination of the percentage of donor or host contribution to hematopoiesis has an error of approximately ±5%. In the setting of donor-recipient sex mismatch, fluorescence in situ hybridization (FISH) analysis using Y- and X-chromosome specific probes permits rapid quantitative chimerism analysis of sex-mismatched donor-recipient pairs.

The diagnosis of graft rejection is confirmed if T lymphocytes are of only host origin in the setting of clinical graft failure. If mixed chimerism of the T-cell compartment is identified in the setting of poor graft function, repeat follow-up assessments are necessary to rule out progression to rejection. In the case of relapse (without rejection), only the malignant cells are host, while T cells are donor. Hence, donor lymphocyte infusions for relapse after marrow transplant may be effective only if T cells of donor origin can be identified. In case of marrow injury due to drugs or viral infection, both myeloid and lymphoid cells are of donor origin.

Blood and marrow should be simultaneously evaluated when attempting to define the cause of graft failure, particularly if relapse of hematologic malignancy is suspected. In relapse, cytogenetic analysis or disease-related FISH probes that are specific for chromosome rearrangements such as translocations [e.g., BCR/ABL t(9:22)(q34;q11) in CML] are useful diagnostic reagents. In addition, flow cytometric phenotype consistent with clonal precursor expansion is a useful marker of relapse.

Causes of graft failure (and see Chapter 12)

Effects of preceding chemotherapy in the autologous HSCT setting

In the autologous transplant setting, previously obtained cryopreserved HSC are infused following myeloablative preparative regimens. Damage to harvested HSC can occur prior to transplantation if patients have been subjected to multiple cycles of conventional-dose chemotherapy or if they have received irradiation that includes significant areas of marrow. The Seattle transplant team reported on factors associated with poor engraftment of autologous PBSC (Bensinger *et al.*, 1995). Two hundred forty-three consecutive patients with malignancies underwent myeloablative conditioning and received PBSC mobilized with granulocyte or granulocyte-macrophage colony-stimulating factor (G-CSF or GM-CSF) ± chemotherapy (predominantly cyclophosphamide [CY]-based). Those patients who received a CD34+ cell dose <2.5 × 10^6/kg (*n* = 23) had delayed engraftment of neutrophils and delayed platelet recovery with 20% of all transplanted patients remaining platelet-transfusion dependent beyond 60 days after transplantation. In multivariate analysis, greater than six chemotherapy cycles before PBSC mobilization, preceding localized irradiation therapy, and the presence of marrow disease at stem cell harvest all predicted lower CD34+ cell collection.

Weaver *et al.* (1995) reported similar results from an analysis of 692 patients who received mobilized autologous PBSC following myeloablative chemotherapy. The single most important predictor of neutrophil and platelet engraftment kinetics was the CD34+ cell content of infused PBSC. Although a minimum threshold CD34+ cell dose could not be defined since all patients studied achieved neutrophil recovery (defined as an ANC >0.5 × 10^9/l) by day +32, those patients who required two mobilization procedures to achieve ≥2.5 × 10^6 CD34+ cells/kg experienced slower platelet recovery. Thus, it is preferable to harvest autologous PBSC for use in high-dose chemotherapy hematopoietic support as early as possible in the course of treatment for the underlying malignancy. Multiple harvests of mobilized PBSC may be required to obtain sufficient CD34+ cells necessary to ensure adequate hematopoietic recovery. In a study of 119 patients who had inadequate collection (≥2.5 × 10^6/kg) of autologous CD34+ cells following initial mobilization, a second attempt at mobilization with G-CSF or chemotherapy plus G-CSF was successful in reaching a total collection of ≥2.5 × 10^6 CD34+/kg in 48% of cases (Weaver *et al.*, 1998).

Bentley *et al.* (1997) reported a series of 51 patients who received autologous PBSC infusion following myeloablative conditioning; seven were considered engraftment failures due to platelet and/or red cell transfusion dependence beyond day 100 posttransplant. Six of these seven long-term engraftment failures received low doses of progenitor cells quantified as <1 × 10^5 colony-forming units-granulocyte macrophage (CFU-GM)/kg. In multivariate analysis, the significant predictors of poor neutrophil engraftment were CFU-GM dose and number of prior chemotherapy regimens. Despite the clinical benefits of mobilized PBSC for use in the autologous transplant setting, with more rapid recovery of neutrophil and platelet counts compared to marrow, these studies confirm that low yields of CFU-GM and CD34+ cells are obtained if PBSC are collected after stem cells have been damaged following exposure to multiple cycles of nadir-inducing chemotherapy.

Degree of donor-recipient histocompatibility in the allogeneic HSCT setting

In the allogeneic transplant setting, the incidence of graft failure has been shown to correlate with the degree of donor HLA incompatibility (Table 70.1 and Fig. 70.3). In a study that assessed engraftment following bone marrow transplantation (BMT) in the 1980s among 930 patients who received unmodified marrow grafts from HLA-identical siblings following CY and total body irradiation (TBI), the incidence of graft failure was 2%. This was compared to results in 269 patients who received comparable preparative regimens followed by unmodified marrow grafts from family members who shared one HLA haplotype but differed to a variable degree for the HLA-A, -B, and -D antigens of the haplotype not shared with the recipient. Graft failure occurred in 3 of 43 transplants (7%) from donors who were phenotypically HLA-matched with their recipient for the nonshared haplotype (HLA antigens similar but not inher-

Table 70.1. *Effect of donor-recipient histocompatibility on graft failure*

Degree of donor-recipient histocompatibility (related donor)	Incidence of graft failure	Patients with graft failure/total number of patients
HLA-identical sibling	2%	19/930
Phenotypic HLA-match	7%	3/43
1-locus mismatch	9%	11/121
2-locus mismatch	21%	18/86
Haploidentical (3-locus)	5%[a]	1/19

[a] Haploidentical recipients were young children conditioned with 15.75 Gy TBI and transplanted with parental marrow.
Adapted from Anasetti *et al.* (1989).

ited from the same parents), in 11 of 121 transplants (9%) from donors incompatible for one HLA locus, in 18 of 86 transplants (21%) incompatible for two loci, and in 1 of 19 transplants (5%) incompatible for three loci. The reasons for the better outcome in the three loci mismatched recipients are most likely increased intensity of preparative regimens used, very young patient age and, consequently, large marrow cell numbers transplanted. Independent risk factors for graft failure were donor incompatibility for HLA-B and -D and a positive crossmatch for anti-donor lymphocytotoxic antibody. Residual host lymphocytes were detected in 11 of 14 patients with graft failure, suggesting the mechanism for graft failure was host-mediated immune rejection (Anasetti *et al.*, 1989).

Improved molecular techniques for characterizing additional class I alleles such as HLA-C have shown that HLA-C mis-

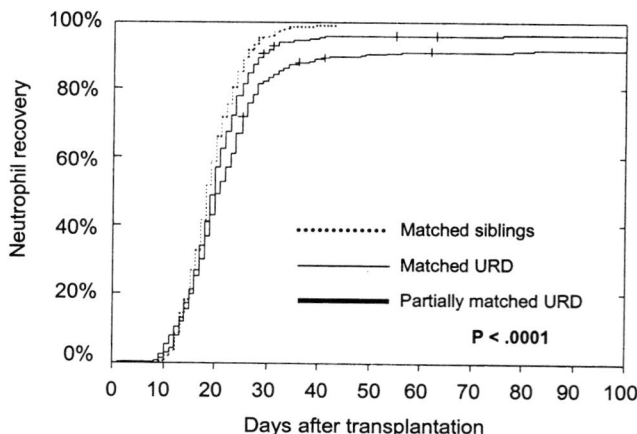

Fig. 70.3. Engraftment of matched sibling and unrelated donor bone marrow. Hematologic recovery to neutrophil count of >0.5 × 10^9/l following bone marrow transplantation for chronic myeloid leukemia in chronic phase. Data from the National Marrow Donor Program Registry for HLA-matched sibling donors (*n* = 364), HLA-matched unrelated donors (*n* = 1,209), and partially HLA-matched unrelated donors (*n* = 386). Graft failure occurred in 1% ± 1% matched sibling donor, 4% ± 1% matched unrelated donor, and 8% ± 2% partially matched unrelated donor recipients (*P* < .0001). Reproduced, with permission, from Weisdorf *et al.* (2002).

matching between unrelated donors and recipients results in an increased risk of graft failure. In a retrospective case-controlled study, the estimated odds ratio of graft failure for HLA-C disparity was 4.0, even after accounting for the contribution of serologically undetectable HLA-A and HLA-B allele disparities (Petersdorf *et al.*, 1997). In support of the biologic importance of HLA-C matching, HLA-C-specific cytotoxic T cells have been detected in a case of rejection of a T-cell-depleted marrow graft (Pei *et al.*, 2001).

Improved DNA-based typing methods for the HLA class I and II alleles have been developed and have been compared with serologically detected polymorphisms in order to determine if there are acceptable disparities between the unrelated donor and recipient. Disparities between HLA sequence polymorphisms that are serologically detectable are termed *antigen mismatches,* whereas those that can be identified only by DNA-based typing methods are termed *allele mismatches.* Based on NMDP and Seattle data analysis, allele mismatches in class II genes have been identified as an independent risk factor for GVHD, while class I allele level mismatching was not associated with GVHD (Petersdorf *et al.*, 1998, 2001b). In the largest and most informative study to date, DNA sequencing was used to define HLA-A, B, and C alleles and class II alleles in 471 patients who received non-T-cell-depleted bone marrow from unrelated donors for the treatment of CML after myeloablative TBI-based conditioning therapy in Seattle from 1985 to 2000 (Petersdorf *et al.*, 2001a). Patients with fully HLA-matched donors had a 0.7% rate of graft failure. A single HLA-allele mismatch did not increase the risk of graft rejection, whereas a single class I antigen mismatch significantly increased the graft rejection rate to 14%. However, if the donor had two or more class I allele mismatches, the graft failure rate was 22%. The risk of graft rejection was 71% if the recipient was homozygous at the mismatched class I locus (with either an allele or antigen mismatched donor). Thus, HLA class I antigen mismatches that are serologically detectable confer an enhanced risk of graft failure after BMT. Transplants from donors with a single class I allele mismatch that are not serologically detectable may be used without an increased risk of graft failure (Petersdorf *et al.*, 2001a). However, serological matching for class I polymorphisms does not exclude the possibility of multiple class I allele mismatches. This study points to the importance of DNA-based typing of class I and II alleles to identify the optimally HLA-matched unrelated donor.

Increased immunosuppression of the recipient with intensified preparative regimens has permitted relative improvement in the rate of successful engraftment of haploidentical, two to three HLA loci mismatched marrow (Anasetti *et al.*, 1989). A decrease in the incidence of graft failure from 17% to 9% was observed when the total hyperfractionated TBI dose was increased from 12 Gy over 6 days to 13.2 or 14.4 Gy (120 cGy, thrice daily, for 11 to 12 doses), respectively. On the other hand, intensive conditioning regimen immunosuppression resulted in increased toxicity and increased risk of infectious complications after transplantation.

Antibodies directed against host T cells to prevent rejection of mismatched HSC have been used as an alternative to increased TBI dose. In Seattle, the addition of antithymocyte globulin (ATG) (10 mg/kg/day, day −2 to day +3) to the standard preparative regimen of CY (120 mg/kg) plus TBI (15.75 Gy) was used for grafts mismatched in the HVG direction (rejection vector). In this setting, ATG did not decrease the incidence of graft failure. Other anti-T-cell antibodies (e.g., Campath-1) (Hale & Waldmann, 1994; Willemze *et al.*, 1992) or anti-leukocyte adhesion molecules (CD18/CD11) (Baume *et al.*, 1989) have been introduced to the preparative regimen with the hope of enhancing engraftment of mismatched donor marrow with limited success.

Recipient sensitization through preceding blood product transfusions in the allogeneic HSCT setting

Patients with aplastic anemia, sickle cell anemia, and beta thalassemia have a much higher rate of allogeneic graft failure than patients with hematologic malignancies such as acute myeloid leukemia (AML) or acute lymphoblastic leukemia (ALL). This may in part be due to the decreased intensity of immunosuppressive conditioning given to these patients. However, to a large extent rejection is due to allosensitization to blood product antigens, given that these patients receive their transfusions in the absence of immunosuppressive chemotherapy.

In 1980 the Seattle group reported that patients with aplastic anemia who had been transfused with blood products prior to transplantation had an increased rate of graft rejection (30%–45%) compared to patients not previously transfused (6%) (Storb *et al.*, 1980). These findings in patients were consistent with previously reported prospective studies in a preclinical canine model of marrow transplantation (Storb *et al.*, 1970, 1971). The long-term benefit of the decreased incidence of rejection was reflected by the 80% 18-year actuarial survival among 53 nontransfused recipients of HLA-identical sibling marrow compared with 64% survival in 115 previously transfused transplant patients (Doney *et al.*, 1997).

Currently used preparative regimens for marrow transplantation of aplastic anemia include combinations of CY and ATG or CY plus total lymphoid irradiation (TLI), or other modifications of TLI. These regimens, in combination with the introduction of cyclosporine and methotrexate for GVHD prevention, have resulted in significantly lower rates of graft failure. In an update of the multicenter experience with the Seattle regimen consisting of CY and ATG conditioning, HLA-identical marrow, and combined cyclosporine and methotrexate postgrafting immunosuppression, 4 of 94 patients rejected their grafts from HLA-matched siblings between 2 and 7 months after transplantation. Of the four patients with graft rejection, three were alive following second HSCT (Storb *et al.*, 2001). Despite these improvements, failing grafts have been observed upon tapering of cyclosporine either due to persistence of the underlying pathologic condition that resulted in the development of aplastic anemia in the first place or to persistence of sensitized host T lymphocytes. Consistent with the latter possibility is the observation that patients with mixed donor-host hematopoietic chimerism after transplant have a higher rejection risk than those who are complete donor chimeras (Hill *et al.*, 1986). In this situation, prolonged cyclosporine use with very gradual taper may rescue hematopoiesis in occasional patients with either donor or recipient hematopoiesis, although this possibility is speculative.

Thalassemia patients undergoing HLA-matched sibling marrow transplantation have a 6% to 25% risk of graft failure with emergence of host hematopoiesis (Lucarelli *et al.*, 1993, 1995). Reasons for graft rejection include (1) insufficient host immunosuppression and/or insufficient myeloablation with busulfan (BU)/CY conditioning, reflected by low serum BU levels, and (2) liver fibrosis associated with iron overload, which can reflect extensive pretransplant transfusion of blood products and allosensitization. Successful engraftment of second marrow transplants has been reported following conditioning with CY/ATG (or CY/anti-lymphocyte globulin) as was used for aplastic anemia patients (Di Bartolomeo *et al.*, 1993; Stucki *et al.*, 1998). Eight of 9 young children with late secondary graft failure and complete autologous reconstitution survived after a second myeloablative BU/CY regimen and marrow transplant with 4 having sustained donor engraftment (Gaziev *et al.*, 1999). Studies using the BU/CY conditioning regimen in patients with other diseases have demonstrated a correlation between BU pharmacokinetics and graft rejection (Slattery *et al.*, 1995) (see Chapter 33). When oral BU doses are not adjusted based on steady-state blood levels, BU/CY-based preparative regimens have been associated with an increased risk of graft failure in recipients of both HLA-mismatched bone marrow transplants (Schultz *et al.*, 1994) and in recipients of HLA-matched unrelated donor transplants (Mehta *et al.*, 1994).

Similarly, there has been a 10% to 20% risk of graft rejection for children undergoing transplantation of HLA-matched sibling marrow for sickle cell anemia (Walters *et al.*, 1996). The cause for this high rate of rejection may also reflect allosensitization to blood products from pretransplant transfusions.

The dog model of marrow transplantation has unambiguously shown the importance of transfusion-induced allosensitization to minor histocompatibility donor antigens (Table 70.2 and Fig. 70.4). Marrow grafts between dog leukocyte antigen (DLA)-identical littermates following 9.2 Gy TBI have an incidence of rejection of less than 5%, while animals given three preceding whole blood transfusions from the DLA-identical marrow donor before transplant become sensitized and have a 100% graft rejection rate. A single transfusion of DLA-matched donor whole blood prior to marrow transplantation resulted in graft rejection in 73% of dogs. Dogs that received blood transfusions from random unrelated donors on days –24, –17, and –10 prior to 9.2 Gy TBI and marrow from a DLA-identical littermate had a 27% incidence of graft rejection (Storb *et al.*, 1979; Storb & Deeg, 1986).

Leukocyte-depletion or irradiation of blood products has been successfully used to prevent allosensitization to donor marrow. Three leukocyte-poor red cell transfusions from a matched littermate donor prior to marrow transplantation resulted in a 36% graft rejection rate (Storb *et al.*, 1979). Irradiation of either DLA-identical or random unrelated whole blood with 20 Gy reduced the incidence of matched littermate graft rejection to 10% and 6%, respectively (Bean *et al.*, 1991, 1994). Irradiation of blood products prevents recipient sensitization to minor histocompatibility antigens and reduces the incidence of graft rejection. Thus, while it is advisable to avoid unnecessary blood product transfusions, the use of leuko-depleted and irradiated blood products for all patients who are candidates for marrow transplantation may help to reduce the risk of subsequent graft rejection.

T-cell depletion of allogeneic grafts

In clinical studies, the use of T-cell-depleted marrow for allogeneic transplantation has been complicated by an increased

Table 70.2. *Effect of pretransplant blood product transfusion on MHC-matched hematopoietic engraftment: outcome of marrow grafts from DLA-identical littermates after 9.2 Gy TBI*

Source of blood product transfused[a]	In vitro blood product treatment		Dogs with donor engraftment	Number engrafted/ total number of dogs studied
	2000 cGy γ-irradiation	Leukocyte depletion		
No preceding transfusion	N/A	N/A	98%	61/62
Marrow donor	–	–	0%	0/27
	+	–	85%	17/20
	–	+	64%	9/14
Platelet transfusion	–	+	53%	8/15
Unrelated dogs (each recipient transfused with blood from 6 different unrelated dogs total)	–	–	37%	10/27
	+	–	94%	15/16

[a] Preceding blood product transfusions on days –24, –17, –10. Fifty ml of heparinized blood per transfusion.
Adapted from Bean *et al.* (1991); Bean *et al.* (1994); Storb *et al.* (1979); Storb & Deeg (1986).

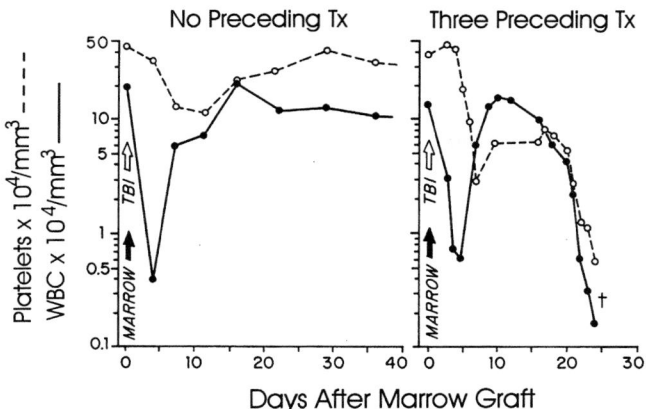

Fig. 70.4. Hematologic changes in dogs following 9.2 Gy TBI and infusion of DLA-identical littermate marrow. (**A,** left) Recipient without prior blood product transfusion shows sustained donor engraftment. (**B,** right) Recipient received three preceding whole blood transfusions days −24, −17, and −10 from the same DLA-identical littermate. This is an example of secondary graft failure due to pretransplant sensitization to donor minor histocompatibility antigens. Adapted from Storb *et al.* (1979).

incidence of graft failure (Table 70.3). Both primary and secondary graft failures have been recognized, as well as an increased incidence of disease relapse. The primary aim of T-cell depletion is prevention of GVHD; however, the increased incidence of subsequent complications of graft failure, relapse, and delayed immune reconstitution has limited the usefulness of this approach. Despite the development of multiple different strategies for less complete or more selective methods of T-cell depletion, no definitive improvement in overall survival outcome has been shown with any of the T-cell depletion strategies.

Results from a multicenter, retrospective International Bone Marrow Transplant Registry (IBMTR) analysis involving 731 leukemia patients who received T-cell-depleted, HLA-identical donor marrow between 1982 and 1987 identified a 10-fold increased incidence of graft failure compared to that among 2,480 patients who received non–T-cell-depleted transplants during the same time period (Marmont *et al.*, 1991). The overall rate of graft failure in the T-cell-depleted cohort was 12%

Table 70.3. *Probability of graft failure with T-cell depletion of donor marrow*[a]

Related donor graft	T-cell-depleted	Non–T-cell-depleted
HLA-identical sibling	12%	2%
Phenotypic match or 1-locus mismatch	18%	8%
2–3 HLA loci mismatch	43%	27%

[a] Multicenter IBMTR data (1980–1987) of 329 leukemia patients receiving related, non-HLA identical marrow grafts (151 T-cell-depleted) and 2,977 leukemia patients receiving HLA-identical sibling marrow (606 T-cell-depleted). Adapted from Ash *et al.* (1991).

and in the non–T-cell-depleted controls was less than 2%. Posttransplant immune suppression with methotrexate and/or cyclosporine reduced the risk of treatment failure. In addition, patient age greater than 20 years and donor-recipient sex mismatch were risk factors for graft failure. The method of T-cell depletion did not affect probability of graft failure. Relapse rates in patients receiving T-cell depletion versus non–T-cell depletion of donor grafts were 37% and 15%, respectively, in patients with early leukemia (including AML or ALL in first remission and CML in chronic phase). Relapse rates were 51% and 34%, respectively, in patients with intermediate leukemia (AML or ALL in ≥ second remission and CML in accelerated phase). Patients with advanced leukemia had 70% versus 51% relapse rates, respectively. Leukemia-free survival was significantly worse in all three risk categories of patients receiving T-cell-depleted grafts. Two-year survival in patients with early leukemia was 44% among recipients of T-cell-depleted grafts and 54% in non–T-cell-depleted grafts. In patients with advanced leukemia, survival was 15% and 30%, respectively.

In another IBMTR analysis, data involving 870 leukemia patients transplanted between 1982 and 1994 receiving either unrelated or HLA-mismatched related donor marrow were compared with data on 998 patients receiving non–T-cell-depleted transplants (Champlin *et al.*, 2000). Fifty-two percent of the T-cell-depleted graft recipients were treated with narrow-specificity antibodies, categorized as antibodies targeting either the αβ T-cell receptor, or up to three combinations of antibodies targeting CD3, CD4, CD5, CD6, CD7, and CD8. The remainder received grafts treated with either broad specificity antibodies targeting a greater range of T-cell antigens, or Campath antibodies, elutriation, or lectin methods for T-cell depletion. Graft failure occurred in 6% ± 2% of non–T-cell-depleted recipients, 10% ± 4% of narrow-specificity antibody-treated recipients, and in 19% ± 5% of other T-cell-depleted recipients. Although the incidence of acute GVHD was higher in the recipients of non–T-cell-depleted grafts, transplant-related mortality was higher in the T-cell-depleted graft recipients. Overall 5-year leukemia-free survival in the non–T-cell-depleted group was 31% ± 4%, 29% ± 5% in the narrow-specificity antibody T-cell-depleted group, and 16% ± 4% in the group with other methods of T-cell depletion. This study confirmed the previous findings of no improvement in overall outcome with T-cell-depletion methods.

Other centers have reported on results of T-cell depletion of marrow, and results were consistent with the IBMTR findings. Although the incidence and mortality of GVHD have been reduced, overall survival has not been improved due to the high rates of graft failure and disease relapse. The following studies are representative of findings with T-cell depletion.

In an early pilot study reported by the Seattle transplant team (Martin *et al.*, 1985), 20 adult patients with leukemia were conditioned with CY plus fractionated TBI (12.0 or 15.75 Gy) and received cyclosporine after infusion of 2- to 3-log T-cell-depleted marrow from HLA-identical donors. Eight patients rejected their grafts, one transiently. Seven with graft rejection received 12.0 Gy TBI; only one out of the nine patients who received 15.75 Gy TBI had graft rejection. T-cell depletion was achieved with a mixture of eight murine anti-T-cell monoclonal antibodies, directed against multiple T-cell antigens, followed by rabbit serum complement-mediated cell lysis. The majority of deaths were due to graft failure and infectious complications. The relapse rate within 1 year after transplant was 35% and overall survival was 20%.

Less stringent T-cell-depleted marrow transplantation was developed as an alternative to complete T-cell depletion. The Milwaukee transplant team results of 55 patients who received either HLA-identical or 1- to 2-HLA antigen mismatched marrow that was treated with the anti-CD3 monoclonal antibody $T_{10}B_9$ followed by rabbit complement with 1.6 log T-cell depletion, showed an overall incidence of graft rejection of 6%. Patients received intensive pretransplantation conditioning regimens including high-dose cytosine arabinoside, CY, 14 Gy TBI, and methylprednisolone (Ash *et al.*, 1990). The incidence of acute GVHD was 17% and 53%, respectively, in HLA-matched and HLA-mismatched recipients of T-cell-depleted marrow. Three-year relapse-free survival was 48% and 32%, respectively, in 15 "good risk" and 32 "poor risk" leukemia patients.

Removal of CD4+ cells and partial depletion of CD8+ cells from donor marrow for HLA-mismatched unrelated donor recipients was explored as a method to prevent graft rejection and avoid GVHD. In a study designed to find a CD8 T-cell marrow dose that prevented both graft rejection and GVHD following a myeloablative 13.2 or 13.5 Gy TBI-based conditioning regimen, 27 adult patients were treated with either HLA-DRB1 allele disparate or HLA-A or -B antigen disparate donor marrow grafts (Martin *et al.*, 1999). Following stringent CD4+ cell depletion, the number of CD8+ cells infused into recipients was decreased in a step-wise manner from one patient cohort to the next. Removal of CD4+ cells did not cause graft rejection nor appreciably decrease the risk of grades II–IV GVHD. More stringent depletion of CD8+ cells was associated with an increased risk of rejection in patients with either an HLA-DRB1 allele disparate or an HLA-A or -B antigen disparate donor. In both groups of patients the risk of grades III–IV GVHD was greater than 15% at any dose of CD8+ cells in the donor marrow associated with less than 5% risk of graft failure. This study showed the importance of donor CD8+ cells for preventing allogeneic marrow graft rejection, but the clinical outcome after HLA-mismatched marrow transplantation was not improved by removing CD4+ cells and some of the CD8+ from the graft. This study pointed to the need for future efforts to find alternative methods for transplantation when optimal matching of the donor and recipients is not possible.

The Hammersmith Hospital transplant center reported a probability of graft failure of 16% among 115 patients undergoing unrelated donor T-cell-depleted marrow transplant for first chronic phase (86 patients) or advanced phase (32 patients) CML (Spencer *et al.*, 1995). T-cell depletion was achieved either in vitro ($n = 28$) with either Campath-1M or Campath-1G monoclonal antibodies or in vivo ($n = 84$) with infusion of varying forms of antilymphocyte therapy after transplantation of donor marrow. T-cell-depleted grafts from donors older than 40 years of age had a failure rate of 22%. The probability of relapse at 3 years was 20% and 36%, respectively, for patients with chronic phase and advanced phase CML. Three-year leukemia-free survival was 41% and 26%, respectively. The incidence of grade III to IV acute GVHD was 24%. The overall survival of CML patients in this study was less favorable than current results from non-T-cell-depleted unrelated donor grafts.

Similar results of increased risk of graft failure were reported in a cohort of 137 children with ALL that received Campath 1-depleted marrow and postgrafting cyclosporine for HLA-matched unrelated donor recipients, or cyclosporine plus methotrexate for recipients of mismatched unrelated donor grafts (Green *et al.*, 1999). Recipients of HLA-matched grafts had 4.8% incidence of graft failure compared with 15.7% rate of graft failure in HLA-mismatched recipients. Although the incidence of acute GVHD was 23% and 20%, the overall 3-year leukemia-free survival was 45% and 40%, respectively.

Hematopoietic cell dose of allogeneic grafts

In the non–T-cell-depleted marrow transplant setting the effect of low marrow cell dose has become an important factor for the improved outcome of patients after allogeneic HSCT. In the 1970s and 1980s it was already recognized that infusion of a low marrow cell dose was associated with an increased risk of allogeneic graft rejection in aplastic anemia patients (Storb *et al.*, 1977; Niederwieser *et al.*, 1988). It was also recognized that a low nucleated bone marrow cell dose of $<2.5 \times 10^8$/kg was a risk factor for delayed engraftment and increased graft failure mortality in patients with hematologic malignancies undergoing allogeneic BMT (Mehta *et al.*, 1997b). In subsequent studies, CD34+ content of marrow, PBSC, and cord blood has been identified as a clinically useful tool to predict transplant outcome. Retrospective studies have indicated that infusion of at least 2×10^6 CD34+ cells/kg is necessary for improved survival after transplant (Singhal *et al.*, 2000). In a retrospective study of 212 patients who received HLA-identical sibling donor unmanipulated bone marrow grafts, a median of 2.4×10^8 marrow nucleated cells and 3.7×10^6 CD34+ cell/kg of recipient body weight were infused. A CD34+ cell dose of $>3 \times 10^6$/kg was strongly associated with improved hematopoietic recovery after transplant, decreased incidence of fungal infection and transplant-related mortality, and improved overall survival (Bittencourt *et al.*, 2002) (Fig. 70.5).

Infusion of a very large number of CD34+ cells is not necessarily associated with an improved transplant outcome. In a study of patients with hematological malignancies who underwent conventional PBSC transplantation from HLA-identical sibling donors, recipients of $>8 \times 10^6$ CD34+ cells/kg of recipient body weight had a 53% risk of extensive chronic GVHD compared with 36% in recipients of $<8 \times 10^6$ CD34+ cells/kg.

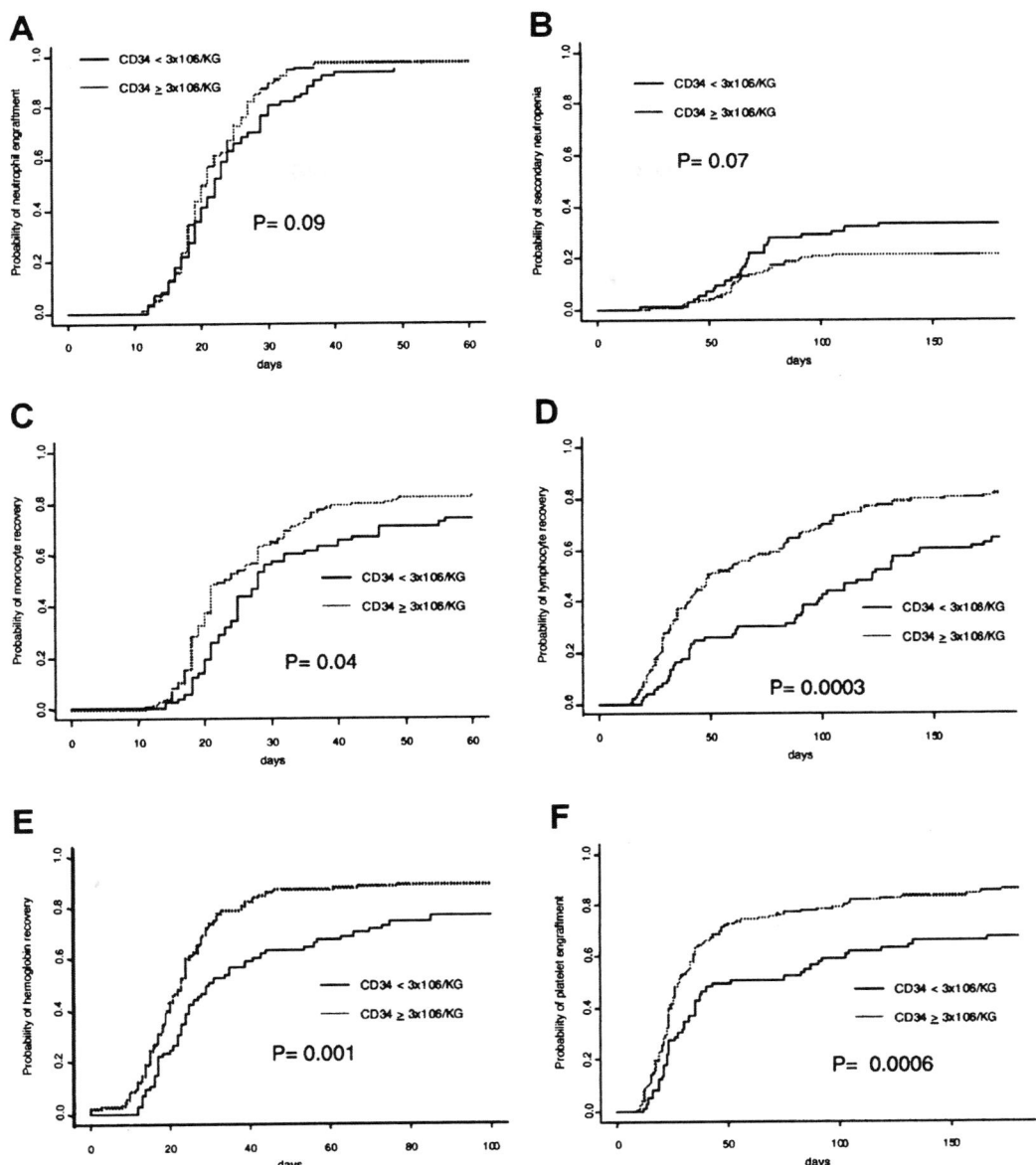

Fig. 70.5. The association of CD34 cell dose with hematopoietic recovery after HLA-identical sibling bone marrow transplantation (*n* = 212). Shown is the cumulative incidence of hematopoietic recoveries according to the transplanted CD34 cell dose. The panels show (**A**) neutrophil, (**B**) secondary neutropenia, (**C**) monocyte, (**D**) lymphocyte, (**E**) hemoglobin, and (**F**) platelet recoveries. Reproduced, with permission, from Bittencourt *et al.* (2002).

To ensure reliable engraftment a target minimum of 4×10^6 CD34+ cells/kg was collected. There was no difference in engraftment kinetics, acute GVHD, disease relapse, and survival between recipients of low versus high CD34+ cell dose grafts. Neither the absolute number nor relative proportion of CD3+ or CD14+ cell dose was associated with transplant outcome (Zaucha *et al.*, 2001). This study suggests that an ideal range of 4 to 8 CD34+ cells/kg of recipient body weight may be the optimal cell dose to transplant. Whether or not other cellular components influence the outcome of non–T-cell-depleted allogeneic HSCT remains to be determined.

G-CSF-mobilized PBSC may not be the only method to obtain increased numbers of CD34+ cells for transplantation. In a randomized prospective trial of HLA-identical sibling conventional transplantation, G-CSF-primed allogeneic bone marrow resulted in significantly less chronic GVHD and comparable engraftment to G-CSF mobilized PBSC (Morton *et al.*, 2001). The number of CD34+ cells was increased threefold in the G-PBSC group, and there were ninefold more CD3+ cells. Median times to neutrophil and platelet engraftment were similar. The incidence of chronic GVHD was 80% in the G-PBSC group and 22% in the recipients of G-primed bone marrow. The 18-month survival estimates were similar for the two groups.

The use of umbilical cord blood from sibling and unrelated donors has been successfully used to treat patients with high-risk or recurrent hematological malignancies or children with selected inherited immunodeficiency states, metabolic disorders, and bone marrow failure syndromes (see Chapter 68). The advantage of cord blood is the potential for decreased risk of GVHD despite HLA-disparity between the donor and recipient. One reason that unrelated donor cord blood transplantation for children has been generally more successful than for adults has been attributed to the increased number of nucleated cells per kilogram of recipient body weight infused in children (Gluckman *et al.*, 1997; Rubinstein *et al.*, 1998). In a retrospective study of 102 unrelated donor cord blood recipients, there was an improved probability of survival if the thawed grafts contained at least 1.7×10^5 CD34+ cells/kg of recipient body weight and if grafts were not greater than 2 HLA-antigens disparate. The incidence of primary graft failure in recipients of $<1.7 \times 10^5$ CD34+/kg was 28% (Fig. 70.6). In this group of low CD34+ cell dose recipients, the 1-year transplant-related mortality rate was 70% (Wagner *et al.*, 2002).

Nonfatal graft failure following non-myeloablative HSCT

Allogeneic HSCT in older patients or medically unfit patients with minimally toxic, non-myeloablative preparative regimens has been an important advance in the field of transplantation. However, the reduced intensity of the conditioning regimen has increased the potential risk of graft rejection. In an initial multicenter study reported by McSweeney *et al.* (2001), a non-myeloablative preparative regimen of 2 Gy TBI, followed by transplantation of HLA-identical sibling donor PBSC and postgrafting immunosuppression with a combination of CSP and

mycophenolate mofetil (MMF), was given to 45 patients with hematologic malignancies and medical contraindications to conventional HSCT. Regimen toxicities and myelosuppression were mild, allowing 53% of patients to have entirely outpatient transplants. Graft rejection occurred in 20% of patients. Reflective of the truly non-myeloablative nature of the preparative regimen, all episodes of graft rejection were nonfatal and were usually associated with transient minor disturbances in blood counts, except for one patient who had 3 weeks of pancytopenia before recovery. Pretransplant factors predictive of graft rejection of graft rejection were a lack of intensive preceding therapy and a diagnosis of CML. Low donor T-cell chimerism at day 28 predicted rejection. To reduce the risk of graft rejection, fludarabine 30 mg/m²/day on days –4, –3, and –2 was added to the 2 Gy conditioning regimen. Since this modification to the non-myeloablative preparative regimen, the incidence of graft rejection following an HLA-identical sibling PBSC graft has been substantially decreased to 3.4% (Sandmaier *et al.*, 2001).

Adverse effects of drugs given in either the allogeneic or autologous HSCT settings

Drugs used after transplantation that have antimetabolite activity, such as methotrexate, trimethoprim-sulfamethoxazole, or ganciclovir, can delay initial engraftment, perhaps by decreasing the proliferation rate of mature hematopoietic precursors (Table 70.4). The antifolate activity of methotrexate inhibits de novo purine synthesis. At high doses, this can result in delayed engraftment. However, considering the modest doses that are used in combination with cyclosporine, methotrexate remains an essential agent for the prevention of GVHD following unmodified allogeneic HSCT. Some HSC transplant centers avoid the day +11 methotrexate dose in order to avoid cumulative toxicity and to promote more rapid engraftment. With the modest standard doses of methotrexate used (15 mg/m² on day +1, 10 mg/m² on days +3, +6, and +11), neutrophil engraftment is slightly delayed, and the benefit of GVHD prevention outweighs the potential delay in engraftment. However, acute renal failure and large pleural effusions or ascites are relative

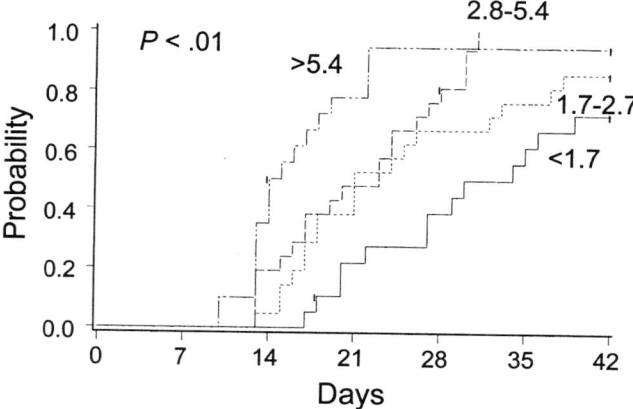

Fig. 70.6. Cumulative incidence of neutrophil engraftment (three consecutive days of neutrophil count $>0.5 \times 10^9$/l) after unrelated donor umbilical cord transplantation ($n = 102$): effect of CD34 cell dose ($\times 10^5$/kilogram recipient body weight). Reproduced, with permission, from Wagner *et al.* (2002).

Table 70.4. *Drugs routinely given after hematopoietic stem cell transplant that may suppress graft function*

Drug	Treatment
Methotrexate (MTX)[a]	Measure blood levels. If $>4 \times 10^{-8}$M 24 hours after last dose, initiate leucovorin (folinic acid) rescue
Ganciclovir (GCV)	Start G-CSF to increase ANC; consider switch to foscarnet
Trimethoprim-sulfamethoxazole (TMP-SMX)	Reduce dose and/or frequency of administration; consider switch to dapsone

[a] Myelosuppressive risk increased if poor renal function or pleural effusion or ascites complicating posttransplant course.

contraindications for methotrexate administration following allogeneic HSCT. This is due to elimination of methotrexate primarily through renal excretion. Accumulated methotrexate is slowly released from extravascular fluid collections, prolonging the terminal half-life of the drug and leading to potentially increased toxicity. Alternatively, methotrexate can be administered in these situations if the dose is adjusted and there is close monitoring of plasma drug concentrations. Leucovorin (folinic acid) rescue is indicated if methotrexate levels exceed 4×10^{-8} molar 24 hours after the last dose. The standard leucovorin dose is 10 mg/m^2 every 6 hours, increased to 100 mg/m^2 for methotrexate levels greater than 10^{-7} molar.

Trimethoprim-sulfamethoxazole (TMP-SMX) is an antibiotic combination used primarily for *Pneumocystis carinii* pneumonia prophylaxis after HSCT. It has also been used as effective prophylaxis for bacterial infections in recipients with chronic GVHD (Lew *et al.*, 1995). The marrow suppressive effects of the drug are presumably related to the weak inhibition of mammalian dihydrofolate reductase activity, decreasing purine production. It has been associated with delayed and engraftment and depressed hematopoiesis after engraftment (Imrie *et al.*, 1995; Lew *et al.*, 1995). Once engraftment has been established, oral dosing of TMP-SMX administered twice daily on two sequential days per week is effective prophylaxis against *P. carinii* and has been well tolerated without significant neutropenia, while daily administration of TMP-SMX results in depressed neutrophil counts. Dapsone has been used as an alternative to TMP-SMX, in cases of allergic reaction not amenable to desensitization, with a lower incidence of neutropenia. However, dapsone has not been shown to be as effective *P. carinii* prophylaxis as TMP-SMX (Souza *et al.*, 1999). Aerosolized pentamidine is significantly inferior to TMP-SMX for *P. carinii* prophylaxis (Vasconcelles *et al.*, 2000).

Ganciclovir is the treatment of choice for patients with evidence of active cytomegalovirus (CMV) infection or disease following transplantation (see Chapters 74 and 78). Early use of this drug at the time of CMV antigenemia and PCR positivity has dramatically decreased the mortality from CMV reactivation (Goodrich *et al.*, 1991). However, at therapeutic doses, ganciclovir, which is a thymidine analogue, can inhibit hematopoiesis in some patients. Ganciclovir administration immediately following marrow infusion results in delayed neutrophil and platelet engraftment in a dog model (Appelbaum *et al.*, 1988). Since CMV reactivation rarely occurs prior to day +30 after transplantation (Limaye *et al.*, 1997), ganciclovir has been routinely used only after initial engraftment. Although prophylaxis with ganciclovir is more effective than preemptive use of ganciclovir for early CMV disease, routine use of prophylactic ganciclovir after neutrophil engraftment in CMV seropositive patients without evidence of CMV antigenemia is no longer recommended due to the substantial risk of neutropenia (Salzberger *et al.*, 1997). Current guidelines for prevention of CMV disease before day +100 after allogeneic HSCT include weekly monitoring for CMV pp65 antigenemia and immediate initiation of ganciclovir treatment when any level of CMV antigenemia or

viremia by culture occurs (Boeckh, 1999) (also see Chapters 74 and 78). If neutropenia (ANC $<1 \times 10^9$/l for 2 or more consecutive days) develops while on ganciclovir therapy, ganciclovir should be held and re-instated when neutrophil counts recover. Foscarnet can be substituted for ganciclovir (Ippoliti *et al.*, 1997) or, alternatively, growth factors such as G-CSF may be helpful to support recovery of neutrophil counts following ganciclovir-induced neutropenia and may be particularly appropriate in settings where toxicity from foscarnet is unacceptable.

Adverse effects of virus infections in both the allogeneic and autologous HSCT settings

There is substantial evidence that certain viral infection may inhibit hematopoiesis in general and megakaryocytopoiesis in particular (Table 70.5). CMV infection has been suspected of causing myelosuppression in a subset of marrow transplant recipients. A retrospective study determined that the relatively rare envelope glycoprotein B (gB) types 3 and 4 are strongly associated with a high incidence of death due to myelosuppression. Of 94 patients with strain type 3 or 4, 20 (21.3%) died of infectious complications of neutropenia, while only 4 of 182 (2.2%) patients with strain type 1 or 2 did so after allogeneic transplantation (Torok-Storb *et al.*, 1997). How exactly CMV gB types 3 and 4 cause marrow suppression is unknown. In addition, occult CMV infection of marrow stroma without detection by blood culture and pp65 antigenemia has been observed in patients with secondary graft failure (Boeckh *et al.*, 1998).

Human herpes virus 6 (HHV-6), the principal causative agent of exanthem subitum (roseola infantum), has been reported to be myelosuppressive. It is an important pathogen after allogeneic transplant as it can cause fatal encephalitis (Drobyski *et al.*, 1994). Long-term, moderately severe suppression of marrow function has been described in patients who have HHV-6B reactivation after marrow transplantation (Carrigan & Knox, 1994). HHV-6 has been associated with delayed platelet recovery after transplant (Imbert-Marcille *et al.*, 2000; Ljungman *et al.*, 2000). However, not all investigators have confirmed myelosuppression due to HHV-6B reactivation (Kadakia *et al.*, 1996; Buchbinder *et al.*, 2000).

Table 70.5. *Virus infections that may suppress graft function*

CMV gB3 and 4	Relatively rare CMV strain posttransplant associated with severe myelosuppression (Torok-Storb *et al.*, 1997)
HHV-6B	Frequent reactivation after BMT (Carrigan & Knox, 1995). Case reports of myelosuppression (Carrigan & Knox, 1994)
Parvovirus B19	Case report of anemia after platelet transfusion (Cohen *et al.*, 1997)
Hepatitis G	Possible association with aplastic anemia (Kiem *et al.*, 1997). No confirmed case of posttransplant myelosuppression (Rodriguez-Inigo *et al.*, 1997)

Hepatitis G virus (HGV) is a recently discovered flavivirus, but it is unclear whether there are illnesses caused by this virus. In studies of HSCT patients, there was no increased incidence of hepatitis in these patients compared with HGV-negative controls, and there was no effect of HGV infection on graft function (Rodriguez-Inigo *et al.*, 1997; Ljungman *et al.*, 1998).

Human parvovirus B19 has been identified as an infectious etiologic agent for pure red cell aplasia (PRCA). Engraftment failure has also been associated with B19 parvovirus infection following peripheral blood stem cell transplantation (Solano *et al.*, 1996). Additional case reports of anemia and thrombocytopenia associated with B19 parvoviral infection responsive to immunoglobulin therapy have been reviewed (Broliden, 2001).

Marrow stroma effects in both the allogeneic and autologous HSCT settings

Hematopoietic reconstitution after marrow transplantation requires surviving marrow stromal cells to provide the appropriate growth and differentiation milieu for the incoming donor cells. Very high doses of irradiation to the marrow have been shown to result in long-term decrease in the ability of the marrow stroma to support hematopoesis. In 1966, Knospe, Blom, and Crosby reported that irradiation of a single extremity in rats with 2,000 to 10,000 r (rads midline tissue dose) was followed by initial marrow regeneration after 7 to 14 days. This suggested an influx of hematopoietic cells from unirradiated areas. There was a subsequent episode of hematopoietic depression with disruption of sinusoidal microcirculation in the irradiated limbs. Only at the 2,000 r dose level did sustained hematopoiesis develop with restoration of sinusoidal microcirculation. In dogs, 4,000 r in divided doses over 4 weeks to one-half of the axial skeleton followed by cryopreserved autologous marrow infusion resulted in prolonged (>4 month) decreased uptake of ^{59}Fe in irradiated marrow, consistent with biopsy findings of sustained hypocellularity (Gerdes & Storb, 1970). Chemotherapy agents such as doxorubicin, busulfan, and BCNU have been associated with injury to the hematopoietic microenvironment (Greenberger, 1991). The mechanism of stromal damage by these agents is unclear. In marrow recipients who have been previously heavily treated with irradiation or chemotherapy, poor graft function may reflect damaged marrow stroma. Additionally, stromal function may be compromised by otherwise occult infection by particular strains of CMV (Torok-Strob *et al.*, 1997; Boeckh *et al.*, 1998).

Treatment of autologous graft failure

Treatment of graft failure in the autologous transplant setting is generally limited to the use of growth factors such as G-CSF or GM-CSF, blood product transfusion support, and discontinuation of marrow suppressive drugs. Due to the high risk of poor graft function, it is not advisable to proceed with autologous transplantation in patients who have less than 2.5×10^6/kg CD34$^+$ cells collected. If autologous engraftment remains poor

following growth factor treatment, effective therapy options are limited. The Toronto transplant group reported on seven patients with persistent delayed engraftment despite 4 weeks of GM-CSF after autologous marrow transplant. Administration of interleukin-3 (IL-3) followed by GM-CSF did not improve graft recovery (Crump *et al.*, 1993). Infusion of autologous bone marrow in patients with slow engraftment after high-dose therapy supported by a suboptimal dose (<1 × 10^6 CD34$^+$ cells/kg) of PBSC was frequently ineffective, probably because poor PBSC mobilization represents poor marrow function (Watts *et al.*, 1998).

Delayed platelet recovery

Between 10% and 20% of patients have delayed platelet recovery after autologous or allogeneic HSCT, and the risks of bleeding and development of platelet transfusion allosensitization remain serious clinical problems. Recombinant human thrombopoietin (TPO) was administered to 38 patients (22 allogeneic graft recipients and 16 autologous graft recipients) with delayed platelet recovery defined as platelet transfusion dependence at 35 days following HSCT and megakaryocyte hypoplasia. Despite TPO dose escalation, only 2 of 38 patients had improvement in platelet recovery (Nash *et al.*, 2000). It remains to be seen if combination cytokine therapy may enhance platelet recovery in this setting.

Treatment of allogeneic graft failure

A rational approach to the treatment of graft failure in allograft patients relies strongly on the results of the peripheral blood and marrow chimerism studies. If hematopoietic graft failure without evidence of relapse occurs, three treatment options are available after discontinuation of marrow suppressive drugs: (1) the administration of a hematopoietic growth factor, such as recombinant human GM-CSF or recombinant human G-CSF; (2) a booster infusion of G-CSF-mobilized donor PBSC or donor marrow with or without additional immunosuppressive conditioning; (3) infusion of previously harvested cryopreserved autologous PBSC. Graft failure due to relapse with evidence of donor T-cell chimerism is managed by either donor lymphocyte infusions (DLI) or a combination of cytoreductive chemotherapy followed by DLI. Alternatively, if the patient is at least 1 year after transplant and in good clinical condition, a second myeloablative conditioning regimen and donor HSC infusion can be considered (Fig. 70.7).

If there is evidence of donor chimerism, the first-line treatment is the use of a hematopoietic growth factor to stimulate neutrophil recovery. If there is no response to growth factors, infusion of additional donor marrow or G-CSF-mobilized PBSC without additional immunosuppressive conditioning is appropriate. However, if there is clear evidence of graft rejection, a second infusion of donor HSC must be preceded by additional immunosuppressive conditioning to prevent repeat rejection of the donor graft. The most successful experience in

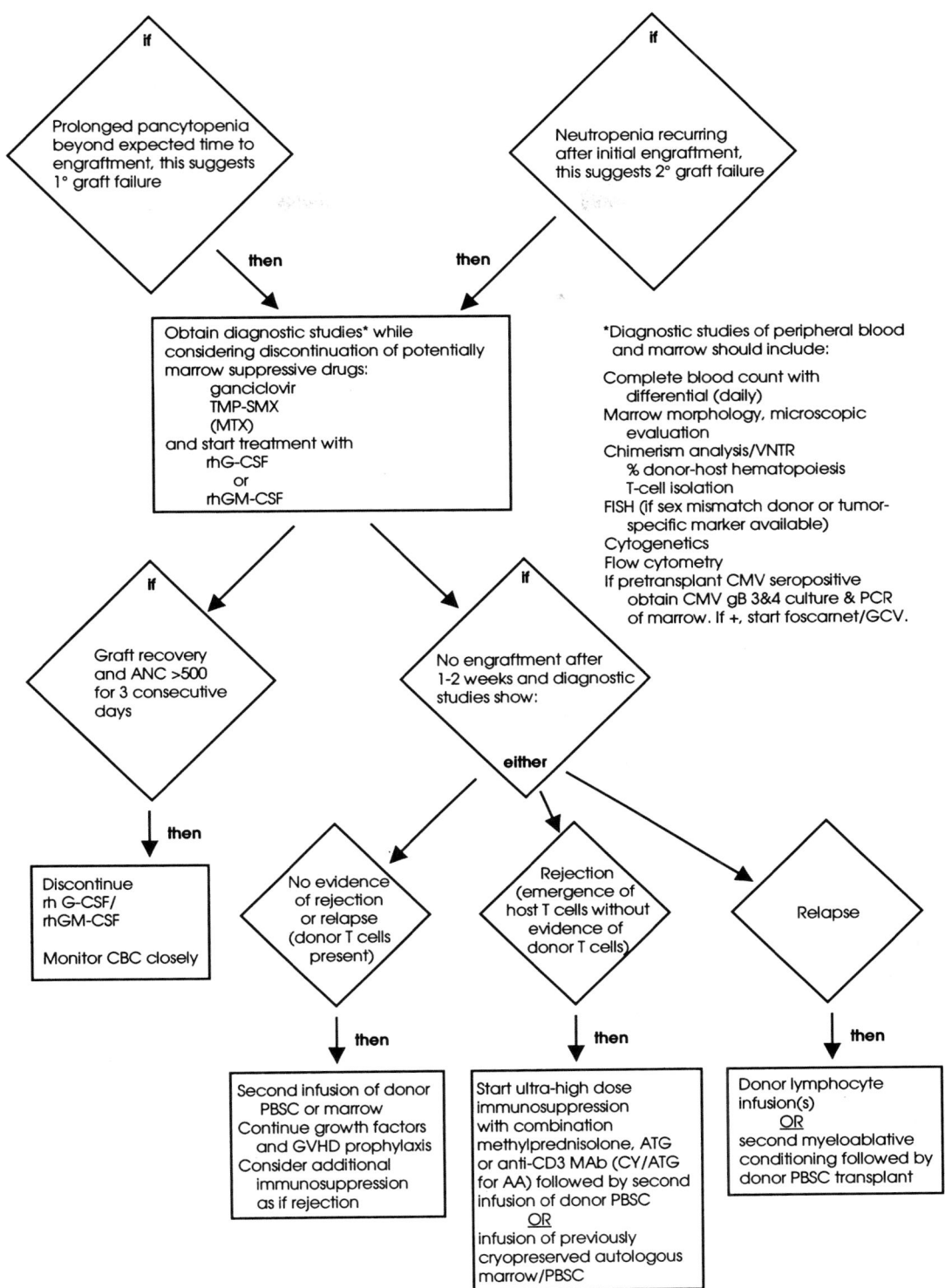

Fig. 70.7. Algorithm to evaluate and treat suspected graft failure. Once graft failure is suspected it is imperative to efficiently coordinate the diagnostic studies and rapidly obtain results. In the allogeneic setting, until results of chimerism analyses are available, initial therapy for graft failure consists of administration of recombinant human (rh) G-CSF (5–32 µg/kg/day intravenously) or rhGM-CSF (250–500 µg/m²/day administered intravenously over 2 hours) until ANC >500 for 3 consecutive days. If results of chimerism analyses indicate that there is evidence of donor hematopoiesis, and in particular donor T lymphocytes, eventual donor engraftment is very likely. In this setting, hematopoietic growth factors are the treatment of choice for their simplicity and effectiveness. If there is no increase in neutrophils after 1 to 2 weeks of administration of growth factors, a booster infusion of donor PBSC along with immunosuppressive drugs for GVHD prevention can be an effective intervention. If chimerism studies confirm early graft rejection, it is unlikely that growth factors will enhance donor engraftment. An infusion of donor PBSC with additional conditioning immunosuppressive agents such as high-dose steroids and anti-thymocyte globulin (ATG) or anti-T-cell antibody to prevent rejection should be promptly arranged. Alternatively, some centers have rescued patients with previously collected cryopreserved autologous stem cells.

second HSCT has been for the treatment of graft failure in patients with severe aplastic anemia (Stucki *et al.,* 1998). Alternatively, infusion of previously harvested cryopreserved autologous HSC may be considered.

Given the limited treatment options for graft failure, the best approach is to optimize the conditions that prevent graft failure from occurring in the first place, as described in the previous section, Causes of Graft Failure.

Hematopoietic growth factors

In 1990 Nemunaitis *et al.* reported on the use of GM-CSF for patients with graft failure after allogeneic BMT. Nine of 15 patients had an increase in ANC to $\geq 0.5 \times 10^9/l$ within 14 days of starting GM-CSF. Although platelet recovery was slow, most patients who responded with increased neutrophil counts eventually recovered to platelet independence. The overall survival of patients treated with GM-CSF for graft failure was improved (1-year actuarial survival of 50%) when compared to an unmatched group of historical controls (1-year actuarial survival of 23%). This study established a role for growth factors as an important therapy for delayed neutrophil recovery after transplantation. Most of the early clinical experience with growth factors for the treatment of graft failure was with GM-CSF (Sierra *et al.,* 1994), but subsequent clinical experience with G-CSF indicates that either growth factor can be used successfully. Sequential use of GM-CSF followed by G-CSF was not shown to improve outcome of patients with graft failure (Weisdorf *et al.,* 1995).

Few other hematopoietic growth factors have been examined as agents to enhance allograft recovery. Interleukin-1β (which stimulates multipotent stem cell growth) had no clinically durable effects on peripheral blood counts in patients with marrow failure after autologous or allogeneic transplantation and had moderate toxicity (Nemunaitis *et al.,* 1994). Recombinant human erythropoietin (rhEpo) has been studied after allogeneic transplantation to enhance recovery from anemia. In a study of 34 patients given rhEpo after allogeneic HSCT, the patients that received rhEpo after day +35 had an improved recovery of hemoglobin concentration and achieved more rapid red blood cell transfusion independence compared to control patients (Baron *et al.,* 2002). This study suggested that for some patients, rhEpo may be useful to decrease transfusion requirements late after allogeneic HSCT, but an adequately powered, randomized prospective study is needed to confirm these results and to evaluate the cost versus potential benefit.

Second allogeneic HSCT without immunosuppressive conditioning

If there is no response to G-CSF or GM-CSF administration, infusion of a donor PBSC "boost" may enhance hematopoietic recovery, as long as there is no evidence of graft rejection, stromal damage, or CMV infection. However, graft failure unresponsive to hematopoietic growth factors and withdrawal of graft-suppressing drugs is often due to graft rejection. For this reason, it is important to obtain chimerism studies prior to and after initiation of growth factors to confirm the presence of donor chimerism. In a report from Huddinge Hospital, booster marrow or blood cells from the same donor were given for primary ($n = 6$) or secondary ($n = 12$) graft failure without additional conditioning. Of the patients with primary graft failure, two had recovery of neutrophil counts attributable to the infusion of additional donor cells. Patients classified as having secondary graft failures were those with adequate donor neutrophil engraftment but low platelet counts. Following non–T-cell-depleted donor cell booster infusion and a variety of regimens for GVHD prophylaxis, 10 of 12 patients had improvement in platelet counts (Remberger *et al.,* 1998). Case reports using donor PBSC to treat graft failure in patients with donor chimerism without reconditioning have also been published (Molina *et al.,* 1995).

Second allogeneic HSCT with immunosuppressive conditioning

If there is evidence of immunologic rejection of the graft documented by the emergence of purely host T lymphocytes by chimerism analysis, reconditioning of the patient for a second donor HSCT is necessary. In this setting, infusion of donor marrow or PBSC without additional immunosuppression does not lead to engraftment. Immunosuppression for second transplants with various combinations of TBI or TLI and CY or cytosine arabinoside resulted in uniformly high toxicity, graft failure, and death, particularly in patients with leukemia who had received a TBI-based myeloablative regimen for the first transplant. Kerman *et al.,* 1989 initially reported on a second transplant-conditioning regimen of ATG plus high-dose methylprednisolone (20 mg/kg/day followed by taper) prior to infusion of T-cell-depleted donor marrow. Three of five patients engrafted, although long-term disease-free survival was poor (one survivor at 3 years). Five of 12 patients with graft failure after unrelated donor transplantation survived at a median of 38 months after second unrelated transplant, although posttransplant complications were considerable (Grandage *et al.,* 1998). Ljungman and colleagues (1996) reported a patient with aplastic anemia who had a second episode of rejection after a second bone marrow transplant and who entered a third durable remission subsequent to treatment with anti-lymphocyte globulin, donor lymphocyte infusions, GM-CSF, and erythropoietin. Five years after this treatment, hematopoiesis was of donor origin.

For patients who have primary graft rejection after allogeneic marrow transplantation and are not responding to growth factor administration, other less toxic immunosuppressive conditioning regimens for second donor marrow infusion have been studied. One potential approach is with the monoclonal antibody OKT3 (anti-CD3) administered in combination with high-dose corticosteroids. Schlegel and colleagues (2000) reconditioned six children with early graft rejection following a highly purified "megadose" CD34+ selected, MHC-disparate

PBSC transplantation. Successful engraftment after second transplant with stem cells from the same donor was achieved in five of the six children. The median time to engraftment after second transplant was day 10 (range 9–13). Chimerism analysis demonstrated complete donor chimerism in 4 of the 5 within the first month after second transplant, and mixed chimerism in the fifth patient, who converted to full donor chimerism after T-cell add-back. The use of the OKT-3 based immunosuppressive regimen appeared to suppress residual host alloreactivity; however, patients remained at risk for infection, relapse, or GVHD after second transplant, and two of the six children survived long term. In a larger series of patients treated for graft failure, successful second allogeneic HSCT involved the use of immunosuppressive conditioning combined with postgrafting immunosuppression (Guardiola *et al.*, 2000).

Second allogeneic transplant for aplastic anemia

For patients with aplastic anemia who have rejected a first HLA-matched sibling graft, improved survival has been shown with the use of a second conditioning regimen using CY/ATG (Storb *et al.*, 1987). The survival from second transplant has dramatically improved with the use of this conditioning regimen, particularly since the introduction of combined cyclosporine/methotrexate GVHD prophylaxis after first and second transplant (Fig 70.8). In Seattle, during the time period 1970 to 1976, 28 patients underwent a second transplant from an HLA-matched sibling after rejecting a first transplant for severe aplastic anemia. The second conditioning regimen included various combinations of CY, ATG, TBI, or procarbazine and long-term survival was 5%. Between 1977 and 1981, 12 patients received a second marrow transplant for graft failure and were conditioned with CY/ATG followed by methotrexate GVHD prophylaxis. Ten-year survival was 20%. Between 1982

and 1994, 13 patients who rejected the first graft received CY/ATG followed by second marrow transplant and combined cyclosporine plus methotrexate GVHD prophylaxis. Ten-year survival was 83% (Fig. 70.9). The use of 6-month cyclosporine plus short-course methotrexate after the first transplant delayed the onset of first graft rejection. The increased time interval to second transplant was associated with decreased mortality and improved engraftment of the second transplant (Stucki *et al.*, 1998). This finding emphasizes the importance of CY/ATG conditioning followed by combined methotrexate/cyclosporine immunosuppression for prevention of rejection and improved survival after first and second marrow transplantation for aplastic anemia.

Autologous HSCT rescue after allogeneic graft failure

The Royal Marsden Hospital group reported on the outcome of a series of 10 patients who were rescued with autologous marrow ($n = 8$) or PBSC ($n = 2$) following failed allogeneic engraftment (Mehta *et al.*, 1996). Seven of 10 patients had received T-cell-depleted marrow from HLA-mismatched related donors following CY/TBI conditioning for hematologic malignancies. The other three patients had failed to engraft after receiving unrelated donor marrow transplants. The decision to proceed with autologous rescue was largely arbitrary and related to immediate availability of previously cryopreserved autologous cells. Days of rescue ranged from 21 to 40 (median 22.5), after which immunosuppression with cyclosporine was rapidly tapered off. The leukocyte counts at the time of rescue were 0.1 to $0.3 \times 10^9/l$ with ANC less than $0.1 \times 10^9/l$. No life-threatening infection preceded or followed rescue with cells, and after rescue, patients recovered uneventfully. There was no evidence of GVHD. Four patients with acute leukemia died of disease relapse, five patients with acute leukemia were alive and in complete remission 9 months to 9 years after autologous rescue, and one patient with CML was in

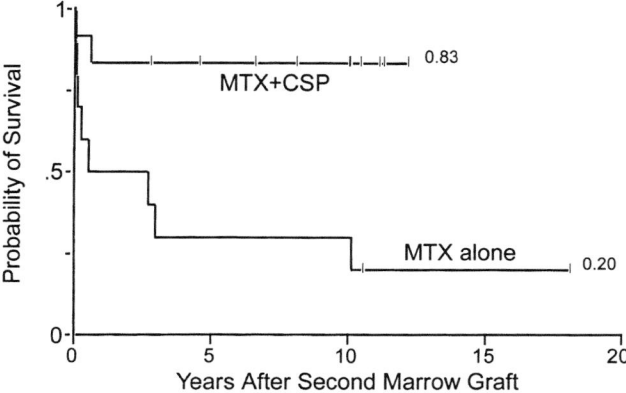

Fig. 70.8. Probability of survival among 22 aplastic anemia patients who were conditioned with cyclophosphamide and anti-thymocyte globulin for their second marrow graft after rejection of the first marrow graft. After the second transplant patients received either methotrexate (MTX) alone or the combination of MTX and cyclosporine (CSP) as postgrafting GVHD prophylaxis. Reproduced, with permission, from Stucki *et al.* (1998).

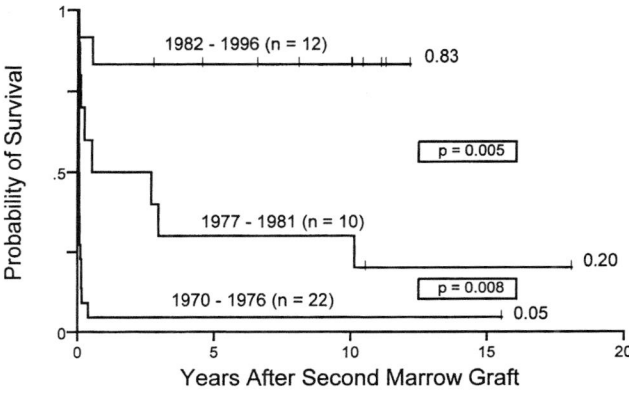

Fig. 70.9. Ten-year probability of survival for 44 patients with aplastic anemia receiving second bone marrow transplants between 1970 and 1976, 1977 and 1981, and 1982 and 1996. Reproduced, with permission, from Stucki *et al.* (1998).

hematologic remission at 7 months after rescue. Thus, infusion of previously cryopreserved autologous PBSC may be a reasonable option for patients who have clearly rejected their grafts with no evidence of donor chimerism and who have previously stored a sufficient amount of CD34+/kg PBSC or bone marrow. In addition, infusion of autologous hematopoietic cells should be considered only in patients who are clinically unstable, for logistical reasons do not have a readily available donor (such as a volunteer unrelated donor), or who have relatively good-risk underlying disease. On the other hand, patients with graft failure that show evidence of surviving donor cells, who are in good clinical condition, who have not stored autologous PBSC or marrow, and who have high-risk disease are better candidates for a second infusion of donor stem cells.

Disease relapse

For the treatment of disease relapse, which can be a late manifestation of graft failure, myeloablative conditioning for second transplant within 6 to 12 months after the first transplant is poorly tolerated and is associated with a very high mortality. If disease relapse is maintained in a less advanced stage, improved survival from a second transplant is achieved if it can be delayed for at least 1 year beyond the first transplant. In patients with CML who relapse after transplantation from an HLA-identical sibling, DLI has been successfully used to achieve complete remission if mixed chimerism is detected. The issue of DLI therapy is more extensively discussed in (Chapters 22 and 65).

Conclusions

Graft failure is a serious complication after HSCT, subjecting patients to a high risk of fatal infection. Graft failure indicates inadequate hematopoietic function at a point in time at which recovery of hematopoiesis should be expected following HSCT. Primary graft failure is the failure to achieve an ANC of greater than 0.2×10^9/l by 21 to 28 days following transplantation of unmodified marrow or PBSC. Secondary graft failure is the loss of peripheral blood counts following initial engraftment. Graft rejection is seen in the allogeneic transplant setting only and represents an immunologically mediated failure of donor hematopoiesis.

Assessment of graft failure includes examination of peripheral blood and marrow aspirate and biopsy, along with molecular analysis of chimerism status in order to distinguish rejection, relapse, or poor donor graft function. Risk factors for graft rejection include donor-recipient histoincompatibility, recipient sensitization to donor antigens through preceding blood transfusions, T-cell depletion, and inadequate immunosuppressive conditioning. Advances in HLA-typing technology using DNA sequencing for both class I and II antigens have made it possible to identify optimally HLA-matched unrelated donors, thereby reducing the risk of graft failure. Other factors resulting in poor graft function include infusion of low numbers of,

or damaged, stem cells, myelosuppressive drugs given after transplant, concurrent viral infection with CMV gB types 3 and 4 and possibly HHV6-B, and damaged marrow stroma.

In aplastic anemia the incidence of graft failure has decreased due to potent immunosuppressive conditioning with CY/ATG, and the combined use of cyclosporine and methotrexate for GVHD prophylaxis. Avoidance of pretransplant blood product transfusions or use of leuko-depleted and irradiated blood products also reduce the risk of HLA-compatible graft rejection for the treatment of nonmalignant diseases.

The outcome of allograft failure is likely to be improved if the diagnosis is considered and treatment initiated early. If graft rejection has been ruled out, the initial treatment for graft failure is administration of G-CSF or GM-CSF for up to 2 weeks or possibly longer. If growth factors are unsuccessful, the treatment is either a second transplant of donor PBSC or infusion of previously cryopreserved autologous PBSC or marrow. In the setting of graft rejection, additional recipient immunosuppression is always necessary prior to second donor PBSC infusion.

References

Alizadeh, M., Bernard, M., Danic, B. et al. (2002). Quantitative assessment of hematopoietic chimerism after bone marrow transplantation by real-time quantitative polymerase chain reaction. Blood, 99, 4618–25.

Anasetti, C., Amos, D., Beatty, P.G. et al. (1989). Effect of HLA compatibility on engraftment of bone marrow transplants in patients with leukemia or lymphoma. New England Journal of Medicine, 320, 197–204.

Appelbaum, F.R., Meyers, J.D., Deeg, H.J. et al. (1988). Toxicity trial of prophylactic 9-[2-Hydroxy-1-Hydroxymethyl)Ethoxymethyl] Guanine (Ganciclovir) after marrow transplantation in dogs. Antimicrobial Agents and Chemotherapy, 32, 271–3.

Ash, R.C., Casper, J.T., Chitambar, C.R. et al. (1990). Successful allogeneic transplantation of T-cell-depleted bone marrow from closely HLA-matched unrelated donors. New England Journal of Medicine, 322, 485–94.

Ash, R.C., Horowitz, M.M., Gale, R.P. et al. (1991). Bone marrow transplantation from related donors other than HLA-identical siblings: effect of T cell depletion. Bone Marrow Transplantation, 7, 443–52.

Baron, F., Sautois, B., Baudoux, E. et al. (2002). Optimization of recombinant human erythropoietin therapy after allogeneic hematopoietic stem cell transplantation. Experimental Hematology, 30, 546–54.

Baume, D., Kuentz, M., Pico, J.-L. et al. (1989). Failure of a CD18/ anti-LFA1 monoclonal antibody infusion to prevent graft rejection in leukemic patients receiving T-depleted allogeneic bone marrow transplantation. Transplantation, 47, 472–4.

Bean, M.A., Graham, T., Appelbaum, F.R. et al. (1994). Gamma-irradiation of pretransplant blood transfusions from unrelated donors prevents sensitization to minor histocompatibility antigens on dog leukocyte antigen-identical canine marrow grafts. Transplantation, 57, 423–6.

Bean, M.A., Storb, R., Graham, T. et al. (1991). Prevention of transfusion-induced sensitization to minor histocompatibility antigens on DLA-identical canine marrow grafts by gamma irradiation of marrow donor blood. *Transplantation*, **52**, 956–60.

Bensinger, W., Appelbaum, F., Rowley, S. *et al.* (1995). Factors that influence collection and engraftment of autologous peripheral-blood stem cells. *Journal of Clinical Oncology*, **13**, 2547–55.

Bentley, S.A., Brecher, M.E., Powell, E. *et al.* (1997). Long-term engraftment failure after marrow ablation and autologous hematopoietic reconstitution: differences between peripheral blood stem cell and bone marrow recipients. *Bone Marrow Transplantation*, **19**, 557–63.

Bittencourt, H., Rocha, V., Chevret, S. *et al.* (2002). Association of CD34 cell dose with hematopoietic recovery, infections, and other outcomes after HLA-identical sibling bone marrow transplantation. *Blood*, **99**, 2726–33.

Boeckh, M. (1999). Current antiviral strategies for controlling cytomegalovirus in hematopoietic stem cell transplant recipients: prevention and therapy (Review). *Transplant Infectious Disease*, **1**, 165–78.

Boeckh, M., Hoy, C., & Torok-Storb, B. (1998). Occult cytomegalovirus infection of marrow stroma. *Clinical Infectious Diseases*, **26**, 209–10.

Broliden, K. (2001). Parvovirus B19 infection in pediatric solid-organ and bone marrow transplantation (Review). *Pediatric Transplantation*, **5**, 320–30.

Buchbinder, S., Elmaagacli, A.H., Schaefer, U.W., & Roggendorf, M. (2000). Human herpesvirus 6 is an important pathogen in infectious lung disease after allogeneic bone marrow transplantation. *Bone Marrow Transplantation*, **26**, 639–44.

Carrigan, D.R. & Knox, K.K. (1994). Human herpesvirus 6 (HHV-6) isolation from bone marrow: HHV-6-associated bone marrow suppression in bone marrow transplant patients. *Blood*, **84**, 3307–10.

Carrigan, D.R. & Knox, K.K. (1995). Bone marrow suppression by human herpesvirus-6: comparison of the A and B variants of the virus (letter; comment). *Blood*, **86**, 835–6.

Champlin, R.E., Passweg, J.R., Zhang, M.J. *et al.* (2000). T-cell depletion of bone marrow transplants for leukemia from donors other than HLA-identical siblings: advantage of T-cell antibodies with narrow specificities. *Blood*, **95**, 3996–4003.

Cohen, B.J., Beard, S., Knowles, W.A. *et al.* (1997). Chronic anemia due to parvovirus B19 infection in a bone marrow transplant patient after platelet transfusion. *Transfusion*, **37**, 947–52.

Crump, M., Couture, F., Kovacs, M. *et al.* (1993). Interleukin-3 followed by GM-CSF for delayed engraftment after autologous bone marrow transplantation. *Experimental Hematology*, **21**, 405–10.

Di Bartolomeo, P., Di Girolamo, G., Angrilli, F. *et al.* (1993). Second marrow transplants in patients with thalassemia major rejecting the first graft. *Bone Marrow Transplantation*, **12** (Suppl 1), 78–80.

Doney, K., Leisenring, W., Storb, R., Appelbaum, F.R. for the Seattle Bone Marrow Transplant Team. (1997). Primary treatment of acquired aplastic anemia: outcomes with bone marrow transplantation and immunosuppressive therapy. *Annals of Internal Medicine*, **126**, 107–15.

Drobyski, W.R., Knox, K.K., Majewski, D., & Carrigan, D.R. (1994). Brief report: fatal encephalitis due to variant B human herpesvirus-6 infection in a bone marrow-transplant recipient. *New England Journal of Medicine*, **330**, 1356–60.

Dufour, C., Dallorso, S., Casarino, L. *et al.* (1999). Late graft failure 8 years after first bone marrow transplantation for severe acquired aplastic anemia. *Bone Marrow Transplantation*, **23**, 743–5.

Gaziev, D., Polchi, P., Lucarelli, G. *et al.* (1999). Second marrow transplants for graft failure in patients with thalassemia. *Bone Marrow Transplantation*, **24**, 1299–306.

Gerdes, A.J. & Storb, R. (1970). The repopulation of irradiated bone marrow by the infusion of stored autologous marrow. *Radiology*, **94**, 441–5.

Gluckman, E., Rocha, V., Boyer-Chammard, A. *et al.* (1997). Outcome of cord-blood transplantation from related and unrelated donors. *New England Journal of Medicine*, **337**, 373–81.

Gmur, J.P., Burger, J., Schaffner, A. *et al.* (1990). Pure red cell aplasia of long duration complicating major ABO-incompatible bone marrow transplantation. *Blood*, **75**, 290–5.

Goodrich, J.M., Mori, M., Gleaves, C.A. *et al.* (1991). Early treatment with ganciclovir to prevent cytomegalovirus disease after allogeneic bone marrow transplantation. *New England Journal of Medicine*, **325**, 1601–7.

Grandage, V.L., Cornish, J.M., Pamphilon, D.H. *et al.* (1998). Second allogeneic bone marrow transplants from unrelated donors for graft failure following initial unrelated donor bone marrow transplantation. *Bone Marrow Transplantation*, **21**, 687–90.

Green, A., Clarke, E., Hunt, L. *et al.* (1999). Children with acute lymphoblastic leukemia who receive T-cell-depleted HLA mismatched marrow allografts from unrelated donors have an increased incidence of primary graft failure but a similar overall transplant outcome. *Blood*, **94**, 2236–46.

Greenberger, J.S. (1991). Toxic effects on the hematopoietic microenvironment (review). *Experimental Hematology*, **19**, 1101–9.

Guardiola, P., Kuentz, M., Garban, F. *et al.* (2000). Second early allogeneic stem cell transplantations for graft failure in acute leukaemia, chronic myeloid leukaemia and aplastic anaemia. French Society of Bone Marrow Transplantation. *British Journal of Haematology*, **111**, 292–302.

Hale, G. & Waldmann, H. (1994). Control of graft-versus-host disease and graft rejection by T cell depletion of donor and recipient with Campath-1 antibodies. Results of matched sibling transplants for malignant diseases. *Bone Marrow Transplantation*, **13**, 597–611.

Hill, R.S., Petersen, F.B., Storb, R. *et al.* (1986). Mixed hematologic chimerism after allogeneic marrow transplantation for severe aplastic anemia is associated with a higher risk of graft rejection and a lessened incidence of acute graft-versus-host disease. *Blood*, **67**, 811–16.

Imbert-Marcille, B.M., Tang, X.W., Lepelletier, D. *et al.* (2000). Human herpesvirus 6 infection after autologous or allogeneic stem cell transplantation: a single-center prospective longitudinal study of 92 patients. *Clinical Infectious Diseases*, **31**, 881–6.

Imrie, K.R., Prince, H.M., Couture, F. *et al.* (1995). Effect of antimicrobial prophylaxis on hematopoietic recovery following autologous bone marrow transplantation: ciprofloxacin versus co-trimoxazole. *Bone Marrow Transplantation*, **15**, 267–70.

Ippoliti, C., Morgan, A., Warkentin, D. *et al.* (1997). Foscarnet for prevention of cytomegalovirus infection in allogeneic marrow transplant recipients unable to receive ganciclovir. *Bone Marrow Transplantation, 20*, 491–5.

Kadakia, M.P., Rybka, W.B., Stewart, J.A. *et al.* (1996). Human herpesvirus 6: infection and disease following autologous and allogeneic bone marrow transplantation. *Blood, 87*, 5341–54.

Kernan, N.A., Bordignon, C., Heller, G. *et al.* (1989). Graft failure after T-cell-depleted human leukocyte antigen identical marrow transplants for leukemia: I. Analysis of risk factors and results of secondary transplants. *Blood, 74*, 2227–36.

Kiem, H.-P., Myerson, D., Storb, R. *et al.* (1997). Prevalence of hepatitis G virus in patients with aplastic anemia (Letter). *Blood, 90*, 1335–6.

Knospe, W.H., Blom, J., & Crosby, W.H. (1966). Regeneration of locally irradiated bone marrow. I. Dose dependent, long-term changes in the rat, with particular emphasis upon vascular and stromal reaction. *Blood, 28*, 398–415.

Lew, M.A., Kehoe, K., Ritz, J. *et al.* (1995). Ciprofloxacin versus trimethoprim/sulfamethoxazole for prophylaxis of bacterial infections in bone marrow transplant recipients: a randomized, controlled trial. *Journal of Clinical Oncology, 13*, 239–50.

Limaye, A., Bowden, R.A., Myerson, D., & Boeckh, M. (1997). Cytomegalovirus disease occurring before engraftment in marrow transplant recipients. *Clinical Infectious Diseases, 24*, 830–5.

Ljungman, P., Halasz, R., Hagglund, H. *et al.* (1998). Detection of hepatitis G virus/GB virus C after allogeneic bone marrow transplantation. *Bone Marrow Transplantation, 22*, 499–501.

Ljungman, P., Lawler, M., Lonnqvist, B. *et al.* (1996). Rejection of the second allogeneic graft in a patient with severe aplastic anemia reversed by antilymphocyte globulin and donor lymphocyte infusions. *Bone Marrow Transplantation, 18*, 1179–81.

Ljungman, P., Wang, F.Z., Clark, D.A. *et al.* (2000). High levels of human herpesvirus 6 DNA in peripheral blood leucocytes are correlated to platelet engraftment and disease in allogeneic stem cell transplant patients. *British Journal of Haematology, 111*, 774–81.

Lucarelli, G., Galimberti, M., Polchi, P. *et al.* (1993). Marrow transplantation in patients with thalassemia responsive to iron chelation therapy. *New England Journal of Medicine, 329*, 840–4.

Lucarelli, G., Giardini, C., & Baronciani, D. (1995). Bone marrow transplantation in thalassemia (Review). *Seminars in Hematology, 32*, 297–303.

Marmont, A.M., Horowitz, M.M., Gale, R.P. *et al.* (1991). T-cell depletion of HLA-identical transplants in leukemia. *Blood, 78*, 2120–30.

Martin, P.J., Hansen, J.A., Buckner, C.D. *et al.* (1985). Effects of in vitro depletion of T cells in HLA-identical allogeneic marrow grafts. *Blood, 66*, 664–72.

Martin, P.J., Rowley, S.D., Anasetti, C. *et al.* (1999). A phase I-II clinical trial to evaluate removal of CD4 cells and partial depletion of CD8 cells from donor marrow for HLA-mismatched unrelated recipients. *Blood, 94*, 2192–9.

McSweeney, P.A., Niederwieser, D., Shizuru, J.A. *et al.* (2001). Hematopoietic cell transplantation in older patients with hematologic malignancies: replacing high-dose cytotoxic therapy with graft-versus-tumor effects. *Blood, 97*, 3390–400.

Mehta, J., Powles, R.L., Mitchell, P. *et al.* (1994). Graft failure after bone marrow transplantation from unrelated donors using busul-

phan and cyclophosphamide for conditioning. *Bone Marrow Transplantation, 13*, 583–7.

Mehta, J., Powles, R., Singhal, S. *et al.* (1996). Outcome of autologous rescue after failed engraftment of allogeneic marrow. *Bone Marrow Transplantation, 17*, 213–17.

Mehta, J., Powles, R., Singhal, S. *et al.* (1997a). Early identification of patients at risk of death due to infections, hemorrhage, or graft failure after allogeneic bone marrow transplantation on the basis of the leukocyte counts. *Bone Marrow Transplantation, 19*, 349–55.

Mehta, J., Powles, R., Treleaven, J. *et al.* (1997b). Number of nucleated cells infused during allogeneic and autologous bone marrow transplantation: an important modifiable factor influencing outcome (Letter to Editor). *Blood, 90*, 3808–10.

Mielcarek, M., Leisenring, W., Torok-Storb, B., & Storb, R. (2000). Graft-versus-host disease and donor-directed hemagglutinin titers after ABO-mismatched related and unrelated marrow allografts: evidence for a graft-versus-plasma cell effect. *Blood, 96*, 1150–6.

Molina, L., Chabannon, C., Viret, F. *et al.* (1995). Granulocyte colony-stimulating factor-mobilized allogeneic peripheral blood stem cells for rescue graft failure after allogeneic bone marrow transplantation in two patients with acute myeloblastic leukemia in first complete remission. *Blood, 85*, 1678–9.

Morton, J., Hutchins, C., & Durrant, S. (2001). Granulocyte-colony-stimulating factor (G-CSF)-primed allogeneic bone marrow: significantly less graft-versus-host disease and comparable engraftment to G-CSF-mobilized peripheral blood stem cells. *Blood, 98*, 3186–91.

Nash, R.A., Kurzrock, R., DiPersio, J. *et al.* (2000). A phase I trial of recombinant human thrombopoietin in patients with delayed platelet recovery after hematopoietic stem cell transplantation. *Biology of Blood and Marrow Transplantation, 6*, 25–34.

Nemunaitis, J., Ross, M., Meisenberg, B. *et al.* (1994). Phase I study of recombinant human interleukin-1 beta (rhIL-1 beta) in patients with bone marrow failure. *Bone Marrow Transplantation, 14*, 583–8.

Nemunaitis, J., Singer, J.W., Buckner, C.D. *et al.* (1990). Use of recombinant human granulocyte-macrophage colony-stimulating factor in graft failure after bone marrow transplantation. *Blood, 76*, 245–53.

Niederwieser, D., Pepe, M., Storb, R. *et al.* (1988). Improvement in rejection, engraftment rate and survival without increase in graft-versus-host disease by high marrow cell dose in patients transplanted for aplastic anemia. *British Journal of Haematology, 69*, 23–8.

Offner, F., Schoch, G., Fisher, L.D. *et al.* (1996). Mortality hazard functions as related to neutropenia at different times after marrow transplantation. *Blood, 88*, 4058–62.

Pei, J., Akatsuka, Y., Anasetti, C. *et al.* (2001). Generation of HLA-C-specific cytotoxic T cells in association with marrow graft rejection: analysis of alloimmunity by T-cell cloning and testing of T-cell-receptor rearrangements. *Biology of Blood and Marrow Transplantation, 7*, 378–83.

Petersdorf, E.W., Gooley, T.A., Anasetti, C. *et al.* (1998). Optimizing outcome after unrelated marrow transplantation by comprehensive matching of HLA class I and II alleles in the donor and recipient. *Blood, 92*, 3515–20.

Petersdorf, E.W., Hansen, J.A., Martin, P.J. *et al.* (2001a). Major-histocompatibility-complex class I alleles and antigens in hematopoietic-cell transplantation. *New England Journal of Medicine,* **345,** 1794–800.

Petersdorf, E.W., Kollman, C., Hurley, C.K. *et al.* (2001b). Effect of HLA class II gene disparity on clinical outcome in unrelated donor hematopoietic cell transplantation for chronic myeloid leukemia: the US National Marrow Donor Program Experience. *Blood,* **98,** 2922–9.

Petersdorf, E.W., Longton, G.M., Anasetti, C. *et al.* (1997). Association of HLA-C disparity with graft failure after marrow transplantation from unrelated donors. *Blood,* **89,** 1818–23.

Remberger, M., Ringden, O., Ljungman, P. *et al.* (1998). Booster marrow or blood cells for graft failure after allogeneic bone marrow transplantation. *Bone Marrow Transplantation,* **22,** 73–8.

Rodriguez-Inigo, E., Tomas, J.F., Gomez-Garcia de Soria, V. *et al.* (1997). Hepatitis C and G virus infection and liver dysfunction after allogeneic bone marrow transplantation: results from a prospective study. *Blood,* **90,** 1326–31.

Rubinstein, P., Carrier, C., Scaradavou, A. *et al.* (1998). Outcomes among 562 recipients of placental-blood transplants from unrelated donors. *New England Journal of Medicine,* **339,** 1565–77.

Salzberger, B., Bowden, R.A., Hackman, R.C. *et al.* (1997). Neutropenia in allogeneic marrow transplant recipients receiving ganciclovir for prevention of cytomegalovirus disease: risk factors and outcome. *Blood,* **90,** 2502–8.

Sandmaier, B.M., Maloney, D.G., Gooley, T. *et al.* (2001). Nonmyeloablative hematopoietic stem cell transplants (HSCT) from HLA-matched related donors for patients with hematologic malignancies: clinical results of a TBI-based conditioning regimen. *Blood,* 98 (Part 1), 742a–743a, #3093 (Abstract).

Schlegel, P.G., Eyrich, M., Bader, P. *et al.* (2000). OKT-3-based reconditioning regimen for early graft failure in HLA-non-identical stem cell transplants. *British Journal of Haematology,* **111,** 668–73.

Schultz, K.R., Ratanatharathorn, V., Abella, E. *et al.* (1994). Graft failure in children receiving HLA-mismatched marrow transplants with busulfan-containing regimens. *Bone Marrow Transplantation,* **13,** 817–22.

Sierra, J., Terol, M.J., Urbano-Ispizua, A. *et al.* (1994). Different response to recombinant human granulocyte-macrophage colony-stimulating factor in primary and secondary graft failure after bone marrow transplantation. *Experimental Hematology,* **22,** 566–72.

Singhal, S., Powles, R., Treleaven, J. *et al.* (2000). A low CD34+ cell dose results in higher mortality and poorer survival after blood or marrow stem cell transplantation from HLA-identical siblings: should 2 × 10(6) CD34+ cells/kg be considered the minimum threshold? *Bone Marrow Transplantation,* **26,** 489–96.

Slattery, J.T., Sanders, J.E., Buckner, C.D. *et al.* (1995). Graft-rejection and toxicity following bone marrow transplantation in relation to busulfan pharmacokinetics. *Bone Marrow Transplantation,* **16,** 31–42.

Solano, C., Juan, O., Gimeno, C., & Garcia-Conde, J. (1996). Engraftment failure associated with peripheral blood stem cell transplantation after B19 parvovirus infection. *Blood,* **88,** 1515–17.

Souza, J.P., Boeckh, M., Gooley, T.A. *et al.* (1999). High rates of pneumocystis carinii pneumonia in allogeneic blood and marrow transplant recipients receiving dapsone prophylaxis. *Clinical Infectious Diseases,* **29,** 1467–71.

Spencer, A., Szydlo, R.M., Brookes, P.A. *et al.* (1995). Bone marrow transplantation for chronic myeloid leukemia with volunteer unrelated donors using ex vivo or in vivo T-cell depletion: major prognostic impact of HLA class I identity between donor and recipient. (Review). *Blood,* **86,** 3590–7.

Storb, R., Blume, K.G., O'Donnell, M.R. *et al.* (2001). Cyclophosphamide and antithymocyte globulin to condition patients with aplastic anemia for allogeneic marrow transplantations: the experience in four centers. *Biology of Blood and Marrow Transplantation,* **7,** 39–44.

Storb, R. & Deeg, H.J. (1986). Failure of allogeneic canine marrow grafts after total body irradiation: Allogeneic "resistance" vs transfusion induced sensitization. *Transplantation,* **42,** 571–80.

Storb, R., Deeg, H.J., Whitehead, J. *et al.* (1986). Methotrexate and cyclosporine compared with cyclosporine alone for prophylaxis of acute graft versus host disease after marrow transplantation for leukemia. *New England Journal of Medicine,* **314,** 729–35.

Storb, R., Epstein, R.B., Rudolph, R.H., & Thomas, E.D. (1970). The effect of prior transfusion on marrow grafts between histocompatible canine siblings. *Journal of Immunology,* **105,** 627–33.

Storb, R., Prentice, R.L., & Thomas, E.D. (1977). Marrow transplantation for treatment of aplastic anemia. An analysis of factors associated with graft rejection. *New England Journal of Medicine,* **296,** 61–6.

Storb, R., Rudolph, R.H., Graham, T.C., & Thomas, E.D. (1971). The influence of transfusions from unrelated donors upon marrow grafts between histocompatible canine siblings. *Journal of Immunology,* **107,** 409–13.

Storb, R., Thomas, E.D., Buckner, C.D. *et al.* (1980). Marrow transplantation in thirty "untransfused" patients with severe aplastic anemia. *Annals of Internal Medicine,* **92,** 30–6.

Storb, R., Weiden, P.L., Deeg, H.J. *et al.* (1979). Rejection of marrow from DLA-identical canine littermates given transfusions before grafting: antigens involved are expressed on leukocytes and skin epithelial cells but not on platelets and red blood cells. *Blood,* **54,** 477–84.

Storb, R., Weiden, P.L., Sullivan, K.M. *et al.* (1987). Second marrow transplants in patients with aplastic anemia rejecting the first graft: use of a conditioning regimen including cyclophosphamide and antithymocyte globulin. *Blood,* **70,** 116–21.

Stucki, A., Leisenring, W., Sandmaier, B.M. *et al.* (1998). Decreased rejection and improved survival of first and second marrow transplants for severe aplastic anemia (a 26-year old retrospective analysis). *Blood,* **92,** 2742–9.

Sullivan, K.M., Witherspoon, R.P., Storb, R. *et al.* (1988). Prednisone and azathioprine compared with prednisone and placebo for treatment of chronic graft-versus-host disease: prognostic influence of prolonged thrombocytopenia after allogeneic marrow transplantation. *Blood,* **72,** 546–54.

Torok-Storb, B., Boeckh, M., Hoy, C. *et al.* (1997). Association of specific cytomegalovirus (CMV) genotypes with death from myelosuppression after marrow transplantation. *Blood,* **90,** 2097–102.

Vasconcelles, M.J., Bernardo, M.V., King, C. *et al.* (2000). Aerosolized pentamidine as pneumocystis prophylaxis after bone marrow transplantation is inferior to other regimens and is associated with decreased survival and an increased risk of other infections. *Biology of Blood & Marrow Transplantation, 6,* 35–43.

Wagner, J.E., Barker, J.N., Defor, T.E. *et al.* (2002). Transplantation of unrelated donor umbilical cord blood in 102 patients with malignant and nonmalignant diseases: influence of CD34 cell dose and HLA disparity on treatment-related mortality and survival. *Blood,* **100,** 1611–18.

Walters, M.C., Patience, M., Leisenring, W. *et al.* (1996). Bone marrow transplantation for sickle cell disease. *New England Journal of Medicine,* **335,** 369–76.

Watts, M.J., Sullivan, A.M., Leverett, D. *et al.* (1998). Back-up bone marrow is frequently ineffective in patients with poor peripheral-blood stem-cell mobilization. *Journal of Clinical Oncology,* **16,** 1554–60.

Weaver, C.H., Hazelton, B., Birch, R. *et al.* (1995). An analysis of engraftment kinetics as a function of the CD34 content of peripheral blood progenitor cell collections in 692 patients after the administration of myeloablative chemotherapy. *Blood,* **86,** 3961–9.

Weaver, C.H., Tauer, K., Zhen, B. *et al.* (1998). Second attempts at mobilization of peripheral blood stem cells in patients with initial low CD34+ cell yields. *Journal of Hematotherapy,* **7,** 241–9.

Weisdorf, D.J., Anasetti, C., Antin, J.H. *et al.* (2002). Allogeneic bone marrow transplantation for chronic myelogenous leukemia: comparative analysis of unrelated versus matched sibling donor transplantation. *Blood,* **99,** 1971–7.

Weisdorf, D.J., Verfaillie, C.M., Davies, S.M. *et al.* (1995). Hematopoietic growth factors for graft failure after bone marrow transplantation: a randomized trial of granulocyte-macrophage colony-stimulating factor (GM-CSF) versus sequential GM-CSF plus granulocyte-CSF. *Blood,* **85,** 3452–6.

Willemze, R., Richel, D.J., Falkenburg, J.H. *et al.* (1992). In vivo use of Campath-1G to prevent graft-versus-host disease and graft rejection after bone marrow transplantation. *Bone Marrow Transplantation,* **9,** 255–61.

Zaucha, J.M., Gooley, T., Bensinger, W.I. *et al.* (2001). CD34 cell dose in granulocyte colony-stimulating factor-mobilized peripheral blood mononuclear cell grafts affects engraftment kinetics and development of extensive chronic graft-versus-host disease after human leukocyte antigen-identical sibling transplantation. *Blood,* **98,** 3221–7.

71 Acute graft-versus-host disease

MARTIN BENESCH AND H. JOACHIM DEEG

Fred Hutchinson Cancer Research Center and the University of Washington, Seattle, USA

Introduction

Hematopoietic stem cell (HSC) transplantation involves the transfer of cells that produce hematopoietic and lymphoid progeny. Aside from treating the patient's disease, the objective is to have these cells accept the environment of the new host as "self." According to our present understanding, this objective requires that the newly developing self-reactive T lymphocytes and mature donor T lymphocytes contained in the transplant inoculum that recognize the transplant recipient as non-self be eliminated or inactivated by central or peripheral mechanisms or both to prevent an adverse graft-versus-host (GVH) reaction. Multiple interactions between donor and host cells take place that contribute to the manifestations of this GVH reaction, leading to the clinical picture of GVH disease (GVHD).

Definition and etiology

Immunologic identity and individuality are expressed in the form of cell surface proteins encoded by genes of the major histocompatibility complex (MHC) and other genes. MHC molecules (termed HLA [human leukocyte antigen] in humans, H-2 in mice, etc.) are critical to the function of the immune system, that is, for the recognition and, generally, destruction of foreign antigens, cells, and tissues, while preserving the individual's integrity. MHC and non-MHC (minor) antigens expressed on transplanted cells and tissues in an immunocompetent individual, are recognized by the recipient's immune system, leading to their rejection (host-versus-graft [HVG] reaction). If, however, the recipient is immunodeficient (or immunosuppressed), immunologically competent cells contained in the graft are able to survive and recognize tissue (transplantation) antigens such as HLA in the recipient, thereby initiating a GVH reaction.

GVH reactions were first described in rodents. Mice given total body irradiation (TBI) and infused with allogeneic spleen or marrow cells recover from radiation injury and radiation-induced marrow aplasia, but, unless other precautions are taken, die with "secondary disease," a syndrome consisting primarily of immunodeficiency, diarrhea, weight loss, skin changes, and liver function abnormalities (van Bekkum & de Vries, 1967), now understood as manifestations of GVHD. These observations led Billingham to formulate in 1966 the requirements for the development of GVHD (Billingham, 1966). In an updated formulation they state:

1. The graft must contain immunocompetent cells, now known as T lymphocytes. The severity of GVHD appears to correlate with the number of T cells transferred.
2. The host must express tissue antigens not expressed in the transplant donor. HLA antigens are potent stimuli for allogeneic T-cell activation. HLA differences between donor and recipient represent the strongest risk factor for the development of GVHD; non-MHC histocompatibility antigens are also recognized as foreign and are responsible for the induction of GVHD after MHC-identical transplantation. Experience has shown that GVH-like reactions can occur between genetically identical individuals or even with the infusion of autologous marrow, either due to modifications of self-antigens or inappropriate self-recognition.
3. The host must be incapable of mounting an effective response to eliminate the transplanted cells. Such an immunocompromise is generally present in allogeneic transplant recipients who have usually received high-dose immunosuppressive chemoradiotherapy before transplantation. This condition may also be met in other situations such as with transfusion support in patients given cytotoxic chemotherapy, after solid organ transplantation, transfusions from donors homozygous for one of the recipient MHC haplotypes, and others (Juji *et al.*, 1989) (Table 71.1). GVHD also develops in recipients prepared with reduced

Table 71.1. *Risk situations for GVHD*

1. Marrow and blood cell transplantation
2. Solid organ transplantation
3. Transfusion of unirradiated blood products in
   a) Neonates and fetuses
   b) Patients with immunodeficiency syndromes
   c) Patients receiving immunosuppressive chemoradiotherapy
   d) Patients given directed blood donations from unidirectionally HLA compatible donors

intensity immunosuppression and the prolonged co-existence of donor and host cells (Mielcarek *et al.*, 2002).

Thus, GVHD in its acute form is a clinical syndrome initiated by a reaction of donor immunocompetent cells against recipient cells and organs. A clear distinction between acute and chronic forms of GVHD as described originally (Glucksberg *et al.*, 1974; Sullivan, 1986a), however, may no longer be tenable (see below).

Clinical spectrum of GVHD

Allogeneic transplants

Acute GVHD generally occurs within 2 to 5 weeks of transplantation; after HLA-nonidentical transplants and in patients not given GVHD prophylaxis, it may develop within days. Dependent upon the degree of histoincompatibility, the number of T lymphocytes transplanted, patient and donor characteristics, and the prophylactic regimen utilized (Chao & Deeg, 1997; Ringden & Deeg, 1997), the incidence of acute GVHD ranges from 10% to 90%.

The immune system, skin, liver, and intestinal tract are the major targets of acute GVHD, but other tissues can be involved (Table 71.2). GVHD is usually observed first and most commonly in the skin as pruritus, erythema, or a maculo-papular rash, often on palms, soles, shoulders and ears and may progress to total body erythroderma. In severe cases, separation at the dermo-epidermal junction results in bullae and desquamation (Fig. 71.1). In milder cases skin lesions remain localized or the skin may clinically be normal, and only biopsies reveal histologic changes typical for GVHD (subclinical GVHD). Mild skin changes may be waxing and waning and may resolve without therapy.

Manifestations of GVHD in liver and gut may appear concurrently with, before, or after the development of skin disease. Symptoms and findings suggesting involvement of the intestinal tract include nausea, vomiting, diarrhea, pain, and paralytic ileus. Liver function impairment includes hyperbilirubinemia, and elevations of alkaline phosphatase and transaminases. However, hepatic failure and metabolic encephalopathy are only infrequently attributable to acute GVHD, and other causes such as veno-occlusive disease and infections must be ruled out. In contrast to veno-occlusive disease, hepatic GVHD only rarely leads to weight gain, capsular pain, or ascites.

Table 71.2.   *Targets of acute GVHD*

Immune system
Skin
Liver
Intestinal tract
Mucous membranes
Airways
Bone marrow
Leukemia/tumor cells

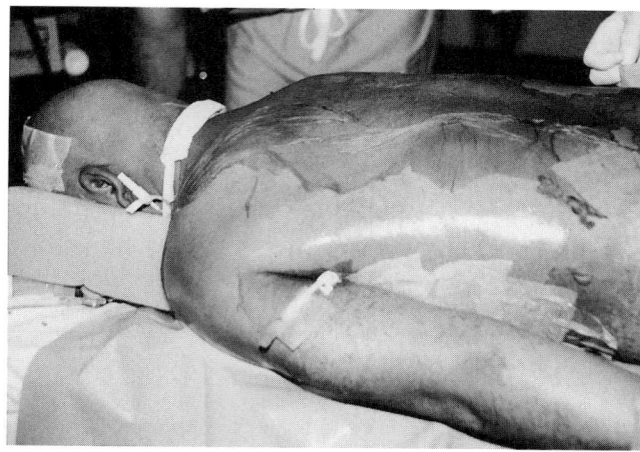

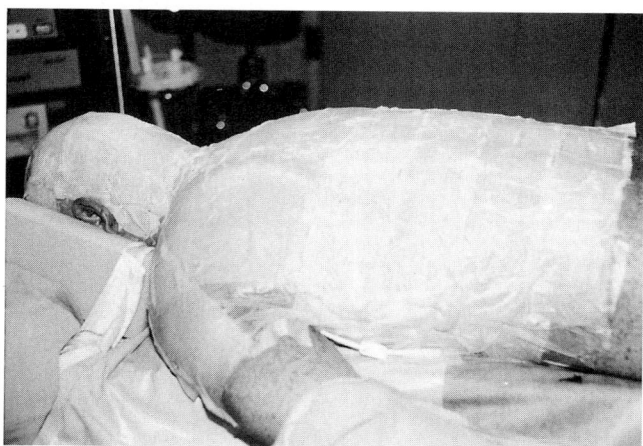

Fig. 71.1. Severe acute GVHD of the skin. **(A)** Diffuse desquamation 24 days after transplantation of marrow from an unrelated donor differing for one HLA-B from the patient. **(B)** Same patient after placement of protective pig skin grafts. (Courtesy Dr. P. Bubak, Seattle.)

Presentation resembling acute hepatitis has been described (Fugii *et al.*, 2001). Coagulopathies (e.g., due to development of factor VIII inhibitor) (Brentjens *et al.*, 2001), thrombocytopenic purpura (TTP), and hemolytic uremic syndrome (HUS) have been observed in patients with GVHD (Ringden & Deeg, 1997). However, in many instances these complications appear to be medication related (cyclosporine [CSP], rapamycin) or associated with intercurrent infections. A cause-effect relationship with GVHD is difficult or impossible to prove.

GVHD also involves the immune system, delays immunologic recovery, and results in prolonged immunodeficiency. Immunodeficiency predisposes to infections, a risk that is further aggravated by immunosuppressive therapy of GVHD and disruption of the mechanical/anatomical barriers of the integument.

Histologic evidence of damage in target tissues, usually apoptotic in nature, establishes the diagnosis of GVHD (Sale *et al.*, 1995). The epidermis and skin appendages lose their integrity. Hepatic small bile ducts may show segmental disruption. Mucosal ulcerations and crypt destruction are present in the intestinal tract. Involvement of other epithelial targets such as the conjunctival, vaginal, oral, and esophageal mucosa is less frequent. Mononuclear cell infiltrates may be subtle, but severe inflammation can develop with disease progression. Target cell destruction may be mediated by soluble factors such as tumor necrosis factor-alpha (TNF-α), perforin, or Fas-ligand (FasL) without direct contact between epithelial target cells and donor lymphocytes. In the skin, damage is prominent at the tips of the rete ridges. In the gut, the most severe damage is seen at the basis of intestinal crypts, and in the liver, in the periductular epithelium. These data suggest that GVHD targets primarily undifferentiated epithelial cells (Sale *et al.*, 1995).

Staging of histologic biopsies is at best semiquantitative, and histologic findings are generally not used in the grading of GVHD. Widely accepted grading systems score clinical manifestations in skin, upper and lower intestinal tract, and liver. In addition to the original grading system proposed by the Seattle Group (Glucksberg *et al.*, 1974), various modifications are in use (Rowlings *et al.*, 1997) (Table 71.3). Opinions differ in regards to the reliability of currently used staging, especially of the intestinal tract and liver (Atkinson *et al.*, 1989; Hings *et al.*, 1994; Martin *et al.*, 1998a, 1998b), and none of the grading schemes is completely satisfactory. This issue is rendered more complex by considerable interobserver variation. Simplified "consensus" schemes for functional GVHD grading (Table 71.4) have been proposed. The International Bone Marrow Transplant Registry (IBMTR) system (Rowlings *et al.*, 1997) has been validated in a retrospective analysis, and, as illustrated in Figure 71.2, the IBMTR severity grade is reflected in transplant-related mortality. Martin *et al.* have shown that for practical purposes IBMTR levels A, B, C, and D roughly correspond to Glucksberg grades I, II, III, and IV, respectively (Martin *et al.*, 1998a).

The reason for intensive efforts at GVHD grading is its prognostic implication. Mild to moderate GVHD (grades I or II by Glucksberg) is associated with only little morbidity, but is a significant risk factor for the development of chronic GVHD (Anasetti *et al.*, 1986). Grades III and IV GVHD carry a grave prognosis. In patients with grade IV, mortality approaches 100%. These observations have led to the proposal of grading acute GVHD on the basis of outcome, that is, taking into account the patient's entire course rather than considering only one time point (Martin *et al.*, 1998b).

An additional challenge, accentuated by observations in patients transplanted with non-myeloablative regimens ("mini-transplants"), are the kinetics of the development of GVHD (Figure 71.3). The historic classification into acute GVHD (onset before day 100) and chronic GVHD (onset after day 100) no longer satisfies clinical needs. GVHD with chronic clinical and histologic characteristics can occur as early as 50 or 60 days after transplantation, and clinical disease with characteristics of acute GVHD may present 5 to 6 months after transplantation or even later. It will be necessary to incorporate these insights into new grading schemes which will, presumably, also consider a time component.

Syngeneic and autologous transplants

Modifications of self-antigens or inappropriate reactions toward self-antigens may also trigger GVH reactions. As a consequence, a GVHD-like syndrome can develop in syngeneic and autologous transplant recipients (Rappeport *et al.*, 1979; Hess, 1997). The disease is often, although not always (Rappeport *et al.*, 1979; Saunders *et al.*, 2000), limited to the skin, and generally resolves promptly without treatment or with administration of corticosteroids. More severe cases have been described (Hwang *et al.*, 2000). Basically, all patients reported to develop syngeneic or autologous (pseudo-) GVHD, were prepared with intensive conditioning regimens, usually involving irradiation. Hess and colleagues have shown that self-reactivity in this context is directed against public MHC class II determinants. Animal models indicate that conditioning (i.e., tissue damage inflicted upon the recipient) is essential for the development of the syndrome (see below, Pathophysiology).

Pathophysiology (see also Chapter 15)

Host environment

According to the model advanced by Ferrara *et al.*, initial damage to host tissue is induced by the transplant conditioning reg-

Table 71.3. *IBMTR criteria for severity index for acute GVHD*

Index[a]	Skin			Liver			Gastrointestinal tract		
	Stage (max)	Extent of rash (%)		Stage (max)	Total bilirubin (mg/100 ml)		Stage (max)	Volume of diarrhea (ml/day)	UGI
A	1	<25		0	<3.4		0	<500	–
B	2	25–50	or	1–2	3.5–7.9	or	1–2	500–1500	Nausea/vomiting or Epigastric pain
C	3	>50	or	3	8.0–15.0	or	3	>1500	Positive histology
D	4	Bullae	or	4	>15.0	or	4	Severe pain and ileus	–

Abbreviations: max, maximum; UGI, upper gastrointestinal tract.
[a] Assign index based on maximum involvement in an individual organ system. Adapted from Rowlings *et al.* (1997).

Table 71.4. *Simplified grading of acute GVHD[a]*

	Organ/extent of involvement					
Grade	Skin		Liver		Intestinal tract	
I	Rash on <50% of skin		None		None	
II	Rash on >50% of skin	or	Bilirubin 2–3 mg/dl	or	Diarrhea >500 ml/day[b] or persistent nausea[c]	
III–IV[d]	Generalized erythroderma with bullous formation	or	Bilirubin >3	or	Diarrhea >1000 ml/day	

[a] Modified from Przepiorka *et al.,* 1995.

[b] Volume of diarrhea applies to adults. For pediatric patients, the volume of diarrhea should be based on body surface area.

[c] Persistent nausea with histologic evidence of GVHD in the stomach or duodenum.

[d] As suggested by this scheme, three severity grades may suffice.

imen (Ferrara, Levy, & Chao, 1999). This is followed by donor cell activation, predominantly involving T cells, adhesion to and interaction with host tissue and costimulatory signals, and amplification of the cytokine network. Finally, the effector phase leads to host cell destruction via inflammatory signals, cytolytic effects, and programmed cell death (apoptosis). According to this hypothesis, the release of inflammatory cytokines occurs primarily in the gut which, when damaged, also allows for transfer of endotoxins/lipopolysaccharides (LPS) into the circulation, and macrophage activation. This, in turn, further enhances the release of cytokines such as TNF-α and interleukin (IL)-1 (Hill *et al.,* 1997; Xun, Tsuchrda, &

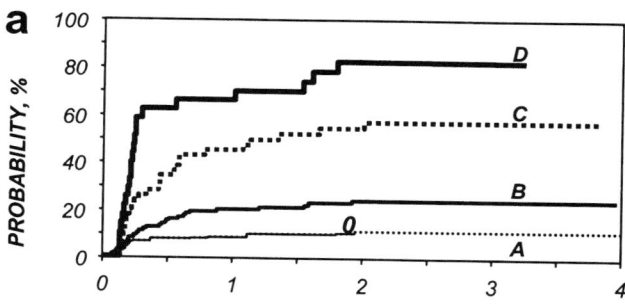

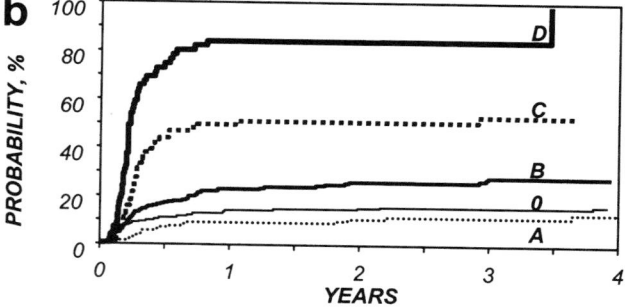

Fig. 71.2. Impact of IBMTR severity grade of GVHD (A, B, C, D) on transplant-related mortality. **a)** patients 16–30 years of age; **b)** patients more than 30 years of age. Reproduced, with permission, from Rowlings *et al.* (1997).

Thompson, 1997; Hill *et al.,* 1999). Those signals may lead to target cell death but also contribute to the expression of costimulatory molecules such as CD80, CD86, and MHC class II antigens on dendritic cells (DC), T cell stimulation and release of TH1 cytokines (IL-2, interferon-γ [IFN-γ]), followed by effector cell expansion and target cell death (Hill & Ferrara, 2000) (Figure 71.4).

The major peripheral targets of GVHD—skin, intestinal tract, and liver—contain high numbers of professional antigen-presenting cells (APC), i.e. macrophages and DC, as originally pointed out by Janossy *et al.* (Janossy *et al.,* 1986). A study by Shlomchik *et al.* strongly supports this notion by showing that host DC play a central role in the development of GVHD (Shlomchik *et al.,* 1999). Studies by other investigators (Baker *et al.,* 1997; Graubert *et al.,* 1997; Hattori *et al.,* 1998) show marked differences, however, particularly in the effector phase, in regard to the signals mediating the GVH effect in different organs (Hiroyasu *et al.,* 1999). For example, Fas/FasL-mediated signals play a central role in hepatic injury, TNF/TNF receptor signals figure prominently in intestinal GVHD, and both pathways contribute to skin manifestations. We have shown that exogenous transferrin interferes in a donor-specific fashion with alloantigen-triggered lymphocyte proliferation, apparently by down-regulating IL-1, IL-2, and TNF-α, and by upregulating IL-10 (Lesnikova *et al.,* 2000). Concurrently, there was a reduction in expression of the co-stimulatory molecules CD80 and CD86. Additional (co-stimulatory) molecules involved in GVHD reactions include CD40L/CD40, CD28, and CTLA4, as well as vascular cellular adhesion molecule-1/intercellular adhesion molecule-1 (VCAM-1/ICAM-1) (CD54), E-selectin, OX40 (CD134)/CD134L and others (Saito *et al.,* 1998; Buhlmann *et al.,* 1999; Tsukada *et al.,* 2000). To what extent B lymphocytes are involved in the pathogenesis of GVHD has remained controversial (Schultz *et al.,* 1995).

The development of acute GVHD requires antigen presentation, which can be direct, by host cells, or indirect, by donor cells. Shlomchik and others have shown that host DC play a pivotal role in the development of GVHD, and β2-microglobulin knock-out mice, unable to express MHC class I antigens fail to develop GVHD (Shlomchik *et al.,* 1999). Interactions of

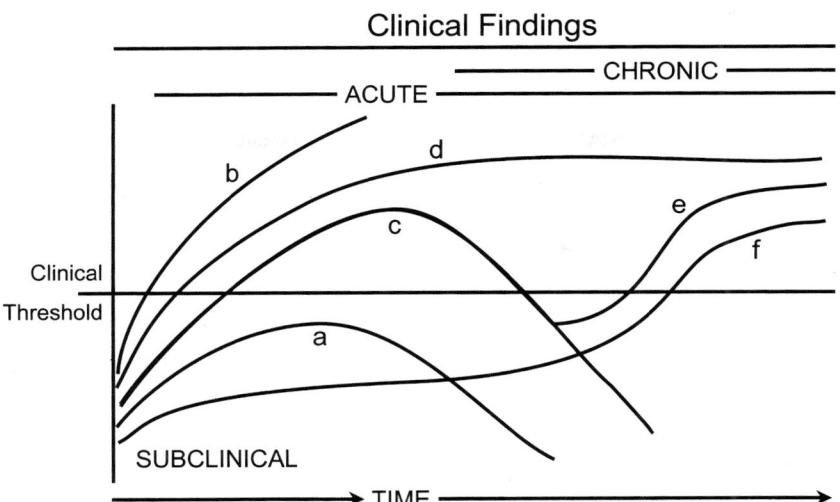

Fig. 71.3. Kinetics of GVHD a) No clinical evidence of GVHD; b) rapidly progressive acute GVHD; c) acute GVHD resolving spontaneously or with therapy; d) acute GVHD progressing to chronic GVHD; e) chronic GVHD after a quiescent phase following acute GVHD; f) de novo onset chronic GVHD or delayed onset acute GVHD.

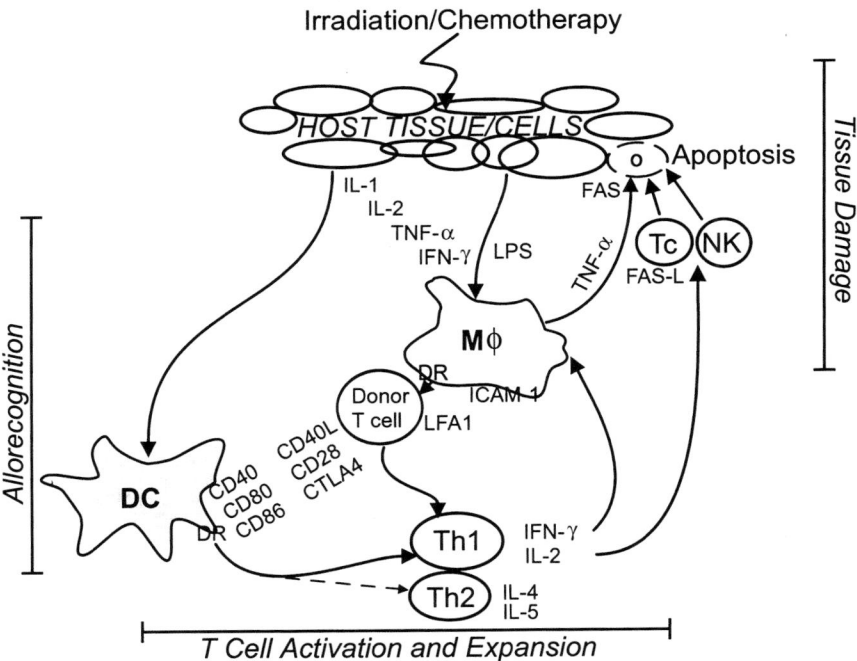

Fig. 71.4. Three components of GVHD immunopathophysiology. (**1**) Conditioning of the patient with cytotoxic regimens results in tissue damage and the release of cytokines. This is the milieu into which donor cells are infused. (**2**) Allorecognition: The antigen-presenting cell, monocyte (Mϕ) or dendritic cell (DC), presents antigen in the form of an HLA-(DR) peptide complex to the donor T cell. The antigen-presenting cell also supplies co-stimulatory signals (e.g. CD80, IL-1). These and additional co-stimulatory interaction (e.g. ICAM-1/LFA-1) lead to (3) T-cell activation, particularly in the direction of Th1 (rather than Th2) cells, and further amplification (in particular by IL-2) and secretion of cytokines (such as IFN-γ), which are able to amplify the function of antigen-presenting cells, in particular monocytes. The function of DC is enhanced by CD40 ligand on activated T cells. The expression of cytokines leads to maturation of cytotoxic T cells (Tc) and activation of NK cells. Along with factors such as TNF-α, these cause and further amplify host-tissue damage (predominantly via apoptosis), and lead to the clinical manifestations of GVHD. IL, interleukin; TNF, tumor necrosis factor; IFN, interferon; DC, dendritic cell; Mϕ, macrophage; DR, HLA-DR; ICAM-1, intercellular adhesion molecule 1; LFA-1, lymphocyte function antigen 1; TH1, CD4+ T cells type 1; TH2, CD4+ T cells type 2; Tc, cytotoxic cell; NK, natural killer cell; LPS, lipopolysaccharide; Fas, death receptor CD95; Fas-L, Fas-ligand.

MHC antigens (with bound peptides, derived from minor histocompatibility antigens) and T-cell receptors lead to activation, clonal expansion, and differentiation of donor T cells. Additional co-stimulatory molecules, in particular CD80 and CD86 on APC interact with antigens on T cells. Signals transmitted via CTLA4 appear to have tolerogenic effects, whereas signals through CD28 will lead to activation (Zhou et al., 2001). Accessory surface molecules such as CD4 or CD8 on T cells also continue to the immunologic synapses between T cells and APC. The genetic make-up of host and donor determine which subset of donor T cells proliferates and differentiates. MHC class II differences stimulate CD4+ T cells; MHC class I differences stimulate CD8+ T cells. In murine models CD4+ cells have been shown to induce GVHD across MHC class II, and CD8+ cells across MHC class I barriers (Korngold & Sprent, 1999). In MHC-identical marrow transplants (non-MHC barriers), GVHD was induced by either subset of T cells or simultaneously by both.

Classically, the efferent arm of acute GVHD involves cytotoxic T cells that cause tissue damage (Ghayur et al., 1990) to target organs such as the skin, liver, gut, and lymphoid organs. The lymphoid organs show reduced cellularity, and in the thymus, diminished proliferative capacity (possibly due to interferon-γ secretion) results in a decrease in CD4+ CD8+ (double-positive) cells (Krenger et al., 2000). Experiments also emphasize the role of other cytokines, in particular, TNF-α, IL-15, and IL-18 (Deeg, 2001a). In mouse models TNF-α is a central mediator of GVHD predominantly in the intestinal tract, and anti-TNF antibody prevents or ameliorates GVHD in mice (Piguet, 1990) and humans (Lichtman et al., 1997; Kobbe et al., 2001). However, the actions of different cytokines and effector cells (e.g., large granular lymphocytes) and regulatory cells is still incompletely understood. The role of regulatory T cells with a CD25+CD4+ phenotype, functionally reminiscent of the classic "suppressor T cell," is currently being defined, but they appear capable of significantly inhibiting GVHD in murine models (Taylor et al., 2002; Johnson et al., 2002).

Data in murine models provide evidence that blockade of LPS-mediated signals (via CD14) is effective in reducing the incidence/severity of GVHD, in part at least by way of reduction of TNF-α levels (Cooke et al., 2001). Additional cytolytic effector pathways involve Fas/FasL which have been implicated in the pathogenesis of murine GVHD particularly in the liver (Mori et al., 1998; Hattori et al., 1998). Elevated serum levels of soluble FasL have been observed in some patients with GVHD (Das et al., 1999), and increased FasL gene expression in circulating mononuclear cells was noted. In contrast to the role of Fas as an apoptosis-inducing molecule in GVHD, perforin-mediated cytotoxicity may be more important in mediating a graft-versus-leukemia (GVL) effect (Schmaltz et al., 2001). However, even T cells from mice doubly deficient in both FasL and perforin/granzyme can cause GVHD when aggressive host conditioning is used (Jiang, Podack, & Levy, 2001).

As indicated above, pathologic/histologic changes of GVHD have also been observed in irradiated and cyclosporine-treated animals transplanted with marrow from genetically identical donors (or even with autologous marrow) (Hess & Jones, 1999). Data show that a syngeneic GVH response is mediated by highly restricted CD8+ cells that recognize MHC class II molecules in association with a peptide from the invariant chain termed CLIP (Hess et al., 2000). Interestingly, only clones responsive to the N-terminal flanking region, producing type 1 cytokines (IL-2, IFN), induce acute GVHD; the C-terminal region-restricted cells appear to be involved in chronic syngeneic GVHD. Regulatory lymphocytes, which would normally inactivate or eliminate autoreactive cells, have been eliminated by the preparative regimen. As a result, autoreactivity and GVHD become prominent after the immunosuppressive effect of CSP has been removed. Syngeneic GVHD, thus, can be seen as an imbalance between autoreactive and autoregulatory lymphocytes, as a direct consequence of thymic dysfunction.

Stem cell source

The kinetics and manifestations of GVHD are dependent upon the source of stem cells. Peripheral blood stem cells (PBSC) mobilized either by means of chemotherapy or hematopoietic growth factors (e.g., granulocyte colony-stimulating factor [G-CSF], stem cell factor) or both, have been used extensively for allogeneic and autologous stem cell rescue and are associated with rapid hematopoietic reconstitution (Powles et al., 2000; Bensinger et al., 2001; Anderson et al., 2001). Furthermore murine studies suggest that G-CSF or IL-4 may polarize donor cells toward TH2 cells and, thereby, favor the development of tolerance (Pan et al., 1995; Krenger et al., 1995). Hence, the use of G-CSF–mobilized PBSC is of considerable interest in the allogeneic transplant setting.

Several clinical studies, some of them in a randomized setting have now been conducted (Powles et al., 2000; Schmitz et al., 2000; Bensinger et al., 2001). While there are some differences, the overall data suggest that the incidence of acute GVHD does not differ significantly between patients transplanted with marrow or PBSC, whereas the incidence of chronic GVHD appears to be increased (Storek et al., 1997). A meta-analysis of five randomized controlled trials and 11 cohort studies on the other hand suggests that, both acute and chronic GVHD are more common after PBSC transplantation than after marrow transplantation (Cutler et al., 2001). This higher incidence of GVHD with PBSC, however, may not be associated with a significant increase in mortality. In fact, results of several trials suggest that in particular in patients with "high risk" disease, survival is improved in comparison to patients given marrow (Powles et al., 2000; Bensinger et al., 2001).

Studies directed at the mechanisms involved in the effects of PBSC show increased production of IL-10, and decreased levels of TNF-α in monocytes from G-CSF–mobilized PBSC along with reduced expression of co-stimulatory molecules and MHC class II antigens. Thus, there may actually be a tolerogenic effect related to monocytes, possibly with a countereffect by increased numbers of T cells. Further studies are needed.

Another less frequently used source of stem cells is cord blood, known to be rich in hematopoietic precursors. Since the fetal immune system is relatively immature, cord blood cells are likely to have a low GVHD potential (Gluckman *et al.*, 1989; Gluckman *et al.*, 1997; Rubinstein *et al.*, 1998; Broxmeyer & Smith, 1999). Cord blood T cells are activated via the T cell receptor, but have a reduced capacity to stimulate (Apperley, 1994). Intracytoplasmatic signaling (following T cell receptor engagement) in cord blood T cells differs from that in adult T cells (Miscia *et al.*, 1999).

Also, cord blood monocytes express lower levels of MHC class II, CD86, and ICAM-1 than monocytes in adult blood, and produce lower levels of IL-10 and IFN-γ. IL-4 and IL-5 are basically absent (Apperley, 1994). Most, if not all, cytotoxicity of cord blood is mediated by natural killer type cells (rather than CD3+ T cells).

Kurtzberg *et al.* (Kurtzberg *et al.*, 1996) reported results on 25 consecutive patients, mostly children transplanted with cord blood. Among these 24 were discordant for 1 to 3 HLA antigens. In 23 of the 25 patients, engraftment was achieved and 11 of 21 evaluable patients developed acute GVHD of grades II–IV. Gluckman *et al.* (Gluckman *et al.*, 1997) presented results on 143 transplants carried out at 45 centers. GVHD of grades II–IV occurred in 9% of HLA-identical, and in 50% of HLA-mismatched transplants. A major challenge in adult patients remains the limited number of cells available for transplantation.

Risk factors

Some risk factors for GVHD in clinical transplantation are listed in Table 71.5. The probability of developing acute GVHD grades II–IV with HLA genotypically identical sibling transplants may be less than 20% to 40%, but with mismatched related and with unrelated transplants it is 60% to 90%. With unrelated transplants, as many as 35% of patients have grades III to IV acute GVHD. However, considerable progress in HLA typing has allowed for selection of unrelated donors on the basis of molecular results (Petersdorf *et al.*, 1998, 2001a, 2001b). This in turn has resulted in improved transplant outcome. In a large cohort study of patients with chronic myeloid leukemia in chronic phase DRB1 allele mismatching was associated with a significant increase in grades III–IV acute GVHD which was reflected in inferior survival (Fig 71.5). HLA-DPB1 also has an effect on GVHD if two alleles are mismatched. MHC class I alleles had a negative impact on engraftment, but did not significantly affect GVHD (Petersdorf *et al.*, 2001b). An effect of HLA matching by molecular criteria on transplant outcome has also been shown in patients with aplastic anemia (Fig. 71.6) (Deeg *et al.*, 1999). Omission of GVHD prophylaxis significantly increases the risk of GVHD. For comparable groups of patients, the incidence of GVHD may be 20% to 30% with state-of-the-art prophylaxis, but 90% to 100% if no prophylaxis is given (Sullivan *et al.*, 1986b).

Use of marrow from allosensitized female donors for male recipients carries a risk of GVHD two- to three-fold higher than with nonsensitized donors for same gender recipients

Table 71.5. *Risk factors for the development of acute GVHD*

Risk factor	Reference
Histoincompatibility	Beatty *et al.*, 1985; Ringdén & Nilsson, 1985; Anasetti *et al.*, 1990; Beatty *et al.*, 1993; Sasazuki *et al.*, 1998; Tseng *et al.*, 1999; Kollman *et al.*, 2001
Allosenzitation of donor	Gale *et al.*, 1987; Flowers *et al.*, 1990; Weisdorf *et al.*, 1991
Patient age	Ringden & Nilsson, 1985; Atkinson *et al.*, 1986; Gale *et al.*, 1987; Anasetti *et al.*, 1990; Weisdorf *et al.*, 1991
Donor age	Atkinson *et al.*, 1986; Weisdorf *et al.*, 1991; Hagglund *et al.*, 1994; Kollman *et al.*, 2001
Gender mismatch	Gale *et al.*, 1987; Weisdorf *et al.*, 1991; Nash *et al.*, 1992
Omission of GVHD prophylaxis	Sullivan *et al.*, 1986; Gale *et al.*, 1987
Type of GVHD prophylaxis	Storb *et al.*, 1986b; Hagglund *et al.*, 1994; Przepiorka *et al.*, 1999
Intensity of conditioning regimen (irradiation)	Deeg *et al.*, 1991; Hagglund *et al.*, 1994; Hill *et al.*, 1997
Infusion of viable donor leukocytes	Collins, Jr. *et al.*, 1997; Lokhorst *et al.*, 1997; Bacigalupo *et al.*, 1997
Stem cell source (PBSC)	Cutler *et al.*, 2001
Number of cells transfused	Przepiorka *et al.*, 1999
Cytokine polymorphisms (IFN-γ, TNF-α, IL-6, IL-10)	Middleton *et al.*, 1998; Cavet *et al.*, 1999; Cavet *et al.*, 2001; Cullup *et al.*, 2001
Serum cytokine levels	Liem *et al.*, 1998; Holler *et al.*, 2000; Imoto *et al.*, 2000; Fujimori *et al.*, 2000; Nakamura *et al.*, 2000
Donor CMV (HSV)-seropositivity	Weisdorf *et al.*, 1991; Hagglund *et al.*, 1994; Broers *et al.*, 2000

Abbreviations: PBSC, peripheral blood stem cells; IFN, interferon; TNF, tumor necrosis factor; IL, interleukin; CMV, cytomegalovirus.

(Gale *et al.*, 1987). The intensity of the GVHD prophylactic regimen inversely correlates with the incidence of acute GVHD (Storb *et al.*, 1986b; Hagglund *et al.*, 1994). Data by the Huddinge team (Remberger *et al.*, 2002) indicate that the incorporation of antithymocyte globulin (ATG) into the transplant conditioning regimen not only facilitates engraftment but also reduces the incidence of GVHD. Russell *et al.* observed an incidence of acute GVHD grades II–IV of 9% in patients with various diagnoses conditioned with fludarabine and busulfan, and given ATG (Russell *et al.*, 2001).

The addition of viable donor buffy coat cells in earlier studies used in patients with aplastic anemia in an attempt to enhance engraftment significantly increased the incidence of chronic GVHD, but had little effect on acute GVHD. This observation has regained interest with the use of viable donor lymphocytes for the re-induction of remission in patients whose leukemia recurs after marrow transplantation (Kolb *et al.*, 1995), and with the use of peripheral blood stem cells

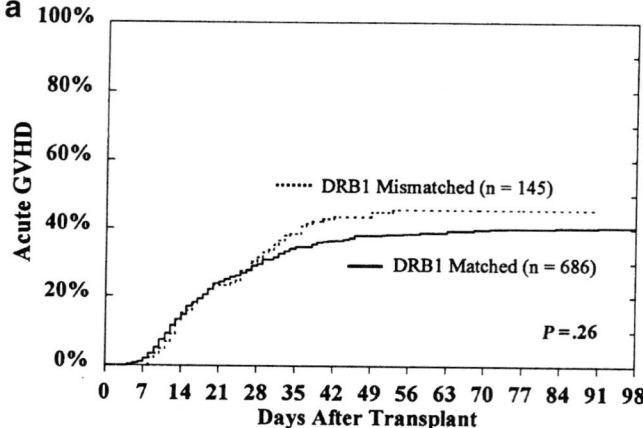

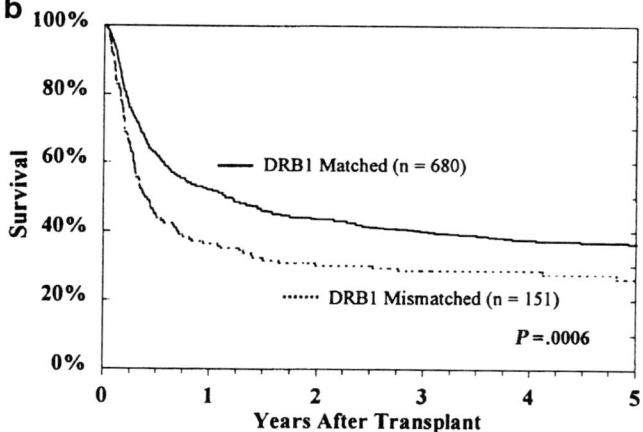

Fig. 71.5. Impact of HLA-DRB1 on severe acute GVHD and survival. **a)** Probability of grades III-IV acute GVHD according to DRB1 match status among patients with CML. **b)** Kaplan-Meier survival among patients with CML. Reproduced, with permission, from Petersdorf *et al.* (2001).

(rather than marrow) for hematopoietic transplantation (Bensinger *et al.*, 1996; Dreger & Schmitz, 1999).

High spontaneous IL-10 production by peripheral blood mononuclear cells immediately pretransplant has been correlated with a low incidence of GVHD (and transplant-related mortality; 8%), compared to patients with low or intermediate levels of IL-10 production (Holler *et al.*, 2000). Recipient gene polymorphisms for IFN-γ, TNF, and IL-10 and donor polymorphism for IL-1Ra have been associated with severe acute GVHD after HLA-identical sibling marrow transplantation, and recipient polymorphisms for IL1-Ra, IL-6 and IL-10 with chronic GVHD (Middleton *et al.*, 1998; Cavet *et al.*, 1999, 2001; Cullup *et al.*, 2001; Rocha *et al.*, 2002). In Japanese children, donor polymorphism for TGF-β1 and recipient polymorphism for TGF-β1 type II receptor were associated with an increased risk of acute GVHD after HLA-identical sibling transplantation (Hattori *et al.*, 2002). In a Japanese study of unrelated donor transplantation, polymorphism for TNF-α was associated with grade III-IV acute GVHD and lower relapse

rate, while polymorphism for TNF receptor 2 was also associated with severe acute GVHD (Ishikawa *et al.*, 2002). Mismatching for CD31 (PECAM-1, platelet-endothelial cell adhesion molecule) has been reported to increase the risk of acute GVHD (Balduini *et al.*, 2001; Grumet *et al.*, 2001).

Other factors including antiviral immunity (Broers *et al.*, 2000) and the role of certain HLA alleles have remained controversial. In a retrospective IBMTR study of 751 patients with CML in chronic phase transplanted from HLA-identical family members, the presence of HLA-A3 increased, and HLA-DR1 decreased, the risk of acute GVHD (Clark *et al.*, 2001). In a Scandanavian study of 493 patients, the presence of HLA-A10 and HLA-B7 increased the risk of acute GVHD, and that of HLA-B27 decreased the risk of chronic GVHD (Remberger *et al.*, 2002). Attempts aimed at determining whether in vitro tests (e.g., skin explant models in which patient skin and donor lymphocytes are co-cultured), identify groups of patients who are at a particular risk of developing GVHD have met with only limited success. In one analysis of risk factors for acute GVHD after allogeneic PBSC transplantation, type of GVHD prophylaxis, and CD34 cell dose were the only two independent variables noted (Przepiorka *et al.*, 1999), although it is currently not clear what the optimal CD34 dose should be. CD34+ cell dose, as well as CD3+ cell dose, were risk factors in patients given CD34-selected HLA-identical sibling PBSC grafts (Urbano-Ispizua *et al.*, 2002) (and see Chapter 124, Breaking News...).

Prophylaxis

Strategies for GVHD prevention have focused mostly on the afferent limb of GVHD, i.e., have been aimed at eliminating donor T cells or blocking T-cell activation. Approaches have included selection of histocompatible donors, in vitro manipulation of the HSC in ocology, gnotobiosis, and in vivo treatment of the patient after transplantation (Table 71.6). However, the deciphering of numerous cytokine- and chemokine-signals, which appear to be involved in the development of clinical GVHD, has drawn attention to the efferent limb as well. When designing and evaluating trials of GVHD prophylaxis, it is important to take into consideration both efficacy and toxicity since net improvements in survival are likely to be achieved only if the effective prevention of GVHD does not negatively affect other endpoints. Overviews of prophylactic and therapeutic trials have been presented (Jacobsohn & Vogelsang, 2002; Chao & Deeg, 1997).

In vivo prophylaxis

In classic studies in mice Uphoff (Uphoff, 1958) used the antimetabolite α-aminopterin for posttransplant GVHD prevention. Methotrexate (MTX) has primarily been shown to be beneficial in dogs and monkeys, and cyclophosphamide showed promise in rats. Corticosteroids and ATG have also acquired a place in the clinical arena. In 1978, CSP was added (Powles *et al.*, 1980), and agents such as tacrolimus (FK-506)

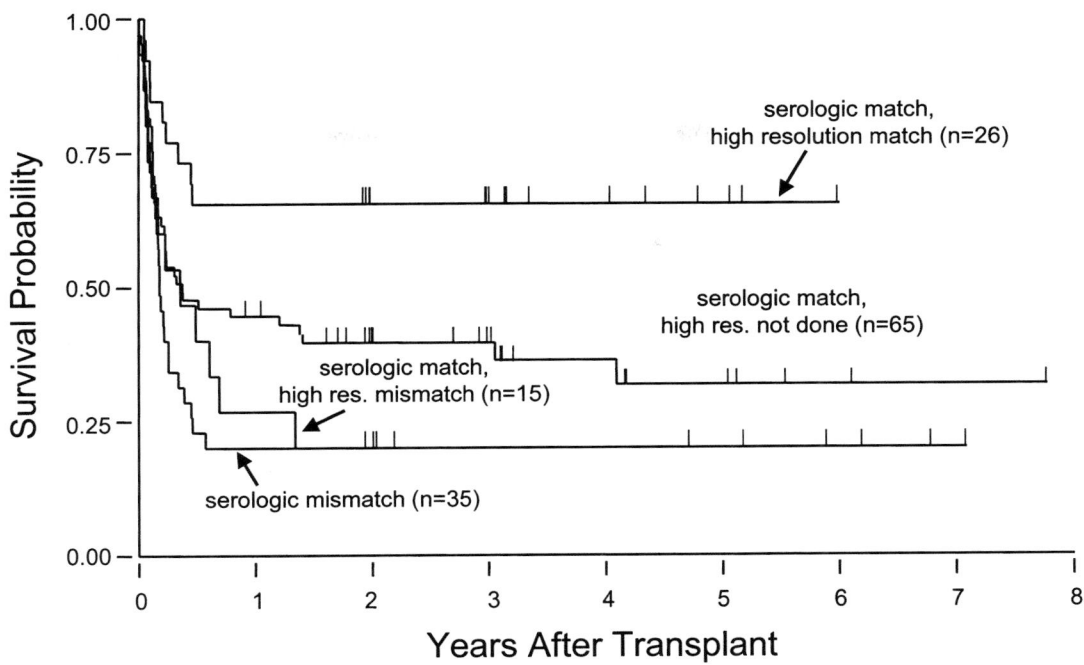

Fig. 71.6. Survival probability among 141 patients with aplastic anemia who had failed to achieve sustained responses to immunosuppressive therapy and were transplanted from unrelated volunteer donors. The figure illustrates the impact of the degree of HLA match between donor and patient on outcome. Thirteen patients died from acute, and 4 from chronic GVHD. HLA matching was a significant factor ($P = .006$) for the risk of death in multivariate analysis. Data from Deeg *et al.* (1999).

(Nash *et al.*, 1996, 2000), thalidomide, mycophenolate mofetil (MMF), and rapamycin (Sirolimus) (Table 71.7) or combinations of them have been added subsequently.

The mechanisms of action of these agents differ (and see Chapter 118). MTX, for example, blocks dihydrofolate reductase and prevents cell division and expansion of T cells already activated. Corticosteroids are lympholytic and mediate their effect via binding to the nucleus and repression of gene transcription; they also block IL-1 synthesis in APC and can induce apoptosis. CSP and tacrolimus bind to cyclophilin and FK binding protein (FKBP), respectively, and the resulting complexes interfere with the serine/threonine phosphatase calcineurin, thereby blocking the activity of transcription factors such as nuclear factor of activated T cells p (NF-ATp). This results in downregulation of IL-2 transcription (Pai *et al.*, 1994). Rapamycin also binds to FKBP (and in vitro, but not in vivo, is a competitive inhibitor of tacrolimus), but its target of interaction is the mammalian TOR protein. This interaction leads to p70 S6 kinase inactivation and inhibition of cell cycle progression in late G1 phase (Vander Woude & Bierer, 1997). MMF is activated to mycophenolic acid, which blocks inosine

Table 71.6. *Modalities of GVHD prevention*

Selection of histocompatible donors
T lymphocyte elimination or inactivation
 – in the donor marrow
 – in the patient posttransplant
Cytokine blockade
Gnotobiosis
Establishment of mixed chimerism (?)

Table 71.7. *Agents and modalities used for prevention and treatment of GVHD*

In Vivo	In Vivo or In Vitro	In Vitro
Methotrexate	Glucocorticoids	Elutriation
Cyclosporine	Monoclonal antibodies	Soybean and sheep red blood cell agglutination
Tacrolimus (FK-506)	Immunotoxins	Column fractionation
Mycophenolate mofetil	Phototherapy	
Rapamycin (Sirolimus)		
Anti-thymocyte globulin (ATG)		
Thalidomide		
Azathioprine		
Immunoglobulin		
Gnotobiosis		
Cytokine antagonists		
Receptor fusion proteins		
CTLA4Ig		
TNFR-Ig		

monophosphate dehydrogenase (IMPDH) and thereby interferes with purine biosynthesis (Hughes & Gruber, 1996).

CTLA4Ig, a fusion protein that interferes with co-stimulatory signals by blocking B7/CD28 and B7/CTLA4 interactions (Lin et al., 1994; Blazar et al., 1994), has been tested in small pilot trials. Blockade of CD28 signals is probably beneficial in the prevention of GVHD, whereas CTLA4 mediated signals facilitate the establishment of tolerance. Monoclonal antibodies to TNF or IL-2 or their receptors as well as the IL-1 antagonist IL-1RA block cytokine signals (Antin et al., 1994), although administration of the latter from day −4 to day +10 posttransplant did not prevent acute GVHD in a randomized double-blind, placebo-controlled tirla (Antin et al., 2002). Potentially

exciting developments involve the use of peptides with high affinity for MHC that block T-cell activation (Schlegel et al., 1996; Ferrara, 2000) and the polarization of CD4+ T cells from a TH1 to a TH2 phenotype (Krenger et al., 1995; Zeng, Dejbaktish–Jones, & Strober, 1997). Anti-CD40L monoclonal antibody (Blazar et al., 1997), anti-CD80 and anti-CD86 monoclonal antibodies (Blazar et al., 1996), anti-CD95L (FasL) monoclonal antibody (Hattori et al., 1998), anti-CD134L monoclonal antibody (Tsukada et al., 2000) (CD134 is an early activation antigen on T cells), TAK-603, a new quinolone that selectively suppresses TH1 cytokine production (Lu et al., 2001), a rationally designed Janus kinase (JAK) 3 inhibitor WHI-P131 (Cetkovic-Cvrlje et al., 2001), selective depletion

Table 71.8. *Drug combinations for GVHD prophylaxis*

Center (references)	Diagnosis	Regimen (no. of patients)	Incidence of acute GVHD[a]	P-value
Minneapolis (Ramsay et al., 1982)	Hematologic malignancies	MTX (35)	48%	$P = .01$
	Aplastic anemia	MTX+PDN+ATG (32)	21%	
Seattle (Storb et al., 1986b)	Acute and chronic myeloid leukemia	CSP (50)	54%	$P = .014$
		MTX+CSP (43)	33%	
Seattle (Storb et al., 1986a)	Aplastic anemia	MTX (24)	53%	$P = .012$
		MTX+CSP (22)	18%	
City of Hope (Forman et al., 1987)	Acute and chronic myeloid leukemia	MTX+PDN (53)	47%	$P \leq .05$
		CSP+PDN (54)	28%	
Baltimore (Santos et al., 1987)	Hematologic malignancies	CY+PDN (40)	68%	$P = .005$
	Aplastic anemia	CSP+PDN (42)	32%	
Stockholm (Tollemar et al., 1988)	Hematologic malignancies	CSP (45)	31%	$P = .02$
	Aplastic anemia	MTX (66)	25%	
		MTX+CSP (29)	8%	
Pesaro (Galimberti et al., 1988)	Thalassemia	CSP (22)	41%	$P \leq .05$
		CSP+CY+MTX (22)	15%	
Seattle (Sullivan et al., 1989)	Hematologic malignancies	Standard MTX (44)	25%	$P = .0001$
		Short MTX (40)	59%	
		Standard MTX+DBC (25)	82%	
Seattle (Storb et al., 1990)	Hematologic malignancies	MTX+CSP (74)	36%	$P = .28$
		MTX+CSP+PDN (73)	45%	
Stanford 1993 (Chao et al., 1993)	Hematologic malignancies	CSP+PDN (74)	23%	$P = .02$
		CSP+PDN+MTX (75)	9%	
Seattle 1997 (Deeg et al., 1997)	Hematologic malignancies	CSP (59)	74%	$P = .01$
		CSP+PDN (61)	60%	
Multicenter (Ratanatharathorn et al., 1998)	Hematologic malignancies	MTX+CSP (164)	44%	$P = .01$
		MTX+FK-506 (165)	32%	
Genoa (Zikos et al., 1998)	Acute myeloid leukemia	Low dose CSP (28)	61%	$P = .02$
		Low dose CSP+low dose MTX (32)	34% (No grade IV GVHD)	
Multicenter (Locatelli et al., 2000a)	Aplastic anemia	CSP (34)	38%	$P = NS$
		CSP+short MTX (37)	30%	
Helsinki (Ruutu et al., 2000)	Hematologic malignancies	MTX+CSP+PDN (53)	13%	$P = .005$
		MTX+CSP (55)	36%	
Multicenter (Nash et al., 2000)	Hematologic malignancies	Short MTX+FK-506 (90)	56%	$P = .0002$
	Aplastic anemia	Short MTX+CSP (90)	74%	
Multicenter (Hiraoka et al., 2001)	Hematologic malignancies	FK-506 (66)+MTX (56)	18%	$P \leq .0001$
	Aplastic anemia	CSP (65)+MTX (56)	48%	

Abbreviations: ATG, anti-thymocyte globulin; CSP, cyclosporine A; CY, cyclophosphamide; DBC, donor buffy coat; MTX, methotrexate; PDN, prednisone or other glucocorticoid; NS, not significant.
[a] GVHD grades II–IV

of host-reactive T cells by a photoactive rhodamine derivative (Chen *et al.*, 2002), donor pretreatment with interleukin-18 (Reddy *et al.*, 2003) and the use of a peptide exhibiting the same molecular surface as a portion of the CDR3-like region in domain 1 of the CD4 molecule (Townsend, Gilbert, & Korngold, 1998) all represent interesting developments.

There has never been a randomized study comparing GVHD prophylaxis with no prophylaxis in allogeneic transplant recipients. However, results of some single-arm studies have been reported, and there is agreement that prophylaxis is necessary and beneficial (Gale *et al.*, 1987). Until the early 1980s, the use of single agent (MTX or CSP) prophylaxis was considered standard (Deeg *et al.*, 1985; Chao & Deeg, 1997). Subsequently, however, two- or even three-drug combinations were tested (Storb *et al.*, 1986a, 1986b, 1989; Nash *et al.*, 1996, 2000) (Table 71.8). The different sites and mechanisms of action provide a rationale for the use of drug combinations, and results indicate that combinations such as MTX + CSP or tacrolimus + MTX offer more effective prophylaxis than any single agent. However, this improvement is not necessarily reflected in superior survival: a combination of MTX, CSP, and corticosteroids, for example, reduced the incidence of acute GVHD grades II to IV to 9%, but survival in this group of patients was identical to that seen in patients given CSP plus prednisone prophylaxis (Chao *et al.*, 1993). Combination regimens have also been associated with more toxicity, and in some trials have resulted in a higher probability of leukemic relapse (Aschan *et al.*, 1991). Conceivably, such an effect can be prevented by utilizing lower drug doses (Bacigalupo *et al.*, 1991; Carlens *et al.*, 1997; Locatelli *et al.*, 2000b). Of interest is also the observation that the addition of corticosteroids to CSP, while reducing

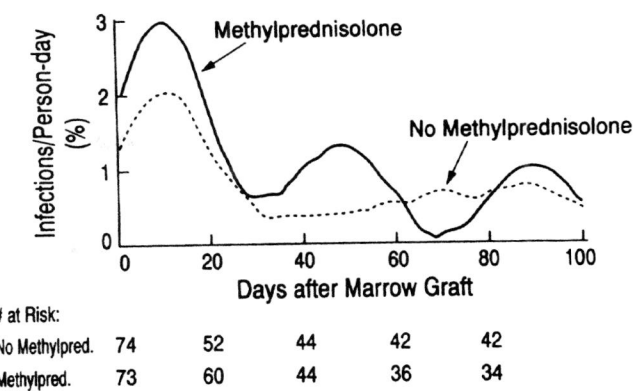

at Risk:

No Methylpred.	74	52	44	42	42
Methylpred.	73	60	44	36	34

Fig. 71.8. Rate of infection in patients receiving cyclosporine and methotrexate with (*n* = 73) and without (*n* = 74) methylprednisone as prophylaxis for acute GVHD. Patients are censored at onset of acute GVHD. A kernal estimator was used with an interval width of 15 days. Reproduced, with permission, from Sayer *et al.* (1994).

only slightly the incidence of acute GVHD, resulted in a substantial increase in the incidence of chronic GVHD (Deeg *et al.*, 1997) (Fig. 71.7). When added prophylactically to CSP + MTX, methylprednisolone was associated with an increased risk of infection (Sayer *et al.*, 1994) (Fig. 71.8). Three randomized trials comparing the combination of CSP + MTX with CSP, MTX, and methylprednisone, observed three different outcomes: in one study the addition of methylprednisolone increased the incidence of acute and chronic GVHD (Storb *et al.*, 1990); in another, there was no difference between the two arms (Atkinson *et al.*, 1991); and in the third, the addition of

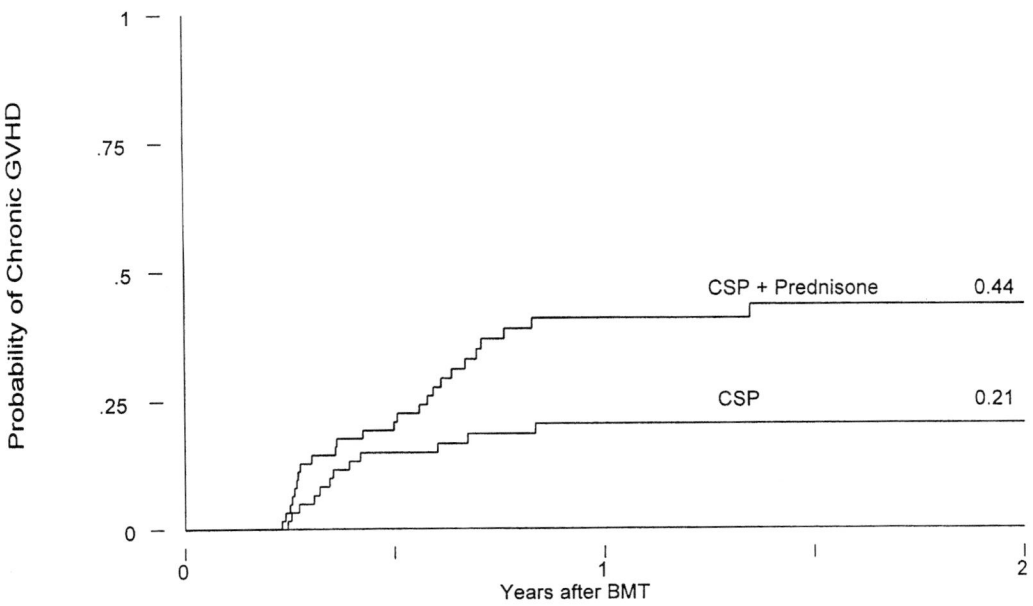

Fig. 71.7. Probability of chronic GVHD if given either cyclosporine (CSP) or CSP plus prednisone for acute GVHD prophylaxis (*P* = .03). Reproduced, with permission, from Deeg *et al.* (1997).

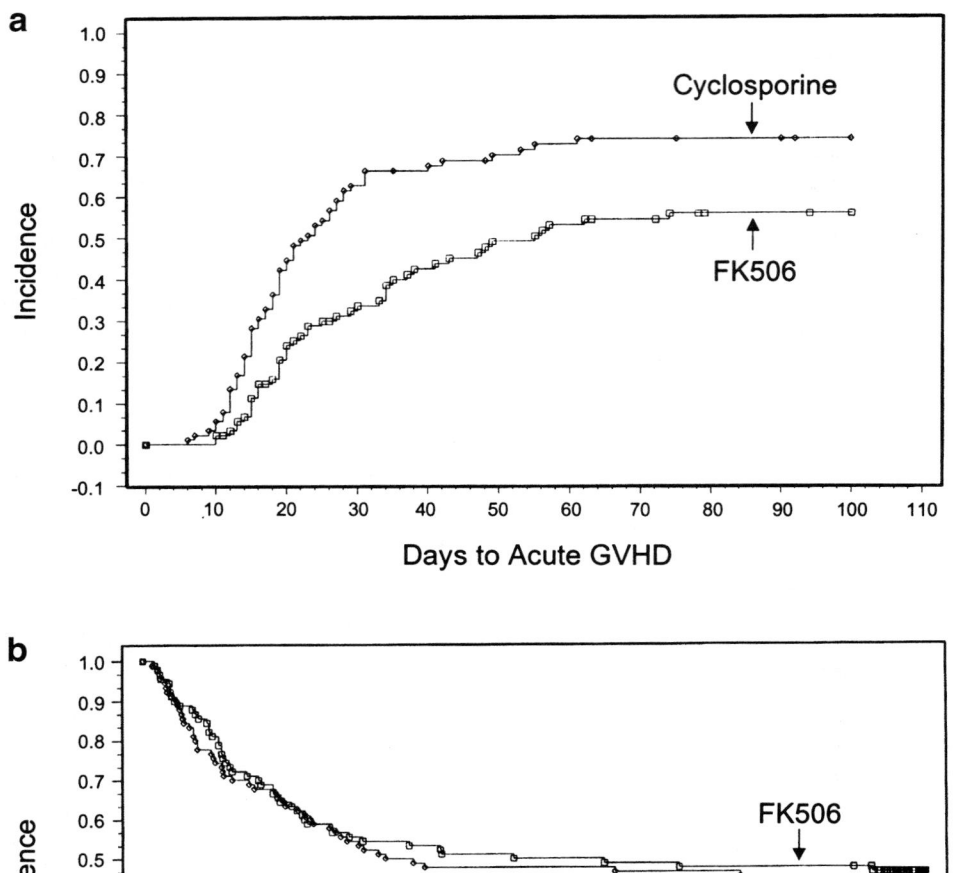

Fig. 71.9. GVHD prophylaxis with MTX combined with tacrolimus or CSP. **a)** Kaplan-Meier estimate of acute GVHD based on site investigator assessment (FK-506 [tacrolimus] + MTX, 56%; CSP + MTX, 74%; P = .0002). **b)** Kaplan-Meier estimate of relapse-free survival (FK-506 [tacrolimus] + MTX, 47%; CSP + MTX, 42%; P = .58). Reproduced, with permission, from Nash *et al.* (2000).

methylprednisolone reduced the incidence of acute GVHD (Ruutu, Volin, & Elonen, 1988). Presumably differences in outcome were related to differences in the timing of methylprednisolone administration (day 0 in the Storb and Atkinson studies versus day 14 in the Ruutu study), and CSP dosing. In a prospective, randomized multicenter trial, the combination of tacrolimus and MTX was significantly superior in preventing acute GVHD grades II–IV compared to CSP and MTX in recipients of T-replete, HLA-identical bone marrow transplants from unrelated donors (56% vs. 74%) (Nash *et al.,* 2000). The former combination also allowed a reduced use of corticosteroids in the management of GVHD. There was no difference

in the incidence of chronic GVHD, and overall survival did not differ between groups (Figure 71.9). A combination of sirolimus, tacrolimus and methotrexate has shown promise in a trial involving mismatched related donors and unrelated donors (Autin *et al.*, 2003).

T-cell depletion

The most effective method of GVHD prevention is the removal of T cells from the donor marrow or peripheral blood cells before infusion into the recipient (Martin & Kernan, 1997; Ho & Soiffer, 2001). T cell depletion is accomplished by physical sep-

Table 71.9. *T-cell depletion for GVHD prophylaxis*

Center (references)	Diagnosis (no. of patients)	Regimen (no. of patients)	Additional immunosuppression (no. of patients)	Incidence of acute GVHD[a]
London (Royal Free) (Prentice *et al.*, 1984)	Hematologic malignancies	Two anti-T cell antibodies + complement (14)	No	0%
London (Royal Free) (Prentice *et al.*, 1985)	Hematologic malignancies Thalassemia (1) Fanconi Anemia (1) Aplastic anemia (1)	Two anti-T cell antibodies + complement (41)	No	6%
Besançon (Hervé *et al.*, 1985)	Hematologic malignancies	OKT3 + OKT11 + complement (10)	MTX (10)	0%
Seattle (Martin *et al.*, 1985)	Hematologic malignancies	Eight anti-T cell antibodies (anti-CD2, CD3, CD4, CD5, CD6, CD8, Tp44) + complement (20)	CSP (20)	23% (No Grade III–IV)
UCLA (Mitsuyasu *et al.*, 1986)	Acute and chronic myeloid leukemia	Anti-T cell antibody (CT-2) + complement (20)	MTX or CSP	15%
		Control (MTX or CSP only) (20)		73% (*P* = .004)
Minnesota 1987 (Filipovich *et al.*, 1987)	Acute and chronic myeloid leukemia	Three anti-T cell antibodies (TA-1, anti-CD3, CD5) conjugated to ricin A (17)	No	24% (No Grade III–IV)
Multicenter (Racadot *et al.*, 1987)	Hematologic malignancies Aplastic anemia (1) Neuroblastoma (1)	Three anti-T cell antibodies (anti-CD2, CD5, CD7) + complement (62)	MTX (16) CSP (10)	8%
Johns Hopkins (Wagner *et al.*, 1988)	Hematologic malignancies	Counterflow elutriation (38)	CSP (38)	14%
Milwaukee (Ash *et al.*, 1990)	Hematologic malignancies Aplastic anemia (4) Immunodeficiency (3) Metabolic disorder (1)	Anti-CD3 + complement (55)	CSP (55)	46%
Multicenter (Hale & Waldmann, 1994)	Hematologic malignancies	Campath-1M, Campath-1G (alone or combined; in vitro and/or in vivo; ± complement) (951)	CSP (334) MTX/CSP (6) MTX (2)	0%–37%
UCLA (Nimer *et al.*, 1994)	Hematologic malignancies	Anti-CD8 + complement (19)	CSP (38)	20%
		Control (CSP only) (19)		80% (*P* = .004)
Columbia (Henslee-Downey *et al.*, 1996)	Hematologic malignancies Aplastic anemia Metabolic disorders (10)	Anti-TCR (in vitro), anti-CD5 ricin A (in vivo) + complement (40)	PDN (included in preparative regimen)	36%
Memorial Sloan Kettering (Papadopoulos *et al.*, 1998)	Acute myeloid leukemia	Soybean lectin agglutination + sheep red blood cell rosette depletion (39)	ATG + PDN (31) PDN (3) (as rejection prophylaxis)	0%
Multicenter (Champlin *et al.*, 2000)	Acute and chronic myeloid leukemia	Narrow-specificity antibodies (450) Broad-specificity antibodies (73) Campath-1 (131) Elutriation (75) Lectins + sheep red blood cell rosetting (141)	CSP ± other drugs (83%)	34%–38%
		Control (No T-cell depletion) (998)		57%
Dana Farber (Soiffer *et al.*, 2001)	Hematologic malignancies	Anti-CD6 + complement (48)	No	42%

Abbreviations: CSP = cyclosporine; MTX = methotrexate; PDN = prednisone or other glucocorticoid; TCR = T-cell receptor.
[a] GVHD grades II–IV.

aration, in the form of either positive (elimination of T cells) or negative selection (enrichment for hematopoietic precursor cells leaving T cells behind: lectin agglutination, counterflow elutriation, column fractionation, CD34 selection) (Ho & Soiffer, 2001). T cells are either killed by a toxin (e.g., ricin A chain) conjugated to anti-T cell antibody, or by incubating donor cells with antibody and complement, which then lyses the antibody-coated T cells. Some rat antibodies (e.g., Campath-1) do not require an exogenous source of complement as they activate the patient's own complement. These depletion procedures allow for 90% to 99.9% T-cell elimination (Table 71.9). A more selective approach involves depletion of donor T cells reactive with host tissues (alloreactive T cells) by sensitizing donor T cells to host tissues, and then depleting activated T cells that have been induced to express activation markers such as IL-2R, CD25, CD69, CD71, or HLA-DR (Harris *et al.*, 1999; van Dijk *et al.*, 1999; Fehse *et al.*, 2000). Another approach has tested the ex vivo incubation of donor marrow in the presence of host cells with CTL4Ig with the objective of blocking B7-mediated costimulation of T cells and to induce host alloantigen-specific anergy (Guinan *et al.*, 1999). A beneficial effect of such an approach was not confirmed in subsequent studies. It is clear now that blockade of CD28 signaling is desirable; however, CTLA4-mediated signals may actually facilitate the establishment of tolerance (Yu, Martin, & Anasetti, 1998; Yu *et al.*, 2000).

Unfortunately intensive GVHD prophylaxis, in particular T-cell depletion, may also cause problems (Fig. 71.10). For one, patients transplanted with donor marrow depleted of T cells by certain methods experience higher rates of graft failure than patients transplanted with unmanipulated cells. Subsets of T cells mediate a graft facilitating effect. A second concern is an increased incidence of relapse. This problem has been most prominent with chronic myeloid leukemia (Papadopoulos *et al.*, 1998). On this background, subsequent trials used selective

depletion of T-cell subsets, specifically CD4, CD6, or CD8 cells (Nimer *et al.*, 1994; Martin *et al.*, 1999; Soiffer *et al.*, 2001). Both approaches were compatible with donor cell engraftment. However, survival among patients so treated was not significantly different from that among patients transplanted with broadly T-cell–depleted marrow. Thus, while T-cell depletion leads to reduced morbidity and mortality related to GVHD, disease-free survival is not improved.

Conversely, patients who experience GVHD have a lower probability of leukemic relapse than patients without GVHD or patients given transplants from syngeneic donors (Sullivan *et al.*, 1989). Importantly, even patients given grafts from allogeneic donors who do not develop GVHD have a lower probability of relapse than patients transplanted from syngeneic donors. However, attempts in clinical trials to separate GVHD from a GVL effect have, so far, been unsuccessful (Truitt & Atasoylu, 1991).

On the other hand, Kolb *et al.* (Kolb, 1999) were the first to show that patients who experienced a relapse of CML after allogeneic marrow transplantation frequently were re-induced into remission with the infusion of viable leukocytes from the original transplant donor. While the development of acute GVHD and marrow aplasia, presumably also a manifestation of GVHD, were frequent problems, remissions were also observed in patients who did not have clinical evidence of GVHD.

Another approach of T-cell engineering is aimed at preserving functional T cells to assure engraftment and provide a GVL effect but then eliminate those cells if evidence of GVHD develops. This involves the transduction of donor lymphocytes with a so-called suicide gene (e.g., the Herpes simplex virus thymidine kinase). GVHD can be abrogated by inactivating the cells via the suicide gene (e.g., by treatment with ganciclovir) (Munshi *et al.*, 1997). Limited clinical results have been reported (Bonini *et al.*, 1997; Tiberghien *et al.*, 2001).

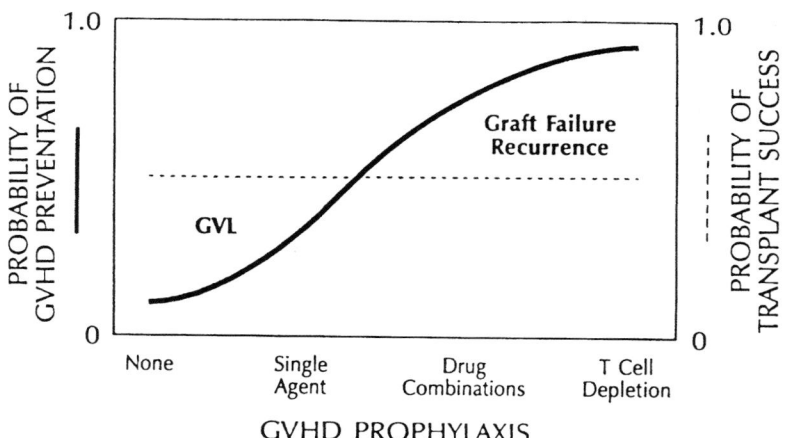

Fig. 71.10. Interrelationship of GVHD, graft-versus-leukemia effect (GVL), GVHD prophylaxis, failure of engraftment, and recurrence of leukemia. With omission of or with only moderately effective GVHD prophylaxis there is a high probability of GVHD (solid line), white failure of engraftment and incidence of leukemic relapse are infrequent; more aggressive regimens provide more effective GVHD prophylaxis, but are associated with an increased probability of graft failure or disease recurrence. The endpoint, survival (broken line), may be similar.

Reduced-intensity conditioning and mixed chimerism

Anecdotal clinical reports suggested that GVHD may be less frequent in patients who transiently or permanently become mixed chimeras (i.e., maintain concurrently normal lymphohematopoietic cells of donor and host origin). Experimental studies in mice showed that mixed chimerism can be achieved by design without jeopardizing the eradication of leukemia (Sykes, 2001). Experiments in a canine model show similarly that mixed chimerism without the development of GVHD is achieved in recipients conditioned with only 200 cGy of TBI, transplanted with histocompatible marrow and given postgrafting immunosuppression with CSP and MMF (Storb et al., 1997). In the clinical arena, this led to the development of transplant regimens which use low-intensity conditioning, with fludarabine and low-dose (200 cGy) TBI or other combinations, and posttransplant immunosuppression, e.g. with CSP or MMF, primarily to avoid early posttransplant toxicity and mortality, but still with the objective of achieving engraftment of donor cells (Maris et al., 2001) (see Chapter 22).

Results to date indicate that this approach does *not* prevent GVHD in humans, with as many as 50% developing the disease. It is of note, however, that the manifestations in many patients are less severe, and may become clinically apparent only 3, 4, or 5 months posttransplant, i.e., later than generally seen in patients conditioned with conventional regimens. It also appears that patients so treated are difficult to taper off steroids. These observations underline the point emphasized earlier, that the historical classification of acute and chronic GVHD requires modifications that consider the kinetics of the disease (Fig. 71.3).

Gnotobiosis

Gnotobiosis, i.e., the maintenance of transplant recipients in a germ-free environment, while extremely successful in mice, has been less effective in clinical studies, presumably because of difficulties with complete decontamination of the patients. Nevertheless, in patients with severe aplastic anemia (conditioned with cyclophosphamide only) (Storb et al., 1983; Vossen, 1990) transplanted in laminar airflow isolation, the incidence of GVHD was reduced, and survival improved. Some investigators have further pursued this technique in larger studies in patients with malignant disorders, and have reported improved outcome (Beelen et al., 1999).

Therapy

Dependent upon numerous factors, including the donor/patient relationship, degree of HLA match, source of stem cells, patient age, intensity of the conditioning regimen, and type of GVHD prophylaxis, some 10% to 90% of patients develop acute GVHD requiring therapy. Effective treatment is important since the probability of survival depends upon the response to therapy (Martin et al., 1990, 1991) (Fig. 71.11). Many drugs used for GVHD prevention also serve for treatment of GVHD (Table 71.7). In fact,

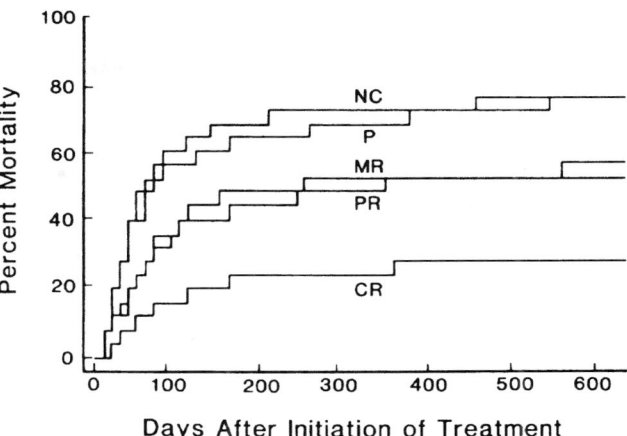

Fig. 71.11. Nonrelapse mortality of patients categorized according to treatment outcome. CR, complete response; PR, partial response; MR, mixed response; NC, no change; P, progression (*P* < .0001 for equality among groups). Reproduced, with permission, from Martin et al. (1990).

many agents were first tested as therapy before being administered as prophylaxis. Generally, these drugs are more effective for prevention, presumably because of limited activation of donor cells in the early phases of GVHD. Furthermore, our understanding of the effector limb of the GVH reaction is rather incomplete, rendering rational design of treatment regimens difficult.

Corticosteroids (for example methylprednisolone, 2 mg/kg/day for 14 days or longer) are the mainstay of acute GVHD therapy. Lysis of lymphocytes during interphase and anti-inflammatory effects may lead to prompt improvement. Complete responses occur in 20%, and useful responses overall in about 40% to 50% of patients with grades II to IV acute GVHD. A prospective randomized study comparing 2 mg/kg/day of methylprednisolone to 10 mg/kg/day failed to show any advantage of the higher dose for any end point studied (Van Lint et al., 1998). "Non-absorbable" oral beclamethasone is effective in a proportion of patients to treat acute intestinal GVHD (McDonald et al., 1998; Bertz et al., 1999).

CSP has been used with some success therapeutically in patients who had not received CSP prophylaxis. Tacrolimus, with a mechanism of action similar to CSP, provides effective therapy in some patients who have failed CSP prophylaxis (Ohashi et al., 1997), although a retrospective analysis suggested a true benefit only in patients who had developed CNS toxicity on CSP (Furlong et al., 2000). A combination of tacrolimus and ATG has yielded promising results in one study (Mollee et al., 2001). MMF and rapamycin (sirolimus), both tested extensively in organ transplant recipients, have been introduced in the treatment of acute GVHD. MMF might be effective in some patients in combination with CSP and prednisolone (Basara et al., 1998). A trial with rapamycin in 21 patients showed a response rate of more than 50%, and suggested improved survival compared to historic controls (Benito et al., 2001).

ATG of horse or rabbit origin are potent anti-T cell agents, achieving responses in 20–30% of patients even after steroid

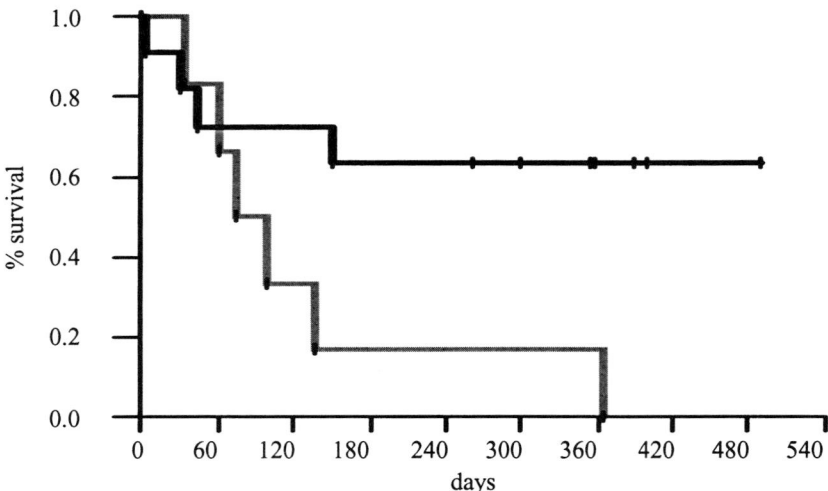

Fig. 71.12. Kaplan-Meier probability of overall survival of patients with acute glucocorticoid-refractory GVHD. Survival after therapy with visilizumab is shown separately for patients treated on a single-dose (solid line, *n* = 11) and on a multidose (striped line [lower curve], *n* = 6) regimen (*P* = .03). Reproduced, with permission, from Carpenter *et al.* (2002).

failure (Storb *et al.,* 1974; Martin *et al.,* 1991; MacMillan *et al.,* 2002). Various different dose regimens have so far been reported (Hsu *et al.,* 2001). However, infections and thrombocytopenia are common complications, and in some trials, patient survival was as low as 5–10% (Khoury *et al.,* 1999; Aral *et al.* 2002).

A broad array of monoclonal antibodies in murine or humanized form, with pan T or T-subset reactivity has been used, often as secondary therapy of GVHD, in patients not responding to corticosteroids. Responses, sometimes sustained, are observed with anti-CD2, anti-CD3, anti-CD5 and other antibodies (Martin *et al.,* 1984; Hebart *et al.,* 1995; Przepiorka *et al.,* 1998). In a trial using the anti-CD147 antibody ABX-CBL, more than half of the patients with steroid-refractory acute GVHD responded, and survival was superior to that observed in a historical comparison group treated with horse ATG (Deeg *et al.,* 2001). Intriguing results have been obtained with a humanized antibody, HuM291 or visilizumab (directed at the T-cell receptor zeta chain), by Carpenter *et al.* (2002). Among 15 patients with steroid-refractory GVHD, 7 and 8 achieved complete and partial response, respectively (Fig 71.12). Of note was that sustained responses were achieved with a single dose of antibody. Many patients experienced a rise in plasma titers of EBV DNA which was controlled following the administration of anti-CD 20 antibody, rituximab.

Another treatment strategy involves antibodies against cytokine receptors. A monoclonal antibody to the IL-2R (B-B10) was found to be effective experimentally and clinically (Hervé *et al.,* 1990). Pilot trials using a genetically engineered humanized monoclonal antibody specific for Tac, the alpha subunit of the IL-2R (anti- Tac, dacluzimab), in patients who had failed to respond to corticosteroids showed responses in about 40% of patients (Anasetti *et al.,* 1994; Przepiorka *et al.,* 2000). A pilot trial with basiliximab, a chimeric antibody to the IL-2 receptor alpha chain, showed a complete response rate of 53% (Masenkell *et al.,* (2002). Experimental data suggest that blockade of other recep-

tors may also be beneficial. One clinical report suggested efficacy of an anti-TNF-α monoclonal antibody (infliximab) in steroid-refractory acute GVHD (Kobbe *et al.,* 2001). This approach should be used cautiously, however, as a high incidence of tuberculosis reactivation was noted in patients with autoimmune diseases treated with this agent (Keane *et al.,* 2001). Toxin-conjugated monoclonal antibodies have also shown encouraging results (van Oosterhout *et al.,* 2000), although only a marginally significant effect was observed in a randomized trial with a ricin A-conjugated anti-CD5 antibody (Martin *et al.,* 1996).

PUVA treatment (photosensitization with 8-methoxypsoralen and UVA irradiation) is effective in the treatment of acute and chronic GVHD of the skin in some patients. Extracorporeal exposure of the recipient's peripheral blood mononuclear cells to the photosensitizing effect of 8-methoxypsoralen and UV light and their subsequent reinfusion is effective in treating acute (and chronic) GVHD refractory to conventional treatment (Besnier *et al.,* 1997; Dall'Amico *et al.,* 1997; Greinix *et al.,* 2000).

Future considerations

Future attempts at prophylaxis and therapy are likely to exploit results derived from ongoing research in cellular and molecular biology. The genetic cloning of receptors for multiple growth factors and for cell surface proteins will allow new insights into cell proliferation (for example, CD28 and CTLA4) and migration. The availability of small molecules that block antigen presentation, lymphocyte activation, or both will be further advanced by the identification of peptides that are critical to receptor function. The discovery of cytosolic proteins that control protein folding and lymphocyte activation is likely to provide the rationale for the use of additional drugs that interfere with these processes. Gene transfer technology may allow the transfer of host histocompatibility genes into donor cells, thereby possibly generating a tool for tolerance induction. The role of CD25$^+$CD4$^+$ regulatory T cells remains to be defined in the clinical setting. Important are also the observations by Ruggeri et al. showing that with appropriate conditioning, T-cell depletion and mismatching for the relevant KIR ligands HLA non-identical stem cells can be transplanted successfully and without the development of GVHD (Ruggeri et al., 1999).

References

Anasetti, C., Beatty, P. G., Storb, R. et al. (1990). Effect of HLA incompatibility on graft-versus-host disease, relapse, and survival after marrow transplantation for patients with leukemia or lymphoma. *Human Immunology*, **29**, 79–91.

Anasetti, C., Doney, K. C., Storb, R. et al. (1986). Marrow transplantation for severe aplastic anemia: long term outcome in fifty "untransfused" patients. *Annals of Internal Medicine*, **104**, 461–466.

Anasetti, C., Hansen, J. A., Waldmann, T. A. et al. (1994). Treatment of acute graft-versus-host disease with humanized anti-Tac: an antibody that binds to the interleukin-2 receptor. *Blood*, **84**, 1320–1327.

Anderson, J. E., Tefferi, A., Craig, F. et al. (2001). Myeloablation and autologous peripheral blood stem cell rescue results in hematologic and clinical responses in patients with myeloid metaplasia with myelofibrosis. *Blood*, **98**, 586–593.

Antin, J. H., Kim, H. T., Cutler, C. et al. (2003). Sirolimus, tacrolimus, and low-dose methotrexate for graft-versus-host disease prophylaxis in mismatched related donor or unrelated donor transplantation. *Blood*, in press.

Antin, J. H., Weinstein, H. J., Guinan, E. C. et al. (1994). Recombinant human interleukin-1 receptor antagonist in the treatment of steroid-resistant graft-versus-host disease. *Blood*, **84**, 1342–1348.

Apperley, J. F. (1994). Umbilical cord blood progenitor cell transplantation. The International Conference Workshop on Cord Blood Transplantation, Indianapolis, November 1993 [see comments]. *Bone Marrow Transplantation*, **14**, 187–196.

Aschan, J., Ringden, O., Sundberg, B. et al. (1991). Methotrexate combined with cyclosporin A decreases graft-versus-host disease, but increases leukemic relapse compared to monotherapy. *Bone Marrow Transplantation*, **7**, 113–119.

Ash, R. C., Casper, J. T., Chitambar, C. R. et al. (1990). Successful allogeneic transplantation of T-cell-depleted bone marrow from closely HLA-matched unrelated donors. *New England Journal of Medicine*, **322**, 485–494.

Atkinson, K., Biggs, J., Concannon, A. et al. (1991). A prospective randomised trial of cyclosporin and methotrexate versus cyclosporin, methotrexate and prednisolone for prevention of graft-versus-host disease after HLA-identical sibling marrow transplantation for haematological malignancy. *Australian and New Zealand Journal of Medicine*, **21**, 850–856.

Atkinson, K., Farrell, C., Chapman, G. et al. (1986). Female marrow donors increase the risk of acute graft-versus-host disease: Effect of donor age and parity and analysis of cell subpopulations in the donor marrow inoculum. *British Journal of Haematology*, **63**, 231–239.

Atkinson, K., Horowitz, M. M., Gale, R. P. et al. (1989). Consensus among bone marrow transplanters for diagnosis, grading and

treatment of chronic graft-versus-host disease. *Bone Marrow Transplantation*, **4**, 247–254.

Bacigalupo, A., Soracco, M., Vassallo, F. et al. (1997). Donor lymphocyte infusions (DLI) in patients with chronic myeloid leukemia following allogeneic bone marrow transplantation. *Bone Marrow Transplantation*, **19**, 927–932.

Bacigalupo, A., Van Lint, M. T., Occhini, D. et al. (1991). Increased risk of leukemia relapse with high-dose cyclosporine A after allogeneic marrow transplantation for acute leukemia. *Blood*, **77**, 1423–1428.

Baker, M. B., Riley, R. L., Podack, E. R., & Levy, R. B. (1997). Graft-versus-host-disease-associated lymphoid hypoplasia and B cell dysfunction is dependent upon donor T cell-mediated Fas-ligand function, but not perforin function. *Proceedings of the National Academy of Sciences of the United States of America*, **94**, 1366–1371.

Balduini, C. L., Frassoni, F., Noris, P. et al. (2001). Donor-recipient incompatibility at CD31-codon 563 is a major risk factor for acute graft-versus-host disease after allogeneic bone marrow transplantation from a human leucocyte antigen-matched donor. *British Journal of Haematology*, **114**, 951–953.

Basara, N., Blau, W. I., Romer, E. et al. (1998). Mycophenolate mofetil for the treatment of acute and chronic GVHD in bone marrow transplant patients. *Bone Marrow Transplantation*, **22**, 61–65.

Beatty, P. G., Clift, R. A., Mickelson, E. M. et al. (1985). Marrow transplantation from related donors other than HLA-identical siblings. *New England Journal of Medicine*, **313**, 765–771.

Beatty, P. G., Anasetti, C., Hansen, J. A. et al. (1993). Marrow transplantation from unrelated donors for treatment of hematologic malignancies: effect of mismatching for one HLA locus. *Blood*, **81**, 249–253.

Beelen, D. W., Elmaagacli, A., Muller, K. D., Hirche, H., & Schaefer, U. W. (1999). Influence of intestinal bacterial decontamination using metronidazole and ciprofloxacin or ciprofloxacin alone on the development of acute graft-versus-host disease after marrow transplantation in patients with hematologic malignancies: final results and long-term follow-up of an open-label prospective randomized trial. *Blood*, **93**, 3267–3275.

Benito, A. I., Furlong, T., Martin, P. J. et al. (2001). Sirolimus (rapamycin) for the treatment of steroid-refractory acute graft-versus-host disease. *Transplantation*, **72**, 1924–1929.

Bensinger, W. I., Clift, R., Martin, P. et al. (1996). Allogeneic peripheral blood stem cell transplantation in patients with advanced hematologic malignancies: a retrospective comparison with marrow transplantation. *Blood*, **88**, 2794–2800.

Bensinger, W. I., Martin, P. J., Storer, B. et al. (2001). Transplantation of bone marrow as compared with peripheral-blood cells from HLA-identical relatives in patients with hematologic cancers. *New England Journal of Medicine*, **344**, 175–181.

Bertz, H., Afting, M., Kreisel, W. et al. (1999). Feasibility and response to budesonide as topical corticosteroid therapy for acute intestinal GVHD. *Bone Marrow Transplantation*, **24**, 1185–1189.

Besnier, D. P., Chabannes, D., Mahé, B. et al. (1997). Treatment of graft-versus-host disease by extracorporeal photochemotherapy: a pilot study. *Transplantation*, **64**, 49–54.

Billingham, R. E. (1966). The biology of graft-versus-host reactions. In *The Harvey Lectures*, pp. 21–78. New York: Academic Press.

Blazar, B. R., Sharpe, A. H., Taylor, P. A. *et al.* (1996). Infusion of anti-B7.1 (CD80) and anti-B7.2 (CD86) monoclonal antibodies inhibits murine graft-versus-host disease lethality in part via direct effects on CD4+ and CD8+ T cells. *Journal of Immunology*, **157**, 3250–3259.

Blazar, B. R., Taylor, P. A., Linsley, P. S., & Vallera, D. A. (1994). In vivo blockade of CD28/CTLA4: B7/BB1 interaction with CTLA4-Ig reduces lethal murine graft-versus-host disease across the major histocompatibility complex barrier in mice. *Blood*, **83**, 3815–3825.

Blazar, B. R., Taylor, P. A., Panoskaltsis-Mortari, A. *et al.* (1997). Blockade of CD40 ligand-CD40 interaction impairs CD4+ T cell-mediated alloreactivity by inhibiting mature donor T cell expansion and function after bone marrow transplantation. *Journal of Immunology*, **158**, 29–39.

Bonini, C., Ferrari, G., Verzeletti, S. *et al.* (1997). HSV-TK gene transfer into donor lymphocytes for control of allogeneic graft-versus-leukemia. *Science*, **276**, 1719–1724.

Brentjens, R. J., Smith, L., Reich, L., & Jakubowski, A. A. (2001). Development of spontaneous factor VIII inhibitor in association with acute graft-versus-host disease. *Bone Marrow Transplantation*, **27**, 887–889.

Broers, A.E.C., van der holt, R., van Esser, J.W.J. *et al.* (2000). Increased transplant-related morbidity and mortality in CMV-seropositive patients despite highly effective prevention of CMV disease after allogeneic T-cell-depleted stem cell transplantation. *Blood*, **95**, 2240–2245.

Broxmeyer, H. E. & Smith, F. O. (1999). Cord blood stem cell transplantation. In *Hematopoietic Cell Transplantation, 2nd Edition*, ed. E. D. Thomas, K. G. Blume & S. J. Forman, pp. 431–443. Boston: Blackwell Science.

Buhlmann, J. E., Gonzalez, M., Ginther, B. *et al.* (1999). Cutting edge: sustained expansion of CD8+ T cells requires CD154 expression by Th cells in acute graft versus host disease. *Journal of Immunology*, **162**, 4373–4376.

Carlens, S., Ringden, O., Remberger, M. *et al.* (1997). Factors affecting risk of relapse and leukemia-free survival in HLA-identical sibling marrow transplant recipients with leukemia. *Transplantation Proceedings*, **29**, 3147–3149.

Carpenter, P. A., Appelbaum, F. R., Corey, L. *et al.* (2002). A humanized non-FcR-binding anti-CD3 antibody, visilizumab, for treatment of steroid-refractory acute graft-versus-host disease. *Blood*, **99**, 2712–2719.

Cavet, J., Dickinson, A. M., Norden, J. *et al.* (2001). Interferon-gamma and interleukin-6 gene polymorphisms associate with graft-versus-host disease in HLA-matched sibling bone marrow transplantation. *Blood*, **98**, 1594–1600.

Cavet, J., Middleton, P. G., Segall, M. *et al.* (1999). Recipient tumor necrosis factor-alpha and interleukin-10 gene polymorphisms associate with early mortality and acute graft-versus-host disease severity in HLA-matched sibling bone marrow transplants. *Blood*, **94**, 3941–3946.

Cetkovic-Cvrlje, M., Roers, B. A., Waurzyniak, B., Liu, X. P., & Uckun, F. M. (2001). Targeting Janus kinase 3 to attenuate the severity of acute graft-versus-host disease across the major histocompatibility barrier in mice. *Blood*, **98**, 1607–1613.

Champlin, R. E., Passweg, J. R., Zhang, M. J. *et al.* (2000). T-cell depletion of bone marrow transplants for leukemia from donors other than HLA-identical siblings: advantage of T-cell antibodies with narrow specificities. *Blood*, **95**, 3996–4003.

Chao, N. J. & Deeg, H. J. (1997). In vivo prevention and treatment of GVHD. In *Graft-vs.-Host Disease, 2nd Edition*, ed. J.L.M. Ferrara, H. J. Deeg & S. Burakoff, pp. 639–666. New York: Marcel Dekker, Inc.

Chao, N. J., Schmidt, G. M., Niland, J. C. *et al.* (1993). Cyclosporine, methotrexate, and prednisone compared with cyclosporine and prednisone for prophylaxis of acute graft-versus-host disease. *New England Journal of Medicine*, **329**, 1225–1230.

Chen, B. J., Cui, X., Liu, C. & Chao, N. J. (2003). Prevention of graft-versus-host disease while preserving graft-versus-leukemia effect after selective depletion of host-reactive T cells by photo-dynamic cell purging process. *Blood*, **99**, 3083–8.

Clark, R. E., Hermans, J., Madrigal, A. *et al.* (2001). HLA-A3 increases and HLA-DR1 decreases the risk of acute graft-versus-host disease after HLA-matched sibling bone marrow transplantation for chronic myelogenous leukaemia. *British Journal of Haematology*, **114**, 36–41.

Collins, R. H., Jr., Shpilberg, O., Drobyski, W. R. *et al.* (1997). Donor leukocyte infusions in 140 patients with relapsed malignancy after allogeneic bone marrow transplantation. *Journal of Clinical Oncology*, **15**, 433–444.

Cooke, K., Olkiewicz, K., Clouthier, S., Liu, C., & Ferrara, J.L.M. (2001). Critical role for CD14 and the innate immune response in the induction of experimental acute graft-versus-host disease. *Blood*, **98** (Suppl. 1), 776a (Abstract).

Cullup, H., Dickinson, A. M., Jackson, G. H. *et al.* (2001). Donor interleukin 1 receptor antagonist genotype associated with acute graft-versus-host disease in human leucocyte antigen-matched sibling allogeneic transplants. *British Journal of Haematology*, **113**, 807–813.

Cutler, C., Giri, S., Jeyapalan, S. *et al.* (2001). Acute and chronic graft-versus-host disease after allogeneic peripheral-blood stem-cell and bone marrow transplantation: A meta-analysis. *Journal of Clinical Oncology*, **19**, 3685–3691.

Dall'Amico, R., Rossetti, F., Zulian, F. *et al.* (1997). Photopheresis in paediatric patients with drug-resistant chronic graft-versus-host disease. *British Journal of Haematology*, **97**, 848–854.

Das, H., Imoto, S., Murayama, T. *et al.* (1999). Levels of soluble FasL and FasL gene expression during the development of graft-versus-host disease in DLT-treated patients. *British Journal of Haematology*, **104**, 795–800.

Deeg, H. J. (2001). Cytokines in graft-versus-host disease and the graft-versus-leukemia reaction. *International Journal of Hematology*, **74**, 26–32.

Deeg, H. J., Blazar, B. R., Bolwell, B. J. *et al.* (2001). Treatment of steroid-refractory acute graft-versus-host disease with anti-CD147 monoclonal antibody, ABX-CBL. *Blood*, **98**, 2052–2058.

Deeg, H. J., Lin, D., Leisenring, W. *et al.* (1997). Cyclosporine or cyclosporine plus methylprednisolone for prophylaxis of graft-versus-host disease: a prospective, randomized trial. *Blood*, **89**, 3880–3887.

Deeg, H. J., Seidel, K., Casper, J. *et al.* (1999). Marrow transplantation from unrelated donors for patients with severe aplastic anemia who have failed immunosuppressive therapy. *Biology of Blood and Marrow Transplantation*, **5**, 243–252.

Deeg, H. J., Spitzer, T. R., Cottler-Fox, M., Cahill, R., & Pickle, L. W. (1991). Conditioning-related toxicity and acute graft-versus-host disease in patients given methotrexate/cyclosporine prophylaxis. *Bone Marrow Transplantation*, **7**, 193–198.

Deeg, H. J., Storb, R., Thomas, E. D. *et al.* (1985). Cyclosporine as prophylaxis for graft-versus-host disease: A randomized study in patients undergoing marrow transplantation for acute nonlymphoblastic leukemia. *Blood*, **65**, 1325–1334.

Dreger, P. & Schmitz, N. (1999). Allogeneic transplantation of peripheral blood stem cells. *Baillière's Best Practice in Clinical Haematology*, **12**, 261–278.

Fehse, B., Frerk, O., Goldmann, M., Bulduk, M., & Zander, A. R. (2000). Efficient depletion of alloreactive donor T lymphocytes based on expression of two activation-induced antigens (CD25 and CD69). *British Journal of Haematology*, **109**, 644–651.

Ferrara, J. L. (2000). Pathogenesis of acute graft-versus-host disease: cytokines and cellular effectors (Review). *Journal of Hematotherapy & Stem Cell Research*, **9**, 299–306.

Ferrara, J. L., Levy, R., & Chao, N. J. (1999). Pathophysiologic mechanisms of acute graft-vs.-host disease (Review). *Biology of Blood and Marrow Transplantation*, **5**, 347–356.

Filipovich, A. H., Vallera, D. A., Youle, R. J. *et al.* (1987). Graft-versus-host disease prevention in allogeneic bone marrow transplantation from histocompatible siblings. *Transplantation*, **44**, 62–69.

Flowers, M.E.D., Pepe, M. S., Longton, G. *et al.* (1990). Previous donor pregnancy as a risk factor for acute graft-versus-host disease in patients with aplastic anaemia treated by allogeneic marrow transplantation. *British Journal of Haematology*, **74**, 492–496.

Forman, S. J., Blume, K. G., Krance, R. A. *et al.* (1987). A prospective randomized study of acute graft-v-host disease in 107 patients with leukemia: methotrexate/prednisone v cyclosporine A/prednisone. *Transplantation Proceedings*, **19**, 2605–2607.

Fujii, N., Takenaka, K., Shinagawa, K. *et al.* (2001). Hepatic graft-versus-host disease presenting as an acute hepatitis after allogeneic peripheral blood stem cell transplantation. *Bone Marrow Transplantation*, **27**, 1007–10.

Fujimori, Y., Takatsuka, H., Takemoto, Y. *et al.* (2000). Elevated interleukin (IL)-18 levels during acute graft-versus-host disease after allogeneic bone marrow transplantation. *British Journal of Haematology*, **109**, 652–657.

Furlong, T., Storb, R., Anasetti, C. *et al.* (2000). Clinical outcome after conversion to FK 506 (tacrolimus) therapy for acute graft-versus-host disease resistant to cyclosporine or for cyclosporine-associated toxicities. *Bone Marrow Transplantation*, **26**, 985–991.

Gale, R. P., Bortin, M. M., van Bekkum, D. W. *et al.* (1987). Risk factors for acute graft-versus-host disease. *British Journal of Haematology*, **67**, 397–406.

Galimberti, M., Polchi, P., Lucarelli, G. *et al.* (1988). A comparative trial of posttransplant immunosuppression in patients transplanted for thalassemia. Cyclosporine alone versus cyclosporine, cyclophosphamide, and methotrexate. *Transplantation*, **45**, 566–569.

Ghayur, T., Seemayer, T. A., & Lapp, W. S. (1990). Histologic correlates of immune functional deficits in graft-vs.-host disease. In *Graft-vs.-Host Disease: Immunology, Pathophysiology, and Treatment*, ed. S. J. Burakoff, H. J. Deeg, J. Ferrara & K. Atkinson, pp. 109–132. New York: Marcel Dekker, Inc.

Gluckman, E., Broxmeyer, H. E., Auerbach, A. D. *et al.* (1989). Hematopoietic reconstitution in a patient with Fanconi's anemia by means of umbilical-cord blood from an HLA-identical sibling. *New England Journal of Medicine*, **321**, 1174–1178.

Gluckman, E., Rocha, V., Boyer-Chammard, A. *et al.* (1997). Outcome of cord-blood transplantation from related and unrelated donors. *New England Journal of Medicine*, **337**, 373–381.

Glucksberg, H., Storb, R., Fefer, A. *et al.* (1974). Clinical manifestations of graft-versus-host disease in human recipients of marrow from HLA-matched sibling donors. *Transplantation*, **18**, 295–304.

Graubert, T. A., DiPersio, J. F., Russell, J. H., & Ley, T. J. (1997). Perforin/granzyme-dependent and independent mechanisms are both important for the development of graft-versus-host disease after murine bone marrow transplantation. *Journal of Clinical Investigation*, **100**, 904–911.

Greinix, H. T., Volc-Platzer, B., Kalhs, P. *et al.* (2000). Extracorporeal photochemotherapy in the treatment of severe steroid-refractory acute graft-versus-host disease: a pilot study. *Blood*, **96**, 2426–2431.

Grumet, F. C., Hiraki, D. D., Brown, B.W.M. *et al.* (2001). CD31 mismatching affects marrow transplantation outcome. *Biology of Blood and Marrow Transplantation*, **7**, 503–512.

Guinan, E. C., Boussiotis, V. A., Neuberg, D. *et al.* (1999). Transplantation of anergic histoincompatible bone marrow allografts. *New England Journal of Medicine*, **340**, 1704–1714.

Hagglund, H., Bostrom, L., Ringden, O., Nilsson, B., & Remberger, M. (1994). Risk factors for acute graft-versus-host disease in 325 consecutive bone marrow recipients. *Transplantation Proceedings*, **26**, 1821–1822.

Hale, G. & Waldmann, H. (1994). Control of graft-versus-host disease and graft rejection by T cell depletion of donor and recipient with Campath-1 antibodies. Results of matched sibling transplants for malignant diseases. *Bone Marrow Transplantation*, **13**, 597–611.

Harris, D. T., Sakiestewa, D., Lyons, C., Kreitman, R. J., & Pastan, I. (1999). Prevention of graft-versus-host disease (GVHD) by elimination of recipient-reactive donor T cells with recombinant toxins that target the interleukin 2 (IL-2) receptor. *Bone Marrow Transplantation*, **23**, 137–144.

Hattori, H., Matsuzuki, A., Suminoe, A. *et al.* (2002). Polymorphisms of transforming growth factor-β 1 and transforming growth factor-β 1 type II receptor genes are associated with acute graft-versus-host disease in children with HLA-matched sibling bone marrow transplantation. *Bone Marrow Transplantation*, **30**, 665–71.

Hattori, K., Hirano, T., Miyajima, H. *et al.* (1998). Differential effects of anti-Fas ligand and anti-tumor necrosis factor alpha antibodies on acute graft-versus-host disease pathologies. *Blood*, **91**, 4051–4055.

Hebart, H., Ehninger, G., Schmidt, H. *et al.* (1995). Treatment of steroid-resistant graft-versus-host disease after allogeneic bone marrow transplantation with anti-CD3/TCR monoclonal antibodies. *Bone Marrow Transplantation*, **15**, 891–894.

Henslee-Downey, P. J., Parrish, R. S., Macdonald, J. S. *et al.* (1996). Combined in vitro and in vivo T lymphocyte depletion for the control of graft-versus-host disease following haploidentical marrow transplant. *Transplantation*, **61**, 738–745.

Hervé, P., Flesch, M., Cahn, J. Y. *et al.* (1985). Removal of marrow T cells with OKT3-OKT11 monoclonal antibodies and complement to prevent acute graft-versus-host disease. A pilot study in ten patients. *Transplantation*, **39**, 138–143.

Hervé, P., Wijdenes, J., Bergerat, J. P. *et al.* (1990). Treatment of corticosteroid resistant acute graft-versus-host disease by in vivo administration of anti-interleukin-2 receptor monoclonal antibody (B-B10). *Blood*, **75**, 1017–1023.

Hess, A. D. (1997). The immunobiology of syngeneic/autologous graft-versus-host disease. In *Graft-vs.-Host Disease, 2nd Edition*, ed. J.L.M. Ferrara, H. J. Deeg & S. J. Burakoff, pp. 561–586. New York: Marcel Dekker, Inc.

Hess, A. D. & Jones, R. J. (1999). Autologous graft-versus-host disease. In *Hematopoietic Cell Transplantation, 2nd Edition*, ed. E.D. Thomas, K. G. Blume & S. J. Forman, pp. 342–348. Boston: Blackwell Science.

Hess, A. D., Thoburn, C. J., Chen, W., & Horwitz, L. R. (2000). Complexity of effector mechanisms in cyclosporine-induced syngeneic graft-versus-host disease. *Biology of Blood and Marrow Transplantation*, **6**, 13–24.

Hill, G. R., Crawford, J. M., Cooke, K. R. *et al.* (1997). Total body irradiation and acute graft-versus-host disease: the role of gastrointestinal damage and inflammatory cytokines. *Blood*, **90**, 3204–3213.

Hill, G. R. & Ferrara, J. L. (2000). The primacy of the gastrointestinal tract as a target organ of acute graft-versus-host disease: rationale for the use of cytokine shields in allogeneic bone marrow transplantation (Review). *Blood*, **95**, 2754–2759.

Hill, G. R., Teshima, T., Gerbitz, A. *et al.* (1999). Differential roles of IL-1 and TNF-alpha on graft-versus-host disease and graft versus leukemia. *Journal of Clinical Investigation*, **104**, 459–467.

Hings, I. M., Severson, R., Filipovich, A. H. *et al.* (1994). Treatment of moderate and severe acute GVHD after allogeneic bone marrow transplantation. *Transplantation*, **58**, 437–442.

Hiraoka, A., Ohashi, Y., Okamoto, S. *et al.* (2001). Phase III study comparing tacrolimus (FK506) with cyclosporine for graft-versus-host disease prophylaxis after allogeneic bone marrow transplantation. Japanese FK506 BMT Study Group. *Bone Marrow Transplantation*, **28**, 181–185.

Hiroyasu, S., Shiraishi, M., Koji, T. *et al.* (1999). Analysis of Fas system in pulmonary injury of graft-versus-host disease after rat intestinal transplantation. *Transplantation*, **68**, 933–938.

Ho, V. T. & Soiffer, R. J. (2001). The history and future of T-cell depletion as graft-versus-host disease prophylaxis for allogeneic hematopoietic stem cell transplantation (Review). *Blood*, **98**, 3192–3204.

Holler, E., Roncarolo, M. G., Hintermeier-Knabe, R. *et al.* (2000). Prognostic significance of increased IL-10 production in patients prior to allogeneic bone marrow transplantation. *Bone Marrow Transplantation*, **25**, 237–241.

Hsu, B., May, R., Carrum, G., Krance, R., & Przepiorka, D. (2001). Use of antithymocyte globulin for treatment of steroid-refractory acute graft-versus-host disease: An international practice survey. *Bone Marrow Transplantation*, **28**, 945–950.

Hughes, S. E. & Gruber, S. A. (1996). New immunosuppressive drugs in organ transplantation (Review). *Journal of Clinical Pharmacology*, **36**, 1081–1092.

Hwang, W.Y.K., Goh, Y. T., Tan, C. H., How, G. F., & Tan, H.C.P. (2000). Severe acute graft-versus-host disease occurring after syngeneic BMT for AML in a patient not given prior cyclosporin A therapy. *Bone Marrow Transplantation*, **25**, 205–207.

Imoto, S., Oomoto, Y., Murata, K. *et al.* (2000). Kinetics of serum cytokines after allogeneic bone marrow transplantation: interleukin-5 as a potential marker of acute graft-versus-host disease. *International Journal of Hematology*, **72**, 92–97.

Ishikawa, Y., Kashiwase, K., Akaza, T. *et al.* (2002). Polymorphisms in *TNFA* and *TNFR2* affect outcome of unrelated bone marrow transplantation. *Bone Marrow Transplantation*, **29**, 569–75.

Jacobsohn, D. A. & Vogelsang, G. B. (2002). Novel pharmacotherapeutic approaches to prevention and treatment of GVHD. *Drugs*, **62**, 879–889.

Janossy, G., Bofill, M., Poulter, L. W. *et al.* (1986). Separate ontogeny of two macrophage-like accessory cell populations in the human fetus. *Journal of Immunology*, **136**, 4354–4361.

Jiang, Z., Podack, E., & Levy, R. B. (2001). Major histocompatibility complex-mismatched allogeneic bone marrow transplantation using perforin and/or Fas ligand double-defective CD4(+) donor T cells: involvement of cytotoxic function by donor lymphocytes prior to graft-versus-host disease pathogenesis. *Blood*, **98**, 390–397.

Johnson, B. D., Konkol, M. C. & Truitt, R. L. (2002). CD25+ immunoregulatory T-cells of donor origin suppress alloreactivity after BMT. *Biology of Blood and Marrow Transplantation*, **8**, 525–35.

Juji, T., Takahashi, K., Shibata, Y. *et al.* (1989). Post-transfusion graft-versus-host disease in immunocompetent patients after cardiac surgery in Japan. *New England Journal of Medicine*, **321**, 56 (Letter).

Keane, J., Gershon, S., Wise, R. P. *et al.* (2001). Tuberculosis associated with infliximab, a tumor necrosis factor alpha–neutralizing agent. *New England Journal of Medicine*, **345**, 1098–1104.

Khoury, H., Kashyap, A., Brewster, C. *et al.* (1999). Anti-thymocyte globulin (ATG) for steroid-resistant acute graft-versus-host disease after allogeneic hematopoietic stem cell transplantation: A costly therapy with limited benefits. *Blood*, **94** (Suppl. 1), 668a (Abstract).

Kobbe, G., Schneider, P., Rohr, U. *et al.* (2001). Treatment of severe steroid refractory acute graft-versus-host disease with infliximab, a chimeric human/mouse antiTNFα antibody. *Bone Marrow Transplantation*, **28**, 47–49.

Kolb, H.-J. (1999). Management of relapse after hematopoietic cell transplantation. In *Hematopoietic Cell Transplantation, 2nd Edition*, ed. E. D. Thomas, K. G. Blume & S. J. Forman, pp. 929–936. Boston: Blackwell Science.

Kolb, H. J., Schattenberg, A., Goldman, J. M. *et al.* (1995). Graft-versus-leukemia effect of donor lymphocyte transfusions in marrow grafted patients. European Group for Blood and Marrow Transplantation Working Party Chronic Leukemia. *Blood*, **86**, 2041–2050.

Kollman, C., Howe, C.W.S., Anasetti, C. *et al.* (2001). Donor characteristics as risk factors in recipients after transplantation of bone marrow from unrelated donors: the effect of donor age. *Blood*, **98**, 2043–2051.

Korngold, R. & Sprent, J. (1999). Murine models for graft-versus-host disease. In *Hematopoietic Cell Transplantation, 2nd Edition*, ed. E. D. Thomas, K. G. Blume & S. J. Forman, pp. 296–304. Boston: Blackwell Science.

Krenger, W., Rossi, S., Piali, L., & Hollander, G. A. (2000). Thymic atrophy in murine acute graft-versus-host disease is effected by impaired cell cycle progression of host pro-T and pre-T cells. *Blood*, **96**, 347–354.

Krenger, W., Snyder, K. M., Byon, J. C., Falzarano, G., & Ferrara, J.L.M. (1995). Polarized type 2 alloreactive CD4+ and CD8+ donor T cells fail to induce experimental acute graft-versus-host disease. *Journal of Immunology, 155*, 585–593.

Kurtzberg, J., Laughlin, M., Graham, M. L. *et al.* (1996). Placental blood as a source of hematopoietic stem cells for transplantation into unrelated recipients. *New England Journal of Medicine, 335*, 157–166.

Lesnikova, M., Lesnikov, V., Arrighi, S. *et al.* (2000). Upregulation of interleukin-10 and inhibition of alloantigen responses by transferrin and transferrin-derived glycans. *Journal of Hematotherapy and Stem Cell Research, 9*, 381–392.

Lichtman, A. H., Krenger, W., & Ferrara, J.L.M. (1997). Cytokine Networks. In *Graft-vs.-Host Disease, 2nd Ed.*, ed. J.L.M. Ferrara, H. J. Deeg, & S. J. Burakoff pp. 179–218. New York: Marcel Dekker, Inc.

Liem, L. M., van Houwelingen, H. C., & Goulmy, E. (1998). Serum cytokine levels after HLA-identical bone marrow transplantation. *Transplantation, 66*, 863–871.

Lin, H., Wei, R. Q., Gordon, D. *et al.* (1994). Review of CTLA4Ig use for allograft immunosuppression. *Transplantation Proceedings, 26*, 3200–3201.

Locatelli, F., Bruno, B., Zecca, M. *et al.* (2000a). Cyclosporin A and short-term methotrexate versus cyclosporin A as graft versus host disease prophylaxis in patients with severe aplastic anemia given allogeneic bone marrow transplantation from an HLA-identical sibling: results of a GITMO/EBMT randomized trial. *Blood, 96*, 1690–1697.

Locatelli, F., Zecca, M., Rondelli, R. *et al.* (2000b). Graft versus host disease prophylaxis with low-dose cyclosporine-A reduces the risk of relapse in children with acute leukemia given HLA-identical sibling bone marrow transplantation: results of a randomized trial. *Blood, 95*, 1572–1579.

Lokhorst, H. M., Schattenberg, A., Cornelissen, J. J., Thomas, L.L.M., & Verdonck, L. F. (1997). Donor leukocyte infusions are effective in relapsed multiple myeloma after allogeneic bone marrow transplantation. *Blood, 90*, 4206–4211.

Lu, Y., Sakamaki, S., Kuroda, H. *et al.* (2001). Prevention of lethal acute graft-versus-host disease in mice by oral administration of T helper 1 inhibitor, TAK-603. *Blood, 97*, 1123–1130.

MacMillan, M. L., Weisdorf, D. J., Davies, S. M. *et al.* (2002). Early antithymocyte globulin therapy improves survival in patients with steroid-resistant acute graft-versus-host disease. *Biology of Blood and Marrow Transplantation, 8*, 40–46.

Maris, M., Niederwieser, D., Sandmaier, B. *et al.* (2001). Nonmyeloablative hematopoietic stem cell transplants (HSCT) using 10/10 HLA antigen matched unrelated donors (URDs) for patients with advanced hematologic malignancies ineligible for conventional HSCT. *Blood, 98* (Suppl 1), 858a (Abstract).

Martin, P., Nash, R., Sanders, J. *et al.* (1998a). Reproducibility in retrospective grading of acute graft-versus-host disease after allogeneic marrow transplantation. *Bone Marrow Transplantation, 21*, 273–279.

Martin, P. J., Hansen, J. A., Buckner, C. D. *et al.* (1985). Effects of in vitro depletion of T cells in HLA-identical allogeneic marrow grafts. *Blood, 66*, 664–672.

Martin, P. J. & Kernan, N. A. (1997). T-cell depletion for GVHD prevention in humans. In *Graft-vs.-Host Disease, Second Ed.*, ed.

J.L.M. Ferrara, H. J. Deeg, & S. J. Burakoff, pp. 615–637. New York: Marcel Dekker, Inc.

Martin, P. J., Nelson, B. J., Appelbaum, F. R. *et al.* (1996). Evaluation of a CD5-specific immunotoxin for treatment of acute graft-versus-host disease after allogeneic marrow transplantation. *Blood, 88*, 824–830.

Martin, P. J., Remlinger, K., Hansen, J. A. *et al.* (1984). Murine monoclonal anti-T cell antibodies for treatment of refractory acute graft-versus-host disease (GVHD). *Transplantation Proceedings, 16*, 1494–1495.

Martin, P. J., Rowley, S. D., Anasetti, C. *et al.* (1999). A phase I–II clinical trial to evaluate removal of CD4 cells and partial depletion of CD8 cells from donor marrow for HLA-mismatched unrelated recipients. *Blood, 94*, 2192–2199.

Martin, P. J., Schoch, G., Fisher, L. *et al.* (1990). A retrospective analysis of therapy for acute graft-versus-host disease: initial treatment. *Blood, 76*, 1464–1472.

Martin, P. J., Schoch, G., Fisher, L. *et al.* (1991). A retrospective analysis of therapy for acute graft-versus-host disease: secondary treatment. *Blood, 77*, 1821–1828.

Martin, P. J., Schoch, G., Gooley, T. *et al.* (1998b). Methods for assessment of graft-versus-host disease. *Blood, 92*, 3479–3481 (Letter).

Massenkeil, G., Rackwitz, S., Genvresse, I. *et al.* (2002). Basiliximab is well tolerated and effective in the treatment of steroid-refractory acute graft-versus-host disease after allogeneic stem cell transplantation. *Bone Marrow Transplantation, 30*, 899–903.

McDonald, G. B., Bouvier, M., Hockenbery, D. M. *et al.* (1998). Oral beclomethasone dipropionate for treatment of intestinal graft-versus-host disease: a randomized, controlled trial. *Gastroenterology, 115*, 28–35.

Middleton, P. G., Taylor, P.R.A., Jackson, G., Proctor, S. J., & Dickinson, A. M. (1998). Cytokine gene polymorphisms associating with severe acute graft-versus-host disease in HLA-identical sibling transplants. *Blood, 92*, 3943–3948.

Mielcarek, M., Sandmaier, B. M., Maloney, D. G. *et al.* (2002). Nonmyeloablative hematopoietic cell transplantation: status quo and future perspectives. *Journal of Clinical Immunology, 22*, 70–74.

Miscia, S., Di Baldassarre, A., Sabatino, G. *et al.* (1999). Inefficient phospholipase C activation and reduced Lck expression characterize the signaling defect of umbilical cord T lymphocytes. *Journal of Immunology, 163*, 2416–2424.

Mitsuyasu, R. T., Champlin, R. E., Gale, R. P. *et al.* (1986). Treatment of donor bone marrow with monoclonal anti-T-cell antibody and complement for the prevention of graft-versus-host disease. *Annals of Internal Medicine, 105*, 20–26.

Mollee, P., Morton, A. J., Irving, I., & Durrant, S. (2001). Combination therapy with tacrolimus and anti-thymocyte globulin for the treatment of steroid-resistant acute graft-versus-host disease developing during cyclosporine prophylaxis [erratum appears in *British Journal of Haematology* (2001), **115**, 235]. *British Journal of Haematology, 113*, 217–223.

Mori, T., Nishimura, T., Ikeda, Y. *et al.* (1998). Involvement of Fas-mediated apoptosis in the hematopoietic progenitor cells of graft-versus-host reaction-associated myelosuppression. *Blood, 92*, 101–107.

Munshi, N. C., Govindarajan, R., Drake, R. *et al.* (1997). Thymidine kinase (TK) gene-transduced human lymphocytes can be highly purified, remain fully functional, and are killed efficiently with ganciclovir. *Blood,* **89,** 1334–1340.

Nakamura, H., Komatsu, K., Ayaki, M. *et al.* (2000). Serum levels of soluble IL-2 receptor, IL-12, IL-18, and IFN-gamma in patients with acute graft-versus-host disease after allogeneic bone marrow transplantation. *Journal of Allergy & Clinical Immunology,* **106,** S45–S50

Nash, R. A., Antin, J. H., Karanes, C. *et al.* (2000). Phase 3 study comparing methotrexate and tacrolimus with methotrexate and cyclosporine for prophylaxis of acute graft-versus-host disease after marrow transplantation from unrelated donors. *Blood,* **96,** 2062–2068.

Nash, R. A., Pepe, M. S., Storb, R. *et al.* (1992). Acute graft-versus-host disease: analysis of risk factors after allogeneic marrow transplantation and prophylaxis with cyclosporine and methotrexate. *Blood,* **80,** 1838–1845.

Nash, R. A., Pineiro, L. A., Storb, R. *et al.* (1996). FK506 in combination with methotrexate for the prevention of graft-versus-host disease after marrow transplantation from matched unrelated donors. *Blood,* **88,** 3634–3641.

Nimer, S. D., Giorgi, J., Gajewski, J. L. *et al.* (1994). Selective depletion of CD8+ cells for prevention of graft-versus-host disease after bone marrow transplantation. A randomized controlled trial. *Transplantation,* **57,** 82–87.

Ohashi, Y., Minegishi, M., Fujie, H., Tsuchiya, S., & Konno, T. (1997). Successful treatment of steroid-resistant severe acute GVHD with 24-h continuous infusion of FK506. *Bone Marrow Transplantation,* **19,** 625–627.

Pai, S. Y., Fruman, D. A., Leong, T. *et al.* (1994). Inhibition of calcineurin phosphatase activity in adult bone marrow transplant patients treated with cyclosporine A. *Blood,* **84,** 3974–3979.

Pan, L., Delmonte, J., Jr., Jalonen, C. K., & Ferrara, J.L.M. (1995). Pretreatment of donor mice with granulocyte colony-stimulating factor polarizes donor T lymphocytes toward type-2 cytokine production and reduces severity of experimental graft versus host disease. *Blood,* **86,** 4422–4429.

Papadopoulos, E. B., Carabasi, M. H., Castro-Malaspina, H. *et al.* (1998). T-cell-depleted allogeneic bone marrow transplantation as postremission therapy for acute myelogenous leukemia: freedom from relapse in the absence of graft-versus-host disease. *Blood,* **91,** 1083–1090.

Petersdorf, E., Anasetti, C., Servida, P., Martin, P., & Hansen, J. (1998). Effect of HLA matching on outcome of related and unrelated donor transplantation therapy for chronic myelogenous leukemia (Review). *Hematology–Oncology Clinics of North America,* **12,** 107–121.

Petersdorf, E. W., Gooley, T., Malkki, M. *et al.* (2001a). The biological significance of HLA-DP gene variation in haematopoietic cell transplantation. *British Journal of Haematology,* **112,** 988–994.

Petersdorf, E. W., Hansen, J. A., Martin, P. J. *et al.* (2001b). Major-histocompatibility-complex class I alleles and antigens in hematopoietic-cell transplantation. *New England Journal of Medicine,* **345,** 1794–1800.

Piguet, P. F. (1990). Tumor necrosis factor and graft-vs.-host disease. In *Graft-vs.-Host Disease: Immunology, Pathophysiology and Treatment,* ed. S. J. Burakoff, H. J. Deeg, J. Ferrara, & K. Atkinson, pp. 255–276. New York: Marcel Dekker, Inc.

Powles, R., Mehta, J., Kulkarni, S. *et al.* (2000). Allogeneic blood and bone-marrow stem-cell transplantation in haematological malignant diseases: A randomised trial. *Lancet,* **355,** 1231–1237.

Powles, R. L., Clink, H. M., Spence, D. *et al.* (1980). Cyclosporin A to prevent graft-versus-host disease in man after allogeneic bone-marrow transplantation. *Lancet, 1,* 327–329.

Prentice, H. G., Blacklock, H. A., Janossy, G. *et al.* (1984). Depletion of T lymphocytes in donor marrow prevents significant graft-versus-host disease in matched allogeneic leukaemic marrow transplant recipients. *Lancet, 1,* 472–476.

Prentice, H. G., Brenner, M. K., Janossy, G. *et al.* (1985). T depletion using MBG6 and RFT8 monoclonal antibody combination and complement lysis prevents significant acute and chronic GVHD in HLA matched allogeneic marrow transplants. *Experimental Hematology,* **13** (Suppl 17), 115–116.

Przepiorka, D., Kernan, N. A., Ippoliti, C. *et al.* (2000). Daclizumab, a humanized anti-interleukin-2 receptor alpha chain antibody, for treatment of acute graft-versus-host disease. *Blood,* **95,** 83–89.

Przepiorka, D., Phillips, G. L., Ratanatharathorn, V. *et al.* (1998). A phase II study of BTI-322, a monoclonal anti-CD2 antibody, for treatment of steroid-resistant acute graft-versus-host disease. *Blood, 92,* 4066–4071.

Przepiorka, D., Smith, T. L., Folloder, J. *et al.* (1999). Risk factors for acute graft-versus-host disese after allogeneic blood stem cell transplantation. *Blood, 94,* 1465–1470.

Racadot, E., Herve, P., Beaujean, F. *et al.* (1987). Prevention of graft-versus-host disease in HLA-matched bone marrow transplantation for malignant diseases: a multicentric study of 62 patients using 3-pan-T monoclonal antibodies and rabbit complement. *Journal of Clinical Oncology, 5,* 426–435.

Ramsay, N.K.C., Kersey, J. H., Robison, L. L. *et al.* (1982). A randomized study of the prevention of acute graft-versus-host disease. *New England Journal of Medicine, 306,* 392–397.

Rappeport, J. M., Mihm, M., Reinherz, E. L., Lopansri, S., & Parkman, R. (1979). Acute graft-vs.-host disease in recipients of bone marrow transplants from identical twin donors. *Lancet, 2,* 717–720.

Ratanatharathorn, V., Nash, R. A., Przepiorka, D. *et al.* (1998). Phase III study comparing methotrexate and tacrolimus (Prograf, FK506) with methotrexate and cyclosporine for graft-versus-host-disease prophylaxis after HLA-identical sibling bone marrow transplantation. *Blood, 92,* 2303–2314.

Reddy, P., Teshima, T., Hildebrandt, G. *et al.* (2003). Pretreatment of donors with interleukin-18 attenuates acute graft-versus-host disease via STAT6 and preserves graft-versus-leukemia effects. *Blood, 101,* 2877–85.

Remberger, M., Storer, B., Ringdén, O., & Anasetti, C. (2002). Association between pretransplant Thymoglobulin and reduced non-relapse mortality rate after marrow transplantation from unrelated donors. *Bone Marrow Transplantation, 29,* 391–397.

Remberger. M. Persson, U., Hauzenberger, D. & Ringden, O. (2002). An association between human leucocyte antigen alleles and acute and chronic graft-versus-host disease after allogeneic haematopoietic stem cell transplantation. *British Journal of Haematology,.* **119,** 751–9.

Ringden, O. & Deeg, H. J. (1997). Clinical spectrum of graft-versus-host disease. In *Graft-vs.-Host Disease, 2nd Edition,* ed. J.L.M.

Ferrara, H. J. Deeg, & S. Burakoff, pp. 525–559. New York: Marcel Dekker, Inc.

Ringden, O. & Nilsson, B. (1985). Death by graft-versus-host disease associated with HLA mismatch, high recipient age, low marrow cell dose, and splenectomy. *Transplantation*, **40**, 39–44.

Rocha, V., Franco, R. F., Porcher, R. *et al.* (2002). Host defense and inflammatory gene polymorphisms are associated with outcomes after HLA-identical sibling bone marrow transplantation. *Blood*, **100**, 3908–18.

Rowlings, P. A., Przepiorka, D., Klein, J. P. *et al.* (1997). IBMTR severity index for grading acute graft-versus-host disease: retrospective comparison with Glucksberg grade. *British Journal of Haematology*, **97**, 855–864.

Rubinstein, P., Carrier, C., Scaradavou, A. *et al.* (1998). Outcomes among 562 recipients of placental-blood transplants from unrelated donors. *New England Journal of Medicine*, **339**, 1565–1577.

Ruggeri, L., Capanni, M., Casucci, M. *et al.* (1999). Role of natural killer cell alloreactivity in HLA-mismatched hematopoietic stem cell transplantation. *Blood*, **94**, 333–339.

Russell, J. A., Duggan, P., Chaudhry, A. M. *et al.* (2001). Low dose antithymocyte globulin incorporated into GVHD prophylaxis for matched related donor stem cell transplantation results in low morbidity and no mortality from acute GVHD. *Blood*, **98** (Suppl 1), 661a (Abstract).

Ruutu, T., Volin, L., & Elonen, E. (1988). Low incidence of severe acute and chronic graft-versus-host disease as a result of prolonged cyclosporine prophylaxis and early aggressive treatment with corticosteroids. *Transplantation Proceedings*, **20**, 491–493.

Ruutu, T., Volin, L., Parkkali, T., Juvonen, E., & Elonen, E. (2000). Cyclosporine, methotrexate, and methylprednisolone compared with cyclosporine and methotrexate for the prevention of graft-versus-host disease in bone marrow transplantation from HLA-identical sibling donor: a prospective randomized study. *Blood*, **96**, 2391–2398.

Saito, K., Sakurai, J., Ohata, J. *et al.* (1998). Involvement of CD40 ligand-CD40 and CTLA4-B7 pathways in murine acute graft-versus-host disease induced by allogeneic T cells lacking CD28. *Journal of Immunology*, **160**, 4225–4231.

Sale, G. E., Shulman, H. M., & Hackman, R. C. (1995). Bone marrow. In *Diagnostic Immunopathology, Second Edition*, ed. R. B. Colvin, A. K. Bhan, & R. T. McCluskey, pp. 435–453. New York: Raven Press, Ltd.

Santos, G. W., Tutschka, P. J., Brookmeyer, R. *et al.* (1987). Cyclosporine plus methylprednisolone versus cyclophosphamide plus methylprednisolone as prophylaxis for graft-versus-host disease: a randomized double-blind study in patients undergoing allogeneic marrow transplantation. *Clinical Transplantation*, **1**, 21–28.

Sasazuki, T., Juji, T., Morishima, Y. *et al.* (1998). Effect of matching of class I HLA alleles on clinical outcome after transplantation of hematopoietic stem cells from an unrelated donor. *New England Journal of Medicine*, **339**, 1177–1185.

Saunders, M. D., Shulman, H. M., Murakami, C. S. *et al.* (2000). Bile duct apoptosis and cholestasis resembling acute graft-versus-host disease after autologous hematopoietic cell transplantation. *American Journal of Surgical Pathology*, **24**, 1004–1008.

Sayer, H. G., Longton, G., Bowden, R., Pepe, M., & Storb, R. (1994). Increased risk of infection in marrow transplant patients given methylprednisolone for graft-versus-host disease prevention. *Blood*, **84**, 1328–1332.

Schlegel, P. G., Aharoni, R., Chen, Y. *et al.* (1996). A synthetic random basic copolymer with promiscuous binding to class II major histocompatibility complex molecules inhibits T-cell proliferative responses to major and minor histocompatibility antigens in vitro and confers the capacity to prevent murine graft-versus-host disease in vivo. [erratum appears in Proceedings of the National Academy of Science United States of America (1996) 93, 8796]. *Proceedings of the National Academy of Sciences of the United States of America*, **93**, 5061–5066.

Schmaltz, C., Alpdogan, O., Horndasch, K. J. *et al.* (2001). Differential use of Fas ligand and perforin cytotoxic pathways by donor T cells in graft-versus-host disease and graft-versus-leukemia effect. *Blood*, **97**, 2886–2895.

Schmitz, N., Beksac, M., Hasenclever, D. *et al.* (2000). A randomised study from the European Group for Blood and Marrow Transplantation comparing allogeneic transplantation of filgrastim-mobilised peripheral blood progenitor cells with bone marrow transplantation in 350 patients (pts) with leukemia. *Blood*, **96** (Suppl 1), 481a (Abstract).

Schultz, K. R., Paquet, J., Bader, S., & Hayglass, K. T. (1995). Requirement for B cells in T cell priming to minor histocompatibility antigens and development of graft-versus-host disease. *Bone Marrow Transplantation*, **16**, 289–295.

Shlomchik, W. D., Couzens, M. S., Tang, C. B. *et al.* (1999). Prevention of graft versus host disease by inactivation of host antigen-presenting cells. *Science*, **285**, 412–415.

Soiffer, R. J., Weller, E., Alyea, E. P. *et al.* (2001). CD6+ donor marrow T-cell depletion as the sole form of graft-versus-host disease prophylaxis in patients undergoing allogeneic bone marrow transplant from unrelated donors. [erratum appears in Journal of Clinical Oncology (2001) 19, 2583]. *Journal of Clinical Oncology*, **19**, 1152–1159.

Storb, R., Deeg, H. J., Farewell, V. *et al.* (1986a). Marrow transplantation for severe aplastic anemia: methotrexate alone compared with a combination of methotrexate and cyclosporine for prevention of acute graft-versus-host disease. *Blood*, **68**, 119–125.

Storb, R., Deeg, H. J., Pepe, M. *et al.* (1989). Methotrexate and cyclosporine versus cyclosporine alone for prophylaxis of graft-versus-host disease in patients given HLA-identical marrow grafts for leukemia: long-term follow-up of a controlled trial. *Blood*, **73**, 1729–1734.

Storb, R., Deeg, H. J., Whitehead, J. *et al.* (1986b). Methotrexate and cyclosporine compared with cyclosporine alone for prophylaxis of acute graft versus host disease after marrow transplantation for leukemia. *New England Journal of Medicine*, **314**, 729–735.

Storb, R., Gluckman, E., Thomas, E. D. *et al.* (1974). Treatment of established human graft-versus-host disease by antithymocyte globulin. *Blood*, **44**, 57–75.

Storb, R., Pepe, M., Anasetti, C. *et al.* (1990). What role for prednisone in prevention of acute graft-versus-host disease in patients undergoing marrow transplants? *Blood*, **76**, 1037–1045.

Storb, R., Prentice, R. L., Buckner, C. D. *et al.* (1983). Graft-versus-host disease and survival in patients with aplastic anemia treated by marrow grafts from HLA-identical siblings. Beneficial effect of a protective environment. *New England Journal of Medicine*, **308**, 302–307.

Storb, R., Yu, C., Wagner, J. L. *et al.* (1997). Stable mixed hematopoietic chimerism in DLA-identical littermate dogs given sublethal total body irradiation before and pharmacological immunosuppression after marrow transplantation. *Blood*, **89**, 3048–3054.

Storek, J., Gooley, T., Siadak, M. *et al.* (1997). Allogeneic peripheral blood stem cell transplantation may be associated with a high risk of chronic graft-versus-host disease. *Blood*, **90**, 4705–4709.

Sullivan, K. M. (1986). Acute and chronic graft-versus-host disease in man (Review). *International Journal of Cell Cloning*, **4** (Suppl 1), 42–93.

Sullivan, K. M., Deeg, H. J., Sanders, J. *et al.* (1986). Hyperacute graft-v-host disease in patients not given immunosuppression after allogeneic marrow transplantation (concise report). *Blood*, **67**, 1172–1175.

Sullivan, K. M., Storb, R., Buckner, C. D. *et al.* (1989). Graft-versus-host disease as adoptive immunotherapy in patients with advanced hematologic neoplasms. *New England Journal of Medicine*, **320**, 828–834.

Sykes, M. (2001). Mixed chimerism and transplant tolerance (Review). *Immunity*, **14**, 417–424.

Taylor, P.A., Lees, C.J. & Blazar, B.R. (2002). The infusion of ex vivo activated and expanded CD4+ CD25+ immune regulatory cells inhibits graft-versus-host disease lethality. *Blood*, **99**, 3493–9.

Tiberghien, P., Ferrand, C., Lioure, B. *et al.* (2001). Administration of herpes simplex-thymidine kinase-expressing donor T cells with a T-cell-depleted allogeneic marrow graft. *Blood*, **97**, 63–72.

Tollemar, J., Ringdén, O., Heimdahl, A., Lonnqvist, B., & Sundberg, B. (1988). Decreased incidence and severity of graft-versus-host disease in HLA matched and mismatched marrow recipients of cyclosporine and methotrexate. *Transplantation Proceedings*, **20**, 470–479.

Townsend, R. M., Gilbert, M. J., & Korngold, R. (1998). Combination therapy with a CD4-CDR3 peptide analog and cyclosporin A to prevent graft-vs-host disease in a MHC-haploidentical bone marrow transplantation model. *Clinical Immunology & Immunopathology*, **86**, 115–119.

Truitt, R. L. & Atasoylu, A. A. (1991). Contribution of CD4+ and CD8+ T cells to graft-versus-host disease and graft-versus-leukemia reactivity after transplantation of MHC-compatible bone marrow. *Bone Marrow Transplantation*, **8**, 51–58.

Tseng, L.-H., Lin, M.-T., Hansen, J. A. *et al.* (1999). Correlation between disparity for the minor histocompatibility antigen HA-1 and the development of acute graft-versus-host disease after allogeneic marrow transplantation. *Blood*, **94**, 2911–2914.

Tsukada, N., Akiba, H., Kobata, T. *et al.* (2000). Blockade of CD134 (OX40)-CD134L interaction ameliorates lethal acute graft-versus-host disease in a murine model of allogeneic bone marrow transplantation. *Blood*, **95**, 2434–2439.

Uphoff, D. E. (1958). Alteration of homograft reaction by A-methopterin in lethally irradiated mice treated with homologous marrow. *Proceedings of the Society for Experimental Biology and Medicine*, **99**, 651–653.

Urbano-Ispizua, A., Rozman, C. Pimentel, P. *et al.* (2002). Risk factors for acute graft-versus-host disease in patients undergoing transplantation with CD34+ selected blood cells from HLA-identical siblings. *Blood*, **100**, 724–7.

van Bekkum, D. W. & de Vries, M. J. (1967). *Radiation Chimaeras*. London: Logos Press Limited.

van Dijk, A. M., Kessler, F. L., Stadhouders-Keet, S. A. *et al.* (1999). Selective depletion of major and minor histocompatibility antigen reactive T cells: towards prevention of acute graft-versus-host disease. *British Journal of Haematology*, **107**, 169–175.

Van Lint, M. T., Uderzo, C., Locasciulli, A. *et al.* (1998). Early treatment of acute graft-versus-host disease with high- or low-dose 6-methylprednisolone: A multicenter randomized trial from the Italian Group for Bone Marrow Transplantation. *Blood*, **92**, 2288–2293.

van Oosterhout, Y. V., van Emst, L., Schattenberg, A. V. *et al.* (2000). A combination of anti-CD3 and anti-CD7 ricin A–immunotoxins for the in vivo treatment of acute graft versus host disease. *Blood*, **95**, 3693–3701.

Vander Woude, A. C. & Bierer, B. E. (1997). Immunosuppression and immunophilin ligands: cyclosporin A, FK506, and rapamycin. In *Graft-vs.-Host Disease, 2nd Edition*, ed. J.L.M. Ferrara, H. J. Deeg, & S. J. Burakoff, pp. 111–149. New York: Marcel Dekker, Inc.

Vossen, J. M. (1990). Gnotobiotic measures for the prevention of acute graft-vs-host disease. In *Graft-Vs-Host Disease: Immunology, Pathophysiology, and Treatment*, ed. S. J. Burakoff, H. J. Deeg, J. Ferrara, & K. Atkinson, pp. 403–414. New York: Marcel Dekker, Inc.

Wagner, J. E., Donnenberg, A. D., Noga, S. J. *et al.* (1988). Lymphocyte depletion of donor bone marrow by counterflow centrifugal elutriation: results of a phase I clinical trial. *Blood*, **72**, 1168–1176.

Weisdorf, D., Hakke, R., Blazar, B. *et al.* (1991). Risk factors for acute graft-versus-host disease in histocompatible donor bone marrow transplantation. *Transplantation*, **51**, 1197–1203.

Xun, C. Q., Tsuchida, M., & Thompson, J. S. (1997). Delaying transplantation after total body irradiation is a simple and effective way to reduce acute graft-versus-host disease mortality after major H2 incompatible transplantation. *Transplantation*, **64**, 297–302.

Yu, X. Z., Bidwell, S. J., Martin, P. J., & Anasetti, C. (2000). CD28-specific antibody prevents graft-versus-host disease in mice. *Journal of Immunology*, **164**, 4564–4568.

Yu, X.-Z., Martin, P. J., & Anasetti, C. (1998). Role of CD28 in acute graft-versus-host disease. *Blood*, **92**, 2963–2970.

Zeng, D., Dejbakhsh-Jones, S., & Strober, S. (1997). Granulocyte colony-stimulating factor reduces the capacity of blood mononuclear cells to induce graft-versus-host disease: Impact on blood progenitor cell transplantation. *Blood*, **90**, 453–463.

Zhou, P., Szot, G., Guo, Z. *et al.* (2001). Role of STAT6 signaling in the induction and long-term maintenance of tolerance mediated by CTLA4-Ig. *Transplantation Proceedings*, **33**, 214–216.

Zikos, P., Van Lint, M. T., Frassoni, F. *et al.* (1998). Low transplant mortality in allogeneic bone marrow transplantation for acute myeloid leukemia: a randomized study of low-dose cyclosporin versus low-dose cyclosporin and low-dose methotrexate. *Blood*, **91**, 3503–3508.

72 Chronic graft-versus-host disease

STEPHANIE J. LEE

Dana-Farber Cancer Center and Harvard University, Boston, USA

Introduction

Chronic graft-versus-host disease (chronic GVHD) is a complex, multi-system disorder with features of autoimmunity and immunodeficiency. The first comprehensive descriptions of this complication were published in 1979–80 (Graze & Gale, 1979; Shulman *et al.*, 1980). Although these early reports described small cohorts of patients, many of the clinical and prognostic observations remain valid and insightful. The limited versus extensive grading scale (intended to reflect need, or lack thereof, for systemic treatment) and the concepts of progressive (arising out of acute GVHD), interrupted (appearing after resolution of acute GVHD), and de novo (no prior acute GVHD) presentation were proposed in 1980 and are still in use today.

Although prevention and treatment of acute GVHD have improved over the past two decades, similar progress in chronic GVHD has remained elusive as it continues to be the leading cause of late nonrelapse mortality following allogeneic hematopoietic stem cell (HSC) transplantation (Socie *et al.*, 1999). Chronic GVHD is also associated with decreased quality of life (QOL), impaired functional status, and continued need for immunosuppressive medication (Duell *et al.*, 1997; Socie *et al.*, 1999; Sutherland *et al.*, 1997; Syrjala *et al.*, 1993). A time-series study of transplantation for aplastic anemia and refractory anemia over the past 30 years suggests that the incidence of chronic GVHD and the case mortality rate (overall 24%) have not significantly changed despite advances in supportive care and transplantation medicine. On a positive note, duration of treatment for chronic GVHD may be shorter, and the most severe organ manifestations are less common (Goerner *et al.*, 2002). The field of HSC transplantation is evolving quickly to embrace alternative graft sources (unrelated donors, peripheral blood stem cells, umbilical cord blood stem cells, and haploidentical donors) and reduced intensity preparative regimens. For the most part, the impact of these modifications on the incidence, organ manifestations, severity, and outcome of chronic GVHD are unknown.

Clinical features

Approximately 30–50% of HLA-matched sibling bone marrow recipients and 50–70% of unrelated donor bone marrow recipients develop chronic GVHD at a median time to onset of 4–6 months posttransplant (Lee *et al.*, 2002b). Traditionally, the diagnosis of acute and chronic GVHD has been distinguished by whether symptoms developed before or after 100 days posttransplantation. More recent debate suggests that this cutoff is too artificial and that clinical manifestations should determine the diagnosis. Chronic GVHD may occur as early as 60 days after allogeneic hematopoietic stem cell transplantation (HSCT) or years later, especially after immunostimulating events such as sunburns or infections (Atkinson, 1990) (Fig. 72.1). Based on data from the International Bone Marrow Transplant Registry (IBMTR), the distribution of chronic GVHD onset for HLA-matched siblings is 20–30% progressive, 30–40% interrupted, and 35% de novo. Data from the National Marrow Donor Program (NMDP) for unrelated donor recipients, where the incidence of acute GVHD is higher, show

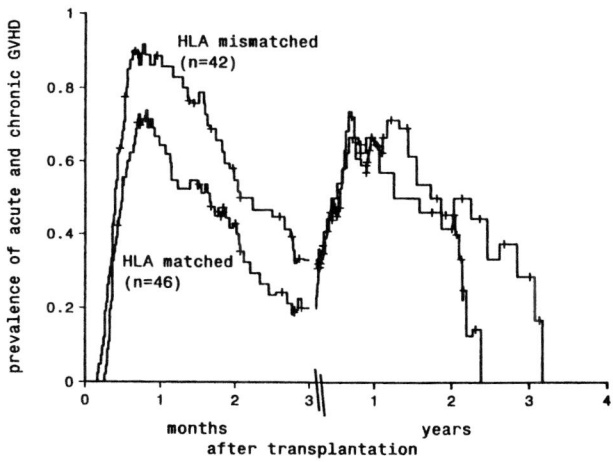

Fig. 72.1. Prevalence of acute GVHD of grades II–IV and clinical extensive chronic GVHD according to HLA compatibility in 88 children undergoing unrelated donor marrow transplantation for malignant hematologic diseases. Resolution of clinical acute GVHD was scored despite continued immunosuppression. Conversely, resolution of chronic GVHD was scored only when patients discontinued immunosuppression indefinitely. Reproduced, with permission, from Balduzzi *et al.* (1995).

the spectrum of onset as 19% progressive, 69% interrupted, and 12% de novo onset (Lee *et al.,* 2002b).

Surprisingly little has been reported about whether the syndrome of chronic GVHD differs if it develops in the context of T cell depletion or peripheral blood grafting. In HLA-matched marrow grafting with primarily methotrexate-based prophylaxis, skin (65%–80%), mouth (48%–72%), liver (40%–73%), and eye (18%–47%) involvement are most commonly reported. Other less frequently involved organs include gastrointestinal tract with accompanying weight loss (16%–26%), lung (10%–15%), esophagus (6%–8%), and joints (2%–12%) (Lee *et al.,* 2002b; Ochs *et al.,* 1994; Sullivan *et al.,* 1991; Jacobsohn *et al.,* 2002) (Fig. 72.2). Table 72.1 outlines the signs, symptoms, and histopathologic findings associated with chronic

GVHD. Because the differential diagnosis for many chronic GVHD manifestations is broad, biopsies and other diagnostic tests should be pursued to rule out alternative etiologies and confirm the diagnosis whenever possible.

Skin

In contrast to acute GVHD which frequently first appears as a salmon-colored, maculopapular rash involving the shoulders, chest, and back, or as erythema involving palms, soles, and ears, chronic GVHD often presents as a lichenoid rash with more variable distribution. Lichenoid lesions are typically violaceous, flat-topped, and usually less confluent than the rash of acute GVHD. Another common chronic GVHD presentation is persistent ery-

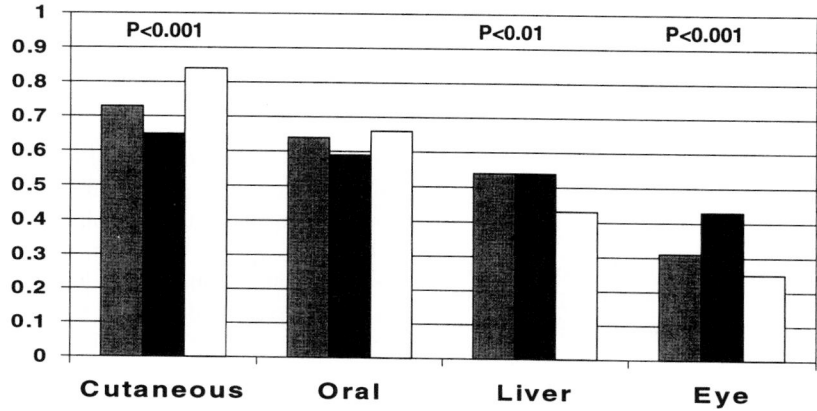

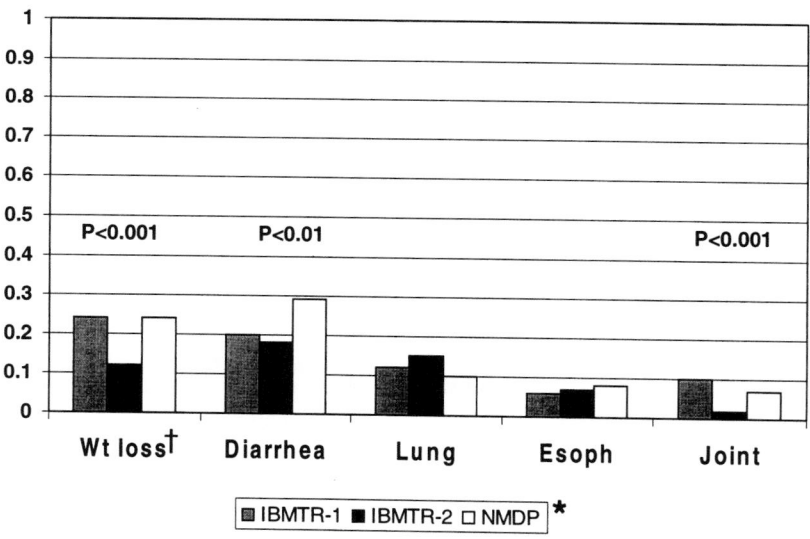

* IBMTR, International Bone Marrow Transplant Registry;
NMDP, National Marrow Donor Program
† Weight loss not collected in IBMTR-2, proportion represents patients with nausea or malabsorption

Fig. 72.2. Frequency of different organ manifestations in two cohorts of HLA-matched sibling (IBMTR-1, *n* = 727; IBMTR-2, *n* = 421) and matched unrelated donor (NMDP, *n* = 378) bone marrow recipients. Reproduced, with permission, from Lee *et al.* (2002b).

Table 72.1. *Signs, symptoms and clinicopathologic findings of chronic graft-versus-host disease*

System	Signs/laboratory findings	Symptoms	Histopathology
Skin (common)	Hyper- and hypopigmentation, lichen planus (violaceous flat-topped papules), poikiloderma (atrophy, telangectasias, dyspigmentation), cutaneous ulcers, scleroderma (thickening due to collagen deposition, may cause decreased range of motion and contractures), icthyosis	Pruritus, lack of flexibility	Lichenoid: hyperkeratosis, focal hypergranulosis, acanthosis, dyskeratotic keratinocytes, vacuolar degeneration, colloid bodies, perivascular and periadnexal lymphoplasmacellular infiltrate Poikiloderma: epidermal atrophy, loss of rete ridges Scleroderma: epidermal atrophy, dermal fibrosis, less inflammation than lichenoid lesion, adnexal structures destroyed Differential diagnosis: drug reaction, eczema
Cutaneous structures	Onchodystrophy, alopecia, loss of sweat glands	Heat sensitivity	Destruction and fibrosis of cutaneous appendages
Liver (common)	Elevated alkaline phosphatase, transaminases, bilirubin	Pruritus	Small bile duct atypia and damage with subsequent necrosis and drop-out, moderate lymphocytic infiltrate, cholestasis, and ballooning Differential diagnosis: drug toxicity (cholestasis, inflammation), veno-occlusive disease, viral infections, gallstones, and infiltrative processes
Mouth (common)	Lichen planus, erythema, ulcers, xerostomia, dental caries, fibrosis, decreased salivary flow	Food sensitivity, pain, dry mouth, decreased oral range of motion from fibrosis	Mucosal atrophy, lymphoplasmacytic inflammation, increased mucopolysaccharides, fibrosis and destruction of minor salivary glands Differential diagnosis: Herpesvirus infection, Sjögren's syndrome[2]
Eyes (common)	Keratoconjunctivitis sicca, corneal ulcerations, Schirmer's[1] test with <5 mm wetting at 5 minutes	Dry eyes, photophobia, pain	Differential diagnosis: post radiation xerophthalmia, Sjögren's syndrome
Esophagus	Esophageal web, desquamation, ulcerations, strictures, submucosal fibrosis, abnormal motility	Odynophagia, dysphagia, heartburn, retrosternal pain	Differential diagnosis: reflux esophagitis, infection
Intestines	Fibrosis, malabsorption	Diarrhea, nausea, anorexia, abdominal pain, weight loss	Differential diagnosis: irritable or inflammatory bowel syndrome, infection
Lung	Restrictive and obstructive abnormalities on pulmonary function testing, bronchiolitis obliterans, pneumothoraces, bronchiectasis, pseudomonal colonization, pulmonary infiltrates	Dyspnea, nonproductive cough, wheezing	Bronchiolitis obliterans with granulation tissue plugs and fibrosis obliterating small airways Interstitial pneumonitis
Musculoskeletal	Polymyositis, arthritis, fasciitis	Arthralgias, myalgias, weakness	
Serous	Pericardial, peritoneal, and pleural effusions	Clinical syndromes of cardiac tamponade, ascites, dyspnea	Usually transudative
Nervous system	Entrapment of nerves, peripheral neuropathy, myasthenia gravis	Pain, paresthesias	
Urologic	Cystitis, phimosis	Pain, hematuria	
Vagina	Erythema, sicca, strictures, stenosis, ulcers	Pain, dyspareunia, difficulty voiding	
Hematopoietic	Thrombocytopenia, neutropenia, eosinophilia, hemolytic anemia		
Immune system	Lymphoid hypocellularity, hyper- or hypogammaglobulinemia	Frequent infections, especially sinus, upper respiratory tract	

[1] Rudolf Schirmer, German opthalmologist, 1831–1896.
[2] Karl Sjögren, Swedish physician, 1896–1974.

thema following acute GVHD. Two later manifestations include scleroderma and poikiloderma. Scleroderma-like thickening due to dermal fibrosis may be highly localized (morphea) or more generalized. Scleroderma over joints can limit mobility, but surgical release of contractures has not been helpful (Beredjiklian et al., 1998). Poikiloderma with thinning of the epidermis and dermis, telangectasia, and mottled pigmentation is often a generalized phenomenon. Total leukoderma has been described with an absence of melanocytes in the epidermis (Jacobsohn et al., 2002) and cytotoxic antimelanocyte antibodies present in serum (Nagler et al., 1996). A follicular papular form has been described (Miyazaki et al., 1993). Later, dermal and subcutaneous fibrosis can cause thickening and hardening of the skin. Clinically this can resemble either the localized morphea form of scleroderma (Van Vloten et al., 1977) or generalized scleroderma, and it can also resemble lichen sclerosus et atrophicus (Cordoba et al., 1999). Unusual distribution has been described, for example, restriction to the field of previous total lymphoid irradiation (Okamoto et al., 1996). Lichenoid cutaneous chronic GVHD occurring in a linear pattern has also been described (Beers et al., 1993; Cohen & Hymes, 1994; Freemer et al., 1994; Wilson & Lockmann, 1994), in some cases thought to be associated with clinical or subclinical herpes zoster infection. It has also been described occurring in Blaschko's lines[1] (Lee, Atkinson, & Kossard, 1996). Hair loss is common in the areas of involved skin and the combined outcome of these cutaneous manifestations can result in a severe cosmetic defect. The fibrosis can result in joint contractures, skin ulceration, poor wound healing and serious difficulty with vascular access, and phimosis (Kami et al., 1998).

In cases of severe ulceration, skin grafts from the donor have been successful and the tissue has remained healthy and uninvolved with chronic GVHD (Graze & Gale, 1979; Knobler et al., 1985). Fasciitis is a rare late manifestation of chronic GVHD that starts with painful edema and progresses to morphea unresponsive to immunosuppression (Janin et al., 1994). Ichthyosis has also been reported (Dilek et al., 1998).

Mouth

Oral pain, atrophy, erythema, and lichenoid lesions of the mucosa are highly associated with chronic GVHD (Schubert et al., 1984). The earliest changes are white striae on the mucosa of the cheeks, lips, or palate and on the epithelium of the external lips, the appearance of which again resembles lichen planus or dyskeratosis congenita. Other common changes are erythema of the mucus membrane and sometimes subsequent progression to ulceration. The ulcers can be painful and can make eating difficult. Such lesions can be further irritated by the sharp edges of carious teeth and extraction may facilitate resolution of such lesions. Destruction of the minor salivary glands results in decreased salivary flow with dryness of the mouth. Additionally, major salivary gland (parotid and submandibular glands) dysfunction also occurs in both acute and chronic GVHD, with

reduction in salivary flow rates as measured by sialometry and salivary gland scintigraphy (Nagler et al., 1996). This can sometimes be the sole feature of chronic GVHD, in which case intraoral psoralen ultraviolet A (PUVA) phototherapy can be effective treatment (Atkinson et al., 1986b). It is important, however, to document the diagnosis by lip biopsy since at least one study has suggested that reduction of salivary flow rate is related to the use of total body irradiation in the pretransplant preparative regimen, rather than to chronic GVHD (Heimdahl et al., 1985).

The combination of mouth pain and decreased salivary gland activity often leads to poor oral hygiene predisposing to dental caries. Fibrosis causing decreased oral range of motion is a very late manifestation. Patients with chronic GVHD undergoing dental work should receive antibiotic prophylaxis.

Liver

Either transaminitis or cholestatic patterns may be seen but are usually asymptomatic, although presentation in acute hepatitis has been described (Strasser et al., 2000; Malik et al., 2001). In cases of isolated liver dysfunction, percutaneous or transvenous liver biopsy should be performed because of the broad differential diagnosis associated with purely laboratory abnormalities. It is especially important to exclude chronic hepatitis B and C and iron overload. The decision of whether or not to treat isolated hepatic chronic GVHD depends on the magnitude and duration of abnormalities since progression to overt liver failure is relatively rare. For mild cholestatic changes only, ursodeoxycholic acid may be beneficial. Liver transplantation has been successfully performed for end-stage hepatic chronic GVHD (Rhodes et al., 1990).

Eye

Eye involvement includes xerophthalmia and keratoconjunctivitis. Severe forms of chronic GVHD result in corneal abrasions and ulcers, and can lead to loss of vision. Symptoms include eye irritation, photophobia, and pain. Protective eye- and sunglasses, frequent lubrication, application of ophthalmic ointment at night, and punctal plugs or cautery can help symptomatically and prevent further damage.

As with dryness of the mouth, however, it should be noted that dry eyes can occur in the absence of chronic GVHD (Tichelli et al., 1996), both in those prepared by a total body irradiation regimen (Calissendorff et al., 1989) and in those prepared by a chemotherapy-only regimen (Abesada-Terk et al., 1990). In an EBMT study (Tichelli et al., 1996), the actuarial probability of developing dry eyes was 21% ± 3% at 15 years posttransplant. Sixty-nine percent of patients with sicca syndrome had GVHD. The probability of developing sicca at 15 years was 38% ± 6% for patients with chronic GVHD and 10% ± 3% for those without chronic GVHD (P < .0001).

Esophagus/gastrointestinal tract

Esophageal symptoms of dysphagia and odynophagia result from desquamation, web and stricture formation, and reflux

---

[1] Alfred Blaschko, German dermatologist, 1858–1922.

esophagitis. Periodic endoscopic dilatations and antacid medications may help symptomatically. Stomach and small intestinal pathology are relatively rare. However, many patients have anorexia, nausea, lower abdominal pain, cramping, and diarrhea. Pancreatic insufficiency without characteristic laboratory and radiographic studies may occur, and this syndrome responds to enzyme supplementation (Akpek et al., 2001b). Weight loss is common and is probably multifactorial from decreased oral intake, poor absorption, and increased resting energy expenditures (Zauner et al., 2001).

Lung

Symptoms of dyspnea and wheezing may herald the diagnosis of bronchiolitis obliterans (BO). In BO, granulation tissue and scarring obliterate the small airways, and pulmonary function testing shows obstructive and restrictive patterns. An underlying autoimmune process is implicated by the association of BO with lung transplantation, collagen-vascular diseases, and viral infections (Holland et al., 1988; Philit et al., 1995). Although low immunoglobulin levels and chronic GVHD are associated with BO, a randomized trial of prophylactic immunoglobulin replacement did not decrease the incidence of BO (Sullivan et al., 1996). Even without BO, pulmonary sicca and bronchiectasis lead to frequent infections and bacterial colonization, often with *Pseudomonas*. These patients may benefit from a treatment program similar to that employed for cystic fibrosis with inhaled antibiotics, aggressive pulmonary hygiene, and prolonged antibiotic courses. Gastric reflux with aspiration may exacerbate symptoms and should be treated with acid inhibitors. Successful lung transplantation has been performed in a small number of patients with end-stage pulmonary chronic GVHD (Boas et al., 1994).

Other rarer pulmonary manifestations include lymphoid interstitial pneumonitis or lymphocytic alveolitis (Leblond et al., 1994; Perrault et al., 1985) and pulmonary fibrosis (Atkinson et al., 1989a; Wolff et al., 2002).

Sinuses

Sinusitis is common in patients with chronic GVHD and results from a combination of the sicca syndrome involving the sinuses together with a predisposition to Gram[2]-positive bacterial infections, particularly with pneumococcus (Bolger et al., 1986). Besides antibiotic therapy, surgical drainage is necessary for the management of recurrent episodes.

Vagina

Vaginal inflammation, sicca, stricture formation, and stenosis have been described with desquamative web formation (Corson et al., 1982; DeLord et al., 1999; Yanai et al., 1999). Treatment may require dilatation together with topical estrogen cream in addition to systemic immunosuppressive therapy.

[2] Hans Gram, Danish pathologist, 1853–1938.

Musculoskeletal system

Occasional cases of polymyositis associated with chronic GVHD have resulted in severe proximal weakness with biopsy showing necrotic muscle fibers, interstitial inflammation, and IgG deposits on immunofluorescent staining (Al-Eid et al., 1983). Additionally, in a larger series (Parker et al., 1996) cytotoxic T cells were demonstrated. A single case report has described successful treatment with intravenous immunoglobulin and methotrexate (Blanche, Dreyfus, & Sicard, 1995). The manifestations are indistinguishable from idiopathic polymyositis. Elevation of serum creatine phosphokinase occurs; it can be the only manifestation of chronic GVHD and it is important to distinguish it from other causes of muscle weakness after allogeneic transplantation since prompt initiation of corticosteroid therapy usually results in rapid improvement, although involvement of the respiratory muscles can be fatal (Oshima et al., 1997). One such case causing respiratory failure, as well as "dropped head syndrome" due to involvement of the extensor muscles of the neck, reqired mechanical ventilation, but recovered following tretment with aggressive immune suppression and intensive rehabilitation (Leano, Miller, & White, 2000). HLA-DRw52 is present in 75% of cases of idiopathic polymyositis, and this association has been noted in two cases of chronic GVHD manifesting as polymyositis (Couriel et al., 2002).

Fasciitis is a rare complication of chronic GVHD and presents with sudden painful skin swelling leading to skin tightness, joint stiffness, contractures, and sores. It often fails to respond adequately to therapy (Janin et al., 1994).

Proximal myopathy secondary to corticosteroid treatment of chronic GVHD is not uncommon (see Chapter 95).

Other side effects occurring in patients receiving prednisone and cyclosporine immunosuppressive treatment for chronic GVHD include a decrease in bone mineral density due to increased collagen and bone turnover, and increased urinary magnesium and calcium excretion leading to a significant risk of osteoporosis (Stern et al., 1996).

Serous surfaces

Shulman et al. (1980) originally used the term serositis to describe the occurrence of pleural and pericardial effusions in patients with extensive chronic GVHD. A subsequent study confirmed the rare occurrence of multiple unexplained effusions involving the pleural, pericardial, or peritoneal cavities in patients in whom other causes of such effusions such as hepatic veno-occlusive disease, cardiac insufficiency, tumor relapse, and granulocyte-macrophage colony-stimulating factor (GM-CSF) toxicity were excluded. This occurred both before and after day 100 posttransplant, but only in recipients of allografts and not autografts, and often associated with cytomegalovirus disease (Seber, Khan, & Kersey, 1996). In one case, antinucleolar antibody was elevated in pleural fluid and blood, and lymphocytes in the pleural fluid were CD8[+]/HLA-DR[+] (Ueda et al., 2000). Constrictive pericarditis has also been described (Silberstein et al., 2001).

Nervous system

Entrapment neuropathy associated with subcutaneous fibrosis has been described (Shulman *et al.*, 1978), as has an incapacitating peripheral neuropathy (Greenspan *et al.*, 1990; Hughes *et al.*, 1999). Vasculitic changes have been reported on biopsy (Hughes *et al.*, 1999). Additionally myasthenia gravis has occurred in association with chronic GVHD posttransplant, the illness including development of antibodies to the acetylcholine receptor (Bolger *et al.*, 1986). Possible central nervous system involvement with focal lymphohistiocytic aggregates has been reported (Vouah *et al.*, 1988), but as with putative renal and urinary bladder involvement, this needs to be substantiated by further case reports.

Vascular system

Capillary leak syndrome, presenting with generalized edema and associated with elevated serum IL-2 levels, has been reported (Funke *et al.*, 1994). The serum level of the soluble form of vascular cell adhesion molecule, sVCAM-1, as well as that of soluble E-selectin, was found to be significantly elevated in patients with extensive chronic GVHD (Matsuda *et al.*, 2001).

Hematopoietic system

Thrombocytopenia (platelet count $<100 \times 10^9$/l) is a poor prognostic sign present in about a third of patients at diagnosis. It is important to rule out classic "autoimmune" thrombocytopenia that might be responsive to antibody therapy such as rituximab or anti-D antibody (Rhogam) (Ratanatharathorn *et al.*, 2000). Eosinophilia, autoimmune neutropenia and hemolytic anemia are also observed, and usually improve with successful treatment of chronic GVHD.

The bone marrow may be hypoplastic (Shulman *et al.*, 1978), and marrow fibrosis resulting in transfusion-dependent anemia, a leukoerythroblastic film, and thrombocytopenia has been reported (Atkinson *et al.*, 1987). With regard to marrow reserve it should be noted that hematopoietic progenitor cells, particularly in the blood, are reduced in patients with chronic GVHD (Atkinson *et al.*, 1986a).

With regard to coagulation abnormalities, the antiphospholipid syndrome has been described (Sohngen *et al.*, 1994), as has acquired factor VIII inhibitor (Seidler *et al.*, 1994).

Lymphoid system

The dominant effect of chronic GVHD on the lymphoid system is severe and consists of persistent lymphoid hypocellularity and atrophy (van Bekkum, 1985). This results in functional asplenia as determined by radioisotope scanning of the spleen (Anderson *et al.*, 1982), which in turn helps explain the predisposition of patients with chronic GVHD to pneumococcal infections (Atkinson *et al.*, 1979; Kulkami *et al.*, 2000). Splenic size may also be monitored in these patients by ultrasonography (Picardi, Selleri, & Rotoli, 1999).

Urologic system

Both renal (Gomez-Garcia *et al.*, 1988) and bladder (Ruutu *et al.*, 1988) involvement have been ascribed to chronic GVHD, but further confirmation is required. The case of bladder involvement presented as severe cystitis. The renal involvement presented clinically and on electron microscopy as minimal change nephrotic syndrome. Other cases occurring at 12 and 27 months after marrow transplant showed membranous nephropathy and focal glumerular sclerosis on biopsy, and responded to cyclosporine therapy but not to initial prednisone treatment (Haseyama *et al.*, 1996; Oliveira *et al.*, 1999).

Growth and development

Growth velocity rate is decreased in patients with chronic GVHD, but reverts to normal and catch-up growth occurs once the chronic GVHD is controlled and therapy stopped (Sanders, 1981). Delayed pubertal development is significantly more frequent among patients with chronic GVHD who have received total body radiotherapy compared to those without chronic GVHD. No significant difference in pubertal development was found with and without chronic GVHD in recipients conditioned for transplant with chemotherapy alone. Likewise, gonadal function after puberty was not affected by chronic GVHD either in males or females given chemotherapy or total body irradiation (Sanders, 1981).

Immunodeficiency

Infections are the leading cause of death among patients with chronic GVHD. Patients are profoundly immunocompromised, both from the innate immunodeficiency associated with chronic GVHD and from the intensive immunosuppressive treatment. Multiple defects in mucosal integrity, depletion of thymic and other lymphoid structures, and reduced number and function of mature T and B cells contribute to the high case fatality rate from bacterial, fungal, and viral pathogens (Siadak & Sullivan, 1994; Storek *et al.*, 1996; Sherer & Shoenfeld, 1998; Maury *et al.*, 2001).

A newer assay for assessment of thymopoietic capacity is the measurement of T cell receptor excision circles (TRECs) among peripheral blood T cells: a by-product of T cell receptor rearrangement includes a circular episome of DNA, which is stable and does not replicate with cellular proliferation. Weinberg *et al.* (2001) measured TREC levels in both CD4+ and CD8+ cells in 56 allograft recipients. TREC levels rose weeks after transplantation and were detected up to 6 years posttransplant. TREC levels correlated with the frequency of phenotypically naïve T cells, indicating that such cells were not expanded progeny of naïve T cells present in the donor graft. Chronic GVHD was the most important factor that predicted low TREC levels, even years posttransplant. Patients with a history of resolved GVHD had decreased numbers of TRECs compared to those with no GVHD.

Chronic GVHD is associated with an increased risk of infection with encapsulated organisms, including *Streptococcus pneumoniae,* and the T cell deficiency and prolonged corticosteroid exposure predispose patients to *Pneumocystis carinii* (Kulkami *et al.,* 2000). Varicella zoster infections occur in approximately 40% of marrow transplant recipients, but in up to 80% of patients with chronic GVHD in whom nonspecific circulating suppressor cells are detectable (Atkinson *et al.,* 1982a). Late interstitial pneumonitis also occurs more frequently in those with chronic GVHD than in those without (Sullivan *et al.,* 1986) and usually has an infectious etiology. Since this can be varied (cytomegalovirus, *Pneumocystis carinii,* and miscellaneous organisms), the importance of adequate tissue procurement (usually by open lung biopsy) is emphasized.

Prolonged prophylactic treatment with one cotrimoxazole double strength tablet twice daily 2 days per week is sufficient to markedly minimize the risk of both bacterial and pneumocystis infection in patients with chronic GVHD, and should be continued while there is clinical evidence of the disease, or while immunosuppression is being administered. Occasional patients will have bacterial infections in spite of prophylactic cotrimoxazole and should receive either prophylactic penicillin or a prophylactic cephalosporin as appropriate, in addition to prophylactic cotrimoxazole.

Other infectious disease recommendations specifically for chronic GVHD include: post-exposure prophylaxis with rifampin for exposure to *Hemophilus influenzae* B; varicella zoster immunoglobulin and acyclovir for exposure to chicken pox if not already immune; immunoglobulin replacement may be beneficial if the total immunoglobulin level is less than 400 mg/dl. Patients with chronic GVHD should not receive live virus vaccinations such as measles, mumps, rubella (MMR), and may fail to generate humoral responses to other vaccines.

Secondary malignancies

A higher incidence of tumors of the skin, buccal cavity, liver, brain/central nervous system, thyroid, bone, and connective tissue is seen after hematopoietic stem cell transplantation (Curtis *et al.,* 1997). While formal screening is not recommended for these tumors, periodic physical examination of the skin, mouth, and thyroid seems prudent. Patients with chronic GVHD have an even higher risk of squamous cell cancers of the buccal cavity and skin. Attention should be paid to these sites on physical exam, and all patients advised to use adequate sun protection and report suspicious lesions.

Prognostic grading schemes

The limited/extensive classification originally proposed by the Seattle group in 1980 is the best established grading system for chronic GVHD. A 1989 survey of transplant physicians concluded these grading criteria were generally reproducible, but a similar, more recent study suggested that agreement about diagnosis, severity, and management was more variable (Atkinson *et al.,* 1989; Lee *et al.,* 2002c). Review of data from HLA-matched sibling recipients reported to the IBMTR suggests that trans-

plant centers are not applying the formal definitions accurately (Lee *et al.,* 2002b), perhaps in part because many patients are unclassifiable by the strict criteria. Seattle has updated the original binary grading scale and labeled the revised scheme as "clinically limited" and "clinically extensive" disease to reflect updated criteria regarding whether or not manifestations require treatment with systemic immunosuppression. However, this revised schema has not been validated (Table 72.2).

Several investigators have tried to develop improved prognostic grading scales based on larger numbers of observed patients. Table 72.3 lists the scales that have been proposed thus far (Shulman *et al.,* 1980; Wingard *et al.,* 1989; Morton *et al.,* 1997; Akpek *et al.,* 2001c; Arora *et al.,* 2001a; Lee *et al.,* 2002b). In aggregate, these studies show that thrombocytopenia (platelet count less than 100×10^9/l), progressive onset, skin involvement, poor performance status, and gastrointestinal involvement portend a poorer prognosis. An overall clinical summary scale of mild, moderate, or severe chronic GVHD has also been used and predicts survival better than the limited/extensive classification (Lee *et al.,* 2002b). However, formal definitions for the mild, moderate, and severe categories have not been established (Gaziev *et al.,* 2001).

Etiology and Pathogenesis

Chronic GVHD animal models exist in the mouse, rat, and dog (Atkinson *et al.,* 1982b; Beschorner *et al.,* 1982; Tutschka *et al.,* 1982; Hamilton & Parkman, 1983; DeClerck *et al.,* 1986; Nonomura *et al.,* 1998; Slayback *et al.,* 2000). In mice, chronic GVHD is associated with a Th2 response with increased interleukin (IL)-4, IL-6, IL-10, and serum immunoglobulin levels (Korholz *et al.,* 1997). In humans, etiology and pathogenesis are less clear, and all branches of the immune system have been implicated. However, direct biological evidence for any of these theories is limited.

The greatest predictor of chronic GVHD is prior acute GVHD. T-cell depletion has been shown to decrease the risk of acute and chronic GVHD in HLA-matched sibling marrow transplantation (Ochs *et al.,* 1994). In addition, increasing severity of acute GVHD is associated with chronic GVHD (Atkinson *et al.,* 1990). These observations are best explained if either (1) alloreactive cells are responsible for both syndromes (donor reactions against host antigens), or (2) if acute GVHD or its treatment causes thymic damage leading to autoimmunity (failure to delete self-reactive clones) (Parkman, 1993; Sherer & Shoenfeld, 1998). Although chronic GVHD is primarily a Th2 phenomenon in mice, both Th1 and Th2 cells have been implicated in humans (Reinherz *et al.,* 1979; Lichtman *et al.,* 1997; Aractingi & Chosidow, 1998; Ratanatharathorn *et al.,* 2001). One study reported that OX40+ (CD134—a member of the tumor necrosis factor superfamily) CD4+ cells predicted onset of chronic GVHD and their decline correlated with response to treatment (Kotani *et al.,* 2001).

Because chronic GVHD is common in the HLA-matched setting, minor antigen mismatches are hypothesized to cause

Table 72.2. *Original and revised Seattle classification for limited and extensive chronic GVHD*

Original Seattle classification	Revised Seattle classification[a]

Limited:
Either or both:
  Localized skin involvement
  Hepatic dysfunction due to chronic GVHD
	Clinical limited:
	  Oral abnormalities consistent with chronic GVHD, a positive skin or lip biopsy, and no other manifestations of chronic GVHD
	  Mild liver test abnormalities (alkaline phosphatase <2 × upper limit of normal, AST or ALT <3 × upper limit of normal and total bilirubin <1.6) with positive skin or lip biopsy, and no other manifestations of chronic GVHD
	  Less than 6 papulosquamous plaques, macular-papular or lichenoid rash involving <20% of body surface area (BSA), dyspigmentation involving <20% BSA, or erythema involving <50% BSA, positive skin biopsy, and no other manifestations of chronic GVHD
	  Ocular sicca (Schirmer's test <5mm with no more than minimal ocular symptoms), positive skin or lip biopsy, and no other manifestations of chronic GVHD
	  Vaginal or vulvar abnormalities with positive biopsy, and no other manifestations of chronic GVHD

Extensive:
Either:
  Generalized skin involvement, or
  Localized skin involvement and/or hepatic dysfunction due to chronic GVHD, plus:
    Liver histology showing chronic aggressive hepatitis, bridging necrosis, or cirrhosis, or
    Involvement of eye (Schirmer's test with <5 mm wetting), or
    Involvement of minor salivary glands or oral mucosa demonstrated on labial biopsy, or
    Involvement of any other target organ
	Clinical extensive:
	  Involvement of two or more organs with symptoms or signs of chronic GVHD, with biopsy documentation of chronic GVHD in any organ
	  >15% base line body weight loss not due to other causes, with biopsy documentation of chronic GVHD in any organ
	  Skin involvement more extensive than defined for clinical limited chronic GVHD, confirmed by biopsy
	  Scleroderma or morphea
	
	  Onycholysis or onychodystrophy thought to represent chronic GVHD, with documentation of chronic GVHD in any organ
	  Decreased range of motion in wrist or ankle extension due to fasciitis caused by chronic GVHD
	  Contractures thought to represent chronic GVHD
	  Bronchiolitis obliterans not due to other causes
	  Positive liver biopsy; or abnormal liver function tests not due to other causes with alkaline phosphatase >2 × upper limit of normal, AST or ALT >3 × upper limit of normal, or total bilirubin >1.6, and documentation of chronic GVHD in any organ
	  Positive upper or lower GI biopsy
	  Fasciitis or serositis thought to represent chronic GVHD and not due to other

causes

[a] Provided by Mary E. D. Flowers and Paul J. Martin, Fred Hutchinson Cancer Research Center, May 2002

Table 72.3. *Prognostic grading schemes*

Reference	n	Platelets	Onset	Skin	Liver	Other poor prognostic factors
Shulman *et al.*, 1980	20	–	–	Generalized involvement	Cirrhosis	"Extensive," poor Karnofsky performance status, recurrent infections, active chronic GVHD after 2 months of therapy
Wingard *et al.*, 1989	85	–	Progressive	Lichenoid involvement	Bilirubin >1.2 mg/dl	
Morton *et al.*, 1997	102	<100 × 10⁹/l	–	–	Bilirubin >2.0 mg/dl	On steroids at onset, interferon-α >6 months duration prior to transplant (CML)
Akpek *et al.*, 2001c	151	<100 × 10⁹/l	Progressive	>50% body surface area	–	Karnofsky score when primary therapy fails
Lee *et al.*, 2000	727	–	–	Involved	–	Karnofsky score, diarrhea, weight loss, lack of oral involvement
Arora *et al.*, 2001 a	159	<100 × 10⁹/l	Progressive	–	–	GI involvement, no response at 6 months

chronic GVHD, although none have yet been directly implicated. Minor antigens are cellular proteins that are processed and presented in the context of MHC class I and II. HA-1, a nonapeptide with a single amino acid difference accounting for its antigenicity, is the best characterized minor antigen (den Haan et al., 1998). However, HA-1 mismatches are associated with an excess of grade III–IV acute GVHD, not chronic GVHD (Gallardo et al., 2001). Minor antigens associated with the Y chromosome (H-Y) are more likely candidates since a parous female donor/male recipient combination is almost uniformly identified as a risk factor for chronic GVHD. However, none of the identified H-Y antigens has yet been linked specifically to an increased incidence of chronic GVHD.

The clinical manifestations of chronic GVHD closely resemble those of several well-recognized autoimmune syndromes including systemic lupus erythematosis, progressive systemic sclerosis, primary biliary cirrhosis, and Sjögren's syndrome. Clinical manifestations resembling those of polyarteritis nodosa have also been described in a patient with chronic GVHD (Ysebaert et al., 2002). Scleroderma, which has cutaneous manifestations similar to late cutaneous chronic GVHD, occurs predominantly in women and has been associated with an increased incidence of circulating fetal male cells, suggesting that persistent microchimerism may play a role (Evans et al., 1999). Other autoimmune hypotheses include loss of specific suppressor cells or expansion of nonspecific suppressor cells.

Given the similarities between chronic GVHD and autoimmune diseases associated with autoantibodies, several studies have tried to link B cells and humoral immunity with chronic GVHD. However, a study of 53 long-term survivors failed to find an association between classic autoantibodies and chronic GVHD (Rouquette-Gally et al., 1988). Another found no association between anti-neutrophil cytoplasmic antibodies and chronic GVHD (Martin et al., 1997). Some antigens, such as promyelocytic leukemia (PML) gene product, are expressed aberrantly in chronic GVHD lesional tissue, but not in uninvolved skin or normal controls (Aractingi et al., 1997). However, circulating antibodies to PML have not been detected.

Finally, cytokine dysregulation has also been implicated through observations that high levels of IL1-β, IL-6, IFN-γ, and TNF-α are associated with more severe chronic GVHD (Barak et al., 1995). High serum TGF-β was also associated with chronic GVHD independent of platelet and white blood cell counts (Liem et al., 1999). Patients with chronic GVHD have low levels of IL-10, an anti-inflammatory cytokine thought to suppress IFN-γ and immunoglobulin production.

In conclusion, there is no consensus about the inciting events and pathogenesis of chronic GVHD in humans. Many studies are contradictory, involve small numbers of patients, and use observational, cross-sectional designs. Larger studies of patients linking clinical status and biologic markers are needed to understand the fundamental biology of the syndrome. Hopefully, this will eventually lead to more effective and less toxic therapies.

Clinical risk factors

A clear understanding of clinical risk factors that predispose individual patients to chronic GVHD is valuable for several reasons. First, it allows physicians to provide better risk assessment for individual patients contemplating allogeneic HSCT. Second, it facilitates the design of clinical studies aimed at decreasing the incidence and severity of chronic GVHD. Finally, it allows comparison between different clinical reports based on the composition of the study populations. Table 72.4 depicts the patient, donor/graft, and procedural factors that have been associated with the development of chronic GVHD. Consistently identified clinical risk factors include older patient age, female donors for male recipients, certain diagnoses (chronic myeloid leukemia and aplastic anemia), use of mismatched or unrelated donors, infusion of donor lymphocytes, use of peripheral blood stem cells (PBSC) instead of bone marrow, lack of T cell depletion, and grade II–IV acute GVHD (Storb et al., 1983; Ringden et al., 1985; Atkinson et al., 1990; Bostrom et al., 1990; Ochs et al., 1994; Carlens et al., 1998; Przepiorka et al., 2001; Zecca et al., 2003). Although acute GVHD is the most powerful predictor of subsequent chronic GVHD, de novo chronic GVHD (no prior acute GVHD)

Table 72.4. *Risk factors for chronic GVHD*

	Patient characteristics	Donor/graft characteristics	Transplant factors
Consistently observed	Older age Male recipient/female donor (especially parous) Chronic myeloid leukemia or aplastic anemia	Mismatched Unrelated Peripheral blood Acute GVHD chemoprophylaxis instead of T-cell depletion Donor lymphocyte infusions	Acute GVHD
Controversial	CMV seropositive Splenectomy	Ethnic diversity between donor and patient	Corticosteroids in the acute GVHD prophylaxis regimen Receiving corticosteroids at time of chronic GVHD diagnosis High CD34+ count (PBSC) Lack of methotrexate in acute GVHD prophylaxis (PBSC)

is associated with similar patient and donor risk factors (Atkinson *et al.*, 1990; Wagner *et al.*, 2000). More controversial risk factors for chronic GVHD include CMV seropositivity, CMV reactivation, splenectomy, steroid prophylaxis for acute GVHD, ethnic diversity between donor and patient, steroid treatment at the time of chronic GVHD diagnosis, high CD34+ cell count in the graft, and absence of methotrexate in PBSC transplantation (Bostrom *et al.*, 1990; Ochs *et al.*, 1994; Przepiorka *et al.*, 2001; Remberger *et al.*, 2001a; Wagner *et al.*, 1998; Zaucha *et al.*, 2001). Administration of contrast medium for CT scanning has been described as triggering skin involvement (Vavricka *et al.*, 2002).

Recipient gene polymorphisms for IFN-γ, TNF, and IL-10, and donor polymorphism for IL-1Ra, have been associated with severe acute GVHD after HLA-identical sibling marrow transplantation, and recipient polymorphisms for IL1-Ra, IL-6 and IL-10 with chronic GVHD (Middleton *et al.*, 1998; Cavet *et al.*, 2001; Cullup *et al.*, 2001; Rocha *et al.*, 2002).

Peripheral blood progenitor cells have been associated with an increased incidence of chronic GVHD (50%–90%) in most studies of HLA-matched sibling transplantation (Storek *et al.*, 1997; Scott *et al.*, 1998; Solano *et al.*, 1998; Vigorito *et al.*,

1998. Champlin *et al.*, 2000; Snowden *et al.*, 2000; Cutler *et al.*, 2001; Morton *et al.*, 2001). Cutler and colleagues performed a meta-analysis using data from 16 studies and reported a pooled relative risk for any chronic GVHD after PBSC of 1.52 (95% CI 1.25–1.88, $P < .001$) and for extensive chronic GVHD (RR 1.66, 95% CI 1.35–2.05, $P < .001$) compared to bone marrow (Fig. 72.3). A randomzied study with a median follow-up 45 months found a 3-year cumulative incidence of chronic GVHD of 65% in the PBSC recipients and 36% in the marrow recipients (Mohty *et al.*, 2002). The incidence of extensive chronic GVHD was 44% and 17% respectively ($p = 0.004$). Prevalence of chronic GVHD was always higher in the PBSC group, ocular involvement was commoner and the PBSC group required more hospitalization. In the long-term follow-up of another randomized trial, the incidence of chronic GVHD was similar in the two arms, but the number of successive treatments needed to control chronic GVHD was higher after PBSC transplantation and the duration of corticosteroid treatment was longer (Flowers *et al.*, 2002). Data suggest that high CD34+ counts may be the most important factor driving this observation, since chronic GVHD did not correlate with CD3+ and CD14+ counts (Zaucha

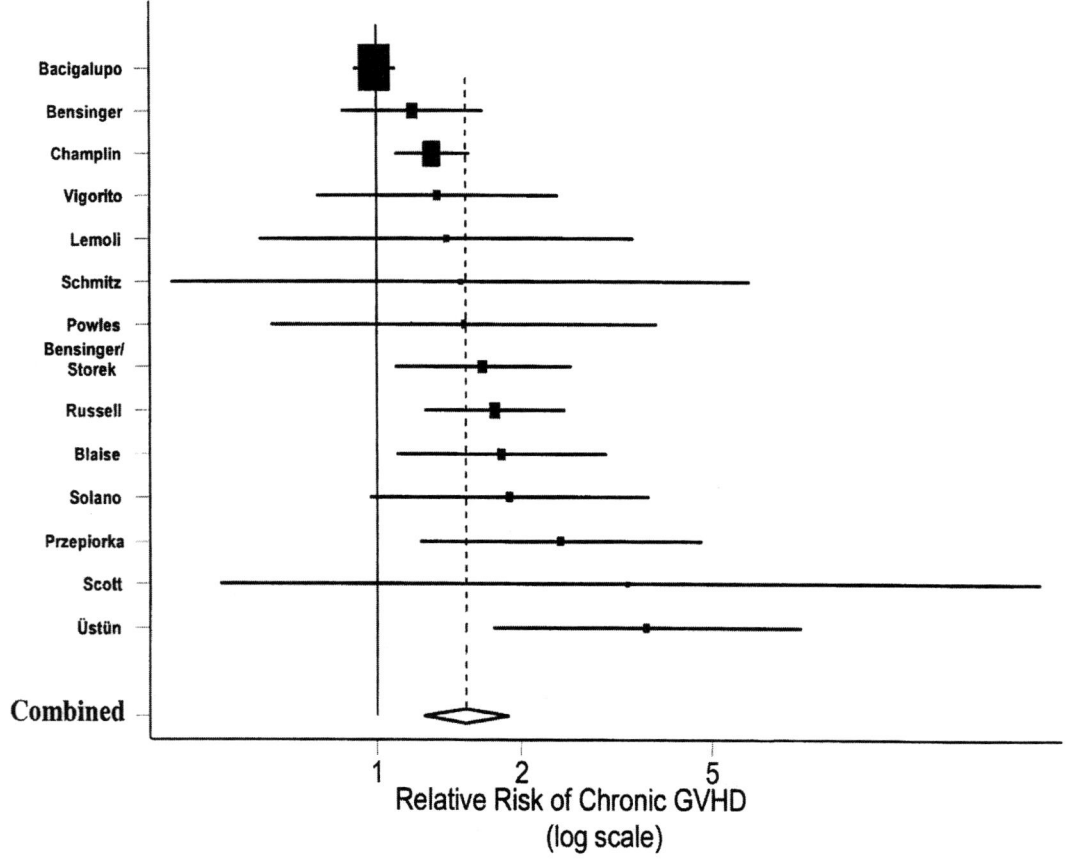

Fig. 72.3. Forest plot for all trials reporting relative risks (RR) of chronic GVHD. Shaded squares reflect individual study sample size and RR, expressed as within-study variance. The solid vertical line denotes a RR of 1.0. The diamond reflects the cumulative RR with confidence intervals for the RR (logarithmic scale). Reproduced, with permission, from Cutler *et al.* (2001).

et al., 2001). An interesting trial performed by Morton and colleagues suggested that donor treatment per se with granulocyte colony-stimulating factor (G-CSF) is not the cause of the higher chronic GVHD incidence. They randomized HLA-matched sibling donors to marrow or PBSC collection after both groups received G-CSF stimulation (*n* = 57). Rates of chronic GVHD were higher in the PBSC arm (80% vs. 22%, *P* < .02) although overall survival was the same (Morton *et al.*, 2001). In the unrelated donor marrow setting, patients have a higher risk for chronic GVHD than HLA-matched siblings (Lee *et al.*, 2002b), but it is not clear whether PBSC further elevates this risk (Remberger *et al.*, 2001b; Elmaagacli *et al.*, 2002).

Finally, several factors have been studied and not found to be associated with chronic GVHD. These include type of myeloablative conditioning regimen, type of calcineurin inhibitor, and whether three or four doses of methotrexate prophylaxis are administered. The reported incidence of chronic GVHD is similar for busulfan/cyclophosphamide and total body irradiation/cyclosphosphamide preparative regimens (Socie *et al.*, 2001a). Use of either tacrolimus or cyclosporine prophylaxis resulted in similar rates of chronic GVHD although there was less extensive chronic GVHD in the tacrolimus group (Ratanatharathorn *et al.*, 1998). Failure to give day 11 methotrexate was not shown to influence rates of chronic GVHD although only a small number of patients was studied (Atkinson & Downs, 1995; Sullivan, 1999).

Prevention

Although acute GVHD is the leading predictor of chronic GVHD, successful efforts to decrease acute GVHD have not meaningfully decreased rates of chronic GVHD. The two notable exceptions are T cell depletion and use of umbilical cord blood as a stem cell source (Kurtzberg *et al.*, 1996; Gluckman *et al.*, 1997), since lower rates of both acute and chronic GVHD are observed with these approaches. However, these conclusions are based on observational studies, and the impact on overall survival is unknown.

Very early studies tried to prevent chronic GVHD with thymic replacement or support. (Witherspoon *et al.*, 1988). Other unsuccessful efforts to prevent chronic GVHD include modification of immunosuppressive tapering schedules, adding immunosuppressive agents, and prophylactic replacement of immunoglobulin (Table 72.5). Many of these randomized studies were well-designed and based on compelling clinical observations. For example, several reports noted that the peak onset of chronic GVHD occurred during the immunosuppression taper (Storb *et al.*, 1989b), and that a lower incidence of chronic GVHD seemed to be associated with prolonged cyclosporine administration (Ruutu *et al.*, 1988; Bacigalupo *et al.*, 1990; Lonnqvist *et al.*, 1990). Based on these observations, the Seattle group performed a large randomized trial (*n* = 162) of 24 months of cyclosporine versus the standard 6 months. Chronic GVHD developed in 39% of patients on the extended cyclosporine arm and 51% in the standard arm (hazard ratio 0.76, 95% CI 0.48–1.21, *P* = .25). However, rates of transplant-

related mortality, relapse-free survival, and overall survival were identical in the two arms (Kansu *et al.*, 2001). In another trial, the intervention studied led to worse outcome: Chao and colleagues (1996) performed a randomized, double-blinded study of 59 patients assigned to thalidomide prophylaxis (starting day +80 post stem cell infusion) or placebo. Interim analysis after 54 evaluable patients showed thalidomide treatment was associated with more chronic GVHD (64% versus 38%, *P* = .06) and higher mortality (92% vs 61% at 18 months, *P* = .006) prompting early closure of the study.

Loughran and colleagues (1990) tried to decrease the morbidity of chronic GVHD through early diagnosis and treatment. Asymptomatic patients were screened with skin and lip biopsies to identify and treat those with subclinical disease, trying to avert clinical chronic GVHD. Outcome was not improved with this approach, and the authors hypothesized that chronic GVHD might be necessary in patients transplanted for advanced malignant disease to prevent relapse. (Sullivan *et al.*, 1988b; Wagner *et al.*, 1998; Loughran *et al.*, 1990).

Treatment

Early unsuccessful attempts to treat chronic GVHD included thymic grafts, donor lymphocyte infusions, and anti-thymocyte globulin (Graze & Gale, 1979; Sullivan *et al.*, 1981). For the last decade, standard therapy has consisted of an alternating daily regimen of corticosteroids and calcineurin inhibitors (cyclosporine or tacrolimus). This approach was based on a phase II study reporting greater than 50% survival compared with 26% seen in historical controls. Eventually 80%–90% of survivors successfully stopped immunosuppressive medications, although treatment lasted a median of 18–36 months (Sullivan *et al.*, 1988a, 1988b). Vogelsang has published excellent guidelines on evaluation, initiation of therapy, and management of the immunosuppressive taper. She recommends starting both steroids and cyclosporine at onset of chronic GVHD, trying to taper the steroids first to every other day, then the cyclosporine to every other day with dose adjustments every 2 weeks. In her experience, 90% of patients who are going to respond do so within 3 months. If disease is stable, therapy is continued and reevaluated every 3 months. (Vogelsang, 2001). Flowers has recently reviewed the success of up-front combination therapy applied in the late 1980s. She reported a nonrelapse mortality of 21% in standard risk patients (*n* = 126) and 39% in high-risk (*n* = 111) patients, defined by progressive onset or thrombocytopenia. Successful discontinuation of all immunosuppressive medications eventually occurred in 60% of standard risk patients and 40% of high-risk patients (Fig. 72.4) (Flowers, 2002).

Table 72.6 shows the clinical trials evaluating primary treatment of chronic GVHD. Two randomized trials (*n* = 52 and *n* = 54) added thalidomide to standard corticosteroid and cyclosporine treatment for newly diagnosed chronic GVHD. Both these trials were closed early after interim analysis suggested that they would not reach statistical significance even if all patients were enrolled (Koc *et al.*, 2000; Arora *et al.*, 2001b). Data from a randomized trial of prednisone with or without

Table 72.5.   *Prevention trials (all patients received bone marrow)*

Intervention	Population	Comment	Chronic GVHD conclusions	Reference
Randomized trials of acute GVHD prophylaxis				
Cyclosporine/steroids versus cyclosporine alone	HLA-matched sibling recipients at high risk of relapse post-transplant, $n = 60$	Decreased incidence of acute GVHD but similar survival	Higher incidence of chronic GVHD (44% versus 21%, $P = .02$) with combination therapy	Deeg et al., 1997
Cyclosporine/metho-trexate versus metho-trexate alone	HLA-matched sibling recipients with aplastic anemia, $n = 46$	Decreased incidence of acute GVHD and better survival	Trend towards higher chronic GVHD in combination (58% vs 36%, $P = .18$)	Storb et al., 1989b
Cyclosporine/metho-trexate versus cyclo-sporine alone	HLA-matched sibling recipients with AML in CR1 or CML, $n = 93$	Decreased incidence of acute GVHD and improved survival	No difference	Storb et al., 1989a
Cyclosporine/metho-trexate ± steroids	HLA matched ($n = 122$) or 1 antigen mismatched ($n = 25$) recipients, heterogeneous diseases		Higher incidence of chronic GVHD (62% versus 40%, $P = .01$) in group receiving steroids independent of acute GVHD	Storb et al., 1990
Cyclosporine/steroids ± methotrexate	HLA-matched sibling recipients with acute leukemia in CR1 or CML, $n = 149$		No difference	Ross et al., 1999
Randomized trials aimed directly at chronic GVHD prevention				
Dose of cyclosporine (high vs. low dose)	HLA-matched sibling recipients with acute leukemia, $n = 81$	Low dose cyclosporine associated with lower relapse rate	No difference	Bacigalupo et al., 1991
Duration of cyclosporine administration (24 months vs. 6 months)	Prior acute GVHD or skin biopsy positive for sub-clinical chronic GVHD, $n = 162$	Incidence of chronic GVHD in 6 month cyclosporine arm lower than historical controls	No difference	Kansu et al., 2001
Duration of cyclosporine administration (6 months vs. 60 days)	No active acute GVHD, $n = 103$	Onset of chronic GVHD more rapid in short cyclosporine arm, higher treatment-related mortality in short cyclo-sporine arm if prior acute GVHD	No difference	Storb et al., 1997
Cyclosporine/metho-trexate ± thalidomide	90% HLA-matched sibling recipients, $n = 54$	Double-blinded, study closed early due to lower survival and more chronic GVHD in the group receiving thalidomide	Thalidomide associated with more chronic GVHD and worse survival	Chao et al., 1996
Immunoglobulin versus no immunoglobulin	Heterogeneous population $n = 250$	Immunoglobulin arm had more total infections in year 2 than control patients	No difference	Sullivan et al., 1996
Different doses of immunoglobulin	Heterogeneous population, $n = 627$	Double-blinded, 3 dose levels of IgG, similar rates of infection and interstitial pneumonitis	No difference	Winston et al., 2001

cyclosporine suggest that cyclosporine does not increase the efficacy of single-agent corticosteroids, although the risk of avascular necrosis is lower with combined therapy. Intriguingly, subset analysis suggested that patients with poor prognosis chronic GVHD (on the basis of progressive onset) had worse disease-free survival with combination therapy (Koc et al., 2002).

If patients fail to respond to, or progress on, corticosteroid-based therapy, then secondary therapy is indicated. Steroid-refractory chronic GVHD is formally defined as either failure to improve after at least two months, or progression after one

month, of standard immunosuppressive therapy including corticosteroids and cyclosporine (Parker et al., 1995; Browne et al., 2000). A number of phase II trials of secondary or salvage regimens have been published, and most report a success rate of 25%–50%. However, most trials contain 40 or fewer patients. Reported response rates are usually based on four categories: complete (resolution of all chronic GVHD manifestations), partial (>50% but less than complete organ responses), no response (<50% response), and progression (worsening while on therapy) (Vogelsang et al., 1992; Parker et al., 1995).

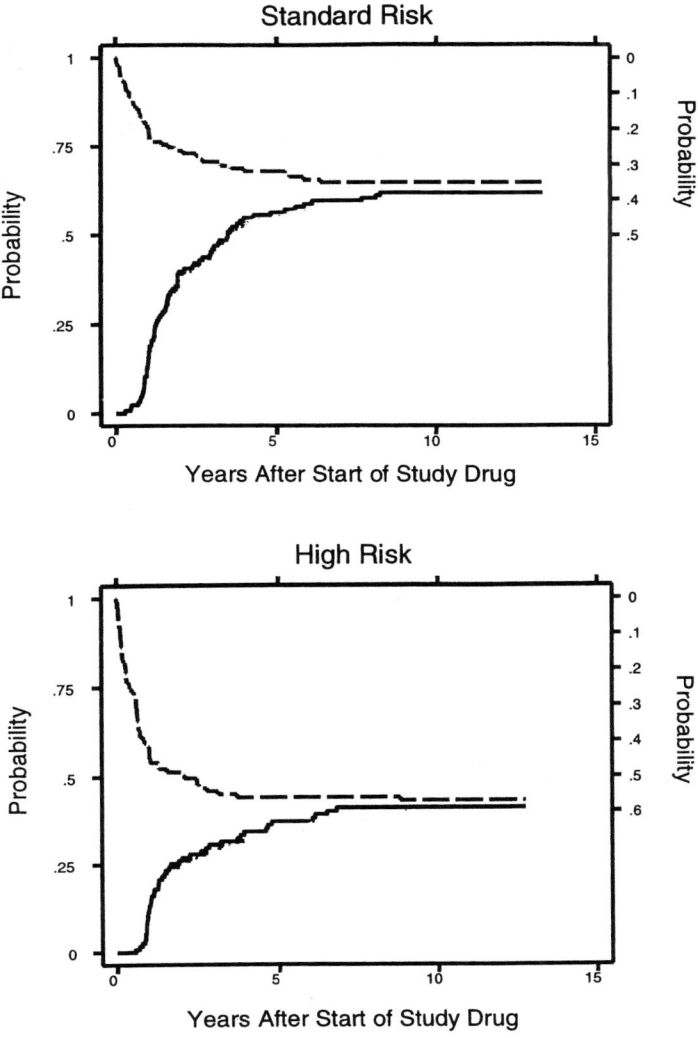

Fig. 72.4. Probability of discontinuation of all systemic immunosuppressive medications (lower curves) and probability of death or relapse during immuno-suppressive therapy (upper curves) in patients with standard risk (*n* = 126) or high-risk (*n* = 111) defined by progressive onset or thrombocytopenia. Reproduced, with permission, from Flowers (2002)

Table 72.7 summarizes agents used as secondary therapy for chronic GVHD, and Figure 72.5 shows the frequency with which they were used in practice in 2001, based on a survey of transplant physicians. Thalidomide and phototherapy (psoralen and ultraviolet A [PUVA] and extracorporeal phototherapy [ECP]) are the best-studied secondary therapies. Vogelsang and colleagues (1992) reported a 32% complete response rate to thalidomide (similar rates in refractory and high-risk patients) and a 27% partial response rate (mostly in previously refractory patients) in 44 patients with either steroid-refractory or untreated high-risk patients. In contrast, Parker reported an 11% complete response rate and 9% partial response rate in 80 patients with refractory chronic GVHD (Parker *et al.*, 1995). Thalidomide has been safely used in children and response rates may be better in this population (Rovelli *et al.*, 1998).

Vogelsang reported satisfactory cutaneous responses in 40 patients treated with PUVA, although 13 subsequently died of chronic GVHD (Vogelsang *et al.*, 1996). Because PUVA is not thought to affect visceral chronic GVHD manifestations, ECP is now favored over PUVA. Greinix reported favorable responses in 16 patients with steroid-refractory chronic GVHD (Greinix *et al.*, 1998). Alcindor and colleagues (2001) studied laboratory correlates of successful ECP in 10 patients treated for steroid-refractory chronic GVHD. Clinical response was correlated with decreases in CD8+ T cells and CD80+ and CD123+ dendritic cells (DC1), and an increase in natural killer cells. In other studies, response of skin GVHD was associated with the presence of amplified populations of clonal T cells (French *et al.*, 2002) and an increase in DC2 numbers (CD83+/CD86+) stimulated Th2 helper T cells to secrete Th2 cytokines, which indirectly inhibited Th1-mediated alloreactivity (Gorgun *et al.*, 2002). ECP has been used successfully in children (Dall'Amico *et al.*, 1997). A randomized trial of ECP versus continued standard therapy for steroid-refractory

Table 72.6. *Primary therapy for chronic GVHD*

Study	Treatment	n	Comments	Conclusions
Sullivan *et al.*, 1981	Group I: Untreated, Group II: cortico-steroids and/or anti-thymocyte globulin, Group III: corticosteroids and cyclophosphamide, procarbazine, or azathioprine	52	Sequential study, alive and free of disability: untreated 15%, corticosteroids and/or ATG 23%, combination therapy 71%	Most effective regimen was corticosteroids and azathioprine
Sullivan *et al.*, 1988b	Corticosteroids ± azathioprine	179	Standard risk patients were randomized, high risk patients given single agent prednisone, 40% of patients in each group had subclinical disease only	Higher mortality from infection if azathioprine part of initial treatment regimen. In high-risk patients (plt <100 K), prednisone alone resulted in 26% survival
Sullivan *et al.*, 1988a	Alternating day corticosteroids and cyclosporine	61	Phase II design, high-risk extensive chronic GVHD, 40 given primary therapy, 21 given salvage, long-term survival >50% compared with historical control of 26%	Alternating day, combination therapy better
Arora *et al.*, 2001b	Cyclosporine, steroids ± thalidomide	54	Randomized, unblinded trial, patients with extensive chronic GVHD.	Closed early (target enrollment n = 134) after interim analysis showed slow accrual and higher response rates in both arms than projected
Koc *et al.*, 2000	Steroids, cyclosporine or tacrolimus, ± thalidomide	51	Randomized, placebo-controlled trial of thalidomide added to standard upfront therapy in higher risk patients with thrombocytopenia or progressive presentation.	Closed early (target enrollment n = 132) after interim analysis showed slow accrual and only 42% probability of reaching statistical significance by enrolling remainder of patients.
Koc *et al.*, 2002	Steroids ± cyclosporine	287	Randomized, unblinded trial, enrolled 1985–1992	Disease-free survival was lower in the combination arm (RR 1.51, 95% CI 1.03–2.21, *P* = .03) in multivariate analysis. Transplant-related mortality, relapse, secondary chronic GVHD therapy rates and discontinuation of all immunosuppressive therapy were not different

Abbreviations: ATG, antithymocyte globulin; plt, platelet count.

chronic GVHD is ongoing, and should provide important comparative data about the effectiveness of this approach.

Impact on other transplantation outcomes

Nonrelapse mortality

Chronic GVHD is the major cause of nonrelapse mortality more than 2 years following allogeneic HSC transplantation, and increasing severity of chronic GVHD is associated with higher nonrelapse mortality rates (Socie *et al.*, 1999; Lee *et al.*, 2002b) (Fig. 72.6). Infection from a broad array of pathogens is the major cause of death, followed by progressive organ failure due to chronic GVHD involvement. De novo chronic GVHD occurs later than the other forms of chronic GVHD and does not seem to adversely affect survival (Weiden *et al.*, 1981). In pre-malignant diseases, such as aplastic anemia and refractory anemias where the risk of relapse and death from the primary disease is low, chronic GVHD has a substantial adverse impact on survival that has not improved significantly over the past 30 years (Deeg *et al.*, 1998; Goerner *et al.*, 2002).

Graft-versus-malignancy effect

As shown in Figs. 72.6 and 72.7, chronic GVHD is associated with lower relapse rates in both early and advanced stage

Table 72.7. *Secondary therapy for chronic GVHD*

Agent	Published success rate	Hypothesized mechanism of action	Side effects	References
High-dose corticosteroids	48% major response rate ($n = 56$)	Lympholytic at these doses	Infection, glucose intolerance, osteoporosis, avascular necrosis, cataracts, psychological effects including psychosis, insomnia	Akpek et al., 2001a
Tacrolimus (Prograf)	35% response rate ($n = 39$)	Binds to FKBP-12 (FK binding protein) and inhibits T lymphocyte activation	Renal dysfunction, neurotoxicity, hypertension	Carnevale-Schianca et al., 2000; Tzakis et al., 1991
Mycophenolate mofetil (Cellcept)	46% objective response ($n = 26$)	Prodrug of mycophenolic acid that is a noncompetitive reversible inhibitor of inosine monophosphate dehydrogenase. Cytostatic for T and B lymphocytes since they lack salvage pathways	Nausea, vomiting, diarrhea, neutropenia	Basara et al., 1998; Mookerjee et al., 1999
Rapamycin (Rapamune)	Not available	Binds to FKBP-12 and mTOR to inhibit cytokine-driven T-cell proliferation	Hyperlipidemia, hypertension, rash	
Extracorporeal photopheresis	33%–80% ($n = 11$–18)	Induces apoptosis in alloreactive T cells, normalization of CD4/CD8 ratios by decreasing CD8+ cells, increases natural killer cells, decreases dendritic cells	GI upset, potential need for central i.v. access	Alcindor et al., 2001; Child et al., 1999; Dall'Amico et al., 1997; Greinix et al., 1998
Psoralen and UVA (PUVA)	40% CR, 38% PR ($n = 11$–40)	Interferes with antigen presentation and inflammatory cytokine production by Langerhans' cells, increases IL10 production by keratinocytes	Increase in skin cancer, phototoxicity, nausea, hepatotoxicity	Eppinger et al., 1990; Jampel et al., 1991; Kapoor et al., 1992; Redding et al., 1998; Vogelsang et al., 1996
UVB radiation	Case series	Treats epidermis only, induces IL-10 in human epidermal cells	Increase in skin cancer, phototoxicity	Enk et al., 1998
Thalidomide	9–42% CR rate ($n = 14$–80)	Anti-inflammatory and immunosuppressive properties	Neuropathy, somnolence, constipation, neutropenia	Browne et al., 2000; Parker et al., 1995; Rovelli et al., 1998; Vogelsang et al., 1992
Etretinate (no longer available), acitretin (Soriatane)	74% improvement ($n = 27$)	Synthetic vitamin A derivative, may affect production of cytokines	Skin scaling, breakdown, nail cracking, xerosis, cheilitis, pruritis, rare pseudotumor cerebri	Marcellus et al., 1999
Azathioprine (Imuran)	Not available	Cleaved to mercaptopurine	Gastrointestinal symptoms, neutropenia, thrombocytopenia	
Hydroxychloroquine (Plaquenil)	9% CR and 44% PR ($n = 40$)	Interferes with antigen processing and presentation, proliferation, TNF-α production, and cytotoxicity	Gastrointestinal symptoms, rare retinal toxicity	Gilman et al., 2000
Ursodeoxycholic acid (Actigal)	33% decrease in bilirubin levels, but not sustained off therapy ($n = 12$)	Replaces native human bile acids, reduces class I HLA expression on hepatocytes	Diarrhea, abdominal pain, headache	Fried et al., 1992
Clofazimine (Lamprene)	55% PR ($n = 22$)	Atypical immunomodulatory effects	Abdominal cramping, hyperpigmentation	Lee et al., 1997
Anti-thymocyte globulin (ATG)	Not available	In vivo T=cell depletion	Anaphylaxis, serum sickness	
Daclizumab (Zenapax)	Not available	Humanized anti-IL-2 receptor antibody	None	
Infliximab (Remicade)	Reported in abstracts	Chimeric IgG monoclonal antibody, binds to TNF-α and prevents binding with receptors	Hypersensitivity reactions, infections	

(continues)

Table 72.7.   *(Continued)*

Agent	Published success rate	Hypothesized mechanism of action	Side effects	References
Etanercept	Letter	Genetically-engineered fusion protein consisting of two identical chains of the extracellular human TNF receptor p75 monomer fused with the Fc domain of human IgG_1 (which binds TNF and lympho-totoxin-A and inhibits their activity)		Andolina *et al.*, 2000
2-deoxyco-formycin (Pentostatin)	Reported in abstracts	Inhibits adenosine deaminase (ADA)	Nausea, vomiting, myelo-suppression, rash, headache	
Rituximab (Rituxan)	Case report	Chimeric anti-CD20 monoclonal antibody	Allergic reactions	Ratanatharathor *et al.*, 2000
Total lymphoid radiation	Case series		Leukopenia	Bullorsky *et al.*, 1993; Socie *et al.*, 1990
Topical azathioprine	Case report	Purine analog metabolized to 6-mercaptopurine	Rash, fever, pancreatitis, arthralgias, malaise, nausea, diarrhea, pancytopenia, hepatitis, infections, malignancy	Epstein *et al.*, 2000
Topical tacrolimus	Case series	0.1% ointment	Localized skin burning, pruritus, irritation	Aoyama *et al.*, 1995
Opthalmic cyclosporine	Case series	1% solution	None	Kiang *et al.*, 1998
Intravenous lidocaine	Case report	Vascular and anti-inflammatory properties	Seizures, drowsiness, tremors, hypotension	Voltarelli *et al.*, 2001

Abbreviations: mTDR, mammalian target of rapamycin; IL, interleukin; TNF, tumor necrosis's factor.

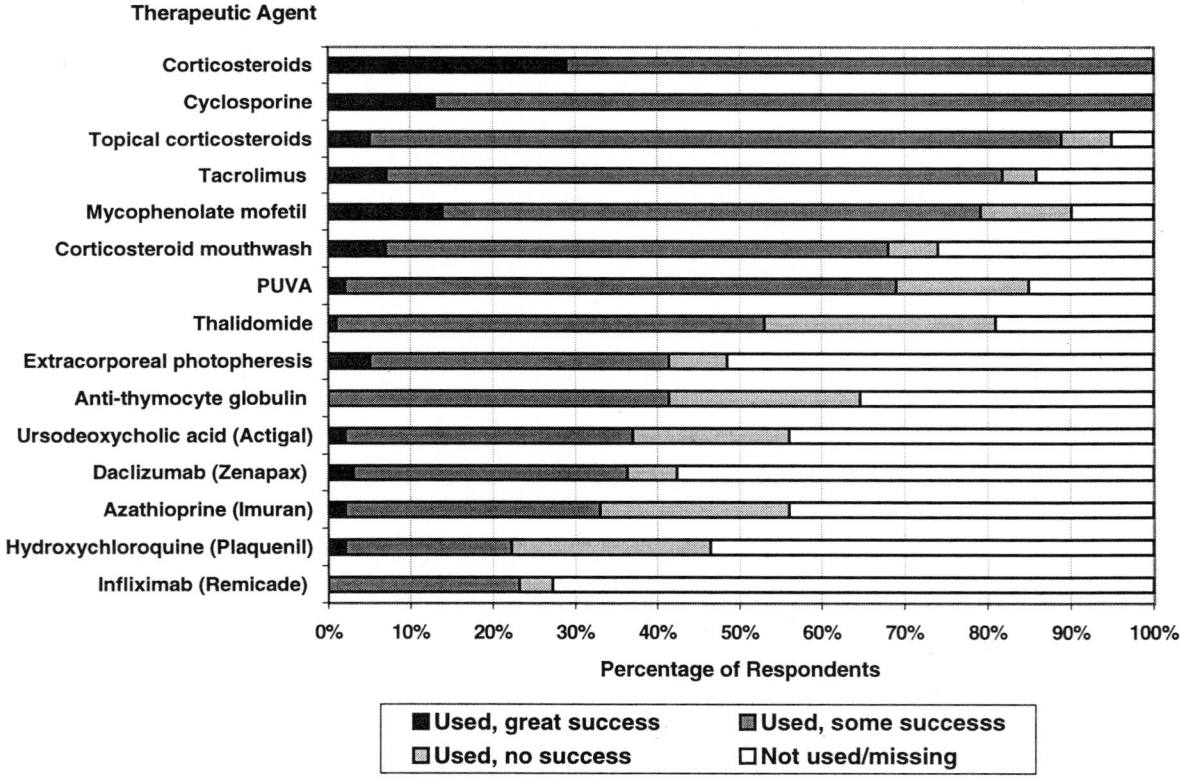

Fig. 72.5. Experience and perceived success with the 15 most common therapies for chronic GVHD. Reproduced, with permission, from Lee *et al.* (2002c).

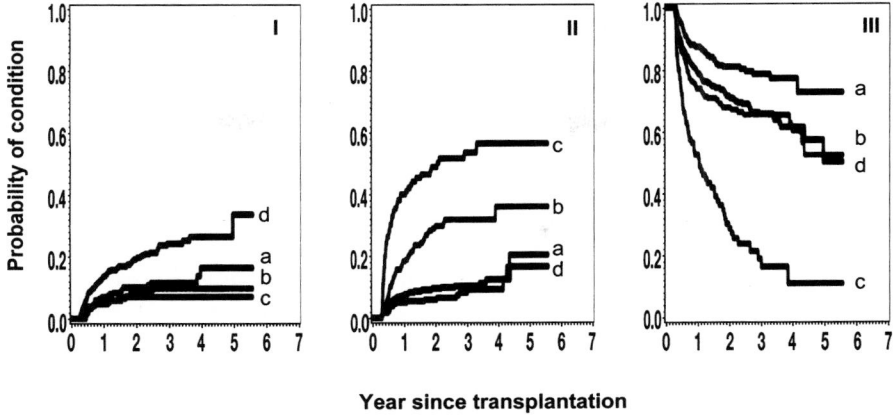

Fig. 72.6. Association of severity of chronic GVHD with relapse (I), treatment-related mortality (II), and disease-free survival (III). Reproduced, with permission, from Lee *et al.* (2002b).

leukemia (Weiden *et al.*, 1979; Weiden *et al.*, 1981; Sullivan *et al.*, 1989; Horowitz *et al.*, 1990; Ringden *et al.*, 1997; Brunet *et al.*, 2001; Lee *et al.*, 2002b). However, the nature of this graft-versus-malignancy effect is poorly understood, and it is not known whether the protective effect relies on development of overt chronic GVHD or is durable once chronic GVHD resolves (Sullivan *et al.*, 1989). Observational data suggest that increased severity of chronic GVHD is not associated with a decreased relapse risk (Fig. 72.6). Nevertheless, studies examining preventive and treatment strategies should carefully follow relapse rates, especially in situations where disease is advanced or cure is thought to be heavily reliant on an intact graft-versus-malignancy effect. For example, eradication of Philadelphia-chromosome positive cells in patients with

chronic myeloid leukemia was correlated with development of chronic GVHD in one study (Pichert *et al.*, 1995).

Impact on functional status and quality of life

Chronic GVHD is associated with substantial quality of life deficits, particularly in the areas of physical and functional status (Syrjala *et al.*, 1993; Chiodi *et al.*, 2000; Heinonen *et al.*, 2001; Lee *et al.*, 2002a; Goerner *et al.*, 2002). (Fig. 72.8). In addition, patients with chronic GVHD report more specific symptoms such as rashes, mouth sores, and frequent infections than unaffected individuals (Schmidt *et al.*, 1993; Sutherland *et al.*, 1997). Social and emotional functioning and satisfaction with transplantation are relatively preserved, although chronic GVHD is asso-

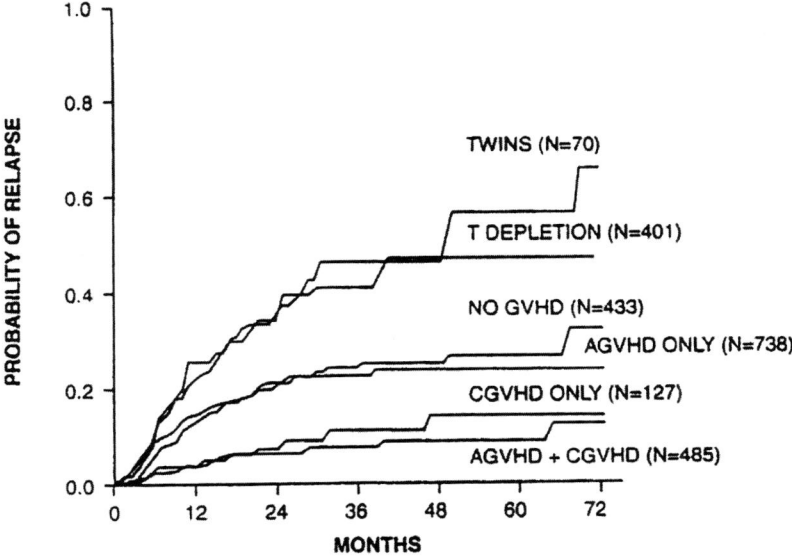

Fig. 72.7. Actuarial probability of relapse after bone marrow transplantation for early leukemia according to type of graft and development of GVHD in recipients of HLA-matched sibling marrow for leukemia, *n* = 2,254. Reproduced, with permission, from Horowitz *et al.* (1990).

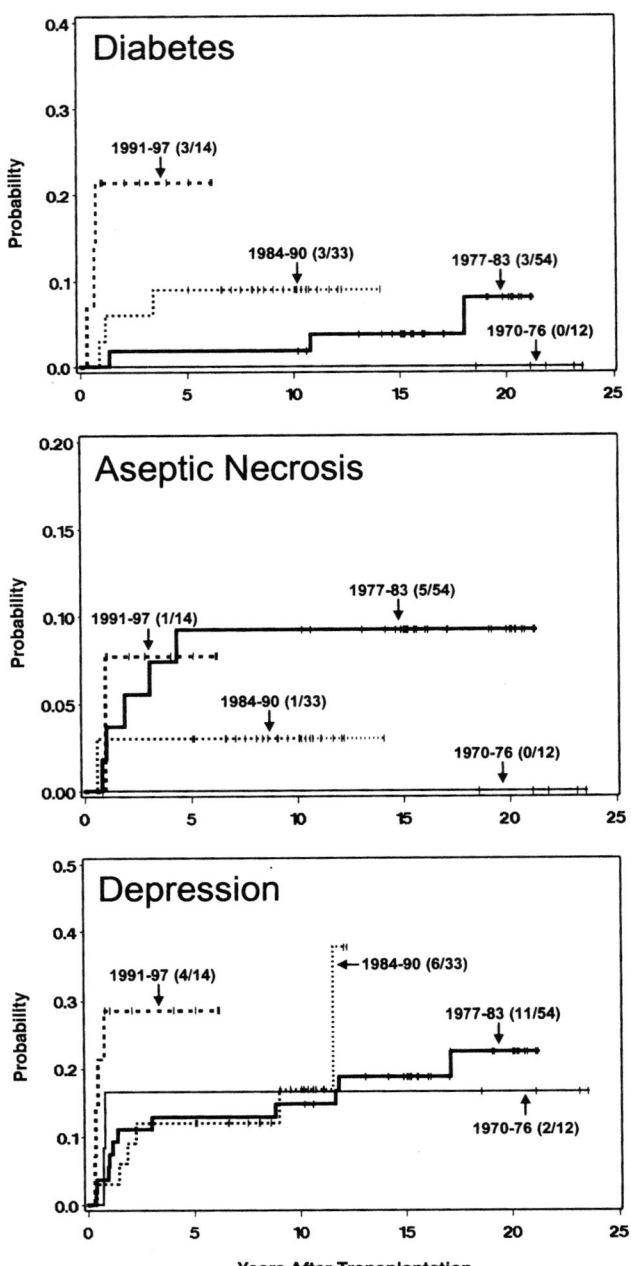

Fig. 72.8. Other complications. Probabilities of developing depression, diabetes mellitus, and aseptic necrosis, all requiring treatment, among 113 patients with extensive chronic GVHD. For any patient, only the first event was considered. Reproduced, with permission, from Goerner *et al.* (2002).

ciated with decreased general health status, sexual inactivity, and loss of employment in long-term survivors (Sullivan *et al.,* 1991; Wingard *et al.,* 1991; Andrykowski *et al.,* 1995; Marks *et al.,* 1999; Socie *et al.,* 2001b; Lee *et al.,* 2002a). Unexpectedly, some studies find that patients with chronic GVHD actually rate their overall quality of life as superior to transplant patients without chronic GVHD (Bush *et al.,* 1995). Authors have attributed this seemingly paradoxical finding to continued reminders of sur-

vivorship, or a shift in expectations emphasizing the positive of survival rather than the negative of functional compromise.

Conclusions

The incidence of chronic GVHD is likely to increase as the field of HSC transplantation embraces greater use of PBSC and mismatched donors. In addition, reduced intensity conditioning regimens are allowing older patients to undergo transplantation, and older age is a recognized risk factor for chronic GVHD. So far, no method can reliably prevent chronic GVHD, although T cell depletion and use of umbilical cord blood seems to decrease the incidence. As we develop a better understanding of the human immune system and the complex cellular and cytokine interactions that regulate it, there is hope that the positive component of chronic GVHD (the graft-versus-malignancy effect) can be separated from the nonspecific morbidity and mortality patients now suffer. Targeted approaches to eliminate or control chronic GVHD would benefit the majority of allogeneic transplant recipients and should be a high priority for the HSCT research community.

References

Abesada-Terk, G., Quintero, M., Przepiorka, D. *et al.* (1990). Diminished tear production in BMT recipients not receiving radiation. *Bone Marrow Transplantation,* **6,** 151 (Letter).

Akpek, G., Lee, S. M., Anders, V., & Vogelsang, G. B. (2001a). A high-dose pulse steroid regimen for controlling active chronic graft-versus-host disease. *Biology of Blood and Marrow Transplantation,* **7,** 495–502.

Akpek, G., Valladares, J. L., Lee, L., Margolis, J., & Vogelsang, G. B. (2001b). Pancreatic insufficiency in patients with chronic graft-versus-host disease. *Bone Marrow Transplantation,* **27,** 163–6.

Akpek, G., Zahurak, M. L., Piantadosi, S. *et al.* (2001c). Development of a prognostic model for grading chronic graft-versus-host disease. *Blood,* **97,** 1219–26.

Alcindor, T., Gorgun, G., Miller, K. B. *et al.* (2001). Immunomodulatory effects of extracorporeal photochemotherapy in patients with extensive chronic graft-versus-host disease. *Blood,* **98,** 1622–5.

Al-Eid, M. A., Tutschka, P. J., Wagner, H. N. *et al.* (1983). Functional asplenia in patients with chronic graft-versus-host disease. *Journal of Nuclear Medicine,* **24,** 1123–6.

Anderson, B. A., Young, P. V., Kean, W. F. *et al.* (1982). Polymyositis in chronic graft-versus-host disease: a case report. *Archives of Neurology,* **39,** 188–90.

Andolina, M., Rabusin, M., Maximova, N., & Di Leo, G. (2000). Etanercept in graft-versus-host disease. *Bone Marrow Transplantation,* **26,** 929 (Letter).

Andrykowski, M. A., Greiner, C. B., Altmaier, E. M. *et al.* (1995). Quality of life following bone marrow transplantation: findings from a multicentre study. *British Journal of Cancer,* **71,** 1322–9.

Anonymous. (2000). Guidelines for preventing opportunistic infections among hematopoietic stem cell transplant recipients. *Biology of Blood and Marrow Transplantation,* **6,** 659–713; 715; 717–27; quiz 729–33.

Aoyama, H., Tabata, N., Tanaka, M., Uesugi, Y., & Tagami, H. (1995). Successful treatment of resistant facial lesions of atopic dermatitis with 0.1% FK506 ointment. *British Journal of Dermatology*, **133**, 494–6.

Aractingi, S. & Chosidow, O. (1998). Cutaneous graft-versus-host disease. *Archives of Dermatology*, **134**, 602–12.

Aractingi, S., de The, H., Gluckman, E., Le Goue, C., & Carosela, E. D. (1997). PML is expressed in chronic graft-versus-host disease lesions. *Bone Marrow Transplantation*, **19**, 1125–8.

Arora, M., Burns, L. J., Davies, S. M. et al. (2001a). Chronic graft versus host disease: a prospective cohort study. *Blood*, 98 (Abstract).

Arora, M., Wagner, J. E., Davies, S. M. et al. (2001b). Randomized clinical trial of thalidomide, cyclosporine, and prednisone versus cyclosporine and prednisone as initial therapy for chronic graft-versus-host disease. *Biology of Blood and Marrow Transplantation*, **7**, 265–73.

Atkinson, K. (1990). Chronic graft-versus-host disease. *Bone Marrow Transplantation*, **5**, 69–82.

Atkinson, K., Bryant, D., Delprado, W. et al. (1989a). Widespread pulmonary fibrosis as a major clinical manifestation of chronic graft-versus-host disease. *Bone Marrow Transplantation*, **4**, 129–32.

Atkinson, K., Dodds, A., Concannon, A. et al. (1987). Late onset transfusion-dependent anemia with thrombocytopenia secondary to marrow fibrosis and hypoplasia associated with chronic graft-versus-host disease. *Bone Marrow Transplantation*, **2**, 445–9.

Atkinson, K. & Downs, K. (1995). Omission of day 11 methotrexate does not appear to influence the incidence of moderate to severe acute graft-versus-host disease, chronic graft-versus-host disease, relapse rate or survival after HLA-identical sibling bone marrow transplantation. *Bone Marrow Transplantation*, **16**, 755–8.

Atkinson, K., Farewell, V., Tsoi, M. S., et al. (1982a). Analysis of late infections after human bone marrow transplantation. Role of non-specific suppressor cells in patients with chronic graft-versus-host disease, and genotypic non identity between marrow donor and recipient. *Blood*, **60**, 714–20.

Atkinson, K., Horowitz, M. M., Gale, R. P. et al. (1989b). Consensus among bone marrow transplanters for diagnosis, grading and treatment of chronic graft-versus-host disease. Committee of the International Bone Marrow Transplant Registry. *Bone Marrow Transplantation*, **4**, 247–54.

Atkinson, K., Horowitz, M. M., Gale, R. P. et al. (1990). Risk factors for chronic graft-versus-host disease after HLA-identical sibling bone marrow transplantation. *Blood*, **75**, 2459–64.

Atkinson, K., Norrie, S., Chan, P. et al. (1986a). Hematopoietic progenitor cell function after HLA-identical sibling bone marrow transplantation: influence of chronic graft-versus-host disease. *International Journal of Cell Cloning*, **4**, 203–20.

Atkinson, K., Shulman, H. M., Deeg, H. J. et al. (1982). Acute and chronic graft-versus-host disease in dogs given hemopoietic grafts from DLA-nonidentical littermates. Two distinct syndromes. *American Journal of Pathology*, **108**, 196–205.

Atkinson, K., Storb, R., Prentice, R. L. et al. (1979). Analysis of late infections in 89 long term survivors of bone marrow transplantation. *Blood*, **53**, 720–31.

Atkinson, K., Weller, P., Ryman, W. et al. (1986b). PUVA therapy for drug-resistant graft-versus-host disease. *Bone Marrow Transplantation*, **1**, 227–36.

Bacigalupo, A., Maiolino, A., Van Lint, M. T. et al. (1990). Cyclosporin A and chronic graft versus host disease. *Bone Marrow Transplantation*, **6**, 341–4.

Bacigalupo, A., Van Lint, M. T., Occhini, D. et al. (1991). Increased risk of leukemia relapse with high-dose cyclosporine A after allogeneic marrow transplantation for acute leukemia. *Blood*, **77**, 1423–8.

Balduzzi, A., Gooley, T., Anasetti, C. et al. (1195). Unrelated donor marrow transplantation in children. *Blood*, **86**, 3247–56.

Barak, V., Levi-Schaffer, F., Nisman, B., & Nagler, A. (1995). Cytokine dysregulation in chronic graft versus host disease. *Leukemia and Lymphoma*, **17**, 169–73.

Basara, N., Blau, W. I., Romer, E. et al. (1998). Mycophenolate mofetil for the treatment of acute and chronic GVHD in bone marrow transplant patients. *Bone Marrow Transplantation*, **22**, 61–5.

Beers, B., Kalish, R. S., Kaye, V. N., & Dahl, M. V. (1993). Linear lichenoid eruption after bone marrow transplantation: an unmasking of tolerance to an abnormal clone? *Journal of the American Academy of Dermatology*, **28**, 888–92.

Beredjiklian, P. K., Drummond, D. S., Dormans, J. P. et al. (1998). Orthopaedic manifestations of chronic graft-versus-host disease. *Journal of Pediatric Orthopedics*, **18**, 572–5.

Beschorner, W. E., Tutschka, P. J., & Santos, G. W. (1982). Chronic graft-versus-host disease in the rat radiation chimera. I. Clinical features, hematology, histology, and immunopathology in long-term chimeras. *Transplantation*, **33**, 393–9.

Blanche, P., Dreyfus, F., & Sicard, D. (1995). Polymyositis and chronic graft-versus-host disease: efficacy of intravenous gammaglobulin and methotrexate. *Clinical and Experimental Rheumatology*, **13**, 377–9.

Boas, S. R., Noyes, B. E., Kurland, G., Armitage, J., & Orenstein, D. (1994). Pediatric lung transplantation for graft-versus-host disease following bone marrow transplantation. *Chest*, **105**, 1584–6.

Bolger, G. B., Sullivan, K. M., Spence, A. M. et al. (1986). Myasthenia gravis after allogeneic bone marrow transplantation: relationship to chronic graft-versus-host disease. *Neurology*, **36**, 1087–91.

Bostrom, L., Ringden, O., Jacobsen, N., Zwaan, F., & Nilsson, B. (1990). A European multicenter study of chronic graft-versus-host disease. The role of cytomegalovirus serology in recipients and donors—acute graft-versus-host disease, and splenectomy. *Transplantation*, **49**, 1100–5.

Browne, P. V., Weisdorf, D. J., DeFor, T. et al. (2000). Response to thalidomide therapy in refractory chronic graft-versus-host disease. *Bone Marrow Transplantation*, **26**, 865–9.

Brunet, S., Urbano-Ispizua, A., Ojeda, E. et al. (2001). Favourable effect of the combination of acute and chronic graft-versus-host disease on the outcome of allogeneic peripheral blood stem cell transplantation for advanced haematological malignancies. *British Journal of Haematology*, **114**, 544–50.

Bullorsky, E. O., Shanley, C. M., Stemmelin, G. R. et al. (1993). Total lymphoid irradiation for treatment of drug resistant chronic GVHD. *Bone Marrow Transplantation*, **11**, 75–6.

Bush, N. E., Haberman, M., Donaldson, G., & Sullivan, K. M. (1995). Quality of life of 125 adults surviving 6–18 years after bone marrow transplantation. *Social Science & Medicine*, (1982) **40**, 479–90.

Calissendorff, B., el Azazi, M., & Lonnqvist, B. (1989). Dry eye syndrome in long term follow-up of bone marrow transplanted patients. *Bone Marrow Transplantation, 4,* 675–8.

Carlens, S., Ringden, O., Remberger, M. *et al.* (1998). Risk factors for chronic graft-versus-host disease after bone marrow transplantation: a retrospective single centre analysis. *Bone Marrow Transplantation, 22,* 755–61.

Carnevale-Schianca, F., Martin, P., Sullivan, K. *et al.* (2000). Changing from cyclosporine to tacrolimus as salvage therapy for chronic graft-versus-host disease. *Biology of Blood and Marrow Transplantation, 6,* 613–20.

Cavet, J., Dickinson, A. M., Norden, J. *et al.* (2001). Interferon-γ and interleukin-6 gene polymorphisms associate with graft- versus-host disease in HLA-matched sibling bone marrow transplantation. *Blood, 98,* 1594–600.

Cavet, J., Middleton, P. G., Segall, M. *et al.* (1999). Recipient tumor necrosis factor-alpha and interleukin-10 gene polymorphisms associate with early mortality and acute graft-versus-host disease in HLA-matched sibling bone marrow transplants. *Blood, 94,* 3941–6.

Champlin, R. E., Schmitz, N., Horowitz, M. M. *et al.* (2000). Blood stem cells compared with bone marrow as a source of hematopoietic cells for allogeneic transplantation. IBMTR Histocompatibility and Stem Cell Sources Working Committee and the European Group for Blood and Marrow Transplantation (EBMT). *Blood, 95,* 3702–9.

Chao, N. J., Parker, P. M., Niland, J. C. *et al.* (1996). Paradoxical effect of thalidomide prophylaxis on chronic graft-versus-host disease. *Biology of Blood and Marrow Transplantation, 2,* 86–92.

Child, F. J., Ratnavel, R., Watkins, P. *et al.* (1999). Extracorporeal photopheresis (ECP) in the treatment of chronic graft-versus-host disease (GVHD). *Bone Marrow Transplantation, 23,* 881–7.

Chiodi, S., Spinelli, S., Ravera, G. *et al.* (2000). Quality of life in 244 recipients of allogeneic bone marrow transplantation. *British Journal Haematology, 110,* 614–9.

Cohen, P. R. & Hymes, S. R. (1994). Linear and dermatomal cutaneous graft-versus-host disease. *Southern Medical Journal, 87,* 758–61.

Cordoba, S., Aragues, M., Fernandez-Herrera, J. *et al.* (1999). Lichen sclerosus et atrophicus in sclerodermatous chronic graft-versus-host disease. *International Journal of Dermatology, 38,* 708–11.

Corson, S. L., Sullivan, K., Batzer, F. *et al.* (1982). Gynecologic manifestations of chronic graft-versus-host disease. *Obstetrics and Gynecology, 60,* 488–92.

Couriel, D. R., Beguelin, G. Z., Giralt, S. *er al.* (2002). Chronic graft-versus-host disease manifesting as polymyositis: an uncommon presentation. *Bone Marrow Transplantation, 30,* 543–6.

Cullup, H., Dickinson, A. M., Jackson, G. H., *et al.* (2001). Donor interleukin 1 receptor antagonist genotype associated with acute graft-versus-host disease in human leucocyte antigen-matched sibling allogeneic transplants. *British Journal of Haematology, 113,* 807–813.

Curtis, R. E., Rowlings, P. A., Deeg, H. J. *et al.* (1997). Solid cancers after bone marrow transplantation. *New England Journal of Medicine, 336,* 897–904.

Cutler, C., Giri, S., Jeyapalan, S. *et al.* (2001). Acute and chronic graft-versus-host disease after allogeneic peripheral-blood stem-cell and bone marrow transplantation: a meta-analysis. *Journal of Clinical Oncology, 19,* 3685–91.

Dall'Amico, R., Rossetti, F., Zulian, F. *et al.* (1997). Photopheresis in paediatric patients with drug-resistant chronic graft-versus-host disease. *British Journal of Haematology, 97,* 848–54.

DeClerck, Y., Draper, V., & Parkman, R. (1986). Clonal analysis of murine graft-vs-host disease. II. Leukokines that stimulate fibroblast proliferation and collagen synthesis in graft-versus host disease. *Journal of Immunology, 136,* 3549–52.

Deeg, H. J., Leisenring, W., Storb, R. *et al.* (1998). Long-term outcome after marrow transplantation for severe aplastic anemia. *Blood, 91,* 3637–45.

Deeg, H. J., Lin, D., Leisenring, W. *et al.* (1997). Cyclosporine or cyclosporine plus methylprednisolone for prophylaxis of graft-versus-host disease: a prospective, randomized trial. *Blood, 89,* 3880–7.

DeLord, C., Treleaven, J., Shepherd, J. *et al.* (1999). Vaginal stenosis following allogeneic bone marrow transplantation for acute myeloid leukemia. *Bone Marrow Transplantation, 23,* 523–5.

den Haan, J. M., Meadows, L. M., Wang, W. *et al.* (1998). The minor histocompatibility antigen HA-1: a diallelic gene with a single amino acid polymorphism. *Science, 279,* 1054–7.

Dilek, I., Demirer, T., Ustun, C. *et al.* (1998). Acquired ichthyosis associated with chronic graft-versus-host disease following allogeneic peripheral blood stem cell transplantation in a patient with chronic myelogenous leukemia. *Bone Marrow Transplantation, 21,* 1159–61.

Duell, T., van Lint, M. T., Ljungman, P. *et al.* (1997). Health and functional status of long-term survivors of bone marrow transplantation. EBMT Working Party on Late Effects and EULEP Study Group on Late Effects. European Group for Blood and Marrow Transplantation. *Annals of Internal Medicine, 126,* 184–92.

Elmaagacli, A. H., Basoglu, S., Peceny, R. *et al.* (2002). Improved disease-free-survival after transplantation of peripheral blood stem cells as compared with bone marrow from HLA-identical unrelated donors in patients with first chronic phase chronic myeloid leukemia. *Blood, 99,* 1130–5.

Enk, C. D., Elad, S., Vexler, A. *et al.* (1998). Chronic graft-versus-host disease treated with UVB phototherapy. *Bone Marrow Transplantation, 22,* 1179–83.

Eppinger, T., Ehninger, G., Steinert, M., Niethammer, D., & Dopfer, R. (1990). 8-Methoxypsoralen and ultraviolet A therapy for cutaneous manifestations of graft-versus-host disease. *Transplantation, 50,* 807–11.

Epstein, J. B., Nantel, S., & Sheoltch, S. M. (2000). Topical azathioprine in the combined treatment of chronic oral graft-versus-host disease. *Bone Marrow Transplantation, 25,* 683–7.

Evans, P. C., Lambert, N., Maloney, S. *et al.* (1999). Long-term fetal microchimerism in peripheral blood mononuclear cell subsets in healthy women and women with scleroderma. *Blood, 93,* 2033–7.

Flowers, M.E.D. (2002). Traditional treatment of chronic graft-versus-host disease. *Blood and Marrow Transplantation Reviews, 12,* 5–8.

Flowers, M.E.D., Parker, P. M., Johnston, L. J. *et al.* (2002). Comparison of chronic graft-versus-host disease after transplantation of peripheral blood stem cells versus bone marrow in allogeneic recipients: long-term follow-up of a randomized trial. *Blood, 100,* 415–9.

French, L. E., Aleindor, T., Shapiro, M. *et al.* (2002). Identification of amplified clonal T cell populations in the blood of patients with chronic graft-versus-host disease: positive correlation with response to photopheresis. *Bone Marrow Transplantation, 30,* 509–15.

Freemer, C. S., Farmer, E. R., Corio, R. L. *et al.* (1994). Lichenoid graft-versus-host disease occurring in a dermatomal distribution. *Archives of Dermatology, 130,* 70–2.

Fried, R. H., Murakami, C. S., Fisher, L. D., Willson, R. A., Sullivan, K. M., & McDonald, G. B. (1992). Ursodeoxycholic acid treatment of refractory chronic graft-versus-host disease of the liver. *Annals of Internal Medicine,* **116,** 624–9.

Funke, I., Prummer, O., Schrezenmeier, H. *et al.* (1994). Capillary leak syndrome associated with elevated IL-2 serum levels after allogeneic bone marrow transplantation. *Annals of Hematology,* **68,** 49–52.

Gallardo, D., Arostegui, J. I., Balas, A. *et al.* (2001). Disparity for the minor histocompatibility antigen HA-1 is associated with an increased risk of acute graft-versus-host disease (GvHD) but it does not affect chronic GvHD incidence, disease-free survival or overall survival after allogeneic human leucocyte antigen-identical sibling donor transplantation. *British Journal of Haematology,* **114,** 931–6.

Gaziev, D., Lucarelli, G., Polchi, P. *et al.* (2001). A three or more drug combination as effective therapy for moderate or severe chronic graft-versus-host disease. *Bone Marrow Transplantation,* **27,** 45–51.

Gilman, A. L., Chan, K. W., Mogul, A. *et al.* (2000). Hydroxychloroquine for the treatment of chronic graft-versus-host disease. *Biology of Blood and Marrow Transplantation,* **6,** 327–34.

Gluckman, E., Rocha, V., Boyer-Chammard, A. *et al.* (1997). Outcome of cord-blood transplantation from related and unrelated donors. Eurocord Transplant Group and the European Blood and Marrow Transplantation Group. *New England Journal of Medicine,* **337,** 373–81.

Goerner, M., Gooley, T., Flowers, M. E. *et al.* (2002). Morbidity and mortality of chronic GVHD after hematopoietic stem cell transplantation from HLA-identical siblings for patients with aplastic or refractory anemias. *Biology of Blood and Marrow Transplantation,* **8,** 47–56.

Gomez-Garcia, P., Herrara-Arroyo, C., Torrez-Gomez, A. *et al.* (1988). Renal involvement in chronic graft-versus-host disease: a report of two cases. *Bone Marrow Transplantation,* **3,** 357–62.

Gorgun, G., Miller, K. B. & Foss, F. M. (2002). Immunologic mechanisms of extracorporeal photochemotherapy in chronic graft-versus-host disease. *Blood,* **100,** 941–7.

Graze, P. R. & Gale, R. P. (1979). Chronic graft versus host disease: a syndrome of disordered immunity. *American Journal of Medicine,* **66,** 611–20.

Greenspan, A., Deeg, H. J., Cottler-Fox, M. *et al.* (1990). Incapacitating peripheral neuropathy as a manifestation of chronic graft-versus-host disease. *Bone Marrow Transplantation,* **5,** 349–52.

Greinix, H. T., Volc-Platzer, B., Rabitsch, W. *et al.* (1998). Successful use of extracorporeal photochemotherapy in the treatment of severe acute and chronic graft-versus-host disease. *Blood,* **92,** 3098–104.

Hamilton, B. L. & Parkman, R. (1983). Acute and chronic graft-versus-host disease induced by minor histocompatibility antigens in mice. *Transplantation,* **36,** 150–5.

Haseyama, K., Watanabe, J., Oda, T. *et al.* (1996). Nephrotic syndrome related to chronic graft-versus-host disease after allogeneic bone marrow transplantation in a patient with malignant lymphoma. *Rinsho Ketsueki,* **37,** 1383–8.

Heimdahl, A., Johnson, G., Danielesson, K. H. *et al.* (1985). Oral condition of patients with leukaemia and severe aplastic amemia. Follow-up one year after bone marrow transplantation. *Oral Surgery, Oral Medicine, and Oral Pathology,* **60,** 498–504.

Heinonen, H., Volin, L., Uutela, A. *et al.* (2001). Quality of life and factors related to perceived satisfaction with quality of life after allogeneic bone marrow transplantation. *Annals of Hematology,* **80,** 137–43.

Holland, H. K., Wingard, J. R., Beschorner, W. E., Saral, R., & Santos, G. W. (1988). Bronchiolitis obliterans in bone marrow transplantation and its relationship to chronic graft-v-host disease and low serum IgG. *Blood,* **72,** 621–7.

Horowitz, M. M., Gale, R. P., Sondel, P. M. *et al.* (1990). Graft-versus-leukemia reactions after bone marrow transplantation. *Blood,* **75,** 555–62.

Hughes, R.A.C., Gabriel, C. M., Goldman, J. M., & Lucas, S. (1999). Vasculitic neuropathy in association with chronic graft-versus-host disease. *Journal of the Neurological Sciences,* **168,** 68–70.

Jacobsohn, D. A., Margolis, J., Doherty, J., Anders, V., & Vogelsang, G. M. (2002). Weight loss and malnutrition in patients with chronic graft-versus-host disease. *Bone Marrow Transplantation,* **29,** 231–6.

Jacobsohn, D. A., Ruble, K., Moresi, J. M. & Vogelsang, G. B. (2002). Rapid-onset leucoderma associated with graft-versus-host disease. *Bone Marrow Transplantation,* **30,** 705–6.

Jampel, R. M., Farmer, E. R., Vogelsang, G. B. *et al.* (1991). PUVA therapy for chronic cutaneous graft-vs-host disease. *Archives of Dermatology,* **127,** 1673–8.

Janin, A., Socie, G., Devergie, A. *et al.* (1994). Fasciitis in chronic graft-versus-host disease. A clinicopathologic study of 14 cases [see comments]. *Annals of Internal Medicine,* **120,** 993–8.

Kami, M., Kanda, Y., Sasaki, M. *et al.* (1998). Phimosis as a manifestation of chronic graft-versus-host disease after allogeneic bone marrow transplantation. *Bone Marrow Transplantation,* **21,** 721–3.

Kansu, E., Gooley, T., Flowers, M. E. *et al.* (2001). Administration of cyclosporine for 24 months compared with 6 months for prevention of chronic graft-versus-host disease: a prospective randomized clinical trial. *Blood,* **98,** 3868–70.

Kapoor, N., Pelligrini, A. E., Copelan, E. A. *et al.* (1992). Psoralen plus ultraviolet A (PUVA) in the treatment of chronic graft versus host disease: preliminary experience in standard treatment resistant patients. *Seminars in Hematology,* **29,** 108–12.

Kiang, E., Tesavibul, N., Yee, R., Kellaway, J., & Przepiorka, D. (1998). The use of topical cyclosporin A in ocular graft-versus-host-disease. *Bone Marrow Transplantation,* **22,** 147–51.

Knobler, H. Y., Sagher, U., Peled, I. J. *et al.* (1985). Tolerance to donor-type skin in the recipient of a bone marrow allograft. Treatment of skin ulcers in chronic graft-versus-host disease with skin grafts from the bone marrow donor. *Transplantation,* **40,** 223–5.

Koc, S., Leisenring, W., Flowers, M. E. *et al.* (2000). Thalidomide for treatment of patients with chronic graft-versus-host disease. *Blood,* **96,** 3995–6.

Koc, S., Leisenring, W., Flowers, M.E.D. *et al.* (2002). Therapy of chronic graft-versus-host disease: a randomized trial comparing cyclosporine plus prednisone versus prednisone alone. *Blood,* **100,** 48–51.

Korholz, D., Kunst, D., Hempel, L. *et al.* (1997). Decreased interleukin 10 and increased interferon-gamma production in patients with chronic graft-versus-host disease after allogeneic bone marrow transplantation. *Bone Marrow Transplantation,* **19,** 691–5.

Kotani, A., Ishikawa, T., Matsumura, Y. *et al.* (2001). Correlation of peripheral blood OX40+(CD134+) T cells with chronic graft-versus-host disease in patients who underwent allogeneic hematopoietic stem cell transplantation. *Blood*, **98**, 3162–4.

Kulkarni, S., Powles, R., Treleaven, J. et al. (2000). Chronic graft versus host disease is associated with long-term risk for pneumococcal infections in recipients of bone marrow transplants. *Blood*, **95**, 3683–6.

Kurtzberg, J., Laughlin, M., Graham, M. L. et al. (1996). Placental blood as a source of hematopoietic stem cells for transplantation into unrelated recipients. *New England Journal of Medicine*, **335**, 157–66.

Leano, A. M., Miller, K., & White, A. C. (2000). Chronic graft-versus-host disease-related polymyositis as a cause of respiratory failure following allogeneic bone marrow transplant. *Bone Marrow Transplantation*, **26**, 1117–20.

Leblond, V., Zouabi, H., Sutton, L. et al. (1994). Late CD8+ lymphocytic alveolitis after allogeneic bone marrow transplantation of chronic graft-versus-host disease. *American Journal of Respiratory and Critical Care Medicine*, **150**, 1056–61.

Lee, M. S., Atkinson, K., & Kossard, S. (1996). Lichenoid graft-versus-host disease occurring in Blaschko's lines. *European Journal of Dermatology*, **6**, 282–3.

Lee, S. J., Cook, E. F., Soiffer, R. J., & Antin, J. H. (2002a). Development and validation of a scale to measure symptoms of chronic graft-versus-host disease. *Biology of Blood and Marrow Transplantation*, **8**, 444–52.

Lee, S. J., Klein, J. P., Barrett, A. J. et al. (2000). Chronic graft-versus-host disease (chronic GVHD) severity score: effects on leukemia-free survival. *Blood*, **96**, 556a.

Lee, S. J., Klein, J. P., Barrett, A. J. et al. (2002b). Severity of chronic graft-versus-host disease: association with treatment-related mortality and relapse. *Blood*, **100**, 406–14.

Lee, S. J., Vogelsang, G., Gilman, A. et al. (2002c). A survey of diagnosis, management, and grading of chronic GVHD. *Biology of Blood and Marrow Transplantation*, **8**, 32–9.

Lee, S. J., Wegner, S. A., McGarigle, C. J., Bierer, B. E., & Antin, J. H. (1997). Treatment of chronic graft-versus-host disease with clofazimine. *Blood*, **89**, 2298–302.

Lichtman, A. H., Krenger, W., & Ferrara, J. L. (1997). Cytokine networks. In *Graft-Versus-Host Disease*, eds. J.L.M. Ferrara, H. J. Deeg, & S. J. Burakoff, pp. 179–218. New York: Marcel Dekker, Inc.

Liem, L. M., Fibbe, W. E., van Houwelingen, H. C., & Goulmy, E. (1999). Serum transforming growth factor-beta1 levels in bone marrow transplant recipients correlate with blood cell counts and chronic graft-versus-host disease. *Transplantation*, **67**, 59–65.

Lonnqvist, B., Aschan, J., Ljungman, P., & Ringden, O. (1990). Long-term cyclosporin therapy may decrease the risk of chronic graft-versus-host disease. *British Journal of Haematology*, **74**, 547–8.

Loughran, T. P., Jr., Sullivan, K., Morton, T. et al. (1990). Value of day 100 screening studies for predicting the development of chronic graft-versus-host disease after allogeneic bone marrow transplantation. *Blood*, **76**, 228–34.

Malik, A. H., Collins, R. H. Saboorian, M. H. & Lee, W. M. (2001). Chronic graft-versus-host disease after hematopoietic cell transplantation presenting as an acute hepatitis. *American Journal of Gastroenterology*, **96**, 588–90.

Marcellus, D. C., Altomonte, V. L., Farmer, E. R. et al. (1999). Etretinate therapy for refractory sclerodermatous chronic graft-versus-host disease. *Blood*, **93**, 66–70.

Marks, D. I., Gale, D. J., Vedhara, K., & Bird, J. M. (1999). A quality of life study in 20 adult long-term survivors of unrelated donor bone marrow transplantation. *Bone Marrow Transplantation*, **24**, 191–5.

Martin, S. J., Audrain, M. A., Oksman, F., Ecoiffier, M., Attal, M., Milpied, N., & Esnault, V. L. (1997). Antineutrophil cytoplasmic antibodies (ANCA) in chronic graft-versus-host disease after allogeneic bone marrow transplantation. *Bone Marrow Transplantation*, **20**, 45–8.

Matsuda, Y., Hara, J., Osugi, Y. et al. (2001). Serum levels of soluble adhesion molecules in stem cell transplantation-related complications. *Bone Marrow Transplantation*, **27**, 977–82.

Maury, S., Mary, J. Y., Rabian, C. et al. (2001). Prolonged immune deficiency following allogeneic stem cell transplantation: risk factors and complications in adult patients. *British Journal of Haematology*, **115**, 630–41.

Middleton, P. G., Taylor, P. R. A., Jackson, G., Proctor, S. J. & Dickinson, A. M. (1998). Cytokine gene polymorphisms associating with severe acute graft-versus-host disease in HLA-identical sibling transplants. *Blood*, **92**, 3943–8.

Mohty, M., Kuentz, M., Michallet, M. et al. (2002). Chronic graft-versus-host disease after allogeneic blood stem cell transplantation: long-term results of a randomized study. *Blood*, **100**, 3128–34.

Mookerjee, B., Altomonte, V., & Vogelsang, G. (1999). Salvage therapy for refractory chronic graft-versus-host disease with mycophenolate mofetil and tacrolimus. *Bone Marrow Transplantation*, **24**, 517–20.

Morton, A., Anasetti, C., Gooley, T. et al. (1997). Chronic graft-versus-host disease (GVHD) following unrelated donor transplantation. *Blood*, **90**, 590a.

Morton, J., Hutchins, C., & Durrant, S. (2001). Granulocyte-colony-stimulating factor (G-CSF)-primed allogeneic bone marrow: significantly less graft-versus-host disease and comparable engraftment to G-CSF-mobilized peripheral blood stem cells. *Blood*, **98**, 3186–91.

Miyazaki, K., Higaki, S., Maruyama, T. et al. (1993). Chronic graft-versus-host disease with follicular involvement. *Journal of Dermatology*, **20**, 242–6.

Nagler, R., Marmary, Y., Kransz, Y. et al. (1996). Major salivary gland dysfunction in human acute and chronic graft-versus-host disease (GVHD). *Bone Marrow Transplantation*, **17**, 219–24.

Nonomura, A., Kono, N., Minato, H., & Nakanuma, Y. (1998). Diffuse biliary tract involvement mimicking primary sclerosing cholangitis in an experimental model of chronic graft-versus-host disease in mice. *Pathology International*, **48**, 421–7.

Okamoto, S., Takahashi, S., Inone, T. et al. (1996). Cutaneous chronic graft-versus-host disease localized to the field of total lymphoid irradiation. *Bone Marrow Transplantation*, **17**, 111–3.

Ochs, L. A., Miller, W. J., Filipovich, A. H. et al. (1994). Predictive factors for chronic graft-versus-host disease after histocompatible sibling donor bone marrow transplantation. *Bone Marrow Transplantation*, **13**, 455–60.

Oliveira, J. S. R., Bahia, D., Franco, M. et al. (1999). Nephrotic syndrome as a clinical manifestation of graft-versus-host disease (GVHD) in a marrow transplant recipient after cyclosporine withdrawal. *Bone Marrow Transplantation*, **23**, 99–101.

Oshima, Y., Takahashi, S., Nagayama, H. et al. (1997). Fatal GVHD demonstrating an involvement of respiratory muscle following donor leukocyte transfusion (DLT). *Bone Marrow Transplantation*, **19**, 737–40.

Parker, P., Chao, N. J., Ben-Ezra, J. *et al.* (1996). Polymyositis as a manifestation of chronic graft-versus-host disease. *Medicine,* **75,** 279–85.

Parker, P. M., Chao, N., Nademanee, A. *et al.* (1995). Thalidomide as salvage therapy for chronic graft-versus-host disease. *Blood,* **86,** 3604–9.

Parkman, R. (1993). Is chronic graft versus host disease an autoimmune disease? *Current Opinion in Immunology,* **5,** 800–3.

Perrault, C., Cousineau, S., D'Angelo, G. *et al.* (1985). Lymphoid interstitial pneumonia after allogeneic bone marrow transplantation. A possible manifestation of chronic graft-versus-host disease. *Cancer,* **55,** 1–9.

Philit, F., Wiesendanger, T., Archimbaud, E. *et al.* (1995). Post-transplant obstructive lung disease ("bronchiolitis obliterans"): a clinical comparative study of bone marrow and lung transplant patients. *European Respiratory Journal,* **8,** 551–8.

Picardi, M., Selleri, C., & Rotoli, B. (1999). Spleen sizing by ultrasound scan and risk of pneumococcal infection in patients with chronic GVHD: preliminary observations. *Bone Marrow Transplantation,* **24,** 173–7.

Pichert, G., Roy, D. C., Gonin, R. *et al.* (1995). Distinct patterns of minimal residual disease associated with graft-versus-host disease after allogeneic bone marrow transplantation for chronic myelogenous leukemia. *Journal of Clinical Oncology,* **13,** 1704–13.

Przepiorka, D., Anderlini, P., Saliba, R. *et al.* (2001). Chronic graft-versus-host disease after allogeneic blood stem cell transplantation. *Blood,* **98,** 1695–700.

Ratanatharathorn, V., Ayash, L., Lazarus, H. M., Fu, J., & Uberti, J. P. (2001). Chronic graft-versus-host disease: clinical manifestation and therapy. *Bone Marrow Transplantation,* **28,** 121–9.

Ratanatharathorn, V., Carson, E., Reynolds, C. *et al.* (2000). Anti-CD20 chimeric monoclonal antibody treatment of refractory immune-mediated thrombocytopenia in a patient with chronic graft-versus-host disease. *Annals of Internal Medicine,* **133,** 275–9.

Ratanatharathorn, V., Nash, R. A., Przepiorka, D. *et al.* (1998). Phase III study comparing methotrexate and tacrolimus (prograf, FK506) with methotrexate and cyclosporine for graft-versus-host disease prophylaxis after HLA-identical sibling bone marrow transplantation. *Blood,* **92,** 2303–14.

Redding, S. W., Callander, N. S., Haveman, C. W., & Leonard, D. L. (1998). Treatment of oral chronic graft-versus-host disease with PUVA therapy: case report and literature review. *Oral Surgery, Oral Medicine, Oral Pathology, Oral Radiology, & Endodontics,* **86,** 183–7.

Reinherz, E. L., Parkman, R., Rappeport, J., Rosen, F. S., & Schlossman, S. F. (1979). Aberrations of suppressor T cells in human graft-versus-host disease. *New England Journal & Medicine,* **300,** 1061–8.

Remberger, M., Aschan, J., Lonnqvist, B. *et al.* (2001a). An ethnic role for chronic, but not acute, graft-versus-host disease after HLA-identical sibling stem cell transplantation. *Transplantation Proceedings,* **33,** 1769–70.

Remberger, M., Ringden, O., Blau, I. W. *et al.* (2001b). No difference in graft-versus-host disease, relapse, and survival comparing peripheral stem cells to bone marrow using unrelated donors. *Blood,* **98,** 1739–45.

Rhodes, D. F., Lee, W. M., Wingard, J. R. *et al.* (1990). Orthotopic liver transplantation for graft-versus-host disease following bone marrow transplantation. *Gastroenterology,* **99,** 536–8.

Ringden, O., Labopin, M., Gluckman, E. *et al.* (1997). Strong antileukemic effect of chronic graft-versus-host disease in allogeneic marrow transplant recipients having acute leukemia treated with methotrexate and cyclosporine. The Acute Leukemia Working Party of the European Group for Blood and Marrow Transplantation (EBMT). *Transplantation Proceedings,* **29,** 733–4.

Ringden, O., Paulin, T., Lonnqvist, B., & Nilsson, B. (1985). An analysis of factors predisposing to chronic graft-versus-host disease. *Experimental Hematology,* **13,** 1062–7.

Rocha, V., Franco, R. F., Porcher, R. *et al.* (2002). Host defense and inflammatory gene polymorphisms are associated with outcomes after HLA-identical sibling bone marrow transplantation. *Blood,* **100,** 3908–18.

Ross, M., Schmidt, G. M., Niland, J. C. *et al.* (1999). Cyclosporine, methotrexate, and prednisone compared with cyclosporine and prednisone for prevention of acute graft-versus-host disease: effect on chronic graft-versus-host disease and long-term survival. *Biology of Blood and Marrow Transplantation,* **5,** 285–91.

Rouquette-Gally, A. M., Boyeldieu, D., Prost, A. C., & Gluckman, E. (1988). Autoimmunity after allogeneic bone marrow transplantation. A study of 53 long-term-surviving patients. *Transplantation,* **46,** 238–40.

Rovelli, A., Arrigo, C., Nesi, F. *et al.* (1998). The role of thalidomide in the treatment of refractory chronic graft- versus-host disease following bone marrow transplantation in children. *Bone Marrow Transplantation,* **21,** 577–81.

Ruutu, T., Ruutu, M., Volin, L. *et al.* (1988). Severe cystitis as a manifestation of chronic graft-versus-host disease after bone marrow transplantation. *British Journal of Urology,* **62,** 612–3.

Ruutu, T., Volin, L., & Elonen, E. (1988). Low incidence of severe acute and chronic graft-versus-host disease as a result of prolonged cyclosporine prophylaxis and early aggressive treatment with corticosteroids. *Transplantation Proceedings,* **20,** 491–3.

Sanders, J. E. (1981). Effects of chronic graft-versus-host disease on growth and development. In *Graft-Versus-Host Disease.* ed. S. Burakoff, H. J. Deeg, J. Ferrara, & K. Atkinson, pp. 665–680. New York: Marcel Dekker Inc.

Schmidt, G. M., Niland, J. C., Forman, S. J. *et al.* (1993). Extended follow-up in 212 long-term allogeneic bone marrow transplant survivors. Issues of quality of life. *Transplantation,* **55,** 551–7.

Schubert, M. M., Sullivan, K. M., Morton, T. H. *et al.* (1984). Oral manifestations of chronic graft-v-host disease. *Archives of Internal Medicine,* **144,** 1591–5.

Scott, M. A., Gandhi, M. K., Jestice, H. K. *et al.* (1998). A trend towards an increased incidence of chronic graft-versus-host disease following allogeneic peripheral blood progenitor cell transplantation: a case controlled study. *Bone Marrow Transplantation,* **22,** 273–6.

Seber, A., Khan, S. P., & Kersey, J. H. (1996). Unexplained effusions: association with allogeneic bone marrow transplantation and acute or chronic graft-versus-host disease. *Bone Marrow Transplantation,* **17,** 207–11.

Seddik, M., Seemayer, T. A., & Lapp, W. S. (1980). T cell functional defect associated with thymic epithelial cell injury induced by a graft-versus-host reaction. *Transplantation,* **29,** 61–6.

Seidler, C. W., Mills, L. E., Flowers, M. E., & Sullivan, K. M. (1994). Spontaneous factor VIII inhibitor occurring in association with chronic graft-versus-host disease. *American Journal of Hematology,* **45,** 240–3.

Serrano, J., Prieto, E., Mazarbeitia, F. *et al.* (2001). Atypical chronic graft-versus-host disease following interferon therapy for chronic myeloid leukaemia after allogeneic BMT. *Bone Marrow Transplantation, 27*, 85–7.

Sherer, Y. & Shoenfeld, Y. (1998). Autoimmune diseases and autoimmunity post-bone marrow transplantation. *Bone Marrow Transplantation, 22*, 873–81.

Shulman, H. M., Sale, G. E ., Lerner, K. G. *et al.* (1978). Chronic cutaneous graft-versus-host disease in man. *American Journal of Pathology, 91*, 545–70.

Shulman, H. M., Sullivan, K. M ., Weiden, P. L. *et al.* (1980). Chronic graft-versus-host syndrome in man. A long-term clinico-pathologic study of 20 Seattle patients. *The American Journal of Medicine, 69*, 204–17.

Siadak, M. & Sullivan, K. M. (1994). The management of chronic graft-versus-host disease. *Blood Reviews, 8*, 154–60.

Silberstein, L., Davies, A., Kelsey, S. *et al.* (2001). Myositis, poly-serositis with a large pericardial effusion and constrictive peri-carditis as manifestations of chronic graft-versus-host disease after non-myeloablative peripheral stem cell transplantation and subsequent donor lymphocyte infusion. *Bone Marrow Transplantation, 27*, 231–3.

Slayback, D. L., Dobkins, J. A ., Harper, J. M., & Allen, R. D. (2000). Genetic factors influencing the development of chronic graft-versus-host disease in a murine model. *Bone Marrow Transplantation, 26*, 931–8.

Snowden, J. A., Nivison-Smith, I., Atkinson, K. *et al.* (2000). Allogeneic PBPC transplantation: an effect on incidence and dis-tribution of chronic graft-versus-host disease without long-term survival benefit? *Bone Marrow Transplantation, 25*, 119–20.

Socie, G., Clift, R. A., Blaise, D. *et al.* (2001a). Busulfan plus cyclophosphamide compared with total-body irradiation plus cyclophosphamide before marrow transplantation for myeloid leukemia: long-term follow-up of 4 randomized studies. *Blood, 98*, 3569–74.

Socie, G., Devergie, A., Cosset, J. M. *et al.* (1990). Low-dose (one gray) total-lymphoid irradiation for extensive, drug-resistant chronic graft-versus-host disease. *Transplantation, 49*, 657–8.

Socie, G., Mary, J. Y., Esperou, H. *et al.* (2001b). Health and func-tional status of adult recipients 1 year after allogeneic haematopoietic stem cell transplantation. *British Journal of Haematology, 113*, 194–201.

Socie, G., Stone, J. V., Wingard, J. R. *et al.* (1999). Long-term sur-vival and late deaths after allogeneic bone marrow transplanta-tion. Late Effects Working Committee of the International Bone Marrow Transplant Registry [see comments]. *New England Journal of Medicine, 341*, 14–21.

Sohngen, D., Heyll, A., Meckenstock, G. *et al.* (1994). Antiphospholipid syndrome complicating chronic graft-versus-host disease after allogeneic bone marrow transplantation. *American Journal of Hematology, 47*, 143–4.

Solano, C., Martinez, C., Brunet, S. *et al.* (1998). Chronic graft-ver-sus-host disease after allogeneic peripheral blood progenitor cell or bone marrow transplantation from matched related donors. A case-control study. Spanish Group of Allo-PBT. *Bone Marrow Transplantation, 22*, 1129–35.

Stern, J. M., Chesnut, C. H., Bruemmer, B. *et al.* (1996). Bone den-sity loss during treatment of chronic GVHD. *Bone Marrow Transplantation, 17*, 395–400.

Storb, R., Deeg, H. J., Pepe, M. *et al.* (1989a). Methotrexate and cyclosporine versus cyclosporine alone for prophylaxis of graft-versus-host disease in patients given HLA-identical marrow grafts for leukemia: long-term follow-up of a controlled trial. *Blood, 73*, 1729–34.

Storb, R., Deeg, H. J., Pepe, M. *et al.* (1989b). Graft-versus-host dis-ease prevention by methotrexate combined with cyclosporin com-pared to methotrexate alone in patients given marrow grafts for severe aplastic anaemia: long-term follow-up of a controlled trial [see comments]. *British Journal of Haematology, 72*, 567–72.

Storb, R., Leisenring, W., Anasetti, C. *et al.* (1997). Methotrexate and cyclosporine for graft-versus-host disease prevention: what length of therapy with cyclosporine? *Biology of Blood and Marrow Transplantation, 3*, 194–201.

Storb, R., Pepe, M., Anasetti, C. *et al.* (1990). What role for pred-nisone in prevention of acute graft-versus-host disease in patients undergoing marrow transplants? *Blood, 76*, 1037–45.

Storb, R., Prentice, R. L., Sullivan, K. M. *et al.* (1983). Predictive factors in chronic graft-versus-host disease in patients with aplas-tic anemia treated by marrow transplantation from HLA-identical siblings. *Annals of Internal Medicine, 98*, 461–6.

Storek, J., Gooley, T., Siadak, M. *et al.* (1997). Allogeneic peripheral blood stem cell transplantation may be associated with a high risk of chronic graft-versus-host disease. *Blood, 90*, 4705–9.

Storek, J., Witherspoon, R. P., Webb, D., & Storb, R. (1996). Lack of B cells precursors in marrow transplant recipients with chronic graft-versus-host disease. *American Journal of Hematology, 52*, 82–9.

Strasser, S. I., Shulman, H. M., Flowers, M. E. *et al.* (2000). Chronic graft-versus-host of the liver: presentation as an acute hepatitis. *Hepatology, 32*, 1265–71.

Sullivan, K. M. (1999). Graft-versus-host disease. In *Hematopoietic cell transplantation*, eds. E. D. Thomas, K. G. Blume, & S. J. Forman, pp. 515–536. Malden Blackwell Science, Inc.

Sullivan, K. M., Agura, E., Anasetti, C. *et al.* (1991). Chronic graft-versus-host disease and other late complications of bone marrow transplantation. *Seminars in Hematology, 28*, 250–9.

Sullivan, K. M., Meyers, J. D., Flournoy, N. *et al.* (1986). Early and late interstitial pneumonia following human bone marrow transplanta-tion. *International Journal of Cell Cloning, 4* (Suppl 1), 107–21.

Sullivan, K. M., Shulman, H. M., Storb, R. *et al.* (1981). Chronic graft-versus-host disease in 52 patients: adverse natural course and successful treatment with combination immunosuppression. *Blood, 57*, 267–76.

Sullivan, K. M., Storek, J., Kopecky, K. J. *et al.* (1996). A controlled trial of long-term administration of intravenous immunoglobulin to prevent late infection and chronic graft-versus-host disease after marrow transplantation: clinical outcome and effect on sub-sequent immune recovery. *Biology of Blood and Marrow Transplantation, 2*, 44–53.

Sullivan, K. M., Weiden, P. L., Storb, R. *et al.* (1989). Influence of acute and chronic graft-versus-host disease on relapse and survival after bone marrow transplantation from HLA-identical siblings as treatment of acute and chronic leukemia [published erratum appears in Blood 1989 Aug 15;74(3):1180]. *Blood, 73*, 1720–8.

Sullivan, K. M., Witherspoon, R. P., Storb, R. *et al.* (1988a). Alternating-day cyclosporine and prednisone for treatment of high-risk chronic graft-v-host disease. *Blood, 72*, 555–61.

Sullivan, K. M., Witherspoon, R. P., Storb, R. *et al.* (1988b). Prednisone and azathioprine compared with prednisone and placebo for treatment of chronic graft-v-host disease: prognostic influence of prolonged thrombocytopenia after allogeneic marrow transplantation. *Blood,* **72,** 546–54.

Sutherland, H. J., Fyles, G. M., Adams, G. *et al.* (1997). Quality of life following bone marrow transplantation: a comparison of patient reports with population norms. *Bone Marrow Transplantation,* **19,** 1129–36.

Syrjala, K. L., Chapko, M. K., Vitaliano, P. P., Cummings. C., & Sullivan, K. M. (1993). Recovery after allogeneic marrow transplantation: prospective study of predictors of long-term physical and psychosocial functioning. *Bone Marrow Transplantation,* **11,** 319–27.

Tichelli, A., Duell, T., Weiss, M. *et al.* (1996). Late-onset keratoconjunctivitis sicca syndrome after bone marrow transplantation: incidence and risk factors. *Bone Marrow Transplantation,* **17,** 1105–11.

Tutschka, P. J., Teasdall, R., Beschorner, W. E., & Santos, G. W. (1982). Chronic graft-versus-host disease in the rat radiation chimera. II. Immunological evaluation in long-term chimeras. *Transplantation,* **34,** 289–94.

Tzakis, A. G., Abu-Elmagd, K., Fung, J. J. *et al.* (1991). FK 506 rescue in chronic graft-versus-host-disease after bone marrow transplantation. *Transplantation Proceedings,* **23,** 3225–7.

Ueda, T., Manabe, A., Kikuchi, A. *et al.* (2000). Massive pericardial and pleural effusion with anasarca following allogeneic bone marrow transplantation. *International Journal of Hematology,* **71,** 394–7.

Valvricka, S. R., Halter, J., Furrer, K. *et al.* (2002). Contrast media triggering cutaneous gtraft-versus-host disease. *Bone Marrow Transplantation,* **29,** 899–901.

van Bekkum, D. W. (1985). Graft-versus-host disease. In *Bone Marrow Transplantation. Biological Mechanisms and Clinical Practice.* ed. D. W. van Bekkum & B. Lowenberg, pp. 147–212. New York: Marcel Dekker Inc.

Van Vloten, W. A., Scheffer, E., Dooren, L. J. *et al.* (1977). Localized scleroderma-like lesions after bone marrow transplantation in man. A chronic graft-versus-host reaction. *British Journal of Dermatology,* **4,** 337–41.

Vigorito, A. C., Azevedo, W. M., Marques, J. F. *et al.* (1998). A randomised, prospective comparison of allogeneic bone marrow and peripheral blood progenitor cell transplantation in the treatment of haematological malignancies. *Bone Marrow Transplantation,* **22,** 1145–51.

Vogelsang, G. B. (2001). How I treat chronic graft-versus-host disease. *Blood,* **97,** 1196–201.

Vogelsang, G. B., Farmer, E. R., Hess, A. D. *et al.* (1992). Thalidomide for the treatment of chronic graft-versus-host disease [see comments]. *New England Journal of Medicine,* **326,** 1055–8.

Vogelsang, G. B., Wolff, D., Altomonte, V. *et al.* (1996). Treatment of chronic graft-versus-host disease with ultraviolet irradiation and psoralen (PUVA). *Bone Marrow Transplantation,* **17,** 1061–7.

Voltarelli, J. C., Ahmed, H., Paton, E. J. *et al.* (2001). Beneficial effect of intravenous lidocaine in cutaneous chronic graft-versus-host disease secondary to donor lymphocyte infusion. *Bone Marrow Transplantation,* **28,** 97–9.

Vouah, E. E., Gruber, R., Shearer, W. *et al.* (1988). Graft-versus-host disease in the central nervous system. A real entity? *American Journal of Clinical Pathology,* **89,** 543–6.

Wagner, J. L., Flowers, M. E., Longton, G. *et al.* (1998). The development of chronic graft-versus-host an analysis of screening studies and the impact of corticosteroid use at 100 days after transplantation. *Bone Marrow Transplantation,* **22,** 139–46.

Wagner, J. L., Seidel, K., Boeckh, M., & Storb, R. (2000). De novo chronic graft-versus-host disease in marrow graft recipients given methotrexate and cyclosporine: risk factors and survival. *Biology of Blood and Marrow Transplantation,* **6,** 633–9.

Weiden, P. L., Flournoy, N., Thomas, E. D. *et al.* (1979). Antileukemic effect of graft-versus-host disease in human recipients of allogeneic-marrow grafts. *New England Journal of Medicine,* **300,** 1068–73.

Weiden, P. L., Sullivan, K. M., Flournoy, N., Storb, R., & Thomas, E. D. (1981). Antileukemic effect of chronic graft-versus-host disease: contribution to improved survival after allogeneic marrow transplantation. *New England Journal of Medicine,* **304,** 1529–33.

Weinberg, K., Blazar, B. R., Wagner, J. E. *et al.* (2001). Factors affecting thymic function after allogeneic hematopoietic stem cell transplantation. *Blood,* **97,** 1458–66.

Wilson, B. B. & Lockmann, D. W. (1994). Linear lichenoid graft-versus-host disease. *Archives of Dermatology,* **130,** 1206–7.

Wingard, J. R., Curbow, B., Baker, F., & Piantadosi, S. (1991). Health, Functional status, and employment of adult survivors of bone marrow transplantation. *Annals of Internal Medicine,* **114,** 113–8.

Wingard, J. R., Piantadosi, S., Vogelsang, G. B. *et al.* (1989). Predictors of death from chronic graft-versus-host disease after bone marrow transplantation. *Blood,* **74,** 1428–35.

Winston, D. J., Antin, J. H., Wolff, S. N. *et al.* (2001). A multicenter, randomized, double-blind comparison of different doses of intravenous immunoglobulin for prevention of graft-versus-host disease and infection after allogeneic bone marrow transplantation. *Bone Marrow Transplantation,* **28,** 187–96.

Witherspoon, R. P., Sullivan, K. M., Lum, L. G. *et al.* (1988). Use of thymic grafts or thymic factors to augment immunologic recovery after bone marrow transplantation: brief report with 2 to 12 years' follow-up. *Bone Marrow Transplantation,* **3,** 425–35.

Wolff, D., Reichenberger, F., Steiner, B. *et al.* (2002). Progressive interstitial fibrosis of the lung in sclerodermoid chronic graft-versus-host disease. *Bone Marrow Transplantation,* **29,** 357–60.

Yanai, N., Shufaro, Y., Or, R., & Meirow, D. (1999). Vaginal outflow tract obstruction by graft-versus-host reaction. *Bone Marrow Transplantation,* **24,** 811–2.

Ysebaert, L., Deconinck, E., Larosa, F. *et al.* (2002). Polyvisceral arteritis in chronic graft-versus-host disease: antiphospholipid-negative thrombiotic syndrome mimicking polyarteritis nodosa. *Bone Marrow Transplantation,* **29,** 873–4.

Zaucha, J. M., Gooley, T., Bensinger, W. I. *et al.* (2001). CD34 cell dose in granulocyte colony-stimulating factor-mobilized peripheral blood mononuclear cell grafts affects engraftment kinetics and development of extensive chronic graft-versus-host disease after human leukocyte antigen-identical sibling transplantation. *Blood,* **98,** 3221–7.

Zauncer, C., Rabitsch, W., Schneeweiss, B. *et al.* (2001). Energy and substrate metabolism in patients with chronic extensive graft-versus-host disease. *Transplantation,* **71,** 524–8.

Zecca, M., Prete, A., Rondelli, R. *et al.* (2003). Chronic graft-versus-host disease in children: incidence, risk factors and impact on outcome. *Blood,* **100,** 1192–1200.

73 Bacterial infections

ADRIAN DEKKER AND DAN ENGELHARD

University Medical Center, Utrecht, The Netherlands and Hadassah University Hospital, Jerusalem, Israel

Introduction

Bacterial infection is a frequent complication of hematopoietic stem cell (HSC) transplantation. Its occurrence is determined by a number of factors including the recipient's pretransplant clinical history and underlying disease, the type and intensity of the pretransplant preparative regimen, the regimen (if any) used for infection prevention, and the microbiological flora of the patient and the individual transplant unit. For example, patients who have been neutropenic long term, such as those with severe aplastic anemia, are likely to have a very different posttransplant experience with bacterial infections than those who come to transplant clinically well, such as those in the first chronic phase of chronic myeloid leukemia. The most important clinical predisposing factors to bacterial infection posttransplant are mucositis of the mouth, pharynx, and gastrointestinal tract induced by high-dose pretransplant chemotherapy or chemoradiation conditioning regimen (resulting particularly in bacteremia due to oral viridans streptococci), and the use of central intravenous catheters (resulting particularly in infection due to coagulase-negative staphylococci) (Donnelly, 1995). Later posttransplant, the most important clinical predisposing factor to bacterial infection is the presence of moderate or severe graft-versus-host disease (GVHD), particularly of the gastrointestinal tract, and its treatment by increased immunosuppressive therapy. Ulceration of the gastrointestinal mucosa provides a ready portal of entry for Gram-negative bacteria[1]. The main immunologic predisposing factors to bacterial infection posttransplant are duration of neutropenia (Mossad *et al.*, 1996; Nosanchuk *et al.*, 1996) and defects of humoral immunity. Even after normal neutrophil numbers recover, neutrophil function, including chemotaxis and killing of intracellular organisms, may remain abnormal. B-cell numbers remain low long term posttransplant and although serum immunoglobulin levels recover relatively quickly with normal IgG and IgM levels by 3 months posttransplant, in vivo antibody production to specific antigens remains defective up to a year in those without chronic GVHD and longer in those who develop chronic GVHD. Infections in general, but particularly fungal and bacterial

infection, appear less common after allogeneic PBSC transplants compared to marrow transplants (Storek *et al.*, 2001), probably related to higher lymphocyte and lymphocyte-subset counts in the PBSC recipients.

Polymorphisms of genes encoding proteins involved in innate immunity and inflammation influence predisposition to infection in HSC allograft recipients (Rocha et al., 2002): the risk of severe bacterial infection in this study was increased if the donor's genotype for myeloperoxidase, an enzyme important in the microbicidal activity of leukocytes, was AG or AA as opposed to GG. Similarly, polymorphisms for mannose-binding lectins (MBL), an important component of the opsonization of pathogens for phagocytosis in the innate immune response are associated with major infection after allogeneic HSC transplantation (Mullighan et al., 2002). Human MBL is encoded by the gene MBL2. MBL2 coding mutations in either the donor or recipient were associated with an increased risk of infection. Recommendations from the Centers for Disease Control and Prevention (USA), the Infectious Diseases Society of America and the American Society of Blood and Marrow Transplantation on preventing opportunistic infection in HSC recipients have been published (Centers for Disease Control and Prevention, 2000), as have guidelines for the use of antimicrobial agents in neutropenic patients with cancer from the Infectious Diseases Society of America (Hughes et al., 2002).

Types of bacterial infection

The site of infection and the type of infecting bacteria in a 10-year survey from a single transplant unit are shown in Table 73.1. During the first 30 days posttransplant (the time when neutropenia was maximal), the three most common types of infection were fever of unknown origin (presumed bacterial), Gram-positive and Gram-negative septicemia, and central venous catheter exit site infection. (Nonbacterial infections that can occur during this time period include those due to herpes simplex, *Candida*, and *Aspergillus*.)

Between day 31 and day 90 posttransplant the three most common types of infection were again fever of unknown origin

---

[1] Hans Christian Joachim Gram, Danish Pathologist, 1853–1938.

Table 73.1. *Most common bacterial infections after bone marrow transplantation*[a]

Time posttransplant					
Days 0–30		Days 31–90		Day ≥ 180	
Cause	No. of episodes	Cause	No. of episodes	Cause	No. of episodes
Fever of unknown origin[b]	171	Fever of unknown origin[b]	64	Bronchopulmonary infection (total = 49)	
				Bronchitis of unknown cause[b]	16
Septicemia (total = 95)		Septicemia (total = 54)		Pneumonia of unknown cause[b]	14
Gram-positive	54	Gram-positive	31	Gram-positive pneumonia	5
Gram-negative	41	Gram-negative	23	Gram-negative pneumonia	5
				Bronchitis due to other bacteria	4
				Gram-positive bronchitis	3
Hickman catheter exit site infection (total = 55)		Bronchopulmonary infection (total = 32)		Gram-negative bronchitis	1
				Pneumonia due to other bacteria	1
Gram-positive	27	Pneumonia of unknown cause[b]	8	Septicemia (total = 15)	
Unknown cause[b]	26	Bronchitis of unknown cause[b]	7	Gram-positive	10
Gram-negative	2	Gram-positive pneumonia	7	Gram-negative	5
		Gram-negative bronchitis	5		
Bronchopulmonary infection (total = 20)		Gram-negative pneumonia	3	Ear, nose, throat infection (total = 14)	
Pneumonia of unknown cause[b]	9	Gram-positive bronchitis	2	Sinusitis of unknown cause[b]	9
Bronchitis of unknown cause[b]	6			Gram-positive sinusitis	4
Gram-positive pneumonia	4	Hickman catheter exit site infection (total = 17)		Otitis media of unknown cause[b]	1
Gram-negative pneumonia	1	Unknown cause[b]	9		
		Gram-positive	7	Hickman catheter exit site infection (total = 5)	
Urinary tract infection (total = 16)		Gram-negative	1	Unknown cause[b]	3
Gram-negative	10	Enteritis (total = 12)		Gram-positive	1
Gram-positive	6	Gram-negative	6	Gram-negative	1
		Gram-positive	3		
		Other bacteria	3	Fever of unknown origin[b]	4
Enteritis (total = 16)					
Gram-positive	12				
Gram-negative	2	Urinary tract infection (total = 10)			
Other bacteria	2	Gram-negative	5		
		Unknown cause[b]	4		
		Gram-positive	1		
		Ear, nose, throat infection; unknown cause (total = 6)			
		Otitis media of unknown cause[b]	3		
		Sinusitis of unknown cause[b]	3		

[a] Data from 274 HLA-identical sibling marrow transplant recipients at St. Vincent's Hospital, Sydney, 1981–91. Infections with less than 4 episodes during this time period not shown.

[b] Presumed bacterial on clinical grounds.

(the majority presumed bacterial), Gram-positive and Gram-negative septicemia, followed by bronchopulmonary infection. (Nonbacterial infections that can occur during this time period include those due to cytomegalovirus, BK virus, adenovirus, varicella zoster, *Candida, Aspergillus, Pneumocystis carinii,* and *Toxoplasma gondii.*)

After day 180 when most patients have normal neutrophil counts, but a portion of whom have chronic GVHD, the three most common types of bacterial infections were bronchopulmonary infection, septicemia, and ear, nose, and throat infections (Table 73.1). (Nonbacterial infections that can occur dur-

ing this latter time period include those due to varicella zoster, *Pneumocystis carinii,* and *Aspergillus.*)

In one study of bacterial pneumonia in 255 consecutive recipients of allogeneic or autologous bone marrow transplants, 37 (15%) patients experienced 52 episodes of bacterial pneumonia: during the first 100 days posttransplant, hospital acquired Gram-negative bacteria were the predominant causative organisms, while after day 100 community-acquired Gram-positive bacteria, particularly pneumococcus, predominated with occasional cases due to *Haemophilus influenzae.* When all episodes of pneumonia were considered, a significant association was found between bacterial pneumonia and hepatic veno-occlusive disease (VOD) and chronic GVHD (Lossos *et al.*, 1995). The association between chronic GVHD and bacterial infection is well known and that between hepatic VOD and pneumonia is likely due to basal atelectasis produced by the presence of tense ascites.

Infections during the neutropenic period

The absolute neutrophil count (ANC) remains low ($<0.5 \times 10^9/l$) for up to 4 weeks after allogeneic transplant with a shorter period among patients receiving cyclosporine alone, compared to those receiving cyclosporine and methotrexate, or methotrexate alone, as posttransplant immune suppression. In one study, the addition of prophylactic methylprednisolone (1 mg/kg intravenously from day 0 to day 22 posttransplant and then 0.5 mg/kg daily from days 22 to 35 posttransplant) increased the risk of infection by 1.5 times during the early posttransplant period (Sayer *et al.*, 1994). Bacteremia or other serious bacterial infections occur in at least one-half of all patients during this period and fevers of unknown origin, assumed to be bacterial, in up to 85%. Both Gram-negative and Gram-positive infections occur, and many of the Gram-positive (*Staphylococcus aureus, Staphylococcus epidermidis*) infections are likely related to the ubiquitous use of long-term central venous indwelling catheters for venous access. In one single institution study, viridans streptococci (oral commensals) were the most common cause of bacteremia in 61 consecutive allograft recipients given myeloablative conditioning (Graber *et al.*, 2001). Twenty isolates from 15 patients were *Streptococcus mitis*. Most were resistant to norfloxacin, used for prophylaxis on this program. Twenty-six percent had severe oral pathology while neutropenic. Septicemia with *Pseudomonas* species or multiresistant *Staphylococcus aureus* represent the most dangerous infections. Although most bacteremias resolve with antibiotic treatment alone (Ender *et al.*, 1996; Engelhard *et al.*, 1996), approximately 10% of central venous catheters must be removed because of persistent bacteremia (Lina *et al.*, 1995) or local subcutaneous "tunnel" infections (Petersen *et al.*, 1986). While many physicians when removing a Hickman catheter leave the Dacron cuff in place, an effort should be made to remove it, since the cuff itself can also be infected and lead to systemic infection (Ruppel *et al.*, 1994). Therapeutic granulocyte transfusions should, if possible, not be used because of the serious risk they pose of introducing cytomegalovirus infection.

Neutropenia can recur later posttransplant, either due to medications, such as contrimoxazole used for prophylaxis of *Pneumocystis carinii* pneumonia, ganciclovir used for prophylaxis or therapy of cytomegalovirus infection, autoimmune neutropenia following bone marrow transplantation (Klumpp *et al.*, 1992), or as a consequence of viral infection or acute GVHD. Recurrent neutropenia again puts the transplant recipient at risk of bacterial (and fungal) infection, and in such circumstances consideration should be given to the therapeutic use of hematopoietic growth factors such as granulocyte-macrophage colony stimulating factor (GM-CSF) or granulo-

cyte colony-stimulating factor (G-CSF) in combination with appropriate antibiotic therapy.

Gram-negative sepsis is common in patients with ulcerative enteritis, most commonly due to acute GVHD involving the gastrointestinal tract. One particularly devastating infection occurring in the immediate posttransplant neutropenic period is necrotizing enterocolitis. Symptoms include severe abdominal pain and diarrhea, often hemorrhagic. This is usually initiated by pretransplant chemotherapy or chemoradiation causing mucositis of the gastrointestinal (GI) tract, thus allowing bacterial invasion of the bowel wall.

Septic shock due to streptococcal infection

In some units up to one-third of bacterial infections posttransplant are due to streptococci and again, while most recover, a small proportion have a fatal outcome (Villablanca *et al.*, 1990). The increasing incidence of streptococcal infections posttransplant is likely related to the use of oral quinolones to produce bacterial decontamination of the gut in order to minimize the risk of Gram-negative bacterial infections. A viridans streptococcal septic shock syndrome has been recognized as a rare but often progressive and fatal complication of this. In one study of 832 patients transplanted between 1976 and 1988, 123 had an episode of *Streptococcus viridans* bacteremia and 10 patients (8%) developed clinical shock within an average of 2 (range 0–4) days of their first positive blood culture. The septic shock occurred at a median of 6 days posttransplant when all 10 patients were neutropenic. Six of the 10 patients died as a consequence. The most frequent of the viridans streptococcal species isolated in the shock patients was *Streptococcus mitis* (Steiner *et al.*, 1993). Other reports have emphasized the danger of this infection because of associated capillary leak syndrome (Funke *et al.*, 1994) or fatal acute rhabdomyolysis (Martino *et al.*, 1994b). In this regard it is encouraging that a prospective, randomized, double-blind, placebo-controlled prophylactic trial has demonstrated that the addition of penicillin V to pefloxacin (a fluoroquinolone) effectively reduced the number of febrile episodes and the incidence of bacteremia in granulocytopenic patients with cancer, especially those infections due to streptococcal species (International Antimicrobial Therapy Cooperative Group of the European Organization for Research and Treatment of Cancer, 1994). In another randomized trial of the addition of penicillin (or vancomycin if penicillin-allergic) to antimicrobial prophylaxis of norfloxacin, fluconazole, and acyclovir, in 43 patients undergoing high-dose chemotherapy with autologous bone marrow transplantation, excessive morbidity in the form of streptococcal septic shock occurred in the group not receiving Gram-positive prophylaxis. There were significantly fewer overall infections as well as streptococcal infections in the group receiving Gram-positive prophylaxis, although there were no significant differences in the number of deaths, duration of broad-spectrum antibiotic therapy, or the incidence of neutropenic fever between the two groups (Broun *et al.*, 1994). In one study, intravenous cephalothin for 10 days after transplantation was used for prevention of streptococcal infections; only 6 out of 170 patients (4%) had an episode of *Streptococcus viridans* bacteremia (van Kraaij *et al.,* 2002).

Late bacterial infections

Most recipients of family member donor transplants do not have bacterial infections beyond 6 months posttransplant. However, those who do usually have chronic GVHD (Atkinson *et al.,* 1979, 1982; Kulkami *et al.,* 2000; Engelhard *et al.,* 2002). This syndrome is accompanied by a severe and persistent combined immune deficiency rendering patients susceptible not only to bacterial infections, but to viral (particularly DNA herpes virus infections) and *Pneumocystis* infection. The lymphoid organs in chronic GVHD are typically hypocellular and atrophic and it is of interest that Gram-positive cocci, particularly pneumococci, are the most common infecting agents late posttransplant (Fig 73.1). This is likely due to the functional asplenia that comprises part of the lymphoid system atrophy in patients with chronic GVHD (Al-Eid *et al.,* 1983; Dahut & Georgiadis, 1995), as well as the prolonged deficiency of IgG, rendering such patients unable to opsonize encapsulated bacteria. Interestingly, in a survey of 358 patients receiving an HLA-identical marrow graft for chronic myeloid leukemia, pretransplant splenectomy did not predispose to an increased incidence of late infectious complications (Kalhs *et al.,* 1995). However, the following should be noted with regard to the risk of infection postsplenectomy (Fielding, 1994):

- Risk of serious infection: up to 5%
- Risk of fatal infection: up to 21%
- Risk of overwhelming postsplenectomy infection [rapidly fatal sepsis with disseminated intravascular coagulation (DIC) and high levels of bacteremia] usually pneumococcal: up to 1% in adults, higher in children
- Organisms: most commonly pneumococcus, also *Haemophilus influenzae,* meningococcus, *Pseudomonas* species, and *Escherichia coli.*
- Febrile episodes in asplenic patients should be treated aggressively with intravenous antibiotics covering the fore-

going organisms (e.g., i.v. ceftriaxone 2 g daily or every 12 hours, and gentamicin 5 mg/kg/day).

The sites and types of late infections in recipients of family member allografts are shown in Table 73.2. Approximately one-third of long-term survivors were shown to have 3 or more infections and such infections were often troublesome. Six percent of patients had 5, 6, 8, 9, and 10 infections during the period analyzed and 9% had fatal infections.

The preponderance of upper respiratory infections is likely due to the occurrence of sinusitis as a complication of chronic GVHD, and the frequency of pulmonary infections is likely due to the bronchopulmonary sicca characteristic of such patients. The organisms responsible for late bacterial infections in these patients are shown in Table 73.3. The main risk factors for bacterial infections after family member donor transplants were active chronic GVHD and HLA nonidentity between donor and recipient (Atkinson *et al.,* 1982). The latter finding suggests that full genotypic identity for HLA antigens

Table 73.2. *Sites and types of late infections*

Site	Type	Number of episodes	Total number
Pulmonary	Bacterial pneumonia	23	
	Interstitial pneumonia	7	
	Fungal pneumonia	4	
	Bronchitis	25	
	Pleurisy	3	62
Cutaneous	Varicella zoster	29	
	Herpes simplex	2	
	Wart	3	
	Cellulitis, boil	8	
	Paronychia	3	
	Fungal	4	49
Ear, nose, and throat	Bacterial pharyngitis/ tonsilitis	11	
	Oral candida	20	
	Esophageal candida	1	
	Otitis media	16	
	Oral herpes simplex	6	
	Gingivitis	1	
	Tooth abscess	2	
	Sinusitis	27	84
Systemic	Bacterial sepsis	11	
	Infectious mononucleosis	1	
	Measles	1	
	"Acute febrile illness"	4	17
Ophthalmic	Purulent conjunctivitis	12	
	Herpes simplex keratitis	3	15
Genitourinary	Cystitis	11	
	Vaginitis	2	13
Central nervous system	Meningitis	2	
	Herpes simplex encephalitis	1	3
Miscellaneous	Hyperalimentation line infection	1	1
TOTAL		244	

Reproduced, with permission from Atkinson *et al.* (1982).

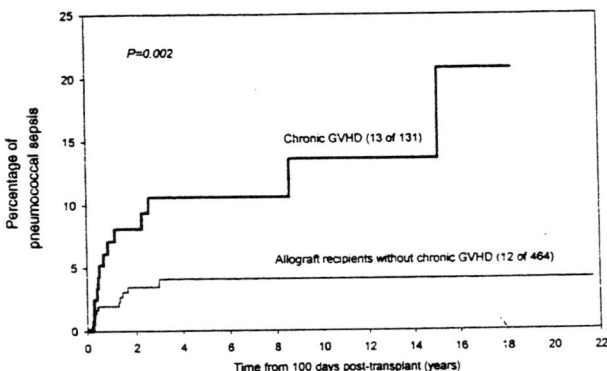

Fig. 73.1. Significantly higher risk for pneumococcal sepsis among allograft recipients with chronic graft-versus-host disease. Reproduced, with permission, from Kulkami *et al.* (2000).

Table 73.3. *Organisms responsible for late infections*

Organism	Number of episodes	Total number
Bacterial		38
Gram-positive cocci		
Pneumococcus	11	
Staphylococcus aureus	10	
β-haemolytic streptococcus	8	
Gram-negative bacilli		
Pseudomonas	3	
Escherichia coli	2	
Klebsiella	1	
Miscellaneous		
Haemophilus influenzae	2	
Mycobacterium fortuitum	1	
Fungal		27
Candida	22	
Nocardia	2	
Aspergillus	2	
Tinea sp.	1	
Viral		49
Varicella zoster[a]	29	
Herpes simplex	15	
Cytomegalovirus	2	
Measles, respiratory syncytial virus, and mycoplasma	1 each	
TOTAL	114	

[a] Not always isolated but presumed to be present on the basis of the clinical findings.

Reproduced, with permission, from Atkinson *et al.* (1982).

between marrow stem cell (and resulting prothymocyte) and recipient (host) thymic epithelial cell is required for optimal reconstitution of the immune system after allogeneic transplantation in humans.

In one study in which 818 autologous and 1,007 allogeneic bone marrow transplant (BMT) recipients from 22 centers in the United Kingdom were surveyed, 6.2% developed severe infections 3 months or later posttransplant that required readmission to the hospital. The most common infections were due to cytomegalovirus ($n = 19$), *Pneumocystis* ($n = 12$), pneumococcus ($n = 15$), *Pseudomonas* ($n = 7$), and *Aspergillus* ($n = 8$) (Hoyle & Goldman, 1994).

In a study that compared the incidence of late infections after allogeneic related and unrelated donor transplant recipients (Ochs *et al.*, 1995), the incidence of any late infection was greater in unrelated donor versus related donor recipients, and multivariate analysis showed advanced GVHD to be the only significantly associated risk factor. However, GVHD was apparent as a risk factor only in related donor recipients whereas unrelated donor recipients, with or without GVHD, had more late infections compared with related donor recipients without GVHD. It should be noted that in this study late infections were defined as those occurring beyond day 50 posttransplant and not as in other studies those infections occurring beyond 3 or 6 months posttransplant. The proportion of infec-

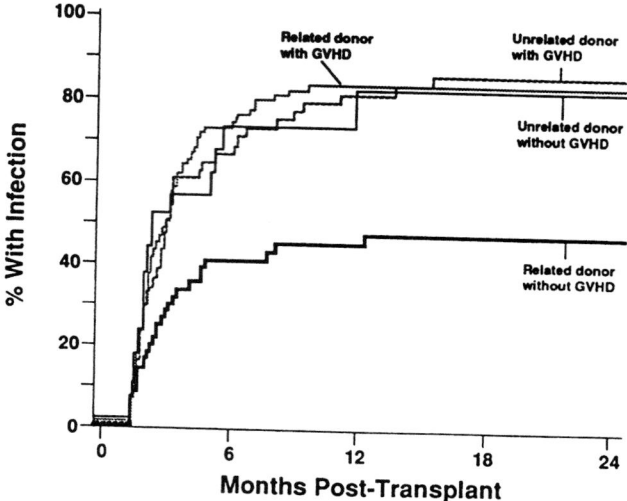

Fig. 73.2. Incidence of late infections. The effect of donor source and GVHD on the incidence of late infection in related donor and unrelated donor BMT recipients considered as a time-dependent covariate. Reproduced, with permission, from Ochs *et al.* (1995).

tions caused by bacteria, viruses, and fungi did not change significantly over time. Within the related and unrelated donor subgroups, the relative frequency of bacterial, viral, and fungal infections was similar in all time periods (Fig. 73.2).

In a study of infections occurring between 6 and 12 months postallografting, Storek and colleagues (1997) found the blood CD4⁺ count the only parameter correlating with infection score (Fig. 73.3).

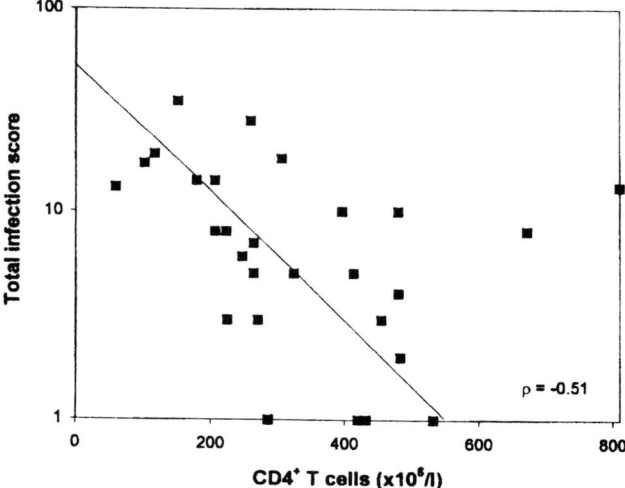

Fig. 73.3. The association between the total infection score (which takes into account the frequency and severity of infections that occurred within 180 days preceding the 1-year-posttransplant exam) and the absolute CD4⁺ T-cell count. The correlation coefficient (*P*) was calculated by the Spearman rank-correlation method. In this graph with log-scale vertical axis, zero values were arbitrarily assigned the value of 1. Reproduced, with permission, from Storek *et al.* (1997).

IgG$_2$ and IgG$_4$ subclass deficiency have been associated with late pneumococcal infection after allogeneic BMT. Interestingly antibodies to capsular polysaccharide antigens have been found to be predominantly restricted to the IgG$_2$ subclass (Aucouturier *et al.*, 1987; Sheridan *et al.*, 1990). In one study, six cases of fatal pneumococcal sepsis were described between 3 and 39 months posttransplant, and represented approximately 2% of the allograft population for the center during the study period who survived 3 months or longer. Five of the six patients had chronic GVHD and were receiving immunosuppressive therapy (Rege, Mehta, & Treleaven, 1994). Pneumococcal pneumonia may present in an atypical fashion after HSC transplantation. One patient given an autologous BMT for Hodgkin's disease presented with anorexia, pallor, weight loss, and right-sided chest pain. Examination revealed marked hepatomegaly and a massive right pleural effusion, an aspirate of which (as well as blood cultures) grew pneumococcus. Complete resolution occurred with imipenem therapy. Late pneumoccocal arthritis has also been described after allogeneic transplantation, again usually in patients with chronic GVHD (Schwella *et al.*, 1993; Dahut & Georgiadis, 1995; Gomez-Casares *et al.*, 1995). Pneumoccocal meningitis can also occur, occasionally due to penicillin-resistant pneumococcus (D'Antonio *et al.*, 1992). Additionally, spontaneous pneumococcal peritonitis has been described in such patients (Julisa *et al.*, 1985).

Prophylactic cotrimoxazole one double strength tablet taken twice daily for 2 to 3 days per week is utilized by most transplant programs to minimize the risk of late bacterial infections as well as that of *Pneumocystis carinii* pneumonia. It should be continued for 6 months after allogeneic transplantation in those without GVHD, and for the duration of active chronic GVHD in those who demonstrate it or for the duration of immunosuppressive therapy to prevent or treat GVHD. In those patients (usually those with chronic GVHD) who get "breakthrough" bacterial infections while receiving prophylactic cotrimoxazole (usually pneumococcal or hemophilus infections) prophylactic oral penicillin can be added to the cotrimoxazole. The role of vaccination for late infections is discussed below.

Management of bacterial infections

Fever of unknown origin

As soon as a marrow transplant recipient's temperature is elevated to a certain arbitrary level (38.5° C in many units), a septic workup should be immediately instituted. This should include:

1. physical examination
2. blood cultures
3. throat swab
4. central venous catheter exit site swab
5. midstream urine sample
6. chest x-ray

As soon as two sets of blood cultures have been drawn, the patient should be started on intravenous broad-spectrum antibacterial antibiotics. The choice of these will vary according to individual transplant units' preferences and the spectrum of infecting bacteria found therein, but a common combination is an aminoglycoside, such as gentamicin 3 to 5 mg/kg/day, together with a semisynthetic penicillin with antipseudomonas activity, such as piperacillin 4 g i.v. every 6 hours or timentin (a combination of ticarcillin and potassium clavulanate) 3.1 g i.v. every 6 hours (adult dosages with normal renal and hepatic function). Other aminoglycosides may be substituted for gentamicin in appropriate circumstances such as tobramycin 3 to 5 mg/kg/day or amikacin 15 mg/kg/day. Alternatives to the semisynthetic penicillins include a third-generation cephalosporin such as ceftazidime 1 to 6 g i.v. daily in 2 or 3 divided doses (ceftazidime has significant activity against *Pseudomonas*) or a carbapenem such as imipenem (with cilastin) 0.5 to 1 g every 6 hours (although imipenem has unreliable activity against *Pseudomonas*). Monotherapy, such as the use of ceftazidime alone, is not generally recommended in this situation because of the risk of the development of bacterial resistance. Once-daily administration regimens, such as the use of ceftriaxone (1–3 g/day), are also not ideal because of potential lack of activity against the unidentified responsible organism. All the above doses quoted are for adults with normal renal and hepatic function.

With a broad-spectrum combination antibiotic approach the majority of fevers during the neutropenic period will resolve within 48 to 72 hours. However, all transplant units should have a clear-cut strategy in place for the management of those fevers that do not, and which have no other ready explanation (such as drug allergy, association with blood product administration, or the underlying hematologic malignancy). A typical approach (see Table 73.4) for such an escalation strategy would be the introduction of vancomycin at 48 hours after the initiation of the primary antibacterial antibiotics, followed 24 hours later by the addition of

Table 73.4. *Management of fever of unknown origin in the neutropenic patient after marrow transplant*

Time from development of fever (hours)	Strategy
0	1. Rapid assessment (physical exam) and culture (blood, urine, throat, central venous catheter exit site). Chest x-ray.
0	2. Start i.v. broad-spectrum antibacterial antibiotics
48	3. Add i.v. vancomycin if no response
72	4. Add antifungal antibiotic
96	5. Remove indwelling catheter
	6. Additional measures if severe infection a) G-CSF or GM-CSF b) Renal dose dopamine/packed cell transfusion (if blood pressure compromised)

Abbreviations: G-CSF, granulocyte colony-stimulating factor; GM-CSF, granulocyte-macrophage colony-stimulating factor.

an antifungal agent, such as fluconazole (to cover *Candida* species) (if not already receiving it prophylactically) or voriconazole or amphotericin (if *Aspergillus* is part of the local microbiological flora), followed 24 to 48 hours later by removal of any indwelling catheter, particularly a right atrial intravenous catheter.

Additional measures for continuing severe fever include the use of G-CSF or GM-CSF to accelerate neutrophil recovery, and possibly the use of renal dose dopamine if the systolic blood pressure is compromised. Packed cell transfusion is the best replacement therapy for septic shock since erythrocytes remain predominantly in the intravascular space, and this will minimize the risk of increased-leak pulmonary edema [acute respiratory distress syndrome (ARDS)] due to the sepsis. Interestingly, septic shock is relatively uncommon in leukopenic patients, possibly because the lack of monocytes prevents release of the monokine mediators of shock such at tumor necrosis factor and interleukin-1. The use of recombinant human activated protein C (drotrenogin alfa) has been shown to significantly reduce mortality in patients with severe sepsis, although the risk of bleeding may be increased (Bernard *et al.*, 2001; Pastores *et al.*, 2002).

If unexplained fever persists, consider the following possibilities:

- cryptic bacterial infection (e.g., sinusitis)
- fungemia (e.g., hepatosplenic candidiasis)
- drug fever (including antibiotic fever)
- viremia (especially with CMV)

Right atrial indwelling intravenous catheter exit site infection (Hickman, Broviac, Groshon, or similar)

Redness and tenderness around the catheter exit site is common in the first 4 weeks posttransplant. An exit site swab should be taken and treatment initiated with flucloxacillin 1 g i.v. every 6 hours or vancomycin 1 g i.v. every 12 hours (minimum infusion period for vancomycin 1 hour to prevent severe skin discomfort and erythema). This approach will allow salvage of the catheter in many cases.

Infection of the right atrial indwelling catheter subcutaneous track ("tunnel" infection)

Redness, tenderness, and edema along and surrounding the subcutaneous part of the catheter can initially be managed as an exit site infection. However, it is a more serious infection, is less readily resolved by intravenous antibiotic treatment, and usually requires removal of the catheter, with continuation of intravenous antibiotics through a new central line. The tip of all intravenous lines removed from HSC transplant patients should be sent to the microbiology laboratory for culture.

Septic thrombophlebitis

Unilateral arm edema with axillary tenderness indicating septic thrombophlebitis is another more serious catheter-associated infection. The catheter should be removed and antibiotic treatment instituted, usually with intravenous vancomycin and an antipseudomonal agent such as a semisynthetic penicillin or a third-generation cephalosporin such as ceftazidime.

Infection in the lumen/tip of the indwelling intravenous catheter (line sepsis)

Any of the following suggest infection of the intravenous portion of the catheter:

1. Temporal relationship between bacteremia and catheter manipulation
2. Positive blood cultures from catheter, but not (or lower colony count) from simultaneous peripheral vein sample
3. Recurrent bacteremia with the same organism
4. Polymicrobial bacteremia
5. Bacteremia occurring in the absence of neutropenia or gut ulceration
6. Bacteremia not responding to appropriate antibiotic therapy in patients with a normal neutrophil count

An attempt to salvage the catheter using appropriate antibiotics with or without hematopoietic growth factors may be made initially. However, infection with multiresistant *Staphylococcus aureus* or *epidermidis*, *Pseudomonas* species, or *Candida* species usually necessitates catheter removal, as does severe infection with systemic "toxic" symptoms (for example rigors) or shock. However, a study of 53 BMT recipients with *Corynebacterium jeikeium* bacteremia (usually due to *C. jeikeium* colonization of an indwelling right atrial catheter) indicated that the majority were successfully managed by vancomycin treatment alone, without a need for catheter removal (Wang, Mattson, & Wald, 2001).

Indwelling catheter-related bacterial endocarditis

Indwelling catheter-related right-sided endocarditis has been described in 5% of marrow transplant recipients due in 4 cases to *Staphylococcus epidermidis*, 1 *Enterococcus faecalis*, 1 *Corynebacterium jeikeium*, 1 *Pseudomonas alcaligenes*, and 1 *Achromobacter xylosoxidans* (Martino *et al.*, 1990). Six of the seven cases recovered with courses of antibacterial antibiotic therapy lasting 3 to 7 weeks. Patients with pre-existing heart valvular disease are at definite risk of bacterial endocarditis, particularly during the neutropenic period and should receive antibacterial antibiotic prophylaxis for all invasive procedures, including bone marrow aspirates, lumbar punctures, insertion of Hickman catheters, and bladder catheterization. Current recommended prophylaxis for adults is ampicillin 1 to 3 g and gentamicin 1.5 mg/kg i.v. immediately before the procedure, followed by ampicillin 1 to 5 g i.v. 6 hours later. For patients allergic to penicillin, vancomycin 1 g i.v. and gentamicin 2.5 mg/kg i.v. 1 hour before the procedure may be substituted.

For patients who develop infective endocarditis, treatment will depend on the infecting organism. A guide is given in Table 73.5.

Table 73.5. *Guide to antibiotic therapy in adult patients with bacterial endocarditis after marrow transplantation*[a]

Infecting organism	Antibiotic therapy	Example of treatment
None (awaiting cultures)	Penicillinase-resistant penicillin + aminoglycoside	Flucloxacillin[b] 2 g i.v. every 6 hours
Staphylococcus aureus		Gentamicin 2.5 mg/kg i.v. every 12 hours
Streptococcus viridans (MIC <0.1 µg/ml)	Penicillin G + aminoglycoside	Penicillin G[b] 20 million units i.v. day.
Enterococcus		Gentamicin 2.5 mg/kg i.v. every 12 hours

[a] On native (not prosthetic) valve.

[b] Substitute vancomycin 1 g i.v. every 12 hours if penicillin-allergic.

Unusual bacterial infections after HSC transplantation

Legionella infection

Legionella are facultative intracellular pathogens that multiply within macrophages and monocytes and are a common cause of community-acquired pneumonia. Like infections caused by other intracellular organisms, an appropriate cellular immune response is a critical component of the host defense against *Legionella*. Many studies have documented that immune-suppressed patients are at an increased risk of acquiring and dying from *Legionella* infection. A number of cases of Legionnaires' disease in BMT patients have been reported (Kugler *et al.*, 1983; Meletis *et al.*, 1987; Schwebke *et al.*, 1990; Benz-Lemoine *et al.*, 1991; Matulonis *et al.*, 1993; Harrington *et al.*, 1996). In a review of legionellosis in a bone marrow transplant center over a 6-year period ending in 1993, Harrington and colleagues (1996) reported 10 cases of culture-proven *Legionella* infection. Infections were caused by four species of *Legionella* with no apparent clustering of cases. Detection of *Legionella* using direct fluorescent antibody assays proved unreliable due to the high proportion of rare *Legionella* species isolated. The clinical presentation, course, and outcome of patients varied and did not correlate with underlying disease, type of transplant, transplant day, or engraftment status. Five of the seven patients infected with non-*pneumophila* species recovered from their pneumonia compared to none of the three patients infected with *Legionella pneumophila*. Persistent or relapsed infection after 3 weeks of appropriate therapy was documented in one case, suggesting that prolonged antibiotic treatment is indicated in these patients. Chest x-ray showed unilateral infiltrates in six of the ten and bilateral infiltrates in four. Pleural effusion occurred in two cases and cavitation in one. All 10 patients had fever ≥ 38.5° C; nine had rales or rhonchi; seven were hypoxemic. Lung tissue, obtained by open biopsy (5 cases) or fine needle aspirate (1 case) gave the highest yield of diagnostic samples, followed by sputum (67%), pleural fluid (50%), and bronchoalveolar lavage fluid (43%). Pericarditis has also been associated with Legionnaires' disease in a BMT recipient (Scerpella *et al.*, 1994). *Legionella micdadei* can occur in patients with septic pulmonary embolism (Schwebke *et al.*, 1990), and this can occur even during periods of severe thrombocytopenia. It should be noted that bacteriologic filters do not ensure absolute security against this organism, and this emphasizes the need for frequent monitoring of the two factors governing *Legionella* growth, namely water temperature, and chlorination and maintenance of the institution's cooling tower (Oren *et al.*, 2002). In one study, 225 patients undergoing BMT (of whom 201 were treated on a new BMT unit) were compared for incidence of *Legionella* infections to 150 neutropenic patients treated in other units of the hospital. The new BMT unit had a multifaceted approach to decontamination of its water system including heating, particulate filtration, ultraviolet sterilization, and a monthly pulse of hyperchlorination of the water. There were only 3 cases of *Legionella* pneumonia among 201 patients undergoing transplantation on the new unit compared to 33 cases detected from 150 patients treated on the general medical floors (Matulonis *et al.*, 1993). Nosocomial cases in hospital units can be completely prevented by heating of the hospital water supply to 60° C and chlorination. While erythromycin remains the treatment of choice for established Legionnaires' disease, the newer quinolone antibiotics are also effective as prophylactic treatment for such patients and are thought to avoid pharmacologic interaction with cyclosporine.

Mycobacterial infection

Both *Mycobacterium tuberculosis* and atypical mycobacterial infections (for example, those caused by *Mycobacterium avium-intracellulare*) can occur after marrow transplantation (Navari *et al.*, 1983; Kurzrock *et al.*, 1984; Sullivan *et al.*, 1985; Ozkaynak *et al.*, 1990; Roy & Weisdorf, 1997), mainly in recipients of T-cell–depleted allografts or those who develop GVHD (Martino *et al.*, 1996). It is commoner after allogeneic than autologous transplantation (de la Camara *et al.*, 2000). In one large retrospective review of 2,241 BMTs, the overall incidence was 0.49% (Roy & Weisdorf, 1997). Other rare mycobacterial species can also cause disease in marrow transplant recipients including *Mycobacterium haemophilum* (Kiehn *et al.*, 1993; Straus *et al.*, 1994; White *et al.*, 1995), *Mycobacterium neoaurum* (Holland *et al.*, 1994) and *Mycobacterium fortuitum* (Okano *et al.*, 2001). Disseminated bacille Calmette-Guérin (BCG)[2] infection has also been reported in children with SCID (Skinner *et al.*, 1996; Ikinciogullari *et al*, 2002). One report demonstrated that functional purified protein derivative (tuberculin) (PPD) spe-

[2] Leon Calmette, French bacteriologist, 1863–1933; Camille Guérin, French bacteriologist, 1872–1961.

cific CD4[+] T cells, transferred with the marrow, restored T-cell immunity to PPD, both in vitro and in vivo in the early period after BMT, while recipients of T-cell–depleted BMT failed to develop this immunity. Three of five nondepleted recipients who developed chronic GVHD also failed to establish a PPD-specific immune response (Rouleau et al., 1993). These data indicate that patients who receive T-cell–depleted grafts and those who develop chronic GVHD are at increased risk of developing active tuberculosis due to a diminished specific T-cell response against Mycobacterium tuberculosis. Total body irradiation has also been identified as a risk factor (Ip et al., 1998).

Most reported infections involve the lung although there are single case reports of meningeal involvement (Martino et al., 1996), disseminated infection (Skinner et al., 1996; Kindler et al., 2001), and intestinal involvement (Inada et al., 1995). It usually occurs late posttransplant—at a median of 324 days posttransplant in one report (de la Camara et al., 2000). Diagnosis may be made not only from sputum, but also from bronchoalveolar lavage samples and marrow aspirate samples. Aggressive multidrug antituberculosis therapy is indicated. A commonly used regimen for pulmonary tuberculosis is shown in Table 73.6. It should be noted that rifampicin can cause a dramatic decrease in cyclosporine blood levels. A high mortality rate in allogeneic recipients (25%) has been reported (de la Camara et al., 2000).

Rare species of mycobacteria that can cause infection in marrow transplant recipients include Mycobacterium haemophilum, Mycobacterium neoaurum, and Mycobacterium fortuitum. Infection with Mycobacterium haemophilum causes disseminated cutaneous lesions, bacteremia, and disease of the bones, joints, lymphatics, and lungs. Improper culture techniques may delay laboratory diagnosis. The organism requires hemin or ferric ammonium citrate and incubation of media at 30° C for optimum growth. Physicians should consider this pathogen when evaluating a patient with ulcerating cutaneous lesions, joint effusions, or osteomyelitis (Kiehn et al., 1993). In one report from a single center, two distinctly different presentations were observed: three patients presented with cutaneous lesions while two others developed pulmonary disease only. Respiratory failure developed in the patients with pneumonia and they died. The remaining three patients survived free of infection (White et al., 1995). Infection with Mycobacterium neoaurum has only been described in two immune-suppressed patients (Holland et al., 1994). One patient developed bacteremia after an allogeneic marrow transplant: Mycobacterium neoaurum was isolated on three separate occasions from blood taken via the Hickman catheter. The patient responded to therapy with ticarcillin/clavulanate and tobramycin, but the Hickman catheter was removed because of the persistence of the organisms in blood cultures taken from the catheter. An association with central venous catheters was also noted by Roy and Weisdorf (1997). Okano et al. (2001) described a case of Mycobacterium fortuitum causing subcutaneous infection, requiring surgical debridement, as well as anti-tuberculous chemotherapy, to effect cure. Five cases were reported in the series of mycobacterial infections occurring after HSC transplantation by Roy and Weisdorf (1997), three of which were associated with the central venous catheter.

Patients with a previous history of pulmonary tuberculosis, or those with a chest x-ray appearance compatible with granulomas and a positive PPD skin test, prior to transplant should receive prophylactic isoniazid 300 mg daily together with pyridoxine 25 mg daily immediately pretransplant and for at least 3 months posttransplant. Prophylaxis against recurrent Mycobacterium avium complex infection in a patient undergoing allografting for chronic myeloid leukemia (CML) successfully utilized ethambutol, cycloserine, and ciprofloxacin given throughout the immediate posttransplant period, but changed at day 25 posttransplant to ciprofloxacin and clarithromycin due to hepatic toxicity; the latter were maintained until day 100 posttransplant (Hermida et al., 1995).

Listeriosis

Listeriosis is a rare infection posttransplant, occurring in approximately 0.4% to 0.6% of transplants (Chang et al., 1995; Nolla-Salas et al., 1997; Safdar et al., 2002), but should always be suspected when meningitis occurs posttransplant. Contaminated food, particularly milk and cheese, is the most common sources of Listeria monocytogenes. In a case report of septicemia occurring in a 6-year-old girl who had received an unrelated donor marrow transplant, Listeria monocytogenes and other Listeria species were found in cooked and chilled foods consumed during the inpatient stay (Want et al., 1993). In another series, three patients presented at 4, 7, and 9 months posttransplant (Long et al., 1993). One patient had had an allograft and two others an autograft. All three patients presented with classical features of meningitis and Listeria monocytogenes was cultured from the cerebrospinal fluid. Response to

Table 73.6. A commonly used regimen for pulmonary tuberculosis

Drug	Dose	Duration
Rifampicin	450 mg (<50 kg) or 600 mg (> 50 kg)	Once daily before breakfast for 2 months[a]
Isoniazid	300 mg	
Pyrazinamide	1.5 g (<50 kg) or 2 g (>50 kg)	
Ethambutol followed by	15–20 mg/kg (up to 1.2 g)	
Rifampicin	Same doses	Once daily for a further 4 months if the organism is susceptible to rifampicin and isoniazid[b]
Isoniazid	Same dose	

[a] Treatment can also be given three times weekly, which may help improve compliance.
[b] If the organism is resistant to isoniazid and rifampicin, specialist consultation should be sought.

Table 73.7. *Rare infections after hematopoietic stem cell transplantation*

Bacterium	Infection site	Comment	Reference
Aeromonas hydrophila	Arm	Hand immersed in sewage water 5 years post-allogeneic BMT. Developed myonecrosis requiring amputation	Moses *et al.* (1995)
Bordatella bronchiseptica	Blood, lung	Persistent, progressive infection	Bauwens *et al.* (1992)
Capnocytophaga (normal oral flora)	Blood	Associated with oral mucositis and neutropenia	Bilgrami *et al.* (1992)
Clostridium botulinum	CNS (motor weakness, respiratory failure—botulism)	3-year-old child 42 days post-ABMT for neuroblastoma. Botulism toxin in stool. Given human botulism immune globulin and recovered.	Shen *et al.* (1994)
Clostridium septicum	Blood, hepatic metastases	ABMT for metastatic breast cancer 1 to 2 months previously; organism in blood cultures and hepatic metastases, prompt recovery with clindamycin and imipenem.	Thel *et al.* (1994)
Comamonas acidovorans	Blood, in-dwelling catheter	Central venous catheter preserved	Ender *et al.* (1996)
Lactobacillus rhamnosus	Blood, pericardial fluid		Kalima *et al.* (1996)
Leptotrichia buccalis (normal oral flora)	Blood	Associated with oral mucositis and neutropenia. On prophylactic ciprofloxacin and vancomycin. 1 of 4 patients developed ARDS.	Schwartz *et al.* (1995)
Morganella morganii	Pericardium	Caused pericarditis after splenectomy for immune cytopenia post-allograft for ALL	Sica *et al.* (1995)
Rahnella aquatilis	Blood	Related to in-dwelling catheter	Hoppe *et al.* (1993)
Plesiomonas shigelloides	Blood	Successfully treated with ciprofloxacin. High mortality rate in literature.	Lee *et al.* (1996)
Stomatococcus mucilaginosus (normal oral flora)	Blood	Associated with oral mucositis and neutropenia	Andstrom *et al.* (1994)
Francisella tularensis (causes tularemia)	Lung	Responded to ciprofloxacin	Naughton *et al.* (1999)
Agrobacterium yellow group	Sepsis and septic arthritis	Responded to broad-spectrum antibiotics	Chalandon *et al.* (2000)
Stenotrophomonas maltophilia	Blood	Associated with mucositis and neutropenia	Labarca *et al.* (2002)

Abbreviations: BMT, bone marrow transplantation; CNS, central nervous system; ARDS, acute respiratory distress syndrome; ALL, acute lymphoblastic leukemia.

treatment with parenteral ampicillin and gentamicin is usually excellent (Safdar *et al.*, 2002).

Hemosiderosis, either idiopathic or caused by transfusion, appears to be another risk factor and *Listeria monocytogenes* septicemia has been reported complicating allogeneic marrow transplantation for transfusion-dependent Diamond-Blackfan[3] syndrome (Lee *et al.*, 1995).

Tetanus

Tetanus has been described after allogeneic marrow transplantation and can be successfully treated by high-dose penicillin G (12 to 24×10^6 U/24 h) in adults with normal renal function.

Rare infections after HSC transplantation

Reports of rare bacterial infections after HSC transplantation continue to grow and are detailed in Table 73.7.

[3] Louis Klein Diamond, U.S. pediatrician, born 1902; Kenneth D. Blackfan, U.S. pediatrician, 1883–1941.

Antimicrobial agents of choice against selected bacteria

These are shown in Table 73.8.

Developments in antibiotics

Several points should be emphasized with regard to marrow transplant recipients:

1. There is an increasing trend to once daily aminoglycoside administration (due to the fact that reduced dosing frequency, while maintaining an equivalent total daily dose, results in higher initial bactericidal activity and a prolonged postantibiotic inhibitory effect).

2. The advent of oral fluoroquinolones has simplified management of conditions such as osteomyelitis and septic arthritis caused by Gram-negative organisms, which, while infrequent posttransplant, occasionally occur. Additionally, the quinolones are active in *Salmonella* and *Shigella* infection, including the increasingly prevalent multiresistant *Salmonella typhi* strains being reported from the Indian subcontinent.

Table 73.8. *Antimicrobial agents of choice against selected microorganisms*[a,b,c]

Organism	First-choice therapy	Second-choice therapy
Branhamella catarrhalis	Amoxicillin clavulanate	Cotrimoxazole
Campylobacter jejuni	Fluoroquinolones	Erythromycin
Chlamydia trachomatis	Tetracycline, doxycycline	Erythromycin
Clostridium perfringens	Penicillin G	Tetracycline
Clostridium difficile	Metronidazole (orally)	Vancomycin (orally)
Corynebacterium JK	Vancomycin	Ciprofloxacin
Enterobacter species	Aminoglycoside	Antipseudomonal penicillin
Enterococci (Group D streptococci)	Penicillin or ampicillin + gentamicin	Vancomycin + gentamicin
Haemophilus influenzae	Amoxicillin	Amoxicillin clavulanate, or cotrimoxazole or third-generation cephalosporin
Legionella pneumophila	Erythromycin	Rifampicin
Listeria monocytogenes	Ampicillin	Cotrimoxazole
Mycoplasma pneumoniae	Erythromycin	Tetracycline
Nocardia asteroides	Cotrimoxazole	Minocycline
Proteus mirabilis	Ampicillin	Cotrimoxazole
Pseudomonas aeruginosa	Aminoglycoside and antipseudomonal penicillin or ceftazidime	Aztreonam or imipenem
Shigella species	Ciprofloxacin, norfloxacin	Cotrimoxazole
Methicillin (or multi) resistant *Staphylococcus aureus*	Vancomycin	Rifampicin and fusidic acid
Methicillin-resistant *Staphylococcus epidermidis*	Vancomycin	Rifampicin + fusidic acid
Xanthomonas maltophilia	Cotrimoxazole	Ticarcillin clavulanate

[a] None of these choices supercede the demonstrated antibiotic sensitivity of a given isolate.

[b] Should usually be administered intravenously to neutropenic patient, except where indicated, and two active agents should normally be given in combination.

[c] Bactericidal agents are preferred to bacteriostatic agents (erythromycin, tetracycline) for neutropenic patients.

They are also the first antibiotics effective in eliminating the *Salmonella typhi* carrier state. It should be noted, however, that resistance to these antibiotics has emerged rapidly in methicillin-resistant staphylococci and to a variable extent in *Pseudomonas aeruginosa* and *Campylobacter jejuni*.

3. Several new macrolide antibiotics are available, including roxithromycin, azithromycin, and clarithromycin. These have varying potential advantages over erythromycin, including better patient tolerance, improved pharmacokinetics (prolonged half-life, higher tissue levels), and in some cases, a broader spectrum, particularly with azithromycin against *Haemophilus influenzae* and some Enterobacteriaciae. Interestingly, some "difficult" organisms appear particularly susceptible, including *Legionella* and *Mycobacterium avium intracellulare* (clarithromycin), and *Toxoplasma gondii* and *Chlamydia trachomatis* (azithromycin).

4. Several recently recognized adverse reactions to antibacterial antibiotics include a severe idiosyncratic prolonged flucloxacillin hepatitis typified by cholestasis, and elevated bilirubin and alkaline phosphatase values; a protracted, but mostly reversible cholestatic jaundice following amoxicillin clavulanate therapy; convulsions in those with a lowered seizure threshold, and confusion in the elderly, as well as anaphylaxis following quinolone use; and convulsions fol-

lowing the use of imipenem, predominantly in those with preexisting urologic or renal impairment.

5. Isolates of *Staphylococcus aureus* have been descibed that are resistant to the glycopeptide antibiotic vancomycin (Smith *et al.,* 1999). These isolates had thicker extracellular matrices on electron microcopy than control methicillin-resistant *S. aureus* isolates. The emergence of such strains emphasizes the importance of the prudent use of antibiotics, the capacity to identify resistant strains and the use of infection-control precautions to minimize transmission. Linezolid, an example of a new class of antibiotics—the oxazolidinones (protein synthesis inhibitors)—is effective against vancomycin-resistant *S. fecalis* as well as Gram-positive organisms such as methicillin-resistant *S. aureus*, although myelosuppression may be problematic. Quinupristin-dalfopristin is also effective against vancomycin-resistant S. fecalis.

Reduction of antibiotic dosage in renal failure

Acute renal failure is common after marrow transplantation, usually occurring in the early posttransplant period and usually multifactorial in etiology (Chapter 90). Predisposing factors include cyclosporine treatment, septicemia, hypotension, and aminoglycoside or amphotericin therapy. The renal failure in such cases is often reversible, and thus it is important to treat

Table 73.9. *Reduction of antimicrobial drug dosage in severe renal failure*

Agents that should not be given	Agents requiring a major dosage reduction	Agents requiring a moderate dosage reduction	Agents requiring no dosage reduction
Nalidixic acid	Amikacin	Acyclovir	Erythromycin
Nitrofurantoin	Gentamicin	Amoxicillin	Methicillin
Norfloxacin	Netilmicin	Ampicillin	
Tetracycline	Tobramycin	Amphotericin	
	Vancomycin	Aztreonam	
		Carbenicillin	
		Cefamandole	
		Cefotaxime	
		Ceftriaxone	
		Ceftazidime	
		Cephalothin	
		Ciprofloxacin	
		Cotrimoxazole	
		Flucloxacillin	
		Fluconazole	
		Ganciclovir	
		Imipenem	
		Moxalactam	
		Penicillin G	
		Piperacillin	
		Ticarcillin	

any complicating infections with adequate, but safe, concentrations of antibiotic.

A guide to antibiotic dosage in adult patients with renal failure is given in Tables 73.9 and 73.10.

Later posttransplant a (usually) asymptomatic elevation of serum creatinine occurs, most commonly due to cyclosporine nephrotoxicity. Again, infections occurring in this setting will need to be treated with appropriately modified antibiotic dosage.

Role of oral hygiene in predisposing to bacterial infections after HSC transplantation

Chronic dental sepsis is not uncommon pretransplant and all prospective marrow transplant recipients should be seen by a dentist several months prior to transplant. Occasionally such sepsis can be sufficiently severe to warrant postponement of the transplant. Posttransplant the mouth serves as a source for systemic infection due to oropharyngeal mucositis, a reduced salivary flow rate, and an increase in caries-related microorganisms (Donnelly *et al.*, 1993; Dens *et al.*, 1996). In one study, 23 of 33 consecutive allogeneic BMT recipients developed bacteremia due to viridans streptococci as mucositis progressed to its peak severity. The addition of clindamycin to the empiric systemic antibiotic regimen of ceftazidime 2 g every 8 hours did not shorten the duration of fever. Not only does the high-dose pretransplant preparative regimen produce a dramatic reduction of

Table 73.10 *Dose reductions of antimicrobial agents in renal impairment*

Drug	Method[a]	Adjustment for renal failure		
		GFR >50 ml/min	GFR = 10–50 ml/min	GFR <10 ml/min
Acyclovir	I,D	q 8 h	q 12–24 h	$\frac{1}{2}$ dose q 24 h
Amikacin[b]	D,I	60–90% q 12 h	30–70% q 12–18 h	20–30% q 24–48 h
or		50–100% q 24 h	50% q 24 h	25% q 48 h
Amoxicillin	I	q 8 h	q 8–12 h	q 24 h
Amphotericin	I	q 24 h	q 24 h	q 24–36 h
Ampicillin	I	q 6 h	q 6–12 h	q 12–24 h
Azlocillin	I	q 4–6 h	q 6–8 h	q 8 h
Aztreonam	D	100%	50–75%	25%
	I	q 8–12 h	q 12–24 h	q 24 h
Benzylpenicillin	D	100%	75%	20–50%
	I	q 6 h	q 8 h	q 12 h
Cefaclor	D	100%	50–100%	50%
	I	q 8 h	q 8 h	q 12 h
Cefamandole	I	q 6 h	q 6–8 h	q 12 h
Cefazolin	I	q 8 h	q 12 h	q 24–48 h
Cefotaxime	I	q 6 h	q 12 h	q 24 h
Cefoxitin	I	q 8 h	q 8–12 h	q 24–48 h
Ceftazidime	I	q 8–12 h	q 24–48 h	q 48–72 h
Ceftriaxone	D	100%	100%	100%
	I	q 24 h	q 24 h	q 24 h
Cephalexin	I	q 6 h	q 6 h	q 8–12 h
Cephalothin	I	q 6 h	q 8 h	q 12 h
Chloramphenicol	D	100%	100%	100%
	I	q 6 h	q 6 h	q 6 h
Ciprofloxacin	D	100%	50%	33%
	I	q 12 h	q 12–24 h	q 24 h

(continues)

Table 73.10   (Continued)

Drug	Method[a]	Adjustment for renal failure		
		GFR >50 ml/min	GFR = 10–50 ml/min	GFR <10 ml/min
Clavulanic acid	D	100%	100%	50–75%
Clindamycin	D	100%	100%	100%
	I	q 6 h	q 6 h	q 6 h
Cotrimoxazole	I	q 12 h	q 18 h	q 24 h
	D,I	q 12 h	¹/₂ dose q 12 h	¹/₂ dose q 24 h
Doxycycline	D	100%	100%	100%
	I	q 12–24 h	q 12–24 h	q 12–24 h
Erythromycin	D	100%	100%	50–75%
	I	q 6 h	q 6 h	q 8 h
Ethambutol	I	q 24 h	q 24	q 48 h
Flucloxacillin	I	q 6 h	q 8 h	q 12 h
Fluconazole	I	q 24 h	q 24–48 h	q 48–72 h
Flucytosine[b]	I	q 6–8 h	q 12–24 h	q 24–48 h
Foscarnet[c]	D	40–100%	Avoid	Avoid
Ganciclovir[c]	I	q 12 h	q 24 h	q 48–96 h
Gentamicin[b]	D, I	60–90% q 12 h	30–70% q 12–18 h	20–30% q 24–48 h
or		70–100% q 24 h	70% q 24 h; 60% q 48 h	40% q 48 h
Griseofulvin	D	100%	100%	100%
	I	q 6 h	q 6 h	q 6 h
Imipenem	D	100%	50%	25%
	I	q 6 h	q 12 h	q 24 h
Isoniazid	D	100%	100%	50%
	I	q 24 h	q 24 h	q 48 h
Ketoconazole	D	100%	100%	100%
	I	q 24 h	q 24 h	q 24 h
Lincomycin	I	q 6 h	q 6–12 h	q 12–24 h
Metronidazole	D	100%	100%	50%
	I	q 6 h	q 6 h	q 12 h
Minocycline	D	100%	100%	100%
Nalidixic acid	D	100%	Avoid	Avoid
Netilmicin[b]	D, I	55–90% q 8–12 h	20–60% q 12 h	10–20% q 24–48 h
or		60–100% q 24 h	60% q 24 h; 40% q 48 h	30% q 48 h
Nitrofurantoin	D	100%	Avoid	Avoid
Norfloxacin	I	q 12 h	q 12–24 h	Avoid
Pentamidine	I	q 24 h	q 24–36 h	q 48 h
Phenoxymethyl penicillin	D	100%	75%	50%
Piperacillin	I	q 4–6 h	q 6–8 h	q 8 h
Pyrimethamine	D	100%	100%	100%
	I	q 24 h	q 24 h	q 24 h
Rifampicin	D	100%	100%	100%
	I	q 24 h	q 24 h	q 24 h
Ribavirin	I,D	q 8 h	8 h	¹/₂ dose 8 h
Sulfadiazine	I	q 6 h	8 h	12 h
Tetracycline	I	q 8–12 h	12–24 h	24 h
Ticarcillin	I	q 4 h	8 h	12 h
Tobramycin[b]	D, I	60–90% q 12 h	30–70% q 12–18 h	20–30% q 24–48 h
or		70–100% q 24 h	70% q 24 h; 60% q 48 h	40% q 48 h
Trimethoprim	I	q 24 h	36 h	48 h
Vancomycin[b]	D, I	500 mg q 6–12 h	125–250 mg q 12 h	500 mg to 1 g q 4–7 days
	I	q 24–72 h	q 70–240 h	q 240 h

[a] Method of dosage adjustment: D, dose adjustment; I, dosage interval adjustment.

[b] Monitoring of concentration is recommended to determine precise dosage requirements.

[c] See Chapter 83.

Abbreviation: GFR, glomerular filtration rate.

salivary flow rate, particularly in the first month posttransplant, but it was also found to decrease the buffer capacity of saliva. In another study sepsis was due to oral organisms in 41% of patients with microbiologicaly proven septicemia (Heimdahl *et al.*, 1989). The routine introduction of acyclovir as prophylaxis against herpes simplex oral infection decreased the incidence of *Streptococcus* viridans septicemia in marrow transplant recipients, presumably by preventing herpetic ulceration as a portal of entry for oral microbes (Ringden *et al.*, 1984).

Role of surveillance cultures

Surveillance cultures taken from nose, throat, and stool or perianal area immediately pretransplant and at weekly intervals posttransplant may be useful in alerting the physician to the possible carriage by transplant recipients of organisms difficult to treat effectively, such as multiresistant *Staphylococcus aureus*, vancomycin-resistant enterococci (VRE) or *Pseudomonas aeruginosa*. One prospective study of the value of surveillance cultures, however, suggested that they were useful only in excluding *Candida albicans* infections (Riley *et al.*, 1995). In this study, all patients were admitted to a laminar airflow or high-efficiency particulate air-filtered (HEPA) room, maintained on reduced microbial diets, and received oral nonabsorbable antibiotics. Pretransplant and weekly posttransplant cultures of the stool, throat, and urine were obtained on all patients. Nasal and vaginal cultures were performed on 26 of the 48 patients. The sensitivity, specificity, positive predictive value, and negative predictive value for *Candida albicans* infections were 100%, 57%, 14%, and 100%, respectively. Those for Gram-positive infections were only 33%, 36%, 11%, and 70%, and for Gram-negative infections were 17%, 88%, 17%, and 88%. Individual transplant units should decide on the cost effectiveness of such a policy.

Role of sterile environment and selective microbial suppression (including gut decontamination)

There is little doubt that total patient decontamination with oral nonabsorbable antibiotics, sterile food, and laminar airflow facilities results in less bacterial infection than either selective decontamination or no gut decontamination combined with simple reverse barrier nursing. The expense involved in running a laminar airflow facility and total bacterial decontamination of the recipient is high and is likely to become less and less realistic with escalating health care costs. In a historically controlled study of 113 consecutive patients undergoing autologous BMT, no benefit of protective isolation was found in 59 patients compared with 54 patients treated without isolation measures (all patients received oral ciproflxacin, oral antifungal prophylaxis, and streptococcal prophylaxis) (Dekker, Verdonck, & Rozenberg-Arska, 1994). However, in a large retrospective IBMTR study of 5,065 patients with leukemia, the risk of treatment-related mortality in the first 150 days after an allogeneic bone marrow transplant was significantly less in

patients treated in HEPA (high-efficiency particulate air) filtration and/or LAF (laminar air flow) units compared to patients nursed in conventional single rooms plus any combination of hand-washing and the use of gloves, masks, or gowns (Passweg *et al.*, 1998). This in turn led to improved survival, especially in recipients of transplants from donors other than HLA-identical siblings. Excellent results have been described without protective isolation (Russell *et al.*, 1992; van Kraaij *et al.*, 2002).

There is current enthusiasm for selective microbial suppression with many studies utilizing prophylactic oral antibiotics (Attal *et al.*, 1991; Gluckman *et al.*, 1991), particularly the quinolones including ciprofloxacin (de Witte *et al.*, 1987; De Pauw *et al.*, 1990; Lew *et al.*, 1991), sometimes combined with rifamipicin (Gilbert *et al.*, 1994; Meisenberg *et al.*, 1996), norfloxacin (Schmeiser *et al.*, 1988; Classen *et al.*, 1990), ofloxacin (Schmeiser *et al.*, 1993), and enoxacin. In one trial, prophylactic ciprofloxacin 750 mg orally twice daily was prospectively compared with cotrimoxazole (trimethoprim/sulfamethoxazole, 160 mg trimethoprim and 800 mg sulfamethoxazole orally twice daily) as prophylaxis for bacterial infections. The two antibiotics were found to be equally safe and effective in the prevention of bacterial infection when the overall infection rate was used as the principal endpoint. However, cotrimoxazole prophylaxis was associated with a higher incidence of *Clostridium difficile* enterocolitis and infections caused by Gram-negative bacteria, as well as a trend toward prolongation of granulocytopenia (Lew *et al.*, 1995). In a meta-analysis (Engels *et al.*, 1998), which included 1408 subjects from 18 studies, it was demonstrated that quinolone prophylaxis substantially reduced the incidence of Gram-negative infections and total infections. However, there was no significant effect of quinolone prophylaxis on infection-related mortality. The trials included in this meta-analysis reported a low incidence (3%) of quinolone-resistant Gram-negative bacterial infections among patients who received quinolone prophylaxis. Nevertheless, several reports on the emergence of quinolone-resistant *E. coli* in neutropenic patients receiving fluoroquinolone prophylaxis are of major concern (Carratala *et al.*, 1996; van Kraaij *et al.*, 1998; Perea *et al.*, 1999; Yeh *et al.*, 1999). It is clear that the benefit of quinolone prophylaxis will be limited in communities with a high prevalence of quinolone-resistant strains. It could be argued that quinolone prophylaxis should be used more cautiously, e.g. restricting its use to the highest risk patients (Sepkowitz, 2002). While the advantage of less bacterial (especially less Gram-negative) infections is demonstrable in some of these studies, fluoroquinolone prophylaxis in patients with profound neutropenia is ineffective against Gram-positive bacterial infections in the bloodstream, particularly those caused by streptococci and coagulase-negative staphylococci, which appear to have emerged as significant causes of morbidity, decreased treatment efficacy, and an increased cost of empiric antimicrobial therapy. For this reason, some programs use additional specific prophylaxis against streptococcal infection during the neutropenic period posttransplant, for example with roxithromycin (Dekker *et al.*, 1994; Kern *et al.*,

1994). In the latter study, patients in a prospective randomized trial received oral roxithromycin 150 mg twice daily as additional prophylaxis to ofloxacin. This indeed did produce a reduced incidence of viridans group streptococcal bacteremia, but the incidence of bacteremia caused by other organisms, the incidence of febrile episodes from any cause, the risk of infection-associated complications including prolonged or secondary fever, pneumonia, septic shock, the need for mechanical ventilation, and/or infection-related deaths, as well as antimicrobial usage were comparable between the two groups.

A further potential disadvantage of the increasing use of prophylactic antibiotic therapy is the encouragement of antimicrobial resistance. Antibiotic use results in the emergence of new mechanisms of antimicrobial resistance, examples of which include the following:

1. In areas of heavily prolonged third-generation cephalosporin use, resistance has occurred. *Pseudomonas, Enterobacter, Serratia,* and *Citrobacter* species may produce stably derepressed mutants, which generate large amounts of chromosomally-mediated beta lactamase capable of destroying many extended-spectrum beta-lactam antibiotics. Single amino acid substitutions have occurred in the beta lactamases of *E. coli* and *klebsiella,* rendering them resistant to broad-spectrum cephalosporins (for example, cefotaxime and ceftazidime) and monobactams (aztreonam). Being located on plasmids, these enzymes have great propensity for hospitalwide epidemics and outbreaks have proven difficult to eradicate. With unrestricted antibiotic usage more are likely to evolve and to further increase the cost burden of antibiotic utilization.

2. Strains of pneumococcus resistant to penicillin (due to chromosomal alterations in target penicillin-binding proteins) are becoming more prevalent worldwide. Pneumococcal meningitis will respond to third-generation cephalosporins, but rare strains with mean inhibitory concentrations above 8.0 mg/l have required treatment with vancomycin. Pneumococcal isolates should be screened for resistance.

3. Increases in enterococcal infection may also relate to increasing use of cephalosporins to which enterococci are intrinsically resistant. Synergy between beta-lactam antibiotics and gentamicin is essential in the treatment of enterococcal endocarditis, for example. Development of plasmid-mediated high-level gentamicin resistance has led to failure of therapy due to loss of synergy and also to potential for rapid spread. In some hospitals in the United States these comprise up to 50% of enterococcal strains. Both vancomycin and penicillin-resistant strains are now also recognized, but remain rare. The majority of penicillin-resistant strains have acquired a beta-lactamase plasmid from a *Staphylococcus aureus* and remain sensitive to the addition of beta-lactamase inhibitors, such as amoxicillin clavulanate.

The new quinolones, such as norfloxacin, however, possess a novel mechanism of action by inhibiting DNA gyrase. This prevents acquisition of plasmid-mediated resistance factors. They also provide broad-spectrum activity against the aerobic pathogens including *Pseudomonas aeruginosa* and preserve the anerobic GI flora, maintaining the colonization that provides resistance against fungal overgrowth or acquisition of new aerobic pathogens. Norfloxacin is poorly absorbed from the bowel, thus providing high concentrations in the GI tract. These properties overcome some limitations associated with the use of earlier nonabsorbable or poorly absorbable prophylactic antibiotic regimens or the use of cotrimoxazole for this purpose (but see the earlier section on streptococcal infections associated with quinolone prophylaxis and the emergence of quinolone-resistant *E. coli* noted above).

One noteworthy beneficial effect of the growth suppression of intestinal anaerobic bacteria is a reduction in the risk of acute GVHD after HLA-identical sibling BMT (Beelen *et al.,* 1992). In a retrospective analysis of 194 predominantly adult patients given HLA-identical sibling marrow transplants under conditions of strict protective isolation and intestinal antimicrobial decontamination, ineffective, as compared with sustained, growth suppression of intestinal anerobic bacteria was found as one of four significant risk factors for grade II to IV acute GVHD. (The other factors were CML as the underlying disease, female marrow donors for male recipients, and methotrexate as the sole prophylactic agent for GVHD.)

Role of prophylactic systemic antibiotics

Prophylactic systemic antibiotics (for example, with an aminoglycoside and a semisynthetic antipseudomonal penicillin), together with laminar airflow facilities, can be shown to result in a decreased incidence of septicemia during neutropenia (Avril *et al.,* 1994), but in no difference in survival. In contrast, some studies failed to show any benefit, including one controlled trial in which patients were randomized to receive vancomycin 10 mg per kilogram i.v. every 6 hours from 5 days pretransplant to 1 day posttransplant to decrease the incidence of Gram-positive infections during the period of neutropenia immediately posttransplant. In this study there was no statistical difference in the occurrence of documented septicemia, documented Gram-positive coccal infection, or fever of unknown origin between the two groups (Teinturier *et al.,* 1995). Again the major argument against such an approach is the very real danger of development of new mechanisms of antimicrobial resistance.

Role of intravenous immunoglobulin

Several nonrandomized and one major prospective controlled randomized study (Sullivan *et al.,* 1990) have shown a reduction in the incidence of postengraftment septicemia in immunoglobulin recipients. In contrast, one randomized, stratified, nonblinded study of 170 patients, treated in three tertiary care university hospitals, failed to show any difference between intravenous immunoglobulin (IVIG) treated patients and control patients in terms of the incidence of Gram-positive or Gram-negative bacteremia or death due to infection. In fact, fewer deaths occurred among the control group due to a higher incidence of fatal hepatic veno-occlusive disease in patients receiving IVIG (Wolff *et al.*, 1993). Furthermore, systemic immunoglobulin preparations remain expensive.

It should be noted that immunoglobulin preparation, antibody titer, and dosing schedule vary widely between institutions.

Role of hematopoietic growth factors

There are currently at least 21 cloned factors that affect human hematopoiesis (Chapter 3), and the first of these have been incorporated into clinical HSC transplantation practice for several years now. They include GM-CSF and G-CSF. Both have been shown to decrease the duration of neutropenia after both autologous and allogeneic transplantation (see Chapters 31 and 32), and at least one prospective randomized trial has shown this to translate to fewer days of infection, although clinical and microbiologically confirmed sepsis was similar between the two groups (Gisselbrecht *et al.*, 1994).

Role of vaccination (reviewed in Ljungman, 1999; Singhal & Mehta, 1999)

Although specific immunity is transferred from the donor to the recipient by allogeneic marrow transplantation (Lum *et al.*, 1986b), most marrow transplant recipients lose their immunity to bacterial (e.g., tetanus, diphtheria) agents, as well as to viruses, over a period of time (Lum *et al.*, 1986a; Ljungman *et al.*, 1991; Parkkali *et al.*, 1996), and systematic reimmunization is necessary after immune reconstitution has occurred (Ljungman *et al.*, 1995), although the response to reimmunization may be poor (Lortan *et al.*, 1992), and qualitative (Gerritsen *et al.*, 1994) as well as quantitative defects of specific antibody responses may be present long-term after vacci-

nation. Factors that can potentially affect response to immunization after transplantation have not been well-characterized, but include the type of transplant (Chan *et al.*, 1997), pretransplant immune status of the recipient and the donor, the source of cells, purging/T-cell depletion, time elapsed from transplant (Avanzini *et al.*, 1995; Parkkali *et al.*, 1997), GVHD (Hammarstrom *et al.*, 1993), and the number of vaccine doses.

Live antibacterial vaccines (e.g. BCG, typhoid Ty$_{21a}$) are contraindicated in patients with GVHD and those receiving immunosuppressive therapy irrespective of the time since transplant, and probably also in all others within 2 years of transplantation. Inactive or subunit vaccines are safe in all transplant recipients, but may fail to elicit a response in immunocompromised individuals or if administered too early.

Blood stem cell transplant recipients may respond to vaccines earlier than marrow recipients as a result of accelerated immune reconstitution (Roberts *et al.*, 1993; Ottinger *et al.*, 1996). However, no data are available on immunization following blood stem cell transplants, and it is probably reasonable to treat both groups in the same way at the present time.

Not all vaccines are required in all transplant recipients, and reimmunization practices vary widely between centers (Ljungman *et al.*, 1995; Henning *et al.*, 1997). (See Table 73.11 for a recommended reimmunization schedule based upon published data.) Other schedules for some of these vaccines, e.g. Hib and tetanus toxoid, have been explored (Vance *et al.*, 1998). In an EBMT survey 65% of responding centers routinely immunized patients who received allogeneic BMT whereas 37% were routinely immunizing recipients of autologous BMT. Tetanus toxoid and inactivated poliovirus vaccine were the most frequently used vaccines in both allogeneic BMT and autologous BMT centers.

Augmentation of immunity to some of the common pathogenic organisms by adoptive transfer could potentially reduce infection-related morbidity and mortality. However, adoptive transfer of antibody responses is possible only for recall anti-

Table 73.12. *Vaccination against bacterial pathogens*

Vaccine	Schedule	Comments
Pneumococcal polysaccharide vaccine	1 dose at 12 months	Likely to be ineffective in patients with chronic GVHD
Pneumococcal conjugate vaccine	Three doses. Starting time not defined.	Contains only 7 serotypes that might not be appropriate according to local epidemiology. Can be considered in young children and in patients with chronic GVHD. Studies are ongoing.
Hemophilus group B conjugate	2–3 doses starting at 6–12 months.	
Meningococcal vaccine	Not routinely indicated	Can be considered in certain epidemiological situations
Tetanus toxoid	3 doses starting at 6–12 months	
Diptheria toxoid	3 doses starting at 6–12 months	
Pertussis	3 doses for children <7 years	Severe infections are rare after SCT
BCG	Should not be used	Risk/benefit ratio does not favor vaccination
Other live bacterial vaccines	Should not be used.	Risk/benefit ratio does not favor vaccination

Abbreviations: GVHD, graft-versus-host disease; SCT, stem cell transplantation; BCG, bacille Calmette-Guérin.
Adapted from Ljungman (1999) and Centers for Disease Control (2000).

gens. Transfer of responses to priming antigens, which would broaden the range of organisms against which patients could be protected, has not been successful (Wimperis *et al.,* 1990). There are circumstances under which immunization of the donor, usually in conjunction with posttransplant immunization of the recipient, may benefit the patient. Donor and recipient immunization with the *Haemophilus influenzae* (Hib)-conjugate vaccine before transplantation has been shown to result in higher antibody concentrations in patients as early as 3 months after transplantation compared with immunization of patients posttransplant (Molrine *et al.,* 1996). Similar findings were made with heptavalent pneumococcal conjugate vaccine (Molrine *et al.,* 2002).

Gottlieb *et al.* (1990) immunized marrow donors and/or recipients pretransplant with a polyvalent *Pseudomonas* O-polysaccharide-toxin A conjugate vaccine. When either donor or recipient alone was vaccinated, no increase in specific antibody titers was observed in the recipient posttransplant. However, when both donor and recipient were vaccinated before transplant, antibody titers increased to levels shown to be protective in animal models of Gram-negative sepsis.

A schedule for vaccination against bacterial pathogens is shown in Table 73.11.

Conclusions

Bacterial infection remains a predictable and serious hurdle to survival after HSC transplantation. Life-threatening bacterial infections, including those facilitated by iatrogenic procedures, occur in a small group of patients, especially in those with prolonged neutropenia or increased immune suppression pre- and/or posttransplant. Bacterial infections should respond increasingly to newer antibiotics, but a major danger exists in the stimulation of new mechanisms of antibacterial resistance by microbes with the use of antibiotics unnecessarily, particularly for prophylaxis.

References

Al-Eid, M. A., Tutschka, P. J., Wagner, H. N. *et al.* (1983). Functional asplenia in patients with chronic graft-versus-host disease: concise communication. *Journal of Nuclear Medicine,* **24,** 1123–26.

Andstrom, E., Bygdeman, S., Ahlen, S. *et al.* (1994). *Stomatococcus mucilaginosus* septicemia in bone marrow transplanted patients. *Scandanavian Journal of Infectious Disease,* **26,** 209–14.

Atkinson, K., Farewell, V., Tsoi, M. S. *et al.* (1982). Analysis of late infections after human bone marrow transplantation. Role of non-specific suppressor cells in patients with chronic graft-versus-host disease, and genotypic non-identity between marrow donor and recipient. *Blood,* **60,** 714–20.

Atkinson, K., Storb, R., Prentice, R. L. *et al.* (1979). Analysis of late infections and 89 long-term survivors of bone marrow transplantation. *Blood,* **53,** 720–31.

Attal, M., Schlaiferd, Rubie, H. *et al.* (1991). Prevention of gram-positive infections after bone marrow transplantations after systemic vancomycin: a prospective randomised trial. *Journal of Clinical Oncology,* **9,** 865–70.

Aucouturier, P., Barra, A., Intrator, L. *et al.* (1987). Long-lasting IgG subclass and antibacterial polysaccharide antibody deficiency after allogeneic bone marrow transplantation. *Blood,* **70,** 779–85.

Avanzini, M. A., Carra, A. M., Moccario, R. *et al.* (1995). Antibody response to pneumococcal vaccine in children receiving bone marrow transplantation. *Journal of Clinical Immunology,* **15,** 137–44.

Avril, M., Hartmann, O., Valteau-Couanet, D. *et al.* (1994). Anti-infective prophylaxis with ceftazidime and teicoplanin in children undergoing high-dose chemotherapy and bone marrow transplantation. *Pediatric Hematology and Oncology,* **11,** 63–73.

Bauwens, J. E., Spach, D. H., Schacker, T. W. *et al.* (1992). *Bordetella bronchiseptica* pneumonia and bacteremia following bone marrow transplantation. *Journal of Clinical Microbiology,* **30,** 2474–5.

Beelen, D. W., Haralambie, E., Brandt, H. *et al.* (1992). Evidence that sustained growth suppression of intestinal anaerobic bacteria reduces the risk of acute graft-versus-host disease after sibling marrow transplantation. *Blood,* **80,** 2668–76.

Bernard, G. R., Vincent, J- L., Laterre, P- F. *et al.* (2001). Efficacy and safety of recombinant human activated protein C for severe sepsis. *New England Journal of Medicine,* **344,** 699–709.

Benz-Lemoine, E., Del Wail, V., Castel, O. *et al.* (1991). Nosocomial Legionnaires' disease in a bone marrow transplant unit. *Bone Marrow Transplantation,* **7,** 61–3.

Bilgrami, S., Bergstrom, S. K., Peterson, D. E. *et al.* (1992). *Capnocytophaga* bacteremia in a patient with Hodgkin's disease following bone marrow transplantation: case report and review. *Clinical Infectious Disease,* **14,** 1045–9.

Broun, R., Wheat, J. L., Kneebon, P. H. *et al.* (1994). A randomized trial of the addition of gram-positive prophylaxis to standard antimicrobial prophylaxis for patients undergoing autologous bone marrow transplantation. *Antimicrobial Agents and Chemotherapy,* **38,** 576–9.

Carratala, J., Fernandez-Sevilla, A., Tubau, F. *et al.* (1996). Emergence of fluoroquinolone-resistant *Escherichia coli* in fecal flora of cancer patients receiving norfloxacin prophylaxis. *Antimicrobial Agents and Chemotherapy,* **40,** 503–5.

Centers for Disease Control and Prevention. (2002). Guidelines for preventing opportunistic infections among hematopoietic stem cell transplant recipients: recommendations of CDC, the Infectious Disease Society of America, and the American Society of Blood and Marrow Transplantation. *MMWR Morbidity and Mortality Weekly Report,* **49,** (RR-10), 1-25 and *Biology of Blood and Marrow Transplantation,* **6,** 659–734.

Chalandon, Y., Roscoe, D. L., & Nantel, S. H. (2000). Agrobacterium yellow group: bacteremia and possible septic arthritis following peripheral blood stem cell transplantation. *Bone Marrow Transplantation,* **26,** 101–4.

Chan, C. Y., Molrine, D. C., Antin, J. H. *et al.* (1997). Antibody responses to tetanus toxoid and *Haemophilus influenzae type b* conjugate vaccines following autologous peripheral blood stem cell transplantation (PBSCT). *Bone Marrow Transplantation,* **20,** 33–8.

Chang, J., Powles, R., Mehta, J. *et al.* (1995). Listeriosis in bone marrow transplant recipients: incidence, clinical features, and treatment. *Clinical Infectious Disease,* **21,** 1289–90.

Classen, D. C., Burke, J. P., Ford, C. D. *et al.* (1990). *Streptococcus mitis* sepsis in bone marrow transplant patients receiving oral antimicrobial prophylaxis. *American Journal of Medicine,* **89,** 441–6.

D'Antonio, D., Dibartolomeo, P., Iacone, A. *et al.* (1992). Meningitis due to penicillin-resistant *Streptococcus pneumoniae* in patients with chronic graft-versus-host disease. *Bone Marrow Transplantation,* **9,** 229–300.

Dahut, W. & Georgiadis, M. (1995). Pneumococcal arthritis and functional asplenia after allogeneic bone marrow transplantation. *Bone Marrow Transplantation,* **15,** 161.

Dekker, A. W., Verdonck, L. F., & Rozenberg-Arska, M. (1994). Infection prevention in autologous bone marrow transplantation and the role of protective isolation. *Bone Marrow Transplantation,* **14,** 89–93.

De la Camara, R., Martino, R., Granados, E. *et al.* (2000). Tuberculosis after hematopoietic stem cell transplantation: incidence, clinical characteristics and outcome. *Bone Marrow Transplantation,* **26,** 291–8.

De Pauw, B. E., Donnelly, J. P., de Witte, T. *et al.* (1990). Options and limitations of long-term oral ciprofloxacin as antibacterial prophylaxis in allogeneic bone marrow transplant recipients. *Bone Marrow Transplantation,* **5,** 179–82.

de Witte, T., Novakova, I., Branolte, J. *et al.* (1987). Long-term oral ciprofloxacin for infection prophylaxis in allogeneic bone marrow transplantation. *Pharmacological Weekly,* **9** (Suppl), 648–52.

Dens, F., Boogaerts, M., Boute, P. *et al.* (1996). Caries-related salivary microorganisms and salivary flow rate in bone marrow recipients. *Oral Surgery, Oral Medicine, Oral Pathology, and Oral Radiology,* **81,** 38–43.

Donnelly, J. P. (1995). Bacterial complications of transplantation: diagnosis and treatment. *Journal of Antimicrobial Chemotherapy,* **36** (Suppl B), 59–72.

Donnelly, J. P., Muus, P., Horrevorts, A. M. *et al.* (1993). Failure of clindamycin to influence the course of severe oral mucositis associated with streptococcal bacteremia in allogeneic bone marrow transplant recipients. *Scandinavian Journal of Infectious Diseases,* **25,** 43–50.

Ender, P. T., Dooley, D. P., Moore, R. H. *et al.* (1996). Vascular catheter-related *Comamonas acidovorans* bacteremia managed with preservation of the catheter. *Pediatric Infectious Diseases Journal,* **15,** 918–20.

Engelhard, D., Cordonnier, C., Shaw, P. J. *et al.* (2002). Early and late invasive pneumococcal infection following stem cell transplantation: a European Bone Marrow Transplantation survey. *British Journal of Haematology,* **117,** 444–450.

Engelhard, D., Elishoov, H., Strauss, N. *et al.* (1996). Nosocomial coagulase-negative staphylococcal infections in bone marrow transplantation recipients with central vein catheters. A five year prospective study. *Transplantation,* **61,** 430–4.

Engels, E. A., Lau, J., Braza, M. (1998). Efficacy of quinolone prophylaxis in neutropenic cancer patients: a meta-analysis. *Journal of Clinical Oncology,* **16,** 1179–87.

Fielding, A. K. (1994). Prophylaxis against late infection following splenectomy and bone marrow transplant. *Blood Reviews,* **8,** 179–91.

Frere, P. Hermanne, J-P., Debouge, M-H. *et al.* (2002). Changing patterns of bacterial susceptibility to antibiotics in hematopoietic stem cell transplantation. *Bone Marrow Transplantation,* **29,** 589–94.

Funke, I., Prummer, O., Schrezenmeier, H. *et al.* (1994). Capillary leak syndrome associated with elevated IL-2 serum levels after allogeneic bone marrow transplantation. *Annals of Hematology,* **68,** 49–52.

Gerritsen, E. J., Van Tol, M. J., Van't Veer, M. B. *et al.* (1994). Clonal dysregulation of the antibody response to tetanus-toxoid after bone marrow transplantation. *Blood,* **84,** 4374–82.

Gilbert, C., Meisenberg, B., Vredenburgh, J. *et al.* (1994). Sequential prophylactic oral and empiric once daily parenteral antibiotics for neutropenia and fever after high-dose chemotherapy and autologous bone marrow support. *Journal of Clinical Oncology,* **12,** 1005–11.

Gisselbrecht, C., Prentice, H. G., Bacigalupo, A. *et al.* (1994). Placebo-controlled phase III trial of lenograstim in bone marrow transplantation. *Lancet,* **343,** 696–700.

Gluckman, E., Roudet, C., Hirsch, I. *et al.* (1991). Prophylaxis of bacterial infections after bone marrow transplantation. A randomised prospective study comparing oral broad-spectrum non-absorbable antibiotics (vancomycin-tobramycin-colistin) to absorbable antibiotics (ofloxacin-amoxicillin). *Chemotherapy,* **37** (Suppl 1), 33–38.

Gomez-Casares, M. T., Naranjo, A., Campo, C. *et al.* (1995). Another case of pneumococcal arthritis after allogeneic bone marrow transplantation (Letter). *Bone Marrow Transplantation,* **15,** 650.

Gottlieb, D. J., Cryz, S. J. Jr, Furer, E. *et al.* (1990). Immunity against *Pseudomonas aeruginosa* adoptively transferred to bone marrow transplant recipients. *Blood,* **76,** 2470–5.

Graber, C. J., de Almeida, K.N.F., Atkinson, J. C. *et al.* (2001). Dental health and viridans streptococcal bacteremia in allogeneic hematopoietic stem cell transplant recipients. *Bone Marrow Transplantation,* **27,** 537–42.

Hammarstrom, V., Pauksen, K., Azinge, J. *et al.* (1993): Pneumococcal immunity and response to immunization with pneumococcal vaccine in bone marrow transplant patients: the influence of graft-versus-host reaction. *Supportive Care of Cancer,* **1,** 195–9.

Harrington, R. D., Woolfrey, A. E., Bowden, R. *et al.* (1996). Legionellosis in a bone marrow transplant center. *Bone Marrow Transplantation,* **18,** 361–8.

Heimdahl, A., Mattson, T., Dahllsof, G. *et al.* (1989). The oral cavity as a port of entry for early infections in patients treated with bone marrow transplantation. *Oral Surgery, Oral Medicine and Oral Pathology,* **68,** 711–16.

Henning, K. J., White, M. H., Sapkowitz, K. A., & Armstrong, D. (1997). A national survey of immunization practices following allogeneic bone marrow transplantation. *Journal of the American Medical Association,* **277,** 1148–51.

Hermida, G., Richard, C., Baro, J. *et al.* (1995). Allogeneic BMT in a patient with CML and prior disseminated infection by *Mycobacterium avium* complex. *Bone Marrow Transplantation,* **16,** 183–5.

Holland, D. J., Chen, S. C., Chew, W. W., & Gilbert, G. L. (1994). *Mycobacterium neoaurum* infection of a Hickman catheter in an immunosuppressed patient. *Clinical Infectious Diseases,* **18,** 1002–3.

Hoppe, J. E., Herter, M., Aleksic, S. *et al.* (1993). Catheter-related *Rahnella aquatilis* bacteremia in a pediatric bone marrow transplant recipient. *Journal of Clinical Microbiology,* **31,** 1911–12.

Hoyle, C. & Goldman, J. M. (1994). Life-threatening infections occurring more than 3 months after BMT. *Bone Marrow Transplantation,* **14,** 247–52.

Hughes, W. T., Armstrong, D., Bodey, G. P. *et al.* (2002). 2002 guidelines for the use of antimircobiral agents in neutropenic patients with cancer. *Clinical Infectious Diseases,* **34,** 730–51.

Ikinciogullari, A., Dogu, F., Ciftci, E. *et al.* (2002). An intensive approach to the treatment of disseminated BCG infection in a SCID patient. *Bone Marrow Transplantation,* **30,** 45–7.

Ilan, Y., Nagler, A., Adler, R. *et al.* (1993). Ablation of persistent hepatitis B by bone marrow transplantation from a hepatitis B-immune donor. *Gastroenterology,* **104,** 1818–21.

Inada, T., Shirono, K., & Tsuda, H. (1995). Intestinal mycobacteriosis in a patient with acute myeloid leukemia after autologous peripheral blood stem cell transplantation. *European Journal of Haematology,* **54,** 205–6.

International Antimicrobial Therapy Cooperative Group of the European Organization for Research and Treatment of Cancer (1994). Reduction of fever and streptococcal bacteremia in granulocytopenic patients with cancer. A trial of oral penicillin V with placebo combined with pefloxacin. *Journal of the American Medical Association,* **272,** 1183–9.

Ip, M. S., Yuen, K. Y., Woo, P. C. *et al.* (1998). Risk factors for pulmonary tuberculosis in bone marrow transplant recipients. *American Journal of Respiratory and Critical Care Medicine,* **158,** 1173–7.

Julisa, A., Acebedo, G., Jornet, J., & Zuazu, J. (1985). Spontaneous pneumococcal peritonitis: late infection after bone marrow transplantation. *New England Journal of Medicine,* **312,** 587.

Kalhs, P., Schwarzinger, I., Anderson, G. *et al.* (1995). A restrospective analysis of the long-term effects of splenectomy on late infections, graft-versus-host disease, relapse, and survival after allogeneic marrow transplantation for chronic myelogenous leukemia. *Blood,* **86,** 2028–32.

Kalima, P., Masterton, R. G., Roddie, P. H., & Thomas, A. E. (1996). *Lactobacillus rhamnosus* infection in a child following bone marrow transplant. *Journal of Infection,* **32,** 165–7.

Kern, W. V., Hay, B., Kern, P. *et al.* (1994). A randomized trial of roxithromycin in patients with acute leukemia and bone marrow transplant recipients receiving fluoroquinolone prophylaxis. *Antimicrobial Agents and Chemotherapy,* **38,** 465–72.

Kiehn, T. E., White, M., Pursell, K. J. *et al.* (1993). A cluster of four cases of *Mycobacterium haemophilum* infection. *European Journal of Clinical Microbiology and Infectious Disease,* **12,** 114–18.

Kindler, T., Schindel, C., Brass, U., & Fischer, T. (2001). Fatal sepsis due to *Mycobacterium tuberculosis* after allogeneic bone marrow transplantation. *Bone Marrow Transplantation,* **27,** 217–8.

Klumpp, T. R., Block, C. C., Caligiuri, M. A. *et al.* (1992). Immune-mediated cytopenia following bone marrow transplantation: Case reports and review of the literature. *Medicine,* **71,** 73–83.

Kugler, J. W., Armitage, J. O., Helms, C. M. *et al.* (1983). Nosocomial Legionnaires' disease. Occurrence in recipients of

bone marrow transplants. *American Journal of Medicine,* **74,** 281–8.

Kulkami, S., Powles, R., Treleaven, J. *et al.* (2000). Chronic graft versus host disease is associated with long-term risk for pneumococcal infections in recipients of bone marrow transplants. *Blood,* **95,** 3683–6.

Kurzrock, R., Zander, A., & Vellekoop, L. (1984). Mycobacterial pulmonary infections after bone marrow transplantation. *American Journal of Medicine,* **77,** 35–40.

Labarca, J. A., Leber, A. L., Kern, V. L. *et al.* (2002). Outbreak of *Stenotrophomonas maltophilia* bacteremia in allogenic bone marrow transplant patients: role of severe neutropenia and mucositis. *Clinical Infectious Diseases,* **30,** 195–97.

Lee, A. C., Ha, S. Y., Yuen, K. Y., & Lau, Y. L. (1995). *Listeria* septicemia complicating bone marrow transplantation for Diamond-Blackfan syndrome. *Pediatric Hematology and Oncology,* **12,** 295–9.

Lee, A. C., Yuen, K. Y., Ha, S. Y. *et al.* (1996). *Plesiomonas shigelloides* septicemia: case report and literature review. *Pediatric Hematology and Oncology,* **13,** 265–9.

Lew, M. A., Kehoe, K., Ritz, J. *et al.* (1991). Prophylaxis of bacterial infections with ciprofloxacin in patients undergoing bone marrow transplantation. *Transplantation,* **51,** 630–5.

Lew, M. A., Kehoe, K., Ritz, J. *et al.* (1995). Ciprofloxacin versus trimethoprim/sulfamethoxazole for prophylaxis of bacterial infections in bone marrow transplant recipients: a randomized, controlled trial. *Journal of Clinical Oncology,* **13,** 239–50.

Lina, B., Forey, F., Tigaud, J. D., & Fleurette, J. (1995). Chronic bacteremia due to staphylococcal epidermidis after bone marrow transplantation. *Journal of Medical Microbiology,* **42,** 156–60.

Ljungman, P. (1999). Immunization of transplant recipients. *Bone Marrow Transplantation,* **23,** 635–6.

Ljungman, P., Cordonnier, C., De Bock, R. *et al.* (1995). Immunisations after bone marrow transplantation: results of a European survey and recommendations from the infectious diseases working party of the European Group for Blood and Marrow Transplantation. *Bone Marrow Transplantation,* **15,** 455–60.

Ljungman, P., Duraj, V., & Magnius, L. (1991). Response to immunization against polio after allogeneic marrow transplantation. *Bone Marrow Transplantation,* **7,** 89–93.

Long, S. G., Leyland, M. J., & Milligan, D. W. (1993). *Listeria* meningitis after bone marrow transplantation. *Bone Marrow Transplantation,* **12,** 537–9.

Lortan, J. E., Vellodi, A., Jurges, E. S., & Hugh-Jones, K. (1992). Class and subclass-specific pneumococcal antibody levels and response to immunization after bone marrow transplantation. *Clinical and Experimental Immunology,* **88,** 512–19.

Lossos, I. S., Breuer, R., Or, R. *et al.* (1995). Bacterial pneumonia in recipients of bone marrow transplantation. A five year prospective study. *Transplantation,* **60,** 672–8.

Lum, L. G., Munn, N. A., Schanfield, M. S., & Storb, R. (1986a). The detection of specific antibody formation to recall antigens after human bone marrow transplantation. *Blood,* **67,** 582–7.

Lum, L. G., Seigneuret, M. C., & Storb, R. (1986b). The transfer of antigen-specific humoral immunity from marrow donors to marrow recipients. *Journal of Clinical Immunology,* **6,** 389–96.

Martino, P., Micozzi, A., Venditti, M. *et al.* (1990). Catheter-related right-sided endocarditis in bone marrow transplant recipients. *Reviews of Infectious Diseases,* **12,** 250–7.

Martino, R., Martinez, C., Brunet, S. *et al.* (1996). Tuberculosis in bone marrow transplant recipients: report of two cases and review of the literature. *Bone Marrow Transplantation,* **18,** 809–12.

Martino, R., Nomdedeu, J., Sureda, A. *et al.* (1994). Acute rhabdomyolysis complicating viridans streptococcal shock syndrome. *Acta Haematologica,* **92,** 140–1.

Matulonis, U., Rosenfeld, C. S., & Shadduck, R. K. (1993). Prevention of *Legionella* infections in a bone marrow transplant unit: multi-faceted approach to decontamination of a water system. *Infection Control and Hospital Epidemiology,* **14,** 571–5.

Meisenberg, B., Gollard, R., Breh, M. *et al.* (1996). Prophylactic antibiotics eliminate bacteria and allow safe outpatient management following high-dose chemotherapy and autologous stem cell rescue. *Supportive Care in Cancer,* **4,** 364–9.

Meletis, J., Arlet, G., Dournon, E. *et al.* (1987). Legionnaires' disease after bone marrow transplantation. *Bone Marrow Transplantation,* **2,** 307–13.

Molrine, D. C., Guinan, E. C., Antin, J. H. *et al.* (1996). Donor immunization with *Haemophilus influenzae type b* (Hib)-conjugate vaccine in allogeneic bone marrow transplantation. *Blood,* **87,** 3012–18.

Molrine, D. C., Antin, J. H. Guinan, E. C. *et al.* (2002). Donor immunization with penumoncoccal vaccine and early protective antibody responses following allogeneic hematopoietic cell transplantation. *Blood,* **101,** 831–6.

Moses, A. E., Leibergal, M., Rahav, G. *et al.* (1995). *Aeromonas hydrophila* myonecrosis acompanying mucormycosis 5 years after bone marrow transplantation. *European Journal of Clinical Microbiology and Infectious Disease,* **14,** 237–40.

Mossad, S. B., Longworth, D. L., Goormastic, M. *et al.* (1996). Early infectious complications in autologous bone marrow transplantation: a review of 219 patients. *Bone Marrow Transplantation,* **18,** 265–71.

Mulligan, C. G., Heatley, S., Doherty, K. *et al.* (2002). Mannose-binding gene polymorphisms are associated with major infection following allogeneic hematopoietic stem cell transplantation. *Blood,* **99,** 3524–9.

Naughton, M. Brown, R., Adkins, D., & DiPersio, J. (1999). Tularemia—an unusual case of a solitary pulmonary nodule in the post-transplant setting. *Bone Marrow Transplantation,* **24,** 197–9.

Navari, R. M., Sullivan, K. M., Springmeyer, S. C. *et al.* (1983). Mycobacterial infections in marrow transplant patients. *Transplantation,* **36,** 509–13.

Nolla-Salas, J., Almela, M., Coll, P., & Gasser, I. (1997). Listeriosis in bone marrow transplant recipients. *Bone Marrow Transplantation,* **19,** 955–8.

Nosanchuk, J. D., Sepkowitz, K. A., Pearse, R. N. *et al.* (1996). Infectious complications of autologous bone marrow and peripheral stem cell transplantation for refractory leukemia and lymphoma. *Bone Marrow Transplantation,* **18,** 355–9.

Ochs, L., Shu, X. O., Miller, J. *et al.* (1995). Late infections after allogeneic bone marrow transplantation: comparison of incidence in related and unrelated donor transplant recipients. *Blood,* **86,** 3979–86.

Okano, A., Shimazaki, C., Ochiai, N. *et al.* (2001). Subcutaneous infection with *Mycobacterium fortuitum* after allogeneic bone marrow transplantation. *Bone Marrow Transplantation,* **28,** 709–11.

Oren, I., Zuckerman, T., Avivi, I. *et al.* (2002). Nosocomial outbreak of Legionella pneumophila serogroup 3 pneumonia in a new bone marrow transplant unit: evaluation, treatment and control. *Bone Marrow Transplantation,* **30,** 175–9.

Ottinger, H. D., Beelen, D. W., Scheulen, B. *et al.* (1996). Improved immune reconstitution after allotransplantation of peripheral blood stem cells instead of bone marrow. *Blood,* **88,** 2775–9.

Ozkaynak, M. F., Lenarsky, C., Kohn, D. *et al.* (1990). *Mycobacterium avium* intracellulare infections after allogeneic bone marrow transplantation in children. *American Journal of Pediatric Hematology and Oncology,* **12,** 220–4.

Parkkali, T., Ölander, R.-M., Ruutu, T. *et al.* (1997). A randomized comparison between early and late vaccination with tetanus toxoid vaccine after allogeneic BMT. *Bone Marrow Transplantation,* **19,** 933–8.

Parkkali, T., Ruutu, T., Stenvik, M. *et al.* (1996). Loss of protective immunity to polio, diphtheria and *Haemophilus influenzae type b* after allogeneic bone marrow transplantation. *APMIS,* **104,** 383–8.

Passweg, J. R., Rowlings, P. A., Atkinson, K. *et al.* (1998). Influence of protective isolation on outcome of allogeneic bone marrow transplantation for leukemia. *Bone Marrow Transplantation,* **21,** 1231–8.

Pastores, S. M., Papadopoulos, E., van den Brink, M. *et al.* (2002). Sectic shock and multiple organ failure after hematopoietic stem cell transplantation: treatment with recombinant human activated protein. *C. Biology of Blood and Marrow Transplantation,* **8,** 131–4.

Perea, S., Hidalgo, M., Arcediano, A. *et al.* (1999). Incidence and clinical impact of fluoroquinolone-resistant *Escherichia coli* in the faecal flora of cancer patients treated with high dose chemotherapy and ciprofloxacin prophylaxis. *Journal of Antimicrobial Chemotherapy,* **44,** 117–20.

Petersen, F. B., Clift, R. A., Hickman, R. *et al.* (1986). Hickman catheter complications in marrow transplant recipients. *Journal of Parenteral and Enteral Nutrition,* **10,** 58–62.

Rege, K., Mehta, J., & Treleaven, J. (1994). Fatal pneumococcal infections following allogeneic bone marrow transplant. *Bone Marrow Transplantation,* **14,** 903–6.

Riley, D. K., Pavia, A. T., Beatty, P. J. *et al.* (1995). Surveillance cultures in bone marrow transplant recipients: worthwhile or wasteful? *Bone Marrow Transplantation,* **15,** 469–73.

Ringden, O., Heimdahl, A., Lonnquist, B. *et al.* (1984). Decreased incidence of viridans streptococcal septicaemia in allogeneic bone marrow transplant recipients after the introduction of acyclovir. *Lancet,* **1,** 744.

Roberts, M. M., To, L. B., Gillis, D. *et al.* (1993). Immune reconstitution following peripheral blood stem cell transplantation, autologous bone marrow transplantation and allogeneic bone marrow transplantation. *Bone Marrow Transplantation,* **12,** 469–75.

Rocha, V., Franco, R F., Porcher, R. *et al.* (2002). Host defense and inflammatory gene polymorphisms are associated with outcomes after HLA-identical sibling bone marrow transplantation. *Blood*, **100**, 3908–18.

Rouleau, M., Senik, A., Leroy, E. *et al.* (1993). Long-term persistence of transferred PPD-reactive T cells after allogeneic bone marrow transplantation. *Transplantation, 55*, 72–6.

Roy, V. & Weisdorf, D. (1997). Mycobacterial infections following bone marrow transplantation: a 20 year retrospective review. *Bone Marrow Transplantation*, **19**, 467–70.

Ruppel, L. J., Brown, R. A., Borson, R. A., & Whitman, E. D. (1994). Retained Hickman catheter cuff as an infection source following allogeneic bone marrow transplant. *Bone Marrow Transplantation*, **14**, 169–71.

Russell, J. A., Poon, M. C., Jones, A. R. *et al.* (1992). Allogeneic bone marrow transplantation without protective isolation in adults with malignant disease. *Lancet, 339*, 38–40.

Safdar, A., Papadopoulos, E. B. & Armstrong, D. (2002). Listeriosis in recipients of allogeneic blood and marrow transplantation: thirteen year review of disease characteristics, treatment outcomes and a new association with human cytomegalovirus infection. *Bone Marrow Transplantation, 29*, 913–16.

Sayer, H. G., Longton, G., Bowden, R. *et al.* (1994). Increase risk of infection in marrow transplant patients receiving methylprednisolone for graft-verus-host disease prevention. *Blood, 84*, 1328–32.

Scerpella, E. G., Whimbey, E. E., Champlin, R. E., & Bodey, G. P. (1994). Pericarditis associated with Legionnaires' disease in a bone marrow transplant recipient [letter] *Clinical Infectious Diseases, 19*, 1168–70.

Schmeiser, T., Kern, W. V., Hay, B. *et al.* (1993). Single-drug oral antibacterial prophylaxis with ofloxacin in BMT recipients. *Bone Marrow Transplantation, 12*, 57–63.

Schmeiser, T., Kurrle, E., Arnold, R. *et al.* (1988). Norfloxacin for prevention of bacterial infections during severe granulocytopenia after bone marrow transplantation. *Scandinavian Journal of Infectious Disease, 20*, 625–31.

Schwartz, D. N., Schable, B., Tenover, F. C., & Miller, R. A. (1995). *Leptotrichia buccalis* bacteremia in patients treated in a single bone marrow transplant unit. *Clinical Infectious Disease, 20*, 762–7.

Schwebke, J. R., Hackman, R., & Bowden, R. (1990). Pneumonia due to *Legionella micdadei* in bone marrow transplant recipients. *Reviews of Infectious Diseases, 12*, 824–8.

Schwella, N., Schwerdtfeger, R., Schmidt-Wolf, I. *et al.* (1993). Pneumococcal arthritis after allogeneic bone marrow transplantation. *Bone Marrow Transplantation, 12*, 165–6.

Sepkowitz, K. A. (2002). Antibiotic prophylaxis in patients receiving hematopoietic stem cell transplant. (Mini-review.) *Bone Marrow Transplantation, 29*, 367–71.

Shen, W. P., Felsing, N., Lang, D. *et al.* (1994). Development of infant botulism in a 3 year old female with neuroblastoma following autologous bone marrow transplantation: potential use of human botulism immune globulin. *Bone Marrow Transplantation, 13*, 345–7.

Sheridan, J. F., Tutschka, P. J., Sedmak, D. D., & Copelan, E. A. (1990). Immunoglobulin G sub-class deficiency and pneumococcal infection after allogeneic bone marrow transplantation. *Blood, 75*, 1583–16.

Siadak, M. & Sullivan, K. M. (1994). The management of chronic graft-versus-host disease. *Blood Reviews, 8*, 154–60.

Sica, S., Di Mario, A., Salutari, P. *et al.* (1995). *Morganella morganii* pericarditis after resolvent splenectomy for immune pancytopenia following allogeneic bone marrow transplantation for acute lymphoblastic leukemia. *Clinical Infectious Disease, 21*, 1052–3.

Singhal, S. & Mehta, J. (1999). Reimmunization after blood or marrow stem cell transplantation. *Bone Marrow Transplantation, 23*, 637–46.

Skinner, R., Appleton, A. L., Sprott, M. S. *et al.* (1996). Disseminated BCG infection in severe combined immune deficiency presenting with severe anemia and associated with gross hypersplenism after bone marrow transplantation. *Bone Marrow Transplantation, 17*, 877–80.

Smith, T. L., Pearson, M. L., Wilcox, K. R. *et al.* (1999). Emergence of vancomycin resistance in *Staphylococcus aureus*. *New England Journal of Medicine, 340*, 493–501.

Steiner, M., Villablanca, J., Kersey, J. *et al.* (1993). Viridans streptococcal shock in bone marrow transplantation patients. *American Journal of Hematology, 42*, 354–8.

Storek, J., Dawson, M. A., Storer, B. *et al.* (2001). Immune reconstitution after allogeneic marrow transplantation compared with blood stem cell transplantation. *Blood, 97*, 3380–9.

Storek, J., Gooley, T., Witherspoon, R. P. *et al.* (1997). Infectious morbidity in long-term survivors of allogeneic marrow transplantation is association with low CD4 T cell counts. *American Journal of Hematology, 54*, 131–8.

Straus, W. L., Ostroff, S. M., Jernigan, D. B. *et al.* (1994). Clinical and epidemiologic characteristics of *Mycobacterium hemophilum*, an emerging pathogen in immuno-compromised patients. *Annals of Internal Medicine, 120*, 118–25.

Sullivan, K. M., Kopecky, K. G., Jokom, J. *et al.* (1990). Immunomodulatory and antimicrobial efficacy of intravenous immunoglobulin in bone marrow transplantation. *New England Journal of Medicine, 323*, 705–12.

Sullivan, K. M., Meyers, J. D., & Clark, J. (1985). Mycobacterial pulmonary infections after allogeneic bone marrow transplantation. *American Journal of Medicine, 79a*, 107.

Teinturier, C., Hartmann, O., Lemerle, J. *et al.* (1995). Prevention of gram-positive infections in patients treated with high-dose chemotherapy and bone marrow transplantation: a randomized controlled trial of vancomycin. *Pediatric Hematology and Oncology, 12*, 73–7.

Thel, M. C., Ciaccia, D., Vredenburgh, J. J. *et al.* (1994). Clostridium septicum abscess in hepatic metastases: successful medical management. *Bone Marrow Transplantation, 13*, 495–6.

van Kraaij, M.G.J., Dekker, A. W., Peters, E. *et al.* (1998). Emergence and infectious complications of ciprofloxacin-resistant *Escherichia coli* in haematological cancer patients. *European Journal of Clinical and Microbiological Infectious Disease, 17*, 591–2.

van Kraaij, M.G.J., Verdonck, L. F., Rozenberg-Arska, M. *et al.* (2002). Early infections in adults undergoing matched related and matched unrelated/mismatched donor stem cell transplantation: a comparison of incidence. *Bone Marrow Transplantation, 30*, 303–9.

Vance, E., George, S., Guinan, E. C. *et al.* (1998). Comparison of multiple immunization schedules for *Haemophilus influenzae type b-*conjugate and tetanus toxoid vaccines following bone marrow transplantation. *Bone Marrow Transplantation,* **22,** 735–41.

Villablanca, J. G., Steiner, M., Kersey, J. *et al.* (1990). The clinical spectrum of infections with viridans streptococci in bone marrow transplant patients. *Bone Marrow Transplantation,* **5,** 387–93.

Wang, C. C., Mattson, D., & Wald, A. (2001). *Corynebacterium jeikeium* bacteremia in bone marrow transplant patients with Hickman catheters. *Bone Marrow Transplantation,* **27,** 445–9.

Want, S. V., Lacey, S. L., Ward, L., & Buckingham, S. (1993). An epidemiological study of listeriosis complicating a bone marrow transplant. *Journal of Hospital Infection,* **23,** 299–304.

White, M. H., Papadopoulos, E. B., Small, T. N. *et al.* (1995). *Mycobacterium hemophilum* infections in bone marrow transplant recipients. *Transplantation,* **60,** 957–60.

Wimperis, J. Z., Brenner, M. K., Prentice, H. G. *et al.* (1986). Transfer of a functioning humoral immune system in transplantation of T lymphocyte-depleted bone marrow. *Lancet,* **1,** 339–43.

Wimperis, J. Z., Gottlieb, D., Duncombe, A. S. *et al.* (1990). Requirements for the adoptive transfer of antibody responses to a priming antigen in man. *Journal of Immunology,* **144,** 541–7.

Wolff, S. N., Fay, J. W., Herzig, R. H. *et al.* (1993). High-dose weekly intravenous immunoglobulin to prevent infections in patients undergoing autologous bone marrow transplantation or severe myelosuppressive therapy. A study of the American Bone Marrow Transplant Group. *Annals of Internal Medicine,* **118,** 937–42.

Yeh, S. P., Hsueh, E. J., Yu, M. S. *et al.* (1999). Oral ciprofloxacin as antibacterial prophylaxis after allogeneic bone marrow transplantation: a reappraisal. *Bone Marrow Transplantation,* **24,** 1207–11.

74 Viral infections

PER LJUNGMAN AND HERMANN EINSELE

Huddinge University Hospital, Stockholm, Sweden and University of Tübingen, Tübingen, Germany

Introduction

Viral infections are important as causes of morbidity and mortality after allogeneic hematopoietic stem cell transplantation (SCT). Severe viral infections are more common after unrelated and HLA-mismatched donor SCT, and, in particular, after haploidentical SCT. Although some viral infections are not infrequent, the risk of severe viral disease is usually lower after autologous SCT.

The most likely explanation for these different presentations of viral infections in patients undergoing different types of transplantation lies in the immune response to viral infections. B-cell function and specific antiviral antibodies are the main defense mechanisms against infection with exogenous viruses, thus reducing the risk for reinfection in seropositive individuals. On the other hand, T-cell function, in particular cytotoxic T-cell function, is the main mechanism for preventing severe viral disease and also for controlling viruses such as herpesviruses that can cause latency and thus reactivate in an immunocompromised individual. Different degrees of T-cell dysfunction in different types of transplant patients, therefore, likely best explain the difference in the impact of viral infections in allogeneic and autologous SCT patients, and also the differences between different groups of allogeneic SCT patients. However, the immune defects in SCT patients are frequently complex with defects in cytotoxic T-lymphocyte, helper T-lymphocyte, NK-cell, and B-lymphocyte functions. T-cell dysfunction is usually most important early after SCT, while deficient B-cell reconstitution can remain for many years after SCT. Furthermore, since loss of specific antibodies occurs frequently over time after allogeneic SCT, this will also increase the risk of reinfection with previously encountered viruses, such as measles or varicella zoster virus, and allow reactivation of viruses controlled by antibodies, such as hepatitis B virus (HBV). This chapter aims to present modern diagnostic techniques and monitoring of viral load, as well as preventive and therapeutic options for virus infections after allogeneic SCT.

Diagnosis of viral infections

The classical ways of detecting viral infections have been by serology and virus isolation. These techniques have been either too insensitive or too slow to be of practical use in transplant recipients. However, during recent years important advances have been made both in improving sensitivity and in speed, making specific diagnosis as well as monitoring of viral infections feasible. Early identification of patients at risk for developing viral disease can reduce virus-related morbidity and mortality, thereby improving overall patient outcome. Cytomegalovirus (CMV) isolation, and in particular CMV viremia, were shown more than a decade ago to be strong predictors for CMV disease, but simultaneous detection of viremia and development of disease occur not infrequently (Meyers, Ljungman, & Fisher, 1990). More sensitive techniques such as antigenemia, polymerase chain reaction (PCR) for CMV DNA, or determination of viral load by quantitative PCR have higher sensitivity than CMV viremia as predictive risk factors for CMV disease (Gor *et al.*, 1998; Emery *et al.*, 2000; Hebart *et al.*, 2001c). The development of techniques allowing monitoring of viral load seems to help in assessing the risk of CMV disease posttransplant, with patients with higher viral loads clearly carrying a higher risk of developing CMV disease (Gor *et al.*, 1998). In addition, an increasing viral load in patients receiving antiviral therapy with ganciclovir was found to be a clear indication for intensifying antiviral maintenance therapy (Nichols *et al.*, 2001b). In patients suspected of having CMV end-organ disease, appropriate diagnostic procedures should be undertaken (Ljungman *et al.*, 2002b).

Specimen Collection

The appropriate collection of specimens is critical for the successful identification of viruses in clinical samples. The source of the specimen, the timing of collection in relation to onset of symptoms, the rapidity and method of delivery to the laboratory, and the clinical and epidemiological data provided to the laboratory are important factors that directly affect the likelihood of successful isolation and/or identification of a viral pathogen (Table 74.1).

Serology

The presence of IgG antibodies against a virus indicates a previous infection and the possibility of reactivation posttransplant. However, serology is usually not useful for diagnosis of active virus infections after SCT, since many patients are

Table 74.1. *The role of the laboratory in testing for viruses in the HSC transplant recipient*

Pretransplant	Test donor and recipient for IgG antibodies to detect patients at risk for reactivation of infection
Posttransplant	Receive regular surveillance samples from the recipient
	Process these samples by methods that
	Are sensitive and specific
	Give rapid results
	Provide prognostic information regarding risk for disease
	Receive samples from patients with conditions where a potential viral etiology is included in the differential diagnosis; for example,
	Broncho-alveolar lavage fluid in cases of pneumonitis
	Biopsies from affected organs
	Receive samples from patients with suspected resistance to antiviral drugs
	Rapid identification or exclusion of resistance
	Advice on alternative drugs to be used

unable to mount antibody responses. Serology should be performed before SCT to determine risk status of patients and donors. Monitoring after transplant with sensitive techniques is indicated in all allogeneic SCT patients.

Electron microscopy

Electron microscopy is probably the most rapid method for identifying herpesviruses in vesicular fluid. On examination by electron microscopy, herpesvirus particles may be seen, but the type of herpesvirus cannot be distinguished because all types look the same. It is also used for the diagnosis of viruses in the stool. Although electron microscopy is quick to perform, it is a labor-intensive method, and a high titer of virus (at least 10^6 viral particles per milliliter) is required.

Immunfluorescence

An alternative method, which is more sensitive and specific than electron microscopy, is immunofluorescence (IF). After the slide is dried and fixed in acetone, the cells can be stained with antibodies to viruses that are directly conjugated to fluorescein isothiocynate.

Cell culture

Many viruses (for example, herpesviruses) can be isolated and propagated easily in many different primary and continuous cell lines. Cell cultures inoculated with a clinical specimen will develop a typical cytopathic effect (CPE) of ballooning, degenerating cells, and occasionally multinucleated giant cells, within 1–7 days. Depending upon the cell line used and the titer of

virus in the specimen, many of the cultures show a CPE within 24 hours. Although the CPE produced by virus replication is usually characteristic, the changes seen may be similar to those produced by other viruses. Therefore CPE should be confirmed by virus-specific assays (e.g., neutralization with specific antibody or IF using monoclonal antibodies). Cell culture is an extremely sensitive method of viral detection, providing the clinical material is collected, transported, and stored correctly.

Shell vial technique

Virus-specific antigens (e.g., the immediate early or early CMV antigens) are produced in tissue culture long before cytopathic effects are detectable, and can be identified with specific antibodies linked to enzymes or other markers, using the shell vial technique. The latter technique takes 24 to 48 hours.

Antigenemia assay

The antigenemia assay (detection of the CMV protein pp65 in the nucleus of circulating neutrophils) correlates with, and is positive earlier than, viremia (Van der Bij *et al.*, 1988; Boeckh *et al.*, 1992), and together with the PCR assays has replaced the shell vial assay as the trigger for initiating pre-emptive ganciclovir administration. The test is rapid and semi-quantitative, but requires that there be no neutropenia and that infection has progressed sufficiently to be detectable in granulocytes. It is inferior to quantitative DNA-based testing for monitoring response to treatment (see below).

Detection of nucleic acid—polymerase chain reaction

Increasing use is now being made of the amplification of viral DNA or RNA. The most commonly used technique is PCR. These techniques have been evaluated and shown to be useful on blood (Einsele *et al.*, 1991) and cerebrospinal fluid (CSF) (Cinque *et al.*, 1992, 1993; Wang *et al.*, 1999), while its use on tissue or on broncho-alveolar lavage fluid (BAL) has yet not been accepted as an indicator of disease. Other techniques to detect viral DNA such as the hybrid capture assay (Hebart *et al.*, 2001b) or the branched DNA assay have been applied and shown good sensitivity and have also allowed quantification of viral load. However their sensitivity is inferior when compared to PCR assays. An assay for measuring CMV-specific messenger RNA, which more directly reflects active viral gene expression and replication, is being assessed (Hebart *et al.*, 2002).

Quantitative PCR

Early identification of patients at risk for developing viral disease could reduce virus-related morbidity and mortality, thereby improving overall patient management. Viral load has been found to be an important risk factor for the development of viral disease. Thus, quantitative PCR assays are increasingly being used to assess viral load in patients with CMV, Epstein-Barr virus (EBV), HBV, hepatitis C virus (HCV) and adenovirus infections. The development of real-time technology has allowed introduction of viral load measurements in routine management. Monitoring of viral load using real-time PCR formats also allows simultaneous assessment of the load of different viruses in the blood, and thus can help individualize antiviral therapy and the study of virus-virus interactions.

Histopathology and immunohistopathology

To diagnose tissue invasive disease, the most common method, and the most rapid, is tissue section examination of tissue biopsies. Results can be available within 6 hours, using microwave oven rapid processing techniques. Tissue sections can also be stained with monoclonal antibodies against viral antigens.

Cytomegalovirus (CMV)

Posttransplant, CMV is most often associated with life-threatening interstitial pneumonitis (IP). Infection can also occur in the gastrointestinal tract, liver, and retina; joint involvement has been described, as has oral and (asymptomatic) ovarian involvement. CMV infection can cause pancytopenia. Serious CMV disease occurs much more commonly after allogeneic than after autologous transplantation. In one series of 795 autograft recipients, 2% developed CMV IP; the frequency was higher among those who were seropositive pretransplant and among those transplanted for hematological malignancies compared to those transplanted for solid tumors (Konoplev et al., 2001). CD34 selection is also a risk factor in autologous transplantation. Prior to the introduction of prophylactic or pre-emptive ganciclovir regimens, the corresponding incidence in allogeneic transplant recipients was commonly 20% or higher.

The median time of first virus isolation, seroconversion, and CMV IP is 8 to 9 weeks after allogeneic transplantion (Fig. 74.1). A CMV seropositive patient may have a reactivation of a latent strain of the virus, receive a new strain with the transplanted HSC if the donor is CMV seropositive, or receive CMV with blood products. The risk of infection among seronegative patients who receive prophylactic granulocyte transfusions increases to 75%, whereas the use of granulocytes in seropositive patients does not affect the incidence of infection. Symptomatic CMV infection (CMV disease) significantly reduces survival posttransplant. Prior to the introduction of prophylactic or pre-emptive antiviral treatment, 10% to 50% of patients developed CMV-associated IP, which was fatal in 50% to 80% (Meyers, Fluornoy, & Thomas, 1980). CMV disease increasingly also occurs later posttransplant—at a median of 169 days in 17% of patients in one study (Boeckh et al., 2003), and associated in another study with ganciclovir-resistant strains; involvement of unusual sites such as the central nervous system was reported (Wolf et al., 2003).

Risk factors

Factors increasing the risk of CMV infection include age, GVHD, GVHD prophylaxis and treatment, and total body irradi-

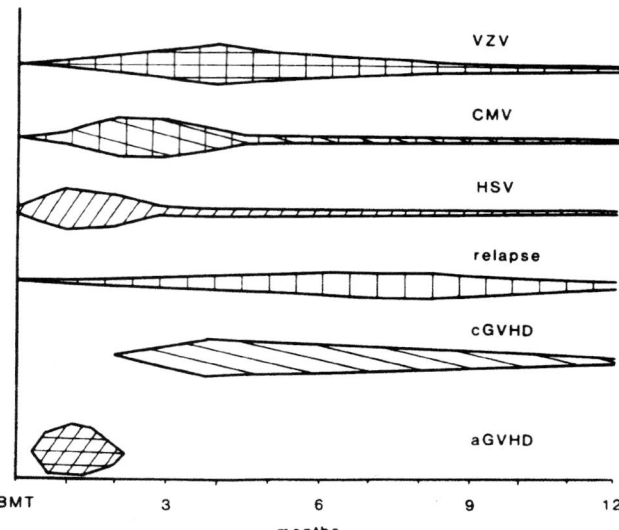

Fig. 74.1. Time frame for different herpes virus infections, relapse, and acute and chronic GVHD in relation to time post-BMT. VZV, varicella zoster; CMV, cytomegalovirus; HSV, herpes simplex virus; CGVHD, chronic GVHD; aGVHD, acute GVHD; relapse, recurrence of hematologic malignancy after allogeneic HSCT.

ation. Nichols and colleagues (2001a) determined the risk factors and outcomes associated with rising CMV antigenemia levels during pre-emptive anti-CMV treatment. Corticosteroid therapy was the primary risk factor. In other studies, CMV viremia, quantitative pp65 antigenemia, and DNA load have been described as risk factors independent of GVHD. Hebart and colleagues (2001a) demonstrated that the risk of disease in patients receiving PCR-based pre-emptive antiviral treatment was dependent on the transplant modality, with different patterns seen in recipients of T-depleted transplants compared to T replete transplants. CMV antigenemia can occur after day 100 and is then often associated with chronic GVHD (Machado et al., 2001). Risk factors for the occurrence of late CMV disease include the presence of chronic GVHD and the prolonged use of ganciclovir prophylaxis (de Medeiros, Moreira, & Pasquini, 2000), as well as preceding detection of CMV pp65 antigenemia, CD4+ T-cell counts lower than 50 cells/mm^3, lymphopenia <100 lymphocytes/mm^3, and undetectable CMV-specific T-cell responses (Boeckh et al., 2003).

In recipients of syngeneic (identical twin) and autologous transplants, there is a zero and low incidence (Ljungman et al., 1994) of, and mortality from, CMV IP, respectively. It appears more common in recipients of unrelated allografts compared to related allografts (Takenaka et al., 1997).

In a case-matched controlled study, the onset of CMV disease was significantly delayed in recipients of non-myeloablative conditioning compared to the controls who received conventional myeloablative conditioning (Junghanss et al., 2002), although the overall one year incidences were similar. It was concluded that CMV surveillance and pre-emptive ganciclovir treatment should extend beyond day 100, at least in recipients of this specific non-myeloablative conditioning regimen (TBI

200cGy with or without fludarabine). Generally, the risk of CMV disease does not appear to be lower after nonmyeloablative conditioning regimens, and, in those utilizing Campath-1H, the incidence is high (see Chapter 22).

Preventing infection/disease in CMV seronegative patients

Patients who are CMV seronegative before SCT should if possible be transplanted from a CMV seronegative donor (Bowden et al., 1991b). If a CMV seronegative donor is used, the risk for CMV transmission is mainly through subsequent blood product transfusion. To reduce the risk of transmission from blood products, blood products from CMV seronegative donors or leukocyte-depleted blood products should be used. These two options were tested in a randomized trial and shown to be comparable (Bowden et al., 1995). A non-randomized, successive cohort study using PCR monitoring showed a similar risk for CMV DNA detection in donor-seronegative/recipient-seronegative (D–/R–) patients receiving CMV negative and leukocyte-depleted compared to leukocyte-depleted blood products (Ljungman et al., 2002c). The use of CMV seronegative blood products does not significantly impact on the risk for R+/D– patients (Bowden et al., 1986). No data exist regarding the possible effectiveness of antiviral prophylaxis in D+/R– patients, although immune globulin has been shown not to be effective (Bowden et al., 1991a; Ruutu et al., 1997).

Preventing CMV disease

Since the prognosis of established CMV disease is still poor, preventive measures are very important. The available strategies can be divided into prevention of a recurrence/reactivation of CMV (prophylaxis) or prevention of development of disease when a reactivation has occurred (pre-emptive therapy) (Table 74.2). In general, recipients of HLA-identical sibling and HLA-identical unrelated transplants are well managed with a pre-emptive approach, while those at higher risk of GVHD may benefit from a prophylactic approach initiated earlier posttransplant (Aaia, 2002).

Prophylactic strategies

Several randomized trials of intravenous immune globulin (IVIG) have been performed, producing divergent results. Bass et al. (1993) summarized these trials in a meta-analysis showing a slight but significant reduction in CMV disease and pneumonia in those receiving IVIG. All these studies were, however, performed, before the introduction of other more effective preventive strategies and therefore, due to the high cost of high-dose IVIG and its modest effect, immune globulin has been replaced in most transplant centers by other more effective strategies.

Acyclovir and valaciclovir have only modest effects in vitro and in vivo on CMV replication. However, two large studies of acyclovir prophylaxis (500 mg/m^2 three times daily during the pancytopenic phase followed by 800 mg orally four times daily) have shown a reduction of CMV infection and an improvement in survival (Meyers et al., 1988; Prentice et al., 1994, 1997). Valaciclovir was shown in a large randomized prospective trial to significantly reduce the risk for CMV viremia above what was achieved with high-dose acyclovir (Ljungman et al., 2002a). There was no survival advantage and no reduction in the (low) risk for CMV disease. Therefore, if either acyclovir or valaciclovir are used as CMV prophylaxis after allogeneic SCT, a strategy of pre-emptive therapy must also be used.

Intravenous ganciclovir was effective for the prevention of CMV disease in two randomized, double-blind, placebo-controlled trials in which slightly different regimens were used (Goodrich et al., 1993a; Winston et al., 1993). Ganciclovir reduced the incidence of CMV infection in both studies, while the incidence of CMV disease was significantly reduced in one study. However, mortality did not differ between the ganciclovir and placebo groups in either study. These studies were performed before the widespread use of growth factors such as G-CSF and ganciclovir-induced neutropenia was a problem in both studies. Furthermore, ganciclovir prophylaxis has also been associated with delayed immune reconstitution to CMV and thereby the development of late CMV disease (Li et al., 1994). An alternative to intravenous ganciclovir is its oral formulation. Oral ganciclovir has been investigated only in a small prophylactic study of 21 recipients, showing a poor tolerability and a high rate of CMV infection (Boeckh et al., 1998). A larger randomized study is ongoing. Valganciclovir is the prodrug of ganciclovir, giving similar blood levels to intravenous ganciclovir, and is currently being evaluated in SCT patients.

Foscarnet has been used in three small trials and although it reduced the risk of CMV infection, no data on survival have been presented. The major side-effects of foscarnet can be reduced with careful monitoring and hydration (Ringden et al., 1989; Reusser et al., 1992; Bacigalupo et al., 1994).

No controlled trial of CMV prophylaxis has been performed in autologous SCT recipients. It would be logical, however, to try to prevent primary infections in autologous SCT recipients, for example with the use of leukocyte-depleted or CMV negative blood products. Boeckh et al. (1995) showed in a retrospective analysis that high-dose acyclovir did not influence the risk of CMV disease.

Pre-emptive therapy

Goodrich et al. (1991) showed that pre-emptive therapy based on the shell vial assay could reduce the risk for CMV disease and improve survival. Since then, pre-emptive therapy based on early detection of CMV has become the most commonly used strategy for prevention of CMV disease after allogeneic SCT (Ljungman et al., 1993b; Avery et al., 2000). Einsele et al. (1995) showed in a randomized trial that the use of PCR monitoring reduced the incidence of CMV disease and the risk for CMV-associated mortality compared to monitoring by rapid isolation. Boeckh et al. (1996a) showed in a randomized study

Table 74.2. *Antiviral agents used for prevention and therapy in hematopoietic stem cell transplant recipients*

Agent	Indications	Dose	Route	Comments	Reference
Acyclovir	Prevention of HSV	400 mg 3×/day	po		Ljungman *et al.*, 1986b
		5 mg/kg 3×/day	i.v.		Saral *et al.*, 1981
	Treatment of HSV	400 mg 5 ×/day	po		Shepp *et al.*, 1985
		5 mg/kg 3 ×/day	i.v.		Meyers *et al.*, 1982
	Prevention of VZV	400 mg 3 ×/day	po		Ljungman *et al.*, 1986b
	Treatment of VZV	800 mg 5 ×/day	po	Local herpes zoster	Ljungman *et al.*, 1989c
		10 mg/kg 3 ×/day	i.v.	Varicella, disseminated	Shepp *et al.*, 1985
	Prevention of CMV	500 mg/m² 3 ×/day	i.v.	zoster, local zoster	Prentice *et al.*, 1994
		800 mg × 4	po		
Valacyclovir	Prevention of HSV	1 g 3 ×/day	po	Prodrug of acyclovir	Höglund *et al.*, 2001
	Treatment of HSV	No published data	po		
	Prevention of VZV	No published data	po		
	Treatment of VZV	No published data	po		
	Prevention of CMV	2 g 4 ×/day	po		Ljungman *et al.*, 2002a
Famciclovir	Treatment of VZV	500 mg 3 ×/day	po	Prodrug of penciclovir	Tyring *et al.*, 2001
Ganciclovir	Prevention of CMV	5 mg/kg 2 ×/day for 5 days followed by 5 mg/kg 1 ×	i.v.		Goodrich *et al.*, 1993b
	Preemptive therapy of CMV	5 mg/kg 2 ×/day for 2 weeks followed by 5 mg/kg 1 ×/day 5 days/ week for 2 weeks or to day 100	i.v.		Boeckh *et al.*, 1999; Einsele *et al.*, 1995; Goodrich *et al.*, 1991; Reusser *et al.*, 2002
	Therapy of CMV disease	5 mg/kg 2 ×/day for at least 2 weeks.	i.v.	+/– immune globulin	Emanuel *et al.*, 1988; Machado *et al.*, 2000; Reed *et al.*, 1988; Schmidt *et al.*, 1988
	Prevention of CMV	1 g 3 ×/day	po	Poor tolerability, high frequency of break-through. Not indicated	Boeckh *et al.*, 1998
Valganciclovir	Prevention of CMV	Studies are ongoing	po	Prodrug of ganciclovir	
Foscarnet	Preemptive treatment of CMV	60 mg/kg 2 ×/day for two weeks followed by 90 mg 1 ×/day 5 days/ week for two weeks.	i.v.	Should be given with hydration	Reusser *et al.*, 2002
	Treatment of CMV disease	60 mg/kg 3 ×/day for at least two weeks	i.v.		Aschan *et al.*, 1992
	Treatment of acyclovir-resistant HSV	40 mg/kg 3 ×/day			Safrin *et al.*, 1990
Cidofovir	Treatment of CMV	3–5 mg/kg once weekly, maintenance every 2 weeks	i.v.	Must be given with probenecid and hydration	Ljungman *et al.*, 2001a
	Treatment of adenovirus	3–5 mg/kg once weekly, maintenance every 2 weeks	i.v.	Must be given with probenecid and hydration	Ljungman *et al.*, 2001b
Ribavirin	Treatment of RSV	2 g 3 ×/day	inhalation	± IVIG	Ljungman *et al.*, 2001c; Whimbey *et al.*, 1995
		15–20 mg/day in 3 doses	i.v.	Avoid staff exposure	Sparrelid *et al.*, 1997

Abbreviations: HSV, herpes simplex virus; VZV, varicella zoster virus; CMV, cytomegalovirus; RSV, respiratory syncytial virus

that antigenemia-based pre-emptive therapy could be used with similar efficacy to ganciclovir prophylaxis in the prevention of CMV disease. This study illustrates the strengths and weaknesses of the two strategies. Ganciclovir prophylaxis was more effective in preventing CMV disease during the time it was given (the first 100 days after SCT), while the risks for late CMV disease, ganciclovir-associated neutropenia, and for invasive fungal disease were higher, equalizing the risk for CMV

disease and survival at 180 days after transplantation. The results of the pre-emptive therapy strategy could be improved during the first 100 days by using a more sensitive antigenemia assay (Boeckh *et al.*, 1999).

Either ganciclovir or foscarnet can be used for pre-emptive therapy. Reusser *et al.* (2002) found no difference in efficacy between the two drugs while the toxicity profiles differed. Ganciclovir caused more neutropenia and foscarnet more electrolyte disturbances, but there was no difference in renal toxicity. The combination of ganciclovir and foscarnet has been used with high efficacy in patients with high-level antigenemia without additional toxicity (Bacigalupo *et al.*, 1996). Cidofovir (3–5 mg/kg per week) might be an effective alternative as second-line pre-emptive therapy, resulting in a 66% success rate when instituted after failure of either ganciclovir or foscarnet (Ljungman *et al.*, 2001a). Cidofovir is associated with significant renal toxicity and controlled prospective studies are necessary. A small prospective study of pre-emptive cidofovir showed a difference in effectiveness when used in patients who had undergone non-myeloablative conditioning (7 of 10 patients) compared to those (0 of 7) who had received standard myeloablative conditioning (Platzbecker *et al.*, 2001).

The duration of pre-emptive therapy has varied in published studies. The two most commonly used approaches have been to continue therapy until day 100 after SCT (Goodrich *et al.*, 1991), or until the indicator test becomes negative, usually resulting in a shorter duration of therapy (Einsele *et al.*, 1995; Reusser *et al.*, 2002). The drawback with shorter courses of therapy is that treatment might have to be restarted but the advantages are lower cost, less risk of side-effects, and potentially better reconstitution of the specific immune response to CMV.

Treatment of established disease

The results of therapy in established CMV disease are still poor. Survival in CMV pneumonia remains approximately 50% when the combination of ganciclovir and immune globulin is used (Emanuel *et al.*, 1988; Reed *et al.*, 1988; Schmidt *et al.*, 1988; Ljungman *et al.*, 1992). Machado *et al.* (2000) have, however, published the results of an uncontrolled study of 139 allogeneic SCT patients showing that the advantage of adding immune globulin is limited, with no improvement in survival in CMV pneumonia over ganciclovir therapy given alone. For patients with CMV disease other than pneumonia, the addition of immune globulin does not seem to be beneficial (Ljungman *et al.*, 1998). It has been suggested that the combination of ganciclovir and foscarnet offers a clinical benefit in the treatment of CMV disease without a significant increase in toxicity (Bacigalupo *et al.*, 1996). A retrospective survey reported that cidofovir salvaged 9 of 16 patients with CMV pneumonia failing therapy with ganciclovir, foscarnet, or the combination (Ljungman *et al.*, 2001a).

Antiviral resistance

Resistance to ganciclovir is usually mediated through mutations in the *UL97* gene. It has been more commonly reported in AIDS patients and in solid organ transplant recipients than in hematopoietic stem cell transplant patients. It has been proposed that prolonged exposure to ganciclovir, a high viral load in the presence of suboptimal concentrations of antiviral drugs, and intense immunosuppression, predisposes to the emergence of resistant strains (Emery & Griffiths, 2000; Limaye *et al.*,

2000). Other therapeutic alternatives are then foscarnet or cidofovir. It should be noted that increasing levels of antigenemia early after initiation of antiviral therapy is not usually a sign of antiviral resistance and does not necessitate change of therapy (Nichols *et al.*, 2001b).

Adoptive immunotherapy

Despite the major advances that have been made in CMV management, several problems still exist including the increased incidence of late CMV disease. The lack of specific immunity to CMV, including both the cytotoxic T-cell (CTL) response and the helper T-cell response, has been associated with a high risk for CMV disease (Reusser *et al.*, 1991; Ljungman *et al.*, 1993a; Krause *et al.*, 1997). Monitoring of specific immunity is therefore likely to become important for routine patient management in the near future. Fluorescent HLA-peptide tetramers containing immunodominant peptides from CMV have been used to monitor the presence of CMV cytotoxic T lymphocytes (CTL) in the stem cell graft (Gratama *et al.*, 2001) and their recovery in the blood posttransplant (Cwynarski *et al.*, 2001; Gratama *et al.*, 2001). When both recipient and donor were CMV-seropositive pretransplant, recovery of CMV-specific CTL was rapid and represented up to 21% of all CD8+ cells (Cwynarski *et al.*, 2001). Recovery was slower in recipients of unrelated transplants compared to that after HLA-identical sibling grafts. CTL numbers increased after episodes of CMV reactivation, but were suppressed by corticosteroid treatment. Recovery of CMV-specific CTL to levels $> 10 \times 10^6/l$ was associated with protection from CMV disease. Furthermore, the number of CMV-specific CD8+ T cells present in the graft pretransplant correlated with the number of courses of pre-emptive ganciclovir administered posttransplant (Gratama *et al.*, 2001). In addition, peptide-specific intracellular cytokine staining was shown to document CMV-specific CD4+ and CD8+ T cell responses. For long-term control of CMV infection posttransplant, CMV-specific T helper cell responses seem to be essential (Ljungman *et al.*, 1993a; Krause *et al.*, 1997; Hebart *et al.*, 2001a). Reconstitution of CMV-specific CD4+ cells follows a similar pattern to that of CD8+ cells (Foster *et al.*, 2002).

Riddell's group has shown that CMV-specific CTL can be cloned in vitro, given safely to the patient, and their activity detected during follow-up (Reusser *et al.*, 1991; Riddell *et al.*, 1992; Walter *et al.*, 1995). A phase II study has been completed but has not been published. Preliminary data indicate that the risk of CMV infection and disease was low and side-effects were rare. New techniques such as the use of peptide-pulsed dendritic cells and tetramer technology have been developed that might allow an easier selection of CMV-specific T-cells and several laboratories are presently testing these strategies in early phase clinical trials (Cwynarski *et al.*, 2001; Kleihauer *et al.*, 2001; Peggs *et al.*, 2001; Szmania *et al.*, 2001). For example, transfer of CMV-specific CD4+ T cells was shown to be effective in inducing CMV-specific CD8+ T cell responses and reducing CMV DNA load (Einsele *et al.*, 2002).

Herpes simplex virus (HSV)

Clinical symptoms

Herpes simplex virus (HSV) can cause both local and disseminated infections after both allogeneic and autologous SCT. The most common manifestation is a local mucous membrane or skin lesion, either oral or genital. The manifestations in HSC transplant patients are frequently atypical, causing generalized inflammation and pain from the mucous membranes without classical vesicular or ulcerative lesions. Therefore, awareness and diagnostic attempts are important to rule out HSV infections in patients with slowly healing or atypical mucositis. Esophagitis presenting as pain and difficulty in swallowing does occur in the absence of prophylaxis. Generalized and invasive disease can occur but is uncommon today when prophylaxis is generally used (see below). Encephalitis does not seem to be more frequent in immunocompromised compared to immune competent individuals, although it is frequently fatal or results in significant sequelae.

Direct testing of suspected lesions by direct IF is rapid and sensitive (Table 74.3). In patients with more diffuse symptoms, virus isolation can be used. PCR is the technique of choice for CNS disease. Serology is useful for determining the risk of reactivation of HSV infection and should be performed before transplantation.

Prevention and therapy

The first controlled studies of prophylaxis and therapy of HSV in allogeneic SCT patients were performed more than 20 years ago, showing that effective antiviral agents can make an important impact on morbidity and mortality (Saral et al., 1981; Hann et al., 1983; Ljungman et al., 1986b). Therefore, acyclovir prophylaxis is indicated in all HSV seropositive SCT recipients and in some autologous patients with a high risk of mucositis (Centers for Disease Control, 2000). The duration of antiviral prophylaxis should last at least during the pancytopenic phase, but a longer duration should be considered in patients with

GVHD or a history of frequent reactivations before the transplant (Centers for Disease Control, 2000). HSV reactivations frequently occur early after prophylaxis is stopped (Saral et al., 1981; Hann et al., 1983; Wade et al., 1984a, 1984b). Valaciclovir, the prodrug of acyclovir, can presumably be used in place of acyclovir as prophylaxis, but no dose-finding study has been performed in SCT patients. However, valaciclovir gives acyclovir serum levels similar to those with the use of i.v. acyclovir in neutropenic patients (Hoglund et al., 2001). Therapy for established HSV disease can be given either orally or intravenously. The most commonly used drug is acyclovir, which should be given intravenously in patients with disseminated HSV or suspected CNS disease.

Acyclovir, valaciclovir, famciclovir, and ganciclovir all require the viral enzyme thymidine kinase for activation. Mutant and resistant virus strains lacking this enzyme can develop. Although acyclovir has now been in extensive use for almost 20 years, there has been only a moderate increase in the detection rate of resistant strains (Wade, McLaren, & Meyers, 1983; Englund et al., 1990; Reusser et al., 1996) although acyclovir-resistant HSV seems to have become more common in particular after unrelated or HLA-mismatched SCT and in patients with GVHD (Darville et al., 1998; Chakrabarti et al., 2000; Chen et al., 2000). Patients in whom HSV is detected despite compliance with prophylaxis, and in patients with mucositis not healing at the expected rate, should be suspected to have resistant virus and appropriate diagnostic procedures performed. Detection of thymidine kinase mutants can be performed in specialized virological laboratories.

The recommended drug for acyclovir-resistant HSV is foscarnet (Safrin et al., 1990; Verdonck et al., 1993; Naik et al., 1995). Two reports have described mutants resistant to both acyclovir and foscarnet (Chakrabarti et al., 2000; Chen et al., 2000). Currently, the only available antiviral drug available for treatment of doubly resistant HSV is cidofovir. However, although HSV strains have been sensitive in vitro, the clinical response in high-risk allogeneic SCT patients treated with cidofovir has been variable (Chakrabarti et al., 2000; Chen et al., 2000).

Table 74.3. *Choice of diagnostic test for the detection of herpesvirus infections in the hematopoietic stem cell transplant recipient*

	Diagnostic technique					
Virus	Serology	EM	IF	qPCR	DEAFF/Shell vial	Cell culture
HSV	+*	++	+++	++ (CSF samples)	−	+
VZV	+*	++	+++	++ (CSF samples)	−	+
CMV	+++*	−	+++ (antigenemia test)	+++	+	+
EBV	+*	−	−	+++	−	−
HHV-6	−	−	−	+++	−	+
HHV-7	−	−	−	+++	−	+
HHV-8	−	−	−	++	−	+/−

Abbreviations: EM, electron microscopy; IF, direct immunofluorescence; q PCR, quantitative polymerase chain reaction; DEAFF, detection of early fluorescent foci.

* Useful pretransplant for risk stratification.

Varicella zoster virus (VZV)

Clinical symptoms

Primary varicella zoster virus (VZV) infection (varicella) is an uncommon but very severe complication in SCT patients (Locksley *et al.,* 1985b). The risk is highest in children, but second cases of varicella-like disease in seropositive adults becoming seronegative after SCT have been described.. Reactivated VZV infection—herpes zoster—is common after both allogeneic and autologous SCT occurring in approximately one third of all patients (Locksley *et al.,* 1985b; Ljungman *et al.,* 1986a; Schuchter *et al.,* 1989; Wacker *et al.,* 1989; Steer *et al.,* 2000). Severe and fatal cases have also been reported after allogeneic SCT with reduced intensity conditioning. Herpes zoster is usually dermatomal in SCT patients, but in the absence of antiviral therapy, disseminated and potentially fatal infections with visceral involvement can occur (Locksley *et al.,* 1985a). The clinical picture can be atypical with gastrointestinal, liver, or CNS disease occurring in the absence of skin lesions, and presenting as severe gastrointestinal pain, rapidly developing hepatitis, or meningoencephalitis, respectively. Schiller and colleagues (1991) described VZV presenting as an abdominal illness with severe abdominal pain, anorexia, vomiting, abdominal tenderness and rigidity, and gastrointestinal hemorrhage preceding the development of a typical vesicular skin rash by up to 5 days. Hepatitis and pancreatitis were present. A case report described a patient with abdominal pain and vomiting who had a VZV infection of the gastric mucosa, diagnosed by PCR, and who made a full recovery after treatment with acyclovir. Inappropriate secretion of antidiuretic hormone can accompany the abdominal pain. Occasionally the brain and bone marrow can be also involved in this disseminated process. Other case reports of presentation with abdominal pain without skin involvement have described a fatal outcome. The onset appears to be delayed by administration of ganciclovir to day 100 posttransplant and in those with limited, as opposed to extensive, chronic GVHD (Koc *et al.,* 2000; Steer *et al.,* 2000) (Figs. 74.2 and 74.3). Diagnosis of primary or reactivated VZV infections is usually made by direct IF. In patients with classical dermatomal lesions, specific diagnostic procedures are frequently unnecessary, but in some patients there might be difficulties in differentiating HSV and VZV. VZV infections in the CNS are diagnosed by PCR on CSF. Serology is useful to determine patients at risk for a primary VZV infection and should be performed in all patients before transplantation, and, at least in allogeneic SCT patients, also at regular intervals after SCT.

Prevention of primary VZV infection

VZV occurs regularly in the general population and is very contagious. Seronegative SCT patients are at risk for developing varicella and preventive measures are therefore indicated. It is frequently difficult to assess with accuracy the grade of exposure in SCT patients, and questions regarding the need for preventive measures in possibly exposed seronegative individuals

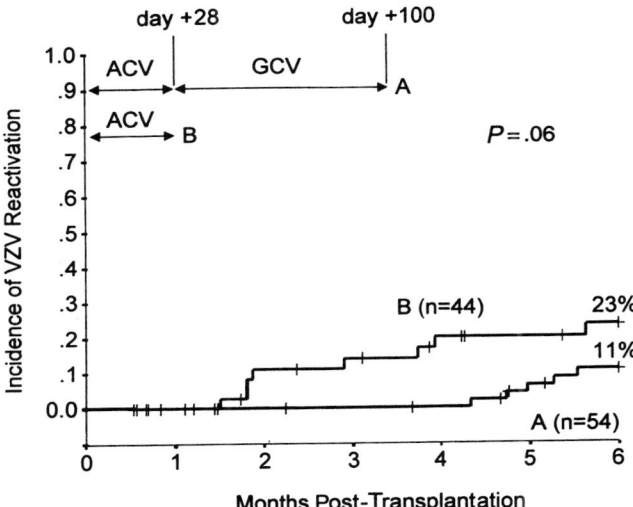

Fig. 74.2. Impact of duration of antiviral prophylaxis on onset of VZV reactivation during the early post-transplantation period. P indicates probability of VZV reactivation, log rank test; ACV, acyclovir; GCV, ganciclovir; VZV, varicella zoster. Reproduced, with permission, from Koc et al. (2000).

are therefore not uncommon. Varicella zoster immune globulin is the recommended prophylactic measure in seronegative SCT recipients after a household or other type of close exposure, if it can be given within 4 days of exposure (Centers for Disease Control, 2000). Another option could be antiviral chemoprophylaxis with acyclovir or valaciclovir, but there are no published data regarding such a strategy's effectiveness. Varicella vaccine has been shown to be safe in children with acute leukemia, but there is no controlled trial published in SCT

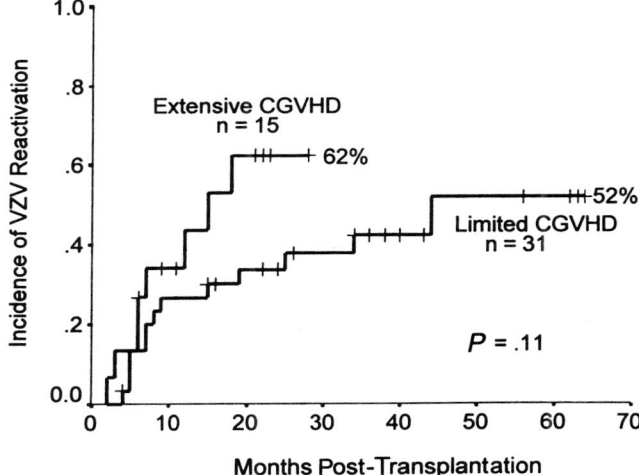

Fig. 74.3. Comparison of estimated incidence of varicella zoster virus (VZV) reactivation at 5 years in patients with limited chronic graft-versus-host disease (CGVHD) versus those with extensive CGVHD. P indicates probability of VZV reactivation, log rank test. Reproduced, with permission, from Koc et al. (2000).

recipients, and its use is not recommended earlier than 24 months after transplantation or in patients with GVHD or in those receiving immunosuppressive therapy (Ljungman, 1999; Centers for Disease Control, 2000).

Prevention of reactivated infection—herpes zoster

The risk of herpes zoster is highest between 3 and 6 months after transplantation. Thus, the duration of antiviral prophylaxis must be long to be effective. Two randomized, controlled studies have been performed comparing 6 months of prophylactic acyclovir with placebo (Ljungman et al., 1986b; Selby et al., 1989). These showed that acyclovir was effective in reducing the risk for herpes zoster during the 6 months of therapy, but at 12 months after transplantation there was no longer any difference. Valaciclovir has not been studied for VZV prophylaxis, but the rate of VZV disease was reduced in a study when valaciclovir was compared to acyclovir as CMV prophylaxis (Ljungman et al., 2002a). Some centers use valaciclovir as long-term prophylaxis against VZV (Centers for Disease Control, 2000).

Treatment of VZV disease

The recommended therapy for primary varicella or disseminated herpes zoster is intravenous acyclovir 10 mg/kg (or 500 mg/m^2) three times daily. For localized dermatomal herpes zoster, oral acyclovir 800 mg given five times daily was compared to i.v. acyclovir in a small randomized study in allogeneic SCT patients and the outcomes were comparable (Ljungman et al., 1989c). Famciclovir 500 mg given three times daily was compared to acyclovir 800 mg five times daily in SCT, solid organ transplant, and oncology patients and the results indicated similar efficacy (Tyring et al., 2001). No controlled study has been performed with valaciclovir given for treatment of herpes zoster in SCT patients, but its efficacy is likely similar to that of acyclovir. Acyclovir-resistant VZV is rare, but has been reported after SCT (Reusser et al., 1996). In such patients, foscarnet or cidofovir is the treatment of choice, since the usual mechanism of resistance in VZV is similar to that in HSV.

Epstein-Barr virus (EBV)[1]

Clinical symptoms of EBV infection

Epstein-Barr virus (EBV) is frequently detected after allogeneic SCT (Gratama et al., 1992; Wang et al., 1996). However, only a few case reports have suggested that it directly causes significant disease such as meningoencephalitis (Dellemijn et al., 1995) or hairy leukoplakia (Epstein et al.,

---

[1] Michael Epstein, British pathologist/virologist, born 1921.
  Yvonne Barr, British scientist, born 1932.

1993). The development of techniques allowing measurement of viral load will likely lead to better understanding of EBV's importance after SCT.

EBV-associated lymphoproliferative disease (EBV-LPD) (and see Chapter 88)

Epstein-Barr virus–associated lymphoproliferative disease (EBV-LPD) is a serious complication of allogeneic SCT and solid organ transplantation (Gross et al., 1998; Micallef et al., 1998). Although the incidence of EBV-LPD is generally less than 2% following allogeneic SCT, it may increase up to 20% in patients with established risk factors such as unrelated donor SCT, T-cell depletion, anti-thymocyte globulin therapy, and other forms of intensified immunosuppression for prevention or treatment of GVHD (Curtis et al., 1999).

EBV-LPD initially presents as a reversible polymorphic polyclonal lymphoproliferation that may result in monoclonal malignant lymphoma if left untreated. EBV-LPD usually presents EBV latency pattern III phenotype. However, at the single cell level the lesions show a heterogeneous EBV protein expression pattern with the presence of different latency types in individual tumor cells. The latent membrane protein (LMP1) of EBV is expressed in the tumor cells of EBV-associated posttransplant lymphomas and the LMP1 genome can also be identified in lymphocytes from most stem cell donors. It was recently shown that CD34$^+$ selection of peripheral blood stem cells does not protect against transfer of donor-type EBV-positive founder cells and also that recipient-type EBV-LPD is not uncommon (Schafer et al., 2001). Outgrowth of recipient-type lymphoma may be favored by LMP1 deletion variant strains present in recipient lymphocytes.

Diagnosis

Early identification of patients at risk could reduce the EBV-LPD-related morbidity and mortality. Previously, patients with EBV-related disorders were mostly identified by qualitative PCR. However, EBV DNA load monitoring in peripheral blood seems to be a better predictor for EBV-LPD. For example, Rooney et al. (1998) found a strong statistically significant correlation between the presence of biopsy-proven EBV-LPD and EBV burden in the peripheral blood of allogeneic SCT recipients.

Different thresholds of EBV DNA load for the development of EBV-LPD have been reported. In one study, the EBV load was positive for all 9 patients with, and for 17 patients without, EBV-LPD (Gartner et al., 2002). The viral loads of patients with manifest EBV-LPD differed from the loads of those without EBV-LPD (median loads, 1.4×10^6 vs. 4×10^4 copies/μg of DNA; $P < .0001$). A threshold value of 10^5 copies/μg of DNA showed the best diagnostic efficacy (sensitivity, 87%; specificity, 91%) (see also Figure 74.4). However, in patients with less than three major risk factors for EBV-LPD, the positive predictive value of this threshold was rather low. The timing of monitoring also seems to be critical. One week prior to the

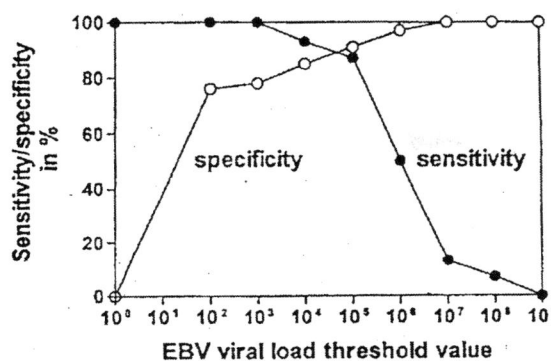

Fig. 74.4. Threshold value calculation for EBV load for diagnosis of EBV-associated lymphoproliferative disease. The corresponding sensitivities (closed symbols) and specificities (open symbols) for different threshold values are shown. Reproduced, with permission, from Gartner *et al.* (2002).

manifestation of EBV-LPD, the EBV load was as low in patients who developed EBV-LPD as in patients without disease (median, 2.2×10^4 copies/µg of DNA). EBV DNA was detected earlier in patients with primary infections than in those with reactivations (33 vs. 79 days; $P = .01$), but the peak levels were similar in the two groups (Gartner *et al.*, 2002). Quantitation of viral load can be used for predicting response to treatment (van Esser *et al.*, 2001b) (Fig. 74.5 and 74.6).

In another large study, 85 EBV-seropositive recipients of T-cell–depleted and 65 EBV-seropositive recipients of an unma-

nipulated graft were monitored by quantitative real-time plasma PCR until day 180 after SCT (van Esser *et al.*, 2001a). Probabilities of developing viral reactivation were high after both unmanipulated and T-cell–depleted SCT ($31\% \pm 6\%$ vs. $65\% \pm 7\%$, respectively). A high CD34$^+$ cell number in the graft appeared as a novel significant predictor ($P = .001$) for EBV reactivation. Recurrent reactivation was observed more frequently in recipients of a T-cell–depleted graft, and EBV-LPD occurred only after T-cell–depleted SCT. High-risk status including T-cell depletion and use of ATG were predictors for developing EBV-LPD. Plasma EBV viral load predicted EBV-LPD after T-cell depleted SCT (Table 74.4). The positive and negative predictive values of a viral load of 1000 gEq/ml were 39% and 100%, respectively.

Thus, monitoring of viral load is recommended in the management of EBV infection in the recipient of an allogeneic (especially T-cell–depleted) SCT. The threshold recommendation for introduction of anti-EBV therapy will depend on the patient population and the assay used, as well as the material analyzed (whole blood vs. plasma vs. serum).

Prevention and therapy

The first option for prevention or treatment of EBV-LPD is, if possible, reduction of immunosuppression. Several antiviral drugs including acyclovir, ganciclovir, foscarnet, and cidofovir have antiviral effects against EBV. However, no study has been performed on the efficacy of these drugs against EBV in SCT recipients. There are data from solid organ transplant recipients indicating a reduction of EBV shedding during antiviral therapy, but rapid rebounds occurred when the antiviral therapy was withdrawn. Instead, most interest during the last few years have been directed to the use of other therapeutic modalities such as therapy with specific or non-specific T-cells, or with monoclonal antibodies.

Cloned EBV-specific donor T-cells (Rooney *et al.*, 1995) and non-specific donor lymphocyte infusions have been used as treatment of EBV-LPD (Papadopoulos *et al.*, 1994). Both strategies reduced the tumor masses, but the use of non-specific donor lymphocyte infusions was associated with an increased risk of severe acute GVHD. EBV-specific T-cell infusions have also been used prophylactically (Rooney *et al.*, 1995). EBV CTL can also reduce the EBV viral load (Gustafsson *et al.*, 2000).

The monoclonal antibody directed against the B-cell antigen CD20 (rituximab) has been used to treat EBV-LPD after both solid organ and SCT. Milpied *et al.* (2000) reported results from 26 solid organ and 6 SCT patients. Four of the latter with high EBV viral load were treated for suspected EBV-LPD; 65% of the solid organ transplant patients and 5 of 6 of the SCT patients responded. Kuehnle *et al.* (2000) reported successful treatment with rituximab in three patients with proven EBV. Haddad *et al.* (2001) reported promising results with the use of an anti-interleukin-6 monoclonal antibody for therapy of EBV-LPD. (Haddad *et al.*, 2001).

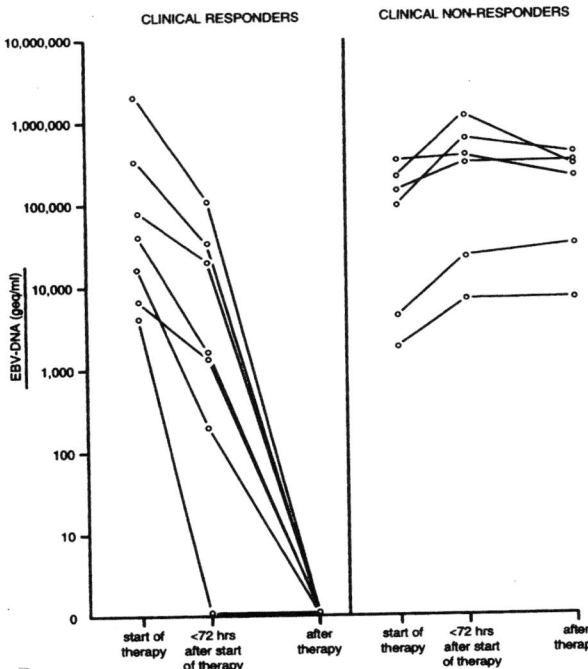

Fig. 74.5. Individual EBV-DNA levels for clinical resonders (left) and clinical non-responders (right) at the start of therapy, after 72 h and at clinical response evaluation. Reproduced, with permission, from van Esser et al. (2001b).

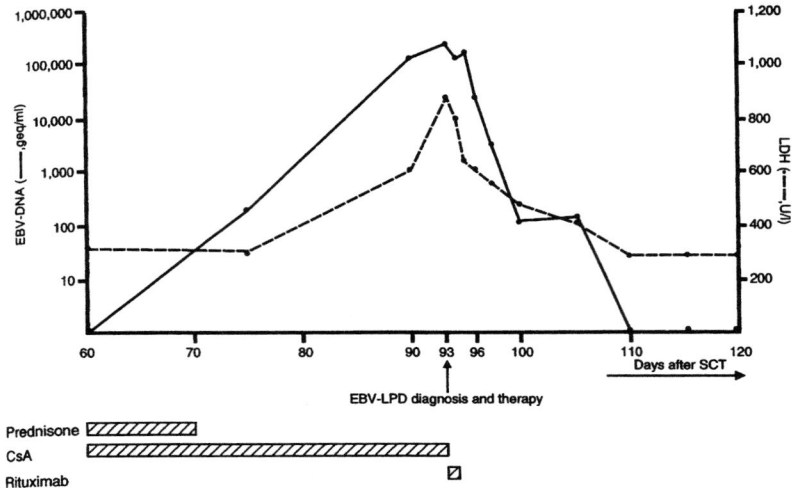

Fig. 74.6. EBV DNA levels and LDH in patient #14 who developed EBV-LPD at d 93 after allogeneic SCT for multiple myeloma and was treated using anti-CD20 immunotherapy. Reproduced, with permission, from van Esser et al. (2001b).

Human herpesvirus type 6 (HHV-6)

Human herpesvirus 6 (HHV-6) exists in two subtypes that differ from each other in 4–8% of their DNA. Subtype B is the cause of exanthem subitum in childhood. It is unclear what if any disease is caused by primary infection of subtype A. Since this infection is very common early in life, the rate of seropositivity in adults is very high (more than 95%).

Clinical picture

HHV-6 reactivates early after transplantation and up to 40% of patients are HHV-6 PCR-positive during the first month after transplant (Wang et al., 1996). The peak in viral load also occurs within the first four weeks (Ljungman et al., 2000). It has been reported that patients receiving peripheral blood stem cell transplants are more frequently PCR-positive than patients receiving bone marrow grafts (Maeda et al., 2000).

HHV-6 has been associated with skin rashes, interstitial pneumonia, encephalitis, hepatitis, and bone marrow suppression after SCT (Carrigan et al., 1991; Drobyski et al., 1993; Carrigan & Knox, 1995; Wang et al., 1999; Ljungman et al., 2000; Zerr et al., 2001). The best documented pathology caused by HHV-6 is encephalitis. HHV-6 has a propensity for the central nervous system (Caserta et al., 1994; Challoner et al., 1995), and although HHV-6 DNA can occasionally be detected in the CSF of asymptomatic SCT recipients (Wang et al., 1999; Zerr et al., 2001), several studies have shown that HHV-6 is an important cause of encephalitis in allogeneic SCT recipients (Drobyski et al., 1994; Mookerjee & Vogelsang, 1997; Bosi et al., 1998; Rieux et al., 1998; Zerr et al., 2001). The symptoms are frequently uncharacteristic including lethargy, confusion, convulsions, and decreased consciousness, but focal neurological changes has also been reported. Analysis of CSF frequently shows increased protein levels but pleocytosis is rare (Zerr et al., 2001). Magnetic resonance imaging can show abnormalities, but it can also be normal. EEG usually

Table 74.4. *Incidence of Epstein-Barr virus lymphoproliferative disease by viral load following allogeneic T-cell depleted SCT*

EBV load (gEq/ml)	No. of patients with specified reactivation	No. of patients with EBV-LPD	Predictive values	
			Positive (%)	Negative (%)
100	41	10	24	100
1,000	26	10	39	100
10,000	14	7	50	
100,000	7	5	71	94
500,000	1	1	100	89

Abbreviations: SCT, stem cell transplantation; gEq/ml, genome equivalents of EBV DNA/ml; EBV-LPD, Epstein-Barr virus lymphoproliferative disease.

Reproduced, with permission, from van Esser *et al.* (2001a).

shows diffuse changes. The prognosis is poor unless the encephalitis is treated with antiviral drugs.

The other common manifestation of HHV-6 is bone marrow suppression. HHV-6 can infect hematopoietic progenitor cells and reduce colony formation (Burd, Knox, & Carrigan, 1993; Isomura *et al.*, 1997) HHV-6 has been associated with bone marrow suppression and graft rejection (Carrigan & Knox, 1994; Wang *et al.*, 1996). Increased levels of HHV-6 DNA are also associated with delayed platelet engraftment (Ljungman *et al.*, 2000).

In one study HHV-6 DNA was detected in the blood of 78% of allogeneic HSC transplant recipients (Ljungman *et al.*, 2000). Using quantitative PCR, the HHV-6 viral load was higher at 4 weeks posttransplant than at 8 or 12 weeks. Three patients had HHV-6 encephalitis and one had hepatitis. Recipients of HLA-mismatched family member or unrelated donor transplants had significantly higher levels than recipients of matched sibling transplants.

Diagnosis

There is no "gold standard" diagnostic test for HHV-6 infection. Serology is not helpful due to the very high rate of seropositivity in the population. The usefulness of virus isolation and qualitative PCR on peripheral blood is limited as a large proportion of patients become positive after transplantation (Wang *et al.*, 1996). Quantifying viral load might be helpful to better define the contribution of HHV-6 to posttransplant complications (Cone *et al.*, 1999; Ljungman *et al.*, 2000). Detection of HHV-6 DNA in CSF can occur, but is rare in immunocompromised patients without CNS symptoms. Therefore, the combination of symptoms of encephalitis with detection of HHV-6 DNA is highly suggestive of HHV-6 disease of the CNS. Detection of HHV-6 in other organs such as lungs or liver is much more difficult to interpret, and proof of invasive infection with detection of virus in tissue by, for example, immunohistochemistry (but not PCR), and pathologic changes consistent with viral infection without any other identified pathogen, is required to support the diagnosis of HHV-6 disease.

Prevention and therapy

There is no prospective published study on the use of antiviral prophylaxis against HHV-6, although in a retrospective study ganciclovir appeared effective (Tokimasa *et al.*, 2002). Wang *et al.* (1996) showed in an epidemiological study that patients who received high-dose acyclovir had lower HHV-6 DNA levels and were less likely to suffer from delayed marrow engraftment. In vitro studies show that ganciclovir, cidofovir, and foscarnet should be effective for treating HHV-6. Both ganciclovir and foscarnet have been reported as being effective against HHV-6 meningoencephalitis after SCT (Wang *et al.*, 1999; Zerr *et al.*, 2002), and ganciclovir for other HHV-6 manifestations including pneumonitis, thrombocytopenia, enterocolitis and/or HHV-6 copy number (Tokimasa *et al.*, 2002).

Respiratory viruses

Respiratory viruses such as respiratory syncytial virus (RSV), parainfluenza viruses, and influenza A and B are widespread in the community with major seasonal variations. Despite the fact that these viruses are so common, it is only in recent years that their role as pathogens in stem cell transplant patients has begun to be appreciated.

The frequency of respiratory virus infections varies between different studies. In a prospective study by the EBMT, the frequency of respiratory virus infections was only 4.3% in allogeneic and 0.4% in autologous transplant patients. This is much lower than has previously been reported from the M.D. Anderson Cancer Center (Whimbey *et al.*, 1996). There are several potential explanations for these differences. One is that the sampling for respiratory viruses might have varied between the participating centers. Another reason for variability is most likely the use of different diagnostic techniques at the participating centers. Virus isolation is more sensitive than antigen tests and it has been previously shown that the RSV viral load in respiratory specimens obtained from the upper airways of adults is frequently low and therefore false-negative antigen tests might result. However, infection in the lower respiratory tract is likely to be more accurately diagnosed, since the false-negativity rate is low when tests are performed on BAL fluid. The epidemiological situation in the local community has also been shown to influence the risk for infection in the SCT patients. It is therefore important to recognize that respiratory viruses can easily be spread nosocomially through immune competent staff and patient relatives, and outbreaks of both RSV and parainfluenza infections have been documented in transplant units (Zambon *et al.*, 1998; Mazzulli *et al.*, 1999; Jones *et al.*, 2000). The infections can be spread through the air by droplets, but are more commonly spread through the hands of staff. Thus, infection control measures are important in the control of respiratory infections.

The influence on transplant-related mortality has been estimated in the EBMT study: 1.1% of allogeneic patients transplanted at the participating centers died of the infection (Ljungman *et al.*, 2001c). It is interesting to compare this figure with the risk of mortality in CMV infection: in a large randomized study comparing valaciclovir to acyclovir, the overall CMV-associated mortality was 2.2% (Ljungman *et al.*, 2002a).

The Centers for Disease Control (2000) in the USA have recommended that healthcare workers and visitors with symptoms of an upper respiratory tract infection be restricted from contact with HSC recipients and candidates undergoing conditioning treatment in order to minimize the risk of CRV transmission. To screen HSC transplant recipients for CRVs, active clinical surveillance for CRV disease should be conducted on all hospitalized HSC patients undergoing conditioning. This should include daily checking for signs and symptoms of CRV infection. (In some centers the transplant is postponed if symptoms are present or if the result of an RSV rapid assay is positive).

Respiratory syncytial virus

Over the last decade RSV has been the cause of several out-breaks of respiratory virus infection in SCT patients, forcing closure of transplant units and enforcement of strict infection control measures (Garcia *et al.*, 1997). Harrington *et al.* (1992) described an outbreak at the Fred Hutchinson Cancer Research Center in which 31 cases of RSV infections were documented and the overall mortality was 45%. Eighteen patients developed pneumonia and the mortality in patients with pneumonia was 78%. Whimbey *et al.* (1996) described 33 patients with an over-all mortality of 37%. In the prospective survey by the EBMT, the overall mortality in patients with a RSV lower respiratory tract infection was 30% and the RSV-associated mortality 17%.

Several studies have analyzed risk factors for progression to lower respiratory tract disease. The outcome is worse after allo-geneic than after autologous transplantation. The group at M.D. Anderson has reported that infections occurring pre-engraft-ment have a worse prognosis (Whimbey *et al.*, 1996). This was not found in other studies (McCarthy *et al.*, 1999; Ljungman *et al.*, 2001c). In the EBMT study the most important risk factor for lower respiratory tract disease was lymphocytopenia (Ljungman *et al.*, 2001c).

Prevention and therapy

No study has been performed regarding prevention of infection with RSV in SCT recipients and no controlled study has been performed with pre-emptive therapy to prevent lower respira-tory tract disease after detection of an upper respiratory tract infection. In a small phase I study of the RSV monoclonal anti-body palivizumab, three patients were treated for an upper res-piratory tract infection and none developed lower respiratory tract disease (Boeckh *et al.*, 2001). Another pre-emptive ther-apy option is ribavirin. No controlled study has been published and results of non-controlled studies are inconclusive. Ghosh *et al.* (2000) treated 14 patients with the combination of ribavirin and high-dose IVIG, and 4 of 14 patients developed pneumo-nia. In a prospective survey, no regimen was superior to any other or to no therapy (Ljungman *et al.*, 2001c), strongly sup-porting the necessity for controlled studies. One such study comparing aerosolized ribavirin with placebo is ongoing.

Only uncontrolled phase II studies of treatment of RSV dis-ease have been performed. In the series by Harrington *et al.* (1992), 13 patients with pneumonia were treated with aerosolized ribavirin and four patients survived. Whimbey *et al.* (1995) combined aerosolized ribavirin with a high titer anti-RSV immune globulin and showed that patients, who were treated with the combination before respiratory failure developed, had a mortality rate of 31%. However, patients who had therapy insti-tuted when ventilatory support was necessary, had a mortality of 100%. DeVincenzo *et al.* (2000) reported 11 children treated with a high-titer anti-RSV immune globulin in combination with ribavirin. Ten of 11 children survived (91%). On the other hand, McCarthy *et al.* (1999) reported 26 patients with RSV infections and no apparent effect on outcome with ribavirin therapy.

Lewinsohn *et al.* (1996) studied intravenous ribavirin in 10 patients in a phase I study but the results were poor. Ljungman *et al.* (2001c) reported in a prospective but non-controlled study similar outcomes with ribavirin given intravenously and as aerosol. Controlled studies are needed to assess the best thera-peutic option for RSV lower respiratory tract infections.

Parainfluenza viruses

Parainfluenza viruses can cause severe and fatal infections after SCT, although the mortality seems to be lower than for RSV (Ljungman *et al.*, 1989b; Wendt *et al.*, 1992; Nichols *et al.*, 2001a). The subtype most associated with severe infections is type 3 (Ljungman *et al.*, 1989b; Wendt *et al.*, 1992; Lews *et al.*, 1996; Nichols *et al.*, 2001a). In a retrospective study from the Seattle group, unrelated donor transplantation was the only identified risk factor for parainfluenza infection (Nichols *et al.*, 2001a). Furthermore, the dose of corticosteroids at the time of parainfluenza infection acquisition was the most important fac-tor associated with the development of parainfluenza type 3 pneumonia, both among allogeneic and autologous HSCT recipients. Parainfluenza infection was also an independent predictor of mortality (Nichols *et al.*, 2001a).

Prevention and therapy

The usefulness of antiviral therapy is still to be determined. The currently available antiviral agent is ribavirin. Wendt *et al.* (1992) and Nichols *et al.* (2001a) both failed to find any effect of ribavirin therapy. Other studies have shown some indication of effectiveness by ribavirin therapy (Lewis *et al.*, 1996; Ljungman, 1997; Sparrelid *et al.*, 1997). Lewis reported five patients treated with aerosolized ribavirin, three before respiratory failure devel-oped; all 3 survived while two patients who required ventilator support both died (Lewis *et al.*, 1996). Sparrelid described sev-eral cases in which ribavirin seemed to be effective in ventilator-dependent patients (Sparrelid *et al.*, 1997).

Influenza viruses

Influenza is an important infection to consider in SCT recipi-ents since it is common and has capacity to cause significant morbidity and mortality. Whimbey *et al.* (1994) reported a mortality of 17% in a series from M.D. Anderson Cancer Center. In a study from the EBMT, the influenza-associated mortality was 15%, with no difference between allogeneic and autologous SCT recipients, confirming that influenza is a potentially serious disease in all SCT recipients (Ljungman *et al.*, 2001c). Fatal influenza infections can occur several years after an allogeneic SCT, in particular in patients with chronic GVHD, and this should be kept in mind when preventive strate-gies are considered.

Prevention and therapy

The primary mode for prevention of influenza is vaccination. The main problem is the poor response to vaccination if given early after transplantation. Vaccination was shown to be ineffective in eliciting a protective antibody response if given earlier than 6 months after allogeneic and autologous SCT (Engelhard *et al.*, 1993). Influenza vaccination is recommended both by the EBMT and the CDC and should be given to all SCT transplant patients at 6 months after transplantation and yearly while patients are immunosuppressed (Ljungman, 1999; Centers for Disease Control, 2000). Pauksen *et al.* (2000) in a randomized trial found a slight but significant advantage for the addition of GM-CSF to vaccination. In the prospective EBMT study, vaccinated patients developed severe and even fatal infections, supporting the consideration that vaccination should also be given to family members and hospital staff, in order to reduce the risk for transmission of influenza (Ljungman *et al.*, 2001c). Seasonal influenza vaccination is strongly recommended for all healthcare workers in contact with HSC transplant patients. Lifelong seasonal influenza vaccination is recommended for all HSC transplant candidates and recipients, beginning with the influenza season before transplant and resuming >6 months posttransplant.

The possibilities for prevention with antiviral agents include amantadine and rimantadine and the new neuramidase inhibitors, zanamivir and oseltamivir. Amantadine and rimantadine have been effective in the elderly (non-transplant) population, but the rate of development of resistance is rapid and, although anecdotal reports exist, it is not possible from these case reports to assess their usefulness. No controlled study has been performed of either prevention or therapy of influenza in SCT patients. However, the CDC recommends amantadine or rimantadine as prophylaxis during community outbreaks to patients less than 6 months after a SCT (Centers for Disease Control, 2000). Amantadine, rimantadine, ribavirin (Hayden *et al.*, 1996), and the neuramidase inhibitors could be used for therapy of severe influenza infections but there is currently no information regarding these drugs' effectiveness after hematopoietic stem cell transplantation.

Adenoviruses

Adenoviruses cause a number of clinical syndromes in immune competent individuals that are usually mild and self-limiting including conjunctivitis, hemorrhagic cystitis, gastroenteritis and upper respiratory tract infections. However, more severe manifestations have also been reported including hepatitis, nephritis, meningoencephalitis and pneumonia. Although 51 distinct Ad serotypes, which have been classified into subgroups A–F, have been identified, most human disease is associated with only one-third of these types. Depending on the serotype, there are considerable differences in the tissue specificity and virulence of adenoviruses.

Adenovirus infections have been associated with morbidity and mortality after allogeneic SCT. The frequency of adenovirus infections has varied greatly between different studies. Shields *et al.* (1985) reported a 5% frequency. Flomenberg *et al.* (1994) reported a frequency of 21%, with a higher frequency in children (31%) than in adults (13.6%). Similarly

Wasserman *et al.* (1998) reported a frequency of 18% in a pediatric population. La Rosa *et al.* (2001) reported a frequency of 3% among 2,889 adult bone marrow transplant patients transplanted at the M.D. Anderson Cancer Center.

The most severe disease manifestations are pneumonia, encephalitis, and fulminant hepatitis, but hemorrhagic cystitis and gastroenteritis are more common. Risk factors for disease are children as compared to adults (Howard *et al.*, 1999), allogeneic transplantation (Howard *et al.*, 1999; La Rosa *et al.*, 2001), total body irradiation (Hale *et al.*, 1999), isolation from more than one site (Flomenberg *et al.*, 1994; Howard *et al.*, 1999), acute GVHD (Flomenberg *et al.*, 1994), unrelated donor transplantation (Baldwin *et al.*, 2000), and in vivo T-cell depletion using Campath-1H (Chakrabarti *et al.*, 2002). In the latter study, severe lymphocytopenia (<300/µl) at the time of first detection of adenovirus was a major risk factor for the development of adenovirus disease, as was failure to reduce immune suppression and a positive adenovirus PCR result in bood. The risk for invasive disease has varied between 1% and 7% in the published studies (Shields *et al.*, 1985; Flomenberg *et al.*, 1994; Baldwin *et al.*, 2000; La Rosa *et al.*, 2001). The mortality has also varied between the different studies. Shields reported a mortality of 8% in patients with documented adenovirus infections, Baldwin of 6%, and La Rosa reported an overall mortality of 26%. There are several problems associated with comparing more recent results with results from older studies. The most important is that more patients today undergo high-risk transplantation with unrelated or haplo-mismatched family member donors. Another problem regarding the reported risks for disease and outcome is that there is no established definition for invasive disease, and different authors have used different definitions. It seems logical to use definitions similar to the established definitions for CMV disease, requiring proof of tissue involvement with adenovirus together with appropriate symptoms and signs for proven invasive disease, and detection of adenovirus from stool or urine together with symptoms, but without proven tissue invasion, as a definition for possible disease.

Diagnostic techniques

Serology is of limited value in the early post-SCT period because of variable ability of patients to mount an antibody response to infection, and passive acquisition of antibody from blood products or intravenous immunoglobulin.

Biopsies, BAL fluid, or CSF should be tested for adenovirus in the setting of disseminated disease. Other specimens that could be tested for adenovirus are blood, urine, and throat secretions, with the aim of providing background for possible pre-emptive therapy with antiviral agents (see below).

Many diagnostic tests for adenoviruses have been developed that are based on conventional culture in epitheloid cell lines, IF, or radioimmunoassay (RIA) (Ray & Minnich, 1987; Torres & Vicente, 1992). However, more specific identification of adenoviruses usually relies, after initial detection by one or more of the above adenovirus genus-specific tests, on cell culture-based type-specific neutralization (Hierholzer *et al.*, 1989) or restriction enzyme analysis of DNA extracted from infected cells (Kajon & Wadell, 1994). These assays have been used successfully to classify adenoviruses, but they can be time-consuming and depend on a sufficient yield of infectious viruses. Consequently, although epidemiologically useful, these assays are not suitable for rapid and sensitive identification of adenoviruses.

PCR assays have now been developed for the rapid and sensitive identification of adenoviruses (Allard et al., 1990, 1994, 2001). Although PCR assays have proved comparable to, or better than, classic cell culture or immunodiagnostic assays for the identification of adenoviruses, each of the assays has its own limitations for clinical and epidemiological purposes.

Prevention and treatment

Currently there is no established effective prophylaxis or therapy for adenovirus infections in SCT recipients. Anecdotal cases have been published of the use of IVIG (Flomenberg et al., 1994). Ribavirin has been used in case reports with varying outcome (Cassano, 1991; Liles et al., 1993; Hromas et al., 1994; Kapelushnik et al., 1995; Mann et al., 1998; Chakrabarti et al., 1999; Baldwin et al., 2000; Miyamura et al., 2000). La Rosa et al. (2001) showed no appreciable impact of ribavirin therapy in 12 patients, of whom only 2 survived. Bordigoni et al. (2001) treated 13 patients with definite (3), probable (5) disease, or asymptomatic infection with ribavirin. Only 3 of these 13 patients survived. Cidofovir might have efficacy against adenovirus infections, but no controlled studies have been performed in SCT recipients. Legrand et al. (2001) reported 7 children treated with cidofovir for adenovirus gastrointestinal disease. The infection resolved in five, one patient died of progressive adenovirus disease, and one patient died of aspergillosis. The Infectious Diseases Working Party of the EBMT, in a retrospective study of 29 patients given cidofovir therapy for proven or possible adenovirus disease, found a success rate of 69% (Ljungman et al., 2001b).

It has been suggested, analogous to the situation for CMV, that detection of adenovirus in blood is a risk factor for development of disseminated disease. Therefore, pre-emptive therapy against adenovirus has been proposed. In the EBMT study, pre-emptive therapy was used in 16 patients with a success rate of 87% (Ljungman et al., 2001b). However, prospective studies are needed.

Since adenovirus disease is associated with severe immune incompetence, the use of adenovirus-specific CTL has been proposed and adenovirus-specific CTL have been produced in vitro (Regn et al., 2001). However, no clinical study has been performed, although the use of donor leucocyte infusions has been reported (Hromas et al., 1994b).

Hepatitis B virus (HBV) (and see Chapter 89)

Hepatitis B virus (HBV) infections are common in many countries and therefore patients or their donors might be HBV antibody- or antigen-positive pretransplant. In patients who are HBsAg-positive before transplantation, there does not seem to be an markedly increased risk of severe liver complications after transplantation (Reed et al., 1991; Locasciulli et al., 1995), and long-term survival is similar in HBV-positive and negative patients (Lau et al., 1997a), although patients are potentially at risk for VOD, fulminant hepatitis and chronic hepatitis (see Table 69.4 and Chapter 69). Patients who are anti-HBs positive at the time of transplant can become HBsAg and HBV-DNA positive during long-term follow-up, because of loss of specific antibodies to HBV. However, long-term data are not available for assessing, for example, the risk of developing hepatocellular carcinoma in SCT patients positive for HBsAg.

Prevention and therapy

In a seronegative recipient, the use of an HBV antigen-positive marrow donor should, if possible, be avoided, since risk of transfer of HBV is high and hepatitis is likely to develop (Lau et al., 2000). However, if a seropositive donor must be used, vaccination of the patient before transplant is logical since Locasciulli et al. (1995) showed that patients who are antibody-positive to HBV before transplant were less likely to develop severe liver complications. HBV specific immune globulin can also be given to the patient before transplantation (Locasciulli et al., 1995).

There are two antiviral agents with efficacy against HBV that can be used for prevention of severe HBV in seropositive SCT patients—famciclovir and lamivudine. In one study of 8 HBV-positive patients and 24 historical controls, famciclovir reduced the risk for posttransplant hepatitis (Lau et al., 1998b). Lamivudine has also been used in SCT patients to prevent reactivation (Picardi et al., 1998; Uchida et al., 2000; Endo et al., 2001; Nakagawa et al., 2002); Ohnishi et al., 2002). However, the long-term outcome is uncertain and additional studies are needed. Another interesting observation, demonstrating the effect of donor immunity in control of viral infections in the recipient, is that the use of HBV-immune donors can result in clearance of HBV in HBsAg positive recipients (Ilan et al., 1993, 1994, 2000; Lau et al., 1997b, 1998a).

Hepatitis C virus (HCV) (and see Chapter 89)

Hepatitis C virus is the major agent causing parenteral non-A, non-B hepatitis. If the marrow donor is HCV RNA positive, the risk for transmission to the patient is very high, although the resulting hepatitis is usually not severe (Shuhart et al., 1994). Patients with HCV and abnormal liver function tests have been reported to have an increased risk for VOD (Locasciulli et al., 1999; Strasser et al., 1999a). HCV-infected patients surviving more than 20 years after allogeneic SCT have a very high risk for development of liver cirrhosis (Strasser et al., 1999b).

Prevention and treatment

The use of an HCV positive donor should be avoided if alternatives exist. Alpha-interferon with the addition of ribavirin is the treatment of choice in immune competent individuals and, if there is time, treatment of the intended donor should be considered. One case report has been published in which an HCV RNA positive donor was treated for 6 months. RNA-negativity was obtained and no transmission to the recipient occurred after transplantation (Vance *et al.*, 1996).

In a small pilot study of four patients who were HCV-positive, ribavirin given orally was given through the pancytopenic phase posttransplant without severe side-effects, and three of these patients became HCV-negative during long-term follow-up (Ljungman *et al.*, 1996).

Since the risk for cirrhosis is high in long-term survivors, therapy with interferon, with or without ribavirin, may be indicated. Two small series have been published, both showing that the therapy is feasible without severe side-effects, and can result in HCV-RNA negativity and a reduction of the inflammatory score in liver biopsies (Ljungman *et al.*, 1995; Giardini *et al.*, 1997). However, whether therapy will change the long-term outcome and thereby reduce the risk for late complications is presently unknown.

Measles

Measles can be fatal in immunocompromised hosts (Kaplan *et al.*, 1992; Breitfeld *et al.*, 1973). Until recently, the good vaccination coverage in the general population in Europe and the USA has reduced the risk of outbreaks. However, during the last few years the vaccination rates of children in several countries have decreased. Recently a large epidemic of 15,000 cases was reported from Italy, and smaller outbreaks have been reported from several countries. This is relevant since occasional severe cases have been reported in SCT recipients (Nakano *et al.*, 1996; Machado *et al.*, 2002). Most patients will lose immunity during extended follow-up and are therefore vulnerable to infection (Ljungman *et al.*, 1994b).

Machado *et al.* (2002) reported eight cases of measles occurring during a large epidemic of measles in São Paolo, Brasil. One of the eight patients developed a severe infection but all survived. Vaccination against measles have been shown to be safe and effective in patients without GVHD or ongoing immunosuppression (Ljungman *et al.*, 1989a).

Parvovirus B19

Parvovirus B19 exhibits a marked tropism for human bone marrow and replicates only in erythroid cells. It is transmissible by the respiratory route or by blood. Infection may cause a number of hematologic complications including aplasia, chronic anemia, and idiopathic thrombocytopenic purpura. Occasional case reports of protracted parvovirus infections have been published after stem cell transplantation (Heegaard & Laub Petersen, 2000; Kaptan *et al.*, 2001).

Human papilloma virus

A case has been described of a recipient of an autologous blood stem cell transplant for non-Hodgkin's lymphoma who had several flat warts on his right hand, which had shown no progression during conventional dose chemotherapy. On day 15 posttransplant the warts began to develop and spread to his forehead and face, neck, and arms over several days. Human papilloma virus type 3 was detected by PCR analysis (Maruyama *et al.*, 1996).

Papovaviruses

Papovaviruses are a group of DNA-viruses with two members—JC virus and BK virus—that can be pathogenic in SCT patients. JC virus is the agent causing progressive multifocal leukoencephalopathy (PML) and BK-virus has been implicated in hemorrhagic cystitis and nephropathy in transplant recipients. Both BK and JC polyoma viruses are excreted in the urine of many patients following transplant. Papoviruria has been associated with hemorrhagic cystitis. In one study, hemorrhagic cystitis occurred in 19 of 38 (50%) with persistent BK viruria, in 1 of 12 (8.3%) with only a single urine sample positive for BK virus, and in none of 45 who did not excrete BK virus ($P < .001$). Shedding of BK virus also had a strong temporal correlation with the onset of hemorrhagic cystitis (R = .95) (Bedi *et al.*, 1995). In another study, quantitative PCR was used to evaluate BK viruria (Leung *et al.*, 2001). When compared with asymptomatic patients, those with hemorrhagic cystitis had a significantly higher peak BK viruria, but no detectable increase in BK viremia. Other studies, however, have not found a relationship with human polyoma virus infection and hemorrhagic cystitis (Azzi *et al.*, 1994; Bogdanovic *et al.*, 1996). Furthermore, several other viruses such as adenovirus and CMV have been shown to cause hemorrhagic cystitis. Thus, the association is still somewhat controversial.

Case reports have been published regarding antiviral therapy of polyomavirus infections with vidarabine or cidofovir. In one case report of polyoma virus–associated hemorrhagic cystitis, a dramatic response occurred with the use of vidarabine 10 mg/kg daily for 5 days given as a 12-hour infusion (Chapman, Flower, & Durrant, 1991). Cidofovir is active in vitro against polyomaviruses such as BK and JC viruses and was reported to be effective against polyoma virus–associated HC (Held *et al.*, 2000).

Rotavirus

Rotaviruses are icosahedral, spherical particles containing double-stranded RNA. They are divided into five groups, A to E, and also into different subtypes. Rotavirus infections mostly affect otherwise normal children less than 3 years of age. Reinfection in adults can occur. The symptoms are usually diarrhea and vomiting. In BMT recipients, gastroenteritis caused by rotavirus has been described (Yolken *et al.*, 1982). Electron microscopy and ELISA (enzyme-linked immunosorbent assay) can confirm the diagnosis. There is no proven effective treatment, although two cases described by Kanfer *et al.* (1994) appeared to respond to oral immunoglobulin (6 g daily for 5 days).

Coxsackie virus

Coxsackie virus is a picornavirus. Different clinical syndromes include meningitis, hand-foot-mouth syndrome, conjunctivitis, herpangina, pleuritis, myalgias, and myocarditis. In BMT patients Coxsackie A1 virus infection with diarrhea and a significant mortality has been reported (Yolken *et al.*, 1982). The diagnosis can be obtained by virus isolation from stool, cerebrospinal fluid, secretions from nose and pharynx, tears, or urine, and by serology. Prolonged enteroviral infection has been described in a BMT recipient who developed pericarditis and heart failure posttransplant. Enterovirus was detected in two samples of pleural fluid antimortem and in lungs, liver, and spleen at postmortem (Galama *et al.*, 1996).

Human immunodeficiency virus

Prior to the era of blood product screening for HIV, several cases of AIDS were reported in marrow transplant recipients. No such infections have been reported since the introduction of routine screening for HIV.

The reservoirs for HIV (T cells, monocytes, macrophages, dendritic cells) are replaced by cells of donor origin posttransplant. Syngeneic and allogeneic bone marrow transplantation, together with concomitant antiviral therapy, has been used therapeutically in AIDS patients but with limited success The advent of highly-active anti-retroviral therapy (HAART) is, however, enabling the re-exploration of such approaches: nine patients with HIV-associated Hodgkin's disease or non-Hodgkin's lymphoma were given a high-dose chemotherapy conditioning regimen of cyclophosphamide, BCNU, and etoposide followed by autologous G-CSF–mobilized peripheral blood stem cells. Seven of the nine remained in remission of the lymphoma at a median of 19 months posttransplant (Krishnan *et al.*, 2001). Non-myeloablative conditioning has been used prior to HLA-identical sibling PBSC transplantation for hematologic malignancies in two patients with concomitant HIV infection (Kang *et al.*, 2002) (see Chapter 121)

Human T-cell leukemia/lymphoma virus

Both human T-cell leukemia/lymphoma virus (HTLV)-1 and HTLV-2 can be transmitted through blood transfusions. HTLV-1 is the causative agent of adult T-cell leukemia/lymphoma (ATLL). In a study using ELISA technology a seroprevalence of HTLV in 1 of 317 patients (0.3%) prior to marrow transplantation was documented (Loughran & Shriver, 1994). A patient given an HLA-matched unrelated donor transplant for aplastic anemia, who acquired HTLV-1 infection from a pretransplant blood transfusion, developed HTLV-associated myelopathy with motor weakness and a neurogenic bladder 3 years posttransplant. HTLV-1 sequences were amplified from the cerebrospinal fluid (Emmanouilides & Territo, 1999). Kikuchi *et al.* (2000) described a case of HTLV-1 infection transmitted by

bone marrow transplantation. Antibodies were detected in the recipient's serum 12 days posttransplant. Allogeneic HSC transplantation has been used successfully to treat ATLL caused by HTLV infection (see Chapter 51).

Vaccination against viral infections

Vaccination is an important tool for protection against viral infections. Pretransplant immunity is frequently lost to many viruses such as measles, mumps, rubella, and poliovirus after SCT. A study of 124 patients who had survived at least 2 years after allogeneic BMT showed that most allogeneic transplant recipients become seronegative for measles, mumps, and rubella during follow-up (Ljungman *et al.*, 1994b). The calculated probabilities of being immune to measles at 3, 5, and 7 years posttransplant were 47%, 27%, and 20%, respectively. The corresponding probabilities for mumps were 37%, 12%, and 6%, respectively; and for rubella 47%, 33%, and 28%, respectively. Thus, long-term B-cell memory function is not maintained, regardless of the immune status of the donor (Ljungman *et al.*, 1994b).

Both the European Group for Blood and Marrow Transplantation and the CDC have developed recommendations for vaccination of stem cell transplant recipients (Ljungman *et al.*, 1995; Ljungman, 1999; Centers for Disease Control, 2000). It is important to weigh risk and benefit of vaccination (Table 74.5). Vaccination containing inactivated viruses, subunit vaccines, and recombinant DNA vaccines can be given safely. Recommended viral vaccines include HBV, influenza, and poliovirus. The effectiveness of vaccination is poor early after transplantation (Engelhard *et al.*, 1993; Pauksen *et al.*, 2000), but starts to improve after approximately 6 months (Parkkali *et al.*, 1997). To achieve an optimal vaccination response, repeated doses usually have to be administered (Ljungman *et al.*, 1991). An interesting option to improve the early vaccination response after SCT is to vaccinate the stem cell donor before transplantation. This strategy has been explored for HBV and it was shown that donor immunity could be transferred to the recipients and then boosted by early posttransplant vaccinations (Ilan *et al.*, 1994).

The risk of severe side effects exists when live, attenuated viral vaccines are used. It is therefore important to weigh risks and potential benefits. Measles, mumps, and rubella (MMR) vaccine has been given safely to patients at two years after SCT without chronic GVHD or ongoing immune suppression (Ljungman *et al.*, 1989a, 1994b; King *et al.*, 1996). Live varicella vaccine has been administered to occasional patients without severe side effects (Sauerbrei *et al.*, 1997), but is currently not recommended by either the CDC or the EBMT. (An inactivated varicella vaccine given before and after autologous transplantation appeared to offer protection from zoster infection [Hata *et al.* 2002]). Live poliovirus vaccine should not be used in stem cell transplant patients. It is also important that hospital staff taking care of SCT patients and family members of SCT patients should not receive live poliovirus vaccine.

Table 74.5. *Recommendations for vaccination against viral infections*

Vaccine	Schedule	Comments
Influenza	Yearly staring at 4–6 months after SCT	Poor effectiveness early after SCT. Family members and staff taking care of SCT patients should be vaccinated.
Inactivated poliovirus	Three doses starting at 6–12 months after SCT	
Hepatitis B virus	Three doses starting at 6–12 months after SCT	The indication for HBV vaccination depends on the epidemiological situation for HBV in the individual country. Donor vaccination may be indicated in certain situations.
Hepatitis A virus	Schedule not defined	Safe, can be considered in patients that might become exposed.
Measles[a]	1–2 doses starting at 24 months after SCT	Only to patients without GVHD or ongoing immunosuppression.
Rubella[a]	1 dose starting at 24 months after SCT	Individual patient consideration, e.g., females with pregnancy potential. Only to patients without GVHD or ongoing immunosuppression.
Mumps[a]	Usually not indicated unless included in the MMR vaccine	Individual patient consideration. Only to patients without GVHD or ongoing immunosuppression
Varicella[a]	Usually not indicated	Not before 24 months after SCT. If used, it should only be given to seronegative patients without GVHD or ongoing immunosuppression.
Other live vaccines	Usually not indicated	Risk/benefit ratio has to favor vaccination.

Abbreviations: SCT, stem cell transplantation; HBV, hepatitis B virus; GVHD, graft-versus-host disease; MMR, measles-mumps-rubella. Adapted from Ljungman (1999) and Centers for Disease Control (2000). [a] Live virus vaccines.

Other live vaccines include yellow fever, but this vaccine is not recommended for immunosuppressed patients.

References

Allard, A., Albinsson, B., & Wadell, G. (2001). Rapid typing of human adenoviruses by a general PCR combined with restriction endonuclease analysis. *Journal of Clinical Microbiology, 39,* 498–505.

Allard, A., Girones, R., Juto, P., & Wadell, G. (1990). Polymerase chain reaction for detection of adenoviruses in stool samples. *Journal of Clinical Microbiology, 28,* 2659–2667.

Allard, A., Kajon, A., & Wadell, G. (1994). Simple procedure for discrimination and typing of enteric adenoviruses after detection by polymerase chain reaction. *Journal of Medical Virology, 44,* 250–257.

Aschan, J., Ringdén, O., Ljungman, P., Lönnqvist, B., & Ohlman, S. (1992). Foscarnet for treatment of cytomegalovirus infections in bone marrow transplant recipients. *Scandinavian Journal of Infectious Diseases, 24,* 143–150.

Avery, R. K., Adal, K. A., Longworth, D. L., & Bolwell, B. J. (2000). A survey of allogeneic bone marrow transplant programs in the United States regarding cytomegalovirus prophylaxis and preemptive therapy. *Bone Marrow Transplantation, 26,* 763–767.

Azzi, A., Fanci, R., Bosi, A. *et al.* (1994). Monitoring of polyomavirus BK viruria in bone marrow transplantation patients by DNA hybridization assay and by polymerase chain reaction: an approach to assess the relationship between BK viruria and hemorrhagic cystitis. *Bone Marrow Transplantation, 14,* 235–240.

Bacigalupo, A., Bregante, S., Tedone, E. *et al.* (1996). Combined foscarnet-ganciclovir treatment for cytomegalovirus infections after allogeneic hemopoietic stem cell transplantation. *Transplantation, 62,* 376–380.

Bacigalupo, A., Tedone, E., Sanna, M. A. *et al.* (1992). CMV infections following allogeneic BMT: risk factors, early treatment and correlation with transplant related mortality. *Haematologica, 77,* 507–513.

Bacigalupo, A., Tedone, E., Van Lint, M. T. *et al.* (1994). CMV prophylaxis with foscarnet in allogeneic bone marrow transplants recipients at high risk of developing CMV infections. *Bone Marrow Transplantation, 13,* 783–788.

Baldwin, A., Kingman, H., Darville, M. *et al.* (2000). Outcome and clinical course of 100 patients with adenovirus infection following bone marrow transplantation. *Bone Marrow Transplantation, 26,* 1333–1338.

Bass, E., Powe, N., Goodman, S. *et al.* (1993). Efficacy of immune globulin in preventing complications of bone marrow transplantation: a meta-analysis. *Bone Marrow Transplantation, 12,* 179–183.

Bedi, A., Miller, C. B., Hanson, J. L. *et al.* (1995). Association of BK virus with failure of prophylaxis against hemorrhagic cystitis following bone marrow transplantation. *Journal of Clinical Oncology, 13,* 1103–9.

Boeckh, M., Bowden, R. A., Goodrich, J. M., Pettinger, M., & Meyers, J. D. (1992). Cytomegalovirus antigen detection in peripheral blood leukocytes after allogeneic marrow transplantation. *Blood, 80,* 1358–1364.

Boeckh, M., Berrey, M. M., Bowden, R. A. *et al.* (2001). Phase 1 evaluation of the respiratory syncytial virus-specific monoclonal antibody palivizumab in recipients of hematopoietic stem cell transplants. *Journal of Infectious Diseases, 184,* 350–354.

Boeckh, M., Gooley, T. A., Myerson, D. *et al.* (1996a). Cytomegalovirus pp65 antigenemia-guided early treatment with ganciclovir versus ganciclovir at engraftment after allogeneic marrow transplantation: a randomized double-blind study. *Blood, 88,* 4063–4071.

Boeckh, M., Leisenring, W., Riddell, S. R. *et al.* (2003). Late cytomegalovirus disease and mortality in recipients of allogeneic hematopoietic stem cell transplants; importance of viral load and T cell immunity. *Blood, 101,* 407–14.

Boeckh, M., Gooley, T. A., Reusser, P., Buckner, C. D., & Bowden, R. A. (1995). Failure of high-dose acyclovir to prevent cytomegalovirus disease after autologous marrow transplantation. *Journal of Infectious Diseases*, **172**, 939–943.

Boeckh, M., Riddell, S., Cunningham, T. *et al.* (1996b). Increased risk of late CMV infection and disease in allogeneic marrow transplant recipients after ganciclovir prophylaxis is due to a lack of CMV-specific T cell responses. *Blood*, 302a.

Boeckh, M., Stevens, A. T., & Bowden, R. A. (1996c). Cytomegalovirus pp65 antigenemia after autologous marrow and peripheral blood stem cell transplantation. *Journal of Infectious Diseases*, **174**, 907–912.

Boeckh, M., Zaia, J. A., Jung, D. *et al.* (1998). A study of the pharmacokinetics, antiviral activity, and tolerability of oral ganciclovir for CMV prophylaxis in marrow transplantation. *Biol Blood Marrow Transplantation*, **4**, 13–19.

Boeckh, M., Bowden, R. A., Gooley, T., Myerson, D., & Corey, L. (1999). Successful modification of a pp65 antigenemia-based early treatment strategy for prevention of cytomegalovirus disease in allogeneic marrow transplant recipients. *Blood*, **93**, 1781–1782 (Letter).

Bogdanovic, G., Ljungman, P., Wang, F., & Dalianis, T. (1996). Presence of human polymavirus DNA in the peripheral circulation of bone marrow transplant patients with and without hemorrhagic cystitis. *Bone Marrow Transplantation*, **17**, 573–576.

Bordigoni, P., Carret, A. S., Venard, V., Witz, F., & Le Faou, A. (2001). Treatment of adenovirus infections in patients undergoing allogeneic hematopoietic stem cell transplantation. *Clinical Infectious Diseases*, **32**, 1290–1297.

Bosi, A., Zazzi, M., Amantini, A. *et al.* (1998). Fatal herpesvirus 6 encephalitis after unrelated bone marrow transplant. *Bone Marrow Transplantation*, **22**, 285–288.

Boström, L., Ringdén, O., Sundberg, B. *et al.* (1989). Pretransplant herpes virus serology and chronic graft-versus-host disease. *Bone Marrow Transplantation*, **4**, 547–552.

Bowden, R., Cays, M., Schoch, G. *et al.* (1995). Comparison of filtered blood (FB) to seronegative blood products (SB) for prevention of cytomegalovirus (CMV) infection after marrow transplant. *Blood*, **86**, 3598–3603.

Bowden, R. A., Fisher, L. D., Rogers, K., Cays, M., & Meyers, J. D. (1991a). Cytomegalovirus (CMV)-specific intravenous immunoglobulin for the prevention of primary CMV infection and disease after marrow transplant [see comments]. *Journal of Infectious Diseases*, **164**, 483–487.

Bowden, R. A., Sayers, M., Flournoy, N. *et al.* (1986). Cytomegalovirus immune globulin and seronegative blood products to prevent primary cytomegalovirus infection after marrow transplantation. *New England Journal of Medicine*, **314**, 1006–1010.

Bowden, R. A., Slichter, S. J., Sayers, M. H. *et al.* (1991b). Use of leukocyte-depleted platelets and cytomegalovirus-seronegative red blood cells for prevention of primary cytomegalovirus infection after marrow transplant. *Blood*, **78**, 246–250.

Breitfeld, V., Hashida, Y., Sherman, F. *et al.* (1973). Fatal measles infection in children with leukemia. *Laboratory Investigation*, **29**, 279–281.

Broers, A. E., van Der Holt, R., van Esser, J. W. *et al.* (2000). Increased transplant-related morbidity and mortality in CMV-seropositive patients despite highly effective prevention of CMV disease after allogeneic T-cell-depleted stem cell transplantation. *Blood*, **95**, 2240–2245.

Burd, E. M., Knox, K. K., & Carrigan, D. R. (1993). Human herpesvirus-6–associated suppression of growth factor-induced macrophage maturation in human bone marrow cultures. *Blood*, **81**, 1645–1650.

Carrigan, D. R., Drobyski, W. R., Russler, S. K. *et al.* (1991). Interstitial pneumonitis associated with human herpesvirus-6 infection after marrow transplantation. *Lancet*, **338**, 147–149.

Carrigan, D. R. & Knox, K. K. (1994). Human herpesvirus 6 (HHV-6) isolation from bone marrow: HHV-6-associated bone marrow suppression in bone marrow transplant patients. *Blood*, **84**, 3307–3310.

Carrigan, D. R. & Knox, K. K. (1995). Bone marrow suppression by human herpesvirus-6: comparison of the A and B variants of the virus. *Blood*, **86**, 835–836 (Letter; comment).

Caserta, M. T., Hall, C. B., Schnabel, K. *et al.* (1994). Neuroinvasion and persistence of human herpesvirus 6 in children. *Journal of Infectious Diseases*, **170**, 1586–1589.

Cassano, W. F. (1991). Intravenous ribavirin therapy for adenovirus cystitis after allogeneic bone marrow transplantation. *Bone Marrow Transplantation*, **7**, 247–248.

Centers for Disease Control (2000). Guidelines for preventing opportunistic infections among hematopoietic stem cell transplant recipients. Recommendations of CDC, the Infectious Disease Society of America, and the American Society of Blood and Marrow Transplantation. MMWR. *Morbidity and Mortality Weekly Report*, **49**, 1–125.

Chakrabarti, S., Collingham, K. E., Fegan, C. D., & Milligan, D. W. (1999). Fulminant adenovirus hepatitis following unrelated bone marrow transplantation: failure of intravenous ribavirin therapy. *Bone Marrow Transplantation*, **23**, 1209–1211.

Chakrabarti, S., Mautner, V., Osman, H. *et al.* (2002). Adenovirus infections following allogeneic stem cell transplantation: incidence and outcome in relation to graft manipulation, immunosuppression and immune recovery. *Blood*, **100**, 1619–27.

Chakrabarti, S., Pillay, D., Ratcliffe, D. *et al.* (2000). Resistence to antiviral drugs in herpes simplex virus infections among allogeneic stem cell transplant recipients: risk factors and prognostic significance. *Journal of Infectious Diseases*, **181**, 2055–2058.

Challoner, P. B., Smith, K. T., Parker, J. D. *et al.* (1995). Plaque-associated expression of human herpesvirus 6 in multiple sclerosis. *Proceedings of the National Academy of Sciences of the United States of America*, **92**, 7440–7444.

Chapman, C., Flower, A. J., & Durrant, S. T. (1991). The use of vidarabine in the treatment of human polyomavirus associated acute haemorrhagic cystitis. *Bone Marrow Transplantation*, **7**, 481–483.

Chen, Y., Scieux, C., Garrait, V. *et al.* (2000). Resistant herpes simplex virus type 1 infection: an emerging concern after allogeneic stem cell transplantation. *Clinical Infectious Diseases*, **31**, 927–935.

Cinque, P., Brytting, M., Vago, L. *et al.* (1993). Epstein-Barr virus DNA in cerebrospinal fluid from patients with AIDS-related primary lymphoma of the central nervous system. *Lancet*, **342**, 398–401.

Cinque, P., Vago, L., Brytting, M. *et al.* (1992). Cytomegalovirus infection of the central nervous system in patients with AIDS: diagnosis by DNA amplification from cerebrospinal fluid. *Journal of Infectious Diseases*, **166**, 1408–1411.

Cone, R. W., Huang, M. L., Corey, L. *et al.* (1999). Human herpesvirus 6 infections after bone marrow transplantation: clinical and virologic manifestations. *Journal of Infectious Diseases*, **179**, 311–318.

Craddock, C., Szydlo, R. M., Dazzi, F. *et al.* (2001). Cytomegalovirus seropositivity adversely influences outcome after T-depleted unrelated donor transplant in patients with chronic myeloid leukaemia: the case for tailored graft-versus-host disease prophylaxis. *British Journal of Haematology*, **112**, 228–236.

Crippa, F., Corey, L., Chuang, E. L., Sale, G., & Boeckh, M. (2001). Virological, clinical, and opthalmologic features of cytomegalovirus retinitis after hematopoietic stem cell transplantation. *Clinical Infectious Diseases*, **32**, 214–219.

Curtis, R. E., Travis, L. B., Rowlings, P. A. *et al.* (1999). Risk of lymphoproliferative disorders after bone marrow transplantation: a multi-institutional study. *Blood*, **94**, 2208–2216.

Cwynarski, K., Ainsworth, J., Cobbold, M. *et al.* (2001). Direct visualization of cytomegalovirus-specific T-cell reconstitution after allogeneic stem cell transplantation. *Blood*, **97**, 1232–1240.

Darville, J. M., Ley, B. E., Roome, A. P., & Foot, A. B. (1998). Acyclovir-resistant herpes simplex virus infections in a bone marrow transplant population. *Bone Marrow Transplantation*, **22**, 587–589.

Dellemijin, P. L., Brandenburg, A., Niesters, H. G. *et al.* (1995). Successful treatment with ganciclovir of presumed Epstein-Barr meningo-encephalitis following bone marrow transplant. *Bone Marrow Transplantation*, **16**, 311–312.

de Medeiros, C. R., Moreira, V. A., & Pasquini, R. (2000). Cytomegalovirus as a cause of very late interstitial pneumonia after bone marrow transplantation. *Bone Marrow Transplantation*, **26**, 443–4.

DeVincenzo, J. P., Hirsch, R. L., Fuentes, R. J., & Top, F. H., Jr. (2000). Respiratory syncytial virus immune globulin treatment of lower respiratory tract infection in pediatric patients undergoing bone marrow transplantation—a compassionate use experience. *Bone Marrow Transplantation*, **25**, 161–165.

Drobyski, W. R., Dunne, W. M., Burd, E. M. *et al.* (1993). Human herpesvirus-6 (HHV-6) infection in allogeneic bone marrow transplant recipients: evidence of a marrow-suppressive role for HHV-6 in vivo. *Journal of Infectious Diseases*, **167**, 735–739.

Drobyski, W. R., Knox, K. K., Majewski, D, & Carrigan, D. R. (1994). Brief report: fatal encephalitis due to variant B human herpesvirus-6 infection in a bone marrow-transplant recipient. *New England Journal of Medicine*, **330**, 1356–1360.

Einsele, H., Ehninger, G., Steidle, M. *et al.* (1991). Polymerase chain reaction to evaluate antiviral therapy for cytomegalovirus disease. *Lancet*, **ii**, 1170–1172.

Einsele, H., Ehninger, G., Steidle, M. *et al.* (1993). Lymphocytopenia as an unfavorable prognostic factor in patients with cytomegalovirus infection after bone marrow transplantation. *Blood*, **82**, 1672–1678.

Einsele, H., Ehninger, G., Hebart, H. *et al.* (1995). Polymerase chain reaction monitoring reduces the incidence of cytomegalovirus disease and the duration and side effects of antiviral therapy after bone marrow transplantation. *Blood*, **86**, 2815–2820.

Einsele, H., Hebart, H., Kauffmann-Schneider, C. *et al.* (2000). Risk factors for treatment failures in patients receiving PCR-based preemptive therapy for CMV infection. *Bone Marrow Transplantation*, **25**, 757–763.

Einsele, H., Roosnek, E., Rufer, N. *et al.* (2002). Infusion of cytomegalovirus (CMV)-specific T cells for the treatment of CMV infection not responding to antiviral chemotherapy. *Blood*, **99**, 3916–3922.

Emanuel, D., Cunningham, I., Jules, E. K. *et al.* (1988). Cytomegalovirus pneumonia after bone marrow transplantation successfully treated with the combination of ganciclovir and high-dose intravenous immune globulin. *Annals of Internal Medicine*, **109**, 777–782.

Emery, V. C. & Griffiths, P. D. (2000). Prediction of cytomegalovirus load and resistance patterns after antiviral chemotherapy. *Proceedings of the National Academy of Sciences of the United States of America*, **97**, 8039–8044.

Emery, V. C., Sabin, C. A., Cope, A. V. *et al.* (2000). Application of viral-load kinetics to identify patients who develop cytomegalovirus disease after transplantation. *Lancet*, **355**, 2032–2036.

Emmanouilides, C. E. & Territo, M. (1999). HTLV-1-associated myelopathy following allogeneic bone marrow transplantation. *Bone Marrow Transplantation*, **24**, 205–6.

Endo, T., Sakai, T., Fujimoto, K. *et al.* (2001). A possible role for lamivudine as prophylaxis against hepatitis B reactivation in carriers of hepatitis B who undergo chemotherapy and autologous peripheral blood stem cell transplantation for non-Hodgkin's lymphoma. *Bone Marrow Transplantation*, **27**, 433–436.

Engelhard, D., Nagler, A., Harden, I. *et al.* (1993). Antibody response to a two-dose regimen of influenza vaccine in allogeneic T cell-depleted and autologous BMT recipients. *Bone Marrow Transplantation*, **11**, 1–5.

Englund, J. A., Zimmerman, M. E., Swierkosz, E. M. *et al.* (1990). Herpes simplex virus resistant to acyclovir. A study in a tertiary care center. *Annals of Internal Medicine*, **112**, 416–422.

Epstein, J. B., Sherlock, C. H., & Wolber, R. A. (1993). Hairy leukoplakia after bone marrow transplantation. *Oral Surgery, Oral Medicine, and Oral Pathology*, **75**, 690–695.

Flomenberg, P., Babbitt, J., Drobyski, W. R. *et al.* (1994). Increasing incidence of adenovirus disease in bone marrow transplant recipients. *Journal of Infectious Diseases*, **169**, 775–781.

Foster, A. E., Gottlieb, D. J., Sartor, M. *et al.* (2002). Cytomegalovirus-specific CD4[+] and CD8[+] T-cells follow a similar reconstitution pattern after allogeneic stem cell transplantation. *Biology of Blood and Marrow Transplantation*, **8**, 501–11.

Galama, J. M., de Leeuw, N., Wittebol, S., Peters, H., & Melchers, W. J. (1996). Prolonged enteroviral infection in a patient who developed pericarditis and heart failure after bone marrow transplantation. *Clinical Infectious Diseases*, **22**, 1004–1008.

Garcia, R., Raad, I., Abi-Said, D. *et al.* (1997). Nosocomial respiratory syncytial virus infections: prevention and control in bone marrow transplant patients. *Infection Control and Hospital Epidemiology*, **18**, 412–416.

Gartner, B. C., Schafer, H., Marggraff, K. *et al.* (2002). Evaluation of use of Epstein-Barr viral load in patients after allogeneic stem cell transplantation to diagnose and monitor posttransplant lymphoproliferative disease. *Journal of Clinical Microbiology,* **40,** 351–358.

Ghosh, S., Champlin, R. E., Englund, J. *et al.* (2000). Respiratory syncytial virus upper respiratory tract illnesses in adult blood and marrow transplant recipients: combination therapy with aerosolized ribavirin and intravenous immunoglobulin. *Bone Marrow Transplantation,* **25,** 751–755.

Giardini, C., Galimberti, M., Lucarelli, G. *et al.* (1997). Alpha-interferon treatment of chronic hepatitis C after bone marrow transplantation for homozygous beta-thalassemia. *Bone Marrow Transplantation,* **20,** 767–772.

Goodrich, J., Bowden, R., Fisher, L. *et al.* (1993a). Ganciclovir prophylaxis to prevent cytomegalovirus disease after allogeneic marrow transplant. *Annals of Internal Medicine,* **118,** 173–178.

Goodrich, J. M., Bowden, R. A., Fisher, L. *et al.* (1993b). Ganciclovir prophylaxis to prevent cytomegalovirus disease after allogeneic marrow transplant. *Annals of Internal Medicine,* **118,** 173–178.

Goodrich, J. M., Mori, M., Gleaves, C. A. *et al.* (1991). Early treatment with ganciclovir to prevent cytomegalovirus disease after allogeneic bone marrow transplantation. *New England Journal of Medicine,* **325,** 1601–1607.

Gor, D., Sabin, C., Prentice, H. G. *et al.* (1998). Longitudinal fluctuations in cytomegalovirus load in bone marrow transplant patients: relationship between peak virus load, donor/recipient serostatus acute GVHD and CMV disease. *Bone Marrow Transplantation,* **21,** 597–605.

Gratama, J. W., Lennette, E. T., Lönnqvist, B. *et al.* (1992). Detection of multiple Epstein-Barr viral strains in allogeneic bone marrow transplant recipients. *Journal of Medical Virology,* **37,** 39–47.

Gratama, J. W., van Esser, J. W., Lamers, C. H. *et al.* (2001). Tetramer-based quantification of cytomegalovirus (CMV)-specific CD8(+) T lymphocytes in T-cell–depleted stem cell grafts and after transplantation may identify patients at risk for progressive CMV infection. *Blood,* **98,** 1358–1364.

Grob, J. P., Grundy, J. E., Prentice, H. G. *et al.* (1987). Immune donors can protect marrow-transplant recipients from severe cytomegalovirus infections. *Lancet,* **1,** 774–776.

Gross, T. G., Hinrichs, S. H., Winner, J. *et al.* (1998). Treatment of posttransplant lymphoproliferative disease (PTLD) following solid organ transplantation with low-dose chemotherapy. *Annals of Oncology,* **9,** 339–340.

Gustafsson, A., Levitsky, V., Zou, J. Z. *et al.* (2000). Epstein-Barr virus (EBV) load in bone marrow transplant recipients at risk to develop posttransplant lymphoproliferative disease: prophylactic infusion of EBV-specific cytotoxic T cells. *Blood,* **95,** 807–814.

Haddad, E., Paczesny, S., Leblond, V. *et al.* (2001). Treatment of B-lymphoproliferative disorder with a monoclonal anti-interleukin-6 antibody in 12 patients: a multicenter phase 1–2 clinical trial. *Blood,* **97,** 1590–1597.

Hale, G. A., Heslop, H. E., Krance, R. A. *et al.* (1999). Adenovirus infection after pediatric bone marrow transplantation. *Bone Marrow Transplantation,* **23,** 277–282.

Hann, I. M., Prentice, H. G., Blacklock, H. A. *et al.* (1983). Acyclovir prophylaxis against herpes virus infections in severely immuno-

compromised patients: randomised double blind trial. *British Medical Journal,* **287,** 384–388.

Harrington, R. D., Hooton, T. M., Hackman, R. C. *et al.* (1992). An outbreak of respiratory syncytial virus in a bone marrow transplant center. *The Journal of Infectious Diseases,* **165,** 987–993.

Hata, A., Asanuma, H., Rinki, M. *et al.* (2002). Use of an inactivated varicella vaccine in recipients of hematopoietic-cell transplants. *New England Journal of Medicine,* **347,** 76–34.

Hayden, F., Sable, C., Connor, J., & Lane, J. (1996). Intravenous ribavirin by constant infusion for serious influenza and parainfluenza infection. *Antiviral Therapy,* **1,** 51–56.

Hebart, H., Brugger, W., Grigoleit, U. *et al.* (2001a). Risk for cytomegalovirus disease in patients receiving polymerase chain reaction-based preemptive antiviral therapy after allogeneic stem cell transplantation depends on transplantation modality. *Blood,* **97,** 2183–2185.

Hebart, H., Wuchter, P., Loeffler, J. *et al.* (2001b). Evaluation of the Murex CMV DNA Hybrid Capture assay (version 2.0) for early diagnosis of cytomegalovirus infection in recipients of an allogeneic stem cell transplant. *Bone Marrow Transplantation,* **28,** 213–218.

Hebart, H., Rudolph, T., Loeffler, J. *et al.* (2002). Evaluation of the NucliSens CMV pp67 assay for detection and monitoring of human cytomegalovirus infection after allogeneic stem cell transplantation. *Bone Marrow Transplantation,* **30,** 181–7.

Heegaard, E. D. & Laub Petersen, B. (2000). Parvovirus B19 transmitted by bone marrow. *British Journal of Haematology,* **111,** 659–661.

Held, T. K., Biel, S. S., Nitsche, A. *et al.* (2000). Treatment of BK virus-associated hemorrhagic cystitis and simultaneous CMV reactivation with cidofovir. *Bone Marrow Transplantation,* **26,** 347–350.

Hierholzer, J. C., Bingham, P. G., Coombs, R. A. *et al.* (1989). Comparison of monoclonal antibody time-resolved fluoroimmunoassay with monoclonal antibody capture-biotinylated detector enzyme immunoassay for respiratory syncytial virus and parainfluenza virus antigen detection. *Journal of Clinical Microbiology,* **27,** 1243–1249.

Höglund, M., Ljungman, P., & Weller, S. (2001). Comparable aciclovir exposures produced by oral valaciclovir and intravenous aciclovir in immunocompromised cancer patients. *Journal of Antimicrobial Chemotherapy,* **47,** 855–861.

Holmberg, L. A., Boeckh, M., Hooper, H. *et al.* (1999). Increased incidence of cytomegalovirus disease after autologous CD34-selected peripheral blood stem cell transplantation [see comments]. *Blood,* **94,** 4029–4035.

Howard, D. S., Phillips, I. G., Reece, D. E. *et al.* (1999). Adenovirus infections in hematopoietic stem cell transplant recipients. *Clinical Infectious Diseases,* **29,** 1494–1501.

Hromas, R., Clark, C., Blanke, C. *et al.* (1994). Failure of ribavirin to clear adenovirus infections in T cell–depleted allogeneic bone marrow transplantation. *Bone Marrow Transplantation,* **14,** 663–664.

Hromas, R., Cornetta, K., Srour, E. *et al.* (1994b). Donor leukocyte infusion as therapy of life-threatening adenoviral infections after T-cell-depleted bone marrow transplantation. *Blood* **84,** 1689–90.

Ilan, Y., Nagler, A., Adler, R. *et al.* (1993). Ablation of persistent hepatitis B by bone marrow transplantation from a hepatitis B-immune donor. *Gastroenterology,* **104,** 1818–1821.

Ilan, Y., Nagler, A., Shoulval, D. *et al.* (1994). Development of antibodies to hepatitis B virus surface antigen in bone marrow transplant recipient following treatment with peripheral blood lymphocytes from immunized donors. *Journal of Clinical and Experimental Immunology,* **97,** 299–302.

Ilan, Y., Nagler, A., Zeira, E. *et al.* (2000). Maintenance of immune memory to the hepatitis B envelope protein following adoptive transfer of immunity in bone marrow transplant recipients. *Bone Marrow Transplantation,* **26,** 633–638.

Isomura, H., Yamada, M., Yoshida, M. *et al.* (1997). Suppressive effects of human herpesvirus 6 on in vitro colony formation of hematopoietic progenitor cells. *Journal of Medical Virology,* **52,** 406–412.

Jacobsen, N., Andersen, H., Skinhöj, P. *et al.* (1986). Correlation between donor cytomegalovirus immunity and chronic graft-versus-host disease after allogeneic bone marrow transplantation. *Scandinavion Journal of Hematology,* **36,** 499–506.

Jones, B. L., Clark, S., Curran, E. T. *et al.* (2000). Control of an outbreak of respiratory syncytial virus infection in immunocompromised adults. *Journal of Hospital Infection,* **44,** 53–57.

Junghanss, C., Boeckh, M., Carter, R. A. *et al.* (2002). Incidence and outcome of cytomegalovirus infections following nonmyeloablative compared with myeloablative allogeneic stem cell transplantation, a matched control study. *Blood,* **99,** 1978–85.

Kajon, A. & Wadell, G. (1994). Genome analysis of South American adenovirus strains of serotype 7 collected over a 7-year period. *Journal of Clinical Microbiology,* **32,** 2321–2323.

Kanfer, E. J., Abrahamson, G., Taylor, J., Coleman, J. C., & Samson, D. M. (1994). Severe rotavirus-associated diarrhoea following bone marrow transplantation: treatment with oral immunoglobulin. *Bone Marrow Transplantation,* **14,** 651–652.

Kang, E. M., de Witte, M., Malech, H. *et al.* (2002). Nonmyeloablative conditioning followed by transplantation of genetically modified HLA-matched peripheral blood progenitor cells for hematologic malignancies in patients with acquired immunodeficiency syndrome. *Blood,* **99,** 698–701.

Kapelushnik, J., Or, R., Delukina, M. *et al.* (1995). Intravenous ribavirin therapy foe adenovirus gastroenteritis after bone marrow transplantation. *Journal of Pediatric Gastroenterology and Nutrition,* **21,** 110–112.

Kaplan, L., Daum, R., Smaron, M., & McCarthy, C. (1992). Severe measles in immunocompromised patients. *JAMA: the Journal of the American Medical Association,* **267,** 1237–1241.

Kaptan, K., Beyan, C., Ural, A. U. *et al.* (2001). Successful treatment of severe aplastic anemia associated with human parvovirus B19 and Epstein-Barr virus in a healthy subject with allo-BMT. *American Journal of Hematology,* **67,** 252–255.

Kikuchi, H., Ohtsuka, E., Ono, K. *et al.* (2000). Allogeneic bone marrow transplantation-related transmission of human T lymphotropic virus type I (HTLV-1). *Bone Marrow Transplantation,* **26,** 1235–7.

King, S. M., Saunders, E. F., Petric, M., Gold, R. (1996). Response to measles, mumps and rubella vaccine in pediatric bone marrow transplant recipients. *Bone Marrow Transplantation,* **17,** 633–6.

Kleihauer, A., Grigoleit, U., Hebart, H. *et al.* (2001). Ex vivo generation of human cytomegalovirus-specific cytotoxic T cells by peptide-pulsed dendritic cells. *British Journal of Haematology,* **113,** 231–239.

Koc, Y., Miller, K. B., Schenkein, D. P. *et al.* (2000). Varicella zoster virus infections following allogeneic bone marrow transplantation: frequency, risk factors, and clinical outcome. *Biology of Blood and Marrow Transplantation,* **6,** 44–9.

Konoplev, S., Champlin, R. E., Giralt, S. *et al.* (2001). Cytomegalovirus pneumonia in adult autologous blood and marrow transplant recipients. *Bone Marrow Transplantation,* **27,** 877–81.

Krause, H., Hebart, H., Jahn, G., Muller, C. A., & Einsele, H. (1997). Screening for CMV-specific T cell proliferation to identify patients at risk of developing late onset CMV disease. *Bone Marrow Transplantation,* **19,** 1111–1116.

Krishnan, A., Molina, A., Zaia, J. *et al.* (2001). Autologous stem cell transplantation for HIV-associated lymphoma. *Blood,* **98,** 3857–9.

Kuehnle, I., Huls, M. H., Liu, Z. *et al.* (2000). CD20 monoclonal antibody (rituximab) for therapy of Epstein-Barr virus lymphoma after hemopoietic stem-cell transplantation. *Blood,* **95,** 1502–1505.

La Rosa, A. M., Champlin, R. E., Mirza, N. *et al.* (2001). Adenovirus infections in adult recipients of blood and marrow transplants. *Clinical Infectious Diseases,* **32,** 871–876.

Larsson, K., Lönnqvist, B., Ringdén, O., Hedquist, B., & Ljungman, P. (2002). CMV retinitis after allogeneic bone marrow transplantation: a report of five cases. *Transplant Infectious Disease,* **4,** 75–79.

Lau, G. K., Liang, R., Chiu, E. K., Lee, C. K., & Lam, S. K. (1997a). Hepatic events after bone marrow transplantation in patients with hepatitis B infection: a case controlled study. *Bone Marrow Transplantation,* **19,** 795–799.

Lau, G. K., Liang, R., Lee, C. K. *et al.* (1998a). Clearance of persistent hepatitis B virus infection in Chinese bone marrow transplant recipients whose donors were anti-hepatitis B core- and anti-hepatitis B surface antibody-positive. *Journal of Infectious Diseases,* **178,** 1585–1591.

Lau, G. K., Liang, R., Wu, P. C. *et al.* (1998b). Use of famciclovir to prevent HBV reactivation in HBsAg-positive recipients after allogeneic bone marrow transplantation. *Journal of Hepatology,* **28,** 359–368.

Lau, G. K., Lie, A. K., Kwong, Y. L. *et al.* (2000). A case-controlled study on the use of HBsAg-positive donors for allogeneic hematopoietic cell transplantation. *Blood,* **96,** 452–458.

Lau, G. K., Lok, A. S., Liang, R. H. *et al.* (1997b). Clearance of hepatitis B surface antigen after bone marrow transplantation: role of adoptive immunity transfer. *Hepatology,* **25,** 1497–1501.

Legrand, F., Berrebi, D., Houhou, N. *et al.* (2001). Early diagnosis of adenovirus infection and treatment with cidofovir after bone marrow transplantation in children. *Bone Marrow Transplantation,* **27,** 621–626.

Lewinsohn, D., Bowden, R., Matsson, D., & Crawford, S. (1996). Phase I study of intravenous ribavirin treatment of respiratory syncytial virus pneumonia after marrow transplantation. *Antimicrobial Agents and Chemotherapy,* **40,** 2555–2557.

Lewis, V. A., Champlin, R., Englund, J. *et al.* (1996). Respiratory disease due to parainfluenza virus in adult bone marrow transplant recipients. *Clinical Infectious Diseases*, **23**, 1033–1037.

Li, C. R., Greenberg, P. D., Gilbert, M. J., Goodrich, J. M., & Riddell, S. R. (1994). Recovery of HLA-restricted cytomegalovirus (CMV)-specific T-cell responses after allogeneic bone marrow transplant: correlation with CMV disease and effect of ganciclovir prophylaxis. *Blood*, **83**, 1971–1979.

Liles, W. C., Cushing, H., Holt, S., Bryan, C., & Hackman, R. C. (1993). Severe adenoviral nephritis following bone marrow transplantation: successful treatment with intravenous ribavirin. *Bone Marrow Transplantation*, **12**, 409–412.

Limaye, A. P., Corey, L., Koelle, D. M., Davis, C. L., & Boeckh, M. (2000). Emergence of ganciclovir-resistant cytomegalovirus disease among recipients of solid-organ transplants. *Lancet*, **356**, 645–649.

Ljungman, P. (1997). Respiratory virus infections in bone marrow transplant recipients: The European perspective. *American Journal of Medicine*, **102**, (Suppl 3A).

Ljungman, P. (1999). Immunization of transplant recipients. *Bone Marrow Transplantation*, **23**, 635–636.

Ljungman, P., Andersson, J., Aschan, J. *et al.* (1996). Oral ribavirin for prevention of severe liver disease caused by hepatitis C virus during allogeneic bone marrow transplantation. *Clinical Infectious Diseases*, **23**, 167–169.

Ljungman, P., Aschan, J., Azinge, J. N. *et al.* (1993a). Cytomegalovirus viraemia and specific T-helper cell responses as predictors of disease after allogeneic marrow transplantation. *British Journal of Haematology*, **83**, 118–124.

Ljungman, P., Biron, P., Bosi, A. *et al.* (1994a). Cytomegalovirus interstitial pneumonia in autologous bone marrow transplant recipients. Infectious Disease Working Party of the European Group for Bone Marrow Transplantation. *Bone Marrow Transplantation*, **13**, 209–12.

Ljungman, P., Björkstrand, B., Ehrnst, A., Forsgren, M., & Lönnqvist, B., eds. (1991). *Cytomegalovirus infection among autologous bone marrow transplant (ABMT) recipients.*

Ljungman, P., Cordonnier, C., Einsele, H. *et al.* (1998). Use of intravenous immune globulin in addition to antiviral therapy in the treatment of CMV gastrointestinal disease in allogeneic bone marrow transplant patients: a report from the European Group for Blood and Marrow Transplantation (EBMT). Infectious Disease Working Party of the EBMT. *Bone Marrow Transplantation*, **21**, 473–476.

Ljungman, P., De Bock, R., Cordonnier, C. *et al.* (1993b). Practices for cytomegalovirus diagnosis, prophylaxis and treatment in allogeneic bone marrow transplant recipients: a report from the Working Party for Infectious Disease of the EBMT. *Bone Marrow Transplantation*, **12**, 399–403.

Ljungman, P., de La Camara, R., Milpied, N. *et al.* (2002a). Randomized study of valaciclovir as prophylaxis against CMV reactivation in allogeneic bone marrow transplant recipients. *Blood*, **99**, 3050–3056.

Ljungman, P., Deliliers, G. L., Platzbecker, U. *et al.* (2001a). Cidofovir for cytomegalovirus infection and disease in allogeneic stem cell transplant recipients. The Infectious Diseases Working Party of the European Group for Blood and Marrow Transplantation. *Blood*, **97**, 388–392.

Ljungman, P., Engelhard, D., Link, H. *et al.* (1992). Treatment of interstitial pneumonitis due to cytomegalovirus with ganciclovir and intravenous immune globulin: experience of European Bone Marrow Transplant Group. *Clinical Infectious Diseases*, **14**, 831–835.

Ljungman, P., Fridell, E., Lönnqvist, B. *et al.* (1989a). Efficacy and safety of vaccination of marrow transplant recipients with a live attenuated measles, mumps, and rubella vaccine. *Journal of Infectious Diseases*, **159**, 610–615.

Ljungman, P., Gleaves, C. A., & Meyers, J. D. (1989b). Respiratory virus infection in immunocompromised patients. *Bone Marrow Transplantation*, **4**, 35–40.

Ljungman, P., Griffiths, P., & Paya, C. (2002b). Definitions of cytomegalovirus infection and disease in transplant recipients. *Clinical Infectious Diseases*, **34**, 1094–1097.

Ljungman, P., Johansson, N., Aschan, J. *et al.* (1995). Long-term effects of hepatitis C virus infection in allogeneic bone marrow transplant recipients. *Blood*, **86**, 1614–1618.

Ljungman, P., Larsson, K., Kumlien, G. *et al.* (2002c). Leukocyte depleted, unscreened blood products give a low risk for CMV infection and disease in CMV seronegative allogeneic stem cell transplant recipients with seronegative stem cell donors. *Scandinavian Journal of Infectious Disease*, **34**, 347–350.

Ljungman, P., Lewensohn-Fuchs, I., Hammarstrom, V. *et al.* (1994b). Long-term immunity to measles, mumps, and rubella after allogeneic bone marrow transplantation. *Blood*, **84**, 657–663.

Ljungman, P., Lonnqvist, B., Gahrton, G. *et al.* (1986a). Clinical and subclinical reactivations of varicella-zoster virus in immunocompromised patients. *Journal of Infectious Diseases*, **153**, 840–847.

Ljungman, P., Lönnqvist, B., Ringdén, O., Skinhöj, P., & Gahrton, G. (1989c). A randomized trial of oral versus intravenous acyclovir for treatment of herpes zoster in bone marrow transplant recipients. Nordic Bone Marrow Transplant Group. *Bone Marrow Transplantation*, **4**, 613–615.

Ljungman, P., Niederwieser, D., Pepe, M. S. *et al.* (1990). Cytomegalovirus infection after marrow transplantation for aplastic anemia. *Bone Marrow Transplantation*, **6**, 295–300.

Ljungman, P., Ribaud, P., Matthes-Martin, S. *et al.* (2001b). Cidofovir for adenovirus infection after allogeneic stem cell transplantion (SCT). A retrospective survey of the Infectious Diseases Working Party of the European Group for Blood and Marrow Transplantation. *Bone Marrow Transplantation*, **27** (Suppl 1), S61.

Ljungman, P., Wang, F. Z., Clark, D. A. *et al.* (2000). High levels of human herpesvirus 6 DNA in peripheral blood leucocytes are correlated to platelet engraftment and disease in allogeneic stem cell transplant patients. *British Journal of Haematology*, **111**, 774–781.

Ljungman, P., Ward, K. N., Crooks, B. N. *et al.* (2001c). Respiratory virus infections after stem cell transplantation: a prospective study from the Infectious Diseases Working Party of the European Group for Blood and Marrow Transplantation. *Bone Marrow Transplantation*, **28**, 479–484.

Ljungman, P., Wilczek, H., Gahrton, G. *et al.* (1986b). Long-term acyclovir prophylaxis in bone marrow transplant recipients and lymphocyte proliferation responses to herpes virus antigens in vitro. *Bone Marrow Transplantation*, **1**, 185–192.

Locasciulli, A., Alberti, A., Bandini, G. *et al.* (1995). Allogeneic bone marrow transplantation from HBsAg+ donors: a multicenter study from the Gruppo Italiano Trapianto di Midollo Osseo (GITMO). *Blood,* **86,** 3236–3240.

Locasciulli, A., Testa, M., Valsecchi, M. G. *et al.* (1999). The role of hepatitis C and B virus infections as risk factors for severe liver complications following allogeneic BMT: a prospective study by the Infectious Disease Working Party of the European Blood and Marrow Transplantation Group. *Transplantation,* **68,** 1486–1491.

Locksley, R., Flournoy, N., Sullivan, K., & Meyers, J. (1985a). Infection with varicella-zoster virus after marrow transplantation. *Journal of Infectious Diseases,* **152,** 1172–1178.

Locksley, R. M., Flournoy, N., Sullivan, K. M., & Meyers, J. D. (1985b). Infection with varicella-zoster virus after marrow transplantation. *Journal of Infectious Diseases,* **152,** 1172–1181.

Lönnqvist, B., Ringdén, O., Wahren, B., Gahrton, G., & Lundgren, G. (1984). Cytomegalovirus infection associated with and preceding chronic graft-versus-host disease. *Transplantation,* **38,** 465–468.

Loughran, R. P. & Shriver, M. K. (1994). Seroprevalence of HTLV-I and HTLV-II in marrow transplant recipients. *Bone Marrow Transplantation,* **14,** 433–6.

Machado, C. M., Dulley, F. L., Boas, L. S. *et al.* (2000). CMV pneumonia in allogeneic BMT recipients undergoing early treatment of pre-emptive ganciclovir therapy. *Bone Marrow Transplantation,* **26,** 413–417.

Machado, C. M., Goncalves, F. B., Pannuti, C. S., Dulley, F. L., & de Souza, V. A. (2002). Measles in bone marrow transplant recipients during an outbreak in Sao Paulo, Brazil. *Blood,* **99,** 83–87.

Machado, C. M., Menezes, R. X., Macedo, M. C. A. *et al.* (2001). Extended antigenemia surveillance and late cytomegalovirus infection after allogeneic BMT. *Bone Marrow Transplantation,* **28,** 1053–9.

Maeda, Y., Teshima, T., Yamada, M., & Harada, M. (2000). Reactivation of human herpesviruses after allogeneic peripheral blood stem cell transplantation and bone marrow transplantation. *Leukemia and Lymphoma,* **39,** 229–239.

Mann, D., Moreb, J., Smith, S., & Gian, V. (1998). Failure of intravenous ribavirin in the treatment of invasive adenovirus infection following allogeneic bone marrow transplantation: a case report. *Journal of Infection,* **36,** 227–228.

Maruyama, F., Miyazaki, H., Matsui, T. *et al.* (1996). Rapid progression of flat warts in a patient with malignant lymphoma after PBSCT. *Bone Marrow Transplantation,* **18,** 1009–11.

Mazzulli, T., Peret, T. C., McGeer, A. *et al.* (1999). Molecular characterization of a nosocomial outbreak of human respiratory syncytial virus on an adult leukemia/lymphoma ward. *Journal of Infectious Diseases,* **180,** 1686–1689.

McCarthy, A. J., Kingman, H. M., Kelly, C. *et al.* (1999). The outcome of 26 patients with respiratory syncytial virus infection following allogeneic stem cell transplantation. *Bone Marrow Transplantation,* **24,** 1315–1322.

Meyers, J. D. (1988). Prevention and treatment of cytomegalovirus infection after marrow transplantation. *Bone Marrow Transplantation,* **3,** 95–104.

Meyers, J. D., Fluornoy, N., & Thomas, E. D. (1980). Cytomegalovirus infection and specific cell-mediated immunity after marrow transplant. *Journal of Infectious Diseases,* **142,** 816–24.

Meyers, J. D., Ljungman, P., & Fisher, L. D. (1990). Cytomegalovirus excretion as a predictor of cytomegalovirus disease after marrow transplantation: importance of cytomegalovirus viremia. *Journal of Infectious Diseases,* **162,** 373–380.

Meyers, J. D., Reed, E. C., Shepp, D. H. *et al.* (1988). Acyclovir for prevention of cytomegalovirus infection and disease after allogeneic marrow transplantation. *New England Journal of Medicine,* **318,** 70–75.

Meyers, J. D., Wade, J. C., Mitchell, C. D. *et al.* (1982). Multicenter collaborative trial of intravenous acyclovir for treatment of mucocutaneous herpes simplex virus infection in the immunocompromised host. *American Journal of Medicine,* **73,** 229–235.

Micallef, I. N., Chhanabhai, M., Gascoyne, R. D. *et al.* (1998). Lymphoproliferative disorders following allogeneic bone marrow transplantation: the Vancouver experience. *Bone Marrow Transplantation,* **22,** 981–987.

Miller, W., Flynn, P., McCullough, J. *et al.* (1986). Cytomegalovirus infection after bone marrow transplantation: an association with acute graft-v-host disease. *Blood,* **67,** 1162–1167.

Milpied, N., Vasseur, B., Parquet, N. *et al.* (2000). Humanized anti-CD20 monoclonal antibody (rituximab) in post transplant B-lymphoproliferative disorder: a retrospective analysis on 32 patients. *Annals of Oncology,* **11,** 113–116.

Miyamura, K., Hamaguchi, M., Taji, H. *et al.* (2000). Successful ribavirin therapy for severe adenovirus hemorrhagic cystitis after allogeneic marrow transplant from close HLA donors rather than distant donors. *Bone Marrow Transplantation,* **25,** 545–548.

Mookerjee, B. P. & Vogelsang, G. (1997). Human herpes virus-6 encephalitis after bone marrow transplantation: successful treatment with ganciclovir. *Bone Marrow Transplantation,* **20,** 905–906.

Naik, H. R., Siddique, N., & Chandrasekar, P. H. (1995). Foscarnet therapy for acyclovir-resistant herpes simplex virus 1 infection in allogeneic bone marrow transplant recipients. *Clinical Infectious Diseases,* **21,** 1514–1515.

Nakagawa, M., Simizu, Y., Suemura, M., & Sato, B. (2002). Successful long-term control with lamivudine against reactivated hepatitis B infection following intensive chemotherapy and autologous peripheral blood stem cell transplantation in non-Hodgkin's lymphoma: experience of 2 cases. *American Journal of Hematology,* **70,** 60–63.

Nakano, T., Shimono, Y., Sugiyama, K. *et al.* (1996). Clinical features of measles in immunocompromised children. *Acta Paediatrica Japanic,* **38,** 212–217.

Nichols, W. G., Corey, L., Gooley, T., Davis, C., & Boeckh, M. (2001a). Parainfluenza virus infections after hematopoietic stem cell transplantation: risk factors, response to antiviral therapy, and effect on transplant outcome. *Blood,* **98,** 573–578.

Nichols, W. G., Corey, L., Gooley, T. *et al.* (2001b). Rising pp65 antigenemia during preemptive anticytomegalovirus therapy after allogeneic hematopoietic stem cell transplantation: risk factors, correlation with DNA load, and outcomes. *Blood,* **97,** 867–874.

Nichols, W. G., Corey, L., Gooley, T., Davis, C., & Boeckh, M. (2002). High risk of death due to bacterial and fungal infection among cytomegalovirus (CMV)-seronegative recipients of stem cell transplants from seropositive donors: evidence for indirect effects of primary CMV infection. *Journal of Infectious Diseases,* **185,** 273–282.

Ohnishi, M., Kanda, Y., Takeuchi, T. *et al.* (2002). Limited efficacy of lamivudine against hepatitis B virus infection in allogeneic hematopoietic stem cell transplant recipients. *Transplantation,* **73,** 812–815.

Papadopoulos, E. B., Ladanyi, M., Emanuel, D. *et al.* (1994). Infusions of donor leukocytes to treat Epstein-Barr virus-associated lymphoproliferative disorders after allogeneic bone marrow transplantation [see comments]. *New England Journal of Medicine,* **330,** 1185–1191.

Parkkali, T., Stenvik, M., Ruutu, T. *et al.* (1997). Randomized comparison of early and late vaccination with inactivated polio vaccine after allogeneic BMT. *Bone Marrow Transplantation,* **20,** 663–8.

Pauksen, K., Linde, A., Hammarstrom, V. *et al.* (2000). Granulocyte-Macrophage Colony-Stimulating Factor as Immunomodulating Factor Together with Influenza Vaccination in Stem Cell Transplant Patients. *Clinical Infectious Diseases,* **30,** 342–348.

Peggs, K., Verfuerth, S., & Mackinnon, S. (2001). Induction of cytomegalovirus (CMV)-specific T-cell responses using dendritic cells pulsed with CMV antigen: a novel culture system free of live CMV virions. *Blood,* **97,** 994–1000.

Picardi, M., Selleri, C., De Rosa, G. *et al.* (1998). Lamivudine treatment for chronic replicative hepatitis B virus infection after allogeneic bone marrow transplantation. *Bone Marrow Transplantation,* **21,** 1267–1269.

Platzbecker, U., Bandt, D., Thiede, C. *et al.* (2001). Successful pre-emptive cidofovir treatment for CMV antigenemia after dose-reduced conditioning and allogeneic blood stem cell transplantation. *Transplantation,* **71,** 880–885.

Prentice, H. G., Gluckman, E., Powles, R. L. *et al.* (1994). Impact of long-term acyclovir on cytomegalovirus infection and survival after allogeneic bone marrow transplantation. European Acyclovir for CMV Prophylaxis Study Group. *Lancet,* **343,** 749–753.

Prentice, H. G., Gluckman, E., Powles, R. L. *et al.* (1997). Long-term survival in allogeneic bone marrow transplant recipients following acyclovir prophylaxis for CMV infection. The European Acyclovir for CMV Prophylaxis Study Group. *Bone Marrow Transplantation,* **19,** 129–133.

Ray, C. G. & Minnich, L. L. (1987). Efficiency of immunofluorescence for rapid detection of common respiratory viruses. *Journal of Clinical Microbiology,* **25,** 355–357.

Reed, E., Myerson, D., Corey, L., & Meyers, J. (1991). Allogeneic marrow transplantation in patients positive for hepatitis B surface antigen. *Blood,* **77,** 195–200.

Reed, E. C., Bowden, R. A., Dandliker, P. S., Lilleby, K. E., & Meyers, J. D. (1988). Treatment of cytomegalovirus pneumonia with ganciclovir and intravenous cytomegalovirus immunoglobulin in patients with bone marrow transplants. *Annals of Internal Medicine,* **109,** 783–788.

Regn, S., Raffegerst, S., Chen, X. *et al.* (2001). Ex vivo generation of cytotoxic T lymphocytes specific for one or two distinct viruses for the prophylaxis of patients receiving an allogeneic bone marrow transplant. *Bone Marrow Transplantation,* **27,** 53–64.

Reusser, P., Cordonnier, C., Einsele, H. *et al.* (1996). European survey of herpesvirus resistance to antiviral drugs in bone marrow transplant recipients. Infectious Diseases Working Party of the European Group for Blood and Marrow Transplantation (EBMT). *Bone Marrow Transplantation,* **17,** 813–817.

Reusser, P., Einsele, H., Lee, J. *et al.* (2002). Randomized multicenter trial of foscarnet versus ganciclovir for preemptive therapy of cytomegalovirus infection after allogeneic stem cell transplantation. *Blood,* **99,** 1159–1164.

Reusser, P., Fisher, L. D., Buckner, C. D., Thomas, E. D., & Meyers, J. D. (1990). Cytomegalovirus infection after autologous bone marrow transplantation: occurrence of cytomegalovirus disease and effect on engraftment. *Blood,* **75,** 1888–1894.

Reusser, P., Gambertoglio, J. G., Lilleby, K., & Meyers, J. D. (1992). Phase I–II trial of foscarnet for prevention of cytomegalovirus infection in autologous and allogeneic marrow transplant recipients [see comments]. *Journal of Infectious Diseases,* **166,** 473–479.

Reusser, P., Riddell, S. R., Meyers, J. D., & Greenberg, P. D. (1991). Cytotoxic T-lymphocyte response to cytomegalovirus after human allogeneic bone marrow transplantation: pattern of recovery and correlation with cytomegalovirus infection and disease. *Blood,* **78,** 1373–1380.

Riddell, S. R., Watanabe, K. S., Goodrich, J. M. *et al.* (1992). Restoration of viral immunity in immunodeficient humans by the adoptive transfer of T cell clones. *Science,* **257,** 238–241.

Rieux, C., Gautheret-Dejean, A., Challine-Lehmann, D. *et al.* (1998). Human herpesvirus-6 meningoencephalitis in a recipient of an unrelated allogeneic bone marrow transplantation. *Transplantation,* **65,** 1408–1411.

Ringden, O., Lonnqvist, B., Aschan, J., & Sundberg, B. (1989). Foscarnet prophylaxis in marrow transplant recipients. *Bone Marrow Transplantation,* **4,** 713 (Letter).

Rooney, C. M., Smith, C. A., Ng, C. Y. *et al.* (1995). Use of gene-modified virus-specific T lymphocytes to control Epstein-Barr-virus-related lymphoproliferation. *Lancet,* **345,** 9–13.

Rooney, C. M., Smith, C. A., Ng, C. Y. *et al.* (1998). Infusion of cytotoxic T cells for the prevention and treatment of Epstein-Barr virus-induced lymphoma in allogeneic transplant recipients. *Blood,* **92,** 1549–1555.

Ruutu, T., Ljungman, P., Brinch, L. *et al.* (1997). No prevention of cytomegalovirus infection by anti-cytomegalovirus hyperimmune globulin in seronegative bone marrow transplant recipients. The Nordic BMT Group. *Bone Marrow Transplantation,* **19,** 233–236.

Safrin, S., Assaykeen, T., Follansbee, S., & Mills, J. (1990). Foscarnet therapy for acyclovir-resistant mucocutaneous herpes simplex virus infection in 26 AIDS patients: preliminary data. *Journal of Infectious Diseases,* **161,** 1078–1084.

Saral, R., Burns, W. H., Laskin, O. L., Santos, G. W., & Lietman, P. S. (1981). Acyclovir prophylaxis of herpes-simplex-virus infections. *New England Journal of Medicine,* **305,** 63–67.

Sauerbrei, A., Prager, J., Hengst. U. *et al.* (1997). Varicella vaccination in children after bone marrow transplantation. *Bone Marrow Transplantation,* **20,** 381–3.

Schafer, H., Berger, C., Aepinus, C. *et al.* (2001). Molecular pathogenesis of Epstein-Barr virus associated posttransplant lymphomas: new insights through latent membrane protein 1 fingerprinting. *Transplantation,* **72,** 492–496.

Schiller, G. J., Nimer, S. D., Gajewski, J. L., & Golde, D. W. (1991). Abdominal presentation of varicella-zoster infection in recipients of allogeneic bone marrow transplantation. *Bone Marrow Transplantation*, **7**, 489–91.

Schmidt, G. M., Kovacs, A., Zaia, J. A. *et al.* (1988). Ganciclovir/immunoglobulin combination therapy for the treatment of human cytomegalovirus-associated interstitial pneumonia in bone marrow allograft recipients. *Transplantation*, **46**, 905–907.

Schuchter, L. M., Wingard, J. R., Piantadosi, S. *et al.* (1989). Herpes zoster infection after autologous bone marrow transplantation. *Blood*, **74**, 1424–1427.

Selby, P. J., Powles, R. L., Easton, D. *et al.* (1989). The prophylactic role of intravenous and long-term oral acyclovir after allogeneic bone marrow transplantation. *British Journal of Cancer*, **59**, 434–438.

Shepp, D. H., Newton, B. A., Dandliker, P. S., Flournoy, N., & Meyers, J. D. (1985). Oral acyclovir therapy for mucocutaneous herpes simplex virus infections in immunocompromised marrow transplant recipients. *Annals of Internal Medicine*, **102**, 783–785.

Shields, A. F., Hackman, R. C., Fife, K. H., Corey, L., & Meyers, J. D. (1985). Adenovirus infections in patients undergoing bone-marrow transplantation. *New England Journal of Medicine*, **312**, 529–533.

Shuhart, M. C., Myerson, D., Childs, B. H. *et al.* (1994). Marrow transplantation from hepatitis C virus seropositive donors: transmission rate and clinical course. *Blood*, **84**, 3229–3235.

Söderberg, C., Larsson, S., Rozell, B. L. *et al.* (1996a). Cytomegalovirus-induced CD13-specific autoimmunity—a possible cause of chronic graft-vs-host disease. *Transplantation*, **61**, 600–609.

Söderberg, C., Sumitran, K. S., Ljungman, P., & Möller, E. (1996b). CD13-specific autoimmunity in cytomegalovirus-infected immunocompromised patients. *Transplantation*, **61**, 594–600.

Sparrelid, E., Ljungman, P., Ekelof-Andstrom, E. *et al.* (1997). Ribavirin therapy in bone marrow transplant recipients with viral respiratory tract infections. *Bone Marrow Transplantation*, **19**, 905–908.

Steer, C. B., Szer, J., Sasadeusz, J. *et al.* (2000). Varicella-zoster infection after allogeneic bone marrow transplantation: incidence, risk factors and prevention with low-dose aciclovir and ganciclovir. *Bone Marrow Transplantation*, **25**, 657–664.

Strasser, S. I., Myerson, D., Spurgeon, C. L. *et al.* (1999a). Hepatitis C virus infection and bone marrow transplantation: a cohort study with 10-year follow-up. *Hepatology*, **29**, 1893–1899.

Strasser, S. I., Sullivan, K. M., Myerson, D. *et al.* (1999b). Cirrhosis of the liver in long-term marrow transplant survivors. *Blood*, **93**, 3259–3266.

Szmania, S., Galloway, A., Bruorton, M. *et al.* (2001). Isolation and expansion of cytomegalovirus-specific cytotoxic T lymphocytes to clinical scale from a single blood draw using dendritic cells and HLA-tetramers. *Blood*, **98**, 505–512.

Takenaka, K., Gondo, H., Tanimoto, K. *et al.* (1997). Increased incidence of cytomegalovirus (CMV) infection and CMV-associated disease after allogeneic bone marrow transplantation from unrelated donors. *Bone Marrow Transplantation*, **19**, 241–8.

Tokimasa, S., Hara, J., Osugi, Y. *et al.* (2002). Ganciclovir is effective for prophylaxis and treatment of human herpesvirus-6 in allogeneic stem cell transplantation. *Bone Marrow Transplantation*, **29**, 259–8.

Torres, G. & Vicente, M. (1992). [Detection of respiratory syncytial and adenovirus in nasopharyngeal aspirates: comparison of cellular cultures and immunofluorescence]. *Revista Medica de Chile*, **120**, 415–419 (Spanish).

Tyring, S., Belanger, R., Bezwoda, W. (2001). A randomized, double-blind trial of famciclovir versus acyclovir for the treatment of localized dermatomal herpes zoster in immunocompromised patients. *Cancer Investigation*, **19**, 13–22.

Uchida, N., Gondo, H., Himeji, D. *et al.* (2000). Lamivudine therapy for a hepatitis B surface antigen (HBsAg)-positive leukemia patient receiving myeloablative chemotherapy and autologous stem cell transplantation. *Bone Marrow Transplantation*, **26**, 1243–1245.

Van der Bij, W., Torensma, R., Van Son, W. *et al.* (1988). Rapid detection and quantification of active cytomegalovirus infection by monoclonal antibody staining of blood leucocytes. *Journal of Medical Virology*, **25**, 179–188.

van Esser, J. W., van der Holt, B., Meijer, E. *et al.* (2001a). Epstein-Barr virus (EBV) reactivation is a frequent event after allogeneic stem cell transplantation (SCT) and quantitatively predicts EBV-lymphoproliferative disease following T-cell–depleted SCT. *Blood*, **98**, 972–978.

van Esser, J. W. J., Niesters, H. G. M., Thijsen, S. F. T. *et al.* (2001b). Molecular quantification of viral load in plasma allows for fast and accurate prediction of response to therapy of Epstein-Barr virus-associated lymphoproliferative disease after allogeneic stem cell transplantation. *British Journal of Haematology*, **113**, 814–21.

Vance, E. A., Soiffer, R. J., McDonald, G. B. *et al.* (1996). Prevention of transmission of hepatitis C virus in bone marrow transplantation by treating the donor with alpha-interferon. *Transplantation*, **62**, 1358–1360.

Verdonck, L. F., Cornelissen, J. J., Smit, J. *et al.* (1993). Successful foscarnet therapy for acyclovir-resistant mucocutaneous infection with herpes simplex virus in a recipient of allogeneic BMT. *Bone Marrow Transplantation*, **11**, 177–179.

Wacker, P., Hartmann, O., Benhamou, E., Salloum, E., & Lemerle, J. (1989). Varicella-zoster virus infections after autologous bone marrow transplantation in children. *Bone Marrow Transplantation*, **4**, 191–194.

Wade, J. C., Day, L. M., Crowley, J. J., & Meyers, J. D. (1984a). Recurrent infection with herpes simplex virus after marrow transplantation: role of the specific immune response and acyclovir treatment. *The Journal of Infectious Disease*, **149**, 750–756.

Wade, J. C., McLaren, C., & Meyers, J. D. (1983). Frequency and significance of acyclovir-resistant herpes simplex virus isolated from marrow transplant patients receiving multiple courses of treatment with acyclovir. *Journal of Infectious Disease*, **148**, 1077–1082.

Wade, J. C., Newton, B., Flournoy, N., & Meyers, J. D. (1984b). Oral acyclovir for prevention of herpes simplex virus reactivation after marrow transplantation. *Annals of Internal Medicine*, **100**, 823–828.

Walter, E. A., Greenberg, P. D., Gilbert, M. J. *et al.* (1995). Reconstitution of cellular immunity against cytomegalovirus in recipients of allogeneic bone marrow by transfer of T-cell clones from the donor [see comments]. *New England Journal of Medicine*, **333**, 1038–1044.

Wang, F. Z., Dahl, H., Linde, A. *et al.* (1996). Lymphotropic herpesviruses in allogeneic bone marrow transplantation. *Blood*, **88**, 3615–3620.

Wang, F. Z., Linde, A., Hagglund, H. *et al.* (1999). Human herpesvirus 6 DNA in cerebrospinal fluid specimens from allogeneic bone marrow transplant patients: does it have clinical significance? *Clinical Infectious Disease*, **28**, 562–568.

Wasserman, R., August, C. S., & Plotkin, S. A. (1988). Viral infections in pediatric bone marrow transplant patients. *Pediatric Infectious Disease Journal*, **7**, 109–115.

Wendt, C. H., Weisdorf, D. J., Jordan, M. C., Balfour, H. H., Jr., & Hertz, M. I. (1992). Parainfluenza virus respiratory infection after bone marrow transplantation. *New England Journal of Medicine*, **326**, 921–926.

Whimbey, E., Champlin, R. E., Couch, R. B. *et al.* (1996). Community respiratory virus infections among hospitalized adult bone marrow transplant recipients. *Clinical Infectious Diseases*, **22**, 778–782.

Whimbey, E., Champlin, R. E., Englund, J. A. *et al.* (1995). Combination therapy with aerosolized ribavirin and intravenous immunoglobulin for respiratory syncytial virus disease in adult bone marrow transplant recipients. *Bone Marrow Transplantation*, **16**, 393–399.

Whimbey, E., Elting, L. S., Couch, R. B. *et al.* (1994). Influenza A virus infections among hospitalized adult bone marrow transplant recipients. *Bone Marrow Transplantation*, **13**, 437–440.

Wingard, J. R., Chen, D. Y., Burns, W. H. *et al.* (1988). Cytomegalovirus infection after autologous bone marrow transplantation with comparison to infection after allogeneic bone marrow transplantation. *Blood*, **71**, 1432–1437.

Winston, D. J., Ho, W. G., Bartoni, K. *et al.* (1993). Ganciclovir prophylaxis of cytomegalovirus infection and disease in allogeneic bone marrow transplant recipients. Results of a placebo-controlled, double-blind trial. *Annals of Internal Medicine*, **118**, 179–184.

Wolf, D. G., Lurain, N. S., Zuckerman, T. *et al.* (2003). Emergence of late cytomegalovirus central nervous system disease in hematopoietic stem cell transplant recipients. *Blood*, **1001**, 463–5.

Yolken, R. H., Bishop, C. A., Townsend, T. R. *et al.* (1982). Infectious gastroenteritis in bone-marrow-transplant recipients. *New England Journal of Medicine*, **306**, 1010–1012.

Zaia, J. A., Gallez-Hawkins, G. M., Tegtmeier, B. R. *et al.* (1997). Late cytomegalovirus disease in marrow transplantation is predicted by virus load in plasma. *Journal of Infectious Diseases*, **176**, 782–785.

Zaia, J. A. (2000). Prevention and management of CMV-related problems after hematopoietic stem cell transplantation. *Bone Marrow Transplantation* **99**, 633–8.

Zambon, M., Bull, T., Sadler, C. J., Goldman, J. M., & Ward, K. N. (1998). Molecular epidemiology of two consecutive outbreaks of parainfluenza 3 in a bone marrow transplant unit. *Journal of Clinical Microbiology*, **36**, 2289–2293.

Zerr, D. M., Gooley, T. A., Yeung, L. *et al.* (2001). Human herpesvirus 6 reactivation and encephalitis in allogeneic bone marrow transplant recipients. *Clinical Infectious Diseases*, **33**, 763–771.

Zerr, D. M., Gupta, D., Huang, M. L., Carter, R., & Corey, L. (2002). Effect of antivirals on human herpesvirus 6 replication in hematopoietic stem cell transplant recipients. *Clinical Infectious Diseases*, **34**, 309–317.

75 Fungal infections

JAN TOLLEMAR

Karolinska Institute and Huddinge University Hospital, Stockholm, Sweden

Introduction

Fungal infections are opportunistic infections, whose pathogenicity is determined by the affected host's immune and clinical status. In immune compromised patients, fungi may cause serious or lethal infections. The incidence of both superficial and invasive disseminated fungal infections is increasing in immune compromised patients such as hematopoietic stem cell (HSC) transplant recipients. The overall incidence ranges between 2% and 40% depending considerably on diagnostic criteria and definition of infection. Autopsy studies, however, report invasive fungal infections contributing to death in 10% to 30% of HSC transplant recipients (Wingard *et al.*, 1987; Tollemar *et al.*, 1989a). In an EORTC/EBMT study on invasive fungal infections from 19 European bone marrow transplant (BMT) centers the incidence was 11.2% (De Bock *et al.*, 1995). With the use of modern antifungal drugs and early institution of treatment, the incidence of fatal fungal infections has been significantly reduced from 11.5% to 6% ($P < .05$) (Andström *et al.*, 1996). There is a difference in the incidence of fungal infections between autologous and allogeneic HSC transplant recipients, with fewer infections after autologous transplantation. This might be explained by the lack of graft-versus-host disease (GVHD), itself immunosuppressive, as is its treatment.

The majority of fungal infections are caused by *Candida* species, followed by *Aspergillus* species; in many centers other species than *Candida albicans* now predominate and many cases of aspergillosis are due to species other than *Aspergillus fumigatus*. Occasionally other fungi such as *Fusarium, Coccidioides, Malassezia, Trichosporon, Scedosporium,* or *Histoplasma,* may occur (Morrison, Haake, & Weisdorf, 1994; Rolston, 2001; Jahagidar & Morrison, 2002; Marr *et al.*, 2002) (Table 75.1). Infections with *Histoplasma* and *Coceidioides* depend on geographical location. Most candida infections occur during the neutropenic phase early after transplant (Fig. 75.1). However, infections may also occur later depending on the patient's clinical and immune status, especially in patients with chronic GVHD. At the Fred Hutchinson Cancer Center, as well as at other institutions, the incidence of invasive aspergillosis (particularly between day 40 and 180 posttransplant) increased in both allograft and autograft recipients during the 1990s, as did that of infection due to Fusarium species and Zygomycetes (Marr *et al.*, 2002a). In two studies from Seattle the onset of aspergillosis was found to be bimodal with peaks at day 16 and 96 after the transplant (Marr *et al.*, 2002a and b); late infections were common also for other molds, including *Zygomycetes, Fusarium,* and *Scedosporium spp.* (Wald *et al.*, 1997; Marr *et al.*, 2002b). Serious fungal infections occurring after engraftment are often due to Aspergillus (Marr *et al.*, 2002a).

The invasive form of a fungal infection represents a serious clinical problem. It is often hard to determine when to start antifungal treatment due to difficulty in diagnosis. The reported mortality from invasive fungal infections has decreased slightly over the last several years: 58% compared to 70% for candidiasis, and 71% compared to 90% for systemic aspergillosis (Shah & Just, 1989; De Bock *et al.*, 1995). However, even in 2002 the one-year patient survival after mold infections was reported to be only 20% (Marr *et al.*, 2002a and b). Widely available antifungal agents have narrow antifungal spectra, and, in some cases, severe adverse effects. There is no consensus on treatment duration; rather, this depends on the patient's immune status. When to stop therapy is also often uncertain.

Defective immunity and risk factors

Early after HSC transplantation patients lack both nonspecific and specific defenses against fungi. Nonspecific defenses

Table 75.1. *Classification of fungal infections occurring in HSC transplant recipients*

Type of fungus	Examples
Opportunistic yeasts	*Candida* species
	Cryptococcus neoformans
Hyaline molds	*Aspergillus* species
	Fusarium species
Dematiaceous molds	*Pseudoallescheria boydii*
Endemic dimorphic fungi	*Histoplasma capsulatum*
	Coccidioides immitis

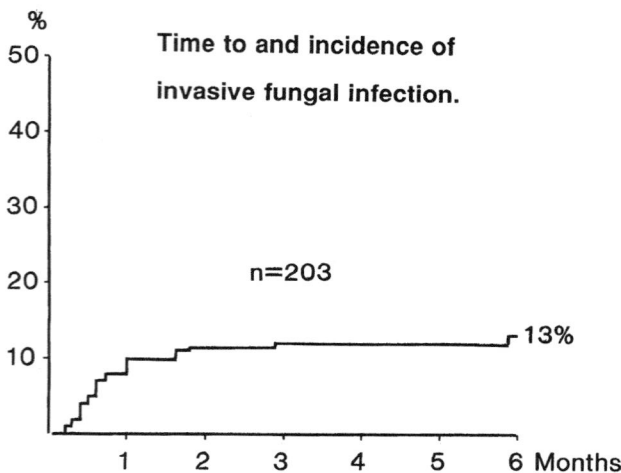

Figure 75.1. Time to and probability of a proven invasive fungal infection in allogeneic bone marrow transplant recipients. Reproduced, with permission, from Tollemar et al. (1989b).

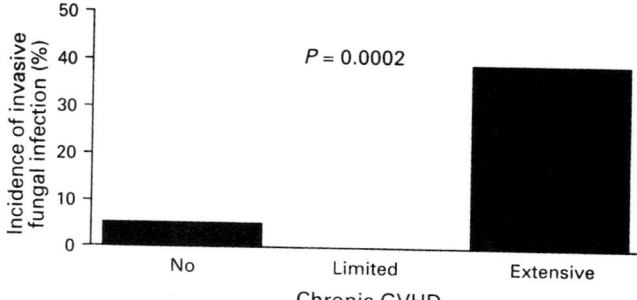

Figure 75.2. Incidence of invasive fungal infections according to the grade of chronic GVHD. Reproduced, with permission, from Jantunen et al. (1997).

include surface barriers; the skin and mucosal membranes of the respiratory, gastrointestinal, and urinary tracts are disrupted by chemotherapy, radiotherapy, indwelling catheters, and herpesvirus lesions. The neutropenic state, as well as the lack of monocytes, during the early posttransplant period increases the risk of invasive candidiasis and aspergillosis. The risk increases daily during the neutropenic state (Martin, Counts, & Thomas, 1977) (Table 75.2). The concomitant lack of T lymphocytes permits the development of superficial Candida infections or, very occasionally, cryptococcal meningitis, but is not considered to be a risk factor for disseminated fungal infection. The impact of the new approach of non-myeloablative conditioning regimens on infectious complications is as yet not well defined. These protocols may lead to faster engraftment with less disruption of mucosal integrity. However, one study of 71 patients receiving reduced conditioning compared to 123 patients receiving standard myeloablative therapy revealed a reduced risk for CMV infection and disease but no change in the risk for fungal infections (Martino et al., 2001).

Although recovery of neutrophils in patients receiving myeloablative conditioning usually occurs within 1 to 2 weeks, full T-cell immune reconstitution takes a year or longer. However, in colonized patients the lymphocyte response to Candida anti-

gens returns within 3 to 6 months of transplant (Tollemar & Ringdén, 1991). GVHD (Jantunen et al., 1997) (Figs. 75.2 and 75.3) and its treatment with corticosteroids, cyclosporine, or antithymocyte globulin (ATG), appears to predispose to late fungal infection. Volpi and colleagues (2001) reported that the use of granulocyte colony-stimulating factor (G-CSF) posttransplant in recipients of T-cell–depleted haploidentical family member transplants was associated with a slower recovery of CD4+ cells in the blood and a long-lasting effect on Th2 immunity in that Th2-inducing dendritic cells did not produce interleukin (IL)-12 and the patients had high frequencies of IL-4- and IL-10-producing CD4+ cells that did not express the IL-12 receptor β_2 chain. This correlated with the recovery rate of antifungal T-cell responses. They have since ceased the use of G-CSF administration posttransplant. The same group has described defective anti-fungal T-helper (Th1) immunity in a murine model of allogeneic T-cell-depleted bone marrow transplantation (impaired production of interferon-γ and IL-12 with high-level production of IL-4 and IL-10) (Mencacci et al., 2001). Attempts are being made to minimize this infection risk clinically by infusing cloned pathogen-specific, non-alloreactive donor T cells posttransplant (Perrucio et al., 2001).

In a survey from our own institution, risk factors for fungal infections were evaluated in 203 consecutive BMT patients, in whom the autopsy-verified incidence of fungal infection was 10% (7.5% Candida species, 2.5% Aspergillus species) (Tollemar et

Table 75.2.   Duration of neutropenia and prevalence of autopsy-proven fungal infection

	Days with neutrophil count $<0.5 \times 10^9/l$		
	1–20	21–40	>41
Number of patients	43	22	7
Incidence of fungal infection (%)	21	41	57

Data from Martin, Counts, & Thomas (1977).

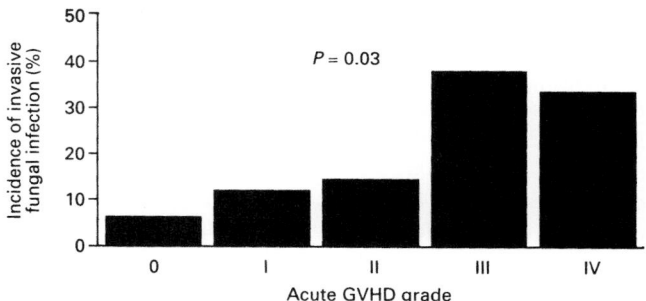

Figure 75.3. Incidence of late invasive fungal infections (diagnosed >100 days posttransplant) according to the severity of acute GVHD. Reproduced, with permission, from Jantunen et al. (1997).

al., 1989a). The infections occurred at a median of 19 (range 5–267) days posttransplant. In multivariate analysis, risk factors at the time of transplant were splenectomy, recipient cytomegalovirus seropositivity, and low bone marrow cell dose. Risk factors during the first 30 days posttransplant were ATG treatment and acute GVHD grade II–IV (bivariate logistic regression analysis). In two other risk factor analyses in 1,506 and 665 BMT recipients, the incidence of fungal infection was 11.4% and 12.5%, respectively (Goodrich *et al.,* 1991; Verfaillie *et al.,* 1991). Additional risk factors were higher age, a conditioning regimen containing total body irradiation, duration of neutropenia, a diagnosis of acute myeloid leukemia, an HLA-mismatched transplant, and *Candida* colonization, especially by *Candida tropicalis*. Infections in general, but particularly fungal and bacterial infection, appear less common after allogeneic PBSC transplants compared to marrow transplants (Storek *et al.,* 2001), probably related to higher lymphocyte and lymphocyte subset counts in the PBSC recipients. In a survey of 395 recipients of HLA-identical sibling PBSC transplants, the incidence of invasive fungal infections was 14%, and the only two significant risk factors for developing a non-*Candida* (mainly *Aspergillus*) invasive fungal infection were acute GVHD grade II–IV and steroid prophylaxis for GVHD (Fig. 75.4), (Martino *et al.,* 2002). Risk factors for aspergillosis were evaluated in 2496 patients, of which 158 had an invasive infection: before day 40, underlying disease, donor type, season and transplant outside laminar air flow rooms were risk factors; after day 40, underlying disease, donor type, age, GVHD, neutropenia, and corticosteroid use were associated with the infection. Although neutropenia was associated with the infection, the majority of patients (69%) were not neutropenic at diagnosis in this study (Wald *et al.,* 1997).

Fungal colonization is encouraged by the prolonged use of broad-spectrum antibacterial antibiotics. In a risk factor analyses of 58 children, the incidence of deep *Candida* infection was 8.7%; all infections occurred before engraftment and were fatal. In this study, risk factors were an HLA-mismatched sibling transplant, donor seropositivity for herpes simplex virus, and positive serology for fungi pretransplant (Klingspor *et al.,* 1996). Factors found to be associated with fungal infection in allogeneic BMT recipients are presented in Table 75.3. In a risk factor analysis for invasive aspergillosis after allogeneic transplantation, Ribaud and colleagues (1999) found GVHD status at the time of infection and the cumulative prednisolone dose taken during the week preceding the diagnosis of infection to be particularly important.

Marr and colleagues (2002b) examined the risk factors for invasive aspergillosis with regard to time post allograft: within the first 40 days of transplant, older patient age and use of cord blood were associated with increased risk, while a diagnosis of CML in first chronic phase (versus other hematologic malignancies and aplastic anemia), and the use of HLA-identical related PBSC (versus marrow) conferred protection. Between days 40 and 180 posttransplant, risk factors included older patient age, a diagnosis of myeloma, receipt of a T-cell-

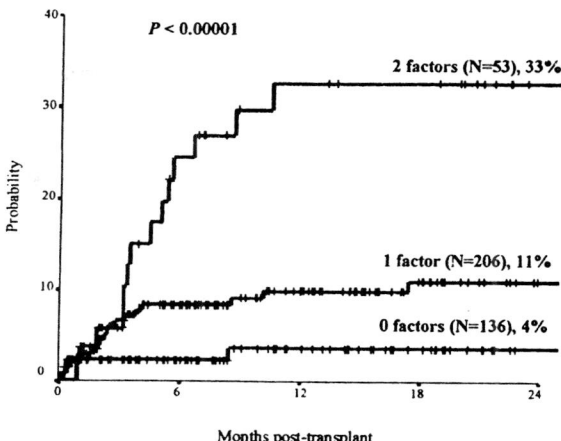

Figure 75.4. Probability of developing a non-*Candida* invasive fungal infection according to the presence of 0, 1, or 2 risk factors (steroid prophylaxis and development of moderate-to-severe graft-versus-host disease). Reproduced, with permission, from Martino *et al.* (2002).

depleted or CD34-selected transplant, receipt of corticoseroids, neutropenia, lymphopenia, GVHD, CMV disease and respiratory virus infections. Beyond day 180, risk factors were chronic GVHD and CMV disease. The mechanism of the association between CMV disease and invasive aspergillosis is unknown; possibilities include the immune-modulating effect of the virus, or neutropenia associated with treatment of the CMV disease with ganciclovir.

Table 75.3. *Risk factors for invasive fungal infection in allogeneic marrow transplant recipients by multivariate analysis from three separate studies, and in one study of children by Fischer's exact test*

Risk factor	*P* value
Splenectomy	.0029
CMV seropositive recipient	.0100
Low bone marrow cell dose	.0154
Acute GVHD grade II–IV[a]	.005
ATG treatment[a]	.006
Higher age	<.0001
Fungal colonization	<.0001
Longer neutropenia	.0005
Total body irradiation	<.05
Acute myeloid leukemia	<.001
HLA-mismatched transplant, adults	<.001
HLA-mismatched transplant, children[b]	.0184
HSV seropositive donor[b]	.0139
IgA anti-*Candida* antibody[b]	.0452

Abbreviations: CMV, cytomegalovirus; GVHD, graft-versus-host disease; ATG, antithymocyte globulin; HSV, herpes simplex virus.

[a] Bivariate analysis.

[b] Fischer's exact test.

Data from Tollemar *et al.* (1989b), Goodrich *et al.* (1991), Verfaillie *et al.* (1991), and Klingspor *et al.* (1996).

Fungal pathogens

Candida

Candida is the most frequent soil-dwelling fungal pathogen. The organism is usually endogenous and gastrointestinal tract colonization has been documented in 70% of normal subjects (Odds, 1988). *Candida* may breach the epithelial barrier and reach the bloodstream through intravenous catheters. Alternatively, *Candida* may enter the bloodstream from a colonized intestinal tract. The damage produced in the gut mucosa by chemotherapy/irradiation further increases the chance of fungi gaining access to the vascular system. It has also been shown that *Candida* can infect through an intact mucous membrane.

A number of species of *Candida* pathogenic in humans are listed in Table 75.4. The two most common causing disseminated infection are *Candida albicans* and *tropicalis*. With the use of prophylactic fluconazole treatment, the incidence of infection due to non-*Candida albicans* strains such as *Candida krusei, glabrata,* and *parapsilosis* has increased (Wingard *et al.,* 1991, 1993; Lòpez-Jiménez *et al.,* 1997).

The most common clinical syndromes in marrow transplant recipients are

1. Superficial mucosal colonization/infection, including oropharyngeal candidiasis, esophageal candidiasis, vaginal candidiasis, and cystitis
2. Candidemia (fungemia)
3. Acute disseminated candidiasis
4. Chronic disseminated (hepatosplenic) candidiasis
5. Single organ candidiasis

Organs most often affected during hematogenous dissemination of *Candida* are the kidneys, brain, heart, lungs, eyes, skin, skeletal muscle, liver, spleen, bone, and joints. In an affected organ, multiple small, micro- or macro-abscesses develop. They seldom become large enough before death for detection by ultrasonography, but can be detected in the liver, spleen, and kidneys by abdominal computed tomography (CT) scanning.

Candidemia (fungemia)

Candidemia is the most common cause of fungemia in HSC transplant recipients. The isolation of *Candida* from the blood of a relatively asymptomatic patient should focus attention on the central venous catheter as a likely source. The longer the duration of candidemia, the more likely is the development of disseminated infection with tissue involvement (Table 75.5). In a retrospective study of vascular catheter-associated fungemia (98% *Candida* spp.) in 155 patients with cancer, the best outcome occurred in patients in whom the line was removed and systemic antifungal drugs were given. The authors concluded that all cases of fungemia should be taken seriously (Lecciones *et al.,* 1992).

Acute disseminated candidiasis

Acute disseminated candidiasis is characterized by persistent fungemia, hypotension, multiorgan failure, skeletal muscle involvement, and cutaneous lesions. In addition to specific antifungal therapy, hemodynamic support and monitoring is often required in these critically ill patients.

Chronic disseminated candidiasis

The most common manifestation of chronic disseminated candidiasis is hepatosplenic candidiasis. Chronic disseminated candidiasis is established during the course of fungemia while the patient is neutropenic, and becomes clinically overt as chronic refractory progressive lesions upon recovery from neutropenia (Pestalozzi *et al.,* 1997). Hepatosplenic and other tissue lesions are radiologically occult during neutropenia but become evident by diagnostic imaging methods upon recovery from neutropenia. Unlike acute disseminated candidiasis, chronic disseminated candidiasis is less often associated with hypotension, fungemia, or multiorgan failure. Earlier studies and more recent reports emphasize the chronicity and refractory nature of this infection.

The clinical manifestations are generally nonspecific. The patient most often presents with fever, but other signs and symptoms are rare, other than abdominal tenderness if intraabdominal organ involvement is present. Signs of sepsis or septic shock including hypotension, tachycardia, and shaking chills may be present in up to 30% of patients. Macronodular cutaneous lesions, pink to red in color and up 1 cm in diameter, may occur as a manifestation of disseminated candidiasis. They may vary from a single nodule to a widespread rash, which can be mistaken for an allergic reaction. However, skin rash or endophthalmitis occurs in fewer than 5% of the patients with disseminated candidiasis (Meunier, 1988). There are reports that the abscesses demonstrable by abdominal CT scanning do not completely resolve radiologically, even when rendered sterile by adequate antifungal therapy.

Table 75.4. *Pathogenic* Candida *species*

C. albicans
C. tropicalis
C. pseudotropicalis
C. guilliermondi
C. krusei
C. parapsilosis
C. stellatoidea
C. lusitaniae
C. glabrata (Torulopsis glabrata)

Table 75.5. *Relationship between the duration of* Candida fungemia *and tissue involvement*

	Days of *Candida* fungemia			
	1	2	3–7	>7
Tissue involvement (% patients)	50	33	57	80

Data from Verfaillie *et al.* (1991).

Aspergillus

Aspergillus species are soil-dwelling fungi that, in contrast to *Candida,* can often be isolated from air samples, dust, food, and plants within hospitals. The most pathogenic species of *Aspergillus* are *fumigatus, flavus,* and *niger.* The infection is nosocomial and usually hospital-acquired by airborne transmission to the respiratory tract. Furthermore, outbreaks of *Aspergillus* infections have been reported when construction works have been carried out in hospital premises (Meunier, 1988; Ansorg *et al.,* 1996). Hospital water distribution systems can serve as a potential indoor reservoir of aspergillus and other molds, leading to aerosolization of fungal spores (Anaissie *et al.,* 2003). Measures to minimize the risk of patient exposure to this include provision of sterile (boiled) water for drinking and sterile sponges for bathing. Additionally, cleaning the floors of the shower facility can significantly reduce the mean air concentration of these organisms.

Clinical syndromes include allergic aspergillosis, parasinusitis, aspergilloma, and invasive aspergillosis. The latter is the common type occurring in immune suppressed patients, and includes hemorrhagic bronchopneumonia, pulmonary infection with cavitation, and/or hemorrhages, which can be fatal (Table 75.6). In one series, the lungs were the most commonly involved organ (90%), followed by the central nervous system (41%) (Jantunen *et al.,* 2000). Obstructing tracheobronchial aspergillosis has also been described in HSC transplant recipients (Angelucci *et al.,* 1991; Choi *et al.,* 1997; Machida *et al.,* 1999), and can mimic the "mosaic attenuation" pattern on high-resolution chest CT scanning normally suggestive of bronchiolitis obliterans (Nusair *et al.,* 2002). Pulmonary or paranasal sinus infections in BMT patients (Siberry, Costarangos, & Cohen, 1997) may be the portal entry for dissemination to other major organs. *Aspergillus* was the most common cause of brain abscess (58%) in HSC transplant patients, followed by *Candida* (33%) (Hagensee *et al.,* 1994). Skin involvement, presenting as red painful nodules with central necrosis (and usually a manifestation of disseminated disease), has been described (Schimmelpfennig *et al.,* 2001). Subcutaneous metastatically spreading infection without necrotizing cutaneous papules or ulcerating lesions has also been reported (Cornely *et al.,* 2001) Clinical presentation is with fever unresponsive to broad-spectrum antibacterial antibiotics, usually with the development of pulmonary infiltrates, sometimes with a typical triangular wedge shape due to blood vessel occlusion with thrombosis. The classical second site for lesions is the central nervous system, where prompt diagnosis by biopsy and initiation of treatment can be lifesaving. Other metastatic sites include heart, kidney, liver, and spleen. With the increasing use of non-myeloablative regimens incorporating intensely immunosuppressive agents such as fludarabine, Campath 1, and ATG, there is an increased likelihood of opportunistic infections including *Aspergillus,* and these may involve unusual sites such as joints (Panigrahi *et al.,* 2001).

Other fungi in HSC transplant recipients

Cryptococcus

Cryptococcus neoformans is distributed worldwide and is found in soil, vegetable matter, and in avian feces. It has a polysaccharide capsule that excludes India ink and that is therefore responsible for the halo seen on smears stained by India ink. *Cryptococcus neoformans* is a common cause of fungal meningitis in some immune compromised patients, especially those with defects of cell-mediated immunity, such as those with human immunodeficiency virus (HIV) infection. Surprisingly, therefore, it is seldom reported in HSC transplant recipients. The onset of infection may be insidious without dramatic neurologic findings other than headache. A presumptive diagnosis may be considered if budding yeast can be demonstrated with India ink staining of cerebrospinal fluid or if cryptococcal antigen is present. Cultures are necessary for confirmation. Other uncommon sites of infection are lung and skin. The treatment of choice consists of amphotericin B with or without 5-flucytosine or fluconazole, followed by suppressive therapy with a triazole (Yao, Liao, & Wen, 2000). There are promising results (mainly in HIV patients) with fluconazole as well as with AmBisome (Ringden *et al.,* 1991; Coker *et al.,* 1993; Powderly, 1996; Chen, 2002). Several new antifungal drugs, including voriconazole, posaconazole, cancidas, and anidulafungin have revealed excellent antifungal activity in animal studies as well as in in vitro studies of isolates (Barchiesi *et al.,* 2001; Roling *et al.,* 2002).

Histoplasma

Histoplasma capsulatum is endemic in the central United States of America. The fungus is soil-dwelling and in endemic areas most people have been infected. The primary infection is in the lung and may be followed by a flu-like illness characterized by fever, myalgia, and cough. In immune compromised patients the infection may disseminate to major organs. The diagnosis can be made on the isolation or identification of the fungus in clinical specimens including blood cultures. Serologic tests are usually not useful. The treatment of choice is amphotericin.

Coccidioides

Coccidioides immitis is a soil-dwelling fungus present endemically in North, Central, and South America. The infection is acquired by airborne transmission, causing pulmonary infection. This may disseminate in immune compromised patients to produce deep organ involvement with a poor prognosis.

Table 75.6. *Respiratory tract manifestations of invasive aspergillosis*

Hemorrhagic bronchopneumonia
Pulmonary infection with hemorrhagic infarction and cavitation
Necrotizing tracheobronchitis
Invasive sinusitis
Local extension to intrathoracic structures
Chronic necrotizing aspergillosis

Diagnostic tests consist mainly of demonstration of the fungus from clinical specimens. The treatment of choice in advanced disease or in immune compromised hosts is amphotericin.

Fusarium infections

Fusarium infections, which typically occur in patients with profound persistent granulocytopenia, produce a pattern similar to that of invasive aspergillosis (Boutati & Anaissie, 1997; Rolston, 2001). At Fred Hutchinson Cancer Research Center *Fusarium* infections increased in frequency during the 1990s, mainly in patients who had multiple transplants. Treatment was amphotericin B or a lipid formulation thereof, but some received investigational triazoles as rescue therapy; mortality was 80% with a median survival of 25 days (Marr *et al.*, 2002). Fusarium infections in neutropenic BMT recipients are characterized by pulmonary infiltrates and sinusitis. Biopsy of the cutaneous lesions often reveals fine, dichotomously branching, acutely angular, septate hyphae. Unlike *Aspergillus* species, *Fusarium* species are frequently detected by advanced blood culture detection systems, such as lysis centrifugation. This emerging fungal pathogen often does not respond to conventional doses of amphotericin B and may require substantially higher doses for successful outcome. Some cases of invasive *Fusarium* infection may be completely refractory to amphotericin B, therefore requiring investigational antifungal compounds; voriconazole has demonstrated in vitro activity (Ghannoum & Kuhn, 2002).

Mucormycosis

Mucormycotic infections are caused by fungi of the family *Rhizopus, Mucor,* or *Absidia* and are rare, usually being associated with diabetes or immunosuppression. Sites of infection can be sinonasal, rhinocerebral, aural, bronchial, pulmonary, and central nervous system. The disease can disseminate via the vascular route rapidly causing death within days. Rhinocerebral mucormycosis is characterized by sinusitis and a painless necrotic black palatal or nasal septal ulcer or eschar. This syndrome is also known as zygomycosis and an identical illness can be caused by *Aspergillus, Fusarium,* and *Pseudoallescheria boydii.* If symptoms and signs of acute fulminant invasive fungal sinusitis are present, urgent surgery should be performed to obtain material for histopathologic evaluation and if appropriate to aggressively debride the devitalized tissue supporting fungal growth (Drakos *et al.,* 1993). Treatment with amphotericin B up to 1.5 mg/kg/day should be initiated immediately without waiting for the results of the fungal cultures and continued for a minimum of 14 days. Total doses of 2.5 to 4 g of ampotericin B may be necessary if the patient is immunocompromised. Liposomal amphotericin B, the azole voriconazole, and combinations of antifungal agents may also prove useful in treatment of this syndrome. Acute invasive sinusitis must be distinguished from noninvasive fungal sinusitis, which may be manifest as allergic sinusitis or sinus mycetoma (fungus ball). These two types of sinusitis can be distinguished clinically using radiologic and histopathologic examination and require close interaction with ear, nose, and throat surgeons (deShazo, Chipin, & Swain, 1997).

Infections reported posttransplant (Jantunen *et al.*, 1996; Oliver *et al.,* 1996) include cutaneous (Trigg, Comito, & Rumelhart, 1996; Leong *et al.,* 1997), vulval (Nomura *et al.,* 1997), aural (Paterson *et al.,* 2000), bony (Oo *et al.,* 1998), and bronchial (Maddox *et al.,* 2001) involvement. In the case reported by Oliver it was concluded that the transplant recipient acquired hepatic mucormycosis from ingestion of a naturopathic medicine that contained the organism. Gaziev and colleagues (1996) described four cases of mucormycosis that occured among 711 patients who underwent transplantation for thalassemia and reviewed an additional 18 cases in the HSC transplant literature. All thalassemia patients were polytransfused and were in an advanced phase of disease with severe acquired hemochromatosis. Mucormycosis was the primary cause of death in three of the four thalassemia patients. Two of the infections were detected within the first 100 days posttransplant. Only one of the four patients had partial resolution of sinonasal mucormycosis following aggressive antifungal therapy combined with hyperbaric oxygen treatment.

Rare fungi in HSC transplant recipients

A small number of case reports dealing with other rare fungal infections in BMT recipients have been published and are listed in Table 75.7. Some are described in more detail below.

Scedosporium apiospermum

This organism, also known as *Pseudoallescheria boydii,* is an uncommon but highly aggressive organism in granulocytopenic patients that produces a pattern of infection similar to that of *Aspergillus* species, with invasion of blood vessels and infection of the respiratory tract. This organism may be completely resistant to amphotericin B. Treatment with miconazole may be successful; however, in neutropenic patients this agent also may not be effective. In vitro studies and limited clinical experience suggest the combination of amphotericin B plus an antifungal azole (e.g., miconazole). In in-vitro testing, both voriconazole and posaconazole have activity and might be considered. However, no treatment data have been presented.

Trichosporon species

Trichosporon beigelii is the most common of the *Trichosporon* species causing invasive infection. Although invasive *Trichosporon* infections are uncommon in immunocompromised patients including HSC transplant recipients (Erer *et al.,* 2000), they often produce a fatal disseminated mycosis in patients with profound granulocytopenia or those receiving coricosteroids. Clinical manifestations include fungemia, funguria, renal dysfunction, cutaneous lesions, pulmonary infiltrates, and chorioretinitis. Despite the administration of amphotericin B, fungemia may persist. In vitro and in vivo studies indicate that the organism is inhibited, but not killed, by safely achievable serum concentrations of amphotericin B. Newer antifungal triazoles, however, have been found to be active in vivo against this organism. The combination of amphotericin B plus an azole may also be effective.

Table 75.7. *Published case reports of rare fungi causing disseminated infection in hematopoietic stem cell transplant recipients*

Fungus	Reference
Pseudoallescheria boydii	Gumbart, 1983
Alternative names:	Guyotat *et al.*, 1987
Petriellidium boydii	Walsh *et al.*, 1992
Allescheria boydii	
Scedosporium apiospermum	
Monosporium apiospermum	
Trichosporon capitatum (beigelii)	Liu *et al.*, 1990
Trichosporon cutaneum	Lowenthal *et al.*, 1987
	Siegert *et al.*, 1988
Fusarium	Blazar *et al.*, 1984
	Bleggi-Torres *et al.*, 1996
Chrysosporium	Warwick *et al.*, 1991
Scopulariopsis	Neglia *et al.*, 1987
Malassezia furfur	Redline *et al.*, 1985
Saccharomyces cervisiae	Cairoli *et al.*, 1993
Paecilomyces varioti	Shing *et al.*, 1996
Paecilomyces lilacinus	Orth *et al.*, 1996
Hansenula anomala	Goss *et al.*, 1994
Penicillium brevicompactum	de la Camara *et al.*, 1996
Cokeromyces recurvatus	Tsai *et al.*, 1997
Neosartorya fischeri	Lonial *et al.*, 1997
Phialophora verrucosa	Lundstrom *et al.*, 1997
Aspergillus ustus	Iwen *et al.*, 1998
Chaetomium atrobrunneum	Guppy *et al.*, 1998;
	Chinnamma *et al.*, 1999
Trichoderma longibrachiatum	Richter *et al.*, 1999
Paecilomyces lilacinus	Chan-Tack *et al.*, 1999
Candida dubliniensis	Meis *et al.*, 1999
Cunninghamella spp.	Darrisaw *et al.*, 2000
Exophiala jeanselmei	Clancy *et al.*, 2000
Rhodotorula spp.	Alliot *et al.*, 2000
Curvularia spp.	Bonduel *et al.*, 2001

Nocardia

Nocardiosis is an infection caused by an aerobic actinomycete that commonly occurs in soil; the infection usually occurs after inhalation of the organism by immune compromised individuals. There have been at least 12 cases of nocardiosis reported posttransplant (Hodohara *et al.*, 1993; Freites *et al.*, 1995; Shearer & Chandrasekar, 1995; Choucino *et al.*, 1996; Elliot *et al.*, 1997; Machado *et al.*, 1997); in a review of the literature by Choucino *et al.* (1996), the rate after allogeneic transplantation was 1.7% and after autologous transplantation 0.2%; all 10 patients had received immunosuppressive medications and all but one of the allogeneic recipients had acute or chronic GVHD. Four patients had had extensive exposure to soil or dust before nocardiosis developed. Seventy percent of the patients died, but death was less often due to progressive nocardial infection than to complications of GVHD and associated invasive infection with *Aspergillus* species. Three patients had nocardiosis despite receiving prophylaxis with cotrimoxazole intermittently 2 or 3 times weekly. The site of disease included lung and subcutaneous tissues.

Malassezia

The genus *Malassezia* consists of 7 species. These dimorphic saprophytic yeasts have unusual lipophilic growth requirements. Most human infections are caused by *Malassezia furfur*, which includes the species previously known as *Pityrosporum ovale* and *Pityrosporum orbicularae*. Infections in HSC recipients have been described (Redline *et al.*, 1985; Bufill *et al.*, 1988; Morrison & Weisdorf, 2000). This fungus colonizes the skin of affected patients, from which it may gain access to a central venous catheter. The commonest manifestation of the skin involvement is Pityriais (tinea) versicolor, which consists of hypo- or hyper-pigmented skin lesions with thin scales and which tends to be truncal in location. The spectrum of infection ranges from asymptomatic catheter colonization to fungemia. Redline and colleagues (1985) noted the association with administration of intralipid therapy. In the series by Bufill, skin infection occurred early posttransplant and resolved with neutrophil engraftment in all cases. In contrast, 5 of the 6 the patients described by Morrison & Weisdorf had neutrophil counts above $0.5 \times 10^6/l$ at the time of infection. Infection occurred in the skin in 3, on the vulva in 1, and in the blood in 2. Treatment includes removal of the indwelling catheter, cessation of intravenous fat emulsions, and topical antifungal therapy for skin involvement. The genus exhibits in vitro susceptibility to imidazole derivatives, is moderately sensitive to amphotericin B, but usually resistant to flucytosine. However, the role of systemic antifungal treatment in HSC transplant recipients is presently unclear.

Diagnostic approaches

Although invasive fungal infection is frequently suspected, accurate diagnosis is difficult in the immune compromised patient. Noninvasive tests such as blood cultures, or tests for antibodies and antigens or metabolites of these organisms, are often insensitive and often negative, although more recently the detection of candidemia has been greatly improved by newer blood culture detection techniques, most notably the lysis centrifugation system and the BacT Alert system. These systems have been able to detect candidemia earlier and more frequently than conventional broth and biphasic systems. The nonradiometric infrared resin broth system (BacTec) may be similar to lysis centrifugation in the detection of fungemia. Nonculture techniques such as polymerase chain reaction, antigen and antibody detection, and measurement of metabolites for *Candida* species remain investigational.

Testing for antibodies is of limited value, because HSC transplant recipients have no ability to produce specific antibodies during the main risk period. However, pretransplant serology before BMT can be useful for indicating which patients will be at risk for a subsequent potentially fatal infection, as was shown in the risk factor analysis in children (Klingspor *et al.*, 1996). Other approaches include testing for fungal antigens or metabolites. At least four antigen tests have been described, three for *Candida* and one for *Aspergillus*. Sensitivity and specificity vary, depending on the patient population and whether random or sequential tests are taken. We found a sensitivity of 53% and a specificity of 100% for the Cand-tec test (Ramco Laboratories, Inc. Houston, USA) in marrow-transplanted patients with proven fungal infection (Tollemar et al., 1989a). Determination of D- and L-arabinitol ratios in urine by gas chromatography have shown promising results as a diagnostic tool for disseminated candidiasis, but clinical trials are needed (Larsson et al., 1994). At some centers prospective panfungal PCR screening has been explored with promising results, especially with regard to invasive aspergillosis with a sensitivity of 100% and specificity of 65% (Hebart et al., 2000). A nested polymerase chain reaction (PCR) test for Aspergillus species large ribosomal subunit genes is under evaluation (Williamson et al., 2000). Serial screening using a commercially available ELISA assay for galactomannan, a major aspergillus cell wall constituent, appears promising (Maertens et al., 2001).

For suspected pulmonary infection, high-resolution CT scanning followed by bronchoscopy may provide an etiology. A "halo" sign is commonly present early in the radiological (CT) course of pulmonary aspergillosis in the neutropenic patient (Cailloit et al., 2001). If other internal organs show radiologic evidence of abscesses, fine needle aspiration under ultrasound or CT control (of, for example, liver or kidney) is one such approach (Jantunen et al., 2000). The aspirate sample should be examined both cytologically and microbiologically. For a definitive diagnosis, histological demonstration of the fungal pathogen invading tissue has to be made.

Prophylaxis and treatment

Prophylaxis

Nonspecific antifungal prophylaxis in HSC transplant recipients does not differ from that provided to other types of patients at risk. It consists mainly of elimination and reduction of risk factors and exposure, optimized hospital care, and finally chemoprophylaxis. Antifungal chemoprophylaxis has mostly been attempted by oral administration of either polyenes, which interfere with the gastrointestinal fungal colonization, or azole compounds, which are absorbed and may have a systemic effect. In two randomized trials of 356 and 300 BMT patients, respectively, fluconazole at a dose of 400 mg given orally or intravenously was successful in reducing fungal colonization, and superficial and deep infections caused by Candida species, but not those caused by Aspergillus species. The incidence of fungal infections decreased from 15.8% to 2.8% and from 17% to 7%, respectively ($P < .01$, $P = .004$) (Goodman et al., 1992; Slavin et al., 1995). There has been controversy as to the optimal duration of such prophylaxis, specifically whether treatment should be given only for the period of engraftment or whether it should be continued through the period of acute GVHD risk. In a long-term follow-up of the study by Slavin et al. (1995), it was found that patients given fluconazole (for 75 days posttransplant) had protection against both early and late disseminated Candida infections (Figs. 75.5 and 75.6) as well as a decreased incidence of gut GVHD, resulting in an overall

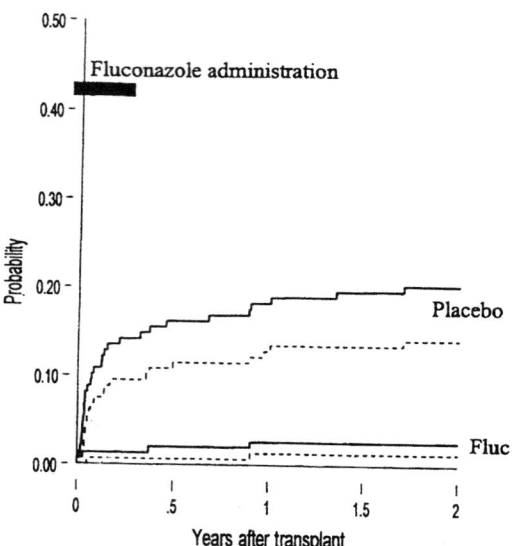

Figure 75.5. The development of invasive candidiasis and candidiasis-related death. Probability of the development of invasive candidiasis (bloodstream and tissue infection, solid lines) and candidiasis-related death (dashed lines) in placebo recipients and fluconazole (fluc) recipients. Compared with fluconazole recipients, more patients in the placebo arm had candidal infection (20% vs. 3%, $P < .001$) and candidiasis-related death (14% vs. 1%, $P < .001$). Also presented is the duration of fluconazole administered (conditioning through day 75, bold line). Reproduced, with permission, from Marr et al. (2000).

survival benefit (Fig. 75.7) compared to those patients receiving placebo (Marr et al., 2000). Lower doses of fluconazole have shown variable results (Alangaden et al., 1994) and cannot be recommended. Indeed, in children the dose of fluconazole should be increased to 8 to 12 mg/kg/day. Furthermore, there is a risk of developing or selecting fluconazole-resistant strains with inadequate dosing (Hoppe, Klingebiel, & Niethammer, 1994).

For prevention of Aspergillus infections, isolation in a laminar airflow room or nasal sprays of amphotericin B seem effective (Meunier, 1988; Trigg, Morgan, & Burns, 1997; Wald et al., 1997). A randomized trial comparing itraconazole oral solution with fluconazole in 445 adult hematological patients of whom 230 underwent autologous or allogeneic bone marrow transplantation, showed the same prophylactic efficacy with regard to candidal infections, but itraconazole afforded greater protection against fatal Aspergillus infections (Morgenstern et al., 1999).

In our own experience in a randomized trial of AmBisome (1 mg/kg/day i.v.) used prophylactically, we observed that it was well tolerated, reduced the number of patients with fungal colonization [33% compared to 64% ($P < .05$)], and reduced the incidence of proven systemic fungal infection from 8% to 3% (not significant). Similar results were found in a study by Kelsey and colleagues (1999).

In a prospective randomized study of 355 recipients of auto- and allografts, low-dose amphotericin (0.2 mg/kg/day iv) was as effective as fluconazole (400 mg/kg/day po or iv) in the prevention of fungal infections posttransplant (Wolff et al., 2000).

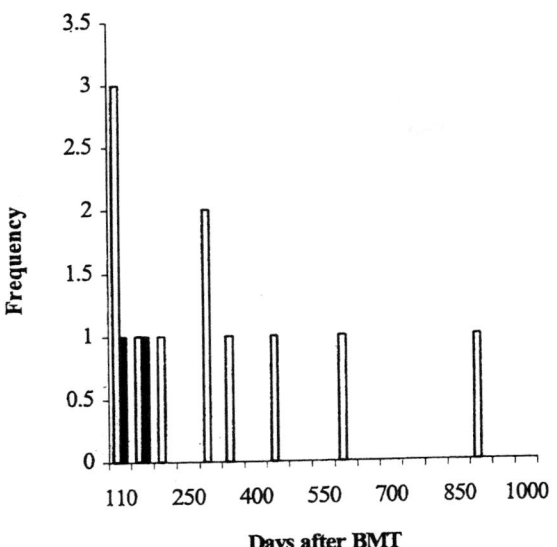

Figure 75.6. Frequency of candidal infection after day 110 of BMT. The number of placebo recipients (□) and fluconazole recipients (■) in whom invasive candidiasis developed after day 110 is shown. Reproduced, with permission, from Marr *et al.* (2000).

Proven fungal infections occurred in 7.5% and 4.1% of amphotericin-treated and fluconazole-treated patients respectively. The corresponding figures were 14.3% and 9.1% for allograft recipients and 5.6% and 2.1% for autograft recipients. However, fluconazole was significantly better tolerated, especially in allograft recipients (19% developed toxicity vs. 0% for fluconazole). A prophylactic trial comparing colloidal suspension amphotericin B (Amphocil) (4 mg/kg/day iv) with fluconazole 200 mg/kg day po was stopped prematurely because of a high incidence of infusion-related toxicity, including chills, fever, and hypotension, in the amphotericin arm (Timmers *et al.*, 2000). Previous studies of aerosolized amphotericin B suggested a possible prophylactic effect (Conneally *et al.*, 1993). However, this was not supported in a recent multicenter trial in 382 patients, excluding patients treated in HEPA-filtered rooms or those receiving amphotericin B or itraconazole treatment. The incidence of proven, probable, or possible invasive aspergillosis in patients receiving amphoteracin by inhalation was 7% versus 4% for untreated patients (P = .37) (Schwartz *et al.*, 1999). Its limited success in HSC transplant recipients might be due to difficulties in administration due to side-effects such as bronchspasm, nausea, and vomiting, resulting in poor compliance (Leather & Wingard, 2002).

For patients who require hospitalization, the Centers for Disease Control (2000) in the United States have issued guidelines for preventing opportunistic infections in HSC transplant recipients. Their recommendations for hospital infection-control measures to minimize exposure to molds include the following: allograft recipients should be placed in rooms with greater than 12 air exchanges per hour and point-of-use high-efficiency (>99%) particulate air (HEPA) filters that are capable of removing particles >0.3 μm in diameter. This is particularly important

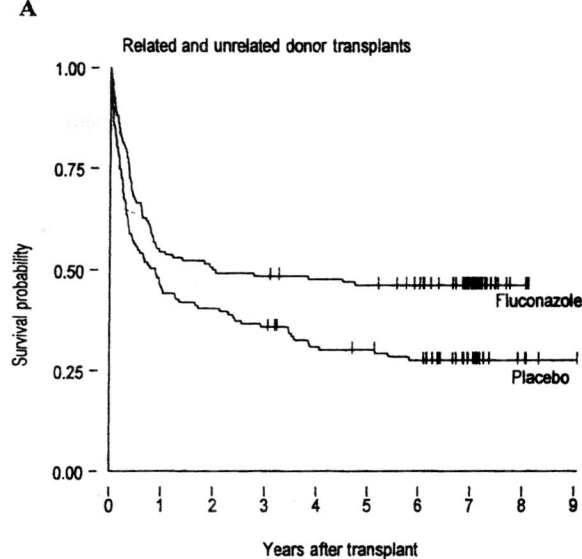

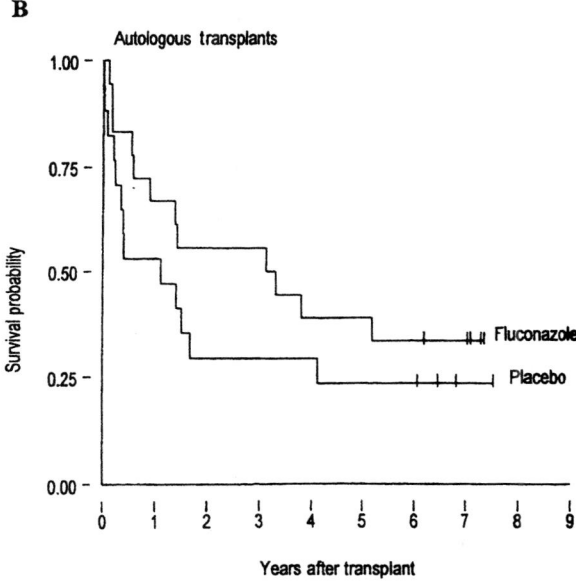

Figure 75.7. The survival probability in allogeneic and autologous BMT patients. Probability of survival in (**A**) 134 allogeneic BMT recipients who received fluconazole and 131 who received placebo (P = .0018) and (**B**) 18 autologous BMT recipients who received fluconazole and 17 who received placebo (P = .6). The allogeneic recipients included 213 patients who received HLA-matched grafts and 52 patients who received mismatched grafts. Tick marks represent patients alive at the last follow-up. Reproduced, with permission, from Marr *et al.* (2000).

during times of hospital construction and renovation. Use of HEPA-filtered rooms should be considered for autologous HSC transplant recipients if they develop prolonged neutropenia, the main risk factor for nosocomial aspergillosis.

Additionally, hospital rooms for HSC transplant recipients should have positive room-air pressure when compared to adjoining hallways, toilets, and anterooms. A consistent pressure differential should be maintained at <2.5 pascals or 0.01

inch by water gauge. Aspergillus can also be waterborne and some programs utilize avoidance of tap water and sponge baths rather than showers.

Although exposure to plants and flowers has not been shown conclusively to be the cause of fungal infections in immuno-compromized patients, most experts strongly recommend that plants and dried or fresh flowers not be allowed in the rooms of hospitalized HSC recipients or candidates.

Other approaches to reduce the risk of fungal infection or improving survival of an infection include administration of hematopoietic growth factors (for example, M-CSF, GM-CSF) (Nemunaitis *et al.,* 1991, 1993; Richardson, Brownlie, & Shankland, 1992; Bodey *et al.,* 1994; Roilides *et al.,* 1994; Moore *et al.,* 1998), or by giving immunoglobulin treatment, which has been reported to result in a low incidence of fungal infection (Milliken & Powles, 1990).

Treatment

There is currently intense development and testing of new anti-fungal drugs (Table 75.8), although, after more than 30 years, intravenous administration of amphotericin B remains the gold standard for the treatment of most invasive fungal infections in the immune compromised host, although this position is being challenged (see voriconazole below). However, this may soon change in favor of new antifungal drugs or a combination of them. Amphotericin B is a polyene antibiotic active against most commonly encountered fungi including *Candida* (with the exception of *Candida parapsilosis*) and *Aspergillus* species. It acts by binding irreversibly to the fungal cell membrane compo-nent, ergosterol, thereby causing a fatal leakage of potassium and other fungal cell products. However, a number of adverse side effects, especially renal impairment when it is used at the same time as cyclosporine, may prevent the use of therapeutic doses (Shulman *et al.,* 1981). This has led to the development of different lipid formulations of the drug as new delivery meth-ods, with reduced toxicity and enhanced efficacy in immune suppressed patients (Meunier, Prentice, & Ringden, 1991; Ringden *et al.,* 1991; Tollemar, 1995; Wingard, 1997).

Table 75.8. *Antifungal agents for systemic use*

Amphotericin B
Lipid formulations of amphotericin B
    Amphotericin B colloidal dispersion (Amphotec; ABCD)
    Amphotericin B lipid complex (Abelcet; ABLC)
    Liposomal amphotericin B (AmBisome)
    (Liposomal Nystatin)
Azoles
    Fluconazole
    Itraconazole
    Voriconazole
    Posaconazole
Echinocandins/Pneumocandins
    Caspofungin
    Micafungin
    Anidulafungin

Presently, three different amphotericin B preparations are com-mercially available: the liposomal form AmBisome, the col-loidal dispersion Amphocil/tec and the lipid complex Abelcet. Each of these preparations differ in size, structure, pharmacoki-netics, antifungal activity, and probably also in clinical efficacy. In general, the lipid formulations are cleared through the reticu-loendothelial system by tissue macrophages at infected sites. Doses up to 4 to 5 mg/kg/day are tolerated. Nephrotoxicity is reduced with all three preparations. However, acute toxicity, such as fever and chills, has been noted frequently with both Abelcet and Amphocil but not with AmBisome. Efficacy has been demonstrated in immune compromised patients with all three lipid formulations (Khoury *et al.,* 1997; Mehta *et al.,* 1997; Pasic, Flannagan, & Cant, 1997; Wingard, 1997). A lipo-somal nystatin preparation is also under development.

Another approach to overcome toxicity, and thereby to increase efficacy, has been to combine amphotericin B with 5-flucytosine (100 mg/kg/day in 4 divided doses). However, 5-flucytosine should be used with caution early after transplant, because of its marrow suppressive effect and propensity for resistance develop-ment. Currently, few centers use this approach.

Empirical therapy

Empirical therapy is used because of the insensitivity of diagnos-tic methods and poor outcome in HSCT patients with established fungal infections. In many transplant centers patients who are neutropenic and still febrile after 72 hours of antibacterial antibi-otic treatment are given amphotericin B until they become afebrile or reach a neutrophil count of $0.5 \times 10^9/l$, or both. The dose used is often 0.3 to 0.5 mg/kg of conventional amphotericin B. At our own institution, AmBisome at a dose of 1 mg/kg/day has been used empirically, and since this approach was started the incidence of autopsy-proven fungal infections has been reduced by 50% (Andström *et al.,* 1996). There are two studies on liposomal amphotericin B compared to conventional ampho-tericin B for fever of unknown origin. The first compared two doses of AmBisome (1 and 3 mg/kg/d) to 1 mg/kg/d of the con-ventional drug. In this study both doses of AmBisome was sig-nificantly safer than conventional amphotericin B in adults and children, as well as showing equivalent or possibly superior effi-cacy with regard to resolution of fever of unknown origin (Prentice *et al.,* 1997). In the second study, a randomized, dou-ble-blind, multicenter study of liposomal amphotericin (3 mg/kg/day) versus amphotericin B (0.6 mg/kg/day) as empirical antifungal therapy in febrile neutropenic patients, there was no difference in efficacy between the two, but the use of the liposo-mal preparation was associated with a significantly lower inci-dence of adverse events (including less fever, chills, nephrotoxic-ity, and hypokalemia) (Walsh *et al.,* 1999).

With regard to azoles with extended fungal spectrum, both itraconazole and voriconazole have been studied in patients with fever of unknown origin. A randomized, controlled multicenter study compared intravenous and oral itraconazole with intra-venous amphotericin B as empirical antifungal therapy for per-sistent fever in neutropenic cancer patients receiving broad-spec-trum antibacterial therapy (Boogaerts *et al.,* 2001). The response rates were 47% and 38%, respectively. Breakthrough fungal infection and mortality rates were similar. However, there were significantly fewer drug-related adverse events in the itraconazole group, including less chills, less nephrotoxicity, and less hypokalemia (Boogaerts *et al.*, 2001). Finally, voriconazole has been compared to liposomal amphotericin B in patients with neutropenia and persistent fever. This study failed to show non-inferiority, but voriconazole had fewer breakthrough infections and was better tolerated (Walsh *et al.*, 2002).

Shortcomings in empirical therapy (such as overtreatment) could be eliminated by a pre-emptive strategy guided by rapid and reliable new diagnostic methods such as PCR. This approach was investigated in one study of 42 febrile neutropenic pediatric cancer patients. Treatment consisted of amphotericin B instituted when 2 consecutive positive PCR tests, repeated every 2–3 days, occurred. Out of 83 febrile episodes, 31 were PCR positive and 84% of these episodes were shown to be due to a fungal infection. Thus, the majority of febrile episodes were of nonfungal origin. The study also showed a reduced mortality from fungal infections compared with historical controls (Lin, Lu, & Chen, 2001). This approach needs further investigation, and at our center a multicenter randomized trial using PCR-guided pre-emptive treatment versus empirical treatment with liposomal amphotericin B in allogeneic HSCT patients is ongoing.

Amphotericin B and amphotericin lipid formulations

Amphotericin B is still considered to be first-line therapy in HSC transplant recipients, although in some centers lipid formulations have more or less replaced it (Meyers & Thomas, 1988; Tollemar, 1995; Andström *et al.*, 1996; Wingard, 1997; Bowden *et al.*, 2002). The usual dose of amphotericin B for systemic infection is 1 mg/kg daily, or alternate daily, depending on renal function. No difference in the incidence of fever (50%–59%) or chills (25%–29%) was found between a rapid (1 hour) infusion compared to a more prolonged infusion (4–6 hours) in one study in which high-pressure liquid chromatography was used to assay serum levels (target serum level 1–2 mg/l) (Emminger *et al.*, 1991). The most commonly used doses with lipid formulations are presented in Table 75.9, but the doses in these studies have not been established in randomized trials; furthermore, they differ between the three preparations. In the early studies of lipid formulation amphotericin that have been described in HSC transplant recipients, Amphocil was found to be safe at doses up to 7.5 mg/kg and had a tolerable infusion-related toxicity and demonstrable antifungal activity with a complete or partial response rate across dose levels and infection types of 52% (Bowden *et al.*, 1996). The complete response rate for fungemia was 53% and the complete or partial response rate for pneumonia was 52%. In a recent randomized trial between Amphocil 6 mg/kg/d and amphotericin B 1–1.5 mg/kg/d in invasive aspergillosis, the same efficacy was seen. Fewer patients had renal toxicity but, interestingly, more infusion-related chills and fever episodes occurred with Amphocil (Bowden *et al.*, 2002). Using AmBisome, Andström *et al.* (1996) reported a significant reduction in autopsy-proven invasive fungal infection (6%) compared to a retrospective comparison with conventional amphotericin B (11%). Survival or cure of mycotic infections occurred in 5 of 13 patients (38%). In a study using liposomal amphotericin B in doses from 3 to 5 mg/kg, Kruger *et al.* (1996) reported a reduced sensitivity for *Candida* species to the liposomal preparation compared to the conventional preparation. In a randomized multicenter study of aspergillosis during neutropenia, Leenders *et al.* (1998) reported that AmBisome at a dose of 5 mg/kg/d was superior to 1 mg/kg/d of amphotericin B both in efficacy and safety. However, that higher doses are better was not shown in a prospective, randomized, multi-center study, in which no difference in efficacy for treating invasive aspergillosis was detected when 1 mg/kg/day of AmBisome was compared to 4 mg/kg/day (Ellis *et al.*, 1998).

Table 75.9. *Antifungal treatment of systemic Candida and Aspergillus infection*

Type of fungal infection	Drug	Dose/day	Total dose	Treatment duration (days)
Candida				
Fungemia[b]	1) Amph.B[a]	0.5–1 mg/kg	0.5–1 g	14 days after last positive blood culture
	or 2) AmBisome	1–3 mg/kg	1–2 g	For at least 10 days
	or 3) Fluconazole	200–400 mg	2–4 g	7–14 days
Acute[b] or chronic disseminated infection	1) Amph.B plus or minus 5-flucytosine	1 mg/kg 100 mg/kg and according to serum levels	≥2 g	Unknown; clinical picture must guide
	or 2) AmBisome	2–3 mg/kg	≥2 g	Unknown; clinical picture must guide
Aspergillus[c]				
Invasive	Amph.B plus or minus 5-flucytosine	1–1.5 mg/kg 100 mg/kg and according to serum levels	≥2.5 g	Unknown; clinical picture must guide
	or AmBisome	3–5 mg/kg	≥2 g	Unknown; clinical picture must guide

[a] Amph.B = Amphotericin B i.v.
[b] Remove vascular catheter when diagnosis made.
[c] Voriconazole is now approved in U.S. and Europe as first-line therapy to invasive aspergillosis. Caspospongin is now approved as second-line therapy for invasive aspergillosis.
Data from Meyers & Thomas (1988) and Tollemar (1995).

Azoles

The azole drugs represent an important part of antifungal therapy. Available agents for treatment include ketoconazole, miconazole, fluconazole, itraconazole, and voriconazole. Ketoconazole has poor efficacy and interacts to produce high cyclosporine blood levels resulting in cyclosporine toxicity. Fluconazole is fungistatic, and has no activity against *Aspergillus* species. Fluconazole has proven to be useful in the treatment of oropharyngeal candidiasis and may have a role in treatment of systemic *Candida* infections. However, experience in disseminated infections, especially in neutropenic patients, is thus far limited. Miconazole 20 to 40 mg/kg/day (plus amphotericin) may be used in the treatment of infections with *Pseudoallescheria boydii*. Itraconazole has activity against *Aspergillus* species. Posttransplant use has been limited partly because of poor oral bioavailability. Doses of up to 400 mg twice daily have been used (4–10 mg/kg/day). Voriconazole is active in vitro against amphotericin B–resistant *Aspergillus* and against azole-resistant *Candida* species, including *C. krusei* and *C. glabrata,* as well as *Cryptococcus, Fusarium,* and *Scedosporium apiospermum.* There is both an oral and an intravenous preparation. Transient visual changes are the only significant toxicities so far described. In a phase III trial of invasive aspergillosis, voriconazole was compared to amphotericin B in 277 patients with proven or probable aspergillosis (Herbrecht *et al.,* 2002). The survival rate at 12 weeks was 70.8% versus 57.9% in favor of voriconazole, which was also safe. Intravenous voriconazole was given as 6 mg/kg twice daily on day 1, followed by a 4 mg/kg twice daily for at least 7 days, followed by 200 mg twice daily orally. As a result of this trial, voriconazole is now licensed as first-line therapy for aspergillosis in both the USA and Europe. Voriconazole has good CNS penetration.

New azoles under development include posaconazole a potent triazole with activity against *Candida* spp. *Aspergillus* spp. and potency in animal models of blastomycosis, cryptococcosis, and coccidiomycosis. It is in phase III testing (Groll, Piscitelli, & Walsh, 1998).

Echinocandins/pneumocandins

The echinocandins/pneumocandins are a new class of antifungal agents and include caspofungin. They act by inhibiting glucan synthesis in the fungal cell wall, a target not present in mammalian cells. They have a broad range of activity, being active against azole-resistant *Candida* and are fungistatic against *Aspergillus.* They are, however, inactive against *Fusarium, Trichosporon,* and *Cryptococcus.* Caspofungin is administered intravenously. Nephrotoxicity has not been described.

In the U.S. caspofungin is approved in the treatment of candidemia, candida esophagitis, candida infections causing intraabdominal abcesses, peritonitis or pleural space infections, and invasive aspergillosis in patients refractory or interolerant to other antifungal therapies. Caspospungin does not have good CNS penetration, A single 70 mg loading dose should be administered by slow IV infusion on day 1, followed by 50 mg daily thereafter. In one study caspofungin reduced the blood AUC_{0-12} of tacrolimus by 20%. In other studies, cyclosporine increased

the AUC of caspofungin by approximately 35%. For patients receiving caspofungin and either cyclosporine or tacrolimus, monitoring the levels of each drug is recommened. Rifampin can cause a 30% decrease in caspofungin trough concentrations.

Other agents in development include micafungin (FK-463) and anidulafungin (LY303366).

Another approach to increase the efficacy of treatment is by improving the patient's hematopoietic status. This has been attempted by giving neutrophil transfusions from donors stimulated with G-CSF and promising results in neutropenic patients with fungal infections have been seen (Feldman *et al.,* 1993; Clarke *et al.,* 1995). Another approach is to administer G-CSF or GM-CSF directly to the patient. Interferon-γ has also been used. In some cases surgical resection or drainage may be needed to effect cure of *Aspergillus* and some other fungal infections.

A summary of the treatment by antifungal agents of systemic candidiasis and aspergillosis is given in Table 75.9, of mucosal candidiasis in Table 75.10, and of treatment approaches additional to the use of antifungal agents in Table 75.11. Table 75.12 shows *Candida* species usually resistant to either amphotericin or to fluconazole.

Fungal infections occurring pretransplant

Candida

In order to determine if a prior history of hepatosplenic candidiasis resulted in an increase in *Candida*-associated morbidity and mortality after marrow transplantation, Bjerke, Myers, and Bowden (1994) prospectively observed 15 consecutive patients with biopsy-proven hepatosplenic candidiasis that developed pretransplant. All patients had received amphotericin B before transplant and this was continued at a dose of 0.5 mg/kg/day from the time of pretransplant conditioning through marrow engraftment, at which time it was discontinued if CT evidence of disease was stable or improved. Seventy-three percent of the patients had persistently abnormal CT scans pretransplant. Posttransplant, 3 of 15 died with evidence

Table 75.10. *Treatment approaches to mucosal candidiasis with antifungal agents*

Site of involvement	Treatment[a]
Oropharynx	Nystatin suspension
	Amphotericin lozenges
	Fluconazole po or i.v.
Esophagus	Fluconazole po or i.v.
	Amphotericin B i.v.
Vagina	Nystatin pessaries/cream
	Clotrimazole troches/cream
	Miconazole cream
	Fluconazole po
Bladder	Fluconazole po or i.v.
	Amphotericin B i.v.

[a] Different agents may be used singly or in combination as clinically indicated.

Table 75.11. *Treatment approaches for systemic fungal infections in addition to the use of antifungal agents*

1. Reversal of immune suppression
    e.g., taper and stop corticosteroid therapy
2. Enhance neutrophil recovery if neutropenic
    e.g., G-CSF/GM-CSF administration
    or G-CSF–mobilized granulocyte transfusions
3. Surgery
    e.g., for invasive aspergillosis, consider if
    i) hemoptysis from a single cavitary lesion
    ii) progression of a cavitary lesion despite antifungal therapy
    iii) infiltration into pericardiuim, great vessels, bone, or thoracic soft tissue while receiving antifungal therapy
    iv) progressive sinusitis

Abbreviations: G-CSF, granulocyte colony-stimulating factor; GM-CSF, granulocyte-macrophage colony-stimulating factor.

of fungal disease, although fungal species differed from those diagnosed pretransplant; this compared historically to a mortality rate of 90% in posttransplant patients documented to have hepatosplenic candidiasis. Comparison of CT scans obtained before and after transplant showed an improvement in 9 of 15, complete resolution in 2 of 15, with none showing progression. The authors concluded that hepatosplenic candidiasis was not an absolute contraindication to HSC transplantation when patients received amphotericin B pretransplant and continued it until engraftment occurred. Martino and colleagues (1994) described a patient who had chronic systemic candidiasis pretransplant and who received prophylactic oral or intravenous fluconazole 200 mg daily throughout the posttransplant period; the transplant proceeded successfully.

Aspergillus

A previous aspergillosis infection is considered by some centers to be an contraindication to HSC stem cell transplantation; however, there are data indicating that such patients can be transplanted successfully. Michailov *et al.* (1996) reported seven adult patients with a prior history of invasive pulmonary aspergillosis prior to autologous transplantation for acute myeloid leukemia (AML). The marrow was purged ex vivo by mafosfamide; all patients received amphotericin B for a median total dose of 1.915 g pretransplant; no patient underwent surgery; the median time from diagnosis of invasive aspergillosis to autologous BMT was 7.3 (range 3–10) months. During the transplant procedure all patients received prophylactic

Table 75.12. *Candida species resistant to antifungal agents*

Resistant to amphotericin B	Resistant to fluconazole
Candida parapsilosis	*Candida krusei*
	Torulopsis glabrata

amphotericin B and itraconazole. No reactivation of aspergillosis posttransplant was noted. Posttransplant itraconazole was continued for a median of 3 (range 3–5) months. In a retrospective survey in 16 European centers, 48 patients with documented or probable aspergillosis prior to the transplant were evaluated. Treatment prior to the transplant was medical in all 48, with the addition of surgery in 20 patients; clinical and radiological resolution was seen in 62%. The incidence of relapse was low—33%, but the mortality in those cases was 88%. Patients receiving systemic prophylaxis either by amphotericin B, liposomal amphotericin B, itraconazole, or a combination of these drugs had less relapses (29%) than non-prophylaxed patients (57%) (Offner *et al.*, 1998). There were two patients in Martino's series (1994) with invasive pulmonary aspergillosis and one of the two underwent partial lobectomy. Both patients received prophylactic intraconazole 400 mg daily orally throughout the transplant procedure; both transplants were performed successfully (Martino *et al.*, 1994). A similar experience was reported by Richard *et al.* (1993) and, after a reduced intensity conditioning regimen/allograft procedure, by Hermann and colleagues (2001).

Other fungal infections

Olalla *et al.* (1996) described a patient with AML who developed an invasive middle ear infection with mucormycosis after consolidation chemotherapy. This resolved successfully with surgery and antifungal therapy and the patient underwent autologous blood stem cell transplantation with antifungal prophylaxis using liposomal amphotericin; there was no indication of reactivation of the mycosis posttransplant.

The fourth patient in Martino's series had pneumonia caused by *Scedosporium apiospermum* during consolidation chemotherapy for acute leukemia, which was successfully treated with itraconazole during the transplant procedure; he also received oral itraconazole 400 mg daily and the transplant was performed successfully.

A patient with AML recovered after treatment for infection with *Curvularia* sp. and was subsequently successfully consolidated with an autologous BMT (Berlanga *et al.*, 1995).

Conclusions

The difficulties the clinician has in dealing with fungal infections are multiple. Noninvasive diagnostic techniques are insensitive and the new PCR tests are not yet fully evaluated or widely available. The clinical presentation of an infection is often occult, although the infection may rapidly progress. Azole therapy has not so far been fully evaluated in neutropenic patients. Amphotericin therapy is often toxic and prolonged with no firm endpoint. However, with access to lipid formulations of amphotericin B, the newer triazoles, and echinocandins we now have the potential to prevent, treat, and cure, not all, but many of the previously fatal infections. An aggressive approach to diagnosis and early institution of treatment at first suspicion must be applied.

References

Alangaden, G., Chandrasekar, P. H., Bailey, E., & Khaliq, Y. (1994). Antifungal prophylaxis with low-dose fluconazole during bone marrow transplantation. *Bone Marrow Transplantation,* **14,** 919–24.

Alliot, C., Desablens, B., Garidi, R., & Tabuteau, S. (2000). Opportunistic infection with *Rhodotorula* in cancer patients treated by chemotherapy: two case reports. *Clinical Oncology,* **12,** 115–7.

Anaissie, E. G., Stratton, S. L., Dignant, M. C. *et al.* (2003). pathogenic molds (including Aspergillus species) in hospital water distribution systems: a 3-year prospective study and clinical implications for patients with hematologic malignancies. *Blood,* **101,** 2542–6.

Andström, E. E., Ringden, O., Remberger, M. *et al.* (1996). Safety and efficacy of liposomal amphotericin B in allogeneic bone marrow transplant recipients. *Mycoses,* **39,** 185–93.

Angelucci, E., Ugolini, M., Lucarelli, G. *et al.* (1991). Endobronchial aspergillosis in marrow transplant patients. *Bone Marrow Transplantation,* **8,** 328–9 (Letter).

Ansorg, R., van den Boom, R., von Heinegg, E. H., & Rath, P. M. (1996). Association between incidents of *Aspergillus* antigenemia and exposure to construction works at a hospital site. *Zentralblatt fur Bakteriologie,* **284,** 146–52.

Barchiesi, F., Schimizzi, A. M., Caselli, F. *et al.* (2001). Activity of new antifungal triazole, posaconazole, against *Cryptococcus neoformans. Journal of Antimicrobial Chemotherapy,* **48,** 769–73.

Berlanga, J. J., Querol, S., Gallardo, D. *et al.* (1995). Successful treatment of *Curvularia* sp infection in a patient with primarily resistant acute promyelocytic leukemia. *Bone Marrow Transplantation,* **16,** 617–19.

Bjerke, J. W., Meyers, J. D., & Bowden, R. A. (1994). Hematosplenic candidiasis: contraindication to transplantation? *Blood,* **84,** 2811–4.

Blazar, B. R., Hurd, D. D., Snover, D. C. *et al.* (1984). Invasive *Fusarium* in bone marrow transplantation recipients: a report of three cases and a review of the literature. *American Journal of Medicine,* **77,** 645–51.

Bleggi-Torres, L. F., de Medeiros, B. C., Neto, J. Z. *et al.* (1996). Disseminated *Fusarium* sp. infection affecting the brain of a child after bone marrow transplantation. *Bone Marrow Transplantation,* **18,** 1013–15.

Bodey, G. P., Anaissie, E., Gutterman, J. *et al.* (1994). Role of granulocyte-macrophage colony-stimulating factor as adjuvant treatment in neutropenic patients with bacterial and fungal infection. *European Journal of Clinical Microbiology and Infectious Diseases,* **13,** (Suppl 2), 18–22.

Bonduel, M., Santos, P., Figueroa Turienzo, C., Chantada, G., & Paganini, H. (2001). Atypical skin lesions caused by *Curvularia* sp. and *Pseudallescheria boydii* in two patients after allogeneic bone marrow transplantation. *Bone Marrow Transplantation,* **27,** 1311–3.

Boogaerts, M., Winston, D. J., Bow, E. J. *et al.* (2001). Intravenous and oral intraconazole versus intravenous amphotericin B deoxycholate as empirical therapy for persistent fever in neutropenic patients with cancer who are receiving broad-spectrum antibacterial therapy. *Annals of Internal Medicine,* **135,** 412–22.

Boutati, E. I. & Anaissie, E. J. (1997). *Fusarium,* a significant emerging pathogen in patients with hematologic malignancy: ten years' experience at a cancer center and implications for management. *Blood,* **90,** 999–1008.

Bowden, R. A., Chandrasekar, P., White, M. *et al.* (2002). A double-blind, randomized, controlled trial of amphotericin B colloidal dispersion versus amphotericin B for treatment of invasive aspergillosis in immunocompromised patients. *Clinical Infectious Diseases,* **35,** 359–66.

Bowden, R. A., Kay, S., Gooley, T. *et al.* (1996). Phase one study of amphotericin B, colloidal dispersion for the treatment of invasive fungal infections after marrow transplant. *Journal of Infectious Diseases,* **173,** 1208–15.

Bufill, J. A., Lum, L. G., Caya, J. G. *et al.* (1988). *Pityrosporum* folliculitis after bone marrow transplantation. Clinical observations in five patients. *Annals of Internal Medicine,* **108,** 560–3.

Caillot, D., Couaillier, J. F., Bernard, A. *et al.* (2001). Increasing volume and changing characteristics of invasive pulmonary aspergillosis on sequential thoracic computed tomography scans in patients with neutropenia. *Journal of Clinical Oncology,* **19,** 253–9.

Cairoli, R., Provisione, M., & Marenco, P. (1993). *Saccharomyces:* possible agent of unexplained fever in BMT patients. *19th Annual Meeting of the EBMT Group,* (Abstract).

Centers for Disease Control and Prevention (2000). Guidelines for preventing opportunistic infections among hematopoietic stem cell transplant recipients: recommendations of CDC, the Infectious Disease Society of America, and the American Society of Blood and Marrow Transplantation. *MMWR Morbidity and Mortality Weekly Report,* **49,** (RR-10), 1–25, and *Biology of Blood and Marrow Transplantation,* **6,** 659–734.

Chan-Tack, K. M., Thio, C. L., Miller, N. S. *et al.* (1999). *Paecilomyces lilacinus* fungemia in an adult bone marrow transplant recipient. *Medical Mycology,* **37,** 57–60.

Chen, S. C. (2002). Cryptococcosis in Australasia and the treatment of cryptococcal and other fungal infections with liposomal amphotericin B. *Journal of Antimicrobial Chemotherapy,* **49** (Suppl 1), 57–61.

Chinnamma, T., Anderson, D., Carey, R. B., Mitchell, K., & Mileusnic, D. (1999). Fatal *Chaematomium* cerebritis in a bone marrow transplant patient. *Human Pathology,* **30,** 874–9.

Choi, J. H., Yoo, J. H., Chung, I. J. *et al.* (1997). Esophageal aspergillosis after bone marrow transplant. *Bone Marrow Transplantation,* **19,** 293–4.

Choucino, G., Goodman, S. A., Greer, J. P. *et al.* (1996). Nocardial infections in bone marrow transplant recipients. *Clinical Infectious Diseases,* **23,** 1012–19.

Clancy, C. J., Nguyen, M. H., & Wingard, J. R. (2000). Subcutaneous phaeohyphomycosis in transplant recipients: review of the literature and demonstration of in vitro synergy between antifungal agents. *Medical Mycology,* **38,** 169–75.

Clarke, K., Szer, J., Shelton, M. *et al.* (1995). Multiple granulocyte transfusions facilitating successful unrelated bone marrow transplantation in a patient with very severe aplastic anemia complicated by suspected fungal infection. *Bone Marrow Transplantation,* **16,** 723–6.

Coker, R. J., Viviani, M., Gazzard, B. G. *et al.* (1993). Treatment of cryptococcosis with liposomal amphotericin B (AmBisome) in 23 patients with AIDS. *AIDS,* **7,** 829–35.

Conneally, E., Cafferkey, M. T., Daly, P. A. *et al.* (1993). Nebulized amphotericin B as prophylaxis against aspergillosis in granulocytic patients. *Bone Marrow Transplantation,* **5,** 403–6.

Cornely, O. A., Pels, H., Bethe, U. *et al.* (2001). A novel type of metastatically spreading subcutaneous aspergillosis without epidermal lesions following allogeneic stem cell transplantation. *Bone Marrow Transplantation*, **28**, 899–901.

Darrisaw, L., Hanson, G., Vesole, D. H., & Kehl, S. C. (2000). *Cunninghamella* infection post bone marrow transplant: case report and review of the literature. *Bone Marrow Transplantation*, **25**, 1213–6.

De Bock, R., Marinus, A., Nagler, A. *et al.* (1995). EBMT/EORTC study on invasive fungal infections (IFI) in bone marrow transplant (BMT) patients. *Bone Marrow Transplantation*, **15** (Suppl 2), 104 (Abstract).

de la Camara, R., Pinilla, I., Munoz, E. *et al.* (1996). *Penicillium brevicompactum* as the cause of a necrotic lung ball in an allogeneic bone marrow transplant recipient. *Bone Marrow Transplantation*, **18**, 1189–93.

deShazo, R. D., Chapin, K., & Swain, R. E. (1997). Fungal sinusitis. *New England Journal of Medicine*, **337**, 254–9.

Drakos, P. E., Nagler, A., Or, R. *et al.* (1993). Invasive fungal sinusitis in patients undergoing bone marrow transplantation (Review). *Bone Marrow Transplantation*, **12**, 203–8.

Elliott, M. A., Tefferi, A., Marshall, W. F., & Lacy, M. Q. (1997). Disseminated nocardiosis after allogeneic bone marrow transplantation. *Bone Marrow Transplantation*, **20**, 425–6.

Ellis, M., Spence, D., de Pauw, B. *et al.* (1998). An EORTC international, multicenter randomized trial (EORTC number 19923) comparing two dosages of liposomal amphotericin B for treatment of invasive aspergillosis. *Clinical Infectious Diseases*, **27**, 1406–12.

Emminger, W., Lang, H.R.M., Emminger-Schidmeier, W. *et al.* (1991). Amphotericin B serum levels in pediatric bone marrow transplant recipients. *Bone Marrow Transplantation*, **7**, 95–9.

Erer, B., Galimberti, M., Lucarelli, G. *et al.* (2000). *Trichosporon beigelii:* a life-threatening pathogen in immunocompromised hosts. *Bone Marrow Transplantation*, **25**, 745–9.

Feldman, E., Hester, J., Vartivarian, S. *et al.* (1993). The use of granulocyte-colony stimulating factor (G-CSF) enhanced granulocyte transfusions from normal donors in patients (pts) with neutropenia-related fungal infections. In Program and Abstracts of the 33rd Interscience Conference on Antimicrobial Agents and Chemotherapy (New Orleans). Washington, DC: American Society for Microbiology.

Freites, V., Sumoza, A., Bisotti, R. *et al.* (1995). Subcutaneous *Nocardia asteroides* abscess in a bone marrow transplant recipient. *Bone Marrow Transplantation*, **15**, 135–6.

Gaziev, D., Baronciani, D., Galimberti, M. *et al.* (1996). Mucormycosis after bone marrow transplantation: report of four cases in thalessemia and review of the literature. *Bone Marrow Transplantation*, **17**, 409–14.

Ghannoum, M. A. & Kuhn, D. M. (2002). Voriconazole—better chances for patients with invasive mycoses. *European Journal of Medical Research*, **7**, 242–56.

Goodman, J. L., Winston, D. J., Greenfield, R. A. *et al.* (1992). A controlled trial of fluconazole to prevent fungal infections in patients undergoing bone marrow transplantation. *New England Journal of Medicine*, **326**, 845–51.

Goodrich, J. M., Reed, E. C., Mori, M. *et al.* (1991). Clinical features and analysis of risk factors for invasive candidal infection after marrow transplantation. *Journal of Infectious Diseases*, **164**, 731–40.

Goss, G., Grigg, A., Rathbone, P., & Slavin, M. (1994). *Hansenula anomala* infection after bone marrow transplantation. *Bone Marrow Transplantation*, **14**, 995–7.

Groll, A. H., Piscitelli, S. C., & Walsh, T. J. (1998). Clinical pharmacology of systyemic antifungal agents: a comprehensive review of agents in clinical use, current investigational compounds, and putative targets for antifungal development. *Advances in Pharmacology*, **44**, 343–500.

Gumbart, C. H. (1983). *Pseudoallescheria boydii* infection after bone marrow transplantation. *Annals of Internal Medicine*, **99**, 193–4.

Guppy, K. H., Thomas, C., Thomas, K., & Anderson, D. (1998). Cerebral fungal infections in the immunocompromised host: a literature review and a new pathogen—*Chaetomium atrobrunneum:* case report. *Neurosurgery*, **43**, 1463–9.

Guyotat, D., Pieus, M. A., Bouvier, R. *et al.* (1987). A case of disseminated *Scedosporium apiospermum* infection after bone marrow transplantation. *Mykosen*, **30**, 151–4.

Hagensee, M. E., Bauwens, J. E., Kjos, B., & Bowden, R. A. (1994). Brain abscess following marrow transplantation: experience at the Fred Hutchinson Cancer Research Center, 1984–92. *Clinical Infectious Diseases*, **19**, 402–8.

Hebart, H., Löffler, J., Meisner, C. *et al.* (2000). Early detection of *Aspergillus* infection after allogeneic stem cell transplantation by polymerase chain reaction screening. *Journal of Infectious Diseases*, **181**, 1713–9.

Herbrecht, R., Denning, D. W., Patterson, T. F. *et al.* (2002). Voriconazole versus amphotericin B for primary therapy of invasive aspergillosis. *New England Journal of Medicine*, **347**, 408–15.

Hermann, S., Klein, S. A., Jacobi, V. *et al.* (2001). Older patients with high-risk fungal infections can be successfully allografted using non-myeloablative conditioning in combination with intensified supportive care regimens. *British Journal of Haematology*, **113**, 446–54.

Hodohara, K., Fujiyama, Y., Hiramitu, Y. *et al.* (1993). Disseminated subcutaneous *Nocardia asteroides* abscesses in a patient after bone marrow transplantation. *Bone Marrow Transplantation*, **11**, 341–3.

Hoppe, J. E., Klingebiel, T., & Niethammer, D. (1994). Selection of *Candida glabrata* in pediatric bone marrow transplant recipients receiving fluconazole. *Pediatric Hematology & Oncology*, **11**, 207–10.

Iwen, P. C., Rupp, M. E., Bishop, M. E. *et al.* (1998). Disseminated aspergillosis caused by *Aspegillus ursus* in a patient following allogeneic peripheral stem cell transplantation. *Journal of Clinical Microbiology*, **36**, 3713–17.

Jahagirdar, B. N., Morrison, V. A. (2002). Emerging fungal pathogens in patients with hematologic malignancies and marrow/stem-cell transplants recipients. *Seminars in Respiratory Infections.* **17**, 113–20.

Jantunen, E., Kolho, E., Ruutu, P. *et al.* (1996). Invasive cutaneous mucormycosis caused by *Absidia corymbifera* after allogeneic bone marrow transplantation. *Bone Marrow Transplantation*, **18**, 229–30.

Jantunen, E., Piilonen, A., Volin, L. *et al.* (2000). Diagnostic aspects of invasive *Aspergillus* infections in allogeneic BMT recipients. *Bone Marrow Transplantation*, **25**, 867–71.

Jantunen, E., Ruutu, P., Niskanen, L. *et al.* (1997). Incidence and risk factors for invasive fungal infections in allogeneic BMT recipients. *Bone Marrow Transplantation*, **19**, 801–8.

Kelsey, S. M., Goldman, J. M., McCann, S. *et al.* (1999). Liposomal amphotericin (AmBisome) in the prophylaxis of fungal infections in neutropenic patients: a randomized, double-blind, placebo-controlled study. *Bone Marrow Transplantation,* **23,** 163–8.

Khoury, H., Adkins, D., Miller, G. *et al.* (1997). Resolution of invasive central nervous system aspergillosis in a transplant recipient. *Bone Marrow Transplantation,* **20,** 179–80.

Klingspor, L., Stintzing, G., Fasth, A. *et al.* (1996). Deep *Candida* infection in children receiving allogeneic bone marrow transplants: incidence, risk factors and diagnosis. *Bone Marrow Transplantation,* **17,** 1043–9.

Kruger, W., Sobottka, I., Stockschlader, M. *et al.* (1996). Fatal outcome of disseminated candidosis after allogeneic bone marrow transplantation under treatment with liposomal and conventional amphotericin B. A report for cases with determination of the MIC values. *Scandinavian Journal of Infectious Diseases,* **28,** 313–16.

Larsson, L., Pehrson, C., Wiebe, T. *et al.* (1994). Gas chromatographic determination of D-arabinitol/L-arabinitol ratios in urine: a potential method for diagnosis of disseminated candidiasis. *Journal of Clinical Microbiology,* **8,** 1855–9.

Leather, H. L. & Wingard, J. (2002). Prophylaxis, empirical therapy, or pre-emptive therapy of fungal infections in immunocompromised patients: which is better for whom? *Current Opinion in Infectious Diseases,* **15,** 369–75.

Lecciones, J. A., Lee, J. W., Navarro, E. E. *et al.* (1992). Vascular catheter-associated fungemia in patients with cancer, an analysis of 55 episodes. *Clinical Infectious Diseases,* **14,** 875–83.

Leenders, A. C., Daenen, S., Jansen, R. L. *et al.* (1998). Liposomal amphotericin B compared with amphotericin B deoxycholate in the treatment of documented and suspected neutropenia-associated invasive fungal infections. *British Journal of Haematology,* **103,** 205–12.

Leong, K. W., Crowley, B., White, B. *et al.* (1997). Cutaneous mucormycosis due to *Absidia corymbifera* occurring after bone marrow transplantation. *Bone Marrow Transplantation,* **19,** 513–5.

Lin, M. T., Lu, H. S., & Chen, W. L. (2001). Improving efficacy of antifungal therapy by polymerase chain reaction–based strategy among febrile patients with neutropenia and cancer. *Clinical Infectious Diseases,* **33,** 1621–7.

Liu, K. L., Herbrecht, R., Bergerat, J. P. *et al.* (1990). Disseminated *Trichosporon capitatum* infection in a patient with acute leukemia undergoing bone marrow transplantation. *Bone Marrow Transplantation,* **6,** 219–21.

Lonial, S., Williams, L., Carrum, G. *et al.* (1997). *Neosartorya fischeri:* an invasive fungal pathogen in an allogeneic bone marrow transplant patient. *Bone Marrow Transplantation,* **19,** 753–5.

Lòpez-Jimenéz, J., Duarte-Palomino., R., Cabezudo., E. *et al.* (1997). *Candida parapsilosis* fungemias in bone marrow transplant recipients: implications for azole prophylactic therapy. *Blood,* **89,** 3491–2.

Lowenthal, R. M., Atkinson, K., Challis, D. R. *et al.* (1987). Invasive *Trichosporon cutaneum* infection: an increasing problem in immunosuppressed patients. *Bone Marrow Transplantation,* **3,** 321–7.

Lundstrom, T. S., Fairfax, M. R., Dugan, M. C. *et al.* (1997). *Phialophora verrucosa* infection in a BMT patient. *Bone Marrow Transplantation,* **20,** 789–91.

Machado, C. M., Macedo, M. C., Castelli, J. B. *et al.* (1997). Clinical features and successful recovery from disseminated nocardiosis after BMT. *Bone Marrow Transplantation,* **19,** 81–2.

Machida, U., Kami, M., Kanda, Y. *et al.* (1999). *Aspergillus* tracheobronchitis after allogeneic bone marrow transplantation. *Bone Marrow Transplantation,* **24,** 1145–9.

Maddox, L., Long, G. D., Vredenburgh, J. J., & Folz, R. J. (2001). *Rhizopus* presenting as an endobrochial obstruction following bone marrow transplant. *Bone Marrow Transplantation,* **28,** 634–6.

Maertens, J., Verhaegen, J., Lagrou, K., Van Eldere, J., & Boogaerts, M. (2001). Screening for circulating galactomannan as a non-invasive diagnostic tool for invasive aspergillosis in prolonged neutropenic patients and stem cell transplantation recipients: a prospective validation. *Blood,* **97,** 1604–10.

Marr, K. A., Carter, R. A., Boeckh, M. *et al.* (2002b). Invasive aspergillosis in allogeneic stem cell transplant recipients: changes in epidemiology and risk factors. *Blood,* **100,** 4358–66.

Marr, K. A., Carter, R. A., Crippa, F. *et al.* (2002a). Epidemiology and outcome of mould infections in haematopoietic stem cell transplant recipients. *Clinical Infectious Diseases,* **34,** 909–17.

Marr, K. A., Seidel, K., Slavin, M. A. *et al.* (2000). Prolonged fluconazole prophylaxis is associated with persistent protection against candidiasis-related death in allogeneic marrow transplant recipients: long-term follow-up of a randomized placebo-controlled trial. *Blood,* **96,** 2055–61.

Martin, D. H., Counts, G. W., & Thomas, E. D. (1977). Fungal infections in human bone marrow transplant recipients. In Seventeenth Interscience Conference on Antimicrobial Agents and Chemotherapy, p. 406. New York: American Society For Microbiology, (Abstract).

Martino, R., Caballero, M. D., Canals, C. *et al.* (2001). Reduced-intensity conditioning reduces the risk of severe infections after allogeneic peripheral blood stem cell transplants. *Bone Marrow Transplantation,* **28,** 341–7.

Martino, R., Nomdedeu, J., Altes, A. *et al.* (1994). Successful bone marrow transplantation in patients with invasive fungal infections; report of four cases. *Bone Marrow Transplantation,* **13,** 265–9.

Martino, R., Subira, M., Rovira, M. *et al.* (2002). Invasive fungal infections after allogeneic peripheral blood stem cell transplantation: incidence and risk factors in 395 patients. *British Journal of Haematology,* **116,** 475–82.

Mehta, J., Kelsey, S., Chu, P. *et al.* (1997). Amphotericin B lipid complex (ABLC) for the treatment of confirmed or presumed fungal infections in immunocompromised patients with hematologic malignancies. *Bone Marrow Transplantation,* **20,** 39–43.

Meis, J. F., Ruhnke, M., De Pauw, B. E. *et al.* (1999). *Candida dubliniensis* candidemia in patients with chemotherapy-induced neutropenia and bone marrow transplantation. *Emerging Infectious Diseases,* **5,** 150–3.

Mencacci, A., Perruccio, K., Bacci, A. *et al.* (2001). Defective anti-fungal T-helper (THl) immunity in a murine model of allogeneic T-cell–depleted bone marrow transplantation and its restoration by treatment with TH2 cytokine antagonists. *Blood,* **97,** 1483–90.

Mendpara, S. D., Ustun, C., Kallab, A. M. *et al.* (2002). Cryptococcal meningitis following autologous stem cell transplantation in a patient with multiple myeloma. *Bone Marrow Transplantation,* **30,** 259–60.

Meunier, F. (1988). Fungal infections in the compromised host. In *Clinical Approach to Infection in the Compromised Host,* ed. R. H. Rubin & L. S. Young, pp. 193–220. New York: Plenum Press.

Meunier, F., Prentice, H. G., & Ringdén, O. (1991). Liposomal amphotericin B (AmBisome): safety data from a phase II/III clinical trial. *Journal of Antimicrobial Chemotherapy,* **28** (Suppl B), 83–91.

Meyers, J. D. & Thomas, E. D. (1988). Infection complicating bone marrow transplantation. In *Clinical Approach to Infection in the Compromised Host,* ed. R. H. Rubin & L. S. Young, pp. 525–56. New York: Plenum Press.

Michailov, G., Laporte, J. P., Lesage, S. *et al.* (1996). Autologous bone marrow transplantation is feasible in patients with a prior history of invasive aspergillosis. *Bone Marrow Transplantation,* **17,** 569–72.

Milliken, S. T. & Powles, R. L. (1990). Antifungal prophylaxis in bone marrow transplantation. *Reviews of Infectious Diseases,* **12** (Suppl 3), 374–9.

Moore, J. J., Herbert, L. C., Berger, L. A. *et al.* (1998). Adjuvant use of GM-CSF in invasive aspergillosis. *Blood,* **92** (Suppl 1), 335b.

Morgenstern, G, R., Prentice, A. G., Prentice, H. G. *et al.* (1999). A randomized controlled trial of itraconazole versus fluconazole for the prevention of fungal infections in patients with hematological malignancies. U.K. multicentre antifungal prophylaxis study group. *British Journal of Haematology,* **105,** 901–11.

Morrison, V. A., Haake, R. J., & Weisdorf, D. J. (1994). Non-*Candida* fungal infections after bone marrow transplantation: risk factors and outcome. *American Journal of Medicine,* **96,** 497–503.

Morrison, V. A., & Weisdorf, D. J. (2000). The spectrum of *Malassezia* infections in the bone marrow transplant population. *Bone Marrow Transplantation,* **26,** 645–8.

Neglia, H., Hurd, D., Ferrieri, P. *et al.* (1987). Invasive scopulariopsis in the immunocompromised host. *American Journal of Medicine,* **83,** 1163–6.

Neumunaitis, J., Meyers, J. D., Buckner, C. D. *et al.* (1991). Phase I trial of recombinant human macrophage colony-stimulating factor in patients with invasive fungal infections. *Blood,* **78,** 907–13.

Neumunaitis, J., Shannon-Dorcy, K., Appelbaum, F. R. *et al.* (1993). Long-term follow up of patients with invasive fungal disease who received adjunctive therapy with recombinant human macrophage colony-stimulating factor. *Blood,* **82,** 1422–7.

Nomura, J., Ruskin, J., Sahebi, F. *et al.* (1997). Mucormycosis of the vulva following bone marrow transplantation. *Bone Marrow Transplantation,* **19,** 859–60.

Nusair, S., Amir, G., Or, R. & Breuer, R. (2002). Invasive airway aspergillosis with new airflow obstruction minicking post-BMT bronchioloitis obliterans. *Bone Marrow Transplantation,* **29,** 711–3.

Odds, F. C. (1988). *Candida and Candidosis. A Review and Bibliography.* 2nd Ed. London, UK: Bailliere Tindall.

Offner, F., Cordonnier, C., Ljungman, P. *et al.* (1998). Impact of previous aspergillosis on the outcome of bone marrow transplantation. *Clinical Infectious Diseases,* **26,** 1098–103.

Olalla, I., Otin, M., Hermida, G. *et al.* (1996). Autologous peripheral blood stem cell transplantation in a patient with previous invasive middle ear mucormycosis. *Bone Marrow Transplantation,* **18,** 1183–4.

Oliver, M. R., Van Voorhis, W. C., Boeckh, M. *et al.* (1996). Hematic mucormycosis in a bone marrow transplant recipient who ingested naturopathic medicine. *Clinical Infectious Diseases,* **22,** 521–4.

Oo, M. M., Kutteh, L. A., Koc, O. N. *et al.* (1998). Mucormycosis of petrous bone in an allogeneic stem cell transplant recipient. *Clinical Infectious Diseases,* **27,** 1546–7.

Orth, B., Frei, R., Itin, P. H. *et al.* (1996). Outbreak of invasive micosis caused by *Paecilomyces lilacinus* from a contaminated skin lotion. *Annals of Internal Medicine,* **125,** 799–806.

Panigrahi, S., Nagler, A., Or, D. *et al.* (2001). Indolent *Aspergillus* arthritis complicating fludarabine-based non-myeloablative stem cell transplantation. *Bone Marrow Transplantation,* **27,** 659–61.

Pasic, S., Flannagan, L., & Cant, A. J. (1997). Liposomal amphotericin (AmBisome) is safe in bone marrow transplantation for primary immunodeficiency. *Bone Marrow Transplantation,* **19,** 1229–32.

Paterson, P. J., Marshall, S. R., Shaw, B. *et al.* (2000). Fatal invasive cerebral *Absidia corymbifera* infection following bone marrow transplantation. *Bone Marrow Transplantation,* **26,** 701–3.

Perrucio, K., Tosti, A., Posati, S. *et al.* (2001). Transfer of functional immune responses to *Aspergillus* and CMV after haploidentical hematopoietic transplantation. *Bone Marrow Transplantation,* **27** (Suppl 1) S23 (Abstract).

Pestalozzi, B. C., Krestin, G. P., Schanz, U. *et al.* (1997). Hepatic lesions of chronic disseminated candidiasis may become invisible during neutropenia. *Blood,* **90,** 3858–64.

Powderly, W. (1996). Recent advances in the management of cryptococcal meningitis in patients with AIDS. *Clinical Infectious Diseases,* **22** (Suppl 2), 119–23.

Prentice, H. G., Hann, I. M., Herbrecht, R. *et al.* (1997). A randomized comparison of liposomal versus conventional amphotericin B for the treatment of pyrexia of unknown origin in neutropenic patients. *British Journal of Haematology,* **98,** 711–18.

Redline, R. W., Redline, S. S., Boxerbaum, B. *et al.* (1985). Systemic *Malassezia furfur* infections in patients receiving intralipid therapy. *Human Pathology,* **16,** 815–22.

Ribaud, P., Chastang, C., Latge, J.-P. *et al.* (1999). Survival and prognostic factors of invasive aspergillosis after allogeneic bone marrow transplantation. *Clinical Infectious Diseases,* **28,** 322–30.

Richard, C., Romon, I., Baro, J. *et al.* (1993). Invasive pulmonary aspergillosis prior to BMT in acute leukemia patients does not predict a poor outcome. *Bone Marrow Transplantation,* **12,** 237–41.

Richardson, M. D., Brownlie, C. E., & Shankland, G. S. (1992). Enhanced phagocytosis and intracellular killing of *Candida albicans* by GM-CSF activated neutrophils. *Journal of Medical and Veterinary Mycology,* **30,** 433–41.

Richter, S., Cormican, M. G., Pfaller, M. A. *et al.* (1999). Fatal disseminated *Trichoderma longibrachiatum* infection in an adult bone marrow transplant patient: species identification and review of the literature. *Journal of Clinical Microbiology,* **37,** 1154–60.

Ringden, O., Meunier, F., Tollemar, J. *et al.* (1991). Efficacy of amphotericin B encapsulated in liposomes (AmBisome) in the treatment of invasive fungal infections in immunocompromised patients. *Journal of Antimicrobial Chemotherapy,* **28** (Suppl B), 73–82.

Roilides, E., Holmes, A., Blake, C. *et al.* (1994). Antifungal activity of elutriated monocytes against *Aspergillus fumigatus* hyphae; enhanced by granulocyte-macrophage colony-stimulating factor and interferon gamma. *Journal of Infectious Diseases,* **170,** 894–99.

Roling, E. E., Klepser, M., E., Wasson, A. *et al.* (2002). Antifungal activities of fluconazole, caspofungin (MK0991), and anidulafungin LY303366 alone and in combination against *Candida* spp and *Cryptococcus neoformans* via time-kill methods. *Diagnostic Microbiology and Infectious Disease,* **43,** 13–7.

Rolston, K. (2001). Overview of systemic fungal infections. *Oncology* (Williston Park, N.Y.), **15** (Suppl 9), 11–4.

Schimmelpfennig, C., Naumann, R., Zuberbier, T. *et al.* (2001). Skin involvement as the first manifestation of systemic aspergillosis after allogeneic hematopoietic cell transplantation. *Bone Marrow Transplantation,* **27,** 753–5.

Schwartz, S., Behre, G., Heinemann, V. *et al.* (1999). Aerolized amphotericin B inhalations as prophylaxis of invasive *Aspergillus* infections during prolonged neutropenia. Results of a prospective multicenter trial. *Blood,* **93,** 3654–612.

Shah, P. M. & Just, G. (1989). Fungal infections in organ transplantation. In *Diagnosis and Therapy of Systemic Fungal Infections,* ed. K. Holmberg & R. Meyer, pp. 71–78. New York: Raven Press.

Shearer, C. & Chandrasekar, P. H. (1995). Pulmonary nocardiosis in a patient with a bone marrow transplant. *Bone Marrow Transplantation,* **15,** 479–81.

Shing, M. M., Ip, M., Li, C. K. *et al.* (1996). *Paecilomyces varioti* fungemia in a bone marrow transplant patient. *Bone Marrow Transplantation,* **17,** 281–3.

Shulman, H., Strikeer, G., Deeg, H. J. *et al.* (1981). Nephrotoxicity of cyclosporine A after allogeneic marrow transplantation. *New England Journal of Medicine,* **305,** 1392–5.

Siberry, G. J., Costarangos, C., & Cohen, B. A. (1997). Destruction of the nasal ceptum by *Aspergillus* infection after autologous bone marrow transplantation. *New England Journal of Medicine,* **337,** 275–6.

Siegert, W., Hensze, G., Wagner, J. *et al.* (1988). Invasive *Trichosporon cutaneum (beigelii)* infection in a patient with relapsed acute myeloid leukemia undergoing bone marrow transplantation. *Transplantation,* **46,** 151–3.

Slavin, M., Osborne, B., Adams, R. *et al.* (1995). Efficacy and safety of fluconazole prophylaxis for fungal infections after marrow transplantation—a prospective, randomized, double-blind study. *Journal of Infectious Diseases,* **171,** 1545–52.

Storek, J., Dawson, M. A., Storer, B. *et al.* (2001). Immune reconstitution after allogeneic marrow transplantation compared with blood stem cell transplantation. *Blood,* **97,** 3380–9.

Timmers, G. J., Zweegman, S., Simoons-Smit, A. M. *et al.* (2000). Amphotericin B colloidal dispersion (Amphocil) vs fluconazole for the prevention of fungal infections in neutropenic patients: data of a prematurely stopped trial. *Bone Marrow Transplantation,* **25,** 879–84.

Tollemar, J. (1995). Diagnosis and treatment of invasive fungal infections in transplant recipients. In *Workshop: Prophylaxis and Treatment of Invasive Fungal Infections,* by the Medical Products Agency of Sweden, **2,** 89–102.

Tollemar, J., Holmberg, K., Ringden, O. *et al.* (1989a). Surveillance test for the diagnosis of invasive fungal infections in bone marrow transplant recipients. *Scandinavian Journal of Infectious Diseases,* **21,** 205–12.

Tollemar, J. & Ringden, O. (1991). Early recovery of lymphocyte response to *Candida* after bone marrow transplantation in colonized patients. *Bone Marrow Transplantation,* **7,** 285–91.

Tollemar, J., Ringdén, O., & Boström, L. (1989b). Variables predicting deep fungal infections in bone marrow transplant recipients. *Bone Marrow Transplantation,* **4,** 635–41.

Trigg, M. E., Comito, M. A., & Rumelhart, S. L. (1996). Cutaneous *Mucor* infection treated with wide incision in two children who underwent marrow transplantation. *Journal of Pediatric Surgery,* **31,** 976–7.

Trigg, M. E., Morgan, D., & Burns, T. L. (1997). Successful program to prevent *Aspergillus* infections in children undergoing marrow transplantation: use of nasal amphotericin. *Bone Marrow Transplantation,* **19,** 43–47.

Tsai, T. W., Hammond, L. A., Rinaldi, M. *et al.* (1997). *Cokeromyces recurvatus* infection in a bone marrow transplant recipient. *Bone Marrow Transplantation,* **19,** 301–2.

Verfaillie, C., Weisdorf, D., Haake, R. *et al.* (1991). *Candida* infections in bone marrow transplant recipients. *Bone Marrow Transplantation,* **8,** 177–84.

Volpi, I., Perrucio, K., Tosti, A. *et al.* (2001). Postgrafting administration of granulocyte colony-stimulating factor impairs functional immune recovery in recipients of human leukocyte antigen haplotype-mismatched hematopoietic transplants. *Blood,* **97,** 2514–21.

Wald, A., Leisenring, W., van Burik, J. A. *et al.* (1997). Epidemiology of *Aspergillus* infections in a large cohort of patients undergoing bone marrow transplantation. *Journal of Infectious Diseases,* **177,** 1775–6.

Walsh, M., White, L., Atkinson, K. *et al.* (1992). Fungal *Pseudoallescheria boydii* lung infiltrates unresponsive to amphotericin B in leukemic patients. *Australian and New Zealand Journal of Medicine,* **22,** 265–8.

Walsh, T. J., Finberg, R. W., Arndt, C. *et al.* (1999). Liposomal amphotericin B for empirical therapy in patients with persistent fever and neutropenia. *New England Journal of Medicine,* **340,** 764–71.

Walsh, T. J., Pappas, P., Winston, D. J. *et al.* (2002). Voriconazole compared with liposomal amphoteracin B for empirical antifungal therapy in patients with neutropenia and persistent fever. *New England Journal of Medicine,* **346,** 225–34.

Warwick, A., Ferrieri, P., Burke, B. *et al.* (1991). Presumptive invasive *Chrysosporium* infection in bone marrow transplant recipients. *Bone Marrow Transplantation,* **8,** 319–22.

Williamson, E.C.M., Leeming, J. P., Palmer, H. M. *et al.* (2000). Diagnosis of invasive aspergillosis in bone marrow transplant recipients by polymerase chain reaction. *British Journal of Haematology,* **108,** 132–9.

Wingard, J. R. (1997). Efficacy of amphotericin B lipid complex injection (ABLC) in bone marrow transplant recipients with life-threatening systemic mycoses. *Bone Marrow Transplantation,* **19,** 343–7.

Wingard, J. R., Beals, S. U., Santos, G. W. *et al.* (1987). *Aspergillus* infections in bone marrow transplant recipients. *Bone Marrow Transplantation,* **2,** 175–81.

Wingard, J. R., Merz, W. G., Rinaldi, M. G. *et al.* (1991). Increase in *Candida krusei* infection among patients with bone marrow transplantation and neutropenia treated prophylactically with fluconazole. *New England Journal of Medicine,* **325,** 1274–7.

Wingard, J. R., Merz, W. G., Rinaldi, M. G. *et al.* (1993). Association of *Torulopsis glabrata* infections with fluconazole prophylaxis in neutropenic bone marrow transplant patients. *Antimicrobial Agents and Chemotherapy,* **37,** 1847–9.

Wolff, S. N., Fay, J., Stevens, D. *et al.* (2000). Fluconazole vs low-dose amphotericin B for the prevention of fungal infections in patients undergoing bone marrow transplantation: a study of the North American Marrow Transplant Group. *Bone Marrow Transplantation,* **25,** 853–9.

Yao, Z., Liao, W., & Wen, H. (2000). Antifungal therapy for treatment of cryptococcal meningitis. *Chinese Medical Journal,* **113,** 178–80.

76 Protozoal and helminthic infections

RODRIGO MARTINO

Hospital la Santa Creu i Sant Pau, Barcelona, Spain

Protozoal diseases

Introduction

Worldwide, human infections with parasitic protozoa account for a major proportion of diseases caused by infectious agents. For example, malaria infects approximately 600 million people and the ever-spreading resistance of the organisms causing malaria and their mosquito vectors to most available compounds is imposing a considerable therapeutic challenge.

The host-parasite relationship in protozoal infections is complex because of the distinctive biological features of the organisms. Protozoa are unicellular pathogens and are microscopic in size, although they are far larger than viruses and bacteria. They multiply within mammalian hosts (as do viruses, bacteria, and fungi). They have developed elaborate mechanisms for evading host-protective responses, for example by antigenic variation.

With the exception of *Pneumocystis carinii* infection and toxoplasmosis, however, protozoal infections are very rare in the hematopoietic stem cell transplant (HSCT) recipient. In fact, most infections have not been described in this patient population or have been reported only as case reports. However, these same parasites produce serious infections in other immunocompromised host populations, and thus knowledge of them is of interest to physicians caring for HSCT recipients.

Pneumocystis carinii infection (and see Chapter 78)

Pneumocystis carinii is a eukaryotic microbe with morphologic features similar to those of protozoa. Lack of growth on fungal culture media, and response to therapies used to treat protozoal infections, have supported the notion that it is a protozoan. However, *Pneumocystis carinii* has an affinity for fungal stains, its ultrastructure is more similar to fungi, and molecular analysis of its 16S ribosomal mRNA and mitochondrial DNA indicates that it is phylogenetically closely related to the Ascomycetes yeasts. Thus, this pathogen is increasingly classified as a yeast-like fungus in clinical mycology textbooks.

Epidemiology and risk factors

Within the first years of life, nearly all children have serologic evidence of exposure to *Pneumocystis carinii*. Thus, a widely accepted hypothesis for its pathogenesis has been that *Pneumocystis carinii* remains latent in the lung and reactivation occurs during severe immune depression. It can be found incidentally in the lungs of immunocompromised individuals. However, case clusters and familial spread have been reported, suggesting that *Pneumocystis carinii* may also be acquired by exposure to coughing by persons with community respiratory infections (Thomas & Limper, 1998).

Risk factors for clinical infection include treatment with corticosteroids or cyclosporine and a low CD4$^+$ cell count. In adults with the acquired immunodeficiency syndrome (AIDS) the risk of developing *Pneumocystis carinii* pneumonia (PCP) increases dramatically when the CD4$^+$ lymphocyte count falls below 200×10^6/l. One such case has been described in a 5-year-old recipient of an autologous bone marrow transplant (BMT) whose CD4$^+$ lymphocyte count fell to 5×10^6/l (Castagnola *et al.*, 1995).

The most common clinical manifestation of *Pneumocystis carinii* infection is interstitial pneumonitis. Rarely pneumothoraces and chronic lung cavitation have been described. Extrapulmonary infection is very rare and is usually seen in those with active pulmonary infection. (Such presentations have included external auditory polyps, mastoiditis, choroiditis, cutaneous lesions, small bowel obstruction, ascites, hepatic or splenic infiltration, hilar or mediastinal lymphadenopathy, thyroiditis, thymic involvement, and cytopenia due to marrow involvement. At autopsy disseminated infection has been documented in other organs including abdominal lymph nodes, pancreas, gastric mucosa, adrenal glands, myocardium, kidneys, and central nervous system.). PCP may present very insidiously with fatigue and low-grade fever, with few respiratory symptoms and minimal x-ray findings. Such insidious onset is particularly common in patients receiving high-dose corticosteroids, while the clinical and radiological picture is more typical in other settings.

Diagnosis

As with other invasive infections in HSCT recipients, the gold standard for the diagnosis of PCP is the histological documentation of tissue invasion of *P. carinii* (PC) cysts or trophozoites in lung tissue obtained by transbronchial biopsy or by open lung biopsy or at autopsy (Thomas & Limper, 1998). Fortunately, in the case of PCP the diagnosis can usually be obtained by the direct visualization of PC trophozoites (trophic form) from bronchoalveolar (BAL) fluid, using either a modified Wright-Giemsa or a Papanicolaou[1] stain, and cysts stained with toluidine blue O stain (Naimey & Wuerker, 1995). Alternatively, a sample of induced sputum can also be processed in the same manner, with high sensitivity in experienced hands, at least in AIDS patients (Naimey & Wuerker, 1995). BAL usually remains positive during the first 96 hours after therapy is started, allowing the test to be performed after empirical therapy has been started. This opportunity for confirming the diagnosis after treatment has started is important, since delayed therapy increases the mortality from PCP to around 60% (Tuan *et al.,* 1992; Hoyle & Goldman, 1994; Lyytikäinen *et al.,* 1996; Pagano *et al.,* 2002). When few or no cysts are seen in tissue, BAL, or even sputum, higher sensitivity can be obtained by the use of immunostaining using monoclonal antibodies for human PC (Kovaks *et al.,* 1998).

The polymerase chain reaction (PCR) has also been successfully used on samples of induced sputum and BAL fluid, using primers for the human PC DNA or RNA. As with PCR techniques for other infectious agents, the techniques described in different studies are not standardized and thus not necessarily reproducible (Ribes *et al.,* 1997; Sing *et al.,* 2000; Torres *et al.,* 2000). Additionally, the level of sensitivity varies widely between techniques. Despite these caveats, it appears that all published tests have a very high sensitivity and negative predictive value, and thus a negative PCR result for PC from a BAL sample virtually excludes the diagnosis of PCP. A positive result in BAL or saliva, however, may represent detection of subclinical infection or colonization. It would be prudent, however, to treat such patients preemptively, since a positive PCR is predictive of later PCP in immunocompromised hosts (Elvin *et al.,* 1996).

Prophylaxis

Historically, 5% to 30% of interstitial pneumonias in BMT recipients were due to PC, occurring in both autologous and allogeneic HSCT recipients (Krowka *et al.,* 1985). The incidence dramatically decreased with the introduction and widespread use of trimethoprim-sulfamethoxazole (TMP-SMX) prophylaxis. The risk of PCP depends on the intensity and duration of immunosuppression and underlying immune deficits. Thus, in HSCT recipients, the risk is greatest in allogeneic HSCT recipients during intensive immunosuppression for graft-versus-host disease (GVHD), a period during which PCP prophylaxis should always be given. This is the reason that cases of PCP occur many months or years after transplant (Tuan *et al.,* 1992; Hoyle *et al.,* 1994; Lyytikäinen *et al.,* 1996). However, autograft recipients and low-risk allograft recipients are also at risk during the first months after the transplant, and it is thus prudent to give prophylaxis for the first 3 to 6 months to all HSCT patients.

The recommended drug for prophylaxis is TMP-SMX, at a dose of 4 to 6 double-strength tablets per week. Besides being the most effective prophylaxis for PCP, TMP-SMX prevents other opportunistic infections, including infection with *Toxoplasma gondii,* and community-acquired respiratory, gastrointestinal, and urinary tract pathogens (Dworkin *et al.,* 2001). Intolerance of TMP-SMX is not very common in HSCT recipients. In such cases, the recommended drug is inhaled pentamidine (300 mg every 2 to 4 weeks) (Link *et al.,* 1993), while dapsone was shown to be less effective in one large study (Souza *et al.,* 1999; Fishman, 2001). Alternatively, desensitization to TMP-SMX may be attempted (see Chapter 78).

Patients who have developed and have fully recovered from PCP before an HSCT can safely undergo the procedure with standard pre- and posttransplant prophylaxis (Martino *et al.,* 1994).

Therapy

The recommended therapy for PCP in HSCT recipients is high-dose intravenous TMP-SMX. Patients who improve after intravenous treatment can continue on oral TMP-SMX therapy. The recommended total duration of therapy is not well established, although successfully treated cases receive a total median duration of treatment (i.v. plus oral) of around 30 days. Patients who are allergic or intolerant to TMP-SMX should receive intravenous pentamidine, although this is an uncommon occurrence in HSCT recipients. A brief course of corticosteroids has been shown to improve the outcome of PCP in AIDS patients and is also recommended for other patient population (Thomas & Limper, 1998). The recommended drug is methylprednisolone (50–80mg/day for 5 to 10 days). Among the new agents with activity against PC are atavaquone, which has been used in patients allergic to TMP-SMX, and the echinocandins (e.g., caspofungin, micofungin), but no clinical information is currently available to recommend their use.

Toxoplasmosis

Toxoplasma gondii is a protozoan that commonly infects animals and birds. Although *T. gondii* infection in humans is usually asymptomatic, clinical disease occurs in the immune suppressed patient. Infection may be acute (recently acquired) or chronic (latent). *T. gondii* exists in three forms during its life cycle: the tachyzoite, which is the asexual invasive form; the tissue cyst (containing bradyzoites), which persists in the tissues of the infected host during the chronic phase of the infection; and the oocyst (containing sporozoites), which is produced during the sexual cycle in the intestine of the definitive host—the cat. Transmission to humans occurs by ingesting tissue cysts or oocysts, or by blood product transfusion or organ transplantation. Following infection by oral ingestion, tachyzoites disseminate from the gastrointestinal tract and can invade virtually any cell or tissue where they proliferate and produce necrotic foci surrounded by inflammation. In immune suppressed patients, acute infection may result in severe damage to multiple organs. Even in individuals with a normal immune response, tissue

---

[1] Nicholas Papanicolaou, Greek-American pathologist, 1883–1962.

cysts form in multiple organs (latent infection), and can subsequently give rise to a severe localized reactivation producing, for example, toxoplasma encephalitis or chorioretinitis.

Toxoplasmosis appears to be a rare opportunistic infection following HSCT. Until recently, only 55 cases had been reported after HSCT (Derouin et al., 1992; Chandrasekar et al., 1997; Sing et al., 1999), which contrasts with the high frequency of this complication in other patient populations with severe cellular immunodeficiencies, mainly advanced AIDS. Table 76.1 summarizes the case series of toxoplasmosis in HSCT, and all other cases have been described as case reports. The seroprevalence for T. gondii varies greately between and even within countries, ranging from less than 15% in some North American studies (Slavin et al., 1994) and in pediatric wards, to 50% to 80% of adult HSCT recipients in countries with high endemicity such as France (Derouin et al., 1992; Foot et al., 1994; Bretagne et al., 1995). This varying seroprevalence is probably the main reason for the great variability in the frequency of diagnosed cases of toxoplasmosis after HSCT, which has been estimated to average 0.8% (O'Driscoll & Holliman, 1991), with < 0.4% in areas of low endemicity to 2% to 3% in those with high antibody prevalence. The disease, however, may be underdiagnosed, since around half of the cases reported in the literature were diagnosed at autopsy (Mele et al., 2002).

Toxoplasmosis occurs mainly in allogeneic transplant recipients, although cases after autologous transplants have been published (Chandrasekar et al., 1992; Geissmann et al., 1994; Yadlapati et al., 1997). Around 95% of patients are seropositive before HSCT, indicating that reactivation of latent tissue cysts in previously infected individuals is the usual mechanism implicated, as has been demonstrated in AIDS patients. It is thus important to determine the patient's serostatus prior to transplant. However, the disease may also develop in seronegative recipients from seronegative donors, suggesting that primary infection after transplant may also occur. The disease usually begins early after transplant with 95% of the cases occurring within the first 6 months after the procedure, although late cases have been reported (Hoyle et al., 1994; Martino et al., 2000a). Acute GVHD has been suggested as a possible predisposing factor for toxoplasma disease, and in a study by the European Group for Blood and Marrow Transplantation (EBMT) (Martino et al., 2000a) 77% of cases occurred in patients with moderate-to-severe acute GVHD or chronic GVHD. The central nervous system (CNS) is the main site of disease, but pneumonitis and myocarditis are also frequent findings, particularly when the diagnosis is made at autopsy. In fact, myocarditis, nephritis, and involvement of other deep organs are rarely made clinically but are frequent findings at autopsy (Slavin et al., 1994; Martino et al., 2000a).

Two large series have added further insight into the importance of not overlooking this infection in this patient population. A study from the Memorial Sloan-Kettering Cancer Center in New York described 10 cases of disseminated toxoplasmosis among 463 patients who received T-cell-depleted allogeneic BMT (2.2% frequency) (Small et al., 2000). When compared with other studies this frequency appears to be high, especially when considering that the pretransplant seroprevalence was only 23% and that these patients had a very low incidence of moderate-to-severe GVHD. This experience suggests that T-cell depletion may be an independent risk factor for this infection, although a case-control study would be needed to confirm this suspicion. Two other studies have been recently published by the EBMT Infectious Diseases Working Party (Martino et al., 2000a; Martino et al., 2000b). The first study summarized the results of a survey among European transplant centers, which showed that this infection occurs almost exclusively after an allogeneic HSCT, with 41 cases diagnosed after 4,391 allogeneic HSCT (frequency 0.93%) and none after 7,097 autologous HSCT (Martino et al., 2000b). However, as previously stated, cases have been described after autologous HSCT. Additionally, we have recently seen a case of pulmonary toxoplasmosis 10 months after a CD34+-cell selected autologous HSCT, suggesting that T-cell depletion may also increase the risk after autologous transplants.

Toxoplasma encephalitis typically presents with focal neurologic abnormalities of subacute onset, frequently accompanied by nonfocal signs and symptoms such as headache, altered mental status, and fever. The most common focal neurologic sign is motor weakness but patients may also present with cranial nerve abnormalities, speech disturbances, visual field defects, sensory disturbances, cerebellar signs, focal seizures, and movement disorders. Meningeal signs are very rare. The cerebral spinal fluid may show slight mononuclear pleocytosis, increased protein, and normal glucose levels. Computed tomography (CT) brain scans often show multiple bilateral cerebral lesions that tend to be located at the corticomedullary junction and the basal ganglia. These lesions are generally hypodense and show ring enhancement after intravenous contrast injection. Magnetic resonance imaging (MRI) scans show lesions as high signal abnormalities on T2-weighted imaging, although other nonspecific space-occupying lesions may be seen (Martino et al., 2000b). MRI is more sensitive than CT in the early diagnosis of this infection. Toxoplasma pneumonitis may develop in the absence of extrapulmonary disease. Its clinical and radiologic features are nonspecific and may mimic interstitial pneumonitis due to other causes (Pendry et al., 1990; Michel et al., 1994; Saad et al., 1996). In a literature review the only significant variable influencing outcome was site of infection: patients with disseminated disease had 5.28 times the odds of dying of toxoplasmosis compared to subjects with cerebral disease (Mele et al., 2002).

Toxoplasma chorioretinitis appears surprisingly rarely compared to the incidence noted in the AIDS population, particularly since many transplant programs utilize eye examination routinely pre- and posttransplant because of the incidence of chronic ocular GVHD posttransplant (Pauleikhoff et al., 1987). Interestingly, two cases of reactivation of toxoplasma chorioretinitis were reported in recipients of autologous transplants (Peacock et al., 1995).

Since toxoplasmosis is difficult to diagnose, various levels of diagnostic certainty have been proposed, which will aid in the

Table 76.1. *Results of published case series of toxoplasmosis after HSCT*

Author	No. cases	No. transplants (% frequency)	Percent seropositivity pretransplant in the entire transplant cohort	Types of transplant	No. patients seropositive pretransplant	Median day onset posttransplant (range)	No. treated for toxoplasmosis	No. survived toxoplasmosis	Comments
Derouin et al.	7	296 alloBMT (2.4)	NS	alloBMT	7	74 (55–180)	2	2	
Slavin et al.	12	3,803 alloBMT (0.31) 509 autoBMT (0)	15	alloBMT	11/11 tested	59 (35–97)	NS	2	
Bretagne et al.	2	550 alloBMT (0.3)	70	alloBMT	NS	NS	NS	NS	
Chandrasekar et al.	3	662 (0.5)	NS	2 alloBMT 1 synBMT	NS	46 (1–90)	1	none	
Maschke et al.	20[a]	655 (3.1)	NS	NS	20/20	73 (14–689)	NS	5	
Martino et al.	41	4,391 alloSCT (0.93) 7,097 autoSCT (0)	Variable	alloSCT	31/33 tested	64 (4–516)	23	14	Late disease (after day +63) and having received therapy were associated with improved survival
Small et al.	10	463 alloBMT (2.2)	23	TCD-alloBMT	7/10	78 (36–155)	5	1	Risk factors for toxoplasmosis were unrelated donor BMT and recipient seropositivity pretransplant

Abbreviations: BMT, bone marrow transplantation; alloSCT, allogeneic stem cell transplantation; autoSCT, autologous SCT; NS, not specified; TCD, T-cell depleted.

[a] 4 definite and 16 possible cases of toxoplasmosis.

interpretation of further studies in this area (Martino et al., 2000a). Histologically defined cases are considered as definite cases of toxoplasma disease, PCR-defined cases as probable, and CNS imaging-defined cases as possible cases.

The prognosis of this infection has been considered to be very poor based on the limited published data, with nearly 90% of patients dying of toxoplasmosis. This contrasts with the 70% to 80% response rates observed in patients with AIDS. However, the results from New York and the EBMT studies suggest that, if appropriately treated, up to 60% of patients may show clinical-radiological improvement or even a complete response. This highlights the importance for a high index of suspicion for toxoplasmosis in immunocompromised patients in order to perform appropriate diagnostic tests and to start therapy as soon as possible. Since toxoplasmosis is so difficult to diagnose histologically in these patients, noninvasive diagnostic tests would be of utmost importance. Isolation of the parasite from blood or body fluids using rodents or cell culture techniques is time-consuming, expensive, and is available only in few routine microbiology laboratories. In the HSCT recipient, the utility of serology is mainly to identify those at risk for developing toxoplasmosis posttransplant, since serologic studies posttransplant are seldom of use. PCR techniques were developed for diagnosis of neonatal infections and for the noninvasive diagnosis of cerebral toxoplasmosis in patients with AIDS (Hohlfeld et al., 1994). These techniques are applicable for blood, CSF, and BAL samples, the usual samples that are available in HSCT recipients with this infection. However, PCR techniques are not standardized, and thus the results of published studies are difficult to interpret. In AIDS patients with brain lesions PCR in blood and CSF has a sensitivity of 50% to 65% and a specificity of 95% to 100% for toxoplasmosis (Ellis, 1998), but there are no data available in HSCT recipients other than case reports. In the EBMT study 46% of the patients with toxoplasma disease and all six with infection had at least one positive PCR result, thus confirming the widespread use of this diagnostic technology in clinical practice (Martino *et al.*, 2000a). Particularly interesting were the patients with positive PCR tests from blood samples without evidence of disease (Bretagne *et al.*, 2000; Held *et al.*, 2000). These patients probably represent a transitional state between the local reactivation of tissue cysts into tachyzoites and the establishment of localized or disseminated tissue destruction by replicating tachyzoites favored by the intense cellular immunosuppression after transplant or during GVHD. This observation may be somewhat similar to the early detection of CMV infection by PCR or the pp65 antigenemia test. Unlike the latter, however, the clinical significance of detecting *Toxoplasma gondii* DNAemia is currently unknown, and it may represent a common phenomenon in seropositive patients. On the other hand, several cases of well-documented disseminated toxoplasmosis with negative serum PCR results have been described (Held *et al.*, 2000), and our patient with pulmonary toxoplasmosis described earlier had a negative PCR in blood samples but positive cytology and PCR in BAL samples. The earlier onset of toxoplasma infection (median day 35, range 13–51) than disease (median day 64, range 4–516) in the EBMT study suggests that infection may indeed precede disease in many cases (Martino *et al.*, 2000a). Thus, research efforts to establish the role of PCR in this setting are clearly warranted. Unfortunately, as with other PCR-based diagnostic tests for infectious diseases, the technique is not standardized, making comparisons between centers difficult unless a quality control is established (Costa *et al.*, 2001). Determining the recipient's pretransplant serostatus for *Toxoplasma gondii* is essential since the risk of toxoplasmosis in seronegative recipients appears to be very low.

Treatment

Initial therapy should be administered for at least 3 weeks and the total therapy duration should be continued until 4 to 6 weeks after all clinical evidence of toxoplasmosis resolves. The dosage of the medications utilized may need to be reduced or the regimen changed if side effects occur (primarily diarrhea or drug rash). Extended therapy is with pyrimethamine and sulfadiazine or pyrimethamine and clindamycin (Table 76.2). Most patients respond to one or another of these regimens and neurologic

improvement of toxoplasma brain involvement usually occurs within 7 days. Because pyrimethamine is a folic acid antagonist the most common side effect is dose-related bone marrow suppression, and patients receiving pyrimethamine should be placed on a daily oral dose of 5 to 10 mg of folinic acid (not folic acid), and have a complete blood count performed twice weekly. Other side effects of sulfonamides include fever, rash, and hepatitis.

Prophylaxis

Data from AIDS patients suggest that prophylactic cotrimoxazole is useful in minimizing the risk of reactivation of toxoplasmosis, although there are well-reported cases of toxoplasmosis breaking through cotrimoxazole prophylaxis in marrow transplant recipients (Slavin *et al.*, 1994). One study in marrow transplant recipients of pyrimethamine and sulfadoxine (Fansidar) described no proven cases of toxoplasmosis in 69 patients receiving this regimen; additionally, no cases of PCP were reported (Foot *et al.*, 1994). Table 76.2 describes the recommended prophylaxis in seropositive patients.

Malaria

Malaria, a disease characterized by recurrent fever and chills associated with the synchronous lysis of parasitized red blood cells, is produced by intra-erythrocytic parasites of the genus *Plasmodium: Plasmodium falciparum, P. vivax, P. ovale,* and *P. malariae.* At least 200 to 300 million cases of malaria occur each year with 1 to 2 million deaths. Most deaths are due to *P. falciparum* infection and occur among children less than 5 years old in sub-Saharan Africa. The major factor responsible for the recent resurgence of malaria is drug resistance, both in terms of the widespread resistance of the vector to economical insecticides such as DDT, and the increasing prevalence of chloroquine resistance in *P. falciparum,* which is now endemic in South America, Southeast Asia, and Africa.

When an infected mosquito bites a human, sporozoites travel via the bloodstream to the liver, where they enter hepatocytes and mature into tissue schizonts, which release merozoites that are infectious for red cells and produce the asexual erythrocytic cycle. During this cycle, the parasites mature from rings to trophozoites to schizonts. Schizonts lyse their host red cells as

Table 76.2. *Suggested treatment and prophylaxis for toxoplasmosis in HSCT recipients*

Treatment	Dose
Pyrimethamine (plus folinic acid) plus one of the following	Oral, 200 mg loading dose, then 50 to 75 mg qd (folinic acid, oral or i.v. 5 to 10 mg qd)
Sulfadiazine or	Oral, 1 to 1.5 g q 6 hr
Clindamycin	Oral or i.v., 600 mg q 6 hr
Prophylaxis	
Trimethoprim plus sulfamethoxazole or	2 double strength tablets per day twice per week
Pyrimethamine plus sulfadoxine (Fansidar)	1 tablet twice per week

they mature and release the next generation of merozoites, which invade previously uninfected red cells. Two of the four species that infect humans (*P. vivax* and *P. ovale*) produce dormant forms in the liver, which mature 6 to 11 months or more after the initial infection, and thus produce relapsing malaria.

The infection produces a microvascular disease involving the brain, lung, and kidney. Most patients manifest recurrent fever and chills (at 48-hour intervals for *P. vivax* and *P. ovale* and at 72-hour intervals for *P. malariae*). By contrast, patients with *P. falciparum* have irregular fever or fever and chills. The most severe manifestations are coma (cerebral malaria); massive hemolysis (Blackwater fever), which may lead to renal failure; and noncardiogenic pulmonary edema.

The most direct way to diagnose malaria is to prepare and examine Giemsa-stained thick or thin smears using oil immersion magnification (×1,000). New diagnostic techniques include fluorescent staining with acridine orange and PCR.

Despite the large worldwide prevalence of malaria, there are only five reported cases of malaria reported in HSCT recipients, two of whom acquired the infection by the transplant procedure (Dharmasena & Gordon-Smith, 1986; O'Donnell, Goldman, & Wagner, 1998). The other three cases occurred early posttransplant. In one case (Lefrere *et al.*, 1996), both donor and recipient had been in an endemic area 2 months and 1 year, respectively, pretransplant. On day 12 posttransplant, while asymptomatic, a blood smear was found to show 12.5% parasitemia. Treatment was with intravenous quinine initially for 3 days followed by halofantrine. In the second patient (Salutari *et al.*, 1996), blood smears revealed 4% parasitemia at day 14 posttransplant. Fever persisted despite neutrophil recovery, broad-spectrum intravenous antibacterial antibiotic therapy, empiric amphotericin therapy, and removal of the central venous catheter. The fever subsided within 48 hours of starting treatment with chloroquine (total of 3 days), followed by primaquine. No recurrence of malaria was described in either of the latter two cases. In the third case (Tran, Tran, & Lin, 1997), fever occurred on days 6 and 11 posttransplant and *P. falciparum* parasites were found on the blood smear on day 11.

Treatment

Successful treatment of malaria depends primarily on effective antimalarial drugs, as well as other measures including infusion of glucose and, if necessary, exchange transfusion. Monitoring the blood glucose level is important because hypoglycemia is a common cause of coma, and because both quinine and quinidine stimulate the release of insulin directly from pancreatic beta cells. Corticosteroids are contraindicated in cerebral malaria because they prolong the duration of coma. The treatment of chloroquine-susceptible malaria is satisfactory with chloroquine as monotherapy (10 mg/kg over 4 hr i.v., followed by 5 mg/kg q 12 hr over 2 hr, total dose not to exceed 25 mg/kg; p.o. 600 mg, followed by an additional 300 mg after 6 hr and 300 mg on days 2 and 3). Patients with chloroquine-resistant strains should be treated as recommended for other patient groups, with special emphasis on possible drug interactions.

Prophylaxis

For prophylaxis, chloroquine and proguanil are generally regarded as the safest drugs available for nonimmune travelers, and are very rarely associated with severe adverse reactions when used at the recommended doses. In areas where multidrug resistant falciparum malaria is prevalent, both mefloquine or the combination of chloroquine and proguanil can be used (Høgh *et al.*, 2000).

Leishmaniasis[2]

Visceral leishmaniasis (or Kala-azar) is an invasive parasitic infection caused by *Leishmania donovani*. The disease is endemic in many parts of the world, including the Mediterranean basin. The parasite is transmitted to humans from infected mammals through sandflies. The usual clinical presentation includes a combination of fever, weight loss, weakness, splenomegaly, hepatomegaly, anemia, leukopenia, hypergammaglobulinemia, and hypoalbuminemia. The diagnosis can theoretically be made serologically, but this is probably of little use in HSCT recipients; a definite diagnosis requires observation of the characteristic amastigotes in macrophages of the spleen, liver, or bone marrow. Although there have been no reported cases of leishmaniasis in HSCT recipients, there have been several reports in solid organ transplant recipients (Hernández-Pérez *et al.*, 1999). Treatment should be as in other patient groups, with antimonials or a preparation of amphotericin B.

Giardiasis

Giardiasis is an infection of the small intestine caused by the flagellated protozoan *Giardia lamblia*. Clinically this disease is characterized by diarrhea, and if prolonged, by malabsorption and weight loss. Infection occurs very easily with ingestion of as few as 10 to 25 cysts, and thus person-to-person spread is well documented; another common source is contaminated water. Infection may be asymptomatic or associated with diarrhea, cramps, flatulence, nausea, tiredness, bloating, anorexia, and occasionally chills. Unlike other parasitic infections, giardiasis occurs occasionally in HSCT recipients in many institutions, and severe gastrointestinal infections have been reported (Bromiker *et al.*, 1989).

The diagnosis is established by observing cysts or trophozoites in stool or trophozoites in small bowel contents. At least three stool specimens should be examined before a negative conclusion is drawn. Therapy is with metronidazole 250 mg 3 times daily for 7 days or quinacrine hydrochloride 100 mg 3 times daily for 7 days. Approximately 10% of patients require a second course of either drug.

Amebiasis

Human amebiasis is due to infection with the protozoan *Entamoeba histolytica*. This parasite infects 1% of the world's

---

[2] William Leishman, Scottish pathologist, 1865–1926.

population, primarily in poor developing areas, where infection results from ingestion of the fecally excreted cyst form from contaminated water or food or by direct fecal-oral contact. Amebiasis can cause acute rectocolitis (dysentery), fulminant colitis with perforation, toxic megacolon, chronic nondysenteric colitis, and ameboma. Outside the gastrointestinal tract, disease manifestations include liver abscess (which may be complicated by peritonitis), empyema, pericarditis, lung abscess, brain abscess, meningoencephalitis, and genitourinary disease. The diagnosis rests on the morphologic identification of trophozoites in fecal specimens, and at least three stool samples are necessary to reach a 90% yield. There are at least four cases of amebiasis reported after BMT (Anderlini *et al.*, 1994; Bavaro *et al.*, 1994; Feingold *et al.*, 1998). Bavaro and colleagues reported a 36-year-old recipient of an allogeneic transplant who developed cramping abdominal pain and diarrhea at day 23 posttransplant. Stool examination demonstrated the presence of trophozoites and cysts of *E. histolytica*; rectosigmoidoscopy showed an edematous mucosa and small flask-shaped ulcers. Initially therapy with metronidazole 250 mg 3 times daily and paromomycin 500 mg 3 times daily failed to clear the infection and the agents were increased to 500 mg 4 times daily each with the addition of rolitetracycline 275 mg 3 times daily. This produced resolution of the infection. The two patients described by Anderlini were unusual in that both presented with fever and nodular pulmonary infiltrates 6 and 9 months after an allogeneic and autologous transplant, respectively. The second patient also had painful subcutaneous nodules that subsequently ulcerated. Both patients developed neurologic involvement with coma and died. Autopsy examination revealed necrotizing meningoencephalitis with amebic trophozoites and cysts consistent with acanthamoeba species. Another fatal case of meningoencephalitis has also been reported (Feingold *et al.*, 1998). There is no treatment known to be efficacious for meningoencephalitis, although there are occasional reports of survival in non-HSCT patients treated with systemic and intrathecal amphotericin.

Cryptosporidiosis and microsporidiosis

Cryptosporidiosis is a gastrointestinal infection characterized by watery diarrhea, abdominal cramps, malabsorption, and weight loss. It is usually a severe, unrelenting illness in immune suppressed patients, especially those with AIDS, while it is a self-limited disease in the immunologically normal host. It is caused by the coccidian protozoan cryptosporidium. The environmentally resistant form is the oocyst that can be identified in fecal specimens. In humans it is spread from person to person, and contaminated water is the most common means of transmission. Clinical manifestations include watery diarrhea, cramping abdominal pain, weight loss, flatulence, nausea, vomiting, and anorexia; myalgias and malaise may also be present. Fecal examination reveals cryptosporidiosis and mucus but no leukocytes or blood. The incubation period is between 2 and 14 days. Biliary cryptosporidiosis has also been documented, but only in immune suppressed patients and is charac-

terized by the classic signs of cholangitis, including severe right upper quadrant pain, nausea, and vomiting.

A number of reports have been described after HSCT (Manivel, Filipovich, & Snover, 1985; Rio *et al.*, 1986; Kibbler *et al.*, 1987; Martino *et al.*, 1988; Gentile *et al.*, 1991; Nachbaur *et al.*, 1997). Most of these cases presented with diarrhea. One case (Kibbler *et al.*, 1987) described pulmonary cryptosporidiosis associated with terminal respiratory failure. One of the two patients in Nachbaur's report died of pulmonary involvement, while the other responded to treatment with paromomycin, azithromycin, and recombinant interleukin-2.

Unfortunately, there is currently no known effective treatment for cryptosporidiosis. Sparamycin has been utilized without success in patients with AIDS, and currently paromomycin and azithromycin are being studied.

At least one case of human microsporidial infection posttransplant has been reported (Kelkar *et al.*, 1997). The patient had pulmonary involvement in association with *Candida tropicalis* infection. The diagnosis was only made at autopsy.

American trypanosomiasis (Chagas' disease)[3]

American trypanosomiasis or Chagas' disease results from infection with the protozoan parasite *Trypanosoma cruzi*. There are species of blood-sucking bugs that become infected when they take a blood meal from animals or humans who have circulating parasites. The ingested parasites transform in the bug and transmission to a second vertebrate host occurs when the infected bug takes a subsequent blood meal and defecates during or after feeding, so that infective forms are deposited on the skin. *T. cruzi* and its arthropod vectors are widely distributed in Central and South America, where the infection is endemic. The disease may occur either as an acute or chronic form.

Acute Chagas' disease

The disease is characterized by a local area of erythema and induration (chagoma) in the skin at the site of parasite entry, with fever, lymphadenopathy, hepatosplenomegaly, and transient skin rashes. Myocarditis and meningoencephalitis can occur. Signs and symptoms of acute disease gradually subside within a few weeks to several months. The acute disease is diagnosed by direct microscopic examination of anticoagulated blood or buffy coat preparation for motile trypanosomes. Additionally, blood or affected tissues can be cultured on special media.

Chronic Chagas' disease

In contrast, chronic Chagas' disease is usually characterized by cardiac signs and symptoms, followed by mega disease of the esophagus or colon. Symptoms include dysphagia, fullness, chest pain, and regurgitation. Aspiration with secondary pneumonia occurs commonly as does weight loss. Chronic chagasic megacolon produces chronic constipation, abdominal pain,

---

[3] Carlos Chagas, Brazilian physician, 1879–1934.

volvulus, obstruction, and sometimes bowel perforation. The diagnosis of chronic Chagas' disease requires demonstration of antibodies to *T. cruzi* in the presence of the characteristic cardiac abnormalities and/or mega disease.

There are at least five reports of Chagas' disease occurring in HSCT recipients (Villalba *et al.*, 1992; Pasternak *et al.*, 1997; Dictar *et al.*, 1998; Altclas *et al.*, 1999), including acute and chronic forms of the disease. Patients with the chronic form can reactivate posttransplant (Dictar *et al.*, 1998; Altclas *et al.*, 1999). Therapy should be with nifurtimox or benznidazole as in other patient groups. Nifurtimox can be used at a dose of 8 to 12 mg/kg/day. Benznidazole is an alternative. Both drugs are administered for 60 to 90 days and have considerable side effects, the most common of which with nifurtimox are gastrointestinal intolerance with anorexia, nausea, vomiting, and abdominal pain. Neurologic symptoms include restlessness, insomnia, disorientation, paresthesias, polyneuritis, and seizures. Skin rashes can also occur. Peripheral neuropathy and bone marrow suppression have been reported with benznidazole. There is no evidence currently that the established pathologic changes of chronic Chagas' disease can be reversed by therapy with either agent.

Trichomoniasis

Trichomonas vaginalis is among the most prevalent of all pathogenic protozoa, infecting as many as 3 million women per year in the United States alone. It is usually spread by sexual contact. As many as half of *T. vaginalis* infections in women are asymptomatic, and the remainder are associated with vaginal discharge, vulvo-vaginal irritation, dyspareunia, or dysuria. The discharge tends to be watery and copious but in some cases it is thick and may be yellow or green. Patients may notice an odor, although this is more common with bacterial vaginosis. Upon pelvic examination there is usually inflammation of the vaginal walls; punctate hemorrhages on the exocervix (the classic "strawberry cervix") are uncommon on gross inspection, but may be observed in approximately half of infected women by colposcopy. Most men with trichomoniasis are asymptomatic, although the organism is sometimes isolated from men with symptoms of urethritis who are negative for other pathogens. Identifying the parasite in vaginal discharge usually makes the diagnosis. The treatment of choice is metronidazole; a single dose of 2 g is effective. All sexual partners must be treated concurrently to prevent reinfection. Metronidazole 250 mg 3 times daily for 7 days is an alternative. A single case report exists of fatal meningoencephalitis due to *Trichomonas fetus* in a recipient of a blood stem cell allograft (Okamoto *et al.*, 1998). This organism had not been previously reported to cause disease in humans.

Other protozoal diseases

There is a single case report from Oman of dysentery due to *Blastocystis hominis* (a parasite with doubtful pathogenicity in immunocompetent hosts), occurring in a patient with acute GVHD of the gastrointestinal tract after an HLA-identical sibling transplant (Ghosh, Ayyaril, & Nirmala, 1998). Prolonged metronidazole treatment was required to eradicate the parasite and cure the diarrhea. African trypanosomiasis (sleeping sickness), filariasis, and babesiosis have not been described in HSCT recipients and will not be dealt with here, although it should be noted that the latter two can be transmitted by blood transfusion.

Helminthic diseases

The only disease caused by helminths that has been reported among HSCT recipients is toxocariasis (Fischmeister *et al.*, 2001), which is caused by the helminths *Toxocara canis* (a natural parasite of dogs and foxes) or *T. cati* (cats). Transmission results from ingestion of embryonated eggs from a contaminated environment such as water or soil. Larvae hatch in the small intestine, penetrate the mucosa, and migrate to the liver, lungs, heart, and other organs. Manifestations include fever, hepatomegaly (visceral larva migrans syndrome), endophthalmitis, myocarditis, rash, and encephalitis. Diagnosis is by detection of specific antibodies to the parasite. Anemia, eosinophilia, and hypergammaglobulinemia occur. Treatment is with antihelminthic agents such as albendazole or mebendazole.

References

Altclas, J., Jaimovich, G., Milovic, V. *et al.* (1996). Chagas' disease after bone marrow transplantation: case report. *Bone Marrow Transplantation,* **18,** 447–8.

Anderlini, P., Przepiorka, D., Luna, M. *et al.* (1994). Acanthamoeba meningoencephalitis after bone marrow transplantation. *Bone Marrow Transplantation,* **14,** 459–61.

Bavaro, P., Di Girolamo, G., Di Bartolomeo, P. *et al.* (1994). Amebiasis after bone marrow transplantation: case report. *Bone Marrow Transplantation,* **13,** 213–14.

Bretagne, S., Costa, J.M., Kuentz, M. *et al.* (1995). Late toxoplasmosis evidenced by PCR in a marrow transplant recipient. *Bone Marrow Transplantation,* **15,** 809–11.

Bretagne, S., Costa, J.M., Foulet, F., Jabot-Lestang, L., Baud-Camus, F., & Cordonnier, C. (2000). Prospective study of toxoplasma reactivation by polymerase chain reaction in allogeneic stem-cell transplant recipients. *Transplant Infectious Diseases,* **2,** 127–32.

Bromiker, R., Korman, S.H., Or, R. *et al.* (1989). Severe giardiasis in two patients undergoing bone marrow transplantation. *Bone Marrow Transplantation,* **4,** 701–3.

Candolfi, E., Derouin, F., & Kien, T. (1987). Detection of circulating antigens in immunocompromised patients during the reactivation of chronic toxoplasmosis. *European Journal of Clinical Microbiology,* **6,** 44–8.

Castagnola, E., Dini, G., Lanino, E. *et al.* (1995). Low CD4 lymphocyte count in a patient with P carinii pneumonia after autologous bone marrow transplantation. *Bone Marrow Transplantation,* **15,** 977–8.

Chandrasekar, P.H., Momin, F., & the Bone Marrow Transplant Team. (1997). Disseminated toxoplasmosis in marrow recipients:

a report of three cases and a review of the literature. *Bone Marrow Transplantation*, **19**, 685–9.

Costa, J.M., Munoz, C., Kruger, D. *et al.* (2001). Quality control for the diagnosis of Toxoplasma gondii reactivation in SCT patients using PCR assays. *Bone Marrow Transplantation*, **28**, 527–8.

Cruciani, M., Marcati, P., Malena, M., Bosco, O., Serpelloni, G., & Mengoli, C. (2002). Meta-analysis of diagnostic procedures for Pneumocystis carinii pneumonia in HIV-1-infected patients. *European Respiratory Journal*, **20**, 982–9.

Derouin, F., Devergie, A., Auber, P. *et al.* (1992). Toxoplasmosis in bone marrow transplant recipients: report of seven cases and review. *Clinical Infectious Diseases*, **15**, 267–70.

Dharmasena, F. & Gordon-Smith, E.C. (1986). Transmission of malaria by bone marrow transplantation. *Transplantation*, **42**, 228.

Dictar, M., Sinagra, A., Verón, M.T. *et al.* (1998). Recipients and donors of bone marrow transplants suffering from Chagas' disease: management and preemptive therapy of parasitemia. *Bone Marrow Transplantation*, **21**, 391–3.

Dworkin, M.S., Williamson, J., Jones, J.L., & Kaplan, J.E. (2001). Prophylaxis with trimethoprim-sulfamethoxazole for human immunodeficiency virus-infected patients: impact on risk for infectious diseases. *Clinical Infectious Diseases*, **33**, 393–8.

Ellis, J.T. (1998). Polymerase chain reaction approaches for the detection of Neospora caninum and Toxoplasma gondii. *International Journal of Parasitology*, **28**, 1053–60.

Elvin, K., Olsson, M., Lidman, C., & Bjorkman, A. (1996). Detection of asymptomatic Pneumocystis carinii infection by polymerase chain reaction: predictive for subsequent pneumonia. *AIDS*, **10**, 1296–7.

Feingold, J.M., Abraham, J., Bilgrami, S. *et al.* (1998). Acanthamoeba meningoencephalitis following autologous peripheral stem cell transplantation. *Bone Marrow Transplantation*, **22**, 297–300.

Fischmeister, G., Holter, W., Matthes-Martin, S. *et al.* (2001). Allogeneic bone marrow transplantation-mediated transfer of specific immunity against Toxocara canis associated with excessive IgE. *Bone Marrow Transplantation*, **28**, 519–21.

Fishman, J.A. (2001). Prevention of infection caused by Pneumocystis carinii in transplant recipients. *Clinical Infectious Diseases*, **15**, 1397–405.

Foot, A.B.M., Gariny, J.F., Ribaud, P. *et al.* (1994). Prophylaxis of toxoplasmosis infection with pyrimethamine/sulfadoxine (Fansidar) in bone marrow transplant recipients. *Bone Marrow Transplantation*, **14**, 241–5.

Geissmann, F., Derouin, F., Marolleau, J.P. *et al.* (1994). Disseminated toxoplasmosis following autologous bone marrow transplantation [letter]. *Clinical Infectious Diseases*, **19**, 800–1.

Gentile, G., Venditti, M., Micozzi, A. *et al.* (1991). Cryptosporidiosis in patients with hematologic malignancies. *Reviews of Infectious Diseases*, **13**, 842–6.

Ghosh, K., Ayyaril, M., & Nirmala, V. (1999). Acute GVHD involving the gastrointestinal tract and infestation with Blastocystis hominis in a patient with chronic myeloid leukemia following allogeneic bone marrow transplantation. *Bone Marrow Transplantation*, **22**, 1115–7.

Held, T.K., Krüger, D., Switala, A.R. *et al.* (2000). Diagnosis of toxoplasmosis in bone marrow transplant recipients: comparison of PCR-based results and immunohistochemistry. *Bone Marrow Transplantation*, **25**, 1257–62.

Hernández-Pérez, J., Yebra-Bango, M., Jiménez-Martínez, E. *et al.* (1999). Visceral leishmaniasis (kala-azar) in solid organ transplantation: report of five cases and review. *Clinical Infectious Diseases*, **29**, 918–21.

Høgh, B., Clarke, P.D., Camus, D. *et al.* (2000). Atovaquone-proguanil versus chloroquine-proguanil for malaria prophylaxis in non-immune travellers: a randomized, double-blind study. *Lancet*, **356**, 1888–94.

Hohlfeld, P., Daffos, F., Costa, J.M. *et al.* (1994). Prenatal diagnosis of congenital toxoplasmosis with a polymerase-chain-reaction test on amniotic fluid. *New England Journal of Medicine*, **331**, 695–9.

Hoyle, C. & Goldman, J.M. (1994). Life-threatening infections occurring more than 3 months after BMT. *Bone Marrow Transplantation*, **14**, 247–52.

Jehn, U., Fink, M., Gundlach, P. *et al.* (1984). Lethal cardiac and cerebral toxoplasmosis in a patient with acute myeloid leukemia after successful allogeneic bone marrow transplantation. *Transplantation*, **38**, 430–3.

Johnson, J.D., Butcher, P.D., Savva, D., & Holliman, R.E. (1993). Application of the polymerase chain reaction to the diagnosis of human toxoplasmosis. *Journal of Infection*, **26**, 147–58.

Kelkar, R., Sastry, P.S.R.K., Kulkarni, S.S. *et al.* (1997). Pulmonary microsporidial infection in a patient with CML undergoing allogeneic marrow transplant. *Bone Marrow Transplantation*, **19**, 179–82.

Kibbler, C.C., Smith, A., Hamilton-Dutoit, S.J. *et al.* (1987). Pulmonary cryptosporidiosis occurring in a bone marrow transplant patient. *Scandinavian Journal of Infectious Diseases*, **19**, 581–4.

Krowka, M.J., Rosenow, E.C., & Hoagland, J.C. (1985). Pulmonary complications of bone marrow transplantation. *Chest*, **87**, 237–46.

Lefrere, F., Besson, C., Datry, A. *et al.* (1996). Transmission of Plasmodium falciparum by allogeneic bone marrow transplantation. *Bone Marrow Transplantation*, **18**, 473–4.

Leyva, W.H. & Santa, Cruz, D.J. (1986). Cutaneous toxoplasmosis. *Journal of the American Academy of Dermatology*, **14**, 600–5.

Link, H., Vöhringer, H.F., Wingen, F. *et al.* (1993). Pentamidine aerosol for prophylaxis of Pneumocystis carinii pneumonia after BMT. *Bone Marrow Transplantation*, **11**, 403–6.

Lowenberg, B., van Gijn, J., Prins, E. *et al.* (1983). Fatal cerebral toxoplasmosis in a bone marrow transplant recipient with leukemia. *Transplantation*, **35**, 30–4.

Lyytikäinen, O., Ruutu, T., Volin, L. *et al.* (1996). Late onset Pneumocystis carinii pneumonia following allogeneic bone marrow transplantation. *Bone Marrow Transplantation*, **17**, 1057–9.

Manivel, C., Filipovich, A., & Snover, D.C. (1985). Cryptosporidiosis as a cause of diarrhea following bone marrow transplantation. *Diseases of the Colon and Rectum*, **28**, 741–2.

Martino, R., Bretagne, S., Rovira, M. *et al.* (2000b). Toxoplasmosis after hematopoietic stem transplantation. Report of a five-year survey from the Infectious Diseases Working Party of the European Group for Blood and Marrow Transplantation (EBMT-IDWP). *Bone Marrow Transplantation*, **25**, 1111–3.

Martino, P., Gentile, G., Caprioli, A. *et al.* (1988). Cryptosporidiosis in a bone marrow transplant unit. *Journal of Infectious Diseases,* **158,** 647–8.

Martino, R., Maertens, J., Bretagne, S. *et al.* (2000a) Toxoplasmosis after hematopoietic stem cell transplantation. A study by the European Group for Blood and Marrow Transplantation (EBMT) Infectious Diseases Working Party (IDWP). *Clinical Infectious Diseases,* **31,** 1188–94.

Martino, R., Martínez, C., Sureda, A., & Brunet, S. (1994). Successful BMT in patients with recent Pneumocystis carinii pneumonia: report of two cases. *Bone Marrow Transplantation,* **16,** 491.

Maschke, M., Dietrich, U., Prumbaum, M. *et al.* (1999). Opportunistic CNS infection after bone marrow transplantation. *Bone Marrow Transplantation,* **23,** 1167–76.

Mele, A., Paterson, P. J., Prentice, H. J., & Kibber, C. C. (2002). Toxoplasmosis in bone marrow transplantation: a report of two cases and systematic review of the literature. *Bone Marrow Transplantation,* **29,** 691–8.

Michel, G., Thuret, I., Chambost, H. *et al.* (1994). Lung toxoplasmosis after HLA-mismatched bone marrow transplantation (case report). *Bone Marrow Transplantation,* **14,** 455–7.

Nachbaur, D., Kropshofer, G., Feichtinger, H. *et al.* (1997). Case report. Cryptosporidiosis after CD34-selected autologous peripheral blood stem cell transplantation (PBSCT). Treatment with paromomycin, azithromycin and recombinant human interleukin-2. *Bone Marrow Transplantation,* **19,** 1261–3.

Naimey, G.L. & Wuerker, R.B. (1995). Comparison of histologic stains in the diagnosis of Pneumocystis carinii. *Acta Cytologica,* **39,** 1124–7.

O'Donnell, J., Goldman, J.M., & Wagner, K. (1998). Donor-derived Plasmodium vivax infection following volunteer unrelated bone marrow transplantation. *Bone Marrow Transplantation,* **21,** 313–4.

O'Driscoll, J.C. & Holliman, R.E. (1991). Toxoplasmosis and bone marrow transplantation. *Reviews in Medical Microbiology,* **2,** 215–22.

Okamoto, S., Wakui, M., Kobayashi, H. *et al.* (1998). Trichomonas foetus meningoencephalitis after allogeneic peripheral blood stem cell transplantation. *Bone Marrow Transplantation,* **21,** 89–91.

Pagano, L., Fianchi, L., Mele, L. *et al.* (2002). Pneumocystis carinii pneumonia in patients with malignant haematological diseases: 10 years' experience of infection in GIMEMA centres. *British Journal of Haematology,* **117,** 379–86.

Pasternak, J., Amato Neto, V., & Hammerschack, N. (1997). Chagas' disease after BMT. *Bone Marrow Transplantation,* **19,** 958.

Pauleikhoff, D., Messmer, E., Beelen, D.W. *et al.* (1987). Bone marrow transplantation and toxoplasmic retinochoroiditis. *Graefes Archives of Clinical and Experimental Ophthalmology,* **225,** 239–43.

Peacock, J.F., Greven, C.M., Couz, J.M., & Hurd, D.D. (1995). Reactivation of toxoplasmic retinochoroiditis in patients undergoing bone marrow transplantation: is there a role for chemoprophylaxis? *Bone Marrow Transplantation,* **15,** 983–7.

Pendry, K., Tait, R.C., McLay, A. *et al.* (1990). Toxoplasmosis after BMT for CML. *Bone Marrow Transplantation,* **5,** 65–7.

Ribes, J.A., Limper, A.H., Espy, M.J., & Smith, T.F. (1997). PCR detection of Pneumocystis carinii in bronchoalveolar lavage specimens: analysis of sensitivity and specificity. *Journal of Clinical Microbiology,* **35,** 830–5.

Rio, B., Le Tourneau, A., Sobahni, I. *et al.* (1986). Cryptosporidiosis in grafting of allogeneic bone marrow. *Presse Medicale,* **15,** 141–6.

Saad, R., Vincent, J.F., Cimon, B. *et al.* (1996). Pulmonary toxoplasmosis after allogeneic bone marrow transplantation: case report and review. *Bone Marrow Transplantation,* **18,** 211–12.

Salutari, P., Sica, S., Chiusolo, P. *et al.* (1996). Plasmodium vivax malaria after autologous bone marrow transplantation: an unusual complication. *Bone Marrow Transplantation,* **18,** 805–6.

Seong, D.C., Przepiorka, D., Bruner, J.M. *et al.* (1993). Leptomeningeal toxoplasmosis after allogeneic marrow transplantation. Case report and review of the literature. *American Journal of Clinical Oncology,* **15,** 105–8.

Shepp, D.H., Hackman, R.C., Conley, F.K. *et al.* (1985). Toxoplasma gondii reactivation identified by detection of parasitemia in tissue culture. *Annals of Internal Medicine,* **103,** 218–21.

Sing, A., Leitritz, L., Roggenkamp, A., Kolb, H.J. *et al.* (1999). Pulmonary toxoplasmosis in bone marrow tranplant recipients: report of two cases and review. *Clinical Infectious Diseases,* **29,** 429–33.

Sing, A., Trebesius, K., Roggenkamp, A. *et al.* (2000). Evaluation of diagnostic value and epidemiological implications of PCR for Pneumocystis carinii in different immunosuppressed and immunocompetent patient groups. *Journal of Clinical Microbiology,* **38,** 1461–7.

Slavin, M.A., Meyers, J.D., Remington, J.S., & Hackman, R.C. (1994). Toxoplasma gondii infection in marrow transplant recipients: a twenty year experience. *Bone Marrow Transplantation,* **13,** 549–57.

Small, T.N., Leung, L., Stiles, J. *et al.* (2000). Disseminated toxoplasmosis following T-cell-depleted related and unrelated bone marrow transplantation. *Bone Marrow Transplantation,* **25,** 969–73.

Souza, J.P., Boeckh, M., Gooley, T.A., Flowers, M.E., & Crawford, S.W. (1999). High rates of Pneumocystis carinii pneumonia in allogeneic blood and marrow transplant recipients receiving dapsone prophylaxis. *Clinical Infectious Diseases,* **29,** 1467–71.

Thomas, C.F., Limper, A.H. (1998). Pneumocystis pneumonia: clinical presentation and diagnosis in patients with and without acquired immune deficiency syndrome. *Seminars in Respiratory Infections,* **13,** 285–95.

Torres, J., Goldman, M., Wheat, L.J. *et al.* (2000). Diagnosis of Pneumocystis carinii pneumonia in human immunodeficiency virus-infected patients with polymerase chain reaction: a blinded comparison to standard methods. *Clinical Infectious Diseases,* **30,** 141–5.

Tran, V-B., Tran, V-B., & Lin, K-H. (1997). Malaria infection after allogeneic bone marrow transplantation in a child with thalassemia. *Bone Marrow Transplantation,* **19,** 1259–60.

Tuan, I.Z., Dennison, D., Weisdorf, D.J. (1992). Pneumocystis carinii following BMT. *Bone Marrow Transplantation,* **10,** 267–72.

Villalba, R., Fornes, G., Alvarez, M.A. *et al.* (1992). Acute Chagas' disease in a recipient of a bone marrow transplant in Spain: case report. *Clinical Infectious Diseases,* **14,** 594–5.

Yadlapati, S., Dorsky, D., Remington, J.S. *et al.* (1997). Ocular toxoplasmosis after autologous peripheral-blood stem-cell transplantation. *Clinical Infectious Diseases,* **25,** 1255–6.

77 Hepatic veno-occlusive disease

PAUL RICHARDSON AND EVA GUINAN

Dana–Farber Cancer Institute, Harvard Medical School, Boston, USA

Introduction

Veno-occlusive disease (VOD) of the liver (Bearman, 1995; Richardson & Guinan, 1999; Bearman, 2001; Richardson & Guinan, 2001) is a clinical syndrome characterized by jaundice, liver enlargement and pain, fluid retention, and weight gain. It is defined histopathologically by narrowing or fibrous obliteration of terminal hepatic venules and small lobular veins with damage to the surrounding centrilobular hepatocytes and sinusoids in zone 3 of the liver acinus (Shulman *et al.*, 1980; Shulman & McDonald, 1984). Its onset is typically within the first month after hematopoietic stem cell transplantation (SCT), although later onset has been described (Lee *et al.*, 1997; Toh *et al.*, 1999). As the diagnosis is based on clinical criteria, the incidence reported and severity seen is variable, ranging from 10% to 60%, and may be influenced by programmatic differences in conditioning regimens and patient characteristics (Bearman, 1995) (Table 77.1). It is more common in the allogeneic setting, as illustrated by a prospective EBMT study of 1,652 patients from 73 centers over a 6-month period, in which the incidence of VOD was 8.9% in 631 allogeneic recipients and 3.1% in 1,010 autologous recipients (Carreras *et al.*, 1998). VOD is now considered to be part of the spectrum of nonmarrow organ injury syndromes that can occur after high-dose therapy and SCT, and which includes idiopathic pneumonitis, diffuse alveo-lar hemorrhage, thrombotic microangiopathy, and capillary-leak syndrome. There is a growing body of evidence indicating that early injury to vascular endothelium either directly by the conditioning regimen, or indirectly through the production of certain cytokines, is a common denominator between these events (Holler *et al.*, 1990; Baglin, 1994; Krenger *et al.*, 1997).

The prognosis of VOD is variable. Mild disease is defined retrospectively by an absence of adverse effects from liver dysfunction with complete resolution of symptoms and signs. Moderate disease is also characterized by eventual complete resolution, but adverse effects of liver dysfunction result in requirement for therapy such as diuresis for fluid retention and analgesia for pain. Although a large proportion of patients fall into the mild to moderate category, a significant fraction of VOD is severe. While some patients with severe disease may be treatable, the larger proportion are essentially incurable with a fatality rate approaching 100% (McDonald *et al.*, 1993; Carreras *et al.*, 1998).

Pathogenesis

Injury from chemo-radiotherapy and cytokines to hepatic sinusoidal/venular endothelium and hepatocytes in zone 3 of the liver acinus are the key initial events in the pathogenesis of VOD, leading to activation of clotting factors (in particular fac-

Table 77.1. *Incidence of VOD among 190 patients based on preparative regimen*

Preparative regimen	Incidence of severe VOD	*P*[a]
Cyclophosphamide (120 mg/kg) + TBI (1,200 cGy)	6/75 (8%)	
Cyclophosphamide (120 mg/kg) + TBI (>1,200 cGy)	27/116 (23%)	.006
Other chemotherapy + TBI (1,200 cGy)	4/25 (16%)	.2
Cyclophosphamide alone	0/4 (0%)	>.2
Busulfan + cyclophosphamide	12/38 (32%)	.001
BCNU + etoposide + cyclophosphamide	5/15 (33%)	.006

[a] Compared with cyclophosphamide (120 mg/kg) + TBI (1,200 cGy).

Reproduced, with permission, from Bearman (1995).

1235

tor VIII, von Willebrand factor and fibrinogen) and their deposition in the subendothelial zone of affected venules and surrounding sinusoids, with extravasation of blood into the space of Disse (Fig. 77.1) (Shulman *et al.*, 1980; Shulman *et al.*, 1987). Unusually large von Willebrand factor (VWF) multimers have been detected in the serum after HSC transplantation and are normally cleaved and degraded into smaller multimers by VWF-capase, identified as a metalloprotease produced in the liver and termed ADAMTS13. In one study this caspase activity was significantly reduced in VOD patients, even before initiation of the conditioning regimen (Park *et al.*, 2002). Congestion and ischemia from decreased sinusoidal blood flow result in additional hepatocyte damage and necrosis.

Later features include intense collagen deposition in the sinusoids, sclerosis of the venular walls, and collagen deposition within the venular lumen and abluminally (Shulman *et al.*, 1987). This progresses to obliteration of the venule and further hepatocyte necrosis. When advanced, VOD histopathology is marked by extensive necrotic tissue and fibrosis (Watanabe *et al.*, 1996).

Recently, the term *sinusoidal obstruction syndrome* (SOS) has been proposed to replace the established terminology of VOD (DeLeve *et al.*, 2002). Although the emergence of sinusoidal obstruction is clearly apparent in rat models of VOD (DeLeve, 1996), and is seen in human disease (DeLeve *et al.*, 2002), the first recognizable histologic change of liver toxicity due to VOD in patients is widening of the subendothelial space between the basement membrane and the lumen of central veins. Accompanying venular changes, dilation and engorge-

ment of the sinusoids with extravasation of red cells and frank necrosis of perivenular hepatocytes follow, and become more widespread as the extent of venular injury increases (Shulman *et al.*, 1994). Correlation of histologic findings in this cohort study of 76 consecutive necropsy patients found the strongest statistical association between the severity of VOD and the extent of hepatocyte necrosis, sinusoidal fibrosis, thickening of the subendothelium, phlebosclerosis, and venular narrowing. Until and unless prospective studies show otherwise, a change in the term VOD to SOS thus seems premature.

Risk factors

Risk factors for developing VOD can be divided into pre-SCT and SCT-related features (Nevill *et al.*, 1991; McDonald *et al.*, 1993; Carreras *et al.*, 1998). Pre-SCT factors include elevation of liver transaminase levels (specifically AST) on admission, older age, poor performance status, female gender, advanced disease, prior hepatic radiation, the number of days on broad-spectrum antibiotics pre-SCT, prior amphotericin B, vancomycin and/or acyclovir therapy, the number of days with fever pre-SCT, and the degree of histocompatibility (Bearman, 1995; Carreras *et al.*, 1998). In an Egyptian study, schistosomiasis causing hepatic periportal fibrosis (detected by ultrasonography) was found to be a predisposing factor to VOD after allogeneic SCT (Mahmoud, 1996).

Reduced pretransplant diffusion capacity of the lung may be an independent risk factor for VOD (Matute-Bello *et al.*, 1998).

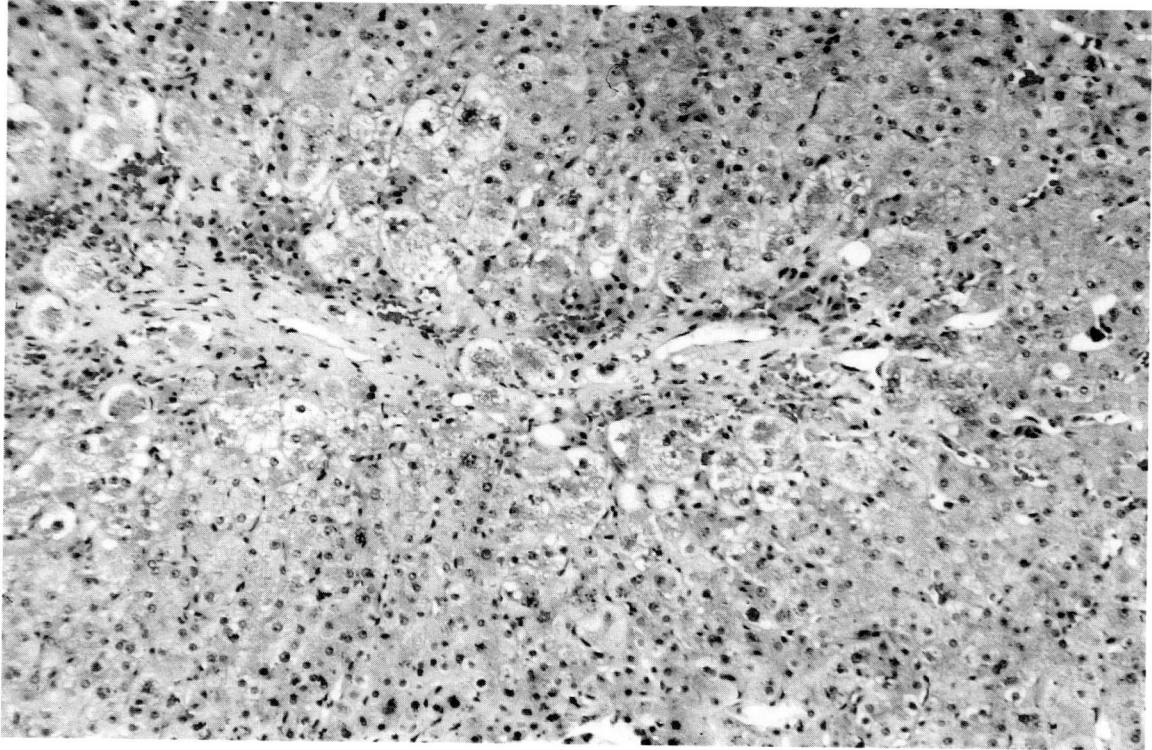

Fig. 77.1. Liver biopsy showing characteristic changes of veno-occlusive disease with terminal venular fibrosis, fibrin deposition, and marked zone 3 hepatocellular damage. Centrilobular hepatocytes show ballooning degeneration, necrosis, and hemosiderin pigment.

Norethisterone treatment, previously used in women to minimize menstrual bleeding during the thrombocytopenic period posttransplant, has been incriminated as a risk factor, possibly by causing microthrombosis in small hepatic veins (Hagglund *et al.,* 1998). Some factors also appear to predict VOD severity; for example, a fourfold elevation of AST above normal and increasing histoincompatibility between donor and recipient are associated with severe VOD and high fatality (McDonald *et al.,* 1993). Conversely, in nonrandomized studies, a low incidence of VOD has been found in patients receiving T-cell-depleted grafts (Soiffer *et al.,* 1991; Moscardo *et al.,* 2001).

SCT-associated factors include total body irradiation (TBI) dose, dose rate, and dose of busulfan (Bearman, 1995; Carreras *et al.,* 1998). A randomized study showed a significantly higher incidence in patients receiving busulfan and cyclophosphamide compared to cyclophosphamide and TBI conditioning (Ringden *et al.,* 1994) (Fig. 77.2) In a study of 350 patients treated with busulfan 16 mg/kg and cyclophosphamide 120 mg/kg the overall incidence of VOD was 27% (Styler *et al.,* 1996). In an IBMTR study of 1,717 recipients of HLA-identical sibling SCT for leukemia between 1988 and 1990, variables associated with an increased risk of VOD were conditioning with busulfan and cyclophosphamide compared to TBI (Rozman *et al.,* 1996). Several groups have reported an association between busulfan levels (i.e. area under the curve measurement during drug administration) and VOD risk (Grochow *et al.,* 1989; Slattery *et al.,* 1995; Dix *et al.,* 1996; Vassal *et al.,* 1996; Ljungman *et al.,* 1997; Copelan *et al.,* 2001).

An important new risk factor for VOD is the administration of gemtuzumab ozogamicin (Mylotarg), an anti-CD33 monoclonal antibody linked to the toxin calicheamycin (Tack *et al.,* 2001; McDonald, 2002). Sinusoidal endothelial cells and stellate cells in zone 3 of the hepatic sinus express CD33, and, as a result, significant toxic liver injury has been reported both when this agent is given to AML patients prior to and after SCT, with resultant severe VOD and a high case fatality rate (McDonald, 2002).

Diagnosis

VOD is a clinical syndrome characterized by hepatomegaly and/or right upper quadrant pain, jaundice, and fluid retention (Bearman, 1995; Richardson & Guinan, 1999, 2001). Other causes of hepatomegaly, weight gain, and jaundice must be excluded (Table 77.2). Symptoms can develop from as early as the day of transplant up to 3 weeks post-SCT (Table 77.3), and occasionally later (Lee *et al.,* 1997; Toh *et al.,* 1999) (Fig 77.3). The first signs of VOD, hepatomegaly and/or right upper quadrant pain and fluid retention, typically occur relatively early posttransplant. Jaundice, ascites, and encephalopathy become apparent later (Table 77.3). Sodium avidity is an early event, contributing to subsequent peripheral edema, worsening ascites, pulmonary infiltration, and a requirement for supplemental oxygen. Progressive oliguric renal failure, as part of hepato-renal syndrome, occurs in half of patients with severe disease (McDonald, 1993) (Table 77.4).

Ultrasound and computed tomography (CT) imaging can be useful in identifying hepatomegaly, confirming the presence of ascites and, together with Doppler studies, in determining whether or not there is attenuation or reversal of venous flow or frank portal vein thrombosis (Brown *et al.,* 1990). These modalities are also useful in excluding pericardial effusion, constrictive pericarditis, extrahepatic venous obstruction, and mass lesions of the liver (Hosoki *et al.,* 1989; Nicolau *et al.,* 1993). Doppler ultrasound has gained popularity because it is noninvasive and can be performed at the bedside. However, pulsatile hepatic venous flow is a relatively nonspecific finding

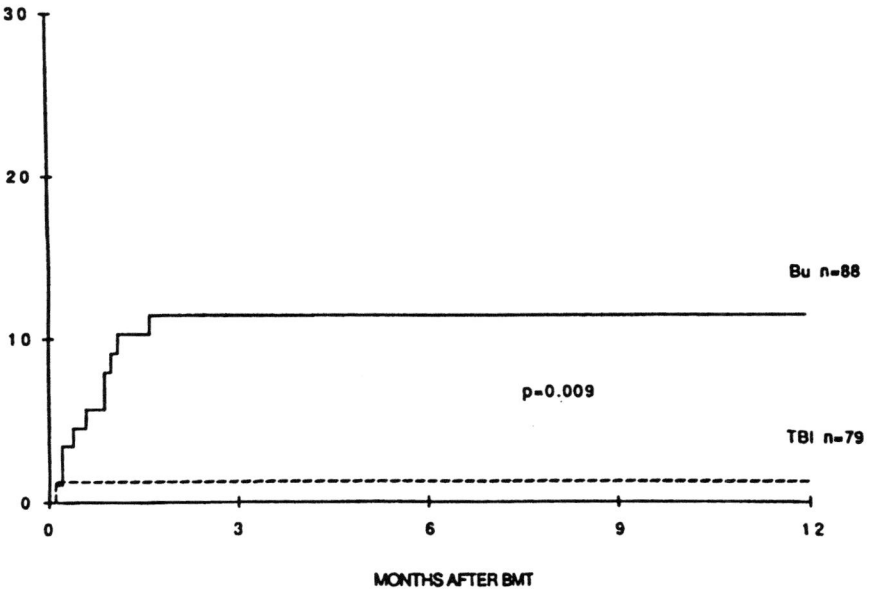

Fig. 77.2. Time to and cumulative incidence of VOD among patients randomized to treatment with busulfan (*n* = 88) or TBI (*n* = 79). The difference was statistically significant (*P* = .009). Reproduced, with permission, from Ringden *et al.* (1994).

Table 77.2. *An approach to the differential diagnosis of hepatic veno-occlusive disease in HSC transplant recipients*

1. Exclude GVHD, but note that
    GVHD can develop early and VOD may occur later than 20 days posttransplant
    GVHD may present with liver enlargement and jaundice
    GVHD may be associated with VOD
2. Rule out other diseases presenting with ascites and/or jaundice and/or sudden weight gain
    Hepatic vein obstruction (for example, due to *Aspergillus*)
    Sepsis (cholangitis lenta)
    Pericardial effusion
    Right heart failure
    Renal failure
    Pancreatic disease

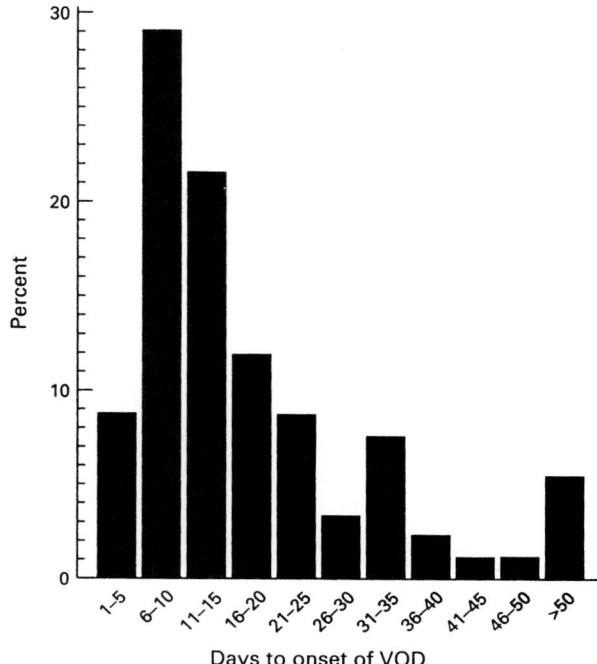

Fig. 77.3. Time to onset of 95 cases of hepatic VOD after HLA-identical sibling transplants for leukemia. Reproduced, with permission, from Rozman *et al.* (1996).

and reversal of portal flow is typically a late feature of VOD. Doppler measurement of hepatic arterial resistance has been studied prospectively in a limited number of patients with VOD as means of providing earlier clues to diagnosis and prognosis (Sonneveld *et al.*, 1998). Magnetic resonance imaging (MRI) has attracted interest but its role remains to be established, other than as a means of excluding other causes of liver dysfunction (van den Bosch & van Hoe, 2000).

Transvenous liver biopsy and hepatic venous pressure measurement remain the gold standards for diagnosis. The high risk of hemorrhage limits the role of percutaneous biopsy in the evaluation of VOD (Carreras *et al.*, 1993). In this setting, the transfemoral or transjugular method is generally preferred. As well as providing tissue, this technique permits measurement of the wedged hepatic venous pressure gradient (WHVPG). A WHVPG of >10 mm of mercury has 91% specificity, 52% sensitivity, and a positive predictive value of 86% (Shulman *et al.*, 1995).

Laboratory parameters are helpful in the diagnosis of VOD. Thrombocytopenia and refractoriness to platelet transfusions

may be an early, albeit nonspecific, sign (Rio *et al.*, 1986). Of interest, it has been shown that plasminogen activator inhibitor-1 (PAI-1), an inhibitor of the fibrinolytic system that is released by sinusoidal endothelial cells and stellate cells, may be an early marker of VOD, being significantly elevated in patients with the syndrome when compared to patients with other liver diseases (Park *et al.*, 1997; Salat *et al.*, 1997). In a prospective study of coagulation/fibrinolysis parameters, the level of N-terminal propeptide for type III procollagen before conditioning and on days 0 and +7, was significantly higher in patients who developed VOD compared to those who did not, as were tissue plasminogen activator (tPA) levels on the day of SCT (Tanikawa *et al.*, 2000). On day 7 post-SCT, levels of protein C were significantly lower in those with VOD compared to those without.

Table 77.3. *Time of onset of VOD and multiorgan failure based on 190 patients with VOD*

Sign or symptom	Mean day of onset
Hepatomegaly or liver tenderness	0.6 ± 7.7
Weight gain >2% of baseline weight	0.7 ± 4.3
Pulmonary infiltrates	5.2 ± 11.3
Serum bilirubin >2 mg/dl	5.9 ± 4.8
Pleural effusion	6.2 ± 9.9
Edema	7.0 ± 7.2
Cardiac failure	7.4 ± 8.3
Oxygen support	7.5 ± 8.3
Bleeding requiring transfusion support	8.2 ± 5.8
Renal insufficiency	10.5 ± 5.0
Ascites	11.5 ± 6.2
Mechanical ventilation	12.0 ± 4.3
Confusion or disorientation	14.0 ± 6.5
Renal failure	14.6 ± 6.1

Reproduced, with permission, from Bearman (1995).

Table 77.4. *Proportion of patients with VOD who develop multiorgan dysfunction*

Variable	No VOD (*n* = 86)	Mild or moderate VOD (*n* = 136)	Severe VOD (*n* = 54)
Renal insufficiency	13%	38%	81%
Renal failure	0%	10%	54%
Cardiac failure	14%	26%	63%
Pulmonary infiltrates	16%	36%	78%
Oxygen support	9%	31%	63%
Mechanical ventilation	1%	4%	43%

Reproduced, with permission, from Bearman (1995).

Whether low protein C and antithrombin 3 (AT III) levels are primary events or secondary events from ongoing vascular injury or leak remains unclear (Faioni *et al.*, 1993; Catani *et al.*, 1996).

As a function of endothelial damage, endothelial stress products including hyaluronic acid, thrombomodulin, transforming growth factor beta (TGF-β), and serum levels of vascular endothelial growth factor (VEGF) have been reported to be elevated in patients with VOD (Anscher *et al.*, 1993; Eltumi *et al.*, 1993; Richardson *et al.*, 1997; Iguchi *et al.*, 2001). While tumor necrosis factor alpha (TNF-α) levels in serum are low in established disease, it has been postulated that high levels of TNF-α and interleukin (IL)-1β may contribute to initial endothelial damage (Scrobohaci *et al.*, 1991; Bianchi & Tracey 1993/1994). Other studies of IL-6, IL-8 as well as TNF-α and IL-1β levels in patients after SCT have suggested a possible relationship between IL-6 and IL-8, but not TNF-α and IL-Iβ, levels with jaundice, renal dysfunction, and pulmonary disease (Ferra *et al.*, 1998). Data showing elevation of plasma levels of C-reactive protein in allo-SCT patients with severe VOD, compared to those without, support a possible role for IL-6 (Schots *et al.*, 1998). It is also of note that preactivated peripheral blood mononuclear cells can induce apoptosis in co-cultured human endothelial cells through a mechanism that is both TNF-α dependent and independent (Lindner *et al.*, 1997). This model and the above data may in part explain why VOD is seen more commonly in recipients of allografts and less frequently in recipients of autografts.

Prognosis

In attempting to develop a model to estimate prognosis, a Cox regression analysis was used to generate risk curves predictive of severe VOD based on a large cohort of patients in whom VOD occurred within the first 16 days post-SCT after preparation with one of three specific regimens: cyclophosphamide and total body irradiation (CyTBI); busulfan and cyclophosphamide (BuCy), or cyclophosphamide, BCNU, and VP-16 (CBV) (Bearman *et al.*, 1993) (Fig. 77.4). Severe VOD was associated with a case fatality rate of 98% by day +100 after SCT. Calculations were based on total serum bilirubin and percentage weight gain at various time points subsequent to SCT, up to day +16. Similar models have yet to be proposed for other temporal or therapeutic settings, and models based on possible surrogates, such as cytokines, endothelial stress products, or markers of fibrosis have also not yet been developed.

In aggregate, however, irrespective of time frame and conditioning regimen, the rates of rise in bilirubin and weight gain are much higher in patients with severe VOD, and the mean maximum bilirubin and percent weight gain are significantly greater in patients with severe VOD compared to those with milder illness (McDonald, 1993) (Table 77.5 and Fig. 77.4). Other clinical features associated with worse outcome include the development of ascites, which occurs in fewer than 20% of patients with mild to moderate VOD, compared to 48% or more in patients with severe disease, and is reflective of increased portal hypertension (McDonald, 1993). WHVPG values in patients

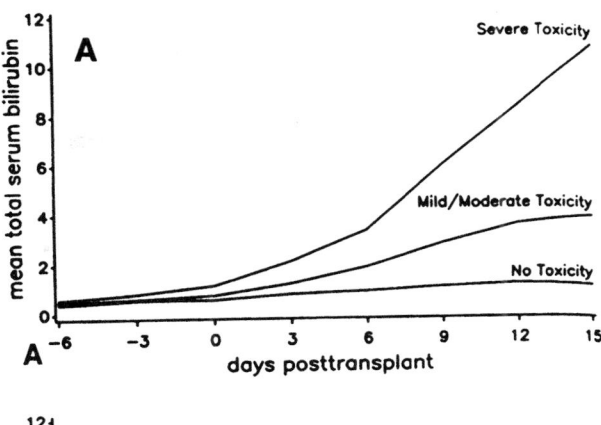

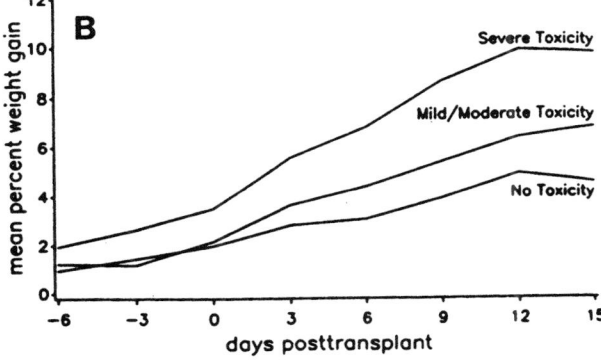

Fig. 77.4. Mean total serum bilirubin (mg/dl) and percent weight gain above baseline in patients who developed mild, moderate, or severe VOD. Reproduced, with permission, from Bearman (1995). Note: In this risk model for VOD, risk is defined by using total serum bilirubin (mg/dl) and percent weight gain above baseline. The model applies between day −1 and day +16 after hematopoietic HSCT for patients who received CY/TBI, CBV, or BU/CY conditioning only.

with VOD beyond 20 mm of mercury are associated with a particularly poor prognosis (Shulman *et al.*, 1995). A cardinal feature predicting high mortality in VOD is the presence of multiorgan failure (MOF) (Tables 77.3 and 77.4). In fact, patients with severe VOD usually die of renal, pulmonary, and/or cardiac failure, rather than from hepatic insufficiency per se.

Preliminary studies of genetic polymorphisms in SCT patients have suggested a possible association between a mutation of glutathione S transferase synthesis and increased VOD risk (Tse *et al.*, 2000; Poonkuzhali *et al.*, 2001). Similarly, in a large, prospective study of allelic variants for TNF-α in SCT patients, a high incidence of MOF was seen in association with a specific allelic variant (TNF d3), which causes increased TNF-α production in response to injury (Haire *et al.*, 2000).

Approaches to therapy

Prevention

Given the lack of effective therapies, the prevention of fatal VOD is an obvious priority. Selection of particular condition-

Table 77.5. *Signs of VOD in patients with moderate, mild, or severe VOD*

Clinical feature	All patients with VOD	Patients with mild VOD	Patients with moderate VOD	Patients with severe VOD
% Weight gain before day 20	10.9 ± 7.1	7.0 ± 3.5	10.1 ± 5.3	15.5 ± 9
Median day on which bilirubin was first >2 mg/dl (range)	6 (2–9)	6.5 (3.5–10)	7 (4–10)	3 (1–6)
Mean maximum total serum bilirubin before day 20	12.3 ± 12.8	4.7 ± 2.9	7.9 ± 6.6	25 ± 15.2
% Patients with edema	63	23	70	85
% Patients with ascites	23	5	16	48

Reproduced, with permission, from Bearman (1995).

ing regimens for patients at high risk is one approach, and this is perhaps best embodied by the emerging field of non-mye-loablative or reduced toxicity conditioning regimens prior to allogeneic transplantation, in which the incidence of VOD is reportedly low. However, depending on the underlying disease, this may or may not be an optimal therapeutic strategy (Barrett & Childs, 2000; Maris *et al.,* 2001). Assessment of risk by virtue of genetic predisposition to VOD, as indicated above, may be possible. The possibility of risk stratification pre-SCT for both the development and the sequelae of VOD exists. Additional, more comprehensive studies to better define such risks are needed. Moreover, the relationship of genetic risk, if able to be defined, to specific regimens and agents will also need to be established.

The most established practice in VOD prevention has been the use of pharmacokinetics to monitor drug levels with the intent of minimizing hepatic injury. This approach is currently best illustrated by the monitoring of busulfan levels. The observed relationship between elevated busulfan levels and VOD may possibly be in part due to busulfan-mediated deple-tion of hepatic glutathione, which in turn predisposes hepato-cytes to additional injury from ensuing cyclophosphamide exposure. This argument is consistent with data suggesting that increased exposure to the toxic metabolites of cyclophos-phamide may contribute to the development of VOD (Slattery *et al.,* 1996). The observation that ursodiol has important antioxidant properties within hepatocytes may explain why ursodiol's protective effect has been most apparent in patients receiving busulfan-based conditioning (Ohashi *et al.,* 2000).

The prophylactic administration of ursodeoxycholic acid, a hydrophilic water-soluble bile acid, has been studied in a num-ber of randomized placebo-controlled prospective trials. Several have shown a statistically significant benefit in patients predicted to be at high risk of VOD (Essell *et al.,* 1998; Ohashi *et al.,* 2000), although a large phase III study by the Nordic Bone Marrow Transplantation group failed to demonstrate sig-nificant benefit (Ruutu *et al.,* 1999).

The supplement of hepatic gluthathione has been tested in experimental models (Teicher *et al.,* 1988; DeLeve, 1998), but this has been difficult to translate into patients due to concerns regarding tumor protection. The feasibility of restoring hepatic glutathione levels to concentrations that are truly effective in humans is also unclear. However, reports of a significant decline in gluthathione and other antioxidants after chemother-apy for SCT, coupled with a report of *N*-acetyl cysteine supple-mentation in the successful treatment of VOD, suggest that fur-ther evaluation of supportive nutrition, including antioxidants, is warranted (Jonas *et al.,* 2000; Ringden *et al.,* 2000). The role of such antioxidants, including vitamin E, remains investiga-tional at this time (Goringe *et al.,* 1998).

Other approaches to VOD prevention, such as the role of cor-ticosteroids, have also attracted interest (Khoury *et al.,* 1998). Given that inflammation does not appear to be a central compo-nent to the pathogenesis of VOD, it is difficult to understand why steroids should be of direct benefit. However, it is possible that they may abrogate other intercurrent or separate forms of liver injury. Modulating inflammation with pentoxifylline and TNF-α neutralization have been unsuccessful to date. Pentoxifylline administration in prospective randomized placebo-controlled trials has been either ineffective or associ-ated with more VOD than placebo (Clift *et al.,* 1993; Ferra *et al.,* 1997).

Treatments targeted at preventing vascular injury have been more extensively examined. Following the initial findings from Besançon, France, in autologous transplantation (Cahn *et al.,* 1985), a small number of randomized trials have studied the effect of low-dose continuous intravenous heparin. Only one ran-domized study has demonstrated a beneficial effect of heparin prophylaxis (Attal *et al.,* 1992). However, this study was con-ducted mainly in low-risk patients and other uncontrolled studies suggested that heparin was ineffective and/or dangerous, because of increased risk of hemorrhage (Bearman *et al.,* 1990; Marsa-Vila *et al.,* 1991; Carreras *et al.,* 1998; Hagglund *et al.,* 1998). The use of ATIII concentrates has been shown to be of no protec-tive value in a prospective study (Budinger *et al.,* 1996). Low-molecular-weight heparins seem to be relatively safe and may have some effect in the prevention of VOD (Lee *et al.,* 1996; Or *et al.,* 1996), but well-designed, randomized studies are needed to confirm these preliminary results.

Prostaglandin E_1 (PGE_1) is a vasodilator with cytoprotective effect on endothelium as well as platelet aggregation inhibitory effect and prothrombolytic activity (Vaughan *et al.,*1989). In one trial, it was given by continuous intravenous infusion from 8 days pretransplant to day 30 posttransplant at a dose of 0.3 µg/kg/hr, and the results in 50 treated patients were compared to 59 historical controls, with both groups receiving low-dose heparin. The incidence of VOD was 12.2% in the PGE$_1$ treated group and 25.5% in the nontreated group, suggesting that prophylactic PGE$_1$ might decrease the incidence and severity of VOD (Gluckman et al., 1990). A randomized trial performed from Buffalo, New York, showed that prophylactic PGE$_1$, heparin, and tPA treatment was associated with an improved survival after day 100 posttransplant, compared to heparin and tPA alone (Schriber et al., 1996). However, a prospective study by the Seattle group using higher doses of PGE$_1$ in a phase I/II study, without concomitant heparin, could not demonstrate any beneficial effect of this drug and was complicated by significant toxicity (Bearman et al., 1993).

Treatment

Based on the histologic observations of microthrombosis, fibrin deposition, and marked factor VIII/vWF staining in patients with VOD, strategies aimed at promoting fibrinolysis with or without concomitant anticoagulant therapy have been developed (Bearman et al., 1992; Leahey & Bunin, 1996). Recombinant human (rh) tPA, in association with low-dose, unfractionated heparin (UFH), was initially reported to be effective in the treatment of VOD by Baglin et al. (1990). Since then, numerous studies and other case reports have been published (Bearman et al., 1993; de Tejada et al., 1994; Simpson et al., 1994; Espigado et al., 1995; Feldman et al., 1995; Goldberg et al., 1996; Leahey & Bunin, 1996; Patton et al., 1996). In the largest study published of patients with established VOD post-SCT, 42 patients received treatment with rh tPA and concomitant UFH for severe disease. Twelve of 42 (29%) patients responded, with response defined as a reduction in pretreatment bilirubin by at least 50%. No patient with renal insufficiency and/or hypoxemia at the time of treatment responded, and 10 (24%) developed severe bleeding secondary to treatment, with a significant number experiencing fatal hemorrhage. The authors concluded that rh tPA/UFH should not be given to patients with MOF and treatment should be given early in the disease course or not at all (Bearman et al., 1997).

The administration of ATIII and activated protein C (APC) has been shown to be ineffective in a number of studies in established VOD (Haire et al., 1996; Strasser & McDonald, 1998), although a trial of ATIII in 10 patients with regimen-related organ dysfunction following SCT suggested some clinical benefit in three patients with VOD (Morris et al., 1997). PGE$_1$ infusions for patients with VOD have been largely unsuccessful (Ibrahim et al., 1991).

Defibrotide (DF), a single-stranded polydeoxyribonucleotide with a molecular weight of 15 to 30 kD (Bianchi et al., 1993), has been identified as an agent that might be able to modulate endothelial cell injury without increasing systemic bleeding, thereby protecting host hepatocytes and sinusoidal endothe-

lium without compromising the antitumor effects of cytotoxic therapy (Richardson et al., 1998). DF has specific aptameric binding sites on vascular endothelium, namely adenosine receptors A1 and A2, which are part of the growing family of nucleotide receptors involved in endothelial cell regulation and response to injury (Bracht & Schror, 1994). Studies have shown that DF increases prostacyclin (PGI-2), prostaglandin E$_2$, and thrombomodulin in vivo. DF also upregulates TFPI and tPA (Berti et al., 1990; Coccheri & Biagi, 1991; Zhou et al., 1994; Fareed, 1997). It decreases thrombin generation and also decreases circulating PAI-1 (Palmer & Goa, 1993). DF inhibits fibrin deposition and may modulate vitronectin and fibronectin release, which as components of extracellular matrix are linked to collagen formation and fibrosis (Coccheri et al., 1988; Ulutin, 1993; Jamieson et al., 1996).

Clinical trials of DF have demonstrated activity in peripheral vascular disease, microvascular thrombotic states, ischemic organ injury, and chemotherapy-related hemolytic-uremic syndrome (HUS) (Bonomini et al., 1984; Coccheri & Biagi, 1991; Ulutin, 1993; Viola et al., 2000). Preclinical studies of human derived, LPS-exposed microvascular and macrovascular endothelium by Falanga et al. (1999, 2000) showed selective and protective effects of DF in LPS-mediated microvascular injury through enhanced fibrinolysis and modulation of sTF and TFPI expression. This differential activity of the drug on microvascular rather than macrovascular endothelium is particularly intriguing in the context of its application to diseases of the microvasculature such as VOD.

A pilot treatment protocol was launched in the United States for patients with severe VOD, defined by a greater than 40% risk according to the Bearman model (Richardson et al., 1998) or by the presence of MOF. DF treatment was given intravenously, typically every 6 hours and infused over 2 hours with a dose range of 10 to 60 mg/kg/day. In the first cohort of 19 evaluable patients, complete responses (defined as a bilirubin less than 2 mg/dl) were seen in 8 of 19 (42%), most of whom had resolution of MOF and survived to day 100 and beyond. Response was typically evident within the first 7 days and the active dose appeared to be approximately 25 mg/kg/day. None of the nonresponders survived beyond day 100, with a median survival of only 36 (range 15–89) days posttransplant (Richardson et al., 1998). Additional trials of DF administration to patients with severe VOD and MOF by other groups have produced similar results (Abecasis et al., 1999; Salat et al., 1999; Zinke et al., 1999; Chopra et al., 2000; Jenner et al.,; 2000). While the natural history of more moderate VOD is certainly less morbid, it is interesting that the complete response rate in the European experience with DF therapy was higher in patients with moderate but significant VOD, suggesting that earlier intervention may be more effective (Chopra et al., 2000).

An analysis of the expanded U.S. experience has confirmed the favorable safety profile of DF when used in a multi-institutional setting following specific treatment guidelines (Richardson et al., 2002). A complete response rate of 36% and an overall survival of 35% was observed in a total of 88 SCT patients with severe VOD and MOF. DF was administered intravenously in doses ranging from 5 to 60 mg/kg/day for a median of 15 days. Predictors of survival included younger age, autologous SCT, and abnormal portal flow, while busulfan-based conditioning and encephalopathy predicted worse outcome. Decreases in mean creatinine and PAI-1 levels during DF therapy also predicted better survival, suggesting that certain features associated with successful outcome could correlate with DF-related treatment effects. Further evaluation of DF therapy for severe VOD may therefore allow better definition of predictors of response or failure (Richardson *et al.*, 2002). Prospective, multi-institutional trials of DF in the treatment of severe VOD are now underway in the United States and Europe (Richardson *et al.*, 2001).

Supportive care

Supportive management of patients with moderate to severe VOD should aim to maintain intravascular volume and renal perfusion without exacerbating extravascular fluid accumulation. Avoiding additional drug toxicity to the liver and the kidney is important. Table 77.6 outlines some recommended measures. As far as additional drug toxicity is concerned, cyclosporine withdrawal is attractive in view of its intrinsic hepatic, renal, and, above all, endothelial toxicity; however, the risk of exacerbating or precipitating graft-versus-host disease (GVHD) makes this difficult. Charcoal hemofiltration, capable of adsorbing bilirubin and other factors from the circulation, has been reported to be useful (Tefferi *et al.*, 2001). Intrahepatic

Table 77.6. *Supportive management of hepatic VOD*

1. Maintain intravascular volume and renal perfusion without increasing extravascular fluid accumulation
   Negative sodium balance
   Vascular filling with hyperoncotic solutions (avoid use of hydroxy-ethyl-starch)
   Very cautious use of diuretics; packed red cells, salt-poor albumin useful
   Paracentesis with fluid replacement (albumin, colloid fluids) if tense ascites problematic
   Dialysis or ultrafiltration if volume overload with hypoxemia
2. Avoid additional drug-induced toxicity
   Methotrexate
   Nephrotoxic drugs (amphotericin B, aminoglycoside, antibiotics, contrast agents, etc.)
   Psychotropic drugs
   Cyclosporine
3. Platelet infusions and coagulation factor replacement as needed
4. Surgical approaches
   Placement of a porta-caval shunt/transjugular intrahepatic portosystemic shunting?[a]
   Liver transplantation?[b]

[a] Fried *et al.*, 1996; Smith *et al.*, 1996; de la Rubia *et al.*, 1996; Levy *et al.*, 1996.
[b] Schlitt *et al.*, 1995; Bunin, *et al.*, 1996; Hagglund *et al.*, 1996.

portosystemic shunting (TIPS) (in which a channel is created between the hepatic vein and the portal vein by a catheter inserted percutaneously and kept patent with a metal stent) can achieve a significant reduction in the hepatic venous pressure gradient and has resulted in improvement in ascites, urinary output, and coagulation parameters in some patients. Most patients died of other complications (de la Rubia *et al.*, 1996; Fried *et al.*, 1996; Smith *et al.*, 1996; Azoulay *et al.*, 2000). As an approach, TIPS should thus probably be reserved for patients with intractable portal hypertension who have large ascites and are unable to mobilize fluid. Liver transplant in those who have been able to undergo the procedure has resulted in clinical improvement in about 30%, as estimated from small cases series, but difficulties with this modality include finding a suitable liver graft, managing the effects of multisystem organ failure, and the prevention of liver graft rejection (Rapoport *et al.*, 1991; Hagglund *et al.*, 1995).

Conclusions

Hepatic VOD is a manifestation of conditioning regimen-related toxicity in SCT patients (with a contribution from previous chemotherapy, including newer agents such as Mylotarg) and is most probably increased by allogeneic effects between donor cells, cytokine release, and recipient tissues. It is currently a limiting factor for improving the efficacy of both auto-SCT and allo-SCT, and better methods of both prophylaxis and treatment are needed. Prevention is clearly a priority, and efforts designed to identify at-risk patients, utilize pharmacokinetics to better individualize chemotherapy administration, and prevent vascular and hepatocyte injury are ongoing. The treatment of severe VOD remains inadequate with a very high fatality rate. Current directions in the investigation of VOD therapy target endothelial injury. The use of rh tPA in conjunction with UFH in low-risk patients has been confounded by the risk of serious toxicity and the likelihood that a significant number of patients would have been expected to improve without therapy. An alternative agent, defibrotide, has shown considerable promise and remarkably little toxicity, although experience remains relatively limited. TIPS, charcoal hemofiltration, and liver transplantation are other approaches currently under investigation in severe disease, but are unlikely to be of benefit to substantial numbers of patients, especially when used alone.

References

Abecasis, M., Ferreira, I. *et al.* (1999). Defibrotide as salvage therapy for hepatic veno-occlusive disease (VOD). *Bone Marrow Transplantation*, **23**, 749 (abstract).

Anscher, M.S., Peters, W.P. *et al.* (1993). Transforming growth factor beta as a predictor of liver and lung fibrosis after autologous bone marrow transplantation for advanced breast cancer. *New England Journal Medicine*, **328**, 1592–8.

Attal, M., Huguet, F. *et al.* (1992). Prevention of hepatic veno-occlusive disease after bone marrow transplantation by continuous infusion of low-dose heparin: a prospective, randomized trial. *Blood*, **79**, 2834–40.

Azoulay, D., Castaing, D. *et al.* (2000). Transjugular intrahepatic portosystemic shunt (TIPS) for severe veno-occlusive disease of the liver following bone marrow transplantation. *Bone Marrow Transplantation*, **25**, 987–92.

Baglin, T.P. (1994). Veno-occlusive disease of the liver complicating bone marrow transplantation. *Bone Marrow Transplantation*, **13**, 1–4.

Barrett, J. & Childs, R. (2000). Non-myeloblative stem cell transplants. *British Journal of Haematology*, **111**, 6–17.

Bearman, S.I. (1995). The syndrome of hepatic veno-occlusive disease after marrow transplantation. *Blood*, **85**, 3005–20.

Bearman, S.I. (2001). Avoiding hepatic veno-occlusive disease: what we know and where are we going? *Bone Marrow Transplantation*, **27**, 1113–20.

Bearman, S.I., Hinds, M.S. *et al.* (1990). A pilot study of continuous infusion heparin for the prevention of hepatic veno-occlusive disease after bone marrow transplantation. *Bone Marrow Transplantation*, **5**, 407–11.

Bearman, S.I., Lee, J.L. *et al.* (1997). Treatment of hepatic venooclusive disease with recombinant human tissue plasminogen activator and heparin in 42 marrow transplant patients. *Blood*, **89**, 1501–6.

Bearman, S.I., Shen, D. *et al.* (1993). A phase 1/2 study of prostaglandin E1 for the prevention of hepatic venocclusive disease after bone marrow transplantation. *British Journal of Haematology*, **84**, 724–30.

Bearman, S.I., Shuhart, M.C. *et al.* (1992). Recombinant human tissue plasminogen activator for the treatment of established severe venocclusive disease of the liver after bone marrow transplantation. *Blood*, **80**, 2458–62.

Berti, F., Rossoni, G. *et al.* (1990). Defibrotide by enhancing prostacyclin generation prevents endothelin-I induced contraction in human saphenous veins. *Prostaglandins*, **40**, 337–50.

Bianchi, G., Barone, D. *et al.* (1993). Defibrotide, a single-stranded polydeoxyribonucleotide acting as an adenosine receptor agonist. *European Journal of Pharmacology*, **238**, 327–34.

Bianchi, M. & Tracey, K.J. (1993/94). The role of TNF in complications of marrow transplantation. *Marrow Transplantation Reviews*, **3**, 57–61.

Bonomini, V., Vangelista, A. *et al.* (1984). A new antithrombotic agent in the treatment of acute renal failure due to hemolytic-uremic syndrome and thrombotic thrombocytopenic purpura. *Nephron*, **37**, 144 (letter).

Bracht, F. & Schror, K. (1994). Isolation and identification of aptamers from defibrotide that act as thrombin antagonists in vitro. *Biochemical and Biophysical Research Communications*, **200**, 933–6.

Brown, B.P., Abu-Yousef, M. *et al.* (1990). Doppler sonography: A noninvasive method for evaluation of hepatic venocclusive disease. *American Journal of Radiology*, **154**, 721–4.

Budinger, M.D., Bouvier, M. *et al.* (1996). Results of a phase 1 trial of anti-thrombin III as prophylaxis in bone marrow transplant patients at risk for venocclusive disease. *Blood*, **88**, 172a (abstract).

Bunin, N., Leahey, A., & Dunn, S. (1996). Related donor liver transplant for veno-occlusive disease following T-depleted unrelated donor bone marrow transplantation. *Transplantation*, **61**, 664–6.

Cahn, J.Y., Flesch, M. *et al.* (1985). Maladie veino-occlusive du foie et autogreffe de moelle osseuse. Role preventif de l'heparine? *Nouvelle Revue d'Hematologie*, **27**, 27–8.

Carreras, E., Bertz, H. *et al.* (1998). Incidence and outcome of hepatic veno-occlusive disease after blood or marrow transplantation: a prospective cohort study of the European Group for Blood and Marrow Transplantation. European Group for Blood and Marrow Transplantation Chronic Leukemia Working Party. *Blood*, **92**, 3599–604.

Carreras, E., Granena, A. *et al.* (1993). Transjugular liver biopsy in BMT. *Bone Marrow Transplantation*, **11**, 21–6.

Catani, L., Gugliotta, L. *et al.* (1996). Endothelium and bone marrow transplantation. *Bone Marrow Transplantation*, **17**, 277–80.

Chopra, R., Eaton, J.D. *et al.* (2000). Defibrotide for the treatment of hepatic veno-occlusive disease: results of the European compassionate-use study. *British Journal of Haematology*, **111**, 1122–9.

Clift, R.A., Bianco, J.A. *et al.* (1993). A randomized controlled trial of pentoxifylline for the prevention of regimen-related toxicities in patients undergoing allogeneic marrow transplantation. *Blood*, **82**, 2025–30.

Coccheri, S. & Biagi, G. (1991). Defibrotide. *Cardiovascular Drug Review*, **9**, 172–96.

Coccheri, S., Biagi, G. *et al.* (1988). Acute effects of defibrotide, an experimental antithrombotic agent, on fibrinolysis and blood prostanoids in man. *European Journal of Clinical Pharmacology*, **35**, 151–6.

Copelan, E.A., Bechtel, T.P. *et al.* (2001). Busulfan levels are influenced by prior treatment and are associated with hepatic veno-occlusive disease and early mortality but not with delayed complications following marrow transplantation. *Bone Marrow Transplantation*, **27**, 1121–4.

de la Rubia, J., Carral, A. *et al.* (1996). Successful treatment of hepatic veno-occlusive disease in a peripheral blood progenitor cell transplant patient with a transjugular intrahepatic portosystemic stent-shunt (TIPS). *Haematologica*, **81**, 536–9.

de Tejada, E., Maldonado, M.S. *et al.* (1994). Fatal hemorrhage after recombinant tissue plasminogen activator therapy for hepatic veno-occlusive disease complicating autologous BMT. *Bone Marrow Transplantation*, **14**, 176–7.

DeLeve, L., Shulman, H.M. *et al.* (2002). Toxic injury to hepatic sinusoids: sinusoidal obstruction syndrome (veno-occlusive disease). *Seminars in Liver Disease*, **22**, 27–42.

DeLeve, L.D. (1996). Cellular target of cyclophosphamide toxicity in the murine liver: role of glutathione and site of metabolic activation. *Hepatology*, **24**, 830–7.

DeLeve, L.D. (1998). Glutathione defense in non-parenchymal cells. *Seminars in Liver Disease*, **18**, 403–13.

Dix, S.P., Wingard, J.R. *et al.* (1996). Association of busulfan area under the curve with veno-occlusive disease following BMT. *Bone Marrow Transplantation*, **17**, 225–30.

Eltumi, M., Trivedi, P. *et al.* (1993). Monitoring of veno-occlusive disease after bone marrow transplantation by serum aminopropeptide of type III procollagen. *Lancet*, **342**, 518–21.

Espigado, H., Rodriguez, J.M. *et al.* (1995). Reversal of severe hepatic veno-occlusive disease by combined plasma exchange and rt-PA treatment. *Bone Marrow Transplantation*, **16**, 313–6.

Essell, J.H., Schroeder, M.T. *et al.* (1998). Ursodiol prophylaxis against hepatic complications of allogeneic bone marrow transplantation. A randomized, double-blind, placebo-controlled trial. *Annals of Internal Medicine*, **128**, 975–81.

Faioni, E.M., Krachmalnicoff, A. *et al.* (1993). Naturally occuring anticoagulants and bone marrow transplantation: Plasma protein C predicts the development of venocclusive disease of the liver. *Blood*, **81**, 3458–62.

Falanga, A., Marchetti, M. *et al.* (1999). Defibrotide (DF) modulates tissue factor expression by microvascular endothelial cells. *Blood*, **94**, 146a.

Falanga, A., Marchetti, M. *et al.* (2000). Impact of defibrotide on the fibrinolytic and procoagulant properties of endothelial cells macro- and mico-vessels. *Blood*, **96**, 53a.

Fareed, J. (1997). Modulation of endothelium by heparin and related polyelectrolytes. In *Advances in Vascular Pathology 1997*, eds. A. Nicolaides & S. Novo. Amsterdam: Elsevier Science B.V.

Feldman, L., Gabai, E. *et al.* (1995). Recombinant tissue plaminogen activator (rTPA) for hepatic veno-occlusive disease after allogeneic BMT in a pediatric patient. *Bone Marrow Transplantation*, **16**, 727–31.

Ferra, C., de Sanjose, S. *et al.* (1998). IL-6 and IL-8 levels in plasma during hematopoietic progenitor transplantation. *Haematologica*, **83**, 1082–7.

Ferra, C., Sanjose, S. *et al.* (1997). Pentoxifylline, ciprofloxacin and prednisone failed to prevent transplant-related toxicities in bone marrow transplant recipients and were associated with an increased incidence of infectious complications. *Bone Marrow Transplantation*, **20**, 1075–80.

Fried, M.W., Connaghan, D.G. *et al.* (1996). Trans jugular intrahepatic protosystemic shunt for the management of severe venocclusive disease following bone marrow transplantation. *Hepatology*, **24**, 588–91.

Gluckman, E., Jolivet, I. *et al.* (1990). Use of prostaglandin E1 for prevention of liver veno-occlusive disease in leukaemic patients treated by allogeneic bone marrow transplantation. *British Journal of Haematology*, **74**, 277–81.

Goldberg, S.L., Shubert, J. *et al.* (1996). Treatment of hepatic veno-occlusive disease with low-dose tissue plasminogen activator: impact on coagulation profile. *Bone Marrow Transplantation*, **18**, 633–6.

Goringe, A.P., Brown, S. *et al.* (1998). Glutamine and vitamin E in the treatment of hepatic veno-occlusive disease following high-dose chemotherapy. *Bone Marrow Transplantation*, **21**, 829–32.

Grochow, L.B., Jones, R.J. *et al.* (1989). Pharmacokinetics of busulfan: correlation with veno-occlusive disease in patients undergoing bone marrow transplantation. *Cancer Chemotherapy Pharmacology*, **25**, 55–61.

Hagglund, H., Remberger, M. *et al.* (1998). Norethisterone treatment, a major risk-factor for veno-occlusive disease in the liver after allogeneic bone marrow transplantation [see comments]. *Blood*, **92**, 4568–72.

Hagglund, H., Ringden, O. *et al.* (1995). No beneficial effects, but severe side effects caused by recombinant human tissue plasminogen activator for treatment of hepatic veno-occlusive disease after allogeneic bone marrow transplantation. *Transplantation*, **27**, 3535.

Hagglund, H., Ringden, O., Ericzon, B.G. *et al.* (1996). Treatment of hepatic veno-occlusive disease with recombinant human tissue plasminogen tissue activator or orthotopic liver transplantation

after allogeneic bone marrow transplantation. *Transplantation*, **62**, 1076–8.

Haire, W.D., Cavet, J. *et al.* (2000). Tumor necrosis factor d3 allele predicts for organ dysfunction after allogeneic blood stem cell transplantation. *Journal of the American Society of Hematology*, (abstract).

Haire, W.D., Stephens, L.C. *et al.* (1996). Antithrombin III (AT3) treatment of organ dysfunction during bone marrow transplantation (BMT)—results of a pilot study. *Blood*, **88**, 458a (abstract).

Holler, E., Kolbe, H.J. *et al.* (1990). Increased serum levels of TNFa precede major complications of bone marrow transplantation. *Blood*, **75**, 1011–6.

Hosoki, T., Kuroda, C. *et al.* (1989). Hepatic venous outflow obstruction: evaluation with pulsed duplex sonography. *Radiology*, **170**, 733–7.

Ibrahim, A., Pico, J.L. *et al.* (1991). Hepatic veno-occlusive disease following bone marrow transplantation treated by prostaglandin E1. *Bone Marrow Transplantation*, **7** (Suppl), 53.

Iguchi, A., Kobayahi, R. *et al.* (2001). Vascular endothelial growth factor (VEGF) is one of the cytokines causative and predictive of hepatic veno-occlusive disease (VOD) in stem cell transplantation. *Bone Marrow Transplantation*, **27**, 1173–80.

Jamieson, A., Alcock, P. *et al.* (1996). The action of polyanionic agents defibrotide and pentosan sulphate on fibrinolytic activity in the laboratory rat. *Fibrinolysis*, **10**, 27–35.

Jenner, M.J., Micallef, I.N. *et al.* (2000). Successful therapy of transplant-associated veno-occlusive disease with a combination of tissue plasminogen activator and defibrotide. *Medical Oncology*, **17**, 333–6.

Jonas, C.R., Puckett, A.B. *et al.* (2000). Plasma antioxidant status after high-dose chemotherapy: a randomized trial of parenteral nutrition in bone marrow transplantation patients. *American Journal of Clinical Nutrition*, **72**, 181–9.

Khoury, H., Adkins, D. *et al.* (1998). Treatment of hepatic veno-occlusive disease with high dose corticosteroids: an update on 28 stem cell transplant recipients. *Blood*, **92**, 1132 (abstract).

Krenger, W., Hill, G.R. *et al.* (1997). Cytokine cascades in acute graft-versus-host disease. *Transplantation*, **64**, 553–8.

Leahey, A.M. & Bunin, N.J. (1996). Recombinant human tissue plasminogen activator for the treatment of severe hepatic veno-occlusive disease in pediatric bone marrow transplant patients. *Bone Marrow Transplantation*, **17**, 1101–4.

Lee, J.H., Lee, K.H. *et al.* (1996). Veno-occlusive disease (VOD) of the liver in Korean patients following allogeneic bone marrow transplantation (BMT): efficacy of recombinant human tissue plasminogen activator (rt-PA) treatment. *Journal of Korean Medical Science*, **11**, 118–26.

Lee, J.L., Gooley, T. *et al.* (1997). Venocclusive disease of the liver after high-dose chemotherapy with alkylating agents: incidence, outcome and risk factors. *Hepatology*, **26**, [pt 2], 149A.

Levy, V., Azoulay, D., Rio, B. *et al.* (1996). Successful treatment of severe hepatic veno-occlusive disease after allogeneic bone marrow transplantation by transjugular intrahepatic portosystemic stent-shunt (TIPS). *Bone Marrow Transplantation*, **18**, 443–5.

Lindner, H., Holler, E. *et al.* (1997). Peripheral blood mononuclear cells induce programmed cell death in human endothelial cells and may prevent repair: role of cytokines. *Blood*, **89**, 1931–8.

Ljungman, P., Hassan, M. et al. (1997). High busulfan concentrations are associated with increased transplant-related mortality in allogeneic bone marrow transplant patients. Bone Marrow Transplantation, 20, 909–13.

Mahmoud, H.K. (1996). Schistosomiasis as a predisposing factor to veno-occlusive disease of the liver following allogeneic bone marrow transplantation. Bone Marrow Transplantation, 17, 401–3.

Maris, M., Sandmaier, B.M. et al. (2001). Non-myeloblative hematopoietic stem cell transplantation. Transfusion Clinique Biologique, 8, 231–4.

Marsa-Vila, L., Gorin, N.C. et al. (1991). Prophylactic heparin does not prevent liver veno-occlusive disease following autologous bone marrow transplantation. European Journal of Haematology, 47, 346–52.

Matute-Bello, G., McDonald, G.D. et al. (1998). Association of pulmonary function testing abnormalities and severe veno-occlusive disease of the liver after marrow transplantation. Bone Marrow Transplantation, 21, 1125–30.

McDonald, G.B. (1993). Venocclusive disease of the liver following marrow transplantation. Marrow Transplantation Reviews, 3, 49–56.

McDonald, G.B. (2002). Management of hepatic sinusoidal obstruction syndrome following treatment with gemtuzumab ozogamicin (mylotarg (r)). Clinical Lymphoma, 2, S35–9.

McDonald, G.B., Hinds, M.S. et al. (1993). Veno-occlusive disease of the liver and multiorgan failure after bone marrow transplantation: a cohort study of 355 patients. Annals of Internal Medicine, 118, 255–67.

Morris, J.D., Harris, R.E. et al. (1997). Antithrombin-III for the treatment of chemotherapy-induced organ dysfunction following bone marrow transplantation. Bone Marrow Transplantation, 20, 871–8.

Moscardo, F., Sanz, G.F. et al. (2001). Marked reduction in the incidence of hepatic veno-occlusive disease after allogeneic hematopoietic stem cell transplantation with CD34+ positive selection. Bone Marrow Transplantation, 27, 983–8.

Nevill, T.J., Barnett, M.J. et al. (1991). Regimen-related toxicity of busulfan-cyclophosphamide conditioning regimen in 70 patients undergoing allogeneic bone marrow transplantation. Journal of Clinical Oncology, 9, 1224–32.

Nicolau, C., Concepcio, B. et al. (1993). Sonographic diagnosis and hemodynamic correlation in veno-occlusive disease of the liver. Journal of Ultrasound in Medicine, 12, 437–40.

Ohashi, K., Tanabe, J. et al. (2000). The Japanese multicenter open randomized trial of ursodeoxycholic acid prophylaxis for hepatic veno-occlusive disease after stem cell transplantation. American Journal of Hematology, 64, 32–8.

Or, R., Nagler, A. et al. (1996). Low molecular weight heparin for the prevention of veno-occlusive disease of the liver in bone marrow transplantation patients. Transplantation, 61, 1067–71.

Palmer, K.J. & Goa, K.L. (1993). Defibrotide: a review of its pharmacodynamic and pharmacokinetic properties, and therapeutic use in vascular disorders. Drugs, 45, 259–94.

Park, J.-D., Yasui, M. et al. (1997). Changes in hemostatic parameters in hepatic veno-occlusive disease following bone marrow transplantation. Bone Marrow Transplantation, 19, 915–20.

Park, J.-D., Yoshioka, A., Kawa, K. et al. (2002). Impaired activity of plasma von Willebrand factor-cleaving protease may predict the occurrence of hepatic veno-occlusive disease after stem cell transplantation. Bone Marrow Transplantation, 29, 789–94.

Patton, D.F., Harper, J.L. et al. (1996). Treatment of veno-occlusive disease of the liver with bolus tissue plasminogen activator and continuous infusion antithrombin III concentrate. Bone Marrow Transplantation, 17, 443–7.

Poonkuzhali, S., Vidya, S. et al. (2001). Glutathione S-transferase gene polymorphism and risk of major complications in patients undergoing allogeneic Bone marrow transplantation. Blood, 98, 852a.

Rapoport, A.P., Doyle, H.R. et al. (1991). Orthotopic liver transplantation for life threatening veno-occlusive disease of the liver after allogeneic bone marrow transplantation. Bone Marrow Transplantation, 8, 421–4.

Richardson, P. & Guinan, E. (2001). Hepatic veno-occlusive disease following hematopoietic stem cell transplantation. Acta Haematologica, 106, 57–68.

Richardson, P., Murakami, C. et al. (2002). Multi-institutional use of defibrotide in 88 patients post stem cell transplant with severe veno-occlusive disease and multi-system organ failure; response without significant toxicity in a high risk population and factors predictive of outcome. Blood, 100, 4337–43.

Richardson, P., Warren, D. et al. (2001). Multi-institutional phase II randomized dose finding study of defibrotide (DF) in patients (pts) with severe veno-occlusive disease (VOD) and multi-system organ failure (MOF) post stem cell transplantation (SCT): promising response rate without significant toxicity in a high risk population. Blood, 98, 853a.

Richardson, P.G., Elias, A.D. et al. (1997). Treatment of severe veno-occlusive disease (VOD) with defibrotide (DF): compassionate use results in efficacy without significant toxicity in a high risk population. Blood, 90, 252a.

Richardson, P.G., Elias, A.D. et al. (1998). Treatment of severe veno-occlusive disease with defibrotide: compassionate use results in response without significant toxicity in a high-risk population. Blood, 92, 737–44.

Richardson, P.G. & Guinan, E.C. (1999). The pathology, diagnosis and treatment of hepatic veno-occlusive disease: current status and novel approaches. British Journal of Haematology, 107, 485–693.

Ringden, O., Remberger, M. et al. (2000). N-acetylcysteine for hepatic veno-occlusive disease after allogeneic stem cell transplantation. Bone Marrow Transplantation, 25, 993–6.

Ringden, O., Ruutu, T. et al. (1994). A randomized trial comparing busulfan with total body irradiation as conditioning in allogeneic marrow transplant recipients with leukemia: a report from the Nordic Bone Marrow Transplantation Group. Blood, 83, 2723–30.

Rio, B., Andreu, G. et al. (1986). Thrombocytopenia in venocclusive disease after bone marrow transplantation or chemotherapy. Blood, 67, 1773–6.

Rozman, C., Carreras, E. et al. (1996). Risk factors for hepatic veno-occlusive disease following HLA-identical sibling bone marrow transplants for leukemia. Bone Marrow Transplantation, 17, 75–80.

Ruutu, T., Eriksson, B. et al. (1999). Ursodiol prevention of hepatic complications in allogeneic stem cell transplantation: results of a prospective, randomized, placebo-controlled trial. Bone Marrow Transplantation, 23, 756 (abstract).

Salat, C., Holler, E. et al. (1997). Plasminogen activator inhibitor-1 confirms the diagnosis of hepatic veno-occlusive disease in patients with hyperbilirubinemia after bone marrow transplant. *Blood*, **89**, 2184–8.

Salat, C., Pihusch, R. *et al.* (1999). Successful treatment of veno-occlusive disease with defibrotide—a report of two cases. *Bone Marrow Transplantation, 23*, 757 (abstract).

Schlitt, H.J., Tischler, H.J., Ringe, B. *et al.* (1995). Allogeneic liver transplantation for hepatic veno-occlusive disease after bone marrow transplantation—clinical and immunological considerations. *Bone Marrow Transplantation, 16*, 473–8.

Schots, R., Kaufman, L. *et al.* (1998). Monitoring of C-reactive protein after allogeneic bone marrow transplantation identifies patients at risk of severe transplant-related complications and mortality. *Bone Marrow Transplantation, 22*, 79–85.

Schriber, J.R., Milk, B.J. *et al.* (1996). A randomized phase II trial comparing heparin (Hep) +/– prostaglandin E1 (PG) to prevent hepatotoxicity (HT) following bone marrow transplantation (BMT): preliminary results. *Blood, 88*, 1642.

Scrobohaci, M.L., Drouet, L. *et al.* (1991). Liver veno-occlusive disease after bone marrow transplantation changes in coagulation parameters and endothelial markers. *Thrombosis Research, 63*, 509–19.

Shulman, H.M., Fisher, L.B. *et al.* (1994). Venoocclusive disease of the liver after marrow transplantation: Histological correlates of clinical signs and symptoms. *Hepatology, 19*, 1171–80.

Shulman, H.M., Gooley, T. *et al.* (1995). Utility of transvenous liver biopsies and wedged hepatic venous pressure measurements in sixty marrow transplant recipients. *Transplantation, 59*, 1015–22.

Shulman, H.M., Gown, A.M. *et al.* (1987). Hepatic veno-occlusive disease after bone marrow transplantation. Immunohistochemical identification of the material within occluded central venules. *American Journal of Pathology, 127*, 549–58.

Shulman, H.M. & McDonald, G.B. (1984). Liver disease after marrow transplantation. In *The Pathology of Bone Marrow Transplantation,* ed. G.E. Sale & H.M. Shulman, pp. 104–35. New York: Masson.

Shulman, H.M., McDonald, G.B. *et al.* (1980). An analysis of hepatic venocclusive disease and centrilobular hepatic degeneration following bone marrow transplantation. *Gastroenterology, 79.*

Simpson, D.R., Browett, P.J. *et al.* (1994). Successful treatment of veno-occlusive disease with recombinant tissue plasminogen activator in a patient requiring peritoneal dialysis. *Bone Marrow Transplantation, 14*, 635–6.

Slattery, J.T., Kalhorn, T.F. *et al.* (1996). Conditioning regimen-dependent disposition of cyclophosphamide and hydroxycyclophosphamide in human marrow transplantation patients. *Journal of Clinical Oncology, 14*, 1484–94.

Slattery, J.T., Sanders, J.E. *et al.* (1995). Graft-rejection and toxicity following bone marrow transplantation in relation to busulfan pharmacokinetics. *Bone Marrow Transplantation, 16*, 31–42.

Smith, F.O., Johnson, M.S. *et al.* (1996). Transjugular intrahepatic portosystemic shunting (TIPS) for the treatment of severe hepatic veno-occlusive disease. *Bone Marrow Transplantation, 18*, 643–6.

Soiffer, R., Dear, K. *et al.* (1991). Hepatic dysfunction follwoing T-cell-depleted allogeneic bone marrow transplantation. *Transplantation, 52*, 1014–9.

Sonneveld, P., Lameris, J.S. *et al.* (1998). Color-flow imaging sonography of portal and hepatic vein flow to monitor fibrinolytic therapy with r-TPA for veno-occlusive disease following myeloablative treatment. *Bone Marrow Transplantation, 21*, 731–4.

Strasser, S.I. & McDonald, G.B. (1998). Gastrointestinal and hepatic complications. In *Hematopoietic Cell Transplantation* (2nd ed.), ed. S.J. Forman, K.G. Blume, & E.D. Thomas. Blackwell Scientific Publications.

Styler, M.J., Crilley, P. *et al.* (1996). Hepatic dysfunction following busulfan and cyclophosphamide myeloblation: a retrospective, multicenter analysis. *Bone Marrow Transplantation, 18*, 171–6.

Tack, D.K., Letendre, L. *et al.* (2001). Development of hepatic veno-occlusive disease after Mylotarg infusion for relapsed acute myeloid leukemia. *Bone Marrow Transplantation, 28*, 895–7.

Tanikawa, S., Mori, S. *et al.* (2000). Predictive markers for hepatic veno-occlusive disease after hematopoietic stem cell transplantation in adults: a prospective single center study. *Bone Marrow Transplantation, 26*, 881–6.

Tefferi, A., Kumar, S. *et al.* (2001). Charcoal hemofiltration for hepatic veno-occlusive disease after hematopoietic stem cell transplantation. *Bone Marrow Transplantation, 28*, 997–9.

Teicher, B.A., Crawford, J.M. *et al.* (1988). Glutathione monoethyl ester can selectively protect liver from high dose BCNU or cyclophosphamide. *Cancer, 62*, 1275–81.

Toh, H.C., McAfee, S.L. *et al.* (1999). Late onset veno-occlusive disease following high-dose chemotherapy and stem cell transplantation. *Bone Marrow Transplantation, 24*, 891–5.

Tse, W.T., Beyer, W. *et al.* (2000). Genetic polymorphisms in glutathione s-transferase and plasminogen activator inhibitor and risk of veno-occlusive disease (VOD). *Journal of the American Society of Hematology.*

Ulutin, O.N. (1993). Antithrombotic effect and clinical potential of defibrotide. *Seminars in Thrombosis and Hemostasis, 19*, 186–91.

van den Bosch, M.A. & van Hoe, L. (2000). MR imaging findings in two patients with hepatic veno-occlusive disease following bone marrow transplantation. *European Radiology, 10*, 1290–3.

Vassal, G., Koscielny, S. *et al.* (1996). Busulfan disposition and hepatic veno-occlusive disease in children undergoing bone marrow transplantation. *Cancer, Chemotherapy and Pharmacology, 37*, 247–53.

Vaughan, D.E., Plavin, S.R. *et al.* (1989). PGE1 accelerates thrombolysis by tissue plasminogen activator. *Blood, 73*, 1213–7.

Viola, F., Marubini, S. *et al.* (2000). Improvement of walking distance by defibrotide in patients with intermittent claudication: results of a randomized, placebo-controlled study (the DICLIS study). *Thrombosis and Haemostasis, 83*, 672–7.

Watanabe, K., Iwaki, H. *et al.* (1996). Veno-occlusive disease of the liver following bone marrow transplantation: a clinical-pathological study of autopsy cases. *Artificial Organs, 20*, 1145–50.

Zhou, Q., Chu, X. *et al.* (1994). Defibrotide stimulates expression of thrombomodulin in human endothelial cells. *Thrombosis and Hemostasis, 71*, 507–10.

Zinke, W., Neumeister, P. *et al.* (1999). Defibrotide—an approach in the treatment of severe veno-occlusive disease? *Bone Marrow Transplantation, 23*, 760 (abstract).

78 Interstitial pneumonitis

CATHERINE CORDONNIER

Henri Mondor Hospital, Creteil, France

Introduction

Interstitial pneumonitis (IP) has long been a major cause of mortality and morbidity after bone marrow transplantation (BMT). Indeed cytomegalovirus (CMV) pneumonitis had been the single most common cause of infectious death after allogeneic transplantation with a case-fatality rate of up to 85%. With the advent of the use of prophylactic or "early intervention" ganciclovir, however, this now appears to be changing.

IP after marrow transplantation is a clinical, radiologic, and histopathologic syndrome with characteristic features and can be due to a number of different etiologies (Table 78.1), including CMV, *Pneumocystis carinii*, fungal infection, and a form of the syndrome in which no infectious etiology can be identified—so-called idiopathic interstitial pneumonitis, or "idiopathic pneumonia syndrome" (Clark *et al.*, 1993). This is most likely due in most cases to the pretransplant chemotherapy or chemoradiation regimen causing pulmonary damage. CMV used to be the most common cause of IP but this is changing, and in most units in which prophylactic or preemptive ganciclovir is routinely utilized to minimize the incidence of CMV disease, idiopathic IP is now the most common form of IP, at least after HLA-identical family member transplantation (Atkinson *et al.*, 1998) (Fig. 78.1 and Table 78.2). Rarer causes include infection with fungi, toxoplasma, and other viruses including herpes simplex, varicella zoster, respiratory viruses, adenovirus, and BK papovavirus (Sandler *et al.*, 1997). IP is much more common in recipients of allogeneic transplants than in those receiving autologous transplants (Wingard *et al.*, 1988b; Reusser *et al.*, 1990). The syndrome is more common in allogeneic transplant recipients receiving total body irradiation (TBI) as part of the conditioning regimen, and it may be more common in recipients of HLA-identical unrelated donor transplants compared to recipients of HLA-identical sibling transplants. IP occurs most commonly in the first 12 weeks posttransplant with a median time of occurrence at 8 weeks posttransplant. IP can also occur late posttransplant, most often in those with chronic GVHD, in which case the etiology is more heterogeneous than in early IP (Table 78.3).

Pathogenesis

IP due to infectious agents

Infective IP results from the severe combined humoral and cellular immune deficiency consistently seen after marrow transplantation (Noel *et al.*, 1978; Brown, Weissman, & Shizuru, 2001). This immune deficiency is due firstly to the fact that the regenerating immune system simply takes time to develop competence and, secondly, to the use of immune suppressive therapy for the prevention or treatment of GVHD. Thirdly, GVHD is of itself immune suppressive,

Table 78.1. *Causes of interstitial pneumonitis early after marrow transplantation*

1. Cytomegalovirus
2. *Pneumocystis carinii*
3. Idiopathic: Most commonly due to pretransplant chemotherapy or chemoradiotherapy. Occasionally possibly due to acute GVHD.
4. Rare miscellaneous causes:
   Fungal infections *(Candida, Aspergillus)*
   Chlamydia trachomatis[a]
   Herpes virus type 6[b]
   Adenovirus[c]
   Legionella
   Mycoplasma
   Respiratory syncytial virus[d]
   Influenza virus
   Parainfluenza virus[e]
Exclude a) Increased pressure pulmonary edema
        b) Increased permeability pulmonary edema (adult respiratory distress syndrome)
        c) Pulmonary hemorrhage

Abbreviation: GVHD, graft-versus-host disease.
[a] Meyers *et al.* (1983).
[b] Carrigan *et al.* (1991).
[c] Shields *et al.* (1985).
[d] Hertz *et al.* (1989).
[e] Wendt *et al.* (1992).

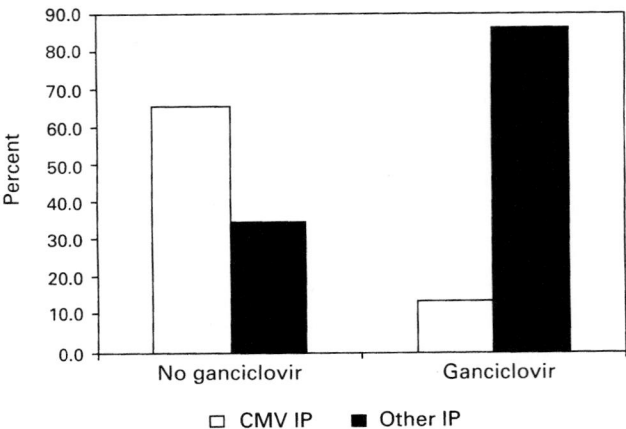

Fig. 78.1. Change in the pattern of interstitial pneumonitis etiology with introduction of propylactic ganciclovir. (Reproduced, with permission, from Atkinson *et al.*, 1998.)

since the lymphoid system is a target organ for this disease. In addition to the systemic immune deficiency, local pulmonary immune deficiency also plays a role. For example, in 25 bone marrow transplant recipients broncho-alveolar lavage fluid differed from that from normal volunteers by the presence of IgG_2 and IgG_3 and the absence of IgG_4 (Milburne, Prentice, & Grundy, 1993). In IP due to CMV infection, both specific T-cell and nonspecific cytotoxic cell responses appear to be important in determining recovery (Quinnan *et al.*,1981). Studies in rat recipients of allogeneic bone marrow transplants showed that CMV induced microvascular damage and congestion of alveolar septa, resulting in interstitial lung disease, independent of concomitant GVHD (Stals *et al.*, 1996).

Idiopathic IP

The pathogenesis of idiopathic IP, also called "idiopathic pneumonia syndrome," is likely to be multifactorial. In the absence of infectious agents, and, until recently, of a demonstrated relationship between IP and GVHD, and consistent with what is known from the lung toxicity of chemotherapy or radiation, idiopathic IP has long been thought to result primarily from the pretransplant high-dose chemotherapy or chemoradiation conditioning regimen. IP after hematopoietic stem cell (HSC) transplantation has been shown to be associ-

Table 78.2. *Cause of interstitial pneumonitis in patients receiving or not receiving prophylactic ganciclovir*

Cause	No ganciclovir (%)	Ganciclovir (%)
Cytomegalovirus	65.5	13.6
Idiopathic	15.4	50.0
Pneumocystis carinii	14.5	4.5
Other	3.6	31.8

Table 78.3. *Causes of interstitial pneumonitis late after marrow transplantation* (n = 31)

1. Idiopathic	7	
2. Cytomegalovirus	6	
3. *Pneumocystis carinii*	6	
4. Miscellaneous	5	
Lymphocytic bronchitis (2)		
Respiratory syncytial virus		
Measles		
Legionella		
5. Varicella zoster	3	
6. Unknown	4	

Reproduced, with permission, from Sullivan *et al.* (1986).

ated with non-specific inflammatory processes, for example increased alveolar expression of cytokines, such as interleukin (IL)-1, IL-2, IL-6, and tumor necrosis factor (TNF)-α (Clark *et al.*, 1999). Similarly, increased alveolar levels of lipopolysaccharide (LPS)-binding protein and of soluble CD14 were found in the alveolar compartment, suggesting that such patients might be at increased risk for LPS-mediated injury through the LBP amplification pathway, even in the absence of GVHD (Clark *et al.*, 1999). Induction in the lung of chemokines that attract both monocytes and T cells has been described (Panoskaltsis-Mortari *et al.*, 2000). [Chemokines are small (8 to 14 kD) proteins that regulate leukocyte function and migration in inflammation They are categorized by the presence and position of conserved cysteine residues. Most chemokines belong either to the CXC (alpha), CC (beta), or C (gamma) family. Members of the alpha family are chemotactic for neutrophils, eosinophils, and basophils; members of the beta family are chemotactic for monocytes and lymphocytes, while members of the gamma family are chemotactic for lymphocytes.] Following tissue injury, upregulation of adhesion molecules on endothelial surfaces causes tethering and rolling of circulating leukocytes. These cells are then activated by chemokines on the luminal surface of endothelium, resulting in diapedesis and entry into the lung. In the study by Panoskaltsis-Mortari, messenger RNA and protein levels of both CC and CXC were elevated in the lung. Most of these findings are consistent with nonspecific injuries and may be independent of GVHD, since they have been documented in both the autologous and allogeneic transplant settings. Damaged or dying cells can also leak cytoplasmic actin, which may be directly toxic to pulmonary endothelium. Actin-scavenging proteins, such as gelsolin, appear to counteract the pathophysiological consequences of extracellular actin. Plasma gelsolin levels were significantly lower in patients with idiopathic IP who subsequently died of the condition compared to patients without serious pulmonary complications (DiNubile *et al.*, 2002).

However, more recently, there has been increasing evidence, both experimental and clinical, that GVHD plays a role in the pathogenesis of idiopathic IP. In a murine allogeneic BMT system, noninfectious pneumonitis and mononuclear cell infiltration around vessels and bronchioles were observed only in mice receiving allogeneic BMT, in which minor histocompatibility antigenic differences existed between donor and recipient (Cooke *et al.,* 1996). This injury was associated with aggravated broncho-alveolar lavage (BAL) fluid levels of endotoxin, neutrophils, and tumor necrosis factor-α. Injection of endotoxin (lipopolysaccharide) 6 weeks posttransplant caused profound lung injury only in mice with moderate GVHD. Using the same model, Cooke *et al.* showed that the occurrence of idiopathic IP was associated with an expansion of host-reactive donor T cells in the BAL fluid. These cells were also present, although reduced in number, in the lung after T-cell depletion of the marrow inoculum, but were not found in the spleen (Cooke *et al.,* 1998). Other studies in mice have shown that IP can occur in mice infected with *Pneumocystis carinii* and conditioned with TBI and given either allogeneic or syngeneic marrow grafts, but was exacerbated by GVHD. The pneumonitis was worse in the allogeneic recipients and was associated with an infiltration of CD4+ T cells (Garvy & Harmsen, 1996). Histologically, IP has been described as part of the spectrum of pulmonary GVHD (Yousem, 1995). Clinically, interstitial pneumonitis has been associated with both acute (Atkinson *et al.,* 1991b) and chronic (Atkinson *et al.,* 1989; Gondo *et al.,* 1993; Leblond *et al.,* 1994) GVHD.

Clinical presentation

Symptoms include shortness of breath, both at rest and on exertion, and sometimes a dry cough. Sputum production is not a feature. Clinical signs on examination of the chest may be minimal or absent. In other cases, rales may be heard. Symptoms and signs reflect the fact that the disease involves the interstitial tissue of the lung (alveolar walls and pulmonary vascular endothelium) rather than alveolar air spaces. Thus air space consolidation is not a feature of the syndrome, at least in its early stages. The chest X-ray typically shows an area or areas of diffuse opacification, often in micronodular form and traversing pulmonary anatomic boundaries. Often both lung fields are involved, although occasionally the appearance may be predominantly unilateral, at least initially, and occasionally the disease can present as a single pulmonary nodule. Blood gases demonstrate hypoxemia with hypocapnea. Pulmonary function tests predominantly show a restrictive defect.

The etiology of the IP cannot be determined from the clinical presentation.

Histologic appearance includes a mononuclear infiltrate of the interstitial tissue with relative sparing of alveolae (fully described in Chapter 104). Occasionally, however, alveolar involvement can occur and polymorphonuclear leukocyte infiltration can be present (Fig. 78.2). The of distinguishing clinical features between an interstitial pneumonitis and a pneumonia characterized by air space consolidation (lobar or otherwise) are detailed in Table 78.4.

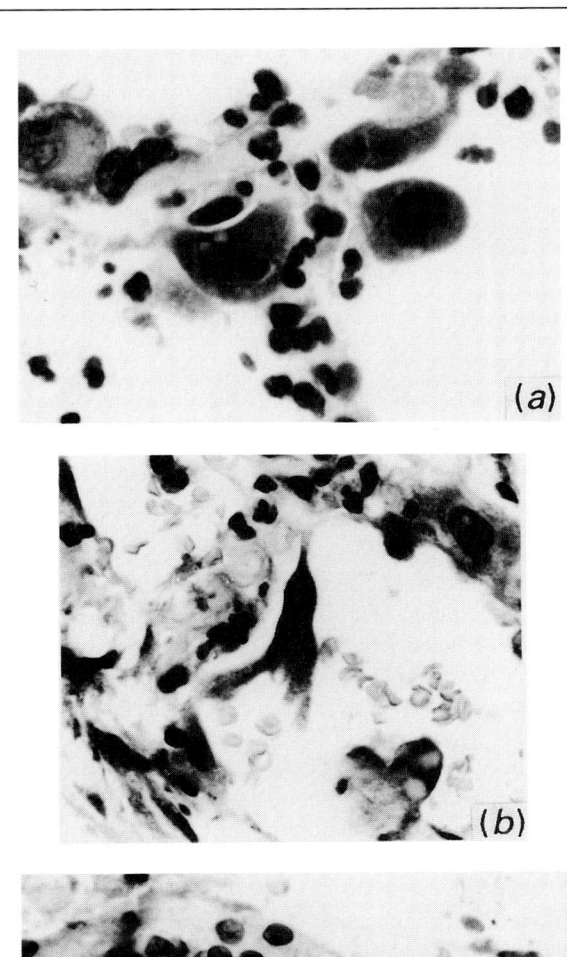

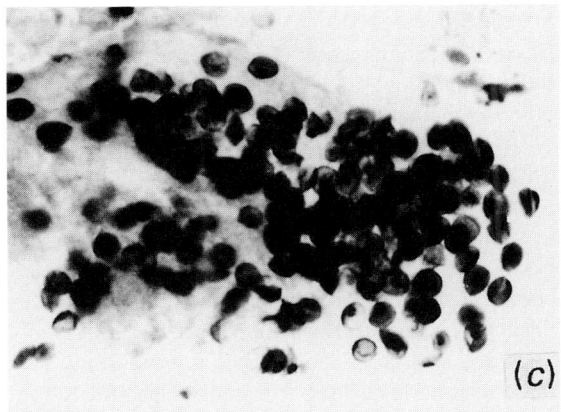

Fig. 78.2. Histologic features of interstitial pneumonitis due to different causes. (**A**) Infected pneumocytes with characteristic nuclear inclusions, diagnostic of CMV disease. (Hematoxylin & eosin ×600.) (**B**) Atypical stellate pneumocyte characteristic of chemotherapy or chemoradiotherapy pulmonary toxicity. (Hematoxylin & eosin ×400.) (**C**) *Pneumocystis carinii* cysts. (Methenamine silver ×600.)

CMV pneumonitis (and see Chapter 74)

Since reactivation and transmission of the virus through the graft are the two mechanisms of acquisition of CMV infection in hematopoietic stem cell transplant recipients, CMV pneumonitis is only observed in CMV seropositive recipients of autologous or allogeneic transplants, or in seronegative recipi-

Table 78.4. *Differences between interstitial pneumonitis (any cause) and bronchopneumonia/lobar pneumonia*

Feature	Interstitial pneumonitis	Broncho/lobar pneumonia
Fever	++	++
Dyspnea/tachypnea	++	+
Cough	+	++
Sputum production	+	++
Rales	+	+
Rhonchi	−	+
Chest X-ray	Diffuse "ground glass" appearance: not restricted to anatomic borders	Air space consolidation restricted to anatomic borders (lobar). Bilateral basal patches (broncho)
Ear lobe blood pO$_2$	Decreased	Decreased
Pulmonary function tests	Restricted	Normal (lobar) Obstructive (broncho)
Optimal diagnostic intervention	Open lung biopsy to obtain tissue	Sputum examination and culture
Histopathology	Abnormal interstitium	Alveolar consolidation/bronchial inflammation

ents transplanted from a seropositive donor. CMV pneumonitis as the manifestation of a primary infection in a seronegative patient transplanted from a seronegative donor is extremely unlikely, and would raise the question of accidental transfusion of CMV-seropositive blood products posttransplant.

Because asymptomatic CMV reactivation may occur in the lung as in other tissues, especially during the first 3 months following transplant, it is important to use accepted definitions for CMV pneumonitis. A definition of CMV pneumonitis was proposed during the first International CMV Worshop in 1993 and recently updated (Ruutu & Volin, 1990; Ljungman & Griffiths, 1993; Ljungman *et al.*, 2002). CMV pneumonitis is defined, in this proposal, as the combination of signs and/or symptoms of pulmonary disease combined with the detection of CMV in BAL fluid or from lung tissue samples. CMV can be detected by virus isolation, histopathology, immunohisto-chemistry, or in situ hybridization. Due to the high sensitivity of the technique and its frequent positivity in asymptomatic, seropositive transplant patients, it is recommended that the detection of CMV by polymerase chain reaction (PCR) alone be considered insufficient evidence for the diagnosis of CMV pneumonia.

CMV pneumonitis is least frequently seen after autologous transplantation and most frequently after unrelated or hap-loidentical family member transplantation. It is generally thought to be an infrequent problem after autologous trans-plantation with the incidence in several reports being between 3% and 5%. In a survey of 2,252 cases of autolo-gous BMT, the incidence was 0.8%, but this varied from 0% to 8.6% between different centers (Ljungman *et al.*, 1994). Survival beyond 30 days from the diagnosis of pneumonitis was 43%, but three patients suffered recurrences that were fatal, giving an overall survival of 28%. Thus, although infre-quent, CMV pneumonitis is a serious complication of autolo-gous BMT.

Until pre-emptive or prophylactic CMV strategies were implemented in routine practice for allogeneic stem cell transplant recipients, CMV pneumonitis was a frequent com-plication, and the cause of death in 10% to 15% of patients. CMV pneumonitis typically occurred around day 60 after transplant, mostly associated with fever, mononucleosis, and acute GVHD. In the absence of effective treatment, CMV pneumonitis had a fatality rate of 80% (Wingard *et al.*, 1988a). CMV was often associated with other infectious causes of pneumonia (i.e., aspergillus or pseudomonas) con-fusing the clinical diagnosis. The routine use of prophylactic or pre-emptive strategies for CMV infection in at-risk allo-geneic recipients has considerably decreased the incidence of the disease—now less than 2% in the overall allogeneic stem cell transplant population in recent studies (Cordonnier *et al.*, 2001; Reusser *et al.*, 2002). In patients given T-cell-depleted bone marrow and blood stem cell haploidentical allogeneic transplants, CMV pneumonitis remains more common and fatal, most likely due to the severe CD4+ cytopenia seen after these transplants (Aversa *et al.*, 1994; Bacigulupo *et al.*, 1997). Of concern is the fact that these patients received CMV prophylactic therapy.

Although less CMV pneumonitis is now observed during the first 3 months following transplant, the use of prophylactic strategies has become associated with late onset CMV pneu-monitis, occurring after day 100, and sometimes more than 1 year after transplant (Li *et al.*, 1994; Nguyen *et al.*, 1999). This development has been attributed to delayed or impaired CMV-specific T-cell lymphocyte response (Li *et al.*, 1994). In the M.D. Anderson experience, the incidence of late CMV pneu-monitis was 6.3%, with a comparable fatality rate in early and late cases (74%) (Nguyen *et al.*, 1999).

Other viral pneumonitis

Herpes simplex virus infection may be associated with lung involvement. However, this is of rare occurrence due to the wide use of prophylactic acyclovir during the early posttrans-plant period. Varicella-zoster virus may also cause interstitial pneumonia and the absence of cutaneous symptoms may make the diagnosis difficult.

High levels of HHV6-DNA have frequently been found in lung tissue of patients with idiopathic or CMV interstitial pneumonitis when compared to controls (Cone *et al.*, 1993), but the role of the virus in the causation of the lung symptoms remains controversial.

Due to the decreased incidence of CMV pneumonitis, community respiratory viral infections are increasingly recognized as an important cause of pneumonitis in stem cell transplant patients, occurring up to four times more frequently than CMV pneumonitis (Whimbey *et al.*, 1997). Many factors may explain differences in incidence between centers, including age, transplant population, study period, prevalence of the infection in the normal population, and diagnostic laboratory methods. In two large prospective series, the incidence of upper and lower respiratory infections together was 3.5% in allogeneic recipients in European centers (Ljungman *et al.*, 2001) and 4% at the Fred Hutchinson Cancer Research Center (Bowden, 1997). Respiratory syncytial (RSV) virus infection is the most frequent, and often occurs during community outbreaks. Pneumonitis is usually preceded by upper respiratory tract infection, manifesting as rhinorrhea, sinus congestion, or sore throat. Once pneumonitis is present, the fatality rate is high, around 80%, regardless of the time posttransplant. Lymphocytopenia was found to significantly increase the risk of pneumonia in infected patients in the European experience (Ljungman *et al.*, 2001). Influenza A and B virus and parainfluenza virus also cause pneumonitis, and have been reported to occur in stem cell transplant units during community outbreaks. Although the mortality rate seems lower than that of RSV, it remains a significant cause of death (Bowden, 1997; Ljungman *et al.*, 2001; Nichols *et al.*, 2001b). Adenovirus infection is now well documented in some HSC transplant populations, especially in children transplanted with haplo-mismatched or unrelated donors, and especially during the first 3 months after transplant. Interstitial pneumonia may be part of a systemic infection, which occurs in about 20% of infected patients (Flomemberg *et al.*, 1994; La Rosa *et al.*, 2001).

Pneumocystis carinii pneumonitis (and see Chapter 76)

Because of the widespread use of prophylactic cotrimoxazole or pentamidine, *Pneumocystis carinii* pneumonitis (PCP) is now a relatively uncommon cause of IP posttransplant. It usually occurs after the first month and within the first 5 months posttransplant. Occasional cases have been reported within 1 month of transplant (Mahon *et al.*, 1991; Tuan, Dennison, & Weisdorf, 1992). Without specific prophylaxis, between 5% and 15% of patients develop PCP and approximately 1% to 2% still experience this complication even when prophylaxis is utilized posttransplant (Tuan, Dennison, & Weisdorf, 1992).

PCP can also occur late posttransplant, after the commonly used 6-month posttransplant prophylaxis period has passed. In a review of late-onset PCP in 110 BMT patients, 16 episodes were documented and only one patient had been receiving PCP prophylaxis at the onset of the pneumonitis (Lyytikäinen *et al.*, 1996). Fourteen of the 16 episodes occurred more than 6 months posttransplant (median 10.5, range 4–42 months). Three occurred beyond 1 year posttransplant. All three had extensive chronic GVHD. Of the 11 patients with an onset between 7 and 12 months posttransplant, all except one were on methylprednisolone as treatment for chronic GVHD (*n* = 7) or cytopenia (*n* = 2), and 5 had relapse of their hematologic malignancy. The risk of developing PCP between 7 and 12 months posttransplant was calculated at 13.4%. It was suggested that PCP prophylaxis be continued until 1 year posttransplant in those receiving corticosteroid treatment as well as for those with hematologic relapse and beyond 1 year in those with extensive chronic GVHD. Mortality rates as high as 40% have been reported for late-onset PCP in marrow transplant recipients.

Since PCP is known to reactivate with further immune suppression, it was encouraging that a report of two cases in which PCP occurred pretransplant showed no recurrence posttransplant. Posttransplant prophylaxis in each case was given with aerosolized pentamidine (Martino *et al.*, 1995).

A case of PCP occurring after autologous transplant was reported in a child with peripheral neuroectodermal tumor and pulmonary metastases who received pulmonary radiation therapy at 60 days posttransplant and who presented with PCP at 90 days posttransplant when her CD4+ T-cell count was 5/microliter (Castagnola *et al.*, 1995). However, despite other anecdotal reports, the relationship between PCP risk and CD4+ T-cell count is not as well established after HSC transplantation as it is in the AIDS population. Other risk factors are likely important, especially corticosteroid therapy.

Toxoplasma pneumonia (and see Chapter 76)

T. gondii is a rare cause of interstitial pneumonitis (Derouin *et al.*, 1992; Martino *et al.*, 2000), usually occurring during the first 6 months posttransplant, but sometimes later (Bretagne *et al.*, 1995). It occurs almost exclusively in allogeneic stem cell transplant recipients who are seropositive for toxoplasma before transplant, and results from reactivation. Neurological symptoms or signs may be absent, which makes the diagnosis difficult. Toxoplasmosis may be identified in broncho-alveolar fluid by immunofluoresence staining or in blood through PCR testing. Many cases of toxoplasmosis after HSC transplantation are only diagnosed at autopsy (Small *et al.*, 2000), underscoring the need for PCR evaluation in order to improve the prognosis (Bretagne *et al.*, 2000).

Idiopathic IP

Idiopathic IP, more recently called the idiopathic pneumonia syndrome (Clark *et al.*, 1993; Kantrow *et al.*, 1997) has been reported after both autologous and allogeneic HSC transplantation, and with conditioning regimens that include or do not include TBI. It may occur at any time, but most frequently occurs 2 and 6 months posttransplant. In a report of 158 consecutive autologous marrow transplant recipients, idiopathic IP occurred within the first 3 months of transplant in 11% of patients treated with TBI (Carlson *et al.*, 1994). In another consecutive series of 271 patients receiving an autologous transplant after a busulfan-containing regimen, the incidence of idiopathic pneumonia was 4% with a median time of onset of 102 days after transplant (Bilgrami *et al.*, 2001). In a series of allogeneic transplant recipients, the incidence of idiopathic IP was 6.3% prior to the regular institution of ganciclovir prophylaxis for CMV disease and 3.2% after its introduction (not significantly different) (Atkinson *et al.*, 1998).

IP associated with chronic GVHD

Seven long-term survivors of bone marrow allografts, all of whom had chronic GVHD, developed IP at a median of 210 (range 120–445) days posttransplant (Leblond *et al.*, 1994). BAL showed lymphocytosis with an overall expansion of the CD8+ subset. Pulmonary function tests revealed a restrictive defect and biopsy samples obtained from two patients showed interstitial lymphoid infiltration with fibrosis of the alveolar walls. Six of the seven patients were cured by starting, or increasing the dosage of immune suppressive medications, with a marked improvement in respiratory symptoms within 1 month.

Diagnosis

Two points should be emphasized regarding obtaining a diagnosis of IP after HSC transplantation. Firstly, a direct procedure to procure lung cells or lung tissue is needed. This may be achieved either by fiberoptic bronchoscopy and BAL, or by lung biopsy. Whatever the first-line procedure, it should be done expeditiously, in order to initiate appropriate treatment as well as to withhold inappropriate treatment. Secondly, on the material obtained, specific tests must be performed in order to detect or exclude the most common causes of IP after transplant. In general, the same tests are done on alveolar cells and on lung tissue.

As at least half the cases of IP after stem cell transplantation are of infectious origin (Table 78.2), and as the most common pathogens are found in the alveolar compartment (CMV or *P. carinii*), it is reasonable to begin the investigative process with BAL. This provides information on a large section of lung, often larger than that provided by surgery. However, the main problem raised by BAL is that, if negative, it does not prove that idiopathic IP is the cause. There is always concern that an infectious agent has not been identified through BAL. Therefore, the diagnosis of idiopathic IP should be established by the documentation of a lung sample showing no evidence of an infectious agent, in combination with the histopathologic presence of either

nonspecific inflammatory features, or changes consistent with chemotherapy or chemoradiation damage.

Sputum examination and culture

The majority of patients with IP after HSC transplantation do not produce sputum and thus this is not usually a useful avenue of diagnostic investigation. Occasionally, however, sputum may be obtained and *Chlamydia trachomatis* has been diagnosed as a rare cause of pneumonia in such circumstances. While induced sputum appears a useful means of diagnosing PCP in patients with AIDS, pneumocysts are much less frequent in number in patients with PCP after HSC transplantation, making this investigation less useful in this setting. In theory, sputum examination could be very helpful for pathogens that are not normal colonizers of the mouth or the throat, such as mycobacteria or *Legionella* sp. In practice, however, the yield provided by sputum examination is extremely low.

BAL and other endoscopic samples

Bronchoscopic sampling with BAL is the first-line approach for diagnosing pulmonary infection in many HSC transplant centers. The diagnostic yield of BAL alone, without concomitant transbronchial biopsy, in the stem cell transplant population with pneumonia, varies between 31% (White *et al.*, 1997) and 66% (Cordonnier *et al.*, 1986). The complication rate with experienced teams is very low. BAL is a safe, noninvasive, and reproducible procedure. It can be performed in thrombocytopenic patients (with platelet transfusion cover) as long as the operator is informed of the risk, and the patient is compliant. Patients who are hypoxemic before the exam need at least nasal oxygen, since lavage will be always followed by a transient worsening of hypoxemia. Close follow-up after the procedure is mandatory.

The samples can be examined by a variety of methods including direct fluorescence with multiple virus-specific monoclonal antibodies after cytospinning the BAL fluid (Emanuel *et al.*, 1986; Cordonnier *et al.*, 1987; Crawford *et al.*, 1988; Gleaves & Meyers, 1989). Additionally, the BAL sample can be centrifuged and cultured using a shell vial technique, which gives a positive result within 24 to 48 hours of inoculation. The list of viruses should include at least HSV, VZV, CMV, respiratory viruses (RSV, influenza A and B, parainfluenza), and adenovirus. Specific stains (Table 78.5) should be systematically performed, including methenamine silver stain for *P. carinii* and fungi.

Protected brushing or protected aspiration are of little help in IP, since bacteria are seldom the cause of the syndrome. The yield of transbronchial biopsy may be additive to the results provided by BAL, but it can also increase the risk of complications, especially bleeding and pneumothorax. Transbronchial biopsy (TBB) provides lung tissue that may be examined for histologic features of idiopathic IP. However,

Table 78.5. *Protocol for processing open lung/transbronchial biopsy specimens for diagnosis of interstitial pneumonitis*

Divide sample/s aseptically	

Histopathology	*Microbiology*
1. Hematoxylin & eosin stain	1. Gram[2] stain (impression slide of a cut edge)
2. CMV early antigen immunoperoxidase stain	2. ZN stain[3,4]
3. Methenamine silver stain for *Pneumocystis*	3. *Legionella* direct fluorescence stain
4. PAS[1] stain for fungi	4. *Pneumocystis* indirect fluorescence stain (make impression slide and send one to histopathology laboratory fixed in formalin)
	5. Bacterial culture including aerobes, anaerobes, AFB, *Legionella*, *Nocardia*
	6. Fungal culture
	7. Viral culture (use shell vial technique) and chlamydial culture. (After normal working hours this sample may be put in viral culture medium in a Nunc tube (freezing-resistant) and placed in liquid nitrogen container)

Abbreviations: CMV, cytomegalovirus; PAS, Periodic-acid-Schiff[1]; ZN, Ziehl[3]-Neelsen[4]

the tissue sample procured is small and the absence of a pathogen does not rule out a possible infection. Thus, TBB has not been shown to greatly supplement the diagnostic yield of BAL in immunocompromised patients, except perhaps for mycobacterial infections.

Few series have prospectively compared BAL and open lung biopsy in immunocompromised patients, including after stem cell transplantation. For multiple reasons, including the noninvasiveness of BAL, it has not been performed prospectively, except in a small study comparing concurrent open lung biopsy with BAL in febrile neutropenic patients with pulmonary infiltrates (Ellis *et al.*, 1995). Ellis *et al.* found that at least one diagnostic finding was obtained in 12 of 13 patients by open lung biopsy, compared to 4 of 13 patients by BAL. Five patients with nonspecific interstitial/alveolar inflammation were diagnosed only by open lung biopsy. This study suggested that open lung biopsy provided superior and more complete diagnostic information in this patient population compared to BAL. However, larger (retrospective) studies

[1] Hugo Schiff, German chemist, 1834–1915.

[2] Hans Gram, Danish pathologist, 1853–1938.

[3] Franz Ziehl, German bacteriologist, 1857–1926.

[4] Friedrich Neelsen, German pathologist, 1854–1894.

have shown a comparable diagnostic yield of BAL and lung biopsy in HSC transplant patients, often with more complications after lung biopsy. Hayes-Jordan *et al.* (2002) reported their experience of a cohort of 528 children, of whom 83 contracted pneumonia. Among them, 19 underwent open lung biopsy and a specific diagnosis was obtained in 17. However, improvement in outcome was seen only in 8 (47.5%) of these patients and the postoperative morbidity was 47% at day 30. Therefore the authors recommended consideration of less invasive procedures, especially BAL, before open lung biopsy, in the investigation of these patients. Ben-Ari *et al.* (2001) compared the diagnostic yield of BAL in 33 ventilated and 30 nonventilated children after bone marrow transplantation. In the nine cases who had an open lung biopsy, BAL and biopsy findings correlated in six patients and discordance was observed in only one.

Tissue biopsy

The classical way of confirming the diagnosis, and, more importantly, of determining the cause of IP after HSC transplantation is to obtain an adequate tissue biopsy. In this regard open lung biopsy is more successful in obtaining a positive diagnosis than transbronchial biopsy (Springmeyer *et al.*, 1982), although the difference in diagnostic yield compared to BAL is not large (Ben Ari *et al.*, 2001; Hayes-Jordan *et al.*, 2002). In a retrospective study that included 87 HSC transplant patients, open lung biopsy yielded a specific diagnosis in only 60% of the patients (Snyder *et al.*, 1990). Independently of whether the procedure is the initial or subsequent diagnostic approach, open lung biopsy should only be proceeded with as long as hemostasis can be maintained by ensuring that the platelet count is at least 30 to $40 \times 10^9/l$ at the time of operation and that no coagulopathy is present (normal prothrombin time and activated partial thromboplastin time). Thus, platelet transfusions or fresh frozen plasma may need to be given to correct a hemorrhagic diathesis prior to surgery. It is important to have a cardiothoracic surgeon experienced in the technique perform such biopsies on a regular basis. The area of lung to be sampled at open lung biopsy should be the one that is most heavily involved radiologically. The only other consideration for open lung biopsy is whether or not the patient can be adequately oxygenated during the general anesthetic. A small (2 to 3 inch) incision is necessary, and a chest drain will need to be kept in situ for 48 hours after the return of the patient from the operating theatre. The main disadvantage of open lung biopsy is incision pain, which may be severe, but usually disappears within 72 hours of the operation. More recently, longer incisions have been used that avoid cutting the latissimus dorsi muscle, and result in less postoperative pain. The pain requires opiate analgesia for its control. An alternative approach currently being explored is to obtain samples using a thoracoscope.

A more conservative, but less useful, alternative to open lung biopsy is transbronchial biopsy. Potential hemorrhage is a serious consideration here since homeostasis is more difficult to achieve should serious bleeding occur. If transbronchial biopsy is utilized, multiple biopsies (at least 6) should be taken, rather than just a single small sample.

In view of the seriousness of the syndrome it is important to process surgically obtained samples as rapidly as possible. In practical terms a member of the medical staff looking after the patient should be deemed responsible for taking the sample from the operating theater to the microbiology and histopathology laboratories. In the microbiology laboratory the sample should be dissected under sterile conditions and portions of one-half of it set up for viral, bacterial, and fungal culture and a Gram stain, ZN stain, PCP indirect fluorescence stain, and a *Legionella* direct fluorescence stain performed. Using the shell vial culture technique and staining with a monoclonal antibody to the CMV early antigen, positive results for CMV can be available within 24 hours (Gleaves *et al.*, 1985; Martin & Smith, 1986).

The second half of the sample should then be processed by the histopathologic laboratory and with current technology (use of microwave ovens) tissue sections can be available within 4 hours of receipt in the laboratory. In addition to hematoxylin and eosin staining of tissue sections, a methenamine silver stain for the presence of *Pneumocystis carinii*, an immunoperoxidase stain using a monoclonal antibody to the early antigen of CMV, and a periodic acid-Schiff stain for fungi should be performed (Table 78.5).

Histopathologic features

Inclusion bodies of CMV in alveolar wall cells or endothelium are characteristic (Fig. 78.2A), as are the presence of pneumocysts and the foamy exudate present in the alveolar spaces in *Pneumocystis pneumonia* (Fig. 78.2C). Chemotherapy or chemoradiation damage is characterized by the presence of abnormal type II pneumocytes (Fig. 78.2B).

Molecular techniques (and see Chapter 74)

Over the past several years, the diagnosis of CMV disease has been remarkably enhanced by the introduction of molecular technology, especially the use of nucleic acid detection by PCR (Einsele *et al.*, 1991; Vlieger *et al.*, 1992). In a prospective study comparing four assays—whole blood PCR, plasma PCR, pp65-antigenemia, and virus culture—in 20 consecutive marrow transplant recipients, 15 of 20 patients were found to be CMV positive by PCR from whole blood, plasma PCR, and pp65 antigenemia, whereas only 9 of 20 developed culture-proven viremia and/or viruria (Hebart *et al.*, 1996). PCR from whole blood, plasma PCR, and pp65 antigenemia revealed identical results in 96 of 109, and discordant results in 13 of 109, blood samples. Thus, all three of these highly sensitive assays seemed to be suitable for screening patients at risk for CMV infection and were superior to viral culture. Similar results were found by

Gozlan *et al.* (1996) in comparing a reverse transcriptase PCR method to detect a late viral mRNA in peripheral blood leukocytes, a PCR method that detected viral DNA in peripheral blood leukocytes, and viral culture from blood leukocytes and urine for the diagnosis of symptomatic CMV infection after marrow transplantation. Forty-five consecutive recipients were prospectively tested at weekly intervals by the four methods. CMV infection demonstrated either by CMV culture or by repeated detection of viral DNA was observed in 28 of the 46 patients although only 14 developed CMV disease. The clinical sensitivity and specificity of each technique for detection of symptomatic infection were, respectively, 71% and 94% for reverse transcription PCR, 100% and 65% for PCR, 43% and 84% for viral culture from leukocytes, and 36% and 74% for viral culture from urine. Another study using reverse transcription nested PCR to detect RNA of a spliced late gene of human CMV was also more sensitive than viral culture from a buffy-coat preparation (Nelson *et al.*, 1996).

Unfortunately, a three-center European external quality control study of PCR for detection of CMV DNA in blood (using the routine in-house PCR assay at each site), found that only 38 of 47 coded peripheral blood samples agreed (35–/3+), while 9 were discrepant. The 9 discrepant samples appeared to contain around 1,000-fold less viral DNA than the 3 concordant positive samples. CMV detection was affected both by the number of leukocytes from which DNA was extracted and by the number of cell equivalents added per PCR. This study suggested it would be valuable to standardize PCR methodology for detection of CMV in blood leukocytes (Grundy *et al.*, 1996).

Several studies have utilized molecular technologies to guide or monitor antiviral therapy. Boeckh *et al.* (1996a) prospectively compared pp65 antigenemia-guided early treatment with ganciclovir versus ganciclovir initiated at engraftment in a randomized double-blind study. Two hundred twenty-six marrow transplant recipients were randomized at engraftment to receive placebo (antigenemia-ganciclovir group) or ganciclovir (ganciclovir group) until day 100 after allogeneic transplantation. In patients with antigenemia of 3 or more positive cells in two slides and/or viremia, the study drug was discontinued and ganciclovir was started for at least 3 weeks or until CMV antigenemia resolved. It was resumed only if antigenemia recurred. More patients in the antigenemia-ganciclovir group developed CMV disease before day 100 compared with the ganciclovir group (14% vs. 2.7%, $P = .002$). Untreated low-grade antigenemia progressed to CMV disease in 19% of patients with grade III–IV acute GVHD compared to 0% of patients with grade 0–II acute GVHD. There was no significant difference in CMV disease by day 180 posttransplant or thereafter. CMV-related deaths, survival, and neutropenia were not significantly different between the two groups. In the ganciclovir group more invasive fungal infections occurred and more ganciclovir was used. The study concluded that delaying the start of ganciclovir until high-grade antigenemia (and discontinuing ganci-clovir based on negative antigenemia), resulted in more CMV disease by day 100 than ganciclovir administered prophylactically at the time of engraftment. However, ganciclovir initiated at engraftment was associated with more early invasive fungal infections and more late CMV disease, resulting in similar survival rates.

Ljungman and colleagues (1996a) conducted a similar study evaluating the efficacy of pre-emptive antiviral therapy based on a semiquantitative nested PCR for CMV DNA in blood leukocytes. Fifty-eight patients were prospectively followed with PCR for CMV DNA and antiviral therapy with ganciclovir was initiated after two consecutive positive tests. The probability of detection of CMV DNA was 48% and the probability of CMV disease by 100 days posttransplant was 6%. Patients with CMV disease had higher CMV DNA levels compared to patients without CMV disease. In comparison to 58 matched historical control patients, detection of CMV DNA was 5 days earlier and antiviral therapy could be initiated 10 days earlier in patients followed by PCR. Pre-emptive antiviral therapy was given to 28 patients for a total of 36 courses. Patients became negative by PCR after 28 of 36 courses (77%). The authors concluded that PCR for CMV DNA could be used for early detection of CMV infection and as a basis for the initiation of pre-emptive antiviral therapy.

Nichols and colleagues (2001a) determined the risk factors and outcomes associated with rising CMV antigenemia levels during pre-emptive anti-CMV treatment. Corticosteroid therapy was the primary risk factor. Overall, rising antigenemia levels did not correlate with development of CMV disease. However, CMV disease did develop in 4 of 47 patients with rising antigenemia levels. All four received maintenance treatment, but 3 died. Re-induction anti-CMV therapy should be considered in this circumstance. Kanda and colleagues (2001) found transplantation from an alternate donor and acute GVHD grades II–IV to be risk factors for developing antigenemia (Fig. 78.3). Declining CMV DNA load in the blood was found to be an indicator for effective antiviral therapy, whereas persistence of a high viral load was associated with fatal CMV disease (Hebart *et al.*, 2001).

In a survey of U.S. BMT centers in 1998–1999, the most commonly used CMV diagnostic tests were CMV-DNA by PCR, shell vial centrifugation culture, tissue culture, pp65 antigenemia, and CMV-DNA by a hybrid capture assay (Avery *et al.*, 2000). In a prospective study, a high degree of concordance was found between the hybrid capture assay and a PCR assay (Hebart *et al.*, 2001).

HLA/CMV peptide tetramers

Fluorescent HLA-peptide tetramers containing immunodominant peptides from CMV have been used to monitor recovery of CMV cytotoxic T cells (CTL) posttransplant (Cwynarski *et al.*, 2001). When both recipient and donor were CMV-seropositive pretransplant, recovery of CMV-specific CTL was rapid

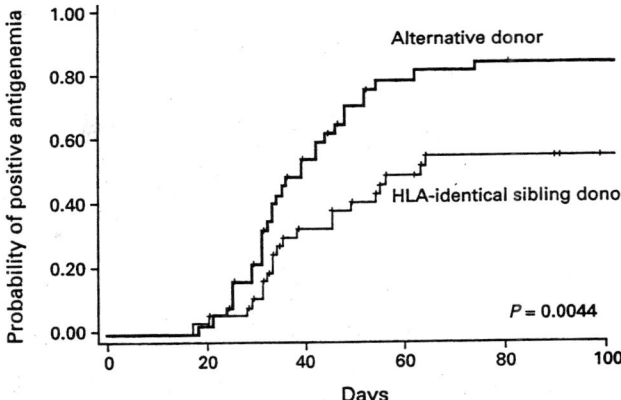

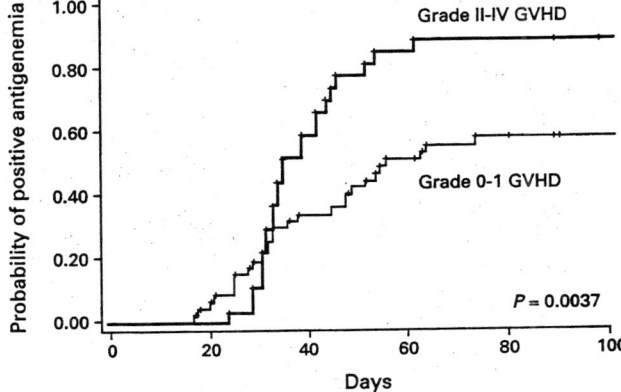

Fig. 78.3. Probability of positive antigenemia in groups divided by the two risk factors are shown by Kaplan-Meier curves. Reproduced, with permission, from Kanda *et al.* (2001).

and reached up to 21% of all CD8[+] cells (Fig. 78.4). Recovery was slower in recipients of unrelated transplants compared to that after HLA-identical sibling grafts. CTL numbers increased after episodes of CMV reactivation, and were suppressed by corticosteroid treatment. Recovery of CMV-specific CTL to levels $> 10 \times 10^6/l$ was associated with protection from CMV disease.

Differential diagnosis

Several other situations may mimic the syndrome of IP in patients who have received HSC transplants.

Adult respiratory distress syndrome

Adult respiratory distress syndrome (ARDS) is best diagnosed by procurement of tissue biopsy when the presence of hyaline membranes will enable the diagnosis to be readily made. The causes of this syndrome are many, but most common after marrow transplantation is sepsis (Table 78.6). It should be noted, however, that pneumonia itself causes ARDS, and that the his-

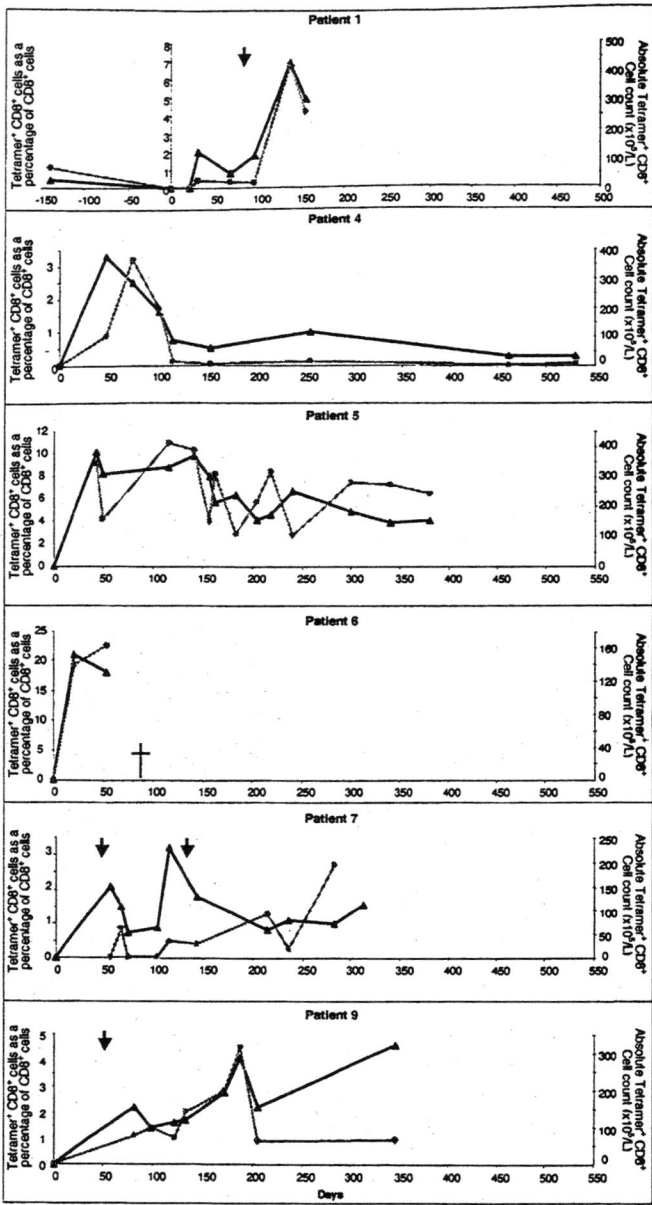

Fig. 78.4. Reconstitution of CMV-specific CTL in CMV-seropositive patients given transplants from CMV-seropositive sibling donors. Results in 6 individual patients are shown. The number of days after transplantation is shown on the x-axis. The percentage of CD8+ T cells binding HLA-peptide tetramer (▲) and the absolute CMV-specific CTL count (●) are shown on the y-axes. Times of CMV reactivation are shown by arrows. Reproduced, with permission, from Cwynarski *et al.* (2001).

tologic changes of ARDS can coexist in the same sections as, for example, those of CMV IP.

Pulmonary edema

An interstitial infiltrate on the chest X ray of a marrow transplant recipient within 14 days of transplant is most commonly

Table 78.6. *Causes of adult respiratory distress syndrome (increased permeability pulmonary edema) related to HSC transplantation*

1. Septic shock
2. Severe pneumonia
3. Oxygen toxicity
4. Disseminated intravascular coagulation
5. Renal failure
6. Pancreatitis
7. Massive blood transfusion
8. Hemodialysis
9. Pulmonary embolism
10. Prolonged hypotension
11. Cerebral injury

due to pulmonary edema (Khouri *et al.*, 1979). Pulmonary edema is not uncommon early posttransplant due to damage to the myocardium from previous anthracycline cytotoxic chemotherapy, from cyclophosphamide in the pretransplant preparative regimen, from the use of high-dose fluid therapy intravenously during the pretransplant preparative regimen to minimize the risk of hemorrhagic cystitis, and from the use of salt-containing medications, such as the semisynthetic antipseudomonal penicillins (ticarcillin and piperacillin). A therapeutic trial of frusemide will normally allow the diagnosis to be made within 12 to 24 hours.

Alveolar hemorrhage (and see Chapter 91)

Alveolar hemorrhage is recognized by the presence of bloody alveolar fluid recovered early after the first episode of hemorrhage. Profound thrombocytopenia, renal failure, smoking history, and fluid overload are risk factors associated with alveolar hemorrhage in immunocompromised hosts (de Lassence *et al.*, 1995). It should be noted that it is usual to observe some degree of hemorrhage in any inflammatory process involving the lung, including ARDS or CMV pneumonitis (de Lassence *et al.*, 1995). Since ARDS can coexist with infectious IP, hemorrhage can occur with these syndromes, including infectious or idiopathic IP. Alveolar hemorrhage has been reported in 10% (Metcalf *et al.*, 1994) to 26% (Jules Elysee *et al.*, 1992) of autologous transplant recipients in series using different definitions of the disease. The presence of alveolar hemorrhage after stem cell transplantation should prompt a vigilant search of an underlying infection, especially aspergillus.

Recurrence of underlying malignancy

Occasionally, recurrence of the underlying malignant disease can occur in the lungs and may mimic IP (Watts & Mroczek-Musulman, 1996; Kottaridis *et al.*, 1999).

Prevention of IP after marrow transplantation

CMV infection

As CMV was the most common cause of IP after stem cell transplantation until recently, the prevention of CMV infection has had a major impact on the incidence of IP. We summarize here the main strategies for the prevention of CMV infection and CMV disease (see also Chapter 74).

Seronegative blood products for recipient/donor pairs seronegative for CMV antibodies pretransplant

In this situation CMV infection can be prevented altogether if blood products are restricted to those obtained from donors also seronegative for CMV (Bowden *et al.*, 1986; Rubie *et al.*, 1993; Winston *et al.*, 1993a). Similarly, if a patient likely to come to transplant requires cellular blood products and his or her CMV serologic status is unknown, he or she should be given CMV seronegative blood products until the CMV status is determined.

Prophylactic or early intervention (pre-emptive) ganciclovir when either the recipient or the donor or both are seropositive for CMV pretransplant

In this situation the recipient is at high risk for developing CMV disease posttransplant (Hersman *et al.*, 1982; Meyers *et al.*, 1986). Several early reports indicated that ganciclovir given either prophylactically (Atkinson *et al.*, 1991a; Yau *et al.*, 1991), or at the first sign of the presence of CMV infection (Goodrich *et al.*, 1991; Schmidt *et al.*, 1991), markedly diminished the risk of CMV disease developing. One protocol (Schmidt *et al.*, 1991) administered ganciclovir or placebo if BAL at day 35 posttransplant revealed evidence of CMV. While this reduced the incidence of subsequent CMV disease it was not completely effective. Moreover, BAL for this purpose was not superior to CMV screening of blood samples, and was much more invasive and time-consuming, so that this approach is not routinely used. In a study of prophylactic ganciclovir, the drug was administered to patients seropositive for CMV starting 8 days pretransplant at a dose of 5 mg/kg 12 hourly until day −1 pretransplant and was then withheld during the period of engraftment. When the white count reached $2.0 \times 10^9/l$, the neutrophil count $0.5 \times 10^9/l$, and the platelet count $20 \times 10^9/l$, ganciclovir was restarted at a dose of 5 mg/kg 3 days weekly. Such a regimen decreased the CMV disease rate from approximately 30% to 3% (Atkinson *et al.*, 1991a). Subsequently, two prospective controlled studies confirmed the efficacy of prophylactic ganciclovir in decreasing the incidence of CMV disease after allogeneic transplantation (Winston *et al.*, 1993b; Goodrich *et al.*, 1993). However, in a nonprospective trial performed in HLA-identical sibling recipients, the effective prevention of CMV disease in seropositive patients by ganciclovir did not translate into superior overall survival when compared to a cohort of CMV seronegative patients transplanted from seronegative donors (Broers *et al.*, 2000).

It should be emphasized that these studies with prophylactic or early intervention ganciclovir were carried out mainly in recipients of family member transplants, and most of the donors were HLA-identical siblings. Prophylactic ganciclovir did not appear as effective in recipients of matched unrelated donor transplants (Atkinson *et al.*, 1995; Canpolat *et al.*, 1996; Einsele *et al.*, 2000), nor was the 3 days per week prophylactic ganciclovir regimen effective in recipients of T-cell-depleted allografts (Przepiorka *et al.*, 1994; Maltazou *et al.*, 1999).

The most common side effect of ganciclovir is hematopoietic toxicity and it can cause leukopenia, thrombocytopenia, or both. This appears to be dose-dependent and is usually reversible over a period of 1 to 2 weeks. However, prolonged or irreversible neutropenia has also occurred. Ganciclovir-induced leukopenia may be reversed with the use of granulocyte colony-stimulating factor (G-CSF) or granulocyte-macrophage colony-stimulating factor (GM-CSF) 5 to 10 µg/kg i.v.i. or subcutaneously daily. In addition adverse neurologic effects occur in 5% to 17% of patients receiving ganciclovir, ranging from headaches to seizure or coma. Confusion is the most common, occurring in 1% to 3% of patients. Other described side effects include thought disorders, dysphoria, hallucinations, abnormal dreams/nightmares, nervousness/anxiety, dizziness, dysesthesia, tremor, ataxia, paresthesiae, psychosis, somnolence, and obtundation.

While effective, prophylactic ganciclovir requires treatment of all patients except CMV seronegative recipients who have CMV seronegative donors, resulting in up to 65% of patients receiving ganciclovir unnecessarily. Since it is associated with considerable toxicity and since it delays reconstitution of protective CMV-specific T-cell responses (Li *et al.*, 1994), other strategies have focused on using sensitive detection methods to identify CMV infection, and to guide pre-emptive ganciclovir therapy. Such methods have included direct detection of CMV pp65 antigen in peripheral blood leukocytes and detection of CMV DNA by PCR in peripheral blood leukocytes as well as in plasma and serum. The CMV antigenemia assay detects CMV in marrow transplant patients with CMV pneumonia on an average of 10 days before the onset of pneumonia. The test can also be quantitated. The details of the approach used at the Fred Hutchinson Cancer Research Center are given in Chapter 20. One study mentioned previously utilized CMV pp65 antigenemia detection to guide early treatment and compared it to prophylactic ganciclovir started at the time of engraftment after allogeneic transplantation (Boeckh *et al.*, 1996a). Delaying the start of ganciclovir until high-grade antigenemia was present and discontinuing ganciclovir based on negative antigenemia, resulted in more CMV disease by day 100 than with ganciclovir administered prophylactically at engraftment, but less early invasive fungal infections and less late CMV disease, resulting in similar survival rates. In a survey of U.S. BMT centers carried out in 1998–1999, 56% of centers utilized a pre-emptive ganciclovir strategy, whereas 21% utilized a prophylactic strategy (Avery *et al.*, 2000).

The use of oral ganciclovir prophylaxis is currently being explored (Boeckh *et al.,* 1998).

Acyclovir

High-dose acyclovir (500 mg/m^2 every 8 hours) given from 5 days before to 30 days after allogeneic transplantation has been reported to be effective in reducing the risk of both CMV infection and CMV disease in seropositive patients given allogeneic marrow transplants (Prentice *et al.,* 1994).

Foscarnet

Foscarnet has been used prophylactically and pre-emptively to minimize the risk of CMV disease after HSC transplantation. In one study, 15 allogeneic transplant recipients were given foscarnet 60 mg/kg twice daily for 14 days as pre-emptive therapy against CMV disease. CMV infection was detected by nested PCR on peripheral blood leukocytes. Of 14 evaluable patients, none developed CMV disease nor did any have to discontinue therapy due to toxicity (Ljungman *et al.,* 1996b). The most common side effects are nausea and nephrotoxicity, especially when given to patients receiving cyclosporine. Sudden severe hypocalcemia can occur and the serum ionized calcium level should be monitored frequently. Foscarnet can give rise to feelings of anxiety and agitation. A dose-finding study for the prophylactic use of foscarnet found the most effective dose for preventing CMV antigenemia and CMV disease to be 120 mg/kg/day (Bregante *et al.,* 2000). It should be noticed that due to the absence of cross-resistance, foscarnet may be given to patients developing CMV~ infection while receiving prophylactic ganciclovir. Recently, a randomized, multicenter trial of the European Blood and Marrow Transplant Group compared ganciclovir (5 mg/kg every 12 hours for 14 days) with foscarnet (60 mg/kg every 12 hours for 14 days) in the pre-emptive therapy of CMV infection after allogeneic stem cell transplantation (Reusser *et al.,* 2002). After 14 days of induction treatment, patients received 14 days of maintenance treatment with the initial study drug (ganciclovir 6 mg/kg/day or foscarnet 90 mg/kg/day 5 days a week) if CMV was still detectable in the blood. Two hundred thirteen patients were treated either with foscarnet (*n* = 110) or ganciclovir (*n* = 103). The occurrence of CMV disease within 180 days after transplant was similar in the two treatment groups. It is noteworthy that impaired renal function was observed in 5% of patients on foscarnet versus 2% of patients on ganciclovir, indicating that extra hydration before and during foscarnet infusion prevents most of the renal toxicity of the drug.

The dosages of both foscarnet and ganciclovir need to be reduced in renal impairment (see Chapter 83, Tables 83.7 and 83.8).

Combination of ganciclovir and foscarnet

A combined foscarnet/ganciclovir pre-emptive treatment approach has been described (Bacigalupo *et al.,* 1996) in patients undergoing allogeneic HSC transplantation with CMV antigenemia defined as 5 or more positive cells/200,000 cells. The prescribed dose was 180 mg/kg/day of foscarnet and 10 mg/kg/day of ganciclovir. The median administered dose in the first 15 days, after adjustments were made for creatinine levels and blood count, was 64% for foscarnet and 53% for ganciclovir. Maintenance was given with foscarnet and ganciclovir on alternate days for an additional 2 weeks. All patients cleared CMV antigenemia by day 15 of treatment although it recurred in 5 patients on maintenance therapy and in 14 patients off maintenance therapy. Of the 32 patients in the trial, 26 survived 119 to 1,051 days posttransplant with a 1-year transplant-related mortality rate of 23%. Eighteen patients who had received unmanipulated bone marrow transplants from HLA-identical siblings were compared with 15 matched controls who had been treated with a single drug (either foscarnet or ganciclovir) for CMV antigenemia of 5 or greater cells. The actuarial 1-year transplant-related mortality rate was 13% for patients receiving combined treatment, compared to 47% for controls receiving a single drug.

Immunoglobulin

CMV immunoglobulin has been shown to be ineffective in reducing the incidence of CMV disease after marrow transplantation in one study (Bowden *et al.,* 1986). A meta-analysis of 12 published studies (incorporating 1,282 patients) of intravenous immunoglobulin (IVIG) indicated that it reduced fatal CMV infection and CMV pneumonitis (Bass *et al.,* 1993). The preliminary results of a double-blind, placebo-controlled, dose-effect study comparing 0, 50, 250, and 500 mg/kg/week of IVIG during the first 3 months of allogeneic HLA-identical transplantation showed a lack of effect of IVIG at any dose on CMV infection, CMV disease, and IP (Cordonnier *et al.,* 2001). The preliminary results of a double-blind, placebo-controlled trial comparing prophylactic IVIG versus placebo, followed by IVIG administration for hypogammaglobulinemia (IgG less than 400 mg/dl) in unrelated donor bone marrow transplantation, also showed no benefit of IVIG on outcome (Sullivan *et al.,* 2000).

CMV-specific T-cell clones

In the future it is possible that CMV immunity may be routinely reconstituted in allogeneic HSC transplant recipients by the adoptive transfer of CMV-specific; T-lymphocyte clones derived from the stem cell donor (Reusser *et al.,* 1991; Walter *et al.,* 1995; Einsele *et al.* 2002), particularly if improvements in the technology of ex vivo generation of such cells occur (Vannuchi *et al.,* 2001; Kleihauer *et al.,* 2001).

Pneumocystis carinii pneumonia

The use of cotrimoxazole has largely eradicated the occurrence of PCP after HSC transplantation. Various prophylactic regimens have been proposed in the literature and much information has been derived from the AIDS population. A suitable regimen for HSC transplant recipients is one double-strength tablet (sulfamethoxazole 800 mg, trimethoprim 140 mg) twice daily 2 days a week once engraftment has taken place. Cotrimoxazole should be continued for the duration of immune suppressive therapy, or for as long as evidence of GVHD is present. Most programs also give one double-strength tablet twice daily for 2 weeks pretransplant. Cotrimoxazole appears significantly superior to alternatives (see below) and if an allergic response to cotrimoxazole occurs, consideration should be given to desensitizing the patient (Table 78.7).

If cotrimoxazole causes pancytopenia, gastrointestinal intolerance, or renal insufficiency and it is felt unwise to further utilize it, an alternative approach is dapsone 100 mg together with trimethoprim 300 mg, both given 2 days per week. Atovaquone, a selective inhibitor of mitochondrial electron transport in a number of parasitic protozoa, was well tolerated in a prospective trial in recipients of autologous peripheral blood stem cells (Colby *et al.*, 1999). Breakthrough PCP can occur in HSC transplant patients given either dapsone 100 mg weekly alone, or pentamidine 300 mg per month intravenously, or by inhalation (Przepiorka *et al.*, 1991; Souza *et al.*, 1999). A dose of 50 mg/m^2 of dapsone alone has been used effectively in children (Maltezou *et al.*, 1997). A retrospective analysis of 327 patients showed aerosolized pentamidine not only to be inferior to cotrimoxazole in preventing PCP, but associated with an increased risk of other infections and a higher mortality at 1 year posttransplant (Vasconelles *et al.*, 2000).

An unexpected possible bonus of prophylactic cotrimoxazole treatment pre– and post–marrow transplant is the rarity of toxoplasmosis posttransplant.

Treatment of established IP

CMV pneumonitis

The treatment of established CMV pneumonitis is difficult with a high (80%) case fatality rate. Some reports (Emanuel *et al.*, 1988; Reed *et al.*, 1988; Schmidt *et al.*, 1988), but not all (Verdonck *et al.*, 1989), have indicated that a combination of ganciclovir 2.5 mg/kg body weight every 8 hours for 14 or 20 days, together with CMV immunoglobulin followed by maintenance ganciclovir and immuno globulin are associated with a better survival rate than in historical series. All efforts should be made to maintain adequate oxygenation; however, a successful outcome is infrequent in adults once mechanical ventilation is required, although better results have been reported in children (Warwick *et al.*, 1998). Noninvasive positive-pressure ventilation, without oro-tracheal intubation, may be appropriate, and preferable, in some patients (Marin *et al.*, 1998). Mortality remains high and prophylactic or pre-emptive therapy (see above) with ganciclovir appears a superior approach.

Foscarnet has also been used to treat CMV pneumonia, including that due to ganciclovir-resistant CMV infection (Drobyski *et al.*, 1991), but has been generally disappointing.

Table 78.7. *Desensitization regimen for cotrimoxazole allergy*

Dosage interval = 3 hours
Solution used = Cotrimoxazole but dose expressed as units of sulfamethoxazole

Dose	Solution Equivalent	
DAY 1		
10 mg =	0.1 ml }	
20 mg =	0.2 ml }	
30 mg =	0.3 ml }	
40 mg =	0.4 ml }	Use 100 mg/ml solution
60 mg =	0.6 ml }	
80 mg =	0.8 ml }	
100 mg =	1 ml }	
200 mg =	2 ml }	
DAY 2		
300 mg =	3 ml }	
500 mg =	5 ml }	Use 100 mg/ml solution
600 mg =	6 ml }	
750 mg =	7.5 ml }	
DAY 3		
400 mg = Half a double strength (DS) tablet		
800 mg = 1 double strength (DS) tablet		
DAY 4		
800 mg =	One DS tablet 4 times daily	
DAY 5		
1,600 mg =	Two DS tablets 3 or 4 times daily depending on patient's weight. Continue at this dosage level for treatment of *Pneumocystis* infection.	

If prophylaxis only required, omit 800 mg dose on Day 3, and commence half a double strength tablet daily on Day 4.

1 double-strength tablet = 800 mg sulfamethoxazole, 160 mg trimethoprim.

Agents shown previously to be ineffective for CMV pneumonitis after marrow transplantation include vidarabine, leukocyte interferon, vidarabine and interferon combined, high-dose acyclovir, recombinant alpha-interferon, and high-dose acyclovir combined with leukocyte interferon.

Respiratory syncytial virus pneumonitis

Pneumonitis due to RSV may be treated by aerosolized ribavirin and intravenous immunoglobulin containing high levels of RSV neutralizing activity. Ten of 11 children with positive nasal swab specimens for RSV antigens, and clinical or radiological evidence of lower respiratory tract involvement were given a single dose of 1.5 g/kg of such immunoglobulin, together with ribavirin. One of them was on mechanical ventilation at the start of treatment. Ten of the 11 survived, only 1 patient dying of RSV illness (De Vincenzo *et al.*, 2000). In another series, five patients with RSV pneumonia were treated with i.v. ribavirin and IVIG and only one died (Ghosh *et al.*, 2001). A sixth patient, who was treated later in the course of respiratory failure, died. In the European experience, there was no clear advantage or disadvantage of adding i.v. ribavirin to either aerosolized ribavirin or to IVIG (Ljungman *et al.*, 2001).

One suggested approach to prevent RSV pneumonia is preemptive treatment for RSV infection before lung involvement (Chakrabarti *et al.,* 2001). However, without a controlled trial, the efficacy of such an approach is unknown.

Pneumocystis carinii pneumonia

Treatment for adults should consist of cotrimoxazole at a dose of 20 mg/kg trimethoprim and 100 mg/kg sulfamethoxazole/day for 14 days; alternatively, pentamidine 4 mg/kg may be given i.v. or i.m. The salvage rate after marrow transplantation is approximately 50%. Side effects of high-dose cotrimoxazole in these patients include marrow suppression and nephrotoxicity. Side effects of pentamidine include sterile abscesses if given intramuscularly, renal impairment, and hypoglycemia. For life-threatening cases of PCP, corticosteroids (prednisolone 2 mg/kg/day) probably have a beneficial effect on outcome, presumably by limiting inflammatory damage (Gagnon *et al.,* 1990; Pareja *et al.,* 1998). However, due to the rarity of *P. carinii* pneumonia after HSC transplantation, no prospective trial has been performed in stem cell transplant patients and all the comparisons are derived from AIDS patient populations.

Fungal pneumonitis

Aspergillus, Candida, and other mold or yeast infections are a rare cause of IP. The treatment is not different whether the pattern of lung involvement is IP or not. The management and treatment of these patients is detailed in Chapter 75.

Other infectious causes

IP due to *Legionella* or mycoplasma may be treated with erythromycin 500 mg i.v. six hourly. Pneumonitis due to *Chlamydia trachomatis* may be treated by tetracycline, doxycycline, or erythromycin.

Chemotherapy or chemoradiation pneumonitis

Anecdotal data suggest that corticosteroids are frequently able to reverse or limit pneumonitis due to pretransplant chemotherapy or chemoradiotherapy (Akasheh *et al.,* 2000; Bilgrami *et al.,* 2001). Prednisolone 2 mg/kg/day may be used initially. If no response is obtained, a limited trial of prednisolone 500 mg daily for 3 days with subsequent rapid dose reduction may be tried. The main problem posed by corticosteroid therapy is the possibility of an underlying, undiagnosed infection that could worsen with steroid therapy. Therefore, open lung biopsy is recommended to document idiopathic IP and rule out an infectious etiology before starting steroids.

Risk factors for IP

IP of any cause, including idiopathic IP, is more common in recipients of allogeneic than autologous transplants, although the incidence is not negligible in recipients of autologous transplants (Pecego *et al.,* 1986; Wingard *et al.,* 1988b, 1990; Reusser *et al.,* 1990; Ljungman *et al.,* 1994; Konoplev *et al.,* 2001). In recipients of allogeneic transplants, the incidence of pneumonitis is higher in patients transplanted for hematologic malignancy compared to those transplanted for severe aplastic anemia (Ljungman *et al.,* 1990), unless those transplanted for severe aplastic anemia are conditioned with a regimen other than cyclophosphamide alone (for example, one containing TBI, procarbazine, or antithymocyte globulin). In a large retrospective study of 1,165 consecutive marrow recipients at the Fred Hutchinson Cancer Center, 85 patients (7.3%) developed idiopathic pneumonia syndrome. The median time of onset was 21 days posttransplant. The incidence in this series was not significantly different in autologous (5.7%) and in allogeneic (7.6%) HSC transplant recipients. Risk factors were identified only for the latter: malignancy other than leukemia (odds ratio: 6.5) and grade IV acute GVHD (odds ratio: 5.4 compared with lower grades).

Interestingly, identical twin transplant recipients have a zero incidence of CMV pneumonitis, but the same incidence of idiopathic IP (presumably due to pretransplant chemotherapy or chemoradiation) as HLA-identical marrow transplant recipients (Appelbaum *et al.,* 1982).

Risk factors for CMV IP

Recipients of autografts have a considerably lower incidence of CMV disease, mainly of CMV pneumonitis, than allograft recipients (Pecego *et al.,* 1986; Wingard *et al.,* 1988a, 1988b; Ljungman *et al.,* 1994; Boeckh *et al.,* 1996b; Bilgrami *et al.,* 1999). In one series of 795 autograft recipients, 2% developed CMV IP: the frequency was higher among those who were seropositive pretransplant and among those transplanted for hematological malignancies compared to those transplanted for solid tumors (Konoplev *et al.,* 2001). An increased risk of CMV disease, however, has been reported in recipients of CD34-selected autologous transplants (Holmberg *et al.,* 1999).

Risk factors for CMV pneumonitis described in a number of reports (Meyers *et al.,* 1986; Weiner *et al.,* 1986; Wingard *et al.,* 1988a, 1988b; Winston, Ho, & Champlin, 1990; Ringden *et al.,* 1993) are increasing recipient age, recipient seropositivity for CMV pretransplant, donor seropositivity for CMV pretransplant, the presence of moderate to severe acute GVHD, and the use of GVHD prophylactic regimens other than cyclosporine. T-cell-depleted prophylactic regimens have been associated with a high incidence of CMV infection, both in recipients of HLA-identical sibling transplants (Couriel *et al.,* 1996), and in recipients of haploidentical family member transplants (Aversa *et al.,* 1994; Bacigalupo *et al.,* 1997). In the study by Couriel and colleagues, 21 patients were at risk for CMV reactivation. This occurred in 19 and 5 developed fatal IP. Median reactivation time was 22 days posttransplant for those developing IP. Twenty of the 21 patients were conditioned with cyclophosphamide 120 mg/kg and TBI 13.7 Gy in 8 fractions and received cyclosporine posttransplant. Donor lymphocytes were infused at 30 and 45 days posttransplant to improve immune reconstitution and to confer graft-versus-leukemia reactivity. Ganciclovir and high-dose intravenous immunoglobulin were given at the first indication of CMV reactivation in blood or bronchial secretions. Nine of the 19 patients reactivated CMV before receiving their first donor lymphocyte transfusion on day 30. These data suggest that patients receiving T-cell-depleted transplants should be protected from CMV disease with prophylactic rather than pre-emptive or early intervention treatments. However, both prophylactic foscarnet and ganciclovir were used in a series of haploidentical transplant recipients described by Bacigalupo and colleagues (1997) and 5 of the 10 patients died of CMV pneumonitis. An important risk factor in these patients appeared to be the prolonged severe CD4+ cytopenia. A reduced risk of persistent CMV pp65 antigenemia and CMV IP has been reported for allogeneic peripheral blood stem cell (PBSC) transplants compared to allogeneic BMTs (Trenschel *et al.*, 2000). Transplantation from alternative donors and occurrence of grade II–IV acute GVHD have been described as independent risk factors for CMV antigenemia (Kanda *et al.*, 2001).

Prolonged use of prophylactic ganciclovir appears to predispose to late CMV IP (Li *et al.*, 1994), with one case occurring at day +811 posttransplant in a patient with chronic GVHD (de Medeiros *et al.*, 2000).

Granulocyte transfusions are also a major source of CMV infection from seropositive donors and should be avoided posttransplant if at all possible (Hersman *et al.*, 1982).

Prognosis

The prognosis of established IP after HSC transplantation depends on its severity. For example, for patients with CMV pneumonitis, clinical features common to surviving patients include good clinical condition at the onset of disease, insidious development of disease, and evidence of normal alveolar gas exchange. The fulminant onset of symptoms, widespread radiographic abnormalities, and marked hypoxemia are characteristics of nonsurvivors (Ettinger *et al.*, 1989). Additionally, lymphocytopenia has been shown to be a bad prognostic factor in patients with CMV infection after marrow transplantation (Einsele *et al.*, 1993; Fries *et al.*, 1993). Finally, in a series of 41 patients given high-dose chemotherapy and autologous BMT for advanced breast cancer, the plasma transforming growth factor-beta concentration measured after induction chemotherapy, but before high-dose chemotherapy and transplant, strongly correlated with the risk of idiopathic IP (and hepatic veno-occlusive disease) posttransplant (Anscher *et al.*, 1993).

Conclusions

CMV disease, and particularly pneumonitis, has been a major hurdle to the improvement of survival results in recipients of allogeneic marrow transplants over the past two decades, particularly those transplanted for hematologic malignancy. In the past several years this has changed with the introduction of either prophylactic or pre-emptive ganciclovir, and now foscarnet, therapy in those at risk for CMV infection. CMV disease is currently much rarer than previously seen in recipients of HLA-identical sibling transplants. It may prove more difficult to eradicate CMV disease in recipients of HLA-disparate family member transplants or matched or mismatched unrelated donor transplants. Respiratory viruses are now the most common viral cause of IP.

Idiopathic IP is likely a multifactorial process, involving at least chemo- and radiotherapy toxicity of the lungs, undocumented infections, and a GVHD-related cytotoxic process. Further studies are needed to more fully understand the pathogenesis of this syndrome.

References

Akasheh, M.S., Freytes, C.O., & Vesole, D.H. (2000). Melphalan-associated pulmonary toxicity folowing high-dose therapy with autologous hematopoietic stem cell transplantation. *Bone Marrow Transplantation, 26,* 1107–9.

Anscher, M.S., Peters, W.P., Reisenbichler, H. *et al.* (1993). Transforming growth factor beta as a predictor of liver and lung fibrosis after autologous bone marrow transplantation for advanced breast cancer. *New England Journal of Medicine, 328,* 1592–8.

Appelbaum, F.R., Meyers, J.D., Fefer, A. *et al.* (1982). Non bacterial, non fungal pneumonia following marrow transplantation in 100 identical twins. *Transplantation, 33,* 265–8.

Aspin, M.M., Gallez-Hawkins, G.M., Giugni, T.D. *et al.* (1994). Comparison of plasma PCR and bronchoalveolar lavage fluid culture for detection of cytomegalovirus infection in adult bone marrow transplant recipients. *Journal of Clinical Microbiology, 32,* 2266–9.

Atkinson, K., Arthur, C., Bradstock, K. *et al.* (1995). Prophylactic ganciclovir is more effective in HLA-identical family member marrow transplant recipients than in more heavily immune suppressed HLA-identical unrelated donor marrow transplant recipients. *Bone Marrow Transplantation, 16,* 401–5.

Atkinson, K., Bryant, D., Delprado, W. *et al.* (1989). Widespread pulmonary fibrosis as a major clinical manifestation of chronic graft-versus-host disease. *Bone Marrow Transplantation, 4,* 129–32.

Atkinson, K., Downs, K., Golenia, M. *et al.* (1991a). Prophylactic use of ganciclovir in allogeneic bone marrow transplantation: absence of clinical cytomegalovirus infection. *British Journal of Haematology, 79,* 57–62.

Atkinson, K., Nivison-Smith, I., Dodds, A. *et al.* (1998). A comparison of the pattern of interstitial pneumonitis following allogeneic bone marrow transplantation before and after the introduction of prophylactic ganciclovir therapy in 1989. *Bone Marrow Transplantation, 21,* 691–5.

Atkinson, K., Turner, J., Biggs, J.C. *et al.* (1991b). An acute pulmonary syndrome possibly representing acute graft-versus-host disease involving the lung interstitium. *Bone Marrow Transplantation*, **8**, 231–4.

Aversa, F., Tabilio, A., Terenzi, A. *et al.* (1994). Successful engraftment of T cell depleted haploidentical "three loci" incompatible transplants in leukemia patients by addition of recombinant human granulocyte colony stimulating factor mobilized peripheral blood progenitor cells to bone marrow inoculum. *Blood*, **84**, 3948–55.

Avery, R.K., Adal, K.A., Longworth, D.L., & Bolwell, B.J. (2000). A survey of allogeneic bone marrow transplant programs in the United States regarding cytomegalovirus prophylaxis and preemptive therapy. *Bone Marrow Transplantation*, **26**, 763–7.

Bacigalupo, A., Bregante, S., Tedone, E. *et al.* (1996). Combined foscarnet-ganciclovir treatment for cytomeglovirus infections after allogeneic hemopoietic stem cell transplantation. *Transplantation*, **62**, 376–80.

Bacigalupo, A., Mordini, N., Pitto, G. *et al.* (1997). Transplantation of HLA-mismatched CD34+ selected cells in patients with advanced malignancies: severe immunodeficiency and related complications. *British Journal of Haematology*, **98**, 760–6.

Bass, E.B., Powe, N.R., Goodman, S.N. *et al.* (1993). Efficacy of immune globulin in preventing complications of bone marrow transplantation: a meta-analysis. *Bone Marrow Transplantation*, **12**, 273–82.

Ben-Ari, J., Yaniv, I., Nahum, E. *et al.* (2001). Yield of bronchalveolar lavage in ventilated and non-ventilared children after bone marrow transplantation. *Bone Marrow Transplantation*, **27**, 191–4.

Bilgrami, S., Aslanzadeh, J., Feingold, J.M. *et al.* (1999). Cytomegalovirus viremia, viruria and disease after autologous peripheral blood stem cell transplantation: no need for surveillance. *Bone Marrow Transplantation*, **24**, 69–73.

Bilgrami, S.F., Metersky, M.L., McNally, D. *et al.* (2001). Idiopathic pneumonia syndrome following myeloablative chemotherapy and autologous transplantation. *Annals of Pharmacotherapy*, **35**, 196–201.

Boeckh, M., Gooley, T.A., Myerson, D. *et al.* (1996a). Cytomegalovirus pp65 antigenemia-guided early treatment with ganciclovir versus ganciclovir at engraftment after allogeneic marrow transplantation: a randomized double-blind study. *Blood*, **88**, 4063–71.

Boeckh, M., Stevens-Ayers, T., Bowden, R.A. *et al.* (1996b). Cytomegalovirus pp65 antigenemia after autologous marrow and peripheral blood stem cell transplantation. *Journal of Infectious Diseases*, **174**, 907–12.

Boeckh, M., Zaia, J.A., Jung, D. *et al.* (1998). A study of the pharmacokinetics, antiviral activity, and tolerability of oral ganciclovir for CMV prophylaxis in marrow transplantation. *Biology of Blood and Marrow Transplantation*, **4**, 13–9.

Bowden, R.A. (1997). Respiratory virus infections after marrow transplant: The Fred Hutchinson Cancer Research Center experience. *American Journal of Medicine*, **102**, (3A), 27–30.

Bowden, R.A., Sayers, M., Fluornoy, N. *et al.* (1986). Cytomegalovirus immune globulin and seronegative blood products to prevent primary cytomegalovirus infection after marrow transplantation. *New England Journal of Medicine*, **314**, 1006–10.

Bregante, S., Bertilson, S., Tedone, E. *et al.* (2000). Foscarnet prophylaxis of cytomegalovirus infections in patients undergoing allogeneic bone marrow transplantation (BMT): a dose-finding study. *Bone Marrow Transplantation*, **26**, 23–9.

Bretagne, S., Costa, J.M., Foulet, F. *et al.* (2000). Prospective study of toxoplasma reactivation by PCR in allogeneic stem cell transplant recipients. *Transplant Infectious Diseases*, **2**, 127–132.

Bretagne, S., Costa, J.M., Kuentz, M. *et al.* (1995). Late toxoplasmosis evidenced by PCR in a marrow transplant recipient. *Bone Marrow Transplantation*, **15**, 809–11.

Broers, A.E.C., van der Holt, R., van Esser, J.W.J. *et al.* (2000). Increased transplant-related morbidity and mortality in CMV-seropositive patients despite highly effective prevention of CMV disease after allogeneic T-cell-depleted stem cell transplantation. *Blood*, **95**, 2240–5.

Brown, J.M., Weissman, I.L., & Shizuru, J.A. (2001). Immunity to infections following hematopoietic cell transplantation. *Current Opinion in Immunology*, **13**, 451–7.

Canpolat, C., Culbert, S., Gardner, M. *et al.* (1996). Ganciclovir prophylaxis for cytomegalovirus infection in pediatric allogeneic bone marrow transplant recipients. *Bone Marrow Transplantation*, **17**, 589–93.

Carlson, K., Backlund, L., Smedmyr, B. *et al.* (1994). Pulmonary function and complications subsequent to autologous bone marrow transplantation. *Bone Marrow Transplantation*, **14**, 805–11.

Carrigan, D.R., Drobyski, W.R., Russler, S.K. *et al.* (1991). Interstitial pneumonitis associated with human herpesvirus-6 infection after marrow transplantation. *Lancet*, **338**, 147–9.

Castagnola, E., Dini, G., Lanino, E. *et al.* (1995). Low CD4 lymphocyte count in a patient with P carinii pneumonia after autologous bone marrow transplantation. *Bone Marrow Transplantation*, **15**, 977–8.

Chakrabarti, S., Collingham, K.E., Holder, K. *et al.* (2001). Preemptive oral ribavirin therapy of paramyxovirus infections after haematopoietic stem cell transplantation: a pilot study. *Bone Marrow Transplantation*, **28**, 759–63.

Clark, J.G., Hansen, J.A., Hertz, M.L. *et al.* (1993). NHLBI Workshop summary. Idiopathic pneumonia syndrome after bone marrow transplantation. *American Review of Respiratory Disease*, **147**, 1601–6.

Clark, J.G., Madtes, D.K., Martin, T.R. *et al.* (1999). Idiopathic pneumonia after bone marrow transplantation: cytokine activation and lipopolysaccharide amplification in the bronchoalveolar compartment. *Critical Care Medicine*, **27**, 1800–6.

Colby, C., McAfee, S.L., Sackstein, R. *et al.* (1999). A prospective randomized trial comparing the toxicity and safety of atovaquone with trimethoprim/sulfamethoxazole as Pneumocystis carinii pneumonia prophylaxis following autologous peripheral blood stem cell transplantation. *Bone Marrow Transplantation*, **24**, 897–902.

Cone, R., Hackman, R., Huang, M. *et al.* (1993). Human Herpesvirus 6 in lung tissue from patients with pneumonitis after bone marrow transplantation. *New England Journal of Medicine*, **329**, 156–61.

Cooke, K.R., Kobzik, L., Martin, T.R. *et al.* (1996). An experimental model of idiopathic pneumonia syndrome after bone marrow transplantation: I. the roles of minor H antigens and endotoxin. *Blood*, **88**, 3230–9.

Cooke, K.R., Krenger, W., Hill, G. *et al.* (1998). Host reactive donor T cells are associated with lung injury after experimental allogeneic bone marrow transplantation. *Blood*, **92**, 2571–80.

Cordonnier, C., Bernaudin, J.F., Bierling, P. *et al.* (1986). Pulmonary complications occurring after allogeneic bone marrow transplantation. *Cancer,* **58,** 1047–54.

Cordonnier, C., Chevret, S., Legrand, M. *et al.* (2001). IV immuneglobulin prophylaxis in allogeneic sibling stem cell transplant patients: a randomized, dose-effect, placebo-controlled, double-blind, multicenter trial. *Blood,* **98,** 779a.

Cordonnier, C., Escudier, E., Nicolas, J.C. *et al.* (1987). Evaluation of three assays on alveolar lavage fluid and the diagnosis of cytomegalovirus pneumonitis after bone marrow transplantation. *Journal of Infectious Diseases,* **155,** 495–500.

Couriel, D., Canosa, J., Engler, H. *et al.* (1996). Early reactivation of cytomegalovirus and high risk of interstitial pneumonitis following T depleted BMT for adults with hematological malignancies. *Bone Marrow Transplantation,* **18,** 347–53.

Crawford, S.W., Bowden, R.A., Hackman, R.C. *et al.* (1988). Rapid detection of cytomegalovirus pulmonary infection by bronchoalveolar lavage and centrifugation and culture. *Annals of Internal Medicine,* **108,** 180–5.

Cwynarski, K., Ainsworth, J., Cobbold, M. *et al.* (2001). Direct visualization of cytomegalovirus-specific T-cell reconstitution after allogeneic stem cell transplantation. *Blood,* **97,** 1232–40.

de Lassence, A., Fleury-Feith, J., Beaune, J. *et al.* (1995). Alveolar hemorrhage: diagnostic criteria and results in 194 immunocompromised hosts. *American Journal of Respiratory and Critical Care Medicine,* **151,** 157–63.

Derouin, F., Gluckman, E., Beauvais, B. *et al.* (1986). Toxoplasma infection after human allogeneic bone marrow transplantation: clinical and serological study of 80 patients. *Bone Marrow Transplantation,* **1,** 67–73.

de Medeiros, C.R., Moreira, V.A., & Pasquini, R. (2000). Cytomegalovirus as a cause of very late interstitial pneumonia after bone marrow transplantation, *Bone Marrow Transplantation,* **26,** 443–4.

DeVincenzo, J.P., Hirsch, R.L., Fuentes, R.J., & Top, F.H. (2000). Respiratory syncytial virus immune globulin treatment of lower respiratory tract infection in pediatric patients undergoing bone marrow transplantation. *Bone Marrow Transplantation,* **25,** 161–5.

DiNubile, M. J., Stossel, T. P., Ljunghusen, O. C. *et al.* (2002). Prognostic implications of declining gelsolin levels after allogeneic stem cell transplantation. *Blood,* **100,** 4367–71.

Drobyski, W.R., Knox, K.K., Carrigan, D.R., & Ash, R.C. (1991). Foscarnet therapy of ganciclovir-resistant cytomegalovirus in marrow transplantation. *Transplantation,* **52,** 155–7.

Einsele, H., Ehninger, G., Steadle, M. *et al.* (1993). Lymphocytopenia as an unfavorable prognostic factor in patients with cytomegalovirus infection after bone marrow transplantation. *Blood,* **82,** 1672.

Einsele, H., Hebart, H., Kauffmann-Schneider, C. *et al.* (2000). Risk factors for treatment failures in patients receiving PCR-based preemptive therapy for CMV infection. *Bone Marrow Transplantation,* **25,** 757–63.

Einsele, H., Steidle, M., Vallbracht, A. *et al.* (1991). Early occurrence of human cytomegalovirus infection after bone marrow transplantation as demonstrated by the polymerase chain reaction. *Blood,* **77,** 1104–10.

Einsele, H., Roosnek, E., Rufer, N. *et al.* (2002). Infusion of cytomegalovirus (CMV)-specific T cells for the treatment of CMV infection not responding to antiviral chemotherapy. *Blood,* **99:** 3916–3922.

Ellis, M.E., Spence, D., Bouchama, A. *et al.* (1995). Open lung biopsy provides a higher and more specific diagnostic yield compared to broncho-alveolar lavage in immunocompromised patients. *Scandinavian Journal of Infectious Disease,* **27,** 157–62.

Emanuel, D., Cunningham, I., Jules-Elysee, K. *et al.* (1988). Cytomegalovirus pneumonia after bone marrow transplantation successfully treated with the combination of ganciclovir and high dose intravenous immunoglobulin. *Annals of Internal Medicine,* **109,** 777–82.

Emanuel, D., Peppard, J., Stover, D. *et al.* (1986). Rapid immunodiagnosis of cytomegalovirus pneumonia by broncho-alveolar lavage using human and murine monoclonal antibodies. *Annals of Internal Medicine,* **104,** 476–81.

Ettinger, N.A., Selby, P., Powles, R. *et al.* (1989). Cytomegalovirus pneumonia: the use of ganciclovir in marrow transplant recipients. *Journal of Antimicrobial Chemotherapy,* **24,** 53–62.

Flomemberg, P., Babbitt, J., Brobyski, W.R. *et al.* (1994). Increasing incidence of adenovirus disease in bone marrow transplant recipients. *Journal of Infectious Diseases,* **169,** 775–81.

Fries, B.C., Khaira, D., Pepe, M.S., & Torok-Storb, B. (1993). Declining lymphocyte counts following cytomegalovirus (CMV) infection are associated with fatal CMV disease in bone marrow transplant patients. *Experimental Hematology,* **21,** 1387–92.

Gagnon, S., Boota, A.M., Fischl, M.A. *et al.* (1990). Corticosteroids as adjunctive therapy for severe Pneumocystis carinii pneumonia in the acquired immunodeficiency syndrome. *New England Journal of Medicine,* **323,** 1444–50.

Garvy, B.A. & Harmsen, A.G. (1996). The role of T cells in infection-driven interstitial pneumonia after bone marrow transplantation in mice. *Transplantation,* **62,** 517–25.

Ghosh, S., Champlin, R.E., Ueno, N.T. *et al.* (2001). Respiratory syncytial viral infections in autologous blood and marrow transplant recipients with breast cancer: combination therapy with aerosolized ribavirin and parenteral immunoglobulins. *Bone Marrow Transplantation,* **28,** 271–5.

Gleaves, C.A. & Meyers, J.D. (1989). Rapid detection of cytomegalovirus in bronchoalveolar lavage specimans for marrow transplant patients: evaluation of a direct fluorescein-conjugated monoclonal antibody reagent. *Journal of Virological Methods,* **26,** 345–9.

Gleaves, C.A., Smith, T.F., Shuster, E.A., & Pearson, G.R. (1985). Comparison of standard tube and shell vial culture techniques for the detection of cytomegalovirus and clinical specimens. *Journal of Clinical Microbiology,* **21,** 217–21.

Gondo, H., Harada, A.M., Hara, N. *et al.* (1993). Idiopathic interstitial pneumonitis possibly associated with chronic graft-versus-host disease. *Rinsho Ketsueki,* **34,** 183–9.

Goodrich, J.M., Bowden, R.A., Fisher, L. *et al.* (1993). Ganciclovir prophylaxis to prevent cytomegalovirus disease after allogeneic marrow transplant. *Annals of Internal Medicine,* **118,** 173–8.

Goodrich, J.M., Mori, M., Gleaves, C.A. *et al.* (1991). Early treatment with ganciclovir to prevent cytomegalovirus disease after allogeneic bone marrow transplantation. *New England Journal of Medicine*, **325**, 1601–7.

Gozlan, J., Laporte, J.P., Lesage, S. *et al.* (1996). Monitoring of cytomegalovirus infection and disease in bone marrow recipients by reverse transcription PCR and comparison with PCR and blood and urine cultures. *Journal of Clinical Microbiology*, **34**, 2085–8.

Grundy, J.E., Ehrnst, A., Einsele, H. *et al.* (1996). A 3-center European external quality control study of PCR for detection of cytomegalovirus DNA in blood. *Journal of Clinical Microbiology*, **34**, 1166–70.

Hayes-Jordan, A., Benaim, E., Richardson, S. *et al.* (2002). Open lung biopsy in pediatric bone marrow transplant patients. *Journal of Pediatric Surgery*, **37**, 446–52.

Hebart, H., Muller, C., Loüffler, J. *et al.* (1996). Monitoring of CMV infection: a comparison of PCR from whole blood, plasma-PCR, pp65-antigenemia and virus culture in patients after bone marrow transplantation. *Bone Marrow Transplantation*, **17**, 861–8.

Hebart, H., Wuchter, P., Loeffler, J. *et al.* (2001). Evaluation of the Murex CMV DNA Hybrid Capture assay (version 2.0) for early diagnosis of cytomegalovirus infection in recipients of an allogeneic stem cell transplant. *Bone Marrow Transplantation*, **28**, 213–8.

Hersman, J., Meyers, J.D., Thomas, E.D. *et al.* (1982). The effect of granulocyte transfusion on the incidence of cytomegalovirus infection after allogeneic marrow transplantation. *Annals of Internal Medicine*, **96**, 149–52.

Hertz, M.I., Englund, Z.A., Snover, D. *et al.* (1989). Respiratory syncytial virus-induced acute lung injury in adult patients with bone marrow transplants: a clinical approach and review of the literature. *Medicine*, **68**, 269–81.

Holmberg, L., Boeckh, M., Hooper, H. *et al.* (1999). Increased incidence of cytomegalovirus disease after autologous CD34-selected peripheral blood stem cell transplantation. *Blood*, **94**, 4029–35.

Jules-Elysee, K.D.E., Stover, D., Yahalom, J. *et al.* (1992). Pulmonary complications in lymphoma patients treated with high dose therapy and autologous bone marrow transplantation. *American Review of Respiratory Diseases*, **146**, 485–91.

Kanda, Y., Mineishi, S., Saito, T. *et al.* (2001). Pre-emptive therapy against cytomegalovirus (CMV) disease guided by CMV antigenemia assay after allogeneic hematopoietic stem cell transplantation: a single-center experience in Japan. *Bone Marrow Transplantation*, **27**, 437–44.

Kantrow, S.P., Hackman, R.C., Boeckh, M. *et al.* (1997). Idiopathic pneumonia syndrome: changing spectrum of lung injury after marrow transplantation. *Transplantation*, **63**, 1079–86.

Khouri, N.S., Saral, R., Armstrong, E.M. *et al.* (1979). Pulmonary interstitial changes following bone marrow transplantation. *Radiology*, **133**, 587–92.

Kleihauer, A., Grigoleit, U., Hebart, H. *et al.* (2001). Ex vivo generation of human cytomegalovirus-specific cytotoxic T cells by peptide-pulsed dendritic cells. *British Journal of Haematology*, **113**, 231–9.

Konoplev, S., Champlin, R.E., Giralt, S. *et al.* (2001). Cytomegalovirus pneumonia in adult autologous blood and marrow transplant recipients. *Bone Marrow Transplantation*, **27**, 877–81.

Kottaridis, P.D., Ketley, N., Peggs, K. *et al.* (1999). An unusual case of intrapulmonary granulocytic sarcoma presenting as interstitial pneumonitis following allogeneic bone marrow transplantation for acute myeloid leukaemia and responding to donor lymphocyte infusion. *Bone Marrow Transplantation*, **24**, 807–9.

La Rosa, A.M., Champlin, R.E., Mirza, R. *et al.* (2001). Adenovirus infections in adult recipients of blood and marrow transplants. *Clinical Infectious Diseases*, **32**, 871–6.

Leblond, V., Zouabi, H., Sutton, L. *et al.* (1994). Late CD8+ lymphocytic alveolitis after allogeneic bone marrow transplantation in chronic graft-versus-host disease. *American Journal of Respiratory and Critical Care Medicine*, **150**, 1056–61.

Li, C.R., Greenberg, P.D., Gilbert, M.J. *et al.* (1994). Recovery of HLA-restricted cytomegalovirus (CMV)-specific T-cell responses after allogeneic bone marrow transplant: correlation with CMV disease and effect of ganciclovir prophylaxis. *Blood*, **83**, 1971–9.

Link, H., Battmer, K., & Stumme, C. (1993). Cytomegalovirus infection in leukocytes after bone marrow transplantation demonstrated by mRNA in situ hybridization. *British Journal of Haematology*, **85**, 573–7.

Ljungman, P., Biron, P., Bosi, A. *et al.* (1994). Cytomegalovirus interstitial pneumonia in autologous bone marrow transplant recipients. *Bone Marrow Transplantation*, **13**, 209–12.

Ljungman, P., & Griffiths, P. (1993). Definitions of cytomegalovirus infection and disease. In: *Multidisciplinary approach to understanding cytomegalovirus disease*, ed. S. Michelson & S. Plotkin, pp. 233–7. Amsterdam: Experta Medica International Congress Series.

Ljungman, P., Griffiths, P., & Paya, C. (2002). Definitions of cytomegalovirus infection and disease in transplant recipients. *Clinical Infectious Diseases*, **34**, 1094–7.

Ljungman, P., Lore, K., Aschan, J. *et al.* (1996a). Use of a semi-quantitative PCR for cytomegalovirus DNA as a basis for pre-emptive antiviral therapy in allogeneic bone marrow transplant patients. *Bone Marrow Transplantation*, **17**, 583–7.

Ljungman, P., Niederwieser, D., Pepe, M.S. *et al.* (1990). Cytomegalovirus infection after marrow transplantation for aplastic anemia. *Bone Marrow Transplantation*, **6**, 295–300.

Ljungman, P., Oberg, G., Aschan, J. *et al.* (1996b). Foscarnet for pre-emptive therapy of CMV infection detected by a leukocyte-based nested PCR in allogeneic bone marrow transplant patients. *Bone Marrow Transplantation*, **18**, 565–8.

Ljungman, P., Ward, K.N., Crooks, B.N.A. *et al.* (2001). Respiratory virus infections after stem cell transplantation: a prospective study from the Infectious Diseases Working Party of the European Group for Blood and Marrow Transplantation. *Bone Marrow Transplantation*, **28**, 479–84.

Lyytikäinen, O., Ruutu, T., Volin, L. *et al.* (1996). Late onset Pneumocystis carinii pneumonia following allogeneic bone marrow transplantation. *Bone Marrow Transplantation*, **17**, 1057–9.

Mahon, F.X., Sadoun, A., Benz-Lemoine, E. *et al.* (1991). Possible prevention of Pneumocystis carinii pneumonia by pentamidine aerosol after bone marrow transplantation. *Bone Marrow Transplantation*, **8**, 64–5.

Maltazou, H., Whimbey, E., Abi-Said, D. *et al.* (1999). Cytomegalovirus disease in adult marrow transplant recipients receiving ganciclovir prophylaxis: a retrospective study. *Bone Marrow Transplantation*, **24**, 665–9.

Maltezou, H.C., Petropoulos, D., Choroszy, M. *et al.* (1997). Dapsone for Pneumocystis carinii prophylaxis in children undergoing bone marrow transplantation. *Bone Marrow Transplantation*, **20**, 879–81.

Marin, D., Gonzalez-Barca, E., Domingo, E. *et al.* (1998). Noninvasive mechanical ventilation in a patient with respiratory failure after hematopoietic progenitor transplantation. *Bone Marrow Transplantation*, **22**, 1123–4.

Martin, W.J. & Smith, T.F. (1986). Rapid detection of cytomegalovirus in broncho-alveolar lavage specimans by monoclonal antibody method. *Journal of Clinical Microbiology*, **23**, 1106–8.

Martino, R., Maertens, J., Bretagne, S. *et al.* (2000). Toxoplasmosis after hematopoietic stem cell transplantation. A study by the European Group for Blood and Marrow Transplantation Infectious Diseases Working Party. *Clinical Infectious Diseases*, **31**(5), 1188–94.

Martino, R., Martinez, C., Brunet, S., & Sureda, A. (1995). Successful bone marrow transplantation in patients with recent Pneumocystis carinii pneumonia: report of two cases. *Bone Marrow Transplantation*, **16**, 491–2.

Metcalf, P., Rennard, S.I., Reed, E.C. *et al.* (1994). Corticosteroids as adjunctive therapy for diffuse alveolar hemorrhage associated with bone marrow transplantation. *American Journal of Medicine*, **96**, 327–34.

Meyers, J.D., Flournoy, N., & Thomas, E.D. (1982). Non bacterial pneumonia after allogeneic marrow transplantation: a review of 10 years' experience. *Reviews of Infectious Diseases*, **4**, 1119–32.

Meyers, J.D., Flournoy, N., & Thomas, E.D. (1986). Risk factors for cytomegalovirus infection after human marrow transplantation. *Journal of Infectious Diseases*, **153**, 478–88.

Meyers, J.D., Hackman, R.C., & Stamm, W.E. (1983). Chlamydia trachomatis infection as a cause of pneumonia after human marrow transplantation. *Transplantation*, **36**, 130–4.

Meyers, J.D., Reid, E.C., Schepp, D.H. *et al.* (1988). Acyclovir for prevention of cytomegalovirus infection and disease after allogeneic marrow transplantation. *New England Journal of Medicine*, **318**, 70–5.

Milburne, H.J., Prentice, H.G., & Grundy, J.E. (1993). IgG subclasses in the lungs of patients with interstitial pneumonitis following bone marrow transplantation. *European Respiratory Journal*, **6**, 944–50.

Nelson, P.N., Rawal, B.K., Boriskin, Y.S. *et al.* (1996). A polymerase chain reaction to detect a spliced late transcript of human cytomegalovirus in the blood of bone marrow transplant recipients. *Journal of Virological Methods*, **56**, 139–48.

Nichols, W.G., Corey, L., Gooley, T. *et al.* (2001a). Rising pp65 antigenemia during preemptive anticytomegalovirus therapy after allogeneic hematopoietic stem cell transplantation: risk factors, correlation with DNA load, and outcomes. *Blood*, **97**, 867–74.

Nichols, W.G., Corey, L., Gooley, T. *et al.* (2001b). Parainfluenza virus infections after hematopoietic stem cell transplantation: risk factors, response to antiviral therapy, and effect on transplant outcome. *Blood*, **98**, 573–8.

Noel, D.R., Witherspoon, R.P., & Storb, R. (1978). Does graft-versus-host disease influence the tempo of immunologic recovery after allogeneic human marrow transplantation? An observation of 56 long-term survivors. *Blood*, **51**, 1087–105.

Nguyen, Q., Champlin, R., Giralt, S. *et al.* (1999). Late cytomegalovirus pneumonia in adult allogeneic blood and marrow transplant recipients. *Clinical Infectious Diseases*, **28**, 618–23.

Panoskaltsis-Mortari, A., Strieter, R.M., Hermanson, J.R. *et al.* (2000). Induction of monocyte - and T-cell-attracting chemokines in the lung during the generation of idiopathic pneumonia syndrome following allogeneic murine bone marrow transplantation. *Blood*, **96**, 834–9.

Pareja, J.G., Garland, R., & Koziel, H. (1998). Use of adjunctive corticosteroids in severe adult non-HIV Pneumocystis carinii pneumonia. *Chest*, **113**, 1215–24.

Pecego, R., Hill, R., Appelbaum, F.R. *et al.* (1986). Interstitial pneumonitis following autologous bone marrow transplantation. *Transplantation*, **42**, 515–7.

Prentice, H.G., Gluckman, E., Powles, R.L. *et al.* (1994). Impact of long-term acyclovir on cytomegalovirus infection and survival after allogeneic bone marrow transplantation. European Acyclovir for CMV Prophylaxis Study Group. *Lancet*, **343**, 749–53.

Przepiorka, D., Ippoliti, C., Panina, A. *et al.* (1994). Ganciclovir 3 times per week is not adequate to prevent cytomegalovirus reactivation after T cell depleted marrow transplantation. *Bone Marrow Transplantation*, **13**, 461–4.

Przepiorka, D., Selvaggi, K., Rosenzweig, P.Q. *et al.* (1991). Aerosolized pentamidine for prevention of pneumocystis pneumonia after allogeneic marrow transplantation. *Bone Marrow Transplantation*, **7**, 324–35.

Quinnan, G.V., Kirmani, N., Esber, E. *et al.* (1981). HLA-restricted cytotoxic T lymphocyte and nonthymic cytotoxic lymphocyte responses to cytomegalovirus infection of bone marrow transplant recipients. *Journal of Immunology*, **126**, 2036–41.

Reed, E.C., Bowden, R.A., Dandliker, P.S. *et al.* (1988). Treatment of cytomegalovirus pneumonia with ganciclovir and intravenous cytomegalovirus immunoglobulin in patients with bone marrow transplants. *Annals of Internal Medicine*, **109**, 783–8.

Reusser, P., Einsele, H., Lee, J. *et al.* (2002). Randomized multicenter trial of foscarnet versus ganciclovir for preemptive therapy of cytomegalovirus infection after allogeneic stem cell transplantation. *Blood*, **99**, 1159–64.

Reusser, P., Fisher, L.D., Buckner, C.D. *et al.* (1990). Cytomegalovirus infection after autologous bone marrow transplantation: occurrence of cytomegalovirus disease and effect on engraftment. *Blood*, **75**, 1888–94.

Reusser, P., Riddell, S.R., Meyers, J.D., & Greenberg, P.D. (1991). Cytotoxic T lymphocyte responses to cytomegalovirus after human allogeneic bone marrow transplantation: pattern of recovery and correlation with cytomegalovirus infection and disease. *Blood*, **78**, 1373–80.

Ringden, O., Horowitz, M.M., Gale, R.P. *et al.* (1993). Outcome after allogeneic bone marrow transplant for leukemia in older adults. *Journal of the American Medical Association*, **270**, 57–60.

Rubie, H., Attal, M., Campardou, A.M. *et al.* (1993). Risk factors for cytomegalovirus infection in BMT recipients transfused exclusively with seronegative blood products. *Bone Marrow Transplantation*, **11**, 209–14.

Ruutu, T. & Volon, L. (1990). Cytomegalovirus is frequently isolated in broncho-alveolar lavage fluid at bone marrow transplant recipients without pneumonia. *Annals of Internal Medicine*, **112**, 913–6.

Sandler, E.S., Aquino, V.M., Gross-Shohet, E. *et al.* (1997). BK papova virus pneumonia following hematopoietic stem cell transplantation. *Bone Marrow Transplantation*, **20**, 163–5.

Schmidt, G.M., Horak, D.A., Niland, J.C. *et al.* (1991). A randomized, controlled trial of prophylactic ganciclovir for cytomegalovirus pulmonary infection in recipients of allogeneic bone marrow transplants. *New England Journal of Medicine*, **324**, 1005–11.

Schmidt, G.M., Kovacs, A., & Zaia, J.A. (1988). Ganciclovir/immunoglobulin combination therapy for the treatment of CMV-associated interstitial pneumonitis in bone marrow allograft recipients. *Transplantation*, **46**, 905–7.

Shields, A.F., Hackman, R.C., Fife, K.H. *et al.* (1985). Adenovirus infections in patients undergoing bone marrow transplantation. *New England Journal of Medicine*, **312**, 529–33.

Small, T.N., Leung, L., Stiles, J. *et al.* (2000). Disseminated toxoplasmosis following T cell-depleted related and unrelated bone marrow transplantation. *Bone Marrow Transplantation*, **25**, 969–73.

Snyder, C.L., Ramsay, N.K., McGlave, P.B. *et al.* (1990). Diagnostic open lung biopsy after bone marrow transplantation. *Journal of Pediatric Surgery*, **25**, 871–7.

Souza, J.P., Boeckh, M., Gooley, T.A. *et al.* (1999). High rates of Pneumocystis carinii pneumonia in allogeneic blood and marrow transplant recipients receiving dapsone prophylaxis. *Clinical Infectious Diseases*, **29**, 1467–71.

Springmeyer, S.C., Silvestri, R.C., Sale, G.E. *et al.* (1982). The role of transbronchial biopsy for the diagnosis of diffuse pneumonias in immunocompromised marrow transplant recipients. *American Review of Respiratory Diseases*, **126**, 763–5.

Stals, F.S., Steinhoff, G., Wagenaar, S.S. *et al.* (1996). Cytomegalovirus induces interstitial lung disease in allogeneic bone marrow transplant recipient rats independent of acute graft-versus-host response. *Laboratory Investigation*, **74**, 343–52.

Sullivan, K.M., Meyers, J.B., Flournoy, N. *et al.* (1986). Early and late interstitial pneumonia following bone marrow transplantation. *International Journal of Cell Cloning*, **4**, 107–21.

Sullivan, K.M., Seidel, K., Jocom, J. *et al.* (2000). Intravenous immunoglobulin prophylaxis in unrelated donor marrow transplantation: a phase III double-blind, placebo-controlled multi-institutional trial. In *Proceedings of the Thirty-sixth Annual Meeting of the American Society of Clinical Oncology*, **19**, (abstract).

Trenschel, R., Ross, S., Husing, J. *et al.* (2000). Reduced risk of persisting cytomegalovirus pp65 antigenemia and cytomegalovirus interstitial pneumonia following allogeneic PBSCT. *Bone Marrow Transplantation*, **25**, 665–72.

Tuan, I.Z., Dennison, D., & Weisdorf, D.J. (1992). Pneumocystis carinii pneumonitis following bone marrow transplantation. *Bone Marrow Transplantation*, **10**, 267–72.

Vannuchi, A.M., Glinz, S., Bosi, A. *et al.* (2001). Selective ex vivo expansion of cytomegalovirus-specific CD4$^+$ and CD8$^+$ T lymphocytes using dendritic cells pulsed with a human leucocyte antigen A 0201-restricted peptide. *British Journal of Haematology*, **113**, 479–82.

Vasconelles, M.J., Bernardo, M.V.P., King, C. *et al.* (2000). Aerosolized pentamidine as pneumocystis prophylaxis after bone marrow transplantation is inferior to other regimens and is associated with decreased survival and an increased risk of other infections. *Biology of Blood and Marrow Transplantation*, **6**, 35–43.

Verdonck, L.F., de Gast, G.C., Dekker, A.W. *et al.* (1989). Treatment of cytomegalovirus pneumonia after bone marrow transplantation with cytomegalovirus immunoglobulin combined with ganciclovir. *Bone Marrow Transplantation*, **4**, 187–9.

Vlieger, A.M., Boland, G.J., Jiwa, N.M. *et al.* (1992). Cytomegalovirus antigemia assay or PCR can be used to monitor ganciclovir treatment in bone marrow transplant recipients. *Bone Marrow Transplantation*, **9**, 247–53.

Walter, E.A., Greenberg, P.D., Gilbert, M.J. *et al.* (1995). Reconstruction of cellular immunity against cytomegalovirus in recipients of allogeneic bone marrow by transfer of T cell clones from the donor. *New England Journal of Medicine*, **333**, 1038–44.

Warwick, A.B., Mertens, A.C., Ou Shu, X. *et al.* (1998). Outcomes following mechanical ventilation in children undergoing bone marrow transplantation. *Bone Marrow Transplantation*, **22**, 787–94.

Watts, R.G. & Mroczek-Musulman, E. (1996). Pulmonary interstitial disease mimicking ideopathic pneumonia syndrome as the initial site of relapse of neuroblastoma following autologous bone marrow transplantation: a case report. *American Journal of Hematology*, **53**, 137–40.

Weiner, R.S., Bortin, M.M., Gale, R.P. *et al.* (1986). Interstitial pneumonitis after bone marrow transplantation. Assessment of risk factors. *Annals of Internal Medicine*, **104**, 168–75.

Wendt, C.H., Weisdorf, D.J., Jordan, M.C. *et al.* (1992). Parainfluenza virus respiratory infection after bone marrow transplantation. *New England Journal of Medicine*, **326**, 921–6.

Whimbey, E., Englung, J.A., & Couch, R.B. (1997). Community respiratory virus infections in immunocompromised patients with cancer. *American Journal of Medicine*, **102**(3A), 10–18.

White, P., Bonacum, J.T., & Miller, C.B. (1997). Utility of fiberoptic bronchoscopy in bone marrow transplant patients. *Bone Marrow Transplantation*, **20**, 681–7.

Wingard, J.R., Mellits, E.D., & Sostrin, M.B. (1988a). Interstitial pneumonitis after allogeneic bone marrow transplantation. Nine year experience at a single institution. *Medicine*, **67**, 175–86.

Wingard, J.R., Mellits, E.D., Sostrin, M.B. *et al.* (1988b). Interstitial pneumonitis following autologous bone marrow transplantation. *Transplantation*, **46**, 61–5.

Wingard, J.R., Piantadosi, S., Burns, W.H. *et al.* (1990). Cytomegalovirus infections in bone marrow transplant recipients given intensive cytoreductive therapy. *Reviews of Infectious Diseases*, **12** (Suppl 7), S793–804.

Winston, D.J., Ho, W.G., Bartoni, K., & Champlin, R.E. (1993a). Intravenous immunoglobulin and CMV-seronegative blood products for prevention of CMV infection and disease in bone marrow transplant recipients. *Bone Marrow Transplantation,* **12,** 283–8.

Winston, D.J., Ho, W.G., & Bartoni, K. *et al.* (1993b). Ganciclovir prophylaxis for cytomegalovirus infection and disease in allogeneic bone marrow transplant recipients. Results of a placebo-controlled double blind trial. *Annals of Internal Medicine,* **118,** 179–84.

Winston, D.J., Ho, W.G., & Champlin, R.E. (1990). Cytomegalovirus infections after allogeneic bone marrow transplantation. *Reviews of Infectious Diseases,* **12**(Suppl 7), S776–92.

Yau, J.C., Dimopoulos, M.A., Huan, S.D. *et al.* (1991). Prophylaxis of cytomegalovirus infection with ganciclovir in allogeneic marrow transplantation. *European Journal of Haematology,* **47,** 371–6.

Yousem, S.A. (1995). The histological spectrum of pulmonary graft-versus-host disease in bone marrow transplant recipients. *Human Pathology,* **26,** 668–75.

79 Hemorrhagic cystitis

DAVID S. RITCHIE AND ANDREW GRIGG

Royal Melbourne Hospital, Melbourne, Australia

Introduction

Hemorrhagic cystitis (HC) refers to the syndrome of hematuria and symptoms of lower urinary tract irritability (dysuria with frequency and urgency) that is seen following high-dose therapy and hematopoietic stem cell (HSC) transplantation. By convention these symptoms are not due to bacterial infection, glomerulopathy, or generalized bleeding diathesis, although the hematuria may be aggravated by thrombocytopenia. There is no universally accepted system that grades the severity of HC; a system proposed by Droller, Saral, and Santos (1982) is outlined in Table 79.1.

Epidemiology

The incidence of HC varies considerably according to definition, the pretransplant conditioning regimen used, preventive measures employed, and the efficacy of graft-versus-host disease (GVHD) prophylaxis. In two large series of autologous or allogeneic transplants, HC occurred in 15% to 20% of patients; of these 5% to 6% had severe HC resulting in urinary obstruction, renal failure, or the need for bladder cauterization (Sencer, Haake, & Weisdorf, 1993; Seber *et al.*, 1999). In the authors' experience, however, HC of this severity is rare. It is difficult to estimate the mortality attributable to HC per se, because of the contribution of comorbidities. Only one patient died of complications solely due to HC in the study by Sencer *et al.*, but Baronciani and colleagues (1995) reported 7 deaths in a series of 73 cases of severe HC. In addition to morbidity and mortality, considerable expense is associated with prolonged hospitalization, and often intense and invasive treatment is required for patients already vulnerable to opportunistic infections and other complications.

Pathogenesis

Although HC can present at any time following transplant, there are two main patterns with early-onset and late-onset disease. The pathogenesis of these two forms appears distinct, and each is associated with a distinct set of risk factors (Table 79.2). Early-onset HC occurs during or shortly after high-dose chemotherapy or chemoradiotherapy, usually containing an oxazophosphorine drug such as cyclophosphamide or ifosfamide. HC is the dose-limiting toxicity of ifosfamide. Acrolein, a urinary by-product of oxazophosphorine metabolism, is thought to be responsible for the urothelial toxicity (Fig. 79.1). Although the entire urinary tract is exposed to this compound, the bladder is most at risk due to prolonged exposure. Acrolein directly damages the bladder mucosa, resulting in sloughing of the epithelium, which is replaced by thin and friable granulation tissue containing telangiectatic subepithelial blood vessels. Macroscopically the bladder mucosa appears edematous and hyperemic with punctate hemorrhagic areas. The risk of HC increases with cyclophosphamide dose, and is higher in patients who have received pelvic irradiation or busulfan (Sencer *et al.*, 1993). The incidence was significantly higher in recipients of HLA-identical sibling transplants prospectively randomized to receive busulfan/cyclophosphamide as conditioning compared to those receiving cyclophosphamide/total body irradiation (TBI) (Fig. 79.2) (Ringden *et al.*, 1994). Additional risk factors identified include

Table 79.1. *Grading of hemorrhagic cystitis*

0 = no irritative symptoms
1 = micoscopic hematuria
2 = macroscopic hematuria
3 = macroscopic hematuria with small clots
4 = massive macroscopic hematuria requiring instrumentation for clot evacuation and/or causing urinary retention

Table 79.2. *Risk factors for hemorrhagic cystitis*

Early onset	Late onset
Cyclophosphamide	Early-onset hemorrhagic cystitis
Prior pelvic irradiation	Adenoviruria
Busulfan in conditioning regimen	Prolonged BK viruria
Previous busulfan therapy	GVHD

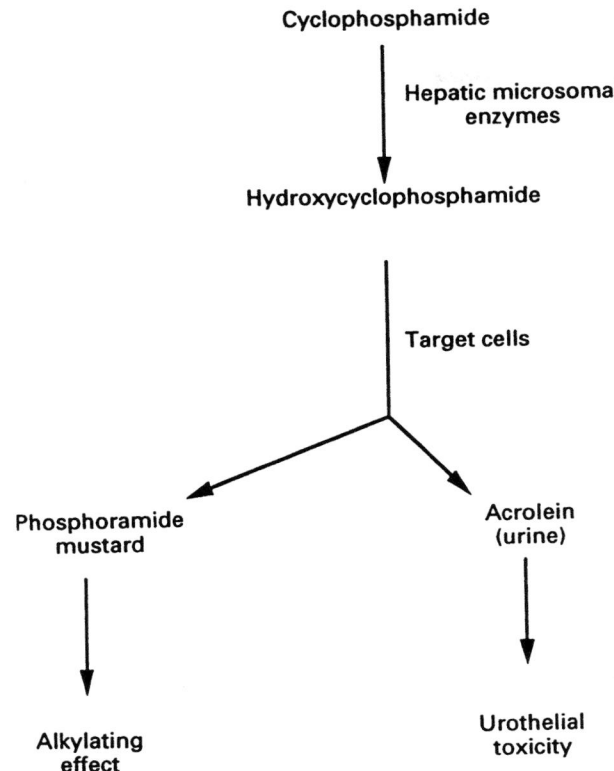

Fig. 79.1. Pathogenesis of cyclophosphamide-induced HC.

and may cause damage either by direct contact with bladder mucosa or via the bloodstream.

Delayed presentation of HC is described, occurring weeks to months posttransplant. The pathogenesis of late-onset HC is less clearly understood. Early-onset HC is a risk factor, along with viruria and GVHD. The viruses most frequently implicated are the BK virus (BKV) and adenovirus 11 (Sencer *et al.*, 1993; Russell, Vowels, & Vale, 1994; Bedi *et al.*, 1995; Childs *et al.*, 1998).

BKV is a polyomavirus, which infects the majority of the population in childhood, usually subclinically. It persists indefinitely in the kidney after primary infection and may be reactivated and excreted in the urine of immunocompromised patients. In two series roughly half of BKV-seropositive patients undergoing allogeneic bone marrow transplantation (BMT) developed BK viruria (Azzi *et al.*, 1994; Bedi *et al.*, 1995). HC has been attributed to polyoma viruses in children, but its role posttransplant is under debate, since BK viruria is also documented in the absence of HC (Bogdanovic *et al.*, 1996. Nonetheless, much circumstantial evidence favors an etiologic role for BKV. Arthur *et al.* (1988) demonstrated a temporal relationship between BK viruria and the onset of symptoms of HC. Late-onset HC lasting more than a week was associated with BKV excretion in 15 of 19 patients. Bedi and colleagues (1995) found that 19 of 38 patients who excreted BKV developed HC compared with none of 45 who did not develop viruria. In another study, quantitative polymerase chain reaction (PCR) was used to evaluate BK viruria and viremia in 50 hematopoietic stem cell transplant recipients (Leung *et al.*, 2001). When compared with asymptomatic patients, those with HC had significantly higher peak BK viruria, but no detectable

grade II–IV GVHD and age greater than 10 years (Seber *et al.*, 1999). Occasional reports exist of HC following high-dose busulfan alone. Busulfan itself is excreted unchanged in urine

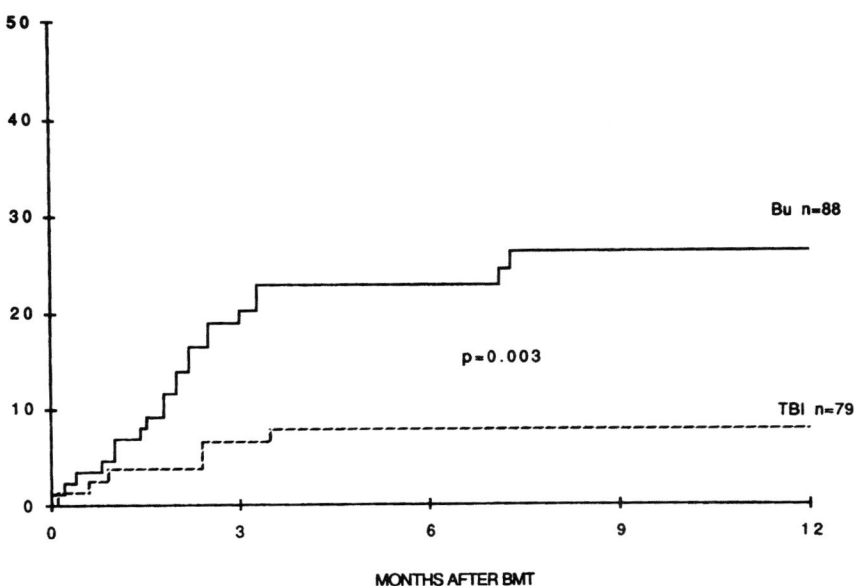

Fig. 79.2.   Time to and cumulative incidence of symptomatic HC among patients randomized to treatment with busulfan (*n* = 88) or TBI (*n* = 79). The difference was statistically significant (*P* = .003). Reproduced, with permission, from Ringden *et al.* (1994).

increase in BK viremia. In regression analysis, BK viruria was the only risk factor. The etiologic role of this agent is further supported by evidence that vidarabine decreases polyoma virus excretion, hastening resolution of symptoms (Kawakami *et al.*, 1997). Additionally, cidofovir, a cytidine nucleoside analogue active against polyomaviruses such as BK and JC viruses, has been used to successfully treat HC (Held *et al.*, 2000).

The frequency with which adenovirus is cultured from urine in patients with HC varies considerably between reports, perhaps reflecting environmental or genetic differences in patient populations. In the study by Leung and colleagues (2001), there was no difference in the degree of adenoviruria in patients with and without hemorrhagic cystitis. The species most commonly isolated has been adenovirus type 11, which has a tropism for the urinary tract. Sencer *et al.* (1993) found adenoviruria prior to hematuria to be the clinical factor most highly associated with HC. In another series, 8 of 12 patients who developed HC excreted adenovirus type 11 in their urine at the onset of cystitis; adenoviruria was rarely detected in asymptomatic patients (Miyamura *et al.*, 1989). Adenovirus-associated HC often occurred in the setting of grade II to IV acute GVHD, suggesting that viral reactivation may be related to profound immunosuppression. Furthermore, occasional reports exist in which response to antiviral therapy (adenine arabinoside and ribavirin) has resulted in resolution of both symptoms and viruria in adenovirus-associated HC (Murphy *et al.*, 1993; Kitayabashi *et al.*, 1994; Kawakami *et al.*, 1997). Cidofovir has been used successfully for the treatment of adenoviral HC in adult allogeneic stem cell transplant recipients (Sato *et al.*, 2002).

Cytomegalovirus (CMV) has been reported to cause HC (Russell *et al.*, 1994), as has HHV-6 and in separate reports have been successfully treated with ganciclovir (Spach *et al.*, 1993; Kim *et al.*, 2002).

The role of GVHD in HC is a subject of debate. The timing and severity of late-onset HC and acute GVHD are closely related. It could be argued that while the immunosuppression associated with GVHD increases the rate of viruria, HC occurs as a result of the bladder epithelium acting as a target organ for GVHD rather than from direct viral injury. Ost *et al.* (1987) have argued that bladder epithelium may be a target for acute GVHD, although the typical mononuclear inflammatory infiltrate seen in chronic GVHD is not seen on biopsy or at autopsy. In a series of 65 children undergoing allogeneic BMT, the frequency of HC among patients with grade II to IV acute GVHD was 40% (Russell *et al.*, 1994). Two other reports have found acute GVHD to be a risk factor (Seber *et al.*, 1999; Trotman *et al.*, 1999). However, in their large series, Sencer and colleagues (1993) did not find GVHD to be independently associated with HC in adults by multivariate analysis. In contrast, Childs *et al.* (1998) found that T-cell depletion was associated with a high incidence of virally induced HC, probably reflecting the poor immune reconstitution that occurs following T-depleted allografts.

Diagnosis

The diagnosis of HC is usually made on clinical grounds. A midstream urine (MSU) sample is necessary to exclude bacterial infection. Urinary cytology may demonstrate characteristic changes in urothelial cells in up to a third of patients with hematuria following transplant. These consist of an increased number of enlarged and abnormally shaped cells containing hyperchromatic nuclei (Stella *et al.*, 1990). Polyomavirus is associated with intranuclear inclusion bodies in uroepithelial cells in urine, detectable with the Papanicolaou[1] stain (Kawakami *et al.*, 1997). The presence of BKV is demonstrable on electron microscopy, by enzyme-linked immunosorbent assay (ELISA) of the supernatant of centrifuged urine, or by detection of BKV genomic sequences by PCR. BKV grows poorly in cell lines normally used for viral culture, and may require special cells (such as HEK cells) for culture. BKV detection in the urine by PCR is the most reliable and rapid means by which to detect infection.

Adenovirus can be demonstrated by standard cell culture or by electron microscopy, and may be distinguished from BKV by the larger diameter of viral particles on transmission electron microscopy of urinary sediment (Kawakami *et al.*, 1997). PCR and in situ hybridization have been used to detect adenovirus DNA in paraffin-embedded lung biopsies from transplant recipients with pneumonitis, nephritis, and cystitis (Matsuse *et al.*, 1994). Similarly PCR of urine samples will reliably detect adenovirus infection. Serologic tests for these viruses are generally not helpful.

Imaging modalities have not traditionally proved helpful in the diagnosis of HC. Radiolabeled leukocyte imaging of the bladder has been evaluated with promising results (Palestro *et al.*, 1993). Ultrasonographic assessment of the bladder may provide prognostically useful information. Gartoni *et al.* (1993) graded patients into three categories:

Type 1: circumscribed thickening of the bladder wall protruding into the lumen
Type 2: diffuse thickening of the bladder wall
Type 3: intraluminal lobulated bulky mass reducing bladder capacity.

The median duration of hematuria for type 3 lesion was 90 days compared with 14 days in combined type 1 and 2 lesions. All five patients with type 3 lesions required endoscopic removal of clots and three patients died of complications related to HC.

Prevention

There is no standard approach to prophylaxis of HC. The two most commonly used methods have been hyperhydration and the chemoprotectant 2-mercaptoethane sodium sulfonate (mesna). Intravenous hyperhydration (usually 3 l/m^2/day) during and after the administration of cyclophosphamide dilutes the concentration

---

[1] George Papanicolaou, Greek-American pathologist, 1183–19672.

of acrolein and reduces the time of exposure to the bladder mucosa. This approach has successfully reduced the incidence of severe HC (Hows *et al.,* 1984), but has the potential to cause fluid overload and hyponatremia, particularly as cyclophosphamide acts on the renal tubule to cause inappropriate water retention.

Mesna has been shown to reduce the incidence of HC in patients receiving oxazophosphorines (Droller *et al.,* 1982). Mesna is converted to inactive di-mesna in serum, but is reactivated in the kidney. In urine, mesna binds to acrolein forming an inactive thioether, which is voided harmlessly. Mesna also reacts with 4-hydroxy metabolites directly, thereby inhibiting the initial formation of acrolein. Mesna appears well tolerated, and does not seem to interfere with the cytotoxicity of chemotherapy or impair HSC engraftment. Mesna may be given intravenously or orally with equal bioavailability and urinary excretion kinetics (Goren *et al.,* 1998).

Randomized trials comparing the efficacy of mesna and hyperhydration in preventing HC posttransplant have yielded variable results. Assessment of these studies is limited by differences in dosage and timing of administration. Mesna has been given as a bolus or continuous infusion, at doses between 60% and 160% of the cyclophosphamide dose, and ceased on the last day of administration or continued for a further 24 hours (reviewed by Haselberger & Schwinghammer, 1995). It is likely that the degree of uroepithelial protection is dose- and time-dependent. Timing errors in the administration of mesna have been significantly associated with the development of symptomatic hematuria. As mesna is excreted rapidly, and thiol levels are related to the frequency of micturition, mesna must be given at least every 3 hours. Only one prospective study (Hows *et al.,* 1984) demonstrated an advantage for mesna over hyperhydration.

Other prophylactic measures include catheterization and continuous bladder irrigation, hourly voiding protocols, and the use of diuretics. Bladder irrigation has been studied with variable results. In a retrospective series of 199 patients undergoing BMT, Turkeri and colleagues (1995) reported that the incidence of HC in patients undergoing continuous bladder irrigation was 23% compared to 53% in patients who did not (*P* <.004). However, Vose *et al.* (1993) prospectively compared mesna to bladder irrigation in 200 transplant patients randomly assigned to each treatment group, and found that the incidence of grade III and IV HC was the same in each group; moreover, bladder irrigation was both uncomfortable and increased the incidence of urinary tract infections. Furthermore bladder irrigation does not protect the upper urinary tract from the effects of acrolein. Frequent voiding is both theoretically useful and inevitable with hyperhydration. Loop diuretics may be useful by both increasing urine flow and acidifying urine, since the formation of acrolein is favored by an alkaline pH.

Studies have suggested protective benefits from a combination of hyperhydration and continuous bladder irrigation (Meisenberg *et al.,* 1994), and bladder irrigation with sorbitol (Rosenzweig, Schaefer, & Rosenfeld, 1994). No patients in these studies developed macroscopic HC. Animal studies have suggested a role for amifostine in protecting the bladder epithelium from acrolein (Srivastava *et al.,* 1999).

Treatment

The treatment of HC depends on its cause and severity. Mild cases with microscopic hematuria and dysuria often resolve of their own accord. Hyperhydration is usually employed for macroscopic hematuria as high fluid throughout is essential to prevent clot formation. Cystoscopy with bladder irrigation may be necessary to remove clots and to cauterize bleeding points; suprapubic cystotomy may make bladder irrigation more effective, but should be reserved for severe cases.

The use of antiviral therapy in individual patients with viruria and HC has proven effective in resolving viruria, and apparently hastening the resolution of symptoms. Vidarabine and ribavirin have been used for both adenovirus- and polyomavirus-associated HC (Murphy *et al.,* 1993; Kitayabashi *et al.,* 1994; Kawakami *et al.,* 1997). Ganciclovir has successfully been used for the treatment of CMV-associated HC (Spach *et al.,* 1993), and adenovirus-associated HC (Chen *et al.,* 1997). Cidofovir, a cytidine nucleoside analogue active against polyomaviruses such as BK and JC viruses, has been used to successfully treat polyoma virus-associated HC (Held *et al.,* 2000) (Fig. 79.3). It should be noted that cidofovir itself can cause HC and may induce renal impairment.

Intravesical instillation of various agents has been used to treat refractory bleeding. The superiority of any one agent has not been demonstrated in randomized studies (reviewed by Efros *et al.,* 1994). Alum acts by precipitating protein over the bleeding surface. Although inexpensive and nontoxic, proteinaceous deposits may obstruct the ureter or indwelling catheters, and it is rarely completely effective. Silver nitrate has been used with good results in children, but repeated instillation is frequently necessary. Formalin is effective, but requires a general anesthetic and may be complicated by vesico-ureteric reflux and renal papillary necrosis, or bladder and ureteric fibrosis. Phenol has been used in refractory severe HC, but application requires the bladder to be surgically opened. Intravesical application of a Helmstein pressure balloon may control bleeding but may result in bladder mucosa necrosis, damage to detrusor function, and bladder rupture.

Intravesical prostaglandins have been used by some groups. These agents may act by promoting vascular smooth muscle contraction in the bladder wall. Prostaglandin $F_{2\alpha}$ ($PGF_{2\alpha}$) is administered by indwelling catheter at the bedside with few systemic effects (for a protocol see Table 79.3). The major side effect is painful bladder spasms, which limit the tolerability of this approach but may be alleviated by the use of antispasmodic agents. A cystoscopy with clot removal should be performed prior to instillation as the presence of clots impairs prostaglandin action. Levine and Jarrard (1993) found that $PGF_{2\alpha}$ produced complete resolution of gross hematuria in 9 of 18 patients with partial responses in another 8. Over 70% experienced painful bladder spasms. Although promising, insuffi-

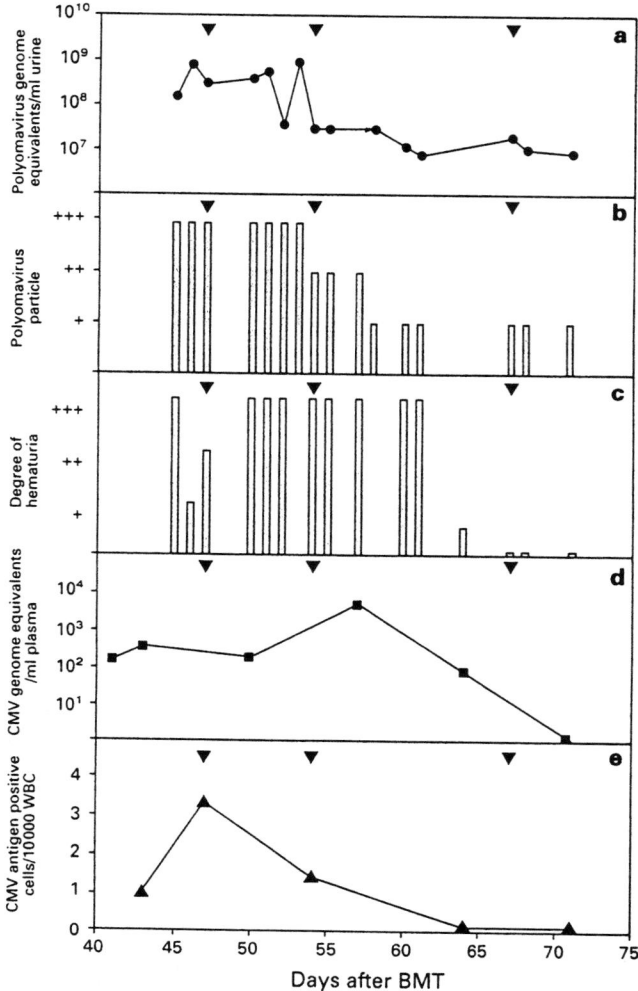

Fig. 79.3. Course of BK virus viruria, hematuria, and CMV reactivation in a patient with simultaneous CMV reactivation and hemorrhagic cystitis. (**a**) Number of BK virus genomic equivalents per ml of urine; (**b**) degree of BK viruria; (**c**) degree of hematuria; (**d**) degree of CMV viruria; (**e**) degree of CMV antigenemia. The triangles in each panel denote the time of cidofovir treatment. Reproduced, with permission, from Held *et al.* (2000).

cient data exist regarding the optimal dosage, dosing schedule, and duration of treatment, and no randomized studies have compared the efficacy of this approach to standard therapies.

A number of other approaches have been used including the use of systemic antifibrinolytic therapy, estrogens, hyperbaric oxygen (HBO) and various cytokines. Aminocaproic acid may be used to decrease hemorrhage (Lakhani *et al.*, 1999), but theoretically increases the risk of intravesical clot formation. Conjugated estrogen, given intravenously initially followed by chronic oral administration, has been reported to be effective in five patients with radiation- or cyclophosphamide-induced HC refractory to other treatment (Liu *et al.*, 1991). Preclinical data in rats demonstrated a potential role for HBO in preventing acrolein-induced bladder injury. There is evidence of efficacy in radiation-induced cystitis and anecdotal reports suggest that

Table 79.3.   *Suggested protocol for prostaglandin F$_2$ administration*

1. Prior cystoscopy with intraoperative clot evacuation with or without a cystogram to determine bladder capacity.
2. Instill 50–100 ml 0.4% prostaglandin F$_{2\alpha}$ analogue, retain for 1–2 hours and follow with 2 hours of continuous bladder irrigation with saline.
3. Concomitant use of oral or rectal antispasmodics.
4. Repeat 4 times per day for 4–5 days.

HBO therapy may hasten resolution of severe HC following BMT (Shameem *et al.*, 1992; Hattori *et al.*, 2001). The use of intravesical granulocyte-macrophage colony-stimulating factor (GM-CSF) has been described (Vela-Ojeda *et al.*, 1999). Animal models of HC have shown a therapeutic role for intravenous keratinocyte growth factor in ameliorating the severity of HC (Ulich *et al.*, 1997).

In severe HC, a multidisciplinary approach will be required. Levine and Richie (1989) developed an algorithm for management of severe HC, which is presented in Table 79.4. If these measures fail to control bleeding, external stents may be used to divert obstructed urine flow, and ligation of the hypogastric arteries with or without cystectomy may be necessary. Favorable outcomes have occasionally been reported with cystectomy (Garderet *et al.*, 2000; Koc *et al.*, 2000), and with selective vesical artery embolization (Rovira *et al.*, 2002) in very severe cases of HC. Other important measures include blood product support, particularly correction of thrombocytopenia. Symptomatic relief can be obtained with the use of antispasmodic agents, with opiate analgesia required in more severe cases.

Outcome

HC is usually self-limited and resolves without sequelae; severe hemorrhage, which may be life-threatening, is fortunately seen rarely. Bladder fibrosis and contracture, ureteric obstruction with renal failure, and bladder cancer are documented complications of HC (Sencer *et al.*, 1993). Adenoviruria and HC may be manifestations of potentially lethal systemic adenovirus infections.

Table 79.4.   *Management of severe hemorrhagic cystitis*

1. High fluid intake
2. Correction of thrombocytopenia
3. Cystoscopic evacuation of clots followed by bladder irrigation with 1–2% alum for 48–72 hours through a large-bore catheter, and continuing 72 hours after bleeding ceases.
4. Intravesical instillation of carboprost tromethamine 0.2% (prostaglandin).
5. Cystoscopy with fulguration of any discrete bleeding sites and instillation of 2.5–4% formalin.
6. Consider selective embolization or cystectomy in the case of life-threatening hemorrhage.

Conclusions

New diagnostic and therapeutic techniques are emerging for HC. Examples of these include the role of ultrasound in assessing the severity of HC and the use of prostaglandins, specific antiviral therapy, and hyperbaric oxygen in treatment. The benefit of these advances requires assessment in prospective trials to better define an optimal approach to prevention and management of HC.

References

Arthur, R.R., Shah, K.V., Charache, P., & Saral, R. (1988). BK and JC virus infections in recipients of bone marrow transplants. *Journal of Infectious Disease*, **158**, 563–9.

Azzi, A., Fanci, R., Bosi, A. *et al.* (1994). Monitoring of polyomavirus BK viruria in bone marrow transplantation patients by DNA hybridization assay and by polymerase chain reaction: an approach to assess the relationship between BK viruria and hemorrhagic cystitis. *Bone Marrow Transplantation*, **14**, 235–40.

Baronciani, D., Angelucci, E., Erer, B. *et al.* (1995). Suprapubic cystotomy as treatment for severe hemorrhagic cystitis after bone marrow transplantation. *Bone Marrow Transplantation*, **16**, 267–70.

Bedi, A., Miller, G.B., Hanson, J.L. *et al.* (1995). Association of BK virus with failure of prophylaxis against hemorrhagic cystitis following bone marrow transplantation. *Journal of Clinical Oncology*, **13**, 1103–9.

Bogdanovic, G., Ljungman, O., Wang, F., & Dalianis, T. (1996). Presence of human polyomavirus DNA, in the peripheral circulation of bone marrow transplant patients with and without hemorrhagic cystitis. *Bone Marrow Transplantation*, **17**, 573–6.

Chen, F.E., Liang, R.H.S., Lo, J.Y. *et al.* (1997). Treatment of adenovirus-associated haemorrhagic cystitis with ganciclovir. *Bone Marrow Transplantation*, **20**, 997–9.

Childs, R., Sanchez, C., Engler, H. *et al.* (1998). High incidence of adeno- and polyomavirus-induced hemorrhagic cystitis in bone marrow transplantation for hematological malignancy following T cell depletion and cyclosporine. *Bone Marrow Transplantation*, **22**, 889–93.

Droller, M.J., Saral, R., & Santos, G. (1982). Prevention of cyclophosphamide-induced hemorrhagic cystitis. *Urology*, **20**, 256–8.

Efros, M.D., Ahmed, T., Goombe, N., & Ghoudhury, M.S. (1994). Urologic complications of high-dose chemotherapy and bone marrow transplantation. *Urology*, **43**, 355–60.

Frustaci, S., Foladore, S., De Pascale, A. *et al.* (1992). Feasibility and efficacy of arginine 2-mercaptoethanesulfonate (argimesna) in the prevention of hemorrhagic cystitis from ifosfamide. *Annals of Oncology*, **3** (Suppl 2), 5115–8.

Garderet, L., Bittencourt, H., Sebe, P. *et al.* (2000). Cystectomy for severe hemorrhagic cystitis in allogeneic stem cell transplant recipients. *Transplantation*, **70**, 1807–11.

Gartoni, G., Arcese, W., Avvisati, G. *et al.* (1993). Role of ultrasonography in the diagnosis and follow-up of hemorrhagic cystitis after bone marrow transplantation. *Bone Marrow Transplantation*, **12**, 463–7.

Goren, M.P., Anthony, L.B., Hande, K.R. *et al.* (1998). Pharmacokinetics of an intravenous-oral versus intravenous-mesna regimen in lung cancer patients receiving ifosfamide. *Journal of Clinical Oncology*, **16**, 616–21.

Haselberger, M.B. & Schwinghammer, T.L. (1995). Efficacy of mesna for prevention of hemorrhagic cystitis after high-dose cyclophosphamide therapy. *Annals of Pharmacotherapy*, **29**, 918–21.

Hattori, K., Yabe, M., Matsumoto, M. *et al.* (2001). Successful hyperbaric oxygen treatment of life-threatening hemorrhagic cystitis after allogeneic bone marrow transplantation. *Bone Marrow Transplantation*, **27**, 1315–7.

Held, T.K., Biel, S.S., Nitsche, A. *et al.* (2000). Treatment of BK virus-associated hemorrhagic cystitis and simultaneous CMV reactivation with cidofovir. *Bone Marrow Transplantation*, **26**, 347–50.

Hows, J.M., Mehta, A., Ward, L. *et al.* (1984). Comparison of mesna with forced diuresis to prevent cyclophosphamide-induced hemorrhagic cystitis in marrow transplantation. *British Journal of Cancer*, **50**, 753–6.

Kawakami, M., Ueda, S., Maeda, T. *et al.* (1997). Vidarabine therapy for virus-associated cystitis after allogeneic bone marrow transplantation. *Bone Marrow Transplantation*, **20**, 485–90.

Kim, Y.-J., Kim, D.-W., Lee, D.-G. *et al.* (2002). Human herpesvirus-6 as a possible cause of encephalitis and hemorrhagic cystitis after allogeneic hematopoietic stem cell transplantation. *Leukemia*, **16**, 958–9.

Kitayabashi, A., Hirokawa, M., Kuroki, J. *et al.* (1994). Successful vidarabine therapy for adenovirus type 11-associated acute hemorrhagic cystitis after allogeneic bone marrow transplantation. *Bone Marrow Transplantation*, **14**, 853–4.

Koc, S., Hagglund, H., Ireton, R.C. *et al.* (2000). Successful treatment of severe hemorrhagic cystitis with cystectomy following matched donor allogeneic hematopoietic cell transplantation. *Bone Marrow Transplantation*, **26**, 899–901.

Lakhani, A., Raptis, A., Frame, D. *et al.* (1999). Intravesicular instillation of E-aminocaproic acid for patients with adenovirus-induced hemorrhagic cystitis. *Bone Marrow Transplantation*, **24**, 1259–60.

Leung, A.Y.H., Suen, C.K.M., Lie, A.K.W. *et al.* (2001). Quantification of polyoma BK viruria in hemorrhagic cystitis complicating bone marrow transplantation. *Blood*, **98**, 1971–8.

Levine, L.A. & Jarrard, D.F. (1993). Treatment of cyclophosphamide-induced hemorrhagic cystitis with intravesical carboprost tromethamine. *Journal of Urology*, **149**, 719–23.

Levine, L.A. & Richie, J.P. (1989). Urological complications of cyclophosphamide. *Journal of Urology*, **141**, 63.

Liu, T.K., Harty, I., Steinbok, G.S. *et al.* (1991). Treatment of radiation or cyclophosphamide induced hemorrhagic cystitis using conjugated estrogen. *Urology*, **144**, 41–3.

Matsuse, T., Matsui, H., Nagase, T. *et al.* (1994). Adenovirus pulmonary infections identified by PCR and in situ hybridization in bone marrow transplant recipient. *Journal of Clinical Pathology*, **47**, 973–7.

Meisenberg, B., Lassiter, M., Hussein, A. *et al.* (1994). Prevention of hemorrhagic cystitis after high-dose alkylating agent chemotherapy and autologous bone marrow support. *Bone Marrow Transplantation*, **14**, 287–91.

Miyamura, K., Takeyama, K., Kojima, S. *et al.* (1989). Hemorrhagic cystitis associated with urinary excretion of adenovirus type 11 following allogeneic bone marrow transplantation. *Bone Marrow Transplantation*, **4**, 533–5.

Murphy, G.F., Wood, D.P. Jr., McRoberts, J.W., & Henslee-Downey, P.J. (1993). Adenovirus-associated hemorrhagic cystitis treated with intravenous ribavirin. *Journal of Urology*, **149**, 565–6.

Ost, L., Lonnqvist, B., Eriksson, L. *et al.* (1987). Hemorrhagic cystitis—a manifestation of GVHD? *Bone Marrow Transplantation*, **2**, 19–25.

Palestro, C.J., Cohen, I.R., & Goldsmith, S.J. (1993). Labeled leukocyte imaging in chemical cystitis. *Clinical Nuclear Medicine*, **18**, 75–6.

Ringden, O., Ruutu, T., Renberger, M. *et al.* (1994). A randomised trial comparing busulphan with total body irradiation as conditioning in allogeneic marrow transplant recipients with leukemia: a report from the Nordic Bone Marrow Transplantation Group. *Blood*, **83**, 2723–30.

Rosenzweig, M.Q., Schaefer, M., & Rosenfeld, C.F. (1994). Prevention of transplant-related hemorrhagic cystitis using bladder irrigation with sorbitol. *Bone Marrow Transplantation*, **14**, 491–2.

Rovira, M., Real, I., Carreras, E. *et al.* (2002). Successful treatment of severe hemorrhagic cystitis by selective embolization of vesical arteries in HCT. *Bone Marrow Transplantation*, **29**, Suppl 2).

Russell, S.J., Vowels, M.R., & Vale, T. (1994). Hemorrhagic cystitis in pediatric bone marrow transplant patients, an association with infective agents, GVHD and prior cyclophosphamide. *Bone Marrow Transplantation*, **13**, 533–9.

Sato, N., Okamoto, S., Sawafuji, K. *et al.* (2002). Cidofovir for the treatment of adenoviral hemorrhagic cystitis in adult allogeneic stem cell transplant recipients. *Bone Marrow Transplantation*, **29**, (Suppl 2).

Seber, A., Shu, X.O., Defor, T. *et al.* (1999). Risk factors for severe hemorrhagic cystitis following BMT. *Bone Marrow Transplantation*, **23**, 35–40.

Sencer, S.F., Haake, R.J., & Weisdorf, D.J. (1993). Hemorrhagic cystitis after bone marrow transplantation. Risk factors and complications. *Transplantation*, **56**, 875–9.

Shameem, I.A., Shimabukuro, T., Shirataki, S. *et al.* (1992). Hyperbaric oxygen therapy for control of intractable cyclophosphamide-induced hemorrhagic cystitis. *European Urology*, **22**, 263–4.

Spach, D.H., Bauwens, J.E., Myerson, D. *et al.* (1993). Cytomegalovirus-induced hemorrhagic cystitis following bone marrow transplantation. *Clinical Infectious Diseases*, **16**, 142–4.

Srivastava, A., Nair, S.C., Srivastava, V.M. *et al.* (1999). Evaluation of uroprotective efficacy of amifostine against cyclophosphamide induced hemorrhagic cystitis. *Bone Marrow Transplantation*, **23**, 463–7.

Stella, F., Battistelli, S., & Marcheggiani, F. *et al.* (1990). Urothelial changes due to busulphan and cyclophosphamide treatment in bone marrow transplantation. *Acta Cytologica*, **34**, 885–90.

Trotman, J., Nivison-Smith, I., & Dodds, A. (1999). Haemorrhagic cystitis: incidence and risk factors in a transplant population using hyperhydration. *Bone Marrow Transplantation*, **23**, 797–801.

Turkeri, L.N., Lum, L.G., Uberti, J.P. *et al.* (1995). Prevention of hemorrhagic cystitis following allogeneic bone marrow transplantation preparative regimens with cyclophosphamide and busulfan: role of continuous bladder irrigation. *Journal of Urology*, **153**, 637–40.

Ulich, T.R., Whitcomb, L., Tang, W. *et al.* (1997). Keratinocyte growth factor ameliorates cyclophosphamide-induced ulcerative hemorrhagic cystitis. *Cancer Research*, **57**, 472–5

Vela-Ojeda, J., Tripp-Villanueva, F., Sanchez-Cortes, E. *et al.* (1999). Intravesical rhGM-CSF for the treatment of late onset hemorrhagic cystitis after bone marrow transplant. *Bone Marrow Transplantation*, **24**, 1307–10.

Vose, J.M., Reed, E.C., Pippert, G.C. *et al.* (1993). Mesna compared with continuous bladder irrigation as uroprotection during high-dose chemotherapy and transplantation: a randomized trial. *Journal of Clinical Oncology*, **11**, 1306–10.

80   Oro-pharyngeal mucositis

MARK M. SCHUBERT

Fred Hutchinson Cancer Research Center, Seattle Cancer Care Alliance, and University of Washington, Seattle, USA

Introduction

While significant strides continue to be made in supportive care for patients undergoing hematopoietic cell transplantation (HSCT), oro-pharyngeal mucositis remains a significant clinical problem for HSCT patients who receive high-dose chemotherapy conditioning regimens with or without total body irradiation (Bellm *et al.*, 2000; Sonis, 1998, 2000; Sonis *et al.*, 2001a; Sonis & Fey, 2002). Oro-pharyngeal mucositis not only causes significant pain and suffering, but can increase the risk for infection, increase hospital stays, and dramatically increase the cost of care (Sonis *et al.*, 2001a).

Simply defined, mucositis can be described as inflammation and ulcerative breakdown of mucosal surfaces that can result from a variety of causes. Oro-pharyngeal mucosal breakdown following HSCT can be associated with conditioning regimen toxicity (cancer chemotherapy or ionizing radiation), infections (viral, fungal, and/or bacterial oral infections), trauma, and/or graft-versus-host disease (GVHD) as well as some agents used to prevent GVHD (methotrexate). Additionally, multiple insults can occur simultaneously. For example, mucositis initially caused by conditioning regimen toxicity can be complicated and worsened by an oral herpes simplex infection. For the sake of clarity, in this chapter, the term *mucositis* will be applied to oro-pharyngeal mucosal damage and breakdown resulting from the direct toxicity of conditioning regimens that is usually noted in the first several weeks posttransplant. The contribution of all currently recognized factors that can contribute to further damage will also be briefly discussed. However, it remains important to realize that the clinical expression of oro-pharyngeal mucositis and reactions that occur during both the early and later periods posttransplant can have a relatively limited clinical range of presentations, even though the etiologies at various times can be quite diverse. This makes it imperative that all oral lesions occurring in the first several weeks after conditioning are carefully assessed and that rigorous diagnostic protocols are utilized in order to identify potential etiologies that can be treated. The clinical presentation should be correlated with known risk factors for mucositis and appropriate diagnostic steps (especially viral, fungal, and bacterial cultures) taken.

Oro-pharyngeal mucositis can vary from mildly symptomatic mucosal inflammation to widespread ulceration and bleeding, causing intense pain, preventing normal oral functioning, and increasing the risk of secondary infections (Schubert, Sullivan, & Truelove, 1986a; Elting *et al.*, 1992; Shoidt *et al.*, 1998). Though the impact on quality of life can be quite evident, mucositis can at times represent a life-threatening complication. For example, severe pharyngeal mucositis can produce epiglottic or pharyngeal edema of such severity that intubation becomes necessary to maintain an adequate airway (Murray *et al.*, 1995). Damaged oro-pharyngeal mucosal surfaces can also increase the risk for systemic bacterial infections and increase the risk for invasive oral fungal infections. In a study reported by Sonis *et al.* (2001a), a one point increase in the severity of mucositis using the Oral Mucositis Assessment Scale (OMAS) resulted in:

- 1 additional day with fever ($P < .01$)
- 2.1-fold increased risk of significant infection ($P < .01$)
- 2.7 additional days of total parenteral nutrition ($P < .0001$)
- 2.6 additional days of i.v. narcotic therapy ($P < .0001$)
- \$25,405 in additional hospital charges ($P < .0001$)
- 3.9-fold increase in 100-day mortality risk ($P < .01$)

Finally, mucositis can also have a significant impact on the cost of care due to extended hospitalization, treatment of secondary infectious complications, and increased need for intensive supportive care (Ruescher *et al.*, 1998). In the study reported by Sonis *et al.* (2001a), hospital charges were \$42,749 higher when ulcerative mucositis was present.

Etiology of oro-pharyngeal mucositis

Significant strides have been made over the past 8 years in elucidating the mechanism and factors associated with the etiology of oral mucositis. For many years, it was felt that mucositis resulted merely from the direct cytotoxic damage to the oro-pharyngeal mucosal basal epithelium cells caused by HSCT conditioning regimens. However, it is becoming increasingly clear that the ultimate clinical expression of mucositis is dependent on the complex physiological cascade and interaction of a number of both

Table 80.1. *Factors contributing to oro-pharyngeal mucositis*

Direct factors	Indirect/secondary factors
Conditioning regimen	Immunosuppression
Chemotherapy	Neutropenia
Total body irradiation	T-cell loss/dysfunction
Total lymphoid irradiation	B-cell loss/dysfunction (IgA)
GVHD prophylaxis	Infections
Methotrexate	Bacterial organisms
	Normal flora
GVHD therapy	Opportunistic pathogens
Steroids	Streptococci/
Cyclosporine	staphylococci
Other immunosuppressants	Acquired pathogens
Salivary gland dysfunction	Gram-negative pathogens
Loss of mucins, secretory IgA	Fungal organisms
Antimicrobial proteins/	*Candida* species
enzymes	*Aspergillus,*
	mucormycosis
Trauma	Viral infections
Physical	Herpes simplex
Eating, mouth breathing	Cytomegalovirus
Chemical	Varicella zoster (rare)
Emesis, medications	

direct and indirect factors (Table 80.1, Fig. 80.1). In 1998, Sonis first proposed a four-step model to explain the manner in which mucositis develops and later resolves (Sonis, 1998). This model has been updated and now identifies five phases of mucositis when viewed relative to the mucosal epithelial compartment (Sonis, personal communication, 2002). Much of this work has been derived from animal models and it is not certain how much directly applies to mucositis in humans, though there is increasing confirmatory evidence being obtained from research involving human studies (Sonis *et al.*, 1992, 1997, 2000, 2001, 2002).

Phase 1—Initial injury: following exposure to chemotherapy and/or radiation, reactive oxygen species are produced along with the upregulation of several key transcription factors and early injury response genes. Cytokines, such as interleukin 1 (IL-1), are released. Il-1 and tumor necrosis factor (TNF) cause an inflammatory response that appears to induce increased subepithelial vascularity and, additionally, endothelial injury is apparent in the immediate submucosal tissue.

Phase 2—Submucosal phase: during this phase, connective tissue deterioration is noted along with the upregulation of additional genes associated with tissue damage responses. Early apoptosis of clonogenic basal epithelial cells is noted along with activation of alternate apoptotic pathways.

Phase 3—Epithelial phase: with upregulation of "healing genes." Localized hyperproliferative activity is noted, but there is also a decreased renewal of epithelial cells. In addition, there is parallel activation of cytotoxic pathways and caspase expression. The reduced rate of epithelial renewal results in mucosal atrophy. Typically, this phase begins approximately 4 to 5 days after conditioning.

Phase 4—Ulceration and bacterial colonization phase: tissue injury is induced, amplified, and prolonged by secondary and tertiary cytotoxic mechanisms. Pro-inflammatory cytokines are maximally expressed, which corresponds to maximum evidence of inflammatory infiltrate. Ulcerated tissue becomes covered with pseudomembranous fibrin exudates that coagulate on the surface. Mixed bacterial flora can colonize damaged mucosal surfaces and can cause further local tissue damage. Gram-negative bacteria can introduce endotoxins (lipopolysaccharides) into tissues that induce tissue-borne mononuclear cells to release additional cytokines and produce nitric oxide. It is important to recognize that patients tend to reach their neutrophil nadir during this phase, approximately 14 days after the start of myeloablative therapy and 3 or 4 days after mucositis peaks. Additionally, there is growing evidence that epithelial cell–derived antimicrobial peptides, such as defensins, may not be secreted, thus increasing the risk for local infection.

Late in Phase 4, balance of activity starts to tip in favor of recovery.

Phase 5—Healing: with the diminished cytotoxic stimuli an overwhelming healing response ensues with elimination of inflammation and epithelial cell proliferation. Conditioning regimen damage can be increased by direct damage from other factors that can be encountered during the first 2 weeks posttransplant and include such things as methotrexate administration for GVHD prophylaxis. Mucosal trauma and irritation, even from normal oral function, can have a profound effect when it is superimposed on conditioning regimen–related damage. Conditioning regimen–induced damage to salivary glands decreases salivary secretion, compromising saliva's local barrier function and promoting dehydration of tissues.

Both local and systemic immune dysfunction early posttransplant increases the risk of oral infections that can secondarily involve oral tissues and thus worsen overall mucosal damage, as well as slow healing. Some oral infections are obvious and the damage they cause can be dramatic (e.g., herpes simplex infections), while other types of infections may be sub-

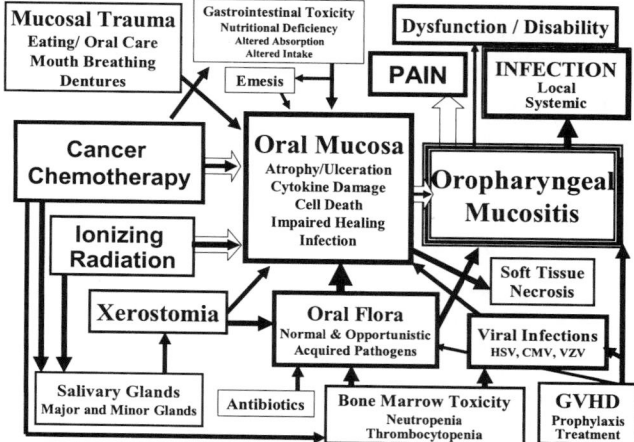

Fig. 80.1. Contributing factors to oro-pharyngeal mucositis and sequelae following HSC transplantation.

tle and far from obvious. Finally, when oral acute GVHD occurs during the second and third weeks posttransplant, the mucosal inflammation and ulceration it causes can essentially continue to induce inflammatory damage that worsens the late stages of conditioning regimen–induced mucositis and prevents healing.

Although it is still not possible to prevent oro-pharyngeal mucositis, certain therapies have clearly shown an ability to decrease the overall degree and duration of oro-pharyngeal mucositis. Most of these treatments aim to prevent or reduce indirect oral toxicities, such as trauma and infection. Included in this approach are the use of prophylactic antiviral regimens to prevent reactivation of herpes simplex virus (HSV) and antifungal regimens to reduce oral fungal colonization, the use of biological response modifiers that improve early neutrophil engraftment [e.g., granulocyte colony-stimulating factor (G-CSF)], and the use of agents or techniques that specifically affect various oral health parameters and/or improve immune recovery.

Mucositis measurement and research

The importance of accurate and consistent measurement of mucositis extends from routine clinical care of HSCT patients to sophisticated clinical research settings. It is important that oral mucositis changes be precisely described, objectively classified, and examiners be able to reproducibly measure the range and severity of subjective and objective oral changes. Over the past decade, there has been a significant activity in clinical research relative to development of agents or treatment to prevent and/or reduce oral mucositis. Commensurate with this research have been efforts to develop mucositis rating scales that provide the most accurate and appropriate measure of oral mucositis (Schubert et al., 1992; Schubert, 1993; Parulekar et al., 1998; Schubert, Peterson, & Lloid, 1999; Sonis et al., 1999). Until fairly recently, the most commonly employed mucositis scoring systems have utilized relatively global clinical assessment scales to measure the severity of "oral toxicity." Scales such as the NCI-CTC, WHO, or SWOG oral mucosal toxicity scales have been those most commonly used. These scales generally use a 0–3 or 4 scale to provide an "overall" score to rate oral status. They often blend objective (e.g., erythema and ulceration) with subjective (e.g., pain) and functional variables (e.g., eating, swallowing), which, while they can give a gross overall impression of oral stature, may not accurately reflect true oral mucosal status. As an example, the WHO scale is as follows:

Grade 0—mucositis absent
Grade I—erythema and sore throat
Grade II—ulcerations present but can eat
Grade III—ulcerations present but cannot eat
Grade IV—total parenteral nutrition needed

It is common for these scales to use "unable to eat" or "requires hyperalimentation" to represent grade III mucositis (severe mucositis), yet patients with severe gut toxicity cannot eat, and a patient could have grade I or II mucositis but be on hyperalimentation for gastrointestinal problems even though they could technically take food by mouth; this patient would score a "IV" (most severe grade) for mucositis. These scales cannot differentiate between patients with a single small ulcer versus a patient with multiple or extensive ulceration. Or, a patient who is displaying significant suffering and may not be eating by mouth may be scored as a "IV" (most severe) when there may be only mild mucosal inflammation and no ulcerations. Consequently, they lack precision. In response, a number of more detailed oral mucositis assessment scales have been developed that attempt to specifically measure objective mucosal variables that represent clinical changes associated with mucosal damage and breakdown caused by the conditioning regimen and other factors (Schubert et al., 1992; Sonis et al., 1999). These scales are especially appropriate for research applications. Currently, the approach taken by many researchers is to score mucosal changes on a mucositis index and rate subjective variables (pain, dryness, etc.) and performance variables (ability to talk, eat, and swallow) with separate measures, using instruments such as visual analog scales.

The variation in available scales to measure mucositis does give examiners a choice of instrument. However, since no one scale is universally applicable, a number of questions should be asked when choosing a scale:

Why is mucositis being measured and what is the scale attempting to measure? If the goal of measuring mucositis is to support direct clinical care, then a global scale that considers numerous patient qualities—objective mucosal changes plus subjective responses—with a global four-point (normal to severe changes/responses) is reasonable. At the other extreme, if the scale is being chosen to rate mucositis as part of a clinical research trial for testing of a mucosal growth factor, then both primary (mucosal status relative to an intervention) and patient subjective (oral pain) and performance status (eating, swallowing, etc.) may need to be measured. For this, a detailed clinical assessment of variables specific to the expression of the expected impact on the etiology would be important and the subjective and performance changes could be measured on separate scales.

Who will be administering the scale and how frequently will the scale be administered? The types and range of changes from normal for oral tissues in an HSCT setting can be significant, and as the complexity of a scale increases, so does the need to have examiners with extensive knowledge of normal appearances and the range of changes relative to the rating scale to be used. As the complexity of the variables being scored by the scale increases, the necessity for training and calibrating (and recalibrating) of examiners increases.

Also, as the complexity of a scale increases, examination and scoring times increase. Thus as scoring goes from a once or twice a week scoring to daily scoring, the time, effort, and cost increase. These logistic issues become more acute if the scores move from a single-center study to a multicenter study.

Under what conditions will the scale be administered? This is more of a practical concern; the more detailed the assessment, the better the examination conditions must be. If the oral tissues cannot be adequately illuminated and visualized, any results will be less accurate and reproducible. For instance, if the rating of the degree of mucosal inflammation (i.e., erythema) is important, the type and spectra of the illumination source is important if the correct interpretation of erythema is to be scored. "White" light sources such as those produced by halogen bulbs are usually the best. Also the convenience and comfort of both the examiner and the patient during the examination can influence the quality of the overall examination.

Design of mucositis research

It is very clear, when reviewing the scientific literature relative to oral mucositis research,that there is significant need to focus carefully on research design for clinical trials. Most studies in the literature today cannot be easily compared with each other due to inconsistent design and varied research techniques. Many studies contain obvious design flaws that even hinder acceptance of the results. Clinical mucositis research is exceedingly complex—all factors that influence the occurrence, severity, and course of mucositis need to be considered and controlled for. The design of clinical mucositis trials requires both good clinical practice (GCP) and consideration of mucositis-specific design. Careful study of the literature can be invaluable in planning.

Mucositis clinical research includes 8 elements:

1. Selection of patients: Subjects need to be representative of the area of cancer therapy and "predictably" at risk for mucositis. Inclusion and exclusion criteria need to be clearly defined and adhered to—with special attention to those elements that can affect the clinical presentation and course of mucositis and subsequently controlling for them. All subjects should receive the same pretransplant stabilizing care. During the study, all subjects should receive the same standards of care. When conducting a multicenter trial, significant effort should be exerted to make certain that there is truly equivalent oral care and support being provided at all centers. Consideration should be given to other elements such as age, other underlying conditions, other medical or oral care subjects could receive, and the subject's ability to comply with study activities.

2. Allocation of patients to treatment groups and subject blinding: Whenever possible, a randomized, double-blind scheme to allocate patients to study groups should be utilized.

3. Therapeutic regimen: Since the single most important contributing factor to mucositis is the chemotherapy and total body irradiation conditioning regimen, investigators should choose a treatment regimen that produces a predictable degree of mucositis (onset, severity, and duration). If multiple regimens are utilized, they need to be truly equivalent, based on research findings and not on a clinician's impression of "being the same." Randomization schemes may want to consider the impact of multiple conditioning regimens. The more variable the treatment protocols (i.e., conditioning regimens), the weaker the study.

4. Study administration: Consistent and firm adherence to study protocol is an obviously important factor.

5. Withdrawals from the study: Document and report withdrawals for whatever reason. Subjects should not be replaced, but additional subjects can be randomized to increase the overall total enrollment to preserve power.

6. Outcome measurement: One of the most critical elements of study design is choice of mucositis scale or scales. This is problematic as there is not a universally accepted mucositis scale that meets all measurement needs. Considerable thought should go into choosing a scale, and it may be appropriate to utilize multiple scales. Examiners need to be trained, calibrated, and recalibrated throughout the study. Scoring of subjective and performance criteria can be performed using separate validated scales.

7. Statistical analysis: A statistician should be involved with the design of the study from the early design stages. Consider stratification schemes where appropriate. It is generally accepted that "intent to treat" analysis be utilized for trials of this nature.

8. Reporting of study design and results: Report how the study was conducted in detail and include all critical elements of study design. Many times it is difficult to determine if a study is flawed or poorly controlled or if the authors failed to inform readers as to what they did. If study design or conduct is compromised, then state in the report what happened.

Risk factors for oro-pharyngeal mucositis

Studies to identify other therapy and patient-related risk factors for oro-pharyngeal mucositis beyond specific cancer therapies have not found consistent factors. Cancer therapy–related factors, along with patient–related factors (age, basic oro-dental health, and functional trauma) have all been shown or proposed as relevant factors. It is important to realize that when assessing studies reporting on the incidence and severity of oral mucositis, a variety of different mucositis scales have been utilized and thus comparison of results between studies may not be possible. Additionally, since other factors than just conditioning regimens will affect mucositis, it is important to consider all potential contributing factors such as patient age, underlying diseases, oral infections (both mucosal and dental), potential incidence for mucosal trauma, etc., when clinically assessing patients. It is clear that standard oral care protocols can vary significantly between institutions and the impact on the expression of oral mucositis may be considerable.

Conditioning regimen toxicity

While it is clear that the etiology of mucositis is generally multifactorial, HSCT conditioning regimens are the single most significant and predictable etiologic factor during the first 21 days posttransplant (Bearman *et al.,* 1988; Kolbinson *et al.,* 1988; Dahllof *et al.,* 1989; Epstein *et al.,* 1999; Blijlevens *et al.,* 2000; Wardley *et al.,* 2000; Sonis & Fey, 2002) The oro-pharyngeal mucosa and submucosa are very susceptible to direct and indirect damage caused by cancer chemotherapy and ionizing radiation. (Lockhart & Sonis, 1981; Squire, 1990; Squire & Kremer, 2001). The combination of direct damage to the proliferating basal cells of the oral epithelium plus indirect damage mediated by inflammatory cytokines causes mucosal atrophy and interferes with cell maturation and, where applicable, subsequent keratinization. This results in the oral mucosa appearing erythematous and atrophic. The associated damage to submucosal connective tissue and vasculature results in hyalinization of collagen and vascular dilation. IL-1 may also increase vascularity and thus result in increased concentrations of cytotoxic drugs in mucosal tissues.

Throughout the history of HSCT, oral mucositis has held a prominent position relative to early toxicity and has remained so, despite efforts to specifically reduce toxicity of conditioning regimens while trying to improve cure rates (Stiff, 2001). In the early years of marrow transplantation, there tended to be a relatively small number of conditioning regimen protocols that often centered on the use of cyclophosphamide alone or in combination with single-dose total body irradiation (TBI). Over the years, a significant number of different protocols have been developed (see Chapter 21). Although single chemotherapy agent protocols are still used (e.g., cyclophosphamide for aplastic anemia, melphalan for multiple myeloma), the number and complexity of multidrug chemotherapy conditioning protocols has grown significantly. Patients conditioned with some single-agent chemotherapy agents (for example, cyclophosphamide alone) have tended to have no or mild to moderate oro-pharyngeal mucositis, while those regimens that utilize combination chemotherapy (e.g., busulfan and cyclophos-

phamide or busulfan and melphalan with or without thiotepa) tend to produce moderate to severe oro-pharyngeal mucositis (Bensinger *et al.,* 1992; Srivastava *et al.,* 1993). In a prospective study comparing the mucositis potential of various HSCT conditioning regimens, Wardley *et al.* (2000) reported the relationship of various conditioning regimens to oral mucositis. (Fig. 80.2). In this study, regimens utilizing melphalan with and without TBI caused both the earliest occurring and worst mucositis when measured with the WHO mucositis scale. Cyclophosphamide plus TBI, busulfan alone, and busulfan-cyclophosphamide regimens caused less mucositis and these regimens produced relatively similar mucositis severity, though the busulfan alone regimen had a slightly later time to peak mean mucositis (Fig 80.2). Regimens that were least toxic to oral mucosa were cyclophosphamide-carmustine and cyclophosphamide-etoposide-carmustine. Unfortunately, the influence of methotrexate for acute GVHD prophylaxis was not analyzed or reported.

The experience for the Seattle group has been somewhat different. While high-dose melphalan protocols do cause mucositis, the frequency and severity have not made it the regimen most likely to cause mucositis (M. Schubert, unpublished results). While we have found that TBI-containing regimens are more predictable in causing mucositis than chemotherapy-only protocols, the Boston group reported that TBI does not increase the risk of mucositis (Woo *et al.,* 1993). Over the years, the use of modified TBI schemes has undergone significant clinical testing. The Seattle group originally utilized a single-dose 10 Gy TBI schedule. However, because it was not possible to increase the single-dose level above 10 Gy due to both early and late serious radiation toxicity, fractionated dosing has been implemented with total doses now ranging from 12 Gy to 17.5 Gy. Additionally, both single-daily dosing regimens and hyperfractionated daily regimens are being studied.

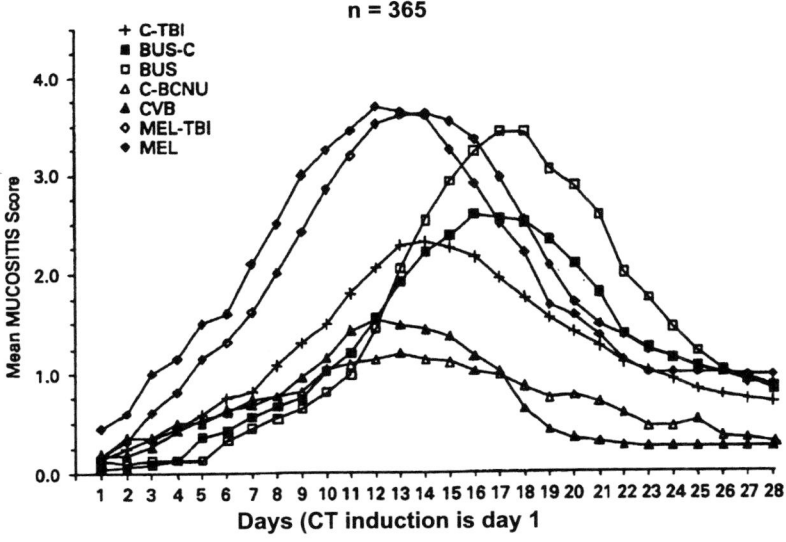

Fig. 80.2. Mean mucositis score associated with each treatment regimen (SEM ± 0.5 grade). Reproduced, with permission, from Wardley *et al.* (2000).

We have found that the addition of TBI to the conditioning regimen significantly increases mucositis due to increased direct mucosal damage and, possibly, indirectly due to xerostomia (Schubert, Sullivan, & Truelove, 1986; Schubert & Izutsu, 1987; Chapko et al., 1989; Borgmann et al., 1994; Schubert, unpublished results). Single dose TBI (e.g., 10 Gy) is more stomatotoxic than daily fractionated doses (200 cGy × 6 days or 225 cGy × 6 days), with mucositis increasing as TBI dose increases (Bearman et al., 1988; Chapko et al., 1989). However, we have also observed that multiple daily fractionated TBI (120–140 cGy 3 ×/day to total doses of 12–15 cGy) tends to increase the risk of oro-pharyngeal mucositis compared to single daily fractions that result in similar total doses. If total lymphoid irradiation (TLI) with fields including the posterior oral and pharyngeal regions is utilized in addition to TBI, the oro-pharyngeal mucositis is severe and risks include frank oro-pharyngeal airway embarrassment.

When considering the potential stomatotoxicity of various conditioning regimens, not only is it important to consider which drugs are being delivered, but also their dose and schedule (Borowski et al., 1994). Similarly, the specifics of TBI conditioning regimens need to be considered: size of dose fractions, frequency of administration and total dose. Finally, certain agents such as methotrexate and etoposide may also be secreted in saliva, which may increase the level of direct mucosal toxicity (Pico et al., 1998).

Patient age

Sonis reported that mucositis tends to be worse in very young patients; however, analysis of mucositis patterns carried out by the Seattle group has found that very young (under 6 years of age) and old patients (55 years old and older) tend to have less mucositis (Sonis & Fey, 2002; Sonis, 2002; Schubert, unreported data). We hypothesize that, despite the fact that children have a higher mucosal epithelial mitotic index that would potentially result in more damage, they would also be able to recover more rapidly from mucosal damage than older patients; this would result in a lower clinical expression of mucosal breakdown. On the other hand, with decreasing mitotic activity of basal mucosal cells in older patients, the number of vulnerable cells is decreased and thus there is less overall expression of mucositis.

Rate of engraftment

The rate of granulocyte engraftment has also been reported to affect mucosal recovery, with the suggested mechanism related to improved clearing of invading microorganisms from tissues (see below). However, in general we have clearly observed consistent mucosal healing despite slow engraftment or failure to engraft. The use of hematopoietic growth factors [G-CSF, granulocyte-macrophage colony-stimulating facor (GM-CSF)] has been reported in some studies to reduce mucositis (see below), but the results have not been consistent and the exact mechanism is not clear. It would seem logical that neutrophil engraftment would improve healing, but not be a prerequisite of healing.

Hepatic veno-occlusive disease

Hepatic veno-occlusive disease has been reported to be associated with more severe mucositis with oro-pharyngeal mucositis being predictive of veno-occlusive disease, and both representing aspects of conditioning regimen toxicity (Wingard et al., 1991). More recently, the association has not been consistently noted, and if present, this is generally interpreted as being related to independent simultaneous toxicity caused by conditioning regimen toxicity.

Trauma

With increased interference with proliferation of mucosal basal epithelial cells, the resulting mucosal thinning and hampered tissue repair make the mouth and throat much more susceptible to physical trauma from oral function (eating, talking, mouth breathing) as well as emesis (Bocca et al., 1999). Thus, when challenged, the compromised mucosa cannot withstand or repair this additional damage, and this results in worse mucositis. It is not uncommon to see areas of most intense mucositis corresponding to mucosal surfaces that directly contact teeth (buccal mucosa, lateral tongue, and lower labial mucosa). Finally, toxicity from conditioning regimens to salivary glands and the immune system results in loss of lubrication and barrier function, and can have a profound effect on mucosal health and integrity (see below), which is ultimately expressed as increased mucositis. Thus strategies to prevent or reduce mucosal trauma will have a beneficial effect in reducing the severity of mucosal breakdown.

Clinical presentation of mucositis

While the cellular events associated with oropharyngeal mucositis begin immediately following the administration of cytotoxic cancer therapies, it will generally take approximately 4 to 7 days for mucosal changes to become clinically evident in patterns recognizable as mucositis (Pico et al., 1998; Sonis, 1998; Bocca et al., 1999; Demarosi et al., 2002). The cellular turnover rate for oral mucosa varies throughout the mouth and ranges from 4 to 5 days for nonkeratinized mucosa surfaces (labial and buccal mucosa, lateral and ventral tongue) and 11 to 14 days for orthokeratinized attached mucosa (hard palate, attached gingivae, etc.)—the less the keratinization and the more rapid the turnover rate, the worse the damage. The rate and severity of involvement for mucositis are clearly influenced by these differences (Squire, 1990; Squire & Kremer, 2001). Clinically, conditioning regimen–induced oro-pharyngeal mucositis will present initially as patchy mucosal atrophy and erythema with nonkeratinized surfaces initially involved (Table 80.2). An exception can be noted with exposure to TBI, which disrupts normal cellular exfoliation and results in more complete keratinization of surface cells

Table 80.2. *Severity of oral mucositis by mucosal surfaces involved*

Oral mucosal surface	Mucositis score[a]
Ventral tongue	30.2
Buccal mucosa	27.8
Labial mucosa	23.7
Gingiva	23.0
Dorsal tongue	15.8
Lips	12.7
Hard palate	7.9
Soft palate	7.7

[a] Summation of scores for erythema, atrophy, ulceration, and pseudomembrane for each site for days 0–14 posttransplant. Adapted from Kolbinson *et al.,* 1988

(Kolbinson *et al.,* 1988), and while atrophic, they will appear to be whiter. As the clinical expression of damage to the basal epithelium and submucosal cells becomes more pronounced, larger areas of moderate to severe atrophy and erythema are noted, again, especially on nonkeratinized mucosal surfaces. If direct mucosal toxicity is more intense or if secondary injury (trauma and infection) occurs, the risk of ulceration increases. However, areas of severe mucosal atrophy and ulceration tend to be covered by pseudomembranous fibrin exudates that are usually white to light yellow in color and tend to be firmly adherent. Compromise of the epithelial mucosal barrier increases the risk of pain, and when combined with the indirect toxicities of granulocytopenia, thrombocytopenia, and salivary gland dysfunction, infectious and bleeding complications are significantly increased (Connolly, Lockhart, & Sonis, 1983; Heimdahl *et al.,* 1989; Mattsson *et al.,* 1991). Mucosal damage from conditioning regimen direct toxicity will usually peak between 7 and 11 days posttransplant, which often corresponds to the nadir of neutrophil counts. Mucosal surfaces show gradual resolution over the next several days to weeks (Kolbinson *et al.,* 1988; Chapko *et al.,* 1989; Schubert, 1992; Sonis, 1998). Uncomplicated mucositis will heal within 14 to 21 days after transplant. Patients receiving methotrexate for GVHD prophylaxis will heal more slowly.

Generally, the symptoms of mucositis begin to be noted toward the end of conditioning and gradually increase to peak during the second week posttransplant (McGuire *et al.,* 1998). As the oral mucosa becomes atrophic and erythematous, patients will often report increasing stinging and burning of the mouth, especially with eating or use of oral care products. Pharyngeal pain often precedes oral pain by 2 to 3 days. More distinct oral pain becomes noticeable 3 to 4 days posttransplant, peaks with the worst mucosal damage, and resolves with mucosal healing. Increasing pain usually parallels the increasing severity of mucosal breakdown. Generally, pain and mucosal breakdown peak together and subside together. Oropharyngeal mucositis pain has been reported to be the most significant and most common pain requiring intervention for the first 100 days posttransplant (Bellm *et al.,* 2000).

Symptoms of oral dryness start late during conditioning and gradually increase as chemo- or chemoradiotherapy-induced salivary gland dysfunction worsens. Saliva tends to be thicker and have a more mucus character as the serous glands are more susceptible to damage initially.

Oral infections

There is a growing body of evidence that supports the contention that oral microflora, including those bacteria associated with dental plaque, can negatively influence oro-pharyngeal mucositis produced by cancer chemotherapy or ionizing radiation (Ferretti *et al.,* 1987; Samaranayake *et al.,* 1988; Raether *et al.,* 1989; Spijkervet *et al.,* 1989; Epstein, 1990; Peterson, 1990; Spijkervet *et al.,* 1990, 1991; Wahlin *et al.,* 1991; Offidani *et al.,* 1999; Shenep, 2000; Graber *et al.,* 2001). Lucas and colleagues (1998) found a significant increase in the mean bacterial plaque score and in the degree of gingival inflammation in children at 7 days posttransplant, which corresponded with peak mucositis scores. However, which organisms are most responsible and the exact nature of the relationship of normal oral flora to mucositis remains to be determined, though local invasion through compromised mucosa barriers as well as stimulation of more intense immune responses does worsen mucositis. While several studies utilizing antibiotic protocols to specifically target certain groups of organisms have reported reduced mucositis, follow-up studies have not produced consistent results. It is reasonable to hypothesize that the oral flora of patients includes many organisms that have relatively low virulence, but are capable of damaging local (i.e., mucosal) tissues and/or inducing local immune responses that result in tissue breakdown. In addition to immune suppression, the use of broad-spectrum antibiotics and xerostomia combine to increase the risk of oral infection due to the emergence of opportunistic pathogens (Driezen *et al.,* 1979; Schubert *et al.,* 1986a, 1986b, 1988; Wingard, 1990). The risk of bacteremia and septicemia from organisms of oral origin, especially in patients with oro-pharyngeal mucositis, is of major concern (Schubert *et al.,* 1988; Wingard, 1990; Valteau *et al.,* 1991). Of particular concern is the risk of viridans group streptococcal bacteremia and infection in patients with severe mucositis, especially in those receiving oral, nonabsorbable quinolone antibiotics (Vilavlanca *et al.,* 1990; Steiner *et al.,* 1993; Schiodt *et al.,* 1998; Offidani *et al.,* 1999; Marron *et al.,* 2000; Shenep, 2000; Graber *et al.,* 2001) (see Chapter 73).

Up until the early 1980s, reactivation of latent HSV was a major contributor to severe oro-pharyngeal mucositis following HSC transplantation, especially during the first 30 days posttransplant (Schubert *et al.,* 1986a, 1990a; Schubert, 1991; Carrega *et al.,* 1994; Hoppe *et al.,* 1997). However, with standard use of acyclovir, and subsequently valacyclovir, for prophylaxis and treatment of HSV infections, the frequency of devastating oral HSV mucositis has been dramatically reduced (Bubley *et al.,* 1989; Bergmann, Mogensen, & Ellegaard, 1990; Woo, Sonis, & Sonis, 1990; Epstein *et al.,* 1996; Dignani *et al.,*

2002). It is common to see oral HSV infections arise when prophylactic acyclovir is discontinued. Cytomegalovirus (CMV) can cause oral lesions after HSCT, even in the absence of CMV disease at other sites (Schubert et al., 1993; Lloid et al., 1994). While other viruses (varicella-zoster, Epstein-Barr, coxsackie, adenovirus, human herpesvirus 6 and 7, and human polyomavirus) have been implicated in oral lesions posttransplant, the frequency and scope of their involvement remains unclear, and, probably, infrequent (Zaia, 1990).

Candida is the fungal organism most frequently isolated from the oral cavity and oro-pharynx and usually presents as white pseudomembranous plaques (Marr & Bowden, 1999; Bodey et al., 2002). The contribution of Candida to the signs and symptoms of oro-pharyngeal mucositis is not clear. Colonization studies show that between 20% and 50% of patients will be colonized with Candida in spite of topical or systemic fungal prophylaxis. While C. albicans has been the yeast most frequently isolated from the mouth, C. glabrata, C. krusei, C. tropicalis, and C dubliniensis are being isolated from neutropenic transplant patients (Meis et al., 1999; Kusne & Krystofiak, 2001; Safdar et al., 2001; Bodey et al., 2002). Other fungal organisms causing invasive oral lesions of considerable concern are Aspergillus, zygomycetes group, and histoplasma (Dreizen et al., 1979; Schubert et al., 1986; Meyers, 1990; Chambers et al., 1995; Schiodt et al., 1998; Marr & Bowden, 1999; Bodey et al., 2002).

Oral graft-versus-host disease

GVHD can cause oral mucosal lesions that range clinically from mucosal atrophy and erythema to oral lichen planus–like striae and plaques to widespread pseudomembranous ulcerations (Schubert et al., 1984; Schubert & Sullivan, 1990; Woo, Lee, & Schubert, 1997). Both acute and chronic GVHD have oral manifestations. Acute oral GVHD lesions generally occur between 18 and 100 days posttransplant and thus do not generally influence oral mucositis significantly, though oral acute GVHD can merge and evolve from mucositis to present as what appears to be a non-healing mucositis that can persist past the normal healing time for mucositis (i.e., after days 18–21 posttransplant). Although oral acute GVHD lesions can influence the clinical presentation of mucositis and slow the rate of healing of oral mucositis in allogeneic patients, oral acute GVHD does not clearly become clinically distinguishable from conditioning regimen–induced oro-pharyngeal mucositis until about 24 to 28 days posttransplant. The diagnosis of oral GVHD can often be confused by the presence of simultaneous infections, especially viral (Schubert & Sullivan, 1990). Patients with hyperacute GVHD occurring in the first 1–2 weeks posttransplant can have oral lesions that manifest as severe mucosal inflammation and breakdown and are clinically indistinguishable from the changes due to conditioning regimen–induced mucositis. Chronic oral GVHD lesions occur much later (70 days posttransplant and later).

In addition to the oral lesions induced by GVHD, GVHD prophylaxis regimens that utilize methotrexate and related agents (e.g., trimetrexate) can clearly increase the severity of oro-pharyngeal mucositis due to the direct damage to oral mucosa caused by these chemotherapy agents (Dahllof et al., 1988; Deeg et al., 1991; Doney et al., 1995).

Xerostomia

Both radiation and chemotherapy can induce major and minor salivary gland dysfunction with decreased salivary flow rates and altered sialochemistry (Chaushu et al., 1995; Kosuda et al., 1999; Buchali et al., 2000). Additionally, salivary gland dysfunction can result from acute GVHD (Nagler et al., 1996). Changes in salivary flow rates and constituents can have a significant effect on oral mucositis. The loss of salivary mucins reduces lubrication of mucosal surfaces, and compromises the ability of these mucins to provide a barrier function and thus allow for increased microbial adherence to mucosal surfaces. The loss of salivary proteins, enzymes, and antibodies (especially IgA) influences oral microbial colonization and increases susceptibility to infection (Levine, Jone, & Loomis, 1987; Wahlin, 1991; Wahlin et al., 1991; Mansson-Rahemtulla et al., 1992). Recovery from conditioning regimen–related xerostomia can vary from a few weeks for patients conditioned with chemotherapy alone, to months or occasionally years, for some patients receiving high-dose TBI plus TLI. Most TBI-related xerostomia resolves at between 3 and 12 months posttransplant, although some instances of salivary dysfunction can be permanent (Schubert & Izutsu, 1987).

While most patients generally recover normal salivary gland function after transplant, or at least remain symptomatically stable, some patients will have persistent complaints of xerostomia. Increased frequency of fluid intake or the use of sugarless candies, mints, or gum can help keep patients comfortable. Secretagogues will often help. In the future it may be possible to use gene therapy and tissue engineering to develop treatments for those with severe salivary dysfunction (Atkinson & Baum, 2001).

Hemorrhage

A number of factors contribute to the risk of oro-pharyngeal bleeding. Conditioning- and/or disease-induced thrombocytopenia is the most common hematologic factor associated with oral bleeding, although coagulopathies also occur. Bleeding can range from ecchymotic lesions to frank spontaneous hemorrhage. Bleeding can be associated with pre-existing periodontal disease, or can occur with severe mucositis (especially when associated with oral HSV infection) (Connolly et al., 1983). Although oral bleeding in this setting is clinically alarming and uncomfortable, it is not usually a serious event, and local control measures along with maintenance of adequate platelet counts will usually provide satisfactory management until mucosal healing occurs. However, oral hemorrhage in the presence of severe oro-pharyngeal mucositis can compromise the oral airway and increase the risk of aspiration (Connolly et al., 1983).

Management of oro-pharyngeal mucositis

Despite significant advances in supportive care in general for patients undergoing HSCT over the past decade, management of oro-pharyngeal mucositis remains marginally effective (Peterson, 1999; Schubert, Peterson, & Lloid, 1999; Biron *et al.*, 2000; Kostler *et al.*, 2001). Currently, a number of promising agents are under clinical development that have promise for being able to prevent or reduce the direct and indirect oro-pharyngeal mucosa damage and/or promote more rapid healing (Peterson, 1999; Stiff, 2001). These include such agents as growth factors, anti-inflammatory agents, and a wide range of antimicrobial agents (see below). In the mean time, the management of oro-pharyngeal mucositis remains dependent on symptomatic management, along with strategies to prevent local infections and trauma (Schubert *et al.*, 1986; Sonis & Clark, 1991) (Table 80.3). Constant diagnostic vigilance must be directed toward determining which factors are responsible for modifying (i.e., worsening) mucositis and then utilizing appropriate preventative and therapeutic measures.

Table 80.3. *Management strategies for oro-pharyngeal mucositis*

Pretransplant oral & dental stabilization	
Elimination:	Active dental caries
	Peridontal disease
	Endodontic infections
	Potential sources of trauma
Patient education and motivation	
Basic oral care:	Routine brushing & flossing
	Routine rinsing
	Normal saline solution
	Sodium bicarbonate solution
Education/motivation:	Patient responsibilities for self-care
	Common oral complications
	Standard care protocols
Mucositis pain management strategies	
Topical anesthetics:	Lidocaine
	Benzocaine
	Diphenhydramine
	Doxepin
	Benzydamine
Mucosal coating agents:	Antacid solutions
	Sucralfate
	Artificial saliva solutions
	Hydroxypropylcellulose gel
Anti-inflammatory agents:	Ice
	(Benzydamine)
Experimental approaches to mucositis management	
Antimicrobials:	Chlorhexidine, Isoganan, other
Anti-inflammatories	Benzydamine, alginate sodium, Fibronectin, Misoprosit
Cytokines and growth factors:	IL-3, IL-6, IL-11, G-CSF, GM-CSF, EGF, TGF-β3, KGF
Other:	Low-energy lasers
	Pilocarpine/cevimeline
	Amifostine

All patients should receive compete oral and dental examinations prior to transplant to determine the presence of dental, periodontal, or oral problems that could negatively impact the post-transplant oral course—most importantly, deep dental decay, abscesses, gingivitis, or periodontitis. Whenever possible, patients should receive care that eliminates active dental caries, periodontal infection, and pulpal disease. Fractured or sharp teeth should be smoothed. All patients should be given instructions on appropriate oral care posttransplant. Routine and effective daily oral care protocols—brushing and flossing—have been shown to have a beneficial effect on oral complications (Borowski *et al.*, 1994; Dodd *et al.*, 1996; Bocca *et al.*, 1999; Dodd et al, 1999; Cheng *et al.*, 2001). Current strategies include the following.

Daily oral care protocols

1. Tooth brushing with a soft or ultra-soft toothbrush; toothpaste is optional since flavors frequently cause burning and stinging. It is important to note that healthy gingival tissues that are not traumatized do not bleed. Allowing dental plaque to build up on the teeth and gingival tissues leads to gingivitis—an infection—and increases the risk of bleeding, local infection, and bacteremia. If gingival tissues are allowed to get healthy and then maintained throughout transplant, the risk of oral complications is decreased.

2. Flossing is necessary to keep the interproximal tissues free of bacterial plaque and thus reduce the risk for infection and bleeding. Flossing needs to be carried out carefully so as to not traumatize tissues.

3. Frequent normal saline or other bland rinses help to keep tissues cleared of debris and moisturized and can help soothe mild to moderate mucositis pain. Eight to 12 ounces of solution should be rinsed every 1 to 4 hours as needed to maintain comfort.

Symptom management/pain management

1. Topical anesthetics can provide short-term pain relief for mild to moderate mucositis (Carnel *et al.*, 1990; Elad *et al.*, 1999). A variety of agents can be used and include such anesthetic agents as lidocaine and benzocaine or antihistamines such as diphenhydramine. A unique agent that can be used in these situations is the liquid form of doxepin: when used as a rinse, it can provide immediate pain relief due to an anesthetic action that lasts for approximately 15 to 20 minutes, but is followed by an analgesic action that provides continued pain relief with an anesthetic effect. Several cautions must be mentioned here. Patients should be warned not to anesthetize the posterior oropharynx in order to avoid reducing or eliminating the gag reflex, which would increase the risk of aspiration. Patients should not numb their mouths and attempt to eat!

2. Mucosal coating agents (alginate sodium, antacid solutions, hydroxypropyl cellulose) have long been recommended for symptomatic relief, but there is little or no research to support their use and their efficacy generally needs to be

assessed on a case by case basis (Rodu & Russel, 1988; Hasagawa et al., 1989; Oshitani et al., 1990; Pfeiffer et al., 1990). Sucralfate has been extensively studied for mucositis management, but results have been conflicting and it is not possible to determine guidelines for its use (Allison et al., 1995; Giorgi et al., 1996; Shenep et al., 1998; Castagna et al., 2001). In general, sucralfate does not appear to have a significant effect on reducing the severity or shortening the course of mucositis, though it may help reduce pain.

3. Oral cryotherapy involves having patients hold ice chips in their mouths during the administration of chemotherapy agents and is based on the hypothesis that the ice will induce local vasoconstriction and thus decrease drug delivery to mucosal tissues (Mahood et al., 1991). However, it is clear that this technique would only work with agents that have a relatively short serum half life (10–15 minutes, e.g., bolus injected 5 FU) (Clarkson et al., 2000). Since these types of agents are not used routinely as part of HSCT conditioning regimens, their use for HSCT patients cannot be justified. It has been hypothesized that there is a potential risk for increased mucositis with cryotherapy if it is not used long enough, due to the fact that a rebound vasodilation could occur after the ice therapy is stopped and this could result in increased drug delivery to tissues and potentially increased mucositis if the blood levels of the chemotherapeutic agents are still high. Sucking ice chips can be used to help reduce mouth pain and provide relief of xerostomia for patients with mucositis.

4. Xerostomia management with the use of artificial salivas or through stimulation of glands (to increase salivary flow rates through taste stimulation) or the use of secretagogues (pilocarpine or cevimeline) can help with patient comfort. The latter may actually have more health benefits due to the properties of saliva.

5. Narcotic analgesics form the core of management strategies for severe mucositis. (Chapman & Hill, 1989; Hill et al., 1991; Coda et al., 1997). These agents can be delivered through intravenous routes, patches, or oral routes if tolerated by the patient. Patient controlled analgesia (PCA) has been shown to provide for the most effective pain relief with less medication and fewer side effects (Hill et al., 1991; Dunbar et al., 1996; Chapman et al., 1997). Often it is important to customize and tailor protocols to assure maximal benefit. When a patient goes on to these protocols, it is important that they continue with standard oral care as much as possible (see Chapter 81).

Infection prophylaxis

The early years of HSCT were plagued by serious infectious complications. Subsequently, prophylactic regimens to prevent viral, fungal, and bacterial infections have significantly reduced the frequency and severity of infectious complications. The mucosal destruction caused by the reactivation of HSV in the first 21 days posttransplant when combined with mucositis can result in very severe mucosal destruction. The routine use of antiviral prophylaxis with acyclovir or valacyclovir has had a profound effect in reducing herpetic stomatitis in HSV-seropostive patients following transplant and the consequent oropharyngeal mucosal damage (Peterson, 1990; Saral, 1990; Wingard, 1990; Dignani et al., 2002). Similarly, prophylactic antifungal therapy has helped reduce the frequency and severity of systemic and oral Candida infections in transplant patients (Marr & Bowden, 1999; Wingard, 2002).

There have been no studies of the impact of prophylactic systemic antibacterial agents on oral mucositis. The efficacy of topical prophylactic antibacterial agents to prevent or reduce mucositis is an area of intense study currently (see below). Opinion delineating effectiveness of rinsing with chlorhexidine solutions to reduce or preventing mucositis is clearly divided (McGaw & Belch, 1985; Ferretti et al., 1987; Epstein et al., 1992; Dodd et al., 1996, 2000). While there have been several studies indicating effectiveness of chlorhexidine, the variable quality of these studies hampers interpretation and acceptance of the results. Several studies have shown no benefit from chlorhexidine rinses. Furthermore, there is clearly a problem with compliance with the alcohol-based chlorhexidine rinses, which can be irritating and painful to use as mucosal thinning increases with evolving mucositis. Additionally, it is possible that the lack of activity of chlorhexidine against Gram-negative organisms may diminish the efficacy of this agent, since Gram-negative organisms have been implicated as being more problematic relative to influencing mucositis (Sonis, 1998).

Management of oral GVHD

Generally stated, the most effective way to manage oral GVHD is effective systemic therapy. Local GVHD treatment strategies, however, can augment and speed stabilization and provide for better symptom management. Treatment with topical steroids (e.g., dexamethasone, clobetasol), and azathioprine solutions are the most reasonable strategies to utilize initially to reduce oral mucosal damage and promote healing (Schubert & Sullivan, 1990; Woo, Lee, & Schubert MM, 1997; Epstein et al., 2001)) For more resistant cases, PUVA therapy or possibly extracorporeal photophoresis may need to be utilized (Atkinson et al., 1986; Menillo et al., 2001; Dall'Amico & Messina, 2002).

Until effective strategies are developed that can clearly prevent mucosal damage and/or speed up healing, mucositis management will depend on the above strategies. It is important to attempt to identify all factors influencing the clinical course and employ appropriate treatments. It is often necessary to utilize a customized approach that tailors treatment to the patient's responses and ability to comply with various agents. It is clear that successful management depends on persistent and frequent use of all strategies.

Future directions in mucositis management

Over the past decade, there has been considerable interest and research activity in the area of mucositis prevention and management. With the evolving elucidation of the pathophysiology of mucositis, new targets for therapy are rapidly evolving and it is possible that within the next decade that mucositis will become a problem of the past (Sonis *et al.*, 2001; Peterson & Sonis, 2001).

Strategies have been investigated to specifically either prevent oral mucosal damage and/or promote healing of mucositis induced by chemotherapy or chemoradiotherapy. Although a number of agents have been reported to reduce the severity of mucositis, most have not been examined by rigorous research efforts and confirmatory evidenced-based analysis is needed. Currently, areas of research can be divided into (1) topical antimicrobials, (2) anti-inflammatory agents, (3) cytokines and growth factors, and (4) other approaches.

Antimicrobial agents

In the late 1980s a clinical trial was conducted that indicated that rinsing with a 0.12% solution of chlorhexidine could reduce the severity of oral mucositis (Ferretti *et al.*, 1987). However, attempts to duplicate these results have met with varying success. Other studies using antimicrobial lozenges (containing polymixin B, tobramycin, and amphotericin B) have been reported to help reduce the severity of mucositis in patients receiving head and neck radiation; this approach has not been studied in HSCT patients (Spijkervet *et al.*, 1990, 1991). In another approach to reduce mucositis, trials have been completed in which an antimicrobial defensins protein (Isoganan HCl®) that was administered during conditioning and for several weeks after transplant and demonstrated the ability to reduce the severity of mucositis (Giles *et al.*, 2002). Phase III trials have been concluded. A number of other topical antimicrobial agents are under investigation in clinical trials.

Anti-inflammatory agents

There have been a number of reports over the years indicating the efficacy of benzydamine rinses for reducing the severity and duration of mucositis (Schubert & Newton, 1987; Epstein *et al.*, 1989). While the exact mode of action is not certain, benzydamine has been noted to produce an initial analgesic effect that diminishes rapidly, although there is a persistent analgesia. Laboratory studies have suggested that benzydamine is able to produce an anti-inflammatory effect by interfering with pro-inflammatory cytokine activity. Favorable results have been reported from a multicenter trial that investigated the use of benzydamine HCl to prevent or reduce mucositis associated with head and neck radiation (Epstein *et al.*, 2001). Further testing is necessary to determine the usefulness of this agent in the HSC transplant setting, but earlier studies were encouraging (Schubert & Newton, 1987).

The potential benefits of a number of different agents have been reported to help prevent or reduce the severity of mucositis and include alginate sodium (Dozono *et al.*, 1989), fibronectin (Matysiak, Klos, & Ochocka, 1988), and

prostaglandin E2 (Matejka *et al.*, 1990). The potential benefit of prostaglandin E1 and E2 remains unclear. While some workers have reported some success with these agents (Porteder *et al.*, 1988; Pretnar *et al.*, 1989), others have reported little or no benefit (Labar *et al.*, 1993; Duenas-Gonzalez *et al.*, 1996). A multicenter pilot trial that tested the potential efficacy of the prostaglandin E2, misoprostol, in reducing mucositis showed potential benefit, but clearly requires more extensive testing (D. E. Peterson, personal communication).

Attempts to utilize the anti-inflammatory effects of topical steroids to improve the course of mucositis have not been demonstrated. A study that utilized oral prednisone along with pentoxifylline and ciprofloxacin not only failed to prevent mucositis, but also demonstrated an increased risk of infection (Ferra *et al.*, 1997). The use of topical or systemic steroids to prevent or reduce oral mucositis cannot be recommended currently.

Cytokines and growth factors

Cytokines and growth factors are proteins that mediate cellular responses (Thomson, 1998). Cytokines and growth factors are released by cells to transmit messages within or between cells by binding to specific receptors on target cells and trigger mechanisms within the targeted cells. Cytokines are generally responsible for mediating inflammatory and immune responses. Classically, growth factors (e.g., epidermal growth factor, fibroblast growth factors, and vascular endothelial growth factor) stimulate cells to proliferate and are produced constitutively (Goldsby, 2000).

IL-2 is a pro-inflammatory cytokine that induces mucositis rather than ameliorates it. Clinical trials in which IL-2 has been used to enhance antitumor effects of chemotherapy have resulted in increased toxicities, including mucositis. Future efforts could potentially target an "anti-IL-2" to reduce mucositis tissue damage.

IL-3 is a cytokine that is involved with the growth and differentiation of hematopoietic cells (Ellitott *et al.*, 1989; Groopman, 1990; Goldsby, 2000). In a clinical trial involving patients undergoing autologous HSCT, individuals who received IL-3 demonstrated less mucositis, but the agent was generally not tolerated well.

IL-6 is another pro-inflammatory cytokine that is produced by a wide variety of cells, including fibroblasts, monocytes, macrophages, and T lymphocytes (Imrie *et al.*, 1997; Goldsby, 2000). IL-6 promotes the terminal differentiation of B lymphocytes into plasma cells, promotes stimulation of antibody secretion, and promotes differentiation of myeloid stem cells. While a correlation between plasma levels for IL-6 and mucositis has been shown, in a phase I clinical toxicity trial conducted by Imrie *et al.* (1997), IL-6 administration demonstrated reduced mucositis.

IL-11 is a cytokine secreted by bone marrow stromal cells and promotes proliferation of hematopoietic cells and production of platelets. There is some evidence that IL-11 may also inhibit proliferation of epithelial cells, downregulate pro-inflammatory mediators such as tumor necrosis factor, and it has been shown to ameliorate mucositis in animal models (Keith *et al.,* 1994; Kaye, 1996; Sonis, Edwards, & Lucey, 1999; Sonis *et al.,* 2000; Stiff, 2001). In a multicenter phase I trial in which patients being transplanted for hematopoietic malignancies conditioned with chemoradiotherapy were given IL-11, severe fluid retention and multiorgan failure occurred and the benefits for mucositis reduction were difficult to determine. There is insufficient evidence to support its use at this time.

Colony-stimulating factors are hematopoietic growth factors that regulate the proliferation of bone marrow progenitor cells and development of mature blood cells (Kanz *et al.,* 1991). G-CSF and GM-CSF specifically target the development of the granulocyte-macrophage lineage (Gabrilove *et al.,* 1988; Kitayama *et al.,* 1989). Additionally, both of these growth factors will activate mature neutrophils. Finally, GM-CSF promotes effector functions of eosinophils, monocytes, and macrophages (Goa & Bryson, 1994). G-CSF and GM-CSF are used to improve hematopoiesis following cancer therapies and for mobilizing donor peripheral blood stem cells. The effect of G-CSF on mucositis has been studied in several trials and results are not conclusive. Two randomized studies have shown some reduction in mucositis, but several cohort studies have failed to show benefit (Karthaus *et al.,* 1998; Crawford *et al.,* 1999; Godder & Henslee-Downey, 2001; Patte *et al.,* 2002). Furthermore, Wardley *et al.* (2000) concluded that the most important determinant of mucositis was the type of cytotoxic conditioning regimen and not the use of myeloid growth factors. It is important to note that G-CSF has shown no benefit for radiation-induced mucositis.

Studies involving GM-CSF have also produced conflicting results relative to their ability to reduce oro-pharyngeal mucositis (Ibrahim & al-Mullhim, 1997; Hejna *et al.,* 2001; van der Lelie *et al.,* 2001; Fung & Ferrill, 2002). Several randomized studies have shown that topical rinses with GM-CSF were able to reduce oral mucositis, but in other randomized studies and cohort studies, no benefit has been realized from topical rinses. Subcutaneous GM-CSF appears to shorten the duration of mucositis, but not the severity.

In general, CSFs have produced inconsistent benefits when used to reduce or prevent oro-pharyngeal mucositis. It is clear that they promote more rapid marrow recovery, especially relative to early neutrophil engraftment and the potential mechanism of action relative to mucositis may be most directly related to this latter event. By decreasing the influence or impact of microflora on damaged mucosal tissues by the more rapid repopulation of mucosal tissues with neutrophils and macrophages, there is accelerated healing of mucosal ulceration (Lieschke *et al.,* 1992).

A variety of epithelial growth factors have been or are currently under study for to their ability to prevent or reduce the severity and duration of oro-pharyngeal mucositis (Hudson-Godman, Girard, & Jones, 1990).

Epidermal growth factor (EGF) promotes cell proliferation and differentiation of a variety of cell types, including oral mucosal epithelium and can be found in saliva, serum, and urine. In an animal study, Sonis *et al.* (1992) demonstrated that administration of EGF concomitant with the administration of cancer chemotherapy increased mucositis. In a clinical study, EGF levels in saliva have been found to correlate inversely with the severity of oral mucositis during oro-pharyngeal radiation therapy (Epstein *et al.,* 2000). Considerably more study is needed to clarify the relationship of EGF to mucositis and whether it could be administered after cytotoxic therapy to allow for more rapid recovery of oral tissues.

Transforming growth factors (TGFs) are a family of growth factors (TGF-β1, -β2, and -β3), that appear to inhibit proliferation of many cells, including epithelial and endothelial cells and lymphoid and hematopoietic cells, and cause growth arrest and apoptosis (Sonis *et al.,* 1994; Hesketh, 1997). TGF-β3 is a known inhibitor of cell division of epithelial cells (Elovic *et al.,* 1990; Sonis *et al.,* 1997; Knox *et al.,* 2000). In a phase I study of TGF-β3, the agent was well tolerated and demonstrated beneficial effects on chemotherapy-induced oral mucositis (Wymenga *et al.,* 1999). However, in a multicenter study, no beneficial effects were found, though the result may have been affected by changes in the formulation of the cytokine (Foncuberta *et al.,* 2001).

Keratinocyte growth factors (KGFs) represent a promising approach to mucositis prevention currently under study (Stiff, 2001). KGFs are members of the fibroblast growth factor (FGF) family that specifically bind to the KGF receptor, a variant of FGF receptor 2 that is found only in epithelial tissues. KGF mediates proliferation and differentiation of a wide variety of epithelial cells, including hepatocytes, gastrointestinal epithelial cells, and keratinocytes in stratified squamous epithelia (Danilenko, 1999). Two KGF molecules are currently being explored: a recombinant human KGF (rHuKGF or KGF-1) and genomically derived KGF (KGF-2); both appear to provide cytoprotection against epithelial tissue damage. Comparative trials between the two molecules have not been conducted. Animal model studies for mucositis caused by radiation- and/or chemotherapy-induced oral and gastrointestinal mucositis have been extremely encouraging and both molecules are currently in clinical trials (Farrell *et al.,* 1999, 2002). The current trials utilize a 3-day induction period prior to commencement of conditioning to induce mucosal proliferation with the objective of making epithelial tissues thicker and more resistant to breakdown. Following conditioning, KGF is administered to re-induce mucosal proliferation to "heal" mucosal damage induced by conditioning regimen–induced mucosal cytotoxicity. The phase III clinical trial for KGF-1 has been concluded and KGF-2 is currently in phase II trials.

Other approaches

Low-energy laser therapy

For over 30 years, reports of the potential benefits of low-energy laser therapy (LELT) to promote wound healing and relieve pain have appeared in the medical literature. Several studies have reported the effectiveness of helium-neon (HeNe) laser therapy to reduce the severity of oro-pharyngeal mucositis in patients undergoing HSCT (Schubert *et al.,* 1994; Barasch *et* al., 1995; Cowen et al., 1997) or head and neck radiation (Bensadoun et al., 1999). The mode of action for LELT is not clear though several theories have been advanced based on laboratory studies. The most prominent proposes that laser energy is absorbed by mitochondrial chromophores and the energy exchange promotes an "intracellular healing" effect at a molecular and enzymatic level. It has also been suggested that LELT may be capable of detoxification of free radicals and/or reduction of free radical formation induced by anticancer chemotherapy and radiation therapy (B. Rossi, personal communication). Laser therapy does not appear to stimulate cell proliferation, inasmuch as LELT can be administered during conditioning and there is no promotion of epithelial cell cytotoxicity.

Helium-neon has been the most studied of the LELT wavelengths, but considerable work is underway with additional wavelengths produced by aluminum-gallium-arsenide (AlGaAs) diode sources that may also be able to provide similar positive effects; diode lasers are considerably less expensive to manufacture and are smaller and more convenient to use clinically. More work is necessary to determine the efficacy of this form of therapy.

Salivary gland dysfunction management strategies

In some instances it has been suggested that some cancer chemotherapy agents used for conditioning may actually be secreted into the saliva and thus increase the toxic effect of that agent on the oral mucosa. In one study, transplant patients receiving etoposide were given propantheline to decrease salivary gland secretion in an attempt to decrease exposure of oral tissues to the agent, to in turn reduce the frequency and severity of mucositis (Ahmed et al., 1993). Atropine can also be given in an attempt to decrease the excessive salivation sometimes associated with oro-pharyngeal mucositis.

Over the past decade attention has been paid to the potential benefits of maintaining salivary flow rates during cancer therapies. Studies in which pilocarpine has been administered to head and neck radiation patients during radiation therapy has produced inconsistent results relative to both mucositis severity and salivary gland function (Valdez et al., 1993; Zimmerman et al., 1997; Nagler et al.,1998; Sangthawan et al., 2001; Warde et al., 2002). It is not certain whether pilocarpine treatment actually protects/preserves salivary gland tissue or whether it merely maximizes function from unirradiated glands. The situation with pilocarpine therapy for patients receiving cancer chemotherapy has not been studied as extensively as it has for head and neck radiation patients. However, in a study conducted by Awidi et al. (2001), prophylactic pilocarpine treatment was found to significantly reduce the mucositis scores.

Finally, management of GVHD-associated xerostomia with secretagogues, pilocarpine, and cevimeline, have shown promise. Not only is there symptomatic relief, but there also appears to be potential benefits relative to normalizing sialochemistry and thus potentially restoring the protective benefits of saliva (Singhal et al., 1997; Nagler et al., 1998; Nagler & Nagler, 1999, 2001).

Pentoxifylline

Oxpentifylline (pentoxifylline) was originally reported to reduce the severity of oral mucositis, presumably due to the downregulation of TNF-mediated mucosal damage (Holler et al., 1990; Bianco et al., 1991). However, subsequent studies have not been able to substantiate this and there appears to be no benefit to its use (Clift et al., 1993; van der Jagt et al., 1994; Ferra et al., 1997).

Amifostine

Amifostine (ethyol) is a phosphorylated aminothiol that is rapidly cleared from the plasma and then metabolized to an active free thiol metabolite that is rapidly taken up into cells. It has been shown to protect normal tissues from radiation toxicity, alkylating agents, and platinum compounds, due both to a modification of the DNA target and to oxygen free radical scavenger activity. It is currently approved in the United States to reduce salivary gland damage for patients undergoing head and neck radiation. In vitro it also protects bone marrow progenitor cells from the cytotoxic activity of a number of drugs. Capelli and colleagues (2000) administered amifostine immediately prior to high-dose melphalan conditioning regimen for autologous PBSC transplantation. The incidence and duration of severe (grade 3–4 on the WHO scale) mucositis was 21% and zero days (range 0–11 days), respectively, in the amifostine group compared to 53% and 7 days (range 0–11 days) in a historical control group. The duration of analgesic therapy was also significantly lower in the amifostine group. However, in a pilot study reported by Chauncey et al. (2000), after 3 days of oral busulfan (12 mg/kg), amifostine was given to 21 patients with a variety of malignancies at a dose of 910 mg/m^2 i.v. for 10 minutes, preceding the infusion of each of 2 doses of melphalan (100 mg/m^2) and thiotepa (500 mg/m^2) for a total of 4 days. Amifostine failed to produce a decrease in mucositis when scored utilizing the OMAS scale, and in fact there was a trend for the treatment group to have slightly higher mucositis scores. Obviously, further randomized clinical trials are required to evaluate amifostine in this setting.

In summary, while mucositis is still a major complication of HSCT, given the level of effort being exerted, the prospect for meaningful prevention and management seems possible. However, it will likely take the combining of several strategies—growth factors with antimicrobials and effective anti-inflammatory agents—to achieve this. In the meantime, consistent and persistent attention to maintaining optimal oral health and conscientiously administered supportive care to manage symptoms does provide benefits and can improve the course of care for patients.

References

Ahmed, T., Engleking, C., Szalyga, J. et al. (1993). Propantheline prevention of mucositis from etoposide. Bone Marrow Transplantation, 12, 131–2.

Allison, R.R., Vongtama, V., Vaughan, J., & Shin, K.H. (1995). Symptomatic acute mucositis can be minimized or prophylaxed by the combination of sucralfate and fluconazole. *Cancer Investigation,* **13,** 16–22.

Atkinson, J.C. & Baum, B.J. (2001). Salivary enhancement: current status and future therapies. *Journal of Dental Education,* **65,** 1096–101.

Atkinson, K., Veller, P., Ryman, W., & Biggs, J. (1986). PUVA therapy for drug-resistant graft-versus-host disease. *Bone Marrow Transplantation,* **1,** 227–36.

Awidi, A., Homsi, U., Kakail, R.I. *et al.* (2001). Double-blind, placebo-controlled cross-over study of oral pilocarpine for the prevention of chemotherapy-induced oral mucositis in adult patients with cancer. *European Journal of Cancer,* **37,** 2010–4. Comment in *European Journal of Cancer,* (2001) **37,** 1971–5.

Barasch, A., Peterson, D.E., Tanzer, J.M. *et al.* (1995). Helium-neon laser effects on conditioning–induced oral mucositis in bone marrow transplantation patients. *Cancer,* **76,** 2550–6..

Bearman, S.I., Appelbaum, F.R., Buckner, C.D. *et al.* (1988). Regimen-related toxicity in patients undergoing bone marrow transplantation. *Journal of Clinical Oncology,* **6,** 1562–8.

Bellm, L.A., Epstein, J.B., Rose-Ped, A. *et al.* (2000). Patient reports of complications of bone marrow transplantation. *Supportive Care in Cancer,* **8,** 33–9.

Bensadoun, R.J., Frnaquin, J.C., Ciais, G. *et al.* (1999). Low-energy Ne/Ne laser in the prevention of radiation-induced mucositis. A multicenter phase III randomized study in patients with head and neck cancer. *Supportive Care in Cancer,* **7,** 244–52.

Bensinger, W.I., Buckner, C.D., Clift, R.A. *et al.* (1992). Phase I study of busulfan and cyclophosphamide in preparation for allogeneic marrow transplant for patients with multiple myeloma. *Journal of Clinical Oncology,* **10,** 1492–7.

Bergmann, O.J., Mogensen, S.C., & Ellegaard, J. (1990). Herpes simplex virus and intraoral ulcers in immunocompromised patients with haematologic malignancies. *European Journal of Clinical Infectious Disease,* **9,** 185–90.

Bianco, J.A., Appelbaum, F.F., Nemunaitis, J. *et al.* (1991). Phase I-II trial of pentoxifylline for the prevention of transplant-related toxicities following bone marrow transplantation. *Blood,* **78,** 205–11.

Biron, P., Sebban, C., Gourmet, R. *et al.* (2000). Research controversies in management of oral mucositis. *Supportive Care in Cancer,* **8,** 68–71.

Blijlevens, N.M., Donnelly, J.P., & De Pauw, B.E. (2000). Mucosal barrier injury: biology, pathology, clinical counterparts and consequences of intensive treatment for haematological malignancy: an overview. *Bone Marrow Transplantation,* **25,** 1269–78.

Bocca, M., Coscia, D., Bottalico, L., & De Stefano, R. (1999). Orodental management in patients with malignant hematologic diseases who are waiting for bone marrow transplantation. *Minerva Stomatologica,* **48,** 615–9.

Bodey, G.P., Mardani, M., Hanna, H.A. *et al.* (2002). The epidemiology of Candida glabrata and Candida albicans fungemia in immunocompromised patients with cancer. *American Journal of Medicine,* **112,** 380–5.

Borgmann, A., Emminger, W., Emminger-Schmidmeier, W. *et al.* (1994). Influence of fractionated total body irradiation on mucosal toxicity in intensified conditioning regimens for autologous bone marrow transplantation in pediatric cancer patients. *Clinical Paediatrics,* **206,** 299–302.

Borowski, B., Benhamou, E., Pico, J.L. *et al.* (1994). Prevention of oral mucositis in patients treated with high-dose chemotherapy and bone marrow transplantation: a randomized controlled trial comparing two protocols of dental care. *European Journal of Cancer,* **30B,** 93–7.

Bubley, G.J., Chapman, B., Chapman, S.K. *et al.* (1989). Effect of acyclovir on radiation- and chemotherapy-induced mouth lesions. *Antimicrobial Agents and Chemotherapy,* **33,** 862–5.

Buchali, A., Feyer, P., Groll, J. *et al.* (2000). Immediate toxicity during fractionated total body irradiation as conditioning for bone marrow transplantation. *Radiotherapy Oncology,* **54,** 157–62.

Capelli, D., Santini, G., De Souza, A. *et al.* (2000). Amifostine can reduce mucosal damage after high-dose melphalan conditioning for peripheral blood progenitor cell autotransplant: a retrospective study. *British Journal of Haematology,* **110,** 300–7.

Camel, S.B., Blakeslee, D.B., Oswald, S.G., & Barnes, M. (1990). Treatment of radiation- and chemotherapy-induced stomatitis. *Otolaryngology, Head and Neck Surgery,* **102,** 326–30.

Carrega, G., Castagnola, E., Canessa, A. *et al.* (1994). Herpes simplex virus and oral mucositis in children with cancer. *Supportive Care in Cancer,* **2,** 266–9.

Castagna, L., Benhamou, E., Pedaza, E. *et al.* (2001). Prevention of mucositis in bone marrow transplantation: a double blind randomized controlled trial of sucralfate. *Annals of Oncology,* **12,** 953–5.

Chambers, M.S., Lyzak, W.A., Martin, J.W. *et al.* (1995). Oral complications associated with aspergillosis in patients with a hematologic malignancy. Presentation and treatment. *Oral Surgery, Oral Medicine, Oral Pathology, Oral Radiology, Endodontics,* **79,** 559–63.

Chapko, M.K., Syrjala, K.L., Schhilter, L. *et al.* (1989). Chemoradiotherapy toxicity during bone marrow transplantation: time course and variation in pain and nausea. *Bone Marrow Transplantation,* **4,** 181–6.

Chapman, C.R., Donaldson, G.W., Jacobson, R.C., & Hautman, B. (1997). Differences among patients in opioid self-administration during bone marrow transplantation. *Pain,* **71,** 213–23.

Chapman, C.R. & Hill, H.F. (1989). Prolonged morphine self-administration and addiction liability. Evaluation of two therories in a bone marrow transplant unit. *Cancer,* **63,** 1636–44.

Chauncey, T.R., Gooley, T.A., Lloid, M.E. *et al.* (2000). Pilot trial of cytoprotection with amifostine given with high-dose chemotherapy and autologous peripheral blood stem cell transplantation. *American Journal of Clinical Oncology,* **23,** 406–11.

Chaushu, G., Itzkovitz-Chaushu, S., Yefenof, E. *et al.* (1995). A longitudinal follow-up of salivary secretion in bone marrow transplant patients. *Oral Surgery, Oral Medicine, Oral Pathology, Oral Radiology, Endodontics,* **79,** 164–9.

Cheng, K.K., Molassiotis, A., Chang, A.M. *et al.* (2001). Evaluation of an oral care protocol intervention in the prevention of chemotherapy-induced oral mucositis in paediatric cancer patients. *European Journal of Cancer,* **37,** 2056–63.

Clarkson, J.E., Worthington, H.V., & Eden, O.B. (2000). Prevention of oral mucositis or oral candidiasis for patients with cancer receiving chemotherapy (excluding head and neck cancer). *Cochrane Database System Review* 2000:CD000978.

Clift, R.A., Bianco, J.A., Appelbaum, F.R. *et al.* (1993). A randomized controlled trial of pentoxifylline for the prevention of regimen-related toxicities in patients undergoing allogeneic marrow transplantation. *Blood*, **82**, 2025–30.

Coda, B.A., O'Sullivan, B., Donaldson, G. *et al.* (1997). Comparative efficacy of patient-controlled administration of morphine, hydromorphone, or sufentanil for the treatment of oral mucositis pain following bone marrow transplantation. *Pain*, **72**, 333–46.

Connolly, S.F., Lockhart, P.B., & Sonis, S.T. (1983). Severe oral hemorrhage and sepsis following bone marrow transplant failure. *Oral Surgery, Oral Medicine, Oral Pathology*, **56**, 483–6.

Cowen, D., Tardieu, C., Schubert, M. *et al.* (1997). Low energy helium-neon laser in the prevention of oral mucositis in patients undrgoing bone marrow transplant: results of a double blind randomized trial. *International Journal of Radiation Oncology, Biology, Physics*, **38**, 697–703.

Crawford, J., Tomita, D.K., Mazanet, R. *et al.* (1999). Reduction of oral mucositis by filgrastim (r-metHuG-CSF) in patients receiving chemotherapy. *Cytokines, Cellular Molecular Therapy*, **5**, 187–93.

Dahllof, G., Heimdahl, A., Bolme, P. *et al.* (1988). Oral condition in children treated with bone marrow transplantation. *Bone Marrow Transplantation*, **3**, 43–51.

Dahllof, G., Heimdahl, A., Modeer, T. *et al.* (1989). Oral mucous membrane lesions in children treated with bone marrow transplantation. *Canadian Journal of Dental Research*, **97**, 268–77.

Dall'Amico, R. & Messina, C. (2002). Extracorporeal photochemotherapy for the treatment of graft-versus-host disease. *Therapeutic Apheresis*, **6**, 296–304.

Danilenko, D.M. (1999). Preclinical and early clinical development of keratinocyte growth factor, an epithelial-specific tissue growth factor. *Toxicologic Pathology*, **27**, 64–71.

Deeg, H.J., Spitzer, T.R., Cottler-Fox, M. *et al.* (1991). Conditioning-related toxicity and acute graft-versus-host disease in patients given ethotrexate/cyclosporine prophylaxis. *Bone Marrow Transplantation*, **7**, 193–8.

Demarosi, F., Bez, C., & Carrassi, A. (2002). Prevention and treatment of chemo- and radiotherapy-induced oral mucositis. *Minerva Stomatologica*, **51**, 173–86.

Dignani, M.C., Mykietiuk, A., Michelet, M. *et al.* (2002). Valacyclovir prophylaxis for the prevention of Herpes simplex virus reactivation in recipients of progenitor cells transplantation. *Bone Marrow Transplantation*, **29**, 263–7.

Dodd, M.J., Larson, P.J., Dibble, S.L. *et al.* (1996). Randomized clinical trial of chlorhexidine versus placebo for prevention of oral mucositis in patients receiving chemotherapy. *Oncology Nursing Forum*, **23**, 921–7.

Doney, K.C., Storb, R., Beach, K. *et al.* (1995). A toxicity study of trimetrexate used in combination with cyclosporine as acute graft-versus-host disease prophylaxis in HLA-mismatched, related donor bone marrow transplants. *Transplantation*, **60**, 55–8.

Dodd, M.J., Dibble, S.L., Miaskowski, C. *et al.* (2000). Randomized clinical trial of the effectiveness of 3 commonly used mouthwashes to treat chemotherapy-induced mucositis. *Oral Surgery, Oral Medicine, Oral Pathology, Oral Radiology, Endodontics*, **90**, 39–47.

Dorr, W., Spekl, K., & Farrell, C.L. (2002). The effect of keratinocyte growth factor on healing of manifest radiation ulcers in mouse tongue epithelium. *Cell Proliferation*, **35** (Suppl 1), 86–92.

Dozono, H., Nakamura, K., Motoya, T. *et al.* (1989). Prevention of stomatitis induced by anti-cancer drugs. *Gan To Kagaku Ryoho*, **16**, 3449–51.

Dreizen, S., McCredie, K.B., Dickie, K.A. *et al.* (1979). Oral complications of bone marrow transplantation in adults with acute leukemia. *Postgraduate Medicine*, **66**, 187–94.

Duenas-Gonzalez, A., Sobrevilla-Calvo, P., Frias-Mendivil, M. *et al.* (1996). Misoprostol prophylaxis for high-dose chemotherapy-induced mucositis: a randomized double-blind study. *Bone Marrow Transplantation*, **17**, 809–12.

Dunbar, P.J., Chapman, C.R., Buckley, F.P., & Gavrin, J.R. (1996). Clinical analgesic equivalence for morphine and hydromorphone with prolonged PCA. *Pain*, **68**, 265–70.

Elad, S., Cohen, G., Zylber-Katz, E. *et al.* (1999). Systemic absorption of lidocaine after topical application for the treatment of oral mucositis in bone marrow transplantation patients. *Journal of Oral Pathology and Medicine*, **28**, 170–2.

Elliott, M.J., Vadas, M.A., Eglinton, J.M. *et al.* (1989). Recombinant human interleukin-3 and granulocyte-macrophage colony-stimuilating factor show common biological effects and binding characteristics on human monocytes. *Blood*, **74**, 2349–59.

Elovic, A., Galli, S.J., Weller, P.F. *et al.* (1990). Production of transforming growth factor alpha by hamster eosinophils. *American Journal of Pathology*, **137**, 1425–34.

Elting, L.S., Bodey, G.P., & Keefe, B.H. (1992). Septicemia and shock syndromes due to viridans streptococci: a case control study of predisposing factos. *Clinical Infectious Diseases*, **14**, 1201–7.

Epstein, J.B. (1990). Infection prevention in bone marrow transplantation and radiation patients. *NCI Monographs*, **9**, 73–85.

Epstein, J.B., Gorsky, M., Epstein, M.S., & Nantel, S. (2001b). Topical azathioprine in the treatment of immune-mediated chronic oral inflammatory conditions: a series of cases. *Oral Surgery, Oral Medicine, Oral Pathology, Oral Radiology, Endodontics*, **91**, 56–61.

Epstein, J.B., Gorsky, M., Guglietta, A. *et al.* (2000). The correlation between epidermal growth factor levels in saliva and the severity of oral mucositis during oropharyngeal radiation therapy. *Cancer*, **89**, 2258–65.

Epstein, J.B., Ransier, A., Sherlock, C.H. *et al.* (1996). Acyclovir prophylaxis of oral herpes virus during bone marrow transplantation. *European Journal of Cancer B: Oral Oncology*, **32B**, 158–62.

Epstein, J.B. & Schubert, M.M. (1999). Oral mucositis in myelosuppressive cancer therapy. *Oral Surgery, Oral Medicine, Oral Pathology, Oral Radiology, Endodontics*, **88**, 273–6.

Epstein, J.B., Silverman, S., Jr, Paggiarino, D.A. *et al.* (2001a). Benzydamine HCl for prophylaxis of radiation-induced oral mucositis: results from a multicenter, randomized, double-blind, placebo-controlled clinical trial. *Cancer*, **15**, 875–85.

Epstein, J.B., Stevenson-Moore, P., Jackson, S. *et al.* (1989). Prevention of oral mucositis in radiation therapy; a controlled study with benzydamine hydrochloride rinse. *International Journal of Radiation Oncology, Biology and Physics*, **16**, 1571–5.

Epstein, J.B., Vickars, L., Spinelli, J., & Reece, D. (1992). Efficacy of chlorhexidine and nystatin rinses in prevention of oral complications in leukemia and bone marrow transplantation. *Oral Surgery, Oral Medicine, Oral Pathology, 73, 682–9.*

Farrell, C.L., Rex, K.L., Chen, J.N. *et al.* (2002). The effects of keratinocyte growth factor in preclinical models of mucositis. *Cell Proliferation, 35, 78–85.*

Farrell, C.L., Rex, K.L., Kaufman, S.A. *et al.* (1999). Effects of keratinocyte growth factor in the squamous epithelium of the upper aerodigestive tract of normal and irradiated mice. *International Journal of Radiation Biology, 75, 609–20.*

Ferra, C., de Sanjose, S., Lastra, C.F. *et al.* (1997). Pentoxifylline, ciprofloxacin, and prednisone failed to prevent transplant-related toxicities in bone marrow transplant recipients and were associated with an increased incidence of infectious complications. *Bone Marrow Transplantation, 201, 1075–80.*

Ferretti, G.A., Ash, R.C., Brown, A.T. *et al.* (1987). Chlorhexidine for prophylaxis against oral infections and associated complications in bone marrow transplant patients. *Journal of the American Dental Association, 114, 461–7.*

Foncuberta, M.C., Cagnoni, P.J., Brandts, C.H. *et al.,* Investigators in TGF-beta3/OM Study Protocols, 203/205. (2001). Topical transforming growth factor-beta3 in the prevention or alleviation of chemotherapy-induced oral mucositis in patients with lymphomas or solid tumors. *Journal of Immunotherapy, 24, 384–8.*

Fung, S.M. & Ferrill, M.J. (2002). Granulocyte macrophage-colony stimulating factor and oral mucositis. *Annals of Pharmacotherapy, 36, 517–20.*

Gabrilove, J.L., Jakubowski, A., Sher, H. *et al.* (1988). Effect of granulocyte colony-stimulating factor on neutropenia and associated morbidity due to chemotherapy for transitional-cell carcinoma of the urothelium. *New England Journal of Medicine, 318, 1414–22.*

Giles, F.J., Redman, R., Yazji, S., & Bellm, L. (2002). Iseganan HCl: a novel antimicrobial agent. *Expert Opinion in Investigational Drugs, 11, 1161–70.*

Giorgi, F., Bascioni, R., De Signoribus, G., & di Saverio, F. (1996). Sucralfate propohylaxis of fluorouracil-induced stomatitis. *Tumori, 82, 585–87.*

Goa, K.L. & Bryson, H.M. (1994). Recombinant granulocyte-macrophage colony-stimulating stimulating factor (rGM-CSF): an appraisal of its pharmacoeconomic status in neutropenia associated with chemotherapy and autologous bone marrow transplant. *Pharmacoeconomics, 5, 56–77.*

Godder, K.T. & Henslee-Downey, P.J. (2001). Colony-stimulating factors in stem cell transplantation: effect on quality of life. *Journal of Hematotherapy Stem Cell Research, 10, 215–28.*

Goldsby, R. (2000). Growth Factors. In *Kuby Immunology,* ed. R.A. Goldsby, T.J. Kindt, & B.A. Osborne, 4th ed. New York: W.H. Freeman.

Graber, C.J., de Almeida, K.N., Atkinson, J.C. *et al.* (2001). Dental health and viridans streptococcal bacteremia in allogeneic hematopoietic stem cell transplant recipients. *Bone Marrow Transplantation, 27, 537–42.*

Groopman, J.E. (1990). Status of colony-stimulating factors in cancer and AIDS. *Seminars in Oncology, 17(Suppl 1), 31–37; discussion 38–41.*

Hasagawa, T., Takahashi, T., Inada, Y. *et al.* (1989). Reparative effects of sodium alginate (Alloid G) on radiation stomatitis (1989). *Nippon Acta Radiologica, 49, 1047–51.*

Heimdahl, A., Mattsson, T., Dahllof, G. *et al.* (1989). The oral cavity as a port of entry for early infections in patients treated with bone marrow transplantation. *Oral Surgery, Oral Medicine, Oral Pathology, 68, 711–16.*

Hejna, M., Kostler, W.J., Raderer, M. *et al.* (2001). Decrease of duration and symptoms in chemotherapy-induced oral mucositis by topical GM-CSF: results of a prospective randomised trial. *European Journal of Cancer, 37(16), 1994–2002. Comment in: 37(16), 1971–5.*

Hesketh, R. (1997). *The Oncogene and Tumor Suppressor Gene Facts Book.* San Diego: Academic Press.

Hill, H.F., Mackie, A.M., Coda, B.A. *et al.* (1991). Patient-controlled analgesic administration. A comparison of steady-state morphine infusions with bolus doses. *Cancer, 67, 873–82.*

Holler, E., Kolb, H.J., Holler, A. *et al.* (1990). Increased serum levels of tumor necrosis factor alpha precede major complications of bone marrow transplantation. *Blood, 75, 1011–16.*

Hoppe, J.E., Klausner, M., Klingebiel, T., & Niethammer, D. (1997). Retrospective analysis of yeast colonization and infections in paediatric bone marrow transplant recipients. *Mycoses, 40, 47–54.*

Hudson-Godman, P., Girard, N., & Jones, M.B. (1990). Wound repair and the potential use of growth factors. *Heart and Lung, 19, 379–84.*

Ibrahim, E.M. & al-Mulhim, F.A. (1997). Effect of granulocyte-macrophage colony-stimulating factor on chemotherapy-induced oral mucositis in non-neutropenic cancer patients. *Medicine, 14, 47–51.*

Imrie, K.R., Sheridan, B., Colwill, R. *et al.* (1997). A phase I study of interleukin-6 after autologous bone marrow transplantation for patients with poor prognosis Hodgkin's disease. *Leukemia Lymphoma, 25, 555–63.*

Kanz, L., Lindemann, A., Oster, W. *et al.* (1991). Hemopoietins in clinical oncology. *American Journal of Clinical Oncology, 14(Suppl 1), s27–3.*

Karthaus, M., Rosenthal, C., Huebner, G. *et al.* (1998). Effect of topical oral G-CSF on oral mucositis: a randomised placebo-controlled trial. *Bone Marrow Transplantation, 22, 781–5.*

Kaye, A. (1996). Clinical development of recombinant human interleukin-11 to treat chemotherapy-induced thrombocytopenia. *Current Opinion in Hematology, 3, 209–15.*

Keith, J.C., Albert, L., Sonis, S.T. *et al.* (1994). IL-11, a pleiotropic cytokine: exciting new effects of IL-11 on gastrointestinal mucosal biology. *Stem Cells, 12, 79–90.*

Kitayama, H., Ishikawa, J., Yamagami, T. *et al.* (1989). Granulocyte colony-stimulating factor in allogeneic bone marrow transplantation. *Japanese Journal of Clinical Oncology, 19, 367–72.*

Knox, J., Pudoziunas, A., & Feld, R. (2000). Chemotherapy-induced oral mucositis, prevention, and management. *Drugs and Aging, 17, 257–67.*

Kolbinson, D.K., Schubert, M.M., Flournoy, N., & Truelove, E.L. (1988). Early oral changes following bone marrow transplantation. *Oral Surgery, Oral Medicine, Oral Pathology, 66, 130–8.*

Kostler, W.J., Hejna, M., Wenzel, C., & Zielinski, C.C. (2001). Oral mucositis complicating chemotherapy and/or radiotherapy: options for prevention and treatment. *CA Cancer Journal for Clinicians, 51, 290–315.*

Kosuda, S., Satoh, M., Yamamoto, F. *et al.* (1999). Assessment of salivary gland dysfunction following chemoradiotherapy using quantitative salivary gland scintigraphy. *International Journal of Radiation, Oncology, Biology, and Physics,* **45**, 379–84.

Kusne, S. & Krystofiak, S. (2001). Infection control issues after bone marrow transplantation. *Current Opinions in Infectious Diseases,* **14**, 427–31.

Labar, B., Mrsic, M., Pavletic, Z. *et al.* (1993). Prostaglandin E2 for prophylaxis of oral mucositis following BMT. *Bone Marrow Transplantation,* **11**, 379–82.

Levine, J.J., Jone, P.C., & Loomis, R.E. (1987). Functions of human saliva and salivary mucins: an overview. In *Oral Mucosal Diseases,* ed. I.C. Mackenzie, C.A. Squier, & E. Dabelsteen, pp. 24–27. Copenhagen: Laegeforenginens.

Lieschke, G.J., Ramenghi, U., O'Connor, M.P. *et al.* (1992). Studies of oral neutrophil levels in patients receiving G-CSF after autologous marrow transplantation. *British Journal of Haematology,* **82**, 589–95.

Lloid, M.E., Schubert, M.M., Myerson, D. *et al.* (1994). Cytomegalovirus infection of the tongue following marrow transplantation. *Bone Marrow Transplantation,* **14**, 99–104.

Lockhart, P.B. & Sonis, S.T. (1981). Alterations in the oral mucosa caused by chemotherapeutic agents. *Journal of Dermatologic Surgery and Oncology,* **7**, 1019–25.

Lucas, V.S., Roberts, G.J., & Beighton, D. (1998). Oral health of children undergoing allogeneic bone marrow transplantation. *Bone Marrow Transplantation,* **22**, 801–8.

Mahood, D.J., Dose, A.M., Loprinzi, C.L. *et al.* (1991). Inhibition of fluorouracil-induced stomatitis by oral cryotherapy. *Journal of Clinical Oncology,* **9**, 449–52.

Marr, K.A. & Bowden, R.A. (1999). Fungal infections in patients undergoing blood and marrow transplantation. *Transplantation and Infectious Diseases,* **1**, 237–46.

Marron, A., Carratala, J., Gonzalez-Barca, E. *et al.* (2000). Serious complications of bacteremia caused by Viridans streptococci in neutropenic patients with cancer. *Clinical Infectious Diseases,* **31**, 1126–30.

Mansson-Rahemtulla, B., Techanitiswaad, T., Rahemtulla, F. *et al.* (1992). Analysis of salivary components in leukemia patients receiving chemotherapy. *Oral Surgery, Oral Medicine, Oral Pathology,* **73**, 35–46.

Matejka, M., Nell, A., Kment, G. *et al.* (1990). Local benefit of prostaglandin E2 in radiochemotherapy-induced oral mucositis. *British Journal of Oral and Maxillofacial Surgery,* **28**, 89–91.

Mattsson, T., Heimdahl, A., Dahllof, G. *et al.* (1991). Variables predicting oral mucosal lesions in allogeneic bone marrow recipients. *Head & Neck,* **13**, 224–9.

Matysiak, M., Klos, M., & Ochocka, M. (1988). Fibronectin—a new drug in the treatment of complications of chemotherapy in children with proliferative diseases of the hematopoietic system. *Pediatria Polska,* **63**, 728–32.

McGaw, W.T. & Belch, A. (1985). Oral complications of acute leukemia: prophylactic impact of a chlorhexidine mouth rinse regimen. *Oral Surgery, Oral Medicine, Oral Pathology,* **60**, 275–80.

McGuire, D.B., Yeager, K.A., Dudley, W.N. *et al.* (1998). Acute oral pain and mucositis in bone marrow transplant and leukemia patients: data from a pilot study. *Cancer Nursing,* **21**, 385–93.

Meis, J.F., Ruhnke, M., De Pauw, B.E. *et al.* (1999). Candida dubliniensis candidemia in patients with chemotherapy-induced neutropenia and bone marrow transplantation. *Emergence of Infectious Diseases,* **5**, 150–3.

Menillo, S.A., Goldberg, S.L., McKiernan, P., & Pecora, A.L. (2001). Intraoral psoralen ultraviolet A irradiation (PUVA) treatment of refractory oral chronic graft-versus-host disease following allogeneic stem cell transplantation. *Bone Marrow Transplantation,* **28**, 807–8.

Meyers, J.D. (1990). Fungal infections in bone marrow transplant patients. *Seminars in Oncology,* **17**, 10–13.

Murray, J.C., Chiu, J.K., Dorfman, S.R., & Ogden, A.K. (1995). Epiglottitis following preparation for allogeneic bone marrow transplantation. *Bone Marrow Transplantation,* **15**, 997–8.

Nagler, R., Marmary, Y., Krausz, Y. *et al.* (1996). Major salivary gland dysfunction in human acute and chronic graft-versus-host disease (GVHD). *Bone Marrow Transplantation,* **17**, 219–24.

Nagler, R.M. & Laufer, D. (1998). Protection against irradiation-induced damage to salivary glands by adrenergic agonist administration. *International Journal of Radiation Oncology, Biology, and Physics,* **40**(2), 477–81.

Nagler, R.M. & Nagler, A. (1999). Pilocarpine hydrochloride relieves xerostomia in chronic graft-versus-host disease: a sialometrical study. *Bone Marrow Transplantation,* **23**(10), 1007–11.

Nagler, R.M. & Nagler, A. (2001). The effect of pilocarpine on salivary constituents in patients with chronic graft-versus-host disease. *Archives of Oral Biology,* **46**(8), 689–95.

Offidani, M., Corvatta, L., Olivieri, A. *et al.* (1999). Infectious complications after autologous peripheral blood progenitor cell transplantation followed by G-CSF. *Bone Marrow Transplantation,* **24**, 1079–87.

Oshitani, T., Okada, K., Kushima, T. *et al.* (1990). Clinical evaluation of sodium alginate on oral mucositis associated with radiotherapy. *Journal of Japanese Society for Cancer Therapy,* **20**, 1129–37.

Parulekar, W., Mackenzie, R., Bjarnason, G., & Jordan, R.C. (1998). Scoring oral mucositis. *Oral Oncology,* **34**, 63–71.

Patte, C., Laplanche, A., Bertozzi, A.I. *et al.* (2002). Granulocyte colony-stimulating factor in induction treatment of children with non-Hodgkin's lymphoma, a randomized study of the French Society of Pediatric Oncology. *Journal of Clinical Oncology,* **20**, 441–8.

Peterson, D.E. (1990). Pretreatment strategies for infection prevention in chemotherapy patients. *NCI Monographs,* **9**, 61–71.

Peterson, D.E. (1999). Research advances in oral mucositis. *Current Opinions in Oncology,* **11**, 261–6.

Peterson, D.E. & Sonis, S.T. (2001). Future research directions. *Journal of the National Cancer Institute Monographs,* **29**, 3–5.

Pfeiffer, P., Madsen, E.L., Hansen, O., & May, O. (1990). Effect of prophylactic sucralfate suspension on stomatitis induced by cancer chemotherapy. A randomized, double-blind cross-over study. *Acta Oncologica,* **29**, 1713.

Pico, J.L., Avila-Garavito, A., & Naccache, P. (1998). Mucositis: its occurrence, consequences, and treatment in the oncology setting. *Oncologist,* **3**, 446–51.

Porteder, H., Rausch, E., Kment, G. *et al.* (1988). Local prostaglandin E2 in patients with oral malignancies undergoing chemo- and radiotherapy. *Journal of Cranio-Maxillo-Facial Surgery,* **16**, 371–4.

Pretnar, J., Glazar, D., Mlakar, U., & Modic, M. (1989). Prostaglandin E2 in the treatment of oral mucositis due to radiochemotherapy in patients with haematological malignancies. *Bone Marrow Transplantation,* **4**(Suppl 3), 106.

Raether, D., Walker, P.O., Bostrum, B., & Weisdorf, D. (1989). Effectiveness of oral chlorhexidine for reducing stomatitis. *Pediatric Dentistry,* **11**, 37–42.

Rodu, B. & Russel, C.M. (1988). Performance of a hydroxypropyl cellulose film former in normal and ulcerated oral mucosa. *Oral Surgery,* **65**, 699–704.

Ruescher, T.J., Sodeifi, A., Scrivani, S.J. *et al.* (1998). The impact of mucositis on alpha-hemolytic streptococcal infection in patients undergoing autologous bone marrow transplantation for hematologic malignancies. *Cancer,* **82**, 2275–81.

Safdar, A., van Rhee, F., Henslee-Downey, J.P. *et al.* (2001). Candida glabrata and Candida krusei fungemia after high-risk allogeneic marrow transplantation, no adverse effect of low-dose fluconazole prophylaxis on incidence and outcome. *Bone Marrow Transplantation,* **28**, 873–8.

Samaranayake, L.P., Robertson, A.G., MacFarlane, T.W. *et al.* (1988). The effect of chlorhexidine and benzydamine mouthwashes on mucositis induced by therapeutic irradiation. *Clinical Radiology,* **39**, 291–4.

Sangthawan, D., Watthanaarpornchai, S., & Phungrassami, T. (2001). Randomized double blind, placebo-controlled study of pilocarpine administered during head and neck irradiation to reduce xerostomia. *Journal of the Medical Association of Thailand,* **84**, 195–203.

Saral, R. (1990). Management of acute viral infections. *NCI Monographs,* **9**, 107–10.

Schiodt, I., Bergmann, O.J., Johnsen, H.E., & Hansen, N.E. (1998). Early infections after autologous transplantation for haematological malignancies. *Medical Oncology,* **15**, 103–8.

Schubert, M.M. (1991). Oral manifestations of viral infections in immunocompromised patients. *Current Opinion in Dentistry,* **1**, 384–97.

Schubert, M.M. (1993). Measurement of oral tissue damage and mucositis pain. In *Current and Emerging Issues in Cancer Pain,* ed. C.R. Chapman & K.M. Foley, pp. 247–265. New York: Raven Press.

Schubert, M.M., Epstein, J.B., Lloid, M.E., & Cooney, E. (1993). Oral infections due to cytomegalovirus in immunocompromised patients. *Journal of Oral Pathology and Medicine,* **22**, 268–73.

Schubert, M.M., Franquin, J., Niccoli-Filo, W. *et al.* (1994). Effects of low-energy laser on oral mucositis: a phase I/II pilot study. *Cancer Researcher Weekly,* **7**, 14–15.

Schubert, M.M. & Izutsu, K.T. (1987). Iatrogenic salivary gland dysfunction. *Journal of Dental Research,* **66** (Special issue): 680–8.

Schubert, M.M. & Newton, R.E. (1987). The use of benzydamine HCl for the management of cancer therapy-induced mucositis: preliminary report of a multicentre study. *International Journal of Tissue Reactions,* **9**, 99–103.

Schubert, M.M., Peterson, D.E., Flournoy, N. *et al.* (1990). Oral and pharyngeal herpes simplex virus infection after allogeneic bone marrow transplantation: analysis of factors associated with infection. *Oral Surgery, Oral Medicine, Oral Pathology,* **70**, 286–93.

Schubert, M.M., Peterson, D.D., Hamilton, D., & Counts, G. (1988). Changes in oral microflora following marrow transplantation. *Journal of Dental Research,* **67**, 249.

Schubert, M.M., Peterson, D.E., & Lloid, M.E. (1999). Oral complications. In *Hematopoietic Cell Transplant,* ed. E.D. Thomas, K.G. Blume, & S.J. Forman, pp. 751–63. Blackwell Scientific Publishers.

Schubert, M.M., Peterson, D.E., Meyers, J.D., & Thomas, E.D. (1986a). Head and neck aspergillosis in patients undergoing bone marrow transplantation. *Cancer,* **57**, 1092–6.

Schubert, M.M. & Sullivan, K.M. (1990). Recognition, incidence, and management of oral graft-versus-host disease. *NCI Monographs,* **9**, 135–43.

Schubert, M.M., Sullivan, K.M., Morton, T.H. *et al.* (1984). Oral manifestations of chronic graft-v-host disease. *Archives of Internal Medicine,* **144**, 1591–5.

Schubert, M.M., Sullivan, K.M., & Truelove, E.L. (1986b). Head and neck complications of bone marrow transplantation. In *Head and Neck Management of the Cancer Patient,* ed. D.E. Peterson, E.G. Elias, & S.T. Sonis, pp. 401–428. Boston:Martinus Nijhoff.

Schubert, M.M., Williams, B.E., Lloid, M.E. *et al.* (1992). Clinical assessment scale for the rating of oral mucosal changes associated with bone marrow transplantation. Development of an oral mucositis index. *Cancer,* **69**, 2469–77.

Shenep, J.L. (2000). Viridans-group streptococcal infections in immunocompromised hosts. *International Journal of Antimicrobial Agents,* **14**, 129–35.

Shenep, J.L., Kalwinsky, D.K., Hutson, P.R. *et al.* (1988). Efficacy of oral sucralfate suspension in prevention and treatment of chemotherapy-induced mucositis. *Journal of Pediatrics,* **113**, 758–63.

Singhal, S., Powles, R., Treleaven, J. *et al.* (1997). Pilocarpine hydrochloride for symptomatic relief of xerostomia due to chronic graft-versus-host disease or total-body irradiation after bone-marrow transplantation for hematologic malignancies. *Leukemia Lymphoma,* **24**(5–6), 539–43.

Sonis, S.T. (1998). Mucositis as a biological process: a new hypothesis for the development of chemotherapy-induced stomatotoxicity. *Oral Oncology,* **34**, 39–43.2

Sonis, S.T. (2002). Oral complications. In *Cancer Medicine,* ed. R.C. Bast, D.W. Kufe, R.E. Pollock *et al.,* pp. 2371–9. Hamilton Ontario: BC Decker.

Sonis, S.T. & Clark, J. (1991). Prevention and management of oral mucositis induced by antineoplastic therapy. *Oncology,* **5**, 11–22.

Sonis, S.T., Costa, J.W., Evitts, S.M. *et al.* (1992). Effect of epidermal growth factor on ulcerative mucositis in hamsters that receive cancer chemotherapy. *Oral Surgery, Oral Medicine, Oral Pathology,* **74**, 749–55.

Sonis, S., Edwards, L., & Lucey, C. (1999). The biological basis for the attenuation of mucositis: the example of interleukin-11. *Leukemia,* **13**, 831–4.

Sonis, S.T., Eilers, J.P., Epstein, J.B. *et al.* (1999). Validation of a new scoring system for the assessment of clinical trial research of oral mucositis induced by radiation or chemotherapy. *Cancer,* **85**, 2103–13.

Sonis, S.T. & Fey, E.G. (2002). Oral complications of cancer therapy. *Oncology,* **16**, 680–6; discussion, 686, 691–2, 695.

Sonis, S.T., Lindquist, L., Van Vugt, A. *et al.* (1994). Prevention of chemotherapy-induced mucositis by transforming growth factor beta 3. *Cancer Research,* **54,** 1135–8.

Sonis, S.T., Oster, G., Fuchs, H. *et al.* (2001a). Oral mucositis and the clinical and economic outcomes of hematopoietic stem-cell transplantation. *Journal of Clinical Oncology,* **19**(8), 2201–5.

Sonis, S.T., Peterson, R.L., Edwards, L.J. *et al.* (2000). Defining mechanisms of action of interleukin-11 on the progression of radiation-induced oral mucositis in hamsters. *Oral Oncology,* **36,** 373–81.

Sonis, S.T., Peterson, D.E., McGuire, D.B., & Williams, D.A. (2001b). Prevention of mucositis in cancer patients. *NCI Monographs,* **29,** 1–2.

Sonis, S.T., Scherer, J., Phelan, S. *et al.* (2002). The gene expression sequence of radiated mucosa in an animal mucositis model. *Cell Proliferation,* **35**(Suppl 1), 93–102.

Sonis, S.T., van Vugt, A.G., Brien, J.P. *et al.* (1997). Transforming growth factor-beta 3 mediated modulation of cell cycling and attenuation of 5-fluorouracil induced oral mucositis. *Oral Oncology,* **33,** 47–54.

Spijkervet, F.K.L., Van Saene, H.K., Panders, A.K. *et al.* (1989). Effect of chlorhexidine rinsing on the oropharyngeal ecology in patients with head and neck cancer who have irradiation mucositis. *Oral Surgery, Oral Medicine, Oral Pathology,* **67,** 165–71.

Spijkervet, F.K.L., Van Saene, H.K.F., Van Saene, J.J. *et al.* (1990). Mucositis prevention by selective elimination of oral flora in irradiated head and neck cancer patients. *Journal of Oral Pathology and Medicine,* **19,** 486–9.

Spijkervet, F.K.L., Van Saene, H.K.F., Van Saene, J.J. *et al.* (1991). Effect of selective elimination of the oral flora on mucositis in irradiated head and neck cancer patients. *Journal of Surgical Oncology,* **46,** 167–73.

Squire, C.A. (1990). Mucosal alterations. *NCI Monographs,* **9,** 169–72.

Squire, C.A. & Kremer, M.J. (2001). Biology of oral mucosa and esophagus. *Journal of the National Cancer Institute Monographs,* **29,** 7–15.

Srivastava, A., Bradstock, K.F., Szer, J. *et al.* (1993). Busulphan and melphalan prior to autologous bone marrow transplantation. *Bone Marrow Transplantation,* **12,** 323–9.

Steiner, M., Villablanca, J., Kersey, J. *et al.* (1993). Viridans streptococcal shock in bone marrow transplantation patients. *American Journal of Hematology,* **42,** 354–8.

Stiff, P. (2001). Mucositis associated with stem cell transplantation: current status and innovative approaches to management. Il-11, KGF. *Bone Marrow Transplantation,* **27**(Suppl 2), S3–S11.

Thomson, A. (1998). *The Cytokine Handbook.* San Diego: Academic Press.

Valdez, I.H., Wolff, A., Atkinson, J.C. *et al.* (1993). Use of pilocarpine during head and neck radiation therapy to reduce xerostomia and salivary dysfunction. *Cancer,* **71,** 1848–51.

Valteau, D., Hartmann, O., & Brugieres, L. (1991). Streptococcal septicemia following autologous bone marrow transplantation in children treated with high-dose chemotherapy. *Bone Marrow Transplantation,* **7,** 415–19.

van der Jagt, R.H., Pari, G., McDiarmid, S.A. *et al.* (1994). Effect of pentoxifylline on regimen related toxicity in patients undergoing allogeneic or autologous bone marrow transplantation. *Bone Marrow Transplant,* **13,** 203–7; Comment in: **14,** 1011–2.

van der Lelie, H., Thomas, B.L., van Oers, R.H. *et al.* (2001). Effect of locally applied GM-CSF on oral mucositis after stem cell transplantation: a prospective placebo-controlled double-blind study. *Annals of Hematology,* **80,** 150–4.

Vilavlanca, J.G., Steiner, M., Kersey, J. *et al.* (1990). The clinical spectrum of infections with viridans streptococci in bone marrow transplant patients. *Bone Marrow Transplantation,* **5,** 387–93.

Wahlin, Y.B. (1991). Salivary secretion rate, yeast cells, and oral candidiasis in patients with acute leukemia. *Oral Surgery, Oral Medicine, Oral Pathology,* **71,** 689–95.

Wahlin, Y.B., Granstrom, S., Persson, S., & Sjostrom, M. (1991). Multivariate study of enterobacteria and pseudomonas in saliva of patients with acute leukemia. *Oral Surgery, Oral Medicine, Oral Pathology,* **72,** 300–8.

Warde, P., O'Sullivan, B., Aslanidis, J. *et al.* (2002). A phase III placebo-controlled trial of oral pilocarpine in patients undergoing radiotherapy for head-and-neck cancer. *International Journal of Radiation Oncology, Biology, and Physics,* **54,** 9.

Wardley, A.M., Jayson, G.C., Swindell, R. *et al.* (2000). Prospective evaluation of oral mucositis in patients receiving myeloablative conditioning regimens and haemopoietic progenitor cell rescue. *British Journal of Haematology,* **110,** 292–9.

Wingard, J.R. (1990). Infectious and noninfectious systemic consequences. *NCI Monographs,* **9,** 21–6.

Wingard, J.R. (2002). Antifungal chemoprophylaxis after blood and marrow transplantation. *Clinical Infectious Diseases,* **10,** 1386–90.

Wingard, J.R., Niehaus, C.S., & Peterson, D.E. (1991). Oral mucositis after bone marrow transplantation: a marker of treatment toxicity and predictor of hepatic veno-occlusive disease. *Oral Surgery, Oral Medicine, Oral Pathology,* **72,** 419–24.

Woo, S.B., Lee, S.J., & Schubert, M.M. (1997). Graft-vs.-host disease. *Critical Reviews in Oral Biology and Medicine,* **8,** 201–16.

Woo, S.B., Sonis, S.T., & Monopoli, M.M., & Sonis, A.L. (1993). A longitudinal study of oral ulcerative mucositis in bone marrow transplant recipients. *Cancer,* **72,** 1612–7.

Woo, W.B., Sonis, S.T., & Sonis, A.L. (1990). The role of herpes simplex virus in the development of oral mucositis in bone marrow transplant recipients. *Cancer,* **66,** 2375–9.

Wymenga, A.N., van der Graaf, W.T., Hofstra, L.S. *et al.* (1999). Phase I study of transforming growth factor-beta3 mouthwashes for prevention of chemotherapy-induced mucositis. *Clinical Cancer Research,* **5,** 1363–8.

Zaia, J.A. (1990). Viral infections associated with bone marrow transplantation. *Hematology/Oncology Clinics of North America,* **4,** 603–23.

Zimmerman, R.P., Mark, R.J., Tran, L.M., & Juillard, G.F. (1997). Concomitant pilocarpine during head and neck irradiation is associated with decreased posttreatment xerostomia. *International Journal of Radiation Oncology, Biology, and Physics,* **37,** 571–5.

81 Pain control

SCOTT A. LANUM AND STEPHANIE B. MAGDANZ

University of Washington Medical Center/Seattle Cancer Care Alliance, Seattle, USA

Introduction

Pain is an experience influenced by the patient's emotions and perceptions of its meaning, making a clear objective definition difficult. The definition of pain proposed by the International Association for the Study of Pain is "an unpleasant sensory and emotional experience associated with actual or potential tissue damage or described in terms of such damage" (IASP, 1980). It is estimated that one-third of cancer patients receiving active therapy and 60% to 90% of cancer patients with advanced disease experience moderate to severe pain (Foley, 2001). Pain in a cancer patient generally implies a pathologic process and should be taken seriously. Cancer-related pain can lead to physical deterioration manifested as sleep disturbances, weakness, fatigue, and emotional reactions such as anxiety and depression (Enck, 2000).

Pain in hematopoietic stem cell transplant (HSCT) recipients is unique. Unlike most cancer-related pain, pain associated with HSCT is most often caused by the procedure itself rather than the underlying disease. Patients undergoing HSCT receive intensive high-dose chemotherapy or chemoradiotherapy as part of the preparative regimen prior to stem cell transplantation. Doses may be several times higher than conventional doses and are, therefore, associated with substantial neurotoxicity, organ toxicity, and tissue toxicity. All of these can contribute to pain (Chapman *et al.*, 1985).

Many patients who come to transplantation, such as patients with multiple myeloma or severe treatment-refractory rheumatoid arthritis, already suffer from chronic pain related to their disease and may be using high doses of long-acting opiates to control their pain. As non-myeloablative HSCT technology widens the population eligible to receive a transplant to include older patients with more medical problems, it is likely that the number of patients presenting to transplant centers with pre-existing chronic pain conditions will increase. Obviously, the management of HSCT-related pain in these patients will be different from that of patients not suffering from a chronic pain state. In addition to having higher tolerance to opioid analgesics, these patients may have different perceptions and expectations of pain and its management.

Another challenging patient population is the patient with a recent or remote history of substance abuse. It is essential that staff do not undertreat pain in these patients for fear of contributing to addiction and abuse. Early consultation with a pain specialist, preferably in the pretransplant evaluation period, is invaluable in these instances.

Undertreatment of pain

Undertreatment of pain in patients with cancer can prolong recovery time and hospitalization, potentiate a chronic pain state, and cause anxiety, depression, or even death (Baumann, 1999). Barriers to pain management include patient reluctance to treat pain aggressively because of fear of addiction or side effects, health care professionals' inadequate knowledge of pain management, the underutilization of existing pain management techniques, concerns about the regulation of controlled substances, fear of tolerance and addiction to narcotic analgesics, and concern about the side effects of analgesics (Baumann, 1999; Jacox *et al.*, 1994).

Health care providers do not always have adequate knowledge of pain management, particularly in patients with complicated cancer-related pain syndromes. Although self-reporting using a pain rating scale is the most reliable means of assessing pain (Jacox *et al.*, 1994), patients undergoing HSCT in one study often reported experiencing pain without being asked to rate their pain (Pederson & Parran, 1997). In a survey of nurses working with both adult and pediatric HSCT patients, 39% felt that correlation of physiologic and behavioral assessments, as well as the patient's report of pain were all required before dosages of pain medications were increased, rather than relying on the patient's self-reported need alone (Pederson & Parran, 1997). Pain is best measured simply by asking the patient (Table 81.1). The patient often knows what has worked in the past and is the only person who can balance acceptable pain control and side effects (Pederson & Parran, 1997).

Analgesics

Moderate nociceptive pain can be controlled with acetaminophen, a nonsteroidal anti-inflammatory drug (NSAID), or an opioid such as codeine, oxycodone, or morphine. NSAIDs

Table 81.1. *Assessment mnemonic (PAINED)*

Mnemonic	Description
Place	Location—may be more than one
Amount	Intensity (using pain assessment scales)—onset, duration, pattern of pain
Intensifiers	What makes the pain worse?—activity, position, time of day, swallowing, etc.
Nullifiers	What makes the pain better?—type and amount of medication, nondrug methods
Effects	Effect of pain on quality of life—functional status, sleep, appetite, social interactions; side effects of analgesics
Descriptors	Description of the quality of the pain—aching, throbbing, burning, stabbing, pressure, etc.

Adapted from Lynch & Abraham (2002).

should be used with caution in patients with renal dysfunction, concomitant diuretic use, or hypovolemia, because these agents can precipitate renal failure. NSAIDs are usually avoided in the HSCT setting because of their inhibitory effects on platelet function and risk of gastric or duodenal ulceration. When prolonged

pain is expected (such as with mucositis) it may be appropriate to use patient-controlled analgesia (PCA). For more information on analgesic medications, see Table 81.2 and Chapter 83.

Routes of administration

There are a variety of delivery options available for analgesics. These options include oral, intravenous, subcutaneous, intramuscular, transdermal, rectal, transmucosal, and perispinal. The oral route should be considered first (Stevens & Ghazi, 2000). HSCT patients often experience diarrhea as a result of conditioning regimen toxicity or lower gastrointestinal tract graft-versus-host disease (GVHD), making rectal administration of analgesics difficult. The rectal route of administration is generally avoided in HSCT patients, especially during the neutropenic period for fear of causing trauma-induced septicemia. Subcutaneous and intramuscular routes are generally avoided because of thrombocytopenia and the risk of infection. The intravenous route is readily available for patients who are unable to swallow oral medications due to severe oro-pharyngeal mucositis or who cannot tolerate anything by mouth because of nausea and vomiting.

Table 81.2. *Comparison of common opioids used in HSCT patients*

Drug	Place in therapy	Dosage forms	Onset of action	Duration	Dosing
Morphine	Moderate–severe pain; "gold standard"	i.v.: epid, i.t., i.m. s.l.: 10 mg tab i.r.: 15, 30 mg Soln: 10 mg/5 ml, 20 mg/1 ml s.r.: 15, 30, 60, 100, 200 mg p.r.: 5, 10, 20 mg	i.v.: 2–5 min s.l.: 5–10 min i.r.: 10–15 min Soln: 15–20 min s.r.: 1–2 hrs p.r.: 30 min	i.v.: 1–4 hrs s.l.: 1–4 hrs i.r.: 1–4 hrs Soln: 1–4 hrs s.r.: 8–12 hrs p.r.: 3–4 hrs	i.v. bolus: 1–5 mg q1–4 hr i.v. cont inf: 1 mg/hr s.l./i.r.: q1–2 hr prn Soln: q2–4 hr prn s.r.: q12 hr, increase to q8hr if requiring high doses
Hydromorphone	Moderate–severe pain; morphine intolerance or morphine failures	i.v. p.o.: 2, 4 mg p.r.: 3 mg	i.v.: 2–5 min p.o.: 20–30 min p.r.: 20–30 min	i.v.: 1–4 hrs p.o.: 2–4 hrs p.r.: 6–8 hrs	i.v. bolus: 0.2–1 mg q1–4 hrs i.v. cont inf: 0.2 mg/hr p.o.: 2–4 mg q2–4 hr p.r.: q6–8 hr
Meperidine	Moderate–severe pain; chilling/rigors; allergy to other opioids	i.v. p.o.: 50 mg Soln: 50 mg/5 ml	i.v.: 2–5 min p.o.: 20–30 min	i.v.: 4 hrs p.o.: 4–5 hrs	i.v.: 50–100 mg q3–4 hr p.o.: 50–100 mg q4–6 hr Soln: 50–100 mg q4–6 hr
Fentanyl	Moderate–severe pain; unable to tolerate p.o.; intolerant of other opioids	i.v., epidural Transdermal: 25, 50, 75, 100 mcg/hr Transmuc: 200, 400, 800, 1,600 mcg	i.v.: 1–5 min Transdermal: 12–18 hrs Transmuc: 5 min	i.v.: 1–2 hrs Transdermal: 72 hrs Transmuc: 1–2 hrs	i.v. bolus: 25–100 mcg q1–2 hr i.v. cont inf: 25–50 mcg/hr Transdermal: q72 hr Transmuc: varies
Oxycodone	Mild–severe pain; initial prescription in narcotic naïve patients	p.o.: 5, 10, 15, 20, 30 mg Soln: 1 mg/ml SR: 10, 20, 40, 80 mg	p.o.: 20–30 min Soln: 15–20 min s.r.: 1–2 hrs	p.o.: 2–6 hrs Soln: 2–6 hrs s.r.: 8–12 hrs	p.o.: 5–20 mg q2–6 hr Soln: 5–20 mg q2–6 hr s.r.: q12hr
Methadone	Moderate–severe pain; intolerance to other opioids; opioid withdrawal	i.v. p.o.: 5, 10 mg Soln: 10 mg/5 ml	i.v.: 5–10 min p.o.: 30–40 min Soln: 30 min	i.v.: 6 hrs p.o.: 6 hrs Soln: 6 hrs	p.o.: 5–10 mg q6 hr Soln: 5–10 mg q6 hr

Abbreviations: i.v., intravenous; i.m., intramuscular; i.t., intrathecal; s.l., sublingual; i.r., immediate release; Soln, solution; s.r., sustained release; p.r., per rectum; p.o., oral; Transmuc, transmucosal; cont inf, continuous infusion.

Adapted from Baumann (1999).

Side effects

Clinically important side effects of opioids include central nervous system (CNS)-related and non-CNS-related effects. CNS-related side effects include drowsiness and sedation, nausea and vomiting, agitation, nightmares, anxiety, euphoria, dysphoria, depression, paranoia, hallucinations, and respiratory depression. Non-CNS-related side effects include dry mouth, constipation, sweating, itching, and urinary retention (Enck, 2000).

Opioid conversion

Patients frequently require a change of medication during opioid therapy due to intolerable side effects, inadequate pain relief, or for cost considerations. When changing from one route of administration to another, or when switching from one opiate to another, it is essential that the clinician be knowledgeable about the relative potency of the opioids as well as the bioavailability of the route chosen. Using equianalgesic dosing charts (Table 81.3) when converting from one opioid to another can lead to overdosing or underdosing in many patients. Interpatient variability is common; therefore dosing should be titrated based on the patient's reported pain and side effects whenever the opioid, route, or dose is changed (Enck, 2000; Stevens & Ghazi, 2000).

Types of pain

HSCT recipients experience pain during pretransplant workup, hospital admission, chemoradiotherapy, stem cell infusion, and engraftment (Table 81.4). Patients undergo a number of painful diagnostic and treatment procedures, such as placement of a central venous access device, bone marrow aspirations, lumbar punctures, biopsies, endoscopy, angiography, and bronchoscopy (Chapman et al., 1985; Lyne et al., 2002).

Regimen-related toxicities that can cause pain include cystitis, which may produce severe pain and distress from bladder spasms. Headaches occur most frequently during chemoradiotherapy and from 7 to 11 days after treatment. Intrathecal methotrexate can cause headache, stiff neck, paraplegia, and leg pains (Chapman et al., 1985).

Corticosteroids are often used in the course of HSCT, usually to treat GVHD. Withdrawal of steroids can result in pseudorheumatism, a syndrome characterized by diffuse pain and tenderness in muscle and joints. These symptoms usually reverse when corticosteroids are resumed. Long-term therapy with corticosteroids, which is sometimes necessary in the HSCT patient with chronic GVHD, can be complicated by aseptic necrosis of the head of the femur or humerus. Patients suffering from this condition may experience constant deep, aching pain that is often severe (Chapman et al., 1985).

Some infectious complications of HSCT can also result in significant pain. Reactivation of varicella zoster infection occurs later in the transplant process resulting in excruciatingly painful lesions in one or more dermatomes. The condition is usually self-limiting with pain resolving after healing of the lesions, but some patients may suffer from postherpetic neuralgia, in which pain and sensory loss persist in the affected dermatome(s) even after the initial skin involvement has cleared.

Table 81.3. *Opiate equianalgesic chart: approximate parenteral and oral doses*

Opioids/Narcotics	Equianalgesic dosing (mg)		Comments
	Parenteral (i.v., i.m., s.c.)	Oral	
Morphine	10	30	(MS Contin, Oramorph)
Codeine	130	200	Doses over 65 mg may produce diminishing analgesia
			Most constipating
Oxycodone	15	30	(Oxycontin, Tylox, Percocet, Roxicodone)
			Percocet tab: 5 mg oxycodone & 650 mg acetaminophen
Hydromorphone	1.5	7.5	(Dilaudid)
			Short half-life; drug of choice for patients with hepatic and renal failure
Hydrocodone	–	30	(Vicodin, Lortab, Lorcet)
			Equianalgesic data not available
			Vicodin tab: 5 mg hydrocodone & 500 mg acetaminophen
Methadone	10	20	(Dolophine)
			Risk of delayed toxicity at onset of dosing or dosing increments due to accumulation
Meperidine	75	300	(Demerol)
			Normeperidine (toxic metabolite) accumulates causing CNS excitation
			Avoid in renal insufficiency
Fentanyl	100 mcg	——	(Duragesic)
			Not typically used for acute pain

Equianalgesic doses are approximate; use only as a guideline.

All doses must be titrated to patient response.

Adapted from Baumann (1999).

Table 81.4. *Common pain syndromes and sequence in HSCT*

Timing	Toxicity	Symptom
Immediate	Local tissue ulceration or inflammation due to chemotherapy line placement	Pain at or around chemotherapy infusion line
	Stimulation of hematopoiesis during stem cell mobilization with growth factors	Bone pain
	Tissue trauma during bone marrow harvest	Pain at site of bone marrow harvest
	Esophageal tears related to severe vomiting	Abdominal or esophageal pain
	Hemorrhagic cystitis following cyclophosphamide	Spasmodic pain in bladder; burning pain with urination
Early	Thrombocytopenia	Painful intramuscular hematoma
	Cyclosporine prophylaxis for GVHD (may also occur late)	Painful dysesthesias of hands and feet
	Leukopenia; infection	Sore throat; perirectal abscesses
Delayed	Acute graft-versus-host disease (GVHD)	Severe diarrhea, abdominal cramps, and tenesmus
	Veno-occlusive disease of the liver	Abdominal pain
	Mouth ulceration and esophagitis occur and agranulocytosis prevents healing for 2–3 weeks	Severe oral pain
	Pancreatitis	Epigastric pain
	Parotid inflammation	Parotid pain
Late	Peripheral neuropathy	Burning pain in extremities
	Reactivation of Herpes zoster	Postherpetic neuralgia
	Pseudorheumatism from withdrawal of corticosteroids	Arthritic bone pain
	Avascular necrosis of bone	Bone pain; loss of joint function
	Chronic GVHD	Persisting abdominal cramps

Adapted from Chapman *et al.* (1985).

Patients may experience painful dysesthesia, intermittent lancinating pain, and constant burning pain. Postherpetic neuralgia is difficult to treat and often does not respond to traditional analgesics (Chapman *et al.*, 1985).

Abdominal pain occurs frequently in patients after HSCT and is associated with a variety of conditions, including chemotherapy-related acute nausea and vomiting, chronic nausea and vomiting, infection in the gastrointestinal (GI) tract, hepatic veno-occlusive disease, and GVHD of the upper or lower GI tract (Pederson & Parran, 1997).

Mucositis pain

The most common source of pain in the HSCT recipient is mucositis. It is estimated that 76% to 90% of patients undergoing HSCT using traditional myeloablative conditioning regimens will develop some degree of mucositis (Chapko *et al.*, 1989; Berger & Kilroy, 2001). The incidence and severity of mucositis following non-myeloablative ("mini") conditioning regimens is significantly less. Mucositis usually begins a few days prior to transplantation and persists until engraftment (2–3 weeks after transplantation). Oro-pharyngeal mucositis first appears as erythema and mild inflammation that is asymptomatic, but soon progresses to white, elevated, desquamated patches that are painful to the touch. These patches can become distinct ulcers covered with pseudomembranes that cause continual pain, even when not touched. Eventually, the ulcers may coalesce. Marked xerostomia is present and mucus becomes thick as the condition progresses. The pain associated with mucositis can be mild and managed adequately with topical analgesics, but often in the HSCT setting, pain is so severe that intravenous narcotics are required. The pain associated with oro-pharyngeal mucositis is often exacerbated by swallowing and patients may prefer to spit out or use a suction device to remove their oral secretions. In a significant number of patients, oral nutritional intake becomes impossible and parenteral nutrition may be required (Berger & Kilroy, 2001).

Treatment of mucositis pain includes topical and systemic analgesics. Meticulous oral hygiene is important in minimizing mucositis pain and preventing infections. Patients are encouraged to frequently rinse the oral mucosa with agents such as saline, sodium bicarbonate solution, or chlorhexidine gluconate (a topical disinfectant). The pain may become so severe, however, that rinsing becomes impossible. During the initial stages of mucositis (or near the end when healing is taking place), the pain may be mild enough to treat adequately with topical anesthetics such as viscous lidocaine, either swished in the mouth or carefully applied to distinct painful lesions. This provides temporary relief of mild pain, but may also numb the tissues, putting the patient at risk of tissue injury from accidental biting due to lack of a pain warning. The patient's taste perception may also be altered. In addition to topical agents, mild to moderate mucositis pain can be managed with orally administered systemic analgesics, provided the patient can swallow oral medications safely. Where possible, it is best to use tablet or capsule formulations of oral systemic analgesics or slurries of these agents made at the bedside by crushing tablets in water. Many commercially available liquid formulations are alcohol-containing elixirs that may exacerbate pain when coming into contact with denuded mucosa. Acetaminophen (paracetamol) in doses ranging from 325 to 1,000 mg every 4 to 6 hours (not to exceed 4 g in 24 hours) may be effective as a single agent in treating mild pain, or as an adjunct to more potent agents such as opioids. There are many products available combining acetaminophen and an opioid in the same tablet or capsule. Some centers may avoid the use of acetaminophen due to fears of suppressing fever. Use of this agent should conform to the institutional policies for antipyretic agents in immunocompromised patients. More severe pain is best treated with orally administered narcotics. Table 81.3 lists the dosage forms, dose ranges, and onset and duration of action for common opiate analgesics. If the patient is unable to take oral medications because of nausea or pain, a number of opioids are available in parenteral formulations for intravenous administration. The incidence of side effects with this route of administration may be increased over that of orally administered opioids.

Once the patient requires frequent administration of intravenous opioids, or the pain cannot be controlled by staff-administered bolus doses, the patient may benefit from an intravenous infusion of opioids via a PCA device. A number of studies have demonstrated the safety and efficacy of opioids delivered via PCA to control the pain associated with oro-pharyngeal mucositis in HSCT patients. Hill *et al.* (1990) randomly assigned 84 adult HSCT patients to receive morphine by a nurse-administered continuous infusion protocol or by PCA and compared pain relief, amount of drug used, severity of mucositis, and side effects (nausea, alertness, and respiratory rate). Fifty-eight of these patients were considered evaluable for the study outcomes. The authors found no differences in patient-reported pain relief, side effects, or severity of mucositis. However, patients in the PCA group used a little more than half as much (53%) morphine as those in the nurse-administered group and were able to discontinue the drug sooner. Another study at the same institution (Mackie *et al.*, 1991) found similar results in adolescent (12–18 years) patients undergoing HSCT. Patient-reported pain relief and side effects were similar between PCA and nurse-administered morphine groups, but total morphine use in the PCA group was about 40% that of the nurse-administered group. Pillitteri and Clark (1998) found similar results using diamorphine. Pain control was deemed equivalent, while less diamorphine and fewer days of diamorphine use were reported in the PCA group. Although less drug was administered via PCA in each of these studies, self-assessed pain relief was similar between PCA and nurse-administered groups. A study by Zucker *et al.* (1998) comparing the use of meperidine (pethidine) by either PCA or staff-administered continuous infusion protocol found that patients in the PCA group not only used less drug (440 mg vs. 641 mg in 24 hours) than the continuous infusion group, but also reported better control of pain (mean pain scores 49.9% vs. 70.9%). Meperidine is a narcotic analgesic that is avoided in many centers because of the potential for toxicity due to accumulation of a renally cleared metabolite, normeperidine. Dunbar *et al.* (1995) evaluated the use of PCA for the administration of morphine or hydromorphone to children aged 4 to 12

years. Ninety-five percent of the evaluable children were able to master use of the PCA device with acceptable control of pain and side effects, as measured by the investigators.

A few studies compared different opioids administered by PCA. Collins *et al.* (1996) compared morphine and hydromorphone delivered via PCA device in 10 children undergoing HSCT and found no differences in side effects or efficacy, although the study was probably underpowered to detect a difference. A much larger randomized, double-blind, parallel-group trial (Coda *et al.*, 1997) compared the efficacy and side effects of morphine, hydromorphone, and sufentanil administered via PCA in 119 adult HSCT patients. One hundred patients were considered evaluable at the end of the study period. No difference was found between the three opiates in level of analgesia; however, the composite side effects score (nausea, pruritus, mood, ability to concentrate, sedation, quality of sleep) was lower in the morphine group. Time to treatment failure, defined as discontinuation of PCA for any reason prior to resolution of mucositis pain, was longer in the morphine group. Treatment failures due to inadequate pain relief were more frequent in the sufentanil group (7 of 36) than either the morphine (1 of 30) or hydromorphone (0 of 34) groups. The authors concluded that morphine should remain the drug of first choice for PCA in the HSCT setting. It is important to note that in all of these studies, mean pain scores reported by patients were generally 40 to 60 on a 100-point visual analogue scale despite analgesic drug treatment. This indicates a need for further study to minimize and treat the pain of oro-pharyngeal mucositis and emphasizes the need for staff and patients to realize that complete resolution of pain is unrealistic at the present time.

Strupp *et al.* (2000) reported the use of continuously applied transdermal fentanyl to treat pain associated with grade IV mucositis in 74 patients undergoing autologous HSCT. Adequate analgesia was achieved with acceptable side effects and no need for supplementary analgesia. This approach offers the advantage of continuous parenteral pain relief while avoiding the intravenous route. However, since fentanyl can persist in the skin reservoir for 12 to 16 hours after removal of the transdermal system, some clinicians would argue that this route of administration might be inadvisable in patients who can develop rapidly fatal complications such as sepsis. Further study is warranted to examine the safety and effectiveness of this approach in the management of oro-pharyngeal mucositis pain.

Bone pain

Bone pain can be a debilitating symptom in patients undergoing HSCT. It may be prevalent in patients with multiple myeloma, a malignancy often treated with HSCT. Mechanisms of bone pain include growth of tumor cells within the bone, pathological fractures, spinal cord compression, bone marrow expansion in patients with hematologic malignancies, and drug-induced bone pain (Mercadante, 1997). Corticosteroid treatment for GVHD can cause osteoporosis and vertebral compression fractures. Osteoporosis is an important cause of bone pain and of pathological fractures after long-term use of steroids in cancer patients. Ribs and vertebrae, bones with a high degree of trabecular structure, are generally the most severely effected (Mercadante, 1997). Typical bone pain is described as sharp, cramplike, throbbing, or pulsating. Movement and weight-bearing acutely increase the intensity of most types of bone pain (Baumann, 1999).

NSAIDs, opioids, and bisphosphonates have all been used to treat metastatic bone pain. Bisphosphonates bind to hydroxyapatite crystals, making it more difficult for osteoclasts to recognize exposed unmineralized bone surfaces. Bisphosphonates are also directly toxic to osteoclasts. Pamidronate is the bisphosphonate most commonly used to alleviate bone pain in cancer patients. In a study conducted in 377 patients with stage III multiple myeloma and more than one lytic bone lesion, patients received pamidronate 90 mg i.v. or placebo every 4 weeks for 9 months. Patients receiving pamidronate experienced fewer pathologic fractures and required less radiation to bone. They also had decreases in pain scores from baseline whereas placebo recipients had worsening quality of life as well as performance status (Berenson et al., 1998).

Third-generation bisphosphonates are currently being investigated for treatment of bone metastases. These bisphosphonates are more potent than pamidronate and can be given with shorter infusion times. Zoledronate 4 mg was shown to be at least as effective as pamidronate 90 mg for decreasing the need for radiation to the bone, improving pain scores, and decreasing the number of skeletal-related events (Berenson et al., 2001).

Bone marrow harvest or peripheral blood stem cell collection pain

Collection of stem cells for HSCT by either bone marrow harvest or mobilization and collection of peripheral blood stem cells is associated with significant pain. Bone marrow harvest is an intrinsically traumatic procedure involving aspiration of marrow from the posterior or anterior iliac crests, or more rarely the sternum (Hill et al., 1989). The procedure has traditionally been carried out under general or regional anesthesia (Hill et al., 1989), although some centers report successful harvesting under local anesthesia (Sim et al., 1996). Donors are typically discharged after recovery from anesthesia and are sent home with analgesics. Typical analgesics include combinations of acetaminophen (paracetamol) with an opioid such as oxycodone (Percocet) or an opioid alone. The pain associated with bone marrow harvesting is mostly from the physical trauma caused during the procedure. The pain tends to be greatest directly after the procedure and gradually gets better over a course of 1 to 2 weeks.

In contrast, pain associated with peripheral blood stem cell collection is mostly related to administration of growth factors such as filgrastim or sargramostim. The pain, typically described as bony pain, headaches, and generalized body aches, starts with the first dose of growth factor, worsens as dosing continues, and resolves soon after completion of the apheresis procedure (Stroncek et al., 1996; Murata et al., 1999). The incidence of bone pain, which is usually described as grade 2 or less, correlates with the dose of filgrastim. Doses greater than 8.8 mcg/kg/day are associated with a higher relative risk of bone pain (Murata et al., 1999).

Several randomized studies compared the incidence of pain between patients having stem cells collected via bone marrow harvest versus leukapheresis of growth-factor-stimulated peripheral blood stem cells. Auquier et al. (1995) reported significantly more pain in the bone marrow harvest group. Interestingly, this group also experienced more anxiety before the procedure, which may have influenced their perception of pain afterwards. In contrast, Rowley et al. (2001) reported equivalent levels of maximal pain, average pain, and pain duration through the day in 68 donors randomized to receive bone marrow harvest of filgrastim mobilization followed by peripheral blood stem cell collection. Pain was the primary complaint of both groups. Pain resolved quickly after filgrastim administration was stopped upon completion of apheresis in the peripheral blood stem cell group, but persisted for up to 14 days in the bone marrow harvest group. Fortanier et al. (2002) reported similar results in another randomized trial of bone marrow harvest versus lenograstim-stimulated peripheral blood stem cell collection, with no difference in maximal pain scores between groups, but different time courses of pain. Maximal pain in the peripheral stem cell collection group occurred during growth-factor administration and diminished quickly after collection; however, maximal pain occurred immediately after harvesting in the bone marrow group. The evidence from these clinical trials indicates that both procedures are associated with a high incidence of mild to moderate (and occasionally severe) pain. All donors should be given adequate supplies of potent analgesics such as oxycodone, morphine, or combinations of acetaminophen with opiates, both during the procedure and for as many days afterwards as is required to return to baseline.

Conclusions

Pain is an almost universal complication of HSCT. Both patients and donors can experience mild to moderate pain, and in many instances pain can be severe and debilitating. It is essential that health care providers are aware of pain and its consequences in the HSCT patient and that they are knowledgeable about the time course and appropriate management of pain. Assessment of pain should be performed routinely and frequently by the staff, and patients should be encouraged to assess, report, and seek proper treatment of pain throughout the transplant course. Routine monitoring for effectiveness of the pain management strategy as well as side effects is essential. Management of pain in HSCT patients is challenging, but in most cases satisfactory control can be attained.

References

Auquier, P., Macquart-Moulin, G., Moatti, J.P. *et al.* (1995). Comparison of anxiety, pain and discomfort in two procedures of hematopoietic stem cell collection: leukacytapheresis and bone marrow harvest. *Bone Marrow Transplantation, 16,* 541–7.

Baumann, T.J. (1999). Pain management. In *Pharmacotherapy: A Pathophysiologic Approach,* 4th Ed., ed. J.T. DiPiro, R.L. Talbert, G.C. Yee *et al.,* pp. 1014–26. Stamford, CT: Appleton & Lange.

Berenson, J., Lichtenstein, A., Porter, L. *et al.* (1998). Long-term pamidronate treatment of advanced multiple myeloma patients reduces skeletal events. Myeloma Aredia Study Group. *Journal of Clinical Oncology, 16,* 593–602.

Berenson, J.R., Rosen, L.S., Howell, A. *et al.* (2001). Zoledronic acid reduces skeletal-related events in patients with osteolytic metastases. *Cancer, 91,* 1191–200.

Berger, A.M. & Kilroy, T.J. (2001). Oral complications. In *Cancer: Principles and Practice of Oncology,* 6th Ed., ed. V.T. DeVita, S. Hellman, & S.A. Rosenberg, pp. 2881–93. Philadelphia: Lippincott Williams & Wilkins.

Chapko, M.K., Syrjala, K.L., Schilter, L. *et al.* (1989). Chemoradiotherapy toxicity during bone marrow transplantation: time course and variation in pain and nausea. *Bone Marrow Transplantation, 4,* 181–6.

Chapman, C.R., Syrjala, K., & Sangur, M. (1985). Pain as a manifestation of cancer treatment. *Seminars in Oncology Nursing, 1,* 100–7.

Coda, B.A., O'Sullivan, B., Donaldson, G. *et al.* (1997). Comparative efficacy of patient-controlled administration of morphine, hydromorphone, or sufentanil for the treatment of oral mucositis pain following bone marrow transplantation. *Pain, 72,* 333–46.

Collins, J.J., Greake, J., Grier, H.E. *et al.* (1996). Patient-controlled analgesia for mucositis pain in children: a three-period crossover study comparing morphine and hydromorphone. *Journal of Pediatrics, 129,* 722–8.

Dunbar, P.J., Buckley, P., Gavrin, J.R. *et al.* (1995). Use of patient-controlled analgesia for pain control for children receiving bone marrow transplant. *Journal of Pain Symptom Management, 10,* 604–11.

Enck, R.E. (2000). Meeting the challenge: earlier use of long-acting opioids in the oncology setting. In *Clinical Dialogues in Pain Management.* Kingston, NJ: Medicom of Princeton, Inc.

Foley, K.M. (2001). Management of cancer pain. In *Cancer: Principles and Practice of Oncology,* 6th Ed., ed. V.T. DeVita, S. Hellman, & S.A. Rosenberg, pp. 2977–3011. Philadelphia: Lippincott Williams & Wilkins.

Fortanier, C., Kuentz, M., Sutton, L. *et al.* (2002). Healthy sibling donor anxiety and pain during bone marrow or peripheral blood stem cell harvesting for allogeneic transplantation: results of a randomized study. *Bone Marrow Transplantation, 29,* 145–9.

Hill, H.F., Chapman, C.R., Jackson, T.L., & Sullivan, K.M. (1989). Assessment and management of donor pain following marrow harvest for allogeneic bone marrow transplantation. *Bone Marrow Transplantation, 4,* 157–61.

Hill, H.F., Chapman, C.R., Kornell, J.A. *et al.* (1990). Self-administration of morphine in bone marrow transplant patients reduces drug requirement. *Pain, 40,* 121–9.

IASP Subcommittee on Taxonomy. (1980). Pain terms: a list with definitions and notes on usage. *Pain, 8,* 249.

Jacox, A.K., Carr, D.B., Payne, R. *et al.* (1994). *Management of Cancer Pain, Clinical Practice Guideline, No. 9.* Rockville, Md: U.S. Department of Health and Human Services, Public Health Service, Agency for Health Care Policy and Research; AHCPR Publication No. 94-0592.

Lynch, M. & Abraham, J. (2002). Ensuring a good death: pain and palliative care in a cancer center. *Cancer Practice, 10*(Suppl 1), S33–38.

Lyne, M.E., Coyne, P.J., & Watson, A.C. (2002). Pain management issues for cancer survivors. *Cancer Practice, 10*(Suppl 1), S27–32.

Mackie, A.M., Coda, B.C., & Hill, H.F. (1991). Adolescents use patient-controlled analgesia effectively for relief from prolonged oro-pharyngeal mucositis pain. *Pain, 46,* 265–9.

Mercadante, S. (1997). Malignant bone pain: pathophysiology and treatment. *Pain, 69,* 1–18.

Murata, M., Harada, M., Kato, S. *et al.* (1999). Peripheral blood stem cell mobilization and apheresis: analysis of adverse events in 94 normal donors. *Bone Marrow Transplantation, 24,* 1065–71.

Pederson, C. & Parran, L. (1997). Bone marrow transplant nurses' knowledge, beliefs, and attitudes regarding pain management. *Oncology Nursing Forum, 24,* 1563–71.

Pillitteri, L.C. & Clark, R.E. (1998). Comparison of a patient-controlled analgesia system with continuous infusion for administration of diamorphine for mucositis. *Bone Marrow Transplantation, 22,* 495–8.

Rowley, S.D., Donaldson, G., Lilleby, K. *et al.* (2001). Experiences of donors enrolled in a randomized study of allogeneic bone marrow or peripheral blood stem cell transplantation. *Blood, 97,* 2541–8.

Sim, K.M., Boey, S.K., & Wong, L.T. (1996). Bone marrow harvesting using local anaesthesia and PCA-alfentanil: a feasible alternative to general or regional anaesthesia. *Bone Marrow Transplantation, 18,* 787–90.

Stevens, R.A. & Ghazi, S.M. (2000). Routes of opioid analgesic therapy in the management of cancer pain. *Cancer Control; JMCC, 7,* 132–41.

Stroncek, D.F., Clay, M.E., Petzoldt, M.L. *et al.* (1996). Treatment of normal individuals with granulocyte-colony-stimulating factor: donor experiences and the effects on peripheral blood CD34+ cell counts and on the collection of peripheral blood stem cells. *Transfusion, 36,* 585–9.

Strupp, C., Sudhoff, T., Germing, U. *et al.* (2000). Transdermal fentanyl during high-dose chemotherapy and autologous stem cell support. *Oncology Reports, 7,* 659–61.

Zucker, T.P., Flesche, C.W., Germing, U. *et al.* (1998). Patient-controlled versus staff-controlled analgesia with pethidine after allogeneic bone marrow transplantation. *Pain, 75,* 305–12.

82 Toxicities of stem cell transplantation regimens

SCOTT I. BEARMAN

University of Colorado Health Sciences Center, Denver, USA

Introduction

Hematopoietic stem cell (HSC) transplantation is the treatment of choice for many hematologic malignancies and selected nonmalignant disorders. The success of treatment must balance treatment-related complications and eradication of disease. Autologous transplants employ lethal doses of chemotherapy or chemoradiotherapy to attempt to eradicate all disease. In this circumstance, assuming the HSC source is not involved at the time it is collected, the stem cell infusion serves to restore hematopoietic activity. Allogeneic transplants also employ lethal chemotherapy or chemoradiotherapy to provide significant cytoreduction. In addition, allotransplants also exploit a graft-versus-tumor effect.

Regimen-related toxicity (RRT) refers to those toxicities that can be attributed directly to the preparative regimen. While this excludes graft-versus-host disease (GVHD), hemorrhage and infection, there are clearly toxicities that can be contributed by the regimen as well as by GVHD prophylaxis. It is often difficult to assign attribution. A toxicity grading system developed 15 years ago continues to be one of the few specifically devised with myeloablative therapy in mind (Table 82.1) (Bearman *et al.*, 1988). This system was devised from patients who were treated with cyclophosphamide plus total body irradiation (TBI), most of whom received cyclosporine and methotrexate as GVHD prophylaxis. With this preparative regimen, life-threatening or fatal RRT occurred more commonly in patients who received higher doses of TBI, who were in relapse, and who underwent allogeneic transplants. It also showed that, for patients whose maximum RRT in any single organ was grade 2, those who suffered grade 2 RRT in three or more organs were much more likely to die by day 100 than those who developed grade 2 RRT in two or fewer organs. Those patients who developed grade 3 RRT were unlikely to survive 100 days from transplant although not all deaths could be attributed to RRT (Fig. 82.1). The toxicities associated with ablative preparative regimens have not changed significantly. However, a number of different regimens are in common use today, and these are amenable to RRT scoring using this approach (Kroger *et al.*, 1998; Donato *et al.*, 2001; Nevil *et al.*, 1991).

A significant difference in the past several years has been the use of reduced intensity regimens to prepare patients for allo-transplantation (see Chapter 22). These regimens are described as being non-myeloablative and they differ significantly in their intensity and in their toxicities. Some, in fact, are quite toxic. This chapter will review the regimen-related toxicities associated with ablative regimens and will discuss some of the toxicities of newer preparative approaches.

Toxicities associated with myeloablative preparative therapy (and see Chapter 21)

Myeloablative regimens typically combine agents that are non-cross-resistant and have nonoverlapping, nonhematopoietic toxicities. For the most part, dose-limiting toxicities of myeloablative regimens are similar among the different regimens. However, differences in toxicity are important. For example, patients who have received prior mediastinal radiotherapy do not tolerate TBI and must receive non-TBI-containing regimens (Appelbaum *et al.*, 1987; Bearman *et al.*, 1989). The major toxicities of common myeloablative preparative regimens are shown in Table 82.2.

Cardiac toxicity (and see Chapter 92)

The oxazophosphorine chemotherapeutic agents cyclophosphamide and ifosfamide were shown more than 30 years ago to produce hemorrhagic pancarditis within 24 hours when lethal doses were given to laboratory animals (Storb *et al.*, 1970; O'Connell & Berenbaum, 1974). Autopsies from patients who die of cardiac toxicity show pericardial effusions and multiple areas of hemorrhagic necrosis (Gottdeiner *et al.*, 1981; Angelucci *et al.*, 1992). Risk factors that have been reported to be associated with severe cardiac toxicity include previous anthracycline dose (Steinherz *et al.*, 1981; Larsen *et al.*, 1992) and reduced pretransplant ejection fraction. While other investigators have not found similar results (Bearman *et al.*, 1990; Ayash *et al.*, 1992; Hertenstein *et al.*, 1994; Carlson *et al.*, 1994), an assessment of the cardiac ejection fraction is routine in patients being considered for transplant.

Table 82.1.   *A regimen-related toxicity grading system for stem cell transplantation*

	Grade 1	Grade 2	Grade 3
Cardiac	Mild ECG abnormalities, not requiring medical intervention OR noted cardiac enlargement on CXR, with no clinical symptoms	Moderate ECG abnormalities requiring and responding to medical intervention OR requiring continuous monitoring without treatment OR congestive heart failure responsive to diuretics or digoxin	Severe ECG abnormalities with no or only partial response to medical intervention OR heart failure with no or only minor response to intervention OR decrease in voltage by > 50%
Bladder	Macroscopic hematuria after 2 days from last chemotherapy, with no subjective symptoms of cystitis and not caused by infection	Macroscopic hematuria after 7 days from last chemotherapy not caused by infection OR hematuria after 2 days with subjective symptoms of cystitis not caused by infection	Hemorrhagic cystitis with frank blood, necessitating invasive local intervention with instillation of sclerosing agents, nephrostomy, or other surgical procedure
Renal	Increase in creatinine up to twice baseline value	Increase in creatinine above twice baseline value but not requiring dialysis	Requirement of dialysis
Pulmonary	Dyspnea without change in CXR, not caused by congestive heart failure or infection OR CXR showing isolated infiltrate or mild interstitial changes without symptoms and not caused by infection or congestive heart failure	CXR with extensive localized infiltrate or moderate interstitial changes combined with dyspnea and not caused by infection or congestive heart failure OR $\geq$ 10% decrease in pO_2 from baseline and not requiring mechanical ventilation OR $\geq$ 50% FiO_2 by mask and not caused by infection or congestive heart failure	Interstitial or alveolar changes requiring mechanical ventilatory support or > 50% FiO_2 and not caused by infection or congestive heart failure
Hepatic	Mild hepatic dysfunction with bilirubin 2–5.9 mg/dl and weight gain 2.5–4.9% from baseline of noncardiac origin OR SGOT increase 2–4.9 times baseline	Moderate dysfunction with bilirubin 6–19.9 mg/dl and weight gain $\geq$ 5% from baseline or ascites > 100 ml, of noncardiac origin OR SGOT increase $\geq$ 5 times baseline	Severe dysfunction with bilirubin $\geq$ 20 mg/dl; hepatic encephalopathy; respiratory compromise due to ascites
CNS	Somnolence but patient is easily arousable and oriented after arousal	Somnolent with confusion after arousal OR other new subjective CNS symptoms with no loss of consciousness not more easily explained by other medication, bleeding, or CNS infection	Seizures or coma not explained by other medication, CNS infection, or bleeding
Stomatitis	Pain or ulceration not requiring continuous i.v. narcotics	Pain or ulceration requiring continuous i.v. narcotics	Severe pain or ulceration requiring protective intubation OR resulting in documented aspiration pneumonia with or without intubation
GI	Watery stools 500–1999 ml/day not related to infection	Watery stools $\geq$ 2 l/day not related to infection OR macroscopic hemorrhagic stools with no effect on cardiovascular status not caused by infection; or subileus not related to infection	Ileus requiring nasogastric suction or surgery and not related to infection OR hemorrhagic enterocolitis affecting cardiovascular status and requiring infection and not related to infection

Grade 4 toxicity is fatal

Subclinical cardiac toxicity has been reported by several investigators to be relatively common (Steinherz *et al.,* 1981; Kupari *et al.,* 1990; Quezado *et al.,* 1993; Morandi *et al.,* 2001;). These include asymptomatic pericardial effusions and echocardiographic findings consistent with left ventricular dysfunction, such as decreased fractional shorting, increased end-diastolic volume, and increased pre-ejection time/ejection time ratios.

The actual mechanism by which cardiac toxicity occurs is unclear. Morandi and colleagues (Morandi *et al.,* 2001) measured troponin I levels in 16 patients with advanced or high-risk breast cancer who received 7 g/m^2 of cyclophosphamide as part of a high-dose chemotherapy program. Cyclophosphamide was given in 5 divided doses every 3 hours over a 13-hour period. Troponin was measured at baseline and at 6, 12, 24, and 48 hours after the first dose of cyclophosphamide. Troponin I levels did not exceed normal values in any patient and was not measurable in 12 of the 16 patients. These results suggest that the pathogenesis of cyclophosphamide-induced cardiac toxicity is not disruption of myocyte membrane stability.

Murdych and Weisdorf (Murdych & Weisdorf, 2001) evaluated the incidence of serious cardiac complications in more than 2,800 patients transplanted over a 20-year period at the

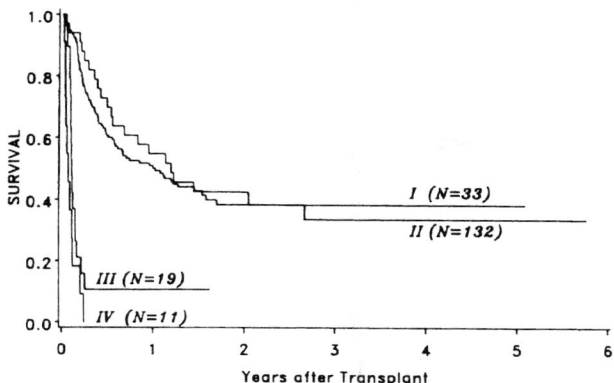

Fig. 82.1. Overall survival for patients undergoing marrow transplant for leukemia grouped according to the highest grade toxicity seen in any single organ. Reproduced, with permission, from Bearman *et al.* (1988).

University of Minnesota. Twenty-six of 2,921 (<1%) patients developed life-threatening complications, half of whom died. Severe cardiac toxicity remains an uncommon complication of high-dose cytoreduction.

Having stated that, mention should be made about cardiac toxicity in AL amyloidosis patients. Cardiac involvement is common in this disease and many patients with AL amyloidosis who have undergone transplant had symptomatic cardiac disease. At Boston University, 20 of 28 patients who died within 3 months of transplant had evidence of amyloid cardiomyopathy prior to transplant (Sanchorawala *et al.*, 2001). At the Mayo Clinic, 5 out of 6 patients with interventricular septal wall thickness greater than 15 mm died after transplant. None of these patients had congestive heart failure and all had left ventricular ejection fractions of 54% or more (Gertz *et al.*, 2000). Cardiac arrthymias are common in patients with cardiac amyloid. Moreau and colleagues reported that 3 of 9 patients who died within 1 month of transplant had fatal cardiac arrthymias. In a study of intermediate-dose melphalan (100 mg/m^2) for patients who were ineligible to receive 200

mg/m^2, 5 of 30 patients died of transplant-related complications by day 100. Two of the 5 had cardiac arrests. Their pre-transplant ejection fractions were 37% and 40% (Comenzo *et al.*, 1999).

Since most patients with AL amyloid who have been transplanted had evidence of cardiac amyloid, although many are asymptomatic, it is difficult to give firm recommendations regarding who is an appropriate candidate. While the Mayo Clinic and Boston University groups differ regarding minimum left ventricular ejection fraction required (55% and 40%, respectively), clinical congestive heart failure, exertional syncope, thromboembolic events due to atrial dysfunction, and symptomatic ventricular tachycardia are absolute contraindications for high-dose therapy (and see Chapter 40).

Renal toxicity (and see Chapter 90)

Renal dysfunction occurs commonly after ablative high-dose preparative therapy. The causes include tumor lysis, infusion of cryopreserved marrow or stem cells, certain chemotherapeutic agents, and nephrotoxins. Ifosfamide, melphalan, and cisplatin are the agents used in high-dose regimens most likely to cause renal dysfunction. Renal dysfunction due to these drugs is usually mild and reversible (Bearman *et al.*, 1988). Severe renal dysfunction occurs most commonly in association with dysfunction of multiple organs.

Renal dysfunction can occur early or late and the presentations are usually quite different. Early renal dysfunction occurs in about 40% of patients. Twenty-five to 50% of these patients may require dialysis (Zager *et al.*, 1989). Early renal dysfunction is more common in recipients of allogeneic transplants, due to the routine use of cyclosporine or tacrolimus. Severe renal dysfunction occurs more commonly in patients receiving nephrotoxic antibiotics and in patients with sepsis. Treatment of early renal dysfunction is supportive and requires the often difficult balancing of intravascular volume with the need for diuretics, hemodialysis, or ultrafiltration. A proportion of patients who require dialysis ultimately die.

Table 82.2. *Commonly used myeloablative regimens and their toxicities.*

Regimen	Primarily used in		Common indications	Major toxicities
	Autologous transplants	Allogeneic transplants		
Cyclophosphamide + total body irradiation	Yes	Yes	AML, ALL, CML	Mucositis, hepatic toxicity, IPS
Busulfan + cyclophosphamide	Yes	Yes	AML, CML	Mucositis, hepatic toxicity, IPS
Etoposide + total body irradiation	Yes	Yes	Lymphoid malignancies	Mucositis
Cyclophosphamide + etoposide + BCNU	Yes	No	Lymphoid malignancies	Mucositis, lung injury
BCNU + etoposide + cytarabine + melphalan	Yes	No	Lymphoid malignancies	Mucositis, lung injury
Cyclophosphamide + cisplatin + BCNU	Yes	No	Breast cancer	Lung injury
Cyclophosphamide + thiotepa + carboplatin	Yes	No	Breast cancer	Mucositis
Melphalan ± total body irradiation	Yes	Yes	Multiple myeloma	Mucositis

Abbreviations: AML, acute myeloid leukemia; ALL, acute lymphoid leukemia; CML, chronic myeloid leukemia; IPS, idiopathic pneumonia syndrome.

Late renal dysfunction usually presents as hemolytic-uremic syndrome (HUS), with microangiopathic hemolytic anemia, hypertension and renal failure and, sometimes, encephalopathy. It can occur in both the autologous and allogeneic settings and is usually attributable to TBI. Partial shielding of the kidneys and fractionation have resulted in a decrease in the incidence of HUS (Zager, 1994; Lawton et al., 1992). Both cyclosporine and tacrolimus can cause HUS (Singh et al., 1996; Woo et al., 1997). Reports state that sirolimus is also associated with HUS (Benito et al., 2001). Unfortunately, switching from cyclosporine to tacrolimus because of HUS usually does not result in improvement in renal function (Furlong et al., 2000).

There are data that suggest that amifostine may protect against chemotherapy-associated toxicities in transplant recipients (Phillips et al., 2001), including renal toxicity. Hartmann and colleagues (Hartmann et al., 2001) conducted a randomized study of amifostine cytoprotection in 40 patients undergoing autologous transplantation after preparation with carboplatin, etoposide, and ifosfamide. There was a significant improvement in maintenance of renal function (as measured by glomerular filtration rate) in patients who received amifostine versus those who did not (10% reduction versus 37% reduction, $P = .01$). Chauncey et al. (2000), however, did not find a benefit from amifostine when compared with historical controls.

Several groups have investigated whether patients with pre-existing renal dysfunction are appropriate candidates for autologous stem cell transplantation (Sanchorawala et al., 2001; Gertz et al., 2000; Badros et al., 2001; San Miguel et al., 2000; Dember et al., 2001). Those most likely to have renal dysfunction as a result of underlying disease are patients with multiple myeloma or AL amyloidosis.

Renal dysfunction in patients with AL amyloidosis is common and manifests as nephrotic syndrome and/or renal insufficiency. Nephrotic syndrome improves in many patients after high-dose melphalan and autologous stem cell transplantation (Sanchorawala et al., 2001; Gertz et al., 2000; Dember et al., 2001; Sezer et al., 1999). Renal function worsens in many of these patients during the immediate peritransplant period and is reversible in most cases (Dember et al., 2001). Unfortunately, the natural history of AL amyloidosis results in further decreases in creatinine clearance over time. It appears that patients who achieve complete hematologic responses after high-dose melphalan have better preservation of renal function than do patients who have persistent disease after transplant. At Boston University Medical Center, which has treated more than 200 patients with AL amyloidosis with high-dose chemotherapy and HSCT, renal failure does not exclude patients provided that they meet other eligibility criteria for cardiac and pulmonary function. These patients have more treatment-related toxicity but their complete remission rate and 1-year survival are comparable to those of patients without end-stage renal disease (Sanchorawala et al., 2001).

San Miguel and colleagues (San Miguel et al., 2000) reviewed 566 patients in the Spanish Autologous Stem Cell Transplantation registry transplanted for multiple myeloma.

Patients were categorized according to renal function (abnormal function at diagnosis but normal at transplant; abnormal at both diagnosis and transplant; normal at both diagnosis and transplant). Although treatment-related mortality (TRM) was significantly greater in patients who had abnormal renal function at both diagnosis and transplant, independent risk factors for TRM were poor performance status, hemoglobin ≤ 9.5 mg/dl, and creatinine ≥ 5 mg/dl. Response to transplant was not influenced by renal function. Independent variables for unfavorable overall survival were poor performance status, high beta$_2$-microglobulin level, and no response to transplant.

Badros et al. (2001) treated 81 multiple myeloma patients with renal failure using high-dose melphalan and autologous stem cell support. Thirty-eight patients were on dialysis. Sixty patients (including 27 on dialysis) received 200 mg/m^2 of melphalan. At this dose, 16 patients developed pulmonary toxicity, 8 of whom required ventilatory support. The remaining 21 patients received 140 mg/m^2. Pulmonary complications and encephalopathy were significantly more common in dialysis patients. Early TRM was 5% for patients who received 140 mg/m^2 and 7% for those who received 200 mg/m^2 of melphalan. Although it was intended that patients undergo a second cycle of high-dose melphalan, only 31 did so. There was no apparent advantage for patients who received tandem transplants in this study.

Hepatic toxicity (and see Chapters 77 and 89)

Hepatic toxicity is the most problematic regimen-related toxicity after ablative preparative therapy. Hepatic toxicity is characterized by fluid retention and painful hepatomegaly early in the course of disease, followed by elevated bilirubin and, sometimes, transaminases (McDonald et al., 1993; Shulman et al., 1994; Strasser et al., 2000). Because clinical signs of portal hypertension follow those of hepatic parenchymal injury and because not all patients with this clinical syndrome have hepatic venular occlusion on biopsy or autopsy material (Shulman et al., 1994) DeLeve and colleague (Deleve et al., 2002) have suggested that a more appropriate name for this toxicity is sinusoidal obstruction syndrome (SOS) rather than the more commonly used veno-occlusive disease (VOD). An excellent review and the rationale for the nomenclature change can be found elsewhere (DeLeve et al., 2000). For the remainder of this chapter, hepatic toxicity after ablative therapy will be referred to as SOS-VOD.

Sinusoidal endothelial cell (SEC) injury appears to precede injury to hepatocytes in SOS-VOD. Plasminogen activator inhibitor-1, an endothelial cell marker, increases early and specifically in patients with SOS-VOD (Salat et al., 1994; Salat et al., 1997). Thrombomodulin, another endothelial marker, also increases after high-dose therapy (Testa et al., 1996). Direct exposure of SEC to cyclophosphamide does not result in endothelial damage (DeLeve, 1996). However, exposure to acrolein or 4-hydroxycyclophosphamide results in significant endothelial injury. When SEC and hepatocytes are co-cultured

Table 82.3. *Histopathologic changes in patients with SOS-VOD*

| | Severity of clinical illness | | | | |
Histologic feature	Severe (n = 32)	Mild/moderate (n = 11)	None (n = 5)	LDUE (n = 28)	P[a]
Occluded hepatic venules	75%	55%	60%	50%	.04
Eccentric luminal narrowing and/or phlebosclerosis	28%	0%	0%	7%	.004
Sinusoidal fibrosis	69%	36%	40%	29%	.001
Hepatocyte necrosis	75%	45%	40%	54%	.03
Sinusoidal congestion	75%	91%	80%	75%	.6
Cholestasis	50%	45%	40%	25%	.1
GVHD	63%	55%	60%	43%	.2
Nodular regenerative hyperplasia	3%	9%	20%	11%	.2

Abbreviations: LDUE, liver dysfunction of uncertain etiology.

[a] Compares severe with all other categories.

and exposed to cyclophosphamide, SEC suffer more damage than do hepatocytes. This is believed to be due to the metabolic activation of cyclophosphamide by hepatocytes and the generation of the toxic metabolite acrolein and can be reversed by supporting intracellular levels of glutathione (DeLeve, 1996). Cyclophosphamide metabolism is affected by busulfan (Slattery *et al.,* 1996), possibly because busulfan reduces glutathione levels in hepatocytes and SEC (DeLeve & Wang, 2000). SOS-VOD occurs less frequently when cyclophosphamide administration precedes busulfan (Meresse *et al.,* 1992). Although busulfan levels are far more consistent after intravenous administration, fatal SOS-VOD can still occur after i.v. busulfan plus cyclophosphamide (Andersson *et al.,* 2002).

Histopathologically, a variety of changes are found (Table 82.3). The number of histologic abnormalities correlates with the severity of the clinical illness (Badros *et al.,* 2001).

The first signs of SOS-VOD, fluid retention and painful hepatomegaly, appear on or around the date of stem cell infusion. Hyperbilirubinemia usually starts a week or so later. Fewer than 20% of patients with mild or moderate disease and about half of patients with severe disease develop ascites (McDonald *et al.,* 1993). Patients who die of SOS-VOD usually do so because of multiorgan failure rather than liver failure (Zager, 1994; McDonald *et al.,* 1993). Patients who demonstrate early rapid increases in weight and bilirubin are likely to die. Mortality can be predicted from a mathematical model based on these clinical signs and can be very helpful in patients who receive cyclophosphamide-based regimens (Bearman *et al.,* 1993).

Risk factors for SOS-VOD include active hepatic parenchymal inflammation pretransplant (elevated transaminases) (McDonald *et al.,* 1993), second transplants using ablative preparation (Radich *et al.,* 1993), and pre-existing hepatic fibrosis (Tanikawa *et al.,* 2000; Rio *et al.,* 1993). Richard *et al.* (1996) found levels of soluble thrombomodulin and von Willebrand factor were increased prior to transplant in patients who went on to develop SOS-VOD, suggesting that endothelial injury prior to the start of preparative therapy may also be a risk factor.

SOS-VOD has been reported to occur in up to 53% of patients who receive myeloablative preparative therapy, with up to two-thirds dying of this complication (McDonald *et al.,* 1993). The incidence of SOS-VOD has decreased significantly in recent years. Carreras *et al.* (1998) reported that 87 of 1,652 (5.3%) consecutive patients transplanted at EBMT Centers during a 6-month period developed SOS-VOD, 16 of whom (18%) died. The decreased incidence and severity of SOS-VOD is probably due to healthier patients, fewer underlying risk factors (for example, chronic hepatitis C), and more transplants being performed using less intensive preparative regimens. In the literature, the great disparity among reports regarding incidence and mortality is also a function of the definition of SOS-VOD and how deaths are attributed to it.

Several investigators have reported an association between hepatic toxicity and treatment with gemtuzumab ozogamicin (Mylotarg®) (Giles *et al.,* 2001; Sievers *et al.,* 2001; Rajvanshi *et al.,* 2002), a humanized anti-CD33 monoclonal antibody conjugated to the antitumor antibiotic calicheamicin. Studies have been conducted both in patients who have and have not had previous HSC transplants. Giles *et al.* (2001) reported that 14 of 119 patients (12%) who received gemtuzumab developed SOS-VOD. Twelve of these 14 patients died, including 5 in whom SOS-VOD was a major contributor to death. Sievers and colleagues (Sievers *et al.,* 2001) treated 142 patients using 1 to 3 doses of gemtuzumab. Of 137 patients who had not undergone previous transplant, 33 developed grade 3 or 4 hyperbilirubinemia (24%). Two patients died of liver failure. Of 27 patients who underwent transplant after receiving gemtuzumab, 3 (11%) died of SOS-VOD.

Rajvanshi *et al.* (2002) reported on the outcome of 23 consecutive patients who received gemtuzumab for relapsed AML after previous stem cell transplant. SOS-VOD developed in 11 patients. The presentation of hepatic toxicity in these patients is shown in Table 82.4. Histologic material was available from 6 patients. One had only evidence of GVHD while the remaining 5 had varying degrees of zone 3 injury. While the number of

Table 82.4. *Presentation of SOS-VOD in 11 patients receiving gemtuzumab ozogamicin for relapsed leukemia after previous hematopoietic stem cell transplant*

Finding	Number of patients with abnormality	Peak value, median (range)	Median time from gemtuzumab infusion, days (range)
Ascites (onset)	7		8 (6–24)
Elevated serum AST	11	242 (86–3091) U/l	8 (3–37)
Weight gain	7	8.9 (5–19.5)%	16 (3–25)
Hyperbilirubinemia	10	5.6 (1.5–13.2) mg/dl	17 (9–41)
Elevated alkaline phosphatase	10	439 (186–964) U/l	22 (5–41)

Abbreviation: AST, aspartate aminotransferase.
From Rajvanshi *et al.*, 2002

samples was very limited, patients who had longer duration from gemtuzumab to liver biopsy had more extensive fibrosis than did patients with shorter intervals. Those with shorter intervals had more venular subendothelial edema and congestion and more hepatocyte necrosis and hemorrhage.

SOS-VOD can only be prevented by avoiding myeloablative preparative regimens. Some nonablative preparative strategies appear to be without hepatic toxicity but others are clearly more intense and more toxic. This will be discussed in more detail below. Several strategies have been employed in an attempt to reduce the incidence and severity of SOS-VOD. Their utility is questionable. Fractionated TBI results in less SOS-VOD than single dose TBI (Grinsky *et al.*, 2000). In BCNU-containing regimens, fractionating the dose also appears to reduce SOS-VOD compared to a single dose (Ayash *et al.*, 1990). Shielding the liver during TBI may reduce hepatic toxicity but may increase the risk of relapse (Anderson *et al.*, 2001). Results of heparin or antithrombin III are mixed (Bearman, 1995). However, neither are routinely used at most institutions, suggesting that confidence in these agents is weak. Ursodeoxycholic acid has been studied in several prospective randomized studies. Essell and colleagues (Essell *et al.*, 1998) and Ohashi *et al.* (2000) reported that the incidence of SOS-VOD was less in patients who received ursodiol prophylaxis. However, in neither study was there a difference in mortality between the treatment and control groups. A trial comparing heparin plus ursodiol versus heparin alone did not show any differences in hepatic toxicity (Park *et al.*, 2002) Bile steroids have been reported to prevent endothelial and hepatocyte injury, possibly by downregulation of inflammatory mediators. Whether ursodiol actually works or results in benefit to transplant patients is unclear.

Most patients with SOS-VOD recover spontaneously and treatment is supportive. Several approaches have been studied in patients with severe illness. Tissue plasminogen activator has

been evaluated by several groups (Bearman *et al.*, 1997; Schriber *et al.*, 1999; Kulkarni *et al.*, 1999; Hagglund *et al.*, 1996). Approximately 30% of patients appear to respond, but almost as many develop significant hemorrhagic complications (Bearman *et al.*, 1997; Schriber *et al.*, 1999; Hagglund *et al.*, 1996). Tissue plasminogen activator has no efficacy in patients who already have multiorgan dysfunction (Bearman *et al.*, 1997; Schriber *et al.*, 1999).

Defibrotide (DF) is a single-stranded polydeoxyribonucleotide with anti-ischemic, antithrombotic, and thrombolytic activity and no significant anticoagulant effects. Richardson and colleagues (Richardson *et al.*, 2002) have studied DF in 88 patients with severe SOS-VOD. Ninety-seven percent of patients had multiorgan dysfunction, including 34% and 31% who were ventilator-dependent and on dialysis, respectively. Complete responses occurred in 36% of patients. Younger patients, autologous stem cell recipients, fall in PAI-1 and creatinine were all associated with improved outcome. No significant adverse events occurred.

There has been one report using *N*-acetylcysteine, a precursor of intracellular reduced glutathione, for treatment of SOS-VOD (Ringden *et al.*, 2000). Three patients were treated, all of whom had gained at least 10% weight gain and moderate elevations in bilirubin. SOS-VOD resolved in all patients. L-glutamine, another glutathione precursor, has been used both therapeutically and prophylactically. The data are limited. Two of two patients treated for SOS-VOD responded (Goringe *et al.*, 1998). Of 18 who received L-glutamine prophylactically, none developed hepatic toxicity (Brown *et al.*, 1998). Clearly, additional studies with sufficient power are needed.

Because animal models of SOS-VOD suggest that sinusoidal vasoconstriction contributes to zone 3 ischemia, administration of nitrates may make sense physiologically (DeLeve & Wang, 1999). Only one patient has been reported (Kajiume *et al.*, 2000). The ability to maintain blood pressure may be difficult in this patient population.

Transjugular intrahepatic portosystemic shunts have been used in patients with severe SOS-VOD, with mixed results (Azoulay *et al.*, 2000; Zenz *et al.*, 2001; Fried *et al.*, 1996; Smith *et al.*, 1996; Meacher *et al.*, 1999). All reports are small series or case reports. Of the 21 patients reported in the literature, all had severe SOS-VOD, 20 had ascites, and most had renal failure. Eleven patients died within 2 weeks of the procedure. Only 2 of the remaining 10 patients were long-term survivors. One patient developed acute respiratory distress, fever, and hypotension 8 hours after the procedure (Meacher *et al.*, 1999). He was noted to have a significant increase in leukocyte count. No infectious etiology could be found and the patient died of multiorgan failure 14 days after the procedure. His physicians suggested that he developed pulmonary leukostasis as a result of the rapid resolution in hypersplenism following the procedure.

A small number of patients with SOS-VOD have undergone surgical portosystemic shunts (Murray *et al.*, 1987) or have received liver transplants (Hagglund *et al.*, 1996; Nimer *et al.*,

1990; Rapaport *et al.*, 1991). Transplantation has been successful in several.

Pulmonary toxicity (and see Chapters 78 and 91)

Pulmonary toxicity includes all diagnoses of noninfectious pneumonia occurring after stem cell transplantation. It presents with variable clinical manifestations and histologic findings, has multiple etiologies, and has been referred to by several names. Idiopathic pneumonia syndrome (IPS) is the preferred term rather than diffuse interstitial pneumonitis, as widespread alveolar injury is a prominent feature (Clark *et al.*, 1993). IPS occurs in fewer than 10% of transplant recipients and with similar frequency after autologous and allogeneic transplant (Kantrow *et al.*, 1997). The median time of onset is 21 days posttransplant. Kantrow and colleagues (Kantrow *et al.*, 1997) reported that the cumulative incidence of IPS is significantly greater in patients who develop grade IV acute GVHD compared with allogeneic patients who develop grades 0–III acute GVHD and in those with malignancies other than leukemia (Kantrow *et al.*, 1997).

The mortality among patients who develop IPS is approximately 75%, most of whom die of respiratory failure (Kantrow *et al.*, 1997; Wingard *et al.*, 1988). A small proportion die of other causes (Bach *et al.*, 2001; Khassawneh *et al.*, 2002). Mechanical ventilation is required in almost 70% of patients, a median of 2 days after the onset of radiographic changes. Rarely do IPS patients who require mechanical ventilation survive to be discharged from the hospital. Most patients with IPS who die, do so due to respiratory failure. Corticosteroids are usually not effective.

The pathogenesis of IPS is poorly understood. Panoskaltsis-Mortari and colleagues (Panoskaltis-Mortari *et al.*, 1997) have studied the proinflammatory events that occur in the peritransplant period that may promote IPS in mice. Recipient B10.BR mice were lethally irradiated on day–1 and received T-depleted C57BL/6 marrow on day 0. Some mice also received NK cell-depleted spleen cells as a source of T cells to produce acute GVHD. Immunoperoxidase stains of recipient lungs from day 7 showed increased numbers of CD3+ cells in perivascular, peribronchial, and interstitial sites in animals who received both marrow and splenocytes. These changes were not seen in mice who received allogeneic (T-depleted) marrow alone or syngeneic marrow. Furthermore, increases in Mac-1+ cells were also seen. Intense staining for B7-1 was observed at sites of Mac-1+ cells. This suggested that colocalization of T cells and macrophages promoted antigen presentation to, and costimulation of, allogeneic T cells in the lung. The authors also evaluated cytokine mRNA expression on day 7 and found that cells that transcribed TGFβ$_1$ were the most frequent. The frequency and intensity were greatest in mice that had received both marrow and splenocytes. Furthermore, addition of cyclophosphamide to the preparative regimen increased the number of TGFβ$_1$-expressing cells. TGFβ is associated with lung fibrosis (Khalil *et al.*, 1991).

Lung injury is also common in regimens that contain BCNU (Table 82.5) (Jones *et al.*, 1993; Wilczynski *et al.*, 1998; Fleming *et al.*, 1998; Alessandrino *et al.*, 2000; Caballero *et al.*, 1997; Grovas *et al.*, 1999). BCNU-induced lung injury occurs in up to 64% of patients treated with cyclophosphamide, cisplatin, and BCNU for high-risk or advanced breast cancer (Jones *et al.*, 1993; Wilczynski *et al.*, 1998). In such patients the area under the curve (AUC) of BCNU was significantly greater in patients who developed lung injury than in patients who did not (Jones *et al.*, 1993) (Fig. 82.2). It has been termed *delayed pulmonary toxicity syndrome* (DPTS) to distinguish it from IPS (Wilczynski *et al.*, 1998). The median onset of DPTS is 10 weeks posttransplant and is characterized by a median DLCO decrease of 42% from baseline, with a less pronounced fall in vital capacity and FEV1. Most patients who develop DPTS present with a dry cough and dyspnea on exertion, with or without fever. A small percentage of patients are asymptomatic and are diagnosed based only on their pulmonary function tests. Patients who develop symptoms have a more rapid presentation, with a more marked fall in DLCO. The median DLCO nadir occurs 15 to 18 weeks posttransplant at 58% of baseline value. Corticosteroid administration results in an improvement in DLCO over time (Wilczynski *et al.*, 1998; Fleming *et al.*, 1998). Death from DPTS is unusual. However, lack of familiarity with this syndrome may result in incorrect treatment and resulting deterioration leading to significant respiratory compromise. McGaughey *et al.* (2001) reported that

Table 82.5. *Pulmonary toxicity after BCNU-containing regimens*

Reference	Regimens	N	Incidence
Wilczynski *et al.*, 1998	Cyclophosphamide (5.625 g/m^2) + cisplatin (165 mg/m^2) + BCNU (600 mg/m^2)	45	64%
Fleming *et al.*, 1998	Cyclophosphamide (7.2 g/m^2) + etoposide (2.4 g/m^2) + BCNU (300–600 mg/m^2)	136	5%[a]
Alessandrino *et al.*, 2000	Cyclophosphamide (4 g/m^2) + etoposide (1 g/m^2) + BCNU (600 mg/m^2)	40	35%
Alessandrino *et al.*, 2000	BCNU (300–600 mg/m^2) + etoposide (1 g/m^2) + melphalan (200 mg/m^2)	25	12%
Caballero *et al.*, 1997	BCNU (300 mg/m^2) + etoposide (800 mg/m^2) + cytarabine (1600 mg/m^2) + melphalan (140 mg/m^2)	148	1%[b]
Grovas *et al.*, 1999	BCNU (600 mg/m^2) + thiotepa (900 mg/m^2) + etoposide (750 mg/m^2)	11	27%

[a] Grade 3/4 RRT.

[b] Fatal RRT.

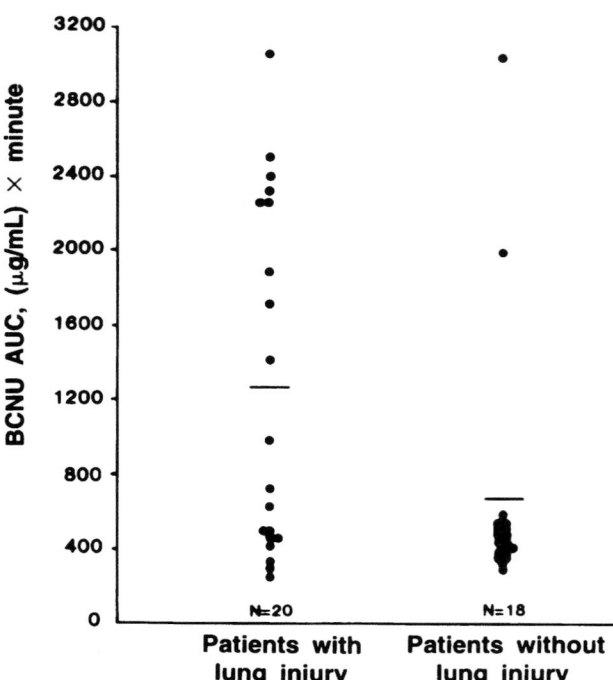

Fig. 82.2. Scatter diagram demonstrating BCNU area under the curve (AUC) of patients who developed lung injury (left column) and those who did not (right column). Reproduced, with permission, from Jones et al. (1993).

inhaled steroids could prevent DPTS. Sixty-three patients were treated with inhaled fluticasone propionate as part of a phase II study in patients receiving high-dose cyclophosphamide, cisplatin, and BCNU. At a median of 44 days and 96 days posttransplant, the DLCO was decreased 8% and 21%, respectively. This compared with decreases of 29% and 33% in historical controls who did not receive fluticasone. Overall 35% of patients developed DPTS, compared to an incidence of 73% in historical controls. No fungal pneumonias occurred and no patients died of DPTS.

Neurotoxicity (and see Chapter 93)

Both central nervous system (CNS) toxicity and peripheral neuropathy can be caused by agents used in transplant preparative regimens. Seizures, which can occur after high-dose busulfan, can be prevented with antiseizure medications provided therapeutic levels are achieved (Vassal et al., 1990; Grigg et al., 1989). Cerebellar and, to a lesser extent, cerebral toxicity can occur in patients who receive high-dose cytarabine (Damon et al., 1989; Rubin et al., 1992). This can be limited by careful attention to renal function and dose adjustment when indicated (Smith et al., 1997). Encephalopathy has been described after high-dose melphalan (Schuh et al., 1999). Acquired pseudocholinesterase deficiency after high-dose cyclophosphamide leading to apnea during general anesthesia has been described (Koeoglu et al., 1999).

In most circumstances, CNS toxicity is subclinical. Extensive white matter changes have been reported in many patients (Brown et al., 1995). Most are asymptomatic and the significance is unclear. These findings are believed to be due to changes in free and bound water fractions rather than neuronal damage. One circumstance in which CNS toxicity is clinically apparent is leukoencephalopathy (Bleyer, 1981; Thompson et al., 1986). Signs and symptoms include seizure, confusion, dysarthria, weakness, and coma; onset is usually several months posttransplant. Leukoencephalopathy usually occurs in patients who receive therapy (radiation and/or intrathecal chemotherapy) after transplant. It is typically progressive and fatal. Leukoencephalopathy can also occur after administration of cyclosporine or tacrolimus (Bechstein, 2000). This tends to present sooner than leukoencephalopathy directed specifically at the CNS, and usually improves after discontinuation of treatment. Neurotoxicity resolves or improves in the majority of patients who develop neurotoxicity on cyclosporine and are switched to tacrolimus (Benito et al., 2001).

Cognitive dysfunction has been reported in some patients after high-dose cytoreductive therapy. In a prospective study of neurocognitive function in children who underwent transplant, Phipps and colleagues (Phipps et al., 2000) found that the single predictor of late neurocognitive sequelae was age at transplant. Patients who were 6 or older had a minimal risk of cognitive sequelae while patients younger than 6 and particularly those younger than 3 years of age had a greater risk (Phipps et al., 2000). A minority of adult transplant recipients experience neuropsychological impairment, characterized by slowed reaction time, difficulty with attention and concentration, and troubles with reasoning and problem solving (Andrykowski et al., 1990). Neuropsychological difficulties correlated with TBI dose. The incidence of cognitive impairment is greater for breast cancer patients who receive high-dose chemotherapy (32%) than those who receive standard dose chemotherapy (17%). Both have a significantly greater incidence than breast cancer patients who receive no systemic treatment (Van Dam et al., 1998).

The risk of peripheral neuropathy in transplant patients has increased, particularly with the incorporation of taxanes in high-dose regimens (Stemmer et al., 1996; Doroshow et al., 1997; Mayordomo et al., 1997; Gluck et al., 1996; Vahdat et al., 1998; Nieto et al., 2000; Papadopoulos et al., 2001). There is some disagreement regarding whether taxane drug levels correlate with neurotoxicity. Stemmer et al. (1996) reported a clear association between paclitaxel AUC and severity of peripheral neuropathy in patients who received paclitaxel, cyclophosphamide, and cisplatin. Papadopoulos et al., (2001) on the other hand, found no correlation between paclitaxel pharmacokinetics and total neuropathy scores after high-dose paclitaxel, although there was a significant correlation between pre- and post-total neuropathy scores in 10 patients who had detailed neurologic evaluations (including nerve conduction studies) performed (Gluck et al., 1996). Neurotoxicity due to taxanes decreases over time. CNS toxicity due to taxanes can occur, although it is rare (Nieto et al., 1999). There are data that suggest that glutamine may reduce taxane-induced neuropathy (Vahdat *et al.*, 2001).

Hemorrhagic cystitis (and see Chapter 79)

Hemorrhagic cystitis is common after stem cell transplantation, particularly in patients who receive cyclophosphamide or ifosfamide. Acrolein, the nonenzymatic metabolite of these agents, causes hyperemia and ulceration of the bladder mucosa, resulting in hemorrhage and focal necrosis. The rate at which acrolein is excreted in the urine appears to be more closely associated with hemorrhagic cystitis than the cumulative amount of acrolein excreted (Al-Rawithi *et al.*, 1998). In addition, patients who have previously received busulfan appear to be at increased risk of hemorrhagic cystitis (Thomas *et al.*, 1987). Prophylaxis for acrolein-associated hemorrhagic cystitis includes either hyperhydration with forced diuresis, bladder irrigation, or mesna. Randomized studies comparing one prophylactic strategy to another have shown mixed results (Hows *et al.*, 1984; Vose *et al.*, 1993; Bedi *et al.*, 1995; Ringden *et al.*, 1994; Ringden *et al.*, 1994).

That hemorrhagic cystitis occurs even with effective urothelial prophylaxis suggests additional etiologies. A great deal of attention has been paid to the role of BK polyoma virus in the etiology of hemorrhagic cystitis (Bedi *et al.*, 1995; Leung *et al.*, 2001; Arthur *et al.*, 1986; Apperly *et al.*, 1987; Chan *et al.*, 1994). Several investigators have demonstrated the presence of BK viruria in patients undergoing transplant. Early reports suggested an etiologic role for BK virus but polymerase chain reaction (PCR) studies showed that many patients without clinical signs of hemorrhagic cystitis also had BK virus in their urine. Leung and colleagues (Leung *et al.*, 2001) performed quantitative PCR on urine samples from 50 patients, 20 of whom developed hemorrhagic cystitis. Hemorrhagic cystitis had two presentations, early microscopic hematuria occurring a median of 4 days posttransplant (14 patients) and late gross hematuria occurring a median of 37 days posttransplant (6 patients) and lasting a median of 18 days. BK viruria was detected in all 50 patients studied. The total and peak numbers of genome copies in patients without hemorrhagic cystitis was significantly lower than in patients with hemorrhagic cystitis. Among 21 patients with more than 10^{10} copies/day, 15 developed hemorrhagic cystitis (including the 6 with gross hematuria), while only 5 of 29 patients with less than 10^{10} copies/day developed microscopic hematuria. However, the number of viral copies did not correlate with the clinical severity of hemorrhagic cystitis (Leung *et al.*, 2001).

To evaluate whether viruria was due to viral reactivation or urothelial damage, quantitative PCR for adenovirus was also performed. All patients had quantifiable adenovirus viruria. Unlike BK virus, the number of copies was similar in patients with or without hemorrhagic cystitis. These observations suggest that neither background viral reactivation nor urothelial damage explain the increase in BK viruria in patients with hemorrhagic cystitis. A logistic regression analysis showed BK viruria to be the only significant independent risk factor for hemorrhagic cystitis (Leung *et al.*, 2001).

Adenovirus has also been associated with late hemorrhagic cystitis. Akiyama and colleagues (Akiyama *et al.*, 2001) cultured urine from 43 patients with hemorrhagic cystitis and found that 26 (60%) were positive for adenovirus (22 of which were type 11). The incidence of PCR-documented adenovirus viruria in patients with hemorrhagic cystitis was similar, 57%. However, in this study, PCR was not quantitative and therefore no information is available regarding the number of viral copies and extent of disease (Akiyama *et al.*, 2001).

Treatment of hemorrhagic cystitis is problematic. Most cases of early microscopic hematuria resolve spontaneously. Late hemorrhagic cystitis can result in significant bleeding and pain. A variety of medical and surgical therapies have been reported, including bladder instillation with formalin, (Shrom *et al.*, 1976) prostaglandin E_1, (Trigg *et al.*, 1990) or alum, (Efros *et al.*, 1994) electrode fulguration, (Lapides, 1970) and suprapubic cystostomy (Baronciani *et al.*, 1995). As these reports are largely anecdotal, it is not possible to assess whether one is superior to another.

Mucositis (and see Chapter 80)

Mucositis occurs in approximately 75% of patients who receive myeloablative preparative therapy (Bearman *et al.*, 1988; Woo *et al.*, 1993; Pico *et al.*, 1998) and is, by far, the most common complaint of transplant patients (Bellm *et al.*, 2000; Stiff, 2001). Mucositis is the result of injury to actively dividing cells in the basal cell layer of the mucosa, ultimately leading to atrophy and ulceration, and local infection contributed to by neutropenia.

A variety of chemotherapeutic regimens and modalities consistently cause mucositis, including TBI, thiotepa, melphalan, etoposide, and paclitaxel. In general, treatment of mucositis includes oral rinsing, topical anesthetics, and systemic narcotic analgesics. Injury to the basal cell layer begins with the first day of treatment and lasts about 10 to 14 days. Rapoport and colleague (Rapoport *et al.*, 1999) found that patients with leukemia who undergo allotransplantation using a TBI-containing regimen are most likely to develop mucositis. They also found that patients with severe mucositis (rated using the Oral Assessment Guide) were more likely to develop bacteremia than patients with less severe mucositis and were more likely to die of treatment-related complications. Horowitz *et al.* (1999) also studied the correlation between mucositis and treatment outcome, using the Oral Mucositis Assessment Scale (OMAS). They found that the mucositis score correlated with infection, number of febrile days, and total hospital charges. They did not find a correlation between mucositis as measured by OMAS and mortality.

Several studies have evaluated various strategies to prevent mucositis. Glutamine supplementation, either parenterally or orally has been studied in several randomized studies. One study found no benefit while two others reported a benefit for patients using glutamine (Anderson *et al.*, 1998; Coghlin *et al.*,

2000; Huang *et al.*, 2000). The largest of these studies evaluated oral glutamine in 193 transplant recipients (Anderson *et al.*, 1998). Autologous stem cell recipients had less oral pain and decreased narcotic use. Allogeneic transplant recipients did not enjoy these same benefits, although survival at day 28 was superior in patients who were randomized to glutamine. It was speculated that the lack of improvement in allotransplant recipients was due to the use of methotrexate for GVHD prophylaxis.

Hematopoietic growth factors have been studied to prevent mucositis. While improvement has been reported in patients receiving conventional dose chemotherapy, (Crawford *et al.*, 1994; Gabrilove *et al.*, 1988) transplant patients did not have a similar benefit (Nemunitis *et al.*, 1995). On the other hand, interleukin-11 may have some benefit, at least in autologous transplant recipients. The results of a randomized, placebo-controlled, dose-escalation study of interleukin-11 in autologous transplant recipients prepared using busulfan, melphalan, and thiotepa suggested potential benefit in this patient group (Schwerkoske *et al.*, 1999). A similar study in allogeneic transplant patients prepared with cyclophosphamide/TBI and receiving cyclosporine and methotrexate as GVHD prophylaxis had to be stopped early due to excessive toxicity, particularly fluid retention and multiorgan failure (Antin *et al.*, 2002).

Keratinocyte growth factor (KGF) has been studied as prophylaxis against mucositis. KGF stimulates the proliferation and differentiation of epithelial cells, including gastrointestinal mucosal cells and was shown in animal models to reduce mucositis in animals receiving chemotherapy and/or radiation (Farrell *et al.*, 1998; Farrell *et al.*, 1999). Furthermore, pretreatment with KGF improved survival in these animals. Spielberger and colleagues (Spielberger *et al.*, 2001) conducted a prospective, randomized, placebo-controlled study of KGF before or before and after TBI, high-dose etoposide, and cyclophosphamide and autologous stem cell transplantation. They found that KGF given before and following high-dose chemoradiotherapy resulted in less oral pain, narcotic analgesics, and duration of total parenteral nutrition compared to patients who received placebo.

The synthetic protegrin antibiotic IB-367 has been studied to prevent mucositis in transplant patients. Protegrins are a class of antibiotics derived from the specific granules of porcine neutrophils with an extremely broad spectrum of activity. Vesole and co-workers (Vesole & Fuch, 1999) conducted a phase II study of IB-367 in 187 transplant patients who received preparative regimens that consistently cause mucositis. IB-367 reduced mucositis by 42% in patients who took this agent for 4 or more days prior to stem cell infusion. A prospective randomized study is currently underway.

Gastrointestinal toxicity (and see Chapter 89)

Nausea and vomiting, abdominal pain, and diarrhea are common complaints in patients undergoing transplant and, while debilitating, are rarely life-threatening. Nausea and vomiting can occur due to effects of cytoreductive agents on the vomiting centers of the brain or because of direct mucosal toxicity. It can also occur secondary to opioid treatment of mucosal pain. A variety of antiemetic agents are available, including the type 3 serotonin antagonists ondansetron, granisetron, and tropisetron, which are effective in about half of patients (Fox-Geiman *et al.*, 2001; Lacerda *et al.*, 2000). Delayed nausea and vomiting, which can be due to gastroparesis, remains problematic (Eagle *et al.*, 2001).

Abdominal pain after transplantation can have many causes. These include acute GVHD and *Clostridium difficile* enterocolitis. Typhlitis may also occur. It usually presents with sudden onset of right-sided abdominal pain, bloody diarrhea, fever, and nausea and vomiting. It is most frequently caused by *Clostridium septicum* and can be life-threatening or fatal.

Diarrhea after transplant can have multiple causes, including GVHD, infection, or medications. While it is usually bothersome, it is uncommon for diarrheal volume to affect hemodynamic parameters.

Recent developments

Reduced-intensity regimens (and see Chapter 22)

The use of reduced-intensity preparative regimens for allogeneic transplantation has been the focus of an enormous research effort by many investigators in the past several years. Reduced-intensity regimens were initially developed in order to include patients who would otherwise not be candidates for typical ablative programs, such as older patients and those with organ dysfunction. In addition, these regimens would reduce or eliminate cytoreduction for patients with nonmalignant diseases. Allotransplantation for malignant disease using reduced-intensity regimens relies on a graft-versus-tumor effect with moderate or minimal cytoreduction. The term "reduced-intensity" rather than "non-myeloablative" is used because some of these regimens can be quite aggressive.

Most reduced-intensity regimens include fludarabine with either additional chemotherapeutic agents, TBI, anti-thymocyte globulin, or monoclonal antibodies (Table 82.6). Sibling donors, unrelated donors, and umbilical cord blood have all been used as the source of stem cells. Unfortunately, most reports include relatively small numbers of patients and only one report specifically addresses regimen-related toxicity.

Flowers *et al.* (Flowers *et al.*, 2000) analyzed RRT in 65 patients who received 200 cGy of TBI with ($n = 19$) or without fludarabine ($n = 46$). Two patients (3%) died of RRT and 16 patients (25%) developed grade 3 RRT in one or more organs. The organ most commonly affected was the liver, with 8 patients (12%) developing grade 3 RRT. How many of these patients had previously received gemtuzumab ozogamicin (Mylotarg®) is unknown.

Tandem regimens

A number of investigators have studied the combination of two or more high-dose regimens, either employing the same agents or non-cross-resistant agents. The rationale for such a tandem approach is that cytoreduction of tumor bulk with one cycle may make a second cycle more effective. This may be particu-

Table 82.6. *Common reduced-intensity regimens for allotransplantation*

Author	Regimen	Indication	N	Nonrelapse mortality	Fatal SOS-VOD	IPS
Nagler et al., 2000	Fludarabine + busulfan + antithymocyte globulin	Lymphoma	23	30%	0%	5%
McSweeney et al., 2001	200 cGy total body irradiation	Hematologic malignancy	45	7%	0%	0%
Khouri et al., 2001	Fludarabine + cyclophosphamide + rituximab	Indolent lymphoma	20	5%	0%	0%
Childs et al., 2000	Cyclophosphamide + fludarabine	Renal cell carcinoma	19	11%	0%	0%

Abbreviations: SOS-VOD, sinusoidal obstruction syndrome/veno-occlusive disease; IPS, idiopathic pneumonia syndrome.

larly true with solid tumors, where tumor heterogeneity may reduce the ability of a single regimen to eradicate all disease. Furthermore, when the second cycle is composed of different and non-cross-resistant agents, the likelihood of induced drug resistance may be less. However appealing this rationale is, success is dependent on the ability of patients to tolerate multiple cycles of high-dose therapy.

Multiple cycles of high-dose therapy with autologous stem cell transplantation have been studied in patients with various malignancies, including metastatic breast cancer, multiple myeloma, poor-prognosis lymphoma, neuroblastoma, and testicular cancer. This approach has generally been found to be well tolerated (Table 82.7) (Bashey *et al.,* 2000; Bitran *et al.,* 1996; Vahdat *et al.,* 1995; Ayash *et al.,* 1994; Ayash *et al.,* 2001; Somlo *et al.,* 2001; Haioun *et al.,* 2001; Barlogie *et al.,* 1999). The reported TRM ranges from 0 to 10%. TRM is due to infection or RRT in similar proportions. In some studies, a number of patients did not undergo their second high-dose cycle due to disease progression, poor tolerance of the first transplant, or an unwillingness by the patient to receive additional treatment.

Barlogie *et al.* (1999) as part of their "total therapy" program for multiple myeloma, treated 14 patients with ablative allografts as their second high-dose regimen. All had achieved partial remissions after the first high-dose cycle. Twenty-one percent of these patients died within 100 days and 50% died within 12 months, usually of treatment-related complications.

To avoid this type of outcome, several investigators have begun to study high-dose cytoreduction with autologous stem cell support, followed by adoptive immunotherapy using reduced-intensity allogeneic transplants (Carella *et al.,* 2000; Bearman *et al.,* 2000; Maloney *et al.,* 2001). In most circumstances, the interval between the two transplants was less than 100 days. These programs have combined several autologous transplant regimens with fludarabine or TBI-based non-myeloablative preparative regimens and have been well tolerated (Table 82.8).

Summary

Regimen-related toxicity continues to be an important cause of morbidity and mortality after myeloablative preparative therapy. New toxicities, in general, only reflect agents that have recently come into practice, such as peripheral neuropathy due to taxanes. There is a growing interest in reduced-intensity allogeneic preparative regimens and in multiple cycles of high-dose therapy supported by autologous hematopoietic progenitor cells. The use of sequential high-dose cytoreduction with autologous progenitor cell support followed by reduced-intensity allografting has the potential to produce significant tumor reduction and improved graft-versus-tumor effects with limited mortality due to the preparative regimen. This approach, combined with improved prevention and treatment of GVHD, could result in greatly improved treatment results.

Table 82.7. *Treatment-related mortality reported after tandem or multiple cycles of high-dose chemotherapy with autologous hematopoietic stem cell support*

Author	Regimen	Indication	N	Treatment-related mortality (n)
Bashey et al., 2000	Cy + Mito + Carbo > Thiotepa + Carbo	Breast cancer	29	Infection (1)
Bitran et al,. 1996	Cy + Thiotepa > Melphalan	Breast cancer	27	Infection (2)
Vahdat et al., 1995	Paclitaxel > Melphalan > Cy + Carbo + thiotepa	Breast cancer	36	None
Ayash et al., 1994	Melphalan > Cy + thiotepa + Carbo	Breast cancer	20	None
Ayash et al., 2001	Carboplatin + Etoposide × 2	Testes cancer	29	Multiorgan failure (3)
Somlo et al., 2001	Melphalan + Carboplatin × 2	Breast cancer	50	None
Haioun et al., 2001	Mitoxantrone + Cy + Etoposide + BCNU > Bu + Carbo + melphalan	Lymphoma	29	VOD-SOS (2), infection (1)
Barlogie et al., 1999	Melphalan > Melphalan ± TBI	Multiple myeloma	195	Not reported

Abbreviations: Cy, cyclophosphamide; Mito, mitoxantrone; Carbo, carboplatin; Bu, busulfan; TBI, total body irradiation.

Table 82.8. *Sequential autologous transplantation and non-myeloablative allotransplantation*

| Author | N | Indication | Transplant preparative regimen | | GVHD prophylaxis | NRM (N)[a] |
			Autologous	Allogeneic		
Carella *et al.*, 2000	38	Hodgkin's and non-Hodgkin's lymphoma	BEAM	Flu + Cy	Methotrexate + cyclosporine	5[b]
Bearman *et al.*, 2000	16	Hematologic malignancy; stage IV breast cancer	Multiple	TBI ± Flu	Cyclosporine + MMF	2[c]
Maloney *et al.*, 2001	32	Multiple myeloma	Melphalan	TBI	Cyclosporine + MMF	1[d]

Abbreviations: Flu, fludarabine; Cy, cyclophosphamide; TBI, total body irradiation; MMF, mycophenolate mofetil; NRM, non-relapse mortality.

[a] Excluding graft-vs.-host disease.

[b] 5 nonrelapse deaths at 1 year (2 infection, 3 GVHD).

[c] One infection; one myocardial infarction.

[d] Cause of death not reported.

References

Akiyama, H., Kurosu, T., Sakashita, C. *et al.* (2001). Adenovirus is a key pathogen in hemorrhagic cystitis associated with bone marrow transplantation. *Clinical Infectious Diseases, 32,* 1325–30.

Alessandrino, E.P., Bernasconi, P., Colombo, A. *et al.* (2000). Pulmonary toxicity following carmustine-based preparative regimens and autologous peripheral blood progenitor cell transplantation in hematological malignancies. *Bone Marrow Transplantation, 25,* 309–13.

Al-Rawithi, S., El-Yazigi, A., Ernst, P. *et al.* (1998). Urinary excretion and pharmacokinetics of acrolein and its parent drug cyclophosphamide in bone marrow transplant patients. *Bone Marrow Transplantation, 22,* 485–90.

Anderson, J.E., Appelbaum, F.R., Schoch, G. *et al.* (2001). Relapse after allogeneic bone marrow transplantation for refractory anemia is increased by shielding lungs and liver during total body irradiation. *Biology of Blood and Marrow Transplantation, 7,* 163–70.

Anderson, P.M., Ramsay, N.K., Shu, X.O. *et al.* (1998). Effect of low-dose oral glutamine on painful stomatitis during bone marrow transplantation. *Bone Marrow Transplantation, 22,* 339–44.

Andersson, B.S., Kashyap, A., Gian, V. *et al.* (2002). Conditioning therapy with intravenous busulfan and cyclophosphamide (IV BuCy2) for hematologic malignancies prior to allogeneic stem cell transplantation: a phase II study. *Biology of Blood and Marrow Transplantation, 8,* 145–54.

Andrykowski, M.A., Altmaier, E.M., Barnett, R.L. *et al.* (1990). Cognitive dysfunction in adult survivors of allogeneic marrow transplantation: relationship to dose of total body irradiation. *Bone Marrow Transplantation, 6,* 269–76.

Angelucci, E., Mariotti, E., Lucarelli, G. *et al.* (1992). Sudden cardiac tamponade after chemotherapy for marrow transplantation in thalassaemia. *Lancet, 339,* 287–9.

Antin, J.H., Lee, S.J., Neuberg, D. *et al.* (2002). A phase I/II double-blind, placebo-controlled study of recombinant human interleukin-11 for mucositis and acute GVHD prevention in allogeneic stem cell transplantation. *Bone Marrow Transplantation, 29,* 373–7.

Appelbaum, F.R., Sullivan, K.M., Buckner, C.D. *et al.* (1987). Treatment of malignant lymphoma in 100 patients with cyclophosphamide, total body irradiation, and marrow transplantation. *Journal of Clinical Oncology, 5,* 1340–7.

Apperly, J.F., Rice, S.J., Bishop, J.A. *et al.* (1987). Late-onset hemorrhagic cystitis associated with urinary excretion of polyomaviruses after bone marrow transplantation. *Transplantation, 43,* 108–12.

Arthur, R.R., Shah, K.V., Baust, S.J. *et al.* (1986). Association of BK viruria with hemorrhagic cystitis in recipients of bone marrow transplants. *New England Journal of Medicine, 315,* 230–4.

Ayash, L.J., Clarke, M., Silver, S.M. *et al.* (2001). Double dose-intensive chemotherapy with autologous stem cell support for relapsed and refractory testicular cancer: the University of Michigan experience and literature review. *Bone Marrow Transplantation, 27,* 939–47.

Ayash, L.J., Elias, A., Wheeler, C. *et al.* (1994). Double dose-intensive chemotherapy with autologous marrow and peripheral-blood progenitor-cell support for metastatic breast cancer: a feasibilty study. *Journal of Clinical Oncology, 12,* 37–44.

Ayash, L.J., Hunt, M., Antman, K. *et al.* (1990). Hepatic venocclusive disease in autologous transplantation of solid tumors and lymphoma. *Journal of Clinical Oncology, 8,* 1699–708.

Ayash, L.J., Wright, J.E., Tretyakov, O. *et al.* (1992). Cyclophosphamide pharmacokinetics: correlation with cardiac toxicity and tumor response. *Journal of Clinical Oncology, 10,* 995–1000.

Azoulay, D., Castaing, D., Lemoine, A. *et al.* (2000). Transjugular intrahepatic portosystemic shunt (TIPS) for severe veno-occlusive disease of the liver following bone marrow transplantation. *Bone Marrow Transplantation, 25,* 987–92.

Bach, P.B., Schrag, D., Nierman, D.M. *et al.* (2001). Identification of poor prognostic features among patients requiring mechanical ventilation after hematopoietic stem cell transplant. *Blood, 98,* 3234–40.

Badros, A., Barlogie, B., Siegel, E. *et al.* (2001). Results of autologous stem cell transplant in multiple myeloma patients with renal failure. *British Journal of Haematology, 114,* 822–9.

Barlogie, B., Jagannath, S., Desikan, K.R. *et al.* (1999). Total therapy with tandem transplants for newly diagnosed multiple myeloma. *Blood, 93,* 55–65.

Baronciani, D., Angelucci, E., Erer, B. *et al.* (1995). Suprapubic cystotomy as treatment for severe hemorrhagic cystitis after bone marrow transplantation. *Bone Marrow Transplantation, 16,* 267–70.

Bashey, A., Corringham, S., Garrett, J. et al. (2000). A phase II study of two cycles of high-dose chemotherapy with autologous stem cell support in patients with metastatic breast cancer who meet eligibility criteria for a single cycle. Bone Marrow Transplantation, 25, 519–24.

Bearman, S.I. (1995). The syndrome of hepatic veno-occlusive disease after marrow transplantation. Blood, 85, 3005–20.

Bearman, S.I., Anderson, G.L., Mori, M. et al. (1993). Venocclusive disease of the liver: development of a model for predicting fatal outcome after marrow transplantation. Journal of Clinical Oncology, 11, 1729–36.

Bearman, S.I., Appelbaum, F.R., Back, A. et al. (1989). Regimen-related toxicity and early posttransplant survival in patients undergoing marrow transplantation for lymphoma. Journal of Clinical Oncology, 7, 1288–94.

Bearman, S.I., Appelbaum, F.R., Buckner, C.D. et al. (1988). Regimen-related toxicity and early posttransplant survival in patients undergoing marrow transplantation. Journal of Clinical Oncology, 6, 1562–8.

Bearman, S.I., Cagnoni, P.J., Nieto, Y. et al. (2000). High-dose chemotherapy and autologous transplantation followed by nonmyeloablative allogeneic transplantation: separating cytoreduction from adoptive immunotherapy. Blood, 96, (Suppl 1), 1767.

Bearman, S.I., Lee, J.L., Baron, A.E., & McDonald, G.B. (1997). Treatment of hepatic venocclusive disease with recombinant human tissue plasminogen activator and heparin in 42 marrow transplant patients. Blood, 89, 1501–6.

Bearman, S.I., Petersen, F.B., Schor, R.A. et al. (1990). Radionuclide ejection fractions in the evaluation of patients being considered for bone marrow transplantation: risk for cardiac toxicity. Bone Marrow Transplantation, 5, 173–7.

Bechstein, W.O. (2000). Neurotoxicity of calcineurin inhibitors: impact and clinical management. Transplant International, 13, 313–26.

Bedi, A., Miller, C.B., Hanson, J.L. et al. (1995). Association of BK virus with failure of prophylaxis against hemorrhagic cystitis following bone marrow transplantation. Journal of Clinical Oncology, 13, 1103–9.

Bellm, L.A., Epstein, J.B., Rose-Ped, A. et al. (2000). Patient reports of complications of bone marrow transplantation. Supportive Care in Cancer, 8, 33–9.

Benito, A.I., Furlong, T., Martin, P.J. et al. (2001). Sirolimus (rapamycin) for the treatment of steroid-refractory acute graft-versus-host disease. Transplantation, 72, 1924–9.

Bitran, J.D., Samuels, B., Klein, L. et al. (1996). Tandem high-dose chemotherapy supported by hematopoietic progenitor cells yields prolonged survival in stage IV breast cancer. Bone Marrow Transplantation, 17, 157–62.

Bleyer, W.A. (1981). Neurologic sequelae of methotrexate and ionizing radiation: a new classification. Cancer Treatment Report, 65(Suppl), 89–98.

Brown, M.S., Simon, J.H., Stemmer, S.M. et al. (1995). MR and proton spectroscopy of white matter disease induced by high-dose chemotherapy with bone marrow transplant in advanced breast cancer. American Journal of Neuroradiology, 16, 2013–20.

Brown, S.A., Goringe, A., Fegan, C. et al. (1998). Parenteral glutamine protects hepatic function during bone marrow transplantation. Bone Marrow Transplantation, 22, 281–4.

Caballero, M.D., Rubio, V., Rifon, J. et al. (1997). BEAM chemotherapy followed by autologous stem cell support in lymphoma patients: analysis of efficacy, toxicity and prognostic features. Bone Marrow Transplantation, 20, 451–58.

Carella, A.M., Cavaliere, M., Lerma, E. et al. (2000). Autografting followed by nonmyeloablative immunosuppressive chemotherapy and allogeneic peripheral-blood hematopoietic stem-cell transplantation as treatment of resistant Hodgkin's disease and non-Hodgkin's lymphoma. Journal of Clinical Oncology, 13, 3918–24.

Carlson, K., Smedmyr, B., Backlund, L., & Simonsson, B. (1994). Subclinical disturbance in cardiac function at rest and in gas exchange during exercise are common findings after autologous bone marrow transplantation. Bone Marrow Transplantation, 14, 949–54.

Carreras, E., Bertz, H., Arcese, W. et al. (1998). Incidence and outcome of hepatic veno-occlusive disease after blood or marrow transplantation: a prospective cohort study of the European Group for Blood and Marrow Transplantation. European Group for Blood and Marrow Transplantation Chronic Leukemia Working Party. Blood, 92, 3599–604.

Chan, P.K., Ip, K.W., Shiu, S.Y. et al. (1994). Association between polyomaviruria and microscopic haematuria in bone marrow transplant recipients. Journal of Infection, 29, 139–46.

Chauncey, T.R., Gooley, T.A., Lloid, M.E. et al. (2000). Pilot trial of cytoprotection with amifostine given with high-dose chemotherapy and autologous peripheral blood stem cell transplantation. American Journal of Clinical Oncology, 23, 406–11.

Childs, R., Chernoff, A., Contentin, N. et al. (2000). Regression of metastatic renal-cell carcinoma after nonmyeloablative allogeneic peripheral-blood stem-cell transplantation. New England Journal of Medicine, 343, 750–8.

Clark, J.G., Hansen, J.A., Hertz, M.I. et al. (1993). Idiopathic pneumonia syndrome after bone marrow transplantation (NHLBI Workshop Summary). American Review of Respiratory Diseases, 147, 1601–6.

Coghlin Dickson, T.M., Wong, R.M., Offrin, R.S. et al. (2000). Effect of oral glutamine supplementation during bone marrow transplantation. Journal of Parenteral and Enteral Nutrition, 24, 61–6.

Comenzo, R.L., Sanchorawala, V., Fisher, C. et al. (1999). Intermediate-dose intravenous melphalan and blood stem cells mobilized with sequential GM + G-CSF or G-CSF alone to treat AL (amyloid light chain) amyloidosis. British Journal of Haematology, 104, 553–9.

Crawford, J., Glaspy, J., Vincent, M. et al. (1994). Effect of filgrastim on oral mucositis in patients with small cell lung cancer receiving chemotherapy (cyclophosphamide, doxorubicin, and etoposide). Proceedings of the American Society of Clinical Oncology, 13, 442.

Damon, L.E., Mass, R., & Linker, C.A. (1989). The association between high-dose cytarabine neurotoxicity and renal insufficiency. Journal of Clinical Oncology, 7, 1563–8.

DeLeve, L.D. (1996). Cellular target of cyclophosphamide toxicity in murine liver: role of glutathione and site of metabolic activation. Hepatology, 24, 830–7.

DeLeve, L.D., Shulman, H.M., & McDonald, G.B. (2002). Toxic injury to hepatic sinusoids: sinusoidal obstruction syndrome (veno-occlusive disease). Seminars in Liver Disease, 22, 27–43.

DeLeve, L. & Wang, X. (1999). Decrease in hepatic nitric oxide production contributes to hepatic veno-occlusive disease (HVOD). Hepatology, 30, 218a.

DeLeve, L.D. & Wang, X. (2000). Role of oxidative stress and glutathione in busulfan toxicity in cultured murine hepatocytes. *Pharmacology*, **60**, 143–54.

Dember, L.M., Sanchorawala, V., Seldin, D.C. *et al.* (2001). Effect of dose-intensive intravenous melphalan and autologous blood stem-cell transplantation on AL amyloidosis-associated renal disease. *Annals of Internal Medicine*, **134**, 746–53.

Donato, M., Gershenson, D.M., Wharton, J.T. *et al.* (2001). High-dose topotecan, melphalan and cyclophosphamide (TMC) with stem cell support: a new regimen for the treatment of advanced ovarian cancer. *Gynecologic Oncology*, **82**, 420–6.

Doroshow, J.H., Synold, T., Somlo, G. *et al.* (1997). High-dose infusional paclitaxel (P), platinum (DDP), cyclophosphamide (CY), and cyclosporine A (CSA) with peripheral blood progenitor cell rescue for high risk primary and responsive metastatic breast cancer. *Proceedings of the American Society of Clinical Oncology*, **16**, 235.

Eagle, D.A., Gian, V., Lauwers, G.Y. *et al.* (2001). Gastroparesis following bone marrow transplantation. *Bone Marrow Transplantation*, **28**, 59–62.

Efros, M.D., Ahmed, T., Coombe, N., & Choudhury, M.S. (1994). Urologic complications of high-dose chemotherapy and bone marrow transplantation. *Urology*, **43**, 355–60.

Essell, J.H., Schroeder, M.T., Harman, G.S. *et al.* (1998). Ursodiol prophylaxis against hepatic complications of allogeneic bone marrow transplantation. *Annals of Internal Medicine*, **128**, 975–81.

Farrell, C.L., Bready, J.V., Rex, K.L. *et al.* (1998). Keratinocyte growth factor protects mice from chemotherapy and radiation-induced gastrointestinal injury and mortality. *Cancer Research*, **58**, 933–9.

Farrell, C.L., Rex, K.L., Kaufman, S.A. *et al.* (1999). Effects of keratinocyte growth factor in the squamous epithelium of the upper aerodigestive tract of normal and irradiated mice. *International Journal of Radiation Biology*, **75**, 609–20.

Fleming, D.R., Wolff, S.N., Fay, J.W. *et al.* (1998). Protracted results of dose-intensive therapy using cyclophosphamide, carmustine, and continuous infusion etoposide with autologous stem cell support in patients with relapse or refractory Hodgkin's disease: a phase II study from the North American Marrow Transplant Group. *Leukemia and Lymphoma*, **35**, 91–8.

Flowers, C.R., Sandmaier, B.M., Maloney, D.G. *et al.* (2000). Regimen related toxicities associated with nonmyeloablative conditioning and postgrafting cyclosporine and mycophenolate mofetil. *Blood*, **96** (Suppl 1), 2242.

Fried, M.W., Connaghan, D.G., Sharma, S. *et al.* (1996). Transjugular intrahepatic portosystemic shunt for the management of severe venoocclusive disease following bone marrow transplantation. *Hepatology*, **24**, 588–91.

Fox-Geiman, M.P., Fisher, S.G., Kiley, K. *et al.* (2001). Double-blind comparative trial of oral ondansetron versus oral granisetron versus IV ondansetron in the prevention of nausea and vomiting associated with highly emetogenic preparative regimens prior to stem cell transplantation. *Biology of Blood and Marrow Transplantation*, **7**, 596–603.

Furlong, T., Storb, R., Anasetti, C. *et al.* (2000). Clinical outcome after conversion to FK506 (tacrolimus) therapy for acute graft-versus-host disease resistant to cyclosporine or for cyclosporine-associated toxicities. *Bone Marrow Transplantation*, **26**, 985–91.

Gabrilove, J.L., Jakubowski, A., Scher, H. *et al.* (1988). Effect of granulocyte colony stimulating factor on neutropenia and associated morbidity due to chemotherapy for transitional cell carcinoma of the urothelium. *New England Journal of Medicine*, **318**, 1414–22.

Gertz, M.A., Lacy, M.Q., Gastineau, D.A. *et al.* (2000). Blood stem cell transplantation as therapy for primary systemic amyloidosis (AL). *Bone Marrow Transplantation*, **26**, 963–9.

Giles, F.J., Kantarjian, H.M., Kornblau, S.M. *et al.* (2001). Mylotarg™ (gemtuzumab ozogamicin) therapy is associated with hepatic venooclusive disease in patients who have not received stem cell transplantation. *Cancer*, **92**, 406–13.

Gluck, S., Arnold, A., Dulude, H., & Gallant, G. (1996). High-dose cyclophosphamide, mitoxantrone and paclitaxel with blood progenitor cell support for the treatment of metastatic breast cancer. *Proceedings of the American Society of Clinical Oncology*, **15**, 137. (Abstract).

Goringe, A.P., Brown, S., O'Callaghan, U. *et al.* (1998). Glutamine and vitamin E in the treatment of hepatic veno-occlusive disease following high-dose chemotherapy. *Bone Marrow Transplantation*, **21**, 829–32.

Gottdeiner, J.S., Appelbaum, F.R., Ferrans, V.J. *et al.* (1981). Cardiotoxicity associated with high-dose cyclophosphamide therapy. *Archives of Internal Medicine*, **141**, 758–63.

Grigg, A.P., Shepherd, J.D., & Phillips, G.L. (1989). Busulphan and phenytoin. *Annals of Internal Medicine*, **111**, 1149–50.

Grinsky, T., Benhamou, E., Bourhis, J-H. *et al.* (2000). Prospective randomized comparison of single-dose versus hyperfractionated total-body irradiation in patients with hematologic malignancies. *Journal of Clinical Oncology*, **18**, 981–6.

Grovas, A.C., Boyett, J.M., Lindsley, K. *et al.* (1999). Regimen-related toxicity of myeloablative chemotherapy with BCNU, thiotepa, and etoposide followed by autologous stem cell rescue for children with newly diagnosed glioblastoma multiforme: report from the Children's Cancer Group. *Medical and Pediatric Oncology*, **33**, 83–7.

Hagglund, H., Ringden, O., Ericzon, B.G. *et al.* (1996). Treatment of hepatic venocclusive disease with recombinant human tissue plasminogen activator or orthotopic liver transplantation after allogeneic bone marrow transplantation. *Transplantation*, **62**, 1076–80.

Haioun, C., Mounier, N., Quesnel, B. *et al.* (2001). Tandem autotransplant as first-line consolidation treatment in poor-risk aggressive lymphoma: a pilot study of 36 patients. *Annals of Oncology*, **12**, 1749–55.

Hartmann, J.T., von Vangerow, A., Fels, L.M. *et al.* (2001). A randomized trial of amifostine in patients with high-dose VIC chemotherapy plus autologous blood stem cell transplantation. *British Journal of Cancer*, **84**, 313–20.

Hertenstein, B., Stefanic, M., Schmeiser, T. *et al.* (1994). Cardiac toxicity of bone marrow transplantation: predictive value of cardiologic evaluation before transplant. *Journal of Clinical Oncology*, **12**, 998–1004.

Horowitz, M.M., Oster, G., Fuchs, H. *et al.* (1999). Oral Mucositis Assessment Scale as a predictor of clinical and economic outcomes in bone marrow transplant patients. *Blood*, **94**,(Suppl 1), 399a.

Hows, J.W., Mehta, A., Ward, L. *et al.* (1984). Comparison of mesna with forced diuresis to prevent cyclophosphamide induced haemorrhagic cystitis in marrow transplantation: a prospective randomized study. *British Journal of Cancer*, **50**, 753–6.

Huang, E.Y., Leung, S.W., Wang, C.J. *et al.* (2000). Oral glutamine to alleviate radiation-induced oral mucositis: a pilot randomized trial. *International Journal of Radiation Oncology, Biology, and Physics*, **46**, 535–9.

Jones, R.B., Matthes, S., Shpall, E.J. *et al.* (1993). Acute lung injury following treatment with high-dose cyclophosphamide, cisplatin, and carmustine: pharmacodynamic evaluation of carmustine. *Journal of the National Cancer Institute*, **85**, 640–7.

Kajiume, T., Yoshimi, S., Nagita, A. *et al.* (2000). Application of nitric oxide for a case of veno-occlusive disease after peripheral blood stem cell transpslantation. *Pediatric Hematology and Oncology*, **17**, 501–4.

Kantrow, S.P., Hackman, R.C., Boeckh, M. *et al.* (1997). Idiopathic pneumonia syndrome. Changing spectrum of lung injury after marrow transplantation. *Transplantation*, **63**, 1079–86.

Khalil, N., O'Connor, R.N., Unruh, H.W. *et al.* (1991). Increased production and immunohistochemical localization of transforming growth factor-beta in idiopathic pulmonary fibrosis. *American Journal of Respiratory Cell and Molecular Biology*, **5**, 155–62.

Khassawneh, B.Y., White, P., Anaissie, E.J. *et al.* (2002). Outcome from mechanical ventilation after autologous peripheral blood stem cell transplantation. *Chest*, **121**, 185–8.

Khouri, I.F., Saliba, R.M., Giralt, S.A. *et al.* (2001). Nonablative allogeneic hematopoietic transplantation as adoptive immunotherapy for indolent lymphoma: low incidence of toxicity, acute graft-versus-host disease, and treatment-related mortality. *Blood*, **98**, 3595–9.

Koeoglu, V., Chiang, J., & Chan, K.W. (1999). Acquired pseudo-cholinesterase deficiency after high-dose cyclophosphamide. *Bone Marrow Transplantation*, **24**, 1367–8.

Kroger, N., Hoffknecht, M., Hanel, M. *et al.* (1998). Busulfan, cyclophosphamide and etoposide as high-dose conditioning therapy in patients with malignant lymphoma and prior dose-limiting radiation therapy. *Bone Marrow Transplantation*, **21**, 1171–5.

Kulkarni, S., Rodriguez, M., Lafuente, A. *et al.* (1999). Recombinant tissue plasminogen activator (rtPA) for the treatment of hepatic veno-occlusive disease (VOD). *Bone Marrow Transplantation*, **23**, 703–7.

Kupari, M., Volin, L., Suokas, A. *et al.* (1990). Cardiac involvement in bone marrow transplantation: electrocardiographic changes, arrhythmias, heart failure and autopsy findings. *Bone Marrow Transplantation*, **5**, 91–8.

Lacerda, J.F., Martins, C., Carmo, J.A. *et al.* (2000). Randomized trial of ondansetron, granisetron, and tropisetron in the prevention of acute nausea and vomiting. *Transplantation Proceedings*, **32**, 2680–1.

Lapides, J. (1970). Treatment of delayed intractable hemorrhagic cystitis following radiation or chemotherapy. *Journal of Urology*, **104**, 707–8.

Larsen, R.L., Barber, G., Heise, C.T., & August, C.S. (1992). Exercise assessment of cardiac function in children and young adults before and after bone marrow transplantation. *Pediatrics*, **89**, 722–9.

Lawton, C.A., Barber-Derus, S.W., Murray, J.K. *et al.* (1992). Influence of renal shielding on the incidence of late renal dysfunction associated with T-lymphocyte depleted bone marrow transplantation in adult patients. *International Journal of Radiation Oncology, Biology Physics*, **23**, 681–6.

Leung, A.Y.H., Suen, C.K.M., Lie, A.K.W. *et al.* (2001). Quantification of polyoma BK viruria in hemorrhagic cystitis complicating bone marrow transplantation. *Blood*, **98**, 1972–8.

Maloney, D.G., Sahebi, F., Stockerl-Goldstein, K.E. *et al.* (2001). Combining an allogeneic graft-vs-myeloma effect with autologous stem cell rescue in the treatment of multiple myeloma. *Blood*, **98** (Suppl 1), 1822.

Mayordomo, J.I., Yubero, A., Cajal, R. *et al.* (1997). Phase I trial of high-dose paclitaxel in combination with cyclophosphamide, thiotepa and carboplatin with autologous peripheral blood stem cell rescue. *Proceedings of the American Society of Clinical Oncology*, **16**, 102.

McDonald, G.B., Hinds, M.S., Fisher, L.B. *et al.* (1993). Venocclusive disease of the liver and multiorgan failure after bone marrow transplantation: a cohort study of 355 patients. *Annals of Internal Medicine*, **118**, 255–67.

McGaughey, D.S., Nikcevich, D.A., Long, G.D. *et al.* (2001). Inhaled steroids as prophylaxis for delayed pulmonary toxicity syndrome in breast cancer patients undergoing high-dose chemotherapy and autologous stem cell transplantation. *Biology of Blood and Marrow Transplantation*, **7**, 274–8.

McSweeney, P.A., Niederwieser, D., Shizuru, J.A. *et al.* (2001). Hematopoietic cell transplantation in older patients with hematologic malignancies: replacing high-dose cytotoxic therapy with graft-versus-tumor effects. *Blood*, **97**, 3390–400.

Meacher, R., Venkatesh, B., & Lipman, J. (1999). Acute respiratory distress syndrome precipitated by transjugular intrahepatic porto-systemic shunting for severe hepatic veno-occlusive disease. Is it due to pulmonary leucostasis? *Intensive Care Medicine*, **25**, 1332–3.

Meresse, V., Hartmann, O., Vassal, G. *et al.* (1992). Risk factors of hepatic venocclusive disease after high-dose busulfan-containing regimens followed by autologous bone marrow transplantation: a study in 136 children. *Bone Marrow Transplantation*, **10**, 135–41.

Morandi, P., Ruffini, P.A., Benvenuto, G.M. *et al.* (2001). Serum cardiac troponin I levels and ECG/echo monitoring in breast cancer patients undergoing high-dose (7 g/m^2) cyclophosphamide. *Bone Marrow Transplantation*, **28**, 277–82.

Moreau, P., Leblond, V., Bourquelot, P. *et al.* (1998). Prognostic factors for survival and response after high-dose therapy and autologous stem cell transplantation in systemic AL amyloidosis: a report on 21 patients. *British Journal of Haematology*, **101**, 766–9.

Murdych, T. & Weisdorf, D.J. (2001). Serious cardiac complications during bone marrow transplantation at the University of Minnesota, 1977–1997. *Bone Marrow Transplantation*, **28**, 283–7.

Murray, J.A., LaBrecque, D.R., Gingrich, R.D. *et al.* (1987). Successful treatment of hepatic venocclusive disease in a bone marrow transplant patient with a side-to-side portacaval shunt. *Gastroenterology*, **92**, 1073–7.

Nagler, A., Slavin, S., Varadi, G. *et al.* (2000). Allogeneic peripheral blood stem cell transplantation using a fludarabine-based low intensity conditioning regimen for malignant lymphoma. *Bone Marrow Transplantation*, **25**, 1021–8.

Nemunitis, J., Rosenfeld, C.S., Ash, R. *et al.* (1995). Phase III randomized, double-blind placebo-controlled trial of rhGM-CSF following allogeneic bone marrow transplantation. *Bone Marrow Transplantation*, **15**, 949–54.

Nevill, T.J., Barnett, M.J., Klingemann, H.G. *et al.* (1991). Regimen-related toxicity of a busulfan-cyclophosphamide conditioning regimen in 70 patients undergoing allogeneic bone marrow transplantation. *Journal of Clinical Oncology*, **9**, 1224–32.

Nieto, Y., Cagnoni, P.J., Bearman, S.I. *et al.* (1999). Acute encephalopathy: a new toxicity associated with high-dose paclitaxel. *Clinical Cancer Research*, **5**, 481–6.

Nieto, Y., Cagnoni, P.J., Shpall, E.J. *et al.* (2000). Phase I trial of docetaxel (DTX) (Taxotere) with peripheral blood progenitor cell (PBPC) support, with melphalan (MEL) and carboplatin (CB), in refractory advanced cancer. *Proceedings of the American Society of Clinical Oncology*, **19**, 217.

Nimer, S.D., Milewicz, A.L., Champlin, R.E. *et al.* (1990). Successful treatment of hepatic venocclusive disease in a bone marrow transplant patient with orthotopic liver transplantation. *Transplantation*, **49**, 819–21.

O'Connell, T.X. & Berenbaum, M.C. *et al.* (1974). Cardiac and pulmonary effects of high-dose cyclophosphamide and isophosphamide. *Cancer Research*, **34**, 1586–91.

Ohashi, K., Tanabe, J., Watanabe, R. *et al.* (2000). The Japanese multicenter open randomized trial of ursodeoxycholic acid prophylaxis for hepatic veno-occlusive disease after stem cell transplantation. *American Journal of Hematology*, **64**, 32–8.

Papadopoulos, K.P., Egorin, M.J., Huang, M. *et al.* (2001). The pharmacokinetics and pharmacodynamics of high-dose paclitaxel monotherapy (825 mg/m^2 continuous infusion over 24 h) with hematopoietic support in women with metastatic breast cancer. *Cancer Chemotherapy and Pharmacology*, **47**, 45–50.

Park, S.H., Lee, M.H., Lee, H. *et al.* (2002). A randomized trial of heparin plus ursodiol vs heparin alone to prevent hepatic veno-occlusive disease after hematopoietic stem cell transplantation. *Bone Marrow Transplantation*, **29**, 137–43.

Panoskaltis-Mortari, A., Taylor, P.A., Yaeger, T.M. *et al.* (1997). The critical early postinflammatory events associated with idiopathic pneumonia syndrome in irradiated murine allogeneic recipients are due to donor T cell infusion and potentiated by cyclophosphamide. *Journal of Clinical Investigation*, **100**, 1015–27.

Phillips, G.L., Meisenberg, B., Hale, G.A. (2001). Amifostine cytoprotection of escalating doses of melphalan and autologous hematopoietic stem cell transplantation: final results of a phase I and II study. *Proceedings of the American Society of Clinical Oncology*, **20**, 24.

Phipps, S., Dunavant, M., Srivastava, D.K. *et al.* (2000). Cognitive and academic functioning in survivors of pediatric bone marrow transplantation. *Journal Clinical of Oncology*, **18**, 1004–11.

Pico, J.L., Avila-Garavito, A., & Naccahie, P. (1998). Mucositis: its occurence, consequences, and treatment in the oncology setting. *Oncologist*, **3**, 446–51.

Quezado, Z.M.N., Wilson, W.H., Cunnion, R.E. *et al.* (1993). High-dose ifosfamide is associated with severe, reversible cardiac dysfunction. *Annals of Internal Medicine*, **118**, 31–6.

Radich, J.P., Sanders, J.E., Buckner, C.D. *et al.* (1993). Second allogeneic marrow transplantation for patients with recurrent leukemia after initial transplantation with total-body irradiation-containing regimens. *Journal of Clinical Oncology*, **11**, 304–13.

Rajvanshi, P., Shulman, H.M., Sievers, E.L., & McDonald, G.B. (2002). Hepatic sinusoidal obstruction after gemtuzumab ozogamicin (Mylotarg) therapy. *Blood*, **99**, 2310–4.

Rapaport, A.P., Doyle, H.R., Starzl, T. *et al.* (1991). Orthotopic liver transplantation for life-threatening veno-occlusive disease of the liver after allogeneic bone marrow transplant. *Bone Marrow Transplantation*, **8**, 421–4.

Rapoport, A.P., Miller, Watelet, L.F., Linder, T. *et al.* (1999). Analysis of factors that correlate with mucositis in recipients of autologous and allogeneic stem cell transplants. *Journal of Clinical Oncology*, **17**, 2446–53.

Richard, S., Seigneur, M., Blann, A. *et al.* (1996). Vascular endothelial lesion in patients undergoing bone marrow transplantation. *Bone Marrow Transplantation*, **18**, 955–9.

Richardson, P.G., Murakami, C., Wei, L.J. *et al.* (2002). Multi-institutional use of defibrotide (DF) in 88 patients post stem cell transplant (SCT) with severe veno-occlusive disease (VOD) and multi-system organ failure (MOF); response without significant toxicity in a high risk population and factors predictive of outcome. *Blood*, **100**, 4337–43.

Ringden, O., Remberger, M., Lehmann, S. *et al.* (2000). N-acetylcysteine for hepatic veno-occlusive disease after allogeneic stem cell transplantation. *Bone Marrow Transplantation*, **25**, 993–6.

Ringden, O., Ruutu, T., Remberger, M. *et al.* (1994). A randomized trial comparing busulfan versus total body irradiation in allogeneic marrow transplant recipients with leukemia: a report from the Nordic Bone Marrow Transplantation Group. *Blood*, **83**, 2723–30.

Ringden, O., Ruutu, T., Remberger, M. *et al.* (1994). A randomized trial comparing busulfan versus total body irradiation in allogeneic marrow transplant recipients with hematological malignancies. *Transplantation Proceedings*, **26**, 1831–2.

Rio, B., Bauduer, F., Arrago, J.P., & Zittoun R. (1993). N-terminal peptide of type III procollagen: a marker for the development of hepatic veno-occlusive disease after BMT and a basis for determining the timing of prophylactic heparin. *Bone Marrow Transplantation*, **11**, 471–2.

Rubin, E.H., Anderson, J.W., Berg, D.T. *et al.* (1992). Risk factors for high-dose cytarabine neurotoxicity: an analysis of a Cancer and Leukemia Group B trial in patients with acute myeloid leukemia. *Journal of Clinical Oncology*, **10**, 948–53.

Salat, C., Holler, E., Kolb, H.-J. *et al.* (1997). Plasminogen activator inhibitor-1 confirms the diagnosis of hepatic veno-occlusive disease in patients with hyperbilirubinemia after bone marrow transplantation. *Blood*, **89**, 2184–8.

Salat, C., Holler, E., Reinhardt, B. *et al.* (1994). Parameters of the fibrinolytic system in patients undergoing BMT: elevation of PAI-1 in veno-occlusive disease. *Bone Marrow Transplantation*, **14**, 747–50.

San Miguel, J.F., Lahuerta, J.J., Garcia-Sanz, R. *et al.* (2000). Are myeloma patients with renal failure candidates for autologous stem cell transplantation? *Hematology Journal*, **1**, 28–36.

Sanchorawala, V., Wright, D.G., Seldin, D.C. *et al.* (2001). An overview of the use of high-dose melphalan with autologous stem cell transplantation for the treatment of AL amyloidosis. *Bone Marrow Transplantation*, **28**, 637–42.

Schriber, J., Milk, B., Shaw, D. *et al.* (1999). Tissue plasminogen activator (tPA) as therapy for hepatotoxicity following bone marrow transplantation. *Bone Marrow Transplantation*, **24**, 1311–14.

Schuh, A., Dandridge, J., Haydon, P., & Littlewood, T.J. (1999). Encephalopathy complicating high-dose melphalan. *Bone Marrow Transplantation*, **24**, 1141–3.

Schwerkoske, J., Schwartzberg, L., Weaver, C. *et al.* (1999). A phase I, double-masked, placebo-controlled study to evaluate tolerability of Neumega (rh IL-11; opreleukin) to reduce mucositis in patient with solid tumor or lymphoma receiving high dose chemotherapy with autologous peripheral blood stem cell reinfusion. *Proceedings of the American Society of Clinical Oncology*, **18**, 584a.

Sezer, O., Schmid, P., Shweigert, M. *et al.* (1999). Rapid reversal of nephrotic syndrome due to primary systemic AL amyloidosis after VAD and subsequent high-dose chemotherapy with autologous stem cell support. *Bone Marrow Transplantation*, **23**, 967–9.

Shrom, S.H., Donaldson, M.H., Duckett, J.W. *et al.* (1976). Formalin treatment for intractable hemorrhagic cystitis. A review of the literature with 16 additional cases. *Cancer*, **38**, 1785–9.

Shulman, H.M., Fisher, L.B., Schoch, H.G. *et al.* (1994). Venocclusive disease of the liver after marrow transplantation: histologic correlates of clinical signs and symptoms. *Hepatology*, **19**, 1171–80.

Sievers, E.L., Larson, R.A., Stadtmauer, E. *et al.* (2001). Efficacy and safety of gemtuzumab ozogamicin in patients with CD33-positive acute myeloid leukemia in first relapse. *Journal of Clinical Oncology,* **19,** 3244–54.

Singh, N., Gayowski, T., & Marino, J.R. (1996). Hemolytic uremic syndrome in solid-organ transplant recipients. *Transplantation International,* **9,** 68–75.

Slattery, J.T., Kalhorn, T.F., McDonald, G.B. *et al.* (1996). Conditioning regimen-dependent disposition of cyclophosphamide and hydroxycyclophosphamide in human marrow transplantation patients. *Journal of Clinical Oncology,* **14,** 1484–94.

Smith, F.O., Johnson, M.S., Scherer, L.R. *et al.* (1996). Transjugular intrahepatic portosystemic shunting (TIPS) for treatment of severe hepatic veno-occlusive disease. *Bone Marrow Transplantation,* **18,** 643–6.

Smith, G.A., Damon, L.E., Rugo, H.S. *et al.* (1997). High-dose cytarabine dose modification reduces the incidence of neurotoxicity in patients with renal insufficiency. *Journal of Clinical Oncology,* **15,** 833–9.

Somlo, G., Chow, W., Hamasaki, V. *et al.* (2001). Tandem-cycle high-dose melphalan and cisplatin with peripheral blood progenitor cell support in patients with breast cancer and other malignancies. *Biology of Blood and Marrow Transplantation,* **7,** 284–93.

Spielberger, R.T., Stiff, P., Emmanouilides, C. *et al.* (2001). Efficacy of recombinant human keratinocyte growth factor in reducing mucositis in patients with hematologic malignancies undergoing autologous peripheral blood progenitor cell transplantation after radiation-based conditioning—results of a phase 2 trial. *Proceedings of the American Society of Clinical Oncology,* **20,** 25.

Steinherz, L.J., Steinherz, P.G., Mangiacasale, D. *et al.* (1981). Cardiac changes with cyclophosphamide. *Medical and Pediatric Oncology,* **9,** 417–22.

Stemmer, S.M., Cagnoni, P.J., Shpall, E.J. *et al.* (1996). High-dose paclitaxel, cyclophosphamide, and cisplatin with autologous hematopoietic progenitor-cell support: a phase I trial. *Journal of Clinical Oncology,* **14,** 1463–72.

Stiff, P. (2001). Mucositis associated with stem cell transplantation: current status and innovative approaches to management. *Bone Marrow Transplantation,* **27** (Suppl 2), S3–S11.

Storb, R., Buckner, C.D., Dillingham, L.A., & Thomas, E.D. (1970). Cyclophosphamide regimens in rhesus monkeys with and without marrow infusion. *Cancer Research,* **30,** 2195–203.

Strasser, S.I., McDonald, G.B., Schoch, H.G. *et al.* (2000). Severe hepatocellular injury after hematopoietic cell transplant: incidence and etiology in 2136 consecutive patients. *Hepatology,* **32,** 299.

Tanikawa, S., Mori, S., Ohhashi, K. *et al.* (2000). Predictive markers for hepatic veno-occlusive disease after hematopoietic stem cell transplantation in adults: a prospective single center study. *Bone Marrow Transplantation,* **26,** 881–6.

Testa, S., Manna, A. Porcellini, A. *et al.* (1996). Increased plasma level of vascular endothelial glycoprotein thrombomodulin as an early indicator of endothelial damage in bone marrow transplantation. *Bone Marrow Transplantation,* **18,** 383–8.

Thomas, A.E., Patterson, J., Prentice, H.G. *et al.* (1987). Haemorrhagic cystitis in bone marrow transplantation patients: possible increased risk associated with prior busulphan therapy. *Bone Marrow Transplantation,* **1,** 347–55.

Thompson, C.B., Sander, J.E., Flournoy, N. *et al.* (1986). The risks of central nervous system relapse and leukoencephalopathy in patients receiving bone marrow transplants for acute leukemia. *Blood,* **67,** 195–9.

Trigg, M.E., O'Reilly, J., Rumelhart, S. *et al.* (1990). Prostaglandin E$_1$ bladder instillations to control severe hemorrhagic cystitis. *Journal of Urology,* **143,** 92–4.

Vahdat, L., Papadopoulos, K., Balmaceda, C. *et al.* (1998). Phase I trial of sequential high-dose chemotherapy with escalating dose paclitaxel, melphalan, and cyclophosphamide, thiotepa, and carboplatin with peripheral blood progenitor support in women with responding metastatic breast cancer. *Clinical Cancer Research,* **4,** 1689–95.

Vahdat, L., Papadopoulos, K., Lange, D. *et al.* (2001). Reduction of paclitaxel-induced peripheral neuropathy with glutamine. *Clinical Cancer Research,* **7,** 1192–7.

Vahdat, L., Raptis, G., Fennelly, D. *et al.* (1995). Rapidly cycled courses of high-dose alkylating agents supported by filgrastim and peripheral blood progenitor cells in patients with metastatic breast cancer. *Clinical Cancer Research,* **1,** 1267–73.

Van Dam, F.S., Schagen, S.B., Muller, M.J. *et al.* (1998). Impairment of cognitive function in women receiving adjuvant treatment for high-risk breast cancer: high-dose versus standard-dose chemotherapy. *Journal of the National Cancer Institute,* **90,** 210–18.

Vassal, G., Deroussent, A., Hartmann, O. *et al.* (1990). Dose-dependent neurotoxicity of high-dose busulfan in children: a clinical and pharmacological study. *Cancer Research,* **50,** 6203–7.

Vesole, D.H. & Fuchs, H.J. (1999). IB-367 reduces the number of days of severe oral mucositis complicating myeloablative chemotherapy. *Blood,* **94** (Suppl 1), 154a.

Vose, J.M., Reed, E.C., Pippert, G.C. *et al.* (1993). Mesna compared with continuous bladder irrigation as uroprotection during high-dose chemotherapy and transplantation: a randomized trial. *Journal of Clinical Oncology,* **11,** 1306–10.

Wilczynski, S.W., Erasmus, J.J., Petros, W.P. *et al.* (1998). Delayed pulmonary toxicity syndrome following high-dose chemotherapy and bone marrow transplantation for breast cancer. *American Journal of Respiratory Critical Care Medicine,* **157,** 565–73..

Wingard, J.R., Mellits, E.D., Sostrin, M.B. *et al.* (1988). Interstitial pneumonitis after bone marrow transplantation. Nine-year experience at a single institution. *Medicine,* **67,** 175–86.

Woo, M., Przepiorka, D., Ippoliti, C. *et al.* (1997). Toxicities of tacrolimus and cyclosporin A after allogeneic blood stem cell transplantation. *Bone Marrow Transplantation,* **20,** 1095–8.

Woo, S.B., Sonis, S.T., Monopoli, M.M. *et al.* (1993). A longitudinal study of oral ulcerative mucositis in bone marrow transplant recipients. *Cancer,* **72,** 1612–17.

Zager, R.A. (1994). Acute renal failure in the setting of bone marrow transplantation. *Kidney International,* **46,** 1443–58.

Zager, R.A., O'Quigley, J., Zager, B.K. *et al.* (1989). Acute renal failure following bone marrow transplantation: a retrospective study of 272 patients. *American Journal of Kidney Disease,* **13,** 210–16.

Zenz, T., Rossle, M., Bertz, H. *et al.* (2001). Severe veno-occlusive disease after allogeneic bone marrow or peripheral stem cell transplantation—role of transjugular intrahepatic portosystemic shunt (TIPS). *Liver,* **21,** 31–6.

83 Drug administration, toxicity, and interactions posttransplant

AMY R. McWILLIAMS, ANNE POON, AND ANIA U. SWEET

University of Washington Medical Center, Seattle Cancer Care Alliance, Seattle, USA

Introduction

This chapter offers a practical guide to drug toxicity, drug administration, and drug-drug interactions encountered after hematopoietic stem cell transplantation (HSCT). The fact that many medications are used concurrently during the posttransplant period requires the health care provider to be aware of possible additive and synergistic drug toxicities, drug-drug interactions, and necessary drug monitoring. In this chapter, an emphasis has been placed on agents used for prevention and treatment of graft-versus-host disease (GVHD) and infectious complications.

Immunosuppressive agents

Methotrexate (MTX)

Methotrexate, a tetrahydrofolate reductase inhibitor, is used in combination with other immunosuppressive agents in order to prevent GVHD in patients undergoing allogeneic HSCT. In several clinical trials, a combination of MTX with cyclosporine (CSP) was superior to either agent alone in reducing early transplant mortality due to acute GVHD and interstitial pneumonia (Storb *et al.*, 1989a, b; Mrsic *et al.*, 1990; Aschan *et al.*, 1991). However, during these trials no significant difference in frequency of chronic GVHD was observed. In the late 1990s several investigators evaluated the efficacy of methotrexate in combination with tacrolimus for GVHD prophylaxis and concluded that this regimen was also effective (Uberti *et al.*, 1997; Ratanatharathorn *et al.*, 1998; Przepiorka *et al.*, 1999a,b).

A short-course MTX regimen consists of four intravenous MTX doses administered on days +1, +3, +6, and +11 posttransplant. The first MTX dose is given 24 hours after the end of the peripheral blood stem cell or bone marrow infusion. When MTX is used in combination with CSP, the following MTX dosing regimen is often used: 15 mg/m^2 on day +1, and 10 mg/m^2 on days +3, +6 and +11. Nash *et al.* (1992) retrospectively evaluated 446 patients who received MTX/CSP in combination for GVHD prophylaxis and identified a reduction of cumulative MTX dose to less than 80% as one of the risk factors for development of acute GVHD. In contrast, the risk of acute GVHD was not increased in patients who received less than 80% of the intended MTX dose when given in combination with tacrolimus (Uberti *et al.*, 1997). This observation was further explored in clinical trials and currently a "mini-methotrexate" regimen (5 mg/m^2 on days +1, +3, +6, and +11) is used in combination with tacrolimus (FK506) in many transplant centers in the United States (Przepiorka *et al.*, 1999a).

Lower MTX doses are associated with less intense damage to the most sensitive tissues such as the bone marrow, oral mucosa, and gastrointestinal tract. In the initial trials, the Seattle group reported longer time to neutrophil recovery in the MTX/CSP group than in the CSP alone group (24 and 19 days, respectively). However, the recovery of platelets and red blood cells was not significantly different between these groups. Transient elevation of liver function tests (LFTs) was also observed (Storb *et al.*, 1989b).

Routine monitoring of MTX levels is not required unless the patient is at high risk for MTX toxicity (i.e., patients with extravascular fluid collections in the lungs and abdomen and/or patients with severe renal impairment). Leucovorin, a folinic acid rescue, is administered to patients with high MTX levels, according to previously published guidelines, to prevent excessive toxicities (Bleyer, 1985) (Fig. 83.1). Occasionally, doses are withheld in patients with severe mucositis requiring intubation, severe liver damage, or severe renal failure.

Calcineurin inhibitors

Calcineurin inhibitors have become the backbone of immunosuppressive regimens used to prevent GVHD. In fact, the combination of a calcineurin inhibitor with short course methotrexate has become the standard regimen for prevention of GVHD following myeloablative allogeneic transplantation in transplant centers around the world (Hiraoka *et al.*, 2001). These agents, which include cyclosporine and tacrolimus, enter T lymphocytes and inhibit calcineurin phosphatase activity with resultant inhibition of T-cell activation (see Chapter 118). They selectively inhibit transcription of interleukin-2 and several other cytokines, mainly in T-helper lymphocytes. They are par-

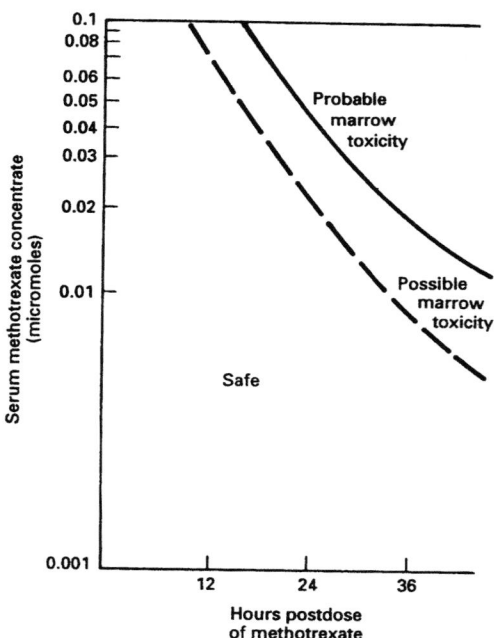

Fig. 83.1. Relationship between serum methotrexate concentration (μmoles) and bone marrow toxicity early posttransplantation. (Reproduced by kind permission of Dr. Archie Bleyer.)

ticularly suited for use in HSCT because they lack clinically significant myelosuppressive effects (Ishida, Matsuda, & Kida, 1995). However, the toxicity profile of calcineurin inhibitors is quite extensive.

One of the most common and troublesome side effects of calcineurin inhibitors is nephrotoxicity. The risk of nephrotoxicity increases with increasing dose and duration of therapy. Cyclosporine causes vasoconstriction of the afferent and efferent glomerular arterioles with resultant reductions of renal blood flow and glomerular filtration rate (Lanese & Conger, 1993). Calcium channel blockers may help protect from cyclosporine-induced nephrotoxicity by reducing renal vasoconstriction (Palmer et al., 1991). Since CSP and tacrolimus are not cleared renally, but rather via metabolism predominantly by the cytochrome P450 enzymes, dosage adjustments for renal dysfunction are not necessary. Dosage reductions should be considered if the renal dysfunction is determined to be caused by CSP or tacrolimus in an effort to reduce this toxicity.

As with nephrotoxicity, the risk of hypertension increases with increasing dose and duration of therapy. Calcineurin inhibitor-induced hypertension is characterized by renal vasoconstriction, sodium retention, increased sympathetic activity, and renin suppression and usually develops within the first few weeks after initiating therapy. Though the exact cause of the vasoconstriction remains to be determined, it is thought to be due to decreased production of natural vasodilators, such as prostaglandins and nitric oxide, and increased secretion of vasoconstrictors, such as endothelin and thromboxane (Lanese & Conger, 1993; Ruggenenti et al., 1993). This hypertension

may respond to dose reduction, but often requires addition of an antihypertensive to the medication regimen. Calcium channel blockers (CCBs), especially dihydropyridines such as amlodipine or nifedipine, are generally considered to be the treatment of choice for CSP-induced hypertension due to their ability to reverse the vasoconstriction (Cifkova & Hallen, 2001). If diltiazem or verapamil is chosen for treatment, close monitoring of the CSP level is required, since the inhibition of CSP metabolism by these agents may cause the level to rise. Since CSP-induced hypertension is initially accompanied by suppression of renin activity, ACE inhibitors may have limited efficacy and may aggravate hyperkalemia and nephrotoxicity (Midtvedt et al., 2001b). Diuretics are generally avoided for treatment of hypertension and are reserved for management of fluid status since they can worsen azotemia. Beta-blockers, combined alpha- and beta-blockers (i.e., labetalol) and clonidine (a centrally acting alpha-2 agonist) may be effective when used alone or in combination with dihydropyridines. For patients unable to take medications by mouth, intravenous labetalol, intravenous hydralazine, and clonidine patches provide alternatives. The onset of the antihypertensive effect of clonidine patches is 2 to 3 days, thus it should not be used for patients requiring rapid reduction of blood pressure. See Table 83.1 for doses, adverse effects, and drug interactions of selected antihypertensive agents found to be useful in treating calcineurin inhibitor-induced hypertension.

Neurotoxicity associated with calcineurin inhibitors may manifest as severe headaches, visual abnormalities, confusion, encephalopathy or seizures. The most frequent neurological effect is tremor, occurring in 20% to 40% of patients taking CSP. This tremor is usually mild and generalized and develops shortly after initiation of CSP therapy (O'Sullivan, 1985; Kahan, 1989; Patchell, 1994). Cyclosporine has been associated with burning palmar and plantar paresthesias. The severity of this side effect may be minimized by slowing the CSP infusion rate. Cyclosporine can cause a posterior leukoencephalopathy, which is a reversible syndrome of headache, altered mental status, seizures, and occasionally cortical blindness (see Chapter 93). Magnetic resonance imaging (MRI) of the brain shows multifocal, bilateral white matter abnormalities. Patients are usually hypertensive and over half of them have high CSP levels, low magnesium levels, and/or low cholesterol levels. Resolution of these neurological abnormalities occurs within weeks of treatment of hypertension and CSP dosage reduction or drug withdrawal (Gijtenbeek, van den Bent, & Vecht, 1999). A change from CSP to tacrolimus (or vice versa) in patients who develop neurotoxicity should be considered since there is evidence that such a change can result in resolution or improvement of the neurotoxicity (Furlong et al., 2000).

Anaphylaxis secondary to calcineurin inhibitors is rare and is believed to be a reaction to the polyoxyethylated castor oil (Cremaphor EL®) vehicle used to dissolve the i.v. formulations of both CSP and tacrolimus. Since i.v. formulations of both agents contain the polyoxyethylated castor oil vehicle, a switch

Table 83.1. *Selected antihypertensive agents useful in HSCT patients*

Medication	Antihyper-tensive dose	Adverse effects	Drug interactions	Comments
Calcium-channel blocking agents				
Amlodipine (Norvasc®)	Initial: 2.5–5 mg p.o. QD Maximum: 10 mg/day	Headache, dizziness, periph-eral edema, reflex tachycar-dia, flushing, fatigue, nau-sea, muscle cramps, mood changes, nasal congestion	β-blockers, cimetidine, digoxin, fentanyl, other hypotensive agents, phenytoin, quinidine, grapefruit juice	Dihydropyridines are the preferred agents for CSP-induced hyperten-sion. They are useful in patients with angina. Avoid in active CAD. Dose-related peripheral edema caused by dihydropyridines responds to diuretics.
Felodipine (Plendil®)	Initial: 2.5–5 mg p.o. QD Maximum: 20 mg/day			
Isradipine (DynaCirc®)	Initial: 1.25–2.5 mg p.o. BID Maximum: 20 mg/day			
Nifedipine XR® (Procardia XL®, Adalat CC®)	Initial: 30–60 mg p.o. QD Maximum: 120 mg/day			
Diltiazem HCl (Cardizem®, Cardizem CD®, Cardizem SR®, Tiazac®)	Initial: 120–240 mg p.o. daily Maximum: 540 mg/day	Bradycardia, ECG changes, first-degree AV block, flushing, peripheral edema, consti-pation, pruritus or burning at the injection site	β-blockers, carbamazepine, cimetidine, cyclosporine, digoxin, sirolimus, tacrolimus	Effective for CSP-induced hyperten-sion. Causes significant elevation of CSP and tacrolimus levels. Useful in treatment of supraven-tricular tachyarrhythmias and angina. Parenteral dosage form is available (ECG monitoring is required).
Specific β₁-adrenergic receptor blocking agents				
Atenolol (Tenormin®)	Initial: 25–50 mg p.o. QD Maximum: 100 mg/day	Bradycardia, coldness of the extremities, dizziness, fatigue, headache, mental depression, nightmares, wheezing, diarrhea, nausea, impotence	Reserpine, other hypotensive agents, nondihydropyridine calcium-channel blockers	Agents of choice in patients with CAD and good LV function. Use with caution in patients with bronchospastic disease, hyperthy-roidism (may mask tachycardia), and diabetes (may mask symptoms of hypoglycemia). Avoid abrupt withdrawal. Parenteral formulations are indicated for MI and arrhythmias.
Metoprolol tartrate (Lopressor®)	Initial: 50 mg p.o. BID Maximum: 450 mg/day			
α/β-adrenergic receptor blocking agents				
Labetalol (Normodyne®, Trandate®)	Initial: 100 mg p.o. BID Maximum: 2400 mg/day Parenteral: Continuous infusion or 20 mg i.v. bolus over 2 minutes	Nausea, dizziness, drowsiness, fatigue, diarrhea, muscle cramps, impotence, mental depression	β-adrenergic agonists, cimetidine, diltiazem, verapamil, TCAs, nitroglycerin	Useful in patients unable to take oral medications. Avoid abrupt withdrawal.
Angiotensin converting enzyme (ACE) inhibitors				
Enalapril maleate (Vasotec®)	Initial: 2.5–5 mg p.o. QD Maximum: 40 mg/day Parenteral: 1.25 mg i.v. q6h	Cough, hyperkalemia, angio-edema, headache, dizziness, abdominal pain, diarrhea, rash	Allopurinol, capsaicin, digoxin, indomethacin, lithium, potassium supplements, potassium-sparing diuretics, rifampin, tetracycline	Agents of choice for treatment of essential hypertension in patients with diabetes and heart failure. May decrease GFR in patients receiving cyclosporine. Consider potential risk of neutropenia, especially in patients with renal function impairment. Photosensitivity may occur.
Lisinopril (Prinivil®, Zestril®)	Initial: 2.5–10 mg p.o. QD Maximum: 40 mg/day			

Medication	Antihypertensive dose	Adverse effects	Drug interactions	Comments
α-Adrenergic receptor agonists				
Clonidine (Catapres®)	*Oral* Initial: 100 mcg p.o. BID Maximum: 2400 mcg/day *Transdermal system* Initial: 0.1 mg/ 24 hr q week Maximum: 0.3 mg/24 hr	Dry mouth, drowsiness, dizziness, sedation, constipation, fatigue, headache	β-blockers, levodopa, prazosin, TCAs, verapamil	Transdermal or sublingual route may be used in patients unable to swallow pills. Avoid abrupt withdrawal of clonidine.
α-1-Adrenergic receptor blocking agents				
Doxazosin (Cardura®)	Initial: 1 mg p.o. QD Maximum: 16 mg/day	Orthostatic effects (dizziness, syncope, vertigo), headache, somnolence, lethargy, nausea, edema, rhinitis	β-blockers, midodrine, oxilofrine, finasteride	Start with the lowest recommended dose because of postural effects. May help in patients with benign prostatic hypertrophy (BPH).
Terazosin (Hytrin®)	Initial: 1 mg p.o. QHS Maximum: 20 mg/day			
Direct vasodilators				
Hydralazine (Apresoline®)	*Oral* Initial: 10 mg p.o. QID Maximum: 400 mg/day *Parenteral:* Initial: 5–10 mg i.v. q6h	Headache, palpitations, tachycardia, GI distress, SLE, rash, blood dyscrasias fever, paresthesias, numbness	Diuretics, other antihypertensive agents, epinephrine, monoamine oxidase inhibitors	Intravenous formulation available for hospitalized patients unable to take oral medications.

Abbreviations: CAD, coronary artery disease; GFR, glomerular filtration rate; GI, gastrointestinal; LV, left ventricle; SLE, systemic lupus erythematosus; TCAs, tricyclic antidepressants.

from one to the other is likely to cause the same reaction and is not recommended. Since Neoral® contains a polyoxyethylated castor oil derivative in the capsules and oral solution, the safety of changing intravenous cyclosporine to Neoral® after an anaphylactic reaction is unclear. A case of anaphylaxis after ingestion of oral Neoral® has been reported. However, switching to oral Sandimmune® has been done safely since it contains no polyoxyethylated castor oil (Takamatsu *et al.*, 2001).

Gastrointestinal side effects are relatively common with both agents, though they are more frequent with tacrolimus than with CSP. These effects are generally mild and include nausea and vomiting, anorexia, diarrhea, and abdominal discomfort (The US multicenter FK506 liver study group, 1994). Increased liver enzymes and bilirubin are rare and usually reversible with reduction of the dose or drug discontinuation (Landewe *et al.*, 1994). Liver toxicity usually occurs within the first month of therapy and with higher doses. Gingival hyperplasia and hirsutism are known to occur with CSP, but are not a side effect of tacrolimus therapy (Dongari, McDonnell, & Langlais, 1993). Electrolyte abnormalities caused by CSP therapy include hyperkalemia, hypomagnesemia, hyperuricemia, metabolic acidosis, and hypophosphatemia.

Whole blood samples should be used to test levels of both drugs. Target tacrolimus steady-state or trough levels are 5 to 15 ng/ml, using an enzyme-linked immunoabsorbent assay (Przepiorka *et al.*, 1999a). In general, CSP trough levels between 150 and 450 ng/ml (using the monoclonal whole blood assay) without evidence of toxicity or GVHD are acceptable. However, most non-myeloablative HSCT protocols target a CSP trough level of 500 ng/ml for the first month posttransplant. Levels for both immunosuppressants should be obtained at least once a week and 3 to 4 days after conversion from i.v. to p.o., changes in dose, or addition/deletion of interacting medications. Steady-state levels are not achieved for at least 72 hours following any change in dosing. When evaluating levels, practitioners should consider that samples drawn earlier than 72 hours after a dose change may not accurately reflect steady-state concentrations. Cyclosporine and tacrolimus levels should be used only as a guide, along with clinical observations, when considering dosage adjustments.

Since CSP and tacrolimus are cleared via metabolism almost entirely by the cytochrome P450 3A4 enzyme, there are a variety of drugs that interact with these agents. Cytochrome P450 3A4 enzymes are located in the lumen of the gastrointestinal tract and in the liver. P-glycoprotein is an efflux pump also located in the gastrointestinal wall that pumps CSP back into the gastrointestinal lumen. Both cytochrome P450 3A4 enzymes and P-glycoprotein can be induced and inhibited. Drugs that interact with CSP and tacrolimus do so primarily via their effect on these elimination methods (Yee & McGuire, 1990a, 1990b). See Table 83.2 for a list of clinically significant drug interactions.

Glucocorticoids

Systemic glucocorticoids

Despite appropriate prophylaxis with methotrexate and a calcineurin inhibitor, acute GVHD still occurs in a majority of allogeneic HSCT patients. Systemic glucocorticoids are the drugs of choice for the initial treatment of grade II–IV acute GVHD. There are many mechanisms by which glucocorticoids exert their actions. Glucocorticoids are lympholytic and have anti-inflammatory properties. They also alter the immune response of lymphocytes and inhibit the release of critical cytokines (IL-1, IL-2, IL-3, IL-6, and TNF-alpha) implicated in the pathophysiology of GVHD (Schimmer & Parker, 1996) (and see Chapter 15).

Methylprednisolone 1 to 2 mg/kg daily is administered intravenously until patients are able to switch to oral prednisone. Methylprednisolone doses greater than 1 mg/kg/day should be

Table 83.2. *Significant drug interactions with immunosuppressive agents*

Immuno-suppressive drug	Interacting agents	Effect
Methotrexate	Aspirin, cisplatin, NSAIDs, piperacillin, probenecid	Decreased renal clearance of methotrexate
	Chloramphenicol, salicylates, sulfonamides, tetracycline, phenytoin	Displacement of MTX from protein-binding sites
Cyclosporine/ tacrolimus (FK506)	Fluconazole, itraconazole, ketoconazole, erythromycin, clarithromycin, verapamil, diltiazem, nicardipine, amlodipine, amiodarone, nefazodone, fluvoxamine, fluoxetine, cimetidine, delavirdine, nevirapine, indinavir, bromocriptine, methylprednisolone, ritonavir, saquinavir, quinupristin-dalfopristin, zafirlukast, zileuton, danazol	Increased CSP/FK506 levels via inhibition of CSP/FK506 metabolism
	Phenytoin, phenobarbital, carbamazepine, rifamycins	Decreased CSP/FK506 levels via induction of CSP/FK metabolism
	Grapefruit juice	Increased CSP/FK506 levels via inhibition of CSP/FK506 metabolism in GI tract
	St. John's Wort	Decreased CSP/FK506 levels via induction of metabolism?
Cyclosporine	H2 blockers, metoclopramide	Increased CSP levels via increased intestinal absorption
	Sulfinpyrazone	Decreased CSP levels
	Orlistat	Decreased CSP absorption
	Digoxin	Increased digoxin levels
	Lovastatin, simvastatin, atorvastatin, cerivastatin	Increased risk of rhabdomyolysis due to competition for metabolism
Tacrolimus	Methotrexate	Reduced absorption of FK506?
	Chloramphenicol	Increased FK506 levels via unknown mechanism
	Antacids containing magnesium or aluminum, sucralfate	Decreased FK506 absorption
Mycophenolate mofetil (MMF)	Antacids containing magnesium or aluminum, cholestyramine, iron	Decreased MMF absorption
	Sulfinpyrazone	Interference with renal tubular secretion of MMF
	Acyclovir/ganciclovir	Competition for renal tubular secretion
	Probenecid	May inhibit renal tubular secretion of MMF
Glucocorticoids	Aminoglutethimide, rifampin, carbamazepine, phenobarbital, phenytoin, primidone	Decreased corticosteroid activity
	Hypoglycemic agents, antihypertensives, diuretics, oral anticoagulants (warfarin)	Decreased efficacy of these agents by corticosteroids
	Acetazolamide, diuretics	Enhanced hypokalemic effects of corticosteroid
	Cyclosporine	Increased cyclosporine levels
	NSAIDs	Increased risk of GI discomfort and/or GI bleeding
Sirolimus	Diltiazem, nicardipine, verapamil, clotrimazole, fluconazole, itraconazole, clarithromycin, erythromycin, troleandomycin, metoclopramide, cimetidine, danazol, protease inhibitors, grapefruit juice	Increased sirolimus levels
	Carbamazepine, phenytoin, phenobarbital, rifampin, St. John's Wort	Decreased sirolimus levels
	HGM-CoA reductase inhibitors	Increased risk for rhabdomyolysis
	Propofol, intravenous lipid preparations	Increased lipid abnormalities

administered in two divided doses. Patients should be converted to prednisone once lack of absorption is no longer a concern, and oral intake and medications are tolerated. The conversion factor between intravenous methylprednisolone and oral prednisone is 4:5. Glucocorticoids are continued until symptoms are controlled, at which point patients are slowly tapered off steroids as per institutional guidelines. Taper schedules vary, however; at the Fred Hutchinson Cancer Research Center, the glucocorticoid dose is typically tapered 10% every 3 to 5 days. During situations where a flare of GVHD occurs while a patient is on the steroid taper, the rate of the taper may be slowed or temporarily stopped until symptoms are controlled. If this is unsuccessful, conversion from oral prednisone to intravenous methylprednisolone at increased doses may be required for acute management.

Various systemic glucocorticoids are available and dosing equivalency between each agent is described in Table 83.3. Oral glucocorticoids should be administered with food to limit the extent of gastrointestinal upset (Schimmer & Parker, 1996). Intravenous administration of methylprednisolone in doses ≤ 125 mg can be administered as an intravenous push; however doses > 125 mg should be given as a 15 to 30 minute infusion since rapid administration of large doses is associated with perineal burning or itching.

Acute and chronic adverse effects of systemic corticosteroids and their management are described in Table 83.4 (Stanbury & Graham, 1998). Clinically relevant drug interactions with glucocorticoid therapy are listed in Table 83.2.

Topical glucocorticoids

Topical glucocorticoids can be used alone or in conjunction with systemic glucocorticoid therapy for management of isolated areas of upper gastrointestinal or skin GVHD. Oral beclomethasone dipropionate, which is not significantly absorbed and thus works via a local effect, may serve as a viable option and/or adjunct to systemic (1 mg/kg) steroid therapy in patients with isolated upper gastrointestinal GVHD (Shanahan, 1998). A commercial oral formulation of beclomethasone is currently unavailable in the United States but can be extemporaneously compounded from bulk crystalline beclomethasone powder into a dietary corn oil-based emulsion. Studies are currently ongoing to investigate the efficacy of immediate and sustained-release oral beclomethasone tablets. In randomized phase I and II controlled studies, oral dosing of beclomethasone is 8 mg daily in four divided doses for 28 days; however optimal duration of therapy remains to be determined (Baehr et al., 1995; McDonald et al., 1998). Oral beclomethasone is well tolerated with the most frequently reported side effects being poor taste and diarrhea. These side effects are attributable to the corn oil vehicle in which the beclomethasone powder is dissolved. In contrast to systemic steroids, topical beclomethasone is not associated with an increased risk of local and/or systemic bacterial and fungal infections, Cushingoid features, or hyperglycemia. Adrenal insufficiency is a concern with chronic oral beclomethasone since subclinical adrenal suppression was documented in patients receiving therapy during the 28-day study period. Therefore, in patients who require therapy beyond 28 days, monitoring for adrenal suppression and appropriate replacement therapy with hydrocortisone may be necessary (Baehr et al., 1995; McDonald et al., 1998). For acute management of adrenal insufficiency, intravenous hydrocortisone 100 mg should be administered. This may be repeated three to four times in a 24-hour period. Hydrocortisone 20 to 60 mg daily in divided doses may be required for chronic replacement therapy, and should be continued until adrenal function has recovered. Oral beclomethasone should be administered with a meal or snack at breakfast, lunch, dinner, and at bedtime whenever possible.

For management of cutaneous GVHD, topical glucocorticoid creams or ointments, such as hydrocortisone, triamcinolone, or clobetasol may be applied locally.

Mycophenolate mofetil (MMF)

Mycophenolate mofetil is hydrolyzed in vivo to its active form, mycophenolic acid (MPA). MPA is a potent, selective, noncompetitive, and reversible inhibitor of inosine monophosphate dehydrogenase, which inhibits the de novo pathway of guanosine nucleotide synthesis without being incorporated into DNA. Since the proliferation of T and B lymphocytes is critically dependent on de novo synthesis of purines, MPA has potent cytostatic effects on lymphocytes. MPA inhibits proliferative responses of T and B lymphocytes to mitogenic and allogeneic stimulation. MPA also suppresses formation of antibody by B lymphocytes. Most of the experience with MMF for

Table 83.3. *Glucocorticoids and dosage equivalency*

Drug	Relative glucocorticoid potency	Relative mineralocorticoid potency	Sodium-retaining capacity	Dose equivalency (mg)	Half-life (hours)
Beclomethasone	25	0	0	0.8	36–72
Dexamethasone	30	0	0	0.8	36–72
Hydrocortisone	1	1	1	20	8–12
Methylprednisolone	5	0.5	0.5	4	12–36
Prednisolone	4	0.8	0.8	5	12–36
Prednisone	4	0.8	0.8	5	12–36
Triamcinolone	5	0	0	4	12–36

Table 83.4. *Management of glucocorticoid adverse effects*

	Adverse effect	Monitoring parameters	Management
Acute effects	Sodium and fluid retention	Serum sodium, weight, intravenous and oral fluid intake	Low salt diet, fluid restriction, diuretics if necessary
	Hypokalemia	Serum potassium	Increase dietary potassium intake, potassium supplements
	Hypertension	Blood pressure	Antihypertensives if drug-related, restrict fluid if fluid related
	Hyperglycemia	Blood sugar	Decrease dietary glucose, insulin or oral hypo-glycemic agents as needed
	Muscle weakness and wasting	Electrolyte abnormalities (calcium, magnesium, potassium)	Weight-bearing exercise, replace or decrease elec-trolyte supplementation, use lowest effective dose
	GI intolerance or bleed	Hematocrit, blood in stool, GI discomfort	Proton pump inhibitor Administer with food
	Weight gain	Fluid intake	Fluid restriction
	Steroid psychosis	Mentation	Use lowest effective dose
	Insomnia	Duration of sleep, ability to fall asleep	Agents for sleep, if twice daily dosing is used, avoid administering second dose late in the evening
Chronic effects	Hypercholesterolemia and/ or hypertriglyceridemia	Cholesterol and triglyceride	Dietary modification, antihyperlipidemic agents if necessary
	Osteoporosis	DEXA scan	Lifestyle changes including: decrease alcohol intake, stop smoking; increase calcium intake (oral calcium supplements may be necessary); weight-bearing exercise; hormonal replacement if applicable, bisphosphonate therapy
	Cataracts	Ophthalmologic exam	Steroid ophthalmic eyedrops, surgery
	Avascular necrosis		Discontinue therapy if possible
	Cushingoid features		

prophylaxis of GVHD in HSCT has been in combination with CSP in the non-myeloablative setting. However, it is currently being studied as a replacement for methotrexate in myeloablative protocols.

Doses range from 30 to 60 mg/kg/day (in 2–4 divided doses). MMF can be administered orally (as capsules, tablets, or suspension) or as an intravenous infusion. Oral absorption in healthy volunteers is 94%. In a pharmacokinetic study of MMF, area under the curve (AUC) and trough levels of MPA were much lower in HSCT patients than values after solid organ transplants or in healthy individuals. This raises the possibility that HSCT patients may have reduced absorption of MMF secondary to intestinal toxicity following high-dose conditioning or impaired enterohepatic circulation (Jenke *et al.*, 2001). Food has been shown to decrease the peak concentration (C_{max}) of MPA by 40%, though it does not alter the extent of absorption. Since nausea, vomiting, and diarrhea are the most common side effects of MMF, it may be difficult for HSCT patients to take MMF on an empty stomach, though this is the preferred method. Thus, MMF may be taken with food if patients are unable to tolerate taking the doses on an empty stomach.

MMF is virtually devoid of nephrotoxicity and hepatotoxicity. The most serious side effect of MMF is bone marrow suppression. Patients may develop leukopenia, anemia, or thrombocytopenia, which occasionally requires dose reduction or drug discontinuation. MMF also increases the risk for serious life-threatening and opportunistic infections and has been associated with an increased incidence of posttransplant lymphoproliferative disorders. MMF drug levels may be measured, but it is unclear at this time what should be used as the target therapeutic range.

Antithymocyte globulin (ATG)

Antithymocyte globulin (ATG) is a pan-antilymphocyte immunoglobulin composed of purified animal polyclonal antibodies directed against human lymphocytes. ATG is an accepted salvage modality for the treatment of steroid-refractory acute GVHD. Currently available intravenous formulations include horse ATG (ATGAM) and rabbit ATG (Thymoglobulin). Dosing of horse and rabbit ATG varies depending on institutional practices, study protocols, and geographical location of each transplant center. In a 2001 international survey of antithymocyte globulin use for steroid-refractory GVHD, Hsu and colleagues reported that the typical daily dosing regimen for horse ATG ranged from 5 to 40 mg/kg, while the daily dose for rabbit ATG ranged from 0.5 to ≥ 10 mg/kg. Higher dosing of both products was used primarily in the pediatric population (Hsu *et al.*, 2001).

The adverse effect profile of both ATG formulations is similar. Most common adverse effects are infusion-related reactions, hypersensitivity, and hematological effects. Infusion-related adverse effects commonly present as fever (50% with horse; 85% with rabbit) and chills/rigors (16% with horse; 85% with rabbit); however, they can also present as hypotension, hypertension, and/or pruritus. These reactions typically occur during the infusions. Antihistamines, acetaminophen, meperidine, and corticosteroids (methylprednisolone or hydrocortisone) are recommended for prophylaxis and treatment of these reactions with either formulation of ATG. In situations where the infusion-related adverse effects are only associated with fever, pruritus, chills, and rigors, therapy should be stopped, followed by symptomatic management. Re-initiation of therapy at a slower rate may be attempted following resolution of the infusion-related events. Therapy, however, should be discontinued when hypotension or hypertension occurs during the infusion as these symptoms may be suggestive of an anaphylactic reaction. Re-initiation of therapy in such situations is not recommended. Hypersensitivity reactions can occur in up to 10% and 28% of patients receiving horse ATG and rabbit ATG, respectively. These reactions can present as serum sickness or dermatological reactions characterized as rash, urticaria, and pruritus, and often require corticosteroid premedication prior to each infusion. The usual time to onset ranges from 6 to 14 days after initial therapy and is reversible upon discontinuation of therapy. Anaphylaxis, manifesting as hypotension, hypertension, respiratory distress, or pain in the chest, flank, or back can occur in up to 1% of patients. The routine practice of skin testing with an intradermal injection of 0.1 ml (1:1000 dilution) of horse ATG and a normal saline control is recommended prior to the initial administration of horse ATG infusions; however, skin test results are not predictive of future adverse reactions. Consequently, drugs used for anaphylaxis treatment should be readily available with each ATG infusion. Routine skin testing prior to rabbit ATG is unnecessary. In cases of serum sickness, hypotension, hypertension, and/or anaphylaxis, the therapy must be discontinued and supportive care initiated (McCaul et al., 2000; Khoury et al., 2001; Remberger et al., 2001).

Major hematological toxicities include leukopenia and thrombocytopenia, with a higher incidence of leukopenia and thrombocytopenia seen with rabbit ATG than horse ATG (57% vs. 14% and 37% vs. 30%). Monitoring for infections is recommended as they are common complications associated with ATG use (Khoury et al., 2001; Remberger et al., 2001).

Administration through a central line is desired, as thrombophlebitis commonly occurs with peripheral administration of horse ATG at concentrations greater than 1 mg/ml. The maximum tolerated concentrations for central and peripheral line administration of horse ATG are 4 mg/ml and 1 mg/ml, respectively. A 0.2 to 1 micron filter must be used with the administration of horse ATG while a 0.22 micron filter must be used for rabbit ATG. Horse ATG infusions must be infused over a minimum of at least 4 hours. The first infusion of rabbit ATG must be delivered over a minimum of 6 hours. The rate of subsequent infusions may be increased to infuse over a minimum of 4 hours if the first infusion is well tolerated.

There are no reported pharmacologic and pharmacokinetic interactions with either ATG formulation. However, when con-current administration of other immunosuppressive agents are used, profound immunosuppression can occur. This can result in an increased incidence of infections, posttransplant lymphoproliferative disorders, and/or secondary malignancies.

Sirolimus (rapamycin)

Sirolimus is a novel immunosuppressive agent approved by the U.S. Food and Drug Administration (FDA) in 1999 for prophylaxis of kidney rejection in renal transplant recipients. The role of sirolimus in prophylaxis and treatment of GVHD is currently being explored in clinical trials (Antin et al., 2003). Sirolimus binds to cytosolic proteins called immunophilins similarly to tacrolimus and CSP; however, its mechanism of action (MOA) is unique from the MOA of the two latter agents. Sirolimus, upon forming a complex with FK-binding protein, binds to a specific cell cycle regulatory protein defined as mTOR (mammalian target of rapamycin). The final result of the activity of this macrolide lactone is inhibition of T-lymphocyte proliferative responses to a variety of cytokines such as IL-2, IL-4, and IL-15 (Ingle, Sievers, & Holt, 2000; MacDonald et al., Zimmerman 2000) (see Chapter 118). Besides a novel MOA and synergistic activity with CSP, sirolimus also offers a different adverse effect profile from calcineurin inhibitors, making combination regimens an attractive immunosuppressive option (MacDonald et al., 2000).

The most common adverse effects associated with sirolimus are dose-dependent, and include hypertriglyceridemia, thrombocytopenia, neutropenia, and transient mild elevation of LFTs (Ingle et al., 2000). Due to sirolimus' metabolic effects on low, intermediate, and high-density lipoproteins, a lipid screen should be obtained before the therapy is initiated and regularly thereafter. In addition, whole blood sirolimus trough levels should be monitored weekly for the first month of therapy and biweekly thereafter to minimize toxicities. The first level should be obtained no earlier than 4 to 6 days into treatment and should be kept in a recommended range of 5 to 15 ng/ml (McDonald et al., 2000; Mahalati & Kahan 2001). This desired blood level may be altered by other agents affecting cytochrome P450 3A enzymes and the P-glycoprotein efflux pump. Drugs interacting with sirolimus are listed in Table 83.2 (MacDonald et al., 2000). Patients should also be advised to take this drug consistently with relation to food, since fatty meals can have a significant effect on sirolimus absorption. In addition, patients taking CSP microemulsion should space sirolimus four hours apart from any cyclosporine dose because concurrent administration increases the sirolimus AUC by 50% (MacDonald et al., 2000; Mahalati & Kahan, 2001).

Monoclonal antibodies

Daclizumab and basiliximab
Daclizumab and basiliximab are immunoglobulin G (IgG) monoclonal antibodies used in the treatment of steroid-resistant

acute GVHD. Daclizumab is a humanized IL-2 receptor antagonist that is composed of 90% human and 10% murine proteins. Basiliximab is a chimera of human and murine genes with the murine genes representing the entire portion of the variable region of the IgG antibody. These agents competitively bind with the IL-2 receptor of activated T cells to inhibit further IL-2-mediated lymphocyte activation. In general, humanization of these murine monoclonal antibodies results in longer half-life for prolonged therapeutic effect and less potential for immunogenicity (Tse & Moore 1998; Berard et al., 1999; Bell & Kamm, 2000).

In clinical studies, both agents appear to be viable alternatives for steroid-resistant GVHD, although more clinical experience exists with daclizumab (Anasetti et al., 1994; Przepiorka et al., 2000; Gero et al., 2001; Wolfgang et al., 2001). Both agents are administered intravenously over 30 to 60 minutes. Dosing of these agents for salvage GVHD treatment varies in the literature and the optimal dosing regimen remains to be determined (Anasetti et al., 1994; Wolfgang et al., 2001). The complete response rate and survival rate were highest with the daclizumab regimen of 1 mg/kg on days 1, 4, 8, 15, and 22 as described by Przepiorka and colleagues. In this study, the complete response rate on day 43 was 47% and survival on day 120 was 53% (Przepiorka et al., 2000). Unlike other monoclonal antibodies such as rituximab, infliximab, and OKT3, these agents are well tolerated with no reports of infusion-related adverse effects. Consequently premedication with acetaminophen and diphenhydramine is unnecessary (Onrust & Wiseman, 1999; Wiseman & Faulds, 1999). An increased incidence of infectious complications and cytomegalovirus (CMV) reactivation was documented when daclizumab therapy was used in HSCT patients. It remains unclear if these infectious complications are related to the underlying GVHD process or the drug, since infection is a common cause of death in patients with acute or chronic GVHD. Since the incidence of bacterial, viral, fungal, and opportunistic infections was not increased when compared to placebo in renal transplant patients, this suggests that the difference in infectious complications seen in HSCT are related to GVHD rather than the antibody therapy (Przepiorka et al., 2000). Regardless, prophylaxis for viral, fungal, and PCP infections is recommended. Immunogenicity and development of posttransplant lymphoproliferative disorders is low with these agents. Drug interactions have not been described with either agent.

Infliximab

Infliximab is a chimeric human/murine IgG monoclonal antibody targeted against tumor necrosis factor-alpha (TNF-alpha), a cytotoxic inflammatory cytokine implicated in the development of GVHD. Infliximab's activity is linked to its ability to bind with TNF-alpha and prevent the latter binding to the TNF-alpha receptor. It is composed of 75% human and 25% murine proteins. Infliximab is FDA-approved for the treatment of rheumatoid arthritis (RA) and Crohn's disease; however, it has been used in some case reports for the treatment of steroid-

refractory acute GVHD (Bell & Kamm, 2000; Couriel et al., 2000; Markham & Lamb, 2000). In these case reports, doses of 5 mg/kg or 10 mg/kg were administered as single infusions for acute GHVD treatment (Kobbe et al., 2001). The optimal dose and duration of treatment remain to be determined.

Compared to placebo, infliximab is associated with a greater incidence of reported adverse effects (84.2% vs. 70.3%). Hypersensitivity reactions have been reported with infliximab use and occur in 7% of patients during the initial infusion and 10% during subsequent infusions. These reactions are characterized by urticaria, dyspnea, pruritus, or hypotension. Formation of human antichimeric antibody (HACA) is concerning with infliximab as 25% of the IgG molecule is composed of murine proteins that can be recognized as foreign. HACA formation is seen in 10% to 20% of patients. HACA positivity, however, may not specifically correlate with higher infusion-related adverse effects. An increased infection risk, especially upper respiratory and urinary tract infections, was noted in patients receiving infliximab versus placebo (Markham & Lamb, 2000; Seymour, Worsley, & Smith, 2001; Taylor, 2001). Consequently, patients receiving infliximab should be routinely monitored for infectious complications.

Alemtuzumab, ABX-CBL, and visilizumab

Alemtuzumab, ABX-CBL, and visilizumab are the newest antibody agents under investigation for steroid-refractory acute GVHD. They function as antibodies to the CD52, CD147, and CD3 receptors, respectively. Unlike the interleukin-2 receptor antagonists and infliximab, the clinical experience with these agents is limited and their role in steroid-resistant acute GVHD remains to be defined. Alemtuzumab is the only agent in this group currently marketed in the United States. These agents are only available for intravenous administration (Veradi et al., 1996; Cole et al., 1999; Flynn & Byrd, 2000; Deeg et al., 2001).

Infusion-related adverse events and infection are common with alemtuzumab and visilizumab. Infusion-related events, characterized by fever, rigors, nausea, hypotension, and diarrhea, typically occur during the initial infusion. This complication is believed to be associated with a cytokine release syndrome that is also commonly seen with other monoclonal antibodies such as rituximab and OKT3. Prophylaxis with acetaminophen and diphenhydramine 30 minutes prior to the administration of alemtuzumab, and hydrocortisone, acetaminophen, and diphenhydramine 30 minutes prior to each infusion of visilizumab may decrease the severity of these effects. Treatment with hydrocortisone may be needed for management of severe reactions and temporary discontinuation of the infusion and symptomatic management with meperidine, inhaled β_2 agonists and volume support may be warranted upon onset of these reactions. Bacterial, fungal, and opportunistic infections are associated with these therapies and prophylaxis with antivirals and PCP medications is recommended (Veradi et al., 1996; Protein Design Labs, 1998; Cole et al., 1999; Flynn & Byrd, 2000).

Myalgia is a reversible, dose-limiting side effect of ABX-CBL. The incidence, severity, and duration of pain increases with increasing doses while the onset of pain is more rapid with increasing dose. The etiology remains undefined; however, based on the previous findings, it may be associated with the pharmacokinetics and pharmacodynamics of the drug. A slower infusion rate may be beneficial to minimize this side effect. Premedication with narcotics is also recommended and additional narcotics may be necessary during the infusion. Discontinuation of the drug may be necessary if myalgias are uncontrolled by narcotics (Deeg et al., 2001). Similar to other monoclonal antibodies, drug interactions have not been reported with these agents.

Thalidomide

Thalidomide (N-phtalidoglutarimide) came back into the clinical arena in the late 1980s, mostly due to its antitumor, anti-inflammatory, and immunomodulatory properties. The proposed mechanism for the immunomodulatory effects of thalidomide involves inhibition of TNF-alpha production, alteration and modification of cytokine activity, reduction in phagocytosis by polymorphonuclear leukocytes, and a decrease in circulating helper T-cell to suppressor T-cell ratio (Hussein, 2000). The use of thalidomide as a salvage treatment for chronic GVHD (cGVHD) was first reported in a rat model, and subsequently the same group of investigators used thalidomide in humans for this indication (Volgelsang et al., 1988, 1992). The overall efficacy reported in the literature with 200 to 1,000 mg of thalidomide per day was 43% with a median time to response of 2 to 3 months (Parker et al., 1995; Rovelli et al., 1998; Poel, Pasman, & Schouten, 2001). The efficacy of thalidomide could not be established by a phase III clinical trial performed at the Fred Hutchinson Cancer Research Center because of a high discontinuation rate. The authors reported a 92% termination rate of thalidomide due to adverse effects such as neutropenia and peripheral neuropathy. However, a high discontinuation rate (65%) was also observed in the placebo group (Koc et al., 2000).

The most common adverse effects reported in patients treated with thalidomide for cGVHD include sedation, dizziness, constipation, rash, peripheral neuropathy, and neutropenia (Parker et al., 1995; Singhal et al., 1999; Hussein, 2000). In order to minimize some of these adverse effects, therapy should be initiated with a low dose and titrated slowly as tolerated to the desired dose (Hussein, 2000). Sensory and motor peripheral neuropathy occurred in 15% to 50% of HSCT patients, and neutropenia was observed in 18% to 64% of HSCT patients (Koc et al., 2000; Poel et al., 2001). True hypersensitivity reactions have not been observed in patients receiving thalidomide for cGVHD (Poel et al., 2001). Thalidomide has high teratogenic potential and all patients require extensive counseling and education about the drug before thalidomide initiation. In addition, appropriate contraceptive measures must be implemented. Major drug interactions with thalidomide are associated with CNS depressants such as barbiturates, alcohol, chlorpromazine, and reserpine. Caution must be exercised

when thalidomide is combined with these agents. Amphetamines and methylphenidate antagonize the sedative effects of thalidomide (Somers, 1960).

Antibacterial agents

Broad-spectrum antibiotics are utilized frequently in HSCT patients, especially during the neutropenic period. The organism causing infections in neutropenic patients is not found in almost 70% of all febrile episodes. Lack of proper antimicrobial coverage is linked to 50% mortality in these patients (Maschmeyer et al., 1997). Currently, the Infectious Diseases Society of America recommends initiation of empiric antibiotic therapy in a neutropenic patient at the onset of first fever or when signs and symptoms of an infectious process are detected in patients who are afebrile (Hughes et al., 2002).

Secondary to the widespread use of prophylactic antibiotics with Gram-negative coverage and the presence of indwelling catheters, Gram-positive bacteria are responsible for approximately 60% to 70% of documented (by culture) infections occurring in neutropenic patients. Some of these infecting Gram-positive organisms may be resistant to methicillin, leaving only vancomycin, quinupristin/dalfopristin, linezolid, and teicoplanin (not available in the United States) as options for treatment. Gram-positive organisms infecting neutropenic patients include coagulase-negative staphylococci, enterococci, Corynebacterium jeikeium, Staphylococcus aureus, viridans streptococci, and pneumococci. The most common Gram-negative bacteria infecting neutropenic patients include Escherichia coli, Klebsiella spp., and Pseudomonas aeruginosa (Hughes et al., 2002).

Aminoglycosides

Aminoglycosides have been available since the 1950s and are still widely utilized in clinical practice. Aminoglycosides have excellent activity against Gram-negative aerobes including Klebsiella, E. coli, H. influenzae, Proteus, Enterobacter, Citrobacter, Pseudomonas aeruginosa, Serratia, and most isolates of Acinetobacter. Amikacin is the aminoglycoside of choice for Stenotrophomonas maltophilia. This group of antibiotics has no to little activity against anaerobes. Aminoglycosides are active against some Gram-positive aerobic bacteria (i.e., staphylococci); however, the toxicity profile of aminoglycosides limits their use to severe infections when synergy between β-lactams and aminoglycosides or glycopeptides and aminoglycosides is desired (Lortholary et al., 1995).

Aminoglycosides must penetrate the outer and inner membranes of Gram-negative bacteria using an oxygen-dependent transport system and then bind to the 30S subunit of the ribosome. This binding disrupts the process of bacterial protein synthesis and eventually leads to bacterial cell death. The lethal effect of aminoglycosides is rapid and is thought to be concentration-dependent. Aminoglycosides have a significant post-antibiotic effect (PAE), defined as persistent killing of bacteria despite an antibiotic concentration below the minimum inhibitory concentration (MIC). The duration of PAE for Gram-negative bacilli ranges from 2 to 4 hours after aminoglycoside administration. The presence of leukocytes prolongs PAE observed with aminoglycosides (Lortholary *et al.,* 1995).

Aminoglycosides are administered parenterally. The recommended initial dosing is listed in Table 83.5. Aminoglycosides are eliminated renally and approximately 85% of the drug is eliminated within 24 hours as unchanged drug. Appropriate dosage adjustments are required in patients with abnormal renal function (Pancoast, 1988). Toxicities seen with aminoglycosides can be minimized if proper monitoring is performed and appropriate dosage adjustments are made in response to measured drug levels. Blood samples for monitoring of the standard dosing regimen should be obtained within 30 minutes of the next infusion (trough) and 30 minutes post aminoglycoside infusion (peak). Peak aminoglycoside levels correlate with aminoglycoside efficacy and ototoxicity, while trough levels correlate with renal toxicity. Desired serum concentrations for standard dosing can be found in Table 83.5. Optimal monitoring for once daily aminoglycoside therapy is still being developed. Nomograms for once daily aminoglycoside monitoring with dosage adjustment guidelines are available (Nicolau *et al.,* 1995).

The most common adverse effects associated with aminoglycoside administration are ototoxicity and nephrotoxicity. Aminoglycoside-induced ototoxicity (vestibular and auditory) is often irreversible. Auditory toxicity presents as tinnitus, while the symptoms of vestibular toxicity include nausea, vomiting, and headache. An increased risk for ototoxicity is associated with coadministration of loop diuretics and other ototoxic agents, prolonged aminoglycoside therapy, and high aminoglycoside serum levels. Gentamicin is the most ototoxic of the aminoglycosides, followed by tobramycin and amikacin. Netilmicin is thought to be least ototoxic. In contrast to ototoxicity, nephrotoxicity is usually reversible; however, the recovery phase may take months. Nephrotoxicity is caused by aminoglycoside accumulation in the proximal tubules. The risk factors for nephrotoxicity include older age, pre-existing renal impairment, recent aminoglycoside therapy, concurrent administration of nephrotoxic agents (i.e., amphotericin, cyclosporine, foscarnet, and vancomycin), volume depletion, liver failure, and prolonged aminoglycoside administration. Less common adverse effects observed with aminoglycosides include skin rash, nausea, vomiting, neuromuscular blockade, and confusion (Pancoast, 1988).

Aminoglycosides should not be administered via the same line as β-lactam antibiotics because of the risk of aminoglycoside inactivation. Potential additive toxicity exists when aminoglycosides are used concurrently with other ototoxic agents (i.e., bumetanide, furosemide, ethacrynic acid, carboplatin, cisplatin) and/or nephrotoxic agents (i.e., amphotericin B, cidofovir, cyclosporine, tacrolimus, vancomycin). The use of these combinations should be avoided whenever possible.

Antipseudomonal cephalosporins

Ceftazidime

Ceftazidime is a third-generation cephalosporin with broad-spectrum antimicrobial activity against Gram-negative and some Gram-positive aerobes. Its activity against *Clostridium perifringes* is fairly good; however, this agent has little activity against other anaerobic bacterial organisms. Ceftazidime is very effective against nosocomial pathogens from the family of Enterobacteriaceae (i.e., *E. coli, K. pneumoniae, P. mirabilis*). Approximately 85% of the strains of *Pseudomonas aeruginosa* remain sensitive to ceftazidime. Its activity against *Citrobacter, Enterobacter,* and *Serratia* is not as predictable and may vary according to geographical location. Other Gram-negative organisms displaying excellent sensitivity to ceftazidime include common respiratory pathogens such as *H. influenzae* and *M. catarrhalis.* This drug has little to no efficacy in the treatment of infections caused by *Stenotrophomonas maltophilia,* methicillin-resistant staphylococci, enterococci, or *Listeria monocytogenes.* In clinical practice, ceftazidime is used to treat lower respiratory tract, intra-abdominal, urinary, skin, and soft tissue infections. Ceftazidime is widely accepted as first-line empiric therapy

Table 83.5. *Dosing and desired drug levels for selected aminoglycosides*

Aminoglycoside	Conventional dosing		Once daily dosing	Comments
	Dosing regimen	Desired serum conc. (mg/l)		
Gentamicin	LD: 2 mg/kg MD: 1.2–1.7 mg/kg q8h	Peak: 4–10 Trough: 0.5–2	5–7 mg/kg q24h	More active than tobramycin against *Serratia marcescens*. Least expensive.
Tobramycin	LD: 2 mg/kg MD: 1.2–1.7 mg/kg q8h		5–7 mg/kg q24h	More active than gentamicin against *Pseudomonas aeruginosa.*
Amikacin	LD: 7.5 mg/kg MD: 7.5 mg/kg q12h or 5 mg/kg q8h	Peak: 20–30 Trough: 1–8	15 mg/kg q24h	Broadest activity among aminoglycosides. Active against *Stenotrophomonas maltophilia.*

Abbreviations: LD, loading dose; MD, maintenance dose.

for neutropenic fever as a single agent (Rains, Bryson, & Peters, 1995).

Ceftazidime is only available as a parenteral preparation in the United States. The recommended dose for adult patients with neutropenic fever is 2 g intravenously every 8 hours. For other indications its dosing may range from 1 to 6 g per day divided into 2 or 3 doses. This drug is cleared renally and dosing adjustments should commence once creatinine clearance falls below 50 ml/min. No dosage adjustments are recommended for patients with liver failure (Rains et al., 1995).

Ceftazidime is generally well tolerated and the most frequent adverse effects include skin rashes, fever, local pain, and phlebitis. Gastrointestinal intolerance is reported infrequently with this antibiotic. Headache, dizziness, and transient paresthesias may occur, but are infrequent. Serious CNS adverse effects have rarely been reported with ceftazidime use, including encephalopathy, seizures, myoclonus, and hallucinations. Hematologic adverse effects, such as eosinophilia, thrombocytosis, thrombocytopenia, and leukopenia, have been documented in patients treated with ceftazidime. Superinfections (i.e., candidiasis, vaginitis, pseudomembranous colitis) are possible after exposure to this broad-spectrum antibiotic (Rains et al., 1995). Anaphylaxis may occur with the use of ceftazidime and potential for cross-sensitivity with penicillins, though low, does exist. In patients with a history of penicillin allergy and positive skin test, the reported frequency of allergic reactions to ceftazidime was 5.6% (Salkind, Cuddy, & Foxworth, 2001). Desensitization protocols for ceftazidime are available.

Cefepime

Cefepime has been classified as a fourth-generation cephalosporin due to its broad spectrum of activity and its resistance to hydrolysis by bacterial β-lactamases. While its aerobic Gram-negative activity is comparable to ceftazidime, cefepime has much better Gram-positive aerobic activity than ceftazidime (Wynd & Paladino, 1996). Cefepime has excellent activity against streptococci and moderate efficacy against methicillin-susceptible Staphylococcus aureus. It has no clinical utility against enterococci (Ennis & Cobbs, 1995). Cefepime is not a very good agent for the treatment of anaerobic infections. Cefepime can be used in the treatment of bacteremia, urinary tract, intra-abdominal, respiratory tract, and skin and soft tissue infections (Wynd & Paladino, 1996).

Cefepime is only available as a parenteral formulation and the intravenous dose can range from 1 to 6 g/day. The higher doses of cefepime (2 g every 8 hours) are used in patients with severe infections and in patients with neutropenic fever. Approximately 85% of cefepime is excreted via the renal pathway as unchanged drug. Dosing adjustments should be undertaken when creatinine clearance falls below 60 ml/min (Wynd & Paladino, 1996).

Cefepime is well tolerated and the most common adverse effects reported with this agent include headache, nausea, diarrhea, and skin rashes. Minor laboratory abnormalities such as hypophosphatemia, eosinophilia, activated partial thrombo-

plastin time, abnormal liver function tests, and false-positive Coombs test have been observed with the administration of cefepime (Wynd & Paladino, 1996).

Carbapenems

Imipenem-cilastatin and meropenem are two carbapenem antibiotics highly utilized for treatment of polymicrobial infections and as empirical therapy in patients with neutropenic fever. The FDA recently approved a third carbapenem named ertapenem. However, the only potential advantage of this agent over the former two drugs in this class is that it is dosed only once daily. Imipenem-cilastatin and meropenem have proven efficacy for the treatment of neutropenic fever, whereas experience with ertapenem is limited. Carbapenems have a broad spectrum of activity and are active against anaerobic organisms and most Gram-positive and Gram-negative aerobic infections, with the exception of Stenotrophomonas maltophilia and Pseudomonas cepacia. These two Gram-negative organisms are able to produce metallo-β-lactamases that have the potential to inactivate imipenem-cilastatin and meropenem. The advantage of carbapenems over other broad spectrum β-lactam antibiotics (i.e., third-generation cephalosporins) is their resistance to hydrolysis by extended spectrum β-lactamases. However, carbapenems have the potential to induce cephalosporinases that may decrease bacterial sensitivity to other antibiotics (Asbel & Levison, 2000). An increase in superinfections (i.e., Enterococcus faecium, Stenotrophomonas maltophilia, and Candida spp.) has been reported with the use of carbapenems. Therefore, these antibiotics should be reserved for treatment of severe nosocomial infections, complicated polymicrobial infections, septic episodes, and febrile neutropenia. Antimicrobial therapy should be streamlined once the responsible organism is identified (Bradley, Garau, & Lode, 1999). Monotherapy with imipenem-cilastatin or meropenem is effective in patients with neutropenic fever; however, gastrointestinal adverse effects and cost of therapy need to be considered when choosing a first-line agent for empiric treatment (Asbel & Levison, 2000).

Imipenem-cilastatin and meropenem are only available as parenteral preparations. Imipenem is combined with cilastatin in order to minimize its degradation by renal peptidases and to prolong its half-life. Meropenem is significantly more stable against renal peptidases and does not require protection with this dehydropeptidase inhibitor. The dosing of imipenem-cilastatin ranges from 250 mg to 1 g every 6 to 8 hours. High doses of 4 g per day are typically utilized for treatment of Pseudomonas aeruginosa infections. The recommended adult dose for meropenem is 1 to 2 g intravenously every 8 hours. Both imipenem-cilastatin and meropenem are renally cleared and appropriate dosage adjustments are required in patients with renal function impairment (Asbel & Levison, 2000). Imipenem-cilastatin requires more frequent dosing and is administered over a longer period of time than meropenem (60 minutes versus 15 to 30 minutes, respectively) (Hurst & Lamb, 2000).

The most serious adverse effect associated with imipenem-cilastatin is seizures. The risk of seizures is dose-dependent and increases in patients with renal failure, patients receiving agents with seizure threshold–lowering potential (i.e., theophylline, cyclosporine), or patients receiving a total dose above 3 to 4 g per day. In patients with renal failure appropriate dosage adjustments should minimize the possibility of this adverse effect. If dosing guidelines for imipenem-cilastatin are followed, the estimated risk of seizures is less than 1% (Alvan & Nord, 1995). Meropenem is not associated with a high risk of seizures; therefore, it is FDA-approved for the treatment of meningitis.

Gastrointestinal adverse effects including nausea, vomiting, and diarrhea are reported by patients receiving carbapenems. Nausea is more common with imipenem-cilastatin and is dose- and infusion rate-dependent (Hurst & Lamb, 2000). Hypersensitivity reactions and cross-reactivity with penicillins have been reported with carbapenems. Blood dyscrasias, although reported, are rather infrequent with carbapenems (Alvan & Nord, 1995). Local reactions at the infusion site, including phlebitis, thrombophlebitis, and vein pain, may occur with the use of imipenem-cilastatin and meropenem (Buckley et al., 1992; Hurst & Lamb, 2000).

Drugs possibly interacting with imipenem-cilastatin are β-lactam antibiotics (decreased efficacy of other β-lactams), ganciclovir (reports of seizures when these two agents are used together), and chloramphenicol (antagonism of imipenem-cilastatin activity).

Monobactams

Aztreonam is a parenteral monobactam antibiotic with activity against Gram-negative aerobic organisms. This agent has no activity against either Gram-positive aerobes or anaerobes. Aztreonam has been used in the treatment of septicemia, lower respiratory, urinary tract, intra-abdominal, gynecological, bone and joint, and skin and soft tissue infections (Alvan & Nord, 1995; Asbel & Levison, 2000). Aztreonam, in combination with vancomycin, has been compared to other antibiotic combinations in clinical trials evaluating its efficacy as treatment for neutropenic fever (Kelsey, Shaw, & Newland, 1992a; Raad et al., 1996). The efficacy of the aztreonam/vancomycin combination has been similar to that reported with gentamicin/piperacillin combination (Kelsey et al., 1992a). Currently, aztreonam plays a major role as an agent of choice in patients with true allergy to penicillins or cephalosporins since it has a different structure than these β-lactams. However, aztreonam is capable of producing hypersensitivity reactions on its own in rare cases (Alvan & Nord, 1995).

Aztreonam dosing ranges from 1 to 2 g every 6 to 8 hours in adults with normal renal function. In patients with neutropenic fever, intravenous doses of 2 g every 8 hours are generally used (Asbel & Levison, 2000). Approximately 65% of aztreonam is eliminated renally as unchanged drug. Dosage adjustments are recommended in patients with renal dysfunction (Alvan & Nord, 1995).

Overall, aztreonam is well tolerated. The most common adverse effects occurring in less than 2% of patients include local reactions around the infusion site, nausea, vomiting, and diarrhea. Pseudomembranous colitis and group D streptococcus colonization can also occur in patients being treated with aztreonam (Brogden & Heel, 1986). Toxic epidermal necrolysis possibly due to aztreonam has been reported in two bone marrow transplant recipients (Alvan & Nord, 1995).

Extended-spectrum penicillins

In the face of increasing bacterial resistance, the invention of a combination of broad-spectrum penicillins with β-lactamase inhibitors (i.e., clavulanic acid, sulbactam, and tazobactam) has improved in vivo and in vitro efficacy of selected penicillins. The antipseudomonal penicillin-β-lactamase inhibitor combinations, such as ticarcillin/clavulanic acid (Timentin®) and piperacillin/tazobactam (Zosyn®), are potential choices for empiric therapy of febrile neutropenia in HSCT patients. Amoxicillin/clavulanic acid (Augmentin®) in combination with a quinolone is acceptable for neutropenic prophylaxis in low-risk patients and can be used in an outpatient regimen (Hughes et al., 2002). Secondary to the risk of severe hypersensitivity reactions associated with the use of penicillin antibiotics, the history of true penicillin allergy must be excluded before therapy with these agents is initiated. Laboratory abnormalities such as eosinophilia, leukopenia, thrombocytopenia, anemia, abnormal lever function tests, and false-positive Coombs test have been observed with the administration of penicillins (Bush, Calmon, & Johnson, 1995).

Amoxicillin/clavulanate potassium (Augmentin®)

The addition of clavulanic acid to amoxicillin broadens amoxicillin's spectrum of activity to include β-lactamase producing strains of methicillin-sensitive *Staphylococcus aureus, Bacteroides* spp., *Haemophilus influenzae,* and some of the Enterobacteriaceae (i.e., *Klebsiella, Escherichia coli*). The addition of clavulanic acid does not alter amoxicillin activity against streptococci, enterococci, *Clostridia, Salmonella,* and *Shigella* strains. This agent has little to no activity against *Citrobacter, Enterobacter, Pseudomonas,* and *Serratia.* Amoxicillin/clavulanic acid has very good activity against β-lactamase-producing oral anaerobes. This antibiotic can be considered for treatment of ear infections, sinusitis, lower respiratory tract, urinary tract, and skin and soft tissue infections (Bush et al., 1995). Many patients are transitioned from intravenous therapy to an outpatient antibiotic regimen containing amoxicillin-clavulanic acid for treatment of these infections.

A parenteral preparation of amoxicillin/clavulanic acid is not available in the United States. When amoxicillin/clavulanic acid is administered orally, it is quickly absorbed from the gastrointestinal tract and food does not affect this process. In order to decrease the incidence of gastrointestinal distress, patients should be advised to take this medication with food. Typical adult dosing for amoxicillin/clavulanic acid is 250 to 500 mg three times a day or 500 to 875 mg twice daily. Amoxicillin/ clavulanic acid is renally eliminated and dosage adjustments are recommended for patients with creatinine clearance less that 30 ml/min (Bush *et al.*, 1995).

Amoxicillin/clavulanic acid is well tolerated and the adverse effects associated with its administration include nausea, vomiting, diarrhea (attributed to the clavulanic acid component), candidal vaginitis, and skin rashes (Bush *et al.*, 1995). Noteworthy drug interactions documented with amoxicillin/clavulinic acid include allopurinol (increased frequency of rash), cimetidine (increased absorption of amoxicillin/clavulanic acid), methotrexate (decreased methotrexate elimination), oral contraceptives (decreased contraceptive efficacy) and probenecid (decreased excretion of amoxicillin/clavulanic acid).

Ampicillin sodium/sulbactam sodium (Unasyn®)

An ampicillin and sulbactam combination enhances the spectrum of antimicrobial activity of ampicillin to include β-lactamase-producing strains of *Staphylococcus aureus, Haemophilus influenzae, Moraxella catarrhalis, Escherichia coli, Klebsiella, Providencia, Proteus,* and anaerobes. This agent has no activity against *Citrobacter, Enterobacter, Pseudomonas,* and *Serratia.* Ampicillin/sulbactam has good antimicrobial activity against sensitive strains of enterococci. Ampicillin/sulbactam, with its broad spectrum of antimicrobial activity, plays a role in the treatment of intra-abdominal infections, gynecologic infections, lower respiratory tract infections, and skin and soft tissue infections (Bush *et al.*, 1995).

In the United States this antibiotic is only available as a parenteral preparation. The recommended dosing regimen for adult patients ranges from 1.5 to 3 g administered every 6 hours. Ampicillin/sulbactam is cleared renally and appropriate dosing adjustments are advised in patients with creatinine clearance below 30 ml/min. The list of drugs interacting with ampicillin/sulbactam is similar to that reported with amoxicillin/clavulanic acid. Aminoglycosides should not be administered concurrently with ampicillin-sulbactam via the same line due to potential aminoglycoside inactivation. Ampicillin/sulbactam is generally well tolerated and the most frequent adverse effects include nausea, vomiting, diarrhea, pain at the injection site, and skin rashes (Bush *et al.*, 1995).

Piperacillin sodium/tazobactam sodium (Zosyn®)

The addition of tazobactam to piperacillin expands the activity of this agent against β-lactamase producing Enterobacteriaceae, *Haemophilus influenzae, Neisseria gonorrhoeae,* and *Moraxella catarrhalis.* In vitro activity of this combination is comparable to imipenem/cilastatin and is better than that of ceftazidime. This agent has excellent activity against Gram-positive and Gram-negative anaerobes. In vitro inhibition of Bush type 1 β-lactamases observed with tazobactam does not translate to significant in vivo activity against the organisms known to produce these enzymes. Activity against *Pseudomonas aeruginosa* is not enhanced by the addition of tazobactam. Piperacillin/tazobactam has little activity against *Stenotrophomonis maltophilia*

(Bush *et al.*, 1995). In patients with febrile neutropenia, the successful use of piperacillin/tazobactam in combination with an aminoglycoside has been documented in several clinical trials (Mackie *et al.*, 1986; Kelsey *et al.*, 1992b; Hazel *et al.*, 1997). In addition, piperacillin/tazobactam is efficacious in the treatment of lower respiratory tract, intra-abdominal, urinary tract, and skin and soft tissue infections (Perry & Markham, 1999).

Piperacillin/tazobactam is only available for parenteral administration. The recommended dosing regimen for adult patients with normal renal function is 3.375 to 4.5 g every 6 hours as an intravenous infusion. Higher doses may be necessary in patients infected with *Pseudomonas aeruginosa.* This agent is eliminated renally and excreted to some extent in the bile. Dosing adjustments for renal function impairment should be initiated if calculated creatinine clearance falls below 40 ml/min; however, no dosage adjustments are necessary in patients with hepatic impairment (Bush *et al.*, 1995).

Piperacillin/tazobactam is usually well tolerated and the most common adverse effects associated with its use include nausea, diarrhea, headache, insomnia, skin rash, pruritus, and fever (Bush *et al.*, 1995). Pseudomembranous colitis may also occur in patients undergoing treatment with piperacillin/ tazobactam (Perry & Markham, 1999).

Ticarcillin disodium/clavulanate potassium (Timentin®)

The addition of clavulanic acid to ticarcillin expands its spectrum of activity to include 60% to 80% of ticarcillin-resistant strains of Enterobacteriaceae and all β-lactamase strains of *Bacteroides* spp., *Haemophilus influenzae,* and methicillin-sensitive *Staphylococcus aureus* (Nathwani & Wood, 1993). However, bacterial strains of *Citrobacter, Enterobacter, Pseudomonas,* and *Serratia* are known to produce Bush group 1 β-lactamases that are not susceptible to inhibition by clavulanic acid (Bush *et al.*, 1995). Therefore, addition of another agent is necessary to effectively eradicate these organisms if treatment with ticarcillin/clavulanic acid is selected. Ticarcillin/clavulanic acid has potential application in the treatment of lower respiratory infections, intra-abdominal infections, pelvic infections, osteomyelitis, skin and soft tissue infections, urinary tract infections, and bacteremia (Bush *et al.*, 1995). In neutropenic patients, empiric therapy with ticarcillin-clavulanic acid has been shown to be effective when it was combined with an aminoglycoside (Krieger *et al.*, 1985; Mackie *et al.*, 1986; Schaison *et al.*, 1986).

Ticarcillin/clavulanic acid is only available as a parenteral preparation. The recommended dosing regimen for adults is 3.1 g every 4 to 6 hours administered intravenously. Less frequent dosing of every 8 hours is recommended for treatment of urinary tract infections. Ticarcillin/clavulanic acid is cleared renally and appropriate dosage adjustments need to be initiated if creatinine clearance (CrCl) is less than 60 ml/min. Aminoglycosides should not be administered concurrently with ticarcillin-clavulanic acid via the same line due to potential aminoglycoside inactivation. In addition, probenecid administration may decrease renal tubular excretion of ticarcillin/

clavulanic acid, prolonging its half-life and increasing its serum concentration (Bush *et al.*, 1995).

Common adverse effects associated with ticarcillin/clavulanic acid include diarrhea, nausea, fever, phlebitis, and skin rashes. The ticarcillin component is associated with hypokalemia and a dose-dependent platelet dysfunction caused by binding of this drug to the adenosine 5'-diphosphate receptors on platelets. Potential prolongation of bleeding time needs to be considered in HSCT patients. In addition, ticarcillin/clavulanic acid contains a relatively high sodium load (4.8 mEq/g) and may contribute to volume overload and fluid retention in predisposed patients. Seizures have been reported with high drug levels of ticarcillin/clavulanic acid (Bush *et al.*, 1995).

Quinolones

Quinolones exhibit their antimicrobial activity in a concentration-dependent manner through their inhibition of DNA gyrase. DNA gyrase is a bacterial enzyme that is essential for bacterial DNA replication (Zhanel & Noreddin, 2001). Nalidixic acid and cinoxacin are the oldest agents of this class; however, the role of these agents in HSCT is limited by their narrow spectrum of activity and rapid development of resistance. The development of ciprofloxacin and ofloxacin represented a significant development for agents of this class. These agents have a broader spectrum of Gram-negative activity that allow for their use in treatment of systemic organisms such as *Pseudomonas* species, *Moraxella catarrhalis,* and *Hemophilus influenza* (Mandell & Petri, 1996). Many additional quinolone agents have been marketed since then, such as levofloxacin, trovafloxacin, sparfloxacin, and grepafloxacin. Postmarketing reports of cardiac toxicity, however, led to the removal of sparfloxacin and grepafloxacin from the market, while reports of hepatotoxicity and death resulted in the restricted availability and use of trovafloxacin. These agents all have a broader spectrum of activity that includes Gram-positive (such as methicillin-susceptible *Staphylococcus aureus* and *S. pneumoniae*) and Gram-negative bacteria. Moxifloxacin and gatifloxacin are the newest agents of this class. The spectrum of activity of these agents is the broadest of the agents in this class and includes activity against Gram-positive, Gram-negative, and anaerobic organisms such as *Actinomyces, Bacteroides* species, *Clostridium* species (excluding *C. difficile*) and *Peptostreptococcus* species (Perry *et al.*, 2002). In one study comparing the in vitro effects of ciprofloxacin, levofloxacin, moxifloxacin, and gatifloxacin, it appeared that moxifloxacin and gatifloxacin have enhanced activity against *S. pneumoniae* (Saravolatz *et al.*, 2001). Ciprofloxacin has less activity against Gram-positive organisms such as *Streptococcus* species, including *Streptococcus pneumoniae,* when compared to the newer quinolones. This suggests that ciprofloxacin may be less effective in eradicating infections caused by these organisms (Zhanel & Noreddin, 2001). As a general rule, as the spectrum of activity broadens with newer generation quinolones (levofloxacin, moxifloxacin, and gatifloxacin), the activity against

Gram-negative organisms (including *Pseudomonas aeruginosa*) decreases.

As a class, quinolones have excellent oral bioavailability and may be taken with or without food. With the exception of moxifloxacin, which is only available in an oral formulation, the other quinolones are available in oral and intravenous dosage forms. These agents undergo hepatic metabolism and renal elimination. Dosage reductions for all quinolones, except moxifloxacin, should be made for renal dysfunction (CrCl <50 ml/min for levofloxacin and ciprofloxacin, and CrCl <30 ml/min for gatifloxacin). Dosage reductions for severe hepatic dysfunction are recommended for moxifloxacin and gatifloxacin; however, specific guidelines for reduction are not available at this time (Rodvold & Neuhauser, 2001).

Quinolones are generally safe and well-tolerated medications. Gastrointestinal and CNS effects are the most frequent adverse effects reported with quinolone use. Nausea and diarrhea are the most frequently described GI effects. CNS effects are most often described as headache, dizziness, and drowsiness. Seizures are rare and associated with patients who have predisposing factors such as an underlying seizure disorder, head trauma, anoxia, metabolic disorders, or concomitant therapy with NSAIDs or theophylline. Of the currently marketed agents, trovafloxacin has the highest incidence, followed by gatifloxacin and moxifloxacin, while levofloxacin has the lowest incidence of CNS effects. Phototoxicity is a class effect and can be concerning with quinolone therapy. These effects vary in presentation, from mild erythema to bullous drug eruptions. They are often delayed (~3 weeks following the initial exposure), but can be acute following the administration of the initial dose. Phototoxic reactions are reversible upon drug discontinuation. Lomefloxacin and sparfloxacin have the highest incidence, while moxifloxacin and gatifloxacin have the lowest incidence, of phototoxicity. Prolongation of the QT interval is another concerning class effect of quinolone therapy. It occurs most commonly with grepafloxacin and sparfloxacin and consequently these agents were withdrawn from the market. Unlike these two agents, the other quinolones do not possess clinically significant cardiac effects. Other less common adverse effects include nephrotoxicity, ocular toxicity, hypersensitivity reactions, and arthropathy. True anaphylaxis reactions and hematologic toxicities are rare with quinolone therapy (Rodvold & Neuhauser, 2001).

Clinically significant drug interactions with quinolone therapy include antacids, mineral supplements, sucralfate, theophylline, caffeine, and warfarin. Multivalent cation (magnesium, aluminum, calcium, iron, zinc)-containing antacids and supplements bind with quinolones and form an insoluble complex that results in decreased drug absorption. Sucralfate also interferes with quinolone absorption, an effect that is attributed to the aluminum component of the drug. Appropriate spacing of dose times of the quinolone and the interacting agent is essential to ensure adequate drug absorption. Quinolones must be taken 2 hours before or 4 to 6 hours following the cation-containing drug. Quinolones can inhibit the clearance of theophylline and caffeine. This interaction is not a class effect but depends on each quinolone's affinity for the cytochrome P450-1A2 isoenzyme. Enoxacin has the strongest affinity for this isoenzyme followed by ciprofloxacin. Consequently, when theophylline is administered with enoxacin or ciprofloxacin, appropriate monitoring of theophylline levels is recommended. In comparison, ofloxacin, levofloxacin, trovafloxacin, gatifloxacin, and moxifloxacin have lower affinities for the 1A2 isoenzyme and do not appear to affect theophylline or caffeine metabolism. Anecdotal case reports suggested that quinolones may inhibit the metabolism of warfarin; however, prospective studies examining this interaction failed to show such interactions. Concomitant administration of cyclosporine and ciprofloxacin may lead to increases in serum creatinine. The exact mechanism is unknown; however, it may be due to synergistic nephrotoxic effects or inhibition of cyclosporine metabolism by ciprofloxacin. Consequently, cyclosporine levels should be monitored when concomitantly administered with ciprofloxacin. Concomitant administration of quinolones with inducers of hepatic cytochrome P450 enzymes, such as rifampin or phenytoin, may increase the metabolism of quinolones (Fish, 2001).

Metronidazole

Metronidazole is a nitroimidazole antibiotic that exerts its activity through a reduction reaction. This reaction deprives bacterial organisms of reduction equivalents and ultimately results in bacterial DNA breakage (Tracy & Webster, 1996). Metronidazole is the drug of choice (over oral vancomycin) for the treatment of pseudomembranous colitis caused by *Clostridium difficile* in immunocompromised and immunocompetent patients. Metronidazole's spectrum of activity also includes various protozoal species such as *Giardia* spp., *Gardnerella* spp., and *Entamoeba histolytica*, and Gram-positive and negative anaerobic organisms such as *Bacteroides* spp., *Fusobacterium* spp., *Peptostreptococci*, and *Clostridium perfringens* (Kasten, 1999).

Oral administration of metronidazole results in rapid and complete absorption that is unaffected by food. Metronidazole is hepatically metabolized and renally excreted and dosage adjustments may be necessary with hepatic and severe renal failure (CrCl < 10 ml/min) (Freeman, Klutman, & Lamp, 1997). Typical dosing for *Clostridium difficile* treatment is 250 mg every 6 hours to 500 mg every 8 hours for 10 to 14 days. The oral route is preferred; however, intravenous administration can be used when patients are unable to take oral medications. For empiric coverage or treatment of documented anaerobic infections, higher doses of 500 mg every 6 hours (up to a daily maximum dose of 4 g) may be necessary (Kasten, 1999).

CNS and GI complaints are the most common adverse effects associated with metronidazole use. CNS side effects, including seizures, encephalopathy, ataxia, and peripheral neuropathy, are reversible upon drug discontinuation. These effects are usually dose-dependent and associated with prolonged use.

GI discomfort and metallic taste in the mouth are also common complaints. Nausea (12% incidence) is frequent, whereas dry mouth, vomiting, and diarrhea are less frequent. Other rare adverse effects include leukopenia, nephrotoxicity, hepatotoxicity, pneumonitis, visual loss, pancreatitis, and dermatologic effects (Freeman *et al.*, 1997).

Metronidazole inhibits the metabolism of carbamazepine, calcineurin inhibitors (cyclosporine and tacrolimus), fosphenytoin, phenytoin, and warfarin. Appropriate monitoring of serum drug levels and INR should occur when these medications are given concomitantly to avoid unwanted toxicities. Enhanced hepatic enzyme metabolism of metronidazole has also been reported when given with fosphenytoin, phenobarbital, or phenytoin. Appropriate monitoring of clinical response to metronidazole is warranted when these medications are given together. Disulfiram-like reactions, characterized by nausea, vomiting, pyschosis, and confusion, have occurred when metronidazole is given with alcohol and alcohol-containing medications (such as intravenous trimethoprim/sulfamethoxazole, cough syrups, and etoposide). Therefore, the combination of metronidazole with alcohol or alcohol-containing medications should be avoided (Williams & Woodcock, 2000).

Vancomycin

Vancomycin is a tricyclic glycopeptide antibiotic that inhibits bacterial cell wall synthesis. It also alters the permeability of bacterial cell membranes and inhibits RNA synthesis. Overuse of vancomycin has resulted in the emergence of microbial resistance, particularly in enterococci. Its use should be restricted to specific indications in order to prevent the spread of resistance. Vancomycin should be withheld from initial empiric treatment of febrile neutropenia unless a patient has:

1. A suspected serious infection related to an indwelling catheter (i.e., bacteremia or tunnel infection);
2. Known colonization with methicillin-resistant *S. aureus* or a penicillin- or cephalosporin-resistant pneumococcus;
3. A positive blood culture for Gram-positive bacteria (therapy should subsequently be changed, when appropriate, based on final identification and susceptibility testing);
4. Hypotension or another symptom of sepsis (Centers for Disease Control and Prevention, 1995).

The normal dose is 10 to 15 mg/kg by intravenous infusion every 12 hours (usually 1g i.v. every 12 hours) for systemic Gram-positive infections. Vancomycin should be infused over at least 1 hour to minimize infusion-related side effects. Vancomycin is eliminated renally and must be adjusted for renal dysfunction. Anuric patients may require as little as 1 g every 7 to 10 days. Monitoring vancomycin serum concentrations can aid the clinician in determining how to adjust doses. Target peak concentrations are between 20 and 35 mcg/ml and target trough concentrations are between 5 and 12 mcg/ml. Vancomycin is bacteriostatic and its efficacy is dependent on maintenance of sufficient trough levels. Since clinical efficacy is not correlated with vancomycin peak concentrations and there is little evidence that toxicity is related to peak levels, many practitioners monitor only trough levels. Patients for whom both peak and trough concentration monitoring is still recommended include:

1. Patients with rapidly changing renal function;
2. Patients with CNS infection, endocarditis or other site of infection that is difficult to penetrate;
3. Patients who are on concomitant nephrotoxic agents (especially aminoglycosides);
4. Patients who are not responding to therapy (Wilhelm & Estes, 1999). Vancomycin is also used orally to treat *Staphylococcus aureus* enterocolitis and *Clostridium difficile* colitis at doses of 125 mg every 6 hours. Doses may be increased to 250 or 500 mg every 6 hours for resistant infections. When administered orally, vancomycin is not significantly absorbed and this route of administration should not be used to treat systemic infections. Likewise, intravenous vancomycin does not reach sufficient levels in the gastrointestinal tract to effectively treat antibiotic-associated colitis and therefore should not be used for this indication (Wilhelm & Estes, 1999).

The most common adverse reaction to vancomycin is red man syndrome. Red man syndrome is an infusion-related, histamine-mediated reaction characterized by flushing of the face, neck, chest, and upper extremities. Though red man syndrome is not a true anaphylactic reaction, in rare cases patients may experience a sudden and profound drop in blood pressure or even cardiac arrest (Newfield & Roizen, 1979; Glicklich & Figura, 1984; Mayhew & Deutsch, 1985; Symons, Hobbes, & Leaver, 1985). Red man syndrome often occurs with the first dose of vancomycin, since it is caused by histamine release. Management of red man syndrome includes slowing the infusion rate and/or premedicating with antihistamines. True IgE-mediated anaphylactic reactions rarely occur secondary to vancomycin, and do not usually occur with the first dose since IgE antibodies to the drug have not yet developed. Some patients who have experienced anaphylactic reactions have successfully undergone desensitization, allowing them to be treated with vancomycin despite their allergy to it (Anne, Middleton, & Reisman, 1994).

Significant nephrotoxicity caused by vancomycin is uncommon, though it may potentiate the renal injury caused by concurrently administered aminoglycosides. The incidence of acute renal failure when vancomycin is given with an aminoglycoside may reach 20% to 30% (Appel *et al.*, 1986; Rybak *et al.*, 1990, 1999).

Linezolid

Linezolid is an oxazolidinone derivative antibiotic that inhibits bacterial protein synthesis by binding to bacterial 23S ribosomal RNA of the 50S subunit. This prevents the formation of the initiation complex with the 70S ribosomal subunit, which is essential for the bacterial translation process. Linezolid is bacteriostatic

against enterococci and staphylococci and bactericidal against most streptococci strains, *Bacteroides fragilis,* and *C. perfringens* (Clemett & Markham 2000). Linezolid has been used to successfully treat infections caused by antibiotic-susceptible and antibiotic-resistant strains of Gram-positive organisms, including vancomycin-resistant enterococci, methicillin-resistant *S. aureus,* and penicillin-resistant *S. pneumoniae* (Rubinstein *et al.*, 2001). The oral bioavalability of linezolid is 100% in normal volunteers, thus linezolid is dosed 600 mg twice daily orally or by intravenous infusion. The pharmacokinetics of linezolid appear to be unaffected by renal or hepatic dysfunction; therefore, no dosage adjustments are necessary for either condition (Batts, 2000).

Myelosuppression, including anemia, leukopenia, thrombocytopenia, and pancytopenia is the most concerning side effect of linezolid in HSCT patients. It appears to be more common in patients who have been on linezolid for >10 to 14 days and is generally reversible (Attassi *et al.*, 2002). Headache, nausea, and diarrhea were the most common side effects seen during phase III trials.

Linezolid is a weak, reversible, nonselective inhibitor of monoamine oxidase. There is a theoretic risk for adrenergic agents (phenylpropanolamine, pseudoephedrine, sympathomimetic agents, vasopressor or dopaminergic agents) used concomitantly to cause hypertension or hypertensive crisis and a risk for serotonergic agents (TCAs, venlafaxine, trazodone, sibutramine, meperidine, dextromethorphan, and SSRIs) used concomitantly to cause serotonin syndrome. To date there are no reports of hypertensive crisis secondary to drug interactions with linezolid; however, there is one case report of a patient developing serotonin syndrome after taking linezolid with sertraline, bupropion, and trazodone for 2 months. This patient's symptoms reportedly resolved upon discontinuation of the serotonergic medications and administration of cyproheptadine, a serotonin antagonist (Lavery *et al.*, 2001). The manufacturer recommends that patients be instructed to avoid foods or drinks that contain tyramine, such as aged cheeses, dried meats, sauerkraut, pickled foods, soy sauce, tap beers, or red wines.

Quinupristin/Dalfopristin

Quinupristin/dalfopristin (Synercid®) is a combination streptogramin product with inhibitory effects against most Gram-positive bacteria including methicillin-resistant *Staphylococcus aureus* (MRSA), vancomycin-resistant *Enterococcus faecium* (VREF), penicillin-resistant *Streptococcus pneumoniae,* other streptococci, *Clostridium perfringens,* and *Peptostreptococcus* spp. It also has activity against *Moraxella catarrhalis, Legionella pneumophilia,* and *Mycoplasma pneumoniae* (Lamb, Figgitt, & Faulds, 1999). *Enterococcus faecalis* is not included in quinupristin/dalfopristin's spectrum of activity. These two streptogramins work synergistically to inhibit bacterial protein synthesis by binding to different sites on the 50S ribosomal subunit. Quinupristin/dalfopristin is only available in a parenteral formulation and must be administered as an intravenous infusion. The dose is 7.5 mg/kg every 8 hours for VREF or 7.5 mg/kg every 12 hours for complicated skin infections. Dose adjustments are not necessary for renal dysfunction, but may be necessary for hepatic dysfunction. Specific recommendations for dosage adjustments in patients with hepatic dysfunction are not available at this time (Lamb *et al.,* 1999).

Quinupristin/dalfopristin should be administered through a central line whenever possible, since it can cause pain and phlebitis when infused through a peripheral vein. The addition of diphenhydramine or hydrocortisone does not prevent or diminish this effect; however, these infusion-related effects are dose- and concentration-dependent (Low, 1995). Arthralgias and myalgias have been reported to occur in up to 47% of patients during therapy with quinupristin/dalfopristin (Olsen, Rebuck, & Rupp, 2001). Occasionally these are severe enough that cessation of therapy is necessary. Arthralgias and myalgias are reversible upon discontinuation of the drug. Hyperbilirubinemia and elevated liver enzymes have been reported to occur in clinical trials (Allington & Rivey, 2001). Monitoring of liver function tests is recommended during therapy with quinupristin/dalfopristin. Other side effects seen with quinupristin/dalfopristin are headache, nausea, vomiting, diarrhea, rash, and pruritus.

Quinupristin/dalfopristin is an inhibitor of cytochrome P450 3A4 enzymes, therefore coadministration with any agent that is primarily metabolized by these enzymes should be avoided (Lamb *et al.,* 1999). Quinupristin/dalfopristin is likely to increase levels of HMG-CoA reductase inhibitors, calcium channel blockers, some benzodiazepines, protease inhibitors, non-nucleoside reverse transcriptase inhibitors, vinca alkaloids, paclitaxel, docetaxel, methylprednisolone, carbamazepine, and quinidine. It significantly increases cyclosporine AUC, half-life, and C_{max}. Careful monitoring of cyclosporine and tacrolimus levels is necessary if quinupristin/dalfopristin is administered concomitantly. Avoid using quinupristin/dalfopristin in patients taking cytochrome P450 substrates that may cause QT prolongation.

Trimethoprim/sulfamethoxazole

Trimethoprim/sulfamethoxazole (TMP-SMX) is a combination antibiotic that exerts its antimicrobial actions through a two-step enzymatic pathway whereby sulfamethoxazole inhibits para-aminobenzoic acid and trimethoprim inhibits dihydrolate reductase. This two-step process results in the inhibition of folic acid synthesis by bacterial cells and the conversion of dihydrofolate to tetrahydrofolate (Mandell & Petri, 1996). TMP-SMX is the agent of choice for the prophylaxis and treatment of *Pneumocystis carinii* pneumonia (PCP). Advantages of TMP-SMX over alternative therapies include a lower incidence of PCP infection, excellent tissue penetration, most rapid clinical response (3 to 5 days in mild to moderate disease), and 100% oral bioavailability (Fishman, 1998). PCP prophylaxis is indicated for all immunosuppressed allogeneic HSCT patients. Routine PCP prophylaxis in all autologous HSCT patients is controversial, since their period of immunosuppression is shorter compared to allogeneic HSCT patients. PCP prophylaxis should be considered in autologous HSCT patients if they

have an underlying hematologic malignancy, are receiving intense conditioning regimens or graft manipulation, or have received fludarabine or cladribine chemotherapy (Souza, Boeckh, & Gooley, 1999; Jarvis, Kaplan, & Edlin, 2001).

PCP prophylaxis with TMP-SMX or alternative agents may be initiated prior to transplant; however, it should be discontinued 48 hours prior to stem cell infusion to prevent delays in engraftment (Tuan, Dennison & Weisdorf, 1992). PCP prophylaxis should be restarted upon engraftment in all allogeneic and qualifying autologous patients. For prophylaxis in allogeneic HSCT patients, TMP-SMX should continue until immunosuppression is discontinued (~6 months posttransplant) unless patients must remain on immunosuppression for GVHD treatment or have chronic GVHD (Fishman, 1998; Dykewicz, 2001; Jarvis *et al.,* 2001). Dosing regimens for prophylaxis include 1 double-strength tablet (160 mg/800 mg) twice daily for two consecutive days of the week, 1 double-strength tablet daily for 3 consecutive days of the week, or 1 single-strength (80 mg/400 mg) tablet daily (Dykewicz, 2001; Jarvis *et al.,* 2001). Dosing for PCP treatment is based on the trimethoprim component and usually consists of 15 to 20 mg/kg/day for 10 to 21 days. Dosing adjustments are recommended in patients with renal dysfunction (CrCl <50 ml/min) (Fishman, 1998).

Most commonly described adverse effects include rash (including Stevens-Johnson syndrome[1]), nausea and vomiting, fever, transaminase elevations, neutropenia, anemia, thrombocytopenia, and renal dysfunction. A majority of these effects are associated with the sulfa component of TMP-SMX and are often reversible upon discontinuation of the agent. Hyperkalemia is uncommon when TMP-SMX is used for prophylaxis; however, it is more common when a higher dose is required for treatment. This is mainly because trimethoprim structurally resembles a potassium-sparing diuretic (Hsu, 1995). In patients with declining neutrophil counts or minor intolerances such as rash, transaminase elevations, and gastrointestinal intolerances secondary to TMP-SMX, alternative TMP-SMX dosing regimens are recommended prior to switching to less effective alternative therapies. In patients with a history of a rash, TMP-SMX desensitization should be considered prior to changing therapies (Cortese, Soucy, & Endy, 1996) (see Chapter 78). Folinic acid supplementation has been investigated in humans and animal models for potential management of TMP-SMX-induced neutropenia. The role of folinic acid is controversial (Heidt, Kieskamp, & Timmersman, 1985; Bjornson *et al.,* 1986; D'Antonio *et al.,* 1986; Bygbjerg, Lund, & Hording, 1988). Consequently, use of folinic acid (leucovorin) is not recommended until greater data for safety and efficacy are available (Nunn & Allistone, 1984; Safrin, Lee, & Sande, 1994). Increased photosensitivity is also associated with TMP-SMX use and sunscreen (SPF 15 or higher) should be applied to sun-exposed areas at least 30 minutes prior to being outdoors to protect the skin.

---

[1] Albert Stevens, American pediatrician, 1884–1945.
Frank Johnson, American pediatrician, 1894–1934.

TMP-SMX is hepatically metabolized and renally excreted. Consequently, hepatic metabolism of warfarin, phenytoin, and fosphenytoin is impaired with concurrent TMP-SMX administration. Renal excretion of procainamide, metformin, methotrexate, and digoxin is also reduced with concurrent TMP-SMX use. Appropriate monitoring of drug levels and INR is warranted when these agents are given with TMP-SMX. Hypoglycemia has been reported when sulfonylureas and TMP-SMX are combined and close monitoring of blood sugars is recommended when these agents are used. Hyperkalemia may be potentiated if TMP-SMX is used concurrently with ACE inhibitors, potassium-sparing diuretics, or potassium supplements. Appropriate monitoring of potassium is warranted when these medications are given in combination. Concomitant administration with cyclosporine may result in an increase in serum creatinine.

Dapsone, pentamidine, and atovaquone

Dapsone, pentamidine, and atovaquone are alternatives for patients who are intolerant to TMP-SMX. Dapsone is the drug of second choice for PCP prophylaxis as a single agent or for treatment in combination with trimethoprim or pyrimethamine (Hughes *et al.*, 1997). It should not be used for PCP prophylaxis in patients who tolerate TMP-SMX, as a higher incidence of PCP infections has been associated with dapsone use (Beumont *et al.*, 1996; Souza *et al.*, 1999). Typical oral dosing for prophylaxis and treatment is 100 mg daily; however, alternative regimens are also effective. Overall, dapsone is better tolerated than TMP-SMX but may be associated with dose-related ($\geq$ 200 mg/day) hemolytic anemia, methemoglobinemia, and peripheral motor weakness. Testing for the presence of glucose-6-phosphate dehydrogenase deficiency should occur prior to initiating dapsone therapy; however, negative results are not reliably predictive, as hemolysis can also occur in patients with normal activity (Pengelly, 1963; DeGowin *et al.*, Carson, 1966; DeGowin, 1967). Other adverse effects include agranulocytosis, aplastic anemia, hypersensitivity, and dermatologic reactions.

Aerosolized pentamidine, when used for PCP prophylaxis, is associated with the highest incidence of PCP infections, increased risk of other infections, decreased survival, medical professional and caregiver exposure, and cumbersome administration (Link *et al.*, 1993; Vasconcelles *et al.*, 2000). Atovaquone use for PCP prophylaxis and treatment has been studied in autologous bone marrow transplantation and HIV patients. Its use is associated with higher treatment failures, lower prevention rates, poor oral bioavailability and higher costs compared to other currently available options for PCP prophylaxis and treatment (Haile & Flaherty, 1993; Chan *et al.*, 1999; Colby *et al.*, 1999). Recommendations for use in the transplant setting are limited at this time.

Macrolides

Erythromycin, clarithromycin, and azithromycin are macrolide antibiotics that inhibit protein synthesis by binding reversibly to the 50S ribosomal subunits (Kapusnik-Uner, Sande, Chambers,

1996). These agents have good activity against Gram-positive organisms such as *Streptococcus,* as well as *Mycoplasma,* and *Legionella* species and limited activity against Gram-negative organisms such as *Hemophilus influenzae;* however, their widespread use posttransplant is limited by the narrow spectrum of activity, safety profile, patient tolerability, and drug interactions seen with these agents (Amsden, 1996).

Clarithromycin and erythromycin share similar spectrum of activities, pharmacokinetics, and pharmacodynamics. Azithromycin, however, differs from these two agents. Erythromycin and clarithromycin undergo hepatic metabolism via the cytochrome P450-3A enzyme system, while azithromycin undergoes biliary metabolism. Consequently, a lower incidence of drug interactions is seen with azithromycin. Dosage adjustment for hepatic impairment is unnecessary with macrolide therapy. Dosage adjustment for renal impairment (CrCl <30 ml/min) is necessary only with clarithromycin (Amsden, 1996; Periti *et al.,* 1992).

Gastrointestional disturbances are the most common side effect reported with macrolide use, the incidence being highest with erythromycin (21%–32%) compared to clarithromycin (13%) and azithromycin (12%). The incidence of nausea associated with oral administration of erythromycin is not improved when it is changed to intravenous administration. Oral erythromycin is associated with reversible allergic reactions, reversible cholestatic hepatitis, and mild AST elevations. Intravenous erythromycin is also associated with pain upon injection and phlebitis. Severity may be decreased with slower rates of infusion and further drug dilution. Rare side effects include QT prolongation with ventricular tachycardia, and dose dependent (> 4 g/day) transient auditory impairment (Amsden, 1996).

Clinically significant drug interactions seen with erythromycin and clarithromycin include warfarin, benzodiazepines, digoxin, penicillins, carbamazepine, theophylline, and cyclosporine through a CYP450 3A-enzyme induction and inhibition. Appropriate monitoring of these drug levels is warranted when these agents are administered with clarithromycin or erythromycin. Azithromycin does not possess these interactions; however, coadministration of azithromycin with antacids is associated with decreased serum azithromycin concentrations. Though these interactions are clinically insignificant, the manufacturer continues to recommend spacing of azithromycin 1 hour before or 2 hours after antacid use (Von Rosensteil *et al.,* 1995; Nahata, 1996; Rapp, 1998). Clarithromycin may be taken without regards to meals; with the exception of enteric-coated erythromycin preparations, all other erythromycin preparations should be taken on an empty stomach. Azithromycin capsules and multidose oral suspension should be administered at least 1 hour before or 2 hours after meals, while azithromycin tablets and single-dose oral suspension can be administered regardless of food (AHFS, 2000).

Antifungal agents

Triazole antifungal agents, including fluconazole, itraconazole, and voriconazole, work by inhibiting the cytochrome P-450 dependent enzyme lanosterol 14-alpha-demethylase, which is responsible for converting lanosterol to ergosterol. Ergosterol is a component of the fungal cell membrane. Disruptions in its biosynthesis caused by triazoles result in significant damage to the cell membrane and increased permeability (Groll et al., 1998; Terrell, 1999). Though this damage ultimately results in cell lysis and cell death, the triazoles are generally considered to be fungistatic at the concentrations that are clinically achievable. Since the most common fungal infection in HSCT patients is candidiasis, allogeneic transplant recipients should be given fluconazole prophylaxis to prevent invasive candidiasis during neutropenia. Autologous transplant recipients who have leukemia or lymphoma, or who are likely to have prolonged neutropenia or significant mucositis from intense conditioning regimens, should also receive fluconazole prophylaxis (Centers for Disease Control and Prevention, 2000)

Fluconazole

Fluconazole is the most widely used triazole antifungal agent. Since its spectrum of activity includes *Candida albicans,* with less activity against *C. glabrata* and no activity against *C. krusei* or aspergillus species, its role in HSCT is primarily as prophylaxis against *C. albicans* infection at doses of 200 to 400 mg orally or by intravenous infusion once daily. It has been shown to be effective in preventing local and systemic *Candida* infections and has been shown to improve survival in patients undergoing HSCT (Marr *et al.,* 2000; Wolff *et al.,* 2000). Fluconazole prophylaxis should be started with the first day of conditioning and continued at least until engraftment. There is evidence that continuing fluconazole until day +75 post allogeneic transplant is associated with persistent protection against disseminated candidiasis and related death; therefore the Seattle group routinely continues fluconazole prophylaxis until day +75 in allogeneic transplant recipients (Marr *et al.,* 2000). It can be given orally, as tablets or liquid, or by intravenous infusion. It is well absorbed orally with a bioavailability of 85% to 90% and absorption is not affected by food or gastric pH (Groll *et al.,* 1998; Terrell, 1999). Fluconazole is primarily excreted unchanged in the urine, therefore doses must be adjusted in patients with renal dysfunction (Fluconazole package insert).

Itraconazole

Itraconazole was the first azole shown to be effective for the treatment of *Aspergillus* infections (Kauffman & Carves, 1997; Sheehan *et al.,* 1999; Terrell, 1999; Luna *et al.,* 2000). In contrast to fluconazole, the bioavailability of itraconazole varies widely from patient to patient. Dissolution and absorption are greatly affected by gastric pH. H2 blockers and proton pump inhibitors may impair absorption. It is recommended that itraconazole capsules be taken with food and an acidic beverage like cola or cranberry juice to maximize absorption. Itraconazole liquid formulation increases bioavailability (over

capsules) by 30% when taken with food, and by another 25% when taken on an empty stomach (Reynes *et al.,* 1997; Barone *et al.,* 1998). Therefore, the Seattle Cancer Care Alliance uses itraconazole liquid as its oral formulation of choice, rather than capsules, and instructs patients to take the liquid on an empty stomach. Oral doses are 200 mg twice daily or can be calculated based on weight (2.5 mg/kg orally BID). The intravenous dose is 200 mg i.v. Q12h × 4 doses, then 200 mg i.v. QD. Plasma itraconazole levels above 250 ng/ml correlate with effective prophylaxis in neutropenic patients (Boogaerts *et al.,* 1989, 2001a,b). Itraconazole is extensively metabolized by the cytochrome P450 3A4 isoenzyme and does not require dose adjustment in renal dysfunction. However, the solubilizer used in the injection (hydroxypropyl-beta-cyclodextrin) is excreted by the kidneys and may accumulate in patients with renal dysfunction. It is recommended that the intravenous formulation of itraconazole not be used in patients with a creatinine clearance >30 ml/min (Itraconazole package insert).

Voriconazole

Voriconazole is a potent azole antifungal with a wide spectrum of activity that was recently approved in the United States. Like the other triazole antifungals, voriconazole works by inhibiting ergosterol biosynthesis. Voriconazole exhibits excellent bioavailability and a broad in vitro spectrum, including activity against *Candida* spp. (including *C. krusei* and *C. glabrata*), *Aspergillus* spp., and *Cryptococcus neoformans.* The antifungal spectrum of voriconazole does not include Zygomycetes. In a trial comparing voriconazole to liposomal amphotericin B for empirical therapy in patients with neutropenia and persistent fever, voriconazole was found to be as effective as liposomal amphotericin B. The doses of voriconazole used in this trial were 6 mg/kg intravenously every 12 hours for two doses (loading dose), then 3 mg/kg intravenously every 12 hours (maintenance dose). After at least 3 days of intravenous therapy, patients were switched to oral voriconazole 200 mg every 12 hours. Voriconazole maintenance dosing could be increased in the study to 4 mg/kg intravenously every 12 hours or 300 mg orally every 12 hours if there was evidence of fungal infection (Walsh *et al.,* 2002).

The triazoles are generally well tolerated, but may cause nausea, abdominal pain, vomiting, and diarrhea. Rash and headache occur fairly frequently with these agents. Decreased libido and impotence have been reported to occur occasionally with itraconazole therapy. Mild elevations in liver function tests occur in 1% to 7% of patients and are generally reversible upon discontinuation of the drug, or sometimes resolve spontaneously without a change in dose. Severe hepatotoxicity to itraconazole, including liver failure and death, has been reported to occur in patients with or without pre-existing liver disease. Clinicians should weigh the benefits versus the risks before initiating therapy with triazole antifungals. In May 2001 the FDA issued a letter warning that rare cases of congestive heart failure (CHF) and pulmonary edema have been reported with itraconazole during postmarketing surveillance. Clinicians should discontinue itraconazole if signs and symptoms of CHF appear during therapy. Side effects to voriconazole reported thus far include transient, reversible visual disturbances, elevated liver enzymes, and skin reactions. The visual disturbances are characterized as an alteration in the perception of light and are seen usually during the first infusion, but resolve with subsequent infusions. Visual hallucinations, distinct from other visual disturbances, have also been reported during treatment with voriconazole (Maschmeyer, 2002; Walsh et al., 2002).

Triazole antifungals are inhibitors of cytochrome P450 3A4 enzymes leading to elevated levels of drugs that are metabolized by these enzymes. Itraconazole and voriconazole are more potent inhibitors of cytochrome P450 enzymes; therefore interactions caused by these two agents are more clinically significant than those caused by fluconazole. Coadministration of itraconazole or voriconazole with terfenadine, astemizole, cisapride, pimozide, or quinidine is contraindicated, since inhibition of metabolism of these agents by itraconazole/voriconazole may lead to life-threatening arrhythmias. Coadministration of voriconazole with ergot alkaloids is contraindicated since voriconazole may increase the plasma concentration of ergot alkaloids and lead to ergotism. Coadministration of itraconazole with HMG Co-A reductase inhibitors metabolized by cytochrome P450 3A4 (i.e., simvastatin and lovastatin) is also contraindicated, since inhibition of their metabolism increases the risk of developing myopathy and rhabdomyolysis. Pravastatin and fluvastatin are least likely to be affected by itraconazole and can be used as alternatives to simvastatin or lovastatin in patients taking itraconazole or voriconazole. Atorvastatin metabolism is significantly inhibited by itraconazole and concomitant use is not recommended. If concomitant use is deemed necessary, dose reduction of atorvastatin and close monitoring of creatine kinase (CK) levels is warranted. If a patient develops any signs or symptoms of myopathy or rhabdomyolysis or CK levels are significantly elevated from baseline, atorvastatin should be discontinued immediately. Caution should be used when coadministering azole antifungals with benzodiazepines, since inhibition of metabolism may increase benzodiazepine concentrations and enhance the intensity and duration of benzodiazepine adverse effects. One study looking at the effect of voriconazole on the pharmacokinetics of cyclosporine in renal transplant recipients found that the mean cyclosporine AUC increased 1.7-fold with concurrent administration of voriconazole. Authors of this study recommended decreasing the cyclosporine dose by 50% and monitoring cyclosporine levels carefully when voriconazole is initiated. The same recommendations have been made for itraconazole. Likewise, the cyclosporine level should be monitored and the dose increased as necessary when voriconazole/itraconazole therapy is discontinued or interrupted (Romero et al., 2002). Concomitant voriconazole and sirolimus administration is contraindicated since sirolimus levels are increased significantly. Coadministration of voriconazole with rifampin, rifabutin, carbamazepine, or long-acting barbiturates (i.e., phenobarbital) is contraindicated since these agents induce the metabolism of voriconazole, leading to potentially subtherapeutic levels of voriconazole.

Amphotericin B

Amphotericin B is a polyene antifungal agent that binds to ergosterol located in the plasma membranes of fungi, altering cell membrane permeability and causing leakage of cell components with subsequent cell death. Amphotericin B is effective against both *Candida* and *Aspergillus,* the two most common invasive fungal infections in neutropenic patients, and its use has long been the standard of care for neutropenic fever unresponsive to broad-spectrum antibiotics (Gallis, Drew, & Pickard, 1990; Grasela et al., 1990; Groll et al., 1996). Trials comparing conventional amphotericin B with some triazoles and with lipid amphotericin B formulations have raised the question of whether conventional amphotericin B should remain the first-line agent (White et al., 1998; Walsh et al., 1999; Winston et al., 2000; Boogaerts et al., 2001a). The doses traditionally used for empiric treatment of febrile neutropenia are 0.5 to 1 mg/kg/day by intravenous infusion. Doses as high as 1.5 mg/kg/day have been used to treat proven *Aspergillus* infections, but this dose should not be exceeded.

Nephrotoxicity is the most common and problematic toxicity of amphotericin B with some degree of renal toxicity occurring in over 80% of patients. Amphotericin B causes renal vasoconstriction resulting in cortical ischemia and a fall in glomerular filtration rate. Renal impairment manifests as an increase in BUN and serum creatinine, and a decrease in creatinine clearance. Renal impairment is often accompanied by increased uric acid secretion, potassium, magnesium, and bicarbonate wasting, and renal tubular acidosis. Sodium loading (150 mEq/day) appears to help prevent amphotericin B-induced nephrotoxicity and should be used routinely. Infusion of 500 ml of normal saline both before and after the amphotericin B dose provides the required amount of salt and helps prevent dehydration. Sodium loading may also be administered orally via dietary changes or oral salt supplements (Anderson, 1995).

Infusion-related reactions are common and include fever, chills, headache, hypotension, rigors, nausea, vomiting, and anorexia. These side effects may be minimized by premedication with acetaminophen 650 to 1,000 mg orally and diphenhydramine 25 to 50 mg orally or intravenously. Meperidine 25 to 50 mg intravenously is frequently used to treat amphotericin B-induced chills and rigors. Other adverse reactions that have been reported with amphotericin B include anemia, likely due to a suppression of erythropoietin production, liver enzyme elevations, and thrombophlebitis when infused though a peripheral vein.

The most significant and well-documented drug interaction with amphotericin B is the increased renal toxicity that results when amphotericin B is combined with cyclosporine, tacrolimus, or another nephrotoxin. Such combinations should be avoided whenever possible. Hypokalemia that accompanies amphotericin B may facilitate digitalis toxicity and may enhance muscle relaxation caused by nondepolarizing neuromuscular blockers. Potassium levels should be monitored and potassium supplements given, if needed, when a patient on amphotericin B is receiving these agents concurrently.

Lipid amphotericin B products

Since amphotericin B causes significant nephrotoxicity (doubling of serum creatinine) in nearly 50% of patients, the need to decrease this serious side effect has led to the development of lipid formulations of amphotericin B (Gallis et al., 1990). Lipid formulations of amphotericin B include amphotericin B colloidal dispersion with a disclike structure (ABCD, Amphocil®, Amphotec®), amphotericin B lipid complex with a ribbonlike shape (ABLC, Abelcet®), and liposomal amphotericin B with amphotericin B encapsulated in a true liposome (AmBisome®). These lipid formulations have the same in vitro spectrum of activity as conventional amphotericin B, but are less nephrotoxic. They all contain amphotericin B, but have different properties with respect to clearance by the reticuloendothelial system, peak concentration (C_{max}), AUC, and volume of distribution (V_d). The clinical significance of these differences remains to be determined (Dupont, 2002).

The incidence and severity of infusion-related side effects varies among the lipid amphotericin products. When compared to conventional amphotericin B, liposomal amphotericin caused a significantly lower incidence of chills, rigors, fevers, dyspnea, hypotension, hypertension and tachycardia (Walsh et al., 1999). In contrast, ABCD and ABLC have an incidence of infusion-related side effects comparable to, if not worse than, conventional amphotericin B (Hann & Prentice, 2001). The significant cost of the lipid amphotericin B products precludes their use for all patients in which amphotericin B is indicated. Patients for which lipid amphotericin products should be considered are those who have failed or are intolerant of conventional amphotericin B. Lipid amphotericin products should be considered for use as a first-line agent in patients with preexisting renal dysfunction or who are receiving other nephrotoxic medications when amphotericin B is necessary for treatment of a suspected or documented fungal infection. Doses of liposomal amphotericin B range from 1 to 5 mg/kg/day administered intravenously. Doses up to 15 mg/kg/day have been used in select cases of resistant fungal infections. The dose of ABLC is 2.5 to 5 mg/kg/day by intravenous infusion. ABCD is usually dosed at 3 to 4 mg/kg/day by intravenous infusion up to a maximum tolerated dose of 7.5 mg/kg/day. The same drug interactions seen with conventional amphotericin B could potentially occur with lipid amphotericin B products as well.

Caspofungin

Caspofungin is an echinocandin derivative that is a noncompetitive inhibitor of β-(1,3)-glucan synthase. This enzyme is responsible for formation of β-(1,3)-glucan, an essential cell wall component in many pathogenic fungi. Inhibition of synthesis of this polysaccharide disrupts the cell wall integrity and osmotic stability, which ultimately leads to cell lysis. Potential toxicity of caspofungin is limited since mammalian cells do not require β(1,3)-D-glucan for formation of cell membranes. Caspofungin has exhibited efficacy in vitro and in vivo against various fungi and yeasts, including Aspergillus and Candida species. It has been approved by the FDA for treatment of invasive aspergillosis in patients who are refractory to, or do not tolerate, conventional antifungal agents.

The dose is a 70 mg loading dose, followed by 50 mg once daily and is given as an intravenous infusion (Keating & Jarvis, 2001). Dosage adjustments are not necessary in patients with renal dysfunction or mild hepatic dysfunction. Dose reductions (from 50 mg/day to 35 mg/day) for patients with moderate hepatic dysfunction are recommended by the manufacturer. Caspofungin use has not been studied in patients with severe liver dysfunction.

Caspofungin is devoid of nephrotoxicity, with its most frequent adverse effects being fever, nausea, vomiting, and thrombophlebitis associated with the infusion. Increased ALT and AST have been reported with caspofungin therapy, but have been transient and have not limited therapy (Keating & Jarvis, 2001).

Drug interactions with caspofungin are not well documented due to the relatively limited number of patients treated thus far in clinical trials. Cyclosporine increases the AUC of caspofungin by 35% when these agents are given concomitantly, though the cyclosporine level is unaffected. Elevated transaminase levels have been seen in healthy volunteers receiving cyclosporine and caspofungin, leading the manufacturer to recommend that these two medications not be used concurrently. Since many patients with fungal infections are receiving cyclosporine, the incidence and severity of this interaction needs to be clarified further. Tacrolimus whole blood concentrations and AUC were decreased by about 20% when administered in combination with caspofungin. Tacrolimus concentrations should be monitored and appropriate dosage adjustments made in patients receiving caspofungin concurrently. Enhanced clearance of caspofungin may occur when administered with hepatic enzyme inducers such as rifampin, carbamazepine, or phenytoin. The manufacturer recommends increasing the caspofungin dose to 70 mg daily in patients not responding to 50 mg daily during combined therapy with hepatic enzyme inducers. No antagonism was seen between caspofungin and amphotericin B in an in vitro study looking at the activity of these agents in combination against Aspergillus and Fusarium species, though some synergistic effects were observed (Arikan et al., 2002). There is significant interest in using caspofungin in combination with amphotericin B, lipid amphotericin B products, or triazole antifungals for treatment of fungal infections resistant to monotherapy. Efficacy of this approach remains to be determined.

Other antifungals

Posaconazole and ravuconazole are two other triazole antifungals under investigation, and micafungin (FK 463) is another echinocandin currently in clinical trials. These agents may offer additional treatment options in the future.

Antiviral agents

Acyclovir

Acyclovir is a nucleoside 2'-deoxyguanosine analog with significant in vivo activity against herpes simplex virus (HSV) and varicella-zoster virus (VZV). Acyclovir needs to be phosphorylated in vivo to be active. The first phosphorylation is accomplished by viral thymidine kinase with subsequent phosphorylations performed by intracellular enzymes (Wagstaff, Faulds, & Goa, 1994). Activated acyclovir inhibits viral DNA polymerase and prevents viral replication. Bone marrow transplant recipients at risk for HSV and VZV infections benefited from prophylactic use of acyclovir in several well-designed clinical trials. The rate of HSV reactivation in seropositive patients was 70% to 80% before the use of prophylactic antiviral agents (Ljungman, 2001). Prophylactic acyclovir use has practically eliminated HSV disease (Saral et al., 1981; Hann et al., 1983). Similarly, long-term prophylaxis (6 to 12 months) with acyclovir successfully suppressed VZV reactivation in seropositive patients in several clinical trials, although a small number of patients developed VZV upon discontinuation of prophylaxis (Ljungman et al., 1986; Selby et al., 1989). CMV is less susceptible to acyclovir in vivo than VZV and HSV because of lower susceptibility of CMV DNA polymerase for triphosphorylated acyclovir. However, use of high prophylactic doses resulted in a delay of CMV infections and was associated with overall increased survival (Meyers et al., 1988; Prentice et al., 1994; Wagstaff et al., 1994).

Oral acyclovir is poorly absorbed with reported bioavailability of 15% to 30%. The half-life of acyclovir is significantly prolonged in patients with renal function impairment; therefore, dose adjustment is recommended in patients with renal dysfunction (Wagstaff et al., 1994). Toxicities with this agent are uncommon, but occasionally patients may report gastrointestinal problems, headache, and rash with oral dosing (Mertz et al., 1988). Intravenous administration of acyclovir may cause local irritation and phlebitis if administered via a peripheral line. Neurotoxicity presenting as confusion, lethargy, hallucinations, tremors, delirium, seizures, and coma has been reported in 1% of patients. If neurotoxicity occurs, the dose of the drug should be decreased or acyclovir should be discontinued. In addition, acute reversible nephrotoxicity occurred in patients secondary to rapid i.v. infusion and/or dehydration. The reduction in rate of administration (recommended rate is 1 hour), dose decrease, and adequate hydration are appropriate maneuvers intended to minimize and prevent nephrotoxicity. Coadministration of acyclovir with probenecid may increase acyclovir levels and prolong its elimination half-life (Morris, 1994; Wagstaff et al., 1994) (Table 83.6).

Valacyclovir

Valacyclovir is a valine-ester of acyclovir that is rapidly converted to acyclovir in the gut mucosa and in the liver. The

Table 83.6. *Selected dosing regimens for acyclovir and valacyclovir in HSCT*

Indication	Acyclovir dose and duration	Valacyclovir dose and duration
Herpes simplex virus (HSV)		
Prophylaxis	800 mg p.o. BID or 250 mg/m² i.v. q12h Duration: 30 days if VZV(−)	500 mg p.o. BID Duration: 30 days if VZV(−)
Treatment	250 mg/m² i.v. q8h or 400 mg PO 5 times/day Duration: 7 days	500–1,000 mg p.o. BID Duration: 7 days
Varicella zoster virus (VZV)		
Prophylaxis	800 mg p.o. BID or 250 mg/m² i.v. q12h Duration: 6–12 months	500 mg p.o. BID Duration: 6–12 months
Treatment	500 mg/m² i.v. q8h Duration: 7 days	1,000 mg p.o. TID Duration: 7 days
Cytomegalovirus (CMV)		
Prophylaxis	500 mg/m² i.v. q8h for 4 weeks followed by 800 mg p.o. QID for 8 months	2,000 mg p.o. QID for 90 days
Treatment	Acyclovir and valacyclovir are not indicated for treatment of CMV infections	

advantage of valacyclovir over acyclovir is its higher bioavailability, reported as 54% after a single 1,000 mg dose (Ormrod, Scott, & Perry, 2000). The effective treatment dose of valacyclovir can be administered less frequently than that recommended for acyclovir, and patient compliance may be improved with less frequent daily dosing. The disadvantage of valacyclovir is its cost, since oral acyclovir is available in a generic form. The mechanism of action, spectrum of activity, pharmacodynamic properties, drug interactions, and tolerability of valacyclovir are similar to acyclovir. Table 83.6 gives recommended dosing guidelines for valacyclovir in HSCT patients.

Ganciclovir

Ganciclovir is another nucleoside analog with activity against DNA viruses such as CMV, VZV, HSV, human herpesvirus type 6 (HHV6), and Epstein-Barr virus (EBV). Ganciclovir undergoes activation via the same pathways as acyclovir, and its phosphorylated form competitively inhibits deoxyguanosine triphosphate halting viral DNA synthesis (Faulds & Heel, 1990). Ganciclovir is used in the posttransplant setting to prevent or treat CMV infection. There are two approaches for prophylaxis of CMV disease: (1) prophylaxis with ganciclovir beginning at the time of engraftment; and (2) pre-emptive therapy with ganciclovir starting only if CMV is detected by a routine, weekly PCR or antigenemia screening. In order to avoid excessive treatment and toxicity with ganciclovir, the pre-emptive therapy is preferred if pp65 antigenemia screening is available (Boeckh, 1999; Ljungman, 2001).

Ganciclovir has been evaluated in several clinical trials and has been shown to decrease development of CMV disease; however, improvement in overall survival has not been shown with its use (Goodrich et al., 1993; Winston et al., 1993; Boeckh et al., 1996).

Oral ganciclovir has poor bioavailability of approximately 6%. Currently, the parenteral formulation is the formulation of choice in clinical practice. Ganciclovir is eliminated by the kidneys and almost 100% of ganciclovir is recovered unchanged in the urine (Markham & Faulds, 1994). The standard induction dosing regimen for patients with normal renal function is 5 mg/kg i.v. every 12 hours for 7 to 10 days. Refer to Table 83.7 for dosing adjustments in patients with renal function impairment.

The most common adverse effect associated with ganciclovir use is bone marrow suppression including neutropenia, thrombocytopenia, and anemia. Reported neutropenia ranged from 31% to 58% in HSCT patients and was associated with several risk factors: (1) liver disease at engraftment; (2) renal function impairment posttransplant; and (3) low marrow cellularity at day 28 (Goodrich et al., 1993, Winston et al., 1993, Boeckh et al., 1996).

If a significant decrease in white blood cell count is observed, hematopoietic growth factors may be initiated and, in general, ganciclovir should be discontinued if the absolute neutrophil count is less than 1,000/mm^3 (Markham & Faulds, 1994). However, in some cases neutropenia is not reversible and has been identified as an independent risk factor for mortality in HSCT patients. In addition, thrombocytopenia may be a potential complication; however, anemia is uncommon (Markham & Faulds, 1994).

Drug interactions with ganciclovir involve agents that can affect rapidly dividing cells and include antineoplastic agents, pentamidine, trimethoprim-sulfamethoxazole, and other nucleoside analogs (i.e., zidovudine). Probenecid can diminish excretion of ganciclovir and increase its toxicity (Morris, 1994; Faulds & Heel, 1990).

Foscarnet

Foscarnet is a pyrophosphate analog with a broad spectrum of antiviral activity against herpesviruses (HSV, VZV, CMV, EBV, HHV6), hepatitis B viruses (HBV) and human immunodeficiency virus (HIV) (Wagstaff & Bryson, 1994). Foscarnet inhibits DNA polymerase and viral DNA chain elongation and it does not need to be phosphorylated by viral enzymes to be active. Foscarnet is indicated for prophylaxis of CMV infection and disease and treatment of acyclovir-resistant HSV infections in HSCT recipients. In clinical practice this antiviral agent is also used for treatment of CMV disease in patients intolerant to ganciclovir. Foscarnet is administered as an intravenous infusion, since its oral absorption is poor. Foscarnet is mainly excreted unchanged in the urine (83%–88%) and the remainder tends to accumulate in bone and cartilage. The unpredictable bone deposition is a possible cause for the wide inter- and intrapatient plasma concentration variability of foscarnet (Wagstaff & Bryson, 1994). Since foscarnet is dependent on the kidneys for elimination, doses should be adjusted in patients with renal function impairment (Table 83.8). Foscarnet is initially administered every 8 to 12 hours in patients requiring induction treatment. After 1 to 3 weeks of induction therapy, patients who respond to treatment can be switched to maintenance dosing (approximately one-half of the induction dose). Foscarnet infusion should be over 60 to 120 minutes.

The major disadvantage of foscarnet is its toxicity profile. In early clinical trials foscarnet was administered as a continuous infusion without adequate hydration and caused nephrotoxicity in 20% to 60% of patients (Chrisp & Clissold, 1991). Tubular necrosis resulting from foscarnet in patients with normal baseline renal function is reversible and may be minimized by adequate hydration pre- and during foscarnet infusion, dose reduction, and avoidance of concurrent use of nephrotoxins (Wagstaff & Bryson, 1994). Foscarnet often leads to severe electrolyte imbalance. Alterations in calcium, magnesium, and potassium have been reported in 15% to 43% of patients (hypocalcemia, hypercalcemia, hypokalemia, and hypomagne-

Table 83.7. *Ganciclovir dosing adjustment for renal function impairment*

Creatinine clearance (ml/min)	Induction		Maintenance	
	Dose (mg/kg)	Dosing interval (hours)	Dose (mg/kg)	Dosing interval (hours)
≥70	5	12	5	24
59–69	2.5	12	2.5	24
25–49	2.5	24	1.25	24
10–24	1.25	24	0.625	24
<10	1.25	3 times per week following hemodialysis	0.625	3 times per week following hemodialysis

Table 83.8. *Foscarnet dosing for treatment of CMV disease in patients with renal function impairment*

Creatinine clearance (ml/min/kg)	Induction		Maintenance	
	Dose (mg/kg)	Dosing interval (hours)	Dose (mg/kg)	Dosing interval (hours)
>1.4	90	12	90	24
≥1–1.4	70	12	70	24
≥0.8–1	50	12	50	24
≥0.6–0.8	80	24	80	48
≥0.5–0.6	60	24	60	48
≥0.4–0.5	50	24	50	48
≥0.4	Not recommended	Not recommended	Not recommended	Not recommended

semia), while changes in phosphate levels occurred in 6% to 8% of patients (hypophosphatemia, hyperphosphatemia) (Wagstaff & Bryson, 1994). Symptomatic hypocalcemia can persist even after drug discontinuation, because foscarnet is stored in the bone matrix and is slowly released over several months (Morris, 1994). Hematologic toxicity of foscarnet differs from that observed with ganciclovir and is most frequently associated with reduction in red blood cells (anemia has been reported in 20% to 50% of patients). Gastrointestinal adverse effects (nausea and vomiting in 20% to 30% of patients), penile and vulval mucosal ulceration (3%–9%), headache, fatigue, and transient neurological and psychological disturbances are also associated with foscarnet administration (Chrisp & Clissold, 1991; Wagstaff & Bryson, 1994). Infusion of undiluted foscarnet via a peripheral line may lead to thrombophlebitis.

Concomitant administration of amphotericin B products, cyclosporine, tacrolimus, aminoglycosides, loop diuretics, intravenous pentamidine, and other nephrotoxins should be avoided if possible. Renal function should be closely monitored in patients treated with foscarnet, especially if concurrent use of nephrotoxins is unavoidable. Serum electrolytes should also be closely monitored, and other drugs known to cause electrolyte imbalances should be used with caution (i.e., intravenous pentamidine use with foscarnet may result in severe hypocalcemia) (Chrisp & Clissold, 1991; Wagstaff & Bryson, 1994).

Cidofovir

Cidofovir is a broad-spectrum antiviral agent active against most herpesviruses and adenovirus. It is approved by the FDA for treatment of CMV retinitis in patients with AIDS (Ljungman, 2001). Cidofovir is a cytidine nucleotide analog able, in its phosphorylated form, to inhibit viral DNA polymerase. In contrast to ganciclovir, the phosphorylation step of cidofovir is mediated by host intracellular enzymes and not by the viral proteins. This major difference plays a role in resistance patterns to antiviral agents (Plosker & Noble, 1999; Safrin, Cherrington, & Jaffe, 1999). Use of cidofovir in HSCT recipients has not been extensively studied and most data come from clinical trials performed in AIDS patients (Ljungman, 2001).

The serum half-life of cidofovir is approximately 2.5 hours; however, the intracellular half-life of cidofovir diphosphate is much longer and is estimated to be approximately 65 hours (Plosker & Noble, 1999). The recommended dosing regimen is 5 mg/kg once weekly for 2 weeks (induction), then 5 mg/kg every other week (maintenance). The oral absorption of cidofovir is poor and this drug is only given intravenously (over 1 hour). Over 90% of cidofovir is eliminated unchanged in the urine within 24 hours postadministration (Plosker & Noble, 1999).

The dose-limiting adverse effect of cidofovir is nephrotoxicity, reported in 20% to 25% of patients. Although renal function impairment is partially reversible in the majority of patients, dependence on hemodialysis and/or death have been reported even after one or two cidofovir doses (Plosker & Noble, 1999). Objective signs of nephrotoxicity include elevation in serum creatinine and/or proteinuria and should be monitored before each cidofovir dose. Cidofovir accumulates in the proximal tubule, the site of cellular injury. Probenecid administration is thought to decrease the concentration of cidofovir within the renal compartment. Oral probenecid 2 g must be administered 3 hours before, and 1 g 2 hours and 1 g 8 hours after, each cidofovir dose (Plosker & Noble, 1999; Safrin et al., 1999). In order to improve probenecid tolerance, it should be taken with food and premedications such as acetaminophen and antihistamines may be helpful. Some of the adverse effects reported with cidofovir (nausea, vomiting, fever, and rash) are being attributed to probenecid. An additional recommended renal-sparing measure involves adequate hydration with normal saline: 1 liter given immediately 1 to 2 hours before cidofovir and additional 1 to 2 liters of normal saline after cidofovir infusion, if the patient can tolerate the additional volume (Plosker & Noble, 1999).

Due to the high risk of nephrotoxicity, the following guidelines should be used to select patients who will qualify for cidofovir:

1. Serum creatinine must be less than 1.5 mg/dl;
2. Calculated creatinine clearance must be greater than 55 ml/min;
3. Less than 2+ proteinuria must be found in the urine (Plosker & Noble, 1999; Safrin et al., 1999).

Nephrotoxic agents should not be administered concomitantly with cidofovir or for a period of 7 days afterwards (Plasker & Noble, 1999). However, in the HSCT population certain nephrotoxic agents cannot be withheld for this duration and their use must be based on clinical judgment.

Immune globulins

The role of immune globulins in HSCT recipients is controversial. Seattle Cancer Care Alliance adheres to recommendations published by Boeckh in 1999. Neither immune globulin (IVIG) nor CMV-specific hyperimmune globulin (CMV-IVIG) is recommended for prophylaxis of CMV disease in HSCT recipients at this point (Boeckh, 1999). There is no benefit with IVIG for prevention of CMV disease in autologous transplant recipients (Wolff et al., 1993). In allogeneic transplant patients the situation is more complicated and the results from several clinical trials are conflicting. Sullivan et al. (1990) reported a decrease in the risk of acute GVHD, CMV interstitial pneumonia, and bacterial infections in patients who received IVIG; however, overall survival was not improved. In contrast, Feinstein et al. (1999) reported no difference in acute GVHD, interstitial pneumonia, or bacterial infections in patients receiving IVIG prophylaxis. In this study the investigators also observed that IVIG recipients had a higher risk for relapse than the controls, 31% versus 18%, respectively, whereas Sullivan et al. did not observe any difference in the relapse rates (Sullivan *et al.,* 1990; Feinstein *et al.,* 1999). Patients who develop CMV pneumonia should receive either IVIG or CMV-IVIG in addition to an appropriate antiviral agent (Boeckh, 1999). In the case of CMV gastritis, immune globulin preparations have not been shown to be beneficial (Ljungman *et al.,* 1998a). Superiority of much more expensive CMV-IVIG over IVIG cannot be concluded from available data at this time (Boeckh, 1999).

Immune globulin (IVIG)

Immune globulin is a solution of IgG antibodies obtained from pooled human plasma. IVIG provides passive immunity to patients. Many preparations of injectable immune globulin are currently available (i.e., Gamimune N®, Gammagard S/D®, Gammar-P®, Iveegam®, Panglobulin®, Polygam S/D®, Sandoglobulin®, Venoglobulin-S®). Since differences between these preparations exist, the reader is advised to determine which preparation is available at his/her particular institution. Due to the limited scope of this review the specific characteristics and differences between these preparations are not described here and the focus is placed on Gamimune N®, since it has been evaluated in clinical trials in HSCT patients.

Most of the adverse effects seen with IVIG are related to the rate of infusion and not the total dose. Patients with hypogammaglobulinemia or who have not received IVIG in the preceding 8 weeks are at the highest risk for infusion-related adverse effects. Patients should be appropriately monitored during IVIG infusion for infusion-related reactions. These unwanted effects may be avoided with premedications such as antihistamines, analgesics, and/or corticosteroids. The adverse effects reported in HSCT patients receiving IVIG include chills, fever, pruritus, headache, and flushing (Sullivan *et al.,* 1990). Occasionally, reactions to IVIG may manifest as anaphylaxis 30 to 60 minutes into the infusion (i.e., hypotension, chest tightness, tachycardia, face flushing, chills, fever, dizziness, nausea, vomiting, or diaphoresis). The proper management involves temporary discontinuation of IVIG and administration of supportive measures. Immune globulin may be restarted at a lower rate once these symptoms resolve. Osmotic injury to the proximal renal tubules resulting in renal function impairment has been linked to IVIG. Renal function should be monitored and the recommended dosage should not be exceeded. The highest risk for renal function impairment has been associated with immune globulin preparations stabilized with sucrose (i.e., Gammar-P®, Panglobulin®, Sandoglobulin®). Gamimune N® 5% contains maltose that may cause mild diuresis. In addition, Gamimune N® administration caused local reactions such as erythema, pain, phlebitis, and eczematous reactions in some patients.

Immune globulin administration may alter response to certain vaccines (i.e., hepatitis A virus vaccine, measles virus vaccine live, mumps virus vaccine live). IVIG should not be administered with other medications or i.v. fluids via the same port. A dose of 500 mg/kg i.v. every other day for 2 weeks is recommended in patients with CMV pneumonia (Boeckh, 1999). Prophylactic dosing of 500 mg/kg (Gamimune N®) every week commencing on day –7 and continued until day +90 posttransplant was proposed by Sullivan *et al.* (1990). The rate of administration of 5% IVIG solution in this study was as follows: start at 0.02 ml/kg/min for 30 minutes; if tolerated increase to 0.04 ml/kg/min; if tolerated increase to maximum rate of 0.08 ml/kg/min. Again, the reader is reminded that the rates will vary based on the IVIG product and manufacturer's recommendations for infusion rate should be followed.

Cytomegalovirus immune globulin (CMV-IG)

CMV-IG is intended to provide passive immunity to CMV. This immune globulin is obtained from the pooled human plasma containing high titers of CMV. The CMV titer in CMV-IVIG is 4 to 8 times higher than that contained in IVIG. The infusion-related adverse effects associated with CMV-IVIG are similar to ones observed with IVIG. The recommended management of infusion-related adverse effects for IVIG is also appropriate for patients receiving CMV-IVIG. This product does not carry a renal function warning; however, it contains 50 mg of sucrose. The dose used in patients with pulmonary CMV disease at Seattle Cancer Care Alliance is 150 mg/kg every other day for 2 weeks followed by 150 mg/kg once weekly for 4 weeks (11 doses total). The recommended administration rate should be followed for the first infusion: start at 15 mg/kg/hr for 30 minutes; if tolerated increase to 30 mg/kg/hr for 30 minutes; if tolerated increase to 60 mg/kg/hr (maximum rate of 75 ml/hr should not be exceeded). For subsequent infusions the rate may be increased every 15 minutes if tolerated by the patient.

Hematopoietic growth factors

Granulocyte colony-stimulating factor (G-CSF)

G-CSF (filgrastim, lenograstim) is generally well tolerated. In patients who receive G-CSF for mobilization of hematopoietic progenitor cells into peripheral blood, mild to moderate musculoskeletal symptoms, principally medullary bone pain, are most frequently reported. Bone pain has been described as pulsating deep pain; mild, nonspecific aches; or pressure in the lower back, pelvis, ribs, or sternum. Bone pain appears to occur at sites containing bone marrow. Mild to moderate nausea, vomiting, and abdominal pain are frequently reported although it is unclear whether these effects are caused by G-CSF. Other less common effects include transient, generalized rash and erythema, swelling, or pruritus at the injection site. Minor bruising, inflammation, or bleeding may occur with subcutaneous administration. Marked leukocytosis and transient decrease in platelet count have been reported occasionally. Anaphylactoid and allergic-type reactions are rare.

There are no clinically important drug interactions reported to date.

The usual dosage posttransplant is 5 µg/kg/day, given by subcutaneous injection or as an intravenous infusion over 4 hours; the usual dose for mobilizing peripheral blood stem cells is 10 µg/kg/day.

Granulocyte-macrophage colony-stimulating factor (GM-CSF)

GM-CSF is generally well tolerated at the recommended dosages. Higher dosages are associated with adverse effects. Some adverse effects reported in clinical studies may be related to the specific GM-CSF formulation used (sargramostim, molgramostim, regramostim). The most frequently reported adverse effects for sarostim are mild to moderate fever, chills, headache, asthenia, nausea, diarrhea, myalgia, and bone pain. Mild to moderate bone pain occurs in the lower back, pelvis, sternum, ribs, spine, or shoulder. Bone pain appears to be related to the leukocyte count. These effects are reversible upon discontinuation of the drug and may be related to dose. In placebo-controlled studies of sargramostim in autologous bone marrow or peripheral blood stem cell transplant recipients, only asthenia, diarrhea, rash, and malaise occurred at a frequency exceeding that of placebo by at least 5%. A "flulike" syndrome is commonly reported consisting of mild to moderate fever, fatigue, malaise, myalgia, chills, headache, asthenia, and GI complaints that are generally controllable by antipyretics and analgesics. An intermittent low-grade fever is common and can be difficult to distinguish from fever due to infection. Adverse GI effects (nausea, vomiting, abdominal cramps) have been reported although it is unclear if these effects are related to sargramostim therapy. Respiratory effects include pulmonary infiltrates, dyspnea, lung disorder, and sequestration of granulocytes in the pulmonary circulation. A first-dose reaction manifested as respiratory distress, hypoxia, hypotension, flushing, syncope, tachycardia, and bone pain has been reported. These signs have resolved with symptomatic treatment and usually do not recur with subsequent doses in the same treatment cycle. Capillary leak syndrome, edema, and pleural and/or pericardial effusion have been reported, especially at higher dosages, usually >20 µg/kg. Transient, reversible, supraventricular arrhythmia has been reported occasionally. Serious allergic or anaphylactoid reactions are rare. Injection site reactions and alterations in LFTs may occur. Sargramostim may cause a rapid rise in leukocyte count with marked leukocytosis reported occasionally. A dose-related eosinophilia and monocytosis may occur.

Specific drug interaction studies have not been performed to date. Drugs that might theoretically potentiate the myeloproliferative effects of sargramostim should be used with caution (e.g., corticosteroids, lithium).

The usual dosage posttransplant is 5 µg/kg/day, given by subcutaneous injection or as an intravenous infusion over 4 hours.

Analgesics

A variety of agents are available for pain management posttransplant. Therapy selection should be based on such factors as pain pathophysiology, the agent's pharmacodynamic and pharmacokinetic profile, dosage form, patient's allergies, and patient's narcotic use history (and see Chapter 81). In general, dosage adjustments of drugs should be made slowly so that certain side effects (i.e., sedation, respiratory depression) are minimized. Rapid and large changes in analgesic doses and analgesic agents should be avoided.

Nonsteroidal anti-inflammatory drugs (NSAIDs) and acetaminophen

NSAIDs and acetaminophen are effective agents for mild to moderate pain. Traditional NSAIDs nonselectively inhibit both isoforms of cyclooxygenase, the enzyme that converts arachidonic acid to prostaglandin and thromboxane. The COX-1 isoform is important for platelet aggregation, renal blood flow regulation, and gastric mucosal cytoprotection, while the COX-2 isoform is present during inflammatory conditions (Jackson & Hawkey, 2000; Lucas & Lipman, 2002). The use of nonselective NSAIDs posttransplant is primarily limited by their undesired adverse effect profile. Development of selective COX-2 inhibitors, celecoxib and rofecoxib, allows for the use of more selective NSAIDs posttransplant. These agents offer comparable efficacy and a lower risk of GI bleeds secondary to their lack of platelet effect when compared to nonselective NSAIDs. COX-2 inhibitors are not devoid of the renal toxicity seen with nonselective NSAIDs (Hawkey, 2001). Dosing for acute pain management with celecoxib is 200 mg twice daily and rofecoxib is 50 mg daily. Use of these agents is contraindicated in patients with aspirin allergies. Structurally, celecoxib contains a sulfonamide moiety and it should be used with caution in patients with a sulfa allergy. Rofecoxib and doses up to 400 mg of celecoxib may be administered without regard to meals. Celecoxib and rofecoxib have similar pharmacodynamic and pharmacokinetic profiles except for their sites of metabolism. Unlike rofecoxib, celecoxib is metabolized via the cytochrome P450 enzyme system. Celecoxib metabolism is inhibited by fluconazole. Consequently, celecoxib therapy should be initiated at the lowest recommended dose when used in conjunction with inhibitors of cytochrome P450 enzymes (Lucas & Lipman, 2002).

Acetaminophen is an effective alternative for mild to moderate pain management. It possesses antipyretic activity; however, it is a weak anti-inflammatory agent. Acetaminophen is hepatically metabolized and is contraindicated in severe hepatic failure. The maximum daily dose is 4 g. Skin rashes, characterized as erythema or urticaria, occur occasionally. Hepatotoxicity secondary to acetaminophen overdose is the most acute and severe adverse effect associated with this drug.

Opioids

Opioids remain the mainstay of therapy for the management of moderate to severe cancer pain. A variety of agents, dosage forms, and routes of delivery are available for pain management. The use of pure mu-receptor agonists, such as fentanyl, hydromorphone, morphine, and oxycodone, is preferred for cancer pain management. Of these agents, morphine is the agent of choice, primarily because of its routes for administration, drug forms, clinical experience, and side effect profile. At equipotent doses, these agents offer equal analgesic effect and similar side effect profiles. Patients may require scheduled dosing regimens with the option of additional medications for breakthrough pain management. When deciding on the dose to give for breakthrough pain management, approximately one-third of the daily scheduled dose to be given in divided doses is an appropriate starting point. If patients require more than this for pain control, the scheduled dose should be increased. Equianalgesic dosages between selected opioids are shown in Table 83.9. To keep dosing regimens simple, the same opiate should be used for scheduled and breakthrough pain management. Agents such as codeine and mixed agonists/antagonists including butorphanol, nalbuphine, and pentazocine should be avoided because of undesirable side effects, decreased analgesic effect, long plasma half-lives, minimal data for cancer pain, ceiling effect, and risk for metabolite accumulation in the setting of organ dysfunction. The risk of narcotic withdrawal is also common in patients receiving mixed agonists/antagonists (Wood, 1996; Walsh, 2000).

The oral and intravenous routes are the traditional routes of administration; however, many other routes of administration are available including transdermal, transmucosal/buccal, rectal, sublingual, and subcutaneous routes. Fentanyl is the only agent that is available for transmucosal/buccal and transdermal administration. The rectal route of administration is undesirable in neutropenic patients because of the risk of local trauma and consequent introduction of bacteria into the blood stream (Walsh, 2000).

The adverse effects of opioids are well described. Gastrointestinal complaints including nausea, vomiting, and constipation are the most frequent adverse effects associated with opioid therapy. Nausea and vomiting result from direct stimula-

tion of the chemoreceptor trigger zone following opioid administration. This effect is dose-related and tolerance usually develops with continued use. Though nausea, vomiting, pruritus, and sedation will diminish with continued use, constipation continues to occur. Patients requiring large doses of opioids should also be prescribed an appropriate bowel regimen to prevent opioid-induced ileus. Other side effects also include CNS effects (i.e., drowsiness, mental status changes, and myoclonus), pruritus, respiratory depression, urinary retention, and psychological effects. True anaphylaxis and hematological effects are rare (Schug, Zech, & Grong, 1992).

Opioids should be administered with food to minimize GI upset. Concomitant use of alcohol and alcohol-containing medications should be avoided, since alcohol can potentiate the CNS effects of narcotics. Sustained-release products should not be crushed or broken as rapid release and absorption may cause signs and symptoms of overdose.

Adjuvant analgesics

Anticonvulsants, antidepressants, alpha-2 adrenergic agonists, and NMDA receptor antagonists are effective adjuvant agents for pain management in specific clinical situations, for example, neuropathic pain. Gabapentin, a gamma-aminobutyric acid analog, is the first-line adjuvant agent used for treatment of neuropathic pain. The starting dose is 300 mg orally three times daily and may be titrated up to a maximum daily dose of 3,600 mg. To prevent rebound pain associated with an abrupt withdrawl of the medication, discontinuation of therapy should be slow (over at least 1 week). Gabapentin is excreted as unchanged drug in the urine; therefore dose adjustment for renal impairment (CrCl ≤ 60 ml/min) is recommended.

The most common side effects of gabapentin include fatigue, somnolence, dizziness, headache, ataxia, and hypertension. Fatigue, somnolence, dizziness, and headache are most commonly reported during the first 3 days of therapy and subside with continued use. Other less common adverse effects

Table 83.9. *Equianalgesic and pharmacokinetic comparison of narcotic analgesic agents*

Agents	Equivalent doses (mg)		$T_{1/2}$(hr)	Site of metabolism	Peak effect (hr)	Duration of analgesia (hr)
	Oral	i.v.				
Codeine	200	120 to 130	3	Liver	1 (p.o.) 15 to 30 (i.m.)	4 to 6
Fentanyl	–	0.1 to 0.2	1 to 6	Liver	<0.5 (i.m.)	0.5 to 2
Hydromorphone	6 to 7.5	1.5 to 2	2 to 4	Liver	1.5 to 2 (p.o.) 0.5 to 1 (i.m.)	4 to 5
Meperidine	300	75 to 100	3 to 5	Liver	1 to 2 (p.o.) 0.5 to 1 (i.m.)	2 to 4
Methadone	15	7.5 to 10	22 to 25	Liver	1 to 2 (p.o.) 0.5 to 1 (i.m.)	4 to 6
Morphine	30 to 40	10	2 to 3.5	Liver	1 to 2 (p.o.) 0.5 to 1 (i.m.)	4 to 7
Oxycodone	15 to 30	–	–	Liver/kidney	0.5 to 1 (p.o.)	4 to 6

included weight gain, diarrhea, abnormal coordination, edema, and diplopia. Use of gabapentin in diabetic patients should be cautious because fluctuations in glucose levels have been reported. Leukopenia (1%) and other hematological effects are rare. Concomitant antacid use results in a 20% decrease in the bioavailability of gabapentin. Administering gabapentin at least 2 hours after antacids avoids this interaction (Farrar & Portenoy, 2001).

Posttransplant use of tricyclic antidepressants (TCAs), and traditional anticonvulsants (i.e., carbamazepine, phenytoin, divalproex) is limited by the potential of these agents to cause bone marrow suppression and therefore is often avoided. Data on the use of alpha-2 adrenergic agonists and NMDA receptor antagonists is limited in HSCT patients. The experience of using serotonin selective reuptake inhibitors such as fluoxetine, sertraline, and paroxetine, for neuropathic pain management in HSCT is also limited.

Antiemetics

Nausea and vomiting is a universal, unpleasant, and distressing complication experienced by patients during their transplant course. The etiologies are numerous and may include regimen-related toxicities, medications (opioid narcotics, cyclosporine, itraconazole), GI infections and acute GVHD. A large armamentarium of agents is available for prophylaxis and symptomatic management of nausea and vomiting. These agents include glucocorticoids, serotonin type III antagonists ($5HT_3$), dopamine antagonists, anticholinergics, benzodiazepines, and cannabinoids. Dexamethasone alone or in combination with $5HT_3$ antagonists is indicated for prophylaxis of mild to moderate and moderate to highly emetogenic regimens, but its use posttransplant is limited. Serotonin type III antagonists have replaced high-dose metoclopramide (2 mg/kg) for prophylaxis, given their improved side effect profile and efficacy for chemotherapy-induced nausea and vomiting. At equipotent doses, all $5HT_3$ antagonists are similar in efficacy and safety with moderately to highly emetogenic chemotherapeutic regimens. In one study, dolasetron was found to be less effective than ondansetron or granisetron in preventing nausea and vomiting associated with high-dose chemotherapy and TBI preceding HSCT; however, the maximum dose of dolasetron was not utilized in this study (Bubalo et al., 2001). Serotonin antagonists are highly efficacious for prophylaxis of nausea and vomiting and for the treatment of breakthrough of nausea and vomiting immediately following chemotherapy; however, they are ineffective for symptomatic management of nausea and vomiting associated with GVHD. These agents are equally as efficacious as traditional agents (such as the dopamine antagonists, anticholinergic antagonists, and benzodiazepines) for nausea and vomiting posttransplant but given the costs of these agents, more traditional agents used alone or in combination with each other, may offer a more economical method for posttransplant nausea and vomiting management.

Benzodiazepines are most effective for anticipatory nausea and vomiting. Dronabinol, a centrally acting agent traditionally used as an appetite stimulant, is also effective for nausea and vomiting. Higher doses (5 mg every 4–6 hours) than those used for appetite stimulation (2.5 mg every 4–6 hours) may be required to achieve antiemetic effects. The use of dronabinol in the elderly population should be cautious, as altered mental status changes and dysphoria may occur. Guidelines for appropriate use of these agents are further described in published guidelines for antiemetic use (American Society of Health-Systems Pharmacists 1999; Gralla et al., 1999). Prototypical agents from each class, their dosing regimens, adverse effects, and management are listed in Table 83.10.

Antidiarrheal agents

The etiology of diarrhea posttransplant is often multifactorial and can result from the effects of the conditioning regimen, medications (i.e., antibiotics), infections (i.e., Clostridium difficile, Cryptosporidium, CMV, adenovirus, etc.) or GVHD (Ippoliti, 1998). Infectious causes should be ruled out before treatment with antisecretory agents is initiated due to potential risk for toxic megacolon. In addition, in order to select a specific agent, the patient's allergies, preference, and adverse effects profile of the particular drug should be considered. Unfortunately, octreotide is the only agent available in an intravenous form. Table 83.11 gives detailed information on agents used most frequently in the HSCT population posttransplant.

Acid-reducing agents

Proton pump inhibitors (PPIs)

PPIs are the drugs of choice for acid suppression and are superior to H2 antagonists in increasing gastric pH for the symptomatic management of acid-related conditions and Helicobacter pylori infections. These agents covalently bind to the exposed cysteine residues found on the H^+K^+ adenosine triphosphatase (ATPase) enzyme system leading to the inhibition of the gastric acid pump. Currently marketed PPIs include esomeprazole, omeprazole, lansoprazole, pantoprazole, and rabeprazole. Pantoprazole is the only PPI available in an intravenous formulation and should be administered using the provided in-line 1.2 micron filter and infused over 15 minutes. Dosing regimens for these agents are as follows: esomeprazole, omeprazole, and rabeprazole 20 to 40 mg daily, lansoprazole 30 to 60 mg daily, and pantoprazole 40 to 80 mg daily. The intravenous to oral conversion of pantoprazole is 1:1. Omeprazole, esomeprazole, and lansoprazole should be administered on an empty stomach because of absorption concerns, while rabeprazole and pantoprazole can be administered without regard to meals. In general, for patients who have difficulty swallowing esomeprazole, omeprazole, and lansoprazole, the contents of the capsules may be emptied on to applesauce and swallowed. The pellets should not be chewed or crushed. Sustained-release or enteric-coated rabeprazole and pantoprazole should be swallowed whole and not be crushed, broken, or chewed. Omeprazole liquid (2 mg/ml) can also be extemporane-

Table 83.10. *Antiemetics for nausea and vomiting management posttransplant*

Drug class	Drugs	Dosing regimens	Adverse effects and management
5HT$_3$ antagonists	Ondansetron	24 mg p.o. (or 8 mg i.v.) 30 minutes prior to chemotherapy (i.v. doses > 24 mg: Give as a 15–30 min infusion) 8 mg p.o. twice to three times daily (delayed nausea/vomiting)	Common: Headache, asymptomatic prolongation of ECG intervals (greater with dolasetron) Less common: Constipation, asthenia, somnolence, diarrhea, fever, tremor or twitching, ataxia, lightheadedness, dizziness, nervousness, thirst, muscle pain, warm or flushing sensation on i.v. administration Infrequent: Transient elevations in serum transaminases
	Granisetron	2 mg p.o. (or 1–2 mg i.v.) 30 minutes prior to chemotherapy	
	Dolesetron	100–200 mg (or 100 mg i.v.) 30 minutes prior to chemotherapy	
	Tropisetron	5 mg p.o./i.v. over 30 minutes prior to chemotherapy 5 mg p.o. every 6–12 hours × 2 OR 5 mg p.o. daily × 7 days postchemotherapy (delayed nausea/vomiting)	
Glucocorticoids	Dexamethasone	10–20 mg p.o./i.v. 30 minutes prior to chemotherapy (prophylaxis) 4–10 mg p.o./i.v. every 6–12 hours (delayed nausea/vomiting)	Common: Gastrointestinal upset, anxiety, insomnia Less common: Hyperglycemia, facial flushing, euphoria, perineal itching or burning (slow rate of infusion)
	Methylprednisolone	40–125 mg i.v. 30 minutes prior to chemotherapy	
Dopamine antagonists	Metoclopramide	0.5–3 mg/kg p.o./i.v. every 4–6 hours or 30 minutes prior to chemotherapy 20 mg (up to 0.5 mg/kg) p.o. for delayed emesis 5–10 mg p.o./i.v. 30 minutes prior to meals (promotility)	Common: Sedation, restlessness, diarrhea, agitation, CNS depression Less common: Extrapyramidal effects (EPS associated more frequently with higher doses), hypotension, neuroleptic syndrome, supraventricular tachycardia (with i.v. administration) EPS management: Diphenhydramine 25–50 mg p.o./i.v. or Benzotropine 1–4 mg i.v./p.o. daily or twice daily (max 6 mg/day) pre antiemetic
	Prochlorperazine	5–20 mg p.o./i.v. every 4–6 hours	Common: Sedation, lethargy, skin sensitization Less common: Cardiovascular effects (hypotension associated with rapid administration of chlorpromazine), EPS, cholestatic jaundice, hyperprolactinemia Infrequent: Neuroleptic malignant syndrome, hematologic abnormalities Hypotension management: Infuse over 30–60 minutes
	Chlorpromazine	10–20 mg i.v. over 30–60 minutes every 4–6 hours	
	Promethazine	25–50 mg p.o./i.v. every 4–6 hours	
Dopamine antagonists	Droperidol	1.25–5 mg i.v. every 4–6 hours	Common: Sedation hypotension, tachycardia, arrhythmias (droperidol) Less common: Extrapyramidal effects, dizziness, increase in blood pressure, chills, hallucinations
	Haloperidol	1–5 mg p.o./i.v. every 6 hours	
Benzodiazepine	Lorazepam	0.5–2 mg p.o./i.v. every 4–6 hours or 30 minutes prior to chemotherapy	Common: Sedation, amnesia Infrequent: Respiratory depression, ataxia, blurred vision, hallucinations, paradoxical reactions
Anticholinergics	Diphenhydramine	25–50 mg p.o./i.v. every 4–6 hours (max: 400 mg daily)	Common: Sedation, dry mouth, constipation Less common: Confusion, blurred vision, and urinary retention
	Scopolamine	1.5 mg topical patch every 72 hours	Common: Dry mouth, drowsiness, impaired eye accommodation Infrequent: Disorientation, memory disturbances, dizziness, hallucinations
Cannabinoid	Dronabinol	5–10 mg p.o. every 4–6 hours or 30 minutes prior to chemotherapy	Most common: Drowsiness, euphoria, somnolence, vasodilation, vision difficulties, abnormal thinking, dysphoria Less common: diarrhea, flushing, tremor, myalgia

Table 83.11. *Selected antidiarrheal agents useful in the HSCT population posttransplant*

Class	Agent	Dose	Adverse effects	Drug interactions
Antimotility agents	Diphenoxylate 2.5 mg/ atropine 25 mcg (Lomotil®)	5 mg/50 mcg QID; max 20 mg/day of diphenoxylate component	Xerostomia, dry skin, blurred vision, tachycardia, urinary retention, flushing, hyperthermia, drowsiness, GI disturbances, HA, skin rash, pancreatitis	CNS depressants (i.e., barbiturates, tranquilizers, alcohol), MAOIs
	Loperamide (Imodium®)	Initially 4 mg, then 2 mg after each loose stool; max 16 mg/day	Xerostomia, dizziness, drowsiness, GI disturbances, HA, skin rash	CNS depressants
	Opium tincture	0.6 ml QID; max 6 ml per day	Adverse effects associated with opioid agonist administration may occur	CNS depressants
Proabsorptive agents	Clonidine (Catapres®)	0.1–0.6 mg q12h	Hypotension, dry mouth, drowsiness, dizziness, sedation, constipation	Alcohol, levodopa, betablockers, TCAs, prazosin, verapamil
Antisecretory agents	Octreotide (Sandostatin®)	100–600 mcg/day in 2–4 divided doses s.c.; max 1,500 mcg/day	Nausea, GI upset, HA, hyper- and hypoglycemia. Long-term therapy: cholelithiasis, tachyphylaxis	Cyclosporine
Adsorbents	Kaolin-pectin mixture (Kaopectate®)	30–120 ml after each loose stool	Constipation	

Abbreviations: CNS, central nervous system; GI, gastrointestinal; HA, headache; MAOIs, monoamine oxidase inhibitors; TCAs, tricyclic antidepressants.

ously compounded by mixing omeprazole 100 mg with 50 ml of 8.4% sodium bicarbonate. This solution is stable for 14 days and should be refrigerated. Lansoprazole oral suspension is commercially available for ease of administration.

PPIs undergo extensive hepatic metabolism via cytochrome P450 3A4 and 2C19 enzyme system. The drug interactions vary, with omeprazole having the most and pantoprazole and esomeprazole having the least. Omeprazole has been shown to slow the metabolism of diazepam and other benzodiazepines, thereby resulting in enhanced and prolonged effects of benzodiazepines. When these agents are concurrently administered, patients should be monitored for CNS depression. The dose of benzodiazepines may need to be adjusted accordingly. Since agents such as lorazepam and temazepam utilize a different route of metabolism, the use of these agents is preferred to avoid the interaction. Omeprazole also alters the metabolism of carbamazepine, digoxin, fosphenytoin, phenytoin, and warfarin. Patients should be monitored for signs of toxicity when omeprazole is administered with any of these agents. As a class, PPIs also interfere with the absorption of drugs that require an acidic medium for optimal absorption. These agents include, but are not limited to, iron supplements, ampicillin, ampicillin/sulbactam, itraconazole, and ketoconazole. Appropriate monitoring of the efficacy of these agents is warranted if PPIs are concurrently administered (Horn, 2000). PPIs are well tolerated. The most common adverse effects include headache, fatigue, dizziness, reversible edema, and gastrointestinal complaints (i.e., diarrhea, abdominal pain, flatulence, and nausea). Hematologic adverse effects are rare with this class of agents (Horn, 2000).

Histamine 2 (H2) receptor antagonists

Currently marketed H2 antagonists include cimetidine, ranitidine, famotidine, and nitazidine. Ranitidine is the preferred agent in this class, since it is available orally and intravenously, has a favorable adverse effect profile, and less drug interactions. Use of H2 antagonists posttransplant should be made with caution, as hematological adverse effects including agranulocytosis, neutropenia, aplastic anemia, and thrombocytopenia have been reported, especially with cimetidine. These hematological adverse effects do not appear to be dose- or duration-related. These effects are usually reversible upon drug discontinuation. Other nonhematological effects include delirium and gastrointestinal side effects. Hypotension and bradycardia are associated with rapid administration. Nephrotoxicity and hepatotoxicity are rare adverse effects. Mild creatinine elevations following H2 antagonist administration are common; however, acute interstitial nephritis (AIN) has been documented. AIN is more commonly seen in men older than 50 years of age with a typical onset within 2 weeks (1 day to 11 months) of therapy. Hepatotoxicity is more common with ranitidine administration. These reactions are reversible upon discontinuation of the offending agent (Fisher & Le Couteur, 2001).

Sucralfate

Sucralfate, a sulfated sucrose aluminum-containing salt, is an oral nonsystemic alternative to currently available PPIs and H2 antagonists for ulcer management. It exerts its actions by adhering to, and forming a protective barrier at, the affected ulcer sites. Sucralfate is generally well tolerated with constipation (2%) and dry mouth (0.7%) being the most common adverse drug effects (Ishimori,1981; Robertson *et al.,* 1989). Systemic absorption of aluminum salt is minimal; however, aluminum accumulation and toxicity has been associated with therapy and aluminum levels should be monitored in patients at increased risk for toxicity (Robertson *et al.,* 1989; Burgess, 1991). The risk of aluminum toxicity is increased in patients with compromised renal function, in patients receiving concomitant aluminum-containing products (i.e., aluminum-containing antacids and phosphate binders) (Ishimori, 1981). Typical dosing is 1 g four times daily. Dosage adjustments in patients with renal and hepatic insufficiency are unnecessary. Food interferes with the bioavailability of sucralfate at the ulcer site and therefore it is recommended that sucralfate be administered on an empty stomach, either 1 hour before or 2 hours after meals (Robertson *et al.,* 1989). Concurrent adminstration of sucralfate with quinolones, cimetidine, antacids, digoxin, lansoprazole, ketoconazole, phenytoin, and warfarin is not recommended because of absorption concerns. Consequently, staggered dosing of at least 2 hours (30 minutes with lansoprazole and antacids) is warranted to avoid loss of effectiveness of either agent (Burgess, 1991).

Antacids

A variety of antacid formulations are available for symptomatic heartburn relief. Many of these agents contain an aluminum, magnesium, or calcium salt alone or in combination with each other. Liquid formulations and suspensions are preferred; however, tablets are equally efficacious if chewed thoroughly. Diarrhea and constipation are the most common adverse effects related to antacid use. Electrolyte abnormalities (calcium, magnesium, phosphate, and sodium) may occur with excessive use. Fluid retention may also be seen with excessive use or large doses. Concurrent administration of antacids with other medications can result in incomplete absorption of the other drugs. Therefore interacting agents should be taken at least 1 to 2 hours before, or 2 to 6 hours after, antacids. Some of these agents

Table 83.12. *Drugs used in HSC transplant recipients optimally requiring administration through a central venous line*

Acyclovir
Amphotericin B
Antithymocyte globulin
Extended spectrum pencillins
Foscarnet
Ganciclovir
Phenytoin
Potassium chloride (in high concentrations)
Quinupristin/dalfopristin
Sulfamethoxazole/trimethoprim
Total parenteral nutrition
Vancomycin

Table 83.13. *Drugs used in HSC transplant recipients that require monitoring of serum or whole blood levels*[a]

Aminoglycosides
Carbamazepine
Cyclosporine
Digoxin
Methotrexate
Phenytoin
Tacrolimus
Vancomycin

[a] See also Chapter 33.

include fluoroquinolones, cyclosporine, atenolol, digoxin, itraconazole, ketoconazole, and mycophenolate mofetil.

Drugs used in HSC transplant recipients requiring administration through a central venous line—see Table 83.12

Drugs used in HSC transplant recipients that require monitoring of serum or whole blood levels—see Table 83.13 (and see Chapter 33)

References

Allington, D.R. & Rivey, M.P. (2001). Quinupristin/dalfopristin: a therapeutic review. *Clinical Therapeutics,* **23,** 24–44.

Alvan, G. & Nord, C.E. (1995). Adverse effects of monobactams and carbapenems. *Drug Safety,* **12,** 305–13.

Ambinder, R.F., Burns, W.H., Lietman, P.S. *et al.* (1984). Prophylaxis: a strategy to minimize antiviral resistance. *Lancet,* **1,** 1154–5.

American Society of Health-System Pharmacists. (1999). ASHP therapeutic guidelines on the pharmacologic management of nausea and vomiting in adult and pediatric patients receiving chemotherapy or radiation therapy or undergoing surgery. *American Journal of Health System Pharmacists,* **56,** 729–64.

Amsden, G.W. (1996). Erythromycin, clarithromycin, azithromycin: are the differences real? *Clinical Therapeutics,* **18,** 56–68.

Anasetti, C., Hansen, J.A., Waldmann, T.A. *et al.* (1994). Treatment of acute graft-versus-host disease with humanized anti-tac: an antibody that binds to the interleukin-2 receptor. *Blood,* **84,** 1320–7.

Anderson, C.M. (1995). Sodium chloride treatment of amphotericin B nephrotoxicity. Standard of care? *Western Journal of Medicine,* **162,** 313–7.

Anne, S., Middleton, E., & Reisman, R.E. (1994). Vancomycin anaphylaxis and successful desensitization. *Annals of Allergy,* **73,** 402.

Antin, J. H., Kim, H. T., Cutler, C. *et al.* (2003). Sirolimus, tacrolimus, and low-dose methotrexate for graft-versus-host disease prophylaxis in mismatched related donor or unrelated donor transplantation. *Blood,* in press.

Appel, G.B., Given, D.B., Levine, L.R., & Cooper, G.L. (1986). Vancomycin and the kidney. *American Journal of Kidney Disease,* **8,** 75.

Arikan, S., Lozano-Chiu, M., Paetznick, V., & Rex, J.H. (2002). In vitro synergy of caspofungin and amphotericin B against Aspergillus and Fusarium spp. *Antimicrobial Agents and Chemotherapy,* **46,** 245–7.

Asbel, L.E. & Levison, M.E. (2000). Cephalosporins, carbapenems, and monobactams. *Infectious Disease Clinics of North America,* **14,** 4335–47.

Aschan, J., Ringden, O., Sundberg, B. *et al.* (1991). Methotrexate combined with cyclosporin A decreases graft-versus-host disease, but increases leukemic relapse compared to monotherapy. *Bone Marrow Transplantation,* **7,** 113–19.

Attassi, K., Hershberger, E., Alam, R., & Zervos, M.J. (2002). Thrombocytopenia associated with linezolid therapy. *Clinical Infectious Diseases,* **34,** 695–8.

Baehr, P.H., Levine, D.S., Bouvier, M.E. *et al.* (1995). Oral beclomethasone dipropionate for treatment of human intestinal graft-versus-host disease. *Transplantation,* **60,** 1231–8.

Barone, J.A., Moskovitz, B.L., Guarnieri, J. *et al.* (1998). Enhanced bioavailability of itraconazole in hydroxypropyl-beta-cyclodextrin solution versus capsules in healthy volunteers. *Antimicrobial Agents and Chemotherapy,* **42,** 1862.

Batts, D.H. (2000). Linezolid—a new option for treating Gram-positive infections. *Oncology,* **14,** S23–9.

Bell, S.J. & Kamm, M.A. (2000). Review article: the clinical role of anti-TNF alpha antibody treatment in Crohn's disease. *Alimentary Pharmacology Therapeutics,* **14,** 501–14.

Berard, J.L., Velez, R.L., Freeman, R.B. *et al.* (1999). A review of interleukin-2 receptor antagonists in solid organ transplantation. *Pharmacotherapy,* **19,** 1127–37.

Beumont, M.G., Graziani, A., Ubel, P.A. *et al.* (1996). Safety of dapsone as Pneumocystis carinii pneumonia in human immunodeficiency virus-infected patients with allergy to trimethoprim/sulfamethoxazole. *American Journal of Medicine,* **100,** 611–6.

Bjornson, B.H., McIntyre, A.P., Harvey, J.M. *et al.* (1986). Studies of the effects of trimethoprim and sulfamethoxazole on human granulopoiesis. *American Journal of Hematology,* **23,** 1–7.

Bleyer, W.A. (1985). Clinical pharmacology and therapeutic drug monitoring of methotrexate. *AACC TDM-T,* **6,** 1–14.

Boeckh, M. (1999). Management of cytomegalovirus infections in blood and marrow transplant recipients. *Advances in Experimental Medicine and Biology,* **458,** 89–109.

Boeckh, M., Gooley, T.A., Myerson, D. *et al.* (1996). Cytomegalovirus pp65 antigenemia-guided early treatment with ganciclovir versus ganciclovir at engraftment after allogeneic marrow transplantation: a randomized double-blind study. *Blood,* **88,** 4063–71.

Boogaerts, M., Winston, D.J., Bow, E.J. *et al.* (2001a). Intravenous and oral itraconazole versus intravenous amphotericin B deoxycholate as empirical antifungal therapy for persistent fever in neutropenic patients with cancer who are receiving broad-spectrum antibacterial therapy: a randomized, controlled trial. *Annals of Internal Medicine,* **135,** 412–22.

Boogaerts, M.A., Maertens, J., Van Der Geest, R. *et al.* (2001b). Pharmacokinetics and safety of a 7-day administration of intravenous itraconazole followed by a 14-day administration of itra-

conazole oral solution in patients with hematologic malignancy. *Antimicrobial Agents and Chemotherapy,* **45,** 981–5.

Boogaerts, M.A., Verhoef, G.E., Zachee, P. *et al.* (1989). Antifungal prophylaxis with itraconazole in prolonged neutropenia: correlation with plasma levels. *Mycoses,* **32,** S103–8.

Bradley, J.S., Garau, J., & Lode, H. (1999). Carbapenems in clinical practice: a guide to their use in serious infection. *International Journal of Antimicrobial Agents,* **11,** 93–100.

Brogden, R.N. & Heel, R.C. (1986). Aztreonam: a review of its antibacterial activity, pharmacokinetic properties and therapeutic use. *Drugs,* **31,** 96–130.

Bubalo, J., Seelig, F., Karbowicz, S. *et al.* (2001). Randomized open-labeled trial of dolesetron for the control of nausea and vomiting associated with hematopoietic stem cell transplantation. *Biology of Blood and Marrow Transplantation,* **7,** 439–45.

Buckley, M.M., Brigden, R.N., Barradell, L.B. *et al.* (1992). Imipenem/cilastatin: A reappraisal of its antimicrobial activity, pharmacokinetic properties and therapeutic efficacy. *Drugs,* **44,** 408–44.

Burgess, E. (1991). Aluminum toxicity from oral sucralfate therapy. *Nephron,* **59,** 523–4.

Bush, L.M., Calmon, J., & Johnson, C.C. (1995). Newer penicillins and beta-lactamase inhibitors. *Infectious Disease Clinics of North America,* **9,** 653–86.

Bygbjerg, I.C., Lund, J.T., & Hording, M. (1988). Effect of folic and folinic acid on cytopenia occuring during cotrimoxazole treatment of Pneumocystis carinii pneumonia. *Scandinavian Journal of Infectious Disease,* **20,** 685–6.

Centers for Disease Control and Prevention. (1995). Recommendations for preventing the spread of vancomycin resistance: recommendations of the Hospital Infection Control Practices Advisory Committee (HICPAC). *Morbidity and Mortality Weekly Report,* **44**(RR-12), 1–13.

Centers for Disease Control and Prevention. (2000). Guidelines for preventing opportunistic infections among hematopoietic stem cell transplant recipients. *Morbidity and Mortality Weekly Report,* **49**(RR-10), 1–125, CE 1–7.

Chan, C., Montaner, J., Lefebvre, E.A. *et al.* (1999). Atovaquone suspension compared with aerosolized pentamidine for prevention of Pneumocystis carinii pneumonia in human immunodeficiency virus-infected subjects intolerant of trimethoprim or sulfonamides. *Journal of Infectious Disease,* **180,** 369–76.

Chrisp, P. & Clissold, S.P. (1991). Foscarnet: a review of its antiviral activity, pharmacokinetic properties and therapeutic use in immunocompromised patients with cytomegalus retinitis. *Drugs,* **41,** 104–29.

Cifkova, R. & Hallen, H. (2001). Cyclosporin-induced hypertension. *Journal of Hypertension,* **19,** 2283–5.

Clemett, D. & Markham, A. (2000). Linezolid. *Drugs,* **59,** 815–27.

Colby, C., McAfee, S.L., Sackstein, R. *et al.* (1999). A prospective randomized trial comparing the toxicity and safety of atovaquone with trimethoprim/sulfamethoxazole as Pneumocystis carinii pneumonia prophylaxis following autologous peripheral blood stem cell transplantation. *Bone Marrow Transplantation,* **24,** 897–902.

Cole, M.S., Stellrect, K.W., Shi, J.D. *et al.* (1999). Visilizumab, a humanized anti-CD3 antibody, is immunosuppressive to T cells while exhibiting reduced mitogenicity in vitro. *Transplantation,* **68,** 563–71.

Cortese, L.M., Soucy, D.M., & Endy, T.P. (1996). Trimethoprim/sulfamethoxazole desensitization. *Annals of Pharmacotherapy,* **30,** 184–6.

Couriel, D.R., Hicks, K., Giralt, S. *et al.* (2000). Role of tumor necrosis factor-alpha inhibition with infliximab in cancer therapy and hematopoeitic stem cell transplantation. *Current Opinion in Oncology,* **12,** 582–7.

D'Antonio, R.G., Johnson, D.B., Winn, R.E. *et al.* (1986). Effect of folinic acid on the capacity of trimethoprim-sulfamethoxazole to prevent and treat Pneumocystis carinii pneumonia in rats. *Antimicrobial Agents and Chemotherapy,* **29,** 327–9.

Deeg, H.J., Blazar, B.R., Bolwell, B.J. *et al.* (2001). Treatment of steroid-refractory acute graft-versus-host disease with anti-CD147 monoclonal antibody ABX-CBL. *Blood,* **98,** 2052–8.

DeGowin, R.L. (1967). A review of therapeutic and hemolytic effects of dapsone. *Archives of Internal Medicine,* **120,** 242–8.

DeGowin, R.L., Eppes, R.B., Powell, R.D., & Carson, P.E. (1966). The hemolytic effects of diaphenylsulfone (DDS) in normal subjects and in those with glucose-6-phosphate-dehydrogenase deficiency. *Bulletin of the World Health Organization,* **35,** 165–79.

Dongari, A., McDonnell, H.T., & Langlais, R.P. (1993). Drug-induced gingival overgrowth. *Oral Surgery Oral Medicine Oral Pathology,* **76,** 543.

Dupont, B. (2002). Overview of the lipid formulations of amphotericin B. *The Journal of Antimicrobial Chemotherapy,* **49,** S31–6.

Dykewicz, C.A. (2001). Summary of the guideline for preventing opportunistic infections among hematopoietic stem cell transplant recipients. *Clinical Infectious Diseases,* **33,** 139–44.

Ennis, D.M. & Cobbs, C.G. (1995). The newer cephalosporins. *Infectious Disease Clinics of North America,* **9,** 687–713.

Farrar, J.T. & Portenoy, R.K. (2001). Neuropathic cancer pain: the role of adjuvant analgesics. *Oncology,* **15,** 1435–42.

Faulds, D. & Heel, C. (1990). Ganciclovir: a review of its antiviral activity, pharmacokinetic properties, and therapeutic efficacy in cytomegalovirus infections. *Drugs,* **39,** 597–638.

Feinstein, L.C., Seidel, K., & Jocum, J. (1999). Reduced dose intravenous immunoglobulin does not decrease transplant-related complications in adults given related donor marrow allografts. *Biology of Blood and Marrow Transplantation,* **5,** 369–78.

Fish, D.N. (2001). Fluroquinolone adverse effects and drug interactions. *Pharmacotherapy,* **21,** 252S–72S.

Fisher, A.A. & Le Couteur, D.G. (2001). Nephrotoxicity and hepatotoxicity of histamine H_2 receptor antagonists. *Drug Safety,* **24,** 39–57.

Fishman, J.A. (1998). Treatment of infection due to Pneumoncystis carinii. *Antimicrobial Agents and Chemotherapy,* **42,** 1309–14.

Flynn, J.M. & Byrd, J.C. (2000). Campath-1H monoclonal antibody therapy. *Current Opinion in Oncology,* **12,** 574–81.

Freeman, C.D., Klutman, N.E., & Lamp, K.C. (1997). Metronidazole: a therapeutic review and update. *Drugs,* **54,** 679–708.

Furlong, T., Storb, R., Anasetti, C. *et al.* (2000). Clinical outcome after conversion to FK 506 (tacrolimus) therapy for acute graft-versus-host disease resistant to cyclosporine or for cyclosporine-associated toxicities. *Bone Marrow Transplantation,* **26,** 985–91.

Gallis, H.A., Drew, R.H., & Pickard, W.W. (1990). Amphotericin B: 30 years of clinical experience. *Reviews of Infectious Diseases,* **12,** 308–29.

Garnett, W.R. (1982). Sucralfate—alternative for peptic ulcer disease. *Clinical Pharmacotherapy,* **1,** 307–14.

Gero, M., Isabelle, G., Stephan, R. *et al.* (2001). The interleukin 2 receptor antagonist basiliximab is well tolerated and effective in the therapy of steroid-resistant acute graft-versus-host disease (GvHD) after allogeneic stem cell transplantation. American Society of Hematology Clinical Meeting. Abstract 2781.

Gijtenbeek, J.M.M., van den Bent, M.J., & Vecht, Ch.J. (1999). Cyclosporine neurotoxicity: a review. *Journal of Neurology,* **246,** 339–46.

Glicklich, D. & Figura, I. (1984). Vancomycin and cardiac arrest. *Annals of Internal Medicine,* **101,** 880.

Gluckman, E., Lotsberg, J., Devergie, A. *et al.* (1983). Prophylaxis of herpes infections after bone-marrow transplantation by oral acyclovir. *Lancet,* **2,** 706–8.

Goodman & Gilman's The Pharmacological Basis of Therapeutics, 9th ed. (1996). New York: The McGraw-Hill Companies, Inc.

Goodrich, J.M., Bowden, R.A., Fisher, L. *et al.* (1993). Ganciclovir prophylaxis to prevent cytomegalovirus disease after allogeneic marrow transplant. *Annals of Internal Medicine,* **118,** 173–8.

Gralla, R.J., Osoba, D., Kris, M.G. *et al.* (1999). Recommendations for the use of antiemetics: evidence-based, clinical practice guidelines. *Journal of Clinical Oncology,* **17,** 2971–94.

Grasela, T.H. Jr., Goodwin, S.D., Walawander, M.K. *et al.* (1990). Prospective surveillance of intravenous amphotericin B use patterns. *Pharmacotherapy,* **10,** 341–8.

Groll, A.H., Piscitelli, S.C., & Walsh, T.J. (1998). Clinical pharmacology of systemic antifungal agents in clinical use, current investigational compounds, and putative targets for antifungal drug development. *Advances in Pharmacology,* **44,** 343.

Groll, A.H., Shah, P.M., Mentzel, C. *et al.* (1996). Trends in the postmortem epidemiology of invasive fungal infections at a university hospital. *Journal of Infection,* **33,** 23–32.

Haile, L.G. & Flaherty, J.F. (1993). Atovaquone: a review. *Annals of Pharmacotherapy,* **12,** 1488–94.

Hann, I.M. & Prentice, H.G. (2001). Lipid-based amphotericin B: a review of the last 10 years of use. *International Journal of Antimicrobial Agents,* **17,** 161–9.

Hann, I.M., Prentice, H.G., Blacklock, H.A. *et al.* (1983). Acyclovir prophylaxis against herpes virus infections in severely immuno-compromised patients: randomized double blind trial. *British Medical Journal,* (Clinical Research Ed.), **287,** 384–8.

Hawkey, C.J. (2001). Gastrointestinal safety of COX-2 specific inhibitors. *Gastroenterology Clinics of North America,* **30,** 921–33.

Hazel, D.L., Graham, J., Dickinson, J.P. *et al.* (1997). Piperacillin-tazobactam as empiric monotherapy in febrile neutropenic patients with haematological malignancies. *Journal of Chemotherapy,* **9,** 267–72.

Heidt, P.J., Kieskamp, M.J., & Timmersman, C.P. (1985). The influence of calcium leucovorin on the co-trimoxazole induced inhibition of leukocyte regeneration after bone marrow transplantation in mice. *Progress in Clinical Biological Research,* **181,** 437–41.

Hemstreet, B.A. (2001). Use of sucralfate in renal failure. *Annals of Pharmacotherapy,* **35,** 360–4.

Hiraoka, A., Ohashi, Y., Okamoto, S. *et al.* (2001). Phase III study comparing tacrolimus (FK506) with cyclosporine for graft-versus-host disease prophylaxis after allogeneic bone marrow transplantation. *Bone Marrow Transplantation,* **28,** 181–5.

Horn, J. (2000). The proton-pump inhibitors: similarities and differences. *Clinical Therapeutics,* **22,** 266–80.

Hsu, B., May, R., Carrum, G. *et al.* (2001). Use of antithymocyte globulin for treatment of steroid refractory acute graft-versus-host disease: an international practice survey. *Bone Marrow Transplantation,* **28,** 945–50.

Hsu, I. (1995). Hyperkalemia and high-dose trimethoprim/sulfamethoxazole. *Annals of Pharmacotherapy,* **29,** 427–9.

Hughes, W.T., Armstrong, D., Body, G.P. *et al.* (2002). 2002 guidelines for the use of antimicrobial agents in neutropenic patients with cancer. *Clinical Infectious Diseases,* **34,** 730–51.

Hurst, M. & Lamb, H.M. (2000). Meropenem: A review of its use in patients in intensive care. *Drugs,* **59,** 653–80.

Hussein, M.A. (2000). Research on thalidomide in solid tumors, hematologic malignancies, and supportive care. *Oncology,* **14,** S9–15.

Ingle, G.R., Sievers, T.M., & Holt, C.D. (2000). Sirolimus: continuing the evolution of transplant immunosuppression. *Annals of Phamacotherapy,* **34,** 1044–55.

Ippoliti, C. (1998). Antidiarrheal agents for the management of treatment-related diarrhea in cancer patients. *American Journal of Health-System Pharmacy,* **55,** 1573–80.

Ishida, Y., Matsuda, H., & Kida, K. (1995). Effect of cyclosporin A on human bone marrow granulocyte-macrophage progenitors with anti-cancer agents. *Acta Paediatrica Japonica,* **37,** 610–3.

Ishimori, A. (1981). Safety experience with sucralfate in Japan. *Journal of Clinical Gastroenterology,* **3,** S169–72.

Jackson, L.M. & Hawkey, C.J. (2000). COX-2 selective nonsteroidal anti-inflammatory drugs: do they really offer any advantages? *Drugs,* **59,** 1207–16.

Jain, A., Brody, D., Hamad, I. *et al.* (2000). Conversion to neoral for neurotoxicity after primary adult liver transplantation under tacrolimus. *Transplantation,* **69,** 172–6.

Jarvis, W.R., Kaplan, J.E., & Edlin, B.R. (2001). Guidelines for preventing opportunistic infections among hematopoietic stem cell transplant recipients. http://www.cdc.gov/preview/mmwrhtml/rr4910al.html.

Jenke, A., Renner, U., Richter, M. *et al.* (2001). Pharmacokinetics of intravenous mycophenolate mofetil after allogeneic blood stem cell transplantation. *Clinical Transplantation,* **15,** 176–84.

Kahan, B.D. (1989). Cyclosporine. *New England Journal of Medicine,* **321,** 1725–38.

Kapusnik-Uner, J.E., Sande, M.A., & Chambers, H.F. (1996). Antimicrobial agents: tetracyclines, chloramphenicol, erythromycin, and miscellaneous antibacterial agents. In *Goodman & Gillman: The Pharmacological Basis of Therapeutics,* ed. J.G. Hardman, L.E. Limbird, P.B. Molinoff, R.W. Ruddon, & A. Goodman-Gillman, pp. 1135–40. New York: The McGraw Hill Companies.

Kasten, M.J. (1999). Clindamycin, metronidazole, and chloramphenicol. *Mayo Clinic Proceedings,* **74,** 825–33.

Kauffman, C.A. & Carver, P.L. (1997). Use of azoles for systemic antifungal therapy. *Advances in Pharmacology,* **39,** 143–89.

Keating, G.M. & Jarvis, B. (2001). Caspofungin. *Drugs,* **61,** 1121–9.

Kelsey, S.M., Shaw, E., & Newland, A.C. (1992a). Aztreonam plus vancomycin versus gentamicin plus piperacillin as empirical therapy for the treatment of fever in neutropenic patients: a randomised controlled study. *Journal of Chemotherapy,* **4,** 107–13.

Kelsey, S.M., Weinhardt, B., Pocock, C.E. *et al.* (1992b). Piperacillin/tazobactam plus gentamicin as empirical therapy for febrile neutropenic patients with haematological malignancy. *Journal of Chemotherapy,* **4,** 281–5.

Khoury, H., Kashyap, A., Adkins, D.R. *et al.* (2001). Treatment of steroid-resistant acute graft-versus-host disease with anti-thymocyte globulin. *Bone Marrow Transplantation,* **27,** 1059–64.

Kobbe, G., Schneider, P., Rohr, U. *et al.* (2001). Treatment of severe steroid refractory acute graft versus host disease with infliximab, a chimeric human/mouse anti-TNF alpha antibody. *Bone Marrow Transplantation,* **28,** 47–9.

Koc, S., Leinsenring, W., Flowers, M.E.D. *et al.* (2000). Thalidomide for treatment of patients with chronic graft-versus-host disease. *Blood,* **96,** 3995–6.

Krieger, O., Bernhart, M., Plohowich, R. *et al.* (1985). Timentin in combination with tobramycin as empirical therapy in febrile neutropenic patients with haematological malignancies. *Journal of Antimicrobial Chemotherapy,* **17,** S211–7.

Lamb, H.M., Figgitt, D.P., & Faulds, D. (1999). Quinupristin/dalfopristin: a review of its use in the management of serious Grampositive infections. *Drugs,* **58,** 1061–97.

Landewe, R.B.M., Goei The, H.S., Rijthoven van, A.W. *et al.* (1994). Cyclosporine in common clinical practice: an estimation of the benefit/risk ratio in patients with rheumatoid arthritis. *Journal of Rheumatology,* **21,** 1631–6.

Lanese, D.M. & Conger, J.D. (1993). Effects of endothelin receptor antagonist on cyclosporine-induced vasoconstriction in isolated rat renal arterioles. *The Journal of Clinical Investigation,* **91,** 2144.

Lavery, S., Ravi, H., McDaniel, W.W., & Pushkin, Y.R. (2001). Linezolid and serotonin syndrome. *Psychosomatics,* **42,** 432–4.

Link, H., Vohringer, H.F., Wingen, F. *et al.* (1993). Pentamidine aerosol prophylaxis of Pneumocystis carinii pneumonia after BMT. *Bone Marrow Transplantation,* **11,** 403–6.

Ljungman, P. (2001). Prophylaxis against herpesvirus infections in transplant recipients. *Drugs,* **61,** 187–96.

Ljungman, P., Cordonnier, C., Einsele, H. *et al.* (1998a). Use of intravenous immune globulin in addition to antiviral therapy in the treatment of CMV gastrointestinal disease in allogeneic bone marrow transplant patients: a report from the European Group for Blood and Marrow transplantation (EBMT). Infectious Disease Working Party of EBMT. *Bone Marrow Transplantation,* **21,** 473–6.

Ljungman, P., De la Camara, R., Milpied, N. *et al.* (1998b). A randomized study of valacyclovir as prophylaxis against CMV infection and disease in BMT recipients. *Bone Marrow Transplantation,* **23,** S80.

Ljungman, P., Wilczek, H., Gharton, G. *et al.* (1986). Long-term acyclovir prophylaxis in bone marrow transplant recipients and lymphocyte proliferation responses to herpes virus antigens in vitro. *Bone Marrow Transplantation,* **1,** 185–92.

Lortholary, O., Tod, M., Cohen, Y., & Petitjean, O. (1995). Aminoglycosides. *Medical Clinics of North America,* **79,** 761–87.

Low, D.E. (1995). Quinupristin/dalfopristin: spectrum of activity, pharmacokinetics, and initial clinical experience. *Microbial Drug Resistance,* **1,** 223–34.

Lucas, L.K. & Lipman, A.G. (2002). Recent advances in pharmacotherapy for cancer pain management. *American Cancer Society,* **10,** S14–20.

Luna, B., Drew, R.H., & Perfect, J.R. (2000). Agents for treatment of invasive fungal infections. *Otolaryngology Clinics of North America,* **33,** 277–99.

MacDonald, A., Scarola, J., Burke, J., & Zimmerman, J.J. (2000). Clinical pharmacokinetics and therapeutic drug monitoring of sirolimus. *Clinical Therapeutics,* **22,** B101–21.

Mackie, M.J., Reilly, J.T., Purohit, S. *et al.* (1986). A randomized trial of Timentin and tobramycin versus piperacillin and tobramycin in febrile neutropenic patients. *Journal of Antimicrobial Chemotherapy,* **17,** S219–24.

Mahalati, K. & Kahan, B.D. (2001). Clinical pharmacokinetics of sirolimus. *Clinical Pharmacokinetics,* **40,** 573–85.

Mandell, G.L. & Petri, W.A. (1996). Antimicrobial agents: sulfonamides, trimethoprim-sulfamethoxazole, quinolones, and agents for urinary tract infections. In *Goodman & Gillman: The Pharmacological Basis of Therapeutics,* ed. J.G. Hardman, L.E. Limbird, P.B. Molinoff, R.W. Ruddon, & A. Goodman-Gillman, pp. 1057–72. New York: The McGraw Hill Companies.

Markham, A. & Faulds, D. (1994). Ganciclovir: an update of its therapeutic use in cytomegalovirus infection. *Drugs,* **48,** 455–84.

Markham, A. & Lamb, H.M. (2000). Infliximab: a review of its use in the management of rheumatoid arthritis. *Drugs,* **59,** 1341–59.

Marr, K.A., Seidel, K., Slavin, M.A. *et al.* (2000). Prolonged fluconazole prophylaxis is associated with persistent protection against candidiasis-related death in allogeneic marrow transplant recipients: long-term follow-up of a randomized, placebo-controlled trial. *Blood,* **96,** 2055–61.

Maschmeyer, G. (2002). New antifungal agents—treatment standards are beginning to grow old. *Journal of Antimicrobial Chemotherapy,* **49,** 239–41.

Maschmeyer, G., Hiddemann, W., Link, H. *et al.* (1997). Management of infections during intensive treatment of hematologic malignancies. *Annals of Hematology,* **75,** 9–16.

Mayhew, J.F. & Deutsch, S. (1985). Cardiac arrest following administration of vancomycin. *Canadian Anaesthetists' Society Journal,* **32,** 65–6.

McCaul, K.G., Nevill, T.J., Barnett, M.J. *et al.* (2000). Treatment of steroid-resistant acute graft-versus-host disease with rabbit antithymocyte globulin. *Journal of Hematotherapy and Stem Cell Research,* **9,** 367–74.

McDonald, G.B., Bouiver, M., Hockenbery, D.M. *et al.* (1998). Oral beclomethasone dipropionate for treatment of intestinal graft-versus-host-disease: a randomized, controlled trial. *Gastroenterology,* **115,** 28–35.

Mertz, G.I., Jones, C.C., Mills, J. *et al.* (1988). Long-term acyclovir suppression of frequently recurring genital herpes simplex viral infection. A multicenter, double-blind trial. *Journal of the American Medical Association,* **260,** 201–6.

Meyers, J.D., Reed, E.C., Shepp, D.H. *et al.* (1988). Acyclovir for prevention of cytomegalovirus infection and disease after allogeneic marrow transplantation. *New England Journal of Medicine,* **318,** 70–5.

Midtvedt, K., Hartmann, A., Foss, A. *et al.* (2001a). Sustained improvement of renal graft function for two years in hypertensive renal transplant recipients treated with nifedipine as compared to lisinopril. *Transplantation,* **72,** 1787–92.

Midtvedt, K., Ihlen, H., Hartmann, A. *et al.* (2001b). Reduction of left ventricular mass by lisinopril and nifedipine in hypertensive renal transplant recipients: a prospective randomized double-blind study. *Transplantation,* **72,** 107–11.

Morris, D.J. (1994). Adverse effects and drug interactions of clinical importance with antiviral drugs. *Drug Safety,* **10,** 281–91.

Mrsic, M., Labar, B., Bogdanic, B. *et al.* (1990). Combination of cyclosporine and methotrexate for prophylaxis of acute graft-versus-host disease after allogeneic bone marrow transplantation for leukemia. *Bone Marrow Transplantation,* **6,** 137–41.

Nahata, M. (1996). Drug interactions with azithromycin and the macrolides: an overview. *Journal of Antimicrobial Chemotherapy,* **37,** C133–42.

Nash, R.A., Pepe, M.S., Storb, R. *et al.* (1992). Acute graft-versus-host disease: analysis of risk factors after allogeneic marrow transplantation and prophylaxis with cyclosporine and methotrexate. *Blood,* **80,** 1838–45.

Nathwani, D. & Wood, M.J. (1993). Penicillins: a current review of their clinical pharmacology and therapeutic use. *Drugs,* **45,** 866–94.

Newfield, P. & Roizen, M.F. (1979). Hazards of rapid administration of vancomycin. *Annals of Internal Medicine,* **91,** 581.

Nicolau, D.P., Freeman, C.D., Belliveau, P.P. *et al.* (1995). Experience with once-daily aminoglycoside proGram administered to 2184 adult patients. *Antimicrobial Agents and Chemotherapy,* **39,** 650–5.

Nunn, P.P. & Allistone, J.C. (1984). Resistance to trimethoprim-sulfamethoxazole in the treatment of Pneumocystis carinii pneumonia: implication of folinic acid. *Chest,* **86,** 149–50.

Olsen, K.M., Rebuck, J.A., & Rupp, M.E. (2001). Arthralgias and myalgias related to quinupristin-dalfopristin administration. *Clinical Infectious Diseases,* **32,** e83–e86.

Onrust, S.V. & Wiseman, L.R. (1999). Basiliximab. *Drugs,* **57,** 207–13.

Ormrod, D., Scott, L.J., & Perry, C.M. (2000). Valacyclovir. A review of its long term utility in the management of genital herpes simplex virus and cytomegalovirus infections. *Drugs,* **59,** 839–63.

O'Sullivan, D.P. (1985). Convulsions associated with cyclosporin A. *British Medical Journal,* **290,** 858.

Palmer, B.F., Dawidson, I., Sagalowsky, A. *et al.* (1991). Improved outcome of cadaveric renal transplantation due to calcium channel blockers. *Transplantation,* **52,** 640.

Pancoast, S.J. (1988). Aminoglycoside antibiotics in clinical use. *Medical Clinics of North America,* **72,** 581–612.

Parker, P., Chao, N., Nademanee, A. *et al.* (1995). Thalidomide as salvage therapy for chronic graft-versus-host disease. *Blood,* **86,** 3604–9.

Pascual, J., Marcen, R., & Ortuno, J. (2001). Anti-interleukin-2 receptor antibodies: basiliximab and daclizumab. *Nephrology Dialysis Transplantation,* **16,** 1756–60.

Patchell, R.A. (1994). Neurological complications of organ transplantation. *Annals of Neurology, 36,* 688–703.

Pengelly, C.D.R. (1963). Dapsone-induced hemolysis. *British Medical Journal, 2,* 662.

Periti, P., Mazzei, T., Mini, E. *et al.* (1992). Pharmacokinetic drug interactions of macrolides. *Clinical Pharmacokinetics, 23,* 106–31.

Perry, C.M. & Markham, A. (1999). Piperacillin/tazobactam: an updated review of its use in the treatment of bacterial infections. *Drugs, 57,* 805–43.

Perry, C.M., Ormrod, D., Hurst, M., & Onrust, S.V. (2002). Gatifloxacin: a review of its use in the management of bacterial infections. *Drugs, 62,* 169–207.

Plosker, G.L. & Noble, S. (1999). Cidofovir: a review of its use in cytomegolovirus retinitis in patients with AIDS. *Drugs, 58,* 325–45.

Poel, M.H.W., Pasman, P.C., & Schouten, H.C. (2001). The use of thalidomide in chronic refractory graft versus host disease. *Netherlands Journal of Medicine, 59,* 45–9.

Prentice, H.G., Gluckman, E., Powels, R.L. *et al.* (1994). Impact of long-term acyclovir on cytomegalovirus infection and survival after allogeneic bone marrow transplantation. European Acyclovir for CMV prophylaxis study group. *Lancet, 343,* 748–53.

Prentice, H.G., Gluckman, E., Powels, R.L. *et al.* (1997). Long-term survival in allogeneic bone marrow transplant recipients following acyclovir prophylaxis for CMV infection. European Acyclovir for CMV prophylaxis study group. *Bone Marrow Transplantation, 19,* 129–33.

Protein Design Labs. (1998). HuM291, Investigator's Brochure.

Przepiorka, D., Kernan, N.A., Ippoliti, C. *et al.* (2000). Daclizumab, a humanized anti-interleukin-2 receptor alpha chain antibody, for treatment of acute graft-versus-host disease. *Blood, 95,* 83–9.

Przepiorka, D., Khouri, I., Ippoliti, C. *et al.* (1999a). Tacrolimus and minidose methotrexate for prevention of acute graft-versus-host disease after HLA-mismatched marrow or blood stem cell transplantation. *Bone Marrow Transplantation, 24,* 763–8.

Przepiorka, D., Petropoulos, D., Mullen, C.A. *et al.* (1999b). Tacrolimus for prevention of graft-versus-host disease after mismatched unrelated donor cord blood transplantation. *Bone Marrow Transplantation, 23,* 1291–5.

Raad, I.I., Whimbey, E.E., Rolstonm, K.V. *et al.* (1996). A comparison of aztreonam plus vancomycin and imipenem plus vancomycin as initial therapy for febrile neutropenic cancer patients. *Cancer, 77,* 1386–94.

Rains, C.P., Bryson, H.M., & Peters, D.H. (1995). Ceftazidime: an update of its antibacterial activity, pharmacokinetic properties and therapeutic efficacy. *Drugs, 49,* 577–617.

Rapp, R.P. (1998). Pharmacokinetics and pharmacodynamics of intravenous and oral azithromycin: enhanced tissue activity and minimal drug interactions. *The Annals of Pharmacotherapy, 32,* 785–93.

Ratanatharathorn, V., Nash, R., & Przepiorka, D. (1998). Phase III study comparing methotrexate and tacrolimus (Prograf, FK506) with methotrexate and cyclosporine for graft-versus-host disease prophylaxis after HLA-identical sibling bone marrow transplantation. *Blood, 92,* 2303–14.

Remberger, M., Aschan, J., Barhlot, L. *et al.* (2001). Treatment of severe acute graft-versus-host disease with antithymocyte globulin. *Clinical Transplantation, 15,* 147–53.

Reynes, J., Bazin, C., Ajana, F. *et al.* (1997). Pharmacokinetics of itraconazole (oral solution) in two groups of human immunodeficiency virus-infected adults with oral candidiasis. *Antimicrobial Agents and Chemotherapy, 41,* 2554.

Robertson, J.A., Salusky, G.B., Goodman, W.G. *et al.* (1989). Sucralfate, intestinal aluminum absorption, and aluminum toxicity in dialysis patients. *Annals of Internal Medicine, 111,* 179–81.

Rodvold, K.A. & Neuhauser, M. (2001). Pharmacokinetics and pharmacodynamics of fluoroquinolones. *Pharmacotherapy, 21,* 232S–52S.

Romero, A.J., Pogamp, P.L., Nilsson, L.G., & Wood, N. (2002). Effect of voriconazole on the pharmacokinetics of cyclosporine in renal transplant patients. *Clinical Pharmacology and Therapeutics, 71,* 226–34.

Rovelli, A., Arrigo, C., Nesi, F. *et al.* (1998). The role of thalidomide in the treatment of refractory chronic graft-versus-host disease following bone marrow transplantation in children. *Bone Marrow Transplantation, 21,* 577–81.

Rubinstein, E., Cammarata, S.K., Oliphant, T.H. *et al.* (2001). Linezolid (PNU-100766) versus vancomycin in the treatment of hospitalized patients with nosocomial pneumonia: a randomized, double-blind, multicenter study. *Clinical Infectious Diseases, 32,* 402–12.

Ruggenenti, P., Perico, N., Mosconi, L. *et al.* (1993). Calcium channel blockers protect transplant patients from cyclosporine-induced daily renal hypoperfusion. *Kidney International, 43,* 706–11.

Rybak, M.J., Abate, B.J., Kang, S.L. *et al.* (1999). Prospective evaluation of the effect of an aminoglycoside dosing regimen on rates of observed nephrotoxicity and ototoxicity. *Antimicrobial Agents and Chemotherapy, 43,* 1549–55.

Rybak, M.J., Albrecht, L.M., Burke, S.C., & Chandrasekar, P.H. (1990). Nephrotoxicity of vancomycin, alone and with an aminoglycoside. *Journal of Antimicrobial Chemotherapy, 25,* 679–87.

Safrin, S., Cherrington, J., & Jaffe, H.S. (1999). Cidofovir. Review of current and potential clinical uses. *Advances in Experimental Medicine and Biology, 458,* 111–20.

Safrin, S., Lee, B.L., & Sande, M.A. (1994). Adjunctive folinic acid with trimethoprim-sulfamethoxazole for Pneumocystis carinii pneumonia in AIDS patients is associated with an increased risk of therapeutic failure and death. *Journal of Infectious Diseases, 170,* 912–7.

Salkind, A.R., Cuddy, P.G., & Foxworth, J.W. (2001). Is this patient allergic to penicillin? An evidence-based analysis of the likelihood of penicillin allergy. *JAMA, 285,* 2498–505.

Saral, R., Burns, W.H., Laskin, O.L. *et al.* (1981). Acyclovir prophylaxis of herpes-simplex-virus infections. *New England Journal of Medicine, 305,* 63–7.

Saravolatz, L., Manzor, O., Check, C. *et al.* (2001). Antimicrobial activity of moxifloxacin, gatifloxacin, and six fluoroquinolones against Streptococcus pneumoniae. *Journal of Antimicrobial Chemotherapy, 47,* 475–7.

Schaison, G., Reinert, P., Leverger, G. *et al.* (1986). Timentin (tivarcillin and clavulanic acid) in combination with aminoglycosides in the treatment of febrile episodes in neutropenic children. *Journal of Antimicrobial Chemotherapy, 17,* 177–81.

Schimmer, B.P. & Parker, K.L. (1996). Adrenocorticotropic hormone-adrenocortical steroids and their synthetic analogs:

inhibitors of the synthesis and actions of adrenocortical hormones. In *Goodman & Gilman's The Pharmacological Basis of Therapeutics,* ed. J.G. Hardman, L.E. Limbird, & P.B. Molinoff, pp. 1459–86. New York: The McGraw-Hill Companies.

Schug, S.A., Zech, D., & Grond, S. (1992). Adverse effects of systemic opioid analgesics. *Drug Safety,* **7,** 200–13.

Selby, P.J., Powles, R.L., Easton, D. *et al.* (1989). The prophylactic role of intravenous and long-term oral acyclovir after allogeneic bone marrow transplantation. *British Journal of Cancer,* **59,** 434–8.

Seymour, H.E., Worsley, A., & Smith, J.M. (2001). Anti-TNF agents for rheumatoid arthritis. *British Journal of Clinical Pharmacology,* **51,** 201–8.

Shanahan, F. (1998). Intestinal graft-versus-host disease. *Gastroenterology,* **115,** 220–2.

Sheehan, D.J., Hitchcock, C.A., & Sibley, C.M. (1999). Current and emerging azole antifungal agents. *Clinical Microbiology Reviews,* **12,** 40–79.

Singhal, S., Mehta, J., Desikan, R. *et al.* (1999). Antitumor activity of thalidomide in refractory multiple myeloma. *New England Journal of Medicine,* **341,** 1565–71.

Somers, G.F. (1960). Pharmacological properties of thalidomide (a-pthalimido glutarimide), a new-sedative hypnotic drug. *British Journal of Pharmacology,* **15,** 111–16.

Souza, J.P., Boeckh, M., & Gooley, T.A. (1999). High rates of Pneumocystis carinii pneumonia in allogeneic blood and marrow transplant recipients receiving dapsone prophylaxis. *Clinical Infectious Diseases,* **29,** 1467–71.

Stanbury, R.M. & Graham, E.M. (1998). Systemic corticosteroid therapy—side effects and their management. *British Journal of Ophthalmology,* **82,** 704–8.

Storb, R., Deeg, H.J., Pepe, M. *et al.* (1989a). Graft-versus-host disease prevention by methotrexate combined with cyclosporin compared to methotrexate alone in patients given marrow grafts for severe aplastic anemia: long-term follow-up of a controlled trial. *British Journal of Haematology,* **72,** 567–72.

Storb, R., Deeg, H.J., Pepe, M. *et al.* (1989b). Methotrexate and cyclosporine versus cyclosporine alone for prophylaxis of graft-versus-host disease in patients given HLA-identical marrow grafts for leukemia: long-term follow-up of a controlled trial. *Blood,* **73,** 1729–34.

Sullivan, K.M., Kopecky, K.J., & Jocom, J. (1990). Immunomodulatory and antimicrobial efficacy of intravenous immunoglobulin in bone marrow transplantation. *New England Journal of Medicine,* **323,** 705–12.

Symons, N.L., Hobbes, A.F., & Leaver, H.K. (1985). Anaphylactoid reactions to vancomycin during anaesthesia: two clinical reports. *Canadian Anaesthetists' Society Journal,* **32,** 178–81.

Takamatsu, Y., Ishizu, M., Ichinose, I. *et al.* (2001). Intravenous cyclosporine and tacrolimus caused anaphylaxis but oral cyclosporine capsules were tolerated in an allogeneic bone marrow transplant recipient. *Bone Marrow Transplantation,* **28,** 421–3.

Taylor, P.C. (2001). Anti-tumor necrosis factor therapies. *Current Opinions in Rheumatology,* **13,** 164–9.

Terrell, C.L. (1999). Antifungal agents. Part II. The azoles. *Mayo Clinic Proceedings,* **74,** 78–100.

The US multicenter FK506 liver study group. (1994). A comparison of tacrolimus (FK506) and cyclosporine for immunosuppression

in liver transplantation. *New England Journal of Medicine,* **331,** 1110–5.

Tracy, J.W. & Webster, L.E. (1996). Drugs used in the chemotherapy of protozoal infections. In *Goodman & Gillman: The Pharmacological Basis of Therapeutics,,* ed. J.G. Hardman, L.E. Limbird, P.B. Molinoff, R.W. Ruddon, & A. Goodman-Gillman, pp. 987–1008. New York: The McGraw Hill Companies.

Tse, J.C. & Moore, T.B. (1998). Monoclonal antibodies in the treatment of steroid-resistant acute graft versus host disease. *Pharmacotherapy,* **18,** 988–1000.

Tuan, I.Z., Dennison, D. & Weisdorf, D.J. (1992). Pneumoncystis carinii pneumonitis after bone marrow transplant. *Bone Marrow Transplantation,* **10,** 267–72.

Uberti, J.P., Silver, S.M., Adams, P.T. *et al.* (1997). Tacrolimus and methotrexate for the prophylaxis of acute graft-versus-host disease in allogeneic bone marrow transplantation in patients with hematologic malignancies. *Bone Marrow Transplantation,* **19,** 1233–8.

Ulrich, C.M., Yasui, Y., Storb, R. *et al.* (2001). Pharmacogenetics of methotrexate: toxicity among marrow transplantation patients varies with the methylenetetrahydrofolate reductase C677T polymorphism. *Blood,* **98,** 231–4.

Vasconcelles, M.J., Bernardo, M.V., King, C. *et al.* (2000). Aerosolized pentamidine as pneumocystis prophylaxis after bone marrow tranplantation is inferior to other regimens and is associated with decreased survival and an increased risk of other infections. *Biology of Blood and Marrow Transplantation,* **6,** 35–43.

Veradi, G., Or, R., Slavin, S. *et al.* (1996). In vivo CAMPATH-1 monoclonal antibodies: a novel mode of therapy for acute graft-versus-host disease. *American Journal of Hematology,* **52,** 236–7.

Volgelsang, G., Farmer, E., Hess, A. *et al.* (1992). Thalidomide for the treatment of chronic graft-versus-host disease. *New England Journal of Medicine,* **326,** 1055–8.

Volgelsang, G., Hess, A., Friedman, K. *et al.* (1988). Therapy of chronic graft-v-host disease in a rat model. *Blood,* **74,** 507–11.

Von Rosenstiel, N.A. & Adam, D. (1995). Macrolide antibacterials: drug interactions of clinical significance. *Drug Safety,* **13,** 105–16.

Wagstaff, A., Faulds, D., & Goa, K. (1994). Acyclovir: a reappraisal of its antiviral activity, pharmacokinetic properties and therapeutic efficacy. *Drugs,* **47,** 153–205.

Wagstaff, A.J. & Bryson, H.M. (1994). Foscarnet: a reappraisal of its antiviral activity, pharmacokinetic properties and therapeutic use in immunocompromised patients with viral infections. *Drugs,* **48,** 199–226.

Walsh, D. (2000). Pharmacological management of cancer pain. *Seminars in Oncology,* **27,** 45–63.

Walsh, T.J., Finberg, R.W., Arndt, C. *et al.* (1999). Liposomal amphotericin B for empirical therapy in patients with persistent fever and neutropenia. *New England Journal of Medicine,* **340,** 764–71.

Walsh, T.J., Pappas, P., Winston, D.J. *et al.* (2002). Voriconazole compared with liposomal amphotericin B for empirical antifungal therapy in patients with neutropenia and persistent fever. *New England Journal of Medicine,* **346,** 225–34.

White, M.H., Bowden, R.A., Sandler, E.S. *et al.* (1998). Randomized, double-blind clinical trial of amphotericin B colloidal dispersion vs. amphotericin B in the empirical treatment of fever and neutropenia. *Clinical Infectious Diseases, 27,* 296–302.

Wilhelm, M.P. & Estes, L. (1999). Vancomycin. *Mayo Clinic Proceedings, 74,* 928–35.

Williams, C.S. & Woodcock, K.R. (2000). Do ethanol and metronidazole interact to produce a disulfiram-like reaction? *Annals of Pharmacotherapy, 34,* 255–7.

Winston, D.J., Hathorn, J.W., Schuster, M.G. *et al.* (2000). A multicenter, randomized trial of fluconazole versus amphotericin B for empiric antifungal therapy of febrile neutropenic patients with cancer. *American Journal of Medicine, 108,* 282–9.

Winston, D.J., Ho, W.G., Bartoni, K. *et al.* (1993). Ganciclovir prophylaxis of cytomegalovirus infection and disease in allogeneic bone marrow transplant recipients. Results of a placebo-controlled, double-blind trial. *Annals of Internal Medicine, 118,* 179–84.

Wiseman, L.R. & Faulds, D. (1999). Daclizumab: a review of its use in the prevention of acute rejection in renal transplant recipients. *Drugs, 58,* 1029–42.

Wolff, S.N., Fay, J.W., Herzig, R.H. *et al.* (1993). High-dose weekly intravenous immunoglobulin to prevent infections in patients undergoing autologous bone marrow transplantation or severe myelosuppressive therapy. A study of the American Bone Marrow Transplant Group. *Annals of Internal Medicine, 118,* 937–42.

Wolff, S.N., Fay, J., Stevens, D. *et al.* (2000). Fluconazole vs low-dose amphotericin B for the prevention of fungal infections in patients undergoing bone marrow transplantation: A study of the North American Marrow Transplant Group. *Bone Marrow Transplantation, 25,* 853–9.

Wolfgang, W., Nadesta, B., Blau, I.G. *et al.* (2001). Treatment of steroid refractory acute and chronic graft-versus-host disease with daclizumab. *British Journal of Haematology, 112,* 820–3.

Wood, A.J. (1996). Pharmacologic treatment of cancer pain. *New England Journal of Medicine, 335,* 1124–32.

Wynd, M.A. & Paladino, J.A. (1996). Cefepime: A fourth-generation parenteral cephalosporin. *Annals of Pharmacotherapy, 30,* 1414–24.

Yee, G.C. & McGuire, T.R. (1990a). Pharmacokinetic drug interactions with cyclosporin (Part I). *Clinical Pharmacokinetics, 19,* 319–32.

Yee, G.C. & McGuire, T.R. (1990b). Pharmacokinetic drug interactions with cyclosporin (Part II). *Clinical Pharmacokinetics, 19,* 400–15.

Zhanel, G.G. & Noreddin, A.M. (2001). Pharmacokinetics and pharmacodynamics of the new fluroquinolones: focus on respiratory infections. *Current Opinion in Pharmacotherapy, 1,* 459–63.

84 Growth and development of the pediatric recipient

MARIE BLEAKLEY AND PETER J. SHAW

The Children's Hospital at Westmead, Sydney, Australia

Introduction

Achieving normal growth and development of the child is a central part of pediatric management. Pediatric oncologists are privileged to treat patients for a number of tumors that have been largely curable since the 1970s. The decade of the eighties was one where increasing numbers of cured patients were seen. Many of these patients are now adults. Although the majority enjoy very good health, problems may occur in almost every organ system. Although hematopoietic stem cell transplantation (HSCT) can be curative, it may cause or exacerbate several problems in the developing child.

Growth

Growth is compromised by a number of factors posttransplant (Table 84.1). In pediatrics short stature is defined as a height less than the third percentile. However, when dealing with short stature, all patients are below this percentile, thus limiting its value. To assess the severity of height reduction, and to be able to monitor the change or response to intervention longitudinally, a more valuable measure is the height standard deviation score (SDS). The SDS is the number of standard deviations the patient's measurement deviates from the mean. So, for example

Table 84.1. *Growth impairment after HSCT: potential contributing factors*

Irradiation
    Cranial radiotherapy
    Total body irradiation
Age
Gender
Transplant type (autologous versus allogeneic)
Graft versus host disease.
Corticosteroids
Endocrine disorders
    Growth hormone deficiency
    Thyroid impairment
    Pubertal disturbance
Skeletal effects

a height of 2, 2.5, or 3 standard deviations below the mean (SDS of -2 to -3) shows an increasing severity of height deficit, although all are less than the third percentile. Final height, the ultimate measure of growth, is typically defined as having been reached when the growth rate is <1 cm/year, or radiologically documented closure of hand/wrist or iliac crest epiphyses. The degree of growth impairment at final height can be assessed as the SDS compared to the normal population and/or the patient's height SDS compared to their parents' SDS (so called "genetic height" SDS, = [mother's SDS + father's SDS]/2).

Evidence of growth impairment

A study by the Late Effects Working Party (LEWP) of the European Blood and Marrow Transplant Group (EBMT) reported the outcome of 181 patients treated in 22 centers who had received HSCT prior to puberty, and who had reached their final height (Cohen *et al.*, 1999c). The patients had been diagnosed with acute lymphoblastic leukemia (ALL, 73), acute myeloid leukemia, (AML, 46), chronic myeloid leukemia (CML) (2), myelodysplastic syndrome (MDS, 2), non-Hodgkin's lymphoma (NHL, 2), or severe aplastic anemia (SAA, 48) and had been transplanted between October 1973 and October 1993 at a mean age of 9.8 years (range 1.5 to 14.9). Transplantation was allogeneic (153 of 181, matched sibling donor (MSD) 149), syngeneic (2), and autologous (25). Total body irradiation (TBI) was administered in 125 of 181 (69%) and was fractionated (fTBI) in 73 patients (40%) (cumulative dose to 13.2 Gy) and single dose (sTBI) in 52 (29%) (3 to 10 Gy). Cranial radiotherapy (CRT) had been given to 28% of patients during previous treatment and 2.2% had received craniospinal irradiation. Chronic extensive graft-versus-host disease (GVHD) was reported in 10%. Growth hormone (GH) had been administered to 15% of patients and 30% had received sex steroid hormones. The mean final height SDS was significantly lower than the genetic height SDS. Height relative to the age standardized general population fell significantly from the time of HSCT (mean -0.15 standard deviation $\pm$ 1.16) to the final height (-1.09 ± 1.45) with a mean decrease in height SDS of 0.94 ± 1.30.

A similar reduction of final height was reported in two smaller studies. Cohen *et al* (1996) reported a mean decrease in height SDS between HSCT and final height of −1.09 ± 0.21 among 28 patients receiving allogeneic HSCT at a mean age of 10 for leukemia or SAA. In a study of 53 children transplanted before 10 years of age, Couto-Silva *et al.* (2000) found a height SDS of −1.2 ± 0.2 at final height compared with −0.3 ± 0.2 at HSCT. In these two studies the final height SDS was also lower than genetic height SDS.

Factors contributing to growth impairment

Factors that have been suggested to contribute to growth impairment after HSCT are outlined in Table 84.1. Among these, exposure to irradiation, young age at HSCT, and the presence of chronic GVHD have been most extensively studied, and are generally considered to have an adverse impact on growth after HSCT.

Radiotherapy effect

Irradiation has been consistently found to have a significant adverse effect on final height. The EBMT LEWP study found that the group of patients who received either sTBI or fTBI, thoraco-abdominal irradiation (TAI), or total lymphoid irradiation (TLI) but had had no prior CRT had a relative risk (RR) of growth deficiency of 6.89 (2.55–18.57) compared with children who received no irradiation (Cohen *et al.*, 1999c). Children who received CRT during first-line therapy with or without subsequent TBI as conditioning for HSCT had an RR of 6.96

(2.11–22.95) of growth deficiency. The effect of CRT and TBI on growth after transplant and final height appeared to be cumulative (Fig. 84.1). Children exposed to both CRT and sTBI had the worst height outcomes with a median delta SDS of −2.07 ± 0.91 and 25% of patients having greater than −3.0 height SDS. Growth deficits were also observed in the following groups: sTBI (median delta SDS −1.37 ± 1.06), CRT + fTBI (−1.11 ± 1.61), fTBI (−0.88 ± 1.25), and TAI/TLI (−0.71 ± 0.72). Children not exposed to irradiation showed no growth deficit. Children with SAA who received irradiation (TBI 3–4 Gy, TAI 5–11 Gy, or TLI 7.5 Gy) had significantly worse growth than children with SAA conditioned without irradiation.

Cranial radiotherapy

Cohen *et al.* (1996) compared the final height SDS of 14 children with leukemia conditioned for alloHSCT with TBI but without exposure to prior CRT with 11 children receiving TBI and exposed to prior CRT (18 Gy in 5 and 24 Gy in 6). They found a greater mean difference in height among those exposed to CRT (mean delta SDS −1.46 ± 0.26 compared with −0.91 ± 0.34). Among 14 children all of whom had received TBI as conditioning for HSCT, Holm *et al.* (1996) observed a greater reduction of final height among the patients who had also received prior CRT (mostly 24 Gy). They also noted a change in height SDS between diagnosis and HSCT among the CRT group.

Several groups have compared growth rate in the first few years following HSCT in patients conditioned with TBI with or without prior exposure to CRT and have found a greater reduction in growth rate following HSCT in children who received

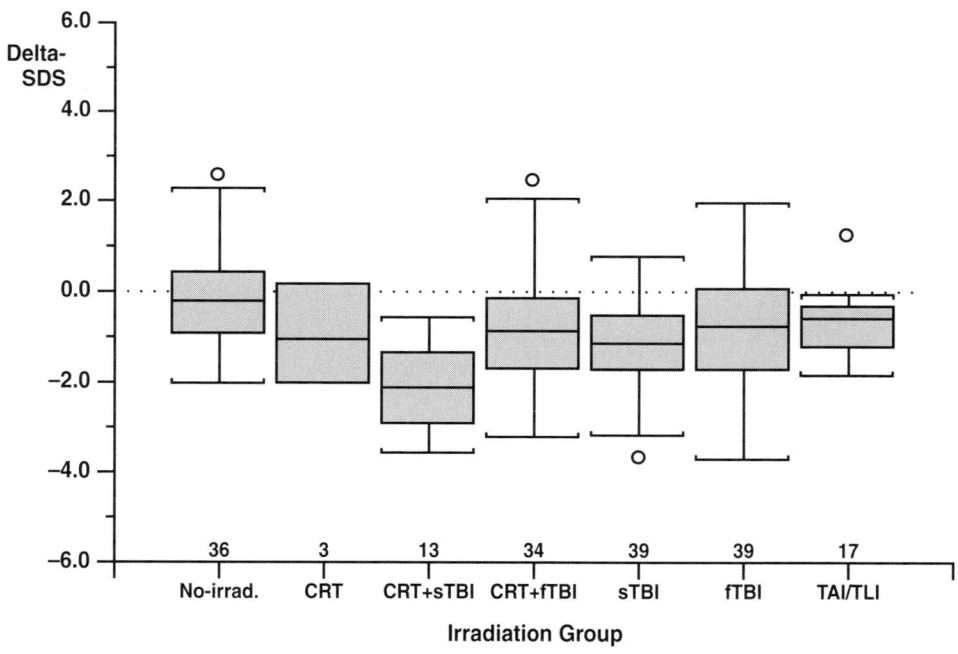

Fig. 84.1. Delta SDS (final height–SDS at BMT) in different irradiation groups. Numerals indicate the number of cases studied in each group. Box plot: the lower line of the box indicates the 25th percentile, the upper line the 75th percentile, and the horizontal lines above and below the boxes represent the 3rd and 97th percentiles, respectively. Reproduced, with permission, from Cohen *et al.* (1999c).

Table 84.2. *Growth rate following HSCT with total body irradiation with or without cranial radiotherapy*

| Study | Follow-up (years) | Diagnosis | | Total body irradiation | | |
				Cranial radiotherapy		No cranial radiotherapy
Arvidson *et al.* (2000)	7.5	Leukemia/NHL	$N = 10$	Delta SDS –0.63 (95% CI –1.0, –0.2)	$N = 7$	No significant change SDS
Cohen *et al.* (1999b)	>5	Leukemia	$N = 23$	Delta SDS –1.46 ± 1.01	$N = 18$	Delta SDS –1.11 ± 0.73
Alter *et al.* (1996)	5	AML	$N = 12$	Pre HSCT htSDS=0.80 ± 0.41, Post HSCT htSDS= –1.75 ± 0.82	$N = 12$	Pre HSCT htSDS = –0.78 ± 0.31 Post HSCT htSDS=–1.05 ± 0.35
Huma *et al.* (1995)[a]	4	Leukemia	$N = 31$	Pre HSCT htSDS=–0.52 ± 0.20 Post HSCT htSDS=–1.83 ± 0.43	$N = 41$	Pre HSCT htSDS = –0.11 ± 0.20 Post HSCT htSDS = –0.73 ± 0.21
Wingard *et al.* (1992)	1	Leukemia/NHL	$N = 21$	Delta SDS=–2.6	$N = 25$	Delta SDS=–0.9

[a] Huma *et al.* (1995) performed a multivariate analysis to determine the effect of CRT on growth in the first 4 years after HSCT among 72 pediatric patients with acute leukemia, all conditioned with radiotherapy. Prior CRT was associated with a greater relative growth impairment independent of the other variables included in the model (diagnosis, age, sex, TBI, and acute and chronic GVHD). The results shown in the table refer to the growth rates for patients with and without CRT controlling for these variables.

CRT (Table 84.2). Giorgiani and colleagues (1995) also found that children receiving TBI and CRT ($N = 17$) had a more marked growth impairment in the first 3 to 4 years post-HSCT than patients receiving TBI without radiotherapy ($N = 37$). Furthermore, growth appeared to slow more quickly after HSCT in patients with prior CRT (Fig. 84.2). The dose effect of prior CRT has not been formally studied in the pediatric HSCT population. However, in a group of 127 long-term survivors of ALL, CRT given for central nervous system (CNS) prophylaxis was associated with reductions in final height. Furthermore, 24

Gy of CRT had a significantly greater detrimental effect on height compared to 18 Gy (SDS –1.38 ± 0.16 versus –0.65 ± 0.15) (Sklar, *et al.*, 1993).

Irradiation of the spine in the initial treatment protocol may also contribute to growth impairment. Very few of the pediatric HSCT recipients reported were exposed to spinal irradiation prior to TBI, so the effect of craniospinal irradiation has not been formally studied within the HSCT cohort. In studies of long-term survivors of pediatric ALL craniospinal irradiation has been confirmed as a risk factor for reduced adult height (Schriock *et al.*, 1991; Schell *et al.*, 1992).

Total body irradiation

The effect of HSCT involving conditioning with TBI is illustrated by a comparison of the growth of monozygotic twins, one the recipient of TBI at the age of 9 years, in Figure 84.3 (Brauner *et al.*, 1993). As stated previously the EBMT LEWP data confirmed the adverse effects of TBI on final height after HSCT independent of CRT in a large cohort (Cohen *et al.*, 1999c). Clement-De Boers *et al.* (1996) also reported on the effect of TBI on final height in a series of 30 patients transplanted prior to ($N = 27$) or during ($N = 3$) early puberty. Sixteen patients with leukemia who had not received prior CRT were conditioned with sTBI (7.5 to 8 Gy except 1 patient, 2 × 6 Gy). Fourteen patients with SAA were conditioned without TBI ($N = 11$) or with sTBI at 4 Gy ($N = 3$). The loss of height SDS between HSCT and final height for patients exposed to TBI was –1.57 ± 0.94. The boys and girls, respectively, reached a final height of 13.2 cm ± 3.5 cm and 6.8 cm ± 5.8 cm below their genetic height. In comparison the SAA patients experienced no significant loss of height (delta SDS –0.06 ± 1.42) and their final height did not differ from their genetic height. On multiple linear regression analysis a higher TBI dose was associated with greater final height deficit.

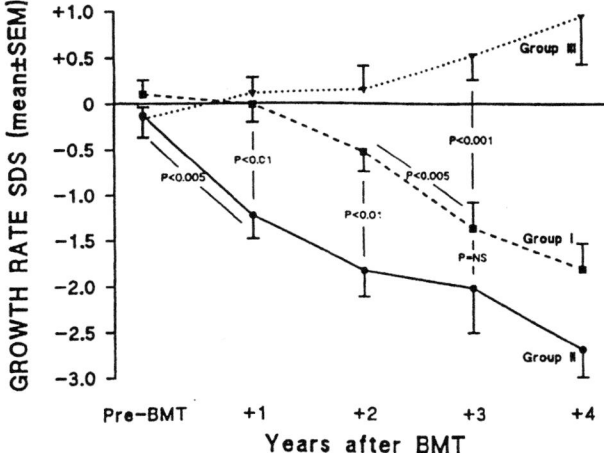

Fig. 84.2. Mean growth rate SDS before and after HSCT in group I, group II, and group III children. In group II, a statistically significant growth rate impairment was observed already during the first year after HSCT, whereas group I children showed a significant decrease in growth rate only between the second and the third year after HSCT. Group III growth rate did not change significantly during the whole observation time. Reproduced, with permission, from Giorgiani *et al.* (1995).

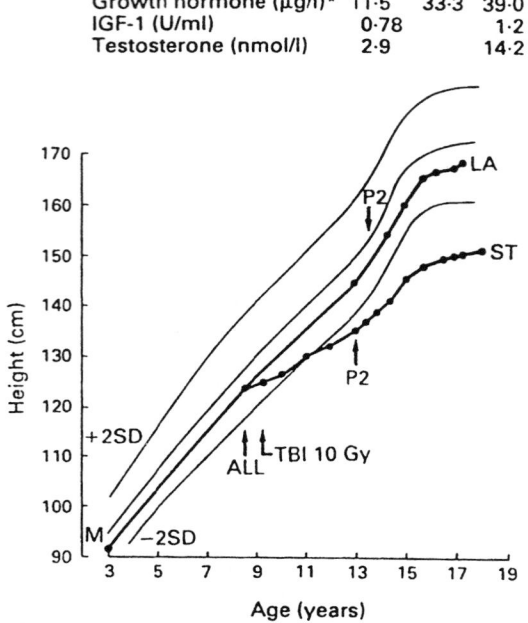

Growth hormone (µg/l)*	11·5	33·3	39·0
IGF-1 (U/ml)		0·78	1·2
Testosterone (nmol/l)		2·9	14·2

Fig. 84.3. Growth of monzygotic twins: case 7 (ST) was given a BMT for ALL from his brother LA. He was conditioned by TBI. The plasma GH peak after the arginine-insulin stimulation test* and the plasma IGF-1 of ST were normal. P2 indicates the onset of puberty. Reproduced, with permission, from Brauner *et al.* (1993).

Single fraction TBI is believed to have a greater detrimental effect on growth after HSCT than fTBI. Brauner *et al.* (1997) compared growth over 5 years after HSCT between 18 children who received six fractions of 2 Gy TBI over a 3-day period for conditioning for autologous HSCT for neuroblastoma or lymphoma, with 14 patients treated with 10 Gy sTBI for leukemia. None of the children had previously received CRT. Both groups had reductions in height SDS after transplant. This was greater in children receiving sTBI at 2 years after transplant, but failed

to achieve statistical significance at 5 years (Fig. 84.4). A similar result was also found in an early paper by the same authors (Brauner *et al.*, 1993). There was a nonsignificant trend toward greater growth impairment 6 years following HSCT in 10 children receiving sTBI (delta SDS –1.12 ± 0.30) compared with 9 children receiving fTBI (delta SDS –0.57 ± 0.32) in a study by Michel *et al.* (1997). In a large cohort of patients all conditioned with TBI for pediatric leukemia, Sanders *et al.* (1986) observed a greater growth deficit at 3 years among 79 patients receiving sTBI 9.2 to 10 Gy compared with 63 patients receiving fTBI over 7 days to a cumulative dose of 12 to 15.75 Gy.

There may potentially be a dose effect of TBI on growth after HSCT in children although this has not clearly been established to date. In a multivariate analysis of growth in the first 4 years after HSCT in 72 pediatric leukemic patients all of whom received fTBI as conditioning for allogeneic HSCT there was no significant difference in height loss found between patients who received 1,375 cGy compared with 1,500 cGy of TBI (Huma *et al.*, 1995). Hovi *et al.* (1999) reported 16 patients with neuroblastoma receiving TBI (sTBI 10 Gy in 11 patients and 12 Gy fTBI in 5 patients) conditioning for autologous HSCT. Five of them had also received prior local irradiation to the skull. There was a trend observed toward greater height decrease in the first 2 years among patients who had received 12 Gy compared with 10 Gy (delta SDS –1.0 for 12 Gy versus delta SDS –0.6 for 10 Gy). Subsequently all of the patients receiving 12 Gy required treatment with GH compared to 1 of 9 patients receiving 10 Gy.

Total abdominal irradiation and total lymphoid irradiation

Total abdominal irradiation as conditioning for SAA may also have an adverse effect on growth after HSCT. Cohen *et al.* (1999b) observed a significant reduction in height SDS over 5 years after HSCT among 11 SAA patients who had received 9 Gy single dose TAI (delta SDS –1.27 ± 1.51), but no growth impairment among 27 children with SAA conditioned with

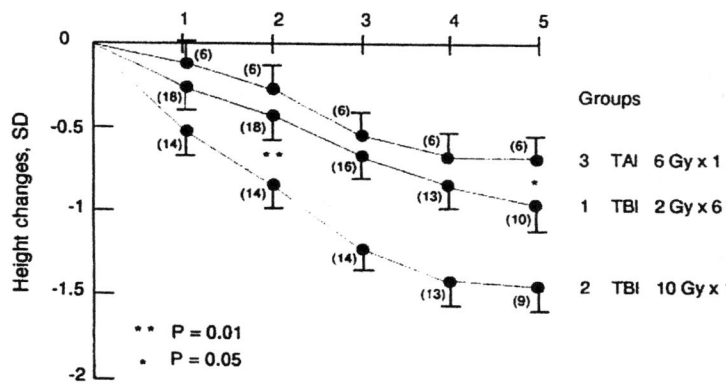

Fig. 84.4. Changes in mean height of patients given TAI or TBI. The number of patients is indicated in parentheses. The *P* value corresponds to group 2 compared with groups 1 and 3 after 2 years, and to group 2 compared with group 3 after 5 years, of conditioning for BMT. Reproduced, with permission, from Brauner *et al.* (1997).

chemotherapy alone. Among 18 patients with SAA conditioned with 7.5 Gy TLI, Bushhouse *et al.* (1989) also observed a fall in height SDS from HSCT to 3 years after HSCT.

Chemotherapy effect

Several studies have now reported the final height of patients receiving bone marrow transplant as children who had not been exposed to irradiation. In the EBMT LEWP analysis 10 patients conditioned with busulfan and cyclophosphamide (BuCy) alone had a similar final height to their genetic height and a delta SDS of 0.05 ± 1.13. Children with SAA conditioned with cyclophosphamide only ($N = 26$) at a median age of 9.8 years had a delta SDS of –0.12 ± 1.08. (Cohen *et al.*, 1999c). Similarly, in the cohort of Clement-De Boers *et al.* (1996) of 14 patients with SAA, 11 of whom received chemotherapy alone, there was no significant growth impairment. Among a group of 47 patients with thalassemia conditioned with busulfan/cyclophosphamide (BuCy), children transplanted at less than 7 years of age were shown to achieve a final height that was normal for the population (height SDS –0.17 ± 0.29 compared with genetic height SDS of 0.05 ± 0.78). Conversely, patients older than 7 at HSCT were growth impaired (height SDS –2.04 ± 0.34 compared with genetic height SDS of 0.42 ± 0.74) (De Simone *et al.*, 2001). Growth rate in the first few years after HSCT among children conditioned with chemotherapy alone has been studied in a number of patient groups (Table 84.3). In the only study that found significant growth impairment among these children, 33% of patients had received prior CRT and the follow-up was relatively short (Wingard *et al.*, 1992). Pretransplant height SDS

did not differ significantly between patients who had and had not received CRT in this study. However, it has been noted that the effects of CRT on GH deficiency may not be apparent for several years after its administration (Clayton & Shalet, 1991). Therefore, the prior CRT may still have been a significant source of bias in the Wingard study. The different pattern of growth following HSCT between children conditioned with BuCy and TBI is shown in Figure 84.5 (Michel *et al.*, 1997).

Chronic GVHD

Chronic GVHD (cGVHD) is believed to impair growth following HSCT, and possibly to reduce final height. However, the difference in growth rate between children with cGVHD and other children has not always been found to be statistically significant, probably because of the limited numbers of children who develop extensive cGVHD. In the EBMT LEWP analysis there was a trend toward a greater reduction of final height after HSCT for the 18 children with extensive cGVHD (delta SDS –1.34 ± 1.85) compared with limited cGVHD (–1.08 ± 1.30) or no cGVHD (–0.84 ± 1.20). Chronic GVHD was not found on multivariate analysis to influence growth after HSCT (Cohen *et al.*, 1999c). However, the analysis may have had insufficient power to detect an effect. Cohen *et al.* (1996) compared the final height of 12 patients with cGVHD with 16 patients without GVHD and also found a trend toward growth impairment among those with GVHD (cGVHD delta SDS –1.36 ± 0.90 vs. no GVHD –0.89 ± 1.2). Clement-De Boers *et al.* (1996) failed to find a significant association between GVHD and change in SDS from HSCT to final height on multiple linear regression analysis, but the analysis was also limited by insufficient sample size.

Table 84.3. *Growth impairment after conditioning without TBI*

Condition	Reference	Number	Age at HSCT	Conditioning	CRT	Outcome
Severe aplastic anemia	Cohen *et al.* (1999c)	26	9.8	Cyclophosphamide	Nil	HSCT height to final height –0.12 ± 1.08
	Cohen *et al.* (1999b)	27	8.1	Cyclophosphamide	Nil	HSCT height to final height –0.44 ± 1.48
Acute myeloid leukemia	Afify *et al.* (2000)	23	10.9	BuCy	Nil	Delta SDS from HSCT to 4 years ($N=16$)+0.20, or 5 years ($N=11$)+0.11
	Michel *et al.* (1997)	26	6.5	BuCy	4/26	Delta SDS from HSCT to 3 years –0.05 ± 0.16 and to 6 years –0.30 ± 0.3
	Shankar *et al.* (1996)	19	7	BuCy	Nil	HSCT height –0.4 ± 1.3 to 1 year ($N=19$) height –0.1 ± 1.2 and 3-year height SDS ($N=7$) –0.2 ± 1.6
	Wingard *et al.* (1992)	24	<12	BuCy	33% 24 Gy median	HSCT height SDS to 2-year post HSCT SDS –1.5 (range –5.0+2.0)
Thalassemia	De Simone *et al.* (2001)	26	5	BuCy	Nil	Final height SDS corrected for parental height SDS +0.49 ± 0.62
Neuroblastoma	Hovi *et al.* (1999)	15	3.0	Melphalan or VP16 carboplatin, thiotepa	Nil	HSCT height SDS –0.7 ± 1.1 10-year post-HSCT height SDS range –0.7 to –0.9
Various	Giorgiani *et al.* (1995) Neuroblastoma 50%	22	<13	BuCy ± melphalan	Nil	Growth rate SDS 4 years post-HSCT +0.95 ± 0.51
	Adan *et al.* (1997) SAA, CID, misc	30	0.2–9	BuCy ± VP16	Nil	Improvement in growth for patients growth retarded prior to HSCT

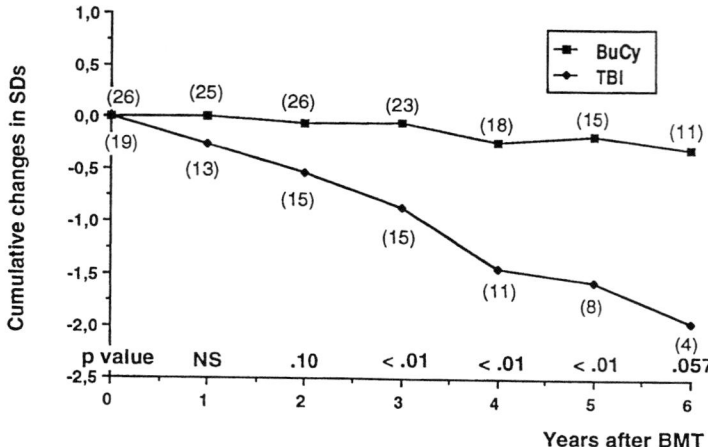

Fig. 84.5. Growth according to preparative regimen. Comparisons are made using the Wilcoxon sum-rank test. Numbers in parentheses indicate number of patients who had height determinations at each time. Reproduced, with permission, from Michel *et al.* (1997).

Some, but not all, of the studies of growth rate in the first few years after HSCT have also suggested that growth impairment is more marked in patients with cGVHD. In multivariate models of the determinants of growth impairment in the first 4 years after HSCT in 72 pediatric patients with acute leukemia, including 15 patients with cGVHD and 4 patients with extensive cGVHD, cGVHD was not of significant prognostic value (Huma *et al.*, 1995). The difference in growth rate over 5 years after HSCT was not significantly different between children with and without cGVHD (delta SDS –0.91 ± 0.40 versus –0.26 ± 0.15) in the study of Michel *et al.* (1997). In a study comparing the growth of 17 patients with nil or limited cGVHD with 7 patients with extensive cGVHD after HSCT with TBI for acute leukemia, a significant difference in growth velocity was found in the first 4 years after HSCT (Alter *et al.*, 1996). In the first year after HSCT the median growth of patients with cGVHD was more than 3.5 SDS below normal. Similarly, among 12 patients undergoing allogeneic HSCT for AML or MDS 4 developed limited cGVHD. These patients had a mean growth velocity SDS at 1 year of –0.9 ± 0.6 compared with –0.2 for the whole cohort (Shankar *et al.*, 1996). Sanders *et al.* (1986) also observed more marked growth impairment in 41 patients with cGVHD in a cohort of 142 patients transplanted for leukemia. This was statistically significant among the 90 boys, but not in the group of 52 girls, although a similar trend was apparent in this later group. The growth of 5 patients who did not receive glucocorticoid treatment did not appear to be different from the growth velocity of the other children with cGVHD. Sanders *et al.* (1991a) have reported that in children conditioned with chemotherapy alone, although growth velocity may be reduced during cGVHD, catch-up growth occurs following the resolution of GVHD and cessation of corticosteroid treatment.

Age
In the EBMT LEWP study (Cohen *et al.,* 1999c) younger age at HSCT was found on multivariate logistic regression analysis

to increase the risk of growth deficiency after HSCT. Children less than 8.8 years at HSCT had an RR of growth deficiency of 5.29 compared to children older than 11 years at transplant. On linear regression, the younger the age at HSCT, the greater the final height delta SDS and the lower the final height SDS. Clement-De Boers *et al.* (1996) also found a negative effect of younger age at HSCT and final height SDS on multiple linear regression analysis, while a correlation between loss of height SDS after HSCT and younger age at HSCT was found by Cohen *et al.* (1996).

One study that evaluated the effect of age on growth in the first few years failed to find a significant effect (Huma *et al.,* 1995). In patients with childhood ALL who do not receive HSCT a pattern of a delayed growth impairment has been observed among patients treated at younger age (Schell *et al.,* 1992). The differences in growth effects of chemotherapy or of HSCT between age groups may not be apparent in short-term studies and longer follow-up may be required.

Whether younger age is a significant risk factor for growth impairment after HSCT may also depend on other variables such as the use of CRT and TBI. In a multivariate analysis of predictors of final height in 109 (non-HSCT) survivors of childhood ALL, CRT and an interaction term for age and CRT were significant predictors of adult height. This indicates that younger children receiving CRT have a greater decrement in final height SDS compared to older children receiving CRT. When the groups who did and did not receive CRT were analyzed separately, age was a significant predictor of final height in the irradiated group but not in the chemotherapy only group (Katz *et al.,* 1993). Interactions between age and other variables following HSCT have not been reported to date.

Other contributing factors
Gender has been found in some studies to influence growth after HSCT. In the EBMT LEWP report male gender was associated with an RR of 4.5 of a negative change in height SDS

between HSCT and final height. Boys had a mean height delta SDS of –1.17 ± 1.34 compared with a height delta SDS for girls of –0.56 ± 1.13 (Cohen et al., 1999c). Gender did not significantly influence final height SDS in multivariate analysis in another study (Clement-De Boers et al., 1996). However, in that study among the subgroup of patients conditioned with TBI the mean loss of height SDS among boys was –1.96 SDS ± 0.82 compared with –0.92 ± 0.71 for girls.

Corticosteroid use has also been proposed as a contributing factor to growth impairment after transplant. The effects of corticosteroids are difficult to separate from the effects of GVHD, for which they are most frequently prescribed. However, in the Seattle cohort it was observed that the growth of 5 patients who did not receive glucocorticoid treatment did not appear to be different from the growth velocity of the other children with chronic GVHD (Sanders et al., 1986). In an univariate analysis of the effects of corticosteroid use on growth after HSCT, Michel et al. (1997) found a trend to greater growth impair-

ment over 3 years among 20 children receiving corticosteroids (delta SDS –0.61 ± 0.28) compared with 25 children not requiring corticosteroid therapy (delta SDS –0.18 ± 0.12).

Other variables that have been examined as potential determinants of growth after HSCT include transplant type and diagnosis. In the EBMT LEWP study no significant influence of type of transplant (autologous compared with allogeneic) or type of leukemia was found (Cohen et al., 1999c).

Mechanisms of growth impairment following HSCT

Endocrine factors

Growth hormone deficiency GH deficiency has been identified as one factor that may mediate growth impairment in pediatric HSCT recipients. GH stimulation tests have been performed in a number of studies with a variable proportion of the subjects found to be GH deficient (Table 84.4). There is little consistency in findings among studies. However, in general, in studies

Table 84.4. *Growth hormone stimulation test results in recipients of pediatric HSCT*

Study	Test type	Criteria	Study population	Time from HSCT	TBI	CRT	Number (%) below lower level normal
De Simone et al. (2001)	Insulin, arginine, clonidine	<10 ng/ml	Unselected	1 and 2 years	No	No	0/47[a] (0)
De Simone et al. (1995)	Clonidine	<8 ng/ml	Unselected	1 and 2 years	No	No	16/22 (73)
Holm et al. (2000)	Arginine	15 mU/l[b]	Unselected	NS[c]	Yes	13/25	8/25 (32) CRT 6/13 (46) No CRT 2/12 (17)
Clement De-Boers et al. (1996)	Arginine Exercise or L-dopa	<10 ng/ml	Growth velocity <25th percentile	NS	19/30	Nil	0/30 (0)
Huma et al. (1995)	Insulin, L-dopa, clonidine	<10 ng/ml	Children with poor growth	3.7 years	Yes	13/18	15/18 (83) CRT 12/13 (92) No CRT 3/5 (60)
Giorgiani et al. (1995)	Insulin, arginine and/or L-dopa	<10 ng/ml on 2 tests	Growth >2 SDS below normal	NS	Yes	14/37	35/37 (95)
Brauner et al. (1997)	Arginine and insulin	<10 mcg/l	Unselected	2.9 years	Yes	No	12/32 (38)
Brauner et al. (1993)	Arginine and insulin	<10 mcg/l	Unselected	3 years	Yes	No	3/11 (27)
Olshan et al. (1993)	Arginine and clonidine	<10 mcg/l two tests	Unselected	NS	Yes	2/6	3/6 2 tests (50) 5/6 ≥ 1 test (83)
Ogilvy-Stuart et al. (1992)	Insulin	<10 mcg/l	Unselected	2.4 years	Yes	4/31	15/29 (52)
Dopfer et al. (1989)	GnRH, TRH, and arginine	NS	Unselected	NS	Yes	19/25	6/25 (24)
Wingard et al. (1992)	Glucagon	NS	Growth > 2 SDS below normal	1	3/7	NS	0/7 (0) lowest 9.1 ng/ml
Sanders et al. (1991b)	Clonidine	NS	NS	NS	Yes	Some	93/118 (79)
Sanders et al. (1986)	L-dopa or insulin	<10 ng/ml	Children not on glucocorticoids	3 median	Yes	25/43	27/43 (63) CRT 21/25 (84) No CRT 6/18 (33)
Leiper et al. (1987)	Insulin	<20 mU/l	Unselected	NS	Yes	8/17	10/17 (59)

[a] 47/102 followed until adulthood. All alive had testing at 12 and 24 months and all normal.

[b] Different assays at different time points therefore different criteria.

[c] Not specified in publication.

of unselected HSCT recipients (i.e., with a range of growth rates) it appears that children who have not been exposed to irradiation are infrequently GH deficient (0–36%), whereas a greater proportion of patients exposed to TBI without CRT (16–38%) and patients exposed to both TBI and CRT (46–84%) are diagnosed with GH deficiency.

GH deficiency as demonstrated by stimulation tests may not be entirely due to the effects of irradiation. Ryalls *et al.* (1992) studied 23 children prior to, and 6 and 12 months following, HSCT with TBI. They found that more than half of the children (both those who had and had not received prior CRT) would have been diagnosed as GH deficient prior to HSCT on the basis of an insulin-induced hypoglycemia test. There was no further reduction in stimulated GH levels at 6 and 12 months post-HSCT.

It is of interest that even within patient groups selected for GH stimulation testing on the basis of poor growth rates, not all patients are found to be GH deficient (Wingard *et al.,* 1992; Giorgiani *et al.,* 1995; Huma *et al.,* 1995). There was no correlation between GH levels measured on GH stimulation tests and growth rates in the only study that has reported results of a correlational analysis (Brauner *et al.,* 1997). This suggests either lack of sensitivity of the tests employed, or the presence of other factors contributing to poor growth following HSCT.

Some of the variability in the findings of studies employing GH stimulation tests may be due to variation in the test protocols, GH assays, and criteria for the diagnosis of GH deficiency. Other factors that may confound the results of GH stimulation studies include (1) the proportion of patients receiving corticosteroids for the treatment of cGVHD; (2) the proportion of patients in the immediate peripubertal period, which is recognized to be associated with low GH levels on provocation tests (GH Research Society, 2000); (3) time after HSCT that GH stimulation tests are performed, allowing for the possibility that GH deficiency develops progressively over time especially in patients exposed to radiation, or conversely that there may be some spontaneous recovery of GH secretion over time. Sanders *et al.* (1991b) noted that of 47 patients who had spontaneous and stimulated GH tests performed, 10 patients had test results that did not agree with each other or reflect the child's growth in the previous 12 months and that these patients all subsequently became GH deficient.

Other methods of studying GH deficiency may prove to be more sensitive in the HSCT population. Holm *et al.* (1996) performed 24-hour monitoring of spontaneous GH secretion involving blood samples every 30 minutes in 9 patients who had undergone HSCT and compared the results to 15 age and sex-matched healthy controls. The HSCT patients had a comparable number of peaks and amplitude of GH secretion but the area under the curve above the calculated baseline was lower in the patients.

IGF1 (somatomedin C) and IGFBP have also been studied in children after HSCT. No consistent relationship between IGF1 or IGFBP and GH or growth after HSCT had been shown (Wingard *et al.,* 1992; Holm *et al.,* 1996; Brauner *et al.,* 1997;

Couto-Silva *et al.,* 2000). In one group of patients who had been exposed to TBI, IGF1 was found to be below the lower level of normal in 7 of 32 and higher than normal in 4 of 32, while IGFBP3 was below the lower level of normal in 11 of 32. In children who had not been exposed to TBI the somatomedin levels were normal or high. It was concluded that the levels of IGF1 and IGFBP reflect the combined effects of reduced GH, acting to reduce levels, and bone refractoriness to the somatomedins, acting to increase levels (Brauner *et al.,* 1997).

Pubertal disorders

Pubertal disorders may contribute to growth impairment. Premature puberty is a recognized complication of CRT in childhood (Ureana *et al.,* 1991). Although it is infrequently seen in pediatric HSCT recipients, if present, premature puberty is likely to lead to a reduced final height. A greater height loss between HSCT and final height has been found in recipients of pediatric HSCT with TBI who reach puberty earlier (boys $r = 0.81$ and girls $r = 0.93$) (Clement-De Boers *et al.,* 1996). More commonly pubertal delay occurs, especially in females (see below) contributing to a prolonged period of reduced growth rate. Patients nearing pubertal age at the time of HSCT have been found to have a significantly greater height decrease over the 3-year posttransplant period than other children (Michel *et al.,* 1997). If a prepubertal reference is used to compensate for the effect of pubertal delay among HSCT recipients, it can be shown that pubertal growth is more impaired than prepubertal growth in children conditioned with TBI for HSCT (Clement-De Boers *et al.,* 1996). The issue of pubertal delay may confound studies of growth rates following HSCT between cohorts of transplant recipients of dissimilar age ranges.

Thyroid hormone status

Hypothyroidism is likely to cause growth impairment in children. Subclinical hypothyroidism with an elevated TSH but normal T4 level, reflecting dysfunction of the hypothalamic-pituitary-thyroid-axis is also considered as a possible contributing factor. Overt hypothyroidism has been reported in 0 to 17% of pediatric HSCT recipients while subclinical hypothyroidism is more common (0–37%) (Table 84.5). No attempt to correlate thyroid abnormalities with growth impairment after pediatric HSCT has been reported.

Limited information is available about the factors contributing to thyroid dysfunction after pediatric HSCT. It is clear that thyroid dysfunction is in some way a direct effect of HSCT, as patients studied prior to HSCT have normal TSH levels and normal TRH test results (Borgstrom & Bolme, 1994). Both overt and subclinical hypothyroidism appear to be more common in cohorts receiving TBI, but have been reported in some series where children have not been exposed to radiation (Boulad *et al.,* 1995; Michel *et al.,* 1997; Afify *et al.,* 2000). No correlation of thyroid abnormalities with previous CRT, sTBI, or fTBI; presence or absence of cGVHD; or patient age or sex was found in the largest cohort reported (Sanders *et al.,* 1986).

Table 84.5. *Thyroid function abnormalities in recipients of pediatric HSCT*

Study	TBI	CRT	TSH elevation with normal T4 (%)	T4 low (%)
Afify *et al.* (2000)	No	No	3/21 (14)	0/21 (0)
Legault & Bony (1999)	Some	NS	4/39 (10)	2/39 (5)
Mathes-Martin *et al.* (1999)	Some	NS	3/73 (4)	0/73 (0)
Michel *et al.* (1997)	Some	Some	3/40 (8)	5/40 (13)
Shankar *et al.* (1996)	No	No	0/19 (0)	0/19 (0)
Katsanas *et al.* (1990)	Some	NS	20/80 (25)	0/80 (0)
Borgstrom *et al.* (1994)	Yes	4/27	10/27 (37)	3/27 (11)
Boulad *et al.* (1995)	Yes	NS	16/100	0/100
Brauner *et al.* (1993)	Some	No	5/29 (17)	3/29 (10)
Ogilvy-Stuart *et al.* (1992)	Yes	4/31	3/31 (10)	2/31 (6)
Wingard *et al.* (1992)	Some	NS	5/17 (29)	0/17 (0)
Sanders *et al.* (1986)	Yes	Some	25/116 (21)	13/116 (11)
Urban *et al.* (1988)	No	Yes	0/10 (0)	0/10 (0)
Leiper *et al.* (1987)	Yes	8/17	NS	3/17 (17)

Abbreviation: NS, not specified.

Dose of TBI (13.75 versus 15 Gy hyperfractionated), gender, type of leukemia, type of HSCT (T-cell depleted or unmodified), or the presence or absence of cGVHD, did not influence the risk of thyroid dysfunction in another cohort (Boulad *et al.*, 1995). Fractionation of TBI may reduce the incidence of thyroid disturbance. With sTBI of 10 Gy, 31% of patients in one series developed subclinical hypothyroidism and 15% overt hypothyroidism; of those given fTBI in doses of 12 to 15.75 Gy, 13% had subclinical and 3% overt hypothyroidism (Sanders *et al.*, 1991a).

Skeletal effects of HSCT

It is believed that HSCT with TBI directly affects bones and cartilage and impairs the ability of these tissues to respond to growth-stimulating factors. Not all patients, even with severely impaired growth, after HSCT have a detectable deficiency of GH or somatomedins, and children may fail to respond to GH replacement. It is well recognized that local radiotherapy to the spine or long bones produces focal growth impairment, and it is assumed that TBI acts in a similar fashion on metaphyseal growth plates throughout the body.

Some studies report disproportionate short stature after HSCT involving TBI. Greater reductions of sitting height, reflecting particularly impaired spinal growth are typically observed (Leiper *et al.*, 1987; Papadimitriou *et al.*, 1991). The effects of radiation on the spine tend to become evident during the pubertal growth spurt. It is only after this is complete that the severity of reduced spinal growth can be assessed. So far, data on sitting height in people who have obtained adult height after pediatric HSCT are lacking. As most of the patients in the series reporting sitting height have not received craniospinal irradiation in addition to TBI, it is thought that spinal growth is reduced because of a greater inherent susceptibility of the spine to the direct effects of TBI, possibly because of the increased number of growth plates. Alternatively, the spine may be more susceptible to GH deficiency, or to the effects of chemotherapy. It is of interest that of 109 children who received cranial irradiation and chemotherapy (without HSCT) for ALL, 88 (81%) had relatively shorter backs compared with legs, with 25 (33%) showing marked disproportion (Davies *et al.*, 1994). Although spinal growth may be relatively more affected, experience with GH therapy suggests that the skeletal effects of HSCT are not limited to the spine. In 13 children who had received cyclophosphamide and TBI for HSCT at a mean of 3.2 years before assessment (8 of 13 also prior CRT), sitting height SDS was found to be more impaired than subischial leg length (sitting SDS -2.26 ± 0.68, subischial SDS -0.87 ± 0.63). Both sitting and subischial SDS failed to improve with GH therapy, suggesting that HSCT directly impaired growth of both the lower limb and vertebral epiphyses (Papadimitriou *et al.*, 1991). In children who do not receive any cranial radiotherapy, but do receive local irradiation to the spine as part of HSCT, skeletal disproportion may be more apparent. Brauner *et al.* (1997) showed that sitting heights at 4 to 6 years after HSCT were reduced in patients receiving fTBI and sTBI and TAI at 2 to 5 years (mean sitting height SDS fTBI -1.3 ± 0.2, sTBI -1.6 ± 0.3, TAI -1.8 ± 0.3). A greater relative reduction of sitting height was seen in the TAI group (difference standing to sitting height SDS fTBI -0.2 ± 0.1, sTBI 0.5 ± 0.1, TAI 1.1 ± 0.5). None of this cohort had received prior cranial irradiation.

Bone age has not generally been found to be significantly retarded after HSCT (Shankar *et al.*, 1996; Arvidson *et al.*, 2000). However, bone age retardation may occur in the presence of overt GH deficiency. Brauner *et al.* (1997) observed that there was a greater difference between bone age and chronological age among 9 HSCT recipients who had subnormal levels of GH at a mean of 3 years after HSCT (1.7 ± 0.3) compared with 13 patients with normal GH levels (0.7 ± 0.1).

Discrete skeletal abnormalities are detectable on radiological imaging in many survivors of pediatric HSCT. Of 10 individuals who had undergone HSCT with TBI for pediatric leukemia, 5 were found to have osteochondromas, 3 had metaphyseal growth abnormalities, 2 had mild scoliosis, 1 a slipped femoral capital epiphysis, 1 had avascular necrosis of the femoral condyles, and 1 had a femoral enchondroma (Fletcher et al., 1994). Avascular necrosis is considered to be related primarily to the use of corticosteroids to treat GVHD, rather than the use of TBI (Mascarin et al., 1991).

The prevalence of reduced bone density after HSCT is controversial. Osteoporosis was detectable radiologically in 7 of 53 (13%) recipients of pediatric HSCT at a median time of 4.6 years after transplant. Approximately half of the patients had received TBI (Matthes-Martin et al., 1999). Whole body bone mass was reported to be reduced 2 years after HSCT in patients with myeloid leukemia (Bhatia et al., 1998). In a detailed analysis of bone mass and bone density at a mean of 7.5 years after HSCT with TBI in children, Nysom et al. (2000), found that, adjusted for sex and age, the mean whole-body mineral content and bone mineral area density ware significantly less than healthy controls. However, the reduced bone mineral content was caused by a significantly reduced height for age, and bone area for height and bone mineral content for bone area were similar to controls. That is, the survivors' bones were smaller, in proportion to their short stature, but there was no actual reduction in bone density accounting for bone size.

TBI has profound effects on craniofacial growth, particularly in children under 6 years old. Dental development is severely disturbed, with dental agenesis, impaired root development, and reduced length of the mandible and height of the alveolar processes (Dahllof et al., 1988). Mandibular growth at least seems responsive to therapy with GH (Dahllof et al., 1991) and orthodontic therapy can be undertaken (Dahllof et al., 2001).

Treatment of growth impairment after HSCT

Growth hormone

There is no evidence to date that the administration of GH to recipients of pediatric HSCT is associated with an increase in final height. The EBMT LEWP reported the outcome of 28 patients who received GH treatment for a median period of 3.5 years (range 0.3 to 7 years) starting at 13.2 ± 2.1 years of age (range 9.8 to 17.9 years), 3.8 ± 2.0 years from HSCT. The mean delta SDS from HSCT to final height for these patients was -1.14 ± 1.24, which was not statistically different from 153 patients not treated with exogenous GH (delta SDS -0.90 ± 1.31). There was also no statistically significant difference in patients who received GH compared with those who did not, within groups stratified by irradiation exposure, and gender (Cohen, 1999c). However, there is an inherent bias in studying this problem in that the patients who receive GH therapy tend to be those with particularly severe growth impairment following HSCT, and it is not clear what the final height outcome of these patients would have been without therapy.

Short-term results of GH therapy in pediatric HSCT recipients show a modest effect at best (Table 84.6). In the first 1 to 3 years after the initiation of therapy growth velocity tends to increase in relation to the year before treatment is commenced (Huma et al., 1995; Brauner et al., 1997). This effect is not always seen in all patients (De Simone et al., 1997). The growth velocity may still remain at or below the age standardized growth velocity of the normal population (Brauner et al., 1997) such that there is no effective "catch-up growth" (Fig. 84.6). It has also been noted that the effect of GH therapy on growth velocity for HSCT patients in some series (e.g., 3.2 cm per year for neuroblastoma patients) is less than the reported average increase of 4.8 cm per year in patients with constitutional delay of growth and development (Olshan et al., 1993). Furthermore the increase in growth velocity may be initially promising but not sustained with prolonged treatment (Papadimitriou et al., 1991; Hovi et al., 1999). There is no consensus about indications for GH therapy for pediatric HSCT recipients. If a child demonstrates a decrease in height SDS of more than 2 SDs, and has documented GH deficiency on two stimulation tests on at least one occasion, a trial of GH therapy does not seem unreasonable. Consideration of GH replacement therapy should particularly be given to children with GH deficiency in whom sex steroid therapy to induce puberty is planned. It is now considered that there is no evidence to support an increase in the risk of leukemic relapse or de novo malignancy with GH therapy (Shalet et al., 1998).

Thyroid hormone replacement

L-thyroxine replacement is indicated for patients with frank hypothyroidism (high TSH and low T4). Indications for treatment of subclinical hypothyroidism are less certain. Treatment of an elevated TSH may reduce the risk of thyroid adenomas and carcinomas, and could potentially be beneficial to growth. However, an increased risk of early osteoporosis has also been reported when TSH is reduced to very low levels with L-thyroxine therapy. In some cases subclinical hypothyroidism is self-resolving (Borgstrom et al., 1994; Boulad et al., 1995; Afify et al., 2000). One appropriate approach is to follow-up patients with subclinical hypothyroidism with twice yearly TSH and T4 levels and to prescribe L-thyroxine only if TSH concentrations remain high or are increasing (Cohen 1999a).

Weight and metabolic disorders

Weight

Change in body composition with an increased adiposity has been observed in several series of long-term survivors of pediatric ALL treated without HSCT (Schell et al., 1992; Birkebaek et al., 1998). There have been a limited number of studies addressing this form of growth disturbance after HSCT in children. In 20 recipients of autologous HSCT transplanted between the ages of 1.9 and 10.9 years weight/height SDS was close to zero at diagnosis, increased significantly from diagnosis to

Table 84.6. *Effect of growth hormone therapy on growth impairment after HSCT*

Study Patient number	Criteria for GH treatment	Growth hormone protocol	Results
Couto-Silva *et al.* (2000) N = 13	Peak GH <10 µg/l and height loss from HSCT > 1 SD or random in 2 pts	0.7 U/kg/week s.c. 6 days/week	Growth rate increased from 4.1 ± 0.4 to 6.1 ± 0.5 cm/year during first year
Brauner *et al.* (1997) N = 7	Peak GH <10 µg/l and height loss from HSCT > 1 SD or random in 1 pt	0.5–0.6 U/kg/week s.c. 6 days/week	Growth rate became normal for age but without catch-up growth –2.1 ± 0.9 SDS before and –0.2 ± 0.4 SDS for the first year
De Simone *et al.* (1997) N = 7	>2 SDs below normal Age at GH 12 years	0.9 U/kg/week s.c. daily	5/7 patients improved—median SDS from –2.42 ± 0.2 to –2.0 ± 0.2 2/7 did not improve—worsening SDS from –3.60 ± 1.13 to –4.85 ± 0.49
Giorgiani *et al.* (1995) N = 23	Peak GH <10 µg/l on 2 stim tests if normal GTT and bone age <12	0.6 U/kg/week s.c. 4–6 days	Growth velocity increased—SDS –2.29 ± 0.27 to +0.86 ± 0.38 1-year and to +1.66 ± 0.56 at 2 years Actual height SDS score not significant –1.44 ± 0.19 to –1.12 ± 0.2 first year and to –0.78 ± 0.40 after 2 years
Huma *et al.* (1995) N = 9	GH treatment of 9/15 dx with peak GH < 10 µg/l. Age at GH 12.4 years	0.2–0.3 mg/kg/week s.c. daily or 3 × week	Growth velocity before SDS –2.7 ± 0.7 Growth velocity after SDS +1.2 ± 0.61 year
Hovi *et al.* (1999) N = 5	Peak GH <10 µg/l. Age 4.3 to 10.5 years	0.7 U/kg/week s.c. s.c. daily	Pretreatment growth velocity 3 to 4.1 cm per year First 3 years mean height SDS increased 0.4 SDS in GH replaced and decreased 0.8 SDS in nonsubstituted Not sustained. Fifth year growth velocity no better than before GH
Olshan *et al.* (1993) N = 4	Peak GH <10 µg/l or short stature with normal test	0.15 mg/kg/week for 6 months then 0.375 mg/kg/week s.c. daily	Modest increases in growth velocity in three quarters but nil significant increase in HSDS of >0.3
Papadimitriou *et al.* (1991) N = 13	Abnormal growth rate. 10/13 peak GH stim < 10 µg/l	13 U/m²/week increasing to a mean of 18 µ/m² week in 2nd and 3rd years s.c. daily	Height SDS mean at HSCT –0.66 ± 0.84 Start GH treatment SDS –1.52 GH did not improve height SDS Height velocity increased from 3.6 ± 0.95 to 5.2 ± 1.5 cm/year 1st year Decreased to 5.0 ± 2.5 in the second year Decreased to 4.6 ± 2.0 in third year

ABMT, and did not change significantly subsequently. However, a large variation in weight for height was observed with 6 of 20 children having a weight/height SDS > 2 at a median time of 3.1 years after transplant (Arvidson *et al.*, 2000). In 79 pediatric HSCT recipients reported by the LEWP of EBMT a significant increase in the body mass index (BMI: weight/height^2) from 17.27 to 19.57 at last follow-up examination is reported. This is appropriate considering the anticipated increase in BMI with normal growth and development. The pattern of variation of BMI between patients with different exposure to irradiation (TBI and CRT, TBI no CRT, TAI, no irradiation) was not significant (Cohen *et al.*, 1999b). In 53 pediatric patients receiving HSCT, BMI SDS appeared to increase over 5 years following chemotherapy conditioning (although no statistically significant difference was found), but not with TBI or TLI (Couto-Silva *et al.*, 2000). BMI was not found to differ significantly between pediatric HSCT recipients at a median of 10.8 years after transplant, and nontransplant leukemia sur-

vivors at least 3 years after completion of therapy or age and sex-matched healthy controls (Taskinen *et al.*, 2000).

BMI may not be an adequate way to determine adiposity in survivors of pediatric HSCT. Nysom *et al.* (2001) measured BMI and whole body percent fat by dual-energy X-ray absorptiometry 8 years after HSCT with TBI conditioning in 25 patients. The individual patient results were quite heterogeneous, with the majority (16) of patients' BMI essentially unchanged from the level prior to diagnosis or BMT, 2 patients increased, and 7 reduced. Age and sex-adjusted mean BMI was not significantly different from population references, but was significantly reduced (BMI SDS –0.4) in comparison to recently examined local controls. Two patients were overweight or obese. Whole body fat percent was significantly increased (SDS +1.1) compared to healthy controls but did not differ significantly from 39 ALL survivors treated with cranial irradiation but not HSCT. A whole body fat percent above the 90 percentile was found in 11 patients. Regression analysis showed cranial irradiation and GH

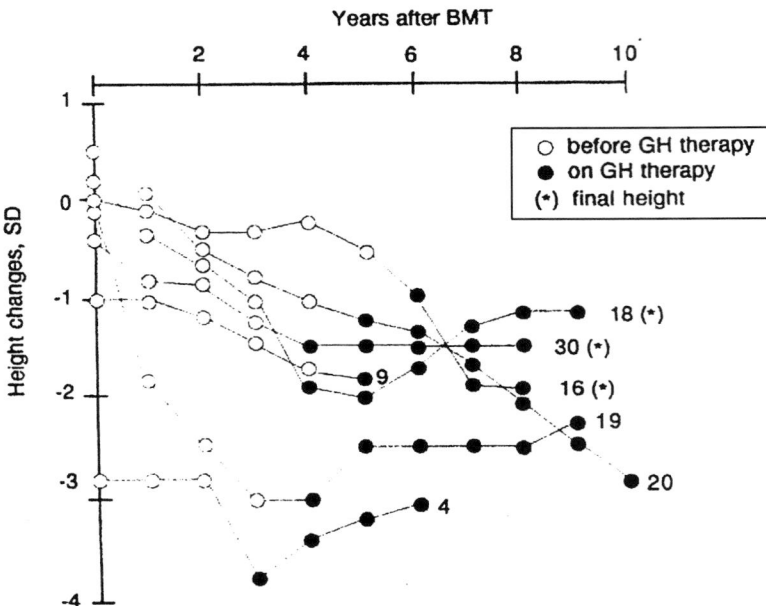

Fig. 84.6. Individual height changes in seven patients with GH therapy for GH deficiency caused by TBI conditioning to BMT. Reproduced, with permission, from Brauner *et al.* (1997).

deficiency to be significant predictors of higher percentage body fat, and these effects were not independent of each other. BMI was also found to be higher in patients treated with cranial irradiation. Multivariate analysis did not show the following factors to be significant predictors of increased total body fat: sex, age at BMT, length of follow-up, use of dexamethasone, cumulative dose of dexamethasone, corticosteroids or anthracyclines, or the cumulative dose of dexamethasone and prednisone. Thus, survivors of pediatric allogeneic HSCT tend to have increased total body fat and decreased lean body mass. This appears to be associated with cranial irradiation possibly mediated by growth insufficiency. Increased adiposity is a risk factor for syndromes of insulin resistance, impaired glucose tolerance, and non-insulin-dependent diabetes. Lorini *et al.* (1995) studied 34 patients between 9 months and 10 years after pediatric HSCT. On intravenous glucose tolerance tests they found normoglycemia, but elevated insulin levels, insulin/glycemia ratio, first-phase insulin release, and levels of C-peptide compared with controls. Taskinen *et al.* (2000) reported the results of 23 patients receiving pediatric HSCT at a median of 10.8 years earlier and found a 52% incidence of hyperinsulinemia, with most patients also having glucose intolerance, dyslipidemia, and/or abdominal obesity.

Puberty and gonadal function (and see Chapters 94 and 97)

HSCT has major effects on progress through puberty and gonadal development. Leahey *et al.* (1999) compared outcome in 52 survivors of AML, 26 treated by chemotherapy alone at a mean age of 6.6 ± 1 years, and 26 with the addition of HSCT (mean age at diagnosis 9.2 ± 1.3 years; 9 given TBI, 17 BuCy).

Of those girls who were then >12 years, 6 of 9 post-HSCT had ovarian failure and were on hormone replacement therapy (HRT). Two girls had a single fraction of 8 Gy TBI and had regular periods with normal estradiol levels. None of the 11 girls treated with chemotherapy had ovarian failure. The adolescent boys treated by chemotherapy or BMT showed normal pubertal progression.

The impact of HSCT in adults has been well described. Kauppila *et al.* (1998) reported results that are typical. All 20 adults receiving TBI-based regimens or BuCy had elevated follicle-stimulating hormone (FSH); all females had elevated luteinizing hormone (LH) and 4 of 10 males had elevated LH. All males had normal testosterone levels and a normal LH response to GnRH. Nine of the 10 females and none of the males required HRT. Mertens *et al.* (1998) reviewed gonadal function in 270 patients undergoing HSCT at 6 to 54 years. Younger patients were slower to reach an elevated FSH and were more likely to have normal FSH at last follow-up.

Spontaneous menarche with TBI

In adults, sustained high gonadotrophins normally indicate hypergonadotrophic hypogonadism, which is usually irreversible. The situation in the pediatric patient is different. In prepubertal children, normal gonadotrophin levels do not predict normal gonadal function and similarly, abnormal gonadotrophins do not predict abnormal gonadal function, in that there is still the possibility of subsequent menstruation or spermatogenesis.

TBI has profound effects on follicular development in the ovary and causes destruction of the germinal epithelium in the testis. There is evidence that younger age and a fractionated schedule reduces the impact on the ovary. Sanders *et al.* (1988) reported that those girls treated with 12 Gy fractionated were 4.8 times more likely to have return of normal ovarian function than either a single fraction of 10 Gy or fractionated total dose of 15.75 Gy. In the majority of cases, TBI leads in boys to small testicular volume, compensatory increase in FSH, an often normal level of luteinizing LH, with normal to low testosterone. Progress through puberty tends to be less severely affected in boys. Although the ovaries are felt to be more radioresistant than testes, the testicular Leydig[1] cells are even more resistant, so most boys will have adequate testosterone levels for normal puberty. Testicular radiation almost always leads to low testosterone, compensatory increased LH, and need for replacement therapy to achieve puberty and maintain secondary sexual characteristics.

In prepubertal children given TBI, 13 of 27 girls and 18 of 45 boys had normal pubertal development, with normal menstruation in the girls. These 13 girls had an onset of menarche at a median of 13 years (Sanders *et al.*, 1991b). Several other authors have described spontaneous onset of menarche in prepubertal girls (Spinelli *et al.*, 1994; Sarafoglou *et al.*, 1997; Bakker *et al.*, 2000). Matsumoto *et al.* (1999) reported ovarian function in 18 girls who underwent HSCT with TBI premenarche (16 were prepubertal). Of 14 transplanted before 10 years, 12 achieved menarche; this was 0 of 4 for girls over 11 years. They also provided serial gonadotrophin levels in individual patients. This illustrated that menarche was often preceded by high FSH values. Gonadotrophins, usually low in the first decade, often rose after 10 years to very high levels, and would return to normal or lower levels in some. Sustained high levels were usually seen in those who did not experience menarche. Menarche could occur while gonadotrophin levels were normal, falling from high levels or remaining high. Thus, the simple finding of elevated gonadotrophins did not indicate that the ovary was incapable of initiating puberty. Perhaps higher gonadotrophin levels are needed to stimulate the remaining undamaged or partially damaged follicles.

Effect of chemotherapy conditioning

Prepubertal patients conditioned with cyclophosphamide alone for SAA have normal puberty. Sanders *et al.* (1991b) reported that 17 of 18 girls and 11 of 12 boys given cyclophosphamide for SAA before puberty had normal pubertal development and normal menstruation in the girls. Although there has been a significant increase in the use of BuCy as conditioning, detailed information regarding recovery of gonadal function is still scanty in the literature. Afify *et al.* (2000) reported sequential gonadotrophin levels and progress through puberty in a cohort of uniformly treated AML patients given BuCy. All girls had elevated gonadotrophins, even those who were very young pre-HSCT. Of 6 pubertal girls 5 are on HRT. Thibaud *et al.* (1998)

and Teinturier *et al.* (1998) compared outcome of ovarian function in a total of 29 girls who received chemotherapy conditioning; the 14 who did not receive busulfan (various regimens) had normal ovarian function, whereas all 15 given busulfan-containing regimens (mainly busulfan/melphalan and cyclophosphamide) had ovarian failure. Data on gonadal function for patients treated with BuCy for thalassemia is still limited. De Sanctis *et al.* (1991) reported 30 thalassemia patients, still prepubertal at 9 to 17 years. Eighty percent of girls showed hypergonadotrophic hypogonadism. Of 22 thalassemic patients reported by De Simone *et al.* (1995), only 2 patients are now postpubertal; one girl and boy were in early puberty at HSCT at 13 years and progressed slowly through puberty. Delayed or absent puberty is the most common endocrine abnormality in conventionally treated thalassemic patients. Even those patients who have undergone successful BMT will continue to have excess toxic iron stores until these are depleted, by regular chelation therapy or venesection, in order to achieve normal iron levels.

Data in boys are still limited, but appear to follow the pattern seen with TBI. Afify *et al.* (2000) reported that, apart from one boy who received testicular irradiation and orchiectomy for a testicular relapse, boys tend to progress normally through puberty, have normal testosterone levels, small testes, and elevated FSH in most and LH in half. De Sanctis *et al.* (1991) also reported that Leydig function seemed normal in boys treated with BuCy for thalassemia.

Potential fertility and offspring

Sanders *et al.* (1996) reported the outcome of fertility and pregnancy in a large cohort of patients. Of 82 prepubertal girls > 12 years, 28% developed normal ovarian function and 9 became pregnant. Of 114 boys, 15 developed normal gonadal function and partners became pregnant in two cases. However, all pregnancies among 5 females who received TBI while prepubertal terminated in spontaneous abortion.

Even if regular menstruation does occur, signaling follicular development, there are many obstacles to potential fertility. Holm *et al.* (1999) performed ultrasound of the uterus and ovaries in 12 females after TBI, at a median of 8 years post-BMT. All had entered puberty, 3 spontaneously and 8 with HRT. In all cases the uterus and ovaries were very small; median volume of both uterus and ovaries was −2.6 SD. Ovarian follicles were detected in 2 or 12, and these were 2 of the 3 youngest, who had progressed through puberty without substitution therapy and had menstruated regularly. A reduced ovarian volume is associated with a reduced number of follicles. The uterus normally continues to grow in volume for several years after menarche. Doses of HRT used to initiate or maintain secondary sexual characteristics and regular periods may not be sufficient to maintain uterine growth. Blood flow was reduced (only 1 of 9 had diastolic flow) and this may also be due to irradiation. There are no similar reported data for patients who received BuCy. Larsen *et al.* (2000) reported on oocyte donation in two patients after TBI. One woman with a

---

[1] Franz von Leydig, German anatomist, 1821–1908.

normal-sized uterus delivered at 37 weeks, whereas one who had a small uterus miscarried at 17 weeks. It is important to assess uterine size for the possibility of supporting a normal pregnancy. This may be most appropriate at such time as it is an issue for the individual patient.

Thibaud et al. (1998) reported a cohort of girls in which FSH was elevated in all 29 when first measured, although it subsequently returned to normal in 4 with regular spontaneous menstruation. They therefore recommended cessation of HRT for 2 months at regular intervals. However, the onset or return of menstruation may be followed by premature menopause. HRT can be used in an attempt to preserve the few remaining follicles, so it may be better to continue such treatment. This will also reduce side effects associated with hypogonadism, assist in uterine growth, and assist in acquisition of adult bone mass.

Neuropsychological effects and quality of life

Investigations of the neuropsychological function of survivors of pediatric transplants are still in their infancy compared to the very extensive data for patients with ALL treated without a transplant. We know that 24 Gy of CRT produce an average 11 point reduction in global IQ, with more severe effects in younger patients (Cousens et al., 1988). Even a dose of 18 Gy results in deficits of attention and short-term memory (Cousens et al., 1991). van Weel-Sipman et al. (1990) tested 17 patients at 4 years posttransplant who were more than 10 years of age at the time of transplant. Psychological testing did not reveal any major differences between cohorts of patients treated for ALL with and without HSCT. However, Smedler et al (1990) used a detailed set of psychological tests on patients and their sibling donors. Patients over 11 years at transplant were normal, but those aged 3 to 11 years had minor abnormalities. Those receiving TBI aged 3 years or less showed major delays in motor function, and low average to subnormal performance in other areas of cognitive function.

Kramer et al. (1997) reported the 1-year and 3-year outcome of a group of children transplanted for a variety of malignant and nonmalignant conditions. Compared to the pre-HSCT assessment, there was a significant reduction in IQ score in 67 children studied at 1 year. The 26 patients also studied at 3 years showed no further reduction in IQ score at the later time point. The numbers (n = 194) were insufficient to define associations between

outcome and age at transplant, use of TBI and/or busulfan. Phipps et al. (2000) have initiated a prospective longitudinal study in a large cohort of patients. Current results reported were on 102 patients at 1 year and 54 patients at 3 years post-HSCT. There were no significant differences at 1 or 3 years, and no differences between patients conditioned with or without TBI. The mean age of this group at HSCT was 10 years. The youngest patients did show a trend to worse results, and are more comparable to the population reported by Kramer et al. (1997; mean age at HSCT 3.5 years). Simms et al. (1998) studied 51 children with no prior cranial irradiation and showed no difference in functioning at 1 year compared to pre-HSCT, for the chemotherapy (mean age at HSCT 8 years) and TBI (mean age 7 years) groups. This evaluation may be too early for us to assess the true impact of the treatment. The lower total doses of radiation used with TBI may be below a threshold dose, compared to the 18 to 24 Gy typically used in the past for CRT in ALL.

The potential interaction between the effect of the disease, the impact of intensive therapy, isolation in hospital, and the altered family dynamics in a young child is uncertain. Pot-Mees (1989) has documented the profound psychosocial effects of transplantation on the child and family, many of whom had received no therapy prior to transplant, which was performed without TBI. Felder-Puig et al. (1999) reported a group of 26 survivors of HSCT, 2 to 13 years post-HSCT (mean 7 years) and suggested that there may be long-term emotional and social problems but the small size and retrospective nature of the study precludes any firm conclusions. When looking at more global measures of survival late after HSCT, Matthes-Martin et al. (1999) reported that, among 73 long-term survivors of HSCT, 75% had an excellent quality of life, with no physical or psychosocial impairment. There was little detectable organ damage in those surviving more than 1 year, and only 2 of 58 had to change school type.

Long-term follow-up

Given the favorable outcome for children surviving more than a year post-HSCT, a regular plan of follow-up is needed. A proposed minimal required battery of screening endocrinological investigations for long-term follow-up of recipients of pediatric HSCT has been outlined in an editorial by Cohen et al. (1999a). A modified version is summarized in Table 84.7.

Table 84.7.   *Suggested evaluation of growth and endocrine function for the pediatric HSCT recipient*

Time	Investigations indicated	
Pre-HSCT	Anthropometric	Height, weight, sitting height, pubertal staging
6 and 12 months	Anthropometric	Height, weight, sitting height
2 years then annual	Anthropometric	Height, weight, sitting height, pubertal staging
	Radiological	Bone age
		Bone mineral densitometry—third yearly
	Endocrine	TSH, T4
		LH, FSH from age 9 years
		Growth hormone stimulation tests for children with growth >2 SDS below HSCT SDS and prior to initiation of sex steroid replacement

References

Adan, L., de Lanversin, M.-L., Thalasinos, C. *et al.* (1997). Growth after bone marrow transplantation in young children conditioned with chemotherapy alone. *Bone Marrow Transplantation,* **19,** 253–6.

Afify, Z., Shaw, P.J., Clavano-Harding, A., & Cowell, C.T., (2000). Growth and endocrine function in children with acute myeloid leukemia after bone marrow transplantation using busulfan/cyclophosphamide. *Bone Marrow Transplantation,* **25,** 1087–92.

Alter, C.A., Thornton, P.S., Willi, S.M. *et al.* (1996). Growth in children after bone marrow transplantation for acute myelogenous leukemia as compared to acute lymphocytic leukemia. *Journal of Pediatric Endocrinology and Metabolism,* **9,** 51–7.

Arvidson, J., Carlson, K., Lannering, B., & Lonnerholm, T. (2000). Prepubertal growth and growth hormone secretion in children after treatment for hematological malignacies, including autologous bone marrow transplantation. *Pediatric Hematology and Oncology,* **17,** 285–97.

Bakker, B., Massa, G.G., Oostdijk, W. *et al.* (2000). Pubertal development and growth after total body irradiation and bone marrow transplantation for haematological malignancies. *European Journal of Pediatrics,* **159,** 31–7.

Bhatia, S., Ramsay, N.K.C., Weisdorf, D. *et al.* (1998). Bone mineral density in patients undergoing bone marrow transplantation for myeloid malignacies. *Bone Marrow Transplantation,* **22,** 87–90.

Birkebaek, N.H. & Clausen, N. (1998). Height and weight pattern up to 20 years after treatment for acute lymphoblastic keukaemia. *Archives of Diseases of Childhood,* **79,** 161–4.

Borgstrom, B. & Bolme, P. (1994). Thyroid function in children after allogeneic bone marrow transplantation. *Bone Marrow Transplantation,* **13,** 59–64.

Boulad, F., Bromley, M., Black, P. *et al.* (1995). Thyroid dysfunction following bone marrow transplantation using hyperfractionated radiation. *Bone Marrow Transplantation,* **15,** 71–6.

Brauner, R., Adan, L., Souberielle, J. *et al.* (1997). Contribution of growth hormone deficiency to the growth failure that follows bone marrow transplantation. *Journal of Pediatrics,* **130,** 785–92.

Brauner, R., Fontoura, M., Zucker, J.M. *et al.* (1993). Growth and growth hormone secretion after bone marrow transplantation. *Archives of Diseases of Childhood,* **68,** 458–63.

Bushhouse, S., Ramsay, N., Pescovitz, O.H. *et al.* (1989). Growth in children following irradiation for bone marrow transplantation. *American Journal of Pediatric Hematology/Oncology,* **11,** 134–40.

Clayton, P.E. & Shalet, S.M. (1991). Dose dependency of time of onset of radiation-induced growth hormone deficiency. *Journal of Pediatrics,* **118,** 226–8.

Clement-De Boers, A., Oostdijk, W., Van Weel-Sipman, M.H. *et al.* (1996). Final height and hormonal function after bone marrow transplantation in children. *Journal of Pediatrics,* **129,** 544–50.

Cohen, A.(1999a). Is endocrinological assessment and follow-up of children after bone marrow transplantation necessary? *Pediatric Transplantation,* **3,** 1–4.

Cohen, A., Duell, T., Socie, G. *et al.* (1999b). Nutritional status and growth after bone marrow transplantation (BMT) during childhood; EBMT Late-Effects Working Party retrospective data. *Bone Marrow Transplantation,* **23,** 1043–7.

Cohen, A., Rovelli, A., Bakker, B. *et al.* (1999c). Final height of patients who underwent bone marrow transplantation for hematological disorders during childhood: a study by the working party for late effects-EBMT. *Blood,* **93,** 4109–15.

Cohen, A., Rovelli, A., Van-Lint, M.T. *et al.* (1996). Final height of patients who underwent bone marrow transplantation during childhood. *Archives of Diseases of Childhood,* **74,** 437–40.

Cousens, P., Ungerer, J.A., Crawford, J.A., & Stevens, M..M. (1991). Cognitive effects of childhood leukemia therapy: a case for four specific deficits. *Journal of Pediatric Psychology,* **16,** 475–88.

Cousens, P., Waters, B., Said, J., & Stevens, M. (1988). Cognitive effects of cranial irradiation in leukemia: a survey and meta-analysis. *Journal of Child Psychology & Psychiatry,* **29,** 839–52.

Couto-Silva, A.C., Trivin, C., Esperou, H. *et al.* (2000). Changes in height, weight and plasma leptin after bone marrow transplantation. *Bone Marrow Transplantation,* **26,** 1205–10.

Dahllof, G., Barr, M., Bolme, P. *et al.* (1988). Disturbances in dental development after total body irradiation in bone marrow transplant recipients. *Oral Surgery, Oral Medicine, Oral Pathology,* **65,** 41–4.

Dahllof, G., Forsberg, C-M., Nasman, M. *et al.* (1991). Craniofacial growth in bone marrow transplant recipients treated with growth hormone after total body irradiation. *Scandinavian Journal of Dental Research,* **99,** 44–7.

Dahllof, G., Jonsson, A., Ulmner, M., & Huggare, J. (2001). Orthodontic treatment in long-term survivors after pediatric bone marrow transplantation. *American Journal of Orthodontics and Dentofacial Orthopedics,* **120,** 459–65.

Davies, H.A., Didcock, E., Didi, M. *et al.* (1994). Disproportionate short stature after cranial irradiation and combination chemotherapy for leukemia. *Archives of Diseases of Childhood,* **70,** 472–5.

De Sanctis, V., Galimberti, M., Lucarelli, G. *et al.* (1991). Gonadal function after allogenic bone marrow transplantation for thalassemia. *Archives of Diseases of Childhood,* **66,** 517–20.

De Simone, M., Di Bartolomeo, P., Olioso, P. *et al.* (1997). Growth after recombinant human growth hormone (rhGH) treatment in transplant thalassemic patients. *Bone Marrow Transplantation,* **20,** 567–73.

De Simone, M., Olioso, P., Di Bartolomeo, P. *et al.* (1995). Growth and endocrine function following bone marrow transplantation for thalassemia. *Bone Marrow Transplantation,* **15,** 227–33.

De Simone, M., Verrotti, A., Iughetti, L. *et al.* (2001). Final height of thalassemic patients who underwent bone marrow transplantation during childhood. *Bone Marrow Transplantation,* **28,** 201–5.

Dopfer, R., Ranke, M.B., Einsele, H. *et al.* (1989). Influence of allogeneic bone marrow transplantation on the endocrine system in children. *Folia Haematologica,* **116,** 3–4.

Felder-Puig, R., Peters, C., Matthes- Martin, S. *et al.* (1999). Psychosocial adjustment of pediatric patients after allogeneic stem cell transplantation. *Bone Marrow Transplantation,* **24,** 75–80.

Fletcher, B.D., Crom, D.B., Krance, R.A., & Kun, L.E. (1994), Radiation-induced bone abnormalities after bone marrow transplantation for childhood leukemia. *Pediatric Radiology,* **191,** 231–5.

GH Research Society. (2000). Consensus guidelines for the diagnosis and treatment of growth hormone (GH) deficiency in childhood and adolescence: summary statement of the GH Research Society. *Journal of Clinical Endocrinology & Metabolism,* **85,** 3990–3.

Giorgiani, G., Bozzola, M., Locatelli, F. *et al.* (1995). Role of busulfan and total body irradiation on growth of prepubertal children receiving bone marrow transplantation and results of treatment with recombinant human growth hormone. *Blood,* **86,** 825–31.

Holm, K., Nyson, K., Brocks, V. *et al.* (1999). Ultrasound B-mode changes in the uterus and ovaries and Doppler changes after total body irradiation and allogeneic bone marrow transplantation in childhood. *Bone Marrow Transplantation,* **23,** 259–63.

Holm, K., Nyson, K., Rasmussen, M.H. *et al.* (1996). Growth, growth hormone and final height after HSCT. Possible recovery of irradiation-induced growth hormone insufficiency. *Bone Marrow Transplantation,* **18,** 163–70.

Hovi, L., Saarinen-Pihkala, U.M., Vettenranta, K. *et al.* (1999). Growth in children with poor-risk neuroblastoma after regimens with or without total body irradiation in preparation for autologous bone marrow transplantation. *Bone Marrow Transplantation,* **24,** 1131–6.

Hovi, L., Rajantie, J., Perkkio, M. *et al.* (1990). Growth failure and growth hormone deficiency in children after bone marrow transplantation for leukemia. *Bone Marrow Transplantation,* **5,** 183–6.

Huma, Z., Boulad, F., Black, P. *et al.* (1995). Growth in children after bone marrow transplantation for acute leukemia. *Blood,* **86,** 819–24.

Katsanis, E., Shapiro, R.S., Robison, L.L. *et al.* (1990). Thyroid dysfunction following bone marrow transplantation: long-term follow-up of 80 pediatric patients. *Bone Marrow Transplantation,* **5,** 335–40.

Katz, J.A., Pollock, B.H., Jarcaruso, D. *et al.* (1993). Final height attained in patients successfully treated for acute lymphoblastic leukemia. *Journal of Pediatrics,* **123,** 546–52.

Kauppila, M., Koskinen, P., Irjala, K. *et al.* (1998). Long-term effects of allogeneic bone marrow transplantation (BMT) on pituitary, gonad, thyroid and adrenal function in adults. *Bone Marrow Transplantation,* **22,** 331–7.

Kirk, J.A., Raghupathy, P., Stevens, M.M. *et al.* (1987). Growth failure and growth-hormone deficiency after treatment for acute lymphoblastic leukemia. *Lancet,* **1,** 190–3.

Kramer, J.H., Crittenden, M.R., DeSantes, K., & Cowan, M.J. (1997). Cognitive and adaptive behavior 1 and 3 years following bone marrow transplantation. *Bone Marrow Transplantation,* **19,** 607–13.

Larsen, E.C., Loft, A., Holm, K. *et al.* (2000). Oocyte donation in women cured of cancer with bone marrow transplantation including total body irradiation in adolescence. *Human Reproduction,* **15,** 1505–8.

Leahey, A., Teunissen, H., Friedman, D.L. *et al.* (1999). Late effects of chemotherapy compared to bone marrow transplantation in the treatment of pediatric acute myeloid leukemia and myelodysplasia. *Medical and Pediatric Oncology,* **32,** 163–9.

Legault, L. & Bonny, Y. (1999). Endocrine complications of bone marrow transplantation in children. *Pediatric Transplantation,* **3,** 60–6.

Leiper, A.D., Stanhope, R., Lau, T. *et al.* (1987). The effect of total body irradiation and bone marrow transplantation during childhood and adolescence on growth and endocrine function. *British Journal of Haematology,* **67,** 419–26.

Lorini, R., Cortona, L., Scaramuzza, A. *et al.* (1995). Hyperinsulinemia in children and adolescents after bone marrow transplantation. *Bone Marrow Transplantation,* **15,** 873–7.

Mascarin, M., Giavitto, M., Zanazzo, G.A. *et al.* (1991). Avascular necrosis of bone in children undergoing allogeneic bone marrow transplantation. *Cancer,* **68,** 655–9.

Matsumoto, M., Shinohara, O., Ishiguro, H. *et al.* (1999). Ovarian function after bone marrow transplantation performed before menarche. *Archives of Diseases in Childhood,* **80,** 452–4.

Matthes-Martin, S., Lamche, M., Laderstein, R. *et al.* (1999). Organ toxicity and quality of life after bone marrow transplantation in pediatric patients: a single centre retrospective analysis. *Bone Marrow Transplantation,* **23,** 1049–53.

Mertens, A.C., Ramsay, N.K.C., Kouris, S., & Neglia, J.P.(1998). Patterns of gonadal dysfunction following bone marrow transplantation. *Bone Marrow Transplantation,* **22,** 345–50.

Michel, G., Socie, G., Gebhard, F. *et al.*(1997). Late effects of allogeneic bone marrow transplantation for children with acute myeloblastic leukemia in first complete remission; the impact of conditioning regimen without total-body irradiation—a report from the Societe Francaise de Greffe de Moelle. *Journal of Clinical Oncology,* **15,** 2238–46.

Nysom, K., Holm, K., Fleischcher Michaelson, K. *et al.* (2000). Bone mass after allogeneic BMT for childhood leukemia or lymphoma. *Bone Marrow Transplantation,* **25,** 191–6.

Nysom, K., Holm., K., Michealson, K.F. *et al.* (2001). Degree of fatness after allogeneic BMT for childhood leukemia or lymphoma. *Bone Marrow Transplantation,* **27,** 817–20.

Oglivy-Stuart, A.L., Clark, D.J., Wallace, W.H.B. *et al.* (1992).Endocrine deficit after fractionated total body irradiation. *Archives of Diseases in Childhood,* **67,** 1107–10.

Olshan, J.S., Wiili, S.M., Gruccio, D., & Moshang, T. (1993). Growth hormone function and treatment following bone marrow transplant for neuroblastoma. *Bone Marrow Transplantation,* **12,** 381–5.

Papadimitriou, A., Uruena, M., Hamill, G. *et al.* (1991). Growth hormone treatment of growth failure secondary to total body irradiation and bone marrow transplantation. *Archives of Diseases of Childhood,* **66,** 689–92.

Phipps, S., Dunavent, M., Srivastava, D.K. *et al.* (2000). Cognitive and academic functioning in survivors of pediatric bone marrow transplantation. *Journal of Clinical Oncology,* **18,** 1004–11.

Pot-Mees, C. (1989). *The Psychosocial Effects of Bone Marrow Transplantation in Children.* The Netherlands: Eburon.

Ryalls, M., Spoudeas, H.A., Hindmarsh, P.C. *et al.* (1993). Short-term endocrine consequences of total body irradiation and bone marrow transplantation in children treated for leukemia. *Journal of Endocrinology,* **136,** 331–8.

Sanders, J., Pritchard, S., Mahoney, P. *et al.* (1986). Growth and development following marrow transplantation for leukemia. *Blood,* **68,** 1129–35.

Sanders, J.E., Buckner, C.D., Amos, D. *et al.* (1988). Ovarian function following marrow transplantation for aplastic anemia or leukemia. *Journal of Clinical Oncology,* **6,** 813–8.

Sanders, J.E., Hawley, J., Levy, W. *et al.* (1996). Pregnancies following high dose cyclophosphamide with or without busulphan or total body irradiation and bone marrow transplantation. *Blood,* **87,** 3045–52.

Sanders, J.E. & the Seattle Marrow Transplant Team. (1991b). The impact of marrow transplant preparative regimens on subsequent growth and development. *Seminars in Hematology,* **28,** 244–9.

Sanders, J.E. & the Long-Term Follow-Up Team. (1991a). Endocrine problems in children after bone marrow transplant for hematologic malignancies. *Bone Marrow Transplantation,* **8** (Suppl 1), 2–4.

Sarafogolou, K., Boulad, F., Gillio, A., & Sklar, C. (1997). Gonadal function after bone marrow transplantation for acute leukemia during childhood. *Journal of Pediatrics,* **130,** 210–6.

Schell, M.J., Ochs, J.J., Schriock, E.A., & Carter, M. (1992). A method of predicting adult height and obesity in long-term survivors of childhood acute lymphoblastic leukemia. *Journal of Clinical Oncology,* **10,** 128–33.

Schriock, E.A., Schell, M.J., Carter, M. *et al.* (1991). Abnormal growth patterns and adult short stature in 115 long-term survivors of childhood leukemia. *Journal of Clinical Oncology,* **9,** 400–5.

Shalet, S.M. & Brennan, B.M.D. (1998). Growth and growth hormone status following treatment for childhood leukaemia. *Hormone Research,* **50,** 1–10.

Shankar, S.M., Bunin, N.J., & Moshang, T. (1996). Growth in children undergoing bone marrow transplantation after busulfan and cyclophosphamide conditioning. *Journal of Pediatric Hematology/ Oncology,* **18,** 362–6.

Simms, S., Kazak, A.E., Gannon, T. *et al.* (1998). Neuropsychological outcome of children undergoing bone marrow transplantation. *Bone Marrow Transplantation,* **22,** 181–4.

Sklar, C., Mertens, A., Walter, A. *et al.* (1993). Final height after treatment for childhood acute lymphoblastic leukemia: Comparison of no cranial irradiation with 1800 and 2400 centigrays of cranial irradiation. *Journal of Pediatrics,* **123,** 59–64.

Smedler, A-C., Ringdén, K., Bergman, H., & Bolme, P. (1990). Sensory-motor and cognitive functioning in children who have undergone bone marrow transplantation. *Acta Pediatrica Scandinavia,* **79,** 613–21.

Spinelli, S., Chiodi, S., Bacigalupo, A. *et al.* (1994). Ovarian recovery after total body irradiation and allogeneic bone marrow transplantation; long term follow-up of 79 females. *Bone Marrow Transplantation,* **14,** 373–80.

Taskinen, M., Saarinen-Pihkala, U.M., Hovi, L., & Lipsanen-Nyman, M. (2000). Impaired glucose tolerance and dyslipidaemia as late effects after bone-marrow transplantation in childhood. *Lancet,* **356,** 993–7.

Teinturier, C., Hartmann, O., Valteau-Couanet, D. *et al.* (1998). Ovarian function after autologous bone marrow transplantation in childhood: high-dose busulfan is a major cause of ovarian failure. *Bone Marrow Transplantation,* **22,** 989–94.

Thibaud, E., Rodriguez-Macias, K., Trivin, C. *et al.* (1998). Ovarian function after bone marrow transplantation during childhood. *Bone Marrow Transplantation,* **21,** 287–90.

Thuret, I., Michel, G., Carla, H. *et al.* (1995). Long term side-effects in children receiving allogeneic bone marrow transplantation in first complete remission of acute leukemia. *Bone Marrow Transplantation,* **15,** 337–41.

Urban, C., Schwingshandl, J., Slavc, I. *et al.* (1988). Endocrine function after bone marrow transplantation without the use of preparative total body irradiation. *Bone Marrow Transplantation,* **3,** 291–6.

Uruena, M., Stanhope, R., Chessells, J.M., & Leiper, A.D. (1991). Impaired pubertal growth in acute lymphoblastic leukemia. *Archives of Diseases of Childhood,* **66,** 1403–7.

van Weel-Sipman, M.H., van't Veer-Korthof, E.Th., van den Berg, H. *et al.* (1990). Late effects of total body irradiation and cytostatic preparative regimen for bone marrow transplantation in children with hematological malignancies. *Radiotherapy and Oncology* (Suppl 1), 155–7.

Wingard, J.R., Plotnick, L.P., Freemer, C.S. *et al.* (1992). Growth in children after bone marrow transplantation: busulfan plus cyclophosphamide versus cyclophosphamide plus total body irradiation. *Blood,* **79,** 1068–73.

85 Recurrence of the underlying malignant disease

SERGIO A. GIRALT AND RICHARD E. CHAMPLIN

The University of Texas M.D. Anderson Cancer Center, Houston, USA

Introduction

Disease relapse after hematopoietic stem cell (HSC) transplantation remains the single most important cause of treatment failure (Bortin, Horowitz, & Rimm, 1992; Bortin *et al.*, 1992). Modifications in the conditioning regimen that have resulted in lower relapse rates have failed to improve disease-free survival because of the higher incidence of regimen-related toxicity associated with more intense preparative regimens (Clift *et al.*, 1990; Aurer & Gale, 1991).

The number of patients relapsing after transplant is increasing with the increasing number of transplants performed worldwide (Bortin *et al.*, 1992). However, the condition of these patients at the time of their relapse has improved, since transplants are being performed earlier in the course of the disease for most hematologic malignancies (Bortin, Horowitz, & Rimm, 1992; Bortin *et al.*, 1992). Therefore, the attitudes concerning the treatment of patients relapsing after HSC transplantation have changed for many patients from one of conservative therapy with palliation, to more aggressive approaches aimed at re-establishing remission and long-term disease control (Kumar, 1994).

The rate of relapse decreases with increasing time elapsed since transplant, such that 82% of patients leukemia-free at 2 years posttransplant will be alive in complete remission at 9 years posttransplant, regardless of the type of leukemia, its status at transplant, or the type of transplant (Frassoni *et al.*, 1994). In this EBMT experience, the latest relapse after an allograft or an autograft for acute myeloid leukemia (AML) was 6.6 and 6 years, respectively, and for acute lymphoblastic leukemia (ALL) was 6.8 and 5.3 years, respectively. A case of chronic myeloid leukemia (CML) relapsing 14 years post-allografting has been described (Yong & Goldman, 1999). Similar data have been reported by the IBMTR (Socie *et al.*, 1999).

Mechanisms of leukemia relapse after allogeneic HSC transplantation

Disease recurrence after allogeneic transplantation is almost always host-derived, although rare reports (20 between 1971 and 2000) of donor cell leukemia have been identified (Fialkow *et al.*, 1971; Boyd, Ramberg, & Thomas, 1982; Cooley *et al.*, 2000). Of these 20, 13 were in ALL and 6 in AML. It has been described in CML also (McCann *et al.*, 1993). All these patients had received an HLA-identical sibling graft, although the phenomenon has also been described after unrelated donor transplantation (Hambach *et al.*, 2001).

The mechanisms of relapse of host-origin leukemia probably involve one or more of the following:

1. Incomplete eradication of the malignant cell.
2. Inadequate graft-versus-leukemia effect, due to lack of immune recognition or development of leukemia tolerance.
3. De novo leukemic transformation of surviving normal recipient cells due to persistence of the original oncogenic stimulus.

Bacigalupo and colleagues (1991, 2001) showed that a dose of cyclosporine of 5 mg/kg/day was associated with a higher risk of relapse than a dose of 1 mg/kg/day, as was a TBI dose of <9.9 Gy (Bacigalupo *et al.*, 2000) (Fig. 85.1).

With the introduction of polymerase chain reaction (PCR) techniques, the definition of leukemia relapse needs reassessment. Leukemia relapse is commonly defined as the resurgence of any leukemic cell following transplantation detected by conventional morphologic or cytogenetic techniques. Evidence of minimal residual disease documented by PCR cannot at this time be considered as synonymous with disease relapse, since progression to overt leukemia may be more related to whether or not the patient received a T-cell-depleted transplant (Radich *et al.*, 1995; Mackinnon, Barnett, & Heller, 1996). Quantitative PCR methods, however, may define thresholds for inevitable disease progression, in which case PCR positivity may be equated with relapse; this will require further study (Cross *et al.*, 1993).

Risk factors for relapse after allogeneic transplantation

The major risk factor for relapse posttransplant is the status of the hematologic malignancy at the time of transplant. Patients transplanted for advanced leukemia have a much increased chance of relapse compared to those transplanted for early leukemia.

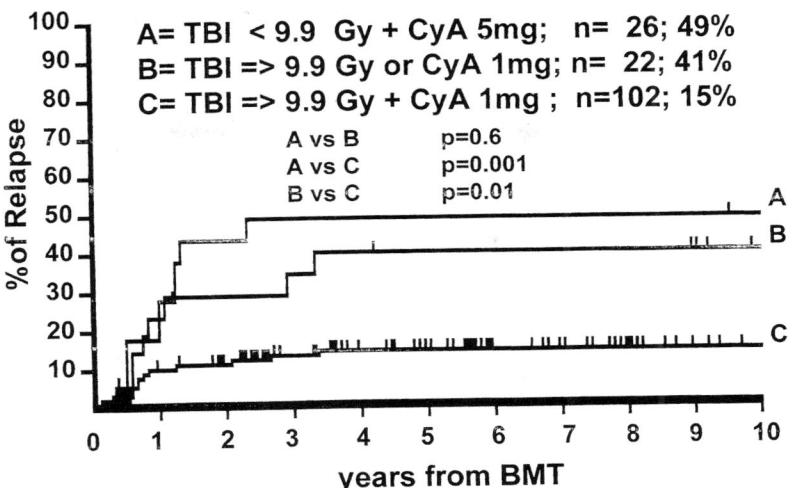

Fig. 85.1. The combined dose effect of cyclosporine A (CyA) and of total body irradiation (TBI) on leukemia relapse: group A received low-dose TBI (<9.9 Gy) and high-dose immunosuppression after transplant (CyA 5 mg/kg); group B received either TBI > 9.9 Gy or 1 mg/kg CyA; and group C received both TBI > 9.9 Gy and 1 mg/kg CyA. The actuarial probability of relapse was higher in group A and group B (49% and 41%) and was significantly lower only in patients in group C. Reproduced, with permission , from Bacigalupo et al. (2000).

Additional factors predisposing to relapse include absence of, or mild, graft-versus-host disease (GVHD) (because of an absence of a graft-versus- leukemia effect (see Chapter 65) and T-cell depletion of the donor stem cells (for the same reason) (see Chapter 26). The use of bone marrow as opposed to peripheral blood stem cells has been associated with a greater risk of relapse, possibly due to the lower number of T cells in marrow (Bensinger et al., 2001). Higher numbers of CD3[-], CD4[bright] type 2 dendritic cells also appear associated with an increased risk of relapse, possibly due to their ability to influence T-cell differentiation post-transplant toward the Th2 pathway (Waller et al., 2001).

Natural history of leukemia relapse after HSC transplantation

The survival of patients who relapse after an allogeneic transplant depends on the type of leukemia, stage of the disease, interval from transplant to recurrence, patient's performance status, and treatment. Patients with acute leukemia who relapse after an allograft and who receive no further treatment have a median survival of 3 to 4 months, with no long-term survivors (Frassoni et al., 1988; Mortimer et al., 1989).

Re-attaining a complete remission is the major prognostic factor for survival for patients with acute leukemia relapsing after an allograft, and the most important factor predicting re-attainment of complete remission is the remission duration after the transplant. Patients with remissions of less than 1 year have a 10% to 30% chance of achieving a complete remission as opposed to 50% to 70% for patients with remissions lasting more than 1 year (Frassoni et al., 1988; Mortimer et al., 1989). Patients with acute leukemia who achieve a complete remission with conventional chemotherapy have a median survival of approximately 10 to 14 months.

Patients with chronic myeloid leukemia relapsing after an allograft have a more benign natural history. Patients with an isolated cytogenetic relapse have a median survival of greater than 6 years compared to 3 years for patients relapsing into a clinical chronic phase (Arcese et al., 1993). Spontaneous cytogenetic remissions have been reported in up to 20% of recipients of unmanipulated allografts, but have not been described in patients receiving T-cell-depleted transplants (Arthur et al., 1988; Hughes et al., 1989). Patients who relapse into a more advanced phase have a median survival duration of less than 6 months, with a poor response to interferon or conventional chemotherapy (Arcese et al., 1993).

Spontaneous complete remission with recovery of donor hematopoiesis after relapse has been described after allogeneic transplantation for myelodysplasia in a patient who experienced two episodes of cytomegalovirus pneumonitis after treatment with ganciclovir (Beguin et al., 1996).

Extramedullary relapse

Extramedullary relapses, such as central nervous system (CNS) and testicular relapses, are frequent and can occur in up to 20% of recipients of allografts for AML and in 6% to 30% of patients with ALL. CNS relapse posttransplant usually occurs in the presence of concurrent marrow relapse. Advanced disease and prior history of CNS involvement are the most important risk factors for CNS relapse post-BMT (Thompson et al., 1986; Frassoni et al., 1988; Ganem et al., 1989; Mortimer et al., 1989; Singhal et al., 1996). Granulocytic sarcoma as the sole manifestation of relapse is uncommon after allogeneic transplantation, with an incidence of less than 1% according to a retrospective review. These lesions appeared between 4 and 56 (median 13) months posttransplant, and presented as single or multiple lesions on the trunk, limbs, or breasts. The risk of progression to overt leukemia and death was related primarily to disease stage at the time of transplant. Eight patients achieved long-term disease control with a variety of treatment strategies (Békássy *et al.*, 1996). In other series, the outcome has been variable. In one study it was poor except for a single patient who underwent a second allograft (Koc *et al.*, 1999). In another, survival after extramedullary relapse was better than after marrow-only relapse (Chong *et al.*, 2000) (Fig. 85.2). Other reports have indicated a more frequent occurrence of extramedullary relapse post-allografting, suggesting the possibility of a less effective graft-versus-leukemia (GVL) effect outside the marrow and bloodstream (Chong *et al.*, 2000; Lee *et al.*, 2000). In the latter series extramedullary relapse occurred later than marrow relapse, and was associated with the presence of chronic GVHD.

Approaches to treatment of leukemia relapse after allogeneic HSC transplantation

Patients relapsing after allogeneic transplant will usually be in a chimeric state in which the recurrent leukemia is of recipient origin, but the residual normal hematopoietic and immune systems are derived from donor cells. Strategies to induce remission should therefore include therapeutic approaches that exploit this unique chimeric situation (Giralt & Champlin, 1994).

Withdrawal of immune suppression

Abrupt cyclosporine withdrawal has been reported to induce complete remissions in patients with CML, AML, and ALL (Odom *et al.*, 1978; Higano *et al.*, 1990; Collins *et al.*, 1992). A retrospective analysis from the Seattle group suggested that patients with CML and two consecutive abnormal cytogenetic tests could benefit from cyclosporine discontinuation without exacerbation of GVHD (Flowers *et al.*, 1994). Although described primarily with cyclosporine, it can be assumed that withdrawal of any immune suppressive agent could reinduce remissions. Therefore, discontinuation of immunosuppressive therapy in patients who relapse after an allogeneic transplant is a reasonable first therapeutic strategy to reinduce remission. Elective early withdrawal of prophylactic immune suppression

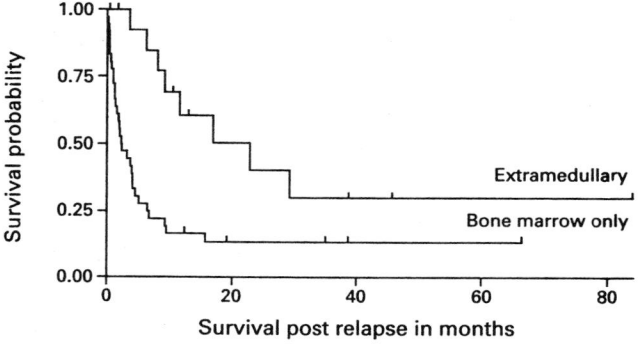

Fig. 85.2. Probability of survival postrelapse according to the site of relapse posttransplant. *P* = .004 on univariate analysis only. Reproduced, with permission, from Chong *et al.* (2000).

(e.g., cyclosporine) (between days 30 and 60 posttransplant) is now being explored in patients at high risk of relapse posttransplant (Abraham *et al.*, 1997).

Conventional chemotherapy and radiotherapy

For patients ineligible or unwilling to receive investigational therapy, conventional chemotherapy can prolong survival and improve quality of life in patients obtaining a complete remission. Patients with AML can be successfully treated with a combination of cytosine arabinoside and anthracyclines, while patients with ALL have responded to combination therapy using vinca alkaloids, corticosteroids, and an anthracycline. Isolated extramedullary relapses can be treated by involved field radiation, which can on occasions result in long-term disease-free survival (Sapozink & Cox, 1983; Bowman *et al.*, 1984; Barrett, Tew, & Joshi, 1985; Bostrom *et al.*, 1987; Frassoni *et al.*, 1988; Mortimer *et al.*, 1989).

Second allogeneic transplant

Second allogeneic transplantation have been successful in selected patients who relapse after a first allogeneic transplant (Table 85.1). Treatment-related mortality is high (up to 70% in some series), but approximately 20% of patients achieve long-term disease control (Champlin *et al.*, 1985; Atkinson *et al.*, 1986; Blume & Forman, 1987; Sanders *et al.*, 1988; Barrett *et al.*, 1991; Mrsic *et al.*, 1992; Wagner *et al.*, 1992; Radich *et al.*, 1993; Chiang *et al.*, 1996; Kishi *et al.*, 1997; Michallet *et al.*, 2000; Bosi *et al.*, 2001) (Fig. 85.3). Patients with early relapse, or those who experienced serious toxic effects during the first transplant, are poor candidates for repeat high-dose chemotherapy and should be offered alternative approaches.

Most second transplants have involved the same donor. Since patients undergoing a second transplant generally retain donor-derived immunity, the preparative regimen is not required to be immunosuppressive (Blume & Forman, 1987). For patients with more than one possible donor, there are no data that support the use of an alternative HLA-compatible donor as a means to achieve a greater GVL effect, but this remains a reasonable alternative.

Allogeneic peripheral blood stem cells are being actively explored as a source of stem cells for both first and second transplants. Advantages include more rapid hematopoietic recovery with less regimen-related toxicity (Nemunaitis *et al.*, 1993). Additionally, the large lymphocyte doses infused could potentially induce a greater antileukemic effect than after a second bone marrow transplant (BMT) (see Chapter 11).

Since acute leukemia relapsing after allogeneic transplantation responds less well, or not at all, to donor lymphocyte infusions (DLI), compared, for example, to CML, an alternative approach to both DLI or a second transplant involving a conventional myeloablative conditioning regimen, is a second transplant preceded by a non-myeloablative regimen. Fourteen patients prepared by the FLAG +/– Ida reduced intensity regi-

Table 85.1. *Second allogeneic transplants for leukemia relapsed after first allogeneic transplant*

Reference	Number of patients	100-day mortality	Relapse rate (%)	Leukemia-free survival at 4 years (%)	Positive prognostic factors
Radich *et al.*, 1993	77	36	70	14	Acute GVHD, younger age, CML
Barrett *et al.*, 1991	87	47	69	11	>18 months remission post BMT1, chronic GVHD
Mrsic *et al.*, 1992	114	40	65	21	>6 months from BMT1, Karnofsky > 80, age < 25, CML

Abbreviations: GVHD, graft-versus-host disease; CML, chronic myeloid leukemia; BMT, bone marrow transplant.

men [fludarabine 150 mg/m^2, cytosine arabinoside 10 g/m^2, idarubicin 8 mg/m^2, and granulocyte colony-stimulating factor (G-CSF)] demonstrated a 60% actuarial survival rate and a 26% disease-free survival rate at 58 months posttransplant (Pawson *et al.*, 2001).

Granulocyte colony-stimulating factor

G-CSF can induce cytogenetic and hematologic remissions in patients relapsing after allogeneic BMT (Giralt *et al.*, 1993). In an update of the initial report, 7 of 23 patients responded. Responders to filgrastim had a lower percentage of peripheral blood (0% vs. 4%) and bone marrow (9% vs. 33%) blast cells. All responding patients relapsed between 1 and 20 (median 12) months after initiation. This therapy represents a nontoxic form of re-induction, which can be used for selected patients with indolent relapses until more definitive therapy is planned or needed (Giralt *et al.*, 1994). In another report the complete response rate was 43% with event-free and overall survival rates of 43% and 73%, respectively (Fig. 85.4) (Bishop *et al.*, 2000). The rate of decrease in bone marrow blast cells and the rise in platelet counts in a patient with AML relapsed 8 months after a second allogeneic transplant and given G-CSF 5 μg/kg/day is shown in Figure 85.5 (Carral, Sanz, & Sanz, 1996).

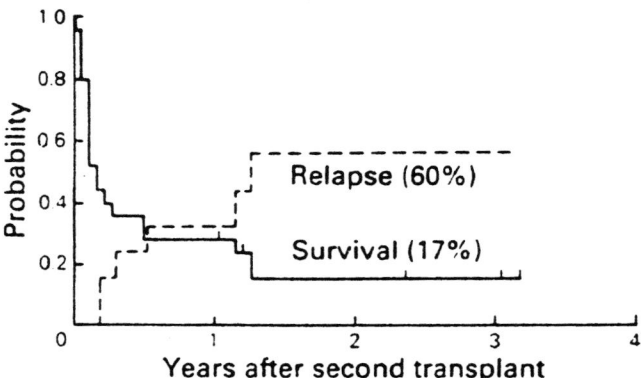

Fig. 85.3. Kaplan-Meier product limit estimates of disease-free survival (*solid line*) and relapse (*dotted line*) for 26 patients measured from the time of second bone marrow transplantation. Surviving patients are represented by tick marks. Reproduced, with permission, from Sanders *et al.* (1988).

Interferon-α

Interferon-α (IFN-α) has direct activity against leukemic cells and important immune-modulatory effects, such as upregulation of MHC antigen expression and stimulation of T-lymphocyte and natural killer (NK) cell activity (Baron *et al.*, 1991). Treatment with IFN-α has been effective in selected patients with CML recurrent after allogeneic BMT (Arcese *et al.*, 1991, 1993; Higano, Raskind, & Singer, 1992) (Fig. 85.6).

The EBMTR reported that the actuarial probability of 6-year survival for patients with CML relapsing after an allograft was 36%. IFN-α therapy emerged as an independent prognostic factor for survival along with CML phase, time from transplant to relapse, and female sex. IFN-α was also associated with a higher cytogenetic response rate and delayed disease progression (Arcese *et al.*, 1993).

Interleukin-2

Interleukin-2 (IL-2) can also enhance the antileukemic and cytotoxic activity of T lymphocytes and NK cells, and has single agent activity in a variety of hematologic malignancies (Rosenberg *et al.*, 1984). The experience with the combination of IFN-α and IL-2 in the setting of relapse after HSC transplantation has been limited and has shown conflicting results (Giralt *et al.*, 1995b; Mehta *et al.*, 1995). In a pilot trial, the M.D. Anderson group used an initial dose of IL-2 of 3.6 × 10^6 IU/m^2 in combination with IFN-α 5.0 × 10^6 U/m^2 three times a week. Nine patients at this dose level required a 50% dose reduction because of toxicity or GVHD. One of five patients with acute leukemia responded, but died of fungal pneumonia. At half of the above dose most patients tolerated therapy well, but no responses were seen in spite of six patients developing clinical signs of GVHD. Thus, cytokine therapy by itself may not be sufficient to reinduce remissions in patients with acute leukemia relapsing after allogeneic transplantation (Giralt *et al.*, 1995b). However, Mehta *et al.*, 1995) reported three patients who received combination cytokine therapy and had long-term remissions.

Other investigators have reported good responses to a combination of cytokine therapy and donor lymphocyte infusions (Slavin *et al.*, 1996). The Hadassah group reported responses in five of six patients receiving combination cytokine and cellular therapy for relapse BMT (Slavin *et al.*, 1996). Further studies are needed to better define the utility of these strategies.

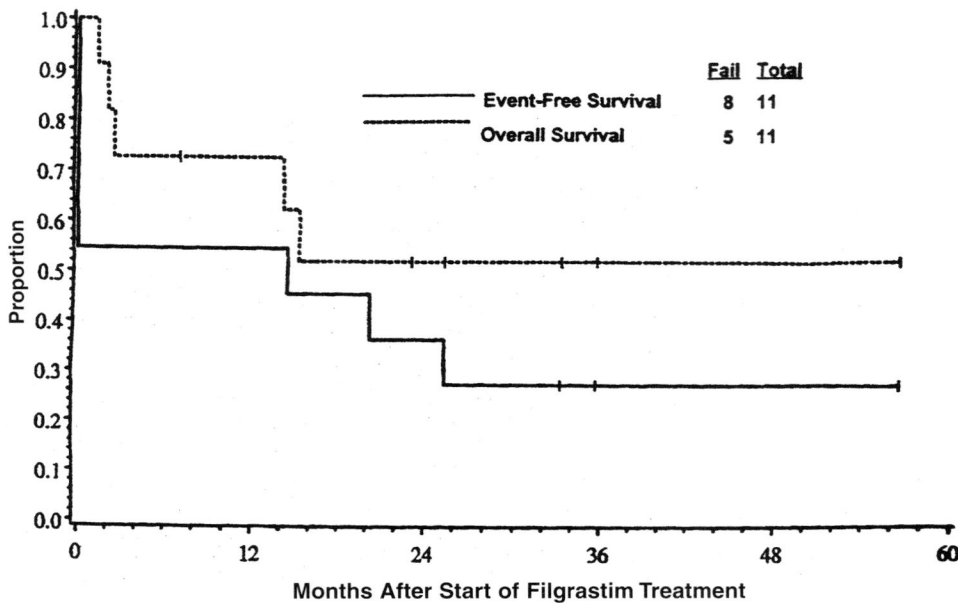

Fig. 85.4. Outcome after treatment with filgrastim among assessable patients. Reproduced, with permission, from Bishop *et al.* (2000).

Thalidomide

Thalidomide has demonstrated activity in patients with relapsed or refractory myeloma, and its use has been described in patients relapsing after allogeneic HSC transplantation (Biagi *et al.*, 2001).

Donor lymphocyte infusions (and see Chapter 65)

The most direct evidence for a GVL effect comes from the observation that DLI can reinduce remissions in patients relapsing after an allogeneic transplant (Kolb *et al.*, 1990). These observations have been confirmed by multiple investigators (Bar *et al.*, 1993; Drobyski *et al.*, 1993; Hertenstein *et al.*, 1993; Porter *et al.*, 1994; van Rhee *et al.*, 1994; Kolb *et al.*, 1995; Collins *et al.*, 1997). Results from the largest reported series suggest that patients with CML recurring as isolated cytogenetic relapse or chronic phase respond better to this treatment than

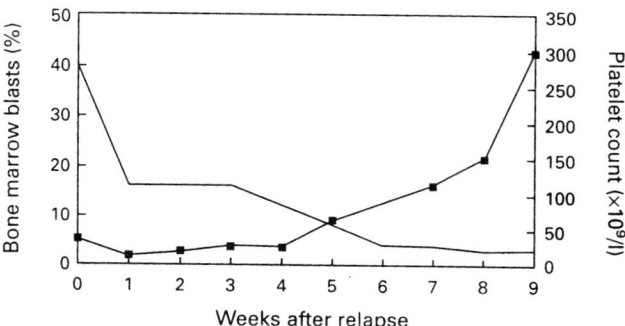

Fig. 85.5. Bone marrow infiltration and platelet count in relation to filgrastim therapy in patient No. 1. Reproduced, with permission, from Carral, Sanz, & Sanz (1996).

patients with more advanced CML or with acute leukemia. The response rates in CML relapsed in chronic phase is approximately 80%. Patients with CML who receive donor lymphocytes have a median survival of greater than 30 months as opposed to less than 1 year for patients with acute leukemia, in which only a handful of patients obtain long-term disease control (Kolb *et al.*, 1995; Collins *et al.*, 1997). All studies to date have shown that there is a lag time between infusion and response, and that pancytopenia occurs primarily in patients with low levels of residual donor hematopoiesis at the time of infusion. GVHD occurs in approximately 50% of patients and, although related to response, remissions can occur without any clinical evidence of GVHD. Two large surveys have identified prognostic factors for response and survival (Table 85.2) (Kolb *et al.*, 1995; Collins *et al.*, 1997).

Use of donor lymphocytes for treatment of relapse posttransplant is hampered by the occurrence of GVHD in CML and the relative lack of effectiveness in acute leukemia. Strategies to decrease the risk of GVHD after DLI in CML have included selective depletion of CD8+ cells, administration of low doses of lymphocytes, and infusion of donor lymphocytes into which the herpes simplex virus thymidine kinase (HSV-TK) gene has been transduced, so as to function as a suicide gene in the event of GVHD (see Chapter 117). Monitoring for molecular evidence of disease (using short tandem repeats) has been used successfully to guide treatment with DLI (de Weger *et al.*, 2000).

Results of CD8-depleted DLI suggest that, at least in CML, CD8+ lymphocytes are not essential for the GVL effect and may be the main subset mediating GVHD. At our center 17 patients have been treated with CD8-depleted donor lymphocyte infusions for CML relapsed after allogeneic BMT. The median age of the patients was 39 (range 23–57) years. The median number of CD8+ cells infused after CD8 depletion was

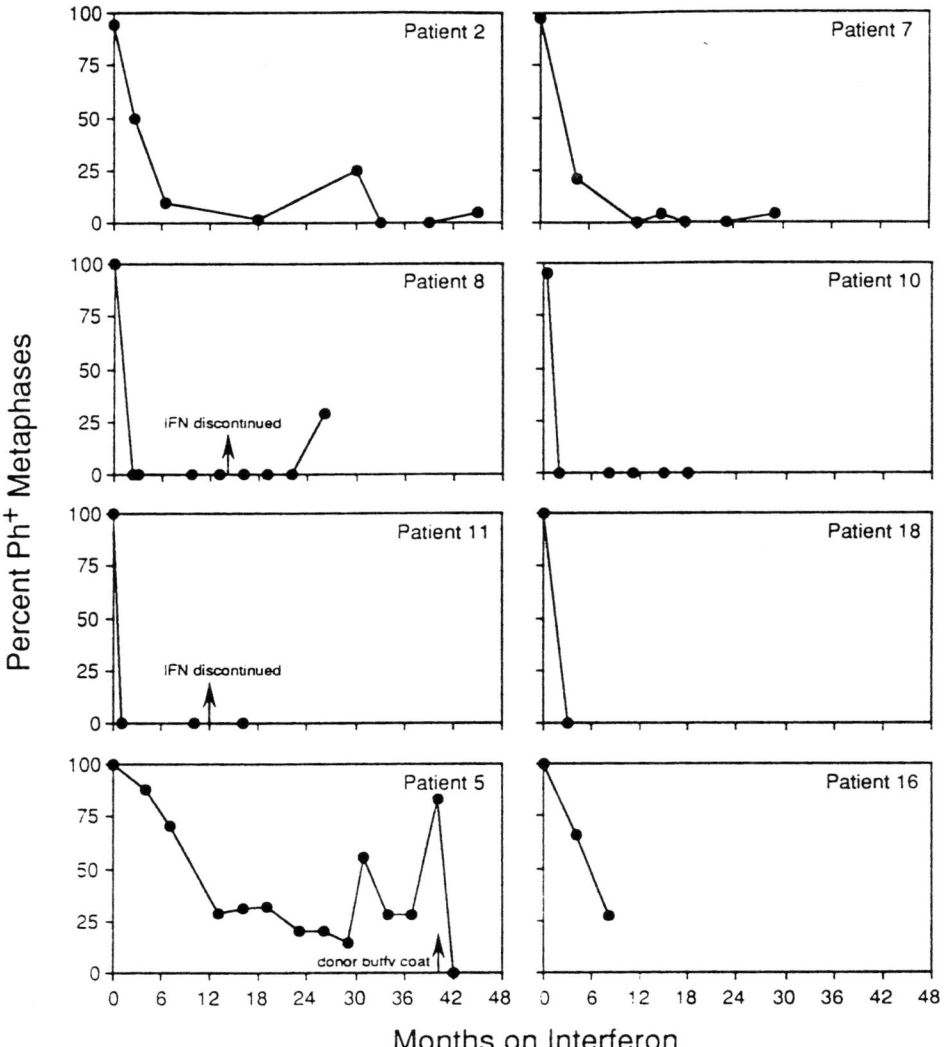

Fig. 85.6. Time course for the eight patients who had cytogenetic responses. Reproduced, with permission, from Higano, Raskind, & Singer (1992).

Table 85.2. *Predictors for response to, and complications after, donor lymphocyte infusions for chronic myeloid leukemia after allogeneic transplantation*

Predictors for response
  Chronic phase at the time of BMT
  T-cell-depleted transplant
  Relapse into chronic phase
  GVHD after donor lymphocyte infusion
  Aplasia after donor lymphocyte infusion
  Lymphocyte dose of < 5.0×10^8/kg
  Less than 2 years from relapse to donor lymphocyte infusion
Predictors for GVHD or aplasia
  T-cell-depleted initial transplant
  Interferon therapy
  Hematologic relapse

0.3×10^6/kg, with a median of 30.8×10^6 CD4+ cells/kg and 4.7×10^6 CD56+ cells/kg. Ten of 11 patients infused during cytogenetic relapse, chronic phase, or chronic phase with clonal evolution, achieved a complete hematologic and cytogenetic remission. Two patients developed acute GVHD, and two patients developed chronic GVHD, one of which was steroid-refractory. Three patients died in remission of Gram-negative sepsis, fungal pneumonia, or steroid-refractory GVHD. Ten patients remain alive (8 in complete remission) at a median of 440 (range, 40–1,200) days postinfusion. One patient who relapsed at 14 months was reinduced into a second cytogenetic complete remission with a second infusion of CD8-depleted donor lymphocytes (Giralt *et al.*, 1995a).

The Dana-Farber group has also reported that CD8-depleted donor lymphocytes are effective in treating CML relapsed postallograft. In their experience CD4+ cell doses of 0.3 to 1.5 × 10^8/kg were administered to 19 patients with CML. The infused product contained between 1% and 6% CD8$^+$ cells and between 43% and 66% CD4$^+$ cells. Five of the 7 patients with nontransformed CML achieved cytogenetic remissions and 2 patients at the higher dose levels developed GVHD (Alyea et al., 1995). This study also supports the hypothesis that at least for CML CD8$^+$ cells are not essential for the graft-versus-tumor effect.

The optimum lymphocyte dose for treatment of relapse posttransplant is unknown. Based on the work of Mackinnon et al. (1995a, 1995b), there seems to be a threshold dose of approximately 1×10^7 CD3$^+$ cells/kg, since lower doses do not regularly induce remissions in patients with CML in hematologic relapse. However, in isolated cytogenetic relapses or molecular relapses the dose of lymphocytes required may be lower.

The incorporation of the HSV-TK gene into lymphocytes allows an alternative therapy of GVHD in the event that this complication occurs after DLI. HSV-TK transduced lymphocytes are sensitive to ganciclovir and are eliminated upon exposure to this drug. This in theory would permit abrogation of GVHD with ganciclovir should this complication occurr. Bonini et al. (1994) reported the results of a clinical trial of HSV-TK transduced donor lymphocytes for treatment of Epstein-Barr virus (EBV)-related lymphoma and leukemia relapse after allogeneic transplantation. Of the six patients reported, two developed GVHD of the skin and liver. Both patients received ganciclovir with rapid elimination of marked lymphocytes and resolution of clinical signs of GVHD. This technology requires further evaluation to determine the extent of transduction necessary to guarantee abrogation of GVHD, whether abrogation of GVHD will result in recurrence of the malignancy, and finally whether the cytokine dysregulation that has already occurred with established GVHD will reverse itself by elimination of the effector cells.

Responses to donor lymphocytes are less frequent and less durable in patients with acute leukemia. The reason for this difference is not understood. Evidence suggests that alterations in the expression of MHC class I and class II antigens, as well as co-stimulatory molecules such as ICAM-1 and B7.1, occur in patients relapsing after allogeneic transplantation, and may allow escape from attempts at immune manipulation (Dermine et al., 1997). The contribution of concomitant chemotherapy, or other maneuvers is uncertain. Chemotherapy is probably beneficial in patients with rapidly proliferating disease in whom disease control is required in order to give time for the donor lymphocyte infusions to exert their effect (Szer et al., 1993; Kolb et al., 1995; Collins et al., 1997). The optimum chemotherapy prior to DLI for leukemia relapse is unknown. G-CSF mobilized donor peripheral blood cells (containing both immune effector cells and CD34$^+$ stem cells) have been reported to facilitate recovery after salvage chemotherapy in such patients (Flowers et al., 1995; Glass et al., 1997).

Imatinib

Preliminary observations suggest that imatinib mesylate is highly active against posttransplant relapse of CML, but long-term safety and efficacy have not been established. The MD Anderson group reported on 28 patients given 400–1000 mg/day for relapse occurring a median of 9 (range 1–137) months posttransplant. Thirteen patients had undergone salvage DLI. Complete hematologic responses occurred in 100% of those in chronic phase, 83% for accelerated phase, and 43% for blast phase. Cytogenetic response rates were 63% for chronic or accelerated phase and 43% for blast phase. The 1-year estimated survival was 74%. Recurrence of GVHD occurred in 5 patients. Severe granulocytopenia occurred in 43% and thrombocytopenia in 27% (Kantarjian et al., 2002). Imatinib has been shown to induce a complete hematologic response and complete restoration of donor-type hematopoiesis in a patient who did not benefit from DLI (Olivarria et al., 2002).

Treatment of relapse of other hematologic malignancies after HSC transplantation

DLI have been reported to be effective in treating relapses of hematologic malignancies other than CML and AML after allogeneic transplantation including multiple myeloma, chronic lymphatic leukemia, and non-Hodgkin's lymphoma (Alyea et al., 1995; Kolb et al., 1996; Rondón et al., 1996; Collins et al., 1997). The Dana-Farber experience with CD8-depleted DLI in 7 patients with myeloma relapsed after allogeneic BMT reported 2 partial remissions and 3 complete remissions. Of the 5 responders, 3 developed evidence of GVHD. Disease progression occurred in 3 patients at 26, 38, and 62 weeks after the infusion. These data suggest that in myeloma, as in CML, the graft-versus-tumor effect does not require CD8$^+$ cells, and may be independent of GVHD (Alyea & Ritz, 1997).

Treatment options for patients with lymphoma relapsing after an allogeneic transplant vary from observation alone (in the case of low-bulk, low-grade lymphoma) to withdrawal of immune suppression (Fig. 85.7), donor lymphocyte infusions, and second transplants (in the case of aggressive lymphoma) (Vose et al., 1992; van Besien et al., 1997). As with other diseases, treatment needs to be individualized and will depend on the extent of the disease, the remission duration posttransplant, performance status, and histologic subtype.

Relapse after autologous HSC transplantation

Patients with various hematologic malignancies who have relapsed after an autologous transplant can respond to salvage therapy and achieve long-term disease control with a second autograft or an allogeneic transplant (Schouten et al., 1989; Schwella et al., 1994; Tsai et al., 1995; de Lima et al., 1997; Hale et al., 2001), although treatment-related mortality can be high, particularly with the use of myeloablative conditioning prior to a conventional allograft (de Lima et al., 1997; Radich et al., 2000). Use of alternative donors in patients without compatible siblings, such as partially HLA-matched related donors or HLA-matched unrelated donors, has been attempted successfully in small numbers of patients with acute leukemia or lymphomas relapsed after an autologous transplant (Godder et al., 1996, 2001; Hale et al., 2001) (Figs. 85.8, 85.9 and 85.10). Patients unwilling or unable to undergo second transplants can

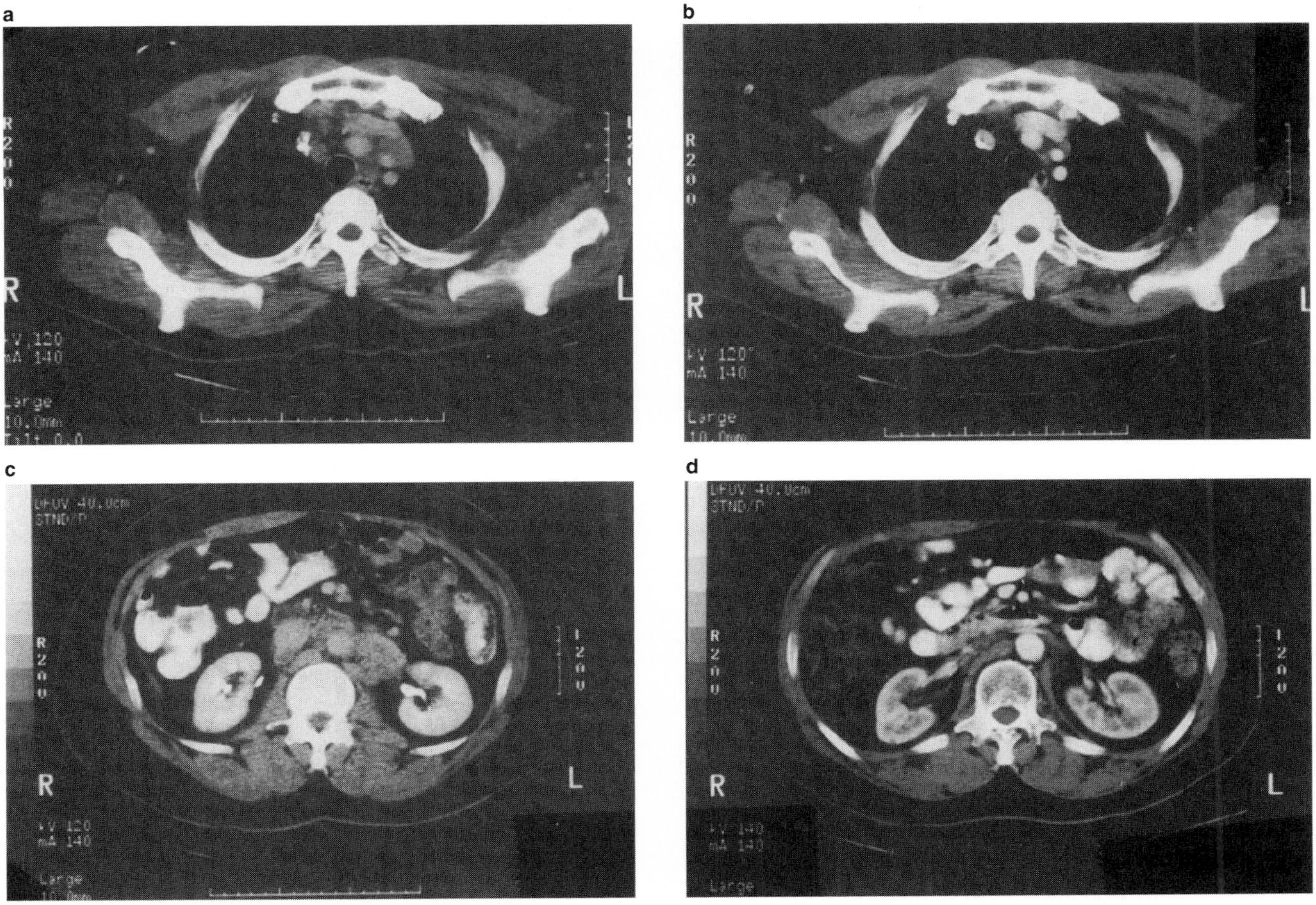

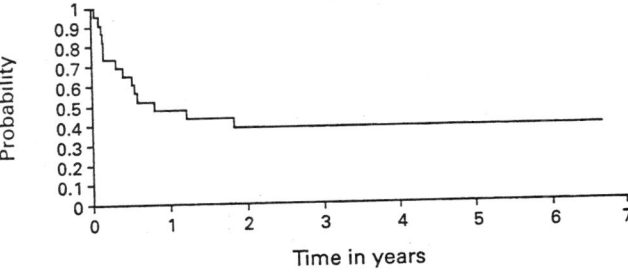

Fig. 85.7. Patient 2. **(a)** Mediastinal adenopathy 88 days after transplantation; **(b)** mediastinal adenopathy 143 days after transplantation and 55 days after withdrawal of tacrolimus; **(c)** retroperitoneal adenopathy 88 days after transplantation. Active disease was demonstrated by fine needle aspiration. **(d)** Retroperitoneal adenopathy 143 days after transplantation and 55 days after withdrawal of tacrolimus. Reproduced, with permission, from van Besien *et al.* (1997).

still obtain benefit from conventional dose chemotherapy or radiotherapy in terms of survival and quality of life, and should be considered for these types of therapy (Vose *et al.,* 1992). This is especially true for patients with multiple myeloma in whom long-term survival can be achieved, especially in patients with a long remission posttransplant and low serum β_2-microglobulin

at the time of relapse. This type of disease control can be achieved in some patients even without the benefit of a second autologous transplant (Hunault *et al.,* 1995; Tricot *et al.,* 1995). In a pair-matched control study, salvage autografting was compared to salvage allografting for myeloma patients relapsing after an initial autograft (Mehta *et al.,* 1998). Autografting appeared superior for overall survival but event-free survival was comparable (Figs. 85.11 and 85.12). The use of reduced

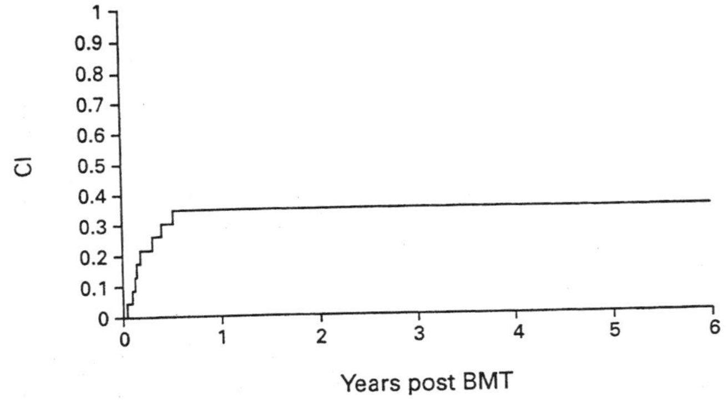

Fig. 85.8. Cumulative incidence of regimen-related mortality in children who underwent alloBMT following ABMT. Reproduced, with permission, from Hale *et al.* (2001).

Fig. 85.9. Kaplan-Meier analysis of disease-free survival among children who underwent alloBMT following ABMT. Reproduced, with permission, from Hale *et al.* (2001).

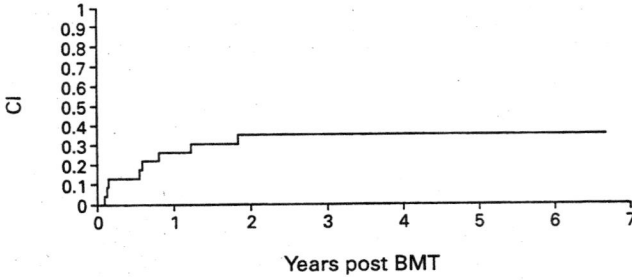

Fig. 85.10. Cumulative incidence of relapse in children who underwent alloBMT following ABMT. Reproduced, with permission, from Hale *et al.* (2001).

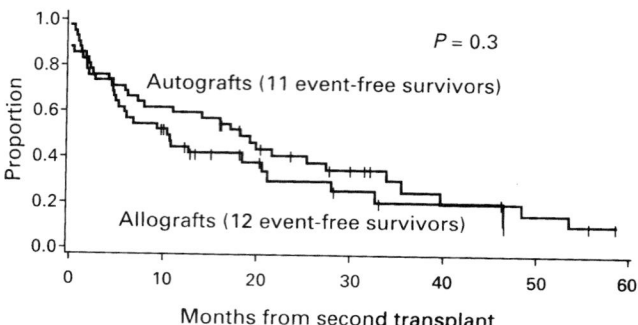

Fig. 85.12. Event-free survival (survival in complete or stable partial remission). Reproduced, with permission, from Mehta *et al.* (1998).

intensity conditioning followed by an allograft ("mini-allograft") is being increasingly explored in this setting (Kottaridis *et al.,* 2000; Dey *et al.,* 2001, Vesole, Simic, & Lazarus, 2001). Martino and colleagues (2002), using fludarabine and melphalan in most patients, reported a 1 year treatment-related mortality of 24% and a progression-free survival at 1 year of 57%.

Conclusions

Relapse of the underlying malignancy will likely remain a major challenge to the success of allogeneic transplantation for hematologic malignancies for some years to come. Better understanding of the biological basis of leukemia tolerance, and mechanisms of resistance to current high-dose chemotherapy are needed in order to devise novel therapies both for the prevention and the treatment of this complication.

In the interim, patients relapsing after transplant should be encouraged to participate in ongoing trials exploring novel immune modulatory and other strategies. Obviously, preservation of quality of life is of utmost importance, but for many patients this goal is best attained through reinduction of a remission and maintenance of this remission for as long as possible.

Figure 85.13 summarizes the current protocols available at M.D. Anderson Cancer Center for treatment of CML relapsed posttransplant. Patients with a molecular relapse only (deter-

mined by the PCR technique) are monitored closely until evidence of progression is confirmed, either by conventional cytogenetic techniques or hypermetaphase fluorescent in situ hybridization (FISH) (Seong *et al.,* 1997). Initial therapy includes withdrawal of immune suppression in all patients; if no response is seen after 2 to 4 weeks then further strategies are explored. Patients with cytogenetic relapses are treated with CD8-depleted DLI if the donor is available; however, it is also reasonable to give a trial of IFN-α in these patients, since the relative benefits of these strategies have never been compared in a randomized fashion, and IFN-α is potentially less toxic. Patients who have relapsed into chronic phase are preferably treated with CD8-depleted donor lymphocytes with or without IFN-α. Patients relapsing into transformed phases are managed as if they had acute leukemia. With accumulating experience (Kantarjian *et al.* (2002), imatinib should now be considered in this algorithm.

Figure 85.14 summarizes treatment strategies at M.D. Anderson Cancer Center for treatment of acute leukemia relapsed posttransplant. Patients relapsing on immune suppressive therapy have this therapy withdrawn; if no effect is seen within 2 to 4 weeks, they then proceed to other therapy. Patients with acute leukemia are offered a second allogeneic transplant with full-dose conditioning regimen, if they are young, have a good performance status, and had a long remission after the initial transplant. Patients with indolent relapses, no peripheral blood blast cells, and less than 30% bone marrow blasts are given a trial of G-CSF; other patients receive either high-dose melphalan or decitabine supported by G-CSF-mobilized allogeneic blood stem cells. Immune suppressive therapy is used after second transplant, but is tapered by 90 days posttransplant if no signs or symptoms of GVHD have developed Patients then receive DLI in an attempt to prevent relapse.

Patients relapsing after an autologous transplant receive a second autologous transplant if they had a long remission after first transplant, remain chemosensitive, and have adequate autologous stem cells collected. Patients ineligible for a second autologous transplant undergo an allogeneic blood stem cell transplant if an HLA-compatible donor is available.

Finally, many patients prefer not to undergo further aggressive therapy: these patients need continued symptomatic and palliative care to ensure an adequate quality of life until death.

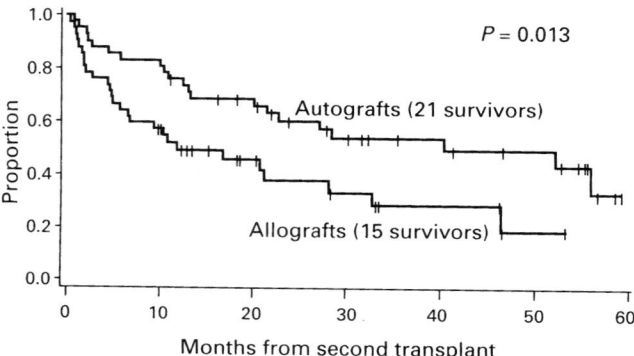

Fig. 85.11. Overall survival. Reproduced, with permission, from Mehta *et al.* (1998).

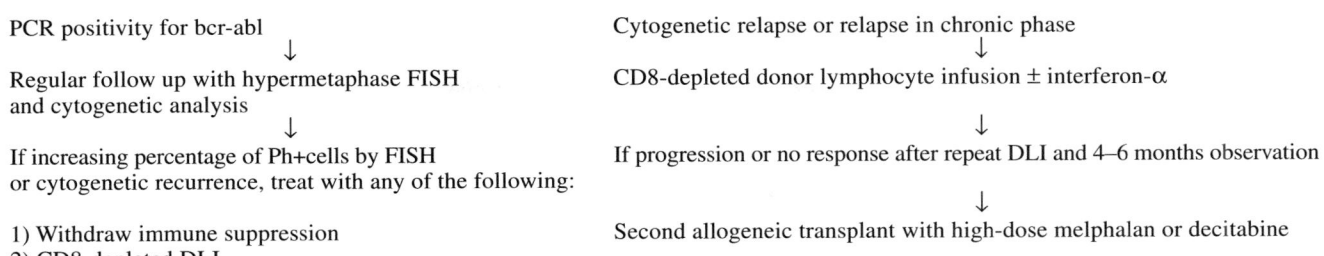

Fig. 85.13. Strategies for treatment of CML relapsed after allogeneic HSC transplantation at M.D. Anderson Cancer Center.

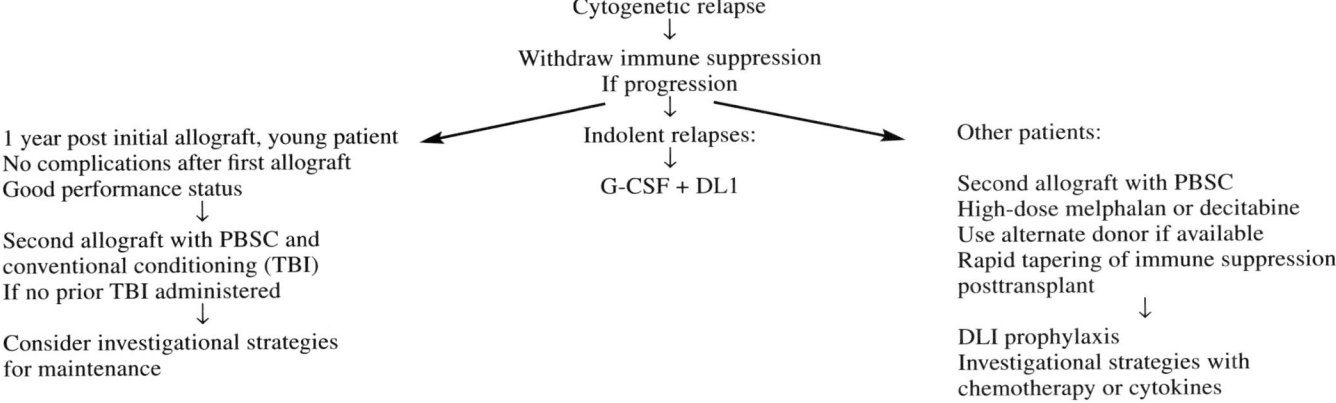

Fig. 85.14. Strategies for treatment of acute leukemia relapsed after allogeneic HSC transplantation at M.D. Anderson Cancer Center.

References

Abraham, R., Szer, J., Bardy, P., & Grigg, A. (1997). Early cyclosporine taper in high-risk sibling allogeneic bone marrow transplants. *Bone Marrow Transplantation*, **20**, 773–7.

Alyea, A. & Ritz, J. (1997). Induction of graft-versus-myeloma by donor lymphocyte infusions following allogeneic bone marrow transplant. Presented at the VI International Workshop on Multiple Myeloma 1997, Boston, Massachusetts.

Alyea, E., Soiffer, R., Murray, C. *et al.* (1995). Adoptive immunotherapy following allogeneic bone marrow transplantation (BMT) with donor lymphocytes depleted of CD8+ T-cells. *Blood*, **86** (Suppl 1), 293a (Abstract).

Arcese, W., Goldman, J., Arcangelo, E. *et al.* (1993). Outcome of patients who relapse after allogeneic bone marrow transplantation for chronic myeloid leukemia. *Blood*, **82**, 3211–9.

Arcese, W., Mauro, F., Alimena, G. *et al.* (1991). Interferon therapy for Ph positive CML patients relapsing after T-cell depleted allogeneic bone marrow transplantation. *Bone Marrow Transplantation*, **5**, 309–15.

Arthur, C., Apperley, J., Guo, A. *et al.* (1988). Cytogenetic events after bone marrow transplantation for chronic myeloid leukemia in chronic phase. *Blood*, **71**, 79–86.

Atkinson, K., Biggs, J., Concannon, A. *et al.* (1986). Second marrow transplants for recurrence of hematological malignancy. *Bone Marrow Transplantation*, **1**, 159–66.

Aurer, I. & Gale, R. (1991). Are new conditioning regimens for transplants in acute myelogenous leukemia better? *Bone Marrow Transplantation*, **7**, 255–611.

Bacigalupo, A., Lamparelli, T., Gualandi, F *et al.* (2001). Increased risk of leukemia relapse with high dose cyclosporine after allogeneic marrow transplantation for acute leukemia: 10 year follow-up of a randomized study. *Blood*, **98**, 3174–5.

Bacigalupo, A., Van Lint, M.T., Occhini, D. *et al.* (1991). Increased risk of leukemia relapse with high-dose cyclosporine A after allogeneic marrow transplantation for acute leukemia. *Blood*, **77**, 1423–8.

Bacigalupo, A., Vitale, V., Corvo, R. *et al.* (2000). The combined effect of total body irradiation (TBI) and cyclosporin A (CyA) on the risk of relapse in patients with acute myeloid leukaemia undergoing allogeneic bone marrow transplantation. *British Journal of Haematology*, **108**, 99–104.

Bar, B., Schattenberg, A., Mensink, E. *et al.* (1993). Donor leukocyte infusions for chronic myelogenous leukemia after allogeneic bone marrow transplantation. *Journal of Clinical Oncology*, **11**, 513–9.

Baron, S., Tyring, S., Fleischmann, W. *et al.* (1991). The Interferons. Mechanism of action and clinical applications. *Journal of the American Medical Association*, **266**, 1375–83.

Barrett, A., Locatelli, F., Treleaven, J. *et al.* (1991). Second transplants for leukemic relapse after bone marrow transplantation: high early mortality but favorable effect of chronic GVHD on continued remission *British Journal of Haematology*, **78**, 561–74.

Barrett, A., Tew, C., & Joshi, R. (1985). How should acute lymphoblastic leukemia relapse after bone-marrow transplantation be treated? *Lancet*, **1**, 1188–91.

Beguin, Y., Collignon, J., Laurent, C., & Fillet, G. (1996). Spontaneous and complete recovery of donor haemopoiesis without GVHD after relapse and apparent marrow graft rejection in poor-prognosis myelodysplastic syndrome. *British Journal of Haematology,* **94,** 507–9.

Bensinger, W.I., Martin, P.J., Storer, B. *et al.* (2001). Transplantation of bone marrow as compared to peripheral-blood cells from HLA-identical relatives in patients with hematologic cancers. *New England Journal of Medicine,* **344,** 175–81.

Békássy, A., Hermans, J., Gorin, N.C., & Gratwohl, A. (1996). Granulocytic sarcoma after allogeneic bone marrow transplantation: a retrospective European multicenter survey. *Bone Marrow Transplantation,* **17,** 801–8.

Biagi, J.J., Mileshkin, L., Grigg, A.P. *et al.* (2001). Efficacy of thalidomide therapy, for extramedullary relapse of myeloma following allogeneic transplantation. *Bone Marrow Transplantation,* **28,** 1145–50.

Bishop, M.R., Tarantolo, S.R., Pavletic, S. *et al.* (2000). Filgrastim as an alternative to donor leukocyte infusion for relapse after allogeneic stem-cell transplantation. *Journal of Clinical Oncology,* **18,** 2269–72.

Blume, K. & Forman, S. (1987). High dose busulfan/etoposide as a preparatory regimen for second bone marrow transplants in hematologic malignancies. *Blut,* **55,** 49–53.

Bonini, C., Verzeletti, S., Servida, P. *et al.* (1994). Transfer of the HSV-TK gene into donor peripheral blood lymphocytes for in vivo immunomodulation of donor anti tumor immunity after allo BMT. *Blood,* **84** (Suppl 1), 110a (Abstract).

Bortin, M., Horowitz, M., Gale, R. *et al.* (1992). Changing trends in allogeneic bone marrow transplantation for leukemia in the 1980s. *Journal of the American Medical Association,* **268,** 607–12.

Bortin, M., Horowitz, M., & Rimm, A. (1992). Increasing utilization of allogeneic bone marrow transplantation: results of the 1988–1990 survey. *Annals of Internal Medicine,* **116,** 505–12.

Bosi, A., Laszlo, D., Labopin, M. *et al.* (2001). Second allogeneic bone marrow transplantation in acute leukemia: results of a survey by the European Cooperative Group for Blood and Marrow Transplantation. *Journal of Clinical Oncology,* **19,** 3675–84.

Bostrom, B., Woods, W., Nesbit, M. *et al.* (1987). Successful reinduction of patients with acute lymphoblastic leukemia who relapse following bone marrow transplantation. *Journal of Clinical Oncology,* **5,** 376–81.

Bowman, W., Aur, R., Hustu, H., & Rivera, G. (1984). Isolated testicular relapse in acute lymphocytic leukemia of childhood: categories and influence on survival. *Journal of Clinical Oncology,* **2,** 924–9.

Boyd, C., Ramberg, R., & Thomas, E. (1982). The incidence of recurrence of leukemia after allogeneic bone marrow transplantation. *Leukemia Research,* **6,** 833–7.

Carral, A., Sanz, G.F., & Sanz, M.A. (1996). Filgrastim for the treatment of leukemia relapse after bone marrow transplantation. *Bone Marrow Transplantation,* **18,** 817–9.

Chak, L., Sapozink, M., & Cox, R. (1983). Extramedullary lesions in non-lymphocytic leukemia; results of radiation therapy. *International Journal of Radiation Oncology, Biology, Physics,* **9,** 1173–6.

Champlin, R., Ho, W., Lenarsky, C. *et al.* (1985). Successful second bone marrow transplantation for AMO or ALL. *Transplantation Proceedings,* **17,** 496–9.

Chiang, K.Y., Weisdorf, D.J., Davies, S.M. *et al.* (1996). Second bone marrow transplantation following a uniform conditioning regimen as therapy for malignant relapse. *Bone Marrow Transplantation,* **17,** 39–42.

Chong, G., Byrnes, G., Szer, J., & Grigg, A. (2000). Extramedullary relapse after allogeneic bone marrow transplantation for haematological malignancy. *Bone Marrow Transplantation,* **26,** 1011–5.

Clift, R., Buckner, C., Appelbaum, F. *et al.* (1990). Allogeneic marrow transplantation in patients with acute myeloid leukemia in first remission: a randomized trial of two irradiation regimens. *Blood,* **76,** 1867–71.

Collins, R., Rogers, Z., Bennett, M. *et al.* (1992). Hematologic relapse of chronic myelogenous leukemia following allogeneic bone marrow transplantation: apparent graft-versus-leukemia effect following abrupt discontinuation of immunosuppresion. *Bone Marrow Transplantation,* **10,** 391–5.

Collins, R., Shpilberg, O., Drobyski, W. *et al.* (1997). Donor leukocyte infusions in 140 patients with relapsed malignancy after allogeneic bone marrow transplantation. *Journal of Clinical Oncology,* **15,** 433–44.

Cooley, D.C., Sears, D.A., Udden, M.M. *et al.* (2000). Donor cell leukemia: report of a case occurring 11 years after allogeneic bone marrow transplantation and review of the literature. *American Journal of Hematology,* **63,** 46–53.

Cross, N., Feng, L., Chase, A. *et al.* (1993). Competitive polymerase chain reaction to estimate the number of BCR-ABL transcripts in chronic myeloid leukemia after bone marrow transplantation. *Blood,* **82,** 1929–36.

de Lima, M., van Besien, K.W., Giralt, S.A. *et al.* (1997). Bone marrow transplantation after failure of autologous transplant for non-Hodgkin's lymphoma. *Bone Marrow Transplantation,* **19,** 121–7.

de Weger, R.A., Tilanus, M.G.J., Scheidel, K.C. *et al.* (2000). Monitoring of residual disease and guided donor leukocyte infusion after allogeneic bone marrow transplantation by chimaerism analysis with short tandem repeats. *British Journal of Haematology,* **110,** 647–53.

Dermine, S., Mavroudis, D., Jiang, Y. *et al.* (1997). Immune escape from a graft-versus-leukemia effect may play a role in the relapse of myeloid leukemias following allogeneic bone marrow transplantation. *Bone Marrow Transplantation,* **19,** 989–99.

Dey, B.R., McAfee, S., Sackstein, R. *et al.* (2001). Successful allogeneic stem cell transplantation with nonmyeloablative conditioning in patients with relapsed hematologic malignancy following autologous stem cell transplantation. *Biology of Blood and Marrow Transplantation,* **7,** 604–12.

Drobyski, W., Keever, C., Roth, M.S. *et al.* (1993). Salvage immunotherapy using donor leukocyte infusions as treatment for relapsed chronic myelogenous leukemia after allogeneic bone marrow transplantation: efficacy and toxicity of a defined T cell dose. *Blood,* **82,** 2310–8.

Fialkow, P.J., Thomas, E.D., Bryant, J.I., & Neiman, P.E. (1971). Leukaemic transformation of engrafted human marrow cells in vivo. *Lancet,* **1,** 251–5.

Flowers, M., Clift, R., Schoch, G. *et al.* (1994). Discontinuation of cyclosporine to induce a graft-versus-leukemia effect in patients with cytogenetic relapse after allogeneic bone marrow transplantation for chronic myelogenous leukemia. *Blood,* **84** (Suppl 1), 540a (Abstract).

Flowers, M., Sullivan, K., Martin, P. *et al.* (1995). G-CSF stimulated donor peripheral blood infusions as immunotherapy in patients with hematologic malignancies relapsing after allogeneic transplantation. *Blood,* **86,** 564a (Abstract).

Frassoni, F., Barrett, J., Granena, A. *et al.* (1988). Relapse after allogeneic bone marrow for acute leukemia. A survey of the EBMTR of 117 cases. *British Journal of Haematology,* **70,** 317–20.

Frassoni, F., Labopin, M., Gluckman, E. *et al.* (1994). Are patients with acute leukaemia, alive and well 2 years post bone marrow transplantation cured? A European survey. Acute Leukaemia Working Party of the European Group for Bone Marrow Transplantation (EBMT). *Leukemia,* **8,** 924–8.

Ganem, G., Kuentz, M., Bernaudin, F. *et al.* (1989). Central nervous system relapses after bone marrow transplantation for acute lymphoblastic leukemia in remission. *Cancer,* **64,** 1796–804.

Giralt, S. & Champlin, R.E. (1994). Leukemia relapse after allogeneic bone marrow transplantation: a review. *Blood,* **84,** 3603–112.

Giralt, S., Escudier, S., Kantarjian, H. *et al.* (1993). Treatment with filgrastim for relapse of leukemia and myelodysplasia after allogeneic bone marrow transplantation. Preliminary observations. *New England Journal of Medicine,* **329,** 757–61.

Giralt, S., Hester, J., Huh, Y. *et al.* (1995a). CD8-depleted donor lymphocyte infusion as treatment for relapsed chronic myelogenous leukemia after allogeneic bone marrow transplantation. *Blood,* **86,** 4337–43.

Giralt, S., Hester, J., Talpaz, M. *et al.* (1994). Cytokine therapy for patients relapsing after allogeneic bone marrow transplantation. *Journal of Cellular Biochemistry,* Suppl 18B, 88a.

Giralt, S., O' Brien, S., Talpaz, M. *et al.* (1995b). Alpha interferon and interleukin-2 as treatment for leukemia relapse after allogeneic bone marrow transplantation. *Cytokines and Molecular Therapy,* **1,** 115–22.

Glass, B., Majolino, I., Dreger, P. *et al.* (1997). Allogeneic peripheral blood progenitor cells for treatment of relapse after bone marrow transplantation. *Bone Marrow Transplantation,* **20,** 533–41.

Godder, K., Pat, A., Abhyarkar, S. *et al.* (1996). Partially mismatched related donor transplants as salvage therapy for patients with refractory leukemia who relapse post bone marrow transplantation. *Bone Marrow Transplantation,* **17,** 49–53.

Godder, K.T., Metha, J., Chiang, K.Y. *et al.* (2001). Partially-mismatched related donor bone marrow transplantation as salvage for patients with AML who failed autologous stem cell transplantation. *Bone Marrow Transplantation,* **28,** 1031–6.

Hale, G.A., Tong, X., Benaim, E. *et al.* (2001). Allogeneic bone marrow transplantation for children failing prior autologous bone marrow transplantation. *Bone Marrow Transplantation,* **27,** 155–62.

Hambach, L., Eder, M., Dammann, E. *et al.* (2001). Donor cell-derived acute myeloid leukemia developing 14 months after matched unrelated bone marrow transplantation for chronic myeloid leukemia. *Bone Marrow Transplantation,* **28,** 705–7.

Hertenstein, B., Wiesneth, M., Novotny, J. *et al.* (1993). Interferon-α and donor buffy coat transfusions for treatment of relapsed chronic myeloid leukemia after allogeneic bone marrow transplantation. *Transplantation,* **56,** 1114–8.

Higano, C., Brixey, M., Bryant, E. *et al.* (1990). Durable complete remission of acute non-lymphocytic leukemia associated with discontinuation of immunosuppression following relapse after allogeneic bone marrow transplantation. A case report of a probable graft-versus-leukemia effect. *Transplantation,* **50,** 175–7.

Higano, C., Raskind, W., & Singer, J. (1992). Use of α-interferon for the treatment of relapse of chronic myelogenous leukemia in chronic phase after allogeneic bone marrow transplantation. *Blood,* **80,** 1437–42.

Hughes, T., Economou, K., Mackinnon, S. *et al.* (1989). Slow evolution of chronic myeloid leukemia relapsing after bone marrow transplantation with T-cell depleted donor marrow. *British Journal of Haematology,* **73,** 462–7.

Hunault, M., Rio, B., Zittoun, R. *et al.* (1995). Pattern of relapse and treatment of multiple myeloma after high dose therapy. *Blood,* **86** (Suppl 1), 835a (Abstract).

Kantarjian, H. M., O'Brien, S., Cortes, J. E. *et al.* (2002). Imatinib mesylate therapy for relapse after allogeneic stem cell transplantation for chornic myelogenous leukemia. *Blood,* **100,** 1590–5.

Kishi, K., Takahashi, S., Gondo, H. *et al.* (1997). Second allogeneic bone marrow transplantation for posttransplant leukemia relapse: results of a survey of 66 cases in 24 Japanese institutes. *Bone Marrow Transplantation,* **19,** 461–6.

Koc, Y., Miller, K.B., Schenkein, D.P. *et al.* (1999). Extramedullary tumors of myeloid blasts in adults as a pattern of relapse following allogeneic bone marrow transplantation. *Cancer,* **85,** 608–15.

Kolb, H., Mittermuller, J., Clemm, C. *et al.* (1990). Donor leukocyte transfusions for treatment of recurrent chronic myelogenous leukemia in marrow transplant patients. *Blood,* **76,** 2462–5.

Kolb, H., Schattenberg, A., Goldman, J. *et al.* (1995). Graft-versus-leukemia effect of donor lymphocyte transfusions in marrow grafted patients. *Blood,* **86,** 2041–50.

Kottaridis, P.D., Milligan, D.W., Chopra, R. *et al.* (2000). In vivo CAMPATH-1H prevents graft-versus-host disease following non-myeloablative stem cell transplantation. *Blood,* **96,** 2419–25.

Kumar, L. (1994). Leukemia: management of relapse after allogeneic bone marrow transplantation. *Journal of Clinical Oncology,* **12,** 1710–7.

Lee, K-H., Lee, J-H., Kim, S. *et al.* (2000). High frequency of extramedullary relapse of acute leukemia after allogeneic bone marrow transplantation. *Bone Marrow Transplantation,* **26,** 147–52.

Mackinnon, S., Barnett, L., & Heller, G. (1996). Polymerase chain reaction is highly predictive of relapse in patients following T cell depleted allogeneic bone marrow transplantation for chronic myeloid leukemia. *Bone Marrow Transplantation,* **17,** 643–7.

Mackinnon, S., Papadopoulos, E., Carabasi, M. *et al.* (1995a). Adoptive immunotherapy evaluating escalating doses of donor leukocytes for relapse of chronic myeloid leukemia following bone marrow transplantation: separation of graft-versus-leukemia responses from graft-versus-host disease. *Blood,* **86,** 1261–8.

Mackinnon, S., Papadopoulos, E., Carabasi, M. *et al.* (1995b). Adoptive immunotherapy using donor leukocytes following bone marrow transplantation for chronic myeloid leukemia: is T cell dose important in determining biologic response? *Bone Marrow Transplantation,* **15,** 591–5.

Martino, R., Caballero, M. D., de la Serna, J. *et al.* (2002). Low transplant-related mortality after second allogeneic peripheral blood stem cell transplant with reduced-intensity conditioning in patients who have failed a prior autologous transplant. *Bone Marrow Transplantation,* **30,** 63–8.

McCann, S.R., Lawler, M., Bacigalupo, A. *et al.* (1993). Recurrence of Philadelphia chromosome-positive leukemia in donor cells after marrow transplantation for chronic granulocytic leukemia. *Leukemia and Lymphoma,* **10,** 419–25.

Mehta, J., Powles, R., Singhal, S. *et al.* (1995). Cytokine-mediated immunotherapy with or without donor leukocytes for poor-risk acute myeloid leukemia relapsing after allogeneic bone marrow transplantation. *Bone Marrow Transplantation,* **16,** 133–7.

Mehta, J., Tricot, G., Jagannath, S. *et al.* (1998). Salvage autologous or allogeneic transplantation for multiple myeloma refractory to or relapsing after a first-line autograft? *Bone Marrow Transplantation, 21,* 887–92.

Michallet, M., Tanguy, M.L., Socie, G. *et al.* (2000). Second allogeneic haematopoietic stem cell transplantation in relapsed acute and chronic leukaemias for patients who underwent a first allogeneic bone marrow transplantation: a survey of the Societe Francaise de Greffe de Moelle (SFGM). *British Journal of Haematology, 108,* 400–7.

Mortimer, J., Binder, M., Schulman, S. *et al.* (1989). Relapse of acute leukemia after marrow transplantation. Natural history and results of subsequent therapy. *Journal of Clinical Oncology, 7,* 50–7.

Mrsic, M., Horowitz, M., Atkinson, K. *et al.* (1992). Second HLA-identical sibling transplants for leukemia recurrence. *Bone Marrow Transplantation, 9,* 269–75.

Nemunaitis, J., Albo, V., Zeigler, Z. *et al.* (1993). Reduction of allogeneic transplant morbidity by combining peripheral blood and bone marrow progenitor cells. *Leukemia and Lymphoma, 10,* 405–6.

Odom, L., Githers, J., Morse, H. *et al.* (1978). Remission of relapsed leukemia during a graft-versus-host reaction. A graft-versus-leukemia reaction in man? *Lancet, 2,* 537–40.

Olivarria, E., Craddock, C., Dazzi, F. *et al.* (2002). Imatinib mesylate (ST1571) in the treatment of relapse of chronic myeloid leukemia after allogeneic stem cell transplantation. *Blood, 99,* 3861–2.

Pawson, R., Potter, M.N., Theocharous, P. *et al.* (2001). Treatment of relapse after allogeneic bone marrow transplantation with reduced intensity conditioning (FLAG +/– Ida) and second allogeneic transplant. *British Journal of Haematology, 115,* 622–9.

Porter, D., Roth, M., McGarigle, C. *et al.* (1994). Induction of graft-versus-host disease as immunotherapy for relapsed chronic myeloid leukemia. *New England Journal of Medicine, 330,* 100–6.

Radich, J., Gooley, T., Sanders, J.E. *et al.* (2000). Second allogeneic transplantation after failure of first autologous transplantation. *Biology of Blood and Marrow Transplantation, 6,* 272–9.

Radich, J., Sanders, J., Buckner, C. *et al.* (1993). Second allogeneic marrow transplantation for patients with recurrent leukemia after initial transplant with total body irradiation containing regimens. *Journal of Clinical Oncology, 11,* 304–10.

Radich, J.P., Gehly, G., Gooley, T. *et al.* (1995). Polymerase chain reaction detection of the BCR-ABL fusion transcript after allogeneic marrow transplantation for chronic myeloid leukemia: results and implications in 346 patients. *Blood, 85,* 2632–42.

Rondón, G., Giralt, S., Huh, Y. *et al.* (1996). Complete remission due to graft-versus-leukemia effect against chronic lymphocytic leukemia. *Bone Marrow Transplantation, 18,* 669–72.

Rosenberg, S., Grimm, E., McGrogan, M. *et al.* (1984). Biological activity of recombinant human interleukin-2. *Science, 223,* 1412–4.

Sanders, J., Buckner, C., Clift, R. *et al.* (1988). Second marrow transplants in patients with leukemia who relapse after allogeneic marrow transplantation. *Bone Marrow Transplantation, 3,* 11–9.

Schouten, H.C., Armitage, J.O., Klassen, L.W. *et al.* (1989). Allogeneic bone marrow transplantation in patients with lymphoma relapsing after autologous transplantation. *Bone Marrow Transplantation, 4,* 119–21.

Schwella, N., Schwerdtfeger, R., Konig, V. *et al.* (1994). Allogeneic bone marrow transplantation for recurrence of leukemia after autologous bone marrow transplantation. *Transplantation, 57,* 1263–5.

Seong, D., Giralt, S., Fischer, H. *et al.* (1997). Usefulness of detection of minimal residual disease by "Hyper Metaphase" fluorescent in situ hybridization after allogeneic BMT for chronic myelogenous leukemia. *Bone Marrow Transplantation, 19,* 565–70.

Singhal, S., Powles, R., Treleaven, J. *et al.* (1996). Central nervous system relapse after bone marrow transplantation for acute leukemia in first remission. *Bone Marrow Transplantation, 17,* 637–41.

Slavin, S., Naparstek, E., Nagler, A. *et al.* (1996). Allogeneic cell therapy with donor peripheral blood cells and recombinant human interleukin-2 to treat leukemia relapse after allogeneic bone marrow transplantation. *Blood, 87,* 2195–204.

Socie, G., Veum Stone, J., Wingard, J.R. *et al.* (1999). Long-term survival and late deaths after allogeneic bone marrow transplantation. *New England Journal of Medicine, 341,* 14–21.

Szer, J., Grigg, A., Phillips, G., & Sheridan, W. (1993). Donor leucocyte infusions after chemotherapy for patients relapsing with acute leukemia following allogeneic BMT. *Bone Marrow Transplantation, 11,* 109–11.

Thompson, C., Sanders, J., Flournoy, N. *et al.* (1986). The risks of central nervous system relapse and leukoencephalopathy in patients receiving marrow transplants for acute leukemia. *Blood, 67,* 195–9.

Tricot, G., Jagannath, S., Vesole, D.H. *et al.* (1995). Relapse of multiple myeloma after autologous transplantation: survival after salvage therapy. *Bone Marrow Transplantation, 6,* 7–11.

Tsai, T., Goodman, S., Schiller, G. *et al.* (1995). Allogeneic bone marrow transplantation for relapse after autologous bone marrow transplantation in lymphomas and acute leukemia. *Blood, 86,* 969a (Abstract).

van Besien, K.W., de Lima, M., Giralt, S.A. *et al.* (1997). Management of lymphoma recurrence after allogeneic transplantation: the relevance of the graft-versus-lymphoma effect. *Bone Marrow Transplantation, 19,* 977–82.

van Rhee, F., Lin, F., Cullis, J. *et al.* (1994). Relapse of chronic myeloid leukemia after allogeneic bone marrow transplant: the case for giving donor leukocyte transfusions before the onset of hematologic relapse. *Blood, 83,* 3377–83.

Vesole, D.H., Simic, A., & Lazarus, H.M. (2001). Controversy in multiple myeloma transplants: tandem autotransplants and mini-allografts. *Bone Marrow Transplantation, 28,* 725–35.

Vose, J., Bierman, P.J., Anderson, J.R. *et al.* (1992). Progressive disease after high-dose therapy and autologous transplantation for lymphoid malignancy: clinical course and patient follow up. *Blood, 80,* 2142–8.

Wagner, J., Vogelsang, G., Zehnbauer, B. *et al.* (1992). Relapse of leukemia after bone marrow transplantation: effect of second myeloablative therapy. *Bone Marrow Transplantation, 9,* 205–9.

Waller, E.K., Rosenthal, H., Jones, T.W. *et al.* (2001). Larger numbers of CD4 bright dendritic cells in donor bone marrow are associated with increased relapse after allogeneic bone marrow transplantation. *Blood, 97,* 2948–56.

Yong, A.S.M. & Goldman, J.M. (1999). Relapse of chronic myeloid leukaemia 14 years after allogeneic bone marrow transplantation. *Bone Marrow Transplantation, 23,* 827–8.

86 Myelodysplasia after autologous stem cell transplantation

JONATHAN W. FRIEDBERG

University of Rochester, Rochester, USA

Introduction

The acute treatment-related mortality with autologous hematopoietic stem cell transplantation (ASCT) is now well below 5% in most single-institution and cooperative group series. (Philip *et al.*, 1995; Freedman *et al.*, 1999; Horning *et al.*, 2001; Vose *et al.*, 2002). With longer survival, late complications of ASCT are significant causes of morbidity and mortality. Myelodysplastic syndrome (MDS) and secondary acute myeloid leukemia (AML) have emerged as the major late complication of ASCT, particularly in patients with non-Hodgkin's lymphoma. (Rohatiner, 1994; Stone *et al.*, 1994). In long-term follow-up of a series of 552 patients undergoing ASCT for Non-Hodgkins lymphoma (NHL) at Dana-Farber Cancer Institute, approximately 17% of the deaths posttransplant were from MDS or complications of therapy for MDS. (Friedberg *et al.*, 2001).

Defining MDS after ASCT is complicated, since many patients have prolonged cytopenias after transplant, without evidence of subsequent transformation to AML. In a prospective study of 53 patients undergoing ASCT, bone marrow cellularity and megakaryocytes were significantly decreased in 38% and 49% of patients, respectively, 6 months posttransplant, and some dysplastic features were almost always present in the bone marrow through 6 months posttransplant (Amigo *et al.*, 1999). It is therefore important to strictly define MDS post-ASCT using either the French-American-British (FAB) or the World Health Organization (WHO) classification system, requiring bone marrow dysplasia in at least two cell lines, peripheral cytopenias, and variable blast counts in the bone marrow on review of aspirate smears (Bennett *et al.*, 1982; Greenberg *et al.*, 1997; Harris *et al.*, 1999). Patients with persistent cytopenias 6 months to 1 year after transplant without significant marrow dysplasia should not be considered as having MDS. Differentiating MDS from AML after ASCT is difficult, and in this chapter the term MDS will refer to both MDS and AML, since the disease course of the two is virtually indistinguishable after ASCT.

Cytogenetic analysis of bone marrow aspirates is another critical step in establishing this diagnosis. When cytogenetics is performed, virtually all patients have abnormalities of chromosome 5 and/or 7, or complex abnormalities (>3 clonal abnormalities), as shown in Figure 86.1 (Darrington *et al.*, 1994; Miller *et al.*, 1994; Stone *et al.*, 1994; Rowley *et al.*, 1996). Longitudinal cytogenetic studies have demonstrated more numerous abnormalities in patients with secondary MDS who received radiation as compared with those who only received chemotherapy prior to developing MDS (Whang-Peng *et al.*, 1988). However, cytogenetic analysis is not sufficient to diagnose MDS in this setting, as not all patients with clonal abnormalities develop a clinical MDS syndrome (Lambertenghi Deliliers *et al.*, 1999). For example, Traweek and colleagues described 10 patients with clonal chromosomal abnormalities that developed after ASCT for Hodgkin's disease and NHL, half of whom did not develop clinical MDS during a relatively short follow-up period (Traweek *et al.*, 1994).

Incidence and risk factors of MDS after stem cell transplantation

Several reported series have examined clinical risk factors for subsequent development of MDS after ASCT (Pedersen-Bjergaard *et al.*, 2000). These are summarized in Table 86.1. Important considerations in the interpretation of single-institution studies are length and quality of patient follow-up, definition of MDS, and uniformity of treatment regimens. As expected, risk factors differ between studies; however, the incidence over time in most studies is strikingly similar. Unlike secondary MDS from chemotherapy alone, the incidence post-ASCT continues to increase over time without evidence of a plateau on the Kaplan-Meier curve, as shown in Figure 86.2. For example, in a series from Johns Hopkins, there was a continuing risk of secondary MDS for at least 12 years after ASCT (Akpek *et al.*, 2001). This is similar to the incidence of solid tumors after curative combined modality therapy for Hodgkin's disease, where even longer follow-up has failed to show a decline in new cases (Ng *et al.*, 2002).

In the above-mentioned series from the Dana-Farber Cancer Institute of 552 patients with NHL receiving a standard conditioning regimen of 1,200 to 1,400 cGy total body irradiation (TBI) and cyclophosphamide, followed by B-cell purged

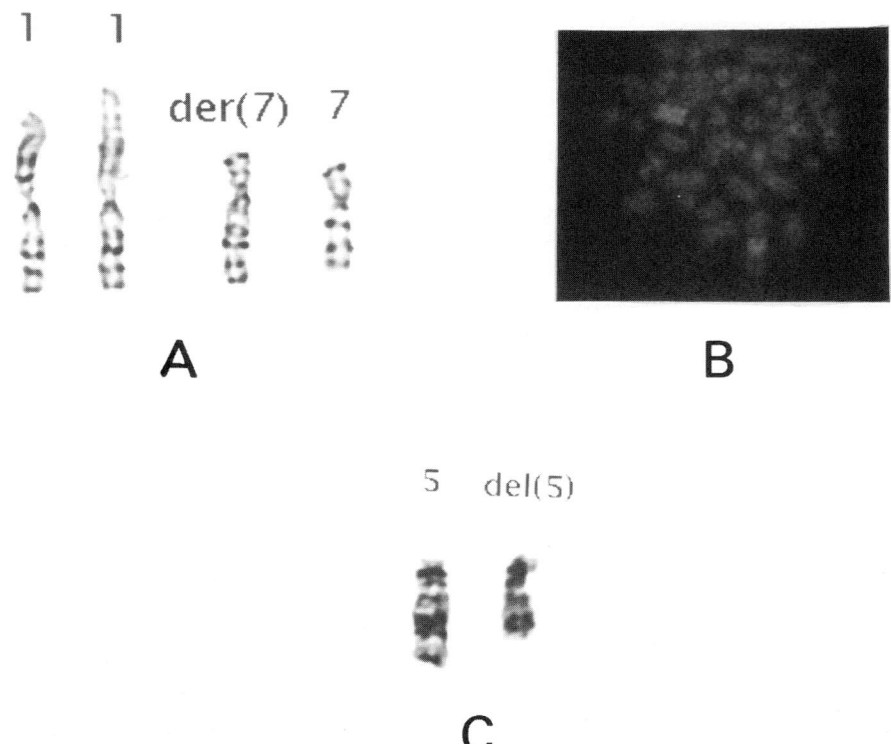

Fig. 86.1. Partial complex karyotype of a patient with MDS after ASCT for NHL, showing typical abnormalities. (A) Deletion of 7q and extra copy of 1q, ie del(7)t(1;7)(p11;q11.2). (B) FISH with the whole chromosome painting probe confirming deletion of 7q identified in A. (C) Interstitial deletion of 5q15 to 5q33, i.e., del(5)(q15q33).

ASCT, 41 patients developed MDS, strictly defined, at a median (range 12–129) of 47 months from transplant (Friedberg *et al.*, 1999). At time of diagnosis of MDS, 29 patients were in remission and 12 patients had relapsed with NHL; the majority of these patients had not received further cytotoxic therapy since transplant. The absolute risk of developing MDS after autologous bone marrow transplantation (ABMT) for NHL was 7.4%. The cumulative risk of development of MDS was 14.5% at 10 years posttransplant (Friedberg *et al.*, 2000). In a logistic regression model, low number of stem cells infused per kilogram and prior localized irradiation were the only significant predictors of developing MDS.

At St. Bartholomew's Hospital, 230 patients with NHL received the same conditioning regimen and purged ASCT as those in the Dana-Farber series, and 27 subsequently developed MDS. The median time to development of MDS was 4.4 years, and on multivariate analysis, prior fludarabine therapy and older age were associated with an increased risk of developing MDS (Micallef *et al.*, 2000). Cytogenetic analysis in 24 of these cases revealed 17 patients with del(5), 15 patients with del(7), and 18 patients with complex karyotypes.

In the City of Hope Cancer Center series, none of these factors were found to be predictive in 22 patients who developed MDS after ASCT for non-Hodgkin's lymphoma or Hodgkin's disease (Krishnan *et al.*, 2000). The incidence of MDS in this series was 8.6% at 6 years. As expected, pre-BMT exposure to topoisomerase II inhibitors increased the risk of MDS with chromosomal 11q23 abnormalities. Pretransplant radiation was independently associated with an increased risk of MDS; however, there was no significant impact on amount or type of pretransplant chemotherapy. A similar finding was noted by Bhatia *et al.* (1996) in a series from Minnesota of patients with both Hodgkin's and non-Hodgkin's lymphoma, where peripheral blood stem cell transplantation with associated mobilization chemotherapy had a higher risk of posttransplant MDS. In contrast, a series from Spain found no impact of source of stem cells and subsequent MDS, and likely previous associations were confounded by mobilization chemotherapy, and extent of chemotherapy pretransplant (Sevilla *et al.*, 2002).

The specific role of TBI conditioning in the development of MDS has been assessed by several studies. Almost 5,000 patients with lymphoma have undergone ASCT and are reported to the European Bone Marrow Transplant Registry: 68 patients have developed MDS (Milligan *et al.*, 1999). While this incidence is lower than in other series, there is a concern about potential for underreporting this complication. The median follow-up from the date of transplant was 6.7 years for patients who developed MDS, but only 2.9 years for the patients without MDS, suggesting that a substantial number of patients remain at risk of developing MDS. Multivariate analy-

Table 86.1. *Selected series of myelodysplasia after autologous hematopoietic stem cell transplantation*

Institution	Diagnosis	Incidence	Median follow-up[a]	Risk factors
Dana-Farber (Friedberg *et al.*, 1999)	NHL	41/552	75 months	Prior XRT Low number of cells infused
St. Bartholomew's (Micallef *et al.*, 2000)	NHL	27/330	72 months	Older patient age Prior fludarabine
City of Hope (Krishnan *et al.*, 2000)	NHL and HD	22/612	Not reported	Etoposide mobilization Prior XRT
Minnesota (Bhatia *et al.*, 1996)	NHL and HD	10/258	37 months	PBSCT Age > 35
Nebraska (Darrington *et al.*, 1994)	NHL and HD	12/511	Not reported	Age > 40 TBI conditioning
MD Anderson (Hosing *et al.*, 2002)	NHL	22/493	21 months	TBI conditioning Prior fludarabine
Beth Israel/Brigham (Wheeler *et al.*, 2001)	NHL and HD	6/300	47 months	Prior XRT Number of prior relapses
Copenhagen (Pedersen-Bjergaard *et al.*, 1997)	NHL and HD	6/76	Not reported	Prior chemotherapy
Arkansas (Govindarajan *et al.*, 1996)	MM	7/188	29 and 36 months	Prior chemotherapy
Duke (Laughlin *et al.*, 1998)	Breast cancer	5/864	44 months	
Registry studies EBMT (Milligan *et al.*, 1999)	NHL and HD	66/4,998	80 months (MDS) 34 months (non-MDS)	Older patient age TBI conditioning Indolent histology Prolonged interval pre-ASCT
Spanish Cooperative Group (Sureda *et al.*, 2001)	HD	12/494	30 months	Prior XRT TBI conditioning Age >40
French Cooperative Group (Andre *et al.*, 1998)	HD	8/467	21 months	Splenectomy PBSCT

[a] Follow-up after ASCT.

Abbreviations: XRT, localized radiotherapy; PBSCT, peripheral blood stem cell transplantation; TBI, total body irradiation; NHL, non-Hodgkin's lymphoma; HD, Hodgkin's disease; EBMT, European Bone Marrow Transplant Group.

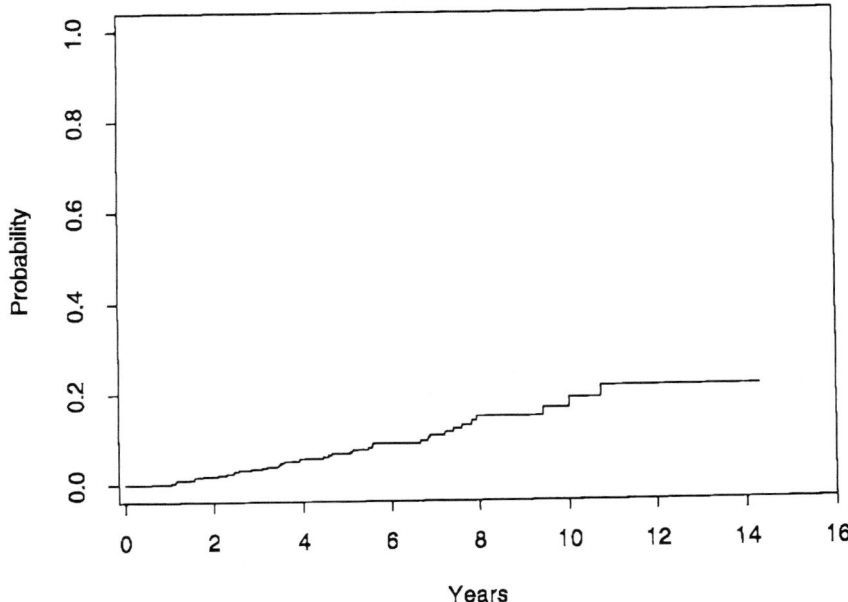

Fig. 86.2. Cumulative incidence of MDS after ASCT in 552 patients transplanted at Dana-Farber Cancer Insitute.

sis revealed age at transplant, exposure to TBI in conditioning, long interval between diagnosis of lymphoma and transplant, and indolent histology as independent variables predicting for subsequent MDS. For patients with Hodgkin's disease, female gender was identified as a risk factor. The amount of previous chemotherapy, including cumulative alkylating agent exposure, was not found to be a significant factor.

A prior, single institution series from the University of Nebraska also determined that TBI-based conditioning was a significant, independent risk factor for the development of MDS after ASCT for both Hodgkin's and non-Hodgkin's lymphoma (Darrington *et al.*, 1994). A series from M.D. Anderson Hospital of 493 patients with NHL identified TBI, particularly when combined with etoposide, as the major risk factor in multivariate analysis (Hosing *et al.*, 2002). Similarly, a retrospective series from France found that both TBI and pretransplant localized radiation appeared to increase the risk of MDS in patients with both Hodgkin's disease and non-Hodgkin's lymphoma (Park *et al.*, 2000).

Further evidence that TBI conditioning is a significant independent risk factor for MDS is the relatively low incidence in patients with breast cancer undergoing ASCT with chemotherapy-only conditioning, where, despite extensive previous alkylating agent exposure, the risk was only 3% at 5 years in two series (Roman-Unfer *et al.*, 1995; Laughlin *et al.*, 1998). Due to the frequency of early disease-related deaths in this population of patients, calculation of cumulative MDS incidence is very difficult. Similarly, Wheeler *et al.* (2001) reported a relatively low incidence of MDS after chemotherapy-only conditioning with cyclophosphamide, carmustine, and etoposide for both Hodgkin's and non-Hodgkin's lymphoma, compared with series using protocols involving TBI.

The risk of MDS following ASCT for multiple myeloma (Govindarajan *et al.*, 1996) and germ cell tumors (Kollmannsberger *et al.*, 1998) also appears to be less than in similar populations of patients with NHL. It is not possible to establish whether the increased risk of MDS in patients with lymphoma is truly a disease-related phenomenon, or secondary to other factors such as a tendency to use more TBI for conditioning, or exposure to high doses of alkylating agents pretransplant. Of note, in a series of patients with multiple myeloma, the risk of MDS post-ASCT increased with more prolonged exposure to chemotherapy prior to stem cell mobilization (Govindarajan *et al.*, 1996).

Reported risks of developing MDS after autotransplantation for Hodgkin's disease are varied, with some studies suggesting a lower risk than similar patients with NHL (Taylor *et al.*, 1997; Andre *et al.*, 1998; Harrison *et al.*, 1999) and others reporting a similarly high risk (Pedersen-Bjergaard *et al.*, 1997). Confounding most of the studies of Hodgkin's disease is the use of MOPP-like chemotherapy regimens prior to transplantation, which may have a more profound effect on development of MDS than the transplant itself (Harrison *et al.*, 1999). In a series from the Spanish Cooperative group of 494 patients undergoing transplantation for Hodgkin's disease with a variety

of conditioning regimens, adjuvant radiotherapy, TBI conditioning, and advanced patient age were predictive factors for secondary malignancies, including 12 patients who developed MDS (Sureda *et al.*, 2001).

An ABMTR case-control series of 56 cases and 168 matched controls within a cohort of 2,739 patients autografted for Hodgkin's disease or non-Hodgkin's lymphoma found the intensity of pretransplant chemotherapy with mechlorethamine (nitrogen mustard) or chlorambucil, compared to cyclophosphamide-based therapy, to be a significant risk factor for posttransplant MDS/AML (Metayer *et al.*, 2003). Additionally, TBI doses of 13.2 Gy in the pretransplant conditioning regimen were associated with increased risk.

In summary, the reported cumulative risk of MDS exceeds 10% in several series of patients undergoing autotransplantion for NHL, and is somewhat lower after transplantation for other diseases. Older patients with extensive prior chemotherapy, patients receiving localized radiotherapy, and those receiving TBI conditioning appear to be at the highest risk for this complication.

Pathogenesis

MDS and AML are well-recognized long-term complications of cytotoxic chemotherapy, specifically DNA-damaging agents (Greaves, 1997). There is a clear positive relationship between the cumulative dose of alkylating agents or topoisomerase II inhibitors and the risk of developing secondary MDS and AML (Tucker *et al.*, 1987; Ratain & Rowley, 1992). An increased incidence of MDS and AML has also been linked to previous radiation exposure (Kodama *et al.*, 1996). In one series of patients treated with low-dose TBI and chemotherapy for NHL, the 15-year estimated cumulative incidence of MDS was 17% (Travis *et al.*, 1996). In general, the peak incidence of MDS occurs 4 to 6 years after the initiation of cytotoxic therapy, although latency periods as short as 12 months (particularly for patients treated with topoisomerase II inhibitors), and as long as 15 to 20 years in the setting of radiation exposure, have been reported. In the setting of conventional chemotherapy, it has been shown that patients with gene deletions of glutathione transferases appear to have an increased risk of developing secondary hematologic malignancies (Haase *et al.*, 2002). Additional study is necessary to determine whether or not such enzymatic polymorphisms play a role in MDS after ASCT.

Although the majority of patients with MDS post-ASCT present with complex karyotypes, deletions of chromosomes 5 and 7 are most common, and several candidate genes that influence hematopoietic growth and differentiation are located in the 5q segment (Karp & Smith, 1997). Aberrant expression of growth factors on this chromosome may promote leukemic transformation, and the entire 5q gene segment appears to be intrinsically unstable, and particularly vulnerable to damage from cytotoxic therapy in the setting of radiation or high-dose chemotherapy (Boultwood *et al.*, 1994).

It remains unknown, and is quite controversial, to what degree MDS after ASCT arises from reinfused damaged stem cells or is a direct result of conditioning therapy (Milligan, 2000; Fung *et al.*, 2001). Clonal hematopoiesis detected by X-linked clonality assays after ASCT has been shown to predict the development of MDS, although a significant proportion of NHL patients have clonal hematopoiesis at the time of transplant (Legare *et al.*, 1997; Mach-Pascual *et al.*, 1998). In an elegant study from St. Bartholomew's Hospital, London, G-banding and fluorescence in situ hybridization (FISH) were used to detect clonal cytogenetic abnormalities from pretransplant bone marrows in patients who subsequently developed MDS. The majority of patients, as expected, had complex abnormalities at the time of diagnosis of MDS. Using single locus-specific FISH probes (del 5q31; del 7q22; del 13q14), the same clonal cytogenetic abnormalities were found in the pretransplant specimens in 20 of 20 patients screened, suggesting MDS arises from reinfused damaged stem cells (Lillington *et al.*, 2001). In this study, 3 of 24 patients screened who did not develop MDS also had clonal cytogenetic abnormalities detected pretransplant, as has been reported by other groups (LaCasce *et al.*, 1999) Similarly, Abruzzese and colleagues (1999) reported that 9 of 12 patients who developed MDS after ASCT had evidence by FISH of the same cytogenetic abnormalities in specimens obtained at the time of bone marrow harvest. Some groups consider the presence of such pretransplant clonal abnormalities a relative contraindication to ASCT (Chao *et al.*, 1991), and advocate cytogenetic assessment of all patients with lymphoma considered for ASCT.

Telomeres are protective structures at the end of chromosomes, which normally shorten as cells divide; thus they represent an index of proliferative stress. Telomere length in stem cells has been shown to be abnormal in primary MDS, as well as after ASCT and alloSCT in a variety of settings (Boultwood *et al.*, 1997; Engelhardt *et al.*, 1998). Critically shortened telomeres result in an increased incidence of cellular cytogenetic abnormalities, and have been hypothesized to increase vulnerability to leukemic transformation (Ball *et al.*, 1998; Engelhardt & Finke, 2001). The impact of shortened telomeres on the development of MDS remains controversial (Rufer *et al.*, 2001), and ongoing laboratory and clinical investigations are addressing this issue.

Although this laboratory evidence suggests a contribution of previous stem cell damage, the evolving consensus is that in many cases of MDS after ASCT, damaged stem cells survive the conditioning regimen (Laporte *et al.*, 1991), and thus may be at higher risk of leukemic transformation. The significantly increased incidence of MDS in TBI-treated patients, and the relatively high incidence of MDS after low-dose (non-myeloablative) TBI for lymphoma, supports this argument. Moreover, 10 patients in the Dana-Farber series who developed MDS after ASCT were treated with only CHOP chemotherapy alone prior to transplantation, a regimen not historically associated with significant stem cell damage in standard dosing (Friedberg *et al.*, 2000).

Disease course, therapy, and prevention

Morphologic analysis and follow-up of these patients has revealed two distinct patterns of MDS after ASCT: an aggressive form, with striking marrow dysplasia, typical cytogenetic changes, and rapid transformation to leukemia; and a more indolent form, associated with transient cytogenetic changes, and minimal intermittent marrow dysplasia (Traweek *et al.*, 1994). Unlike the aggressive form, "indolent" MDS changes do not necessarily progress to leukemic transformation even after

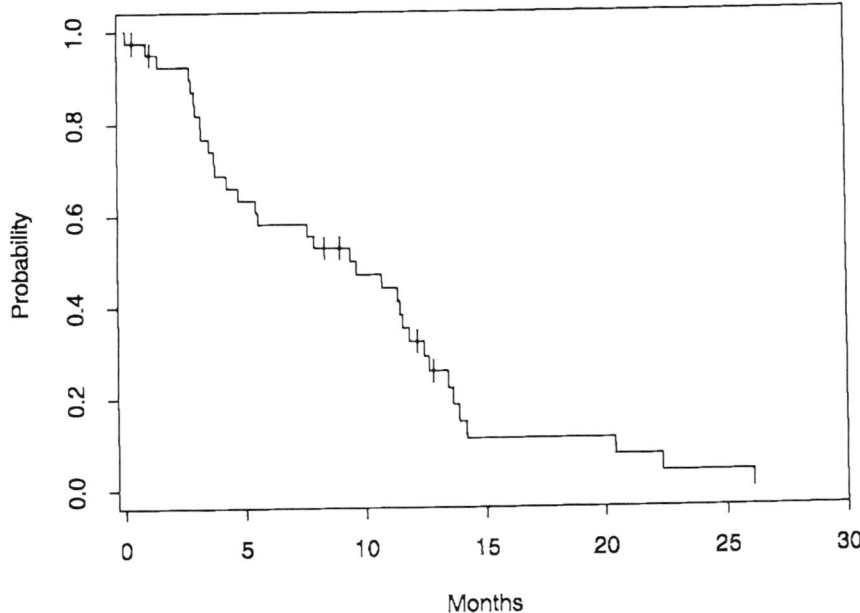

Fig. 86.3. Kaplan-Meier curve of overall survival after diagnosis of MDS after ASCT for NHL at Dana-Farber Cancer Institute.

years of follow-up and, in fact, revert to normal in some cases (Wilson *et al.*, 1997). Often, these cytogenetic changes are not the typical del(5) or del(7) seen in aggressive MDS. The focus of this chapter and of the vast majority of studies is on the "aggressive" form of MDS.

The median survival of patients with "aggressive" MDS after ASCT is generally measured in months, and very few patients survive after 1 year (Fig. 86.3). The disease generally progresses rapidly to acute leukemia, which is poorly responsive to standard chemotherapy induction regimens. Unlike primary MDS, a subset of which is generally responsive to supportive therapy with growth factors and transfusions, MDS after ASCT, even when it presents without circulating blasts, has an extremely poor prognosis. In the Dana-Farber series, there was no significant difference in survival from diagnosis of MDS in patients with refractory anemia, refractory anemia with ringed sideroblasts, and refractory anemia with excess blasts compared with refractory anemia with excess blasts in transformation and AML.

The International Prognostic Scoring System (see Chapter 54) has found the prognosis of patients with primary MDS to depend on several factors, including karyotype, percentage of bone marrow blasts, and number of peripheral cytopenias (Greenberg *et al.*, 1997). This has not been predictive in patients with secondary MDS. Although the majority of patients post-ASCT present with high-risk features, even those with low-risk features by the International Prognostic Scoring System have a very limited survival (Friedberg *et al.*, 1999).

Allogeneic hematopoietic stem cell transplantation (alloSCT) is the only potentially curative therapy for patients with primary MDS (Castro-Malaspina *et al.*, 2002). Cytogenetic findings, according to the International Prognostic Scoring System, have been found to strongly predict outcome of alloSCT in patients with primary MDS. In a series from Vancouver, only 6% of patients with primary MDS and poor-risk cytogenetics were alive and in remission 7 years after alloSCT (Nevill *et al.*, 1998). Data on alloSCT for patients with secondary AML from previous chemotherapy exposure are very limited, but in the largest series from Seattle, the 5-year disease-free survival was less than 10% (Witherspoon *et al.*, 2001). The vast majority of patients with MDS after ASCT have complex and high-risk cytogenteic abnormalities, and as expected, the outcome of conventional alloSCT is poor. Of 13 patients undergoing alloSCT for MDS after ASCT at Dana-Farber, all died, and the majority of deaths were from complications of transplant, with only 2 due to relapsed AML (Friedberg *et al.*, 1999). Thus, conventional alloSCT does not represent a viable salvage option for MDS occurring after ASCT, due to conditioning-related mortality. Thus, these patients may be good candidates for non-myeloablative conditioning regimens and subsequent donor lymphocyte infusions to immunologically ablate residual malignant clones (Corradini *et al.*, 2002). Such therapy is currently under investigation at many centers.

Since standard therapy is dismal at the present time, alternative strategies need to be considered in order to minimize the development of MDS. Chemotherapy-only conditioning regi-

mens have similar response rates to TBI-containing regimens in most subtypes of NHL (Berglund *et al.*, 2000), and may decrease risk of MDS, particularly for those patients treated with localized radiotherapy (Armitage, 2000; Mounier & Gisselbrecht, 1998). Radiolabeled monoclonal antibodies theoretically can deliver higher doses of radiation to tumor sites while sparing normal tissues, and could potentially replace external beam irradiation or TBI (Kaminski *et al.*, 1993; Witzig *et al.*, 2002). Twenty-nine patients with relapsed B-cell lymphoma have been treated at the Fred Hutchinson Cancer Research Center with ablative doses of [131]Iodine anti-CD20 antibody as conditioning followed by ASCT (Liu *et al.*, 1998). No MDS was reported, although the median follow-up was only 42 months. However, in a subsequent series of 52 patients treated in Seattle with a combination of chemotherapy and radiolabeled antibody as conditioning, several patients had prolonged chromosomal abnormalities, and one patient thus far has developed MDS (Press *et al.*, 2000). Further follow-up of this cohort is needed to determine whether the cumulative incidence of MDS is less with radioimmunotherapy conditioning.

As discussed, clonal hematopoiesis pretransplant appears to increase the risk of subsequent MDS. There are at least 5 methods for assessing this risk based on the presence of clonal abnormalities in hematopoietic cells, including standard cytogenetics, interphase FISH, analysis for loss of heterozygosity, polymerase chain reaction for point mutations, and X-inactivation-based clonality assays (Gilliland & Gribben, 2002). Abnormalities in one of these assessments pretransplant may represent relative contraindications to transplant. However, since no single mutation or gene rearrangement is sufficient for the development of MDS after transplant, and not all patient with cytogenetic abnormalities develop clinical MDS, these are imperfect assessments. The optimal "screening" modality has yet to be determined, and prospective studies are ongoing.

Finally, it is prudent to limit exposure to known stem cell toxins, including prolonged exposure to alkylating agents, purine analogs, and topoisomerase-II inhibitors, as much as possible in patients for whom ASCT is considered a treatment option. The introduction of novel treatment options for NHL, particularly unlabeled monoclonal antibody therapy (McLaughlin *et al.*, 1998), allows minimization of such toxic therapy in many circumstances.

Conclusions

MDS has emerged as a major complication of ASCT, and has an extremely poor prognosis. The appreciation of this syndrome emphasizes the importance of long-term follow-up of patients treated with ASCT, and is a testimony to the value of both single-institution databases, and registries in this field. Although non-myeloablative transplantation offers hope as potential treatment for this disease, prevention is obviously the ultimate goal. With increased recognition of the scope of this complication, refinements in conditioning regimens and pretransplant therapy will hopefully begin to impact the incidence, and attention to risk factors may allow more appropriate patient selection for ASCT.

References

Abruzzese, E., Radford, J.E., Miller, J.S. *et al.* (1999). Detection of abnormal pretransplant clones in progenitor cells of patients who developed myelodysplasia after autologous transplantation. *Blood,* **94,** 1814–9.

Akpek, G., Ambinder, R.F., Piantadosi, S. *et al.* (2001). Long-term results of blood and marrow transplantation for Hodgkin's lymphoma. *Journal of Clinical Oncology,* **19,** 4314–21.

Amigo, M.L., del Canizo, M.C., Rios, A. *et al.* (1999). Diagnosis of secondary myelodysplastic syndromes (MDS) following autologous transplantation should not be based only on morphological criteria used for diagnosis of de novo MDS. *Bone Marrow Transplantation,* **23,** 997–1002.

Andre, M., Henry-Amar, M., Blaise, D. *et al.* (1998). Treatment-related deaths and second cancer risk after autologous stem-cell transplantation for Hodgkin's disease. *Blood,* **92,** 1933–40.

Armitage, J.O. (2000). Myelodysplasia and acute leukemia after autologous bone marrow transplantation. *Journal of Clinical Oncology,* **18,** 945.

Ball, S.E., Gibson, F.M., Rizzo, S. *et al.* (1998). Progressive telomere shortening in aplastic anemia. *Blood,* **91,** 3582–92.

Bennett, J.M., Catovsky, D., Daniel, M.T. *et al.* (1982). Proposals for the classification of the myelodysplastic syndromes. *British Journal of Haematology,* **51,** 189–99.

Berglund, A., Enblad, G., Carlson, K. *et al.* (2000). Long-term follow-up of autologous stem-cell transplantation for follicular and transformed follicular lymphoma. *European Journal of Haematology,* **65,** 17–22.

Bhatia, S., Ramsay, N.K., Steinbuch, M. *et al.* (1996). Malignant neoplasms following bone marrow transplantation. *Blood,* **87,** 3633–9.

Boultwood, J., Fidler, C., Kusec, R. *et al.* (1997). Telomere length in myelodysplastic syndromes. *American Journal of Hematology,* **56,** 266–71.

Boultwood, J., Lewis, S., & Wainscoat, J.S. (1994). The 5q-syndrome. *Blood,* **84,** 3253–60.

Castro-Malaspina, H., Harris, R.E., Gajewski, J. *et al.* (2002). Unrelated donor marrow transplantation for myelodysplastic syndromes: outcome analysis in 510 transplants facilitated by the National Marrow Donor Program. *Blood,* **99,** 1943–51.

Chao, N.J., Nademanee, A.P., Long, G.D. *et al.* (1991). Importance of bone marrow cytogenetic evaluation before autologous bone marrow transplantation for Hodgkin's disease. *Journal of Clinical Oncology,* **9,** 1575–9.

Corradini, P., Tarella, C., Olivieri, A. *et al.* (2002). Reduced-intensity conditioning followed by allografting of hematopoietic cells can produce clinical and molecular remissions in patients with poor-risk hematologic malignancies. *Blood,* **99,** 75–82.

Darrington, D.L., Vose, J.M., Anderson, J.R. *et al.* (1994). Incidence and characterization of secondary myelodysplastic syndrome and acute myelogenous leukemia following high-dose chemoradiotherapy and autologous stem-cell transplantation for lymphoid malignancies. *Journal of Clinical Oncology,* **12,** 2527–34.

Engelhardt, M. & Finke, J. (2001). Does telomere shortening count? *Blood,* **98,** 888–90.

Engelhardt, M., Ozkaynak, M.F., Drullinsky, P. *et al.* (1998). Telomerase activity and telomere length in pediatric patients with malignancies undergoing chemotherapy. *Leukemia,* **12,** 13–24.

Freedman, A.S., Neuberg, D., Mauch, P. *et al.* (1999). Long-term follow-up of autologous bone marrow transplantation in patients with relapsed follicular lymphoma. *Blood,* **94,** 3325–33.

Friedberg, J., Neuberg, D., & Freedman, A.S. (2000). Myelodysplasia after autotransplantation. *Journal of Clinical Oncology,* **18,** 3446–7.

Friedberg, J.W., Neuberg, D., Monson, E. *et al.* (2001). The impact of external beam radiation therapy prior to autologous bone marrow transplantation in patients with non-Hodgkin's lymphoma. *Biology of Blood and Marrow Transplantation,* **7,** 446–53.

Friedberg, J.W., Neuberg, D., Stone, R.M. *et al.* (1999). Outcome in patients with myelodysplastic syndrome after autologous bone marrow transplantation for non-Hodgkin's lymphoma. *Journal of Clinical Oncology,* **17,** 3128–35.

Fung, H.C., Nademanee, A.P., Bhatia, S., & Forman, S.J. (2001). Is there an association between total-body irradiation and secondary acute myelogenous leukemia/myelodysplastic syndrome in patients with relapsed/refractory Hodgkin's disease treated with autologous stem-cell transplantation? *Journal of Clinical Oncology,* **19,** 3585–8.

Gilliland, D.G. & Gribben, J.G. (2002). Evaluation of the risk of therapy-related MDS/AML after autologous stem cell transplantation. *Biology of Blood and Marrow Transplantation,* **8,** 9–16.

Govindarajan, R., Jagannath, S., Flick, J.T. *et al.* (1996). Preceding standard therapy is the likely cause of MDS after autotransplants for multiple myeloma. *British Journal of Haematology,* **95,** 349–53.

Greaves, M.F. (1997). Aetiology of acute leukaemia. *Lancet,* **349,** 344–9.

Greenberg, P., Cox, C., LeBeau, M.M. *et al.* (1997). International scoring system for evaluating prognosis in myelodysplastic syndromes. *Blood,* **89,** 2079–88.

Haase, D., Binder, C., Bunger, J. *et al.* (2002). Increased risk for therapy-associated hematologic malignancies in patients with carcinoma of the breast and combined homozygous gene deletions of glutathione transferases M1 and T1. *Leukemia Research,* **26,** 249–54.

Harris, N.L., Jaffe, E.S., Diebold, J. *et al.* (1999). World Health Organization classification of neoplastic diseases of the hematopoietic and lymphoid tissues: report of the Clinical Advisory Committee meeting, Airlie House, Virginia, November 1997. *Journal of Clinical Oncology,* **17,** 3835–49.

Harrison, C.N., Gregory, W., Hudson, G.V. *et al.* (1999). High-dose BEAM chemotherapy with autologous haemopoietic stem cell transplantation for Hodgkin's disease is unlikely to be associated with a major increased risk of secondary MDS/AML. *British Journal of Cancer,* **81,** 476–83.

Horning, S.J., Negrin, R.S., Hoppe, R.T. *et al.* (2001). High-dose therapy and autologous bone marrow transplantation for follicular lymphoma in first complete or partial remission: results of a phase II clinical trial. *Blood,* **97,** 404–9.

Hosing, C., Munsell, M., Yazji, S. *et al.* (2002). Risk of therapy-related myelodysplastic syndrome/acute leukemia following high-dose therapy and autologous bone marrow transplantation for non-Hodgkin's lymphoma. *Annals of Oncology,* **13,** 450–9.

Kaminski, M.S., Zasadny, K.R., Francis, I.R. *et al.* (1993). Radioimmunotherapy of B-cell lymphoma with [131I]anti-B1 (anti-CD20) antibody. *New England Journal of Medicine,* **329,** 459–65.

Karp, J.E. & Smith, M.A. (1997). The molecular pathogenesis of treatment-induced (secondary) leukemias: foundations for treatment and prevention. *Seminars in Oncology*, **24**, 103–13.

Kodama, K., Mabuchi, K., & Shigematsu, I. (1996). A long-term cohort study of the atomic bomb survivors. *Journal of Epidemiology*, **6**, 95–105.

Kollmannsberger, C., Beyer, J., Droz, J.P. *et al.* (1998). Secondary leukemia following high cumulative doses of etoposide in patients treated for advanced germ cell tumors. *Journal of Clinical Oncology*, **16**, 3386–91.

Krishnan, A., Bhatia, S., Slovak, M.L. *et al.* (2000). Predictors of therapy-related leukemia and myelodysplasia following autologous transplantation for lymphoma: an assessment of risk factors. *Blood*, **95**, 1588–93.

LaCasce, A., Neuberg, D., Janosova, A. *et al.* (1999). Clonal karyotypic abnormalities after autologous bone marrow transplantation for non-Hodgkin's lymphoma are common and not always associated with myelodysplastic syndrome. *Blood*, **94**, 344a.

Lambertenghi Deliliers, G., Annaloro, C., Pozzoli, E. *et al.* (1999). Cytogenetic and myelodysplastic alterations after autologus hemopoietic stem cell transplantation. *Leukemia Research*, **23**, 291–7.

Laporte, J.P., Fouillard, L., Douay, L. *et al.* (1991). GM-CSF instead of autologous bone-marrow transplantation after the BEAM regimen. *Lancet*, **338**, 601–2.

Laughlin, M.J., McGaughey, D.S., Crews, J.R. *et al.* (1998). Secondary myelodysplasia and acute leukemia in breast cancer patients after autologous bone marrow transplant. *Journal of Clinical Oncology*, **16**, 1008–12.

Legare, R.D., Gribben, J.G., Maragh, M. *et al.* (1997). Prediction of therapy-related acute myelogenous leukemia (AML) and myelodysplastic syndrome (MDS) after autologus bone marrow transplant (ABMT) for lymphoma. *American Journal of Hematology*, **56**, 45–51.

Lillington, D.M., Micallef, I.N., Carpenter, E. *et al.* (2001). Detection of chromosome abnormalities pre-high-dose treatment in patients developing therapy-related myelodysplasia and secondary acute myelogenous leukemia after treatment for non-Hodgkin's lymphoma. *Journal of Clinical Oncology*, **19**, 2472–81.

Liu, S.Y., Eary, J.F., Petersdorf, S.H. *et al.* (1998). Follow-up of relapsed B-cell lymphoma patients treated with iodine-131-labeled anti-CD20 antibody and autologous stem-cell rescue. *Journal of Clinical Oncology*, **16**, 3270–8.

Mach-Pascual, S., Legare, R.D., Lu, D. *et al.* (1998). Predictive value of clonality assays in patients with non-Hodgkin's lymphoma undergoing autologous bone marrow transplant: a single institution study. *Blood*, **91**, 4496–503.

McLaughlin, P., Grillo-Lopez, A.J., Link, B.K. *et al.* (1998). Rituximab chimeric anti-CD20 monoclonal antibody therapy for relapsed indolent lymphoma: half of patients respond to a four-dose treatment program. *Journal of Clinical Oncology*, **16**, 2825–33.

Metayer, C., Curtis, R., Vose J. *et al.* (2003). Myelodysplastic syndrome and acute myeloid leukemia after autotransplantation for lymphoma: a multicenter case-control study. *Blood*, **101**, 2915–23.

Micallef, I.N., Lillington, D.M., Apostolidis, J. *et al.* (2000). Therapy-related myelodysplasia and secondary acute myelogenous leukemia after high-dose therapy with autologous

hematopoietic progenitor-cell support for lymphoid malignancies. *Journal of Clinical Oncology*, **18**, 947.

Miller, J.S., Arthur, D.C., Litz, C.E. *et al.* (1994). Myelodysplastic syndrome after autologous bone marrow transplantation: an additional late complication of curative cancer therapy [see comments]. *Blood*, **83**, 3780–6.

Milligan, D.W. (2000). Secondary leukaemia and myelodysplasia after autografting for lymphoma: is the transplant to blame? *Leukemia and Lymphoma*, **39**, 223–8.

Milligan, D.W., Ruiz De Elvira, M.C., Kolb, H.J. *et al.* (1999). Secondary leukaemia and myelodysplasia after autografting for lymphoma: results from the EBMT. EBMT Lymphoma and Late Effects Working Parties. European Group for Blood and Marrow Transplantation. *British Journal of Haematology*, **106**, 1020–6.

Mounier, N. & Gisselbrecht, C. (1998). Conditioning regimens before transplantation in patients with aggressive non-Hodgkin's lymphoma. *Annals of Oncology*, **9**, S15–21.

Nevill, T.J., Fung, H.C., Shepherd, J.D. *et al.* (1998). Cytogenetic abnormalities in primary myelodysplastic syndrome are highly predictive of outcome after allogeneic bone marrow transplantation. *Blood*, **92**, 1910–7.

Ng, A.K., Bernardo, M.P., Weller, E. *et al.* (2002). Long-term survival and competing causes of death in patients with early-stage Hodgkin's disease treated at age 50 or younger. *Journal of Clinical Oncology*, **20**, 2101–8.

Park, S., Brice, P., Noguerra, M.E. *et al.* (2000). Myelodysplasias and leukemias after autologous stem cell transplantation for lymphoid malignancies. *Bone Marrow Transplantation*, **26**, 321–6.

Pedersen-Bjergaard, J., Andersen, M.K., & Christiansen, D.H. (2000). Therapy-related acute myeloid leukemia and myelodysplasia after high-dose chemotherapy and autologous stem cell transplantation. *Blood*, **95**, 3273–9.

Pedersen-Bjergaard, J., Pedersen, M., Myhre, J., & Geisler, C. (1997). High risk of therapy-related leukemia after BEAM chemotherapy and autologous stem cell transplantation for previously treated lymphomas is mainly related to primary chemotherapy and not to the BEAM-transplantation procedure. *Leukemia*, **11**, 1654–60.

Philip, T., Guglielmi, C., Hagenbeek, A. *et al.* (1995). Autologous bone marrow transplantation as compared with salvage chemotherapy in relapses of chemotherapy-sensitive non-Hodgkin's lymphoma [see comments]. *New England Journal of Medicine*, **333**, 1540–5.

Press, O.W., Eary, J.F., Gooley, T. *et al.* (2000). A phase I/II trial of iodine-131-tositumomab (anti-CD20), etoposide, cyclophosphamide, and autologous stem cell transplantation for relapsed B-cell lymphomas. *Blood*, **96**, 2934–42.

Ratain, M.J. & Rowley, J.D. (1992). Therapy-related acute myeloid leukemia secondary to inhibitors of topoisomerase II: from the bedside to the target genes. *Annals of Oncology*, **3**, 107–11.

Rohatiner, A. (1994). Myelodysplasia and acute myelogenous leukemia after myeloablative therapy with autologous stem-cell transplantation. *Journal of Clinical Oncology*, **12**, 2521–3.

Roman-Unfer, S., Bitran, J.D., Hanauer, S. *et al.* (1995). Acute myeloid leukemia and myelodysplasia following intensive chemotherapy for breast cancer. *Bone Marrow Transplantation*, **16**, 163–8.

Rowley, J.D., Vignon, C., Gollin, S.M. *et al.* (1996). Chromosomal translocations in secondary acute myeloid leukemia. *New England Journal of Medicine,* **334,** 601–3.

Rufer, N., Brummendorf, T.H., Chapuis, B. *et al.* (2001). Accelerated telomere shortening in hematological lineages is limited to the first year following stem cell transplantation. *Blood,* **97,** 575–7.

Sevilla, J., Rodriguez, A., Hernandez-Maraver, D. *et al.* (2002). Secondary acute myeloid leukemia and myelodysplasia after autologous peripheral blood progenitor cell transplantation. *Annals of Hematology,* **81,** 11–5.

Stone, R.M. (1994). Myelodysplastic syndrome after autologous transplantation for lymphoma: the price of progress [editorial]. *Blood,* **83,** 3437–40.

Stone, R.M., Neuberg, D., Soiffer, R. *et al.* (1994). Myelodysplastic syndrome as a late complication following autologous bone marrow transplantation for non-Hodgkin's lymphoma. *Journal of Clinical Oncology,* **12,** 2535–42.

Sureda, A., Arranz, R., Iriondo, A. *et al.* (2001). Autologous stem-cell transplantation for Hodgkin's disease: results and prognostic factors in 494 patients from the Grupo Espanol de Linfomas/Transplante Autologo de Medula Osea Spanish Cooperative Group. *Journal of Clinical Oncology,* **19,** 1395–404.

Taylor, P.R., Jackson, G.H., Lennard, A.L. *et al.* (1997). Low incidence of myelodysplastic syndrome following transplantation using autologous non-cryopreserved bone marrow. *Leukemia,* **11,** 1650–3.

Travis, L.B., Weeks, J., Curtis, R.E. *et al.* (1996). Leukemia following low-dose total body irradiation and chemotherapy for non-Hodgkin's lymphoma. *Journal of Clinical Oncology,* **14,** 565–71.

Traweek, S.T., Slovak, M.L., Nademanee, A.P. *et al.* (1994). Clonal karyotypic hematopoietic cell abnormalities occurring after autologous bone marrow transplantation for Hodgkin's disease and non-Hodgkin's lymphoma. *Blood,* **84,** 957–63.

Tucker, M.A., Meadows, A.T., Boice, J.D., Jr. *et al.* (1987). Leukemia after therapy with alkylating agents for childhood cancer. *Journal of the National Cancer Institute,* **78,** 459–64.

Vose, J.M., Sharp, G., Chan, W.C. *et al.* (2002). Autologous transplantation for aggressive non-Hodgkin's lymphoma: results of a randomized trial evaluating graft source and minimal residual disease. *Journal of Clinical Oncology,* **20,** 2344–52.

Whang-Peng, J., Young, R.C., Lee, E.C. *et al.* (1988). Cytogenetic studies in patients with secondary leukemia/dysmyelopoietic syndrome after different treatment modalities. *Blood,* **71,** 403–14.

Wheeler, C., Khurshid, A., Ibrahim, J. *et al.* (2001). Incidence of post transplant myelodysplasia/acute leukemia in non-Hodgkin's lymphoma patients compared with Hodgkin's disease patients undergoing autologous transplantation following cyclophosphamide, carmustine and etoposide (CBV). *Leukemia and Lymphoma,* **40,** 499–509.

Wilson, C.S., Traweek, S.T., Slovak, M.L. *et al.* (1997). Myelodysplastic syndrome occurring after autologous bone marrow transplantation for lymphoma. Morphologic features. *American Journal of Clinical Pathology,* **108,** 369–77.

Witherspoon, R.P., Deeg, H.J., Storer, B. *et al.* (2001). Hematopoietic stem-cell transplantation for treatment-related leukemia or myelodysplasia. *Journal of Clinical Oncology,* **19,** 2134–41.

Witzig, T.E., Gordon, L.I., Cabanillas, F. *et al.* (2002). Randomized controlled trial of yttrium-90-labeled ibritumomab tiuxetan radioimmunotherapy versus rituximab immunotherapy for patients with relapsed or refractory low-grade, follicular, or transformed B-cell non-Hodgkin's lymphoma. *Journal of Clinical Oncology,* **20,** 2453–63.

87 New solid tumors following hematopoietic stem cell transplantation

MICHAEL R. BISHOP AND P. JEAN HENSLEE-DOWNEY

National Cancer Institute, Bethesda, and South Carolina Cancer Center, Columbia, USA

Introduction

Over the past 30 years the number of, indications for, and eligibility for both autologous and allogeneic hematopoietic stem cell transplantation (HSCT) have steadily increased (Bortin *et al.*, 1992; Gratwohl *et al.*, 2000). As the success of HSCT continues to increase, so does the number of long-term survivors (Socie *et al.*, 1999). It is important to realize that the overwhelming majority (93%) of long-term survivors after transplantation remain in good health (Duell *et al.*, 1997) and in this study 89% had returned to full-time work or school. However, this group of patients is subject to a unique set of problems such as chronic graft-versus-host disease (GVHD), recurrence of their original disease, complications of the chemotherapy and radiation administered as part of the preparative regimen and/or therapy administered posttransplant (e.g., cyclosporine, glucocorticoids) (Atkinson, 1990; Kolb & Bender-Goetze, 1990; Socie *et al.*, 1999), and the development of secondary or new malignancies (Kolb & Bender-Goetze, 1990; Sanders *et al.*, 1991; Kolb, Guenther, & Duel, 1992; Curtis *et al.*, 1997; Kolb *et al.*, 1999; Socie *et al.*, 2000; Bhatia *et al.*, 2001). Often these problems are interrelated, and it sometimes becomes difficult to distinguish them, and their etiologies, from each other.

One specific problem that occurs with a relatively increased frequency in the posttransplant setting is the occurrence of new or secondary malignancies as detailed in Table 87.1 (Curtis *et al.*, 1997). The incidence of new malignancies following HSCT is approximately 1% to 3%, but this number takes on greater significance as both the number of transplants performed and the follow-up time posttransplant continue to increase (Witherspoon, Deeg, & Storb, 1994). A significant percentage of these secondary malignancies are hematologic [lymphoproliferative dis-

Table 87.1. *Primary causes of death among patients who were disease-free 2 years after transplantation.*[a]

Cause of death	AML (*N* = 214)	ALL (*N* = 167)	CML (*N* = 238)	Aplastic anemia (*N* = 60)	Total (*N* = 679)
Relapse	117 (56)	79 (48)	108 (47)	0	304 (46)
GVHD	47 (23)	38 (23)	81 (36)	38 (66)	204 (31)
Infection without GVHD	11 (5)	7 (4)	14 (6)	7 (12)	39 (6)
Bacterial	5	2	5	3	15
Viral	2	1	3	2	8
Fungal	0	1	0	0	1
Protozoal	0	1	0	0	1
Infectious pneumonia[b]	2	0	4	1	7
Other infection[b]	2	2	2	1	7
New cancer	15 (7)	16 (10)	8 (4)	1 (2)	40 (6)
Organ failure	11 (5)	14 (9)	10 (4)	5 (9)	40 (6)
Other[c]	7 (3)	10 (6)	7 (3)	7 (12)	31 (5)
Unknown	6	3	10	2	21

Data shows number of patients (percent).

[a] Percentages shown are of deaths with known causes. Because of rounding, not all percentages total 100.

[b] The type of infection was not otherwise specified.

[c] Other causes of death were hemorrhage in 10 patients (3, 1, 3, and 3 in patients with AML, ALL, CML, and aplastic anemia, respectively), interstitial pneumonitis in 6 patients (3, 1, and 2 in patients with ALL, CML, and aplastic anemia, respectively), drug reaction in 1 patient with aplastic anemia, and miscellaneous causes in 14 patients (4, 6, 3, and 1 in patients with AML, ALL, CML, and aplastic anemia, respectively).

Reproduced, with permission, from Curtis *et al.* (1997).

orders, lymphomas, myelodysplasias and acute leukemias], which occur early (3 months to 5 years). This chapter will focus on the development of new solid tumors after HSCT.

Pathogenesis of new solid tumors

In attempting to understand the pathogenesis of new solid tumors associated with HSCT, several issues should be considered. First, the majority of patients are already at risk for the development of a secondary malignancy either due to a primary or secondary immunodeficiency related to their primary disease or its treatment. Second, the literature on the pathogenesis of new solid tumors following stem cell transplantation is relatively small, although data continue to accumulate (Curtis et al., 1997; Kolb et al., 1999). Of interest, the literature on new malignancies in general and solid tumors specifically following HSCT shares many similar clinical and therapeutic characteristics with the same events occurring after solid organ transplantation, an alternative but instructive data set (Weintraub & Warnke, 1982; Starzl et al., 1984; Penn, 1993; Jonas et al., 1997; Cardillo et al., 2001; Winkelhorst et al., 2001). Finally, one can draw information from a more extensive literature that examines the occurrence of secondary malignancies following the treatment of a primary malignancy using chemotherapy and/or radiation without HSCT (Borek, 1979; Coleman, 1982; Meadows et al., 1985; Michels et al., 1985; Blayney et al., 1987; Hawkins et al., 1987; Land, 1987; Tucker et al., 1987, 1988; Pui et al., 1989; Urba & Longo, 1992; Bhatia et al., 1996; van Leeuven, 1997; Dores et al., 2002).

The exact etiology of secondary malignancy is not well understood and is influenced by multiple factors including alteration in immune function, oncogenic viruses, carcinogenic effects of chemotherapy and ionizing radiation, and a host of other environmental factors, which play either individual or interrelated roles in the development of primary and secondary malignancies (Coleman, 1982; van Leeuven, 1997). While the development of secondary malignancies is most probably multifactorial, the components will be segregated and assimilated to more readily understand their interrelationship.

Alterations in immune function have been associated experimentally and clinically with the development of malignancy (Penn, 1994). A thorough understanding of this association is relevant to secondary malignancies following HSCT, since the primary disease itself and its treatment may result in an alteration in immune function. Prolonged immunosuppression in laboratory animals results in an increased incidence of cancer (Krueger et al., 1971). There is also an increased incidence of cancers in a number of immunodeficiency states, most notably in the acquired immunodeficiency syndrome (Zeigler et al., 1984). Both the diversity and the associated defects of the various immunodeficient states make it apparent that more than one mechanism is involved in the development of malignancy.

One of the first theories regarding the role of the immune system in tumor development was that of immune surveillance (Thomas, 1959). A major function of the immune system is the recognition of altered cells, leading to the inhibition of their growth and their destruction (Burnet, 1971). Suppression of immune surveillance would permit uncontrolled growth and proliferation, which might result in a malignant transformation. If this theory is correct, an increase in all types of malignancies might be expected. However, after HSCT the majority of secondary malignancies are of hematologic origin, and the majority of secondary solid tumors originate in the skin and thyroid gland. This suggests that other factors must contribute to, or result in, the development of new solid tumors. Accelerated neoplastic development has been observed in irradiated animals injected with a mixture of tumor cells and lymphocytes that results in a low lymphocyte to tumor burden ratio (Weintraub & Warnke, 1982). These observations served as the basis for the immune stimulation theory. Unfortunately, similar to the immune surveillance theory, it does not explain the disproportionate occurrence of certain malignancies. In other animal models it has been shown that the repeated or constant administration of foreign antigens results in a high incidence of malignant lymphoma (Gleichmann et al., 1975). Dysregulation of cellular and humoral immune functions may allow the unregulated growth of cell subsets that may evolve into a malignancy. The majority of chemotherapeutic agents in use today, as well as radiation therapy, are capable of suppressing both humoral and cell-mediated immune functions (Harris et al., 1976). The iatrogenic immunosuppression associated with cardiac, renal, and hepatic transplantation (Jonas et al., 1997; Cardillo et al, 2001; Winkelhorst et al., 2001) is associated with an increased incidence of skin, cervical, lung, and oral cancers. It is clear that a single hypothesis is incapable of explaining the observed clinical events; however, loss of normal regulatory mechanisms of the immune system appears to be a common denominator.

The association of exposure to ionizing radiation and the development of malignancy have been well documented (Kohn & Fry, 1984). The exact mechanism(s) by which radiation induces carcinogenesis is not entirely clear. Radiation is known to be capable of producing gene alterations (e.g., chromosome translocation), which may result in oncogene activation. Whether these alterations increase the incidence of particular cancers has not been clearly demonstrated. The interaction of radiation and multiple host factors determines the susceptibility of a particular tissue to tumor development. Both physical (dose, dose rate, and fractionation) and biological factors (age, sex, and genetic features) influence the risk of secondary malignancy from ionizing radiation (Hall, 1997). Attempts to correlate a particular radiation dose with a defined risk of secondary malignancy have not been totally accurate. At lower doses of radiation the risk appears to increase with dose; however, at higher doses the risk actually decreases as dose is increased. This is attributed to a higher percentage of cell kill rather than cell damage. The time interval of therapy also has an impact on the induction of carcinogenesis, in that a reduction in dose rate appears to be associated with a marked reduction in the development of malignancy (Han et al., 1980). Fractionation of radiotherapy has been used extensively in HSCT in attempts to reduce radiation-associated toxicity and increase leukemia cell kill, but fractionation can still result in the development of malignancy at certain dose levels (Borek, 1979). Generally, the risk of cancer increases with age, but the incidence of breast cancer and certain other solid tumors is increased with exposure at a younger age (Tokunaga et al., 1985). The latent period for these tumors appears to be inversely related to age at exposure (Land, 1987).

Secondary solid tumors have been well documented as potential complications of standard dose chemotherapy and radiation in the treatment of Hodgkin's disease (Blayney et al., 1987), breast cancer, childhood cancers, and a variety of other malignancies (Hawkins et al., 1987; Tucker et al., 1987, 1988; Pui et al., 1989). The incidence, risk factors, and clinical features of these secondary malignancies are extremely relevant, since the vast majority of patients coming to transplant have received some form of such prior therapy. There are now large population bases, especially in Hodgkin's disease and pediatric malignancies, from which data related to this subject can be examined. Hodgkin's disease is extremely interesting in that patients are treated with multiple chemotherapeutic agents, radiation, or various combinations of the two (Urba & Longo, 1992). Patients with Hodgkin's disease are also unique in that they have inherent immunologic abnormalities including anergy, decreased in vitro lymphocyte responsiveness, and a depressed CD4:CD8 T-cell ratio (Brown et al., 1967; Lauria et al., 1983). Stanford University Medical Center reported a relative risk of 5.2 for developing a second malignancy compared to the general population in 1,507 patients with Hodgkin's disease observed over a 15-year period (Tucker et al., 1988). The mean 15-year actuarial risk of all secondary malignancies was 17.6%, of which 13.2% were due to solid tumors. The risk of a secondary malignancy was observed to increase over time for all tumor types with the exception of leukemias, which appeared to reach a plateau level at 10 years. In contrast the risk for solid tumors continued to rise after 10 years.

In an extensive analysis of 32,591 Hodgkin's disease patients, including 1,111 who had survived over 25 years, there were 2,153 observed second cancers (Dores et al., 2002). Cancers of the lung, digestive tract, and female breast accounted for the majority of the secondary malignancies. The actuarial risk of developing a secondary solid tumor 25 years after the diagnosis of Hodgkin's disease was 21.9%. The relative risk of a second cancer decreased with increasing age at the time of Hodgkin's disease diagnosis. The site-specific burden of cancer varied according to age at time of Hodgkin's disease diagnosis. For patients diagnosed before age 21 the greatest risk was for the development of breast cancer. For patients diagnosed after age 30, the greatest risk was for lung cancer. The risk of solid tumors did not increase until 10 years after the diagnosis of Hodgkin's disease. The risk of solid tumor development was increased after treatment with either chemotherapy or radiation alone; however, the greatest risk was in patients who received combined modality treatment.

A second patient population at relatively high risk for secondary malignancies are childhood cancer survivors. The Late Effects Study Group (LTGS) has been collecting data on secondary malignancies, therapy, and predisposing factors in children since 1972, and has previously reported a 10-fold increase of secondary malignancies in children with a primary malignancy compared to age-matched populations (Meadows et al., 1985). The LTGS reported 88 cases of secondary malignancies including breast cancer, bone sarcomas, soft tissue sarcomas, brain tumors, colorectal cancers, and thyroid carcinoma (Bhatia et al., 1996). Older age (10–16 years), exposure to radiation, and exposure to alkylating agents were all associated with an increased risk of developing secondary cancers. The risk of secondary malignancies was evaluated in a retrospective cohort of 13,581 children diagnosed with common cancers before age 21 years and surviving at least 5 years. In 298 individuals, 314 secondary malignancies were identified. The largest observed excess of secondary cancers was of bone and breast cancers. A statistically significant excess of new solid tumors followed all childhood cancers. In multivariate regression models adjusted for therapeutic radiation exposure, new solid tumors of any type were independently associated with female sex, childhood cancer at a younger age, childhood Hodgkin's disease or soft-tissue sarcoma, and exposure to alkylating agents. Twenty years after the childhood cancer diagnosis, the cumulative estimated incidence of secondary malignancies was 3.2%.

Secondary solid tumors following HSCT

Incidence

The incidence of new malignancies, either hematologic or solid, developing after HSCT is relatively low. The probability of a new solid tumor after allogeneic HSCT is approximately 2%, as shown in Figure 87.1 (Kolb et al., 1999; Socie et al., 2000). One of the first reports on the development of secondary malignancies after HSCT was by Witherspoon and colleagues (1989), who reviewed the data on 2,246 transplant recipients at the Fred Hutchinson Cancer Research Center (FHCRC) in Seattle. They reported a rate of 1.2 secondary cancers per 100 exposure-years during the first year after transplantation. The rate declined to 0.4 per 100 between years 2 and 5 after transplantation and to 0.3 per 100 beyond 6 years. Since that time there have been additional reports on solid tumors following HSCT (Lowsky et al., 1994; Curtis et al., 1997; Kolb et al., 1999; Socié et al., 1999, 2000).

In a joint analysis by the International Bone Marrow Transplantation Registry (IBMTR), the FHCRC, and the National Cancer Institute in the United States, a retrospective analysis was performed on 19,229 patients who received either an allogeneic or a syngeneic transplant between 1964 and 1992, in order to determine the likelihood of developing a secondary solid tumor (Curtis et al., 1997). The cumulative incidence of secondary solid cancers at 5, 10, and 15 years after transplantation was 0.7%, 2.2%, and 6.7%, respectively. The risk was 8.3 times higher among those who survived 10 or more years after transplantation as compared to the general population. The most commonly observed secondary solid tumors were cutaneous and mucosal malignancies, primarily melanoma and buccal or pharyngeal carcinoma. Other secondary solid tumors reported in this series, in order of prevalence, included central nervous system cancers, thyroid cancer, breast cancer, bone cancers,

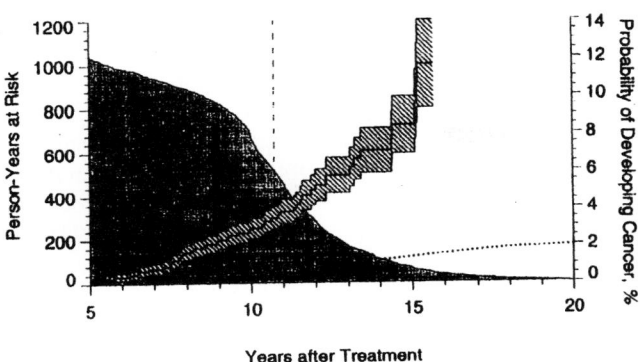

Fig. 87.1. Cumulative probability of developing a malignant neoplasm as a function of time after bone marrow transplantation. Patients (n = 1,036) underwent transplantation before 1986 and had survived at least 5 years; data were collected until March 1996. The gray shaded area shows the number of patients under observation as a function of time after transplantation (person-years at risk). The step function with the hatched range of SEs represents the observed cumulative tumor incidence: that is, the probability of developing malignant disease up to the specified time. The dotted line shows values according to the age-specific incidence rates from the Saarland Cancer Registry and the Danish Cancer Registry. The vertical dashed line shows the median observation time after transplantation. Reproduced with permission from Kolb *et al.* (1999)

connective tissue cancers, hepatic cancer, rectal cancer, and lung cancer. When these data were compared to the general population, there was an increased risk for the development of buccal mucosal cancers, liver cancer, CNS cancers, thyroid cancers, bone cancers, and connective tissue cancers. There was a strong correlation of younger age at the time of transplantation with an increased risk for the development of secondary solid tumors (Table 87.2). Over half the tumors in patients transplanted under the age of 10 years were either brain or thyroid cancers. The risk of solid cancer varied with the primary disease, with the highest incidence observed in those who were transplanted for acute leukemia. There was an association between a higher incidence of melanoma and buccal mucosa cancers and the use of total body irradiation or T-cell depletion of marrow grafts. The authors concluded that recipients of allogeneic or syngeneic

HSC transplants, particularly those receiving transplants at a young age, have an increased incidence of new solid cancers and that the excess risk of cancer rises sharply with time.

The Late Effects Working Party of the European Cooperative Group for Blood and Marrow Transplantation looked at the incidence of secondary malignancies in 1,036 consecutive patients, who survived at least 5 years after transplantation (Kolb *et al.*, 1999). This patient group included 70 patients who had received either a syngeneic or an autologous HSCT. The actuarial incidence of secondary malignancies was 3.5% at 10, and 12.8% at 15 years posttransplant. The rate of new malignant disease was 3.8-fold higher than that of an age-matched control population. The most frequent malignancies were neoplasms of the skin, oral cavity, uterus and cervix, thyroid, breast and glial tissue. In contrast to the results observed by Curtis and colleagues (1997), older patient age at transplant was a significant factor for the development of a secondary malignancy. This factor was observed only in female recipients. The most significant risk factor for a secondary malignancy was treatment of chronic GVHD with immunosuppressive agents, especially cyclosporine. The risk for a secondary malignancy was higher for patients who received an allogeneic as compared to either a syngeneic or autologous HSCT, although it did not reach statistical significance.

Socié and colleagues (2000) looked specifically at the incidence of secondary malignancies in children who underwent allogeneic transplant for acute leukemias. Using data from the IBMTR and FHCRC, 3,182 patients under the age of 17 were analyzed. Forty-five new cancers were identified; approximately half were posttransplant lymphoproliferative disorders and the other half were solid tumors. The solid tumors identified included squamous cell carcinoma of the tongue, papillary thyroid carcinoma, melanoma, osteosarcoma, and brain cancers. The median time from transplant to the development of a solid tumor was 6 years. There was a strong association between younger age at transplant (<5 years) and the development of a solid cancer, which were primarily brain and thyroid cancers in this age group. In contrast to studies in adults, there was a decreased risk of new solid tumors in patients who developed chronic GVHD.

Approximately 5% of patients have been observed to develop new malignancies following autologous transplanta-

Table 87.2. *Ratio of observed to expected cases and absolute excess risk of new invasive solid cancers according to age at transplantation[a]*

Age at transplantation	No. of patients	Person years at risk	Obs	Exp	Obs:Exp (95% CI)	Excess risk[b]
<10 yr	2,745	7,989	22	0.6	36.6 (22.9–55.4)	26.8
10–19 yr	4,178	12,008	8	1.7	4.6 (2.0–9.1)	5.2
20–29 yr	4,948	11,996	21	4.6	4.6 (2.8–7.0)	13.7
30–39 yr	4,474	8,914	13	9.4	1.4 (0.7–2.4)	4.1
≥40 yr	2,884	4,457	16	13.5	1.2 (0.7–1.9)	5.7

[a] Obs denotes observed cases, Exp expected cases, and CI confidence interval.

[b] The absolute excess risk is the number of observed cases minus the number of expected cases per 10,000 patients per year.

Reproduced, with permission, from Curtis *et al.* (1997).

tion (Darrington *et al.*, 1994; Miller *et al.*, 1994; Stone *et al.*, 1994). However, these secondary malignancies were almost exclusively myeloid leukemias and myelodysplastic disorders (Chapter 86). Bhatia and colleagues (2001) at the City of Hope National Medical Center in Duarte looked at the posttransplant incidence of new solid tumors in 2,129 patients, including 759 patients who received an autologous HSCT. Twenty-nine new solid tumors were observed with an actuarial incidence of 6.4% at 10 years. However, only two new solid tumors were identified among recipients of autografts.

In most studies of new solid tumors occurring after HSCT, the patients were transplanted for hematologic malignancy. The FHCRC and Hôpital St. Louis in Paris analyzed 700 patients who received an allogeneic transplant for aplastic anemia or Fanconi anemia, to examine the incidence of secondary malignancies in patients without a primary malignancy (Deeg *et al.*, 1996). The overall incidence of malignancy following transplantation was 14%, indicating that this complication might be more common in patients transplanted for nonmalignant disorders, particularly Fanconi anemia. Eighteen solid tumors (17 squamous cell and one mucoepidermoid carcinoma) were identified, presenting 30 to 221 months (median, 99 months) posttransplant. The hazard for solid tumors increased progressively with time posttransplant.

Bordigoni and colleagues (2002) reported a cumulative incidence of 20% for development of osteochondromas in patients less than 18 years transplanted between 1981 and 1997 with myeloablative conditioning regiments for acute leukemia or neuroblastoma.

Treatment

Long-term follow-up is critical to the detection of secondary solid tumors following transplantation (Antin, 2002). The continuing risk for the development of new solid tumors necessitates that patients be closely followed for the remainder of their lives. It has been suggested that at a minimum patients undergo

Table 87.3. *Ratio of observed to expected cases of new invasive solid cancers according to the time since transplantation[a]*

Site of cancer	Time after transplantation										
	<1 yr 19,229 (12,476)		1–4 yr 9,501 (22,778)		5–9 yr 3,234 (8386)		≥10 yr 690 (1,724)		Total 19,229 (45,364)		
No. of patients (person-yr)	Obs	Obs:Exp	Obs	Obs:Exp	Obs	Obs:Exp	Obs	Obs:Exp	Obs	Obs:Exp	95% CI
All solid tumors	9	1.2	34	2.3[b]	24	4.1[b]	13	8.3[b]	80	2.7[b]	2.1–3.3
Buccal cavity or pharynx	0	0.0	3	3.9	9	32.4[b]	5	77.9[b]	17	11.1[b]	6.5–17.8
Lip	0	0.0	1	19.5	1	51.7	0	0.0	2	18.9[b]	2.1–68.2
Tongue	0	0.0	1	6.4	2	35.8	3	238.2[b]	6	19.5[b]	7.1–42.4
Salivary gland	0	0.0	0	0.0	3	117.2[b]	0	0.0	3	23.2[b]	4.7–67.7
Gum or other site in mouth	0	0.0	1	5.1	2	26.9[b]	2	107.4[b]	5	12.5[b]	4.0–29.2
Pharynx	0	0.0	0	0.0	1	9.7	0	0.0	1	1.7	0.0–9.5
Colon	0	0.0	1	1.4	0	0.0	0	0.0	1	0.7	0.0–3.8
Rectum	0	0.0	1	2.3	0	0.0	1	20.6	2	2.2	0.3–7.9
Liver	1	9.2	1	5.0	0	0.0	1	54.4	3	7.5[b]	1.5–22.0
Lung	1	1.3	1	0.8	0	0.0	0	0.0	2	0.7	0.1–2.6
Breast (female)	1	0.6	4	1.2	1	0.8	1	2.9	7	1.1	0.4–2.2
Cervix	0	0.0	1	1.4	0	0.0	0	0.0	1	0.7	0.0–3.9
Uterine corpus	0	0.0	0	0.0	1	6.8	0	0.0	1	1.4	0.0–7.9
Testis	0	0.0	2	2.5	0	0.0	0	0.0	2	1.2	0.1–4.4
Brain or other CNS site	1	2.5	3	4.2	7	26.0[b]	0	0.0	11	7.6[b]	3.8–13.5
Thyroid	1	3.2	2	3.4	2	8.1	3	42.1[b]	8	6.6[b]	2.8–12.9
Bone	0	0.0	3	16.0[b]	1	14.0	1	77.7[b]	5	13.4[b]	4.3–31.3
Connective tissue	1	7.3	2	8.2	1	10.7	0	0.0	4	8.0[b]	2.2–20.5
Melanoma of the skin	2	3.5	7	6.7[b]	1	2.2	1	7.4	11	5.0[b]	2.5–8.9
Other[c]	1	0.4	3	0.9	1	0.8	0	0.0	5	0.8	0.2–1.8

[a] Data include all invasive solid tumors except nonmelanoma skin cancer. The analysis included patients receiving allogeneic or syngeneic transplants; patients with a primary disease of Fanconi's anemia or an immunodeficiency disease were excluded. Obs denotes observed cases, Exp expected cases, CI confidence interval, and CNS central nervous system.

[b] $P < .05$.

[c] Other new cancers included cancer of the penis (in one patient), Kaposi's sarcoma (in one), neuroblastoma of the nasal passages (in one), and metastatic cancer with an unknown primary site (in two).
Reproduced, with permission, from Curtis *et al.* (1997).

screening procedures (e.g., testing of stool for occult blood, mammograms) as suggested for the general public. In addition, special attention should be given to the skin, thyroid, and buccal mucosa in light of the relatively high incidence of these malignancies in long-term transplant survivors. Transplant recipients should be advised to avoid sunlight and wear sunscreen, be instructed on how to identify early cancer and precursor lesions (e.g., dysplastic nevi, actinic keratoses, and oral leukoplakia), and avoid carcinogenic exposures (e.g., exposure to tobacco), which may potentiate the risk of solid cancers.

In contrast to secondary hematologic malignancies, the majority of secondary solid tumors are not fatal. In patients who are found to have new solid tumors, conventional chemotherapy and/or radiotherapy for each respective tumor type are the treatments of choice. In one single institution experience, four of five patients, who developed a total of six second tumors posttransplant (endometrial, cervical, ovarian, and thyroid carcinomas, osteosarcoma and sarcoma of the small intestine) were alive at the time of the report (Favre-Schmuziger et al., 2000). They were treated as intensively as if they had not had a prior HSC transplant. Reduction of immunosuppression is of questionable benefit, but should be initiated, especially if its continuation compromises conventional antineoplastic therapy. There is the theoretical possibility that reduction of immunosuppression may benefit tumor eradication by improvement in immune function.

Conclusions

The leading cause of death in long-term HSCT survivors is recurrence of disease. In long-term survivors of allogeneic HSCT, the second leading cause of death is chronic GVHD (Socie et al., 1999). Secondary solid tumors account for approximately 6% of deaths after allogeneic HSCT. Secondary solid tumors are rare after autologous HSCT. As the risk of new solid tumors continues over time posttransplant, it is imperative that these patients are continuously monitored and that preventive measures are initiated and maintained. Data collection on this complication should be incorporated into all treatment protocols in order that it may be available for future trial planning. Furthermore, as information regarding the incidence, prevention, and treatment of secondary tumors becomes available it should be incorporated into the informed consent of patients considering HSCT. The International Bone Marrow Transplant Registry, the European Bone Marrow Transplant Group, and the North American Autologous Blood and Marrow Transplant Registry continue to monitor the long-term side effects of HSCT including secondary solid tumors. It is hoped that data from these studies will give a clearer understanding of this difficult and concerning problem.

References

Antin, J. (2002). Long-term care after hematopoietic-cell transplantation in adults. *New England Journal of Medicine*, **347**, 36–42.

Atkinson, K. (1990). Chronic graft-versus-host disease. *Bone Marrow Transplantation*, **5**, 69–82.

Bhatia, S., Louie, A.D., Bhatia, R. et al. (2001). Solid cancers after bone marrow transplantation. *Journal of Clinical Oncology*, **19**, 464–71.

Bhatia, S., Robison, L.L., Oberlin, O. et al. (1996). Breast cancer and other second neoplasms after childhood Hodgkin's disease. *New England Journal of Medicine*, **334**, 745–51.

Blayney, D.W., Longo, D.L., Young, R.C. et al. (1987). Decreasing risk of leukemia with prolonged follow-up after chemotherapy and radiotherapy for Hodgkin's disease. *New England Journal of Medicine*, **316**, 710–14.

Bordigoni, P., Turello, R., Clement, L. et al. (2002). Osteochondroma after pediatric hematopoietic stem cell transplantation: report of eight cases. *Bone Marrow Transplantation*, **29**, 611–4.

Borek, C. (1979). Neoplastic transformation following split doses of X rays. *British Journal of Radiology*, **52**, 845–6.

Bortin, M.M., Horowitz, M.M., & Rimm, A.A. (1992). Increasing utilization of allogeneic bone marrow transplantation: results of the 1988–1990 survey. *Annals of Internal Medicine*, **116**, 505–12.

Brown, R.S., Haynes, H.A., Foley, H.J. et al. (1967). Hodgkin's disease. Immunological, clinical and histological features of 50 untreated patients. *Annals of Internal Medicine*, **67**, 291–302.

Burnet, F.M. (1971). Immunological surveillance in neoplasia. *Transplantation Reviews*, **7**, 3–25.

Cardillo, M., Rossini, G., Scalamogna, M. et al. (2001). Tumor incidence in heart transplant patients: report of the North Italy Transplant Program Registry. *Transplantation Proceedings*, **33**, 1840–3.

Coleman, C.N. (1982). Adverse effects of cancer therapy: risk of secondary neoplasms. *American Journal of Pediatric Hematology and Oncology*, **4**, 103–11.

Curtis, R.E., Rowlings, P.A., Deeg, H.J. et al. (1997). Solid cancers after bone marrow transplantation. *New England Journal of Medicine*, **336**, 897–904.

Darrington, D.L., Vose, J.M., Anderson, J.R. et al. (1994). Incidence and characterization of secondary myelodysplastic syndrome and acute myelogenous leukemia following high-dose chemoradiotherapy and autologous stem cell transplantation for lymphoid malignancies. *Journal of Clinical Oncology*, **12**, 2527–34.

Deeg, H.J., Socie, G., Schoch, G. et al. (1996). Malignancies after marrow transplantation for aplastic anemia and Fanconi anemia: a joint Seattle and Paris analysis of results in 700 patients. *Blood*, **87**, 386–92.

Dores, G.M., Metayer, C., Curtis, R.E. et al. (2002). Second malignant neoplasms among long-term survivors of Hodgkin's disease: a population-based evaluation over 25 years. *Journal of Clinical Oncology*, **20**, 3484–94.

Duell, T., van Lint, M.T., Ljungman, P. et al. (1997). Health and functional status of long term survivors of bone marrow transplantation. EBMT Working Party on Late Effects and EULEP Study Group on Late Effects. European Group for Blood and Marrow Transplantation. *Annals of Internal Medicine*, **126**, 184–92.

Favre-Schmuziger, G., Hofer, S., Passweg, J. et al. (2000). Treatment of solid tumors following allogeneic bone marrow transplantation. *Bone Marrow Transplantation*, **25**, 895–8.

Gleichmann, E., Gleichmann, H., Schwartz, R.S. et al. (1975). Immunologic induction of malignant lymphoma: identification of donor and host tumors in the graft-versus-host model. *Journal of the National Cancer Institute*, **54**, 107–16.

Gratwohl, A., Passweg, J., Baldomero, H. et al. (2000). Hematopoietic stem cell transplantation in Europe 1998. *Hematology Journal, 1,* 333–50.

Hall, E.J. (1997). Etiology of cancer: physical factors. In *Cancer: Principles and Practice of Oncology,* ed. V.T. DeVita Jr, S. Hellman, & S.A. Rosenberg, 5th ed., pp. 203–18. Philadelphia: JB Lippincott.

Han, A., Hill, C.K., & Elkind, M.M. (1980). Repair of cell killing and neoplastic transformation at reduced dose rates of 60Co gamma rays. *Cancer Research, 40,* 3328–32.

Harris, J., Sengar, D., Stewart, T. et al. (1976). The effect of immunosuppressive chemotherapy on immune function in patients with malignant disease. *Cancer, 37,* 1058–69.

Hawkins, M.M., Draper, G.J., & Kingston, J.E. (1987). Incidence of second primary tumours among childhood cancer survivors. *British Journal of Cancer, 56,* 339–47.

Jonas, S., Rayes, N., Neumann, U. et al. (1997). De novo malignancies after liver transplantation using tacrolimus-based protocols or cyclosporine-based quadruple immunosuppression with an interleukin-2 receptor antibody or antithymocyte globulin. *Cancer, 80,* 1141–50.

Kohn, H.I. & Fry, R.J.M. (1984). Radiation carcinogenesis. *New England Journal of Medicine, 310,* 504–11.

Kolb, H.J. & Bender-Goetze, C. (1990). Late complications after allogeneic bone marrow transplantation for leukemia. *Bone Marrow Transplantation, 6,* 61–72.

Kolb, H.J., Guenther, W., & Duell, T. (1992). Cancer after bone marrow transplantation. IBMTR and EBMT/EULEP Study Group on Late Effects. *Bone Marrow Transplantation, 10* (Suppl 1), 135–8.

Kolb, H.J., van Weel, M., Apperly, J.F. et al. (1999). Malignant neoplasms in long-term survivors of bone marrow transplantation. *Annals of Internal Medicine, 131,* 738–44.

Krueger, C.R.F., Malmgren, R.A., & Berard, C.R. (1971). Malignant lymphomas and plasmacytomas in mice under prolonged immunosuppression and persistent antigenic stimulation. *Transplantation, 11,* 138–44.

Land, C.E. (1987). Temporal distributions of risk for radiation-induced cancers. *Journal of Chronic Diseases, 40* (Suppl 2), 45S–57S.

Lauria, F., Foa, R., Gobbi, M. et al. (1983). Increased proportion of suppressor/cytotoxic (OKT8+) cells in patients with Hodgkin's disease in long-lasting remission. *Cancer, 52,* 1385–8.

Lowsky, R., Lipton, J., Fyles, G. et al. (1994). Secondary malignancies after bone marrow transplantation in adults. *Journal of Clinical Oncology, 12,* 2187–92.

Meadows, A.T., Baum, E., Fossati-Bellani, F. et al. (1985). Second malignant neoplasms in children: an update from the Late Effects Study Group. *Journal of Clinical Oncology, 3,* 532–8.

Michels, S.D., McKenna, R.W., Arthur, D.C. et al. (1985). Therapy-related acute myelogenous leukemia and myelodysplastic syndrome: a clinical and morphological study of 65 cases. *Blood, 65,* 1364–72.

Miller, J.S., Arthur, D.C., Litz, C.E. et al. (1994). Myelodysplastic syndrome after autologous bone marrow transplantation: an additional late complication of curative cancer therapy. *Blood, 83,* 3780–6.

Penn, I. (1993). Tumors after renal and cardiac transplantation. *Hematology/Oncology Clinics of North America, 7,* 431–45.

Penn, I. (1994). Depressed immunity and the development of cancer. *Cancer Detection and Prevention, 18,* 241–52.

Pui, C.H., Behm, F.G., Raimondi, S.C. et al. (1989). Secondary acute myeloid leukemia in children treated for acute lymphoid leukemia. *New England Journal of Medicine, 321,* 136–42.

Sanders, J.E. & the Seattle Marrow Transplant Team. (1991). The impact of marrow transplant preparative regimens on subsequent growth and development. *Seminars in Hematology, 28,* 244–9.

Socié, G., Curtis, R.E., Deeg, H.G. et al. (2000). New malignant disease after allogeneic marrow transplantation for childhood acute leukemia. *Journal of Clinical Oncology, 18,* 348–57.

Socié, G., Veum Sone, J., Wingard, J.R. et al. (1999). Long-term survival and late deaths after allogeneic bone marrow transplantation. *New England Journal of Medicine, 341,* 14–21.

Starzl, T.E., Porter, K.A., Iwatsuki, S. et al. (1984). Reversibility of lymphomas and lymphoproliferative lesions developing under cyclosporine-steroid therapy. *Lancet, 1,* 583–7.

Stone, R.M., Neuberg, D., & Soiffer, R. (1994). Myelodysplastic syndrome as a late complication following autologous bone marrow transplantation for non-Hodgkin's lymphoma. *Journal of Clinical Oncology, 12,* 2535–42.

Thomas, L. (1959). Discussion of Medawar P.B.: reaction to homologous tissue antigens in relation to hypersensitivity. In *Cellular and Humoral Aspects of the Hypersensitive States,* ed. H.S. Lawrence, pp. 529–32. New York: Paul Hober.

Tucker, M.A., Meadows, A.T., Boice, J.D. et al. (1987). Leukemia after therapy with alkylating agents for childhood cancer. *Journal of the National Cancer Institute, 78,* 459–64.

Tucker, M.A., Coleman, C.A., Cox, R.S. et al. (1988). Risk of second cancers after treatment for Hodgkin's disease. *New England Journal of Medicine, 318,* 76–81.

Tokunaga, M., Land, C.E., Yamamoto, T. et al. (1985). Incidence of female breast cancer among atomic bomb survivors, Hiroshima and Nagasaki 1950–1980. *Radiation Effects Research Foundation Technical Report,* 15–84. Hiroshima, RERF.

Urba, W.J. & Longo, D.L. (1992). Hodgkin's disease. *New England Journal of Medicine, 326,* 678–87.

van Leeuven, F.E. (1997). Second cancers. In *Cancer: Principles and Practice of Oncology,* ed. V.T. DeVita Jr, Hellman, S., & S.A. Rosenberg, 5th ed, pp. 2778–95. Philadelphia: JB Lippincott.

Weintraub, J. & Warnke, R.A. (1982). Lymphoma in cardiac allotransplant recipients. *Transplantation, 33,* 347–55.

Winkelhorst, J.T., Brokelman, W.J., Tiggeler, R.G., & Wobbes, T. (2001). Incidence and clinical course of de-novo malignancies in renal allograft recipients. *European Journal of Surgical Oncology, 27,* 409–13.

Witherspoon, R.P., Deeg, H. J., & Storb, R. (1994). Secondary malignancies after marrow transplantation for leukemia or aplastic anemia. *Transplantation, 57,* 1413–8.

Witherspoon, R.P., Fisher, L.D., Schoch, G. et al. (1989). Secondary cancers after bone marrow transplantation for leukemia or aplastic anemia. *New England Journal of Medicine, 321,* 784–9.

Ziegler, J.L., Beckstead, J.A., Volberding, P.A. et al. (1984). Non-Hodgkin's lymphoma in 90 homosexual men. *New England Journal of Medicine, 311,* 565–70.

88 Posttransplant lymphoproliferative disease

CATHERINE M. BOLLARD, CLIONA M. ROONEY, AND HELEN E. HESLOP

Baylor College of Medicine, Houston, USA

Introduction

Epstein-Barr virus (EBV)[1]-associated lymphoproliferative disorder (LPD) is a potentially life-threatening consequence of immune suppression after hematopoietic stem cell transplantation (HSCT). Persistence and reactivation of EBV infection within the cells of the immune system is a unique characteristic of gamma herpesviruses and is fundamental to the pathogenesis of this EBV-associated disease, which is due to outgrowth of donor derived EBV-infected B cells. The risk of this complication varies with different donor sources and HSCT product manipulation, with the highest incidence seen in recipients of unrelated donor or mismatched family member transplants where selective T-cell depletion is used (Curtis et al., 1999; Aguilar et al., 1999). Over the past 10 years immunotherapy strategies aimed at reconstituting T cell responses to EBV or targeting B cells have improved the outcome of EBV-LPD posttransplant. In addition techniques to detect the disease early have been developed, allowing pre-emptive therapy.

Biology of Epstein-Barr virus infection

EBV is an enveloped herpesvirus with a 172 kb double-stranded DNA genome (Rickinson & Kieff, 1996). In the immunocompetent host, EBV infection results in a mild self-limiting illness (Rickinson, 1994). Over 95% of the adult population worldwide are seropositive for EBV, primarily after developing the infection during childhood (Henle et al., 1974). Like other herpesviruses, EBV is then able to maintain a latent infection with the virus genome retained in the host cells without production of infectious virions. EBV targets oral epithelial cells and B cells. The CD21 receptor of the B lymphocyte allows the EBV to enter the cell and establish latent infection in vivo with the expression of latency-associated transforming proteins (Qu & Rowe, 1992). There are three types of EBV latency defined by the number and type of latent protein expressed on the host's B cells (Fig. 88.1).

[1]Michael Epstein, British pathologist/virologist, born 1921. Yvonne Barr, British scientist, born 1932.

During acute infectious mononucleosis, between 1 in 100 and 1 in 1000 circulating B cells in the peripheral blood are infected with EBV and express a type 3 latency pattern of transcription (Tierney et al., 1994).Type 3 latency involves the expression of EBV nuclear antigens (EBNA)-1, -2, -3A, -3B, -3C, the leader protein (LP), latent membrane proteins (LMP) -1, -2A, -2B, and the cytosolic protein RK-BARFO (the product of the BamH1 open reading frame) (Rickinson & Moss, 1997). In addition, abundantly expressed small non-polyadenylated RNAs termed EBV early RNA (EBER) 1 and 2 are transcribed but not translated (Hopwood & Crawford, 2000). The expression of the 9 viral antigens and the presence of cell adhesion and co-stimula-

Types of EBV Latency

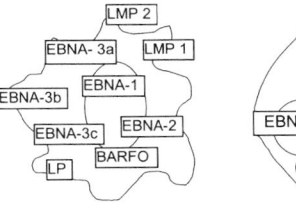
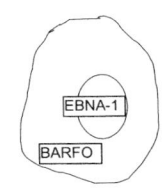

Type 3
EBL lymphoma post transplant
Lymphoblastoid cell lines

Type 2
Hodgkin's disease
Nasopharyngeal carcinoma

Type 1
Burkitt's lymphoma

Figure 88.1. Infected B cells express EBV-latency associated transforming proteins. The three types of EBV latency shown in this figure depend on the number and type of latent proteins expressed on the host's B cells. Type 3 latency as seen in lymphoblastoid cell lines (LCL) as well as posttransplant lymphoproliferative disease (PTLD), involves the expression of all the latency-associated viral proteins. The expression of these viral antigens and the presence of cell adhesion and costimulatory molecules make these B cells highly immunogenic and in the immunocompetent host susceptible to immune-mediated killing by EBV-specific cytotoxic T cells. In contrast, in type 1 and 2 latency, only a limited array of EBV antigens are expressed, allowing the infected cells to escape immune regulation by CTLs, resulting in proliferation and malignant transformation as seen in EBV-related Burkitt's lymphoma (type 1 latency), or nasopharyngeal carcinoma and Hodgkin's disease (type 2 latency).

tory molecules make these B cells highly immunogenic and in the immunocompetent host, susceptible to immune mediated killing by EBV-specific cytotoxic T cells (Rickinson & Moss, 1997). Further, type 3 latency is demonstrated in vitro by the establishment of immortalized EBV-transformed lymphoblastoid B-cell lines (LCL). In the immunocompetent host, once the type 3 latency expressing B cells are eliminated by the cellular immune response, around 1 in 10^6 infected B cells persist which express a more restricted pattern of EBV genes. This viral gene expression in resting infected B cells in normal seropositive individuals is limited to the immunosubdominant LMP-2A antigen, BARFO, EBNA-1 (which possesses gly-ala repeat sequences that inhibit HLA class I antigen processing), and EBERs (Qu & Rowe, 1992). This expression of a minimal subset of genes, which are weak targets for CTL activity, allows infected cells to evade the immune system and maintain a low level persistent infection (Lewin *et al.*, 1987).

Pathogenesis of EBV-driven lymphoproliferative disease (LPD)

In seropositive individuals, EBV-infected cells may undergo lytic replication usually with a transient expression of the full panel of type 3 latent antigens, followed by immune recognition and elimination by EBV-specific CTL. In contrast, type 1 and type 2 latency express only a limited array of EBV antigens as seen in nasopharyngeal carcinoma, Hodgkin's disease,[2] and Burkitt's lymphoma[3] (Fig. 88.1) (Sample *et al.*, 1991; Brook *et al.*, 1992; Deacon *et al.*, 1993).

An ongoing balance exists in normal seropositive individuals between the EBV viral load and the immune defense mechanisms. However, following transplantation where cytotoxic T cell numbers and/or activity are suppressed, the EBV-infected B cells expressing a type 3 latency are able to proliferate

unchecked (d'Amore *et al.*, 1991). This leads to accumulation of EBV-infected B cells in the body and enhanced viral replication as demonstrated by elevated levels of EBV DNA detected in the peripheral blood by polymerase chain reaction (PCR) (Riddler *et al.*, 1994; Rowe *et al.*, 1997; Rooney *et al.*, 1995; Lucas *et al.*, 1998). These changes reflect the loss of CTL activity and in some patients, uncontrolled EBV-driven B-cell lymphoproliferation occurs leading to development of lymphoma.

Incidence and risk factors

The reported incidence of LPD after hematopoietic stem cell transplantation ranges from 1% to 25% of transplant recipients (Table 88.1). The incidence is highest in the first six months posttransplant (120 cases/10,000patients/year) (Curtis *et al.*, 1999). In a multivariate analysis, risk of LPD at <12 months post HSCT was shown to be strongly associated with patients receiving HSCT from HLA mismatched family donors or unrelated donors (Curtis *et al.*, 1999). Moreover, risk is increased if the marrow is depleted of T cells to prevent graft-versus-host disease (Chiang *et al.*, 2001; Skinner *et al.*, 1988; Shapiro *et al.*, 1988; Lucas *et al.*, 1996; Gerritsen *et al.*, 1996; Heslop & Rooney, 1997; Hale &Waldmann, 1998). However if both T and B-cells are depleted simultaneously, the incidence is much lower. In a large review of HSCT recipients treated with the Campath-1 antibody, which removes mature T and B cells (Hale & Waldmann, 1998) the incidence of LPD was less than 2%. Other methods of B-cell depletion, such as elutriation, which removes over 90% of B cells from the donor graft, (Gross *et al.*, 1998) or the addition of monoclonal antibodies for B cell depletion to the T-cell depletion regimen (Cavazzana-Calvo *et al.*, 1998; Liu *et al.*, 1999) are also associated with a low risk. An analysis of 272 unrelated-donor umbilical cord blood transplants also revealed a low incidence of 2% (±3.7%)

Table 88.1.   *Incidence of LPD after bone marrow transplantation*

Type of transplant	Incidence of EBV-LPD	References
Allogeneic HSCT (all types)	1%–1.8%	Micallef *et al.*, 1998 Curtis *et al.*, 1999 Gross *et al.*, 1999
Mismatched-related donor HSCT and T-cell depletion	5.7%–31%	Heslop & Rooney, 1997 Cavazzana-Calvo *et al.*, 1998 Chiang *et al.*, 2001
Unrelated-donor HSCT and T-cell depletion	5%–29%	Heslop & Rooney, 1997 Lucas *et al.*, 1998 Micallef *et al.*, 1998 O'Reilly *et al.*, 1998 Curtis *et al.*, 1999 Gross *et al.*, 1999
Unrelated donor HSCT and Campath depletion	1.3%	Hale *et al.*, 1998
Unrelated donor cord blood transplant	2%	Barker *et al.*, 2001

[2]Thomas Hodgkin, English physician and pathologist, 1798-1866.
[3]Denis Burkitt, British surgeon, 1911-1993.

at 2 years (Barker *et al.*, 2001). Taken together, these data suggest that the incidence of EBV-LPD may depend on the balance between EBV-infected B cells and EBV-specific T-cell precursors in the infused product.

An additional risk factor is the posttransplant immunosuppression regimen employed (Swinnen *et al.*, 1990; Sokal *et al.*, 1997). In one study the relative risk of developing LPD after treatment with antithymocyte globulin (ATG) or anti-CD3 was 6.4 and 43.2 respectively (Curtis *et al.*, 1999). One study looked at the incidence of EBV reactivation in 17 patients post allogeneic stem cell transplant who were treated with visilizumab for glucocorticoid-refractory graft-versus-host-disease (GVHD) (Carpenter *et al.*, 2002). Visilizumab is a humanized anti-CD3 monoclonal antibody characterized by its ability to selectively induce apoptosis in activated T cells. In 12 of 16 evaluable patients, EBV DNA levels increased in the plasma post visilizumab and 9 patients had reactivation of >1,000 copies plasma EBV DNA/ml. In 4 patients the rise was transient lasting a range of 1–39 days, and in 5 patients the elevations in EBV DNA levels persisted and patients were treated pre-emptively with anti-CD20 monoclonal antibody. However, in 3 patients, progressive rises of plasma EBV DNA to > 10,000 copies/ml were seen and 2 of these patients developed rapidly fatal LPD, demonstrating an 11% incidence of EBV lymphoma in this patient group.

LPD is rare after autologous stem cell transplantation with only sporadic case reports (Lones *et al.*, 2000; Heath *et al.*, 2002; Anderson *et al.*, 1990; Hauke *et al.*, 1998; Peniket *et al.*, 1998), although more cases have been reported recently perhaps reflecting increased awareness or alternately increased use of more immunoablative preparatory regimens used in conjunction with transplantation of stem cells depleted of T cells by procedures such as CD34 selection (Peniket *et al.*, 1998) or in vitro purging (Briz *et al.*, 1997). In particular, several cases have been reported after CD34-selected autologous transplantation for autoimmune disease (Openshaw *et al.*, 2002).

Finally, HSC transplant recipients with underlying immunodeficiencies such as Wiskott-Aldrich syndrome (WAS) represent an independent risk group for EBV-LPD (Bhatia *et al.*, 1996). Even in the absence of the transplant setting, patients with immunodeficiency syndromes are at increased risk of developing EBV-associated LPD (Okano, 2001). In the presence of disturbed T-cell function, EBV may induce not only prolonged proliferation but also transformation of B-cells. One group demonstrated that patients with primary, congenital immunodeficiency have an incidence of LPD ranging from 0.7% for patients with X-linked agammaglobulinemia to 12–15% in patients with ataxia-telangiectasia (Oertel & Riess, 2002). Given this underlying increased risk pretransplant, the outcome of 28 transplants performed in 26 WAS patients at a single center over a 15-year period, were retrospectively analyzed (Ozsahin *et al.*, 1996). Ten transplants were from an HLA genetically identical donor, one from a matched unrelated donor, and 17 from a related HLA-mismatched donor. All but one of the HLA mismatched marrow samples were T-cell depleted. EBV-associated LPD occurred in 7 of 16 recipients of HLA-mismatched versus no occurrences among 11 recipients of HLA-identical BMT. LPD was observed 2 to 4 months post BMT, was fatal in four patients, and resolved in four patients after treatment with monoclonal anti-B-cell antibodies (Ozsahin *et al.*, 1996).

Pathology and clinical presentation

Ablation of the recipient's bone marrow before transplantation and reconstitution of the recipient's immune system with donor lymphocytes means that LPD is usually of donor B-cell origin (Shapiro *et al.*, 1988). In the HSC transplant setting, LPD usually presents early posttransplant and without treatment is usually rapidly fatal (Shapiro *et al.*, 1988). EBV-associated LPD that arises in allogeneic HSCT recipients is characterized by high-grade histologic subtype (Orazi *et al.*, 1997) and the majority of the tumor cells express a type 3 latency pattern of gene expression and are phenotypically identical to LCL derived in vitro (Orazi *et al.*, 1997; Rea *et al.*, 1994). The diagnosis of LPD post HSCT is usually established within the first year following transplant when profound deficiencies of EBV-specific cytotoxic T lymphocytes are observed (Lucas *et al.*, 1996). In these patients with early-onset LPD, the EBV-infected cells are almost always donor-derived. There is a small subset of HSCT patients who develop "late-onset" LPD up to 4 years posttransplant (Gratama *et al.*, 1988). Generally these patients have underlying immunodeficiency syndromes and/or incomplete engraftment posttransplant. In contrast to the early-onset group, the EBV-infected cells may be of host origin.

The clinical presentation of LPD post HSCT is variable with a diverse spectrum of clinical symptoms and signs. It may present as a generalized systemic illness not unlike infectious mononucleosis with prominent B symptoms (fevers, sweats, anorexia) and rapid enlargement of the tonsils and cervical nodes, or it may present with nodular deposits in other organs including lung, liver, spleen, kidneys, small intestine, bone marrow, or the central nervous system. It may also present as fulminant disease with diffusely infiltrative multiorgan involvement difficult to distinguish from sepsis or severe GVHD (Swinnen, 2000). Retrospective analyses of several case reports and studies reported that LPD emerged as an incidental finding, discovered at autopsy, in nearly 20% of patients (Gratama *et al.*, 1991; Gross *et al.*, 1999; Claviez *et al.*, 2000). These different presentations emphasize the need for a high index of suspicion in considering the diagnosis.

Diagnosis

The diversity of clinical and histological presentation of LPD can therefore make diagnosis difficult. Any patient suspected of LPD based on clinical symptoms should undergo total body imaging to assess for radiographical evidence of lymphoma. If there is any suspicion of tumor infiltration of any organ or lymph node, then biopsy is warranted. Immunohistochemical analysis of tumor biopsy material is essential to provide a definitive diagnosis of LPD, and in situ hybridization for detection of the

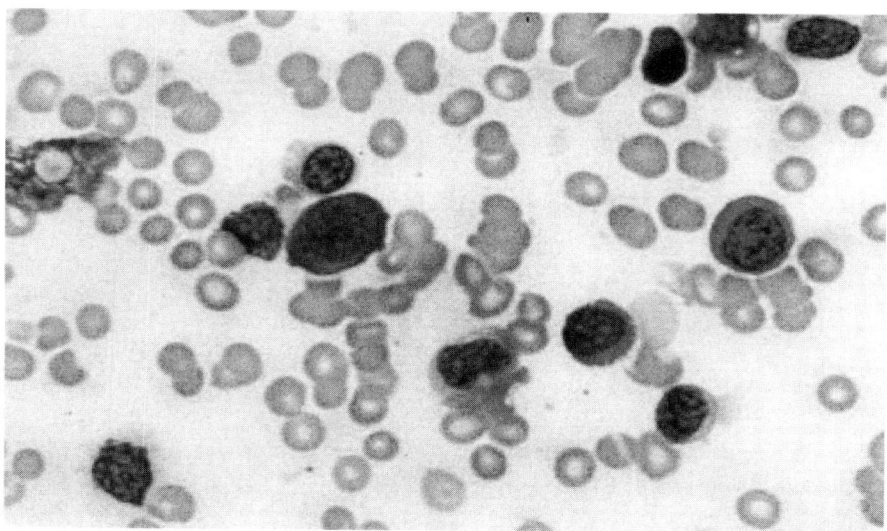

Figure 88.2. Circulating EBV-infected B cells in a patient who presented with fevers following a T-cell-depleted matched unrelated donor transplant.

EBER and/or LMP-1 is routinely used to determine EBV involvement (Figs. 88.2 and 88.3) (Harris *et al.,* 1997). Detection of elevated EBV DNA levels is not diagnostic of EBV-associated lymphoproliferative disease, but as discussed below, may provide useful information to detect patients at risk for developing LPD post BMT. Serological analysis is of little value in the diagnosis of LPD as false negatives may be seen as a result of the severe immune dysfunction in patients post BMT (Hopwood & Crawford, 2000) and false positives as a result of blood transfusion or administration of intravenous immunoglobulin (IVIG). Assessment of tumor cell clonality is of limited use in providing clear prognostic information in LPD, although monoclonal tumors can be more aggressive possibly due to additional cellular genetic mutations (Micallef *et al.,* 1998). Most cases of LPD

probably arise as polyclonal proliferations, with some lesions progressing to oligoclonal or monoclonal tumors (Nalesnik *et al.,* 1988). When clonality is assessed, the preferred method is by PCR to detect immunoglobulin gene rearrangements, as there is risk of sampling error in determining clonality by immunohistochemistry (Trainor *et al.,* 1991).

Early detection of LPD using PCR

As prompt diagnosis and intervention are likely to improve outcome, many bone marrow transplant centers have evaluated whether monitoring patients' EBV-DNA levels posttransplant can predict onset of LPD (Table 88.2) (Rowe *et al.,* 1997; Rooney *et al.,* 1995a; Rooney *et al.,* 1998; Stevens *et al.,* 1999; Stevens *et*

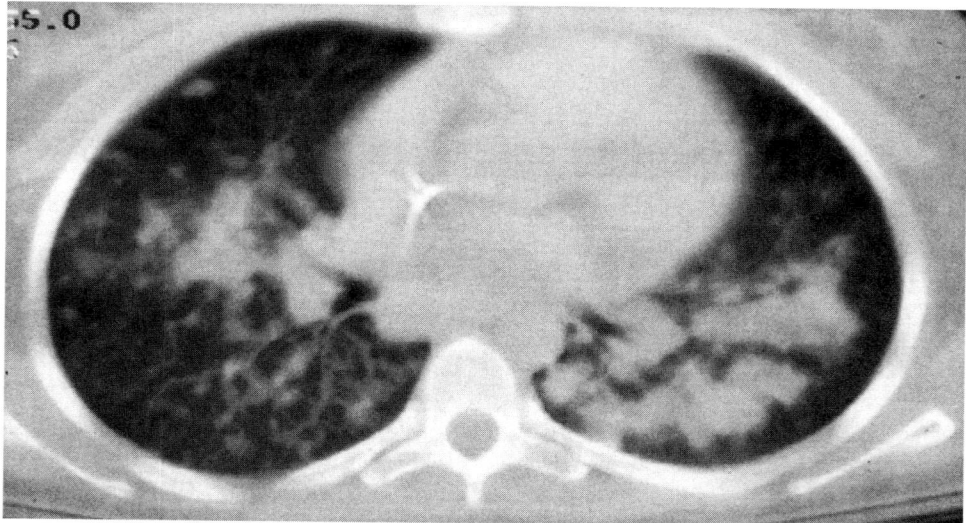

Figure 88.3. CT scan showing multiple pulmonary nodules in a patient who presented with fevers, pharyngitis, and increased EBV DNA levels 45 days after a T-cell-depleted 5/6 HLA-matched unrelated donor transplant. Biopsy of a cervical lymph node confirmed the diagnosis of EBV lymphoproliferative disorder.

Table 88.2.   *Published reports assessing utility of quantitative EBV DNA assays in patients post BMT*

Reference	EBV DNA "cut-off" level predictive for disease	EBV DNA level detection method	Number of patients with PTLD	Number (%) of patients with PTLD and ↑ EBV DNA	Number of patients without PLTD	Number of patients without PTLD with EBV DNA levels > cut-off
Rooney *et al.*, 1995	2,000 copies/µg DNA	Semi-quantitative PCR	5	4 (80%)	14	0 (0%)
Lucas *et al.*, 1998	40,000 copies/ml	Semi-quantitative PCR	7	5	34	2 (6%)
Stevens *et al.*, 2001	>2000 genome copies/ml	Quantitative competitive PCR	6	5 (83%)	8	2 (25%)
Van Essen *et al.*, 2001	>50 genomes/ml (reactivation)	Quantitative real-time PCR	10	10 (100%)	140	44 (31%)
Wagner *et al.*, 2001	>4000 EBV copies/µg DNA	Quantitative real-time PCR	3	3(100%)	76	18 (24%)
Gartner *et al.*, 2002	10,000 copies EBV/µg DNA	Quantitative competitive PCR	9	9 (100%)	50	17 (34%)
Lankester *et al.*, 2002	$\geq 10^2$ gEq/ml	Quantitative real-time PCR	6	6 (100%)	20	1 (0.5%)

Abbreviations: PTLD, posttransplant lymphoproliferative disease; PCR, polymerase chain reaction.

al., 2001). Several groups demonstrated by semiquantitative PCR analysis, that an increase in EBV load in peripheral blood mononuclear cells (PBMC) precedes the onset of LPD in recipients of T-cell-depleted HSCT (Rooney *et al.*, 1995; Lucas *et al.*, 1998; Gustafsson *et al.*, 2000). More recently we and others have developed a quantitative real-time PCR (RQ PCR) assay specific for the conserved viral EBER 1 gene. In healthy individuals, the EBV load in PBMC analyzed by RQ PCR ranges from 0–200 EBV copies/µg PBMC DNA. We have shown that using quantitative PCR, EBV DNA levels >4000 copies/µg DNA are highly predictive for the development of EBV lymphoma in recipients of T-cell–depleted marrow and therefore serve as a guide to commence treatment (Wagner *et al.*, 2001). However, the correlation between elevated EBV DNA level and development of lymphoma was less strong in patients after HSCT who did not receive a T-cell–depleted product, where many individuals developed elevated levels of EBV load, but did not develop LPD (Lucas *et al.*, 1998; Wagner *et al.*, 2001). Other groups have also reported that while EBV reactivation is a frequent event after both T-cell–depleted and unmanipulated transplantation, high EBV loads only have a high correlation with development of EBV lymphoma after T-cell-depleted transplants (Wagner *et al.*, 2001; van Esser *et al.*, 2001). The ability to identify patients who can mount an immune response, and therefore do not require anti-EBV therapy, would greatly aid the management of PTLD and several groups are looking at developing functional assays of EBV-specific T-cell function for this purpose.

Therapeutic management

A variety of therapeutic approaches to LPD post HSCT have been explored. The use of radiotherapy or surgical resection for anatomically localized LPD can result in complete eradication of the disease, especially for the treatment of EBV lymphoma after solid organ transplantation (Armitage *et al.*, 1991). While withdrawal of immunosuppression is often effective in solid organ recipients, this strategy is not usually effective in HSCT recipients because the developing donor-derived immune system cannot provide sufficient immune recovery to eradicate EBV-infected B cells in HSC transplant patients. Occasional responses have been observed when the immune response is already recovering (Heslop *et al.*, 1994).

Drug therapies

Chemotherapy, primarily using CHOP-based regimens (cyclophosphamide, doxorubicin, vincristine, and prednisone) has been used to treat LPD post HSCT, but mortality is high (up tp 70%) secondary to significant toxicity (Swinnen, 1999; Morrison *et al.*, 1994). One group of patients who developed LPD after cardiac transplantation were treated with the regimen Pro-MACE-CytaBOM, consisting of prednisone, doxorubicin, cyclophosphamide, etoposide, cytarabine, bleomycin, vincristine, methotrexate, and leucovorin. In this group, the overall mortality rate was 25%, and none of the patients who survived had relapsed at 65 months follow-up (Swinnen *et al.*, 1995). Nevertheless, the use of chemotherapy in patients with LPD post HSCT is associated with significantly higher mortality rates, primarily due to infective complications (Swinnen, 2000). For this reason, other drugs including interferon-α2b and antiviral agents such as acyclovir have been used to treat LPD in this setting. Therapy with interferon-α plus IVIG has been used in solid organ, and a small number of hematopoietic stem cell, transplant recipients with some responses (Swinnen, 1998).

High doses of acyclovir, ganciclovir, or cidofovir have been used in combination treatment protocols that included immunosuppression reduction, monoclonal antibodies, and/or interferon (Davis, 1998; Schaar *et al.*, 2001; Hanel *et al.*, 2001). A limitation with this approach is that EBV cells are latently infected and these antiviral agents only block active herpesvirus replication and do not affect the growth of cells that are already transformed. One center developed an antiviral strategy using a combination of ganciclovir and arginine butyrate, which is a selective activator of the EBV thymidine kinase (TK) gene in latently EBV-infected lymphoid cells and tumor cells. A phase I/II trial has been initiated in patients who develop LPD after lung transplantation. Six patients, all with LPD resistant to conventional radiation and/or chemotherapy, were treated with the arginine butyrate/ganciclovir combination and complete clinical responses were seen in four patients, with a partial response occurring in a fifth patient (Mentzer et al., 2001). Hydroxyurea has also been shown to have anti-EBV activity in vitro and promising results were reported in 2 patients with HIV-related EBV-associated primary central nervous system lymphoma (Slobod et al., 2000).

Monoclonal antibodies

The use of monoclonal anti-B-cell antibodies has also been investigated for the treatment of this disease. A mixture of anti-CD21 and anti-CD24 antibodies was found to be effective in a European multicenter trial, which included HSCT recipients with LPD. Twenty-seven patients post HSCT were treated, with an overall survival rate of 46% at a median follow-up of 61 months (Fischer et al., 1991; Benkerrou et al., 1998). The toxicity was mild, but these antibodies are no longer available clinically. Our group and others have investigated the feasibility of treating LPD with the humanized murine anti-CD20 antibody rituximab (Rituxan) (Table 88.3) (Skoda-smith et al., 2001; Ifthikharuddin et al., 2000; Kuehnle et al., 2001; Milpied et al., 2000; McGuirk et al., 1999). Although follow-up is relatively short and the number of patients in each series is relatively small, the overall response rates ranged from 69% to 100% and this agent therefore represents a promising strategy for LPD post HSCT. The reported toxicity of rituximab as treatment for LPD in small single center reports has generally been mild. However there are potential hazards of CD20 therapy. The profound B-cell depletion may further exacerbate immunodeficiency in transplant recipients, although eventual recovery should occur as CD20 is not expressed on B-cell precursors. Nevertheless in solid organ transplant recipients, hypogammaglobulinemia associated with fatal invasive aspergillosis and CMV reactivation has been reported (Verschuuren et al., 2002; Suzan et al., 2001). In addition, CD20 therapy may result in selection of a CD20-negative population of proliferating B cells (Davis et al., 1999).

Adoptive immunotherapy

Because EBV is normally controlled by a CTL response, adoptive immunotherapy approaches using T cells to restore EBV-specific immunocompetence, and therefore to control EBV-LPD post HSCT have been used by several groups (Table 88.4). In the first reported study from Sloan Kettering, unse-

lected populations of donor lymphocytes were administered to HSC transplant recipients (Papadopoulos et al., 1994). The rationale for this strategy was that most EBV-seropositive individuals have a high frequency of EBV-specific precursors, so that transfer of unmanipulated donor lymphocyte populations should be able to restore the immune response to EBV. In the Sloan Kettering experience the overall response rate was high with 20 of 22 patients attaining complete remissions (O'Reilly et al., 1998). Other centers have seen lower response rates to donor leukocyte infusions (Lucas et al., 1998), which may reflect different patient populations or better outcome with early diagnosis and treatment.

While donor lymphocyte infusion does have therapeutic activity (Papadopoulos et al., 1994; Heslop et al., 1994), such therapy is limited by potentially fatal complications that arise from alloreactive T cells also present in the lymphocyte infusion (Lucas et al., 1998; Heslop et al., 1994). One solution to the problem of alloreactivity when administering donor leukocyte infusions is to transduce the T cells with a suicide gene. The suicide gene used most frequently is the herpes simplex virus 1-thymidine kinase (HSV-Tk) gene, which renders transduced cells sensitive to ganciclovir so that they can be subsequently ablated should signs of GVHD develop. Several studies suggest that the use of such cells early or late after transplantation is associated with no acute toxicity, persistent circulation of the gene-modified cells occurs, and alloreactive T cells appear to be sensitive to gancyclovir (Bonini et al., 1997; Tiberghien et al., 2001). However, two concerns with this approach are that the transgene may be immunogenic (Ridell et al., 1996) and that the ex vivo activation necessary for retroviral transduction may inhibit virus-reactive cells (Sauce et al., 2002). An alternative "suicide gene" is a chimeric human protein expressing the Fas intracellular domain, with 2 copies of an FK-506-binding protein. In vitro, transduced primary human T lymphocytes retrovirally transduced to express the Fas/FK-506 chimeric protein functioned the same as untransduced cells. However, transduced cells rapidly underwent apoptosis with the addition of subnanomolar concentrations of AP1903, a bivalent "dimerizer" drug that binds FK-506 binding protein and induces Fas crosslinking. T cells were eliminated regardless of their proliferation state; this AP1903/Fas system contains only human components suggesting it may be a promising alternative to HSV-Tk for the removal of alloreactive T cells and prevention/treatment of GVHD (Thomis et al., 2001).

Another approach to overcome the risk of GVHD with T-cell therapy is the generation of donor-derived, EBV-specific cytotoxic T lymphocytes (CTLs) (Gustafsson et al., 2000; Rooney et al., 1995b; Regn et al., 2001; O'Reilly et al., 1997). In the majority of EBV-LPD cases that occur in hematopoietic stem cell recipients, the transformed cells are of donor origin and express all latent cycle virus-associated antigens, providing excellent targets for virus-specific T cells. EBV-transformed lymphoblastoid cell B lines (LCL) likewise express all latent cycle virus-associated antigens and several co-stimulatory molecules that facilitate CTL generation (Fig. 88.1). They can be

Table 88.3. *Published reports on use of anti-CD20 for treatment of PTLD post HSCT*

Reference	Patient number	Pathological diagnosis?	Anti-CD20 dose	Additional treatment	Number (%) complete response	Side-effects	Comments
McGuirk *et al.*, 1999	2	No	375 mg/m² 3–4 infusions	Irradiated DLI	2 (100%)	1 patient subsequently died of multiple infections	
Milpied *et al.*, 2000	6	Yes in 2 patients	375 mg/m² 2–8 infusions	Nil	5 (83%)	Nil reported	4 pts treated preemptively based on fever, lymphadenopathy and ↑EBV DNA
Kuehnle *et al.*, 2000	3	Yes in 1 patients	375 mg/m² 1 infusion	1 patient received EBV-specific cytotoxic T lymphocytes (CTL)	3 (100%)	1 patient: hypogammaglobulinemia & B cell deficiency > 7 months	2 pts treated preemptively based on ↑EBV DNA ± ↑liver function tests
Hanel *et al.*, 2001	1	Yes	375 mg/m² 4 infusions	Cidofovir	1 (100%)	Nil reported	Case report of patient with PTLD of CNS
Skoda-Smith *et al.*, 2001	1	Yes	375 mg/m² 4 infusions	Chemotherapy and second transplant with CD34⁺ and CD3⁺ donor cells	1 (100%)	Nil reported	
Faye *et al.*, 2001	12	Yes in 8 patient	375 mg/m² 1–9 infusions	Nil	8 (66%)	None	8 patients with tumors and 4 with fever and increased EBV load
van Esser *et al.*, 2002	17	Yes in 3 patients	375 mg/m² 1–2 infusions	1 patient and donor leukocyte infusion	17 (100%)	B cells ↓ in 14/17 pts. Opportunistic infections seen. No deaths.	15 pts treated preemptively based on ↑EBV DNA with one dose. 2 patients treated for PTLD with 2 doses anti-CD20.

Abbreviations: CNS, central nervous system; SCID, severe combined immunodeficiency; DLI, donor lymphocyte infusions; PTLD, posttransplant lymphoproliferative disease.

readily prepared from any donor and provide a source of antigen-presenting cells that endogenously express the appropriate antigens for presentation of HLA class I-restricted epitopes. Our group generated EBV-specific T-cell lines from donor lymphocytes and used them as prophylaxis and treatment for EBV-induced lymphoma in patients post HSCT (Rooney *et al.*, 1995b). CTLs were generated by initiating an LCL line from infecting donor PBMC with a laboratory strain of EBV. These LCL were irradiated and then used as antigen-presenting cells to stimulate and expand EBV-specific CTLs from the donor lymphocyte population. The resultant EBV-specific CTL were polyclonal and contained both CD4⁺ and CD8⁺ EBV-specific T cells, which is considered advantageous since the presence of

antigen-specific CD4⁺ helper T cells is important for in vivo survival of cytotoxic CD8⁺ T cell populations. Since 1993, 60 patients who received a T-cell-depleted HSCT were given EBV-CTLs prophylactically. The first 26 patients enrolled on to the study received CTL that were genetically modified with the neomycin resistance gene. None of the 57 patients who received the EBV-CTL as prophylaxis developed LPD compared with an incidence of 11.5% in a comparable group who did not receive CTLs (Heslop & Rooney, 1997). Nine of these patients had high EBV DNA levels in peripheral blood, predictive of the imminent onset of EBV-LPD, prior to receiving CTLs and had a rapid decrease in EBV-DNA levels that correlated with an increase in EBV-specific CTL precursor fre-

Table 88.4. *Published reports on use of EBV-cytotoxic T cells as prophylaxis or treatment for PTLD post HSCT*

Study	Patient number (patient age range)	Type of transplant	Pathological evidence of PTLD	CTL lines and dose	Results
Rooney et al., 1998	39 (9 mths–20yr)	T-depleted HSCT (mismatched related donor or matched unrelated donor)	No—prophylaxis study	Allogeneic (donor-derived) EBV-CTL Minimum dose of 4 × $10^7/m^2$ and maximum dose of 12 × $10^7/m^2$	No patients developed PTLD compared with 11.5% controls. No toxicity
Rooney et al., 1998 and Gottschalk et al., 2001	3 (12–17 yrs)	T-depleted HSCT	Yes—lymphoblastic lymphoma	Allogeneic (donor-derived) EBV-CTI 2–4 × $10^7/m^2$	2 compete remissions, 1 died (no response to CTL secondary to tumor mutation resistant to CTL)
Gustafsson et al., 2000	9 (1–39 yrs)	T depleted HSCT or unmanipulated HSCT with ATG/OKT3 conditioning (mismatched or matched unrelated donor or matched related donor)	No—treatment based on ↑EBV DNA levels	Allogeneic (donor-derived) EBV-CTL 4 × $10^7/m^2$	8 patients had ↓EBV DNA levels. 1 patient subsequently died of PTLD (CTL showed poor specificity for EBV targets on cyto toxicity assay)

Abbreviations: PTLD, posttransplant lymphoproliferative disease; CTL, cytotoxic T lymphocytes.

quency. Using conventional PCR and real-time PCR, the marker gene was identified in the peripheral blood at least 69 months post CTL (Bollard et al., 2001). Although toxicity was low in this prophylaxis group, inflammatory responses were seen in three of the nine patients with elevated EBV DNA levels who had incipient disease.

Three patients who declined or were ineligible for our prophylaxis study were treated for established EBV lymphoma. The EBV-specific CTL therapy induced a remission in 2 patients, although in one case significant inflammation occurred at sites of disease after CTL administration (Rooney et al., 1998). The patient who failed treatment was found to have an escape mutant in her EBV lymphoma cells. Therefore, although the donor EBV-CTL line recognized two immunodominant HLA-A 11-restricted epitopes in EBNA-3B, the patient's tumor cells had a mutation in the EBNA-3B epitope, thereby rendering the tumor resistant to the donor CTLs (Gottschalk et al., 2001). Although polyclonal CTL lines were used, such lines may have target restriction after only one week of culture (Gottschalk et al., 2001) and a restricted pattern of T- cell antigen receptor usage on spectratyping has been observed (Musk et al., 2001), which is likely due to immunodominance of particular EBV-derived peptides presented in the context of different HLA types (Rickinson & Moss, 1997). Therefore, the risk of tumor escape mutants remains a concern, as it does with the use of monoclonal antibody therapies. In addition, the infusion of CTLs to patients with incipient or established disease warrants caution because of the inflammatory response at disease sites. However, adoptively transferred EBV-CTLs do persist long-term and can prevent, as well as effectively treat, EBV-driven LPD.

A study from Sweden has confirmed the efficacy of EBV-specific CTLs in reducing the viral load in patients with high EBV DNA levels after hematopoietic stem cell transplantation (Gustafsson et al., 2000). However, one out of six patients who received EBV-specific CTLs subsequently developed overt EBV-LPD and died of progressive disease. In vitro testing of the donor CTL line of this patient showed that it lacked a strong EBV-specific component, which may explain this failure of CTL therapy.

An additional limitation of CTL therapy is that since LPD requires immediate treatment, CTLs must be available at diagnosis. The generation of EBV-specific CTLs requires 2 to 3 months, although this time can be reduced by using EBV antigen-loaded dendritic cells as antigen-presenting cells. Another strategy described by Koehne et al. (2000) is to select virus-specific cells early in culture by their susceptibility to transduction with a retroviral vector (Koehne et al., 2000) Another concern is that if used prophylactically, recipients are only protected from one of the many viruses that may cause morbidity and mortality during the period of immunosuppression posttransplant. Several groups have investigated approaches for modifying the LCLs used as antigen-presenting cells to generate multispecific CTLs. Transduction of LCL with a retroviral vector encoding pp65 has allowed generation of CTLs specific for both CMV and EBV (Sun et al., 1999), while infection of LCL with adenovirus results in generation of CTLs specific for both adenovirus and EBV (Regn et al., 2001). An alternative strategy to generate broad antiviral immunity is to culture donor mononuclear cells with recipient cells and then deplete populations expressing activation markers such as CD25, which should contain alloreactive cells (Montagna et al.,

1999). The residual allodepleted T cell product will contain CTLs specific for multiple viruses and potentially residual tumor cells.

Conclusions and future directions

The introduction of modified methods of graft manipulation along with the availability of antibody- and cellular-based therapies should substantially reduce future mortality from EBV lymphoma in BMT recipients. The current challenges are learning how to use monitoring tests to diagnose this complication early and determining how to identify which patients should receive pre-emptive treatment. It is obviously preferable to treat patients with early or incipient disease as treatment of bulky disease is associated with significant morbidity (Lucas et al., 1998; Rooney et al., 1998; Papadopoulos et al., 1994) and a higher likelihood of generating escape mutants (Gottschalk et al., 2001). However, as donor T cells have the risk of alloreactivity and rituximab may increase the risk of infections, it is important to identify which patients have sufficient endogenous EBV-specific immune function to control reactivation. Preemptive treatment should be considered in patients with high EBV load and a strong likelihood of developing LPD, such as recipients of T-cell–depleted transplants or patients who have received anti-T-cell antibodies in vivo for the prophylaxis or treatment of GVHD.

References

Aguilar, L. K., Rooney, C. M., & Heslop, H. E. (1999). Lymphoproliferative disorders involving Epstein-Barr virus after hematopoietic stem cell transplantation. *Current Opinion in Oncology,* **11,** 96–101.

Anderson, K. C., Soiffer, R., DeLage, R. et al. (1990). T-cell-depleted autologous bone marrow transplantation therapy: analysis of immune deficiency and late complications. *Blood,* **76,** 235–244.

Armitage, J. M., Kormos, R. L., Stuart, R. S. et al. (1991). Posttransplant lymphoproliferative disease in thoracic organ transplant patients: ten years of cyclosporine-based immunosuppression. *Journal of Heart and Lung Transplantation,* **10,** 877–886.

Barker, J. N., Martin, P. L., Coad, J. E. et al. (2001). Low incidence of Epstein-Barr virus-associated posttransplantation lymphoproliferative disorders in 272 unrelated-donor umbilical cord blood transplant recipients. *Biology of Blood and Marrow Transplantation,* **7,** 395–399.

Benkerrou, M., Jais, J. P., Leblond, V. et al. (1998). Anti-B-cell monoclonal antibody treatment of severe posttransplant B-lymphoproliferative disorder: prognostic factors and long-term outcome. *Blood,* **92,** 3137–3147.

Bhatia, S., Ramsay, N. K., Steinbuch, M. et al. (1996). Malignant neoplasms following bone marrow transplantation. *Blood,* **87,** 3633–3639.

Bollard, C., Onishi, H., Huls, M. et al. (2001). Long-term follow-up of patients who received EBV-specific CTLs for the prevention or treatment of EBV-associated lymphoproliferative disease. *Biology of Blood and Marrow Transplantation,* **7,** 61 (Abstract).

Bonini, C., Ferrari, G., Verzeletti, S. et al. (1997). HSV-TK gene transfer into donor lymphocytes for control of allogeneic graft versus leukemia. *Science,* **276,** 1719–1724.

Briz, M., Fores, R., Regidor, C. et al. (1997). Epstein-Barr virus associated B-cell lymphoma after autologous bone marrow transplantation for T-cell acute lymphoblastic leukemia. *British Journal of Haematology,* **98,** 485–487.

Brooks, L., Yao, Q. Y., Rickinson, A. B., & Young, L. S. (1992). Epstein-Barr virus latent gene transcription in nasopharyngeal carcinoma cells: coexpression of EBNA1, LMP1, and LMP2 transcripts. *Journal of Virology,* **66,** 2689–2697.

Carpenter, P. A., Appelbaum, F. R., Corey, L. et al. (2002). A humanized non-FcR-binding anti-CD3 antibody, visilizumab, for treatment of steroid-refractory acute graft-versus-host disease. *Blood,* **99,** 2712–2719.

Cavazzana-Calvo, M., Bensoussan, D., Jabado, N. et al. (1998). Prevention of EBV-induced B-lymphoproliferative disorder by ex vivo marrow B-cell depletion in HLA-phenoidentical or non-identical T-depleted bone marrow transplantation. *British Journal of Haematology,* **103,** 543–551.

Chiang, K. Y., Hazlett, L. J., Godder, K. T. et al. (2001). Epstein-Barr virus-associated B cell lymphoproliferative disorder following mismatched related T cell-depleted bone marrow transplantation. *Bone Marrow Transplantation,* **28,** 1117–1123.

Claviez, A., Tiemann, M., Wagner, H. J., Dreger, P., & Suttorp, M. (2000). Epstein-Barr virus-associated post-transplant lymphoproliferative disease after bone marrow transplantation mimicking graft-versus-host disease. *Pediatric Transplantation,* **4,** 151–155.

Curtis, R. E., Travis, L. B., Rowlings, P. A. et al. (1999). Risk of lymphoproliferative disorders after bone marrow transplantation: a multi-institutional study. *Blood,* **94,** 2208–2216.

d'Amore, E. S. G., Manivel, J. C., Gajl-Peczalska, K. J. et al. (1991). B-Cell Lymphoproliferations after bone marrow transplant. *Cancer,* **68,** 1285–1294.

Davis, C. L. (1998). The antiviral prophylaxis of post-transplant lymphoproliferative disorder. *Springer Seminars in Immunopathology,* **20,** 437–453.

Davis, T. A., Czerwinski, D. K., & Levy, R. (1999). Therapy of B-cell lymphoma with anti-CD20 antibodies can result in the loss of CD20 antigen expression [In Process Citation]. *Clinical Cancer Research,* **5,** 611–615.

Deacon, E. M., Pallesen, G., Niedobitek, G. et al. (1993). Epstein-Barr virus and Hodgkin's disease: transcriptional analysis of virus latency in the malignant cells. *The Journal of Experimental Medicine,* **177,** 339–349.

Faye, A., Quartier, P., Reguerre, Y. et al. (2001). Chimaeric anti-CD20 monoclonal antibody (rituximab) in post-transplant B-lymphoproliferative disorder following stem cell transplantation in children. *British Journal of Haematology,* **115,** 112–118.

Fischer, A., Blanche, S., LeBidois, J. et al. (1991). Anti-B-cell monoclonal antibodies in the treatment of severe B-cell lymphoproliferative syndrome following bone marrow and organ transplantation. *New England Journal of Medicine,* **324,** 1451–1456.

Gartner, B. C., Schafer, H., Marggraff, K. et al. (2002). Evaluation of use of Epstein-Barr viral load in patients after allogeneic stem cell transplantation to diagnose and monitor posttransplant lymphoproliferative disease. *Journal of Clinical Microbiology,* **40,** 351–358.

Gerritsen, E. J., Stam, E. D., Hermans, J. *et al.* (1996). Risk factors for developing EBV-related B cell lymphoproliferative disorders (BLPD) after non-HLA-identical BMT in children. *Bone Marrow Transplantation,* **18,** 377–382.

Gottschalk, S., Ng, C. Y. C., Smith, C. A. *et al.* (2001). An Epstein-Barr virus deletion mutant that causes fatal lymphoproliferative disease unresponsive to virus-specific T cell therapy. *Blood,* **97,** 835–843.

Gratama, J. W., Oosterveer, M. A. P., Zwaan, F. E. *et al.* (1988). Eradication of Epstein-Barr virus by allogeneic bone marrow transplantation: implications for sites of viral latency. *Proceedings of the National Academy of Sciences USA,* **85,** 8693–8696.

Gratama, J. W., Zutter, M. M., Minarovits, J. *et al.* (1991). Expression of Epstein-Barr virus-encoded groowth-transformation-associated proteins in lymphoproliferations of bone marrow transplant recipients. *International Journal of Cancer,* **47,** 188–192.

Gross, T. G., Hinrichs, S. H., Davis, J. R. *et al.* (1998). Depletion of EBV-infected cells in donor marrow by counterflow elutriation. *Experimental Hematology,* **26,** 395–399.

Gross, T. G., Steinbuch, M., DeFor, T. *et al.* (1999). B cell lymphoproliferative disorders following hematopoietic stem cell transplantation: risk factors, treatment and outcome. *Bone Marrow Transplantation,* **23,** 251–258.

Gustafsson, A., Levitsky, V., Zou, J. Z. *et al.* (2000). Epstein-Barr virus (EBV) load in bone marrow transplant recipients at risk to develop posttransplant lymphoproliferative disease: prophylactic infusion of EBV-specific cytotoxic T cells. *Blood,* **95,** 807–814.

Hale, G. & Waldmann, H., for CAMPATH users. (1998). Risks of developing Epstein-Barr virus-related lymphoproliferative disorders after T-cell-depleted marrow transplants. *Blood,* **91,** 3079–3083.

Hanel, M., Fiedler, F., & Thorns, C. (2001). Anti-CD20 monoclonal antibody (rituximab) and cidofovir as successful treatment of an EBV-associated lymphoma with CNS involvement. *Onkologie,* **24,** 491–494.

Harris, N. L., Ferry, J. A., & Swerdlow, S. H. (1997). Posttransplant lymphoproliferative disorders: summary of Society for Hematopathology Workshop. *Seminars in Diagnostic Pathology,* **14,** 8–14.

Hauke, R. J., Greiner, T. C., Smir, B. N. *et al.* (1998). Epstein-Barr virus-associated lymphoproliferative disorder after autolgous bone marrow transplantation: report of two cases. *Bone Marrow Transplantation,* **21,** 1271–1274.

Heath, J. A., Broxson, E. H., Jr., Dole, M. G. *et al.* (2002). Epstein-Barr virus-associated lymphoma in a child undergoing an autologous stem cell rescue. *Journal of Pediatric Hematology/Oncology,* **24,** 160–163.

Henle, G., Henle, W., & Horwitz, C. (1974). Antibodies to Epstein-Barr virus-associated antigens in infectious mononucleosis. *Journal of Infectious Diseases,* **130,** 231–239.

Heslop, H. E., Brenner, M. K., & Rooney, C. M. (1994). Donor T cells to treat EBV-associated lymphoma. *New England Journal of Medicine,* **331,** 679–680.

Heslop, H. E., Li, C., Krance, R. A., Loftin, S. K., & Rooney, C. M. (1994). Epstein-Barr infection after bone marrow transplantation. *Blood,* **83,** 1706–1708.

Heslop, H. E. & Rooney, C. M. (1997). Adoptive immunotherapy of EBV lymphoproliferative diseases. *Immunological Reviews,* **157,** 217–222.

Hopwood, P., & Crawford, D. H. (2000). The role of EBV in posttransplant malignancies: a review. *Journal of Clinical Pathology,* **53,** 248–254.

Ifthikharuddin, J. J., Mieles, L. A., Rosenblatt, J. D., Ryan, C. K., & Sahasrabudhe, D. M. (2000). CD-20 expression in posttransplant lymphoproliferative disorders: treatment with rituximab. *American Journal of Hematology,* **65,** 171–173.

Koehne, G., Gallardo, H. F., Sadelain, M., & O'Reilly, R. J. (2000). Rapid selection of antigen-specific T lymphocytes by retroviral transduction. *Blood,* **96,** 109–117.

Kuehnle, I., Huls, M. H., Liu, Z. *et al.* (2000). CD20 monoclonal antibody (rituximab) for therapy of Epstein-Barr virus lymphoma after hematopoietic stem-cell transplantation. *Blood,* **95,** 1502–1505.

Lankester, A. C., van Tol, M. J., Vossen, J. M., Kroes., A. C., & Claas, E. (2002). Epstein-Barr virus (EBV)-DNA quantification in pediatric allogeneic stem cell recipients: prediction of EBV-associated lymphoproliferative disease. *Blood,* **99,** 2630–2631.

Lewin, N., Aman, P., Masucci, M. G. *et al.* (1987). Characterization of EBV-carrying B-cell populations in healthy seropositive individuals with regard to density, release of transforming virus and spontaneous outgrowth. *International Journal of Cancer,* **39,** 472–476.

Liu, Z., Wilson, J. M., Jones, M. C. *et al.* (1999). Addition of B cell depletion of donor marrow with anti-CD20 antibody to a T cell depletion regimen for prevention of EBV lymphoma after bone marrow transplant. *Blood,* **94,** 638a (Abstract).

Lones, M. A., Kirov, I., Said, J. W., Shintaku, I. P., & Neudorf, S. (2000). Post-transplant lymphoproliferative disorder after autologous peripheral stem cell transplantation in a pediatric patient. *Bone Marrow Transplantation,* **26,** 1021–1024.

Lucas, K., Small, T., Heller, G., Dupont, B., & O'Reilly, R. J. *et al.* (1996). The development of cellular immunity to Epstein-Barr virus after allogeneic bone marrow transplantation. *Blood,* **87,** 2594–2603.

Lucas, K. G., Burton, R. L., Zimmerman, S. E. *et al.* (1998). Semiquantitative Epstein-Barr virus (EBV) polymerase chain reaction for the determination of patients at risk for EBV-induced lymphoproliferative disease after stem cell transplantation. *Blood,* **91,** 3654–3661.

McGuirk, J. P., Seropian, S., Howe, G. *et al.* (1999). Use of rituximab and irradiated donor-derived lymphocytes to control Epstein-Barr virus-associated lymphoproliferation in patients undergoing related haplo-identical stem cell transplantation. *Bone Marrow Transplantation,* **24,** 1253–1258.

Mentzer, S. J., Perrine, S. P., & Faller, D. V. (2001). Epstein-Barr virus post-transplant lymphoproliferative disease and virus-specific therapy: pharmacological re-activation of viral target genes with arginine butyrate. *Transplant Infectious Disease,* **3,** 177–185.

Micallef, I. N., Chhanabhai, M., Gascoyne, R. D. *et al.* (1998). Lymphoproliferative disorders following allogeneic bone marrow transplantation: the Vancouver experience. *Bone Marrow Transplantation,* **22,** 981–987.

Milpied, N., Vasseur, B., Parquet, N. *et al.* (2000). Humanized anti-CD20 monoclonal antibody (rituximab) in posttransplant B-lymphoproliferative disorder: a retrospective analysis on 32 patients. *Annals of Oncology,* **11** (Suppl 1), 113–116.

Montagna, D., Yvon, E., Calcaterra, V. *et al.* (1999). Depletion of alloreactive T cells by a specific anti-interleukin-2 receptor p55 chain immunotoxin does not impair in vitro antileukemia and antiviral activity. *Blood,* **93,** 3550–3557.

Morrison, V. A., Dunn, D. L., Manivel, J. C., Gajl-Peczalska, K. J., & Peterson, B. A. (1994). Clinical characteristics of post-transplant lymphoproliferative disorders. *American Journal of Medicine,* **97,** 14–24.

Musk, P., Szmania, S., Galloway, A. T. *et al.* (2001). In vitro generation of Epstein-Barr virus-specific cytotoxic T cells in patients receiving haplo-identical allogeneic stem cell transplantation. *Journal of Immunotherapy,* **24,** 312–322.

Nalesnik, M. A., Locker, J., Jaffe, R. *et al.* (1988). Clonal characteristics of posttransplant lymphoproliferative disorders. *Transplantation Proceedings,* **20,** 280–283.

Oertel, S. H. & Riess, H. (2002). Immunosurveillance, immunodeficiency and lymphoproliferations. *Recent Results in Cancer Research,* **159,** 1–8.

Okano, M. (2001). Epstein-Barr virus in patients with immunodeficiency disorders. *Biomedicine & Pharmacotherapy-Biomedecine & Pharmacotherapie,* **55,** 353–361.

Openshaw, H., Nash, R. A., & McSweeney, P. A. (2002). High-dose immunosuppression and hematopoietic stem cell transplantation in autoimmune disease: clinical review. *Biology of Blood and Marrow Transplantation,* **8,** 233–248.

Orazi, A., Hromas, R. A., Neiman, R. S. *et al.* (1997). Posttransplantation lymphoproliferative disorders in bone marrow transplant recipients are aggressive diseases with a high incidence of adverse histologic and immunobiologic features. *American Journal of Clinical Pathology,* **107,** 419–429.

O'Reilly, R. J., Small, T. N., Papadopoulos, E. *et al.* (1997). Biology and adoptive cell therapy of Epstein-Barr virus-associated lymphoproliferative disorders in recipients of marrow allografts. *Immunological Reviews,* **157,** 195–216.

O'Reilly, R. J., Small, T. N., Papadopoulos, E. *et al.* (1998). Adoptive immunotherapy for Epstein-Barr virus-associated lymphoproliferative disorders complicating marrow allografts. *Seminars in Immunopathology,* **20,** 455–491.

Ozsahin, H., Le Deist, F., Benkerrou, M. *et al.* (1996). Bone marrow transplantation in 26 patients with Wiskott-Aldrich syndrome from a single center. *Journal of Pediatrics,* **129,** 238–244.

Papadopoulos, E. B., Ladanyi, M., Emanuel, D. *et al.* (1994). Infusions of donor leukocytes to treat Epstein-Barr virus-associated lymphoproliferative disorders after allogeneic bone marrow transplantation. *New England Journal of Medicine,* **330,** 1185–1191.

Peniket, A. J., Perry, A. R., Williams, C. D. *et al.* (1998). A case of EBV-associated lymphoproliferative disease following high-dose therapy and CD34-purified autologous peripheral blood progenitor transplantation. *Bone Marrow Transplantation,* **22,** 307–309.

Qu, L., & Rowe, D. T. (1992). Epstein-Barr virus latent gene expression in uncultured peripheral blood lymphocytes. *Journal of Virology,* **66,** 3715–3724.

Rea, D., Fourcade, C., Leblond, V. *et al.* (1994). Patterns of Epstein-Barr virus latent and replicative gene expression in Epstein-Barr virus B cell lymphoproliferative disorders after organ transplantation. *Transplantation,* **58,** 317–324.

Regn, S., Raffegerst, S., Chen, X. *et al.* (2001). Ex vivo generation of cytotoxic T lymphocytes specific for one or two distinct viruses for the prophylaxis of patients receiving an allogeneic bone marrow transplant. *Bone Marrow Transplantation,* **27,** 53–64.

Rickinson, A. B. (1994). EBV infection and EBV-associated tumors. In *Viruses and Cancer,* ed. A. C. Minson, J. C. Neil, & M. A. McRae, pp. 81–100. Cambridge: Cambridge University Press.

Rickinson, A. B. & Kieff, E. (1996). Epstein-Barr virus. In *Fields Virology,* ed. B. N. Fields, D. M. Knipe, & P. M. Howley, pp. 2397–2446. Philadelphia: Lipincott-Raven.

Rickinson, A. B., & Moss, D. J. (1997). Human cytotoxic T lymphocyte responses to Epstein-Barr virus infection. *Annual Review of Immunology,* **15,** 405–431.

Riddler, S. A., Breinig, M. C., & McKnight, J.L.C. (1994). Increased levels of circulating Epstein-Barr virus (EBV)-infected lymphocytes and decreased EBV nuclear antigen antibody responses are associated with the development of posttransplant lymphoproliferative disease in solid-organ transplant recipients. *Blood,* **84,** 972–984.

Riddell, S. R., Elliot, M., Lewinsohn, D. A. *et al.* (1996). T-cell mediated rejection of gene-modified HIV-specific cytotoxic T lymphocytes in HIV-infected patients. *Nature Medicine,* **2,** 216–223.

Rooney, C. M., Loftin, S. K., Holladay, M. S. *et al.* (1995a). Early identification of Epstein-Barr virus-associated post-transplant lymphoproliferative disease. *British Journal of Haematology,* **89,** 98–103.

Rooney, C. M., Smith, C. A., Ng, C. *et al.* (1995b). Use of gene-modified virus-specific T lymphocytes to control Epstein-Barr virus-related lymphoproliferation. *Lancet,* **345,** 9–13.

Rooney, C. M., Smith, C. A., Ng, C.Y.C. *et al.* (1998). Infusion of cytotoxic T cells for the prevention and treatment of Epstein-Barr virus-induced lymphoma in allogeneic transplant recipients. *Blood,* **92,** 1549–1555.

Rowe, D. T., Qu, L., Reyes, J. *et al.* (1997). Use of quantitative competitive PCR to measure Epstein-Barr virus genome load in the peripheral blood of pediatric transplant patients with lymphoproliferative disorders. *Journal of Clinical Microbiology,* **35,** 1612–1615.

Sample, J., Brooks, L., Sample, C. *et al.* (1991). Restricted Epstein-Barr virus protein expression in Burkitt lymphoma is due to a different Epstein-Barr nuclear antigen 1 transcriptional initiation site. *Proceedings of the National Academy of Sciences USA,* **88,** 6343–6347.

Sauce, D., Bodinier, M., Garin, M. *et al.* (2002). Retrovirus-mediated gene transfer in primary T lymphocytes impairs their anti-Epstein-Barr virus potential through both culture-dependent and selection process-dependent mechanisms. *Blood,* **99,** 1165–1173.

Schaar, C. G., van der Pijl, J. W., van Hoek, B. *et al.* (2001). Successful outcome with a "quintuple approach" of posttransplant lymphoproliferative disorder. *Transplantation,* **71,** 47–52.

Shapiro, R. S., McClain, K., Frizzera, G. *et al.* (1988). Epstein-Barr virus associated B cell lymphoproliferative disorders following bone marrow transplantation. *Blood,* **71,** 1234–1243.

Skinner, J. C., Gilbert, E. F., Hong, R. *et al.* (1988). B cell lymphoproliferative disorders following T cell depleted allogeneic bone marrow transplantation. *American Journal of Pediatric Hematology/Oncology,* **10,** 112–119.

Skoda-Smith, S., Douglas, V. K., Mehta, P., et al. (2001). Treatment of post-transplant lymphoproliferative disease with induction chemotherapy followed by haploidentical peripheral blood stem cell transplantation and rituximab. *Bone Marrow Transplantation,* **27,** 329–332.

Slobod, K. S., Taylor, G. H., Sandlund, J. T. *et al.* (2000). Epstein-Barr virus-targeted therapy for AIDS-related primary lymphoma of the central nervous system. *Lancet,* **356,** 1493–1494.

Sokal, E. M., Antunes, H., Beguin, C. *et al.* (1997). Early signs and risk factors for the increased incidence of Epstein-Barr virus-related posttransplant lymphoproliferative diseases in pediatric liver transplant recipients treated with tacrolimus. *Transplantation,* **64,** 1438–1442.

Stevens, S. J., Verschuuren, E. A., Pronk, I. *et al.* (2001). Frequent monitoring of Epstein-Barr virus DNA load in unfractionated whole blood is essential for early detection of posttransplant lymphoproliferative disease in high-risk patients. *Blood,* **97,** 1165–1171.

Stevens, S. J., Vervoort, M. B., van den Brule, A. J. *et al.* (1999). Monitoring of Epstein-Barr virus DNA load in peripheral blood by quantitative competitive PCR. *Journal of Clinical Microbiology,* **37,** 2852–2857.

Sun, Q., Pollok, K. E., Burton, R. L. *et al.* (1999). Simultaneous ex vivo expansion of cytomegalovirus and Epstein-Barr virus-specific cytotoxic T lymphocytes using B-lymphoblastoid cell lines expressing cytomegalovirus pp65. *Blood,* **94,** 3242–3250.

Suzan, F., Ammor, M., & Ribrag, V. (2001). Fatal reactivation of cytomegalovirus infection after use of rituximab for a post-transplantation lymphoproliferative disorder. *New England Journal of Medicine,* **345,** 1000.

Swinnen, L. J. (1998). Treatment of organ transplant-related lymphoma. *Hematology/Oncology Clinics of North America,* **11,** 963–973.

Swinnen, L. J. (1999). Overview of posttransplant B-cell lymphoproliferative disorders. *Seminars in Oncology,* **26,** 21–25.

Swinnen, L. J. (2000). Diagnosis and treatment of transplant-related lymphoma. *Annals of Oncology,* **11** (Suppl 1), 45–48.

Swinnen, L. J., Costanzo-Nordin, M. R., Fisher, S. G. *et al.* (1990). Increased incidence of lymphoproliferative disorder after immunosuppression with the monoclonal antibody OKT3 in cardiac-transplant recipients. *New England Journal of Medicine,* **323,** 1723–1728.

Swinnen, L. J., Mullen, G. M., Carr, T. J., Costanzo, M. R., & Fisher, R. I. (1995). Aggressive treatment for postcardiac transplant lymphoproliferation. *Blood,* **86,** 3333–3340.

Thomis, D. C., Marktel, S., Bonini, C. *et al.* (2001). A Fas-based suicide switch in human T cells for the treatment of graft-versus-host disease. *Blood,* **97,** 1249–1257.

Tiberghien, P., Ferrand, C., Lioure, B. *et al.* (2001). Administration of herpes simplex-thymidine kinase-expressing donor T cells with a T-cell-depleted allogeneic marrow graft. *Blood,* **97,** 63–72.

Tierney, R. J., Steven, N., Young, L. S., & Rickinson, A. B. (1994). Epstein-Barr virus latency in blood mononuclear cells: analysis of viral gene transcription during primary infection and in the carrier state. *Journal of Virology,* **68,** 7374–7385.

Trainor, K. J., Brisco, M. J., Wan, J. H. *et al.* (1991). Gene rearrangement in B-and T-lymphoproliferative disease detected by the polymerase chain reaction. *Blood,* **78,** 192–196.

van Esser, J. W., Niesters, H. G., van der, H. B. *et al.* (2002). Prevention of Epstein-Barr virus-lymphoproliferative disease by molecular monitoring and preemptive rituximab in high-risk patients after allogeneic stem cell transplantation. *Blood,* **99,** 4364–4369.

van Esser, J. W., van der, H. B., Meijer, E. *et al.* (2001). Epstein-Barr virus (EBV) reactivation is a frequent event after allogeneic stem cell transplantation (SCT) and quantitatively predicts EBV-lymphoproliferative disease following T-cell–depleted SCT. *Blood,* **98,** 972–978.

Verschuuren, E. A., Stevens, S. J., van Imhoff, G. W. *et al.* (2002). Treatment of posttransplant lymphoproliferative disease with rituximab: the remission, the relapse, and the complication. *Transplantation,* **73,** 100–104.

Wagner, H. J., Cheng, Y. C., Liu, Z. *et al.* (2001). Monitoring of transplanted patients at risk of Epstein-Barr virus (EBV)-induced lymphoproliferative disorder (LPD) by real time PCR quantification of EBV DNA in peripheral blood. *Blood,* **98** (Suppl 1), 480a (Abstract).

PART X ORGAN-SPECIFIC COMPLICATIONS

89 Gastrointestinal, hepatic, gallbladder, pancreatic, and perianal complications

RAYMOND McCRUDDEN, DAVID B. WILLIAMS, TERENCE O'CONNOR, AND CHRISTOPHER R. VICKERS

St. Vincent's Hospital and University of New South Wales, Sydney, Australia

Introduction to gastrointestinal complications

The impact of the gastroenterologist assessing patients pre and post hematopoietic stem cell (HSC) transplant has been poorly defined. In one study the commonest problems where gastroenterology consultation was sought included the possibility of graft-versus-host disease, diarrhea, vomiting, upper and lower gastrointestinal bleeding, dysphagia, abdominal pain, and anorexia (Fallows, Rubinger, & Bernstein, 2001). Out of 79 patients reviewed for GI problems a change in management was noted in 54%. Gastrointestinal disease was a cause of death in 2.5%.

Virtually all patients develop a disturbance of the gastrointestinal (GI) tract following hematopoietic stem cell (HSC) transplantation. The main problems experienced by patients can be grouped as follows:

1. Graft-versus-host disease (GVHD)
2. Opportunistic infection
3. Toxicity due to drugs, radiation, or total parenteral nutrition (TPN)

These are not exclusive and some or all may be present concurrently. Most patients experience oral mucositis, nausea or vomiting, and some degree of diarrhea especially during the first month posttransplant. The underlying causes require early diagnosis and specific antimicrobial/antiviral treatment or increased immunosuppression may be required. There is an overlap between risk of infection, GVHD, and immunosuppression. Severe intestinal or hepatic damage can result in significant morbidity and mortality, even when the donor stem cells have engrafted and are functioning.

GI symptoms prior to transplantation should be investigated as the opportunity early posttransplant may be restricted by thrombocytopenia and neutropenia. A history of peptic ulcer disease or recent dyspepsia requires exclusion of active ulceration. Prior GI or biliary sepsis needs careful evaluation. Oral cavity lesions prior to transplant should be addressed. In a small study of 88 patients, the incidence of oral *Candida albicans* was 15.5% and correlated with mouth dryness or reduced basal saliva secretion (Herman *et al.*, 2002).

Common GI problems early after HSC transplantation

The major problems after marrow transplantation are shown in Table 89.1. These normally occur early after transplant (within the first 2 months).

Nausea/vomiting

Nausea and vomiting after HSC transplantation can be caused by the following:

1. Chemoradiotherapy
2. Medications, particularly nystatin or amphotericin oral suspension, cotrimoxazole, oxpentifylline, methotrexate, and occasionally cyclosporine
3. GVHD of the GI tract, especially of the upper GI tract
4. Hepatic disease including GVHD and viral hepatitis
5. Infection involving the esophagus, stomach, or intestine (usually viral or fungal, occasionally bacterial)
6. Occasionally pancreatitis, abdominal abscess

During the first 14 to 21 days posttransplant severe nausea or vomiting, abdominal pain, and watery diarrhea may develop as a result of pretransplant chemotherapy or chemoradiation. Prolonged or intractable retching, vomiting, and hiccuping are distressing complaints and symptomatic treatment with conventional antiemetic therapy may be required. The vomiting should be minimized for symptomatic relief and to reduce the risk of an esophageal tear (Mallory-Weiss syndrome)[1] or gastric mucosal hemorrhage. There is evidence that inflammation of the stomach and upper intestine may alter the pharmacokinetics of cyclosporine (Schultz *et al.*, 1998, 2000). In a series of 82 patients the incidence of antiemetic outcome was prospectively evaluated following HSC transplantation (Ballen *et al.*, 2001). Following the initiation of chemotherapy the percentage of patients with emesis was day 1: 13%, day 2: 21%,

---

[1] Kenneth Mallory, American pathologist, born 1900. Soma Weiss, American physician, 1898–1942.

day 3: 30%, day 4: 38%, day 5: 44%, day 6: 39%, and day 7: 18%. A previous history of emesis, use of total body irradiation, type of transplant, or use of dexamethasone did not affect emesis control. Most patients receiving high-dose chemotherapy experienced emesis that was difficult to control, suggesting that new treatment approaches are needed to improve emesis control in this group of patients. With regard to toxicity from myeloablative therapy, the gut mucosa barrier may also play a role in the efficacy of HSC transplantation. There is accumulating evidence too that disruption to the mucosal surface can be detected prior to clinical findings (Johansson & Ekman, 1997). In a group of 17 patients the gastrointestinal wall permeability was assessed through nuclear imaging techniques (^{51}Cr-EDTA absorption test) before the start of cytotoxic therapy and again at days 4, 7, and 14 post HSC transplant (Johansson, Brune, & Ekman, 2001). Myeloablative therapy significantly increased intestinal permeability in contrast to those who received reduced intensity conditioning (RIC). It is possible that GI tract damage may, through myeloablative therapy, be an important factor in the initiation of GVHD. A randomized pilot study examining the efficacy of an oral immunological preparation (IgA-IgG) administered from day 1 to one week after chemotherapy found that there was significantly less permeability in the treatment group compared to the placebo group (Johansson & Ekman, 1999), signifying that IgA-IgG had a protective effect on the gut mucosa which would normally be damaged during the myeloablative regimen.

Persistent vomiting or retching after day 14 may be due to acute GVHD or opportunistic intestinal infection, or a combination of both (Wu *et al.*, 1998). Posttransplantat lymphoproliferative disorder of the stomach has also been described (Jacobson, Paterson, & Carr-Locke, 2000). Care must be taken to provide fluid and electrolyte replacement in order to prevent metabolic alkalosis and the development of paralytic ileus. Gastroparesis can cause nausea, vomiting, and bloating. In a retrospective analysis it was confirmed by scintigraphic study in 26% of allografted patients but in no autograft recipients (Eagle *et al.*, 2001). The median day of onset was 54 (range 34–113) days posttransplant. GVHD and CMV infection did not appear to play a role. Patients usually respond to prokinetic agents.

Diarrhea

Causes of diarrhea after marrow transplantation include the following:

1. Chemotherapy or chemoradiotherapy
2. Intestinal GVHD
3. Intestinal infections—viral [e.g. cytomegalovirus (CMV)], parasites [e.g., *Giardia, Strongyloides* (Chim *et al.*, 1997)], fungal (e.g., *Candida*)
4. Drugs (e.g., nonabsorbable antibiotics)
5. Pseudomembranous colitis, secondary to antibiotic therapy and caused by *Clostridium difficile*

Diarrhea usually develops after day 4 posttransplant and may be associated with abdominal pain. Stool cultures should always be taken. Mild symptoms can usually be controlled by conventional antidiarrheal and antispasmodic medication. A profuse watery or hemorrhagic diarrhea is most likely due to acute GVHD or infective enteritis and can be a significant management problem. In a prospective study, 150 acute diarrheal episodes developed in 126 patients posttransplant (Cox *et al.*, 1994). Acute GVHD was responsible for 48%, and an infection for 13%, of these episodes. Intestinal infection was found in 20 of the 150 episodes and the agents involved included viruses (astrovirus, adenovirus, CMV, and rotavirus) in 12 patients, hospital-acquired bacteria (*Clostridium difficile* and *Aeromonas*) in 7 patients, and mixed infection in one patient. In 39% of episodes no clear etiology could be found for self-limited diarrhea. *C. difficile* infection accounts for about 15%–25% of antibiotic-associated diarrhea occurring in approximately 5%–7% of autologous transplant recipients and 5%–15% of allograft recipients (Tomblyn *et al.*, 2002). In one study a strong association was found with grade II–IV acute GVHD (Chakrabarti *et al.*, 2000). In another study of infectious diarrhea posttransplant in 60 adult allogeneic and autologous recipients, 31 out of 48 patients had acute diarrheal episodes, occuring in 79% of allogeneic patients and 47% of autologous recipients (van Kraaij *et al.*, 2000). Infectious diarrhea was found in 6% of cases. Interestingly intestinal pathogens were isolated in 13 out of 172 stool specimens in asymptomatic individuals and included: rotavirus (4), adenovirus (3), *C. difficile* toxin (2), and others. In 40 of 48 (83%) episodes of diarrhea no clear cause was found. In terms of symptoms, large volume secretory diarrhea (liters per day) may be difficult to control, but usually settles with specific therapy of the underlying cause and adequate fluid replacement. Octreotide can substantially reduce stool output in both acute gut GVHD and chemoradiation-related toxicity (Ely *et al.*, 1991; Morton & Durrant, 1995; Crouch *et al.*, 1996; Wasserman *et al.*, 1997). It is essential to perform endoscopy, in conjunction with stool culture, if a cause other than chemoradiotherapy toxicity is considered possible. Multiple biopsies should be taken as long as the platelet count is greater than 50×10^9/l and coagulation parameters are normal at the time of biopsy. Diarrhea of any cause markedly interferes with absorption of oral cyclosporine and can be an indication for institution, or continuation, of the intravenous preparation (Atkinson *et al.*, 1984).

Bleeding

In contrast to the general population, HSC transplant patients are often younger and without cardiovascular disease. They do, however, suffer from intestinal necrosis, ablation of immunity, and thrombocytopenia in relation to cytoreductive therapy (Schwartz *et al.*, 2001). Minor GI bleeding occurs not infrequently in the early posttransplant period. It settles with correction of thrombocytopenia and abnormal clotting factor profiles.

Table 89.1. *Major common GI complaints early after HSC transplantation and respective causes*

Nausea and vomiting	Dysphagia and odynophagia	Diarrhea	Abdominal pain	Large volume bleeding	Ileus
Chemoradiotherapy	Esophageal mucositis from the conditioning regimen	Chemotherapy Chemoradiotherapy	Duodenal/gastric ulcer	Duodenal/gastric ulcer	Drugs, especially opiate analgesics
Medications e.g., nystatin, amphotericin, cotrimoxazole, oxpentifylline, methotrexate, cyclosporine	Antibiotic esophagitis (doxycycline, tetracycline)	Drugs e.g., nonabsorbable antibiotics, mycophenolate	Hemorrhagic cystitis	Small bowel or colonic ulcer (often secondary to CMV)	Sepsis
GVHD of the upper GI tract	GVHD involving the esophagus	Intestinal GVHD	Intestinal GVHD	Acute GVHD	Acute intestinal GVHD
Hepatic disease including GVHD and viral hepatitis	Reflux esophagitis		Liver disease: viral hepatitis veno-occlusive disease abscess	Previous rectal biopsy site	Electrolyte abnormalities, especially hypokalemia
Infection: esophagus, stomach, or intestine (usually viral or fungal, occasionally bacterial)	Esophageal infection (viral, fungal)	Infections Viral e.g., CMV Parasites e.g., *Giardia*, *Strongyloides* Fungal e.g., *Candida*	Intestinal infection (CMV, *Candida*, *Clostridium difficile*)	Viral of fungal ulcers (rare)	Intestinal infection, including CMV enteritis, *Candida* enteritis
Occasionally pancreatitis abdominal abscess		Pseudomembranous colitis	Pancreatitis Gall bladder disease	Post HSCT for systemic amyloid	Pancreatitis Abdominal abscess
Post transplantation lymphoproliferative disorder of the stomach			Herpes zoster Bleeding into rectus sheath Neutropenic colitis	Gastric erosions	Pneumonia

Abbreviations: GVHD, graft-versus-host disease; CMV, cytomegalovirus.

Causes include esophagitis (viral, fungal, or peptic), acute GVHD, viral enteritis, and perianal fissures or hemorrhoids. Rarely bleeding may be large volume and the more likely causes are

1. Duodenal or gastric ulcer
2. Small bowel or colonic ulcer (often CMV)
3. Previous rectal biopsy site
4. Acute GVHD
5. Gastric erosions

Appropriate endoscopic investigation is essential if bleeding is significant. Kaur and colleagues (1996) investigated overt GI bleeding in a series of 579 consecutive bone marrow transplant recipients. Bleeding manifestations included hematemesis ($n = 24$), melena ($n = 8$), hematochezia ($n = 7$), and combinations ($n = 4$). The median time from bone marrow infusion to the onset of overt GI bleeding was 7.5 (range 0–45) days. Fourteen patients had evidence of orthostatic hypotension attributable to GI bleeding. Upper endoscopy was performed in 26 patients; 18 had diffuse esophagitis and gastritis. Two patients with bleeding ulcers underwent electrocautery. Colonoscopy was performed in five patients and revealed a cecal ulcer on one subject, tumor recurrence in one person, and colitis in another. No patient underwent surgical intervention. One patient died as a result of GI bleeding.

The incidence of acute bleeding was investigated in 1,402 patients receiving transplants between 1986 and 1995 (Nevo et al., 1998). Ten percent had minor GI bleeding; 14% of patients had a moderate to severe GI tract heamorrhage during the first 100 days. Bleeding was noted more frequently after allogeneic transplants than autologus transplants and may have been related to GVHD-related bleeding and bleeding due to infections. An overall decrease in survival was noted in those who developed bleeding. Other studies have also demonstrated an association between poorer survival and incidence of GI bleeding in HSC transplant patients (Price et al., 1998). It is possible that bleeding may act as a surrogate marker for the extent of the conditioning regimen-related tissue damage (Kumar et al., 2001) and other major transplant-related complications such as GHVD, but in the case of the latter, few studies have set out to examine this in detail (Nevo et al., 1999). Nevo and colleagues examined a cohort of allogeneic HSC transplant patients specifically with the intention of documenting the timing of bleeding in relation to GVHD. The incidence of GVHD was 27.4% and that of bleeding overall was 40.2%. Out of 143 patients with moderate to severe bleeding episodes the incidence of GI bleeding was 92 (64.3%). The incidence of bleeding was higher in those with GVHD and correlated with GVHD severity. In GI hemorrhage, median survival of 26 patients with GVHD was 3.4 months which was statistically significantly reduced compared to 9.1 months in the non-GVHD group; this has been documented previously (Nevo et al., 1998). There was a significant delay in the onset of GI bleeding in those with acute GVHD with a mean time of onset of 54 days compared to 29 days in the non GVHD group. There was no correlation with thrombocy-topenia in the GVHD group. In the non-GVHD group, bleeding severity correlated with outcome; in the GVHD group any bleeding, however minor, was a poor prognosistic sign in GVHD stages 2–4. Late GI hemorrhage may be related to slow epithelial recovery after GVHD or late infections (Fox, Vogelsang, & Beschorner, 1996).

The incidence of severe GI bleeding, causes, and outcome was investigated in a case series of 1,102 patients (Schwartz et al., 2001). All HSC transplant patients were followed up during the period of 1986–1987 and again in 1996–1997 to examine for any changes in prevalence of bleeding. The incidence of severe GI bleeding over this decade fell significantly from 50 of 467 (10.7%) to 15 of 635 (2.4%). The overall mortality fell from 3.9% to 0.9%, but the mortality in those with bleeding remained high (34% vs. 40%) especialy in those with GVHD. The time of onset was the same for both groups (around a median of 42 vs. 47 days) but the causes of bleeding were remarkably different. For the period 1986–1987, 27 of 50 cases bled from multiple GI sites, viral and fungal ulcers, or GVHD. In the later group, the incidence of GVHD was decreased by 80% and the incidence of viral and fungal ulcers had all but disappeared. GVHD was still the most common underlying cause, accounting for 7 of 15 cases with other causes being duodenal diverticula, gastric antral vascular ectasia, and, in one case, a Dieulafoy[2] lesion. In 12 of 15 cases the causes were in the upper GI tract, of whom two stopped bleeding spontaneously with platelet transfusions. Of the three patients who bled from lower GI tract lesions, 2 stopped spontaneously with platelet transfusions.

GI bleeding occurring as a complication of autologous transplantation has been reported in the setting of amyoidosis (for review see Gertz, Lacy, & Dispenzieri, 2000). In a series of 23 patients GI tract bleeding was noted in 5 patients after high dose melphalan and stem cell rescue for amyloidosis (Comenzo et al., 1998). The same authors noted an incidence of 7% after modification of the chemotherapy (Comenzo et al., 1999). In a series of 45 patients who underwent HSC transplantation for systemic amyloidosis, 9 patients (20%) had GI bleeding in the immediate posttransplantation period (median 9.5 days range 1–48) (Kumar et al., 2001), which is earlier than that seen for other HSC transplant patients (Schwartz et al., 2001). Kumar reported that patients with multiorgan failure and those on hemodialysis tended to have a higher incidence of gastrointestinal blood loss. Upper GI tract endoscopy revealed diffuse esophagitis and gastritis in most cases, with 1 case of hemorrhagic mucosa, 1 patient with internal hemorrhoids and 1 with a Mallory-Weiss tear in combination with a duodenal ulcer and adherent clot. In two cases interventional endoscopy was required to stop bleeding and achieve hemostasis. The reason for the increased incidence of GI bleeding post HSC transplantation remains unclear in these patients. Intensive care stay was prolonged with the overall hospital stay being more than

---

[2] Georges Dieulafoy, French physician, 1839–1911.

doubled among those in whom bleeding developed. One case report described gastrointestinal perforation early after peripheral blood stem cell transplantation for AL amyloidosis leading to death at 4 days (Schulenburg et al., 1998). Persistent upper GI bleeding has been treated with somatostatin when platelet transfusion support was not effective (Sambresqui et al., 1995).

Sudden massive GI hemorrhage has been noted in one case report of CMV enteritis causing segmental ischemia of the duodenum and jejunum (Keates et al., 2001). In rare cases complications can arise from endoscopy itself, for example from duodenal biopsy leading to duodenal hematoma (Wolford & McDonald, 1988; Ramakrishna & Treem, 1997; Worynski et al., 1998), bleeding from endoscopic cautery or injection therapy site leading to more extensive mucosal injury (Schwartz et al., 2001), and subconjunctival hemorrhage (Rajvanshi & McDonald, 2001). In 1993 the role of endoscopy leading to clinical sepsis in HSC transplant patients was examined (Kaw, Przepiorka, & Sekas, 1993): 25 patients received prophylactic antiobiotics and 28 did not. No evidence of bacteremia was noted in either group attributable to endoscopic procedures and the investigators concluded that not all HSC transplant recipients require routine antibiotic prophylaxis prior to endoscopic procedures. No trials have examined the efficacy of proton pump inhibitors over H_2 antagonists in the HSC transplant setting.

The following recommendations can be made for the management of acute GI bleeding:

1. Restore hemodynamic parameters with blood and give platelets if the platelet count is <50,000/μl
2. Prompt upper gastroscopy to rule out treatable causes (such as viral ulcers or vascular ectasia) with, for example, adrenaline injection, electrocautery, or argon plasma coagulation, and to rule out viral infections or GVHD with antral biopsies
3. Consider an omeprazole infusion if there is an acute ulcer with signs of early risk of re-bleeding such as a spurting vessel or visible vessel (Lau et al., 2000b).
4. Consider a proton pump inhibitor such as omeprazole or lanzoprazole for ulcerative lesions or esophagitis/gastritis over a histamine$_2$ antagonist.
5. Continue platelet transfusions if there is generalized mucosal ooze from gastric/duodenal erosions secondary to acute intestinal GVHD.

Dysphagia/odynophagia

Causes of dysphagia/odynophagia after HSC transplantation are shown in Table 89.1 and include the following:

1. Esophageal mucositis from the conditioning regimen
2. Esophageal infection (viral, Candida)
3. Reflux esophagitis
4. GVHD involving the esophagus
5. Antibiotic esophagitis (doxycycline, tetracycline)

Esophageal discomfort is not uncommon early after HSC transplantation as a consequence of conditioning regimen-related toxicity and usually resolves by day 21. Esophageal symptoms developing after this time require investigation by means of endoscopy and mucosal biopsy to diagnose herpes simplex, CMV, or Candida esophagitis, after which appropriate treatment can be instituted. Reflux esophagitis can be treated with H_2 receptor antagonists such as ranitidine. Proton proton pump inhibitors such as omeprazole can be utilized for persistent symptoms.

Abdominal pain

Causes of abdominal pain after HSC transplantation are shown in Table 89.1 and include the following:

1. Intestinal GVHD
2. Intestinal infection (CMV, Candida, Clostridium difficile)
3. Liver disease—viral hepatitis, veno-occlusive disease, abscess
4. Pancreatitis
5. Duodenal/gastric ulcer
6. Hemorrhagic cystitis
7. Herpes zoster (Schiller et al., 1991)
8. Bleeding into rectus sheath
9. Gall bladder disease
10. Neutropenic colitis

Erect and supine abdominal x-rays, together with appropriate endoscopic examination or computed tomography (CT) scanning, should be considered to evaluate abdominal pain. Ultrasound and Doppler flow studies may be useful in assessing hepatobiliary disease.

Ileus

Causes of ileus after marrow transplantation are shown in Table 89.1. and include the following:

1. Drugs, especially opiate analgesics
2. Sepsis
3. Acute intestinal GVHD
4. Electrolyte abnormalities, especially hypokalemia
5. Intestinal infection, including CMV enteritis, Candida enteritis
6. Pancreatitis
7. Abdominal abscess
8. Pneumonia

Supportive management of ileus requires correction of fluid and electrolyte deficits, and attention to nutritional status. Cessation of oral intake is advisable and nasogastric tube decompression may be necessary. Caution in passing a tube should be taken in the patient with significant thrombocytopenia or coagulopathy. Specific therapy of the underlying problem usually results in resolution of ileus, but recovery may be prolonged.

Nutrition

Maintenance of nutrition, fluid, and electrolyte balance is vital during the critical first 3 to 4 weeks posttransplant (Muscaritoli *et al.*, 2002). Oral intake may be negligible because of nausea, vomiting, and anorexia. Significant protein and fluid losses can occur through diarrhea. TPN must be initiated early to maintain weight and nutrition and to reduce catabolism. TPN allows for modulation of fluid, electrolyte, and macronutrient administration, which is important when complications occur such as GVHD or hepatic veno-occlusive disease (VOD) occur. For example, in the case of VOD complicated by hepatic encephalopathy, the need for enriching the feed with branched chain amino acids has been emphasized. A lipid-based TPN preparation may be associated with a lower incidence of lethal acute GVHD in allogeneic HSC transplant patients (Muscaritoli *et al.*, 1998). In one study TPN appeared to be superior to partial parenteral nutrition during the early posttransplant period (Hwang, Chiang, & Wang, 2001). Naso-jejunal feeding appears to be effective in children (Sefcick *et al.*, 2001). Nasogastric tube feeding in children has also been successful, but requires intensive multidisciplinary input to ensure success (Langdana *et al.*, 2001). Vitamin B12 1,000 μg is recommended for all patients pretransplant, together with a multivitamin preparation/folic acid 5 mg daily and Vitamin K 10 mg subcutaneously weekly during intravenous feeding. Conversion to oral feeding should be instituted as soon as possible to stimulate bile flow and reduce the risk of gall bladder sludge syndrome. Severe hypophasphatemia during hematopietic reconstitution after allogeneic HSC transplantation has been reported (Steiner *et al.*, 2000), suggesting that regular phosphate monitoring and replacement, in addition to electrolyte surveillance, may be useful around this time.

A number of observations have been made regarding low body mass index in HSC transplant recipients (Nysom *et al.*, 2000; Schimmer *et al.*, 2001; Kananen *et al.*, 2002), though it remains to be proven that nutrional status has an impact on this. Weight loss and malnutrition do occur post HSC transplantation (Iestra *et al.*, 2002; Jacobsohn *et al.*, 2002): elevated resting energy expenditure and elevated TNF-α levels may play a part. A lowered body mass index (BMI) may be an independent risk factor for mortality (Jacobsohn *et al.*, 2002). In one prospective study, despite intensive nutritional and dietitics input in patients who had received total body irradiation, body weight could not be restored to 95% of the pretreatment level within 1 year of the transplant. Anorexia, dry mouth, altered taste, nausea, and tiredness are generally the most common symptoms associated with eating difficulties (Iestra *et al.*, 2002).

Obesity has been shown to be an independent risk factor for complications posttransplant (Tarella *et al.*, 2000; Meloni *et al.*, 2001).

GI problems presenting later posttransplant

Once the patient has recovered from the early acute complications of marrow transplant, GI tract symptoms become consid-

erably less common. However, up to 50% of HLA-identical sibling marrow transplant recipients may develop chronic GVHD, which can occasionally cause malnutrition, intestinal strictures, or malabsorption (Sullivan *et al.*, 1981). Opportunistic infection (e.g., CMV enteritis) can recur, but usually within the first year posttransplant, and often when moderate-to-severe chronic GVHD (not necessarily of the GI tract) is present (Atkinson *et al.*, 1995).

Major GI organ complications

The major GI organ complications following bone marrow transplantation are summarized in Table 89.2.

Mouth

In the posttransplant period the oral cavity can be a source of distressing symptoms. Careful daily examination is required for opportunistic infection. Prophylactic fluconazole, antifungal lozenges or oral suspension are prescribed daily, as oral candidiasis is common. Mucositis and mouth ulceration are frequent, due to the pretransplant conditioning regimen and the use of methotrexate as GVHD prophylaxis. Stomatitis from herpes simplex virus I (HSV-1) is particularly painful, and may extend into the laryngopharynx and upper esophagus. Prophylactic acyclovir is effective in minimizing the occurrence of HSV infection.

Various studies have demonstrated that significant oral mucositis occurs in about 75% of patients who undergo an HSC transplant after myeloablative conditioning (Pico, Avila-Garavito, & Naccache, 1998; for reviews see Blijlevens Donnelly, & De Pauw, 2000; Stiff, 2001): In two surveys, 42%–65% of patients felt it was the most debilitating transplant experience (Bellm *et al.*, 2000; Stiff, 2001). Two major events appear to produce mucositis: direct injury caused by the ablative regimen and local infections of the damaged mucosal surface, which is then exacerbated by neutropenia (Sonis, 1998; Wilkes, 1998; Cairncross *et al.*, 2000). Significant risk factors for mucositis include a diagnosis of leukemia, the use of total body irradiation in the preparative regimen, and allogeneic HSC transplant (Rapoport *et al.*, 1999). Recent research has focused on intervention in aspects of mucosal ulceration and infection. Keratinocyte growth factor and interleukin-11 have activity in increasing basal cell proliferation, preventing apoptosis in the region and ameliorating the mucositis seen with high-dose chemotherapy regimens (Stiff, 2001). It has been suggested that mucositis be renamed mucosal barrier injury (Blijlevens, Donnelly, & De Pauw, 2000). Sucralfate may have a role in reducing mucosal injury if given prophylactically (Castagna *et al.*, 2001). Dental care must be optimized prior to transplant (Borowski *et al.*, 1994: Carl, 1995; Barker, 1999; Yeager *et al.*, 2000). Caries or dental abscesses must be treated. Gingivitis requires expert attention to dental hygiene.

Acute GVHD may rarely affect the mouth and cause a painful glossitis and stomatitis. Chronic GVHD with mucositis

Table 89.2. *Major GI organ complications*

Organ	<21 days posttransplant	>21 days posttransplant
Mouth	Conditioning regimen–induced mucositis Infection: *Candida*, HSV	Infection: *Candida*, HSV Acute GVHD Chronic GVHD Xerostomia due to conditioning regimen
Esophagus	Conditioning regimen–induced mucositis Reflux esophagitis	Infection: HSV, CMV, *Candida* Reflux esophagitis Acute GVHD "Pill" ulceration Chronic GVHD
Stomach	Mallory-Weiss tear Conditioning regimen–induced gastritis	CMV gastritis Peptic ulceration Acute GVHD
Duodenum	Conditioning regimen–induced duodenitis	CMV duodenitis Peptic ulceration Acute/chronic GVHD
Small intestine/colon	Conditioning regimen–induced enteritis Neutropenic colitis	CMV enteritis/colitis Pseudomembranous colitis

Abbreviations: HSV, herpes simplex virus; GVHD, graft-versus-host disease; CMV, cytomegalovirus.

and xerostomia can lead to dysphagia and weight loss (Schubert *et al.*, 1984). Rarely, fibrous webs in the oro- and laryngopharynx can form, and need excision or dilatation (McDonald *et al.*, 1986b). Dental caries can progress rampantly in the presence of xerostomia. Xerostomia may also be a consequence of the pretransplant conditioning regimen.

Later posttransplant, gingival hyperplasia can occur and is a side effect of cyclosporine. Gingival hyperplasia normally resolves with reduction in dosage, or cessation, of cyclosporine. Nongingival soft tissue growths in the mouth have also been described, arising as lumps from the buccal mucosa or tongue (Woo *et al.*, 1996).

Esophagus

In the first few days following transplant, endoscopy can reveal areas of epithelial desquamation, a cytotoxic effect of the conditioning regimen. The patient may experience retrosternal discomfort, dysphagia from transient esophageal hypomotility, or symptoms of gastroesophageal reflux. Prophylactic oral antifungal treatment should be maintained, together with acid suppression therapy such as proton pump inhibitors. Oral cytoprotective agents, such as sucralfate dissolved in water, are also effective.

Opportunistic viral infection may be present when symptoms persist or occur for the first time after day 14, usually coinciding with recovery of granulocyte counts. Severe odynophagia and ulceration of the esophagus can occur, CMV and HSV-1 being the usual pathogens (McDonald *et al.*, 1985). Endoscopy and biopsy should always be performed as specific

therapy is warranted. Endoscopic appearances range from discrete vesicles to large coalescent ulcers in the distal esophagus. Perforation into the pleural or peritoneal cavity is rare. Biopsies should be taken of both ulcerated and nonulcerated regions since virus may not be found in necrotic areas. HSV infection usually responds to acyclovir, whereas CMV is best treated with ganciclovir or foscarnet.

Esophageal candidiasis can present with acute odynophagia in the absence of oral infection. Endoscopic features range from superficial erosions to large ulcers. Brushings and culture of biopsy material can be useful in cases seemingly refractory to antifungal therapy. Esophageal aspergillosis is rare (Choi *et al.*, 1997).

Acute GVHD may present with symptoms of dysphagia and odynophagia, although the esophageal mucosa usually appears normal despite extensive intestinal disease. Esophageal ulceration may also result from local toxicity due to delayed transit of certain drugs ("pill esophagitis"); the most common are tetracycline, ketoconazole, and erythromycin. They should be taken in a sitting position with liberal fluids.

Esophageal involvement with chronic GVHD is uncommon and may rarely result in a scleroderma-like esophagus with hypomotility, dysphagia, and reflux (McDonald *et al.*, 1986b) or with dysphagia and odynophagia (Sodhi, Srinivasan, & Thomas, 2000). Lesions usually involve the upper to midesophagus with desquamation, webs, and tapering strictures. Esophageal clearing is often poor and the occasional patient will develop distal stricturing due to acid peptic reflux (McDonald, Sullivan, & Plumely, 1984). Symptomatic relief may be achieved with acid suppression therapy and prokinetic agents such as cisapride. Dilatation of webs and strictures may be beneficial. Even with generalized desquamation of the esophageal epithelium, complete resolution can be obtained with high-dose immunosuppression (Sodhi, Srinivasan, & Thomas, 2000). Severe esophagitis documented by endoscopy has been reported in lymphoma patients receiving autologous HSC transplantation (Vishny et al., 1994). Severe esophagitis also occurring both early and late after allogeneic transplantation (and not associated with GVHD) has been described in patients transplanted for Fanconi anemia (Yakoub-Agha et al., 2000). In all five cases there was subsequent stricture formation. Severe esophageal strictures have also been described after autologous bone marrow transplantation (Memoli et al., 1988; Stemmelin et al., 1995; Ghavamzadeh et al., 1999), though in the most recent report this may have been due to the underlying disease (dyskeratosis congenita).

Stomach and duodenum

Nausea and epigastric discomfort associated with an erosive antral gastritis or duodenitis is relatively common early post-transplant and is often related to the conditioning regimen, gastric infection with CMV, occasionally HSV (Kingreen et al., 1997) and, in one case report, varicella zoster (Rivera-Vaquerizo et al., 2001); infection may also be found in conjunction with gastric or duodenal ulceration. Protein-losing gastritis associated with CMV infection has been described (Pinho et al., 1996).

GVHD was originally thought to affect the stomach less commonly than the lower GI tract, although an acute upper gastrointestinal GVHD syndrome had been recognized (Weisdorf et al., 1990). In a study of 76 patients with 78 episodes of nausea and vomiting after HSC transplantation the diagnosis was found to be acute GVHD of the stomach in 63 patients (81%), with an additional 4 patients (5%) who had concurrent causes. Infection by herpes simplex virus, CMV, or Candida was found in 6 patients, three of whom had concurrent GVHD. Lymphocytic gastritis causing nausea, vomiting, and anorexia has been described in recipients of autologous transplants (Tzung et al., 1998). All patients responded to oral prednisolone. Its pathogenesis is currently unclear.

Few studies have evaluated the correlation between endoscopic and histological diagnosis. In a small case series from Seattle, 10 patients with acute upper intestinal GVHD were studied with endoscopic abnormalities compared to histological assessments (Ponec, Hackman, & McDonald, 1999). No correlation was found with endoscopic signs and histological diagnosis. Histological findings included crypt epithelial cell apoptosis, crypt destruction, and variable lymphocytic infiltration of the epithelium and lamina propria. Extent of involvement was also variable ranging from diffuse and uniform to focal areas in the stomach and duodenum, highlighting the necessity of obtaining adequate gastric biopsies. Antral biopsies alone (as opposed to antral and duodenal) were adequate to make the diagnosis, though endoscopic

assessment and histology of gastric specimens could not accurately grade the severity of acute GVHD elsewhere in the intestine unless extensive mucosal sloughing was seen. The histological diagnosis of intestinal GVHD is not straightforward (Bombi et al., 1995; Wakui et al., 1999). The reproducibility of diagnosis and recognition of gastric GVHD was examined in a blinded study of 56 gastric biopsy specimens (24 allotransplants, 32 controls) (Washington et al., 1997). The blinded histological diagnosis of gastric GVHD had a false-positivity rate of 24% and this was due to CMV gastritis, HIV infection, primary immunodeficiency, and status after renal transplantation. In view of these findings, guidelines for endoscopists and histologists have been proposed (Ponec, Hackman, & McDonald, 1999).

Small intestine and colon

The most serious complication involving the small intestine and colon is acute GVHD, occurring in 20% to 50% of patients given HLA-identical sibling marrow. It develops within 2 to 10 weeks of transplantation and usually in conjunction with skin and/or liver involvement (for review see Iqbal et al., 2000). Intestinal GVHD is predominantly specific to allogeneic transplantation (Wakui et al., 1999). One case report exists of intestinal GVHD in a syngeneic HSC transplant recipient (Spaner et al., 1998). Clinical grading is based on the extent and severity of target organ damage (McDonald et al., 1986b; van Bekkum, 1991; Ferrara & Deeg, 1991). Risk factors for development of acute GVHD include HLA-identical unrelated donor, HLA mismatch, increasing donor parity, donor-recipient sex mismatch, increasing donor or patient age, ineffective GVHD prophylaxis, intensity of the conditioning regimen, and prior herpes virus infection (Nash et al., 1992; Tabbara, 1996).

Although anorexia, nausea, and high-volume diarrhea are common, there is a wide overlap of symptoms and signs of other intestinal disease such as opportunistic infection, C. difficile infection, chemoradiation toxicity, medication-induced side effects, or other lesions such as gastric or duodenal ulceration (Spencer et al., 1986; Weisdorf et al., 1990; Roy et al., 1991; Cox et al., 1994; Wu et al., 1998). Roy reported that there was no significant difference in clinical presentation in those patients undergoing endoscopy with or without GVHD (Roy et al., 1991). Diagnosis on clinical grounds alone can therefore be difficult. However, with evidence that GVHD is a progressive disease and that early intervention changes outcome, a rapid and accurate diagnosis is imperative (Nash et al., 1992).

Wu prospectively evaluated 78 patients with persistent nausea and anorexia after HSC transplantation with endoscopy and found acute intestinal GVHD in 81%. With early intervention a high response rate to prednisolone was noted (Wu et al., 1998). A retrospective analysis of clinical, endoscopic, histological, and microbiological data was obtained during the evaluation and treatment of 61 distinct episodes of unexplained gastrointestinal complaints in 37 adult allogeneic bone marrow transplant recipients. Twelve of the 61 events (20%) were due to acute intestinal GVHD. Gastrointestinal infections were found in 14 of the 61 episodes (23%); and were due to herpesviruses (8 of 61) and fungi (9 of 61) (Terdiman *et al.,* 1996). Patients with and without GVHD were similar in terms of their age, sex, underlying illness, clinical symptoms and signs, physical examination, laboratory values, and endoscopic findings. Small-bowel biopsy had a sensitivity of 90% for detecting the pathological changes of acute intestinal graft-versus-host disease in this series. It was concluded that gastrointestinal GVHD cannot be accurately diagnosed from its clinical presentation and that endoscopic small-bowel biopsy is an essential tool in evaluating patients with upper GI symptoms.

Symptoms produced by intestinal injury may be the most disabling. Fluid, protein, and mineral depletion resulting from diarrhea and malabsorption can produce severe nutritional deficits (Papadopoulou *et al.,* 1996), requiring prolonged TPN or isoosmotic enteral feeding. In a prospective study of GI function after transplant, acute GVHD produced severe protein-losing enteropathy and resulted in greater decline in nutritional status and sense of well-being (Papadopoulou *et al.,* 1996). Profuse diarrhea is usually accompanied by abdominal cramps, nausea, and vomiting. Diarrheal volumes of up to 15 l/day may occur.

Fecal fluid that is greenish and watery with exfoliated debris is characteristic. Diarrhea may be either secretory or exudative (Ghilain *et al.,* 1990). Frank hemorrhage or perforation can ensue from deep ulceration. Signs of peritonism can be found in severe cases, indicating full thickness inflammation of the intestinal wall with serositis. Although this clinical presentation suggests acute GVHD, other diagnoses for consideration include infection and toxic effects of chemoradiation therapy. CMV enteritis can mimic acute GVHD in its clinical features and frequently coexists (Einsele *et al.,* 1994). The diagnosis of concurrent CMV infection is important, since dissemination may follow immunosuppression administered for GVHD. Jejunal vasculitis and necrotizing enteritis have been reported (Jafri *et al.,* 1990). Stool should be examined for bacterial pathogens, fungi, parasites (e.g. *Giardia, Cryptosporidium*) and *Clostridium difficile* toxin. Rotavirus or other enteroviruses have been described as a cause of diarrhea posttransplant (Townsend *et al.,* 1982).

Endoscopic appearances in acute GVHD may range from normal to frank mucosal ulceration (Terdiman *et al.,* 1996). Endoscopic features that may suggest the presence of intestinal GVHD include hyperemia and diffuse mucosal loss. Although mucosal edema is a common and non-specific finding sloughing of the mucosa is infrequent but highly specific (Ponec, Hackman, & McDonald, 1999). Since GVHD most prominently involves the ileum and right colon, the rectal mucosa is often macroscopically normal. There is accumulating evidence that the single most useful marker of intestinal GVHD is epithelial cell apoptosis (Epstein *et al.,* 1980; Gallucci *et al.,* 1982; Snover *et al.,* Snover, 1990; Bombi *et al.,* 1995). Identical histologic findings before day 20 can also be induced by the pretransplant conditioning regimen (McDonald *et al.,* 1986b).

Imaging has a role in the diagnosis of intestinal GVHD particularly in those patients who are too unwell to undergo endoscopy. Abdominal x-ray appearances may be normal or reveal extensive changes throughout the gut. Mucosal edema can be suggested by thumb printing and luminal irregularity, most noticeable in the distal small intestine. Pneumatosis cystoides intestinalis may be present. Radiologic barium follow-through studies show rapid transit with dilatation and coarse thickening of valvulae conniventes and the intestinal wall (Fisk *et al.,* 1981). Technetium (^{99m}Tc)-labeled white cell scanning and intestinal permeability studies using ^{51}Cr-EDTA and ^{14}C-mannitol have been used to assess extent and severity of disease (Mahendra *et al.,* 1994). Severe ulcerative acute GVHD may heal with submucosal fibrosis and the development of luminal strictures or webs. Increased bowel wall thickness associated with substantial bowel wall enhancement with gadolinium chelate can be documented with magnetic resonance imaging (MRI) (Worawartanakul *et al.,* 1996). More experience and improvements with software are warranted in the context of prospective trials to determine if MRI is reliable in determining severity of GVHD and in distinguishing it from infections. Bowel wall thickening and an additional echogenic double layer in a patient with severe intestinal GVHD has been reported with the use of ultrasound (Haber *et al.,* 2000). The latter finding may signify severe mucosal ulceration with coating of the mucosal surface with sloughed membranes. High resolution ultrasound (HRU) and color Doppler imaging (CDI) have been incorporated in a small series of 12 patients suspected of having intestinal GVHD and/or severe cutaneous GVHD (Klein *et al.,* 2001). All patients showed thickened bowel wall segments, especially in the ileocecal areas. Even in patients with no clinical features of intestinal GVHD, intestinal involvement in 3 of 12 cases was noted. In 4 of 12 cases an increased arterial blood flow in the bowel wall could be demonstrated, which correlated with evidence of inflammation at endoscopic biopsy. In 4 of 12 cases ischemic bowel wall lesions with a high resistance flow pattern in the superior mesenteric artery was noted. In these patients there was no response to immunosuppression and they subsequently died. It is possible therefore that HRU and CDI are useful imaging parameters, not only in the early diagnosis of intestinal GVHD, but also in predicting the severity of acute GVHD and identifying patients with a poor prognosis. Severity of intestinal GVHD may be assessed by assays of leukotriene B4 and other cytokines such as tumour necrosis factor-α (TNE-α) and interferon-γ (Takatsuka *et al.,* 2000).

Treatment of severe acute GVHD can prove difficult. Severe disease is associated with reduced survival and a higher risk of infectious complications. Studies suggest a clinical response rate of about 40% using high-dose corticosteroids and second-line therapy of cyclosporine and antithymocyte globulin (ATG) (Martin *et al.,* 1990, 1991; Nishi *et al.,* 2001). A similar response rate was seen in steroid-refractory disease treated with monoclonal interleukin-2 receptor antibody (Anasetti *et al.,* 1994). The use of direct intramesenteric artery injection with steroids for severe intestinal GVHD has been reported (Sato et al., 1997). To counteract the systemic effects of corticosteroids, promising results have been obtained with different preparations of steroids such as beclomethasone diprionate (McDonald et al., 1998), budesonide capsules (Bertz et al., 1999), and betamethasone enemas (Wada et al., 2001). Other agents that have been examined include thalidomide (Browne et al., 2000), colostrum (Inoue et al., 1998), and lactoferrin (Inoue et al., 2001).

Infection should be ruled out in the work-up for any patient with suspected intestinal GVHD. Stool cultures can reveal a variety of agents. There is one case report of intestinal GVHD being made on stool smears revealing detached intestinal cells with apoptosis detected by the DNA nick end labeling method (Hirano et al., 1999).

Management requires urgent diagnosis by endoscopic tissue biopsy. Exclusion of CMV infection by means of immunoperoxidase staining for CMV early antigen or polymerase chain reaction (PCR) techniques should be made. Vigilance for Gram-negative sepsis and concurrent CMV infection is mandatory. Reinstitution of prophylactic ganciclovir during severe gut GVHD, even if CMV is not demonstrated to be present, should be considered. Maintenance of antifungal and PCP prophylaxis during severe GVHD and its treatment is strongly recommended. Occasionally, surgical resection may be necessary, for example for massive bleeding (Evans et al., 1998).

Chronic GVHD is a complex, autoimmune-like multisystem disorder. Gut involvement can result in mucosal atrophy, malabsorption, and rarely, segmental fibrotic strictures of the small intestine. In a series of 232 children, where 17 symptomatic individuals (7.3%) had evidence of chronic intestinal GVHD, the clinical, histological, and immunohistochemical features of the disease were reported (Patey-Mariaud de Serre et al., 2002). Chronic GVHD was part of a systemic syndrome in 88% of cases and was preceded by acute intestinal GVHD in 88% of cases. Complete recovery occurred in only 58% cases and death due to GVHD occurred in 17% of cases. Histological features included villous atrophy, glandular lesions (mainly apoptotic with variable intesity), and lamina propria infiltrate with cytotoxic T lymphocytes (CD3+, CD8+, TiA1+, granzyme B−), which were significantly increased compared to non-GVHD controls. The intensity of the histological features correlated poorly with the severity of the disease. As with acute intestinal GVHD, the best marker for disease was epithelial cell apoptosis. A bacterial overgrowth syndrome can develop and responds to broad-spectrum antibiotics (McDonald et al., 1986b). Specific therapy of chronic GVHD early in the course of the disease with immunosuppression is often effective, more than 50% of patients being able to discontinue treatment after 9 to 12 months (Tabbara, 1996). Treatment of intestinal injury is also directed at maintaining body weight with protein, vitamin, and mineral supplementation. A low-disaccharide, high-caloric, and low-fat diet may be required to reduce malabsorption. Medium-chain triglycerides and pancreatic exocrine replacement can be tried empirically. Stricturoplasty or surgical

resection may be necessary for obstructive symptoms (Evans et al., 1998).

Neutropenic colitis

This uncommon disorder is seen in severely neutropenic patients whose peripheral leukocyte count is less than 0.5×10^9/l (Kliegman & Fanaroff, 1984; Kliegman, Walker, & Yolken, 1993). It thus occurs early after transplantation, and has a considerable mortality rate. It occurs most commonly in the cecum and ascending colon and is characterized by a direct toxic mucosal necrosis, which may spread throughout all layers of the intestinal wall and results in perforation of the colon. It is most likely due to direct bacterial invasion of the colon with local release of enterotoxin. The patient usually develops pain and tenderness in the right iliac fossa (typhlitis). Signs of peritonism may be present but may not necessarily indicate perforation. Close clinical review is necessary for the development of progressive signs, and daily erect chest x-ray for evidence of pneumoperitoneum. CT scans are useful when abdominal films are unhelpful (Boggio et al., 2000). An edematous cecum and/or right colon, spiculation, and inflammation of the pericolic fat, and pneumatosis are diagnostic of typhlitis. Intensive broad-spectrum antibiotic therapy is indicated. Granulocyte transfusions may be necessary, but the risk of introducing CMV disease should be weighed carefully. An alternative to granulocyte transfusions is the use of a hematopoietic growth factor, such as granulocyte colony-stimulating factor G-CSF or granulocyte-macrophage colony-stimulating factor (GM-CSF), to accelerate neutrophil recovery. The colon will recover once the peripheral neutrophil count is reconstituted. Surgery requires subtotal colectomy and defunctioning ileostomy and has a high mortality. Nevertheless, it may be the only option in a patient who is acutely unwell and septic. Gas-forming clostridial species often supervene in neutropenic colitis, and produce an intense acute necrotizing fasciitis through adjacent tissue planes. Wide surgical debridement of necrotic fascia may be required, with high-dose penicillin and hyperbaric oxygen treatment.

Infective colitis

CMV infection commonly involves the small intestine and colon, typically occurring 1 to 3 months after transplantation. The risk of infection is enhanced by the occurrence and severity of acute GVHD (Tabbara, 1996). Presentation can be similar to acute GVHD, with diarrhea, pain, ulceration, and protein-losing enteropathy. The right colon and ileum appear most often involved, with deep ulceration sometimes leading to massive bleeding and perforation (Goodman, Boitnott, & Yardley, 1979; West et al., 1982). Colonoscopy can generally be undertaken with safety as long as bleeding parameters are satisfactory, but care regarding perforation must be taken if focal deep ulcers are found. Biopsy specimens from both ulcerated and grossly normal mucosa can reveal typical CMV inclusions or CMV RNA using PCR technology (Einsele et al., 1994).

Colitis due to herpes simplex infection has also been described posttransplant (Naik & Chandrasekar, 1996).

Other causes of diarrhea in the posttransplant population include antibiotic-associated diarrhea (*C. difficile* infection), bacillary dysentery, or opportunistic infection with *Cryptosporidium* or *Candida*. Stool cultures and colonoscopy or sigmoidoscopy should be performed. The endoscopic findings of yellow plaques of mucosal edema typical of *Clostridium difficile* infection are often not found in granulocytopenic patients, and empirical treatment with oral vancomycin or metronidazole may be required (Bartlett, 2002). There is an association with *C. difficile* infection and GVHD with increased nonrelapse mortality (Chakrabarti *et al.*, 2000). It is possible that *C. difficile* toxin may predispose to a more severe grade of GVHD and therefore worsening outcome. Pneumatosis cystoides intestinalis, a poorly understood phenomenon thought to result from mucosal injury, with free air mimicking intestinal perforation has been described after allogeneic marrow transplantation (Navari *et al.*, 1983; Lipton *et al.*, 1994; Kurbegov & Sondheimer, 2001; Zülke *et al.*, 2002).

Endoscopy in HSC transplant recipients

The role of endoscopy was examined in patients undergoing autologous HSC transplantation for relapsed Hodgkin's and non-Hodgkin's lymphoma in 65 consecutive patients (Vishny *et al.*, 1994). 41 patients (38 of whom had chest irradiation) underwent 48 endoscopies for upper GI bleeding (12 of 48), persistent nausea and (7 of 48), odynophagia (25 of 48), and dysphagia (14 of 48). All patients who had dysphagia or odynophagia had endoscopic evidence of severe esophagitis, with confluent erosions or ulcerations. Gastrointestinal bleeding, which presented as melena or hematemesis, was caused by severe esophagitis in 11 of 12 patients. Yeasts were detected in 11 of 42 histological, or cytological specimens and were isolated in 4 of 26 cultures. No bleeding or infectious complications occurred in any patient as a result of the endoscopy procedure.

Screening endoscopy before and after HSC transplantation is a safe procedure and detects a high number of GI abnormalities. A prospective study of screening upper gastrointestinal endoscopy before HSC transplantation was undertaken in 24 allogeneic and 17 autologous patients (Forbes *et al.*, 1995) and repeated on two occasions at day 30 and day 120 posttransplant: 21 of 41 patients (51%) had an abnormality which necessitated a change in treatment; 10 of the 41 had abnormalities pretransplant, 10 of 32 (31%) at day 30 posttransplant, and 7 of 22 (32%) at day 120. Pathology included mucosal erosions or ulcers (22), infections (5), and previously undiagnosed GVHD (3). In 8 of 28 endoscopies, erosions or ulceration was present despite patients being on regular antacid therapy.

With regard to colonoscopy or sigmodoscopy, patients are often too unwell to tolerate a large volume oral bowel preparation In the sick patient with diarrhea the procedure can usually be performed without preparation. Due to risk of perforation, care should be taken to limit air insufflation in cases of severe viral colitis, severe GVHD, or neutropenic colitis. Perforation, with subsequent death, occurred in 1.8% of patients in one series (Fallows, Rubinger, & Bernstein, 2001).

Introduction to hepatic complications

Abnormalities of liver function tests are commonly seen after hematopoietic stem cell transplantation (McDonald *et al.*, 1986a, 1986b; Liatsos *et al.*, 2001). Determination of the cause of the liver dysfunction is helped by the fact that some liver diseases tend to occur within certain intervals following transplantation.

The most common cause of serious dysfunction within the first 20 days is VOD, in which acute liver toxicity occurs as a result of pretransplant chemotherapy or chemoradiotherapy. Jaundice from day 20 to day 100 may be due to acute GVHD. Bacterial and fungal infection of the liver is more common within the first 50 days, when the peripheral leukocyte count is often low. Viral infections tend to occur later in the posttransplant period as a result of immune suppression. Hepatotoxicity due to drugs, total parenteral nutrition, and the biliary sludge syndrome may occur at any time; perhaps the most common single cause of hepatic dysfunction posttransplant, however, is cyclosporine hepatotoxicity. The liver function test profile can be helpful in distinguishing the different hepatic disorders that occur posttransplant.

The type of donor, pretransplant viral serology, transfusion history, and extent of immunosuppression also assist in establishing a diagnosis. In many cases the cause is multifactorial. Because these factors may vary from center to center and country to country, the relative frequency of different causes of hepatic dysfunction may vary (Kim *et al.*, 2000). A time course of liver complications after HSC transplantation is shown in Table 89.3.

Pre-existing liver disease in candidates for HSC transplantation

It is important to carefully evaluate the presence of liver disease prior to HSC transplantation, as there is potentially an increased risk of hepatic VOD, chronic hepatitis, or fungemia. The clinical assessment should take into consideration the underlying hematological disease, family history, transfusion history, drug history, liver function and clotting tests, viral serology, liver imaging and histology of any liver biopsy undertaken (Liatsos *et al.*, 2001).

Pretransplant liver biopsy may be required in patients with abnormal liver enzymes or clinical stigmata of chronic liver disease for assessment of fibrosis or cirrhosis (Strasser & McDonald, 1999b), but may not always be practicable. If coagulation or ascites prevents a transthoracic approach then the transjugular route is a suitable alternative; this latter approach also allows multiple passes, measurement of hepatic venography, and, in some centers, CO_2 portography, wedged hepatic venous and caval pressure measurements (Papatheodoridis *et al.*, 1999; Vlachogiannakos *et al.*, 2000).

Table 89.3. *Major hepatic complications posttransplant*

0–20 days posttransplant	21–100 days posttransplant	>100 days posttransplant
Acute GVHD	Acute GVHD	GVHD
Drug-induced toxicity	Drug-induced toxicity	Drug induced toxicity
Bacterial sepsis	HBV and HCV infection	HBV and HCV infection
Fungal infection	Veno-occlusive disease	Sepsis
Veno-occlusive disease	CMV, HSV, VZV infection	Nodular regenerative hyperplasia
	Adenovirus infection	
	Children around day 40	
	Adults around day 90	
Viral hepatitis	EBV-PTLD	
	Sepsis	
	Veno-occlusive disease	

Abbreviations: CMV, cytomegalovirus; EBV-PTLD, Epstein-Barr virus posttransplant lymphoproliferative disease; GVHD, graft-versus-host disease; HBV, hepatitis B virus; HCV, hepatitis C virus; HSV, herpes simplex virus; VZV, varicella zoster virus.

Viral hepatitis (and see Chapter 74)

Assessment of hepatitis B virus (HBV) in both donor and recipient pretransplant

Hepatitis B virus (HBV) serology should be ascertained for both recipient and donor prior to transplant. In addition to HBV surface antigen (HbsAg) and anti-HBs, total antibody to hepatitis B core (anti-HBc) should be assessed as it may confirm recent infection or ongoing infection during the window period when HbsAg disappears and anti-HBs has not yet appeared. Anti-HBc IgM is helpful in delineating acute infection. If these screening tests are positive, the following additional tests should be obtained: E antigen markers (HBeAg and anti-HBe) provide information regarding level of viremia, but it is the detection of HBV DNA that confirms active viral replication. HBV DNA should always be measured, therefore, in both recipient and donor even if HbeAg is absent, as this may signify precore genetic mutants. If HBV DNA is positive in either donor or recipient, then appropriate prophylactic antiviral treatment should be considered pretransplant (this is discussed in the discussion of hepatitis B posttransplant below). An interpretation of serum hepatitis markers in recipients and potential donors prior to HSC transplantation is outlined in Table 89.4.

Hepatitis B infection in the recipient

HBV infection in the recipient should not be a contraindication to transplant per se; however, the recipient should be screened for evidence of pre-existing cirrhosis or fibrosis, as this may be a risk factor for subsequent VOD (Strasser & McDonald, 1999b). While evidence of viral replication may be low pretransplant there is a risk of reactivation during the period of impaired cellular immunity seen in the first 3–6 months posttransplant. Reconstitution of cellular immunity posttransplant, consequent to tapering or withdrawal of immunosuppressive therapy, can lead to a hepatitis which in some patients may progress to fulminant hepatic failure (see below). The risk of reactivation may be particularly high in those with chronic GVHD (Seth *et al.*, 2002).

Hepatitis B infection in the donor

There is clear evidence that hepatitis B infection can be transferred from donor to recipient (Strasser & McDonald, (1999b). The subsequent infection may have a worse prognosis in recipients who have never been exposed to the virus compared to those who have previously been infected and are now immune (Chen *et al.*, 1995; Locasciulli *et al.*, 1995a; Ustun *et al.*, 1997). If the donor is HBV DNA negative then the risk of transfer of infection is low (Strasser & McDonald, 1999b). For donors who are currently infected (HBV DNA positive), prophylactic treatment should be considered with antiviral therapy (see below).

Assessment of hepatitis C virus (HCV) in both donor and recipient pretransplant

It is not uncommon for patients who have had hematologic disease to come to transplant with active hepatitis C virus (HCV) infection especially if they were recipients of a blood transfusion prior to routine blood donor screening for HCV (Strasser *et al.*, 1999a; Leung *et al.*, 2000). Although the incidence of transfusion-associated infection has declined, injection drug use and high-risk sexual behavior continue to be major risk factors in the general population (Alter *et al.*, 1999). Serological testing alone for HCV may be inadequate to exclude infection in immunocompromised patients, therefore some recommend that testing should include PCR for HCV RNA (Locasciulli *et al.*, 1998). A guide to serological assessment for hepatitis C is presented in Table 89.4.

Hepatitis C in recipient pretransplant. It is important to identify HCV infected individuals before transplant, so that any underlying liver disease may be fully investigated. In addition to an assessment for signs of chronic liver disease and biochemical markers of hepatitis, a liver biopsy should be considered, particularly if there is evidence, or a clinical suspicion, of fibrosis/cirrhosis, length of infection over 10 years or a history of concurrent high alcohol intake (Strasser & McDonald, 1999b). Individuals with evidence of fibrosis or cirrhosis are at significant risk of VOD posttransplant (Strasser *et al.*, 1999a).

Table 89.4. *Guidelines for the management of patients and/or donors who have serum markers of viral hepatitis during pretransplant evaluation*

Virus	Recipient (patient) result	Donor result	Interpretation	Guidelines
Hepatitis A virus	HAV IgG antibody positive	Negative	Recipient has had remote infection	No impact on HSCT
	HAV IgG antibody negative	HAV IgG antibody positive	Donor has had remote infection	No impact on HSCT
	HAV IgM antibody positive	HAV IgM antibody negative	Recipient has recently acquired infection with HAV	Delay HSCT, possible risk of VOD
	HAV IgM antibody negative	HAV IgM antibody positive	Donor has recently acquired infection with HAV	Delay HSCT, potential risk of transmission of HAV to recipient
Hepatitis B virus	Positive antibody to HBsAg	All HBV tests negative	Recipient has had prior exposure to HBV (may also have antibodies to HBcAg) or has been vaccinated (no antibodies to HBcAg); immunity is present	No impact on HSCT
	All HBV tests negative	Positive antibody to HBsAg	Donor has had prior exposure to HBV or has been vaccinated; immunity is present	No impact on transplant; recipient may develop antibodies to HBsAg+ post HSCT (passive immunity)
	Positive antibody to HBcAg (negative HBsAg and no antibody to HBsAg)	All HBV tests negative	Recipient has had prior exposure to HBV; can indicate presence of latent HBV	Risk of activation of HBV post HSCT; if so, there is a risk of severe hepatitis B
				Test recipient for HBV DNA at day 14; consider lamivudine immediately if HBV DNA positive
				Consider immunizing the allogeneic donor with recombinant HBV vaccine
	All HBV tests negative	Positive antibody to HBcAg (negative HBsAg and no antibody to HBsAg)	Donor has had prior exposure to HBV; can indicate presence of latent HBV	Test donor for HBV DNA; if negative, little risk to the recipient post HSCT
				If HBV DNA positive consider lamivudine
	HBsAg positive or HBeAg positive or HBV DNA positive	All HBV tests negative	Recipient has HBV infection currently; remote or recent acquisition; may have normal liver, chronic hepatitis, or cirrhosis	3 potential risks for the recipient post HSCT
				VOD (if hepatitis or cirrhosis present)
				Fulminant hepatitis B (10–15%)
				Chronic hepatitis
				Consider immunizing the allogeneic donor with recombinant hepatitis B vaccine
	HBsAg positive or HBeAg positive or HBV DNA positive	Positive antibody to HBsAg	Recipient has HBV infection currently; remote or recent acquisition; may have normal liver, chronic hepatitis, or cirrhosis	3 potential risks for the recipient post HSCT
			Donor has had prior exposure to HBV or has been vaccinated; immunity is present	VOD (if hepatitis or cirrhosis present)
				Fulminant hepatitis B (10–15%)
				Chronic hepatitis
				Donor may confer cellular and humeral immunity to recipient posttransplant
				Treat recipient pre HSCT if HBV DNA positive with lamivudine

(continues)

Table 89.4. (continued)

Virus	Recipient (patient) result	Donor result	Interpretation	Guidelines
	HBsAg positive or HBeAg positive or HBV DNA positive	HBVcAb positive	Recipient has HBV infection currently; remote or recent acquisition; may have normal liver, chronic hepatitis, or cirrhosis. Donor has had prior exposure to HBV; can indicate presence of latent HBV	3 potential risks for the recipient post HSCT: VOD (if hepatitis or cirrhosis present); Fulminant hepatitis B (10–15%); Chronic hepatitis. Treat recipient pre HSCT if HBV DNA positive with lamivudine
	HBsAg positive or HBeAg positive or HBV DNA positive	HBsAg positive or HBeAg positive or HBV DNA positive	Both recipient and donor have HBV infection or remote acquisition; may have normal liver, chronic hepatitis, or cirrhosis	3 potential risks for the recipient post HSCT: VOD (if hepatitis or cirrhosis present); Fulminant hepatitis B (10–15%); Chronic hepatitis. Theoretical risk for the donor during anesthesia if cirrhosis is present. Treat recipient pre HSCT if HBV DNA positive with lamivudine
	All HBV tests negative	HBsAg positive or HBeAg positive or HBV DNA positive	Donor has HBV infection currently; remote or recent acquisition; may have normal liver, chronic hepatitis, or cirrhosis	Theoretical risk for the donor during anesthesia if cirrhosis is present. Risk of transmission of HBV to the patient; risks of fulminant hepatitis or chronic hepatitis posttransplant. Consider treating the HBV-infected donor with antiviral medications, e.g., with lamivudine, to reduce the risk of transmission of HBV (up to 6 months prescription)
	Positive antibody to HBsAg	HBsAg positive or HBeAg positive or HBV DNA positive	Recipient has had prior exposure to HBV or has been vaccinated; immunity is present. Donor has HBV infection currently; remote or recent; may have normal liver, chronic hepatitis, or cirrhosis	Potential risk for the donor during anesthesia if cirrhosis is present. Recipient's immunity to HBV may be ablated by conditioning therapy. Risk of transmission of HBV to the patient; risks of fulminant hepatitis: monitor HBV DNA at day 14 post HSCT in recipient

	Positive antibody to HBcAg	HBsAg positive or HBeAg positive or HBV DNA positive	Recipient has had prior exposure to HBV; can indicate occult infection (i.e., risk of reactivation HBV) Donor has HBV infection currently; remote or recent; may have normal liver, chronic hepatitis, or cirrhosis	Potential risk for the donor during anesthesia if cirrhosis is present Risk of acquiring the donor's HBV or activation of the patient's latent HBV post HSCT or both; monitor HBV DNA at day 14 post HSCT in recipient Consider using another equally HLA-matched donor if one is available Consider treating the HBV-infected donor with antiviral medications to reduce the risk of transmission of HBV (up to 6 month prescription)
Hepatitis C virus	Positive antibody to HCV but HCV RNA negative	All HCV tests negative	Patient has acquired antibodies by passive transfer or has been previously infected by HCV or is still infected by HCV but a relatively insensitive test for HCV RNA was used	Likely no impact on HSCT Possibility of appearance of HCV posttransplant Consider repeating PCR for HCV RNA
	Positive antibody to HCV and HCV RNA positive	All HCV tests negative	Recipient has HCV infection currently. Recipient may have normal liver, chronic hepatitis, or cirrhosis	Three potential risks for the patient post HSCT: VOD (if hepatitis or cirrhosis is present); fulminant hepatitis C (<1% risk); and chronic hepatitis
	All HCV tests negative	Positive antibody to HCV and HCV RNA positive	Donor has HCV infection currently. Donor may have normal liver, chronic hepatitis, or cirrhosis	Potential risk for the donor during anesthesia if cirrhosis is present Very high risk of transmission of HCV to the patient; risks of fulminant hepatitis (1%) or chronic hepatitis post HSCT. Consider using another equally HLA-matched donor, if one is available. Consider treating the HCV-infected donor with interferon alpha and ribavirin combination therapy until HCV RNA in serum is negative, to reduce risk of transmission of HCV to the patient (1–3 months may be needed).

Abbreviations: HAV, hepatitis A virus; HSCT, hematopoietic stem cell transplantation; VOD, veno-occlusive disease; HBsAg, hepatitis B surface antigen; HBV, hepatitis B virus; HBcAg, hepatitis B core antigen; HBeAg, hepatitis Be antigen; HCV, hepatitis C virus.

In those without evidence of cirrhosis or fibrosis there is as yet no consensus regarding treatment pretransplant (interferon itself may be hazardous to the patient), but HCV infection per se should not be considered a contraindication to HSC transplantation (Ribas & Gale, 1997).

Hepatitis C in the donor pretransplant.   Hepatitis C virus is invariably transmitted from infected donors to recipients (see below). This transmission may be preventable if the donor is considered for combination therapy prior to transplant and if time is available (Vance *et al.*, 1996; Di Bisceglie, McHutchison, & Rice, 2002), bearing in mind that the optimal treatment time to obtain eradication of HCV in an individual is of the order of six to twelve months. Undetectable viremia can be obtained after 3 months of treatment; therefore, HSC harvest can be obtained at this time (with interferon stopped one week prior in order to avoid problems with engraftment in the recipient); combination therapy can then be recommenced for the donor to complete the treatment regimen (Strasser & McDonald, 1999b).

Other causes of viral hepatitis

In aplastic anemia a viral etiology has been implicated as a causitive factor, with unidentified types of viral hepatitis being the most common cause for hepatitis-associated aplastic anemia (HAAA) (Safadi *et al.*, 2001). In a prevalence study of 68 patients with aplastic anaemia who underwent HSC transplantation, the prevalence of biochemical markers of hepatitis pretransplant was 17 out of 68. In 15 cases where serological samples were available, none had evidence of active hepatitis A, B, C, D, E, G, or TTV virus infection at the time of diagnosis. Two cases of parvovirus were identified, though in both this was following blood transfusion. Relapsing hepatitis was not observed in any patients posttransplant. The etiological agent associated with HAAA remains unclear.

Hepatitis G (GB/C) or HGV has been identified in 1.5%–4% of routine blood donors (Strasser & McDonald, 1999b) and is readily transmitted by blood product transfusion (Wang *et al.*, 1996). Thirty-one percent to 65% of HSC transplant recipients have evidence of HGV infection (Rodriguez-Inigo *et al.*, 1997; Skidmore *et al.*, 1997). There is accumulating evidence that it has no role in either acute or chronic liver disease (Corbi *et al.*, 1997; Tomas *et al.*, 1997; Akiyama *et al.*, 1998; Maruta *et al.*, 1999).

Fungal liver disease

Immunosuppressed patients may harbor fungi that, following transplantation, may disseminate during the granulocytopenic stage. Fungal liver disease is usually heralded by fever, tender hepatomegaly, and an elevated serum alkaline phosphatase. Fungal microabcesses may not be detectable on standard imaging studies, but hepatosplenic candidiasis characteristically shows small lucent areas in liver, spleen, and kidneys on abdominal computed tomography (CT) scanning. Even with effective antifungal treatment, these lucent areas do not always resolve radiologically. Liver biopsy or fine needle aspiration is usually required for confirmation.

Biliary disease

An upper abdominal ultrasound should be performed during the transplant assessment for gallstones in patients with an appropriate history. Patients with asymptomatic gallstones are managed conservatively. Symptomatic gallstones should be removed prior to transplantation, for example by laparascopic cholecystectomy. Biliary-type pain, a dilated common bile duct on ultrasound, or cholestatic liver enzymes should always be investigated and treated prior to transplantation. Bacterial cholangitis in the posttransplant patient may be rapidly fatal. Surgical or endoscopic clearance of bile duct stones posttransplant may be hazardous because of thrombocytopenia. Temporary biliary drainage can usually be achieved with an endoscopically placed stent. It is strongly advised, however, that biliary stents be removed prior to the initiation of the pretransplant conditioning regimen, because of the associated high risk of Gram-negative, particularly *Pseudomonas,* sepsis. Percutaneous transhepatic biliary procedures are generally inadvisable because of the risk of hemobilia and bleeding from the liver capsule.

Liver disease following transplantation: the first 100 days

A diagnostic algorithm is presented in Table 89.5 for cases of abnormal liver function.

Veno-occlusive disease (and see Chapters 77 and 82)

The most serious early primary liver complication posttransplant is VOD or "sinusoidal obstruction syndrome" (for review see Bearman, 2001) and represents regimen-related toxicity after high-dose cytoreductive conditioning therapy. It is the main reason for the dose limitation of current cytoreductive protocols for HSC transplantation (Atkinson *et al.*, 1987; Brodsky *et al.*, 1990; Ozkaynak *et al.*, 1991). VOD is usually seen by day 20 posttransplant, characterized clinically by jaundice, painful hepatomegaly, weight gain more than 2% above baseline, ascites, and histologically by diffuse damage in the centrilobular zone of the liver (McDonald *et al.*, 1986a, 1986b). Sudden severe thrombocytopenia can be a striking feature, as can dyspnea due to tense ascites and concomitant pleural effusions. Clinical features can occur prior to the infusion of stem cells or may develop later than day 20 (Toh *et al.*, 1999).

The incidence of VOD ranges up to 54% in several large series (Jones *et al.*, 1987; McDonald *et al.*, 1993). There may be an increased incidence with the utilization of more intense conditioning protocols (McDonald *et al.*, 1993). Severe disease occurs in up to 27% of cases and is frequently followed by progressive multiorgan failure (McDonald *et al.*, 1993). Mortality rates of 98% by day 100 have been reported for severe VOD. Predictive models based on jaundice and weight gain to estimate probability of severe VOD and fatality have high specificity but only moderate sensitivity (Bearman *et al.*, 1993a).

Table 89.5. *Diagnostic algorithm in cases of abnormal liver function tests post bone marrow transplantation*

Hepatitis picture		Cholestatic picture			
Viral hepatitis (> Day 40 usually)	Drugs (Day 0–40)	GVHD (Acute > Day 15, Chronic > Day 100)	Drugs (Day 0–40)	Sepsis (Day 0–40)	VOD (Day 0-30 usually)
HBV DNA HCV PCR Serology/PCR for CMV, HSV, VZV Adenovirus	Exclude other causes	Diagnose clinically or consider liver biopsy	Exclude other causes	Consider tuberculosis and cholangitis lenta	Diagnose clinically or consider liver biopsy Ultrasound

Abbreviations: CMV, cytomegalovirus; GVHD, graft-versus-host disease; HBV, hepatitis B virus; HCV, hepatitis C virus; HSV, herpes simplex virus; PCR, polymerase chain reaction; VOD, veno-occlusive disease; VZV, varicella zoster virus.

Risk factors for the development of VOD have been identified: elevated transaminases prior to conditioning, vancomycin therapy (as a marker for persistent fever), cytoreductive therapy with a high-dose regimen; gemtuzumab ozogamicin (Mylotarg) therapy (Rajvanshi *et al.*, 2002), HLA-mismatched or unrelated donor (McDonald *et al.*, 1993), second transplant procedure (Sanders *et al.*, 1988), raised serum C reactive protein (CRP) levels (Schots *et al.*, 1998), raised serum hyaluronic acid (Fried, *et al.*, 2001), neuroblastoma in children (Horn *et al.*, 2002), and busulfan pharmacokinetics (area under curve, AUC) (Grochow *et al.*, 1989; Slattery *et al.*, 1995; Dix *et al.*, 1996; Vassal *et al.*, 1996; Ljungman *et al.*, 1997). Serum tumor necrosis factor-alpha (TNF-α) levels have been found to be significantly elevated prior to development of clinical VOD (Holler *et al.*, 1990; Tanaka *et al.*, 1993). Low plasma protein C levels prior to cytoreductive therapy has been reported to predict VOD (Faioni *et al.*, 1993). Several groups have reported that elevated levels of procollagen-III peptide (PIIIP) can also precede clinical disease, thereby suggesting usefulness as a marker for VOD and allowing differentiation from acute GVHD (Eltumi *et al.*, 1993; Schuler *et al.*, 1996).

Multivariate analyses suggest that autologous transplants are not associated with a lower incidence of VOD compared to allogeneic transplants (Jones *et al.*, 1987; McDonald *et al.*, 1993). Increased platelet transfusion requirements also appear to be associated with the severity of VOD (Gordon *et al.*, 1998). CD34$^+$ positively selected peripheral blood stem cells (PBSC) could result in a marked reduction in the incidence of VOD following HSC transplantation (Moscardo *et al.*, 2001).

Histopathology reveals a constellation of lesions involving hepatic venules and structures in zone 3 of the hepatic acini. These include hepatic venular occlusion, eccentric luminal narrowing and eventual fibrosis of central hepatic venules, sinusoidal fibrosis, phlebosclerosis, and pericentral hepatocyte necrosis. The severity of disease is proportional to the number of zone 3 changes (Shulman *et al.*, 1994). Studies suggest that the primary site of the toxic injury is sinusoidal endothelial cells, followed by a series of biologic processes resulting in cytokine activation and disordered local coagulation that lead to circulatory compromise of centrilobular hepatocytes, fibrosis, and obstruction of liver blood flow. A new name for VOD has therefore been proposed: sinusoidal obstruction syndrome (DeLeve, Shulman, & McDonald 2002). There are no specific sonographic findings strongly associated with VOD in the early stages (Hommeyer *et al.*, 1992). However, Doppler studies of the hepatic veins and directional portal blood flow may be useful as a baseline measure and allow exclusion of major hepatic vein thrombosis.

To date in the published literature there are no treatment strategies proven in prospective, randomized, controlled studies. Prophylactic strategies have been proposed concentrating on reducing glutathione depletion, modifying inflammatory mediators, coagulation and fibrogenesis markers (Bearman, 2001). Prostaglandin E1 has also been reported to be beneficial (Gluckman *et al.*, 1990), but a later study was limited by severe toxicity (Bearman *et al.*, 1993b). Three patients with VOD have been treated successfully with N-acetyl-cysteine with a view to replacing depleted stores of glutathione (Ringden *et al.*, 2000). Other successful case reports have included glutamine plus vitamin E (Goringe *et al.*, 1998) and high-dose steroids (Khoury *et al.*, 2000). Ursodeoxycholic acid (UDCA) has been shown to be associated with less disease (Essell *et al.*, 1992; Ohashi *et al.*, 2000), but no difference was observed in long-term survival between the two groups. With regard to anticoagulation, the efficacy of heparin remains in dispute. Only one randomized study documented an effective reduction in VOD with continuous infusion of low-dose heparin, commenced prior to transplant, which was without added risk of bleeding (Attal *et al.*, 1992). Patients in the heparin group had less VOD than those in the nonheparin treated group; however, severe VOD was not different in either group. In a single arm study heparin was ineffective (Bearman *et al.*, 1990). In a randomized trial of low molecular weight heparin (LMWH), the duration of clinical signs of VOD was reduced in the LMWH treated patients (Or *et al.*, 1996). In a nonrandomized retrospective cohort study of 462 consecutive adult HSC transplant recipients, three prophylactic regimens were incorporated: low-dose heparin, heparin and prostaglandin E1 (PGE1), or LMWH. The prophylactic group was compared to a historical cohort receiving no VOD prophylaxis. By multivariate analysis unrelated donors, decreased performance status and altered AST levels were significant risk factors for developing VOD: the incidence of VOD was lower in the prophylaxis group and LMWH was more effective than unfractionated heparin. PGE1 showed no additional effect. No prospective randomized trials of heparin versus LMWH versus placebo exist in the literature to assess the efficacy of heparin compounds in the prevention of VOD.

In a randomized trial of heparin plus UDCA versus heparin alone in the treatment of VOD, no difference was seen in efficacy between the two groups (Park *et al.*, 2002). Recombinant tissue plasminogen activator (rTPA) has been used to treat severe VOD and appeared promising initially (Baglin, Harper, & Marcus, 1990; Bearman *et al.*, 1992; Yu *et al.*, 1994). One group also reported the successful use of rTPA in conjunction with plasma exchange (Espigado *et al.*, 1995). However, there are reports of severe bleeding complications related to rTPA therapy (Hagglund *et al.*, 1995; Bearman *et al.*, 1997; Schriber *et al.*, 1999).

Encouraging results have been reported with the use of defibrotide in the treatment of patients with severe VOD (Richardson *et al.*, 1998; Abecasis *et al.*, 1999). Defibrotide is a large single-stranded polydeoxyribonucleotide known to have antithrombotic, anti-inflammatory, and thrombolytic properties. It is an adenosine receptor agonist that results in thrombin antagonism in vitro with little toxicity (Richardson *et al.*, 2002). In a small treatment group resolution of VOD was seen in 42%. There was no significant toxicity associated with its use. Orthotopic liver transplantation has been tried in several cases but did not result in long-term survival (Rapoport *et al.*, 1991; Hagglund *et al.*, 1995). Transjugular intrahepatic portosystemic shunting has been performed safely, but resulted in limited clinical benefit (Fried *et al.*, 1992; Azoulay *et al.*, 2000; Zenz *et al.*, 2001). In cases refractory to other treatment, charcoal hemofiltration has had some efficacy for adsorbing circulating bilirubin and other protein bound toxins (Tefferi *et al.*, 2001).

Portal vein thrombosis

Acute portal vein thrombosis (PVT) has been described after autologous HSC transplantation (Grigg *et al.*, 1996). Three patients developed abdominal pain and abnormal liver enzymes without hyperbilirubinemia early after autografting. Doppler ultrasound demonstrated thrombosis of the main portal vein and its branches in all three cases. One case resolved spontaneously and two after treatment with LMWH. Risk factors for PVT include cirrhosis, neoplasm, intra-abdominal sepsis, myeloproliferative disorders and acquired and inheritable hypercoagulable forms of protein C deficiency, antithrombin III deficiency, and factor V Leiden (Egesel *et al.*, 2000). In patients undergoing HSC transplantation, decreased levels of protein C and antithrombin III have been documented, usually

in the clinical context of veno-occlusive disease (Gordon *et al.*, 1991; Bierman & Armitage, 1993; Haire *et al.*, 1995). Few other isolated cases of PVT have been described posttransplant (Grigg *et al.*, 1996). A retrospective review in one center of 1,847 HSC transplants, 8 patients were noted to have PVT (Kikuchi *et al.*, 2002). Four received autologous, and 4 allogeneic, grafts. All had evidence of VOD and concurrent ascites. Median levels of antithrombin III and protein C were low; 4 died due to VOD and multiorgan failure; PVT did not appear to contribute to death. It is possible that the incidence of PVT, although rare, is directly related to diminished portal venous flow secondary to hepatic sinusoidal obstruction (VOD) as well as to a hypercoagulable state related to low levels of antithrombin III and protein C.

Acute GVHD

Liver involvement usually occurs in association with skin and intestinal GVHD. Immunologic mechanisms mediate the injury, which is predominantly directed at biliary epithelial cells. The frequency of acute GVHD increases with the degree of donor-recipient histoincompatibility. The incidence in HLA-identical sibling marrow recipients is up to 35%, rising to 90% in recipients of family member transplants mismatched for two or three HLA antigens. An unrelated HLA-identical marrow recipient has a risk of up to 70%. Other identified risk factors include sex mismatch between donor and recipient (female donor to male recipient), increasing donor parity, increased radiation dose, and dose reduction of prophylactic methotrexate or cyclosporine (Nash *et al.*, 1992).

Acute hepatic GVHD appears from day 15 to beyond day 45 posttransplant. Skin and intestinal manifestations of acute GVHD are usually apparent before the onset of jaundice (McDonald *et al.*, 1986a). However, a hyperacute form can occur as early as day 6 and can be confused with VOD. Cholestatic liver injury develops with jaundice, hepatomegaly, and elevation of the serum alkaline phosphatase, gamma glutamyl transpeptidase, and 5′-nucleotidase values up to 20 times normal (Yasmineh, Filipovich, & Killeen, 1989). Elevation of transaminases rarely exceeds 10 times normal, although a biopsy-confirmed case of acute hepatic GVHD has been reported in which an elevation of serum transaminase levels (with normal or near-normal serum bilirubin values) was the primary presentation (Fujii *et al.*, 2001). The height of the serum bilirubin concentration correlates with the severity and mortality of the disease, but can be influenced by renal insufficiency, intravascular hemolysis, or prior VOD. It is unusual for acute GVHD to present with symptoms or signs of liver failure such as encephalopathy, hypoglycemia, coagulopathy, or ascites. If these are present, additional factors are likely involved. Acute GVHD tends to be associated with profound immunosuppression, with subsequent susceptibility to infection, further compounding liver injury. Cholestasis induced by acute GVHD may impair absorption of drugs such as cyclosporine. Liver biopsy is not usually necessary, but may be so if liver dysfunction persists despite improvement in skin and intestinal GVHD, or when a change of direction in treatment is considered. Biopsy can exclude other causes of liver disease such as VOD, drug hepatotoxicity, viral or fungal infection, and TPN-induced cholestasis.

The histologic pattern of disease is similar to that seen in acute rejection following liver transplantation (Snover *et al.,* 1987a). Histopathology is variable, depending on when in the disease course the biopsy is taken. In very early disease, hepatocyte necrosis may be present with only a mild lobular infiltrate (Snover *et al.,* 1984; Snover, 1984; Shulman *et al.,* 1988). The histologic features at this stage are similar to that seen in acute viral hepatitis. Later the presence of portal tract changes help to distinguish GVHD from other diseases. Biliary epithelial cells develop severe atypia with vacuolation, nuclear pleomorphism, and ballooning. Only a modest lymphocytic infiltrate is present and shows a prevalence of CD4+ cells. With disease progression there is destruction of small bile ducts accompanied by ductular proliferation. Endothelialitis affecting the central veins is also seen. Apoptotic and dysmorphic bile duct epithelial cell changes, resembling those seen in acute GVHD, have been reported in biopsies of recipients of autologous HSC transplants (Saunders *et al.,* 2000).

Patients with severe acute GVHD usually die of infection rather than liver failure. Less severe disease may respond to immunosuppression with high-dose steroids or antithymocyte globulin, but resolution of liver enzyme abnormalities can take months. Clinical improvement has been reported in steroid-refractory (acute) GVHD with use of a monoclonal antibody specific for the IL-2 receptor (Herve *et al.,* 1990; Anasetti *et al.,* 1994).

Infection

Bacterial and fungal infections are common during the early posttransplant phase. Usually by day 20 there is repair of mucosal injury and recovery of the granulocyte count. Recovery of lymphocyte-mediated function can be delayed for months to years and viral infections occur during this period. Chronic GVHD delays immune reconstitution further.

Bacterial infection

Bacterial sepsis (Collin *et al.,* 2001) can seriously impair liver function. Cholangitis lenta, as the name suggests, is a form of chronic sepsis in conjunction with biliary tract inflammation without any obvious extrinsic obstruction (Lefkowitch, 1982). It most typically occurs in the neutropenic period posttransplant with or without jaundice and systemic illness. The diagnosis is usually one of exclusion and resolution following antibiotic treatment. Kupffer cell function and endotoxin clearance is diminished in liver disease. Severe sepsis can result in acute liver failure with encephalopathy, hypoglycemia, and coagulopathy. Protracted hyperbilirubinemia can follow, despite a fall in liver enzymes and successful antibiotic therapy. Liver biopsy is not usually required.

Fungal infection

More than 50% of cases of disseminated fungal infection have liver involvement (Lewis, Patel, & Zimmerman, 1982), often not recognized during life. To determine the prevalence of fungal infection at post mortem in bone marrow transplant patients, case records were reviewed in one hospital for the period 1980–1989 (Rossetti *et al.,* 1995). Fungal infection, predominantly *Candida albicans* was noted in 67 cases (9% of 731 patients). Of the 67, hepatic fungal infection was noted in 34 cases. Risk factors for fungal liver infection were deep fungal infection after HSC transplantation, colonization or superficial infection, severe liver dysfunction secondary to VOD, and/or GVHD. No correlation was noted in this series with protective isolation, prophylactic oral antifungal drugs, antibiotic therapy, or immunosuppression. Many cases are seen in patients with poor marrow function receiving high-dose immunosuppression as treatment for acute GVHD. Liver biopsy may be valuable in patients with unexplained fever, elevated serum alkaline phosphatase values, or tender hepatomegaly. A high index of clinical suspicion is needed (Thaler *et al.,* 1988). With the introduction of fluconazole as prophylactic therapy in the early 1990s, two placebo-controlled trials showed that the incidence of positive blood cultures and superficial infection with *C. albicans* was reduced (Ozsahin *et al.,* 1992; Slavin *et al.,* 1995). The prevalence study on post mortem records was therefore repeated at the same center in a cohort of 355 marrow transplant recipients who died from 1990 through 1994 (van Burik *et al.,* 1998); 50% of the cohort had received fluconazole prophylaxis; 141 (40%) cases had disseminated fungal infection; 31 cases (9%) had histological evidence of fungal infection within the liver with a higher incidence in those who had no prophylaxis (26 cases (16%) vs. 5 cases in those who did (3%)). Only 4 cases did not involve *Candida* species, 3 of whom did not receive fluconazole. The number of patients with mold infections found at autopsy was significantly increased in those who had received fluconazole. Reports are emerging of the changing epidemiology of mold infections, including those involving the liver (Marr *et al.,* 2002).

Viral infection (and see also Chapter 74)

Hepatitis C. Hepatitis C virus (HCV) RNA testing by PCR is preferable to antibody evaluation for identifying HCV infection in HSC transplant recipients, due to impairment of the immune response with reduced reactivity to HCV antigens and reduced antibody formation (Lok *et al.,* 1993). HCV RNA positivity in donors is an accurate predictor of HCV infection in recipients though the resulting acute infection is often subclinical. (Shuhart *et al.,* 1994, 1996). HCV infection is not an uncommon problem in HSC transplantation (Liang, Lau, & Kwong, 1999; Strasser & McDonald, 1999b). Although there are contradictory reports as to the risk of development of severe liver disease, consensus is emerging that patients with HCV infection can receive HSC transplantation without significantly added risk in the short to mid term (Ribas & Gale, 1997). The prevalence of HCV has been reported to range up to 48%

(Norol et al., 1994; Ljungman et al., 1995; Ochocka et al., 1995). These same studies suggested that HCV RNA positivity was neither a predictor of VOD/GVHD nor a marker for liver failure. Similarly, HCV infection did not appear to influence the outcome of transplantation. Viral genotype did not appear to affect the severity of liver disease when it occurred (Locasciulli et al., 1995c).

In the immediate posttransplant period, regardless of whether the recipient comes to transplant infected with HCV or acquires the infection at the time of transplantation, there will be little or no biochemical evidence of an active viral infection (Chen et al., 1995). Biochemical evidence of hepatitis (that usually remains subclinical) only occurs around the time of the return of cellular immunity and the tapering of immunosuppressive therapy (around day 60–120) (Locasciulli et al., 1995b). The main difficulty may be in distinguishing hepatic GVHD from an acute flare of HCV. Unfortunately no biochemical test or PCR for HCV can distinguish this, and if there is a genuine dilemma a liver biopsy may be required. While fulminant liver injury is rare with HCV infection posttransplant, there are reports highlighting serious consequences. In one series, 7 of 9 patients who became viremic posttransplant died of liver failure, with viremia correlating with the onset of hepatic decompensation (Locasciulli et al., 1995b). Another group reported a high risk of early fatal VOD in patients with HCV infection prior to transplant (Frickhofen et al., 1994). It has been noted that a late and even fatal hepatitis can occur with reduction in the dose, or discontinuation, of immunosuppression (Fan et al., 1991; Ljungman et al., 1995), suggesting an immune-mediated mechanism as well as cytopathic effect in HCV liver injury. In a prospective study, 193 consecutive patients undergoing HSC transplantation were evaluated for the role of HCV virus infections pre- and posttransplant; 43 patients died with liver disease being the main cause of death (13 of 43, 30%). Severe VOD occurred in 8% of cases, fulminant hepatic failure in 0.5%, and 12% of cases had ALT >500 U/l (normal <42 U/l). Predictive risk factors for life threatening liver disease were unrelated donors and abnormal ALT levels in the donor pretransplant (Locasciulli et al., 1999).

Following an acute flare of HCV infection posttransplant, the biochemical picture invariably normalizes but will then often adopt a pattern of chronic hepatitis with periodic biochemical flares. Once all immunosuppressive therapy has been ceased in the recipient, therapy should be considered (Strasser & McDonald, 1999b). Although progression to chronic hepatitis is more likely with ongoing HCV infection, the incidence is similar to that in patients with HCV infection not undergoing transplantation (Alter et al., 1999). Long-term follow-up will be necessary to evaluate the risk of progression to cirrhosis; an initial study suggests that, although cirrhosis is rare for all HSC transplant patients overall, there is a significant risk of progression for those infected with HCV (Strasser et al., 1999c). Interferon-α therapy has been used for treatment posttransplant with a report of long-term responders (Ljungman et al., 1995). Reassuringly, there was no development or exacerbation of chronic GVHD during

therapy. Though few case reports exist, combination therapy with interferon-α and ribavirin should be considered in any long-term survivors with chronic hepatitis C (Liatsos et al., 2001); ribavirin appears to be well tolerated in HSC transplant recipients (Ljungman et al., 1996). Treatment of acute hepatitis C with interferon-α 2b has been shown to prevent chronic infection in non-transplant patients (Jaeckel et al., 2001; Hoofnagle, 2001). It remains to be seen whether combination therapy with ribavirin offers an advantage in the acute setting.

Hepatitis B.   Reactivation of HBV infection in HBsAg carriers with increased viral replication is recognized as a complication of immunosuppression (Liang, Lau, & Kwong, 1999; Strasser & McDonald, 1999b). There are several reports of fulminant hepatitis following HSC transplantation after immune reconstitution occurred (Pariente et al., 1988; Van Dam et al., 1990). The use of HBsAg+ donors increases the risk of severe liver disease in recipients (Locasciulli et al., 1995c; Lau et al., 2000a). However, McDonald et al., (1987) reported on 50 HBsAg+ carriers who were successfully transplanted without progression to serious liver disease. Locasciulli et al., (1990) reported similar results in 30 HbsAg+ patients, none of whom developed acute liver failure and 21 of whom cleared HBsAg during follow-up. In contrast, in a case-controlled study by Lau and colleagues (2000a), 44% of recipients of marrow from HbsAg+ donors developed HBV-related hepatitis posttransplant versus 11% in the control group who received HbsAg− marrow ($P = .03$). Furthermore, HBV-related hepatic failure was seen in 6 of 18 recipients of positive marrow versus none of 18 in the control group ($P = .07$). Five of the nine HbsAg-− recipients in the experimental group became positive after receiving HBsAg+ marrow, and serum HBV DNA was positive in all five donors, indicative of a high viral load. The patients in the experimental group who developed HBV-related hepatitis posttransplant were more likely to have a donor carrying a precore A_{1896} and/or core promoter T_{1762}/A_{1764} HBV variant. These virus variants are associated with rapid replication of HBV DNA. Adoptive transfer of immunity to HBV can be achieved through passive immunization of the donor (Ilan et al., 1993; Lau et al., 1998a, 2002). Active immunization of recipients around the time of transplant has been reported, although seroconversion may be transient and antibody titers low (Nagler et al., 1995).

Management of the HBsAg+ patient after transplantation can be difficult and requires close monitoring of HBsAg, HBeAg, and HBV DNA. Case reports confirm the disappearance of HBsAb and HBeAb after transplant with the later emergence of HBsAg with viral reactivation (Chen et al., 1993). There is usually no clinical evidence of a hepatitis following cytoreductive therapy and before the return of cellular immunity although HBV DNA titres may increase to very high levels (Strasser & McDonald, 1999b). The level of viremia may rise further still with corticosteroid therapy. At the time of immune reconstitution a clinical flare may occur. Twelve percent of flares culminate in hepatic failure and death (Webster et al., 1989; Liang, Lau, & Kwong, 1999). Those harboring pre-core mutants

(HBeAg⁻ mutants) are at particular risk (Omata *et al.,* 1994; Miura *et al.,* 1997). The differential diagnosis in a hepatitis B-infected allograft recipient with progressive elevations of AST, ALT, and bilirubin at the time of tapering immunosupressive therapy is hepatic GVHD, HBV reactivation, a herpesvirus infection or drug-induced liver injury (Strasser & McDonald, 1999a). A liver biopsy may be necessary to outline the dominant process.

Several agents are known to reduce HBV replication (Bain, 2000; Strasser & McCaughan, 2000; Liatsos *et al.,* 2001). There are an increasing number of case reports on the use of antiviral therapy to control HBV after HSC transplantation including with gancyclovir (Mertens *et al.,* 1996) and, more successfully with lamivudine (Dienstag *et al.,* 1995, 1999; Picardi *et al.,* 1998; Uchida *et al.,* 2000; Hashino *et al.,* 2002). Lamivudine decreases fibrogenesis as measured by immunohistochemical markers (Kweon *et al.,* 2001). It is likely that future therapies for HBV infection will focus on combination agents (such as adefovir and lamivudine). For an introduction to combination therapy for HBV infection, see Strasser and McCaughan (2000) and Di Bisceglie (2002). Markers of increasing HBV viremia usually occur within 1–2 weeks posttransplant, and it is at this stage that therapy should be considered, i.e., prior to a clinical flare of hepatitis—with the aim of suppressing viral replication and minimizing viral mutation (Endo *et al.,* 2001). Recipients with a viremia from a precore mutant HBV, as suggested by negative HBeAg but positive HBV DNA, are at particular risk (Omata *et al.,* 1994; Miura *et al.,* 1997).

Other viruses causing hepatitis. A severe and often fatal hepatitis can occur after infection with adenovirus (Shields *et al.,* 1985; Johnson *et al.,* 1990), herpes simplex 1 virus, echovirus (Biggs *et al.,* 1990) or varicella zoster virus (VZV) (Schiller *et al.,* 1991). Fulminant liver failure and death can ensue within a few days. A rapidly rising transaminase level above 600 IU/l is characteristic. Hepatitis due to cytomegalovirus (CMV) tends to be low grade, usually occurring in conjunction with infection in other sites such as lung or intestinal tract (Snover *et al.,* 1987b; Finny *et al.,* 2001). The risk of developing CMV infection and disease increases with the occurrence and severity of GVHD. Endoscopic biopsy of the intestinal tract can be diagnostic. Rarely diffuse intra- and extrahepatic duct strictures can occur, as well as ampulla of Vater[3] obstruction (Murakami, Chan, & McDonald, 2002). Adenovirus has been reported in approximately 6% of pediatric HSC transplant recipients, which is similar to the incidence in adults (Hale *et al.,* 1999). The time of onset, however, differs: usually occurring around day 30 in children and day 90 in adult recipients. Liver manifestations include hepatomegaly, coagulopathy, hepatitis, and rarely fulminant hepatic failure (Somervaille *et al.,* 1999).

Diagnosis can be made by PCR on samples of blood, sputum, urine, bronchoalveolar lavage, and liver tissue (Echavarria

et al., 1999). Liver biopsy shows extensive necrosis with irregular, dark intranuclear viral inclusions in surviving hepatocytes. Herpes simplex virus (HSV) usually occurs systemically after day 45. Hepatitis is rare but is severe on presentation with progressive jaundice and coagulopathy. The incidence has declined with the use of prophylactic acyclovir posttransplant (Hayashi *et al.,* 1991). Fulminant hepatic failure has been reported with HSV type 2 despite prophylactic use of acyclovir (Gruson *et al.,* 1998). Epstein-Barr virus (EBV) usually presents as a low grade hepatitis, but may also be associated with posttransplant lymphoproliferative disease (PTLD). Detection of the virus can be made by PCR for EBV DNA (Beck *et al.,* 1999). There may be an association with PTLD onset and the severity of GVHD (Chiang *et al.,* 2001). Liver biopsy demonstrates portal infiltration with small round lymphocytes (immunoblastic B cells) (Zutter *et al.,* 1988) (see Chapter 88). Other rare hepatic complications have been reported with VZV (David *et al.,* 1998), human herpesvirus 6 (HHV-6) (Lau *et al.,* 1998b), human parvovirus (B19 virus) (Schleuning *et al.,* 1999), and transfusion-transmitted virus (TTV) (Kanda & Hirai, 2001).

Drug-induced liver disease

Drug hepatotoxicity is probably more common than appreciated, but severe liver damage is rare (Strasser *et al.,* 1999b). The drugs most commonly used in the posttransplant period and their potential liver toxicities are shown in Table 89.6. Cyclosporine is the most common cause of conjugated hyperbilirubinemia in the posttransplant period, occurring in up to 48% of patients in one study (Anasetti *et al.,* 1994). It is not usually associated with marked elevations of transaminase or alkaline phosphatase levels. The cholestatic effect may be secondary to a decrease in bile flow and bile salt secretion (Chan & Shaffer, 1997). Total parenteral nutrition can induce cholestasis, but does not usually require cessation of treatment. Liver enzymes and serum bilirubin settle when the patient resumes normal eating. Liver biopsy is not usually helpful in drug-induced hepatotoxicity, but may be important in excluding other causes of liver disease. The usual histologic features of drug hepatotoxicity, such as portal tract eosinophilia or lobular granulomata, are rarely seen because of immunosuppression and low white blood cell numbers.

Nodular regenerative hyperplasia

This unusual and rare condition is characterized by a noncirrhotic nodular regeneration of liver lobules. Its incidence after HSC transplantation has been reported at 22.5% (Snover *et al.,* 1989), although other groups have not confirmed this (Shulman *et al.,* 1994; Bertheau *et al.,* 1995). Periportal areas undergo nodular regeneration with compression and atrophy of the adjacent centilobular areas. Variable sinusoidal dilatation and congestion can occur, but there is no obliterative venulitis, as is seen

---

[3] Abraham Vater, German anatomist and botanist, 1684-1751.

Table 89.6. *Drugs commonly used posttransplant and their potential effects on the liver*

Drug	Potential liver toxicity
Antilymphocyte/antithymocyte globulin	Hepatitis
Augmentin/clavulanic acid	Hepatitis, cholestasis
Azathioprine	Cholestasis
Clotrimazole	Hepatitis
Cyclosporine	Hyperbilirubinemia
	Dose-dependent hepatitis
Ketoconazole/itraconazole	Hepatitis
Methotrexate (long term)	Transient hepatitis, liver fibrosis
Penicillin derivatives	Hepatitis
Phenothiazines	Cholestasis
Total parenteral nutrition	Hepatitis, cholestasis
Trimethoprim-sulfamethoxazole	Hepatitis, cholestasis
GM-CSF	Hepatitis, cholestasis

Abbreviation: GM-CSF, granulocyte-macrophage colony-stimulating factor.

in VOD. Liver biopsy is essential for diagnosis and reticulin staining shows characteristic histopathology. The etiology is unknown but a disturbance of liver blood flow from obliteration of portal venules or arterioles is thought to be the most likely cause, with the better perfused periportal areas undergoing regeneration (Wanless *et al.,* 1980). The condition is also seen in other patients on immune suppressive treatment or with connective tissue diseases (Stromeyer & Ishak, 1981; Wanless, 1990).

Nodular regenerative hyperplasia may lead to portal hypertension and esophageal varices because of the profound disturbance of liver architecture. It does not lead to liver failure and the synthetic function of the liver remains intact. Rarely it may present with ascites and can mimic VOD, although usually appearing later than 2 to 5 weeks after transplant. No specific treatment exists, although it is wise to cease or substitute potentially hepatoxic medications.

Idiopathic hyperammonemia

This rare syndrome presents with an onset of encephalopathy and rapid development of coma. The serum ammonia concentration is usually greatly elevated (>200 μmol/l). It is most commonly seen 25 to 50 days or later posttransplant, without any obvious evidence of liver disease (Tse, Cederbaum, & Glaspy, 1991; Ho *et al.,* 1997). The course is usually rapidly fatal. One study identified 12 patients out of a 21-year BMT database of 2,358 patients (0.005%) (Davies *et al.,* 1996). Eight of these patients received marrow from an HLA-matched sibling donor, three from an unrelated donor, and one autologous marrow. Patients presented most frequently with symptoms of metabolic encephalopathy with lethargy and confusion evolving into unresponsiveness, coma, and, in eight cases, seizures. Ten of the 12 patients died 1 to 9 (median 3.5) days after the diagnosis. Hyperventilation and respiratory alkalosis can occur.

Liver biopsy shows microvesicular steatosis. Rapid diagnosis and institution of treatment is important. Therapy includes discontinuation of parenteral alimentation to lower protein intake, together with agents such as lactulose, omeprazole, and metronidazole or neomycin. Success in promoting urea production has been obtained with carnitene and intravenous flumazanil, an antagonist of endogenous benzodiazepines (Frere *et al.,* 2000). Mechanical ventilation is sometimes necessary for the management of respiratory alkalosis. Dialysis may also be effective for reducing ammonia concentration. Infusions of sodium benzoate have been attempted with variable success. The etiology is not known, but it is most likely due to the expression of a defect in the urea cycle pathway induced by chemotherapy or irradiation.

Non-alcoholic steatohepatitis

The diagnosis of non-alcoholic steatohepatitis (NASH) requires exclusion of alcohol abuse and histological demonstration of steatosis in association with necro-inflammatory foci, ballooning degeneration of hepatocytes with or without Mallory bodies, and pericellular fibrosis. The pathogenesis is still debated but the disease is associated with a number of conditions including obesity, insulin resistance, TPN, and exposure to a wide range of drugs including corticosteroids and synthetic estrogens. While most individuals with hepatic steatosis within the general population do not develop serious liver disease, a proportion develop NASH, which may lead to fibrosis, cirrhosis, and hepatic failure. One report identified NASH in 2.8% of 106 allogeneic BMT recipients (Tomas *et al.,* 2000). A case that led to rapidly progressive liver failure has been described in a patient allografted for Schwachman-Diamond syndrome (Ritchie *et al.,* 2002).

Liver disease after day 100

Chronic GVHD (and see Chapter 72)

Chronic GVHD may follow, or progress from, acute GVHD or can develop de novo in approximately 20% of cases. It is a complex multisystem disorder that develops 3 to 6 months posttransplant and can affect 50% or more of long-term survivors (McDonald *et al.,* 1986a, 1986b). Clinical features include keratoconjunctivitis sicca, sclerodermatous skin changes, chronic oral mucositis, and ongoing immune deficiency (Sullivan *et al.,* 1981). Chronic liver disease is seen in 90% of patients with chronic GVHD. Most have fluctuating jaundice with elevations of serum alkaline phosphatase 5 to 10 times normal. Obliteration of interlobular bile ducts (vanishing bile duct syndrome) sometimes develops with progressive rise in serum bilirubin and alkaline phosphatase. Rarely, progression to biliary cirrhosis (Knapp *et al.,* 1987; Stechschulte *et al.,* 1990) or variceal bleeding may occur (Yau *et al.,* 1986). As with acute GVHD, presentation resembling acute hepatitis has been described (Strasser *et al.,* 2000; Malik *et al.,* 2001).

Histologic findings are predominantly confined to the portal tracts, with an intense portal infiltrate, disorganized or absent bile ductules, inflammatory piecemeal necrosis, and eventually fibrous bridges and cirrhosis. Remaining bile ductules show atypical epithelium with a coagulative appearance. These features are similar to those seen in chronic rejection of a liver allograft.

Most cases respond to an increase in immunosuppression early in the course of disease. Ursodeoxycholic acid can improve symptoms of pruritus and significantly reduce elevations of serum bilirubin and transaminases in refractory cases (Fried *et al.*, 1992). Treatment with orthotopic liver transplantation has been reported (Rhodes *et al.*, 1990).

Viral hepatitis

Viral hepatitis can manifest clinically both early and late posttransplant, and is dealt with above.

Iron overload (siderosis)

Iron overload has been found to be a common contributor to liver dysfunction later posttransplant (Kornreich *et al.*, 1997), both in patients transplanted for thalassemia (Kami, Hamaki, & Kishi, 2000) (see Chapter 60), as well as those transplanted for hematologic malignancy (Tomas *et al.*, 2000). Iron status can be assessed by measuring serum ferritin levels, and, if indicated, by grading stainable iron on liver biopsy sections with a Perls' stain.[4] In any patient with a raised ferritin, it is important to screen for the heriditary hemochromatosis gene before starting any kind of transfusion therapy, in order to avoid the development of gross iron-overload (Liatsos *et al.*, 2001). Venesection and/or chelation using desferrioxamine can be utilized to reverse hepatic dysfunction due to siderosis (Angelucci *et al.*, 1997; Porter, 2001). Iron depletion prior to HSC transplantation has been undertaken successfully, suggesting that iron depletion in the pretransplant period may contribute to reduced transplant-related toxicity in selected cases (de la Serna *et al.*, 1999).

Recurrence of underlying malignancy

Tumor recurrence may occur in the liver of patients who have been transplanted for hematologic malignancy or solid tumors. Patients usually present with hepatomegaly, malaise, and abnormal liver enzymes. Fungal infection requires exclusion. Fine needle aspiration or liver biopsy is required for diagnosis.

Cirrhosis

In a study by Strasser *et al.* (1999c), cirrhosis was identified in 31 of 3,721 patients who had survived 1 or more years posttransplant, in 23 of 1,850 who had survived 5 years or more, and in 19 of 860 who had survived 10 years or more. The cumulative incidence after 10 years was estimated to be 0.6%

[4]Max Perls, German pathologist, 1843-1881.

and after 20 years it was 3.8%. The median time from transplant to diagnosis of cirrhosis was 10.1 (range 1.2–24.9) years. Twenty-three patients presented with complications of portal hypertension, and one with hepatocellular carcinoma. At the time of the report 13 patients had died from hepatic disease and 2 of other causes. Hepatitis C virus infection was present in 81% of patients with cirrhosis compared to 45% of controls. Cirrhosis was attributable to hepatitis C infection in 15 of 16 patients presenting more than 10 years posttransplant. Long-term survivors should clearly be evaluated for the presence of abnormal liver function tests and hepatitis virus infection.

Liver biopsy in HSC transplant recipients

Percutaneous liver biopsy in experienced hands is generally a safe procedure (Grant & Neuberger, 1999; Bravo, Sheth, & Chopra, 2001). In the early posttransplant period, thrombocytopenia, coagulopathy, and platelet transfusion refractoriness can make biopsy relatively hazardous. Careful assessment of risk and benefit must be made. Bleeding after biopsy is unlikely if the platelet count is greater than $50 \times 10^9/l$ though it is still advisable to utilize platelet transfusion immediately before and during the procedure if the platelet count is less than $100 \times 10^9/l$.

Several groups have reported on transvenous liver biopsy in HSC transplant recipients (Carreras *et al.*, 1993; Shulman *et al.*, 1995; Iqbal *et al.*, 1996). Adequate tissue specimens can be obtained by means of biopsy needle or forceps, although multiple passes may be required. Using a balloon-tipped catheter, hepatic venous pressure gradient (HVPG) can be determined by subtracting wedged hepatic vein pressure from free hepatic vein pressure. In a significant number of cases, diagnosis and treatment are modified as a consequence of biopsy findings. Both of the above studies suggested that HVPG >10 mmHg was associated with a diagnosis of VOD, and that such a measure could be used to follow the clinical course. Serious complications such as intra-abdominal bleeding and liver capsule perforation were noted.

Liver biopsy is perhaps most useful in determining unexplained liver dysfunction (e.g., exclusion of fungal infection), or where a change of treatment is contemplated (e.g., in a patient with acute GVHD and deteriorating liver function despite clinical improvement of skin and intestinal disease).

Gall bladder disease

In a review of 7,412 marrow transplant recipients, 9 cases of biliary obstruction were identified (0.12%) (Murakami *et al.*, 1999). The presentation was bimodal, with 7 cases occurring before day 100 and 2 occurring between 2 and 4 years posttransplant. In this series the causes of obstruction were gallbladder sludge ($n = 1$), duodenal hematoma ($n = 1$), choledocholithiasis with biliary pancreatitis ($n = 1$), bile duct infection ($n = 2$), recurrent malignancy ($n = 1$), choledocholithiasis associated with a benign stricture ($n = 1$), EBV-related lymphoproliferative disease ($n = 1$), and a benign stricture of unknown etiology ($n = 1$). Biliary obstruction is thus a rare cause of jaundice posttransplant.

The gall bladder sludge syndrome causes biliary-type pain, nausea, and vomiting. Biliary sludge accumulates in over 50% of patients during the first 21 days, while they are eating poorly or being fed intravenously. One study found a large proportion of the sludge (84.6%) to be unmeasurable residue. Calcium bilirubinate crystals were present in large amounts in all samples, while cholesterol crystals were almost absent (Ko *et al.*, 1996; Ko, Sekijima, & Lee, 1999). With resumption of eating and stimulation of gall bladder contraction, passage of sludge or minute calculi causes symptoms of biliary colic. Symptomatic treatment only is usually required. The symptoms usually settle after a few days (Messing *et al.*, 1983; Roslyn *et al.*, 1983; Messing, 2000).

Acute acalculous cholecystitis occurs rarely, but may produce florid clinical signs. Ultrasound shows an edematous gall bladder wall. HIDA (hydroxyiminodiacetic acid) radionuclide scanning may show no opacification of the gall bladder when the cystic duct is occluded. Mild abnormalities of liver enzymes and serum bilirubin may be present. Due to the risk of a gangrenous gall bladder, cholecystectomy is usually required if hematologic parameters allow.

Pancreatic disease

Pancreatitis has been reported in 3.5%–4.4% of pediatric and adult HSC transplant patients (Werlin *et al.*, 1992; Washington, Peters, & Gottfried, 1993; Gossage, & Gottfried, 1994; Shore *et al.*, 1996; Salomone *et al.*, 1999), with an even higher incidence at autopsy—up to 27% in one study (Ko *et al.*, 1997) suggesting an additional impact of acute pancreatitis on morbidity and mortality in severely ill transplant patients. Causes include transplant-related toxicity (conditioning chemotherapy and irradiation), acute GVHD, bacterial and viral infections [e.g., varicella zoster (Ladriere *et al.*, 2001) or CMV], cyclosporine, and other immunosuppression (Nieto *et al.*, 2000) including corticosteroids (Ko *et al.*, 1997). The major risk factors appear to be severe acute GVHD (grade III–IV) and hepatic GVHD with a high prevalence of gall bladder sludge and gall stones in one study (Jacobson *et al.*, 1993; Ko *et al.*, 1996); however, it is likely that pancreatitis cannot be attributable to a single pathogenetic factor (Salomone *et al.*, 1999). Two cases have been reported of the treatment of acute pancreatitis after HSC transplantation with C1 esterase inhibitor, leading to a successful outcome in both children (Schneider *et al.*, 1999).

Pancreatic insufficiency has been described in patients with chronic GVHD (Akpek *et al.*, 2001). Patients presented with unexplained diarrhea (steatorrhea) and weight loss in the presence of an adequate caloric intake; GI biopsies and D-xylose absorption tests were normal; stool cultures were negative, but a CT scan showed an atrophic pancreas in one case. All four patients responded well to pancreatic enzyme supplements. Dose and duration of the replacement therapy was adjusted according to the clinical response.

The development of a pancreatic pseudocyst in an immune compromised patient may require surgical drainage, since pseudocysts are not drained adequately by radiologically guided techniques. An autopsy study of 184 patients found an incidence of 28%, indicating this to be a relatively common, but often subclinical, complication (Ko *et al.*, 1997).

Introduction to perianal complications

The hematopoietic stem cell (HSC) transplant recipient is at particular risk for the development of perianal infection (Handler *et al.*, 1994). Already debilitated from the underlying hematologic disease, the patient often undergoes further intensive chemotherapy or chemoradiotherapy immediately prior to transplant. This invariably produces gastrointestinal ulceration and diarrhea. The white count is very low in the period immediately following transplantation, and gastrointestinal GVHD may occur, leading to further diarrhea. Posttransplant immune suppression leads to increased susceptibility to infection. In this setting the moist, excoriated, intertrigonous perianal area is susceptible to minor trauma, with a breach of the anoderm acting as a portal of entry for bacteria. For this reason digital rectal examination and sigmoidoscopy should be avoided in the neutropenic phase. Table 89.7 indicates measures to minimize the development of perianal infection.

Perianal infection in the leukemic patient

Such perianal septic lesions are well recognized in patients with acute leukemia not undergoing HSC transplantation and may be life-threatening (Sehdev *et al.*, 1973; Chirletti *et al.*, 1988; Grewal *et al.*, 1994). The incidence of perianal infection in the acute leukemic, granulocytopenic patient was 5.7% with a 25% mortality in one series (Carlson, Ferguson, & Amerson, 1988). The mortality rate rises significantly if the patient is not in remission (69%) versus 0% if in remission (Musa, Katakkar, & Khaliq, 1975). Over half of all patients with acute leukemia have a history of previous anorectal problems (Musa, Katakkar, & Khaliq, 1975), and such a history should be carefully sought from the HSC transplant patient. Indeed, in one series of leukemic patients with anal septic problems, the anal lesion was the first manifestation of hematologic disease in 20% of cases (Vanhueverzwyn *et al.*, 1980). It has been noted in the leukemic patient that anal infection will often follow the passage of a constipated motion, which is associated with a little bright blood per

Table 89.7. *Prevention of perianal infection*

Avoid rectal examination, suppositories, enemas
Avoid constipation
Keep anal area clean and dry—if diarrhea use soft disposable material, not toilet paper
Minimize diarrhea
Weekly stool culture

rectum, suggesting the initiating event to be a minor traumatic anal tear (Givler, 1969). Pus is absent from the septic anal lesions due to the neutropenia. Instead the discharge is serous. Additionally, subepithelial leukemic infiltrates of perianal connective tissue are well documented (Carle, 1982). A small biopsy may be indicated, but the risk of thereby producing perianal infection must be carefully weighed.

In the majority of neutropenic patients with septicemia the responsible organism can be isolated from the feces, sometimes in pure culture before the onset of septicemia (Daw *et al.*, 1988). Daw and colleagues concluded that fecal culture is the most useful approach in the bacteriologic surveillance of neutropenic patients. The most common organisms in Daw's series were *E. coli, Pseudomonas aeruginosa,* and *Enterobacter cloacae.* In one Japanese series of infected patients with hematologic disorders, half the Gram-negative bacteria were *Pseudomonas* species.

Necrotizing lesions and *Pseudomonas* infection

The extreme danger of necrotizing anorectal lesions associated with *Pseudomonas* infection in leukemic patients is well documented (Givler, 1969; Wolf, Liu, & Rabinowitz, 1989; Gucluer, Ergun, & Demircay, 1999). Givler reported five cases of *Pseudomonas* septicemia and necrotizing anorectal ulcers in leukemic patients, all of whom died (Givler, 1969). In Givler's series the ulcers were large, up to 8 cm in diameter, involving the distal rectum and extending on to the anus and perianal skin. The surrounding tissues were indurated, erythematous, and markedly edematous. Bullous vesicles containing thin dark fluid were present on the perineum in some cases. Histology revealed ulcer margins and bases composed of necrotic tissue, which extended deeply into perianal adipose tissue. Myriads of Gram-negative rods were present, particularly concentrated within the walls of arteries and veins. Givler commented that inflammatory cell infiltrates were either totally absent or limited to a few small foci of lymphocytes. No leukemic infiltrates were present. Granulation tissue and scarring were absent regardless of the clinical duration of the lesions. Typical skin lesions were present in these patients (usually ecthyma gangrenosum) and foci of nodular hemorrhagic necrosis were found in other tissues. The perianal lesion was thought to be the portal of entry for the *Pseudomonas* septicemia in two of Givler's patients and in two others it was thought to be a secondary invader. In one case a positive throat culture for *Pseudomonas* preceded the anorectal lesion. Givler stated that the virulence of the *Pseudomonas* was dependent on the production of toxin. Hemorrhagic necrosis appears to be due to a protease component, whereas the edema is due to a lecithinase component.

In leukemic patients with perianal infection the most important prognostic indicator of outcome is said to be the number of days of neutropenia during the infectious episode (Glenn *et al.*, 1988).

Treatment

The majority of these infections (88% in Glenn's series) settle with conservative measures and intensive intravenous antibi-

Table 89.8. *Conservative treatment of perianal sepsis*

Appropriate systemic antibiotics with Gram-negative and anaerobe coverage
Hematopoietic growth factor (G-CSF, GM-CSF) to accelerate neutrophil recovery
Consider granulocyte transfusions
Fastidious local care of lesion (clean, dry)
Stool softeners
Analgesia

Abbreviations: G-CSF, granulocyte colony-stimulating factor; GM-CSF, granulocyte-macrophage colony-stimulating factor.

otics including an aminoglycoside. Conservative measures include Sitz baths, warm compresses soaked in Betadine or aqueous chlorhexidine, stool softeners, and analgesics (Table 89.8). Surgical intervention is reserved for fluctuance, development of necrotic tissue, progression of infection, and failed medical treatment. When possible, surgery is withheld until the white cell count increases, as an incision into an indurated area in the neutropenic phase can lead to progression of the necrotic process, and widespread sloughing of the buttock area, with subsequent fecal incontinence (Walsh & Stickley, 1934; Blank, 1955). Hemorrhage due to thrombocytopenia is also a significant risk. The risk of surgical intervention during the neutropenic phase, outside of the above guidelines, was demonstrated in one series where operative intervention had a mortality of 44.4% compared with 9% for conservative management (Carlson, Ferguson, & Amerson, 1988). In the operative group three further patients had progression of infection, two requiring colostomy.

Perianal complications in the HSC transplant recipient

In the HSC transplant recipient, perianal complications may occur during or after remission-induction chemotherapy (when they may well delay the transplant) or during the neutropenic phase of the immediate posttransplant period (Hilbe *et al.*, 2000). Complications include perianal ulceration, anal fissure with or without fistula and abscess, thrombosed external haemorrhoids, perineal furuncle, *Pseudomonas aeruginosa* infection (locally and systemically), and acute necrotizing fascitis. Acute necrotizing fasciitis, also known as Fournier's[5] gangrene, is a symbiotic infection usually composed of a Gram-positive[6] coccus and a Gram-negative rod. The coccus is usually *Streptococcus* and its protease component opens a plane of least resistance along muscle fascial planes, which are then invaded by Gram-negative rods. Acute necrotizing fasciitis can also be produced by a pure streptococcal infection. *Pseudomonas* is frequently the responsible Gram-negative organism. Acute necro-

---

[5] Jean Alfred Fournier, French dermatologist, 1832–1914.
[6] Hans Gram, Danish pathologist, 1853-1938.

tizing fasciitis can occur following minor gynecologic and anorectal surgical procedures in otherwise perfectly fit patients or in young children undergoing chemotherapy (Murphy *et al.,* 1995). The immunosuppressed HSC transplant recipient is particularly susceptible to this complication (Martinelli *et al.,* 1998). Acute necrotizing fasciitis usually begins as a refractory cellulitis in the non-immunosuppressed patients. Given the absence of white cells in the early posttransplant period, it will usually present as an area of tissue necrosis, whereas skin necrosis and vesicle formation are late signs in the non-immunosuppressed patient. In the non-immunosuppressed patient the infection involves the muscle fascial planes early. The muscle fascia becomes an edematous, thick, grey necrotic membrane with sparing of skin, muscle, and subcutaneous fat until late in the process. It is essential that a definitive diagnosis be made immediately. This requires a biopsy of the necrotic grey membrane or the necrotic tissue, which usually reveals tissues full of Gram-positive cocci and Gram-negative rods (although, as stated above, either alone can sometimes produce the complete clinical picture). The infection often spreads relentlessly to cause death from uncontrolled septicemia despite intensive antibiotic therapy, although there are case reports of complete resolution in BMT recipients (Martinelli *et al.,* 1998).

In the non-immunosuppressed patient wide excisional surgery with frequent returns to the operating theater for excisional debridement can salvage these patients. This is accompanied by intensive broad-spectrum intravenous antibiotics, but these are supportive only and will not solve the problem alone. Hyperbaric oxygen therapy can play a useful supportive role.

In the HSC transplant recipient wide excisional surgery is usually out of the question, due to the absence of white cells and platelets, and the only hope of salvaging this situation is to recognize the problem immediately when it occurs and perform very local excision of the necrotic tissue accompanied by intensive intravenous antibiotic support, hyperbaric oxygen, and hydrogen peroxide irrigation. Irrespective of the treatment, the mortality rate for this condition in the immunosuppressed HSC transplant patient will be extremely high. In the case of sepsis of the perianal region the same guidelines for surgical intervention stated above hold, but the problem must be definitively resolved prior to transplant. To commence further chemoradiotherapy and proceed to transplantation with a residual non-healed breach in the anal epithelium is to court disaster.

An anal abscess can be drained by a minimally invasive technique in the neutropenic phase and then the fistula-in-ano laid open when the white cell count returns to a safe level. Cohen and colleagues (1996) reviewed the records of 963 bone marrow transplants performed at the City of Hope National Medical Center. They found 24 patients who were diagnosed as having perianal infections following their transplants. Fifteen patients did not have purulent collections requiring drainage and were treated with antibiotics and supportive measures alone. Nine patients (37.5%) underwent surgical intervention between 10 and 380 days posttransplant. At the time of surgical intervention 7 patients had purulent collections and 2 patients

had acute and chronic inflammation, tissue necrosis, and fibrosis. Interestingly, 2 patients had an absolute neutrophil count of less than $1 \times 10^9/l$ at the time of surgery and a purulent collection was found in one of these patients. Cultures taken from perianal abscesses were almost all polymicrobial and the most common organisms were *E. coli, Bacteroides, Enterococcus,* and *Klebsiella.* The mean time to complete wound closure in those undergoing surgical intervention was lengthy at 37.6 days. While 5 patients healed in less than 15 days, 2 patients took 93 and 114 days, respectively. Two allograft recipients described by Gucluer and colleagues (1999) had resolution of ecthyma gangrenosum, with perirectal or vulval/groin ulceration growing *Pseudomonas aeruginosa,* within 3 and 8 weeks respectively.

References

Abecasis, M. M., Conceicao, Silva, J. P., Ferreira, I., Guimaraes, A., & Machado, A. (1999). Defibrotide as salvage therapy for refractory veno-occlusive disease of the liver complicating allogeneic bone marrow transplantation. *Bone Marrow Transplantation,* **23,** 843–846.

Akiyama, H., Nakamura, N., Tanikawa, S. *et al.* (1998). Incidence and influence of GB virus C and hepatitis C virus infection in patients undergoing bone marrow transplantation. *Bone Marrow Transplantation,* **21,** 1131–1135.

Akpek, G., Valladares, J. L., Lee, L., Margolis, J., & Vogelsang, G. B. (2001). Pancreatic insufficiency in patients with chronic graft-versus-host disease. *Bone Marrow Transplantation,* **27,** 163–166.

Alter, M. J., Kruszon-Moran, D., Nainan, O. V. *et al.* (1999). The prevalence of hepatitis C virus infection in the United States, 1988 through 1994. *New England Journal of Medicine,* **341,** 556–562.

Anasetti, C., Hansen, J. A., Waldmann, T. A. *et al.* (1994). Treatment of acute graft-versus-host disease with humanized anti-Tac: an antibody that binds to the interleukin-2 receptor. *Blood,* **84,** 1320–1327.

Angelucci, E., Muretto, P., Lucarelli, G. *et al.* (1997). Phlebotomy to reduce iron overload in patients cured of thalassemia by bone marrow transplantation. Italian Cooperative Group for Phlebotomy Treatment of Transplanted Thalassemia Patients. *Blood,* **90,** 994–998.

Atkinson, K., Arthur, C., Bradstock, K. *et al.* (1995). Prophylactic ganciclovir is more effective in HLA-identical family member marrow transplant recipients than in more heavily immune-suppressed HLA-identical unrelated donor marrow transplant recipients. Australasian Bone Marrow Transplant Study Group. *Bone Marrow Transplantation,* **16,** 401–405.

Atkinson, K., Biggs, J. C., Britton, K. *et al.* (1984). Oral administration of cyclosporin A for recipients of allogeneic marrow transplants: implications of clinical gut dysfunction. *British Journal of Haematology,* **56,** 223–231.

Atkinson, K., Biggs, J., Noble, G. *et al.* (1987). Preparative regimens for marrow transplantation containing busulphan are associated with hemorrhagic cystitis and hepatic veno-occlusive disease but a short duration of leucopenia and little oro-pharyngeal mucositis. *Bone Marrow Transplantation,* **2,** 385–394.

Attal, M., Huguet, F., Rubie, H. et al. (1992). Prevention of hepatic veno-occlusive disease after bone marrow transplantation by continuous infusion of low-dose heparin: a prospective, randomized trial. *Blood*, **79**, 2834–2840.

Azoulay, D., Castaing, D., Lemoine, A., Hargreaves, G. M., & Bismuth, H. (2000). Transjugular intrahepatic portosystemic shunt (TIPS) for severe veno-occlusive disease of the liver following bone marrow transplantation. *Bone Marrow Transplantation*, **25**, 987–992.

Baglin, T. P., Harper, P., & Marcus, R. E. (1990). Veno-occlusive disease of the liver complicating ABMT successfully treated with recombinant tissue plasminogen activator (rt-PA). *Bone Marrow Transplantation*, **5**, 439–441.

Bain, V. G. (2000). Hepatitis B in transplantation. *Transplant Infectious Disease*, **2**, 153–165.

Ballen, K. K., Hesketh, A. M., Heyes, C. et al. (2001). Prospective evaluation of antiemetic outcome following high-dose chemotherapy with hematopoietic stem cell support. *Bone Marrow Transplantation*, **28**, 1061–1066.

Barker, G. J. (1999). Current practices in the oral management of the patient undergoing chemotherapy or bone marrow transplantation. *Supportive Care in Cancer*, **7**, 17–20.

Bartlett, J. G. (2002). Clinical practice. Antibiotic-associated diarrhea. *New England Journal of Medicine*, **346**, 334–339.

Bearman, S. I. (2001). Avoiding hepatic veno-occlusive disease: what do we know and where are we going? *Bone Marrow Transplantation*, **27**, 1113–1120.

Bearman, S. I., Anderson, G. L., Mori, M. et al. (1993a). Venoocclusive disease of the liver: development of a model for predicting fatal outcome after marrow transplantation. *Journal of Clinical Oncology*, **11**, 1729–1736.

Bearman, S. I., Hinds, M. S., Wolford, J. L. et al. (1990). A pilot study of continuous infusion heparin for the prevention of hepatic veno-occlusive disease after bone marrow transplantation. *Bone Marrow Transplantation*, **5**, 407–411.

Bearman, S. I., Lee, J. L., Baron, A. E., & McDonald, G. B. (1997). Treatment of hepatic venocclusive disease with recombinant human tissue plasminogen activator and heparin in 42 marrow transplant patients. *Blood*, **89**, 1501–1506.

Bearman, S. I., Shen, D. D., Hinds, M. S., Hill, H. A., & McDonald, G. B. (1993b). A phase I/II study of prostaglandin E1 for the prevention of hepatic venocclusive disease after bone marrow transplantation. *British Journal of Haematology*, **84**, 724–730.

Bearman, S. I., Shuhart, M. C., Hinds, M. S., & McDonald, G. B. (1992). Recombinant human tissue plasminogen activator for the treatment of established severe venocclusive disease of the liver after bone marrow transplantation. *Blood*, **80**, 2458–2462.

Beck, R., Westdorp, I., Jahn, G. et al. (1999). Detection of Epstein-Barr virus DNA in plasma from patients with lymphoproliferative disease after allogeneic bone marrow or peripheral blood stem cell transplantation. *Journal of Clinical Microbiology*, **37**, 3430–3431.

Bellm, L. A., Epstein, J. B., Rose-Ped, A., Martin, P., & Fuchs, H. J. (2000). Patient reports of complications of bone marrow transplantation *Supportive Care in Cancer*, **8**, 33–39.

Bertheau, P., Hadengue, A., Cazals-Hatem, D. et al. (1995). Chronic cholestasis in patients after allogeneic bone marrow transplantation: several diseases are often associated. *Bone Marrow Transplantation*, **16**, 261–265.

Bertz, H., Afting, M., Kreisel, W. et al. (1999). Feasibility and response to budesonide as topical corticosteroid therapy for acute intestinal GVHD. *Bone Marrow Transplantation*, **24**, 1185–1189.

Bierman, P. J. & Armitage, J. O. (1993). Bone marrow transplantation at the University of Nebraska Medical Center. *Nebraska Medical Journal*, **78**, 272–277.

Biggs, D. D., Toorkey, B. C., Carrigan, D. R., Hanson, G. A., & Ash, R. C. (1990). Disseminated echovirus infection complicating bone marrow transplantation. *The American Journal of Medicine*, **88**, 421–425.

Blank, W. A. (1995). Anorectal complications in leukaemia. *American Journal of Surgery*, **90**, 738–741.

Blijlevens, N. M., Donnelly, J. P., & De Pauw, B. E. (2000). Mucosal barrier injury: biology, pathology, clinical counterparts and consequences of intensive treatment for haematological malignancy: an overview. *Bone Marrow Transplantation*, **25**, 1269–1278.

Boggio, L., Pooley, R., Roth, S. I., & Winter, J. N. (2000). Typhlitis complicating autologous blood stem cell transplantation for breast cancer. *Bone Marrow Transplantation*, **25**, 321–326.

Bombi, J. A., Nadal, A., Carrears, E. et al. (1995). Assessment of histopathologic changes in the colonic biopsy in acute graft-versus-host disease. *American Journal of Clinical Pathology*, **103**, 690–695.

Borowski, B., Benhamou, E., Pico, J. L. et al. (1994). Prevention of oral mucositis in patients treated with high-dose chemotherapy and bone marrow transplantation: a randomised controlled trial comparing two protocols of dental care. *European Journal of Cancer. Part B, Oral Oncology*, **30B**, 93–97.

Bravo, A. A., Sheth, S. G., & Chopra, S. (2001). Liver biopsy. *New England Journal of Medicine*, **344**, 495–500.

Brodsky, R., Topolsky, D., Crilley, P., Bulova, S., & Brodsky, I. (1990). Frequency of veno-occlusive disease of the liver in bone marrow transplantation with a modified busulfan/cyclophosphamide preparative regimen. *American Journal of Clinical Oncology*, **13**, 221–225.

Browne, P. V., Weisdorf, D. J., Defor, T. et al. (2000). Response to thalidomide therapy in refractory chronic graft-versus-host disease. *Bone Marrow Transplantation*, **26**, 865–869.

Cairncross, G., Swinnen, L., Bayer, R. et al. (2000). Myeloablative chemotherapy for recurrent aggressive oligodendroglioma. *Neurooncology*, **2**, 114–119.

Carl, W. (1995). Oral complications of local and systemic cancer treatment. *Current Opinion in Oncology*, **7**, 320–324.

Carle, G. (1982). Anorectal involvement in leukemia. *Journal of the Royal College of Surgeons of Edinburgh*, **27**, 118–

Carlson, G. W., Ferguson, C. M., & Amerson, J. R. (1988). Perianal infections in acute leukemia. Second place winner: Conrad Jobst Award. *The American Surgeon*, **54**, 693–695.

Carreras, E., Granena, A., Navasa, M. et al. (1993). Transjugular liver biopsy in BMT. *Bone Marrow Transplantation*, **11**, 21–26.

Castagna, L., Benhamou, E., Pedraza, E. et al. (2001). Prevention of mucositis in bone marrow transplantation: a double blind randomised controlled trial of sucralfate. *Annals of Oncology*, **12**, 953–955.

Chakrabarti, S., Lees, A., Jones, S. G., & Milligan, D. W. (2000). *Clostridium difficile* infection in allogeneic stem cell transplant recipients is associated with severe graft-versus-host disease and non-relapse mortality. *Bone Marrow Transplantation,* **26,** 871–876.

Chan, F. K. & Shaffer, E. A. (1997). Cholestatic effects of cyclosporine in the rat. *Transplantation,* **63,** 1574–1578.

Chen, P. M., Fan, S., Liu, J. H. *et al.* (1993). Reactivation of hepatitis B virus in two chronic GVHD patients after transplant. *International Journal of Hematology,* **58,** 183–188.

Chen, P. M., Liu, J. H., Fan, F. S. *et al.* (1995). Liver disease after bone marrow transplantation—the Taiwan experience. *Transplantation,* **59,** 1139–1143.

Chiang, K. Y., Hazlett, L. J., Godder, K. T. *et al.* (2001). Epstein-Barr virus-associated B cell lymphoproliferative disorder following mismatched related T cell-depleted bone marrow transplantation. *Bone Marrow Transplantation,* **28,** 1117–1123.

Chim, C. S., Luk, W. K., & Yuen, K. Y. (1997). Trichostrongylus infestation masquerading as conditioning toxicity of the gut bone marrow transplantation. *Bone Marrow Transplantation,* **19,** 955–6.

Chirletti, P., Beverati, M., Apice, N. *et al.* (1988). Prophylaxis and treatment of inflammatory anorectal complications in leukemia. *Italian Journal of Surgical Sciences,* **18,** 45–48.

Choi, J. H., Yoo, J. H., Chung, I. J. *et al.* (1997). Esophageal aspergillosis after bone marrow transplant. *Bone Marrow Transplantation,* **19,** 293–294.

Cohen, J. S., Paz, I. B., O'Donnell, M. R., & Ellenhorn, J. D. (1996). Treatment of perianal infection following bone marrow transplantation. *Diseases of the Colon and Rectum,* **39,** 981–985.

Collin, B. A., Leather, H. L., Wingard, J. R., & Ramphal, R. (2001). Evolution, incidence, and susceptibility of bacterial bloodstream isolates from 519 bone marrow transplant patients. *Clinical Infectious Diseases,* **33,** 947–953.

Comenzo, R. L., Sanchorawala, V., Fisher, C. *et al.* (1999). Intermediate-dose intravenous melphalan and blood stem cells mobilized with sequential GM+G-CSF or G-CSF alone to treat AL (amyloid light chain) amyloidosis. *British Journal of Haematology,* **104,** 553–559.

Comenzo, R. L., Vosburgh, E., Falk, R. H. *et al.* (1998). Dose-intensive melphalan with blood stem-cell support for the treatment of AL (amyloid light-chain) amyloidosis: survival and responses in 25 patients. *Blood,* **91,** 3662–3670.

Corbi, C., Traineau, R., Esperou, H. *et al.* (1997). Prevalence and clinical features of hepatitis G virus infection in bone marrow allograft recipients. *Bone Marrow Transplantation,* **20,** 965–968.

Cox, G. J., Matsui, S. M., Lo, R. S. *et al.* (1994). Etiology and outcome of diarrhea after marrow transplantation: a prospective study. *Gastroenterology,* **107,** 1398–1407.

Crouch, M. A., Restino, M. S., Cruz, J. M., Perry, J. J., & Hurd, D. D. (1996). Octreotide acetate in refractory bone marrow transplant-associated diarrhea. *Annals of Pharmacotherapy,* **30,** 331–336.

David, D. S., Tegtmeier, B. R., O'Donnell, M. R., Paz, I. B., & McCarty, T. M. (1998). Visceral varicella-zoster after bone marrow transplantation: report of a case series and review of the literature. *American Journal of Gastroenterology,* **93,** 810–813.

Davies, S. M., Szabo, E., Wagner, J. E., Ramsay, N. K., & Weisdorf, D. J. (1996). Idiopathic hyperammonemia: a frequently lethal complication of bone marrow transplantation. *Bone Marrow Transplantation,* **17,** 1119–1125.

Daw, M. A., Munnelly, P., McCann, S. R. *et al.* (1988). Value of surveillance cultures in the management of neutropenic patients. *European Journal of Clinical Microbiology & Infectious Diseases,* **7,** 742–747.

de la Serna, J., Bornstein, R., Garcia-Bueno, M. J., & Lahuerta-Palacios, J. J. (1999). Iron depletion by phlebotomy with recombinant erythropoietin prior to allogeneic transplantation to prevent liver toxicity. *Bone Marrow Transplantation,* **23,** 95–97.

DeLeve, L. D., Shulman, H. M., & McDonald, G. B. (2002). Toxic injury to hepatic sinusoids: sinusoidal obstruction syndrome (veno-occlusive disease). *Seminars in Liver Disease,* **22,** 27–42.

Di Bisceglie, A. M. (2002). Combination therapy for hepatitis B. *Gut,* **50,** 443–445.

Di Bisceglie, A. M., McHutchison, J., & Rice, C. M. (2002). New therapeutic strategies for hepatitis C. *Hepatology,* **35,** 224–231.

Dienstag, J. L., Perrillo, R. P., Schiff, E. R. *et al.* (1995). A preliminary trial of lamivudine for chronic hepatitis B infection. *New England Journal of Medicine,* **333,** 1657–1661.

Dienstag, J. L., Schiff, E. R., Mitchell, M. *et al.* (1999). Extended lamivudine retreatment for chronic hepatitis B: maintenance of viral suppression after discontinuation of therapy. *Hepatology,* **30,** 1082–1087.

Dix, S. P., Wingard, J. R., Mullins, R. E. *et al.* (1996). Association of busulfan area under the curve with veno-occlusive disease following BMT. *Bone Marrow Transplantation,* **17,** 225–230.

Eagle, D. A., Gian, V., Lauwers, G. Y. *et al.* (2001). Gastroparesis following bone marrow transplantation. *Bone Marrow Transplantation,* **28,** 59–62.

Echavarria, M. S., Ray, S. C., Ambinder, R., Dumler, J. S., & Charache, P. (1999). PCR detection of adenovirus in a bone marrow transplant recipient: hemorrhagic cystitis as a presenting manifestation of disseminated disease. *Journal of Clinical Microbiology,* **37,** 686–689.

Egesel, T., Buyukasik, Y., Dundar, S. V. *et al.* (2000). The role of natural anticoagulant deficiencies and factor V Leiden in the development of idiopathic portal vein thrombosis. *Journal of Clinical Gastroenterology,* **30,** 66–71.

Einsele, H., Ehninger, G., Hebart, H. *et al.* (1994). Incidence of local CMV infection and acute intestinal GVHD in marrow transplant recipients with severe diarrhoea. *Bone Marrow Transplantation,* **14,** 955–963.

Eltumi, M., Trivedi, P., Hobbs, J. R. *et al.* (1993). Monitoring of veno-occlusive disease after bone marrow transplantation by serum aminopropeptide of type III procollagen. *Lancet,* **342,** 518–521.

Ely, P., Dunitz, J., Rogosheske, J., & Weisdorf, D. (1991). Use of a somatostatin analogue, octreotide acetate, in the management of acute gastrointestinal graft-versus-host disease. *American Journal of Medicine,* **90,** 707–710.

Endo, T., Sakai, T., Fujimoto, K. *et al.* (2001). A possible role for lamivudine as prophylaxis against hepatitis B reactivation in carriers of hepatitis B who undergo chemotherapy and autologous peripheral blood stem cell transplantation for non-Hodgkin's lymphoma. *Bone Marrow Transplantation,* **27,** 433–436.

Epstein, R. J., McDonald, G. B., Sale, G. E., Shulman, H. M., & Thomas, E. D. (1980). The diagnostic accuracy of the rectal biopsy in acute graft-versus-host disease: a prospective study of thirteen patients. *Gastroenterology,* **78,** 764–771.

Espigado, I., Rodriguez, J. M., Parody, R. *et al.* (1995). Reversal of severe hepatic veno-occlusive disease by combined plasma exchange and rt-PA treatment. *Bone Marrow Transplantation,* **16,** 313–316.

Essell, J. H., Thompson, J. M., Harman, G. S. *et al.* (1992). Pilot trial of prophylactic ursodiol to decrease the incidence of veno-occlusive disease of the liver in allogeneic bone marrow transplant patients. *Bone Marrow Transplantation,* **10,** 367–372.

Evans, J., Percy, J., Eckstein, R., Ma, D., & Schnitzler, M. (1998). Surgery for intestinal graft-versus-host disease: report of two cases. *Diseases of the Colon and Rectum,* **41,** 1573–1576.

Faioni, E. M., Krachmalnicoff, A., Bearman, S. I. *et al.* (1993). Naturally occurring anticoagulants and bone marrow transplantation: plasma protein C predicts the development of venocclusive disease of the liver. *Blood,* **81,** 3458–3462.

Fallows, G., Rubinger, M., & Bernstein, C. N. (2001). Does gastroenterology consultation change management of patients receiving hematopoietic stem cell transplantation? *Bone Marrow Transplantation,* **28,** 289–294.

Fan, F. S., Tzeng, C. H., Hsiao, K. I. *et al.* (1991). Withdrawal of immunosuppressive therapy in allogeneic bone marrow transplantation reactivates chronic viral hepatitis C. *Bone Marrow Transplantation,* **8,** 417–420.

Ferrara, J. L. & Deeg, H. J. (1991). Graft-versus-host disease. *New England Journal of Medicine,* **324,** 667–674.

Finny, G. J., Mathews, V., Abraham, P. *et al.* (2001). A pilot study on the role of cytomegalovirus & human herpesvirus-6 infections in Indian bone marrow transplant recipients. *The Indian Journal of Medical Research,* **114,** 39–46.

Fisk, J. D., Shulman, H. M., Greening, R. R. *et al.* (1981). Gastrointestinal radiographic features of human graft-versus-host disease. AJR. *American Journal of Roentgenology,* **136,** 329–336.

Forbes, G. M., Rule, S. A., Herrmann, R. P., Davies, J. M., & Collins, B. J. (1995). A prospective study of screening upper gastrointestinal (GI) endoscopy prior to and after bone marrow transplantation (BMT). *Australian and New Zealand Journal of Medicine,* **25,** 32–36.

Fox, R. J., Vogelsang, G. B., & Beschorner, W. E. (1996). Denuded bowel after recovery from graft-versus-host disease. *Transplantation,* **62,** 1681–1684.

Frere, P., Canivet, J. L., Gennigens, C. *et al.* (2000). Hyperammonemia after high-dose chemotherapy and stem cell transplantation. *Bone Marrow Transplantation,* **26,** 343–345.

Frickhofen, N., Wiesneth, M., Jainta, C. *et al.* (1994). Hepatitis C virus infection is a risk factor for liver failure from veno-occlusive disease after bone marrow transplantation. *Blood,* **83,** 1998–2004.

Fried, M. W., Duncan, A., Soroka, S. *et al.* (2001). Serum hyaluronic acid in patients with veno-occlusive disease following bone marrow transplantation. *Bone Marrow Transplantation,* **27,** 635–639.

Fried, R. H., Murakami, C. S., Fisher, L. D. *et al.* (1992). Ursodeoxycholic acid treatment of refractory chronic graft-versus-host disease of the liver. *Annals of Internal Medicine,* **116,** 624–629.

Fujii, N., Takenaka, K., Shinagawa, K. *et al.* (2001). Hepatic graft-versus-host disease presenting as an acute hepatitis after allo-

geneic peripheral blood stem cell transplantation. *Bone Marrow Transplantation,* **27,** 1007–1010.

Gallucci, B. B., Sale, G. E., McDonald, G. B. *et al.* (1982). The fine structure of human rectal epithelium in acute graft-versus-host disease. *American Journal of Surgical Pathology,* **6,** 293–305.

Gertz, M. A., Lacy, M. Q., & Dispenzieri, A. (2000). Myeloablative chemotherapy with stem cell rescue for the treatment of primary systemic amyloidosis: a status report. *Bone Marrow Transplantation,* **25,** 465–470.

Ghavamzadeh, A., Alimoghadam, K., Nasseri, P. *et al.* (1999). Correction of bone marrow failure in dyskeratosis congenita by bone marrow transplantation. *Bone Marrow Transplantation,* **23,** 299–301.

Ghilain, J. M., Martiat, P., Fiasse, R., Ferrant, A., & Michaux, J. L. (1990). [Exudative enteropathy caused by an acute graft-vs-host reaction. Apropos of a case report]. *Acta Gastro-enterolica Belgica,* **53,** 488–498.

Givler, R. L. (1969). Necrotizing anorectal lesions associated with *Pseudomonas* infection in leukemia. *Diseases of the Colon and Rectum,* **12,** 438–440.

Glenn, J., Cotton, D., Wesley, R., & Pizzo, P. (1988). Anorectal infections in patients with malignant diseases. *Reviews of Infectious Diseases,* **10,** 42–52.

Gluckman, E., Jolivet, I., Scrobohaci, M. L. *et al.* (1990). Use of prostaglandin E1 for prevention of liver veno-occlusive disease in leukaemic patients treated by allogeneic bone marrow transplantation. *British Journal of Haematology,* **74,** 277–281.

Goodman, Z. D., Boitnott, J. K., & Yardley, J. H. (1979). Perforation of the colon associated with cytomegalovirus infection. *Digestive Diseases and Sciences,* **24,** 376–380.

Gordon, B., Haire, W., Kessinger, A., Duggan, M., & Armitage, J. (1991). High frequency of antithrombin 3 and protein C deficiency following autologous bone marrow transplantation for lymphoma. *Bone Marrow Transplantation,* **8,** 497–502.

Gordon, B., Tarantolo, S., Ruby, E. *et al.* (1998). Increased platelet transfusion requirement is associated with multiple organ dysfunctions in patients undergoing hematopoietic stem cell transplantation. *Bone Marrow Transplantation,* **22,** 999–1003.

Goringe, A. P., Brown, S., O'Callaghan, U. *et al.* (1998). Glutamine and vitamin E in the treatment of hepatic veno-occlusive disease following high-dose chemotherapy. *Bone Marrow Transplantation,* **21,** 829–832.

Grant, A. & Neuberger, J. (1999). Guidelines on the use of liver biopsy in clinical practice. British Society of Gastroenterology. *Gut,* **45,** (Suppl 4), IV1–IV11.

Grewal, H., Guillem, J. G., Quan, S. H., Enker, W. E., & Cohen, A. M. (1994). Anorectal disease in neutropenic leukemic patients. Operative vs. nonoperative management. *Diseases of the Colon and Rectum,* **37,** 1095–1099.

Grigg, A., Gibson, R., Bardy, P., & Szer, J. (1996). Acute portal vein thrombosis after autologous stem cell transplantation. *Bone Marrow Transplantation,* **18,** 949–953.

Grochow, L. B., Jones, R. J., Brundrett, R. B. *et al.* (1989). Pharmacokinetics of busulfan: correlation with veno-occlusive disease in patients undergoing bone marrow transplantation. *Cancer Chemotherapy and Pharmacology,* **25,** 55–61.

Gruson, D., Hilbert, G., Le Bail, B. *et al.* (1998). Fulminant hepatitis due to herpes simplex virus-type 2 in early phase of bone marrow transplantation. *Hematology and Cell Therapy,* **40,** 41–44.

Gucluer, H., Ergun, T., & Demircay, Z. (1999). Ecthyma gangrenosum. *International Journal of Dermatology,* **38,** 299–302.

Haber, H. P., Schlegel, P. G., Dette, S. *et al.* (2000). Intestinal acute graft-versus-host disease: findings on sonography. *American Journal of Roentgenology,* **174,** 118–120.

Hagglund, H., Ringden, O., Ljungman, P. *et al.* (1995). No beneficial effects, but severe side effects caused by recombinant human tissue plasminogen activator for treatment of hepatic veno-occlusive disease after allogeneic bone marrow transplantation. *Transplantation Proceedings,* **27,** 3535.

Haire, W. D., Ruby, E. I., Gordon, B. G. *et al.* (1995). Multiple organ dysfunction syndrome in bone marrow transplantation. *Journal of the American Medical Association,* **274,** 1289–1295.

Hale, G. A., Heslop, H. E., Krance, R. A. *et al.* (1999). Adenovirus infection after pediatric bone marrow transplantation. *Bone Marrow Transplantation,* **23,** 277–282.

Handler, B. S., Longo, W. E., Vernava, A. M., Herrmann, V. M., & Dunphy, F. R. (1994). Gastrointestinal disease in patients receiving salvage chemotherapy or bone marrow transplantation. *Missouri Medicine,* **91,** 637–640.

Hashino, S., Nozawa, A., Izumiyama, K. *et al.* (2002). Lamivudine treatment for reverse seroconversion of hepatitis B 4 years after allogeneic bone marrow transplantation. *Bone Marrow Transplantation,* **29,** 361–363.

Hayashi, M., Takeyama, K., Takayama, J. *et al.* (1991). Severe herpes simplex virus hepatitis following autologous bone marrow transplantation: successful treatment with high dose intravenous acyclovir. *Japanese Journal of Clinical Oncology,* **21,** 372–376.

Herman, P., Krivan, G., Maszzi, T. *et al.* (2002). Evaluation of fungal colonization of oral cavity before and after stem cell transplantation (SCT) in the context of basal saliva secretion. *Bone Marrow Transplantation,* **27,** S337–S338.

Herve, P., Wijdenes, J., Bergerat, J. P. *et al.* (1990). Treatment of corticosteroid resistant acute graft-versus-host disease by in vivo administration of anti-interleukin-2 receptor monoclonal antibody (B-B10). *Blood,* **75,** 1017–1023.

Hilbe, W., Nussbaumer, W., Bonatti, H. *et al.* (2000). Unusual adverse events following peripheral blood stem cell (PBSC) mobilisation using granulocyte colony stimulating factor (G-CSF) in healthy donors. *Bone Marrow Transplantation,* **26,** 811–813.

Hirano, K., Kondo, F., Kondo, Y. *et al.* (1999). Stool smears for diagnosis of intestinal acute graft-versus-host disease. *Bone Marrow Transplantation,* **24,** 799–801.

Ho, A. Y., Mijovic, A., Pagliuca, A., & Mufti, G. J. (1997). Idiopathic hyperammonaemia syndrome following allogeneic peripheral blood progenitor cell transplantation (allo-PBPCT). *Bone Marrow Transplantation,* **20,** 1007–1008.

Holler, E., Kolb, H. J., Moller, A. *et al.* (1990). Increased serum levels of tumor necrosis factor alpha precede major complications of bone marrow transplantation. *Blood,* **75,** 1011–1016.

Hommeyer, S. C., Teefey, S. A., Jacobson, A. F. (1992). Venocclusive disease of the liver: prospective study of US evaluation. *Radiology,* **184,** 683–686.

Hoofnagle, J. H. (2001). Therapy for acute hepatitis C. *New England Journal of Medicine,* **345,** 1495–1497.

Horn, B., Reiss, U., Matthay, K., McMillan, A., & Cowan, M. (2002). Veno-occlusive disease of the liver in children with solid tumors undergoing autologous hematopoietic progenitor cell transplantation: a high incidence in patients with neuroblastoma. *Bone Marrow Transplantation,* **29,** 409–415.

Hwang, T. L., Chiang, C. L., & Wang, P. N. (2001). Parenteral nutrition support after bone marrow transplantation: comparison of total and partial parenteral nutrition during the early posttransplantation period. *Nutrition,* **17,** 773–775.

Iestra, J. A., Fibbe, W. E., Zwinderman, A. H., van Staveren, W. A., & Kromhout, D. (2002). Body weight recovery, eating difficulties and compliance with dietary advice in the first year after stem cell transplantation: a prospective study. *Bone Marrow Transplantation,* **29,** 417–424.

Ilan, Y., Nagler, A., Adler, R. *et al.* (1993). Adoptive transfer of immunity to hepatitis B virus after T cell-depleted allogeneic bone marrow transplantation. *Hepatology,* **18,** 246–252.

Inoue, M., Okamura, T., Sawada, A., Kawa, K. (1998). Colostrum and severe gut GVHD. *Bone Marrow Transplantation,* **22,** 402–403.

Inoue, M., Okamura, T., Yasui, M. *et al.* (2001). Lactoferrin for gut GVHD. *Bone Marrow Transplantation,* **28,** 1091–1092.

Iqbal, M., Creger, R. J., Fox, R. M. *et al.* (1996). Laparoscopic liver biopsy to evaluate hepatic dysfunction in patients with hematologic malignancies: a useful tool to effect changes in management. *Bone Marrow Transplantation,* **17,** 655–662.

Iqbal, N., Salzman, D., Lazenby, A. J., & Wilcox, C. M. (2000). Diagnosis of gastrointestinal graft-versus-host disease. *The American Journal of Gastroenterology,* **95,** 3034–3038.

Jacobsohn, D. A., Margolis, J., Doherty, J., Anders, V., & Vogelsang, G. B. (2002). Weight loss and malnutrition in patients with chronic graft-versus-host disease. *Bone Marrow Transplantation,* **29,** 231–236.

Jacobson, A. F., Teefey, S. A., Lee, S. P. *et al.* (1993). Frequent occurrence of new hepatobiliary abnormalities after bone marrow transplantation: results of a prospective study using scintigraphy and sonography. *American Journal of Gastroenterology,* **88,** 1044–1049.

Jacobson, B. C., Paterson, J. M., & Carr-Locke, D. L. (2000). Posttransplantation lymphoproliferative disorder of the stomach. *Gastrointestinal Endoscopy,* **51,** 595.

Jaeckel, E., Cornberg, M., Wedemeyer, H. *et al.* (2001). Treatment of acute hepatitis C with interferon alfa-2b. *New England Journal of Medicine,* **345,** 1452–1457.

Jafri, F. M., Mendelow, H., Shadduck, R. K., & Sekas, G. (1990). Jejunal vasculitis with protein-losing enteropathy after bone marrow transplantation. *Gastroenterology,* **98,** 1689–1692.

Johansson, J. E., Brune, M., & Ekman, T. (2001). The gut mucosa barrier is preserved during allogeneic, haemopoietic stem cell transplantation with reduced intensity conditioning. *Bone Marrow Transplantation,* **28,** 737–742.

Johansson, J. E. & Ekman, T. (1997). Gastro-intestinal toxicity related to bone marrow transplantation: disruption of the intestinal barrier precedes clinical findings. *Bone Marrow Transplantation,* **19,** 921–925.

Johansson, J. E. & Ekman, T. (1999). Gut mucosa barrier preservation by orally administered IgA-IgG to patients undergoing bone marrow transplantation: a randomised pilot study. *Bone Marrow Transplantation*, **24**, 35–39.

Johnson, P. R., Yin, J. A., Morris, D. J. *et al.* (1990). Fulminant hepatic necrosis caused by adenovirus type 5 following bone marrow transplantation. *Bone Marrow Transplantation*, **5**, 345–347.

Jones, R. J., Lee, K. S., Beschorner, W. E. *et al.* (1987). Venoocclusive disease of the liver following bone marrow transplantation. *Transplantation*, **44**, 778–783.

Kami, M., Hamaki, T., & Kishi, Y. (2000). Hepatic iron concentration and total body iron stores in thalassemia major. *New England Journal of Medicine*, **343**, 1657.

Kananen, K., Volin, L., Tahtela, R. *et al.* (2002). Recovery of bone mass and normalization of bone turnover in long-term survivors of allogeneic bone marrow transplantation. *Bone Marrow Transplantation*, **29**, 33–39.

Kanda, Y. & Hirai, H. (2001). TT virus in hematological disorders and bone marrow transplant recipients. *Leukemia and Lymphoma*, **40**, 483–489.

Kaur, S., Cooper, G., Fakult, S., & Lazarus, H. M. (1996). Incidence and outcome of overt gastrointestinal bleeding in patients undergoing bone marrow transplantation. *Digestive Diseases and Sciences*, **41**, 598–603.

Kaw, M., Przepiorka, D., & Sekas, G. (1993). Infectious complications of endoscopic procedures in bone marrow transplant recipients. *Digestive Diseases and Sciences*, **38**, 71–74.

Keates, J., Lagahee, S., Crilley, P., Haber, M., & Kowalski, T. (2001). CMV enteritis causing segmental ischemia and massive intestinal hemorrhage. *Gastrointestinal Endoscopy*, **53**, 355–359.

Khoury, H., Adkins, D., Brown, R. *et al.* (2000). Does early treatment with high-dose methylprednisolone alter the course of hepatic regimen-related toxicity? *Bone Marrow Transplantation*, **25**, 737–743.

Kikuchi, K., Rudolph, R., Murakami, C., Kowdley, K., & McDonald, G. B. (2002). Portal vein thrombosis after hematopoietic cell transplantation: frequency, treatment and outcome. *Bone Marrow Transplantation*, **29**, 329–333.

Kim, B. K., Chung, K. W., Sun, H. S. *et al.* (2000). Liver disease during the first post-transplant year in bone marrow transplantation recipients: retrospective study. *Bone Marrow Transplantation*, **26**, 193–197.

Kingreen, D., Nitsche, A., Beyer, J., & Siegert, W. (1997). Herpes simplex infection of the jejunum occurring in the early post-transplantation period. *Bone Marrow Transplantation*, **20**, 989–991.

Klein, S. A., Martin, H., Schreiber-Dietrich, D. *et al.* (2001). A new approach to evaluating intestinal acute graft-versus-host disease by transabdominal sonography and colour Doppler imaging. *British Journal of Haematology*, **115**, 929–934.

Kliegman, R. M. & Fanaroff, A. A. (1984). Necrotizing enterocolitis. *New England Journal of Medicine*, **310**, 1093–1103.

Kliegman, R. M., Walker, W. A., & Yolken, R. H. (1993). Necrotizing enterocolitis: research agenda for a disease of unknown etiology and pathogenesis. *Pediatric Research*, **34**, 701–708.

Knapp, A. B., Crawford, J. M., Rappeport, J. M., & Gollan, J. L. (1987). Cirrhosis as a consequence of graft-versus-host disease. *Gastroenterology*, **92**, 513–519.

Ko, C. W., Gooley, T., Schoch, H. G. *et al.* (1997). Acute pancreatitis in marrow transplant patients: prevalence at autopsy and risk factor analysis. *Bone Marrow Transplantation*, **20**, 1081–1086.

Ko, C. W., Murakami, C., Sekijima, J. H. *et al.* (1996). Chemical composition of gallbladder sludge in patients after marrow transplantation. *The American Journal of Gastroenterology*, **91**, 1207–1210.

Ko, C. W., Sekijima, J. H., & Lee, S. P. (1999). Biliary sludge. *Annals of Internal Medicine*, **130**, 301–311.

Kornreich, L., Horev, G., Yaniv, I. *et al.* (1997). Iron overload following bone marrow transplantation in children: MR findings. *Pediatric Radiology*, **27**, 869–872.

Kumar, S., Dispenzieri, A., Lacy, M. Q., Litzow, M. R., & Gertz, M. A. (2001). High incidence of gastrointestinal tract bleeding after autologous stem cell transplant for primary systemic amyloidosis. *Bone Marrow Transplantation*, **28**, 381–385.

Kurbegov, A. C. & Sondheimer, J. M. (2001). Pneumatosis intestinalis in non-neonatal pediatric patients. *Pediatrics*, **108**, 402–406.

Kweon, Y. O., Goodman, Z. D., Dienstag, J. L. *et al.* (2001). Decreasing fibrogenesis: an immunohistochemical study of paired liver biopsies following lamivudine therapy for chronic hepatitis B. *Journal of Hepatology*, **35**, 749–755.

Ladriere, M., Bibes, B., Rabaud, C. *et al.* (2001). [Varicella zoster virus infection after bone marrow transplant. Unusual presentation and importance of prevention]. *Presse Medicale (Paris, France: 1983)*, **30**, 1151–1154.

Langdana, A., Tully, N., Molloy, E., Bourke, B., & O'Meara, A. (2001). Intensive enteral nutrition support in paediatric bone marrow transplantation. *Bone Marrow Transplantation*, **27**, 741–746.

Lau, G. K., Liang, R., Lee, C. K. *et al.* (1998a). Clearance of persistent hepatitis B virus infection in Chinese bone marrow transplant recipients whose donors were anti-hepatitis B core-and anti-hepatitis B surface antibody-positive. *Journal of Infectious Diseases*, **178**, 1585–1591.

Lau, G. K., Lie, A. K., Kwong, Y. L. *et al.* (2000a). A case-controlled study on the use of HBsAg-positive donors for allogeneic hematopoietic cell transplantation. *Blood*, **96**, 452–458.

Lau, G. K., Suri, D., Liang, R. *et al.* (2002). Resolution of chronic hepatitis B and anti-HBs seroconversion in humans by adoptive transfer of immunity to hepatitis B core antigen. *Gastroenterology*, **122**, 614–624.

Lau, J. Y., Sung, J. J., Lee, K. K. *et al.* (2000b). Effect of intravenous omeprazole on recurrent bleeding after endoscopic treatment of bleeding peptic ulcers. *New England Journal of Medicine*, **343**, 310–316.

Lau, Y. L., Peiris, M., Chan, G. C. *et al.* (1998b). Primary human herpes virus 6 infection transmitted from donor to recipient through bone marrow infusion. *Bone Marrow Transplantation*, **21**, 1063–1066.

Lefkowitch, J. H. (1982). Bile ductular cholestasis: an ominous histopathologic sign related to sepsis and "cholangitis lenta." *Human Pathology*, **13**, 19–24.

Leung, W., Hudson, M. M., Strickland, D. K. *et al.* (2000). Late effects of treatment in survivors of childhood acute myeloid leukemia. *Journal of Clinical Oncology*, **18**, 3273–3279.

Lewis, J. H., Patel, H. R., & Zimmerman, H. J. (1982). The spectrum of hepatic candidiasis. *Hepatology*, **2**, 479–487.

Liang, R., Lau, G. K., & Kwong, Y. L. (1999). Chemotherapy and bone marrow transplantation for cancer patients who are also chronic hepatitis B carriers: a review of the problem. *Journal of Clinical Oncology,* 17, 394–398.

Liatsos, C., Mehta, A. B., Potter, M., & Burroughs, A. K. (2001). The hepatologist in the haematologists' camp. *British Journal of Haematology,* 113, 567–578.

Lipton, J., Patterson, B., Mustard, R. *et al.* (1994). Pneumatosis intestinalis with free air mimicking intestinal perforation in a bone marrow transplant patient. *Bone Marrow Transplantation,* 14, 323–326.

Ljungman, P., Anderson, J., Aschan, J. *et al.* (1996). Oral ribavirin for prevention of severe liver disease caused by hepatitis C virus during allogeneic bone marrow transplantation. *Clinical Infectious Diseases,* 23, 167–169.

Ljungman, P., Hassan, M., Bekassy, A. N., Ringden, O., & Oberg, G. (1997). High busulfan concentrations are associated with increased transplant-related mortality in allogeneic bone marrow transplant patients. *Bone Marrow Transplantation,* 20, 909–913.

Ljungman, P., Johansson, N., Aschan, J. *et al.* (1995). Long-term effects of hepatitis C virus infection in allogeneic bone marrow transplant recipients. *Blood,* 86, 1614–1618.

Locasciulli, A., Alberti, A., Bandini, G. *et al.* (1995a). Allogeneic bone marrow transplantation from HBsAg+ donors: a multicenter study from the Gruppo Italiano Trapianto di Midollo Osseo (GITMO). *Blood,* 86, 3236–3240.

Locasciulli, A., Bacigalupo, A., van Lint, M. T. *et al.* (1990). Hepatitis B virus (HBV) infection and liver disease after allogeneic bone marrow transplantation: a report of 30 cases. *Bone Marrow Transplantation,* 6, 25–29.

Locasciulli, A., Bacigalupo, A., van Lint, M. T. *et al.* (1995b). Hepatitis C virus infection and liver failure in patients undergoing allogeneic bone marrow transplantation. *Bone Marrow Transplantation,* 16, 407–411.

Locasciulli, A., Nava, S., Sparano, P., & Testa, M. (1998). Infections with hepatotropic viruses in children treated with allogeneic bone marrow transplantation. *Bone Marrow Transplantation,* 21, (Suppl 2), S75–S77.

Locasciulli, A., Pontisso, P., Alberti, A. *et al.* (1995c). The genotype of hepatitis C virus does not affect severity of liver disease after bone marrow transplantation. *Blood,* 85, 2640.

Locasciulli, A., Testa, M., Valsecchi, M. G. *et al.* (1999). The role of hepatitis C and B virus infections as risk factors for severe liver complications following allogeneic BMT: a prospective study by the Infectious Disease Working Party of the European Blood and Marrow Transplantation Group. *Transplantation,* 68, 1486–1491.

Lok, A. S., Chien, D., Choo, Q. L. *et al.* (1993). Antibody response to core, envelope and nonstructural hepatitis C virus antigens: comparison of immunocompetent and immunosuppressed patients. *Hepatology,* 18, 497–502.

Mahendra, P., Bedlow, A. J., Ager, S. *et al.* (1994). Technetium (^{99m}Tc)-labelled white cell scanning, ^{51}Cr-EDTA and ^{14}C-mannitol-labelled intestinal permeability studies: non-invasive methods of diagnosing acute intestinal graft-versus-host disease. *Bone Marrow Transplantation,* 13, 835–837.

Marr, K. A., Carter, R. A., Crippa, F., Wald, A., & Corey, L. (2002). Epidemiology and outcome of mould infections in hematopoietic stem cell transplant recipients. *Clinical Infectious Diseases,* 34, 909–917.

Martin, P. J., Schoch, G., Fisher, L. *et al.* (1990). A retrospective analysis of therapy for acute graft-versus-host disease: initial treatment. *Blood,* 76, 1464–1472.

Martin, P. J., Schoch, G., Fisher, L. *et al.* (1991). A retrospective analysis of therapy for acute graft-versus-host disease: secondary treatment. *Blood,* 77, 1821–1828.

Martinelli, G., Alessandrino, E. P., Bernasconi, P. *et al.* (1998). Fournier's gangrene: a clinical presentation of necrotizing fasciitis after bone marrow transplantation. *Bone Marrow Transplantation,* 22, 1023–1026.

Maruta, A., Tanabe, J., Hashimoto, C. *et al.* (1999). Long-term liver function of recipients with hepatitis G virus infection after bone marrow transplantation. *Bone Marrow Transplantation,* 24, 359–363.

McDonald, G. B., Bouvier, M., Hockenbery, D. M. *et al.* (1998). Oral beclomethasone dipropionate for treatment of intestinal graft-versus-host disease: a randomized, controlled trial. *Gastroenterology,* 115, 28–35.

McDonald, G. B., Hinds, M. S., Fisher, L. D. *et al.* (1993). Veno-occlusive disease of the liver and multiorgan failure after bone marrow transplantation: a cohort study of 355 patients. *Annals of Internal Medicine,* 118, 255–267.

McDonald, G. B., Sharma, P., Hackman, R. C., Meyers, J. D., & Thomas, E. D. (1985). Esophageal infections in immunosuppressed patients after marrow transplantation. *Gastroenterology,* 88, 1111–1117.

McDonald, G. B., Shulman, H. M., Sullivan, K. M., & Spencer, G. D. (1986a). Intestinal and hepatic complications of human bone marrow transplantation. Part I. *Gastroenterology,* 90, 460–477.

McDonald, G. B., Shulman, H. M., Sullivan, K. M., & Spencer, G. D. (1986b). Intestinal and hepatic complications of human bone marrow transplantation. Part II. *Gastroenterology,* 90, 770–784.

McDonald, G. B., Shulman, H. M., Wolford, J. L., & Spencer, G. D. (1987). Liver disease after human marrow transplantation. *Seminars in Liver Disease,* 7, 210–229.

McDonald, G. B., Sullivan, K. M., & Plumley, T. F. (1984). Radiographic features of esophageal involvement in chronic graft-vs.-host disease. *American Journal of Roentgenology,* 142, 501–506.

Meloni, G., Proia, A., Capria, S. *et al.* (2001). Obesity and autologous stem cell transplantation in acute myeloid leukemia. *Bone Marrow Transplantation,* 28, 365–367.

Memoli, D., Spitzer, T. R., Cottler-Fox, M. *et al.* (1988). Acute esophageal stricture after bone marrow transplantation. *Bone Marrow Transplantation,* 3, 513–516.

Mertens, T., Kock, J., Hampl, W. *et al.* (1996). Reactivated fulminant hepatitis B virus replication after bone marrow transplantation: clinical course and possible treatment with ganciclovir. *Journal of Hepatology,* 25, 968–971.

Messing, B. (2000). [Parenteral nutrition: indications and techniques]. *Annals de medicine interne,* 151, 652–658.

Messing, B., Bories, C., Kunstlinger, F., & Bernier, J. J. (1983). Does total parenteral nutrition induce gallbladder sludge formation and lithiasis? *Gastroenterology,* 84, 1012–1019.

Miura, Y., Takamatsu, H., Okumura, H. *et al.* (1997). Allogeneic bone marrow transplantation for a patient complicated by chronic hepatitis due to precore mutant hepatitis B virus: failure of management with interferon-alpha therapy. *American Journal of Hematology*, **54**, 344–345.

Morton, A. J. & Durrant, S. T. (1995). Efficacy of octreotide in controlling refractory diarrhea following bone marrow transplantation. *Clinical Transplantation*, **9**, 205–208.

Moscardo, F., Sanz, G. F., de La Rubia, J. *et al.* (2001). Marked reduction in the incidence of hepatic veno-occlusive disease after allogeneic hematopoietic stem cell transplantation with CD34(+) positive selection. *Bone Marrow Transplantation*, **27**, 983–988.

Murakami, C. S., Chan, G. S. & McDonald, G. B. (2002). Incidence and etiology of extrahepatic biliary obstruction in bone marrow transplant patients. *Gastroenterology*, **112**, 1340a.

Murakami, C. S., Louie, W., Chan, G. S. *et al.* (1999). Biliary obstruction in hematopoietic cell transplant recipients: an uncommon diagnosis with specific causes. *Bone Marrow Transplantation*, **23**, 921–927.

Murphy, J. J., Granger, R., Blair, G. K. *et al.* (1995). Necrotizing fasciitis in childhood. *Journal of Pediatric Surgery*, **30**, 1131–1134.

Musa, M. B., Katakkar, S. B., & Khaliq, A. (1975). Anorectal and perianal complications of hematologic malignant neoplasms. *Canadian Journal of Surgery*, **18**, 579–583.

Muscaritoli, M., Conversano, L., Torelli, G. F. *et al.* (1998). Clinical and metabolic effects of different parenteral nutrition regimens in patients undergoing allogeneic bone marrow transplantation. *Transplantation*, **66**, 610–616.

Muscaritoli, M., Grieco, G., Capria, S., Iori, A. P., & Fanelli, F. R. (2002). Nutritional and metabolic support in patients undergoing bone marrow transplantation. *American Journal of Clinical Nutrition*, **75**, 183–190.

Nagler, A., Ilan, Y., Adler, R. *et al.* (1995). Successful immunization of autologous bone marrow transplantation recipients against hepatitis B virus by active vaccination. *Bone Marrow Transplantation*, **15**, 475–478.

Naik, H. R. & Chandrasekar, P. H. (1996). Herpes simplex virus (HSV) colitis in a bone marrow transplant recipient. *Bone Marrow Transplantation*, **17**, 285–286.

Nash, R. A., Pepe, M. S., Storb, R. *et al.* (1992). Acute graft-versus-host disease: analysis of risk factors after allogeneic marrow transplantation and prophylaxis with cyclosporine and methotrexate. *Blood*, **80**, 1838–1845.

Navari, R. M., Sharma, P., Degg, H. J. *et al.* (1983). Pneumatosis cystoides intestinalis following allogeneic marrow transplantation. *Transplantation Proceedings*, **25**, 1720–4.

Nevo, S., Enger, C., Swan, V. *et al.* (1999). Acute bleeding after allogeneic bone marrow transplantation: association with graft versus host disease and effect on survival. *Transplantation*, **67**, 681–689.

Nevo, S., Swan, V., Enger, C. *et al.* (1998). Acute bleeding after bone marrow transplantation (BMT)-incidence and effect on survival. A quantitative analysis in 1,402 patients. *Blood*, **91**, 1469–1477.

Nieto, Y., Russ, P., Everson, G. *et al.* (2000). Acute pancreatitis during immunosuppression with tacrolimus following an allogeneic umbilical cord blood transplantation. *Bone Marrow Transplantation*, **26**, 109–111.

Nishi, T., Okazaki, K., Fujii, S. *et al.* (2001). Successful treatment with steroids of upper gastrointestinal acute graft vs. host disease after hematopoietic stem cell transplantation. *Endoscopy*, **33**, 985–987.

Norol, F., Roche, B., Girardin, M. F. *et al.* (1994). Hepatitis C virus infection and allogeneic bone marrow transplantation. *Transplantation*, **57**, 393–397.

Nysom, K., Holm, K., Michaelsen, K. F. *et al.* (2000). Bone mass after allogeneic BMT for childhood leukaemia or lymphoma. *Bone Marrow Transplantation*, **25**, 191–196.

Ochocka, M., Karwacki, M., Matysiak, M. *et al.* (1995). [Results of treatment for severe acquired aplastic anemia in children]. *Pediatria Polska*, **70**, 205–211.

Ohashi, K., Tanabe, J., Watanabe, R. *et al.* (2000). The Japanese multicenter open randomized trial of ursodeoxycholic acid prophylaxis for hepatic veno-occlusive disease after stem cell transplantation. *American Journal of Hematology*, **64**, 32–38.

Omata, F., Ueno, F., Kushibiki, Y., & Takahashi, H. (1994). Fulminant hepatitis following bone marrow transplantation in hepatitis B virus carrier siblings. *Journal of Gastroenterology*, **29**, 653–655.

Or, R., Nagler, A., Shpilberg, O. *et al.* (1996). Low molecular weight heparin for the prevention of veno-occlusive disease of the liver in bone marrow transplantation patients. *Transplantation*, **61**, 1067–1071.

Ozkaynak, M. F., Weinberg, K., Kohn, D. *et al.* (1991). Hepatic veno-occlusive disease post-bone marrow transplantation in children conditioned with busulfan and cyclophosphamide: incidence, risk factors, and clinical outcome. *Bone Marrow Transplantation*, **7**, 467–474.

Ozsahin, M., Pene, F., Touboul, E. *et al.* (1992). Total-body irradiation before bone marrow transplantation. Results of two randomized instantaneous dose rates in 157 patients. *Cancer*, **69**, 2853–2865.

Papadopoulou, A., Lloyd, D. R., Williams, M. D., Darbyshire, P. J., & Booth, I. W. (1996). Gastrointestinal and nutritional sequelae of bone marrow transplantation. *Archives of Disease in Childhood*, **75**, 208–213.

Papatheodoridis, G. V., Patch, D., Watkinson, A., Tibbals, J., & Burroughs, A. K. (1999). Transjugular liver biopsy in the 1990s: a 2-year audit. *Alimentary Pharmacology & Therapeutia*, **13**, 603–608.

Pariente, E. A., Goudeau, A., Dubois, F. *et al.* (1988). Fulminant hepatitis due to reactivation of chronic hepatitis B virus infection after allogeneic bone marrow transplantation. *Digestive Diseases and Science*, **33**, 1185–1191.

Park, S. H., Lee, M. H., Lee, H. *et al.* (2002). A randomized trial of heparin plus ursodiol vs heparin alone to prevent hepatic veno-occlusive disease after hematopoietic stem cell transplantation. *Bone Marrow Transplantation*, **29**, 137–143.

Patey-Mariaud de Serre, N., Reijasse, D., Verkarre, V. *et al.* (2002). Chronic intestinal graft-versus-host disease: clinical, histological and immunohistochemical analysis of 17 children. *Bone Marrow Transplantation*, **29**, 223–230.

Picardi, M., Selleri, C., De Rosa, G. *et al.* (1998). Lamivudine treatment for chronic replicative hepatitis B virus infection after allogeneic bone marrow transplantation. *Bone Marrow Transplantation*, **21**, 1267–1269.

Pico, J. L., Avila-Garavito, A., & Naccache, P. (1998). Mucositis: Its Occurrence, Consequences, and Treatment in the Oncology Setting. *Oncologist*, **3**, 446–451.

Pinho, V. C., Ibrahim, A., Avila, G. A. *et al.* (1996). Protein-losing gastropathy associated with cytomegalovirus: a rare and late complication of allogeneic bone marrow transplantation. *Bone Marrow Transplantation,* **17,** 887–889.

Ponec, R. J., Hackman, R. C., & McDonald, G. B. (1999). Endoscopic and histologic diagnosis of intestinal graft-versus-host disease after marrow transplantation. *Gastrointestinal Endoscopy,* **49,** 612–621.

Porter, J. B. (2001). Practical management of iron overload. *British Journal of Haematology,* **115,** 239–252.

Price, K. J., Thall, P. F., Kish, S. K., Shannon, V. R., & Andersson, B. S. (1998). Prognostic indicators for blood and marrow transplant patients admitted to an intensive care unit. *American Journal of Respiratory and Critical Care Medicine,* **158,** 876–884.

Rajvanshi, P. & McDonald, G. B. (2001). Subconjunctival hemorrhage as a complication of endoscopy. *Gastrointestinal Endoscopy,* **53,** 251–253.

Rajvanshi, P., Shulman, H. M., Sievers, E. L. & McDonald, G. B. (2002). Hepatic sinusoidal obstruction after gemtuzumab ozogamicin (Mylotarg) therapy. *Blood,* **99,** 2310–2314.

Ramakrishna, J. & Treem, W. R. (1997). Duodenal hematoma as a complication of endoscopic biopsy in pediatric bone marrow transplant recipients. *Journal of Pediatric Gastroenterology and Nutritron,* **25,** 426–429.

Rapoport, A. P., Doyle, H. R., Starzl, T. *et al.* (1991). Orthotopic liver transplantation for life-threatening veno-occlusive disease of the liver after allogeneic bone marrow transplant. *Bone Marrow Transplantation,* **8,** 421–424.

Rapoport, A. P., Miller Watelet, L. F., Linder, T. *et al.* (1999). Analysis of factors that correlate with mucositis in recipients of autologous and allogeneic stem-cell transplants. *Journal of Clinical Oncology,* **17,** 2446–2453.

Rhodes, D. F., Lee, W. M., Wingard, J. R. *et al.* (1990). Orthotopic liver transplantation for graft-versus-host disease following bone marrow transplantation. *Gastroenterology,* **99,** 536–538.

Ribas, A. & Gale, R. P. (1997). Should people with hepatitis C virus infection receive a bone marrow transplant? *Bone Marrow Transplantation,* **19,** 97–99.

Richardson, P. G., Elias, A. D., Krishna, A. *et al.* (1998). Treatment of severe veno-occlusive disease with defibrotide: compassionate use results in response without significant toxicity in a high-risk population. *Blood,* **92,** 737–744.

Richardson, P. G., Murakami, C., Warren, D. L. *et al.* (2002). Multi-institutional emergency use of defibrotide in 75 patients post SCT with severe VOD and multisystem organ failure: Response without significant toxicity in a high risk population. *Blood,* **96,** 2510.

Ringden, O., Remberger, M., Lehmann, S. *et al.* (2000). N-acetylcysteine for hepatic veno- occlusive disease after allogeneic stem cell transplantation. *Bone Marrow Transplantation,* **25,** 993–996.

Ritchie, D. S., Angus, P. W., Bhathal, P. S., & Grigg, A. P. (2002). Liver failure complicating non-alcoholic steatohepatitis following allogeneic bone marrow transplantation for Schwachman-Diamond syndrome. *Bone Marrow Transplantation,* **29,** 931–3.

Rivera-Vaquerizo, P. A., Gomez-Garrido, J., Vicente-Gutierrez, M. *et al.* (2001). Varicella zoster gastritis 3 years after bone marrow transplantation for treatment of acute leukemia. *Gastrointestinal Endoscopy,* **53,** 809–810.

Rodriguez-Inigo, E., Tomas, J. F., Gomez-Garcia, d.S.V. *et al.* (1997). Hepatitis C and G virus infection and liver dysfunction after allogeneic bone marrow transplantation: results from a prospective study. *Blood,* **90,** 1326–1331.

Roslyn, J. J., Pitt, H. A., Mann, L. L., Ament, M. E., & DenBesten, L. (1983). Gallbladder disease in patients on long-term parenteral nutrition. *Gastroenterology,* **84,** 148–154.

Rossetti, F., Brawner, D. L., Bowden, R. *et al.* (1995). Fungal liver infection in marrow transplant recipients: prevalence at autopsy, predisposing factors, and clinical feature. *Clinical Infectious Diseases,* **20,** 801–811.

Roy, J., Snover, D., Weisdorf, S. *et al.* (1991). Simultaneous upper and lower endoscopic biopsy in the diagnosis of intestinal graft-versus-host-disease. *Transplantation,* **51,** 642–646.

Safadi, R., Or, R., Ilan, Y. *et al.* (2001). Lack of known hepatitis virus in hepatitis-associated aplastic anemia and outcome after bone marrow transplantation. *Bone Marrow Transplantation,* **27,** 183–190.

Salomone, T., Tosi, P., Raiti, C. *et al.* (1999). Clinical relevance of acute pancreatitis in allogeneic hemopoietic stem cell (bone marrow or peripheral blood) transplants. *Digestive Diseases and Sciences,* **44,** 1124–1127.

Sambresqui, A., Zylberman, M., Foncuberta, C. *et al.* (1995). Somatostatin for the treatment of upper gastrointestinal bleeding (UGIB) in patients undergoing autologous bone marrow transplantation (ABMT). *Bone Marrow Transplantation,* **16,** 323.

Sanders, J. E., Buckner, C. D., Clift, R. A. *et al.* (1988). Second marrow transplants in patients with leukemia who relapse after allogeneic marrow transplantation. *Bone Marrow Transplantation,* **3,** 11–19.

Sato, T., Sakamaki, S., Nagaoka, Y. *et al.* (1997). Intra-mesenteric artery steroid administration relieved severe refractory gastrointestinal graft-vs.-host disease in an allogeneic bone marrow transplantation patient. *American Journal of Hematology,* **56,** 277–280.

Saunders, M. D., Shulman, H. M., Murakami, C. S. *et al.* (2000). Bile duct apoptosis and cholestasis resembling acute graft-versus-host disease after autologous hematopoietic cell transplantation. *The American Journal of Surgical Pathology,* **24,** 1004–1008.

Schiller, G. J., Nimer, S. D., Gajewski, J. L., & Golde, D. W. (1991). Abdominal presentation of varicella-zoster infection in recipients of allogeneic bone marrow transplantation. *Bone Marrow Transplantation,* **7,** 489–491.

Schimmer, A. D., Mah, K., Bordeleau, L. *et al.* (2001). Decreased bone mineral density is common after autologous blood or marrow transplantation. *Bone Marrow Transplantation,* **28,** 387–391.

Schleuning, M., Jager, G., Holler, E. *et al.* (1999). Human parvovirus B19-associated disease in bone marrow transplantation. *Infection,* **27,** 114–117.

Schneider, D. T., Nurnberger, W., Stannigel, H., Boning, H., & Gobel, U. (1999). Adjuvant treatment of severe acute pancreatitis with C1 esterase inhibitor concentrate after haematopoietic stem cell transplantation. *Gut,* **45,** 733–736.

Schots, R., Kaufman, L., Van, R. *et al.* (1998). Monitoring of C-reactive protein after allogeneic bone marrow transplantation identifies patients at risk of severe transplant-related complications and mortality. *Bone Marrow Transplantation,* **22,** 79–85.

Schriber, J., Milk, B., Shaw, D. *et al.* (1999). Tissue plasminogen activator (tPA) as therapy for hepatotoxicity following bone marrow transplantation. *Bone Marrow Transplantation,* **24,** 1311–1314.

Schubert, M. M., Sullivan, K. M., Morton, T. H. *et al.* (1984). Oral manifestations of chronic graft-v-host disease. *Archives of Internal Medicine,* **144,** 1591–1595.

Schulenburg, A., Kalhs, P., Oberhuber, G. *et al.* (1998). Gastrointestinal perforation early after peripheral blood stem cell transplantation for AL amyloidosis. *Bone Marrow Transplantation,* **22,** 293–295.

Schuler, U., Subat, S., Schmidt, H., Schneider, A., & Ehninger, G. (1996). Evaluation of procollagen-III peptide as a marker for veno-occlusive disease after bone marrow transplantation. *Annals of Hematology,* **73,** 25–28.

Schultz, K. R., Nevill, T. J., Balshaw, R. F. *et al.* (2000). Effect of gastrointestinal inflammation and age on the pharmacokinetics of oral microemulsion cyclosporin A in the first month after bone marrow transplantation. *Bone Marrow Transplantation,* **26,** 545–551.

Schultz, K. R., Nevill, T. J., Toze, C. L. *et al.* (1998). The pharmacokinetics of oral cyclosporin A (Neoral) during the first month after bone marrow transplantation. *Transplantation Proceedings,* **30,** 1668–1670.

Schwartz, J. M., Wolford, J. L., Thornquist, M. D. *et al.* (2001). Severe gastrointestinal bleeding after hematopoietic cell transplantation, 1987–1997: incidence, causes, and outcome. *The American Journal of Gastroenterology,* **96,** 385–393.

Sefcick, A., Anderton, D., Byrne, J. L., Teahon, K., & Russell, N. H. (2001). Naso-jejunal feeding in allogeneic bone marrow transplant recipients: results of a pilot study. *Bone Marrow Transplantation,* **28,** 1135–1139.

Sehdev, M. K., Dowling, M. D., Jr., Seal, S. H., & Stearns, M. W., Jr. (1973). Perianal and anorectal complications in leukemia. *Cancer,* **31,** 149–152.

Seth, P. Alrajhi, A. A., Kagevi, I. *et al.* (2002). Hepatitis B reactivation with clinical flare in allogneic stem cell transplants with chronic graft-versus-host disease. *Bone Marrow Transplantation,* **30,** 189–94.

Shields, A. F., Hackman, R. C., Fife, K. H., Corey, L., & Meyers, J. D. (1985). Adenovirus infections in patients undergoing bone-marrow transplantation. *New England Journal of Medicine,* **312,** 529–533.

Shore, T., Bow, E., Greenberg, H. *et al.* (1996). Pancreatitis post-bone marrow transplantation. *Bone Marrow Transplantation,* **17,** 1181–1184.

Shuhart, M. C., Myerson, D., Childs, B. H. *et al.* (1994). Marrow transplantation from hepatitis C virus seropositive donors: transmission rate and clinical course. *Blood,* **84,** 3229–3235.

Shuhart, M. C., Myerson, D., Spurgeon, C. L. *et al.* (1996). Hepatitis C virus (HCV) infection in bone marrow transplant patients after transfusions from anti-HCV-positive blood. *Bone Marrow Transplantation,* **17,** 601–606.

Shulman, H. M., Fisher, L. B., Schoch, H. G., Henne, K. W., & McDonald, G. B. (1994). Veno-occlusive disease of the liver after marrow transplantation: histological correlates of clinical signs and symptoms. *Hepatology,* **19,** 1171–1181.

Shulman, H. M., Gooley, T., Dudley, M. D. *et al.* (1995). Utility of transvenous liver biopsies and wedged hepatic venous pressure measurements in sixty marrow transplant recipients. *Transplantation,* **59,** 1015–1022.

Shulman, H. M., Sharma, P., Amos, D., Fenster, L. F., & McDonald, G. B. (1988). A coded histologic study of hepatic graft-versus-host disease after human bone marrow transplantation. *Hepatology,* **8,** 463–470.

Skidmore, S. J., Collingham, K. E., Harrison, P. *et al.* (1997). High prevalence of hepatitis G virus in bone marrow transplant recipients and patients treated for acute leukemia. *Blood,* **89,** 3853–3856.

Slattery, J. T., Sanders, J. E., Buckner, C. D. *et al.* (1995). Graft-rejection and toxicity following bone marrow transplantation in relation to busulfan pharmacokinetics. *Bone Marrow Transplantation,* **16,** 31–42.

Slavin, M. A., Osborne, B., Adams, R. *et al.* (1995). Efficacy and safety of fluconazole prophylaxis for fungal infections after marrow transplantation-a prospective, randomized, double-blind study. *Journal of Infectious Diseases,* **171,** 1545–1552.

Snover, D. C. (1984). Acute and chronic graft versus host disease: histopathological evidence for two distinct pathogenetic mechanisms. *Human Pathology,* **15,** 202–205.

Snover, D. C. (1990). Graft-versus-host disease of the gastrointestinal tract. *American Journal of Surgical Pathology,* **14,** (Suppl 1), 101–108.

Snover, D. C., Freese, D. K., Sharp, H. L. *et al.* (1987a). Liver allograft rejection. An analysis of the use of biopsy in determining of rejection. *American Journal of Surgical Pathology,* **11,** 1–10.

Snover, D. C., Hutton, S., Balfour, H. H., Jr., & Bloomer, J. R. (1987b). Cytomegalovirus infection of the liver in transplant recipients. *Journal of Clinical Gastroenterology,* **9,** 659–665.

Snover, D. C., Weisdorf, S., Bloomer, J., McGlave, P., & Weisdorf, D. (1989). Nodular regenerative hyperplasia of the liver following bone marrow transplantation. *Hepatology,* **9,** 443–448.

Snover, D. C., Weisdorf, S. A., Ramsay, N. K., McGlave, P., & Kersey, J. H. (1984). Hepatic graft versus host disease: a study of the predictive value of liver biopsy in diagnosis. *Hepatology,* **4,** 123–130.

Snover, D. C., Weisdorf, S. A., Vercellotti, G. M. *et al.* (1985). A histopathologic study of gastric and small intestinal graft-versus-host disease following allogeneic bone marrow transplantation. *Human Pathology,* **16,** 387–392.

Sodhi, S. S., Srinivasan, R., & Thomas, R. M. (2000). Esophageal graft versus host disease. *Gastrointestinal Endoscopy,* **52,** 235.

Somervaille, T. C., Kirk, S., Dogan, A., Landon, G. V., & Mackinnon, S. (1999). Fulminant hepatic failure caused by adenovirus infection following bone marrow transplantation for Hodgkin's disease. *Bone Marrow Transplantation,* **24,** 99–101.

Sonis, S. T. (1998). Mucositis as a biological process: a new hypothesis for the development of chemotherapy-induced stomatotoxicity. *Oral Oncology,* **34,** 39–43.

Spaner, D., Lowsky, R., Fyles, G. *et al.* (1998). Acute intestinal graft-versus-host disease in a syngeneic bone marrow transplant recipient. *Transplantation,* **66,** 1251–1253.

Spencer, G. D., Hackman, R. C., McDonald, G. B. *et al.* (1986). A prospective study of unexplained nausea and vomiting after marrow transplantation. *Transplantation,* **42,** 602–607.

Stechschulte, D. J., Jr., Fishback, J. L., Emami, A., & Bhatia, P. (1990). Secondary biliary cirrhosis as a consequence of graft-versus-host disease. *Gastroenterology, 98,* 223–225.

Steiner, M., Steiner, B., Wilhelm, S., Freund, M., & Schuff-Werner, P. (2000). Severe hypophosphatemia during hematopoietic reconstitution after allogeneic peripheral blood stem cell transplantation *Bone Marrow Transplantation, 25,* 1015–1016.

Stemmelin, G. R., Pest, P., Peters, R. A. *et al.* (1995). Severe esophageal stricture after autologous bone marrow transplant. *Bone Marrow Transplantation, 15,* 1001–1002.

Stiff, P. (2001). Mucositis associated with stem cell transplantation: current status and innovative approaches to management. *Bone Marrow transplantation, 27* (Suppl 2), S3–S11.

Strasser, S. I. & McCaughan, G. W. (2000). Therapies for chronic hepatitis B: emerging roles for nucleoside analogues. *Australian and New Zealand Journal of Medicine,* 30: 556–558.

Strasser, S. I. & McDonald, G. B. (1999a). Gastrointestinal and hepatic complications. In *Hematopoietic Cell Transplantation,* eds. E. D. Thomas, K. G. Blume, & S. J. Forman, pp. 627–645. Cambridge, MA: Blackwell.

Strasser, S. I. & McDonald, G. B. (1999b). Hepatitis viruses and hematopoietic cell transplantation: a guide to patient and donor management. *Blood, 93,* 1127–1136.

Strasser, S. I., Myerson, D., Spurgeon, C. L. *et al.* (1999a). Hepatitis C virus infection and bone marrow transplantation: a cohort study with 10-year follow-up. *Hepatology, 29,* 1893–1899.

Strasser, S. I., Shulman, H. M., & McDonald, G. B. (1999b). Cholestasis after hematopoietic cell transplantation. *Clinics in Liver Disease, 3,* 651–68. x.

Strasser, S. I., Schulman, H. M., Flowers, M. E.. *et al.* (2000). Chronic graft-versus-host of the liver: presentation as an acute hepatitis. *Hepatology, 32,* 1265–71.

Strasser, S. I., Sullivan, K. M., Myerson, D. *et al.* (1999c). Cirrhosis of the liver in long-term marrow transplant survivors. *Blood, 93,* 3259–3266.

Stromeyer, F. W. & Ishak, K. G. (1981). Nodular transformation (nodular "regenerative" hyperplasia) of the liver. A clinicopathologic study of 30 cases. *Human Pathology, 12,* 60–71.

Sullivan, K. M., Shulman, H. M., Storb, R. *et al.* (1981). Chronic graft-versus-host disease in 52 patients: adverse natural course and successful treatment with combination immunosuppression. *Blood, 57,* 267–276.

Tabbara, I. A. (1996). Allogeneic bone marrow transplantation: acute and late complications. *Anticancer Research, 16,* 1019–1026.

Takasuka, H., Yamada, S., Okamoto, T. *et al.* (2000). Predicting the severity of intestinal graft-versus-host disease from leukotriene B4 levels after bone marrow transplantation. *Bone Marrow Transplantation, 26,* 1313–1316.

Tanaka, J., Imamura, M., Kasai, M. *et al.* (1993). Rapid analysis of tumor necrosis factor-alpha mRNA expression during venooclusive disease of the liver after allogeneic bone marrow transplantation. *Transplantation, 55,* 430–432.

Tarella, C., Caracciolo, D., Gavarotti, P. *et al.* (2000). Overweight as an adverse prognostic factor for non-Hodgkin's lymphoma patients receiving high-dose chemotherapy and autograft. *Bone Marrow Transplantation, 26,* 1185–1191.

Tefferi, A., Kumar, S., Wolf, R. C. *et al.* (2001). Charcoal hemofiltration for hepatic veno-occlusive disease after hematopoietic stem cell transplantation. *Bone Marrow Transplantation, 28,* 997–999.

Terdiman, J. P., Linker, C. A., Ries, C. A. *et al.* (1996). The role of endoscopic evaluation in patients with suspected intestinal graft-versus-host disease after allogeneic bone-marrow transplantation. *Endoscopy, 28,* 680–685.

Thaler, M., Pastakia, B., Shawker, T. H., O'Leary, T., & Pizzo, P. A. (1998). Hepatic candidiasis in cancer patients: the evolving picture of the syndrome. *Annals of Internal Medicine, 108,* 88–100.

Toh, H. C., McAfee, S. L., Sackstein, R. *et al.* (1999). Late onset veno-occlusive disease following high-dose chemotherapy and stem cell transplantation. *Bone Marrow Transplantation, 24,* 891–895.

Tomas, J. F., Pinilla, I., Garcia-Buey, M. L. *et al.* (2000). Long-term liver dysfunction after allogeneic bone marrow transplantation: clinical features and course in 61 patients. *Bone Marrow Transplantation, 26,* 649–655.

Tomas, J. F., Rodriguez-Inigo, E., Bartolome, J. *et al.* (1997). Detection of hepatitis G virus from serum and liver of a patient with long-term liver dysfunction after autologous bone marrow transplantation. *Bone Marrow Transplantation, 19,* 1053–1057.

Tomblyn, M., Gordon, L., Singhal, S. *et al.* (2002). Rarity of toxigenic *Clostridium difficile* infections after hematopoietic stem cell transplantation: implications for symptomatic management of diarrhoea. *Bone Marrow Transplantation, 30,* 517–9.

Townsend, T. R., Bolyard, E. A., Yolken, R. H. *et al.* (1982). Outbreak of Coxsackie A1 gastroenteritis: a complication of bone-marrow transplantation. *Lancet, 1,* 820–823.

Tse, N., Cederbaum, S., & Glaspy, J. A. (1991). Hyperammonemia following allogeneic bone marrow transplantation. *American Journal of Hematology, 38,* 140–141.

Tzung, S. P., Hackman, R. C., Hockenbery, D. M. *et al.* (1998). Lymphocytic gastritis resembling graft-vs.-host disease following autologous hematopoietic cell transplantation. *Biology of Blood and Marrow Transplantation, 4,* 43–48.

Uchida, N., Gondo, H., Himeji, D. *et al.* (2000). Lamivudine therapy for a hepatitis B surface antigen (HBsAg)-positive leukemia patient receiving myeloablative chemotherapy and autologous stem cell transplantation. *Bone Marrow Transplantation, 26,* 1243–1245.

Ustun, C., Koc, H., Karayalcin, S. *et al.* (1997). Hepatitis B virus infection in allogeneic bone marrow transplantation. *Bone Marrow Transplantation, 20,* 289–296.

van Bekkum, D. W. (1991). What is graft versus host disease? *Bone Marrow Transplantation, 7* (Suppl 2), 110–111.

van Burik, J. H., Leisenring, W., Myerson, D. *et al.* (1998). The effect of prophylactic fluconazole on the clinical spectrum of fungal diseases in bone marrow transplant recipients with special attention to hepatic candidiasis. An autopsy study of 355 patients. *Medicine, 77,* 246–254.

Van Dam, J., Farraye, F. A., Gale, R. P., & Zeldis, J. B. (1990). Fulminant hepatic failure following bone marrow transplantation for hepatitis-associated aplastic anemia. *Bone Marrow Transplantation, 5,* 57–60.

van Kraaij, M. G., Dekker, A. W., Verdonck, L. F. *et al.* (2000). Infectious gastro-enteritis: an uncommon cause of diarrhoea in adult allogeneic and autologous stem cell transplant recipients. *Bone Marrow Transplantation, 26,* 209–303.

Vance, E. A., Soiffer, R. J., McDonald, G. B. *et al.* (1996). Prevention of transmission of hepatitis C virus in bone marrow transplantation by treating the donor with alpha-interferon. *Transplantation, 62,* 1358–1360.

Vanhueverzwyn, R., Delannoy, A., Michaux, J. L., & Dive, C. (1980). Anal lesions in hematologic diseases. *Diseases of the Colon and Rectum,* **23,** 310–312.

Vassal, G., Koscielny, S., Challine, D. *et al.* (1996). Busulfan disposition and hepatic veno-occlusive disease in children undergoing bone marrow transplantation. *Cancer Chemotherapy and Pharmacology,* **37,** 247–253.

Vishny, M. L., Blades, E. W., Creger, R. J., & Lazarus, H. M. (1994). Role of upper endoscopy in evaluation of upper gastrointestinal symptoms in patients undergoing bone marrow transplantation. *Cancer Investigation,* **12,** 384–389.

Vlachogiannakos, J., Patch, D., Watkinson, A., Tibballs, J., & Burroughs, A. K. (2000). Carbon-dioxide portography: an expanding role? *Lancet,* **355,** 987–988.

Wada, H., Mori, A., Okada, M. *et al.* (2001). Treatment of intestinal graft-versus-host disease using betamethasone enemas. *Transplantation,* **72,** 1451–1453.

Wakui, M., Okamoto, S., Ishida, A. *et al.* (1999). Prospective evaluation for upper gastrointestinal tract acute graft-versus-host disease after hematopoietic stem cell transplantation. *Bone Marrow Transplantation,* **23,** 573–578.

Walsh, G. & Stickley, C. S. (1934). Acute leukaemia with primary symptoms in the rectum. *Southern Medical Journal,* **96,** 684–689.

Wang, J. T., Tsai, F. C., Lee, C. Z. *et al.* (1996). A prospective study of transfusion-transmitted GB virus C infection: similar frequency but different clinical presentation compared with hepatitis C virus. *Blood,* **88,** 1881–1886.

Wanless, I. R. (1990). Micronodular transformation (nodular regenerative hyperplasia) of the liver: a report of 64 cases among 2,500 autopsies and a new classification of benign hepatocellular nodules. *Hepatology,* **11,** 787–797.

Wanless, I. R., Godwin, T. A., Allen, F., & Feder, A. (1980). Nodular regenerative hyperplasia of the liver in hematologic disorders: a possible response to obliterative portal venopathy. A morphometric study of nine cases with an hypothesis on the pathogenesis. *Medicine (Baltimore),* **59,** 367–379.

Washington, K., Bentley, R. C., Green, A. *et al.* (1997). Gastric graft-versus-host disease: a blinded histologic study. *American Journal of Surgical Pathology,* **21,** 1037–1046.

Washington, K., Gossage, D. L., & Gottfried, M. R. (1994). Pathology of the pancreas in severe combined immunodeficiency and DiGeorge syndrome: acute graft-versus-host disease and unusual viral infections. *Human Pathology,* **25,** 908–914.

Washington, K., Peters, W., & Gottfried, M. R. (1993). Pathology of the pancreas in bone marrow transplant patients. *Human Pathology,* **24,** 152–159.

Wasserman, E., Hidalgo, M., Hornedo, J., & Cortes-Funes, H. (1997). Octreotide (SMS 201-995) for hematopoietic support-dependent high-dose chemotherapy (HSD-HDC)-related diarrhoea: dose finding study and evaluation of efficacy. *Bone Marrow Transplantation,* **20,** 711–714.

Webster, A., Brenner, M. K., Prentice, H. G., & Griffiths, P. D. (1989). Fatal hepatitis B reactivation after autologous bone marrow transplantation. *Bone Marrow Transplantation,* **4,** 207–208.

Weisdorf, D. J., Snover, D. C., Haake, R. *et al.* (1990). Acute upper gastrointestinal graft-versus-host disease: clinical significance and response to immunosuppressive therapy. *Blood,* **76,** 624–629.

Werlin, S. L., Casper, J., Antonson, D., & Calabro, C. (1992). Pancreatitis associated with bone marrow transplantation in children. *Bone Marrow Transplantation,* **10,** 65–69.

West, J. C., Armitage, J. O., Mitros, F. A. *et al.* (1982). Cytomegalovirus cecal erosion causing massive hemorrhage in a bone marrow transplant recipient. *World Journal of Surgery,* **6,** 251–255.

Wilkes, J. D. (1998). Prevention and treatment of oral mucositis following cancer chemotherapy. *Seminars in Oncology,* **25,** 538–551.

Wolf, J. E., Liu, H. H., & Rabinowitz, L. G. (1989). Ecthyma gangrenosum in the absence of *Pseudomonas* bacteremia in a bone marrow transplant recipient. *The American Journal of Medicine,* **87,** 595–597.

Wolford, J. L. & McDonald, G. B. (1988). A problem-oriented approach to intestinal and liver disease after marrow transplantation. *Journal of Clinical Gastroenterology,* **10,** 419–433.

Woo, S. B., Allen, C. M., Orden, A., Porter, D., & Antin, J. H. (1996). Non-gingival soft tissue growths after allogeneic marrow transplantation. *Bone Marrow Transplantation,* **17,** 1127–1132.

Worawattanakul, S., Semelka, R. C., Kelekis, N. L., & Sallah, A. S. (1996). MR findings of intestinal graft-versus-host disease. *Magnetic Resonance Imaging,* **14,** 1221–1223.

Worynski, A., Zimmerman, M., Herrmann, R. P., & Forbes, G. M. (1998). Intramural duodenal haematoma following endoscopic biopsy in a bone marrow transplant patient. *Australian and New Zealand Journal of Medicine,* **28,** 843–844.

Wu, D., Hockenberry, D. M., Brentnall, T. A. *et al.* (1998). Persistent nausea and anorexia after marrow transplantation: a prospective study of 78 patients. *Transplantation,* **66,** 1319–1324.

Yakoub-Agha, I., Damaj, G., Garderet, L. *et al.* (2000). Severe esophagitis after allogeneic bone marrow transplantation for Fanconi's anemia. *Bone Marrow Transplantation,* **26,** 215–218.

Yasmineh, W. G., Filipovich, A. H., & Killeen, A. A. (1989). Serum 5′nucleotidase and alkaline phosphatase—highly predictive liver function tests for the diagnosis of graft-versus-host disease in bone marrow transplant recipients. *Transplantation,* **48,** 809–814.

Yau, J. C., Zander, A. R., Srigley, J. R. *et al.* (1986). Chronic graft-versus-host disease complicated by micronodular cirrhosis and esophageal varices. *Transplantation,* **41,** 129–130.

Yeager, K. A., Webster, J., Crain, M., Kasow, J., & McGuire, D. B. (2000). Implementation of an oral standard for leukemia and transplantation patients. *Cancer Nursing,* **23,** 40–47.

Yu, L. C., Malkani, I., Regueira, O., Ode, D. L., & Warrier, R. P. (1994). Recombinant tissue plasminogen activator (rt-PA) for veno-occlusive liver disease in pediatric autologous bone marrow transplant patients. *American Journal of Hematology,* **46,** 194–198.

Zenz, T., Rossle, M., Bertz, H. *et al.* (2001). Severe veno-occlusive disease after allogeneic bone marrow or peripheral stem cell transplantation—role of transjugular intrahepatic portosystemic shunt (TIPS). *Liver,* **21,** 31–36.

Zülke, C., Ulbrich, S., Graeb, C. *et al.* (2002). Acute pneumatosis cystoides intestinalis following allogeneic transplantation—the surgeon's dilemma. *Bone Marrow Transplantation,* **29,** 795–8.

Zutter, M. M., Martin, P. J., Sale, G. E. *et al.* (1988). Epstein-Barr virus lymphoproliferation after bone marrow transplantation. *Blood,* **72,** 520–529.

90 Renal complications

YIMING LIT AND JULIAN SEIFTER

Harvard University, Boston, USA

Introduction

Allogenic or autologous hematopoietic stem cell transplantation (HSCT) has been increasingly used as a therapy for patients with a wide range of hematologic and other diseases. HSCT usually involves the use of pretransplant myeloablative chemotherapy with or without total body irradiation, and posttransplant immune suppression, such as cyclosporine, to prevent or treat graft-versus-host disease (GVHD). The inherent toxicities of HSCT have been known to cause a variety of complications, including both acute and chronic renal failure. Many patients receiving HSCT develop acute renal function impairment (Kone *et al.,* 1988; Gruss *et al.,* 1995), and between 5% and 20% of long-term survivors develop some degree of chronic renal function impairment (Cohen, 2001). Causes are shown in Table 90.1.

Pre-existing renal disease

Extant kidney conditions, particularly when associated with renal impairment, are a relative contraindication to stem cell grafting. Clearly, the major problem with renal impairment is that it will severely hamper the facility and flexibility with which drugs are administered, especially in the areas of GVHD prophylaxis and the treatment of infection; this applies both to nephrotoxic and renally excreted drugs. A diminished renal reserve at the outset will also increase the susceptibility of a recipient to renal damage from other causes such as sepsis and obstruction.

Of interest here is multiple myeloma, where stem cell transplantation may also provide effective therapy and perhaps cure.

Table 90.1. *Causes of renal dysfunction in bone marrow transplant recipients*

1. Cyclosporine and tacrolimus (FK-506)
2. Other nephrotoxic drugs
3. Irradiation
4. Sepsis, especially when septic shock present
5. Urinary tract obstruction
6. Pre-existing renal disease, including myeloma kidney

Myeloma kidney, which is mostly a toxic nephropathy due to tubular injury from precipitated light chains, can be a chronic process with permanent fibrosis and renal impairment. In at least one center, however, this has not been a contraindication to autologous HSC transplantation in this patient population (see Chapter 40). Likewise, allogeneic HSC transplantation has been performed for aplastic anemia in a patient on long-term dialysis (Hamaki *et al.,* 2002). The conditioning regimen consisted of melphalan (reduced to 60 mg/m^2, ATG, and total lymphoid irradiation).

Early renal complications

Early renal complications often result from the side effects of the pretransplant conditioning and posttransplant immune suppression. Nausea, vomiting, and diarrhea can cause prerenal azotemia. Sepsis, hypotension, and the use of nephrotoxic antibiotics, such as aminoglycosides and amphotericin B, can cause severe impairment of renal function, including acute tubular necrosis. Allergic interstitial nephritis from antibiotics or allopurinol may also be a factor. Other disease entities that occur during this posttransplant period include tumor lysis syndrome, marrow infusion toxicity, and hepatic veno-occlusive disease (Zager, 1994).

The commonest cause of impaired renal function in HSCT recipients is drug toxicity, most commonly from cyclosporine or tacrolimus.

Drug toxicity

Cyclosporine and tacrolimus

Cyclosporine can cause three forms of nephrotoxicity: acute renal function impairment, hemolytic uremic syndrome, and chronic renal function impairment. It can also cause electrolyte disturbances (Table 90.2).

The toxicity from cyclosporine is thought to be due to its mediation of afferent arteriolar vasoconstriction and decreased glomerular filtration rate (Lanese & Conger, 1993). The increase in vascular resistance may be reflected clinically by a rise in serum creatinine level and hypertension (Remuzzi &

1454

Table 90.2. *Clinical spectrum of renal and electrolyte disturbances associated with cyclosporine toxicity*

1. Azotemia: ranging from asymptomatic biochemical abnormality to acute renal failure
2. Glomerular capillary thrombosis in association with hemolytic-uremic syndrome
3. Hypertension
4. Hyperkalemia
5. Hyperuricemia
6. Impaired urinary concentrating ability
7. Hypomagnesemia

Perico, 1995; English *et al.,* 1987). Acute cyclosporine nephrotoxicity is usually reversible with discontinuation of therapy.

Patients who receive cyclosporine for longer than 6 months are at risk for developing chronic nephrotoxicity. Chronic cyclosporine nephrotoxicity has been carefully studied in patients after cardiac transplantation and in those treated for autoimmune diseases (Myers & Newton, 1991; Bertani *et al.,* 1991; Feutren & Mihatsch, 1992; Deray *et al.,* 1992; Wilkinson & Cohen, 1999). These patients have a 35% to 45% reduction in glomerular filtration rate (GFR) compared to patients not treated with cyclosporine. Some patients may eventually progress to end-stage renal failure and require renal replacement therapy (Goldstein *et al.,* 1997; Frimat *et al.,* 1998).

The pathology of cyclosporine nephropathy is an obliterative arteriolopathy (Figs. 90.1, 90.2, and 90.3). It is characterized by ischemic collapse or scarring of the glomeruli, vacuolization of the tubules, and focal areas of tubular atrophy and interstitial

fibrosis, showing a striped pattern, beginning in the medulla and progressing to the medullary rays of the cortex (Bennett *et al.,* 1996). The changes are not necessarily dose-related. It is associated with degenerative hyaline changes in the walls of afferent arteriolar-sized blood vessels extending from the preglomerular area proximally up the afferent arteriole. Dieterle *et al.* reported renal pathology in autopsied or biopsied bone marrow transplant recipients (Dieterle *et al.,* 1990). Striped interstitial fibrosis was present in 25 patients and arteriolopathy was present in 36 of the 51 patients studied. Serum creatinine levels increased 40% to 80% by three months posttransplant. The renal pathology seemed to be worse when total body radiation was used to condition the recipient for transplant, even when the kidneys were shielded. Mihatsch *et al.* observed obliterative arteriolopathy with downstream glomerulosclerosis in cyclosporine-treated patients (Mihatsch *et al.,* 1988). They proposed that the arteriolopathy with ultimate vascular occlusion produces a pattern of striped interstitial fibrosis with nephron dropout, tubular atrophy, and if progressive, compromised renal function. Myers *et al.* also suggested that chronic afferent vascular injury leads to compromise in the integrity of afferent arterioles, leading to the irreversible changes observed (Myers & Newton, 1991).

In addition to deterioration in renal function, a number of electrolyte disturbances have been described. Hyperkalemia can result from cyclosporine-induced inhibition of the renin-angiotensin-aldosterone system, or cyclosporine-induced tubular unresponsiveness to aldosterone. Hyperuricemia can occur, possibly caused by decreased uric acid excretion from tubular dysfunction. Renal tubular acidosis may be seen due to a decrease in aldosterone effect, and a decrease in ammonium

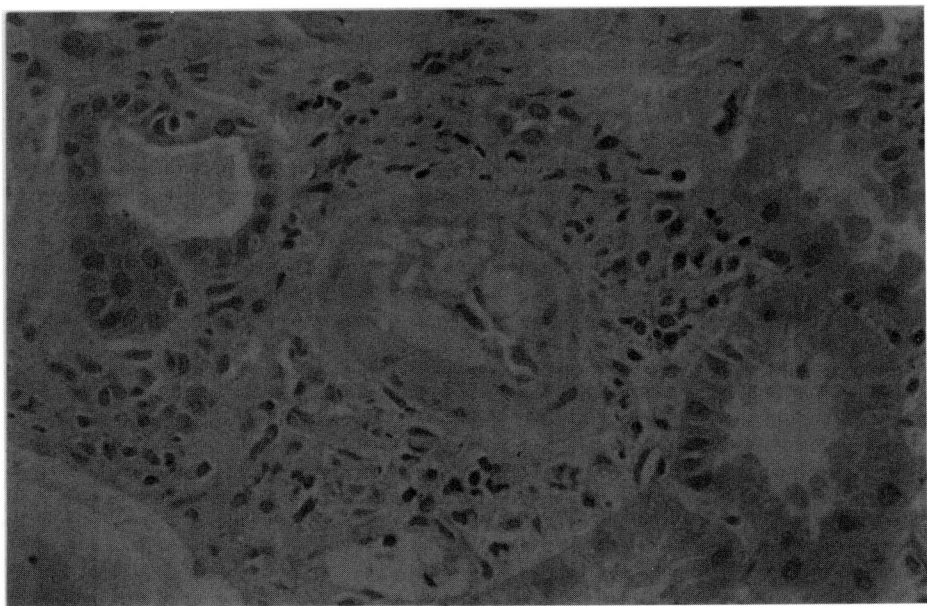

Fig. 90.1. Cyclosporine arteriolopathy. The arteriole (between two tubules) shows severe mucoid endothelial swelling, protein insudation, and luminal narrowing. (Hematoxylin & eosin ×200). Slide courtesy of Dr. S. Rainer.

production. Hypophosphotemia and hypomagnesemia have also been associated with cyclosporine use.

Tacrolimus has a similar nephrotoxic effect to cyclosporine. It can also cause hyperkalemia and hyperuricemia (Porayko *et al.*, 1994; European FK506 Multicentre Liver Study Group, 1994; The U.S. Multicenter FK506 Liver Study Group, 1994). The most effective treatment is reduction in dose or withdrawal of drug (Table 90.3). Studies in renal and liver transplant recipients suggest that substituting cyclosporine with non-nephrotoxic immunosuppressive agents may ameliorate renal dysfunction (Ducloux *et al.*, 1998; Hueso *et al.*, 1998; Schlitt *et al.*, 2001). Fish oils, calcium channel blockers, and pentoxifylline have been suggested to have beneficial effect on patients with chronic cyclosporine nephropathy. However, studies so far have been conflicting (van der Heide *et al.*, 1993; Kooijmans-Coutinho *et al.*, 1996; Chrysostomou *et al.*, 1993; Ladefoged *et al.*, 1994; Rahn *et al.*, 1999; Frantz *et al.*, 1997).

Aminoglycoside antibiotics
Aminoglycosides are commonly used for Gram-negative infections posttransplant. The incidence of nephrotoxicity is 10%–20% (Humes, 1988). Acute tubular necrosis can occasionally occur. Aminoglycosides are reabsorbed in the proximal tubule, and have a long tissue half-life. Renal injury can persist for several days after the discontinuation of the drug. Several risk factors have been identified that increase aminoglycoside nephrotoxicity (Kapoor & Chan, 2001). They include

duration of therapy
concurrent renal ischemia due to volume depletion
high peak dose levels
concurrent sepsis

concurrent administration of other nephrotoxic agents
concurrent liver disease
pre-existing renal insufficiency

The degree of toxicity of aminoglycosides is determined by the number of cationic amino groups per molecule (Bennett *et al.*, 1986). Studies suggest that cationic aminoglycosides bind to the anionic phospholipids on the luminal membrane of the proximal tubule (Moestrup *et al.*, 1995). Streptomycin is the least nephrotoxic with three cationic amino groups. Amikacin, gentamicin, and neomycin have increasing toxicity with four, five, and six per molecule, respectively. Acute tubular necrosis (ATN) induced by aminoglycosides is usually non-oliguric. Patients may also have glycosuria and ammoaciduria due to tubular defects. Nephrogenic diabetes insipidus may occasionally occur. Discontinuation of the drug usually leads to complete recovery within a few weeks.

Amphotericin B
Amphotericin B is a polyene antifungal agent. Amphotericin B causes renal impairment in 60%–80% of patients (Kapoor & Chan, 2001). Clinical manifestation includes urinary magnesium and potassium wasting, hyperchloremic metabolic acidosis due to renal tubular acidosis, nephrogenic diabetes insipidus, and renal insufficiency (Kapoor & Chan, 2001). The mechanism by which amphotericin B causes renal dysfunction is incompletely understood. Renal vasoconstriction is believed to cause a reduction in glomerular filtration rate. Amphotericin B works by inserting itself into the cell membrane and thus increasing its permeability (Zager *et al.*, 1992). The increase in membrane permeability of the macula densa cells, enhancing influx of sodium chloride into the

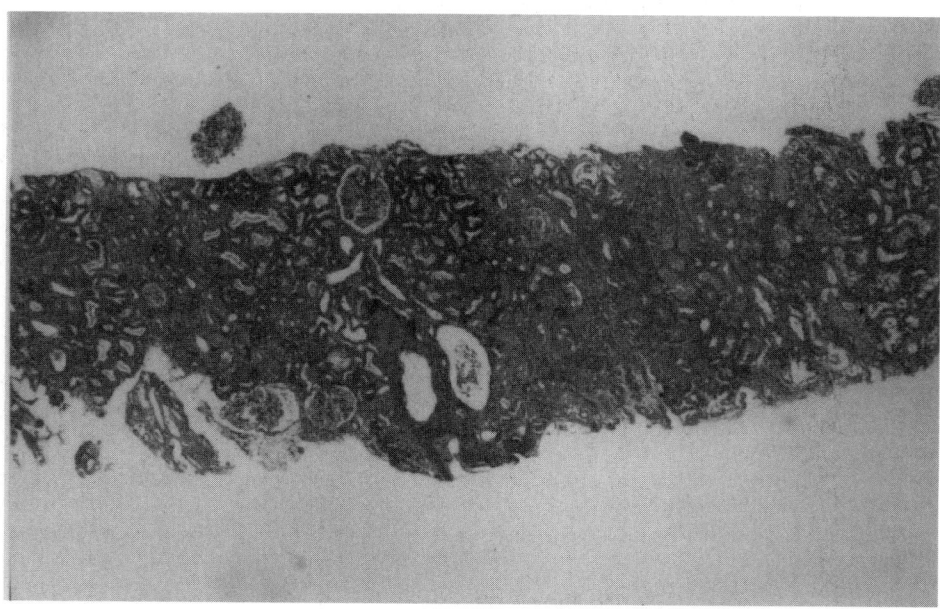

Fig. 90.2. Chronic cyclosporine nephropathy. Focal areas of fibrosis and tubular atrophy in a "striped pattern" (Masson's trichrome ×4).

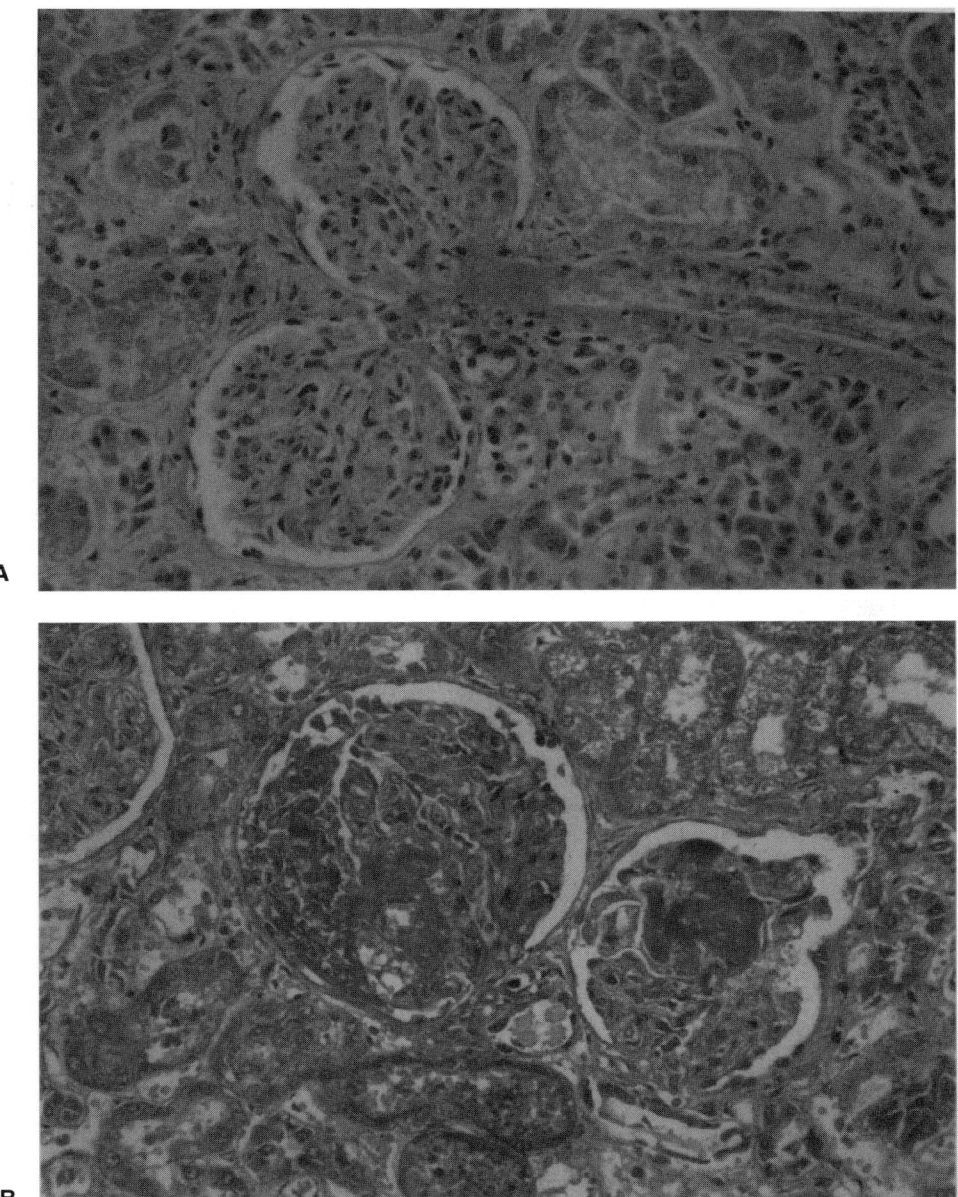

Fig. 90.3. Cyclosporine associated arteriolar [(**A**) hematoxylin & eosin ×100] and glomerular capillary [(**B**) Masson's trichrome ×100] thrombi in the recipient of a mismatched family member bone marrow transplant.

cells, may activate the tubuloglomerular feedback system and lead to afferent arteriolar vasoconstriction (Branch, 1988; Heidemann *et al.*, 1983). This increase in membrane permeability also accounts for the electrolyte disorders in amphotericin B nephrotoxicity. It promotes passive distal potassium secretion down the favorable gradient from intracellular space to the tubular lumen, causing urinary potassium wasting. The hypokalemia may be partially controlled with potassium-sparing diuretics such as amiloride. Amphotericin also decreases hydrogen secretion, causing hyperchloremic metabolic acidosis (Douglas & Healy, 1969). Decreased magne-

sium reabsorption leads to hypomagnesemia, and resistance to antidiuretic hormone leads to nephrogenic diabetes insipidus. An in vitro study suggested that deoxycholate, a detergent used as a solubilizing agent for amphotericin B, contributes, at least partly, to the tubular toxicity (Zager *et al.*, 1992). Plasma creatinine concentration usually only rises moderately, up to 2.5 mg/dl. Severe renal failure caused by amphotericin B is uncommon, unless another nephrotoxic agent is used concurrently, such as an aminoglycoside or cyclosporine, or volume depletion is also present. The nephrotoxicity caused by amphotericin B is dose-dependent.

Table 90.3. *Management of a raised serum creatinine level due to cyclosporine nephrotoxicity (in an otherwise well patient)*

1. If creatinine is above upper limit of normal range, cease cyclosporine administration for 48 hours
2. Restart at two-thirds previous dose if serum creatinine level is normalizing
3. Continue to monitor cyclosporine dose at least twice weekly until day 84 posttransplant

There is a low risk at doses less than 0.5 mg/kg/day, and a cumulative dose of less than 600 mg (Fisher *et al.,* 1989). Amphotericin B nephrotoxicity can be prevented at least in part by salt loading. Llanos *et al.* performed a controlled study of patients receiving a 10-week course of amphotericin B, at an average dose 50 mg/day, three times a week. The group of patients given 1 liter of isotonic saline prior to amphotericin B had stable renal function. In the other group that only received water, serum creatinine level rose from 0.6 to 1.0 mg/dl (Llanos *et al.,* 1991).

Lipid formulations of amphotericin have been developed to reduce amphotericin B nephrotoxicity (see Chapter 75).

Vancomycin

Vancomycin is used in the treatment of Gram-positive infections. Early reports suggested that its nephrotoxicity arose from impurities in its preparation (Appel *et al.,* 1986). Current technology has enhanced vancomycin purification greatly. Renal failure caused by vancomycin alone is uncommon. Most studies showed that 5%–15% of patients on vancomycin alone develop only mild renal dysfunction (Downs *et al.,* 1989). Concurrent use of aminoglycoside can increase the risk of developing significant renal impairment to 30% (Rybak *et al.,* 1990).

Acyclovir

Acyclovir is commonly used to prevent or treat herpes simplex virus (HSV) infection in HSCT recipients. Acyclovir is both filtered and secreted in the kidney. Intravenous administration of acyclovir may lead to the deposition of acyclovir crystals in the tubules causing intratubular obstruction and interstitial inflammation (Sawyer *et al.,* 1988). Birefringent needle-shaped acyclovir crystals can sometimes be seen in the urine. Acute renal impairment develops shortly after in the infusion. The nephrotoxicity can both be prevented and treated by hydration. Slower drug infusion over 1 to 2 hours also can reduce the risk of renal impairment. Oral acyclovir has much lower nephrotoxic effect.

Ifosfamide

Ifosfamide is an alkylating agent used for conditioning before autologous stem cell transplantation. Renal toxicities include hypokalemia, hyperchloremic metabolic acidosis, nephrogenic diabetes insipidus, natriuresis, and hypophosphatemic rickets or osteomalacia. Glomerular toxic effects leading to chronic renal failure are less common than tubular dysfunction, but have been described. Irreversible renal failure seems to be caused by damage to the renal tubular epithelium and microvasculature (Kramer *et al.,* 2001). Nephrotoxicity can be caused by ifosfamide itself or its metabolite. It may be caused by the production of chloracetaldehyde, a toxin to epithelial cells. Damage can be seen in glomeruli, interstitium, and proximal and distal tubules. Proximal tubular damage is the most prominent. Risk factors for developing nephrotoxicity from ifosfamide include young age, previous exposure to cisplatin, pre-existing renal insufficiency, and a total dose of greater than 50 g/m^2 (Kapoor & Chan, 2001).

Tumor lysis syndrome

The tumor lysis syndrome is a potentially life-threatening complication that can develop within the first several days of the pretransplant conditioning chemo- or chemoradiotherapy. It usually occurs in patients with highly sensitive tumors. It results from massive release of intracellular constituents into the circulation, causing hyperuricemia, hyperphosphatemia, anion gap metabolic acidosis, and acute renal failure (ARF). ARF is thought to be secondary to intratubular obstruction from precipitation of uric acid, xanthine, and phosphate. Treatment includes vigorous volume expansion, urinary alkalinization, allopurinol, and sometimes hemodialysis. Because many patients undergoing HSCT are in remission of their disease and widespread recognition of this syndrome has led to appropriate preventive treatment, tumor lysis syndrome is now a fairly uncommon complication post-HSCT.

Marrow infusion toxicity

The hematopoietic stem cells of patients receiving autologous HSCT are usually cryopreserved at −156 to −196°C and with 10% dimethylsulfoxide (DMSO). During the process of freezing and thawing, many granulocytes and red blood cells are lysed (Davis *et al.,* 1990). When patients are receiving the marrow infusion, they are exposed to the cell lysis products and DMSO. Some of these patients develop overt hemoglobinuria, along with other side effects including nausea, vomiting, bradycardia, dyspnea, headache, abdominal pain, fever, chills, and hyper- or hypotension. In one study a small percentage (9%) were observed to develop ARF (Smith *et al.,* 1987), thought to be induced by hemoglobin nephrotoxicity. Due to the prophylactic volume expansion that these patients receive prior to therapy, ARF in this setting has become uncommon. The solute and bicarbonate diuresis prevents hemoglobin cast formation (Zager *et al.,* 1994).

Hepatic veno-occlusive disease

One of the most serious acute renal complications of HSCT is a hepatorenal-like syndrome resulting from hepatic veno-occlusive disease (VOD) (Zager *et al.,* 1994; Leblond *et al.,* 1995). VOD is caused by endothelial cell injury of hepatic venules from the pretransplant conditioning regimen, leading to venular thrombosis and sinusoidal and portal hypertension (Zager *et al.,*

1994). It is characterized by progressive hyperbilirubinemia, and clinically manifested as a salt-retentive state with weight gain, ascites, peripheral edema, azotemia, progressive jaundice, right upper quadrant pain, and encephalopathy. Weight gain can occur 1 to 7 days posttransplant, whereas ARF begins after the onset of hyperbilirubinemia, about 10 to 16 days posttransplant. The fractional excretion of sodium typically remains below 1%. Urinalysis usually shows muddy brown granular casts. A serum bilirubin of >7 mg/dl generally predicts the likelihood for dialysis (Zager, 1994). In a study done by Fink et al., (1995), urinary excretion of N-acetyl-beta-D-glucosaminidase (NAG), a presumed marker of proximal tubular cell damage, was measured. It was found that NAG excretion was increased in all HSCT patients, but was markedly increased in patients with VOD, with and without ARF. It therefore, appears that proximal tubular damage, though present, does not contribute to the development of ARF. Renal hypoperfusion more likely plays a predominant role in the pathogenesis of ARF associated with VOD. Although hepatic VOD is regarded as the primary cause of the renal failure, a superimposed event, such as sepsis, is often observed to trigger the renal deterioration (Zager et al., 1989). Concomittant use of amphotericin B has also been associated with the development of the hepatorenal-like syndrome (Sawaya et al., 1991). It is unclear whether the drug itself contributes to the development of ARF or it merely acts as a marker for infection.

Once ARF develops, treatment is mainly supportive. Hemodialysis remains the main modality of treatment.

Hypophosphatemia

Hypophosphatemia is usually caused by decreased dietary intake, decreased intestinal reabsorption, increased urinary phosphate excretion, and shifting of phosphate from the extracellular into the intracellular space. It is sometimes reported in patients receiving HSCT. The mechanism of hypophosphatemia in HSCT patients is presumably due to phosphate uptake by the replicating hematopoietic cells. Severe hypophosphatemia, defined as a serum level less than 1.0 mg/dl (0.32 mmol/l), can cause a variety of symptoms involving multiple systems: central nervous system—metabolic encephalopathy, manifesting as irritability and paresthesias (it can progress to confusion, delirium, seizures, and coma (Subramanian & Khardori, 2002); cardiovascular system—decreased myocardial contractility; musculo-skeletal system—proximal myopathy; it can also lead to rhabdomyolysis (Knochel, 1992; Desroches et al., 1992).

In one retrospective study in HSCT recipients by Crook et al., (1996) 77% of the 17 patients had a low serum phosphate level; 2 had severe hypophosphatemia (Crook et al., 1996). Raanani et al. performed a study on the relationship between cytokine release and hypophosphatemia in HSCT patients (Raanani et al., 2001). They noted that the development of hypophosphatemia in the engraftment period preceded the rise in WBC by 2 days. There was a concurrent rise in interleukin (IL)-6 and IL-8 levels. Phosphate levels should be monitored in the post-HSCT period.

Later renal complications

Thrombotic thrombocytopenic purpura (TTP) and hemolytic-uremic syndrome (HUS)

The acute presentation of this syndrome in HSC transplant recipients was first reported by Powles et al. (1980) and Shulman et al. in 1981. Clinically, it is characterized by arterial hypertension, microangiopathic hemolytic anemia, thrombocytopenia, elevated LDH level, proteinuria, microscopic hematuria, and severe renal failure within 6 weeks of HSCT (Zager et al., 1994). More recently a spectrum of related and overlapping syndromes has been described: multifactorial fulminant thrombotic microangiopathy (TMA), conditioning regimen-associated hemolytic-uremic syndrome (HUS), CEP-associated nephrotoxicity with microangiopathic hemolytic anemia (MAHA), and CSP-associated neurotoxicity with MAHA (Petitt & Clark, 1994; Iacopino et al., 1999). Posttransplant, it is referred to as transplantation-associated thrombotic microangiopathy (TA-TMA), to distinguish it from other thrombotic microangiopathies (Daly et al., 2002). A grading system has been proposed (Table 90.4), which appears to have prognostic value (Fig. 90.4). The reports of the incidence of TTP-HUS post-HSCT have been extremely variable, 2%–76% following allogeneic HSCT, and 0%–27% following autologous HSCT (Pettitt & Clark, 1994). The variation may be due to inconsistency in diagnostic criteria used in different studies (Iacopino et al., 1999). Because HSCT causes complications that mimic different components of TTP-HUS, it makes the diagnosis of this syndrome difficult. For example, microangiopathic changes are frequently found in post-HSCT patients. Anemia and thrombocytopenia are often present as well. Fever and neurologic changes are also not uncommon in these patients without TTP. Also to be considered in the differential diagnosis is hemophagocytic syndrome, which has been noted after HSC transplantation (Sato et al., 1998; Ishikawa et al., 2000; Abe et al., 2002), and which is characterized by fever, cytopenia, and the presence of more than 3% mature activated macrophages in the marrow. Involvement of the central nervous system has been described. Marked and acute elevations of serum ferritin and soluble IL-1 receptor support the diagnosis. The diagnosis of TTP-HUS in post-HSCT patients, therefore, relies on the clinical suspicion of the treating physician. High-dose pretransplant conditioning regimen, severe acute GVHD,

Table 90.4. *Grading system for bone marrow transplant thrombotic microangiopathy (BMT-TM)*

Grade	LD(U/l)	% Fragmented cells	Clinical BMT-TM
0	Normal or increased	≤1.2	None
1	Normal	≥1.3	Subclinical
2	Increased	1.2~4.8	Mild
3	Increased	4.9~9.6	Moderate
4	Increased	≥9.7	Severe

Reproduced, with permission, from Zeigler et al. (1995).

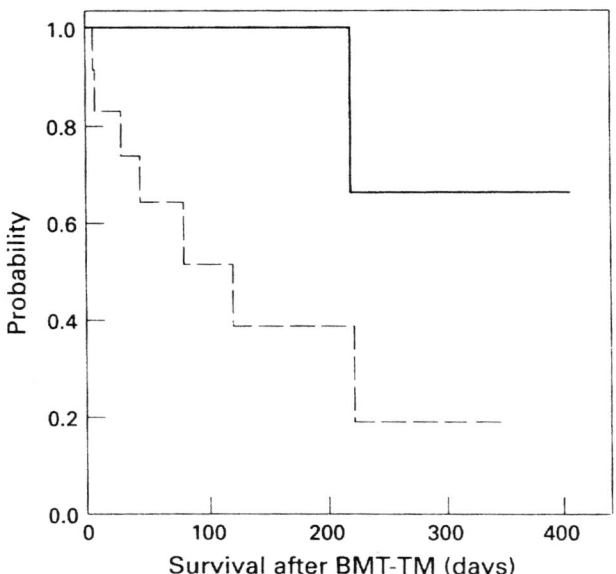

Fig. 90.4. Kaplan-Meier plot of survival from day of diagnosis of bone marrow transplant thrombotic microangiopathy (BMT-TM). (—) patients with grade 2 BMT-TM (*n* = 10); (—) patients with grades 3–4 BMT-TM (*n* = 12); *P* = .018 by log-rank test. Reproduced, with permission, from Zeigler *et al.* (1995).

systemic infection, and cyclosporine are risk factors in the development of TTP-HUS post-HSCT (Roy *et al.,* 2001). Currently, the pathogenesis of classical TTP is thought to involve a plasma factor leading to endothelial cell apoptosis, as the plasma from patients with TTP can cause microvascular endothelial cell apoptosis. These patients have a deficiency in a von Willebrand's factor cleaving metalloprotease, leading to larger than normal von Willebrand's factor multimers which cause platelet aggregation (Mitra *et al.,* 1997; Dang *et al.,* 1999;

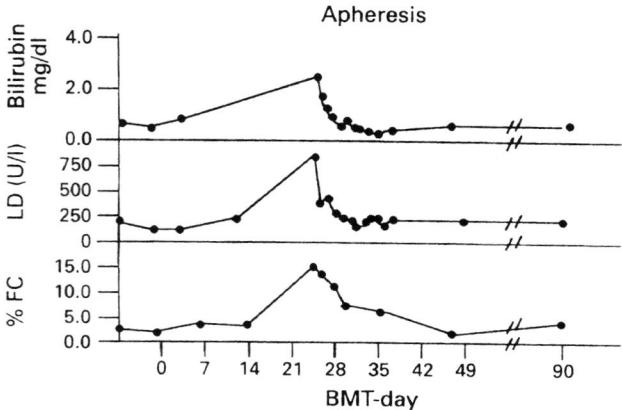

Fig. 90.5. The time course of response to apheresis (with combined cryosupernatant and PAI exchange) is depicted for a patient with grade 4 bone marrow transplant thrombotic microangiopathy (BMT-TM). LD, lactic dehydrogenase; FC, fragmented cells. Reproduced, with permission, from Zeigler *et al.* (1996).

Furlan *et al.,* 1998; Tsai & Lian, 1998). However, in TA-TMA the vWF cleaving metalloprotease activity is generally preserved (Van der Plas *et al.,* 1999; Elliott *et al.,* 2001), although abnormalities of the vascular endothelium have been described on ultrastructural examination, and are thought to be central to the pathogenesis (Cohen *et al.,* 1989). Also described at the onset of TTP and HUS following allotransplantation is elevation of serum levels of IL-8, thrombomodulin, and plaminogen activator inhibitor-1 (Takatsuka *et al.,* 2002).

The outcome of patients diagnosed with TTP-HUS is poor. Mortality ranges from 50% to 75% (Holler *et al.,* 1989; Zeigler *et al.,* 1995; Busca & Uderzo, 2000; Kondo *et al.,* 1998; Uderzo *et al.,* 2000; Cohen *et al.,* 1993). Three risk factors have been identified by Schriber *et al.* for prediction of mortality: time to diagnosis (<120 days post-HSCT), the use of cyclosporine or tacrolimus, and the presence of neurological signs or symptoms (Schriber & Herzig, 1997). The high-risk group commonly consists of patients given an allogeneic HSCT, who have received cyclosporine or tacrolimus for GVHD prophylaxis, and who have had a superimposed event such as hepatic VOD, CMV infection, or GVHD. Treatment of this form of TTP-HUS-like syndrome with plasmapheresis has not generally been found to be very effective (Sarode *et al.,* 1995). However, there have been case reports of successful treatment with aggressive plasmaphoresis (Chown *et al.,* 1996) (Fig. 90.5). A proposed algorithm for the management of patients with TTP-HUS is

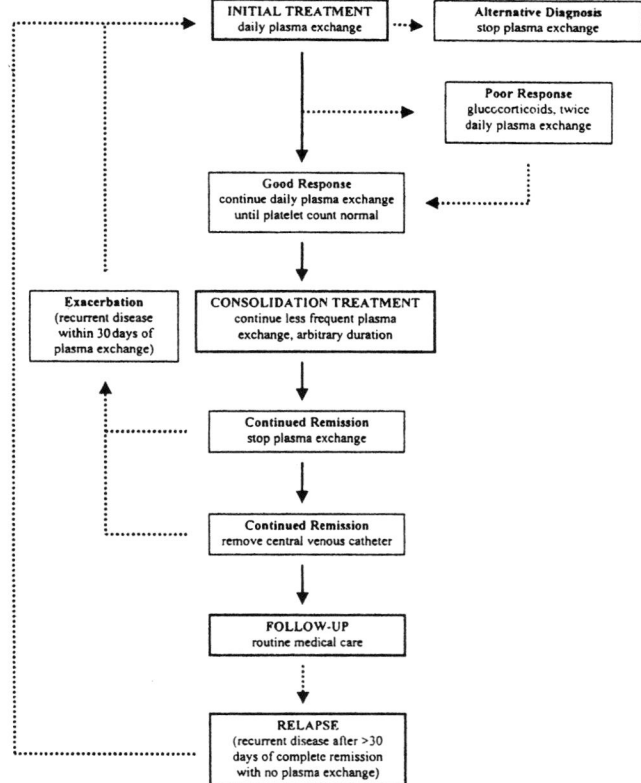

Fig. 90.6. Algorithm for the management of patients with TTP-HUS. Reproduced, with permission, from George (2000).

shown in Figure 90.6. Because cyclosporine or tacrolimus has been linked to its pathogenesis, many physicians choose to reduce the dose of, or discontinue, the drugs. However, no proof exists so far that this strategy is effective in halting or reversing renal dysfunction. There is a case report of using transdermal isosorbide tape as a nitric oxide source to a patient with HUS after HSCT who had improvement in renal function and increase in platelet numbers (Kajiume *et al.*, 2000).

Nitric acid is a free radical that is protective of endothelial cells within blood vessels. Interestingly, high-dose chemotherapy followed by autologous blood stem cell (CD34-selected) support has been used to treat TTP/HUS refractory to conventional therapy (Musso *et al.*, 1999). The use of defibrotide has been reported in one study with some promise (Corti *et al.*, 2002). Converting the patient from cyclosporine to tacrolimus has not been of benefit (Furlong *et al.*, 2000).

Bone marrow transplantation (BMT) nephropathy

In adults, the incidence of this syndrome has been reported as between 0.6% and 13%, and in children up to 45% (Cruz *et al.*, 1997). It has been somewhat arbitrarily divided into an acute form and a chronic form. The acute form resembles TTP-HUS and is relatively rare. The more common presentation is a subacute to chronic nephropathy that manifests typically between 3 to 12 months posttransplant. In both the acute and chronic form of BMT nephropathy, histologic findings include arteriolar and glomerular capillary intramural fibrin thrombi, tubular dilation with intraluminal debris, red blood cell casts, mesangiolysis, and focal tubular necrosis (Cruz *et al.*, 1997). Electron

microscopy may show endothelial cell injury and accumulation of clear heterogenous material in the subendothelial space and mesangial areas. The histologic appearance is very similar to both HUS and radiation nephritis (Guinan *et al.*, 1988).

The pathogenesis of BMT nephropathy is not completely understood. It was initially thought to be induced by cyclosporine toxicity. Over the past two decades, numerous cases of this syndrome have been reported. It has become more apparent that cyclosporine exposure is not a prerequisite. Increasing evidence has pointed to the pretransplant myeloablative therapy as a major cause of this disease entity, particularly total body irradiation. Lawton *et al.* found that partial renal shielding during total body irradiation reduced the incidence of BMT nephropathy (Lawton *et al.*, 1997). A late decline in renal function was observed in patients treated with total body irradiation, but not in those who received chemotherapy alone (Leblond *et al.*, 1995). Many believe now that BMT nephropathy is a form of radiation nephritis; however, BMT nephropathy has been described in patients who did not receive total body irradiation. Alkylating agents such as cyclophosphamide have also been implicated in the pathogenesis (Hebert *et al.*, 1994).

In patients developing the syndrome more than 3 months after HSCT, the presentation is usually less aggressive. The most common period of presentation for this chronic form is 8–12 months post-HSCT. Hypertension is mild to moderate, and hemolytic anemia is less severe. Renal function deterioration is also slower. Proteinuria is usually >1 g/24 hour, and microscopic hematuria may be present. Anemia is often disproportional to the degree of renal failure. Hyperkalemia, meta-

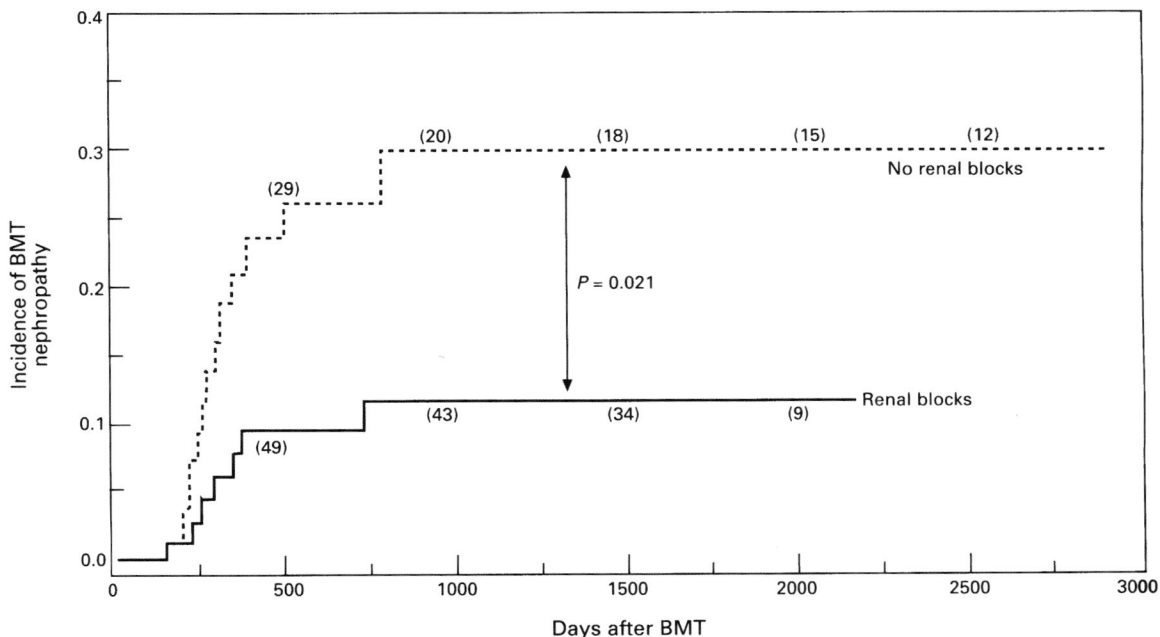

Fig. 90.7. Actuarial incidence of BMT nephropathy (Np) for patients treated with and without renal blocks. The number of patients at risk are shown in parentheses. Plotting of curves stops when there are less than six patients at risk. There is a statistically significant (*P* = .021) decrease in the development of BMT Np via the use of renal blocking. Reproduced, with permission, from Lawton *et al.* (1997).

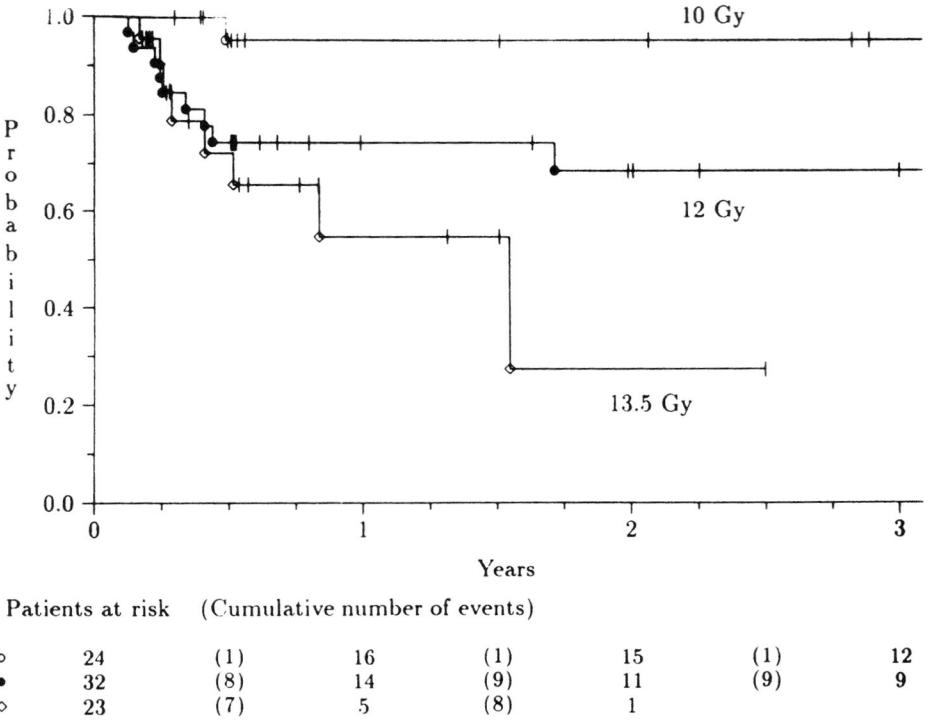

Fig. 90.8. Renal dysfunction-free survival and TBI dose. Reproduced, with permission, from Miralbell *et al.* (1996).

bolic acidosis, and low erythropoietin levels are frequently found. Most patients demonstrate a biphasic pattern in deterioration in renal function, with steady decline in the first 12 to 24 months, then stabilization with no recovery afterward (Kapoor & Chan, 2001).

Treatment for HSCT nephropathy currently is largely supportive. If patients progress to end-stage renal disease, dialysis or renal transplantation may be required. Measures, however, can be taken to prevent the development of HSCT nephropathy. As mentioned earlier, partial renal shielding during total body irradiation can greatly reduce the risk of developing HSCT nephropathy (Lawton *et al.*, 1997; Lawton *et al.*, 1992). In a study by *Lawton et al.* patients underwent 14 Gy total body irradiation (TBI): 29% of 72 patients with no renal shielding developed HSCT nephropathy, whereas 14% of 68 patients with 15% renal shielding had HSCT nephropathy, and none developed HSCT nephropathy in group of 17 patients with 30% renal shielding (Fig. 90.7) (Lawton *et al.*, 1997). Lower dose of TBI, hyperfractionation of the total radiation dose, and slow radiation administration has also been recommended for reducing the risk of developing HSCT nephropathy. In a study by Miralbell *et al.* (1996), it was found that TBI dose and the presence of GVHD were significantly correlated with renal dysfunction: 79 patients with malignant hematologic diseases received an allogeneic HSCT after conditioning with high-dose chemotherapy and TBI. All had normal renal function before conditioning. The 18-month probability of renal dysfunction-free survival for the whole group was 77%. For those condi-

tioned with 10, 12, or 13.5 Gy the probabilities were 95%, 74%, and 55%, respectively (Fig. 90.8). For patients with and without GVHD they were 61% and 88% respectively. Angiotensin-converting enzyme (ACE) inhibitors have been found to preserve renal function and improve survival in a rat model of total body irradiation (Cohen *et al.*, 1997; Moulder *et al.*, 1997). Juckett *et al.* (2001) studied the influence of ACE gene polymorphism in the development of HSCT nephropathy. ACE genotype did not seem to influence survival, but the DD genotype may be protective against renal injury after HSCT.

References

Abe, Y, Hara, K., Matsushima, T. *et al.* (2002). Hemophagocytic syndrome: a rare complication of allogeneic nonmyeloablative hematopoietic stem cell transplantation. *Bone Marrow Transplantation*, **29,** 799–801.

Appel, G. B. *et al.* (1986). Vancomycin and the kidney. *American Journal of Kidney Diseases*, **8,** 75–80.

Bearman, S. I. *et al.* (1990). A pilot study of continuous infusion heparin for the prevention of hepatic veno-occlusive disease after bone marrow transplantation. *Bone Marrow Transplantation*, **5,** 407–11.

Bearman, S. I. *et al.* (1992). Recombinant human tissue plasminogen activator for the treatment of established severe venocclusive disease of the liver after bone marrow transplantation. *Blood,* **80,** 2458–62.

Bearman, S. I. *et al.* (1993). A phase I/II study of prostaglandin E1 for the prevention of hepatic venocclusive disease after bone marrow transplantation. *British Journal of Haematology,* **84,** 724–30.

Bennett, W. M. *et al.* (1986). Modification of experimental aminoglycoside nephrotoxicity. *American Journal of Kidney Disease,* **8,** 292–6.

Bennett, W. M. *et al.* (1996). Chronic cyclosporine nephropathy: the Achilles' heel of immunosuppressive therapy. *Kidney International,* **50,** 1089–100.

Bertani, T. *et al.* (1991). Nature and extent of glomerular injury induced by cyclosporine in heart transplant patients. *Kidney International,* **40,** 243–50.

Branch, R. A. (1988). Prevention of amphotericin B-induced renal impairment. A review on the use of sodium supplementation. *Archives of Internal Medicine,* **148,** 2389–94.

Busca, A. & Uderzo, C. (2000). HSCT: bone marrow transplant associated thrombotic microangiopathy. *Hematology,* **5,** 53–67.

Chown, S. R. *et al.* (1996). The role of plasma exchange for TTP/HUS post-bone marrow transplant. *Bone Marrow Transplantation,* **17,** 898–9.

Chrysostomou, A. *et al.* (1993). Diltiazem in renal allograft recipients receiving cyclosporine. *Transplantation,* **55,** 300–4.

Cohen, E. P. *et al.* (1993). Clinical course of late-onset bone marrow transplant nephropathy. *Nephron,* **64,** 626–35.

Cohen, E. P. (2001). Renal failure after bone-marrow transplantation. *Lancet,* **357,** 6–7.

Cohen, E. P., Fish, B. L., & Moulder, J. E. (1997). Successful brief captopril treatment in experimental radiation nephropathy. *The Journal of Laboratory and Clinical Medicine,* **129,** 536–47.

Cohen, H., Bull, H. A., & Seddon, A. *et al.* (1989). Vascular endothelial cell function and ultrastructure in thrombotic microangiopathy following allogeneic bone marrow transplantation. *European Journal of Hematology,* **43,** 207–14.

Corti, P., Uderzo, C., Tagliabue. A. *et al.* (2002). Defibrotide as a promising treatment for thrombotic thrombocytopenic purpura in patients undergoing bone marrow transplantation. *Bone Marrow Transplantation,* **29,** 542–3 (letter).

Crook, M., Swaminathan, R., & Schey, S. (1996). Hypophosphataemia in patients undergoing bone marrow transplantation. *Leukemia & Lymphoma,* **22,** 335–7.

Cruz, D. N., Perazella, M. A., & Mahnensmith, R. L. (1997). Bone marrow transplant nephropathy: a case report and review of the literature. *Journal of the American Society of Nephrology: JASN,* **8,** 166–73.

Daly, A. S., Xenacostas, A., & Lipton, J. H. (2002). Transplantation-associated thrombotic microangiopathy: twenty-two years later. *Bone Marrow Transplantation,* **30,** 709–15.

Dang, C. T. *et al.* (1999). Enhanced endothelial cell apoptosis in splenic tissues of patients with thrombotic thrombocytopenic purpura. *Blood,* **93,** 1264–70.

Davis, J. M. *et al.* (1990). Clinical toxicity of cryopreserved bone marrow graft infusion. *Blood,* **75,** 781–6.

Deray, G. *et al.* (1992). Renal function and blood pressure in patients receiving long-term, low-dose cyclosporine therapy for idiopathic autoimmune uveitis. *Annals of Internal Medicine,* **117,** 578–83.

Desroches, L. *et al.* (1992). Rhabdomyolysis and acute renal failure following prolonged driving. *Annals of Emergency Medicine,* **21,** 346.

Dieterle, A. *et al.* (1990). Chronic cyclosporine-associated nephrotoxicity in bone marrow transplant patients. *Transplantation,* **49,** 1093–100.

Douglas, J. B. & Healy, J. K. (1969). Nephrotoxic effects of amphotericin B, including renal tubular acidosis. *The American Journal of Medicine,* **46,** 154–62.

Downs, N. J. *et al.* (1989). Mild nephrotoxicity associated with vancomycin use. *Archives of Internal Medicine,* **149,** 1777–81.

Ducloux, D. *et al.* (1998). Mycophenolate mofetil in cyclosporine-associated nephrotoxicity. *Transplantation Proceedings,* **30,** 2825–7.

Elliott, M., Nichols, W., Plumhoff, E. *et al.* (2001). Post-transplant thrombotic thrombocytopenic purpura (TTP), a complication of high-risk myeloablative and non-myeloablative transplantation, is not associated with von Willebrand factor cleaving protease (vWF-CP) deficiency. *Blood,* **98,** 193a (abstract).

English, J. *et al.* (1987). Cyclosporine-induced acute renal dysfunction in the rat. Evidence of arteriolar vasoconstriction with preservation of tubular function. *Transplantation,* **44,** 135–41.

European FK506 Multicentre Liver Study Group. (1994). Randomised trial comparing tacrolimus (FK506) and cyclosporin in prevention of liver allograft rejection. *Lancet,* **344,** 423–8.

Feutren, G. & Mihatsch, M. J. (1992). Risk factors for cyclosporine-induced nephropathy in patients with autoimmune diseases. International Kidney Biopsy Registry of Cyclosporine in Autoimmune Diseases. *New England Journal of Medicine,* **326,** 1654–60.

Fink, J. C. *et al.* (1995). Marked enzymuria after bone marrow transplantation: a correlate of veno-occlusive disease-induced "hepatorenal syndrome". *Journal of the American Society of Nephrology: JASN,* **6,** 1655–60.

Fisher, M. A. *et al.* (1989). Risk factors for amphotericin B-associated nephrotoxicity. *The American Journal of Medicine,* **87,** 547–52.

Frantz, R. P. *et al.* (1997). Effects of pentoxifylline on renal function and blood pressure in cardiac transplant recipients: a randomized trial. *Transplantation,* **63,** 1607–10.

Frimat, L. *et al.* (1998). Treatment of end-stage renal failure after heart transplantation. *Nephrology, Dialysis, Transplantation,* **13,** 2905–8.

Furlan, M. *et al.* (1998). von Willebrand factor-cleaving protease in thrombotic thrombocytopenic purpura and the hemolytic-uremic syndrome. *New England Journal of Medicine,* **339,** 1578–84.

Furlong, T., Storb, R., Anasetti, C. *et al.* (2000). Clinical outcome after conversion to FK 506 (tacrolimus) therapy for acute graft-versus-host disease resistant to cyclosporine or for cyclosporine-associated toxicities. *Bone Marrow Transplantation,* **26,** 1005–9.

George, J. N. (2000). How I treat patients with thrombotic thrombocytopenic purpura-hemolyic uremic syndrome. *Blood,* **96,** 1223–9.

Goldstein, D. J. *et al.* (1997). Cyclosporine-associated end-stage nephropathy after cardiac transplantation: incidence and progression. *Transplantation,* **63,** 664–8.

Gruss, E. *et al.* (1995). Acute renal failure in patients following bone marrow transplantation: prevalence, risk factors and outcome. *American Journal of Nephrology,* **15,** 473–9.

Guinan, E. C. *et al.* (1988). Intravascular hemolysis and renal insufficiency after bone marrow transplantation. *Blood,* **72,** 451–5.

Hamaki, T., Katori, H., Kami, M. *et al.* (2002). Successful allogeneic blood stem cell transplantation for aplastic anemia in a patient with renal insufficiency requiring dialysis. *Bone Marrow Transplantation*, **30**, 195–8.

Hebert, M. J. *et al.* (1994). Mesangiolysis associated with bone marrow transplantation: new insights on possible etiogenic factors. *American Journal of Kidney Diseases*, **23**, 882–3.

Heidemann, H. T. *et al.* (1983). Amphotericin B nephrotoxicity in humans decreased by salt repletion. *American Journal of Medicine*, **75**, 476–81.

Holler, E. *et al.* (1989). Microangiopathy in patients on cyclosporine prophylaxis who developed acute graft-versus-host disease after HLA-identical bone marrow transplantation. *Blood*, **73**, 2018–24.

Hueso, M. *et al.* (1998). Low-dose cyclosporine and mycophenolate mofetil in renal allograft recipients with suboptimal renal function. *Transplantation*, **66**, 1727–31.

Humes, H. D. (1988). Aminoglycoside nephrotoxicity. *Kidney International*, **33**, 900–11.

Iacopino, P. *et al.* (1999). Severe thrombotic microangiopathy: an infrequent complication of bone marrow transplantation. Gruppo Italiano Trapianto Midollo Osseo (GITMO). *Bone Marrow Transplantation*, **24**, 47–51.

Ishikawa, J., Maeda, T., Miyazaki, T. *et al.* (2000). Early onset of hemophagocytic syndrome following allogeneic bone marrow transplantation. *International Journal of Hematology*, **72**, 243–6.

Juckett, M. B. *et al.* (2001). Loss of renal function following bone marrow transplantation: an analysis of angiotensin converting enzyme D/I polymorphism and other clinical risk factors. *Bone Marrow Transplantation*, **27**, 451–6.

Kajiume, T. *et al.* (2000). Application of nitric oxide for a case of veno-occlusive disease after peripheral blood stem cell transplantation. *Pediatric Hematology and Oncology*, **17**, 601–4.

Kapoor, M. & Chan, G. Z. (2001). Malignancy and renal disease. *Critical Care Clinics*, **17**, 571–98, viii.

Knochel, J. P. (1992). Hypophosphatemia and rhabdomyolysis. *American Journal of Medicine*, **92**, 455–7.

Kondo, M. *et al.* (1998). Hemolytic uremic syndrome after allogeneic or autologous hematopoietic stem cell transplantation for childhood malignancies. *Bone Marrow Transplantation*, **21**, 281–6.

Kone, B. C. *et al.* (1988). Hypertension and renal dysfunction in bone marrow transplant recipients. *Quarterly Journal of Medicine*, **69**, 985–95.

Kooijmans-Coutinho, M. F. *et al.* (1996). Dietary fish oil in renal transplant recipients treated with cyclosporin-A: no beneficial effects shown. *Journal of the American Society of Nephrology: JASN*, **7**, 513–8.

Kramer, A., Andrassy, K., & Ho, A. D. (2001). Renal failure after bone marrow transplantation. *Lancet*, **358**, 149.

Ladefoged, S. D. *et al.* (1994). Influence of diltiazem on renal function and rejection in renal allograft recipients receiving triple-drug immunosuppression: a randomized, double-blind, placebo-controlled study. *Nephrology, Dialysis, Transplantation*, **9**, 543–7.

Lanese, D. M. & Conger, J. D. (1993). Effects of endothelin receptor antagonist on cyclosporine-induced vasoconstriction in isolated rat renal arterioles. *Journal of Clinical Investigation*, **91**, 2144–9.

Lawton, C. A. *et al.* (1992). Influence of renal shielding on the incidence of late renal dysfunction associated with T-lymphocyte

depleted bone marrow transplantation in adult patients. *International Journal of Radiation Oncology, Biology, and Physics*, **23**, 681–6.

Lawton, C. A. *et al.* (1997). Long-term results of selective renal shielding in patients undergoing total body irradiation in preparation for bone marrow transplantation. *Bone Marrow Transplantation*, **20**, 1069–74.

Leblond, V. *et al.* (1995). Evaluation of renal function in 60 long-term survivors of bone marrow transplantation. *Journal of the American Society of Nephrology: JASN*, **6**, 1661–5.

Llanos, A. *et al.* (1991). Effect of salt supplementation on amphotericin B nephrotoxicity. *Kidney International*, **40**, 302–8.

Marsa-Vila, L. *et al.* (1991). Prophylactic heparin does not prevent liver veno-occlusive disease following autologous bone marrow transplantation. *European Journal of Haematology*, **47**, 346–54.

Mihatsch, M. J., Thiel, G., & Ryffel, B. (1988). Morphologic diagnosis of cyclosporine nephrotoxicity. *Seminars in Diagnostic Pathology*, **5**, 104–21.

Miralbell, R. *et al.* (1996). Renal toxicity after allogeneic bone marrow transplantation: the combined effects of total-body irradiation and graft-versus-host disease. *Journal of Clinical Oncology*, **14**, 579–85.

Mitra, D. *et al.* (1997). Thrombotic thrombocytopenic purpura and sporadic hemolytic-uremic syndrome plasmas induce apoptosis in restricted lineages of human microvascular endothelial cells. *Blood*, **89**, 1224–34.

Moestrup, S. K. *et al.* (1995). Evidence that epithelial glycoprotein 330/megalin mediates uptake of polybasic drugs. *Journal of Clinical Investigation*, **96**, 1404–13.

Moulder, J.E. Fish, B. L., & Cohen, E. P. *et al.* (1997). Noncontinuous use of angiotensin converting enzyme inhibitors in the treatment of experimental bone marrow transplant nephropathy. *Bone Marrow Transplantation*, **19**, 729–35.

Musso, Poretto, F., & Crescimanno, A. *et al.* (1999). Successful treatment of resistant thrombotic thrombocytopenic purpura/hemolytic uremic syndrome with autologous peripheral blood stem and progenitor (CD34+) cell transplantation. *Bone Marrow Transplantation*, **24**, 207–9.

Myers, B. D. & Newton, L. (1991). Cyclosporine-induced chronic nephropathy: an obliterative microvascular renal injury. *Journal of the American Society of Nephrology: JASN*, **2** (Suppl 1), S45–52.

Noskin, G. *et al.* (1999). Treatment of invasive fungal infections with amphotericin B colloidal dispersion in bone marrow transplant recipients. *Bone Marrow Transplantation*, **23**, 697–703.

Pettitt, A. R. & Clark, R. E. (1994). Thrombotic microangiopathy following bone marrow transplantation. *Bone Marrow Transplantation*, **14**, 495–504.

Porayko, M. K. *et al.* (1994). Nephrotoxic effects of primary immunosuppression with FK-506 and cyclosporine regimens after liver transplantation. *Mayo Clinic Proceedings*, **69**, 105–11.

Powles, R. L., Clink, H. M., Spence, D. *et al.* (1980). Cyclosporine to prevent graft-versus-host disease in man after allogeneic bone marrow transplantation. *Lancet*, **1**, 327–9.

Raanani, P. *et al.* (2001). Engraftment-associated hypophosphatemia—the role of cytokine release and steep leukocyte rise post stem cell transplantation. *Bone Marrow Transplantation, 27,* 311–7.

Rahn, K. H. *et al.* (1999). Effect of nitrendipine on renal function in renal-transplant patients treated with cyclosporin: a randomised trial. *Lancet,* **354,** 1415–20.

Remuzzi, G. & Perico, N. (1995). Cyclosporine-induced renal dysfunction in experimental animals and humans. *Kidney International Supplement,* **52,** S70–4.

Roy, V. *et al.* (2001). Thrombotic thrombocytopenic purpura-like syndromes following bone marrow transplantation: an analysis of associated conditions and clinical outcomes. *Bone Marrow Transplantation, 27,* 641–6.

Rybak, M. J. *et al.* (1990). Nephrotoxicity of vancomycin, alone and with an aminoglycoside. *Journal of Antimicrobial Chemotherapy,* **25,** 679–87.

Sarode, R. *et al.* (1995). Therapeutic plasma exchange does not appear to be effective in the management of thrombotic thrombocytopenic purpura/hemolytic uremic syndrome following bone marrow transplantation. *Bone Marrow Transplantation,* **16,** 271–5.

Sato, M., Matsushima, T., Takada, S. *et al.* (1998). Fulminant, CMV-associated haemophagocytic syndrome following unrelated bone marrow transplantation. *Bone Marrow Transplantation,* **29,** 1219–22.

Sawaya, B. P. *et al.* (1991). Direct vasoconstriction as a possible cause for amphotericin B-induced nephrotoxicity in rats. *The Journal of Clinical Investigation,* **87,** 2097–107.

Sawyer, M. H. *et al.* (1988). Acyclovir-induced renal failure. Clinical course and histology. *American Journal of Medicine,* **84,** 1067–71.

Schlitt, H. J. *et al.* (2001). Replacement of calcineurin inhibitors with mycophenolate mofetil in liver-transplant patients with renal dysfunction: a randomised controlled study. *Lancet,* **357,** 587–91.

Schriber, J. R. & Herzig, G. P. (1997). Transplantation-associated thrombotic thrombocytopenic purpura and hemolytic uremic syndrome. *Seminars Hematology,* **34,** 126–33.

Shulman, H. *et al.* (1981). Nephrotoxicity of cyclosporin A after allogeneic marrow transplantation: glomerular thromboses and tubular injury. *New England Journal of Medicine,* **305,** 1392–5.

Smith, D. M. *et al.* (1987). Acute renal failure associated with autologous bone marrow transplantation. *Bone Marrow Transplantation,* **2,** 195–201.

Subramanian, R. & Khardori, R. (2000). Severe hypophosphatemia. Pathophysiologic implications, clinical presentations, and treatment. *Medicine,* **79,** 1–8.

Takatsuka, H., Wakae, T., Mori, A. *et al.* (2002). Thrombotic thrombocytopenic purpura and hemolytic uremic syndrome following allogeneic bone marrow transplantation. *Bone Marrow Transplantation,* **29,** 907–11.

The U.S. Multicenter FK506 Liver Study Group. (1994). A comparison of tacrolimus (FK 506) and cyclosporine for immunosuppression in liver transplantation. *New England Journal of Medicine,* **331,** 1110–5.

Tsai, H. M. & Lian, E. C. (1998). Antibodies to von Willebrand factor-cleaving protease in acute thrombotic thrombocytopenic purpura. *New England Journal of Medicine,* **339,** 1585–94.

Uderzo, C. *et al.* (2000). Impact of thrombotic thrombocytopenic purpura on leukemic children undergoing bone marrow transplantation. *Bone Marrow Transplantation,* **26,** 1005–9.

van der Heide, J. J. *et al.* (1993). Effect of dietary fish oil on renal function and rejection in cyclosporine-treated recipients of renal transplants. *New England Journal of Medicine,* **329,** 769–73.

van der Plas, R. M., Schiphorst, M. & Huizinga, E. (1999). Von Willebrand factor proteolysis is deficient in classic, but not in bone marrow transplantation-associated thrombotic thrombocytopenic purpura. *Blood,* **93,** 3798–802.

Wilkinson, A. H. & Cohen, D. J. (1999). Renal failure in the recipients of nonrenal solid organ transplants. *Journal of the American Society of Nephrology: JASN,* **10,** 1136–44.

Zager, R. A. *et al.* (1989). Acute renal failure following bone marrow transplantation: a retrospective study of 272 patients. *American Journal of Kidney Diseases,* **13,** 210–6.

Zager, R. A. (1994). Acute renal failure in the setting of bone marrow transplantation. *Kidney International,* **46,** 1443–58.

Zager, R. A., Bredl, C. R., & Schimpf, B. A. (1992). Direct amphotericin B-mediated tubular toxicity: assessments of selected cytoprotective agents. *Kidney International,* **41,** 1588–94.

Zeigler, Z. R. *et al.* (1995). Bone marrow transplant-associated thrombotic microangiopathy: a case series. *Bone Marrow Transplantation,* **15,** 247–53.

91 Pulmonary complications

DAVID BRYANT

St. Vincent's Hospital and University of New South Wales, Sydney, Australia

Introduction

Hematopoietic stem cell (HSC) transplantation results in lung dysfunction in at least 50% of patients and pulmonary diseases are among the most common causes of morbidity and mortality after HSC transplantation (Krowka, Rosenow, & Hoagland, 1985) (Tables 91.1 and 91.2). In the majority of patients, symptoms are scarce, even in advanced disease, emphasizing the need for care in assessment and for repeated testing of subjects at risk. In a study of 339 patients, the incidence of severe pulmonary complications (defined as diffuse pulmonary hemorrhage or need for mechanical ventilation or death from respiratory failure) was 24% in allograft recipients but only 2.9% in autograft recipients (Ho *et al.*, 2001). The incidence in recipients of T-replete allografts immunosuppressed with cyclosporine and methotrexate was 33% compared with 8% in recipients of T-cell-depleted allografts (Fig. 91.1). It is important for physicians involved in the care of such patients to arrange for pulmonary function testing prior to transplant, to have a high index of clinical suspicion concerning pulmonary complications posttransplant, and to arrange for their early and appropriate investigation. It should be noted that interstitial pneumonitis is dealt with separately in Chapter 78. Infectious and non-infectious complications can occur both early and late posttransplant. The time course of some of the non-infectious complications is shown in Figure 91.2.

Pretransplant pulmonary function

Before attempting to assess the effects of transplantation on pulmonary function, it should be stressed that, despite the absence of clinical disease, patients may have abnormal pretransplant pulmonary function. Candidates have usually had varying degrees of exposure to cytotoxic drugs and/or radiation, may have had episodes of both septicemia and pneumonia, and may have had blood component administration as well

Table 91.1. *Pulmonary complications of hematopoietic stem cell transplantation*

Early (before day 100)	Late (after day 100)	At any time
Increased pressure pulmonary edema (fluid overload)	Restrictive lung disease	Acute bacterial, fungal, or viral infections
Oro-pharyngeal mucositis	Relapse of underlying malignancy	URTI
Pulmonary hemorrhage	Associated with chronic GVHD	Acute bronchitis
Pulmonary vascular disease	Sinusitis and bronchopulmonary sicca with	Lobar pneumonia
Bone marrow emboli	acute bronchitis or pneumonia	Bronchopneumonia
Thromboembolism	Obliterative bronchiolitis	Lung abscess/coin lesion on chest x-ray
Veno-occlusive disease	Lymphoid interstitial pneumonitis	Pneumothorax secondary to fine needle
Lymphocytic bronchitis	Pulmonary fibrosis	aspirate/pleural tap
Aspiration pneumonia		Increased leak pulmonary edema (ARDS)
Atelectasis/pleural effusion secondary to hepatic veno-occlusive disease		Allergic bronchospasm
		Organizing pneumonia
Recall radiation pneumonitis		Pulmonary fibrosis secondary to previous pneumonia
Acute GVHD of lung		
Previous history of infective pulmonary disease		

Abbreviations: URTI, upper respiratory tract infection; GVHD, graft-versus-host disease; ARDS, adult respiratory distress syndrome.

Table 91.2. *Frequency, mortality rate, and timing of some pulmonary complications posttransplant*

	Incidence	Mortality	Median time of onset after transplant
Early complications (in first 100 days)			
Pulmonary edema	10–40%	Low	1–3 weeks
Oro-pharyngeal mucositis	90–100%	<1%	1–3 weeks
Pulmonary hemorrhage	10–20%	50–80%	1–3 weeks
Pulmonary vascular disease			
Bone marrow emboli	?	Nil	Day of transplant
Thromboembolism	Rare	Minimal	4–12 weeks
Veno-occlusive disease	Rare	Unclear but low	6–8 weeks
Lymphocytic bronchitis	Up to 25%	Nil	4–8 weeks
Late complications (after 100 days)			
Restrictive lung disease	<10%	Rare	?
Leukemia recurrence	Lung involvement uncommon	High unless successful therapy	Any time, but 95% within 2 years of transplant
Obliterative bronchiolitis	5–10%	High if rapidly progressive	6–12 months

as a variety of antibiotics. The extent and nature of these events varies between the different disorders that necessitate HSC transplantation, and may help to explain some of the reported difference in pretransplant pulmonary function testing (Link *et al.,* 1986), as well as serving to emphasize the importance of obtaining pretransplant pulmonary function studies not only to detect significant nonmalignant disease, but to serve as a baseline for comparison after the transplant.

The majority of transplant candidates have no obvious pulmonary symptoms and have pulmonary function measurements that are either normal or show a minimal reduction in diffusing capacity (DLCO) (Prince *et al.,* 1989).

A pretransplant forced expiratory volume in 1 second (FEV) <80% has been associated with a higher risk of severe posttransplant pulmonary complications (Ho *et al.,* 2001).

Posttransplant pulmonary function

In long-term survivors, there is an initial decline in pulmonary function with complete or partial subsequent recovery. Posttransplant lung volumes and DLCO are lower than pretransplant values up to 1 year posttransplant, with some degree of subsequent recovery. The DLCO is significantly lower at all posttransplant intervals, although some increase does occur 6 to 12 months posttransplant. After both allogeneic (Kaplan *et al.,* 1994; Nysom *et al.,* 1996) and autologous (Arvidson *et al.,* 1994; Nenadov Beck *et al.,* 1995)

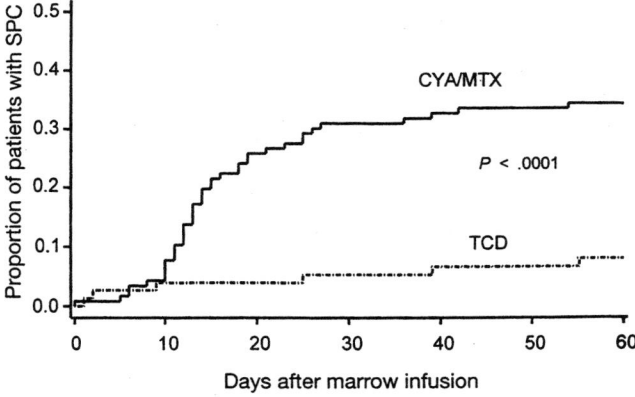

Fig. 91.1. Kaplan-Meier curves showing time to onset of severe pulmonary complication (SPC) stratified by type of graft-versus-host disease prophylaxis. Time to onset is defined as day of the first abnormal chest x-ray that subsequently led to a diagnosis of SPC. TCD indicates T-cell depletion alone; CYA/MTX, cyclosporine/methotrexate. Reproduced, with permission, from Ho *et al.* (2001).

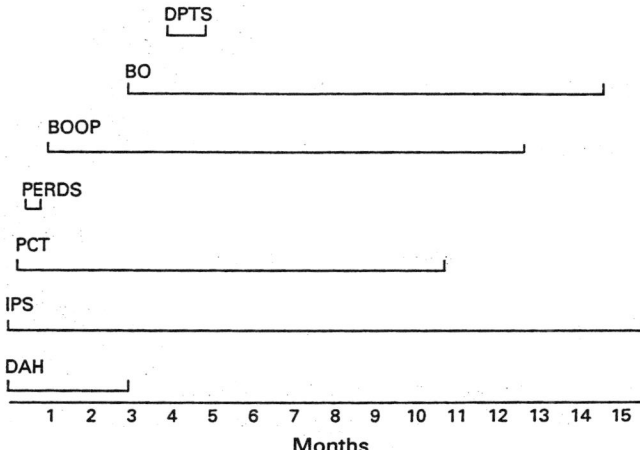

Fig. 91.2. Approximate time of onset of non-infectious pulmonary complications following hematopoietic stem cell transplant. BO = Bronchiolitis obliterans; BOOP = Bronchiolitis obliterans organizing pneumonia; DAH = diffuse alveolar hemorrhage; DPTS = delayed pulmonary toxicity syndrome; IPS = idiopathic pneumonia syndrome; PERDS = periengraftment respiratory distress syndrome; PCT = pulmonary cytolytic thrombi. Reproduced, with permission, from Afessa *et al.* (2001).

transplants in children, posttransplant values for total lung capacity, vital capacity, and FEV_1 showed a significant decrease posttransplant with some recovery with time. A restrictive effect was absent in some patients from each study except that of Arvidson *et al*. Factors associated with delayed or incomplete recovery are graft-versus-host disease (GVHD), posttransplant pulmonary infection, and higher radiation dose to the lungs (Gore *et al*., 1996).

Early complications (first 100 days)

Increased pressure pulmonary edema

One of the earliest pulmonary complications is the rapid onset of pulmonary edema for which two groups of factors are of pathogenetic importance. Firstly, cardiac or renal function may be abnormal as a result of previous chemotherapy. In patients with leukemia, prior anthracycline therapy may have produced impaired cardiac function. In the immediate pretransplant preparative regimen, high-dose cyclophosphamide is toxic to the myocardium. In addition, previous platinum chemotherapy and also previous sepsis may have produced renal impairment. Secondly, large volumes of fluid (4–6 l/day in adults) are often infused in the peritransplant period in order to administer drugs, give parenteral nutrition, and minimize the toxicity of the conditioning regimen. The pulmonary edema generally has a rapid onset, and is most common in the first 2 to 3 weeks after transplantation. This complication has been reported in 13 of 30 (43%) consecutive marrow transplant recipients, with 13% of affected individuals requiring temporary mechanical ventilation (Dickout *et al*., 1987). However, in a subsequent prospective trial, aggressive diuresis and a reduction in fluid administration at the first sign of weight gain or edema eliminated this complication. This condition needs to be distinguished from the interstitial changes described by Wise *et al*. (1984), who reported a form of nonspecific interstitial pneumonia that, on radiographic criteria, strongly resembled pulmonary edema. The disorder developed during the first 2 weeks after transplantation, was histologically characterized by diffuse alveolar damage, and was self-limited with resolution or improvement occurring within 1 to 3 weeks.

A sensible practical measure is to have a standing order for frusemide 20 to 40 mg daily, should the 24-hour fluid balance exceed 1 liter positive, or the daily weight rise by more than 1 kg.

Oro-pharyngeal mucositis

Inflammation of the oral and nasopharyngeal mucosa is one of the earliest pulmonary tract problems to arise posttransplant. It is usually the result of the mucosal toxicity of the conditioning regimen and, in extreme cases, may result in the aspiration of secretions, or the development of laryngeal edema, both requiring emergency attention. It is more fully described in Chapters 80 and 82.

Engraftment syndrome (and see Chapter 13)

The occurrence of a potentially lethal syndrome accompanying prompt hematologic recovery after autologous or (less commonly) allogeneic marrow or blood stem cell transplantation has been reported and is known as the engraftment syndrome (Lee *et al*., 1995; reviewed in Spitzer, 2001). Characteristic clinical findings include noninfectious fever, skin rash, capillary leak, and pulmonary infiltrates (Ravenel *et al*., 2000) occurring during the early engraftment period soon after infusion of the stem cells. Distinction from GVHD in the allogeneic setting can be difficult. It can occur after non-myeloablative conditioning regimens. A proposal for a uniform definition of engraftment syndrome (Spitzer, 2001) included the following as major criteria: temperature >38.5°C with no identifiable infectious etiology; erythematous skin rash involving >25% of body surface area and not attributable to medication; noncardiogenic pulmonary edema manifested by diffuse pulmonary infiltrates consistent with this diagnosis; and hypoxia.

The incidence of the syndrome varies widely in different reports at the present time. In one study of 248 patients, 59% had both skin rash and noninfectious neutropenic fever, and were thought to have the syndrome. The median time of onset was 7 (range 4–22) days posttransplant with a median duration of 11 (range 4–28) days (Lee *et al*., 1995). In another series of 61 patients, only 6 developed a syndrome of noninfectious fever, fluid retention, and pulmonary infiltrates during the early phase of neutrophil recovery (Ravoet *et al*., 1996). The clinical condition of one patient improved spontaneously while the syndrome resolved within 48 hours after initiation of corticosteroid therapy in four others. In Lee's series, prompt defervescence of fever occurred in >90% patients within a median of 1 day after initiating corticosteroid treatment. The reported mortality rate after autologous transplantation has also been variable, but is higher in those with a capillary leak component. Most deaths have occurred as a result of respiratory failure (Capizzi *et al*., 2001).

Diffuse alveolar hemorrhage

Diffuse alveolar hemorrhage (DAH) has been reported in 2.5% to 20% of patients after HSC transplantation with a mortality ranging from 50% to 80% (Ettinger & Trulock, 1991; Metcalf *et al*., 1994; Lewis, Defor, & Weisdorf, 2000). The onset is usually within the first few weeks of transplant. Patients with DAH are usually thrombocytopenic and more commonly have respiratory tract infection or more severe mucositis than those without the syndrome. It is thought that DAH arises as a result of nonspecific injury to the lung during the conditioning regimen, with aggravation by any associated infection or thrombocytopenia, and it has been reported in association with microangiopathic disease (Srivastava, Gottlieb, & Bradstock, 1995).

Hemoptysis is unusual in DAH and patients commonly have clinical and radiographic findings (including fever, dyspnea, nonproductive cough, hypoxemia, crackles, and diffuse alveolar infiltrates) that suggest infection (Khan, Jones, & England, 1987). The diagnosis of DAH is usually made via bronchoscopy. A progressive, more heavily blood-stained return on sequential lavage is the characteristic finding, together with hemorrhagic changes on lung biopsy and an elevation of the alveolar macrophage hemosiderin content (Khan, Jones, & England, 1987). However, the lavage fluid appearance may be grossly normal in the presence of other indices of DAH and the macroscopic appearance of the fluid alone should therefore not be used to exclude DAH. Treatment is supportive with correction of any associated abnormalities. High-dose corticosteroids (more than 30 mg of methylprednisolone or its equivalent daily) are reported to improve survival (Metcalf *et al.,* 1994; Raptis *et al.,* 1999). Some centers have used up to 1 g of methylprednisolone daily for 3 days with subsequent rapid taper (e.g., by 50% every 3 days). A single case report has described successful treatment with recombinant Factor VIIa (Hicks, Peng, & Gajewski, 2002). The prognosis is usually better in those who do not have associated infection.

Pulmonary vascular disease

Pulmonary vascular abnormalities are identified histologically in up to 50% of autopsy specimens of lungs from patients who have had an HSC transplant, but the clinical significance of most of these changes is minimal. The specific syndromes which have been described are as follows.

Bone marrow emboli

Some fat and bone fragments may escape the initial filtering of harvested marrow and be subsequently transfused, but they do not appear to cause either clinical or pathologically significant change (Abrahams & Catchatourian, 1983).

Pulmonary thromboembolism

Endothelial swelling and thrombi are frequent findings in some series, occurring in up to 50% of transplant patients at autopsy, but it is uncertain whether or not these changes result in any significant alteration in pulmonary function. Pulmonary embolism is rare posttransplant, but can occur even early posttransplant and in the presence of marked thrombocytopenia (see Chapter 100). When it does occur, heparin anticoagulation is indicated, although lower doses than normal should be used if the platelet count is low, and therapy monitored at least twice daily initially to obtain an activated partial thromboplastin time (APTT) of at least 1.5 to 2 times baseline value. In the presence of marked thrombocytopenia, such a policy is dangerous but must be weighed against the significant danger of recurrent pulmonary embolism. Platelet transfusions should be given as normally indicated.

Pulmonary veno-occlusive disease

Patients with hepatic veno-occlusive disease have a high risk of subsequent pulmonary veno-occlusive disease. Pulmonary veno-occlusive disease has been described in both children and adults with symptoms usually beginning between 6 and 8 weeks after transplant (Williams *et al.,* 1996; Or *et al.,* 1997). These patients present with dyspnea and signs of pulmonary hypertension. The diagnosis is supported by the exclusion of thromboemboli, the absence of radiographic evidence of interstitial pneumonia, and the lack of primary cardiac disease. However, lung biopsy, demonstrating the typical fibrinous occlusion of small pulmonary venules, is needed to confirm the diagnosis in patients presenting with posttransplant pulmonary hypertension. The syndrome has been described after both autologous and allogeneic transplantation (Salzman *et al.,* 1996) but there are only very few cases reported after autologous transplantation (Seguchi, 2000). One case was accompanied by microangiopathic hemolytic anemia 1 year after a second transplant (Kuga *et al.,* 1996). One reported case showed diffuse endothelial injury that involved pulmonary arteries, venules, and capillaries (Musani *et al,* 2001). Prompt recognition of the disorder and the administration of corticosteroids have proved helpful in some cases.

Lymphocytic bronchitis

This has been reported in up to 25% of marrow recipients at autopsy (Ettinger & Trulock, 1991). The majority of patients had a nonproductive cough and dyspnea occurring between 4 and 8 weeks posttransplant. It is characterized by lymphocytic infiltration of the bronchial epithelium, with loss of cilia together with mucosal necrosis. Distal infection was three times greater in affected patients, probably due to the loss of mucociliary defense mechanisms. It is not thought to result in death, but symptomatic treatment is required, especially for any associated infection.

Aspiration pneumonia

Aspiration pneumonia may occur in HSC transplant recipients whose level of consciousness is impaired. The risk is exacerbated by thick tenacious sputum or oro-pharyngeal secretions associated with oro-pharyngeal mucositis. The tenacity of oro-pharyngeal secretions may be exacerbated by use of phenothiazine antiemetic therapy. As always in the HSC transplant recipient, a high index of suspicion for aspiration pneumonia should be maintained when these circumstances obtain.

Atelectasis and/or pleural effusion secondary to hepatic veno-occlusive disease

When ascites becomes tense from any cause after HSC transplantation, but most commonly with hepatic veno-occlusive disease, bilateral basal atelectasis is common as well as basal pleural effusions. The development of atelectasis in these circumstances should be prevented by frequent chest physiotherapy. Ascites should be drained daily if it causes respiratory embarrassment.

Recall radiation pneumonitis

While idiopathic interstitial pneumonitis (Chapter 78) may in some circumstances represent a response to the pretransplant chemotherapy or chemoradiotherapy, "recall" radiation pneumonitis may occur in the first several weeks posttransplant in patients who have had previous local radiotherapy to the thorax (e.g., mantle irradiation for Hodgkin's disease). Diagnosis is as for interstitial pneumonitis in general. Treatment with high-dose methylprednisolone may be useful, but the syndrome can be fatal. Radiation pneumonitis can also occur because of radiotherapy given after the transplant. Four of 34 patients who underwent high-dose chemotherapy and autologous blood stem cell transplantation for high-risk breast cancer with local post-transplant radiation given to the chest wall, developed radiation pneumonitis. All responded favorably to prednisone treatment (van der Wall *et al.*, 1996).

Acute GVHD involving lung parenchyma

One report suggested that occasionally lung parenchyma may be a target of acute GVHD (Atkinson *et al.*, 1991). Presenting features were cough, dyspnea, and an asymmetric infiltrate on chest x-ray. Lung biopsy demonstrated an interstitial and peri-bronchial lymphocytic infiltrate and acute bronchial epithelial degeneration. A response to glucocorticosteroids was seen.

Pulmonary cytolytic thrombi

A syndrome characterized by fever and pulmonary nodules which histopathologically show a pattern of necrotic, basophilic thromboemboli has been described in children at a median of 72 (range 8–343) days after allogeneic stem cell transplantation (Gulbahce *et al.*, 2000; Woodard *et al.*, 2000) (Figs. 91.3 and 91.4) Immunohistochemical staining revealed entrapped leukocytes and disrupted endothelium. Biopsy tissue was sterile on culture. Empiric therapy included corticosteroids and amphotericin. Eleven of 13 patients were receiving treatment for GVHD at the time of development of the syndrome.

Previous history of infective pulmonary disease

Patients coming to transplant with a history of pulmonary tuberculosis should receive prophylaxis with isoniazid 300 mg daily (together with pyridoxine 25 mg daily to minimize the risk of isoniazid-induced peripheral neuropathy) for 3 to 6

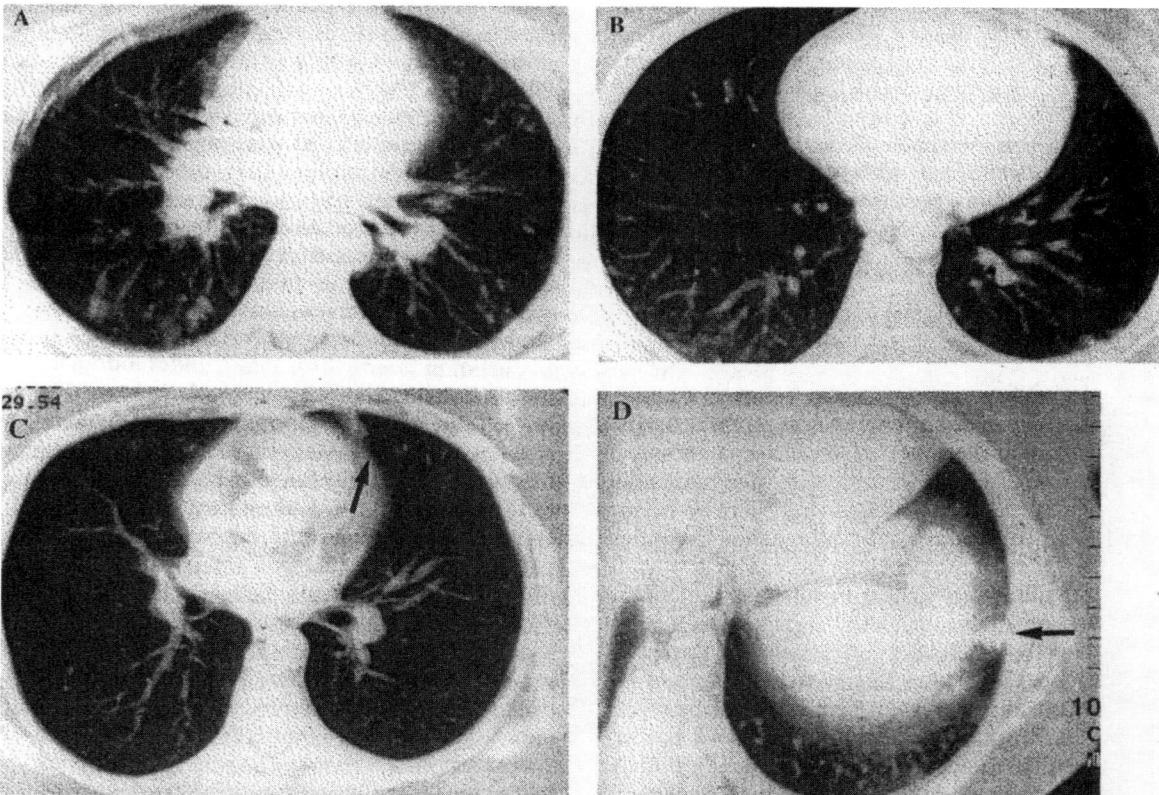

Fig. 91.3. Computed tomography in pulmonary cytolytic thrombi. (**A**) Small, discrete peripheral pulmonary nodules at the left lung base (arrow). (**B**) Multiple hazy, ill-defined nodules of varying size (arrow). (**C**) Peripheral, pleural nodules of varying size (arrow). (**D**) Discrete, left-sided anterior nodule (arrow). Reproduced, with permission, from Woodard *et al.* (2000).

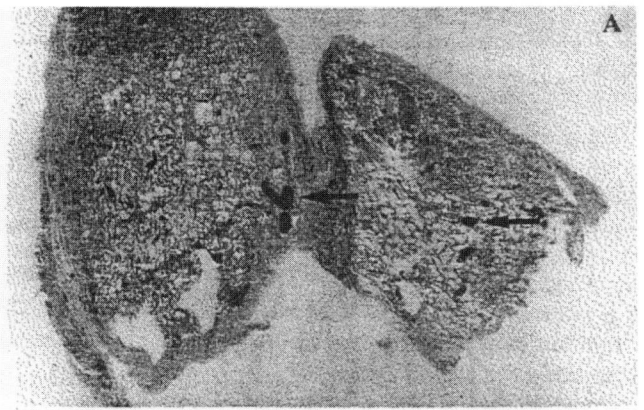

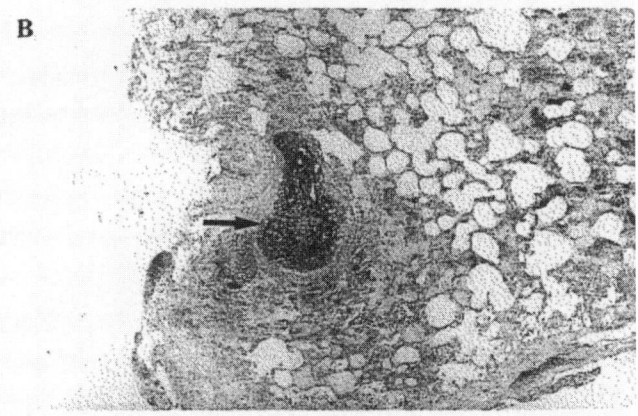

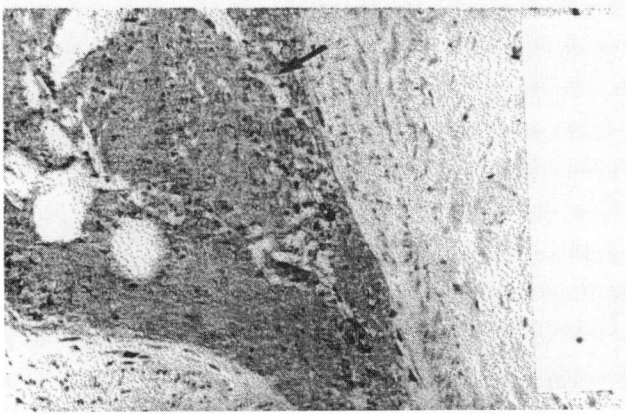

Fig. 91.4. Histology of pulmonary cytolytic thrombi (PCT). (A) Lung biopsy specimen of a patient with PCT. Arrow demonstrating thrombi in small and medium-sized vessels (hematoxylin and eosin, 5×). (B) Cellular thrombus with surrounding hemorrhage and edema and more distant normal lung tissue (arrow, hematoxylin and eosin, 10×). (C) Thrombus showing cellular debris with few intact cells staining positively (black-stained cells in mid-field) for CD45 (immunohistochemical stain for CD45, 250×). Reproduced, with permission, from Woodard *et al.* (2000).

months posttransplant. Patients coming to transplant with a previous history of fungal infection of the respiratory tract, in particular by *Aspergillus* involving sinuses or lung tissue, should ideally have received at least 2 g of amphotericin intra-

venously as primary treatment and should receive itraconazole 200 mg twice daily throughout the early posttransplant period until at least 3 to 6 months posttransplant. Voriconazole is also effective against *Aspergillus* (see Chapter 75).

Late complications (after day 100)

Restrictive lung disease

Restrictive ventilatory changes are characteristic posttransplant, but are asymptomatic in the majority of cases. These changes are thought to be related to the acute effects of irradiation/cytotoxic drugs and/or infection and tend to improve 1 year or more posttransplant (Table 91.3).

Granulomatous pneumonitis

Granulomatous pneumonitis occurred in a patient 18 months after an HLA-identical sibling bone marrow transplant for non-Hodgkin's lymphoma (Sundar *et al.*, 2001) The patient presented with dry cough, fever, and exertional dyspnea, 6 months after ill-defined nodules were detected by chest x-ray and computed tomography (CT) scanning at a time when she was asymptomatic. The changes progressed to multiple opacities with associated ground glass change. Open lung biopsy showed interstitial granulomatous inflammation with a histologic pattern suggestive of hypersensitivity pneumonitis. Special stains and cultures for acid-fast bacilli (AFB) and fungi were negative. The patient had a dramatic response to methylprednisolone 2 mg/kg/day. The donor was diagnosed with sarcoidosis involving his mediastinal lymph nodes 10 months after donating marrow and also responded well to corticosteroids. (Transmission of sarcoidosis by allogeneic marrow transplantation has been previously described—see Chapter 119).

Table 91.3. *Longitudinal changes in restrictive lung disease after bone marrow transplantation*

Reference	Time after transplant	Pattern of change
Sorensen *et al.*, 1984	1 year	Progressive decline in VC and DLCO
Springmeyer *et al.*, 1983	Up to 4 years	Early small fall in VC and DLCO, then improvement over next 3 years
Prince *et al.* (1989)	2 years	VC unaltered but a progressive fall in DLCO (as % of predicted value) 12%/year in group as a whole 28%/year in those with CML

Abbreviations: VC, vital capacity; DLCO, single breath diffusing capacity; CML, chronic myeloid leukemia.

Late complications associated with chronic GVHD

Sinusitis and bronchopulmonary sicca

Sinusitis is a common component of chronic GVHD and is predisposed to both by the infection susceptibility of these patients and by the generalized sicca of the bronchopulmonary tree that is also a common feature. Acute episodes of sinusitis should be managed in the normal way with culture of nasal discharge, decongestant therapy, and appropriate antibiotic treatment. A similar strategy applies to episodes of acute bronchitis or pneumonia. Repeated episodes of sinusitis may seed the bronchopulmonary tree and be responsible for recurrent episodes of bronchitis or pneumonia. In these circumstances, antibiotic prophylaxis additional to cotrimoxazole may be required such as cephalexin 250 mg twice daily or penicillin 250 mg twice daily. Finally, repeated episodes of sinusitis should be evaluated by an ear, nose, and throat surgeon for the possibility of surgical drainage of the sinuses (Chapter 99).

Obliterative bronchiolitis (bronchiolitis obliterans)

The onset of this syndrome is usually 6 to 12 months posttransplant. Pathologic examination of lung tissue shows obliterative bronchiolitis, the clinical severity of which ranges from asymptomatic to fulminant and fatal. There is an association with chronic GVHD (Table 91.4). The lack of a precise definition and of uniform diagnostic criteria has led to variations in the reported incidence which varies between 5% and 20% of patients posttransplant (Schultz et al., 1994; Philit et al., 1995). The pathogenesis of this change remains obscure, but there are recognized risk factors including chronic GVHD, increased donor age, acute GVHD, and either HLA-mismatched related or HLA-matched unrelated donor transplants (Table 91.5). Similar long-term complications have been reported after lung transplantation, suggesting that obliterative bronchiolitis may be a manifestation of lung rejection, as well as part of the chronic GVHD syndrome after allogeneic HSC transplantation. However, obliterative bronchiolitis after HSC transplantation is an earlier and less common complication than in patients after lung transplantation (Philit et al., 1995).

In all cases, pulmonary symptoms consist of dyspnea and a progressively productive cough. The chest radiograph is usually normal at the time of presentation, but may show hyperinflation as the disorder progresses. Areas of parenchymal hypoattenuation, bronchial dilatation, bronchiolectasis and expiratory air trapping are seen in the majority of cases on

Table 91.4. *Changes in spirometry in patients after HSC transplantation related to presence of chronic GVHD*

Reference	Change in FEV$_1$	
	Chronic GVHD	No chronic GVHD
Schultz et al., 1994	30% had fall	3% had fall
Prince et al., 1989	4% fall/year	4% rise/year

Table 91.5. *Risk factors for airflow obstruction in recipients of HSC transplants*

Increased age
Male gender
Cigarette smoking
Lower FEV/VC before transplantation
HLA-nonidentical grafts
Acute or chronic GVHD
Use of methotrexate
Viral respiratory tract infections

high-resolution CT scanning of the lungs (Sargent et al., 1995). A definitive diagnosis requires video-assisted thoracoscopic lung biopsy which shows small airway involvement with fibrinous obliteration of the lumen (Afessa et al., 2001), but is suggested by pulmonary function tests showing the development of airflow limitation (usually without any significant reversibility with bronchodilators) and the exclusion of infection by lung biopsy and lavage. Transbronchial lung biopsy is unlikely to assist with the diagnosis both because of the patchy distribution of the disease and because of the peripheral nature of the affected airways (Afessa et al., 2001). Improved control of chronic GVHD will decrease the incidence of this airway disorder. The causes are probably multifactorial and donor T-lymphocyte interaction with host cells is a likely contributor in many cases. The clinical course is variable, but the process is usually fatal in cases with rapid progression or severe obstruction. Treatment is directed at immune suppression, and at diagnosing and treating the infections that frequently occur in association with the airflow obstruction (Crawford & Clark, 1993). Double lung transplantation may offer a therapeutic option for the treatment of chronic GVHD pulmonary disease in selected patients (Boas et al., 1994).

Lymphoid interstitial pneumonitis and pulmonary fibrosis

Lymphoid interstitial pneumonitis has been reported as a late complication of allogeneic bone marrow transplantation, possibly associated with chronic GVHD (Perrault et al., 1985), and this may progress to pulmonary fibrosis (Atkinson et al., 1989). Diagnosis is best made by open lung biopsy. High doses of corticosteroids may favorably influence the course of this disease.

Pleural effusion

Shulman et al. (1980) originally used the term serositis to describe the occurrence of pleural and pericardial effusions in patients with extensive chronic GVHD. One study confirmed the rare occurrence of multiple unexplained effusions involving the pleural, pericardial, or peritoneal cavities in patients in whom other causes of such effusions such as hepatic veno-occlusive disease, cardiac insufficiency, tumor relapse, and GM-CSF (granulocyte-macrophage colony-stimulating factor) toxicity were excluded. This occurred both before and after day 100 posttransplant, but only in recipients of allografts and not autografts, and was often associated with cytomegalovirus disease (Seber, Khan, & Kersey, 1996). In one case, antinucleolar antibody was elevated in pleural fluid and blood, and lymphocytes in the pleural fluid were CD8+ HLA-DR+ (Ueda *et al.*, 2000).

Delayed pulmonary toxicity syndrome

A delayed pulmonary toxicity syndrome occurring months to years after autologous stem cell transplantation in patients with breast cancer conditioned with high-dose cyclophosphamide, cisplatin, and carmustine has been described (Wilczynski *et al.*, 1998). It is characterized by interstitial pneumonitis (IP) and fibrosis but is distinguished from other types of IP by a low mortality and responsiveness to corticosteroid treatment. It seems primarily related to the carmustine (BCNU) dose (see chapter 82).

Hepatopulmonary syndrome

There is a single case report of chronic hypoxemia and intrapulmonary vascular dilatations in association with liver disease occurring in a 10-year-old girl with chronic GVHD after allogeneic transplantation (Griese & Bender-Gotze, 1999). She had reduced diffusion capacity but normal spirometric lung function.

Relapse of underlying malignancy

Occasionally, the underlying malignancy may recur with parenchymal or pleural involvement. This may manifest radiologically as a parenchymal infiltrate, pleural shadowing, or pleural effusion. As with any cause of diffuse lung disease after HSC transplantation, diagnosis of a parenchymal infiltrate is best made by open lung biopsy. Pleural fluid should be examined cytologically for the presence of malignant cells. Marrow involvement is likely to be present concurrently. Management of relapse after transplant is described in Chapter 85.

Complications occurring at any time posttransplant

Acute bacterial, fungal, or viral infections

Upper respiratory tract infection
Surprisingly, viral upper respiratory tract infections do not appear to occur with increased frequency or severity in HSC transplant recipients, regardless of the presence or absence of acute or chronic GVHD, and despite the universal severe combined immune deficiency that occurs posttransplant.

Acute bronchitis, lobar pneumonia, and bronchopneumonia
Each of these infections may occur early or late posttransplant. Management should be vigorous and must include culture of

sputum, institution of appropriate antibiotic therapy, and chest physiotherapy.

The risk of developing *Pneumocystis carinii* pneumonia (PCP) between 7 and 12 months posttransplant is 13% (Lyytikainen *et al.*, 1996) and PCP prophylaxis should therefore be continued until 1 year posttransplant. Long-term prophylaxis (beyond 1 year) should be given to patients with extensive chronic GVHD or those receiving continued immune suppression.

Bacterial pneumonia is an important complication of HSC transplantation (Losses *et al.*, 1995). It occurs in both the early and late posttransplant period. During the first 100 days, hospital-acquired Gram-negative bacteria are the predominant pathogens, whereas after day 100, community-acquired Gram-positive bacteria predominate (Martino *et al.*, 1995). The mortality due to hospital-acquired pneumonia is significantly higher than that of community-acquired pneumonia (29% vs. 3%).

Due to improved prophylaxis and therapy, lethal pneumonia due to *Pneumocystis carinii* and cytomegalovirus are becoming rare events. *Aspergillus* species, on the other hand, have emerged as frequent causative pathogens during the last few years. Prolonged granulocytopenia and prolonged administration of corticosteroids are major risk factors of pulmonary aspergillosis, which is often fatal. In institutions where there is a significant incidence of this complication, it may be necessary to reduce the *Aspergillus* count in the air in the rooms where patients are being nursed by supplying sterile air and by using prophylactic amphotericin B (Quabeck, 1994).

Careful monitoring of patients with major chest infections after transplantation is mandatory as these patients' condition can deteriorate quickly and without warning. It is essential to obtain complete diagnostic information as early as possible and this may necessitate microbiological examination of sputum induced by the inhalation of hypertonic saline, broncho-alveolar lavage samples obtained at bronchoscopy, or open lung biopsy in selected cases.

Coin lesion on chest X-ray/lung abscess
These may occur pre- or posttransplant and require careful investigation. They are most commonly due to fungal infections, but bacterial infections can produce an identical radiologic picture, and even cytomegalovirus can occasionally produce such an appearance. Fine needle aspirate should performed under CT or ultrasound control, providing coagulation parameters (normal prothrombin and APTT times, platelet count 50×10^9/l or greater) are satisfactory. The sample should be processed for both microbiology and cytology. Patients should be observed for several hours postaspirate and a chest x-ray performed to check for pneumothorax. The risk of pneumothorax with fine needle aspirate is approximately 10%. Fine needle aspirate may be repeated within 1 week if initial reports are not helpful. In this situation,

empirical therapy with antifungal as well as antibacterial antibiotics are indicated, and, if occurring pretransplant, it is important to have resolution of the coin lesion before the start of the pretransplant preparative regimen. The possibility of surgical resection should be considered for fungal infections with *Aspergillus* or other relatively antibiotic-refractory species (see Chapter 75).

Not all coin lesions occurring posttransplant are infective in nature. Pulmonary malignancies have been reported, as well as rarer abnormalities including a solitary pulmonary cholesteroloma (Token & Angler, 1996).

Pneumothorax secondary to fine needle aspirate of lung or aspiration of pleural fluid

This should be treated in the normal way and, if more than one-third of the lung is deflated, an underwater, sealed chest drain should be inserted. As with any pneumothorax, mediastinal and subcutaneous emphysema may occur.

Acute mediastinitis associated with central venous catheter complications

Central venous catheters can migrate into the mediastinum and cause mediastinitis. In one case it was thought due to extravasation of lipid-containing hyperalimentation fluid (Keung *et al.*, 1996).

Interstitial pneumonitis

Although most cases occur within the first 100 days posttransplant, interstitial pneumonitis may occur later, and in the past it has been a major factor limiting the success of allogeneic HSC transplantation. It is the commonest cause of respiratory failure posttransplant. If requiring oro-tracheal intubation and mechanical ventilation, the prognosis is poor. Noninvasive positive-pressure ventilation may be an alternative in some patients (Marin *et al.*, 1998). It is discussed fully in Chapter 78 .

Adult respiratory distress syndrome (increased leak pulmonary edema)

There are many causes for this syndrome. After HSC transplantation, the most common cause is septicemia or pneumonia, as well as hepatic veno-occlusive disease or acute renal failure.

Allergic bronchospasm

Asthma occurring in the allogeneic donor can be transferred by the stem cell inoculum. Additionally, acute or chronic bronchospasm may occur in response to a number of therapeutic agents (e.g., amphotericin), and may require treatment with nebulized salbutamol or even systemic aminophylline.

Organizing pneumonia and bronchiolitis obliterans organizing pneumonia (BOOP)

Occasionally, an episode of pneumonia or pneumonitis (e.g., PCP) may not resolve normally. This can produce symptoms resembling the primary infection. Biopsy shows an organizing pneumonia without evidence of microorganisms. The syndrome is often responsive to corticosteroid treatment. Bronchiolitis obliterans organizing pneumonia (BOOP) has also been described after marrow transplantation (Mathew *et al.*, 1994; Kanda *et al.*, 1997; Kleinau *et al.*, 1997). In contrast to bronchiolitis obliterans, BOOP (or cryptogenic organizing pneumonia) is a proliferative lesion characterized by the appearance of bronchiolitis with granulation tissue in small airways, alveolar ducts and some alveoli, and areas of organizing pneumonia (Fig. 91.5). Patients usually present with cough, fever, and dyspnea with a clinical spectrum ranging from a mild illness to respiratory failure. Radiologic imaging studies show bilateral airspace consolidation for small nodular opacities (Fig. 91.6) and pulmonary function tests show a restrictive pattern. In the series described by Mathew *et al.* (1994), all three patients were treated with corticosteroids and in two the syndrome resolved in 1 to 2 months. The third patient developed progressive pulmonary failure and died 2 weeks after diagnosis. A combination of prednisolone and low-dose erythromycin (10 mg/kg) has also been used (Ishii *et al.*, 2000).

Pulmonary fibrosis secondary to previous pneumonia

This may occur after both bacterial and viral pneumonias and can produce long-term pulmonary impairment. It is not usually amenable to treatment.

Chest radiography

Most of the pulmonary complications that have been described have a nonspecific radiographic appearance. The most crucial information for proper interpretation of the chest x-ray is the chronologic onset of radiographic abnormalities after transplantation (Winer-Muram *et al.*, 1996). Before and just after engraftment, localized peripheral opacities with a surrounding rim of edema are usually due to fungal infections, and therapy with antifungal agents, with or without measures to accelerate or enhance neutrophil recovery and function, is indicated. After engraftment, diffuse interstitial change is the most common abnormality. In allogeneic transplant patients who are serologically positive for cytomegalovirus or who receive stem cells from serologically positive donors, pneumonitis caused by this virus used to be the most common lung infection. Idiopathic interstitial pneumonia has a similar radiographic appearance, and, with the current success of prophylactic or pre-emptive therapeutic measures to combat cytomegalovirus disease, now represent the most common type of interstitial pneumonitis (see Chapters 74 and 78). Nodular opacities may be due to a number of disorders, including opportunistic infection, organizing

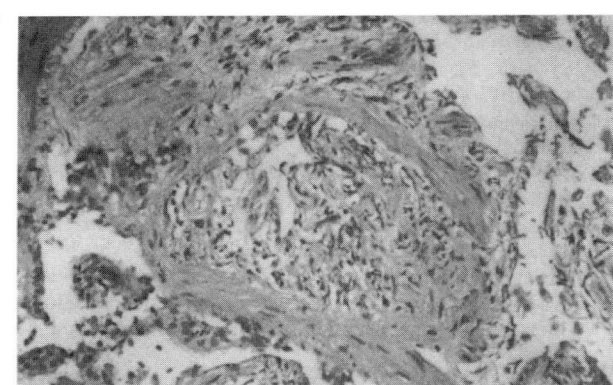

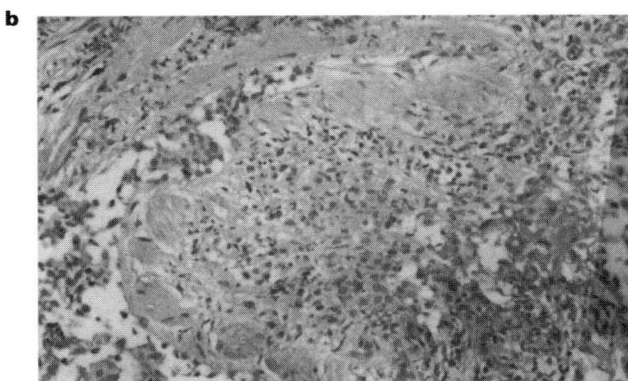

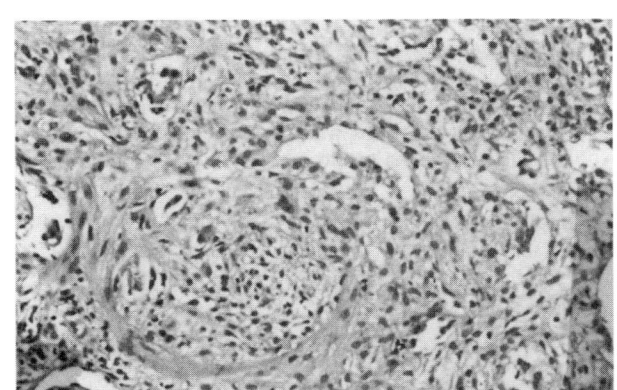

Fig. 91.5. (A) Bronchiolus almost completely occluded by loose connective tissue (hematoxylin & eosin, original magnification ×150). (B) Small bronchiolus filled with cellular granulation tissue with some lymphocytes (hematoxylin & eosin, original magnification ×200). (C) Bronchiolitis obiterans with severe interstitial pneumonia, narrowing of the alveoli, and focal disruption of granulation tissue in small air spaces (PAS, original magnification ×200). Reproduced, with permission, from Kleinau *et al.* (1997).

pneumonia, and neoplasia. Fine needle aspiration or open lung biopsy is usually required for a definitive diagnosis. High-resolution computed tomography has been recommended for febrile neutropenic patients who have a normal chest x-ray (Heussel *et al.*, 1999). It appears to be especially sensitive at diagnosing invasive aspergillosis.

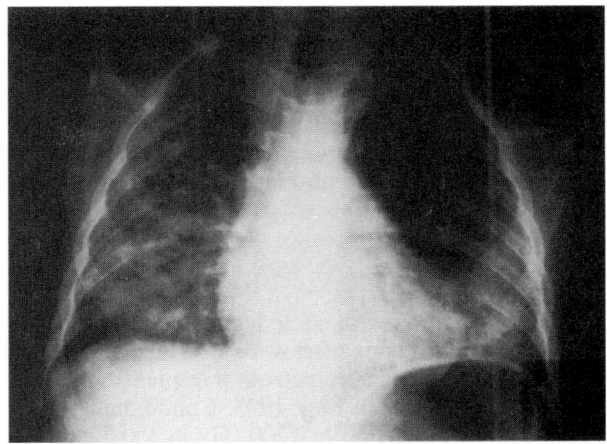

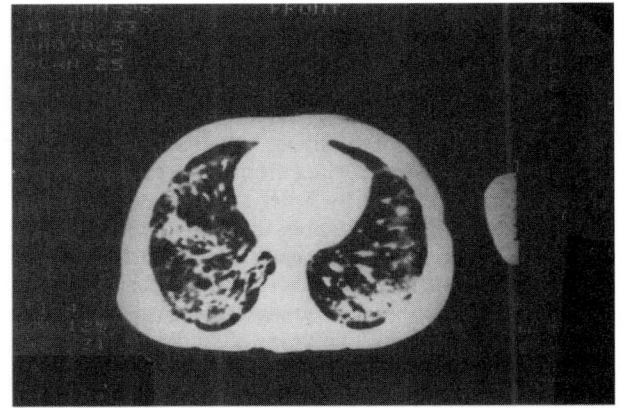

Fig. 91.6. Imaging before therapy: (A) chest radiograph with bilateral patchy infiltrates; (B) lung CT scan with peribronchiolar thickening and marked irregular-shaped infiltrates distributed over all lung zones. Reproduced, with permission, from Kleinau *et al.* (1997).

Other investigations

Bronchoscopy with broncho-alveolar lavage (BAL) is a safe diagnostic procedure that should be considered early after the onset of pulmonary complications in HSC transplant recipients. Morbidity is uncommon (2%) and a causative agent is identified in between 36% (Cazzadori *et al.*, 1995; Murray *et al.*, 2001) and 70% of immunosuppressed patients (Campbell *et al.*, 1993; Lanino *et al.*, 1996). This will result in a change in treatment in at least two-thirds of subjects. However, in patients in whom the diagnosis remains uncertain, and in whom there is a lack of clinical progress, early consideration should be given to thoracoscopic lung biopsy. This is associated with a higher complication rate than BAL alone, mainly due to bleeding.

An algorithm for the investigation of non-infectious complications of HSC transplantation is shown in Figure 91.7.

Mechanical ventilation

Pulmonary complications are common after HSC transplantation and are responsible for up to 40% of posttransplant mortal-

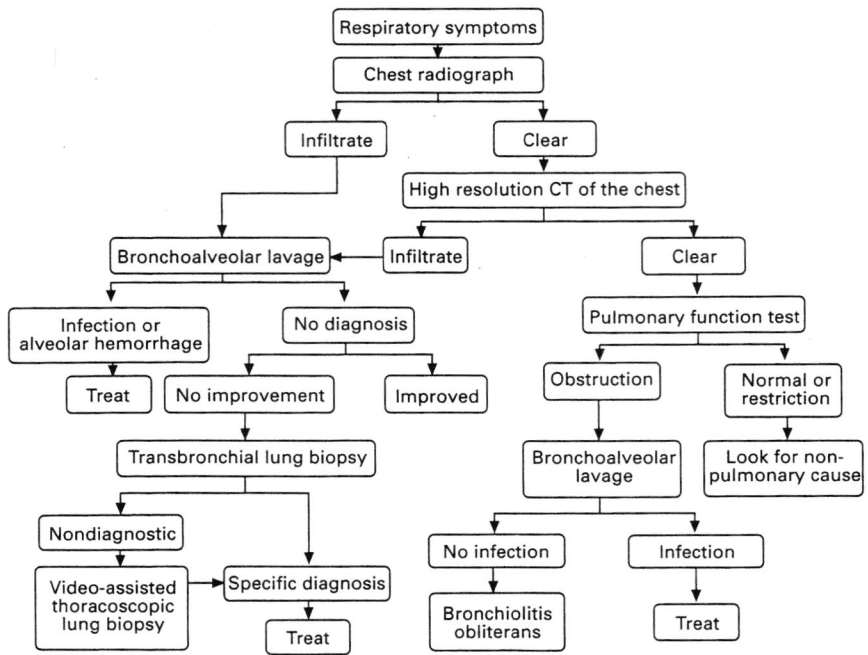

Fig. 91.7. An algorithmic approach to non-infectious pulmonary complications of HSCX. Reproduced, with permission, from Afessa *et al.* (2001).

ity (Krowka *et al.*, 1985). A substantial number of such patients develop respiratory failure and require mechanical ventilation. Their outcome remains poor (Afessa *et al.*, 1992; Paz *et al.*, 1993). A number of features have been implicated as conferring a particularly poor prognosis, including prolonged ventilation (>4 days), lung injury (FiO$_2$ >60% or PEEP >5), vasopressor support (>1 hour of a continuous infusion of dopamine at a dose of >3 μg/kg/min, norepinephrine, epinephrine, phenylephrine, dobutamine, amrinone, or milrinone) and simultaneous elevation of serum bilirubin (>68 μmol/l or 4 mg/dl) and serum creatinine (>177 μmol/l or 2 mg/dl). Of these, the concurrent presence of hepatic and renal dysfunction was the most predictive of death in one analysis (Bach *et al.*, 2001). The management of these patients requires close coordination between the BMT team, the pulmonary physician and the staff of the intensive care unit (Faber-Langendoen *et al.*, 1993; Rubenfeld & Crawford, 1996). For those patients who recover from mechanical ventilation, survival may be considerable and quality of life may be good (Bach *et al.*, 2001).

References

Abrahams, C. & Catchatourian, R. (1983). Bone fragment emboli in the lungs of patients undergoing bone marrow transplantation. *American Journal of Clinical Pathology*, **79**, 360–3.

Afessa, B., Litzow, M. R., & Tefferi, A. (2001). Bronchiolitis obliterans and other late onset non-infectious complications in hematopoietic stem cell transplantation. *Bone Marrow Transplantation*, **28**, 425–34.

Afessa, B., Tefferi, A., Hoagland, H. C. *et al.* (1992). Outcome of recipients of bone marrow transplants who require intensive-care

unit support. *Mayo Clinic Proceedings*, **67**, 117–22.Arvidson, J., Brattereby, I.-E, Carlson, K. *et al.* (1994). Pulmonary function after autologous bone marrow transplantation in children. *Bone Marrow Transplantation*, **14**, 117–23.

Atkinson, K., Bryant, D., Delprado, W., & Biggs, J. C. (1989). Widespread pulmonary fibrosis as a major clinical manifestation of chronic graft-versus-host disease. *Bone Marrow Transplantation*, **4**, 129–32.

Atkinson, K., Turner, J., Biggs, J. C. *et al.* (1991). An acute pulmonary syndrome possibly representing acute graft-versus-host disease involving the lung intersitium. *Bone Marrow Transplantation*, **8**, 231–4.

Bach, P. B., Schrag, D., Nierman, D. M. *et al.* (2001). Identification of poor prognostic features among patients requiring mechanical ventilation after hematopoietic stem cell transplantation. *Blood*, **98**, 3234–40.

Boas, S. R., Noyes, B. E., Kurland, G. *et al.* (1994). Pediatric lung transplantation for graft-versus-host disease following bone marrow transplantation. *Chest*, **105**, 1584–6.

Campbell, J. H., Blessing, N., Burnett, A. K., & Stevenson, R. D. (1993). Investigation and management of pulmonary infiltrates following bone marrow transplantation: an eight-year review. *Thorax*, **48**, 1248–51.

Capizzi, S. S., Kumar, S., Huneke, N. E. *et al.* (2001). Peri-engraftment respiratory distress syndrome during autologous hematopoietic stem cell transplantation. *Bone Marrow Transplantation*, **27**, 1299–1303.

Cazzadori, A., Di Perri, G., Todeschini, G. *et al.* (1995). Transbronchial biopsy in the diagnosis of pulmonary infiltrates in immunocompromised patients. *Chest*, **107**, 101–6.

Crawford, S. W. & Clark, J. G. (1993). Bronchiolitis associated with bone marrow transplantation. *Clinics in Chest Medicine*, **14**, 741–9.

Dickout, W. J., Chan, C. K., Hyland, R. H. *et al.* (1987). Prevention of acute pulmonary edema after bone marrow transplantation. *Chest,* **92,** 303–9.

Ettinger, N. A. & Trulock, E. P. (1991). Pulmonary considerations of organ transplantation. *American Review of Respiratory Disorders,* **144,** 213–23.

Faber-Langendoen, K., Caplan, A. L., & McGlave, P. B. (1993). Survival of adult bone marrow transplant patients receiving mechanical ventilation: a case for restricted use. *Bone Marrow Transplantation,* **12,** 501–7.

Griese, M. & Bender-Gotze, C. (1999). Hepatopulmonary syndrome after allogeneic bone marrow transplantation. *Bone Marrow Transplantation,* **24,** 1249–52.

Gore, E. M., Lawton, C. A., Ash, R. C., & Lepchik, R. J. (1996). Pulmonary function changes in long-term survivors of bone marrow transplantation. *International Journal of Radiation Oncology, Biology, Physics,* **36,** 67–75.

Gulbahce, H. E., Manivel, J. C., & Jessurun, J. (2000). Pulmonary cytolytic thrombi: a previously unrecognized complication of bone marrow transplantation. *American Journal of Surgical Pathology,* **24,** 1147–52.

Hicks, K., Peng, D., & Gajewski, J. L. (2002). Treatment of diffuse alveolar hemorrhage afer allogeneic bone marrow transplant with recombinant factor VIIa.. *Bone Marrow Transplantation,* **30,** 975–8.

Ho, V. T., Weller, E., Lee, S. J. *et al.* (2001). Prognostic factors for early severe pulmonary complications after hematopoietic stem cell transplantation. *Biology of Blood and Marrow Transplantation,* **7,** 223–9.

Heussel, C. P., Kauczor, H.-H., Heussel, G. E. *et al.* (1999). Pneumonia in febrile neutropenic patients and in bone marrow and blood stem cell transplant recipients: use of high-resolution computed tomography. *Journal of Clinical Oncology,* **17,** 796–805.

Ishii, T., Manabe, A., Ebihara, Y. *et al.* (2000). Improvement in bronchiolitis obliterans organizing pneumonia after allogeneic bone marrow transplantation by a combination of oral prednisolone and low dose erythromycin. *Bone Marrow Transplantation,* **26,** 907–10.

Kanda, Y., Takahashi, T., Imai, Y. *et al.* (1997). Bronchiolitis obliterans organizing pneumonia after syngeneic bone marrow transplantation for acute lymphoblastic leukemia. *Bone Marrow Transplantation,* **19,** 1251–3.

Kaplan, E. B., Wodell, R. A., Wilmott, R. W. *et al.* (1994). Late effects of bone marrow transplantation on pulmonary function in children. *Bone Marrow Transplantation,* **14,** 613–21.

Keung, Y.-K., Gendreau, J., Barber, A., & Cobos, E. (1996). Acute mediastinitis secondary to leakage of parenteral nutrition from a migrated central venous catheter in a patient undergoing autologous bone marrow transplant. *Bone Marrow Transplantation,* **17,** 871–2.

Khan, E. W., Jones, J. M., & England, D. M. (1987). Diagnosis of pulmonary hemorrhage in the immuno-compromised host. *American Review of Respiratory Disorders,* **36,** 155–60.

Kleinau, I., Perez-Canto, A., Schmid, H. J. *et al.* (1997). Bronchiolitis obliterans organizing pneumonia and chronic graft-versus-host disease in a child after allogeneic bone marrow transplantation. *Bone Marrow Transplantation,* **19,** 841–4.

Krowka, M. J., Rosenow, E. C. & Hoagland, H. C. (1985). Pulmonary complications of bone marrow transplantation. *Chest,* **87,** 237–46.

Kuga, T., Kohda, K, Hirayama, Y. *et al.* (1996). Pulmonary veno-occlusive disease accompanied by microangiopathic hemolytic anemia one year after a second bone marrow transplantation for acute lymphoblastic leukemia. *International Journal of Hematology,* **64,** 143–50.

Lanino, E., Sacco, O., Kotitsa, Z. *et al.* (1996). Fiberoptic bronchoscopy and bronchialveolar lavage for the evaluation of pulmonary infiltrates after BMT in children. *Bone Marrow Transplantation,* **18** (Suppl 2), 117–20.

Lee, C.-K., Gingrich, R. D., Hohl, R. I., & Ajram, K. A. (1995). Engraftment syndrome in autologous bone marrow and peripheral stem cell transplantation. *Bone Marrow Transplantation,* **16,** 175–82.

Lewis, I. D., DeFor, T., & Weisdorf, D. J. (2000). Increasing incidence of diffuse alveolar hemorrhage following allogeneic bone marrow transplantation: cryptic etiology and uncertain therapy. *Bone Marrow Transplantation,* **26,** 539–43.

Link, H., Reinhard, U., Blaurock, M., & Ostendorf, P. (1986). Lung function changes after allogeneic marrow transplantation. *Thorax,* **41,** 508–12.

Losses, I. S., Breuer, R., Or, R. *et al.* (1995). Bacterial pneumonia in recipients of bone marrow transplantation. A five-year prospective study. *Transplantation,* **60,** 672–8.

Lyytikainen, O., Rwtu, T., Volin, L. *et al.* (1996). Late onset *Pneumocystis carinii* pneumonia following allogeneic bone marrow transplantation. *Bone Marrow Transplantation,* **17,** 1057–9.

Marin, D., Gonzalez-Barca, E., Domingo, E., Berlanga, J., & Granena, A. (1998). Noninvasive mechanical ventilation in a patient with respiratory failure after hematopoietic progenitor transplantation. *Bone Marrow Transplantation,* **22,** 1123–4.

Martino, R., Manteiga, R., Sanchez, I. *et al.* (1995). Viridans streptococcal shock syndrome during bone marrow transplantation. *Acta Haematologica,* **94,** 69–73.

Mathew, P., Bozeman, T., Krance, A. *et al.* (1994). Broncholitis obliterans organizing pneumonia (BOOP) in children after allogeneic bone marrow transplantation. *Bone Marrow Transplantation,* **13,** 221–3.

Metcalf, J. P., Rennard, S. I., Reed, E. C. *et al.* (1994). Corticosteroids as adjunctive therapy for diffuse alveolar hemorrhage associated with bone marrow transplantation. *American Journal of Medicine,* **96,** 327–34.

Murray, P. V., O'Brien, M. E. R., Padhani, A. R. *et al.* (2001). Use of first line bronchoalveolar lavage in the immunosuppressed oncology patient. *Bone Marrow Transplantation,* **27,** 967–71.

Musani, A., Pascual, R., & Farber, J. (2001); Pulmonary vaso-occlusive disease associated with autologous bone marrow transplantation and high-dose melphalan. *Chest,* **120** (Suppl), 337–8.

Nenadov Beck, M., Meresse, V., Hartmann, O., & Gaultier, C. (1995). Long-term pulmonary sequelae after autologous bone marrow transplantation in children without total body irradiation. *Bone Marrow Transplantation,* **16,** 771–5.

Nysom, K., Holm, K., Hesse, B. *et al.* (1996). Lung function after allogeneic bone marrow transplantation for leukaemia or lymphoma. *Archives of Diseases of Childhood,* **74,** 432–6.

Or, R., Nagler, A., Elad, S. *et al.* (1997). Non-cardiogenic pulmonary congestion following bone marrow transplantation. *Respiration,* **64,** 170–2.

Paz, H. L., Crilley, P., Weinar, M., & Brodsky, I. (1993). Outcome of patients requiring medical ICU admission following bone marrow transplantation. *Chest,* **104,** 527–31.

Perreault, C., Cousineau, S., D'Angelo, G. *et al.* (1985). Lymphoid interstitial pneumonia after allogeneic bone marrow transplantation. *Cancer,* **55,** 1–9.

Philit, F., Wiesendanger, T., Archimbaud, E. *et al.* (1995). Post-transplant obstructive lung disease. *European Respiratory Journal,* **8,** 551–8.

Prince, D. D., Wingard, J. R., Saral, R. *et al.* (1989). Longitudinal changes in pulmonary function following bone marrow transplantation. *Chest,* **96,** 301–6.

Raptis, A., Mavroudis, D., Suffredini, A. F. *et al.* (1999). High-dose corticosteroid therapy for diffuse alveolar hemorrhage in allogeneic bone marrow stem cell transplant recipients. *Bone Marrow Transplantation,* **24,** 879–83.

Ravenel, J. G., Scalzetti, E. M., & Zamkoff, K. W. (2000). Chest raduographic features of engraftment syndrome. *Journal of Thoracic Imaging,* **15,** 56–60.

Ravoet, C., Feremans, W., Husson, B. *et al.* (1996). Clinical evidence for an engraftment syndrome associated with early and steep neutrophil recovery after autologous blood stem cell transplantation. *Bone Marrow Transplantation,* **18,** 943–7.

Rubenfeld, G. D. & Crawford, S. W. (1996). Withdrawing life support from mechanically ventilated recipients of bone marrow transplants: a case for evidence-based guidelines. *Annals of Internal Medicine,* **125,** 625–33.

Quabeck, K. (1994). The lung as a critical organ in marrow transplantation. *Bone Marrow Transplantation,* **14** (Suppl 4), 19–28.

Salzman, D., Adkins, D. R., Craig, F. *et al.* (1996). Malignancy-associated pulmonary veno-occlusive disease: report of a case following autologous bone marrow transplantation and review. *Bone Marrow Transplantation,* **18,** 755–60.

Sargent, M. A., Cairns, R. A., Murdoch, M. J. *et al.* (1995). Obstructive lung disease in children after allogeneic bone marrow transplantation; evaluation of high resolution CT. *American Journal of Roentgenology,* **164,** 693–6.

Schultz, K. R., Green, G. J., Wensley, D. *et al.* (1994). Obstructive lung disease in children after allogeneic bone marrow transplantation. *Blood,* **84,** 3212–20.

Seber, A., Khan, S. P., & Kersey, J. H. (1996). Unexplained effusions: association with allogeneic bone marrow transplantation and acute or chronic graft-versus-host disease. *Bone Marrow Transplantation,* **17,** 207–11.

Seguchi, M., Hirabayashi, N., Fujii, Y. *et al.* (2000). Pulmonary hypertension associated with pulmonary occlusive vasculopathy after allogeneic bone marrow transplantation. *Transplantation,* **69,** 177–79.

Shulman, H. M., Sullivan, K. M., Weiden, P. L. *et al.* (1980). Chronic graft-versus-host syndrome in man. A long term clinico-pathological study of 20 Seattle patients. *American Journal of Medicine,* **69,** 204–17.

Sorensen, P. G., Ernst, P., Panduro, J., & Moller, J. (1984). Reduced lung function in leukemia patients undergoing bone marrow transplantation. *Scandinavian Journal of Haematology,* **32,** 353–7.

Spitzer, T. R. (2001). Engraftment syndrome following hematopoietic stem cell transplantation. *Bone Marrow Transplantation,* **27,** 893–8.

Springmeyer, S. C., Flournoy, N., Sullivan, K. M. *et al.* (1983). Pulmonary function changes in long term survivors of allogeneic marrow transplantation. In *Recent Advances in BoneMarrow Transplantation,* ed. R. P. Gale, pp. 343–353. New York: Alan R. Liss.

Srivastava, A., Gottlieb, D., & Bradstock, K. F. (1995). Diffuse alveolar hemorrhage associated with microangiopathy after allogeneic bone marrow transplantation. *Bone Marrow Transplantation,* **15,** 863–7.

Sundar, K. M., Carveth, H. J., Gosselin, M. V. *et al.* (2001). Granulomatous pneumonitis following bone marrow transplantation. *Bone Marrow Transplantation,* **28,** 627–30.

Toren, A. & Nagler, A. (1996). Solitary pulmonary cholesteroloma, multiple xanthelasmas and lipemia retinalis complication hypercholesterolemia after bone marrow transplantation. *Bone Marrow Transplantation,* **18,** 457–9.

Ueda, T., Manabe, A., Kikuchi, A. *et al.* (2000). Massive pericardial and pleural effusion with anasarca following allogeneic bone marrow transplantation. *International Journal of Hematology,* **71,** 394–7.

van der Wall, E., Schaake-Koning, C. C., van Zandwijk, N. *et al.* (1996). The toxicity of radiotherapy following high-dose chemotherapy with peripheral blood stem cell support in high-risk breast cancer: a preliminary analysis. *European Journal of Cancer,* **32a,** 1490–7.

Wilczynski, S. W., Erasmus, J. J., Petros, W. P. *et al.* (1998). Delayed pulmonary toxicity syndrome following high-dose chemotherapy and bone marrow transplantation for breast cancer. *American Journal of Respiratory and Critical Care Medicine,* **157,** 565–73.

Williams, L. M., Fussell, S., Veith, R. W. *et al.* (1996). Pulmonary veno-occlusive disease in an adult following bone marrow transplantation. *Chest,* **109,** 1388–91.

Winer-Muram, H. T., Gurney, J. W., Bozeman, P. M., & Krance, R. A. (1996). Pulmonary complications after bone marrow transplantation. *Radiology Clinics of North America,* **34,** 97–117.

Wise, R. H., Shin, M. S., Gockerman, J. P. *et al.* (1984). Pneumonia in bone marrow transplant patients. *American Journal of Roentgenology,* **143,** 707–11.

Woodard, J. P., Gulbace, E., Shreve, M. *et al.* (2000). Pulmonary cytolytic thrombi: a newly recognized complication of stem cell transplantation. *Bone Marrow Transplantation,* **25,** 293–300.

92 Cardiac complications

MICHAEL FENELEY

St. Vincent's Hospital and University of New South Wales, Sydney, Australia

Introduction

The major cardiac complications of hematopoietic stem cell (HSC) transplantation are related to the cardiotoxic effects of conditioning therapy given prior to transplantation, particularly cyclophosphamide, as well as associated volume overload, sepsis, and pre-existing cardiac disease, including anthracycline-induced cardiomyopathy. Although once common (Cazin *et al.,* 1986; Goldberg *et al.,* 1986), more recent evidence indicates that clinically significant cardiac complications now occur in 5% to 10% of patients (Baello *et al.,* 1986; Bearman *et al.,* 1990; Kupari *et al.,* 1990a, Hertenstein *et al.,* 1994). The major reason for this change appears to be the reduction in the dose of cyclophosphamide administered prior to transplantation. Significant cardiac complications were observed in 5% of our own series of 500 bone marrow transplants (Table 92.1). Long-term cardiac complications were noted in 4% of patients in another report. Fatal or life-threatening cardiac complications are much less common, however, occurring in only 0.9% of 2,821 patients treated in one center from 1977 to 1997

Table 92.1. *Cardiac complications in 500 bone marrow transplants*

Complications	Number of cases	%
Pulmonary edema	8	1.6
Pericarditis	5	1
Atrial fibrillation	4	0.8
Recurrent supraventricular tachycardia (Wolff-Parkinson-White syndrome)	1	0.20
Infective endocarditis		
Definite (left-sided)	2	0.40
Probable[a]	1	0.20
Staphylococcal myocarditis	1	0.20
Cardiac toxoplasmosis	1	0.20
Angina pectoris	2	0.40
Nontransmural myocardial infarction	1	0.20
Right atrial thrombus (at autopsy)	1	0.20
Total	27	5.0

[a] Patient with systemic aspergillosis, pericarditis, and adherent right atrial mass on echocardiography.

(Murdych & Weisdorf, 2001). Similarly, none of 57 pediatric patients were found to have symptomatic long-term cardiac complications (Uderzo *et al.,* 2000).

Cardiac toxicity due to conditioning therapy

Relationship to cyclophosphamide dose

A wide variety of myeloablative conditioning regimens for HSC transplantation have been described, but most allogeneic transplant recipients currently receive either cyclophosphamide and total body irradiation (TBI) or busulfan and cyclophosphamide. Two randomized trials have compared these two combinations, with one demonstrating lower overall toxicity and graft-versus-host disease with the busulfan combination (Clift *et al.,* 1994) and the other demonstrating the opposite (Ringden *et al.,* 1999). The available evidence indicates that cyclophosphamide exerts the major cardiotoxic effects of conditioning therapy, that these effects are dose-dependent (Baello *et al.,* 1986; Cazin *et al.,* 1986; Goldberg *et al.,* 1986; Kupari *et al.,* 1990a; Carlson *et al.,* 1994; Hertenstein *et al.,* 1994), and that they are potentially reversible (Kupari *et al.,* 1990b). Cyclophosphamide cardiotoxicity is thought to result from a direct toxic effect on the endothelium, resulting in capillary microthromboses and increased capillary permeability, with extravasation into the myocardium and pericardium, and hemorrhagic myocardial necrosis in severe cases (Buja *et al.,* 1976). Pulmonary toxicity may result from the same mechanisms.

Acute cardiac failure, with or without pericarditis and pericardial effusion, is the most severe clinical manifestation of cardiotoxicity, which usually occurs within 10 days of cyclophosphamide administration. The antidiuretic hormone-like effect of cyclophosphamide, iatrogenic volume overload, increased pulmonary capillary permeability, and the high output load imposed by pyrexia and sepsis may in addition contribute to the clinical syndrome of pulmonary venous congestion and edema (Cazin *et al.,* 1986). Sepsis may be a particularly important factor in fatal childhood cases (Riley *et al.,* 1999).

Approximately 30 fatal cases of cyclophosphamide cardiotoxicity have been reported since the first report in 1971 (Santos *et al.,* 1971). Notably, the total dose of cyclophosphamide exceeded 120 mg/kg in all but one fatal case, and in most cases was 180 mg/kg or greater. At these high doses, cardiac toxicity has been viewed as "the most important limiting factor in marrow transplantation" (Cazin et al., 1986) with a 43% morbidity and 9% mortality in a series of 63 patients. However, "little evidence of short-term cardiac toxicity" (Baello et al., 1986) was reported in 28 patients given 90 mg/kg cyclophosphamide and 9 Gy TBI. Similarly, clinically significant cardiac complications were observed in less than 10% of 45 patients given 120 mg/kg cyclophosphamide and TBI (10 to 12 Gy) (Kupari et al., 1990a). Similar conditioning therapy was employed in most of our own patients, and significant cardiac complications were observed in 5% (Table 92.1). It has been suggested that the dose of cyclophosphamide might be selected more appropriately on the basis of body surface area rather than weight: clinically significant cardiac toxicity was observed in only 1 of 32 patients given ≤ 1.55 g/m^2/day for 4 days but in 13 of 52 patients given a higher dose (Goldberg et al., 1986). More recently, Hertenstein et al. (1994) reported that in 134 patients receiving cyclophosphamide conditioning, serious cardiac toxicity was limited to two patients with a dose higher than this level. Although they reported no signs of cardiac toxicity in 15 other patients who received this high dose, three of these patients died of interstitial pneumonia ($n = 2$) or hepatitis ($n = 1$). Nevertheless, cyclophosphamide is still most commonly administered in a total dose of 120 mg/kg of adjusted ideal body weight, with the dose split over two successive days.

Other chemotherapeutic agents, such as cytosine arabinoside, administered with cyclophosphamide in some conditioning regimens, while not known to be cardiotoxic themselves, have been postulated to enhance cyclophosphamide cardiotoxicity (Baello et al., 1986; Cazin et al., 1986). The incidence of serious cardiotoxicity appears, however, to be determined predominantly by the cyclophosphamide dose (Goldberg et al., 1986). The addition of high-dose doxorubicin and etoposide to cyclophosphamide does not appear to increase cardiac toxicity (Somlo et al., 1994). Similarly, the usual doses of TBI administered with cyclophosphamide for conditioning therapy (8 to 12 Gy) are well below those known to be cardiotoxic (Stewart & Fajardo, 1984), and there is little evidence that such irradiation increases the incidence of cardiotoxicity (Cazin et al., 1986; Carlson et al., 1994). Significant cardiac toxicity (congestive heart failure, transient left ventricular dysfunction, pericardial effusion, ST-T abnormalities, arrhythmias, and atrio-ventricular block) has been reported with, conditioning regimens containing the combination of cyclophosphamide and thiotepa (Alidina et al., 1999; Ando et al., 2000) and with the combination of melphalan and fludarabine (Ritchie et al., 2001).

Subclinical evidence of cardiac toxicity

More subtle evidence of cardiac toxicity is quite common at total cyclophosphamide doses not exceeding 120 mg/kg, including electrocardiographic (ECG) ST segment and T-wave changes in approximately one-third of patients, significant reductions in total QRS voltage in approximately one-quarter of patients, and ECG evidence of increased left ventricular mass (edema) and impaired systolic and diastolic function, although the latter was subclinical in most cases (Kupari et al., 1990a, 1990b). Importantly, these changes are reversible, with complete resolution documented in those surviving 1 year after transplantation (Kupari et al., 1990b).

On the other hand, mild depression of left ventricular ejection fraction persisted for up to 5 years in lymphoma patients conditioned with cyclophosphamide doses of 140 to 180 mg/kg (Carlson et al., 1994). In the same study, neither TBI nor mediastinal irradiation was found to be implicated in the depression of left ventricular ejection fraction. Abnormally prolonged left ventricular time to peak filling has been documented 1 year after marrow transplantation in 25 patients in one study (Lele et al., 1996). A recent report suggests that this abnormality might be predicted by an elevated brain natiuretic peptide level 14 days after transplantation, but the ejection fraction was unchanged in these patients (Niwa et al., 2001). Asymptomatic reductions of left ventricular ejection fraction and impaired diastolic relaxation have been documented 0.5 to 10 (median 5) years after marrow transplantation (20 allogeneic, 10 autologous) in 30 pediatric patients (Pihkala et al., 1994). In contrast, a 5- to 10-year follow-up study of 35 children after autologous marrow transplantation found no long-term effects on echocardiographic left ventricular dimensions or the ejection fraction of either ventricle at rest (Lonnerholm et al., 1999). Stress testing, however, might unmask more subtle cardiac abnormalities. In a cross-sectional study of 63 patients 1 to 16 years after marrow transplantation in childhood or adolescence, only 1 patient had a resting ejection fraction <50%, but 23 of 31 patients tested (74%) had borderline or abnormal responses to exercise, and 8 of these were symptomatic (Eames et al., 1997).

Loss of QRS voltage, particularly when associated with ST segment or T-wave changes, and weight gain (>2 kg persisting for >48 hours) have been reported to predict clinically significant cardiac toxicity (Cazin et al., 1986; Kupari et al., 1990a).

Arrhythmias

Significant cardiac arrhythmias are infrequent at total cyclophosphamide doses of 120 mg/kg (Kupari et al., 1990a), or even at higher doses (Cazin et al., 1986), and may reflect the influence of pyrexia, sepsis, electrolyte disturbances, increased sympatho-adrenal drive, and pre-existing cardiac disease, in addition to the cardiotoxic effects of the conditioning therapy. The most frequently reported abnormalities are atrial or ventricular ectopic beats, atrial fibrillation, and supraventricular tachycardia. One case of complex ventricular arrhythmias associated with a long QT syndrome has been reported (Kupari et al., 1990a). Our own experience (Table 92.1) suggests that arrhythmias requiring specific antiarrhythmic therapy can be expected in approximately 1% of patients when the total dose of cyclophosphamide is 120 mg/kg.

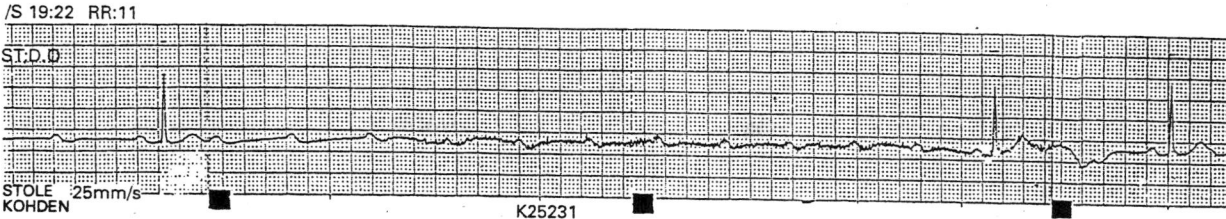

Fig. 92.1. ECG monitoring recorded on day −5 showing advanced atrioventricular (AV)-block with a 9 s asystolic pause. Reproduced, with permission, from Ando *et al.* (2000).

Considerable cardiotoxicity was seen in a series of 39 women with breast cancer receiving cyclophosphamide and thiotepa (200 mg/m^2) conditioning before autologous stem cell transplantation, all of whom had received anthracyclines previously (Ando *et al.*, 2000). One patient developed chronic congestive heart failure, two had transient left ventricular dysfunction, three had pericardial effusion, and two developed ST-T abnormalities during the high-dose chemotherapy. Arrhythmias were observed in nine patients, four of which occurred during stem cell infusion (Figs. 92.1 and 92.2): three atrial arrhythmias, two ventricular arrhythmias, and 4 atrio-ventricular block episodes, including two with complete atrio-ventricular block with an asystolic

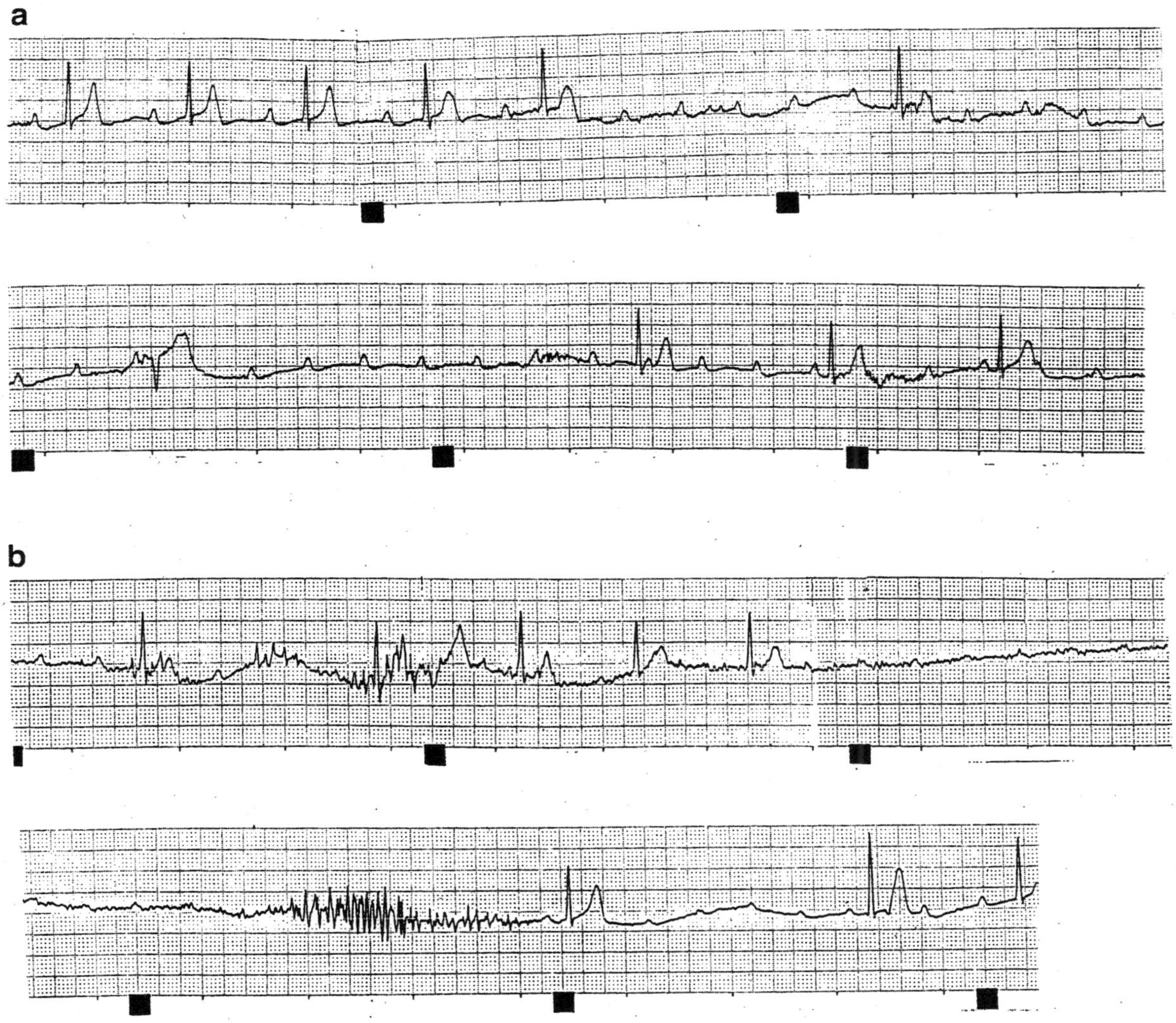

a

b

Fig. 92.2. (a) ECG monitoring on day −1 showing first-degree and advanced AV-block. The PR interval was prolonged to 0.32 s. An advanced AV block with escape beats followed first-degree block. (b) The event shown in (a) progressed to complete AV-block with an 11 s asystolic pause associated with AV junctional beats and a loss of consciousness, which was induced by vomiting. Reproduced, with permission, from Ando *et al.* (2000).

pause. The fact that three patients developed atrio-ventricular block with uncontrolled vomiting suggests that vagal stimulation during emesis may be an important precipitant of atrio-ventricular block due to high-dose chemotherapy.

Transient sinus bradycardia, usually asymptomatic, and hypertension have been reported to be frequently observed during infusion of autologous, cryopreserved bone marrow (Davis *et al.*, 1990; Styler *et al.*, 1992; Keung *et al.*, 1994), and heart block was detected in 10% of these patients in one study (Styler *et al.*, 1992). In the study by Keung *et al.* (1994), 14 of 17 patients receiving unpurged cryopreserved autologous bone marrow and/or peripheral blood stem cells developed a cardiac arrhythmia (82%), of which 11 (65%) developed sinus bradycardia, 4 (24%) second-degree heart block (Fig. 92.3), and one patient complete heart block. The onset of sinus bradycardia occurred at a median of 56 (range 15–513) minutes postinfusion and the onset of heart block a median of 234 (range 30–680) minutes. Hypertension was noted in 7 patients (41%) in this series and usually occurred within 2 hours of infusion. These findings appeared to be related to the total volume of cryopreserved marrow infused, possibly reflecting the total dose of the cryoprotectant dimethylsulfoxide (DMSO) administered. Two fatal cases of cardiac arrest following autologous, cryopreserved marrow infusions have been reported (Rapoport *et al.*, 1991; Hertenstein *et al.*, 1994). More recently, however, no differences in heart rate or blood pressure responses were observed between those receiving autologous, cryopreserved grafts and a control group of allogeneic graft recipients (Lopez-Jimenez *et al.*, 1994). A slight decrease in heart rate was observed in both groups (median 11 to 12 beats per minute), but no patient developed a heart rate of less than 55 beats per minute, and no significant blood pressure changes were observed in either group, although there was a trend to an increase in the ratio of ventricular ectopic beats to supraventricular ectopic beats before and after marrow infusion in the autologous recipients (Fig. 92.4).

Possible reasons for the differences between the latter and former studies, despite the same total volume of marrow and DMSO infused, were a slower infusion rate (duration 95 minutes versus 30–40 minutes), breaks between infusion aliquots, graft infusion through a standard transfusion filter (170 μm),

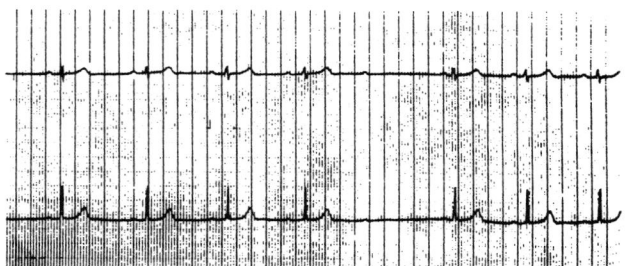

Fig. 92.3. ECG showing second-degree heart block in a 36-year-old Caucasian female with metastatic breast carcinoma 1 hour after receiving stem cell reinfusion. Reproduced, with permission, from Keung *et al.* (1994).

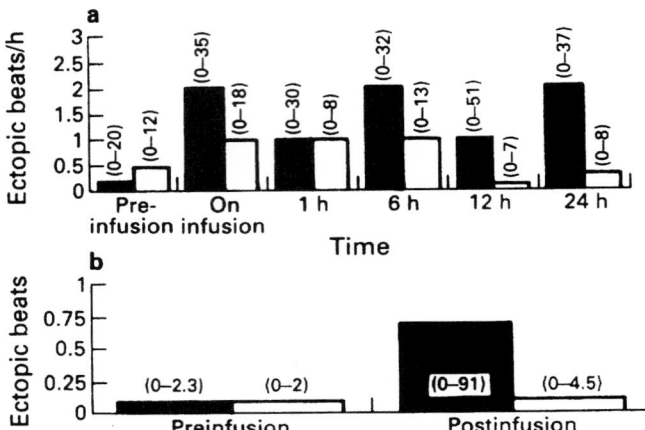

Fig. 92.4. **(A)** Median number of ectopic beats/hour during the period of study. Range is expressed between brackets in each column. No differences were statistically significant at any point. ABMT (■) = autologous recipients; Allo-BMT (□) = allogeneic recipients. **(B)** Ratio of ventricular ectopic beats/supraventricular ectopic beats before and after marrow infusion. Range is expressed between brackets in each column. Reproduced, with permission, from Lopez-Jimenez *et al.* (1994).

and prophylactic use of diuretics in 40% of patients (Lopez-Jimenez *et al.*, 1994).

Previous anthracycline administration and pretransplant ejection fraction

Many patients coming to transplant have undergone prior treatment for hematologic malignancies with anthracycline chemotherapeutic agents, which have well-documented and irreversible cardiotoxic effects. Anecdotal evidence based on the small number of patients who develop serious cardiotoxicity in most series, including our own, does suggest that patients pretreated with anthracyclines are at higher risk (Baello *et al.*, 1986; Cazin *et al.*, 1986; von Herbay *et al.*, 1988; Kupari *et al.*, 1990a). This impression was not confirmed, however, by a systematic study by Bearman *et al.* (1990), but this possibly reflected patient selection bias because very few of the patients who had received anthracyclines in that study had left ventricular ejection fractions less than 50% before bone marrow transplantation.

More recently, Hertenstein *et al.* (1994) reported that 18 of 22 patients with left ventricular ejection fractions less than 55% before marrow transplantation had received anthracyclines. In the same study, cardiac toxicity posttransplant occurred more commonly in those with ejection fractions less than 55% before transplantation, but this was mainly due to minor or subclinical abnormalities in those with ejection fractions between 50% and 54%. Only 8 of 170 patients had ejection fractions less than 50%, and none of these had any sign of cardiac toxicity. The lowest ejection fraction pretransplant was 42%. There is very little information on the incidence of significant cardiotoxicity in patients with more severe left ventricular dysfunction before transplantation because such patients are not accepted for HSC transplantation in many centers.

Similarly, Lehmann and colleagues (2000) found that patients who had received anthracyclines pretransplant had significantly lower left ventricular ejection fractions pretransplant, but no increased risk of decline in cardiac function posttransplant. Although patients with CML had significantly higher pretransplant ejection fractions than those with acute leukemia or myeloma, posttransplant ejection fractions were not significantly different from pretransplant values in any diagnostic group.

Left ventricular fractional shortening by echocardiography was always within normal limits before, and up to 4 years after, bone marrow transplantation in 41 children surviving at least 2 years posttransplant, but was slightly lower in those with higher cumulative previous anthracycline doses (Rovelli et al., 1995).

A multivariate logistic regression analysis of patients undergoing high-dose chemotherapy with autologous stem cell rescue for lymphoma or breast cancer suggested that lymphoma, older age, a low ejection fraction, and higher doses of previous anthracycline exposure predict increased cardiac toxicity (Brockstein et al., 2000). The cumulative anthacycline dose did not appear to be a major predictor of subsequent cardiac toxicity with high-dose chemotherapy in another study (Ando et al., 2000).

Other pre-existing heart disease

A wide variety of pre-existing cardiac disorders may increase the propensity to cardiac complications following HSC transplantation. One of our patients with recurrent supraventricular tachycardia after transplantation had previously documented Wolff-Parkinson-White syndrome,[1] while another patient with thalassemia major had impaired left ventricular function before transplantation due to myocardial iron overload. The latter problem might also be expected in patients with aplastic anemia, but most such patients are transplanted before they have received sufficient blood transfusions to produce hemosiderosis (Goldberg et al., 1986). Sudden cardiac tamponade after chemotherapy that included cyclophosphamide for marrow transplantation in patients with thalassemia has been described (Angelucci et al., 1992, 1994). In a series of 400 consecutive thalassemic patients, cardiac tamponade occurred in eight (2%) during the conditioning regimen or within 1 month of transplantation. Six cases were fatal, and these represented 9% of all causes of death and 29% of those deaths occurring between the start of the conditioning regimen and 1 month posttransplant. The syndrome was characterized by sudden onset of circulatory shock and cardiac arrest. The only effective treatment was

[1] Louis Wolff, American cardiologist, born 1898. Sir John Parkinson, English physician, 1885–1976. Paul Dudley White, American cardiologist, 1886–1973.

immediate drainage of the pericardial fluid. Three of the eight affected patients had bacteremia and it was felt that either bacteremia or the drugs used for the conditioning regimen, particularly cyclophosphamide, were responsible. Fatal cardiac tamponade despite pericardiocentesis due to hemorrhagic myocarditis was described in a patient one day after bone marrow transplantation for aplastic anemia with hemosiderosis (Miura et al., 1997), perhaps due to the high total cyclophosphamide dose (200 mg/kg).

Conversely, the cardiac wall thickening and restrictive filling pattern associated with the lysosomal storage diseases have been shown to improve or stabilize after HSC transplantation (Gatzoulis et al., 1995; Hoogerbrugge et al., 1995).

Cardiac complications due to infection

Despite the high prevalence of bacteremia associated with profound immune suppression and neutropenia following HSC transplantation, infective endocarditis is quite rare. Quinn, Counts, and Meyers (1986) observed right-sided endocarditis due to coagulase-negative staphylococci associated with Hickman catheter infections in only 1.2% of 246 patients. Martino et al. (1990) reported 8 cases of a syndrome compatible with right-sided endocarditis, possibly related to Hickman catheter infections (Staphylococcus epidermidis in 4 cases) in 141 patients, but the diagnosis was definite or probable in only 4 of these cases (2.8%). In 123 cases of viridans streptococcal infection of the blood and/or cerebrospinal fluid, none had infective endocarditis (Villablanca et al., 1990). In our own series (Table 92.1), definite infective endocarditis was diagnosed in only two patients, which was left-sided in both cases and involved valves previously damaged by rheumatic fever. In a third patient with systemic aspergillosis and a pericardial effusion, a lesion observed on the right atrial wall by echocardiography was consistent with an aspergilloma. Fungal endocarditis has been reported after HSC transplantation in only six patients in the literature (Chim et al., 1998).

Pericarditis due to Aspergillus fumigatus after bone marrow transplantation has been reported by others also (Guerin et al., 1989; Le Moing et al., 1998). It appears to result from contiguous spread from the lung or myocardium, and is frequently fatal. We observed only one other patient with septic pericarditis, a patient with staphylococcal microabscesses of the myocardium documented at autopsy. Another patient in our series had cardiac involvement with acute disseminated toxoplasmosis resulting in cardiac arrest. A single case of pneumococcal pericarditis in a 13-year old patient 8 months after allogeneic marrow transplantation complicated by chronic graft-versus-host disease has been reported (Perez Retortillo et al., 1998).

In an autopsy review of 56 patients who had died after marrow transplantation (43 within 2 months) (Chandrasekar et al., 1995), infection of the heart and multiple other systems with Aspergillus (n = 2) or Pseudomonas (n = 1) was demonstrated in only three patients, and only the Pseudomonas infection was recognized antemortem. In contrast, nonbacterial thrombotic (marantic) endocarditis was demonstrated in five patients (right heart valves in four patients and all cardiac valves in one patient). Of particular note, no viral cardiac infections were demonstrated. An enterovirus similar to Coxsackie B was identified recently in multiple organs of a single patient who died with heart failure, pericarditis, and pneumonia, but there was no evidence of the virus in the heart (Galama *et al.*, 1996).

Other pericardial abnormalities

Pericarditis has been noted as a complication of granulocyte-macrophage colony-stimulating factor (GM-CSF) therapy in doses exceeding 15 µg/kg daily to accelerate neutrophil recovery (Lieschke *et al.*, 1989), but this dose is appreciably higher than the currently recommended dose of 3 to 10 µg/kg daily. Constrictive pericarditis has been described recently in two patients after conditioning for allogeneic marrow transplantation with melphalan and a total body irradiation dose substantially lower than that previously associated with constrictive pericarditis, following thoracic radiotherapy to treat malignancy (Cavet *et al.*, 2000). Pericardiectomy in both patients produced marked improvement in left ventricular filling, but a degree of right heart failure persisted secondary to restrictive cardiomyopathy. Pericardial effusion and constrictive pericarditis have also been described as complications of chronic graft-versus-host disease. Unexplained multiple effusions involving two or more of the pericardial, pleural, and peritoneal cavities have been associated with acute or chronic graft-versus-host disease, often in association with CMV disease, after allogeneic marrow transplantation (Seber *et al.*, 1996).

Other cardiac complications

Chest pain

Chest pain consistent with angina pectoris or myocardial infarction may occur after HSC transplantation (Table 92.1). While these occurrences may well reflect pre-existing coronary artery disease, a clinical diagnosis of nontransmural myocardial infarction was associated with normal coronary angiographic findings in at least one reported case (Bearman *et al.*, 1990). A more recent case of fatal acute transmural myocardial infarction posttransplant has been reported (Wang *et al.*, 1996), but the state of the coronary arteries was not documented. Given that cyclophosphamide cardiotoxicity can cause hemorrhagic myocardial necrosis that might result in release of cardiac enzymes, is often associated with pericarditis, and can cause significant ST segment, T wave, and QRS voltage changes, its clinical distinction from ischemic myocardial injury may be difficult in the absence of documented coronary artery disease. Pathologic changes of acute myocardial infarction were detected at autopsy in 2 of 56 patients dying after marrow transplantation (Chandrasekar *et al.*, 1995). Successful autologous bone marrow transplantation has been performed in

a patient known to have single vessel coronary artery disease pretransplant (Schechter, Drakos, & Nagler, 1994).

Thrombosis

Pulmonary thromboembolism, intracardiac thrombus formation, and major vein occlusion are potential complications of indwelling central venous catheters (Ahmed & Payne, 1976), but are relatively rare after HSC transplantation, and are discussed further in Chapter 100. We have documented only one case of right atrial thrombus at autopsy, and this did not contribute to the patient's death. Pulmonary arterial occlusive disease has been reported shortly after bone marrow transplantation in an 8-year old patient (Vaksmann *et al.*, 2002).

Graft-versus-host disease

Two case reports have suggested the possible occurrence of cardiac graft-versus-host disease (GVHD) posttransplant (Gilman *et al.*, 1998; Platzbecker *et al.*, 2001), although the heart is not normally recognized as a target organ in GVHD. In the first reported, reversible complete heart block occurred. The second reported case was a 17 year-old man with acute myeloid leukemia who relapsed 4 months after myeloablative conditioning and an unrelated donor peripheral blood stem cell (PBSC) transplant. He was re-conditioned with a non-myeloablative regimen and received a second infusion of unmanipulated PBSC from the original donor. To maximize a graft-versus-leukemia effect, no immunosuppressive treatment to prevent GVHD was given. He developed skin, liver, and gut GVHD at days 7–10 posttransplant. At the same time, he developed signs of low cardiac output, with orthostatic failure and hypotension. Echocardiography revealed global dysfunction with a left ventricular ejection fraction <30% (>60% before first transplant). On the same day, ventricular fibrillation developed and CPR was initiated. The ECG confirmed electromechanical dissociation and the attempted resuscitation failed. Autopsy examination of the heart revealed severe damage with cytolysis (Fig. 92.5) and massive infiltration by CD3$^+$ T cells, most of which were CD8$^+$. Chimerism analysis showed more than 70% of all nucleated cells in the myocardium to be of donor origin. Molecular testing for a wide range of viruses was negative. It is possible that anthracycline toxicity played a role in the pathogenesis, but the temporal association with GVHD in other organs and the autopsy findings at least raise the possibility of a role for a GVH reaction.

Steroid-induced hypertrophic cardiomyopathy

Hypertrophic cardiomyopathy is a well-known complication of corticosteroid treatment in premature infants, developing with steroid courses of 2–3 weeks duration or longer. It is less common, but has been reported, in full-term infants and children. It is characterized by concentric thickening of the interventricular septum and freewalls of the ventricles and reduction in the

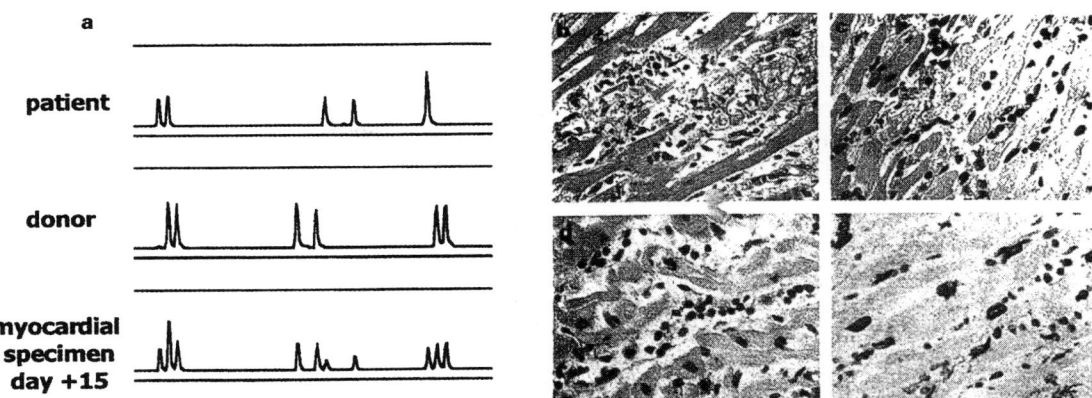

Fig. 92.5. (a) Donor chimerism in the myocardial biopsy on day +15 after second PBSCT revealed that more than 70% of all nucleated cells were of donor origin, (b) Myocardial cytolysis (hematoxylin & eosin, 360×). (c) Massive myocardial infiltration by CD3-positive T cells (hematoxylin & eosin, 360×). (d) Most of the infiltrating CD3-positive cells were CD8-positive cytotoxic T cells of donor origin (hematoxylin & eosin, 360×). (e) A minority of cells were CD68-positive macrophages (hematoxylin & eosin, 360×). Reproduced, with permission, from Platzbecker *et al.* (2001).

intra-cavitary dimensions. Prolonged steroid treatment in young infants and premature neonates induces increased protein synthesis in cardiac myocytes, leading to the hypertrophy. With the increasing availability of pre- and peri-natal diagnosis, and of cord blood as a source of stem cells, very young patients are more frequently undergoing stem cell transplantation. A case has been reported of severe left ventricular outflow tract obstruction complicating steroid therapy in an infant who had undergone allogeneic transplantation for Krabbe's disease at 10 days of age after a 38 week gestation (Lesnik *et al.*, 2001). Methylprednisolone treatment was initiated on the day of transplant (as GVHD prophylaxis with cyclosporine). On day 25 the child presented unwell and a new grade II/VI systolic ejection murmur at the left sternal edge, gallop rhythm, and cardiomegaly on chest x-ray were noted. Echocardiogram demonstrated left ventricular outflow tract obstruction with a peak pressure gradient of 145 mmHg (normal <5 mmHg) (Fig. 92.6). Response was rapid when prednisolone was discontinued, although treatment was initially required for congestive cardiac failure. GVHD subsequently developed and was treated by adding anti-interleukin-2 receptor monoclonal antibody treatment to the cyclosporine.

Tacrolimus-associated myocardial hypertrophy

The use of tacrolimus (but not of cyclosporine) as GVHD prophylaxis has been associated with a significant increase over baseline in left ventricular mass, although this was not associated with any significant clinical events (Espino *et al.*, 2001).

Management of cardiac complications

Serious cardiotoxicity can be prevented in most cases by ensuring that the dose of cyclophosphamide does not exceed 1.55 g/m^2/day (although many commonly used protocols do exceed this), and by avoidance of iatrogenic fluid overload. Serial

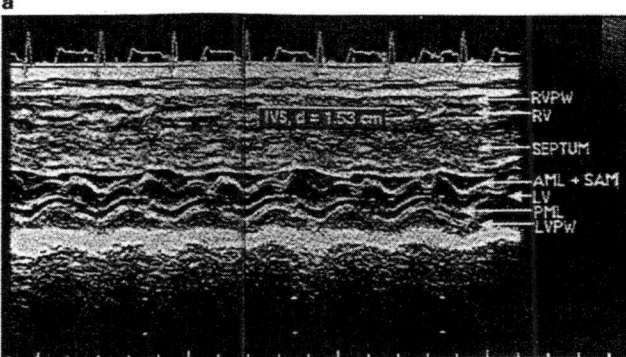

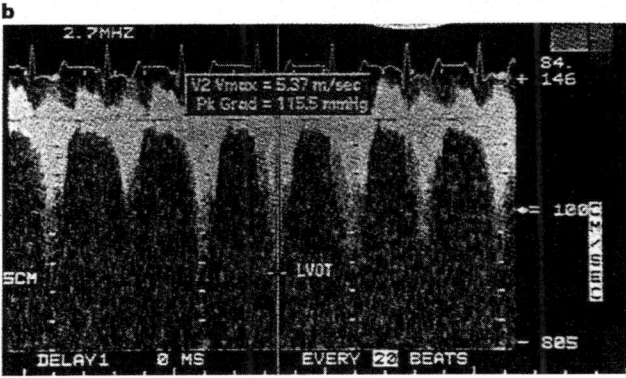

Fig. 92.6. (a) A posttransplant M-mode echocardiography 27 days after steroid therapy, showing gross thickening of the intraventricular septum (1.53 cm, normal for age <4 mm), reduction in the cavity dimensions of the left and right ventricles, and mild thickening of the left ventricle posterior wall. The anterior and posterior leaflets of the mitral valve are separated during systole due to systolic anterior motion of the anterior leaflet. (b) The dynamic pressure gradient across the left ventricular outflow tract is of severe degree and is depicted by the characteristic tapering spectral profile. AML and PMI, anterior and posterior mitral leaflets; SAM, systolic anterior motion of the anterior mitral leaflet; AW, anterior wall; IVS, intraventricular septum; LV, left ventricle; LVOT, left ventricular outflow tract; PW, posterior wall; RV, right ventricle. Reproduced, with permission, from Lesnik *et al.* (2001).

ECGs before and during the conditioning regimen, together with daily measurement of body weight, aid identification of those patients likely to develop serious cardiotoxicity. There are no data to support the routine pretransplant evaluation of all patients with exercise testing, echocardiography, or radionuclide assessment of ejection fraction (Hertenstein *et al.*, 1994; Jain, Floreani, & Anderson, 1996), but full pretransplant evaluation of patients with a prior history, symptoms or signs of cardiac disease, or a history of anthracycline exposure, remains prudent. Closer attention to cyclophosphamide dosage and fluid balance, and consideration of the prophylactic use of diuretics may be warranted in those with a depressed ejection fraction pretransplant.

Once documented radiologically, pulmonary venous congestion should be treated with diuretics in the first instance, with the addition of an angiotensin-converting enzyme (ACE) inhibitor if there is echocardiographic or radionuclide evidence of impaired left ventricular contraction and the patient is not hypotensive. Oral digoxin therapy may also be considered if heart failure persists. Fulminant cardiac failure may necessitate the addition of parenteral inotropic support (e.g., dobutamine), afterload-reducing (e.g., nitroprusside), and/or preload-reducing agents (e.g, nitroglycerin) and artificial ventilatory support. Sustained or recurrent cardiac arrhythmias should be treated with appropriate antiarrhythmic agents and correction of possible precipitating factors, including sepsis and electrolyte disturbances. There is one report of the use of the ACE inhibitor enalapril prophylactically in patients with left ventricular dysfunction pretransplant (Kakavas *et al.*, 1995). Six patients with left ventricular ejection fractions of less than 50% (42% ± 7%) were treated with enalapril 5 mg orally twice daily starting 48 hours prior to conditioning therapy. Left ventricular ejection fraction increased in all patients to 54% ± 6%. No patient experienced clinical deterioration during a follow-up period of 18 ± 11 months.

Infective endocarditis should be excluded in pyrexic patients by blood cultures from sources other than the Hickman catheter and by echocardiography, particularly in patients with a cardiac murmur or previously documented valvular or congenital heart disease. The latter patients should also receive prophylactic antibiotics during any procedure more invasive than a simple venipuncture (e.g., central venous cannulation, bone marrow examination, lumbar puncture, tissue biopsy, urethral catheterization, or dental work) (Table 92.2). For most such procedures, intravenous ampicillin 1 g (or intravenous vancomycin 1 g over 60 minutes if allergic to penicillin) and gentamicin 1.5 mg/kg, administered immediately before the procedure, provide adequate adult cover, with ampicillin 0.5 g being administered 6 hours later, especially for prolonged procedures (and see Chapter 73). Transesophageal echocardiography increases the diagnostic yield in suspected endocarditis.

Although most pericardial effusions occurring after HSC transplantation are not infective, diagnostic aspiration and culture (together with blood cultures) are indicated in pyrexic patients provided that the platelet count is at least 50 × 10⁹/l

Table 92.2. *Indications for prophylactic antibiotics in HSC transplant recipients with valvular or congenital heart disease*

Any procedure more invasive than a simple venipuncture, including:
Central venous cannulation
Bone marrow aspirate or trephine examination
Lumbar puncture
Any tissue biopsy (skin, lip, liver, kidney, gastrointestinal tract, lung)
Urethral catheterization
Upper and lower endoscopy, bronchoscopy, cystoscopy
Fine needle aspirate
Dental work
Any surgical procedure

and coagulation parameters are normal. Therapeutic aspiration is indicated if there is evidence of cardiac tamponade. Echocardiography is particularly valuable in the diagnosis and management of such patients.

References

Ahmed, N. & Payne, R. F. (1976). Thrombosis after central venous cannulation. *Medical Journal of Australia*, **1**, 217–20.

Alidina, A., Lawrence, D., Ford, L. A. *et al.* (1999). Thiotepa-associated cardiomyopathy during blood or marrow transplantation: association with the female sex and cardiac risk factors. *Biology of Blood and Marrow Transplantation*, **5**, 322–7.

Ando, M., Yokozawa, T., Sawada, J. *et al.* (2000). Cardiac conduction abnormalities in patients with breast cancer undergoing high-dose chemotherapy and stem cell transplantation. *Bone Marrow Transplantation*, **25**, 185–9.

Angelucci, E., Mariotti, E., Lucarelli, G. *et al.* (1992). Sudden cardiac tamponade after chemotherapy for marrow transplantation in thalassemia. *Lancet*, **339**, 287–90.

Angelucci, E., Mariotti, E., Lucarelli, G. *et al.* (1994). Cardiac tamponade in thalassemia. *Bone Marrow Transplantation*, **13**, 827–9.

Baello, E. B., Ensberg, M. E., Ferguson, D. W. *et al.* (1986). Effect of high-dose cyclophosphamide and total-body irradiation on left ventricular function in adult patients with leukemia undergoing allogeneic bone marrow transplantation. *Cancer Treatment Reports*, **70**, 1187–93.

Bearman, S. I., Petersen, F. B., Schor, R. A. *et al.* (1990). Radionuclide ejection fractions in the evaluation of patients being considered for bone marrow transplantation: risk for cardiac toxicity. *Bone Marrow Transplantation*, **5**, 173–7.

Brockstein, B. E., Smiley, C., Al-Sadir, J. *et al.* (2000). Cardiac and pulmonary toxicity in patients undergoing high-dose chemotherapy for lymphoma and breast cancer: prognostic factors. *Bone Marrow Transplanation*, **25**, 885–94.

Buja, L. M., Ferrans, B. J., Graw, R. G. Jr., & Blitt, C. D. (1976). Cardiac pathologic findings in patients treated with bone marrow transplantation. *Human Pathology*, **7**, 15–45.

Carlson, K., Smedmyr, B., Backlund, L., & Simonsson, B. (1994). Subclinical disturbances in cardiac function at rest and in gas exchange during exercise are common findings after autologous bone marrow transplantation. *Bone Marrow Transplantation*, **14**, 949–54.

Cavet, J., Lennard, A., Gascoigne, A. *et al.* (2000). Constrictive pericarditis post allogeneic bone marrow transplant for Philadelphia-positive acute lymphoblastic leukaemia. *Bone Marrow Transplantation*, **25**, 571–3.

Cazin, B., Gorin, N. C., Laporte, J. P. *et al.* (1986). Cardiac complications after bone marrow transplantation: a report on a series of 63 consecutive transplantations. *Cancer*, **57**, 2061–9.

Chandrasekar, P. H., Weinmann, A., & Shearer, C. (1995). Autopsy-identified infections among bone marrow transplant recipients: a clinico-pathologic study of 56 patients. *Bone Marrow Transplantation*, **16**, 675–81.

Chim, C. S., Ho, P. L., Yuen, S. T. *et al.* (1998). Fungal endocarditis in bone marrow transplantation: case report and review of literature. *Journal of Infection*, **37**, 287–91.

Clift, R. A., Buckner, C. D., Thomas, E. D. *et al.* (1994). Marrow transplantation for chronic myeloid leukemia: A randomized study comparing cyclophosphamide and total body irradiation with busulfan and cyclophosphamide. *Blood*, **84**, 2036.

Davis, J. M., Rowley, S. D., Braine, H. G. *et al.* (1990). Clinical toxicity of cryopreserved bone marrow graft infusion. *Blood*, **75**, 781–6.

Eames, G. M., Crosson, J., Steinberger, J. *et al.* (1997). Cardiovascular function in children following bone marrow transplant: a cross-sectional study. *Bone Marrow Transplantation*, **19**, 61–6.

Espino, G., Denney, J., Furlong, T., Fitzsimmons, W., & Nash, R. A. (2001). Assessment of myocardial hypertrophy by echocardiography in adult patients receiving tacrolimus or cyclosporine therapy for prevention of acute GVHD. *Bone Marrow Transplantation*, **28**, 1097–1103.

Galama, J. M. D., De Leeuw, N., Wittebol, S. *et al.* (1996). Prolonged enteroviral infection in a patient who developed pericarditis and heart failure after bone marrow transplantation. *Clinical Infectious Diseases*, **22**, 1004–8.

Gatzoulis, M. A., Vellodi, A, Redington, A. N. (1995). Cardiac involvement in mucopolysaccharidoses: effects of allogeneic bone marrow transplantation. *Archives of Diseases of Childhood*, **73**, 259–60.

Gilman, A. L., Kooy, N. W., Atkins, D. L. *et al.* (1988). Complete heart block in association with graft-versus-host disease. *Bone Marrow Transplantation*, **21**, 85–8.

Goldberg, M. A., Antin, J. H., Guinan, E. C., & Rappeport, J. M. (1986). Cyclophosphamide cardiotoxicity: an analysis of dosing as a risk factor. *Blood*, **68**, 1114–18.

Guerin, C., Billard, J. L., Jaubert, J., & Berthoux, F. (1989). Pericardial aspergillosis in a bone marrow transplant recipient. *Intensive Care Medicine*, **15**, 330.

Hertenstein, B., Stefanic, M., Schmeiser, T. *et al.* (1994). Cardiac toxicity of bone marrow transplantation: predictive value of cardiologic evaluation before transplant. *Journal of Clinical Oncology*, **12**, 998–1004.

Hoogerbrugge, P. M., Brouwer, O. F., Bordigoni, P. *et al.* (1995). Allogeneic bone marrow transplantation for lysosomal storage disease. The European Group for Bone Marrow Transplantation. *Lancet*, **345**, 1398–402.

Jain, B., Floreani, A. A., & Anderson, J. R. (1996). Cardiopulmonary function and autologous bone marrow transplantation: results and predictive value for respiratory failure and mortality. *Bone Marrow Transplantation*, **17**, 561–8.

Kakavas, P. W., Ghalie, R., Parrillo, J. E. *et al.* (1995). Angiotensin converting enzyme inhibitors in bone marrow transplant recipients with depressed left ventricular function. *Bone Marrow Transplantation*, **15**, 859–61.

Keung, Y. K., Lau, S., Elkayam, U. *et al.* (1994). Cardiac arrhythmia after infusion of cryopreserved stem cells. *Bone Marrow Transplantation*, **14**, 363–7.

Kupari, M., Volin, L., Suokas, A. *et al.* (1990a). Cardiac involvement in bone marrow transplantation: electrocardiographic changes, arrhythmias, heart failure and autopsy findings. *Bone Marrow Transplantation*, **5**, 91–8.

Kupari, M., Volin, L., Suokas, A. *et al.* (1990b). Cardiac involvement in bone marrow transplantation: serial changes in left ventricular size, mass and performance. *Journal of Internal Medicine*, **227**, 259–66.

Lehmann, S., Isberg, B., Ljungman, P., & Paul, C. (2000). Cardiac systolic function before and after hematopoietic stem cell transplantation. *Bone Marrow Transplantation*, **26**, 187–92.

Lele, S. S., Durrant, S. T. S., Atherton, J. J. *et al.* (1996). Demonstration of late cardiotoxicity following bone marrow transplantation by assessment of exercise diastolic filling characteristics. *Bone Marrow Transplantation*, **17**, 1113–18.

Le Moing, V., Lortholary, O., Timsit, J. F. *et al.* (1998). *Aspergillus* pericarditis with tamponade: report of a successfully treated case and review. *Clinical Infectious Diseases*, **26**, 451–60.

Lesnik, J. J., Singh, G. K., Balfour, I. C., & Wall, D. A. (2001). Steroid-induced hypertrophic cardiomyopathy following stem cell transplantation in a neonate: a case report. *Bone Marrow Transplantation*, **27**, 1105–8.

Lieschke, G. J., Maher, D., Cebon, J. *et al.* (1989). Effects of bacterially synthesized recombinant human granulocyte-macrophage colony-stimulating factor in patients with advanced malignancy. *Annals of Internal Medicine*, **110**, 357–64.

Lonnerholm, G., Arvidson, J., Andersson, L. G. *et al.* (1999). Myocardial function after autologous bone marrow transplantation in children: a prospective long-term study. *Acta Paediatrica*, **88**, 186–92.

Lopez-Jimenez, J., Cervero, C., Munoz, A. *et al.* (1994). Cardiovascular toxicities related to the infusion of cryopreserved grafts: results of a controlled study. *Bone Marrow Transplantation*, **13**, 789–93.

Martino, P., Micozzi, A., Venditti, M. *et al.* (1990). Catheter-related right-sided endocarditis in bone marrow transplant recipients. *Reviews of Infectious Diseases*, **12**, 250–7.

Miura, Y., Ueda, M., Kondou, Y. *et al.* (1997). Sudden cardiac tamponade due to hemorrhagic myocarditis after preconditioning marrow transplantation with cyclophosphamide in a patient with aplastic anemia. *Rinsho Ketsueki*, **38**, 526–31.

Murdych, T. & Weisdorf, D. J. (2001). Serious cardiac complications during bone marrow transplantation at the University of Minnesota, 1977–1997. *Bone Marrow Transplantation*, **28**, 283–7.

Niwa, N., Watanabe, E., Hamaguchi, M. *et al.* (2001). Early and late elevation of plasma atrial and brain natriuretic peptides in patients after bone marrow transplantation. *Annals of Hematology,* **80,** 460–5.

Perez Retortillo, J. A., Marco, F., Richard, C. *et al.* (1998). Pneumococcal pericarditis with cardiac tamponade in a patient with chronic graft-versus-host disease. *Bone Marrow Transplantation,* **21,** 299–300.

Pihkala, J., Saarinen, U. M., Lundstrom, M. *et al.* (1994). Efects of bone marrow transplantation on myocardial function in children. *Bone Marrow Transplantation,* **13,** 149–55.

Platzbecker, U., Klingel, K., Thiede, C. *et al.* (2001). Acute heart failure after allogeneic blood stem cell transplantation due to massive myocardial infiltration by cytotoxic T cells of donor origin. *Bone Marrow Transplantation,* **27,** 107–9.

Quinn, J. P., Counts, G. W., & Meyers, J. D. (1986). Intracardiac infections due to coagulase-negative *Staphylococcus* associated with Hickman catheters. *Cancer,* **57,** 1079–82.

Rapoport, A. P., Rowe, J. M., Packman, C. H. *et al.* (1991). Cardiac arrest after autologous marrow infusion. *Bone Marrow Transplantation,* **7,** 401–3.

Riley, L. C., Hann, I. M., Wheatley, K. *et al.* (1999). Treatment-related deaths during induction and first remission of acute myeloid leukaemia in children treated on the Tenth Medical Research Council acute myeloid leukaemia trail (MRCAML10). The MRC Childhood Leukaemia Working Party. *British Journal of Haematology,* **106,** 436–44.

Ringden, O., Remberger, M., Ruutu, T. *et al.* (1999). Increased risk of chronic graft-versus-host disease, obstructive bronchiolitis, and alopecia with busulfan versus total body irradiation: long-term results of a randomized trial in allogeneic marrow recipients with leukemia. Nordic Bone Marrow Transplantation Group. *Blood,* **93,** 2196.

Ritchie, D. S., Seymour, J. F., Roberts, A. W., Szer, J., & Grigg, A. P. (2001). Acute left ventricular failure following melphalan and fludarabine conditioning. *Bone Marrow Transplantation,* **28,** 101–3.

Rovelli, A., Pezzini, C., Silvestri, D. *et al.* (1995). Cardiac and respiratory function after bone marrow transplantation in children with leukaemia. *Bone Marrow Transplantation,* **16,** 571–6.

Santos, G. W., Sensenbrenner, L. L., Burke, P. J. *et al.* (1971). Marrow transplantation in man following cyclophosphamide. *Transplantation Proceedings,* **3,** 400–4.

Schechter, D., Drakos, P., & Nagler, A. (1994). Underlying coronary artery disease and successful bone marrow transplantation: a case report. *Bone Marrow Transplantation,* **13,** 665–6.

Seber, A., Khan, S. P., & Kersey, J. H. (1996). Unexplained effusions: association with allogeneic bone marrow transplantation and acute or chronic graft-versus-host disease. *Bone Marrow Transplantation,* **17,** 207–11.

Somlo, G., Doroshow, J. H., Forman, S. J. *et al.* (1994). High-dose doxorubicin, etoposide, and cyclophosphamide with stem cell reinfusion in patients with metastatic or high-risk primary breast cancer. City of Hope Bone Marrow Oncology Team. *Cancer,* **73,** 1678–85.

Stewart, J. R. & Fajardo, L. F. (1984). Radiation-induced heart disease: an update. *Progress in Cardiovascular Diseases,* **27,** 173–94.

Styler, M. J., Topolsky, D. L., Crilley, P. A. *et al.* (1992). Transient high grade heart block following autologous bone marrow infusion. *Bone Marrow Transplantation,* **10,** 435–8.

Uderzo, C., Biagi, E., Rovelli. A. *et al.* (2000). Bone marrow for childhood hematological disorders: a global pediatric approach in a twelve year single center experience. *La Pediatra medica e chirurgica.,* **21,** 157–63.

Vaksmann, G., Nelken, B., Deshukdre, A. *et al.* (2002). Pulmonary arterial occlusive disease following, chemotherapy and bone marrow for leukaemia. *European Journal of Pediatrics,* **161,** 247–9.

Villablanca, J. G., Steiner, M., Kersey, J. *et al.* (1990). The clinical spectrum of infections with viridans streptococci in bone marrow transplant patients. *Bone Marrow Transplantation,* **6,** 387–93.

von Herbay, A., Dsorken, B., Mall, G., & Korbling, M. (1988). Cardiac damage in autologous bone marrow transplant patients: an autopsy study. Cardiotoxic pretreatment as a major risk factor. *Klinische Wochenschrift,* **66,** 1175–81.

Wang, B., Cao, L. X., Liu, H. L. *et al.* (1996). Myocardial infarction following allogeneic bone marrow transplantation. *Bone Marrow Transplantation,* **18,** 479–86.

93 Neurologic complications

RAYMOND GARRICK

St. Vincent's Hospital and University of New South Wales, Sydney, Australia

Introduction

Neurologic complications can occur in more than 50% of all hematopoietic stem cell (HSC) transplant recipients, contributing to morbidity or mortality in 60% of allogeneic hematopoietic stem cell (HSC) transplant recipients and are the main cause of death in 10% to 15% (Wiznitzer *et al.,* 1984; Snider, Bashir, & Bierman, 1994; Patchell, 1994; Gallardo *et al.,* 1996; Graus *et al.,* 1996; Bleggi-Torres *et al.,* 2000; de Brabander *et al.,* 2000). With increasing experience, the recognition of early signs of neurologic toxicity from the conditioning treatment or immunosuppressive therapy allows prompt adjustment of treatment, with significant reduction in neurologic complication rates in experienced centers. The introduction of new immunosuppressive agents and the expansion of uses of allogeneic and autologous HSC transplantation have resulted in the introduction of new complications that require continuing vigilance.

Complications involving the nervous system (Table 93.1) arise from the following:

1. The underlying disease, which may itself involve the nervous system and which may predispose the patient to neurologic infection, central nervous system (CNS) hemorrhage, or degeneration.
2. The initial treatment for the underlying disease, which may amplify this risk.
3. The pretransplant preparative regimen as well as incidental medication for nausea, sedation, analgesia, or antibiotic therapy, which may induce iatrogenic complications.
4. Posttransplant immune suppression, which constitutes a major infection risk as well as a risk of toxicity.
5. Posttransplant immune deficiency as well as graft-versus-host disease (GVHD) and its therapy, and late failure of other organs, which continue the neurologic risk beyond the immediate posttransplant period.

Pre-existing involvement of the CNS by the underlying malignancy

The CNS may be involved by the underlying hematologic malignancy at the time of transplant or during the prior course of the disease, particularly in patients with acute lymphoblastic leukemia (ALL), high-grade non-Hodgkin's lymphoma, and lymphoid transformation of chronic myeloid leukemia (CML). All such patients should have their spinal fluid examined prior to initiation of the pretransplant conditioning regimen and, for

Table 93.1. *Neurologic complications of bone marrow transplantation*

Disorder	Usual cause
Metabolic encephalopathy	Systemic organ failure
	Drug toxicity
Cerebrovascular lesions	Hematoma
	Hemorrhage/necrosis
	Infarct
	Cerebral vein and venous sinus thrombosis
	Vasculitis
Infection	Focal or disseminated herpes zoster
	Acute bacterial, viral, or fungal meningitis
	Toxoplasmosis
	Progressive multifocal leukoencephalopathy
Leukoencephalopathy	Cyclosporine
	Prior treatment including cranial irradiation
	PMLE
CNS malignancy	Glioblastoma
	Posttransplant lymphoproliferative disorder
	Leukemic recurrence
	Metastasis
Peripheral nerve lesions	Herpes zoster
	Prior chemotherapy
	GVHD-related acute and subacute neuropathy
	Thalidomide
Myopathy and myasthenia	GVHD especially after transplant for aplastic anemia
Postural headache syndrome	Intracranial hypotension
Cognitive dysfunction	Late postirradiation and chemotherapy

Abbreviations: PMLE, progressive multifocal leukoencephalopathy; GVHD, graft-versus-host disease.

The common groups of neurologic complications are listed in order of frequency. Tremor, confusion, seizures, or focal deficits may occur as dominant symptoms in each group.

those found to have active CNS disease, an attempt should be made to clear the cerebrospinal fluid (CSF) of malignant cells prior to initiation of the conditioning regimen (see Chapter 20). Active CNS disease at the time of transplant or a history of prior CNS disease has been associated with an inferior outcome after transplantation in 373 patients with hematologic malignancies who underwent allogeneic or autologous BMT and who were prepared with high-dose thiotepa, busulfan, and cyclophosphamide. Four patients had active disease at the time of transplant, and 20 with a history of prior CNS disease were identified. Of the four patients with active CNS disease at the time of transplant, two had CNS recurrences posttransplant and one recurred in the marrow. At 2 years posttransplant the disease-free survival of the 20 patients with prior CNS involvement was 23% ± 19% compared to 39% ± 24% for a matched control group. An increased rate of treatment-related toxicity and especially grades 2 to 4 CNS toxicity accounted for the poorer outcome of patients who had a history of CNS disease. Relapse rates were not significantly different between the two groups.

For those with CNS disease at the time of transplant, clearance of the CSF of malignant cells with intrathecal chemotherapy pretransplant and a course of consolidation intrathecal chemotherapy posttransplant will often provide long-term CNS remission.

Neurologic complications of pretransplant conditioning and hematopoietic progenitor cell harvesting

In addition to toxicity from the chemotherapy regimen and metabolic encephalopathy that may occur during the conditioning regimen, patients may develop encephalopathy several weeks after administration of chemotherapeutic agents including carmustine, carboplatin, and etosposide (Burger et al., 1981; Tahsildar et al., 1996). Transient global amnesia and focal cerebral ischemia have occasionally been described following infusion of cryopreserved bone marrow or peripheral blood stem cells (Hoyt, Szer, & Grigg, 2000).

Occasional focal brachial plexus and lower cranial nerve injuries, Horner's syndrome, and cerebral ischemia episodes may occur with internal jugular vein cannulation (Sylvestre et al., 1991).

Hematopoietic stem cell collection from peripheral blood may activate pre-existing autoimmune disorders such as multiple sclerosis (Openshaw et al., 2000). This problem is diminished if mobilization of stem cells by hematopoietic growth factors is combined with immunosuppressive therapy.

Donor sciatic nerve compression following marrow harvest may occur as a result of retroperitoneal hematoma formation from the marrow harvest procedure (Irving, Cooper, & Durrant, 2000). This results in severe prolonged, but reversible, sciatic nerve pain and is effectively identified by MRI scan.

Bone marrow harvest by multiple iliac crest punctures may rarely produce sudden headache from intracranial hypotension due to inadvertent subarachnoid space puncture (Lieberman & Gulati, 1996).

Seizures

Partial and generalized seizures occur in more than 10% of HSC transplant recipients (Patchell, 1994; Patchell et al., 1985) and represent a major CNS dysfunction based on causes that are usually identifiable. Drugs, particularly cyclosporine, but also tacrolimus (FK-506) and OKT3 are the most common causes of seizures; metabolic disorders and hypoxic-ischemic injury, infarction, and infection, are less frequent causes.

The origin of the seizure may be suspected from the presence of corresponding neurologic deficits or focal epileptic manifestations, but cerebral infarction or hemorrhage, infection, and metabolic and drug effects can each provoke either focal or generalized seizures.

The principles of seizure management overlap HSC transplantation management; detailed evaluation of both systemic and CNS status allows removal or modification of the cause, and more effective antiepileptic drug (AED) management. In HSC transplant patients, specific guidelines relating to choice of AED apply. By careful evaluation, long-term AED therapy may possibly be avoided (Table 93.2).

Investigation and seizure assessment

Specific neurologic investigation is advised once metabolic and systemic organ function has been assessed and corrected where

Table 93.2. *Causes of seizures in HSC transplant patients*

Metabolic	Hypoglycemia
	Hyperglycemia
	Hypocalcemia
	Hypomagnesemia
	Hyponatremia
	Hypoxia
Drugs	Busulfan
	L-asparaginase
	High-dose cytosine arabinoside
	Methotrexate
	Cyclophosphamide?
	Irradiation
Immune suppressive agents	Cyclosporine
	Tacrolimus (FK-506)
	OKT3
	Rapamycin
	Corticosteroids
	Azathioprine?
Cerebral vascular event	Infarct
	Hemorrhage
Infection	Meningoencephalitis
	Focal infection (unusual)
Malignancy	Relapse of primary disease
	New CNS malignancy
Pre-existing epilepsy	

possible. The time posttransplant (with associated thrombocytopenia or leukopenia) may preclude some specific investigations. Cranial imaging with computed tomography (CT) or magnetic resonance imaging (MRI) scans is particularly advisable for focal or recurrent seizures and repeated scanning may be necessary to identify a structural cause.

Partial seizures do not always indicate a focal or structural lesion and metabolic disorders frequently produce focal seizure activity.

The electroencephalogram (EEG) is particularly useful for delineating background rhythms as an index of encephalopathy, as well as to identify epileptiform discharges. The EEG may provide information on the underlying epileptic pattern and assist in choice of AED therapy. Acute cerebral events including vascular, inflammatory, or leukoencephalopathic lesions frequently provoke identifiable specific focal EEG discharges—periodic lateralized epileptiform discharges (PLEDS), which are temporary indicators of acute cerebral injury and are relatively refractory to AED therapy.

CSF analysis is usually desirable but may not always be possible. Lumbar puncture should not be attempted unless the platelet count at the time of puncture is $50 \times 10^9/l$ or higher. It is important to recognize that normal CSF does not completely exclude infection. For example, fungal necrotizing encephalitis may have a minimal meningeal reaction (Hotson & Pedley, 1976), and metabolic encephalopathies may be accompanied by markedly disordered CSF protein and glucose and may have an associated pleocytosis.

Seizures associated with conditioning and immune suppressive agents

High-dose busulfan (4 mg/kg/day × 4 days) was reported by Marcus and Goldman (1984) to result in seizures within 2 to 4 days of initiation in the absence of metabolic disturbance. Prophylactic anticonvulsant therapy was recommended; however, seizures did not persist and some other investigators have not experienced seizures using similar doses (Hugh-Jones & Shaw, 1985). A common protocol of short-term phenytoin for several days to cover busulfan conditioning is commonly employed (Murphy, Harden, & Thompson, 1992); alternatively, temporary prophylactic cover with clonazepam 1 mg to 2 mg three times daily or lorazepam 2.5 mg three times daily is advised. We have not experienced neurologic complications with busulfan using this approach; however, somnolence is common and the dosage may need to be reduced in some patients.

Seizures may occur especially in young patients with combined high-dose methylprednisolone and cyclosporine therapy, related to metabolic shifts, hypertension, and fluid retention, as well as to direct cyclosporine-related toxicity with cerebral edema.

Cyclosporine is a highly lipophilic cyclic endecapeptide of fungal origin that suppresses T-lymphocyte function without suppression of B-cell, macrophage, granulocyte, or natural killer cell functions and without myelosuppression. Cyclosporine neurotoxicity occurs with concurrent high-dose steroid therapy or lactam antibiotic therapy and is usually, but not universally, dose-related. Seizure activity may occur with therapeutic levels (whole blood trough concentration 200–1,200 ng/ml) usually in the presence of uremia or other metabolic disturbance (de Groen et al., 1987; Kahan, 1989). Seizures occur in approximately 25% of patients with cyclosporine-induced leukoencephalopathy syndromes. These patients show diffuse slowing and focal abnormalities that are not always epileptiform on EEG. Experimental studies have identified epileptiform EEG activity in 23% to 42% of cyclosporine-treated animals, with generalized seizures seen as preterminal events at high doses (Famigilo et al., 1987). Cyclosporine-related seizures in HSC transplant recipients have been related to a number of factors including:

1. "Capillary leak" related to hypertension and fluid retention (Sloane et al., 1985; Hinchey et.al., 1996; Small et al., 1996).
2. Specific direct nerve toxicity mediated by calcineurin inhibition resulting in depressed neurotransmitter release, synaptic vesicle processing, and susceptibility to glutamate neurotoxicity. Demyelination may be also be related to calcineurin inhibition (Famiglio et al., 1987; Sharkey & Butcher, 1994; Small et al., 1996).
3. Hypomagnesemia with seizure control not necessarily achieved with supplementation (Thompson et al., 1984; June et al., 1985).
4. Hypocholesterolemia (de Groen et al., 1987) and hypertriglyceridemia (Valbonesi et al., 1988) which have been identified as correlates of neurotoxicity in some patients, presumably via alterations in cyclosporine concentration in lipoproteins. Cyclosporine binds to low-density lipoprotein (LDL) and cyclosporine toxicity is more likely to occur with low magnesium and low cholesterol levels, since LDL and lipid tissues bind more cyclosporine without cholesterol competing for binding. Plasma exchange has been used successfully to block CNS disease progression in hypertriglyceridemia-related cyclosporine toxicity (Valbonesi et al., 1988).

Total body irradiation (TBI) or high-dose steroid therapy alone may occasionally be associated with seizures. Azathioprine is not generally associated with neurotoxicity, but generalized seizures have occasionally been reported in association with possible azathioprine-induced raised intracranial pressure.

Acute seizure management in HSC transplant patients

Acute management requires support of the cardiac and respiratory state so that generalized seizures lasting more than 1 to 2 minutes (recurring seizures) are best treated with intravenous benzodiazepine (diazepam 5–10 mg, lorazepam 2–5 mg, or clonazepam 1–2 mg are suitable). Benzodiazepines are not likely to suppress marrow engraftment and are least likely to induce hepatic microsomal enzymes responsible for metabolism of glucocorticosteroids and cyclosporine.

Once life support and convulsion control is achieved, assessment and removal of the underlying cause is important. Seizures are associated with terminal metabolic derangement in patients with infection, organ failure, and some drug toxic states; the majority of these do not have structural pathology identified at autopsy, but seizures associated with L-asparaginase treatment for ALL have been associated with cerebral venous thrombosis with hemorrhage.

Prophylactic/maintenance therapy

Once the etiology of the seizure has been established, and the provocative cause eliminated, maintenance therapy may be advised for recurrent seizures. Standard guidelines modified by HSC transplant considerations often make the choice of AED difficult.

Metabolism of phenytoin, carbamazepine, and phenobarbitone is solely via cytochrome P450 oxygenase in the liver microsomal oxidase enzyme system, which also biodegrades cyclosporine; therefore concurrent usage will reduce trough cyclosporine levels by enzyme induction, with phenobarbitone being a more potent inducer than phenytoin, which, in turn, is more potent than carbamazepine. Valproic acid does not induce hepatic enzyme systems but it, with phenytoin and carbamazepine, may suppress bone marrow activity during engraftment. There is sufficient evidence to recommend caution with these latter three agents during this period. Thus, during the first 4 to 6 weeks posttransplant, clonazepam or lorazepam are most suitable, but have relatively limited anticonvulsant effect and may slightly increase liver enzyme activity. Phenobarbitone does not influence engraftment but has moderate efficacy, and it is necessary to increase cyclosporine doses with careful monitoring to maintain immune suppression; steroid doses should be increased by up to 30%.

The introduction of new anticonvulsant agents has been encouraging; lamotrigine and gabapentin have negligible hepatic enzyme-inducing activity and few serious systemic or neurologic side effects. Lamotrigine may increase blood levels of other medications, but gabapentin has the greatest potential for use in HSC transplant recipients. It has little interaction with any other commonly used drug and in some centers gabapentin has become the agent of choice for chronic seizure management. Its efficacy as monotherapy is comparable with other first-line agents for control of simple partial, complex partial, and secondary generalized seizures for at least short-term therapy over months. Common side effects include variable drowsiness, weight gain, and mood irritability, which are mainly transient. Only oral preparations are available at present but intravenous preparations are currently being evaluated. Seizure control generally requires a dosage between 1,200 and 2,400 mg daily; there is good absorption and tolerance up to a maximum dose of 4,800 mg daily, after which gastrointestinal absorption is reduced. Gabapentin may be underabsorbed in patients with concurrent gastrointestinal disease, particularly GVHD. Dosage reduction is required in patients with renal impairment.

Cerebrovascular events

Cerebrovascular complications are common in HSC transplant recipients with subdural hematomas, infarcts, hemorrhagic necrosis associated with nonbacterial endocarditis, and subarachnoid hemorrhage identified in up to 27% of patients in autopsy series (Mohrmann, Mah, & Vinters, 1990). The extension of HSC transplantation to the treatment of multiple myeloma, lymphoma, and solid tumors may be associated with an increase in cerebrovascular complications, particularly hemorrhagic in myeloma, and thrombotic events following transplantation for lymphoma and breast cancer (Wall et al., 1989; Gordon et al., 1991; Ansari, Schmidley, & Marak, 1997). Hypercoagulable states associated with deficiencies in circulating anticoagulant protein C occur after chemotherapy for malignant diseases, and also posttransplant, resulting in thrombotic and veno-occlusive complications. L-asparaginase therapy for ALL is a well-recognized cause of venous thrombosis and cerebral hemorrhage in pediatric patients (Priest et al., 1982; Feinberg & Swenson, 1988) (Fig. 93.1). Adult patients receiving L-asparaginase prior to HSC transplant are also at risk of this complication. However, in one report none of 3 patients with ALL who developed cerebral venous thrombosis after allogeneic transplantation had received asparaginase in the peritransplant period (Harvey et al., 2000). (Magnetic resonance imaging with angiography was necessary to make the diagnosis in each of the three). Wiznitzer et al. (1984) noted an increased frequency of cerebrovascular events in patients with acute leukemia excluding events related to prior asparaginase therapy. In two of the five patients, prior chemotherapy or radiation-induced vascular injury was likely. Patchell and co-workers (1985) noted that only 6% of patients dying posttransplant had cerebrovascular pathology: two of five patients had cerebral infarcts associated with nonbacterial endocarditis, and one had bacterial endocarditis; two patients had cerebellar hemorrhages associated with normal coagulation parameters but extremely low platelet counts (1×10^9/l) in one patient. Similar rates of cerebrovascular complications have been confirmed by Mohrmann et al. (1990) and Hinchey et al. (1996). The induction of capillary endothelial damage by cyclophosphamide in pretransplant conditioning may be a contributing factor.

Nonbacterial thrombotic endocarditis is four times more common in HSC transplant recipients than in the general autopsy population. It is related to fibrin and platelet deposition on cardiac valves due to disseminated intravascular coagulation and other hypercoagulable states including deficiency in protein C (Diez-Martin et al., 1988; Gordon et al., 1991) (Fig. 93.2).

Parenchymal hemorrhages are rare despite prolonged low platelet counts seen in all HSC transplant patients (Davis &

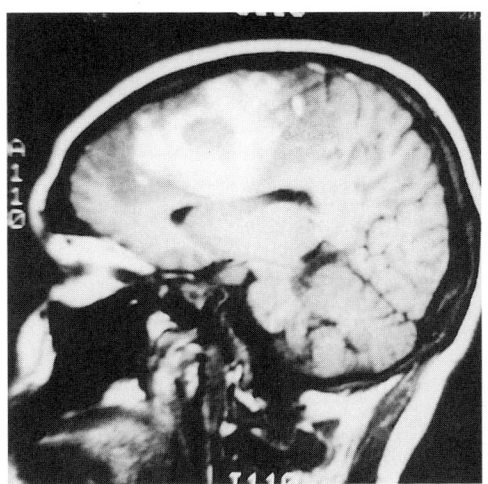
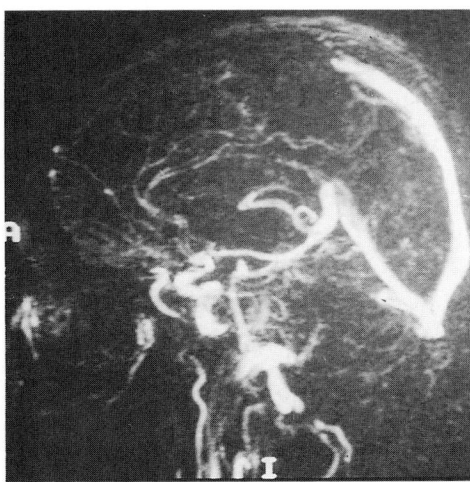

Fig. 93.1. Superior sagittal sinus thrombosis occurring in a 17-year-old male 6 weeks after L-asparaginase treatment for ALL and 1 week after BMT. The CT scan shows a typical area of hemorrhagic ischemic change in the cerebral cortex. Magnetic resonance angiography shows complete obstruction of the anterior portion of the superior sagittal sinus. The patient developed acute left hemiparesis with focal seizures, but made a good clinical recovery after treatment with intravenous heparin.

Patchell, 1988). Intraparenchymal brain hemorrhage is less frequent than subdural hematoma and is almost always observed in patients with myeloid leukemia and allogeneic HSC transplantation (Pomeranz *et al.*, 1994; Graus *et al.*, 1996). Leukapheresis to harvest hematopoietic cells for autologous transplantation may produce acute neurologic compromise (particularly with hypotension at the end of the collection phase), due to subdural or intracerebral hemorrhage (Smith *et al.*, 1990) and bilateral subdural hematomas have been described following lumbar puncture before HSC transplantation (Hentscke *et al.*, 1999). In a retrospective review of 657 consecutive patients, the incidence of subdural hematoma/ hygroma was 2.6% (Colosimo *et al.*, 2000). This was particularly noted following lumbar puncture with the development of post-lumbar puncture headache. Conservative management with platelet support and correction of coagulopathy achieved

resolution in all but four cases. Surgical intervention should be reserved for neurological deterioration.

Cerebrovascular complications in 350 consecutive patients receiving a marrow transplant at St. Vincent's Hospital, Sydney, occurred in 4.3% of patients (Table 93.3). In the majority, the cerebrovascular complication was associated with

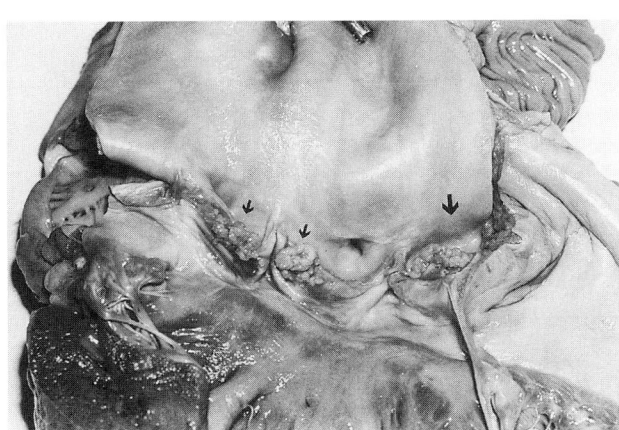

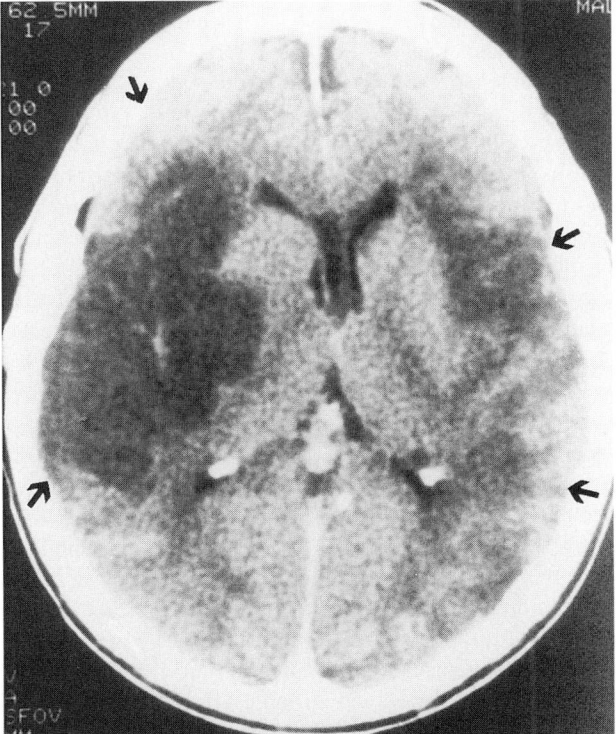

Fig. 93.2. Nonbacterial thrombotic endocarditis in a male with ALL awaiting BMT who developed a series of acute stroke episodes as terminal events. **(A)** Vegetations involving the aortic valve (arrowed); **(B)** unenhanced CT brain scan illustrating typical multiple embolic appearance (arrowed).

Table 93.3. *Cerebrovascular complications of bone marrow transplantation: experience in 350 consecutive patients at St. Vincent's Hospital, Sydney*

Patient	Sex/age	Primary disease	Cerebral lesion	Presumed cause	Outcome
1	M/25	Aplastic anemia	Focal infarct	Sepsis	Died day 24
2	M/41	ALL	Focal infarct	Cyclosporine-induced hypertension	Died day 40
3	F/36	ALL	Infarct	Systemic embolism	Died day 17
4	F/42	CML blast crisis	Capsular infarct	Uncertain sepsis?	Recovery
5	F/17	ALL with CNS involvement	Hematoma	Metabolic failure	Died day 5
6	M/45	CML accelerated phase	Multiple hematomas	Thrombocytopenia	Died day 40
7	F/27	Aplastic anemia	Capsular hematoma	Cyclosporine-induced hypertension	Recovery
8	M/37	AML with CNS involvement	Hematoma	Hypertension; sepsis?	Recovery (surgical evacuation)
9	F/37	AML	Massive hematoma + SDH	Prolonged thrombocytopenia	Died day 56
10	M/47	AML	Late SDH	Uncertain	Recovery (surgical evacuation)
11	F/38	AML (second BMT)	Late SDH	Sepsis	Died day 15
12	F/30	AML with CNS involvement	SDH	Sepsis, thrombocytopenia	Died day 49
13	F/36	CLL	Small SDH	Sepsis	Died day 28
14	M/44	AML	Bilateral late SDH	Sepsis	Recovery
15	F/35	CML blast crisis	SDH	Sepsis and leukemic relapse	Died day 152

Abbreviations: ALL, acute lymphoblastic leukemia; AML, acute myeloid leukemia; CLL, chronic lymphatic leukemia; CML, chronic myeloid leukemia; SDH, subdural hematoma; CNS, central nervous system.

terminal multiple system failure, overwhelming sepsis, or sudden severe hypertension with thrombocytopenia. Nevertheless, with cautious management of infection and surgical evacuation of circumscribed hematomas, recovery with little or no neurologic deficit may be achieved. Evacuation, however, will require a platelet count of at least $50 \times 10^9/l$ at the time of the procedure to allow hemostasis to be secured.

Stroke may occur following herpes zoster or, rarely, generalized varicella infection. This usually occurs within four to eight weeks of the cutaneous infection and is characterized by abrupt onset of focal deficit, lethargy, headache, or seizures. The pathogenesis is varicella virus-mediated necrotizing vasculopathy of large and medium sized arteries. Angiography may show segmental narrowing. Most involve the anterior circulation in relation to herpes zoster ophthalmicus (Bourdette, Rosenberg, & Yatsu, 1983; Hilt *et al.*, 1983; Karlin, 1993).

Patients given allogeneic transplants for sickle cell disease present a unique patient from the neurologic standpoint. In a report of 21 patients treated by HLA-matched sibling marrow transplantation for sickle cell anemia, 7 developed neurologic complications at a median of 1 month posttransplant (Walters *et al.*, 1995). Seizures were the most common complication occurring in six patients, but three patients suffered an intracranial hemorrhage posttransplant. Of eight patients with a history of stroke prior to transplant, four developed a neurologic complication posttransplant. At the present time a stroke or nervous system event is considered an indication for transplant while severe residual functional neurologic impairment (other than hemiplegia alone) is considered an exclusion criterion for transplantation (Walters *et al.*, 1996) (and see Chapter 61).

Infections

Life-threatening infections in the CNS occur in 7% to 14% of HSC transplant recipients with up to 77% of infected immune compromised patients dying (Wiznitzer *et al.*, 1984; Patchell *et al.*, 1985; Mohrmann, Mah, & Vinters, 1990; Patchell, 1994; Snider *et al.*, 1994). Septic embolism from *Aspergillus* species has been reported to be the most common infectious complication in the leukopenic posttransplant period accounting for 15% of neurologic complications in an autopsy series of 180 patients (Bleggi-Torres *et al.*, 2000). Mortality results from delays in diagnosis caused by suppression of typical symptoms and by the large variety of pathogens.

Guidelines for management are based on:

1. The degree of immune compromise with metabolic derangement amplifying the effects of immune suppressant drugs
2. The time frame of different infections from the time of transplant
3. The clinical presentation and rate of progression
4. Results of serial physical and imaging examinations, EEG, biochemical estimations, CSF examination, blood and cannula cultures with polymerase chain reaction (PCR) amplification of specific organism DNA, and stereotactic biopsy.

The pathogenic agents include varicella zoster virus, papova viruses, adenoviruses, atypical bacteria particularly *Listeria monocytogenes*, *Nocardia asteroides,* and mycobacteria, although tuberculous meningitis is distinctly uncommon. Specific fungal species include *Aspergillus* species, mucoraceae, *Candida* species, and *Crytococcus neoformans.* Infection due to rarer fungal species such as *Cladophialophora bantiana* (Emmens *et al.,* 1996), *Histoplasma,* and *Coccidiodes* are restricted to certain geographic locations. Protozoan infections with *Toxoplasma gondii* and *Strongyloides stercoralis* may occur after HSC transplantation.

Help in determining the predominant organism causing CNS infection may be provided by the following:

1. Infection outside the nervous system should raise suspicion of a possible neurologic infection
2. Skin lesions may harbor the pathogenic organism, particularly *Cryptococcus* and persisting lung lesions suggest *Aspergillus, Nocardia,* or *Cryptococcus*
3. Acute meningitis is frequently caused by *Listeria monocytogenes;* the CSF gives abnormal results but not necessarily a positive culture
4. A progressive multifocal syndrome with ataxia, dysarthia, dementia, and focal neurologic deficits raises the suspicion of progressive multifocal leukoencephalopathy caused by the JC polyoma virus
5. A localized mass lesion on brain imaging may contain multiple organisms with predominant organisms being *Aspergillus, Nocardia,* or *Toxoplasma*
6. There may be a geographic or hospital-based predilection to certain infections
7. Acute meningitis within 30 days of transplant is usually bacterial; beyond 30 days *Listeria* or fungus is more likely

A specific time frame for presentation of infection in HSC transplant patients is based on two periods of immune suppression (Winston, Gale, & Meyer, 1979). The first month posttransplant is characterized by absolute or relative granulocytopenia and the most common CNS infections are bacterial. Bacterial infections of the CNS occur in between 1.3% and 5.3% (Wiznitzer *et al.,* 1984; Patchell *et al.,* 1985; Mohrmann, Mah, & Vinters, 1990; Sable & Donowitz, 1994); bacteria gain entry from intravenous lines, paranasal sinuses, or an ulcerated lower gastrointestinal tract. Bacterial meningitis in this early phase may be from *Pseudomonas* or *Haemophilus influenzae,* staphylococci, streptococci, or coliforms, sometimes originating from infected intravenous cannulae or catheters. Bacterial abscess formation is uncommon. During the period of granulocytopenia signs of meningeal irritation are infrequent and headache is only present in approximately half the patients. Additionally, organisms present in the recipient pretransplant can cause disease during this time, including herpes simplex virus, cytomegalovirus, varicella zoster virus, and *Mycobacterium tuberculosis.*

The second window of susceptibility occurs from 1 month to approximately 1 year after transplantation, when passive immunity produced by the transplanted stem cells begins to decrease, and immunity mediated by cells derived from the transplant is not yet optimal. In this period the risk of CNS infection is highest, with viral, fungal, and parasitic infections occurring. Cytomegalovirus and varicella zoster infections are the most common. Opportunistic bacteria include *Listeria monocytogenes* and *Nocardia asteroides. Aspergillus fumigatus* has been isolated in approximately 50% of fungal intracranial infections and is almost always due to hematogenous spread from the lung. This agent demonstrates vascular wall invasion with lumen thrombosis resulting in focal infarction, often hemorrhagic. Depending upon localization of lesions, the CSF may be normal or unremarkable. MRI generally discloses multiple lesions with little contrast enhancement, preferentially involving the basal ganglia, cerebral hemispheres, and corpus callosum. Microbiological diagnosis may be difficult and treatment should be commenced on the basis of clinical and MRI findings. The prognosis, even with rapid treatment, is poor (DeLone *et al.,* 1999; Jantunen *et al.,* 2000a, 2000b; Patterson *et al.,* 2000). Candidiasis and *Torulopsis glabrata* are closely related infections arising from infected central venous catheters or rarely from bowel or genitourinary colonization.

Cryptococcus neoformans is commonly seen in other organ transplant recipients, but has seldom been reported in HSC transplant recipients (Davis & Patchell, 1988). No cases have been identified in our institution.

Bacterial and fungal infections require antibiotic therapy according to conventional guidelines based on sensitivity testing (Chapters 73 and 75). Aggressive antifungal therapy is warranted, but significant neurological toxicity may occasionally occur. Progressive akinetic mutism has been identified in association with amphotericin therapy (Devinsky *et al.,* 1987). Neurotoxicity of fluconazole is uncommon with headache occurring in 1.9% of 4,000 subjects treated. Data regarding the interaction of fluconazole and cyclosporine are inconclusive: a doubling of whole blood cyclosporine level has been described in renal transplant recipients with or without renal impairment, but a prospective trial in HSC transplant recipients receiving 2 weeks of fluconazole treatment showed no change in cyclosporine blood concentration (Kruger *et al.,* 1988; Sugar *et al.,* 1989). Fluconazole consistently results in elevations of plasma phenytoin levels.

Itraconazole, likewise, appears not to cause major changes to cyclosporine concentrations in HSC transplant patients. Itraconazole and amphotericin may be combined, especially for *Aspergillus* infections.

CNS infection with *Toxoplasma gondii* is occasionally identified in HSC transplant recipients (Fig. 93.3) (Chapter 76). Subclinical infection is common in the general population and the encysted bradyzoitic form may be dormant for many years. Overt infection ranges from 1.4% in centers with intermediate or high seroprevalence (greater than 60%) to 0% in centers with low seroprevalence (less than 30%) (Chandrasekar *et al.,* 1997; Martino *et al.,* 2000). Either diffuse meningoencephalitis or focal masses may occur. Solitary spinal intramedullary lesions may occur with CSF PCR differentiating the lesion from neoplastic infiltration (Straathof *et al.,* 2001). Clinical signs may be suppressed by immune suppression and accurate diagnosis may require repeated culture of centrifuged CSF or

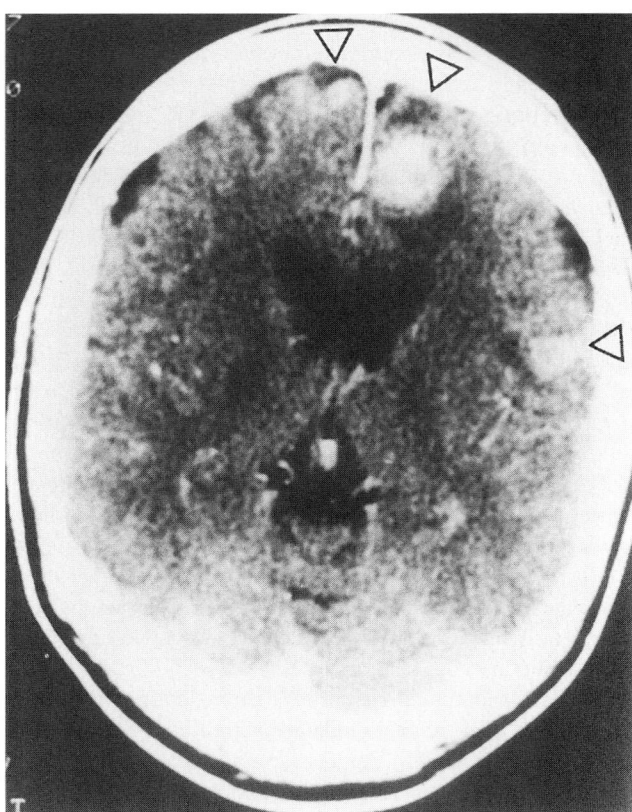

Fig. 93.3. Enhanced CT brain scan demonstrating localized frontal enhancing lesions (arrowed) with typical appearance of toxoplasmosis.

stereotactic biopsy. Polymerase chain reaction (PCR) may identify *T. gondii* DNA in the CSF. This technique combined with magnetic resonance imaging should provide accurate early diagnosis (Roemer *et al.*, 2001). Typically the magnetic scan shows focal contrast-enhancing toxoplasma lesions; however, in leukopenic patients usually in the first month post HSC transplantation or where high corticosteroid intake is present, the MR lesions may not enhance with contrast (Maschke *et al.*, 1999).

The clinical features of viral encephalitis are not specific although meningoencephalitis may be discriminated from limbic encephalitis. CSF inflammatory reactions may be blunted by immunosuppression. MRI may be normal or may show focal, usually multiple, nonenhancing lesions on T2-weighted images. MR spectroscopy may be specifically useful in discriminating viral leukoencephalopathy from leukemic cell infiltration.

A number of viruses can affect the CNS during and after HSC transplantation:

1. Adenovirus meningoencephalitis may arise from transfused blood products. This has mainly been identified on post-mortem studies. No effective therapy is available for this progressive terminal encephalitis.

2. Cytomegalovirus (CMV). Although systemic CMV infection is sufficiently common in allogeneic HSC transplant patients to warrant prophylactic or pre-emptive treatment with ganciclovir, CNS disease has been uncommon. However, Patchell and co-workers (1985) noted CMV encephalitis in 2 of 78 patients dying after BMT, and a further seven patients, all with systemic CMV infection, had viral glial inclusions: three of these patients had nonfocal encephalopathies not explained by metabolic disturbance. It must be noted that CNS complications of ganciclovir, although unusual (5% of reported adverse events), include headache, confusion, coma, paresthesia, tremor, and dysphasia. Concurrent treatment with cyclosporine may result in compounded toxicity.

3. Herpes simplex encephalitis has been identified in two major clinical reviews of CNS complications of HSC transplantation, but appears uncommonly and generally in the setting of diffuse systemic viral infection (Wiznitzer *et al.*, 1984; Patchell *et al.*, 1985).

4. Fatal herpesvirus 6 encephalitis has been reported in a BMT recipient, in whom the diagnosis was confirmed at autopsy by DNA amplification techniques (Drobyski *et al.*, 1994). Successful treatment with ganciclovir has been recorded (Mookerjee *et al.*, 1997). Herpesvirus 6 encephalitis with a subtle presentation of short-term memory loss, insomnia, and temporal lobe seizure activity has been identified in 5 patients with autopsy or CSF identification of herpesvirus 6 DNA on PCR (Wainwright *et al.*, 2001). More diffuse widespread meningoencephalitis due to herpesvirus 6 reactivation may be related to allogeneic mismatched stem cell transplantation, with incomplete response on CSF viral DNA assessment following treatment with acyclovir or ganciclovir (Rieux *et al.*, 1998; Kawano *et al.*, 2000; Tiacci *et al.*, 2000).

5. In contrast, varicella zoster virus infection (VZV) occurs in up to 50% of allogeneic HSC transplant (HSCT) recipients who survive beyond 6 months (Atkinson *et al.*, 1980). In addition, VZV infection occurred in 28% of patients undergoing autologous BMT, with a median onset of infection in the fifth month and 9% occurring after the first year (Schuchter *et al.*, 1989; Koc *et al.*, 2000). Twenty-nine percent of allogeneic, and 5% of autologous, BMT recipients developed diffuse VZV dissemination, with an 8% mortality in the allogeneic group but no mortality in the autologous group. (Many of the infections in the allogeneic patient series described occurred, however, before the availability of acyclovir.) Clinical management is based on administration of high-dose intravenous acyclovir therapy (10–15 mg/kg five times daily or 800 mg orally five times daily for 7 to 10 days). Stroke due to necrotizing vasculitis occasionally occurs within eight weeks of cranial nerve or upper cervical VZV (see above).

6. CNS effects of the Epstein-Barr virus (EBV), another herpesvirus, are usually indirect: B-cell proliferative malignancies with a CNS propensity appear to transform from benign

EBV-dependent polyclonal B-cell hyperplasia: this almost always appears after allogeneic HSC transplantation and the intensity of T-cell depletion and posttransplant immune suppression are the major risk factors (see Chapter 88). Presumed EBV meningoencephalitis, successfully treated with ganciclovir, has been described after allogeneic transplantation (Dellemijn et al., 1995) as has EBV-induced transverse myelitis (Gruhn et al., 1999).

7. The JC papova virus is present in normal individuals and manifests in immunocompromised patients as progressive multifocal leukoencephalopathy (PMLE). PMLE presents as a subacute or chronic evolution of focal and long tract deficits with a decline in cognitive function. MRI provides helpful diagnostic support with increased signal in patchy distribution in white matter just below the cerebral grey matter convolutions or in the brain stem. Definitive diagnosis is made by stereotactic biopsy with confirmation by in situ hybridization for JC papova virus. The clinical course is usually progression to death within 1 month, but the disease sometimes follows a relapsing and remitting form with longer survival. JC virus-related PMLE associated with demyelinating peripheral neuropathy has been reported (Coppo et al., 1999). Apart from reducing immune suppression there is no effective treatment (Richardson, 1988), although recent case reports have shown responses to low-dose cytosine arabinoside and interleukin-2 (5×10^5 units per m^2 per day intravenously) (Jaecle et al., 1997; Re et al., 1999).

8. Ljungman et al. (1994) described a patient transplanted for adult T-cell leukemia who died of acute encephalitis posttransplant. HTLV-1 was detected in brain tissue and in donor-derived lymphocytes. A patient given an HLA-matched unrelated donor transplant for aplastic anemia, who acquired HTLV-1 infection from a pretransplant blood transfusion, developed HTLV-associated myelopathy with motor weakness and a neurogenic bladder 3 years posttransplant. HTLV-1 sequences were amplified from the cerebrospinal fluid (Emmanouilides & Territo, 1999).

9. Acute disseminated encephalomyelitis (ADEM) is a demyelinating disorder of the CNS with an acute clinical onset and a wide variability and severity. It is considered to be immunologically mediated and usually follows viral infection or immunization. Re & Giachetti (1999) described a patient with ADEM occurring several days after a possibly viral febrile episode in the early stage post autologous blood stem cell transplantation for non-Hodgkin's lymphoma. No definite alternative cause for encephalopathy or specific viral agent has been identified.

Encephalopathies

Metabolic disturbances including hyperammonemia

Metabolic encephalopathy is commonly seen in HSC transplantation, occurring in 8% to 37% of patients (Wiznitzer et al., 1984; Patchell et al., 1985; Furlong & Galluci, 1994; Patchell,

Table 93.4. *Causes of metabolic encephalopathy in HSC transplant patients*

Listed in decreasing frequency
1. Hypoxia
2. Hepatic failure
3. Electrolyte imbalance
4. Hypoglycemia/hyperglycemia
5. Renal failure
6. Calcium/magnesium/phosphate depletion
7. Hyperammonemia

1994). While potentially reversible causes are usually present, the majority of cases have multiple interacting pathologies and clinical encephalopathy may occur at a terminal stage. Clinical features include delirium, stupor or coma, partial or generalized seizures, tremor, and ataxia. Causes are listed in Tables 93.4 and 93.5. Clinical evaluation requires knowledge of recent medication intake, since delirium is commonly related to drug therapy. Encephalopathy most commonly occurs during the period of aplasia or leukopenia following transplantation, with confusion, delirium, and seizures. In this situation, the neurological examination may be insufficiently sensitive to identify focal or structural brain disturbance and the majority of patients require further evaluation. EEG may be useful to identify nonconvulsive status epilepticus (Dixit et al., 2000). Vitamin deficiency or electrolyte imbalance may be present (Bleggi-Torres et al., 1997; Gordon et al., 2000). Imaging, preferably with MRI, provides a management approach where an absence of focal signs on examination and a normal magnetic scan points to systemic metabolic abnormality or drug toxicity (Table 93.6). The contribution of antibiotic therapy to encephalopathy and seizures should be considered in each case (Dixit et al., 2000). Hypoactive delirium may be subtle with dyscalculia, memory impairment, and psychomotor slowing as the main encephalopathic features. Hyperactive delirium produces insomnia, vigilance, rapid speech with disorientation, hallucinations, and delusions. Asterixis is common. Ten percent of HSC transplant patients with delirium experience seizures. The combination of metabolic disturbance with administration of medications, usually opioids and especially meperidine (pethidine), corticosteroids, H$_2$ antagonists, and benzodiazepines and the combination of tramadol with selective serotonin reuptake inhibitor (SSRI) antidepressants particularly predisposes to delirium. Electroencephalography is particularly useful in assessment of encephalopathy. Specific metabolic patterns may be identified. The background rhythm is a qualitative marker of encephalopathy and the presence of focal or lateralized epileptiform discharges enhances management. For instance, the presence of triphasic waves is characteristic of hepatic and metabolic disorders, often with good prognosis. Delirium is usually associated with a paucity of alpha activity. The presence of PLEDS is usually associated with an acute cerebral event, most frequently ischemic, and is usually a temporary pattern lasting for several days.

Table 93.5. *Antineoplastic and immune suppressive therapy associated with neurotoxicity*

Busulfan	Seizures, Wernicke-like syndrome with ataxia, confusion and diplopia, responding to thiamine
Carboplatin and cisplatin	Microangiopathic changes with secondary focal and diffuse cerebral ischemia
Chlorambucil pattern	Rare seizures in children with EEG typically 3 H_z spike-wave
Corticosteroids	Dysphoria, psychosis, hiccups, headache, lethargy, papilloedema (raised ICP), increased epidural fat
Cranial irradiation	Leukoencephalopathy, late cognitive dysfunction
Cyclophosphamide	Synergistic effect with cyclosporine toxicity (endothelial damage)
Cyclosporine and tacrolimus	Tremor, seizures, ataxia, leukoencephalopathy, blindness, headaches, predilection for reversible posterior hemispheric white matter changes
Cytosine arabinoside	10% prevalence of encephalopathy; progressive optic atrophy, myelopathy, encephalopathy, cerebellar ataxia, seizures, neuropathy, extrapyramidal dystonias
Etoposide (VP16)	Sudden severe encephalopathy, somnolence, seizures, confusion, motor deficits
Fludarabine	Reversible encephalopathy
5-Fluorouracil with levamisole	Late onset (15 to 19 weeks), ataxia, confusion with focal white matter abnormalities on CT and MRI
Ifosfamide	Early onset, severe ischemia with seizures
L-asparaginase	Delayed onset, cerebral vein and dural sinus thrombosis
Leukapheresis	Hemorrhage, infarction, activation of occult metastasis
Methotrexate	Meningoencephalitis, myelopathy, encephalopathy (transient), leukoencephalopathy, stroke-like syndromes (microangiopathy)
OKT3 monoclonal antibody	Headache, aseptic meningitis (reversible and generally benign)
Paclitaxel (Taxol)	Rapid onset, cumulative peripheral and optic neuropathy
Procarbazine	Synergistic effect with cyclosporine toxicity (endothelial damage)

Abbreviations: ICP, intracranial pressure; PML, progressive multifocal leukoencephalopathy.

Idiopathic hyperammonemia is a rare complication of intensive chemotherapy and has been described after BMT (Davies *et al.*, 1996). It is defined as an elevated plasma ammonia concentration (>200 μmol/l) in the absence of significant liver function abnormality. In a database of 2,358 patients, 12 were identified with this syndrome (0.5%). Eight received marrow from an HLA-matched sibling donor, 3 from an unrelated donor, and 1 autologous marrow. It occurred between 14 and 106 days posttransplant with a median of 25 days. Ten of the 12 patients died 1 to 9 (median 3.5) days after diagnosis, despite treatment with combinations of dialysis and ammonia-trapping therapy. Hyperventilation and respiratory alkalosis can occur. Liver biopsy shows microvesicular steatosis (thus differing from Reye's syndrome or inherited defects of urea synthesis). Rapid diagnosis and institution of treatment is important. Therapy includes discontinuation of parenteral alimentation to lower protein intake, together with agents such as lactulose, omeprazole, and metronidazole or neomycin. Frere and colleagues (2000) used carnitine 50 mg/kg/day to promote urea production. Because their patient responded dramatically to flumazenil, an antagonist of endogenous benzodiazepines, she was also given a continuous infusion of this drug. Mechanical ventilation is sometimes necessary for the management of respiratory alkalosis. Dialysis may also be effective for reducing ammonia concentration.

Reversible leukoencephalopathy has been described in two patients with renal insufficiency and high levels of dimethylsulfoxide (DMSO) after infusion of cryopreserved autologous PBSC (Dhodapkar *et al.*, 1994). In another patient, MRI revealed white matter changes, which resolved over two months (Higman *et al.*, 2000).

Treatment-induced leukoencephalopathy

Delayed transient encephalopathy not associated with cyclosporine or tacrolimus toxicity has been reported to occur

Table 93.6. *Causes of encephalopathy with normal MR imaging during the posttransplant leukopenic period*

Cause	Features
Nonconvulsive status epilepticus	Antibiotic (Cefepime, Imipenem), cyclosporine
Drug-related	Acyclovir, amphotericin B, opioids, sedatives (cyclosporine frequently has abnormal MRI features; early cyclosporine toxicity may have normal MRI)
Systemic organ dysfunction	Encephalopathy may ante-date markers of specific organ failure
Infection (bacterial endocarditis, *Listeria* meningitis, viral meningoencephalitis)	Uncommon
Cytomegalovirus, Wernicke's encephalopathy	Uncommon

within 1 to 2 months of high-dose chemotherapy or chemoradiotherapy and bone marrow or blood stem cell transplantation. Encephalopathy is characterized by confusion, lethargy, somnolence, and seizures (Goldberg *et al.,* 1992). High-grade pyrexia has also been described (Murphy, Parker, & Hutchinson, 1994). Magnetic scans demonstrate multifocal symmetric white matter lesions that settle gradually over 2 to 3 months. CT scans and CSF are normal, but the EEG shows diffuse dysrhythmia. Treatment is supportive with exclusion of specific metabolic abnormalities and infection, and anticonvulsant treatment of seizures (Tahsildar *et al.,* 1996).

Progressive or potentially progressive leukoencephalopathy is a well-recognized complication of treatment for CNS malignancies and leukemia and was first described after BMT by Atkinson *et al.,* in 1977. It has subsequently been recognized in 1% to 2% of BMT recipients.

Leukoencephalopathy usually follows combination therapy with intrathecal methotrexate (MTX) and cranial irradiation, with the most severe sequelae noted when MTX is administered with, or following, radiotherapy, so that posttransplant MTX constitutes a significant risk, particularly when six or more MTX doses are used. The underlying disease in the majority of patients with leukoencephalopathy ALL, but cases with acute myeloid leukemia (AML) are occasionally seen (Fig. 93.4).

Leukoencephalopathy may occur days to many months posttransplant; most cases occur within the first 5 months. An unusual case of multifocal remitting-relapsing cerebral demyelination has been reported in a female who received an allogeneic BMT from a related male donor and who, after a 20-year interval, developed an acute fulminant biopsy-proven demyelinating disorder of cerebral white matter that followed a chronic remitting-relapsing course. In situ hybridization studies revealed Y-chromosome-positive mononuclear cells in biopsy samples of white matter. Intriguingly, MRI studies of the asymptomatic healthy male donor showed multiple white matter lesions (Kelly *et al.,* 1996).

Since HSC transplant patients are exposed to several potential sources of CNS damage, including both the primary treatment of the underlying disease and the immediate pretransplant preparative regimen (as well as subsequent metabolic and cyclosporine-related encephalopathies), the finding of cognitive dysfunction in long-term recipients is common. Direct correlation with the dosage of TBI has been identified (Wiznitzer *et al.,* 1984; Andrykowski *et al.,* 1990). As well as psychometric test abnormalities, clinical observations indicate mood and affective disturbance, and minor memory and concentration difficulties are common (Tables 93.5, 93.6 and 93.7).

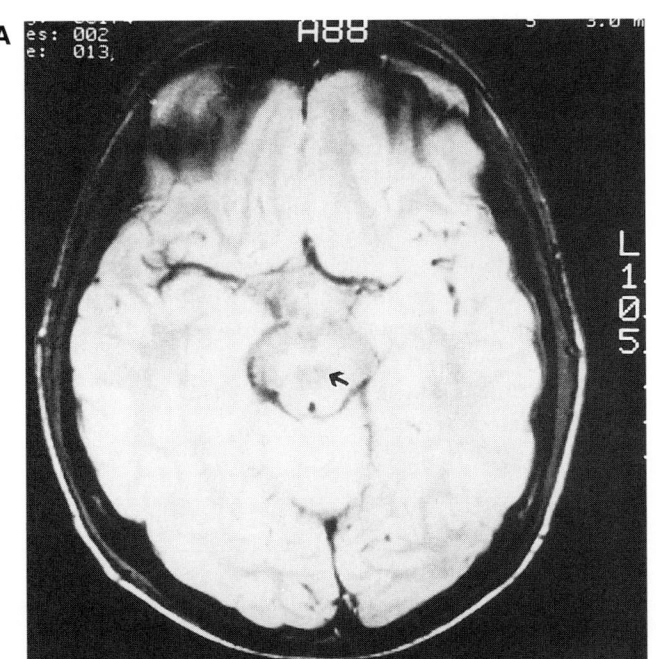
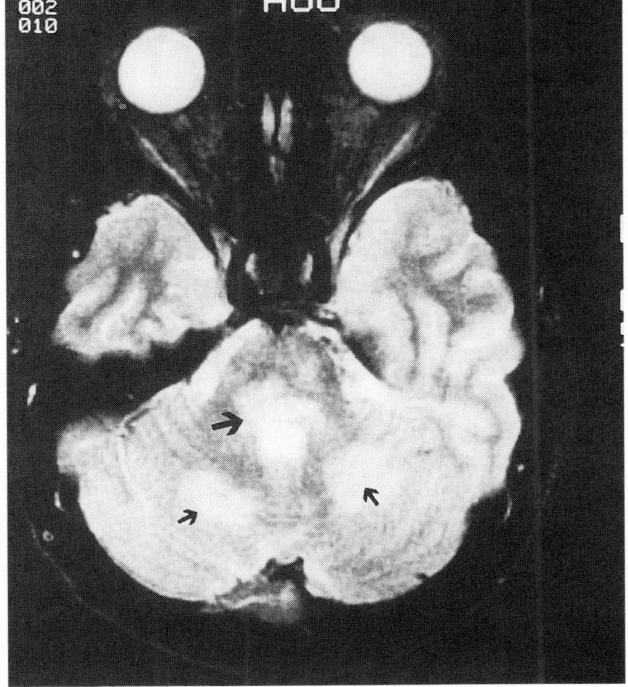

Fig. 93.4. MRI scans demonstrating treatment-induced encephalopathy. A 28-year-old male had previously received successful mantle field irradiation for Hodgkin's disease 6 years before developing acute myeloid leukemia (AML). CNS relapse of the AML was treated with intrathecal cytosine arabinoside and later methotrexate (MTX); cranial irradiation was given with full resolution of neurologic deficit and no cognitive dysfunction. Allogeneic BMT was successful and cyclosporine and corticosteroid therapy were discontinued after 12 months. Intrathecal MTX 12.5 mg second monthly was continued during this period. At this time, he developed progressive ataxia, diplopia, nystagmus, and dysarthria. CSF cytology and stereotactic biopsy of a MRI-identified lesion did not suggest leukemic or infectious pathology. The MRI images demonstrate patchy areas of altered signal intensity (arrowed) in the cerebellum (**A**) and upper brain stem (**B**), which were inconsistent with hemorrhagic lesions.

Antineoplastic and immune suppressive therapy associated with neurotoxicity

Methotrexate

The neurotoxicity of MTX is well described after oral, intravenous, or intrathecal administration and has both acute and chronic forms, generally identified as dose-related toxicity, particularly in the treatment of ALL. In addition, a specific stroke-like syndrome is described in juvenile and adult HSC transplant patients in which fluctuating aphasia, hemiparesis, and mental state change occurs. Symptoms typically evolve 5 to 7 days after a second or subsequent course of MTX therapy without toxic serum levels. Further treatment is allowable (Walker *et al.,* 1986). The CSF and CT scans are unremarkable, but EEG shows focal abnormalities. The pathogenesis may be associated with a focal mineralizing microangiopathy and neuroaxonal dystrophy (Phanthumchinda, Intragumtornchai, & Kasantikul, 1991).

Cytosine arabinoside

High-dose cytosine arabinoside is sometimes used as part of the pretransplant preparative regimen. Neurotoxicity occurs in between 12% to 50% of patients given doses greater than 3 g/m^2/24 hours or cumulative doses of 24 g to 36 g. Symptoms generally evolve within 24 hours of the last dose and may be irreversible with high cumulative doses (Hwang *et al.,* 1985). The majority of affected patients develop a cerebellar syndrome with dysarthria, nystagmus, incoordination, and tremor. Encephalopathy with somnolence, confusion, incontinence, cognitive loss, and with grasp and snout reflexes, is associated with diffuse EEG slowing. Reversible extrapyramidal syndromes and aphasia occasionally occur. At least partial recovery is usual with subjects over age 50 more severely affected. Lower doses are recommended in this group. Autopsy reveals specific Purkinje cell loss in the depths of sulci and reactive astrocytosis. Therapy should be immediately discontinued at the first sign of cerebellar dysfunction. Both diffuse sensorimotor neuropathy and acute demyelinating neuropathy may occur independently of the effects of other peripheral neurotoxic agents such as vincristine or cisplatin. However, potentiation may well occur (Borgeat, De Muralt, & Stalder, 1986). Since recovery is slow and incomplete, extreme caution must be exercised with potentially neurotoxic posttransplant therapy such as thalidomide.

OKT3

OKT3 is a monoclonal antibody directed against T-cells. Aseptic meningitis may occur in about 5% of patients, usually in the first few days of drug exposure. Cerebrospinal fluid shows normal glucose values and mild protein elevation with lymphocytic pleocytosis. This is a benign, self-limiting meningitis which is difficult to separate from other forms of meningitis without careful analysis. An inflammatory or allergic reaction has been considered and is similar to the minor aseptic meningitis occasionally seen with intravenous immunoglobulin. Seizures occasionally occur and cerebral edema has been noted. This generally settles even with continuing OKT3 therapy (Parizel *et al.,* 1997).

Cyclosporine

Neurologic toxicity associated with cyclosporine can be severe (Berden *et al.,* 1985) and occurs in 10% to 25% of allogeneic HSCT patients treated with cyclosporine (Memon *et al.,* 1995; Edwards, Wszolek, & Normand, 1996; Erer *et al.,* 1996; Teshima, Miyoshi, & Ono, 1996; Wasserstein & Honig, 1996). The relationship with seizures and antiepileptic drugs has been previously discussed; isolated seizures are reported in up to 5% of patients and may be associated with hypomagnesemia. Common neurologic symptoms of tremor (30%), distal dysesthesia (11%), ataxia, incoordination, and cognitive disturbance as well as specific encephalopathy are outlined in Table 93.7, which illustrates the spectrum of common neurologic symptoms associated with cyclosporine, in which rapid improvement follows dosage adjustment and cor-

Table 93.7. *Cyclosporine-related neurotoxicity: common and reversible syndromes*

Syndrome	Approximate frequency	Comments
Tremor	16–20%	Dose-related, reversible, direct neurotoxicity
Seizures	5%	Dose-related direct neurotoxicity. Capillary leak? hypomagnesemia? hypocholesterolemia? hyperlipidemia? hypertension; concurrent steroid therapy; prior chemotherapy
Ataxia/incoordination	5%	As above
Mental state change/somnolence	5%	Direct neurotoxicity
Mania	Rare alone	Direct neurotoxicity
Dysesthesia/subclinical neuropathy	Up to 11%	Uncertain mechanism; lipid changes?
Deltoid paralysis	Uncommon	Direct peripheral neurotoxicity?
Headache	20%	May be relieved by propranolol

Table 93.8. *Drug interactions with cyclosporine*

Increased cyclosporine levels (P450IIIA inhibitors)	Decreased cyclosporine levels (P450IIIA increase)	Synergistic toxicity
Androgenic and estrogenic steroids	Carbamazapine	Aminoglycosides
Calcium channel blockers	Phenobarbitone	Amphotericin B
H$_2$ antagonists (especially cimetidine)	Phenytoin	Diuretics
Corticosteroids	Dexamethasone	Melphalan
Danazol	Rifampicin	NSAIDs
Erythromycin	Sulfhinpyrazone	Trimethoprim
Ketoconazole		Digoxin
Norfloxacin		

rection of metabolic derangement and diastolic hypertension. The hypertension is due in part to renal toxicity, but to a large extent is provoked by the tendency of cyclosporine to stimulate the sympathetic nervous system by an unknown mechanism. Much of cyclosporine's neurologic toxicity is due to the production of hypertension, and encephalopathy is roughly correlated with blood levels, but is better correlated with the rate of change of blood pressure from the patient's baseline level. Table 93.8 lists the drug interactions that influence the development of neurotoxicity.

Table 93.9 lists more serious neurologic syndromes associated with cyclosporine. There is a significant overlap of symptoms and signs. Focal white matter alterations on imaging and at autopsy show a major predilection for the occipital cortex.

A reversible posterior leukoencephalopathy syndrome characterized by headaches, confusion, delirium, seizures, motor signs, cortical blindness and other visual abnormalities, including oculogyric crisis has been identified with MRI studies showing extensive bilateral white matter abnormalities, abnormalities in the posterior regions of the cerebral hemispheres suggestive of edema without mass effect and with changes which also involve the brain stem and cerebellar white matter and other cerebral areas. MRI scans show a dramatic recovery over 1 to 2 days, but in some patients white matter changes do not completely resolve and autopsy studies have confirmed laminar changes with gliosis, particularly in the occipital gyri (Antunes et al., 1999). CT scans are usually abnormal with white matter hypodensity in vascular territory in frontal and particularly occipital poles (Fig. 93.5). EEG demonstrates diffuse slow wave dysrhythmia (Shah, 1997). CSF is unremarkable with the only reported abnormalities being nonspecific minor elevations of protein. At least one fatal case has been described (Gopal, Thorning, & Back, 1999).

This syndrome is thought to be a forme fruste of hypertensive encephalopathy: the findings are similar to those in tox-emia of pregnancy and it is emphasized that the patient's blood pressure need not be very high for this syndrome to occur. Encephalopathy with cortical blindness progressing to coma is well described (Rubin & Kang, 1987; Bhatia et al., 1988; Reece et al., 1991; Hinchey et al., 1996). While cyclosporine neurotoxicity typically produces this syndrome, it does occur in other disorders where endothelial dysfunction has been induced (Hinchey et al., 1996; Delanty et al., 1997), and tacrolimus has also been associated with a syndrome including cortical blindness (Shutter et al., 1993; Devine et al., 1996). The MRI is usually abnormal with multiple white matter lesions, most commonly, but not necessarily confined to, the occipital lobes. Cortical gray matter involvement is less common. Patients with mild encephalopathy or mild occipital lobe dysfunction may have a normal MRI scan (Casey et al., 2000). Single photon emission computed tomography (SPECT) identifies a decrease in radionuclide uptake in these areas, suggesting a vasoconstrictive mechanism (Uoshima et al., 2000), a finding confirmed by magnetic resonance angiography (Shbarou, Chao, & Morgenlander, 2000) (Figs. 93.6 and 93.7).

A syndrome of predominant ataxia and tremor together with confusion, mild weakness, hyporeflexia, and extensor plantar responses was noted by Atkinson and co-workers (1984) in 5 of 64 BMT patients, in whom all symptoms resolved when cyclosporine dosage was reduced or stopped. Toxicity was char-

Table 93.9. *Cyclosporine-related neurotoxicity: rare and more serious syndromes*

Syndrome	Approximate frequency	Comment
Paraparesis/ quadriparesis	Uncommon	Dose-related hypomagnesemia? Hypocholesterolemia? Demyelination; prostaglandin-mediated vascular leakage
Leukoencephalopathy, cerebellar syndrome	5%	As above (partial dose relationship)
Akinetic mutism, extrapyramidal syndrome with pseudobulbar palsy	Unusual	Dose-related, potentially reversible
Dysarthria, speech ataxia	Unusual	
Visual hallucinations, cortical blindness	Unusual	Dose related, reversible
Ocular flutter	Unusual	Reversible (Apsner et al., 1997)
Sixth cranial nerve palsy	Unusual	Reversible (Openshaw et al., 1997)
Seizures and thrombotic microangiopathy		Changes in brain, kidney, and lung similar to thrombotic thrombocytopenic purpura. Primarily in allogeneic transplants from donors other than HLA-identical siblings

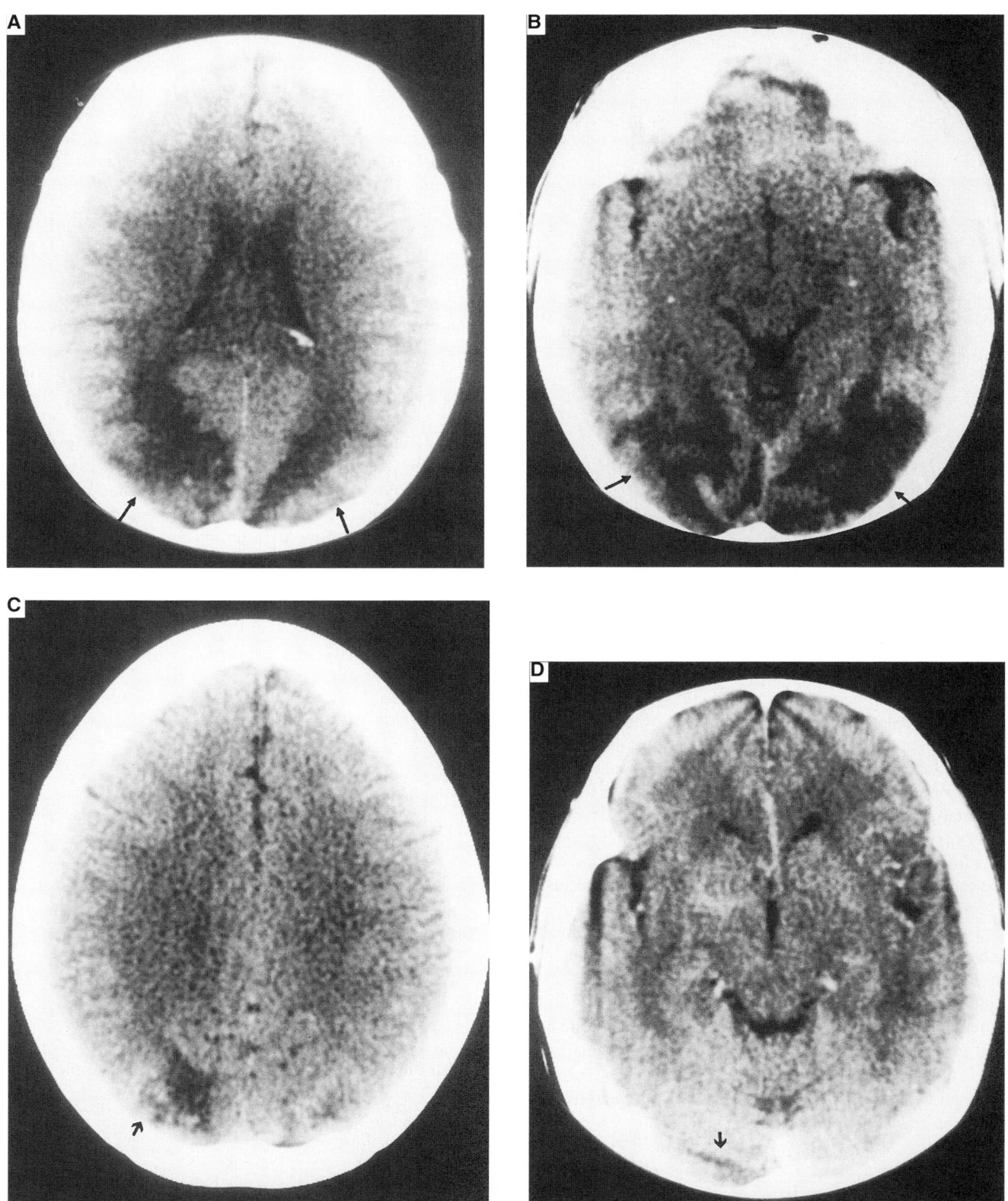

Fig. 93.5. Cortical blindness associated with cyclosporine treatment. CT scans obtained during the acute phase [scans (**A**) and (**B**)] in a 38-year-old woman who underwent allogeneic BMT for AML.She developed acute encephalopathy with vascular throbbing headache, nuchal rigidity, and cortical blindness. Full clinical recovery occurred over 2 weeks after withdrawal of cyclosporine although some residual CT lucency remained [scans (**C**) and (**D**)].

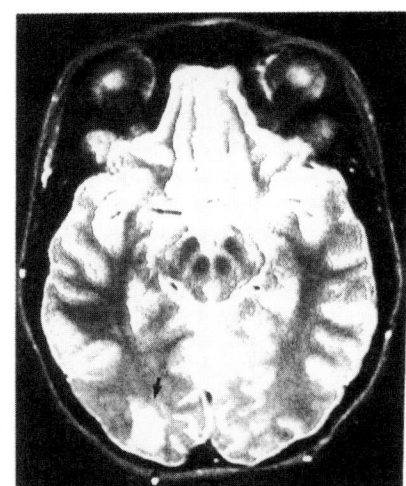

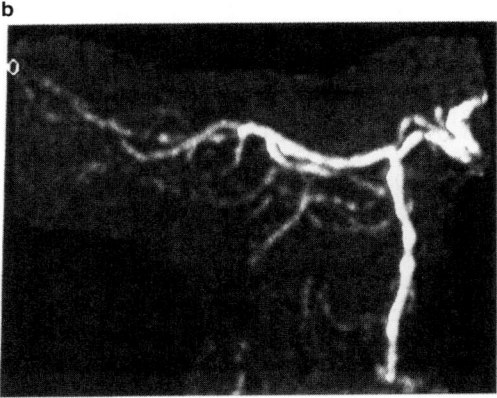

Fig. 93.6. Magnetic resonance imaging, case 2. (a) T_2-weighted image showing the right occipital white matter hyperintensity; (b) MR angiography showing the multiple areas of narrowing of intracranial arteries, with beaded appearance, in particular the basilar artery. Reproduced, with permission, from Shbarou et al. (2000).

acterized in three by a predominantly cerebellar syndrome in which confusion and amnesia were prominent, and in two by a predominantly myelopathic syndrome with urinary retention, quadriparesis, and a spinal sensory level with only minor intention tremor and drowsiness. Cranial neuropathy did not occur. A number of studies have identified potentially pathogenic mechanisms: conditioning therapy with craniospinal irradiation and intrathecal MTX may be a predisposing factor. Hypomagnesemia associated with cyclosporine-induced renal tubular dysfunction has been identified in patients with both major and minor CNS signs and with seizures. Magnesium replacement may reverse symptoms (Thompson et al., 1984). However, not all patients with cyclosporine toxicity have either hypomagnesemia or reduced total body magnesium, and cyclosporine-related hypocholesterolemia (de Groen et al., 1987), hyperlipidemia (Valbonesi et al., 1988), hypertension, and concurrent high-dose steroid have also been identified with severe CNS toxicity.

Pathologic studies have identified a blood-brain barrier disruption with edema and focal necrosis with a specific occipital white matter predominance (Sloane et al., 1985). More florid necrosis was noted in a liver transplant patient with similar toxic encephalopathy (Boon et al., 1988); focal demyelination especially in the spinal cord (with normal brain tissue) was identified in patients who developed a cyclosporine-associated cerebellar ataxia/spinal syndrome (Lind et al., 1989). Evolving and resolving radiographic and electromyographic signs of demyelination have been observed; diffuse edema without other brain pathology was noted after cyclosporine-induced seizures (Velu, Debusscher, & Stryckmans, 1985). Reece and co-workers (1991) described autopsy findings in eight patients in a retrospective review of 239 BMT recipients. In addition to fungal and CMV infections in three patients, findings included occipital, cortical, and anoxic neurones and reactive astrocytes, small hemorrhagic foci in the inferior occipital poles, and diffuse pallor of myelin associated with widespread gliosis of the white matter. Specific stains for micro-organisms were negative. Subarachnoid hemorrhage associated with cyclosporine neurotoxicity has been reported (Teksam, Casey, Michel, & Truwit, 2001).

Cyclosporine-related reversible akinetic mutism with florid dyskinesia, pseudobulbar palsy, and MRI changes consistent with central pontine myelinolysis has been reported in three liver transplant recipients, in whom no significant electrolyte or hepatic dysfunction was present: cholesterol levels were normal or borderline low, and in one patient correction of mild hypomagnesemia did not alter the clinical pattern. Slow resolution of MRI abnormalities occurred in each and judicious reintroduction of cyclosporine did not reproduce symptoms (Bird et al., 1990). The time course of development of severe cyclosporine-related leukoencephalopathy is variable and has been reported from 1.5 to 7 months after ini-

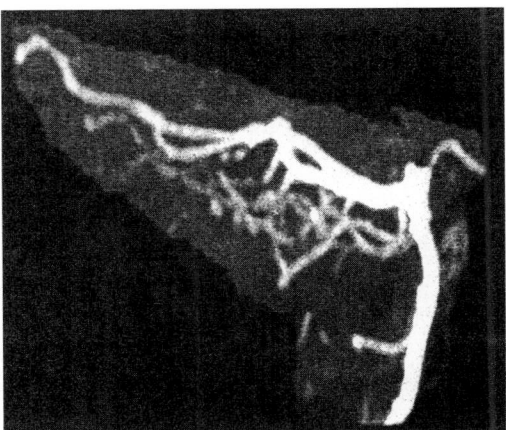

Figure 93.7. Magnetic resonance imaging, case 2. MR angiography showing the marked improvement in the appearance of the basilar artery, approximately 1 month following discontinuation of cyclosporin A. Reproduced, with permission, from Shbarou et al. (2000).

tiation of cyclosporine. Specific therapies directed at reversing deficits have not been identified. The most important management is lowering of blood pressure by any means. Withdrawal or reduction in dosage is usually required to reverse a syndrome. Correction of possible nutritional disorders and metabolic abnormalities is appropriate. Reduction of cerebral edema with intravenous mannitol may be appropriate, whereas steroid therapy may have a mixed effect with possible enhancement of toxic effects. Cytoprotective therapies have not yet been evaluated, but intravenous nimodipine used for this reason, and to lower blood pressure and prevent possible vasospasm, appears to be quite safe (personal observations), and should be considered for cyclosporine-associated cortical blindness. Oral low-dose propranolol has been effective treatment as an alternative to high-dose narcotic usage in patients with cyclosporine-induced headache (Gryn, Goldberg, & Viner, 1992). Interestingly, conversion from cyclosporine to tacrolimus for cyclosporine-associated neurotoxicity has been reported to be successful (Furlong *et al.*, 2000). An acute Parkinsonian syndrome with spasticity and myoclonus has been reported to respond to high-dose methylprednisolone with complete clinical recovery (Lockman, Sung, & Krivit 1991).

Tacrolimus

Tacrolimus (FK-506) is an immunosuppressive agent whose cellular effects are similar to those of cyclosporine. Almost identical encephalopathic syndromes have been described with similar toxicity management (Shutter *et al.*, 1993; Boeve *et al.*, 1996; Small *et al.*, 1996; Mizawa *et al.*, 2000). Neurotoxicity restricted to the brain stem has been reported in a patient presenting with diplopia, nystagmus, visual hallucinations, and internuclear ophthalmoplegia (Oliverio *et al.*, 2000). MR imaging showed bilaterally symmetrical regions of signal abnormality with abnormal contrast enhancement in the brain stem. Symptoms and MRI abnormalities resolved with discontinuation of tacrolimus. Myopathy and rhabdomyolysis induced by tacrolimus have also been reported (Hibi *et al.*, 1995; Campellone *et al.*, 1998). Demyelinating neuropathy may also occur with both cyclosporine and tacrolimus (Bronster *et al.*, 1995).

Cellular mechanisms of cyclosporine neurotoxicity

Cyclosporine and tacrolimus are highly selective inhibitors of cyclophilin, which is a prolyl isomerase or rotamase that influences the folding of proteins. Each agent potently inhibits rotamase activity but immunosuppression does not primarily involve the folding of a protein crucial to the immune response. Instead cyclosporine and similar agents form a drug-protein complex that inhibits the calcium-dependent and calmodulin-dependent protein phosphatase calcineurin. Thus, cyclosporine bound to cyclophilin or immunophilin inhibits calcineurin activity. Calcineurin inhi-

bition mediates immunosuppression by regulation of interleukin-2 gene transcription.

Calcineurin is widely distributed through the CNS and its distribution parallels that of cyclophilin and the binding protein for tacrolimus. The amount of these substances in the nervous system greatly exceeds that in the immune system, so it is expected that calcineurin regulates physiologic processes in the CNS including transmitter release, synaptic vesicle processing, and neuroprotection against glutamate neurotoxicity in ischemia. Additional cyclosporine effects on vascular endothelial cells are mediated by release of endothelin, prostacyclin, and thromboxane A_2 by direct cytotoxic effect. Endothelin is a potent vasoconstrictor and increases in thromboxane and prostacyclin may cause microthrombi. Immunosuppressive drug damage of the blood-brain barrier by various means, together with the hypertension, vasoconstriction with focal hypoperfusion and fluid overload best explains the acute reversible white matter changes in the immunosuppressive CNS syndromes (Benigni *et al.*, 1992; Dawson, 1996).

Thalidomide

Symptomatic sensory peripheral neuropathy is the most prominent complication of thalidomide treatment (see below); however, sedation is an almost universal side-effect and is moderate to severe in 10%–15% of patients.

Interferon-alpha

Neurologic side effects, predominantly mental state changes, drowsiness, and dizziness, occur in mild form in 27% and severely in 6% of patients receiving interferon-alpha (Valentine *et al.*, 1998; Kantarjian *et al.*, 1999). Interferon-alpha therapy following autologous stem cell transplantation may provoke a delayed, slowly evolving sensory motor neuropathy which reverses on cessation of interferon (Emir *et al.*, 1999).

Radiation effects including myelitis

A syndrome similar to the severe neurologic effects of cyclosporine and tacrolimus with confusion, tremor, and parkinsonism may be caused by amphotericin B as a consequence of disruption by radiotherapy of the blood brain barrier, allowing entry of amphotericin B into the brain (Balmaceda *et al.*, 1994; Mott *et al.*, 1995). The combination of drug therapies which alter myelin susceptibility to radiotherapy may be a factor in radiation myelitis production.

Myelitis is a rare but well-documented complication of therapeutic radiation exposure to the spinal cord and is characterized by delayed development of paresthesias, sensory changes and, in severe cases, progressive paresis and paralysis. Although accepted radiation tolerance limits for the spinal cord have successfully limited the incidence of this problem (45–50 Gy in daily 1.8–2 Gy fractions), aggressive systemic therapy may render patients more susceptible to radiation-related neurotoxicity. Schwartz and colleagues (2000) described a patient who received cyclophosphamide 120 mg/kg and TBI 120 cGy × 11 fractions followed by an HLA-identical sibling PBSC transplant for non-Hodgkin's lymphoma. This was followed by delivery of 30.6 Gy involved field radiation to the mediastinum and left supraclavicular fossa for residual tumor. Although the maximum cumulative dose to the spinal cord was less than 45 Gy, the patient subsequently developed progressive lower extremity weakness and MRI abnormalities of the spinal cord limited to the radiation field.

Second malignancy and leukemia recurrence in the CNS

Long-term survivors of hematopoietic stem cell transplantation are at increased risk of new CNS malignancies. The risk of malignant brain tumor was 4.3 times higher in recipients of allogeneic HSC transplantation when total body irradiation was part of the conditioning regimen, with a higher risk in patients with acute leukemia compared with those with lymphoma (Curtis et al., 1997; Socie et al., 2000). Our own experience as well as three other studies indicate glioblastoma as the only primary CNS neoplasm (Sanders et al., 1982; Deeg, 1984; Curtis et al., 1997).

CNS lymphoma associated with organ transplantation is a component of the posttransplant lymphoproliferative disorder (PTLD). This description covers a spectrum of abnormal B-lymphocyte proliferations ranging from benign diffuse polyclonal lymphoid hyperplasia to malignant monoclonal lymphoma (Chapter 88). CNS involvement occurs in 15% to 25% of patients with PTLD and in most of these cases the CNS is the only site of detectable disease. The prevalence of PTLD with CNS involvement is much lower after HSC transplantation than after other types of transplants, presumably because less immunosuppression is used. Evidence of PTLD is noted in 0.075% of HSC transplantation compared with 0.277% of cardiac transplants, 0.55% of liver transplants, and 1% of heart/lung transplants (Patchell, 1994). In the HSC transplant population this syndrome occurs primarily in heavily immune-suppressed T-cell-depleted allogeneic transplant recipients. PTLD is closely associated with EBV infection (whereas primary CNS lymphoma in immunocompetent subjects is not associated with EBV infection). CNS lymphoma in BMT patients is distinguished from progressive multifocal leukoencephalopathy (PMLE) by the prominence of mass effect and gadolinium enhancement on MRI scans.

The mechanism of pathogenesis is selective infection of B lymphocytes by EBV with resultant proliferation; under normal conditions the immune system suppresses the polyclonal B-cell proliferation predominantly by cell-mediated immunity. In the transplant recipient both cellular and humoral immune mechanisms are abnormal and allow proliferation of EBV, which results in an initial polyclonal lymphoproliferation. In the absence of EBV suppressor cells or specific cyto-

toxic T cells, the lymphoproliferation is not influenced by immunologic control mechanisms. The predilection of lymphoproliferations to become established in the CNS is unclear, but the immunologically "privileged" state of the CNS and less intense immune responses may reduce further the control of EBV-induced cell proliferation. Diagnosis is by stereotactic biopsy or identification of a mass lesion elsewhere in the body. In the allogeneic HSC transplant recipient, the disease can be cured by infusion of EBV-specific donor cytotoxic T cells (Chapter 88).

Leukemic recurrence in the CNS after HSC transplantation occurs predominantly in patients transplanted for ALL and develops in between 5% and 20% of patients. Recurrence in AML is uncommon (2% to 5%) (Wiznitzer et al., 1984; Patchell et al., 1985; Thompson et al., 1986; Mohrmann, Mah, & Vinters, 1990; Bhatia et al., 1996).

The clinical features of a second malignancy or leukemic recurrence are not specific. Radiographic findings are likely to be of multicentric mass lesions that may not be clearly seen on a noncontrast CT scan. Symmetric bilateral or callosal deposits suggest glioma or lymphoma. Diagnosis is by CSF cytologic examination if the risk of brain stem herniation is considered minimal.

Peripheral and cranial nerve disorders

The bulk of HSC transplant patients with cranial and peripheral nerve or dermatomal deficits have varicella zoster infection, predominantly involving trigeminal divisions or truncal dermatomes. The frequency and management of this complication have been addressed above.

Isolated or multiple cranial nerve palsies may occur with focal primary disease recurrence, focal infection including toxoplasmosis, and with aminoglycoside toxicity affecting the auditory nerves. Occasional patients demonstrate reversible cranial neuropathies particularly involving facial and auditory nerves in which no underlying infection or disease recurrence is identified. In these cases prominent GVHD is present and improvement is noted with short-term increase in steroid therapy (personal observations).

Peroneal and ulnar nerve palsies associated with debility, compression and GVHD are sometimes identified and require electrophysiologic evaluation to differentiate possible subclinical neuropathies. Mononeuropathies may be the result of intraneural hemorrhage in patients with persistent thrombocytopenia (Graus et al., 1996). Lateral femoral cutaneous nerve involvement with severe GVHD has been reported (Wiznitzer et al., 1984).

As well as diffuse neuropathy from prior vincristine, etoposide (Imrie et al., 1994), or cytosine arabinoside therapy, diffuse neuropathies related to cyclosporine therapy occur after allogeneic HSC transplantation. Occasional cases of severe polyneuropathy occurring late after successful transplantation appear in two forms: one related to chronic GVHD (Greenspan et al., 1990; Amato et al., 1993), the other to disordered T-cell function resulting in Guillain-Barré[1] type acute inflammating polyneuropathy (Eliashiv et al., 1991). In the former condition, a progressive sensorimotor neuropathy with axonal degeneration-type abnormalities on nerve conduction testing, and chronic demyelination with negative immunofluorescence in nerve and muscle biopsy, was noted. Slow clinical and electrophysiologic recovery occurred with suppression of the GVHD process by increasing immune suppressive therapy. In the latter condition clinical progression followed the course of typical acute monophasic inflammatory polyneuropathies with resolution after progression to profound flaccid paresis. The diagnosis is supported by CNS findings of elevated protein levels without major pleocytosis (Hagensee et al., 1994; Myers & Williams, 1994; Perry et al., 1994). This condition responds to plasma exchange or intravenous immunoglobulin (Wen et al., 1997).

Concurrent chemotherapy-related neuropathy, possible CMV infection of peripheral nerves, or the chance occurrence of a nonspecific viral postinfectious neuropathy must be considered in such acute incapacitating neuropathies. Although plasma exchange failed to alter the course of one reported patient (Eliashiv et al., 1991), this mode of management, as well as high-dose intravenous immunoglobulin, may be appropriate. Recurrent acute inflammatory demyelinating polyradiculitis has been described after allogeneic transplantation, possibly related to administration of cyclosporine (Liedtke et al., 1994).

Isolated autonomic neuropathy with intractable postural hypotension and impaired sympathetic sudomotor function in the extremities is occasionally identified in HSC transplant recipients; subclinical neuropathy from prior vincristine or other chemotherapy is usually the underlying cause. In these patients, adrenal insufficiency should be excluded and symptomatic relief is obtained with elastic support stockings, tilting the foot of the bed downward, and oral fludrocortisone, dihydroergotamine, or rarely, midodrine.

A selective autonomic neuropathy with dizziness, syncopal attacks, postural hypotension, and profound impairment of tests of sympathetic, but not parasympathetic, function unassociated with GVHD has also been described after HSC transplantation (Roskrow et al., 1992). The exact mechanism of this disorder has not been identified.

In patients receiving thalidomide therapy for chronic GVHD, treatment-induced sensorimotor neuropathy occurs at varying times but often well beyond 1 month of treatment and evolves with painful paresthesia in the hands and feet. This is followed by sensory loss in the lower limbs. Neurological symptoms do not correlate with either duration of treatment or daily dose. Women and older patients are at greatest risk (Ochonisky et al., 1994). There may be individual susceptibility and possible genetic predisposition. Estimates of the incidence of neuropathy from thalidomide range from 4%–70% (Tseng et al., 1996); however, neuropathy of clinical signifi-

cance occurs in over 10% of treated patients. Openshaw and co-workers (1996) identified clinical polyneuropathy in 14% of patients treated with thalidomide for GVHD, with changes commencing after 1 month of treatment with doses varying from 400 to 1,200 mg daily. Clinical symptoms and a decline in the sensory nerve action potential amplitudes occur concurrently. Reports of slow resolution or irreversible damage (Fullerton & O'Sullivan, 1968) relate to prolonged treatment after the appearance of neurological symptoms. In order to reduce the risk of neuropathy, patients must be educated about the early symptoms including paresthesia or prickling in the lower limbs and should be instructed to report symptoms immediately. Histories of diabetes mellitus or previous treatment with neurotoxic agents including vincristine, high-dose cytosine arabinoside, or prolonged metronidazole are contraindications to thalidomide treatment.

Examination for signs of neuropathy should be performed monthly for the first 3 months after starting treatment and periodically thereafter. Sensory nerve action potentials are recommended as baseline electrophysiological assessment and this should be repeated at 3–6 monthly intervals and more frequently if the amplitude of sensory action potential diminishes by more than 30%. A reduction of 50% requires cessation of therapy (Gardner-Medwin, Smith, & Powell, 1994; Molloy et al., 2001). Generally, there is minimal or no change in motor nerve conduction velocity but F-wave latencies may be delayed as an early motor nerve conduction change even before the development of sensory abnormalities (Sadoh et al., 1999). Thalidomide therapy may be restarted cautiously at a lower dose once symptoms of peripheral neuropathy resolve. The decision to permanently discontinue thalidomide treatment requires consideration of the benefits of controlling the underlying disease. Thalidomide-induced perioral neuropathy, characterized by unpleasant oral dysesthesia, has been recognized as a thalidomide complication in a patient with graft-versus-host disease after allogeneic peripheral blood stem cell transplantation for breast cancer (Elad et al., 1997).

Autologous HSC transplantation has been used in the treatment of aggressive immune-mediated demyelinating polyneuropathy associated with Waldenström's macroglobulinemia, with antibodies directed to myelin-associated glycoprotein (MAG). After a successful transplant, clinical neuropathy symptoms may subside, but patients remain affected by residual neuropathy, which may show improvement only after several years (Rudnicki & Harik, 1997).

Graft-versus-host disease

Neurologic and neuromuscular complications associated or possibly associated with GVHD are listed in Table 93.10.

Peripheral neuropathy

Direct neurologic manifestations of GVHD are uncommon, if indeed they occur at all. Delineation of direct pathogenesis is

[1] Georges Guillain, French neurologist, 1876–1951; Jean Alexander Barré, French neurologist, 1880–1967.

inconclusive. Indirect evidence of GVHD-induced mononeuropathies and diffuse sensory neuropathy is based on temporal association with, and improvement with immune suppression of, GVHD (Greenspan *et al.*, 1990; Wiznitzer *et al.*, 1991; Hughes *et al.*, 1999). Other immune suppressive effects may be active and the causes for neuropathy (particularly infection with CMV and other postinfectious or paraneoplastic states) require consideration. Until additional case reports or reproducible animal models are available, an association between peripheral neuropathy and GVHD remains speculative.

Central nervous system

Findings of cerebellar biochemical and morphologic changes in several animal models of GVHD have been reviewed (Nelson & McQuillen, 1988), with the mechanisms underlying these changes being unclear. Systemic GVHD has been shown to induce the expression of major histocompatibility complex molecules in the CNS, so that some form of CNS GVHD is theoretically possible (Corriveau, Huh, & Shatz, 1998). Proof that such a process causes a clinical syndrome is not available. However, an angiitis syndrome has been reported in 5 patients with GVHD following BMT (Padovan *et al.*, 1999), and subsequent murine BMT models with induced GVHD have confirmed a mild cerebral angiitis in allogeneic transplant recipient animals but not in syngeneic controls (Padovan *et al.*, 2001). One human study in a 3-week-old infant, who developed systemic GVHD after an unsuccessful BMT for severe combined immunodeficiency, identified focal histiocytic aggregates in the brain (Rouah *et al.*, 1988). Two cases of immune-mediated myelopathy, one with optic neuropathy, have been described in patients with chronic GVHD (Openshaw *et al.*, 1995). Reversible leukoencephalopathy occurring 10 weeks posttransplant and manifested by disorientation, tremor, and myoclonus have been observed in the context of GVHD. MRI showed an abnormal signal primarily within the brain stem and deep white matter that resolved almost completely after treatment of the GVHD

(Provenzale & Graham, 1996; Padovan *et al.*, 1998). The described MR changes were associated with chronic GVHD and treatment with corticosteroids and cyclosporine, so that the independent role of each variable is difficult to determine. While these studies raise speculation, direct evidence for the CNS as a target organ of GVHD after HSC transplantation has not been forthcoming, and in large clinical studies the incidence of CNS dysfunction was no higher in patients with GVHD than in those without (Wiznitzer *et al.*, 1984; Patchell *et al.*, 1985). Incomplete CNS development may account for nonspecific histologic findings in transplanted neonates with GVHD.

Myositis

Myositis is a well-established complication of chronic GVHD and occurs in approximately 8% of patients with established chronic GVHD. It has not been reported in large studies of autologous or identical twin HSC transplantation. However, Schmidley & Galloway (1990) reported one patient who underwent autologous BMT for Hodgkin's disease, in whom myositis was identified by typical histologic changes and an unequivocal clinical response to steroids. The majority of patients with myositis have received allogeneic HSC transplantation for aplastic anemia, although in one reported case the myositis predated the transplant. A predilection for older patients correlates with the tendency for chronic GVHD to occur more frequently in older patients. The time from transplant to onset of myositis is usually between 4 months and 4 years and almost all patients experience an initial episode of acute GVHD (Nelson & McQuillen, 1988). Myositis is occasionally the sole manifestation of chronic GVHD. Clinical and electromyographic features are identical to idiopathic polymyositis, and the response to corticosteroids and azathioprine is similar. There are no distinctive biopsy features and immune fluorescence staining is not specific. Electron microscopy suggests a lymphocytotoxic mechanism, supporting the notion of myositis as a direct manifestation of chronic

Table 93.10. *Graft-versus-host disease-related neurologic and neuromuscular complications*

Disorder	Frequency in presence of GVHD	Specific features
Polymyositis	8%	Not seen in autologous or identical twin marrow transplant recipients; mostly in patients transplanted for aplastic anemia. May be sole manifestation of GVHD; possible infective pathogenesis
Myasthenia gravis	Rare (less than 0.5%)	Electrophysiologically and clinically is classic MG; anti-Ach-R antibodies correlate with disease course. No thymic abnormality. Most have had allogeneic transplants for aplastic anemia. Occasionally in patients transplanted for hematologic malignancies. None had HLA-B8
Peripheral neuropathies	Occasional reports	Direct link with GVHD inconclusive
Central nervous system lesions	Not identified	Isolated case reports of minor histologic change. Speculative animal studies

Abbreviations: MG, myasthenia gravis; Ach-R, acetylcholine receptor.

GVHD (Urbano-Marquez *et al.*, 1986). Prognosis relates to the activity of the chronic GVHD.

Myasthenia gravis

Myasthenia gravis (MG) occurs rarely after HSC transplantation, with the majority of cases also occurring after allogeneic transplantation for aplastic anemia. The onset of weakness is late (26 to 39 months posttransplant). Neuromuscular weakness is frequently severe with bulbar weakness and respiratory insufficiency, resulting in low-grade inhalational interstitial pneumonitis, which may be confused on chest x-ray with pulmonary fibrosis or interstitial changes directly due to chronic GVHD involving the lung. Responses to edrophonium and oral pyridostigmine and clinical response to plasma exchange resemble those in classical autoimmune MG; clinical improvement is maintained with immune suppressive therapy, which may directly affect the acetylcholine receptor site as well as controlling chronic GVHD. All patients have elevated anti-acetylcholine receptor antibody titers that correlate with the disease course. Some patients exhibit antibodies to striated muscle, but other tissue autoantibodies common in autoimmune MG are rarely seen. Unlike the majority of patients with autoimmune MG, chronic GVHD-related MG patients are not HLA-B8 positive. In all cases studied, the cells responsible for anti-acerylcholine receptor antibody production have been of donor origin (Bolger *et al.*, 1986; Nelson & McQuillen, 1988). Anti-acetylcholine receptor antibodies develop from donor cells, rather than by transfer of already activated B-cell clones. The mechanism of mediation of GVHD-related MG remains unclear, IgM and IgG anti-acetylcholine receptor antibodies may be elevated for long periods before clinical manifestations occur (Smith *et al.*, 1983). The occurrence of MG in HSC transplant patients only in association with chronic GVHD suggests that the GVHD triggers the development of B cells making anti-acetylcholine receptor antibody (Bolger *et al.*, 1986).

Benign and iatrogenic neurologic syndromes

Postlumbar puncture headache

Postlumbar puncture headache is common and often occurs when CSF is obtained pretransplant or for investigation of encephalopathy with headache. This low CSF pressure headache may be protracted over several days to 2 weeks and is characterized by prompt improvement on lying flat and a satisfactory response to routine analgesia. Treatment is conservative with fluid supplementation and rest. Traditional therapy with short periods of high-dose steroids (risk of avascular necrosis of bone) or epidural injection with autologous venous blood (risk of leukemic seeding) should be avoided. The possibility of subdural hematoma induced by lumbar puncture must be considered (Hentschke *et al.*, 1999).

Other causes of headache include ondansetron and cyclosporine treatment.

Persisting intracranial hypotension

A syndrome of intracranial hypotension characterized by headache, nausea, tinnitus, vertigo, diplopia, and lethargy is recognized in association with spontaneous dural tear, multiple lumbar punctures, or without an obvious precipitating cause. The suspicion of meningeal infection or tumor recurrence is raised by this syndrome. However, a characteristic magnetic scan finding of diffuse meningeal thickening involving the interhemispheric fissure, the tentorium, and the peripheral meninges is noted. There is a characteristic diffuse gadolinium enhancement and some patients have subdural fluid collections or downward displacement of the cerebellar tonsils. Meningeal biopsy performed in affected patients reveals nonspecific inflammatory change or no abnormality.

Effective treatment comprises bed rest, analgesia, antiemetics, and intravenous hydration. In HSC transplant patients a search for an epidural tear and epidural venous blood injection should be avoided. Corticosteroid therapy may be effective by encouraging fluid retention or decreasing the inflammatory response to the presence of cells or protein in the spinal fluid. This syndrome is clearly recognizable on magnetic scanning and consideration of this possibility during clinical assessment may prevent unnecessary investigation (Panullo *et al.*, 1993; Lay, Mokri, & Campbell, 1996) (Fig. 93.8).

Migraine

There is some evidence that migraine is mediated by platelets, and at least one case report of severe classical migraine first developing within 1 month of marrow transplant from a maternal donor who had long-standing migraine (Williams & Franklin, 1989).

Corticosteroid myopathy

Corticisteroid-related myopathy is not uncommon during protracted treatment for GVHD and requires differentiation from GVHD-related myositis. Biochemical assessment with creative phosphokinase (CPK) levels may not differentiate the two, since steroid myopathy is associated with normal biochemistry, but sometimes myositis patients have normal CPK levels. Electromyography provides differentiation in some patients. The exact incidence is uncertain but is probably significantly higher than the 2% to 12% reported incidence (Patchell, 1994). The clinical evolution is with an initially subtle hip girdle weakness, first noted as difficulty in rising from the squatting position. Recovery with steroid reduction is extremely slow over months. The myopathy of extreme illness (intensive care myopathy) results in muscle with reduced electrical excitability; therefore, neuropathic electrophysiologic changes are seen. Prolonged weakness in HSC transplant patients with organ failure may occur, particularly after general anesthesia, since metabolites of relaxant agents, particularly pancuronium, may remain active for days. In some patients differentiation of the cause of myopathy may only be obtained by muscle biopsy.

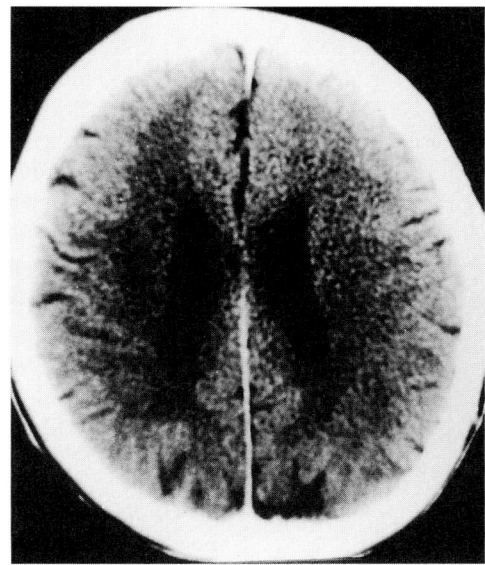 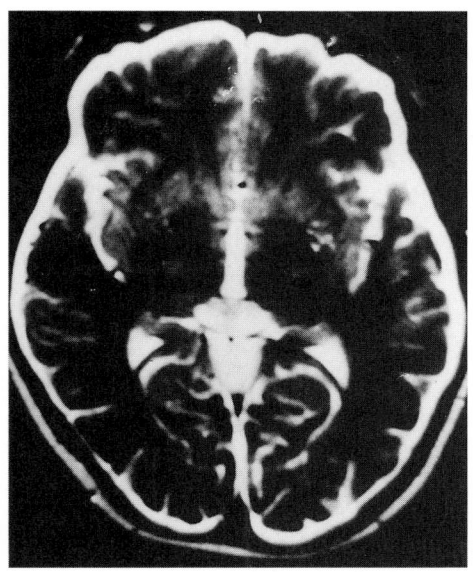

Fig. 93.8. CT and MRI scans obtained in a 54-year-old male patient 4 months after BMT for non-Hodgkin's lymphoma who had received intrathecal methotrexate pretransplant. Investigation of persistent postural headache failed to identify infection or tumor recurrence. The CT scan is unhelpful with no obvious dural or subdural abnormality but the MRI scan shows a diffuse thickening of the entire leptomeninges, typical of persisting low CSF pressure syndrome.

Maintenance of physical activity and weight bearing during high-dose steroid therapy significantly reduces the evolution of steroid-induced myopathy. It occurs more frequently after treatment with halogenated steroids (such as dexamethasone) than after prednisolone or hydrocortisone.

Extrapyramidal disorders

Extrapyramidal disorders are frequently seen with antiemetics, particularly prochlorperazine, metoclopramide, haloperidol, and occasionally with repeated doses of serotonin $5HT_3$ antagonist antiemetics including ondansetron. Dystonic reactions (either focal or generalized), motor restlessness, dyskinesia, or extrapyramidal tremors are frequently seen, usually with prompt resolution upon medication withdrawal or following centrally acting anticholinergic therapy (benztropine 0.5–2 mg i.v.). Failure of resolution raises the possibility of cyclosporine or amphotericin-related progressive extrapyramidal syndrome.

Confusional states

Corticosteroid-related psychosis may commence as acute confusion and evolve to an affective disorder with mania, a schizophrenic syndrome with hallucinations and delusions, or to a delirium that is more common is older patients. Steroid psychosis is significantly less likely with halogenated steroids.

Acute confusion, agitation, hallucinations, and apparent dysphasia may occur with high-dose narcotic analgesic therapy (codeine or morphine) alone, or in combination with antiemetics including ondansetron, SSRI's, antiviral agents (acyclovir or ganciclovir), or cyclosporine. Dysarthria and stupor may occur in HSC transplant patients with phenothiazine, butyrophenone, or benzodiazepine therapy at moderate doses.

Hiccups and myoclonic jerks

Hiccups and myoclonic jerks are symptomatic of brain stem and spinal focal lesions, but may occur as benign entities following sedative withdrawal, or, in the case of hiccups, with esophageal or gastric irritation, or with prolonged steroid therapy. Myoclonic jerks usually respond to clonazepam, but hiccups are more refractory to simple drug therapy. Hiccups occur commonly in HSC transplant patients. Therapy with prochlorperazine or chlorpromazine is generally sufficient. Alternative treatment with benzodiazepines, metoclopramide, ondansetron, or with butyrophenone (haloperidol) may also be effective. Clonazepam or valproic acid may occasionally be helpful if the hiccups have a central origin. Bowel-specific agents such as cisapride are generally ineffective, but antacids and H_2 receptor antagonists are sometimes helpful in abolishing local gastric irritation. A small proportion of patients have intractable hiccups.

Epilepsia partialis continua with prolonged focal myoclonus, has been described in a 6-year-old recipient of an HLA-identical sibling transplant (Antunes et al., 2000). Myoclonic jerks of both hands developed at 5 months posttransplant. MRI showed bilateral subcortical, non-enhancing lesions in the posterior frontal lobes. There was no improvement with phenytoin and valproic acid, nor with the later addition of clonazepam and trials of antibiotic and anti-toxoplasma treatment. Brain biopsy showed gliosis and vascular endothelial hypertrophy, as well as isolated necrotic or degenerating cells, some exhibiting nuclear alterations suggestive of a viral cytopathic effect. Despite no specific infectious agent being identified, cidofovir, a broad spectrum antiviral agent, was given for a total of 4 doses over 6 weeks, with rapid improvement.

Restless legs syndrome

Occasionally, treatment with agents such as promethazine may cause an uncomfortable restless legs syndrome, which may last for several hours.

Benign intracranial hypertension

Steroid withdrawal occasionally provokes headache and papilledema related to benign intracranial hypertension. Detailed investigation is required in these cases to exclude intracranial infection or recurrence of the underlying malignancy. Resolution with cautious readjustment of steroid dosage or repeated lumbar puncture is usual. Steroid-induced epidural fat deposition occurs rarely, but is clearly identified on magnetic resonance scanning.

Neuroleptic malignant syndrome

Neuroleptic malignant syndrome, a severe adverse effect of psychotropic drugs, is characterized by hyperthermia, extrapyramidal symptoms, autonomic instability, alterations in conciousness, elevated creatinine phosphokinase in serum, and leukocytosis (Pope *et al.*, 1983). Several cases have been described after HSC transplantation (Garrido & Chauncey, 1998; Onose, *et al.*, 2002).

Pre-existing neurologic disease other than the underlying malignancy

Patients with pre-existing epilepsy or prior neurovascular disturbances require particular consideration with detailed baseline evaluation and stabilization prior to transplantation, utilizing EEG, CT, or MRI scanning and possibly angiography in the case of subjects with a thrombotic predisposition. Revising anticonvulsant therapy may be advisable as discussed above, but may not be practical, thus necessitating appropriate adjustment of steroid and immune suppressive doses. For the management of patients with sickle cell neurological complications, see Chapter 61.

Conclusions

Neurologic complications of HSC transplantation are common and are seen in over half of all patients. The causes range from minor, self-limiting or benign drug side-effects to life-threatening fulminant syndromes. Encephalopathies (either metabolic or drug-induced) are common, and seizures and seizure management constitute the major requirement for acute neurologic evaluation. Infections and vascular disorders, particularly related to nonthrombotic endocarditis, are not uncommon, and require detailed and often serial investigation for identification and management. Less common but well-delineated problems relate to treatment side-effects, recurrence of malignancy, or neuromuscular manifestations of GVHD. Apart from dermatomal and cranial varicella zoster infection, peripheral neuropathies are uncommon. Prompt informed neurologic assessment and familiarity with the neurologic effects of immunosuppressive agents and ancillary treatments are paramount in preventing mortality and long-term morbidity.

References

Amato, A. A., Barohn, R. J., Sahenk, Z. *et al.* (1993). Polyneuropathy complicating bone marrow and solid organ transplantation. *Neurology,* **43,** 1513–1518.

Andrykowski, M. A., Altmaier, E. M., Barnett, R. L. *et al.* (1990). Cognitive dysfunction in adult survivors of allogeneic marrow transplantation: relationship to dose of total body irradiation. *Bone Marrow Transplantation,* **6,** 269–79.

Ansari, M. K., Schmidley, J. W., & Marak, R. (1997). Neuropathological complications of bone marrow transplantation for multiple myeloma. *Neurology,* **48** (Suppl 2), A309 (Abstract).

Antunes, N. L., Boulad, F., Prasad, V. *et al.* (2000). Rolandic encephalopathy and epilepsia partialis continua following bone marrow transplant. *Bone Marrow Transplantation,* **26,** 917–9.

Antunes, N. L., Small, T. N., George, D., Boulad, F., & Lis, E. (1999). Posterior leukoencephalopathy syndrome may not be reversible. *Pediatric Neurology,* **20,** 241–243.

Apsner, R., Schulenburg, A., Steinhoff, N. *et al.* (1997). Cyclosporin A-induced ocular flutter after marrow transplantation. *Bone Marrow Transplantation,* **20,** 255–6.

Atkinson, K., Biggs, J., Darveniza, P. *et al.* (1984). Cyclosporine-associated central nervous system toxicity after allogeneic bone marrow transplantation. *Transplantation,* **38,** 34–7.

Atkinson, K., Clink, H., Lawler, S. *et al.* (1977). Encephalopathy following bone marrow transplantation. *European Journal of Cancer,* **13,** 623–5.

Atkinson, K., Meyers, J. D., Storb, R. *et al.* (1980). Varicella zoster virus infection after marrow transplantation for aplastic anemia or leukemia. *Transplantation,* **29,** 47–50.

Balmaceda, C. M., Walker, R. W., Castro-Malaspina, H., Dalmau, J. (1994). Reversal of amphotericin-B-related encephalopathy. *Neurology,* **44,** 1183–1184.

Benigni, A., Morigi, M., Perico, N. *et al.* (1992). The acute effects of FK506 and cyclosporine on endothelial cell function and renal vascular resistance. *Transplantation,* **54,** 775–80.

Berden, J.H.M., Hoitsma, A. J., Merx, J. L., & Keyser, A. (1985). Severe central nervous system toxicity associated with cyclosporin. *Lancet,* **1,** 219–20 (Letter).

Bhatia, S., Ramsay, N.K.C., Steinbuch, M. *et al.* (1996). Malignant neoplasms following bone marrow transplantation. *Blood,* **87,** 3633–9.

Bird, G.L.A., Meadows, J., Goka, J. *et al.* (1990). Cyclosporine-associated akinetic mutism and extrapyramidal syndrome after liver transplantation. *Journal of Neurology, Neurosurgery and Psychiatry*, **53**, 1068–71.

Bleggi-Torres, L. F., de Medeiros, B. C., Werner, B. *et al.* (2000). Neuropathological findings after bone marrow transplantation: an autopsy study of 180 cases. *Bone Marrow Transplantation*, **25**, 301–307.

Bleggi-Torres, L. F., Medeiros, B. C., Ogasawara, V.S.A. *et al.* (1997). Iatrogenic Wernicke's encephalopathy in allogeneic bone marrow transplantation: a study of eight cases. *Bone Marrow Transplantation*, **20**, 391–395.

Boeve, B. F., Kimmel, D. W., Aronson, A. E., & de Groen, P. C. (1996). Dysarthria and apraxia of speech associated with FK-506 (tacrolimus). *Mayo Clinic Proceedings*, **71**, 969–72.

Bolger, G. B., Sullivan, K. M., Spence, A. M. *et al.* (1986). Myasthenia gravis after allogeneic bone marrow transplantation: relationship to chronic graft-versus-host disease. *Neurology*, **36**, 1087–91.

Boon, A. P., Adams, D. H., Carey, C. M. *et al.* (1988). Cyclosporin-associated cerebral lesions in liver transplantation. *Lancet*, **1**, 1457 (Letter).

Borgeat, A., De Muralt, B., & Stalder, M. (1986). Peripheral neuropathy associated with high-dose Ara-C therapy. *Cancer*, **58**, 852–4.

Bourdette, D., Rosenberg, N., & Yatsu, F. (1983). Herpes zoster ophthalmicus and delayed ipsilateral cerebral infarction. *Neurology*, **33**, 1428–1432.

Bronster, D., Yonover, P., Stein, J. *et al.* (1995). Demyelinating sensory motor polyneuropathy after administration of FK506. *Transplantation*, **59**, 1006–1068.

Burger, P., Kamenar, E., Schold, C. *et al.* (1981). Encephalomyelopathy following high-dose BCNU therapy. *Cancer*, **48**, 1818–1827.

Campellone, J., Lacomis, D., Kramer, D. *et al.* (1998). Acute myopathy after liver transplantation. *Neurology*, **50**, 46–53.

Casey, S. O., Sampaio, R. C., Michel, E., & Truwit, C. L. (2000). Posterior reversible encephalopathy syndrome: utility of fluid-attenuated inversion recovery MR imaging in the detection of cortical and subcortical lesions. *American Journal of Neuroradiology*, **21**, 1199–1206.

Chandrasekar, P. H. & Momin, F. (1997). Disseminated toxoplasmosis in marrow transplant recipients: a report of three cases and review of the literature. *Bone Marrow Transplantation*, **19**, 685–689.

Colosimo, M., McCarthy, N., Jayasinghe, R. *et al.* (2000). Diagnosis and management of subdural haematoma complicating bone marrow transplantation. *Bone Marrow Transplantation*, **25**, 549–52.

Coppo, P., Laporte, J. P., Aoudjhane, M. *et al.* (1999). Progressive multifocal leucoencephalopathy with peripheral demyelinating neuropathy after autologous bone marrow transplantation for acute myeloblastic leukemia (FAB5). *Bone Marrow Transplantation*, **23**, 401–403.

Corriveau, R. A., Huh, G. S., & Shatz, C. J. (1998). Regulation of class I MHC gene expression in the developing and mature CNS by neural activity. *Neuron*, **21**, 505–20.

Curtis, R. E., Rowlings, P. A., Deeg, H. J. *et al.* (1997). Solid cancers after bone marrow transplantation. *New England Journal of Medicine*, **336**, 897–904.

Davis, D. G. & Patchell, R. A. (1988). Neurologic complications of bone marrow transplantation. *Neurologic Clinics*, **6**, 377–87.

Davies, S. M., Szabo, E., Wagner, J. E. *et al.* (1996). Idiopathic hyperammonemia: a frequently lethal complication of bone marrow transplantation. *Bone Marrow Transplantation*, **17**, 1119–25.

Dawson, T. M. (1996). Immunosuppressants, Immunophilins and the nervous system. *Annals of Neurology*, **40**, 559–60.

de Brabander, C., Cornelissen, J., Smitt, P. A., Vecht, C. J., & van den Bent, M. J. (2000). Increased incidence of neurological complications in patients receiving an allogenic bone marrow transplantation from alternative donors. *Journal of Neurology, Neurosurgery & Psychiatry*, **68**, 36–40.

de Groen, P. C., Aksamit, A. J., Rakela, J. *et al.* (1987). Central nervous system toxicity after liver transplantation: the role of cyclosporine and cholesterol. *New England Journal of Medicine*, **317**, 861–6.

Deeg, H. J. (1984). Bone marrow transplantation: a review of delayed complications. *British Journal of Haematology*, **57**, 185–208.

Delanty, N., Vaughan, C., Frucht, S., & Stuebgen, P. (1997). Erythropoietin-associated hypertensive posterior leukoencephalopathy. *Neurology*, **48** (Suppl 2), A308 (Abstract).

Dellemijn, P.L.I., Brandenburg, A., Niesters, H.G.M. *et al.* (1995). Successful treatment with ganciclovir of presumed Epstein-Barr meningo-encephalitis following bone marrow transplant. *Bone Marrow Transplantation*, **16**, 311–12.

DeLone, D. R., Goldstein, R. A., Petermann, G. *et al.* (1999). Disseminated aspergillosis involving the brain: Distribution and imaging characteristics. *American Journal of Neuroradiology*, **20**, 1597–1604.

Devine, S. M., Newman, N. J., Siegel, J. L. *et al.* (1996). Tacrolimus (FK506)-induced cerebral blindness following bone marrow transplantation. *Bone Marrow Transplantation*, **18**, 569–72.

Devinsky, O., Lemann, W., Evans, A. C. *et al.* (1987). Akinetic mutism in a bone marrow transplant recipient following total-body irradiation and amphotericin B chemoprophylaxis: a positron emission tomographic neuropathologic study. *Archives of Neurology*, **44**, 414–17.

Dhodapkar, M., Goldberg, S. L., Tefferi, A., & Gertz, M. A. (1994). Reversible encephalopathy after cryopreserved peripheral stem cell infusion. *American Journal of Hematology*, **45**, 187–8.

Diez-Martin, J. L., Habermann, T. M., Gastineau, D. A. *et al.* (1988). Non-bacterial thrombotic endocarditis in autologous bone marrow transplantation. *American Journal of Medicine*, **85**, 742–4.

Dixit, S., Kurle, P., Buyan-Dent, L., & Sheth, R. D. (2000). Status epilepticus associated with cefepime. *Neurology*, **54**, 2153–2155.

Drobyski, W. R., Knox, K. K., Majewski, D., & Carrigan, D. R. (1994). Fatal encephalitis due to variant B human herpes virus-6 infection in a bone marrow transplant recipient. *New England Journal of Medicine*, **330**, 1356–60.

Edwards, L. L., Wszolek, Z. K., & Normand, M. M. (1996). Neurophysiologic evaluation of cyclosporine toxicity associated with bone marrow transplantation. *Acta Neurologica Scandinavica*, **94**, 358–64.

Elad, S., Galili, D., Garfunkel, A., & Or, R. (1997). Thalidomide induced perioral neuropathy. *Oral Surgery, Oral Medicine, Oral Pathology, Oral Radiology & Endodontics*, **84**, 362–364.

Eliashiv, S., Brenner, T., Abramsky, O. *et al.* (1991). Acute inflammatory demyelinating polyneuropathy following bone marrow transplantation. *Bone Marrow Transplantation, 8,* 315–17.

Emir, S., Kutluk, T., Chan, K. W. *et al.* (1999). Peripheral neuropathy during alpha-interferon therapy in a child with Hodgkin's disease. *Pediatric Hematology & Oncology, 16,* 557–560.

Emmanouilides, C. E. & Territo, M. (1999). HTLV-1-associated myelopathy following allogeneic bone marrow transplantation. *Bone Marrow Transplantation, 24,* 205–6.

Emmens, R. K., Richardson, D., Thomas, W. *et al.* (1996). Necrotizing cerebritis in an allogeneic bone marrow transplant recipient due to *Cladophialophora bantiana. Journal of Clinical Microbiology, 34,* 1330–2.

Erer, B., Polchi, B., Lucarelli, G. *et al.* (1996). CsA-associated neurotoxicity and ineffective prophylaxis with clonazepam in patients transplanted for thalassemia major: analysis of risk factors. *Bone Marrow Transplantation, 18,* 157–62.

Famiglio, L. M., Racusen, L. C., Fivush, B. A. *et al.* (1987). Mechanism of cyclosporine-associated central nervous system effects in the rat. *Annals of Neurology, 22,* 454 (Abstract).

Feinberg, W. M. & Swenson, M. R. (1988). Cerebrovascular complications of L-asparaginase therapy. *Neurology, 38,* 127–33.

Frere, P., Canivet, J. L., Gennigens, C. *et al.* (2000). Hyperammonemia after high-dose chemotherapy and stem cell transplantation. *Bone Marrow Transplantation, 26,* 343–5.

Fullerton, P. & O'Sullivan, D. (1968). Thalidomide neuropathy: a clinical, electrophysiological, and histological follow-up study. *Journal of Neurology, Neurosurgery & Psychiatry, 31,* 543–551.

Furlong, T., Storb, R., Anasetti, C. *et al.* (2000). Clinical outcome after conversion to FK 506 (tacrolimus) therapy for acute graft-versus-host disease resistant to cyclosporine or for cyclosporine-associated toxicities. *Bone Marrow Transplantation, 26,* 1005–9.

Furlong, T. G. & Galluci, B. (1994). Patterns of occurrence and clinical presentation of neurological complications in bone marrow transplant patients. *Cancer Nursing, 17,* 27–36.

Gallardo, D., Ferra, C., Berlanga, J. J. *et al.* (1996). Neurologic complications after allogeneic bone marrow transplantation. *Bone Marrow Transplantation, 18,* 1135–9.

Gardner-Medwin, J., Smith, N., & Powell, R. (1994). Clinical experience with thalidomide in the management of severe oral and genital ulceration in conditions such as Behcet's disease: use of neurophysiological studies to detect thalidomide neuropathy. *Annals of Rheumatic Diseases, 53,* 828–832.

Garrido, S. M., & Chauncey, T. R. (1998). Neuroleptic malignant syndrome following autologous peripheral blood stem cell transplantation. *Bone Marrow Transplantation, 21,* 427–8.

Goldberg, S. L., Tefferi, A., Rummans, T. A. *et al.* (1992). Post-irradiation somnolence in an adult patient following allogeneic bone marrow transplantation. *Bone Marrow Transplantation, 9,* 499–501.

Gopal, A. K., Thorning, D. R., & Back, A. L. (1999). Fatal outcome due to cyclosporine neurotoxicity with associated pathological findings. *Bone Marrow Transplantation, 23,* 191–3.

Gordon, B., Lyden, E., Lynch, J. *et al.* (2000). Central nervous system dysfunction as the first manifestation of multiple organ dys-

function syndrome in stem cell transplant patients. *Bone Marrow Transplantation, 25,* 79–83.

Gordon, B. G., Saving, K. L., McCallister, J. A. *et al.* (1991). Cerebral infarction associated with protein C deficiency following allogenic bone marrow transplantation. *Bone Marrow Transplantation, 8,* 323–5.

Graus, F., Saiz, A., Sierra, J. *et al.* (1996). Neurologic complications of autologous and allogeneic bone marrow transplantation in patients with leukemia: a comparative study. *Neurology, 46,* 1004–9.

Greenspan, S., Deeg, H. J., Cottler-Fox, M. *et al.* (1990). Incapacitating peripheral neuropathy as a manifestation of chronic graft-versus-host disease. *Bone Marrow Transplantation, 5,* 349–52.

Gruhn, B., Meerbach, A., Egerer, R. *et al.* (1999). Successful treatment of Epstein-Barr virus-induced transverse myelitis with ganciclovir and cytomegalovirus hyperimmune globulin following unrelated bone marrow transplantation. *Bone Marrow Transplantation, 24,* 1355–8.

Gryn, J., Goldberg, J., & Viner, E. (1992). Propanolol for the treatment of cyclosporin-induced headaches. *Bone Marrow Transplantation, 9,* 211–12.

Hagensee, M. E., Benyunes, M., Miller, J. A., & Spach, D. H. (1994). *Campylobacter jejuni* bacteremia and Guillain-Barré syndrome in a patient with GVHD after allogeneic BMT. *Bone Marrow Transplantation, 13,* 349–51.

Harvey, C. J., Peniket, A. J., Miszkiel, K. *et al.* (2000). MR angiographic diagnosis of cerebral venous sinus thrombosis following allogeneic bone marrow transplantation. *Bone Marrow Transplantation, 25,* 791–5.

Hentschke, P., Hagglund, H., Mattsson, J. *et al.* (1999). Bilateral subdural haematomas following lumbar puncture in three haematopoietic stem cell transplant recipients. *Bone Marrow Transplantation, 24,* 1033–5.

Hibi, S., Misawa, A., Tamai, M. *et al.* (1995). Severe rhabdomyolysis associated with tacrolimus. *Lancet, 346,* 702 (Letter).

Higman, M. A., Port, J. D., Beauchamp, N. J., & Chen, A. R. (2000). Reversible leukoencephalopathy associated with re-infusion of DMSO preserved stem cells. *Bone Marrow Transplantation, 26,* 797–800.

Hilt, D., Buchholz, D., Krumholz, A. *et al.* (1983). Herpes zoster ophthalmicus and delayed contralateral hemiparesis caused by cerebral angiitis; diagnosis and management approaches. *Annals of Neurology, 14,* 543–553.

Hinchey, J., Chaves, C., Appignani, B. *et al.* (1996). A reversible posterior leucoencephalopathy syndrome. *New England Journal of Medicine, 334,* 494–500.

Hotson, J. R. & Pedley, T. A. (1976). The neurological complications of cardiac transplantation. *Brain, 99,* 673–94.

Hoyt, R., Szer, J., & Grigg, A. (2000). Neurological events associated with the infusion of cryopreserved bone marrow and/or peripheral blood progenitor cells. *Bone Marrow Transplantation, 25,* 1285–1287.

Hugh-Jones, K. & Shaw, P. J. (1985). No convulsions in children on high-dose busulphan. *Lancet, 1,* 220 (Letter).

Hughes, R.A.C., Gabriel, C. M., Goldman, J. M., & Lucas, S. (1999). Vasculitic neuropathy in association with chronic graft-versus-host disease. *Journal of the Neurological Sciences,* **168,** 68–70.

Hwang, T.-L., Yung, W.K.A., Estey, E. H., & Fields, W. S. (1985). Central nervous system toxicity with high-dose Ara-C. *Neurology,* **35,** 1475–9.

Imrie, K. R., Couture, F., Turner, C. C. *et al.* (1994). Peripheral neuropathy following high-dose etoposide and autologous bone marrow transplantation. *Bone Marrow Transplantation,* **13,** 77–9.

Irving, I., Cooper, M. & Durrant, S. (2000). Sciatic nerve compression following bone marrow harvest. *Bone Marrow Transplantation,* **26,** 705–6.

Jaecle, K. A., Przepiorka, D., Birdwell, R. R. *et al.* (1997). Favourable response of progressive multifocal leucoencephalopathy (PML) to treatment with interleukin-2. *Neurology,* **48** (Suppl 2), A82 (Abstract).

Jantunen, E., Piilonen, A., Volin, L. *et al.* (2000a). Diagnostic aspects of invasive *Aspergillus* infections in allogeneic BMT recipients. *Bone Marrow Transplantation,* **25,** 867–871.

Jantunen, E., Ruutu, P., Piilonen, A. *et al.* (2000b). Treatment and outcome of invasive *Aspergillus* infections in allogeneic BMT recipients. *Bone Marrow Transplantation,* **26,** 759–762.

June, C. H., Thompson, C. B., Kennedy, M. S. *et al.* (1985). Profound hypomagnesemia and renal magnesium wasting associated with the use of cyclosporine for marrow transplantation. *Transplantation,* **39,** 620–4.

Kahan, D. B. (1989). Cyclosporine. *New England Journal of Medicine,* **321,** 1725–38.

Kantarjian H, O'Brien, Smith, T. *et al.* (1999). Treatment of Philadelphia-chromosome positive early chronic phase myelogenous leukemia with daily doses of interferon and low-dose cytarabine. *Journal of Clinical Oncology,* **17,** 284–292.

Karlin, J., (1993). Herpes zoster ophthalmicus; the virus strikes back. *Annals of Ophthalmology,* **25,** 208–215.

Kawano, Y., Miyazaki, T., Watanabe, T. *et al.* (2000). HLA-mismatched CD34-selected stem cell transplant complicated by HHV-6 reactivation in the central nervous system. *Bone Marrow Transplantation,* **25,** 787–790.

Kelly, P., Staunton, H., Lawler, M. *et al.* (1996). Multifocal remitting-relapsing cerebral demyelination 20 years following allogenic bone marrow transplantation. *Journal of Neuropathology and Experimental Neurology,* **55,** 992–998.

Koc, Y., Miller, K. B., Schenkein, D. P. *et al.* (2000). Varicella zoster virus infections following allogeneic bone marrow transplantation: frequency, risk factors, and clinical outcome. *Biology of Blood and Marrow Transplantation,* **6,** 44–49.

Kruger, H. U., Schuler, U., Zimmerman, R., & Ehninger, G. (1988). No severe drug interaction of fluconazole, a triazole anti fungal agent, with cyclosporin. *Bone Marrow Transplantation,* **3** (Suppl 1), 271.

Lay, C. L., Mokri, B., & Campbell, J. K. (1996). Clinical features of spontaneous low pressure headache. *Neurology,* **46,** A204 (Abstract).

Lieberman, F., Gulati, S. (1996). Intracranial hypotension following bone marrow 'donation'. *Neurology,* **42,** 163.

Liedtke, W., Quabeck, K., Beelen, D. W. *et al.* (1994). Recurrent acute inflammatory demyelinating polyradiculitis after allo-

geneic bone marrow transplantation. *Journal of Neurological Science,* **125,** 110–11.

Lind, M. J., Mcwilliam, L., Jip, J. *et al.* (1989). Cyclosporine-associated demyelination following allogeneic bone marrow transplantation. *Hematological Oncology,* **7,** 49–52.

Ljungman, P., Lawler, M., Asjo, B. *et al.* (1994). Infection of donor lymphocytes with human T lymphotrophic virus type 1 (HTLV-1) following allogeneic bone marrow transplantation for HTLV-1 positive adult T-cell leukaemia. *British Journal of Haematology,* **88,** 403–5.

Lockman, L. A., Sung, J. H., & Krivit, W. (1991). Acute parkinsonian syndrome with demyelinating leukoencephalopathy in bone marrow transplant recipients. *Pediatric Neurology,* **7,** 457–463.

Marcus, R. E. & Goldman, J. M. (1984). Convulsions due to high-dose busulphan. *Lancet,* **2,** 1463 (Letter).

Martino, R., Bretagne, S., Rovira, M. *et al.* (2000). Toxoplasmosis after hematopoietic stem cell transplantation. Report of a 5-year survey from the Infectious Disease Working Party of the European Group for Blood and Marrow Transplantation. *Bone Marrow Transplantation,* **25,** 1111–1113.

Maschke, M., Dietrich, U., Prumbaum, M. *et al.* (1999). Opportunistic CNS infections after bone marrow transplantation. *Bone Marrow Transplantation,* **23,** 1167–1176.

Memon, M., deMagalhaes-Silverman, M., Bloom, E. J. *et al.* (1995). Reversible cyclosporine-induced cortical blindness in allogeneic bone marrow transplant recipients. *Bone Marrow Transplantation,* **15,** 283–6.

Mizawa, A., Takeuchi, Y., Hibi, S. *et al.* (2000). FK506-induced intractable leukoencephalopathy following allogeneic bone marrow transplantation. *Bone Marrow Transplantation,* **25,** 331–4.

Mohrmann, R. L., Mah, V., & Vinters, H. V. (1990). Neuropathologic findings after bone marrow transplantation: an autopsy study. *Human Pathology,* **21,** 630–9.

Molloy, F., Floeter, M., Syed, N. *et al.* (2001). Thalidomide neuropathy in patients treated for metastatic prostate cancer. *Muscle & Nerve,* **24,** 1050–1057.

Mookerjee, B. O. & Vogelsang, G. (1997). Human herpes virus-6 encephalitis after bone marrow transplantation: successful treatment with ganciclovir. *Bone Marrow Transplantation,* **20,** 905–906.

Mott, S. H., Packer, R. J., Vezine, L. G. *et al.* (1995). Encephalopathy with parkinsonian features in children following bone marrow transplantations and high dose amphotericin B. *Annals of Neurology,* **37,** 810–814.

Murphy, C. P., Harden, E. A., & Thompson, J. M. (1992). Generalized seizure secondary to high-dose busulfan therapy. *Annals of Pharmacology,* **26,** 30–1.

Murphy, P., Parker, A., & Hutchinson, R. M. (1994). High-grade pyrexia following bone marrow transplantation as a neurotoxic complication of high-dose chemotherapy and radiotherapy in the UKALL XII trial. *Bone Marrow Transplantation,* **13,** 229–31.

Myers, S. E. & Williams, S. F. (1994). Guillian-Barré syndrome after autologous bone marrow transplantation for breast cancer: report of 2 cases. *Bone Marrow Transplantation,* **13,** 341–4.

Nelson, K. R. & McQuillen, M. P. (1988). Neurologic complications of graft-versus-host disease. *Neurologic Clinics*, **6**, 389–403.

Ochonisky, S., Verroust, J., Bastuji-Garin, S. *et al.* (1994). Thalidomide neuropathy incidence and clinicoelectrophysiologic findings in 42 patients. *Archives of Dermatology*, **130**, 66–69.

Oliverio, P. J., Frankel, S. R., Mitchell, S. A., Restrepo, L., & Tornatore, C. S. (2000). Reversible tacrolimus-induced neurotoxicity to the brain stem. *American Journal of Neuroradiology*, **21**, 1251–4.

Onose, M., Kawanishi, C., Onishi, H. *et al.* (2002). Neuroleptic malignant syndrome following BMT. *Bone Marrow Transplantation*, **29**, 803–4 (letter).

Openshaw, H., Slatkin, N. E., Parker, P. M., & Forman, S. J. (1995). Immune-mediated myelopathy after allogeneic marrow transplantation. *Bone Marrow Transplantation*, **15**, 633–6.

Openshaw, H., Stuve, O., Antel, J. P. *et al.* (2000). Multiple sclerosis flares associated with recombinant granulocyte colony stimulating factor. *Neurology*, **54**, 2147–2150.

Openshaw, H. O., Slatkin, N. E., & Parker, P. (1996). Thalidomide neuropathy in bone marrow transplantation. *Neurology*, **46**, A232 (Abstract).

Openshaw, H. O., Slatkin, N. E., & Smith, E. (1997). Eye movement disorders in bone marrow transplant patients on cyclosporin and ganciclovir. *Bone Marrow Transplantation*, **19**, 503–5.

Padovan, C. S., Bise, K., Hahn, J. *et al.* (1999). Angiitis of the central nervous system after allogeneic bone transplantation? *Stroke*, **30**, 1651–1656.

Padovan, C. S., Gerbitz, A., Sostak, P. *et al.* (2001). Cerebral involvement in graft-versus-host disease after murine bone marrow transplantation. *Neurology*, **56**, 1106–1108.

Padovan, C. S., Yousry, T. A., Schleuning, M. *et al.* (1998). Neurological and neuroradiological findings in long-term survivors of allogeneic bone marrow transplantation. *Annals of Neurology*, **43**, 627–633.

Panullo, S. C., Reich, J. B., Krol, G. *et al.* (1993). MRI changes in intracranial hypotension. *Neurology*, **43**, 919–26.

Parizel, P. M., Snoeck, H., van den Hauwe, L. *et al.* (1997). Cerebral complications of murine monoclonal CD3 antibody (OKT3): CT and MR findings. *American Journal of Neuroradiology*, **18**, 1935–1938.

Patchell, R. A. (1994). Neurological complications of organ transplantation. *Annals of Neurology*, **36**, 688–703.

Patchell, R. A., White, C. L. III, Clark, A. W. *et al.* (1985). Neurologic complications of bone marrow transplantation. *Neurology*, **35**, 300–6.

Patterson, T. F., Kirkpatrick, W. R., White, M. *et al.* (2000). Invasive aspergillosis. Disease spectrum, treatment practices, and outcomes. *Medicine*, **79**, 250–260.

Perry, A., Mehta, J., Iveson, T. *et al.* (1994). Guillain-Barré syndrome after bone marrow transplantation. *Bone Marrow Transplantation*, **14**, 165–7.

Phanthumchinda, K., Intragumtornchai, T., & Kasantikul, V. (1991). Stroke-like syndrome, mineralizing microangiopathy, and neuroaxonal dystrophy following intrathecal methotrexate therapy. *Neurology*, **41**, 1847–8.

Pomeranz, S., Naparstek, E., Ashkenazi, E. *et al.* (1994). Intracranial hematomas following bone marrow transplantation. *Journal of Neurology*, **241**, 252–256.

Priest, J. R., Ramsay, N.K.C., Steinberg, P. G. *et al.* (1982). A syndrome of thrombosis and hemorrhage complicating L-asparaginase therapy for childhood acute lymphoblastic leukemia. *Journal of Pediatrics*, **100**, 984–9.

Provenzale, J. M. & Graham, M. L. (1996). Reversible leukoencephalopathy associated with graft-versus-host disease: MR findings. *American Journal of Neuroradiology*, **17**, 1290–4.

Re, A. & Giachetti, R. (1999). Acute disseminated encephalomyelitis (ADEM) after autologous peripheral blood stem cell transplant for non-Hodgkin's lymphoma. *Bone Marrow Transplantation*, **24**, 1351–1354.

Re, D., Bamborschke, S., Feiden, W. *et al.* (1999). Progressive multifocal leukoencephalopathy after autologous bone marrow transplantation and alpha-interferon immunotherapy. *Bone Marrow Transplantation*, **23**, 295–298.

Reece, D. E., Frei-Lahr, D. A., Shepherd, J. D. *et al.* (1991). Neurological complications in allogeneic bone marrow transplant patients receiving cyclosporine. *Bone Marrow Transplantation*, **8**, 393–401.

Richardson, E. P., Jr. (1988). Progressive multifocal leukoencephalopathy 30 years later. *New England Journal of Medicine*, **318**, 315–16.

Rieux, C., Gautheret-Dejean, A., Challine-Lehmann, D. *et al.* (1998). Human herpesvirus-6 meningoencephalitis in a recipient of an unrelated allogeneic bone marrow transplantation. *Transplantation*, **65**, 1408–1411.

Roemer, E., Blau, I., Basara, N., Kiehl, M. *et al.* (2001). Toxoplasmosis, a severe complication in allogeneic hematopoietic stem cell transplantation: successful treatment strategies during a 5-year single-center experience. *Clinical Infections Diseases*, **32**, E1–8.

Roskrow, M. A., Kelsey, S. M., McCarthy, M. *et al.* (1992). Selective autonomic neuropathy as a novel complication of BMT. *Bone Marrow Transplantation*, **10**, 469–70.

Rouah, E., Gruber, R., Shearer, W. *et al.* (1988). Graft-versus-host disease in the central nervous system: a real entity? *American Journal of Clinical Pathology*, **89**, 543–6.

Rubin, A. M. & Kang, H. (1987). Cerebral blindness and encephalopathy with cyclosporine A toxicity. *Neurology*, **37**, 1072–6.

Rudnicki, S. A. & Harik, S. I. (1997). Peripheral and central nervous system dysfunction in a patient with Waldenström's macroglobulinemia. *Neurology*, **48** (Suppl 2), A309 (Abstract).

Sable, G. A. & Donowitz, G. R. (1994). Infections in bone marrow transplant recipients. *Clinical Infectious Diseases*, **18**, 273–81.

Sadoh, D., Hawk, J., & Panayiotopoulos, C. (1999). Chronodispersion in patients on thalidomide. *Clinical Neurophysiology*, **110**, 735–739.

Sanders, J., Sale, F. E., Ramberg, R. *et al.* (1982). Glioblastoma multiforme in a patient with acute lymphoblastic leukemia who received a marrow transplant. *Transplantation Proceedings*, **14**, 770–4.

Schmidley, J. W. & Galloway, P. (1990). Polymyositis following autologous bone marrow transplantation in Hodgkin's disease. *Neurology*, **40**, 1003–4.

Schuchter, L. M., Wingard, J. R., Piantadosi, S. *et al.* (1989). Herpes zoster infection after autologous bone marrow transplantation. *Blood,* **74,** 1424–7.

Schwartz, D. L., Schechter, G. P., Seltzer, S., & Chauncey, T. R. (2000). Radiation myelitis following allogeneic stem cell transplantation and consolidation radiotherapy for non-Hodgkin's lymphoma. *Bone Marrow Transplantation,* **26,** 1355–63.

Shah, A. K. (1997). Cyclosporine (CSA) neurotoxicity in bone marrow transplant (BMT) recipients: clinical neuro-imaging and electro physiological characteristics. *Neurology,* **48** (Suppl 2), A82 (Abstract).

Sharkey, J. & Butcher, S. P. (1994). Immunophilins mediate the neuro-protective effects of FK506 in focal cerebral ischemia. *Nature,* **371,** 336–9.

Shbarou, R.J.M., Chao, N. J., & Morgenlander, J. C. (2000). Cyclosporin A-related cerebral vasculopathy. *Bone Marrow Transplantation,* **26,** 801–4.

Shutter, L. A., Green, J. P., Neuman, N. J. *et al.* (1993). Cortical blindness and white matter lesions in a patient receiving FK506 after liver transplantation. *Neurology,* **43,** 2417–18.

Sloane, J. P., Lwin, K. Y., Gore, M. E. *et al.* (1985). Disturbance of blood-brain barrier after bone marrow transplantation. *Lancet,* **2,** 280–281.

Small, S. L., Fukui, M. B., Bramblett, G. T. *et al.* (1996). Immunosuppression induced leukoencephalopathy from tacrolimus (FK506). *Annals of Neurology,* **40,** 575–80.

Smith, C.I.E., Aarli, J. A., Biverfeld, P. *et al.* (1983). Myasthenia gravis after bone marrow transplantation evidence for a donor origin. *New England Journal of Medicine,* **309,** 1565–8.

Smith, D. M., Ness, M. J., Landmark, J. D. *et al.* (1990). Recurrent neurologic symptoms during peripheral stem cell apheresis in two patients with intracranial metastases. *Journal of Clinical Apheresis,* **5,** 70–3.

Snider, S., Bashir, R., & Bierman, P. (1994). Neurologic complications after high-dose chemotherapy and autologous bone marrow transplantation for Hodgkin's disease. *Neurology,* **44,** 681–4.

Socie, G., Curtis, R. E., Deeg, H. J. *et al.* (2000). New malignant diseases after allogeneic marrow transplantation for childhood acute leukemia. *Journal of Clinical Oncology,* **18,** 348–357.

Straathof, C.S.M., Kortbeek, L. M., Roerdink, H. *et al.* (2001). A solitary spinal cord toxoplasma lesion after peripheral stem-cell transplantation. *Journal of Neurology,* **248,** 814–815.

Sugar, A. M., Saunders, C., Sidelson, B. A., & Bernard, D. B. (1989). Interaction of fluconazole and cyclosporine. *Annals of Internal Medicine,* **110,** 844 (Letter).

Sumikuma, T., Kikuta, T., Hirai, H., Sudo, Y. *et al.* (1999). Discrimination of leukoencephalopathy from leukemic cell invasion by MR spectroscopy in a patient with acute lymphoblastic leukemia. *Rinsho-Ketsueki—Japanese Journal of Clinical Hematology,* **40,** 305–310.

Sylvestre, D. L., Sandson, T. A., & Nachmanoff, D. B. (1991). Transient brachial plexopathy as a complication of internal jugular vein cannulation. *Neurology,* **41,** 760.

Tahsildar, H. I., Remler, B. F., Creger, R. J. *et al.* (1996). Delayed, transient encephalopathy after marrow transplantation: case reports and MRI findings in four patients. *Journal of Neuro-oncology,* **27,** 241–50.

Teksam, M., Casey, S. O., Michel, E., & Truwit, C. L. (2001). Subarachnoid hemorrhage associated with cyclosporine A neurotoxicity in a bone-marrow transplant recipient. *Neuroradiology,* **43,** 242–245.

Teshima, T., Myoshi, T., & Ono, M. (1996). Cyclosporine-related encephalopathy following allogeneic bone marrow transplantation. *International Journal of Hematology,* **63,** 161–4.

Thompson, C. B., June, C. H., Sullivan, K. M., & Thomas, E. D. (1984). Association between cyclosporin neurotoxicity and hypomagnesemia. *Lancet,* **2,** 1116–20.

Thompson, C. B., Sanders, J. E., Flournoy, N. *et al.* (1986). The risks of central nervous system relapse and leukoencephalopathy in patients receiving bone marrow transplantation for acute leukemia. *Blood,* **67,** 195–9.

Tiacci, E., Luppi, M., Barozzi, P. *et al.* (2000). Fatal herpes virus-6 encephalitis in a recipient of a T-cell-depleted peripheral blood stem cell transplant from a 3-loci mismatched related donor. *Haematologica,* **85,** 94–97.

Tseng, S., Pak, G., Washenik, K. *et al.* (1996). Rediscovering thalidomide: a review of its mechanism of action, side effects and potential uses. *American Academy of Dermatology,* **35,** 969–979.

Uoshima, N., Karasuno, T., Yagi, T. *et al.* (2000). Late-onset cyclosporine-induced cerebral blindness with abnormal SPECT imaging in a patient undergoing unrelated bone marrow transplantation. *Bone Marrow Transplantation,* **26,** 105–8.

Urbano-Marquez, A., Estruch, R., Grau, J. M. *et al.* (1986). Inflammatory myopathy associated with chronic graft-versus-host disease. *Neurology,* **36,** 1091–3.

Valbonesi, M., Occhini, D., Frisoni, R. *et al.* (1988). Plasma exchange for the management of cyclosporin A-induced hypertriglyceridemia. *International Journal of Artificial Organs,* **11,** 209–11.

Valentine, A., Meyers, C., Kling, M. *et al.* (1998). Mood and cognitive side effects of interferon-alpha therapy. *Seminars in Oncology,* **25,** 39–47.

van Besien, K., Prezepiorka, D., Mehra, R. *et al.* (1996). Impact of preexisting CNS involvement on the outcome of bone marrow transplantation in adult hematologic malignancies. *Journal of Clinical Oncology,* **14,** 3036–42.

Velu, T., Debusscher, L., & Stryckmans, P. A. (1985). Cyclosporine-associated fatal convulsions. *Lancet,* **1,** 219 (Letter).

Wainright, M.., Martin, P., Morse, R. *et al.* (2001). Human herpesvirus 6 limbic encephalitis after stem cell transplantation. *Annals of Neurology,* **50,** 612–619.

Walker, R. W., Allen, J. C., Rosen, G. *et al.* (1986). Transient cerebral dysfunction secondary to high-dose methotrexate. *Journal of Clinical Oncology,* **4,** 1845–50.

Wall, J. G., Weiss, R. B., Norton, L. *et al.* (1989). Arterial thrombosis associated with adjuvant chemotherapy for breast carcinoma—a cancer and leukemia group B study. *American Journal of Medicine,* **87,** 501–4.

Walters, M. C., Patience, M., Leisenring, W. *et al.* (1996). Bone marrow transplantation for sickle cell disease. *New England Journal of Medicine,* **335,** 369–76.

Walters, M. C., Sullivan, K. M., Bernaudin, R. *et al.* (1995). Neurologic complications of allogeneic marrow transplantation for sickle cell anemia. *Blood,* **85,** 879–84.

Wasserstein, P. H. & Honig, L. S. (1996). Parkinsonism during cyclosporine treatment. *Bone Marrow Transplantation,* **18,** 649–50.

Wen, P. Y., Alyea, E. P., Simon, D. *et al.* (1997). Guillain-Barré syndrome following allogeneic bone marrow transplantation. *Neurology,* **49,** 1711–1714.

Williams, A. C. & Franklin, I. (1989). Migraine after bone marrow transplantation. *Lancet,* **2,** 1286–7.

Winston, D. J., Gale, R. P., & Meyer, D. V. (1979). Infectious complications of human bone marrow transplantation. *Medicine,* **58,** 1–31.

Wiznitzer, M., Packer, R. J., August, C. S., & Burkey, E. D. (1984). Neurological complications of bone marrow transplantation in childhood. *Annals of Neurology,* **16,** 569–76.

94 Endocrine complications

DONALD J. CHISHOLM

St. Vincent's Hospital and University of New South Wales, Sydney, Australia

Introduction

A variety of endocrine complications can occur during or after the period of intensive management of patients undergoing hematopoietic stem cell (HSC) transplantation. Arbitrarily these complications can be divided into early complications occurring during or close to the period of hospitalization for transplant, or late complications occurring months to years after the transplantation event. These complications vary from being quite common (e.g., steroid-induced diabetes mellitus) to very rare (e.g., hypoadrenalism).

Early complications

Disturbances of blood glucose control

Hyperglycemia

Significant hyperglycemia is uncommon in children or young adults undergoing HSC transplantation, but is a relatively frequent occurrence in patients in the middle-aged or older age group. The hyperglycemic state generally conforms to the pattern of non–insulin–dependent or type 2 (maturity onset) diabetes, although insulin therapy is nearly always required. The major factor in development of the hyperglycemia is the use of glucocorticosteroids (prednisolone or dexamethasone), but stress and infective or inflammatory processes may contribute significantly. Glucocorticosteroids act by enhancing hepatic glucose output and causing insulin resistance; inflammatory and infective processes cause insulin resistance by mechanisms that are still not well understood but include "stress hormone" responses (Flier & Moses, 1989); increased levels of tumor necrosis factor-α (TNF-α) due to inflammation or infection may also be important in generating insulin resistance via effects on insulin receptor substrate I (Hotamisligil *et al.,* 1996). Lorini and colleagues (1995) reported increased insulin and C-peptide levels in patients with normoglycemia after autologous or allogeneic transplantation, particularly evident in patients prepared with a conditioning regimen that contained total body irradiation (TBI), and interpreted as a state of insulin resistance. A rare contributor to the development of hyper-glycemia is the use of pentamidine for treatment for pneumocystis pneumonitis, which may cause direct pancreatic beta cell damage (Bouchard *et al.,* 1982) (see also below).

Treatment In the presence of corticosteroid therapy, inflammation, or infection, insulin is usually needed to adequately control hyperglycemia. In the early stages after transplantation when nutrition is being given parenterally, it is usually best to use a constant rate intravenous infusion of insulin, titrating the dose to the blood glucose level and aiming for blood glucose levels of approximately 6 to 10 mmol/1. Blood glucose monitoring at this time poses a problem, as one generally wishes to avoid fingerprick or cutaneous puncture in the presence of a low platelet count, and frequent disconnection of the central line for blood sampling is undesirable. It is generally possible to achieve satisfactory, if not ideal, blood glucose control on the basis of two or three blood glucose measurements every 24 hours, when the delivery of intravenous glucose is maintained constant, and the insulin is administered in the glucose-containing solution. This arrangement offers the safeguard that interruption of intravenous glucose delivery will also be associated with interruption of insulin administration. The required insulin infusion rate is quite variable and may range from 1 to greater than 20 units per hour. In fact, a situation is sometimes experienced where the insulin resistance is so great, and the insulin dose-response curve so shifted to the right (see Fig. 94.1), that further increases in insulin dosage will not reduce blood glucose levels, and the desired result must be achieved by reducing the glucose content of the parenteral fluids.

Once the patient has returned to oral nutrition, it is usually appropriate to introduce subcutaneous insulin injections. As these patients normally retain some endogenous insulin secretion, a single prebreakfast injection of combined quick-acting (neutral) and intermediate-acting insulin will often achieve adequate glycemic control. During periods of infection or stress it may be necessary to give supplementary injections of quick-acting insulin according to a sliding scale, based on blood glucose levels. Administration of glucocorticosteroids seems to have its greatest hyperglycemic effect after meals, so that it is important to use an insulin regimen that maintains

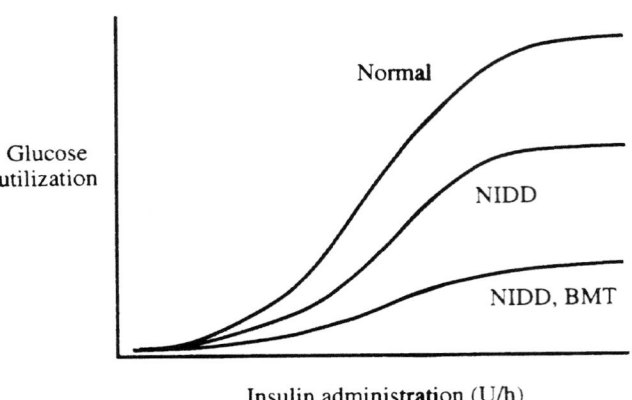

Fig. 94.1. A diagrammatic illustration of the insulin dose-response curve showing the relative insulin resistance of non–insulin-dependent diabetes (NIDD) and the greater insulin resistance, due to steroids, inflammation, with or without infection, in subjects with diabetes after HSC transplantation.

high insulin levels from breakfast through to the evening meal, with lower levels during the night. A morning dose of neutral plus intermediate-acting insulin usually achieves this objective.

It is important to make anticipatory reductions in insulin dosage when steroid doses are reduced, or when treatment of an infection is effective, otherwise hypoglycemia may occur.

Rarely, patients for HSC transplant have pre-existing insulin-dependent (Type 1) diabetes. As these patients have a complete lack of endogenous insulin secretion, there is a tendency for greater fluctuations of blood glucose levels, necessitating more intensive blood glucose monitoring and more intensive insulin administration regimens. Pre-existing Type 2 diabetes can be dealt with on the same basis as for steroid/stress-induced diabetes, but may confer an added risk of morbidity (Schouten *et al.*, 1990).

Hypoglycemia

Hypoglycemia seen in HSC transplant patients is usually the result of an imbalance between insulin, or other hypoglycemic medication, and nutrition or steroid dosage. However, the agent pentamidine may cause an acute release of insulin believed to be associated with beta cell damage, and result in significant hypoglycemia, which may be followed later by hyperglycemia (Bouchard *et al.*, 1982).

Corticosteroid side effects (iatrogenic Cushing's[1] syndrome)

Cushingoid features are not prominent in the early stages after allogeneic transplant, but may begin to make their appearance toward the end of hospitalization. Reduced host defense against infection is an inevitable consequence of high-dose steroid therapy, as with other immune suppressive agents.

[1] Harvey Cushing, American neurosurgeon, 1869–1939.

Abnormal thyroid function tests (sick euthyroid state)

As with any severe illness, and with high-dose steroid therapy, circulating levels of triiodothyronine (T3) are usually very low. The thyroxine level may also be mildly or moderately depressed, owing to reduced thyroid-binding proteins. However, the free thyroxine level is usually within the normal range, and a normal or below normal thyroid-stimulating hormone (TSH) level is a clear indicator that the patient does not have primary hypothyroidism (Turnbridge, 1987). Levels of the biologically inert product of thyroxine, reverse T3, are likely to be elevated, but are not usually measured, as reverse T3 levels do not generally have diagnostic significance.

Inappropriate antidiuretic hormone syndrome

A state of water overload with hyponatremia and relatively low urea and creatinine levels with relatively high urinary sodium excretion may occur as an uncommon side effect of cyclophosphamide, and possibly other cytotoxic agents used at high-dosage, as a consequence of an infective process or due to a perturbation of brain or lung function. It has also been described accompanying abdominal pain and preceding the development of skin rash in patients with varicella zoster infection posttransplant (Drakos *et al.*, 1993; Szabo *et al.*, 2000). Mild to moderate fluid restriction will usually rectify the problem, but if the condition is severe or prolonged, demeclocycline may be used to oppose the effects of antidiuretic hormone (ADH) on the kidney.

Hypoadrenalism

This is a rare occurrence but has been encountered twice in our experience: once due to adrenal hemorrhage associated with septicemia and once in a patient with prior bilateral adrenalectomy. When high doses of glucocorticosteroids are being used, mineralocorticoid (fludrocortisone) requirement is likely to be minimal. But when glucocorticosteroids are reduced to a low maintenance level, a small dose of mineralocorticoid (fludrocortisone 0.05–0.2 mg) may be required to avoid hyponatremia, hypotension, and hyperkalemia.

Sex hormone levels

As with any severe illness, circulating levels of gonadotrophins and estrogen (in females) or testosterone (in males) may be depressed.

Late complications

Impaired glucose tolerance and dyslipidemia

When 23 long-term survivors of HSC transplantation in childhood were studied 3–18 years posttransplant, significant abnormalities of glucose and lipid metabolism were found (Table 94.1 and Fig. 94.2) (Taskinen *et al.*, 2000). Twelve (52%) had

Table 94.1. *Manifestations of the metabolic syndrome*

| | Number of participants with characteristic | | | |
Characteristic	BMT group (n = 23)	ALL group (n = 13)	Healthy controls (n = 23)	Pa
Hyperinsulinemia	12 (52%)	4 (31%)	0	.0002
Abnormal glucose metabolism	10 (43%)	1 (8%)	0	.001
Hypertriglyceridemia	9 (39%)	1 (8%)	1 (4%)	.01
Low HDL-cholesterol	6 (26%)	1 (8%)	1 (4%)	.10
Hyperuricemia	7 (30%)	1 (8%)	2 (9%)	.14
Microalbuminuria	4 (17%)	0	1 (4%)	.34
Overweight	6 (26%)	1 (8%)	1 (4%)	.10
Abdominal obesity	8 (35%)	2 (15%)	2 (9%)	.07

Abbreviations: BMT, bone marrow transplantation; ALL, acute lymphoblastic leukemia.
a Fisher's exact test.
Reproduced, with permission, from Taskinen *et al.* (2000).

insulin resistance, including impaired glucose tolerance in 6 and type 2 diabetes in 4. The core signs of the metabolic syndrome (sometimes known as syndrome X)—hyperinsulinemia and hypertryglyceridemia combined—were present in 9. The frequency of insulin-resistance increased with time posttransplant. Abdominal obesity, though not excess weight, was common in the patients with insulin resistance. We are not aware of a systematic assessment of the features of the insulin resistance syndrome after HSC transplantation in adult life. Measurement of serum lipids, fasting blood glucose and serum insulin is recommended, particularly for those undergoing transplantation in childhood.

Iatrogenic Cushing's syndrome

Cushingoid features tend to develop progressively depending on the steroid dose required to achieve suppression of graft-versus-host disease (GVHD); they include central obesity, moonface, buffalo hump, fragile skin, higher blood pressure levels, and bone demineralization. These side effects tend to be less troublesome and probably more reversible in younger people, and may be slightly less prominent if, when a chronic maintenance dose is reached, the dosage is given as a single morning dose or a second daily dose. Proximal myopathy and psychological problems may also be significant; rarely patients can develop an acute steroid psychosis when on high doses of steroids.

If high doses of steroids have been used for many months and are then withdrawn abruptly, hypoadrenalism may be evidenced by malaise, lethargy, nausea, hypotension, and musculoskeletal pains; as the renin-angiotensin-aldosterone axis is relatively intact in this situation, hyponatremia or hyperkalemia are usually absent. A Synacthen test may be performed if there is doubt about the diagnosis. In this situation, reintroduction of a physiologic replacement dose of steroid (for example, 7.5 mg/day of prednisolone) is appropriate, followed by a gradual reduction of dosage to achieve withdrawl over 5 to 10 weeks.

Gonadal dysfunction (see also Chapters 84 and 97)

Disturbance of gonadal function is a common consequence of TBI or of chemotherapy with such agents as cyclophosphamide or busulfan (Shalet *et al.*, 1995). In general, the greatest damage occurs to germ cells, resulting in a substantial elevation of follicle-stimulating hormone (FSH) levels in both sexes, although in males severe damage has been reported to the Leydig[1] cell (LC) compartment as well (Chattergee *et al.*, 2001). In the male, testosterone and luteinizing hormone (LH) levels tend to remain fairly normal, although in Chattergee's study (2001), two types of LC dysfunction were described: a compensated type with high LH and normal testosterone levels, and an uncompensated type (premature andropause) with high LH and low testosterone levels. However, in the female, estrogen production is low and LH levels are elevated, but to a lesser degree than follicle stimulating hormone (FSH). In general, the impairment of gonadal function is less, and the likelihood of recovery greater, in younger people and in people treated with cytotoxic chemotherapy alone, rather than TBI and chemotherapy. The dosage of irradiation or chemotherapy is also important.

In prepubescent girls, delayed puberty will occur in more than 50% of cases, the delay being related to the dosage of irradiation or chemotherapy and to the age at which treatment takes place.

In prepubescent males, one must expect delayed puberty in 70% to 90% of cases, and spermatogenesis may be severely impaired even after puberty progresses.

Precocious puberty, probably related to disturbed hypothalamic function after irradiation, is an occasional but rare occurrence after HSC transplantation in young children.

In postpubertal females HSC transplantation with TBI or intensive chemotherapy inevitably leads to anovulation, low

[1] Franz von Leydig, German zoologist and comparative anatomist, 1821-1908.

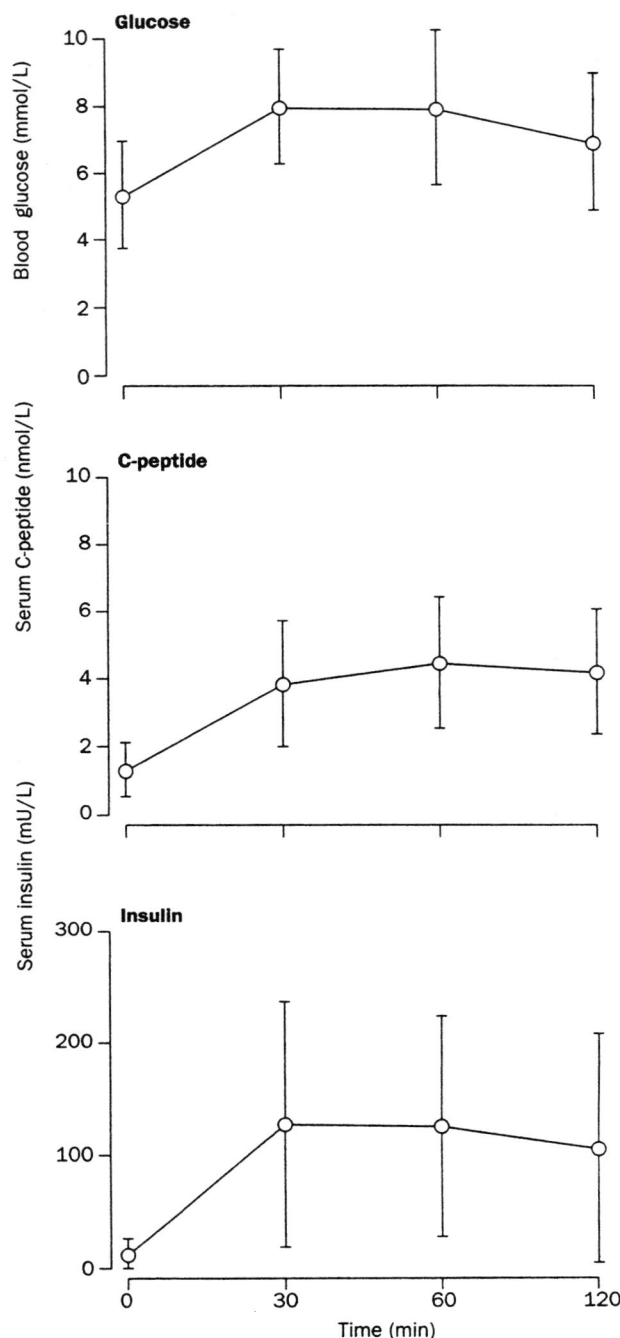

Fig. 94.2. Mean blood glucose, serum C-peptide, and serum insulin concentrations during oral glucose tolerance testing in bone marrow transplantation patients. Reproduced, with permission, from Taskinen *et al.* (2000).

estrogen levels, and substantial elevation of gonadotrophins. Clinically these findings may be associated with menopausal symptoms in a majority of patients and a reduced libido in about half (Heimpel *et al.*, 1991); the onset of these problems appears to be similar whether chemotherapy or TBI is used (Chatterjee *et al.*, 1994a).

Erectile dysfunction is a well-recognized complication of SCT transplantation and major contributory factors include hypogonadism, psychogenic factors, and cavernosal arterial insufficiency (Chattergee *et al.*, 2000).

Recovery of gonadal function may occur after a period of some years: 9 of 41 patients treated with TBI recovered gonadal function in 3 to 7 years in one series (Sanders, 1991), although gonadal function deteriorated in two of these. In women a number of pregnancies have occurred posttransplant, but fertility is less likely after TBI than after chemotherapy (summarized by Lipton *et al.*, 1993). Sanders and colleagues (1996) reviewed the experience of the Fred Hutchinson Cancer Center in Seattle. Records of 1,326 postpubertal and 196 prepubertal patients more than 12 years of age after marrow transplantation performed between 1971 and 1992 were reviewed. Among 708 postpubertal women, 110 recovered normal ovarian function and 32 became pregnant. In addition, 9 formerly prepubertal girls with normal gonadal function became pregnant.

Among 618 postpubertal men, 157 recovered testicular function and partners of 33 became pregnant. An additional two formerly prepubertal men had partners who became pregnant.

There were 115 live births among 146 pregnancies (79%). Spontaneous abortion terminated 4 of 56 (7%) pregnancies for 28 female recipients conditioned with cyclophosphamide only and 6 of 16 (37%) pregnancies for 13 recipients conditioned with a TBI-containing regimen ($P = .02$).

In partners of 28 male cyclophosphamide recipients 4 of 62 (6.4%) pregnancies terminated with spontaneous abortion, but there were no spontaneous abortions among 8 pregnancies of 5 partners of TBI recipients (Fig. 94.3).

Preterm delivery occurred for 8 of 44 (18%) and 5 of 8 (63%) live births for 24 cyclophosphamide and 8 TBI female recipients ($P = .01$). This 25% incidence among all female

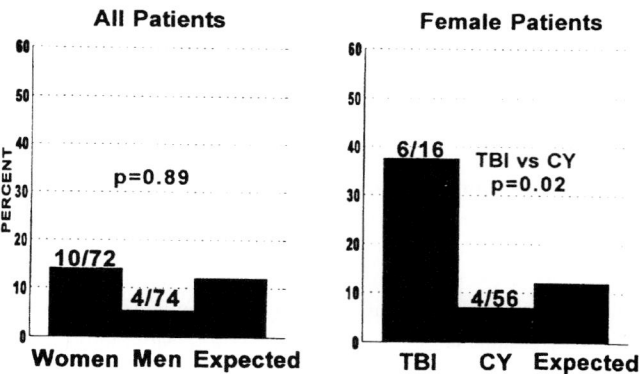

Fig. 94.3. Spontaneous abortion. Incidence of spontaneous abortion for all patients and for female patients. Female patients who received TBI had a significantly greater incidence that those who received cyclophosphamide (CY) ($P = .02$) or the reported (expected) incidence for spontaneous abortion of clinically known pregnancies among the general population. Reproduced, with permission, from Sanders *et al.* (1996).

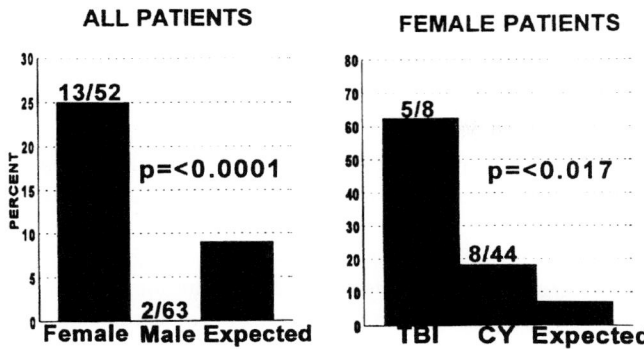

Fig. 94.4. Preterm labor and delivery for live births. Incidence of preterm labor and delivery for 115 live births. Incidence of 25% for all female patients versus incidence among 63 male patients or reported expected incidence in the white population (P = .0001), and 62.5% for female patients who received TBI versus 18% among female cyclophosphamide (CY) recipients (P = .017). Reproduced, with permission, from Sanders *et al.* (1996).

patient pregnancies is higher than the expected incidence of 8%–10% (Fig. 94.4).

The 13 preterm deliveries resulted in 10 low birth weight (LBW, 1.8 to 2.24 kg) and 3 very low birth weight (VLBW, <1.36 kg) infants, for an overall incidence of 25%, which is higher than the expected incidence of 6.5% for the general population (Fig. 94.5). Twelve of the 13 infants were alive at the time of the report. Congenital anomalies were seen among 2 of 52 (3.8%) live-born of female and 6 of 63 (9.5%) live-born of male patients, which is not different from the 13% rate of single congenital anomalies in the general population. These data demonstrated that pregnancies among women who had received a marrow transplant incorporating TBI were likely to be accompanied by an increased risk of spontaneous abortion. Pregnancies among all women who received a marrow transplant were likely to be accompanied by preterm labor and delivery of a low birth weight or very low birth weight baby, who did not seem to be at an increased risk of congenital anomalies. It is possible that there is a long-term adverse effect of TBI on the uterus which may explain these events (Larsen *et al.*, 2000).

Several case reports have been published documenting paternity by men who had undergone transplantation with either myeloablative chemotherapy as conditioning (Shepherd *et al.*, 1996) or a TBI-containing regimen (Jacob, Goodman, & Holmes, 1995).

Treatment A review of the physical, psychological, and social consequences of functional castration consequent on high-dose myeloablative therapy, indicated that involvement of a reproductive endocrinologist is ideal in the management of patients of reproductive potential undergoing HSC transplantation. Ideally this should occur from presentation, but is certainly necessary pretransplant and for long-term follow-up in order to provide endocrine assessment, counseling, and fertility management essential for adequate transplant care (Chatterjee & Goldstone, 1996).

Once the female patient is beyond the early posttransplant period, it is appropriate to consider cyclic estrogen/progesterone therapy to avoid symptoms of estrogen deficiency, and to reduce accelerated atherosclerosis or loss of bone mineral density, which may occur with "early menopause" (and, for bone mineral density, with corticosteroid use). There is no useful therapy to induce ovulation or fertility in this situation and one must hope for spontaneous return of ovarian function (which is unlikely except in younger women not treated with TBI). Although there is no effective therapy for this problem, we are now living in an era where it is possible to harvest and store embryos or ovarian tissue prior to transplant, which could be used for in vitro fertilization at a later time (Meirow, 2000). The use of a gonadotrophin-releasing hormone (GnRH) analogue prior to TBI or cytotoxic therapy has been proposed to suppress gonadotrophins and gonadal function, and to render the gonads less susceptible to damage. Although this could be useful on theoretical grounds, its practicality and likelihood of success are doubtful (Da Cunha, Meistrich, & Nader, 1987).

In postpubertal males, after the early posttransplant phase, LH and testosterone levels will remain normal in the majority of HSC transplantation patients (Heimpel *et al.*, 1991), and normal androgenization, libido, and potency should be maintained, although some male patients will suffer from severe hypogonadism, as evidenced by depressed libido, low testicular volume, elevated FSH and LH levels, and low testosterone levels (Chattergee *et al.*, 2001). Testosterone replacement therapy is often effective for diminished libido. However, a severe impairment of spermatogenic function is invariable and most postpubertal males will be completely azoospermic. Thus, most such recipients will be infertile. A late spontaneous recovery of spermatogenesis occurs in a small percentage of subjects, and is more likely in younger patients and where cyto-

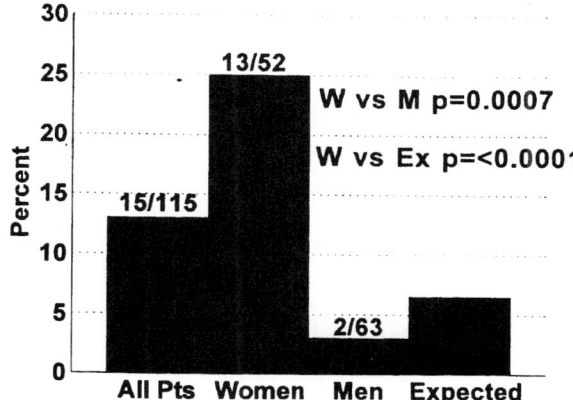

Fig. 94.5. Incidence of neonatal complications of low birth weight (LBW) and very low birth weight (VLBW) infants for all patients, female patients, male patients, and expected rate for general white population. Female patients had a significantly increased incidence of LBW or VLBW babies than did partners of male patients (P = .0007) or the general population (P = .0001). Reproduced, with permission, from Sanders *et al.* (1996).

toxic chemotherapy has been used alone, rather than in combination with TBI (Shalet *et al.,* 1995).

An elevated FSH level is a very strong indication that the patient is azoospermic or has a major impairment of spermatogenic function with a very low chance of fertility. However, there may be a fairly substantial defect in sperm production, even when the FSH level is within normal limits. In general, it is probably unnecessary to undertake a semen analysis if the FSH level is elevated, but if the FSH level returns to normal, semen analysis may be a good guide to prospects of fertility.

There is no effective therapy to improve spermatogenesis after cytotoxic therapy or TBI, and one must simply hope for spontaneous improvement. If there is oligospermia, but a lack of fertility, it may be possible to concentrate motile sperm or use other procedures (such as intracytoplasmic sperm injection, ICSI) to achieve fertility by in vitro fertilization techniques (see Chapter 97).

Cryopreservation of sperm (Redman *et al.,* 1987) should always be considered prior to HSC transplantation, if possible, and can be used for artificial insemination at a later time.

An additional reason for erectile dysfunction in male recipients is cavernosal arterial insufficiency (Chattergee *et al.,* 2000). Patients with erectile dysfunction responded well to a combination of testosterone cypionate 250 mg i.m. monthly for 6 months and sildenafil 50-100 mg orally once or twice weekly (Chattergee, *et al.,* 2002).

Gynecomastia

Gynecomastia (sometimes tender) is an occasional occurrence in males after HSC transplantation (Harris *et al.,* 2001). For reasons that are poorly understood, it may be associated with impaired spermatogenesis and an elevated FSH level, but it may also be associated with the use of therapeutic agents for associated or coincidental conditions (e.g., spironolactone, cimetidine).

Treatment   The condition may respond to withdrawal of causative agent or rectification of testosterone deficiency, when present. However, in many cases, where discomfort or appearance are of concern, surgery is the most useful approach.

Growth (see also Chapter 84)

Impaired growth velocity and impaired growth hormone secretion may occur after chemotherapy, and are a common occurrence after TBI (Sanders, 1991; Shalet *et al.,* 1995). The reduced growth rate after TBI may be due to multiple factors. Impaired growth hormone secretion is often a major factor (Sanders, 1991), and may become more pronounced some years after the irradiation. Growth hormone generates growth mainly by enhancing production of growth factors; impaired growth hormone secretion leads to impaired production of growth factors, especially insulin-like growth factor 1 (IGF-1). It is possible that irradiation of the liver and other tissues also contributes to defective production of IGF-1, and it is

also likely that irradiation of bones impairs skeletal growth. In addition, untreated hypothyroidism, a lack of gonadal steroids, continuing GVHD, poor nutrition, and glucocorticosteroid therapy can all contribute to a reduced growth velocity. There is some evidence that fractionated TBI may cause less subsequent impairment of growth than single-dose irradiation, although this is not clearly established (Shalet *et al.,* 1995).

In a child with impairment of growth after HSC transplantation one should ensure there is adequate nutrition, check for hypothyroidism, and try to establish the lowest acceptable dose of glucocorticosteroids (although not at the expense of increased graft-versus-host activity). Estrogen in females or testosterone levels in males should be checked, as very low levels can contribute to impaired growth velocity; however, gonadal steroid therapy should be approached with great caution as it can accelerate epiphysial fusion and further reduce the eventual adult stature. Once these issues have been dealt with, it may be appropriate to undertake a stimulatory test, such as insulin hypoglycemia, of growth hormone secretion. If there is substantial impairment of the response, growth hormone therapy should be considered. Even if the response to the stimulatory test is relatively normal, in the presence of a very subnormal growth velocity it may be worth undertaking a trial of growth hormone therapy. Alternatively, some authorities recommend a 24-hour assessment of growth hormone secretion to see if the normal spontaneous peaks of growth hormone are present (Blatt *et al.,* 1984), prior to deciding whether growth hormone therapy should be introduced.

Although growth hormone therapy offers the hope of improved growth to children with impaired growth hormone secretion after HSC transplantation, one must anticipate that the response will be less satisfactory than in children with growth hormone deficiency and no other complicating disease process. The reasons for the less satisfactory response relate to the other contributing factors mentioned above; in particular, it has been shown that children treated with growth hormone after spinal irradiation have substantially less linear spinal growth than other children treated with growth hormone.

Other abnormalities of hypothalamic-pituitary and adrenal function

Other abnormalities of hypothalamic-pituitary function may occur after irradiation to this region with a progressively increasing frequency according to radiation dosage. With doses up to 7,500 cGy local irradiation to the hypothalamic-pituitary area, given for cerebral tumors, the risk of pituitary hormone abnormalities may be up to 90% (Samaan *et al.,* 1987), and the majority of children receiving 2,400 cGy to the cranial cavity for treatment of acute lymphoblastic leukemia showed defects of growth and growth hormone secretion (Kirk *et al.,* 1987). However, with doses of 1,000 to 1,400 cGy TBI given routinely immediately prior to HSC transplantation, significant pituitary disturbances, apart from growth hormone deficiency, do not appear to be frequent; hyperprolactinemia is the most likely abnormality, but gonadotrophin deficiency, secondary hypothyroidism, and adrenocorticotropic hormone (CTH) adrenal deficiency may occur in decreasing order of frequency. Mills and colleagues (1994) reported partial hypopituitarism documented at 6 and 8 months after chemotherapy and single-fraction TBI (10.5 Gy) followed by autologous bone marrow transplantation. Hormone profiles demonstrated severe somatotroph insufficiency and impaired adrenocorticotroph secretory capacity, but sparing of the gonadotroph compartment. The patients presented with nonspecific symptoms of malaise, fatigue, nausea, diarrhea, and postural presyncope. One patient had loss of body, but not axillary or pubic, hair. A prospective study of pituitary-gonadal function to evaluate short-term effects of myeloablative chemotherapy or TBI with autologous or allogeneic marrow transplantation in postmenarchal females aged 17 to 30 years found that all patients had evidence of gonadal insufficiency prior to transplant in that their basal and gonadotrophin-stimulated estradiol (E2) levels were significantly lower than those of control subjects and that the myeloablative regimen caused further damage with FSH levels rising further into the menopausal range, their E2 secretion becoming further diminished, and their ovaries almost unresponsive 3 to 4 months posttransplant. Pelvic ultrasound undertaken before and after transplant demonstrated a reduction in ovarian size associated with follicular depletion (Chatterjee et al., 1994a). In contrast thyrotrophic, lactotrophic, and adrenocorticotrophic secretions were unaffected, indicating that the ovary suffers an acute insult during pretransplant conditioning, but that the anterior pituitary gland retains its trophic hormone reserve and secretory capacity. The same authors performed a similar study in 13 postpubertal male patients before and after autologous BMT for lymphoma. All had multiagent cytotoxic treatment prior to transplant and 30% were found to have germ cell dysfunction with abnormal semen parameters before high-dose therapy, indicating damage to the germinal epithelium (Chatterjee et al., 1994b). They also had evidence of reduced LC reserve pretransplant.

The conditioning regimen used was the BEAM regimen (carmustine, etoposide, cytosine arabinoside, melphalan). Posttransplant all patients sustained gonadal injury, the effect on their germ cells being more pronounced than that on the Leydig cells. Fifty percent had reduction in testicular volume and all had azoospermia 2 to 3 months posttransplant. Again, no overt injury to the pituitary gland was detected.

The adrenal gland itself is rarely affected in a manner that requires therapy, although reduced secretion of adrenal androgens may follow TBI (Bolme et al., 1995).

Treatment Replacement of the target gland hormone (thyroxine, cortisone) is appropriate in the case of thyroid-stimulating hormone (TSH) or ACTH deficiency. Hyperprolactinemia may cause suppression of the gonadotrophin-gonadal axis, loss of libido and potency, and a mild degree of fluid retention. It can usually be easily controlled by a small dose of a dopamine agonist, such as bromocriptine or cabergoline.

Thyroid abnormalities

Hypothyroidism

Hypothyroidism is the most common thyroid abnormality after HSC transplantation, but is very much related to the use of TBI. With chemotherapy alone, hypothyroidism is an occasional occurrence. However, after TBI in children, approximately 15% become hypothyroid and twice this number may have compensated hypothyroidism (an elevated TSH with normal thyroid hormone levels) (Borgström & Bolme, 1994; Boulad et al., 1995); the incidence may be significantly lower after fractionated TBI (Sanders, 1991). In adults who had received 3,500 to 4,500 cGy local irradiation for lymphomas or head and neck cancer, one series showed that two-thirds of subjects had an elevated TSH level, and 20% to 25% had definite hypothyroidism (Schimpff et al., 1980).

Treatment Thyroxine replacement in sufficient dosage to return the TSH level to the normal range and maintain a free thyroxine level in the upper normal range is appropriate when there is definite hypothyroidism. If there is compensated hypothyroidism (an elevated TSH with normal thyroid hormone levels), it is less clear whether one should institute thyroxine therapy. Spontaneous improvement with a return of TSH to the normal range will occur in some patients, so one would probably not initiate therapy if the elevation of TSH level is borderline. However, there would be a greater motivation to introduce a small dose of thyroxine if the TSH elevation was substantial. In growing children it is nearly always advisable to introduce thyroxine if the TSH is elevated, because of concern that a marginal deficiency of thyroid hormones may contribute to impaired growth.

Hyperthyroidism

Hyperthyroidism, occasionally accompanied by Graves[2] ophthalmopathy, occurs rarely after HSC transplantation, presumably due to disturbed functioning of the immune system and probably mostly in patients with a predisposing HLA haplotype (Au et al., 2001). Sometimes clinical and biochemical hyperthyroidism occurs in conjunction with chronic (Hashimoto's[3]) thyroiditis or with subacute thyroiditis (de Quervain's[4] disease) (Samaan et al., 1987; Redman & Bajouranas, 1989); the former may be associated with slight discomfort and tenderness of the thyroid, and is recognized by moderate to high titers of thyroglobulin or microsomal antibodies in the blood; the latter disease is associated with pronounced pain and tenderness of the gland, absence of antibodies, a very low thyroid uptake of ^{131}I or technetium, and a high erythrocyte sedimentation rate. "Silent thyroiditis" does not have the pain or tenderness of subacute thyroiditis, but it may

---

[2] Robert Graves, Irish physician, 1796–1853.
[3] Japanese surgeon, 1881–1934.
[4] Fritz de Quervain, Swiss surgeon, 1868–1940.

also be associated with hyperthyroidism and its course, diagnosis (low ^{131}I uptake), and therapy are similar.

Treatment Any of the conventional modalities of therapy (radioactive iodine, a prolonged course of antithyroid drugs, or partial thyroidectomy) may be used, with or without the addition of propranolol to reduce sympathetic overactivity while other measures take effect. However, one may wish to avoid surgery in this group of patients, and it may also be advisable to avoid prolonged use of drugs (such as carbimazole or propylthiouracil) that can cause impaired granulocyte function or rarely, agranulocytosis. Thus, treatment with radioactive iodine is often the preferred option. The amount of irradiation to tissues other than the thyroid, using conventional doses of ^{131}I, is very small, and would certainly not be contraindicated by prior TBI.

If coincident Hashimoto's disease is present, the conventional approach is to use antithyroid drugs until the destructive process naturally terminates the hyperthyroidism; however, our experience has been that this approach often leads to prolonged and relatively difficult therapy, and we therefore tend to recommend early definitive therapy, e.g. ^{131}I, anticipating rapid development of hypothyroidism.

When hyperthyroidism is associated with subacute thyroiditis or "silent thyroiditis," the high thyroid hormone levels are due to inflammatory damage to thyroid cells and are transient. Thus all forms of antithyroid therapy are inappropriate. Propranolol may be used to control the manifestations of transient hyperthyroidism, and corticosteroids will cause a dramatic improvement if pain or systemic symptoms are severe.

Thyroid nodules, neoplasms, or abnormal morphology

Palpable thyroid nodules or abnormalities may occur in 20% to 30% of a population who have received local neck irradiation, and adenomas, colloid nodules, chronic lymphocytic thyroiditis, and fibrosis are well documented (Shalet, 1983). There is a small but definite incidence of thyroid carcinoma, usually well-differentiated papillary carcinoma. The incidence would appear to be up to 0.5%, with an increasing incidence associated with increasing irradiation dosage up to approximately 1,100 cGy, and with a higher incidence when irradiation has been given in childhood. Higher dosage irradiation may be associated with a lesser occurrence of tumors. It should be noted that the mean latent period to the time of detection of a tumor is approximately 10 years (Maxon *et al.*, 1977).

Thyroid ultrasound, to determine whether cystic or solid, and scanning, to determine whether "warm" or "cold," are useful in the assessment of thyroid nodules. If there is a question of possible malignancy, aspiration cytology, in experienced hands, often yields valuable information.

Parathyroid hormone disturbances

Primary hyperparathyroidism has been reported to occur in up to 11% of patients who have received local neck irradiation and appears more frequent with low dose (less than 750 cGy) neck irradiation (Redman & Bajorunas, 1989), although the reason for the increased incidence of this condition is not clear. It is therefore appropriate to check a calcium and/or ionized calcium level annually and, if elevated, to determine the parathyroid hormone level.

Hypoparathyroidism is a rare occurrence after neck irradiation (Glazebrook, 1987) and should also be detected by an annual check on calcium levels.

References

Au, W. Y., Hawkins, B. R., Chan, E.T.Y. *et al.* (2001). Association of the HLA A2-B46-DR9 haplotype with autoimmune thyroid dysfunction after bone marrow transplantation in Chinese patients. *British Journal of Haematology*, **115**, 660–3.

Blatt, J., Bercu, B. B., Gillin, J. C. *et al.* (1984). Reduced pulsatile growth hormone secretion in children after therapy for acute lymphoblastic leukemia. *Journal of Pediatrics*, **104**, 82–6.

Bolme, P., Borgstrom, B., & Carlstrom, K. (1995). Longitudinal study of adrenocortical function following allogeneic bone marrow transplantation in children. *Hormone Research*, **43**, 279–85.

Borgström, B. & Bolme, P. (1994). Thyroid function in children after allogeneic bone marrow transplantation. *Bone Marrow Transplantation*, **13**, 59–64.

Bouchard, P., Sai, P., Reach, G. *et al.* (1982). Diabetes mellitus following pentamidine-induced hypoglycemia in humans. *Diabetes*, **31**, 40–5.

Boulad, F., Bromley, M., Black, P. *et al.* (1995). Thyroid dysfunction following bone marrow transplantation using hypofractionated radiation. *Bone Marrow Transplantation*, **15**, 71–6.

Chattergee, R., Andrews, H. O., McGarrigle, H. H. *et al.* (2000). Cavernosal arterial insufficiency is a major component of erectile dysfunction in some recipients of high-dose chemotherapy/chemoradiotherapy for haematological malignancies. *Bone Marrow Transplantation*, **25**, 1185–9.

Chatterjee, R. & Goldstone, A. H. (1996). Gonadal damage and effects on fertility in adult patients with haematological malignancy undergoing stem cell transplantation. *Bone Marrow Transplantation*, **17**, 5–11.

Chattergee, R., Kottaridis, P. D., McGarigle, H. M. *et al.* (2001). Patterns of Leydig cell insufficiency in adult males following bone marrow transplantation for haematological malignancies. *Bone Marrow Transplantation*, **28**, 497–502.

Chattergee, R., Kottaridis, P. D., McGarigle, H.H., & Linch, D. C. (2002). Management of erectile dysfunction by combination therapy with testosterone and sildenafil in recipients of high-dose therapy for haematological malignancies. *Bone Marrow Transplantation*, **29**, 607–1.

Chatterjee, R., Mills, W., Katz, M. *et al.* (1994a). Prospective study of pituitary-gonadal function to evaluate short-term effects of ablative chemotherapy or total body irradiation with autologous or allogeneic marrow transplantation in post-menarchial female patients. *Bone Marrow Transplantation*, **13**, 511–17.

Chatterjee, R., Mills, W., Katz, M. *et al.* (1994b). Germ cell failure and Leydig cell dysfunction in postpubertal males after autologous bone transplantation with BEAM for lymphoma. *Bone Marrow Transplantation*, **13**, 519–22.

Da Cunha, M. F., Meistrich, M. L., & Nader, S. (1987). Absence of testicular protection by a gonadotropin releasing hormone analogue against cyclophosphamide induced testicular cytotoxicity in the mouse. *Cancer Research, 47,* 1093–7.

Drakos, P., Weinberg, M., Delukina, M. *et al.* (1993). Inappropriate antidiuretic hormone secretion (SIADH) preceding skin manifestations of disseminated varicalla zoster virus infection. *Bone Marrow Transplantation, 11,* 407–8.

Flier, J. S. & Moses, A. C. (1989). Diabetes in acromegaly and other endocrine disorders. In *Endocrinology,* vol. 2, ed. L. J. DeGroot, pp. 1389–99, Philadelphia: W. B. Saunders.

Glazebrook, G. A. (1987). Effect of decicurie doses of radioactive iodine 131 on parathyroid function. *American Journal of Surgery,* **1S4,** 368.

Harris, E., Mahendra, P., McGarrigle, H. H., Linch, D. C., & Chattergee, R. (2001). Gynaecomastia with hypergonadotrophic hypogonadism and Leydig cell insufficiency in recipients of high-dose chemotherapy or chemoradiotherapy. *Bone Marrow Transplantation,* **28,** 1141–4.

Heimpel, H., Arnold, R., Hertzel, W. D. *et al.* (1991). Gonadal function after bone marrow transplantation in adult male and female patients. *Bone Marrow Transplantation,* **8** (Suppl 1), 21–4.

Hotamisligil, G. S., Peraldi, P., Budavari, A. *et al.* (1996). IRS-1 mediated inhibition of insulin receptor tyrosine kinase activity in TNF-α and obesity-induced insulin resistance. *Science,* **271,** 665–7.

Jacob, A., Goodman, A., & Holmes, J. (1995). Fertility after bone marrow transplantation following conditioning with cyclophosphamide and total body irradiation. *Bone Marrow Transplantation,* **15,** 483–4.

Kirk, J. A., Stevens, M. A., Menser, M. A. *et al.* (1987). Growth failure and growth-hormone deficiency after treatment for acute lymphoblastic leukaemia. *Lancet,* **1,** 190–3.

Larsen, E. C., Loft, A., Holm, K., Muller, J., Brocks, V., Andersen A. N. (2000). Oocyte donation in women cured of cancer with bone marrow transplantation including total body irradiation in adolescence. *Human Reproduction,* **15,** 1505–8.

Lipton, J. H., Derzko, C., Fyles, G. *et al.* (1993). Pregnancy after BMT: three case reports. *Bone Marrow Transplantation,* **11,** 415–18.

Lorini, R., Cortona, L., Scaramuzza, A. *et al.* (1995). Hyperinsulinemia in children and adolescents after bone marrow transplantation. *Bone Marrow Transplantation,* **15,** 873–7.

Maxon, H. R., Thomas, S. R., Saenger, E. L. *et al.* (1977). Ionizing irradiation and the induction of clinically significant disease in the human thyroid gland. *American Journal of Medicine,* **63,** 967–78.

Meirow, D. (2000) Reproduction post chemotherapy in young patients. *Molecular & Cellular Endocrinology,* **169,** 123–131.

Mills, W., Chatterjee, R., McGarrigle, H. H. G. *et al.* (1994). Partial hypopituitarism following total body irradiation in adult patients with hematological malignancy. *Bone Marrow Transplantation,* **14,** 471–3.

Redman, J. R. & Bajorunas, D. R. (1989). Therapy related thyroid and parathyroid dysfunction in patients with Hodgkin's disease. In *Hodgkin's Disease: The Consequences of Survival,* ed. M. J. & J. R. Redman, p. 222, Philadelphia: Lea & Febiger.

Redman, J. R., Bajorunas, D. R., Goldstein, M. C. *et al.* (1987). Semen cryopreservation and artificial insemination for Hodgkin's disease. *Journal of Clinical Oncology,* **5,** 233–8.

Samaan, N. A., Schultz, P. N., Yang, K. P. *et al.* (1987). Endocrine complications after radiotherapy for tumours of the head and neck. *Journal of Laboratory and Clinical Medicine,* **109,** 364–72.

Sanders, J. E. (1991). Endocrine problems in children after bone marrow transplant for haematological malignancies. *Bone Marrow Transplantation,* **8** (Suppl 1), 2–4.

Sanders, J. E., Hawley, J., Levy, W. *et al.* (1996). Pregnancies following high-dose cyclophosphamide with or without busulfan or total body irradiation and bone marrow transplantation. *Blood,* **87,** 3045–52.

Schimpff, S. C., Diggs, C. H., Wiswell, J. G. *et al.* (1980). Radiation-related thyroid dysfunction: implications for the treatment of Hodgkin's disease. *Annals of Internal Medicine,* **92,** 91–98.

Schouten, H. C., Maragos, D., Vose, J. *et al.* (1990). Diabetes mellitus or an impaired glucose tolerance as a potential complicating factor in patients treated with high-dose therapy and autologous bone marrow transplantation. *Bone Marrow Transplantation,* **6,** 333–5.

Shalet, S. M. (1983). Disorders of the endocrine system due to radiation and cytotoxic chemotherapy. *Clinical Endocrinology,* **18,** 637–59.

Shalet, S. M., Didi, M., Ogilvy-Stuart, A. L. *et al.* (1995). Growth and endocrine function after bone marrow transplantation. *Clinical Endocrinology,* **42,** 333–9.

Shepherd, J. D., Hoar, D. I., Keown, P. A., & Phillips, G. L. (1996). Successful paternity of twins following transplantation with busulfan, melphalan and cyclophosphamide conditioning. *Bone Marrow Transplantation,* **17,** 461–2.

Szabo, F., Horvath, N., Seimon, S., & Hughes, T. (2000). Inappropriate antidiuretic hormone secretion, abdominal pain and disseminated varicella-zoster virus infection: an unusual triad in a patient 6 months post mini-allogeneic peripheral stem cell transplant for chronic myeloid leukemia. *Bone Marrow Transplantation,* **26,** 231–3.

Taskinen, M., Saarinen-Pihkala, U. M., Hovi, L., & Lisanen-Nyman, M. (2000). Impaired glucose tolerance and dyslipidaemia as late effects after bone-marrow transplantation in childhood. *Lancet,* **356,** 993–7.

Turnbridge, W.M.G. (1987). Thyroid physiology and hypothyroidism. In *Clinical Endocrinology,* ed. G. Besser & A. Cudworth, p. 13. **12,** Philadelphia: Lippincott.

95 Musculoskeletal complications

JACOB M. VAN LAAR AND MILTON L. COHEN

Leiden University Medical Center, Leiden, The Netherlands, and St. Vincent's Hospital and University of New South Wales, Sydney, Australia

Introduction

The usual diseases for which hematopoietic stem cell (HSC) transplantation is performed are uncommonly associated with musculoskeletal manifestations. The obvious exception is drug-induced marrow aplasia in rheumatoid arthritis. Additionally, there is developing interest in the still novel role of autologous HSC transplantation for rheumatoid arthritis itself, based on the notion that it is fundamentally a disease of bone marrow stem cells or an autoimmune disease whose course can be altered by immune system ablation and subsequent reconstitution with autologous or allogeneic stem cells (Brooks, Atkinson, & Hamilton, 1995) (see Chapter 119). The major musculoskeletal complications of the transplantation process itself are infection (septic arthritis and osteomyelitis) and osteonecrosis (Table 95.1). The overall prevalence of these in a cohort of 500 allogeneic transplant recipients at St. Vincent's Hospital, Sydney, was approximately 5%. No such complications have been recorded in a cohort of 300 autologous transplant recipients.

Infective complications

Septic arthritis

Considering the profound immune suppression involved in HSC transplantation, as well as the high relative incidence of

Table 95.1 *Etiology of musculoskeletal complications after HSC transplantation*

Attributable to the disease for which transplantation is
   performed (e.g., rheumatoid arthritis)
Attributable to the process of transplantation itself
   Osteonecrosis
   Infection
   Arthralgia/arthropathy (related to changes in corticosteroid dose)
   Graft-versus-host disease
Not attributable to either, that is, indistinguishable from
   problems in the nontransplant population (e.g., mechanical
   spinal pain)

infection in previously normal joints (Cooper & Cawley, 1986), the low occurrence of septic arthritis (6 patients) in the St. Vincent's population is surprising. Two of these patients developed *Candida* arthritis. One presented with septic arthritis of a knee in the context of *Candida tropicalis* septicemia, which was ultimately fatal. In the other, hip pain was clinically and radiologically attributed to osteonecrosis. Only later was *Candida albicans* cultured from the joint; systemic candidiasis was never confirmed. Although infrequent, *Candida* arthritis usually occurs as part of disseminated disease (Murray, Fialk, & Roberts, 1976; Bayer & Guze, 1978).

A third patient developed septic arthritis of a knee with local osteomyelitis due to *Staphylococcus* epidermidis after a second bone marrow transplant. The infections resolved leaving a badly damaged joint that required total arthroplasty. Septic arthritis should always be suspected when a joint effusion occurs in the context of HSC transplantation. The standard of diagnosis is culture of joint aspirate; in particular, *Candida* is rarely a contaminant (Campen, Kaufman, & Beardmore, 1990). The treatment of septic arthritis is an urgent medical matter, as joint destruction may be rapid. Principles of therapy include the combination of appropriate antibiotics, joint drainage (by closed needle aspiration with the exception of the hip), and early mobilization (Hedström & Lidgren, 1998).

Cytomegalovirus has also been identified as a cause of polyarticular arthritis after autologous marrow transplantation (Burns & Gingrich, 1993).

Osteomyelitis

In addition to the case mentioned above, there was one case of *Candida* osteomyelitis associated with knee joint infection, and one instance of finger osteomyelitis associated with *Nocardia* in the St. Vincent's cohort. A singular instance of vertebral osteomyelitis due to an unidentified organism, associated with a paravertebral abscess, resulted in the collapse of the eleventh and twelfth thoracic vertebra, but with no long-term adverse sequelae.

Corticosteroid-associated complications

Arthralgia

Polyarthralgia, affecting the knees in particular, was frequently experienced in the context of reduction of glucocorticosteroid dosage. This phenomenon, which is occasionally associated with transient acellular joint effusion, is essentially benign and self-limited, although often distressing and difficult to treat (Bennett & Strong, 1975; Weinstein, 1980; Kahl & Medsger, 1986). It usually affects the distal lower limbs, and often occurs at night. Its pathogenesis, whether or not associated with joint effusion, is unknown. It remains unclear whether arthralgia predicts later osteonecrosis: such an association was seen in only one of our patients. Nonetheless it is important that joint effusions be aspirated and examined for cytology and culture. Treatment with analgesics in regular, sufficient doses can relieve distress while resolution is awaited. Narcotic analgesia is sometimes required.

Steroid myopathy

Proximal muscle weakness associated with corticosteroid therapy and considered attributable to it is not infrequent in this patient population, especially those receiving corticosteroid treatment over a prolonged period, for example, for chronic graft-versus-host disease (GVHD). Recovery with steroid dose reduction is slow, often taking a number of months.

Osteonecrosis

One of the most prevalent serious musculoskeletal complications in this population is osteonecrosis, most frequently of the femoral head and commonly bilateral. It is a late event, occurring most commonly in the second year after transplantation, for a cumulative prevalence of approximately 5%–10% (Atkinson, Cohen, & Biggs, 1987; Enright, Haake, & Weisdorf, 1990; Socie et al., 1994; Wiesmann et al., 1998). Of the factors known to be associated with nontraumatic osteonecrosis (Mazières, 1998; Lavernia, Sierra, & Grieco, 1999), corticosteroid therapy poses the greatest risk to transplant patients. Furthermore, steroid dose itself appears to be the major predictor of this risk (Felson & Anderson, 1987). Other risk factors that have been identified in large cohorts include conditioning with total body irradiation (TBI) (Fink et al., 1998), older age, and an initial diagnosis of aplastic anemia or acute leukemia (Socie et al., 1997).

Osteonecrosis should be suspected when joint pain develops insidiously, especially on weight-bearing, typically in the groin when a hip is involved, often with referral to the knee. When associated with painful, limited, passive joint movement and, in the case of the knee or shoulder, joint effusion, the conditions for an arthrosis are fulfilled. Diagnostic attention must exclude infection, which can be achieved only by joint aspiration.

Magnetic resonance imaging (MRI) is the most sensitive and most specific technique for detecting osteonecrosis (Conway, Totty, & McEnery, 1996). However, the degree of bone or joint involvement so demonstrated may be discordant with the clinical features. Bilateral changes may be seen when only one side has been affected clinically. Once there is evidence of osteonecrosis on plain radiology, any chance of prevention of joint damage has been lost. Although collapse of subchondral bone following osteonecrosis is not inevitable, in the case of the femoral head the probability of collapse is of the order of 80% (Fig. 95.1).

Specific management of early osteonecrosis [clinical findings and MRI positive; plain radiography or computed tomography (CT) negative] remains a challenge. Drug treatment with calcitonin or bisphosphonates (to inhibit osteoclast activity) may be rational, but has not been determined to be of benefit. The effectiveness of core decompression of the femoral head, designed to limit ischemic damage, remains controversial, although the larger series report results superior to those obtained with conservative management (Colwell, 1989; Hungerford, 1989; Lavernia, Sierra, & Grieco, 1999). Vascularized bone grafting procedures are technically difficult, but may be preferable in the younger patient (Urbaniek & Harvey, 1999).

Established osteonecrosis (plain radiography or CT positive) is essentially the clinical problem of joint damage, which, perhaps surprisingly, does not necessarily imply either pain or disability. Hence, the management at this stage is adequate pain control plus correction of mechanical factors (such as leg length discrepancy, isometric retraining of antigravity muscles, and use of walking aids). Persistent pain, especially nocturnal, alone or with a significant mechanical disability, is an indication for joint replacement surgery, which carries a good prognosis (Atkinson, Cohen, & Biggs, 1987; Socie et al., 1994; Garino & Steinberg, 1997).

The principles of primary prevention of osteonecrosis in the HSC transplant population include early mobilization of the patient and attempts to minimize total exposure to corticosteroid drugs (Atkinson et al., 1991).

Osteoporosis

Osteoporosis after HSC transplantation is common (Kauppila et al., 1999; Schulte et al., 2000; Schimmer et al., 2001) and may be associated with two situations: prolonged corticosteroid treatment and, in women, with chemo/radiotherapy-induced ovarian failure (Kelly et al., 1990; Castelo Branco et al., 1996; Castaneda et al., 1997; Bhatia et al., 1998; Ebeling et al., 1999; Valimaki et al., 1999). The latter is preventable by ovarian hormone replacement therapy. In a prospective series, both men and women experienced significant loss of hip bone mineral density (BMD) at 12 months posttransplant (Stern et al., 2001). The cumulative dose and numbers of days of glucocorticosteroid therapy and the number of days of cyclosporine or tacrolimus therapy showed significant associ-

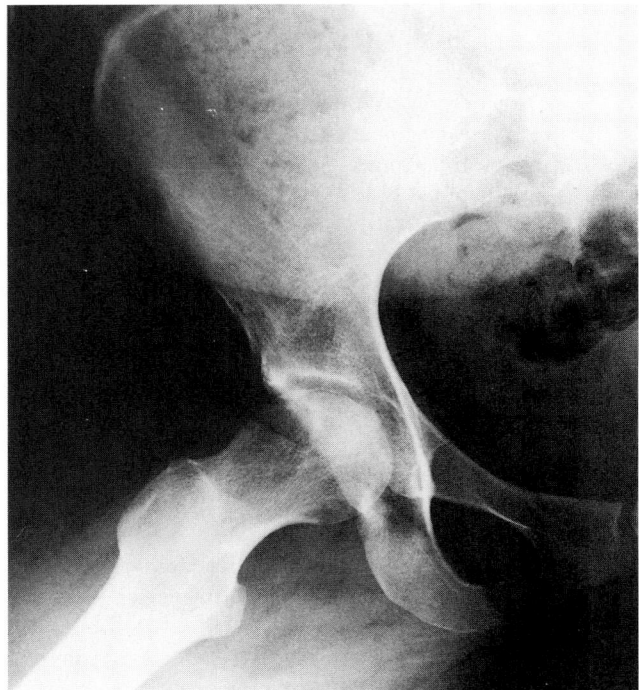
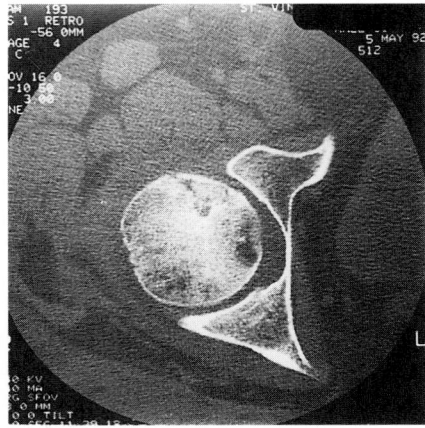
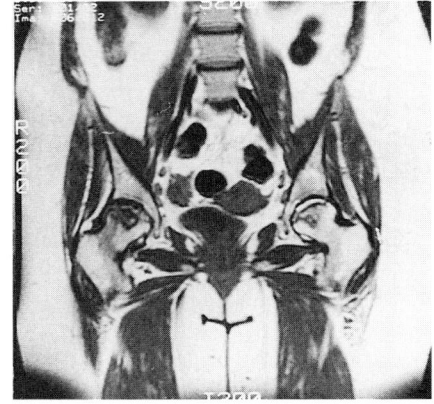

Figure 95.1. Osteonecrosis of the hip. The left-hand panel is a plain radiograph, illustrating a mildly deformed femoral head with patchy osteosclerosis and the typical "crescent" sign, an area of radiolucency just below the superior margin of the femoral head. The acetabulum is intact. The upper right-hand panel is a CT scan of the same region, again showing the patchy osteosclerosis and osteoporosis in the femoral head with a triangular "fragment" in the process of demarcation in its upper part. The lower right-hand panel is an MRI scan, coronal view, of the hip joints. The typical wedge-shaped areas of abnormal signal within the femoral heads, extending to the articular margins, can be seen bilaterally, more severe on the symptomatic right side.

ations with loss of BMD. In a series of children allografted for acute lymphoblastic leukemia (ALL), bone mass at 8 years posttransplant was significantly less compared with healthy controls, but only slightly reduced compared to children with ALL who had not been transplanted (Nysom *et al.*, 2000).

This suggests that underlying disease may pose an independent risk factor for premature osteoporosis, a notion that was corroborated by a recent study showing osteopenia and osteoporosis before HSC transplantation in 21 of 41 adult patients with acute myeloid leukemia (AML) and ALL, but in only 5 of 20 patients with chronic myeloid leukemia (CML) (Massenkeil *et al.*, 2001). Additional factors predisposing to bone loss posttransplant include the high-dose conditioning regimen (particularly TBI), cyclosporine and tacrolimus, granulocyte colony-stimulating factor (G-CSF), long-term heparin administration, and hypothyroidism (Weilbaecher, 2000).

Osteopenia (defined as a reduction in bone mineral density) is common posttransplant (Kashyap *et al.*, 2000), frequent after prolonged glucocorticosteroid treatment, and predisposes to clinical osteoporosis defined as a fracture occurring in osteopenic bone. The so-called T score has been used to quantitate the degree of reduction in bone mass (Schimmer, Minden, & Keating, 2000) This score relates a patient's bone mass to the peak bone mass of a healthy young adult. Thus, a T score of 0 represents mean peak adult bone mass, and a T score of −1 represents bone mass of 1 standard deviation below this mean. Using this scoring system, osteopenia has been further defined as a T score between −1 and −2.5, while osteoporosis has been defined as a score below −2.5. The T score can be translated into risk of fracture. The relative risk of fracture doubles for every standard deviation below adult peak bone mass. Thus, a T score of −1 indicates a two-fold increase in fracture risk.

Table 95.2. *Treatment approach for osteopenia and osteoporosis.*

T score −1 to −2.5
   Lifestyle modification
   Calcium and vitamin D supplements
   Hormone replacement therapy if hypogonadal
     (estrogen, testosterone, raloxifene)
T score ≤ 2.5
   As above and
   Biophosphonates

Reproduced, with permission, from Schimmer, Minden, & Keating (2000).

Radiographs, such as of the thoracic spine as seen on a lateral chest film, may reveal evidence of vertebral fracture. The diagnosis is confirmed by measurement of bone mineral density in the spine and hip and by serum osteocalcin and urinary hydroxyproline levels (measurements of bone turnover). Stern and colleagues (1996) prospectively evaluated nine patients undergoing prednisone and cyclosporine treatment for chronic GVHD for biochemical factors associated with skeletal turnover at the initiation of treatment and 9 months later. They found increased collagen turnover, increased urinary magnesium and calcium excretion, and a significant decrease in bone mineral density in three of five evaluable males and in all three females.

In long-term survivors of allogeneic HSC transplantation, bone mineral density recovers (starting as early as 12 months posttransplant), and bone turnover normalizes (Kananen et al., 2002).

Prevention of osteopenia follows the same principles with respect to corticosteroid treatment as for prevention of osteonecrosis, plus ovarian hormone replacement therapy in women. Recommended modifications of lifestyle risk factors include smoking cessation or avoidance, reduction of alcohol consumption if excessive, instructions in weight-bearing exercise and dietary measures. In addition, drug therapy with calcium supplementation, vitamin D analogues, and bisphosphonate preparations (etidronate and alendronate) is used for prevention and treatment of osteoporosis (Sambrook & Lane, 2001; American College of Rheumatology Ad Hoc Committee on Glucocorticoid-induced Osteoporosis, 2001). A treatment approach based on the patient's T score is shown in Table 95.2. It should be noted that if activated forms of vitamin D (e.g., calcitriol) are used, patients should be carefully monitored for the development of hypercalcemia and hypercalcuria, in which case the dosage of the activated vitamin D supplement needs to be reduced. Treatment of an acute vertebral fracture, or of spinal pain consequent to altered spinal mechanics following vertebral fracture, consists of adequate analgesia, which may require long-term, low-dose opioid drugs, and early mobilization of the patient.

Other problems

Other causes of arthralgia

Polyarthralgia occurring in the context of serum sickness may occur with the use of antilymphocyte or antithymocyte globulin and, rarely, with administration of monoclonal antibody (Varadi et al., 1995); such episodes, being due to circulating immune complexes, run a predictable self-limited, benign course, although severe cases may require a short course of corticosteroids.

Pre-existing arthropathy may become symptomatic during the course of HSC transplantation. Inflammatory diseases, such as rheumatoid arthritis, will be well suppressed by concurrent immunosuppression, although problems due to established joint damage may present. These are likely to be mechanical, requiring local therapy and adequate analgesia. Again, any joint effusion should be aspirated. HLA-B27–associated spondylarthropathies presenting for the first time after autologous stem cell transplantation for hematologic malignancy have been reported (Koch et al., 2000). Clinical manifestations included arthralgias, lower back pain due to sacro-iliitis, and heel spurs.

Mechanical spinal pain

Spinal pain was reported uncommonly in the St. Vincent's Hospital cohort. Spinal pain is an inevitable consequence of the human condition, the majority of such episodes being mechanical, that is, due to altered intervertebral movement patterns (Cohen, 1996). As such, they are benign and reversible. Radiculopathy is not only not a cause of spinal pain, but also does not occur without appropriate neurologic signs. In the context of HSC transplantation, although spinal pain is most likely to be mechanical, suspicion of spinal infection must be high. Here clinical signs are the best guide: progressive pain, uninfluenced by posture, well-localized with corresponding local hyperalgesia (tenderness), and often accompanied by fever and rigors raise the possibility of vertebral osteomyelitis or discitis. CT scanning, prior to needle aspiration, is the diagnostic method of choice.

Acute episodes of pain due to fracture of osteopenic vertebrae have not been seen to date in our population; this may represent the ages and lengths of follow-up of patients.

Mechanical spinal pain may occur secondarily to disease (osteonecrosis, infection) affecting lower limb joints, thus interfering with gait, or secondary to poor muscle control from the relative immobility that may occur with a dire illness. Clinically, having excluded problems attributable to the transplant process itself, the approach to management is, first, reassurance regarding the benign prognosis; second, adequate simple analgesia; and, third, identification and correction of mechanical factors.

Rhabdomyolysis

There are several reports of rhabdomyolysis occurring after allogeneic (Jackson *et al.*, 1995; Tabata *et al.*, 1996) and autologous (Maruyama *et al.*, 1994) transplantation. One developed shortly after the administration of cyclophosphamide as part of the preparative regimen, one on day 23 posttransplant, and one at 4 months posttransplant following the institution of antibacterial and antituberculous medications. Another case report described its development after a generalized seizure induced by an overdose of cyclosporine. The patients presented with severe muscle pain and weakness and acute renal failure. Creatine kinase levels were markedly elevated, in one case peaking at 81,080 U/l. Myoglobinemia and myoglobinuria were present. Hemodialysis was required and two of the three patients survived. A third had myocardial necrosis as well as skeletal muscle damage and did not survive.

Treatment of rheumatoid arthritis and other connective tissue diseases by immune ablation and HSC transplantation

Although not a complication, it has been interesting to note the apparent cure of rheumatoid arthritis in two patients from the St. Vincent's cohort who required bone marrow transplantation for severe aplastic anemia induced by gold and D-penicillamine, respectively. In both patients symptoms attributable to residual joint damage have been minimal (Lowenthal *et al.*, 1993), well over a decade after transplantation. This experience contrasts to a more recent report of mild recurrence of synovitis following allogeneic marrow transplantation for gold-induced aplasia, despite complete donor lymphohematopoiesis (McKendry, Huebsch, & Leclair, 1996). Such observations have given rise to considerable current interest in the treatment of severe rheumatoid arthritis and other connective tissue diseases, including systemic sclerosis (scleroderma) and systemic lupus erythematosus, by immune ablative chemotherapy or chemoradiation, followed by either autologous or allogeneic HSC transplantation (see Chapter 119).

Conclusions

Arthralgia in the absence of joint effusion is commonly experienced in the context of change in glucocorticosteroid dosage, and is benign and self-limited. Joint effusions must be aspirated and cultured, specifically for *Candida*. Painful limited movements of a hip joint should prompt suspicion of osteonecrosis of the femoral head; diagnostic aspiration should be performed to exclude infection. MRI scanning is the most sensitive technique for detecting osteonecrosis. Prevention of osteoporosis, especially in the context of high-dose glucocorticosteroid treatment, requires life-style counseling, calcium supplementation, vitamin D analogues, and bisphosphonates.

References

American College of Rheumatology Ad Hoc Committee on Glucocorticoid-induced Osteoporosis (2001). Recommendations for the prevention and treatment of glucocorticoid-induced osteoporosis. *Arthritis and Rheumatism*, **44**, 1496–1503.

Atkinson, K., Biggs, J., Concannon, A. *et al.* (1991). A prospective randomized trial of cyclosporine and methotrexate versus cyclosporine, methotrexate and prednisolone for prevention of graft-versus-host disease after HLA-identical sibling marrow transplantation for hematological malignancy. *Australian and New Zealand Journal of Medicine*, **21**, 850–6.

Atkinson, K., Cohen, M., & Biggs, J. (1987). Avascular necrosis of the femoral head secondary to corticosteroid therapy for graft-versus-host disease after marrow transplantation: effective treatment with hip arthroplasty. *Bone Marrow Transplantation*, **2**, 421–6.

Bayer, A. S. & Guze, L. B. (1978). Fungal arthritis. I. *Candida* arthritis: diagnostic and prognostic implications and therapeutic considerations. *Seminars in Arthritis and Rheumatism*, **8**, 142–50.

Bennett, W. M. & Strong, D. (1975). Arthralgia after high-dose steroids. *Lancet*, **1**, 332.

Bhatia, S., Ramsey, N. K., Weisdorf, D. *et al.* (1998). Bone mineral density in patients undergoing bone marrow transplantation for myeloid malignancies. *Bone Marrow Transplantation*, **22**, 87–90.

Brooks, P. M., Atkinson, K., & Hamilton, J. A. (1995). Stem cell transplantation in autoimmune disease. *Journal of Rheumatology*, **22**, 1809–11.

Burns, L. J. & Gingrich, R. D. (1993). Cytomegalovirus infection presenting as polyarticular arthritis after autologous BMT. *Bone Marrow Transplantation*, **11**, 77–9.

Campen, D. H., Kaufman, R. L., & Beardmore, T. D. (1990). *Candida* septic arthritis in rheumatoid arthritis. *Journal of Rheumatology*, **17**, 86–8.

Castaneda, S., Carmona, L. Carvajal, I. *et al.* (1997). Reduction of bone mass in women after bone marrow transplantation. *Calcified Tissue International*, **60**, 343–7.

Castelo Branco, C., Rovira, M., Pons, F. *et al.* (1996). The effect of hormone replacement therapy on bone mass in patients with ovarian failure due to bone marrow transplantation. *Maturitas*, **23**, 307–12.

Cohen, M. L. (1996). Cervical and lumbar pain. *Medical Journal of Australia*, **165**, 504–8.

Colwell, C. W., Jr. (1989). The controversy of core decompression of the femoral head for osteonecrosis. *Arthritis and Rheumatism*, **32**, 797–800.

Conway, W. F., Totty, W. G., & McEnery, K. W. (1996). CT and MR imaging of the hip. *Radiology*, **198**, 297–307.

Cooper, C. & Cawley, M.I.D. (1986). Bacterial arthritis in an English health district: a 10 year review. *Annals of the Rheumatic Diseases*, **45**, 458–63.

Ebeling, P. R., Thomas, D. M., Erbas, B. *et al.* (1999). Mechanisms of bone loss following allogeneic and autologous hemopoietic stem cell transplantation. *Journal of Bone Mineralization Research,* **14,** 342–50.

Enright, H., Haake, R., & Weisdorf, D. (1990). Avascular necrosis of bone: a common serious complication of allogeneic bone marrow transplantation. *American Journal of Medicine,* **89,** 733–8.

Felson, D. T. & Anderson, J. J. (1987). Across-study evaluation of association between steroid dose and bolus steroids and avascular necrosis of bone. *Lancet,* **1,** 902–5.

Fink, J. C., Leisenring, W. M., Sullivan, K. M. *et al.* (1998). Avascular necrosis following bone marrow transplantation: a case-control study. *Bone,* **22,** 67–71.

Garino, J. P. & Steinberg, M. E. (1997). Total hip arthroplasty in patients with avascular necrosis of he femoral head: a 2- to 10-year follow-up. *Clinical Orthopaedics,* **334,** 108–115.

Hedström, S. A. & Lidgren, L. (1998). Septic arthritis and osteomyelitis. In *Rheumatology, Second Edition,* ed. J. H. Klippel & P. A. Dieppe, pp. 6.2.1–6.2.10. London; Philadelphia: Mosby.

Hungerford, D. S. (1989). The role of core decompression in the treatment of ischemic necrosis of the femoral head. *Arthritis and Rheumatism,* **32,** 801–6.

Jackson, S. R., Barnett, M. J., Keller, O. *et al.* (1995). Recovery from rhabdomyolysis after allogeneic BMT: report of a case with speculation on causation. *Bone Marrow Transplantation,* **15,** 803–4.

Kahl, L. & Medsger, T. A., Jr. (1986). Severe arthralgias after wide fluctuation in corticosteroid dosage. *Journal of Rheumatology,* **13,** 1063–5.

Kananen, K., Volin, L., Tähtelä, R. *et al.* (2002). Recovery of bone mass and normalization of bone turnover in long-term survivors of allogeneic bone marrow transplantation. *Bone Marrow Transplantation,* **29,** 33–9.

Kashyap, A., Kandeel, F., Yamauchi, D. *et al.* (2000). Effects of allogeneic bone marrow transplantation on recipient bone mineral density. *Biology of Blood and Marrow Transplantation,* **6,** 344–51.

Kauppila, M., Irjala, K., Koskinen, P. *et al.* (1999). Bone mineral density after allogeneic bone marrow transplantation. *Bone Marrow Transplantation,* **24,** 885–9.

Kelly, P. J., Atkinson, K., Ward, R. L. *et al.* (1990). Reduced bone mineral density in men and women with allogeneic bone marrow transplantation. *Transplantation,* **50,** 881–3.

Koch, B., Kranzhöfer, N., Pfreundschu, M., Pees, H. W., & Trümper, L. (2000). First manifestations of seronegative spondylarthropathy following autologous stem cell transplantation in HLA-B27-positive patients. *Bone Marrow Transplantation,* **26,** 673–5.

Lavernia, C. J., Sierra, R. J., & Grieco, F. R. (1999). Osteonecrosis of the femoral head. *Journal of the American Academy of Orthopaedic Surgeons,* **7,** 250–261.

Lowenthal, R. M., Cohen, M. L., Atkinson, K., & Biggs, J. C. (1993). Apparent cure of rheumatoid arthritis following bone marrow transplantation. *Journal of Rheumatology,* **20,** 137–40.

Maruyama, F., Miyazaki, H., Ezaki, K. *et al.* (1994). Severe rhabdomyolysis as a complication of peripheral blood stem cell transplantation. *Bone Marrow Transplantation,* **14,** 481–2.

Massenkeil, G., Fiene, C., Rosen, O. *et al.* (2001). Loss of bone mass and vitamin D deficiency after hematopoietic stem cell transplantation: standard prophylactic measures fail to prevent osteoporosis. *Leukemia,* **15,** 1701–5.

Mazières, B. (1998). Osteonecrosis. In *Rheumatology, Second Edition,* ed. J. H. Klippel & P. A. Dieppe, pp. 8.47.1–8.47.10. London; Philadelphia: Mosby.

McKendry, R. J., Huebsch, L., & Leclair, B. (1996). Progression of rheumatoid arthritis following bone marrow transplantation. A case report with a 13-year followup. *Arthritis and Rheumatism,* **39,** 1246–53.

Murray, H. W., Fialk, M. A., & Roberts, R. B. (1976). *Candida* arthritis. A manifestation of disseminated candidiasis. *American Journal of Medicine,* **60,** 587–95.

Nysom, K., Holm, K., Michaelsen, K. F. *et al.* (2000). Bone mass after allogeneic BMT for childhood leukaemia or lymphoma. *Bone Marrow Transplantation,* **25,** 191–6.

Sambrook, P. & Lane, N. E. (2001). Corticosteroid osteoporosis. *Best Practice and Research Clinical Rheumatology,* **15,** 401–13.

Schimmer, A. D., Mah, K., Bordeleau, L. *et al.* (2001). Decreased bone mineral density is common after autologous blood or marrow transplantation. *Bone Marrow Transplantation,* **28,** 387–91.

Schimmer, A. D., Minden, M. D., & Keating, A. (2000). Osteoporosis after blood and marrow transplantation: clinical aspects. *Biology of Blood and Marrow Transplantation,* **6,** 175–81.

Schulte, C., Beelen, D. W., Schaefer, U. W., & Mann, K. (2000). Bone loss in long-term survivors after transplantation of hematopoietic stem cells: a prospective study. *Osteoporosis International,* **11,** 344–53.

Socie, G., Cahn, J. Y., Carmelo, J. *et al.* (1997). Avascular necrosis of bone after allogeneic bone marrow transplantation: analysis of risk factors for 4388 patients by the Société Francaise de Greffe Moelle (SFGM). *British Journal of Haematology,* **97,** 865–70.

Socie, G., Sfelini, F., Sedel, F. *et al.* (1994). Avascular necrosis of bone after allogeneic bone marrow transplantation: clinical findings, incidence and risk factors. *British Journal of Haematology,* **86,** 624–8.

Stern, J. M., Chestnut, C. H., Bruemmer, B. *et al.* (1996). Bone density loss during treatment of chronic GVHD. *Bone Marrow Transplantation,* **17,** 395–400.

Stern, J. M., Sullivan, K. M., Ott, S. M. *et al.* (2001). Bone density loss after allogeneic hematopoietic stem cell transplantation: a prospective study. *Biology of Blood and Marrow Transplantation,* **7,** 257–64.

Tabata, N., Tanaka, R., Suga, S. *et al.* (1996). Rhabdomyolysis following administration of cyclophosphamide: a case report in a BMT recipient. *Bone Marrow Transplantation,* **17,** 1167–9.

Urbaniek, J. R. & Harvey, E. J. (1999). Revascularization of the femoral head in osteonecrosis. *Journal of the American Academy of Orthopedic Surgeons,* **6,** 44–54.

Varadi, G., Or, R., Rund, D. *et al.* (1995). Severe migratory polyarthritis following in vivo CAMPATH-1G. *Bone Marrow Transplantation,* **16,** 843–5.

Valimaki, M. J., Kinnunen, K., Volin, I. *et al.* (1999). A prospective study of bone loss and turnover after allogeneic bone marrow transplantation: effect of calcium supplementation with or without calcitonin. *Bone Marrow Transplantation*, **23**, 355–61.

Weilbaecher, K. N. (2000). Mechanisms of osteoporosis after hematopoietic cell transplantation. *Biology of Blood and Marrow Transplantation*, **6**, 165–74.

Weinstein, J. (1980). Benign joint effusion associated with glucocorticosteroid therapy. *Journal of Rheumatology*, **7**, 245–7.

Wiesmann, A., Pereira, P., Bohm, P. *et al.* (1998). Avascular necrosis of bone following allogeneic stem cell transplantation: MR screening and therapeutic options. *Bone Marrow Transplantation*, **6**, 565–9.

96 Dermatologic complications

STEVEN KOSSARD

Skin and Cancer Foundation and University of New South Wales, Sydney, Australia

Introduction

Patients undergoing hematopoietic stem cell (HSC) transplantation may experience a wide range of dermatologic complications (Table 96.1). The skin, together with the gastrointestinal tract and liver, represent the major target organs for graft-versus-host-disease (GVHD). The cutaneous component represents an important gauge for GVHD as cutaneous signs usually precede other organ dysfunction and the skin changes can be easily monitored and readily sampled (Farmer, 1985; Mauduit & Claudy, 1988; Tanaka *et al.,* 1991, Aractingi & Chosidow, 1998). However, the diagnosis of GVHD may be complicated by skin reaction to drugs, including those used in the conditioning regimen, prior radiotherapy, as well as immunosuppressive agents and medications used to deal with infections occurring as a consequence of immune suppression.

The recognition of skin changes identical to GVHD in recipients of syngeneic and autologous HSC transplants (Hood *et al.,* 1987) raises the question of the contributory role of drugs, infections, and genetic predisposition to autoimmune reactions in the final expression of GVHD. A survey of chronic cutaneous GVHD in Japanese patients after bone marrow transplantation revealed a lower incidence and milder disease, indicating that the genetic makeup in certain racial groups may also influence this event (Fujii *et al.,* 1992). Some of the cutaneous reactions after syngeneic and autologous transplantation may represent the phenomenon termed cutaneous eruption of lymphocyte recovery. These reactions were initially observed in a group of patients undergoing marrow ablation with cytoreductive therapy for leukemia and consisted of a widespread maculopapular rash coinciding with the return of lymphocytes to the peripheral circulation (Horn *et al.,* 1989; Horn, 1994). Most of the dermatologic complications of bone marrow transplantation can be ascribed to GVHD, lymphocyte recovery, drug reactions, or infections.

Cutaneous GVHD

Both acute and chronic patterns of cutaneous reactions are recognized in GVHD. Acute and chronic GVHD skin reactions show clinical and histologic differences, although their time course may overlap.

Acute GVHD (see also Chapter 71)

Acute cutaneous GVHD rashes appear usually 1 to 8 weeks after grafting, initially as a maculopapular erythema often localized to the face, eyelids (Fig. 96.1), shoulders and upper chest, posterior forearms and anterior thighs, as well as the palms (Fig. 96.2) and soles (Farmer, 1985; Mauduit & Claudy, 1988; Tanaka *et al.,* 1991). The acute reaction may become generalized and resemble a viral exanthem. The rash is pruritic and is associated with a burning sensation that may be particularly troublesome on the palms and soles. Oral mucosal involvement is associated with fine white papules or pale reticular streaks that eventually desquamate (Barrett & Bilous, 1984).

Mild reaction may be associated with minimal macular erythema, which is transitory. Widespread macular and papular eruptions may also develop in autologous and syngeneic transplant recipients. Some of these may represent reactions due to lymphocyte recovery (Horn *et al.,* 1989; Horn, 1994), particularly as the histologic features of both events overlap (Bauer, Hood, & Horn, 1993). While the rash of lymphocyte recovery is usually self-limited, recipients of autologous or syngeneic transplants may rarely develop limited sclerodermoid (Pimpinelli, Santucci, & Bosi, 1992) or lichenoid reactions seen in chronic GVHD (Martin *et al.,* 1995). Autologous cutaneous GVHD occurs in only 10% of patients (Hood *et al.,* 1987) and is seen more frequently after the administration of low-dose cyclosporine possibly due to the capacity of cyclosporine to abrogate the normal intrathymic process of clonal deletion of autoreactive T-cell clones (Jenkins, Schwarz, & Pardoll, 1988; Jones *et al.,* 1989; Hess, Fisher, & Beschorner, 1990; Horn, 1994). Severe reactions are associated with epidermal necrosis and flaccid blisters, identical to that seen in toxic epidermal necrolysis (TEN). In addition to the acute signs of erythema and edema, there may be variable purpura if thrombocytopenia is present.

Acute reactions may be delayed and only appear as immunosuppressive therapy is modified (Valks *et al.,* 2001). As the

Table 96.1. *Dermatological complications of hematopoietic stem cell transplantation*

1. Graft-versus-host disease	Acute Chronic
2. Treatment-related	Rash of lymphocyte recovery Immediate type hypersensitivity, for example, urticaria with ATG Drug allergy, for example, to penicillins, cortrimoxazole, allopurinol Chemotherapy-induced acral dermatitis Skin reactions to recombinant cytokines Busulfan-induced erythema/hyperpigmentation in axillae and groins TBI-induced erythema Nifedipine erythema Vancomycin erythema (too rapid i.v. infusion) Corticosteroid acne Cyclosporine hypertrichosis and facial coarsening Alopecia secondary to chemotherapy/TBI/chronic GVHD Neutrophilic eccrine hidradenitis due to preparatory chemotherapy Roquinimex-related GVHD Leg ulcers with thalidomide
3. Infections	Bacterial: cellulitis/boils/i.v. site infection/septic emboli/paronychia Blistering dactylitis, staphylococcal scalded skin syndrome Fungal: Dermatophyte, *Candida, Aspergillus, Fusarium, Nocardia* Viral: HSV; VZV; CMV (very rare) Mites: scabies, crusted scabies
4. Immunologically mediated	Erythema multiforme (for example, response to HSV infection) Eczema Transfer of contact sensitivity from donor

5. Neoplastic	Recurrence of underlying malignancy, for example, subcutaneous
	  chloromas in AML/CML
	BCC, SCC, solar keratosis (especially in severely immune
	  compromised patients with chronic GVHD). Porokeratosis

6. Miscellaneous	Pityriasis rosea–like reaction Acquired ichthyosis

Abbreviations: ATG, antithymocyte globulin; TBI, total body irradiation; GVHD, graft-versus-host disease; HSV, herpes simplex virus; VZV, varicella zoster virus; CMV, cytomegalovirus; AML, acute myeloid leukemia; CML, chronic myeloid leukemia; BCC, basal cell carcinoma, SCC, squamous cell carcinoma.

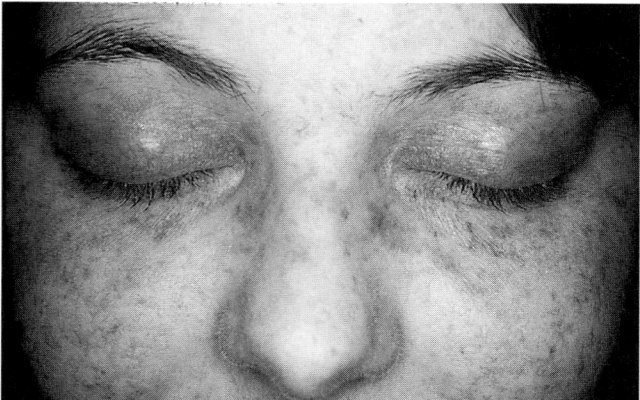

Fig. 96.1. Macular rash of acute GVHD concentrated on eyelids simulating dermatomyositis. For color reproduction, see Color Plate 96.1.

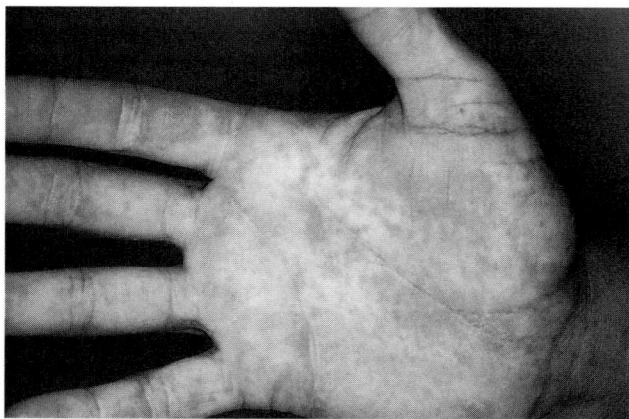

Fig. 96.2. Acute GVHD involving palms characterized by patchy tender erythema. For color reproduction, see Color Plate 96.2.

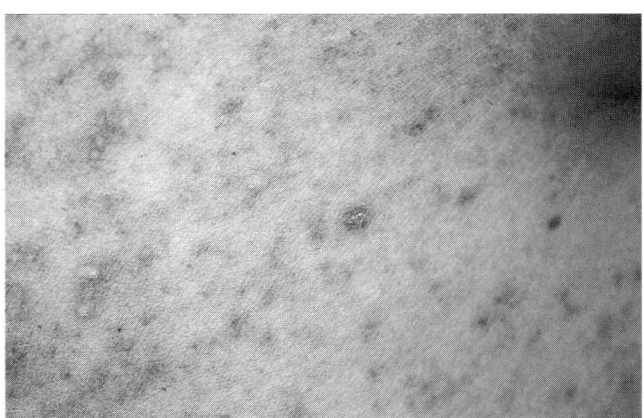

Fig. 96.3. Acute GVHD of the skin with micropapular element reflecting appendageal involvement. For color reproduction, see Color Plate 96.3.

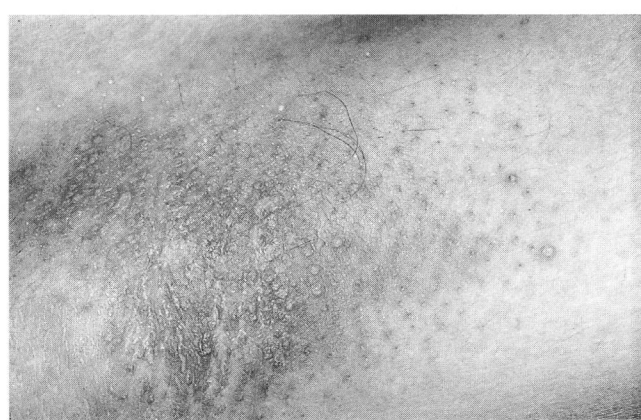

Fig. 96.4. Lichenoid rash seen with early chronic GVHD in the skin. For color reproduction, see Color Plate 96.4.

acute reaction subsides, widespread scaling and desquamation occurs, as well as mottled postinflammatory hyperpigmentation. An increased rate of acute cutaneous GVHD has been reported when roquinimex immunotherapy was added to the management of acute or chronic myeloid leukemia (Ohsuga *et al.*, 2000).

A papular follicular element (Friedman, Le Boit, & Farmer, 1988) or punctate erythema (Fig. 96.3) may be seen with acute reactions, reflecting follicular or eccrine duct involvement (Akosa & Lampert, 1990), and this may lead to follicular hyperkeratinization and keratin plugs resembling follicular lichen planus or miliaria. Icthyosiform features have been described (Chao *et al.*, 1998). One case has been described in which changes of acute GVHD occurred solely within an area affected by congenital piebaldism (Chow, Stewart, & Ho, 1996).

The degree of acute cutaneous GVHD is graded according to the extent and severity of skin involvement:

Grade 1: Less than 25% of skin involvement
Grade 2: 25–50% involvement
Grade 3: Erythroderma
Grade 4: Blistering or toxic epidermal necrolysis reactions

All but the most minimal acute GVHD skin rash should be treated early and vigorously to prevent skin progression (and GVHD development in other organs). A common initial regimen is methylprednisolone 1 mg/kg every 12 hours for 1 week, with a subsequent halving of dose for a further 7 days should resolution be occurring. Prophylactic immunosuppression (usually with cyclosporine) should be continued throughout this time period. For severe acute cutaneous GVHD (grade 3 and 4), a course of antithymocyte globulin may be required if no response occurs to the above dosage of methylprednisolone or to higher dose methylprednisolone (e.g., 500 mg daily for 3 days with subsequent halving every 3 days). Extra corporeal photochemotherapy may also be useful in severe steroid-refractory acute GVHD (Greinix *et al.*, 2000). Further discussion of the treatment of acute GVHD is given in Chapter 71.

Chronic GVHD (see also Chapter 72)

Chronic GVHD may develop in the wake of a continuing acute reaction, but may also emerge after a latent interval during which the skin appears morphologically normal. In some individuals, signs of chronic GVHD may appear without a clinically evident preceding acute phase (de novo chronic GVHD).

Established chronic GVHD usually occurs after 100 days posttransplant, but may appear as early as day 45 (Saurat *et al.*, 1975; Farmer, 1985; Atkinson *et al.*, 1989; Aractingi & Chosidow, 1998).

Early chronic GVHD is associated with the appearance of violaceous papules (Fig. 96.4) resembling lichen planus (Saurat *et al.*, 1975), that are generalized and coalesce to form plaques. Oral, and occasionally genital, mucous membrane involvement is associated with erosions and with white reticular patches (Fig. 96.5), that need to be distinguished from candidiasis. Mild chronic lichenoid GVHD affecting the skin and mucous membranes has also occurred after autologous bone

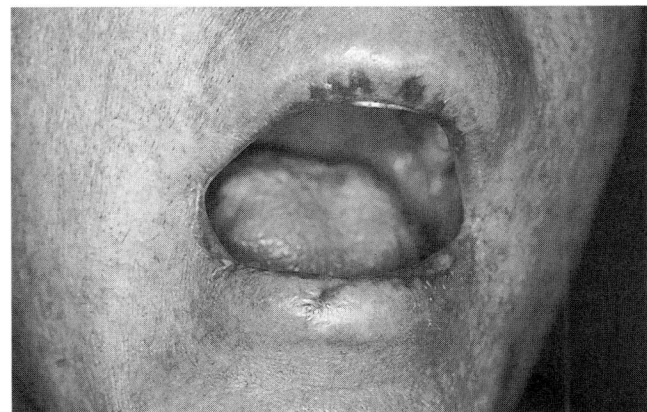

Fig. 96.5. Mucous membrane erosions and white patches seen with chronic GVHD. For color reproduction, see Color Plate 96.5.

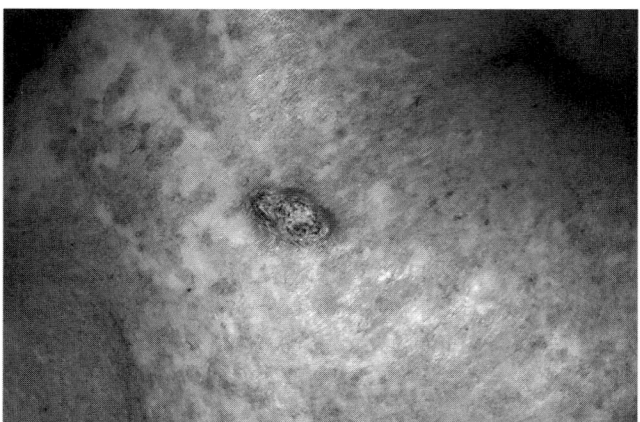

Fig. 96.6. Advanced cutaneous chronic GVHD demonstrating sclerosis, patchy pigmentation, and focal ulceration. For color reproduction, see Color Plate 96.6.

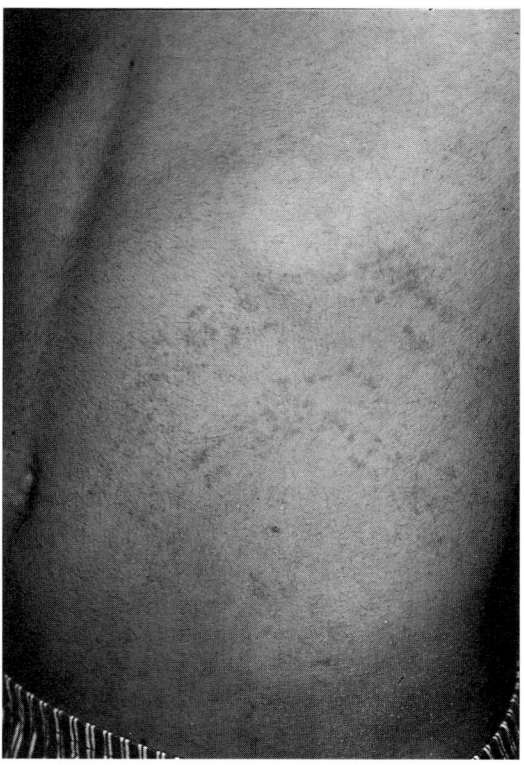

Fig. 96.7. V-shaped lichenoid pattern seen in unilateral chronic GVHD along Blaschko's lines on back. For color reproduction, see Color Plate 96.7.

marrow transplantation (Martin et al., 1995). The lichenoid papular eruption is associated with scaling and may have a photosensitive element as well as associated cutaneous atrophy mimicking connective tissue disease, particularly lupus erythematosus. Prominent follicular involvement may occur in chronic GVHD (Miyazaki, Higaki, & Maruyama, 1993). Continuing chronic GVHD gives way to epidermal atrophy, telangiectasia, and mottled skin color changes (Fig. 96.6), resulting in a poikilodermatous appearance to the skin, similar to that seen in dermatomyositis. Lichenoid reactions are superimposed on this background, reflecting continuing inflammation of the skin. Progressive hair loss with scarring alopecia can occur (Vowels et al., 1993).

Lichenoid GVHD may also occur in a unilateral distribution. A dermatomal distribution may follow prior varicella zoster infection (Cohen & Hymes, 1994; Freemer et al., 1994; Baselga et al., 1996) or the reaction may present in an S- and V-shaped pattern of Blaschko's lines[1] (Fig. 96.7) as a result of cellular mosaicism of the host's skin (Beers et al., 1993; Wilson & Lockman, 1994; Lee, Atkinson, & Kossard, 1996).

Long-standing chronic GVHD leads to progressive sclerosis of the skin, often complicated by joint contractures mimicking severe scleroderma (Spilvogel, Goltz, & Kersey, 1977). However, there is usually no acrosclerosis or Raynaud phenomenon[2] associated with GVHD sclerosis. The sclerosis can be complicated by persistent skin ulceration and loss of skin appendages, resulting in both alopecia and anhidrosis. Persistent severe pain of the lower extremities due to localized polyneuropathy may accompany scleroderma-like lesions on the legs (Aracting et al., 1993). Severe mucous membrane involvement may lead to a Sjögren's-like syndrome[3] with xerophthalmia and xerostomia, due to the destruction of the

mucous glands of the conjunctiva and the minor salivary glands, respectively (Rodu & Gockerman, 1983; Janin-Mercier et al., 1987).

Although chronic GVHD is usually generalized about 20% of the cases may have localized disease confined to a few areas of skin. These patches may be hyperpigmented and indurated resembling localized scleroderma, or consist of small lesions that are hypopigmented with superficial sclerosis, giving a lichen sclerosis-like appearance (Cordoba et al., 1999). Both diffuse melanoderma (Aracting et al., 1996) and total leukoderma (Nagler et al., 1996) have been described. Chronic GVHD may also be localized to the fields of prior radiotherapy (Socie et al., 1989; Okamoto et al., 1996).

Prior virus infection may play a role in localizing clinical cutaneous GVHD. Apart from dermatomal GVHD in areas of previous herpes zoster (Cohen & Hymes, 1994; Freemer et al., 1994; Baselga et al., 1996), sclerodermatous GVHD has developed in areas of a previous measles exanthem (Fenyk et al., 1978). Chronic GVHD may also occur with increased frequency in individuals with preceding cytomegalovirus infection (Lomquist et al., 1984).

The combination of immunosuppression and chronic lichenoid reactions with scarring has resulted in the appearance of isolated skin tumors, particularly squamous and basal cell carcinomas (Howe & Lang, 1988; Lishner et al., 1990), which

[1] Alfred Blaschko, German dermatologist, 1858–1922.
[2] Maurice Raynaud, French physician, 1834–1881.
[3] Henrik Samuel Conrad Sjögren, Swedish ophthalmologist, born 1899.

need to be differentiated from vascular lesions resembling pyogenic granuloma that may also develop on a background of poikiloderma (Garnis, Billick, & Srolvitz, 1984). Whether the rate of skin cancers and their severity in bone marrow transplant patients is lower than that in organ transplants remains to be evaluated. It is possible that the graft-versus-host reaction in the skin may destroy aberrant sun-damaged keratinocytes and reduce the risk of cutaneous malignancy in this group. However, a large study of solid cancers developing after bone marrow transplantation revealed an excess risk of squamous cell carcinoma of the buccal mucosa and skin associated with chronic GVHD and male sex (Curtis *et al.*, 1997). Despite the severity of the sclerosis seen with long-standing chronic GVHD, it may eventually soften and resolve.

Limited chronic GVHD (skin or hepatic involvement only) may not need to be treated, although skin involvement producing cosmetic deformity is an indication for therapy, as is extensive cutaneous involvement. If the appearance of chronic GVHD has followed cessation of prophylactic immunosuppression (usually with cyclosporine), this should be restarted at full therapeutic dosage. If after 4 weeks, no improvement has been made, prednisolone 1 mg/kg on alternate days should be started, and the combination of cyclosporine and prednisolone continued for up to 9 months. Chronic cutaneous GVHD refractory to this combination regimen may be treated with thalidomide, in addition, starting at 100 mg four times a day, increasing to 300 mg four times a day. Side effects are peripheral neuropathy, constipation, and somnolence. Severe leg ulceration may also develop as a complication of thalidomide treatment for GVHD (Schlossberg *et al.*, 2001). Baseline nerve conduction studies should be performed before starting thalidomide. In a number of patients thalidomide has produced resolution of severe subcutaneous and cutaneous fibrosis refractory to cyclosporine and prednisone treatment. An additional treatment modality for chronic GVHD involving either skin or mouth is psoralen and ultraviolet A (PUVA) phototherapy (Hymes *et al.*, 1985; Atkinson *et al.*, 1986; Eppinger *et al.*, 1990; Volc-Platzer *et al.*, 1990; Aubin *et al.*, 1995). In patients unable to tolerate psoralens, UVB alone has been used successfully (Van Dooren-Greebe, Schattenberg, & Koopman, 1991; Enk *et al.*, 1998). Extracorporeal photochemotherapy utilizing leukaphoresis and oral psoralen has also been used as single therapy for chronic cutaneous GVHD (Rossetti *et al.*, 1995). Bath PUVA therapy has been used successfully to treat pediatric patients with drug-resistant cutaneous GVHD (Bonanomi *et al.*, 2001). Occasionally, chronic oral GVHD produces symptomatic dryness of the mouth only. If the diagnosis is confirmed by lip biopsy, oral PUVA therapy is a useful nonsystemic and often effective method of treatment (discussed further in Chapter 72). Etretinate, or its substitute acitretin, may induce improvement in cutaneous sclerosis in refractory sclerodermatous GVHD (Marcellus *et al.*, 1999). Intravenous pulses of lidocaine have also been used to treat refractory sclerodermatous GVHD (Voltarelli *et al.*, 2001). Tacrolimus ointment may be useful for localized chronic GVHD (Choi & Nghiem, 2001).

Cutaneous drug reactions

HSC transplant recipients are exposed to a wide range of drugs in the preparatory phase for transplantation, and subsequently to agents used to secure immune suppression and to deal with infections (Table 96.1). Drug reactions may be seen, particularly with cotrimoxazole, allopurinol, amoxycillin, and other penicillins. Although the majority of drug reactions are self-limited, they may complicate the assessment of GVHD of the skin during the transplant period. This is compounded by the fact that both radiotherapy (Le Boit, 1989) and chemotherapy may result in individual cell necrosis and lichenoid changes in skin biopsies, which may histologically mimic GVHD. The subsequent clinical time course and associated evidence of gut and liver involvement may be required to isolate the relative contribution of a drug reaction and GVHD in the skin, Antithymocyte globulin (ATG) or antilymphocyte globulin (ALG) can cause both erythema and urticaria. When urticaria occurs, no further drug should be given unless a different species of ATG or ALG can be utilized.

Several distinct pharmacologic and toxic cutaneous drug reactions due to chemotherapy have been recognized in patients undergoing HSC transplantation after preparatory high-dose chemotherapy or chemoradiotherapy. Chemotherapy-induced acral erythema (Crider *et al.*, 1986; Kerker & Hood, 1989; Baack & Burgdorf, 1991) is characterized by well-demarcated, painful dusky erythematous patches involving the palms (Fig. 96.8) and soles, as well as the extensor surface of the digits. Severe reactions may be associated with blister formation and subsequent desquamation. Acral erythema has been seen, particularly with cytosine arabinoside and daunorubicin used in the treatment of acute myeloid leukemia, and busulfan in the treatment of chronic myeloid leukemia. Similar reactions have been reported less frequently with hydroxyurea, methotrexate, 6-mercaptopurine, cyclophosphamide, and mitoxantrone. The skin reaction associated with

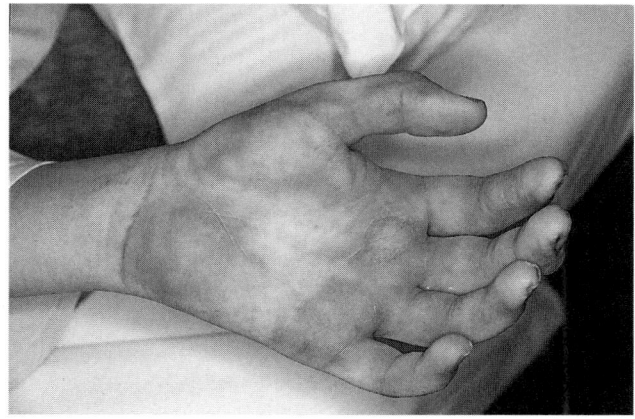

Fig. 96.8. Well-demarcated dusky acral erythema with early blister formation induced by chemotherapy. For color reproduction, see Color Plate 96.8.

GVHD tends to be a more diffuse process with a brighter erythema and simultaneous involvement of the face and upper trunk.

Cutaneous erythematous plaques and nodules may develop after preparatory chemotherapy and on skin biopsy reveal neutrophilic eccrine hidradenitis (Bailey, Barron, & Lucky, 1989).

Flexural erythema localized to the axillary and inguinal folds, with involvement of the scrotum in men, can be seen in association with busulfan therapy. In severe episodes, there may be ulceration, and the reaction characteristically heals with hyperpigmentation.

More diffuse erythematous reactions may be seen as a consequence of preparatory chemotherapy or total body irradiation (TBI), although this is now uncommon with the widespread use of fractionated, as opposed to single-dose TBI. Nifedipine, used commonly to control cyclosporine-associated hypertension, can frequently cause skin erythema and warming and may need to be replaced by a different antihypertensive agent, such as atenolol if this occurs. If vancomycin is infused more rapidly than over a 1-hour infusion period, it can cause painful erythema. This is not an allergic, but rather a physical, reaction to the antibiotic, which can be eliminated by prolonging the duration of the infusion to 1 to 2 hours.

Corticosteroids are associated with the development of acneiform lesions, which can be distinguished from follicular graft-versus-host reactions by their clinical appearance, distribution (forehead, rest of face, anterior upper chest) and histopathology.

Drug-induced TEN may need to be excluded in patients undergoing severe GVHD (McDonald, Singer, & Bianco, 1992).

Cyclosporine can cause coarsening of the facial features, a side effect that, like all other cyclosporine side effects, is reversible on lowering the dose of the drug or stopping its administration.

Skin reactions to recombinant cytokine therapy, particularly granulocyte-macrophage colony-stimulating factor (GM-CSF), may produce discrete papules and plaques or bullous lesions (Horn et al., 1991; Asnis & Gaspari, 1995; Glass, Fotopoulos, & Messina, 1996; Mori et al., 2000).

Busulfan combined with cyclophosphamide as conditioning treatment prior to transplantation may lead to permanent alopecia (Baker et al., 1991) in the absence of GVHD. In contrast, cyclophosphamide combined with TBI results in a transient alopecia, but with hair regrowing by 3 to 4 months posttransplant often darker and curlier than pretransplant.

Cutaneous infections

Immunosuppression is associated with a marked risk of skin infection and this is reflected by the frequent occurrence of *Candida* and dermatophyte infection. Prophylaxis with acyclovir has reduced the frequency of cutaneous, oral, genital, and disseminated herpes simplex infection. Herpes simplex infection may be complicated by the development of ery-

thema multiforme and may require acyclovir to prevent recurrent episodes. Herpes zoster occurs not uncommonly after HSC transplantation (Atkinson et al., 1980), but appears less frequently than previously, possibly due to a decreased incidence of severe chronic GVHD. At the first sign of the typical cutaneous dermatomal involvement, acyclovir 10 mg/kg five times daily for 7 days should be initiated orally or intravenously.

Cultures, if necessary by fine needle aspirate, should be obtained from any areas of cellulitis, hemorrhagic blisters, or tender nodules as these may reveal the presence of *Aspergillus* (Schimmelpfennig et al., 2001), *Pseudomonas,* or a variety of unusual opportunistic organisms such as disseminated *Fusarium* (Mowbray et al., 1988) or subcutaneous *Nocardia* (Freites et al., 1995). Skin involvement by *Aspergillus* may occur at the entry site of indwelling right atrial catheters (Allo et al., 1987).

Immunosuppression also may result in the development of a crusted form of scabies that may not be readily recognized but is highly contagious (Barnes, McCallister, & Lucky, 1987; Magee, Hebert, & Rapini, 1991). Acral bullae due to staphylococci may present as a blistering dactylitis (Kossard & Atkinson, 1994) or as a staphylococcal scalded skin syndrome that may mimic acute GVHD (Goldberg et al., 1989).

Miscellaneous skin manifestations

Both acute and chronic myelold leukemia can present with cutaneous and subcutaneous chloromas and diagnosis should be confirmed by biopsy.

Eczema appearing for the first time posttransplant occurs more frequently than would be expected by chance, but responds to topical corticosteroid cream application. Passive transfer of contact sensitivity has occurred as a complication of allogeneic bone marrow transplantation (Olaguibel et al., 1989).

As with other autoimmune disorders (e.g., rheumatoid arthritis), psoriasis (Eddy et al., 1990) in the recipient can be eradicated by the transplant procedure and represents an unexpected bonus for the recipient (Chapter 119). In some patients psoriasis may be passively transferred (Gardembas-Pain et al., 1990).

Permanent alopecia has been reported as a side effect associated with both chronic GVHD (Vowels et al., 1993) and busulfan as part of the conditioning therapy (Vowels et al., 1993; Ljungman et al., 1995). In the study by Ljungman and colleagues the mean busulfan blood concentration was significantly higher in patients who developed alopecia than in those who did not. In the study by Vowels and colleagues the highest frequency of alopecia was in patients conditioned with busulfan who had received prior cranial irradiation and/or developed chronic GVHD. In this cohort the frequency of alopecia was 75%. Transplantation of hair from the original HSC donor has been used successfully to treat baldness posttransplant, with no evidence of rejection of the hair allograft (Rosati & Bergamo, 1999).

Nail changes occur after both conventional dose chemotherapy and after the conditioning regimen for HSC transplantation. The treatment causes the nails to grow slowly or even to stop growing for short intervals, resulting in characteristic Beau's lines[4] (sometimes knows as Beau-Reil lines).

Generalized granuloma annulare has been described developing 3 weeks after an autologous transplant for Hodgkin's disease (Nevo *et al.*, 1994). A papular erythematous skin rash appeared at day 22 posttransplant and skin biopsy showed dense inflammatory cell infiltrates in the epidermis composed of epithelioid histiocytes in nodular aggregates with a tendency to palisading. Some histiocytic giant cells were observed. Histiocytic cytophagic panniculitis has also been described in a 46 year old patient occurring 32 months after an allogeneic bone marrow transplant for chronic myeloid leukemia. This proliferative histiocytic disorder has involvement confined to the skin. On examination the patient had hyperpigmentation, xerosis, and scaling skin on both legs; skin biopsy showed hemorrhage and an inflammatory infiltrate in the subcutaneous fat involving both septa and lobules extended into the reticular dermis with a perivascular distribution. It was mainly composed of histiocytes, many containing red blood cells, and some lymphocytes. An intense degree of lipophagia was observed (Galende *et al.*, 1994). It should be noted, however, that this patient's chronic myeloid leukemia had relapsed prior to the development of the skin rash and had been treated with hydroxyurea and interferon.

Pityriasis rosea–like eruptions may also develop after HSC transplantation (Spelman *et al.*, 1994). This reaction appears to be distinct from true pityriasis rosea and a drug basis could not been implicated in the patients reported. Acquired ichthyosis may also be seen as a complication of bone marrow transplantation (Spelman *et al.*, 1996). Disseminated superficial actinic porokeratosis may emerge after the pretransplant conditioning regimen (Fields *et al.*, 1995).

Giant cell lichenoid dermatitis has been described occurring in the site of scars from previous varicella zoster infection (Bartolome *et al.*, 2000). Clinically, this appeared as flat violaceous lichenoid papules and confluent plaques. Histopathologic examination showed an inflammatory infiltrate in the papillary dermis with granulomatous aggregates formed by histiocytes, multinucleated giant cells and lymphocytes.

Cryofibrinogenemia, with associated thrombotic vasculopathy, producing skin necrosis of the ears and extremities has been described after autologous HSC transplantation and posttransplant interleukin-2 treatment (Shimoni *et al.*, 2000).

Finally, several cases of bullous pemphigoid have been described after allogeneic marrow transplantation, and may be causally related to preceding cutaneous GVHD (Mikio *et al.*, 1986; Delbaldo *et al.*, 1992).

[4] Joseph Honoré Simon Beau, French physician, 1806–1865.

References

Akosa, A. B. & Lampert, L. A. (1990). The sweat gland in graft-versus-host disease. *Journal of Pathology*, **161**, 261–6.

Allo, M. D., Miller, J., Townsend, T. *et al.* (1987). Primary cutaneous aspergillosis associated with Hickman intravenous catheters. *New England Journal of Medicine*, **317**, 1105–8.

Aracting, I. S., Janin, A., Devergie, A. *et al.* (1996). Histochemical and ultrastructural study of diffuse melanoderma after bone marrow transplantation. *British Journal of Dermatology*, **134**, 325–31.

Aracting, I. S., Socie, G., Devergie, A. *et al.* (1993). Localized scleroderma-like lesions on the legs in bone marrow transplant recipients: association with polyneuropathy in the same distribution. *British Journal of Dermatology*, **129**, 201–3.

Aracting, S. & Chosidow, O. (1998). Cutaneous graft-versus-host disease. *Archives of Dermatology*, **134**, 602–12.

Asnis, L. A. & Gaspari, A. A. (1995). Cutaneous reactions to recombinant cytokine therapy. *Journal of the American Academy of Dermatology*, **33**, 393–410.

Atkinson, K., Horowitz, M. M., Gale, R. P. *et al.* (1989). Consensus among bone marrow transplanters for diagnosis, grading and treatment of chronic graft-versus-host disease. *Bone Marrow Transplantation*, **4**, 247–54.

Atkinson, K., Meyers, J. D., Storb, R. *et al.* (1980). Varicella-zoster virus infection after marrow transplantation for aplastic anemia or leukemia. *Transplantation*, **29**, 47–50.

Atkinson, K., Weller, P., Ryman, W., & Biggs, J. (1986). PUVA therapy for drug-resistant graft-versus-host disease. *Bone Marrow Transplantation*, **1**, 227–36.

Aubin, F., Brion, A., Deconinck, E. *et al.* (1995). Phototherapy in the treatment of cutaneous graft-versus-host disease: our preliminary experience in resistant patients. *Transplantation*, **59**, 151–5.

Baack, B. R. & Burgdorf, W. H. C. (1991). Chemotherapy induced acral erythema. *Journal of the American Academy of Dermatology*, **24**, 457–61.

Bailey, D. L., Barren, D., & Lucky, A. W. (1989). Neutrophilic eccrine hidradenitis: a case report and review of the literature. *Paediatric Dermatology*, **6**, 33–8.

Baker, B. W., Wilson, C. L., Davis, A. L. *et al.* (1991). Busulphan/cyclophosphamide conditioning for bone marrow transplantation may lead to failure of hair regrowth. *Bone Marrow Transplantation*, **7**, 43–7.

Barnes, L., McCallister, R. E., & Lucky, A. W. (1987). Crusted (Norwegian) scabies occurrence in a child undergoing a bone marrow transplant. *Archives of Dermatology*, **123**, 95–7.

Barrett, A. P. & Bilous, M. (1984). Oral patterns of acute and chronic graft-versus-host disease. *Archives of Dermatology*, **120**, 1461–5.

Bartolome, B., Cordoba, S., Fernandez-Herrera, J. *et al.* (2000). Giant cell lichenoid dermatitis within herpes zoster scars in a bone marrow recipient. *Journals of Cutaneous Pathology*, **27**, 255–7.

Baselga, E., Drolet, B. A., Segura, A. D. *et al.* (1996). Dermatomal lichenoid chronic graft-versus-host disease following varicella-zoster infection despite absence of viral genome. *Journal of Cutaneous Pathology*, **23**, 576–81.

Bauer, D. J., Hood, A. F., & Horn, T. D. (1993). Histological comparison of autologous graft-versus-host reaction and cutaneous eruptions of lymphocyte recovery. *Archives of Dermatology*, **129**, 855–8.

Beers, B., Kalish, R. S., Kaye, V. N., & Dahl, M. V. (1993). Unilateral linear lichenoid eruption after bone marrow transplantation: an unmasking of tolerance to an abnormal keratinocyte clone? *Journal of the American Academy of Dermatology*, **28**, 888–92.

Bonanomi, S., Balduzzi, A., Tagliabue, A. *et al.* (2001). Bath PUVA therapy in pediatric patients with drug resistant cutaneous graft-versus-host disease. *Bone Marrow Transplantation*, **6**, 631–2.

Chao, S. C., Tsao, C. J., Liu, C. L., & Lee, J. Y. (1998). Acute cutaneous graft-versus-host disease with icthyosiform features. *British Journal of Dermatology*, **139**, 553–5 (Letter).

Choi, C. J. & Nghiem, P. (2001). Tacrolimus ointment in the treatment of chronic cutaneous graft-versus-host disease: a case series of 18 patients. *Archives of Dermatology*, **137**, 1202–6.

Chow, R. K., Stewart, W. D., & Ho, V. C. (1996). Graft-versus-host reaction affecting lesional skin, but not normal skin in a patient with piebaldism. *British Journal of Dermatology*, **134**, 134–7.

Cohen, P. R. & Hymes, S. R. (1994). Linear and dermatomal cutaneous graft-versus-host disease. *Southern Medical Journal*, **87**, 758–61.

Cordoba, S., Aragues, M., Fernandez-Herrera, J. *et al.* (1999). Lichen sclerosus et atrophicus in sclerodermatous chronic graft-versus-host disease. *International Journal of Dermatology*, **38**, 708–11.

Crider, M. K., Jansen, J., Norins, A. L. *et al.* (1986). Chemotherapy induced acral erythema in patients receiving bone marrow transplantation. *Archives of Dermatology*, **122**, 1023–7.

Curtis, R. E., Rowlings, P. A., Deeg, H. J. *et al.* (1997). Solid cancers after bone marrow transplantation. *New England Journal of Medicine*, **336**, 897–904.

Delbaldo, C., Rieckhoff-Cantoni, L., Helg, C. *et al.* (1992). Bullous pemphigoid associated with acute graft-versus-host disease after allogeneic bone marrow transplantation. *Bone Marrow Transplantation*, **10**, 377–9.

Eddy, D. J., Burrows, D., Bridges, J. M., & Jones, F. G. (1990). Clearance of severe psoriasis after allogeneic bone marrow transplantation. *British Medical Journal*, **300**, 908.

Enk, C. D., Elad, S., Vexler, A. *et al.* (1998). Chronic graft-versus-host disease treated with UVB Phototherapy. *Bone Marrow Transplantation*, **3**, 1179–83.

Eppinger, T., Ehninger, G., Steinert, M. *et al.* (1990). 8-methoxypsoralen and ultraviolet A therapy for cutaneous manifestation of graft-versus-host disease. *Transplantation*, **50**, 807–11.

Farmer, E. R. (1985). Human cutaneous graft-versus-host disease. *Journal of Investigative Dermatology*, **85** (Suppl), 1245–85.

Fenyk, J. R., Smith, C. M., Warkentin, P. I. *et al.* (1978). Sclerodermatous graft-versus-host disease limited to an area of measles exanthem. *Lancet*, **1**, 472–3.

Fields, L. L., White, C. R., & Mazaiarz, R. T. (1995). Rapid development of disseminated superficial porokeratosis after transplant induction therapy. *Bone Marrow Transplantation*, **15**, 993–5.

Freemer, C. S., Farmer, E. R., Corio, R. L. *et al.* (1994). Lichenoid graft-versus-host disease occurring in a dermatomal distribution. *Archives of Dermatology*, **130**, 70–2.

Freites, V., Sumoza, A., Bisotti, R. *et al.* (1995). Subcutaneous *Nocardia asteroides* abscess in bone marrow transplant recipient. *Bone Marrow Transplantation*, **15**, 135–6.

Friedman, K. J., Le Boit, P. E., & Farmer, E. R. (1998). Acute follicular graft-versus-host reaction. *Archives of Dermatology*, **124**, 688–91.

Fujii, H., Hiketa, T., Matsumoto, Y. *et al.* (1992). Clinical characteristics of chronic cutaneous graft-versus-host disease in Japanese leukemia patients after bone marrow transplantation: low incidence and mild manifestations of skin lesions. *Bone Marrow Transplantation*, **10**, 331–5.

Galende, J., Vazquez, M. L., Almeida, J. *et al.* (1994). Histiocytic cytophagic panniculitis: a rare late complication of allogeneic bone marrow transplantation. *Bone Marrow Transplantation*, **14**, 637–9.

Gardembas-Pain, M., Ifrah, N., Foussard, C. *et al.* (1990). Psoriasis after allogeneic bone marrow transplantation. *Archives of Dermatology*, **126**, 1523.

Garnis, S., Billick, R. C., & Srolvitz, H. (1984). Eruptive vascular tumours associated with chronic graft-versus-host disease. *Journal of the American Academy of Dermatology*, **10**, 918–21.

Glass, L. F., Fotopoulos, T., & Messina, J. L. (1996). A generalised cutaneous reaction induced by granulocyte colony stimulating factor. *Journal of the American Academy of Dermatology*, **34**, 455–9.

Goldberg, N. S., Ahmed, T., Robinson, B. *et al.* (1989). Staphylococcal scalded skin syndrome mimicking acute graft-versus-host disease in a bone marrow transplant recipient. *Archives of Dermatology*, **125**, 85–7.

Greinix, H. T., Volc-Platzer, B., Kahls, P. *et al.* (2000). Extracorporeal photochemotherapy in the treatment of severe steroid refractory acute graft-versus-host disease: a pilot study. *Blood*, **96**, 2426–31.

Hess, A. D., Fisher, A. C., & Beschorner, W. E. (1990). Effector mechanisms in cyclosporine A induced syngeneic graft versus host disease. Role of CD4$^+$ and CD8$^+$ T lymphocyte subsets. *Journal of Immunology*, **145**, 526–33.

Hood, A. F., Vogelsand, G. B., Black, L. P. *et al.* (1987). Acute graft-versus-host disease: development following autologous and syngeneic bone marrow transplantation. *Archives of Dermatology*, **123**, 745–50.

Horn, T. D. (1994). Acute cutaneous eruptions after marrow ablation: roses by other names. *Journal of Cutaneous Pathology*, **21**, 385–92.

Horn, T. D., Burke, P. J., Karp, J. E., & Hood, A. F. (1991). Intravenous administration of recombinant human granulocyte-macrophage colony stimulating factor causes a cutaneous eruption. *Archives of Dermatology*, **127**, 49–52.

Horn, T. D., Redd, J. V., Karp, J. E. *et al.* (1989). Cutaneous eruptions of lymphocyte recovery. *Archives of Dermatology*, **125**, 1512–17.

Howe, N. R. & Lang, P. G. (1988). Squamous cell carcinoma of the sole in a patient with chronic graft-versus-host disease. *Archives of Dermatology*, **124**, 1244–5.

Hymes, S. R., Morison, W. L., Farmer, E. R. *et al.* (1985). Methoxsalen and ultraviolet A radiation in treatment of chronic graft versus host reaction. *Journal of the American Academy of Dermatology*, **12**, 30–7.

Janin-Mercier, A., Devergie, A., Arrago, J. P. *et al.* (1987). Systemic evaluation of Sjogren-like syndrome after bone marrow transplantation in man. *Transplantation*, **43**, 677–9.

Jenkins, M. K., Schwartz, R. H., & Pardoll, D. M. (1988). Effects of cyclosporine A on T cell development and clonal deletion. *Science,* **241,** 1655–8.

Jones, R. J., Hess, A. D., Mann, R. B. *et al.* (1989). Induction of graft-versus-host disease after autologous bone marrow transplantation. *Lancet,* **1,** 754–7.

Kerker, B. J. & Hood, A. F. (1989). Chemotherapy induced cutaneous reactions. *Seminars in Dermatology,* **8,** 173–81.

Kossard, S. & Atkinson, K, (1994). Tender acral blister in a bone marrow transplant patient. *Australasian Journal of Dermatology,* **35,** 107–9.

Le Boit, P. E. (1989). Subacute radiation dermatitis: a histologic imitator of acute cutaneous graft-versus-host disease. *Journal of the American Academy of Dermatology,* **20,** 236–41.

Lee, M. S., Atkinson, K., & Kossard, S. (1996). Lichenoid graft-versus-host disease occurring in Blaschko's lines. *European Journal of Dermatology,* **6,** 282–3.

Lishner, M., Patterson, B., Kandel, R. *et al.* (1990). Cutaneous and mucosal neoplasms in bone marrow transplant recipients. *Cancer,* **65,** 473–6.

Ljungman, P., Hassan, M., Bekasssy, A. N. *et al.* (1995). Busulfan concentration in relation to permanent alopecia in recipients of bone marrow transplants. *Bone Marrow Transplantation,* **15,** 869–71.

Lomquist, B., Ringden, O. L., Wahren, B. *et al.* (1984). Cytomegalovirus infection associated with and preceding chronic graft-versus-host disease. *Transplantation,* **38,** 465–8.

Magee, K. L., Hebert, A. A., & Rapini, R. P. (1991). Crusted scabies in a patient with chronic graft-versus-host disease. *Journal of the American Academy of Dermatology,* **25,** 889–91.

Marcellus, D. C., Altomonte, V. L., Farmer, E. R. *et al.* (1999). Etretinate therapy for refractory sclerodermatous chronic graft-versus-host disease. *Blood,* **93,** 66–70.

Martin, R. W., Farmer, E. R., Altomonte, V. L. *et al.* (1995). Lichenoid graft-versus-host disease in an autologous bone marrow transplant recipient. *Archives of Dermatology,* **131,** 333–5.

Mauduit, G. & Claudy, A. (1988). Cutaneous expression of graft-versus-host disease in man. *Seminars in Dermatology,* **7,** 149–55.

McDonald, B. J., Singer, J. W., & Bianco, J. A. (1992). Toxic epidermal necrolysis possibly linked to aztreonam in bone marrow transplant patients. *Annals of Pharmacotherapeutics,* **26,** 34–5.

Mikio, U., Takao, M., Shintaro, S. *et al.* (1986). Development of bullous pemphigoid after allogeneic bone marrow transplantation. *Transplantation,* **42,** 420–2.

Miyazaki, K., Higaki, S., & Maruyama, T. (1993). Chronic graft-versus-host disease with follicular involvement. *Journal of Dermatology,* **20,** 242–6.

Mori, T., Sato, N., Watanabe, R. Okamoto, S., & Ikeda, Y. (2000). Erythema exsudativum multiforme induced by granulocyte colony-stimulating factor in an allogeneic peripheral blood stem cell donor. *Bone Marrow Transplantation,* **26,** 239–40.

Mowbray, D. N., Paller, A. S., Nelson, P. E., & Kaplan, R. L. (1988). Disseminated *Fusarium solani* infection with cutaneous nodules in a bone marrow transplant patient. *International Journal of Dermatology,* **27,** 698–701.

Nagler, A., Goldenhersh, M. A., Levi-Schaffer, F. *et al.* (1996). Total leucoderma: a rare manifestation of cutaneous chronic graft-versus-host disease. *British Journal of Dermatology,* **134,** 780–3.

Nevo, S., Drakos, P., Goldenhersh, M. A. *et al.* (1994). Generalized granuloma annulare post autologous bone marrow transplantation in a Hodgkin's disease patient. *Bone Marrow Transplantation,* **14,** 631–3.

Ohsuga, Y., Rowe, J. M., Liesveld, J., Burns, R. P., & Gaspari, A. A. (2000). Dermatologic changes associated with roquinimex immunotherapy after autologous bone marrow transplant. *Journal of the American Academy of Dermatology,* **42,** 437–4.

Okamoto, S., Takahashi, S., Inoue, T. *et al.* (1996). Cutaneous chronic graft-versus-host disease localised to the field of total lymphoid irradiation. *Bone Marrow Transplantation,* **17,** 111–13.

Olaguibel, J., Almodovar, A., Girer, A. *et al.* (1989). Passive transfer of contact sensitivity to colophony as a complication of allogeneic bone marrow transplant. *Contact Dermatitis,* **20,** 182–4.

Pimpinelli, N., Santucci, M., & Bosi, A. (1992). Localised scleroderma-like lesion in autologous bone marrow transplantation. *Journal of Dermatology,* **2,** 12–14.

Rodu, B. & Gockerman, J. P. (1983). Oral manifestations of the chronic graft-versus-host reaction. *Journal of the American Medical Association,* **249,** 504–7.

Rosati, P. & Bergamo, A. (1999). Allogeneic hair transplant in a bone marrow transplant recipient. *Dermatological Surgery,* **25,** 664–5.

Rossetti, F., Zulian, F., Dall'Amico, R. *et al.* (1995). Extracorporeal photochemotherapy as single therapy for extensive cutaneous chronic graft-versus-host disease. *Transplantation,* **59,** 149–51.

Saurat, J. A., Gluckman, E., Buseell, A. *et al.* (1975). Lichen planus-like eruption after bone marrow transplantation. *British Journal of Dermatology,* **92,** 675–81.

Schimmelpfennig, C., Naumann, R., Zuberbier, T. *et al.* (2001). Skin involvement as the first manifestation of systemic aspergillosis after allogeneic hematopoietic cell transplantation. *Bone Marrow Transplantation,* **27,** 753–5.

Schlossberg, H., Klumpp, T., Sabol, P., Herman, J., & Mangan, K. (2001). Severe cutaneous ulceration following treatment with thalidomide for GVHD. *Bone Marrow Transplantation,* **6,** 229–30.

Shimoni, A., Körbling, M., Champlin, R., & Molldrem, J. (2000). Cryofibrinogenemia and skin necrosis in a patient with diffuse large cell lymphoma after high-dose chemotherapy and autologous stem cell transplantation. *Bone Marrow Transplantation,* **26,** 1343–5.

Socie, G., Gluckman, E., Cosset, J. M. *et al.* (1989). Unusual localisation of cutaneous chronic graft-versus-host disease in the radiation fields in four cases. *Bone Marrow Transplantation,* **4,** 133–5.

Spelman, L. J., Robertson, I. M., Strutton, G. M., & Weedon, D. (1994). Pityriasis rosea–like eruption after bone marrow transplantation. *Journal of the American Academy of Dermatology,* **31,** 348–51.

Spelman, L. J., Strutton, G. M., Robertson, I. M., & Weedon, D. (1996). Acquired ichthyosis in bone marrow transplant recipients. *Journal of the American Academy of Dermatology,* **35,** 17–20.

Spilvogel, R. L., Goltz, R. W., & Kersey, J. H. (1977). Scleroderma-like changes in chronic graft-versus-host disease. *Archives of Dermatology,* **133,** 1424–8.

Tanaka, K., Sullivan, K. M., Shulman, H. M. *et al.* (1991). A clinical review: cutaneous manifestations of acute and chronic graft-versus-host disease following bone marrow transplantation. *Journal of Dermatology,* **18,** 11–17.

Valks, R., Fernandez-Herrera, J., Bartolome, B. *et al.* (2001). Late appearance of acute graft-versus-host disease after suspending or tapering immunosuppressive drugs. *Archives of Dermatology,* **137,** 61–5.

Van Dooren-Greebe, R. J., Schattenberg, A., & Koopman, R. J. (1991). Chronic cutaneous graft-versus-host disease: successful treatment with UVB. *British Journal of Dermatology,* **125,** 498–9.

Volc-Platzer, B., Honigsmann, H., Hinterberger, W., & Wolff, K. (1990). Phototherapy improves chronic cutaneous graft-versus-host disease. *Journal of the American Academy of Dermatology,* **23,** 220–8.

Voltarelli, J. C., Ahmed, H., Paton, E, *et al.* (2001). Beneficial effect of intravenous lidocaine in cutaneous chronic graft-versus-host disease secondary to donor lympohcyte infusion. *Bone Marrow Transplantation,* **6,** 97–9.

Vowels, M., Chan, L. L., Giri, N. *et al.* (1993). Factors affecting hair regrowth after bone marrow transplantation. *Bone Marrow Transplantation,* **12,** 347–50.

Wilson, B. D. & Lockman, D. W. (1994). Linear lichenoid graft versus host disease. *Archives of Dermatology,* **130,** 1206–7.

97 Gynecologic complications

CHRISTOPHER BRADBURY

St. Vincent's Hospital, Sydney, Australia

Introduction

The gynecologic complications seen after high-dose chemotherapy or chemoradiation and hematopoietic stem cell (HSC) transplantation are listed in Table 97.1. Of these the most common is ovarian failure since this will be present in almost all female recipients of HSC transplants for hematologic malignancy due to the dose of chemotherapy or chemoradiotherapy utilized immediately pretransplant in the conditioning regimen (Schimmer *et al.*, 1998). Genital tract infections are the second most common gynecologic problem, most frequently *Candida vulvo-vaginitis*.

Chemotherapy-induced ovarian failure

Chemotherapeutic agents and ionizing radiation with or without an HSC transplant have an adverse effect on ovarian function (Kumar, Biggart, & McEvoy, 1972). The effect of cytotoxic chemotherapeutic agents on the oocyte probably occurs before meiosis with progressive depletion of follicles and oocytes. Ovarian biopsy specimens in patients treated with cyclophosphamide (CY) show an absence of theca and ova (Warne *et al.*, 1973). The ovarian failure due to chemotherapeutic agents is characterized by rising levels of follicle-stimulating hormone (FSH) and luteinizing hormone (LH) together with falling levels of estrogen. Uldall and co-workers (1972) reported that approximately half of all menstruating women treated with high doses of CY became amenorrheic within 7 months, the majority developing cessation of ovarian cycles within the first month of treatment. Other alkylating agents have been shown to have similar histologic and physi-

ologic effects on the ovary. Some cytotoxic agents produce ovarian atrophy.

The factors that determine the effect of cytotoxic agents on ovarian function include (1) mechanism of action of the cytotoxic agent, (2) patient's age, and (3) dose of cytotoxic agent used. Shalet (1980) demonstrated the dose effect on the induction of amenorrhea and the dependency of this dose on patient age (Table 97.2).

Susceptibility of the ovaries to cytotoxic chemotherapy and subsequent ovarian failure appears to depend on the number of potential oocytes as well as oocyte age. Natural aging and loss of germ cells within the ovary is maximal before puberty. Germ cell numbers reach their maximum in the fetus and fall from 7 million at 6 months gestation to 2 million at birth. At puberty, there are 200,000 and there is a gradual fall thereafter until menopause (Fig. 97.1).

The potential for ovarian failure can be assessed by measuring FSH/LH and estradiol levels and by examining ovarian biopsy tissue for the presence of healthy oocytes with development of follicular maturation.

The prepubertal ovary is much less susceptible than the postpubertal ovary to damage by alkylating agents. For example, it was shown by Siris and colleagues (1976) that ovarian function returned to normal in over 90% of prepubertal girls treated with combination chemotherapy for acute leukemia. Similarly, pubertal girls are less susceptible to the effect of CY than older women, and if the total dose of CY can be kept to less than 525 mg/kg, prognosis for subsequent ovulation is good.

Table 97.1. *Gynecologic problems after transplantation*

Ovarian failure
Abnormal uterine bleeding
Genital tract infections
GVHD of the vagina

Abbreviation: GVHD, graft-versus host disease.

Table 97.2. *Relationship between patient age and cyclophosphamide dose in production of amenorrhea*

Patient age (years)	Cyclophosphamide dose required to produce amenorrhea (g)
20–29	20.4
30–39	9.3
>40	5.2

Reproduced, with permission, from Shalet (1980).

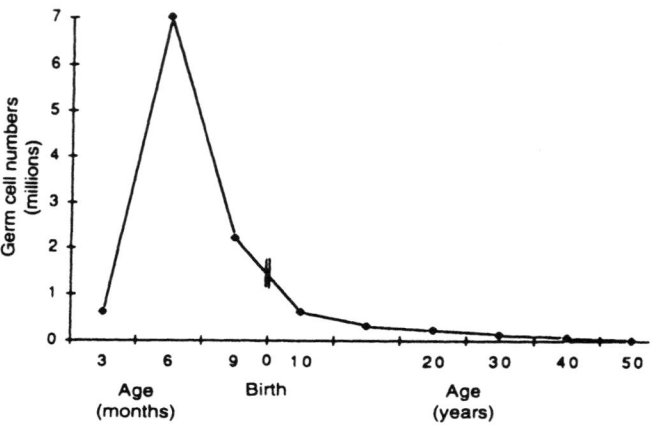

Fig. 97.1. Total number of germ cells in the human ovary from the prenatal to postmenopausal era.

Radiation-induced ovarian failure

Ionizing radiation effects on the ovary depend on oocyte meiotic activity. Again impairment is related to patient age at the time of treatment, which in turn is a function of the number of oocytes in the ovary. Doses of 1.5 Gy do not appear to affect women in the 20 to 35 year age range, while women of all ages have menstrual disturbance with doses of 2.5 to 5 Gy. Over 50% of such women will be rendered infertile. When the dose exceeds 8 Gy 100% will be permanently anovulatory.

Spinelli and colleagues (1994) prospectively followed 79 female recipients of allogeneic bone marrow transplants who had been conditioned with total body irradiation (TBI) during the first year posttransplant (Fig. 97.2–97.4). Most adult women complained of vasomotor and/or genitourinary symptoms. These were associated with decreased plasma levels of 17-beta estradiol (E2) and increased LH and FSH plasma levels, and deterioration in their sexual life. Forty-nine adult women were selected to receive systemic hormonal replacement therapy (HRT), consisting of cyclic transdermal estrogens plus medroxyprogesterone acetate (MPA) or cyclic oral therapy with low doses of conjugated estrogens and MPA. A total of 65% of women never stopped taking the HRT. Vasomotor problems resolved in 91% of patients and improvement of genitourinary symptoms was seen both with local and systemic hormonal therapy. Sexual symptoms were reduced in 21 of 26 women (81%) given HRT compared with 8 of 19 (42%) given local treatment.

In the study the actuarial chance of having a menstrual period at 10 years posttransplant was 43%. It was 100% in premenarchal females and 36% in postmenarchal females ($P = .003$). In the latter group it was 100% if less than 18 years of age and 50% if greater than 18 years. The likelihood was also increased by taking HRT (Fig. 97.4). Blood levels of LH and FSH before and after ovarian recovery are shown in Fig. 97.5 and 97.6, respectively.

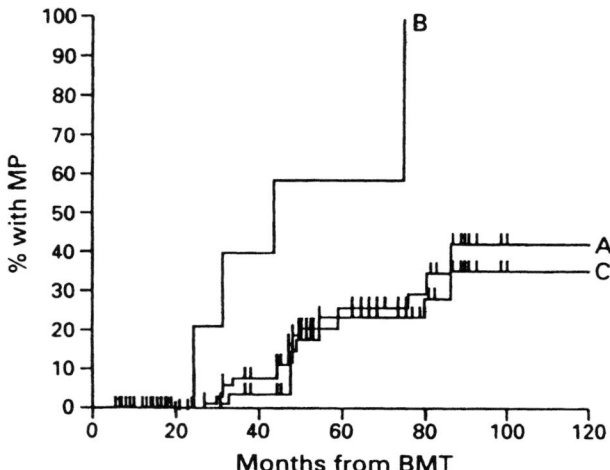

Fig. 97.2. Actuarial chance of having a menstrual period post-BMT at 10 years in premenarchal and postmenarchal females. A = All females, 79 patients., 43%; B = premenarche, 5 patients., 100%; C = postmenarche, 74 patients, 36%. Reproduced, with permission, from Spinelli *et al.* (1994).

Prospects for pregnancy

While pregnancy has been not uncommon in younger women given CY 200 mg/kg over 4 days as conditioning regimen for HLA-identical sibling transplantation for severe aplastic anemia (Cord *et al.*, 1980) and also in two women with leukemia prepared for allogeneic transplant by high-dose melphalan (Milliken *et al.*, 1990), very few women have become pregnant who have received combination chemotherapy or chemoradiotherapy (incorporating TBI) prior to allogeneic HSC transplant

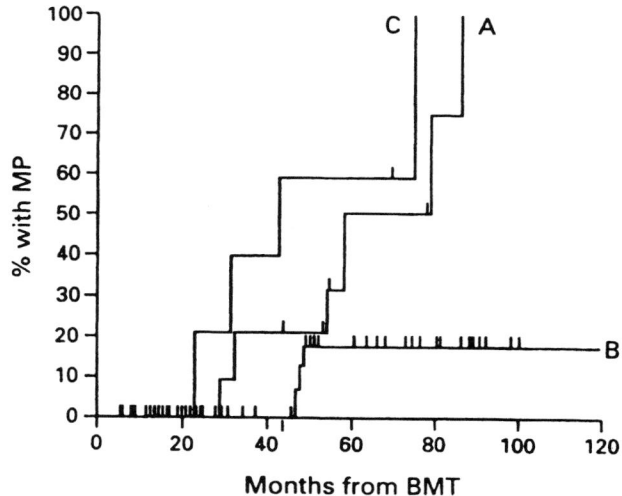

Fig. 97.3. Actuarial chance of having a menstrual period post-BMT at 10 years in postmenarchal females under or over 18 years of age. A = postmenarche, ≤18 years, 14 patients., 100%; B = postmenarche >18 years, 60 patients, 15%; C = premenarche, 5 patients, 100%. Reproduced, with permission, from Spinelli *et al.* (1994).

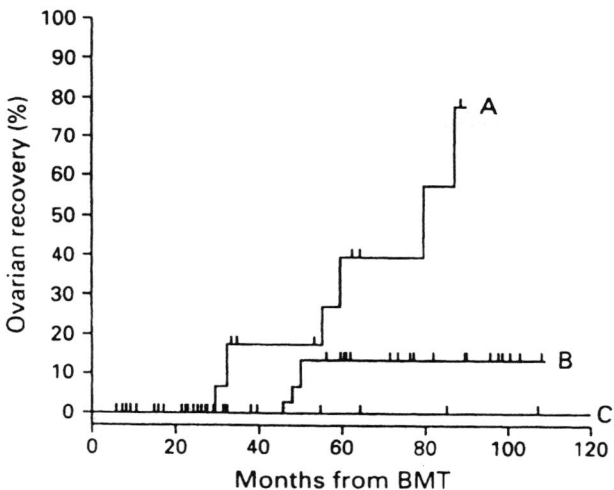

Fig. 97.4. Actuarial chance of having a menstrual period post-BMT at 10 years in postmenarchal females receiving or not receiving HRT. A = ≤18 years, postmenarche, HRT, 12 patients., 80%; B = >18 years, postmenarche, HRT, 31 patients, 13%; C = >18 years, postmenarche, no HRT, 24 patients, 0%. A Versus B, $P < .003$, B Versus C, $P < .3$. Reproduced, with permission, from Spinelli *et al.* (1994).

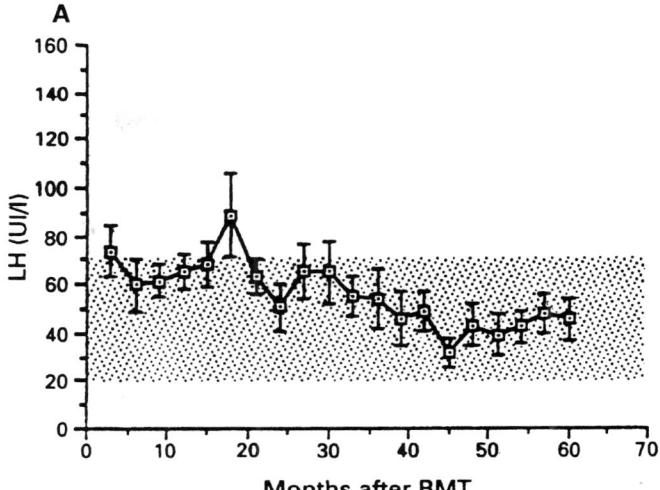

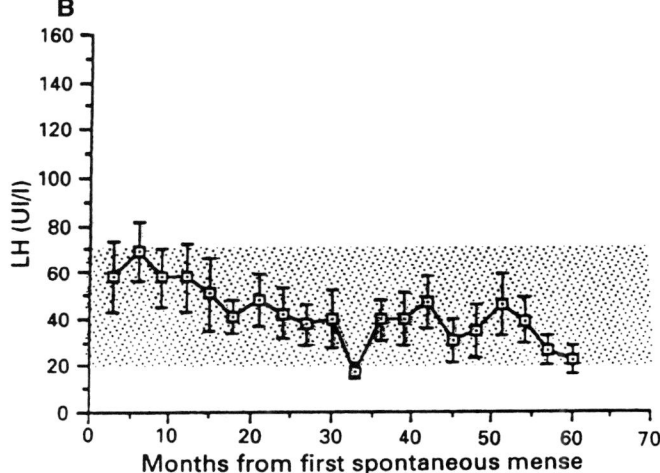

Fig. 97.5. Average ± SE of LH 3-monthly levels evaluated on the patients before (**A**) and after (**B**) ovarian recovery. The difference in LH levels between A and B, tested by the $\chi 2$ test, is statistically significant ($P = .02$). The shaded area represents the indicative range of menopause. Reproduced, with permission, from Spinelli *et al.* (1994).

for hematologic malignancy (Buskard *et al.*, 1988; Giri *et al.*, 1992; Letendre *et al.*, 1997).

Borgna-Pignatti and colleagues (1996) described a delivery of a full-term normal infant in a woman prepared with busulfan and CY prior to an allogeneic transplant for thalassemia. Ashida and colleagues (1996) described delivery of a healthy child to a woman who had been prepared with CY, antilymphocyte globulin, and total lymphoid irradiation 5 Gy prior to an allograft for severe aplastic anemia. Salooja and colleagues (1994) described delivery of three full-term pregnancies out of 22 evaluable women conditioned for autologous transplantation for acute myeloid leukemia with CY in combination with carmustine, cytosine arabinoside, 6-thioguanine, and daunorubicin. Several additional pregnancies have been described in women prepared with TBI-containing regimens (Maruta *et al.*, 1995; Milpied *et al.*, 1996). In a large review of the records of 1,326 postpubertal and 196 prepubertal patients receiving marrow transplants in Seattle from 1971 to 1992, Sanders *et al.* (1996) found that among 708 postpubertal women, 110 recovered normal ovarian function and 32 became pregnant. Some of these had received high-dose chemotherapy alone as conditioning and some had received a TBI-containing regimen. In addition nine formerly prepubertal girls with normal gonadal function became pregnant. Spontaneous abortion terminated 4 of 56 (7%) pregnancies for 28 female CY recipients and 6 of 16 (37%) pregnancies for 13 TBI recipients ($P = .02$). Preterm delivery occurred for 8 of 44 (18%) and 5 of 8 (63%) live births for 24 CY and 8 TBI female recipients ($P = .01$). The 13 preterm deliveries resulted in 10 low birth weight (LBW) of 1.8 to 2.4 kg and 3 very low birth weight (VLBW) infants (<1.37 kg), for an overall incidence of 25%, which is higher than the expected incidence of 6.5% for the general population. Twelve of the 13 premature infants survived at the time of the report. Congenital anomalies were seen among 2 of 51 (3.8%) live-born infants of female patients, which is not different from the 13% of single congenital anomalies reported for the general population. These data demonstrated that pregnancies among women who have received a marrow transplant incorporating TBI conditioning are likely to be accompanied by an increased risk of spontaneous abortion.

Pregnancies among all women who have received a marrow transplant are likely to be accompanied by preterm labor and delivery of LBW or VLBW babies, who do not seem to be at an increased risk of congenital anomalies.

In patients who have received combination cytotoxic chemotherapy (without a subsequent HSC transplant) for

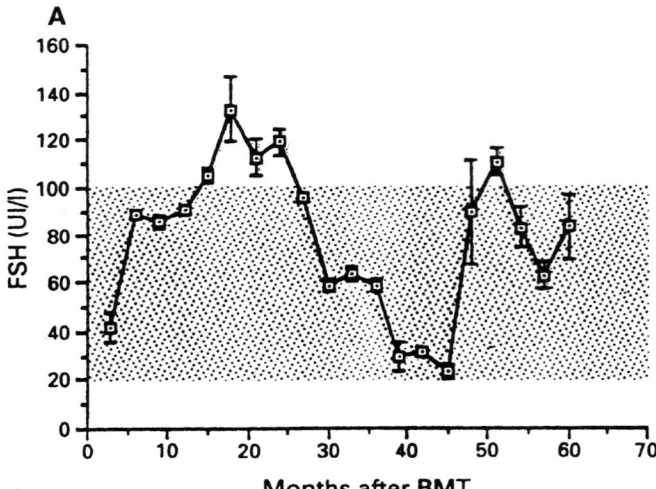

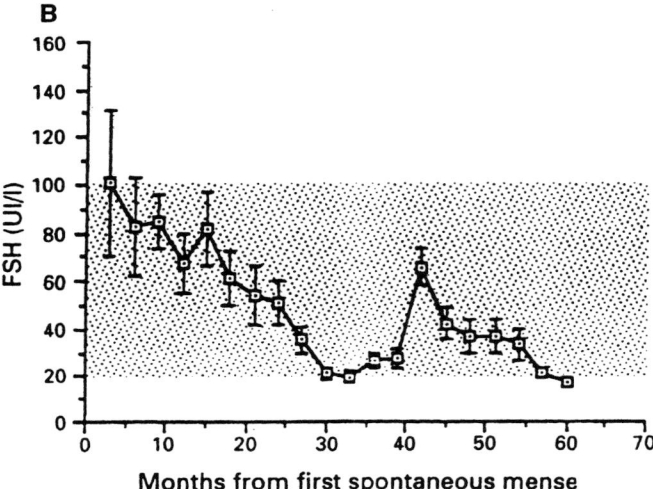

Fig. 97.6. Average ± SE of FSH 3-monthly levels evaluated on the eight patients before (**A**) and after (**B**) ovarian recovery. The difference in FSH levels between A and B, tested by the $\chi2$ test, is statistically significant (P = .015). The shaded area represents the indicative range of menopause. Reproduced, with permission, from Spinelli *et al.* (1994).

leukemia, lymphoma, and other neoplasia, concern of an increased risk of chromosomal abnormalities or congenital abnormalities in the fetus and for an increased rate of spontaneous abortion, have not been substantiated (Ross, 1976; Holmes & Holmes, 1978; Li *et al.,* 1979).

Management of the infertile woman

Patients undergoing elective transplants may choose to have a cycle of ovarian stimulation followed by ultrasound-guided follicle aspiration and oocyte collection. Fertilization of these oocytes with sperm from the woman's partner and cryostorage of the resulting embryo may be performed. Technical development of oocytes storage is not yet satisfactory (Chattergee and Kottaridis, 2002) as the ovulated oocyte is held in the second

meiotic division and the chromosomes are suspended in heat-labile spindles that cannot survive a reduction in temperature.

Posttransplant transfer into the fallopian tube of donor eggs or in vitro fertilization of donor eggs both give a couple opportunity to parent children after successful treatment by HSC transplantation, should embryo cryopreservation not have been feasible pretransplant.

In vitro fertilization techniques in current usage are listed in Table 97.3.

Rio and colleagues (1994) reported a case of a full-term pregnancy arising from donated oocytes in a 36-year-old woman with chronic myeloid leukemia (CML) who had undergone allogeneic bone marrow transplantation 6 years previously. Prior to transplant she underwent controlled ovarian hyperstimulation. The first regimen (Table 97.4A) failed to produce any oocytes. The second (Table 97.4B) resulted in two oocytes, which produced one embryo. This embryo was cryopreserved. She then underwent marrow transplantation with preparation using CY and fractionated TBI 12 Gy. Three and a half years later implantation of her own embryo failed. An embryo transfer of donated oocytes was performed 9 months later. She became pregnant after receiving the hormonal

Table 97.3. *IVF techniques in current use*

Cryo-ET (cryostored embryo transfer): transfer of embryos that were derived in a previous IVF or GIFT cycle and stored in liquid nitrogen.

ET (embryo transfer): unless otherwise qualified, the transfer of IVF embryos through the vagina and cervix into the uterus.

GIFT (gamete intrafallopian transfer): transfer of unfertilized oocytes plus prepared sperm into the fallopian tubes, usually at laparoscopy, but also vaginally, by ultrasound-guided catheterization of the fallopian tube. *Requirement:* at least one normal fallopian tube and more than 100,000 recovered motile spermatozoa.

ICSI (intracytoplasmic sperm insertion): a type of IVF in which a single sperm cell is injected into each oocyte using a micromanipulator. *Requirement:* several motile sperm cells (an elevated serum FSH concentration due to testicular failure is not itself a contraindication).

IVF (in vitro fertilization): a procedure in which oocytes are obtained and fertilized in vitro; conventionally, the embryos are transferred to the uterus, but if the fallopian tubes are normal, embryos can be transferred to the tubes (i.e., ZIFT). *Requirement:* more than 10,000 motile spermatozoa.

MESA (microsurgical epididymal sperm aspiration): aspiration of immature sperm cells from the epididymis or rete testis, above an obstruction that is causing an absence of sperm in the ejaculate; the recovered sperm can be used for ICSI, either immediately or after cryogenic storage. *Requirement:* recovery of motile sperm cells.

ZIFT (zygote intrafallopian transfer): introduction of fertilized oocytes (zygotes) into the fallopian tube; like GIFT, usually done at laparoscopy, but also possible transvaginally. *Requirement:* same as for IVF, and at least one normal fallopian tube.

Table 97.4. *Ultrashort protocol for oocyte harvesting*

A. First attempt
Triptoreline (Decapeptyl, Ipsen, Biotech, Paris, France)
    0.1 mg s.c. from days 1 to 8 of the menstrual cycle
FSH (Metrodine, Serono, Levallois-Perret, France)
    150 IU i.m. from days 4 to 6
Menotrophin (Neo-Pergonal, Serono, France)
    2 vials i.m. from days 7 to 10
Failure
B. Second attempt
Busereline (Suprefact, Hoechst, Puteaux, France)
    0.3 mg × 2/day sc for 13 days
Days 1–5: FSH 300 IU/day + menotrophin 2 vials/day
Days 6–7: FSH 225 IU/day + menotrophin 3 vials/day
Days 8–15: FSH 225 IU/day + menotrophin 2 vials/day
Days 16–19: FSH 225 IU/day + menotrophin 4 vials/day
Days 20–24: FSH 375 IU/day + menotrophin 5 vials/day
Day 25: 5,000 IU human chorionic gonadotrophin
            (HCG 'Endo', Organon, Saint-Denis, France)
Laparoscopy under general anesthesia.
Two ovocytes collected producing 1 embryo, which was
    cryopreserved.

Reproduced, with permission, from Rio *et al.* (1994).

Table 97.5. *Hormonal replacement for nidation and early pregnancy*

Estraderm TTS 100, CIBA-Geigy, Rueil-Malmaison, France
    (estradiol 0.1 mg)
Utrogestan, Besins-Iscoveco, Paris, France (progesterone 100 mg)
Progesterone-Retard Pharlon, Schering, Lys-lez-Lannoy, France
    (hydroxyprogesterone lexanoate 500 mg)
Estradiol 0.2 mg every other day during 14 days
Estradiol 0.4 mg/day + progesterone 300 mg from days –3 to
    day 0 (day of implantation)
Estradiol 0.4 mg/day + progesterone 300 mg from days + 1 to + 7
Estradiol 0.4 mg/day + progesterone 400 mg/day + hydro-
    xyprogesterone valproate 500 mg every other day from
    days + 8 to + 21
Estradiol 0.6 mg/day + progesterone 600 mg/day + hydro-
    xyprogesterone valproate 500 mg every other day from
    days + 22 to + 42
Estradiol 0.8 mg/day + progesterone 500 mg + hydroxyproges-
    terone valproate 500 mg every other day from day + 43 to the
    eighth week of theoretical amenorrhea
Doses of estradiol and progesterone were slowly decreased as
    described in Letur-Konirsch *et al.* 1992.

Reproduced, with permission, from Rio *et al.* (1994).

regimen shown in Table 97.5. The course of the pregnancy was unremarkable; she delivered a 3.3 kg baby girl.

Management of hypoestrogenism

As well as troublesome symptomatology from rapidly induced estrogen deficiency, long-term deleterious effects of bone demineralization and accelerated vascular disease may reduce the quality of life for the female HSC transplant recipient who develops ovarian failure. Hot flushing, vaginal dryness, diminished libido, irritability, insomnia, poor concentration, and other symptoms can readily be reversed by adequate ovarian hormone replacement. Pre- and posttreatment FSH/LH estradiol levels should be measured to ensure adequate replacement treatment. Concomitant progesterone therapy for 12 to 14 days each month will protect against development of adenocarcinoma of the endometrium. A suitable dose of medroxyprogesterone is 10 mg daily. Oral, vaginal, or percutaneous methods of administration of estrogen may be preferred and details of dosage are shown in Table 97.6. The transdermal administration of estrogen has the added advantage of bypassing the gut-liver first phase of metabolism. Thus dosage levels can be reduced to achieve effective concentration of estradiol in the blood. Sixty percent to 90% of natural estrogens administered orally are converted within the gut wall and liver to estrone and to pharmacologically inactive metabolites such as estrone sulfate. Orally administered estrogens makes the liver a first target organ with resultant excessive production of some coagulation factors, angiotensinogen, sex-binding, globulin, and cortisol-binding

globulin. These may contribute to the development of hypertension, gall bladder disease, and thrombosis. Skin application of estrogen will largely bypass these effects (Geola *et al.,* 1980; Mandel *et al.,* 1982). Such application is useful, for example, for the occasional person with a history of deep venous thrombosis or pulmonary embolism.

Table 97.6. *Adult dosages of estrogen preparations by different routes*[a]

Route	Dose
Oral	Piperazine estrone sulfate 1.25 mg/day or conjugated equine estrogens 0.625 mg/day.
Percutaneous[b]	Patches equivalent to 0.3, 0.625, or 1.25 mg of oral conjugated estrogens available. Replace every 3–4 days.
Intravenous	Conjugated equine estrogen 25 mg.
(emergency use only)	Repeat in 6–12 hours if necessary. Follow-up with oral estrogen/progesterone indicated.

[a] Accompanied by progesterone treatment for 12–14 days per month. A typical regimen is Premarin, 0.625 mg po daily, and Provera, 5–10 mg on days 1–14. An alternative convenient approach is to use a low-dose estrogen contraceptive pill such as Triphasil, 1 daily, which contains both estrogen (ethinyl estradiol) and progestogen (levonorgestrel).
[b] An estrogen patch can be used short term, in lieu of systemic treatment, for oral estrogen intolerance or liver function test (LFT) abnormalities. Transdermal estrogen may not convey cardiovascular benefits.

Abnormal uterine bleeding

Menstrual disturbances are common in the female HSC transplant recipient. Ovarian failure, cycle irregularity, and estrogen deficiency cause irregular shedding and endometrial atrophy with a varying degree of blood loss. Sometimes abnormal bleeding is exacerbated by thrombocytopenia or by leukopenia predisposing to endometritis. If bleeding is totally irregular, routine gynecologic assessment should be undertaken with (1) accurate cervical cytology; (2) colposcopy; and (3) cervical swabs for microbiological culture (to include chlamydia).

If high-risk persistent bleeding is present, endometrial sampling with hysteroscopy should be considered. Management of the bleeding will depend on the cause with correction of thrombocytopenia and treatment of infection being important as well as replacement of estrogen. Atrophic and hypoplastic endometrial states secondary to ovarian failure will respond immediately to oral or intravenous estrogen (Table 97.6). Maintenance of a normal ovarian hormone profile will prevent further troublesome bleeding. Combined estrogen and progesterone administration will achieve this effectively. Adjustment of dosage may be necessary to prevent breakthrough bleeding, remembering that other drug regimens may have an effect on estrogen and progesterone metabolism, and, vice versa, that estrogens and progestogens interact with other medications often being taken by the transplant recipient such as cyclosporine (see Chapter 83).

Genital tract infections

Fungal infections

Altered vaginal flora secondary to ovarian failure, low estrogen states, and antibiotic therapy will cause a reduction in *Lactobacillus acidophilus* activity (reduced glycogen and thus less lactic acid production), thereby increasing vaginal pH. *Candida albicans* and other fungi will take advantage of this and with the immune deficiency consistently seen posttransplant, fungal vulvo-vaginitis may become quite troublesome. Antifungal cream such as nystatin or clotrimazole applied to the external genitalia, and vaginal pessaries such as nystatin or miconazole will enable control to be achieved. Attention needs to be given to infestation sources such as bowel and clothes. Estrogen replacement is essential.

Bacterial infections

In the immune suppressed patient, nonpathogenic commensal bacteria such as beta-hemolytic *Streptococcus, Staphylococcus epidermidis,* and *Haemophilus vaginalis* can cause infections as well as more common pathogens such as *Proteus, Klebsiella,* and *E. coli.* Loss of vaginal acidity assists colonization. Vaginal and cervical swabs should be taken to identify the causative organism. Removal of intrauterine contraceptive devices, safe sex practices, and patient awareness will reduce the risk of subsequent pelvic inflammatory disease.

Viral infections

Herpes simplex virus 1 and 2
Primary and secondary attacks are likely to be more severe in patients undergoing HSC transplantation. Acyclovir 200 mg five times daily for 5 days will normally cause resolution of the acute episode and in some patients low-dose prophylaxis (200 mg two or three times daily) is required to prevent repeated attacks.

Human papillomavirus
Immune suppression allows the wart virus to become more aggressive than normal; rapidly spreading wart growth in the vulva, vagina, and cervix may occur. Treatment with cautery or laser together with local 5-fluorouracil cream may be necessary to control an episode. Recurrence is common.

Associated cervical intraepithelial neoplastic changes may become evident, in which case more regular cervical cytology and colposcopy (every 6 months) will be necessary.

Graft-versus-host disease of the vagina

Chronic graft-versus-host disease (GVHD) occasionally involves the vagina but virtually only when chronic GVHD in other organs is present (Corson *et al.,* 1982; DeLord *et al.,* 1999; Yanai *et al.,* 1999). Dryness with resultant dyspareunia can occur and occasionally stricture formation due to fibrosis. Treatment is with topical estrogen cream, systemic estrogen treatment, and immune suppression for the underlying GVHD.

Cervical cytology

In a retrospective review of 347 Pap smears from 64 women who underwent autologous or allogeneic HSC transplantation between 1990 and 1998, the rate of cytological abnormalities was significantly higher than in the general population, both before and after transplant (Sasadeusz *et al.,* 2001). Posttransplant, allograft recipients had a higher rate of abnormalities than autograft recipients. These observations suggest that pretransplant disease and treatment factors increase the risk of cytologic abnormalities and that transplant-related factors such as the conditioning treatment and immunosuppression further increase this risk. Frequent screening may be required, especially in allograft recipients.

References

Ashida, T., Tsubaki, K., Hazu, S. *et al.* (1996). Delivery after bone marrow transplantation with total lymphoid irradiation for severe aplastic anemia. *International Journal of Hematology,* **64,** 279–81.

Borgna-Pignatti, C., Marradi, P., Rugolotto, S., & Marcolongo, A. (1996). Successful pregnancy after bone marrow transplantation for thalassemia. *Bone Marrow Transplantation,* **18,** 235–6.

Buskard, N., Ballem, P., Hill, R., & Fryer, C. (1988). Normal fertility after total body irradiation and chemotherapy in conjunction with a bone marrow transplant for acute leukemia. *Clinical Investigation*, 2 (Suppl), C57 (Abstract).

Chattergee, R., & Kottaridis, P. D. (2002). Treatment of gonadal damage in recipients of allogeneic or autologous transplantation for haematological malignancies. *Bone Marrow Transplantation*, 30, 629–35.

Cord, R., Holmes, I., Sugarman, R. *et al.* (1980). Successful pregnancy after high dose chemotherapy and marrow transplantation for treatment of aplastic anemia. *Experimental Hematology*, 8, 57–60.

Corson, S. L., Sullivan, K., Batzer, F. *et al.* (1982). Gynecological manifestations of graft-versus-host disease. *Obstetrics and Gynecology*, 60, 488–92.

DeLord, C., Treleaven, J., Shepherd, J. *et al.* (1999). Vaginal stenosis following allogeneic bone marrow transplantation for acute myeloid leukemia. *Bone Marrow Transplantation*, 23, 523–5.

Geola, F. L., Fruman, A. M., Tataryn, I. V. *et al.* (1980). Biological effects of various doses of conjugated equine oestrogns in postmenopausal women. *Journal of Clinical Endocrinology*, 51, 620–625.

Giri, N., Vowels, M. R., Barr, A. L. *et al.* (1992). Successful pregnancy after total body irradiation and bone marrow transplantation for acute leukemia. *Bone Marrow Transplantation*, 10, 93–5.

Holmes, G. E. & Holmes, F. F. (1978). Pregnancy outcome of patients treated for Hodgkin's disease. *Cancer*, 41, 1317–22.

Kumar, R., Biggart, J. D., & McEvoy, J. (1972). Cyclophosphamide and reproductive function. *Lancet*, 1, 1212–4.

Letendre, L. & Moore, S. B. (1997). Successful pregnancy after conditioning with cyclophosphamide and fractionated total body irradiation. *Medical Pediatric Oncology*, 28, 147–8.

Letur-Konirsch, H., Cornel, C., Taieb, J. *et al.* (1992). Endocrinology of early pregnancy in women without ovarian function. *Reproduction, Fertility, and Development*, 4, 703–11.

Li, F. P., Fine, W., Jaffe, N. *et al.* (1979). Offspring of patients treated for cancer in childhood. *Journal of the National Cancer Institute*, 62, 1193–7.

Mandel, F. P., Geola, F. L., Lu, J. K. H. *et al.* (1982). Biological effect of various doses of ethenyl oestradiol in post menopausal women. *Obstetrics and Gynecology*, 59, 673–4.

Maruta, A., Matsuzaki, M., Miyashita, H. *et al.* (1995). Successful pregnancy after allogeneic bone marrow transplantation following conditioning with total body irradiation. *Bone Marrow Transplantation*, 15, 637–8.

Milliken, S., Powles, R., Parikh, P. *et al.* (1990). Successful pregnancy following bone marrow transplantation for leukaemia. *Bone Marrow Transplantation*, 5, 135–7.

Milpied, N., Moreau, P., Cuillere, J. C. *et al.* (1996). Successful pregnancy after allogeneic bone marrow transplantation following conditioning including 10-Gy single exposure total body irradiation. *Bone Marrow Transplantation*, 17, 467 (Letter).

Rio, B., Letur-Könirsch, H., Ajchenbaum-Cymbalista, F. *et al.* (1994). Full-term pregnancy with embryos from donated oocytes in a 36 year old woman allografted for chronic myeloid leukemia. *Bone Marrow Transplantation*, 13, 487–8.

Ross, G. T. (1976). Congenital anomalies among children born of mothers receiving chemotherapy for gestational trophoblastic neoplasms. *Cancer*, 37, 1043–7.

Salooja, N., Chatterjee, R., McMillan, A. K. *et al.* (1994). Successful pregnancies in women following single autotransplant for acute myeloid leukemia with a chemotherapy ablation protocol. *Bone Marrow Transplantation*, 13, 431–5.

Sanders, J. E., Hawley, J., Levy, W. *et al.* (1996). Pregnancies following high-dose cyclophosphamide with or without high-dose busulfan or total body irradiation and bone marrow transplantation. *Blood*, 87, 3045–52.

Sasadeusz, J., Kelly, H., Szer, J. *et al.* (2001). Abnormal cervical cytology in bone marrow transplant recipients. *Bone Marrow Transplantation*, 28, 393–7.

Schimmer, A. D., Quatermain, M., Imrie, V. *et al.* (1998). Ovarian function after autologous bone marrow transplantation. *Journal of Clinical Oncology*, 16, 2359–63.

Shalet, S. M. (1980). Effects of cancer chemotrophy on gonadal function of patients. *Cancer Treatment Reports*, 7, 141–52.

Siris, E. S., Levathal, B. G., & Vaitukaitis, J. L. (1976). Effects of childhood leukemia and chemotherapy on puberty and reproduction function in girls. *New England Journal of Medicine*, 294, 1143–6.

Spinelli, S., Choidi, S., Bacigalupo, A. *et al.* (1994). Ovarian recovery after total body irradiation and allogeneic bone marrow transplantation: long-term follow-up of 79 females. *Bone Marrow Transplantation*, 14, 373–80.

Uldall, P. R., Kerr, D. N., & Tacchi, D. (1972). Sterility and cydophosphamide. *Lancet*, 1, 693–4.

Warne, G. L., Fairley, K. F., Hobbs, J. B., & Martin, F. R. (1973). Cyclophosphamide-induced ovarian failure. *New England Journal of Medicine*, 289, 1159–62.

Yanai, N. Shufaro, Y., Or, R., & Meirow, D. (1999). Vaginal outflow tract obstruction by graft-versus-host disease. *Bone Marrow Transplantation*, 24, 811–2.

98   Eye complications

ABHA GULATI AND M. REZA DANA

Schepens Eye Research Institute, Massachusetts Eye and Ear Infirmary and Harvard Medical School, Boston, USA

Introduction

Hematopoietic stem cell (HSC) transplantation is a treatment of choice for a variety of malignant and nonmalignant disorders that has improved the survival for many patients. However, it is associated with systemic and organ-specific complications. Eye complications are common following HSC transplantation (Jack *et al.*, 1983; Jabs *et al.*, 1989; Coskuncan *et al.*, 1994) (Table 98.1). With careful monitoring and treatment, the vast majority of long-term survivors can have normal vision; however, a small proportion of patients may develop significant corneal disease, ulceration and even perforation, and loss of the eye.

Ocular involvement following HSC transplantation is usually multifactorial in etiology and due to such factors as the pretransplantation regimen, pancytopenia, posttransplant immunosuppression, and graft-versus-host disease (GVHD). Pretransplant conditioning regimens are necessary to suppress the recipient's immune system, prevent rejection of graft, and eliminate the patient's own diseased marrow (Storb & Donall Thomas, 1994). Such conditioning regimens typically consist of various chemotherapeutic agents (e.g., cyclophosphamide, busulfan) with or without total body irradiation (TBI). There is an association between TBI and cataract formation (Deeg *et al.*, 1984a). Moreover, pancytopenia caused by the ablation of the recipient's bone marrow, and posttransplant immune suppression can lead to various hemorrhagic complications as well as infections.

GVHD is a major complication of allogeneic HSC transplantation. Ocular involvement occurs in 45% to 60% of GVHD patients (Franklin *et al.*, 1983; Coskuncan *et al.*, 1994). The ocular manifestations of GVHD include keratoconjunctivitis sicca, sterile conjunctivitis, cicatricial lagophthalmos, corneal epithelial defects, corneal ulceration, and corneal melting (Franklin *et al.*, 1983; Hirst *et al.*, 1983; Jacks *et al.*, 1983). Some of these complications are due to direct involvement of conjunctiva or lid skin by GVHD, and others are as a result of involvement of the lacrimal gland by GVHD.

Acute GVHD of the eye

GVHD developing within the first 3 months posttransplant is termed acute GVHD. Acute GVHD primarily affects the skin,

Table 98.1.   *Eye complications of hematopoietic stem cell transplantation*

Acute graft-versus-host disease
Chronic graft-versus-host disease
Ocular surface disease
   KCS, conjunctivitis, MGD, blepharitis, lagophthalmos, ectropion
Cataract
Uveitis
Retinal microvasculopathy
   Cotton-wool spots, microaneurysms, blot and flame hemorrhages, macular edema, neovascularization
Optic neuropathy
   Optic disc edema
Hemorrhage
   Retinal
   Vitreal
   Subconjunctival
Infection
   Bacterial
      Conjunctivitis, keratitis, endophthalmitis, orbital cellulitis
   Fungal
      Corneal ulcer, endophthalmitis
   Viral
      HSV keratitis, VZV keratitis, CMV retinitis
   Protozoal
      Toxoplasma gondii chorioretinitis
Drug toxicity
Involvement of the eye by the underlying disease

Abbreviations: KCS, keratoconjunctivitis sicca; MGD, meibomian gland dysfunction; HSV, herpes simplex virus; VZV, varicella zoster virus; CMV, cytomegalovirus.

liver, gastrointestinal tract, and other mucous membranes such as conjunctiva. The primary clinical manifestation of acute GVHD involving the eye is conjunctivitis, which may be mild or severe (Jack & Hicks, 1981; Franklin *et al.*, 1983; Hirst *et al.*, 1983; Jabs *et al.*, 1983, 1989) (Table 98.2). Although rare, both conjunctival and corneal findings have been described in acute GVHD. Jabs *et al.* (1989) reported the frequency of conjunctival involvement by acute GVHD to be 7.2%. Milder cases simply show hyperemia of the conjunctival mucosa and

Table 98.2. *Manifestations of GVHD of the eye*

Tissue	Acute GVHD	Chronic GVHD
Eyelid	Mild erythema to severe bullae formation, desquamation	Erythema (often violaceous), lichenoid change, scleroderma, madarosis, lagophthalmos, cicatricial ectropion
Conjunctiva	Follicular reaction, chemosis, hemorrhagic conjunctivitis, pseudomembrane formation, ulceration of tarsal conjunctiva	Conjunctival injection, conjunctival epithelial thinning, keratinization and scarring
Cornea	Mild to severe corneal stippling, corneal epithelial thinning, filamentary keratitis, keratinization, sloughing of corneal epithelium, KCS	KCS, corneal epithelial defects, wasting, ulceration, melting, perforation
Lens		Cataract
Lacrimal apparatus	Dacroadenitis, cellular infiltration and blockage of acini with PAS-positive staining material resulting in stasis, KCS	Fibrosis and obliteration of lumen of acini resulting in KCS, canalicular and NLD obstruction
Sclera	Icterus from liver GVHD, episcleritis	
Uvea	Uveitis, choroidal infiltrates with histiocyte-like cells	Uveitis
Retina	Optic disc edema	Retinal microvasculopathy
Orbit	Periorbital GVHD	

Abbreviations: GVHD, graft-versus-host disease; KCS, keratoconjunctivitis sicca; PAS, periodic acid-Schiff[1]; NLD, nasolacrimal duct.

occasionally chemosis. Severe involvement may include fulminant conjunctivitis associated with eye pain, photophobia, blurred vision, subconjunctival hemorrhage, a sterile mucopurulent discharge, pseudomembrane formation of the lower tarsal conjunctivae, and ulceration of the upper tarsal conjunctivae (Spiro *et al.*, 1996). Furthermore, massive filamentary keratitis and sloughing of the corneal epithelium, similar to that seen in massive recurrent corneal erosion, can occur in patients with acute GVHD (Jack *et al.*, 1983). Cultures for bacteria, fungi, and virus are consistently negative. It has been found that the degree of severity of the conjunctival disease corresponds with the systemic disease (Hirst *et al.*, 1983; Jabs *et al.*, 1989; Janin *et al.*, 1996). The eye involvement usually resolves with resolution of the other organ involvement.

Jabs *et al.* (1989) have proposed a system for clinical staging of conjunctival and ocular surface GVHD. Stage I is characterized by conjunctival hyperemia; stage II, by conjunctival hyperemia with the additional findings of a chemotic response or serosanguinous exudates; stage III, by pseudomembranous conjunctivitis; and stage IV, pseudomembranous conjunctivitis with corneal epithelial sloughing (Fig. 98.1). Although pseudomembranous conjunctivitis is uncommon in GVHD, its presence is considered a marker for systemic involvement (Jabs *et al.*, 1989) and is associated with a poor prognosis (Janin *et al.*, 1996).

Histologically, the changes seen in conjunctival biopsy in ocular acute GVHD are similar to those seen in skin GVHD (Farmer, 1986). These changes include mononuclear, mostly lymphocytic, infiltration into the conjunctiva, the presence of dyskeratotic cells and even subepithelial microvesicle formation, and in severe cases total separation of the epithelium from

the subjacent stroma (Fig. 98.2). Autopsy examination often reveals that other ocular tissues may be affected by acute GVHD; the choroid may show cellular infiltrates of large eosinophilic cells resembling histiocytes, with occasional inflammatory cells. Examination of the lacrimal gland may show accumulation of periodic acid-Schiff (PAS) positive material in the acini of ductules, suggesting a stasis phenomenon (Jabs *et al.*, 1989).

Lacrimal gland hypofunction and stasis is believed to be the cause of dry eye seen in patients with acute GVHD (Jabs *et al.*, 1983). Hirst and colleagues (1983) demonstrated a strong correlation between the occurrence of acute GVHD and decrease in tear secretion by clinical tear-function testing. Periorbital involvement by acute GVHD has also been reported (Cole *et al.*, 1997).

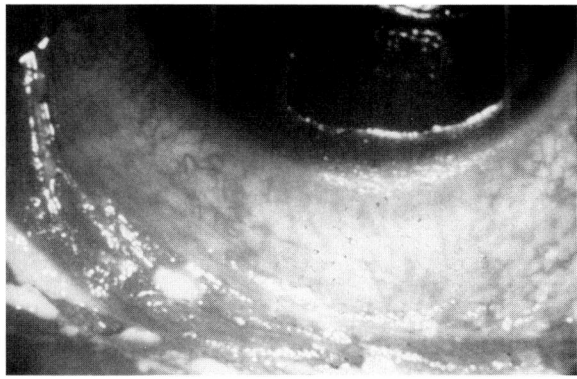

Fig. 98.1. Stage IV ocular GVHD showing intense conjunctival injection, edema, and exudation associated with intense keratopathy and epithelial loss. For color reproduction, see Color Plate 98.1.

[1] Hugo Schiff, German chemist, 1834–1915.

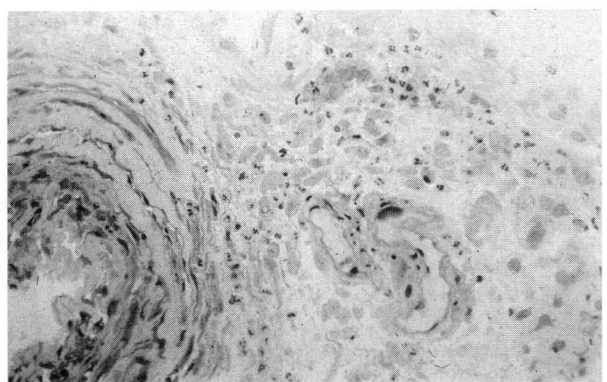

Fig. 98.2. Conjunctival biopsy in acute GVHD showing perivascular inflammation. For color reproduction, see Color Plate 98.2.

Various strategies have been used for prophylaxis of systemic acute GVHD, including selection of a histocompatible donor and immunosuppression. Once ocular GVHD develops, treatment is aimed primarily at the systemic GVHD with immunosuppressive agents such as corticosteroids, cyclosporine, and antithymocyte globulin. Ahmad and colleagues (2002) reported a case of acute GVHD with extensive ocular involvement that responded dramatically to systemic tacrolimus (FK506).

Local measures to protect the eye are most important and are aimed at preventing infection and keeping the eyes lubricated. This is done with wetting agents, lubricants, locally instilled antibiotics, and if necessary patching (Jack & Hicks, 1981; Franklin et al., 1983; Hirst et al., 1983; Jabs et al., 1989; Calissendorff, el Azazi, & Lonnqvist, 1989; Livesey, Homes, & Whittaker, 1989; West, Szer, & Pedersen, 1991). Occasionally surgical intervention may be necessary with performance of conjunctival flaps, tarsorrhaphy, or penetrating keratoplasty.

Chronic GVHD of the eye

GVHD developing or persisting beyond 100 days posttransplant is termed chronic GVHD. However, clinical manifestations typical of chronic GVHD can occur as early as 70 days or as late as 15 months or more post–HSC transplantation. Chronic GVHD differs from acute GVHD in its distribution of target organs and its clinical presentation (Bron, 1994). It is a multiorgan syndrome that clinically bears some resemblance to collagen vascular diseases (Graze & Gale, 1979; Shulman et al., 1980). Chronic GVHD has similarities to various autoimmune disorders, including scleroderma-like involvement of the skin, dacryoadenitis, chronic liver dysfunction, and profound immunodeficiency with recurrent bacterial infections (Jack et al., 1983). Distinct abnormalities that are found on microscopic examination of tissues involved in chronic GVHD are epithelial injury, mononuclear cell infiltrate, and fibrosis. Chronic GVHD may arise as a continuation of acute GVHD, after the resolu-

tion of acute GVHD, or without preceding acute GVHD (Shulman et al., 1978).

In contrast to the situation with acute GVHD, ocular manifestations occur in a high percentage of patients with chronic GVHD and can have severe visual consequences (Arocker-Mettinger et al., 1991). Ocular involvement by chronic GVHD occurs in approximately 40% of all long-term survivors (Jack & Hicks, 1981; Franklin et al., 1983; Deeg, Storb, & Thomas, 1986; Livesey et al., 1989). The primary ocular target tissue is the lacrimal gland producing an obliterative sialadenitis and dacroadenitis. This results in keratoconjunctivitis sicca (KCS) or dry eye syndrome. The histopathologic feature most often identified is keratinization of conjunctival and corneal epithelium caused by the chronic dry eye (Jabs et al., 1983).

There is a close correlation between the severity of the underlying GVHD and the severity of the degree of sicca (Lawley et al., 1977; Jack & Hicks, 1981; Franklin et al., 1983). In fact, Sjögren-like lacrimal insufficiency syndrome,[2] characterized by decreased lacrimation, has been considered one of the diagnostic criteria for chronic GVHD (Lerner et al., 1974; Janin-Mercier et al., 1987). However, Ogawa and associates (2001b) reported substantial differences in the pathogenic process between chronic GVHD and Sjögren's syndrome. They studied the histopathologic characteristics of lacrimal gland involvement and found that in patients with chronic GVHD, there was a predominant infiltration of T cells into the periductal area, an increased number of stromal fibroblasts, and excessive fibrosis in the extracellular matrix. In contrast, Sjögren's syndrome was associated with significant infiltration of B cells (in addition to T cells), clusters of plasma cells in the interlobular areas, and less prominent fibrosis of the extracellular matrix. Ultrastructural studies in chronic GVHD have shown primitive contacts between fibroblasts and lymphocytes, which may reflect functional interactions between fibroblasts and T cells. It has been demonstrated that fibroblasts express HLA class I and class II molecules, as well as co-stimulatory molecules such as CD40 ligand and CD80 under certain conditions (Pechhold et al., 1997; Smith et al., 1997). Based on these findings, it has been suggested that fibroblasts may act as antigen-presenting cells in the lacrimal glands of patients with chronic GVHD and thus play a role in regulating the immune response (Ogawa et al., 2001b).

Conjunctival involvement also occurs in patients with chronic GVHD (Jabs et al., 1989). The changes in conjunctiva represent mucositis and may be distinct from dry eye problems typically described with chronic GVHD. Nasolacrimal duct obstruction as a manifestation of chronic GVHD has also been reported (Hanada & Ueoka, 1989).

Treatment is that of systemic chronic GVHD (Chapter 72). Prednisolone with or without cyclosporine remains the treatment of choice, and some studies suggest that combination improves survival in high-risk patients (Sullivan et al., 1981). Local treatment depends on the nature and extent of the ocular surface disease.

---

[2] Henrik Sjögren, Swedish opthalmologist, 1899–1986.

Ocular surface disease

The ocular surface is composed of the cornea, conjunctiva, and accessory lacrimal glands. A layer of tear film composed of a superficial lipid layer, an aqueous middle layer, and a basal mucin layer covers the normal ocular surface. Ocular surface disease (OSD) characterized by KCS or dry eye syndrome, results from any condition that decreases tear secretion or increases tear film evaporation sufficient to result in increased tear film osmolarity. The lacrimal glands (both the main lacrimal glands in the bony orbit and the accessory lacrimal glands in the conjunctiva) produce the aqueous component of the tear film, and thus, lacrimal gland disease leads to a tear deficient form of dry eye. Most studies implicate GVHD and secondary lacrimal insufficiency as the primary causative factor in OSD following HSC transplantation (Hirst et al., 1983; Jabs et al., 1983; Suh et al., 1999).

However, OSD following HSC transplantation appears not to be due merely to lacrimal insufficiency, as dry eye in these patients is often accompanied by inflammation of both kerato-conjunctival and adnexal tissues. In addition to lacrimal insufficiency, the mucosal lining of the lids and globe can come under direct leukocyte-mediated attack in GVHD (Franklin et al., 1983; Jabs et al., 1989). Cicatricial lagophthalmos, ectropion, and eyelid stiffening due to the cutaneous manifestations of GVHD (Franklin et al., 1983) also contribute to the OSD in HSC transplant recipients.

In addition to the tear deficient type, the evaporative type of dry eye may be associated in HSC transplant recipients. Meibomian glands are specialized sebaceous glands in the tarsal plate of the eyelid that produce the most superficial lipid layer of the tear film. The major function of this lipid layer is to retard evaporation of tears. Meibomian gland dysfunction (MGD) leads to increased evaporation from tear film, and thus dry eye disease. Ogawa and associates (1999) reported severe MGD in patients with severe dry eye and chronic GVHD. It is thought that MGD occurs as a result of destruction of the hair follicles located below the openings of sebaceous ducts by donor T cells in chronic GVHD (Sale, Beauchamp, & Akiyama, 1994).

The majority of patients with OSD also have chronic systemic GVHD; however, severe OSD may occur without systemic involvement. In one study on patients with allogeneic bone marrow transplantation (BMT), we found that 58% of patients had severe OSD; 87% of these patients had coexisting systemic GVHD. However, severe OSD also occurred in several patients (N = 8) who had no systemic GVHD (M. Balaram & M.R. Dana, unpublished data, 2002).

KCS after HSC transplantation has been documented in recipients of both syngeneic and autologous transplants, implying a cause beyond a simple alloreactive immune reaction (Livesey et al., 1989). TBI, ocular toxicity from chemotherapy, infections, and immunosuppressive therapy may be the other contributing factors to KCS after HSC transplantation (Hirst et al., 1983; Atkinson et al., 1990; Bray et al., 1991; Ferrara & Deeg, 1991; Mencucci et al., 1997). Direct irradiation of the lacrimal gland and orbit can cause dry eye syndrome (Parsons et al., 1983). The incidence of KSC is much lower in patients who do not receive TBI as a pre-conditioning regimen (Kerty et al., 1999).

Clinical features of KCS depend on its severity and include symptoms such as grittiness, ocular discomfort, red eye, photophobia, blurred vision, mucus discharge, and eye pain. Diagnosis is made on clinical ophthalmologic examination including vital dye (fluorescein or Rose bengal) staining of the ocular surface, measurement of tear break-up time, and Schirmer testing.[3]

In mild cases, the eye is white and quiet on examination. The most severe manifestation of chronic ocular GVHD with dry eye is a sterile corneal ulcer or nonhealing epithelial defect. Various corneal abnormalities identified may include peripheral corneal vascularization, punctate staining, keratitis, keratinization, and corneal perforation. A pathognomonic sign of chronic conjunctival GVHD is the presence of fibrous-scurvy Arlt[4] lines of the tarsal conjunctiva (Kasmann & Reprecht, 1993).

Treatment includes systemic treatment of chronic GVHD. Systemic immunosuppressive therapy should be considered concurrently with conventional local measures for the management of the coexisting ocular surface inflammation. Systemic administration of tacrolimus (FK506) can be an effective treatment of severe dry eye in patients with chronic GVHD, but long-term administration may be required to achieve a curative response (Ogawa et al., 2001a).

The objectives of local treatment in these patients are twofold, namely supplementation of the preocular tear film and treatment of inflammation. The use of nonpreserved tear supplements is helpful in the amelioration of dry eye symptoms to some extent. Most patients are fairly comfortable using tear substitutes and ocular lubricants, mucolytic agents, and spectacles with sidepieces (to keep out dust particles that may scratch the cornea). A majority of patients with moderate or severe disease also require punctal occlusion. Occlusion of the inferior and/or superior punctum of the eyelid is done to decrease tear drainage. This helps in increasing tear volume and decreasing tear osmolarity. Silicone punctal plugs are used for reversible punctal occlusion. We found a much higher punctal plug failure rate in HSC transplant recipients compared to that found in dry eye syndrome due to other causes. Perhaps the underlying conjunctival inflammation and subconjunctival fibrosis influences plug retention in these patients (Balaram, Schaumberg, & Dana, 2001). HSC transplant patients must be educated regarding this potential complication at the time of punctal plug placement in order to avoid the risk of worsening of OSD due to plug loss. Punctal cauterization may be attempted for permanent and irreversible closure of the punctum.

Use of topical methyl prednisolone has been indicated as an effective treatment option for patients suffering from severe KCS who continue to experience bothersome eye irritation

---

[3] Rudolf Schirmer, German opthalmologist, 1831–1896.
[4] Carl Ferdinand Ritter von Arlt, Austrian opthalmologist, 1812-1887.

despite maximum aqueous enhancement therapies (Marsh & Pflugfelder, 1999), as inflammation is a key pathogenic factor in this condition. Topical steroids should be used judiciously supplemented with appropriate antibiotics to protect the compromised epithelium. In addition to suppressing innate immune responses and therefore increasing the risk of infection, steroids can also increase ocular pressure. Hence, careful monitoring is essential in patients treated with topical steroids. Topical cyclosporine is an appropriate modality in managing ocular surface abnormalities after conventional treatments have been tried (Kiang et al., 1998). We have successfully used topical tacrolimus to treat severe conjunctival inflammation in a patient following allogeneic HSC transplantation with severe OSD (Balaram & Dana, 2001). Topical retinoic acid (Murphy et al., 1996) and autologous serum tears (Rocha et al., 2000) are other modalities that have been used in patients who have not responded to conventional treatment.

In severe cases of GVHD, conjunctival and corneal epithelial defects may progress, and symblepharon and corneal perforation may occur. In one study, treatment of the corneal ulcers with daily collagen shields and hourly polyvinyl-pyrrolidon eye drops resulted in healing of the corneal ulcers within 2 to 3 weeks (Spraul, Lang, & Lang, 1994). Large nonhealing epithelial defects can be managed with bandage contact lenses, and patients who have severe dry eye associated with corneal thinning may require tarsorrhaphy (Table 98.3). Multilayer amniotic membrane transplantation has been used successfully in treating corneal perforation in a patient with severe GVHD (Peris-Martinez et al., 2001). Limbal stem cell transplantation may be performed in patients with severe ocular surface disease (Kenyon & Tseng, 1989). In rare cases of severe ocular

Table 98.3. *Treatment of ocular surface disease*

1. Treatment of systemic GVHD	
2. Eye treatment	
Medical	*Surgical*
Lubricants	Conjunctival flaps
Mucolytic agents	Autograft
Antibiotics	Allograft
Punctal occlusion	Tarsorrhaphy
Silicone punctal plugs	Lateral
Heat cautery	Complete
Laser cautery	Amniotic membrane graft
Topical retinoic acid	Keratoplasty
Autologous serum tears	Limbal stem cell transplantation
Topical steroids	Lid surgery for ectropion
Topical cyclosporine	
Topical tacrolimus	
Spectacles with side pieces	
(to keep out irritants and	
retard evaporation)	
Moist chambers	
Collagen shields	
Bandage soft contact lenses	
Patching	
Lid scrubs and warm compresses	

GVHD, penetrating keratoplasty may be required (Heath, Acheson, & Schulenburg, 1993).

The course of OSD following HSC transplantation is marked by recurrences. However long-term visual prognosis can be good with optimal therapy and close follow-up.

Cataract

After GVHD, cataract is the next most common ocular complication following HSC transplantation. There have been a number of recent studies that have reported the occurrence of cataract in patients undergoing HSC transplantation (Tichelli et al., 1993; Benyunes et al., 1995; Calissendorff, Lonnqvist, & el Azazi, 1995; Belkacemi et al., 1996; Van Kempen-Harteveld et al., 2002). In one large study, posterior subcapsular cataract developed in 10% of patients after BMT (Dunn et al., 1993).

Transplant patients are at considerable risk of developing cataracts as a result of their exposure both to TBI (Deeg et al., 1984; Livesey et al., 1989) and to systemic corticosteroids (Dunn et al., 1993). Deeg and colleagues (1984) reported the incidence of cataracts to be 80% after single-dose TBI as compared to 19% in patients given fractionated TBI. In another study conducted by Bray and colleagues (1991), the incidence of cataract was 63% in patients who received fractionated TBI as compared to 9% in nonirradiated patients. It has been suggested that the incidence of cataract following fractionated TBI is influenced not only by the total dose of radiation but also by its rate of administration (defined by midline tissue dose rate and fractionation schedule) (Bray et al., 1991). A preventive measure, such as lens shielding during TBI, is common practice in many centers (Tichelli, 1994).

The other major factor predisposing to cataract formation is corticosteroid therapy that is given as prophylaxis or treatment for acute or chronic GVHD. Deeg and colleagues (1984) reported a higher incidence of cataract after HSC transplantation in patients with acute lymphoblastic leukemia (ALL) and chronic myeloid leukemia as compared to patients with acute myeloid leukemia or aplastic anemia. It should be noted that nearly all patients with ALL receive corticosteroids as part of their remission induction chemotherapy.

There is no difference biomicroscopically between radiation and corticosteroid-induced cataracts involving the posterior segment of the lens, in contrast to the more diffuse involvement of the core of the lens that occurs in nuclear sclerotic age-related cataracts. The cataracts after HSC transplantation are predominantly posterior subcapsular and bilateral. A significant number of patients who develop cataracts after HSC transplantation have a visual disability. If this is significant, cataract surgery is indicated. Such surgery may be carried out under assisted local anesthesia (peribulbar or retrobulbar), general anesthesia in children, or topical anesthesia.

Extracapsular cataract surgery with insertion of a posterior chamber lens implant into the capsular bag is the treatment of choice. Advances in surgical instrumentation and the use of foldable lenses, allowing cataract extraction through a much smaller incision than was possible earlier, have resulted in lower rates of intraoperative complications. Phacoemulsification is a form of extracapsular cataract extraction in which cataract removal is achieved by ultrasonic fragmentation and aspiration of the lens material requiring a smaller surgical wound, resulting in a shorter healing process and more rapid visual recovery. In our experience, clear-cornea phacoemulsification is an excellent approach in patients with cataract after HSC transplantation (Balaram & Dana, 2001). Clear-cornea approach has an advantage of not manipulating the conjunctiva, which is already compromised in these patients.

The visual prognosis after cataract surgery is good (Calissendorff & Bolme, 1993; Calissendorff et al., 1995; Lureau, Binaghi, & Coscas, 1996; Balaram & Dana, 2001). However, associated OSD may complicate visual rehabilitation after cataract surgery. Coexisting ocular surface disease must be recognized and aggressively treated both before and after surgery to ensure good visual outcome (Balaram & Dana, 2001; Penn & Soong, 2002).

Uveitis

Rarely, HSC transplantation recipients may present with uveitis, which is thought to be a form of GVHD and a result of direct immunologic attack of donor lymphocytes against cells bearing host histocompatibility antigens (Franklin et al., 1983). The incidence of acute anterior uveitis following HSC transplantation was reported to be 3.1% in a study conducted by Kerty and colleagues (1999). Treatment consists of topical steroids. Most cases resolve quickly but some may require systemic corticosteroids or other immunomodulatory medications.

Posterior segment complications

Posterior segment complications following HSC transplantation range from mild transient phenomena to proliferative retinopathy and optic disc edema (Bernauer & Gratwohl, 1992). They may be divided into the following categories (Coskuncan et al., 1994):

1. hemorrhagic
2. BMT retinopathy
3. optic disc edema
4. infections
5. other complications

Hemorrhagic complications occur in the period immediately after HSC transplantation and are presumably related to iatrogenic bone marrow aplasia (Coskuncan et al., 1994), as well as anemia and hyperviscosity state. Retinal and vitreous hemorrhages can be associated with transient visual loss, which usually clear. Fortunately, short-term vision loss due to vitreous or preretinal hemorrhages is not common, occurring in only approximately 1% of patients, and these patients do not experience long-term sequelae (Coskuncan et al., 1994). In a prospective study by Hirst and colleagues (1983), only 2 out of

45 patients suffered transient visual loss as a result of single or repeated retinal or subhyaloid hemorrhages, and in both cases the hemorrhages cleared with resolution of the underlying thrombocytopenia.

BMT retinopathy is an occlusive microvasculopathy and is a well-recognized complication following HSC transplantation (Lopez et al., 1991; Tichelli, 1994; Cunningham, Irvine, & Rugo, 1996; Khawley et al., 1996; Johnson et al., 1999; Gray, Tighe, & Russell, 2000). Clinical manifestations include cotton-wool spots, areas of capillary nonperfusion, retinal telangiectases, microaneurysms, blot and flame hemorrhages, macular edema, and neovascularization. The etiology of BMT retinopathy is uncertain but is probably multifactorial. TBI is thought to be important in the pathogenesis of this disorder and the clinical appearance is similar to that seen in radiation retinopathy. However BMT retinopathy typically occurs at lower radiation dosages than those reported to cause radiation retinopathy (Lopez et al., 1991). Chemotherapeutic agents such as high-dose cytarabine and cyclophosphamide may also contribute to the development of BMT retinopathy, by radiosensitization of the retinal vasculature (Lopez et al., 1991). Other factors that may be involved in the pathogenesis of BMT retinopathy include the use of cyclosporine and the development of GVHD (Bernauer et al., 1991; Lopez et al., 1991).

Most patients with BMT retinopathy have a good prognosis. The ischemic fundus lesions due to occlusive retinal microvasculopathy occur in the first 6 months posttransplant and tend to be reversible in the majority of patients. The retinopathy usually resolves within 2 to 4 months after the withdrawal of cyclosporine or the initiation of corticosteroids. Resolution of retinopathy is associated with recovery of vision. As a result of such favorable findings, treatment is typically not indicated. Macular edema in BMT retinopathy is typically diffuse and may require treatment if visual loss occurs. Lopez and associates (1991) recommended grid photocoagulation for visually significant macular edema. Patients with macular edema have been successfully treated with corticosteroids injected into the sub-Tenon's[5] (episcleral) space (Walton, Vick, & Greenwald, 1999). A case of retinal neovascularization has been treated with early panretinal photocoagulation, with good results (Lopez et al., 1991). However, the efficacy of this intervention needs to be verified with a larger number of patients.

Optic disc edema is another finding in patients following HSC transplantation. Coskuncan et al. (1994) reported that 11 out of 397 patients (2.8%) developed bilateral optic disc edema following transplant. In 8 of these patients, the optic disc swelling resolved after discontinuation of cyclosporine. Optic disc edema was attributed to the presumed neurotoxic effects of cyclosporine. Khawly and associates (1996) observed optic neuropathy in 6 of 9 patients with advanced breast cancer who underwent autologous BMT and hence received no cyclosporine. Optic neuropathy was presumed to arise from the high-dose chemotherapy regimen. Kerty and colleagues (1999)

---

[5] Jacques René Tenon, French surgeon, 1724–1816.

suggested that a causal relationship exists between optic disc edema and acute GVHD. Irreversible visual loss may occur if there is permanent damage to the optic nerve.

Central serous chorioretinopathy has also been described following HSC transplantation (Fawzi & Cunningham, 2001), and is thought to be due to breakdown of the blood-ocular barrier in the choroid due to endothelial dysfunction in the choriocapillaris.

Infections

Infectious complications in HSC transplant recipients are due to leukopenia and the relative lack of granulocytes and lymphocytes following ablation by the pretransplant conditioning regimen. Because full recovery of these two major elements of the immune system occurs separately following transplantation, the risk of infection can be separated into three distinct phases. The first and most dangerous phase is the 2 to 4 week period posttransplant, prior to engraftment, when few circulating leukocytes are present. During this time, patients are at risk for both bacterial and fungal infections, which can advance rapidly and cause death. The second phase of potential infectious complications is from the paucity and immaturity of lymphocytes, and the greatest risk is of fungal and viral infections during the second and third posttransplant months. The third phase of infectious complications occurs after the third month and lasts until lymphocyte maturation occurs. This takes 6 to 18 months. During this period, the ratio of CD4+ to CD8+ T cells is abnormal, T cells respond poorly to antigens, and immunoglobulin production is low. This leads to a risk of infection by encapsulated bacteria such as pneumococci because of a lack of opsonic immunoglobulins. The higher risk of viral infection diminishes as T-cell function gradually improves. The majority of surviving patients recover full immunity and lead lives free from infection.

Ocular bacterial infections include conjunctivitis, orbital cellulitis, and endophthalmitis. Appropriate intravenous antibacterial antibiotics are the primary treatment, although local measures such as vitrectomy and intravitreal antibiotics for endophthalmitis may be required. Fungal infections can cause corneal ulcers and endophthalmitis; treatment is with intravenous amphotericin or the newer azoles, and may include vitrectomy for endophthalmitis.

Peacock and colleagues (1995) reported two cases of posttransplant reactivation of chorioretinitis due to *Toxoplasma gondii*. These patients were seropositive for *T. gondii* pretransplant. The reactivated ocular lesions responded to treatment with sulfadiazine, pyrimethamine, and prednisone. Brinkman and colleagues (1998) reported a patient who developed toxoplasma retinitis/encephalitis 9 months after BMT. They emphasized the possibility of toxoplasma retinitis as a very late disease manifestation in HSC transplant recipients.

Herpes simplex virus (HSV) keratitis is characterized by dendritic corneal ulcers. Treatment is with topical antivirals together with local antibacterial antibiotics to avoid secondary infection. Ocular HSV is not common after HSC transplanta-

tion. Herpes zoster virus (HZV) infection is frequent after allogeneic marrow transplantation, occurring in approximately 40% of long-term survivors (Atkinson et al., 1980). Again, however, ophthalmic involvement (trigeminal nerve) is unusual. In a series of 572 children transplanted at St. Jude Children's Research Hospital between 1983 and 1997, 7 developed herpes zoster opthalmicus at a median of 150 days posttransplant (Walton & Reed, 1999). Complications included keratitis in 6, anterior uveitis in 3, and scleritis in 1. Keratitis was an early complication, developing within the first 4 weeks. Treatment is with oral or intravenous acyclovir or other antivirals, together with local antibacterial antibiotics to the eye to avoid secondary bacterial infection. Local treatment with corticosteroid drops may also be required. Herpes zoster infection is thought to be the most common cause of progressive outer retinal necrosis after HSC transplantation (Lewis, Nagae, & Tano, 1996). Herpetic (HSV, HZV) infections of the eye can lead to significant complications, and the management of these cases requires the involvement of an ophthalmologist, preferably a cornea-external disease specialist.

Cytomegalovirus (CMV) disease used to be a serious cause of morbidity and mortality after HSC transplantation (Meyers, Flournoy, & Thomas, 1982). Typical infection occurs 30 to 100 days after transplantation if no ganciclovir prophylaxis or pre-emptive treatment is given. CMV retinitis occurs in immunosuppressed patients due to hematological dissemination from reactivation of latent CMV as well as exogenously acquired strains. While occurring commonly in patients with acquired immunodeficiency syndrome (AIDS), CMV ocular involvement (retinitis) has been reported only infrequently in HSC transplant recipients (Coskuncan et al., 1994; Okamoto et al., 1997; Miyamoto et al., 1998) in spite of the marked cellular and humoral immune deficiency characteristic of the first year posttransplant. However, with the institution of pre-emptive ganciclovir therapy early after transplantation (Boeckh et al., 1996), most patients survive episodes of CMV infection during the first 3 months after transplantation, and late onset of CMV disease is being recognized more frequently. CMV retinitis in HSC transplant recipients is reported to have an association with chronic extensive GVHD, CMV-positive results of serologic testing before transplantation, pre-existing CMV infection or disease, and delayed lymphocyte engraftment (Crippa et al., 2001). Patients present with symptoms such as blurred vision and floaters. The characteristic ophthalmoscopic picture is that of necrotizing retinitis with or without hemorrhage. CMV retinitis has been described after autologous as well as after allogeneic transplantation. In a report of 20 cases from the EBMT Registry, the median day of diagnosis was 174 (range 19–537) days posttransplant (Larsson et al., 2001). It was bilateral in half the cases. It healed completely in 5, caused permanent impairment of vision in 8, and almost total unilateral or bilateral blindness in 4 patients. Foscarnet has been used successfully to treat ganciclovir-resistant CMV retinitis (Ohta et al., 2001).

Drug toxicity

The most common ocular symptom due to drugs in HSC transplant recipients is the complaint of blurred vision due to corticosteroid treatment, usually as prophylaxis or treatment for GVHD. This resolves rapidly on tapering the dose, or stopping the corticosteroids.

Cyclosporine has been associated with retinal microvascular changes (O'Riordan et al., 1994). Pseudotumor cerebri presenting with diplopia, esotropia, and bilateral optic disc edema has been reported with cyclosporine use after allogeneic transplantation. Improvement occurred within 5 days of discontinuing cyclosporine and the optic disc edema resolved within 3 months (Cruz, Fogg, & Roper-Hall, 1996). The most serious and frightening (for all concerned) ocular drug toxicity is acute cortical blindness associated with cyclosporine (Reece et al., 1991; Memon et al., 1995). This is due to posterior occipital infarction and is considered to be due to cerebral arterial vasospasm. Fortunately it appears generally to be reversible fairly quickly. A strikingly similar syndrome, as described by Devine and associates (1996), occurred with the use of tacrolimus. Acute cortical blindness developed in three patients 5 to 47 days posttransplant but reversal occurred within 1 to 2 weeks.

Cyclosporine-induced ocular flutter has been reported after HSC transplantation (Apsner et al., 1997). Cyclosporine has been postulated to produce transient brain stem or neuromuscular dysfunction with eye movement abnormality in occasional patients (Openshaw, Slatkin, & Smith, 1997). Unusual corneal deposits have been reported after topical use of cyclosporine eye drops in patients with GVHD (Kachi et al., 2000).

Acute iritis (Parkkali et al., 1996), as well as episcleritis, has been described as a complication of granulocyte colony-stimulating factor used for mobilization of blood stem cells. A history of prior inflammatory eye disease probably constitutes a contraindication to the use of this agent.

Ocular toxicity induced by cancer chemotherapy is not uncommon. Cyclophosphamide has been reported to cause blurred vision, KCS, blepharoconjunctivitis, and pinpoint pupils (Fraunfelder & Meyer, 1983). Posterior subcapsular cataract with a polychromatic sheen is a well-established ocular side effect of busulfan (Podos & Canellos, 1969). Methotrexate can cause periorbital edema, ocular pain, blurred vision, photophobia, conjunctivitis, blepharitis, and decreased reflex tear production (Fraunfelder & Meyer, 1983). Cytosine arabinoside has been shown to cause keratitis with high doses and prolonged treatment (Hopen et al., 1981).

Involvement of the eye by the underlying disease

Ocular manifestations are not uncommon in leukemia. Rosenthal (1983) surveyed 657 children with leukemia and found ophthalmic involvement in 9%. In HSC transplant patients, this would likely only occur in those coming to transplant with refractory or relapsed leukemia or at the time of

Table 98.4. *Ocular manifestations of leukemia*

Retina	1. Tortuosity, dilatation and sheathing of vessels 2. Leukemic infiltrates 3. Hemorrhages (dot and blot, flame-shaped, white-centred)
Optic nerve	Leukemic infiltrates manifesting as optic disc edema
Uveal tract	Leukemic infiltrates manifesting as shallow subretinal detachments
Anterior chamber	Hypopyon, pseudohypopyon, spontaneous hyphema
Cornea	Leukemic infiltrates of limbus, sterile ring ulcer, pannus formation
Sclera	Perivascular leukemic infiltration
Orbit and adnexa	Leukemic infiltrates resulting in proptosis, ecchymosis, chemosis, diplopia, visual disturbances, motility disturbances
Glaucoma	1. Leukemic infiltration of trabecular meshwork 2. Angle closure glaucoma secondary to choroidal infiltration and hemorrhage

recurrence of leukemia posttransplant. The ocular manifestations of leukemia are summarized in Table 98.4. Cases of anterior segment masquerade syndrome, in which anterior chamber paracentesis and iris biopsy allowed definitive diagnosis of leukemic relapse, have been reported (Schachat et al., 1988).

Complications in children

HSC transplantation has increasingly become an accepted treatment for many childhood diseases (Abramovitz & Senner, 1995). Advances in supportive care have improved survival rates, contributing to a rapidly growing population of HSC transplant survivors (Sanders, 1991). Suh and associates (1999) performed a retrospective study on 104 pediatric patients who required HSC transplantation, and found that ocular changes developed in 51% of patients. Most frequent findings included dry eye syndrome (12.5%), cataract (23.0%), and posterior segment complications (13.5%). A final visual acuity of 20/40 or better was achieved in 95.7% of eyes. In a study conducted by Ng and colleagues (1999), abnormal tear film was the most important ocular manifestation among children following HSC transplatation.

Cataract formation is a complication that occurs in all age groups, but in the pediatric population, development of amblyopia (lazy eye) is a real risk and concern. Therefore, early cataract detection and timely management are essential in pediatric patients, as delay in treatment may cause irreversible visual loss if amblyopia is detected only after the visual system has matured.

Regular ophthalmic assessment is recommended for early detection and treatment of these potentially problematic complications in the growing eyes of pediatric patients. Yearly surveillance should include an ophthalmology exam. Bi-annual communication with the child's teacher can assist in surveillance, should the child experience visual difficulties in school (Fisher, 1999). Long-term survivors of pediatric HSC transplantation often have complex psychosocial and physical problems that require understanding, evaluation, and management by skilled health care providers. A pediatric ophthalmologist is an integral part of the long-term follow-up process.

Conclusions

HSC transplantation is a lifesaving procedure for an increasing number of children and adults. With the advent of histocompatibility testing, immunomodulatory therapy, and good supportive care, there has been, and will be, an increasing number of long-term survivors who need special management for the various posttransplant ocular complications. Familiarity with the potential complications is important in the successful treatment of these patients. The presence of GVHD increases ocular involvement and its severity. The high prevalence of ocular involvement in GVHD patients necessitates ocular evaluation prior to the onset of significant problems. Occasionally, ocular symptoms may be the first presentation of GVHD and they may be seen in the absence of systemic manifestations. Further, the possibility of recurrence of ocular GVHD after stopping the immunosuppressive therapy requires long-term ocular follow-up. Because these patients often have other life-threatening conditions, management of these patients requires a team effort between transplant physicians and ophthalmologists. However, despite multiple ocular problems, there is generally a good long-term visual prognosis with optimal therapy and close follow-up. Thus, the ocular surveillance plan for HSC transplant recipients should include patient education and periodic eye evaluation in order to facilitate prompt diagnosis and treatment of the various ocular complications.

References

Abramovitz, L.Z. & Senner, A.M. (1995). Pediatric bone marrow transplantation update. *Oncology Nursing Forum, 22,* 107–15.

Ahmad, S.M., Stegman, Z., Fructhman, S., & Asbell, P.A. (2002). Successful treatment of acute ocular graft-versus-host disease with tacrolimus (FK506). *Cornea, 21,* 432–3.

Apsner, R., Schulenberg, A., Steinhoff, N. *et al.* (1997). Cyclosporin A induced ocular flutter after marrow transplantation. *Bone Marrow Transplantation, 20,* 255–6.

Arocker-Mettinger, E., Skorpick, F., Grabner, G. *et al.* (1991). Manifestations of graft-versus-host disease following allogeneic bone marrow transplantation. *European Journal of Ophthalmology, 1,* 28–32.

Atkinson, K., Meyers, J.D., Storb, R. *et al.* (1980). Varicella zoster virus infection after marrow transplantation for aplastic anemia and leukemia. *Transplantation, 29,* 47–50.

Atkinson, K. (1990). Chronic graft-versus-host disease. *Bone Marrow Transplantation, 5,* 69–82.

Balaram, M. & Dana, M.R. (2001). Phacoemulsification in patients with allogeneic bone marrow transplantation. *Ophthalmology, 108,* 1682–7.

Balaram, M., Schaumberg, D.A., & Dana, M.R. (2001). Efficacy and tolerability outcomes after punctal occlusion with silicone plugs in dry eye syndrome. *American Journal of Ophthalmology, 131,* 30–6.

Belkacemi, Y., Ozsahin, M., Pene, F. *et al.* (1996). Cataractogenesis after total body irradiation. *International Journal of Radiation Oncology, Biology, Physics, 35,* 53–60.

Benyunes, M.C., Sullivan, K.M., Deeg, H.J. *et al.* (1995). Cataracts after bone marrow transplantation: long term follow-up of adults treated with fractionated total body irradiation. *International Journal of Radiation Oncology, Biology, Physics, 32,* 661–70.

Bernauer, W. & Gratwohl, A. (1992). Bone marrow transplant retinopathy. *American Journal of Ophthalmology, 113,* 604–5.

Bernauer, W., Gratwohl, A., Keller, A., & Daicker, B. (1991). Microvasculopathy in the ocular fundus after bone marrow transplantation. *Annals of Internal Medicine, 115,* 925–30.

Boeckh, M., Gooley, T.A., Myerson, D. *et al.* (1996). Cytomegalovirus pp65 antigenemia-guided early treatment with ganciclovir versus ganciclovir at engraftment after allogeneic marrow transplantation: a randomized double-blind study. *Blood, 88,* 4063–71.

Bray, L.C., Carey, P.J., Proctor, S.J. *et al.* (1991). Ocular complications of bone marrow transplantation. *British Journal of Ophthalmology, 75,* 611–4.

Brinkman, K., Debast, S., Sauerwein, R. *et al.* (1998). Toxoplasma retinitis/encephalitis 9 months after allogeneic bone marrow transplantation. *Bone Marrow Transplantation, 21,* 635–6.

Bron, D. (1994). Graft-versus-host disease. *Current Opinion in Oncology, 6,* 358–64.

Calissendorff, B.M. & Bolme, P. (1993). Cataract development and outcome of surgery in bone marrow transplanted children. *British Journal of Ophthalmology, 77,* 36–8.

Calissendorff, B., el Azazi, M., & Lonnqvist, B. (1989). Dry eye syndrome in long term follow-up of bone marrow transplant patients. *Bone Marrow Transplantation, 4,* 675–8.

Calissendorff, B.M., Lonnqvist, B., & el Azazi, M. (1995). Cataract development in adult bone marrow transplant recipients. *Acta Ophthamologica Scandinavica, 73,* 152–4.

Cole, J.W., Quint, D.J., Hutchinson, R.J., & Yanik, G.A. (1997). CT demonstration of periorbital graft-versus-host disease. *American Journal of Neuroradiology, 18,* 730–2.

Coskuncan, N.M., Jabs, D.A., Dunn, J.P. *et al.* (1994). The eye in bone marrow transplantation. VI. Retinal complications. *Archives of Ophthalmology, 112,* 372–9.

Crippa, F., Corey, L., Chuang, E.L. *et al.* (2001). Virological, clinical, and ophthalmologic features of cytomegalovirus retinitis after hematopoietic stem cell transplantation. *Clinical Infectious Disease, 32,* 214–9.

Cruz, O.A., Fogg, S.G., & Roper-Hall, G. (1996). Pseudotumor cerebri associated with cyclosporine use. *American Journal of Ophthalmology, 122,* 436–7.

Cunningham, E.T. Jr., Irvine, A.R., & Rugo, H.S. (1996). Bone marrow transplantation retinopathy in the absence of radiation therapy. *American Journal of Ophthalmology, 122,* 268–70.

Deeg, G.J., Storb, R., & Thomas, E.D. (1984). Bone marrow transplantation: a review of delayed complications. *British Journal of Haematology, 57,* 185–208.

Deeg, H.J., Flournoy, N., Sullivan, K.M. *et al.* (1984). Cataracts after total body irradiation and marrow transplantation: a sparing effect of dose fractionation. *International Journal of Radiation Oncology, Biology, Physics, 10,* 957–64.

Devine, S.M., Newman, N.J., Siegel, J.L. *et al.* (1996). Tacrolimus (FK506)-induced cerebral blindness following bone marrow transplantation. *Bone Marrow Transplantation, 18,* 569–72.

Dunn, J.P., Jabs, D.A., Wingard, J. *et al.* (1993). Bone marrow transplantation and cataract development. *Archives of Ophthalmology, 111,* 1367–73.

Farmer, E.R. (1986). The histopathology of graft-versus-host disease. *Advances in Dermatology, 1,* 173–88.

Fawzi, A.A. & Cunningham, E.T. Jr. (2001). Central serous chorioretinopathy after bone marrow transplantation. *American Journal of Ophthalmology, 131,* 804–5.

Ferrara, J.L. & Deeg, H.J. (1991). Graft-versus-host disease. *New England Journal of Medicine, 324,* 667–74.

Fisher, V.L. (1999). Long-term follow-up in hematopoietic stem-cell transplant patients. *Pediatric Transplantation, 3,* 122–9.

Franklin, R.M., Kenyon, K.R., Tutschka, P.J. *et al.* (1983). Ocular manifestation of graft-versus-host disease. *Ophthalmology, 901,* 4–13.

Fraunfelder, F.T. & Meyer, S.M. (1983). Ocular toxicity of antineoplastic agents. *Ophthalmology, 90,* 1–3.

Gray, R.H., Tighe, M., & Russell, N.H. (2000). Rapid onset retinopathy in a diabetic patient following bone marrow transplantation. *Bone Marrow Transplantation, 26,* 695–6.

Graze, P.R. & Gale, R.P. (1979). Chronic graft-versus-host disease: a syndrome of disordered immunity. *American Journal of Medicine, 66,* 611–20.

Hanada, R. & Ueoka, Y. (1989). Obstruction of nasolacrimal ducts closely related to graft-versus-host disease after bone marrow transplantation. *Bone Marrow Transplantation, 4,* 125–6.

Heath, J.D., Acheson, J.F., & Schulenburg, W.E. (1993). Penetrating keratoplasty in severe ocular graft versus host disease. *British Journal of Ophthalmology, 77,* 525–6.

Hirst, L.W., Jabs, D.A., Tutschka, P.J. *et al.* (1983). The eye in bone marrow transplantation. I. Clinical study. *Archives of Ophthalmology, 101,* 580–4.

Hopen, G., Mondino, B.J., Johnson, B.L., & Chervenick, P.A. (1981). Corneal toxicity with systemic cytarabine. *American Journal of Ophthalmology, 91,* 500–4.

Jabs, D.A., Hirst, L.W., Green, W.R. *et al.* (1983). The eye in bone marrow transplantation. II. Histopathology. *Archives of Ophthalmology, 101,* 585–90.

Jabs, D.A., Wingard, J., Green, W.R. *et al.* (1989). The eye in bone marrow transplantation. III. Conjunctival graft-versus-host disease. *Archives of Ophthalmology, 107,* 1343–8.

Jack, M.K. & Hicks, J.D. (1981). Ocular complications in high dose chemoradiotherapy and marrow transplantation. *Annals of Ophthalmology, 13,* 709–11.

Jack, M.K., Jack, G.M., Sale, G.E. *et al.* (1983). Ocular manifestations of graft-versus-host disease. *Archives of Ophthalmology, 101,* 1080–4.

Janin, A., Facon, T., Castier, P. *et al.* (1996). Pseudomembranous conjunctivitis following bone marrow transplantation: immunopathological and ultrastructural study of one case. *Human Pathology, 27,* 307–9.

Janin-Mercier, A., Devergie, A., Arrago, J. *et al.* (1987). Systemic evaluation of Sjogren-like syndrome after bone marrow transplantation in man. *Transplantation, 43,* 677–9.

Johnson, D.W., Cagnoni, P.J., Schossau, T.M. *et al.* (1999). Optic disc and retinal microvasculopathy after high-dose chemotherapy and autologous hematopoietic progenitor cell support. *Bone Marrow Transplantation, 24,* 785–92.

Kachi, S., Hirano, K., Takesue, Y., & Miura, M. (2000). Unusual corneal deposit after the topical use of cyclosporine as eyedrops. *American Journal of Ophthalmology, 130,* 667–9.

Kasmann, B. & Reprecht, K.W. (1993). [Ophthalmologic findings in graft versus host disease (GVHD)]. [German] *Klinische Monatsblatter fur Augenheilkunde, 202,* 491–9.

Kenyon, K.R. & Tseng, S.C. (1989). Limbal autograft transplantation for ocular surface disorders. *Ophthalmology, 96,* 709–23.

Kerty, E., Vigander, K., Flage, T., & Brinch, L. (1999). Ocular findings in allogeneic stem cell transplantation without total body irradiation. *Ophthalmology, 106,* 1334–8.

Khawly, J.A., Rubin, P., Petros, W. *et al.* (1996). Retinopathy and optic neuropathy in bone marrow transplantation for breast cancer. *Ophthalmology, 103,* 87–95.

Kiang, E., Tesavibul, N., Yee, R. *et al.* (1998). The use of topical cyclosporin A in ocular graft-versus-host-disease. *Bone Marrow Transplantation, 22,* 147–51.

Larsson, K., Ljungman, P., Rovira, M. *et al.* (2001). CMV retinitis after allogeneic SCT. Report on an EBMT Infectious Diseases Working Party Survey. *Bone Marrow Transplantation, 27,* (Suppl 1), S61 (abstract).

Lawley, T.J., Peck, G.L., Moutsopoulos, H.M. *et al.* (1977). Scleroderma. Sjogren-like syndrome and chronic graft-versus-host disease. *Annals of Internal Medicine, 87,* 707–9.

Lerner, K.G., Kao, G.F. Storb, R. *et al.* (1974). Histopathology of graft-vs.-host reaction (GvHR) in human recipients of marrow from HL-A-matched sibling donors. *Transplantation Proceedings, 6,* 367–71.

Lewis, J.M., Nagae, Y., & Tano, Y. (1996). Progressive outer retinal necrosis after bone marrow transplantation. *American Journal of Ophthalmology, 122,* 892–5.

Livesey, S.J., Homes, J.A., & Whittaker, J.S. (1989). Ocular complications of bone marrow transplantation. *Eye, 3,* 271–6.

Lopez, P.F., Sternberg, P.Jr., Dabbs, C.K. *et al.* (1991). Bone marrow transplant retinopathy. *American Journal of Ophthalmology, 112,* 635–46.

Lureau, M.A., Binaghi, M., & Coscas, G. (1996). [Cataract surgery after bone marrow transplantation. Apropos of 86 cases]. [French] *Journal Francais d'Ophthalmologie, 19,* 164–9.

Marsh, P. & Pflugfelder, S.C. (1999). Topical non-preserved methyl prednisolone therapy for keratoconjunctivitis sicca in Sjogren's syndrome. *Ophthalmology, 106,* 811–6.

Memon, M., de Magalhaes-Silverman, M., Bloom, E.J. *et al.* (1995). Reversible cyclosporine-induced cortical blindness in allogeneic bone marrow transplant recipients. *Bone Marrow Transplantation, 15,* 283–6.

Mencucci, R., Rossi Ferrini, C., Bosi, A. *et al.* (1997). Ophthalmological aspect in allogeneic bone marrow transplantation: Sjogren-like syndrome in graft-versus-host disease. *European Journal of Ophthalmology, 7,* 13–8.

Meyers, J.D., Flournoy, N., & Thomas, E.D. (1982). Nonbacterial pneumonia after allogeneic marrow transplantation: a review of ten years' experience. *Reviews of Infectious Diseases, 4,* 1119–32.

Miyamoto, T., Gondo, H., Miyoshi, Y. *et al.* (1998). Early viral complications following CD34– selected autologous peripheral blood stem cell transplantation for non-Hodgkin's lymphoma. *British Journal of Haematology, 100,* 348–50.

Murphy, P.T., Sivakumaran, M., Fahy, G., & Hutchinson, R.M. (1996). Successful use of topical retinoic acid in severe dry eye due to chronic graft-versus-host disease. *Bone Marrow Transplantation, 18,* 641–2.

Ng, J.S., Lam, D.S., Li, C.K. *et al.* (1999). Ocular complications of pediatric bone marrow transplantation. *Ophthalmology, 106,* 160–4.

Ogawa, Y., Okamoto, S., Kuwana, M. *et al.* (2001a). Successful treatment of dry eye in two patients with chronic graft-versus-host disease with systemic administration of FK506 and corticosteroids. *Cornea, 20,* 430–4.

Ogawa, Y., Okamoto, S., Wakui, M. *et al.* (1999). Dry eye after hematopoietic stem cell transplantation. *British Journal of Ophthalmology, 83,* 1125–30.

Ogawa, Y., Yamazaki, K., Kuwana, M. *et al.* (2001b). A significant role of stromal fibroblasts in rapidly progressive dry eye in patients with chronic GVHD. *Investigative Ophthalmology and Visual Science, 42,* 111–19.

Ohta, H., Matsuda, Y., Tokimasa, S. *et al.* (2001). Foscarnet therapy for ganciclovir-resistant cytomegalovirus retinitis after stem cell transplantation: effective monitoring of CMV infection by quantitative analysis of CMV mRNA. *Bone Marrow Transplantation, 27,* 1141–5.

Okamoto, T., Okada, M., Mori, A. *et al.* (1997). Successful treatment of severe cytomegalovirus retinitis with foscarnet and intraocular injection of ganciclovir in a myelosuppressed unrelated bone marrow transplant patient. *Bone Marrow Transplantation, 20,* 801–3.

Openshaw, H., Slatkin, N.E., & Smith, E. (1997). Eye movement disorders in bone marrow transplant patients on cyclosporin and ganciclovir. *Bone Marrow Transplantation, 19,* 503–5.

O'Riordan, J.M., FitzSimon, S., O'Connor, M., & McCann, S.R. (1994). Retinal microvascular changes following bone marrow transplantation: the role of cyclosporine. *Bone Marrow Transplantation, 13,* 101–4.

Parkkali, T., Volin, Siren, M.K., & Ruutu, T. (1996). Acute iritis induced by granulocyte colony-stimulating factor used for mobilization in a volunteer unrelated peripheral blood progenitor cells donor. *Bone Marrow Transplantation, 17,* 433–4.

Parsons, J.T., Fitzgerald, C.R., Hood, C.I. *et al.* (1983). The effects of irradiation on the eye and optic nerve. *International Journal of Radiation Oncology, Biology, Physics, 9,* 609–22.

Peacock, J.E., Greven, C.M., Cruz, J.M. *et al.* (1995). Reactivation toxoplasmic retinchoroiditis in patients undergoing bone marrow transplantation: is there a role for chemoprophylaxis? *Bone Marrow Transplantation, 15,* 983–7.

Pechhold, K., Patterson, N.B., Craighead, N. *et al.* (1997). Inflammatory cytokines IFN-gamma plus TNF-alpha induce regulated expression of CD80 (B7-1) but not CD86 (B7-2) on murine fibroblasts. *Journal of Immunology, 158,* 4921–9.

Penn, E.A. & Soong, H.K. (2002). Cataract surgery in allogeneic bone marrow transplant recipients with graft-versus-host disease (1). *Journal of Cataract and Refractive Surgery, 28,* 417–20.

Peris-Martinez, C., Menezo, J.L., Diaz-Llopis, M. *et al.* (2001). Multilayer amniotic membrane transplantation in severe ocular graft versus host disease. *European Journal of Ophthalmology, 11,* 183–6.

Podos, S.M. & Canellos, G.P. (1969). Lens changes in chronic granulocytic leukemia. Possible relationship to chemotherapy. *American Journal of Ophthalmology, 68,* 500–4.

Reece, D.E., Frei-Lahr, D.A., Shepherd, J.D. *et al.* (1991). Neurological complications in allogeneic bone marrow transplant patients receiving cyclosporin. *Bone Marrow Transplantation, 8,* 393–401.

Rocha, E.M., Pelegrino, F.S.A., de Paiva, C.S. *et al.* (2000). GVHD dry eyes treated with autologous serum tears. *Bone Marrow Transplantation, 25,* 1101–3.

Rosenthal, R.A. (1983). Ocular manifestations of leukemia. *Ophthalmology, 90,* 899–905.

Sale, G.E., Beauchamp, M.D., & Akiyama, M. (1994). Parafollicular bulges, but not hair bulb keratinocytes, are attacked in graft-versus-host disease of human skin. *Bone Marrow Transplantation, 14,* 411–13.

Sanders, J.E. (1991). Long-term effects of bone marrow transplantation. *Pediatrician, 18,* 76–81.

Schachat, A.P., Jabs, D.A., Graham, M.L. *et al.* (1988). Leukemic iris infiltration. *Journal of Pediatric Ophthalmology and Strabismus, 25,* 135–8.

Shulman, H.M., Sale, G.E., Lerner, K.G. *et al.* (1978). Chronic cutaneous graft-versus-host disease in man. *American Journal of Pathology, 91,* 545–70.

Shulman, H.M., Sullivan, K.M., Weiden, P.L. *et al.* (1980). Chronic graft-versus-host syndrome in man. A long term clinicopathological study of 20 Seattle patients. *American Journal of Medicine, 69,* 204–17.

Smith, T.J., Sempowski, G.D., Cao, H.J. *et al.* (1997). Human thyroid fibroblasts exhibit a distinctive phenotype in culture: characteristic ganglioside profile and functional CD40 expression. *Endocrinology, 138,* 5576–88.

Spiro, T.P., O'Day, D.G., Bardenstein, D. *et al.* (1996). Severe acute graft-versus-host disease of conjunctivae after allogeneic blood progenitor cell infusion. *Bone Marrow Transplantation, 17,* 1179–80.

Spraul, C.W., Lang, G.E., & Lang, G.K. (1994). [Corneal ulcer in chronic graft-versus-host disease treatment with collagen shields]. [German] *Klinische Monatsblatter fur Augenheilkunde, 205,* 161–6.

Storb, R., & Donall Thomas, E. (1994). The scientific foundation of marrow transplantation based on animal studies. In *Bone Marrow Transplantation,* ed. S.J. Forman, K.G. Blume, & E.D. Thomas, pp.3–11. Boston: Blackwell Scientific Publications.

Suh, D.W., Ruttum, M.S., Stuckenschneider, B.J. *et al.* (1999). Ocular findings after bone marrow transplantation in a pediatric population. *Ophthalmology, 106,* 1564–70.

Sullivan, K.M., Shulman, H.M., Storb, R. *et al.* (1981). Chronic graft-versus-host disease in 52 patients: adverse natural course and successful treatment with combination immunosuppression. *Blood,* **57,** 267–76.

Tichelli, A. (1994). Late ocular complications after bone marrow transplantation. *Nouvelle Revue Française d'Hematologie,* **36** (Suppl 1), S79–82.

Tichelli, A., Gratwohl, A., Egger, T. *et al.* (1993). Cataract formation after bone marrow transplantation. *Annals of Internal Medicine,* **119,** 1175–80.

Van Kempen-Harteveld, M.L., Struikmans, H., Kal, H.B. *et al.* (2002). Cataract after total body irradiation and bone marrow transplantation: degree of visual impairment. *International Journal of Radiation Oncology, Biology, Physics,* **1,** 1375–80.

Walton, R.C. & Reed, K.L. (1999). Herpes zoster opthalmicus following bone marrow transplantation in children. *Bone Marrow Transplantation,* **23,** 1317–20.

Walton, R.C., Vick, V.L., & Greenwald, M.A. (1999). Sub-Tenon's corticosteroids for the treatment of macular edema in bone marrow transplant retinopathy. *Retina,* **19,** 171–3.

West, R.H., Szer, J., & Pedersen, J.S. (1991). Ocular surface and lacrimal disturbances in chronic graft-versus-host disease: the role of conjunctival biopsy. *Australian and New Zealand Journal of Ophthalmology,* **19,** 187–91.

99 Ear, Nose, and Throat Complications

SHYAN VIJAYASEKARAN, PHILLIP CHANG, AND MARCUS D. ATLAS

Sir Charles Gairdner Hospital, Perth, and St Vincent's Hospital, Sydney, Australia

Introduction

Hematopoietic stem cell (HSC) transplantation is currently the treatment of choice for rescuing patients from the consequences of intensive antitumor therapy for a variety of diseases. These include hematologic and some solid tumors. Infective and hemorrhagic complications commonly arise and are often related to the ear, nose, and throat.

There are three mechanisms by which patients undergoing HSC transplantation are made more susceptible to infection. These include altered host resistance from the underlying malignant disease process, altered host resistance resulting from immunosuppressive therapy, and increased inocula of organisms resulting from therapy and the hospital environment (Armstrong *et al.*, 1971).

The source of the infection is often difficult to document in the febrile neutropenic patient, with as many as 40% of cases never having a culture-proven focus (Talcott *et al.*, 1988). Schimpff *et al.* (1972) reported that 22 of 111 demonstrable infections in a group of 48 patients with acute myeloid leukemia originated in the head and neck. For these reasons, the otorhinolaryngologist may be consulted to assess the risk for head and neck infection before prolonged myelosuppression. This allows the early identification and treatment of infectious complications prior to HSC transplantation.

Two-thirds of patients who underwent bone marrow transplantation developed otolaryngologic complications in a report from the University of Pennsylvania (DiNardo & Hendrix, 1991). Infectious complications were most frequent (66%), followed by hemorrhagic (21%), and drug-induced side effects (18%). There were three deaths from otolaryngologic complications in the 50 patients in this series.

Levine found that 21% of deaths in patients with hematologic malignancies resulted from hemorrhage (Levine, Gaw, & Young, 1972). The most common otolaryngologic hemorrhagic complication is epistaxis. Epistaxis has the potential to be fatal especially in the coagulopathic patient and is certainly associated with substantial morbidity.

Pretreatment evaluation of patients prior to HSC transplantation is important for the diagnosis and treatment of pre-existing otorhinolarynologic conditions. These conditions have the potential to be significantly more refractory once myelosuppressive treatment is commenced, and have the potential for greater morbidity and mortality. Furthermore, these conditions left unrecognized may be severe enough to compromise the continuation of the pretransplant conditioning regimen. Surveillance cultures may be useful (Schimpff, 1990). Pretreatment otolaryngologic conditions diagnosed on otolaryngologic review in the series reported by DiNardo and Hendrix included dental impaction, chronic bacterial sinusitis, herpetic stomatitis, and thrombocytopenic epistaxis. All of these conditions were medically treated and had completely resolved prior to myelosuppressive treatment. None of these conditions complicated subsequent therapy (DiNardo & Hendrix, 1991).

Oral manifestations

During chemotherapy the oropharynx is the most common site of otolaryngologic complications. Common complications include oropharyngeal candidiasis, herpetic lesions, oral mucositis, and gingival bleeding.

Myelosuppressive or myeloablative treatment produces unavoidable toxicity to normal, rapidly proliferating cells. The mucosal lining of the oral mucosa is a prime target for treatment-related toxicity because of its rapid cell turnover rate. Oral complications of cancer therapy occur in approximately 40% of patients receiving chemotherapy (Lockhart & Sonis, 1979).

Mucositis and stomatitis (and see Chapter 80)

Gastrointestinal tract epithelial cells have a cell turnover rate similar to that of leukocytes, so the period of greatest damage to the oral mucosa frequently correlates with the white blood cell nadir (Lockhart & Sonis, 1979). Resolution of oral toxicity generally coincides with resolution of the leukopenia. The lips, tongue, floor of the mouth, buccal mucosa, and soft palate are more severely affected by chemo-or chemoradiation toxicity than the hard palate and gingiva. This may be due to their faster rate of epithelial cell turnover (Barrett, 1984).

Chemotherapeutic agents likely to cause mucositis include busulfan, cyclophosphamide, cytosine arabinoside, dactinomycin, daunorubicin, doxorubicin, etoposide, melphalan, methotrexate, mitomycin, and vinblastine.

The terms mucositis and stomatitis are often used interchangeably. However, mucositis generally describes a toxic inflammatory reaction affecting the gastrointestinal tract from mouth to anus, which results from exposure to chemotherapeutic agents or total body irradiation (TBI). Mucositis typically manifests as erythematous or ulcerative lesions.

Stomatitis refers to any inflammatory reaction affecting the oral mucosa, with or without ulceration, and may be caused or exacerbated by local factors. Pre-existing oral conditions such as dental calculus, broken teeth, faulty dentures, periodontal disease, and gingivitis contribute to the development of local infections and may serve as a focus for systemic infection.

Erythematous mucositis may appear as early as 3 days after exposure to chemotherapy, but more typically within 5 to 7 days. Progression to ulcerative mucositis typically occurs within 7 days of the start of chemotherapy. Mucositis is self-limited when uncomplicated by infection and typically heals completely within 2 to 4 weeks (Ziga, 1983).

Systematic assessment of the oral cavity before, during, and after the conditioning regimen permits early identification of toxicity and initiation of oral hygiene measures designed to prevent or decrease further complications (Beck, 1979; Daeffler, 1980).

Once mucositis has developed, meticulous oral hygiene and palliation of symptoms become the focus of care. In the absence of controlled clinical trials, many management recommendations are empirical. Some established guidelines for oral care include oral assessments twice daily for hospitalized patients and frequent oral care (minimum of every 4 hours and at bedtime), increasing in frequency as the severity of mucositis increases.

Oral mucositis can be complicated by infection in the immunocompromised patient. Not only can the mouth itself become infected, but the loss of the oral epithelium as a protective barrier provides a portal of entry for microorganisms into the circulation. Once mucosal integrity is breached, local and systemic infections can be caused by endogenous oral flora, as well as nosocomial and opportunistic organisms. As the absolute neutrophil count falls below $1 \times 10^9/l$ the incidence and severity of infection rises. Patients with prolonged neutropenia are at higher risk for the development of serious infectious complications.

Antibiotics used during neutropenia alter oral flora, creating a favorable environment for fungal overgrowth that may be exacerbated by concurrent steroid therapy (Ostchega, 1980).

Oral care protocols generally include atraumatically cleansing the oral mucosa, moisturizing the lips and oral cavity, and relieving pain and inflammation (Beck, 1979). A soft toothbrush or foam swab cleans teeth effectively and atraumatically. Options for cleansing and debriding agents include "salt and soda" normal saline, sodium bicarbonate, sterile water, and

hydrogen peroxide solution. Indications for use of hydrogen peroxide include crusting and need for gentle debridement. Use should be limited since chronic use may impair timely healing of stomatitis.

Moisturizing can be achieved with water-soluble lubricating jelly, Diclonine hydrochloride 0.5% or 1%, lidocaine 2% viscous, or carbamide peroxide 10% (urea peroxide 10%).

Agents that produce symptoms or injure the mucosa should not be used. Patients may use toothpaste if tolerated; however, over-the-counter mouthwashes generally contain alcohol and should be avoided. Glycerin is hygroscopic and may dry tissues. Topical anesthetics may minimize pain temporarily, but are frequently formulated with additives that can intensify and prolong mucositis.

Chlorhexidine is a broad-spectrum antimicrobial agent with activity against Gram-positive and Gram-negative organisms, yeast, and other fungal organisms. Its use in the prophylaxis of oral infections shows promise in reducing inflammation and ulceration, as well as in reducing oral microorganisms in high-risk patient groups (Ostchega, 1980; Dreizen et al., 1983).

Oral cavity hemorrhage

Hemorrhage may occur during treatment-induced thrombocytopenia and coagulopathy. Periodontal disease may bleed spontaneously or from minimal trauma. Oral bleeding may be minimal, with petechiae located on the lips, soft palate, or floor of the mouth. More severe oral hemorrhage may occur especially from gingival crevices. Spontaneous gingival oozing may occur when platelet counts drop to less than $50 \times 10^9/l$.

The use of toothbrushes and dental floss in patients with platelet counts of less than $50 \times 10^9/l$ is controversial because of the potential to induce bleeding. Occasionally, dental extraction (full or partial) is indicated in patients with severe periodontal disease who require HSC transplantation on an urgent basis.

Oral candidiasis (also see Chapters 75 and 80)

Oral candidiasis is a common complication of HSC transplantation. It is a yeast infection that is generally an overgrowth of the fungus *Candida albicans,* and it may be overlooked because of the range of clinical appearances. The classical description of candidiasis is white, curdlike flecks of material that can be wiped off, leaving a raw bleeding surface. This describes only the pseudomembranous form of the disease, more commonly known as thrush. Less frequently encountered forms of candidiasis include the chronic hyperplastic and erythematous atrophic forms. Immunosuppression, particularly if increased by the concomitant use of corticosteroids or the elimination of competing bacteria by broad-spectrum antibiotics, is the cause of the overgrowth.

The diagnosis can be confirmed by examining a potassium hydroxide preparation of a scraping of the lesion. The dimorphic organism will be seen with ovoid yeast mixed with the hyphal form. These studies can be confirmed by culture.

Although topical antifungal treatment may clear superficial oropharyngeal infections, topical agents are not well absorbed and are ineffective against more deeply invasive fungal infections, which typically involve the esophagus and lower gastrointestinal tract. For this reason, systemic agents are indicated for treating all except superficial fungal infections in the oral cavity.

Treatment of oral candidiasis consists of 7 to 10 days of topical antifungal therapy, such as nystatin or clotrimazole, or systemic drug therapy, such as fluconazole. Signs and symptoms should abate in 1 to 3 days. Recurrence is common in the HSC transplantation population, and therefore prophylactic measures are vital.

Prophylaxis against fungal superinfections includes the use of topical antifungal agents such as nystatin-containing mouthwashes and clotrimazole troches in addition to oral or intravenous fluconazole. Patients with candidiasis should be instructed to clean the oral cavity prior to taking antifungal medication. Irrigation and mechanical plaque removal may be necessary. Disinfection of both dentures and the mouth is necessary. Toothbrushes should be discarded and replaced with a new one after each use. Dentures should be removed while sleeping and soaked in sodium hypochlorite solution.

In some experimental trials, the use of bovine anti-candida immunoglobulin has shown some promise in reducing candida colonization in bone marrow recipients (Tollemar *et al.*, 1999).

In HSC transplant recipients, candidiasis has an increased propensity to spread to the esophagus and supraglottis. It is also more likely to cause sepsis, carrying a significant mortality rate (DiNardo & Hendrix, 1991).

Herpetic gingivostomatitis (also see Chapters 74 and 80)

Herpetic oral lesions are common in HSC transplant recipients unless antiviral prophylaxis is utilized. The herpes simplex virus is responsible for the primary infection and its reactivation in the oral cavity. While either type 1 or type 2 herpes simplex virus may cause a primary infection, type 1 is frequently more common for oral lesions.

The disease course is variable, ranging from a few mild painful ulcers to fever, malaise, sore throat, cervical lymphadenopathy, and multiple ulcerations covering the whole of the oral cavity and orophaynx. Vesicles appear 1 or 2 days after the commencement of symptoms, and persist for another 1 or 2 days. Usually the surrounding gingiva becomes inflamed as well.

Often the otolaryngologist does not have the chance to see the patient during the vesicular phase. When examined, there are numerous 2 to 4 mm ulcers. The base is tan-yellow with an erythematous halo (Fig. 99.1). At this stage the oral lesions are identical to those seen with recurrent aphthous ulcers or ulcers associated with neutropenia. A diagnosis of herpes simplex can be confirmed by exfoliative cytology, viral culture, and

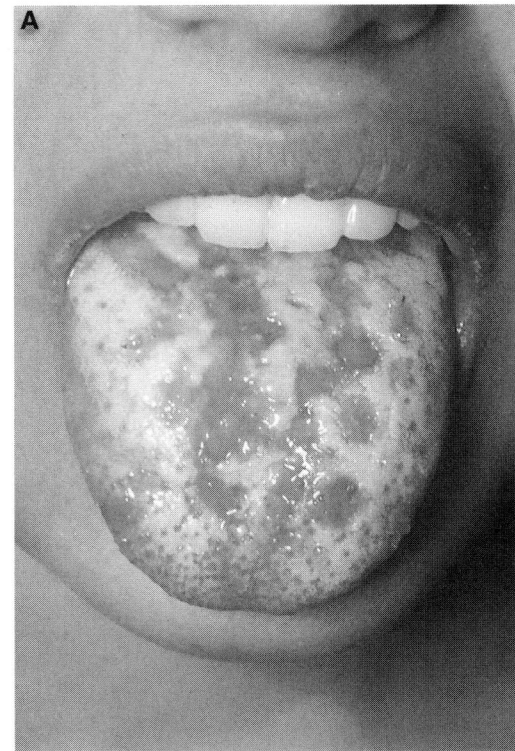

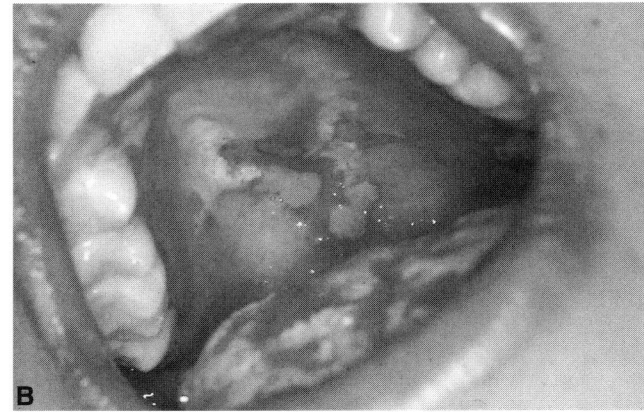

Fig. 99.1. **(A)** Oral herpetic gingivostomatitis in a 19-year-old female bone marrow transplant recipient. Multiple aphthous ulcerations are present on the dorsum of the tongue. **(B)** Similar herpetiform aphthous ulceration is present on the hard palate. Herpes simplex virus was identified on immunofluorescence of the lesions. For full color reproduction, see Color Plate 99.1.

immunofluorescence for the herpes antigen. The clinical course usually lasts 1 to 2 weeks.

Treatment is supportive with intravenous fluid for rehydration, adequate topical and oral analgesia, and intravenous acyclovir for 2 to 3 days, then oral acyclovir for 1 week. Because of the frequency of reactivation of infection in the HSC transplant population, antiviral prophylaxis, usually with acyclovir, is strongly recommended.

Epiglottitis

Epiglottitis in the HSC transplant recipient is a rare complication. Both bacterial and fungal epiglottitis require early recognition so that aggressive antimicrobial chemotherapy can be instituted. Bacterial and fungal epiglottitis have distinct clinical presentations.

Bacterial epiglottitis is more common than its fungal counterpart, and is most often caused by *Haemophilus influenzae*. This fulminant infection presents with rapid airway compromise, typically within hours. The patient is toxic, pale, drooling, and has the stigmata of impending airway obstruction. These patients require examination of the larynx by flexible nasendoscopy or indirect laryngoscopy, emergency airway management, and administration of an appropriate intravenous antibiotic such as a third-generation cephalosporin. The concurrent use of intravenous steroids is more controversial. A high dependency setting is warranted even if intubation is not required.

Fungal epiglottitis has a less fulminant presentation. Colman (1986) reviewed three patients who presented with epiglottitis secondary to *Candida albicans*. These patients had remarkably similar presentations: all had profound bone marrow suppression, with absolute white blood cell counts ranging from 0.08 to 0.5 × 10^9/l. Otolaryngologic consultation was obtained because of the presenting symptoms of severe odynophagia and neck pain, on occasions refractory to narcotic analgesics. The epiglottis and supraglottis were noted to be significantly erythematous and edematous. Concurrent fungal involvement of the upper aerodigestive tract was found in all three patients. No patients experienced airway obstruction. Management consisted of early topical and systemic antifungal chemotherapy, and daily re-examination of the larynx.

Recovery directly depends on immune function. In patients who recover a degree of immune competence, resolution is rapid. In those in whom immune function does not recover, fungal epiglottitis often heralds fatal disseminated fungemia (Cochran & Fee, 1979; Lawson *et al.*, 1980; Colman, 1986).

Nasal and paranasal disorders

Infections of the external nose

Infections of the skin of the external nose occur in the immunosuppressed population in more florid forms. Relatively minor infections of the skin of the external nose and vestibule spread more rapidly and extensively. Early topical and intravenous treatment is therefore more urgent than it is in the immunocompetent host.

Nasal vestibulitis is a chronic staphylococcal infection of the skin and hair follicles of the nasal vestibule. Vestibulitis frequently results from local trauma to the skin of the nasal vestibule from repeated nose picking or nasogastric tubes. Crusting occurs at the base of the vibrissae and the adjacent skin of the nostril is often inflamed (cellulitis). The nasal

vestibule of the HSC transplant recipient is more likely to be colonized by more resistant hospital-acquired pathogens.

In HIV-infected patients *Staphylococcus aureus* is the most common pathogen and has a significant propensity to cause serious infections such as endocarditis and pneumonia (Nguyen *et al.*, 1999).

Topical antibiotic ointment and systemic antibiotics are warranted. The patient is advised to avoid further nasal trauma and to wash his or her hands regularly with chlorhexidine-based hand wash.

Furuncles are tiny abscess cavities that may develop on the skin of either the external nose or vestibule (Fig. 99.2). Single or multiple, these lesions are often very tender. In the immunosuppressed, multiple furuncles may result in folliculitis. As with all infections of the external nose, this condition must be treated aggressively to avoid the infection spreading via the ophthalmic veins to the cavernous sinus and producing cavernous sinus thrombosis.

Rhinitis

Patients undergoing conditioning with high-dose cyclophosphamide frequently report symptoms of nasal congestion that can be distressing and accompanied by significant frontal headache. Inhaled beclomethasone diproprionate has been used effectively to control these symptoms, given as two applications (100 mg) to each nostril twice daily for the duration of cyclophosphamide administration.

Sinusitis

Sinusitis complicates 8% to 21% of those patients undergoing myelosuppressive chemotherapy and bone marrow transplantation (DiNardo & Hendrix, 1991; Shibuya *et al.*, 1995; Thompson *et al.*, 2002). It accounts for 10% of otolaryngologic infections. The most common sites are the maxillary and ethmoid sinuses (Savage *et al.*, 1997) (Table 99.1). In the latter study, the risk of sinusitis increased with increasing doses of TBI. The presence of graft-versus-host disease has also been described as a predisposing factor (Thompson *et al.*, 2002). Sinusitis is very uncommon in recipients of autografts.

In the immunocompromised HSC transplant recipient, sinusitis is more complex for a number of reasons. First, the muted immune capacity means that the clinical presentation may be subtle or unimpressive. Second, the response to topical treatment and antibiotic therapy is less brisk, due to a combination of factors including poor immune response, hospital-acquired pathogens, and poor ciliary function of the nasal mucosa (Cordonnier *et al.*, 1996). Third, more fulminant forms of sinusitis tend to occur when the patient is leukopenic. This is associated with significantly higher morbidity and is a potentially fatal disease with a mortality rate ranging from 50% to 100% (Yee *et al.*, 1994).

The neutropenic patient may not have the typical clinical presentation of sinusitis as seen in the immunocompetent host.

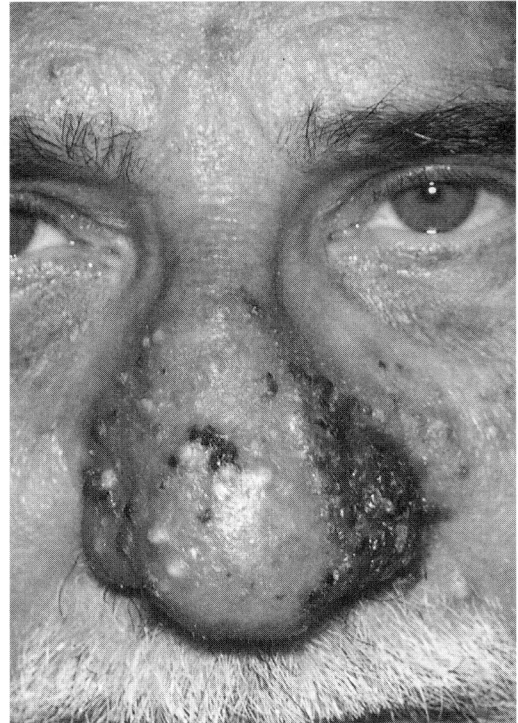

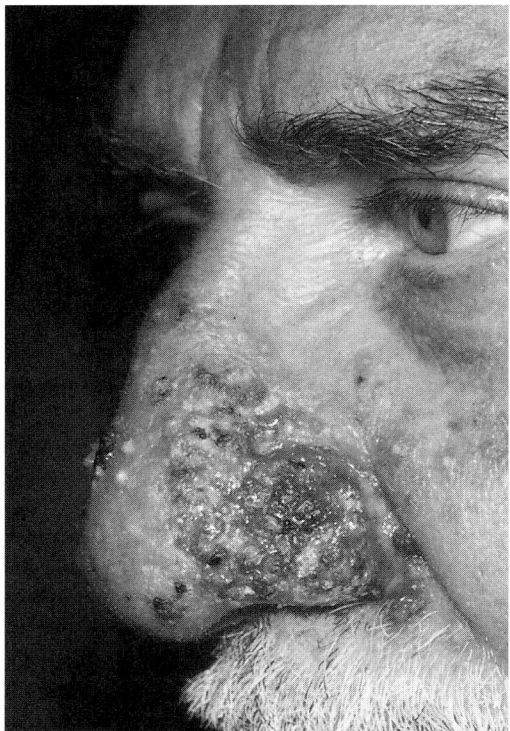

Fig. 99.2. (**A**) Frontal view of a 43-year-old male bone marrow transplant recipient with furunculosis of the external nose and the malar region. (**B**) Side view of the same patient. *Staphylococcus aureus* was isolated on microbiological culture.

Table 91.1. *Characteristics of 44 patients with sinusitis following allogeneic BMT*

Patient characteristics	Number	%
Diagnoses at BMT		
CML chronic phase	32	72.7
CML advanced phase	9	20.4
Acute leukemia	2	4.5
Multiple myeloma	1	2.3
Donors		
Unrelated	27	56.9
Sibling	17	38.6
Other family members[a]	2	4.5
Symptoms[b]		
Nasal congestion	35	79.5
Cough	27	61.4
Fever	19	43.2
Headache	8	18.2
Radiologic findings		
Fluid levels	38	86.4
Opacification	4	9.1
Mucosal thickening[c]	2	4.5
Sinus involvement		
Maxillary	44	100.0
Ethmoid	7	15.9
Frontal	6	13.6
Sphenoid	2	4.5
Leukocyte counts ($\times 10^9$)/l)		
Total WBC <4	27	62.8
Total WBC <1	7	16.3
Neutrophils <0.5	8	18.6
Monocytes <0.5	30	69.8
Lymphocytes <0.5	25	58.1
Low serum Ig levels		
Total Ig <6.7 g/l	14	40.6
IgG <5 g/l	8	25.0
IgA < 1.3 g/l	26	78.8
IgM <0.5 g/l	16	48.5
Acute GVHD		
Grades I–II	26	66.7
Grades III–IV	10	25.6
None	3	7.7
Chronic sinusitis	31	72.1

[a] Included a father in one procedure and first cousin in a second.
[b] Other symptoms included profuse rhinorrhea (7, 15.9%), postnasal drip (3, 6.8%), epistaxis (3, 6.8%), and ear congestion (3, 6.8%).
[c] Maxillary sinuses in both cases.
Reproduced, with permission, from Savage *et al.* (1997).

Symptoms that are seen in the immunocompetent patient include rhinnorhea, postnasal drip, nasal obstruction, epistaxis, and anosmia. The physical findings may include anatomic abnormalities such as a deviated septum, enlarged turbinate, tenderness of the sinuses, and mucopurulent drainage. The neutropenic patient may not have any of these symptoms or signs due to a decrease in the immune response and fever may be the only sign. The paucity of symptoms and signs means that sinusitis may be underdiagnosed and that the clinician needs to have a high index of suspicion.

Although the clinical and radiologic signs may be minimal, management needs to be aggressive. Fulminant fungal sinusitis often requires surgical debridement for control. Sinusitis due to *Aspergillus,* phycomycetes, or *Pseudomonas* may be fulminant and fatal.

In a review of 27 cases of sinusitis in the immunosuppressed host, Berlinger (1985) reported organisms that included *Staphylococcus, Haemophilus influenzae, Corynebacterium,* atypical mycobacterium, *Aspergillus,* phycomycetes, *Fusarium,* and cytomegalovirus; one patient had mucormycosis and five had fulminant aspergillosis. In addition another patient had necrotizing *Pseudomonas* sinusitis, which behaved clinically like malignant otitis externa, but, unlike fulminant fungal sinusitis, there was no soft tissue component. In another series the most common agents were Gram-negative bacteria (56.7%), Gram-positive bacteria (26.7%), and fungi (16.6%) (Imamura *et al.,* 1999).

Sinusitis in those undergoing HSC transplantation tends to occur during periods of severe leukopenia, the period of bone marrow ablation prior to transplantation, or during the first few weeks after the transplant. A review of pretransplant sinus computed tomography (CT) scans in children found that 48% had no evidence of sinus disease, 26% had mild disease, 9% had moderate disease and 17% had severe disease: Two-thirds of those with severe disease pretransplant developed clinical sinusitis posttransplant, compared to 21% of those with mild disease (Billings *et al.,* 2000).

The clinical presentation of bacterial sinusitis and early fuminant fungal sinusitis is usually fever without an obvious source. Early characteristic clinical features are often present, but are subtle and can easily be overlooked. They include rhinnorhea, malar or frontal fullness, and facial or periorbital swelling. In the transplant patient, the pathologic processes of edema, hyperemia, inflammation, pus formation, and abscess formation are all muted due to the leukopenic state. Even in the later stages of fulminant sinusitis characterized by fever and tissue infarction and necrosis within the nose, on the palate, or on the face, this condition is not painful. The telltale necrosis of the sinonasal tract may well be hidden without adequate rhinoscopic examination. For these reasons, physical examination is the most important diagnostic procedure. Examination of the patient by an otorhinolaryngologist includes anterior rhinoscopy and examination with either rigid or flexible nasendoscopy.

On examination of the nasal cavity, the rhinnorhea is rarely frankly turbid as seen in the immunocompetent patient. It is often not blood-stained. Meticulous examination of the mucosa is mandatory, and can only be achieved with nasendoscopy. The earliest sign of tissue infection is a pale-gray mucosa. This indicates fungal invasion of the underlying vasculature. The more classical sign is black mucosa of the inferior or middle turbinate. These lesions are insensate when touched with an instrument, indicating incipient mucosal necrosis. This tissue is friable and often there may be no bleeding from this devitalized tissue, even in the thrombocytopenic patient. An attempt should be made to determine if there is exposed underlying perichondrium of the nasal septum or periosteum of the nasal vault. Specimens should be taken and processed for microbiological culture and light microscopy.

If the nasal mucosal ulcer is painful, cultures are taken for viruses, bacteria, and fungi, and light microscopy of a potassium hydroxide preparation is performed. Nasal ulcers that are painful are usually due to herpes simplex virus, and are usually associated with oral lesions.

If the ulcers are insensitive, do not bleed when brushed or scraped, or are frankly necrotic, this is more suspicious of fulminant fungal sinusitis and an immediate biopsy is indicated. A routine hematoxylin and eosin stain will demonstrate fungal hyphae invading mucosa. The pathologic diagnosis of fulminant fungal sinusitis requires the demonstration of tissue invasion (not only a positive culture result). Gomori[1] methenamine silver stain allows the histopathologist to better visualize the hyphae and determine their configuration. Nonseptate hyphae represents mucormycosis, whereas septate hyphae are more typical of *Aspergillus.*

Advanced fungal rhinosinusitis is fulminant with a frightening rate of tissue loss by progressive necrosis. Often beginning on the lateral nasal wall, floor, and nasal septum, the black necrotic stigmata of this disease may rapidly spread to the mucosa of the palate, especially the upper alveolus, and then involve the maxillary, ethmoid, frontal, and sphenoid sinuses. The thin bony septa of the lamina papyracea provide poor resistance to invasion of the orbital cavity, and within days this may lead to intracranial spread (Fig. 99.3).

Imaging of HSC transplant patients with suspected sinusitis is insensitive for the earliest manifestations of this mucosal condition. By the time there is opacification on the plain sinus film or soft tissue and bony destruction on paranasal CT scans, the clinical diagnosis of fulminant fungal sinusitis should be obvious on inspection by nasendoscopy.

Plain sinus films may be misleading. The pathologic processes responsible for the classical radiologic stigmata of sinusitis (mucosal thickening, air-fluid levels, or opacification of the paranasal sinuses) are minimized in these immunosuppressed patients. Any of these findings on a plain sinus film in the context of mucormycosis or invasive fungal sinusitis indicates advanced disease (Berlinger, 1985).

Paranasal CT scans with axial and coronal cuts and administration of intravenous contrast medium are more sensitive than plain X-rays in the diagnosis of sinusitis. The scan is used to determine the extent of disease, including orbital and intracranial involvement.

Treatment of fulminant fungal sinusitis involves surgical debridement, irrigation of the sinus cavity, and systemic antifungal therapy with amphotericin B, currently the drug of choice for most systemic mycoses. More recently, new preparations of amphotericin B have been evaluated. These include liposomal amphotericin B and amphotericin B colloidal dispersion (see Chapter 75). Measures to enhance neutrophil recovery (hematopoietic growth factors with or without granulocyte transfusions) should be utilized if the patient is neutropenic.

---

[1] George Gomori, Hungarian/U.S. histochemist, 1906–1957.

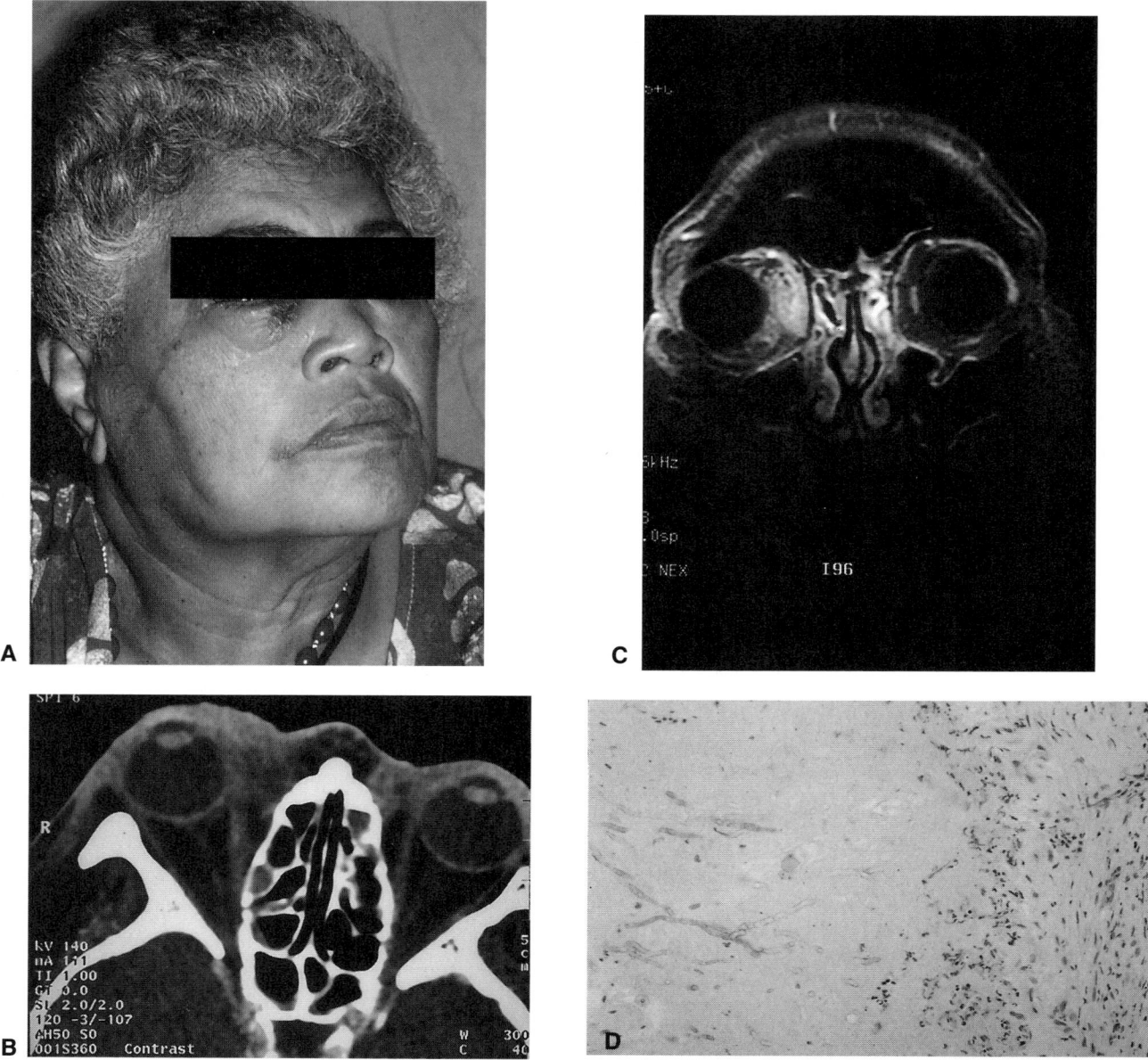

Fig. 99.3. **(A)** A 50-year-old female, immunocompromised after bone marrow transplantation, with acute fulminant fungal sinusitis. She presented with rapidly progressive right periorbital swelling and cutaneous necrosis at the medial canthus. **(B)** An axial CT of the orbit and the ethmoidal sinuses. Soft tissue swelling of the medial orbit is displacing the globe anterolaterally. The ethmoidal air cells demonstrate only minimal mucosal thickening. **(C)** On MRI, a coronal T1-weighted image demonstrates a homogeneous intraorbital mass and inflamed lining of the ethmoid sinuses. **(D)** Photomicrograph of a nasal biopsy, stained with hematoxylin and eosin. Biopsies of necrotic lateral nasal wall demonstrated invasive *Aspergillus*. The *Aspergillus* hyphae are identifiable on the left side of the photomicrograph.

However, medical treatment alone is seldom successful (Malani & Kauffman, 2000).

Surgical debridement is tailored to the location and extent of the disease. Nasal septum and the lateral nasal wall may need to be debrided, either through an intranasal or external approach. Frontal and ethmoidal sinus disease warrants an external frontoethmoidectomy and sphenoidotomy. Soft tissue involvement of the nose and upper lip is not unusual and to achieve adequate debridement, mutilating surgery is often required. Orbital aspergillosis in a bone marrow transplant patient has been successfully treated with surgical excision (without visual compromise), local amphotericin irrigation with an indwelling catheter, and systemic amphotericin B (Harris & Will, 1989).

Insertion of irrigation catheters following the debridement component of the surgical procedure offers a number of advantages in the postoperative management of these patients.

Regular irrigation prevents clot and crust formation and allows the direct instillation of amphotericin (Berlinger, 1985; Harris & Will, 1989).

In addition to the usual risks associated with sinus surgery, the pancytopenic patient has a very high risk of bleeding (Malani & Kauffman, 2000).

Despite adequate surgical debridement and intravenous and topical amphotericin B, fulminant fungal sinusitis may continue to progress if the patient's neutropenia does not recover. Cardinal to cessation of the progression of the necrosis is a white cell count above $1 \times 10^9/l$ (Berlinger, 1985). Granulocyte transfusion or administration of hematopoietic growth factors remains as important in the treatment of this disease as the surgery and antimicrobial agents (Gercovich et al., 1975; Winston et al., 1979; Sinclair et al., 1978).

Given the extreme difficulty faced in treating this disease, prevention is strongly preferred. Preventive measures include decreasing exposure to pathogenic fungi most likely to cause sinusitis—high efficiency filtration air-conditioning, avoiding potted plants and flowers in hospital units, avoiding ground pepper as a seasoning, and avoiding building construction in or near transplant units. Secondly, prophylactic antifungal agents may be used to diminish the invasion rates by fungal pathogens in selected patients.

Early diagnosis and treatment of sinus infections prior to an anticipated neutropenic event may reduce the risk of invasive rhinosinusitis (Mirza & Lamza, 2000).

Epistaxis

Up to 14% of patients undergoing HSC transplantation experience epistaxis necessitating treatment by an otorhinolaryngologist (DiNardo & Hendrix, 1991). Freireich (1966) found that gross hemorrhage in immunocompromised patients is infrequently observed with platelet counts above $20 \times 10^9/l$.

Most epistaxis responds to bedrest, nasal ointment to prevent crusting, and platelet transfusion. The threshold for application of an anterior nasal pack in an immunosuppressed patient is higher than that for an immunocompetent patient. However, a nasal pack may be necessary in refractory epistaxis associated with severe thrombocytopenia, coagulopathy, or vasculitis. Nasal packs have the potential to damage the nasal mucosa and obstruct the drainage and ventilation of the paranasal sinuses via their ostia in the lateral nasal wall. Should a nasal pack be warranted to achieve control of an epistaxis, the lubricated nasal pack should be inserted and removed as atraumatically as possible. Prophylactic antibiotic cover is recommended for as long as the nasal pack remains in place.

Ear disorders

Otitis externa and otitis media

Otitis externa is also a common manifestation in this population, and, as in the non-immunocompromised patient, is usually caused by *Pseudomonas aeruginosa*. Treatment involves meticulous aural toilet, bacteriological assessment, topical and systemic therapy, and vigilance with respect to the development of osteomyelitis of the temporal bone.

Immunocompromised patients have increased rates of otitis media and greater risk of serious complications such as septicemia and recalcitrant infection (Shapiro & Novelli, 1998). Prophylactic antibiotics and early aggressive therapy is recommended. Otherwise treatment is similar to that for the non-immunocompromised person.

Surgery in the immunocompromised patient raises concerns with respect to wound healing and infection. This has been examined prospectively in a small group of HIV-positive patients who underwent tympanomastoid surgery for chronic suppurative otitis media, where a mortality rate of 14% and serious postoperative infection rate of 21% was recorded (Kohan & Giacchi, 1999).

Hearing loss and ototoxicity

HSC transplant recipients are at risk of conductive or sensorineural hearing loss. Immunocompromised patients are more prone to developing external and middle ear infections with or without effusions, all of which contribute to a conductive hearing loss. Sensorineural hearing loss may arise from inner ear or retrocochlear infections such as herpes zoster, but more often arises from ototoxicity secondary to chemotherapy or antibiotic therapy.

In the stem cell transplant population, two of the more commonly used and culpable agents that cause sensorineural hearing loss are the platinum drugs: cisplatin and carboplatin.

Cisplatin results in a high-tone sensorineural hearing loss accompanied by tinnitus. These symptoms may be accompanied by vestibular symptoms in the acute setting. Although the tinnitus is usually temporary, the sensorineural hearing loss is permanent. The incidence of cisplatin ototoxicity varies widely, from 11% to 100% (Schweitzer, 1993).

Cisplatin ototoxicity results in injury to the hair cells of the Organ of Corti[2] (Stadnicki et al., 1975) as well as to the stria vascularis (Kohn et al., 1988).

Freilich and colleagues (1996) reviewed a number of identifiable risk factors for cisplatin ototxicity. These include:

1. Prior or concomitant irradiation to the cranium (Granowetter et al., 1983; Sexauer et al., 1985)
2. Pre-existing hearing loss (Schweitzer, 1993)
3. Decreased renal function (Schweitzer, 1993)
4. The concurrent use of other ototoxics such as aminoglycoside antibiotics (Schweitzer, 1993)
5. Faster infusion rates and higher peak plasma concentrations (Reddel et al., 1982; Kopelman et al., 1988; Laurell & Jungnelius, 1990)
6. Very young age (Brock et al., 1991; Weatherley et al., 1991)
7. Older age (Helson et al., 1978)
8. Higher cumulative doses (Reddel et al., 1982; Brock et al., 1991; Weatherley et al., 1991)

---

[2] Alfonso Corti, Italian anatomist, 1822–1888.

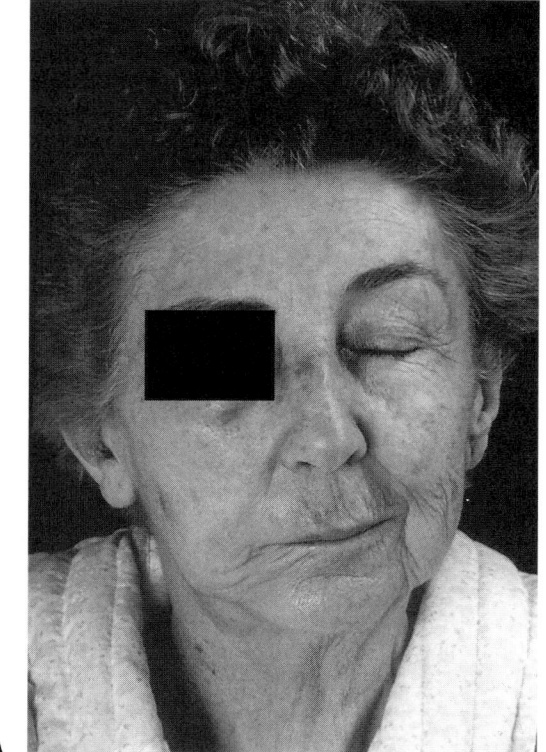

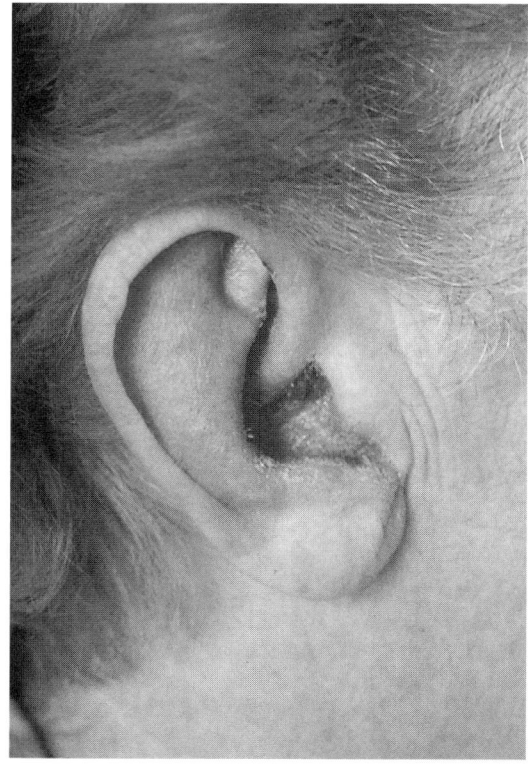

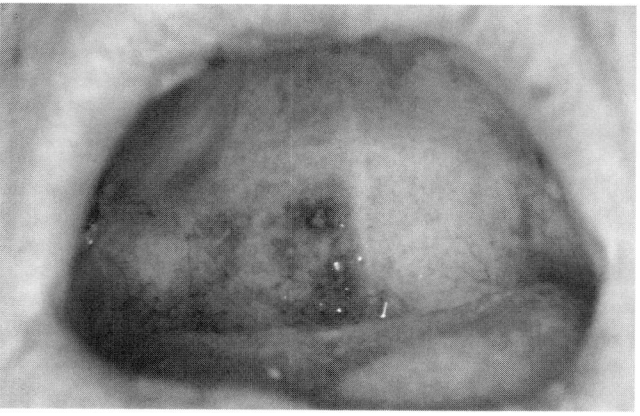

Fig. 99.4. **(A)** A 65-year-old female immunocompromised after bone marrow transplantation with herpes zoster oticus. She presented with a right lower facial nerve palsy. **(B)** Vesicles with crusting were noted in the conchal bowl of the right ear. **(C)** Right palatal vesicles were also noted. She was successfully treated with systemic acyclovir. For color reproduction, see Color Plate 99.4.

Carboplatin is less ototoxic than cisplatin. The incidence of carboplatin ototoxicity ranges from 0 to 19% (Canetta *et al.,* 1987; Gaynon *et al.,* 1990; Kennedy *et al.,* 1990). Ototoxicity may be more likely in those given carboplatin in higher doses, or those treated concomitantly with cisplatin. While animal experiments have demonstrated that carboplatin causes high-tone sensorineural loss, the integrity and function of the hair cells is better preserved (Saito *et al.,* 1989).

Herpes zoster oticus (Ramsay-Hunt Syndrome[3])

The appearance of a varicelliform rash, facial palsy/paralysis, and otalgia are the key features for the diagnosis of herpes zoster oticus (Fig. 99.4). Hunt's classification is as follows:

Class I: Sensory portion of cranial nerve VII with vesicular rash

[3] James Ramsay-Hunt, U.S. neurologist, 1869–1939.

Class II: Sensory and motor cranial nerve VII involved

Class III: Sensory and motor cranial nerve VII with auditory involvement

Class IV: Sensory and motor cranial nerve VII with both auditory and vestibular symptoms

Other cranial nerves involved, in order of occurrence, are IX, V, X, and VI (Carroll & Mastaglia, 1979; Proctor *et al.*, 1979). The varicella zoster virus belongs to the herpes family. It is a double-stranded DNA virus that causes both chickenpox (varicella) and zoster infections. Reactivation of virus stored in sensory ganglia from previous varicella infection results in clinical herpes zoster infection.

Multinucleated giant cells obtained from lesion scrapings and cytopathic effects seen on human diploid fibroblasts from vesicular fluid can verify the clinical diagnosis. These studies, however, require 5 days or more to produce results. Immunofluorescence of varicella antigen obtained from exfoliated cells from lesions can provide a more expedient verification of clinical suspicion.

The pathologic change seen in herpes zoster oticus is geniculate ganglionitis (Hunt, 1907). The temporal bones from a patient with motor involvement of the seventh cranial nerve showed varicella zoster virus infiltration of Schwann cells[4] inducing inflammatory changes in the fallopian canal and neural sheath disruption (Zajtchuk *et al.*, 1972).

The natural history of the disease includes eruption of vesicles occurring simultaneously with motor facial nerve dysfunction. Ten percent of patients with total facial nerve paralysis and 66% of those with partial paralysis recover completely. Recovery is better in those cases in which vesicles appear prior to nerve paralysis (Devriese & Moesker, 1988).

Evaluation includes audiometry and electrodiagnostic tests provide additional information in selected patients. CT to rule out intracranial neoplasia or other infective complications is now being replaced with magnetic resonance imaging, which can identify tumors in the internal auditory canal and cranial vault, and can localize the area of neural inflammation (LaBagnara *et al.*, 1989; Korzec *et al.*, 1991).

Nonspecific management directed at protection of the ipsilateral cornea includes prescribing artificial tears, nocturnal eye patching, and when needed, gold weight insertion in the eyelid or tarsorrhaphy. Oral corticosteroids are recommended at 80 mg of prednisone per day for an adult tapered over no less than 3, and no more than 6, weeks (Gelfand, 1954).

Acyclovir inhibits viral DNA replication. The dose is 10 to 15 mg/kg every 8 hours intravenously for 3 to 5 days, followed by oral dosages for a total of 7 to 10 days of therapy. Renal function should be monitored since the drug can crystallize in renal tubules.

Aspergillus of the temporal bone

External auditory canal *Aspergillus* infection in the immunocompetent host is usually a benign disease with organisms growing

[4] Theodor Schwann, German anatomist/physiologist, 1810–1882.

without invasion. However, in HSC transplant recipients, *Aspergillus* can spread to involve the tympanomastoid cavity with bone destruction (Mielke *et al.*, 1978; Schubert *et al.*, 1986). As with its sinonasal counterpart, pathogenicity depends on the demonstration of tissue invasion, not just a positive fungal culture. The treatment follows similar principles; debridement in the form of a mastoidectomy, and early aggressive antifungal therapy. Again, attention should be directed to accelerating neutrophil recovery in the neutropenic patient.

References

Armstrong, D., Young, L.S., Meyer, R.D., & Blevins, A.H. (1971). Infectious complications of neoplastic disease. *Medical Clinics of North America*, **55**, 729–45.

Barrett, A.P. (1984). Gingival lesions in leukemia: a classification. *Journal of Periodontology*, **55**, 585–8.

Beck, S. (1979). Impact of a systematic oral care protocol on stomatitis after chemotherapy. *Cancer Nursing*, **2**, 185–99.

Berlinger, N.T. (1985). Sinusitis in immunodeficient and immunosuppressed patients. *Laryngoscope*, **95**, 29–34.

Billings, K.R., Aquino, V.M., Biavati, M.J., & Lowe, L.H. (2000). Screening sinus CT scans in pediatric bone marrow transplant patients. *International Journal of Pediatric Otorhinolaryngology*, **52**, 253–60.

Brock, P.R., Bellman, S.C., Yeomans, E.C. *et al.* (1991). Cisplatin ototoxicity in children: a practical grading system. *Medical Pediatric Oncology*, **19**, 295–300.

Canetta, R., Franks, C., Smaldone, L. *et al.* (1987). Clinical status of carboplatin. *Oncology*, **1**, 61–70.

Carroll, S.M. & Mastaglia, F.L. (1979). Optic neuropathy and ophthalmoplegia in herpes zoster oticus. *Neurology*, **29**, 726–9.

Cochran, J. & Fee, W. (1979). Epiglottitis in an immunosuppressed host. *Western Journal of Medicine*, **131**, 150–2.

Colman, M.F. (1986). Epiglottitis in immunocompromised patients. *Head and Neck Surgery*, **8**, 466–8.

Cordonnier, C., Gilain, L., Ricolfi, F. *et al.* (1996). Acquired ciliary abnormalities of nasal mucosa in marrow recipients. *Bone Marrow Transplantation*, **17**, 611–16.

Daeffler, R. (1980). Oral hygiene measures for patients with cancer: I. *Cancer Nursing*, **3**, 347–56.

Devriese, P.P. & Moesker, W.H. (1988). The natural history of facial paralysis in herpes zoster. *Clinical Otolaryngology*, **13**, 289–98.

DiNardo, L.J. & Hendrix, R.A. (1991). The infectious and hematologic complications of myelosuppressive cancer chemotherapy. *Otolaryngology – Head and Neck Surgery*, **105**, 101–6.

Dreizen, S., Bodey, G.P., & Valdivieso, M. (1983). Chemotherapy-associated oral infections in adults with solid tumors. *Oral Surgery, Oral Medicine, and Oral Pathology*, **55**, 113–20.

Freilich, R.J., Kraus, D.H., Budnick, A.S. *et al.* (1996). Hearing loss in children with brain tumors treated with cisplatin and carboplatin-based high-dose chemotherapy with autologous bone marrow rescue. *Medical Pediatric Oncology*, **26**, 95–100.

Freireich, E.J. (1966). Effectiveness of platelet transfusion in leukemia and aplastic anemia. *Transfusion*, **6**, 50–4.

Gaynon, P.S., Ettinger, L.J., Baum, E.S. *et al.* (1990). Carboplatin in childhood brain tumors: a Children's Cancer Study Group phase II trial. *Cancer,* **66,** 2465–9.

Gelfand, M.L. (1954). Treatment of herpes zoster with cortisone. *Journal of the American Medical Association,* **154,** 911–12.

Gercovich, F.G., Richman, S.P., Rodriguez, V. *et al.* (1975). Successful control of systemic *Aspergillus* niger infections in two patients with acute leukemia. *Cancer,* **36,** 2271–6.

Granowetter, L., Rosenstock, J.G., & Packer, R.J. (1983). Enhanced cis-platinum neurotoxicity in pediatric patients with brain tumors. *Journal of Neuro-Oncology,* **1,** 293–7.

Harris, G.J. & Will, B.R. (1989). Orbital aspergillosis—conservative debridement and local amphotericin irrigation. *Ophthalmic Plastic and Reconstructive Surgery,* **5,** 207–11.

Helson, L., Okonkwo, E., Anton, L., & Cvitkovic, E. (1978). Cis-platinum ototoxicity. *Clinical Toxicology,* **13,** 469–78.

Hunt, J.R. (1907). Herpetic inflammations of the geniculate ganglion. A new syndrome and its complications. *Journal of Nervous and Mental Diseases,* **34,** 73–96.

Imamura, R., Voegels, R., Sperandio, F. *et al.* (1999). Microbiology of sinusitis in patients undergoing bone marrow transplantation. *Otolaryngology – Head and Neck Surgery,* **120,** 279–82.

Kennedy, I.C.S., Kitzharris, B.M., Collis, B.M., & Atkinson, C.H. (1990). Carboplatin is ototoxic. *Cancer Chemotherapeutic Pharmacology,* **26,** 232–4.

Kohan, D. & Giacchi, R.J. (1999). Otologic surgery in patients with HIV and AIDS. *Otolaryngology – Head and Neck Surgery,* **121,** 355–60.

Kohn, S., Fradis, M., Pratt, H. *et al.* (1988). Cisplatinum ototoxicity in the guinea pig with special reference to toxic effects in the stria vascularis. *Laryngoscope,* **98,** 865–71.

Kopelman, J., Budnick, A.S., Sessions, R.B. *et al.* (1988). Ototoxicity in high-dose cisplatin by bolus administration in patients with advanced cancer and normal hearing. *Laryngoscope,* **98,** 858–64.

Korzec, K., Sobol, S.M., Kubal, W. *et al.* (1991). Gadolinium-enhanced magnetic resonance imaging of the facial nerve in herpes zoster oticus and Bell's palsy: clinical implications. *American Journal of Otology,* **12,** 163–8.

LaBagnara, J., Jahn, A.F., Habif, D.V., & Solomon, E.M. (1989). MRI findings in two cases of acute facial paralysis. *Otolaryngology – Head and Neck Surgery,* **101,** 562–5.

Laurell, G. & Jungnelius, U. (1990). High-dose cisplatin treatment: hearing loss and plasma concentrations. *Laryngoscope,* **100,** 724–34.

Lawson, R., Bodey, G., & Lura, M. (1980). Candida infection presenting as laryngitis. *American Journal of Medical Science,* **280,** 173–6.

Levine, A.S., Graw, R.G., & Young, R.C. (1972). Management of infections in patients with leukemia and lymphoma: current concepts and experimental approaches. *Seminars in Haematology,* **9,** 141–79.

Lockhart, P.B. & Sonis, S.T. (1979). Relationship of oral complications to peripheral blood leukocyte and platelet counts in patients receiving cancer chemotherapy. *Oral Surgery, Oral Medicine, and Oral Pathology,* **48,** 21–8.

Malani, N.P. & Kauffman, C.A. (2000). Prevention and prophylaxis of invasive fungal rhinosinusitis in the immunocompromised patient. *Otolaryngologic Clinics of North America,* **33,** 301–11.

Mielke, B., Weir, B., Oldring, D., & von Westarp, C. (1978). Fungal aneurysm: case report and review of the literature. *Neurosurgery,* **9,** 578–82.

Mirza, N. & Lamza, D.C. (2000). Diagnosis and management of rhinosinusitis before scheduled immunosuppression. *Otolaryngological Clinics of North America,* **33,** 313–21.

Nguyen, M.H., Kauffman, C., Goodman, R. *et al.* (1999). Nasal carriage and infection with *Staphylococcus aureus* in HIV infected patients. *Annals of Internal Medicine,* **30,** 221–5.

Ostchega, Y. (1980). Preventing and treating cancer chemotherapy's oral complications. *Nursing,* **10,** 47–52.

Proctor, L., Lindsay, J., Perlman, H., & Matz, G. (1979). Acute vestibular paralysis in herpes zoster oticus. *Annals of Otology,* **88,** 303–9.

Reddel, R.R., Kefford, R.F., Grant, J.M. *et al.* (1982). Ototoxicity in patients receiving cisplatin: importance of dose and method of drug administration. *Cancer Treatment Reports,* **66,** 19–23.

Saito, T., Saito, H., Saito, K. *et al.* (1989). Ototoxicity of carboplatin in guinea pigs. *Auris, Nasus, Larynx,* **16,** 13–21.

Savage, D.G., Taylor, P., Blackwell, J. *et al.* (1997). Paranasal sinusitis following allogeneic bone marrow transplant. *Bone Marrow Transplantation,* **19,** 55–9.

Schimpff, S.C., Young, M.V., Greene, W.H. *et al.* (1972). Origin of infection in acute nonlymphocytic leukemia. *Annals of Internal Medicine,* **77,** 707–14.

Schimpff, S.C. (1990). Oral complications of cancer therapies. Surveillance cultures. *Journal of the National Cancer Institute Monograph,* **9,** 37–42.

Schubert, M.M., Peterson, D.E., Meyers, J.D. *et al.* (1986). Head and neck aspergillosis in patients undergoing bone marrow transplantation. *Cancer,* **57,** 1092–6.

Schweitzer, V.G. (1993). Ototoxicity of chemotherapeutic agents. *Otolaryngologic Clinics of North America,* **27,** 759–89.

Sexauer, C.L., Khan, A., Burger, P.C. *et al.* (1985). Cisplatin in pediatric patients with recurrent brain tumors. *Cancer,* **56,** 1497–501.

Shapiro, N.L. & Novelli, V. (1998). Otitis media in children with vertically-acquired HIV infection: the Great Ormond Street Hospital experience. *International Journal of Pediatric Otorhinolaryngology,* **45,** 69–75.

Shibuya, T.Y., Momin, F., Abella, E. *et al.* (1995). Sinus disease in the bone marrow transplant population: incidence, risk factors, and complications. *Otolaryngology – Head and Neck Surgery,* **113,** 705–11.

Sinclair, A.J., Rossof, A.H., & Coltman, C.A. (1978). Recognition and successful management in pulmonary aspergillosis in leukemia. *Cancer,* **42,** 2019–24.

Stadnicki, S.W., Fleischman, R.W., Schaeppi, U., & Merriam, P. (1975). Cisdichlorodiammineplatinum (II): Hearing loss and other toxic effects in rhesus monkeys. *Cancer Chemotherapy Reports,* **59,** 467–80.

Talcott, J.A., Finberg, R., Mayer, R.J., & Goldman, L. (1988). The medical course of cancer patients with fever and neutropenia. *Archives of Internal Medicine,* **148,** 2561–8.

Thompson, A.M., Crouch, M., Zahurak, M.L. *et al.* (2002). Risk factors for post-stem cell transplant sinusitis. *Bone Marrow Transplantation,* **29,** 257–61.

Tollemar, J., Gross, N., Dolgiras, N. *et al.* (1999). Fungal prophylaxis by reduction of fungal colonization by oral administration of bovine anti-candida antibodies in bone marrow transplant recipients. *Bone Marrow Transplantation,* **23,** 283–90.

Weatherley, R.A., Owens, J.J., Catlin, F.I., & Mahoney, D.H. (1991). Cis-platinum ototoxicity in children. *Laryngoscope,* **101,** 917–24.

Winston, D.J., Gale, R.P., Meyer, D.V., & Young, L.S. (1979). Infectious complications of bone marrow transplantation. *Medicine,* **58,** 1–31.

Yee, S., Stern, S.J., Hearnsberger, H.G., & Suen, J.Y. (1994). Sinusitis in bone marrow transplantation. *Southern Medical Journal,* **87,** 522–4.

Zajtchuk, J.T., Matz, G.J., & Lindsay, J.R. (1972). Temporal bone pathology in herpes oticus. *Annals of Otology,* **81,** 331–8.

Ziga, S. (1983). Stomatitis/mucositis. In *Guidelines for Cancer Care: Symptom Management,* ed. J. Yasko, pp. 212–223. Reston, VA: Reston Publishing Company, Inc.

100 Vascular complications

DAVID REES AND MICHAEL A. McGRATH

St Vincent's Hospital and University of New South Wales, Sydney, Australia

Introduction

Vascular complications, particularly those related to central venous access catheters, are a frequent cause of morbidity in hematopoietic stem cell (HSC) transplant recipients. In general these complications are underdiagnosed, and their investigation and management has often assumed a subsidiary role to other major complications of transplantation.

Procoagulant abnormalities in HSC transplant recipients

Pre-existing thrombotic complications

The relationship between hypercoagulability and malignancy has been recognized for more than 125 years. A markedly increased incidence of venous thrombosis and thromboembolic disease in these patients has been repeatedly emphasized since Trousseau's observations in the nineteenth century.[1] The mechanism involves complex molecular effects of certain cancers on the coagulation and fibrinolytic pathways, in addition to the stasis-promoting effects of immobility or venous obstruction by tumor. Tumor cells and their products have also been shown to interact with platelets, monocytes, and other leukocytes, and with the endothelium (Silverstein & Nachman, 1992). Patients with pre-existing thrombotic disorders can also benefit from bone marrow transplantation, as described in the resolution of Budd–Chiari syndrome secondary to paroxysmal nocturnal hemoglobinuria (Graham *et al.*, 1996).

Coagulation abnormalities

Due to thrombocytopenia and/or hepatic disease, marrow transplant recipients are commonly predisposed to a hemorrhagic diathesis. In contrast, however, hemostatic abnormalities have been described in the blood of marrow transplant recipients that potentially constitute a hypercoagulable state (Lokich & Becker, 1983; Harper *et al.*, 1990; Kaufman *et al.*,

1990; Conlan *et al.*, 1991a, 1991b; Sletnes *et al.*, 1996) (Table 100.1).

Studies in patients with malignant lymphoma have demonstrated that a hypercoagulable state can develop during bone marrow harvesting; therefore, insertion of a central intravenous catheter should ideally be avoided immediately after marrow harvesting in order to prevent thrombotic complications at that time (Sletnes *et al.*, 1996).

Significant reductions in the level of the naturally occurring anticoagulant factors protein C, protein S, and antithrombin III have been described following marrow transplantation (Harper *et al.*, 1990; Gordon *et al.*, 1993; Grigg *et al.*, 1996). However, there does not appear to be any predictive relationship between the posttransplant levels and the patient's underlying disease, type of conditioning regimen, age, or sex (Harper *et al.*, 1990).

Table 100.1. *Hypercoagulable abnormalities in HSC transplantation*

Hematologic	Reduced endogenous anticoagulants	Protein C Protein S Antithrombin III Heparin cofactor II
	Raised acute-phase reactants	e.g., Plasma fibrinogen
	Disease-related	Leukostasis Paraprotein Disseminated intravascular coagulation
	Iatrogenic	Cyclosporine
Vessel wall damage	Trauma related to vascular access catheters	
	Irritant intravenous solutions	Potassium Phenytoin Vancomycin
	Distortion	Hematoma Lymphadenopathy Bulky soft tissue disease
Venous stasis	Immobilization	
	Hypoperfusion	Dehydration Septicemia

---

[1] Armand Trousseau, French physician, 1801–1867.

Other procoagulant abnormalities described in these patients include increased plasminogen activator inhibitor, anti-cardiolipin antibodies (Lokich & Becker, 1983; Conlan et al., 1991a, 1991b), reduced factor XII levels, and raised levels of acute phase reactants, notably plasma fibrinogen. In a retrospective analysis of 1,292 patients undergoing HSC transplantation at the University of Minnesota over a 10-year period, Greeno and colleagues (1995) detected newly recognized lupus inhibitors in 3% of the patients. These inhibitors were usually detected in the first 1 to 2 months posttransplant, more frequently in children, particularly those transplanted for Hurler syndrome. Thrombotic complications were rare. Increases in blood viscosity may occur in association with these acute phase changes or as a result of the underlying disease process when accompanied by extreme leukocytosis or macromolecular abnormalities such as the presence of a paraprotein.

Disseminated intravascular coagulation can occur as a complication of septicemia or as a complication peculiar to the underlying hematologic disease, for example, acute promyelocytic leukemia. Sepsis can predispose to thrombosis as a result of the hypoperfusion accompanying shock or by the microbial colonization of vascular catheters with resultant platelet activation and fibrin deposition.

As indicated above, the hypercoagulable state predisposed to by these hematologic changes is offset to a large extent by a reduction in the level of procoagulant blood factors in most patients. Of particular importance is the posttransplant thrombocytopenia that occurs in all patients. A significant reduction in the level of vitamin K dependent clotting factors has also been described (Rio et al., 1986).

Changes in the levels of naturally occurring anticoagulant, especially during acute graft-versus-host disease (GVHD), might reflect activation of, and/or damage to, endothelial cells during GVHD (Leblond et al., 1993).

Endothelium and vessel wall injury

Vessel wall abnormalities are usually the result of trauma accompanying the insertion of catheters or the infusion of chemotherapeutic agents that have direct toxic effects on the endothelium due to the high concentrations present in the region of the infusion. Damage to the vascular endothelium might occur under a number of circumstances related to HSC transplantation. For example, widespread endothelial cell injury might be the pivotal predisposition to intravascular platelet aggregation and the thrombotic microangiopathy that has been associated with the use of cyclosporine, mitomycin C, combinations of other chemotherapeutic and immunosuppressive agents, and total body irradiation (Moake & Byrnes, 1996). Richard and colleagues (1996) found lymphovascular endothelium damaged prior to conditioning and this damage was enhanced posttransplant. They measured the plasma endothelial cell markers von Willebrand[2] factor, soluble thrombomodulin, and soluble

[2] Erik von Willebrand, Finnish physician, 1870–1939.

ICAM-1. In contrast, however, Catani and colleagues (1996) found elevated thrombomodulin to be very rare posttransplant and indeed was only elevated in one patient who developed severe hepatic veno-occlusive disease. Widespread endothelial injury can also occur in septicemia, thereby predisposing to the syndrome of disseminated intravascular coagulopathy. There is also evidence that endothelial cell damage is an important step in the pathogenesis of GVHD (Leblond et al., 1993).

A large hematoma, lymphadenopathy, or bulky soft tissue disease can cause compression of major veins such as the vena cava, subclavian, jugular, iliac, or other major limb veins. In these situations it can be difficult to distinguish between extrinsic compression of a vein and the periphlebitic process that accompanies venous thrombosis. However, ultrasound imaging that includes both B-mode scanning and Doppler (i.e., Duplex study) can provide a reliable diagnosis.

Catheter and infusion-related complications

The mechanisms involved in catheter-associated thrombosis can include one or more of the following: trauma to the vessel wall at the site of the venipuncture; trauma to the endothelium by the catheter; perivascular hematoma formation; the foreign body thrombogenic properties of the catheter itself; chemical irritation of the endothelium and vessel wall by the infusate; and immobilization of the limb, and indeed of the whole patient, during an infusion. Catheter-related complications are reviewed in Peterson et al. (1986) and Sanders et al. (1982).

Pivotal to the successful management of central catheters in patients undergoing HSC transplantation is a skilled team approach that includes a clinician experienced in catheter placement, a clinical nurse specialist in intravenous management, and an alert and fastidious awareness of wound care (Keohane et al., 1983).

To minimize the risk of catheter-associated complications in bone marrow transplant recipients, the duration of use specified in Table 100.2 should not be exceeded.

Management of catheter-related thrombosis is controversial and as yet there are no established guidelines. Anticoagulation and thrombolytic therapy are relatively contraindicated in many HSC transplant patients who may already be endogenously anticoagulated as a result of thrombocytopenia and

Table 100.2. *Recommended duration of use of different i.v. cannulae/catheters*

Peripheral cannula	48 hours
Upper limb central line	
Lower limb central line	
Jugular central line	
Subclavian central line	Indefinite
Hickman/Broviac/Groshong line (jugular or subclavian)	
Hickman/Broviac/Groshong line (femoral)	

impairment of hepatic synthesis of coagulation factors. There are also concerns about anticoagulation of patients who could have septic foci in the brain or viscera. Finally, difficulty may be encountered in monitoring therapy using standard parameters of activated partial thromboplastin time (APTT) and international normalized ratio (INR) in patients with severe sepsis, disseminated intravascular coagulation, hepatic complications, or anti-cardiolipin antibodies.

The following investigations are recommended before commencing any anticoagulant or thrombolytic therapy in this patient population: platelet count, bleeding time, INR, APTT, liver function test, renal function, and plasma fibrinogen.

It is emphasized that hemorrhagic complications are much more likely to occur in patients who are severely anemic or septic, or during the pancytopenic phase posttransplant.

In discussing the management of catheter-related complications in these patients we will consider five specific situations: superficial thrombophlebitis, venous thrombosis and pulmonary embolism, catheter-related thrombosis of the upper extremity, catheter occlusion, and other mechanical complications of venous access catheters.

Superficial thrombophlebitis

Superficial thrombophlebitis commonly results from the infusion of irritant agents via peripheral cannulae. Commonly implicated agents in our experience have included antibiotics, especially flucloxacillin and vancomycin, antithymocyte globulin, the anticonvulsant phenytoin, and solutions with a high potassium concentration. (See Chapter 83 for a list of medications that should be given via a central venous line for this reason.) The clinical symptoms and signs of thrombophlebitis include severe pain and tenderness, erythema, swelling, and a bandlike induration along the course of the vein. Management (Table 100.3) includes immediate cessation of the infusion, removal of the cannula, and elevation of the limb. A local heparinoid cream and gentle support with an elastic compression bandage can relieve the pain and tenderness of superficial thrombophlebitis. Difficulty is often encountered in neutropenic subjects in distinguishing chemical phlebitis from infection at the cannula site, especially as fever can accompany both situations. A culture should always be taken from the

Table 100.3. *Management of superficial thrombophlebitis in HSC transplant recipients*

1. Cease infusion and remove cannula/catheter
2. Send catheter/cannula tip for microbial culture
3. Ultrasound scanning to determine proximal limit of thrombus
4. Heparinoid cream
5. Elastic compression bandage
6. Elevate limb
7. If considered infected as opposed to inflamed, broad-spectrum i.v. antibacterial antibiotics

insertion site and in all cases both the tip of the cannula or catheter as well as blood cultures should be sent for microbiological culture.

Venous thrombosis and pulmonary embolism

Catheter-related thrombosis is usually asymptomatic and is underdiagnosed in the transplant patient (Leiby et al., 1989; Conlan et al., 1991a, 1991b). With venographic surveys, thrombosis rates have ranged from 4% to 42% (Haire et al., 1990), while symptomatic thrombosis in the transplant group has been reported in only 0% to 1.3% of patients. Despite the relative frequency of this complication, it seldom results in long-term sequelae. Potential risk factors for the development of thrombosis include the presence of large compressing mediastinal masses, radiotherapy, multiple previous central venous insertions, patient manipulations of the catheter, improper home care, and small vessel size. The latter factor is an important consideration in the pediatric population (Thomas & Sinnet, 1988).

Thrombosis appears to be more common with catheters inserted in the femoral and internal jugular sites rather than the subclavian vein. There are no consistent data on thrombosis rates associated with double- versus single-lumen catheters (Moosa et al., 1991), although insertion of multiple catheters may be associated with an increased risk (Haire et al., 1991). No relationship has been proven between any particular catheter type and predisposition to thrombosis. In addition to thrombotic occlusion, fibrin sheathing of venous catheters can occur with concomitant venous obstruction.

Thrombocytopenia at the time of catheter insertion may protect against thrombosis, although many HSC transplant recipients will have normal platelet counts at the time of catheter insertion pretransplant. Nevertheless, activation of coagulation has been demonstrated in patients undergoing bone marrow harvesting and therefore catheter-related deep vein thrombosis may be more likely to occur shortly after harvesting (Sletnes et al., 1996).

There is general consensus that catheter-induced thrombosis is less common in transplant patients than in solid tumor patients not undergoing transplantation (Hickman et al., 1979), although this has not been proven in other studies (Haire et al., 1990).

Inability to aspirate blood from the catheter is not a definite indication of thrombosis, but may indicate abutment of the catheter against the vein wall. This is more likely to occur if the end of the catheter has been bevelled for ease of surgical insertion (Thomas & Sinnet, 1988). (We recommend that the tips of venous catheters not be bevelled prior to insertion, for this reason.) Difficulty with both the aspiration of blood and the infusion of fluids should be regarded with suspicion and investigated further (Cassidy et al., 1987).

Complications of catheter-related thrombosis include the superior vena cava syndrome and pulmonary thromboembolism, in addition to persistent arm swelling and discomfort.

The incidence of pulmonary embolism in relation to central access catheters is again likely underestimated in this particular group of patients (Rockoff, Gang, & Vacanti, 1984; Kronborg, 1989; Uderzo et al., 1993).

Pulmonary embolism with bony microfragments has also been described following bone marrow transplantation (Fernandez et al., 1996).

Catheter-related venous thrombosis of the upper extremity

Catheter-related subclavian vein thrombosis should be suspected in any patient who complains of pain or swelling in the supraclavicular fossa, ipsilateral arm, or axilla at rest or on exercise. Physical signs (Table 100.4) include warmth, swelling and discoloration of the limb, and tenderness in the supraclavicular fossa or apex of the axilla. There may be prominent venous collateral vessels over the anterior aspect of the shoulder or chest wall and the axillary vein may be palpated as a tender cord if it is thrombosed. Extension of thrombosis into the superior vena cava is suggested by nonpulsatile distension of the jugular veins and facial swelling with suffusion, periorbital edema, and conjunctival congestion.

Headache, drowsiness, focal neurologic signs, seizures, and loss of central retinal venous pulsation are signs of serious intracranial extension of the venous thrombosis.

Many patients remain asymptomatic and most others appear to have no long-term sequelae. Thus, removal of the catheter is not mandatory. Therapy can continue to be administered through the catheter. Catheter removal is indicated for total occlusion, associated infective phlebitis, superior vena cava syndrome, and for pulmonary embolism.

Systemic thrombolytic therapy may be used to treat catheter occlusions, superior vena cava obstruction, and pulmonary embolism, although there is a substantial risk of hemorrhage with this treatment (Lokich & Becker, 1983), especially in the thrombocytopenic patient.

Table 100.4. *Clinical features of major upper body venous thrombosis*

Subclavian/axillary vein thrombosis
  Pain in arm or axilla or supraclavicular fossa
  Warmth, swelling, discoloration of arm, supraclavicular fossa
  Tenderness in supraclavicular fossa/axilla
  Palpable axillary vein
  Venous collateral vessels over shoulder/chest wall
Internal jugular vein thrombosis
  Pain and tenderness deep to anterior border of sternomastoid muscle
Superior vena cava thrombosis
  Nonpulsatile distension of jugular vein
  Facial swelling
  Conjunctival congestion
  Periorbital edema

The preferred treatment of upper extremity venous thrombosis in this group of patients is subcutaneous low-molecular-weight heparin, followed by warfarin for 3 months, maintaining the INR in the range 1.5 to 2.0. In patients whose platelet count is less than 50×10^9/l, it is our practice not to use anticoagulation, although danaparoid is an option in this situation. In our experience enoxaparin (Clexane) 1.5 mg/kg/day s.c. or dalteparin sodium (Fragmin) 150 units/kg/day s.c. is sufficient to maintain the anti-Xa level in the range 0.3 to 0.8 units/ml.

Other authors have also managed these complications by catheter removal without anticoagulation and this has not resulted in an adverse outcome (Lokich & Becker, 1983).

Catheter occlusion

This complication has been reviewed by Hurtubise et al. (1990), and Lazarus, Lowder, and Herzig (1983). Treatment of occluded catheters with low-dose intraluminal thrombolytic therapy (urokinase 5,000 units in 2 ml) is safe and restores patency in many cases (Rubin, 1983). The volume of thrombolytic instilled should be equivalent to the calculated dead space of the vascular catheter. The urokinase may be left in place for 30 to 60 minutes and the procedure may be repeated several times until successful. Those that remain blocked require removal. Occluded catheters may be rewired and a fresh catheter inserted through the same site. This technique may also be used to change a single-lumen to a double-lumen catheter. Complications include pulmonary thromboembolism, transient bacteremia, and occasionally cardiac arrhythmias.

Low-dose warfarin therapy may have a role in the prophylactic management of catheters in an attempt to prevent thrombosis in patients requiring long-term vascular access. The dosage recommendation is 1 mg a day (Bern et al., 1990). However, monitoring of the INR should be undertaken, even at this low dose level, with adjustments made to maintain the INR at approximately 1.5.

Other mechanical complications

A number of other mechanical complications of central catheters have been described and tend to be less remediable than thrombosis. Such complications occur in 10% to 20% of insertions (Moosa et al., 1991).

Insertion-related complications are mainly the result of percutaneous approaches to the subclavian vein (Madero et al., 1997; Muhm et al., 1997), and include puncture of the subclavian artery and other vascular structures including the heart or trachea, hematoma formation, hemothorax, chylothorax, pneumothorax, and failure of venous cannulation (Pessa & Howard, 1985). Catheter insertion via cephalic vein radicals identified in the delto-pectoral groove at cut-down can avoid many of these complications (Thomas & Sinnet, 1988). Tip malposition occurring at the time of insertion can be corrected by catheter manipulation or by percutaneous manipulation using transvenous snares. Ideally, the catheter tip should lie in the superior vena cava near its junction with the right atrium. In contrast to primary malposition, "secondary migration" indicates catheter tip migration to neighboring veins after satisfactory initial placement (Muhm *et al.,* 1996). This too is amenable to repositioning.

Some complications are largely uncorrectable and include catheter dislodgement out of the vein into the surrounding soft tissue, abutment of the catheter tip against the vein wall, erosion of the dacron cuff at the skin, or retention of the cuff, which can act as a source of infection (Ruppel *et al.,* 1994).

Sutures at the site of insertion into the vein may constrict a catheter that has been inserted by cut-down. Catheter leaks can arise from perforation of the catheter during maintenance and can be repaired using standard kits. Perforation of the catheter in the subcutaneous canal will require removal.

Deep vein thrombosis

Prophylaxis

Prophylactic measures to prevent venous thrombosis should be considered for all high-risk patients, especially during hospitalization. Of particular concern are patients undergoing treatment for malignancy, patients with a previous history of venous thrombosis, and immobilized patients who have recently undergone surgery. Knee-length graduated compression stockings that provide 20 to 25 mmHg compression at ankle level are a routine recommendation. Intermittent pneumatic sequential calf-thigh compression devices are an effective option for high-risk circumstances, such as prolonged immobilization or previous deep vein thrombosis. Subcutaneous heparin prophylaxis complements antistasis prophylaxis in selected patients.

Diagnosis

Clinical assessment of deep venous thrombosis is known to be unreliable. Accurate diagnosis is essential to avoid inappropriate anticoagulation treatment and complications of pulmonary embolism in the short term, and post-phlebitic syndrome in the long term. Contrast venography has been the investigation of choice for some time (Cassidy *et al.,* 1987), but has the disadvantage of being invasive, is often painful, has the potentially serious complication of allergy, and may even induce venous thrombosis.

Ultrasound imaging is now the investigation of choice for the diagnosis of deep vein thrombosis provided that the scan is performed by an experienced vascular technologist (Fletcher *et al.,* 1990). Ultrasound imaging can diagnose other conditions such as calf hematoma, superficial thrombophlebitis, and Baker[3] cyst, which can mimic the clinical presentation of a deep vein thrombosis.

Venous thromboses can occur at unusual sites after HSC transplantation. For example, portal vein thrombosis should be

[3] William Morrant Baker, English surgeon, 1839–1896.

considered in the differential diagnosis of abdominal pain and abnormal liver function after bone marrow transplantation (Grigg *et al.,* 1996).

Management

Patients with venous thrombosis require treatment to prevent propagation of the thrombosis and thromboembolism. The importance of immediate treatment with anticoagulants or thrombolytic agents is unquestioned (Hyers *et al.,* 1995). Inadequate anticoagulant therapy carries a risk of recurrent thromboembolism that can be as high as 25% (Hull *et al.,* 1979; Schulman *et al.,* 1997) (Table 100.5). However, prolonged anticoagulant therapy is associated with a higher risk of hemorrhage (Schulman *et al.,* 1997). Thus, at some point the risk of treatment may outweigh the potential benefit.

Heparin treatment for venous thrombosis may be given as a continuous intravenous infusion or by subcutaneous injection. An APTT value 1.5 to 2.5 times the control value is usually recommended as the target therapeutic range for intravenous heparin (Hyers *et al.,* 1995). Some of the variability in patient response to heparin is a consequence of different plasma concentrations of factor VIII and heparin-binding proteins (Young *et al.,* 1992; Levine *et al.,* 1994).

Low-molecular-weight heparins have several advantages over unfractionated heparin. Their half-lives are longer; the dose response is more predictable; there is less binding to heparin-binding proteins; there is probably less bleeding; and they are more effective than unfractionated heparin in preventing recurrence of thrombosis (Leizorovicz *et al.,* 1994; Lensing *et al.,* 1995; Levine *et al.,* 1996; Siragusa *et al.,* 1996). Furthermore, in two large randomized trials of patients with proximal deep vein thrombosis, outpatient treatment with low-molecular-weight heparin was as effective and as safe as inpatient treatment with an intravenous infusion of unfractionated heparin (Koopman *et al.,* 1996; Levine *et al.,* 1996). Therefore, it is now reasonable to manage deep vein thrombosis with subcutaneous low-molecular-weight heparin, at least until the INR on warfarin has been in the therapeutic range for 2 consecutive days.

The risk of bleeding in patients on anticoagulants not only correlates with the APTT and INR values, but also with factors such as increased age of the patient, previous stroke or gastrointestinal bleeding, thrombocytopenia, anemia, renal disease, liver disease, recent surgery, and concomitant antiplatelet therapy (Levine *et al.,* 1995). Therefore, the dose of the anticoagulant and the target level of anticoagulation needs to be individualized and modified if such conditions are present. For patients with deep vein thrombosis or pulmonary embolism whose platelet count is less than $50 \times 10^9/l$, it is our practice to anticoagulate with lower dose heparin to maintain an APTT of one to two times above baseline, or reduced doses of low-molecular-weight heparin.

Thrombocytopenia occurs in approximately 3% of patients on heparin, and can be transient and reversible or accompanied by new venous or arterial thrombotic events. If this serious complication, heparin-induced thrombocytopenia and thrombosis syndrome (HITTS), is suspected, the treatment of choice is cessation of heparin, and commencement of danaparoid and warfarin. Because there is significant cross-reactivity between low-molecular-weight and unfractionated heparins, we believe that both are contraindicated in patients suspected of having HITTS.

Pulmonary embolism

Diagnosis

The most common symptoms and signs of pulmonary embolism are nonspecific and include dyspnea, tachypnea, tachycardia, pleuritic chest pain, and low-grade fever. Major pulmonary embolism affecting more than one-third of the pulmonary artery circulation is usually accompanied by tachycardia, hypotension, and clinical and ECG signs of acute cor pulmonale. Central cardiac-type chest pain and syncope are indications for urgent management.

The first step to confirmation of a clinical diagnosis of pulmonary embolism is radionuclide pulmonary ventilation and perfusion scanning. If the lung perfusion scan is normal, then pulmonary embolism is excluded, whereas a high-probability pattern (e.g., multiple segmental perfusion defects with normal ventilation) is strong evidence of pulmonary embolism. Unfortunately, however, more than 50% of patients will have nondiagnostic imaging results and need further evaluation. There are two options in seeking diagnostic support in this situation: either testing for the presence of a deep vein thrombosis (e.g., Duplex ultrasound examination of the lower limb deep veins), or pulmonary angiography (Stein, 1996). It would be reasonable to withhold anticoagulant therapy if these tests are normal, although ongoing surveillance by repeating the lung scan and retesting for deep vein thrombosis 5 to 7 days later is indicated in patients considered to be at a continuing high risk of venous thromboembolism.

Other investigations usually performed when pulmonary embolism is suspected include chest X-ray, electrocardiography, and blood gas analysis, the latter by ear lobe capillary sampling if severe thrombocytopenia contraindicates arterial puncture (Fig. 100.1).

Management

Pulmonary embolism is initially managed by a continuous intravenous infusion of heparin with emphasis on achieving therapeutic APTT values (1.5 to 2.5 times control) as quickly as possible (Hyers et al., 1995). Persistently subtherapeutic APTT values are associated with a very high risk of recurrent embolic events.

Thrombolytic therapy is an option in selected patients, but, because of the increased potential for hemorrhagic complications, should be restricted to those HSC transplant recipients who have severe hemodynamic instability due to the pulmonary embolism.

If anticoagulation is contraindicated (e.g., by severe thrombocytopenia), or, if there is recurrent pulmonary embolism despite anticoagulation, then consideration should be given to placement of an inferior vena caval filter after confirmation that the source of the pulmonary embolism is thrombus distal to the inferior vena cava (Hyers et al., 1995).

Heparin treatment for pulmonary embolism is usually combined with warfarin therapy, with the latter being continued for 3 to 6 months. A longer course of oral anticoagulation therapy should be considered if longer lasting, so-called permanent risk factors predominate, or if there is a second episode of venous thromboembolism (Diuguid, 1997; Schulman et al., 1997).

Recurrent venous thromboembolism, or treatment failure despite therapeutic levels of anticoagulation, can occur under a number of circumstances (see Table 100.5).

Patients who remain shocked following pulmonary embolism should be considered for pulmonary embolectomy after angiography to demonstrate the lesion. All patients who have pulmonary embolectomy should have an inferior vena caval filter inserted. Pulmonary embolectomy may be performed as an open surgical procedure or by using a number of more recently developed percutaneous, catheter-based techniques.

Arterial complications

Arterial complications are uncommon in HSC transplant recipients. Iatrogenic injuries to the subclavian artery, and, less commonly the aorta and heart, have been documented as complications of percutaneous central line insertions (Pessa & Howard, 1985). Macrovascular arterial embolism has been encountered, particularly as complications of fungal cardiac infections or noninfective, thrombotic marantic endocarditis. Cardiac aspergillosis has caused coronary embolism (Laszenski et al., 1988) and more extensive embolization throughout the peripheral arterial tree. This organism is noted for its propensity to invade and occlude blood vessels (Schwartz, 1989).

The prognosis following such events is grave, and a high index of suspicion is required in any patient complaining of sudden onset of pain, motor weakness, or sensory loss in a limb. Cardinal physical findings are those of a cold, pulseless limb with tenderness and swelling of ischemic muscle compartments. Diagnosis in other sites, particularly the mesenteric vascular bed, is more problematic and is frequently missed antemortem.

Table 100.5. *Recurrent venous thromboembolism*

Subtherapeutic anticoagulation
Heparin allergy (HITTS)
Hypercoagulable states
Malignancy
Vasculitis

Abbreviation: HITTS, heparin-induced thrombocytopenia and thrombosis syndrome.

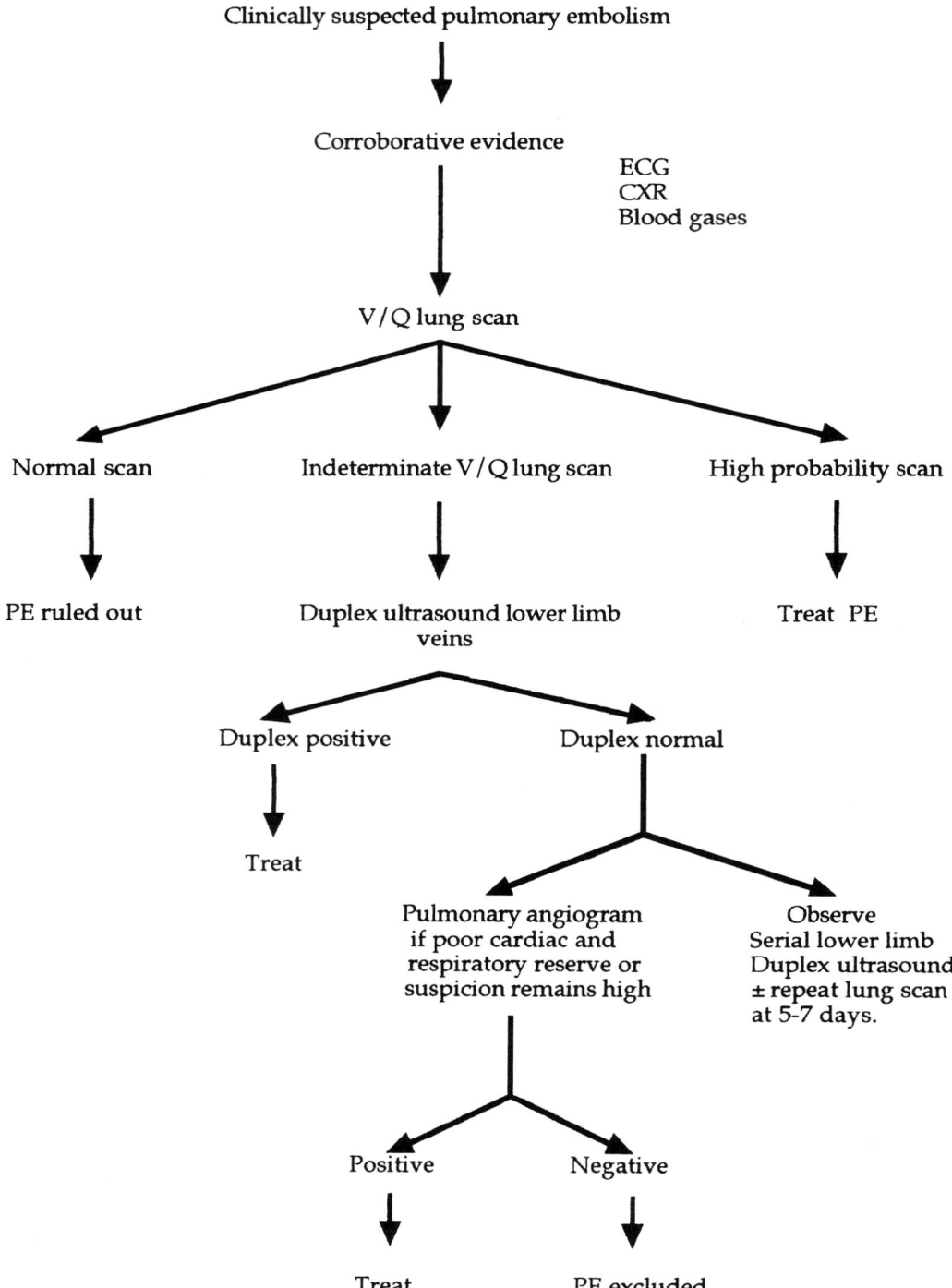

Fig. 100.1. Clinical investigations algorithm for diagnosis of pulmonary embolism. ECG, electrocardiogram; CXR, chest X-ray; V/Q, ventilation-perfusion; PE, pulmonary embolism.

Management of suspected arterial embolism should include prompt anticoagulation with intravenous heparin and urgent angiography to confirm the diagnosis. Surgical embolectomy constitutes definitive management and material removed from the vessel lumen should always be submitted for histology and culture to identify a possible infectious agent, with appropriate antimicrobial treatment instituted as soon as possible.

Microvascular arterial obstruction may be seen in the setting of disseminated intravascular coagulation, although the more typical picture is one of hemorrhage. Thrombotic thrombocytopenic purpura with microvascular obstruction and renal failure has been described in the HSC transplant population (Tschuchnigg *et al.*, 1990; Moake & Byrnes, 1996) (see Chapter 90).

References

Bern, M.M., Lokich, J.J., Wallach, S.R. *et al.* (1990). Very low doses of warfarin can prevent thrombosis in central venous catheters. A randomized prospective trial. *Annals of Internal Medicine,* **112,** 423–8.

Cassidy, F.P., Zajko, A.B., Bron, K.M. *et al.* (1987). Non-infectious complications of long-term central venous catheters: radiologic evaluation and management. *American Journal of Roentgenology,* **149,** 671–5.

Catani, L., Gugliotta, L., & Vianelli, N. (1996). Endothelium and bone marrow transplantation. *Bone Marrow Transplantation,* **17,** 277–80.

Conlan, M.G., Haire, W.D., Kessinger, A., & Armitage, J.O. (1991a). Prothrombotic haemostatic abnormalities in patients with refractory malignant lymphoma presenting for autologous stem cell transplantation. *Bone Marrow Transplantation,* **7,** 475–9.

Conlan, M.G., Haire, W.D., Lieberman, R.P. *et al.* (1991b). Catheter-related thrombosis in patients with refractory lymphoma undergoing autologous stem cell transplantation. *Bone Marrow Transplantation,* **7,** 235–40.

Diuguid, D.L. (1997). Oral anticoagulation therapy for venous thrombo-embolism. *New England Journal of Medicine,* **336,** 433–4.

Fernandez, L.A., Romaguera, R., Viciana, A.L. *et al.* (1996). Pulmonary embolism with bone fragments following vertebral bone marrow infusion for tolerance induction. *Cell Transplantation,* **5,** 513–16.

Fletcher, J.P., Kershaw, L.Z., Barker, D.S. *et al.* (1990). Ultrasound diagnosis of lower limb deep venous thrombosis. *Medical Journal of Australia,* **153,** 453–5.

Gordon, B.G., Haire, W.D., Patton, D.F. *et al.* (1993). Thrombotic complications of BMT: associated with protein C deficiency. *Bone Marrow Transplantation,* **11,** 61–5.

Graham, M.L., Rosse, W.F., Halperin, E.C. *et al.* (1996). Resolution of Budd-Chiari syndrome following bone marrow transplantation for paroxysmal nocturnal haemoglobinuria. *British Journal of Haematology,* **92,** 707–10.

Greeno, E.W., Haarke, E.P., Weisdorf, D., & Verfaillie, C. (1995). Lupus inhibitors following bone marrow transplant. *Bone Marrow Transplantation,* **15,** 287–91.

Grigg, A., Gibson, R., Bardy, P., & Szer, J. (1996). Acute portal vein thrombosis after autologous stem cell transplantation. *Bone Marrow Transplantation,* **18,** 949–53.

Haire, W.D., Lieberman, R.P., Edney, J. *et al.* (1990). Hickman catheter-induced thoracic vein thrombosis. Frequency and long-term sequelae in patients receiving high dose chemotherapy and marrow transplantation. *Cancer,* **66,** 900–8.

Haire, W.D., Lieberman, R.P., Lund, C.B. *et al.* (1991). Thrombotic complications of silicone rubber catheters during autologous marrow and peripheral stem cell transplantation: prospective comparison of Hickman and Groshong catheters. *Bone Marrow Transplantation,* **7,** 57–9.

Harper, P.L., Jarvis, J., Jennings, I. *et al.* (1990). Changes in the natural anticoagulants following bone marrow transplantation. *Bone Marrow Transplantation,* **5,** 39–42.

Hickman, R.O., Buckner, C.D., Clift, R.A. *et al.* (1979). A modified right atrial catheter for access to the venous system in marrow transplant recipients. *Surgery, Gynaecology and Obstetrics,* **148,** 871–5.

Hull, R., Delmore, T., Genton, E. *et al.* (1979). Warfarin sodium versus low-dose heparin in the long term treatment of venous thrombosis. *New England Journal of Medicine,* **301,** 855–8.

Hurtubise, M.R., Bottino, J.C., Lawson, M., & McCredie, K.B. (1990). Restoring patency of occluded central venous catheters. *Archives of Surgery,* **115,** 212–13.

Hyers, T.M., Hull, R.D., & Weg, J.G. (1995). Antithrombotic therapy for venous thromboembolic disease. *Chest,* **108,** (Suppl), 351S–5S.

Kaufman, P.A., Jones, R.B., Greenberg, C.S., & Peters, W.B. (1990). Autologous bone marrow transplantation and factor XII, factor VII and protein C deficiencies. Report of a new association and its possible relationship to endothelial cell injury. *Cancer,* **66,** 515–21.

Keohane, P.P., Jones, B.J., Attrill, H. *et al.* (1983). Effect of catheter tunneling and a nutrition nurse on catheter sepsis during parenteral nutrition. A controlled trial. *Lancet,* **2,** 1388–90.

Koopman, M.M.W., Prandoni, P., Piovella, F. *et al.* (1996). Treatment of venous thrombosis with intravenous unfractionated heparin administered in the hospital as compared with subcutaneous low-molecular-weight heparin administered at home. *New England Journal of Medicine,* **334,** 682–7.

Kronborg, C. (1989). Septic pulmonary embolism caused by *Candida albicans*: a fatal complication of bone marrow transplantation. *Scandinavian Journal of Infectious Disease,* **21,** 113–15.

Laszenski, M., Trigg, M., De Alarcon, P., & Giller, R. (1988). *Aspergillus* coronary embolism causing acute myocardial infarction. *Bone Marrow Transplantation,* **3,** 229–33.

Lazarus, H.M., Lowder, J.N., & Herzig, R.H. (1983). Occlusion and infection in Broviac catheters during intensive cancer therapy. *Cancer,* **52,** 2342–8.

Leblond, V., Salehian, B.D., Borel, C. *et al.* (1993). Alterations in natural anticoagulation levels during allogeneic bone marrow transplantation: a prospective study in 27 patients. *Bone Marrow Transplantation,* **11,** 299–305.

Leiby, J.M., Purcell, H., Demaria, J.J. *et al.* (1989). Pulmonary embolism as a result of Hickman catheter-related thrombosis. *American Journal of Medicine,* **86,** 228–31.

Leizorovics, A., Simonneau, G., Decousus, H., & Boissel, J.P. (1994). Comparison of efficacy and safety of low molecular weight heparins and unfractionated heparin in initial treatment of deep venous thrombosis: a meta-analysis. *British Medical Journal,* **309,** 299–304.

Lensing, A.W.A., Prins, M.H., Davidson, B.L., & Hirsh, J. (1995). Treatment of deep venous thrombosis with low-molecular-weight heparins: a meta-analysis. *Archives of Internal Medicine,* **155,** 601–7.

Levine, M., Gent, M., Hirsh, J. *et al.* (1996). A comparison of low-molecular-weight heparin administered primarily at home with unfractionated heparin administered in the hospital for proximal deep-vein thrombosis. *New England Journal of Medicine,* **334,** 677–81.

Levine, M.N., Hirsh, J., Gent, M. *et al.* (1994). A randomized trial comparing activated thromboplastin time with heparin assay in patients with acute venous thromboembolism requiring large daily doses of heparin. *Archives of Internal Medicine,* **154,** 49–56.

Levine, M.N., Raskob, G., Landefeld, S., & Hirsh, J. (1995). Haemorrhagic complications of anticoagulant treatment. *Chest,* **108** (Suppl), 276S–90S.

Lokich, J.J. & Becker, B. (1983). Subclavian vein thrombosis in patients treated with infusion chemotherapy for advanced malignancy. *Cancer,* **52,** 1586–9.

Madero, L., Ruano, D., Villa, M. *et al.* (1997). Non-tunneled catheters in children undergoing bone marrow transplantation. *Bone Marrow Transplantation,* **17,** 87–9.

Moake, J.L. & Byrnes, J.J. (1996). Thrombotic microangiopathies associated with drugs and bone marrow transplantation. *Hematology-Oncology Clinics of North America,* **10,** 485–97.

Moosa, H.H., Julian, T.B., Rosenfeld, C.S., & Shadduck, R.K. (1991). Complications of indwelling central venous catheters in bone marrow transplant recipients. *Surgery, Gynaecology and Obstetrics,* **172,** 275–9.

Muhm, M., Carl, H.S.P., Sunder-Plassmann, G. *et al.* (1997). Percutaneous nonangiographic insertion of Hickman catheters in marrow transplant recipients by anesthesiologists and intensivists. *Anesthesia and Analgesia,* **84,** 80–4.

Muhm, M., Sunder-Plassmann, G., Kührer, I. *et al.* (1996). Secondary migration: a complication of Hickman central venous catheters. *Bone Marrow Transplantation,* **18,** 651–4.

Pessa, M.E. & Howard, R.J. (1985). Complications of Hickman-Broviac catheters. *Surgery, Gynaecology and Obstetrics,* **161,** 257–60.

Peterson, F.B., Clift, R.A., Hickman, R.O. *et al.* (1986). Hickman catheter complications in marrow transplant recipients. *Journal of Parenteral and Enteral Nutrition,* **10,** 58–62.

Richard, S., Seigneur, M., Blann, A. *et al.* (1996). Vascular endothelial lesion in patients undergoing bone marrow transplantation. *Bone Marrow Transplantation,* **18,** 955–9.

Rio, B., Andreu, G., Nicod, A. *et al.* (1986). Thrombocytopenia in veno-occlusive disease after bone marrow transplantation or chemotherapy. *Blood,* **67,** 1773–6.

Rockoff, M.A., Gang, D.L., & Vacanti, J.P. (1984). Fatal pulmonary embolism following removal of a central venous catheter. *Journal of Pediatric Surgery,* **19,** 307–9.

Rubin, R.N. (1983). Local instillation of small doses of streptokinase for treatment of thrombotic occlusions of long term access catheters. *Journal of Clinical Oncology,* **1,** 572–3.

Ruppel, L.J., Brown, R.A., Borson, R.A., & Whitman, E.D. (1994). Retained Hickman catheter cuff as an infection source following allogeneic bone marrow transplant. *Bone Marrow Transplantation,* **14,** 169–71.

Sanders, J.E., Hickman, R.O., Aker, S. *et al.* (1982). Experience with double lumen right atrial catheters. *Journal of Parenteral and Enteral Nutrition,* **6,** 95–9.

Schulman, S., Granquist, S., Holstrom, M. *et al.* (1997). The duration of oral anticoagulant therapy after a second episode of venous thromboembolism. *New England Journal of Medicine,* **336,** 393–8.

Schwartz, D.A. (1989). Aspergillus pancarditis following bone marrow transplantation for chronic myelogenous leukaemia. *Chest,* **95,** 1338–9.

Silverstein, R.L. & Nachman, R.L. (1992). Cancer and clotting—Trousseau's warning. *New England Journal of Medicine,* **327,** 1163–4.

Siragusa, S., Cosmi, B., Piovella, F. *et al.* (1996). Low-molecular-weight heparins and unfractionated heparin in the treatment of patients with acute venous thromboembolism: results of a meta-analysis. *American Journal of Medicine,* **100,** 269–77.

Sletnes, K.E., Holte, H., Halvorsen, S. *et al.* (1996). Activation of coagulation and deep vein thrombosis after bone marrow harvesting and insertion of a Hickman catheter in ABMT patients with malignant lymphoma. *Bone Marrow Transplantation,* **17,** 577–81.

Stein, P.D. (1996). Diagnosis and management of pulmonary embolism. *Current Opinion in Cardiology,* **11,** 543–9.

Thomas, P.R.S. & Sinnet, H.D. (1988). An evaluation of prolonged venous access catheters in patients with leukaemia and other malignancies. *European Journal of Surgical Oncology,* **14,** 63–8.

Tschuchnigg, M., Bradstock, K.F., Koutts, J. *et al.* (1990). A case of thrombotic thrombocytopenic purpura following allogeneic bone marrow transplantation. *Bone Marrow Transplantation,* **5,** 61–3.

Uderzo, C., Marraro, G., Riva, A. *et al.* (1993). Pulmonary thromboembolism in leukaemic children undergoing bone marrow transplantation. *Bone Marrow Transplantation,* **11,** 201–3.

Young, E., Prins, M., Levine, M.N., & Hirsh, J. (1992). Heparin binding to plasma proteins, an important mechanism for heparin resistance. *Thrombosis and Haemostasis,* **67,** 639–43.

101 Hematologic complications

ANTHONY DODDS

St Vincent's Hospital and University of New South Wales, Sydney, Australia

Introduction

The most common hematologic complication after hematopoietic stem cell (HSC) transplantation is the development of cytopenia prior to, and sometimes beyond, the normal time of engraftment. If persistent, this represents a serious risk to the recipient due to the failure of hematopoietic function. Hemostatic disturbances also occur routinely after HSC transplantation and are usually due to thrombocytopenia, although other alterations leading to both a bleeding tendency and a thrombotic tendency have been described. Finally, secondary hematologic neoplasms, although rare, do occur with greater frequency after HSC transplantation than in an age-matched control population.

Cytopenias

Profound cytopenia is a universal early accompaniment of HSC transplantation following myeloablative conditioning (see Chapter 13). Its duration is variable and related to the dose of stem cells infused, the source of stem cells, the underlying disease [particularly in autologous bone marrow transplantation (BMT)], the posttransplant immune suppression used, and the presence of splenomegaly. Occasionally cytopenias extend beyond the normal time of engraftment; the resulting failure of engraftment is dealt with in Chapters 12 and 70. Allogeneic HSC transplantation is unique in that a new hematopoietic and immune system develops in the presence of the host's residual hematopoietic and immune system. Host elements can persist for months to years after transplant. The resulting mixed chimerism can result in immunologic reactions of either the "host-versus-graft" or the "graft-versus-host" types.

There are a number of possible mechanisms for transient, reversible cytopenia later posttransplant or for prolongation of the obligatory cytopenia immediately posttransplant. There may be suppression of hematopoiesis by drug treatments such as methotrexate or ganciclovir; both viral and bacterial infections especially septicemia are suppressive of marrow function, as are intercurrent complications such as graft-versus-host disease (GVHD). A further cause of pancytopenia is marrow hypoplasia or aplasia resulting from the infusion of allogeneic donor lymphocytes to treat relapse of the original hematologic malignancy occurring postallografting. This is thought to represent a graft-versus-host effect and may require the infusion of additional donor hematopoietic stem cells (see Chapter 65). Second, there may be suppression of hematopoiesis by other immune mechanisms, acting either on bone marrow progenitors, or peripherally leading to a more rapid destruction of hematopoietic cells such as platelets (De Lord *et al.,* 1996).

Failure of sustained engraftment, including graft rejection is dealt with separately (Chapters 12 and 70).

Anemia

Anemia can result from inadequate production or excessive loss of red cells. This may be due to hemolysis, bleeding, or increased pooling and destruction of red cells in an enlarged spleen (Table 101.1).

Table 101.1. *Causes of anemia after bone marrow and blood stem cell transplantation*

Inadequate marrow production of red cells
    Marrow suppression by drugs, microbial agents, or coexistent disease
    Delayed erythroid engraftment associated with ABO incompatibility
    Pure red cell aplasia associated with ABO incompatibility
    Sideroblastic anemia associated with pyridoxine deficiency
    Impaired erythropoietin production
    Marrow involvement by GVHD (including that occurring after donor lymphocyte infusions)
Excessive loss of red cells
    Bleeding
    Hemolysis
        Alloimmune (associated with ABO incompatibility)
        Autoimmune
        Microangiopathic, for example TTP or HUS
    Hypersplenism

Abbreviations: GVHD, graft-versus-host disease; TTP, thrombotic thrombocytopenic purpura; HUS, hemolytic-uremic syndrome.

Inadequate production of red cells can be due to a relative insufficiency of marrow stem cells or a relative lack of erythropoietin production, resulting in insufficient stimulus to red cell production. Relative lack of erythropoietin production has been described after allogeneic, but not autologous BMT (Ireland *et al.*, 1990; Bosi *et al.*, 1991). This may result in an increase in red cell transfusion requirements. While the mechanism for this failure of erythropoietin (EPO) production is uncertain, impaired EPO production has been demonstrated in anemic mice treated with cyclosporine (CSP) (Vannucchi *et al.*, 1991a). The renal toxicity produced by CSP may have a role in the impairment of EPO production. Randomized studies of recombinant human EPO administration given after allogeneic BMT have shown enhanced erythroid engraftment and a variable reduction in transfusion requirements (Klaesson *et al.*, 1994; Miller & Mills, 1994; Biggs *et al.*, 1995) (and see Chapter 32). Suppression of bone marrow production may be caused by drugs; microbial agents, especially viruses including parvovirus B19 (Corbett *et al.*, 1995; Broliden, 2001); or other coexistent disease, such as renal or liver disease.

Primary marrow disorders such as sideroblastic anemia may occur, resulting in late transfusion dependence (Nicholls *et al.*, 1984). Although transient dyserythropoiesis early after HSC transplantation is relatively common, ineffective erythropoiesis due to sideroblastic anemia is rare but may respond to pyridoxine administration. Its cause is uncertain. Another cause of late packed cell transfusion dependence is GVHD involving the marrow (Atkinson *et al.*, 1987).

Immune hemolytic anemia is an important cause of anemia after HSC transplantation, particularly when there is a mismatch of red cell antigens between donor and recipient (see Chapter 69). Such immune hemolytic anemias can be alloimmune, after allogeneic transplantation, or, less commonly, autoimmune (Klumpp, 1991). The syndrome of alloimmune hemolytic anemia most commonly results from an ABO mismatch between the marrow donor and recipient. This subject is covered in more detail in Chapter 69, and is an example of "host-versus-graft" and "graft-versus-host" effects. With a major ABO mismatch, anemia results from persistence of host isoagglutinin, directed against contaminating red cells in the stem cell inoculum (immediate hemolysis) or engrafting red cells (delayed hemolysis) (host-versus-graft effect). Minor ABO mismatches are incompatible in the opposite direction with host red cells destroyed by isoagglutinins present in the stem cell inoculum or produced by the engrafting immune system (graft-versus-host effect). A number of cases of pure red cell aplasia after ABO mismatched allogeneic transplantation have been described (see Chapter 69). These now include allografts preceded by non-myeloablative conditioning regimens (Veelken *et al.*, 2000). Delay of erythroid engraftment, however, is more common than aplasia. It has been seen in most studies of major ABO mismatched BMT. True autoimmune hemolytic anemia is much less common and occurs after autologous, and occasionally allogeneic, transplantation. (Klumpp, 1991; Sloop *et al.*, 1994; Tamura *et al.*, 1994; Azuma *et al.*,

1996; Drobyski *et al.*, 1996; Chen *et al.*, 1997), and may require treatment with immune suppressive agents, plasmapheresis, intravenous immunoglobulin infusions, anti-CD20 monoclonal antibody (Rovelli *et al.*, 2001), or splenectomy (Fig. 101.1). Autoimmune hemolytic anemia occurring posttransplant can be fatal. Richard and colleagues (2000) reported a patient who developed both immune hemolytic anemia and immune thrombocytopenia (Evans' syndrome),[1] as well as transverse myelitis, pulmonary infiltrates, eosinophilia, muscle cramps, and lichenoid dermatitis after an unrelated transplant—all possibly a manifestation of GVHD.

Thrombocytopenia

Prolonged thrombocytopenia after HSC transplantation is a serious complication (Table 101.2). Its presence, coupled with refractoriness to platelet transfusions, results in increased mortality and morbidity from bleeding. The time of onset of bleeding associated with thrombocytopenia after marrow transplantation is shown in Fig. 101.2. Twenty-five percent of the episodes had started by day 12, 50% by day 22, and 75% by day 42 (Nevo *et al.*, 2001). Sixty-one percent of bleeding episodes, in this study had one bleeding site, while 31% had 2 or more sites. Gastrointestinal hemorrhage occurred in 62% of bleeding episodes, hemorrhagic cystitis in 27%, intracranial hemorrhage in 9%, and other sites in 13%. The duration of bleeding was less than 1 week in 24%, 8 to 14 days in 28%, 15 to 28 days in 27%, 29 to 60 days in 15%, and more than 60 days in 3%.

Thrombocytopenia posttransplant has been classified into two types: (1) transient benign thrombocytopenia and (2) chronic persistent thrombocytopenia (First *et al.*, 1985). Patients with the first type usually attain a normal platelet count, but the platelet count subsequently falls, although eventually returns to normal. The transient syndrome has been related to drug therapy, particularly trimethoprim-sulfamethoxazole or ganciclovir administration. A similar syndrome can also be seen after cytomegalovirus (CMV) infections. In one study CMV seropositive recipients of allogeneic BMT had a significant delay in platelet recovery (Verdonck *et al.*, 1991). After autologous BMT this delay was only seen in patients receiving transplants for lymphoma. The mechanism by which CMV interferes with platelet recovery is probably direct cytotoxicity on megakaryocytes or their progenitors. Damage to marrow stromal cells is an alternative possibility. Two specific genotypes of CMV, gB3 and gB4, have recently been associated with severe myelosuppression (Torok-Storb *et al.*, 1997).

In patients with the chronic persistent thrombocytopenia syndrome, a normal platelet count is usually not achieved, despite normal granulocyte and reticulocyte counts. After allogeneic transplantation this syndrome is strongly associated with severe acute GVHD and chronic GVHD, and has a high mortality (Anasetti *et al.*, 1989). Risk factors for delayed

---

[1] Robert Evans, U.S. physician, 1912–1974.

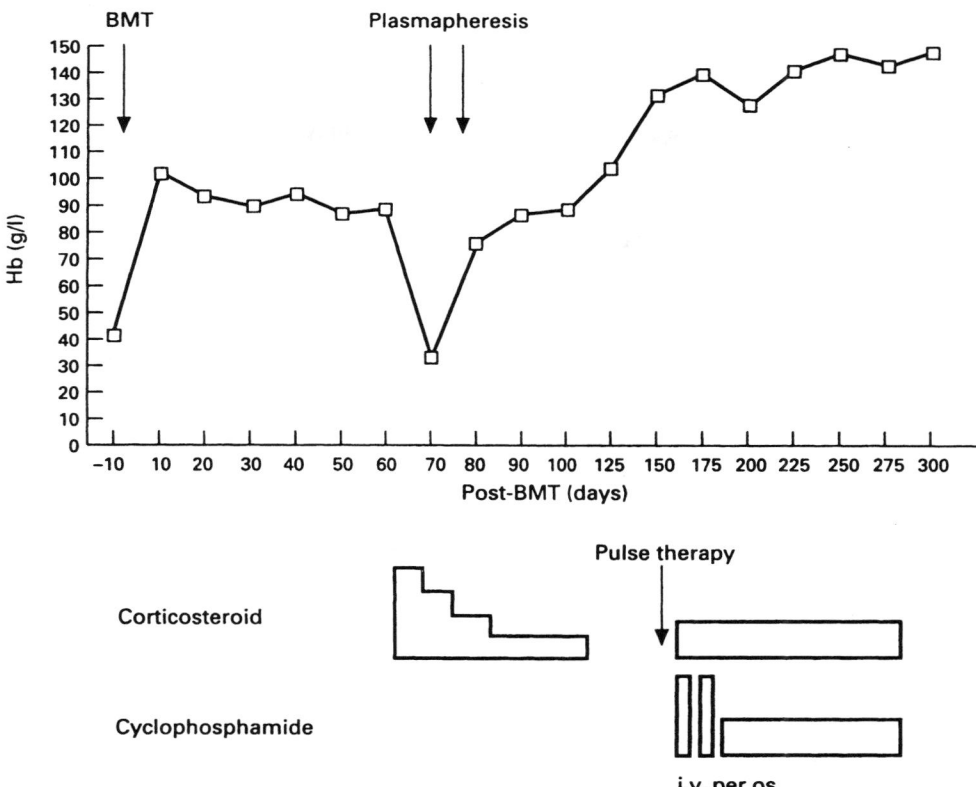

Fig. 101.1. Cold hemagglutinin disease following allogeneic bone marrow transplantation for severe aplastic anemia. Acute hemolysis was reversed by plasmapheresis, corticosteroid, and cyclophosphamide. Reproduced, with permission, from Azuma *et al.* (1996).

platelet recovery in a study of 342 patients included donor type (unrelated donor transplant recipients had slower recovery than HLA-identical sibling recipients); acute GVHD; CMV infection; and the number of nucleated cells infused in the graft (Dominietto *et al.*, 2001).

Other causes of thrombocytopenia include autoimmune and alloimmune mechanisms. The diagnosis of immune thrombocytopenia posttransplant is difficult to make with certainty, because of the frequent occurrence of false-positive and false-negative antiplatelet antibody tests, and because there are often

Table 101.2. *Causes of thrombocytopenia after bone marrow and blood stem cell transplantation*

Inadequate production of platelets
    Delayed megakaryocyte engraftment
    Marrow suppression
        Drugs
        Antimicrobial agents
        Graft-versus-host disease
Excessive loss of platelets
    Autoimmune destruction
    Graft-versus-host disease
    Hypersplenism
    Disseminated intravascular coagulation
    Thrombotic microangiopathies

other reasons for thrombocytopenia in these patients. Despite this, there have been a number of convincing cases of immune thrombocytopenia mediated by platelet-specific antibodies. These have been reported in patients undergoing allogeneic,

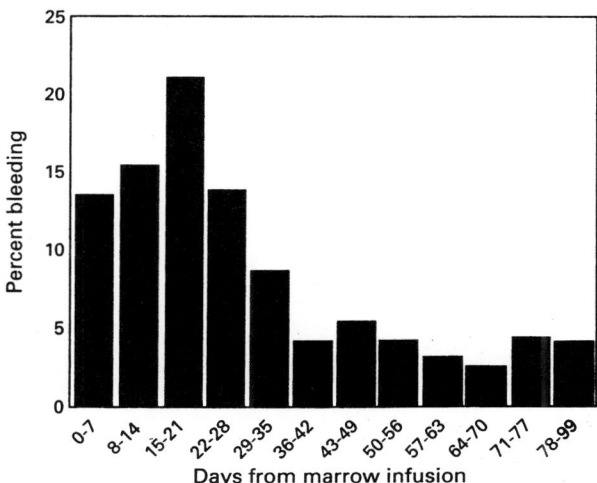

Fig. 101.2. The onset of bleeding within 100 days from marrow infusion. Twenty-five percent of bleeding had started by day 12, 50% by day 22, and 75% by day 42, defining weeks 2–6 post BMT to be the period of "high risk for bleeding." Reproduced, with permission, from Nevo *et al.* (2001).

autologous (Sivakumaran *et al.*, 1995; Jillella, Kallab, & Kutlar, 2000), and syngeneic BMT. In many of the allogeneic patients, it has not been certain whether the thrombocytopenia was alloimmune or autoimmune, although in one case it was clearly autoimmune and was derived from the marrow donor who had an identical platelet autoantibody (Minchinton *et al.*, 1982). In another report the antibody was an alloantibody of recipient origin (Bierling *et al.*, 1994). Immune-mediated thrombocytopenia associated with chronic GVHD, and responsive to treatment with anti-CD20 chimeric monoclonal antibody administration, has been reported (Ratanatharathon *et al.*, 2000).

After autologous BMT prolonged thrombocytopenia can occur, particularly in those transplanted for acute myeloid leukemia (Roberts *et al.*, 1996) (Fig. 101.3). The mechanism for this is uncertain, but may reflect the underlying stem cell disorder in these patients. It appears to be less common in patients receiving autologous blood stem cells. One study suggested that the persistent thrombocytopenia after autologous BMT was due to decreased numbers of available megakaryocytic precursors (Adams *et al.*, 1990). Autoimmune mechanisms have also been described. Heparin-induced thrombocytopenia (observed in 5% to 20% of heparin-treated patients and due to heparin-dependent antiplatelet antibodies) has also been

described as a cause of thrombocytopenia after autologous and allogeneic BMT (Tezcan *et al.*, 1994).

Refractoriness to platelet transfusions after HSC transplantation is common and a major problem of management. Klumpp and colleagues (1996) studied 526 consecutive posttransplant platelet transfusions to determine the factors associated with response to platelet transfusion in the BMT setting. In their study, poor responses to platelet transfusions occurred frequently, with 310 of the 484 evaluable resulting in a postinfusion corrected platelet count increment of $<7.5 \times 10^9/l$. Factors associated with poor response to platelet transfusion in multivariate analysis included the presence of serum lymphocytotoxic antibodies, male sex, body surface area >1.7 m^2, transfusion of red cells on the day of the platelet infusion, concurrent administration of corticosteroids, a major ABO mismatch between the recipient and the platelet product, and, in women, a history of one or more pregnancies prior to transplant. Suprisingly, a history of more than 25 blood product exposures prior to transplant and evidence for prior CMV infection were associated with higher increments to platelet transfusion. Factors that showed little correlation with response to platelet transfusion included the age of the infused platelet product, concurrent fever, recent administration of intravenous

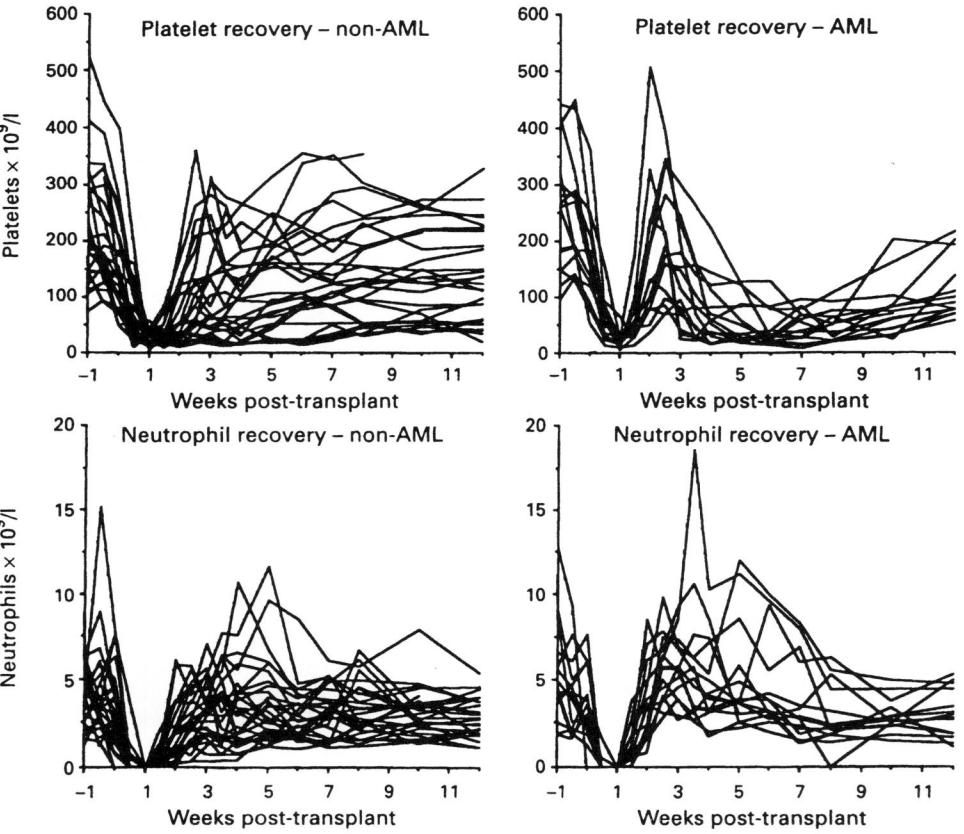

Fig. 101.3. Platelet and neutrophil recovery after peripheral blood stem cell transplantation. Platelet and neutrophil counts for all patients from 1 week before to 12 weeks after PBSC transplant, showing a markedly different pattern of platelet recovery in acute myeloid leukemia patients. Reproduced, with permission, from Roberts *et al.* (1996).

immunoglobulin, and the absolute neutrophil count at the time of the infusion. The authors concluded that the factors associated with response to platelet transfusion in BMT patients appeared to be different from those observed in the nontransplant setting. Anti-PLA1 antibodies have been demonstrated to be associated with platelet refractoriness and platelet responsiveness has been restored by the use of transfusion of PLA1-negative blood products.

Neutropenia

The most frequent cause of neutropenia postengraftment is drug-induced suppression, again most commonly seen with ganciclovir and trimethoprim-sulfamethoxazole. A small number of cases of immune-mediated neutropenia have been reported following allogeneic BMT. These appear to be mainly autoimmune in nature. In one report, a 26-year-old male with chronic myeloid leukemia (CML) received an HLA-compatible unrelated donor transplant and showed good platelet engraftment but poor neutrophil recovery. On day 33 posttransplant surface-bound, anti-neutrophil antibodies were detected by immunofluorescence (Fig. 101.4). In contrast to other reported cases, the white blood cell count and neutrophil count subsequently improved without specific treatment. Neither red blood cells nor platelets were affected (Tosi *et al.,* 1994). Alloimmune neutropenia, although theoretically possible, appears to be even less common. Anti-neutrophil antibodies are not specific for these syndromes, as they may be present posttransplant in the absence of neutropenia, or may be absent in the presence of presumed immune neutropenia. Immune-mediated neutropenia may occur concurrently with other immune cytopenias. In one case where anti-human neutrophil antigen-2a (NB1) antibodies were present, the use of granulocyte colony-stimulating factor (G-CSF) appeared to perpetuate the immune neutopenia (Pocock *et al.,* 2001).

Disorders of hemostasis

Bleeding is a cause of both mortality and morbidity following HSC transplantation. It is usually due to thrombocytopenia or to problems with platelet transfusion therapy, especially platelet refractoriness. Occasionally disseminated intravascular coagulation (DIC) develops during conditioning treatment for acute leukemia in relapse. This is particularly seen in cases of acute promyelocytic leukemia. DIC can also occur with overwhelming sepsis and as an agonal event. Severe hepatic dysfunction such as that due to hepatic veno-occlusive disease (VOD) can result in a coagulopathy with prolongation of the prothrombin time and the partial thromboplastin time. Additionally, vitamin K deficiency may result in a coagulopathy. This can develop in patients with poor nutrition and on prolonged antibiotic treatment. Thus, prophylactic vitamin K should be part of the routine care of these patients.

Clinical thrombosis is not usually a problem following HSC transplantation except in intravenous lines (see Chapter 100), where local mechanisms predominate, and in the liver as part of

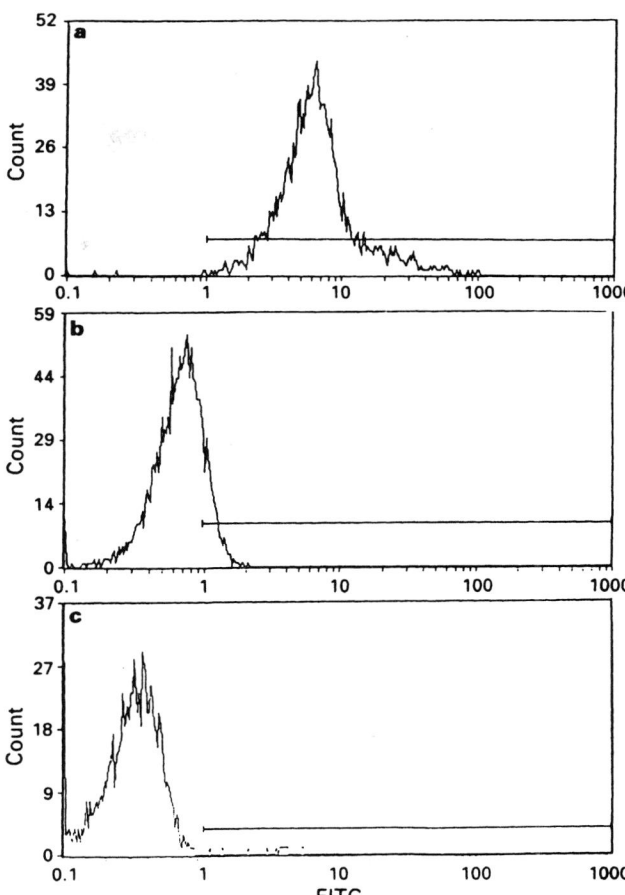

Fig. 101.4. Cytofluorimetric evaluation of surface-bound anti-neutrophil antibodies on day +33 (**a**), +39 (**b**), and +42 (**c**). The horizontal bar indicates the positive range. Strong positivity is shown in (**a**), low positivity in (**b**), and negativity is shown in (**c**). Reproduced, with permission, from Tosi *et al.* (1994).

the syndrome of VOD. Nonbacterial thrombotic endocarditis is another thrombotic complication of BMT (Gordon *et al.,* 1991). Cyclosporine is known to alter the levels of clotting factors, increase mononuclear cell procoagulant activity, reduce prostaglandin synthesis, and produce glomerular thrombosis and infarction (Gruber *et al.,* 1988). This supports the local arteriolopathy-based mechanism of cyclosporine nephrotoxicity. The endothelial damage produced results in intrarenal thrombosis. Cyclosporine may also be a contributing factor to the uncommon complication of microangiopathic damage resulting in the hemolytic-uremic syndrome or the more generalized thrombotic thrombocytopenic purpura (Gruber *et al.,* 1988). These thrombotic microangiopathies, and the coagulation abnormalities associated with them (Kanamori *et al.,* 1998; Natazuka *et al.,* 1998), have been described after both autologous and allogeneic transplants (see Chapter 90). Other contributing factors to their etiology include total body irradiation and high-dose chemotherapy regimens leading to widespread endothelial damage. The most effective therapy for these syndromes has not been determined.

Plasma exchange does not appear to be as effective as in de novo cases (Teruya *et al.*, 2001). Anti-cardiolipin antibodies and associated thromboembolism have also been described posttransplant (Qasim *et al.*, 1998). Cryofibrinogenemia, with associated thrombotic vasculopathy, producing skin necrosis has been described after autologous HSC transplantation and posttransplant interleukin-2 treatment (Shimoni *et al.*, 2000).

Low levels of the natural anticoagulants, protein C, protein S, and antithrombin III have been described after BMT (Harper *et al.*, 1990; Gordon *et al.*, 1991, 1996). Gordon *et al.* (1996) studied 71 adults undergoing HSC transplantation and found low protein C antigen and activity in 21% and 20% of patients, respectively. Protein C reached a nadir 14 days after the preparative regimen and then began to increase toward normal levels. Low levels, however, have been seen months posttransplant. The incidence of deficiency at day 100 was lower in patients receiving blood stem transplantation compared to those receiving bone marrow transplantation. The mechanism for this is uncertain. The drop in levels of protein C and protein S may reflect liver damage from the conditioning or vitamin K deficiency. Low levels of these anticoagulants are known to be associated with an increased risk of thrombosis. The fall in natural anticoagulant levels seen in some patients may be a factor in the genesis of VOD. Patients with a pre-existent laboratory risk factor for thrombosis may be especially at risk for the development of VOD.

Laboratory hemostatic abnormalities have been described after the infusion of stem cells, especially cryopreserved stem cells (Vannucchi *et al.*, 1991b). If heparin has been used as an anticoagulant for fresh stem cells, this may also have a short-term effect. However, the other laboratory alterations described do not appear to result in a clinical thrombotic or hemorrhagic disorder.

Neoplasia

Secondary neoplasms are well recognized as complications of HSC transplantation (Witherspoon *et al.*, 1989). Of the hematologic neoplasms, lymphoma [associated with Epstein-Barr virus (EBV)] after allogeneic transplantation (see Chapter 88), and myelodysplasia and acute myeloid leukemia after autologous transplantation (see Chapter 86), are the most important. Donor cell leukemia is a rare but well-documented event. One possible explanation for this intriguing complication is the transfer of a dormant oncogene from a virus or persisting host cell after transplant.

Myelodysplasia and acute myeloid leukemia are also recognized complications of conventional dose chemotherapy. They have been described following autologous transplantation for lymphoid and other malignancies. Data from the Minneapolis group (Bhatia *et al.*, 1996) suggested that in autotransplants for lymphoma, the cumulative incidence for these complications was 13.5%. They also occur after autotransplants for myeloma and breast cancer. Risk factors have yet to be fully defined but the extent and type of pretransplant conditioning regimen is likely to be important.

Lymphoma occurring early after allogeneic transplantation is better classified as B-cell lymphoproliferative disorder. It is usually an EBV-related disorder, which occurs in donor cells. The cumulative incidence is 1.6% at 4 years (Bhatia *et al.*, 1996). Risk factors include T-cell depletion, HLA mismatch, use of antithymocyte globulin, and a diagnosis of primary immunodeficiency (Gross *et al.*, 1999). This disorder responds poorly to traditional treatments. Alpha interferon may have some efficacy. The use of donor-derived, EBV-specific cytotoxic T lymphocytes as a treatment appears promising (Papadopoulos *et al.*, 1994), as does the use of the monoclonal anti-CD20 antibody, rituxan.

References

Adams, J.A., Gordon, A.A., Jiang, Y.Z. *et al.* (1990). Thrombocytopenia after bone marrow transplantation for leukemia: changes in megakaryocyte growth and growth-promoting activity. *British Journal of Haematology*, **75**, 195–201.

Anasetti, C., Rybka, W., Sullivan, K.M. *et al.* (1989). Graft-v-host disease is associated with autoimmune-like thrombocytopenia. *Blood*, **73**, 1054–8.

Atkinson, K., Dodds, A., Concannon, A., & Biggs, J. (1987). Late onset transfusion-dependent anemia with thrombocytopenia secondary to marrow fibrosis and hypoplasia associated with chronic graft-versus-host disease. *Bone Marrow Transplantation*, **2**, 445–9.

Azuma, E., Nishihara, H., Hanada, M. *et al.* (1996). Recurrent cold hemagglutinin disease following allogeneic bone marrow transplantation successfully treated with plasmapheresis, corticosteroids and cyclophosphamide. *Bone Marrow Transplantation*, **18**, 243–6.

Bhatia, S., Ramsay, N.K.C., Steinbuch, M. *et al.* (1996). Malignant neoplasms following bone marrow transplantation. *Blood*, **87**, 3633–9.

Bierling, T., Pigjon, J-M., Kuentz, M. *et al.* (1994). Thrombocytopenia after bone marrow transplantation caused by a recipient origin Br^a allo-antibody: presence of mixed chimerism 3 years after the graft without hematologic relapse. *Blood*, **83**, 274–9.

Biggs, J.C., Atkinson, K., Booker, V. *et al.* (1995). A prospective randomised double blind trial of the in vivo use of recombinant human erythropoietin in bone marrow transplantation from HLA-identical sibling donors. *Bone Marrow Transplantation*, **15**, 129–34.

Bosi, A., Vannucchi, A.M., Grossi, A. *et al.* (1991). Serum erythropoietin levels in patients undergoing autologous bone marrow transplantation. *Bone Marrow Transplantation*, **7**, 421–5.

Broliden, K. (2001). Parvovirus B19 infection in pediatric solid-organ and bone marrow transplantation. *Pediatric Transplantation*, **5**, 323–30.

Chen, F.E., Owen, I., Savage, D. *et al.* (1997). Late onset hemolysis and red cell autoimmunisation after allogeneic bone marrow transplant. *Bone Marrow Transplantation*, **19**, 491–5.

Corbett, T.J., Saw, H., Popat, U. *et al.* (1995). Successful treatment of parvovirus B19 infection and red cell aplasia occurring after an allogeneic bone marrow transplant. *Bone Marrow Transplantation*, **16**, 711–3.

De Lord, C., Marsh, J.C.W., Smith, J.G. *et al.* (1996). Fatal autoimmune pancytopenia following bone marrow transplantation for aplastic anaemia. *Bone Marrow Transplantation*, **18**, 237–9.

Dominietto, A., Raiola, A.M., van Lint, M.T. *et al.* (2001). Factors influencing haematological recovery after allogeneic haematopoietic stem cell transplants: graft-versus-host disease, donor type, cytomegalovirus infections and cell dose. *British Journal of Haematology*, **112**, 219–27.

Drobyski, W.R., Potluri, J., Sauer, D., & Gottschall, J.L. (1996). Autoimmune hemolytic anemia following T cell-depleted allogeneic bone marrow transplantation. *Bone Marrow Transplantation*, **17**, 1093–9.

First, L.R., Smith, B.R., Lipton, J. *et al.* (1985). Isolated thrombocytopenia after allogeneic bone marrow transplantation. Existence of transient and chronic thrombocytopenic syndromes. *Blood*, **65**, 368–74.

Gordon, B., Haire, W., Kessinger, A. *et al.* (1991). High frequency of antithrombin 3 and protein C deficiency following autologous bone marrow transplantation for lymphoma. *Bone Marrow Transplantation*, **8**, 497–502.

Gordon, B., Haire, W., Ruby, E. *et al.* (1996). Prolonged deficiency of protein C following hematopoietic stem cell transplantation. *Bone Marrow Transplantation*, **17**, 415–19.

Gross, T.G., Steinbuch, M., DeFor, T. *et al.* (1999). B-cell lymphoproliferative disorders following hemopoietic stem cell transplantation: risk factors, treatment and outcome. *Bone Marrow Transplantation*, **23**, 251–8.

Gruber, S.A., Fryd, D.S., Chavers, B. *et al.* (1988). The thrombogenicity of cyclosporine. *Clinical Transplantation*, **2**, 99–101.

Harper, P.L., Jarvis, J., Jennings, I. *et al.* (1990). Changes in the natural anticoagulants following bone marrow transplantation. *Bone Marrow Transplantation*, **5**, 39–42.

Ireland, R.M., Atkinson, K., Concannon, A.J. *et al.* (1990). Serum erythropoietin changes in autologous and allogeneic bone marrow transplant patients. *British Journal of Haematology*, **76**, 128–34.

Jillella, A.P., Kallab, A.M., & Kutlar, A. (2000). Autoimmune thrombocytopenia following autologous hematopoietic cell transplantation: review of literature and treatment options. *Bone Marrow Transplantation*, **26**, 925–7.

Kanamori, H., Maruta, A., Sasaki, S. *et al.* (1998). Diagnostic value of hemostatic parameters in bone marrow transplant-associated thrombotic microangiopathy. *Bone Marrow Transplantation*, **21**, 705–9.

Klaesson, S., Ringden, O., Ljungman, P. *et al.* (1994). Reduced blood transfusion requirements after allogeneic transplantation: results of a randomized, double-blind study with high-dose erythropoietin. *Bone Marrow Transplantation*, **13**, 397–402.

Klumpp, T.R. (1991). Immunohematologic complications of bone marrow transplantation. *Bone Marrow Transplantation*, **8**, 159–70.

Klumpp, T.R., Herman, J.H., Innis, S. *et al.* (1996). Factors associated with response to platelet transfusion following hematopoietic stem cell transplantation. *Bone Marrow Transplantation*, **17**, 1035–41.

Miller, C.B. & Mills, S. (1994). Erythropoietin after bone marrow transplantation. *Haematology-Oncology Clinics of North America*, **8**, 975–92.

Minchinton, R.M., Waters, A.H., Kendra, J., & Barrett, A.J. (1982). Autoimmune thrombocytopenia acquired from an allogeneic bone marrow graft. *Lancet*, **2**, 627–9.

Natazuka, T., Kajimoto, K., Ogawa, R. *et al.* (1998). Coagulation abnormalities and thrombotic microangiopathy following bone marrow transplantation from HLA-matched unrelated donors in patients with hematological malignancies. *Bone Marrow Transplantation*, **21**, 815–19.

Nevo, S., Enger, C., Hartley, E. *et al.* (2001). Acute bleeding and thrombocytopenia after bone marrow transplantation. *Bone Marrow Transplantation*, **27**, 65–72.

Nicholls, M.D., Atkinson, K., Biggs, J.C. *et al.* (1984). Late onset pyridoxine-responsive sideroblastic anemia after allogeneic bone marrow transplantation. *British Journal of Haematology*, **56**, 153–6.

Papadopoulos, E.B., Ladanyi, M., Louie, D.C. *et al.* (1994). Infusions of donor leukocytes to treat Epstein-Barr virus-associated lymphoproliferative disorders after allogeneic bone marrow transplantation. *New England Journal of Medicine*, **330**, 1185–91.

Pocock, C.F., Lucas, G.F., Giles, C. *et al.* (2001). Immune neutropenia associated with anti-human neutrophil antigen-2a (NB1) antibodies following unrelated donor stem cell transplantation for chronic myeloid leukaemia: perpetuation by granulocyte colony-stimulating factor. *British Journal of Haematology*, **113**, 483–5.

Qasim, W., Gerritsen, B., & Veys, P. (1998). Case report. Anticardiolipin antibodies and thromboembolism after BMT. *Bone Marrow Transplantation*, **21**, 845–7.

Ratanatharathon, V., Carson, E., Reynolds, C. *et al.* (2000). Anti-CD20 chimeric monoclonal antibody treatment of refractory immune-mediated thrombocytopenia in a patient with chronic graft-versus-host disease. *Annals of Internal Medicine*, **133**, 275–9.

Richard, S., Fruchtman, S., Scigliano, E. *et al.* (2000). An immunological syndrome featuring transverse myelitis, Evan's syndrome and pulmonary infiltrates after unrelated bone marrow transplant in a patient with severe aplastic anemia. *Bone Marrow Transplantation*, **26**, 1225–8.

Roberts, M.M., Dyson, P.G., Willson, K. *et al.* (1996). Peripheral blood stem cells mobilized from patients with acute myeloid leukaemia have different platelet repopulating abilities compared with those mobilized from patients with other diseases. *Bone Marrow Transplantation*, **18**, 41–5.

Rovelli, A., Vallinoto, C., Castellano, M. *et al.* (2001). Rituximab for immune hemolytic anemia following T- and B-cell-depleted bone marrow Transplantation. *Bone Marrow Transplantation*, **27** (Suppl 1), S34 (abstract).

Shimoni, A., Körbling, M., Champlin, R., & Molldrem, J. (2000). Cryofibrinogenemia and skin necrosis in a patient with diffuse large cell lymphoma after high-dose chemotherapy and autologous stem cell transplantation. *Bone Marrow Transplantation*, **26**, 1343–5.

Sivakumaran, M., Hutchinson, R.M., Pringle, H. *et al.* (1995). Thrombocytopenia following autologous bone marrow transplantation: evidence for autoimmune aetiology and B cell clonal involvement. *Bone Marrow Transplantation*, **15**, 531–6.

Sloop, G.D., Friedberg, R.C., & Vaughan, W.P. (1994). Cryoglobulin with cold agglutinin activity complicating allogeneic bone marrow transplantation. *Bone Marrow Transplantation*, **14**, 659–61.

Tamura, T., Kanamori, H., Yamazaki, E. *et al.* (1994). Cold agglutinin disease following allogeneic bone marrow transplantation. *Bone Marrow Transplantation*, **13**, 321–3.

Teruya, J., Styler, M., Verde, S. *et al.* (2001). Questionable efficacy of plasma exchange for thrombotic thrombocytopenic purpura after bone marrow transplantation. *Journal of Clinical Apheresis*, **16**, 169–74.

Tezcan, A.Z., Tezcan, H., Gastineau, D.A. *et al.* (1994). Heparin-induced thrombocytopenia after bone marrow transplantation: report of two cases. *Bone Marrow Transplantation*, **14**, 487–90.

Torok-Storb, B., Boeckh, M., Hoy, C. *et al.* (1997). Association of specific cytomegalovirus (CMV) genotypes with death from myelosuppression after marrow transplantation. *Blood*, **90**, 2097–102.

Tosi, P., Bandini, G., Tazzari, P. *et al.* (1994). Autoimmune neutropenia after unrelated bone marrow transplantation. *Bone Marrow Transplantation*, **14**, 1003–4.

Vannucchi, A.M., Grossi, A., Bosi, A. *et al.* (1991a). Impaired erythropoietin production in mice treated with cyclosporin A. *Blood*, **78**, 1615–18.

Vannucchi, A.M., Longo, G., Bosi, A. *et al.* (1991b). Early hemostatic modifications following cryopreserved graft infusion. *Bone Marrow Transplantation*, **8**, 171–6.

Veelken, H., Wäsch, R., Behringer, D. *et al.* (2000). Pure red cell aplasia after allogeneic stem cell transplantation with reduced conditioning. *Bone Marrow Transplantation*, **26**, 911–5.

Verdonck, L.F., De Gast, G.C., Van Heugten, H.G. *et al.* (1991). Cytomegalovirus infection causes delayed platelet recovery after bone marrow transplantation. *Blood*, **78**, 844–8.

Witherspoon, R.P., Fisher, L.D., Schoch, G. *et al.* (1989). Secondary cancers after bone marrow transplantation for leukemia or aplastic anemia. *New England Journal of Medicine*, **321**, 784–9.

102 Psychosocial complications

RICHARD P. MCQUELLON AND MICHAEL A. ANDRYKOWSKI

Wake Forest University School of Medicine, Winston-Salem, and University of Kentucky College of Medicine, Lexington, USA

Introduction

Hematopoietic stem cell (HSC) transplantation is a physically demanding, life-threatening medical procedure that is highly stressful under the best of circumstances. Major life adjustments are often necessary including geographic dislocation, job interruption, and changes in social and family roles. A lengthy period of hospitalization may be required. Furthermore, the use of physically taxing marrow-ablative therapy, often including total body irradiation (TBI), produces a range of acute and chronic physical complications. Given this number of stressors, it is not surprising that a wide variety of psychosocial complications of HSC transplantation have been documented in the literature (Andrykowski, 1994a, 1994b; Wellisch & Wolcott, 1994; Andrykowski *et al.*, 1995a, 1995b; Hjermstad & Kaasa, 1995; McQuellon *et al.*, 1998; Carlson & MacRae, 2002).

Much of the research related to psychosocial complications with HSC transplant patients is nested within studies that focus on quality of life (QOL). We will not survey the QOL literature in its entirety for this chapter. However, we will make reference to specific studies when they include measures that address psychosocial complications with HSC transplantation (HSCT). Several fine reviews of the QOL literature (Nietzert *et al.*, 1998; Grant, 1999; Carlson & MacRae, 2002) and excellent empirical QOL articles are available (Chiodi *et al.*, 2000). There is also a growing body of literature on late effects for children who have undergone HSC transplantation (Cohen *et al.*, 1998; Cohen *et al.*, 1999; Fisher, 1999). However, there are few studies examining psychosocial complications or QOL in the pediatric HSC transplant setting, a state of affairs largely attributable to difficulties in measuring these constructs in the pediatric setting (Parsons *et al.*, 1999). The focus of this chapter will be on psychosocial complications in adult HSC transplant recipients.

Psychosocial complications: definition and scope

The word *complicate* is made up of the Latin *com* (together) plus *plicare* (to fold). To complicate means to entangle one (problem) with another. A complication in the context of HSC transplantation is defined as any additional physical or psychosocial problem that occurs as a direct result of the treatment itself. Additional problems burden the patient and make recovery that much more difficult. Physical complications of HSC transplantation, such as oropharyngeal mucositis, can cause debilitating pain. Complications can precipitate additional psychological problems such as helplessness, anxiety, or depression. A psychosocial complication is a problem that arises related to the psychological and/or social functioning of the patient. In general, we consider a psychosocial problem a complication of transplant if the patient identifies it as such, if it is associated temporally with the transplant, or if it is identified by the medical team as related to the treatment process.

Psychosocial complications may stem from several sources. First, a formal psychiatric disorder may develop during the course of HSC transplantation. This would constitute a serious treatment-related psychosocial complication (Andrykowski, 1994a). For example, a patient may develop a major depressive episode associated with use of chemotherapeutic or immunosuppressive drugs, sleep deprivation, nutritional compromise, and/or the experience of loss with regard to work or valued social activities. Approximately 20% to 30% of patients experience significant depressive symptoms during or after transplantation (Syrjala *et al.*, 1993; McQuellon *et al.*, 1998; Prieto *et al.*, 2002). Second, a psychosocial complication may stem from interruption of patients' normal developmental tasks of living. This in itself will be more or less problematic depending on a host of factors (Rowland, 1990). For example, a mother with young children will have to give up some of her mothering role, at least temporarily, as she recovers from the effects of the transplant. An adolescent patient may miss enough school to delay promotion. A middle-aged man may need to interrupt his career trajectory in order to recover over the course of an entire year following treatment. A college student will need to drop out of school for one or two semesters. A young couple contemplating starting a family may have to alter their plans in light of infertility resulting from the transplant. Third, patients typically possess certain implicit expectations regarding the likelihood and speed with which they will return to "normal" following transplant (Andrykowski *et al.,* 1995a, 1998a). Psychosocial complications can stem from failure to meet these expectations. For example, frustration and/or depression might result when the patient, who does not understand that profound fatigue is a likely treatment-related side effect of HSC transplant, experiences the debilitating symptoms of fatigue. In this case, frustration and depression are not direct complications of the transplant, but rather stem from the patient's unrealistic expectations for posttransplant recovery. In nearly every study reporting on psychosocial outcomes following HSC transplantation, significant psychosocial complications are identified for a subgroup of patients (Andrykowski, 1994b; Hjermstad & Kaasa, 1995; Baker *et al.,* 1997; Jacobsen *et al.,* 1998; Broers *et al.,* 2000). These include depression, anxiety, fatigue, nausea, pain, posttraumatic stress symptoms, sleep difficulties, employment problems, sexual and relationship problems, financial pressures, family disruption, cognitive dysfunction, decreased self-esteem, and changes in physical appearance affecting social life and recreational pursuits. These psychosocial complications may be reported as mild to severe. Even helpful devices such as Hickman catheters can be very disruptive to some patients (e.g., the long-distance swimmer forced to abandon her primary coping mechanism of swimming) while hardly noticeable to other patients (e.g., the patient who exercises little). It should be noted that these psychosocial complications often occur irrespective of whether or not the transplant can be judged as an objective, medical "success." Thus, patients evidencing good engraftment and no evidence of the underlying disease that necessitated transplant can nevertheless experience a variety of psychosocial complications. Conversely, patients with significant medical complications may evidence few psychosocial complications or even report enhanced psychosocial adjustment and functioning following the procedure (Fromm *et al.,* 1996; Somerfield *et al.,* 1996).

Psychosocial complications across the course of transplantation and recovery

There is a significant amount of empirically based information regarding psychosocial complications associated with HSC transplantation. Much of this information can be found in an extensive and growing literature investigating QOL and psychological adjustment of patients before and after transplantation (see reviews by Andrykowski, 1994a, 1994b; Hjermstad & Kaasa, 1995; Carlson & MacRae, 2002). Review of this literature is facilitated by organization around a set of chronologic stages the patient proceeds through during the transplant process. Specific transplant stages have been identified by a number of authors and have varied from 5 to 11 in number (Brown & Kelly, 1976; Pfefferbaum *et al.,* 1978; Andrykowski & McQuellon, 1998b). Additionally, a sequence of eight "emotional barriers" to HSC transplantation has been described (Jones, 1994). However, for simplicity sake, we have divided the transplant process into three stages: before, during, and after transplant. The sections that follow will highlight the psychosocial complications typically associated with each of these three stages of the transplant process, which are summarized in Table 102.1.

Table 102.1. *Psychosocial complications associated with the different stages of HSC transplantation*

Stage	Complications
Prior to HSC transplant	1. Debilitating existential anxiety and depressive symptoms associated with the possibility of death. 2. Commitment to HSC transplantation prior to obtaining detailed information regarding risk and benefits resulting in posttransplant anger and frustration. 3. Distress associated with formal consent. 4. Misunderstanding of the risks/benefits of HSC transplantation. 5. Spiritual crisis, being "deserted" by God.
Preparative regimen and hospitalization	1. Psychological stress associated with isolation and separation from family, preparative regimen side effects, e.g. mucositis and lengthy hospitalization. 2. Disruption of social and family life. 3. Loss of employment status. 4. Risk for depression associated with fatigue, weakness, unanticipated side effects, and reduced human touch. 5. Demoralization associated with prolonged hospitalization. 6. Emergence of neurocognitive problems, e.g. poor concentration and memory.
Posttransplant; long-term recovery	1. Increased anxiety associated with loss of intensive emotional support of medical team. 2. Caregiver stress associated with necessary home care activities, e.g. catheter care. 3. Noncompliance with self-care requirements. 4. Grief and distress associated with permanent losses, e.g. fertility, job aspirations. 5. Depressive symptoms and discouragement associated with fatigue. 6. Fear of recurrence exacerbated by follow-up visits.

Psychosocial complications prior to HSC transplantation

In contrast to physical complications, psychosocial complications can develop well before initiation of the treatment process itself. Patients may become depressed or anxious when they are initially informed that HSC transplantation is a life-threatening treatment associated with high morbidity risk and is the only potentially curative treatment available for their disease. Trask and colleagues (2002) assessed 50 candidates for HSC transplantation at an initial consultation where it was determined that transplant may be an appropriate treatment option. Approximately 50% reported clinically significant levels of emotional distress and anxiety, while about 20% reported clinically significant levels of depression. For the most part, however, research has focused on the distress experienced by patients in closer temporal proximity to their transplant. In this regard, it has been reported that a significant proportion of adult recipients report depressive symptoms and psychological distress immediately prior to transplantation (Leigh et al., 1995; Grassi et al., 1996; Baker et al., 1997; Broers et al., 2000; Fife et al., 2000). For example, Grassi et al., found that 30% to 50% of their sample evidenced moderate to severe symptoms of anxiety and depression at the time of hospital admission for autologous HSC transplantation. Similarly, Baker et al. reported that 31% of their sample of 437 HSC transplant candidates (both autologous and allogeneic) showed clinically significant levels of depressive symptoms at a pretransplant assessment. In two separate studies, McQuellon and colleagues also reported high levels of pretransplant psychological distress in a significant portion of patients (McQuellon et al., 1996, 1998). In one of these studies, 52 breast cancer patients treated with autologous bone marrow transplantation (BMT) were assessed prior to transplant on the Profile of Mood States—Short Form (POMS-SF), a measure of psychological distress (Cella et al., 1987). Mean scores of BMT patients were significantly higher than a sample of newly diagnosed cancer patients (Cella et al., 1989). Also, scores on the emotional well-being subscale of the Functional Assessment of Cancer Therapy (a measure of QOL) were significantly lower (indicating poorer emotional well-being) than a sample of disease-free breast cancer patients (McQuellon et al., 1995). In a second study of 86 BMT recipients (both allogeneic and autologous), 24% reported significant depressive symptoms at a pre-BMT baseline assessment. Furthermore, mean mood disturbance scores (POMS-SF) at baseline were similar to those of newly diagnosed cancer patients (McQuellon et al., 1998).

Prior to the initiation of pretransplant conditioning therapy, informed consent for the transplant procedure is obtained. This involves a thorough and formal review and discussion of the risks and benefits associated with transplantation, as well as any alternative course of therapy. Significant elevations in psychological distress have been observed in both adult recipients (Dermatis & Lesko, 1991) and in parents of pediatric recipients (Dermatis & Lesko, 1990) within the 48 hours following the provision of informed consent. This is not surprising given that standard consent forms contain detailed descriptions and listings of potential side effects and morbidities associated with the procedure. This suggests that the consent process is likely conducted in the context of distress. Certainly this is the case when a patient is consented on the day of hospital admission for HSC transplantation, the most common procedure for transplant centers. This can negatively impact upon patients' decision-making capabilities, as well as subsequent recall of specific details from the consent discussion (Andrykowski et al., 1995a).

In summary, the period prior to HSC transplantation is one of great psychosocial vulnerability. Research suggests that one-fourth to one-third of HSC transplant patients may evidence clinically significant levels of psychological distress during the period of time immediately prior to initiation of the transplant. Longitudinal studies have suggested that psychological distress might be greatest during the pretransplant period (Fife et al., 2000). However, it is important to recognize that distress at this time is not necessarily directly attributable to patients' anticipation of their impending transplant. Distress prior to transplant is multifactorial in origin. Reports of distress can be attributable to other existing problems unrelated to transplant or may be long-term sequelae associated with prior diagnosis and treatment of their disease. Finally, the physical demands of conditioning regimens may heavily influence the measurement of distress prior to transplant. Psychological assessment during intensive pretransplant conditioning treatment is complicated by the presence of debilitating symptoms such as mucositis, diarrhea, and general malaise.

Regardless of its source, assessment and recognition of pretransplant distress level is important for both the planning of psychosocial support services during the transplant procedure, as well as interpretation of distress evidenced during posttransplant recovery. In addition, distress levels at or near the time of transplant may be linked to survival following transplant. For example, Loberiza and colleagues (2002) reported an association between depressive syndrome and survival in a prospective study of 193 transplant recipients. Prior to transplant, 35% of patients met criteria for a depressive syndrome. There was a significant difference in the 1-year probability of survival for the depressed (85%) and nondepressed patients (94%). Similarly, Molassiotis and colleagues (1997) reported that a shorter survival time following transplant was significantly associated with less hopefulness, higher symptom distress during transplant hospitalization, and greater "acceptance" of the situation. They speculated that these psychosocial variables may negatively impact immune function, directly affecting survival, or they may act indirectly by producing other behaviors known to affect survival in cancer patients. In contrast to the results of these two studies, Murphy and colleagues (1996) reported no relationship between posttransplant survival and the presence of depression at the time of transplant. While reports of a relationship between psychosocial variables, such as depression or distress, and posttransplant survival are intriguing, the research is far from definitive. It is likely that any existing relationship between psychological stress and survival is relatively weak and difficult to detect. Tumor biology and posttransplant medical complications are likely to be the most powerful factors in determining survival in HSC transplant recipients.

Psychosocial complications during HSC transplantation

This phase begins with initiation of the pretransplant conditioning. It continues through hospital discharge or, in the instance of HSC transplantation delivered in an outpatient setting, until the patient is no longer under the continuous monitoring and care of the transplant medical staff. Our clinical experience suggests that the principal psychosocial complications that emerge at this time revolve around four issues:

1. tolerance of the acute side effects of treatment;
2. coping with infection control procedures and a prolonged period of hospitalization;
3. the emergence of neurologic symptoms that are organic in origin;
4. coping with the eventual withdrawal of the round-the-clock medical monitoring and care characteristic of the HSC transplant setting.

Pretransplant conditioning therapy causes a host of acute side effects including nausea and vomiting, fatigue, hair loss, and painful mouth ulceration. These side effects typically continue for a few days to even a few weeks after the conditioning treatment has been completed (Chapko et al., 1989). Side effects can be severe, even when supportive care is optimal. If severe and prolonged, these side effects can result in anxiety and depression. Even though not life-threatening, hair loss or other appearance changes stemming from treatment can diminish self-esteem. Demoralization can result, sapping the patients' psychological strength and ability to cope with additional stressors.

Many patients hold unrealistic expectations for their recovery and may anticipate only a short period of hospitalization and a quick return to their homes and routine activities (Andrykowski et al., 1998a). Medical complications may arise, however, necessitating a prolonged period of hospitalization. Violation of patients' expectations for posttransplant recovery can be profoundly demoralizing. This is particularly true if a tentative discharge date has been set, only to be postponed. Some patients respond to this disappointment with depression and lethargy, while others respond with anger and agitation. In extreme cases patients may threaten or attempt to leave the transplant unit against medical advice, when they are highly vulnerable to infection or other life-threatening medical complications.

In addition to the potential for stress-related anxiety and depressive reactions, patients are at risk for a variety of neurocognitive or neurologic problems during and following transplantation (Ahles et al., 1996; and see Chapter 93). Episodes of delirium can occur and may last for several hours or several days. During these episodes patients might evidence alterations of consciousness, distorted sensory or perceptual function (e.g., hallucinations), mood swings, impaired social judgment, sleep disturbance, or impaired memory and concentration. The occurrence of these symptoms can be frightening to both the patient and family. Many factors in the HSC transplant setting can underlie these symptoms including central nervous system (CNS) disease, infection, immunosuppressive medications, liver or renal dysfunction, and respiratory compromise (Wellisch & Wolcott, 1994; Gallardo et al., 1996). Symptom resolution often occurs when the underlying organic pathology is identified and addressed.

Finally, while prolonged hospitalization and strict infection control procedures can produce distress and feelings of isolation, the fact that the medical team is immediately available to provide medical assistance and support can also be quite comforting. As a result, hospital discharge can be both an eagerly anticipated milestone as well as a source of anxiety and insecurity. Fears that life-threatening problems might arise when appropriate medical assistance is not readily available can temper the excitement and positive anticipation associated with hospital discharge and the return home. A similar stressor occurs for the patient and family when the patient is transferred out of the protective, familiar environment of the specialized transplant unit into a "step-down bed" in a general oncology unit.

In one of the more ambitious studies of psychosocial complications during the actual transplant phase, HSC transplant patients participated in a structured psychiatric assessment at the time of pretransplant hospital admission and weekly thereafter until hospital discharge (Prieto et al., 2002). The presence of a psychiatric disorder was identified on the basis of the *Diagnostic and Statistical Manual of Mental Disorders, Fourth Edition (DSM-IV)*. An overall prevalence rate of 44% for psychiatric disorders during hospitalization was reported. Adjustment disorders were evident in 22.7% of patients, mood disorders in 14.1%, and anxiety disorders in 8.2%. Delirium was diagnosed in 7.3% of patients. Importantly, a diagnosis of any mood, anxiety, or adjustment disorder was associated with increased length of stay in the hospital, even after adjusting for risk factors at admission. The authors concluded that psychiatric morbidity is associated with increased length of hospital stay in the transplant setting. Given the financial pressures evident in modern medicine, this information is critically important and it suggests that adequate attention be devoted to prevention and management of psychosocial complications during the period of transplant hospitalization.

Psychosocial complications following HSC transplantation

Discharge from the hospital and the return home signals the beginning of an often lengthy process of recovery and life reintegration. The major psychosocial complications characteristic of this phase revolve around coping with the physical aftermath of HSC transplantation as well as managing the uncertainty associated with the ever-present possibility of disease recurrence. While most patients anticipate that they will eventually "return to normal" following transplant, both physically and psychosocially, only a minority actually do (Andrykowski et al., 1995a). A variety of physical late effects of HSC transplantation have been recognized, including pulmonary problems, cataracts, sterility, joint pain, chronic graft-versus-host disease (GVHD), secondary malignancies, and weakness and fatigue (e.g., Kolb & Poetscher, 1997; Kauppila et al., 1998; Niethammer & Mayer, 1998; Kolb et al., 1999; Thomas et al., 2001). While some of these late effects eventually resolve, others are permanent. These physical late effects can have a profound impact on the patient's ability to resume a normal lifestyle following the transplant. Occupational, educational, and recreational activities can be disrupted. The patient's ability to function in the role of parent or spouse can be impaired. Maintenance or establishment of satisfying interpersonal relationships with family and friends can also be negatively impacted. Coping with these changes and losses following transplant constitutes a singular challenge and is the primary source of the psychosocial complications associated with the posttransplant recovery phase.

What is known about psychosocial complications associated with posttransplant recovery can be gleaned from a now rather large body of research, which has examined QOL and psychological adjustment following HSC transplantation. These complications will be reviewed with particular emphasis on the most frequently reported complications: depressive symptoms, anxiety, fatigue and energy depletion, and sexual difficulties. Sleep difficulties can also have a profound effect on mood and they are most likely the result of a variety of physical assaults including various medications and constant disruptions of the sleep cycle during hospitalization. We consider sleep difficulties as a causative factor in mood disturbance and social disruption and not necessarily a separate psychosocial complication.

Syrjala et al. (1993) conducted the first prospective study of long-term recovery after transplant. A total of 67 adult allogeneic transplant recipients were assessed at several points in time: prior to hospital admission, 90 days posttransplant, and 1 and 2 years posttransplant. Prior to transplant, 21% of patients scored in the mildly depressed range and 6% in the moderately depressed range. Significant numbers of patients still evidenced high levels of anxiety (48%) or mild to moderate depression (37%) at the 1-year follow-up. More marked emotional distress at the 1-year follow-up was associated with the presence of family conflict at baseline and nonmarried status. The authors concluded that the psychological issues facing transplant recipients after 1 year are very similar to those faced by other young adult survivors of less aggressive, conventional cancer therapies. These include fear of recurrence, fertility and employment-related concerns, energy loss, and family disruption.

The majority of research relevant to understanding the psychosocial complications associated with the posttransplant recovery phase has been retrospective and cross-sectional in design. For example, Andrykowski et al. (1995b) assessed 200 autologous and allogeneic BMT recipients a mean of approximately 3 years posttransplant. Respondents were recruited from five different transplant centers. Specific areas of common difficulty included energy level, occupational functioning, sleep, and sexual relationships and functioning. Patients tended to evidence significant difficulty with weakness, fatigue, and the ability to engage in vigorous activities. Health difficulties resulted in one-third of the sample being unemployed or retired. Approximately 12% of respondents were considered to be experiencing serious dysfunction in their sexual relationships.

Follow-up data from two prospective, longitudinal studies also shed light on the psychosocial complications experienced following transplant. In the first study (McQuellon et al., 1996), women (n = 24) were assessed from 3 to 17 months after autologous BMT for breast cancer. About one-third reported significant levels of depressive symptoms at this time. Additionally, 25% or more reported concerns in the following areas: job or work situation, finances, general physical health, general frame of mind, appearance, health or life insurance, personal and/or physical relations, and planning for the future. The second study included both autologous and allogeneic BMT recipients (McQuellon et al., 1998). Patients were assessed at discharge (n = 74) and at 100 (n = 64) days and 1 year posttransplant (n = 45). The proportion of patients reporting significant levels of depressive symptoms at these three assessments was 28%, 32%, and 20%, respectively. Slightly less than one-half of the sample (43%) reported significant levels of depressive symptoms during at least one of the three post-BMT assessment points. Finally, patients reported their current energy level as a percentage of their "normal" energy level (normal = 100%) at each of the three posttransplant assessments. Results indicated that energy level increased across the three points of assessment with mean percentages at hospital discharge, 100 days post-BMT, and 1-year post-BMT of 46%, 58%, and 70%, respectively.

Leigh et al. (1995) assessed 31 BMT patients prior to transplant and again approximately 4 and 8 months after the procedure. Prior to transplant, about one-fourth (22%) of the sample were diagnosed as suffering from an anxiety state and 19% from depressive illness as measured by the Hospital Anxiety and Depression Scale (HAD) and the Present State Examination scale (PSE). At 4 months, 9% of the sample were diagnosed with anxiety states and 31% with significant depressive symptoms. At the 8-month follow-up, 6% were diagnosed as suffering from an anxiety state while 19% were described as having depressive illnesses.

Prieto et al. (1996) surveyed 117 allogeneic and autologous HSC transplant survivors a mean of 55 months posttransplant. Patients reported poor functioning in areas of physical ability, work, and sex life when compared with a British reference population. Psychiatric case rates in the HSCT recipients were significantly higher (22%) than the general reference population utilized (9%). Cross-sectional analyses suggested that QOL and psychosocial distress improved with increased time posttransplant.

Bush et al. (1995) surveyed 125 adults surviving 6 to 18 years (mean of 10.1 years) after autologous or allogeneic BMT. Incidence rates for various difficulties as measured by the European Organization for Research and Treatment of Cancer questionnaire (EORTC QLQ-C30) were as follows: emotional dysfunction (63.3%), sleep disturbance (42.7%), cognitive dysfunction (38.9%), fear of relapse and dying (38.7%), social dysfunction (32.3%), and fatigue (55.9%). Ninety-six percent of the recipients indicated people were less supportive over time and that this was the single most distressing hardship of long-term survival. Twenty-seven percent of survivors were dissatisfied with their appearance and between 28% and 36% of respondents were dissatisfied with their sexual appeal, ability to share warmth and intimacy, or interest in sexual thoughts or feelings. More than 26% of patients said that they had physical problems that reduced their satisfaction with sex and intimacy.

Molassiotis et al. (1995) assessed QOL in a sample of 50 autologous and allogeneic recipients a mean of 42 months posttransplant. Twenty-five percent of patients in both groups had failed to return to work or student status and nearly 10% had difficulty in carrying out daily tasks. Among autologous recipients, 22% had clinical signs of anxiety and 10% clinical signs of depression. No cases of clinical depression were identified in the allogeneic patients with 10% evidencing clinical signs of anxiety.

In a detailed study of sexuality in survivors of BMT, the sexual satisfaction of 126 allogeneic and autologous BMT patients from 6 to 149 months posttransplant was examined (Wingard et al., 1992). Twenty-two percent of respondents indicated dissatisfaction with their sexual life. Reported satisfaction was associated with gonadal hormonal levels in both men and women, restoration of menses in women, and freedom from erectile or ejaculatory problems in men. Satisfaction with appearance and overall life satisfaction was associated with sexual satisfaction. The authors reported that one-third of the sample was not happy with their ability to obtain sexual satisfaction. Other studies have also reported difficulties in the area of sexuality following transplantation (Molassiotis et al., 1995; Marks et al., 1996; McQuellon et al., 1996, 1998).

Hann et al. (1997) examined fatigue, sleep quality, and psychological distress in 44 women from 3 to 62 months after autologous BMT for breast cancer. BMT patients reported significantly more frequent and severe fatigue than a comparison group of healthy women with no history of cancer. About one-third of BMT patients reported depressive symptoms, considerably higher than the 5% incidence rate for depressive symptoms in the healthy comparison group. Finally, BMT recipients reported significantly longer sleep latency and poorer sleep efficiency relative to the healthy comparison group.

The extent to which illness intruded on survivors' lives following autologous BMT was evaluated by Schimmer et al.

(2001). Forty-four consecutive autologous BMT survivors seen at a long-term follow-up clinic completed a series of questionnaires. Mean time post BMT treatment to the evaluation point was 4.6 years (± 2.8 years). Mean illness intrusive ratings scale scores for BMT patients were higher than lung or liver transplant recipients and comparable to kidney and heart transplant recipients. Higher scores among these groups were related to increase of disruption in health, work, financial situation, and active recreation. Even after long-term remission following BMT, recipients continued to experience intrusiveness of their illness that compromised subjective well-being.

One other study reported on patient survivorship 3 years after treatment (McQuellon et al., 1999). A total of 30 patients who had participated in an earlier study (McQuellon et al., 1998) were assessed. The following number and percentage of patients reported a lack of energy, $n = 12$ (40%); being bothered by side effects of treatment, $n = 14$ (47%); or tiring easily, $n = 20$ (67%). Five patients (16%) scored greater than 16 on the Center for Epidemiologic Studies–Depression (CES-D) scale, indicating the presence of significant depressive symptoms. However, in spite of these problems the majority of recipients (87%), reported satisfaction with their current quality of life. While instrumental social support (e.g., help with daily tasks) declined over the course of survivorship, in contrast to the findings of Bush et al. (1995), overall social support was reported as high relative to general population norms.

Several studies have investigated the possibility that posttraumatic stress disorder (PTSD) symptoms might be a psychosocial complication following the treatment of breast cancer (Cordova et al., 1995) and after transplantation (Jacobsen et al., 1998, 2002). Estimates of prevalence rates among transplant recipients ranged from 12% to 19%. While this is not a common complication, PTSD does warrant some attention since the presence of PTSD can be debilitating and may interfere with appropriate medical follow-up.

Psychosocial concerns following HSC transplantation

The documentation of the nature and extent of psychosocial complications associated with the posttransplant recovery phase is critical. However, this approach may yield a somewhat misleading picture of the salient psychosocial problems and difficulties experienced by the transplant recipient. Psychosocial complications likely vary in the degree of concern that they generate from the perspective of the transplant recipient. For example, while difficulties in sexual functioning might be rather common in transplant recipients and their origin might be traced directly to the transplant itself, sexual functioning might not be of great *concern* to the transplant recipient. Clearly, clinical management efforts should be targeted toward those psychosocial complications that are of greatest concern at the time that these issues are most salient to the recipient. In light of this, several studies have examined recipients' concerns following transplantation. Andrykowski and colleagues (1999) examined the psychosocial concerns of 110 SCT recipients (87% autologous). Participants ranged from 3 to 62 months posttransplantation with a mean of 17 months. The authors concluded that some concerns are salient over the entire posttransplant course. These included the threat of disease recurrence, reduced energy level and fatigue, and questioning whether they would ever "return to normal." In contrast to these more ubiquitous concerns, some concerns appeared to be more salient early in the course of posttransplant recovery. These included the quality of medical care received and overprotectiveness of the recipient by family and friends. Still other concerns seemed to emerge only later in the course of posttransplant recovery. These included issues regarding feelings of tension or anxiety, as well as concerns regarding sleep difficulties, sexual functioning, relationship with their spouse or partner, and their ability to be affectionate. McQuellon *et al.* (1998) surveyed transplant recipients' concerns at hospital discharge and again at 100 days and 1 year posttransplant. A significant relationship was observed between time since transplant and the specific concerns voiced by recipients. With increased time posttransplant, patients reported increasing concerns regarding finances, insurance status, employment, intimate relationships, including changes in their relationships with family and friends, physical health, their "frame of mind," and their ability to plan for the future. The investigators hypothesized that as the active care of physical difficulties associated with transplantation lessened over the course of time, patients may become "freed up" psychologically to address other areas of their life such as job functioning and interpersonal relationships. If true, this has clear implications for clinical management of the psychosocial complications and concerns of transplant recipients: monitoring and care must be continuous, recognizing that recipient concerns are an evolving phenomenon with many concerns emerging and becoming salient only after considerable time has passed following transplant.

Factors moderating the development of psychosocial complications

The nature and extent of psychosocial complications actually experienced by HSC recipients varies widely. There are a number of factors that can influence the nature and extent of psychosocial complications that may arise over the course of HSC transplantation and recovery. Patient-related factors, such as the extent to which patients possess an optimistic versus pessimistic outlook, flexibility, fighting spirit, hardiness, and a host of other characteristics may reduce the likelihood of psychosocial complications. Such characteristics can be seen as "buffering" the HSC recipient from the stresses associated with the transplant experience, resulting in fewer psychosocial complications. In addition, there is some evidence to suggest that distancing and cognitive escape-avoidance coping styles may be associated with greater mood disturbance and poorer QOL outcomes (Biesecker *et al.*, 2000; Jacobsen *et al.*, 2002).

Potential resources that reduce the likelihood of developing psychosocial complications are listed in Table 102.2.

In addition to the dispositional factors cited in the preceding paragraph, there are social-environmental factors that may reduce risk for psychosocial complications in the HSC transplant recipient. Chief among these is the social support afforded the recipient. This includes not only support from the recipient's family but also support provided by physicians, nurses, housekeeping and food service workers, and clerical personnel. Allied health care providers (recreation therapy, social work services, pastoral care, and psychosocial services) also play a pivotal supportive role during the transplant process. While support from spouse and family is critical throughout the course of HSC transplant and recovery, support from clinic and hospital personnel plays a crucial role during the transplant hospitalization. It is important to recognize that HSC transplant recipients will vary with regard to their utilization and engagement of the support offered by different providers of supportive services. Social support during the HSC transplant process has been reported as excellent relative to the general population (McQuellon *et al.*, 1998). However, some survivors report reduced social support over time as a source of distress (Bush *et al.*, 1995). Both the timing, extent, and nature of supportive services may differ, depending largely on recipient preference. For example, some transplant recipients request frequent prayer with the chaplain on duty in the transplant unit, while others may seek relaxation and imagery training.

The impact of both dispositional and social-environmental factors in reducing (or increasing) risk for psychosocial complications in the HSC transplant setting has been not been systematically studied to any great degree. Thus the extent to which each class of factors moderates distress associated with the transplant procedure is unknown. There is a clear need for research that can expand understanding of the factors that moderate risk for development of psychosocial complications in the HSC transplant recipient. To a large degree, understanding of

Table 102.2. *Potential resources that reduce the likelihood of the development of psychosocial complications*

1. The extent to which referral source and medical team prepare the patient with realistic expectations with regard to HSC transplantation.
2. The degree of psychosocial support provided by the medical team and allied health team professionals before, during, and after hospitalization.
3. The coping resources of the individual patient, e.g., optimism, psychological flexibility, use of meditation and relaxation techniques.
4. The presence of a primary support person, e.g., spouse, parent, sibling, friend, throughout hospitalization and home care.
5. The accessibility of professional psychosocial support resources before, during, and after transplantation.
6. The extent to which the patient has been prepared for follow-up care postdischarge.

these "buffering" factors provides a foundation for enhanced efforts to improve and focus supportive care services in the transplant setting.

Psychosocial assessment prior to HSC transplantation

Prospective identification of patients at greatest risk for psychosocial complications following HSC transplant remains an important, yet elusive, goal. As a first step toward accomplishing this, current standard of care for all HSC transplant patients includes completion of a psychosocial or psychiatric assessment immediately prior to transplantation (Phillips *et al.*, 1997). Assessment at this time is generally not for the purpose of "screening out" poor transplant candidates. Most potential recipients at this point in time are unlikely to possess a major psychiatric disorder or other psychological or social problems that would preclude transplantation. Rather, assessment at this time is for the purpose of identifying those patients who are more likely to develop psychosocial complications pursuant to transplantation and thus might merit additional clinical attention. Several structured clinical assessment tools have been developed for use prior to HSC transplant. These include the Psychosocial Level System (PLS) (Futterman *et al.*, 1991) and a revision of the PLS called the Transplant Evaluation Rating Scale (TERS) (Twillman *et al.*, 1993). The PLS was validated on HSC transplant patients while the TERS was validated on liver transplant patients. Both the PLS and TERS employ psychosocial information such as psychiatric history, current support network, and history of substance abuse and coping style to categorize transplant patients as at either low, medium, or high risk for psychosocial complications during active treatment as well as during posttransplant follow-up (Table 102.3). While the approach is intuitively appealing, there has been little systematic investigation of the utility of the PLS and TERS for identifying patients at high risk for psychosocial complica-

tions in the HSC transplant setting. For the most part, the information gathered by the PLS and TERS is that which a mental health professional would routinely gather during the course of a thorough clinical interview. In this context, an informal prediction of risk for psychosocial complications during the inpatient stay, as well as during the course of posttransplant recovery, could be made in light of the risk factors identified in the clinical interview. No systematic effort has been made to determine whether or not structured approaches such as the TERS or PLS allow for better identification of patients at high risk for psychosocial complications than a standard clinical interview.

A number of standardized assessment instruments have proven useful as an adjunct to the clinical interview in the HSC transplant setting. Some representative instruments are listed and described in Table 102.4. The rationale for the use of these instruments is to gather more comprehensive data in addition to the clinical interview. This information can then be used to guide judgments regarding likely clinical service requirements of patients over the course of the transplant and recovery process. Additionally, these assessments can then constitute an appropriate and useful baseline for research efforts examining the long-term impact of HSC transplantation. Conducting the clinical interview and requesting completion of additional specific assessment instruments communicates to the patient the importance of their psychological well-being. This process also "normalizes" the presence of trained mental health personnel as part of the on-site clinical management team. Many transplant patients and family members view the pretransplant psychosocial assessment as comforting and indicative of a comprehensive concern for the HSC transplant recipient's well-being.

Psychosocial complications and the stem cell donor

Allogeneic HSC transplantation requires that normal marrow or blood stem cells be collected from a living donor and infused into the patient recipient. Clinical experience suggests

Table 102.3. *Predicting level of psychosocial adjustment with the transplant evaluation rating scale (Twillman et al., 1993)*

Level of risk	Psychosocial characteristics
Level One: Patients at low risk for developing psychosocial complications	No prior psychiatric history or substance use/abuse history. Good health behaviors and appropriate compliance during treatment. Excellent family support and history of coping. Appropriate fears and sadness but excellent history of coping with the disease and excellent mental status including cognitive functioning.
Level Two: Patients at moderate risk for developing psychosocial complications	Some psychiatric symptoms and a history of significant substance use/abuse. Partial compliance with previous treatment and some change in health behaviors only after diagnosis was made. Family, social support, and individual coping history only fair. Some denial and lack of clarity over the illness. Moderate fears, anxiety, and depressive symptoms. Some impairment in cognitive functions.
Level Three: Patients at high risk for developing psychosocial complications	Current diagnosis of psychiatric disorder and extensive history of substance use/abuse. History of noncompliance with medical care and poor health behaviors. Poor social/family support and coping skills. Extreme denial over the illness and ambivalence about treatment. Generalized anxiety, severe depressive symptoms, and global disorder of cognitive functions.

Table 102.4. *Self-report psychological assessment instruments*

Instrument	Description
Symptom Specific	
Center for Epidemiologic Studies–Depression (CES-D) scale (Radloff, 1977)	Developed as a 20-item screening instrument; useful in identifying degree of depressive symptoms in patients who may need further clinical evaluation. Two items measure physical well-being reducing overall impact of physical functioning on diagnosis of depression.
Beck Depression Inventory (BDI) (Beck & Steer, 1987)	21-item questionnaire designed to assess severity of depression; includes items that measure physical symptoms which may be common in a medical population.
Brief Symptom Inventory (BSI) (Derogatis & Mellsaratos, 1983)	53 items, 9 scales measuring somatization, anxiety, depression, hostility, phobic anxiety, interpersonal sensitivity, obsessive compulsiveness, etc. and 3 indices of global distress.
Hospital Anxiety and Depression Scale (HADS) (Ford *et al.*, 1995)	14-item questionnaire that assesses anxiety and depression in medical patients. Somatic items have been removed. Cutoff scores identified for nonclinical, subclinical, and clinical levels of anxiety and depression.
National Cancer Center Network (NCCN) Distress Thermometer (DT) (Holland, 1997)	A modified visual analog scale depicted as a thermometer ranging from 0 (no distress) to 10 (extreme distress). Patients rate their general distress level.
General Quality of Life Instruments	
Functional Assessment of Cancer Therapy–G (FACT-G) (Cella *et al.*, 1993)	27 items assess physical, functional, social/family, and emotional well-being and provide a total overall score. Disease site, treatment, and symptom-specific modules available including a BMT module (McQuellon *et al.*, 1996). Translated into over 40 languages.
The European Organization for Research and Treatment of Cancer Quality of Life Questionnaire (EORTC-QLQ) (Aaronson *et al.*, 1993)	49 items assess physical, functional, emotional, family, social and occupational functioning and treatment satisfaction. Includes disease-specific modules and has been translated into many different languages for international use.
Cancer Rehabilitation Evaluation System (CARES)(Ganz *et al.*, 1986)	139 items measure physical, functional, family, emotional, sexual, social, occupational, and treatment satisfaction. Identifies problem areas and asks if patient wants to address.
Social Support Medical Outcome Study – Social Support Survey (Sherbourne & Stewart, 1991)	21 items measure perceived social support. Includes subscales for emotional/informational, tangible, positive interaction affection, and an overall index.

that the allogeneic donor might evidence a wide range of psychosocial complications following donation. The nature and extent of these complications is largely dependent on the outcomes experienced by the transplant recipient and the psychological characteristics of the donor. We have encountered donors who have been traumatized by the experience and describe symptoms suggestive of PTSD. We have also encountered donors who viewed the donation experience as no different than donating blood. Fortunately, while it appears that there are some "donor casualties," the vast majority of HSC donors adjust well to the procedure and its aftermath. Most of the research in this area has examined the experience of unrelated marrow donors recruited through the United States National Marrow Donor Program. In one study, 50 donors were interviewed prior to marrow donation and again at 1 to 2 weeks and at 1 year postdonation (Butterworth *et al.*, 1993). At the 1 to 2 week postdonation interview, a sizable minority of donors described the donation as stressful and inconvenient. Twelve percent reported some degree of worry about their own health. However, at the 1-year assessment, 91% of donors said that they would be willing to

donate again in the future. In an important study investigating unrelated donors' experience following the death of the recipient, researchers found that few donors reported feelings of guilt and responsibility regarding the recipient's death (Butterworth, 1992). However, most donors experienced grief that was surprisingly intense, given that the recipient was unknown to them prior to donation.

While limited by its small sample size, a study by Wolcott *et al.* (1986) provided important information regarding the donation experience from the standpoint of the related donor. In this study, 18 adult related donors whose recipient was alive were surveyed. Significantly, 10% to 20% of donors reported negative feelings and/or experiences associated with their donation of bone marrow. Current quality of the donor-recipient relationship was positively correlated with the health and psychosocial status of the recipient.

It is likely that the extent of psychosocial complications for the HSC transplant donor varies as a function of the donor-recipient relationship. For unrelated donors who do not know the recipient and do not choose to meet the recipient following donation, it is unlikely that negative sequelae will develop. However, even if the outcome is unknown, the donor may have some distress and a sense of incompleteness with regard to donation. When recipients are known to the donor or are a relative, complex dynamics can be set in motion. For example, for the relative who is the only match for their sibling, there may be pressure to donate, even in the face of overwhelming fears and concerns for the procedure. A donor entering the process under pressure may feel resentment and anger at "being trapped." In highly publicized cases, parents have been known to conceive in order to produce a donor for a sick child in the family. No research has been conducted to investigate the postdonation sequelae or impact on the family of this unusual situation.

Additionally, at the present time, there are no data regarding psychosocial complications in donors who have given blood stem cells (by apheresis) as opposed to bone marrow (by percutaneous punctures), the former being a less invasive procedure.

Psychosocial complications and the caregiver: medical and nursing staff

Provision of medical and nursing care for the HSC transplant patient can be both physically and psychologically taxing. The need to work long hours, the often volatile physical condition of patients, the need to provide emotional care and support for both patients and family as they cope with their fears and anxieties, and the realization that things may take a sudden turn for the worse despite excellent provision of care, all contribute to the likelihood that medical and nursing staff may experience considerable distress as a result of the day-to-day performance of their duties. Despite this, there has been little research examining the psychological impact of providing medical and nursing care upon professional caregivers in the HSC transplant setting. A study by Molassiotis and colleagues represents the state-of-the art in this area (1995b). A sample of both HSC transplant physicians and nurses was queried regarding types and sources of occupational stress, the perceived consequences of such occupational stress, and strategies employed to reduce occupational stress. Results indicated that the main occupational stresses for doctors and nurses on an HSC transplant unit were interpersonal staff conflicts (22% and 20%, respectively), excessive responsibility (15% and 24%), and highly demanding patients and families (12% and 20%). Other occupational stresses identified by both groups were advances in transplant technology (5% and 12%) and long work shifts (7% and 8%). Primary sources of stress in both nurses and doctors were regular work with dying patients (41% and 20%, respectively), ethical and moral problems (19% and 13%), and managing intensive care and emergency situations (14% and 22%). Regarding the perceived consequences of these occupational stresses, nurses and physicians most frequently cited increased illness (37% and 19%, respectively), reduced productivity (29% and 31%), and increased clinical errors (23% and 27%). Importantly, the majority of nurses and physicians reported difficulties in their personal or social lives as a result of work-

related stress (74% and 56%, respectively). Finally, it was noteworthy that most nurses reported utilizing stress-reducing techniques while few physicians reporting doing so. Nurses attempted to reduce their stress through informal gatherings with colleagues, formal support meetings, consultation with multidisciplinary teams, workshops or inservice training, psychosocial meetings, private consultations with a psychologist, and new staff orientation/support programs. Both nurses and physicians agreed that the most effective means of reducing occupational stress were informal gatherings or formal support meetings. Clearly there is a strong need for developing effective means for enabling HSC transplant medical and nursing staff to cope with the many stresses associated with their work. Innovative programs for providing HSC transplant staff with psychosocial support have been described (Sarantos, 1988) but their effectiveness remains largely unevaluated.

In some respects, the lack of research interest regarding the psychosocial impact of the HSC transplant caregiving experience upon medical and nursing staff is surprising. The HSC transplant unit essentially functions with all of the stressors characteristic of an intensive care unit (ICU), yet with few of the psychological safeguards typically associated with ICUs. In an ICU, nursing staff typically rotate to care for different patients, so that they do not spend long periods of time with specific patients. This reduces the likelihood of an intense attachment developing with patients who are generally at a high risk for dying. This strategy is seen as reducing the stress experienced by ICU staff. In contrast, in the HSC transplant unit, nursing staff are often assigned to focus on providing care to a specific patient or small set of patients. Provision of such care day after day can result in the development of significant attachment to patients, with a consequently enhanced risk for intense bereavement should a patient die (Kelly *et al.*, 2000). Furthermore, recent developments in the HSC transplant field have placed additional burdens on professional staff. The recent near elimination of HSC transplant as a viable treatment option for breast cancer has resulted in a pronounced reduction in the number of patients that are seen at many transplant centers, at least in the United States. This has necessitated administrative changes that place additional stress on nursing staff. Specifically, since HSC transplant units can function as intensive care units, they are increasingly called upon to house and care for patients who are very seriously ill but have not undergone HSC transplantation. A decreased demand for HSC transplantation can result in frequent shuffling of staff, which disrupts the development of team cohesiveness on the transplant unit. This can have a negative effect on morale.

Psychosocial complications and the caregiver: spouse and family

During and following HSC transplant, the patient typically relies on his or her spouse, partner, or another family member for help with medical care, as well as many routine activities of daily living. The family caregiver is often at the bedside day in and day out, weeks on end, suffering along with the recipient without the benefits of direct physical and emotional care from staff members. Following hospitalization, the family caregiver becomes the primary caregiver for the patient and support for the caregiver may be even less, as attention is generally focused on the recovering recipient's needs and concerns. It is nearly axiomatic among health care professionals that the family caregiver of the HSC transplant recipient will be taxed to their psychological and physical limits by the caregiving process.

Despite this assumption, only a few studies have examined the impact of the HSC transplant experience on the family caregiver. Grimm and colleagues (2000) studied 43 caregivers of patients undergoing either autologous or allogeneic transplantation. Their primary research question was whether an inpatient/outpatient (IPOP) approach to transplant was more or less stressful to the caregiver than a strictly inpatient approach to transplant. Data were collected at six different points in time beginning with a baseline prior to transplant and continuing on through 12 months posttransplant. The authors concluded that the IPOP model of care was less emotionally distressing for family caregivers. Keogh and colleagues (1998) examined the psychological adaptation of both HSC transplant patients and family members using a prospective, longitudinal research design. Twenty-eight transplant patients and their relatives were interviewed prior to transplant and at 3, 6, and 12 months posttransplant. Eighty-eight percent of relatives reported considerable psychological distress at both the pretransplant and 3 month posttransplant assessments. This distress had largely dissipated by 12 months posttransplant. Interestingly, patients' physical and psychological well-being was largely unrelated to relatives' distress levels except at the 3-month posttransplant assessment. This suggests that distress in family caregivers should be closely monitored, even when the patient is doing well both physically and psychologically.

The impact of the HSC transplant experience on family caregivers is profound. The combination of psychological and physical stressors, when experienced in the context of often inadequate social support, may be equally as toxic as that experienced by the recipient. Given these circumstances, it is all the more remarkable to us how well family caregivers function. This is clearly a neglected area for research, although some progress is being made. Weitzner and colleagues (1998) have developed a Caregiver Quality of Life–Cancer (CQOLC) scale. While not utilized to date in the transplant setting, this scale is a promising tool for examining what family caregivers encounter in the process of helping their loved one to heal.

Conclusions

Psychosocial complications can develop at any time over the course of HSC transplantation, beginning with the initial recognition of transplantation as a treatment option, through the acute hospitalization and treatment phase, and continuing through long-term recovery. Most psychosocial complications lessen as the physical symptoms, psychological distress, and

social effects associated with disease and treatment themselves diminish. While most disease-free patients probably re-establish a comfortable psychosocial equilibrium within 1 to 3 years of transplant, some patients never recover emotionally and socially from their transplant experience (Andrykowski et al., 1995a). This is true even when the transplant has been successful from a medical standpoint. Why some patients remain psychosocially scarred several years or more after HSC transplant is perplexing. Such patients are likely those for whom the physical complications of transplantation have been the most severe and most limiting. They are also likely those patients who have the greatest difficulty in coping with the ever-present fear of disease recurrence, fears that may be triggered with each unexplained pain or follow-up physician appointment and round of medical tests. There is also some evidence to suggest that family conflict and lack of social support may inhibit psychosocial recovery in these patients (Syrjala et al., 1993).

Several additional issues are important to consider with regard to the psychosocial complications of HSC transplantation. First, little to nothing is known regarding psychosocial complications in relapsed patients. This is a glaring omission in view of the stress associated with recurrent illness (Cella et al., 1990), and the implications of disease recurrence when the best curative treatment procedure has been expended. It is likely that the incidence of emotional problems (e.g., existential anxiety and depression) is very high in relapsed patients confronting a limited lifespan and no available curative treatment. Second, a psychosocial complication for the recipient is almost always a problem for family members and immediate caregivers. The little research that is available suggests that financial burdens, insurance and employment difficulties, and sexual and role-resumption difficulties all pose significant obstacles to the optimal functioning of the recipient's family (Zabora et al., 1992). This may be especially true when the full financial burden of the transplant comes due during the extended recovery, when the recipient is unable to return to work as anticipated and/or significant medical bills accumulate. There is even some evidence suggesting that the transplant procedure is so stressful for caregivers that it can alter their own immune functioning (Futterman et al., 1996).

HSC transplantation is a continually evolving medical and technical procedure. As a result, the nature and extent of psychosocial complications associated with HSC transplantation is also likely evolving. Recent developments in transplant technology have the potential to produce fewer psychosocial complications and consequently improved QOL in transplant recipients. Colony-stimulating factors (CSFs) are now widely used in the transplant setting to facilitate engraftment. Several studies have examined the impact of CSFs on the QOL of HSC transplant recipients. A recent review of this literature (Godder & Henslee-Downey, 2001) concluded that use of CSFs, specifically sargramostim and filgrastim, was associated with better QOL in the early posttransplant period. By reducing time to engraftment, CSFs are likely to reduce psychosocial complications such as anxiety, depressive symptoms, and/or general malaise associated with lengthy and prolonged hospitalization. Similarly, non-myeloablative conditioning regimens are being used with increasing frequency in the transplant setting. These so-called "mini" transplants require less intensive chemotherapy prior to transplant (Shimoni & Nagler, 2002). As a result, they should be associated with less toxicity and fewer attendant physical complications. This in turn should result in fewer psychosocial complications and better QOL. Finally, increasing emphasis is currently being placed on provision of HSC transplantation in an outpatient setting. A recent comparison of inpatient and outpatient autologous HSC transplant recipients suggested that psychological, physical, social, and financial outcomes of outpatient recipients were comparable or better than those receiving inpatient care (Summers *et al.*, 2000). The authors concluded that outpatient autologous HSC transplantation was efficient and effective and an acceptable alternative for patients with sufficient physical and psychological resilience and motivation. However, while shifting more and more of the transplant procedure to the outpatient setting may not diminish and may even improve patient outcomes, this trend may have serious implications for spouses or family members who function as the patient's primary caregiver. These individuals may be at increased risk for psychosocial complications as responsibility for daily monitoring of health status, medication management, and catheter care is increasingly shifted from nurses in the hospital to family caregivers in the home. In short, as HSC transplant technology evolves over time, new sets of psychosocial complications affecting patients, caregivers, and/or stem cell donors will emerge. These new psychosocial complications will require continuing research and sensitive clinical management by both medical and psychosocial team members.

References

Aaronson, N.K., Ahmedzai, S., Bergman, B. *et al.* (1993). The European Organization for Research and Treatment of Cancer QLQ-C30: a quality-of-life instrument for use in international clinical trials in oncology. *Journal of the National Cancer Institute,* **85**(5), 365–76.

Ahles, T.A., Tope, D.M., Furstenberg, C. *et al.* (1996). Psychologic and neuropsychologic impact of autologous bone marrow transplantation. *Journal of Clinical Oncology,* **14,** 1457–62.

Andrykowski, M.A. (1994a). Psychiatric and psychosocial aspects of bone marrow transplantation. *Psychosomatics,* **35,** 13–24.

Andrykowski, M.A. (1994b). Psychosocial factors in bone marrow transplantation: a review and recommendations for research. *Bone Marrow Transplantation,* **13,** 357–75.

Andrykowski, M.A., Brady, M.J., Greiner, C.B. *et al.* (1995a). Returning to normal following bone marrow transplantation: outcomes, expectations and informed consent. *Bone Marrow Transplantation,* **15,** 573–81.

Andrykowski, M.A., Cordova, M.J., Hann, D.M. *et al.* (1999). Patients' psychosocial concerns following stem cell transplantation. *Bone Marrow Transplantation,* **24,** 1121–29.

Andrykowski, M.A., Greiner, C.B., Altmaier, E.M. *et al.* (1995b). Quality of life following bone marrow transplantation: findings from a multicenter study. *British Journal of Cancer,* **71,** 1322–9.

Andrykowski, M.A. & McQuellon, R.P. (1998a). Readaptation to normal life following bone marrow transplantation. In *The Clinical Practice of Stem Cell Transplantation,* ed. J. Barrett & J. Treleaven, Oxford: Isis Medical Media.

Andrykowski, M.A. & McQuellon, R.P. (1998b) Psychological issues in hematopoietic cell transplantation. In *Hematopoietic Cell Transplantation,* ed. S.J. Forman, K.G. Blume, & E.D. Thomas, Boston: Blackwell Science.

Baker, F. (1997). Psychosocial sequelae of bone marrow transplantation. *Oncology,* **8,** 87–92.

Baker, F., Marcellus, D., Zabora, J. *et al.* (1997). Psychological distress among adult patients being evaluated for bone marrow transplantation. *Psychosomatics,* **38,** 10–19.

Beck, A.T. & Steer, R.A. (1987). *Beck Depression Inventory Manual,* New York: The Psychological Corporation, Harcourt Brace Jovanovich, Inc.

Biesecker, A.C., McQuellon, R.P., Russell, G.B. *et al.* (2000). Coping with bone marrow transplantation (BMT). *Annals of Behavioral Medicine,* **22** (Suppl), 63.

Broers, S., Kaptein, A.A., Le Cessie, S. *et al.* (2000). Psychological functioning and quality of life following bone marrow transplantation: a 3-year follow-up study. *Journal of Psychosomatic Research,* **48,** 11–21.

Brown, H.N. & Kelly, M.J. (1976). Stages of bone marrow transplantation: a psychiatric perspective. *Psychosomatic Medicine,* **38,** 439–46.

Bush, N.E., Haberman, M., Donaldson, G., & Sullivan, K.M. (1995). Quality of life of 125 adults surviving 6–18 years after bone marrow transplantation. *Social Science & Medicine,* **40,** 479–90.

Butterworth, V.A. (1992). When altruism fails: reactions of unrelated bone marrow donors when the recipient dies. *Omega,* **26,** 161–73.

Butterworth, V.A., Simmons, R.G., Bartsch, G. *et al.* (1993). Psychosocial effects of unrelated bone marrow donation: experiences of the National Marrow Donor Program. *Blood,* **81,** 1947–59.

Carlson, L.E. & MacRae, J.H. (2002). Quality of life issues following autologous bone marrow transplantation. *Expert Review of Pharmacoeconomics & Outcomes Research,* **2,** 129–46.

Cella, D.F., Jacobsen, P.B., Orav, E.J. *et al.* (1987). A brief POMS measure of distress for cancer patients. *Journal of Chronic Diseases,* **40,** 939–42.

Cella, D.F., Mahon, S.M., & Donovan, M.I. (1990). Cancer recurrence as a traumatic event. *Behavioral Medicine,* **16,** 15–22.

Cella, D.F., Tross, S., Orav, E.J. *et al.* (1989). Mood states of patients after the diagnosis of cancer. *Journal of Psychosocial Oncology,* **7,** 45–54.

Chapko, M.K., Syrjala, K.L., Schilter, L. *et al.* (1989). Chemoradiotherapy toxicity during bone marrow transplantation: time course and variation in pain and nausea. *Bone Marrow Transplantation,* **4,** 181–6.

Chiodi, S., Spinelli, S., Ravera, G. *et al.* (2000). Quality of life in 244 recipients of allogeneic bone marrow transplantation. *British Journal of Haematology,* **110,** 614–9.

Cohen, A., Duell, T., Socie, G. *et al.* (1999). Nutritional status and growth after bone marrow transplantation (BMT) during childhood: EBMT Late Effects Working Party retrospective data.

European Group for Blood and Marrow Transplantation. *Bone Marrow Transplantation*, **23**, 1043–7.

Cohen, A., Rovelli, R., Zecca, S. *et al.* (1998). Endocrine late effects in children who underwent bone marrow transplantation: a review. *Bone Marrow Transplantation*, **21** (Suppl 2), S64–S67.

Cordova, M.J., Andrykowski, M.A., Kenady, D.E. *et al.* (1995). Frequency and correlates of posttraumatic-stress-disorder-like symptoms after treatment for breast cancer. *Journal of Consulting and Clinical Psychology*, **63**, 981–6.

Dermatis, H. & Lesko, L.M. (1990). Psychological distress in parents consenting to child's bone marrow transplantation. *Bone Marrow Transplantation*, **6**, 411–17.

Dermatis, H. & Lesko, L.M. (1991). Psychosocial correlates of physician-patient communication at time of informed consent for bone marrow transplantation. *Cancer Investigation*, **9**, 621–8.

Derogatis, L.R. & Melisaratos, N. (1983). The Brief Symptom Inventory: an introductory report. *Psychological Medicine*, **13**, 595–605.

Fife, B.L., Huster, G.A., & Cornetta, K.G. (2000). Longitudinal study of adaptation to the stress of bone marrow transplantation. *Journal of Clinical Oncology*, **18**, 1539–49.

Fisher, V.L. (1999). Long-term follow-up in hematopoietic stem-cell transplant patients. *Pediatric Transplant*, **3** (Suppl 1), 122–9.

Ford, S., Lewis, S., & Fallowfield, L. (1995). Psychological morbidity in newly referred patients with cancer. *Journal of Psychosomatic Research*, **39**, 193–202.

Fromm, K., Andrykowski, M.A., & Hunt, J. (1996). Positive and negative psychosocial sequelae of bone marrow transplantation: implications for quality of life assessment. *Journal of Behavioral Medicine*, **19**, 221–40.

Futterman, A.D., Wellisch, D.K., Bond, G., & Carr, C.R. (1991). The Psychosocial Levels System. A new rating scale to identify and assess emotional difficulties during bone marrow transplantation. *Psychosomatics*, **32**, 177–86.

Futterman, A.D., Wellisch, D.K., Zighelboim, J. *et al.* (1996). Psychological and immunological reactions of family members to patients undergoing bone marrow transplantation. *Psychosomatic Medicine*, **58**, 472–80.

Gallardo, D., Ferra, C., Berlanga, J.J. *et al.* (1996). Neurologic complications after allogeneic bone marrow transplantation. *Bone Marrow Transplantation*, **18**, 1135–9.

Ganz, P.A., Rofessart, J., & Polinsky, M.L. (1986). A comprehensive approach to the assessment of cancer patients' rehabilitation needs: The Cancer Inventory of Problem Situations and a companion interview. *Journal of Psychosocial Oncology*, **4**, 27–32.

Godder, K.T. & Henslee-Downey, P.J. (2001). Colony-stimulating factors in stem cell transplantation: effect on quality of life. *Journal of Hematotherapeutic Stem Cell Research*, **10**, 215–28.

Grant, M. (1999). Assessment of quality of life following hematopoietic cell transplantation. In *Hematopoietic Cell Transplantation*, 2nd Ed., ed. Thomas, K.G. Blume, & S.J. Forman, pp. 407–13, London: Blackwell Sciences.

Grassi, L., Rosti, G., Albertazzi, L., & Marangolo, M. (1996). Psychological stress symptoms before and after autologous bone marrow transplantation in patients with solid tumors. *Bone Marrow Transplantation*, **17**, 843–7.

Grimm, P.M., Zawacki, K.L., & Mock, V. (2000). Caregiver responses and needs. An ambulatory bone marrow transplant model. *Cancer Practice*, **8**, 120–8.

Hann, D.M., Jacobsen, P.B., Martin, S.C. *et al.* (1997). Fatigue in women treated with bone marrow transplantation for breast cancer: a comparison with women with no history of cancer. *Supportive Care in Cancer*, **5**, 44–52.

Hjermstad, M.J. & Kaasa, S. (1995). Quality of life in adult cancer patients treated with bone marrow transplantation—a review of the literature. *European Journal of Cancer*, **31A**, 163–73.

Holland, J.C. (1997). Preliminary guidelines for the treatment of distress. *Oncology*, **11**, 109–14.

Jacobsen, P.B., Sadler, I.J., & Booth-Jones, M. (2002). Predictors of posttraumatic stress disorder symptomatology following bone marrow transplantation for cancer. *Journal of Consulting and Clinical Psychology*, **70**, 235–40.

Jacobsen, P.B., Widows, M.R., Hann, D.M. *et al.* (1998). Posttraumatic stress disorder symptoms after bone marrow transplantation for breast cancer. *Psychosomatic Medicine*, **60**, 366–71.

Jones, B. (1994). Psychosocial complications of bone marrow transplantation. In *Clinical Bone Marrow Transplantation: A Reference Textbook*, ed. K. Atkinson, pp. 539–42. Cambridge: Cambridge University Press.

Kaupilla, M., Koskinen, P., Irjala, K. *et al.* (1998). Long-term effects of allogeneic bone marrow transplantation (BMT) on pituitary, gonad, thyroid, and adrenal function in adults. *Bone Marrow Transplantation*, **22**, 331–7.

Kelly, D., Ross, S., Gray, B. *et al.* (2000). Death, dying and emotional labour: problematic dimensions of the bone marrow transplant nursing role? *Journal of Advanced Nursing*, **32**, 952–60.

Keogh, F., O'Riordan, J., McNamara, C. *et al.* (1998). Psychosocial adaptation of patients and families following bone marrow transplantation: a prospective, longitudinal study. *Bone Marrow Transplantation*, **22**, 905–11.

Kolb, H.J. & Poetscher, C. (1997). Late effects after allogeneic bone marrow transplantation. *Current Opinions in Hematology*, **4**, 401–7.

Kolb, H.J., Socie, G., Duell, T. *et al.* (1999). Malignant neoplasms in long-term survivors of bone marrow transplantation. Late Effects Working Party of the European Cooperative Group for Blood and Marrow Transplantation and the European Late Effect Project Group. *Annals of Internal Medicine*, **131**, 738–44.

Leigh, S., Wilson, K.C., Burns, R., & Clark, R.E. (1995). Psychosocial morbidity in bone marrow transplant recipients: a prospective study. *Bone Marrow Transplantation*, **16**, 635–40.

Loberiza, F.R. Jr., Rizzo, J.D., Bredeson, C.N. *et al.* (2002). Association of depressive syndrome and early deaths among patients after stem-cell transplantation for malignant diseases. *Journal of Clinical Oncology*, **20**, 2118–26.

Marks, D.I., Crilley, P., Nezu, C.M., & Nezu, A.M. (1996). Sexual dysfunction prior to high-dose chemotherapy and bone marrow transplantation. *Bone Marrow Transplantation*, **17**, 595–9.

McQuellon, R.P., Craven, B., Russell, G.B. *et al.* (1996). Quality of life in breast cancer patients before and after autologous bone marrow transplantation. *Bone Marrow Transplantation*, **18**, 579–84.

McQuellon, R.P., Muss, H.B., Hoffman, S.L. *et al.* (1995). Patient preferences for treatment of metastatic breast cancer: a study of women with early-stage breast cancer. *Journal of Clinical Oncology*, **13**, 858–68.

McQuellon, R.P., Russell, G.B., Biesecker, A.C. *et al.* (1999). Survivorship following bone marrow transplantation (BMT): a follow-up study at three years. *Psycho-Oncology,* **8,** 6–17.

McQuellon, R.P., Russell, G.B., Cella, D.F. (1997). Quality of life measurement in bone marrow transplantation: development of the Functional Assessment of Cancer Therapy–Bone Marrow Transplant (FACT-BMT) scale. *Bone Marrow Transplantation,* **19,** 357–68.

McQuellon, R.P., Russell, G.R., Rambo, T.D. *et al.* (1998). Quality of life and psychological distress of bone marrow transplantation recipients: the "time trajectory" to recovery over the first year. *Bone Marrow Transplantation,* **21,** 477–86.

Molassiotis, A., Boughton, B.J., Burgoyne, T., & Van Den Akker, O.B. (1995). Comparison of the overall quality of life in 50 long-term survivors of autologous and allogeneic bone marrow transplantation. *Journal of Advanced Nursing,* **22,** 509–16.

Molassiotis, A., van den Akker, O.B., & Boughton, B.J. (1995). Psychological stress in nursing and medical staff on bone marrow transplant units. *Bone Marrow Transplantation,* **15,** 449–54.

Molassiotis, A., van den Akker, O.B.D., & Milligan, W. (1997). Symptom distress, coping style and biological variables as predictors of survival after bone marrow transplantation. *Journal of Psychosomatic Research,* **42,** 275–85.

Murphy, K.C., Jenkins, P.L., & Whittaker, J.A. (1996). Psychosocial morbidity and survival in adult bone marrow transplant recipients—a follow-up study. *Bone Marrow Transplantation,* **18,** 199–201.

Neitzert, C.S., Ritvo, P., Dancey, J. *et al.* (1998). The psychosocial impact of bone marrow transplantation: a review of the literature. *Bone Marrow Transplantation,* **22,** 409–22.

Niethammer, D. & Mayer, E. (1998). Long-term survivors: An overview on late effects, sequelae, and second neoplasias. *Bone Marrow Transplantation,* **21,** (Suppl 2), S61–63.

Parsons, S.K., Barlow, S.E., Levy, S.L. *et al.* (1999). Health-related quality of life in pediatric bone marrow transplant survivors: according to whom? *International Journal of Cancer,* **12** (Suppl), 46–51.

Pfefferbaum, B., Lindamood, M., & Wiley, F.M. (1978). Stages in pediatric bone marrow transplantation. *Pediatrics,* **61,** 625–8.

Phillips, G., Armitrage, J., Bearman, S. *et al.* (1997). American Society for Blood and Marrow Transplantation: guidelines for clinical centers. *Biology of Blood and Marrow Transplantation,* **1,** 22–3.

Prieto, J.M., Blanch, J., Atala, E. *et al.* (2002). Psychiatric morbidity and impact on hospital length of stay among hematologic cancer patients receiving stem-cell transplantation. *Journal of Clinical Oncology,* **20,** 1907–17.

Prieto, J.M., Saez, R., Carreras, E. *et al.* (1996). Physical and psychosocial functioning of 117 survivors of bone marrow transplantation. *Bone Marrow Transplantation,* **17,** 1133–42.

Radloff, L.S. (1977). The CES-D Scale: a self-report depression scale for research in the general population. *Applied Psychological Measurement,* **1,** 385–401.

Rowland, J.H. (1990). Developmental stage and adaptation: adult model. In *Handbook of Psycho-oncology: Psychological Care of the Patient with Cancer,* ed. J.C. Holland & J.H. Rowland, pp. 25–43. New York: Oxford University Press.

Sarantos, S. (1988). Innovations in psychosocial staff support: a model program for the marrow transplant nurse. *Seminars in Oncology Nursing,* **4,** 69–73.

Schimmer, A. D., Elliott, M. E., Abbey S. E. *et al.* (2001). Illness intrusiveness among survivors of autologous blood and marrow transplantation. *Cancer,* **92,** 3147–54.

Sherbourne, C.D. & Stewart, A.L. (1991). The MOS social support survey. *Social Science and Medicine,* **32,** 705–14.

Shimoni, A. & Nagler, A. (2002). Non-myeloablative hematopoietic stem cell transplantation (NST) in the treatment of human malignancies: from animal models to clinical practice. *Cancer Treatment and Research,* **110,** 113–36.

Somerfield, M.R., Curbow, B., Wingard, J.R. *et al.* (1996). Coping with the physical and psychosocial sequelae of bone marrow transplantation among long-term survivors. *Journal of Behavioral Medicine,* **19,** 163–84.

Stetz, K.M., McDonald, J.C., & Compton, K. (1996). Needs and experiences of family caregivers during marrow transplantation. *Oncology Nursing Forum,* **23,** 1422–7.

Summers, N., Dawe, U., & Stewart, D.A. (2000). A comparison of inpatient and outpatient ASCT. *Bone Marrow Transplantation,* **26,** 389–95.

Syrjala, K.L., Chapko, M.K., Vitaliano, P.P. *et al.* (1993). Recovery after allogeneic marrow transplantation: prospective study of predictors of long-term physical and psychosocial functioning. *Bone Marrow Transplantation,* **11,** 319–27.

Thomas, O., Mahe, M., Campion, L. *et al.* (2001). Long-term complications of total body irradiation in adults. *International Journal of Radiation Oncology Biology and Physics,* **49,** 125–131.

Trask, P.C., Paterson, A., Riba, M. *et al.* (2002). Asessment of psychological distress in prospective bone marrow transplant patients. *Bone Marrow Transplantation,* **29,** 917–25.

Tross, S., Herndon, J., & Korzun, A. (1996). Psychological symptoms and disease-free and overall survival in women with stage II breast cancer. Cancer and Leukemia Group B. *Journal of the National Cancer Institute,* **88,** 661–7.

Twillman, R.K., Manetto, C., Wellisch, D.K. *et al.* (1993). The Transplant Evaluation Rating Scale. A revision of the psychosocial levels system for evaluating organ transplant candidates. *Psychosomatics,* **34,** 144–53.

Weitzner, M.A., Jacobsen, P.B., Wagner, J.J. *et al.* (1998). The Caregiver Quality of Life Index–Cancer (CQOLC): development and validation of an instrument to measure quality of life of the family caregiver of patients with cancer. *Quaity of Life Research,* **7,** 3–9.

Wellisch, D.K. & Wolcott, D.L. (1994). Psychological issues in bone marrow transplantation. In *Bone Marrow Transplantation,* ed. S.J. Forman, K.B. Blume, & E.D. Thomas, pp. 556–71. Boston: Blackwell Scientific Publications.

Wingard, J.R., Curbow, B., Baker, F. *et al.* (1992). Sexual satisfaction in survivors of bone marrow transplantation. *Bone Marrow Transplantation,* **9,** 185–90.

Wolcott, D.L., Wellisch, D.K., Fawzy, F.I., & Landsverk, J. (1986). Psychological adjustment of adult bone marrow transplant donors whose recipient survives. *Transplantation,* **41,** 484–8.

Zabora, J.R., Smith, E.D., Baker, F. *et al.* (1992). The family: the other side of bone marrow transplantation. *Journal of Psychosocial Oncology,* **10,** 35–46.

PART XI LABORATORY SERVICES

103 Cytogenetic aspects of hematopoietic stem cell transplantation

MARILYN L. SLOVAK AND JOYCE L. MURATA-COLLINS

City of Hope National Medical Center, Duarte, USA

Introduction

Examination of chromosome alterations associated with malignancy has led to greater understanding of the genetic changes central to initiation and progression of human neoplasia. The effects of these aberrations may increase cellular proliferation, diminish differentiation, or result in the loss of normal apoptotic mechanisms. The presence of multiple pathogenetic events within a single tumor phenotype supports Knudson's theory (1971) that cancers develop through sequential acquisition of gene mutations. Inherited or germline mutations in known tumor suppressor genes such as *RB, TP53,* or *BRCA1* are implicated as a "first hit" in familial cancer. Somatic mutations acquired by gain or loss of whole or partial chromosomes result in altered dosage effects, gene amplification, or deletion. Chromosomal rearrangements may result in aberrant chimeric gene protein products or overexpression, activation, or inactivation of normal cellular proteins.

The hematopoietic disorders are heterogeneous. Detection of genomic alterations provides important pathogenetic information for diagnosis, prognosis, and management, as exemplified by the standard Philadelphia (Ph+) chromosomal translocation t(9;22)(q34.1;q11.2) and its molecular counterpart, *BCR/ABL,* in chronic myeloid leukemia (CML) or the t(15;17)(q22;q21.1) and its chimeric fusion gene, *PML/RARα,* in acute promyelocytic leukemia (APL). Studies have clearly shown that underlying genetic alterations of disease have associated morphologic/immunological profiles and influence the patient's response to cytotoxic therapy. These parameters are now major elements of the recently published World Health Organization classification of tumors of hematopoietic and lymphoid tissues (Jaffe *et al.,* 2001). Distinct gene expression profiles for known cytogenetic subgroups of leukemia are providing the framework and the validation considerations necessary to improve prognostic-risk stratification in the hematopoietic disorders (Yeoh *et al.,* 2002). Furthermore, genetic studies examining clonal evolution of disease not only contribute to our understanding of disease progression, and their association with sensitive minimal residual disease (MRD) assays, but are now defining the timing of clinical management decisions.

Because of its increasing rate of success, hematopoietic stem cell transplantation (HSCT) is becoming the treatment of choice for an increasing variety of genetic, immunologic, and malignant diseases. Advances in genetic methodologies can provide both diagnostic/prognostic information and clinical monitoring tools following chemotherapy and HSCT. The most common genetic tools used in HSCT are classic cytogenetics, fluorescence in situ hybridization (FISH), immunophenotyping or flow cytometry, and molecular genetic studies. Sensitivity of these assays varies from 10^{-1} to 10^{-6} and is limited by the number of cells available for analysis, availability of analytical probes, and sampling or technical error. Each assay, whether polymerase chain reaction (PCR), FISH, flow cytometry, or classic cytogenetics, has advantages and disadvantages. Currently, a multifold laboratory approach is recommended as no single testing procedure presently fulfills the various needs of transplant clinicians. However, with an immediate need to provide pathology and genetic testing procedures in a quantitative, reliable, precise, timely, cost effective, and standardized package, our contemporary laboratory methods must evolve toward a more robust single platform approach, such as described by Yeoh *et al.* (2002), allowing for the accurate identification of high-risk patient subgroups who will most likely benefit from HSCT.

Commonly used genetic methods in bone marrow transplantation (BMT) and peripheral blood stem cell transplantation (PBSCT)

Classic cytogenetics

Classic cytogenetics is a pan genomic screening tool, allowing identification of individual chromosomes and detection of abnormalities of both number and structure within a single test procedure. It is essential to perform cytogenetic studies at disease presentation for diagnostic and prognostic information, to monitor clinical effects during treatment, whenever clonal evolution of disease is suspected, to monitor for MRD or relapse posttransplant, and to rule out therapy-related myelodysplasia/acute myeloid leukemia (MDS/AML) as a

Table 103.1. *Utility and suggested monitoring protocol of cytogenetic studies in HSC transplantation*

Time	Utility
At disease presentation and pretransplant	Diagnostic, staging, and prognostic information
At time of stem cell harvest	Detection of abnormalities in autologous or donor stem cells
Posttransplant at day 30, 90 or 180, 365, and annually	Monitoring effect of treatment for MRD or relapse for origin of relapse for therapy-related MDS/AML for chimerism evaluation

Abbreviations: MRD, minimal residual disease; MDS, myelodysplasia; AML, acute myeloid leukemia.

late complication (Table 103.1). Detection of chromosomal anomalies associated with specific disease types, such as t(9;22)(q34.1;q11.2) in CML, 11q23/MLL gene rearrangements in acute leukemia, t(8;14)(q24.1;q32.33) in Burkitt's lymphoma, t(11;14)(q13;q32.33) in mantle cell lymphoma, *NMYC* amplification in neuroblastoma, and *HER2/neu* amplification in breast cancer, has significant prognostic implications. Cytogenetic analysis is also useful in the diagnosis of Fanconi anemia using chromosome instability studies, in the diagnosis of lymphoma using lymph nodes, in the staging of lymphoma in the marrow, in the differential diagnosis of solid tumors using tumor tissue (especially the round cell tumors of childhood), and for the detection of bone marrow metastasis of solid tumors. Additionally, karyotypic correlation with disease processes pinpoints important regions of the genome for further analysis with emerging molecular biological methodologies.

Cytogenetic analysis permits identification of spontaneously mitotic cells within a tumor population. However, it may not necessarily demonstrate the entire neoplastic cell population and cannot be performed on terminally differentiated cells, such as segmented neutrophils; thus, its sensitivity is limited to cycling cells (Anastasi *et al.*, 1990). The oncology specimen of choice is bone marrow; however, peripheral blood is acceptable whenever numbers of spontaneously mitotic cells (ranging from myelocytes through blasts) are greater than 1×10^9/l. In chronic lymphatic leukemia (CLL), peripheral blood has been reported the tissue of choice, with either B-cell or T-cell mitogens added at culture initiation to induce blast transformation of the well-differentiated leukemic cells, or with the use of unstimulated cell cultures in poorly differentiated anaplastic cases. For a complete analysis, specimen processing requires a minimum of two cultures with 1×10^6 mononuclear cells per ml of culture medium using various culture conditions. For solid tumors, cells from collagenase-disaggregated tissue are cultured short term (<7 days) and harvested depending on their mitotic rate. A complete analysis requires a minimum of 20 fully analyzed metaphases for chromosome number and structural abnormalities. Thus, classic cytogenetic analyses are labor intensive and technically complex assays. Advantages of clas-

sic cytogenetics include the ability to detect a wide range of abnormalities, which may provide diagnostic information for a patient with a clinically nonspecific disease presentation. Commonly used genetic techniques are shown in Table 103.2.

Karyotypic description includes information regarding both chromosome number and structure. A normal diploid (2n) constitution contains 46 chromosomes. Pseudodiploidy describes a karyotype with 46 chromosomes, but is abnormal due to the presence of acquired numerical or structural anomalies. If the numerical chromosome constitution differs from 46 chromosomes, the karyotype is referred to as aneuploid. Clones with fewer than 46 chromosomes are hypodiploid, whereas those containing greater than 46 chromosomes are hyperdiploid. The modal number is the most common chromosome number in a heterogeneous tumor cell population. Additionally, in cancer, variations of haploidy (n), such as triploidy (3n), tetraploidy (4n), and so on, are possible. Commonly used cytogenetic terminology is further described in Table 103.3.

Karyotypic aberrations, resulting in two cells with the same chromosomal gain or structural abnormality, or three cells with loss of the same chromosome, define a clone. Recurrence of the same chromosomal abnormality in two successive analyses is evidence for an abnormal clone, even though this point is not directly addressed in the International System for Human Cytogenetic Nomenclature (ISCN) (1995). The "stemline" is commonly used to describe the most basic clone of the tumor cell population, whereas all clonal deviations of the stemline are designated as "sidelines." Sidelines are commonly associated with clonal evolution of disease. The Latin term, *idem,* for "same" indicates that stemline aberrations are also present in the sideline. When a second clone represents a doubling of the stemline, idemx2 may be used. In many instances, significant karyotypic heterogeneity may exist within a tumor, although the aberrant metaphases share some consistent abnormal cytogenetic characteristics. When this occurs, a composite karyotype (cp) will be reported that describes all clonally occurring abnormalities. For a more detailed guide describing human cytogenetic nomenclature, the reader is referred to ISCN (1995).

Table 103.2. *Commonly used genetic assays in HSC transplantation*

Assay	Common usage	Advantages	Limitations
Flow cytometry	Ploidy and immunophenotype data	Defines tumor's immunophenotype Used in conjunction with other MRD genetic assays	Low sensitivity
Classic cytogenetics	Screen for non random clonal aberrations –acquired –constitutional –chromosome instability syndromes –clonal evolution of disease	Identifies frequent, and rare abnormalities Diagnostic and prognostic markers	Low sensitivity with a 20-cell study Limited to cycling cells
24-color karyotyping	Identify chromosomal markers and cryptic aberrations Spiked with M-TEL probes will increase resolution of the telomeric regions	Refines karyotypic designation in complex karyotypes Identifies "cryptic" anomalies	Research tool Requires expensive instrumentation Does not detect intrachromosomal anomalies Limited sensitivity
Fluorescence in situ hybridization (FISH)	Identifies translocations, deletions, amplification, and engraftment in sex-mismatched HSCT by sex chromosome content	Used in metaphase (dividing) and interphase (nondividing) cells	Requires specific probes for each target area
Probes Enumeration or centromere Whole chromosome paints Locus-specific probes	Confirms suspected clonality Identifies "masked" or cryptic Ph+/MLL rearrangements	Quick and quantitative clinical management tool Amenable for all pathology specimens including paraffin-embedded material	Usually limited to 1–3 probes per hybridization Sensitivity depends on number of probes and number of cells scored Automation desirable for MRD detection
Hypermetaphase FISH	Quantitation of 500+ mitotic cells for specific aberrations	Highly reliable and sensitive	Over contracted metaphase cells provide limited information Compromised analysis with the simultaneous use of multiple probes with varying hybridization conditions
Fiber FISH	Physical mapping tool to characterize translocations with scattered breakpoints	Defines relative order of multi-colored probes within ~50 kb	Labor intensive Research tool
Spectral FISH	Detects 3–10 (multiple) genetic aberrations with a single hybridization in a single cell hybridization	Screen apheresis samples for specific aberrations or when tissue samples are limited	Labor intensive Requires z-axis stacking software
Comparative genomic hybridization	Comprehensive screen for the detection of chromosomal deletions and amplification (chromosomal imbalances)	Does not require any probes Amplification or deletions of 1 to 20 megabases detected Enabling technology behind DNA arrays– matrix-based protocols	Sensitivity depends on tumor cell enrichment—tumor cells must be sorted by flow or microdissected
FICTION or FISH/ immunophenotype	Genotype/phenotype correlation MRD detection Detects chimerism	Detects MRD by cell lineage	Technically difficult Flow sorted cells may be used but adds to expense
PCR Qualitative Quantitative	Detects submicroscopic nonrandom cytogenetic aberrations MRD detection Detects chimerism	Highly specific and quantitative	Requires known DNA sequence; selected primers may not reliably detect variable or rearrangements with widely spanning breakpoint sites
Gene arrays	Defines genetic signature of the tumor	Potential to improve risk-adapted therapy subgroups	Requires validation to define clinical utility

Table 103.3. *Commonly used terms in human cytogenetics*

	Change to chromosomal material	Abbreviation	Example
Structural abnormality			
Translocation	Exchange of material from one chromosome to another	t	t(9;22)(q34.1;q11.2) in CML (also in AML and ALL)
Duplication	Repetition of a segment of chromosome	dup	dup(1)(q12->q31) seen in some cases of B-ALL
Deletion	Loss of a segment of a chromosome	del	del(5)(q13q33) seen in myelodysplasia
Inversion	Reversal of chromosome segment between two breakpoints	inv	inv(16)(p13q22) seen in AML M4Eo
Insertion	Breakage of a chromosome followed by transfer of a segment of the same or another chromosome into that chromosome at the breakpoint	ins	ins(3;5)(q25;q31.1q35) insertion of segment of chromosome 5 into chromosome 3—seen in AML
Isochromosome	A chromosome in which both arms are identical, resulting from transverse rather than longitudinal separation of the centromere during mitosis	i	i(17q) commonly seen in CML-AP
Ring	A circular chromosome formed by breakage at two points within the chromosome, followed by rejoining of the broken ends	r	r(22)(p11q13)
Numerical abnormality			
Aneuploidy	Numerical deviation from the normal cell chromosome content (the latter known as diploidy: 46 chromosomes)		48,XY,+8,+21
Hyperdiploidy	More than 46 chromosomes		55,XX,+4,+6,+7,+14,+14,+18, +20,+21,+21 reported in ALL
Hypodiploidy	Less than 46 chromosomes		44,X,–Y,–21
Pseudodiploidy	46 chromosomes with clonal abnormalities present		46,XY,t(4;11)(q21;q23) reported in AL
Monosomy	Loss of a single individual chromosome	–	45,XY,–7 seen in AML
Trisomy	Gain of a single individual chromosome	+	47,XX,+8 seen in AL

Abbreviations: CML, chronic myeloid leukemia; CML-AP, chronic myeloid leukemia in accelerated phase; AL, acute leukemia; AML, acute myeloid leukemia; ALL, acute lymphoblastic leukemia.

Classic cytogenetics permits unambiguous identification of mitotic leukemic cells, corresponding to a reliable predictor of eventual relapse approaching 10^{-1}, assuming a 20 to 50 cell analysis and based on Hook's (1977) statistical formula. Despite time and cell culturing limitations, classic cytogenetics remains the current method of choice to identify and monitor –5/del(5q), –7/del(7q), inv(3q), or del(20q) and the less frequent translocations observed in leukemia. Additionally, following sex-mismatched allografts, classic cytogenetics or FISH can determine donor engraftment by identifying the gonosomal complement in the marrow. In sex-matched allografts, newer molecular approaches using restriction fragment length polymorphisms (RFLPs), or variations in short tandem repeats (STRs), provide sensitive detection of donor versus recipient cells.

Cytogenetic data for the solid malignancies are limited compared to those for hematopoietic tumors, due to greater technical difficulties in specimen processing and culturing, lower mitotic indices, and the inability to define specific aberrations in a highly rearranged chromosome complement. Often a highly complex karyotype is observed with structural rearrangements that include not only tumor-specific translocations, but also characteristic gene amplification or chromosomal deletions. Solid tumor studies led to conceptual development of tumor suppressor genes, wherein loss of function is a critical step in oncogenesis. Investigations of familial cases of retinoblastoma and of Wilms tumor initially found an association with constitutional chromosomal deletions involving bands 13q14 and 11p13, respectively (Knudson, 1971), followed by gene mapping of tumor suppressor gene loci for RB and WT1. Gene amplification may be intrachromosomal, in the form of homogeneous staining regions (hsr), or extrachromosomal, in the form of small, paired-bodies named double minutes (dmin). These cytogenetic anomalies may harbor multiple copies of oncogenes or genes associated with acquired drug resistance. For example, poor-risk neuroblastoma cases are frequently characterized by extrachromosomal amplification of *NMYC* (Fig. 103.1A) and *HER2/NEU* is amplified in high-risk breast cancer (Fig. 103.1B). Chromosomal anomalies associated with specific myeloid, lymphoid, and solid neoplasms are shown in Tables 103.4 to 103.7.

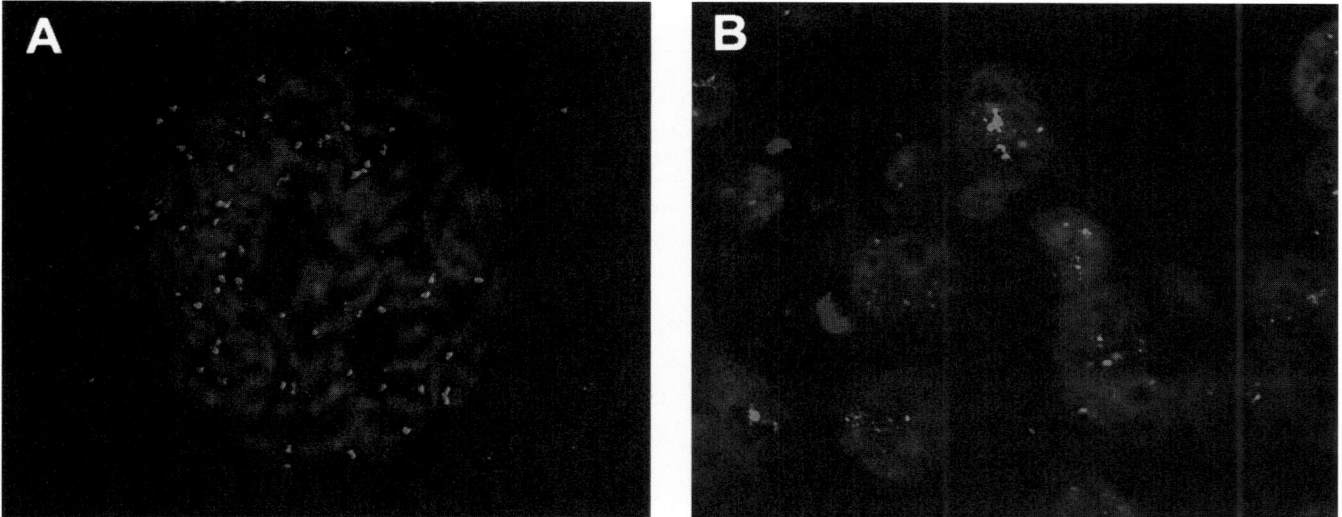

Fig. 103.1. **(A)** *NYMC* amplification in neuroblastoma. Amplified *NMYC* gene sequences are visible in the form of multiple double minute (dmin) chromosomes in this mitotic neuroblastoma cell. *NMYC* amplification correlates with both advanced disease stage and rapid tumor growth. **(B)** *HER2/NEU* amplification detected by dual-color FISH in a paraffin-embedded breast cancer specimen. Four-micron tissue sections were hybridized using a cosmid probe for *HER2/NEU* [spectrum orange (red) signal] and a chromosome 17 centromere control reference probe (spectrum green signal). Clusters of red signals in the presence of 2 to 4 chromosome 17 centromeric signals [indicating diploid (G1) or tetraploid (G2) cells] indicate amplified *HER2/NEU* gene sequences. *HER2/NEU* amplification is observed in ~25% of breast cancers and has been associated with high-grade disease and short disease-free survival. For color reproduction, see Color Plate 103.1.

Table 103.4. *Common cytogenetic abnormalities in myeloid disorders*

Disease	Cytogenetic abnormality	Molecular targets	Detection methods
CML chronic phase	t(9;22)(q34.1;q11.2)	*ABL;BCR*	CC, FISH, PCR
CML accelerated or blast crisis	t(9;22) plus others	*ABL;BCR*	CC, FISH, PCR
	t(3;21)(q26.2;q22.3)	*EVI1;AML1*	
	(i.e., +8, i(17)(q10), +19, +der(22)t(9;22)	plus *TP53* and others to be determined	
AML	t(9;22)(q34.1;q11.2)	*ABL;BCR*	CC, FISH, PCR
	t(16;21)(p11.2;q22.3)	*FUS;ERG*	CC, PCR
	+4		CC, FISH
AML with maturation	t(8;21)(q22;q22.3) with or without loss of X or Y	*ETO;AML1*	CC, FISH, PCR
	t(7;11)(p15;p15)	*HOXA9;NUP98*	CC, FISH
APL (FAB-M3)	t(15;17)(q22;q21.1)	*PML;RARα*	CC, FISH, PCR
	t(11;17)(q23;q21.1)	*PLZF;RARα*	CC, FISH, PCR
	t(11;17)(q13.1;q21.1)	*NUMA1;RARα*	CC
AML with abnormal eosinophils (FAB-M4Eo)	inv(16)(p13.1q22) t(16;16)(p13.1;q22)	*MYH11;CBFβ*	CC, FISH, PCR
Acute monocytic leukemia	t/del 11q23	*MLL(ALL1/HTX)*	CC, FISH, PCR
AML with basophils	t(6;9)(p23;q34.1)	*DEK;CAN*	CC, PCR
AML with increased platelets	inv(3)(q21q26.2) t(3;3)(q21;q26.2) t(3;5)(q26.2;q34)	*EVI1*	CC, FISH
AML/MDS de novo or t-MDS/AML	−5/del(5q)−7/del(7q),+8, +21, other clonal numerical changes	Unknown	CC, FISH
	t(11;V)(q23;V)	*MLL*	CC, FISH, PCR
	t(V;21)(V;q22.3)	*AML1*	CC, FISH, PCR
	t(3;21)(q26;q22.3)	*EVI1;EAP;AML1;MDS*	CC, FISH
	t(3;5)(q25;q35) ins(3;5)(q25;q31.1q35)	*MLF1; NPM*	CC, FISH, PCR
MDS/CMML	t(5;12)(q31-q32;p13)	*PDGFRβ;TEL*	CC

Abbreviations: CML, chronic myeloid leukemia; AML, acute myeloid leukemia; APL, acute promyelocytic leukemia; MDS, myelodysplasia; CMML, chronic myelomonocytic leukemia; CC, classic cytogenetics; FISH, fluorescence in situ hybridization; PCR, polymerase chain reaction, V, variable partner chromosome.

Table 103.5. *Cytogenetic risk categories for AML (SWOG and MRC) and MDS (IPSS)*

Risk status	SWOG coding, AML	MRC coding, AML	IPSS, MDS
Favorable	inv(16)/t(16;16)/del(16q), t(15;17) with/without secondary aberrations; t(8;21) lacking del(9q) or complex karyotypes	inv(16)/t(16;16)/del(16q), t(15;17), t(8;21) with/without secondary abnormalities	As sole aberrations del(5q) del(20q) −Y
Intermediate	Normal, +8, +6, −Y, del(12p)	Normal, 11q23 abn, +8, del(9q), del(7q), +21, +22, all others	All other aberrations not listed in favorable or unfavorable
Unfavorable	del(5q)/−5, −7/del(7q), abn of 3q, 9q, 11q, 20q, 21q, 17p, t(6;9), t(9;22) and complex karyotypes (≥3 unrelated abn)	del(5q)/−5, −7, abn(3q), complex karyotypes (≥5 unrelated abn)	Chromosome 7 aberrations Complex karyotypes (≥3 aberrations)
Unknown	All other abnormalities	Category not recognized	

Modified with permission from Slovak *et al.* (2000). MRC data published by Grimwade *et al.* (1997). IPSS data from Greenberg *et al.* (1997).

Flow cytometry

Flow cytometry is a practical and widely used pathology assay to measure the ploidy level of a tumor and monitor MRD by tumor immunophenotype. Flow cytometry involves the measurement of fluorescence or other characteristics (i.e., light scatter or absorbency) performed on single cells in suspension as they pass through a laser illumination and detection point. DNA measurements ranging from 1.00 up to 1.04 are considered normal. In studies of acute lymphoblastic leukemia (ALL), the cytogenetic cutoff for the favorable hyperdiploidy subgroup has been established at 50 chromosomes. In flow cytometry, a cutoff of 1.16 has been established to discriminate between favorable and unfavorable (Trueworthy *et al.*, 1992). The relative quality of flow cytometric measurements is dependent on the cell preparation, staining, and instrument calibration measurements. The DNA index estimation corresponds to a difference of two to four chromosomes, with a sensitivity of ±5%. Thus, depending on the size of the additional chromosomes in hyperdiploid ALL, even hyperdiploid cases with 52 to 53 chromosomes may have a DNA index below 1.16 (Haas *et al.*, 1998). For more complete flow cytometry instruction, the reader is referred to the publication of Shapiro (1995). For the detection of MRD by flow cytometry, the reader is referred to Chapter 106.

Molecular cytogenetics or FISH

FISH protocols increase the scope of diagnosis and prognosis by allowing determination of specific DNA sequence copy number in both metaphase chromosomes and interphase (nondividing) cells. Chromosome-specific or locus-specific DNA probes are nonisotopically labeled by incorporation of a fluorescently tagged reporter molecule. A nonfluorescing version of FISH, commonly termed ISH, uses a biotin-streptavidin-polyalkaline-phosphatase complex that does not require a fluo-

rescent microscope. For the purposes of this chapter, FISH and ISH are used interchangeably.

Clinical applications of FISH technology take advantage of the molecular probes that are specific for defined regions of cytogenetic interest. Alpha-satellite DNA probes, unique for centromeric regions of each chromosome, are used to detect gains or losses of specific chromosomes, such as trisomy 8 or monosomy 7. Unique sequence or cosmid probes (~40–50 kilobases) can detect deletions [e.g., TP53, RB, or del(5)(q31), Fig. 103.2A] or well-established recurrent translocations [e.g., t(15;17), t(8;21) or t(9;22), Fig. 103.2B]. In addition, whole chromosome "painting" probes, which hybridize to unique sequences spanning an entire chromosome or specific chromosomal regions, aid in determining the chromosomal origin of complex or cryptic translocations (as illustrated in 24-color karyotyping, Fig 103.3).

Because FISH allows rapid screening of unbalanced or aberrant genetic alterations in nondividing cells, this quantitative technique is invaluable when tissue culture fails, mitotic indices are low, and chromosome morphology is suboptimal, as well as establishing clonality when only a single abnormal metaphase is observed by standard cytogenetics. FISH studies supplement standard cytogenetics in the monitoring of patients with specific known chromosomal aberrations. The use of X and Y chromosome-specific probes provides a quick marker of donor engraftment in sex-mismatched transplant recipients, allowing assessment of donor cells in either mitotic, interphase, or in terminally differentiated cells.

Classic cytogenetic studies are hampered in the hypoproliferative lymphoid neoplastic disorders, in particular, well-differentiated CLL and multiple myeloma (MM). In lymphoma, the lymph nodes are generally directed immediately to pathology for fixation and paraffin-embedding, precluding classic cytogenetics but usually remaining amenable for targeted FISH analysis. Newer isolation techniques for individual nuclei from tissue cores have lessened the problems associated with scoring

Table 103.6. *Common numerical and structural cytogenetic alterations in lymphoid diseases*

Disease	Cytogenetic abnormality	Molecular targets	Detection methods
Acute lymphoblastic leukemia/ lymphoma, B cell or T cell	t(7q35), t(14q11.2), t/inv(14q32.1), t(14q32.33)	Antigen receptor gene rearrangements for *TCRβ, TCRα/δ, TCLI, IGH*	CC, FISH, PCR
	del or t(11q23)	*MLL (ALL1/HTX)*-various	CC, FISH, PCR
	del(6q)	Unknown	CC, FISH
	t/del(9q21)	*MTS1/MTS2 (p16/p15)*	CC, FISH, PCR
ALL, pre B-cell lineage	t(9;22)(q34.1;q11.2)	*ABL;BCR*	CC, FISH, PCR
	t(1;19)(q23;p13.3)	*PBX1;E2A*	CC, PCR
	t(4;11)(q21;q23)	*AF4;MLL*	CC, FISH, PCR
	t(12;21)(p13;q22.3)	*TEL;AML1*	CC, FISH
ALL with B-lineage	>50 chromosomes/cell Most commonly: +X,+4,+6,+10,+14,+17,+18,+20,+21	Whole chromosome gains	CC, FISH
ALL with eosinophilia	t(5;14)(q31.1;q32.33)	*IL3;IGH*	CC
Pre or pro-B-ALL	t(17;19)(q22;p13.3)	*BCL5;E2A*	CC, PCR
Burkitt's lymphoma/leukemia	t(8;14)(q24.1;q32.33)	*MYC;IGH*	CC, FISH, PCR
	t(8;22)(q24.1;q11)	*MYC;IGL*	CC
	t(2;8)(p12;q24.1)	*IGK;MYC*	CC
ALL, T-cell lineage	inv(14)(q11.2q32.1)/t(14;14)	*TCRα/δ;TCL1*	CC, PCR for all listed
	t(1;14)(p32;q11.2)	*TAL1/SCL;TCRα/δ*	
	t(8;14)(q24.1;q11.2)	*MYC;TCRα*	
	t(10;14)(q24;q11.2)	*HOX11/TCL3;TCRδ*	
	t(7;9)(q35;q34.3)	*TCRβ;TAN1*	
	t(7;9)(q35;q31)	*TCRβ;TAL2*	
	t(11;14)(p13;q11.2)	*RBTN2;TCRδ*	
	t(11;14)(p15;q11.2)	*RBTN1;TCRα*	
	t(7;19)(q35;p13.1-2)	*TCRβ;LYL1*	
	t(7;10)(q35;q24)	*TCRβ;HOX11/TCL3*	
CLL, B cell	+12	cen 12 or MDM2	CC, FISH
	del(17p)	*TP 53*	CC, FISH, PCR
	del(6q)	*MYB*	CC, FISH
	del(11q)	*ATM*	CC, FISH
	del(13)(q12q14)	Unknown/D13S319	CC, FISH
CLL, T cell	inv(14) (q11.2q32.1)/t(14;14)	*TCRα/δ;TCL1*	CC
Lymphoma All cases	Variable	Antigen receptor gene rearrangements	CC, FISH, PCR
	t(10;14)(q24;q32.33)	*HOX11;IGH*	CC
	t(3;4)(q27;p11)	*BCL6(LAZ3);TTF*	CC
Follicular NHL	t(14;18)(q32.33;q21)	*IGH;BCL2*	CC, FISH, PCR
Mantle cell lymphoma	t(11;14)(q13;q32.33)	*CCND1/BCL1;IGH*	CC, FISH, PCR
Anaplastic large cell lymphoma	t(2;5)(p23;q35)	*ALK;NPM1*	CC, FISH, PCR
Diffuse large B-cell lymphoma	t(3;V)(q27;V)	*BCL6*	CC
T-cell lymphoma	t(4;16)(q26;p13.1)	*IL2;BCM*	CC
MALT lymphoma	t(11;18)(q22;q22)	*PAI2;MALT1*	CC, FISH, PCR
Multiple myeloma	t(11;14)(q13;q32.33)	*CCND1;IgH*	CC, FISH
	t(4;14)(p16.3;q32.33)	*FGFR3;IgH*	FISH
	t(6;14)(p25;q32.33)	*IRF4;IgH*	FISH
	t(14;16)(q32.33;q23)	*IgH;MAF*	FISH
	del(17p)	*TP 53*	CC, FISH
	del(13)(q12q14)	Unknown	CC, FISH

Abbreviations: ALL, acute lymphoblastic leukemia; NHL, non-Hodgkin's lymphoma; CC, classic cytogenetics; FISH, fluorescence in situ hybridization; PCR, polymerase chain reaction; MALT, mucosa-associated lymphoid tissue; PCR for all 14q32.3 aberrations is possible.

Table 103.7.   *Common cytogenetic abnormalities in solid tumors*

Disease	Cytogenetic abnormality	Molecular targets	Detection methods
Myxoid liposarcoma	t(12;16)(q13.3;p11.2)	*FUS;CHOP*	CC
Ewing sarcoma/peripheral neuroepithelioma/Askin's tumor/PNETs[1]	t(11;22)(q24;q12) t(21;22)(q22.3;q12)	*FLI1;EWS* *ERG;EWS*	CC, FISH
Desmoplastic small round cell tumor	t(11;22)(p13;q12)	*WT1;EWS*	CC
Synovial sarcoma	t(X;18)(p11.2;q11.2)	*SSX;SYT*	CC, FISH
Extraskeletal myxoid chondrosarcoma	t(9;22)(q22;q12)	*TEC;EWS*	CC
Clear cell sarcoma	t(12;22)(q13–14;q12)	*ATF1;EWS*	CC
Alveolar rhabdomyosarcoma	t(2;13)(q35;q14) t(1;13)(p36.1;q14)	*PAX3;FKHR* *PAX7;FKHR*	CC, FISH, PCR
Neuroblastoma	dims/hsrs del(1p)(p32->p36)	*NMYC* amplification Unknown	CC, FISH
Colon cancer	del(5q)/(17p)/(18q)	*APC, TP53, DCC*	CC, FISH, PCR
Breast cancer	17q21/13q12 17q21.2/dmin/hsr 17p13.1	*BRCA1;BRCA2* *HER2/NEU (ERBB2)* *TP53*	CC, FISH, PCR
Ovarian cancer	17q21.2/dmin/hsr 17q21	*HER2/NEU (ERBB2)* *BRCA1*	CC, FISH, PCR
Papillary thyroid carcinoma	inv(10)(q11.2q21)	*RET;10S170*	CC
Melanoma of soft parts	t(12;22)(q13;q12)	*ATF1;EWS*	CC
Germ cell tumors	i(12)(p10)	Unknown	CC, FISH

Abbreviations: dmins, double minutes; hsrs, homogeneous staining regions; CC, classic cytogenetics; FISH, fluorescence in situ hybridization; PCR, polymerase chain reaction.

truncated cells from thin paraffin-embedded sections (Paternoster *et al.,* 2002). In this respect, interphase FISH studies represent a major advance allowing for the reliable detection of specific aberrations, independent of the in vitro proliferative activity of the neoplastic cells. Disease-specific FISH probe panels targeting recurrent aberrations in the lymphoid malignancies (Table 103.6) are not only defining the frequency of selected aberrations, but additionally FISH can distinguish atypical CLL from the leukemic phase of t(11;14) mantle cell lymphoma (Remstein *et al.,* 2000), and provides the groundwork to reliably define cytogenetic-based, risk-adapted prognostic groups (Dohner *et al.,* 2000; Facon *et al.,* 2001). However, targeted FISH panels are limited to the specific aberrations being evaluated and without tumor enrichment, accurate detection requires ≥10% tumor cells. Furthermore, for candidates undergoing HSCT, classic cytogenetics prior to transplantation is recommended to rule out any pre-existing chromosome anomalies associated with therapy-related leukemia, especially in heavily pretreated patients.

Many factors can influence false positive and false negative rates for quantitative FISH, including scoring criteria, number of cells scored, nucleus size, probe robustness, ploidy, and chance co-localization of signals in interphase cells. Of particular concern is that a small number of residual host cells may be

found in the bone marrow of allogeneic HSCT (allo-HSCT) recipients in continuous clinical remission for many years posttransplant (Durnam *et al.,* 1989) and observed for several months after non-myeloablative HSCT. This finding does not indicate imminent relapse but relates to the presence of host stromal cells. These factors must all be taken into account when interpreting results and evaluating sensitivity and specificity of a given FISH assay (Chase *et al.,* 1997). As such, tumor-specific FISH probes, in combination with enumeration probes, are preferable to enumeration probes alone to study and monitor MRD.

MRD analyses, using tumor-specific probes such as the *BCR/ABL* fusion gene, are rapid quantitative molecular cytogenetic tools to monitor therapy. FISH is especially useful to identify a cytogenetically cryptic "masked" Philadelphia chromosome translocation, reported to occur in ~5% of CML patients. Sensitivity of a 200 cell, one-probe FISH study nears 10^{-1} to 10^{-2} (Dewald *et al.,* 1997), similar to classic cytogenetics. Because of both intra- and interlaboratory technical variations, each laboratory must perform validation studies to establish sensitivity and specificity ranges for all non–FDA-approved FISH probes used in clinical testing.

For MRD detection, increased sensitivity comparable to PCR techniques in the range of 10^{-3} to 10^{-4} has been reported by use of either a double fusion FISH probe, which detects chimeric sequences on both derivative chromosomes from a reciprocal translocation, or by a pooled three-color/triple-

[1] Frederick Barton Askins, 20th Century U.S. pathologist.

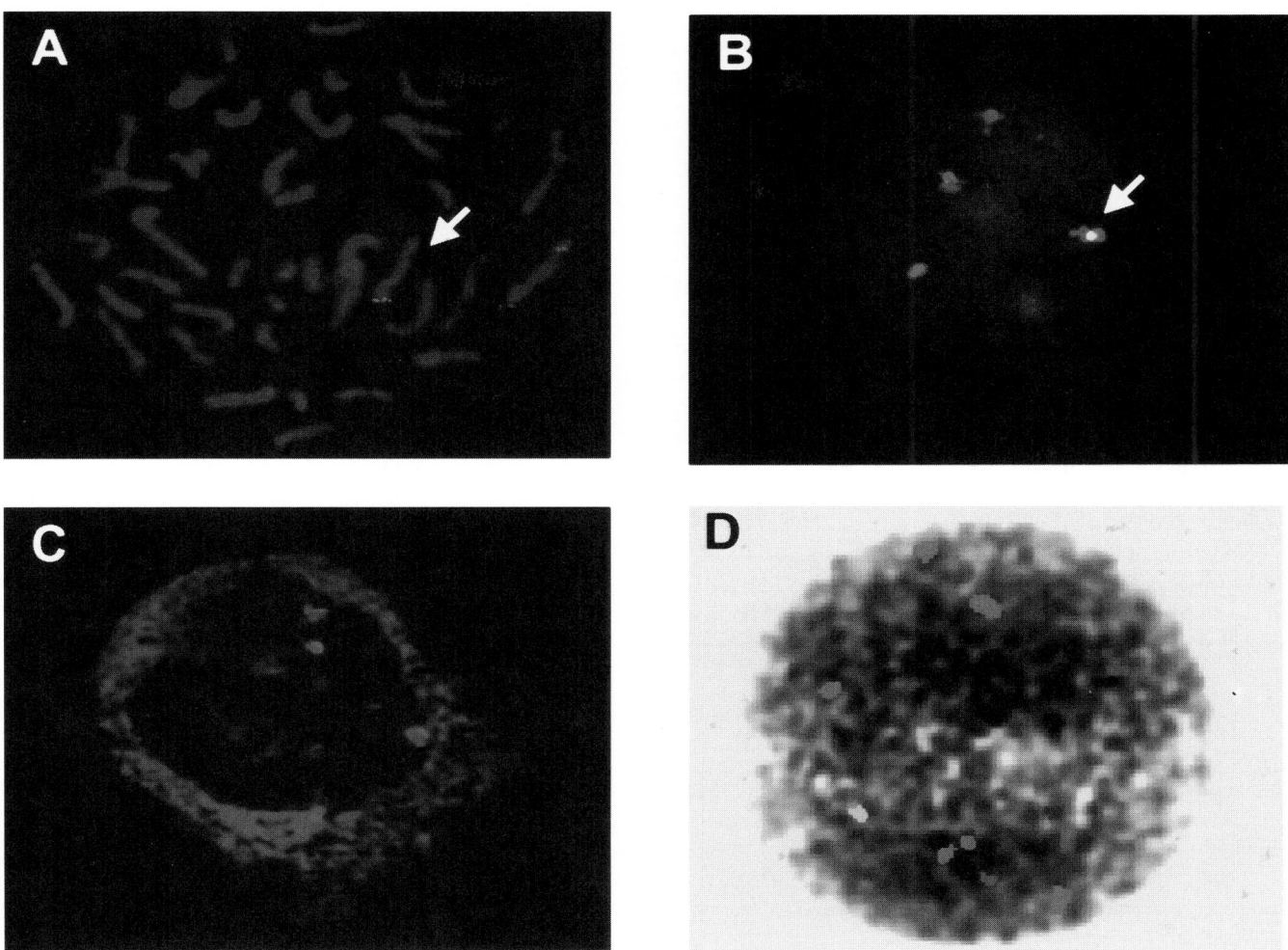

Fig. 103.2. Various fluorescence in situ hybridization (FISH) techniques. (A) Dual color FISH exhibiting a deletion of the long arm of one chromosome 5 (arrow), specifically band 5q31 (spectrum green), in a patient with AML. The spectrum orange chromosome 5 p arm probe identifies the two chromosomes 5 in this metaphase cell. The normal chromosome 5 is seen on the far right. (B) Triple-color/triple-probe FISH detecting the Philadelphia chromosome rearrangement. The normal chromosome 22 is represented by the green signal. The red/aqua fusion represents the normal 9. The red/green fusion is the derivative 22 chromosome (arrow) and the lone aqua signal is the derivative 9 chromosome. Samples without the sole aqua signal would identify deletions in the derivative 9 chromosome. (C) Fluorescence Immunophenotyping and Interphase Cytogenetics as a Tool for Investigation of Neoplasms (FICTION) detection in acute myelogenous leukemia. Trisomy 8 (three blue-green signals) is detected in a CD15 negative cell (right) and a CD15 positive cell (left). FICTION characterizes karyotypically aberrant cells with immunophenotype to allow cell lineage analysis of single cells. (D) Spectral FISH cell with MDS/AML probe panel. This cell shows two 5p15 signals (red) with loss of EGR1 (5q31) (one yellow signal). The patient has two copies of chromosome 7 indicated by two centromeric 7 signals (aqua) and two CULT 1 signals (blue). The patient also has four copies of chromosome 8 indicated by four magenta signals that hybridize to the centromeric region of chromosome 8. For color reproduction, see Color Plate 103.2.

probe approach (Bentz et al., 1994; Kasprzyk & Secker-Walker, 1997; Sinclair et al., 1997; Tanaka et al., 1997; Dewald et al., 1998). Since the limit of sensitivity for interphase FISH is dependent on false positive values, one way to decrease false positivity and increase sensitivity is to target more than one chromosomal abnormality. Kasprzyk and Secker-Walker (1997) studied MRD in 16 high hyperdiploid ALL patients using an interphase FISH approach that simultaneously targeted three chromosomal gains. Dilution experiments mixing control blood lymphocytes with bone marrow

from a patient with greater than 85% blasts and probing with single, dual, and triple probes revealed levels of sensitivity for clonal detection to be 10^{-1}, 10^{-3}, and 10^{-4}, respectively. Of interest, the authors reported extremely low levels of clonal cells (0.01%–0.06%) at the end of treatment. Serial samples showed a tendency for the clone to diminish or disappear over time, with the exception of two patients who relapsed 6 and 30 months posttreatment. FISH, for the detection of MRD in hyperdiploid ALL, showed heterogeneity between patients in clonal elimination. In eight patients, chemotherapy or transplantation apparently eliminated the clone. This approach to MRD detection is technically simple, leukemia-specific, quantitative, and sensitive to 10^{-4}. A double fusion *BCR/ABL* FISH (D-FISH) probe used to monitor response to CML therapy found MRD detection corresponded to ≥3.83% abnormal cells in a 200-cell analysis; however, the limits of detection could be reduced to 0.79% with a 6000 nuclei screen (Dewald *et al.*, 1998). When coupled with automation, multiplex FISH will be a useful MRD assay to monitor early detection of a re-emerging clone, allowing early therapeutic intervention before full relapse.

Detection of the >50 hyperdiploid ALL subgroup can be accomplished by classic cytogenetics, DNA index measurements by flow cytometry, or by FISH. A panel of enumeration probes specific for several recurrent trisomies in ALL (i.e., chromosomes X, 4, 6, 10, 17, 18, 21, and 22) creates a reliable, quick screening tool to identify the ~30% of pediatric patients with this favorable karyotypic picture (Ritterbach *et al.*, 1998). A comparison of flow cytometric studies and a four-probe ALL FISH panel, showed concordance in 208 of 234 (88.8%) cases. Of the discrepant results, 11 children with a DNA index of 1.00 displayed more than two FISH signals for at least one of the probed chromosomes. Cytogenetic studies confirmed the presence of a small hyperdiploid (2%–28%) clone in eight cases. This latter finding is below the limits of detection by flow cytometry. Of the remaining 15 discrepant cases, the FISH panel either did not include the trisomic chromosomes or cytogenetic studies failed to confirm either flow or FISH results. Similar results have been reported in myeloma (Perez Simon *et al.*, 1998). These data underscore the usefulness of FISH to screen for extreme hyperdiploidy in childhood ALL using a specified panel of enumeration probes.

Fiber-FISH is a powerful physical mapping research tool used to characterize translocations with scattered breakpoints, such as the t(11;14) observed in mantle cell lymphoma (Vaandrager *et al.*, 1997). This FISH technique hybridizes multicolored fluorescent probes on stretched DNA fibers to assess the relative order within a ≥50 kb chromosomal region. A misalignment between germline and tumor cells indicates that a chromosomal aberration has occurred; a translocation is confirmed by aligning the "skewed" segment to the suspected partner chromosome.

Spectral karyotyping (also known as multiplex or M-FISH) is based on hybridization of 24 different fluorescently labeled chromosome painting probes specific for each chromosome pair. The technique identifies suspected or cryptic karyotypic aberrations in tumors not adequately resolvable by classic cytogenetics (Fig. 103.3) (Veldman *et al.*, 1997; Rao *et al.*, 1998; Sawyer *et al.*, 1998; Zhang *et al.*, 2001). Unfortunately, this technique is limited in the detection of small deletions, intrachromosomal rearrangements, and detection of telomeric rearrangements, and is dependent on obtaining abnormal metaphases, thus providing limited data in the evaluation of hypoproliferative tumors. Combinatorial labeling of DNA FISH probes and spectral imaging has also led to the development of spectral FISH, allowing for the simultaneous detection of 3 to 10 genetic aberrations in a single cell in a single hybridization, which holds great promise in detecting disease-specific aberrations when tissue samples are limited (Slovak *et al.*, 2001) (Fig. 103.2D). Newer molecular cytogenetic protocols, such as matrix-based comparative genomic hybridization, 2-color multiplex telomeric (M-TEL) assays, and computationally defined, custom-designed, sequence-specific single copy genomic probes, are in development for improved detection of

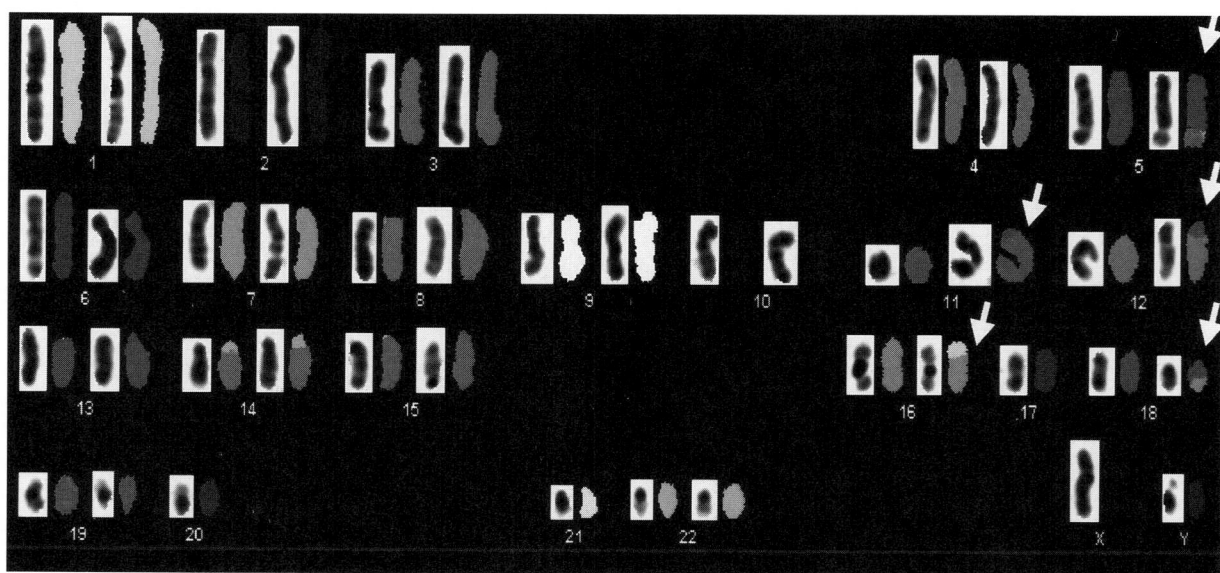

Fig. 103.3. Example of spectral (24-color) karyotyping of chromosomes prepared from a AML bone marrow sample. The DAPI-banded image (left) and spectrally classified chromosomes (right) are shown. Abnormalities of chromosomes 1, 5, 11, 12, 16, 17, 18, 20, and 21 are identified by their classification colors. For color reproduction, see Color Plate 103.3.

genetic rearrangements in both rare and common chromosome alterations within a single cell (Solinas-Toldo *et al.*, 1997; Brown *et al.*, 2001; Rogan *et al.*, 2001).

Combined techniques

Hypermetaphase FISH

This blending of classic cytogenetics and FISH is performed on cells cultured for 12 hours in the presence of a high concentration of colcemid, resulting in collection of cytogenetically aberrant cells at a much higher frequency than with classic cytogenetics (Seong *et al.*, 1995). Prolonged exposure to the mitotic spindle poison allows visualization and quantitation of chromosomal aberrations in 500 to 2,000+ overly contracted mitotic cells, with high reliability and increased sensitivity (Seong *et al.*, 1995; El-Rifai *et al.*, 1997a). Using hypermetaphase FISH in AML, leukemic cells were found during clinical remission in 9 of 22 (41%) patients (median follow-up, 21 months). Detection of abnormal cells was uncommon in the good to intermediate prognosis cytogenetic subgroups [t(8;21), t(15;17), +8], but frequent in the poor prognosis cytogenetic subgroup [−7/del(7q)] (El-Rifai *et al.*, 1997a). With one exception, AML and ALL patients with an increasing and/or persisting level of abnormal cells in two or more subsequent samples, or whose initial samples contained more than 1% abnormal cells, relapsed (El-Rifai *et al.*, 1997a, 1997b). These data suggest that variations in the presence of residual leukemia cells are dependent on the initial cytogenetic findings. Based on Hook's statistical formula (1977), a 2,000 hypermetaphase analysis rules out mosaicism nearing 10^{-3} with 95% confidence, or two logs higher than that of standard cytogenetics (El-Rifai *et al.*, 1997a). This technique is most useful for monitoring leukemias characterized by a translocation, trisomy, or deletions, for which FISH probes are available. Recently, the introduction of second generation, multi-fluorophore DNA FISH probes for detection of *BCR/ABL* has defined potential poor-risk CML patients that may benefit from early transplantation (Huntly *et al.*, 2001; Sinclair *et al.*, 1999; Cohen *et al.*, 2001). These assays coupled with overly contracted chromosomes and poorly spread metaphases, make this approach suitable for MRD detection of monosomy, subtle deletions, or assessing clonal evolution of disease. Compromised hybridization conditions with simultaneous use of small and large probes is the major limitation of this technique.

Comparative genomic hybridization

Comparative genomic hybridization (CGH) was introduced by Kallioniemi *et al.* (1992) to improve detection of chromosomal deletions and amplifications in solid tumors. This technique generates a copy number karyotype by competitive hybridization between tumor and normal DNA sequences on to a normal metaphase chromosome template to provide a comprehensive screen to detect chromosomal imbalances in a tumor. Genomic tumor DNA is isolated from a tumor using flow cytometric sorting or microdissection to minimize cellular contamination

by normal stromal cells and enrich the tumor cell population. Genomic control DNA from normal lymphocytes is also isolated. An equimolar mixture of differentially labeled genomic tumor and control DNA is used for chromosome in situ suppression hybridization on normal metaphases. Because fluorescently labeled tumor and control DNA sequences compete for the same target chromosome sequences, the relative copy number of homologous sequences is reflected as a ratio of the two fluorescence intensities. Individual chromosomes are identified by DAPI staining and the signal intensities of each fluorochrome are captured microscopically using cooled CCD cameras and quantitated by specially designed software (Kallioniemi *et al.*, 1992, 1994; Joos *et al.*, 1993).

In contrast to FISH, neither intact tumor cells nor high-quality metaphases are needed, nor is it restricted to known FISH probes. Amplifications or deletions of 1 to 20 megabases are detectable by this method. Fresh, frozen, or paraffin-embedded tumor tissue samples may be used. The limitations of this method include the inability to detect ploidy, balanced translocations, inversions, point mutations, or small changes involving centromeric or telomeric regions. However, CGH has delineated genomic regions of interest in tumors allowing for selection of locus-specific DNA probes for rapid FISH screening. The sensitivity of CGH is dependent on tumor cell enrichment methods but is comparable to RFLP and targeted FISH analyses. Interestingly, CGH technology is the enabling technology behind the development of DNA array systems. Due to the overall complexity of CGH, this technique has remained in the research setting; however, matrix-based CGH protocol improvements promise the development of biochips with increased resolution to screen for genomic imbalances to meet clinical needs in the near future (Solinas-Toldo *et al.*, 1997).

Molecular cytogenetics in combination with immunophenotyping

Correlative interphase cytogenetic analysis with immune detection on a single cell basis is now possible, using a variation of FISH named FICTION (*F*luorescence *I*mmunophenotyping and interphase *C*ytogenetics as a *T*ool for *I*nvestigations *o*f *N*eoplasms) or MAC (*M*onoclonal *A*ntibody *C*ytogenetics). This combined fluorescence technique is useful in detection of clone-specific aberrations in malignant cells and MRD (Fig. 103.2C). The technique holds promise for studying cell lineage and clonality in hematopoietic disorders by direct visualization of chromosomal changes with cellular phenotype, nuclear morphology, cytoplasmic features, and immunophenotype. Histologic features, proliferative index, or protein markers in solid tumors are also discernible using a variety of specimens, including fresh, frozen, or paraffin-embedded tissue sections. For example, immature cells in bone marrow aspirates present a diagnostic problem. In AML, neoplastic myeloblasts present in small numbers often cannot be distinguished morphologically from regenerating blasts after myelosuppressive therapy. In pediatric ALL patients, neoplastic lymphoblasts may be morphologically similar to immature lymphoid cells (hematogones), which can also be TdT positive and express CD10 and surface markers of immature lymphocytes (Anastasi *et al.,* 1991a, 1991b). To increase detection of cytogenetically aberrant plasma cells, FISH methods to either isolate plasma cells by CD138-labeled magnetic bead sorting or to identify plasma cells with fluorescent-labeled antibodies for cytoplasmic immunoglobulin (cIg-FISH), have been carried out (Fonseca *et al.,* 2001b). In those cases where a few suspicious cells are identified and clonal abnormalities have been detected, this time-consuming and technically sophisticated technique has proven to be beneficial in detecting rare malignant residual/recurrent cells.

Using the MAC technique, morphologic analysis of most hematologic neoplasias can indicate involvement of one or more cell lineages, while ruling out simultaneous involvement of all lineages. MAC studies have given conclusive evidence for involvement of specific lineages in a series of 65 patients with hematologic neoplasms. In MDS and AML, cytogenetic aberrations of del(5q), del(20q), and i(17q) appear to occur in a pluripotent stem cell capable of maturing into granulocytic/monocytic, erythrocytic, or megakaryocytic cells. Additionally, the highly specific 8;21 and 15;17 translocations in AML are seen in granulocytes or monocytic mitoses, not in erythrocytic mitoses. Furthermore, cytogenetic examination of FACS-isolated CD34+/CD38−/CD117+/− stem cell subpopulations has revealed clonal leukemia-specific cytogenetic abnormalities (Haase *et al.,* 1995; Mehrotra *et al.,* 1995; Haase *et al.,* 1997). In one exceptional case of AML (FAB-M3) MAC studies showed the leukemogenic event did not take place in CD34+/CD38− stem cells, but occurred in a more committed CD34+/CD38+ population (Turhan *et al.,* 1995). Preliminary results also suggest that malignant transformation in most cases of ALL occurs in immature CD34+/Lin− stem cells (Quijano *et al.,* 1997). These results have substantial implication for monitoring of residual disease in acute leukemia. Because the majority of patients are mosaic in this HSC subcompartment, additional sorting and genotyping research should focus on strategies for accurate discrimination between normal and abnormal stem cells collected for autografts and MRD parameters.

Molecular genetics (and see Chapter 105)

PCR and RT-PCR assays are useful for submicroscopic identification of an increasing number of characteristic nonrandom chromosomal rearrangements associated with various leukemias, lymphomas, and solid tumors. RT-PCR assays assume that an acquired chimeric fusion gene is constitutively expressed in all translocation-bearing cells. Once the DNA sequence surrounding translocation breakpoints has been elucidated, PCR assays are rapid and may use specimens currently unsatisfactory for other genetic testing methods. Well-designed PCR assays typically demonstrate high degrees of concordance with traditional cytogenetics and automated PCR provides reliable sequential quantitative measurements. Discrepant results

frequently reflect the higher sensitivity of PCR methodologies, which appears to make them suitable for identification of MRD.

Despite these advantages, PCR-based tests have several drawbacks including the requirement for a known DNA sequence, the inability to demonstrate translocations or other cytogenetic aberrations not anticipated in the assay design, the inability to detect translocations in cases where the breakpoint is highly variable and spans large DNA sequences, and difficulty in detecting homozygous loss when tumor cells are "contaminated" with normal tissue (the latter is easily detected by FISH). In contrast, standard cytogenetics may demonstrate unanticipated, clinically significant cytogenetic abnormalities. An increase in sensitivity and ability to detect early disease recurrence must also be weighed against an inability to detect evolving chromosomal changes related to disease progression or secondary disease.

Hematopoietic disorders

Acute myeloid leukemia

Prognostic implications of nonrandom cytogenetic aberrations in myeloid disorders (Table 103.4) treated by chemotherapy have been described (Schiffer *et al.,* 1989; Marosi *et al.,* 1992; Dastugue *et al.,* 1995). The question remains, however, as HSCT strategies for leukemia evolve, whether karyotype at diagnosis and other prognostic factors previously recognized to predict response to chemotherapy also predict response to transplantation. Most reports describing the importance of karyotypic changes in AML within a transplant setting are retrospective, pooled from multiple testing centers using varying treatment regimens, plagued by small sample size or low numbers of detectable cytogenetic abnormalities in the test population (<50%), and lack central review of the karyotypic data and failure to correspond to a uniform classification system for comparability (Ferrant *et al.,* 1995, 1997; Gale *et al.,* 1995; Slovak *et al.,* 2000). In addition, the frequency by which cytogenetic analyses were performed, the techniques used, the number of cells analyzed, and success rates, varied considerably within and among the different centers. Despite the sample size of larger studies from the International Bone Marrow Transplantation Registry (IBMTR), the European Group for Blood and Marrow Transplantation (EBMT), and the North American Study (Southwest Oncology Group or SWOG/Eastern Cooperative Oncology Group or ECOG), the impact of individual cytogenetic abnormalities cannot be assessed due to the small numbers in specific karyotypic groups. Nevertheless, these studies provide direction for future randomized prospective studies addressing the comparative value of dose-intensive chemotherapy and allogeneic or autologous HSCT, to ultimately stratify patients by genotype and optimize treatment modality.

A prospective AML study evaluating the influence of karyotype in 134 consecutive patients assigned to either autologous or allogeneic BMT in first remission, depending on donor availability was reported by Ferrant et al. (1995). Of the 118 patients who obtained a complete remission, 25 received allogeneic and 43 received autologous BMT. The karyotypes were categorized as follows: good, t(15;17), inv(16) ($n = 10$); intermediate, normal, $-X$, $-Y$, t(8;21) ($n = 49$); or unfavorable, all other abnormalities ($n = 44$) (Keating et al., 1988). The 5-year leukemia-free survival (LFS) probabilities for patients with good, intermediate, and unfavorable karyotypes were 65%, 32%, and 11%, respectively. This study was the first to demonstrate that cytogenetics retains its prognostic value when the clinical intention is to treat AML patients in first remission with BMT. In the autologous BMT group, LFS was 100%, 33%, and 10%, respectively ($P = .04$), implying that autologous BMT was best suited for the good-risk cytogenetics subgroup.

The three largest retrospective AML studies correlating karyotype at disease presentation with BMT outcome have been reported (Gale et al., 1995; Ferrant et al., 1997; Slovak et al., 2000). Comparison of the published data on outcome after chemotherapy suggests the prognostic implication of leukemia characterized by chromosome 16 abnormalities was similar in both groups; however, patients with diploid karyotypes, hyperdiploidy, and pseudodiploidy had a better outcome with BMT.

The 13-year EBMT study included 999 patients from 75 EBMT centers with de novo AML, treated by autologous or allogeneic BMT in first complete remission, and in whom a cytogenetic report was available (Ferrant et al., 1997). Karyotypes were classified according to specific chromosomal aberrations reported in the Sixth International Workshop on Chromosomes in Leukemia (Arthur et al., 1989). Karyotype subgroups were further subdivided based on transplant outcome. In the allogeneic subgroup, three cytogenetic categories were defined: good prognosis, abnormalities of chromosome 16 and t(8;21); intermediate prognosis, t(15;17), normal diploid, pseudodiploid, or a hyperdiploid karyotype; and poor prognosis, rearrangements of 11q, abnormalities of chromosomes 5 and 7 or hypodiploidy. In the autologous subgroup, two categories were defined: abnormalities of chromosomes 5 and 7 and hypodiploidy constituted the poor prognosis group whereas all other karyotypes, including abnormalities of chromosome 16 and t(8;21), were associated with a standard or intermediate prognosis. In the poor prognostic karyotype subgroup, no significant difference was observed between allogeneic and autologous transplant recipients for relapse, LFS, or overall survival. In the chromosome 16 abnormality subgroup, allo-BMT patients fared better than auto-BMT patients for relapse and LFS. Allo-BMT patients with t(8;21) and hyperdiploidy (most commonly +8) had a lower relapse probability than auto-BMT patients; however, no significant difference was observed in overall survival. For t(15;17) leukemia, auto-BMT gave a better overall survival probability, confirming an earlier EBMT report by Mandelli et al. (1994).

Regarding relapse in the allo-BMT setting, the good, standard, and poor risk cytogenetic groups had a 9%, 25%, and 61% relapse rate, respectively. In the auto-BMT population,

relapse rates were higher, 46% in the standard group and 77% in the poor risk group. Patients with poor-risk cytogenetics appeared to have an unacceptable relapse rate with either allo- or auto-BMT. Concerns associated with this study are low numbers of karyotypic aberrations at presentation (<55%), no review of karyotypes, questionable lumping of known poor-risk cytogenetics, such as t(9;22) and t(6;9) AML into the standard risk group, and better survival probability in allo-BMT patients treated after the ninth year of the study (January, 1989). The cytogenetic aberrations associated with drug resistance, poor risk, or therapy-related disease, such as monosomy 7, inv(3q), and complex karyotypes remain high-risk factors associated with leukemia relapse and transplant failure in a North American Study (Slovak et al., 1995a).

In a SWOG/ECOG Intergroup clinical trial, associations of cytogenetics were compared with three intensive postremission therapies: intensive chemotherapy, auto-BMT, or allo-BMT from matched related donors in 609 previously untreated AML patients <56 years old (Slovak et al., 2000). Patients were categorized into favorable, intermediate, unfavorable, and unknown cytogenetic risk groups based on pretreatment karyotypes (Table 103.5). Among postremission patients, survival from CR varied significantly among favorable, intermediate, and unfavorable groups ($P = .0003$), with significant evidence of interaction ($P = .017$) between the effects of treatment and cytogenetic risk status on survival (Fig. 103.4A), even though no difference in survival was observed when patients were examined by treatment arm alone (Fig. 103.4B). In this exploratory analysis, patients with favorable cytogenetics did significantly better following auto-BMT and allo-BMT than with chemotherapy alone (Fig. 103.4C), whereas patients with unfavorable cytogenetics did better with allo-BMT (Fig. 103.4D). Unfortunately, in this intent-to-treat study, 26% of the patients on study did not receive their assigned treatment, and the breakdown into the cytogenetic risk groups by three treatment arms once again resulted in small subgroups with limited power.

Although a karyotypic comparison was attempted with published outcome data from the MRC AML 10 trial (Grimwade et al., 1998), the analysis was imperfect, suggesting the need for a more robust and perhaps internationally accepted karyotypic classification scheme to tighten treatment correlates in genetically defined AML subsets. Unquestionably, cytogenetics play an important role in both induction and postremission therapy; however, in order to identify patients by karyotype who will maximally benefit from HSC transplants as well as those who may fail, future prospective studies should be evaluated using larger cohorts and an internationally accepted classification system.

Myelodysplastic syndrome

Early myelodysplastic syndrome (MDS) studies agreed that karyotypic analysis provided relevant clinical information at diagnosis, and patients with normal karyotypes had the most

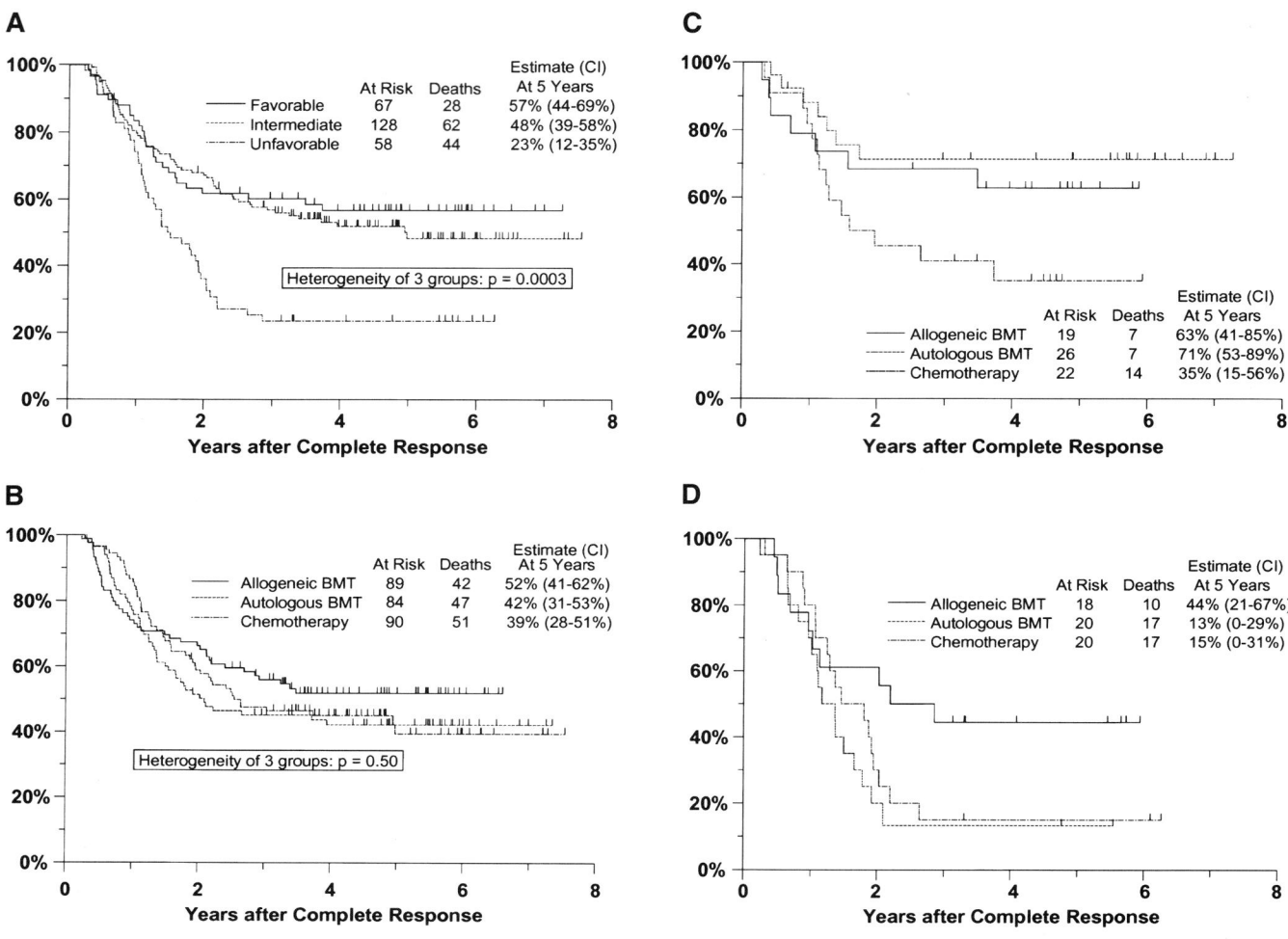

Fig. 103.4. Estimated distributions of survival from complete response by treatment arm and cytogenetic risk status in the North American Study. Survival was measured from date complete response was achieved until death from any cause; tick marks indicate censored observations. 95% CIs are shown in parentheses. (**A**) By cytogenetic risk status (heterogeneity of 3 groups: $P = .0003$). (**B**) By treatment arm (heterogeneity of 3 groups: $P = .50$). (**C**) By treatment arm for the favorable cytogenetic risk group. (**D**) By treatment arm for the unfavorable cytogenetic risk group. From Slovak *et al.* (2000). Copyright American Society of Hematology, used by permission.

favorable outcome after dose-intensive chemotherapy (Fenaux *et al.,* 1991; Morel *et al.,* 1993; Toyama *et al.,* 1993; de Witte *et al.,* 1995; Passmore *et al.,* 1995). Analogous to the AML transplant karyotypic studies, direct comparison of cytogenetics and other prognostic features with clinical outcome was compromised by the lack of a globally accepted systematic MDS prognostic scoring system. The newly established International Prognostic Scoring System (IPSS) facilitates comparisons of future therapeutic choices, based on systematic evaluation of cytogenetics, morphology, demographics, and clinical variables (Greenberg *et al.,* 1997). Using data from seven large previously reported studies, three cytogenetic MDS risk subgroups were established (Table 103.5). Good-risk cytogenetics includes normal bone marrow karyotypes and del(5q), del(20q), or loss of the Y chromosome as sole abnormalities. Poor-risk cytogenetics includes patients with chromosome 7 or complex (≥ 3) abnormalities. All other cytogenetic aberrations

are classified as intermediate risk. When cytogenetic subgroups are combined with percentage of blasts and number of cytopenias in multivariate analysis, four independent risk groups for overall survival and risk for evolution to AML are identified. This improved IPSS risk scoring system provides the guiding framework for future large, randomized transplant trials and companion biological correlative studies to address issues of timing, donor options, and the role of molecular determinants in leukemia evolution in MDS.

Fanconi anemia

Fanconi anemia (FA) is an autosomal recessive disorder characterized by progressive pancytopenia, and diverse congenital abnormalities with an actuarial risk of developing myelodysplasia or AML of greater than 50% by age 40 (Butturini *et al.,* 1994). Complementation studies suggest the genetic basis of

FA is heterogeneous with six different cloned genes identified to date in the pathway that leads to marrow failure in FA patients (Garcia-Higuera *et al.*, 2001). Patients show a wide variation in age of onset of hematologic symptoms and in disease course. Although variable phenotypes make accurate diagnosis on the basis of clinical manifestations unreliable, especially for adult-onset type, study of cultured FA lymphocytes shows higher than normal levels of spontaneous chromosome breakage, that is greatly enhanced following treatment with bifunctional alkylating agents such as mitomycin C (MMC) (Sasaki & Tonomura, 1973) or diepoxybutane (DEB) (Auerbach *et al.*, 1989). Due to a DNA repair defect, chromosomal instability is observed as chromosomal gaps, breaks, fragmentation, exchanges, dicentrics, or radial formations. The combination of increased spontaneous and induced chromosome breakage is pathognomonic for this disorder. Unfortunately, FA heterozygotes (obligate carriers) cannot be differentiated from normal individuals on the basis of spontaneous, DEB, or MMC-induced chromosome breakage (Rosendorff & Bernstein, 1988).

The actuarial risk of clonal cytogenetic abnormalities during bone marrow failure in FA patients by age 30 is 67%, with frequent aberrations of chromosomes 1, 7, and 11 (Butturini *et al.*, 1994; Maarek *et al.*, 1996). However, clonal cytogenetic abnormalities in FA patients lacking morphologic evidence of leukemia are not solely predictive of rapid evolution toward leukemia and shorter survival. Regardless, allo-HSCT remains the sole effective therapy for FA, assuming early intervention and availability of a suitable donor before the onset of AML (Socie *et al.*, 1998).

Acute lymphoblastic leukemia

Durable remission rates for ALL approximate 65% in children and 25% in adults. Cytogenetic classification of ALL identifies low-risk ALL patients from high-risk patients who should be offered intensive treatment with HSCT (Table 103.6). In childhood ALL, trisomy 6, combination trisomy 4 and 10, t(12;21)(p13;q22.3), and extreme hyperdiploidy (>50 chromosomes) indicate a favorable response to conventional therapy (Jackson *et al.*, 1990; Harris *et al.*, 1992; Romana *et al.*, 1995); however, extreme hyperdiploidy does not portend a favorable prognosis in adult ALL (Groupe Francais de Cytogenetique Hematologique, 1996). Childhood leukemia characterized by t(1;19)/E2A-PBX1 responds poorly to conventional antimetabolite-based treatment, but approaches 80% cure rates with dose-intensive therapies (Hunger, 1996), whereas the poor cure rate of Ph+/BCR-ABL and 11q23/MLL ALL with conventional therapy highlights the need for allo-HSCT with an HLA-matched sibling donor (Arico *et al.*, 2000; Biondi *et al.*, 2000; Nishimura *et al.*, 1999). Gains of chromosomes X, 4, 6, 10, and 21 are most common; whole or partial deletions of chromosomes 6, 9, and 12 are also recurrent. An unusual feature of certain high hyperdiploid clones is the apparent ability to remain dormant for many years. Approximately 25% of chil-

dren and 35% of adults relapse in this subgroup (Dastugue *et al.*, 1992). Previously, the presence of any structural rearrangement was felt to compromise the good prognosis of high hyperdiploid patients; however, subsequent studies failed to confirm this. Currently, there is no way to identify the patients in this subgroup who are destined to relapse; however, predictive gene expression arrays appear to be forthcoming (Yeoh *et al.*, 2002).

Regardless of age, the presence of a Ph+/BCR-ABL translocation, t(4;11)(q21;q23) or any other 11q23 rearrangement, Burkitt lymphoma translocations, and hypodiploidy has been associated with a poor prognosis and constitute a relative indication for transplantation (Forman *et al.*, 1987; Pui *et al.*, 1990a, 1990b; Barrett *et al.*, 1992; Raimondi, 1993; Raimondi *et al.*, 1993; Copelan & McGuire, 1995; Groupe Francais de Cytogenetique Hematologique, 1996; Snyder, 2000). A recent prospective CALGB study reporting on the prognostic impact of karyotype for 256 ALL patients with evaluable cytogenetics concluded that trisomy 8 and monosomy 7 should be also be included in the poor-risk ALL cytogenetic subgroup (Wetzler *et al.*, 1999). PCR assays may be used to detect previously cloned and sequenced cytogenetic translocations or immunoglobulin gene rearrangements; however, a caveat of PCR monitoring assays in ALL has been the reported appearance of different cytogenetic clones at relapse in approximately 10% of cases of ALL (Raimondi *et al.*, 1993), and, as true for all nonrandom aberrations in cancer, variant rearrangements may not be detected with the commonly employed amplification primers. Because poor in vitro growth is characteristic of ALL samples, no technique has been able to reveal a detailed picture of all genetic aberrations (Raimondi, 1993). A combined technique of flow cytometry, classic cytogenetics, FISH, and CGH in 14 childhood ALL samples revealed that all 14 cases had at least one karyotypic discrepancy (Haas *et al.*, 1998). Distinct gene expression profiles have been identified for ALL blasts with T-lineage, hyperdiploid >50 chromosomes, t(9;22)/BCR-ABL, t(1;19)/E2A-PBX1, t(12;21)/TEL-AML1, and 11q23/MLL gene rearrangements (Yeoh *et al.*, 2002; Armstrong *et al.*, 2002; Ferrando *et al.*, 2002). Interestingly, further study by FISH and other molecular techniques indicated the "misclassified" gene array cases were variant rearrangements of specific leukemia subgroups, suggesting a common underlying pathogenetic mechanism. These data underscore the need for detailed karyotypic/gene expression definition in ALL cases to refine prognostic impact and future MRD monitoring techniques, most particularly in adult ALL where the prognostic data are sorely lacking.

Chronic myeloid leukemia

Curative CML therapy, defined by the failure to detect *BCR/ABL* transcripts by molecular methods, is possible only with allogeneic HSC transplantation (van Rhee *et al.*, 1997; Weisdorf *et al.*, 2002), with patients in chronic phase exhibiting a greater than 60% and 55% disease-free survival after HLA-matched sibling donor or matched unrelated donor transplant, respectively (Weisdorf et al., 2002). The curative potential of the tyrosine kinase inhibitor imatinib (STI 571; Gleevec) is not yet known. The best outcome after HSCT in patients with CML has been associated with the standard t(9;22)/BCR-ABL Ph+ chromosome translocation. Secondary chromosome aberrations, such as +8, i(17q), +19 and duplication of the Philadelphia chromosome, are reliable indicators of accelerated or blast phase of CML. Few studies have examined the effect of additional chromosomal aberrations in patients undergoing HSC transplant for CML for predicting transplant outcome (Przepiorka & Thomas, 1988; Slovak et al., 1995b; Konstantinidou et al., 2000); however, comparisons among the studies are hampered by phase of CML studied and variation in the cytogenetic categories. Przepiorka and Thomas (1988) examined the cytogenetics of 126 patients in accelerated or blast phase prior to allogeneic or syngeneic HSCT. The authors found a higher risk of relapse posttransplant in those with variant Ph+ chromosome rearrangements and those with trisomy 8 or duplication of the Ph+ chromosome, with a median time to relapse of 19 months and a 73% risk of relapse at 3 years, compared to cases with other or no additional clonal abnormalities [median, not reached; 3-year risk of relapse of 31% (P = .002)]. Interestingly, the presence of an i(17q) alone did not correlate with relapse. In a SWOG study, 31 CML patients in accelerated or blast phase were evaluated by "favorable" cytogenetics (standard or variant Ph+ translocations, as the sole abnormality) or "unfavorable" (all other cytogenetic aberrations) (Slovak et al., 1995a). This small study indicated that the presence of trisomy 8, i(17q) and duplication of the Philadelphia chromosome did not have a negative impact on successful HSCT.

In the largest study to date, Konstantinidou and colleagues (2000) analyzed 418 patients in first or second chronic phase or in accelerated phase and divided them into five categories: standard t(9;22); Ph negative/BCR-ABL positive; variant Ph+ translocations; t(9;22) with +8 or duplication of the Ph chromosome or chromosome 17 abnormalities; and other abnormalities in addition to the Ph chromosome. In comparison to the standard t(9;22) group, Ph negative/BCR-ABL positive had a better LFS with no relapses (76.9% vs. 51.8%). Patients with variant translocations did not show a higher risk of relapse, as observed by Przepiorka and Thomas (1988); however, they were associated with an LFS similar to the group with other additional abnormalities (22.1% and 16%, respectively) and higher relative risk of treatment failure. In agreement with the SWOG study, those with +8, +Ph, or i(17q) as additional aberrations did not show a worse outcome compared to those with no additional abnormalities.

FISH analysis has confirmed that approximately 40% to 50% of variant Ph+ translocations and 10% to 15% of standard t(9;22) have large deletions adjacent to the translocation breakpoint on the derivative 9 chromosome, on the additional partner chromosome, or on both (Dewald et al., 1998; Grand et al., 1999; Sinclair et al., 2000; Cohen et al., 2001). Preliminary evidence suggests derivative 9 deletions are associated with a more rapid onset of blast crisis, resistance to interferon therapy (Cohen et al., 2001; Huntly et al., 2001) and perhaps to imatinib (Cuthbert et al., 2001), with a overall poor median survival [38 months in patients with deletions compared to 88 months in patients without deletions (P = .0001)] (Huntly et al., 2001). Because these deletions appear at disease presentation (Huntly et al., 2001), current studies using second-generation BCR/ABL FISH probes, either alone or in conjunction with expression array studies, will soon identify "high risk" CML patients in whom early HSCT is justified. Although the use of tyrosine kinase inhibitors is a promising alternative to reverse the clinical manifestations of CML, their impact on time to blast crisis, survival, and optimal timing of transplant remains unknown.

Interphase FISH can detect the t(9;22) in CML as well as monitor MRD after transplantation or alpha-interferon (IFN) therapy, regardless of whether a standard or variant translocation is present. Signals from 46 CML patients treated with IFN (n = 17) or allo-BMT (n = 29) were 0.5% to 15% positive for the 9;22 translocation (Dewald et al., 1997; Tanaka et al., 1997). Cut-off levels for detection of the BCR/ABL fusion gene range from 3.8% to 6.0%. False-positive signals are caused by randomly overlapping green and red signals in the nucleus. Using BCR/ABL hypermetaphase FISH combined with a whole chromosome Y paint probe, 0.1% to 0.6% positive Ph+ host cells were identified in seven sex-mismatched allotransplant recipients, suggesting this combination of FISH probes identified MRD at the 10^{-3} level, a level powerful enough to detect minor cell populations. Tanaka et al. (1997) demonstrated that CML patients had a similar percentage of translocation-positive cells in bone marrow and peripheral blood neutrophils. These data indicate that noninvasive monitoring is feasible and reliable. Although interphase FISH is less sensitive than RT-PCR, FISH is an easily quantitatable tool for monitoring residual leukemic cells in patients during therapy. Changes in residual disease that correlate with true response to therapy have not been established in large clinical trials for FISH and quantitative PCR. Nevertheless, MRD testing is guiding therapy in CML.

Chronic lymphatic leukemia

Classic cytogenetic analysis in CLL has a disappointing 40% to 50% clonal cytogenetic abnormality rate due to the low mitotic activity of this lymphoproliferative disorder. Thus, earlier reports attempting to correlate the most common aberrations detected in CLL with clinical characteristics and survival were inconsistent, and the aberrations were not found to be independent prognostic variables. Interestingly, the primary chromosome anomaly of CLL is not yet known, but aberrations of chromosomes 6, 11, 12, 13, and 17 are common (Juliusson et al., 1990). The introduction of interphase FISH studies represents a major advance for these tumors by detecting specific aberrations independent of their poor in vitro proliferative activity. Analyzing mononuclear cells from the blood of 325 CLL patients by a panel of disease-specific

FISH probes, Dohner et al. (2000) identified chromosomal aberrations in 82% of cases allowing for the definition of five major prognostic categories: 17p/TP53 deletions, 11q/ATM deletions, trisomy 12, normal karyotype and 13q deletion as the sole anomaly (Table 103.6). The 17p/TP53 and 11q/ATM deleted subgroups are frequently associated with another poor prognostic factor, unmutated immunoglobulin V genes, and have more advanced disease ($P < .001$) compared to the other groups, with a median treatment-free interval of only 9 and 13 months, respectively (Dohner et al., 2000; Stilgenbauer et al., 2000). In contrast, trisomy 12 CLL patients have a reported 114 months (median) survival, a finding comparable to those CLL patients with normal karyotypes (median, 111 months). CLL patients with 13q abnormalities have a benign clinical course and survive as long as age- and sex-matched controls (median, 133 months) with 33% never requiring therapy. The difference between the poor prognosis of chromosome 13 abnormalities in multiple myeloma (discussed below) and the clinically benign chromosome 13 abnormalities in CLL appears to be related to the extent of the deletion, with submicroscopic deletions in CLL and large deletions/monosomy in myeloma (Fonseca et al., 2001a). Although confirmation in a large prospective trial is needed, these data suggest risk-adapted management: for example, younger B-CLL patients with 17p/TP53 and 11q/ATM deletions may benefit from conventional HSCT approaches, whereas non-myeloablative transplantation may offer potentially curative options for elderly CLL patients with aggressive disease.

Multiple myeloma

Like CLL, hypoproliferative multiple myeloma (MM) has a reported 20% to 60% clonal abnormality rate detected by classic cytogenetics. The addition of cytokines, such as interleukin (IL)-4, IL-6, and GM-CSF, improved detection from a range of 11% to 42% in unstimulated cultures to a range of 18% to 53% in cytokine-stimulated cultures; however, the higher frequency of chromosomal abnormalities is usually observed in advanced clinical stages with highly complex karyotypes (Sawyer et al., 1995; Brigaudeau et al., 1997; Hernandez et al., 1998; Fonseca et al., 1999). Regardless, these limited data identified several recurring aberrations in MM with prognostic importance: translocations involving 14q32/IgH, deletion/monosomy 13, 11q abnormalities, and TP53/17p deletions (Tricot et al., 1995; Drach et al., 1998; Fonseca et al., 1999, 2001; for review of 14q32 translocations see Willis & Dyer, 2000). FISH studies using IgH-specific probes indicated 14q32 translocations occur in approximately 65% of patients with the majority of primary IgH translocations involving 11q13/CCND1, 4p16/FGFR3/MMSET, 6p25/IRF4, and 16q23/CMAF (Table 103.6). The other MM cases most likely involve rearrangements involving the light chain genes (kappa and lambda); however, this assumption remains to be confirmed. IgH rearrangements involving 8q24.1/CMYC, detected in advanced disease and myeloma

cell lines, are considered secondary changes associated with tumor progression (Shou et al., 2000). Of interest, FISH has confirmed that the nonrandom aberrations observed in MM also occur in monoclonal gammopathy of undetermined significance (MGUS). The incidence of 70% monosomy 13 in patients whose myeloma evolved from MGUS, compared to 31% in de novo MM, suggests that genes on chromosome 13 are important in the evolution of MGUS to MM (Avet-Loiseau et al., 1999). Because MGUS and MM cells have low proliferative activity, standard cytogenetic analysis often cannot detect the karyotypic changes characterizing the malignant cells. FISH studies are necessary to assess 11q, 13q, and 14q aberrations, particularly if classic cytogenetics reveals a normal karyotype.

Tricot et al. (1995) were the first to report an adverse prognosis in MM patients with chromosome 13 or 11q aberrations after receiving autologous transplantation. In an Eastern Cooperative Oncology Group (ECOG) study using interphase FISH, chromosome 13 abnormalities were detected in 176 of 325 (54%) of evaluable patients. Patients with a 13q abnormality were less likely to respond to treatment and had a significantly shorter median overall survival (34.9 versus 51 months; $P = .021$) (Fonseca et al., 2002). In fact, the poor prognosis associated with chromosome 13 has now been confirmed regardless if the patient was treated with conventional therapy, thalidomide, or dose-intensive treatments, including HSCT (Desikan et al., 2000; Koninsberg et al., 2000; Zojer et al., 2000; Facon et al., 2001). The myeloma staging system proposed by Facon et al. (2001) recommended that patients with chromosome 13 aberrations and $\beta_2$microglobulin of 2.5 mg/l or greater be offered tandem auto/non-myeloablative transplant regimens, depending on age and availability of an HLA-identical sibling. This risk-adapted proposal will determine if chromosome 13 aberrant myeloma patients will benefit from tandem transplant HST or should be referred for other innovative therapeutic approaches.

Other cytogenetic aberrations that appear to correlate with a poor prognosis include those with a 14q32 abnormality, in particular t(11;14), t(4;14) (which is strongly associated with chromosome 13 aberrations), and t(14;16), whereas patients lacking 14q32 aberrations usually fall into a "good" prognostic category, especially if they lack 13q anomalies and have a β_2-microglobulin level of less than 2.5 mg/l (Drach et al., 1998; Fonseca et al., 2001). Furthermore, MM patients with TP53/17p deletions and stage III disease have a 13.9 month median survival, compared to 38.7 months for patients without deletions of TP53/17p ($p < 0.0001$) (Drach et al., 1998).

Non-Hodgkin's lymphoma

Histology and morphology are important determinants of both treatment outcome and prognosis in non-Hodgkin's lymphoma. Chromosomal abnormalities and molecular rearrangements correlate with histology and immunophenotype, and thus are key to proper disease management and treatment modalities. The most familiar chromosomal rearrangements are t(14;18) (q32.33;q21) in follicular lymphoma, t(3;V)(q27;V) in diffuse large cell lymphomas (DLCL), t(11;14)(q13;q32.33) in mantle cell lymphoma, 8q24.1 translocations in Burkitt's and Burkitt's-like lymphomas, t(11;18)(q22;q22) in mucosa-associated lymphoid tissue (MALT), and t(2;5)(p23;q35) associated with anaplastic large cell lymphoma (Table 103.6) (Cuneo 2000). Due to the variability of breakpoints in the t(11;14), FISH is the most sensitive assay for this aberration. Additionally, lymphomas with abnormalities involving chromosomes 1, 7, and 17 have a worse prognosis than other lymphomas of similar stage and grade without these changes. Preliminary gene expression arrays have revealed two distinct genetic profiles in DLCL with median survival inferior for patients with an activated B-cell pattern compared to cases with the germinal center pattern (Alizadeh et al., 2000). With advances in individual tumor cell isolation methods from paraffin-embedded tissues, FISH technology, and global gene array technology, a comprehensive genetic analysis of lymphoma tissue will become an invaluable aid to the diagnosis and identification of patients who would benefit from HSCT.

Chimerism posttransplant (and see Chapter 30)

Persistence of host cell hematopoiesis after allogeneic HSC transplantation may lead to coexistence of donor and recipient cells, commonly referred to as mixed chimerism. The influence of hematopoietic cell chimerism on clinical outcome posttransplant has received considerable attention, particularly with regard to issues such as risk of relapse, intensity of conditioning regimens, graft-versus-host disease (GVHD), and graft-versus-leukemia (GVL). Thus, it becomes imperative to determine the significance of finding residual host cells posttransplant and to determine what constitutes "stable" versus "unstable" chimerism. The most common techniques used to detect host cells include cytogenetics if nonrandom karyotypic markers are present at diagnosis, FISH in sex-mismatched transplants, or PCR using short tandem repeats (STRs).

Studies have shown that mixed chimerism is not necessarily associated with an increased risk for leukemic relapse; however, close serial monitoring is recommended. In an ISH-based study of 30 sex-mismatched transplants, host cells were detected by interphase cytogenetics in all patients posttransplant, at times varying from 28 to 1,825 days, whereas classic cytogenetic studies detected host cells in only four patients, three of whom were found to be in clinical relapse (Vrazas et al., 1995). These results are corroborated by others who reported >1% of host cells at 1 year posttransplant in more than 50% of transplanted patients in continuous clinical remission (Przepiorka et al., 1991; Wessman et al., 1993). These cells are most likely nondividing host stromal cells persisting in the marrow, irrespective of time of transplant. These data suggest that persistence of host cells, if stable, nonmitotic, or decreasing over time, does not appear to herald

impending relapse. Therefore, to detect MRD, probes that are tumor specific or FICTION studies combining immunophenotyping with FISH are necessary in order to reveal the true nature of residual recipient cells.

Palka et al. (1996) studied 33 allogeneic transplant recipients with a variety of hematologic neoplasms using FISH probes, specific for X and Y chromosomes as well as the BCR/ABL fusion gene. Their findings support the contention that stable mixed chimerism was related to clinical and hematologic remission; however, a progressive increase of host cells was consistently related to clinical and hematologic disease relapse. Elmaagacli et al. (1995) followed 28 male CML patients after sex-mismatched, non-T-cell-depleted allografts by PCR assays. Nineteen patients were monitored for chimeric status between 2 and 11 years posttransplant. Four patients converted from mixed chimerism to complete chimerism and 10 patients (53%) remained mixed. Six patients with mixed chimerism were BCR-ABL + (MRD+); four of these patients relapsed. Detection of MRD, with or without subsequent relapse, occurred exclusively among patients with mixed chimerism. This study, as well as others, suggests that the chimeric state may be closely associated with development of, or the regimen used to prevent, GVHD (Forbes et al., 1995).

Using the combined FICTION technique of immunophenotype (CD3, CD4, CD8, CD20, CD34, CD10) and genotypic analysis (for X and Y), Kogler et al. (1995) analyzed mixed chimerism in different subpopulations of cells from eight sex-mismatched transplants in order to detect leukemic relapse early. In two patients (with ALL and MM), host cell neoplastic relapse expressing the original immunophenotype, was detected at day +176 and day +294, respectively. Interestingly, results in the MM case predicted relapse 9 days before clinical manifestations of relapse became apparent. Such technologies are providing new opportunities to investigate the kinetics of mixed chimerism and the early detection of relapse posttransplant.

Two cases reported by Abeliovich et al. (1996) illustrate the limitation of using molecular analysis of Y-specific sequences as the sole means to document engraftment in women after receipt of a T-cell-depleted allograft from an HLA-matched brother. In both women, the predominant clone posttransplant was 45,X with loss of a sex chromosome. PCR using oligonucleotide primers for the SRY gene, a chromosome Y-specific marker, showed no evidence of male donor cell engraftment. However, the combined use of classic cytogenetics documenting marked chromosome instability in the 46,XX population, a 9q heteromorphism in the 45,X cells previously observed in male donor cells prior to BMT, and DNA polymorphic STRs confirmed the 45,X clones in both patients were derived from male donor cells and should have been designated as 45,X,-Y. Y chromosome loss may have occurred in the donors as a minor clone in their marrow, or could have arisen after transplantation. The use of multiparameter testing remains necessary in such unusual case presentations.

Donor cell leukemia

Approximately 30% of allo-HSCT patients have recurrence of disease posttransplant, making leukemia the single most frequent cause of death following HLA-identical sibling transplantation. Most recurrences are relapses presenting with immunophenotypes and cytogenetic aberrations similar to that observed before transplantation. On rare occasions, leukemia in donor cells has been reported [reviewed in Cooley et al. (2000)].

Identification of donor cell leukemia is dependent on accuracy in determining leukemic cell lineage. Methods frequently used to delineate donor-derived relapse in allograft recipients rely on either cytogenetic tumor markers, FISH, RFLPs, or STRs to distinguish donor and recipient cells. The most convincing studies have used several of these techniques. In one case of Ph+ CML, the male patient received a transplant from his HLA-matched sister who had previously received two courses of dacarbazine (DTIC) and Bacille-Calmette-Guerin for successful treatment of stage 2B malignant melanoma. Two years later, therapy-related AML developed, characterized by a stemline karyotype of 45,XX,−7. FISH analysis, using chromosome 7 specific DNA probes, on archival Wright-stained bone marrow slides detected monosomy 7 in the blast cells, confirming donor origin of the leukemic relapse (Lowsky et al., 1996). These data are consistent with chemotherapy-related cytogenetic abnormalities; however, additional transplant-specific hits must also have occurred because the donor remained well, with a normal female karyotype and a normal peripheral blood count. A similar report by Mouratidou et al. (1993) described a 16-year-old female who presented with AML-M5, but relapsed 1 year later with ALL. She responded well to ALL remission induction chemotherapy, followed by a T-cell-depleted allograft from her HLA-matched brother, but relapsed 1 year later with ALL. Both cytogenetic analysis and FISH using a chromosome Y specific probe identified a Y chromosome in 88% of the blast cells, providing definitive evidence of disease in donor cells. In a third case, a female in second relapse of T-cell ALL posttransplant, presented with two leukemic clones: a stemline 46,XY,del(6)(q23q25) and sideline of 45,X,−4,del(6)(q23q25),+8,−15,−21,+i(21)(q10),+mar. The stemline clearly indicated that male donor cells were involved in the malignant process (Schmitz et al., 1987); however, due to sex chromosome loss and lack of differing chromosome polymorphisms between donor and recipient, the origin of the hypodiploid sideline could not be unequivocally established.

Molecular genetic tools provide a powerful approach to study engraftment and leukemic relapse when cytogenetic studies are equivocal. Stein et al. (1989) performed cytogenetic and RFLP analyses. At diagnosis, the patient's bone marrow cells had a karyotype of 46,XY,t(18;21). A pretransplant marrow identified a normal 46,XY male karyotype in 14 cells and a 45,X,-Y karyotype in one cell. The female donor had a normal 46,XX karyotype with a G-banded polymorphism in the heterochromatic region of chromosome 9 (9qh+). At clinical relapse 19 months posttransplant, normal 46,XX donor cells were observed among a smaller population (~20%) of ill-defined polyploid cells with suboptimal morphology that precluded karyotyping. The patient achieved a 6-month remission, but at second relapse, the polyploid population now represented 68% of all cells collected for analysis. An abnormality of chromosome 6 was identified; however, the X chromosome number was variable with between 2 and 4 copies per cell, with no evidence of a Y chromosome. Molecular analysis, using seven informative DNA probes localized to chromosome X, Y, 5, and 21, identified a significant increase in host cells at relapse not detectable in remission samples. These data strongly suggest the patient suffered from relapse of his ALL, rather than donor cell leukemia.

Donor cell leukemia after allogeneic transplantation for severe aplastic anemia has also been reported (Browne et al., 1991). A male, who failed equine antithymocyte globulin treatment, received an allograft from his fully HLA-compatible female cousin 14 months after initial diagnosis. At day 30 posttransplant, engraftment was confirmed by cytogenetic analysis and at day 122, using a panel of seven STRs, by PCR. Nine months posttransplant, the patient was diagnosed with FAB-M5a leukemia, with a female (donor) karyotype of 46,XX,t(9;11)(p22;q23) and only donor hematopoiesis by PCR testing. Because 11q23 leukemia is commonly observed in de novo as well as therapy-related AML, the occurrence of this secondary hematopoietic leukemia of donor cell origin was of concern for both donor and recipient.

Due to technical limitations of the various assays used to determine origin of recurrence, caution must be exercised. Cytogenetic analysis alone is limited by the requirement of mitotic cells. Determination of a donor cell karyotype in a leukemic specimen posttransplant may reflect the inability to detect mitoses of recurrent host disease. Several reports describe what would have been erroneous assignment of a donor origin to a secondary leukemia, had cytogenetic data alone been used (Minden et al., 1985; Anastasi et al., 1991b). Interpretation of molecular analyses may also be incorrect if the selected DNA probes used do not detect both donor-specific and recipient-specific RFLPs. In addition, molecular analyses may be complicated by loss of specific chromosomes (Stein et al., 1989; Abeliovich et al., 1996), or by emergence of non-leukemic cells of recipient origin (Blazar et al., 1985; Petz et al., 1987). Thus, it is essential to use multiple informative DNA probes localized to more than one chromosome, and to establish that a relapse is associated with a shift in the RFLPs of the transplanted stem cells from a donor to a recipient pattern. Accurate assessment of frequency and possible mechanisms of donor cell relapse requires long-term follow-up using both cytogenetic and molecular analyses.

Indolent clonal cytogenetic aberrations posttransplant

Clinical remission in acute leukemia has been defined as the elimination of leukemic cells to levels undetectable by conventional morphologic review, and restoration of normal poly-clonal hematopoiesis. Elimination of clonal cytogenetic abnormalities is also a hallmark of clinical remission. Thus, persistence or re-emergence of a recurring cytogenetic clone usually correlates with the presence of residual, or relapse of, disease. In the absence of clinical, morphologic, or molecular relapse, the presence of a clonal abnormality must be viewed with caution and close clinical follow-up is required. Using serial cytogenetic studies, reports indicate that clonal and nonclonal cytogenetic aberrations occur in upwards of 20% to 50% of patients treated with high-dose chemotherapy, with or without stem cell rescue (Raynaud et al., 1994; Testoni et al., 1996). Raynaud et al. (1994) found clonal cytogenetic aberrations typically associated with myeloid disorders, such as monosomy 7, del(20)(q11), partial trisomy 1q and 6p abnormalities, in 7 of 39 adult patients after dose-intensive chemotherapy for de novo AML. These new clonal cytogenetic aberrations expanded over time, apparently due to a selective growth advantage, and were observed 10 to 35 months prior to clinical manifestation of recurrent disease. Testoni et al. (1996) and Perot et al. (1993) identified cytogenetic abnormalities after autologous BMT in 13 of 30 (41%) and 20 of 66 (30%) AML patients, respectively. Clonal aberrations corresponded with hematologic relapse. Mild chromosome instability, in the form of nonclonal (found in a single cell) or transitory karyotypic aberrations, were not associated with risk of relapse, but were attributed to the conditioning chemotherapy.

Similarly, clonal karyotypic hematopoietic cell abnormalities occurring after auto-HSCT for advanced stage Hodgkin's disease and non-Hodgkin's lymphomas have also been reported (Traweek et al., 1994). Cytogenetic changes were first detected 1.8 to 6.5 years after induction chemotherapy and 0.5 to 3.1 years posttransplant. Of interest, in 9 of 10 patients the clonal aberrations found were those commonly observed in therapy-related MDS, including abnormalities of chromosomes 5 and 7, aberrations affecting chromosome bands 11q23 and 21q22.3, or a combination of these abnormalities. All 10 patients had morphologically and cytogenetically normal bone marrow at the time of stem cell harvest. In six patients, posttransplant cytogenetic aberrations were associated with recognizable MDS (n = 4) or AML (n = 2). One patient remained cytopenic and three patients had expansion of the clone to comprise the majority of metaphases 3 to 6 years posttransplant. These studies imply that the risk of developing clonal cytogenetic changes after auto-HSCT for malignant lymphoma approaches 9% at 3 years and the majority of these develop therapy-related MDS over time. The exact significance of clonal cytogenetic aberrations in the absence of clinical MDS is not known; longer follow-up is needed in order to understand their possible role in the development of secondary leukemia.

Sex chromosome loss is a normal age-related phenomenon in both females and males (Guttenbach et al., 1995). In males, loss of the Y chromosome increases to a frequency of 1.34% in men aged 76 to 80 years. In females, the rate of X chromosome loss rises to nearly 5% in women older than 75 years of age. Therefore, loss of a sex chromosome, as the sole aberration in

neoplasia, may not represent a clonal aberration per se. However, because some leukemias are characterized by a normal karyotype, the loss of a sex chromosome could represent a monoclonal population in a setting of an acquired 45,X,–(X or Y)/46,XX or 46,XY age-related mosaicism.

Therapy-related MDS/AML (t-MDS/AML) posttransplant (and see Chapter 86)

Secondary hematopoietic disease, manifesting as t-MDS or t-AML with clonal cytogenetic aberrations, is a serious late complication of auto-HSCT. In patients treated by auto-HSCT for malignant lymphoma, the cumulative probability of t-MDS/AML reported in the literature ranges from 4% at 5 years to 18% at 6 years after transplant (Darrington et al., 1994; Miller et al., 1994; Stone et al., 1994; Traweek et al., 1994; Laughlin et al., 1998; Krishnan et al., 2000) and appears to be associated with the use of high-dose etoposide in the conditioning regimen (Krishnan et al., 2000), radiotherapy (Darrington et al., 1994; Stone et al., 1994), and older age at transplantation (Andre et al., 1988; Bhatia et al., 1996). Close scrutiny of the malignant lymphoma population further indicates a high-risk subgroup of patients who have failed initial induction and salvage therapeutic regimens. These patients have been treated on multiple occasions before marrow or blood stem cell harvest, and any permanent insult sustained by normal HSC, as a consequence of previous therapy, could potentially result in t-MDS/AML posttransplant. Cytogenetics, coupled with accurate documentation of the time interval from initial exposure to chemotherapy and development of t-MDS/AML, has been an invaluable aid in determining the mutagenic effect of chemotherapy. Chromosome 5 and 7 deletions are strongly associated with the use of alkylating agents, especially when administered in multicycle, multidrug regimens with or without radiation. The latency period for alkylator-induced t-MDS/AML ranges from 4 to 7 years after initial exposure. The second group of t-MDS/AML changes involves balanced chromosomal rearrangements involving chromosome bands 11q23 or 21q22.3, the normal cellular loci for MLL and AML1, respectively. These latter chromosomal aberrations have been reported in MDS/AML following use of DNA topoisomerase inhibitors such as the epipodophyllotoxins and doxorbicin, with a short latency period, ranging from 6 months to 2 years (Pedersen-Bjergaard et al., 1995). However, many other balanced rearrangements, including those frequently found in de novo disease, commonly occur in t-MDS/AML (Andersen et al., 1998; Rowley & Olney, 2002). In a retrospective single institutional study of 612 patients who had undergone high-dose chemotherapy with autologous stem cell rescue for lymphoma, 22 patients developed t-MDS/AML. Patients primed with etoposide for stem cell mobilization were at a 12.3-fold increased risk of developing t-AML with 11q23/21q22.3 abnormalities (P = .006) (Krishnan et al., 2000). An evaluation of patient characteristics and cytotoxic exposure in 511 cases of t-MDS/AML with balanced chromosome aberrations revealed exposure to

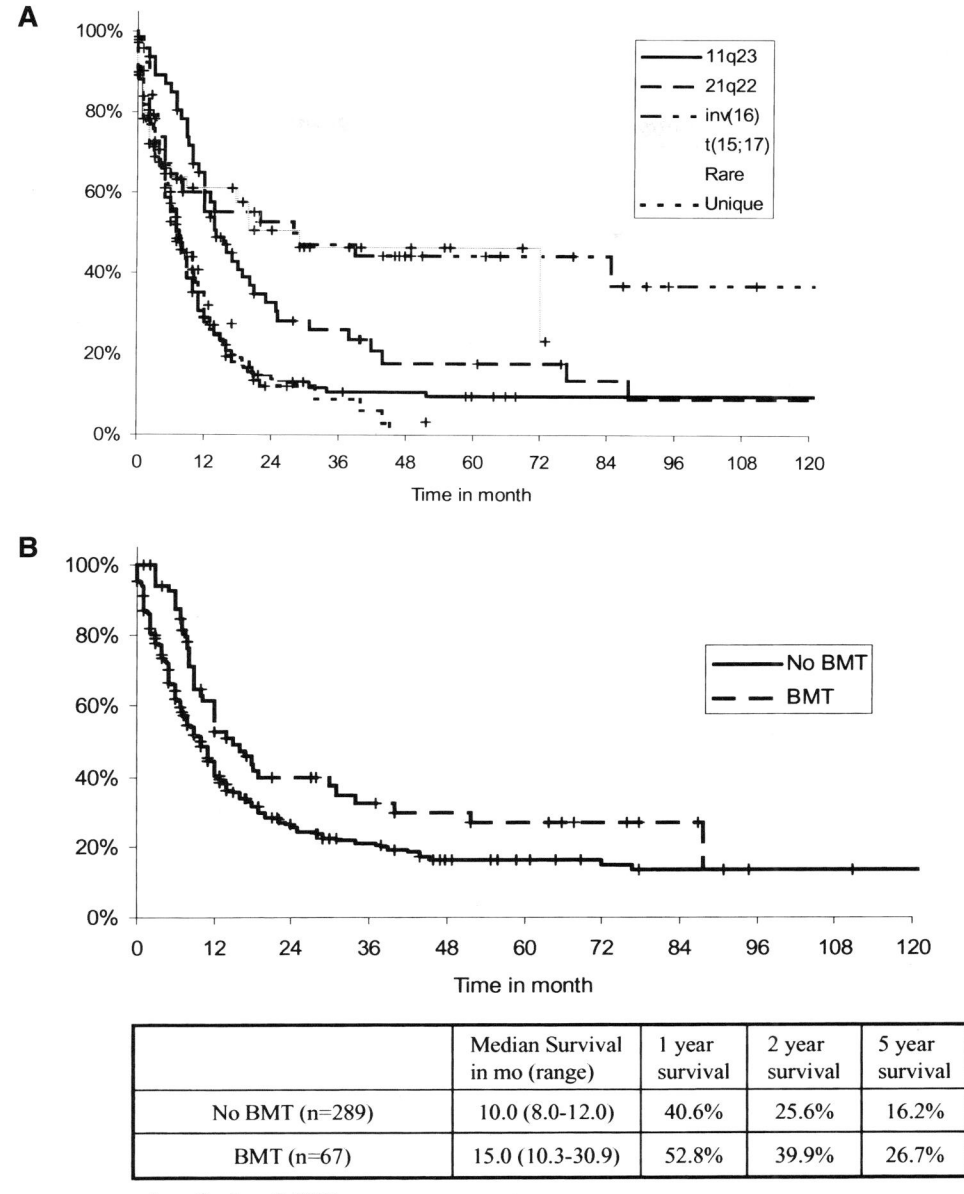

Fig. 103.5. Estimated distribution of survival for therapy-related MDS/AML. **(A)** Crude overall survival by six t-MDS/AML subgroups in months based on data submitted to the International Workshop on the Relationship of Prior Therapy to Balanced Translocations in Treatment-Related Myelodysplasia and Acute Leukemia disease of Workshop, Chicago, IL (Kaplan-Meier estimates). Tick marks indicate censored observations. **(B)** Overall survival of 356 Workshop patients treated with intensive treatment strategies. There is an overall survival advantage in patients who underwent HSCT compared to intensive nontransplant treatment protocols (Kaplan-Meier estimates); tick marks indicate censored observations. CI, confidence interval. From Rowley & Olney (2002). Reprinted by permission of Wiley-Liss, Inc.

topoisomerase agents, age, primary diagnosis, presentation of t-MDS versus t-AML, and latency as predictive factors for six cytogenetic subgroups of t-MDS/AML: 11q23, 21q22.3, inv(16), t(15;17), 11p15, and other rare rearrangements too unique or infrequent to be described in any particular subgroup (Rowley & Olney, 2002) (overall survival data by subgroup, Fig. 103.5A). Importantly, the findings of this large retrospective International Workshop indicated the 67 patients who were treated for their t-MDS/AML with an HSCT had a

significantly better survival than did the 289 patients treated with dose-intensive, nontransplant regimens ($P = .0078$), with median survival of 10.0 mo (95% CI, 8.0–12.0) compared to 15 mo (95% CI, 10.3–30.9), and 5-year survival of 16.2% versus 26.7% for non-HSCT versus HSCT, respectively (Fig. 103.5B). For a detailed discussion, the reader is referred to the Workshop report (Rowley & Olney, 2002).

The importance of performing bone marrow cytogenetic analyses in patients who have been previously heavily treated prior to transplant has been reported by Chao *et al.* (1991b). In this study, pretransplant cytogenetic analysis spared some patients the experience of a therapeutic procedure destined to fail due to an evolving secondary malignancy. These data suggest that pretransplant cytogenetic analysis might indeed be useful in identifying patients with established bone marrow damage who might benefit from an allograft, rather than an autologous transplant. Two retrospective studies have reported the detection of abnormal pretransplant clones in banked progenitor cells of patients who developed t-MDS/AML after autologous transplantation using FISH probes specific for the aberrations identified in the therapy-related disease (Abruzzese *et al.*, 1999; Lillington *et al.*, 2001). These two independent studies indicate the need for improved detection of evolving t-MDS/AML at the time of apheresis. Furthermore, a poor prognosis has been reported when clonal cytogenetic abnormalities persist at marrow harvest while in morphologic remission (Grimwade *et al.*, 1997). These data suggest the treatment given prior to conditioning for transplant, and possibly predisposition, rather than the myeloablative conditioning itself, is most responsible for development of therapy-related MDS/AML. Resolution of this dilemma may be forthcoming with development of predictive clonal hematopoiesis assays such as the HUMARA (human androgen receptor) (Figure 103.6) assay (Mach-Pascual *et al.*, 1998), or the intriguing possibility of defining a genetic signature that could identify patients at high risk of developing t-AML at initial diagnosis (Yeoh *et al.*, 2002). The reproducibility and predictive value of these assays await confirmation.

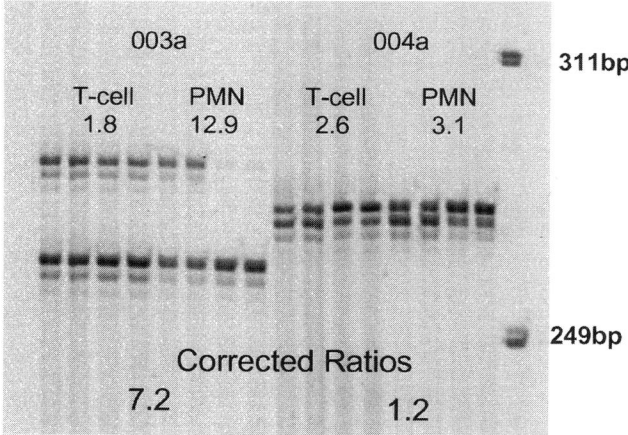

Fig. 103.6. HUMARA (human androgen receptor) assay. Example of clonal hematopoiesis (left) and polyclonal (right) hematopoiesis. Each sample contains eight lanes. The first four lanes are composed of T-cell somatic control DNA with lanes 1 and 2 defining the different parental alleles and lanes 3 and 4 defining the status of the inactive allele only. The PMN or experimental fraction shows loss of upper allele indicating clonal hematopoiesis in sample 003 whereas sample 004 exhibits polyclonal hematopoiesis.

Future directions

Potential strategies to improve the prognosis of high-risk hematopoietic disorders emphasize unequivocal determination of the disease karyotype in order to translate the associated pathobiological significance. Comprehensive genetic characterization of the malignant clone is required for patient care. This is underscored by the use of combined chemotherapy and retinoids in the treatment of acute promyelocytic leukemia, antimetabolite-based therapy in hyperdiploid (>50 chromosomes) ALL, and the use of HSCT in first remission for patients with poor-risk cytogenetics. New molecular genetic technologies, such as spectral karyotyping, FISH probe panels, and global gene expression arrays, promise improved sensitivity to describe specific genetic alterations in individual tumors. Chromosome-specific telomere probes, in association with M-FISH technology, offer the possibility of detecting cryptic translocations, such as the t(4;14) observed in 20% of MM, that are not resolvable by standard G-banding. These technologies have the extraordinary potential to define all the genetic aberrations in an individual tumor cell population. Defining the unique tumor pathogenetic basis for each individual should aid in identifying those patients who would best benefit from dose-intensive chemotherapy followed by autologous or allogeneic HSC transplantation. Future randomized clinical trials using internationally accepted cytogenetic scoring systems will refine the timing of transplantation, donor options, GVHD treatment, and the role of molecular determinants in successful transplantation management of neoplasia. Further genetic-based efforts should establish the role of the individual, disease, treatment, and molecular mechanisms in the pathogenesis of the late effect complication of t-MDS/AML.

References

Abeliovich, D., Yehuda, O., Nagler, A. *et al.* (1996). Predominant 45,X,-Y karyotype in donor cells after allogeneic BMT. *Cancer Genetics and Cytogenetics,* **86,** 1–7.

Abruzzese, E., Radford, J.E. Miller, J.S. *et al.* (1999). Detection of abnormal pretransplant clones in progenitor cells of patients who developed myelodysplasia after autologous transplantation. *Blood,* **94,** 1814–19.

Alizadeh, A.A., Elsen, M.B., Davis, R.E. *et al.* (2000). Distinct types of diffuse large B-cell lymphoma identified by gene expression profiling. *Nature,* **403,** 503–11.

Anastasi, J., Le Beau, M.M., Vardiman, J.W., & Westbrook, C.A. (1990). Detection of numerical chromosomal abnormalities in neoplastic hematopoietic cells by in situ hybridization with a chromosome-specific probe. *American Journal of Pathology,* **136,** 131–9.

Anastasi, J., Thangavelu, M., Vardiman, J.W. *et al.* (1991a). Interphase cytogenetic analysis detects minimal residual disease in a case of acute lymphoblastic leukemia and resolves the question of relapse after allogeneic bone marrow transplantation. *Blood,* **77,** 1087–91.

Anastasi, J., Vardiman, J.W., Rudinsky, R. *et al.* (1991b). Direct correlation of cytogenetic findings with cell morphology using in situ hybridization: an analysis of suspicious cells in bone marrow specimens of two patients completing therapy for acute lymphoblastic leukemia. *Blood, 77,* 2456–62.

Andersen, M.K., Johannson, B., Larsen, S.O., & Pedersen-Bjergaard, J. (1998). Chromosomal abnormalities in secondary MDS and AML. Relationship to drugs and radiation with specific emphasis on the balanced rearrangements. *Haematology, 83,* 483–8.

Andre, M., Henry-Amar, M., Blaise, D. *et al.* (1998). Treatment-related deaths and second cancer risk after autologous stem cell transplantation for Hodgkin's disease. *Blood, 92,* 1933–40.

Arico, M., Valsecchi, M.G., Camitta, B. *et al.* (2000). Outcome of treatment in children with Philadelphia chromosome-positive acute lymphoblastic leukemia. *New England Journal of Medicine, 342,* 998–1006.

Arthur, D.C., Berger, R., Golomb, H.M. *et al.* (1989). The clinical significance of karyotype in acute myelogenous leukemia. *Cancer Genetics and Cytogenetics, 40,* 203–16.

Auerbach, A.D., Rogatko, A., & Schroeder-Kurth, T.M. (1989). International Fanconi Anemia registry: relation of clinical symptoms to diepoxybutane sensitivity. *Blood, 73,* 391–6.

Avet-Loiseau, H., Li, J.Y., Morineau, N. *et al.* (1999). Monosomy 13 is associated with the transition of monoclonal gammopathy of undetermined significance to multiple myeloma. Intergroupe Francophone du Myelome. *Blood, 94,* 2583–89.

Barrett, A.J., Horowitz, M.M., Ash, R.C. *et al.* (1992). Bone marrow transplantation for Philadelphia chromosome-positive acute lymphoblastic leukemia. *Blood, 79,* 3067–70.

Bentz, M., Cabot, G., Moos, M. *et al.* (1994). Detection of chimeric bcr-abl genes on bone marrow samples and blood smears in chronic myeloid and acute lymphoblastic leukemia by in situ hybridization. *Blood, 83,* 1922–8.

Bhatia, S., Ramsey, N.K., Steinbuch, M. *et al.* (1996). Malignant neoplasms following bone marrow transplantation. *Blood, 87,* 3633–9.

Biondi, A., Cimino, G., Pieters, R., & Pui, C.H. (2000). Biological and therapeutic aspects of infant leukemia. *Blood, 96,* 24–33.

Blazar, B.R., Orr, H.T., Arthur, D.C. *et al.* (1985). Restriction fragment length polymorphisms as markers of engraftment in allogeneic marrow transplantation. *Blood, 66,* 1437–44.

Bolwell, B., Kalaycio, M., Andresen, S. *et al.* (2000). Autologous peripheral blood progenitor cell transplantation for transformed diffuse large-cell lymphoma. *Clinical Lymphoma, 1,* 226–31.

Brown, J., Saracoglu, K., Uhrig, S. *et al.* (2001). Subtelomeric chromosome rearrangements are detected using an innovative 12-color FISH assay (M-TEL). *Nature Medicine, 7,* 497–501.

Browne, P.V., Lawler, M., Humphries, P., & McCann, S.R. (1991). Donor-cell leukemia after bone marrow transplantation for severe aplastic anemia. *New England Journal of Medicine, 325,* 710–13.

Butturini, A., Gale, R.P., Verlander, P.C. *et al.* (1994). Hematologic abnormalities in Fanconi anemia: an International Fanconi Anemia Registry Study. *Blood, 84,* 1650–5.

Chao, N.J., Nademanee, A.P., Long, G.D. *et al.* (1991). Importance of bone marrow cytogenetics evaluation before autologous bone marrow transplantation for Hodgkin's disease. *Journal of Clinical Oncology, 9,* 1575–9.

Chase, A., Grand, F., Zhang, J.G. *et al.* (1997). Factors influencing the false positive and negative rates of BCR-ABL fluorescence in situ hybridization. *Genes Chromosomes and Cancer, 18,* 246–53.

Cohen, N., Rozenfeld-Granot, G., Hardan, I. *et al.* (2001). Subgroup of patients with Philadelphia-positive chronic myelogenous leukemia characterized by a deletion of 9q proximal to ABL gene: expression profiling, resistance to interferon therapy, and poor prognosis. *Cancer Genetics and Cytogenetics, 128,* 114–9.

Cooley, L.D., Sears, D.A., Udden, M.M. *et al.* (2000). Donor cell leukemia: report of a case occuring 11 years after allogeneic bone marrow transplantation and review of the literature. *American Journal of Hematology, 63,* 46–53.

Copelan, E.A. & McGuire, E.A. (1995). The biology and treatment of acute lymphoblastic leukemia in adults. *Blood, 85,* 1151–68.

Cuneo, A. (2000). Classification of B-cell non-Hodgkin lymphomas (NHL). *Atlas of Genetics and Cytogenetics in Oncology and Haematology.* http://www.infobiogen.fr

Cuthbert, G.D., Freeman-Edward, J.C., Lennard, A.L. *et al.* (2001). Der(9) deletions and response to ST1571(Glivec®) treatment in chronic phase CML patients. *Blood, 98,* Abstract 4756.

Darrington, D.L., Vose, J.M., Anderson, J.R. *et al.* (1994). Incidence and characterization of secondary myelodysplastic syndrome and acute myelogeneous leukemia following high-dose chemoradiotherapy and autologous stem-cell transplantation for lymphoid malignancies. *Journal of Clinical Oncology, 12,* 2527–34.

Dastugue, N., Payen, C., Lafage-Pochitaloff, M. *et al.* (1995). Prognostic significance of karyotype in de novo adult acute myeloid leukemia. *Leukemia, 9,* 1491–8.

Dastugue, N., Robert, A., Payen, C. *et al.* (1992). Prognostic significance of karyotype in a 12-year follow-up in childhood acute lymphoblastic leukemia. *Cancer Genetics and Cytogenetics, 64,* 49–55.

de Witte, T., Suciu, S., Peetermans, M. *et al.* (1995). Intensive chemotherapy for poor prognosis myelodysplasia (MDS) and secondary acute myeloid leukemia (SAML) following MDS of more than 6 months duration. A pilot study by the Leukemia Cooperative Group of the European Organization for Research and Treatment in Cancer (EORTC-LCG). *Leukemia, 9,* 1805–11.

Desikan, R., Barlogie, B., Sawyer, J. *et al.* (2000). Results of high-dose therapy for 1000 patients with multiple myeloma: durable complete remissions and superior survival in the absence of chromosome 13 abnormalities. *Blood, 95,* 4008–10.

Dewald, G.W., Juneau, A.L., Schad, C.R., & Tefferi, A. (1997). Cytogenetic and molecular genetic methods for diagnosis and treatment response in chronic granulocytic leukemia. *Cancer Genetics and Cytogenetics, 94,* 59–66.

Dewald, G.W., Wyatt, W.A., Juneau, A.L. *et al.* (1998). Highly sensitive FISH method to detect double BCR/ABL fusion and monitor response to therapy in chronic myeloid leukemia. *Blood, 91,* 3357–65.

Dohner, H., Stilgenbauer, S., Benner, A. *et al.* (2000). Genomic aberrations and survival in chronic lymphocytic leukemia. *New England Journal of Medicine, 343,* 1910–6.

Dohner, H., Stilgenbauer, S., Dohner, K. *et al.* (1999). Chromosome aberrations in B-cell chronic lymphocytic leukemia: reassessment based on molecular cytogenetic analysis. *Journal of Molecular Medicine, 77,* 266–31.

Durnam, D.M., Anders, K.R., Fisher, L. *et al.* (1989). Analysis of the origin of marrow cells in bone marrow transplant recipients using a Y-chromosome specific in situ hybridization assay. *Blood,* **74,** 2220–6.

El-Rifai, W., Ruutu, T., Elonen, E. *et al.* (1997a). Prognostic value of metaphase-fluorescence in situ hybridization in follow-up of patients with acute myeloid leukemia in remission. *Blood,* **89,** 3330–4.

El-Rifai, W., Ruutu, T., Vettenranta, K. *et al.* (1997b). Follow-up of residual disease using metaphase-FISH in patients with acute lymphoblastic leukemia in remission. *Leukemia,* **11,** 633–8.

Elmaagacli, A.H., Becks, H.W., Beelen, D.W. *et al.* (1995). Detection of minimal residual disease and persistence of host-type hematopoiesis: a study in 28 patients after sex-mismatched, non-T-cell-depleted allogeneic bone marrow transplantation for Philadelphia chromosome positive chronic myelogenous leukemia. *Bone Marrow Transplantation,* **16,** 823–9.

Facon, T., Avet-Loiseau, H., Guillerm, G. *et al.* (2001). Chromosome 13 abnormalities identified by FISH analysis and serum B2-microglobulin produce a powerful myeloma staging system for patients receiving high-dose therapy. *Blood,* **97,** 1566–71.

Fenaux, P., Morel, P., Rose, C. *et al.* (1991). Prognostic factors in adult de novo myelodysplastic syndromes treated by intensive chemotherapy. *British Journal of Haematology,* **77,** 497–501.

Ferrant, A., Doyen, C., Delannoy, A. *et al.* (1995). Karyotype in acute myeloblastic leukemia: prognostic significance in a prospective study assessing bone marrow transplantation in first remission. *Bone Marrow Transplantation,* **15,** 685–90.

Ferrant, A., Labopin, M., Frassoni, F. *et al.* (1997). Karyotype in acute myeloblastic leukemia: prognostic significance for bone marrow transplantation in first remission: a European group for blood and marrow transplantation study. *Blood,* **90,** 2931–8.

Fonseca, R., Coignet, L.J.A., & Dewald, G.W. (1999). Cytogenetic abnormalities in multiple myeloma. *Hematology Oncology Clinics of North America,* **13,** 1169–80.

Fonseca, R., Harrington, D., Oken, M.M. *et al.* (2002). Biological and prognostic significance of interphase fluorescence in situ hybridization detection of chromosome 13 abnormalities (delta 13) in multiple myeloma: an Eastern Cooperative Oncology group study. *Cancer Research,* **62,** 715–20.

Fonseca, R., Oken, M.M., & Greipp, P.R. (2001a). The t(4;14)(p16.3;q32) is strongly associated with chromosome 13 abnormalities in both multiple myeloma and monoclonal gammopathy of undetermined significance. *Blood,* **98,** 1271.

Fonseca, R., Oken, M.M., Harrington, D. *et al.* (2001b). Deletions of chromosome 13 in multiple myeloma identified by interphase FISH usually denote large deletions of the q arm or monosomy. *Leukemia,* **15,** 981–6.

Forbes, G.M., Fogarty, J., Meyer, B. *et al.* (1995). Intestinal mucosal mononuclear cell chimaerism after sex-mismatched allogeneic bone marrow transplantation. *Bone Marrow Transplantation,* **16,** 589–93.

Forman, S.J., O'Donnell, M.R., Nademanee, A.P. *et al.* (1987). Bone marrow transplantation for patients with Philadelphia chromosome-positive acute lymphoblastic leukemia. *Blood,* **70,** 587–8.

Gale, R.P., Horowitz, M.M., Weiner, R.S. *et al.* (1995). Impact of cytogenetic abnormalities on outcome of bone marrow trans-

plants in acute myelogenous leukemia in first remission. *Bone Marrow Transplantation,* **16,** 203–8.

Garcia-Higuera, I., Taniguchi, T., Ganesan, S. *et al.* (2001). Interaction of the Fanconi anemia proteins and BRCA1 in a common pathway. *Molecular Cell,* **7,** 249–62.

Grand, F., Kulkarni, S., Chase, A. *et al.* (1999). Frequent deletions of hSNF5/INI1, a component of the SWI/SNF complex, in chronic myeloid leukemia. *Cancer Research,* **59,** 3870–4.

Greenberg, P., Cox, C., Lebeau, M.M. *et al.* (1997). International scoring system for evaluating prognosis in myelodysplastic syndromes. *Blood,* **89,** 2079–88.

Grimwade, D., Walker, H., Oliver, F. *et al.* (1997). What happens subsequently in AML when cytogenetic abnormalities persist at bone marrow harvest? Results of the 10th UK MRC AML Trial. *Bone Marrow Transplantation,* **19,** 1117–23.

Grimwade, D., Walker, H., Oliver, F. *et al.* (1998). The importance of diagnostic cytogenetics on outcome in AML: analysis of 1,612 patients entered into the MRC AML 10 trial. *Blood,* **92,** 2322–33.

Groupe Francais De Cytogenetique Hematologique. (1996). Cytogenetic abnormalities in adult acute lymphoblastic leukemia: correlations with hematologic findings and outcome. A collaborative study of the Groupe Francais de Cytogenetique Hematologique. *Blood,* **87,** 3135–42.

Guttenbach, M., Koschorz, B., Bernthaler, U. *et al.* (1995). Sex chromosome loss and aging: in situ hybridization studies on human interphase nuclei. *American Journal of Human Genetics,* **57,** 1143–50.

Haas, O.A., Henn, T., Romanakis, K. *et al.* (1998). Comparative genomic hybridization as part of a new diagnostic strategy in childhood hyperdiploid acute lymphoblastic leukemia. *Leukemia,* **12,** 474–81.

Haase, D., Feuring-Buske, M., Konemann, S. *et al.* (1995). Evidence for malignant transformation in acute myeloid leukemia at the level of early hematopoietic stem cells by cytogenetic analysis of CD34+ subpopulations. *Blood,* **86,** 2906–12.

Haase, D., Feuring-Buske, M., Schafer, C. *et al.* (1997). Cytogenetic analysis of CD34+ subpopulations in AML and MDS characterized by the expression of CD38 and CD117. *Leukemia,* **11,** 674–9.

Harris, M.B., Shuster, J.J., Carroll, A. *et al.* (1992). Trisomy of leukemic cell chromosome 4 and 10 identifies children with B-progenitor cell acute lymphoblastic leukemia with a very low risk of treatment failure: a Pediatric Oncology Group Study. *Blood,* **79,** 3316–24.

Hernandez, J.M., Gutierrez, N.C., Almeida, J. *et al.* (1998). IL-4 improves the detection of cytogenetic abnormalities in multiple myeloma and increases the proportion of clonally abnormal metaphases. *British Journal of Haematology,* **103,** 163–7.

Hook, E.B. (1977). Exclusion of chromosomal mosaicism: Tables of 90%, 95%, and 99% confidence limits and comments on use. *American Journal of Human Genetics,* **29,** 94–7.

Hunger, S.P. (1996). Chromosomal translocations involving the E2A gene in acute lymphoblastic leukemia: clinical features and molecular pathogenesis. *Blood,* **87,** 1211–24.

Huntly, B.J., Reid, A.G., Bench, A.J. *et al.* (2001). Deletions of the derivative chromosome 9 occur at the time of the Philadelphia translocation and provide a powerful and independent prognostic indicator in chronic myeloid leukemia. *Blood*, **98**, 1732–8.

ISCN. (1995). *An International System for Human Cytogenetic Nomenclature*, ed. F. Mitelman. Basel: S. Karger.

Jackson, J.F., Boyett, J., Pullen, J. *et al.* (1990). Favorable prognosis associated with hyperdiploidy in children with acute lymphocytic leukemia correlates with extra chromosome 6. A Pediatric Oncology Group study. *Cancer*, **66**, 1183–9.

Jaffee, E.S., Harria, N.L., Stein, H., & Vardiman, J.W. (Eds.). (2001). *World Health Organization Classification of Tumors. Pathology and Genetics of Tumors of Hematopoietic and Lymphoid Tissues.* Lyon: IARC Press.

Joos, S., Scherthan, H., Speicher, M.R. *et al.* (1993). Detection of amplified DNA sequences by reverse chromosome painting using genomic tumor DNA as probe. *Human Genetics*, **90**, 584–9.

Juliusson, G., Oscier, D.G., Fitchett, M. *et al.* (1990). Prognostic subgroups of B-cell chronic lymphocytic leukemia defined by specific chromosomal abnormalities. *New England Journal of Medicine*, **323**, 720–4.

Kallioniemi, A., Kallioniemi, O.-P., Sudar, D. *et al.* (1992). Comparative genomic hybridization for molecular cytogenetic analysis of solid tumors. *Science*, **258**, 818–21.

Kallioniemi, O.-P., Kallioniemi, A., Piper, J. *et al.* (1994). Optimizing genomic hybridization for analysis of DNA sequence copy number changes in solid tumors. *Genes Chromosomes and Cancer*, **1**, 231–43.

Kasprzyk, A. & Secker-Walker, L.M. (1997). Increased sensitivity of minimal residual disease detection by interphase FISH in acute lymphoblastic leukemia with hyperdiploidy. *Leukemia*, **11**, 429–35.

Keating, M.J., Smith, T.L., Kantarjian, H. *et al.* (1988). Cytogenetic pattern in acute myelogenous leukemia: a major reproducible determinant of outcome. *Leukemia*, **2**, 403–12.

Knudson, A.G. Jr. (1971). Mutation and cancer: statistical study of retinoblastoma. *Proceedings of the National Academy of Sciences USA*, **68**, 820–3.

Kogler, G., Wolf, H.H., Heyll, A. *et al.* (1995). Detection of mixed chimerism and leukemic relapse after allogeneic bone marrow transplantation in subpopulations of leukocytes by fluorescent in situ hybridization in combination with the simultaneous immunophenotypic analysis of interphase cells. *Bone Marrow Transplantation*, **15**, 41–8.

Kolomietz, E., Al-Maghrabi, J., Brennan, S. *et al.* (2001). Primary chromosomal rearrangements of leukemia are frequently accompanied by extensive submicroscopic deletions and may lead to altered prognosis. *Blood*, **97**, 3581–8.

Koninsberg, R., Zojer, N., Ackerman, J. *et al.* (2000). Predictive value of interphase cytogenetics for survival of patients with multiple myeloma. *Journal of Clinical Oncology*, **18**, 804–12.

Konstantinidou, P., Szydlo, R.M., Chase, A., & Goldman, J.M. (2000). Cytogenetic status pre-transplant as a predictor of outcome post bone marrow transplantation for chronic myelogenous leukaemia. *Bone Marrow Transplantation*, **25**, 143–6.

Krishnan, A., Bhatia, S., Slovak, M.L. *et al.* (2000). Predictors of therapy-related leukemia and myelodysplasia following autologous transplantation for lymphoma: an assessment of risk factors. *Blood*, **95**, 1588–93.

Laughlin, M., McGaughey, D., Crews, J. *et al.* (1998). Secondary myelodysplasia and acute leukemia in breast cancer patients after autologous bone marrow transplant. *Journal of Clinical Oncology*, **16**, 1008–12.

Lillington, D.M., Micallef, I.N.M., Carpenter, E. *et al.* (2001). Detection of chromosome abnormalities pre-high-dose treatment in patients developing therapy-related myelodysplasia and secondary acute myelogenous leukemia after treatment for non-Hodgkin's lymphoma. *Journal of Clinical Oncology*, **19**, 2472–81.

Lowsky, R., Fyles, G., Minden, M. *et al.* (1996). Detection of donor cell derived acute myelogenous leukaemia in a patient transplanted for chronic myelogenous leukaemia using fluorescence in situ hybridization. *British Journal of Haematology*, **93**, 163–5.

Maarek, O., Jonveaux, P., Le Coniat, M. *et al.* (1996). Fanconi anemia and bone marrow clonal chromosome abnormalities. *Leukemia*, **10**, 1700–4.

Mach-Pascual, S., Legare, R.D., Lu, D. *et al.* (1998). Predictive value of clonality assays in patients with non-Hodgkin's lymphoma undergoing autologous bone marrow transplant: a single institution study. *Blood*, **91**, 4496–503.

Mandelli, F., Labopin, M., Granena, A. *et al.* (1994). European survey of bone marrow transplantation in acute promyelocytic leukemia (M3). *Bone Marrow Transplantation*, **14**, 293–8.

Marosi, C., Koller, U., Koller-Weber, E. *et al.* (1992). Prognostic impact of karyotype and immunologic phenotype in 125 adult patients with de novo AML. *Cancer Genetics and Cytogenetics*, **61**, 14–25.

Mehrotra, B., George, T.I., Kavanau, K. *et al.* (1995). Cytogenetically aberrant cells in the stem cell compartment (CD34+lin–) in acute myeloid leukemia. *Blood*, **86**, 1139–47.

Miller, J.S., Arthur, D.C., Litz, C.E. *et al.* (1994). Myelodysplastic syndrome after autologous bone marrow transplantation: an additional late complication of curative cancer therapy. *Blood*, **83**, 3780–6.

Minden, M., Messner, H., & Belch, A. (1985). Origin of leukemic relapse after bone marrow transplantation detected by restriction fragment length polymorphism. *Journal of Clinical Investigation*, **75**, 91–3.

Morel, P., Hebbar, M., Lai, J.-L. *et al.* (1993). Cytogenetic analysis has strong independent prognostic value in de novo myelodysplastic syndromes and can be incorporated in a new scoring system: a report on 408 cases. *Leukemia*, **7**, 1315–23.

Mouratidou, M., Sotiropoulos, D., Deremitzaki, K. *et al.* (1993). Recurrence of acute leukemia in donor cells after bone marrow transplantation: documentation by in situ DNA hybridization. *Bone Marrow Transplantation*, **12**, 77–80.

Nishimura, S., Kobayashi, M., Ueda, K. *et al.* (1999). Treatment of infant acute lymphoblastic leukemia in Japan. *International Journal of Hematology*, **69**, 244–52.

Palka, G., Stuppia, L., Di Bartolomeo, P. *et al.* (1996). FISH detection of mixed chimerism in 33 patients submitted to bone marrow transplantation. *Bone Marrow Transplantation*, **17**, 231–6.

Passmore, S.J., Hann, I.M., Stiller, C.A. *et al.* (1995). Pediatric myelodysplasia: a study of 68 children and a new prognostic scoring system. *Blood*, **85**, 1742–50.

Paternoster, S.F., Brockman, S.R., McClure, R.F. *et al.* (2003). A new method to extract nuclei from paraffin-embedded tissue to study lymphoma using interphase FISH. *American Journal of Pathology* (in press).

Pedersen-Bjergaard, J., Pedersen, M., Roulston, D., & Philip, P. (1995). Different genetic pathways in leukemogenesis for patients presenting with therapy-related myelodysplasia and therapy-related acute myeloid leukemia. *Blood,* **86,** 3542–52.

Perez Simon, J.A., Garcia-Sanz, R., Tabernero, M.D. *et al.* (1998). Prognostic value of numerical chromosome aberrations in multiple myeloma: a FISH analysis of 15 different chromosomes. *Blood,* **91,** 3366–71.

Perot, C., Van Den Akker, J., Laporte, J.P. *et al.* (1993). Multiple chromosome abnormalities in patients with acute leukemia after autologous bone marrow transplantation using total body irradiation and marrow purged with mafosfamide. *Leukemia,* **7,** 509–15.

Petz, L.D., Yam, P., Wallace, R.B. *et al.* (1987). Mixed hematopoietic chimerism following bone marrow transplantation for hematological malignancies. *Blood,* **70,** 1331–7.

Przepiorka, D. & Thomas, E.D. (1988). Prognostic significance of cytogenetic abnormalities in patients with chronic myelogenous leukemia. *Bone Marrow Transplantation,* **3,** 113–9.

Przepiorka, D., Thomas, E.D., Durnham, D.M., & Fisher, L. (1991). Use of a probe to repeat sequence of the Y chromosome for detection of host cells in peripheral blood of bone marrow transplant recipients. *American Journal of Clinical Pathology,* **95,** 201–6.

Pui, C.-H., Carroll, A.J., Raimondi, S.C. *et al.* (1990a). Clinical presentation, karyotypic characterization, and treatment outcome of childhood acute lymphoblastic leukemia with a near-haploid or hypodiploid <45 line. *Blood,* **75,** 1170–7.

Pui, C.-H., Crist, W.M., & Look, A.T. (1990b). Biology and clinical significance of cytogenetic abnormalities in childhood acute lymphoblastic leukemia. *Blood,* **76,** 1449–63.

Quijano, C.A., Moore, D., Arthur, D. *et al.* (1997). Cytogenetically aberrant cells are present in the CD34+Cd33–38–19–marrow compartment in children with acute lymphoblastic leukemia. *Leukemia,* **11,** 1508–15.

Raimondi, S.C. (1993). Current status of cytogenetic research in childhood acute lymphoblastic leukemia. *Blood,* **81,** 2237–51.

Raimondi, S.C., Pui, C.H., Head, D.R. *et al.* (1993). Cytogenetically different leukemic clones at relapse of childhood acute lymphoblastic leukemia. *Blood,* **82,** 576–80.

Raynaud, S.D., Brunet, B., Chischportich, M. *et al.* (1994). Recurrent cytogenetic abnormalities observed in complete remission of acute myeloid leukemia do not necessarily mark preleukemic cells. *Leukemia,* **8,** 245–9.

Remstein, E.D., Kurtin, P.J., Buno, I. *et al.* (2000). Diagnostic utility of fluorescence in situ hybridization in mantle-cell lymphoma. *British Journal of Haematology,* **110,** 856–62.

Ritterbach, J., Hiddemann, W., Beck, J.D. *et al.* (1998). Detection of hyperdiploid karyotypes (>50 chromosomes) in childhood acute lymphoblastic leukemia (ALL) using fluorescence in situ hybridization (FISH). *Leukemia,* **12,** 427–33.

Robouts, W.J., Lowenberg, B., van Putten, W.L., & Ploemacher, R.E. (2001). Improved prognostic significance of cytokine-induced proliferation in vitro in patients with de novo acute myeloid leukemia of intermediate risk: impact of internal tandem duplications in the Flt3 gene. *Leukemia,* **15,** 1046–53.

Rogan, P.K., Cazcarro, P.M., & Knoll, J.H.M. (2001). Sequence-based design of single-copy genomic DNA probes for fluorescence in situ hybridization. *Genome Research,* **11,** 1086–94.

Romana, S.P., Mauchauffe, M., Le Coniat, M. *et al.* (1995). The (12;21) of acute lymphoblastic leukemia results in a TEL-AML1 gene fusion. *Blood,* **85,** 3662–7.

Rosendorff, J. & Bernstein, R. (1988). Fanconi's anemia—chromosome breakage studies in homozygotes and heterozygotes. *Cancer Genetics and Cytogenetics,* **33,** 175–83.

Rowley, J.D. & Olney, H.J. (2002). International Workshop on the relationship of prior therapy to balanced chromosome aberrations in therapy-related myelodysplastic syndromes and acute leukemia: overview report. *Genes, Chromosomes & Cancer,* **33,** 331–45.

Sasaki, M.S. & Tonomura, A. (1973). A high susceptibility of Fanconi anemia to chromosome breakage by DNA cross-linking agents. *Cancer Research,* **33,** 1829–36.

Schiffer, C.A., Lee, E.J., Tomiyasu, T. *et al.* (1989). Prognostic impact of cytogenetic abnormalities in patients with de novo acute nonlymphocytic leukemia. *Blood,* **73,** 263–70.

Schmitz, N., Johannson, W., Schmidt, G. *et al.* (1987). Recurrence of acute lymphoblastic leukemia in donor cells after allogeneic marrow transplantation associated with a deletion of the long arm of chromosome 6. *Blood,* **70,** 1099–104.

Seong, D.C., Kantarjian, H.M., & Ro, J.Y. (1995). Hypermetaphase fluorescence in situ hybridization for quantitative monitoring of Philadelphia chromosome-positive cells in patients with chronic myelogenous leukemia during treatment. *Blood,* **86,** 2343–9.

Shapiro, H. (1995). *Practical Flow Cytometry.* New York: John Wiley.

Shou, Y., Martelli, M.L., Gabrea, A. *et al.* (2000). Diverse karyotypic abnormalities of the c-myc locus associated with c-myc dysregulation and tumor progression in multiple myeloma. *Proceedings of the National Academy of Sciences, USA,* **97,** 228–33.

Sinclair, P., Green, A., Grace, C., & Nacheva, E. (1997). Improved sensitivity of BCR-ABL detection: a triple-probe three-color fluorescence in situ hybridization system. *Blood,* **90,** 1395–1402.

Sinclair, P.B., Nacheva, E.P., Leversha, M. *et al.* (2000). Large deletions at the t(9;22) breakpoint are common and may identify a poor-prognosis subgroup of patients with chronic myeloid leukemia. *Blood,* **95,** 738–43.

Slovak, M.L., Kopecky, K.J., Cassileth, P.A. *et al.* (2000). Karyotypic analysis predicts outcome of preremission and postremission therapy in adult acute myeloid leukemia: a Southwest Oncology Group/Eastern Cooperative Oncology Group study. *Blood,* **96,** 4075–83.

Slovak, M.L., Kopecky, K.J., Wolman, S.R. *et al.* (1995a). Cytogenetic correlation with disease status and treatment outcome in advanced stage leukemia post bone marrow transplantation: a Southwest Oncology Group study (SWOG-8612). *Leukemia Research,* **19,** 381–8.

Slovak, M.L., Tcheurekdjian, L., Zhang, F.F., Murata-Collins, J.L. (2001). Simultaneous detection of multiple genetic aberrations in single cells by spectral fluorescence in situ hybridization. *Cancer Research,* **61,** 831–6.

Slovak, M.L., Traweek, S.T., Willman, C.L. *et al.* (1995b). Trisomy 11: an association with stem/progenitor cell immunophenotype. *British Journal of Haematology,* **90,** 266–73.

Smadja, N.V., Bastard, C., Brigaudeau, C. *et al.* (2001). Hypodiploidy is a major prognostic factor in multiple myeloma. *Blood,* **98,** 2229–38.

Snyder, D.S. (2000). Allogeneic stem cell transplantation for Philadelphia chromosome-positive acute lymphoblastic leukemia. *Biology and Blood Marrow Transplantation,* **6,** 597–603.

Socie, G., Devergie, A., Girinski, T. *et al.* (1998). Transplantation for Fanconi's anaemia: long-term follow-up of fifty patients transplanted from a sibling donor after low-dose cyclophosphamide and thoraco-abdominal irradiation for conditioning. *British Journal of Haematology,* **103,** 249–55.

Solinas-Toldo, S., Lampei, S., Stilgenbauer, S. *et al.* (1997). Matrix-based comparative genomic hybridization: biochips to screen for genomic imbalances. *Genes, Chromosomes & Cancer,* **20,** 399–407.

Stein, J., Zimmerman, P.A., Kochera, M. *et al.* (1989). Origin of leukemic relapse after bone marrow transplantation: comparison of cytogenetic and molecular analyses. *Blood,* **73,** 2033–40.

Stilgenbauer, S., Lichter, P., & Dohner, H. (2000). Genetic features of B-cell chronic lymphocytic leukemia. *Review of Clinical Experimental Hematology,* **4,** 48–72.

Stone, R.M., Neuberg, D., Soiffer, R. *et al.* (1994). Myelodysplastic syndrome as a late complication following autologous bone marrow transplantation for non-Hodgkin's lymphoma. *Journal of Clinical Oncology,* **12,** 2535–42.

Tanaka, K., Arif, M., Eguchi, M. *et al.* (1997). Application of fluorescence in situ hybridization to detect residual leukemic cells with 9;22 and 15;17 translocation *Leukemia,* **11,** 436–40.

Taylor, P.R.A., Jackson, G.H., Lennard, A.L. *et al.* (1997). Low incidence of myelodysplastic syndrome following transplantation using autologous non-cryopreserved bone marrow. *Leukemia,* **11,** 1650–3.

Testoni, N., Martinelli, G., Zaccaria, A. *et al.* (1996). Detection of occasional and clonal chromosome aberrations in patients with acute non-lymphocytic leukemia after autologous bone marrow transplantation. *Bone Marrow Transplantation,* **18,** 1141–5.

Toyama, K., Ohyashiki, K., Yoshida, Y. *et al.* (1993). Clinical implications of chromosomal abnormalities in 401 patients with myelodysplastic syndromes: a multicentric study in Japan. *Leukemia,* **7,** 499–508.

Traweek, S.T., Slovak, M.L., Nademanee, A.P. *et al.* (1994). Clonal karyotypic hematopoietic cell abnormalities occurring after autologous bone marrow transplantation for Hodgkin's disease and non-Hodgkin's lymphoma. *Blood,* **84,** 957–63.

Tricot, G., Barlogie, B., Jagannath, S. *et al.* (1995). Poor prognosis in multiple myeloma is associated only with partial or complete deletions of chromosome 13 or abnormalities involving 11q and not with other karyotype abnormalities. *Blood,* **86,** 4250–6.

Tricot, G., Spencer, T., Sawyer, J. *et al.* (2002). Predicting long-term (> or = 5 years event-free survival in multiple myeloma patients following planned tandem autotransplants. *British Journal of Haematology,* **116,** 211–7.

Trueworthy, R., Shuster, J., Look, T. *et al.* (1992). Ploidy of lymphoblasts is the strongest predictor of treatment outcome in B-progenitor cell acute lymphoblastic leukemia of childhood: a Pediatric Oncology Group study. *Journal of Clinical Oncology,* **10,** 606–13.

Turhan, A.G., Lemoine, F.M., Debert, C. *et al.* (1995). Highly purified primitive hematopoietic stem cells are PML-RARA negative and generate nonclonal progenitors in acute promyelocytic leukemia. *Blood,* **85,** 2154–61.

Vaandrager, J.W., Kluin, P., & Schuuring, E. (1996). Direct visualization of dispersed 11q13 chromosomal translocations in mantle cell lymphoma by multicolor DNA fiber fluorescence in situ hybridization. *Blood,* **88,** 1177–82.

Van Rhee, F., Szydlo, R.M., Hermans, J. *et al.* (1997). Long term results after allogeneic bone marrow transplantation for chronic myelogenous leukemia in chronic phase: a report from the chronic leukemia working party of the European Group for Blood and Marrow Transplantation. *Bone Marrow Transplantation,* **20,** 553–60.

Veldman, T., Vignon, C., Schrock, E. *et al.* (1997). Hidden chromosome abnormalities in hematological malignancies detected by multicolor spectral karyotyping. *Nature Genetics,* **15,** 406–10.

Vesole, D.H., Tricot, G., Jagannath, S. *et al.* (1996). Autotransplants in multiple myeloma: what have we learned? *Blood,* **88,** 838–47.

Vrazas, V., Ooms, L.M., Rudduck, C. *et al.* (1995). Application of interphase cytogenetics to monitor bone marrow transplants. *American Journal of Hematology,* **49,** 15–20.

Weisdorf, D.J., Anasetti, C., Antin, J.H. *et al.* (2002). Allogeneic bone marrow transplantation for chronic myelogenous leukemia: comparative analysis of unrelated versus matched sibling donor transplantation. *Blood,* **99,** 1971–7.

Wessman, M., Popp, S., Ruutu, T. *et al.* (1993). Detection of residual host cells after bone marrow transplantation using non-isotopic in situ hybridization and karyotype analysis. *Bone Marrow Transplantation,* **11,** 279–84.

Wetzler, M., Dodge, R.K., Mrozek, K. *et al.* (1999). Prospective karyotype analysis in adult acute lymphoblastic leukemia: the Cancer and Leukemia Group B Experience. *Blood,* **93,** 3983–93.

Willis, T.G. & Dyer, M.J.S. (2000). The role of immunoglobulin translocations in the pathogenesis of B-cell malignancies. *Blood,* **96,** 808–22.

Yeoh, E.-J., Ross, M.E., Shurtleff, S.A. *et al.* (2002). Classification, subtype discovery, and prediction of outcome in pediatric acute lymphoblastic leukemia by gene expression profiling. *Cancer Cell,* **1,** 133–43.

Zhang, F.F., Murata-Collins, J.L., Gaytan, P. *et al.* (2000). 24-color spectral karyotyping reveals chromosome aberrations in "cytogenetically normal" acute myeloid leukemia. *Genes, Chromosomes & Cancer,* **28,** 318–28.

Zojer, N., Koninsberg, R., Ackerman, J. *et al.* (2000). Deletions of 13q14 remains an independent adverse prognostic variable in multiple myeloma despite its frequent deletion by interphase fluorescence in situ hybridization. *Blood,* **95,** 1925–30.

104 Histopathology of hematopoietic stem cell transplantation

ANDREW FIELD, ADRIENNE MOREY, STEPHEN RAINER, JENNIFER TURNER, AND VINCENT MUNRO

St Vincent's Hospital, Sydney, Australia

Introduction

The procedure of hematopoietic stem cell transplantation (HSCT) for malignant conditions uses combinations of chemotoxic agents and radiation to destroy the malignant cells of the underlying disease and to ablate the bone marrow, while in nonmalignant conditions the bone marrow alone is ablated. Immune suppression is then induced to promote engraftment of the infused hemopoietic cells and to suppress graft-versus-host disease (GVHD). Failure to eradicate the tumor cells may result in relapse; failure to eradicate the patient's immune system may result in rejection of the allograft. These factors interacting with the recipient's underlying disease, as well as infections, produce a diversity of pathology that can be grouped pathogenically as: (1) effects of chemoradiation; (2) effects of immune suppression including infections; (3) effects of GVHD. GVHD also occurs in other circumstances such as heart-lung transplants that include mediastinal lymphoid tissue and in liver transplants, but in HSCT GVHD is sufficiently common and serious that it limits the wider application of the overall HSCT procedure.

The processes of GVHD in HSCT and rejection in solid organ transplantation share histological features. Both show lymphocytes indenting, injuring and destroying other cells. In GVHD the cells affected are the basal keratinocytes of the epidermis, the basal cells of the stratified squamous epithelium of the oral mucosa and esophagus, the bile ductular cells of the smaller bile ducts, the epithelial cells at the base of the intestinal crypts in the large and small bowel, and the gastric glandular cells in the stomach. The effects of this process produce acute and chronic changes in the affected tissues.

The histopathologic appearances of GVHD are a product of the process and the medications that modify it. The degree to which cellular injury is produced by an infiltrating cellular infiltrate, and by interleukin and cytokine production, is governed by the degree and nature of the immunosuppression. As these medications are varied over time so the histology varies with occasional major shifts, as occurred in solid organ rejection with the advent of cyclosporine.

The presence of GVHD itself is immune suppressive by its effects on the lymphoid system, and infections, such as cytomegalovirus (CMV) which occur because of the immunosuppression, induce further immunosuppression. The pathological processes in HSCT due to chemoradiation, immune suppression, infection, and GVHD are interrelated with factors from each influencing the final histopathological appearances.

The diagnostic problems of an HSCT unit also undergo continual change. The incidence of a prevalent infection such as *Pneumocystis carinii* declines with the introduction of effective prophylaxis, but it next appears in its granulomatous, organism-poor form, partially suppressed by the prophylactic medication. Similarly, the degree of routine immune suppression is adjusted upwards to combat a high incidence of GVHD in alternate donor transplants, which ameliorates the GVHD but causes an increase in the incidence of opportunistic infections. A recent diagnostic challenge has been the need to identify and classify posttransplant lymphoproliferative disorders, which may involve a number of organ systems.

The histopathologist within an HSCT unit has a critical role to play in the effort to optimize treatment so that GVHD, immune suppression, and chemoradiation effects are held in a dynamic balance that produces the best possible outcomes for the unit and for the individual patients.

Skin

Skin rashes are frequently encountered, especially in allogeneic HSC transplant recipients (see Chapter 96), and because of the skin's accessibility and the low morbidity of biopsying it, the skin has been the most extensively evaluated target organ. The onset of a rash is the most common, and usually the earliest manifestation of GVHD (Glucksberg *et al.*, 1974). However, the cutaneous appearance may be variable and can be simulated by a number of skin disorders including drug eruptions, erythema multiforme, and the toxic effects of chemotherapeutic agents and irradiation (Sale *et al.*, 1977; Farmer & Hood, 1983; Benjamin, Deeg, & Shulman, 1985), thus sometimes making a definitive clinical diagnosis of GVHD difficult. Less frequently cutaneous candidiasis or viral exanthems may mimic the clinical presentation of GVHD, but often the identification of a specific infectious agent or characteristic morphologic changes differentiate these disorders (Lever *et al.*, 1986).

Cutaneous GVHD

Cutaneous GVHD may cause significant morbidity in transplant recipients and its early recognition and treatment is essential for patient management. It may be classified into acute (early) and chronic (late) phases. While day 100 posttransplant has been arbitrarily proposed as the cut-off day for distinguishing between acute and chronic GVHD (Shulman *et al.*, 1978), the histologic appearances are usually sufficiently distinctive to make this temporal division excessively restrictive. For example, the histologic changes of early phase chronic GVHD may develop prior to day 100 posttransplantation (Saurat, 1981).

Acute cutaneous GVHD

Acute cutaneous GVHD usually develops between 2 and 6 weeks posttransplant and frequently presents with an erythematous maculopapular eruption. Initially, this may be confined to the palms and soles, but commonly progresses to involve the face, trunk, and limbs. In severe cases the principal clinical manifestations include diffuse erythroderma, bulla formation, and desquamation.

Histopathologically, acute cutaneous GVHD has the appearance of an interface dermatitis. The earliest sign of epidermal injury is nonspecific vacuolar degeneration of basal cells. With progressive lesions focal necrosis of basal keratinocytes is the most characteristic finding. Some of these necrotic cells show pyknotic hyperchromatic nuclei surrounded by intensely eosinophilic cytoplasm while others are represented by homogeneous eosinophilic bodies or colloid bodies (Lerner *et al.*, 1974). The latter may also be found in the upper papillary dermis. In early lesions individual necrotic keratinocytes may be localized to the tips of rete ridges and the infundibulum of hair follicles, where epidermal stem cells are thought to be concentrated (Sale *et al.*, 1985), but usually they are seen in a more generalized distribution within the lower stratum malpighii.[1] Satellitosis or satellite cell necrosis are terms used to describe an appearance characterized by the juxtaposition of lymphocytes to necrotic keratinocytes, frequently within spongiotic vesicles (Slavin & Santos, 1973; Woodruff *et al.*, 1976) (Fig. 104.1). This is a variable finding and, more important, is no longer considered essential for the diagnosis of acute cutaneous GVHD (Sale *et al.*, 1977). In the most severe lesions clefts appear at the dermoepidermal junction. These may coalesce to form vesicles and bullae (Fig. 104.2). With extensive epidermal necrosis desquamation occurs. A sparse band-like lymphatic infiltrate may be seen in the upper dermis with exocytosis into the lower epidermis. While this feature can be difficult to identify, the presence of lymphocytes within the epidermis improves the specificity of diagnosis during the early posttransplant phase (Elliott *et al.*, 1987; Sviland *et al.*, 1988). Less spe-

cific abnormalities found in the skin include hyperkeratosis, epidermal atrophy, disordered keratinocyte maturation, a nonspecific perivascular lymphatic infiltrate (as distinct from the diffuse infiltrate at the dermoepidermal junction), and pigmentary incontinence secondary to basal layer damage.

Involvement of skin appendages is common. Abnormalities of hair follicles are most prominent in the infundibulum and to a lesser extent the isthmus, and parallel those of the surface epithelium. Isolated follicular involvement has been reported and may represent an early manifestation of acute GVHD (Friedman, Le Boit, & Farmer, 1988) (Fig. 104.3). Although early studies stressed the relative sparing of sweat glands, another study documented frequent abnormalities with similar degenerative changes to those of the surface epithelium present most commonly in the intraepidermal and distal excretory ducts (Fig. 104.4). In addition, there may be an accompanying proliferative lesion characterized by basal cell hyperplasia of duct epithelium. The sweat gland coil is rarely directly involved (Akosa & Lampert, 1990).

The morphologic changes in acute cutaneous GVHD can be extremely variable. To improve diagnostic accuracy and precision, Lerner *et al.* (1974) devised a histologic grading system that was primarily dependent on the degree of epidermal abnormalities (Table 104.1). Although the general use of this grading system has facilitated uniformity in reporting among transplant units, several limitations of this system have become apparent. Firstly, the early feature of vacuolar degeneration is now considered to be nonspecific and alone insufficient for a definitive diagnosis of acute GVHD (Sale *et al.*, 1977). Furthermore, this change has been seen in pretransplant biopsies (Elliott *et al.*, 1987; Sviland *et al.*, 1988). Secondly, early epidermal changes have no predictive value for the development of more severe acute GVHD, and finally, while the original observations of Lerner *et al.* recognized the presence of an epidermal and/or dermal lymphatic infiltrate, it was not considered to be of diagnostic significance. This observation contrasts with more recent studies, which have shown that the presence of an epidermal and upper dermal lymphatic infiltrate improves the specificity for the diagnosis of acute GVHD, and has even been considered by some authors to be necessary for a definite diagnosis (Elliott *et al.*, 1987). Extending this observation, it has also been proposed that the density of the infiltrate is predictive of GVHD progression (Hymes *et al.*, 1985b), although further

Table 104.1. *Histopathologic grading system for cutaneous GVHD*

Grade I	Vacuolar degeneration of basal epidermal cells
Grade II	Grade I plus scattered necrosis of epidermal cells with "eosinophilic" (colloid) bodies and spongiosis
Grade III	Grade II plus focal dermo-epidermal separation and cleft formation
Grade IV	Extensive desquamation

Adapted from Lerner *et al.* (1974).

---

[1] Marcello Malpighi, Italian anatomist, 1628–1694.

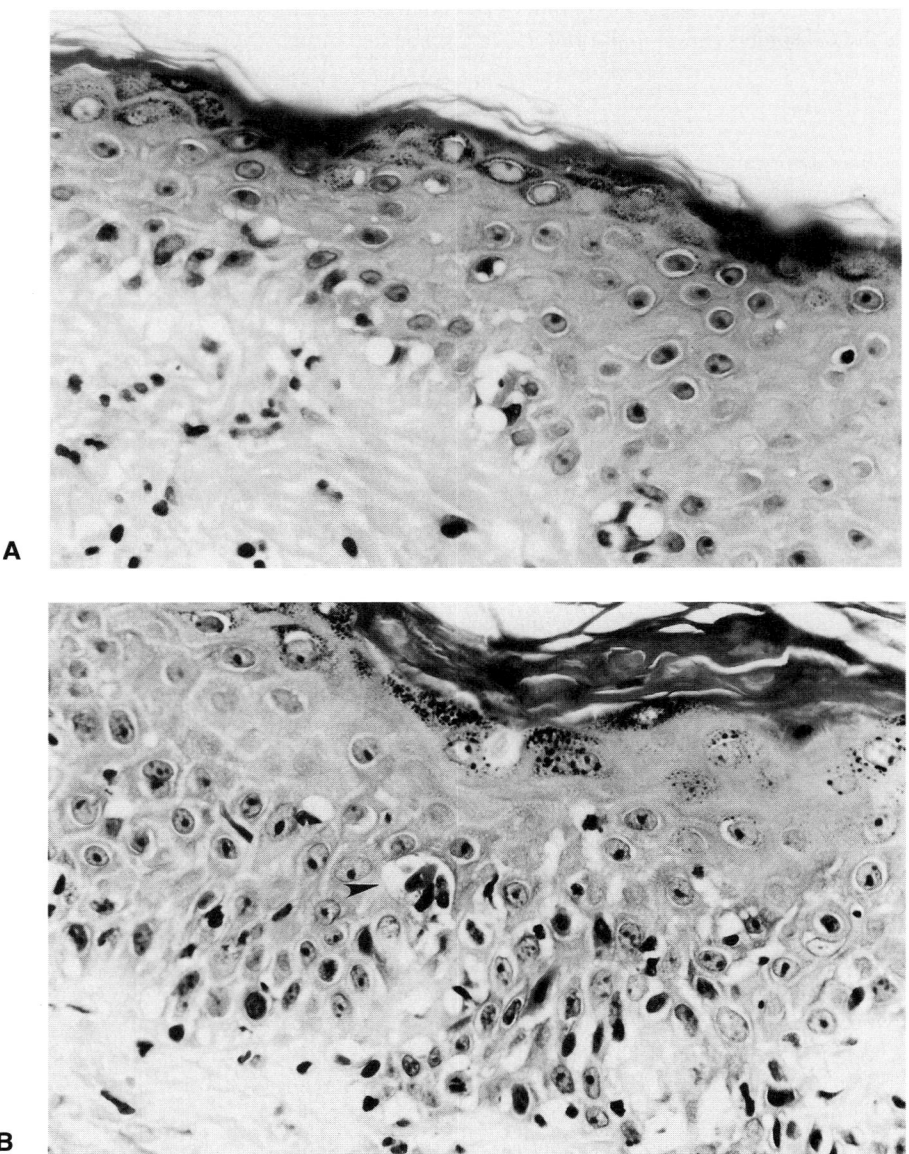

Fig. 104.1. (**A**) Acute cutaneous GVHD, Grade II. The earliest changes characteristic of GVHD are present. There is vacuolar degeneration of the basal layer associated with several necrotic keratinocytes. There is a sparse lymphocytic infiltrate in the papillary dermis (hematoxylin & eosin ×400). (**B**) Florid acute GVHD with multiple necrotic keratinocytes (one small collection is present within a spongiotic vesicle, arrowhead). In addition there is a sparse lymphocytic infiltrate within the epidermis (hematoxylin & eosin ×400).

studies are needed to confirm this. Despite these refinements the clinical utility of the current histologic grading system is undercut by the greater prognostic significance of the clinical staging system for acute GVHD (Thomas *et al.*, 1975). Nevertheless, its continued application is encouraged because it provides confirmation of the clinical diagnosis and defines relatively strict criteria that may be applied to future clinical and pathologic studies.

In addition to the above observations, discrepancies may occur between clinical and histologic diagnoses. A number of explanations have been offered. One interesting report has detailed a significant rate of discrepancies when skin biopsies were performed within 24 hours of the onset of a rash. The authors concluded that the development of histologic changes may lag behind the clinical recognition of a rash (Elliott *et al.*, 1987), an important point to recognize when considering a biopsy specimen. Uncommonly, sampling error due to the focal nature of acute GVHD, or processing artifact, may be misleading (Sale *et al.*, 1977). In such circumstances extensive sampling of the biopsy specimen or rebiopsy may be necessary. Despite these few limitations there is in general good correlation between the clinical and histologic findings.

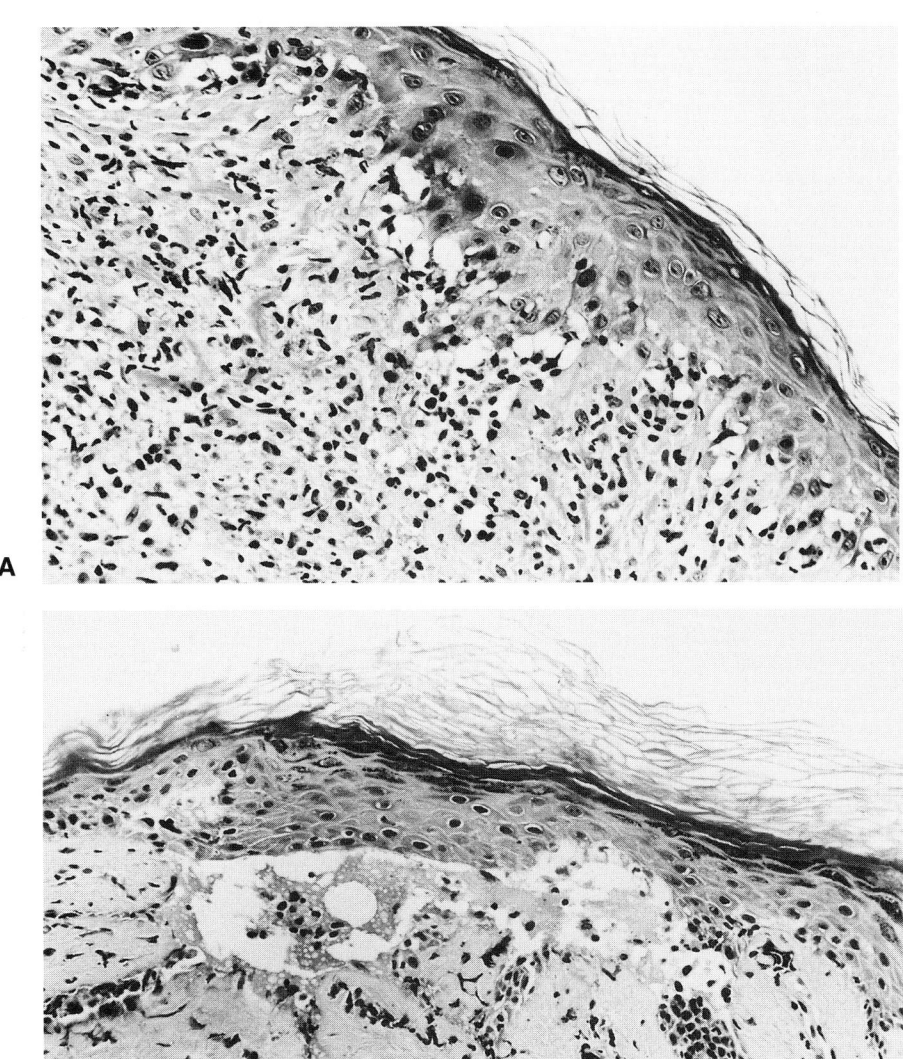

Fig. 104.2. Acute cutaneous GVHD, Grade III. (A) There is marked degeneration of the basal layer leading to cleft formation at the dermo-epidermal junction. There is an unusually heavy mononuclear infiltrate in the dermis with exocytosis into the epidermis. Several lymphocytes adjacent to necrotic keratinocytes (satellite cell necrosis) can be seen in the lower right-hand corner (hematoxylin & eosin ×200). (B) Microvesicle formation (hematoxylin & eosin ×200).

Differential diagnosis

None of the histologic features of acute cutaneous GVHD are pathognomonic for the disease and may be seen in a wide range of skin disorders. In the clinical context of allogeneic HSCT the major dilemma facing the pathologist is the difficulty in distinguishing the changes of mild to moderate acute GVHD from the toxic effects of chemotherapeutic agents and irradiation used in conditioning regimens, and, to a lesser extent, from drug reactions.

Cyclophosphamide/total body irradiation (TBI) and busulfan/cyclophosphamide are two commonly used pretransplant conditioning regimens. The effects of cyclophosphamide and TBI have been well characterized. When administered separately mild and transient epidermal atypia is seen with resolution by 7 to 14 days. However, when the combination is utilized a synergistic effect is seen with moderate epidermal atypia (increased nuclear/cytoplasmic ratio, nuclear pleomorphism, and occasional multinucleation) and focal necrosis of keratinocytes lasting up to 21 days (Sale et al., 1977) (Fig. 104.5). When the busulfan/cyclophosphamide combination is used as pretransplant conditioning the epidermal atypia is reported to be more prominent, a feature attributed to busulfan rather than

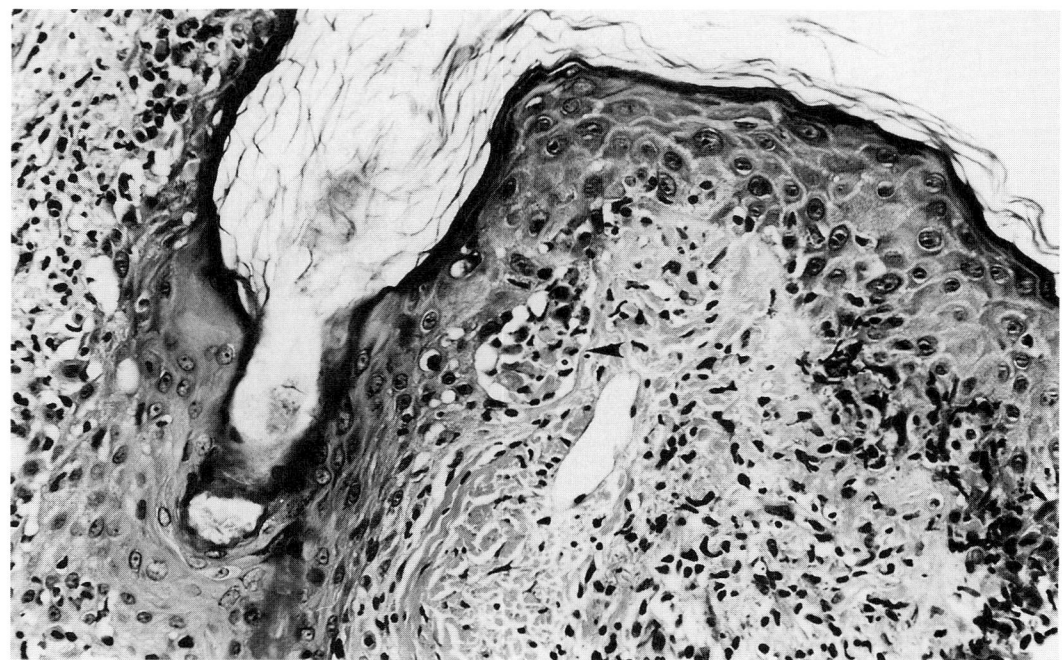

Fig. 104.3. Acute cutaneous GVHD showing predominantly hair follicle involvement. There is extensive degeneration of the basal layer of the follicular infundibulum with vacuolar degeneration and necrotic keratinocytes. There is an aggregate of colloid bodies in a spongiotic vesicle extending into the infundibulum (arrowhead) (hematoxylin & eosin ×400).

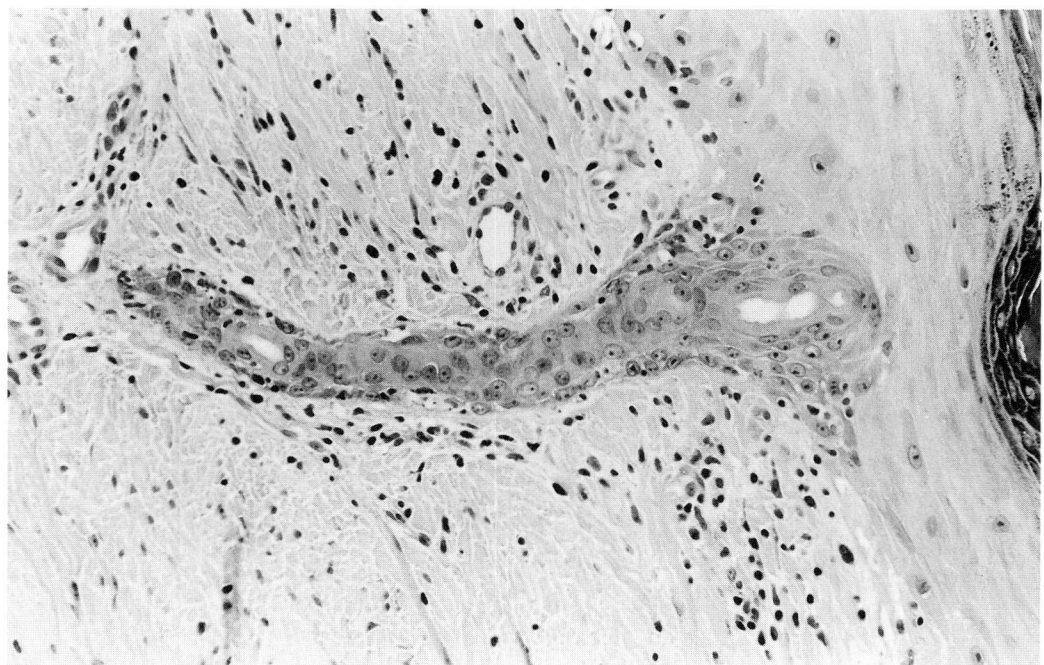

Fig. 104.4. Acute cutaneous GVHD. There is focal destruction of the basal cells in the distal portion of the excretory duct of a sweat gland. The overlying surface epithelium showed similar changes (hematoxylin & eosin ×100).

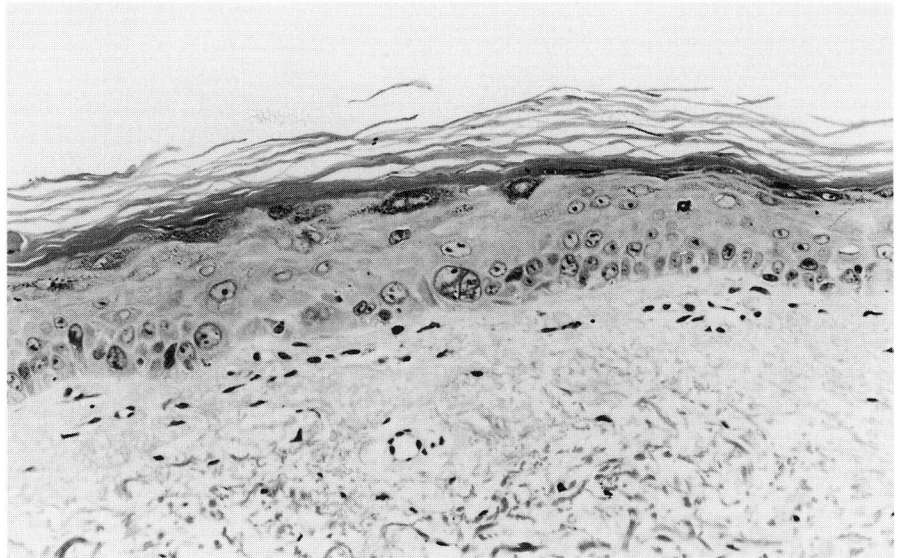

Fig. 104.5.   Skin biopsy showing chemoradiotherapy toxicity. There is marked nuclear pleomorphism, multinucleation, and scattered necrotic keratinocytes. The absence of an epidermal and dermal lymphocytic infiltrate is a characteristic finding (hematoxylin & eosin ×100).

cyclophosphamide. A characteristic finding seen in this latter group includes scattered large keratinocytes often with nuclear irregularity and bizarre chromatin patterns. These features may appear up to 6 weeks posttransplant (Hymes *et al.,* 1985c). Similar findings have been described in cervical and bronchial epithelium (Obermann *et al.,* 1999).

Chemotherapy-induced acral erythema is a distinct clinical syndrome with a median onset of 1 to 2 weeks posttransplant and is characterized by a painful, well-demarcated erythematous macular eruption on the palms, soles, and knuckles, which in its most severe form may blister. This syndrome has been described in patients receiving high-dose chemotherapy and irradiation without HSC transplantation, particularly protocols containing the cytotoxic agent cytosine arabinoside (Herzig *et al.,* 1983; Levine *et al.,* 1985; Crider *et al.,* 1986). We have seen this complication most commonly in patients receiving busulfan/cyclophosphamide conditioning (Morgan *et al.,* 1991). Histologically this syndrome is difficult to differentiate from acute GVHD; however, the clinical picture is distinctive and spontaneous resolution is usual (see Chapter 96).

In general, features that may help distinguish chemoradiotherapy effects from acute GVHD include the absence of an epidermal lymphatic infiltrate and the diffuse epidermal atypia and distribution of necrotic keratinocytes seen in the former compared to the usually basally oriented changes seen in the latter. However, in practice, the histologic features of chemoradiotherapy toxicity are usually not reliably distinguished from mild to moderate acute GVHD during the first 3 to 4 weeks posttransplant. A cautious approach utilizing clinicopathologic correlation, continued observation, and if necessary repeat skin biopsy, is recommended, and in most instances will resolve any difficulties, particularly as the effects of chemoradiotherapy resolve with time, in contrast to the effects of GVHD, which may worsen.

The histologic features of drug eruptions can simulate those of acute GVHD. Distinguishing between the two disorders may be difficult since most transplant recipients are usually on multiple drug therapy. The temporal relationship between the commencement of a drug and the onset of rash may be the only indicator of a possible drug-induced eruption. The presence of significant numbers of eosinophils in a biopsy may also be an indicator, but is not present in all cases. Toxic epidermal necrolysis (TEN) is a distinct clinical syndrome, although there may be overlap with severe erythema multiforme (Goldstein, Wintroub, & Elias, 1987; Heng & Allen, 1991). Histologically TEN is characterized by epidermal necrosis with dermoepidermal cleft formation and extensive desquamation. There are numerous causes but drugs, particularly sulfonamides, are the most commonly implicated etiologic agents. However, reports supported by animal models have proposed common pathogenetic mechanisms for acute GVHD and TEN, and have suggested that TEN may also be a manifestation of severe acute cutaneous GVHD (Peck, Herzig, & Elias 1972; Friedman *et al.,* 1984). This hypothesis is supported by a report of nine cases of TEN occurring in HSCT recipients, in which approximately half the cases were thought due to acute GVHD, while the other half were due to suspected adverse drug reactions, predominantly to sulfonamide therapy. In this report no histologic features could be identified to distinguish the two patient groups (Villada *et al.,* 1990).

Rarely, staphylococcal scalded skin syndrome may clinically mimic severe cutaneous GVHD but morphologically the characteristic subcorneal cleft allows differentiation in almost all cases (Goldberg *et al.,* 1989).

Chronic cutaneous GVHD

Cutaneous abnormalities are the most prominent manifestation of chronic GVHD and have characteristic histopathologic features that allow distinction from acute GVHD. Chronic GVHD may arise as a continuation of acute GVHD, after the resolution of acute GVHD, or without preceding acute GVHD (Shulman *et al.,* 1978). Two phases are recognized, an "early" chronic phase lesion and a characteristic "late" chronic phase lesion. The disease presents clinically with rash, induration, and patchy hyper- or hypopigmentation (Saurat *et al.,* 1975; Shulman *et al.,* 1978).

Histologically, the "early" chronic phase lesion is characterized by lichenoid changes indistinguishable from lichen planus. The variable epidermal hyperplasia with "sawtooth" acanthosis and denser lymphatic infiltrate help differentiate this phase from acute GVHD. The "late" chronic phase lesion is characterized by sclerodermoid changes with involution of the florid epidermal abnormalities accompanied by dermal fibrosis. More specifically the epidermis becomes atrophic, and basal vacuolation, necrotic keratinocytes, and eosinophilic bodies are rarely identified (Fig. 104.6). The epidermal and dermal inflammatory infiltrate is sparse and fibrosis usually begins in the papillary dermis, progressively replacing normal dermal tissue including skin appendages. Residual arrector pili muscles can usually be identified. The final appearance closely resembles scleroderma, but subtle differences exist. For example, the epidermis is usually normal in scleroderma, unlike that in chronic GVHD where residual minor epidermal damage, atrophy, and pigment incontinence may persist (Farmer & Hood, 1983).

It has also been suggested that fibrosis begins higher in the dermis in chronic GVHD (Saurat, 1981). Bulla formation has been reported in sclerodermoid lesions. Morphologically this

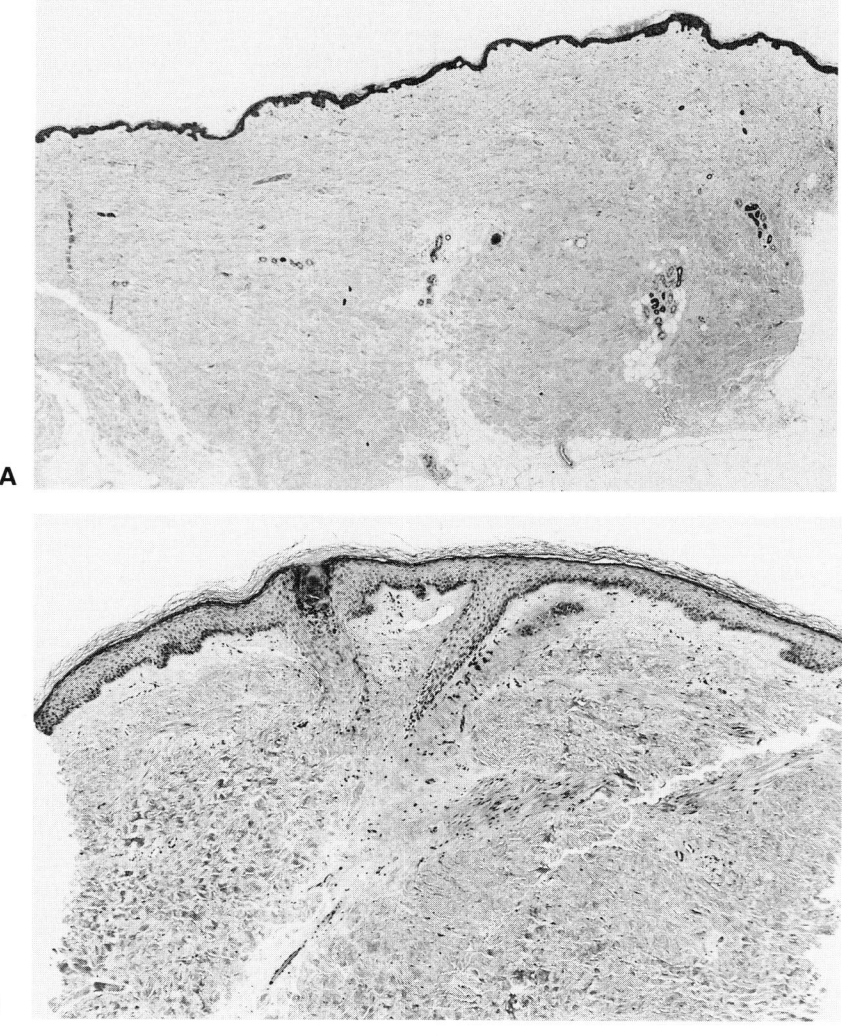

Fig. 104.6. Chronic cutaneous GVHD, late phase. (**A**) Forearm biopsy showing extensive dermal fibrosis and loss of dermal appendages (hematoxylin & eosin ×40). (**B**) In this view there is epidermal atrophy and a sparse dermal infiltrate with loss of hair follicles. Residual arrector pili muscle is surrounded by fibrous tissue (hematoxylin & eosin ×100).

lesion is characterized by a subepidermal cleft associated with dilated lymphatics and dermal edema, features thought to be due to collections of lymphedema (Hymes *et al.*, 1985a). Rarely, chronic scabies producing a lichenoid skin eruption has been clinically mistaken for chronic GVHD (Magee, Herbert, & Rapini, 1991).

Immunopathology of cutaneous GVHD

Numerous immunohistologic studies have been performed on skin from HSC transplant recipients with GVHD. The aims have been, firstly, to determine possible immunopathogenic mechanisms and, secondly, to identify features that may be specific or predictive for early acute GVHD. Three major observations are summarized.

Firstly, the density of the dermal and epidermal lymphatic infiltrate is extremely variable (Lampert *et al.*, 1982) and is composed of a mixture of CD4+ and CD8+ T lymphocytes (Sloane *et al.*, 1984). A feature not always appreciated is the varying composition of the infiltrate depending on the interval posttransplantation (Atkinson *et al.*, 1986). Early on, CD8+ cells tend to predominate. CD4+ cells have been reported to be either increased or decreased when compared to pretransplant levels, but the overall feature is a reduction in the CD4:CD8 ratio (Elliott *et al.*, 1988). One report suggested a predominance of CD4+ cells in the dermis and CD8+ cells in the epidermis (Favre *et al.*, 1997).

Secondly, there is a marked reduction in epidermal Langerhans cells in the immediate posttransplant phase, usually returning to normal levels by the end of the first month. This initial depletion is thought to be due to direct toxicity of the conditioning protocol (Lever *et al.*, 1986). It has been postulated that Langerhans cells are targets for the effector cells of GVHD, which may have an additional depleting effect accounting for delayed recovery posttransplant (Suitters & Lampert, 1983). An alternative hypothesis suggests that the effects of GVHD may be indirect and that epidermal basal layer damage may inhibit migration of Langerhans cells into the epidermis (Elliott *et al.*, 1988).

Thirdly, in the presence of GVHD, keratinocytes aberrantly express the MHC class II antigen HLA-DR. The significance of this finding is unclear as it has been observed in a number of immunologically induced dermatoses including drug eruptions (Breathnach & Katz, 1987). This finding may represent an epiphenomenon associated with T-cell-mediated cytotoxicity (Kasahara *et al.*, 1983).

In summary, while helpful in elucidating possible pathogenetic mechanisms, no immunohistologic features have been found sufficiently discriminating to be clinically applicable.

Mouth

Acute oral GVHD

Occasionally the mouth is involved by acute GVHD, usually manifested clinically as erythema of the mucosa.

Histologically the mucosal surface lesion of acute GVHD is similar to that found in skin, although the mucosal and submucosal lymphatic infiltrate is usually denser and the epithelium is often thicker. The salivary gland lesion is similar to that found in early chronic oral GVHD (see below), except that chronic acinar damage is infrequently found.

Oro-pharyngeal mucositis

More commonly, a severe debilitating nonspecific mucositis develops secondary to the effects of high-dose pretransplant chemoradiotherapy, posttransplant methotrexate used for GVHD prophylaxis, and agranulocytosis. This usually resolves with neutrophil engraftment; however, superinfection with herpes simplex or *Candida albicans* may complicate recovery. In a small number of patients transient enlargement of major salivary glands may develop secondary to chemoradiotherapy, but usually subsides within 14 days. Histologically this lesion is characterized by reversible diffuse acinar damage.

Chronic oral GVHD

The oral cavity is commonly involved in chronic GVHD. Patients usually present with oral discomfort and xerostomia, while common findings include erythema, mucosal atrophy, and a reticulate pattern of white striae (Schubert *et al.*, 1984). Lip biopsies are frequently performed to confirm the presence of chronic GVHD, since decisions regarding continuation or reinitiation of immune suppressive treatment may hinge on its presence. The histologic findings in the mucosal squamous epithelium are similar to those found in the skin (Fig. 104.7). Early lesions of the salivary glands consist of a "nonspecific" lymphatic infiltration of the glandular interstitium consistent with sialadenitis. Characteristic lesions are centered on intralobular and major secretory ducts, and show focal necrosis of ductal epithelium with intraepithelial lymphocytes, duct ectasia, and epithelial atypia. Acinar damage is minimal in the early stages; however, progression of the primary ductal lesion leads to ductal obliteration and secondary atrophy and fibrosis of salivary lobules (Sale *et al.*, 1981) (Fig. 104.8). The histologic changes are similar to those of Sjögren's syndrome,[2] but the lymphoid infiltrate is sparser and epimyoepithelial islands are not seen (Gratwohl *et al.*, 1977). Similar changes are seen in the lacrimal gland. The current minimum criteria for chronic mucosal GVHD include the presence of a lichenoid infiltrate plus focal epithelial necrosis. For salivary gland involvement the minimum criteria include either lymphatic infiltration, atypia and necrosis of ductal epithelium, or extensive inflammation or fibrosis of acini (Schubert *et al.*, 1984). Immunopathologic studies on oral lesions show similar results to those of cutaneous studies (Fujii, Ohashi, & Nagura, 1988).

---

[2] Henrik Sjögren, Swedish opthalmologist, 1896–1974.

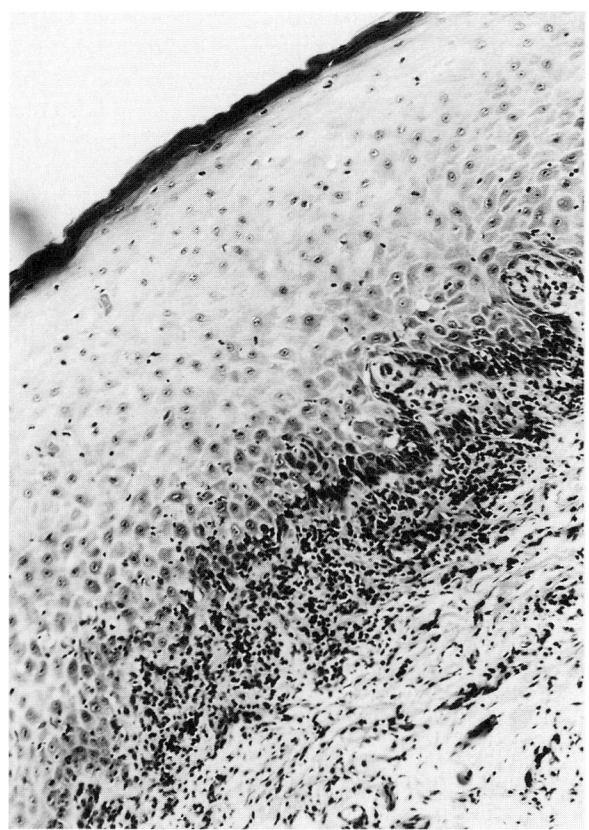

Fig. 104.7. Oral mucosa involved by chronic GVHD showing a moderately heavy mononuclear infiltrate within the corium and invading the epithelium. Focal necrotic basal cells are present (hematoxylin & eosin ×100).

Gastrointestinal system

Acute and chronic gastrointestinal GVHD

Gastrointestinal complications are frequent after HSCT and are mainly due to the effects of GVHD, chemoradiotherapy, opportunistic infections, and drug therapy (see Chapter 89). The clinical manifestations such as anorexia, nausea, vomiting, abdominal discomfort, watery diarrhea, and rarely hemorrhage are relatively nonspecific, but may suggest the gastrointestinal tract (GIT) site is severely affected. For the purposes of this discussion the GIT will be divided into two compartments, esophagus and stomach/intestine, based on the differing mucosal epithelial surfaces and morphologic response to the effects of GVHD.

The number of GIT biopsies in HSC transplant recipients has decreased in recent years due to effective CMV prophylaxis. However, GIT biopsies still play an important diagnostic role in patients with suspected opportunistic infections and GVHD. With the increasing use of HSCT in developing countries, enteric pathogens including *Cryptosporidium parvum* and adenovirus need to be excluded by screening (Kang *et al.,* 2002), and specifically sought in GIT biopsies from HSCT patients (Field, 2002).

Esophagus

The esophagus is uncommonly involved by acute GVHD and the changes may be mimicked by chemoradiotherapy effects in the first 20 days posttransplantation (McDonald *et al.,* 1986). When acute GVHD is suspected, the histologic features and grading are the same as for skin (Sale *et al.,* 1979).

More commonly, nonspecific esophagitis or infective esophagitis is seen, the latter usually caused by herpes simplex virus (HSV), CMV, or fungal organisms including *Candida* species (McDonald *et al.,* 1985) and *Aspergillus* species (Choi *et al.,* 1997). There are several diagnostic pitfalls in assessing biopsies for infective causes. Firstly, CMV inclusions occur in endothelial and stromal cells of the papillary and deeper lamina propria, often missing in esophageal biopsies. Secondly, the diagnosis of fungal esophagitis requires fungal elements within the superficial epithelium or within keratotic or necrotic debris attached to epithelial biopsies. Fungal elements in unattached debris may represent oro-pharyngeal contamination. Thirdly, herpetic inclusions occur in the squamous epithelium especially in the margins of ulcers, and may be scant. Biopsies from the center of ulcers have a low diagnostic yield and should be discouraged. Fourthly, infections and GVHD cannot be excluded in biopsies consisting only of granulation tissue of ulcer base without epithelium.

Later in the posttransplant period chronic GVHD can occur in the esophagus, with changes resembling those seen in chronic skin GVHD. These changes include individual necrotic keratinocytes scattered through the basal layer, mucosal infiltration with lymphocytes, and epithelial desquamation. In severe cases, focal submucosal fibrosis has been found (McDonald *et al.,* 1981).

Stomach and intestine

The earliest histological lesion in these sites that suggests acute GVHD is necrosis of individual epithelial cells (Epstein *et al.,* 1980; Snover *et al.,* 1985) in the base of intestinal crypts and in the isthmus of gastric glands, characterized by the accumulation of karyorrhectic debris in clear spaces within the epithelium or adjacent to the sides and base of crypts (Slavin & Santos, 1973; Lerner *et al.,* 1974). In early and mild acute GVHD, individual cell necrosis can be extremely focal and surrounded by otherwise normal mucosa. In more severe GVHD multiple epithelial cells within a single crypt may show karyorrhexis leading to the descriptive term "exploding crypt" (Sale *et al.,* 1979). The surface epithelium is relatively spared in early lesions with only mild degenerative changes Acute GVHD is marked by dysregulation of inflammatory cytokines (the "cytokine storm") (Ferrara *et al.,* 1996), and it is cytokines that largely cause the GIT injury, which in turn, by the release of endotoxins and other agents, amplifies further cytokine release, worsening systemic GVHD pathology (Hill & Ferrara, 2000).

Progressive degeneration of the epithelium leads to dilatation of intestinal crypts and gastric glands, which are lined by attenuated and often atypical cells, and to crypt abscesses con-

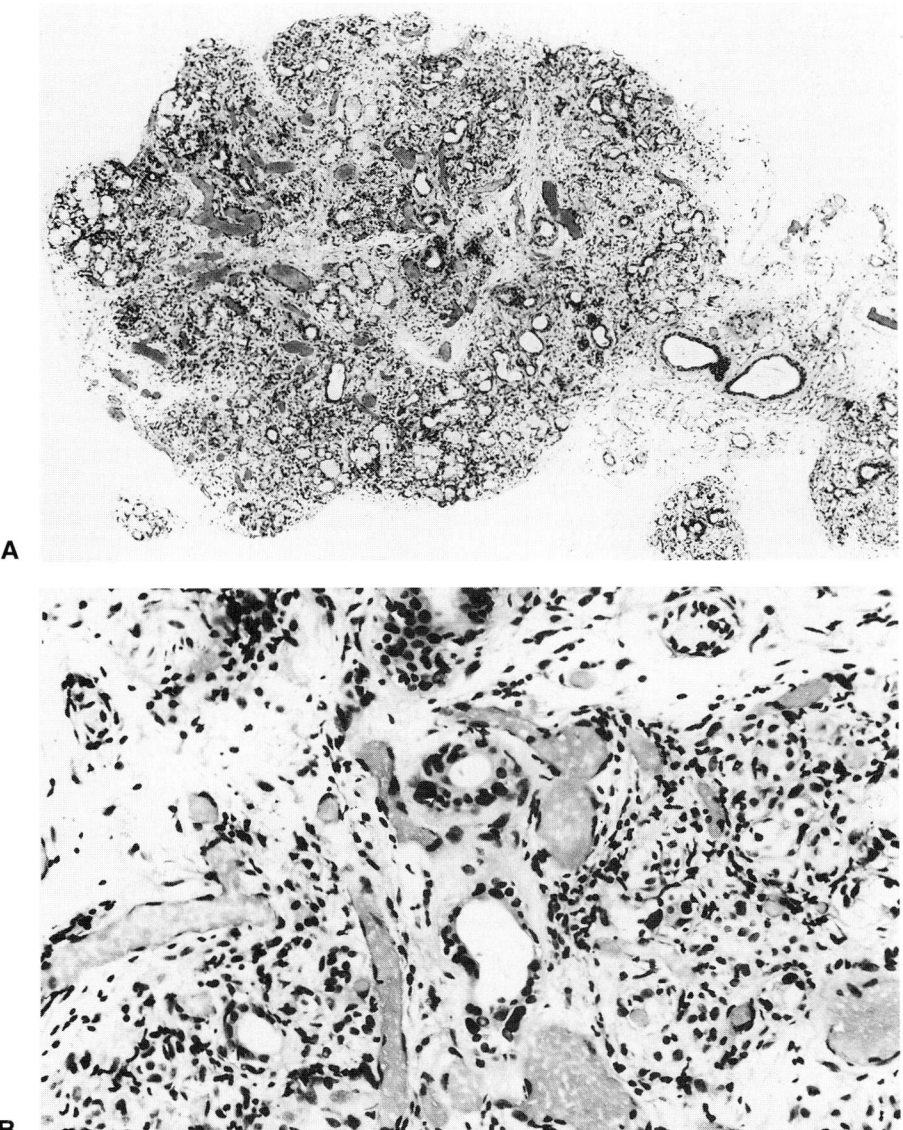

Fig. 104.8. Chronic GVHD involving a minor salivary gland. (A) There is a moderately heavy mononuclear infiltrate within the glandular interstitium associated with lobular atrophy, duct ectasia, and fibrosis (hematoxylin & eosin ×40). (B) Detailed view of an intralobular duct showing intraepithelial lymphocytes, necrosis, degeneration, and attenuation of duct epithelium. There is atrophy of glands with a surrounding mononuclear infiltrate; however, no epimyoepithelial islands are present (hematoxylin & eosin ×200).

taining cellular debris, neutrophils, and eosinophils. Severe lesions show obliteration and loss of entire crypts, and focal and eventually extensive ulceration. Intestinal metaplasia can accompany these changes in the stomach, and in the small intestine partial or total villous atrophy can be seen (Fig. 104.9). Enterochromatin cells and Paneth[3] cells may be spared in the large bowel and appear singly or in small aggregates in areas of obliterated crypts (Lampert *et al.*, 1985). No consistent changes are seen in the composition of the cellular infiltrate within the lamina propria although intraepithelial lymphocytes may be seen adjacent to necrotic crypt epithelium, and one study suggested a correlation between the presence of

eosinophils and the severity of the GVHD (Daneshpouy *et al.*, 2002). The severity of the histologic changes in acute GVHD of the stomach and intestine may be graded according to the modified histologic grading system of Lerner *et al.* (1974) (Table 104.2). In the appropriate clinical context the diagnostic utility of this grading system has been proven (Epstein *et al.*, 1980). However, as in the esophagus, biopsies showing severe mucosal damage or ulceration may be difficult to classify, particularly if no early diagnostic crypt changes are present.

[3] Joseph Paneth, Austrian physician, 1857–1890.

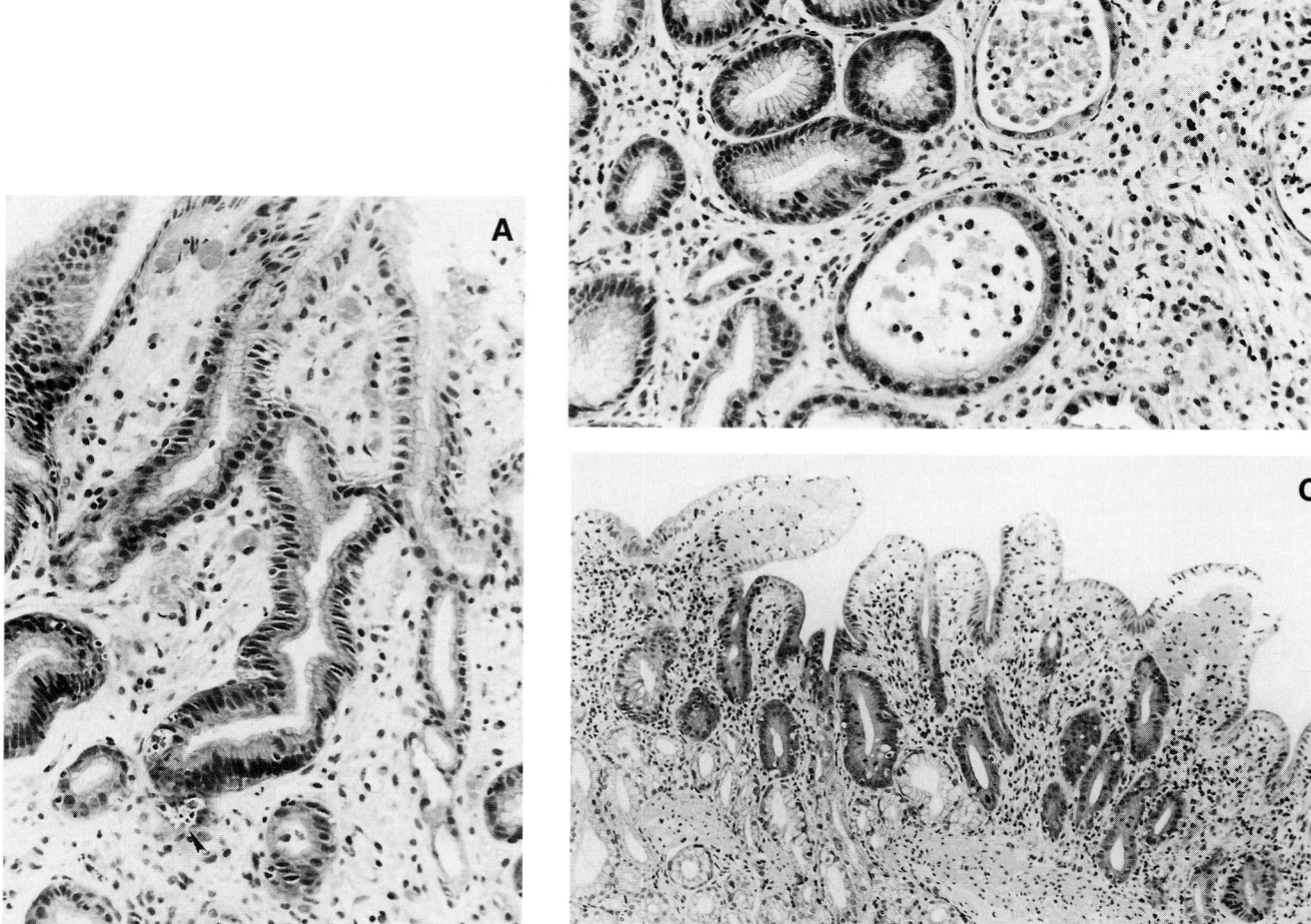

Fig. 104.9. Series of gastrointestinal biopsies demonstrating the spectrum of histologic changes found in acute GVHD. (**A**) Gastric biopsy with mild GVHD, Grade I, showing focal epithelial necrosis localized to the base of a gastric pit (arrowhead). The adjacent epithelium shows minimal changes (hematoxylin & eosin ×200). (**B**) Gastric biopsy with severe acute GVHD showing dilated glands lined by attenuated epithelium and containing cellular debris within their lumen (hematoxylin & eosin ×200). (**C**) Duodenal biopsy showing partial villous atrophy. There are intraepithelial lymphocytes and focal necrosis of epithelium in the adjacent intestinal crypts consistent with acute GVHD (hematoxylin & eosin ×100). (*Figure continues*)

Early series documented more severe involvement of ileum and large intestine in acute GVHD, and rectal biopsy was recommended to obtain a higher diagnostic yield (Sale *et al.,* 1979). Studies then demonstrated the generalized nature of

Table 104.2. *Histopathologic grading system for gastrointestinal GVHD*

Grade I	Single cell necrosis of crypt gland epithelium with focal dilatation of glands
Grade II	Grade I plus focal or diffuse loss of glands/crypts
Grade III	Grade II plus focal mucosal ulceration
Grade IV	Diffuse ulceration

Adapted from Lerner *et al.* (1974).

gastrointestinal GVHD, particularly the involvement of the upper GIT and the general correlation of the degree of rectal, stomach, and duodenal involvement (Snover *et al.,* 1985). However, significant disparity in biopsy findings has been reported in up to 30% of cases (Roy *et al.,* 1991); acute GVHD is often focal, introducing potential sampling problems (Spencer *et al.,* 1986), and in the presence of persistent GIT symptoms, negative rectal biopsies do not exclude acute GVHD or infection. Upper GIT endoscopy and biopsy should always be performed (Weisdorf *et al.,* 1990). Small bowel biopsies offer a 90% sensitivity in detecting GVHD (Terdiman *et al.,* 1996).

Recently, bleeding from gastric antral vascular ectasia, characterized by telangiectatic capillaries, occasional fibrin thrombi in capillaries, and muscularis mucosa hypertrophy, has been

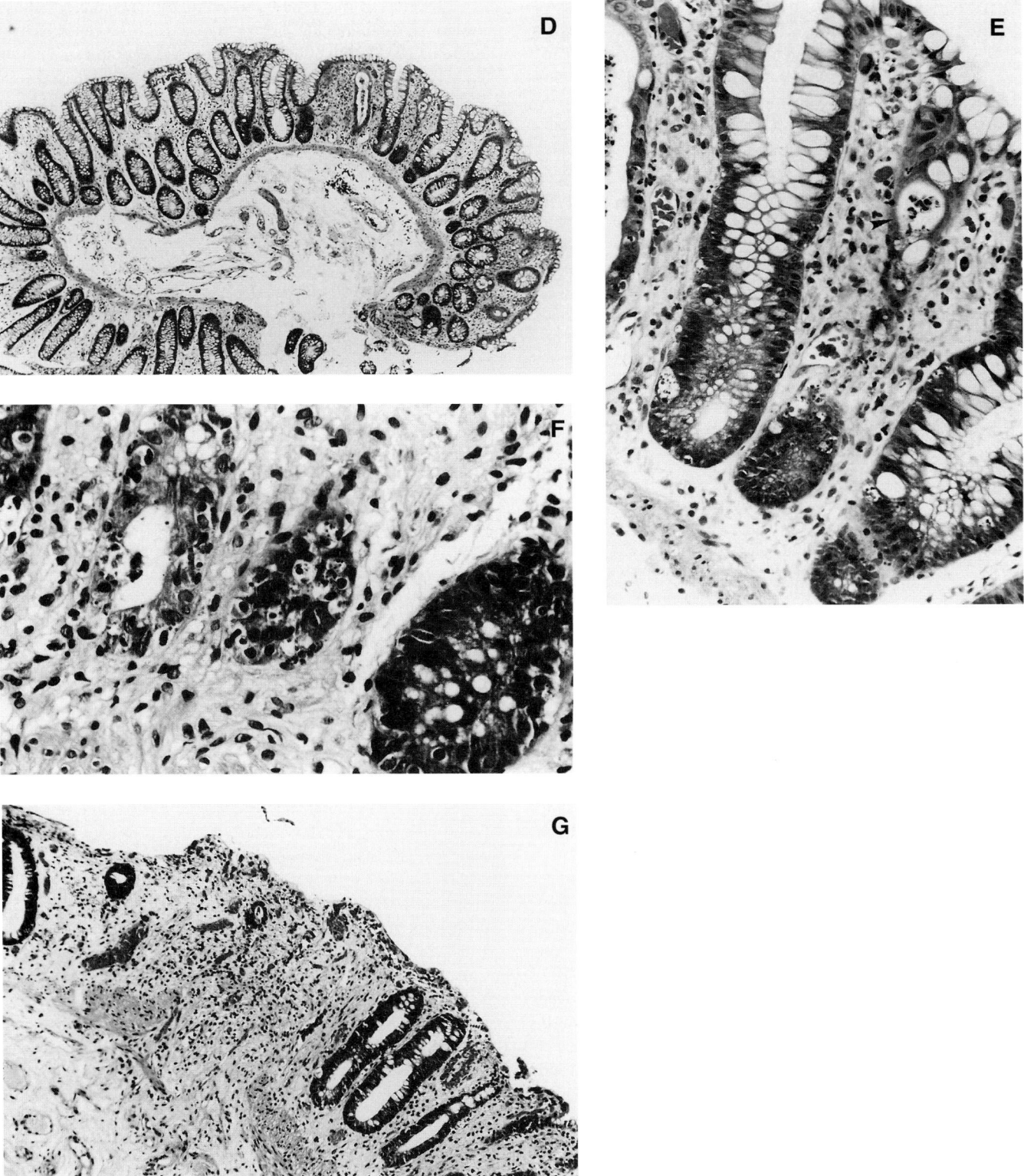

Fig. 104.9. (*continued*)   **(D)** Lower power view of colonic mucosa showing focal GVHD with preservation of the majority of crypts (hematoxylin & eosin ×40). **(E)** High power view of **(D)** showing focal epithelial necrosis and crypt abscess (arrowhead) (hematoxylin & eosin ×400). **(F)** Colonic biopsy showing characteristic appearance of exploding crypt with multiple necrotic cells with karyorrhectic debris (hematoxylin & eosin ×600). **(G)** Colonic biopsy with severe acute (Grade III) GVHD showing focal loss of crypts and ulceration of surface epithelium (hematoxylin & eosin ×100).

described in HSCT patients, possibly related to veno-occlusive disease and busulfan therapy (Tobin *et al.*, 1997).

The histologic features of GVHD of the stomach and small and large intestine are not specific, leading to difficulty distinguishing the effects of chemoradiotherapy and opportunistic infections from acute GVHD. The histologic features of chemoradiotherapy toxicity persist for up to 20 days and may be indistinguishable from mild to moderate GVHD (Epstein *et al.*, 1980). However, the effects of chemoradiotherapy tend to be diffuse in comparison to the focal nature of acute GVHD, and crypt nuclear atypia is more prominent than epithelial necrosis. Considerable overlap is found and a definite diagnosis of GVHD should be made with caution prior to day 20 posttransplant (McDonald *et al.*, 1986).

Active CMV disease is a frequent cause of nonspecific symptoms in allogeneic transplant recipients and can also be superimposed on acute GVHD (McDonald *et al.*, 1986). CMV infection can produce single cell necrosis with karyorrhectic debris occurring in intestinal crypts and gastric glands, with crypt or gastric pit abscesses resembling those found in acute GVHD (Snover, 1985). However, in CMV infection these changes are more commonly associated with intraepithelial neutrophils and a mixed inflammatory cell infiltrate in the adjacent lamina propria; typical intranuclear inclusions and smaller eosinophilic cytoplasmic inclusions in epithelial, endothelial, and stromal cells are diagnostic. In some biopsy specimens characteristic CMV inclusions may be rare and immunoperoxidase stains for CMV, particularly directed against CMV early antigens, enhance the sensitivity of detecting infected cells. A larger number of infected cells suggests clinical significance. In the presence of active CMV infection, it has been said that acute gastrointestinal GVHD cannot be reliably diagnosed (Snover *et al.*, 1985). However, if multiple biopsies from multiple sites in stomach or in bowel show some regions in which early crypt lesions characteristic of acute GVHD are present with no accompanying neutrophilic infiltrate or CMV inclusions, we feel confident in diagnosing coexisting acute GVHD and CMV infection. Other groups appear to utilize this approach in diagnostic assessment (Sale *et al.*, 1979).

The GIT distal to the esophagus is infrequently involved in chronic GVHD and usually sequential biopsies of stomach, duodenum, and especially colon, may show nonspecific degenerative changes usually associated with chronic inflammation best regarded as the sequelae of previous episodes of acute GVHD. These changes in the colon include patchy loss of crypts and irregular, shortened, or even branched crypts, similar to changes normally associated with quiescent chronic inflammatory bowel disease. Rarely segmental focal fibrosis of the lamina propria and submucosa may be seen extending throughout the GIT and may lead to severe scarring of the rectal mucosa (Fox *et al.*, 1996).

Hepatobiliary system

Hepatic abnormalities are common after HSC transplantation and are caused by the toxic effects of chemoradiotherapy, GVHD, infection, and hepatotoxic agents (including cyclosporine and total parenteral nutrition) (Farthing *et al.*, 1982; Snover *et al.*, 1984). Clinical and biochemical findings are not specific, making precise diagnosis of the cause of liver dysfunction difficult, although the interval after transplantation and the liver function test profile may be helpful in distinguishing clinical syndromes. Laparoscopic and transvenous liver biopsies have increased the number of patients with liver and clotting problems who can undergo liver biopsy, yielding useful diagnostic results (Iqbal *et al.*, 1996).

Hepatic GVHD

Involvement of the liver by GVHD usually develops after day 20 posttransplant and usually follows the onset of skin and GIT symptoms. GVHD is rarely an isolated manifestation, although liver dysfunction may be the first and only sign of increasing activity once treatment for GVHD is reduced or ceased. Liver function tests show a cholestatic pattern, with elevations of bilirubin and serum alkaline phosphatase values reflecting the severity of disease. Occasionally, both acute and chronic hepatic GVHD can present as an acute hepatitis, both biochemically and histopathologically (Strasser *et al.*, 2000; Malik *et al.*, 2001: Fujii *et al.*, 2001; Akpek *et al.*, 2002).

The characteristic lesion is injury to small to medium-sized interlobular bile ducts (Sloane, Farthing, & Powles, 1980). Larger bile ducts are relatively spared. Specific features include nuclear multilayering, enlargement and pleomorphism, cytoplasmic vacuolation, eosinophilic focal necrosis and loss of epithelial cells and disruption of ductal walls. Cellular debris may accumulate within the duct lumen and exocytosis of lymphocytes into duct epithelium may be seen. Damaged bile ducts tend to have irregular outlines (Fig. 104.10). With progression to chronic disease there is reduction in the number of small ducts, bile ductular proliferation, and portal fibrosis. Other abnormalities include lobular disorganization with focal hepatocellular necrosis, cholestasis, and a portal and lobular inflammatory infiltrate composed predominantly of lymphocytes, that is usually sparse but may increase with chronicity of the disease (Shulman *et al.*, 1988). Rarely, cirrhosis may supervene (Knapp *et al.*, 1987). Hepatic GVHD may be graded histologically according to the proportion of involved ducts (Lerner *et al.*, 1974) (Table 104.3). Biopsies typical of hepatic GVHD usually show extensive (greater than 50%) bile duct damage (Snover *et al.*, 1984).

Biopsies performed in the early posttransplant period (before day 35) tend to show less specific histologic features with only minimal bile duct changes and relatively greater hepatocellular necrosis, and can cause problems in diagnosing hepatic GVHD. Later biopsies (beyond day 35) show more florid bile duct lesions including progression to bile duct drop-out and portal fibrosis (Shulman *et al.*, 1988). During the assessment of chronic GVHD it has been suggested that the presence of significant hepatocellular necrosis should raise the possibility of an alternative diagnosis (Snover *et al.*, 1984), but biopsies performed soon after the onset of liver dysfunction, irrespective of the interval posttransplantation, may show changes similar to early acute GVHD. Furthermore, there is no significant difference in the dis-

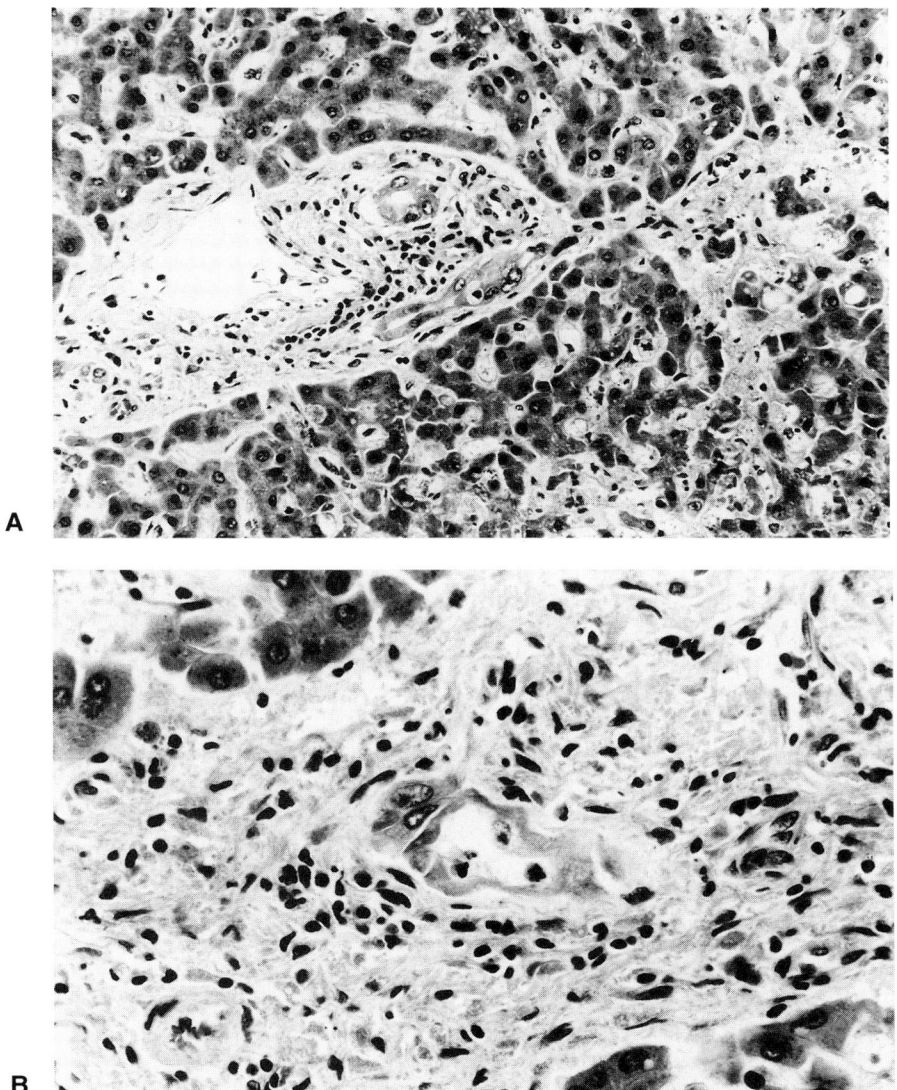

Fig. 104.10. Hepatic GVHD. **(A)** Portal tract showing characteristic injury to bile ducts. The ducts are irregular in outline with focal necrosis and loss of nuclei. The remaining epithelial nuclei show marked pleomorphism (hematoxylin & eosin ×200). **(B)** High power view of small bile duct showing marked irregularity, cell drop-out, and luminal debris. The adjacent hepatic lobules showed prominent centrilobular cholestasis (not shown) (hematoxylin & eosin ×400).

Table 104.3. *Histopathologic grading system for hepatic GVHD*

Grade I	Less than 25% of small bile ducts showing degenerate epithelium ± necrosis
Grade II	25%–49% of small bile ducts involved
Grade III	50%–74% of small bile ducts involved
Grade IV	Greater than or equal to 75% of small bile ducts involved

Adapted from Lerner *et al.* (1974).

tribution or density of portal and lobular inflammatory infiltrates between acute and chronic hepatic GVHD, and endothelialitis, defined as the attachment of lymphocytes to the luminal surface of the endothelium of central and portal veins, has proven of little discriminatory value in identifying acute hepatic GVHD. Endothelialitis was reported in 40% of patients with acute GVHD and in none with chronic GVHD, and was initially thought to be a useful distinguishing feature (Snover *et al.,* 1984). Subsequently, this lesion was identified in a number of disorders, including orthotopic liver transplant rejection.

Oncocytic metaplasia of interlobular bile duct epithelium has been described as part of the histopathologic spectrum of hepatic GVHD (Bligh *et al.,* 1995).

Similar to other target organs, the histologic features of hepatic GVHD are nonspecific and have been found in disorders such as bile duct obstruction, viral hepatitis, and drug toxicity, and this creates diagnostic problems. Distinguishing transfusion-associated hepatitis (hepatitis C) was a significant problem, solved for all practical purposes by the development of specific serologic markers (Choo et al., 1989). CMV hepatitis may be indistinguishable from GVHD, but usually is associated with disseminated CMV infection. Nonetheless, GVHD and viral hepatitis may coexist. Significant atypia of bile duct epithelium, extensive involvement of bile ducts, and bile duct drop-out associated with a sparse inflammatory infiltrate are features that favor the presence of GVHD (Beschorner et al., 1980). Apoptotic and dysmorphic bile duct epithelial cell changes, resembling those seen in acute GVHD, have been reported in biopsies of recipients of autologous HSC transplants (Saunders et al., 2000). Liver pathology present prior to transplant, such as chronic hepatitis B or C or iron overload, contributes to hepatic changes in the post-transplant period (Angelucci et al., 2002).

Cyclosporine used as an effective immune suppressive agent for the prevention and treatment of GVHD produces hepatotoxicity manifested clinically as hyperbilirubinemia without significant elevation of transaminase or serum alkaline phosphatase levels. It can also be distinguished from GVHD by the self-limiting nature of the liver dysfunction demonstrated by withdrawing the drug or reducing the dose (Atkinson et al., 1983). It should be noted that in humans there has been a paucity of studies assessing the hepatic histologic lesions produced by chronic cyclosporine administration, but in animal studies chronic administration has been reported to induce centrilobular ballooning degeneration, cholestasis, fatty change, and focal hepatocyte necrosis (Ryffel et al., 1983). The lack of bile duct abnormalities reported appears to be a distinguishing feature from established GVHD. Other drugs may cause changes indistinguishable from GVHD, although the presence of eosinophils in portal tracts may suggest an allergic reaction. Methotrexate can cause steatosis and centrilobular fibrosis, although it is rarely given for an extended period after transplantation. Corticosteroids have been implicated in the pathogenesis of nodular regenerative hyperplasia and steatosis (Stromeyer & Ishak, 1981). The hepatic effects of total parenteral nutrition are controversial, but have included centrilobular degeneration and cholestasis (Cohen & Olsen, 1981).

Veno-occlusive disease

High-dose chemotherapy or chemoradiotherapy used to condition patients prior to transplant is the major etiologic factor in the development of hepatic veno-occlusive disease (VOD), along with pre-existing liver dysfunction and other factors (McDonald et al., 1984; Bearman, 1995; Tabbara et al., 2002) (see Chapters 77, 82, and 89). The disorder is a significant cause of morbidity and mortality (Jones et al., 1987; Morgan et al., 1991). Clinically, the classical syndrome is characterized by the rapid onset of jaundice, tender hepatomegaly, ascites, and sudden weight gain prior to day 20 posttransplant.

VOD is postulated to be primarily due to injury to the endothelium of the terminal hepatic venules (THVs) and sinusoids with secondary ischemia leading to hepatocyte necrosis, although direct chemotherapy-induced toxicity may contribute to centrilobular hepatocyte necrosis. Histologically, early lesions are characterized by edematous widening of the intima of the THVs and sublobular veins with narrowing or obliteration of the lumen. The surrounding centrilobular zone shows marked congestion and hemorrhage with hepatocyte necrosis (Fig. 104.11). Lesions in patients that have survived the acute phase show concentric fibrous obliteration of the THVs with surrounding centrilobular fibrosis, atrophy of hepatocytes, and dilated sinusoids (Shulman et al., 1980a) (Fig. 104.12). There is deposition of fibrin within the wall of THVs, implicating activation of the coagulation cascade in the pathogenesis of VOD (Shulman, Gown, & Nugent, 1987).

Snover et al. (1989) have questioned the true incidence of VOD in transplant recipients, particularly those diagnosed on clinical grounds alone. In this retrospective study of 103 patients only 9 (8.8%) patients had VOD compared to 23 (22.5%) who were reported to have nodular regenerative hyperplasia (NRH). Furthermore, approximately 50% of patients fulfilling the clinical criteria for VOD in fact had NRH. Because of the relatively low mortality of NRH, this patient group would have been classified as having "mild" VOD in other series. Histologically, NRH shows "slit-like" compression of THVs with areas of periportal hepatocyte regeneration alternating with midzonal (zone II) atrophy. Reticulin staining characteristically shows no fibrosis, although condensation of reticulin is present in atrophic areas.

Respiratory system

Pulmonary complications are a significant factor in the management of HSCT patients (see Chapter 91) (Hamilton & Pearson, 1986). The conditioning period induces profound neutropenia in all patients that lasts 2 to 3 weeks, and a profound immune suppression that affects both humoral and cellular immune function. Cellular immune responses are impaired for 3 months or longer, although nonspecific proliferative and cytotoxic properties recover over this time. Immunoglobulin secretion is also impaired with restoration of partial immune function by 12 months (Ettinger & Trulock, 1991). The restoration is partial because immune suppression medications are often continued to treat GVHD. Local lung defense mechanisms are also impaired following transplantation. Lavage studies show that early after transplantation the majority of cells in the lavage fluid are of donor origin, and alveolar macrophages demonstrate impaired killing of bacteria and fungi and defective phagocytosis and chemotaxis, that gradually recovers over 6 to 12 months (Winston et al., 1982).

Both restrictive and obstructive ventilatory changes occur after HSCT, which are mostly asymptomatic. Restrictive changes often accompany changes in lung diffusing capacity and are presumed to be related to the acute effects of chemora-

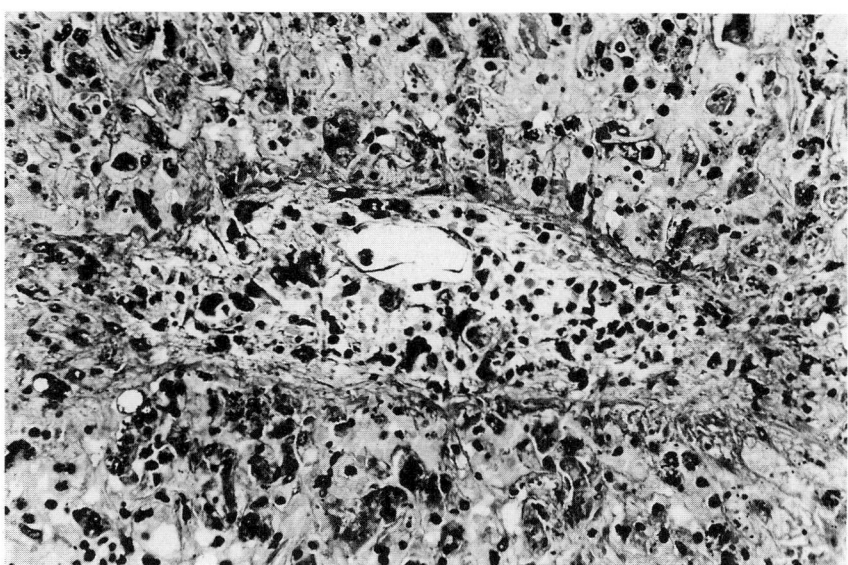

Fig. 104.11. Hepatic veno-occlusive disease, acute phase. There is marked widening of the intima of the terminal hepatic venule (THV) with almost complete occlusion of the lumen. The intima is edematous and contains cellular debris including red blood cells (Masson ×400).

diation. Later a proportion of patients develop progressive obstructive airways changes.

The histological processes occurring in the lung can be studied via lavage, aspiration techniques, bronchial and transbronchial biopsies, and by thorascopic and open lung biopsy procedures. These studies are augmented at the unit level by the intermittent quality control material of the autopsy. The particular profile of the investigative procedures employed varies from unit to unit, reflecting variability of expertise and resource availability.

Lavage and aspiration techniques are relatively low morbidity procedures that allow excellent infection screening and may allow either a specific diagnosis or, by the absence of a cellular response, may suggest the class of process that is occurring, once the period of profound neutropenia has passed (Cordonnier et al., 1986). Bronchial biopsies provide airways lung tissue that may be specifically diagnostic and transbronchial biopsies provide in addition small fragments of the alveolar bed that can be compared lobe to lobe. Open and thorascopic lung biopsies have a high diagnostic yield, provided

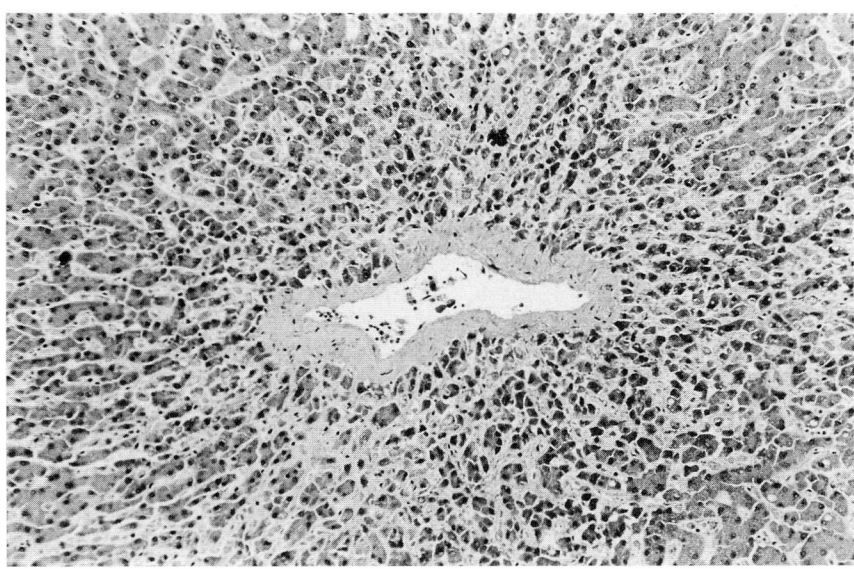

Fig. 104.12. Hepatic veno-occlusive disease, chronic phase, showing concentric fibrosis surrounding THV with surrounding atrophy of hepatocytes and dilated sinuses (hematoxylin & eosin ×200).

that the biopsy is directed to the particular area of the lung of interest; pathological processes in the lung can be focal, and poorly directed open procedures may miss lesions entirely. These invasive procedures carry a high morbidity that must be justified by the potential diagnostic yield. A thoroscopic biopsy performed by a skilled practitioner can require only an overnight hospital stay and may leave only two small access incisions. These tissue biopsies may provide specific diagnoses or may allow the recognition of a lung injury pattern.

Any lung injury pattern identified may have more than one cause and any one pathological process, such as GVHD, may produce more than one lung injury pattern. Close clinico-pathological discussion will help to establish the likely causes of any lung injury and will help to design the most appropriate clinical management response. Determining the precise identity of the original cause of the lung injury may be less important to management than identification and minimization of the injurious influences presently acting on the lung.

Chemoradiation

Chemotherapeutic agents affect the lung from the time of their administration. The precise details of the agents used need consideration. For example, busulfan produces marked atypia of the type II pneumocytes but the degree of atypia overlaps into the atypias produced by other agents.

TBI used in the pretransplant conditioning regimen produces subclinical lung function changes, particularly in the diffusing capacity of the lung. Additionally, radiation at these doses may potentiate the toxic effects of the other agents used and may render the lung particularly sensitive to the injurious effects of shock and inhalation damage. Direct progressive lung radiation damage at these dose ranges is uncommon, but occasionally higher radiation doses may be used for tumor eradication. Radiation doses at these higher levels may produce gradually evolving fibrosing lung damage that evolves slowly over months and carries a poor prognosis.

Chemoradiation produces a lung injury pattern of a type of diffuse alveolar damage. It is often cell-poor with faint, fine granular hyaline membranes and early fibrosis. It contrasts with the congested cellular appearance of diffuse alveolar damage seen following shock in an immune competent host. The lung appearances of diffuse alveolar damage are seldom specific in identifying the initiating agent. Other factors such as shock, infections, and inhalants can also produce diffuse alveolar damage (Fig. 104.13).

Overall the basic approach is to match the observed lung damage to the time course of the various lung injuries that are operative, to carefully exclude infections, and to consider whether GVHD may be present.

Infections

During the 2 to 3 week period of profound neutropenia, bacterial and fungal infections are common. Over the more extended period while the immune system is gradually reconstituting, CMV infections are increased in incidence. *Pneumocystis carinii* has become relatively uncommon with the advent of prophylactic treatment regimens, but it has not disappeared and needs to be considered in any situation where compliance with, or administration of, the prophylactic medication is suboptimal (Fig. 104.14).

The histological appearances of any infection are the product of the infecting organism and the host response. A range of appearances occurs for each organism determined by the degree of immune suppression. Many of the organisms involved such as CMV and *Pneumocystis carinii,* have an organism-rich form in the profoundly immunosuppressed patient, an organism-poor form that is often granulomatous in the partially suppressed patient, and seldom occur in the fully immune competent host.

Many comprehensive accounts of pulmonary infections in the immune compromised host are available together with general consideration of the immune deficient states (Milled & Chapel, 1987). In general, virtually any organism can be a pathogen in a profoundly immunosuppressed host, but in practice, once the immediate posttransplant period with its risks of bacterial and fungal infection has passed, CMV is the main pulmonary infection risk over the first year.

CMV appears to initially infect patches of the lung parenchyma. The characteristic nuclear and cytoplasmic inclusions can be seen in the endothelial cells of capillaries, the alveolar lining cells, and in the smooth muscle cells of the bronchial wall (Fig. 104.15). It can elicit a bronchitis, a chronic interstitial pneumonia, or it can be the cause of diffuse alveolar damage. Alternatively, the inclusions can represent an incidental finding eliciting no inflammation. The presence of inclusions, the nature of the inflammatory response, the presence of other organ involvement and diagnostic blood tests, such as CMV antigenemia or PCR, all contribute information upon which management decisions are made.

Graft-versus-host disease

GVHD in general has a spectrum of appearances with classical acute and chronic GVHD representing the polar extremes. Histopathologically, the transition between these is continuous, with increasing degrees of fibrosis gradually developing in the more long-standing forms and the cellular vacuolar lymphocytic cell apposition of the acute form becoming more sparse and patchy, but often remaining focally intense if the process remains active. The division of GVHD into acute and chronic forms has clinical utility.

Aspects of GVHD in the lung depart from these general appearances. The lung is a highly specialized organ representing a vast alveolar capillary bed aerated by a complex network of air conduction channels, maintained in its functional form by the local lung defense mechanism of the mucociliary clearance mechanism, a balance of the proteases and anti-proteases and the effects of the alveolar macrophage pool. The lung

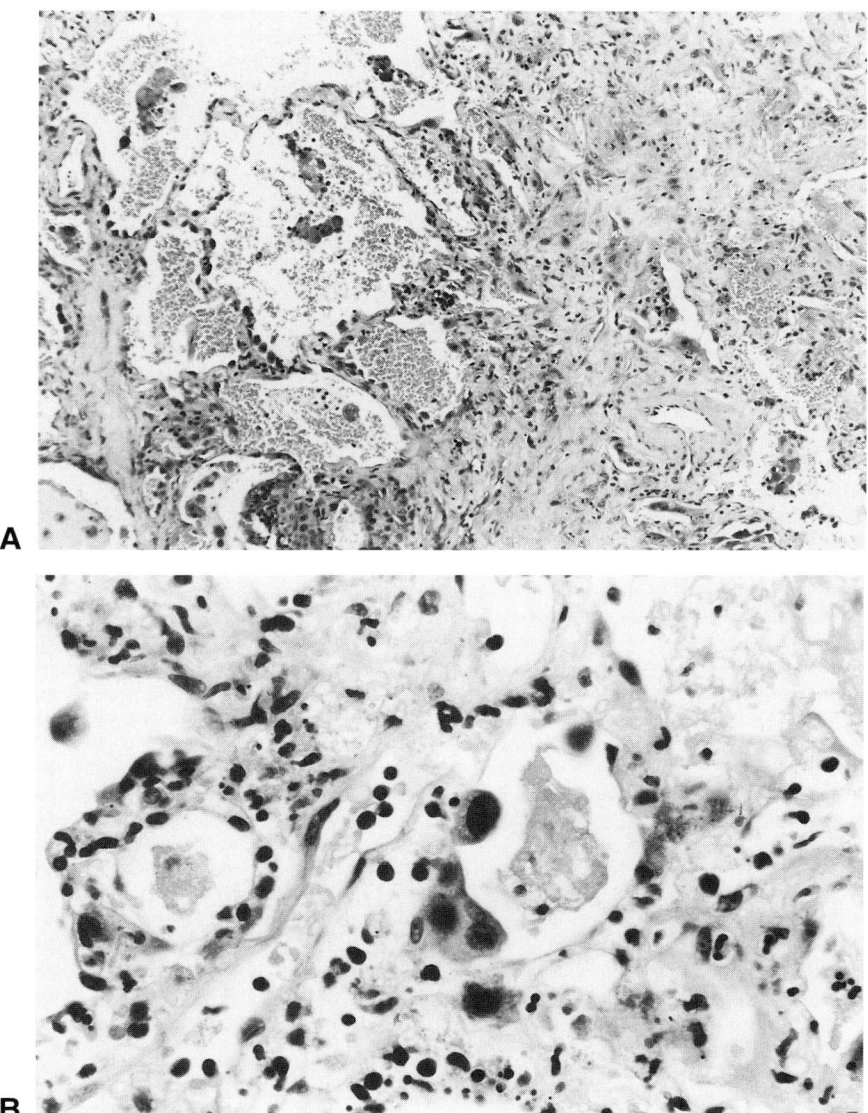

Fig. 104.13. Diffuse alveolar damage secondary to chemoradiotherapy toxicity. (A) Marked distortion of normal parenchymal architecture with fibrous obliteration of alveolar spaces (hematoxylin & eosin ×200). (B) Enlarged and atypical pneumocyte with vacuolated cytoplasm and nucleolar-like inclusion characteristic of chemoradiotherapy toxicity (hematoxylin & eosin ×400).

reacts in a specialized way to other generalized processes such as vasculitis and to rejection. The full nature and range of the changes in the lung in GVHD have not yet been defined (Wojno *et al.,* 1994; Yousem, 1995). Consideration of the general appearances of acute solid organ lung rejection may illustrate aspects of the somewhat allied process of GVHD. In acute lung rejection the standard appearances of rejection are modified by lung injury patterns. A pattern of chronic interstitial pneumonia marks moderate acute rejection, while severe rejection produces a pattern of diffuse alveolar damage. Only in mild acute rejection (the lowest treatable grade) do the perivascular collections of lymphocytes resemble the appearances seen in other organs. The airway wall and mucosal changes that accompany rejection, however, do resemble the more general

pattern and these also resemble the airway changes seen in GVHD in the lung. In many respects these changes also resemble the cutaneous changes described above in acute cutaneous GVHD.

The airways changes are: (1) submucosal lymphocytic infiltrate with indentation of the basement membrane of the respiratory epithelium by lymphocytes; (2) lymphocytic infiltrate within the respiratory epithelium; (3) epithelial cell necrosis and apoptosis; and (4) evidence of epithelial injury and regeneration, including epithelial denudation, squamous metaplasia, and the "up and down" epithelial lesion (alternating regions of basal cell regeneration and hyperplasia with regions of intact normal epithelium) (Beschorner *et al.,* 1978; Workman & Clancy, 1994; Yousem, 1995).

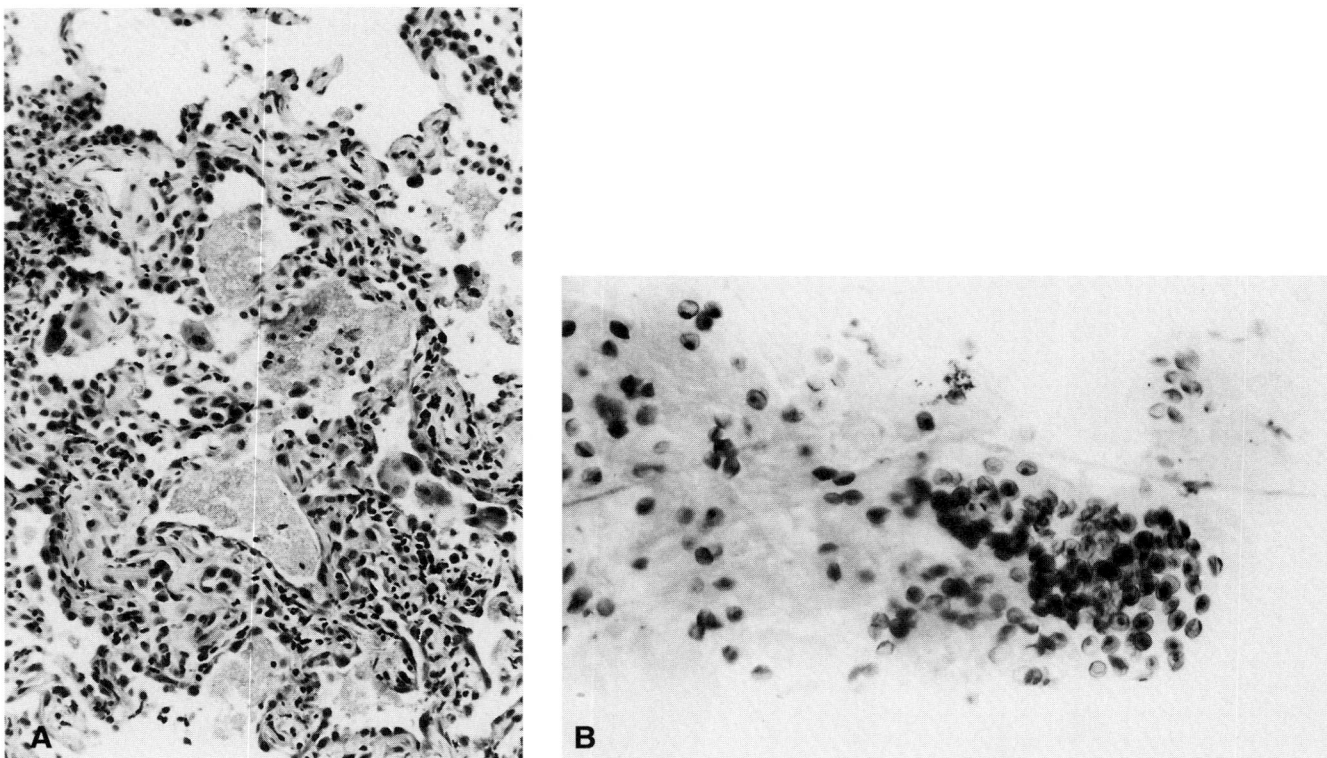

Fig. 104.14. *Pneumocystis carinii* pneumonia. **(A)** Characteristic picture with "foamy" intra-alveolar exudate and interstitial lymphocytic infiltrate (hematoxylin & eosin ×200). **(B)** Methenamine silver stain demonstrating characteristic pneumocystis cysts (hematoxylin & eosin ×600).

There is strong circumstantial evidence for ascribing a proportion of cases of organizing pneumonia (BOOP) to a GVHD reaction, particularly when the alveolar bed changes are accompanied by the airways wall changes described. Whether a proportion of cases presenting with the lung injury pattern of diffuse alveolar damage can be ascribed directly to GVHD or whether GVHD mechanisms join with other lung insults to produce this damage is unclear. It remains to be determined how specific these distinctive but subtle airways changes are for GVHD, and whether they ever accompany chemotherapeutic or radiation lung damage.

Obliterative bronchiolitis

Obliterative bronchiolitis is considered by some to represent chronic GVHD. Its precise cause is unknown and multiple factors may contribute. In general, processes such as CMV infection that injure the bronchiolar lining epithelium lead to a greater incidence of obliterative bronchiolitis. The disorder also occurs outside of the transplantation setting as a late sequel of infections and as a complication of collagen vascular diseases, conditions in which processes damaging the airway mucosa may also be operative. The process can affect the airway from the bronchi to the respiratory bronchioles. It is a pan-airways process of mucosal ulceration and fibrosis that for physiological reasons presents as obliterative bronchiolitis of the terminal bronchioles (Urtbanski *et al.*, 1987; Yousem, 1991). Terminal bronchioles are

the smallest, most peripheral air movement channels. Beyond them gases are conducted by diffusion through an anastomosing network of respiratory bronchioles and alveolar ducts. The terminal bronchioles are unbranched and conduct air to supply the lobules of the alveolar bed where gas exchange occurs. The histological process of obliterative bronchiolitis in its early stages appears to be marked by repeated mucosal shedding evidenced by basement membrane thickening of the airways mucosa and mucosal ulceration, often followed by plugging of the ulcers by macrophages and the development of luminal plugs of fibrous tissue that eventually come to occlude the terminal bronchioles (Fig. 104.16). Blockage of a terminal bronchiole disconnects the lobule it supplies from gas exchange. The disorder may be detected prior to the onset of symptoms by a change in the profile of the lung function tests indicating obstruction. Clinical symptoms do not develop until the majority of the lung's 30,000 terminal bronchioles have been occluded, by which time the disorder is already at a late stage.

Posttransplant lymphoproliferative disease (and see Chapter 88)

Although posttransplant lymphoproliferative disease (PTLD) is less frequent after allogeneic bone marrow transplantation than after solid organ transplantation, it tends to develop early (Curtis *et al.*, 1999), with a high incidence of disseminated disease at presentation and an aggressive clinical course. The dis-

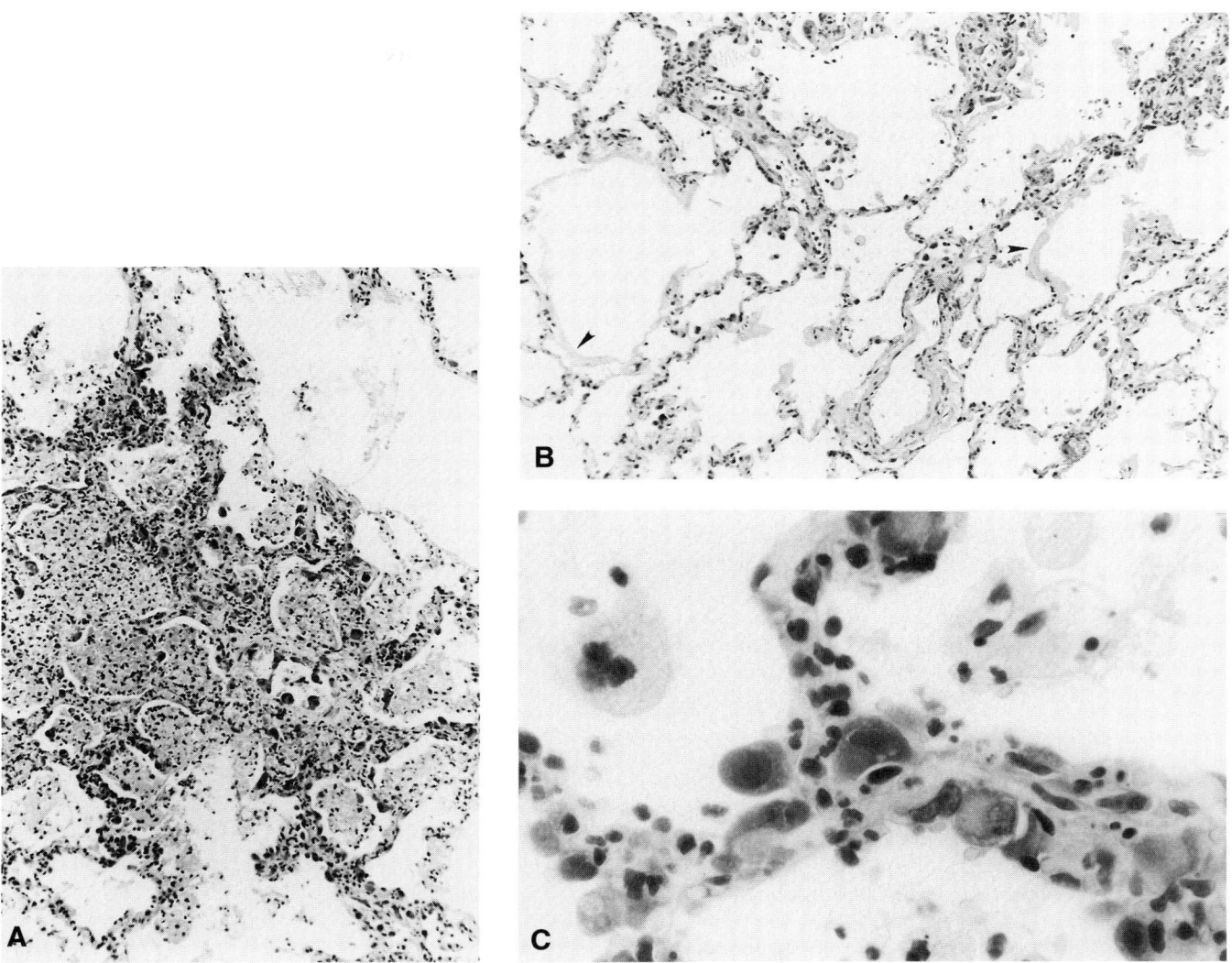

Fig. 104.15. CMV interstitial pneumonitis. (A) Low power view showing a focal collection of intra-alveolar inflammatory cells and cellular debris. The presence of neutrophils is highly suggestive of CMV infection (hematoxylin & eosin ×100). (B) Adjacent parenchyma showing exudative phase of diffuse alveolar damage with hyaline membrane formation (arrowheads) (hematoxylin & eosin ×100). (C) Enlarged infected alveolar pneumocytes with nuclear inclusions diagnostic of CMV infection (hematoxylin & eosin ×600).

ease in HSC transplant recipients is usually of donor origin, and generally represents uncontrolled EBV-induced lymphocyte proliferation in the severely immunocompromised host. Rare cases are of host origin, involve the T-cell lineage, or are EBV-negative. Multiple organ sites are often involved, including upper aerodigestive tract, liver, spleen, GIT, and lymph nodes (Zutter *et al.*, 1988; Micallef *et al.*, 1998). The overall incidence in several large studies is around 1%, with risk factors including HLA mismatch, T-cell depletion of donor marrow, and use of anti-T-cell therapies for severe GVHD (Hale *et al.*, 1998; Curtis *et al.*, 1999). The incidence is up to 20% in patients with more than one risk factor.

The classification recommended by WHO (Jaffe *et al.*, 2001) based on previous work (Knowles *et al.*, 1995; Harris *et al.*, 1997) divides the condition into four main categories histopathologically:

1. Early lesions: plasmacytic hyperplasia or resembling infectious mononucleosis, without tissue architectural effacement
2. Polymorphous PTLD: a destructive heterogeneous proliferation of B cells of varying morphology (from intermediate-sized lymphoid cells to plasmacytoid cells to immunoblasts)
3. Monomorphic PTLD: a monotonous destructive lymphoid proliferation, which most frequently has the appearance of a blastic, diffuse large cell lymphoma, but which should be classified according to the standard WHO lymphoma classification, although specified in the report to be PTLD
4. Hodgkin's lymphoma or Hodgkin's-like PTLD

Polymorphic lesions should be evaluated for clonality by immunophenotyping (preferably by flow cytometry). Analysis of the presence of EBV by in situ hybridization for latency-associated mRNA (EBER) can be useful in establish-

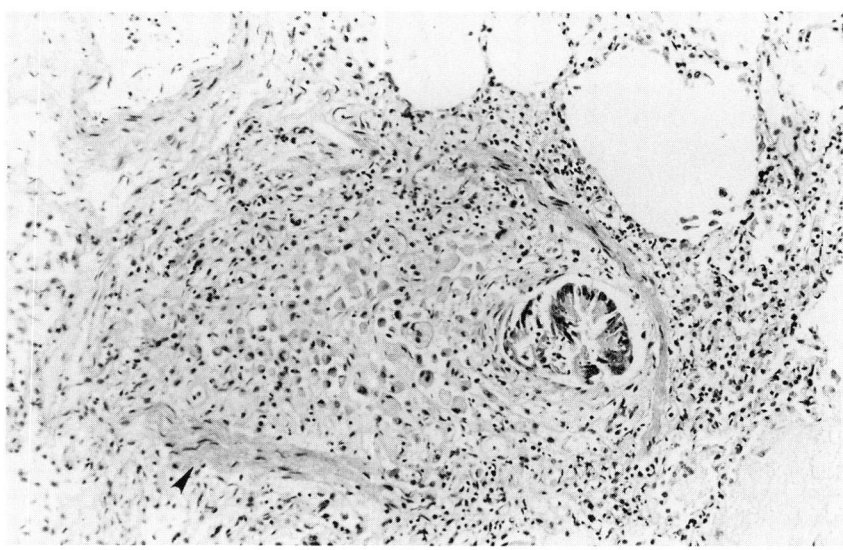

Fig. 104.16. Obliterative bronchiolitis showing almost complete obliteration of the lumen of a terminal bronchiole. The mucosa is thickened by edema, inflammatory cells, and fibrous proliferation (arrowhead: residual muscularis of bronchiole outlining original lumen) (hematoxylin & eosin ×200).

ing the diagnosis in early or equivocal lesions. Early lesions may regress with reduction of immunosuppression, infusion of donor T cells, or administration of anti-CD20 antibodies.

References

Akosa, A.B. & Lampert, I.A. (1990). The sweat gland in graft-versus-host disease. *Journal of Pathology*, **161**, 261–6.

Akpek, G., Boltnott, J. K., Lee, L. A. *et al.* (2002). Hepatic variant of graft-versus-host disease after donor lymphocyte infusion. *Blood*, **1003**, 3903–7.

Angelucci, E., Muretto, P., Nicolucci, A. *et al.* (2002). Effects of iron overload and hepatitis C virus positivity in determining progression of liver fibrosis in thalassemia following bone marrow transplantation. *Blood*, **100**, 17–21.

Atkinson, K., Biggs, J., Dodds, A., & Concannon, A. (1983). Cyclosporine-associated hepatotoxicity after allogeneic marrow transplantation in man: differentiation from other causes of post-transplant liver disease. *Transplantation Proceedings*, **15** (Suppl 1), 2761–7.

Atkinson, K., Bryant, D., Biggs, J. *et al.* (1984). Obstructive airways disease: a rare but serious manifestation of chronic graft-versus-host disease after allogeneic marrow transplantation in humans. *Transplantation Proceedings*, **16**, 1030–3.

Atkinson, K., Bryant, D., Delprado, W., & Biggs, J. (1989). Widespread pulmonary fibrosis as a major clinical manifestation of chronic graft-versus-host disease. *Bone Marrow Transplantation*, **4**, 129–32.

Atkinson, K., Munro, V., Vasak, E., & Biggs, J. (1986). Mononuclear cell subpopulations in the skin defined by monoclonal antibodies after HLA-identical sibling marrow transplantation. *British Journal of Dermatology*, **114**, 145–60.

Atkinson, K., Turner, J., Biggs, J.C. *et al.* (1991). An acute pulmonary syndrome possibly representing acute graft-versus-host disease involving the lung interstitium. *Bone Marrow Transplantation*, **8**, 231–4.

Bearman, S. (1995). The syndrome of hepatic veno-occlusive disease after marrow transplantation. *Blood*, **85**, 3005–20.

Beecroft, D.M.O. (1967). Histopathology of fatal adenovirus infection of the respiratory tract in young children. *Journal of Clinical Pathology*, **20**, 561–9.

Benjamin, S., Deeg, H.J., & Shulman, H.M. (1985). Erythema multiforme-like skin eruptions localized to marrow aspiration sites after autologous marrow transplantation. *Transplantation Proceedings*, **17**, 2029–32.

Beschorner, W.E., Pino, J., Boitnott, J.K. *et al.* (1980). Pathology of the liver with bone marrow transplantation. *American Journal of Pathology*, **99**, 369–82.

Beschorner, W.E., Saral, R., Hutchins, G.M. *et al.* (1978). Lymphocytic bronchitis associated with graft-versus-host disease in recipients of bone-marrow transplants. *New England Journal of Medicine*, **229**, 1030–6.

Bligh, J., Morton, J., Durrant, S., & Walker, N. (1995). Oncocytic metaplasia of bile duct epithelium in hepatic GVHD. *Bone Marrow Transplantation*, **16**, 317–19.

Bradstock, K.F., Coles, R., Despas, P. *et al.* (1984). Fatal obstructive airways disease after bone marrow transplantation. *Transplantation Proceedings*, **16**, 1034–6.

Breathnach, S.M. & Katz, S.C. (1987). Immunopathology of cutaneous graft-versus-host disease. *The American Journal of Dermatopathology*, **9**, 343–8.

Choi, J., Yoo, J., Chung, I. *et al.* (1997). Esophageal aspergillosis after bone marrow transplantation. *Bone Marrow Transplantation*, **19**, 293–4.

Choo, Q.L., Kuo, G., Werner, A.J. *et al.* (1989). Isolation of a cDNA clone derived from a blood borne non-A, non-B viral hepatitis genome. *Science*, **244**, 359–62.

Clark, J.G. & Crawford, S.W. (1987). Diagnostic approaches to pulmonary complications of marrow transplantation. *Chest,* **94,** 477–8.

Cohen, C. & Olsen, M.M. (1981). Pediatric total parenteral nutrition. Liver histopathology. *Archives of Pathology and Laboratory Medicine,* **105,** 152–6.

Cooper, J.A.D., White, D.A., & Matthay, R.A. (1986). Drug-induced pulmonary disease. *American Review of Respiratory Diseases,* **133,** 321–40 (part 1) and 488–505 (part 2).

Cordonnier, C., Bernaudin, J.F., Bierling, P. et al. (1986). Pulmonary complications occurring after allogeneic bone marrow transplantation. *Cancer,* **58,** 1047–54.

Crawford, S.W., Hackman, R.C., & Clark, J.G. (1988). Open lung biopsy diagnosis of diffuse pulmonary infiltrates after marrow transplantation. *Chest,* **95,** 949–53.

Crider, M.K., Jansen, J., Norins, A.L., & McHale, M.S. (1986). Chemotherapy-induced acral erythema in patients receiving bone marrow transplantation. *Archives of Dermatology,* **122,** 1023–7.

Curtis, R.E., Travis, L.B., Rowlings, P.A. et al. (1999). Risk of lymphoproliferative disorders after bone marrow transplantation: a multi-institutional study. *Blood,* **94,** 2208–16.

Daneshpouy, M., Socie, G., Lemann, M. et al. (2002). Activated eosinophils in upper gastrointestinal tract of patients with graft-versus-host disease. *Blood,* **99,** 3033–40.

Elliott, C.J., Sloane, J.P., Pallett, C.D., & Sanderson, K.V. (1988). Cutaneous leukocyte composition after human allogeneic bone marrow transplantation: relationship to marrow purging, histology and clinical rash. *Histopathology,* **12,** 1–6.

Elliott, C.J., Sloane, J.P., Sanderson, K.V. et al. (1987). The histological diagnosis of cutaneous graft-versus-host disease: relationship of skin changes to marrow purging and other clinical variables. *Histopathology,* **11,** 145–55.

Epstein, R.J., McDonald, G.B., Sale, G.E. et al. (1980). The diagnostic accuracy of the rectal biopsy in acute graft-versus-host disease: a prospective study of thirteen patients. *Gastroenterology,* **78,** 764–71.

Ettinger, N.A. & Trulock, E.P. (1991). Pulmonary considerations of organ transplantation (Part 2). *American Review of Respiratory Diseases,* **144,** 213–23.

Farmer, E.R. & Hood, A.F. (1983). Graft-versus-host disease. In *Update: Dermatology in General Medicine,* ed. T. Fitzpatrick, A. Elsen, K. Wolff, I. Freedberg, & K. Austin, pp. 28–39. New York: McGraw-Hill.

Farthing, M.J., Clark, M.L., Sloane, J.P. et al. (1982). Liver damage after bone marrow transplantation. *Gut,* **23,** 465–74.

Favre, A., Cerri, A., Bacigalupo, A. et al. (1997). Immunohistochemical study of skin lesions in acute chronic graft-versus-host disease following bone marrow transplantation. *American Journal of Surgical Pathology,* **21,** 23–34.

Ferrara, J.L., Cooke, K., Pan, L., & Krenger, W. (1996). The immunopathology of acute GVHD. *Stem Cells,* **14,** 473–89.

Field, A.S. (2002). Light microscopic and electron microscopic diagnosis of gastrointestinal opportunistic infections in HIV-positive patients. *Pathology,* **34,** 21–35.

Fox, R., Vogelsang, G., & Beschomev, W. (1996). Denuded bowel after recovery from GVHD. *Transplantation,* **62,** 1681–4.

Friedman, H.Z., Arias, A.M., Catchatourian, R., & Fretzin, D.F. (1984). Toxic epidermal necrolysis following bone marrow transplantation. *Cutis,* **34,** 158–62.

Friedman, K.J., Le Boit, P.E., & Farmer, E.R. (1988). Acute follicular graft versus host reaction. *Archives of Dermatology,* **124,** 688–91.

Fujii, H., Ohashi, M., & Nagura, H. (1988). Immunohistochemical analysis of oral lichen-planus-like eruption in graft-versus-host disease after allogeneic bone marrow transplantation. *American Journal of Clinical Pathology,* **89,** 177–86.

Fujii, N., Takenaka, K., Shinagawa, K. et al. (2001). Hepatic graft-versus-host disease presenting as an actue hepatitis after allogeneic peripheral blood stem cell transplantation. *Bone Marrow Transplantation,* **27,** 1007–10.

Glucksberg, H., Storb, R., Fefer, A. et al. (1974). Clinical manifestations of graft-versus-host disease in human recipients of marrow from HLA-matched sibling donors. *Transplantation,* **18,** 295–304.

Goldberg, N.S., Ahmed, T., Robinson, B. et al. (1989). Staphylococcal scalded skin syndrome mimicking acute graft-versus-host disease in a bone marrow transplant recipient. *Archives of Dermatology,* **125,** 85–7.

Goldstein, S.M., Wintroub, B.W., & Elias, P.M. (1987). Toxic epidermal necrolysis: unmuddying the waters. *Archives of Dermatology,* **123,** 1153–6.

Gratwohl, A.A., Moutsopoulos, H.M., Chused, T.M. et al. (1977). Sjogren-type syndrome after allogeneic bone marrow transplantation. *Annals of Internal Medicine,* **87,** 703–6.

Gross, N.J. (1981). The pathogenesis of radiation-induced lung damage. *Lung,* **159,** 115–25.

Hackman, R.C. & Sale, G.E. (1981). Large airway inflammation as a possible manifestation of a pulmonary graft versus host reaction in bone marrow allograft recipients. *Laboratory Investigations,* **44,** 26A.

Hale, G. & Waldmann, H. (1998). Risks of developing Epstein-Barr virus-related lymphoproliferative disorders after T-cell-depleted marrow transplants. CAMPATH Users. *Blood,* **91,** 3079–83.

Harris, N.L., Ferry, J.A., & Swerdlow, S.H. (1997). Posttransplant lymphoproliferative disorders: Summary of Society for Hematopathology Workshop. *Seminars in Diagnostic Pathology,* **14,** 8–14.

Hamilton, P.J. & Pearson, A.D. (1986). Bone marrow transplantation and the lung. *Thorax,* **41,** 497–502.

Heard, B.E. & Cooke, R.A. (1968). Busulphan lung. *Thorax,* **23,** 193–7.

Heng, M.C.Y. & Allen, S.G. (1991). Efficacy of cyclophosphamide in toxic epidermal necrolysis. *Journal of the American Academy of Dermatology,* **25,** 778–86.

Herzig, R.H., Wolff, S.N., Lazarus, H.M. et al. (1983). High-dose cytosine arabinoside therapy for refractory leukemia. *Blood,* **62,** 361–9.

Hill, G.R. & Ferrara, J.L. (2000). The primacy of the gastrointestinal tract as a target organ of acute graft versus host disease: rationale for the use of cytokine shields in allogeneic bone marrow transplantation. *Blood,* **95,** 2754–9.

Hymes, S.R., Farmer, E.R., Burns, W.H. *et al.* (1985a). Bullous scleroderma-like changes in chronic graft-versus-host disease. *Archives of Dermatology,* **121,** 1189–92.

Hymes, S.R., Farmer, E.R., Lewis, P.G. *et al.* (1985b). Cutaneous graft-versus-host reaction: prognostic features seen by light microscopy. *Journal of the American Academy of Dermatology,* **12,** 468–74.

Hymes, S.R., Simonton, S.C., Farmer, E.R. *et al.* (1985c). Cutaneous busulfan effect in patients receiving bone marrow transplantation. *Journal of Cutaneous Pathology,* **12,** 125–9.

Iqbal, M., Creger, R., Fox, R. *et al.* (1996). Laparoscopic liver biopsy to evaluate hepatic dysfunction in patients with hematologic malignancies. *Bone Marrow Transplantation,* **17,** 655–62.

Jaffe, E.S., Harris, N.L., Stein, H., & Vardiman, J.W. (eds.) (2001). *World Health Organization Classification of Tumours: Tumours of Haematopoietic and Lymphoid Tissues,* pp. 264–9. Lyon: IARC Press.

Jiwa, M., Renske, D., Steenbergen, M. *et al.* (1990). Three sensitive methods for the detection of cytomegalovirus in lung tissue of patients with interstitial pneumonitis. *American Journal of Clinical Pathology,* **93,** 491–4.

Jones, R.J., Lee, K.S.K., Beschorner, W.E. *et al.* (1987). Veno occlusive disease of the liver following bone marrow transplantation. *Transplantation,* **44,** 778–83.

Kang, G., Srivastava, A., Pulimood, A.B. *et al.* (2002). Etiology of diarrhea in patients undergoing allogeneic bone marrow transplantation in South India. *Transplantation,* **73,** 1247–51.

Kasahara, T., Hooks, J.J., Dougherty, S.F., & Oppenheim, J.J. (1983). Interleukin 2 mediated immune interferon (IFN-gamma) production by human T cells and T cell subsets. *Journal of Immunology,* **130,** 1784–9.

Katzenstein, A.A. & Askin, F.B. (1980). Interpretation and significance of pathologic findings in transbronchial lung biopsy. *American Journal of Surgical Pathology,* **4,** 223–34.

Knapp, A.B., Crawford, J.M., Rappeport, J.M., & Gollan, J.L. (1987). Cirrhosis as a consequence of GVHD. *Gastroenterology,* **92,** 513–19.

Knowles, D.M., Cesarman, E., Chadburn, A. *et al.* (1995). Correlative morphologic and molecular analysis demonstrates three distinct categories of post transplant lymphoproliferative disorders. *Blood,* **85,** 552–65.

Lampert, I.A., Janossy, G., Suitters, A.J. *et al.* (1982). Immunological analysis of the skin in graft-versus-host disease. *Clinical and Experimental Immunology,* **50,** 123–31.

Lampert, I.A., Thorpe, P., van Noorden, S. *et al.* (1985). Selective sparing of enterochromatin cells in graft-versus-host disease affecting the colonic mucosa. *Histopathology,* **9,** 875–86.

Lerner, K.G., Kao, G.F., Storb, R. *et al.* (1974). Histopathology of graft-versus-host reaction (GVHR) in human recipients of marrow from HLA-matched sibling donors. *Transplantation Proceedings,* **6,** 367–71.

Lever, R., Turbitt, M., Mackie, R. *et al.* (1986). A prospective study of the histological changes in the skin in patients receiving bone marrow transplants. *British Journal of Dermatology,* **114,** 161–70.

Levine, L.E., Medenica, M.M., Lorincz, A.L. *et al.* (1985). Distinctive acral erythema occurring during therapy for severe myelogenous leukemia. *Archives of Dermatology,* **121,** 102–4.

Magee, K.L., Herbert, A.A., & Rapini, R.P. (1991). Crusted scabies in a patient with chronic graft-versus-host disease. *Journal of the American Academy of Dermatology,* **25,** 889–91.

Malik, A. H., Collins, R. H., Saboorian, M. H., & Lee, W. M. (2001). Chronic graft-versus-host disease after hematopoietic cell transplantation presenting as an acute hepatitis. *American Journal of Gastroenterology,* **96,** 588–90.

McDonald, G.B., Sharma, P., Matthews, D.E. *et al.* (1984). Veno-occlusive disease of the liver after bone marrow transplantation: diagnosis, incidence, and predisposing factors. *Hepatology,* **4,** 116–22.

McDonald, G.B., Sharma, P., Hackman, R.C. *et al.* (1985). Esophageal infections in immuno-suppressed patients after marrow transplantation. *Gastroenterology,* **88,** 1111–17.

McDonald, G.B., Shulman, H.M., Sullivan, K.M., & Spencer, G.D. (1986). Intestinal and hepatic complications of human bone marrow transplantation. *Gastroenterology,* **90,** 460–77 (part 1) and 770–84 (part 2).

McDonald, G.B., Sullivan, K.M., Schuffler, M.D. *et al.* (1981). Esophageal abnormality in chronic graft-versus-host disease in humans. *Gastroenterology,* **80,** 914–21.

Micallef, I.N., Chhanabhai, M., Gascoyne, R.D. *et al.* (1998). Lymphoproliferative disorders following allogeneic bone marrow transplantation: the Vancouver experience. *Bone Marrow Transplantation,* **22,** 981–7.

Morgan, M., Dodds, A., Atkinson, K. *et al.* (1991). The toxicity of busulfan and cyclophosphamide as the preparative regimen for bone marrow transplantation. *British Journal of Haematology,* **77,** 529–34.

Nakhleh, R.E., Snover, D.C., Weisdorf, S., & Platt, J.L. (1989). Immunopathology of graft-versus-host disease in the upper gastrointestinal tract. *Transplantation,* **48,** 61–5.

Neiman, P., Wasserman, P.B., Wentworth, B.B. *et al.* (1973). Interstitial pneumonia and cytomegalovirus infection as complications of human marrow transplantation. *Transplantation,* **15,** 478–85.

Obermann, E.C., Meidenbauer, N., Zeltner, R. *et al.* (1999). Multifocal reversible epithelial dysplasia mimicking carcinoma in situ after conditioning therapy with busulfan and cyclophosphamide. *Bone Marrow Transplantation,* **24,** 446–8.

O'Brien, K.D., Hackman, R.C., Sale, G.E. *et al.* (1984). Lymphocytic bronchitis unrelated to acute graft-versus-host disease in canine marrow graft recipients. *Transplantation,* **37,** 233–8.

Peck, G.L., Herzig, G.P., & Elias, P.M. (1972). Toxic epidermal necrolysis in a patient with graft versus host reaction. *Archives of Dermatology,* **105,** 561–9.

Perreault, C., Cousineau, S., D'Angelo, G. *et al.* (1985). Lymphoid interstitial pneumonia after allogeneic bone marrow transplantation: a possible manifestation of chronic graft-versus-host disease. *Cancer,* **55,** 1–9.

Piguet, P.F., Grau, G.E., Collart, M.A. *et al.* (1989). Pneumopathies of the graft-versus-host reaction. Alveolitis associated with an increased level of tumour necrosis factor mRNA and chronic interstitial pneumonitis. *Laboratory Investigations,* **61,** 37–45.

Ramsey, P.G., Fife, K.H., Hackman, R.C. *et al.* (1982). Herpes simplex virus pneumonia—clinical, virologic and pathologic features in 20 patients. *Annals of Internal Medicine,* **97,** 813–20.

Roy, J., Snover, D., Wetsdorf, S. *et al.* (1991). Simultaneous upper and lower endoscopic biopsy in the diagnosis of intestinal graft-versus-host disease. *Transplantation*, **51**, 642–6.

Ryffel, B., Donatsch, P., Madorin, M. *et al.* (1983). Toxicological evaluation of cyclosporin A. *Archives of Toxicology*, **53**, 107–41.

Sale, G.E., Lerner, K.G., Barker, E.A. *et al.* (1977). The skin biopsy in the diagnosis of acute graft-versus-host disease in man. *American Journal of Pathology*, **89**, 621–34.

Sale, G.E., McDonald, G.B., Shulman, H.M., & Thomas, E.D. (1979). Gastrointestinal graft-versus-host disease in man. A clinicopathological study of the rectal biopsy. *American Journal of Surgical Pathology*, **3**, 291–9.

Sale, G.E., Shulman, H.M., Gallucci, B.B., & Thomas, E.D. (1985). Young rete ridge keratinocytes are preferred targets in cutaneous graft-versus-host disease. *American Journal of Pathology*, **118**, 278–87.

Sale, G.E., Shulman, H.M., Schubert, M.M. *et al.* (1981). Oral and ophthalmic pathology of graft-versus-host disease in man: predictive value of the lip biopsy. *Human Pathology*, **12**, 1022–30.

Saunders, M.D., Shulman, H.M., Murakami, C.S. *et al.* (2000). Bile duct apoptosis and cholestasis resembling acute graft-versus-host disease after autologous hematopoietic cell transplantation. *American Journal of Surgical Pathology*, **24**, 1004–8.

Saurat, J.H. (1981). Cutaneous manifestations of graft-versus-host disease. *International Journal of Dermatology*, **20**, 249–56.

Saurat, J.H., Gluckman, E., Bussel, A. *et al.* (1975). The lichen planus-like eruption after bone marrow transplantation. *British Journal of Dermatology*, **92**, 675–81.

Schubert, M.M., Sullivan, K.M., Morton, T.H. *et al.* (1984). Oral manifestations of chronic graft-v-host disease. *Archives of Internal Medicine*, **144**, 1591–5.

Shulman, H.M., Gown, A.M., & Nugent, D.J. (1987). Hepatic veno-occlusive disease after bone marrow transplantation. Immunohistochemical identification of the material within occluded central venules. *American Journal of Pathology*, **127**, 549–58.

Shulman, H.M., McDonald, G.B., Matthews, D. *et al.* (1980a). An analysis of hepatic veno-occlusive disease and centrilobular hepatic degeneration following bone marrow transplantation. *Gastroenterology*, **79**, 1178–90.

Shulman, H.M., Sale, G.E., Lerner, K.G. *et al.* (1978). Chronic cutaneous graft-versus-host disease in man. *American Journal of Pathology*, **91**, 545–64.

Shulman, H.M., Sharma, P., Amos, D. *et al.* (1988). A coded histological study of hepatic graft-versus-host disease after bone marrow transplantation. *Hepatology*, **8**, 463–70.

Shulman, H.M., Sullivan, K.M., Weiden, P.L. *et al.* (1980b). Chronic graft-versus-host disease syndrome in man. A long term clinicopathological study of 20 Seattle patients. *American Journal of Medicine*, **69**, 204–17.

Slavin, R.E., Millian, J.C., & Mullins, C.M. (1975). Pathology of high-dose intermittent cyclophosphamide therapy. *Human Pathology*, **6**, 693–709.

Slavin, R.E. & Santos, G.W. (1973). The graft versus host reaction in man after bone marrow transplantation: pathology, pathogenesis, clinical features and implication. *Clinical Immunology and Immunopathology*, **1**, 472–98.

Sloane, J.P., Depledge, M.H., Powles, R.L. *et al.* (1983). Histopathology of the lung after bone marrow transplantation. *Journal of Clinical Pathology*, **36**, 546–54.

Sloane, J.P., Farthing, M.J.G., & Powles, R.L. (1980). Histopathological changes in the liver after allogeneic bone marrow transplantation. *Journal of Clinical Pathology*, **33**, 344–50.

Sloane, J.P., Thomas, J.A., Imrie, S.F. *et al.* (1984). Morphological and immunohistological changes in the skin in allogeneic bone marrow recipients. *Journal of Clinical Pathology*, **37**, 919–30.

Snover, D.C. (1985). Mucosal damage simulating acute graft versus host reaction in cytomegalovirus colitis. *Transplantation*, **39**, 699–70.

Snover, D.C., Weisdorf, S., Bloomer, J. *et al.* (1989). Nodular regenerative hyperplasia of the liver following bone marrow transplantation. *Hepatology*, **9**, 443–8.

Snover, D.C., Weisdorf, S.A., Ramsay, N.K. *et al.* (1984). Hepatic graft-versus-host disease: a study of the predictive value of liver biopsy in diagnosis. *Hepatology*, **4**, 123–30.

Snover, D.C., Weisdorf, S.A., Vercellotti, G.M. *et al.* (1985). A histopathological study of gastric and small intestinal graft-versus-host disease following allogeneic bone marrow transplantation. *Human Pathology*, **16**, 387–92.

Spencer, G.D., Hackman, R.C., McDonald, G.B. *et al.* (1986). A prospective study of unexplained nausea and vomiting after marrow transplantation. *Transplantation*, **42**, 602–7.

Stein-Streilein, J., Lipscomb, M.F., Hart, D.A., & Darden, A. (1981). Graft-versus-host reaction in the lung. *Transplantation*, **32**, 38–44.

Strasser, S. I., Shulman, H. M., Flowers, M. E. *et al.* (2000). Chronic graft-versus-host of the liver: presentation as an acute hepatitis. *Hepatology*, **32**, 1265–71.

Stromeyer, F.W. & Ishak, K.G. (1981). Nodular transformation (nodular regenerative hyperplasia) of the liver. *Human Pathology*, **12**, 60–71.

Suitters, A.J. & Lampert, I.A. (1983). The loss of IA⁺ Langerhans cells during graft-versus-host disease in rats. *Transplantation*, **36**, 540.

Sullivan, K.M., Meyers, J.D., Flournoy, N. *et al.* (1986). Early and late interstitial pneumonia following human bone marrow transplantation. *International Journal of Cell Cloning*, **4** (Suppl 1) 107–21.

Sviland, L., Pearson, A.D.J., Eastham, E.J. *et al.* (1988). Histological features of skin and rectal biopsy specimens after autologous and allogeneic bone marrow transplantation. *Journal of Clinical Pathology*, **41**, 148–54.

Tabbara, I.A., Zimmerman, R.N., Morgan, C., & Nahleh, Z. (2002). Allogeneic hematopoietic stem cell transplantation. *Archives of Internal Medicine*, **162**, 1558–66.

Terdiman, J., Linker, C., Ries, C. *et al.* (1996). The role of endoscopic evaluation in patients with suspected interstitial GVHD after allogeneic bone marrow transplantation. *Endoscopy*, **28**, 680–5.

Thomas, E.D., Storb, R., Clift, R.A. *et al.* (1975). Bone marrow transplantation (second of two parts). *New England Journal of Medicine*, **292**, 895–902.

Tobin, R., Hackman, R., Kimmey, M. *et al.* (1997). Bleeding from gastric antral vascular ectasia in bone marrow transplantation patients. *Gastrointestinal Endoscopy*, **44**, 229–39.

Urbanski, S.J., Kossakowska, A.E., Curtis, J. *et al.* (1987). Idiopathic small airways pathology in patients with graft-versus-host disease following allogeneic bone marrow transplantation. *American Journal of Surgical Pathology,* **11,** 965–71.

Villada, G., Roujeau, J.C., Cordonnier, C. *et al.* (1990). Toxic epidermal necrolysis after bone marrow transplantation: study of nine cases. *Journal of the American Academy of Dermatology,* **23,** 870–5.

Weisdorf, D.J., Snover, D.C., Haake, R. *et al.* (1990). Acute upper gastrointestinal graft-versus-host disease: clinical significance and response to immunosuppressive therapy. *Blood,* **76,** 624–9.

Wilkinson, M.J. & Maclennan, K.A. (1989). Vascular changes in irradiated lungs: a morphometric study. *Journal of Pathology,* **158,** 229–32.

Winston, D.J., Territo, M.C., Ho, W.G. *et al.* (1982). Alveolar macrophage dysfunction in human bone marrow transplant recipients. *American Journal of Medicine,* **73,** 859–66.

Wojno, K.J., Vogelsang, G.B., Beschorner, W.E., & Santos, G.W. (1994). Pulmonary hemorrhage as a cause of death in allogeneic bone marrow recipients with severe acute graft-versus-host disease. *Transplantation,* **57,** 88–92.

Woodruff, J.M., Hansen, J.A., Good, R.A. *et al.* (1976). The pathology of the graft-versus-host reaction (GVHR) in adults receiving bone marrow transplants. *Transplantation Proceedings,* **8,** 675–84.

Workman, D.L. & Clancy, J. (1994). Interstitial pneumonitis and lymphocytic bronchiolitis as a direct result of acute lethal graft-versus-host disease duplicate the histopathology of lung allograft rejection. *Transplantation,* **58,** 207–13.

Yousem, M.D. (1995). The histological spectrum of pulmonary graft-versus-host disease in bone marrow transplant recipients. *Human Pathology,* **26,** 668–74.

Yousem, S.A. (1991). Small airways disease. In *Pathology Annual* (Part II), **1991,** 109–44.

Zutter, M.M., Martin, P.J., Sale, G.E. *et al.* (1988). Epstein-Barr virus lymphoproliferation after bone marrow transplantation. *Blood,* **72,** 520–9.

105 Detection of minimal residual disease in hematologic malignancies by molecular technology

HARRY J. ILAND

Royal Prince Alfred Hospital, Sydney, Australia

Introduction

Modern chemotherapeutic regimens, and the advent of allogeneic and autologous stem cell transplantation, have made cure a realistic goal for many patients with hematologic malignancies. As a result, the development of strategies for the detection of minimal residual disease (MRD) and incipient relapse has assumed increasing importance. The ability to identify, and in some cases quantify, the presence of submicroscopic levels of malignant cells has been used to address many important questions in the pre- and posttransplant management of patients with leukemia, lymphoma, and myeloma. The applications of MRD detection are summarized in Table 105.1.

What actually constitutes clinically significant MRD is a difficult question, and varies for different disease entities. This variability arises partly because the concept and definition of remission is itself disease-dependent, and partly because the kinetics and regulation of malignant cell regrowth are certainly not equivalent across the spectrum of hematologic malignancies. For the purposes of this chapter, MRD will be regarded as the persistence of tumor cells at levels below the limits of conventional detection methods (e.g., morphology in leukemia and radiologic imaging in lymphoma), but in numbers sufficient to eventually cause disease recurrence. The ultimate benefit of reliable MRD detection will be the tailoring of therapy for individual patients so as to maximize cure rates, while at the same time minimizing unnecessary toxicity.

Since the ability to distinguish malignant hematopoietic cells from their normal counterparts by morphologic differences is quite limited at the single cell level, the identification of MRD requires the presence of a clonal marker that is unique to the tumor cells, and the ability to recognize this marker when cells bearing it are vastly outnumbered by normal cells. Candidate tumor markers have been identified by surface immunophenotypic analysis, in vitro culture systems, flow cytometric assessment of DNA ploidy, and karyotypic identification of nonrandom cytogenetic abnormalities. In general, the limited sensitivity of these techniques has restricted their incorporation into the routine surveillance programs of patients during remission. One exception is the finding that certain combinations of differentiation antigens are expressed on leukemia blast cells and are absent or extremely rare among their normal counterparts. Thus, in some situations double marker immunofluorescence assays are effectively leukemia-specific and are capable of identifying leukemic cells at approximately the 10^{-4} level (0.01%) (Campana *et al.*, 1990; Drach *et al.*, 1992).

Table 105.1. *Applications of MRD detection*

1. Select patients most likely to benefit from stem cell transplantation
   (a) Patients with detectable MRD after conventional therapy
   (b) Patients at risk of incipient relapse after conventional therapy, demonstrated by the reappearance of MRD or by increasing levels of MRD
2. Assess autologous stem cell harvests for contamination by MRD (including the effectiveness of purging)
3. Compare eradication of MRD following different conditioning regimens for stem cell transplantation
4. Identify patients most likely to relapse after stem cell transplantation
5. Evaluate posttransplant strategies designed to enhance GVL (e.g., donor lymphocyte infusions)

Abbreviations: MRD, minimal residual disease; GVL, graft-versus-leukemia effect.

Fluorescence in situ hybridization (and see Chapter 103)

The increasing recognition of nonrandom cytogenetic abnormalities in hematologic malignancies has been a major catalyst for research into the pathogenesis of these disorders. Continuing identification of new chromosomal lesions is contributing to improved classification systems, particularly as these abnormalities are now widely appreciated as one of the most important predictors of prognosis (Harris *et al.*, 1999). Unfortunately, the sensitivity of cytogenetic analysis using conventional banded preparations is limited by the number of metaphases that are analyzed, and is rarely of use in MRD studies. Thus, while the finding of leukemia-associated cytogenetic abnormalities in remission reliably predicts relapse, their absence does not reliably predict freedom from relapse (Freireich *et al.*, 1992). Furthermore, cytogenetic analysis is time-consuming, labor-intensive, requires highly skilled observers, and is often limited by reduced sample quality (Najfeld, 1997).

Fluorescence in situ hybridization (FISH) provides a more specific, sensitive, and flexible extension of cytogenetic analysis, and is evolving from being purely a research tool to becoming a supplementary diagnostic technique in many routine laboratories. FISH involves the hybridization of fluorescent-labeled DNA probes to chromosomal targets in individual cells, and can be adapted to both dividing (metaphase FISH) and nondividing (interphase FISH) cell preparations. While both metaphase and interphase FISH are useful for the analysis of numerical and structural chromosome abnormalities, interphase FISH has several additional advantages: cell culture is not required, simultaneous assessment of immunophenotype and genotype is possible, and a more reliable estimate of the true proportion of cells with a given cytogenetic abnormality can be obtained. For example, comparative studies have shown that cells containing monosomy 7 are underrepresented in metaphase preparations due to their relative inability to enter mitosis, whereas cells containing trisomy 8 have a proliferative advantage and are therefore overrepresented (Najfeld, 1997).

When compared with conventional cytogenetic analysis, both metaphase and interphase FISH provide improved sensitivity (Garcia-Isidoro *et al.*, 1997), but the sensitivity must be validated for each particular probe set. Depending on the application, the sensitivity of FISH ranges from approximately 0.1% (i.e., it can reliably predict an increased risk of relapse when abnormal cells are visualized at levels of more than one per 1,000 normal cells) (Nylund *et al.*, 1994) to more than 3% (i.e., relapse is predictable only when abnormal cells are visualized at levels of more than three per 100 normal cells) (Garcia-Isidoro *et al.*, 1997).

Several types of DNA probes are now available, and are summarized in Table 105.2. Whereas paint probes target whole chromosomes, and repetitive sequence probes are used to identify major structural regions within chromosomes, sequence-specific probes allow the detection of genomic targets as small as one kilobase in length when used in concert with enhanced

Table 105.2. *DNA probes for use in FISH*

1. Whole chromosome paint probes (chromosome-specific)
2. Repetitive sequence probes
    (a) Alpha satellite centromere probes (chromosome-specific)
    (b) Telomere probes (chromosome-nonspecific)
3. Sequence-specific probes (locus- or gene-specific)

Abbreviations: FISH, fluorescence in situ hybridization.

imaging and signal amplification techniques. When applied to the detection of gene rearrangements, paint probes and repetitive sequence probes, which normally span an intragenic breakpoint, generate a split signal (Liu *et al.*, 1993a). In contrast, combinations of differentially labeled, gene-specific probes in dual-color FISH techniques can reveal gene rearrangements by co-localization of signals (Garcia-Isidoro *et al.*, 1997; Mancini *et al.*, 2000).

Over the past few years a range of advanced molecular cytogenetic strategies have been developed that will eventually enable the characterization of virtually all cancer-associated chromosomal abnormalities (Popescu & Zimonjic, 1997). These techniques include primed in situ labeling (PRINS), multi-fluor FISH, and comparative genomic hybridization. At the present time they are primarily suitable for the characterization of chromosome abnormalities, but technical improvements and conceptual adaptations are likely to enhance their application to the study of MRD in the future.

Genetic lesions in hematologic malignancies

Oncogenesis in solid tumors is characterized by the accumulation of several genetic lesions that involve members of several cancer-associated gene families, such as oncogenes, tumor suppressor genes, and DNA mismatch repair genes. The molecular events that give rise to these lesions include point mutations, gene amplifications, gene deletions, and gene rearrangements, and the karyotypes observed in solid tumors are correspondingly complex. In contrast, the karyotypes seen most commonly in leukemias and lymphomas are relatively simple, and frequently reflect a critical disease-specific gene rearrangement event. As a result, reciprocal translocations are most commonly observed, but gene rearrangements can also result from inversions and interstitial deletions.

Recently, there has been an explosive increase in the number of gene rearrangements that have been characterized at the molecular level (Drexler *et al.*, 1995). Broadly speaking, gene rearrangements arising from chromosomal translocations disrupt normal cell behavior by one of two alternative scenarios (Table 105.3). In some cases, the rearrangement event disrupts the protein-coding regions of two genes, which are then erroneously reunited with each other, thereby generating actively transcribed novel fusion genes, whose associated novel protein products have abnormal functions. In other cases, the rearrangement process disrupts the regulatory control of a specific gene rather than its coding region. Following the rearrangement, the control of the disrupted gene's expression is deregulated either quantitatively or by virtue of its expression in an inappropriate cell lineage. In addition to these abnormal gene rearrangement events, the immunoglobulin heavy and light chain genes, as well as the α, β γ, and δ T-cell-receptor genes, undergo an obligatory gene rearrangement process during normal lymphoid ontogeny. These rearranged antigen-receptor genes provide particularly useful clonal markers in lymphoproliferative disorders.

Table 105.3. *Gene rearrangements in hematological malignancies*

1. Abnormal rearrangements resulting from structural cytogenetic lesions
   (a) Novel fusion genes
   (b) Deregulated gene expression
2. Normal rearrangements occurring during lymphoid ontogeny
   (a) Immunoglobulin heavy and light chain genes
   (b) T-cell-receptor genes

Polymerase chain reaction

Conventional analysis of gene rearrangements has involved the technique of Southern blotting and hybridization with gene-specific probes, but the sensitivity for detection of MRD (1% to 5%) is little better than morphologic assessment alone. In contrast, the ability of the polymerase chain reaction (PCR) to exponentially amplify specific DNA sequences of interest, which are unique to the malignant clone, has improved the sensitivity of residual disease detection by several orders of magnitude.

PCR was originally developed by Mullis, Saiki, Ehrlich, and colleagues at the Cetus Corporation (Saiki *et al.*, 1988). Two flanking oligonucleotide primers, complementary to opposite strands of the DNA sequence of interest, are extended by a thermostable DNA polymerase. Repetitive cycles of denaturation, primer annealing, and primer extension, mediated by cyclical temperature variations, result in an exponential accumulation of PCR products. The major limitation of PCR technology, namely contamination, is a direct consequence of its sensitivity. Elaborate precautions are required to prevent false-positive results due to contamination (Kwok & Higuchi, 1989), particularly that resulting from carryover of previously amplified material. A further limitation of PCR-based detection systems is that the residual cells containing amplifiable clone-specific sequences may not necessarily be tumorigenic, and hence the need for clinical studies to establish the relevance of MRD detection.

Measurement of WT1 gene transcripts by reverse transcriptase PCR appears useful as "panleukemic MRD marker" for predicting and managing relapse following allogeneic HSC transplantation for a variety of acute leukemias and chronic myeloid leukemia (Ogawa *et al.*, 2003).

Chronic myeloid leukemia

The prototypic example of novel fusion genes generated by gene rearrangements, and the most widely studied for the detection of MRD, is the BCR-ABL rearrangement associated with the Philadelphia chromosome, referred to cytogenetically as t(9;22). This abnormality occurs in 95% of patients with chronic myeloid leukemia (CML) and in about 25% of patients with adult acute lymphoblastic leukemia (ALL) (Gale, 1987). At the molecular level, a reciprocal translocation between chromosomes 9 and 22 generates a BCR-ABL fusion gene on the Philadelphia chromo-

some (derivative 22), resulting in expression of a fusion protein with markedly enhanced tyrosine kinase activity. The fundamental role that the BCR-ABL protein plays in the pathogenesis of the disease is exemplified by the dramatic hematological and cytogenetic responses observed with imatinib mesylate, a specific tyrosine kinase inhibitor (Kantarjian *et al.*, 2002).

The breakpoint on chromosome 9 usually occurs in the first intron of the ABL proto-oncogene, whereas the breakpoint on chromosome 22 occurs in a gene of poorly understood function, known as BCR. In CML and in 25% to 50% of patients with Philadelphia chromosome positive ALL, the BCR breakpoint is clustered in a 5.8 kb region known as the major breakpoint cluster region (M-bcr), usually in the intron following either the second or the third M-bcr exon (referred to as b2 and b3, respectively). In the remaining patients with ALL, the BCR breakpoint occurs in one of two minor breakpoint cluster regions (m-bcr-1 and m-bcr-2) in the intron following the first BCR exon (referred to as e1). Although DNA is unsuitable for analysis of BCR-ABL rearrangements by PCR, the chimeric BCR-ABL mRNA generated by the rearrangement provides an excellent template, provided a cDNA copy is first synthesized by reverse transcriptase (RT)-PCR (Kawasaki *et al.*, 1988). For M-bcr breakpoints, PCR primers that target b2 and the second ABL exon (a2) are used (Fig. 105.1). The length of the PCR product obtained indicates if b3 is present in the fusion transcript. For m-bcr-1 and m-bcr-2 breakpoints, primers that target e1 and a2 are employed (Fig. 105.1). To improve specificity and sensitivity, nested primers are generally incorporated in a two-step PCR reaction, and most reports have demonstrated successful amplification of BCR-ABL rearrangements from as few as one leukemic cell in 10^5 to 10^6 normal cells (Delfau *et al.*, 1990).

A large number of reports have attempted to correlate PCR analysis of BCR-ABL rearrangements following allogeneic hematopoietic stem cell (HSC) transplantation for CML with clinical outcome. Early reports suggested that a large proportion of patients exhibited detectable BCR-ABL RNA for prolonged periods posttransplant in the absence of cytogenetic and clinical relapses, implying that PCR positivity was of no prognostic value (Pignon *et al.*, 1990). The contribution of contamination to these results is difficult to assess, but subsequent studies, which have expended considerable effort to prevent contamination, have provided support for the role of molecular monitoring in identifying patients at greatest risk of relapse. Despite highly sensitive two-step PCR assays, most studies demonstrate complete and persistent disappearance of PCR positivity in a significant proportion of patients, and these patients have an extremely low likelihood of relapse (Kohler *et al.*, 1990). Similarly, patients who exhibit transient PCR positivity, usually for no more than 6 months posttransplant, generally remain disease-free. The transient PCR positivity in these patients may be a result of long-lived nonclonogenic cells derived from the original leukemic population, or may reflect a slowly evolving graft-versus-leukemia effect.

In contrast, patients who remain persistently PCR-positive, and patients in whom PCR-detectable BCR-ABL fusion transcripts reappear after more than 6 months posttransplant,

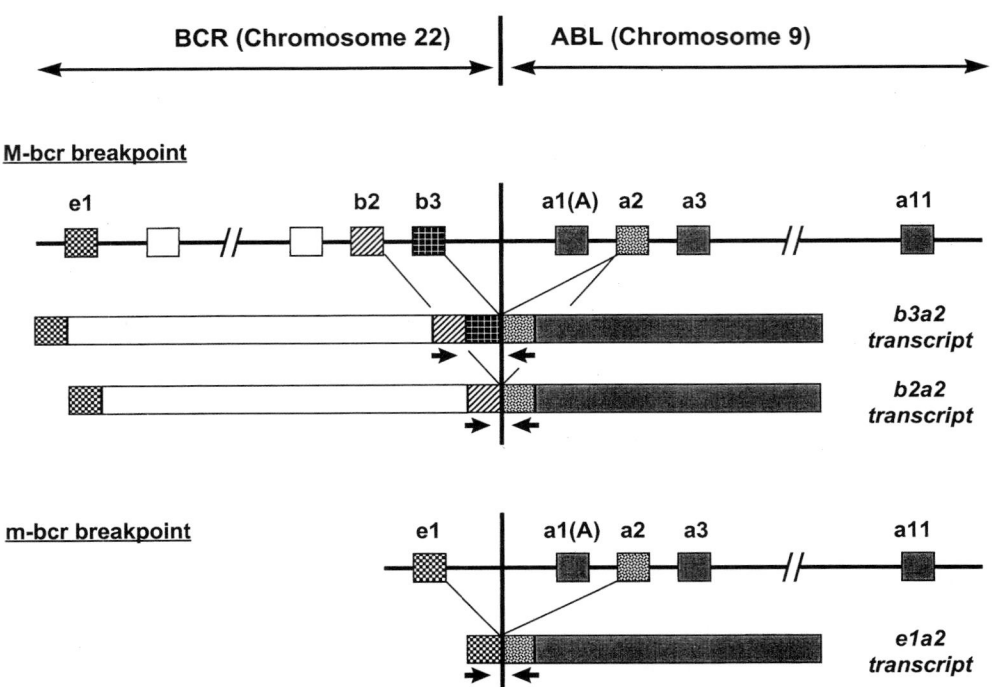

Fig. 105.1. RT-PCR strategy for amplification of BCR-ABL fusion transcripts derived from the BCR-ABL fusion gene in CML and ALL. Arrows indicate location and direction of PCR primers. The figure is not drawn to scale. Although al (A), one of the two alternative first ABL exons, is present within the fusion gene, it is spliced out during processing of the primary fusion transcript.

appear to be at increased risk of cytogenetic and, in some cases, clinical relapse (Cross *et al.,* 1993b). Although less sensitive than RT-PCR, analogous observations have also been made with metaphase FISH in the post–allogeneic transplant setting (el-Rifai *et al.,* 1996). In addition to differences in sensitivity, FISH and RT-PCR provide different perspectives on cells derived from the original leukemic clone by virtue of differences in the nature of their respective target sequences. For example, BCR-ABL fusion genes may persist posttransplant (DNA detected by FISH), but are not necessarily expressed (using quantitative RT-PCR detection of RNA). Thus, FISH may be more accurate in identifying the presence of residual leukemic cells, while quantitative RT-PCR may be more accurate for predicting the risk of relapse (Chomel *et al.,* 2000).

Support for the concept that PCR analysis is of prognostic value comes from studies of patients who received T-cell-depleted grafts, and from patients transplanted beyond chronic phase. Both these categories of patients have an increased likelihood of remaining PCR-positive and a greater incidence of clinical relapse (Delage *et al.,* 1991; Mackinnon *et al.,* 1994, 1996; Pichert *et al.,* 1995). The logistics of molecular monitoring in CML have been simplified by the observation that peripheral blood and bone marrow give entirely concordant results when analyzed simultaneously following HSC transplantation (Lin *et al.,* 1994). Additionally, it has been shown that genomic DNA and cDNA give concordant results for the detection of residual disease after treatment of CML by allografting (Zhang *et al.,* 1996).

Advances in quantitative PCR techniques, such as competitive PCR (Fig. 105.2) and real-time PCR, have further improved the distinction between those patients with decreasing residual leukemic burdens due to a graft-versus-leukemia effect and those with increasing residual leukemic burdens due to incipient clinical relapse (Thompson *et al.,* 1992; Cross *et*

COMPETITOR MOLECULES ADDED

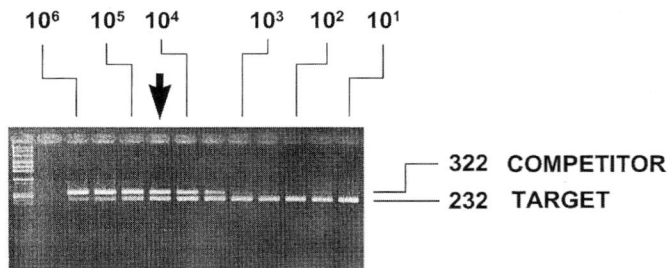

Fig. 105.2. Competitive RT-PCR in CML. Serial dilutions of a synthetic BCR-ABL template (competitor) are added to constant amounts of patient RNA that has been reverse transcribed to cDNA (target). The reaction mixtures are amplified by PCR and then subjected to size separation by electrophoresis. Since the number of competitor molecules added to each reaction is known, the number of initial target molecules can be deduced from the lane in which the competitor and target templates generate equal amounts of PCR product (indicated by arrow; approximately 3×10^4 molecules). Gel photo kindly provided by Tao Zeng, Kanematsu Laboratories, Royal Prince Alfred Hospital.

al., 1993a). The inability of conventional qualitative PCR assays to make this distinction has been formally recognized by the European Investigators on Chronic Myelogenous Leukemia (EICML) Group, which has recommended the routine use of quantitative RT-PCR for the monitoring of MRD following allogeneic transplantation (Lion, 1994) (Fig. 105.3). Studies of the kinetics or increasing numbers of BCR-ABL transcripts correlate with relapse post-BMT (Lin *et al.,* 1996); of 69 patients who had persistently undetectable, decreasing, or low BCR-ABL levels (<50 transcripts per microgram of RNA) on sequential analysis, only 1% subsequently relapsed. Of 29 patients who had increasing or persistently high levels (>50 transcripts per microgram of RNA) on sequential analysis, 72%, relapsed. In 19 patients studied sequentially, a constant increase in the number of transcripts was found before relapse, indicating a constant BCR-ABL transcript doubling time. The doubling time for patients relapsing cytogenetically or into chronic phase (median 24.7 days) was significantly longer than

for patients relapsing into advanced phases (median 14.7 days). These findings have been reinforced by more recent studies employing real-time methods of BCR-ABL quantitation. In a study of 138 patients allografted for CML, Olavarria *et al.* (2001) used quantitative PCR at 3 to 5 months posttransplant to classify the recipients as either being negative for BCR-ABL transcripts, or being positive at a low level (<100 transcripts/μg RNA and/or a BCR-ABL/ABL ratio of <0.02%), or being positive at a high level. The 3-year cumulative incidence of relapse in these three groups was 16.7%, 42.9%, and 86.4%, respectively (*P* = .001; Fig. 105.4). This relationship was apparent regardless of whether the transplants were T-cell-depleted or not, and regardless of whether a sibling or an unrelated donor was used. Similarly, Radich and colleagues (2001) examined the significance of BCR-ABL positivity in 379 patients at 18 months or later posttransplant. Ninety of the 379 had at least one positive test, and 13 relapsed (14%) compared to 3 relapses in the 289 BCR-ABL-negative patients (1%). The median time from BCR-ABL detection to relapse was 916 (range 251–2,654) days. Using quantitative PCR the median BCR-ABL level at relapse was 40,443 copies/μg of RNA compared to a median value of 24 copies/μg in BCR-ABL-positive patients who did not relapse. A correlation has also been reported between the amount of BCR-ABL fusion transcript determined by quantitative RT-PCR and clinical relapse stage after allografting (Elmaagacli *et al.,* 2001).

The identification of molecular relapse by RT-PCR has been accepted as a basis for therapeutic intervention with, for example, donor leukocyte infusions (DLI). Since the potential for DLI to re-establish PCR negativity is related to the extent of relapse (molecular versus cytogenetic versus hematologic) (van

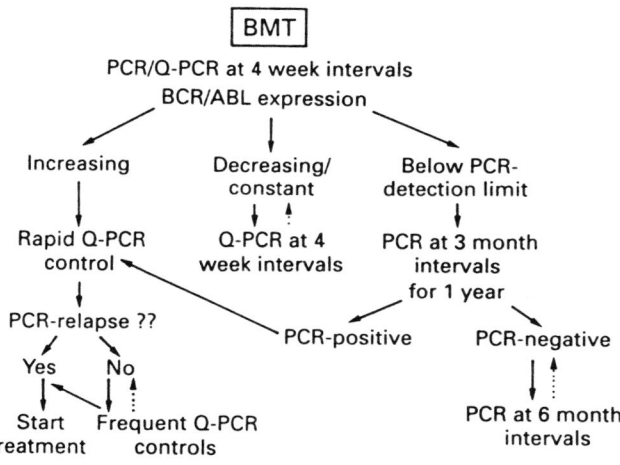

Fig. 105.3. Guidelines for clinical use of PCR analyses in CML patients after BMT. In patients with detectable residual disease after BMT, the monitoring by PCR/Q-PCR analyses should be performed at intervals of 4 weeks. The intervals between PCR analyses indicated are advisable provided that the detection of PCR relapse will be regarded as an indication for therapeutic intervention. As long as the relative BCR-ABL expression is decreasing or constant, the initial frequency of Q-PCR analyses may be maintained. If residual disease is no longer amenable to detection by PCR, the intervals between PCR analyses could be extended to 3 months. After 1 year of continuous PCR negativity, the intervals could be further increased to a maximum of 6 months. Reappearance of BCR-ABL rearranged cells after a previously PCR negative status should prompt frequent follow-up by Q-PCR to permit an early detection of clonal expansion. Similarly, a rapid control by Q-PCR is needed on observation of an increase in BCR-ABL expression. If the presence of increasing marker gene expression is confirmed, it should be assessed whether the findings meet the criteria for PCR relapse. As long as it is not the case, Q-PCR analyses should be performed at a frequency of 1 to 4 weeks to permit early assessment of further clonal proliferation. The progression to PCR relapse should provide a basis for therapeutic considerations. Reproduced, with permission, from Lion (1994).

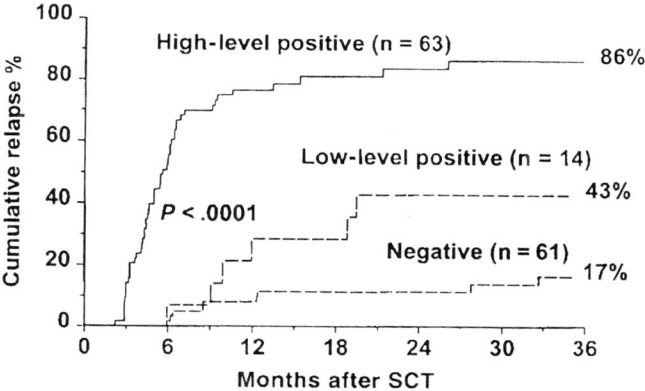

Fig. 105.4. Cumulative incidence of relapse after stem cell transplant (SCT) for CML according to results of an early RT-PCR test. Cumulative incidence of disease recurrence at any (molecular, cytogenetic, or hematologic) level for patients with negative, low-level positive, and high-level positive RT-PCR at 3 to 5 months after SCT, respectively. The *P* value shown has been pooled over strata. The pairwise over strata *P* values are negative versus low positive, *P* = .01; negative versus high positive, *P* < .0001; and low positive versus high positive, *P* = .001. Reproduced, with permission, from Olavarria *et al.* (2001).

Rhee *et al.,* 1994), it is imperative that relapse be detected when the burden of recurrent leukemia is at its lowest. However, detection of leukemia-specific fusion transcripts is not the only method available; monitoring for molecular evidence of disease by analyzing chimerism using short tandem repeats to discriminate between donor and recipient cells has also been used successfully to guide treatment with DLI (de Weger *et al.,* 2000).

BCR-ABL positive acute lymphoblastic leukemia

Data on the use of PCR for assessing MRD in Philadelphia-positive ALL patients have been reported less frequently, but the results illustrate clearly the prognostic value of postchemotherapy (Preudhomme *et al.,* 1997) and posttransplant PCR monitoring (Gehly *et al.,* 1991; Miyamura *et al.,* 1992; Radich *et al.,* 1997) (Fig. 105.5). A large proportion

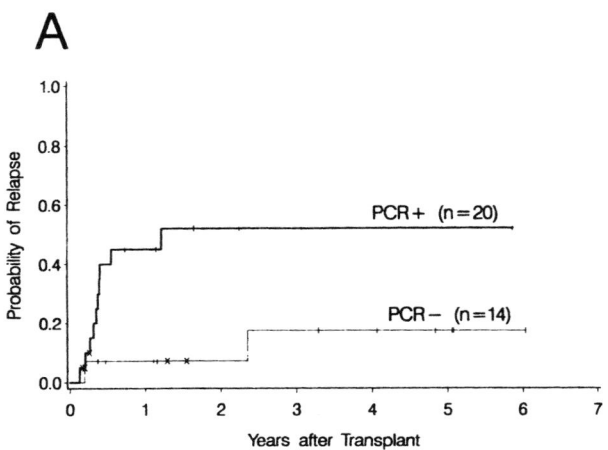

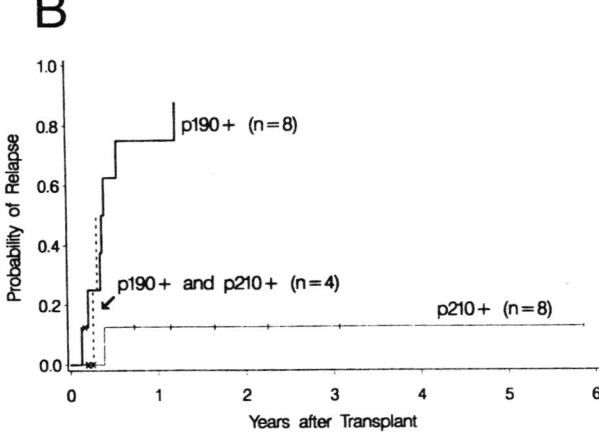

Fig. 105.5. Upper curves **(A)** show the cumulative incidence of relapse by the presence or absence of bcr-abl detected by PCR before day 100 post-BMT. Lower curves **(B)** show the cumulative incidence of relapse by the type of bcr-abl transcript found after transplant. Ticks indicate patients alive without relapse and "x" denote patients who died without relapse. Reproduced, with permission, from Radich *et al.* (1997).

remain PCR-positive after chemotherapy-induced complete remission, reflecting the poor prognosis associated with this clinical entity. Persistent PCR positivity posttransplant is highly predictive of relapse, whereas persistent PCR negativity, particularly extending more than 6 months posttransplant, is associated with prolonged disease-free survival and probable cure. Conversion from posttransplant negativity to positivity appears to be an excellent predictor of incipient relapse. Quantitative RT-PCR for BCR-ABL in ALL has also been used to demonstrate that leukemic cell contamination is 10- to 100-fold higher in remission bone marrow samples than in paired peripheral blood samples (Martin *et al.,* 1994), suggesting that the latter is the preferred source for stem cell harvests.

Acute promyelocytic leukemia

Acute promyelocytic leukemia (APL), the FAB-M3 subtype of acute myeloid leukemia (AML), is uniquely associated with the t(15;17) translocation (Larson *et al.,* 1984). Considerable interest has been generated by the observation that the majority of APL patients achieve complete remission when treated with all-*trans* retinoic acid (ATRA) alone (Huang *et al.,* 1988). ATRA appears to induce an initial proliferation, followed by terminal differentiation, senescence, and eventually cell death. Numerous reports have now established that the retinoic acid receptor alpha gene (RARα) at chromosome 17q21 is rearranged and translocated to chromosome 15. The PML gene (previously referred to as MYL) at chromosome 15q22 is also rearranged (de The *et al.,* 1990), and actively transcribed fusion genes are generated on both derivative chromosomes. The RARα protein is a member of the steroid/thyroid hormone receptor superfamily of nuclear transcription factors, and both sequence and in vitro functional data suggest that the PML protein is also a DNA-binding transcriptional regulator (Kakizuka *et al.,* 1991) with anti-proliferative activity. The bulk of evidence implicates dominant negative effects of the PML-RARα fusion protein as the critical factor in promyelocytic leukemogenesis. First, it has been shown to possess abnormal transcriptional regulatory activity when compared with that of the normal RARα protein (de The *et al.,* 1991; Kakizuka *et al.,* 1991), and it retains a retinoic acid responsive domain that is consistent with the in vivo responsiveness of APL cells to ATRA. Second, PML-RARα disrupts the macromolecular nuclear structures known as nuclear bodies, in which normal PML is localized. Third, mice transgenic for PML-RARα (Brown *et al.,* 1997) are characterized by a partial block of hematopoietic differentiation in the neutrophil lineage. Some of these mice then develop a leukemia that closely resembles human APL, including responsiveness to retinoic acid manifest by myeloid differentiation.

The breakpoint on chromosome 17 consistently occurs in the second intron of the RARα gene, whereas the breakpoint on chromosome 15 is more variable, and is localized within one of three breakpoint cluster regions in the third intron, the sixth exon, or the sixth intron, respectively (Pandolfi *et al.,* 1992). As a result, RNA rather than DNA is more suitable as a template for PCR detection of the rearrangement.

Perhaps more than any other molecular abnormality, the PML-RARα fusion transcript provides an accurate marker of response to therapy and a reliable guide to relapse risk. The clinical reports, though fewer in number than those available for CML, consistently demonstrate correlations between persistent or recurrent RT-PCR positivity and clinical relapse on the one hand, and between persistent RT-PCR negativity and continuing remission on the other (Huang *et al.*, 1993; Miller *et al.*, 1993; Fukutani *et al.*, 1995). The average window period between molecular and hematological relapse is approximately 3 months, although this figure is clearly influenced by the sensitivity of the assay, which in most series is at least 10^{-4}. Even more important than prediction of relapse, the value of molecular monitoring in actually determining outcome has been demonstrated in APL. In a study by Lo Coco *et al.* (1999), 14 patients were given salvage therapy at the time of first molecular relapse. The 2-year Kaplan-Meier survival estimate from time of relapse was 92% in this series, compared with 44% in a previous series of 37 patients who received the same treatment at the time of hematologic relapse ($P < .05$, by log-rank test).

The data relevant to transplantation are even fewer, but those that are available reinforce the importance of RT-PCR testing in selecting patients at risk for relapse and for monitoring the response to myeloablative therapy and transplantation (Martin *et al.*, 1996; Perego *et al.*, 1996; Román *et al.*, 1997) (Fig. 105.6). The presence or absence of MRD after salvage therapy for relapse has also been identified as an important predictor of the duration of remission following a subsequent autologous transplant (Meloni *et al.*, 1997).

Quantitative RT-PCR assays for PML-RARα are still at the developmental stage, utilizing either Taqman™ probes (Cassinat *et al.*, 2000; Slack *et al.*, 2001), or dnazymes in DzyNA™ RT-PCR assays (Applegate *et al.*, 2002a) (Fig. 105.7). Preliminary data suggest that serial quantitative assays can reliably identify incipient relapse (Applegate *et al.*, 2002a, 2002b) (Fig. 105.8).

Acute myeloid leukemia (other than APL)

There is now widespread appreciation of the prognostic importance of nonrandom cytogenetic abnormalities in patients with AML, with both good and bad prognostic subgroups recognized. Recognition of genetic markers that can be exploited in sensitive PCR-based assays for the detection of MRD is particularly important in good-prognosis subtypes of AML, since a more selective approach to myeloablative therapy and transplantation is required in patients who have an intrinsically lower risk of relapse after conventional chemotherapy.

In addition to APL, two other relatively common subtypes of AML are associated with a better than average prognosis. Both the t(8;21) translocation and the inv(16) (i.e., inversion of chromosome 16) produce abnormal chimeric transcription factors that are derived from different DNA-binding subunits of a nor-

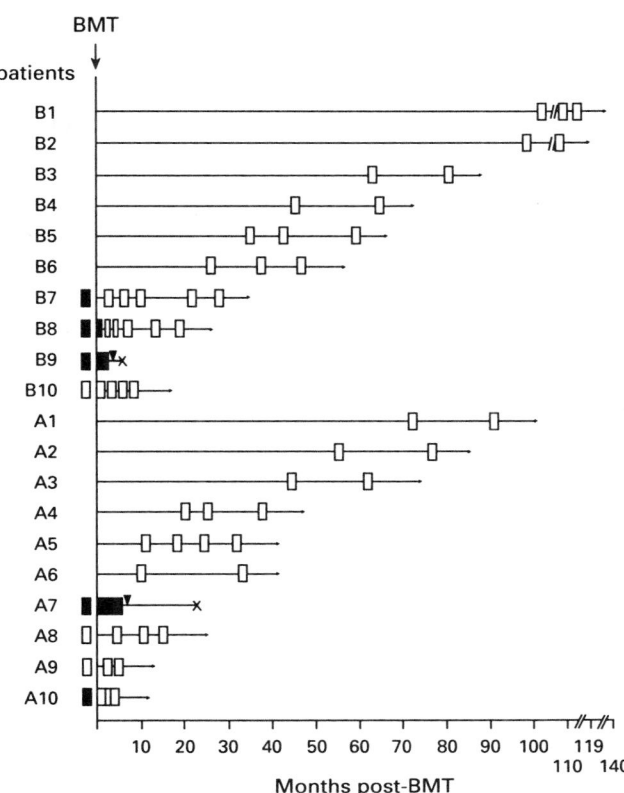

Fig. 105.6. RT-PCR results. White boxes: samples that were negative for the presence of PML-RARα transcript; black boxes: samples that were positive for the presence of PML-RARα transcript; triangle: relapse; X: died. Arrows indicate the time of clinical remission. Reproduced, with permission, from Román *et al.* (1997).

mal transcriptional regulator known as core binding factor (CBF). CBFA1 is encoded by the AML1 gene, which is rearranged with the MTG8 gene (also known as ETO) in t(8;21) leukemias (Nucifora *et al.*, 1993), and the gene encoding the CBFB chain is rearranged with the MYH11 gene in inv(16) leukemias (Liu *et al.*, 1993b). Leukemias carrying t(15;17), t(8;21), or inv(16) account for approximately 30% of all cases of AML.

In contrast to APL, virtually all patients with t(8;21) AML remain positive for fusion transcripts by RT-PCR, despite evidence of polyclonal hematopoiesis (Guerrasio *et al.*, 1995). This long-term persistence has been documented after both chemotherapy and autologous transplantation (Kusec *et al.*, 1994; Miyamoto *et al.*, 1996), and has also been described several years after allogeneic transplantation (Jurlander *et al.*, 1996). Thus, standard RT-PCR does not appear to be clinically useful in determining the subset of t(8;21) patients who are most likely to relapse. Changes in AML1-MTG8 transcript levels detectable by quantitative RT-PCR assays, however, appear to correlate well with remission and relapse, and suggest that the degree of leukemic cytoreduction with myeloablative chemotherapy is greater than that achieved with conventional

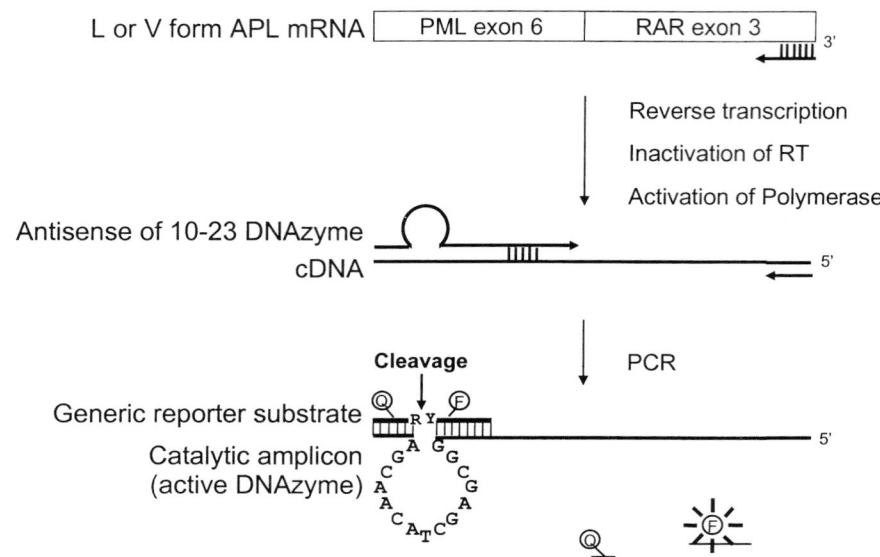

Fig. 105.7. DzyNA RT-PCR strategy for amplification of PML-RARα mRNA transcripts. Reverse transcription of the transcript from total RNA and amplification of cDNA occur sequentially in a single tube. Reverse transcription is achieved using a standard RARα primer, followed by cDNA amplification employing both the standard RARα primer, and a DzyNA primer containing both target sequences (PML) and 5′ tag sequences that are complementary (antisense) to 10–23 deoxyribozymes (DNAzymes). During PCR, PML-RARα amplicons are synthesised which contain the target sequences linked to catalytic (sense) DNAzymes that cleave reporter substrates included in the PCR mix. The accumulation of amplicons is monitored in real-time during PCR by changes in fluorescence produced by separation of fluorophore and quencher moieties incorporated into opposite sides of DNAzyme cleavage sites within the generic substrates. Cleavage of the substrates results in an increase in fluorescence that indicates successful amplification of the target nucleic acid. Adapted, with permission, from Applegate et al. (2002a).

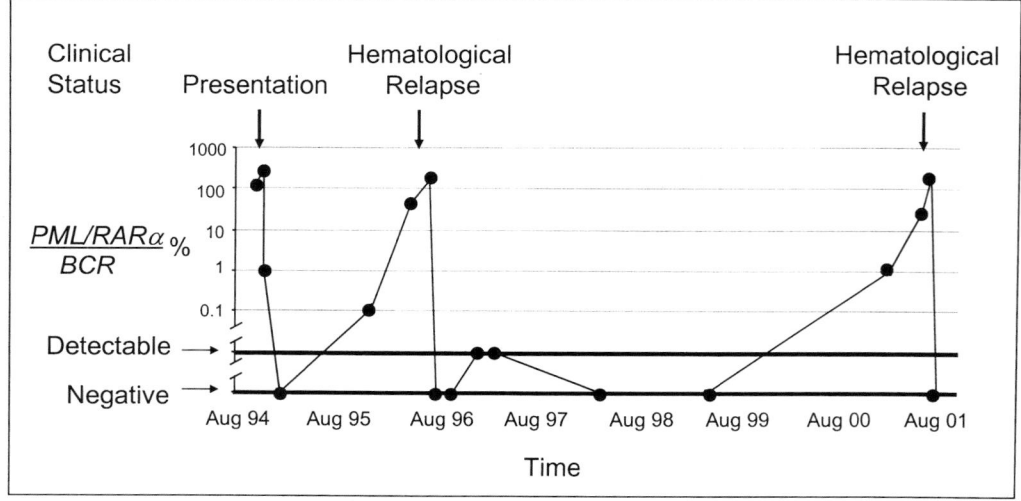

Fig. 105.8. Monitoring of PML/RARα transcripts during the course of APL for over 7 years in one patient. The expression levels of PML/RARα and BCR (control transcript) were estimated from calibration curves, and the ratios of PML-RARα transcripts to control transcripts (%) were calculated and plotted against time. Positive samples that could not be quantified (values below the range covered by the calibration curve) were classified as detectable. Adapted, with permission, from Applegate et al. (2002a).

therapy (Sugimoto *et al.,* 2000). Quantitative analysis of AML1-MTG8 transcripts in serial peripheral blood samples is also possible (Fujimaki *et al.,* 2000).

A CBFB-MYH11 fusion transcript is found in cases of AML associated with a pericentric inversion of chromosome 16, and also in the cytogenetically distinct but molecularly identical t(16;16) translocation. Although these cytogenetic abnormalities are seen in virtually all patients with acute myelomonocytic leukemia with abnormal eosinophils (FAB-M4Eo), molecular assays have demonstrated that this gene rearrangement is also found in other subtypes of AML. In a review of 321 patients entered into U.K. MRC AML trials, 21 had inv(16). All of these, as well as an additional 12 patients who lacked chromosome 16 abnormalities, were RT-PCR-positive for CBFB-MYH11 fusion transcripts, thus highlighting the importance of molecular assessment at diagnosis (Langabeer *et al.,* 1997). RT-PCR assays are more complex than for AML1-ETO, since breakpoints in both the CBFB and the MYH11 genes vary. Contradictory data about long-term RT-PCR positivity have been reported (Tobal *et al.,* 1995; Evans *et al.,* 1997), and therefore quantitative assays are likely to be more informative (Laczika *et al.,* 1998).

Deregulated gene expression in lymphoproliferative disorders

As with AML, some gene rearrangements in lymphoproliferative disorders produce novel chimeric proteins with modified functions (e.g., ETV6-AML1, E2A-PBX1, and MLL-AF4 fusions in ALL with t(12;21), t(1;19), and t(4;11) translocations, respectively), and their applicability to MRD detection has been demonstrated (Cayuela *et al.,* 1996; Cimino *et al.,* 1996). However, the majority of abnormal rearrangements in lymphoid malignancies place one gene under the transcriptional control of another. Although novel fusion transcripts are occasionally generated, the coding region of the deregulated gene is not disrupted, and hence a normally functioning protein is produced. Deregulation may be quantitative, or may be manifested by aberrant expression in cells of an inappropriate lineage. These types of rearrangements usually arise as a result of recombination errors during the process of normal immunoglobulin and T-cell-receptor gene rearrangements (see below).

MYC and Burkitt lymphoma

The MYC oncoprotein is a member of the helix-loop-helix family of transcription factors, and plays a central role in the progression of cells through the cell cycle. Recombination errors during normal immunoglobulin gene rearrangements generate chromosomal translocations that fuse all or part of the MYC gene on chromosome 8 with either the immunoglobulin heavy chain (IgH) or light chain (IgL) genes, resulting in deregulated MYC expression (Cory, 1986). These rearrangements are found in B-cell non-Hodgkin's lymphomas, particularly the small, noncleaved (Burkitt and non-Burkitt) varieties,

as well as the closely related B-cell ALL. Rearrangements involving the IgH genes are associated with t(8;14) translocations (75%), whereas κ-light chain (9%) and λ-light chain (16%) rearrangements are characterized by t(2;8) and t(8;22) translocations, respectively.

PCR detection of MYC-IgH rearrangements has been described, although the variability of the breakpoints on both chromosomes 8 and 14 has necessitated the use of several primer systems (Shiramizu & Magrath, 1990). Despite the high relapse rate of Burkitt lymphoma with conventional chemotherapy, which has justified the use of aggressive therapeutic regimens ± HSC transplantation, no studies of MRD detection posttransplant have been reported. This is presumably a reflection of the need to first localize the breakpoints in individual patients by multiple PCR primer combinations. The situation is likely to be improved by the application of high-fidelity thermostable DNA polymerases (long-range PCR) to MRD detection of MYC rearrangements, with sensitivities in the range of 10^{-3} to 10^{-4} reported by several investigators (zur Stadt *et al.,* 1997; Basso *et al.,* 1999).

BCL-2 and follicular lymphoma

The most common cytogenetic abnormality in B-cell non-Hodgkin's lymphomas is the t(14;18) translocation, occurring in 85% of follicular and 20% of diffuse large cell lymphomas. This translocation is characterized by the rearrangement of the BCL-2 gene on chromosome 18 into the IgH gene locus on chromosome 14 (Weiss *et al.,* 1987), resulting in high-level deregulated expression of BCL-2. Since the protein product of the BCL-2 gene inhibits the normal phenomenon of programmed cell death (apoptosis), it seems likely that the increased BCL-2 expression prolongs survival of B lymphocytes, rendering them susceptible to additional mutations associated with lymphomagenesis.

The majority of BCL-2 gene breakpoints are clustered in a 150 base pair major breakpoint region (mbr) of the 3′ untranslated portion of the third BCL-2 exon (Tsujimoto *et al.,* 1985). Many, but not all, of the remaining breakpoints occur in a second minor cluster region (mcr) some 30 kilobases downstream of the BCL-2 gene (Cleary *et al.,* 1986). The use of long range PCR indicates that a significant number of breakpoints can also be found between the mbr and the mcr, with some clustering approximately 16 kb downstream from the BCL-2 gene (Albinger-Hegyi *et al.,* 2002). Rearrangements involving mbr produce a novel BCL-2-IgH fusion transcript, but the coding sequences for BCL-2 are uninterrupted; hence a normal BCL-2 protein is translated. Deregulated expression is a consequence of both transcriptional activation and abnormal posttranscriptional regulation of BCL-2-IgH RNA. In contrast, mcr rearrangements result in deregulated expression of normal BCL-2 transcripts. The breakpoint on chromosome 14 is located within the 5′ portions of one of the six J_H segments of the IgH gene locus (see below). Thus, two PCR primer systems are sufficient for the identification of the vast majority of BCL-

2 rearrangements; both utilize a common 3′ J$_H$ primer, but different mbr and mcr 5′ primers are required (Stetlet-Stevenson et al., 1988; Ngan et al., 1989).

Minor variations in the precise location of chromosome 18 breakpoints within mbr and mcr ensure that small differences in the size of the PCR product can be utilized both as clone-specific and patient-specific markers, thus minimizing false-positive results due to contamination. Although t(14;18) and BCL-2 rearrangements have been described in nonmalignant lymphoid tissue, minimal residual lymphoma can be unambiguously identified in individual patients by the use of clone-specific probes derived from the unique DNA sequence present at the junction of the BCL-2 and IgH regions (Galoin et al., 1996). As with MYC gene rearrangements, sequence data suggest that BCL-2 rearrangements are mediated, at least in part, by illegitimate recombinase activity (Tsujimoto et al., 1985).

PCR amplification of the t(14;18) translocation is now a well-established technique, with clinical applications encompassing confirmation of diagnosis, refinement of staging, assessment of purging, and MRD detection. The clinical value of PCR detection in the transplant setting has also been convincingly demonstrated. Gribben et al. (1991) used PCR to monitor the efficiency of autograft purging prior to transplantation. In a multivariate analysis, successful conversion of PCR-positive autografts to PCR negativity by purging was the only significant predictor of prolonged posttransplant relapse-free survival in 114 patients with BCL-2 rearranged non-Hodgkin's lymphomas. This group subsequently showed that disease-free survival was also highly correlated with persistent postauto-graft PCR negativity of bone marrow samples, whereas all relapsed patients were PCR-positive prior to relapse (Gribben et al., 1993). As with CML, transient positivity in the early posttransplant period was not a reliable indicator of subsequent relapse. Comparable results indicating that PCR negativity in stem cell harvests and following transplantation correlates with clinical outcome have been reported by Corradini et al. (1997). Gribben's group (1994) also showed that bone marrow was a more informative tissue source than peripheral blood for detecting residual disease by this method at the time of or after autologous transplantation (Fig. 105.9), and that contamination of blood early posttransplant appeared to be the consequence of reinfusion of lymphoma cells within the autologous marrow inoculum.

BCL-1 and mantle cell lymphoma

Mantle cell lymphoma (MCL, centrocytic lymphoma) is a poor prognosis lymphoma associated with t(11;14) or less commonly t(11;22) translocations and rearrangements of the BCL-1 (cyclin D1/PRAD-1) proto-oncogene. BCL-1 breakpoints usually occur within a major translocation cluster, and the gene is rearranged into the immunoglobulin heavy chain gene (or lamda light chain gene) in a comparable manner to BCL-2 rearrangements in follicular lymphomas. Both BCL-1 and IgH gene rearrangements have been used to assess the effectiveness

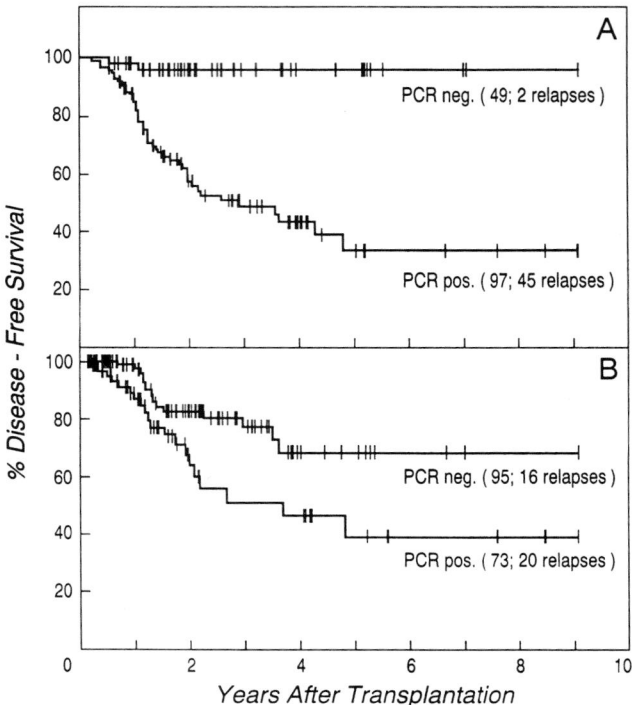

Fig. 105.9. Actuarial probability of disease-free survival after ABMT of patients with a PCR-amplifiable BCL2/IgH translocation. PCR neg refers to those patients in whom PCR did not detect any residual lymphoma cells after transplantation. PCR pos refers to those patients in whom PCR-detectable residual lymphoma cells were found at some time after ABMT. (**A**) Assessment of BM samples from 146 patients; (**B**) assessment of PB samples from 168 patients. Reproduced, with permission, from Gribben et al. (1994).

of purging and the presence of MRD following autologous bone marrow transplantation for MCL (Andersen et al., 1997). Since MCL expresses lambda light chains more frequently than other non-Hodgkin's lymphomas, and since lambda-producing B cells usually delete one or both alleles of their kappa immunoglobulin light chain genes, rearrangement between the kappa deletion element (kappa de) and recombinant signal sequences can also be exploited in PCR-based MRD assays (Bertoni et al., 1999).

SCL and childhood T-cell ALL

The stem cell leukemia (SCL, also known as TAL-1) gene was originally identified in a patient with a T-cell precursor ALL that underwent a lineage switch to myeloid leukemia following treatment with deoxycoformycin. A t(1;14) translocation was present, and the molecular consequences of the translocation included rearrangement of SCL, a novel transcription factor gene on the short arm of chromosome 1 (1p), and disruption of the TCRδ complex on chromosome 14 (Begley et al., 1989). Whereas t(1;14) translocations are observed in only a small proportion of T-ALL patients, a much more common rearrangement of SCL has now been identified (Aplan *et al.*, 1992). An interstitial deletion of chromosome 1p, undetectable by cytogenetic analysis, results in loss of the untranslated 5′ regulatory sequences of SCL and its juxtaposition with the 5′ untranslated region of a gene of unknown function on 1p known as SIL (SCL interrupting locus). SIL expression normally occurs in T cells, whereas SCL expression is predominantly found in erythroid and megakaryocytic cells. Although an SIL-SCL chimeric RNA transcript is generated, its coding regions are composed entirely of SCL sequences, and aberrant SCL expression in T cells is thought to be of major pathogenetic significance in the development of T-ALL. Three types of molecular rearrangement have been described, requiring two sets of PCR primers for elucidation. However, the chimeric transcript in all three types is identical, the first SIL exon being fused to the third SCL exon (Aplan *et al.*, 1992). Consequently, a single PCR primer combination will identify SIL-SCL rearrangements in all patients using RNA as a template in an RT-PCR system analogous to that required for BCR-ABL and PML-RARα amplification. SIL-SCL rearrangements are the most common molecular abnormality associated with T-ALL, and clinical T-ALL studies have demonstrated the identification of MRD prior to hematological relapse (Huang *et al.*, 1995), especially when combined with analysis of T-cell receptor gene rearrangements (Nirmala *et al.*, 2002). A real-time quantitative PCR assay for detection of leukemic cells that harbor the TAL-1 deletion has been developed (Chen *et al.*, 2001), and is capable of detecting MRD at levels of ≥0.001%.

Other gene rearrangements in lymphoma, acute lymphoblastic leukemia, and multiple myeloma

Many more examples of deregulated gene expression have been identified, and are detailed in an excellent review (Drexler *et al.*, 1995). In multiple myeloma, several genes including BCL-1, FGFR3, MMSET, and c-MAF have been implicated in rearrangements into the IgH region, but in contrast to lymphomas, the rearrangements involve illegitimate switch region recombinations rather than mistakes in VDJ joining (Bergsagel *et al.*, 1996; Chesi *et al.*, 2000). In up to 50% of childhood T-cell ALL, deregulated expression is manifested predominantly by rearrangement of transcription factor genes into T-cell-receptor loci.

Immunoglobulin and T-cell-receptor gene rearrangements in lymphoid malignancies

The ability of the immune system to recognize a diverse range of antigens stems from a series of immunoglobulin and T-cell-receptor (TCR) gene rearrangements that occur normally during B-cell and T-cell ontogeny. The immunoglobulin heavy chain (IgH) locus consists of ~100 variable (V_H) gene segments, ~30 diversity (D) segments, and six joining (J_H) segments. Rearrangement at this locus requires a recombinase system comprising lymphoid-specific, recombination-activating

gene proteins 1 and 2 (RAG1 and RAG2), DNA ligase, XRCC4, and components of DNA-dependent protein kinase (Weaver & Alt, 1997). After rearrangement, a unique VDJ sequence is present and this codes for the variable region of the IgH polypeptide chain. The κ and λ immunoglobulin light chain (IgL) genes, as well as the α/δ, β, and γ gene loci whose products constitute the TCR, undergo a comparable series of rearrangements. Further diversity arises from small deletions (exonucleolytic nibbling), nontemplated additions mediated by terminal deoxynucleotidyl transferase (TdT), and somatic hypermutation. The final DNA sequence is unique to the lymphocyte in which these events occur, and also to all the progeny of that cell, and can therefore be utilized as a clone-specific marker in lymphoproliferative malignancies. Although Southern blotting has traditionally been used to demonstrate monoclonal rearrangement of immunoglobulin and TCR genes, PCR strategies are becomingly increasingly popular, and have been exploited for both diagnosis and detection of MRD, particularly in patients with B- and T-lineage ALL. Using TCR-specific consensus primers, monoclonal populations can be identified by PCR in most cases of T-ALL. In B-lineage ALL, IgH-based primers demonstrate monoclonality in approximately 75%, but since TCRγ/δ rearrangements also occur in the majority of these patients, PCR is informative in over 90% if TCR genes are also targeted. When antigen receptor PCR systems are combined with detection of leukemia-specific fusion transcripts, almost 100% of patients have markers suitable for subsequent MRD detection (Kuang *et al.*, 1996).

The rearranged IgH VDJ sequence can be subdivided into four relatively conserved framework regions (FR), and three hypervariable complementarity determining regions (CDR). Several PCR strategies have been devised, the most common being known as CDR3-PCR since the primers flank the most variable portion (CDR3), which contains the D region and the V_HD and DJ_H junctions (Fig. 105.10). CDR3-PCR can detect monoclonal B-cell populations when present at 0.1% to 1% in a background of polyclonal cells. By sequencing the CDR3 region, more sensitive clone-specific PCR systems can be developed that are suitable for the study of MRD. Most of these involve determining the unique DNA sequence at the V_HD and DJ_H junctions, followed by the synthesis of clone-specific oligonucleotide probes and/or PCR primers. The sensitivity of these methods ranges from 10^{-4} to 10^{-6}. Attempts to simplify MRD detection by generating clone-specific probes/primers directly from PCR products, thereby bypassing the requirement for sequencing, are currently under investigation.

Although TCR genes exhibit a more limited germline structure than immunoglobulin genes, clone-specific PCR strategies are still feasible due to extensive junctional diversity generated during TCR rearrangements. In T-ALL, most studies have utilized TCRγ and TCRδ rearrangements as clonal markers. Fortuitously, specific members of these TCR genes are employed preferentially, thereby simplifying primer system design. In T-ALL, Vδ1-Dδ-Jδ1 rearrangements predominate, whereas Vδ2-Dδ3 rearrangements are most common in B-cell

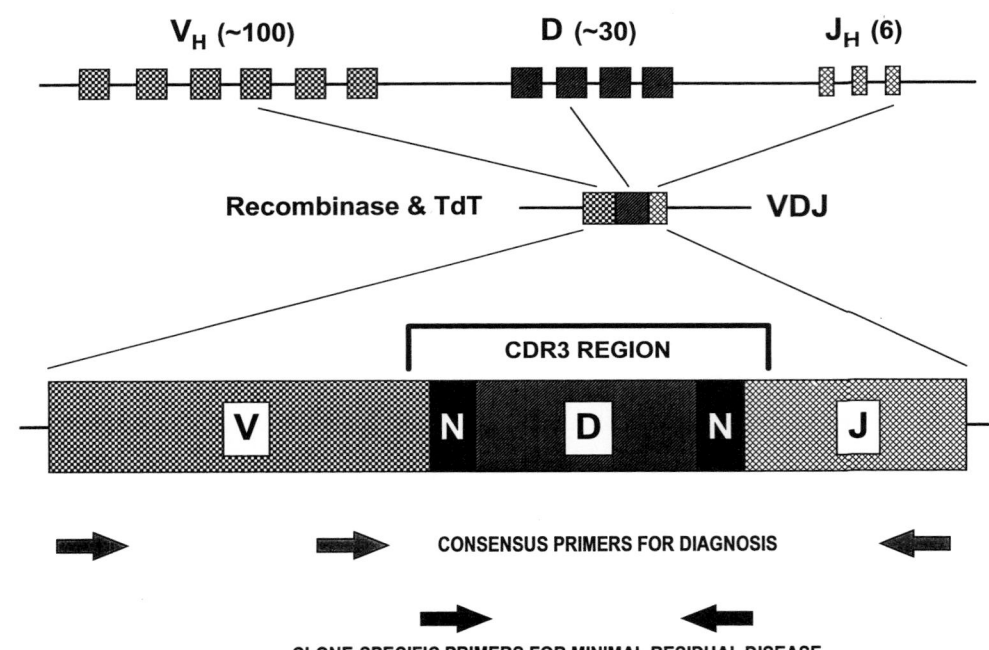

Fig. 105.10. PCR strategies for amplification of IgH gene rearrangements. One each of the V_H, D, and J_H genes are juxtaposed by enzymes of the recombinase system. Diversity is enhanced by exonucleolytic nibbling and TdT-mediated addition of nucleotides at the V_H-D and D-J_H junctions (the "N" regions). The CDR3 region encompasses these junctions, and is the target of amplification in CDR3-PCR systems for the demonstration of monoclonality in B-cell lymphoproliferative disorders. Alternative consensus primers from the most 5' end of the V_H genes are sometimes used (framework 1). Clone-specific primers are generated from the V_H-N-D and the D-N-J_H segments. The figure is not drawn to scale, and PCR primers are indicated by arrows.

precursor ALL. For amplification of TCRγ genes, most investigators have used varying mixtures of Vγ primers in combination with one set of mixed Jγ primers.

Two approaches have been promoted for the prediction of outcome after conventional chemotherapy in ALL. One school relies on quantitation of MRD in early remission to identify both children and adults who are most likely to relapse (Brisco et al., 1994, 1996). The other utilizes serial monitoring with PCR negativity as the endpoint, aiming to recognize those at greatest risk of relapse by either persistence or reappearance of PCR positivity (Yamada et al., 1990; Scholten et al., 1995). While both approaches provide reasonably good correlations between PCR data and long-term outcome in retrospective analyses, prospective studies in which therapeutic decisions are based on molecular analyses have not yet been reported.

Persistence of PCR-detectable MRD in the majority of childhood ALL cases for at least 6 months, and in many for at least 12 months, appears to be common (Roberts et al., 1995), and up to one-third of patients who discontinue therapy after 24 months may still have detectable MRD. In a recent multi-center study of 178 patients (Cave et al., 1998), 42% were still PCR positive at the end of induction therapy, and the number who remained PCR positive fell progressively at later time points after consolidation and late intensification. At all time points tested, the risk of relapse was related to the level of detectable MRD ($P < .001$), and multivariate analysis showed that in com-

parison with immunophenotype, age, risk group (standard or very high risk), and white-cell count at diagnosis, the presence or absence and level of residual disease were the most powerful independent prognostic factors. Since not all patients with PCR-detectable MRD will relapse, it is likely that increased reliance on quantitative methods will be necessary in order to avoid overtreatment of patients who may already be cured, but still have small numbers of amplifiable leukemic genomes. Preliminary evidence suggests that detection of MRD by PCR may be useful for predicting the outcome of subsequent transplantation after relapse in childhood ALL (Steenbergen et al., 1995; Knechtli et al., 1998a). In the study by Knechtli et al. (1998a), outcomes were strongly correlated with the level of detectable MRD assessed in remission marrows 6 to 81 days before transplant. The 2-year event-free survival was 0% in patients with high-level MRD (10^{-2} to 10^{-3}), 36% in those with low-level MRD (10^{-3} to 10^{-5}), and 73% in those with undetectable MRD ($P < .001$, Fig. 105.11). Furthermore, persistence of MRD following allogeneic bone marrow transplantation in patients with acute lymphoblastic leukemia is strongly correlated with an increased likelihood of relapse (Radich et al., 1995; Knechtli et al., 1998b). Clone-specific IgH PCR has also been applied to MRD detection following transplantation in non-Hodgkin's lymphoma (Zwicky et al., 1996), multiple myeloma (Bird et al., 1993; Bjorkstrand et al., 1995), and chronic lymphatic leukemia (Provan et al., 1996).

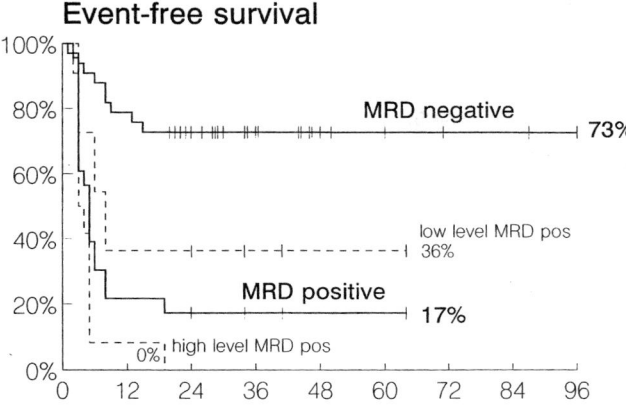

Event-free survival

Time from transplantation (months)

Fig. 105.11. Kaplan-Meier plots comparing event-free survival of patients with MRD ($n = 23$), divided into high level ($n = 12$) and low level ($n = 11$), and negative MRD ($n = 33$), but excluding those who had relapsed in an isolated extramedullary site before BMT. Two-year EFS is given for each MRD category at the end of each curve. Reproduced, with permission, from Knechtli *et al.* (1998a).

There are theoretical reasons why clone-specific PCR may not always be successful in identifying MRD; for example, sanctuary sites such as the central nervous system often escape detection when only bone marrow is used to monitor MRD. In addition, the phenomena of oligoclonality and clonal evolution, which occur in approximately 25% of patients with ALL, may render primers that were specific for the initial dominant clone inappropriate. Instability of antigen receptor gene rearrangements affects IgH loci more than TCR loci, and results from V_H–V_H replacements and from alternate V_H rearrangements with a common DJ_H precursor (Wasserman *et al.*, 1992). The combined use of both IgH and TCR markers, and reliance on the more stable DJ_H region for synthesis of clone-specific primers, should reduce the false negativity rate for detection of MRD to less than 10% (Steward *et al.*, 1994; Marshall *et al.*, 1995; Szczepanski *et al.*, 2002). The necessity for the use of multiple PCR targets in monitoring MRD has been reinforced by the observation that subclones detected either at diagnosis or during induction therapy may exhibit differential chemosensitivity (de Haas *et al.*, 2001). Not surprisingly, subsequent relapses were derived from the slowest-responding clones.

Conclusions

The last few years have witnessed dramatic increases in our understanding of the molecular basis underlying cytogenetic translocations and gene rearrangements in hematologic malignancies. Together with the advent of PCR, this information has revolutionized our approach to the detection of MRD. Studies in CML, APL, and ALL have most clearly demonstrated the value of molecular monitoring. While the technical aspects of this research are well advanced, the clinical studies are still in their infancy, and the precise contribution of PCR to the overall management of patients, particularly with respect to transplantation, requires further clarification. Nevertheless, it is likely that management decisions will one day be guided by the results of these endeavors, ultimately to the benefit of patients.

References

Albinger-Hegyi, A., Hochreutener, B. *et al.* (2002). High frequency of t(14;18)-translocation breakpoints outside of major breakpoint and minor cluster regions in follicular lymphomas: improved polymerase chain reaction protocols for their detection. *American Journal of Pathology*, **160**, 823–32.

Andersen, N.S., Donovan, J.W. *et al.* (1997). Failure of immunologic purging in mantle cell lymphoma assessed by polymerase chain reaction detection of minimal residual disease. *Blood*, **90**, 4212–21.

Aplan, P.D., Lombardi, D.P. *et al.* (1992). Involvement of the putative hematopoietic transcription factor SCL in T-cell acute lymphoblastic leukemia. *Blood, 79*, 1327–33.

Applegate, T.L., Iland, H.J. *et al.* (2002a). Diagnosis and molecular monitoring of acute promyelocytic leukemia (APL) using DzyNA RT-PCR to quantify PML/RARa fusion transcripts. *Cancer Diagnostics: Discovery and Clinical Applications Clinical Chemistry* (in press).

Applegate, T.L., Iland, H.J. *et al.* (2002b). Molecular monitoring of APL using DzyNA RT-PCR. Proceedings of the 34th Annual Oak Ridge Conference. *Clinical Chemistry* (in press).

Basso, K., Frascella, E. *et al.* (1999). Improved long-distance polymerase chain reaction for the detection of t(8;14)(q24;q32) in Burkitt's lymphomas. *American Journal of Pathology*, **155**, 1479–85.

Begley, C.G., Aplan, P.D. *et al.* (1989). Chromosomal translocation in a human leukemic stem-cell line disrupts the T-cell antigen receptor delta-chain diversity region and results in a previously unreported fusion transcript. *Proceedings of the National Academy of Sciences USA*, **86**, 2031–5.

Bergsagel, P.L., Chesi, M. *et al.* (1996). Promiscuous translocations into immunoglobulin heavy chain switch regions in multiple myeloma. *Proceedings of the National Academy of Sciences USA*, **93**, 13931–6.

Bertoni, F., Zucca, E. *et al.* (1999). Immunoglobulin light chain kappa deletion rearrangement as a marker of clonality in mantle cell lymphoma. *Leukemia and Lymphoma, 36*, 147–50.

Bird, J.M., Russell, N.H. *et al.* (1993). Minimal residual disease after bone marrow transplantation for multiple myeloma: evidence for cure in long-term survivors. *Bone Marrow Transplantation, 12*, 651–4.

Bjorkstrand, B., Ljungman, P. *et al.* (1995). Double high-dose chemoradiotherapy with autologous stem cell transplantation can induce molecular remissions in multiple myeloma. *Bone Marrow Transplantation, 15*, 367–71.

Brisco, J., Hughes, E. *et al.* (1996). Relationship between minimal residual disease and outcome in adult acute lymphoblastic leukemia. *Blood, 87*, 5251–6.

Brisco, M.J., Condon, J. *et al.* (1994). Outcome prediction in childhood acute lymphoblastic leukaemia by molecular quantification of residual disease at the end of induction. *Lancet, 343*, 196–200.

Brown, D., Kogan, S. *et al.* (1997). A PMLRAR-alpha transgene initiates murine acute promyelocytic leukemia. *Proceedings of the National Academy of Sciences USA*, **94**, 2551–6.

Campana, D., Coustan-Smith, E. *et al.* (1990). The immunologic detection of minimal residual disease in acute leukemia. *Blood*, **76**, 163–71.

Cassinat, B., Zassadowski, F. *et al.* (2000). Quantitation of minimal residual disease in acute promyelocytic leukemia patients with t(15;17) translocation using real-time RT-PCR. *Leukemia*, **14**, 324–8.

Cave, H., van der Werff ten Bosch, J. *et al.* (1998). Clinical significance of minimal residual disease in childhood acute lymphoblastic leukemia. European Organization for Research and Treatment of Cancer–Childhood Leukemia Cooperative Group. *New England Journal of Medicine*, **339**, 591–8.

Cayuela, J.M., Baruchel, A. *et al.* (1996). TEL-AML1 fusion RNA as a new target to detect minimal residual disease in pediatric B-cell precursor acute lymphoblastic leukemia. *Blood*, **88**, 302–8.

Chen, X., Pan, Q. *et al.* (2001). Quantification of minimal residual disease in T-lineage acute lymphoblastic leukemia with the TAL-1 deletion using a standardized real-time PCR assay. *Leukemia*, **15**, 166–70.

Chesi, M., Kuehl, W.M. *et al.* (2000). Recurrent immunoglobulin gene translocations identify distinct molecular subtypes of myeloma. *Annals of Oncology*, **11** (Suppl 1), 131–5.

Chomel, J-C., Brizard, F., Veinstein, A. *et al.* (2000). Persistence of BCR-ABL genomic rearrangement in chronic myeloid leukemia patients in complete and sustained remission after interferon-α therapy or allogeneic bone marrow transplantation. *Blood*, **95**, 404–9.

Cimino, G., Elia, L. *et al.* (1996). Clinical relevance of residual disease monitoring by polymerase chain reaction in patients with ALL-1/AF-4 positive-acute lymphoblastic leukemia. *British Journal of Haematology*, **92**, 659–64.

Cleary, M.L., Galili, N. *et al.* (1986). Detection of a second t(14;18) breakpoint cluster region in human follicular lymphomas. *Journal of Experimental Medicine*, **164**, 315–20.

Corradini, P., Astolfi, M. *et al.* (1997). Molecular monitoring of minimal residual disease in follicular and mantle cell non-Hodgkin's lymphomas treated with high-dose chemotherapy and peripheral blood progenitor cell autografting. *Blood*, **89**, 724–31.

Cory, S. (1986). Activation of cellular oncogenes in hematopoietic cells by chromosome translocation. *Advances in Cancer Research*, **47**, 189–234.

Cross, N.C., Feng, L. *et al.* (1993a). Competitive polymerase chain reaction to estimate the number of BCR-ABL transcripts in chronic myeloid leukemia patients after bone marrow transplantation. *Blood*, **82**, 1929–36.

Cross, N.C., Hughes, T.P. *et al.* (1993b). Minimal residual disease after allogeneic bone marrow transplantation for chronic myeloid leukemia in first chronic phase: correlations with acute graft-versus-host disease and relapse. *British Journal of Haematology*, **84**, 67–74.

de Haas, V., Verhagen, O.J. *et al.* (2001). Quantification of minimal residual disease in children with oligoclonal B-precursor acute lymphoblastic leukemia indicates that the clones that grow out

during relapse already have the slowest rate of reduction during induction therapy. *Leukemia*, **15**, 134–40.

de The, H., Chomienne, C. *et al.* (1990). The t(15;17) translocation of acute promyelocytic leukemia fuses the retinoic acid receptor alpha gene to a novel transcribed locus. *Nature*, **347**, 558–61.

de The, H., Lavau, C. *et al.* (1991). The PML-RAR alpha fusion mRNA generated by the t(15;17) translocation in acute promyelocytic leukemia encodes a functionally altered RAR. *Cell*, **66**, 675–84.

de Weger, R.A., Tilanus, M.G.J., Scheidel, K.C. *et al.* (2000). Monitoring of residual disease and guided donor leukocyte infusion after allogeneic bone marrow transplantation by chimaerism analysis with short tandem repeats. *British Journal of Haematology*, **110**, 647–53.

Delage, R., Soiffer, R.J. *et al.* (1991). Clinical significance of bcr-abl gene rearrangement detected by polymerase chain reaction after allogeneic bone marrow transplantation in chronic myelogenous leukemia. *Blood*, **78**, 2759–67.

Delfau, M.H., Kerckaert, J.P. *et al.* (1990). Detection of minimal residual disease in chronic myeloid leukemia patients after bone marrow transplantation by polymerase chain reaction. *Leukemia*, **4**, 1–5.

Drach, J., Drach, D. *et al.* (1992). Flow cytometric determination of atypical antigen expression in acute leukemia for the study of minimal residual disease. *Cytometry*, **13**, 893–901.

Drexler, H.G., Borkhardt, A. *et al.* (1995). Detection of chromosomal translocations in leukemia-lymphoma cells by polymerase chain reaction. *Leukemia and Lymphoma*, **19**, 359–80.

Elmaagacli, A.H., Freist, A., Hahn, M. *et al.* (2001). Estimating the relapse stage in chronic myeloid leukemia patients after allogeneic stem cell transplantation by the amount of BCR-ABL fusion transcripts detected using a new real-time polymerase chain reaction method. *British Journal of Haematology*, **113**, 1072–5.

el-Rifai, W., Ruutu, T. *et al.* (1996). Minimal residual disease after allogeneic bone marrow transplantation for chronic myeloid leukemia: a metaphase-FISH study. *British Journal of Haematology*, **92**, 365–9.

Evans, P.A., Short, M.A. *et al.* (1997). Detection and quantitation of the CBFbeta/MYH11 transcripts associated with the inv(16) in presentation and follow-up samples from patients with AML. *Leukemia*, **11**, 364–9.

Freireich, E.J., Cork, A. *et al.* (1992). Cytogenetics for detection of minimal residual disease in acute myeloblastic leukemia. *Leukemia*, **6**, 500–6.

Fujimaki, S., Funato, T. *et al.* (2000). A quantitative reverse transcriptase polymerase chain reaction method for the detection of leukaemic cells with t(8;21) in peripheral blood. *European Journal of Haematology*, **64**, 252–8.

Fukutani, H., Naoe, T. *et al.* (1995). Prognostic significance of the RT-PCR assay of PML-RARA transcripts in acute promyelocytic leukemia. The Leukemia Study Group of the Ministry of Health and Welfare (Kouseisho). *Leukemia*, **9**, 588–93.

Gale, R.P. (1987). Chronic myelogenous leukemia: a model for human cancers. *Baillieres Clinical Haematology*, **1**, 869–86.

Galoin, S., al Saati, T. *et al.* (1996). Oligonucleotide clonospecific probes directed against the junctional sequence of t(14;18): a new tool for the assessment of minimal residual disease in follicular lymphomas. *British Journal of Haematology*, **94**, 676–84.

Garcia-Isidoro, M., Tabernero, M.D. *et al.* (1997). Detection of the Mbcr/abl translocation in chronic myeloid leukemia by fluorescence in situ hybridization: comparison with conventional cytogenetics and implications for minimal residual disease detection. *Human Pathology*, **28**, 154–9.

Gehly, G.B., Bryant, E.M. *et al.* (1991). Chimeric bcr-abl messenger RNA as a marker for minimal residual disease in patients transplanted for Philadelphia chromosome-positive acute lymphoblastic leukemia. *Blood*, **78**, 458–65.

Gribben, J.G., Freedman, A.S. *et al.* (1991). Immunologic purging of marrow assessed by PCR before autologous bone marrow transplantation for B-cell lymphoma. *New England Journal of Medicine*, **325**, 1525–33.

Gribben, J.G., Neuberg, D. *et al.* (1993). Detection by polymerase chain reaction of residual cells with the bcl-2 translocation is associated with increased risk of relapse after autologous bone marrow transplantation for B-cell lymphoma. *Blood*, **81**, 3449–57.

Gribben, J.G., Neuberg, D., Barber, M. *et al.* (1994). Detection of residual lymphoma cells by polymerase chain reaction in peripheral blood is significantly less predictive for relapse than detection in bone marrow. *Blood*, **83**, 3800–7.

Guerrasio, A., Rosso, C. *et al.* (1995). Polyclonal hemopoiesis associated with long-term persistence of the AML1-ETO transcript in patients with FAB M2 acute myeloid leukemia in continuous clinical remission. *British Journal of Haematology*, **90**, 364–8.

Harris, N.L., Jaffe, E.S. *et al.* (1999). World Health Organization Classification of Neoplastic Diseases of the Hematopoietic and Lymphoid Tissues: Report of the Clinical Advisory Committee Meeting. Airlie House, Virginia, November 1997. *Journal of Clinical Oncology*, **17**, 3835–49.

Huang, M.E., Ye, Y.C. *et al.* (1988). Use of all-trans retinoic acid in the treatment of acute promyelocytic leukemia. *Blood*, **72**, 567–72.

Huang, W., Kuang, S.Q. *et al.* (1995). RT/PCR detection of SIL-TAL-1 fusion mRNA in Chinese T-cell acute lymphoblastic leukemia (T-ALL). *Cancer Genetics and Cytogenetics*, **81**, 76–82.

Huang, W., Sun, G.L. *et al.* (1993). Acute promyelocytic leukemia: clinical relevance of two major PML-RAR alpha isoforms and detection of minimal residual disease by retrotranscriptase/polymerase chain reaction to predict relapse. *Blood*, **82**, 1264–9.

Jurlander, J., Caligiuri, M.A. *et al.* (1996). Persistence of the AML1/ETO fusion transcript in patients treated with allogeneic bone marrow transplantation for t(8;21) leukemia. *Blood*, **88**, 2183–91.

Kakizuka, A., Miller, W.H., Jr. *et al.* (1991). Chromosomal translocation t(15;17) in human acute promyelocytic leukemia fuses RAR alpha with a novel putative transcription factor, PML. *Cell*, **66**, 663–74.

Kantarjian, H., Sawyers, C. *et al.* (2002). Hematologic and cytogenetic responses to imatinib mesylate in chronic myelogenous leukemia. *New England Journal of Medicine*, **346**, 645–52.

Kawasaki, E.S., Clark, S.S. *et al.* (1988). Diagnosis of chronic myeloid and acute lymphocytic leukemias by detection of leukemia-specific mRNA sequences amplified in vitro. *Proceedings of the National Academy of Sciences USA*, **85**, 5698–702.

Knechtli, C.J., Goulden, N.J. *et al.* (1998a). Minimal residual disease status before allogeneic bone marrow transplantation is an important determinant of successful outcome for children and adolescents with acute lymphoblastic leukemia. *Blood*, **92**, 4072–9.

Knechtli, C.J., Goulden, N.J. *et al.* (1998b). Minimal residual disease status as a predictor of relapse after allogeneic bone marrow transplantation for children with acute lymphoblastic leukaemia. *British Journal of Haematology*, **102**, 860–71.

Kohler, S., Galili, N. *et al.* (1990). Expression of bcr-abl fusion transcripts following bone marrow transplantation for Philadelphia chromosome-positive leukemia. *Leukemia*, **4**, 541–7.

Kuang, S., Gu, L. *et al.* (1996). Long-term follow-up of minimal residual disease in childhood acute lymphoblastic leukemia patients by polymerase chain reaction analysis of multiple clone-specific or malignancy-specific gene markers. *Cancer Genetics and Cytogenetics*, **88**, 110–17.

Kusec, R., Laczika, K. *et al.* (1994). AML1/ETO fusion mRNA can be detected in remission blood samples of all patients with t(8;21) acute myeloid leukemia after chemotherapy or autologous bone marrow transplantation. *Leukemia*, **8**, 735–9.

Kwok, S. & Higuchi, R. (1989). Avoiding false positives with PCR. *Nature*, **339**, 237–8.

Laczika, K., Novak, M. *et al.* (1998). Competitive CBFbeta/MYH11 reverse-transcriptase polymerase chain reaction for quantitative assessment of minimal residual disease during postremission therapy in acute myeloid leukemia with inversion(16): a pilot study. *Journal of Clinical Oncology*, **16**, 1519–25.

Langabeer, S.E., Walker, H. *et al.* (1997). Frequency of CBF beta/MYH11 fusion transcripts in patients entered into the U.K. MRC AML trials. The MRC Adult Leukemia Working Party. *British Journal of Haematology*, **96**, 736–9.

Larson, R.A., Kondo, K. *et al.* (1984). Evidence for a 15;17 translocation in every patient with acute promyelocytic leukemia. *American Journal of Medicine*, **76**, 827–41.

Lin, F., Goldman, J.M. *et al.* (1994). A comparison of the sensitivity of blood and bone marrow for the detection of minimal residual disease in chronic myeloid leukemia. *British Journal of Haematology*, **86**, 683–5.

Lin, F., van Rhee, F., Goldman, J.M., & Cross, N.C.P. (1996). Kinetics of increasing BCR-ABL transcript numbers in chronic myeloid leukemia patients who relapse after bone marrow transplantation. *Blood*, **87**, 4473–8.

Lion, T. (1994). Clinical implications of qualitative and quantitative polymerase chain reaction analysis in the monitoring of patients with chronic myelogenous leukemia. The European Investigators on Chronic Myeloid Leukemia Group. *Bone Marrow Transplantation*, **14**, 505–9.

Liu, P., Claxton, D.F. *et al.* (1993a). Identification of yeast artificial chromosomes containing the inversion 16 p-arm breakpoint associated with acute myelomonocytic leukemia. *Blood*, **82**, 716–21.

Liu, P., Tarle, S.A. *et al.* (1993b). Fusion between transcription factor CBF beta/PEBP2 beta and a myosin heavy chain in acute myeloid leukemia. *Science*, **261**, 1041–4.

Lo Coco, F., Diverio, D. *et al.* (1999). Therapy of molecular relapse in acute promyelocytic leukemia. *Blood,* **94,** 2225–9.

Mackinnon, S., Barnett, L., & Heller, G. (1996). Polymerase chain reaction is highly predictive of relapse in patients following T cell depleted allogeneic bone marrow transplantation for chronic myeloid leukemia. *Bone Marrow Transplantation,* **17,** 643–7.

Mackinnon, S., Barnett, L., Heller, G., & O'Reilly, R.J. (1994). Minimal residual disease is more common in patients who have mixed T-cell chimerism after bone marrow transplantation for chronic myelogenous leukemia. *Blood,* **83,** 3409–16.

Mancini, M, Cedrone, M. *et al.* (2000). Use of dual-color interphase FISH for the detection of inv(16) in acute myeloid leukemia at diagnosis, relapse and during follow-up: a study of 23 patients. *Leukemia,* **14,** 364–8.

Marshall, G.M., Kwan, E. *et al.* (1995). Characterization of clonal immunoglobulin heavy chain and T cell receptor gamma gene rearrangements during progression of childhood acute lymphoblastic leukemia. *Leukemia,* **9,** 1847–50.

Martin, C., Román, J. *et al.* (1996). Absence of detectable PML-RARa fusion transcripts in long-term remission patients after BMT for acute promyelocytic leukemia. *Blood,* **88** (Suppl 1), 366a (Abstract).

Martin, H., Atta, J. *et al.* (1994). In patients with BCR-ABL-positive ALL in CR peripheral blood contains less residual disease than bone marrow: implications for autologous BMT. *Annals of Hematology,* **68,** 85–7.

Meloni, G., Diverio, D., Vignetti, M. *et al.* (1997). Autologous bone marrow transplantation for acute promyelocytic leukemia in second remission: prognostic relevance of pretransplant minimal residual disease assessment by reverse-transcription polymerase chain reaction of the PML/RARα fusion gene. *Blood,* **90,** 1321–5.

Miller, W.H., Jr., Levine, K. *et al.* (1993). Detection of minimal residual disease in acute promyelocytic leukemia by a reverse transcription polymerase chain reaction assay for the PML/RAR-alpha fusion mRNA. *Blood,* **82,** 1689–94.

Miyamoto, T., Nagafuji, K., Akashi, K. *et al.* (1996). Persistency of multipotent progenitors expressing AML 1/ETO transcripts in long term remission patients with t(8;21) acute myelogenous leukemia. *Blood,* **87,** 4789–96.

Miyamura, K., Tanimoto, M. *et al.* (1992). Detection of Philadelphia chromosome-positive acute lymphoblastic leukemia by polymerase chain reaction: possible eradication of minimal residual disease by marrow transplantation. *Blood,* **79,** 1366–70.

Najfeld, V. (1997). FISHing among myeloproliferative disorders. *Seminars in Hematology,* **34,** 55–63.

Ngan, B.Y., Nourse, J. *et al.* (1989). Detection of chromosomal translocation t(14;18) within the minor cluster region of bcl-2 by polymerase chain reaction and direct genomic sequencing of the enzymatically amplified DNA in follicular lymphomas. *Blood,* **73,** 1759–62.

Nirmala, K., Rajalekshmy, K.R. *et al.* (2002). PCR-heteroduplex analysis of TCR gamma, delta and TAL-1 deletions in T-acute lymphoblastic leukemias: implications in the detection of minimal residual disease. *Leukemia Research,* **26,** 335–43.

Nucifora, G., Birn, D.J. *et al.* (1993). Detection of DNA rearrangements in the AML1 and ETO loci and of an AML1/ETO fusion mRNA in patients with t(8;21) acute myeloid leukemia. *Blood,* **81,** 883–8.

Nylund, S.J., Ruutu, T. *et al.* (1994). Detection of minimal residual disease using fluorescence DNA in situ hybridization: a follow-up study in leukemia and lymphoma patients. *Leukemia,* **8,** 587–94.

Ogawa, H., Tamaki, H., Ikegame, K. *et al.* (2002). The usefulness of monitoring WT1 gene transcripts for the prediction and management of relapse following allogeneic stem cell transplantation in acute type leukemia. *Bood,* **101,** 1698–1704.

Olavarria, E., Kanfer, E., Szydlo, R. *et al.* (2001). Early detection of BCR-ABL transcripts by quantitative reverse transcriptase-polymerase chain reaction predicts outcome after allogeneic stem cell transplantation for chronic myeloid leukemia. *Blood,* **97,** 1560–5.

Pandolfi, P.P., Alcalay, M. *et al.* (1992). Genomic variability and alternative splicing generate multiple PML/RAR alpha transcripts that encode aberrant PML proteins and PML/RAR alpha isoforms in acute promyelocytic leukemia. *EMBO Journal,* **11,** 1397–407.

Perego, R.A., Marenco, P., Bianchi, C. *et al.* (1996). PML/RARα transcripts monitored by polymerase chain reaction in acute promyelocytic leukemia during complete remission, relapse and after bone marrow transplantation. *Leukemia,* **10,** 207–12.

Pichert, G., Roy, D.C. *et al.* (1995). Distinct patterns of minimal residual disease associated with graft-versus-host disease after allogeneic bone marrow transplantation for chronic myelogenous leukemia. *Journal of Clinical Oncology,* **13,** 1704–13.

Pignon, J.M., Henni, T. *et al.* (1990). Frequent detection of minimal residual disease by use of the polymerase chain reaction in long-term survivors after bone marrow transplantation for chronic myeloid leukemia. *Leukemia,* **4,** 83–6.

Popescu, N.C. & Zimonjic, D.B. (1997). Molecular cytogenetic characterization of cancer cell alterations. *Cancer Genetics and Cytogenetics,* **93,** 10–21.

Preudhomme, C., Henic, N., Cazin, B. *et al.* (1997). Good correlation between RT-PCR analysis and relapse in Philadelphia (Ph1)-positive acute lymphoblastic leukemia (ALL). *Leukemia,* **11,** 294–8.

Provan, D., Bartlett-Pandite, L. *et al.* (1996). Eradication of polymerase chain reaction-detectable chronic lymphocytic leukemia cells is associated with improved outcome after bone marrow transplantation. *Blood,* **88,** 2228–35.

Radich, J., Gehlyt, G., & Lee, A. (1997). Detection of bcr-abl transcripts in Philadelphia chromosome-positive acute lymphoblastic leukemia after marrow transplantation. *Blood,* **89,** 2602–9.

Radich, J., Ladne, P. *et al.* (1995). Polymerase chain reaction-based detection of minimal residual disease in acute lymphoblastic leukemia predicts relapse after allogeneic BMT. *Biology of Blood and Marrow Transplantation,* **1,** 24–31.

Radich, J.P., Gooley, T., Bryant, E. *et al.* (2001). The significance of bcr-abl molecular detection in chronic myeloid leukemia patients "late," 18 months or more after transplantation. *Blood,* **98,** 1701–7.

Roberts, W.M., Zipf, T.F. *et al.* (1995). Monitoring residual disease in acute lymphoblastic leukemia: therapeutic implications. *Cytokines and Molecular Therapy,* **1,** 65–9.

Román, J., Martín, C., Torres, A. et al. (1997). Absence of detectable PML-RARα fusion transcripts in long-term remission patients after BMT for acute promyelocytic leukemia. *Bone Marrow Transplantation, 19,* 679–83.

Saiki, R.K., Gelfand, D.H. et al. (1988). Primer-directed enzymatic amplification of DNA with a thermostable DNA polymerase. *Science, 239,* 487–91.

Scholten, C., Fodinger, M. et al. (1995). Kinetics of minimal residual disease during induction/consolidation therapy in standard-risk adult B-lineage acute lymphoblastic leukemia. *Annals of Hematology, 71,* 155–60.

Shiramizu, B. & Magrath, I. (1990). Localization of breakpoints by polymerase chain reactions in Burkitt's lymphoma with 8;14 translocations. *Blood, 75,* 1848–52.

Slack, J.L., Bi, W. et al. (2001). Pre-clinical validation of a novel, highly sensitive assay to detect PML-RARalpha mRNA using real-time reverse-transcription polymerase chain reaction. *Journal of Molecular Diagnostics, 3,* 141–9.

Steenbergen, E.J., Verhagen, O.J. et al. (1995). Prolonged persistence of PCR-detectable minimal residual disease after diagnosis or first relapse predicts poor outcome in childhood B-precursor acute lymphoblastic leukemia. *Leukemia, 9,* 1726–34.

Stetlet-Stevenson, M., Raffeld, M. et al. (1988). Detection of occult follicular lymphoma by specific DNA amplification. *Blood, 72,* 1822–5.

Steward, C.G., Goulden, N.J. et al. (1994). A polymerase chain reaction study of the stability of Ig heavy-chain and T-cell receptor delta gene rearrangements between presentation and relapse of childhood B-lineage acute lymphoblastic leukemia. *Blood, 83,* 1355–62.

Sugimoto, T., Das, H. et al. (2000). Quantitation of minimal residual disease in t(8;21)-positive acute myelogenous leukemia patients using real-time quantitative RT-PCR. *American Journal of Hematology, 64,* 101–6.

Szczepanski, T., Willemse, M.J. et al. (2002). Comparative analysis of Ig and TCR gene rearrangements at diagnosis and at relapse of childhood precursor-B-ALL provides improved strategies for selection of stable PCR targets for monitoring of minimal residual disease. *Blood, 99,* 2315–23.

Thompson, J.D., Brodsky, I. et al. (1992). Molecular quantification of residual disease in chronic myelogenous leukemia after bone marrow transplantation. *Blood, 79,* 1629–35.

Tobal, K., Johnson, P.R. et al. (1995). Detection of CBFB/MYH11 transcripts in patients with inversion and other abnormalities of chromosome 16 at presentation and remission. *British Journal of Haematology, 91,* 104–8.

Tsujimoto, Y., Gorham, J. et al. (1985). The t(14;18) chromosome translocations involved in B-cell neoplasma result from mistakes in VDJ joining. *Science, 229,* 1390–3.

van Rhee, F., Lin, F. et al. (1994). Relapse of chronic myeloid leukemia after allogeneic bone marrow transplant: the case for giving donor leukocyte transfusions before the onset of hematologic relapse. *Blood, 83,* 3377–83.

Wasserman, R., Yamada, M. et al. (1992). VH gene rearrangement events can modify the immunoglobulin heavy chain during progression of B-lineage acute lymphoblastic leukemia. *Blood, 79,* 223–8.

Weaver, D.T. & Alt, F.W. (1997). From RAGs to stitches. *Nature, 388,* 428–9.

Weiss, L.M., Warnke, R.A. et al. (1987). Molecular analysis of the t(14;18) chromosomal translocation in malignant lymphomas. *New England Journal of Medicine, 317,* 1185–9.

Yamada, M., Wasserman, R. et al. (1990). Minimal residual disease in childhood B-lineage lymphoblastic leukemia. Persistence of leukemic cells during the first 18 months of treatment. *New England Journal of Medicine, 323,* 448–55.

Zhang, J.G., Lin, F., Chase, A. et al. (1996). Comparison of genomic DNA and cDNA for detection of residual disease after treatment of chronic myeloid leukemia with allogeneic bone marrow transplantation. *Blood, 87,* 2588–93.

zur Stadt, U., Reiter, A. et al. (1997). Detection of translocation t(8;14)(q24;132) in pediatric Burkitt's lymphomas using "long distance" polymerase chain reaction: a new method for diagnosis of Burkitt's lymphomas. *Klinische Padiatrie, 209,* 165–71.

Zwicky, C.S., Maddocks, A.B. et al. (1996). Eradication of polymerase chain reaction detectable immunoglobulin gene rearrangement in non-Hodgkin's lymphoma is associated with decreased relapse after autologous bone marrow transplantation. *Blood, 88,* 3314–22.

106 Detection of minimal residual disease by immunologic techniques

MARTIN ANDREANSKY AND DARIO CAMPANA

Departments of Hematology-Oncology and Pathology, St. Jude Children's Research Hospital, and University of Tennessee College of Medicine, Memphis, USA

Introduction

Measurements of residual tumor cells are important in the clinical management of patients with cancer, but identification of tumor cells by morphology is inherently subjective and imprecise (Campana & Pui, 1955; Szczepanski et al., 2001). In patients with acute leukemia, for example, the morphology of malignant cells and that of normal hematopoietic cells is similar and the lower limit of leukemia detection by morphology is generally considered to be 5% of the bone marrow cell population. Therefore, patients with acute leukemia in remission by this criterion may have as many as 10^{10} undetectable neoplastic cells (Campana & Pui, 1995). The sensitivity of detection of bone marrow metastases in patients with solid tumors by routine histology and cytology is also limited, and single tumor cells and/or small clumps of malignant cells may easily go unappreciated. Detection of neoplastic cells in patients with solid tumors or leukemia with patchy disease distribution may be improved by increasing the number of bone marrow sites sampled (Mathe et al., 1966; Franklin & Pritchard, 1983), but significant improvements can only be achieved by more sensitive and objective methods.

Methods for detecting minimal (submicroscopic) residual disease (MRD) have multiple potential clinical applications. In patients with acute lymphoblastic leukemia (ALL) and acute myeloid leukemia (AML), these assays provide powerful and independent prognostic information. MRD studies before and/or after allogeneic hematopoietic stem cell transplantation can predict the risk of relapse after transplant in patients with acute leukemia and chronic myeloid leukemia (CML). In patients with lymphoma and solid tumors, MRD assays can help clinical staging and detection of tumor dissemination. Finally, in patients with hematologic and nonhematologic malignancies, MRD assays provide a powerful tool for assessing bone marrow or peripheral blood that has been harvested for autologous hematopoietic stem cell transplantation and for determining the efficacy of "purging" procedures.

Cancer cells can be distinguished from normal bone marrow and peripheral blood cells by genetic and immunophenotypic features. The following sections review the methodologic and clinical advances in the detection of MRD in oncology with emphasis on the use of immunologic techniques.

Methods for detecting MRD in hematologic malignancies

Overview of methods

Numerous methods to study MRD in hematologic malignancies have been developed (Table 106.1). Methods proven to be useful in ALL include flow cytometric profiling of aberrant immunophenotypes, polymerase chain reaction (PCR) amplification of fusion transcripts, and PCR amplification of antigen-receptor genes (Campana & Pui, 1995; Szczepanski et al., 2001). In AML, only the first two can be applied, since most cases lack antigen-receptor gene rearrangements (Campana & Pui, 1995). In CML, RT-PCR amplification of BCR-ABL is the method of choice (Goldman et al., 1999). In follicular B-cell lymphoma, PCR amplification of the juxtaposed BCL2 and immunoglobulin heavy chain (IGH) genes or of IGH gene rearrangements is typically used (Gribben, 2002), whereas PCR amplification of clonally rearranged IGH genes and flow cytometry are the most widely applicable methods to monitor MRD in B-cell lymphoproliferative disorders and multiple myeloma (Gribben, 2002; Ladetto et al., 2002; San Miguel et al., 2002). Conventional karyotyping and fluorescence in situ hybridization can occasionally clarify the nature of morphologically suspicious malignant cells, but their sensitivity is limited (1% at most) (Gray et al., 1990; Mancini et al., 2000).

Flow cytometry

Flow cytometry allows the simultaneous analysis of multiple cellular parameters such as cell morphology, viability, and immunophenotype. In addition, a large numbers of cells can be rapidly screened (typically 10,000 cells or more per minute). Additional capabilities of flow cytometry, such as cell sorting followed by fluorescence in situ hybridization (Engel et al., 1997), or analysis of phenotype and DNA content (Nowak et

Table 106.1. *Methodologic options for detecting MRD in patients with hematologic malignancies*

Diagnosis	Method	Potentially suitable cases (%)	Sensitivity
B-lineage ALL	PCR on translocation breakpoints	30–40	0.1%–0.0001%
	PCR on TCRγ and TCRδ genes	40–60	0.1%–0.001%
	PCR on IgH genes	85–95	0.1%–0.001%
	Flow cytometry	85–95	0.01%
T-lineage ALL	PCR on translocation breakpoints and TAL-1	25–35	0.1%–0.0001%
	PCR on TCRγ and TCRδ genes	40–60	0.1%–0.001%
	Flow cytometry	>95	0.01%
AML	PCR on translocation breakpoints	20–30	0.1%–0.0001%
	Flow cytometry	80–90	0.1%–0.01%
CML	PCR on BCR-ABL	100	0.1%–0.0001%
Follicular lymphoma	PCR on BCL2-IGH	85	0.0.%–0.0001%
	PCR on IgH genes	>90	0.1%–0.001%
B-CLL	PCR on IgH genes	>90	0.1%–0.001%
	Flow cytometry	>90	0.01%
Multiple myeloma	PCR on IgH genes	>90	0.1%–0.001%
	Flow cytometry	>90	0.01%

al., 1997), may also aid MRD studies, but these are rarely, if ever, used in routine studies.

Flow cytometers equipped with two lasers are the best instruments currently available for MRD studies because they allow the discrimination of several fluorochromes (Fig. 106.1). For example, the FACSCalibur instrument used in our laboratory is equipped with a 488 nm argon-ion laser and a 655 nm red diode second laser. Among commonly available fluorochromes, the argon-ion laser excites fluorescein isothiocyanate (FITC; 495 nm), phycoerythrin (PE; 480 and 565 nm), and peridinin chlorophyll protein (PerCP; 488 nm), while the red diode laser excites allophycocyanin (APC; 650 nm). The different emission wavelength of each of these fluorochromes (512, 578, 670, and 659 nm, respectively) can be detected as a

Normal bone marrow

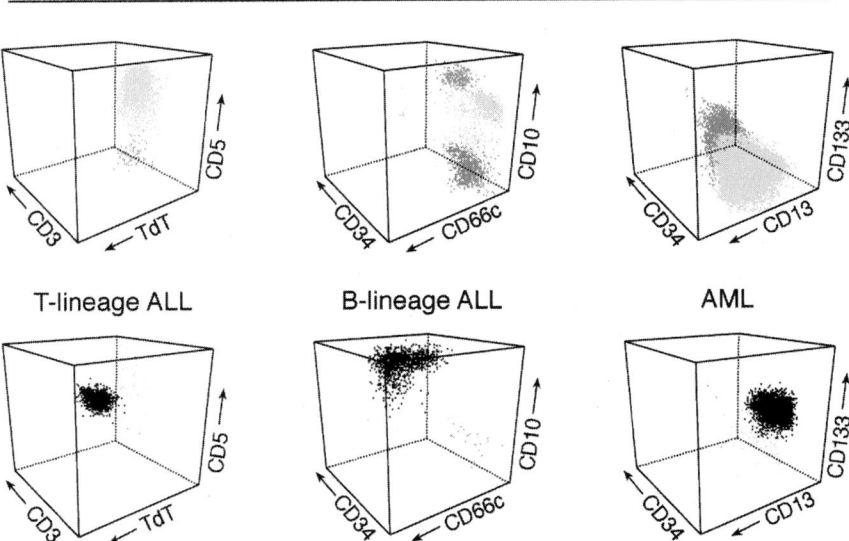

Fig. 106.1. Immunophenotyic differences between normal and leukemic cells demonstrated by 4-color flow cytometry. Three-dimensional dot plots illustrate expression of the indicated markers on bone marrow cells obtained from healthy individuals (top row) and on bone marrow cells obtained from patients with leukemia at diagnosis (bottom row). The analysis was selectively performed on cells with lymphoblast morphology and lacking expression of HLA-DR, CD19, and CD33 (left panels), cells with lymphoblast morphology and expressing CD19 (center panels), and cells with myeloblast morphology and CD33 expression (right panels). For color reproduction, see Color Plate 106.1.

separate signal, thus allowing the simultaneous detection of four markers. Many laboratories have instruments equipped with only the argon-ion laser, allowing detection of only three markers. Although three-color analysis can be used effectively (Coustan-Smith et al., 1998; Lucio et al., 2001), four-color analysis is significantly more informative and allows a more efficient use of cells by reducing the number of tubes required to analyze each sample. Analyzers equipped with an additional ultraviolet laser might further facilitate MRD investigations by allowing the use of five or six markers simultaneously.

The sensitivity of MRD studies by flow cytometry depends on the number of cells that can be analyzed and the degree of morphologic and phenotypic difference between target cells and the remaining cells. Under ideal conditions, that is, a large number of cells (1×10^7 or more) available and phenotypically distinct target cells, one target cell in 10^6 normal cells can be detected (Gross et al., 1993). When MRD is studied in clinical samples, however, the number of cells that can be analyzed for each set of markers is typically lower. Considering that a definite cluster of at least 10 to 20 dots is required to interpret flow cytometric signals, a sensitivity of 1 in 10^4 is probably the maximum that can be expected during routine MRD testing (Campana & Coustan-Smith, 2002).

Markers for MRD studies in ALL

The marker combinations used in our laboratory to detect MRD in children with ALL are summarized in Table 106.2. T-lineage ALL cells express the immunophenotype of normal immature T cells that reside in the thymus and do not normally migrate to the peripheral blood or the bone marrow until they mature and stop expressing terminal deoxynucleotidyl transferase (TdT) and other markers of immaturity (Bradstock et al., 1980; Greaves, 1986). The most useful immunophenotypes for MRD studies in T-ALL are a combination of T-cell markers, such as CD3 and CD5, with TdT or CD34 (Campana & Coustan-Smith, 2002). In a recent multicenter study, expression of T-cell markers with TdT was found in 58 of 64 T-ALL cases, and expression of T-cell markers with CD34 was found in 23 of 58 cases; no cells with these phenotypes were observed in the bone marrow of healthy individuals or nonleukemic patients (Porwit-MacDonald et al., 2000).

B-lineage ALL cells must be distinguished from B-cell progenitors that normally reside in the bone marrow (Janossy et al., 1980; Greaves, 1986), and can also be found in low proportions in the peripheral blood (Froehlich et al., 1981). Several molecules whose expression becomes dysregulated during the leukemic process can be used for this purpose. For example, the human homolog of the rat chondroitin sulfate proteoglycan (NG2), is expressed in B-lineage ALL cells with 11q23 abnormalities (Behm et al., 1996), and CD66c is expressed in approximately 30% to 40% of B-lineage ALL cases (Hanenberg et al., 1994; Mori et al., 1995; Sugita et al., 1999; Carrasco et al., 2000), but neither marker is expressed in normal B-cell progenitors (Campana & Coustan-Smith,

Table 106.2. *Main marker combinations used to study MRD in childhood ALL*

Cell lineage	Marker combination	Applicability (%)[a]
T-lineage ALL	TdT/CD5/CD3	90–95
	CD34/CD5/CD3	20–25
B-lineage ALL	CD19/CD34/CD10/CD38	40–60
	CD19/CD34/CD10/CD58	40–60
	CD19/CD34/CD10/CD45	40–60
	CD19/CD34/CD10/TdT	40–50
	CD19/CD34/CD10/CD66c	30–40
	CD19/CD34/TdT/IgM	10–20
	CD19/CD34/CD10/CD22	10–15
	CD19/CD34/CD10/CD13	10–15
	CD19/CD34/CD10/CD15	10–15
	CD19/CD34/CD10/NG-2	5–10

[a] Percentage of patients within each type of leukemia in whom MRD could be studied with the listed antibody combination. Percentages were calculated by including only cases in which intensity of antigen expression was sufficiently different from that of normal bone marrow cells to afford a sensitivity of detection of 1 in 10^4 for ALL.

2002). Other molecules may be expressed at abnormally high or low levels in B-lineage ALL cells (Hurwitz et al., 1988; Reading et al., 1993; Wells et al., 1998; Dworzak et al., 1998; Campana & Coustan-Smith, 1999; Ciudad et al., 1999; Lucio et al., 2001). This is the case for CD19, CD10, TdT and CD34 (Lavabre-Bertrand et al., 1994; Farahat et al., 1998; Campana & Coustan-Smith, 1999), and CD38 and CD45 (Dworzak et al., 1998; Campana & Coustan-Smith, 1999). The myeloid-associated markers CD13, CD15, and CD65 can be expressed by CD19+CD34+ B-lineage ALL cells, whereas normal CD19+CD34+ B-cell progenitors do not express these markers or express them very weakly (Campana & Coustan-Smith, 1999).

The identification of markers useful to distinguish leukemic cells from normal hematopoietic progenitors requires extensive studies of normal bone marrow cells collected under a variety of different conditions, including active proliferation following chemotherapy or hematopoietic cell transplantation (Campana & Coustan-Smith, 2002). In general, the larger the number of normal cells analyzed, the larger the confines of immunophenotypic normality becomes (Fig. 106.2). This type of analysis may reveal that immunophenotypes thought to be leukemia-specific are also expressed by rare subsets of normal cells.

Markers for MRD studies in AML

AML cells may express markers normally not expressed on myeloid cells, co-express markers normally expressed at different stages of maturation, or express markers at different levels of intensity than normal myeloid cells (Bradstock et al., 1986; Campana et al., 1990; Terstappen & Loken, 1990; Terstappen et al., 1992; Adriaansen et al., 1993; Reading et al., 1993).

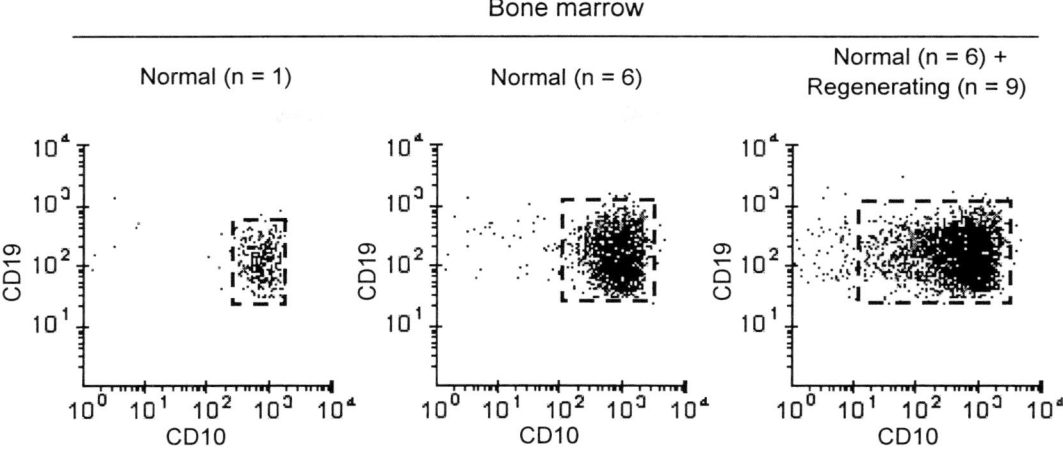

Fig. 106.2. The limits of normality expand when increasing numbers of normal and regenerating bone marrow samples are studied. Bone marrow mononuclear cells were collected from healthy individuals and patients with leukemia recovering from chemotherapy but MRD-negative by flow cytometry and PCR. Cells were labeled with CD19-allophycocyanin, CD10-phycoerythrin, and CD34-fluorescein isothyocyanate. Expression of CD19 and CD10 on selectively gated CD19+CD34+ lymphoid cells is shown. The left panel is a dot plot of 1 sample from a healthy individual. The middle and right panels are overlaid dot plots, illustrating the collective results of 6 samples from healthy individuals (middle), and of 15 samples (6 from healthy individuals and 9 from leukemia patients after chemotherapy). Dot plot overlaying was done with the FCS Express software (DeNovo Software, Thornhill, Ontario, Canada). Dashed rectangles limit areas of normality as defined by each set of samples.

However, only a fraction of cells may be phenotypically abnormal with a given marker combination (Campana & Coustan-Smith, 1999). Although this may reduce the sensitivity of the assay in some cases, reliable MRD detection in AML is possible. In recent studies with four-color flow cytometry, we have identified immunophenotypic combinations that allow measurement of MRD with a sensitivity of 1 leukemic cell among 10,000 or more normal cells in at least 40% of children, and 1 leukemic cell among 1,000 cells in an additional 40% (Table 106.3). One study reported that leukemic cells expressed abnormal immunophenotypes in 175 of 233 adult patients with AML (San Miguel et al., 2001). In another study, cells with abnormal immunophenotypes, sufficiently distinctive to allow detection of 1 leukemic cell in 10,000 normal cells, were found in 65 of 93 patients (Venditti et al., 2000).

The percentage of patients that can be studied is proportional to the degree of specificity of the markers used. For example, a study in which leukemic cells in all 39 children with AML expressed a phenotype suitable for flow cytometric studies of MRD used an assay that only allowed detection of 1 leukemic cell in 100 to 1,000 normal bone marrow cells (Sievers et al., 1996).

Markers for MRD studies in lymphoproliferative disorders and multiple myeloma

Detection of tumor cells in patients with T-cell lymphoblastic lymphoma can be accomplished with an approach identical to that used to study MRD in T-lineage ALL. That is, lymphoma cells can be identified by the expression of nuclear TdT and T cell markers such as CD3 or CD5.

Immunologic detection of MRD in B-cell lymphoproliferative disorders may be attempted by searching for a B-cell clonal excess based on the expression of either kappa or lambda immunoglobulin light chains. This approach, however, has limited sensitivity, typically around 1% (Bagwell et al., 1988). More recently, expression of other markers has been used to distinguish neoplastic from normal B cells. For example, CD19 expression is usually lower in cells from mature B-cell disorders (except prolymphocytic leukemia), whereas the intensity of CD5 is significantly higher in B-CLL cells, and

Table 106.3. *Main marker combinations used to study MRD in childhood AML*

Marker combination	Applicability (%)[a]
CD33/CD34/CD117/CD15	20–40
CD33/CD34/CD117/CD13	20–40
CD13/CD33/CD34/CD56	20–30
CD13/CD33/CD34/CD133	20–30
CD13/CD33/CD34/CD7	20–30
CD13/CD33/CD34/CD38	15–20
CD33/CD34/CD117/HLA-Dr	15–20
CD13/CD33/CD34/CD15	15–20
CD33/CD34/CD117/CD11b	10–15
CD13/CD33/CD34/CD19	5–10

[a] Percentage of patients within each type of leukemia in whom MRD could be studied with the listed antibody combination. Percentages were calculated by including only cases in which intensity of antigen expression was sufficiently different from that of normal bone marrow cells to afford a sensitivity of detection of 1 in 10^3 or greater for AML.

CD79b is generally expressed at lower levels in all types of mature leukemic cells compared to normal B-lymphocytes (Cabezudo *et al.*, 1999; Garcia *et al.*, 1999). A flow cytometric assay relying on CD19/CD5/CD20/CD79b expression could reportedly detect one B-CLL cell in 10^4 to 10^5 leukocytes in all patients (Rawstron *et al.*, 2001).

Flow cytometry can also be used to detect MRD in multiple myeloma. Simultaneous measurement of DNA content and myeloma-related antigens (B-B4 or CD38) could detect aneuploid plasma cells in peripheral blood stem cell harvests and in bone marrow after therapy (Nowak *et al.*, 1999). In 13 of 23 harvests aneuploid myeloma cells were detectable ranging from 0.02% to 0.63%. In the bone marrow of 30 patients aneuploid plasma cells were detectable in all samples after chemotherapy, ranging from 0.12% to 35.7%. Almeida *et al.* (1999) used 21 antibodies to study 61 bone marrow samples from untreated multiple myeloma patients and found aberrant phenotypes in 87%. The most important aberrant parameters were overexpression of CD56 (62%), CD28 (16%), and CD33 (6%) and asynchronous expression of CD117 (28%), surface immunoglobulin (21%), and CD20 (10%). DNA aneuploidy was found in 62% of cases. The simultaneous use of these two techniques in combination with the selective analysis of cells expressing CD38 and CD138 allowed the detection of aberrant/aneuploid plasma cells in 95% of the cases with a sensitivity of 1 in 10^4–10^5.

Clinical relevance of MRD in hematologic malignancies

Acute lymphoblastic leukemia

Detection of MRD by immunologic or molecular techniques in patients with ALL in clinical remission is independently associated with treatment outcome (Coustan-Smith *et al.*, 1998; Ciudad *et al.*, 1998; Cave *et al.*, 1998; Farahat *et al.*, 1998; van Dongen *et al.*, 1998; Szczepanski *et al.*, 2001). We prospectively studied MRD in 629 bone marrow aspirates collected from 195 children with newly diagnosed ALL after remission-induction therapy and at three intervals thereafter (Coustan-Smith *et al.*, 1998, 2000). Detectable MRD (i.e., ≥0.01% leukemic mononuclear cells) at any of these time points was associated with a significantly higher rate of relapse; patients with high levels of MRD after the induction phase (≥1%) or at week 14 of continuation therapy (≥0.1%) had a particularly poor outcome. The predictive strength of MRD remained significant even after considering known adverse presenting features.

We also prospectively quantified residual leukemic cells among bone marrow mononuclear cells collected at day 19 of remission induction chemotherapy from 248 children with newly diagnosed ALL (Coustan-Smith *et al.*, 2002a). In 134 samples (54.0%) we indentified ≥0.01% leukemic cells. Of these, only 32 (12.9%) had leukemic lymphoblasts identifiable by morphology; in 21 (8.5%) samples lymphoblasts rep-

resented ≥5% of bone marrow mononuclear cells, and in 11 lymphoblasts ranged from 1% to 4% (Fig. 106.3). MRD negativity at day 19 identified patients with excellent treatment outcome. The prognostic strength of day 19 bone marrow status defined by flow cytometry was superior to that defined by morphology, and remained significant after adjusting for other clinical and biologic parameters. Lack of detectable leukemic cells at day 19 was more closely associated with relapse-free survival than lack of detectable residual disease at the end of remission induction (day 46). Because of these results, MRD testing during treatment is being used to guide the intensity of therapy in the current clinical protocols for children with ALL at our institution.

MRD measurements in ALL patients have also been shown to be informative in the context of hematopoietic stem cell transplantation. MRD monitoring of BCR-ABL fusion transcripts predicted treatment outcome in patients with t(9;22) who underwent allogeneic or autologous bone marrow transplantation (Radich *et al.*, 1997). MRD detected by PCR amplification of antigen receptor genes in children with ALL prior to

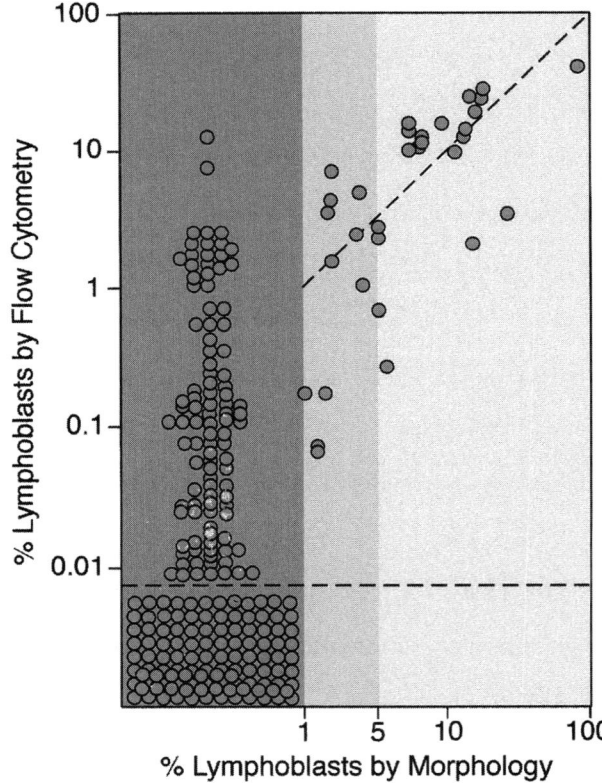

Fig. 106.3. Comparison between morphologic and flow cytometric assessment of residual disease at day 19 of remission induction therapy in children with ALL. Each dot corresponds to the percentage of leukemic cells identified by morphology (x axis) and by flow cytometry (y axis) in bone marrow samples collected at day 19 from 248 children with newly diagnosed ALL. Reproduced, with permission, from Coustan-Smith *et al.* (2002a).

allogeneic bone marrow transplantation was predictive of subsequent relapse (Knechtli *et al.,* 1998). The same group also found that MRD detected after transplantation was indicative of unfavorable outcome (Goulden *et al.,* 1998).

Acute myeloid leukemia

Antigen-receptor genes are rearranged in leukemic cells of less than 10% of patients with AML, and less than half of all patients with AML have nonrandom genetic abnormalities that can be detected by RT-PCR (Liu & Grimwade, 2002). Therefore, studies to detect a correlation between MRD and treatment outcome have been performed only in selected groups of patients, almost exclusively adults. In acute promyelocytic leukemia, PCR detection of PML-RARA transcripts during remission is associated with a high risk of relapse (Grimwade, 1999; Lo Coco *et al.,* 1999). The significance of detecting AML1-ETO transcripts in patients with t(8;21) AML in clinical remission is less clear. Early studies showed that expression of this transcript persists for as long as 12 years of remission after the completion of treatment (Nucifora *et al.,* 1993; Miyamoto *et al.,* 1996; Guerrasio *et al.,* 1995). An explanation for these findings is provided by the finding of AML1-ETO transcripts in apparently normal monocytes, B cells, and hematopoietic colony-forming cells (Miyamoto *et al.,* 2000). Despite the lack of strict association between AML1-ETO transcripts and AML cells, careful quantitation of these transcripts might help to predict overt relapse in patients with t(8;21) AML (Tobal *et al.,* 2000; Morschhauser *et al.,* 2000 Sugimoto *et al.,* 2000).

Several studies have indicated that detection of MRD by flow cytometry during clinical remission is associated with a higher incidence of relapse in patients with AML (Reading *et al.,* 1993; Sievers *et al.,* 1996; Venditti *et al.,* 2000; San Miguel *et al.,* 2001). One study showed that cut-off levels during MRD monitoring of 2–5 leukemic cells in 10^3 normal cells yielded good correlations with outcome, suggesting that a sensitivity of 1 in 10^3 would be sufficiently informative in such patients (San Miguel *et al.,* 1997). In another study, the informative cut-off level was lower (3.5–4.5 in 10^4) (Venditti *et al.,* 2000). A report from San Miguel's group indicated that patients with less than 1 leukemic cell in 10^4 after induction treatment had an excellent response to therapy suggesting that a highly sensitive technique would be most informative (San Miguel *et al.,* 2001). Of note, in patients with AML receiving autologous bone marrow transplantation, levels of cells expressing aberrant immunophenotype in the autograft correlated with disease recurrence (Reichle *et al.,* 1999).

Lymphoproliferative disorders and multiple myeloma

In patients with B-cell lymphoma, detection of residual disease in the bone marrow by PCR amplification of BCL2/IGH is predictive of outcome in the context of autologous bone marrow transplantation (Gribben, 2002). For example, in two studies including 83 patients (with advanced stage, previously untreated, follicular lymphoma) and 153 patients (with relapsed indolent follicular lymphoma) who underwent myeloablative therapy and anti-B-cell monoclonal antibody-purged autologous bone marrow transplantation, patients whose marrow was PCR-negative after purging experienced significantly longer freedom from recurrence than those whose marrow remained PCR-positive (Freedman *et al.,* 1996, 1999). Continued PCR negativity in follow-up samples was also strongly predictive of continued remission.

A study that investigated the significance of MRD detected by flow cytometry in 21 patients with B-CLL in complete or partial remission found that persistence of MRD was a predictor of time to progression (Cabezudo *et al.,* 1997). However, only two patients, who underwent allogeneic bone marrow transplantation, achieved "immunological" remission, defined as percentage of CD5+ CD19+/total CD19+ cells <25% in peripheral blood and <15% in bone marrow. Another study compared flow cytometry to conventional assessment in 104 patients with B-CLL treated with CAMPATH-1H and/or autologous transplantation (Rawstron *et al.,* 2001). During CAMPATH-1H therapy, circulating CLL cells were rapidly depleted in responding patients, but remained detectable in nonresponders. In 25 out of 104 patients achieving complete remission, residual bone marrow disease at levels higher than 0.05% was detected in 6 out of 25 patients, a finding that predicted a significantly poorer event-free and overall survival.

In a study of 87 patients with multiple myeloma, bone marrow samples were evaluated by flow cytometry 3 months after autologous stem cell transplantation or after 12 cycles of chemotherapy (San Miguel *et al.,* 2002). Patients with low levels of residual disease after treatment (<0.12% myeloma plasma cells) had a trend toward improved progression-free survival. Patients in whom at least 30% of plasma cells had a normal phenotype had a significantly longer progression-free survival than patients with less than 30% normal plasma cells (median 60 ± 6 months versus 34 ± 12 months; $P = .02$). Other investigators compared samples of peripheral blood and "backup" bone marrow from 13 patients using PCR amplification of IGH genes (Vescio *et al.,* 1996). The percentage of myeloma cells in marrow (median, 0.74%) was higher than in the blood (median, 0.0024%).

Methods for detecting MRD in nonhematologic malignancies

Microscopy: immunocytochemistry and immunofluorescence

Immunocytochemistry has been extensively used to detect residual disease in patients with solid tumors. The method has high sensitivity and allows detection of 1 tumor cell among 10^5–10^6 normal cells (Moss *et al.,* 1991; Osborne *et al.,* 1991; Franklin *et al.,* 1996). A study that directly compared the sensitivity of immunocytochemistry to that of standard histology and of RT-PCR targeting GAGE and tyrosine hydroxylase (TH) in 259 bone marrow samples from 99 patients with neuroblastoma found that immunocytochemistry and GAGE RT-PCR had a similar sensitivity, superior to that of the other two techniques (Cheung & Cheung, 2001). Immunocytochemistry is labor-intensive, but improvements in computerized image analysis promise to significantly curb this limitation. A study of residual breast cancer cells in bone marrow specimens found that in 17 of the 39 cases specimens were classified by a pathologist as positive for tumor cells after automated cellular image analysis, whereas the same pathologist failed to identify tumor cells on the same slides after analysis by manual microscopy (Bauer et al., 2000).

Analysis of multiple markers by immunocytochemistry requires sequential enzymatic reactions. These are cumbersome and difficult to reproduce in a routine pathology laboratory setting. Therefore, only single marker analysis is usually feasible. The use of immunofluorescence should be advantageous in this regard because multiple markers can be analyzed simultaneously, thus refining the immunophenotypic identification of tumor cells. In principle, sensitivity should be comparable to that of immunocytochemistry (Osborne et al., 1989). In one study, it was found that two-color immunofluorescence was superior to immunocytochemistry and consistently detected one breast cancer cell contaminating 10^6 normal bone marrow cells (Vredenburgh et al., 1996). However, the lack of permanent results and the difficulties in determining the morphology of the cells with a given immunophenotype have limited the popularity of this technology. An interesting application of immunofluorescence was proposed by Mehes et al. (2001), who identified residual neuroblastoma cells by immunofluorescence labeling with a monoclonal antibody specific for ganglioside GD2, searched for GD2+ and obtained the coordinates of their location on the microscope slide using a fluorescence microscope-based automatic image analysis system, then performed fluorescence in situ hybridization and examined cytogenetic aberrations in GD2+ cells using the recorded coordinates.

Flow cytometry

As outlined for hematologic malignancies, the advantages of flow cytometry include objectivity and ability to rapidly analyze a large number of cells. Sensitivity under well-controlled experimental conditions can be extremely high. However, during analysis of MRD in clinical samples, conditions may be not as favorable as in an experimental setting. Authors have reported detection of one breast cancer cell mixed with 2×10^5 peripheral blood cells using two-color analysis (Simpson et al., 1995), and of one breast cancer cell mixed with 10^7 peripheral blood cells using four-color analysis (Gross et al., 1995). Other investigators could detect one breast carcinoma cell in 10^4 bone marrow cells using five monoclonal antibodies reactive against epithelial cell surface determinants (Leslie et al., 1990).

Flow cytometric methods to detect neuroblastoma cells are being progressively refined. In two studies, staining with a combination of antibodies to CD9 (or CD81), CD56 and CD45 identified one neuroblastoma cell in 10^4–10^5 bone marrow or peripheral blood cells (Komada et al., 1998; Nagai et al., 2002). An example of this type of analysis is shown in Fig. 106.4.

Immunomagnetic enrichment of tumor cells

In efforts to increase the sensitivity of tumor cell detection by immunologic or molecular methods, samples can be subjected to an enrichment step, in which antibody-labeled tumor cells are separated by magnetic cell sorting. One study applied cell staining of cytokeratin 8 (after cell permeabilization) followed by magnetic selection of antibody-labeled cells to mixtures of 5–5,000 breast cancer cells with 1.2×10^8 peripheral blood leukocytes and found that tumor cells were enriched by a factor of $10,477 \pm 4,242$ ($n = 25$) (Martin et al., 1998). With the same method, these authors could detect 1–6.8×10^4 cytokeratin-expressing tumor cells in the peripheral blood of 21 of 34 patients with advanced carcinomas of the breast, prostate, colon, rectum, or lung.

From the literature, it is not entirely clear to what extent the enrichment step is beneficial in practice. The enrichment step enhanced detection of breast cancer cells approximately three- to fourfold over direct immunocytochemistry in one study (Naume et al., 1997) and fivefold in another (Berois et al., 1997). In a study of 104 bone marrow or peripheral blood samples obtained from breast cancer patients, cancer cells were enriched by using conjugates directed against the human epithelial antigen and then labeled with anti-cytokeratin (Kruger et al., 2000). The cytokeratin-positive rate increased significantly, from 29.9% before selection to 54.8% after enrichment. Others found that immunomagnetic enrichment with a panel of antibodies afforded a sensitivity of detection of breast cancer cells that was approximately 50-fold greater than that of standard immunocytochemistry (Umiel et al., 2000). In 26 peripheral blood stem cell harvests from 14 patients, breast cancer cells were found in 19 samples from 12 patients using immunomagnetic enrichment. If the enrichment was omitted, breast cancer cells were detected in only 2 specimens from 1 patient. Other investigators, however, found no significant advantage in using an enrichment technique, consisting of an antibody (BerEp4) targeting the 17-1A antigen coupled to magnetic beads, prior to immunocytochemistry in a study of bone marrow aspirates from 70 patients with breast cancer (Kasimir-Bauer et al., 2001).

In efforts to further refine detection of tumor cells, some authors have used a combination of immunomagnetic enrichment with multiparameter flow cytometric and immunocytochemical analysis (Racila et al., 1998). Peripheral blood from 30 patients with breast cancer and 3 patients with prostate cancer, and from 13 healthy individuals were studied. While the average number of epithelial cells per blood sample was 1.5 in healthy controls, the number was 15.9 to 122 in breast cancer patients at various stages of disease, and 16 per blood sample in 3 patients with localized prostate cancer. A similar methodology

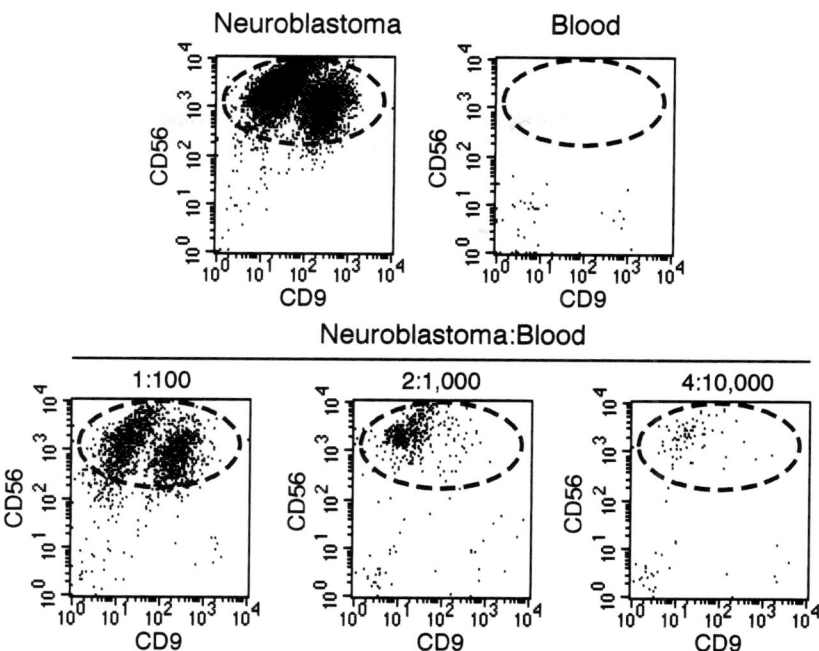

Fig. 106.4. Detection of neuroblastoma cells by flow cytometry. The neuroblastoma cell line SKNSH and normal peripheral blood mononuclear cells were labeled with antibodies to CD45, CD9, and CD56. Mixtures of neuroblastoma cells with peripheral blood at the ratios indicated were also studied. Flow cytometric dot plots show CD9 and CD56 staining after excluding CD45$^+$ cells from the analysis. The dashed line encloses an area consistently empty in studies of normal peripheral blood.

was used to compare 20 patients with localized and metastatic prostate cancer to 22 healthy male controls for the presence of circulating tumor cells (Moreno *et al.*, 2001). In healthy individuals, an average of 0.8 cells per blood sample were detected, whereas 10 patients with localized prostate cancer averaged 5.9 cells per blood sample, and 10 patients with metastatic prostate cancer averaged 46.6 cells per blood sample.

Markers to detect MRD in nonhematologic malignancies

Markers currently used to identify nonhematologic cancer cells are generally expressed in cell types not normally found in bone marrow or peripheral blood. For example, cytokeratins (CK) are integral components of the cytoskeleton of epithelial cells (Pantel & von Knebel, 2000). Ectopic expression of cytokeratins is widely used to detect neoplastic epithelial cells among hematopoietic cells in bone marrow and blood (Schlimok *et al.*, 1987, 1990, 1991; Diel *et al.*, 1992; Pantel *et al.*, 1993; Harbeck *et al.*, 1994; Pantel & von Knebel, 2000). Some antibodies (e.g., A45-B/B3) react with common epitopes of different cytokeratins. Some investigators have pointed out that, among the markers used to track breast cancer cells, only maspin and mammoglobin met the criteria of sensitivity and specificity required for the detection of residual disease: they were expressed in 80% and 97% of breast cancer specimens, respectively, and not expressed in normal controls (Corradini *et*

al., 2001). By contrast, CK19, MUC-1, and CEA were sometimes expressed in normal blood cells and/or hematological tumors.

Table 106.4 lists markers that have been used to identify tumor cells by immunologic or molecular techniques. Several researchers have found it advantageous to use multiple antibodies in "cocktail" combination rather than rely on a single antibody for the detection of occult tumor cells (Cote *et al.*, 1988; Moss *et al.*, 1991; Franklin *et al.*, 1996). This approach takes into consideration the fact that tumor cells often have antigen heterogeneity. In addition, antigen expression can be altered by factors such as chemotherapy, radiotherapy, or the natural progression of the disease. Therefore, the use of multiple antibodies may lead to increased sensitivity.

Clinical relevance of MRD in nonhematologic malignancies

Occult bone marrow metastasis

With the use of more sensitive methods of tumor detection, it has become apparent that occult bone marrow metastases occur frequently, regardless of the malignancy (Osborne *et al.*, 1989; Leslie *et al.*, 1990; Schlimok *et al.*, 1990; Moss *et al.*, 1991; Riesenberg *et al.*, 1993; Franklin *et al.*, 1996; Braun *et al.*, 2000, 2001). Using an anti-cytokeratin antibody and cytopreparations of mononuclear cells isolated from bone marrow aspi-

Table 106.4.   *Markers for detecting disseminated cancer cells*

Cancer	Marker	Detection method	References[a]
Breast	Maspin	RT-PCR	Luppi *et al.*, 1996
	Mammoglobin	RT-PCR	Zach *et al.*, 1999
	CK19	ICC/RT-PCR	Traystman *et al.*, 1997
	Pan-CK	ICC	Braun *et al.*, 2000
	CK, MUC1, CEA	RT-PCR	Berois *et al.*, 2000
	CK, EpCAM	ICC	Kasimir-Bauer *et al.*, 2001
Non-small-cell lung	CK18	ICC	Pantel *et al.*, 1996
	EpCAM	ICC	Kubuschok *et al.*, 1999
	MUC1	RT-PCR	Salerno *et al.*, 1998
Gastric	CK18, u-PAR	ICC	Heiss *et al.*, 2002
Colorectal	CK18	ICC	Schlimok *et al.*, 1990
	CK20	ICC	Yokoyama *et al.*, 2002
		RT-PCR	Weitz *et al.*, 1999
Prostate	PSA, CK18	ICC	Riesenberg *et al.*, 1993
	CK18	ICC	Pantel *et al.*, 1995
	PSA	RT-PCR	Deguchi *et al.*, 1997
Thyroid	TG	RT-PCR	Ditkoff *et al.*, 1996
	TG,TP	RT-PCR	Tallini *et al.*, 1998
	CK20	RT-PCR	Weber *et al.*, 2002
Melanoma	Tyrosinase	RT-PCR	Smith *et al.*, 1991
	MAGE	RT-PCR	Brasseur *et al.*, 1995
Neuroblastoma	GD2	ICC	Cheung *et al.*, 1986
	GD2 + others	ICC	Moss *et al.*, 1991
	GD2 + others	ICC	Seeger *et al.*, 2000
	TH, GAGE, MAGE	RT-PCR	Cheung & Cheung, 2000
Germ cell	β-HCG	RT-PCR	Fan *et al.*, 1998
	β-HCG, FN-EDB, AP, CD44 (v8-10), EGFR, XIST	RT-PCR	Bokemeyer *et al.*, 2001

Abbreviations: CK, cytokeratin; CEA, carcinoembryonic antigen; EpCAM, epithelial cellular adhesion molecule; u-PAR, urokinase plasminogen activator receptor; PSA, prostate-specific antigen; TG, thyroglobulin; TP, thyroid peroxidase; TH, tyroxine hydroxylase; β-HCG, human chorionic gonadotrophin; FN-EDB, fibronectin (EDB variant); AP, germ cell and placental alkaline phosphatase; EGFR, epidermal growth factor receptor; RT-PCR, reverse transcriptase polymerase chain reaction; ICC, immunocytochemistry.
[a] Examples of studies where the markers listed were used.

rates, disseminated tumor cells were found in approximately 25% to 60% of patients with nonmetastatic carcinomas, but tumor cells were generally in very low numbers (around 1 in 10^5 mononuclear bone marrow cells or fewer) (Pantel & von Knebel, 2000). Several studies have indicated the prognostic value of detecting disseminated epithelial tumor cells in the bone marrow in patients with breast (Diel *et al.*, 1996; Mansi *et al.*, 1999; Braun *et al.*, 2000; Kasimir-Bauer *et al.*, 2002), colorectal (Lindemann *et al.*, 1992), gastric (Schlimok *et al.*, 1991), pancreatic (Roder *et al.*, 1999), esophagus (Thorban *et al.*, 1996), and non-small-cell lung carcinoma (Pantel *et al.*, 1996).

Recently, three different studies, using different techniques, showed that in patients with high-risk neuroblastoma, detection of tumor cells in bone marrow correlated with a significantly worse outcome. In a study by the Children's Cancer Group, immunocytology was used to assess bone marrow for neuroblastoma cells (Seeger *et al.*, 2000). A study by another group used RT-PCR to detect tyrosine hydroxylase expression

(Fukuda *et al.*, 2001), whereas a third group used RT-PCR to detect GAGE expression (Cheung *et al.*, 2000). While the first two studies showed correlation between poor outcome and persistence of bone marrow disease after induction therapy, the third study showed correlation of poor outcome with bone marrow disease 24 months after chemotherapy.

Residual tumor cells in peripheral blood stem cell products

Investigators have used peripheral blood instead of bone marrow as a source of hematopoietic stem cells in patients with bone marrow metastases, believing that peripheral blood grafts would contain fewer tumor cells than the contaminated marrow. Studies of MRD, however, have revealed that contamination of peripheral blood with malignant cells is common (Shpall *et al.*, 1997). Studies in breast cancer patients have shown that approximately 20% to 25% of patients with disseminated disease have contamination of the peripheral blood stem cell product (Moss & Ross, 1992; Shpall et al., 1994). In a study of 133 such specimens obtained from 48 patients, tumor contamination was found in 13 specimens from 9 women by immunocytochemistry (Ross et al., 1993). Another study evaluated the contamination of peripheral blood stem cell products in over 100 breast cancer patients with stage II and III disease and reported a 12% incidence (Weaver et al., 1998). The presence of marrow disease is associated with a high rate of positive peripheral blood stem cell samples in patients with stage IV breast cancer (Shpall et al., 1997; Moss, 1999).

A study of 35 patients with stage III, stage IV, and stage IVS neuroblastoma evaluated 51 concomitant paired peripheral blood and bone marrow samples for the presence of neuroblastoma cells using monoclonal anti-GD2 antibody (Faulkner et al., 1998). Twenty-eight patients had evidence of bone marrow disease. Of the 18 patients with less than 10^4 neuroblastoma cells per 10^6 mononuclear cells, six patients had detectable neuroblastoma cells in the peripheral blood. However, of 10 patients with more than 10^4 neuroblastoma cells per 10^6 mononuclear cells in bone marrow, concomitant blood sample was positive for neuroblastoma cells in 9 patients. Another study evaluated paired bone marrow and peripheral blood stem cell harvests in 198 samples from 11 patients with Ewing's sarcoma or neuroblastoma for the presence of tumor cells using RT-PCR assay for PGP 9.5 and immunohistochemistry for neuroblastoma-specific antigens (Leung et al., 1998). Tumor cells were detected in peripheral blood stem cells in 9 of 11 patients and bone marrow harvests in 8 of 9 patients, although bone marrow of all patients was negative for tumor by clinical histology.

The number of contaminating cells in peripheral blood stem cell harvests may increase with increasing number of phereses. In a study in which 101 patients with stage IV breast cancer were evaluated by immunocytochemistry, patients who had positive stem cell products had a median number of four phereses, compared to two for the negative group (Weaver et al., 1998). It has also been shown that the percentage of patients with breast cancer cells in peripheral blood harvests markedly increases following mobilization with chemotherapy and growth factors (Brugger et al., 1994).

The most direct evidence that tumor-contaminated grafts contribute to relapse has been from studies with patients with leukemia and neuroblastoma (Rill et al., 1992; Brenner et al., 1993). In these studies, gene-transfected tumor cells from reinfused harvested marrow were found in patients who relapsed posttransplant. There are data in other neoplasms that suggest tumor contamination is associated with a poor clinical outcome (Table 106.5). In breast cancer, for example, a number of studies have found an association between the presence of marrow disease and poor clinical outcome after autologous HSC transplantation (Fields et al., 1996; Vredenburgh et al., 1995, 1997). However, presence of neuroblastoma cells in peripheral blood stem cells at the time of harvest, as determined by tyrosine hydroxylase RT-PCR, appeared to be associated with clinical outcome but was not clearly predictive (Burchill et al., 2001).

Future perspectives

Over the past two decades there has been great progress in methodologies suitable for MRD detection and in the understanding of the clinical significance of MRD. This progress has propelled MRD investigation to the forefront of the clinical arena and MRD assays are now used by many investigators to select a treatment strategy. There is, however, considerable room for improvement in the methodological aspects of MRD

Table 106.5. *Prognostic value of MRD detection at the time of stem cell collection in patients undergoing autologous HSC transplantation*

Cancer	Marker	Method	No. of patients	Autologous stem cell source	Prognostic value	Reference
Breast Stage II–IV	CK19	RT-PCR	83	Bone marrow	No (stage II–III) Yes (stage IV)	Fields et al., 1996
Breast Stage II–III	CK[a]	ICC	114	Peripheral blood	No	Weaver et al., 1998
Breast Stage IV	CK[a]	ICC	57	Peripheral blood and/or bone marrow	No	Cooper et al., 1998
Breast Stage II–IV	CK	ICC	43	Peripheral blood	No (stage II–III) Yes (stage IV)	Kasimir-Bauer et al., 2001
Neuroblastoma Stage IV	GD2[b]	ICC	195	Bone marrow	Yes	Seeger et al., 2000
Neuroblastoma Stage III–IV	TH	RT-PCR	18	Peripheral blood	No	Burchill et al., 2001
Germ cell	Various[c]	RT-PCR	50	Peripheral blood	No	Bokemeyer et al., 2001

Abbreviations: CK, cytokeratin; TH, tyrosine hydroxylase, RT-PCR, reverse-transcriptase polymerase chain reaction.
[a] CK and other breast cancer-associated markers.
[b] GD2 and other neuroblastoma markers.
[c] Various markers were used (see Table 106.4).

detection, particularly in the identification of specific and robust markers.

Immunologic techniques for detecting MRD rely on phenotypic differences between cancer cells and normal hematopoietic cells. These phenotypic differences are particularly difficult to identify in hematologic malignancies. We used microarrays that allow genome-wide analysis of gene expression to identify new markers for MRD studies in B-lineage ALL (Chen et al., 2001). By this approach, we could compare expression of ~4,000 genes in B-lineage ALL cells and purified normal B-cell progenitors, thus identifying several molecules overexpressed in leukemic cells. These studies led to the identification of CD58 as a useful marker for MRD in B-lineage ALL (Chen et al., 2001), and promise to identify several others. These results suggest that a comparison of the gene profiles of normal and leukemic cells will identify new, widely applicable markers for MRD studies, and should ultimately allow the design of simple antibody panels for practical, reliable, and universal monitoring of MRD.

Another methodological aspect to resolve is the relative clinical significance of detecting MRD in peripheral blood versus bone marrow. We determined that findings in marrow and blood were completely concordant in 150 paired samples from patients with T-lineage ALL (Coustan-Smith et al., 2002). In B-lineage ALL, however, only 37 of the 104 positive marrow samples had a corresponding positive blood samples, and peripheral-blood MRD in these patients was associated with a very high risk of disease recurrence. These results indicate that disease distribution may be different in different malignancies, and findings regarding disease distribution should not be generalized.

There are several aspects of the application of MRD assays the clinical usefulness of which requires further clarification, including the impact of changing therapy on the basis of MRD in patients with acute leukemia, the value of disease staging based on MRD findings in lymphomas and nonhematologic cancers, and the value of MRD studies in the context of autologous stem cell transplantation. Finally, the testing of new treatment approaches, such as small inhibitor molecules, cytokines, immunotoxins, adoptive T cells, compounds interfering with oncogenic molecular aberrations, and inhibitors of angiogenic growth factors may necessitate modifying the way in which anticancer treatments have traditionally been tested. Assaying MRD should be a powerful tool to rapidly evaluate efficacy of novel therapies.

References

Adriaansen, H.J., Jacobs, B.C., Kappers-Klunne, M.C. et al. (1993). Detection of residual disease in AML patients by use of double immunological marker analysis for terminal deoxynucleotidyl transferase and myeloid markers. Leukemia, 7, 472–81.

Almeida, J., Orfao, A., Ocqueteau, M. et al. (1999). High-sensitive immunophenotyping and DNA ploidy studies for the investigation of minimal residual disease in multiple myeloma. British Journal of Haematology, 107, 121–31.

Bagwell, C.B., Lovett, E.J., & Ault, K.A. (1988). Localization of monoclonal B-cell populations through the use of Komogorov-Smirnov D-value and reduced chi-square contours. Cytometry, 9, 469–76.

Bauer, K.D., de la Torre-Bueno, J., Diel, I.J. et al. (2000). Reliable and sensitive analysis of occult bone marrow metastases using automated cellular imaging. Clinical Cancer Research, 6, 3552–9.

Behm, F.G., Smith, F.O., Raimondi, S.C. et al. (1996). Human homologue of the rat chondroitin sulfate proteoglycan, NG2, detected by monoclonal antibody 7.1, identifies childhood acute lymphoblastic leukemias with t(4;11)(q21;q23) or t(11;19)(q23;p13) and MLL gene rearrangements. Blood, 87, 1134–9.

Berois, N., Varangot, M., Aizen, B. et al. (2000). Molecular detection of cancer cells in bone marrow and peripheral blood of patients with operable breast cancer. Comparison of CK19, MUC1 and CEA using RT-PCR. European Journal of Cancer, 36, 717–23.

Berois, N., Varangot, M., Osinaga, E. et al. (1997). Detection of rare human breast cancer cells. Comparison of an immunomagnetic separation method with immunocytochemistry and RT-PCR. Anticancer Research, 17, 2639–46.

Bokemeyer, C., Gillis, A.J., Pompe, K. et al. (2001). Clinical impact of germ cell tumor cells in apheresis products of patients receiving high-dose chemotherapy. Journal of Clinical Oncology, 19, 3029–36.

Bradstock, K.F., Janossy, G., Pizzolo, G. et al. (1980). Subpopulations of normal and leukemic human thymocytes: an analysis with the use of monoclonal antibodies. Journal of the National Cancer Institute, 65, 33–42.

Bradstock, K.F., Kerr, A., Kabral, A. et al. (1986). Coexpression of p165 myeloid surface antigen and terminal deoxynucleotidyl transferase: a comparison of acute myeloid leukemia and normal bone marrow cells. American Journal of Hematology, 23, 43–50.

Brasseur, F., Rimoldi, D., Lienard, D. et al. (1995). Expression of MAGE genes in primary and metastatic cutaneous melanoma. International Journal of Cancer, 63, 375–80.

Braun, S., Pantel, K., Muller, P. et al. (2000). Cytokeratin-positive cells in the bone marrow and survival of patients with stage I, II, or III breast cancer. New England Journal of Medicine, 342, 525–33.

Braun, S., Schindlbeck, C., Hepp, F. et al. (2001). Occult tumor cells in bone marrow of patients with locoregionally restricted ovarian cancer predict early distant metastatic relapse. Journal of Clinical Oncology, 19, 368–75.

Brenner, M.K., Rill, D.R., Moen, R.C. et al. (1993). Gene-marking to trace origin of relapse after autologous bone-marrow transplantation. Lancet, 341, 85–6.

Brugger, W., Bross, K.J., Glatt, M. et al. (1994). Mobilization of tumor cells and hematopoietic progenitor cells into peripheral blood of patients with solid tumors. Blood, 83, 636–40.

Burchill, S.A., Kinsey, S.E., Picton, S. et al. (2001). Minimal residual disease at the time of peripheral blood stem cell harvest in patients with advanced neuroblastoma. Medical and Pediatric Oncology, 36, 213–9.

Cabezudo, E., Carrara, P., Morilla, R., & Matutes, E. (1999). Quantitative analysis of CD79b, CD5 and CD19 in mature B-cell lymphoproliferative disorders. Haematologica, 84, 413–8.

Cabezudo, E., Matutes, E., Ramrattan, M. *et al.* (1997). Analysis of residual disease in chronic lymphocytic leukemia by flow cytometry. *Leukemia,* **11**, 1909–14.

Campana, D. & Coustan-Smith, E. (1999). Detection of minimal residual disease in acute leukemia by flow cytometry. *Cytometry,* **38**, 139–52.

Campana, D. & Coustan-Smith, E. (2002). Advances in the immunological monitoring of childhood acute lymphoblastic leukaemia. *Best Practices Research Clinical Haematology,* **15**, 1–19.

Campana, D., Coustan-Smith, E., & Janossy, G. (1990). The immunologic detection of minimal residual disease in acute leukemia. *Blood,* **76**, 163–71.

Campana, D. & Pui, C.H. (1995). Detection of minimal residual disease in acute leukemia: methodologic advances and clinical significance. *Blood,* **85**, 1416–34.

Cave, H., van der Werff ten Bosch, Suciu, S. *et al.* (1998). Clinical significance of minimal residual disease in childhood acute lymphoblastic leukemia. European Organization for Research and Treatment of Cancer—Childhood Leukemia Cooperative Group. *New England Journal of Medicine,* **339**, 591–8.

Chen, J.S., Coustan-Smith, E., Suzuki, T. *et al.* (2001). Identification of novel markers for monitoring minimal residual disease in acute lymphoblastic leukemia. *Blood,* **97**, 2115–20.

Cheung, I.Y. & Cheung, N.K. (2001). Detection of microscopic disease: comparing histology, immunocytology, and RT-PCR of tyrosine hydroxylase, GAGE, and MAGE. *Medical and Pediatric Oncology,* **36**, 210–2.

Cheung, I.Y., Chi, S.N., & Cheung, N.K. (2000). Prognostic significance of GAGE detection in bone marrows on survival of patients with metastatic neuroblastoma. *Medical of Pediatric Oncology,* **35**, 632–4.

Cheung, N.K., Von Hoff, D.D., Strandjord, S.E., & Coccia, P.F. (1986). Detection of neuroblastoma cells in bone marrow using GD2 specific monoclonal antibodies. *Journal of Clinical Oncology,* **4**, 363–9.

Ciudad, J., San Miguel, J.F., Lopez-Berges, M.C. *et al.* (1999). Detection of abnormalities in B-cell differentiation pattern is a useful tool to predict relapse in precursor-B-ALL. *British Journal of Haematology,* **104**, 695–705.

Ciudad, J., San Miguel, J.F., Lopez-Berges, M.C. *et al.* (1998). Prognostic value of immunophenotypic detection of minimal residual disease in acute lymphoblastic leukemia. *Journal of Clinical Oncology,* **16**, 3774–81.

Cooper, B.W., Moss, T.J., Ross, A.A. *et al.* (1998). Occult tumor contamination of hematopoietic stem-cell products does not affect clinical outcome of autologous transplantation in patients with metastatic breast cancer. *Journal of Clinical Oncology,* 3509–17.

Corradini, P., Voena, C., Astolfi, M. *et al.* (2001). Maspin and mammaglobin genes are specific markers for RT-PCR detection of minimal residual disease in patients with breast cancer. *Annals of Oncology,* **12**, 1693–8.

Cote, R.J., Rosen, P.P., Hakes, T.B. *et al.* (1988). Monoclonal antibodies detect occult breast carcinoma metastases in the bone marrow of patients with early stage disease. *American Journal of Surgical Pathology,* **12**, 333–40.

Coustan-Smith, E., Behm, F.G., Sanchez, J. *et al.* (1998). Immunological detection of minimal residual disease in children with acute lymphoblastic leukaemia. *Lancet,* **351**, 550–4.

Coustan-Smith, E., Sancho, J., Behm, F.G. *et al.* (2002a). Prognostic importance of measuring early clearance of leukemic cells by flow cytometry in childhood acute lymphoblastic leukemia. *Blood,* **100**, 52–8.

Coustan-Smith, E., Sancho, J., Hancock, M.L. *et al.* (2000). Clinical importance of minimal residual disease in childhood acute lymphoblastic leukemia. *Blood,* **96**, 2691–6.

Coustan-Smith, E., Sancho, J., Hancock, M.L. *et al.* (2002b). Use of peripheral blood instead of bone marrow to monitor residual disease in children with acute lymphoblastic leukemia. *Blood,* **100**, 2399–402.

Deguchi, T., Yang, M., Ehara, H. *et al.* (1997). Detection of micrometastatic prostate cancer cells in the bone marrow of patients with prostate cancer. *British Journal of Cancer,* **75**, 634–8.

Diel, I.J., Kaufmann, M., Costa, S.D. *et al.* (1996). Micrometastatic breast cancer cells in bone marrow at primary surgery: prognostic value in comparison with nodal status. *Journal of the National Cancer Institute,* **88**, 1652–8.

Diel, I.J., Kaufmann, M., Goerner, R. *et al.* (1992). Detection of tumor cells in bone marrow of patients with primary breast cancer: a prognostic factor for distant metastasis. *Journal of Clinical Oncology,* **10**, 1534–9.

Ditkoff, B.A., Marvin, M.R., Yemul, S. *et al.* (1996). Detection of circulating thyroid cells in peripheral blood. *Surgery,* **120**, 959–64.

Dworzak, M.N., Fritsch, G., Fleischer, C. *et al.* (1998). Comparative phenotype mapping of normal vs. malignant pediatric B-lymphopoiesis unveils leukemia-associated aberrations. *Experimental Hematology,* **26**, 305–13.

Engel, H., Goodacre, A., Keyhani, A. *et al.* (1997). Minimal residual disease in acute myelogenous leukaemia and myelodysplastic syndromes: a follow-up of patients in clinical remission. *British Journal of Haematology,* **99**, 64–75.

Fan, Y., Einhorn, L., Saxman, S. *et al.* (1998). Detection of germ cell tumor cells in apheresis products using polymerase chain reaction. *Clinical Cancer Research,* **4**, 93–8.

Farahat, N., Morilla, A., Owusu-Ankomah, K. *et al.* (1998). Detection of minimal residual disease in B-lineage acute lymphoblastic leukaemia by quantitative flow cytometry. *British Journal of Haematology,* **101**, 158–64.

Faulkner, L.B., Tintori, V., Tamburini, A. *et al.* (1998). High-sensitivity immunocytologic analysis of neuroblastoma cells in paired blood and marrow samples. *Journal of Hematotherapy,* **7**, 361–6.

Fields, K.K., Elfenbein, G.J., Trudeau, W.L. *et al.* (1996). Clinical significance of bone marrow metastases as detected using the polymerase chain reaction in patients with breast cancer undergoing high-dose chemotherapy and autologous bone marrow transplantation. *Journal of Clinical Oncology,* **14**, 1868–76.

Franklin, I.M. & Pritchard, J. (1983). Detection of bone marrow invasion by neuroblastoma is improved by sampling at two sites with both aspirates and trephine biopsies. *Journal of Clinical Pathology,* **36**, 1215–8.

Franklin, W.A., Shpall, E.J., Archer, P. *et al.* (1996). Immunocytochemical detection of breast cancer cells in marrow and peripheral blood of patients undergoing high dose chemotherapy with autologous stem cell support. *Breast Cancer Research Treatment*, JID-8111104 41, 1–13.

Freedman, A.S., Gribben, J.G., Neuberg, D. *et al.* (1996). High-dose therapy and autologous bone marrow transplantation in patients with follicular lymphoma during first remission. *Blood*, **88**, 2780–6.

Freedman, A.S., Neuberg, D., Mauch, P. *et al.* (1999). Long-term follow-up of autologous bone marrow transplantation in patients with relapsed follicular lymphoma. *Blood*, **94**, 3325–33.

Froehlich, T.W., Buchanan, G.R., Cornet, J.A. *et al.* (1981). Terminal deoxynucleotidyl transferase-containing cells in peripheral blood: implications for the surveillance of patients with lymphoblastic leukemia or lymphoma in remission. *Blood*, **58**, 214–20.

Fukuda, M., Miyajima, Y., Miyashita, Y., & Horibe, K. (2001). Disease outcome may be predicted by molecular detection of minimal residual disease in bone marrow in advanced neuroblastoma: a pilot study. *Journal of Pediatric Hematology and Oncology*, **23**, 10–13.

Garcia, V.J., Delgado, I., Benito, L. *et al.* (1999). CD79b expression in B cell chronic lymphocytic leukemia: its implication for minimal residual disease detection. *Leukemia*, **13**, 1501–5.

Goldman, J.M., Kaeda, J.S., Cross, N.C. *et al.* (1999). Clinical decision making in chronic myeloid leukemia based on polymerase chain reaction analysis of minimal residual disease. *Blood*, **94**, 1484–6.

Goulden, N.J., Knechtli, C.J., Garland, R.J. *et al.* (1998). Minimal residual disease analysis for the prediction of relapse in children with standard-risk acute lymphoblastic leukaemia. *British Journal of Haematology*, **100**, 235–44.

Gray, J.W., Kuo, W.L., Liang, J. *et al.* (1990). Analytical approaches to detection and characterization of disease-linked chromosome aberrations. *Bone Marrow Transplantation*, **6**(Suppl 1), 14–19.

Greaves, M.F. (1986). Differentiation-linked leukemogenesis in lymphocytes. *Science*, **234**, 697–704.

Gribben, J.G. (2002). Monitoring disease in lymphoma and CLL patients using molecular techniques. *Best Practice in Research in Clinical Haematology*, **15**, 179–95.

Grimwade, D. (1999). The pathogenesis of acute promyelocytic leukaemia: evaluation of the role of molecular diagnosis and monitoring in the management of the disease. *British Journal of Haematology*, **106**, 591–613.

Gross, H.J., Verwer, B., Houck, D. *et al.* (1995). Model study detecting breast cancer cells in peripheral blood mononuclear cells at frequencies as low as 10(–7). *Proceeding of the National Academy of Sciences USA*, **92**, 537–41.

Gross, H.J., Verwer, B., Houck, D., & Recktenwald, D. (1993). Detection of rare cells at a frequency of one per million by flow cytometry. *Cytometry*, **14**, 519–26.

Guerrasio, A., Rosso, C., Martinelli, G. *et al.* (1995). Polyclonal haemopoieses associated with long-term persistence of the AML1-ETO transcript in patients with FAB M2 acute myeloid leukaemia in continous clinical remission. *British Journal of Haematology*, **90**, 364–368.

Hanenberg, H., Baumann, M., Quentin, I. *et al.* (1994). Expression of the CEA gene family members NCA-50/90 and NCA-160

(CD66) in childhood acute lymphoblastic leukemias (ALLs) and in cell lines of B-cell origin. *Leukemia*, **8**, 2127–33.

Harbeck, N., Untch, M., Pache, L., & Eiermann, W. (1994). Tumour cell detection in the bone marrow of breast cancer patients at primary therapy: results of a 3-year median follow-up. *British Journal of Cancer*, **69**, 566–71.

Heiss, M.M., Simon, E.H., Beyer, B.C. *et al.* (2002). Minimal residual disease in gastric cancer: evidence of an independent prognostic relevance of urokinase receptor expression by disseminated tumor cells in the bone marrow. *Journal of Clinical Oncology*, **20**, 2005–16.

Hurwitz, C.A., Loken, M.R., Graham, M.L. *et al.* (1988). Asynchronous antigen expression in B lineage acute lymphoblastic leukemia. *Blood*, **72**, 299–307.

Janossy, G., Bollum, F.J., Bradstock, K.F., & Ashley, J. (1980). Cellular phenotypes of normal and leukemic hemopoietic cells determined by analysis with selected antibody combinations. *Blood*, **56**, 430–41.

Kasimir-Bauer, S., Mayer, S., Bojko, P. *et al.* (2001). Survival of tumor cells in stem cell preparations and bone marrow of patients with high-risk or metastatic breast cancer after receiving dose-intensive or high-dose chemotherapy. *Clinical Cancer Research*, **7**, 1582–9.

Kasimir-Bauer, S., Oberhoff, C., Schindler, A.E., & Seeber, S. (2002). A summary of two clinical studies on tumor cell dissemination in primary and metastatic breast cancer: methods, prognostic significance and implication for alternative treatment protocols. *International Journal of Oncology*, **20**, 1027–34.

Knechtli, C.J.C., Goulden, N.J., Hancock, J.P. *et al.* (1998). Minimal residual disease status before allogeneic bone marrow transplantation is an important determinant of successful outcome for children and adolescents with acute lymphoblastic leukemia. *Blood*, **92**, 4072–9.

Komada, Y., Zhang, X.L., Zhou, Y.W. *et al.* (1998). Flow cytometric analysis of peripheral blood and bone marrow for tumor cells in patients with neuroblastoma. *Cancer*, **82**, 591–9.

Kruger, W., Datta, C., Badbaran, A. *et al.* (2000). Immunomagnetic tumor cell selection—implications for the detection of disseminated cancer cells. *Transfusion*, **40**, 1489–93.

Kubuschok, B., Passlick, B., Izbicki, J.R. *et al.* (1999). Disseminated tumor cells in lymph nodes as a determinant for survival in surgically resected non-small-cell lung cancer. *Journal of Clinical Oncology*, **17**, 19–24.

Ladetto, M., Omede, P., Sametti, S. *et al.* (2002). Real-time polymerase chain reaction in multiple myeloma: quantitative analysis of tumor contamination of stem cell harvests. *Experimental Hematology*, **30**, 529–536.

Lavabre-Bertrand, T., Janossy, G., Ivory, K. *et al.* (1994). Leukemia-associated changes identified by quantitative flow cytometry: I. CD10 expression. *Cytometry*, **18**, 209–17.

Leslie, D.S., Johnston, W.W., Daly, L. *et al.* (1990). Detection of breast carcinoma cells in human bone marrow using fluorescence-activated cell sorting and conventional cytology. *American Journal of Clinical Pathology*, **94**, 8–13.

Leung, W., Chen, A.R., Klann, R.C. *et al.* (1998). Frequent detection of tumor cells in hematopoietic grafts in neuroblastoma and Ewing's sarcoma. *Bone Marrow Transplantation*, **22**, 971–9.

Lindemann, F., Schlimok, G., Dirschedl, P. et al. (1992). Prognostic significance of micrometastatic tumour cells in bone marrow of colorectal cancer patients. Lancet, 340, 685–9.

Liu, Y.J. & Grimwade, D. (2002). Minimal residual disease evaluation in acute myeloid leukaemia. Lancet, 360, 160–2.

Lo Coco, F., Diverio, D., Falini, B. et al. (1999). Genetic diagnosis and molecular monitoring in the management of acute promyelocytic leukemia. Blood, 94, 12–22.

Lucio, P., Gaipa, G., van Lochem, E.G. et al. (2001). BIOMED-I concerted action report: flow cytometric immunophenotyping of precursor B-ALL with standardized triple-stainings. BIOMED-1 Concerted Action Investigation of Minimal Residual Disease in Acute Leukemia: International Standardization and Clinical Evaluation. Leukemia, 15, 1185–92.

Luppi, M., Morselli, M., Bandieri, E. et al. (1996). Sensitive detection of circulating breast cancer cells by reverse-transcriptase polymerase chain reaction of maspin gene. Annals of Oncology, 7, 619–24.

Mancini, M., Cedrone, M., Diverio, D. et al. (2000). Use of dual-color interphase FISH for the detection of inv(16) in acute myeloid leukemia at diagnosis, relapse and during follow-up: a study of 23 patients. Leukemia, 14, 364–8.

Mansi, J.L., Gogas, H., Bliss, J.M. et al. (1999). Outcome of primary-breast-cancer patients with micrometastases: a long-term follow-up study. Lancet, 354, 197–202.

Martin, V.M., Siewert, C., Scharl, A. et al. (1998). Immunomagnetic enrichment of disseminated epithelial tumor cells from peripheral blood by MACS. Experimental Hematology, 26, 252–64.

Mathe, G., Schwarzenberg, L., Mery, A.M. et al. (1966). Extensive histological and cytological survey of patients with acute leukaemia in "complete remission". British Medical Journal, 5488, 640–2.

Mehes, G., Luegmayr, A., Ambros, I.M. et al. (2001). Combined automatic immunological and molecular cytogenetic analysis allows exact identification and quantification of tumor cells in the bone marrow. Clinical Cancer Research, 7, 1969–75.

Miyamoto, T., Nagafuji, K., Akashi, K. et al. (1996). Persistence of multipotent progenitors expressing AML1/ETO transcripts in long-term remission patients with t(8;21) acute myelogenous leukemia. Blood, 87, 4789–96.

Miyamoto, T., Weissman, I.L., & Akashi, K. (2000). AML1/ETO-expressing nonleukemic stem cells in acute myelogenous leukemia with 8;21 chromosomal translocation. Proceedings of the National Academy of Sciences, USA, 97, 7521–6.

Moreno, J.G., O'Hara, S.M., Gross, S. et al. (2001). Changes in circulating carcinoma cells in patients with metastatic prostate cancer correlate with disease status. Urology, 5158, 386–92.

Morschhauser, F., Cayuela, J.M., Martini, S. et al. (2000). Evaluation of minimal residual disease using reverse-transcription polymerase chain reaction in t(8;21) acute myeloid leukemia: a multicenter study of 51 patients. Journal of Clinical Oncology, 18, 788–94.

Moss, T.J. (1999). Clinical relevance of minimal residual cancer in patients with solid malignancies. Cancer Metastasis Review, 18, 91–100.

Moss, T.J., Reynolds, C.P., Sather, H.N. et al. (1991). Prognostic value of immunocytologic detection of bone marrow metastases in neuroblastoma. New England Journal of Medicine, 324, 219–26.

Moss, T.J. & Ross, A.A. (1992). The risk of tumor cell contamination in peripheral blood stem cell collections. Journal of Hematotherapy, 1, 225–32.

Nagai, J., Ishda, Y., Koga, N. et al. (2000). A new sensitive and specific combination of CD81/CD56/CD45 monoclonal antibodies for detecting circulating neuroblastoma cells in peripheral blood using flow cytometry. Journal of Pediatric Hematology and Oncology, 22, 20–6.

Naume, B., Borgen, E., Beiske, K. et al. (1997). Immunomagnetic techniques for the enrichment and detection of isolated breast carcinoma cells in bone marrow and peripheral blood. Journal of Hematotherapy, 6, 103–14.

Nowak, R., Oelschlagel, U., Range, U. et al. (1999). Flow cytometric DNA quantification in immunophenotyped cells as a sensitive method for determination of aneuploid multiple myeloma cells in peripheral blood stem cell harvests and bone marrow after therapy. Bone Marrow Transplantation, 23, 895–900.

Nowak, R., Oelschlaegel, U., Schuler, U. et al. (1997). Sensitivity of combined DNA/immunophenotype flow cytometry for the detection of low levels of aneuploid lymphoblastic leukemia cells in bone marrow. Cytometry, 30, 47–53.

Nucifora, G., Larson, R.A., & Rowley, J.D. (1993). Persistence of the 8;21 translocation in patients with acute myeloid leukemia type M2 in long-term remission. Blood, 82, 712–15.

Osborne, M.P., Asina, S., Wong, G.Y. et al. (1989). Immunofluorescent monoclonal antibody detection of breast cancer in bone marrow: sensitivity in a model system. Cancer Research, 49, 2510–13.

Osborne, M.P., Wong, G.Y., Asina, S. et al. (1991). Sensitivity of immunocytochemical detection of breast cancer cells in human bone marrow. Cancer Research, 51, 2706–9.

Pantel, K., Aignherr, C., Kollermann, J. et al. (1995). Immunocytochemical detection of isolated tumour cells in bone marrow of patients with untreated stage C prostatic cancer. European Journal of Cancer, 31A, 1627–32.

Pantel, K., Izbicki, J., Passlick, B. et al. (1996). Frequency and prognostic significance of isolated tumour cells in bone marrow of patients with non-small-cell lung cancer without overt metastases. Lancet, 347, 649–53.

Pantel, K., Izbicki, J.R., Angstwurm, M. et al. (1993). Immunocytological detection of bone marrow micrometastasis in operable non-small cell lung cancer. Cancer Research, 53, 1027–31.

Pantel, K. & von Knebel, D.M. (2000). Detection and clinical relevance of micrometastatic cancer cells. Current Opinion in Oncology, 12, 95–101.

Porwit-MacDonald, A., Bjorklund, E., Lucio, P. et al. (2000). BIOMED-1 concerted action report: flow cytometric characterization of CD7+ cell subsets in normal bone marrow as a basis for the diagnosis and follow-up of T cell acute lymphoblastic leukemia (T-ALL). Leukemia, 14, 816–25.

Racila, E., Euhus, D., Weiss, A.J. et al. (1998). Detection and characterization of carcinoma cells in the blood. Proceedings of the National Academy of Science, USA, 95, 4589–94.

Radich, J., Gehly, G., Lee, A. et al. (1997). Detection of bcr-abl transcripts in Philadelphia chromosome-positive acute lymphoblastic leukemia after marrow transplantation. Blood, 89, 2602–9.

Rawstron, A.C., Kennedy, B., Evans, P.A. *et al.* (2001). Quantitation of minimal disease levels in chronic lymphocytic leukemia using a sensitive flow cytometric assay improves the prediction of outcome and can be used to optimize therapy. *Blood*, **98**, 29–35.

Reading, C.L., Estey, E.H., Huh, Y.O. *et al.* (1993). Expression of unusual immunophenotype combinations in acute myelogenous leukemia. *Blood*, **81**, 3083–90.

Reichle, A., Rothe, G., Krause, S. *et al.* (1999). Transplant characteristics: minimal residual disease and impaired megakaryocytic colony growth as sensitive parameters for predicting relapse in acute myeloid leukemia. *Leukemia*, **13**, 1227–34.

Riesenberg, R., Oberneder, R., Kriegmair, M. *et al.* (1993). Immunocytochemical double staining of cytokeratin and prostate specific antigen in individual prostatic tumour cells. *Histochemistry*, **99**, 61–6.

Rill, D.R., Buschle, M., Foreman, N.K. *et al.* (1992). Retrovirus-mediated gene transfer as an approach to analyze neuroblastoma relapse after autologous bone marrow transplantation. *Human Gene Therapy*, **3**, 129–36.

Roder, J.D., Thorban, S., Pantel, K., & Siewert, J.R. (1999). Micrometastases in bone marrow: prognostic indicators for pancreatic cancer. *World Journal of Surgery*, **23**, 888–91.

Ross, A.A., Cooper, B.W., Lazarus, H.M. *et al.* (1993). Detection and viability of tumor cells in peripheral blood stem cell collections from breast cancer patients using immunocytochemical and clonogenic assay techniques. *Blood*, **82**, 2605–10.

Salerno, C.T., Frizelle, S., Niehans, G.A. *et al.* (1998). Detection of occult micrometastases in non-small cell lung carcinoma by reverse transcriptase-polymerase chain reaction. *Chest*, **113**, 1526–32.

San Miguel, J.F., Almeida, J., Mateo, G. *et al.* (2002). Immunophenotypic evaluation of the plasma cell compartment in multiple myeloma: a tool for comparing the efficacy of different treatment strategies and predicting outcome. *Blood*, **99**, 1853–6.

San Miguel, J.F., Martinez, A., Macedo, A. *et al.* (1997). Immunophenotyping investigation of minimal residual disease is a useful approach for predicting relapse in acute myeloid leukemia patients. *Blood*, **90**, 2465–70.

San Miguel, J.F., Vidriales, M.B., Lopez-Berges, C. *et al.* (2001). Early immunophenotypical evaluation of minimal residual disease in acute myeloid leukemia identifies different patient risk groups and may contribute to postinduction treatment stratification. *Blood*, **98**, 1746–51.

Schlimok, G., Funke, I., Bock, B. *et al.* (1990). Epithelial tumor cells in bone marrow of patients with colorectal cancer: immunocytochemical detection, phenotypic characterization, and prognostic significance. *Journal of Clinical Oncology*, **8**, 831–7.

Schlimok, G., Funke, I., Holzmann, B. *et al.* (1987). Micrometastatic cancer cells in bone marrow: in vitro detection with anti-cytokeratin and in vivo labeling with anti-17-1A monoclonal antibodies. *Proceedings of the National Academy of Sciences, USA*, **84**, 8672–6.

Schlimok, G., Funke, I., Pantel, K. *et al.* (1991). Micrometastatic tumour cells in bone marrow of patients with gastric cancer: methodological aspects of detection and prognostic significance. *European Journal of Cancer*, **27**, 1461–5.

Seeger, R.C., Reynolds, C.P., Gallego, R. *et al.* (2000). Quantitative tumor cell content of bone marrow and blood as a predictor of outcome in stage IV neuroblastoma: a Children's Cancer Group Study. *Journal of Clinical Oncology*, **18**, 4067–76.

Shpall, E.J., Cagnoni, P.J., Bearman, S.I. *et al.* (1997). Peripheral blood stem cells for autografting. *Annual Review of Medicine*, **48**, 241–51.

Shpall, E.J., Jones, R.B., Bearman, S.I. *et al.* (1994). Transplantation of enriched CD34-positive autologous marrow into breast cancer patients following high-dose chemotherapy: influence of CD34-positive peripheral-blood progenitors and growth factors on engraftment. *Journal of Clinical Oncology*, **12**, 28–36.

Sievers, E.L., Lange, B.J., Buckley, J.D. *et al.* (1996). Prediction of relapse of pediatric acute myeloid leukemia by use of multidimensional flow cytometry. *Journal of the National Cancer Institute*, **88**, 1483–8.

Simpson, S.J., Vachula, M., Kennedy, M.J. *et al.* (1995). Detection of tumor cells in the bone marrow, peripheral blood, and apheresis products of breast cancer patients using flow cytometry. *Experimental Hematology*, **23**, 1062–8.

Smith, B., Selby, P., Southgate, J. *et al.* (1991). Detection of melanoma cells in peripheral blood by means of reverse transcriptase and polymerase chain reaction. *Lancet*, **338**, 1227–9.

Sugimoto, T., Das, H., Imoto, S. *et al.* (2000). Quantitation of minimal residual disease in t(8;21)-positive acute myelogenous leukemia patients using real-time quantitative RT-PCR. *American Journal of Hematology*, **64**, 101–6.

Sugita, K., Mori, T., Yokota, S. *et al.* (1999). The KOR-SA3544 antigen predominantly expressed on the surface of Philadelphia chromosome-positive acute lymphoblastic leukemia cells is nonspecific cross-reacting antigen-50/90 (CD66c) and invariably expressed in cytoplasm of human leukemia cells. *Leukemia*, **13**, 779–85.

Szczepanski, T., Orfao, A., van der Velden, V.H. *et al.* (2001). Minimal residual disease in leukaemia patients. *Lancet Oncology*, **2**, 409–17.

Tallini, G., Ghossein, R.A., Emanuel, J. *et al.* (1998). Detection of thyroglobulin thyroid peroxidase, and RET/PTC1 mRNA transcripts in the peripheral blood of patients with thyroid disease. *Journal of Clinical Oncology*, **16**, 1158–66.

Terstappen, L.W. & Loken, M.R. (1990). Myeloid cell differentiation in normal bone marrow and acute myeloid leukemia assessed by multi-dimensional flow cytometry. *Analytical Cellular Pathology*, **2**, 229–40.

Terstappen, L.W., Safford, M., Konemann, S. *et al.* (1992). Flow cytometric characterization of acute myeloid leukemia. Part II. Phenotypic heterogeneity at diagnosis. *Leukemia*, **6**, 70–80.

Thorban, S., Roder, J.D., Nekarda, H. *et al.* (1996). Immunocytochemical detection of disseminated tumor cells in the bone marrow of patients with esophageal carcinoma. *Journal of the National Cancer Institute*, **88**, 1222–7.

Tobal, K., Newton, J., Macheta, M. *et al.* (2000). Molecular quantitation of minimal residual disease in acute myeloid leukemia with t(8;21) can identify patients in durable remission and predict clinical relapse. *Blood*, **95**, 815–9.

Traystman, M.D., Cochran, G.T., Hake, S.J. *et al.* (1997). Comparison of molecular cytokeratin 19 reverse transcriptase polymerase chain reaction (CK19 RT-PCR) and immunocytochemical detection of micrometastatic breast cancer cells in hematopoietic harvests. *Journal of Hematotherapy*, **6**, 551–61.

Umiel, T., Prilutskaya, M., Nguyen, N.H. *et al.* (2000). Breast tumor contamination of peripheral blood stem cell harvests: increased sensitivity of detection using immunomagnetic enrichment. *Journal of Hematotherapy and Stem Cell Research,* **9,** 895–904.

van Dongen, J.J., Seriu, T., Panzer-Grumayer, E.R. *et al.* (1998). Prognostic value of minimal residual disease in acute lymphoblastic leukaemia in childhood. *Lancet,* **352,** 1731–8.

Venditti, A., Buccisano, F., Del Poeta, G. *et al.* (2000). Level of minimal residual disease after consolidation therapy predicts outcome in acute myeloid leukemia. *Blood,* **96,** 3948–52.

Vescio, R.A., Han, E.J., Schiller, G.J. *et al.* (1996). Quantitative comparison of multiple myeloma tumor contamination in bone marrow harvest and leukapheresis autografts. *Bone Marrow Transplantation,* **18,** 103–10.

Vredenburgh, J.J., Peters, W.P., Rosner, G. *et al.* (1995). Detection of tumor cells in the bone marrow of stage IV breast cancer patients receiving high-dose chemotherapy: the role of induction chemotherapy. *Bone Marrow Transplantation,* **16,** 815–21.

Vredenburgh, J.J., Silva, O., Broadwater, G. *et al.* (1997). The significance of tumor contamination in the bone marrow from high-risk primary breast cancer patients treated with high-dose chemotherapy and hematopoietic support. *Biology of Blood and Marrow Transplantation,* **3,** 91–7.

Vredenburgh, J.J., Silva, O., Tyer, C. *et al.* (1996). A comparison of immunohistochemistry, two-color immunofluorescence, and flow cytometry with cell sorting for the detection of micrometastatic breast cancer in the bone marrow. *Journal of Hematotherapy,* **5,** 57–62.

Weaver, C.H., Moss, T., Schwartzberg, L.S. *et al.* (1998). High-dose chemotherapy in patients with breast cancer: evaluation of infusing peripheral blood stem cells containing occult tumor cells. *Bone Marrow Transplantation,* **21,** 1117–24.

Weber, T., Amann, K., Weckauf, H. *et al.* (2002). Detection of disseminated medullary thyroid carcinoma cells in cervical lymph nodes by cytokeratin 20 reverse transcription-polymerase chain reaction. *World Journal of Surgery,* **26,** 148–52.

Weitz, J., Kienle, P., Magener, A. *et al.* (1999). Detection of disseminated colorectal cancer cells in lymph nodes, blood and bone marrow. *Clinical Cancer Research,* **5,** 1830–6.

Wells, D.A., Hall, M.C., Shulman, H.M., & Loken, M.R. (1998). Occult B cell malignancies can be detected by three-color flow cytometry in patients with cytopenias. *Leukemia,* **12,** 2015–23.

Yokoyama, N., Shirai, Y., Ajioka, Y. *et al.* (2002). Immunohistochemically detected hepatic micrometastases predict a high risk of intrahepatic recurrence after resection of colorectal carcinoma liver metastases. *Cancer,* **94,** 1642–7.

Zach, O., Kasparu, H., Krieger, O. *et al.* (1999). Detection of circulating mammary carcinoma cells in the peripheral blood of breast cancer patients via a nested reverse transcriptase polymerase chain reaction assay for mammaglobin mRNA. *Journal of Clinical Oncology,* **17,** 2015–9.

PART XII   STATISTICAL ANALYSIS

107 Statistical analysis in hematopoietic stem cell transplantation

JOHN P. KLEIN

Medical College of Wisconsin, Milwaukee, USA

Introduction

The aim of this chapter is to provide an introduction to the statistical techniques that are used most frequently in the analysis of outcome of hematopoietic stem cell (HSC) transplantation, and to provide reference to the statistical literature that more fully describes these methods. Before discussing the specific techniques that are most commonly used in this area of application, a brief review of the basic concepts of statistical inference is given.

The type of analysis that is used in analyzing HSC transplantation studies depends on the type of data encountered. Table 107.1 gives a brief overview of the types of analyses that would be used when the response of interest is either categorical, continuous, or the time to some event. Many of these techniques are documented in the text books by Altman (1991) or Dawson-Saunders and Trapp (1994). Other excellent introductory books for the techniques most often applied in analyzing HSC transplant data, are the self-learning texts on logistic regression (Kleinbaum, 1994) and survival analysis (Kleinbaum, 1996). A reference to the methods on time to event data is Klein and Moeschberger (1997).

Statistical tests of hypothesis

A statistical hypothesis test decides between one of two contrasting hypotheses: a null hypothesis that is assumed to be true unless there is overwhelming evidence to the contrary and an alternative hypothesis that is the complement of the null hypothesis. In most cases the null hypothesis is that there is no difference between the two treatments and the alternative is that there is. On the basis of the data, we need to decide between these two hypotheses. Two types of errors can be made: a type I error where we falsely conclude the null hypothesis is false (and thus the alternative is true) when in fact it is true, and a type II error when we falsely conclude the null hypothesis is true when in fact it is false. When comparing two treatments, a type I error corresponds to falsely concluding that the two treatments are different, and a type II error occurs when it is falsely concluded there is no difference between the two treatments. The type I error is considered more serious and is

protected against by assigning a small probability to its occurrence. This probability is called the significance level of the test. Typically this is a small number like .05 or .01.

Associated with most tests is a *P* value. The *P* value of a test is the smallest significance level for which the null hypothesis

Table 107.1. *Statistical methods commonly used in the analysis of outcome of HSC transplants*

Discrete or categorical data
1. Chi-squared test on categorical data (for example, tests of association between a categorical risk factor such as race and type of disease)
2. Exact tests for comparing incidence rates (for example, comparison of 100 day mortality rates between males and females)
3. Logistic regression for modeling a dichotomous response variable as a function of covariates (for example, modeling the probability a patient will respond to treatment as a function of age, disease stage, treatment, etc.)

Continuous data
1. T-tests on the difference between mean responses between two groups of patients
2. Analysis of variance to compare differences in means between three or more groups of patients
3. Simple linear regression for modeling a continuous response as a function of covariates (for example, modeling days from diagnosis to transplant as a function of age, gender, disease, etc.)
4. Correlation analysis (Kendall's, Spearman's, Pearson's) to determine the strength of association between two variables
5. Nonparametric tests for comparing two or more groups (Sign test, Kruskal-Wallis test, Wilcoxon-Mann-Whitney test)

Time to event data
1. Actuarial estimates of survival or disease-free survival
2. Cumulative incidence curves for competing risks such as relapse or death in remission
3. Current disease-free survival curves for current status data where a second remission following a post therapy is possible
4. Estimation and comparison of the rate of occurrence of events (weighted log rank tests, smoothed hazard rates)
5. Multivariate Cox regression analysis and relative risk analysis on time to event data (for example, assessment of prognostic factors for survival)

would be rejected for the observed data. It is roughly the chance of seeing a set of data as extreme (in terms of the null hypothesis) as we saw. Small P values are evidence against the null hypothesis, while large values are evidence in favor of the null hypothesis. Common practice is to say the result is significant when the P value is less than .05 (and highly significant when the P value is less than .01). The P value is used to decide whether the null hypothesis is true while the strength of evidence is measured by a confidence interval.

Once the significance level is fixed a good test will also have a small probability of making a type II error. This probability is called the operating characteristic of the test and the probability of not making a type II error is called the power of the test. That is, the power of the test is the likelihood of correctly deciding there is a difference between the two treatments. The power is a function of the sample sizes in the two groups, the variability in response from patient to patient, and the true magnitude of the difference between the treatments. For a fixed sample size, a test will have lower power for small differences between treatments than for big differences. What is meant by small or large differences between treatments depends on the variability of the response being measured.

Point and interval estimation

Point and interval estimates are used as summary measures that describe the outcome of an experiment. The point estimate is a single number that is the best guess, based on the sample data, of the value of the quantity of interest in the population. Associated with any point estimate is the standard error of the point estimate, which is a measure of how well the point estimate is approximating the population quantity it is estimating.

A confidence interval is a random interval that has the property that, with a specified probability, the true value of the parameter lies in the interval. For example, if a 95% confidence interval for the 100 day mortality rate based on a sample of patients given a transplant is (0.05, 0.17), then we can predict with 95% confidence that, if we looked at, say, all patients with acute myeloid leukemia (AML) treated in the same way, between 5% and 17% would not survive 100 days.

Survival curves

Survival analysis techniques are used to draw an inference about the time to an event. Two types of events are commonly found in transplant analyses. The first are terminal events such as death, or treatment failure. Here some patients may be censored in that at the end of the study they have not experienced the event or they may have been lost to follow-up prior to the end of the study. The reason for censoring is assumed to be independent of the event under study.

The survival curve, which is the probability that an individual has yet to experience the event of interest at a given point in time, is commonly used to describe the time to a terminal event. The usual estimator of this quantity is the Kaplan-Meier product-limit estimator or the actuarial estimate of the survival rate (Kaplan & Meier, 1958). This estimate has the advantage over crude estimates based on the number of survivors in that it accounts for the partial information on survival given by censored individuals. This is done by calculating, at each event time, the proportion surviving out of those at risk at that time. The resulting estimate is a step function with jumps at the death times. Standard errors of the estimated survival function are found using Greenwood's formula (see Klein & Moeschberger, 1997, Chapter 4).

To illustrate the Kaplan-Meier estimator, consider a multicenter study of patients prepared for transplantation with a radiation-free conditioning regimen (details of the study are found in Copelan et al., 1991). The preparative regimen used in this study of allogeneic marrow transplantation for patients with AML and acute lymphoblastic leukemia (ALL) was a combination of 16 mg/kg of oral busulfan (BU) and 120 mg/kg of intravenous cyclophosphamide (CY). The categories of patients transplanted were: ALL (38 patients), AML-low-risk (first remission, 54 patients), and AML-high-risk (second remission or untreated first relapse, 15 patients), or second or greater relapse or never in remission (30 patients). Figure 107.1 shows the Kaplan-Meier estimates of leukemia-free survival for the three disease categories. Here the event of interest is relapse or death, whichever comes first.

Two types of interval estimates are available for expressing the uncertainty in the estimate of the survival function. The first is a pointwise confidence interval for the survival function. Here the inference is to the survival probability at a fixed, predetermined point in time. The second is a confidence band, where the inference is to the survival probabilities over a range of time points. Confidence bands are wider than pointwise confidence intervals since one is making a guarantee of containing the entire survival curve in the interval with the desired confidence level rather than the value of the curve at a single point. Techniques for computing confidence bands and pointwise confidence intervals are found in Chapter 4 of Klein and Moeschberger (1997). Figure 107.2 depicts a 95% pointwise confidence interval and a 95% confidence band for the disease-free survival function for the AML patients in the study. The inner band could be used, for example, to make an inference about the disease-free survival rate at 1 year posttransplant. At 1 year one can be 95% confident the disease-free survival probability is between 0.39 and 0.70. The outer band is used when inference is to the entire survival curve.

Cumulative incidence analysis and competing risks

A second type of event encountered in HSC transplant analyses are competing risks. These are a collection of events where the occurrence of one event precludes the observation of another event. Examples are relapse and death in remission or graft-versus-host disease and death. The incidence of these events is represented by a cumulative incidence curve (Gooley et al., 1999), which tells us at each point in time how likely it is that the event has occurred.

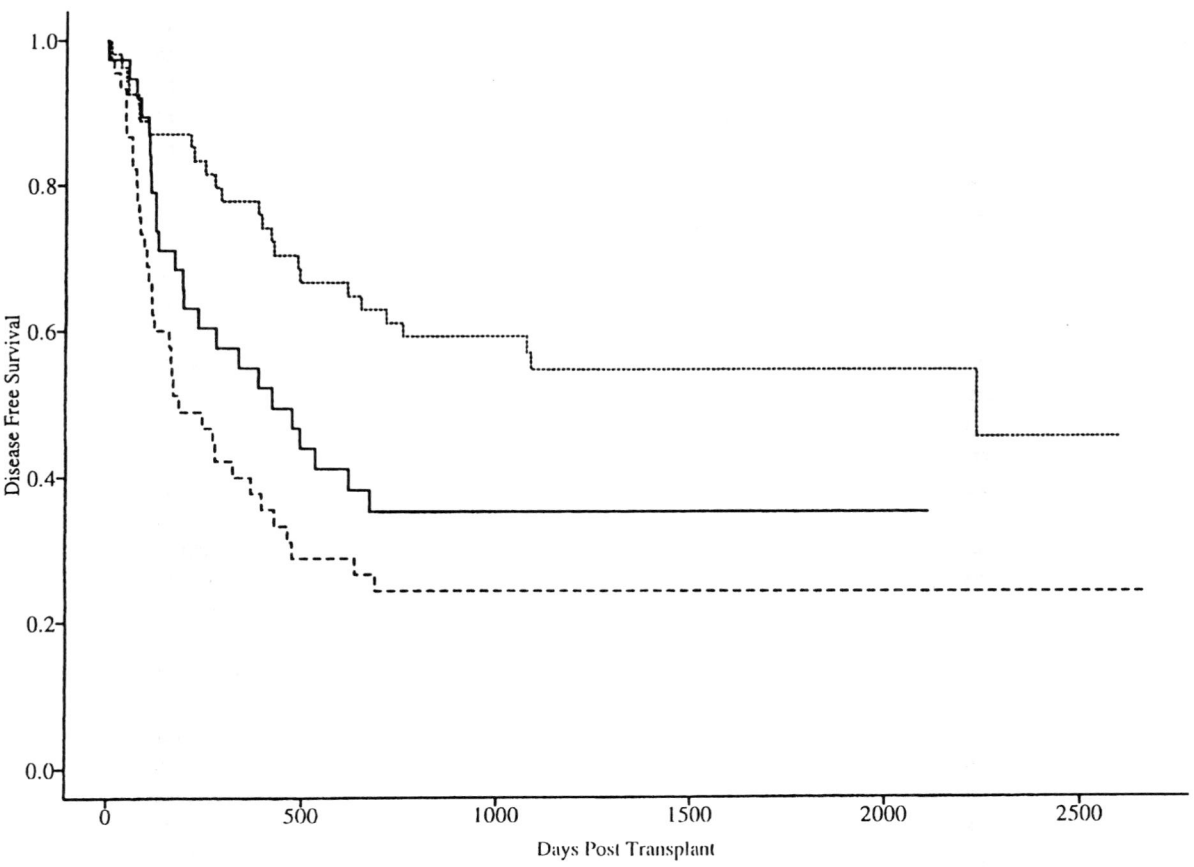

Fig. 107.1. Comparison of disease-free curves. ALL, solid line; AML-low risk, dotted line; AML-high risk, dashed line.

The incidence of competing risks is often represented incorrectly by 1 – the Kaplan-Meier estimate of the event obtained by treating all other events as censored observations. This quantity provides an estimate of the chance of the competing risk occurring in an imaginary patient who cannot experience the other events and it is an over-estimate of the probability of the event happening in a patient who could experience any of the competing risks. Figure 107.3 shows the two curves for relapse for the 54 AML low-risk patients. Here the cumulative incidence curve is the likelihood a patient who is at risk of death or relapse will relapse prior to time t, while the complement of the Kaplan-Meier curve is the chance a hypothetical patient who is not at risk of death will relapse prior to time t. For further discussion see Klein *et al.* (2002a).

Current disease-free survival curves

For survival data a patient is considered a failure when the event of interest occurs. All survival curves are proper curves in that they are non-increasing and all cumulative incidence curves are non-decreasing. With the advent of, for example, posttransplant therapies, such as donor leukocyte infusions (DLI), there is a need for a summary curve which expresses the likelihood that a patient will be alive and in remission at any time after transplant. This curve, called a current disease-free survival function, may go up or down over time, reflecting that patients may move from a poor to good health situation, depending on how they respond to either the initial or posttransplant therapy. Techniques for calculation of the current leukemia-free survival function can be found in Klein *et al.*, 2000 or Klein *et al.*, 2002a. Figure 107.4 shows a typical current disease-free survival curve based on a study of the effectiveness of DLI. Note that as opposed to the leukemia-free survival curve where patients are considered failures at first relapse, this curves shows that about 20% of all patients can be salvaged by DLI.

Hazard rates

An alternative summary curve is the hazard rate. This quantity, also known as the force of mortality in demography, and the age-specific failure rate in epidemiology, may be viewed as the "approximate" probability of an individual of a particular age experiencing the event in the next instant of time. This function is particularly useful in determining the appropriate failure distributions utilizing qualitative information about the mechanism of failure and for describing the way in which the chance

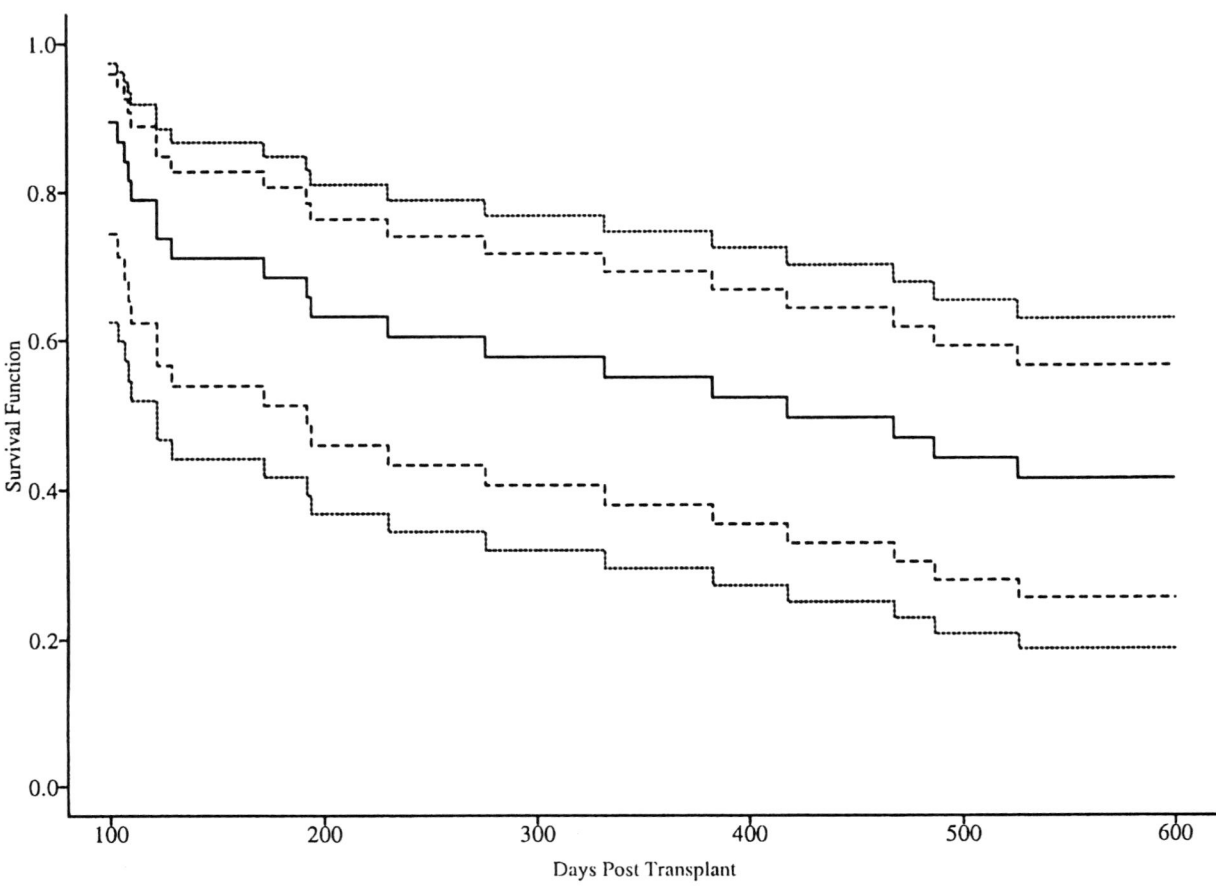

Fig. 107.2. Comparison of 95% pointwise confidence intervals and 95% confidence bands for the disease-free survival of ALL patients. Kaplan-Meier estimate, solid line; pointwise confidence interval, dashed lines; confidence band, dotted lines.

of experiencing the event changes with time. The shape of the hazard rate gives insight into the failure mechanism. Models with increasing hazard rates may arise when there is natural aging. Decreasing hazard functions are much less common, but find occasional use when there is a very early likelihood of failure, such as in patients experiencing certain types of surgical procedures. Most often a bathtub-shaped hazard is appropriate in populations followed from birth. Most population mortality data follow this type of hazard function where, during an early period, deaths result primarily from infant diseases after which the death rate stabilizes followed by an increasing hazard rate due to the natural aging process. Finally, if the hazard rate is increasing early and eventually begins declining, then the hazard is termed hump-shaped. This type of hazard rate is typical of bone marrow or blood stem cell transplantation, where early after transplant there is an initial increase in risk due to rejection, infection, and graft-versus-host disease, followed by a steady decline in risk as the patient recovers.

Hazard rates are estimated by using a kernel smoothing procedure discussed in Chapter 6 of Klein and Moeschberger (1997). Figure 107.5 shows the estimated hazard rates for the three disease classifications of patients described previously.

Here we see the hazard rates initially increase for all three disease types reflecting an increasing risk of death or relapse for about the first 100 to 150 days posttransplant, after which the hazard rate declines and eventually becomes roughly constant.

Comparison of survival curves

There are several tests that can be used to compare two or more survival curves (Fleming & Harrington, 1981; Klein & Moeschberger, 1997, Chapter 7). Most of these tests compare weighted differences between the observed number of deaths in each group and what is expected if there is no difference between the groups. The most common tests are the log rank test, which gives equal weight to all differences occurring over time, and the Wilcoxon test, which gives larger weight to differences that occur early in time. When the null hypothesis that there is no difference in the survival rates of the groups is the same, then all these tests have a chi-squared distribution. As an example, for the BU/CY transplant study example cited previously, the log rank test of the equality of the three disease-type survival curves has a P value of .0010 and the Wilcoxon test has a P value of .0003. Both tests suggest there is evidence of at

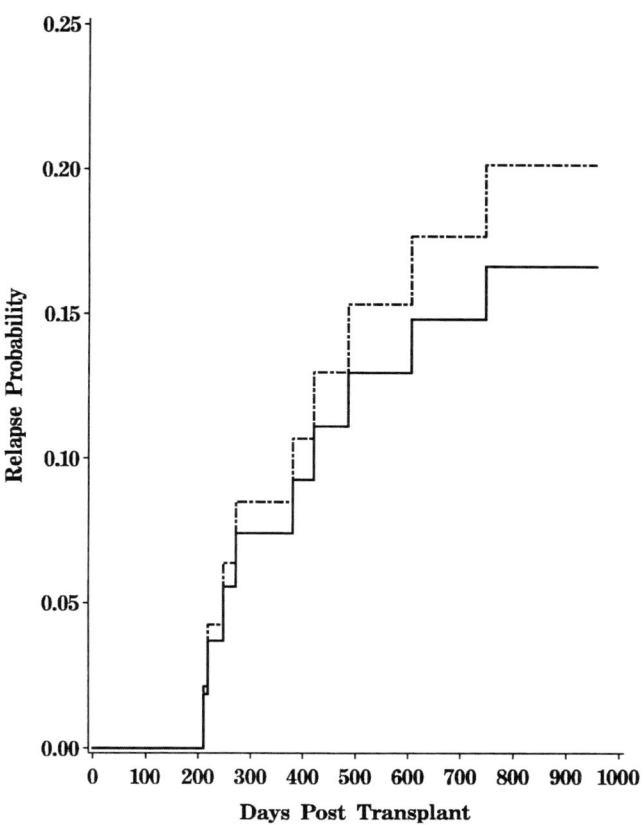

Fig. 107.3. Comparison of cumulative incidence of relapse (solid line) and 1-Kaplan-Meier estimate of relapse (dashed line) for AML-low risk patients.

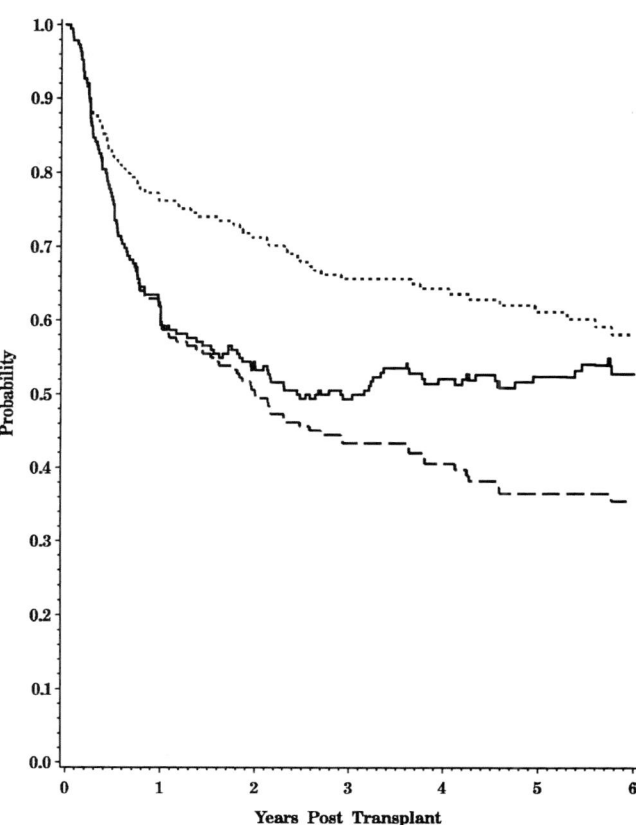

Fig. 107.4. Comparison of overall (dotted line), disease-free (dashed line) and current disease-free survival (solid line) functions.

least one of the three survival curves being different from the other.

Cox regression

A common question in analyzing outcome after HSC transplants is "what factors influence survival?" To answer this question a proportional hazards regression model, first suggested by Cox (1972), is often used. The basic model assumes that the hazard rate for an individual with a given set of risk factors is the product of a baseline hazard function and a regression model for the risk factors. The model is often called a semiparametric model, since no functional form is assumed for the baseline hazard rate but a parametric model is used for the risk factors.

Cox regression models are used in two situations. In the first situation, several groups are compared (main effects) after an adjustment for other risk factors. Here the Cox model is used to make adjustments to the main comparison for difference in the distribution of the risk factors between the groups. The second situation is where Cox models are used to produce a set of prognostic risk factors that are predictive of survival. Examples

of these two approaches can be found in Barrett *et al.* (1994) and Gluckman *et al.* (1995).

The simplest Cox regression model makes several strong statistical assumptions. The most important assumption is that the effects of the risk factors are the same at any point in time. When this is not true, then models that allow for different baseline hazard rates for some risk factors (stratified Cox models) can be used. Another approach is to use time-dependent risk factors in the model that allow for different effects of the factors in distinct time intervals after transplant. Time-dependent covariates can be used to model intermediate events, such as graft-versus-host disease, which occur after transplant. It is important when building a model to distinguish between risk factors that are fixed at the time of transplant, and factors that are only known after transplant. Factors that are known after transplant must be treated as time-dependent factors.

There are a number of diagnostic plots that can be used to check that the Cox model is appropriate. This includes plots to check the proportionality of the hazard rates for individuals with different risk factors, plots to check for possible outliers, plots to check the influence of a particular individual on the estimated magnitude of the estimated effect of a given risk, and plots to determine the correct functional form that a given risk

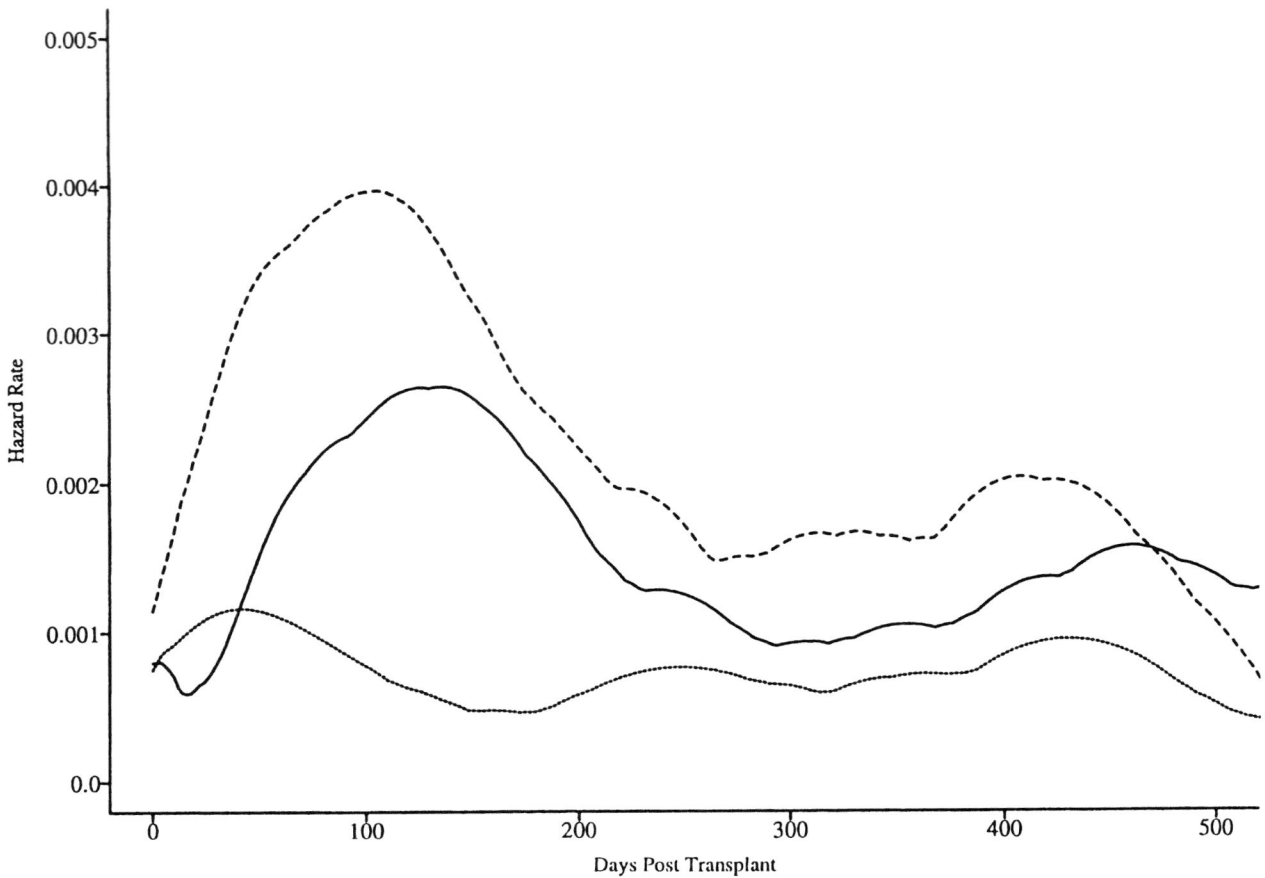

Fig. 107.5. Smoothed estimates of the hazard rate. ALL, solid line; AML-low risk, dotted line; AML-high risk, dashed line.

will have on survival. Examples and details of these plots can be found in Chapter 11 of Klein and Moeschberger (1997).

Relative risk

The relative risk is the ratio, at a given point after transplant, of the chance of experiencing a given event, for an individual in one group as compared to an individual in another group. When the Cox model is used, this quantity is assumed to be the same at any point in time. A relative risk of one, with regards to dying, for example, means that individuals in both groups, who could have died at any point in time, are dying at the same rate and there is no difference in survival between the two groups. Relative risks obtained from a multivariate Cox model are adjusted for other factors (see Klein *et al.*, 2002b, for further discussion of relative risk)

In the BU/CY example, a Cox model was fitted with the factor "disease type at transplant" (AML-low risk, AML-high risk, ALL). After analysis, it was found that other factors that should be adjusted for, when comparing disease groups, were the FAB type for AML patients, and donor and recipient ages. An adjusted test of the hypothesis of no difference between disease groups had a *P* value of .003. To compute relative risks for the

disease groups, one of the groups (ALL) is selected as the baseline (denominator) for the calculation. The relative risk of treatment failure for an AML-low risk patient relative to an ALL patient is 0.33 (95% confidence interval 0.23–0.67). This says that AML low-risk patients are failing about one-third as fast as ALL patients.

Logistic regression

An alternative to the Cox regression model, logistic regression, is available for some endpoints following a bone marrow or blood stem cell transplant. Logistic regression is used to model binary response data. For this technique it is necessary that the outcome be known for each patient. For example, if one wished to model 100 day mortality, each patient would need to be classified as either a 100 day survivor or as dying in the first 100 days. A patient who was lost to follow-up prior to 100 days or did not have the potential of 100 days of follow-up would be excluded from the analysis.

If one calls one of the binary outcomes a success and one a failure, then logistic regression models the log odds in favor of a success as a function of the risk factors (the logit of a success). The odds in favor of a success is the probability of a success divided by the probability of a failure. For the logistic model the logit is assumed to be a linear function of the risk factors. Kleinbaum (1994) presents a very readable description of this technique.

Clinical trials

Randomized clinical trials are considered the gold standard for comparing different therapeutic treatments. These trials are based on randomly assigning patients to treatments and are typically blinded to either patient, physician, or both. The proper and ethical design of randomized trials requires a sound statistical design (Peto *et al.*, 1976, 1977), and a statistician should be involved in the design phase of the study to ensure that these issues are addressed.

Clinical trial designs include parallel group designs (where independent groups of patients are used for each treatment), crossover designs (where each patient is given both treatments), and other longitudinal designs. Designs may be based on a fixed sample size or they may be group sequential designs, where after each block of patients a decision is made as to whether to continue the trial or to stop and make an inference. Good, readable, books on clinical trial design and analysis include Pocock (1983), Meinert (1986), and Buyse, Staquet, and Sylvester (1984).

Interim analysis and stopping rules

Having established the required sample sizes, randomization and stratification schemes and commenced the trial, the situation may occur before the estimated sample size is reached where investigators want to "take a look," (i.e., perform an interim analysis and see how the trial is progressing). Ideally, the number of "looks" should have been established in the design stage of the trial, keeping in mind that each look affects the significance level that can be applied in the analysis. The commonly applied alpha level of .05 implies that in any test on the differences between two samples from a certain population, one would expect to find a significant result purely by chance 5% of the time (i.e., in 1 out of 20 tests). Performing two or more tests on the same set of data therefore increases this probability, and so some adjustment has to be made to the overall significance level to allow for the fact that the data are being analyzed more than once (McPherson, 1974; Pocock, 1982).

In some instances when stopping rules are applied (Armitage, 1975; Whitehead, 1991) a trial may be stopped before reaching the original sample size estimates, for instance if a higher than expected difference between treatments is found. Ethically this is appealing, since it avoids the situation of assigning patients to an ineffective treatment, and allows investigators to proceed with the effective treatment on all patients earlier than expected. However, there are precautions to be considered in stopping a trial too early, such as those addressed in Friedman, Furberg, and Demets (1985) and Whitehead (1991). For example, there is a possibility, if a trial is stopped early, when the sample sizes are small, that the perceived differences could be due simply to sampling variations rather than to an actual difference between treatments.

Databases

Any serious HSC transplant program requires the service of a data collector and a data analyst. Credible statistical analysis relies on accurate data collection and this is best achieved by diligent maintenance of, and transcription from, patient records. In addition, it is strongly recommended that the data collector talks with a physician attached to the program on a regular basis. The statistician is often responsible for designing and maintaining a database to store the large amounts of data generated by an HSC transplant program—data that includes patient background information, daily vital signs, hematologic and biochemical values, and details of the pretransplant preconditioning regimen, posttransplant treatments, infections, and other complications such as graft-versus-host disease, relapse, survival, and causes of death. For any posttransplant event it is important that the timing of the event be recorded, not just whether the event has occurred or not. A well-designed database that allows for complicated retrieval of data subsets will allow the statistician the freedom to perform the most appropriate analysis for a given study.

References

Altman, D. G. (1991). *Practical Statistics for Medical Researcher.* New York: Chapman-Hall.

Armitage, P. (1975). *Sequential Medical Trials. 2nd ed.* Oxford: Blackwell.

Barrett, A. J., Horowitz, M. M., Pollock, B. H. *et al.* (1994). Bone marrow transplants from HLA-identical siblings as compared with chemotherapy for children with acute lymphoblastic leukemia in a second remission. *New England Journal of Medicine,* **331,** 1253–8.

Buyse, M. E., Staquet, M. J., & Sylvester, R. J. (1984). *Cancer Clinical Trials: Methods and Practice.* New York: Oxford University Press.

Copelan, E. A., Biggs, J. C., Thompson, J. M. *et al.* (1991). Treatment for acute myelocytic leukemia with allogeneic bone marrow transplantation following preparation with Bu/CY. *Blood,* **78,** 838–43.

Cox, D. R. (1972). Regression models and life-tables (with discussion). *Journal of the Royal Statistical Association B,* **34,** 187–220.

Dawson-Saunders, B. & Trapp, R. G. (1994). *Basic & Clinical Biostatistics, Second Edition.* East Norwalk, CT: Appleton & Lange.

Fleming, T. R. & Harrington, D. P. (1981). A class of hypothesis tests for one and two samples of censored survival data. *Communications in Statistics,* **10,** 763–94.

Friedman, L. M., Furberg, D. C., & Demets, D. L. (1985). *Fundamentals of Clinical Trials. 2nd ed.* Littleton, Mass: PSG Publishing.

Gluckman, E., Auerbach, A. D., Horowitz, M. M. *et al.* (1995). Bone marrow transplantation for Fanconi anemia. *Blood,* **86,** 2856–62.

Gooley, TA, Leisenring, W, Crowley, J, & Storer, B. (1999). Estimation of failure probabilities in the presence of competing risks: new representations of old estimators. *Statistics in Medicine,* **18,** 695–706.

Kaplan, E. L. & Meier, P. (1958). Non-parametric estimation from incomplete observations. *Journal of the American Statistical Association,* **53,** 457–81.

Klein, J. P., Keiding, N, Shu, Y., Szydlo, R. M., & Goldman, J. M. (2000). Summary curves for patients transplanted for chronic myeloid leukaemia salvaged by a donor lymphocyte infusion: the current leukaemia-free survival curve. *British Journal of Haematology,* **109,** 148–52.

Klein, J. P. & Moeschberger, M. L. (1997). *Survival Analysis—Techniques for Censored and Truncated Data.* New York: Springer-Verlag

Klein, J. P., Rizzo, J. D., Zhang, M. J., & Keiding, N. (2002a). Statistical methods for the analysis and presentation of the results of bone marrow transplants. Part I: unadjusted analysis. *Bone Marrow Transplantation,* **28,** 909–915.

Klein, J. P., Rizzo, J. D., Zhang, M. J., & Keiding, N. (2002b). Statistical methods for the analysis and presentation of the results of bone marrow transplants. Part II: Regression modeling. *Bone Marrow Transplantation,* **28,** 1001–1011.

Kleinbaum, D. G. (1994). *Logistic Regression: A Self Learning Text.* New York: Springer-Verlag.

Kleinbaum, D. G. (1996). *Survival Analysis: A Self Learning Text.* New York: Springer-Verlag.

Kleinbaum, D. G., Kupper, L. L., Morgenstern, H. (1982). *Epidemiologic Research.* New York: Van Nostraud Reinhold.

McPherson, K. (1974). Statistics: the problem of examining accumulating data more than once. *New England Journal of Medicine,* **290,** 501–2.

Meinert, C. L. (1986). *Clinical Trials: Design, Conduct and Analysis.* New York: Oxford University Press.

Peto, R., Pike, M. C., Armatage, P. *et al.* (1976). Design and analysis of randomized clinical trials requiring prolonged observation of each patient. I. Introduction and design. *British Journal of Cancer,* **34,** 585–612.

Peto, R., Pike, M. C., Armatage, P. *et al.* (1977). Design and analysis of randomized clinical trials requiring prolonged observation of each patient. II. Analysis and examples. *British Journal of Cancer,* **35,** 1–17.

Pocock, S. (1982). Statistical aspects of clinical trial design. *Statistician,* **31,** 1–17.

Pocock, S. J. (1983). *Clinical Trials: A Practical Approach.* New York: John Wiley & Sons.

Whitehead, J. (1991). *The Design and Analysis of Sequential Clinical Trials. 2nd ed.* Chichester, England: Ellis Horwood.

PART XIII   DEVELOPING AREAS IN HEMATOPOIETIC STEM CELL TRANSPLANTATION

108 Monoclonal antibodies as antileukemia and antilymphoma drugs

KATHERINE L. RUFFNER AND DANA C. MATTHEWS

Vanderbilt University Medical Center, Nashville, and Fred Hutchinson Cancer Research Center and University of Washington, Seattle, USA

Introduction

Over the last two decades, monoclonal antibodies reactive with discrete subsets of normal and malignant hematopoietic cells have been produced and tested as potential therapeutic agents in patients with lymphohematopoietic malignancies. Two of these antibodies have subsequently received U.S. Food and Drug Administration (FDA) approval for the treatment of lymphoma (rituximab, Rituxan, MabThera) and chronic lymphatic leukemia (CLL) (alemtuzumab, Campath-1H). Following intravenous administration, the antibodies bind to tumor cells and recruit the host immune system against antibody-bound cells, thus inducing antibody- and complement-mediated apoptosis. Conjugates of monoclonal antibodies and cytotoxic drugs have also been produced and evaluated clinically, and one such conjugate has been approved by the FDA for treatment of relapsed acute myeloid leukemia (AML) in the elderly (gemtuzumab ozogamicin, CMA-676, Mylotarg). Drug-antibody conjugates are able to effect cytotoxicity by delivering a cytotoxic drug to target cells and thus are not dependent on the host immune system for elimination of disease. Conjugates of monoclonal antibodies and radionuclides offer an additional advantage in their ability to radiate not only those cells to which they bind directly, but also any antigen-negative target cells lying within the pathlength of the radionuclide (Pagel *et al.*, 2002). The fact that leukemic cells exist in close physical proximity to normal marrow progenitors, which are also radiosensitive, places constraints on this form of therapy for the treatment of leukemia, but is less of a concern in lymphoma, where extensive marrow involvement is less common. Recently, a radioimmunoconjugate (ibritumomab tiuxetan, IDEC-Y2B8, Zevalin) was approved by the FDA for the treatment of rituximab-refractory non-Hodgkin's lymphoma, but patients must have no more than 25% lymphoma involvement of the bone marrow in order to meet criteria for treatment with ibritumomab tiuxetan. In 2003, a second radioimmunoconjugate, ^{137}I-tositamomab (Bexxar) was approved by the FDA for use in non-Hodgkin's lymphoma. One setting in which radioimmunoconjugates may prove to be useful for the treatment of either leukemia or lymphoma is in hematopoietic stem cell (HSC) transplantation, where toxicity to normal hematopoietic progenitors is reversed by the subsequent transplant. The use of radioim-munoconjugates may allow for the delivery of more radiotherapy to sites of disease than can be delivered using the more conventional approach of external beam total body irradiation (TBI), and several clinical trials of radioimmunotherapy as an adjunct to HSC transplantation for the treatment of either disease are currently ongoing. In this chapter, the basis for trials evaluating monoclonal antibodies in the treatment of lymphohematopoietic malignancies will be reviewed, their current status will be summarized, and future research directions discussed.

Use of unmodified antibodies in the treatment of leukemia and lymphoma

The first monoclonal antibodies studied as antileukemia and antilymphoma therapies were murine antibodies directed against human cell surface antigens (Table 108.1). Because most murine antibodies are weak mediators of human antibody-dependent cytotoxicity, minimal effects on tumor burden were seen in clinical trials, although binding of the infused antibodies to tumor cells in the peripheral circulation, bone marrow, and lymph nodes was demonstrated. Subsequently, chimeric or "humanized" versions of several of these antibodies were engineered and evaluated in clinical trials. Chimeric antibodies consist of the variable regions of a murine antibody grafted onto the constant regions of human IgG; humanized antibodies retain only the complementarity-determining region of the original murine antibody grafted onto a human IgG. Chimeric and humanized antibodies have both been shown to effect antibody-dependent cytotoxicity complement-dependent cytotoxicity, and apoptosis of target cells in vitro, presumably because of the presence of a human Fc portion. Collectively, murine, chimeric, and humanized antibodies are referred to as "unmodified antibodies" to distinguish them from antibody-radionuclide or antibody-cytotoxic drug conjugates.

The FDA-approved monoclonal antibody rituximab (C2B8, Rituxan, MabThera) is a chimeric antibody directed against the B-cell surface antigen CD20. In the pivotal phase II multi-institutional trial, 48% of 116 patients with relapsed low grade or follicular lymphoma responded to a course of four weekly doses of rituximab 375 mg/m^2 dose, and the median time to progression for responders was 13 months (McLaughlin *et al.*,

Table 108.1.   *Early trials of unmodified monoclonal antibodies in the treatment of leukemia and lymphoma*

Disease	Investigators	Antibody
AML	Ball *et al.*, 1983 Scheinberg *et al.*, 1991 Caron *et al.*, 1994	Several M195 (anti-CD33) HuM195 (humanized anti-CD33)
CALLA⁺ ALL	Ritz *et al.*, 1981	J5 (anti-CD10)
T cell ALL	Kreitman 1991	Anti-Tac (anti-CD25)
CLL	Dillman *et al.*, 1986; Foon *et al.*, 1984 Osterborg *et al.*, 1997	T101 (anti-CD5) Alemtuzumab, Campath-1H (anti-CD52)
NHL	Press *et al.*, 1987 Maloney *et al.*, 1994 Goldenberg *et al.*, 1991	IF5 (anti-CD20) C2B8 (anti-CD20) LL2 (anti-CD22)

Abbreviations: AML, acute myeloid leukemia; CALLA, common acute lymphoblastic leukemia antigen; ALL, acute lymphoblastic leukemia; CLL, chronic lymphocytic leukemia; NHL, non-Hodgkin's lymphoma

1998). Based on these results, rituximab was initially approved only for use as a single agent given in four doses for the treatment of relapsed indolent non-Hodgkin's lymphoma, but in May 2001 the FDA expanded the label to include use of eight weekly doses, treatment of patients with bulky disease, and retreatment of patients who had previously responded to rituximab (Grillo-Lopez *et al.*, 2002).

Rituximab has also been evaluated in combination with conventional chemotherapy for the treatment of both indolent and aggressive lymphomas and has proven both safe and efficacious. A large (*n* = 399) randomized clinical trial comparing cyclophosphamide, doxorubicin, vincristine, and prednisone (CHOP) chemotherapy plus rituximab to CHOP chemotherapy alone as first-line treatment of diffuse large B-cell lymphomas in patients aged 60–80 demonstrated significant improvements in complete remission rate (76% vs. 63%, *P* = .005), 2-year event-free survival (57% vs. 38%, *P* < .001) and 2-year survival (70% vs. 57%, *P* = .007) in the CHOP plus rituximab arm (Coiffier *et al.*, 2002). Clinical studies evaluating the role of rituximab in combination with conventional chemotherapy in autologous hematopoietic stem cell transplant preparative regimens are currently ongoing.

Alemtuzumab (Campath-1H), the other FDA-approved unmodified antibody, is a humanized antibody directed against CD52, an antigen found on benign and malignant B and T lymphocytes, NK (natural killer) cells, monocytes and macrophages. Although alemtuzumab has been studied in patients with either lymphoid leukemias or lymphomas, it is currently approved only for the treatment of alkylator- and fludarabine-resistant CLL. Its approval for this indication was based on a response rate of 33% with a complete response rate of 2% and a mean time to progression of 9 months seen in 93 patients with CLL who had previously received alkylators and had failed fludarabine (Keating *et al.*, 2002). Alemtuzumab is currently being evaluated in conjunction with standard chemotherapeutic agents and as a component of HSCT preparative regimens for the treatment of lymphoid malignancies, as well as being a component of non-myeloablative conditioning regimens for a wide variety of disorders.

A third unmodified antibody that has been evaluated for the treatment of lymphoid malignancies is epratuzumab (hLL2), a humanized antibody directed against CD22. A single small phase I/II trial of epratuzumab demonstrated objective responses in 6 and complete remissions in 3 of 13 patients with follicular lymphoma, and objective responses in 5 and complete responses in 3 of 22 heavily pretreated patients with diffuse large B cell lymphoma (Leonard *et al.*, 2000). Currently, clinical trials evaluating either epratuzumab as a single agent in rituximab-refractory patients with indolent lymphoma, or the combination of epratuzumab and rituximab for both indolent and aggressive lymphomas, are ongoing.

Both the murine anti-CD33 antibody M195 and its humanized derivative HuM195 have been extensively evaluated at Memorial Sloan Kettering Cancer Center (MSKCC) for the treatment of advanced myeloid malignancies. The cell-surface glycoprotein CD33 is expressed on all normal myeloid cells from the myeloblast to the myelocyte/metamyelocyte stage and on malignant blast cells in greater than 90% of AML patients (Table 108.2). M195 antibody was initially studied as single agent in the treatment of 10 patients with relapsed or refractory AML, blast-phase chronic myeloid leukemia (CML), or chronic myelomonocytic leukemia (CMML). Whole-body gamma camera scanning of patients following administration of a dose of M195 antibody trace-labeled with iodine-131 (¹³¹I) demonstrated localization of antibody to bone marrow, spleen, and sites of extramedullary disease, but no tumor responses were seen following subsequent administration of unlabeled M195 antibody (Scheinberg *et al.*, 1991). In an effort to improve the cytotoxicity of M195 antibody, the humanized derivative HuM195 antibody was produced and evaluated as a single agent in 10 patients with advanced AML or CML. Three patients experienced a reduction in percentage of bone marrow blasts, and a fourth patient entered a complete remission lasting four years (Caron, Dumont, & Scheinberg, 1998). A trial of HuM195 antibody for 35 patients with refractory AML was then conducted, and two patients on this trial achieved com-

Table 108.2.   *Target antigens and characteristics*

	Distribution	Modulation after antibody binding?
Myeloid antigens		
CD33	All normal myeloid cells from the myeloblast to the metamyelocyte; malignant blasts of >90% AML pts	Yes; antigen-antibody complex internalized
CD66	Mature myeloid cells	No
CD45	All nucleated hematopoietic cells; malignant blasts of 85%–95% AML and ALL	No
Lymphoid antigens		
HLA-DR	B cells	No
CD45	All nucleated hematopoietic cells	No
CD20	Normal and malignant B cells	No
CD19	Normal and malignant B cells	Yes; antigen-antibody complex internalized
CD22	Normal and malignant B cells	Yes; antigen-antibody complex internalized
CD25 (Tac)	Activated or malignant T cells	No
CD52	Benign and malignant B cells, T cells, NK cells, monocytes, macrophages	No

Abbreviations: AML, acute myeloid leukemia; ALL, acute lymphoblastic leukemia; NK, natural killer.

plete remission with HuM195 antibody alone (Feldman *et al.*, 1999). The patients entering complete remission had fewer than 30% bone marrow blasts, suggesting that HuM195 antibody may be most effective when given to patients with relatively low disease burdens.

Several other trials have since been conducted evaluating HuM195 antibody in combination with conventional leukemia therapies. In a clinical trial conducted at MSKCC, HuM195 antibody was studied as consolidation therapy following induction with all-*trans* retinoic acid (ATRA) and chemotherapy for patients with acute promyelocytic leukemia (APL), and the results of these trials suggest that HuM195 antibody in combination with ATRA may be superior to ATRA alone for elimination of minimal residual disease in patients with APL (Jurcic, 2001). HuM195 antibody has also been given in combination with interleukin-2 (IL-2) for the treatment of advanced myeloid malignancies, but only one of 13 patients studied achieved a complete remission with this regimen (Kossman *et al.*, 1999), and the toxicity observed has tempered enthusiasm for further investigation of this combination approach.

Use of antibody-toxin and antibody-drug conjugates in the treatment of leukemia and lymphoma

Chimeric and humanized antibodies must remain on the cell surface after binding in order to effect substantial host-mediated cytotoxicity. If a target antigen is internalized or shed following antibody binding, unmodified antibodies against this antigen will be largely ineffective as cytotoxic drugs (Table 108.2), which may partially explain the relatively weak antileukemic efficacy of HuM195 antibody as a single agent in advanced disease. However, if an antibody is conjugated to a toxic moiety that is internalized along with the antibody, cytotoxicity can be effected without participation of the host

immune system. Several such antibody-toxin and antibody-drug conjugates have been produced and tested as therapies for lymphoid or myeloid malignancies, including gemtuzumab ozogamicin (CMA-676, Mylotarg), a humanized anti-CD33 antibody conjugated to the potent antitumor antibiotic calicheamicin, which is now FDA-approved for the treatment of relapsed AML in elderly patients. Once bound to a target cell, the antibody-calicheamicin conjugate is internalized, and the small calicheamicin molecules are cleaved from the antibody and enter the nucleus, where they bind in a sequence-specific manner to the minor groove of DNA and cause double-stranded breaks, thus inducing apoptosis. Of 142 patients with AML in untreated first relapse who were enrolled in several phase II studies, 30% achieved complete remission following two doses of gemtuzumab ozogamicin given at 9 mg/m^2 two weeks apart (Sievers *et al.*, 2001). Trials evaluating the efficacy of gemtuzumab ozogamicin in combination with conventional chemotherapy as either first-line therapy or salvage therapy are currently under way.

Two different toxin conjugates of B43, a murine antibody directed against the B-cell surface antigen CD19, have been evaluated as therapy for acute lymphoblastic leukemia (ALL). Like CD33, CD19 is rapidly internalized following antibody binding. B43-genistein is a conjugate of B43 antibody and the tyrosine kinase inhibitor genistein that induces apoptosis in target cells by binding CD19 and inhibiting the Src-family protein tyrosine kinase associated with CD19. Seven children and eight adults with B-lineage ALL and one adult with CLL were treated with B43-genistein on a phase I/II trial conducted at the Parker Hughes Cancer Center (Uckun *et al.*, 1999). Four ALL patients demonstrated clinical responses, although two later suffered extramedullary relapses. B43-PAP, a conjugate of B43 antibody and pokeweed antiviral antigen, which effects apoptosis by poisoning ribosomes upon internalization into target cells, was evaluated in addition to chemotherapy in a

Children's Cancer Group trial for the treatment of high-risk B-lineage ALL (Seibel *et al.,* 2000). Twenty-eight children were randomized to receive chemotherapy with or without B43-PAP, and bone marrow disease status at day 14 of treatment was compared between the two randomized groups and with a third group of 255 nonrandomized children who received chemotherapy alone. The percentage of children with M1 marrows (<5% blasts) at day 14 was significantly higher in the group randomized to B43-PAP (93%) than in either the group randomized to no B43-PAP (43%, P = .02) or the nonrandomized group (57%, P = .04).

To date, clinical trials of unmodified monoclonal antibodies as single agents have shown the most promising results in the treatment of either indolent disease or substantially debulked aggressive disease, presumably because antibody- and complement-dependent cytotoxicity are relatively ineffective against large-burden aggressive disease. However, unmodified antibodies given along with conventional chemotherapy for the treatment of more aggressive disease have demonstrated superior response rates and time to disease progression compared to conventional chemotherapy alone. Antibody-toxin conjugates have demonstrated some success at controlling recurrent or high-risk acute leukemia, but are reliant on internalization after antibody binding, and appear to be vulnerable to the same cellular mechanisms responsible for disease resistance to chemotherapy (Matsui *et al.,* 2002). Furthermore, both unmodified antibodies and antibody-toxin conjugates are capable of killing only cells to which they bind directly.

Rationale for radioimmunoconjugates

Some of the limitations of unmodified antibodies and antibody-toxin conjugates can be overcome by radioimmunoconjugates, which consist of a radionuclide linked to a monoclonal antibody. If radionuclides that deposit energy locally over several cell diameters are used, antibodies are provided with an effector mechanism that has the capacity to kill not only antigen-positive cells to which the antibodies actually bind, but also antigen-negative variants in the immediate vicinity of the targeted cell (Table 108.3). Also, antigenic modulation following antibody binding might be less of a problem if the radionuclide is retained in the target cell following internalization.

Radiation is a widely used and effective form of therapy for leukemia or lymphoma when used either as a single treatment modality for focal bulky disease or when given systemically (i.e., as TBI) in the context of HSC transplantation. However, the doses at which radiation demonstrates an optimum anticancer effect may approach or exceed normal organ tolerance. Two prospective randomized allogeneic transplant trials, one in acute myeloid leukemia (AML) in first remission and a second in a chronic myeloid leukemia (CML) in chronic phase, comparing conditioning regimens containing cyclophosphamide plus either 12 Gy or 15.75 Gy TBI have been reported (Clift *et al.,* 1990, 1991). In both studies, the higher TBI dose was associated with a decrease in the leukemia recurrence rate post-transplant, from 35% to 13% in the case of AML (P = .06), and from 30% to 7% in the case of CML (P = .008), thus demonstrating the steep dose-response of leukemia to irradiation. However, increasing the TBI dose did not improve overall survival, since the higher dose regimens were associated with an increase in severe or fatal toxicities, principally involving the lung, liver, and mucous membranes. Methods to deliver radiotherapy more specifically to leukemic cells might dramatically improve the outcome of HSC transplantation, particularly in those settings where relapse rates are high, by decreasing relapse rates without increasing toxicity to normal organs.

Table 108.3. *Isotopes for radioimmunotherapy*

Radioisotope	$t^{1/2}$	Energy of decay (MeV)	Path length (mm)	Comments	Antibodies studied as conjugates of this isotope
β and γ emitters					
Iodine[131]	8.1 days	0.6	0.8	Radiation isolation required because of high-energy emissions	Anti-HLA-DR (Lym-1) Anti-CD33 (M195, HuM195, p67) Anti-CD22 (LL2, HLL2) Anti-CD20 (tositumomab) Anti-CD45 (BC8)
Rhenium[188]	17 hr	2.1	4.4	Low-energy γ component permits imaging for biodistribution	Anti-CD66
β emitters					
Yttrium[90]	2.5 days	1.1	5.3	No radiation isolation, but co-administration of a surrogate isotope (^{111}In) required for biodistribution determination	Anti-CD20 (ibritumomab tiuxetan) Anti-CD33 (HuM195) Anti-Tac Anti-CD22 (HLL2)
α emitters					
Bismuth[213]	46 min	8.0	0.06	High-energy, short pathlength, but very short half-life	Anti-CD33 (HuM195)

Use of antibody-radionuclide conjugates in the treatment of myeloid leukemia

Clinical trials of radioimmunotherapy in myeloid leukemia have involved antibodies directed at several different antigenic determinants (Table 108.3). The first clinical trials in AML explored the use of radioimmunoconjugates of M195 antibody and another murine anti-CD33 antibody, p67. Following completion of the phase I study of trace-labeled ^{131}I-M195 antibody followed by multiple doses of unmodified antibody described above, the group from MSKCC performed a dose escalation trial in which antibody labeled with increasing amounts of ^{131}I was administered (Schwartz et al., 1993). Twenty-four patients with recurrent myeloid leukemia were treated with 50 mCi/m^2 to 210 mCi/m^2 in two to four divided doses to allow for re-expression of CD33 following antigen-antibody internalization. Significant leukemic cytoreduction occurred in all patients treated with more than 90 mCi/m^2, and at doses greater than 135 mCi/m^2, pancytopenia was profound and lasted longer than 2 weeks. Because of concerns that higher doses of ^{131}I would be marrow-ablative, delivery of 160 mCi/m^2 or more was only permitted in patients with a suitable source of replacement stem cells. Most patients given doses of 160 mCi/m^2 or more received marrow in an effort to limit the period of pancytopenia after treatment. Three of the 24 patients achieved a complete remission and all of them required stem cell rescue.

Iodine-131-M195 antibody has also been evaluated as an adjunct to allogeneic transplantation for the treatment of advanced myeloid leukemia. Nineteen patients with relapsed or refractory myeloid leukemia were given 120 to 230 mCi/m^2 ^{131}I-M195 antibody followed by busulfan, cyclophosphamide, and stem cell infusion (Jurcic et al., 1995). All patients engrafted, and 18 achieved complete remission, although 10 (53%) died in remission of transplant-related causes. Six patients eventually relapsed, and three (16%) remained alive and disease-free 18 to 29 months posttransplant.

Lastly, ^{131}I-M195 antibody has been studied for the eradication of minimal residual disease. Seven patients with acute promyelocytic leukemia (APL) in morphological second complete remission were given 50 or 70 mCi/m^2 ^{131}I-M195 antibody. Six patients had marrows positive for PML-RARα by polymerase chain reaction (PCR) prior to receiving ^{131}I-M195 antibody, and two of theses patients became transiently PCR-negative following radiolabeled antibody treatment. Median disease-free survival was 8 months, and overall survival was 28 months (Jurcic et al., 1995).

At the Fred Hutchinson Cancer Research Center (FHCRC), Appelbaum and colleagues (1992) explored the use of an ^{131}I-conjugate of the anti-CD33 antibody p67. In this trial, nine patients were first given doses of trace-labeled antibody followed by serial gamma camera scans to determine in vivo localization of ^{131}I-antibody over time or "biodistribution," and the four patients (44%) with "favorable biodistribution," meaning those in which more radiation would be delivered by ^{131}I-p67 antibody to bone marrow than to any normal organ,

received high doses (110–330 mCi) of ^{131}I-p67 antibody followed by a conventional preparative regimen and marrow transplantation. This study demonstrated the feasibility of the approach but highlighted a major limitation of using conventionally labeled anti-CD33 antibody, namely the short residence time of ^{131}I in the marrow, presumably a result of internalization of the antigen-antibody complex with subsequent digestion and release of ^{131}I from the marrow space.

Because of the short residence time of ^{131}I in the marrow demonstrated in studies of ^{131}I-anti-CD33 antibodies, Scheinberg's group developed both yttrium-90 (^{90}Y) and bismuth-213 (^{213}Bi) conjugates of the anti-CD33 antibody HuM195. Unlike ^{131}I, both ^{90}Y and ^{213}Bi are metals, and both are linked to antibodies by means of a bifunctional chelate, which prevents digestion of the radioimmunoconjugate and expulsion of the radionuclide upon internalization into the target cell. Also, ^{90}Y is a pure β emitter and its β particle has both a longer pathlength and a higher energy of decay than the γ particle of ^{131}I, thus allowing for a greater "bystander effect", wherein antigen-negative target cells in the vicinity of the antibody-bound cells are irradiated (Table 108.3). While the lack of a γ component obviates the necessity for radiation isolation following treatment with high doses of ^{90}Y-immunoconjugates, it also makes determination of biodistribution more difficult, because gamma camera imaging cannot be used. Biodistribution of ^{90}Y-labeled antibodies must be estimated by administration of antibody labeled with a combined γ and electron-emitting "surrogate" radiometal such as indium-111 (^{111}In). Bismuth-213 is an α emitter with a very high energy of decay and a very short pathlength, making it ideal for use with an antibody that is internalized into the target cell after binding. However, the half-life of ^{213}Bi is very short (46 minutes), making it difficult to work with as a radioimmunoconjugate. Still, enough γ radiation is released by ^{213}Bi to permit use of gamma cameras for biodistribution determination, and the period of radiation isolation needed is very short because of the short physical half-life of the radionuclide.

In the phase I trial of ^{90}Y-HuM195 conjugate, 19 patients with relapsed or refractory AML received doses of 0.1 to 0.3 mCi/kg of ^{90}Y-HuM195 antibody as a single dose. At 0.3 mCi/kg, grade 4 neutropenia lasting more than 35 days was seen and was considered the dose-limiting toxicity. Half of the 10 patients receiving 0.275 or 0.3 mCi/kg ^{90}Y-HuM195 had hypocellular marrows without evidence of leukemia at two or four weeks post-treatment, and one patient achieved a complete remission lasting five months (Jurcic, 2000). Because of the degree of myelosuppression demonstrated in this trial, further trials of ^{90}Y-HuM195 antibody are including only patients with autologous or HLA-matched allogeneic bone marrow or peripheral blood stem cells available for marrow rescue.

In the phase I trial of ^{213}Bi-HuM195 antibody, 18 patients with relapsed or refractory AML or CML were given 0.28 to 1.0 mCi/kg (16 to 95 mCi) of ^{213}Bi-HuM195 antibody. As with ^{90}Y-HuM195 antibody, prolonged myelosuppression was the dose-limiting toxicity. Biodistribution studies determined by gamma camera scanning revealed rapid uptake of ^{213}Bi-HuM195 antibody in bone marrow, liver, and spleen within 10 minutes of infusion, and the estimated absorbed radiation dose ratios of target organs to whole body were 1000–10,000 times greater than those seen with ^{90}Y-HuM195 or ^{131}I-HuM195 antibodies. Fourteen of the 18 patients treated demonstrated decreases in bone marrow blast percentages, and 14 of 15 evaluable patients demonstrated decreases in circulating blasts (Jurcic, 2001, and personal communication). Currently, a trial is under way evaluating the combination of cytosine arabinoside and ^{213}Bi-HuM195 antibody for the treatment of relapsed or refractory AML, myelodysplasia (MDS), or accelerated or myeloid blast phase CML in patients that are ineligible for allogeneic HSCT.

Radiolabeled antibodies against the CD66 antigen, which is present on normal myeloid cells but is not expressed by blast cells, have also been evaluated for the treatment of myeloid malignancies. Bunjes and colleagues (2001) coupled an anti-CD66 antibody to rhenium-188 (^{188}Re), a combined β and γ-emitter with a physical half-life of 17 hours. Thirty-six patients with AML or MDS received trace-labeled doses of ^{188}Re-anti-CD66 antibody followed by gamma camera scanning to estimate biodistribution. All 36 patients had favorable biodistribution and received therapy doses of ^{188}Re-anti-CD66 antibody delivering a mean of 15.3 Gy radiation to bone marrow followed by one of several conventional myeloablative conditioning regimens and either allogeneic or autologous stem cell infusion. The relapse rate after a median follow-up of 18 months was 26% (9 of 35 evaluable patients), and disease-free survival at 18 months was 45%. When the patients were divided between those in remission ($n = 15$) and those not in remission ($n = 21$) at the time of transplant, disease-free survival at 18 months was 67% and 31%, respectively, suggesting that ^{188}Re-anti-CD66 antibody may be most useful in the treatment of minimal residual disease.

CD45 is an antigen expressed on all nucleated hematopoietic cells and is on 85% to 95% of acute myeloid and lymphoblastic leukemias. Unlike CD33, CD45 is maintained on the cell surface after ligand binding and is also expressed at a higher copy number than CD33 (approximately 200,000 copies/cell vs. 10,000 copies/cell, respectively). Following the disappointing results of the phase I ^{131}I-p67 antibody trial, researchers at FHCRC evaluated the use of ^{131}I-anti-CD45 antibody as an adjunct to HSCT for the treatment of both AML and ALL. Matthews and colleagues (1999) at FHCRC conducted a phase I trial of an ^{131}I-conjugate of the murine anti-CD45 antibody BC8 followed by autologous or matched related donor HSCT for patients with AML, advanced MDS, or ALL. As in the phase I ^{131}I-p67 antibody trial, patients first received a trace-labeled dose of BC8 antibody followed by serial gamma camera scanning to determine the biodistribution of the radionuclide over time, and those with favorable biodistribution were treated with increasing doses of radiation delivered by ^{131}I-BC8 antibody combined with a standard transplant preparative regimen of cyclophosphamide and TBI. Forty-four patients

received trace-labeled doses of antibody, and of these, 37 (84%) had favorable biodistribution, thus demonstrating a substantially higher success rate than seen previously with the internalizing anti-CD33 antibody ^{131}I-p67 (44% with favorable biodistribution) (Fig. 108.1). Thirty-four patients went on to

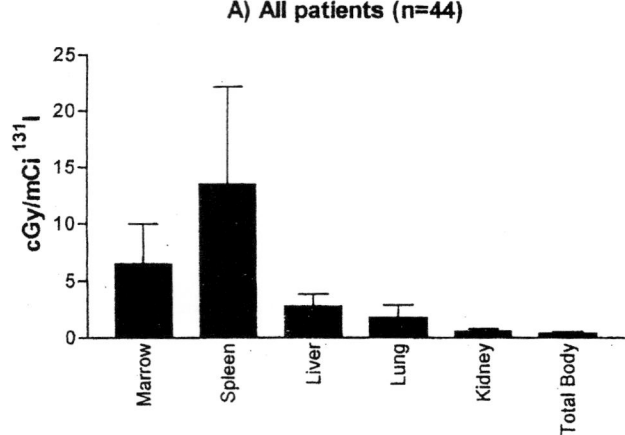

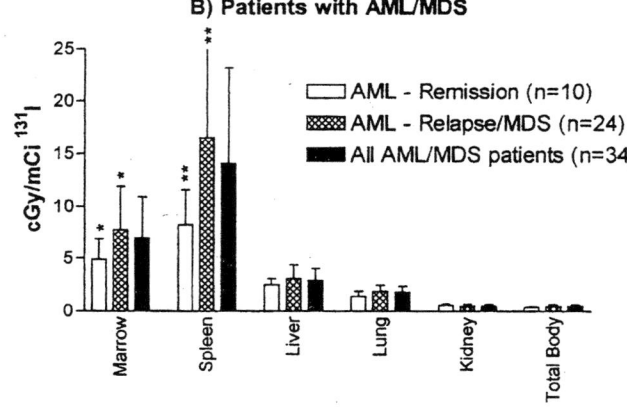

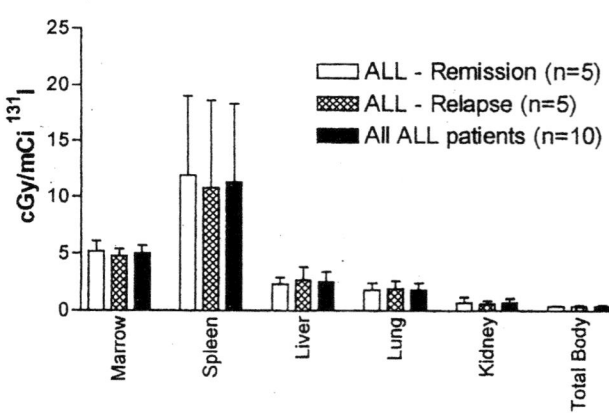

Figure 108.1. Estimated radiation absorbed doses per millicurie of ^{131}I administered for (A) all patients, (B) patients with AML or MDS, and (C) patients with ALL. Reproduced, with permission, from Matthews et al. (1999).

the treatment phase of the study, receiving doses of ^{131}I-BC8 antibody delivering 3.5 Gy to 12.25 Gy to liver (the normal organ receiving the most radiation from antibody) and 10 Gy to 28 Gy to bone marrow. The maximum tolerated dose of ^{131}I-BC8 antibody that could be combined with cyclophosphamide/TBI and autologous or matched related donor HSCT in this trial was 10.5 Gy to liver, which could deliver, on average, 24 Gy to bone marrow and 50 Gy to spleen. This trial demonstrated that ^{131}I-BC8 antibody delivers more radiation to bone marrow and spleen than to liver in most patients with advanced AML, MDS, or ALL, and can be safely combined with a conventional HSCT regimen. Furthermore, 7 of 25 patients (28%) with AML or MDS treated on this study survive disease-free 26 to 100 months posttransplant, and 3 of 9 patients (33%) with ALL survive 34 to 82 months posttransplant (Fig. 108.2).

A phase I/II study for patients with AML in first remission has subsequently been initiated at FHCRC (Ruffner & Matthews, 2000), in which radiation delivered by ^{131}I-BC8 is combined with a standard regimen of busulfan 16 mg/kg and cyclophosphamide 120 mg/kg followed by matched related donor stem cell infusion. Eighty-nine percent of patients enrolled to date have had favorable biodistribution, and 43 patients have subsequently received therapy doses of ^{131}I-BC8 antibody delivering a maximum of 5.25 Gy to liver and an average of 11.0 Gy to bone marrow followed by busulfan/cyclophosphamide and stem cell infusion. After a median follow-up of almost 4 years, 8 patients (19%) have relapsed, 8 (19%) have died of transplant-related mortality, and 27 (63%) are surviving disease-free. Since all but one patient had intermediate or high-risk cytogenetics by Southwest Oncology Group criteria, these results are encouraging, and the study continues accrual with a goal of treating 60 patients.

A phase II trial using ^{131}I-BC8 antibody combined with 120 mg/kg cyclophosphamide and 12 Gy TBI followed by matched related or unrelated donor transplant for patients with advanced AML or MDS has also been opened at FHCRC. Fourteen patients have been enrolled, 13 (93%) had favorable biodistribution, and 12 have proceeded to therapy doses of ^{131}I-BC8 antibody delivering a median of 19 Gy to bone marrow (range 8.9 to 33 Gy) followed by cyclophosphamide/TBI and related-donor ($n = 4$) or unrelated donor ($n = 8$) transplant (Rosario et al., 2001). Three patients (25%) survive disease-free 11 to 19 months posttransplant, four (33%) have relapsed, and five (42%) died of transplant-related toxicity.

Use of antibody-radionuclide conjugates in the treatment of lymphoid leukemia and lymphoma

One of the first radiolabeled antibodies evaluated in clinical trials for the treatment of lymphoid malignancies was ^{131}I-Lym-1 antibody, which targets an epitope on the HLA-DR antigen expressed by B cells. Gerald and Sally DeNardo and colleagues at UC Davis studied ^{131}I-Lym-1 antibody as a single agent in 5 patients with CLL (1994) and in 21 patients with advanced

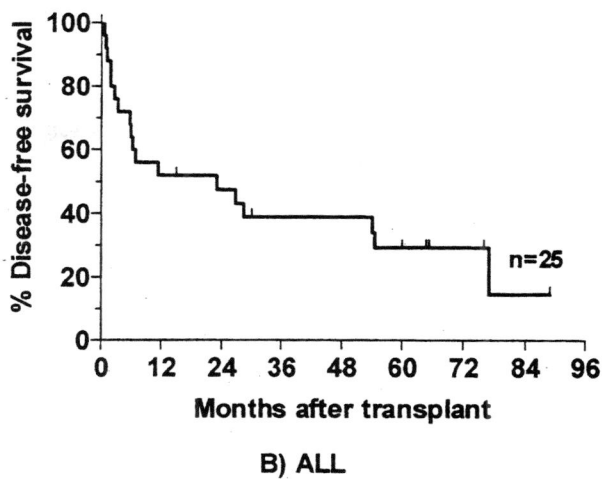

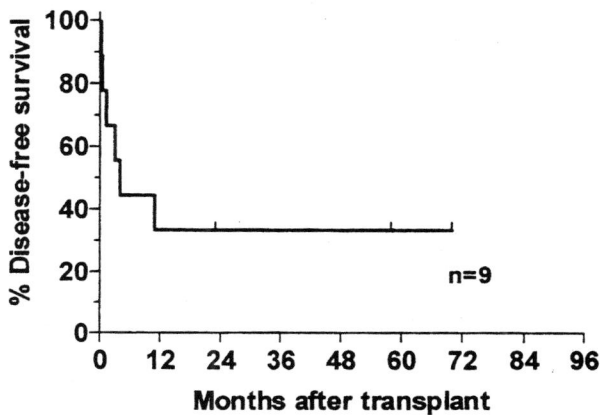

Figure 108.2. Kaplan-Meier analysis of disease-free survival for patients receiving therapeutic dose of ^{131}I-BC8 antibody followed by cyclophosphamide/TBI. (**A**) Patients with AML or MDS. (**B**) Patients with ALL. Reproduced, with permission, from Matthews et al. (1999).

non-Hodgkin's lymphoma (1998). Responses observed included decreased lymphadenopathy in all 5 CLL patients and normalization of leukocyte counts in 2 CLL patients. Also, objective responses were seen in 11 of 21 non-Hodgkin's lymphoma (NHL) patients, including complete responses in 7 patients.

A second target that has been explored in radioimmunotherapy of lymphoid malignancy takes advantage of the fact that the inducible alpha chain of the interleukin-2 receptor (Tac or CD25) is not expressed on resting T cells, but only on activated or abnormal cells. Adult T-cell leukemia (ATL) is a malignancy of mature lymphocytes caused by the retrovirus HTLV-1, and ATL cells express high levels of Tac. Accordingly, Waldmann et al. (1995) studied the use of an anti-Tac antibody radiolabeled with ^{90}Y in 18 patients with ATL. The first 9 patients were treated in a dose escalation trial and the second 9 in a phase II study at a uniform 10 mCi dose of [90]Y. Doses of ^{90}Y anti-Tac could be repeated at 6-week intervals and bone marrow transplant support was not employed. At doses above 10 mCi significant thrombocytopenia and granulocytopenia developed 4 to 5 weeks after therapy, with nadir counts occurring between weeks 5 and 7. Nine of 18 patients responded with either a partial (7) or complete (2) remission. The two complete remissions have lasted longer than 2 years. A third cell surface antigen that has been studied as a target for radiolabeled antibodies in the treatment of lymphoma is CD22, a B-cell restricted adhesion molecule that is broadly expressed by both normal and malignant B cells. Like CD19 and CD33, CD22 is rapidly internalized following binding by antibody. LL2 antibody, the murine parent antibody of hLL2 (epratuzumab), has been evaluated as an ^{131}I-conjugate (^{131}I-LL2, LymphoCide), for the treatment of lymphoma. Juweid et al. (1995) administered ^{131}I-LL2 antibody to 21 patients with B-cell NHL and observed 4 responses, including one complete response, among the 17 evaluable patients. The same investigators (Juweid et al., 1999) have administered both [131]I- and ^{90}Y-conjugates of the humanized antibody hLL2 to patients with B-cell NHL. Biodistribution was performed prior to administration of therapy doses of antibody, and the ^{90}Y-conjugate demonstrated higher ratios of radiation to tumor compared to bone marrow, lung, liver, or kidney, than the ^{131}I-hLL2 conjugate, presumably because of longer retention of ^{90}Y following antibody internalization. Objective tumor responses were seen in 2 of 13 patients given ^{131}I-hLL2 and 2 of 7 patients given ^{90}Y-hLL2.

To date, the most extensively studied radioimmunotherapy target for the treatment of lymphoma is the B-cell specific antigen CD20, against which both ^{131}I-tositumomab (^{131}I-anti-B1 antibody, Bexxar,) and ^{90}Y-ibritumomab tiuxetan (IDEC-Y2B8, Zevalin) are directed. With both ^{131}I-tositumomab and ^{90}Y-ibritumomab tiuxetan, a trace-labeled dose of either ^{131}I-tositumomab or ^{111}In-ibritumomab tiuxetan is administered followed by gamma camera scanning to calculate biodistribution, and the therapeutic dose is chosen based on a maximum calculated radiation dose to total body or to the non-target organ receiving the most radiation from antibody. Prior to each radiolabelled antibody dose, a dose of unlabeled antibody is given to increase the efficiency of tumor uptake of the radiolabelled antibody.

Iodine-131-tositumomab was initially studied at non-myeloablative doses as a single agent for the treatment of B-cell NHL by Kaminski and colleagues. In an update of the University of Michigan experience with ^{131}I-tositumomab, Kaminski et al. (2000) reported the results of 59 patients with relapsed or refractory CD20-positive NHL treated with doses of ^{131}I-tositumomab calculated to deliver a maximum total body dose of either 45 cGy for patients with a prior history of autologous HSCT or 75 cGy for patients who had not undergone previous transplantation. Forty-two (71%) responded and 20 (34%) went into complete remission following treatment with ^{131}I-tositumomab. The median time to disease progression was 12 months for all responders and 20.3 months for complete responders.

In a subsequent multi-center non-randomized trial, 60 patients with CD20-positive, refractory low-grade or transformed low-grade NHL were treated with ^{131}I-tositumomab as a single agent,

and disease responses were compared to those seen following the patients' most recent chemotherapy regimen (Kaminski et al., 2001). Objective responses were seen in 39 (65%) patients following treatment with ^{131}I-tositumomab, compared to objective responses in 17 (28%) patients following last qualifying chemotherapy ($P < .001$). Furthermore, the median duration of response was significantly longer following treatment with ^{131}I-tositumomab (6.5 months) than that achieved with last qualifying chemotherapy (3.4 months, $P < .001$).

Iodine-131-tositumomab has also been studied by Press and colleagues at the University of Washington/FHCRC at myeloablative doses in the setting of autologous HSCT for the treatment of relapsed B-cell NHL. In a phase I/II trial, 52 patients with relapsed or refractory CD20-positive NHL received therapy doses of ^{131}I-tositumomab delivering 20 to 27 Gy to the target organ receiving the most radiation from antibody (determined by individual biodistribution studies) followed by etoposide 60 mg/kg, cyclophosphamide 100 mg/kg, and infusion of autologous peripheral blood stem cells (Press et al., 2000). The maximum tolerated dose of ^{131}I-tositumomab that could be combined with cyclophosphamide/etoposide and autologous transplant on this trial was found to be the dose delivering 25 Gy to lung (the non-target organ receiving the most radiation from radiolabeled antibody in most patients). Twenty-seven (87%) of 31 evaluable patients responded, including 24 (77%) complete remissions and 3 (10%) partial remissions. Estimated overall survival at 2 years for all 52 patients was 83% (95% confidence interval (CI), 72%–94%), and progression-free survival was 68% (95% CI, 53%–83%). Both overall survival and progression-free survival of the patients treated with ^{131}I-tositumomab, cyclophosphamide/ etoposide and autologous transplant were superior to a non-randomized control group of 105 patients with NHL treated with TBI/cyclophosphamide/etoposide and autologous transplantation alone in a multivariate analysis which included disease stage, disease grade (indolent versus aggressive), and disease chemosensitivity (Fig. 108.3).

A study performed at the University of Washington/ FHCRC evaluating the responses of 16 patients with relapsed mantle cell lymphoma (MCL) following treatment with a dose of ^{131}I-tositumomab delivering 20 Gy (one patient), 23 Gy (one patient), or 25 Gy (14 patients) to lung followed by cyclophosphamide, etoposide, and autologous stem cell transplantation was published by Gopal et al. (2002). Patients were required to undergo debulking of disease prior to transplant if splenomegaly was present or the estimated disease burden exceeded 500 cc, and as a result, 5 patients had no measurable disease prior to ^{131}I-tositumomab treatment and transplant. Of the remaining 11 patients who were evaluable for response, 8 (73%) were in complete remission, 1 (9%) was in partial remission, and 2 (18%) had stable disease at the initial one-month follow-up posttransplant. The two patients with stable disease at one month posttransplant were later found to be in complete remission at 3 months and 1 year posttransplant, respectively, without any further chemother-

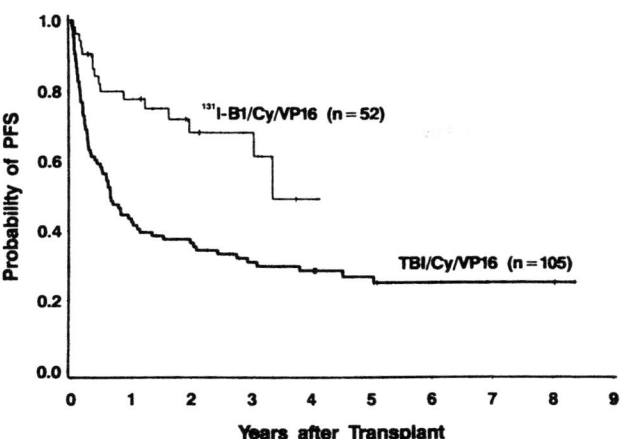

Figure 108.3. Progression-free survival in patients with B-cell lymphomas. Fifty-two patients were treated with ^{131}I-tositumomab, etoposide, cyclophosphamide, and ASCT (thin line), and 105 patients were treated with external beam TBI (1.5 Gy twice a day for 4 days), etoposide (60 mg/kg), cyclophosphamide (100 mg/kg), and ASCT (thick line). Reproduced, with permission, from Press *et al.* (2000).

apy or radiation. Thus, the overall response rate in these 11 patients was 100%, with 10 patients (91%) attaining complete remission. Yttrium-90-ibritumomab tiuxetan (IDEC-Y2B8, Zevalin), which consists of the murine parent anti-CD20 antibody of rituximab (2B8, ibritumomab) covalently bound to ^{90}Y via the chelate tiuxetan, is the first radioimmunoconjugate approved by the FDA for the treatment of hematologic malignancy. Currently, ^{90}Y-ibritumomab tiuxetan is indicated for treatment of relapsed or refractory low-grade, follicular, or transformed B-cell NHL, including disease that is refractory to rituximab. The initial study conducted by Witzig and colleagues (1999) was a phase I/II trial wherein 51 patients with relapsed or refractory low-grade NHL or relapsed intermediate-grade or MCL were treated with 0.2 mCi/kg (5 patients), 0.3 mCi/kg (15 patients), or 0.4 mCi/kg (30 patients) of ^{90}Y-ibritumomab tiuxetan following biodistribution determination using ^{111}In-ibritumomab tiuxetan. (One patient was not treated.) Objective responses were seen in 34 of the 51 patients (67%), with complete responses seen in 13 (26%) patients. Twenty-eight of 34 patients (82%) with low-grade NHL responded, including 9 (26%) complete remissions, 6 of 14 patients (43%) with intermediate-grade NHL responded with 4 (29%) complete remissions, and 0 of 3 patients with MCL responded. Among the 34 responders, the median time to disease progression was 12.9 months. Myelosuppression was seen following therapy with ^{90}Y-ibritumomab tiuxetan, but the study demonstrated that doses of 0.4 mCi/kg could be safely administered to patients without subsequent stem cell support. However, a dose reduction to 0.3 mCi/kg ^{90}Y-ibritumomab tiuxetan is recommended for patients with platelet counts less than 100,000/mm[3], and all patients receiving ^{90}Y-ibritumomab tiuxetan must have no more than 25% involvement of bone marrow by NHL.

The results of a randomized, controlled trial comparing ^{90}Y-ibritumomab tiuxetan to rituximab for the treatment of relapsed or refractory low-grade NHL or transformed B-cell NHL has been published by Witzig and colleagues (2002). One hundred forty-three patients from 27 institutions were enrolled, with 73 randomized to receive ^{90}Y-ibritumomab tiuxetan and 70 randomized to rituximab. The overall response rate in the ^{90}Y-ibritumomab group was significantly superior to that of the rituximab group (80% vs. 56%, $P = .002$), although the duration of response was not (median 14.2 months vs. median 12.1 months, respectively, $P = .644$). Toxicities were similar in the two groups of patients, although incidence of cough, bronchospam, nausea, and vomiting were higher in the ^{90}Y-ibritumomab group. Myelosuppression was seen following treatment with ^{90}Y-ibritumomab tiuxetan, and 57% patients in this group developed grade 3 or 4 neutropenia, but there were no septic deaths.

Current research directions

Monoclonal antibodies have proven promising for the treatment of several types of cancer, including leukemia and lymphoma. Although nearly all antibodies studied to date have demonstrated some anti-tumor efficacy when given as single agents, the optimum use of antibodies is likely to be as components of multi-agent regimens given with or without subsequent stem cell transplantation. In this way, malignancies can be simultaneously treated with several different cytotoxic effectors, presumably minimizing the necessary doses and associated toxicities of each agent. To this end, clinical trials combining either rituxmab, gemtuzumab ozogamicin, or [213]Bi-HuM195 antibody with other chemotherapeutic agents are currently ongoing.

The work of Press, Matthews, Scheinberg, and others has demonstrated that radiolabeled antibodies can be used alone as a preparative regimen for autologous transplantation, or as a component of full-dose myeloablative regimens for allogeneic stem cell transplantation. However, when targeted radiotherapy is given in addition to a myeloablative preparative regimen, the toxicity of allogeneic transplantation may be increased, thus minimizing the benefit obtained from decreased posttransplant relapse rates. If radioimmunotherapy could be substituted for a portion of the TBI or chemotherapy in a preparative regimen, then both relapse risk and posttransplant mortality may be lowered. To this end, two studies combining radioimmunotherapy with non-myeloablative allogeneic transplant for the treatment of advanced myeloid malignancies have been opened: an ^{131}I-BC8 antibody trial at FHCRC, and a ^{90}Y-HuM195 antibody trial at MSKCC. In both studies, the immunosuppression necessary to allow engraftment of allogeneic stem cells is provided by three doses of fludarabine, a small dose (2 Gy) of TBI, and posttransplant cyclosporine and mycophenolate mofetil. The only antileukemic therapy patients receive is 2 Gy TBI and radiolabeled antibody. McSweeney and colleagues (2001) have previously shown that the non-myeloablative regimen of fludarabine/2 Gy TBI/cyclosporine/mycophenolate mofetil enables engraftment of allogeneic stem cells with very little associated toxicity, but is largely ineffective in eradicating aggressive malignancies such as relapsed or refractory AML. By combining radioimmunotherapy with this non-myeloablative regimen, investigators hope to develop a treatment strategy that offers a disease response rate comparable to a conventional allogenic transplant with a toxicity profile comparable to a non-myeloablative transplant.

Another avenue being evaluated to increase the anti-tumor efficacy and decrease the toxicity of radioimmunoconjugates is the pre-targeting approach, which makes use of the high affinity between the proteins biotin and streptavidin. Non-radioactive antibodies labeled with streptavidin are given to patients in doses intended to saturate the antigen present on target cells, followed 24 hours later by the administration of a "clearing agent" consisting of a large biotinylated molecule that serves to clear any unbound antibody-streptavidin from the circulation. Three hours after the clearing agent is administered, a biotin-radionuclide is infused, which by virtue of its small size, rapidly binds to the target cells that are coated with strepavidin-antibody. Pre-clinical experiments have demonstrated up to 10-fold higher tumor:whole body ratios of radiation delivered by pre-targeted antibody compared to conventional radioimmunotherapy, and a clinical trial conducted by Weiden and colleagues (2000) demonstrated a tumor:whole body ratio of 38:1 in seven patients with B-cell NHL given ^{90}Y-biotin following pretargeting with streptavidin-labeled rituximab.

In the 20 years since Ball and colleagues (1983) first administered monoclonal antibodies to patients with leukemia, the field of immunotherapy for the treatment of hematologic malignancies has expanded in multiple directions. New target antigens are being sought, more cytotoxic antibodies are being developed, and new cytotoxic moieties, be they drugs or radionuclides, are being evaluated as antibody conjugates. Given the large body of promising data that has been generated to date, it is likely that antibodies will continue to develop more prominent roles in the treatment of leukemia and lymphoma in the future.

References

Appelbaum, F. R., Matthews, D. C., Eary, J. F. *et al.* (1992). The use of radiolabeled anti-CD33 antibody to augment marrow irradiation prior to marrow transplantation for acute myelogenous leukemia. *Transplantation,* **54,** 829–33.

Ball, E. D., Bernier, G. M., Cornwell, G. G. *et al.* (1983). Monoclonal antibodies to myeloid differentiation antigens: in vivo studies of three patients with acute myelogenous leukemia. *Blood,* **62,** 1203–10.

Bunjes, D., Buchmann, I., Duncker, C. *et al.* (2001). Rhenium 188-labelled anti-CD66 (a, b, c, e) monoclonal antibody to intensify the conditioning regimen prior to stem cell transplantation for patients with high-risk acute myeloid leukemia or myelodysplastic syndrome: results of a phase I-II study. *Blood,* **98,** 565–72.

Caron, P. C., Dumont, L., & Scheinberg, D. A. (1998). Supersaturating infusion humanized anti-CD33 monoclonal antibody HuM195 in myelogenous leukemia. *Clinical Cancer Research,* **4,** 1421–8.

Caron, P. C., Jurcic, J. G., Scott, A. M. *et al.* (1994). A phase 1b trial of humanized monoclonal antibody HuM195 (anti-CD33) in

myeloid leukemia: specific targeting without immunogenicity. *Blood,* **83,** 1760–8.

Clift, R. A., Buckner, C. D., Appelbaum, F. R. *et al.* (1990). Allogeneic marrow transplantation in patients with acute myeloid leukemia in first remission. A randomized trial of two irradiation regimens. *Blood,* **76,** 1867–71.

Clift, R. A., Buckner, C. D., Appelbaum, F. R. *et al.* (1991). Allogeneic marrow transplantation in patients with chronic myeloid leukemia in the chronic phase. A randomized trial of two irradiation regimens. *Blood,* **77,** 1660–5.

Coiffier, B., Lepage, E., Briere, J. *et al.* (2002). CHOP chemotherapy plus rituximab compared with CHOP alone in elderly patients with diffuse large-B-cell lymphoma. *New England Journal of Medicine,* **346,** 235–42.

DeNardo, G. L., DeNardo, S. J., Goldstein, D. S. *et al.* (1998). Maximum tolerated dose, toxicity, and efficacy of ^{131}I-LYM-1 antibody for fractionated radioimmunotherapy of non-Hodgkin's lymphoma. *Journal of Clinical Oncology,* **16,** 3246.

DeNardo, G. L., Lewis, J. P., DeNardo, S. J., & O'Grady, L. F. (1994). Effect of Lym-1 radioimmunoconjugate on refractory chronic lymphocytic leukemia. *Cancer,* **73,** 1425–32.

Dillman, R. O., Beauregard, J., Shawler, D. L. *et al.* (1986). Continuous infusion of T101 monoclonal antibody in chronic lymphocytic leukemia and cutaneous T cell lymphoma. *Journal of Biological Response Modifiers,* **5,** 394–410.

Feldman, E., Kalaycio, M., Schulman, P. *et al.* (1999). Humanized monoclonal anti-CD33 antibody HuM195 in the treatment of relapsed/refractory acute myelogenous leukemia (AML): Preliminary report of a phase II study. *Proceedings of the American Society of Clinical Oncology,* **18,** 4a (Abstract).

Finkelstein, J. B. (2001). FDA panel recommends two new cancer drugs for approval. *Journal of the National Cancer Institute,* **93,** 175–6.

Foon, K. A., Schroff, R. W., Bunn, P. A. *et al.* (1984). Effects of monoclonal antibody therapy in patients with chronic lymphocytic leukemia. *Blood,* **64,** 1085–93.

Goldenberg, D. M., Horowitz, J. A., Sharkey, R. M. *et al.* (1991). Targeting, dosimetry and radioimmunotherapy of B cell lymphomas with iodine-131-labeled LL2 monoclonal antibody. *Journal of Clinical Oncology,* **9,** 548–64.

Gopal, A. K., Rajendran, J. G., Petersdorf, S. H. *et al.* (2002). High-dose chemo-radioimmunotherapy with autologous stem cell support for relapsed mantle cell lymphoma. *Blood,* **99,** 3158–62.

Grillo-Lopez, A. J., Hedrick, E., Rashford, M., & Benyunes, M. (2002). Rituximab: ongoing and future clinical development. *Seminars in Oncology,* **29** (Suppl 2), 105–12.

Jurcic, J. G. (2000). Antibody therapy of acute myelogenous leukemia. *Cancer Biotherapy and Radiopharmaceuticals,* **15,** 319–26.

Jurcic, J. G. (2001). Antibody therapy for residual disease in acute myelogenous leukemia. *Critical Reviews in Oncology/Hematology,* **38,** 37–45.

Jurcic, J. G., Caron, P. C., Nikula, T. K. *et al.* (1995). Radiolabeled anti-CD33 monoclonal antibody M195 for myeloid leukemias. *Cancer Research,* **55** (Suppl), 5908s–10s.

Juweid, M., Sharkey, R. M., Markowitz, A. *et al.* (1995). Treatment of non-Hodgkin's lymphoma with radiolabeled murine, chimeric, or humanized LL2, an anti-CD22 monoclonal antibody. *Cancer Research,* **55,** 5899s–907s.

Juweid, M., Stadtmauer, E., Hajjar, G. *et al.* (1999). Pharmacokinetics, dosimetry, and initial therapeutic results with 131I-and (111)In-/90Y-labeled humanized LL2 anti-CD22 monoclonal antibody in patients with relapsed, refractory non-Hodgkin's lymphoma. *Clinical Cancer Research,* **5,** 3292s–303s.

Kaminski, M. S., Estes, J., Zasadny, R. *et al.* (2000). Radioimmunotherapy with iodine 131 tositumomab for relapsed or refractory B-cell non-Hodgkin lymphoma: updated results and long-term follow-up of the University of Michigan experience. *Blood,* **96,** 1259–66.

Kaminski, M. S., Zelenetz, A. D., Press, O. W. *et al.* (2001). Pivotal study of iodine 131 tositumomab for chemotherapy-refractory low-grade or transformed low-grade B-cell non-Hodgkin's lymphomas. *Journal of Clinical Oncology,* **19,** 3918–28.

Keating, M. J., Flinn, I., Jain, V. *et al.* (2002). Therapeutic role of alemtuzumab (Campath-1H) in patients who have failed fludarabine: results of a large international study. *Blood,* **99,** 3554–61.

Kossman, S. E., Scheinberg, D. A., Jurcic, J. G. *et al.* (1999). A phase I trial of humanized monoclonal antibody HuM195 (anti-CD33) with low-dose interleukin 2 in acute myelogenous leukemia. *Clinical Cancer Research,* **5,** 2748–55.

Leonard, J. P., Coleman, M., Chadburn, A. *et al.* (2000b). Epratuzumab (HLL2, anti-CD22 humanized monoclonal antibody) is an active and well-tolerated therapy for refractory/relapsed diffuse large B cell non-Hodgkin's lymphoma (NHL). *Blood,* **96,** 578a (Abstract).

Leonard, J. P. Coleman, M. Schuster, M. W. *et al.* (2000a). Immunotherapy of non-Hodgkin's lymphoma with epratuzumab (anti-CD22 monoclonal antibody): excellent tolerability with objective responses. *Proceedings of the American Society of Clinical Oncology,* **19,** 17a (Abstract).

Matsui, H., Takeshita, A., Naito, K. *et al.* (2002). Reduced effect gemtuzumab ozogamicin (CMA-676) on P-glycoprotein and/or CD34-positive leukemia cells and its restoration by multidrug resistance modifiers. *Leukemia,* **16,** 813–9.

Matthews, D. C., Appelbaum, F. R., Eary, J. F. *et al.* (1999). Phase I study of 131-anti-CD45 antibody plus cyclophosphamide and total body radiation for advanced acute leukemia and myelodysplastic syndrome. *Blood,* **94,** 1237–47.

McLaughlin, P., Grillo-Lopez, A. J., Link, B. K. *et al.* (1998). Rituximab chimeric anti-CD20 monoclonal antibody therapy for relapsed indolent lymphoma: half of patients respond to a four-dose treatment program. *Journal of Clinical Oncology,* **16,** 2825–33.

McSweeney, P. A., Niederweiser, D., Shizuru, J. A. *et al.* (2001). Hematopoietic cell transplantation in older patients with hematologic malignancies: replacing high-dose cytotoxic therapy with graft-versus-tumor effects. *Blood,* **97,** 3390–400.

Maloney, D. G., Liles, T. M., Czerwinski, D. K. *et al.* (1994). Phase I clinical trial using escalating single-dose infusion of chimeric anti-CD20 monoclonal antibody (IDEC-C2B8) in patients with recurrent B-cell lymphoma. *Blood,* **84,** 2457–66.

Osterborg, A., Dyer, M. J., Bunjes, D. *et al.* (1997). Phase II multicenter study of human CD52 antibody in previously treated chronic lymphocytic leukemia. European Study Group of CAMPATH-1H Treatment in Chronic Lymphocytic Leukemia. *Journal of Clinical Oncology,* **15,** 1567–74.

Pagel, J. M., Matthews, D. C., Appelbaum, F. R. *et al.* (2002). The use of radioimmunoconjugates in stem cell transplantation. *Bone Marrow Transplantation,* **29,** 807–16.

Press, O. W., Appelbaum, F., Ledbetter, J. A. *et al.* (1987). Monoclonal antibody 1F5 (anti-CD20) serotherapy of human B cell lymphomas. *Blood,* **69,** 584–91.

Press, O. W., Eary, J. F., Gooley, T. *et al.* (2000). A phase I/II trial of iodine-131-tositumomab (anti-CD20), etoposide, cyclophosphamide, and autologous stem cell transplantation for relapsed B-cell lymphomas. *Blood,* **96,** 2934–42.

Ritz, J., Pesando, J. M., Sallan, S. E. *et al.* (1991) Serotherapy of acute lymphoblastic leukemia with monoclonal antibody. *Blood,* **58,** 141–52.

Rosario, E., Rajendran, J., Ruffner, K. L. *et al.* (2001). Phase II study of radiolabeled anti-CD45 antibody with cyclophosphamide (CY) and total body irradiation (TBI) followed by allogeneic hematopoietic stem cell transplantation (HSCT) for patient with advanced acute myeloid leukemia (AML) or myelodysplastic syndrome (MDS). *Blood,* **98,** 857a (Abstract).

Ruffner, K. L. & Matthews, D. C. (2000). Current uses of monoclonal antibodies in the treatment of acute leukemia. *Seminars in Oncology,* **27,** 531–9.

Scheinberg, D. A., Lovett, D., Divgi, C. R. *et al.* (1991). A phase I trial of monoclonal antibody M195 in acute myelogenous leukemia: specific bone marrow targeting and internalization of radionuclide. *Journal of Clinical Oncology,* **9,** 478–90.

Schwartz, M. A., Lovett, D. R., Redner, A. *et al.* (1993). Dose-escalation trial of M195 labeled with iodine 131 for cytoreduction and marrow ablation in relapsed or refractory myeloid leukemias. *Journal of Clinical Oncology,* **11,** 294–303.

Seibel, N. L., Sather, H., Steinherz, P. G. *et al.* (2000). Upfront treatment with B43-PAP immunotoxin in newly-diagnosed children with high-risk ALL-Children's Cancer Group 1961. *Blood,* **96,** 721a (Abstract).

Sievers, E. L., Larson, R. A., Stadtmauer, E. A. *et al.* (2001). Efficacy and safety of gemtuzumab ozogamicin in patients with CD33-positive acute myeloid leukemia in first relapse. *Journal of Clinical Oncology,* **19,** 3244–54.

Uckun, F. M., Messinger, Y., Chen, C. L. *et al.* (1999). Treatment of therapy-refractory B-lineage acute lymphoblastic leukemia with an apoptosis-inducing CD19-directed tyrosine kinase inhibitor. *Clinical Cancer Research,* **5,** 3906–13.

Waldmann, T. A. (1991). Monoclonal antibodies in diagnosis and therapy. *Science,* **252,** 1657–62.

Waldmann, T. A., White, J. D., Carrasquillo, J. A. *et al.* (1995). Radioimmunotherapy of interleukin-2Rα-expressing adult T-cell leukemia with Yttrium-90-labeled anti-Tac. *Blood,* **86,** 4063–75.

Weiden, P. L., Breitz, H. B., Press, O. *et al.* (2000). Pretargeted radioimmunotherapy (PRIT) for treatment of non-Hodgkin's lymphoma (NHL): initial phase I/II study results. *Cancer Biotherapy and Radiopharmaceuticals,* **15,** 15–29.

Witzig, T. E., Gordon, L. I., Cabanillas, F. *et al.* (2002). Randomized controlled trial of yttrium-90-labeled ibritumomab tiuxetan radioimmunotherapy versus rituximab immunotherapy for patients with relapsed or refractory low-grade, follicular, or transformed B-cell non-Hodgkin's lymphoma. *Journal of Clinical Oncology,* **20,** 2453–63.

Witzig, T. E., White, C. A., Wiseman, G. A. *et al.* (1999). Phase I/II trial of IDEC-Y2B8 radioimmunotherapy for treatment of relapsed or refractory CD20+ B-cell non-Hodgkin's lymphoma. *Journal of Clinical Oncology,* **17,** 3793–803.

109 Use of monoclonal antibodies for preventing graft rejection and inducing graft-host tolerance

GEOFF HALE AND HERMAN WALDMANN

University of Oxford, Oxford, UK

Introduction

Hematopoietic stem cell (HSC) transplantation is perhaps the most intriguing and complex form of therapy from the point of view of the immunologist. It offers the possibility of a cure for many inborn and acquired defects of the hematopoietic system and permits the delivery of otherwise lethal doses of chemoradiotherapy for the treatment of malignant diseases. A long-term goal in experimental animal models and now beginning to be applied in humans, is that HSC can be used to induce tolerance to other tissues and thus enable the acceptance of other transplanted organs and even be used for the radical treatment of autoimmune disease.

Graft-versus-host disease (GVHD) is a major complication that can be virtually eliminated by removal of donor T lymphocytes from the stem cell inoculum (see Chapter 26). Historically, this has been accomplished by various means, but most of the techniques were relatively complex or hard to reproduce (Dicke, Van Hooff, & Van Bekkum, 1968; Reisner *et al.*, 1981; Noga *et al.*, 1986). When monoclonal antibodies were discovered, in vitro purging of donor T cells was seen as one of the more obvious applications and became the test bed for many different specificities and effector mechanisms. Not all were successful but a handful emerged that were relatively widely used (O'Reilly, 1987). One of these was Campath-1M, a rat IgM antibody directed against the CD52 antigen, a small, abundant, GPI-anchored glycoprotein expressed on virtually all human lymphocytes (Hale *et al.*, 1983; Hale, 2001). It is unusually lytic with human complement and was used with donor serum in a very simple, effective protocol (Waldmann *et al.*, 1984). This has been done in over 1,900 allogeneic marrow transplants throughout the world and the results, along with those from similar studies using other methods of T-cell depletion, showed us that there are rather clear advantages and drawbacks to this maneuver.

Consequences of T-cell depletion of donor bone marrow

It is clear that the risk of both acute and chronic GVHD is diminished by T-cell depletion. Even when no posttransplant immunosuppression was given, the incidence of severe (grade III–IV) acute GVHD was only 8% and of severe chronic GVHD only 2% (Hale & Waldmann, 1994a) (Protocol 01, Fig. 109.1, Table 109.1). However, the price to be paid was an increase in the risk of graft failure (to about 21%) and an increase in the risk of leukemia relapse, most notably in patients with chronic myeloid leukemia (CML) (Apperley *et al.*, 1988). There is little doubt that graft failure was caused by residual host resistance (rejection) since it was very rare when the same protocol was used for purging autografts. In several cases, host T cells with specificity for the donor have been isolated from patients with graft failure (Bunjes *et al.*, 1987; Kernan *et al.*, 1987). This phenomenon was predictable from animal experiments and it seems clear that conventional conditioning regimens are unable to completely eradicate host immune function. In unmanipulated grafts the donor T cells gain the upper hand and GVHD is the likely outcome—by removing donor T cells we had tipped the balance in favor of rejection.

The effects of T-cell depletion in leukemia relapse were less expected. Early reports (Weiden *et al.*, 1979) indicated that patients with acute leukemia who suffered GVHD were at lower risk of relapse, suggesting that donor T cells could exert an antileukemic (graft-versus-leukemia, GVL) effect. There was support for this concept in the experimental literature (e.g., Weiss *et al.*, 1983; Truitt, Shih, & LeFever, 1986). However, observations on patients with T-cell-depleted grafts show only a small increase in relapse risk in acute leukemia but a much bigger effect in CML, disproportionate to the effect of GVHD in unmanipulated transplants (Horowitz *et al.*, 1990). Most people would interpret this as evidence for a specific cytotoxic effect of donor T cells on the leukemia cells separate from GVHD, but we suggested another mechanism where alloreactivity may determine the balance between host and donor hematopoiesis (Waldmann, Hale, & Cobbold, 1987). As CML is a stem cell disease, factors that favor host hematopoiesis (autologous recovery), would also favor relapse. Probably both mechanisms operate to some extent, but their relative importance may determine the best strategy for overcoming the problem of relapse.

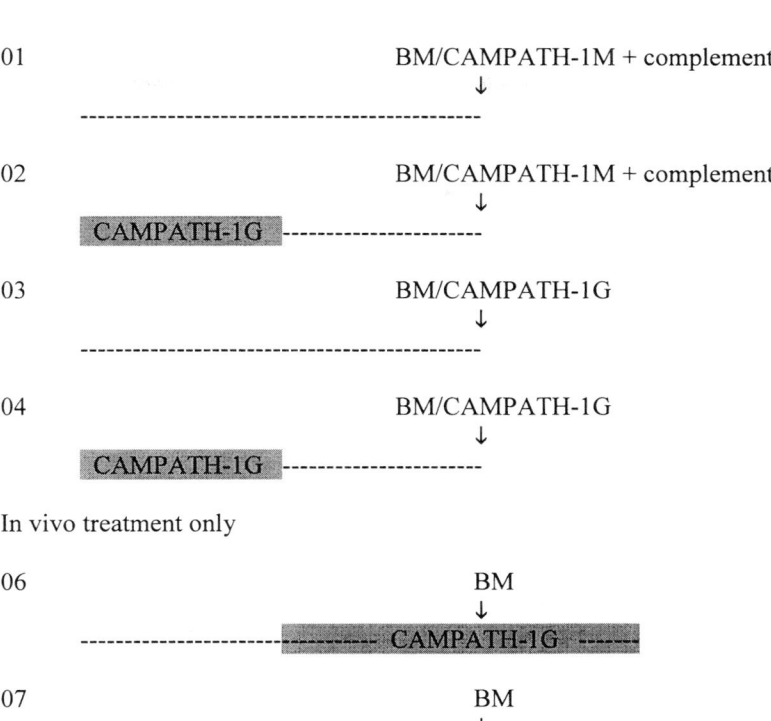

In vitro depletion of bone marrow

01   BM/CAMPATH-1M + complement
                                                   ↓
     ----

02   BM/CAMPATH-1M + complement
                                                   ↓
     CAMPATH-1G ----------------------

03   BM/CAMPATH-1G
                                                   ↓
     ----

04   BM/CAMPATH-1G
                                                   ↓
     CAMPATH-1G ----------------------

In vivo treatment only

06   BM
                                             ↓
     ----------------------- CAMPATH-1G ------

07   BM
                                             ↓
     -------------- CAMPATH-1G ---------

Day   -10   -5   0   +5

Figure 109.1. Methods of using Campath-1 antibodies in hematopoietic stem cell transplantation. Timings are only approximate.

Antibodies for prevention of graft rejection

The first problem that concerned us was how to prevent rejection in the context of T-cell depletion. If this could be solved, it would be of great benefit to patients with nonmalignant diseases as well as considerably widening the scope of marrow transplantation. Efforts to escalate the conditioning regimen, or re-introduce posttransplant immunosuppression, had some success (Hale & Waldmann, 1994a). Some groups tried to perform partial T depletion or to add back a small number of donor T cells, but this tended to result in more GVHD (e.g., Poynton *et al.*, 1988; Potter *et al.*, 1991). Instead we explored the use of monoclonal antibodies to ablate the residual host T cells.

In mice this was relatively easy. Using a combination of CD4 and CD8 antibodies that could deplete the bulk of the recipient's T cells, it was possible to infuse T-cell purged marrow and secure engraftment across major histocompatibility barriers. Where irradiation was lethal the resulting hematopoiesis was virtually 100%

Table 109.1.   *Graft failure and GVHD in HLA-matched sibling transplants*

Protocol number	Antibody treatment		Number of patients	Graft failure	Severe acute GVHD	Severe chronic GVHD
	In vivo	In vitro				
01	none	CP1M	306	20%	7%	2%
02	CP1G	CP1M	195	9%	1%	0%
03	none	CP1G	128	7%	3%	6%
04	CP1G	CP1G	95	20%	1%	0%

Results from three different protocols using Campath-1G (CP1G) to control rejection are compared with historical results using Campath-1M (CP1M) plus complement for T-cell depletion. None of the patients received any posttransplant immunosuppression. The data are pooled from many different centers contributing to the CAMPATH users group (Hale *et al.*, 2001).

donor in origin. Even at sublethal doses (6 Gy) donor engraftment dominated (Cobbold & Waldmann, 1986). Recipients were also able to accept skin grafts from the same donors. They were, in other words, tolerant. Conditioning with lower doses of irradiation (3 Gy) together with the best antibodies was sufficient to permit chimerism, albeit at a low level, but was not permissive for tolerance (Waldmann *et al.*, 1990). Sharabi and Sachs (1989) extended these studies further by adding thymic irradiation at high doses. This gave tissue graft tolerance with minimal damage to the host. Since then, Sykes, Sachs, and co-workers have developed this protocol in incremental stages towards completely non-myeloablative conditioning protocols which have combined a reduction in irradiation with the use of nonlytic "blocking" antibodies and high doses of hematopoietic stem cells (Sykes, 2001). They have consequently been able to achieve mixed chimerism and tolerance with relatively low-impact therapies. However, the transfer of such protocols to the clinic is constrained by many issues, not least of which is the age of the human recipients in whom alloreactive memory T-cell populations are relatively enriched compared to the young specific pathogen–free (SPF) mice on which the protocols are modeled; consequently, any chimerism achieved has only been transient.

Leong *et al.* (1992) investigated the contribution made by irradiation to the conditioning process. As irradiation is both myeloablative and immunosuppressive, one cannot easily determine which of the two properties are important to tolerance induction. By using the specifically myeloablative drug dimethylmyleran (DMM), it was shown that the mere creation of adequate hematopoietic space was sufficient to replace the effects of irradiation. This suggests that extra "space" allows more donor marrow engraftment, which in turn allows more effective induction of tolerance in the few T cells that survive and repopulate after antibody therapy. Subsequent studies showed that the greater the degree of myeloablation, the less the extent of immunosuppression needed.

Where marrow transplantation was tried across minor histocompatibility barriers, it was apparent that no new "space" was needed if sufficient antibody immunosuppression was given. In some strain combinations nondepleting CD4 and CD8 monoclonal antibodies were the only conditioning required to obtain chimerism and transplantation tolerance (Qin *et al.*, 1989). Therefore, if one could guarantee significant donor-type chimerism after allogeneic transplantation, then transplantation tolerance should be possible. There still remains a real issue as to whether "tolerance" requires permanent chimerism or whether temporary chimerism is sufficient to allow initiation of the tolerance processes, which are consolidated on subsequent transplantation of an organ graft. There is also the requirement that one find a conditioning regimen for solid organ graft recipients that is safe (see Chapter 122).

One of the first problems in humans was to identify suitable antibodies that could deplete T cells in vivo. Campath-1M, although it was so efficient at complement activation in vitro, could give only transient depletion of lymphocytes. However, a rat IgG$_{2b}$ antibody, Campath-1G, which had the same specificity, was able to activate cell-mediated killing (ADCC) as well as complement, and it was much more potent for lymphocyte depletion in vivo (Dyer *et al.*, 1989). We reasoned that administration of this antibody during the conditioning regimen for a marrow transplant could help to ablate host T cells and reduce the risk of rejection. In 1988 a study was started to test this concept (Protocol 02, Fig. 109.1, Table 109.1).

Because of the serious consequences of graft rejection, a prospective randomized trial was unethical, and so we compared the results with historical controls. The method of T-cell depletion (with Campath-1M in vitro) remained the same, as did other components of the conditioning regimen. The new feature was Campath-1G administered at 20 mg per day for 5 days prior to total body irradiation (Fig. 109.1). It was given this early so that its lymphotoxic and other effects could be more easily evaluated, and to reduce the risk that residual IgG antibody could contribute to the depletion of donor T cells. Measurement of recipient lymphocyte numbers and proliferative capacity after the in vivo purging showed depletion comparable with that obtained by whole body irradiation or treatment with cyclophosphamide (Theobald *et al.*, 1990). No posttransplant immunosuppression was given. A relatively homogeneous group of 70 patients transplanted for AML in first remission was analyzed in this case-control study, although the same design was used for higher risk patients as well. Final analysis showed a graft rejection rate of 6%, an incidence of acute GVHD grade II–IV of 4%, and an incidence of chronic GVHD of 3% (Hale *et al.*, 1998). Transplant-related mortality was 15% at 6 months, survival at 6 months was 92% and at 5 years was 62%. These results were significantly better than control groups who received T depletion in vitro alone (more rejection), or unmanipulated grafts with conventional prophylaxis using cyclosporine and methotrexate (more GVHD).

A single antibody for prevention of both graft rejection and GVHD

The above study showed that immunologic complications of marrow transplants could largely be overcome by effective depletion of both donor and recipient lymphocytes. Campath-1M was used for depletion of the donor T cells for historical reasons, but it would be more logical to use the same antibody for both treatments. However, earlier attempts with OKT3 as an opsonizing antibody had not been successful (Filipovitch *et al.*, 1982; Prentice *et al.*, 1982), and it was not clear whether the necessary cellular effector mechanisms would be sufficiently intact at the time of marrow transplant. Studies by other transplant teams have shown that this is not a problem and that Campath-1G can also be used to prevent GVHD.

Two approaches have been used: Campath-1G has been administered either in vitro (mixed with the bone marrow) (Protocol 03, Fig. 109.1) or in vivo (before and up to or beyond the day of transplantation) (Protocols 06 and 07, Fig. 109.1). In either approach, the antibody can potentially deplete both donor and host T cells, but the relative efficiency may not be the same.

A priori, we would expect that antibody mixed with the bone marrow would completely opsonize the donor T cells whereas the recipient T cells would be exposed to a much lower concentration. When the antibody is administered in vivo, both donor and recipient will be exposed to a similar (relatively low) concentration and so the impact on GVHD might be less. It was hard to judge in advance what the exact effect would be on the balance of host-versus-graft (HVG) and GVH reactions.

Two teams (Haddassah University Hospital, Jerusalem and University Hospital, Cape Town) pioneered the use of Campath-1G (approximately 20 mg) to treat the bone marrow (Protocol 03). The treated marrow was not washed before infusion, so excess antibody would potentially be available to deplete residual host T cells. In the absence of posttransplant immunosuppression they found a low incidence of GVHD proving that the opsonization of donor T cells was effective (Jacobs et al., 1993). Furthermore, the incidence of graft rejection was significantly less than when T cells were depleted only from the donor bone marrow.

The Campath-1G (in vivo) method (Protocols 04 and 06, Fig. 109.1) was tested at various centers in both HLA-matched sibling transplants (Willemze et al., 1992; Hamblyn et al., 1996) and unrelated donor transplants (Cullis et al., 1991; Spencer et al., 1995). In the absence of posttransplant immunosuppression the incidence of graft failure and acute GVHD was low, but there were several cases of severe chronic GVHD. Therefore in most subsequent cases, cyclosporine was given posttransplant, usually for three months, resulting in good control of rejection and GVHD.

Humanized antibody

All of the studies described were carried out by academic groups and unfortunately, there has never been serious commercial interest in the development of Campath-1G. However, a humanized antibody was created from it by genetic engineering (Riechmann et al., 1988) and this antibody, Campath-1H (alemtuzumab) has been commercially developed and is now approved for the treatment of chronic lymphatic leukemia resistant to chemotherapeutic agents. Therefore, various groups have evaluated Campath-1H in the hematopoietic stem cell transplant setting and compared it with Campath-1G (Hale et al., 2000, 2001). This change has coincided with the widespread use of peripheral blood as a source of stem cells. Both antibodies give very similar control of rejection and GVHD, whether given "in the bag" (i.e., mixed with the stem cells) or administered in vivo. However, the humanized antibody has a significantly longer half-life of approximately 2–3 weeks, which means that it persists for longer in the patients (Rebello et al., 2001). This allows effective control of GVHD even when the antibody is administered well before the transplant, but also raises the possibility of interference with immune reconstitution, delaying the recovery of lymphocytes even beyond that normally seen, and rendering the patients vulnerable to viral infections in the immediate posttransplant period (Davison et al., 2000; Chakrabarti et

al., 2001, 2002). It remains to be seen whether these complications can be minimized by reducing the dose of antibody, or whether an antibody with a shorter half-life such as Campath-1G will be preferable in this type of situation.

It should be noted that the Campath antibodies may prevent GVHD not only by depleting T cells, but also by removing monocyte-derived dendritic cells and their precursors, thus minimizing presentation of host-derived antigens to donor T cells (Klangsinsirikul et al., 2002; Ratzinger et al., 2003).

Reduced intensity conditioning regimens

The use of non-myeloablative conditioning regimens to promote donor engraftment and exploit a graft-versus-leukemia effect, while minimizing regimen-related morbidity and mortality, is being increasingly explored (see Chapter 22). The powerful immunosuppressive effects of Campath-1H may be especially useful in this context, both to promote engraftment and to prevent GVHD, since this would greatly increase the scope of allogeneic transplantation in older patients with more indolent diseases such as chronic lymphatic leukemia and non-Hodgkin's lymphoma. In a study by Kottaridis and colleagues (2000), Campath-1H at a dose of 20 mg/kg/day from day –8 to day –4 was added to the combination of fludarabine and melphalan. This was a poor risk group and 19 of the 44 patients had received a prior HSC transplant. The incidence of acute GVHD grade II or higher was low—occurring in only 2 patients, and the estimated probability of treatment-related mortality was 11%. This type of approach is now being studied a number of other centers, using a range of non-myeloablative conditioning regimens and confirming the significant reduction in risks of GVHD with excellent engraftment.

A rational approach for the use of stem cell transplants to treat leukemia

For many years, workers have tried to balance on the tightrope between GVHD, rejection, relapse, and infection. Some hoped that a small number of donor T cells would restore equilibrium. We think it unlikely that this will work, but even if it does, the critical number will likely vary unpredictably according to the biological diversity of donors and recipients. A better alternative is to deal with the problems individually. GVHD and rejection can largely be eliminated by depletion of lymphocytes. Antibody therapy using Campath-1G or Campath-1H is a particularly simple and effective method. Rapid and stable engraftment can be achieved by giving a large number of stem cells and procedure-related toxicity can be reduced by the use of non-myeloablative conditioning regimens. Donor T cells should be collected for use in the event of relapse or major immunologic problems. Patients whose disease is eradicated by the conditioning can be spared the risks of GVHD, and the need for long-term immunosuppressive drugs, but all patients should be monitored regularly for any sign of relapse, using the most sensitive and appropriate methods. Once the donor stem cells are accepted, it may be much safer to administer small numbers of donor T cells in order to induce an antileukemic effect when required. There will inevitably be a risk of GVHD at this stage, but it may be reduced by starting with small numbers of cells and by administering them after the patient has recovered from the effects of the original conditioning regimen (Mackinnon *et al.*, 1995). A similar approach could be used to introduce T cells specific for viral pathogens like CMV, if they were required.

Selective expansion of regulatory T cells

Immune reconstitution is a significant problem when T cells are ablated with antibodies. There is a need to find ways of removing alloreactive T-cell activity, while leaving within the donor stem cell inoculum sufficient donor T cells to mediate antimicrobial and antitumor immunity. A novel approach to this has been the ex vivo use of antibodies to expand alloreactive regulatory T cells to block potentially damaging alloreactivity, while sparing all other T cells for normal immune function. Regulatory CD4$^+$ T-cells were shown to operate in vivo by Qin *et al.* (1993), who used blockading CD4 antibodies to induce tolerance to transplanted tissues. Since that time such regulatory T cells have been shown to operate in tolerance induced by a range of other therapeutic antibodies (Graca *et al.*, 2000). It was inevitable that attempts would be made to selectively expand these regulatory T cells ex vivo for control of GVHD. In rodent studies, Taylor *et al.* (2002) demonstrated that CD154 antibodies added to cultures of bone marrow stimulated with recipient type alloantigens can selectively expand alloreactive regulatory T cells that can prevent GVHD. This may offer an option for safe T-cell replenishment to be given after marrow purging.

Conclusions

Although we have focused mainly on anti-CD52 antibodies, it is clear that there are several ways of achieving substantial immunosuppression through antibody therapy. Besides using antibodies for cell depletion (which requires the right combination of specificity and isotype), it is possible to obtain reagents that block any one of a number of critical T-cell functions. As we have shown in animal models, the most profound effects are obtained by combination of different antibodies. In human trials it is necessary to proceed stepwise, evaluating the safety and efficacy of each component. This is not easy in hematopoietic stem cell transplantation because the potential complications are so interrelated. T-cell depletion enjoyed an initial euphoric phase, followed by rather deep skepticism, when the rate of graft rejection and leukemia relapse became apparent. Since the first edition of this book there have been four important developments that now result in a more optimistic outlook:

1. The demonstration that antibodies can be used to prevent rejection
2. The use of peripheral blood stem cells to speed engraftment
3. The use of graded doses of donor T cells to treat relapse

4. The development of non-myeloablative conditioning regimens to reduce toxicity but with sufficient immunosuppression to promote engraftment

Now that we have powerful tools for tackling the immunologic complications of stem cell transplants, it is not surprising that transplant physicians are turning their attention to the treatment of a wider range of diseases including severe autoimmune disease.

References

Apperley, J. F., Mauro, F. R., Goldman, J. M. *et al.* (1988). Bone marrow transplantation for chronic myeloid leukemia in first chronic phase: importance of a graft-versus-leukemia effect. *British Journal of Haematology,* **9,** 239–45.

Bunjes, D., Heit, W., Arnold, R. *et al.* (1987). Evidence for the involvement of host-derived OKT8-positive T cells in the rejection of T-depleted HLA-identical bone marrow grafts. *Transplantation,* **43,** 501–5.

Chakrabarti, S., Collingham, K. E., Marshall, T. *et al.* (2001). Respiratory virus infections in adult T cell-depleted transplant recipients: the role of cellular immunity. *Transplantation,* **72,** 1460–3.

Chakrabarti, S., Mackinnon, S., Chopra, R. *et al.* (2002). High incidence of cytomegalovirus infection after non-myeloablative stem cell transplantation: potential role of CAMPATH-1H in delaying immune reconstitution but limiting transplant-related mortality. *Blood,* **99,** 4357–63.

Cobbold, S. P & Waldmann, H. (1986). Skin allograft rejection by L3T4 and Lyt-2 T cell subsets. *Transplantation,* **41,** 634–9.

Cullis, J. O., Goldman, J. M., Hale, G., & Waldmann, H. (1991). Bone marrow transplantation using unrelated donors for CML in chronic phase. *Experimental Hematology,* **19,** 540 (Abstract).

Davison, G. M., Novitzky, N., Kline, A. *et al.* (2000). Immune reconstitution after allogeneic bone marrow transplantation depleted of T-cells. *Transplantation,* **69,** 1341–7.

Dicke, K. A., Van Hooff, J., & Van Bekkum, D. W. (1968). The selective elimination of immunologically competent cells from bone marrow and lymphatic cell mixtures. *Transplantation,* **6,** 562–70.

Dyer, M.J.S., Hale, G., Hayhoe, F.G.I., & Waldmann, H. (1989). Effects of CAMPATH-1 antibodies in vivo in patients with lymphoid malignancies: influence of antibody isotype. *Blood,* **73,** 1431–9.

Fibbe, W. E., Hale, G., Velders, G. J. *et al.* (1997). T-cell depletion of allogeneic blood cell grafts using CAMPATH-IG "in the bag" results in accelerated marrow reconstitution without severe GVHD. *Bone Marrow Transplantation,* **19** (Suppl 1), S47 (Abstract).

Filipovitch, A. H., Ramsay, N.K.C., Warkentin, P. I. *et al.* (1982). Pretreatment of donor bone marrow with monoclonal antibody OKT3 for prevention of acute graft versus host disease in allogeneic histocompatible bone marrow transplantation. *Lancet,* **1,** 1266–9.

Graca, L., Honey, K., Adams, E., Cobbold, S. P., & Waldmann, H. (2000). Anti-CD154 therapeutic antibodies induce infectious transplantation tolerance. *Journal of Immunology,* **165,** 4783–6.

Hale, G. (2001). The CD52 antigen and development of the CAM-PATH antibodies. *Cytotherapy,* **3**, 137–44.

Hale, G., Bright, S., Chumbley, G. *et al.* (1983). Removal of T cells from bone marrow for transplantation: a monoclonal antilympho-cyte antibody that fixes human complement. *Blood,* **62**, 873–82.

Hale, G., Cobbold, S., Novitzky, N. *et al.* (2001). Meeting Report: CAMPATH-1 antibodies in stem-cell transplantation. *Cyto-therapy,* **3**, 145–64.

Hale, G., Jacobs, P., Wood, L. *et al.* (2000). CD52 antibodies for pre-vention of graft versus host disease and graft rejection following transplantation of allogeneic periphoal blood stem cells. *Bone Marrow Transplantation,* **26**, 69–76.

Hale, G. & Rebello, P. (1997). CD52 Workshop Panel report. In *Leucocyte Typing VI,* ed. T. Kishimoto & H. Kikutami, pp. 514–17. New York: Garland Publishing, Inc.

Hale, G. & Waldmann, H., for CAMPATH users. (1994a). Control of graft-versus-host disease and graft rejection by T cell depletion of donor and recipient with Campath-1 antibodies; results of matched sibling transplants for malignant diseases. *Bone Marrow Transplantation,* **13**, 597–611.

Hale, G. & Waldmann, H. for CAMPATH users. (1994b). CAM-PATH-1 monoclonal antibodies in bone marrow transplantation. *Journal of Hematotherapy,* **3**, 15–31.

Hale, G., Zhang, M.-J., Bunges, D. *et al.* (1998). Improving the out-come of bone marrow transplantation by using CD52 monoclonal antibodies to prevent graft-versus-host disease and graft rejec-tion. *Blood,* **92**, 4581–90.

Hamblyn, M., Marsh, J.C.W., Lawler, M. *et al.* (1996). CAMPATH-1G in vivo confers a low incidence of graft-versus-host disease associated with a high incidence of mixed chimerism after BMT for severe aplastic anaemia using HLA-matched sibling donors. *Bone Marrow Transplantation,* **17**, 819–24.

Horowitz, M. M., Gale, R. P., Sondel, P. *et al.* (1990). Graft-versus-leukemia reactions after bone marrow transplantation. *Blood,* **75**, 555–62.

Jacobs, P., Wood, L., Fullard, L. *et al.* (1993). T-cell depletion by exposure to CAMPATH-1G in vitro prevents graft-versus-host disease. *Bone Marrow Transplantation,* **13**, 763–9.

Kernan, N. A., Flomenberg, N., Dupont, B., & O'Reilly, R. I. (1987). Graft rejection in recipients of T-cell-depleted HLA-identical mar-row transplants for leukemia. Identification of host-derived anti-donor allocytotoxic T lymphocytes. *Transplantation,* **43**, 842–7.

Klangsinsirikul, P., Carter, G. I., Byrne, J. L. *et al.* (2002). Campath-1G causes rapid depletion of circulating host dendritic cells (DCs) before allogeneic transplantation but does not delay donor DC reconstitution. *Blood,* **99**, 2586–91.

Kottaridis, P. D., Milligan, D. W., Chopra, R. *et al.* (2000). In vivo CAMPATH-1H prevents graft-versus-host disease following non-myeloablative stem cell transplantation. *Blood,* **96**, 2419–25.

Leong, L. W., Qin, S., Cobbold, S. P., & Waldmann, H. (1992). Classical transplantation tolerance in the adult. The interaction between myeloablation and immunosuppression. *European Journal of Immunology,* **22**, 2825–30.

MacKinnon, S., Papadopoulos, E. P., Capabasi, M. H. *et al.* (1995). Adoptive immunotherapy evaluating escalating dose of donor leukocytes for relapse of chronic myeloid leukemia following bone marrow transplantation: separation of graft-versus-leukemia responses from graft-versus-host disease. *Blood,* **86**, 1261–8.

Noga, S. I., Donnenberg, A. P., Schwartz, C. L. *et al.* (1986). Development of a simplified counterflow centrifugation elutria-tion procedure for depletion of lymphocytes from human bone marrow. *Transplantation,* **41**, 214–19.

Oakhill, A., Pamphilon, D. H., Potter, M. N. *et al.* (1996). Unrelated donor bone marrow transplantation for children with relapsed acute lymphoblastic leukemia in second complete remission. *British Journal of Haematology,* **94**, 574–8.

O'Reilly, R. I. (1987). Current developments in marrow transplanta-tion. *Transplantation Proceedings,* **19**, 92–102.

Potter, M. N., Pamphilon, D. H., Cornish, J. M., & Oakhill, A. (1991). Graft-versus-host disease in children receiving HLA-identical allogeneic bone marrow transplants with a low adjusted T lymphocyte dose. *Bone Marrow Transplantation,* **8**, 357–61.

Poynton, C. H., Whittaker, J. A., Bailey-Wood, R. *et al.* (1988). Mismatched family and unrelated donors for bone marrow trans-plantation using fixed low numbers of T cells. *Bone Marrow Transplantation,* **3** (Suppl 1), 223.

Prentice, H. G., Blacklock, H. A., Janossy, G. *et al.* (1982). Use of anti-T cell monoclonal antibody OKT3 to prevent acute graft ver-sus host disease in allogeneic bone marrow transplantation for acute leukemia. *Lancet,* **1**, 700–3.

Qin, S., Cobbold, S. P., Pope, H. *et al.* (1993). "Infectious" trans-plantation tolerance. *Science,* **259**, 974–7.

Qin, S.-X., Cobbold, S. P., Benjamin, R., & Waldmaan, H. (1989). Induction of classical transplantation tolerance in the adult. *Journal of Experimental Medicine,* **169**, 779–94.

Ratzinger, G., Reagan, J. L., Heller, G. *et al.* (2003). Differential CD52 expression by distinct myeloid dendritic cell subsets: implications for alemtuzumab activity at the level of antigen pre-sentation in allogeneic graft-host interactions in transplantation. *Blood,* **101**, 1422–9.

Reisner, Y., Kapoor, N., Kirkpatrick, D. *et al.* (1981). Transplantation for acute leukemia with HLA-A and B noniden-tical parental marrow cells fractionated with soybean agglutinin and sheep red blood cells. *Lancet,* **2**, 327–31.

Sharabi, Y. & Sachs, D. H. (1989). Mixed chimerism and permanent specific transplantation tolerance induced by a non-lethal prepar-ative regimen. *Journal of Experimental Medicine,* **169**, 493–502.

Spencer, A., Szydlo, R. M., Brookes, P. A. *et al.* (1995). Bone mar-row transplantation for chronic myeloid leukemia with volunteer unrelated donor using ex vivo or in vivo T cell depletion: major prognostic impact of HLA class I identity between donor and recipient. *Blood,* **86**, 3590–7.

Sykes, M. (2001). Mixed chimerism and transplant tolerance. *Immunity,* **14**, 417–24.

Taylor, P. A., Friedman, T. M., Korngold, R., Noelle, R. J., & Blazar, B. R. (2002). Tolerance induction of alloreactive T cells via ex vivo blockade of the CD40:CD40L costimulatory pathway results in the generation of a potent immune regulatory cell. *Blood,* **99**, 4601–9.

Theobald, M., Hoffmann, T., Bunjes, D., & Heit, W. (1990). Comparative analysis of in vivo T cell depletion with radiother-apy, combination chemotherapy and the monoclonal antibody CAMPATH-1G, using limiting dilution methodology. *Transplantation,* **49**, 553–9.

Truitt, R. L., Shih, C. C., & Lefever, A. V. (1986). Manipulation of graft-versus-host disease for a graft-versus-leukemia effect after allogeneic bone marrow transplantation in AKR mice with spontaneous leukemia/lymphoma. *Transplantation, 41,* 301–10.

Waldmann, H., Hale, G., & Cobbold, S. (1987). The immunobiology of bone marrow transplantation. In *Leucocyte Typing III White Cell Differentiation Antigens,* eds. A. J. McMichael *et al.,* pp. 932–7. Oxford: Oxford University Press.

Waldmann, H., Hale, G., Cobbold, S. P. *et al.* (1990). Monoclonal antibody therapy for the prevention of GVHD. In *Graft Versus Host Disease,* eds. S. I. Burakoff, H. G. Deeg, J. Ferrara, & K. Atkinson, pp. 277–92. New York: Marcel Dekker, Inc.

Waldmann, H., Or, R., Hale, G. *et al.* (1984). Elimination of graft versus host disease by in vitro depletion of alloreactive lympho-cytes using a monoclonal rat anti-human lymphocyte antibody (CAMPATH-1). *Lancet, 2,* 483–6.

Weiden, P. L., Flournoy, N., Thomas, E. D. *et al.* (1979). Antileukaemic effect of graft-versus-host disease in human recipients of allogeneic marrow grafts. *New England Journal of Medicine,* **300,** 1068–73.

Weiss, L., Morecki, S., Vitetta, E. S., & Slavin, S. (1983). Suppression and elimination of BCL1 leukemia by allogeneic bone marrow transplantation. *Journal of Immunology,* **130,** 2452–5.

Willemze, R., Richel, D. I., Falkenberg, J.H.F. *et al.* (1992). In vivo use of CAMPATH-1G to prevent graft-versus-host disease and graft rejection after bone marrow transplantation. *Bone Marrow Transplantation,* **9,** 255–61.

110 Ex vivo expansion of hematopoietic stem and progenitor cells

IAN McNIECE

University of Colorado Health Sciences Center, Denver, USA

Introduction

During the past years, sophisticated hematopoietic stem and progenitor cell culture techniques have been devised that allow for the ex vivo amplification of early hematopoietic cells, as well as the generation of large numbers of more differentiated cells of the various hematopoietic lineages (e.g., granulocytic, megakaryocytic, or antigen-presenting dendritic cells). This novel form of cellular manipulation, referred to as ex vivo expansion (reviewed in McNiece & Briddell, 2001), became possible by the development of current stem and progenitor cell selection methods in combination with rapid achievements in hematopoietic growth factor research and development. Whereas the feasibility of an effective ex vivo generation of progenitor cells (using various cytokine combinations), as well as their successful clinical application has been convincingly demonstrated, ex vivo amplification of undifferentiated early hematopoietic cells [e.g., long-term culture initiating cells (LTC-IC)] remains problematic.

Cytokines can be used to induce differentiation into a specific lineage, thus enabling the production of large numbers of more differentiated myeloid and megakaryocytic post-progenitor cells. Clinical studies have demonstrated faster engraftment of neutrophils with expanded cells. Ex vivo expansion can also be utilized to generate professional antigen-presenting dendritic cells (DC) from $CD34^+$ progenitor cells. These might represent ideal cells for immunotherapeutic approaches such as tumor-antigen vaccination trials. This chapter aims to briefly review the current state-of-the-art of the various aspects of the ex vivo expansion of hematopoietic cells and to give an overview of recent developments in this field.

Blood cell production

Bone marrow is the principal site for blood cell formation in humans. In normal adults the body produces about 2.5 billion red blood cells (RBC), 2.5 billion platelets, and 10 billion granulocytes per kilogram of body weight per day (Williams *et al.,* 1990). The production of mature blood cells is a continual process that is the result of proliferation and differentiation of stem cells, committed progenitor cells, and differentiated cells

(Figure 110.1). Within these three stages, extensive expansion of cell numbers occurs through cell division. A single stem cell has been proposed to be capable of more than 50 cell divisions or doublings and has the capacity to generate up to 10^{15} cells, or sufficient cells for up to 60 years (Kay, 1965). The proliferation and differentiation of cells is controlled by a group of proteins called hematopoietic growth factors (HGFs). Many of the HGFs have been isolated and cloned, and large amounts of recombinant proteins are available for clinical use or the ex vivo manipulations of cells. If we could replicate this cell amplification in vitro with HGFs, it might be possible to generate large numbers of cells that could be used for a variety of clinical applications. These clinical applications include:

1. Supplementing stem cell grafts with more mature precursors to shorten or potentially prevent chemotherapy-induced pancytopenia

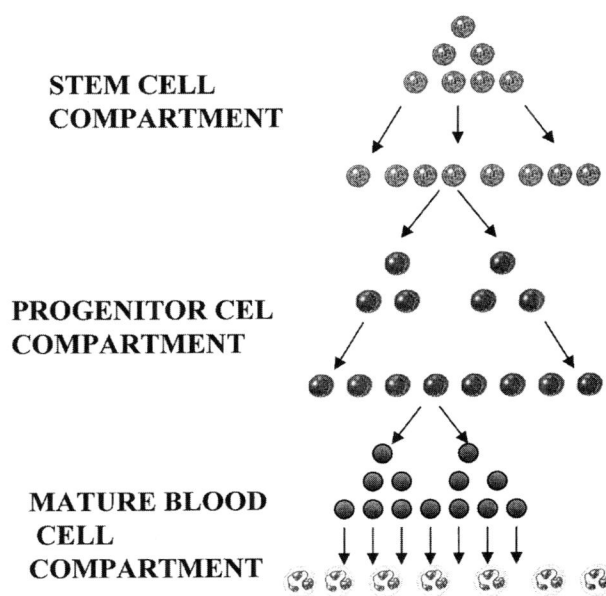

STEM CELL COMPARTMENT

PROGENITOR CEL COMPARTMENT

MATURE BLOOD CELL COMPARTMENT

Fig. 110.1. Model of cellular expansion with differentiation of hematopoietic cells.

2. Increasing the number of primitive progenitor cells to ensure hematopoietic support for multiple cycles of high-dose chemotherapy

3. Obtaining a sufficient number of stem cells from a single marrow aspirate or apheresis procedure, thus reducing the need for large-scale harvesting of marrow or multiple leukaphereses

4. Generating sufficient cells from a single umbilical cord blood to reconstitute an adult following high-dose chemotherapy

5. Purging stem cell products of contaminating tumor cells

6. Generating large volumes of immunologically active cells with antitumor activity to be used in immunotherapeutic regimens

7. Increasing the pool of stem cells which could be targets for the delivery of gene therapy

It is important, therefore, to consider the clinical application when discussing ex vivo expansion approaches, and to define culture conditions that are relevant to the particular cell type being expanded. The relevant properties of the cells in each of the different hematopoietic compartments are summarized below:

– Stem Cells   Long-term engraftment; targets for gene replacement therapy
– Progenitor Cells   Intermediate and short term engraftment
– Mature Cells   Short-term engraftment immune therapy

Hematopoietic growth factors

Numerous reports can be found in the literature that describe the effects of hematopoietic growth factor (HGF) combinations on hematopoietic stem and progenitor cell expansion; however, the optimal growth factor combination has yet to be defined. Brugger and colleagues have previously reported that an HGF combination that included stem cell-factor (SCF), interleukin (IL)-1, IL-3, IL-6, and erythropoietin (EPO), provided optimum expansion of progenitor cells starting from positively selected CD34+ peripheral blood progenitor cells (PBPC) (Brugger et al., 1993). Using this cytokine cocktail, committed progenitor cells [granulocyte-macrophage colony-forming units (CFU-GM), erythrocyte burst-forming units (BFU-E)], as well as multipotential progenitors [colony-forming unit granulocyte-erythrocyte-monocyte-macrophage (CFU-GEMM)] were increased approximately 190-fold (range 46–930 and 250-fold), respectively. Moreover, CD34+/Lin−, as well as mafosfamide-resistant cells, were found to be considerably increased, whereas input LTC-IC were maintained but not expanded (Henschler et al., 1994). Several other groups have also reported on the role of various cytokine-bone marrow combinations involving early as well as late acting growth factors on the ex vivo expansion of progenitor cells (Jacobsen et al., 1995; Keller et al., 1995; Mayani et al., 1995). Certainly SCF has been convincingly demonstrated to be essential for progenitor cell expansion, and fur-

thermore it was shown to be one of the most important survival factors for hematopoietic progenitor cells, even in the absence of cell division (Keller et al., 1995). Further research addressed the role of co-culture systems (utilizing stromal cells, endothelial cells, or osteoblasts), that either involve direct cellular contact or allow diffusion of critical growth factors from accessory cells for effective ex vivo expansion (Dexter et al., 1977; Verfaillie, 1992; Davis et al., 1995; Fennie et al., 1995; Raffi et al., 1995; Gupta et al., 1996; Moore et al., 1997; Taichman et al., 1996; Young et al., 1995; Kawano et al., 2003). In view of possible clinical application, other studies aimed to optimize ex vivo expansion by making use of gas-permeable culture bags (Shapiro et al., 1994) or replacing commonly used static cultures systems by perfusion systems [Sandstrom et al., 1995; Stiff et al., 2000; Engelhardt et al., 2001; Pecora et al., 2001].

Clinical application of ex vivo generated progenitor cells

One of the first clinical studies was by Naparstek and colleagues (Naparstek et al., 1992), who performed a short culture of bone marrow in the presence of granulocyte-macrophage colony-stimulating factor (GM-CSF) and IL-3. Patients undergoing allogeneic bone marrow transplantation (BMT) for malignant hematological diseases were transplanted with two-thirds of the bone marrow on the scheduled day of transplant and one-third of the bone marrow following incubation in GM-CSF plus IL-3 (100 ng/ml) on day 4. The bone marrow was cultured in RPMI plus pooled inactivated human AB serum (7% to 10%) for 4 days. There was no significant acceleration of the time to neutrophil recovery; however, the study suggested faster platelet recovery in patients transplanted with expanded bone marrow cells. The median time to reach an unsupported platelet count of 25,000/µl was 17 days for patients receiving expanded cells, compared to 23 days for the control group (Naparstek et al., 1992). No data were provided in the report on the fold expansion of nucleated cells or granulocyte-macrophage colony forming cells (GM-CFC), although the increase in the number of GM-CFC correlated with the rapid platelet recovery in 12 patients with durable engraftment ($P = .02$). The authors concluded from this study that in vitro culture of bone marrow cells with IL-3 plus GM-CSF may provide a cell product capable of enhancing marrow recovery.

Brugger and colleagues (Brugger et al., 1995) expanded 10% of a PBPC product in the combination of SCF, IL-1β, IL-3, IL-6 and EPO for 12 days in culture and reinfused the cells to the patients after high-dose chemotherapy. Ten cancer patients were mobilized with chemotherapy plus G-CSF and 11 million CD34+ cells were selected on the Ceprate CD34 selection system and incubated in RPMI plus 2% autologous plasma plus growth factors as described above for 12 days in five 175 cm² tissue culture flasks with 30,000 cells per m for a total volume of 100 ml per flask. The median number of of cells generated ex vivo was 2.4 to 23.1 million, which corresponded to a median increase of

62.4 fold (range 33.4–115.5) in the number of total nucleated cells. A median increase in CFC of 50.3 fold (range 14.4–92.5) was obtained. The patients had rapid and sustained engraftment; however, the time to recovery of hematopoiesis was no different than historical controls. No toxic effects were observed with the infusion of the expanded cells. The contribution of the expanded cells is difficult to assess in this study as the chemotherapy used may not be totally myeloablative and so the contribution of endogenous recovery is unknown.

In a second study of expanded PBPC, Williams and colleagues (Williams *et al.*, 1996) infused cells expanded in PIXY321 (a GM-CSF/IL-3 fusion protein) for 12 days. Nine patients with metastatic breast cancer were mobilized with chemotherapy plus G-CSF and one pheresis product from each patient was selected using the Isolex 300i CD34 selection device. The CD34$^+$ cells were cultured in gas-permeable bags containing serum-free X-VIVO 10 medium supplemented with 1% human serum albumin and 100 ng/ml PIXY321. At day 12 of culture the median fold expansion was 26 (range 6–64). The final product contained an average of 29.3% CD15$^+$ neutrophil precursors with a range of 18.5%–48.1%. The patients received the cryopreserved unmanipulated PBPC products on day 0 and the expanded cells on day +1. The median number of expanded cells reinfused was 44.6 million per kg with a range of 0.8–156.6 × 10^6 cells/kg. Although the infusion of the expanded cells was well tolerated, no clinical effect of the expanded cells was observed.

Alcorn and colleagues (Alcorn *et al.*, 1996) expanded CD34$^+$ cells from cryopreserved PBPC. This study is difficult to interpret as there were significant losses of total cells and progenitors after thawing and selection. The recovery of cells post cryopreservation was 58% for total cells and only 21% for GM-CFC. The CD34$^+$ cells were selected using the Isolex 300i and the CD34$^+$ cells cultured for 8 days in Progenitor-34 media supplemented with 5% to 10% autologous serum and SCF (10 ng/ml), IL-3 (10 ng/ml), IL-6 (20 ng/ml), IL-1β (10 ng/ml) and EPO (2 U/ml). The mean increase in total cell number was 21 fold and 139 fold for GM-CFC. Ten patients with nonmyeloid malignancy were reinfused with the expanded cells without any adverse effect. The time to neutrophil and platelet recovery was identical to that of historical controls.

In more recent studies, three groups using similar culture conditions have reported decreased time to neutrophil recovery with ex vivo expanded PBPC (Reiffers *et al.*, 1999; McNiece *et al.*, 2000; Paquette, 2000). Two groups cultured CD34$^+$ cells in Defined Media (Amgen Inc) supplemented with the growth factors SCF, G-CSF, and megakaryocyte growth and development factor (MGDF) at 100 ng/ml for 10 days in Teflon bags (American Fluoroceal) (Reiffers *et al.*, 1999; McNiece *et al.*, 2000), while the third group cultured a mononuclear fraction in the same media and growth factors (Paquette, 2000).

Reiffers and colleagues (Reiffers *et al.*, 1999) reported the results of a phase I/II study in myeloma patients (*n* = 14) using ex vivo expanded PBPC. A median of 4.1 × 10^6 CD34$^+$ cells were expanded for 10 days, after which time the cells were

washed and reinfused into patients. Unexpanded PBPC were also transplanted into patients on day +1 and the patients received G-CSF until neutrophil engraftment was achieved. The posttransplant neutropenia period was markedly reduced in these patients compared to historical controls. The median days of neutropenia (absolute neutrophil count [ANC] >500/μl) was 1.5 days with a range of 0 to 7 days. Nine of the 14 patients never had a neutrophil count below 500/μl. In a comparable group of myeloma patients (*n* = 242) receiving unexpanded PBPC, the median duration of severe neutropenia was 6 days (range 2–24).

Paquette and colleagues (Paquette, 2000) cultured unselected PBPCs in teflon bags in SCF, G-CSF, and MGDF for 9 days. Twenty-four breast cancer patients received between 2 and 24 × 10^9 PBPCs cultured at 1, 2, or 3 × 10^6 cells/ml following STAMP I chemotherapy and infusion of at least 5 × 10^6 CD34$^+$ unexpanded PBPC/kg. The fold expansion of CD34$^+$ cells in culture was reported to be inversely proportional to the initial cell density. No toxicity resulted from infusion of the expanded cells. Eleven patients (46%) recovered neutrophils to >500/μl by days 5 or 6 posttransplant. None of 78 historical control breast cancer patients had neutrophil recovery by the sixth day. Eight patients (33%) had 3 or fewer days of neutropenia and 11 patients did not experience neutropenic fevers or require broad-spectrum antibiotics (Fig. 110.2 and 110.3, Table 110.1).

At the University of Colorado we treated patients (*n* = 21) with high risk stage II, III, or IV breast cancer with ex vivo expanded PBPC (McNiece *et al.*, 2000). All patients were mobilized with G-CSF (filgrastim, 10 μg/kg/day) for 9 days

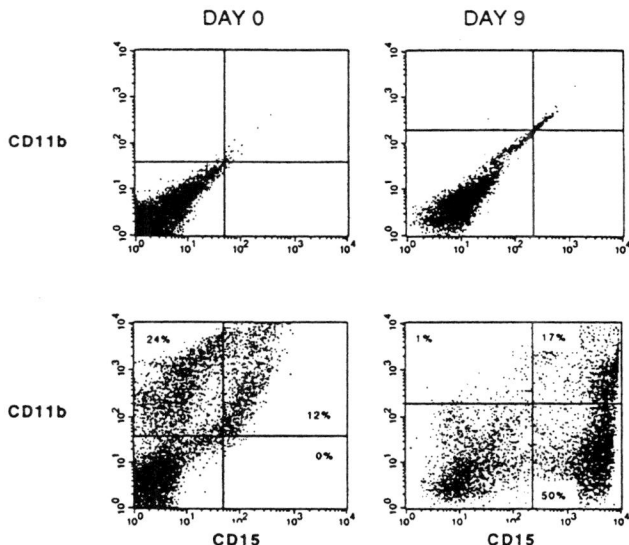

Fig. 110.2. Immunophenotype of ex vivo expanded cells. PBPC were subjected to immunofluorescent staining on days 0 and 9 of culture using FITC-conjugated anti-CD15 and phycoerythrin-conjugated anti-CD11b, or isotype controls, then analyzed by flow cytometry. Reproduced, with permission, from Paquette *et al.* (2000).

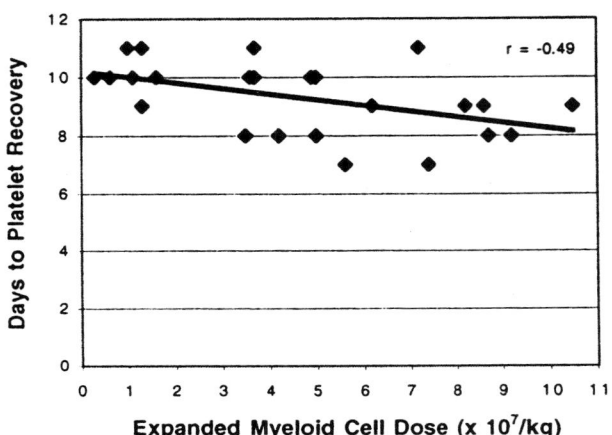

Fig. 110.3. Effect of expanded cell dose on the time to platelet recovery. The number of ex vivo expanded cells administered was correlated with the time to platelet recovery after cell infusion (r = –0.49). Reproduced, with permission, from Paquette *et al.* (2000).

and were leukapheresed on days 5 through 9. Following mobilization all patients received high-dose chemotherapy. A group of historical control patients were identified with similar stage of disease, prior therapy, and high-dose chemotherapy regimens. Leukapheresis products (LP) were harvested on days 5 through 9, with CD34+ cell selection preformed on the first four LPs. The fifth LP was frozen unselected as a backup product. CD34+ selection was performed using the Isolex 300i. After selection, each product was frozen in liquid nitrogen. On day –10 of treatment, two LPs were thawed and placed into ex vivo expansion culture. The cells were diluted in Defined Media (DM) supplemented with 100 ng/ml each of recombinant human (rh) SCF, rhMGDF and rhG-CSF to 20,000 cells per ml in 800 ml of media and transferred into Teflon bags. The bags were incubated at 37° C for 10 days in a 5% CO_2 incubator. On day 0 of treatment the cultures were harvested using a Cobe cell washer, and the media and growth factors removed with washing. Following ex vivo expansion of the CD34 selected cells, patients in cohort 1 (*n* = 10) were reinfused with

Table 110.1   *Outcomes of study and control patients*

Variables	Study[a]	Control[a]	*P*[b]
No. patients	24	48	
Prior chemotherapy cycles	5.7 (2.9)	4.0 (2.1)	.010
CD34+ cells infused	8.4 (5.3)	11.2 (7.9)	.010
Days to ANC > 500/μL	7.3 (1.4)	8.8 (0.7)	.0001
Days to platelet recovery	9.3 (1.2)	10.3 (1.6)	.010
Platelet units transfused	2.7 (2.1)	2.8 (1.6)	.25
Red cell units transfused	3.5 (2.0)	4.2 (1.4)	.02
Days of hospitalization	15.4 (2.6)	16.9 (2.1)	.0005

Abbreviation: ANC, absolute neutrophil count.
[a] Values are mean (± SD).
[b] Probability determined by the Wilcoxon rank sum test.
Reproduced, with permission, from Paquette *et al.* (2002).

expanded cells on day 0 followed by the unexpanded CD34+ cells. Patients in cohort 2 (*n* = 10) received only ex vivo expanded cells and the unexpanded CD34+ cells were maintained frozen in liquid nitrogen as a backup source of hematopoietic cells. Transplantation of ex vivo expanded PBPC resulted in rapid engraftment of neutrophils (ANC >500/μl) with one patient engrafting on day 4 and a number of patients engrafting on days 5 and 6. The median time of neutrophil engraftment was day 6 in the first 15 patients. Historical controls had a median time to neutrophil engraftment of 9 days, with a range of 7 to 30 days (Figure 110.4). The infused total nucleated cell dose/kg had a significant correlation with the days to an ANC >500/μl (r^2 = .785), but there was no significant correlation of the number of infused CD34+ cells/kg (r^2 = .239). Cytospin preparations of the ex vivo expanded cells demonstrated the generation of mature neutrophil cells (Figure 110.5), and we propose that mature neutrophil precursors and mature neutrophils are responsible for the more rapid recovery of neutrophil levels in the patients.

The patients in cohort 2 were transplanted with only expanded cells and these patients have been followed for more than 2 years posttransplant. No patients have experienced late graft failure suggesting that sufficient stem cells are maintained in the expansion conditions to provide long-term engraftment. However, it is possible that the long-term engraftment is provided by endogenous stem cells that survived the high-dose chemotherapy and in the absence of gene marking this cannot be elucidated.

Ex vivo expansion of cord blood (CB) cells

Hematopoietic stem cell (HSC) transplantation from HLA-matched related and unrelated donors has been used successfully to treat patients with hematological malignancies. The major limitation to such transplantation is the availability of a suitable donor. The National Marrow Donor Program (NDMP) has identified a pool of over 4 million potential donors and facilitated many thousands of unrelated donor HSC transplants. However, access to an unrelated HSC transplant donor is still limited due to: 1) the length of time for the donor search process (range 1 month to 6 years (Williams *et al.,* 1990), 2) donor availability at the time of request and, 3) limited availability of donors in certain racial and ethnic populations. Because of these reasons less than 40% of patients who could benefit from HSC transplantation have a suitable donor identified and of those who have a donor identified, less than 40% receive a transplant. Over the past 10 years, CB has been clinically investigated as an alternative source of hematopoietic tissue for allogeneic transplantation of patients lacking an HLA-matched marrow or PBPC donor (Cairo & Wagner, 1997) (and see Chapter 68). The first transplant using CB was performed by Gluckman and colleagues in 1988 (Gluckman *et al.,* 1989).

The ease of collection and potential availability to ethnic groups currently under-represented in the NMDP Registry are the main advantages of CB. Additionally, it has been proposed

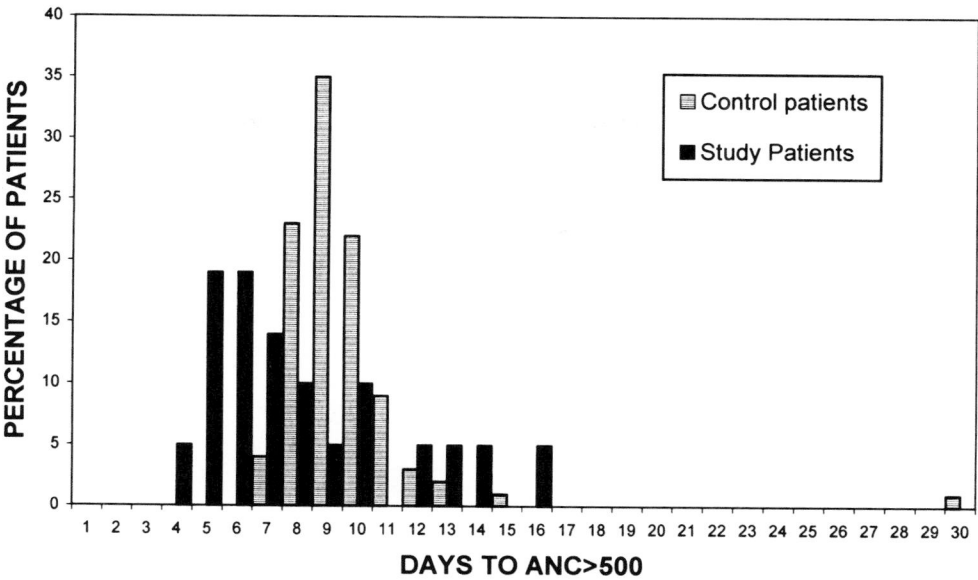

Fig. 110.4. Neutrophil engraftment (time to ANC >500/µl) for patients receiving ex vivo expanded PBPC (study patients) compared to historical control patients matched for disease and prior therapy.

that CB contains fewer T cells and/or more naive T cells than marrow and may permit a greater degree of HLA mismatch with less graft-versus-host disease (GVHD) (De La Selle *et al.*, 1996). The total number of cells in a CB unit is low compared to marrow or PBPC harvests, and because of this the vast majority of CB recipients have been children with an average weight of 20 kg. The progression-free survival rates reported thus far are comparable to the results achieved with allogeneic marrow transplantation, with a suggestion of decreased GVHD (Gluckman *et al.*, 1997). However, the time to neutrophil and platelet engraftment in CB recipients has been delayed compared to that with marrow.

Kurtzberg and colleagues reported on 25 patients who received unrelated donor CB transplants (Kurtzberg *et al.*, 1996). Twenty-three of the 25 transplant patients had evidence of donor engraftment achieving an ANC >500/µl at a median of 22 days (range 14–37) with platelet engraftment at a median of 56 days (range 35–89). The overall event-free survival rate was 48% with a median follow-up of 12.5 months. In another report by Wagner and colleagues (Wagner *et al.*, 1996), 18 patients with malignant and non-malignant diseases received unrelated CB transplants. All patients demonstrated donor engraftment with an ANC >500/µl at a median of 24 days (range 16–53) with platelet engraftment at a median of 54 days (range 39–130). The probability of survival was 65% with a median follow-up of 6 months.

Cord blood nucleated cell dose correlates with neutrophil engraftment

Studies by Gluckman and colleagues have reported on the importance of the nucleated cell dose of the transplanted CB

products (Gluckman *et al.*, 1997). A higher nucleated cell dose was reported to have a positive impact upon neutrophil engraftment and one of the factors which predicted for better survival included a nucleated cell dose >3.7 × 10⁷/kg. These results have led to the recommendation of only transplanting CB units in which the nucleated cell dose is >3.7 × 10⁷/kg. Obviously this limits the size of patients who have an adequate CB unit and therefore the majority of CB transplants to date have been limited primarily to small pediatric patients.

Clinical studies utilizing ex vivo expanded cord blood cells

There have been several studies performed using different culture conditions for the ex vivo expansion of CB cells. Shpall and colleagues have transplanted cancer patients (CML, $n = 3$; CLL, $n = 3$; NHL, $n = 4$; ALL, $n = 5$; AML, $n = 1$, HD, $n = 1$, breast cancer, $n = 2$) who were appropriate candidates for high-dose chemotherapy requiring cellular support (Shpall *et al.*, 1998). The CB products were frozen as a single product ($n = 11$), or divided into aliquots of 2 × 50% ($n = 2$) or 40% and 60% aliquots ($n = 6$), and each fraction frozen separately. The CB products frozen in a single product were thawed on day 0 and 60% was reinfused unmanipulated, while the remaining 40% was CD34-selected and placed into ex vivo expansion culture. The other CB products were thawed at different times with a 50% or 40% aliquot thawed on day −10 for expansion culture and the remaining aliquot thawed on day 0 and reinfused without manipulation. All fractions for expansion were CD34-selected using the Nexell Isolex 300i and the CD34-selected cells were placed into a single Teflon bag containing 800 ml of Defined Media (Amgen Inc.) containing 100 ng/ml each of rhSCF, rhG-CSF and rhMGDF. The bags were incubated for 10 days in a 5% CO_2 incubator, after which time the cells were harvested, washed and reinfused. Following transplantation all patients received GVHD prophylaxis consisting of either cyclosporine 5 mg/kg i.v. every 12 hours starting day –2 and high-dose corticosteroids ($n = 8$), or cyclosporine 5 mg/kg i.v. every 12 hours starting day –2 and moderate dose steroids ($n = 11$).

All patients achieved neutrophil engraftment at a median time of 25 (range 15–35) days and platelet engraftment at 58 days (range 27–91). Considering the low numbers of cells infused per kg in these patients, the time to neutrophil engraftment was faster than previous reports in patients with weights greater than 45 kg (Gluckman *et al.*, 1997). In particular, these data suggest that a potential benefit of expanded CB cells may be lack of graft failure compared to the use of unexpanded CB. Gluckman and colleagues reported that only 48% of patients (>45 kg body weight) had engrafted neutrophils by day 60 posttransplant (Gluckman *et al.*, 1997). Thus, a significant number of patients receiving low numbers of cells/kg are at risk of extended neutropenia and potential neutropenic complications. The use of ex vivo expanded cells may eliminate this potential risk of extended neutropenia.

Several investigators have performed studies of ex vivo expansion of CB using the Aastrom Cell Production System. Jaroscak and colleagues (Jaroscak *et al.*, 1998) described the expansion of CB products that were transplanted into 21 patients. Each patient received unmanipulated CB cells on days 0 and the expanded cells on day +12. No significant effects on engraftment kinetics were observed in these patients. Stiff and colleagues (Stiff *et al.*, 1998) also reported on expansion of CB cells using the Aastrom system for 9 patients. The median weight of the patients was 74 kg with a range of 47 to 117 kg. The median time to neutrophil engraftment was 26 days with a range of 14 to 36 days. Engraftment of platelets was delayed in these patients. The authors concluded that ex vivo expanded CB cells may be useful in adults with otherwise incurable hematologic disorders.

Conclusions

In summary, it has been clearly demonstrated that current ex vivo expansion techniques allow for the generation of cells that mediate rapid short-term engraftment following high-dose therapy. Whether or not ex vivo expanded human CD34+ cells are capable of stable long-term engraftment has yet to be determined, and a definitive answer can only be provided by genetic marking studies in humans (Dunbar *et al.*, 1995) or the use of ex vivo expanded cells for allogeneic transplantation. Among other controversial issues in the field of ex vivo expansion, the identification of the hematopoietic cell population(s) responsible for long-term engraftment, as opposed to those mediating short-term engraftment, is currently a matter of intense discussion.

Ex vivo generated cells offer enormous potential for treating devastating malignant and non-malignant diseases, such as Parkinson's disease, diabetes, chronic heart disease, end-stage kidney disease, liver failure, and cancer. A number of groups have recently reported that stem cells derived from adults may be capable of surprising plasticity or versatility. In the future it may be possible to generate cells of various tissues in vitro and hematopoietic stem cells (HSC) offer the ideal starting population due to the simple access to large numbers of HSC from mobilized peripheral blood progenitor products. In addition, hematopoietic cells have been grown ex vivo and reinfused into patients receiving high-dose chemotherapy and these clinical studies have demonstrated both the safety and clinical efficacy of the expanded cells.

References

Alcorn, M. J., Holyoake, T. L., Richmond, L. *et al.* (1996). CD34-positive cells isolated from cryopreserved peripheral-blood progenitor cells can be expanded ex vivo and used for transplantation with little or no toxicity. *Journal of Clinical Oncology*, **14**, 1839.

Brugger, W., Heimfeld, S. Berenson, R. I., Mertelsmann, R., & Kanz, L. (1995). Reconstitution of hematopoiesis after high-dose chemotherapy by autologous progenitor cells generated ex vivo. *New England Journal of Medicine*, **333**, 283.

Brugger, W., Mocklin, W., Heimfeld, S. *et al.* (1993). Ex vivo expansion of enriched peripheral blood CD34+ progenitor cells by stem cell factor, interleukin-1 beta (IL-1 beta), IL-6, IL-3, interferon-gamma, and erythropoietin. *Blood*, **81**, 2579–84.

Cairo, M. S. & Wagner, J. E. Placental and/or umbilical cord blood: an alternative source of hematopoietic stem cells for transplantation. *Blood*, **90**, 4665–4678.

Davis, T. A., Robinson, D. H., Lee, K. P., & Kessler, S. W. (1995). Porcine brain microvascular endothelial cells support the in vitro expansion of human primitive hematopoietic bone marrow progenitor cells with a high replating potential: requirement for cell-to-cell interactions and colony-stimulating factors. *Blood*, **85**, 1751–61.

De La Selle, V., Gluckman, E., & Bruley-Rosset, M. (1996). Newborn blood can engraft adult mice without inducing graft versus host disease across non H-2 antigens. *Blood*, **87**, 3977–3783.

Dexter, T. M., Moore, M. A., & Sheridan, A. P. (1977). Maintenance of hemopoietic stem cells and production of differentiated progeny in allogeneic and semiallogeneic bone marrow chimeras in vitro. *Journal of Experimental Medicine*, **145**, 1612–16.

Dunbar, C. E., Cottler, F. M., O'Shaughnessy, J. A. *et al.* (1995). Retrovirally marked CD34-enriched peripheral blood and bone marrow cells contribute to long-term engraftment after autologous transplantation. *Blood*, **85**, 3048–57.

Engelhardt, M., Douville, J., Behringer, D. *et al.* (2001). Hematopoietic recovery of ex vivo perfusion culture expanded after bone marrow and unexpanded peripheral blood progenitors after myeloablative chemotherapy. *Bone Marrow Transplantation*, **27**, 249–59.

Fennie, C., Cheng, J., Dowbenko, D. *et al.* (1995). CD34+ endothelial cell lines derived from murine yolk sac induce the proliferation and differentiation of yolk sac CD34+ hematopoietic progenitors. *Blood*, **86**, 4454–67.

Gluckman, E., Broxmeyer, H. E., Auerbach, A. D. et al. (1989). Hematopoietic reconstitution in a patient with Fanconi's anemia bu means of umbilical cord blood from an HLA-identical sibling. New England Journal of Medicine, 321, 1174.

Gluckman, E., Rocha, V., Boyer-Chammard, A. et al. (1997). Outcome of cord-blood transplantation from related and unrelated donors. New England Journal of Medicine, 337, 373.

Gupta, P., McCarthy, J. B., & Verfaillie, C. M. (1996). Stromal fibroblast heparan sulfate is required for cytokine-mediated ex vivo maintenance of human long-term culture-initiating cells. Blood, 87, 3229–36.

Henschler, R., Brugger, W., Luff, T. et al. (1994). Maintenance of transplantation potential ex vivo expanded CD34(+)-selected human peripheral blood progenitor cells. Blood, 84, 2898–903.

Jacobsen, F. W., Keller, J. R., Ruscetti, F. W. et al. (1995). Direct synergistic effects of IL-4 and IL-11 on proliferation of primitive hematopoietic progenitor cells. Experimental Hematology, 23, 990–5.

Jaroscak, J., Martin, P. L., Waters-Pick, B. et al. (1998). A phase I trial of augmentation of unrelated umbilical cord blood transplantation with ex-vivo expanded cells. Blood, 92 (Suppl. 1), 646a.

Kawano, Y., Kobune, M., Yamaguchi, M. et al. (2003). Ex vivo expansion of human umbilical cord hematopoietic progenitor cells using a co-culture system with human telomerase catalytic subunit (hTERT)-transfected human stromal cells. Blood, 101, 532–40.

Kay, H.E.M. (1965). How many cell-generations? Lancet, August 28.

Keller, J. R., Ortiz, M., & Ruscetti, F. W. (1995). Steel factor (c-kit ligand) promotes the survival of hematopoietic stem/progenitor cells in the absence of cell division. Blood, 86, 1757–64.

Kurtzberg, J., Laughlin, M., Graham, M. L. et al. (1996). Placenta blood as a source of hematopoieticstem cells for transplantation into unrelated recipients. New England Journal of Medicine, 335, 57.

Mayani, H., Little, M. T., Dragowska, W. et al. (1995). Differential effects of the hematopoietic inhibitors MIP-1 alpha, TGF-beta, and TNF-alpha on cytokine-induced proliferation of subpopulations of CD34+ cells purified from cord blood and fetal liver. Experimental Hematology, 23, 422–7.

McNiece, I. & Briddell, R. (2001). Ex vivo expansion of hematopoietic progenitor cells and mature cells. Experimental Hematology, 29, 3–11.

McNiece, I., Jones, R., Bearman, S. et al. (2000). Ex vivo expanded peripheral blood progenitor cells provide rapid neutrophil recovery in breast cancer patients following high-dose chemotherapy. Blood, 96, 3001–7.

Moore, K. A., Ema, H., & Lemischka, I. R. (1997). In vitro maintenance of highly purified, transplantable hematopoietic stem cells. Blood, 89, 4337–47.

Naparstek, E., Hardan, Y., Ben-Shahar, M. et al. (1992). Enhanced marrow recovery by short preincubation of marrow allografts with human recombinant interleukin-3 and granulocyte-macrophage colony-stimulating factor. Blood, 80, 1673.

Paquette, R. (2000). Clinical experience with ex vivo expanded unselected peripheral blood progenitor cells. International

Conference on Hematopoietic Stem Cell Biology and Transplantation. Paris, France.

Pecora, A. L., Stiff, P., Lemaistre, C. F. et al. (2001). A phase II trial evaluating the safety and effectiveness of the AastromReplicell system for augmentation of low-dose blood stem cell transplantation. Bone Marrow Transplantation, 28, 295–303.

Raffi, S., Shapiro, F., Pettengell, R. et al. (1995). Human bone marrow microvascular endothelial cells support long-term proliferation and differentiation of myeloid and megakaryocytic progenitors. Blood, 86, 3353–63.

Reiffers, J., Cailliot, C., Dazey, B. et al. (1999). Abrogation of post-myeloablative chemotherapy neutropenia by ex-vivo expanded autologous CD34-positive cells. Lancet, 354, 1092.

Sandstrom, C. E., Bender, J. G., Papoutsakis, E. T., & Miller, W. M. (1995). Effects of CD34+ cell selection and perfusion on ex vivo expansion of peripheral blood mononuclear cells. Blood, 86, 958–70.

Shapiro, F., Yao, T. J., Raptis, G. et al. (1994). Optimization of conditions for ex vivo expansion of CD34+ cells from patients with stage IV breast cancer. Blood, 84, 3567–74.

Shpall, E. J., Quinones, R., Hami, L. et al. (1998). Transplantation of cancer patients receiving high-dose chemotherapy with ex vivo expanded cord blood cells. Blood, 92 (Suppl. 1), 646a.

Stiff, P., Chen, B., Franklin, W. et al. (2000). Autologous transplantation of ex vivo expanded bone marrow cells grown from small aliquots after high-dose chemotherapy for breast cancer. Blood, 95, 2169–74.

Stiff, P., Pecora, A., Parthasarathy, M. et al. (1998). Umbilical cord blood transplants in adults using a combination of unexpanded and ex vivo expanded cells: preliminary clinical observations. Blood, 92 (Suppl. 1), 646a.

Taichman, R. S., Reilly, M. J., & Emerson, S. G. (1996). Human osteoblasts support human hematopoietic progenitor cells in vitro bone marrow cultures. Blood, 87, 518–24.

Verfaillie, C. M. (1992). Direct contact between human primitive hematopoietic progenitors and bone marrow stroma is not required for long-term in vitro hematopoiesis. Blood, 79, 2821–6.

Wagner, J. E., Rosenthal, J., Sweetman, R. et al. (1996). Successful transplantation of HLA-matched and HLA-mismatched umbilical cord blood from unrelated donors: analysis of engraftment and acute graft-versus-host disease. Blood, 88, 795.

Williams, S. F. Lee, W. J., Bender, J. G. et al. (1996). Selection and expansion of peripheral blood CD34+ cells in autologous stem cell transplantation for breast cancer. Blood, 87, 1687.

Williams, W. I., Beutler, E., Erslev, A. I., & Lichtman, M. A., eds. (1990). Hematology 4th edition New York: McGraw-Hill Inc.

Young, J. C., Varma, A., DiGiusto, D., & Backer, M. P. (1996). Retention of quiescent hematopoietic cells with high proliferative potential during ex vivo stem cell culture. Blood, 87, 545–56.

Young, J. W., Szabolcs, P., & Moore, M. A. (1995). Identification of dendritic cell colony-forming units among normal human CD34+ bone marrow progenitors that are expanded by c-kit-ligand and yield pure dendritic cell colonies in the presence of granulocyte/macrophage colony-stimulating factor and tumor necrosis factor alpha. Journal of Experimental Medicine, 182, 1111–19.

111 In utero hematopoietic stem cell transplantation

ROBERTSON PARKMAN

Childrens Hospital, Los Angeles, USA

Introduction

Histocompatible hematopoietic stem cell transplantation (HSCT) is the treatment of choice for genetic diseases involving HSC and their progeny (Parkman, 1986). Diverse diseases including α- and β-thalassemia, osteopetrosis, Hurler's disease, and adrenoleukodystrophy can be corrected and/or stabilized following the ablation of the abnormal recipient HSC and their replacement by normal donor HSC (Krivit *et al.*, 1984, 1990; Lucarelli *et al.*, 1990). However, the majority of patients with genetic diseases treatable by HSCT do not have histocompatible donors.

Alternative sources of HSC have included T-cell-depleted histoincompatible related bone marrow and unrelated bone marrow/cord blood. These alternative sources of HSC have an increased likelihood of transplantation-related mortality/morbidity, principally due to the increased incidence and severity of graft-versus-host disease (GVHD) and/or a decreased incidence of sustained engraftment. Acute GVHD may accelerate the tempo of some genetic diseases (i.e. adrenoleukodystrophy). In addition, diseases such as α-thalassemia and some central nervous system (CNS) storage diseases may have significant morbidity, if not mortality, before birth. Therefore, an alternative approach for the treatment of genetic diseases by HSCT is the in utero transplantation of histoincompatible HSC.

The treatment of a genetic disease by HSCT requires that the recipient be unable to immunologically reject the donor HSC and that the engrafted donor HSC produce adequate levels of progeny to have a clinical impact on the primary disease. In postnatal HSC transplantation, patients are prepared with busulfan to eliminate their abnormal HSC and cyclophosphamide to eliminate their normal immune systems [except in the case of patients with severe combined immune deficiency (SCID)] (Kapoor *et al.*, 1981). Thus, at the time of transplantation, the recipient is unable to immunologically reject the transplanted donor cells and adequate "space" is present to permit the engraftment of the donor HSC.

It has been known since the initial transplants of patients with SCID that the administration of drugs to eliminate recipient HSC is not always required to achieve donor HSC engraftment. Children with SCID who have been transplanted with histocompatible HSC without pretransplant chemotherapy develop T lymphocytes, and in some cases B cells, of donor origin (O'Reilly *et al.*, 1989). Thus, low levels of donor HSC engraftment can be achieved without the administration of marrow-ablative drugs. Based on the study of patients transplanted with autologous genetically modified HSC, the frequency of human HSC engraftment without the administration of pretransplant chemotherapy is 1 in 1,000 (Kohn *et al.*, 1995). The ability to achieve donor HSC engraftment without the administration of pretransplant chemotherapeutic agents has been confirmed in mice (Stewart *et al.*, 1993; Wu & Keating, 1993). When adequate numbers of HSC are transplanted, greater than 50% donor engraftment can be achieved when there are no immunological barriers. These results indicated that there is adequate "space" to permit donor HSC engraftment if large numbers of HSC are transplanted and that the frequency of donor HSC engraftment is directly related to the number of donor cells transplanted. However, the engraftment of donor HSC has not been documented in non-SCID patients without pretransplant immunosuppression—the transplanted donor HSC are rejected by the recipient's immune system.

During the last two decades, investigators working with monkeys, sheep, and mice have demonstrated that it is possible to engraft donor HSC if they are transplanted in utero late in the first trimester (Flake *et al.*, 1986; Harrison *et al.*, 1989; Zanjani *et al.*, 1992; Jones *et al.*, 1996). The engraftment of syngeneic, allogeneic, and xenogeneic HSC has been reproducibly achieved. As in the case of post-natal HSC transplantation, the inability of the recipient to immunologically reject the donor HSC is a prerequisite for sustained donor HSC engraftment.

In humans the thymus first becomes populated with lymphoid cells at 8 weeks of gestation and phytohemagglutinin (PHA)-responsive thymocytes can be identified at 12 weeks of gestation (Parkman & Merler, 1973). Between 12 and 16 weeks of gestation circulating CD3+ T lymphocytes can be identified, and PHA-responsive T lymphocytes can be identified in peripheral lymphoid organs including the spleen by 16 weeks of gestation. Between 12 and 16 weeks there is a logarithmic increase in the number of peripheral lymphoid cells. Until 15 or 16 weeks of gestation, human fetuses may be relatively immunoincompetent and, therefore, incapable of rejecting allogeneic cells.

In most mammals, fetal hematopoiesis originates in the fetal liver. During the latter part of the first trimester, the primary site of hematopoiesis moves from the fetal liver to the developing bone marrow cavity. Studies in sheep and monkeys have demonstrated that the intraperitoneal transplantation of HSC from fetal livers early during the first trimester does not result in donor engraftment, but that transplantation during the latter part of the first trimester reproducibly results in donor hematopoietic engraftment. The lack of engraftment during the first half of the first trimester may be due to the fact that an anatomic marrow space does not exist. When HSC are transplanted during the second trimester, donor engraftment is not achieved because of immunologically mediated rejection of the transplanted cells (Zanjani et al., 1993).

When fetal monkeys and sheep are transplanted with fetal liver cells, recipients have 1% to 5% donor engraftment at birth. However, when adult bone marrow cells are transplanted, most fetuses die in utero and those animals that survive to birth have GVHD (Crombleholme et al., 1990). The removal of T lymphocytes from the adult bone marrow inoculum eliminates GVHD, but also decreases the frequency and the extent of donor engraftment. Thus, the presence of donor T lymphocytes increases the likelihood of donor HSC engraftment possibly due to the inhibition of natural killer cells and other non-specific mechanisms that may inhibit donor HSC engraftment.

Preclinical studies have demonstrated that the intraperitoneal route is superior to the intravenous route, results that are the opposite to those seen in human postnatal transplantation (Huang et al., 1973). In SCID patients the intravenous route was superior to the intraperitoneal route. The superiority of the intraperitoneal route for in utero transplantation may be due to the fact that donor HSC are lost in the placenta following intravenous administration. Additionally, repeated transplants at intervals of 1 to 3 days can result in higher levels of donor engraftment than a single transplant with the same total number of cells (Flake & Zanjani, 1997). These results suggest that there is a limited number of HSC that can engraft at any one time. Once the transplantable sites are saturated, further increases in the number of transplanted HSC do not result in greater donor engraftment. These results are also in contrast to those of postnatal transplants in mice, where increasing the number of donor cells results in increased donor engraftment.

Because of the immunological immaturity of animals during the first trimester, it has been possible to perform xenogeneic transplants. Human HSC have reproducibly engrafted in fetal sheep (Kawashima et al., 1996). The transplantation of positively selected CD34+ cells has resulted in the establishment of human hematopoiesis without GVHD. Of interest is that, while human hematopoiesis was detectable after birth, prenatal sampling showed no evidence of donor engraftment. Thus, the preclinical studies have established that it is possible to achieve donor hematopoietic engraftment late in the first trimester without the development of fatal GVHD if a HSC source devoid of mature T lymphocytes is used. These observations have led investigators to explore the potential clinical use of in utero HSCT to treat genetic diseases (Jones et al., 1996).

Clinical in utero transplantation

The first human in utero transplant was an attempt to treat a child with severe erythroblastosis fetalis by transplantation of parental bone marrow at 17 weeks of gestation (Linch et al., 1986). No evidence of donor hematopoietic engraftment was detected. Multiple other attempts to treat fetuses by in utero transplantation were made during the late 1980s and early 1990s (Cowan & Golbus, 1994). The first unambiguous engraftment in a human fetus of allogeneic HSC was achieved in the mid 1990s when two fetuses with X-linked severe combined immune deficiency due to defects in the common γ-chain were transplanted (Flake et al., 1996; Wengler et al, 1996). X-linked severe combined immune deficiency is characterized by the absence of mature T lymphocytes and the presence of phenotypic but dysfunctional B lymphocytes [due to a defective interleukin (IL)-4 receptor]. The first fetus was transplanted intraperitoneally with positively selected CD34+ cells isolated from paternal bone marrow that contained 0.5% CD3+ T lymphocytes. The fetus was initially transplanted with 14.8×10^6 cells at 16 weeks of gestation, followed by 2×10^6 cells at 17.5 weeks, and 1.8×10^6 cells at 18.5 weeks. At birth the child had a mild macular rash which was diagnosed as GVHD and treated with methylprednisolone for 1 week. A skin biopsy, however, did not confirm the diagnosis of GVHD. At birth the patient's hematological counts were normal. Using dual color immunofluorescence the T lymphocytes were demonstrated to be of donor origin whereas the B lymphocytes and monocytes were of recipient origin. By 1 month of age a low but detectable PHA response was present. Tolerance to the paternal histocompatibility antigens was demonstrated by an absence of a proliferative response to paternal cells, but normal proliferation to third party cells and reduced proliferation to maternal cells. The patient has continued to do well clinically with all T lymphocytes being of donor origin. Although most B lymphocytes continue to be of recipient origin, at 1 year of age some B lymphocytes were of donor origin. The patient continues to receive intermittent immunoglobulin therapy and has not been immunized with a neo-antigen (ψX174) to determine if normal T/B cell collaboration is possible.

A second patient with X-linked SCID was transplanted with paternal cells that were positively selected for CD34 followed by E-rosette formation to remove residual T lymphocytes. Fourteen million cells were transplanted intraperitoneally at 21 weeks of gestation followed by 4×10^6 cells at 22 weeks. The CD34+ cells used for transplantation contained 0.06% CD3+ T

Table 111.1. *Clinical experience with in utero HSC transplantation*

Gest age (wk)[a]	Donor cell source	Disease treated	No. Cases	Postnatal outcome
11	Fetal BM	Rh-disease	1	Postnatal death 32 wk, no engraftment
17	Maternal TCD BM	Rh-disease	1	Survived, no engraftment
28		Bare lymphocyte syndrome	1	Clinically normal, 26% donor HLA expression at 1 yr
	Fetal liver and fetal thymus			
26		SCID	1	Alive, engrafted by PCR for Y
12		β-Thalassemia major	1	Alive, not engrafted
19	Fetal liver	β-Thalassemia major	1	Intrauterine death
14		Nieman-Pick type A	1	? Engraftment without benefit
18		CGD	1	Intrauterine death
34, 23, 25	Paternal TCD BM	MCLD	2	No evidence of engraftment, clinical status c/w primary disease
	Sibling TCD BM	β-Thalassemia	1	
19		SCID	1	Terminated at 24 wk, no peripheral expression, no autopsy
26	Maternal TCD BM	Chediak-Higashi	1	No engraftment at birth
18		α-Thalassemia	1	Terminated at 24 wk, donor + cells in extramedullary hematopoiesis
12	Maternal TCD BM	Rh-disease	1	No detectable engraftment, ? tolerance
14	Fetal liver	β-Thalassemia major	1	Septic abortion
14	Fetal liver	Hurler's disease	1	Low level engraftment, death at age 2
15	Paternal CD34 enriched	CGD	1	Alive, no detectable engraftment
15		α-Thalassemia	1	
	Cryopreserved			
13	Fetal liver	Sickle cell disease	1	No detectable engraftment
18		β-Thalassemia major	1	
13	Paternal CD34 enriched	Globoid leukodystrophy	1	Intrauterine death at 20 wk, extensive donor cell infiltration
16	Paternal CD34 enriched	X-linked SCID	1	Alive at 40 mo, normal immune function, split chimerism
20	Paternal CD34 enriched	X-linked SCID	1	Alive at 3.5 mo, split chimerism
13	Paternal CD34 enriched	α-Thalassemia	1	Alive at 1 yr. Microchimerism, tolerant by MLR
13	CD34, THY-1-enriched BM	CGD	1	Alive, no detectable engraftment

Abbreviations: BM, bone marrow; Rh, rhesus; TCD, T-cell depleted; HLA, human leukocyte antigen; SCID, severe combined immune deficiency; PCR, polymerase chain reactions; CGD, chronic granulomatous disease; MLR, mixed lymphocyte reaction; MCLD, metachromatic leukodystrophy; c/w, consistent with.

[a] Gestational age at first in utero HSC transplantation. In many cases more than one transplant was performed.

Reproduced, with permission, from Flake and Zanjani (1999).

lymphocytes. The child was delivered at 38 weeks by Cesarean section with no clinical evidence of GVHD. At birth the patient had 21% CD3+ cells with 13% CD4+ and 14% CD8+ T lymphocytes. Ninety-two percent of the CD4+ T lymphocytes co-expressed CD45RA demonstrating that they were recent thymic emigrants and were not derived from the transplanted mature donor T lymphocytes. The PHA response was normal. In a fetus with T−B+ NK+ SCID given CD34-selected paternal cells, split chimerism (T cells of donor origin, monocytes, B and NK cells of host origin) allowed humoral immune reconstitution including a 7.8 fold increase in serum antibody to HbsAg after immunization with recombinant HBV vaccine (Bartolome *et al.,* 2002).

These cases conclusively demonstrate that it is possible to engraft children with X-linked SCID in utero with either HSC or committed progenitors cells. Further follow-up studies will

be necessary to establish if there is the long-term ability to generate T lymphocytes and whether significant B lymphocyte differentiation can occur.

The clinical results of these initial in utero transplants for X-linked SCID are similar to those of postnatal T-cell-depleted haploidentical transplants in that T lymphocyte engraftment is readily achieved, whereas B lymphocyte engraftment is difficult to detect (O'Reilly *et al.,* 1989). Following postnatal haploidentical transplantation, most patients require ongoing immunoglobulin replacement therapy due to the lack of significant numbers of B lymphocytes unless marrow-ablative conditioning is given pretransplant (O'Reilly *et al.,* 1989). If significant donor B lymphocyte engraftment is achieved following in utero transplantation, and if the patients do not require ongoing immunoglobulin therapy, in utero transplantation would be superior to postnatal HSCT.

Two other cases of engraftment have occurred following in utero HSCT; one was in a child transplanted for the bare lymphocyte syndrome, a form of SCID (Touraine *et al.*, 1989). The child was transplanted with multiple fetal livers and thymuses both in utero and following birth. Since multiple HSC transplants (including postnatal transplants) occurred, it is difficult to determine the origin of the observed engraftment. The second transplant was in a fetus with globoid cell leukodystrophy given 1.4×10^8 CD34-selected paternal bone marrow cells/kg and 7×10^6 T cells/kg at 13 weeks of gestation. Full donor engraftment occurred but the fetus died at 20 weeks. Paternal hematopoietic cells were infiltrating most tissues (Bambach *et al.*, 1997).

There has been no evidence of sustained donor HSC engraftment in fetuses who did not have SCID. Multiple fetuses have been transplanted for hemoglobinopathies (α- or β-thalassemia) (Westgren *et al.*, 1996) and metabolic disorders (Hurler's disease) (Cowan & Golbus, 1994). It must be noted, however, that in many of these cases the fetuses were transplanted later than 16 to 17 weeks of gestation, a time at which their immunological competence would be adequate to reject allogeneic cells. Therefore, the lack of sustained donor hematopoietic engraftment that has been observed in these fetuses is expected. This experience has been summarized by Flake and Zanjani (1999) (Table 111.1).

The Future

In utero transplantation may have advantages for the treatment of children with primary immunodeficiencies, especially SCID, if it can be demonstrated that multilineage (T and B lymphocyte) engraftment is achieved. The engrafted donor HSC will have longer (5 months) to differentiate before the fetus is born and the developing immune system is challenged by opportunistic organisms. When patients are transplanted postnatally, they have to be maintained in isolation until the recapitulation of their immunological ontogeny is complete since it usually takes 3 months for HSC to differentiate through the recipient thymus and become phenotypic T lymphocytes (O'Reilly *et al.*, 1989). Thus, in utero transplantation for SCID may reduce the costs of HSCT.

The real potential for the use of in utero transplantation is for hematologic and metabolic diseases. Based upon animal experiments, only low levels of donor HSC engraftment can be expected at present. The limited HSC engraftment will not lead to clinical benefit unless there is a selective advantage for the progeny of the donor HSC. One percent to 5% donor HSC engraftment would give rise to only 1% to 5% circulating erythrocytes or 1% to 5% tissue macrophages of donor origin, which would not provide clinical benefit to patients with thalassemia or Hurler's disease, respectively.

However, tolerance to paternal histocompatibility antigens is anticipated following donor HSC engraftment. Thus, it could be possible to treat recipients after birth with busulfan or low dose (1 Gy) total body irradiation without the need for immunosuppression. Thus, patients with either hematologic or metabolic diseases might be transplanted in utero to establish tolerance to paternal histocompatibility antigens. Following birth their abnormal HSC would be reduced, and they could be transplanted with CD34$^+$ paternal cells that would engraft without the danger of an immunologically mediated rejection. Because the recipient would not have to be immunosuppressed, the risks associated with posttransplant infections would be reduced.

Attempts to increase the efficacy of in utero transplantation

The greatest limitation to the use of in utero transplantation to treat hematologic and metabolic diseases is the low level of donor HSC engraftment that is presently expected. Based upon murine studies, however, increases in the number of HSC transplanted could result in increased levels of donor HSC engraftment (Stewart *et al.*, 1993; Wu & Keating, 1993). The number of cells that can be transplant in utero is limited by the volume that can be safely placed into the fetal peritoneal cavity. The usual volumes used for intraperitoneal in utero transplantation have been 0.5 to 1 ml. The use of CD34$^+$ selected bone marrow cells has resulted in 100-fold increase in the number of HSC that can be transplanted compared to whole bone marrow. Further purification of HSC using flow cytometry to isolate CD34$^+$, CD38$^-$ cells would allow further increases in the numbers of HSC that could be transplanted in utero (Terstappen *et al.*, 1991). However, a fetus transplanted with purified CD34$^+$ Thy-1$^+$ (CD90) paternal bone marrow cells for chronic granulomatous disease at 14 weeks of gestation showed no evidence of donor engraftment 6 months after birth (Muench *et al.*, 2001).

A continuing concern is whether the trafficking pattern of adult HSC in the fetal environment is the same as that of fetal HSC (Shaaban *et al.*, 1999). Studies in fetal sheep have shown no significant difference between the engraftment of adult and fetal hematopoietic cells. Nevertheless the inability to engraft fetuses during the first half of the first trimester when fetal hematopoiesis is ongoing suggests that defects in the engraftment of allogeneic HSC may exist. It is also possible that the trafficking of the transplanted cells is not physiological and that the transplanted HSC will engraft in sites that are not optimal for hematopoiesis. Therefore, the co-transplantation of marrow stroma that will anatomically co-migrate with the allogeneic HSC may result in improved donor hematopoietic engraftment (Almeida-Porada *et al.*, 2000).

Successful in utero HSCT has been performed with haploidentical CD34$^+$ cells. The increased availability of unrelated cord blood and the increased frequency of HSC in cord blood suggests that unrelated cord blood may be an alternative source of HSC for in utero transplantation (Wang *et al.*, 1997). Based upon the histocompatibility antigens of the fetus, a greater degree of histocompatibility may be achieved with unrelated cord blood than with haploidentical parental bone marrow (Kurtzberg *et al.*, 1996). The increased number of HSC in cell cycle in cord blood may improve engraftment.

The recent demonstration that a disease (osteogenesis imperfecta) involving the progeny of mesenchymal stem cells can be modified by allogeneic bone marrow transplantation suggests that such diseases could be treated by the prenatal transplantation of mesenchymal stem cells (Horwitz *et al.*, 1999; Liechty *et al.*, 2000).

Conclusions

Only two patients have been successfully engrafted following in utero transplantation with allogeneic HSC. Both patients had severe X-linked combined immune deficiency and were, therefore, unable to reject allogeneic cells. In both cases donor T lymphocytes were detected at birth; the extent of donor B lymphocyte engraftment is uncertain. Additional improvements in the level of donor HSC engraftment will be necessary before the in utero transplantation of allogeneic HSC has a clinical role in the treatment of patients with hematologic or metabolic diseases.

References

Almeida-Porada, G., Porada, C. D., Tran, N., & Zanjani, E. D. (2000). Cotransplantation of human stromal cell progenitors into preimmune fetal sheep results in early appearance of human donor cells in circulation and boosts cell levels in bone marrow at later time points after transplantation. *Blood, 95,* 3620–7.

Bambach, B. J., Moser, H. W., Blakemore, K. *et al.* (1997). Engraftment following in utero bone marrow transplantation for globoid cell leukodystrophy. *Bone Marrow Transplantation, 19,* 399–402.

Bartolome, J., Porta, F., Lafranchi, A. *et al.* (2002). B cell function after haploidentical in utero bone marrow transplantation in a patient with severe combined immunodeficiency. *Bone Marrow Transplantation, 29,* 625–8.

Cowan, M. & Golbus, M. (1994). In utero hematopoietic stem cell transplants for inherited disease. *American Journal of Pediatric Hematology/Oncology, 16,* 35–42.

Crombleholme, T. M., Harrison, M. R., & Zanjani, E. D. (1990). In utero transplantation of hematopoietic stem cells in sheep: the role of T cells in engraftment and graft-vs-host disease. *Journal of Pediatric Surgery, 25,* 885–2.

Flake, A. W., Harrison, M. R., Adzick, N. S., & Zanjani, E.D. (1986). Transplantation of fetal hematopoietic stem cells in utero: the creation of hematopoietic chimeras. *Science, 233,* 766–78.

Flake, A. W., Roncarolo, M.-G., Puck, J. M. *et al.* (1996). Treatment of X-linked severe combined immunodeficiency by in utero transplantation of paternal bone marrow. *New England Journal of Medicine, 355,* 1806–10.

Flake, A. W. & Zanjani, E. D. (1997). In utero hematopoietic stem cell transplantation: A progress report. *JAMA: the Journal of the American Medical Association, 278,* 932–37.

Flake, A. W., & Zanjani, E. D. (1999). In utero hematopoietic stem cell transplantation: ontogenic opportunities and biologic barriers. *Blood, 94,* 2179–91.

Harrison, M. R., Slotnick, R. N., Crombleholme, T. M. *et al.* (1989). I utero transplantation of fetal liver hematopoietic stem cells in monkeys. *Lancet, 2,* 1425–7.

Huang, S. W., Ammann, A. J., Levy, R. L. *et al.* (1973). Treatment of severe combined immunodeficiency by a small number of pre-treated nonmatched marrow cells. *Transplantation, 15,* 174–5.

Horwitz, E. M., Prockup, D. J., Fitzpatrick, L. A. *et al.* (1999). Transplantability and therapeutic effects of bone marrow-derived mesenchymal cells in children with osteogenesis imperfecta. *Nature Medicine, 5,* 309–13.

Jones, D.R.E., Bui, T.-H., Anderson, E. M. *et al.* (1996). In utero haematopoietic stem cell transplantation: current perspective and future potential. *Bone Marrow Transplantation, 18,* 831–7.

Kapoor, N., Kirkpatrick, D., Blaese, R. M. *et al.* (1981). Reconstitution of normal megakaryocytopoiesis and immuno-logic functions in Wiskott-Aldrich syndrome by marrow trans-plantation following myeloablation and immunosuppression with busulfan and cyclophosphamide. *Blood, 57,* 692–6.

Kawashima, I., Zanjani, E., Almaida-Porada, G. *et al.* (1996). CD34+ human marrow cells that express low levels of Kit protein are enriched for long-term marrow-engrafting cells. *Blood, 87,* 4136–42.

Kohn, D. B., Weinberg, K. I., Nolta, J. A. *et al.* (1995). Engraftment of gene-modified umbilical cord blood cells in neonates with adenosine deaminase deficiency. *Nature Medicine, 1,* 1017–23.

Krivit, W., Pierpoint, M. E., Ayza, K. *et al.* (1984). Bone marrow transplantation in the Maroteaux Lamy syndrome (mucopolysac-charidosis VI). *New England Journal of Medicine, 311,* 1606–11.

Krivit, W., Shapiro, E., Kennedy, W. *et al.* (1990) Treatment of late infantile metachromatic leukodystrophy by bone marrow trans-plantation. *New England Journal of Medicine, 322,* 28–32.

Kurtzberg, J., Laughlin, M., Graham, M. L. *et al.* (1996). Placental blood as a source of hematopoietic stem cells for transplantation into unrelated recipients. *New England Journal of Medicine, 335,* 157–66.

Liechty, K. W., MacKenzie, T. C., Shaaban, A. F. *et al.* (2000). Human mesenchymal stem cells engraft and demonstrate site-specific differentiation after in utero transplantation in sheep. *Nature Medicine, 6,* 1282–6.

Linch, D. C, Rodeck, C. H., Nicolaides, K. *et al.* (1986). Attempted bone marrow transplantation in a 17 week fetus. *Lancet, 2,* 1821–2.

Lucarelli, G., Galimberti, M., Polchi, P. *et al.* (1990). Bone marrow transplantation in patients with thalassemia. *New England Journal of Medicine, 322.* 417–21

Muench, M. O., Rae, J., Barcena, A. *et al.* (2001). Transplantation of a fetus with paternal Thy-1+ CD34+ cells for chronic granuloma-tous disease. *Bone Marrow Transplantation, 27,* 355–64.

O'Reilly, R. J., Keever, C. A, Small, T. N., & Brochstein, J. A. (1989). The use of HLA-non-identical T-cell depleted marrow transplants for correction of severe combined immunodeficiency disease. *Immunodeficiency Review, 1,* 273–309.

Parkman, R. (1986). The application of bone marrow transplantation to the treatment of genetic diseases. *Science, 232,* 1373–8.

Parkman, R. & Merler, E. (1973). Discontinuous density gradient analysis of the developing human thymus. *Cellular Immunology, 8,* 382–31.

Shaaban, A.F.T., Kim, H. B., Milner, R., & Flake, A. W. (1999). A kinetic model for the homing and migration of prenatally trans-planted marrow. *Blood, 94,* 3251–7.

Stewart, F. M., Crittenden, R. B., Lowry, P. A. *et al.* (1993). Long-term engraftment of normal and post-5-fluorouracil murine marrow into normal nonmyeloablated mice. *Blood,* **81,** 2566–71.

Terstappen, L.W., Huang, S., Safford, M. *et al.* (1991). Sequential generations of hematopoietic colonies derived from single nonlineage-committed CD34+ CD38– progenitor cells. *Blood,* **77,** 1218–27.

Touraine, J. L., Raudrant, D., Royo, C. *et al.* (1989). In-utero transplantation of stem cells in bare lymphocyte syndrome. *Lancet,* **1,** 1382 (Letter).

Wang, J. C., Doedens, M., & Dick, J. E., (1997). Primitive human hematopoietic cells are enriched in cord blood compared with adult bone marrow or mobilized peripheral blood as measured by the quantitative in vivo SCID-repopulating cell assay. *Blood,* **89,** 3919–24.

Wengler, G. S., Lanfranchi, A., Frusca, T. *et al.* (1996). In utero transplantation of parental CD34 hematopoietic progenitor cells in a patient with X-linked severe combined immunodeficiency (SCIDXI). *Lancet,* **348,** 1484–7.

Westgren, M., Ringden, O., Eik-Nes, S. *et al.* (1996). Lack of evidence of permanent engraftment after in utero fetal stem cell transplantation in congenital hemoglobinopathies. *Transplantation,* **61,** 1176–9.

Wu, D. D. & Keating, A. (1993). Hematopoietic stem cells engraft in untreated transplant recipients. *Experimental Hematology,* **21,** 251–6.

Zanjani, E. D., Ascensao, J. L., & Tavassoli, M. (1993). Liver derived fetal hematopoietic stem cells selectively and preferentially home to the fetal bone marrow. *Blood,* **81,** 399–404.

Zanjani, E. D., Pallavicini, M. G., Ascensao, J. L. *et al.* (1992). Engraftment and long-term expression of human fetal hematopoietic cells in sheep following transplantation in utero. *Journal of Clinical Investigation,* **89,** 1178–88.

112 Dendritic cell immunotherapy

DEREK N. J. HART, ALISON M. RICE, AND JAMES W. YOUNG[1]

Mater Medical Research Institute and Mater Misericordiae Hospitals, Brisbane, Australia and Memorial Sloan-Kettering Cancer Center and The Weill Medical College of Cornell University, New York, USA

Introduction

The ability of hematopoietic stem cell transplantation (HSCT) as a therapeutic procedure to cure malignant disease is unquestioned. The challenge now is to improve our understanding of the mechanisms, enabling clinicians to develop ways to reduce the treatment-related mortality and to prevent subsequent disease relapse. Our rapidly expanding knowledge of the dendritic cell (DC) in health and disease is providing other options. HSCT using either autologous or allogeneic (HLA-matched sibling and matched unrelated donor) bone marrow, cord blood, or peripheral blood stem cells reinfused after myeloablative or non-myeloablative preparative regimens, provides different options for achieving disease control. The results of syngeneic transplantation indicate that chemotherapy and radiotherapy administered during myeloablative conditioning play major roles in eradicating or controlling the malignant disease present at the start of treatment. It is equally clear, however, that malignant disease persists at varying levels after transplantation and that other immune-mediated mechanisms contribute to the ultimate elimination of cancer in long-term survivors. A variety of protocols are testing these mechanisms for efficacy after non-myeloablative conditioning.

There are good data to indicate that there is a significant graft-versus-leukemia (GVL) effect after allogeneic stem cell transplantation for chronic myeloid leukemia (CML), acute myeloid leukemia (AML), and possibly acute lymphoblastic leukemia (ALL) (Kolb *et al.*, 1995; Mavroudis & Barrett, 1996; Jiang & Barrett, 1997; Papadopoulos *et al.*, 1998; Passweg *et al.*, 1998). There have been considerably fewer allogeneic transplants performed for multiple myeloma (MM) and non-Hodgkin's lymphoma (NHL) but here too there is early evidence for a graft anti-rumor effect (Tricot *et al.*, 1996; Khouri *et al.*, 2001). The situation after autologous transplantation is far less clear. Relapse of malignant disease is more common and this may result either from malignant disease that persists

after conditioning, or from malignant cells that contaminate the graft. The procedure of autologous HSCT undeniably perturbs the immune system (e.g., increasing natural killer [NK] activity and probably activating DC, and some would therefore attribute at least a component of the procedure's efficacy to this posttransplant immune stimulation. Indeed, enhancing the natural immune response by using interleukin (IL)-2 therapy after autologous transplantation has generated encouraging results in otherwise poor prognosis patients (Lopez-Jimenez *et al.*, 1997; Meehan *et al.*, 1997).

The now widespread application of donor leukocyte infusion (DLI) to treat relapses after allogeneic stem cell transplantation has confirmed the power of the immune system to eradicate many malignant diseases (Kolb *et al.*, 1995; Mackinnon *et al.*, 1995; Imamura *et al.*, 1996; Perry & Mackinnon, 1996; Peggs & Mackinnon, 2001). These infusions of unselected donor cells, in which T lymphocytes are assumed, but still not proven, to be the effectors, target incompatible host antigens, often eradicate the disease but can cause significant and not infrequently lethal graft-versus-host disease (GVHD) depending on how universally the target antigen is expressed. Non-myeloablative preparative regimens are now including these approaches as a component of the transplantation procedure, because the lesser conditioning used is certain to leave some residual malignant disease. This adoptive immunotherapy approach represents one strategy for cancer treatment; other immunologic approaches include the now familiar "passive" immunization with antibodies (e.g., anti CD20 and anti-HER2neu) as well as "active" immunization of the host against malignant cell antigens (Rosenberg, 1999). Autologous HSCTs provide an opportunity for exploring a new range of biological approaches to cancer treatment in a minimal residual disease (MRD) state.

Immunotherapy as a strategy for treating malignant disease now justifies the current high level of interest because of recent basic scientific and now clinical advances, which indicate that tumor-specific immunotherapy is an achievable option (Hart & Hill, 1999; Rosenberg, 1999; Fong & Engleman, 2000; Lopez & Hart, 2002). Investigators have identified a growing number of tumor-associated antigens (TAA) that are capable of provoking an anti-tumor immune response. These include oncogenic

---

[1] The authors would like to acknowledge Simon Stanworth for his original contribution to this chapter in the previous edition.

viral proteins, recombinant gene-derived proteins, mutated oncogene or tumor suppressor products, oncofetal antigens, other aberrantly expressed molecules, immunoglobulin (Ig) and T-cell receptor (TCR) idiotypes, tissue-specific antigens, and even autoantigens (Shu et al., 1997; Rosenberg, 1999). T lymphocytes have been shown to recognize small differences, even one amino acid, in peptides derived from proteins. Crucial to thinking in this area is the understanding that all cell proteins, whether nuclear, cytoplasmic, or membrane in origin, have the potential to be recognized on the cell surface, when expressed in the context of major histocompatibility complex (MHC) antigens. There is an extensive literature accruing to indicate that specific T lymphocyte anti-TAA responses can be generated, both in vitro and in vivo. In preclinical animal models, anti-TAA responses are associated with tumor regression and these are proving invaluable in refining potential technology for clinical trials. Effective immune responses require that the relevant antigen be presented via an antigen-presenting cell (APC) to the responding T lymphocytes. DC are now recognized as a family of leukocytes that play the key role in generating primary and probably secondary immune responses against specific antigens (Hart, 1997; Banchereau et al., 2000). DC may also play a role in generating self-tolerance and determining the type of immune response that evolves after T and B lymphocyte priming. It is for these reasons that DC have become of great interest to groups attempting to generate cancer immunotherapy schedules. As immunotherapy is likely to be most effective in the context of MRD, the prospect of using DC immunotherapy as HSCT consolidation therapy is particularly appealing (Hart & Hill, 1999). DC may be useful either to prime in vitro for adoptive therapy or for administration in vivo as a vaccine. Antibody-mediated therapy may also have its place and may contribute to pretransplant cytoreduction aimed at debulking disease or enhancing DC function in stimulating cellular immunity against MRD after transplantation (Khouri et al., 2001).

Current immunotherapy contributions in transplantion

Despite the original conceptual enthusiasm for applying the magic bullet of immunotherapy to cancer therapy, early attempts were disappointing. T-lymphocyte (cellular), antibody-targeted (humoral), and (NK)-mediated therapies have all met variable success. Even the first attempts at DC vaccination against tumors in a mouse model produced mixed results (Knight et al., 1985). Indeed it is noteworthy that tumor extracts, when used alone as vaccines, sometimes had the opposite effect, enhancing tumor survival (Hewitt et al., 1976). Recent work also indicates that immature DC may stimulate immunoregulatory CD4+ or CD8+ T cells that dampen rather than enhance immune responses (Dhodapkar et al., 2001).

The use of monoclonal antibodies (Mab) and other physical methods to deplete T lymphocytes in an effort to avoid life-threatening acute GVHD achieved that aim. The loss of the GVL effect outweighed that benefit, however, especially in malignancies like CML (Goldman, Apperley, & Jones, 1986; Apperley et al., 1988) but not in others like AML in first or second remission (Papadopoulos et al., 1998). Laboratory data confirmed that donor-cell-derived T lymphocytes in allogeneic recipients exert anti-host leukemic activity (Datta, Barrett, & Jiang, 1994), but there may also be a role for early NK cell mediated lysis of MRD after transplantation.

CML has proved to be a particularly instructive model for studying clinical GVL responses. The ability to monitor the malignant Philadelphia (Ph) chromosome [t (9;22) translocation] clone using cytogenetic and semi-quantitative polymerase chain reaction (PCR) techniques after transplantation has shown that the disease can survive the myeloablative conditioning protocol, and that the success of the treatment depends on immunologic mechanisms eradicating the disease thereafter (Roth et al., 1992). Subsequent reports have confirmed that similar processes occur in a proportion of AML patients (Mehta et al., 1995; Papadopoulos et al., 1998). Specific responses in the laboratory also support other clinical data, indicating graft-versus-lymphoma (Khouri et al., 2001) and myeloma (Alyea et al., 2001; Badros et al., 2002) activity. Indeed ALL, which was thought to lack potential as an immune target is now being reconsidered as an immunotherapy option (Passweg et al., 1998), as potential new TAAs are defined (Porter et al., 2000).

The histocompatibility antigens on the malignant cells in allogeneic HSCT recipients are the potential targets for T-lymphocyte recognition. In HLA-matched sibling allografts, the evidence suggests that the minor histocompatibility antigens (mHag) act as targets for T-lymphocyte-mediated responses (Perreault, Roy, & Fortin, 1998). In adult recipients of bone marrow from HLA-identical donors, a mismatch of one mHag (HA-1) has been reported to be associated with an increased risk of GVHD (Goulmy et al., 1996). Minor histocompatible antigen-specific T cells have been shown to inhibit leukemic cell growth in vitro (Falkenburg et al., 1991) and in vivo (Pion et al., 1995). The relative expression of mHag, i.e., their degree of expression on hematopoietic cells or additional expression on non-hematopoietic tissues, determines whether the cellular immune responses targeting mHags result in specific GVL or cause the additional potentially devastating complications of acute and chronic GVHD (Goulmy et al., 1996; Takahashi et al., 1996; den Haan et al., 1998). It may also be possible to direct an immune response away from GVHD to an effective GVL response (Mackinnon et al., 1995; Yang et al., 1998; Fontaine et al., 2001), and this approach is receiving much attention, even establishing a paradigm that donor CD8+ cells may mediate GVHD, whereas CD4+ cells may mediate GVL.

Despite the potential risks, the results of donor leukocyte immunotherapy, presumably directed against mHags have been very good. DLI in the absence of immunosuppression generates a very effective response against CML, which has relapsed after HLA-matched sibling allografting (Kolb et al., 1995; Mackinnon et al., 1995; Guglielmi et al., 2002). This is now standard treatment. It is not yet known whether the antigens expressed on CML cells or their leukemic stem cell progenitors are different, present in higher densities, or otherwise more immunologically susceptible (e.g., adhesion molecules, lack of fas ligand, chemokines) compared with other apparently less susceptible leukemias (Porter & Antin, 1998). Tetramer staining has shown that a major part of the T lymphocyte response targets proteinase 3 and that the presence of proteinase 3–specific cytotoxic T lymphocytes (CTL) correlates with allogeneic transplant outcomes (Molldrem et al., 2000). Alternatively, the biology of CML, which involves a relatively slow leukemic progenitor cell proliferation, may render it more susceptible. The latter certainly seems to play a part, as other diseases with relatively slow turnovers, like MM and low-grade NHL, also appear susceptible to DLI (Huang & Vitetta, 1995; Hart & Hill, 1999).

The immune response after autologous stem cell transplantation has been studied in some detail. There is a profound and rapid rise in NK activity immediately following reinfusion of cryopreserved bone marrow. Tumor glycolipids, presented in the context of CD1 molecules may also stimulate NKT cells. Both NK and NKT cells can target leukemic cells (Cervantes et al., 1996). NK cells use a specific receptor system and this type of cytotoxic activity may be particularly effective against tumor targets which lack MHC class I antigens, as class I MHC antigens can give a negative signal to NK cells (Moretta & Moretta, 1997). T lymphocytes would not lyse these cells in the absence of the appropriate MHC restricting element, and such cells would probably also escape NKT cells unless they expressed a CD1 isoform. Specific T-lymphocyte activity against malignant cells has been more difficult to identify in patients, who have received autologous grafts. This may well reflect the major technical difficulties involved in detecting either proliferative or cytotoxic T lymphocytes with a very low precursor frequency, even with new tools such as tetramer staining applied to a specific antigenic peptide and known restricting MHC molecule.

Immunotherapeutic responses against nonhematologic malignancies after allogeneic transplantation have been observed. Allogeneic HSCT for renal cell carcinoma and some other solid tumors have yielded encouraging initial results (Childs et al., 2000; Childs & Barrett, 2002) consistent with the established susceptibility of this malignancy to immunologic treatment modalities, including IL-2 therapy (Belldegrun et al., 1993). Longer follow up, however, has not been as promising, owing to the challenges of balancing the competing need for graft-versus-tumor activity against GVHD that does not prove life-threatening at the same time. The disease control and immunological recovery after non-myeloablative therapy may still represent opportunities for such "bolt-on" immune therapies after autologous HSCT. Immunotherapy in the absence of HSCT has been applied most widely. Another urologic malignancy, transitional cell carcinoma, has been treated with immunotherapy in the form of adjuvant bacille Calmette-Guérin (BCG) for some time with evidence of limited but real efficacy (Prescott et al., 1992).

Malignant melanoma has also been the subject of much effort from immunotherapists. This history and some of the molecular advances identifying several TAA (Houghton, 1994; Rosenberg, 1999), along with the poor prognosis of stage III and IV disease, has made melanoma the leading disease target for international immunotherapy protocols.

Although antibody-mediated antitumor effects are not thought to play a major role in any natural antitumor response, induced by current transplant protocols, antibody-mediated antitumor effects are relevant. Passive antibody therapy can be very successful. Monoclonal antibodies (Mabs) to certain target antigens, notably the CD20 epitope restricted to B-lymphoid lineage cells, may trigger an apoptotic or bystander reaction that results in tumor cell death (Kaminski et al., 1996). Indeed, vaccination strategies that attempt to generate cellular responses using intact antigen rather than peptides may generate significant antibody responses (Small et al., 2000).

Target antigens for transplantation-related immunotherapy

Before addressing how best to generate an effective immune response, it is essential to determine the optimal target antigens. The answer depends on the transplant strategy adopted. One of the attractions of allogeneic transplantation is that the mHags can be exploited as targets. These may have the advantage of generating higher frequency T-cell responses but with the risk of GVHD, if the mHag is not tumor target-restricted. By contrast, autologous immunotherapy targets must exploit tissue-restricted antigens or TAA. Many or most of these are self differentiation antigens to which the host is normally tolerant, and these may stimulate either no or low frequency T lymphocyte responses.

A long program of careful cellular cytotoxicity studies has elaborated the genetics and recently the biochemistry of some of the minor histocompatibility antigens (Goulmy et al., 1996; Mutis et al., 2002). Components of these molecules are processed and presented, just as other antigens are, in the context of MHC molecules. The extent to which these minor histocompatibility antigens are restricted to tumors or shared with normal tissues becomes the key determinant of their suitability as immunotherapeutic targets.

The male-specific H-Y encoded mHag provides a theoretical target for a female allogeneic response (Wang et al., 1995). The SMCY gene is homologous to SMCX (located on the X chromosome), and both share sequence homology with the gene encoding the retinoblastoma-binding protein. Human T cell clones can recognize peptides encoded by SMCY. Functional studies as well as SMCY gene expression studies confirm that this molecule is widely expressed. To date cytotoxic T-cell clones have identified at least eight other mHag, and the phenotype frequency has been determined on an HLA-A2 background (Goulmy et al., 1996). The HA-2 antigen was the first one to be biochemically identified as derived from a class I myosin gene that is also diallelic (Pierce et al., 2001). The amino acid sequence of the HA-1 antigen has also been elucidated (Mutis *et al.,* 2002). These two antigens are expressed on hematopoietic cells and represent target antigens for therapy against hematopoietic malignancies. Other antigens like HA-3 and HA-4 have a broader distribution and may be relevant targets for therapy against nonhematologic malignancies. HA-8 results from a polymorphism of a gene of as yet unknown function (Brickner *et al.,* 2001). As predicted, the genetic background, notably the HLA type and polymorphism in the class I or II antigen-processing systems, will influence their suitability as target antigens (Brickner *et al.,* 2001).

The most promising target antigens for tumor immunotherapy are the viral proteins expressed by tumors that result from the transforming effects of an oncogenic virus. These often generate strong proliferative and cytotoxic T-lymphocyte responses. Indeed, Epstein-Barr viral (EBV) components generate massive cytotoxic responses in normal individuals. EBV-driven lymphomas that express these antigens and develop in immunosuppressed individuals are ideal targets for EBV-specific therapy (Papadopoulos *et al.,* 1994). Nasopharyngeal carcinoma and a proportion of Hodgkin's disease cases express only some of the Epstein-Barr nuclear antigens (EBNA) and latent membrane proteins (LMP), but these are still potential targets (Rooney *et al.,* 2001). Cervical carcinoma expresses antigens derived from human papilloma virus, which are also excellent targets for immunotherapy strategies (Frazer *et al.,* 1999). Human T-cell leukemia/lymphoma virus (HTLV-1) generates T-lymphocyte responses and is a theoretical target for HTLV-1 leukemia/lymphoma immunotherapy. It is unclear whether Kaposi's sarcoma-associated herpesvirus (KSHV/HHV-8) is a relevant target antigen for myeloma immunotherapy. The presence of KSHV/HHV-8 in the bone marrow DC of these patients is contentious; and its role in the oncogenic process, if any, is unclear (Berenson, Vescio, & Said, 1998). Finally, one need scarcely restate the major interest in defining stable human immunodeficiency virus (HIV) protein epitopes that might be targeted in infected patients (McMichael & Hanke, 2002).

Perhaps the most logically appealing targets are the novel oncogenic proteins created by recombination events in certain tumor types (Table 112.1). The *bcr-abl* recombination between chromosomes 9 and 22 occurs in two forms, each of which results in the production of a novel fusion protein in CML and ALL respectively. Human CD4+ and CD8+ T lymphocytes with specificity for the fusion gene product have been isolated (Mannering *et al.,* 1997). As these abnormal proteins are critical to the oncogenic event in CML, the leukemic precursors (Childs *et al.,* 1999) remain a target despite immunologic selection pressures. The practical stumbling block may be the low precursor frequency of peptide-specific T lymphocytes in the patient, and expansion in vitro may be required. There are similar challenges to targeting the ras family of oncogenic proteins (Peace *et al.,* 1993) or mutations in tumor suppressor genes that express products like retinoblastoma protein or p53 (Houbiers *et al.,* 1993). Of course immune-based therapies for diseases like CML must now compete with drugs, e.g., the pro-

Table 112.1. *Potential TAA for DC immunotherapy*

Viral antigens
  EBV
  HTLV-1
  Papilloma virus
  HSV-6
Recombined proteins
  BCR/ABL (chronic myeloid leukemia)
  DEK/CAN (acute myeloid leukemia)
  PML/RARα (promyelocytic leukemia)
  TLS-FUS/ERG (acute myeloid leukemia)
  NPM/ALK (large cell NHL)
  IL-2/BCM (T-NHL)
  ETV6-AML1 (acute lymphoblastic leukemia)
Mutated oncogenes
  H-*ras*
  K-*ras*
  p53
Oncofetal antigens
  MAGE-1 (melanoma)
  MAGE-2 (melanoma)
  NY-ESO (multiple)
  CEA (bowel)
Molecules abnormally expressed
  MUC 1 (breast and other)
  Telomerase (multiple)
  Survivin (multiple)
Idiotype
  Ig (B-NKL, myeloma)
  TCR (T-NHL)
Tissue-specific antigens
  PSM (prostate)
  PAP (prostate)
  PSA (prostate)
  MART-1 (melanoma)
  gp 100
  gp75 (melanoma)
  CD33 (acute myeloid leukemia)
  Proteinase 3 (myeloid leukemia)

tein kinase inhibitor imatinib, that target the same fusion protein resulting from the t(9;22) translocation. Drugs like this may never eradicate the leukemic clone entirely when used alone, whereas there is clear evidence that the immune system does eradicate the malignant clone.

Attempts to define tumor-specific antigens have identified a number of oncofetal antigens. These include carcinoembryonic antigen (CEA) (Nair *et al.,* 1999), MAGE (Thurner *et al.,* 1999a), sperm protein 17 (Chiriva-Internati *et al.,* 2001), and NY-ESO (Zeng *et al.,* 2002). The wider tissue distribution of some of these molecules, however, may render them more toxic as tumor immunotherapy targets.

Aberrantly expressed molecules may be more accessible as targets. Mucin 1 (MUC-1), which may be poorly glycosylated in malignant cells, is expressed as a protein with a repetitive epitope backbone structure. For whatever mechanistic reason, such as increased generation of peptides and association with MHC molecules, this form of the MUC-1 protein is more accessible on malignant cells to T-lymphocyte recognition (Barratt-Boyes, 1996). Although MUC-1 has quite a wide tissue distribution including normal hematopoietic cells and DC (Wykes *et al.*, 2002), animal data (Tanaka *et al.*, 2001) and early human data continue to encourage its investigation. There may be some normal molecules, which are overexpressed in a wide variety of malignancies as part of the general response to cell activation and frequent division. These potentially generic TAA include molecules like telomerase (Vonderheide *et al.*, 2001) and survivin (Andersen *et al.*, 2001), both of which generate CTL responses that lyse tumor targets. We are exploring an RNA binding protein, overexpressed in breast cancer, as another potential generic TAA.

Perhaps the classic TAA in hematologic terms are the immunoglobulin idiotypes, associated with the B-lymphoid neoplasms, notably NHL and MM (Apostolopoulos, McKenzie, & Pieterz, 1996). Likewise, the TCR idiotypes may represent ideal targets for T-lymphoid neoplasms.

In certain circumstances, tissue-specific molecules expressed by the malignant tissue might be exploited as targets. In melanoma, Melan-A/Mart-1, gp100, tyrosinase, and other products associated with normal melanocytes have provided potential targets for "auto-immune" therapy (Houghton, 1994; Rosenberg & White, 1996). In this case, loss of normal tissue may be an acceptable risk to pay for an effective response. A similar logic has led to investigation of prostate-specific membrane antigen (PSMA), prostatic acid phosphatase (PAP), and prostate-specific antigen (PSA) as targets for prostate cancer immunotherapy. Investigators should soon define other breast tissue specific antigens (Nacht *et al.*, 1999). Tissue expressing antigen(s) shared with malignant tissues is an acceptable risk, whereas that may not be the case in other malignancies. Interestingly, the "side effect" of vitiligo in melanoma only occurs in a minority of responders. Although, serious autoimmune responses have been surprisingly few (Gilboa, 2001), this may reflect a paucity of high frequency CTL responses. It may also reflect the fact that tissue-specific proteasome processing differences may account for the differential sensitivity of tissue targets to auto antigen-directed CTL (Kuckelkorn *et al.*, 2002).

The use of whole tumor lysates that may or may not include apoptotic bodies has also been promoted as a source of antigen for engineering immune rsponses against cancer. This has the theoretical advantage of bypassing the need to define antigens and MHC restrictions a priori, thus allowing an immune response to target undefined antigenic peptides. Investigators have not yet conclusively proven that this approach has merit for mainstream therapy, especially with the weak, nonviral, self differentiation antigens common to most tumors. Nonetheless, it is an approach that may help define the potential target tumor antigens recognized by a cellular immune response.

Dendritic cells

DC are specialized or "professional" APCs (Hart *et al.*, 1997; Banchereau & Steinman, 1998; Banchereau *et al.*, 2000) that are critical to the generation of primary and probably secondary immune responses against specific antigens. Their features are listed in Table 112.2. DC have unique migratory properties (Flores-Romo, 2001) and the capacity to acquire, process, and present antigens in association with the requisite accessory signals for activation of naïve and resting T and B lymphocytes (Hart, 1997). They react to inflammatory signals and foreign material providing a link between the innate and acquired immune systems. DC also stimulate resting NK cells (Ferlazzo *et al.*, 2002). The role played by DC in immune responses generated during and after HSCT has therefore become an important area for investigating and understanding immune responses against cancer.

DC were identified originally as having unique morphologic features (Fig. 112.1) and remarkable potency as APC, notably in the mixed leukocyte reaction (MLR) (Fig. 112.2). They lack most of the markers typical of other leukocyte populations; however they express MHC molecules, particularly the class II products, in high density. Only recently have more specific DC surface markers become available that help

Table 112.2.   *Dendritic cell properties*

Major distinguishing criteria
1. The ability to stimulate a primary T lymphocyte response (this may require differentiation/activation of the DC population)
2. Marked cell motility and the ability to extend and retract cell membrane processes freely at 37° C in vitro; the ability to migrate through tissues and track to the T lymphocyte–dependent areas of the lymph node
3. Relatively specialized phagocytic activity (in vitro): DC uptake of extracellular material is greater than hitherto realized in vivo. Active fluid-phase endocytosis is a feature of DC
4. Spontaneous initial and rapid clustering with T lymphocytes at 37° C in vitro
5. A cell surface antigenic phenotype distinguishing it from other leukocytes, notably monocytes/macrophages and B lymphocytes
6. Expression of certain DC-associated molecules according to their differentiation/activation state, e.g., CD83, CMRF-44, DC-LAMP.
7. Cytochemical reactions, which differ from those of monocytes/macrophages

Minor distinguishing criteria
1. High density expression of MHC molecules
2. Dendritic cell morphology

Other APC such as B cells and macrophages are also effective stimulators of primed T lymphocytes, but the DC is special in its ability to stimulate naïve T lymphocytes and hence it is predicted to be critical in driving any initial response against TAA.

A notable feature of DC relevant to their therapeutic use is that their ability to take up and process antigen declines as they become differentiated/activated into co-stimulatory cells.

Abbreviations: DC, dendritic cells; MHC, major histocompatability complex; APC, antigen-presenting cells; TAA, tumor-associated antigens.

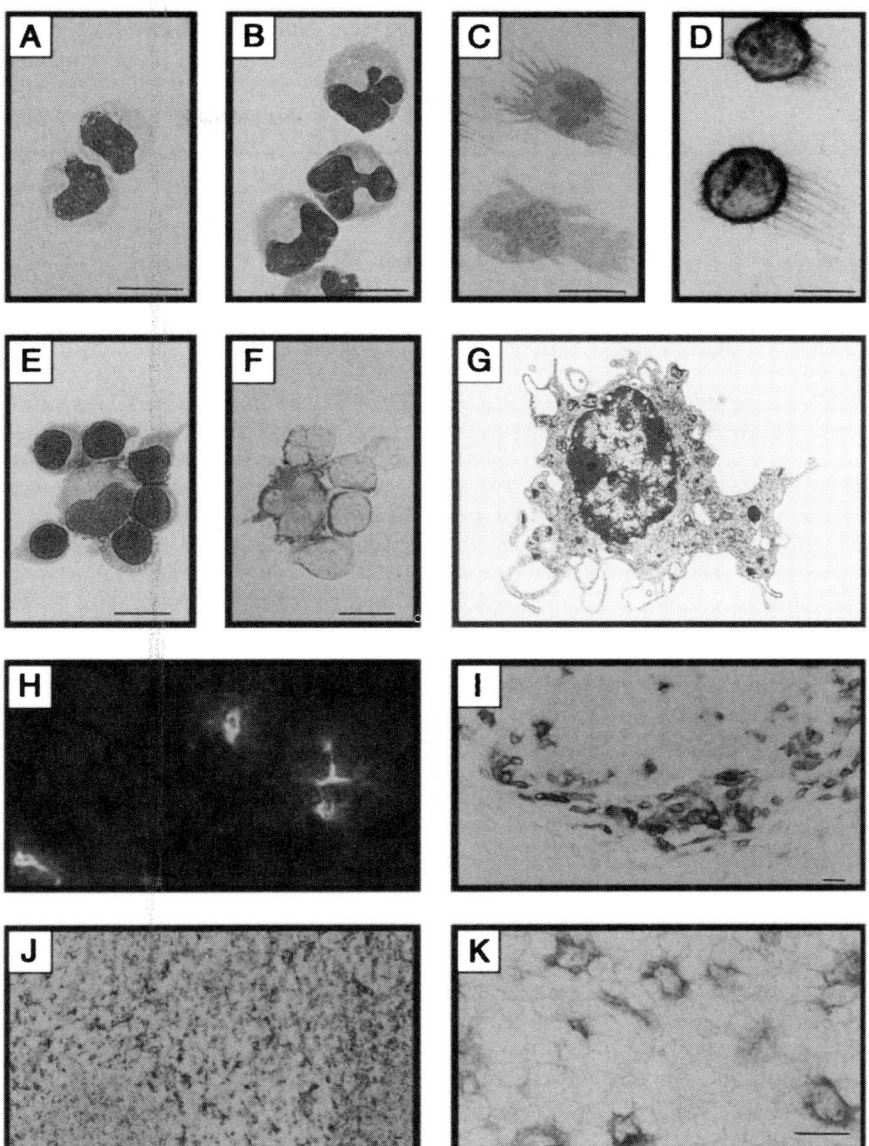

Fig. 112.1. The morphology of human DC. (A) Fresh "lineage negative" blood DC, isolated without a period of tissue culture, using immunoselection (May-Grünwald-Giemsa [MGG], original magnification [OM] × 1,433). (B) CMRF-44 sorted, Nycodenz gradient purified cultured blood DC (MGG, OM × 1,433). (C) Tonsil low-density cultured DC stained with anti-HLA-DR. The veils and dendritic processes are more obvious in these preparations (OM × 1,433). (D) Mo-derived DC preparation stained with CMRF-44 using an immunoenzyme (brown, peroxidase-DAB) technique (in preparation) (OM × 1,433). (E and F) Fresh "lineage negative" blood DC clustered with CD4+ purified autologous T lymphocytes in the presence of staphylococcal enterotoxin A (SEA) and MGG stained. The DC is stained in another cluster (F) for the co-stimulator molecule CD86 using an immunoenzyme (alkaline phosphatase-fast blue) technique (OM × 1,197). (G) EM appearances of a CMRF-44-positive cultured blood DC. Note the mitochondria endosomes and lysosomal vacuoles (OM × 17,000). (H) DC in the interstitial tissues of rat heart identified by anti-MHC class II staining (immunofluorescence) (OM × 479). (I) Dermal CMRF-44+ DC (red, peroxidase-AEC) and T lymphocytes (blue, alkaline phosphatase-fast blue) within a section of normal skin adjacent to a hair follicle (OM × 479). (J) Lymph node interfollicular (T lymphocyte) area containing CMRF-44+ IDC (brown, peroxidase-DAB) compared with CD14 Mo and CD20 B lymphocytes (blue, alkaline phosphatase-fast blue) (OM × 143). (K) Lymph node interfollicular region with CMRF-44+ IDC (blue, alkaline phosphatase-fast blue) showing nuclear labeling for the transcription factor Rel B (brown, peroxidase-DAB) (OM × 1,197). Bar, 10 μm. Reproduced, with permission, from Hart (1997). For color reproduction, see Color Plate 112.1.

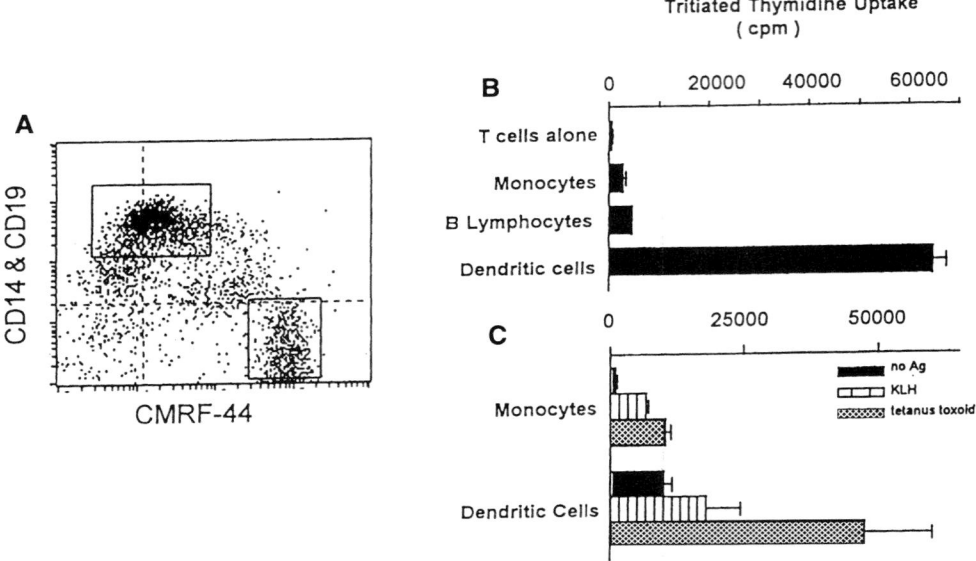

Fig. 112.2. The co-stimulatory capacity of blood-derived CMRF-44 purified DC compared with CD14 Mo and CD19+ B lymphocytes. (A) The flow cytometry labeling of Nycodenz low-density cells is shown before sorting CMRF-44+ CD14– DC and C MRF-44– CD14+ Mo. (B) Allogeneic T-lymphocyte proliferative responses measured with ^{3}H thymidine, are shown using each FACS purified cell populations as stimulators. The allostimulatory capacity of sorted DC, Mo, and B lymphocytes (CD19+ sorted) are compared at a ratio of 1 APC to 50 allogeneic T lymphocytes. (C) DC and Mo are compared in their ability to process and present the soluble protein antigens to KLH and tetanus toxid to autologous T lymphocytes at an APC: T lymphocyte ratio of 1:20. Reproduced, with permission, from Hart (1997).

define them more accurately. These include CD11c (Metlay et al., 1990), CD205 (Jiang et al., 1995), and CD8a (Wu et al., 1995) in mice. CD83 (Zhou & Tedder, 1995), CMRF-44 (Hock et al., 1994), CMRF-56 (Hock et al., 1999), CD1a, and Langerin (CD207) (Valladeau et al., 2000) have proved to be useful markers in man. Human DEC-205 (Kato et al., 1998) appears to have a broader haematopoietic cell distribution. More recent reagents such as BDCA-2 BDCA-3 (Dzionek et al., 2000) and DC-SIGN (Geijtenbeek et al., 2000) define further human DC subsets.

DC develop from bone marrow-derived precursor cells and enter the circulation in an immature form. These myeloid precursor-derived cells migrate into the tissues and establish sentinel networks of epithelial and interstitial DC. After exposure to perturbing or inflammatory stimuli, comprising either bacterial, viral, or possibly tumor-derived products, or alternatively, other inflammatory mediators like IL-1 and tumor necrosis factor-α (TNF-α), these tissue DC migrate to secondary lymphoid organs via the draining lymphatics (Flores-Romo, 2001). Antigen captured at these peripheral sites is processed by the DC and presented on MHC molecules. At the same time, the DC undergo a series of phenotypic and functional changes before interacting with T lymphocytes in the T-cell rich areas of the lymph node. This may involve DC-secreted chemokines like DC-CK1, which attract naive T lymphocytes (Adema et al., 1997). The differentiation and activation of DC during this process in humans can be detected by their expression of the CD83 (Zhou & Tedder, 1995) and CMRF-44 (Fearnley et al.,

1997a) antigens, as well as intracellular molecules such as DC-LAMP (de Saint-Vis et al., 1998).

Although our understanding of DC has improved immensely, there is much to be clarified in terms of DC growth and differentiation. There appear to be several subpopulations of DC, and some of these may develop along separate DC differentiation pathways (Hart, 1997; Banchereau & Steinman, 1998; Shortman & Liu, 2002) (Fig. 112.3). In human blood, there are three CD11c+ "myeloid" DC precursors (MacDonald et al., 2002a). The other human blood CD4+ CD123+ lineage^{neg} subset, originally identified as the interferon-producing cell, is now the subject of intense investigation. These cells have attracted three different terms, which are used variably to describe them as lymphoid, plasmacytoid, or monocytoid DC subsets. The recent identification of a similar DC subset in the mouse, with properties akin to the human CD123+ DC (Traver et al., 2000; Asselin-Paturel et al., 2001; Nakano et al., 2001; Martin et al., 2002) has been a step forward. The CD8a+ IL-12 producing DC subset (described in the previous mouse literature as lymphoid DC) appears to be more like an activated human myeloid DC and can be derived from myeloid progenitors (Traver et al., 2000).

At a tissue level human myeloid DC appear to be divided into epithelial-associated CD1a-positive and non-epithelial-associated CD1a-weak/negative networks, which may be derived from separate hematopoietic precursors and display different turnover kinetics in the tissues. These are the cells which have been studied as DC over the last two decades.

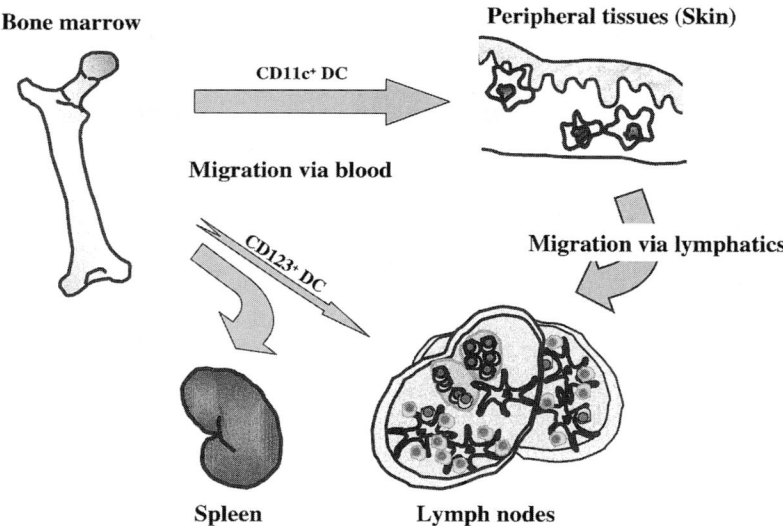

Fig. 112.3. DC physiology: DC subset tissue distribution and migration

Monocytes can, after in vitro exposure to cytokines, evolve characteristics very reminiscent of purified DC (Zhou & Tedder, 1996), including the expression of CD1 isoforms. In vivo, differentiation of mouse monocytes into DC-like cells has been described (Randolph et al., 1999). A recent report even suggests that granulocytes can evolve DC-like characteristics (Oehler et al., 1998). The precursors of CD123+ lymphoid DC are uncertain—they may be derived from common lymphoid progenitors (Blom et al., 2000) or curiously enough, from a CD14+ CD16+ precursor (Ho et al., 2002). The CD123+ DC is thought to migrate via an entirely different route, namely directly via the blood stream across the high endothelial venule into the paracortical area of the lymph node (Cella et al., 1999). There is limited evidence to suggest they may also be attracted to inflammatory sites (Jahnsen et al., 2000).

The analysis of human tonsil (Summers et al., 2001), spleen (McIlroy et al., 2001), and thymus (Bendriss-Vermare et al., 2001) has identified several similar DC subpopulations. Thus, it appears that the precursor subsets described in blood, may be matched by their progeny in central lymphoid tissues. It is notable that despite expectations otherwise, the majority of myeloid DC in tonsil are not activated.

It is possible that, in certain circumstances, these myeloid-derived DC may provide down regulatory, even tolerizing, signals to T lymphocytes (Hackstein et al., 2001). It seems highly likely that normal trafficking of surveillance DC contributes to peripheral tolerance. DC contribute to thymic central tolerance, an outcome still most likely determined by the state of T lymphocyte differentiation. However, DC that lack the co-stimulatory phenotype may tolerize or anergize antigen-specific T lymphocytes both in vitro (Steinbrink et al., 1997) or in vivo (Dhodapkar et al., 2001; Chang et al., 2002). DC exposed to tumor derived IL-10 or TGF-β may generate tumor tolerance/anergy. Similar cells are being investigated for their ability to generate transplantation tolerance (Hackstein et al., 2001).

The hematopoietic growth factors that drive the growth and differentiation of DC are slowly being clarified. Interleukin-3, c-kit-ligand (stem cell factor, SCF), and Flt-3L recruit and expand stem cell-derived precursors into the various DC differentiation pathways. Flt-3L appears to drive both plasmacytoid and myeloid DC differentiation (some effects on monocytic and NK cells also occur). As such, it has been used to increase DC yields (Maraskovsky et al., 1996; Lynch et al., 1997; Hackstein et al., 2001) as has ProGP, a Flt-3L/G-CSF recombinant protein (Bjorck et al., 2002). Granulocyte-macrophage colony-stimulating factor (GM-CSF) and TNF-α differentiate relatively committed DC precursors into DC, and IL-4 suppresses the alternative differentiation of common precursors into macrophages (Jansen et al., 1989), especially in serum or plasma-replete conditions in vitro (Sallusto & Lanzavecchia, 1994; Romani et al., 1996). TGF-β supports the specific differentiation of epithelial type Langerhans cells (Borkowski et al., 1996; Strobl et al., 1996). Chemokines and chemokine receptor expression control DC migration and are likely to have a role in vaccination protocols (Adema et al., 1997; Sallusto & Lanzavecchia, 2000). All DC generated in vitro require some terminal exposure to inflammatory cytokines or activating molecules like CD40L for terminal maturation, activation, and irreversible differentiation (Jonuleit et al., 1997; Albert, Jegathesan, & Darnell, 2001).

Dendritic cells in tumors

As a professional APC, the DC could be expected to play an important role in the initiation of a host's immune response against a developing tumor and consequently have an impact on prognosis. Whether tumors trigger DC recruitment, antigen uptake, and migration is clearly important.

The first studies examining DC in tumors used antibody to S-100 to stain and identify DC. Several studies were summarized recently (Troy & Hart, 1997); the majority suggested that S-100$^+$ DC infiltration in tumors generally correlated with a favorable prognosis. The S-100 marker is not specific for DC and provides little information about the phenotype and function of tumor-infiltrating DC (Kahn et al., 1983). Langerhans' cells have also been studied in a smaller number of epithelial tumors using CD1a staining, but the results have been inconclusive (Fox et al., 1989; Papadimitriou et al., 1992; Troy & Hart, 1997). A study using rats as models investigated DC migration into subcutaneously injected colon carcinomas (Chaux et al., 1993). The DC distribution was heterogeneous but became more abundant as the tumor progressed. This contrasted with the finding of very few macrophages and T cells within the tumor. DC isolated from the tumors were efficient stimulators of T lymphocytes, particularly those isolated from rats immunized against the tumor cells.

In a clinical study of DC within renal cell carcinoma, DC represented only a small proportion of the infiltrating leukocytes. Of these, only a small subset of DC was found to display an activated phenotype (Troy et al., 1998). Similar studies showed that only a proportion of DC in breast tumors had an activated phenotype (Bell et al., 1999; Coventry et al., 2002). These activated DC, when isolated, proved to be significantly stronger stimulators of T lymphocytes than either the nonactivated DC or the tumor macrophages. These novel findings suggest that the tumor environment inhibits DC maturation and activation, providing a possible explanation for the paradox that antigen-expressing tumor cells can be recognized by T lymphocytes in vitro, yet escape tumor surveillance and grow into lethal tumors in immunocompetent hosts.

Other phenotypic studies on malignancies including carcinoma of the prostate (Troy et al., 1998), and bladder (Troy et al., 1999) support the concept that, as a general rule, human tumors may not actively recruit DC as part of the response to a tumor. There is also little evidence to suggest that the DC present in these cancers were being activated, as defined by their relative lack of staining with the antibodies to CMRF-44 and CD83 epitopes. APCs in colorectal carcinoma have likewise been reported to lack CD80 and CD86 expression (Chaux et al., 1996) with fewer activated DC present (Schwaab et al.; 2001) but as in other tumors, a subset of CD83 activated DC is present at the invasive margin (Suzuki et al., 2002). In addition to the failure to recruit and activate DC, it appears that tumors may actively suppress DC function. Vascular endothelial growth factor (VEGF), which is produced by most solid tumors, may directly inhibit maturation of DC from precursor cells (Gabrilovich et al., 1996a). IL-10, also produced by many tumors (Sato et al., 1996), inhibits upregulation of the CD80/86 co-stimulatory molecules on APCs (Willems et al., 1994), and their expression is essential for effective DC–T-lymphocyte interaction. Activation of T lymphocytes by APCs, in the presence of IL-10, leads to long-term anergy in the T lymphocytes (Groux et

al., 1996). Transforming growth factor-β (TGF-β) has also been shown to inhibit indirectly the activation of T lymphocytes by DC (Summers et al., 2001) and may account for poor DC function in multiple myeloma patients (Brown et al., 2001). IL-6 is also reported to have a negative influence on human DC differentiation (Ratta et al., 2002). Prostanoids may also play a major role in tumor inhibition of DC differentiation (Sombroek et al., 2002). Ovarian cancer secretes stroma-derived factor 1 (SDF-1), which recruits lymphoid DC but affects their function (Zou et al., 2000).

The effects of malignancy on DC function may not be confined to the tumor. A study in mice found that mature blood DC from tumor-bearing animals were ineffective at inducing antitumor CTL, whereas DC generated from bone marrow precursors remained fully functional (Gabrilovich et al., 1996b). Breast cancer patients may also have lower numbers of mature DC, and these had reduced stimulating activity perhaps because other suppressive cells were present (Almand et al., 2001). Our own studies in breast cancer indicate that changes in DC numbers and function are only detectable in advanced disease. The cytokine-generated DC derived from circulating precursors, however, were again fully functional (Gabrilovich et al., 1997). DC counts in advanced prostate cancer appear to be reduced (unpublished). Interestingly, cytokine-generated DC from patients with renal cell carcinoma (Radmayr et al., 1995) and prostate cancer (Tjoa et al., 1995) were also fully functional.

DC counts in chronic myelomonocytic leukemia (CMML) are normal—an interesting distinction between DC precursors and CMML monocytes (Vuckovic et al., 1999). DC counts in multiple myeloma are preserved but functional changes occur as mentioned above. Cyclophosphamide/G-CSF stem cell mobilization regimens recruit DC in MM patients, but interestingly, much less so in low grade non-Hodgkin's lymphoma patients. DC can be generated in CML (Choudhury et al., 1997) and DC counts and differentiation may reflect the clonal abnormalities in acute myeloid leukemia (Roddie, Horton, & Turner, 2002; Tsuchiya et al., 2002).

These data provide an argument (Fig. 112.4) to remove DC from the host, to arm them with TAA and return them to the patient in an effort to generate an effective immune response (Nestle, Banchereau, & Hart, 2001).

Dendritic cell preparations

The preparation of DC was formerly labor-intensive and yielded too few cells for clinical or large scale experimental applications. The advent of cytokine-supported cultures ex vivo, and other methodologies has changed the practicalities and several reliable methods have evolved that yield DC conforming to well-established phenotypic and functional criteria for maturation and activation. Each of these DC preparations has the potential for use in immunotherapy.

DC may be derived from purified hematopoietic stem cells. There are established methods for purifying stem cells using

IN VIVO   IN VITRO

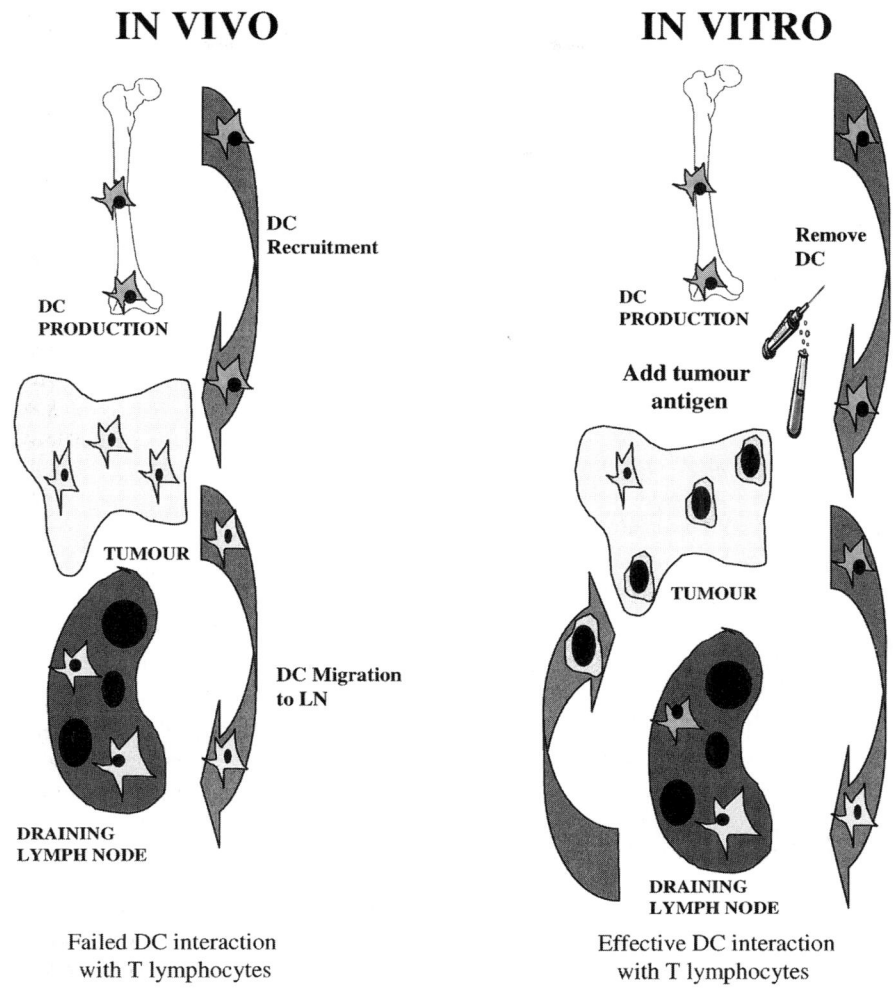

Fig. 112.4. Rationale for DC immunotherapy

CD34 or CD133 reagents for antibody-based cell selection, but this, plus the G-CSF mobilization, are significant preliminary steps before the in vitro culture and generation of DC (Ardeshna *et al.,* 2000; Banchereau *et al.,* 2001; Monji *et al.,* 2002). However, despite the physical resources and patience required these expanded DC products are effective (Banchereau *et al.,* 2001).

Blood monocyte-derived DC (Mo-DC) are readily available and if purified monocyte subpopulations are used (Romani *et al.,* 1994; Sallusto & Lanzavecchia, 1994; Thurner *et al.,* 1999b), produce a more homogeneous precursor population than CD34⁺ hematopoietic progenitor cells (HPCs). One of the attractive features of Mo-DC to investigators is that venesection may provide enough cells (Jonuleit *et al.,* 1997); however, there is an increasing trend to use apheresis procedures to obtain larger number of mononuclear cells for the in vitro cultures (Panelli *et al.,* 2000). Even though Mo-DC have many of the properties of classic DC, they have yet to be identified in vivo and they differ in some aspects

from circulating blood myeloid DC (Osugi, Vuckovic, & Hart, 2002). Mo-DC are very effective if antigen loading and their maturation are optimized.

Some investigators continue to isolate DC directly from circulating blood using modifications of earlier physical methods (Young & Steinman, 1988; Freudenthal & Steinman, 1990) and minimal if any cytokine exposure (Hsu *et al.,* 1996; Fong & Engleman, 2000; Fong *et al.,* 200la). A pre-clinical model for Mab-based blood DC purification may make for a very simple method of clinical blood DC purification (Lopez *et al.,* 2003a).

Apheresis will certainly be essential if blood DC are to be used but recent data suggest that they "mobilize" during the procedure (Lopez *et al.,* 2003b) and that sufficient numbers will be available even without mobilization in cancer patients.

Quality control of these various DC preparations will become a big issue as raised elsewhere (Nestle, Banchereau, & Hart 2001). Assessing their functional migration capacity remains one of the key issues.

Antigen loading into dendritic cells

There is still much to be learned as to how DC take up and process antigen. Despite this, different strategies are already being investigated for loading DC preparations for tumor immunotherapy programs (Table 112.3). Exogenous antigens enter the DC via phagocytosis, endocytosis, or macropinocytosis (Watts, 1997) and are degraded in low pH endosomal compartments into peptide fragments that complex with class II MHC molecules for surface presentation to CD4$^+$ T-helper cells (Kleijmeer *et al.*, 1995; Nijman *et al.*, 1995). It has become apparent that this classic dichotomy between exogenous (MHC II restricted) and endogenous (MHC I restricted) antigen presentation does not account for all antigen processing, particularly in DC. Exogenously acquired antigens are also processed and cross-presented on MHC class I molecules (Watts, 1997). Thus, antigens taken up by macropinocytosis can be released as peptides to bind with TAP proteins in the cytosol for delivery to the MHC class I compartment (Norbury *et al.*, 1997). Peptides when present in high concentrations externally, as occurs in immunotherapy, may exchange with incumbent peptides on surface MHC molecules, thus bypassing intracellular processing. Endogenous antigens (often autologous) can also enter the MHC class II pathway and generate significant CD4$^+$ responses (Lechler, Aichinger, & Lightstone, 1996).

The DC probably uses a series of so-called innate receptors to take up antigen from the environment. The macrophage mannose receptor (MMR) has been described on Mo-DC (Sallusto *et al.*, 1995). Another related C type lectin DEC-205 had been identified, which is more selectively expressed on DC (Kato *et al.*, 2000). The latter has been shown to target antigen very efficiently into DC (Mahnke *et al.*, 2000). Langerin (CD207), another C type lectin identified on Langerhans cell series, also appears to be involved in antigen uptake (Valladeau *et al.*, 2000). Other C type lectins BDCA-2 (Dzionek *et al.*, 2000) and DC-SIGN have been described on various DC populations. BDCA-2 is also another potential antigen-loading receptor (Geijtenbeek *et al.*, 2000). Identification of the relevant carbohydrate ligands for these molecules is being undertaken with a view to using these for antigen delivery. DC also express Fc receptors and work indicates that these may be used to target antigen delivery to the DC (Fanger *et al.*, 1997). Other molecules, such as CD36, act as receptors for apoptotic cells (Albert, Sauter, & Bhardwaj, 1998). The Toll family of receptors represents a key set of molecules, which are differentially expressed on DC subtypes (Kadowaki *et al.*, 2001). These deliver key activity signals to DC but may also act as antigen delivery systems.

It is almost a truism to state that any vaccination protocol will utilize the DC as the "common" pathway for cellular communication with T, and probably B, lymphocytes. In vitro loading of the DC with tumor lysate, protein, and peptides have all proved workable. DNA and RNA loading are also being exploited. However, some critical differences in the ability of DC to process intact antigen effectively have been highlighted. The state of DC maturation, the media, the presence and type of serum/protein additives all make a difference (Jonuleit *et al.*, 1997; Panelli *et al.*, 2000). However, perhaps one of the more important variables is the time of incubation—this not only influences antigen loading but may also determine the type of immune responses initiated. These variables are also important for blood DC preparations (Mannering, McKenzie, & Hart, 1998; Osugi, Vuckovic, & Hart, 2002).

TAA peptides, which bind class I and class II are now readily predicted and validated. They are easy to manufacture and produce under GMP conditions. They can be linked to include multiple (including helper and cytotoxic) epitopes and different structures investigated (Zeng *et al.*, 2001) to optimize delivery. Mouse models validate the role of DC in delivering effective antitumor responses (reviewed in Troy & Hart, 1997). Comparative data in a mouse model suggest that DC peptide administration is more effective than naked DNA vaccination (Bellone *et al.*, 2000).

An alternative, which bypasses the need to consider HLA restricting elements, is to use recombinant proteins—these can of course be engineered if necessary to remove any potentially harmful epitopes. Cost is a consideration but the quantities required may be relatively small. Engineering targeting components as described for the GM-CSF/prostatic acid phosphatase fusion protein may be very effective (Valone *et al.*, 2001).

New strategies have also seen a revival of whole cell vaccine approach in the form of pulsing DC with apoptotic bodies. Necrotic material from tumors may be relevant as it is likely that DC have sophisticated mechanisms to distinguish necrosis from apoptosis, theoretically with different outcomes. DC/tumor cell hybrids are also being explored. The injection of DC tumor hybrids in mice generated cure of advanced metastatic disease (Gong *et al.*, 1997). Tumor fusions have now been generated with human cells, and hybrids produced in the presence of polyethylene glycol (PEG) yielded measurable specific responses against breast cancer cells (Gong *et al.*, 2000a, 2000b). Moreover, striking clinical responses have been reported with the use of electroporated hybrid preparations

---

Table 112.3. *Means of loading antigens into DC*

Conventional delivery
  Incubation with crude tumor lysate
  Protein (intact)
  Protein (degraded)
  Peptide
Assisted uptake
  Tumor cell fusions
  Liposomes
  Mannan (oxidized) conjugated protein/peptides
  Antibody bound TAA
Nucleic acid delivery
  DNA for TAA
  RNA for TAA

Abbreviation: TAA, tumor-associated antigens.

(Kugler *et al.*, 2000). A number of clinical trials using both allogeneic and autologous DC are currently under way in various centers and the initial results should emerge soon (Walden P., personal communication). Interestingly, data suggest that co-incubation of DC with malignant cells is sufficient and cell fusion is not essential (Celluzzi & Falo, 1998).

DNA or RNA constructs may be used to deliver polytopes (multiple peptide epitopes) or recombinant protein to DC. These techniques have been very effective in mouse models. RNA loading is also capable of eliciting human CTL specific responses in vitro (Nair *et al.*, 1999, 2000; Heiser *et al.*, 2001). Total tumor RNA may be used (Nair *et al.*, 1999) and autoimmune responses may be minimal (Gilboa, 2001; Heiser *et al.*, 2001). Electroporated RNA may be superior to DNA plasmid expression of RNA (Van Tendeloo *et al.*, 2001). Clinical trials in patients with prostate cancer using this technique are underway (Heiser *et al.*, 2002).

Recombinant viruses are perhaps now less attractive options. Retroviral vectors have been used to deliver both class I and class II epitopes (Lapointe *et al.*, 2001). Adenovirus (Wan *et al.*, 1997) and canarypox (Engelmayer *et al.*, 2001) virus, known to replicate poorly in humans, have also been used.

Further modifications to antigen loading include delivering the antigens by targeting DC surface antigen receptors (Mahnke *et al.*, 2000) or by using intracellular locations signals such as HIV Tat (Fawell *et al.*, 1994). Various liposomal preparations are also being investigated and peptides may also be made more efficient by lipidation (Jackson *et al.*, 2002).

In vivo loading of antigens into DC may be achieved by DNA vaccination (e.g., by direct targeting of DC in the skin using a gene gun) or by intramuscular DNA vaccination that probably delivers the expressed protein indirectly to the DC. GM-CSF administration plus tumor cell vaccination probably recruits DC to the site and renders tumor cell processing more efficacious (Simons *et al.*, 1997, 1999). Flt-3L may increase DC in lymph nodes and increase the efficacy of vaccination (Pawlowska *et al.*, 2001).

Uptake of antigen into DC only represents one part of a critical set of events in the role of the APC. As well as processing the antigen to present it as a peptide-MHC complex, the DC must migrate to the T lymphocyte area of lymph nodes. To interact effectively with T lymphocytes, the DC must express co-stimulator molecules, chemokines, and cytokines, which initiate, control, and direct the type of T-lymphocyte response. In turn, the DC expression of chemokine receptors will regulate their migration (Sallusto & Lanzavecchia, 2000).

Expression of one or both of the co-stimulator molecules B7-1 (CD80) and B7-2 (CD86) on the APC is essential for the effective activation of T lymphocytes (Guinan *et al.*, 1994), for example, for IL-2 production. These co-stimulator molecules bind the CD28 molecule on T lymphocytes, providing a cyclosporine-independent co-stimulatory signal. If this fails to occur at the time of antigen recognition by the TCR, an alternative T-lymphocyte functional state, such as anergy, may be induced (Guinan *et al.*, 1994; Schwartz, 1996). Another

CD80/86 ligand, CTLA-4, is also induced on activated T lymphocytes, and this may contribute a negative regulatory signal (Gribben *et al.*, 1996). Other DC surface molecules, including CD40, probably contribute to T-lymphocyte activation, and CD40 signaling into DC has a major influence on DC function (McLellan *et al.*, 1996). Indeed CD40 stimulation of DC appears to be essential if DC are to generate an effective CD8 cytotoxic response. DC also express other co-stimulator molecules eg, 4-1BBL (DeBenedette *et al.*, 1997), OX40L (Chen *et al.*, 1999), RANKL (Anderson *et al.*, 1997) and this "apparent redundancy" gives DC great flexibility. It is also possible that the overall DC co-stimulatory molecule repertoire partially defines the resulting type of T-lymphocyte response. For example, CD80 may generate Th1 and CD86 may generate Th2-based responses (Kuchroo *et al.*, 1995).

DC also produce key cytokines, such as IL-1 (Heufler *et al.*, 1992), IL-4 (Rissoan *et al.*, 1999), IL-7 (Sorg *et al.*, 1998) and IL-12, (Heufler *et al.*, 1996), which contribute to T-lymphocyte activation and the differentiation of Th1/TC1 and Th2/TC2 responses. The CD123+ DC produces significant amounts of IFN-α (Cella *et al.*, 1999), but its production is rapidly down regulated as it differentiates into a more co-stimulatory cell (Cella *et al.*, 2000). The co-stimulatory phenotype of both DC types (cell membrane and cytokine expression) differs with the stimulus and notably over time.

DC are very responsive to T lymphocyte-mediated feedback and this conceptually provides a surrogate (T cell–mediated) antigen-specific control of DC activity. DC are also very responsive to other environmental signals. Thus, factors such as IL-10 expressed by macrophages drive an alternative DC phenotype more likely to down regulate T lymphocyte responses (Steinbrink *et al.*, 1997; Hackstein, Morelli, & Thomson, 2001).

Indeed, DC almost certainly play a major role in maintaining tolerance. Most DC probably migrate to draining lymph nodes without being fully activated (Summers *et al.*, 2001). DC isolated from rat mesenteric lymph node contain apoptotic bodies (Huang *et al.*, 2000), suggesting that natural apoptosis in gut epithelial cells results in potential self antigen presentation in draining nodes. DC that present antigen in the absence of inflammatory upregulation of the co-stimulator phenotype appear to have tolerogenic potential in several systems both in vitro (Steinbrink *et al.*, l999) and in vivo (Dhodapkar *et al.*, 2001).

Dendritic cell counts

A significantly improved understanding of DC biology would follow if an accurate means of identifying and counting DC in blood and other tissues were available. It is also a prerequisite to plan DC mobilization and therapeutic procedures. Fortunately, modern flow cytometry techniques allow these relatively rare cells to be tracked in the blood (Fearnley *et al.*, 1999: Ho *et al.*, 2001). Most laboratories prepare human blood DC using a mixture of Mab to lineage antigens (the choice is critical), and then a variety of immunoselection procedures to remove these cells prior to further analysis or use in functional assays. How the cells are prepared and just what subsets of blood DC are present is being redefined at present as a result of recent studies (Hart *et al.*, 2000; MacDonald *et al.*, 2002). Although it is still convenient to describe a CD11c⁺ (CD123ˡᵒ) myeloid subset and CD11⁻ CD123ʰⁱ lymphoid subset, it is clear that other (perhaps even functionally distinct) myeloid subsets can be defined (MacDonald *et al.*, 2002). Laboratories, used to counting rare cell populations, are now starting to analyse blood DC in whole blood or peripheral blood mononuclear cell populations. One can predict a steady expansion of this activity as clinically relevant DC counts are obtained.

Blood DC represent (depending on the phenotypic definition) 0.5%–1.5% of PBMC. Using the Mab CMRF-44 a range of 0.15%–0.70% or $3-17 \times 10^6$ DC/l was obtained (Fearnley *et al.*, 1999). Studies on patients undergoing surgery show an acute rise in absolute blood DC counts, which peak before monocytes (Ho *et al.*, 2001). The influence of blood DC regulation is also emphasized by the normal counts in patients with chronic myelomonocytic leukemia (Vuckovic *et al.*, 1999). Physical exercise also increases blood DC counts and both subsets, i.e., CD11c⁺ and CD123⁺, increase. Analysis in disease is in its infancy—the counts are altered in inflammatory bowel disease and phenotypic changes have also been documented (Vuckovic *et al.*, 2001). Blood DC counts in autoimmune diseases may also show changes. In cancer patients, various influences may or may not include reduced circulating blood DC numbers (Gabrilovich *et al.*, 1997; Brown *et al.*, 2001) and further studies are required. Other data are accruing to suggest blood DC counts are generally maintained in malignancy and that the defects may be more subtle (see below). As disease progresses, DC counts may decline in conjunction with, or related to, other altered leucocyte counts. How these might correlate with any DC changes in cancers themselves remains to be explored.

Blood DC counts have been studied following stem cell mobilization (Fearnley *et al.*, 1999). In normal controls, G-CSF mobilization appears to increase CD123⁺ DC counts selectively over the CD11c⁺ population (Arpinati *et al.*, 2000). This effect is less obvious in cyclophosphamide/G-CSF mobilized patients. Myeloid DC counts increase approximately 40-fold with a 10-fold increase in the lymphoid subset after Flt-3L mobilization. Monocytes also increase in numbers but there is little apparent DC activation (Maraskovsky *et al.*, 2000; Pulendran *et al.*, 2000). Changes in blood DC counts during acute graft-versus-host disease (GVHD) have been noted (Fearnley *et al.*, 1999; Vuckovic, Clark, & Hart, 2002).

Dendritic cells in HSC transplantation

DC are at the center of the immune response and can confidently be predicted to play a significant role in the immunologic phenomena associated with HSC transplantation. Some of the data derived from solid organ transplantation are helpful in this regard. Animal experiments have established that DC associated with transplanted organs stimulate a direct allo-geneic interaction (McKenzie, Beard, & Hart, 1984a, 1984b). Clustering of T lymphocytes around DC was observed in acute rejection. Depleting donor DC ablates this response and may prolong graft survival. This effect can be achieved by direct DC depletion from the graft (Hart & Fabre, 1981a) or passively by in vivo antibody administration (Hart & Fabre, 1981b, 1981c). Conversely, increasing donor DC by Flt-3L stimulation leads to accelerated liver allograft rejection (Qian *et al.*, 1998). Clinical studies using CD45 antibodies to perfuse human kidneys before allografting appeared to reduce the severity of acute rejection (Brewer *et al.*, 1989). Additional indirect processing of the organ graft antigens by recipient APC drives another host DC-mediated allogeneic response. No attempts to control clinical rejection by targeting the patient's DC have been reported although investigators have suggested that cyclosporine, corticosteroids, and other commonly used immunosuppressive agents will affect DC function. A recent publication described the upregulation of inhibitory receptors on Dc correlated with rejection-free episodes in heart transplant recipients (Chang *et al.*, 2002).

It was predicted that similar phenomena might operate in allogeneic HSCT (Hart, 1997). Recent animal data confirm this. The DC remaining in the recipient after conditioning stimulated an acute GVHD response (i.e., via the direct pathway) (van Lochem *et al.*, 1996). An intriguing mouse study (Shlomchik *et al.*, 1999) provided clear evidence that the residual APC population, presumed to be DC, was essential in causing acute GVHD. Although host DC disappear rapidly after conditioning they are able to prime donor T lymphocytes before disappearing (Zhang *et al.*, 2002). Interestingly, the administration of Flt-3L to the recipient before or after transplantation exacerbates GVHD (Blazar *et al.*, 2001). The animal data suggest that conditioning, notably irradiation and gut-derived LPS, generates a cytokine storm that exacerbates acute GVHD (Ferrara, 1994). This is entirely consistent with an activating effect on host DC. Removing DC from the stem cell inoculum also reduced the acute GVHD reaction (i.e., attenuated the indirect pathway). The latter process may provide a significant opportunity for encouraging donor engraftment and subsequent evolution of a T-lymphocyte repertoire that is tolerant to the recipient Studies using Flt-3/G-CSF fusion protein-mobilized donors (MacDonald *et al.*, 2003) have shown that these spleen cell preparations result in less acute GVHD. This effect is consistent with other data obtained with Flt-3L (Blazar *et al.*, 2001), which appears to be a G-CSF–mediated effect on T lymphocytes rather than a DC-mediated effect.

At a clinical level it is interesting to note that GVHD involves tissues associated with epithelial surfaces (i.e., skin, gut, and the liver). It is tempting to speculate that this may involve the CD1a⁺ lineage of epithelial-associated DC, although we failed to detect significant activation of either epidermal or dermal DC in skin biopsy material in patients with GVHD. An in vitro model of GVHD (Dickinson *et al.*, 2002) is now being exploited to examine the role of DC in humans. There is early data indicating that some epithelial-associated

DC survive the conditioning prior to an allogeneic HSC transplant. The repopulation of the epidermis appears to be relatively slow (Perreault, Roy, & Fortin, 1998). However, data on nonepithelial DC from animal studies would suggest they repopulate relatively rapidly (Hart & Fabre, 1981d; Shortman & Liu, 2002). Blood DC counts are altered by stem cell mobilization (Fearnley et al., 1999). G-CSF mobilized allogeneic stem cell harvests include an increased number of CD123+ DC (Arpinati et al., 2000) and this may be due to altered CD62L and CCR7 expression (Vuckovic, Clark, & Hartz, 2002). It has been hypothesized that this accounts for the lack of the expected increase in acute GVHD in the recipients. The animal data only in part support this. The ability to count DC has allowed them to be monitored in allogenic and autologous HSCT recipients. The first data suggest that blood DC counts recover early after allogeneic HSCT (Vuckovic, Clark, & Hart, 2002). Indeed, high counts seemed to precede episodes of acute GVHD in two patients who received mobilized allogeneic stem cells (Vuckovic, Clark, & Hart, 2002). Studies on the origin of the reconstituting DC are under way (Klangsinsirikul et al., 2002) in an effort to substantiate the hypothesis that persistent host DC, which survive conditioning are a trigger to acute GVHD. DC mixed chimerism may predict acute GVHD.

As immunosuppressive regiments to control acute (and chronic) GVHD evolve, it becomes increasingly necessary to ascertain their effects on DC biology. CD52 is expressed on DC (Hart et al., 1997) and Campath-1 administered as an immunosuppressive agent may well be achieving its effect in part via an effect of DC (Klangsinsirikul et al., 2002). Antibodies directed against DC may become therapeutic. CMRF-44, an IgM antibody (Fearnley et al., 1997b) that lyses activated human DC, inhibits an allogeneic MLR but preserves memory immune responses in vitro. An anti-CD83 reagent (Hock et al., 2001) is also immunosuppressive in vitro but curiously enough appears to operate via an unexpected route—NK mediated lysis of activated CD83+ T lymphocytes as well as DC. Finally, drugs targeting key DC molecular pathways such as NF-κB pathways (Yoshimura et al., 2001) may herald a new approach to immunosuppression.

Dendritic cell stimulated responses in vitro

The initial studies defining DC depended heavily on the allogeneic MLR. This response is atypical in that it detects preformed "alloantigens" (i.e., incompatible MHC + peptide). Furthermore, the responding T lymphocytes may not be responding in a true primary fashion, as at least an element of the response may be due to cross-reactivating memory T lymphocytes. For this reason and more importantly because it does not assess antigen processing, the allogeneic MLR may be less relevant for assessing therapeutic DC preparations. In animal models the ability of DC to process and present antigens is tested readily by initial in vivo priming and a second in vitro readout step. Investigation of the mechanisms of primary APC function in humans is much more difficult. It necessitates in

vitro priming with test antigens or TAA (Mannering, McKenzie, & Hart, 1998), and this area has not received much attention because it is very demanding technically. However, it is vital to develop in vitro systems for assessing human DC function.

Human DC have been reported to stimulate primary T-lymphocyte responses to keyhole limpet hemocyanin (KLH) and HIV proteins. Both of these appear to be recognized by a relatively high precursor frequency T-lymphocyte responder population. The ability of DC to prime for other true primary antigens (e.g., pigeon cytochrome C or sperm whale myoglobin) appears to be dominated by the responding T-lymphocyte precursor frequency (Hart, 1997). When the BCR-ABL fusion peptide was tested, the low responding T-lymphocyte frequency appeared to negate any in vitro advantage of priming with purified human DC as opposed to whole blood mononuclear cells (Mannering, McKenzie, & Hart, 1998). KLH processing and presentation appears to differ between CD11c+ blood DC and Mo-DC preparations (Osugi, Vuckovic, & Hart, 2002). The latter appeared to generate greater T lymphocyte IFN-γ responses in the absence of proliferation. The time it takes to generate an in vitro T lymphocyte response is considerable compared to priming in vivo (Ingulli et al., 1997), indicating the inefficacy of the current in vitro priming systems.

A range of DC preparations have now been used to generate in vitro CD8+ T cell (cytotoxic T-lymphocyte; CTL) responses to TAA. Repetitive stimulation is the norm with IL-2 (and often IL-7) used to nurture evolving T lymphocyte responses (Vonderheide et al., 1999; Heiser et al., 2001b). The use of fetal serum (FCS) increases background. The introduction of enzyme-linked immuno spot (EliSpot assay) of IFN-α producing CD8+ T lymphocytes has been used as a surrogate for CTL activity in ⁵¹Cr release assays. The clearest results appear when selected cell populations are analyzed, and again low precursor frequencies are common. Tetramer analysis is also proving invaluable, and not surprisingly some of the high frequency T-cell responses to certain tumor or cancer antigens, e.g., MART-1, may be contributed to by cross reactive antigens (Dutoit et al., 2002). Many investigators restimulate T lymphocytes from patients who have received an in vivo vaccination (Thurner et al., 1999a; Banchereau et al., 2001). Fortunately many aspects of human DC biology, e.g., antigen uptake and presentation, can be assessed by using T-lymphocyte clones in "recall" responses.

Assessing DC priming of naïve T-lymphocyte responses remains difficult. Nonetheless, comparison is essential to assess the multiplicity of improvements possible in DC preparations prior to clinical trials.

Dendritic cell stimulated responses in animals

There is now an extensive body of animal data (Troy & Hart, 1997) to encourage clinical trials. One of the initial studies (Knight et al., 1985) using a mouse sarcoma model demonstrated a 50% survival rate in mice given splenic DC 18 days after tumor inoculation, compared with no survival in animals not receiving DC. However, mice receiving DC pulsed with tumor antigens did not have improved survival—this may have been an early indicator that the DC population or state of activation was crucial. Activated T cells are found in the draining lymph nodes (Nelson et al., 2001).

Contrasting with these findings, Grabbe and colleagues (1991) demonstrated that murine epidermal cells pulsed with tumor fragments, given subcutaneously weekly for 3 weeks before a tumor challenge, prevented its subsequent growth. In a similar study, preimmunization with splenic DC pulsed with idiotype IgM enhanced subsequent rejection of a B-cell tumor challenge (Flamand et al., 1994). The DC used in all these studies were prepared from normal mice with no immunologic impairment. It has subsequently been shown that splenic DC taken from tumor-bearing mice retain normal function (Ardavin et al., 1996). Furthermore, these DC, which were pulsed in vivo with TAA, when transferred from a tumor-bearing host conferred protective immunity to naive syngeneic mice.

Animal studies suggest that a strong, effective antitumor response is likely to require both a CD4+ helper and a CD8+ cytotoxic response (Schoenberger et al., 1998). Exogenously acquired tumor lysates may generate a predominant class II driven CD4+ response. Langerhans' cells, when pulsed with whole tumor lysate, produced proliferative responses in CD4+ T cells, especially primed cells, but no significant response from CD8+ cells (Cohen et al., 1994). MHC class II peptide presentation in mouse tumor models for tumor immunotherapy has not been explored. However, the essential role of CD4+ help in generating CD8+ CTL responses has been established and the use of DC avoids peptide-induced tumor tolerance (Toes et al., 1998).

Generation of CD8+ CTL immunity has been tested experimentally in several models (Young & Inaba, 1996). DC pulsed with an OVA (ovalbumin) peptide that constitutes a strong CTL epitope were able to protect mice against a challenge with an OVA-transduced tumor cell line (Celluzzi & Falo, 1998). Depletion of CD8+ cells dramatically reduced survival. The CD4+ help for these responses may well be nonspecific, although its role was not tested in vivo. Class I–restricted responses have also been produced in sarcoma and lung tumor models (Mayordomo et al., 1995).

Defined class I–restricted epitopes of TAA have been identified for only a limited number of mouse tumors, particularly melanoma (Golumbek et al., 1993). By using unfractionated acid-eluted peptides, Zitvogel et al., 1996) have shown that it is possible to induce an MHC class I–restricted, T-cell–mediated antitumor response using DC that could suppress or slow the growth of established tumors. Using Mab to deplete either the cytotoxic or helper T-lymphocyte subsets, they demonstrated that although the CD8+ cells provided the main response, CD4+ cells were an important contributor. The authors suggested that MHC class II–bound peptides were also eluted and stimulated the CD4+ help. Acid elution of peptides yielded a superior immunogenic source than freeze-thaw lysis, which also pre-

sumably releases intracellular enzymes, such as proteases. DC loaded with acid-eluted peptides generate Th1 responses and subsequent CD8+ CTL responses.

As both CD4+ and CD8+ responses play a significant role in tumor rejection, it would appear that generation of both responses could produce a synergistic response. Therefore, the ideal material for pulsing DC may be a combination of peptides or lysate/whole protein antigens, together with other signals such as CD40L, which enable DC to stimulate both helper and cytotoxic T-lymphocyte responses. Recent in vivo experiments in CD40−/− mice emphasize the importance of CD40-mediated DC activation to drive a T-lymphocyte response (Miga et al., 2001). Mouse studies have helped to clarify the route of administration. The data favor s.c. or i.d. over i.v. administration (Eggert et al., 1999; Serody et al., 2000). It also makes it clear that repetitive vaccination at short intervals may achieve little, as CTL responses rapidly destroy the injected DC (Harris et al., 2002). It has also allowed other methods of loading antigen, e.g., bacterial expression of TAA, to be explored (Radford et al., 2002). The immunological outcome and clinical outcome and, of course, correlations between the two are being keenly sought.

Some interesting data describing the direct inoculation of malignant lesions with DC in mice suggested that DC could influence tumor growth and, if co-inoculated, prevent tumor growth (Candido et al., 2001; Mendoza et al., 2002).

Dendritic cell stimulated responses in humans

The enthusiasm for DC-based tumor immunotherapy has resulted in several trials being initiated. An understanding of several key variables is essential. Firstly, in terms of DC therapeutics the type of DC preparation, dose, site of delivery, and vaccination schedule are critical. Clearly the TAA preparation is a major variable. Assessing outcome at present requires careful disease assessment and extensive immunological assessment until surrogate markers are clarified.

Dose finding studies in DC vaccination have been limited. A potential but unsatisfactory way is to titrate DC numbers injected against a T cell response to a strong test immunogen by measuring HLA-peptide tetramer (which binds to specific T cell receptors) responses or possibly delayed-type hypersensitivity (DTH) reactions in vivo. Empirical dosing of DC and schedules suggest a minimal cell number is required, currently accepted as approximately 10^6 but 10-fold less may suffice. The few dose escalation studies have not shown a clear cell dose effect (Fong & Engleman, 2000), although there are suggestions that this is a relevant variable (Small et al., 2000). Given the critical influence of T-lymphocyte doses in DLI (Guglielmi et al., 2002), it seems likely that a dose effect will become evident.

The issue is further complicated by the choice of the DC injection site. Predictably, DC injected into a lymph node appear to produce a different outcome to the same number of DC injected intradermally or intravenously. Currently available migration studies (Morse et al., 1999a; Thomas et al.,

1999) predict that about 1% of Mo-DC injected into the skin will reach a draining lymph node. Rapid migration of CD34+ DC into lymph nodes occurred following intralymphatic injection, but DC administered i.v. located in lung and liver and ultimately the spleen, but not lymphnodes (Mackensen *et al.*, 1999). Migration is likely to differ accordingly to the type of DC preparation, as they have different chemokine receptors and adhesion-mediating properties. Intranodal injection under ultrasound guidance was used in the first melanoma vaccination study (Nestle, Banchereau, & Hart, 1998). One paper (Fong *et al.*, 2001b) compared T-lymphocyte and antibody responses to blood DC loaded with recombinant mouse prostatic acid phosphatase injected i.v., i.d. or into cannulated lymphatics. Only the latter two routes resulted in T lymphocyte IFN-γ production (T proliferation occurred in each) and the i.v. route resulted in more antibody responses. There appears to be a trend for better outcomes at least in immunological responses in those studies utilizing delivery via the skin (i.d. is predicted to be better than s.c.). The method of injection may be a highly relevant variable, as the degree of traumatic release of inflammatory mediators and DC activation could be very relevant.

Some studies have combined routes but adding i.v. administration to dermal administration might be postulated to compromise the efficacy of the latter route. Injection schedules to date are derived from experiences in animal models and human vaccination studies in infectious diseases. Weekly injections with monthly boosting or monthly injection schedules are currently performed. Again data optimizing these are urgently required, given suggestions that too frequent administration may be counter-productive (Serody *et al.*, 2000). Since DC are critical for priming responses, it may be that alternative vehicles for revaccinating may be possible, improving the feasibility of the procedure.

The type of DC preparation used varies according to institution. CD34-derived DC, Mo-DC, and blood DC have all been used. Mo-DC generated in GM-CFS/IL-4, i.e., the immature form are probably not effective in practice. The clinical data suggest this and recent key experiments involving two patients suggest that these cells may even switch off established responses (Dhodapkar *et al.*, 2001). In the absence of maturing factors, these cells may de-differentiate into macrophages. Of interest for other therapeutic reasons, their exposure to IL-10 may even tolerize anti-TAA responses (Steinbrink *et al.*, 1999).

GM-CSF/IL-4 Mo-DC matured in a variety of factors are clearly efficacious. It is noticeable, however, that individual laboratory protocols differ and the methodology (e.g., media supplements, etc.), as well as the TAA preparation they are exposed to, may have a major effect. For example, the inclusion of FCS (and the intranodal injection) may have been key components of the first reported successes in melanoma (Nestle, Bancherau, & Hart, 1998). Again, a variety of blood DC preparations have been used, but most experience has been gained with a preparation, which includes T lymphocytes and combines these same instances with TAA modified by GM-

CSF. Exactly which components in these cocktails are critical will require significant analysis.

Phase I/II clinical trials

A summary is provided in Table 112.4. The initial clinical trial, involving four patients with relapsed low-grade NHL produced encouraging results without side-effects (Hsu *et al.*, 1996). The most encouraging feature was that this was the first time immunized patients produced a T-lymphocyte response to the idiotype protein antigen. The excellent results in low-grade NHL patients with minimal residual disease (MRD) using GM-GSF and KLH-conjugated idiotype indicated the potential in this disease (Bendandi *et al.*, 1999). Longer term follow-up has shown a variable outcome but it is now recognised that ongoing vaccination may be necessary to maintain immunity.

Multiple myeloma has also attracted attention. Again there are data to suggest patients can mount T-cell–mediated anti-idiotype responses (Osterborg *et al.*, 1998). In vitro studies confirm the ability of autologous Mo-DC to generate such responses (Dabadghao *et al.*, 1998; Wen *et al.*, 1998), and one clinical study suggested that DC generated anti-idiotype responses after autologous stem cell transplantation (Reichardt *et al.*, 1999). Multiple myeloma patients may be more immunosuppressed and idiotype may be a weak TAA, but as all these studies have employed the i.v. route of immunization this may account for the relatively low frequency of anti-idiotype responses (4 of 26 vs. 24 of 26 in the KLH controls [Liso *et al.*, 2000]). Interestingly, 3 of 4 responders in the later study were in complete disease remission. Another study performed in the posttransplant setting (Valone *et al.*, 2001) remains to be fully reported; however, it too suggests responses may occur in the MRD setting after autologous stem cell transplantation for multiple myeloma. Although there were confounding factors, a remarkable 9 of 18 clinical responses (5 complete remissions [CR] and 4 partial remission [PR]) were seen in this context (F. Valone, personal communication).

It is perhaps in melanoma that greatest interest was aroused, and there are a plethora of trials in progress. Few have been formally reported, but the follow-up from the first description of the use of Mo-DC and melanoma peptides/tumor lysates (Nestle, Banchereau, & Hart, 1998) shows 2 CR and 3 PR in 21 patients with metastatic disease, indicating an ongoing control of disease in a proportion of patients, with a mean survival of over 47 months in responder patients. This protocol induced peptide-specific T-cell responses in 10 out of 10 HLA-A2 patients. A second trial (Thurner *et al.*, 1999a) used Mo-DC matured in monocyte-conditioned medium that were injected s.c. and i.d. and induced specific CTL expansion in 8 of 11 HLA-A1 patients, but notably these responses declined after further i.v. injections. Regression of metastases occurred in 6 of 11 patients. The same group has reported poor clinical results (no regressions in 8 evaluable patients) in a third study involving HLA-A2 individuals, using the same MAGE-3 antigen but delivering the DC s.c. Curiously, the later patient group had

Table 112.4. *Reports on the use of dendritic cells for cancer immunotherapy*

Type of cancer	Antigen	DC type	Route	n	Immune response	Clinical response	(Y/N)[a]	Reference
Non-Hodgkin's lymphoma	Idiotype	Blood	i.v. (& then s.c. Ag)	4	4/4 Id specific proliferative	1 CR, 1 PR		Hsu et al., 1996
Multiple myeloma	Idiotype protein	Im Mo	i.v.	1	Id specific proliferative, Ab	Paraprotein fall		Wen et al., 1998
Multiple myeloma (post auto-HSCT)	Idiotype protein + KLH	Blood (i)	i.v.	12	11/12 KLH, 2/12 Id-specific proliferative 1/3 treated Id specific CTL	9/12 alive, minimum follow up 16 months	−	Reichardt et al., 1999
		Blood (ii)	i.v.	14	24/26 KLH, 4/26 Id-specific proliferative	17/26 alive, median follow up 34 months	−	Liso et al., 2000
Multiple myeloma	Idiotype protein + KLH	Im Mo	i.v.	6	6/6 KLH specific proliferative, 3/6 Id specific CTL increase 4/5 Id specific proliferative (2 IFN-γ) 3/6 Id specific CTL increase	1 Paraprotein fall, 2 SD, 2 PD 1 death Better immune response if no pretreatment	Y	Lim & Bailey-Wood, 1999
Multiple myeloma	Idiotype protein	CD34+	s.c. (& s.c. Ag & GM-CSF)	11	4/10 Id specific EliSpot 3/10 Id Ab increase	1 SD, 10 PD		Titzer et al., 2000
Multiple myeloma	Idiotype	Ma Mo	s.c. & i.v. (IL-2)	5	2/5 Id specific proliferative 3/5 EliSpot 0/5 DTH	1 PR, 3 SD, 1 PD		Yi et al., 2002
Leukemia (relapsed post allo-HSCT)	Apoptotic	Allo-Ma Mo	i.v.	4	2/3 Tumor specific CTL	2/4 reduced leukemia count	−	Fujii et al., 2001
Chronic myeloid leukemia (chronic phase, post IFN-α + autologous HSCT)	Leukemic (Ph+) DC + PPD	Ma Mo	i.v.	1	PPD DTH Ph specific CTL	Hematological response Partial cytogeneic response	−	Fujii et al., 1999
Melanoma (pretreated stage IV)	Lysate or mix + KLH peptide (HLA-A1: MAGE-1/MAGE-3; HLA-A2: Melan-A, tyrosinase gp100)	Im Mo (+ FCS)	i.n.	16	16/16 DTH to KLH 11/16 DTH to peptide	2 CR, 3 PR, met regression	Y	Nestle et al. 1998
Melanoma (stage IV)	MAGE-3A1 (HLA-A1) peptide	Ma Mo	s.c. + i.d. then i.v.	11	0/11 DTH to peptide 2/11 EliSpot 8/11 Peptide specific CTL	6/11 met regression Decline in immune response after i.v.	Y	Thurner et al., 1999a
Melanoma (metastatic)	Tumor/Allo-PBMC hybrid	Act. PBMC	s.c.	16	4/14 DTH tumor	1 CR, 1 PR, 5 SD No response in immune compromised	Y	Trefzer et al., 2000
Melanoma (metastatic)	Mart-1; gp100 peptides	Im Mo	i.v. (±IL-2)	10	1/5 Increased CTL	1 PR (met regression)	N	Panelli et al. 2000
Melanoma (stage IV)	MAGE-1, MAGE-3 (HLA-A1), Melan-A, gp100, Tyrosinase (HLA-A2)	CD34+	i.v.	14	4/10 DTH to HLA-2 peptide 1/4 Tetramer specific, 0/5 EliSpot	1 PR, 7 SD, 6 PD	Y	Mackensen et al., 2000
Melanoma (stage IV)	MAGE-3 (HLA-A1 or HLA-A2 peptide)	Ma Mo	s.c., then i.v.	8	2/2 Tetramer specific 8/8 EliSpot 7/8 CTL	1 SD, 7 PD, 4 died Decline in immune response after i.v.		Schuler-Thurner et al., 2000
Melanoma (stage IV)	Melan-A, tyrosinase, MAGE-3 + Flu MP + KLH	CD34+	i.d.	18	10/14 DTH to peptides 16/18 Ag specific EliSpot	3 CR, 4 PR (Met regression; delayed progression) 7 PD, 3 SD	Y	Banchereau et al., 2001
Melanoma	MAGE (A1/A3 peptide) + KLH	Im Mo	i.v. s.c. + in	23	12/23 Peptide specific CTL increase No difference with KLH	2 PR, 7 SD Decreased immune response with time	−	Toungouz et al. 2001
Melanoma	Tumor lysate + KLH	Im Mo	i.d.	11	8/9 KLH EliSpot 3/9 tumor lysate proliferative 4/9 tumor EliSpot 4 DTH to tumor lysate	4 limited SD, 7 PD	−	Chang et al. 2002
Melanoma (stage IV)	Mart-1, Tyrosinase, gp100 peptides	Im Mo	i.v.	16	2/16 DTH to peptides 5/16 IFNγ ELISA response	1CR, 2SD	Y	Lau et al. 2001

Cancer	Antigen/Vaccine	Cell	Route	N	Immune response	Clinical response		Reference
Melanoma (stage IV)	Melan-A or MAGE-1	Im Mo vs. Ma Mo	i.n.	11	1/7 EliSpot Im Ma 5/7 EliSpot Ma Mo (2/4 CTL) (0/4 CTL)	3 PR, 2 SD, 3PD, 3 deaths	Y	Jonuleit et al., 2001
Melanoma (stage IV)	MAGE-3 Melan-A/ MART-1 gp100 and/or tumor lysate	Ma Mo	s.c. (+ IL-2 + Temozolomide)	2	2/2 EliSpot responses	2 PD. Loss of EliSpot response associated with disease progression	Y	Andersen et al., 2001
Breast cancer	CEA (CAP-1) peptide	Ma Mo	i.v.	5/21	DTH to KLH	1 SD, 4 PD	–	Morse et al., 1999
Breast cancer (pretreated stage IV)	Tumor lysate + KLH	Im Mo	i.n.	1	No DTH to lysate	Met regression	–	Kobayashi et al., 2001
Breast cancer (pretreated stage IV)	HER2neu or MUC-1 peptides	Ma Mo	s.c.	7/10	3/7 Peptide specific CTL	1 PR	–	Brossart et al., 2000
Ovarian cancer (pretreated stage IV)	CEA (CAP1) peptide HER2neu or MUC-1 peptides	Ma Mo Ma Mo	i.v. s.c.	3/21 3/10	2/3 peptide specific CTL	1 PR, 2 PD 1 SD, 1 short SD	–	Morse et al., 1999 Brossart et al., 2000
Ovarian cancer (progressive or recurrent)	Tumor lysate		s.c./i.d.	6	5/5 DTH to KLH 1/5 DTH to tumor lysate 5/6 proliferative to KLH 2/6 proliferative to lysate	1 PR, 2 SD, 3 PD	–	Hernando et al., 2002
Uterine cancer (sarcoma)	Tumor lysate + KLH	Ma Mo	s.c./i.d.	2	1/1 DTH to KLH not tumor lysate 1/2 proliferative to KLH 0/2 proliferative to tumor lysate	2 PD	–	Hernando et al., 2002
Prostate cancer (metastatic, hormone refactory)	PSMA P1 and P2 peptides (HLA-A2)	Im Mo	i.v.	51	Proliferative to peptide in HLA-A2	Peptide alone: 2 PR 6 SD 12 PD DC alone: 0 PR 2SD 10PD DC/peptide: 5 PR 3 SD 10 PD (some responders not HLA-A2)	–	Murphy et al., 1996
				33 A1 (retreated) 33 (25) A2 (new cohort)–	–	9 PR, 11 SD, 13 PD (7 deaths) 2 CR, 6 PR	–	Tjoa et al., 1998 Murphy et al., 1999
						10% PSA fall Recall DTH and cytokine response relates to clinical response	–	Tjoa et al., 1999 Lodge et al., 2000
Prostate cancer (recurrence after primary treatment)	PMSA P1 and P2 peptides	Im Mo 50% + GM-SCF	i.v.	37 (B)	–	1 CR, 10 PR	–	Murphy et al., 1999
				37 (B)	–	11 responders 5% PSA fall	–	Tjoa et al., 1999
						Recall DTH and cytokine specific response CR, pre-existing.	–	Lodge et al., 2000 (95)
Prostate cancer	Fusion protein GM-CSF + PAP	Blood	i.v. + s.c. sc, GM-CSF + Ag	31	10/26 Proliferative to PAP Proliferative to GM-CSF and 16/31 Ab PAP	CTL PRs 2 + peptide specific 3/31 ≥ 50% + 3/31 > 25% PSA fall; no objective regression DC dose effect?	Y	Small et al., 2000
Prostate cancer	Fusion protein GM-CSF + PAP	Blood	i.d., s.c. GM-CSF Ag	13	9 proliferative to PAP 11 Ab to PAP + GM-CSF	4/12 PSA or PAP fall	–	Burch et al., 2000
Prostate cancer	mPAP	Blood	i.v. i.d. i.v.	9 6 6	0/9 EliSpot, 5/9 Ab 4/6 EliSpot, 1/6 Ab 3/6 EliSpot, 2/6 Ab 21/21 T proliferative	6/21 clinical stabilization; correlation with T proliferation not route/Ab	Y	Fong et al., 2001a, 2001b
Prostate cancer	PSA mRNA	Im Mo	i.v. + i.d.	13	8/8 EliSpot 9/9 CTL	6/7 decrease log slope PSA 3/3 temporary clearance blood tumor cells.	–	Heiser et al., 2002

(table continues)

Table 112.4. *(Continued)*

Type of cancer	Antigen	DC type	Route	n	Immune response	Clinical response	(Y/N)[a]	Reference
Renal cell carcinoma (metastatic)	Cell lysate + KLH	Ma Mo	i.v.	12	RCC, normal kidney and KLH proliferative	–	–	Holt et al., 1999
				4	1/4 DTH to KLH IFN-γ responses to KLH 4/4 IgM and IgG responses to KLH	1 PR, 2 SD, 1 PD	Y	Rieser et al., 2000
Renal cell carcinoma (metastatic)	Tumor/Allo-DC hybrid (200 Cy)	Ma Mo	i.v.	17	11/17 DTH to tumor	4 CR, 2 PR, 1 mixed	–	Kugler et al., 2000
Metastatic CEA expressing cancer	CAP-1 peptide (HLA-A2)/RNA (HLA-A2⁻)	Im Mo	i.v.	9/8	2/4 HLA-2 MUC-1 Peptide specific IFN-γ CEA specific CTL 9/9 in peptide and 7/8 in RNA cohort	–	–	Nair et al., 1999
Parathyroid carcinoma	Tumor lysate + PTH + KLH	Ma Mo / Im Mo (FCS)	s.c. + i.n.	1	T proliferative, DTH (not to PTH)	No clinical response	–	Schott et al.,1999, 2000
Thyroid medullary carcinoma	CEA Calcitonin + KLH	Ma Mo	i.d.	7	7/7 DTH 1/7 proliferative (partial response)	1 partial 2 mixed responses	Y	Schott et al., 2001
Esophageal cancer	MAGE peptide	Im Mo	i.v.	3	2/3 Peptide specific CTL	2/3 Reduced tumor marker 2PR	N	Sadanga et al., 2001
Stomach cancer	MAGE peptide	Im Mo	i.v.	6	2/3 Peptide specific CTL	4/6 Reduced tumor marker	–	Sadanga et al., 2001
Colorectal cancer	MAGE peptide	Im Mo	i.v.	3	0/3 Peptide specific CTL	1/3 Reduced tumor marker 1 PR	N	Sadanga et al., 2001
Colorectal cancer	CEA (CAP-1) peptide	Im Mo	i.v.	11/21	11/14 DTH to KLH	11 PD	–	Morse et al., 1999
Colorectal cancer	Tumor RNA & KLH	Im Mo	i.v.	15	2/2KLH EliSpot	Minimal changes in CEA?	–	Rains et al., 2001
Colorectal cancer	Tumor lysate + KLH	Im Mo	i.d.	2	1 tumor lysate proliferative 1 tumor EliSpot 1 DTH to tumor lysate	Limited SD, PD	–	Chang et al., 2002
Pancreatic cancer (neuroendocrine)	CEA (CAP-1) peptide	Im Mo	i.v.	1/21	Vaccine DTH, proliferative	1 PD	Y	Morse et al., 1999
Pancreas (neuroendocrine)	Tumor lysate + KLH	Ma Mo	s.c.	1		Decreased marker; met regression	–	Schott et al., 1999, 2001
Glioma	Acid eluted peptide	Ma Mo	s.c.	7	4/7 CTL 4/7 CTL infiltrate in tumor	Prolonged survival (MST 455 days vs. control 257 days)	–	Yu et al., 2001
Glioma (post-radiation and/or chemotherapy)	Tumor/Auto DC fusion	Ma Mo	i.d.	8	6/6 PBMC IFN-γ	2 PR	–	Kikuchi et al., 2001
Glioma	Tumor/IL-4 transduced fibroblasts	Im Mo	i.d.	0	–	–	–	Okada et al., 2001
Solid tumors (pediatric)	Tumor lysate + KLH	Im Mo	i.d.	10	7/10 DTH to KLH 3/10 DTH to tumor	1 PR Tumor regression	–	Geiger et al., 2000
Neuroblastoma	Tumor lysate + KLH	Im Mo	i.d.	1	DTH to tumor lysate	Limited SD	–	Chang et al., 2002

Abbreviations: Ag, antigen; Id, idiotype; CR, complete response; PR, partial response; Im Mo, immature monocyte-derived DC; Ab, antibody; HSCT, hematopoietic stem cell transplantation; KLH, keyhole limpet hemocyanin; CTL, cytotoxic T lymphocytes; SD, stable disease; PD, progressive disease; GM-CSF, granulocyte-macrophage colony-stimulating factor; IL, interleukin; EliSpot, enzyme-linked immuno spot assay; Ma Mo, mature monocyte-derived DC; DTH, delayed-type hypersensitivity; IFN, interferon; PPD, purified protein derivative; DC, dendritic cells; FCS, fetal calf serum; PBMC, peripheral blood mononuclear cells; ELISA, enzyme-linked immunosorbent assay; PSMA, prostate-specific membrane antigen; PSA, prostate-specific antigen; PAP, prostatic acid phosphatase; MPAP, ; CC, renal cell carcinoma; MST, median survival time.

[a] Correlation with immune response Yes/No

active melanoma peptide-specific IFN-γ effector CD8⁺T cells (confirmatory cytotoxic studies were not performed) present.

However, a fourth published study (Panelli *et al.*, 2000) using immature Mo-DC administered i.v. produced poor cytotoxic responses and had only one partial clinical response in 7 patients evaluated. A protocol, which used CD34⁺-derived DC administered s.c. enhanced immunity in at least one assay (EliSpot or proliferation) in 16 of 18 patients —DTH responses were independent of these results (Banchereau *et al.*, 2001). During a ten week evaluation, four patients with multiple lesions experienced regression at one or more disease sites and three with limited disease cleared evidence of the disease. In broad terms, immunological responses predicted for disease response. Another trial made use of CD34⁺-derived DC but gave them i.v.: the monitoring of immunological responses was limited but these patients had a lesser clinical response, again suggesting that perhaps the i.v. route is less effective (Mackensen *et al.*, 2000b).

A consensus (including unpublished studies) is emerging despite the different approaches, that in advanced melanoma some 20%–30% of patients have a significant clinical response. The use of immature Mo-DC may be associated with a lesser outcome (Mackensen *et al.*, 2000b; Toungouz *et al.*, 2001) in melanoma unless their preparation and antigen loading involves activation, as may have occurred in the first trial. Immunological tests may predict for the group with some clinical response (Lau *et al.*, 2001). A formal comparison of immature versus mature Mo-DC used different DC preparations and antigens in the same patients (Jonuleit *et al.*, 2001); it was not possible to allocate the positive clinical outcomes to a particular preparation although, as commented earlier, differences in T cell responses were seen.

Other most encouraging results have been obtained in renal cell carcinoma (Thurnher *et al.*, 1998; Holtl *et al.*, 1999; Rieser *et al.*, 2000). The use of allogeneic tumor cell–DC hybrids was pioneered in this area (Kugler *et al.*, 2000); the excellent results are being investigated further. Again, it is perhaps relevant that this is a disease in which immune responses are known to occur, e.g., following IL-2/LAK therapy. There has been a large cohort of prostate cancer patients studied using two approaches (Table 112.4) (Salgaller *et al.*, 1998; Tjoa *et al.*, 1998, 1999; Murphy *et al.*, 1996, 1999a, 1999b, 2000; Burch *et al.*, 2000; Lodge *et al.*, 2000; Small *et al.*, 2000; Tjoa & Murphy, 2000; Fong *et al.*, 2001a, 2001b), perhaps in part because prostate has organ-specific antigens (e.g., prostate specific membrane antigen [PSMA] and prostatic acid phosphatase [PAP]), which can also be considered as potential TAA. Mo-DC used in conjunction with PSMA peptides have been used in a phase II trial, which described one complete and ten partial responders amongst 37 patients with presumed local recurrence (Murphy *et al.*, 1999b). There was a strong association between clinical responders and pre-existing immune competence (Lodge *et al.*, 2000). A protocol which uses blood DC and the novel DC activating GM-CSF–PAP compound has been show to generate T-cell responses to PAP (Burch *et al.*, 2000). Decreases in PSA

levels as a tumor marker stimulated a phase III study of patients with progressive metastatic disease. A study, which used Mo-DC transfected with mRNA encoding PSA, had no significant toxicity and generated PSA-specific responses in all patients— initial changes in PSA increments need further follow up (Heiser *et al.*, 2002).

Other cancers are also being addressed. Immune responses have resulted following DC vaccination with carcinoembryonic antigen as RNA (Nair *et al.*, 1999) or peptide (Morse *et al.*, 1999b). Peptide-pulsed DC have now been reported to produce cytotoxic responses in breast and ovarian cancer patients (Brossart *et al.*, 2000), and a single case report described a clinical response in breast cancer (Kobayashi *et al.*, 2001). A single CML patient produced cytotoxic T lymphocytes after DC vaccination (Fujii *et al.*, 1999). DC vaccination with tumor lysates showed some benefits in children with fibrosacroma (Geiger *et al.*, 2000).

Results in renal cell carcinoma appear to be promising, but perhaps more unexpected have been the responses noted in patients with brain tumours (Kikuchi *et al.*, 2001; Yu *et al.*, 2001). As gliomas break the classic blood/brain barrier, the ability to deliver effector T lymphocytes to this site is probably unimpaired.

Key issues such as the timing of DC collection or Mo-DC generation, disease status then and at the time of vaccination, confound interpretation.

Phase III clinical trials

A phase III study (Valone *et al.*, 2001) has been completed in patients with hormone-refactory, progressive metastatic prostatic cancer and analysis showed promising outcome in a subset of patients. A second phase III trial in hormone-sensitive patients is being initiated.

Further phase II studies are being explored in multiple myeloma (Valone *et al.*, 2001).

A phase III study performed by the Dermato-Oncology Working Group in melanoma (Nestle, Banchereau, & Hart, 2001) will compare Mo-DC vaccination with melanoma peptides with conventional treatment with dacarbazine. Other phase II studies are establishing protocols, which will encourage phase III studies.

Adverse events have been limited. Minor discomfort at injection sites, minor febrile reactions, hypotension (with infusions), and myalgia have been reported. No definite treatment-related hematological, hepatic, or renal toxicity has resulted. The greatest concern has been the possibility of life-threatening or debilitating autoimmune reactions, which would undo the benefits of the beneficial antitumor response. One view is that this problem has been minimal because relatively weak immune responses have been generated. The alternative view is that where patients have been at risk, the natural tolerance or regulating mechanisms have prevented such detrimental self-reactivity. In the case of melanoma, vaccination against melanoma differentiation antigens might lead to destruction of melanocyte-containing tissue compartments such as the brain or the eye. To date, no serious autoimmune events have been reported, although an allergic reaction to exogenous protein has (Mackensen *et al.,* 2000b). A few patients presented with antinuclear antibodies or antithyroid antibodies without evolving further. Interestingly, the use of melanoma tumor lysates as antigens will induce widespread vitiligo in a significant proportion of patients with metastasizing melanoma. These data demonstrate the power of immune activation against self-antigens using DC pulsed with tumor lysates, and emphasise that careful selection of target antigens will continue to be a major issue.

Given the animal model predictions, the paucity of autoimmune problems is most intriguing. As most TAA generate low affinity CTL responses, it is argued that this may be protective (Gilboa, 2001). An interesting experiment attempting to generate a deliberate auto-antigen response in vitro suggested that the RNA loading system preserved tolerance (Heiser *et al.,* 2001).

Monitoring immune responses and tumor escape

There is an urgent need to identify credible surrogate markers of an immune response that will correlate with clinical responses. Until these techniques are identified or validated, the encouraging results to date can only be progressed via careful trial design, notably by selecting homogenous patient groups to study and documenting their clinical response by well accepted clinical monitoring using current radiological or laboratory (tumor marker) methods. If and when surrogate immunological markers are validated these may be used to test the multiplicity of variables discussed, which have yet to be optimized. These can be incorporated into phase III trials. At present, it is essential that DC vaccination studies are carried out in association with laboratory facilities that can provide a full range of immunological laboratory studies.

It is assumed, but not yet proven (given the limited phase I/II clinical data showing a correlation), that DC vaccination should be optimized to produce maximal TAA specific CTL responses (Table 112.5). DC vaccination may be able to boost the frequency of an existing CTL precursor pool but maintaining this as a memory response appears to be difficult (Thurner *et al.,* 1999a; Toungouz *et al.,* 2001). Again, it is hoped that the crucial high affinity responses (Zeh *et al.,* 1999) will be developed by DC vaccination. Chromium release assays using tumor cell targets is a laudable goal; however, this is clearly not widely achievable. Nonetheless, the ability to isolate and amplify tumor RNA allows autologous tumor target substitutes to be created from patients' Epstein-Barr Virus–transformed B cells or other cell sources (Nair *et al.,* 1999; Heiser *et al.,* 2001). The EliSpot technique is now being widely applied and with observer-independent counting methodology now available, this is providing useful information regarding interferon-γ producing CD8+ T lymphocyte responses providing that sensitization in vitro is performed first; flow cytometry detection of cytokine-producing

cells may also be as sensitive. This technique can also be combined with specific T cell receptor analysis. Analysis of specific TCR receptors for HLA class I restricted peptides is now possible using biotinylated soluble HLA-A2 (i.e., locus allele-specific) TAA peptide–loaded tetramers and these can be detected by flow cytometry. Alternative technology uses a different recombinant soluble (Fc-HLA-A2) dimer loaded with TAA peptide. Data in melanoma, chronic myeloid leukemia, and bowel cancer suggests that the pre-existing TAA-specific T cell frequency is of the order of 0.1%–2.0%. (Lee *et al.,* 1999; Molldrem *et al.,* 2000) and this can be expanded. However, it is very clear that TAA-specific T lymphocytes do not necessarily have antitumor activity. The functional contribution of the tetramer positive cells may even be a negative one. Most studies necessarily sample the blood but it is a valid point that direct tumor sampling may be required, as effective CTL may traffic from the blood to the tumor site.

There is good evidence that CD4+ helper T-lymphocyte responses driven by DC contribute to CTL development. CD4+ TAA specific responses have also be shown to contribute to antitumor responses, not only as direct cytotoxic (class II restricted effectors), but also indirectly via recruitment and activation of other cells types. Classically, this is considered to be measured as part of the delayed-type hypersensitivity (DTH) response. An increase in the DTH response has been documented after DC vaccination and there may be some correlation with clinical outcome (Nestle *et al.,* 1998; Banchereau *et al.,* 2001). DC are also capable of activating NK responses (Fernandez *et al.,* 1999) and Flt-3L effects have been shown to be at least in part due to a direct NK-activating effect (Lynch *et al.,* 1997).

Cancers evolve other methods of immune evasion apart from avoiding DC initiation and presentation of the immune response. Thus, they must be monitored too. In patients whose disease has progressed through conventional therapy there has been extensive opportunity for selective pressure to evolve tumor variants. The malignant cells may produce a host of factors, which directly compromise immune cell function, e.g., TGF-β, VEGF, and even products such as PSA, which has only

Table 112.5. *Optimization of dendritic cells for therapy*

- Isolate of DC with minimal perturbation
- Avoid exposure to foreign proteins
- Optimize antigen uptake capacity, i.e., expression of innate receptors
- Provide optimal antigen for optimal period
- Store (cryopreserve) cells
- Incubate (thaw) with cytokines/chemokines, which optimize migratory capacity
- Consider administration of molecular ligands/cytokines/chemokines which direct co-stimulation phenotype and the type of T lymphocyte response

Abbreviation: DC, dendritic cells.

recently been shown to have immunosuppressive qualities (Kennedy-Smith *et al.,* 2002). More importantly in terms of CTL effectors and defects in tumor antigen processing, antigen display and the TAA tumors display, it is a moot point whether this merits individualizing therapy at this juncture. However, loss of MHC antigens in advanced disease may reflect a hopeless situation and some would argue that rational trial design would exclude such patients rather than waste resources in uninformative cases.

There is clear consensus that the best results will be obtained in patients with MRD. This not only minimizes the risk of tumor escape, but may provide an optimal immune environment for DC initiation of an effective immune response. As with chemotherapy protocols, the aim must be tumor eradication and not just control. Careful study design is required for this population, and integrating DC immunotherapy into an overall treatment program involving other modalities (with a functional immune system) can be challenging. Common diseases susceptible to immunotherapy without standard curative protocols, such as multiple myeloma and low grade NHL, should be investigated early (Hart & Hill, 1999).

Clinical prospects for dendritic cell therapy after HSC transplantation

One of the fundamental assumptions in regard to tumor immunotherapy is that it will operate in support of conventional surgery, radiotherapy, and chemotherapy. Thus, DC immunotherapy in any form is most likely to be applied to patients who have achieved a MRD state after either autologous or allogeneic HSCT (Fig. 112.5).

Allogeneic HSC transplantation

The ability to target DC and influence their function may well contribute significantly to facilitating allogeneic HSCT across currently accepted, and perhaps even greater, antigenic disparities. Immunosuppressive therapies directed against host DC may include antibody-targeted reagents (e.g., CMRF-44 or CD83), or pharmacologic compounds designed to inhibit DC function. This, combined with T-lymphocyte depletion of allogeneic HSC grafts, should result in an immunologic paralysis, which will allow engraftment without significant acute GVHD. It remains to be shown whether DC depletion from donor HSCT will also contribute to reduce acute GVHD. Subsequent T-cell reconstitution may be delayed. Alternative use of DC preparations may facilitate allogeneic HSCT. Thus, certain mouse DC preparation are capable of generating allogeneic tolerance. These may be used as a means of tolerizing allospecific T lymphocytes—a variation on current tolerance anergy inducing protocols (Tzachanis *et al.,* 2002). Initial mouse data appear to rule out the possibility that cytokine-modified donor DC reduce, rather than stimulate, acute GVHD (MacDonald *et al.,* 2003), despite alternative suggestions in solid organ transplants (Hackstein *et al.,* 2001).

Having achieved a MRD state, two approaches to DC tumor immunotherapy might be considered in both allograft and autograft recipients. The first would involve in vivo administration of DC loaded in vitro with antigen. The second would be to evolve a more completely engineered in vitro DC-stimulated T-lymphocyte product for reinfusion as appropriate to the patient. At a practical level, the former is preferable. The use of DC to generate tumor-specific T lymphocytes for passive T-cell therapy may provide more control over the immune response. Ultimately, both cellular components may need to be given to patients as part of ongoing protocols for several years to provide sufficient T-lymphocyte memory. Applying DC immunotherapy after allogeneic HSCT will be challenging. Some options may be readily achieveable subject to ethical considerations. Thus, vaccinating donors with TAA to maximize T-cell precursor frequency prior to transplantation, as has been done with immunoglobulin idiotype (Kwak *et al.,* 1995), is one option. Expanding T cells in a normal non-immunosuppressed environment has much to commend it.

For DC vaccination of patients after allo-HSCT, irradiated donor DC might be considered an alternative to DLI. The same outcome is predicted—an allogeneic T-lymphocyte response which might be antileukemia or antitumor, but with the attendant risk of acute GVHD. Dose titrations of DC will need to be

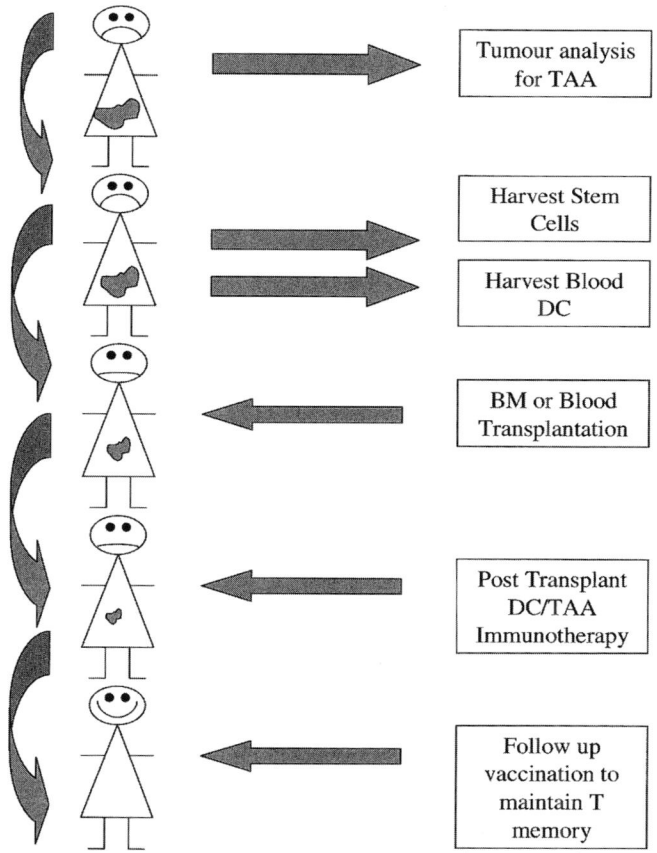

Figure 112.5. A strategy for using DC therapy after HSCT

explored as for DLI. There is no reason to expect this will be more effective or easier than DLI. Optimal timing and the management of immunosuppression will be key issues to clarify. More appropriately, donor DC might be exposed to recipient TAA in one of the antigenic forms described earlier. This has been attempted in four patients and some antileukemic activity was observed with minimal GVHD (Fujii *et al.*, 2001).

Autologous HSC transplantation

The strategy after autologous HSCT is likely to be a development of current DC immunotherapy schedules. Immunotherapy is, as stated, likely to be most effective in a MRD state. Therefore, applying it in patients after autologous HSCT may generate the best results. Two key issues must be considered. Harvesting or producing DC may not be simple. It is possible to harvest them pretransplant. Alternatively, as they appear to reconstitute fairly readily after HSCT, they may be harvested then, when, theoretically, malignant cell contamination is minimized. The second issue yet to be established is the time at which there is sufficient T-lymphocyte reconstitution to allow the optimal response to DC vaccination. Two reports from Stanford University (Reichardt *et al.*, 1999; Liso *et al.*, 2000) describe the results of DC Ig idiotype vaccination after autologous HSCT for myeloma. The results were disappointing but this may reflect the TAA chosen. This area will benefit greatly from optimized use of TAA preparations. In this context, there is no obstacle to the use of tumor lysates or whole cell RNA in an investigational program capable of recognizing new TAA.

References

Adema, G. J., Hartgers, F., Verstraten, R. *et al.* (1997). A dendritic-cell-derived C-C chemokine that preferentially attracts naive T cells. *Nature,* **387,** 713–715.

Albert, M. L., Jegathesan, M., & Darnell, R. B. (2001). Dendritic cell maturation is required for the cross-tolerization of CD8+ T cells. *Nature Immunology,* **2,** 1010–1017.

Albert, M. L., Sauter, B., & Bhardwaj, N. (1998). Dendritic cells acquire antigen from apoptotic cells and induce class I-restricted CTLs. *Nature,* **392,** 86–89.

Almand, B., Clark, J. I., Nikitina, E. *et al.* (2001). Increased production of immature myeloid cells in cancer patients: a mechanism of immunosuppression in cancer. *Journal of Immunology,* **166,** 678–689.

Alyea, E., Weller, E., Schlossman, R. *et al.* (2001). T-cell–depleted allogeneic bone marrow transplantation followed by donor lymphocyte infusion in patients with multiple myeloma: induction of graft-versus-myeloma effect. *Blood,* **98,** 934–939.

Andersen, M. H., Keikavoussi, P., Brocker, E. B. *et al.,* (2001). Induction of systemic CTL responses in melanoma patients by dendritic cell vaccination: cessation of CTL responses is associated with disease progression. *International Journal of Cancer,* **94,** 820–824.

Andersen, M. H., Pedersen, L. O., Becker, J. C. *et al.* (2001). Identification of a cytotoxic T lymphocyte response to the apoptosis inhibitor protein survivin in cancer patients. *Cancer Research,* **61,** 869–872.

Anderson, D. M., Maraskovsky, E., Billingsley, W. L. *et al.* (1997). A homologue of the TNF receptor and its ligand enhance T-cell growth and dendritic-cell function. *Nature,* **390,** 175–179.

Apostolopoulos, V., McKenzie, I.F.C., & Pieterz, G. A. (1996). Breast cancer immunotherapy: current status and future prospects. *Immunology and cell Biology,* **74,** 457–464.

Apperley, J., Mauro, F., & Goldman, J. (1988). Bone marrow transplantation for chronic myeloid leukaemia in first chronic phase: importance of a graft-versus-leukaemia effect. *British Journal of Haematology,* **69,** 239–245.

Ardavin, C., Waanders, G., Ferrero, I. *et al.* (1996). Expression and presentation of endogenous mouse mammary tumor virus superantigens by thymic and splenic dendritic cells and B cells. *Journal of Immunology,* **157,** 2789–2794.

Ardeshna, K. M., Corney, C. P., Ings, S. J. *et al.* (2000). A clinically applicable method for the ex vivo generation of antigen-presenting cells from CD34+ progenitors. *Vox Sanguinis,* **79,** 46–52.

Arpinati, M., Green, C. L., Heimfeld, S. *et al.* (2000). Granulocyte-colony stimulating factor mobilizes T helper 2-inducing dendritic cells. *Blood,* **95,** 2484–2490.

Asselin-Paturel, C., Boonstra, A., Dalod, M. *et al.* (2001). Mouse type I IFN-producing cells are immature APCs with plasmacytoid morphology. *Nature Immunology,* **2,** 1144–1150.

Badros, A., Barlogie, B., Siegel, E. *et al.* (2002). Improved outcome of allogeneic transplantation in high-risk multiple myeloma patients after nonmyeloablative conditioning. *Journal of Clinical Oncology,* **20,** 1295–1303.

Banchereau, J., Briere, F., Caux, C. *et al.* (2000). Immunobiology of dendritic cells. *Annual Review of Immunology,* **18,** 767–811.

Banchereau, J., Palucka, A. K., Dhodapkar, M. *et al.* (2001). Immune and clinical responses in patients with metastatic melanoma to CD34(+) progenitor-derived dendritic cell vaccine. *Cancer Research,* **61,** 6451–6458.

Banchereau, J. & Steinman, R. M. (1998). Dendritic cells and the control of immunity. *Nature,* **392,** 245–252.

Barratt-Boyes, S. M.(1996). Making the most of mucin: a novel target for tumor immunotherapy. *Cancer Immunology Immunotherapy: CII,* **43,** 142–151.

Bell, D., Chomarat, P., Broyles, D. *et al.* (1999). In breast carcinoma tissue, immature dendritic cells reside within the tumor, whereas mature dendritic cells are located in peritumoral areas. *Journal of Experimental Medicine,* **190,** 1417–1426.

Belldegrun, A., Pierce, W., Kaboo, R. *et al.* (1993). Interferon-α primed tumor-infiltrating lymphocytes combined with interleukin-2 and interferon-α as therapy for metastatic renal cell carcinoma. *Journal of Urology,* **150,** 1384–1390.

Bellone, M., Cantarella, D., Castiglioni, P. *et al.* (2000). Relevance of the tumor antigen in the validation of three vaccination strategies for melanoma. *Journal of Immunology,* **165,** 2651–2656.

Bendandi, M., Gocke, C. D., Kobrin, C. B. *et al.* (1999). Complete molecular remissions induced by patient-specific vaccination plus granulocyte-monocyte colony-stimulating factor against lymphoma. *Nature Medicine,* **5,** 1171–1177.

Bendriss-Vermare, N., Barthelemy, C., Durand, I. *et al.* (2001). Human thymus contains IFN-alpha-producing CD11c(−), myeloid CD11c(+), and mature interdigitating dendritic cells. *Journal of Clinical Investigation*, **107**, 835–844.

Berenson, J. R., Vescio, R. A., & Said, J. (1998). Multiple myeloma: the cells of origin—a two way street. (Review). *Leukemia*, **12**, 121–127.

Bjorck, P., Lie, W. R., Woulfe, S. L. *et al.* (2002). Progenipoietin-generated dendritic cells exhibit anti-tumor efficacy in a therapeutic murine tumor model. *International Journal of Cancer*, **100**, 586–591.

Blazar, B. R., McKenna, H. J., Panoskaltsis-Mortari, A. *et al.* (2001). Flt3 ligand (FL) treatment of murine donors does not modify graft-versus-host disease (GVHD) but FL treatment of recipients post-bone marrow transplantation accelerates GVHD lethality. *Biology of Blood and Marrow Transplantation*, **7**, 197–207.

Blom, B., Ho, S., Antonenko, S. *et al.* (2000). Generation of interferon alpha-producing predendritic cell (Pre-DC)2 from human CD34(+) hematopoietic stem cells [In Process Citation]. *Journal of Experimental Medicine*, **192**, 1785–1796.

Borkowski, T. A., Letterio, J. J., Farr, A. G. *et al.* (1996). A role for endogenous transforming growth factor beta 1 in Langerhans cell biology: the skin of transforming growth factor beta 1 null mice is devoid of epidermal Langerhans cells. *Journal of Experimental Medicine*, **184**, 2417–2422.

Brewer, Y., Bewick, M., Palmer, A. *et al.* (1989). Prevention of renal allograft rejection by perfusion with antileukocyte common monoclonal antibodies is dependent on good uptake of antibody by interstitial dendritic cells. *Transplantation Proceedings*, **21**, 1772–1773.

Brickner, A. G., Warren, E. H., Caldwell, J. A. *et al.* (2001). The immunogenicity of a new human minor histocompatibility antigen results from differential antigen processing. *Journal of Experimental Medicine*, **193**, 195–206.

Brossart, P., Wirths, S., Stuhler, G. *et al.* (2000). Induction of cytotoxic T-lymphocyte responses in vivo after vaccinations with peptide-pulsed dendritic cells. *Blood*, **96**, 3102–3108.

Brown, R. D., Pope, B., Murray, A. *et al.* (2001). Dendritic cells from patients with myeloma are numerically normal but functionally defective as they fail to up-regulate CD80 (B7-1) expression after huCD40LT stimulation because of inhibition by transforming growth factor-beta(1) and interleukin-10. *Blood*, **98**, 2992–2998.

Burch, P. A., Breen, J. K., Buckner, J. C. *et al.* (2000). Priming tissue-specific cellular immunity in a phase I trial of autologous dendritic cells for prostate cancer. *Clinical Cancer Research*, **6**, 2175–2182.

Candido, K. A., Shimizu, K., McLaughlin, J. C. *et al.* (2001). Local administration of dendritic cells inhibits established breast tumor growth: implications for apoptosis-inducing agents. *Cancer Research*, **61**, 228–236.

Cella, M., Facchetti, F., Lanzavecchia, A. *et al.* (2000). Plasmacytoid dendritic cells activated by influenza virus and CD40L drive a potent TH1 polarization. *Nature Immunology*, **1**, 305–310.

Cella, M., Jarrossay, D., Facchietti, F. *et al.* (1999). Plasmacytoid monocytes migrate to inflamed lymph nodes and produce large amounts of type I interferon. *Nature Medicine*, **8**, 919–929.

Celluzzi, C. M. & Falo, D. L. (1998). Cutting edge: physical interaction between dendritic cells and tumor cells results in an immunogen that induces protective and therapeutic tumor rejection. *Journal of Immunology*, **160**, 3081–3085.

Cervantes, F., Verfaillie, C., McGlave, P. B. *et al.* (1996). Autologous activated natural killer cells (ANK) suppress CML progenitors but spare normal hematopoiesis in long term bone marrow cultures (LTC). *Blood*, **87**, 2476.

Chang, A. E., Redman, B. G., Whitfield, J. R. *et al.* (2002a). A phase I trial of tumor lysate–pulsed dendritic cells in the treatment of advanced cancer. *Clinical Cancer Research*, **8**, 1021–1032.

Chang, C. C., Ciubotariu, R., Manavalan, J. S. *et al.* (2002b). Tolerization of dendritic cells by T(S) cells: the crucial role of inhibitory receptors ILT3 and ILT4. *Nature Immunology*, **3**, 237–243.

Chaux, P., Hammann, A., Martin, F. *et al.* (1993). Surface phenotype and functions of tumor-infiltrating dendritic cells: CD8 expression by a cell subpopulation. *European Journal of Immunology*, **23**, 2517–2525.

Chaux, P., Moutet, M., Faivre, J. *et al.* (1996). Inflammatory cells infiltrating human colorectal carcinomas express HLA class II but not B7-1 and B7-2 costimulatory molecules of the T-cell activation. *Laboratory Investigation*, **74**, 975–983.

Chen, A. I., McAdam, A. J., Buhlmann, J. E. *et al.* (1999). Ox40-ligand has a critical costimulatory role in dendritic cell: T cell interactions. *Immunity*, **11**, 689–698.

Childs, R. & Barrett, J. (2002). Nonmyeloablative stem cell transplantation for solid tumors: expanding the application of allogeneic immunotherapy. *Seminars in Hematology*, **39**, 63–71.

Childs, R., Chernoff, A., Contentin, N. *et al.* (2000). Regression of metastatic renal-cell carcinoma after nonmyeloablative allogeneic peripheral-blood stem-cell transplantation. *New England Journal of Medicine*, **343**, 750–758.

Childs, R., Epperson, D., Bahceci, E. *et al.* (1999). Molecular remission of chronic myeloid leukaemia following a non-myeloablative allogeneic peripheral blood stem cell transplant: in vivo and in vitro evidence for a graft-versus-leukaemia effect. *British Journal of Haematology*, **107**, 396–400.

Choudhury, A., Gajewski, J. L., Liang, J. C. *et al.* (1997). Use of leukemic dendritic cells for the generation of antileukemic cellular cytotoxicity against Philadelphia chromosome-positive chronic myelogenous leukemia. *Blood*, **89**, 1133–1142.

Cohen, P. J., Cohen, P. A., Rosenberg, S. A. *et al.* (1994). Murine epidermal Langerhans cells and splenic dendritic cells present tumor-associated antigens to primed T cells. *European Journal of Immunology*, **24**, 315–319.

Coventry, B. J., Lee, P. L., Gibbs, D. *et al.* (2002). Dendritic cell density and activation status in human breast cancer—CD1a, CMRF-44, CMRF-56 and CD-83 expression. *British Journal of Cancer*, **86**, 546–551.

Dabadghao, S., Bergenbrant, S., Anton, D. *et al.* (1998). Anti-idiotypic T cell activation in multiple myeloma induced by M-component fragments presented by dendritic cells. *British Journal of Haematology*, **100**, 647–654.

Datta, A., Barret, A., & Jiang, Y. (1994). Distinct T cell population distinguish chronic myeloid leukaemia cells from lymphocytes in the same individual: a model for separating GVHD from GVL reactions. *Bone Marrow Transplantation,* **14,** 517–524.

de Saint-Vis, B., Vincent, J., Vandenabeele, S. *et al.* (1998). A novel lysosome-associated membrane glycoprotein, DC-LAMP, induced upon DC maturation, is transiently expressed in MHC Class II compartment. *Immunity,* **9,** 325–336.

DeBenedette, M. A., Shahinian, A., Mak, T. W. *et al.* (1997). Costimulation of CD28– T lymphocytes by 4-1BB ligand. *Journal of Immunology,* **158,** 551–559.

den Haan, J. M., Meadows, L. M., Wang, W. *et al.* (1998). The minor histocompatibility antigen HA-1: a diallelic gene with a single amino acid polymorphism. *Science,* **279,** 1054–1057.

Dhodapkar, M. V., Steinman, R. M., Krasovsky, J. *et al.* (2001). Antigen-specific inhibition of effector T cell function in humans after injection of immature dendritic cells. *Journal of Experimental Medicine,* **193,** 233–238.

Dickinson, A. M., Wang, X. N., Sviland, L. *et al.* (2002). In situ dissection of the graft-versus-host activities of cytotoxic T cells specific for minor histocompatibility antigens. *Nature Medicine,* **8,** 410–414.

Dutoit, V., Rubio-Godoy, V., Pittet, M. J. *et al.* (2002). Degeneracy of antigen recognition as the molecular basis for the high frequency of naive A2/Melan-a peptide multimer(+) CD8(+) T cells in humans. *Journal of Experimental Medicine,* **196,** 207–216.

Dzionek, A., Fuchs, A., Schmidt, P. *et al.* (2000). BDCA-2, BDCA-3, and BDCA-4: three markers for distinct subsets of dendritic cells in human peripheral blood. *Journal of Immunology,* **165,** 6037–6046.

Eggert, A., Schreurs, M., Boerman, O. *et al.* (1999). Biodistribution and vaccine efficiency of murine dendritic cells are dependent on the route of administration. *Cancer Research,* **59,** 3340–3345.

Engelmayer, J., Larsson, M., Lee, A. *et al.* (2001). Mature dendritic cells infected with canarypox virus elicit strong anti-human immunodeficiency virus CD8+ and CD4+ T-cell responses from chronically infected individuals. *Journal of Virology,* **75,** 2142–2153.

Falkenburg, J. H., Goselink, H. M., van der Harst, D. *et al.* (1991). Growth inhibition of clonogenic leukemic precursor cells by minor histocompatibility antigen-specific cytotoxic T lymphocytes. *Journal of Experimental Medicine,* **174,** 27–33.

Fanger, N. A., Voigtlaender, D., Liu, C. *et al.* (1997). Characterization of expression, cytokine regulation, and effector function of the high affinity IgG receptor FcγRI (CD64) expressed on human blood dendritic cells. *Journal of Immunology,* **158,** 3090–3098.

Fawell, S., Seery, J., Daikh, Y. *et al.* (1994). Tat-mediated delivery of heterologous proteins into cells. *Proceedings of the National Academy of Sciences USA,* **91,** 664–668.

Fearnley, D. B., McLellan, A. D., Mannering, S. I. *et al.* (1997a). Isolation of human blood dendritic cells using the CMRF-44 monoclonal antibody: implications for studies on antigen presenting cell function and immunotherapy. *Blood,* **89,** 3708–3716.

Fearnley, D. B., McLellan, A. D., Troy, A. J. *et al.* (1997b). Non-lineage antigens and dendritic cells functional studies: the CMRF-44 antibody identifies blood precursor and functionally mature dendritic cells. In *Leucocyte Typing VI,* ed. T. Kishimoto, pp. 601–602. New York: Garland Publishing Inc.

Fearnley, D. B., Whyte, L. F., Carnoutsos, S. A. *et al.* (1999). Monitoring human blood dendritic cell numbers in normal individuals and in stem cell transplantation. *Blood,* **93,** 728–736.

Ferlazzo, G., Tsang, M. L., Moretta, L. *et al.* (2002). Human dendritic cells activate resting natural killer (NK) cells and are recognized via the NKp30 receptor by activated NK cells. *Journal of Experimental Medicine,* **195,** 343–351.

Fernandez, N. C., Lozier, A., Flament, C. *et al.* (1999). Dendritic cells directly trigger NK cell functions: cross-talk relevant in innate anti-tumor immune responses in vivo. *Nature Medicine,* **5,** 405–411.

Ferrara, J.L.M. (1994). Paradigm shift for graft-versus-host disease. *Bone Marrow Transplantation,* **14,** 183–184.

Flamand, V., Sornasse, T., Thielemans, K. *et al.* (1994). Murine dendritic cells pulsed in vitro with tumor antigen induce tumor resistance in vivo. *European Journal of Immunology,* **24,** 605–610.

Flores-Romo, L. (2001). In vivo maturation and migration of dendritic cells. *Immunology,* **102,** 255–262.

Fong, L., Brockstedt, D., Benike, C. *et al.* (2001a). Dendritic cell-based xenoantigen vaccination for prostate cancer immunotherapy. *Journal of Immunology,* **167,** 7150–7156.

Fong, L., Brockstedt, D., Benike, C. *et al.* (2001b). Dendritic cells injected via different routes induce immunity in cancer patients. *Journal of Immunology,* **166,** 4254–4259.

Fong, L. & Engleman, E. G. (2000). Dendritic cells in cancer immunotherapy. *Annual Review of Immunology,* **18,** 245–273.

Fontaine, P., Roy-Proulx, G., Knafo, L. *et al.* (2001). Adoptive transfer of minor histocompatibility antigen-specific T lymphocytes eradicates leukemia cells without causing graft-versus-host disease. *Nature Medicine,* **7,** 789–794.

Fox, S. B., Jones, M., Dunnill, M. S. *et al.* (1989). Langerhans cells in human lung tumors: immunohistological study. *Histopathology,* **14,** 269–275.

Frazer, I. H., Thomas, R., Zhou, J. *et al.* (1999). Potential strategies utilised by papillomavirus to evade host immunity. *Immunological Reviews,* **168,** 131–142.

Freudenthal, P. S. & Steinman, R. M. (1990). The distinct surface of human blood dendritic cells, as observed after an improved isolation method. *Proceedings of the National Academy of Sciences USA,* **87,** 7698–7702.

Fujii, S., Shimizu, K., Fujimoto, K. *et al.* (1999). Analysis of a chronic myelogenous leukemia patient vaccinated with leukemic dendritic cells following autologous peripheral blood stem cell transplantation. *Japanese Journal of Cancer Research: Gann,* **90,** 1117–1129.

Fujii, S., Shimizu, K., Fujimoto, K. *et al.* (2001). Treatment of post-transplanted, relapsed patients with hematological malignancies by infusion of HLA-matched, allogeneic-dendritic cells (DCs) pulsed with irradiated tumor cells and primed T cells. *Leukemia & Lymphoma,* **42,** 357–369.

Gabrilovich, D. I., Chen, H. L., Girgis, K. R. *et al.* (1996a). Production of vascular endothelial growth factor by human tumors inhibits the functional maturation of dendritic cells. *Nature Medicine,* **2,** 1096.

Gabrilovich, D. I., Corak, J., Ciernik, I. F. *et al.* (1997). Decreased antigen presentation by dendritic cells in patients with breast cancer. *Clinical Cancer Research,* **3,** 483–490.

Gabrilovich, D. I., Nadaf, S., Corak, J. *et al.* (1996b). Dendritic cells in antitumor immune responses. *Cellular Immunology, 170,* 111–119.

Geiger, J., Hutchinson, R., Hohenkirk, L. *et al.* (2000). Treatment of solid tumours in children with tumor-lysate-pulsed dendritic cells (In Process Citation). *Lancet, 356,* 1163–1165 (Letter).

Geijtenbeek, T. B., Torensma, R., van Vliet, S. J. *et al.* (2000). Identification of DC-SIGN, a novel dendritic cell-specific ICAM-3 receptor that supports primary immune responses. *Cell, 100,* 575–585.

Gilboa, E. (2001). The risk of autoimmunity associated with tumor immunotherapy. *Nature Immunology, 2,* 789–792.

Goldman, J., Apperley, J., & Jones, L. (1986). Bone marrow transplantation for patients with chronic myeloid leukaemia. *New England Journal of Medicine, 314,* 202–207.

Golumbek, P., Levitsky, H., Jaffee, L. *et al.* (1993). The antitumor immune response as a problem of self-nonself discrimination: Implications for immunotherapy. *Immunological Reviews, 12,* 183–192.

Gong, J., Avigan, D., Chen, D. *et al.* (2000a). Activation of antitumor cytotoxic T lymphocytes by fusions of human dendritic cells and breast carcinoma cells [published erratum appears in Proc Natl Acad Sci USA 2000 Apr 25;97(9):5011]. *Proceedings of the National Academy of Sciences USA, 97,* 2715–2718.

Gong, J., Chen, D., Kashiwaba, M. *et al.* (1997). Induction of antitumour activity by immunization with fusions of dendritic and carcinoma cells. *Nature Medicine, 3,* 558–561.

Gong, J., Nikrui, N., Chen, D. *et al.* (2000b). Fusions of human ovarian carcinoma cells with autologous or allogeneic dendritic cells induce antitumor immunity. *Journal of Immunology, 165,* 1705–1711.

Goulmy, E., Schipper, R., Pool, J. *et al.* (1996). Mismatches of minor histocompatibility antigens between HLA-identical donors and recipients and the development of graft-versus-host disease after bone marrow transplantation. *New England Journal of Medicine, 334,* 281–285.

Gribben, J. G., Guinan, E. C., Boussiotis, V. A. *et al.* (1996). Complete blockade of B7 family-mediated costimulation is necessary to induce human alloantigen-specific anergy: a method to ameliorate graft-versus-host disease and extend the donor pool. *Blood, 87,* 4887–4893.

Groux, H., Bigler, M., de Vries, J. E. *et al.* (1996). Interleukin-10 induces a long-term antigen-specific anergic state in human CD4+ T cells. *Journal of Experimental Medicine, 184,* 19–29.

Guglielmi, C., Arcese, W., Dazzi, F. *et al.* (2002). Donor lymphocyte infusion for relapsed chronic myelogenous leukemia: prognostic relevance of the initial cell dose. *Blood, 100,* 397–405.

Guinan, E. C., Gribben, J. G., Boussiotis, V. A. *et al.* (1994). Pivotal role of the B7:CD28 pathway in transplantation tolerance and tumor immunity. *Blood, 84,* 3261.

Hackstein, H., Morelli, A. E., & Thomson, A. W. (2001). Designer dendritic cells for tolerance induction: guided not misguided missiles. *Trends in Immunology, 22,* 437–442.

Harris, N. L., Watt, V., Ronchese, F. *et al.* (2002). Differential T cell function and fate in lymph node and nonlymphoid tissues. *Journal of Experimental Medicine, 195,* 317–326.

Hart, D. N. & Hill, G. R. (1999). Dendritic cell immunotherapy for cancer: application to low-grade lymphoma and multiple myeloma. *Immunology and Cell Biology, 77,* 451–459.

Hart, D.N.J. (1997). Dendritic cells: unique leucocyte populations which control the primary immune response. *Blood, 90,* 3245–3287.

Hart, D.N.J., Clark, G. J., MacDonald, K. *et al.* (2000). 7th leucocyte differentiation antigen workshop DC section summary. In *Leucocyte Typing VII,* ed. D. Mason. Oxford: Oxford University Press.

Hart, D.N.J. & Fabre, J. W. (1981a). Localisation of MHC antigens in long surviving rat renal allografts: probable implication of passenger leucocytes in graft adaptation. *Transplantation Proceedings, 13,* 95–99.

Hart, D.N.J. & Fabre, J. W. (1981b). The mechanism of induction of passive enhancement: evidence for an interaction of enhancing antibody with donor interstitial dendritic cells. *Transplantation, 32,* 431–436.

Hart, D.N.J. & Fabre, J. W. (1981c). Passive enhancement of rat renal allografts using monoclonal xenoantibodies. *Transplantation, 32,* 431–436.

Hart, D.N.J. & Fabre, J. W. (1981d). Demonstration and characterization of Ia-positive dendritic cells in the interstitial connective tissues of rat heart and other tissues, not brain. *Journal of Experimental Medicine, 154,* 347–361.

Hart, D.N.J., Fearnley, D. B., Sorg, R. V. *et al.* (1997). Non-lineage antigens and dendritic cell studies: the CMRF-56 mononuclear antigen identifies dendritic cells after brief culture of human peripheral blood mononuclear cells. In *Leucocyte Typing VI,* ed. T. Kishimoto, pp. 599–601. New York: Garland Publishing Inc.

Heiser, A., Coleman, D., Dannull, J. *et al.* (2002). Autologous dendritic cells transfected with prostate-specific antigen RNA stimulate CTL responses against metastatic prostate tumors. *Journal of Clinical Investigation, 109,* 409–417.

Heiser, A., Maurice, M. A., Yancey, D. R. *et al.* (2001a). Human dendritic cells transfected with renal tumor RNA stimulate polyclonal T-cell responses against antigens expressed by primary and metastatic tumors. *Cancer Research, 61,* 3388–3393.

Heiser, A., Maurice, M. A., Yancey, D. R. *et al.* (2001b). Induction of polyclonal prostate cancer-specific CTL using dendritic cells transfected with amplified tumor RNA. *Journal of Immunology, 166,* 2953–2960.

Hernando, J. J., Park, T. W., Kubler, K. *et al.* (2002). Vaccination with autologous tumour antigen–pulsed dendritic cells. In advanced gynaecological malignancies: clinical and immunological evaluation of a phase I trial. *Cancer Immunology, Immunotherapy: CII, 51,* 45–52.

Heufler, C., Koch, F., Stanzl, U. *et al.* (1996). Interleukin-12 is produced by dendritic cells and mediates T helper 1 development as well as interferon-gamma production by T helper 1 cells. *European Journal of Immunology, 26,* 659–668.

Heufler, C., Topar, G., Koch, F. *et al.* (1992). Cytokine gene expression in murine epidermal cell suspensions: interleukin 1b and macrophage inflammatory protein 1a are selective expressed in Langerhans cells but are differentially regulated in culture. *Journal of Experimental Medicine, 176,* 1221–1226.

Hewitt, H. B., Blake, E. R., & Walder, A. S. (1976). A critique of the evidence for active host defense against cancer, based on personal studies of 27 murine tumours of spontaneous origin. *British Journal of Cancer, 33,* 241–259.

Ho, C. S., Lopez, J. A., Vuckovic, S. *et al.* (2001): Surgical and physical stress increases circulating blood dendritic cell counts independently of monocyte counts. *Blood,* **98,** 140–145.

Ho, C. S., Munster, D., Pyke, C. M. *et al.* (2002). Spontaneous generation and survival of blood dendritic cells in mononuclear cell culture without exogenous cytokines. *Blood,* **99,** 2897–2904.

Hock, B. D., Fearnley, D. B., Boyce, A. *et al.* (1999). Human dendritic cells express a 95 kDa activation/differentiation antigen defined by CMRF-56. *Tissue Antigens,* **53,** 320–334.

Hock, B. D., Kato, M., McKenzie, J. L. *et al.* (2001). A soluble form of CD83 is released from activated dendritic cells and B lymphocytes, and is detectable in normal human sera. *International Immunology,* **13,** 959–967.

Hock, B. D., Starling, G. C., Daniel, P. B. *et al.* (1994). Characterisation of CMRF-44, a novel monoclonal antibody to an activation antigen expressed by the allostimulatory cells within peripheral blood, including dendritic cells. *Immunology,* **83,** 573–581.

Holtl, L., Rieser, C., Papesh, C. *et al.* (1999). Cellular and humoral immune responses in patients with metastatic renal cell carcinoma after vaccination with antigen pulsed dendritic cells. *Journal of Urology,* **161,** 777–782.

Houbiers, J.G.A., Nijman, H. W., van der Burg, S. H. *et al.* (1993). In vitro induction of human cytotoxic T lymphocyte responses against peptides of mutated and wild type p53. *European Journal of Immunology,* **23,** 2072–7.

Houghton, A. N. (1994). Cancer antigens: immune recognition of self and altered self. *Journal of Experimental Medicine,* **180,** 1–4.

Hsu, F. J., Benike, C., Fagnoni, F. *et al.* (1996). Vaccination of patients with B-cell lymphoma using autologous antigen-pulsed dendritic cells. *Nature Medicine,* **2,** 52–58.

Huang, F. P., Platt, N., Wykes, M. *et al.* (2000). A discrete subpopulation of dendritic cells transports apoptotic intestinal epithelial cells to T cell areas of mesenteric lymph nodes. *Journal of Experimental Medicine,* **191,** 435–444.

Huang, Y. W. & Vitetta, E. S. (1995). Immunotherapy of multiple myeloma (Review). *Stem Cells,* **13,** 123–134.

Imamura, M., Hashino, S., & Tanaka, J. (1996). Graft-versus-leukemia effect and its clinical implications. *Leukemia and Lymphoma,* **23,** 477–492.

Ingulli, E., Mondino, A., Khoruts, A. *et al.* (1997). In vivo detection of dendritic cell antigen presentation to CD4+ T cells. *Journal of Experimental Medicine,* **185,** 2133–2141.

Jackson, D. C., Purcell, A. W., Fitzmaurice, C. J. *et al.* (2002). The central role played by peptides in the immune response and the design of peptide-based vaccines against infectious diseases and cancer. *Current Drug Targets,* **3,** 175–196.

Jahnsen, F. L., Lund-Johansen, F., Dunne, J. F. *et al.* (2000). Experimentally induced recruitment of plasmacytoid (CD123high) dendritic cells in human nasal allergy. *Journal of Immunology,* **165,** 4062–4068.

Jansen, J. H., Wientjens, G.-J.H.M., Fibbe, W. E. *et al.* (1989). Inhibition of human macrophage colony formation by interleukin 4. *Journal of Experimental Medicine,* **170,** 577–582.

Jiang, W., Swiggard, W. J., Heufler, C. *et al.* (1995). The receptor DEC-205 expressed by dendritic cells and thymic epithelial cells is involved in antigen processing. *Nature,* **375,** 151–154.

Jiang, Y. Z. & Barrett, J. (1997). The allogeneic CD4+ T-cell–mediated graft-versus-leukemia effect. *Leukemia and Lymphoma,* **28,** 33–42.

Jonuleit, H., Giesecke-Tuettenberg, A., Tuting, T. *et al.* (2001). A comparison of two types of dendritic cell as adjuvants for the induction of melanoma-specific T-cell responses in humans following intranodal injection. *International Journal of Cancer,* **93,** 243–251.

Jonuleit, H., Kuhn, U., Muller, G. *et al.* (1997). Pro-inflammatory cytokines and prostaglandins induce maturation of potent immunostimulatory dendritic cells under fetal calf serum-free conditions. *European Journal of Immunology,* **27,** 3135–3142.

Kadowaki, N., Ho, S., Antonenko, S. *et al.* (2001). Subsets of human dendritic cell precursors express different toll-like receptors and respond to different microbial antigens. *Journal of Experimental Medicine,* **194,** 863–869.

Kahn, H. J., Marks, A., Thom, H. *et al.* (1983). Role of antibody to S100 protein in diagnostic pathology. *American Journal of Clinical Pathology,* **79,** 341–347.

Kaminski, M. S., Zasadny, K. R., & Francis, I. R. (1996). Iodine-131-anti-B1 radioimmunotherapy for B-cell lymphoma. *Journal of Clinical Oncology,* **14,** 1974–1981.

Kato, M., Neil, T. K., Clark, G. J. *et al.* (1998). cDNA cloning of human DEC-205, a putative antigen-uptake receptor on dendritic cells. *Immunogenetics,* **47,** 442–450.

Kato, M., Neil, T. K., Fearnley, D. B. *et al.* (2000). Expression of multilectin receptors and comparative FITC-dextran uptake by human dendritic cells. *International Immunology,* **12,** 1511–1519.

Kennedy-Smith, A. G., McKenzie, J. L., Owen, M. C. *et al.* (2002). Prostate specific antigen inhibits immune responses in vitro: a potential role in prostate cancer. *Journal of Urology,* **168,** 741–747.

Khouri, I. F., Saliba, R. M., Giralt, S. A. *et al.* (2001). Nonablative allogeneic hematopoietic transplantation as adoptive immunotherapy for indolent lymphoma: low incidence of toxicity, acute graft-versus-host disease, and treatment-related mortality. *Blood,* **98,** 3595–3599.

Kikuchi, T., Akasaki, Y., Irie, M. *et al.* (2001). Results of a phase I clinical trial of vaccination of glioma patients with fusions of dendritic and glioma cells. *Cancer Immunology, Immunotherapy: CCI,* **50,** 337–344.

Klangsinsirikul, P., Carter, G. I., Byrne, J. L. *et al.* (2002). Campath-1G causes rapid depletion of circulating host dendritic cells (DCs) before allogeneic transplantation but does not delay donor DC reconstitution. *Blood,* **99,** 2586–91.

Kleijmeer, M. J., Ossevoort, M. A., van Veen, C.J.H. *et al.* (1995). MHC class II compartments and the kinetics of antigen presentation in activated mouse spleen dendritic cells. *Journal of Immunology,* **154,** 5715–5724.

Knight, S. C., Hunt, R., Dore, C. *et al.* (1985). Influence of dendritic cells in tumor growth. *Proceedings of the National Academy of Sciences USA,* **82,** 4495–4497.

Kobayashi, T., Shinohara, H., Toyoda, M. *et al.* (2001). Regression of lymph node metastases by immunotherapy using autologous breast tumor-lysate pulsed dendritic cells: report of a case. *Surgery Today,* **31,** 513–516.

Kolb, H.-J., Schattenburg, A., Goldman, J. M. et al. (1995). Graft-versus-leukemia effect of donor lymphocyte transfusions in marrow grafted patients. Blood, 86, 2041–2072.

Kuchroo, V. K., Das, M. P., Brown, J. A. et al. (1995). B7.1 and B7.2 costimulatory molecules activate differentially the Th1/Th2 developmental pathways: application to autoimmune disease therapy. Cell, 80, 707–718.

Kuckelkorn, U., Ruppert, T., Strehl, B. et al. (2002). Link between organ-specific antigen processing by 20S proteasomes and CD8(+) T cell-mediated autoimmunity. Journal of Experimental Medicine, 195, 983–990.

Kugler, A., Stuhler, G., Walden, P. et al. (2000). Regression of human metastatic renal cell carcinoma after vaccination with tumor cell–dendritic cell hybrids. Nature Medicine, 6, 332–336.

Kwak, L. W., Taub, D. D., Duffey, D. L. et al. (1995). Transfer of myeloma idiotype-specific immunity from an acutely immunised marrow donor. Lancet, 345, 1016–1020.

Lapointe, R., Royal, R. E., Reeves, M. E. et al. (2001). Retrovirally transduced human dendritic cells can generate T cells recognizing multiple MHC class I and class II epitopes from the melanoma antigen glycoprotein 100. Journal of Immunology, 167, 4758–4764.

Lau, R., Wang, F., Jeffery, G. et al. (2001). Phase I trial of intravenous peptide-pulsed dendritic cells in patients with metastatic melanoma. Journal of Immunotherapy, 24, 66–78.

Lechler, R., Aichinger, G., & Lightstone, L. (1996). The endogenous pathway of MHC class II antigen presentation. Immunological Reviews, 151, 51–79.

Lee, P. P., Yee, C., Savage, P. A. et al. (1999). Characterization of circulating T cells specific for tumor-associated antigens in melanoma patients. Nature Medicine, 5, 677–685.

Lim, S. H. & Bailey-wood, R. (1999). Idiotypic protein-pulsed dendritic cell vaccination in multiple myeloma. International Journal of Cancer, 83, 215–22.

Lim, S. H., Wang, Z., Chiriva-Internati, M., & Yue, Y. (2001). Sperm protein 17 is a novel cancer-testis antigen in multiple myeloma. Blood, 97, 1508–1510.

Liso, A., Stockerl-Goldstein, K. E., Auffermann-Gretzinger, S. et al. (2000). Idiotype vaccination using dendritic cells after autologous peripheral blood progenitor cell transplantation for multiple myeloma. Biology of Blood and Marrow Transplantation, 6, 621–627.

Lodge, P. A., Jones, L. A., Bader, R. A. et al. (2000). Dendritic cell-based immunotherapy of prostate cancer: immune monitoring of a phase II clinical trial. Cancer Research, 60, 829–833.

Lopez, J. A., Bioley, G., Turtle, C. et al. (2003a). Single step enrichment of blood DC by positive immunoselection. Journal of Immunological Methods, 274, 47–61.

Lopez, J. A., Crosbie, G. V., Kelly, C. et al. (2003b). Monitoring and Isolation of Blood Dendritic Cells from Apheresis Products in Healthy Individuals: A Platform for Cancer Immunotherapy. Journal of Immunological Methods,

Lopez, J. A. & Hart, D.N.J. (2002). Current issues in Dendritic Cell Cancer Immunotherapy. Current Opinion in Molecular Therapy, 4, 54–63.

Lopez-Jimenez, J., Perez-Oteyza, J., Munoz, A. et al. (1997). Subcutaneous versus intravenous low-dose IL-2 therapy after autologous transplantation: results of a prospective, non-randomized study. Bone Marrow Transplantation, 19, 429–434.

Lynch, D. H., Andreasen, A., Maraskovsky, E. et al. (1997). Flt3 ligand induces tumor regression and antitumor immune responses in vivo. Nature Medicine, 3, 625–630.

MacDonald, K.P.A., Munster, D., Clark, G. C. et al. (2002). Characterization of human blood dendritic cell subsets. Blood, 100, 4512–4520.

MacDonald, K.P.A., Rowe, V., Filippich, C. et al. (2003). Donor pre-treatment with progenipoietin-1 is superior to G-CSF in preventing graft-versus-host disease after allogeneic stem cell transplantation. Blood, 101, 2033–2042.

Mackensen, A., Drager, R., Schlesier, M. et al. (2000a). Presence of IgE antibodies to bovine serum albumin in a patient developing anaphylaxis after vaccination with human peptide-pulsed dendritic cells. Cancer Immunology, Immunotherapy: CCI, 49, 152–156.

Mackensen, A., Herbst, B., Chen, J. L. et al. (2000b). Phase I study in melanoma patients of a vaccine with peptide-pulsed dendritic cells generated in vitro from CD34(+) hematopoietic progenitor cells. International Journal of Cancer, 86, 385–392.

Mackensen, A., Krause, T., Blum, U. et al. (1999). Homing of intravenously and intralymphatically injected human dendritic cells generated in vitro from CD34+ hematopoietic progenitor cells. Cancer Immunology, Immunotherapy: CCI, 48, 118–122.

Mackinnon, S., Papadopoulos, E., & Carabasi, M. (1995). Adoptive immunotherapy evaluating escalating doses of donor leukocytes for relapse of chronic myeloid leukemia after bone marrow transplantation: separation of graft-versus-leukemia responses from graft-versus-host disease. Blood, 86, 1261–1268.

Mahnke, K., Guo, M., Lee, S. et al. (2000). The dendritic cell receptor for endocytosis, DEC-205, can recycle and enhance antigen presentation via major histocompatibility complex class II-positive lysosomal compartments. Journal of Cell Biology, 151, 673–684.

Mannering, S. I., McKenzie, J. L., Fearnley, D. B. et al. (1997). HLA-DR1-restricted bcr-abl (b3a2)-specific CD4+ T lymphocytes respond to dendritic cells pulsed with b3a2 peptide and antigen-presenting cells exposed to b3a2 containing cell lysates. Blood, 90, 290–297.

Mannering, S. I., McKenzie, J. L., & Hart, D. N. (1998). Optimisation of the conditions for generating human DC initiated antigen specific T lymphocyte lines in vitro. Journal of Immunological Methods, 219, 69–83.

Maraskovsky, E., Brasel, K., Teepe, M. et al. (1996). Dramatic increase in the numbers of functionally mature dendritic cells in Flt3 ligand-treated mice: multiple dendritic cell subpopulations identified. Journal of Experimental Medicine, 184, 1953–1962.

Maraskovsky, E., Daro, E., Roux, E. et al. (2000). In vivo generation of human dendritic cell subsets by flt3 ligand [In Process Citation]. Blood, 96, 878–884.

Martin, P., Del Hoyo, G. M., Anjuere, F. et al. (2002). Characterization of a new subpopulation of mouse CD8alpha(+) B220(+) dendritic cells endowed with type 1 interferon production capacity and tolerogenic potential. Blood, 100, 383–390.

Mavroudis, D. & Barrett, J. (1996). The graft-versus-leukemia effect. Current Opinion in Hematology, 3, 423–429.

Mayordomo, J. I., Zorina, T., Storkus, W. J. *et al.* (1995). Bone marrow-derived dendritic cells pulsed with synthetic tumor peptides elicit protective and therapeutic antitumour immunity. *Nature Medicine,* **1,** 1297–1302.

McIlroy, D., Troadec, C., Grassi, F. *et al.* (2001). Investigation of human spleen dendritic cell phenotype and distribution reveals evidence of in vivo activation in a subset of organ donors. *Blood,* **97,** 3470–3477.

McKenzie, J. L., Beard, M.E.J., & Hart, D.N.J. (1984a). Depletion of donor kidney dendritic cells prolongs graft survival. *Transplantation Proceedings,* **16,** 948–951.

McKenzie, J. L., Beard, M.E.J., & Hart, D.N.J. (1984b). Effective depletion of donor dendritic cells prolongs rat cardiac allograft survival. *Transplantation,* **38,** 371–376.

McLellan, A. D., Sorg, R. V., Williams, L. A. *et al.* (1996). Human dendritic cells activate T lymphocytes via a CD40:CD40 ligand-dependent pathway. *European Journal of Immunology,* **26,** 1204–1210.

McMichael, A. & Hanke, T. (2002). The quest for an AIDS vaccine: is the CD8+ T-cell approach feasible? *Nature Reviews Immunology,* **2,** 283–291.

Meehan, K. R., Badros, A., Frankel, S. R. *et al.* (1997). A pilot study evaluating interleukin-2-activated hematopoietic stem cell transplantation for hematologic malignancies. *Journal of Hematotherapy,* **6,** 457–464.

Mehta, J., Powles, R., Singhal, S. *et al.* (1995). Cytokine-mediated immunotherapy with or without donor leukocytes for poor-risk acute myeloid leukemia relapsing after allogeneic bone marrow transplantation. *Bone Marrow Transplantation,* **16,** 133–137.

Mendoza, L., Bubenik, J., Simova, J. *et al.* (2002). Tumor-inhibitory effects of dendritic cells administered at the site of HPV 16-induced neoplasms. *Folia Biologica,* **48,** 114–119.

Metlay, J. P., Witmer-Pack, M. D., Agger, R. *et al.* (1990). The distinct leucocyte integrins of mouse spleen DC as identified with new hamster mAb. *Journal of Experimental Medicine,* **171,** 1753–1771.

Miga, A. J., Masters, S. R., Durell, B. G. *et al.* (2001). Dendritic cell longevity and T cell persistence is controlled by CD154-CD40 interactions. *European Journal of Immunology,* **31,** 959–965.

Molldrem, J. J., Lee, P. P., Wang, C. *et al.* (2000). Evidence that specific T lymphocytes may participate in the elimination of chronic myelogenous leukemia. *Nature Medicine,* **6,** 1018–1023.

Monji, T., Petersons, J., Saund, N. K. *et al.* (2002). Competent dendritic cells derived from CD34+ progenitorsexpress CMRF-44 antigen early in the differentiation pathway. *Immunology and Cell Biology,* **80,** 216–225.

Moretta, A. & Moretta, L. (1997). HLA class I specific inhibitory receptors. *Current Opinion in Immunology,* **9,** 694–701.

Morse, M. A., Coleman, R. E., Akabani, G. *et al.* (1999a). Migration of human dendritic cells after injection in patients with metastatic malignancies. *Cancer Research,* **59,** 56–58.

Morse, M., Deng, Y., Coleman, D. *et al.* (1999b). A phase 1 study of active immunotherapy with carcinoembryonic antigen peptide (CAP-1)-pulsed, autologous human cultured dendritic cells in patients with metastatic cultured dendritic cells in patients with metastatic malignancies expressing carcinoembryonic antigen. *Clinical Cancer Research,* **5,** 1331–1338.

Murphy, G., Tjoa, B., Ragde, H. *et al.* (1996). Phase I clinical trial: T-cell therapy for prostate cancer using autologous dendritic cells pulsed with HLA-A0201-specific peptides from prostate-specific membrane antigen. *Prostate,* **29,** 371–380.

Murphy, G. P., Snow, P., Simmons, S. J. *et al.* (2000). Use of artificial neural networks in evaluating prognostic factors determining the response to dendritic cells pulsed with PSMA peptides in prostate cancer patients. *Prostate,* **42,** 67–72.

Murphy, G. P., Tjoa, B. A., Simmons, S. J. *et al.* (1999a). Infusion of dendritic cells pulsed with HLA-A2-specific prostate-specific membrane antigen peptides: a phase 2 prostate cancer vaccine trial involving patients with hormone-refractory metastatic disease. *Prostate,* **38,** 73–78.

Murphy, G. P., Tjoa, B. A., Simmons, S. J. *et al.* (1999b). Phase II prostate cancer vaccine trial: report of a study involving 37 patients with disease recurrence following primary treatment. *Prostate,* **39,** 54–59.

Mutis, T., Blokland, E., Kester, M. *et al.* (2002). Generation of minor histocompatibility antigen HA-1-specific cytotoxic T cells restricted by nonself HLA molecules: a potential strategy to treat relapsed leukemia after HLA-mismatched stem cell transplantation. *Blood,* **100,** 547–552.

Nacht, M., Ferguson, A. T., Zhang, W. *et al.* (1999). Combining serial analysis of gene expression and array technologies to identify genes differentially expressed in breast cancer. *Cancer Research,* **59,** 5464–5470.

Nair, S. K., Heiser, A., Boczkowski, D. *et al.* (2000). Induction of cytotoxic T cell responses and tumor immunity against unrelated tumors using telomerase reverse transcriptase RNA transfected dendritic cells [see comments]. *Nature Medicine,* **6,** 1011–1017.

Nair, S. K., Hull, S., Coleman, D. *et al.* (1999). Induction of carcinoembryonic antigen (CEA)-specific cytotoxic T-lymphocyte responses in vitro using autologous dendritic cells loaded with CEA peptide or CEA RNA in patients with metastatic malignancies expressing CEA. *International Journal of Cancer,* **82,** 121–124.

Nakano, H., Yanagita, M., & Gunn, M. D. (2001). CD11c(+)B220(+)Gr-1(+) cells in mouse lymph nodes and spleen display characteristics of plasmacytoid dendritic cells. *Journal of Experimental Medicine,* **194,** 1171–1178.

Nelson, D. J., Mukherjee, S., Bundell, C. *et al.* (2001). Tumor progression despite efficient tumor antigen cross-presentation and effective "arming" of tumor antigen-specific CTL. *Journal of Immunology,* **166,** 5557–5566.

Nestle, F. O., Alijagic, S., Gilliet, M. *et al.* (1998). Vaccination of melanoma patients with peptide- or tumor lysate-pulsed dendritic cells. *Nature Medicine,* **4,** 328–332.

Nestle, F. O., Banchereau, J., & Hart, D. (2001). Dendritic cells: On the move from bench to bedside. *Nature Medicine,* **7,** 761–765.

Nijman, H. W., Kleijmeer, M. J., Ossevoort, M. A. *et al.* (1995). Antigen capture and major histocompatibility class II compartments of freshly isolated with cultured human blood dendritic cells. *Journal of Experimental Medicine,* **182,** 163–174.

Norbury, C. C., Chambers, B. J., Prescott, A. R. *et al.* (1997). Constitutive macropinocytosis allows TAP-dependent major histocompatibility complex class I presentation of exogenous soluble antigen by bone marrow-derived dendritic cells. *European Journal of Immunology,* **27,** 280–288.

Oehler, L., Majdic, O., Pickl, W. F. *et al.* (1998). Neutrophil granulocyte-committed cells can be driven to acquire dendritic cell characteristics. *Journal of Experimental Medicine,* **187**, 1019–1028.

Okada, H., Pollack, I. F., Lieberman, F. *et al.* (2001). Gene therapy of malignant gliomas: a pilot study of vaccination with irradiated autologous glioma and dendritic cells admixed with IL-4 transduced fibroblasts to elicit an immune response. *Human Gene Therapy,* **12**, 575–595.

Osterborg, A., Yi, Q., Henriksson, L. *et al.* (1998). Idiotype immunization combined with granulocyte-macrophage colony-stimulating factor in Myeloma patients induced typel, major histocompatibility complex-restricted, Cd8- and Cd4-specific T cell responses. *Blood,* **91**, 2549.

Osugi, Y., Vuckovic, S., & Hart, D.N.J. (2002). Myeloid blood CD11c+ dendritic cells and monocyte derived dendritic cells differ in their ability to stimulate T lymphocytes. *Blood,* **100**, 2858–2866.

Panelli, M. C., Wunderlich, J., Jeffries, J. *et al.* (2000). Phase 1 study in patients with metastatic melanoma of immunization with dendritic cells presenting epitopes derived from the melanoma-associated antigens MART-1 and gp100. *Journal of Immunotherapy,* **23**, 487–498.

Papadimitriou, C. S., Datseris, G., Costopoulos, J. S. *et al.* (1992). Langerhans cells and lymphocyte subsets in human gastrointestinal carcinomas. An immunohistological study on frozen sections. *Pathology, Research, and Practice,* **188**, 989–994.

Papadopoulos, E. B., Carabasi, M. H., Castro-Malaspina, H. *et al.* (1998). T-cell-depleted allogeneic bone marrow transplantation as postremission therapy for acute myelogenous leukemia: freedom from relapse in the absence of graft-versus-host disease. *Blood,* **91**, 1083–1090.

Papadopoulos, E. B., Ladanyi, M., Emanuel, D. *et al.* (1994). Infusions of donor leukocytes to treat Epstein-Barr virus-associated lymphoproliferative disorders after allogeneic bone marrow transplantation. *New England Journal of Medicine,* **330**, 1185–1191.

Passweg, J. R., Tiberghien, P., Cahn, J. Y. *et al.* (1998). Graft-versus-leukemia effects in T lineage and B lineage acute lymphoblastic leukemia. *Bone Marrow Transplantation,* **21**, 153–158.

Pawlowska, A. B., Hashino, S., McKenna, H. *et al.* (2001). In vitro tumor-pulsed or in vivo Flt3 ligand-generated dendritic cells provide protection against acute myelogenous leukemia in nontransplanted or syngeneic bone marrow-transplanted mice. *Blood,* **97**, 1474–1482.

Peace, D. J., Smith, J. W., Disis, M. L. *et al.* (1993). Induction of T cells specific for the mutated segment of oncogenic p21ras protein by immunization in vivo with the oncogenic protein. *Journal of Immunotherapy,* **14**, 10–14.

Peggs, K. S. & Mackinnon, S. (2001). Cellular therapy: donor lymphocyte infusion. *Current Opinion in Hematology,* **8**, 349–354.

Perreault, C., Roy, D. C., & Fortin, C. (1998). Immunodominant minor histocompatibility antigens: the major ones. *Immunology Today,* **19**, 69–74.

Perry, A. R. & Mackinnon, S. (1996). Adoptive immunotherapy post bone marrow transplantation. *Blood Reviews,* **10**, 237–241.

Pierce, R. A., Field, E. D., Mutis, T. *et al.* (2001). The HA-2 minor histocompatibility antigen is derived from a diallelic gene encoding a novel human class I myosin protein. *Journal of Immunology,* **167**, 3223–3230.

Pion, S., Fontaine, P., Baron, C. *et al.* (1995). Immunodominant minor histocompatibility antigens expressed by mouse leukemic cells can serve as effective targets for T cell immunotherapy. *Journal of Clinical Investigation,* **95**, 1561–1568.

Porter, D. L. & Antin, J. H. (1998). Infusion of donor peripheral blood mononuclear cells to treat relapse after transplantation for chronic myelogenous leukemia. In *Biology and Therapy of Chronic Myelogenous Leukemia,* eds. P. McGlave & C. M. Verfaillie, pp. 123–150. Philadelphia: WB Saunders Company.

Porter, D. L., Collins, R. H., Jr., Hardy, C. *et al.* (2000). Treatment of relapsed leukemia after unrelated donor marrow transplantation with unrelated donor leukocyte infusions. *Blood,* **95**, 1214–1221.

Prescott, S., James, K., Hargreave, T. B. *et al.* (1992). Intravesical Evans strain BCG therapy: quantitative immunohistochemical analysis of the immune response within the bladder wall. *Journal of Urology,* **147**, 1636–1642.

Pulendran, B., Banchereau, J., Burkeholder, S. *et al.* (2000). Flt3-ligand and granulocyte colony-stimulating factor mobilize distinct human dendritic cell subsets in vivo. *Journal of Immunology,* **165**, 566–572.

Qian, S., Lu, L., Fu, F. *et al.* (1998). Donor pretreatment with Flt-3 ligand augments antidonor cytotoxic T lymphocyte, natural killer, and lymphokine-activated killer cell activities within liver allografts and alters the pattern of intragraft apoptotic activity. *Transplantation,* **65**, 1590–1598.

Radford, K. J., Higgins, D. E., Pasquini, S. *et al.* (2002). A recombinant *E. coli* vaccine to promote MHC class I-dependent antigen presentation: application to cancer immunotherapy. *Gene Therapy,* **9**, 1455–1463.

Radmayr, C., Bock, G., Hobisch, A. *et al.* (1995). Dendritic antigen-presenting cells from the peripheral blood of renal-cell-carcinoma patients. *International Journal of Cancer,* **63**, 627–632.

Rains, N., Cannan, R. J., Chen, W., & Stubbs, R. S. (2001). Development of a dendritic cell (DC)-based vaccine for patients with advanced colorectal cancer. *Hepatogastroenterology,* **48**, 347–351.

Randolph, G. J., Inaba, K., Robbiani, D. F. *et al.* (1999). Differentiation of phagocytic monocytes into lymph node dendritic cells in vivo. *Immunity,* **11**, 753–761.

Ratta, M., Fagnoni, F., Curti, A. *et al.* (2002). Dendritic cells are functionally defective in multiple myeloma: the role of interleukin-6. *Blood,* **100**, 230–237.

Reichardt, V. L., Okada, C. Y., Liso, A. *et al.* (1999). Idiotype vaccination using dendritic cells after autologous peripheral blood stem cell transplantation for multiple myeloma—a feasibility study. *Blood,* **93**, 2411–2419.

Rieser, C., Ramoner, R., Holtl, L. *et al.* (2000). Mature dendritic cells induce T-helper type-1-dominant immune responses in patients with metastatic renal cell carcinoma. *Urologia Internationalis,* **63**, 151–159.

Rissoan, M., Soumelis, V., Kadowaki, N. *et al.* (1999). Reciprocal control of T helper cell and dendritic cell differentiation. *Science,* **283**, 1183–1186.

Roddie, P. H., Horton, Y., & Turner, M. L. (2002). Primary acute myeloid leukaemia blasts resistant to cytokine-induced differentiation to dendritic-like leukaemia cells can be forced to differentiate by the addition of bryostatin-1. *Leukemia,* **16**, 84–93.

Romani, N., Gruner, S., Brang, D. *et al.* (1994). Proliferating dendritic cell progenitors in human blood. *Journal of Experimental Medicine,* **180,** 83–93.

Romani, N., Reider, D., Heuer, M. *et al.* (1996). Generation of mature dendritic cells from human blood. An improved method with special regard to clinical applicability. *Journal of Immunological Methods,* **196,** 137–151.

Rooney, C. M., Aguilar, L. K., Huls, M. H. *et al.* (2001). Adoptive immunotherapy of EBV-associated malignancies with EBV-specific cytotoxic T-cell lines. *Current Topics in Microbiology and Immunity,* **258,** 221–229.

Rosenberg, R. A. & White, D. E. (1996). Vitiligo in patients with melanoma: normal tissue antigens can be targets for cancer immunotherapy. *Journal of Immunotherapy,* **19,** 81–84.

Rosenberg, S. A. (1999). A new era for cancer immunotherapy based on the genes that encode cancer antigens. *Immunity,* **10,** 281–287.

Roth, M., Antin, J., Ash, R. *et al.* (1992). Prognostic significance of Philadelphia chromosome-positive cells detected by the polymerase chain reaction after allogeneic bone marrow. *Blood,* **79,** 276–282.

Sadanaga, N., Nagashima, H., Mashino, K. *et al.* (2001). Dendritic cell vaccination with MAGE peptide is a novel therapeutic approach for gastrointestinal carcinomas. *Clinical Cancer Research,* **7,** 2277–2284.

Salgaller, M. L., Lodge, P. A., McLean, J. G. *et al.* (1998). Report of immune monitoring of prostate cancer patients undergoing T-cell therapy using dendritic cells pulsed with HIA-A2-specific peptides from prostate-specific membrane antigen (PSMA). *Prostate,* **35,** 144–151.

Sallusto, F., Cella, M., Danieli, C. *et al.* (1995). Dendritic cells use macropinocytosis and the mannose receptor to concentrate macromolecules in the major histocompatibility complex class II compartment: downregulation by cytokines and bacterial products. *Journal of Experimental Medicine,* **182,** 389–400.

Sallusto, F. & Lanzavecchia, A. (1994). Efficient presentation of soluble antigen by cultured human dendritic cells is maintained by granulocyte/macrophage colony-stimulating factor plus interleukin 4 and downregulated by tumor necrosis factor-α. *Journal of Experimental Medicine,* **179,** 1109–1118.

Sallusto, F. & Lanzavecchia, A. (2000). Understanding dendritic cell and T-lymphocyte traffic through the analysis of chemokine receptor expression. *Immunological Reviews,* **177,** 134–140.

Sato, T., McCue, P., Masuoka, K. *et al.* (1996). Interleukin 10 production by human melanoma. *Clinical Cancer Research,* **2,** 1383–1390.

Schoenberger, S. P., Toes, R. E., van der Voort, E. I. *et al.* (1998). T-cell help for cytotoxic T lymphocytes is mediated by CD40-CD40L interactions. *Nature,* **393,** 480–483.

Schott, M., Feldkamp, J., Lettman, M. *et al.* (2001a). Dendritic cell immunotherapy in a neuroendocrine pancreas carcinoma. *Clinical Endocrinology,* **55,** 271–277.

Schott, M., Feldkamp, J., Schattenberg, D. *et al.* (2000). Induction of cellular immunity in a parathyroid carcinoma treated with tumor lysate-pulsed dendritic cells. *European Journal of Endocrinology,* **142,** 300–306.

Schott, M., Seissler, J., Feldkamp, J. *et al.* (1999). Dendritic cell immunotherapy induces antitumour response in parathyroid carcinoma and neuroendocrine pancreas carcinoma. *Hormone and Metabolic Research,* **31,** 662–664.

Schott, M., Seissler, J., Lettman, M. *et al.* (2001b). Immunotherapy for medullary thyroid carcinoma by dendritic cell vaccination. *Journal of Clinical Endocrinology and Metabolism,* **86,** 4965–4969.

Schuler-Thurner, B., Dieckmann, D., Keikavoussi, P. *et al.* (2000). Mage-3 and influenza-matrix peptide-specific cytotoxic T cells are inducible in terminal stage HLA-A2.1$^+$ melanoma patients by mature monocyte-derived dendritic cells. *Journal of Immunology,* **165,** 3492–3496.

Schwaab, T., Weiss, J. E., Schned, A. R. *et al.* (2001). Dendritic cell infiltration in colon cancer. *Journal of Immunotherapy,* **24,** 130–137.

Schwartz, R. H. (1996). Models of T cell anergy: is there a common molecular mechanism? *Journal of Experimental Medicine,* **184,** 1–8.

Serody, J. S., Collins, E. J., Tisch, R. M. *et al.* (2000). T cell activity after dendritic cell vaccination is dependent on both of the type of antigen and the mode of delivery. *Journal of Immunology,* **164,** 4961–4967.

Shlomchik, W. D., Couzens, M. S., Tang, C. B. *et al.* (1999). Prevention of graft versus host disease by inactivation of host antigen-presenting cells. *Science,* **285,** 412–415.

Shortman, K. & Liu, Y. J. (2002). Mouse and human dendritic cell subtypes. *Nature Reviews. Immunology,* **2,** 151–161.

Shu, S., Plautz, G. E., Krauss, J. C. *et al.* (1997). Tumor immunology (Review). JAMA: the *Journal of the American Medical Association,* **278,** 1972–1981.

Simons, J. W., Jaffee, E. M., Weber, C. E. *et al.* (1997). Bioactivity of autologous irradiated renal cells carcinoma vaccines generated by ex vivo granulocyte-macrophage colony-stimulating factor gene transfer. *Cancer,* **57,** 1537–1546.

Simons, J. W., Mikhak, B., Chang, J. F. *et al.* (1999). Induction of immunity to prostate cancer antigens: results of a clinical trial of vaccination with irradiated autologous prostate tumor cells engineered to secrete granulocyte-macrophage colony-stimulating factor using ex vivo gene transfer. *Cancer Research,* **59,** 5160–5168.

Small, E. J., Fratesi, P., Reese, D. M. *et al.* (2000). Immunotherapy of hormone-refractory prostate cancer with antigen-loaded dendritic cells. *Journal of Clinical Oncology,* **18,** 3894–3903.

Sombroek, C. C., Stam, A. G., Masterson, A. J. *et al.* (2002). Prostanoids play a major role in the primary tumor-induced inhibition of dendritic cell differentiation. *Journal of Immunology,* **168,** 4333–4343.

Sorg, R. V., McLellan, A. D., Hock, B. D. *et al.* (1998). Human dendritic cells express functional interleukin-7. *Immunobiology,* **198,** 514–526.

Steinbrink, K., Jonuleit, H., Muller, G. *et al.* (1999). Interleukin-10 treated human dendritic cells induce a melanoma antigen-specific anergy in CD8+ T cells resulting in a failure to lyse tumor cells. *Blood,* **93,** 1634–1642.

Steinbrink, K., Wolfl, M., Jonuleit, H. *et al.* (1997). Induction of tolerance by IL-10-treated dendritic cells. *Journal of Immunology,* **159,** 4772–4780.

Strobl, H., Riedl, E., Scheinecker, C. *et al.* (1996). TGF-beta 1 promotes in vitro development of dendritic cells from CD34+

hemopoietic progenitors. *Journal of Immunology,* **157,** 1499–1507.

Summers, K. L., Hock, B. D., McKenzie, J. L. *et al.* (2001). Phenotypic characterization of five dendritic cell subsets in human tonsils. *American Journal of Pathology,* **159,** 285–295.

Suzuki, A., Masuda, A., Nagata, H. *et al.* (2002). Mature dendritic cells make clusters with T cells in the invasive margin of colorectal carcinoma. *Journal of Pathology,* **196,** 37–43.

Takahashi, H., Nakagawa, Y., Leggatt, G. R. *et al.* (1996). Inactivation of human immunodeficiency virus (HIV)-1 envelope-specific CD8+ cytotoxic T lymphocytes by free antigenic peptide: a self-veto mechanism? *Journal of Experimental Medicine,* **183,** 879–889.

Tanaka, Y., Koido, S., Chen, D. *et al.* (2001). Vaccination with allogeneic dendritic cells fused to carcinoma cells induces antitumor immunity in MUC1 transgenic mice. *Clinical Immunology,* **101,** 192–200.

Thomas, R., Chambers, M., Boytar, R. *et al.* (1999). Immature human monocyte-derived dendritic cells migrate rapidly to draining lymph nodes after intradermal injection for melanoma immunotherapy. *Melanoma Research,* **9,** 474–481.

Thurner, B., Haendle, I., Roder, C. *et al.* (1999a). Vaccination with mage-3A1 peptide-pulsed mature, monocyte-derived dendritic cells expands specific cytotoxic T cells and induces regression of some metastases in advanced stage IV melanoma. *Journal of Experimental Medicine,* **190,** 1669–1678.

Thurner, B., Roder, C., Dieckmann, D. *et al.* (1999b). Generation of large numbers of fully mature and stable dendritic cells from leukapheresis products for clinical application. *Journal of Immunological Methods,* **223,** 1–15.

Thurnher, M., Rieser, C., Holtl, L. *et al.* (1998). Dendritic cell-based immunotherapy of renal cell carcinoma. *Urologia Internationalis,* **61,** 67–71.

Titzer, S., Christensen, O., Manzke, O. *et al.* (2000). Vaccination of multiple myeloma patients with idiotype-pulsed dendritic cells: immunological and clinical aspects. *British Journal of Haematology,* **108,** 805–16.

Tjoa, B., Erickson, S., Barren, R. *et al.* (1995). In vitro propagated dendritic cells from prostate cancer patients as a component of prostate cancer immunotherapy. *Prostate,* **27,** 63–69.

Tjoa, B. A. & Murphy, G. P. (2000). Development of dendritic-cell based prostate cancer vaccine. *Immunology Letters,* **74,** 87–93.

Tjoa, B. A., Simmons, S. J., Bowes, V. A. *et al.* (1998). Evaluation of phase I/II clinical trials in prostate cancer with dendritic cells and PSMA peptides. *Prostate,* **36,** 39–44.

Tjoa, B. A., Simmons, S. J., Elgamal, A. *et al.* (1999). Follow-up evaluation of a phase II prostate cancer vaccine trial. *Prostate,* **40,** 125–129.

Toes, R. E., van der Voort, E. I., Schoenberger, S. P. *et al.* (1998). Enhancement of tumor outgrowth through CTL tolerization after peptide vaccination is avoided by peptide presentation on dendritic cells. *Journal of Immunology,* **160,** 4449–4456.

Toungouz, M., Libin, M., Bulte, F. *et al.* (2001). Transient expansion of peptide-specific lymphocytes producing IFN-gamma after vaccination with dendritic cells pulsed with MAGE peptides in patients with mage-A1/A3-positive tumors. *Journal of Leukocyte Biology,* **69,** 937–943.

Traver, D., Akashi, K., Manz, M. *et al.* (2000). Development of CD8α positive dendritic cells from a common myeloid progenitor. *Science,* **290,** 2152–2154.

Trefzer, U., Weingart, G., Chen, Y. *et al.* (2000). Hybrid cell vaccination for cancer immune therapy: first clinical trial with metastatic melanoma. *International Journal of Cancer,* **85,** 618–26.

Tricot, G., Vestole, D. H., Jagannath, S. *et al.* (1996). Graft-versus-myeloma effect: proof of principle. *Blood,* **87,** 1196–1198.

Troy, A., Davidson, P., Atkinson, C. *et al.* (1998a). Phenotypic characterisation of the dendritic cell infiltrate in prostate cancer. *Journal of Urology,* **160,** 214–219.

Troy, A. J., Davidson, P. J., Atkinson, C. H. *et al.* (1999). CD1a dendritic cells predominate in transitional cell carcinoma of bladder and kidney but are minimally activated. *Journal of Urology,* **161,** 1962–1967.

Troy, A. J. & Hart, D.N.J. (1997). Dendritic cells in cancer: progress towards a new cellular therapy. *Journal of Hematotherapy,* **6,** 523–533.

Troy, A. J., Summers, K. L., Davidson, P. J. *et al.* (1998b). Minimal recruitment and activation of dendritic cells within renal cell carcinoma. *Clinical Cancer Research,* **4,** 585–593.

Tsuchiya, T., Hagihara, M., Shimakura, Y. *et al.* (2002). The generation of immunocompetent dendritic cells from CD34+ acute myeloid or lymphoid leukemia cells. *International Journal of Hematology,* **75,** 55–62.

Tzachanis, D., Berezovskaya, A., Nadler, L. M. *et al.* (2002). Blockade of B7/CD28 in mixed lymphocyte reaction cultures results in the generation of alternatively activated macrophages, which suppress T-cell responses. *Blood,* **99,** 1465–1473.

Valladeau, J., Ravel, O., Dezutter-Dambuyant, C. *et al.* (2000). Langerin, a novel C-type lectin specific to Langerhans cells, is an endocytic receptor that induces the formation of Birbeck granules. *Immunity,* **12,** 71–81.

Valone, F. H., Small, E., MacKenzie, M. *et al.* (2001). Dendritic cell-based treatment of cancer: closing in on a cellular therapy. *Cancer Journal,* **7,** Suppl 2, S53–61.

van Lochem, E., van der Keur, M., Mommaas, A. M. *et al.* (1996). Peptide-pulsed dendritic cells induce tumoricidal cytotoxic T lymphocytes from healthy donors against stably HLA-A* 0201-binding peptides from the melan-A/MART-self antigen. *European Journal of Immunology,* **26,** 1683–9.

Van Tendeloo, V. F., Ponsaerts, P., Lardon, F. *et al.* (2001). Highly efficient gene delivery by mRNA electroporation in human hematopoietic cells: superiority to lipofection and passive pulsing of mRNA and to electroporation of plasmid cDNA for tumor antigen loading of dendritic cells. *Blood,* **98,** 49–56.

Vonderheide, R. H., Hahn, W. C., Schultze, J. L. *et al.* (1999). The telomerase catalytic subunit is a widely expressed tumor-associated antigen recognized by cytotoxic T lymphocytes. *Immunity,* **10,** 673–679.

Vonderheide, R. H., Schultze, J. L., Anderson, K. S. *et al.* (2001). Equivalent induction of telomerase-specific cytotoxic T lymphocytes from tumor-bearing patients and healthy individuals. *Cancer Research,* **61,** 8366–8370.

Vuckovic, S., Clark, G. J., & Hart, D.N.J. (2002). Growth factors, cytokines and dendritic cell development. *Current Pharmaceutical Design,* **8,** 405–418.

Vuckovic, S., Fearnley, D. B., Gunningham, S. P. *et al.* (1999). Dendritic cells in chronic myelomonocytic leukaemia. *British Journal of Haematology,* **105,** 974–985.

Vuckovic, S., Florin, T.H.J., Khalil, D. *et al.* (2001). CD40 and CD86 upregulation with divergent CMRF-44 expression on blood dendritic cells in inflammatory bowel diseases. *American Journal of Gastroenterology,* **96,** 2946–2956.

Wan, Y., Bramson, J., Carter, R. *et al.* (1997). Dendritic cells transduced with an adenoviral vector encoding a model tumor-associated antigen for tumor vaccination. *Human Gene Therapy,* **8,** 1355–1363.

Wang, W., Meadows, L. R., den Haan, J. M. *et al.* (1995). Human H-Y: a male-specific histocompatibility antigen derived from the SMCY protein. *Science,* **269,** 1588–1590.

Watts, C. (1997). Capture and processing of exogenous antigens for presentation on MHC molecules. *Annual Reviews of Immunology,* **15,** 821–850.

Wen, Y. J., Ling, M., Bailey-Wood, R. *et al.* (1998). Idiotype protein pulsed adherent peripheral blood mononuclear cell-derived dendritic cells prime immune system in multiple myeloma. *Clinical Cancer Research,* **4,** 957.

Willems, F., Marchant, A., Delville, J. -P. *et al.* (1994). Interleukin-10 inhibits B7 and intercellular adhesion molecule-1 expression on human monocytes. *European Journal of Immunology,* **24,** 1007–1009.

Wu, L., Vremec, D., Ardavin, C. *et al.* (1995). Mouse thymus dendritic cells: kinetics of development and changes in surface markers during maturation. *European Journal of Immunology,* **25,** 418–425.

Wykes, M., MacDonald, K.P.A., Tran, M. *et al.* (2002). MUC1 epithelial mucin (CD227) is expressed by activated dendritic cells. *Journal of Leukocyte Biology,* **72,** 692–701.

Yang, Y. G., Sergio, J. J., Pearson, D. A. *et al.* (1998). Interleukin-12 preserves the graft-versus-leukemia effect of allogeneic CD8 T cells while inhibiting CD4-dependent graft-versus-host disease in mice. *Blood,* **90,** 4651–4660.

Yi, Q., Desikan, R., Barlogie, B., & Munshi, N. (2002). Optimizing dendritic cell–based immunotherapy in multiple myeloma. *British Journal of Haematology,* **117,** 297–305.

Yoshimura, S., Bondeson, J., Brennan, F. M. *et al.* (2001). Role of NFkappaB in antigen presentation and development of regulatory T cells elucidated by treatment of dendritic cells with the proteasome inhibitor PSI. *European Journal of Immunology,* **31,** 1883–1893.

Young, J. W. & Inaba, K. (1996). Dendritic cells as adjuvants for class I major histocompatibility complex-restricted antitumor immunity. *Journal of Experimental Medicine,* **183,** 7–11.

Young, J. W. & Steinman, R. M. (1988). Accessory cell requirements for the MLR and polyclonal mitogens, as studied with a new technique for enriching blood dendritic cells. *Cellular Immunology,* **111,** 167–182.

Yu, J. S., Wheeler, C. J., Zeltzer, P. M. *et al.* (2001). Vaccination of malignant glioma patients with peptide-pulsed dendritic cells elicits systemic cytotoxicity and intracranial T-cell infiltration. *Cancer Research,* **61,** 842–847.

Zeh, H. J., Perry-Lalley, D., Dudley, M. E. *et al.* (1999). High avidity CTLs for two self-antigens demonstrate superior in vitro and in vivo antitumor efficacy. *Journal of Immunology,* **162,** 989–994.

Zeng, G., Li, Y., El-Gamil, M. *et al.* (2002). Generation of NY-ESO-1-specific CD4+ and CD8+ T cells by a single peptide with dual MHC class I and class II specificities: a new strategy for vaccine design. *Cancer Research,* **62,** 3630–3635.

Zeng, W., Ghosh, S., Macris, M. *et al.* (2001). Assembly of synthetic peptide vaccines by chemoselective ligation of epitopes: influence of different chemical linkages and epitope orientations on biological activity. *Vaccine,* **19,** 3843–3852.

Zhang, Y., Louboutin, J. P., Zhu, J. *et al.* (2002). Preterminal host dendritic cells in irradiated mice prime CD8+ T cell- mediated acute graft-versus-host disease. *Journal of Clinical Investigation,* **109,** 1335–1344.

Zhou, L. J. & Tedder, T. F. (1995). Human blood dendritic cells selectively express CD83, a member of the immunoglobulin superfamily. *Journal of Immunology,* **154,** 3821–3835.

Zhou, L. J. & Tedder, T. F. (1996). CD14+ blood monocytes can differentiate into functionally mature CD83+ dendritic cells. *Proceedings of the National Academy of Sciences USA,* **93,** 2588–2592.

Zitvogel, L., Mayordomo, J. I., Tjandrawan, T. *et al.* (1996). Therapy of murine tumors with tumor peptide-pulsed dendritic cells: dependence on T cells, B7 costimulation and T helper cell 1-associated cytokines. *Journal of Experimental Medicine,* **183,** 87–97.

Zou, W., Borvak, J., Marches, F. *et al.* (2000). Macrophage-derived dendritic cells have strong Th1-polarizing potential mediated by beta-chemokines rather than IL-12. *Journal of Immunology,* **165,** 4388–4396.

113 Antigen-specific T cells in cancer immunotherapy

MICHAEL KALOS

Corixa Corporation, Seattle, USA

Introduction

A role for the immune system in the eradication of tumors was suggested early in the 20th century by Ehrlich (Ehrlich, 1909). Subsequently, Burnet (Burnet, 1970) and others gradually expanded the initial hypothesis to reflect an increased understanding both of neoplasia and the immune system. A landmark in the field of antigen-specific immunotherapy of cancer was the identification by Boon and colleagues of MAGE-1, a tumor-specific gene product that was recognized by T cells derived from a melanoma patient (VanderBruggen, 1991). The discovery of MAGE-1 established the potential for vaccine-based treatment of cancer by the demonstration that T cells existed in the peripheral circulation that were capable of recognizing specific proteins expressed and processed by tumor cells. The subsequent identification and characterization of a number of gene products that were expressed aberrantly by tumor cells and continued progress in unraveling the intricacies of the immune system, have precipitated the development of a number of antigen-specific vaccination strategies for the activation of tumor antigen-specific T cells.

A critical role for antigen-specific T cells in the eradication of cancer has been established in numerous animal models. Results from both in vitro systems and human clinical trials indicate that T cells can be identified that recognize antigenic fragments derived from gene products expressed by tumors. Furthermore, analysis of cancer patients that have been treated with tumor-specific vaccines have provided evidence for the in vivo stimulation of tumor-specific T cells, both de novo and as a result of vaccination strategies. However, results from clinical trials have been for the most part disappointing, since the majority of patients undergoing cancer treatment do not mount successful antitumor responses. The relative ineffectiveness of cancer vaccines can be attributed at least in part to the facts that tumors that arise in vivo develop and expand both as a consequence of immune evasion and because they are essentially self tissues to which the immune system is to a large extent tolerized.

In the context of the above observations, the fundamental questions that need to be addressed with regard to the ultimate efficacy of tumor antigen-specific T cells for cancer immunotherapy are (1) Do tumor antigen-specific T cells exist in the peripheral circulation that can recognize and effectively eliminate tumors? (2) If the appropriate T cells exist, what methodologies can be employed to effectively activate them? The objectives of this chapter are to summarize what is known about the interaction of T cells and tumors, highlight current strategies for the identification and activation of tumor-specific T cells, and finally provide insight into potential future strategies for the successful activation of T cells for the immunotherapy of cancer.

Development and activation of antigen-specific T cells

The antigen-specific T-cell compartment is composed of two main subtypes of T cells that are classified based on the expression of surface molecules. CD8+ T cells are defined by expression of the CD8 molecule, and CD4+ T cells by expression of the CD4 molecule. CD8+ T cells generally express effector functions that include cytolysis (thus also referred to as cytotoxic T lymphocytes or CTL) and cytokine production that result in target cell destruction, while CD4+ T cells generally express helper functions that include cytokine production and result in immune system activation. Both CD8+ and CD4+ T cells recognize antigen via a multicomponent surface receptor complex termed the T-cell receptor (TCR). The TCR is composed of at least six chains ($\alpha,\beta,\gamma,\delta,\varepsilon$, and ζ) that assemble on the surface of T cells. Antigen recognition is mediated by the α and β chains (or γ and δ chains on certain epithelial T cells), while the main signal-transmitting component is the ζ chain. The α/β TCR recognizes a bipartite complex on the surface of target cells. For CD8+ T cells, the complex is composed of peptides generally 8 to 11 amino acids long and the MHC class I surface molecule expressed on most cell types. For CD4+ T cells, the complex is composed of peptides generally 8 to 15 amino acids long and the MHC class II surface molecule expressed on professional APC. In general terms, peptides that are destined for association with class I complexes are preferentially processed from proteins expressed in the cytoplasm

(York & Rock, 1996), and peptides destined for association with class II complexes are preferentially processed from proteins that have been internalized by professional antigen-presenting cells (APC) via cellular uptake processes (Watts, 1997). Recognition of MHC:peptide complexes at the appropriate threshold results in a productive TCR engagement with the consequent activation of T-cell effector functions. Productive T-cell engagement is ultimately an integration of signaling events that involve both engagement of the TCR and also interactions between co-stimulatory and adhesive molecules expressed on T cells and target cells or APC. As discussed in more detail below, recognition of complexes at suboptimal levels leads to T-cell death, anergy, or simply lack of activation (Weiss, 1991).

T-cell genesis and maturation occurs primarily in the thymus. A fundamental concept for T-cell immunology is the process of negative selection, during which T cells that recognize peptide:MHC complexes in the thymus are eliminated by the induction of apoptotic pathways (Kappler et al., 1987). As a result of negative selection, essentially all T cells that recognize peptides derived from self antigens expressed in the thymus with high affinity are eliminated. The corollary process, positive selection, also occurs in the thymus. As a result of positive selection, T cells with a basal degree of affinity for self-MHC molecules are selected for survival and maturation (von Boehmer, 1994). Thus, T cells that survive the thymus and migrate to the periphery have the potential to recognize, in the context of self MHC, peptides derived from non-self proteins, self proteins not expressed in the thymus, or with significantly lower affinity, self proteins expressed in the thymus.

T cells that circulate in the periphery and have not encountered antigen are defined as naïve, whereas T cells that have previously encountered antigen can exist in an activated, memory, or anergized/tolerized state. As described initially by Jenkins and Schwartz (1987), naïve T cells require two signals for effective activation: the first signal is antigen-dependent and is provided by engagement of TCR by antigen:MHC, and the second (co-stimulatory) signal is antigen-independent and is provided by specialized molecules expressed on professional APC. In the absence of co-stimulation, engagement of TCR on naïve T cells results in a state defined as anergy or tolerance, during which T cells become functionally impaired and nonresponsive to antigen-expressing cells. Activated T cells express effector functions, and require a lower threshold of TCR engagement to recognize target cells. Following activation, expansion, and expression of effector functions, the majority of antigen-specific T cells die, and a small subset differentiates into long-term memory cells, which can be re-activated at a lower threshold compared to naïve cells following re-exposure to antigen (Dutton et al., 1998).

A number of molecules, expressed by both T cells and APC, have been described that are involved in the co-stimulatory process. Two classes of molecules have been shown to be critically involved in the co-stimulation of T cells. The first class of molecules involves members of the B7 family of molecules, specifically B7.1 (CD80) and B7.2 (CD86), expressed by dendritic cells (DC), activated B cells as well as T cells (reviewed in Carreno & Collins, 2002). A large body of literature has demonstrated that B7.1 and/or B7.2 are critical for T-cell co-stimulation. T cells express at least two molecules on their surface that serve as ligands for B7 molecules. CD28, expressed constitutively on the surface of the majority of CD8[+] and CD4[+] T cells, has been shown to be critical for activation of T cells. CTLA-4, a closely related family member to CD28, is expressed on the surface of T cells following activation. CTLA-4 has been shown to be involved in the subsequent down-modulation of the immune response. The second class of molecules that are expressed by T cells belong to the TNF-receptor family, and include CD40L (reviewed in Grewal & Flavell, 1996). CD40, the receptor for CD40L, is expressed on activated macrophages, monocyte- and bone marrow-derived as well as follicular DC, thymic epithelial cells, endothelial cells, and B cells. Following T-cell activation, CD40L is markedly upregulated in CD4[+] and a subset of CD8[+] cells. Ligation of CD40 by CD40L results in DC maturation, and has been shown to induce upregulation of B7 family members thus enhancing the T-cell APC interaction.

Immune evasion mechanisms for tumors

Based on the prevalence and outgrowth of cancers in both immune compromised animal models and patients, it is clear that tumors arise with a reasonable frequency in vivo. However, most tumors are eliminated by a functional immune system. Tumor cells that expand and develop into life-threatening masses generally do so as a result of some form of immune evasion. As reviewed recently by Marincola, tumors accomplish immune evasion via multiple mechanisms (Marincola et al., 2000). A driving force in the ability of tumors to evade the immune system is their inherent genetic instability. Heterogeneity in antigen expression by tumors, both spontaneously and following immunotherapy, has been documented in a number of cases (Jager et al., 1996b, 1997; Riker et al., 1999; Ohnmacht et al., 2001; Saleh et al., 2001). Tumors have been shown to directly downregulate expression of class I MHC molecules (Garrido et al., 1993; Ferrone & Marincola, 1995) or downregulate surface expression of MHC molecules through mutations that affect biochemical pathways involved in antigen processing and surface MHC complex assembly (Cromme et al., 1994; Kaklamanis et al., 1995; Chen et al., 1996; Korkolopoulou et al., 1996; Kurokohchi et al., 1996; Singal et al., 1996; Johnsen et al., 1998, 1999; Vitale et al., 1998). Loss of antigen and MHC surface expression have been associated with tumor progression in vaccinated patients (Jager et al., 1997; Mendez et al., 2001). A recent report demonstrated that treatment of tumor cells that had lost HLA class I surface expression with 5-aza-2'-deoxycytidine resulted in re-expression of surface class I alleles, suggesting that, in addition to mutational events, tumor-specific hypermethylation events may be important for modulating tumor escape mechanisms (Serrano et al., 2001).

Tumors have been shown to directly kill T cells by expression of Fas-Ligand (FasL) on their surface (Didenko *et al.*, 2002), or secretion of soluble FasL (Song *et al.*, 2001), and ligation of the apoptosis inducing receptor Fas on the surface of T cells (Walker *et al.*, 1998; O'Connell *et al.*, 1999) while simultaneously developing resistance to the effects of Fas-L through multiple mechanisms including expression of antagonistic receptors, deletion or mutation of Fas, and mutations in components of the Fas transduction pathway (Moller *et al.*, 1994; Knipping *et al.*, 1995; Natoli *et al.*, 1995; Tachibana *et al.*, 1995).

Tumors have also been shown to both directly produce and stimulate the production of a number of immunosuppressive factors that inhibit T-cell activity (Chouaib *et al.*, 1997; Elgert *et al.*, 1998). The primary immunosuppressive factor produced by tumors is transforming growth factor-β (TGF-β). This factor is produced by a number of tumors and has been shown to dramatically affect T-cell activation, proliferation, differentiation, and production of cytokines by both T cells and DC (Espevik *et al.*, 1987; Moses *et al.*, 1990; Ruegemer *et al.*, 1990; Pazdrak *et al.*, 1995; Gorelik & Flavell, 2002). It was recently shown that genetic modification of T cells to express a dominant-negative TGF-β receptor rendered those T cells resistant to the immunosuppressive effects of TGF-β (Bollard *et al.*, 2002).

Another important factor produced by tumors and involved in immunosuppression is vascular endothelial growth factor (VEGF). VEGF is produced by most solid tumors and has been shown to block DC maturation (Gabrilovich *et al.*, 1996), and is implicated as a major contributor to the immunosuppression associated with tumor growth (reviewed in Carbone & Ohm, 2002).

Interleukin (IL)-10 has been shown to be secreted by a number of tumor types (Gastl *et al.*, 1993). As discussed below, although IL-10 has been shown to exert immunosuppressive effects on T cells, at least in part by inhibiting cytokine secretion by Th1 cells, it also has been shown to play a role in tumor rejection.

Cytokines critical for T-cell antitumor immunity

Cells of the immune and hematopoietic systems produce a multitude of soluble cytokines that are critical for the transmission of differentiation, activation, and suppressive signals to immune cells. In the complex microenvironment of tumors, effective modulation of the antitumor response is accomplished by the integration of multiple cytokine signals produced by and transmitted to T cells, APC, and tumors.

Based on their cytokine secretion profiles, CD8$^+$ and CD4$^+$ T cells can each be categorized into two subtypes. CD4$^+$ T cells are divided into Th1 or Th2 T subtypes. In general terms, Th1 cells are defined by the production of IL-2, γ-IFN, and TNF-α, and are critical for the development of cellular (i.e., T cell) immunity, and Th2 cells are defined by the production of IL-4, IL-10, and TGF-β and mediate the development of a humoral (i.e., antibody-mediated) immune response. CD8$^+$ T cells are divided into Tc1 or Tc2 T sub-

types. Tc1 cells produce γ-IFN and TNF-α, while Tc2 cells secrete IL-4, IL-5, and IL-10. Antitumor immunity is thought to be mediated primarily by Th1 and Tc1 cells (Nishimura *et al.*, 1999; Kemp & Ronchese, 2001).

Among the large number of cytokines a subset have been identified that appear to be critical for T-cell activation and function:

IL-2, secreted primarily by Th1 CD4$^+$ cells, is a potent growth factor for T cells, B cells, and macrophages. Adoptive transfer experiments in mice have demonstrated the critical requirement for IL-2 for the maintenance of CD8$^+$ T cells in vivo and the eradication of disseminated leukemia (Greenberg *et al.*, 1985; Cheever *et al.*, 1986; Greenberg, 1986; Thompson *et al.*, 1986; Klarnet *et al.*, 1987). The critical role for IL-2 in the development and maintenance of antitumor CD8$^+$ T responses has been demonstrated in multiple animal models (Lee *et al.*, 1998; Geutskens *et al.*, 2000; Lee *et al.*, 2001). Although IL-2 administered to cancer patients, either alone or with vaccines, has been demonstrated to result in tumor regression, the associated toxicity due to general immune activation precludes the use of this approach for cancer therapy (Atkins *et al.*, 1999; Fischer *et al.*, 2000; Fisher *et al.*, 2000). Finally, tumor cells genetically modified to express IL-2 have been used in vaccination protocols (Palmer *et al.*, 1999; Osanto *et al.*, 2000).

IL-4, secreted primarily by Th2 CD4$^+$ T cells, has been shown to be critical for the development of effective antitumor immunity. Several animal models have demonstrated an important role for IL-4 in tumor eradication (Tepper *et al.*, 1989; Bosco *et al.*, 1990; Golumbek *et al.*, 1991; Schuler *et al.*, 1999). Knockout mice that lack IL-4 display impaired CTL and Th1 responses and fail to develop systemic tumor immunity (Schuler *et al.*, 1999). By adoptive transfer of purified CD4$^+$ and CD8$^+$ T cells from IL-4 defective mice, it was demonstrated that the generation of tumor-specific CTL activity was associated with IL-4 production from CD8$^+$ and not CD4$^+$ T cells (Schuler *et al.*, 2001). Although IL-4 has been shown to inhibit the growth of tumor cell lines (Topp *et al.*, 1995), to date it has not been shown to be effective in clinical trials (Arienti *et al.*, 1999).

IL-10 is produced primarily by Th2 CD4$^+$ T cells but also by a number of immune cells including B cells, macrophage, and NK cells. IL-10 is generally associated with immunosuppressive effects such as the inhibition of IL-2, GM-CSF, and γ-IFN production and Th1 T-cell proliferation (Fiorentino *et al.*, 1991a, 1991b; Taga *et al.*, 1993). IL-10 has also been shown to negatively affect DC functions (Macatonia *et al.*, 1993; Beissert *et al.*, 1995; Faulkner *et al.*, 2000) and affect expression of co-stimulatory molecules on DC (Chang *et al.*, 1995). Paradoxically, IL-10 has also been shown to enhance cytokine production by Th1 cells, in concert with IL-2 enhance proliferation of activated CD8$^+$ T cells (Groux *et al.*, 1998), and promote the maintenance of tumor-specific CD8$^+$ T cells (Fujii *et al.*, 2001). In a mouse model for experimental glioma, it was shown that tumor rejection was associated with production of

IL-10 by CD4+ T cells and IL-10 that was highly expressed in the tumor bed of animals that rejected tumors, while IL-10 deficient mice were unable to reject tumors (Segal *et al.*, 2002).

γ-IFN is produced by both CD4+ and CD8+ T cells as well as NK cells and is considered to be a critical cytokine in mediating antitumor effector functions. γ-IFN has been shown to be involved in tumor rejection (Dighe *et al.*, 1994). The effects of γ-IFN in tumor rejection are pleiotropic; γ-IFN has been shown to upregulate expression of MHC and adhesion molecules on both tumor cells and APC, thus increasing the avidity of the T cell:tumor/APC interaction (Dighe *et al.*, 1994). In concert with TNF-α, γ-IFN has been shown to have direct cytotoxic effects on tumors (Williamson *et al.*, 1983; Fransen *et al.*, 1986). High levels of γ-IFN production have been correlated with regression in a number of tumor types (Lowes *et al.*, 1997; Wong *et al.*, 2000). γ-IFN has been shown to affect tumor growth indirectly by the inhibition of angiogenesis (Qin & Blankenstein, 2000). Using a tumor variant that was unresponsive to γ-IFN, Beatty *et al.* demonstrated that the anti-angiogenic effects of γ-IFN required tumor responsiveness to the cytokine (Beatty & Paterson, 2001). Paradoxically, γ-IFN has also been demonstrated recently to enhance tumor evasion of the immune system both by downregulating expression and altering the processing of tumor antigens (Beatty & Paterson, 2000; Morel *et al.*, 2000).

GM-CSF is a cytokine produced by T cells, B cells, and macrophages as well as a variety of nonimmune cells such as endothelial cells and fibroblasts. The role of GM-CSF in the immune response against tumors has been examined primarily using gene transfer experiments. By introducing GM-CSF into a number of mouse tumors, it has been demonstrated that GM-CSF secreted by tumors mediates the rejection of tumors (Dranoff *et al.*, 1993; Jaffee *et al.*, 1995; Thomas *et al.*, 1998; Yoshida *et al.*, 1998; Kinoshita *et al.*, 2001). Based on these results, the use of GM-CSF transduced tumors as vaccines has been evaluated in a number of human clinical trials. Promising results have been obtained using both allogeneic as well as autologous tumors (Soiffer *et al.*, 1998; Simons *et al.*, 1999; Jaffee *et al.*, 2001). Although the mechanism of action for GM-CSF in these settings is unclear, it is likely to involve its critical role in the differentiation and maintenance of DC function.

IL-12 is produced primarily by APC such as DC, monocytes, and macrophages. IL-12 has been shown to be involved in the development of Th1 type immune responses (Trinchieri, 1993), and also to be involved in the activation of CD8+ T cells (Trinchieri, 1994). The relevance of IL-12 in tumor rejection has been demonstrated in animal tumor rejection models in which infusion of anti-IL-12 antibodies was shown to inhibit the rejection of highly immunogenic tumor (Fallarino *et al.*, 1996, 1999).

The critical role of cytokines for the development of robust T-cell responses has resulted in their inclusion in vaccine protocols to enhance vaccine efficacy. Cytokines have been co-administered with vaccines in a soluble form, or have been expressed in whole tumor vaccines by gene transfer, with observed clinical efficacy in some cases. Given the complexity of the cytokine networks involved in modulating the immune system, it is clear that further understanding of cytokine biology will facilitate the application of these molecules in cancer immunotherapy.

The role of dendritic cells and the development of a T-cell antitumor response

Since the original description of the potent ability of DC to stimulate primary T-cell responses, dendritic cells have received considerable attention for use in immunotherapeutic strategies against cancer. Several comprehensive reviews have been published on the biology of DC and their use in cancer immunotherapy (Esche *et al.*, 1999; Timmerman & Levy, 1999; Nouri-Shirazi *et al.*, 2000; Meidenbauer *et al.*, 2001).

For clinical applications DC have typically been generated from PBMC-derived monocytes or CD34+ precursor cells, following apheresis. Treatment of monocytes with GM-CSF and IL-4 results in their differentiation, over a period of 5 to 7 days, into immature DC (Romani *et al.*, 1994); DC differentiation from CD34+ cells requires additional cytokines. Immature DC are very potent in terms of taking up antigens by micropinocytosis, receptor-mediated endocytosis, and phagocytosis (Fanger *et al.*, 1996; Albert *et al.*, 1998) and are very effective in terms of antigen processing, but do not express high levels of co-stimulatory molecules and rapidly turn over surface MHC: peptide complexes. Upon removal of cytokines, immature DC de-differentiate into precursor cells. Immature DC can be induced to further differentiate into mature DC by combinations of cytokines, or by the addition of CD40L (Caux *et al.*, 1994). Mature DC have a stable phenotype, lose the capacity to take up and process antigen, but express high levels of stable surface MHC:peptide, co-stimulatory molecules, and cytokines that induce T-cell activation (Cella *et al.*, 1997; Bancbereau *et al.*, 2000).

A number of reports have demonstrated that immature DC are very efficient at uptake of apoptotic bodies (Rubartelli *et al.*, 1997; Albert *et al.*, 1998). The uptake of apoptotic bodies appears to result in processing of antigens and presentation through both class II and class I pathways. DC that take up apoptotic bodies appear to be potent for induction of CTL activity; this observation may reflect a physiological role for this pathway in the efficient stimulation of the immune system against cells that are apoptotic as a consequence of viral or microbial infection.

An additional mechanism for the presentation of tumor antigens by DC to T cells is cross-priming. Originally described by Bevan (1976), cross-priming describes the ability of specialized APC such as DC to take up and process tumor-derived proteins and present epitopes from these proteins to CD8+ T cells in the context of class I molecules. Cross-priming results in the activation of T cells that can then mediate antitumor effects either through cytolysis or, in the case of class I–negative tumors, through secretion of effector cytokines such as γ-IFN and

TNF-α. Cross-priming has been shown to require the presence of cognate CD4[+] T cells (Bennett *et al.*, 1997), with the role of the CD4[+] T cell being the activation of the DC via CD40-CD40L interactions (Bennett *et al.*, 1998; Ridge *et al.*, 1998; Schoenberger *et al.*, 1998). The effect of CD40L on DC maturation at least in part reflects the requirement for a CD40L:CD40 interaction between activated CD4[+] T cell and DC.

In most DC-based clinical protocols to date, immature DC have been the choice of APC. However, as discussed above, immature DC take up and process antigens very efficiently, whereas mature DC are poised to present antigens in an optimal fashion to T cells. In this regard, it is reasonable to conclude that vaccine antigens in the form of cell lysates, recombinant protein or virus infection should be delivered to immature DC that are matured ex vivo prior to infusion into patients, and peptide antigens should be loaded onto mature DC prior to infusion. Since DC precursors represent less than 1% of PBMC, methodologies to expand the frequency of DC in vivo such as treatment with flt-3 ligand (Lynch, 1998; McKenna, 1999) are likely to be critical for future clinical use.

Role of antigen-specific T cells in the eradication of cancer

Animal models

A large number of mouse experimental tumor models have been developed to examine the role of T cells in the eradication of tumors. In the vast majority of these settings, tumors were modified to express an allo-antigen to which a potent immune response could be generated (Pardoll, 1995; Svane *et al.*, 1999). In most models, both CD8[+] and CD4[+] T cells have been shown to play a role for the effective eradication of tumors (Goedegebuure & Eberlein, 1995; Ossendorp *et al.*, 1998; Cohen *et al.*, 2001). Historically, CD8[+] T cells have been considered to be the primary mediators of T-cell antitumor effects, at least in part because the great majority of tumors do not express class II MHC molecules. In the seminal work of Greenberg and colleagues, it has been demonstrated through adoptive transfer that CD8[+] T cells were capable of eradicating disseminated leukemia in mice (Greenberg *et al.*, 1985; Greenberg, 1991). Importantly, complete tumor eradication in these models required either exogenous IL-2 or the presence of CD4[+] T-cell help. A number of additional T-cell transfer–based experimental systems have demonstrated a role for CD8[+] T cells in the eradication or inhibition of tumor cell growth (Rosenberg *et al.*, 1986; Barth *et al.*, 1991; Lynch & Miller, 1994). Removal of CD8[+] T cells has been shown to enhance tumor growth (Svane *et al.*, 1999). More recently, transgenic mouse models have been developed to critically examine the contributions of CD8[+] and CD4[+] T cells in the eradication of tumors. Hanson *et al.* generated a TCR transgenic mouse in which CD8[+] T cells expressed a TCR specific for the syngeneic CMS5 fibrosarcoma rejection antigen mutated ERK2(136–144) (Hanson *et al.*, 2000). In this model,

animals were capable of specifically eliminating lethal doses of CM5S cells, and adoptively transferred splenocytes from TCR transgenic mice conferred protection to both established and inoculated tumor burdens.

The importance of CD4[+] T cells in tumor eradication has been shown in a number of mouse model systems. Kern *et al.* showed that adoptive transfer of CD4[+] T cells, in the absence of detectable tumor-specific CTL, resulted in the eradication of disseminated leukemia (Kern *et al.*, 1990). Adoptive transfer of activated (i.e., L-selection-low) purified CD4[+] T cells from tumor bearing mice into syngeneic mice bearing the same tumor has been shown to result in the rejection of tumor (Kagamu & Shu, 1998). Tumor-specific CD4[+] T cells have been identified in tumor infiltrating lymphocyte (TIL) populations (Goedegebuure & Eberlein, 1995). The role of CD4[+] T cells in mediating tumor rejection has been thought to be indirect, in part because most tumor cells express class I but not class II molecules. CD4[+] T cells were thought to act primarily through the provision of cytokines (T-cell help) to activate and maintain the CD8[+] T-cell compartment and also recruit inflammatory-responsive cells such as macrophages, granulocytes, and NK cells to directly kill tumor cells (Pardoll, 1995; Hung *et al.*, 1998; Qin & Blankenstein, 2000). Evidence suggests that CD4[+] T cells may play a more direct role in tumor rejection. In a mouse model it was shown that if CD4[+] T cells were depleted following vaccination but before tumor challenge (thus allowing for helper function in response to the vaccine), mice were unable to reject tumors, suggesting an effector role for the tumor-specific CD4[+] T-cell population (Dranoff *et al.*, 1993). Additionally, vaccination of mice against class I–negative tumor cells has been shown to result in the complete rejection of tumor cells, with both CD4[+] and NK T cells critical to the rejection (Levitsky *et al.*, 1994). Hung *et al.* showed that, in addition to CD8[+] T cells, CD4[+] T cells were important for the recruitment of additional antitumor effector cells, perhaps through the secretion of cytokines in response to specific stimulation by APC at the tumor site (Hung *et al.*, 1998). Using a class II–negative mesothelioma cell line transfected with the influenza hemagglutinin (HA) gene and two lines of transgenic mice that expressed CD8[+] and CD4[+] TCR specific for HA, Marzo *et al.* showed that tumor-specific CD4[+] cells enhanced tumor eradication, particularly when CTL numbers were suboptimal, demonstrating the importance for presentation of tumor antigens to class II-restricted cells (Marzo *et al.*, 1999). In an extension of that work, Marzo *et al.* have demonstrated that CD4[+] T cells were required for the maintenance of CD8[+] T cell and infiltration of the tumor mass by CD8[+] cells (Marzo *et al.*, 2000).

As discussed above, an important role for CD4[+] T cells in the generation of effective antitumor immunity has been shown to involve the maturation of DC with subsequent activation of CD8[+] T-cell effector functions. This effect of CD4[+] T cells, referred to as "DC licensing" has been shown to be mediated at least in part by the interaction of CD40 on DC with CD40L on activated CD4[+] T cells (Bennett *et al.*, 1998; Ridge *et al.*, 1998;

Schoenberger *et al.*, 1998). The critical role of the CD40:CD40L interaction for effective T-cell activation was recently shown by Albert and colleagues, with the demonstration that while CD40 ligation as a result of the interaction of mature DC with activated CD4$^+$ T cells leads to the effective activation of the CD8$^+$ T-cell compartment, in the absence of the DC:CD4$^+$ T-cell interaction DC induced tolerance in the CD8$^+$ T cells (Albert *et al.*, 2001).

Clinical trials

A number of clinical trials have been conducted based on the potential to activate tumor antigen-specific T cells through vaccination (see Nestle, 2000, for review). To date, most trials have been directed toward the therapy of melanoma, primarily because tumor-associated antigens that contain defined CD8$^+$ T-cell epitopes have been most commonly described for this tumor type. Vaccination strategies have involved the use of tumor antigen-derived peptides, recombinant tumor antigens, or tumor lysates either administered alone, in the context of adjuvants, or loaded onto DC (Nestle *et al.*, 1998; Thurner *et al.*, 1999; Geiger *et al.*, 2000; Banchereau *et al.*, 2001; Sadanaga *et al.*, 2001; Toungouz *et al.*, 2001) as well as irradiated whole tumor, gene modified to express immunostimulatory cytokines such as GM-CSF or IL-2 (Soiffer *et al.*, 1998; Simons *et al.*, 1999; Jaffee *et al.*, 2001).

In general, therapeutic outcomes in clinical trials to date have been disappointing (for review see Bodey *et al.*, 2000). Although in vivo expansion of antigen-specific T cells has been observed in numerous cases following vaccination, there is a poor correlation between T-cell responses and measurable clinical effects. Conversely, when remissions are observed they often occur in the absence of measurable T-cell activity. Nonetheless, pre- and prospective analyses of patients with early stage cancers have revealed evidence of a role for T cells in the control of tumor growth. The presence of TIL in early primary tumors as well as in lymph node metastases has been associated with reduced mortality and metastatic disease (Clemente *et al.*, 1996; Mihm *et al.*, 1996). Nakano *et al.* demonstrated that in renal cell carcinoma patients, increases in the proliferative capacity of CD8$^+$ T cells at the tumor site were associated with prolonged survival while simply increases in number of CD8$^+$ and CD4$^+$ T cells at the tumor mass were associated with decreased survival (Nakano *et al.*, 2001). In melanoma patients, Jager *et al.* analyzed Melan A/MART-1-specific T-cell responses in the skin and PBMC of an HLA-A2-positive melanoma patient immunized with Melan A/MART-1 HLA-A2 binding peptides (Jager *et al.*, 2000). Major regression of metastatic melanomas were observed, and a monoclonal population of Melan A/MART-1-specific CTL could be detected following in vitro stimulation, with the same monoclonal population detectable in skin biopsies taken from areas with vitiligo. Coulie *et al.* recently reported on the characterization of CD8$^+$ T-cell response in melanoma patients that had received a MAGE-3 derived peptide vaccine. By using HLA-A1 tetramers loaded with the immunizing peptide, these investigators were able to show that, in a melanoma patient that had demonstrated a partial rejection of a large metastatic lesion, a monoclonal CD8$^+$ T-cell population specific for the immunizing peptide could be detected following, but not before, immunization (Coulie *et al.*, 2001).

Strategies to detect antigen-specific T cells

Because a vaccine will only be successful if there exist precursor antigen-specific T cells that can be stimulated by administration of the immunogen, demonstrating the presence of antigen-specific T cells is generally considered to be a prerequisite for establishing an antigen as a vaccine candidate. A number of strategies, discussed and summarized by Clay, Hobeika, and co-workers (Clay *et al.*, 2001; Hobeika *et al.*, 2001), have been developed to detect antigen-specific T cells.

The principal in vivo assay has been the DTH test, in which soluble antigen is injected intradermally and the diameter of erythema, a measure of local inflammation, is measured 48 to 72 hours later. DTH responses usually reflect the presence of antigen-specific CD4^{++} T cells; however, they have also been reported to be mediated by CD8$^+$ T cells (Puccetti *et al.*, 1994). Although the DTH test is one of the most widely used tests performed to measure successful vaccination (Schreiber *et al.*, 1999; Simons *et al.*, 1999), it suffers from a lack of standardization.

A number of in vitro assays have been developed to measure antigen-specific T cells. Each of these assays depends on the ability to detect T cells from PBMC, the only practical, reproducibly available source of T cells. Since the frequency of circulating tumor antigen-specific T cells is exceedingly low, such protocols generally involve a T-cell expansion step prior to the assay. In vitro assays suffer from two caveats that might result in an underestimation of the frequency of tumor antigen-specific T cells: First, it is possible that only a subset of antigen-specific T cells are amenable to in vitro stimulation and expansion, either due to the T-cell activation status or the use of in vitro stimulation regimens, and thus particular cells might be missed. Second, a number of experiments indicate that activated antigen-specific T cells may be localized to tumor masses and proximal lymph nodes and are not circulating. In vitro assays to identify antigen-specific T cells rely on the ability to either measure a T-cell effector function (cytolysis, cytokine production, or proliferation) or alternatively, the ability to physically detect T cell (TCR binding to MHC tetramers loaded with relevant peptides, TCR typing). Table 113.1 presents a summary of current methodologies to detect antigen-specific T cells. Among the assays, the ELISPOT, ICC-flow cytometric analysis, and MHC tetramer appear to be the best in terms of both sensitivity and information generated, with good concordance among them.

The ELISPOT assay measures cytokine (typically γ-IFN) production by T cells in response to antigen. The ELISPOT assay is essentially an ELISA assay where the readout is enu-

Table 113.1. *Summary of methodologies to detect antigen-specific T cells*

Assay	Measurement	Comments
DTH	Cytokine-mediated inflammation	In vivo, qualitative
Limit dilution assay (LDA)	Cytotoxicity	In vitro, quantitative, cumbersome, requires in vitro stimulation
Lymphoproliferation	Antigen-specific T-cell proliferation	In vitro, qualitative, occasionally can be measured directly from blood
Direct cytotoxicity	Cytotoxicity	In vitro, qualitative, insensitive, often requires in vitro stimulation
RT-PCR	Cytokine mRNA levels	In vitro, quantitative, no in vitro stimulation required, needs to be further validated
Intracellular staining (ICC)	Intracellular cytokine protein levels	In vitro, quantitative, sensitive, rapid, information rich, expensive
ELISA/ELISPOT	Cytokine secretion	In vitro, quantitative, sensitive, separate assay for each cytokine
Tetramer binding	TCR binding to MHC:peptide	In vitro, quantitative, requires knowledge of peptide: MHC, does not measure only functional cells
TCR typing	Clonotypic T cells	In vitro, requires knowledge of TCR usage, not functional

merated on the basis of spots on a solid support. The ELISPOT assay has received wide use to quantitate antigen-specific CD8+ and CD4+ T cells (for reviews see Schmittel *et al.*, 2000; Bennouna *et al.*, 2002).

Flow cytometry has been applied to estimate precursor frequencies of antigen-specific cells as low as $1/10^5$ cells (Given *et al.*, 1999). Suni *et al.* described a straightforward approach to quantitate antigen-specific T-cell responses in whole blood (Suni *et al.*, 1998). DeRosa and colleagues recently described the development of an 11-color 13-parameter flow cytometric assay to identify very specific T-cell subsets directly from blood (De Rosa *et al.*, 2001). Further refinement of this type of multiparameter assay will certainly be of value for characterization of tumor antigen-specific T-cell responses following vaccination.

MHC tetramers, originally described by Altman and colleagues (Altman *et al.*, 1996), are rapidly becoming a methodology of choice to analyze antigen-specific vaccine responses. MHC tetramer methodology is based on the use of soluble MHC tetramers, either covalently bound or with the potential to bind peptides of interest, linked to a fluorescent moiety, and engineered to form tetrameric complexes. The formation of tetrameric complexes allows for very high sensitivity for detecting, via FACS analysis, T cells that express TCR with affinity for MHC tetramer:peptide complexes. MHC tetramers have been used to monitor T-cell responses in a number of early clinical trials (Yee *et al.*, 1999, 2000; Jager *et al.*, 2000; Coulie *et al.*, 2001; Dutoit *et al.*, 2001; Speiser *et al.*, 2002).

Strategies to expand antigen-specific T cells

A number of in vitro strategies to stimulate and expand cancer antigen-specific CD8+ and CD4+ T cells in vitro have been described (Yee *et al.*, 1996; Correale *et al.*, 1997; Kim *et al.*, 1997; Correale *et al.*, 1998; Perez-Diez *et al.*, 1998; Peshwa *et al.*, 1998; Chaux *et al.*, 1999a; Huang *et al.*, 1999; Butterfield

et al., 2001). Because tumor antigen-specific precursor T cells exist at very low frequencies in the peripheral circulation, such strategies have typically focused on the identification of responses in patients, where responses may be amplified. Despite this fact, in vitro stimulation protocols have generally required amplification of antigen-specific T cells to demonstrate the presence of tumor antigen-specific effector T cells. In vitro stimulation protocols have involved the use of APC, pulsed with recombinant protein, peptides derived from the primary amino acid sequence of candidate antigen and predicted to bind desired HLA molecules, or APC modified to express tumor antigens as a result of recombinant virus infection or plasmid transfection.

Protocols based on the use of recombinant peptides have generally relied on the use of computer algorithms to identify tumor antigen-derived peptide sequences predicted to bind to particular HLA molecules. Although peptide-based protocols have been shown to be successful in terms of expanding antigen-specific CD8+ and CD4+ T cells, peptides selected on the basis of computer algorithms often do not represent naturally processed epitopes and thus resulting T cells are often peptide but not protein-specific. An additional major limitation of the peptide-based approach is the requirement for detailed knowledge of the peptide-binding requirements for particular HLA class I or class II molecules. Hural *et al.* have recently described an in vitro approach that utilizes overlapping peptide pools to expand tumor antigen-specific CD4+ T cells that recognized naturally processed epitopes without knowledge of MHC binding requirements (Hural *et al.*, 2002). The general applicability of this approach may enable rapid assessment of potential immunogenicity of vaccine candidates.

In vitro approaches that involve pulsing recombinant whole protein on to DC have been developed to generate antigen-specific CD4+ T cells (Chaux *et al.*, 1999b, 2001; Schultz *et al.*, 2000). These approaches suffer from the requirement for very highly purified protein preparations to minimize expansion of CD4$^+$ T cells specific for contaminants present in the protein preparations.

Whole-gene based in vitro stimulation protocols have been recently developed for expanding antigen-specific CD8$^+$ T cells. These strategies utilize either viral or plasmid vectors to introduce genes into APC. These approaches result in the expansion of T cells that, by definition, recognize naturally processed epitopes. Among the virus systems, vaccinia, canarypox, and adenovirus vectors appear to be most promising. The use of recombinant vaccinia viruses expressing tyrosinase or MART-1 to expand antigen-specific CTL from melanoma patients has been reported (Yee *et al.*, 1996; Valmori *et al.*, 2000). Chaux *et al.* have recently reported the use of the ALVAC (canarypox) delivery vector to introduce genes into DC and expand MAGE-A1 reactive CTL from the blood of healthy individuals (Chaux *et al.*, 1999a). Adenovirus has also been shown to be an effective means to deliver and express transgenes in PBMC-derived DC (Zhong *et al.*, 1999). Adenovirus-infected DC have been used in a number of instances to stimulate T-cell activity against tumor antigens (Butterfield *et al.*, 1998; Wan *et al.*, 1997; Diao *et al.*, 1999; Kaplan *et al.*, 1999; Ranieri *et al.*, 1999; Friedman *et al.*, 2002) and adenovirus infection of DC has been shown to enhance the stimulatory capacity of these APC (Morelli *et al.*, 2000; Rouard *et al.*, 2000).

An intriguing approach to introduce antigens into DC has involved RNA transfection. Pioneered by Gilboa and colleagues (Boczkowski *et al.*, 1996), this approach has been validated extensively in animal models in vitro (for review see Mitchell & Nair, 2000). Encouraging preliminary results have been obtained from early stage clinical trials using RNA loaded DC in colon, and prostate cancer patients (Heiser *et al.*, 2002; Nair *et al.*, 2002).

Naked DNA transfection has been shown to have promise as an alternative methodology to introduce genes for vaccination. Naked DNA can be delivered intradermally or intramuscularly, using injection or through the use of projectile-based approaches such as the GeneGun (Harrison *et al.*, 2002) or micro-enhancer arrays (Mikszta *et al.*, 2002). DNA immunization has been shown to elicit both humoral as well as T-cell responses (Tuting *et al.*, 1997; Haupt *et al.*, 2002), as well as long-lasting cellular immunity (Gurunathan *et al.*, 2000). Naked DNA immunization offers a number of potential advantages over viral-mediated transduction. DNA production is inexpensive, there is an absence of immune responses against DNA backbone, and there is the potential to co-introduce multiple DNA species that encode co-stimulatory factors or immunostimulatory cytokines. On the basis of animal models, it has been suggested that the best strategy for achieving a robust immune response may involve an initial immunization with naked DNA followed by boosting with viral vectors. Recent clinical trials in prostate and colorectal cancer using naked DNA immunization followed by adenovirus boosts have shown promise, particularly in patients with minimal residual disease and no metastases (Mincheff *et al.*, 2001).

Tumor antigens under consideration for T-cell vaccines

A large body of literature exists on the identification of gene products with potential for use as cancer vaccines. The vast majority of gene products that are expressed by tumors are also expressed at significant levels by normal cells and thus are not reasonable candidates for the development of T-cell-based immunotherapy protocols. However, tumor cells also express a number of gene products that are not expressed by normal tissues and therefore serve as attractive targets for the T-cell arm of the immune system. The neoplastic phenotype is associated with expression of viral antigens expressed by viruses such as HPV, EBV, HBV, and HCV, differentiation antigens, as well as gene products whose expression is normally restricted to fetal and/or privileged tissues (cancer/testis antigens). Specific mutational events in normal cellular genes such as CDK-4 (Wolfel *et al.*, 1995) and bcr-abl (Mannering *et al.*, 1997), that result in point mutations, deletions, and translocations of normal cellular genes have also been associated with specific tumor types. Tumor cells have been shown in a number of instances to overexpress specific gene products (Her-2/neu, p53), as well as transcribe unique RNA species derived from intronic sequences or from alternative reading frames of known genes (NYESO-1Rf2, TRP-2). Finally, tumor cells can aberrantly modify and glycosylate proteins (MUC-1), and such proteins have the potential to be differentially processed and presented to the immune system. Tumor antigen targets have been identified by a number of methodologies, including T-cell and serological expression cloning (Tureci *et al.*, 1997), genome based (Schultze & Vonderheide, 2001), and microarray analysis (Xu *et al.*, 2000, 2001) as well as proteomics (Le Naour, 2001).

In a few cases, the presence of CD8$^+$ and or CD4$^+$ T cells that recognize tumors that present naturally processed epitopes derived from the antigen candidates has been demonstrated, supporting the use of those antigens as vaccines. Renkvist and colleagues have recently compiled a comprehensive listing of human tumor antigens recognized by T cells (Renkvist *et al.*, 2001). Table 113.2 presents a summary of tumor antigens for which data exist for the presence of a T-cell response that recognizes naturally processed antigen-derived epitopes. Excluded from this table are reports on unique antigens, that is, antigens that are uniquely expressed by a single tumor as a result of a mutational event. Although the presence of T cells specific for such antigens reflects the development of T-cell antitumor immunity, these antigens are not of general utility since the antigenic epitope is unique to the original tumor and is not expressed by other tumors.

Current clinical strategies to activate antigen-specific T cells

Over the past 10 years, a number of clinical trials have been initiated to examine the potential for the activation of tumor

Table 113.2. *Summary of tumor antigens to which CD8 and/or CD4 T-cell responses have been identified*

Antigen	Tumor expression	Other tissue expression	T cells (references)
I: Cancer testis-oncofetal			
MAGE-A1	Melanoma, multiple others	Spermatocytes, spermatogonia	CD8 (van der *et al.*, 1994b; Chaux *et al.*, 1999a; Fujie *et al.*, 1999; Tanzarella *et al.*, 1999; Luiten van der, 2000; Pascolo *et al.*, 2001)
			CD4 (Chaux *et al.*, 2001)
MAGE-A2	Melanoma, multiple others	Spermatocytes, spermatogonia	CD8 (Visseren *et al.*, 1997; Kawashima *et al.*, 1998; Tahara *et al.*, 1999; Tanzarella *et al.*, 1999; Keogh *et al.*, 2001)
MAGE-A3	Melanoma, multiple others	Spermatocytes, spermatogonia, placenta	CD8 (van der *et al.*, 1994a; Gaugler *et al.*, 1994; Herman *et al.*, 1996; Kawashami *et al.*, 1998; Oiso *et al.*, 1999; Tanzarella *et al.*, 1999; Kobayashi *et al.*, 2001b; Schultz *et al.*, 2001)
			CD4 (Chaux *et al.*, 1999b; Schultz *et al.*, 2000)
MAGE-A4, 6, 10, 12	Melanoma, multiple others	Spermatocytes, spermatogonia, placenta	CD8 (Duffour *et al.*, 1999; Huang *et al.*, 1999; Tanzarella *et al.*, 1999; Zorn & Hercend, 1999; Heidecker *et al.*, 2000; Panelli *et al.*, 2000; Schultz *et al.*, 2000)
BAGE	Melanoma, multiple others	Spermatocytes, spermatogonia	CD8 (Boel *et al.*, 1995)
GAGE-1, -2, -8	Melanoma, multiple others	Spermatocytes, spermatogonia, placenta	CD8 (Van den *et al.*, 1995; De Backer *et al.*, 1999)
NY-ESO-1	Melanoma, multiple others	Spermatocytes, spermatogonia, ovary	CD8 (Jager *et al.*, 1998; Chen *et al.*, 2000)
			CD4 (Zarour *et al.*, 2000; Zeng *et al.*, 2000, 2001)
NY-ESO-1 ORF2	Melanoma, multiple others	Spermatocytes, spermatogonia	CD8 (Jager *et al.*, 1998; Wang *et al.*, 1998a)
DAM-6, -10	Melanoma, multiple others	Spermatocytes, spermatogonia	CD8 (Fleischhauer *et al.*, 1998)
NA88-A	Melanoma, multiple others	Spermatocytes, spermatogonia	CD8 (Moreau-Aubry *et al.*, 2000)
SSX-2 (HOM-Mel-40)	Melanoma, multiple others	Testis, thyroid	CD8 (Ayyoub *et al.*, 2002)
II: Shared tumor-specific			
G250	Cervical, colon, ovarian, renal	None	CD8 (Vissers *et al.*, 1999)
GnT-V	Brain, melanoma, sarcoma	Breast, brain (low)	CD8 (Guilloux *et al.*, 1996)
RAGE	Bladder, colon, head/neck, mammary, melanoma, mesothelioma, renal, sarcoma	Retina	CD8 (Gaugler *et al.*, 1996)
SART-1	Esophageal, head/neck, lung, uterine	Fetal tissue/testis	CD8 (Kikuchi *et al.*, 1999; Yang *et al.*, 1999)
SART-2	Brain, esophageal, head/neck, lung, adenocarcinoma, melanoma, renal, uterine	None	CD8 (Nakao *et al.*, 2000)
ART-4	Cervical, esophageal, endometrial, gastric, head/neck, leukemia, lung, ovarian	Testis, placenta, fetal tissue	CD8 (Kawano *et al.*, 2000)
III: Widely expressed antigens			
CEA	Breast, colon, gastric, lung, melanoma, pancreas, rectal	Heart, pancreas, placenta, skeletal muscle	CD8 (Tsang *et al.*, 1997; Kawashima *et al.*, 1999; Nukaya *et al.*, 1999; Keogh *et al.*, 2001; Huarte *et al.*, 2002)
Her-2/neu	Breast, melanoma, ovarian	Multiple, primarily epithelial tissues	CD8 (Fisk *et al.*, 1995; Peoples *et al.*, 1995; Kawashima *et al.*, 1998, 1999; Kono *et al.*, 1998; Rongcun *et al.*, 1999; Scardino *et al.*, 2001; Tanaka *et al.*, 2001)
			CD4 (Kobayashi *et al.*, 2000; Keogh *et al.*, 2001; Sotiriadou *et al.*, 2001; Perez *et al.*, 2002)
MUC-1	Breast, B-cell lymphoma, ovarian	Epithelial tissues	CD8 (Domenech *et al.*, 1995; Brossart *et al.*, 2001)
MUC-2	Breast, colon, ovarian, pancreas	Bronchus, cervix, colon, gall bladder, small intestine	CD8 (Bohm *et al.*, 1998)

(Table continues)

Table 113.2. *(Continued)*

Antigen	Tumor expression	Other tissue expression	T cells (references)
III: Widely expressed antigens *(continued)*			
PRAME	Adenocarcinoma, renal, lung, head/neck, melanoma	Adrenals, brain, kidney, skin, ovary, endometrium	CD8 (Ikeda *et al.*, 1997; Kessler *et al.*, 2001)
WT-1	Leukemia, colon, gastric, breast, lung, ovary, uterine, thyroid	Kidney, overy, testis, spleen	CD8 (Oka *et al.*, 2000; Azuma *et al.*, 2002)
Cyclophilin-B	Epithelial cancer, leukemias	All normal tissues	CD8 (Gomi *et al.*, 1999)
Human chorionic gonadotrophin	Colon, breast, prostate, bladder	Multiple	CD8 (Dangles *et al.*, 2002) CD4 (Dangles *et al.*, 2002)
Teomerase (htert)	Widely	Multiple	CD8 (Vonderheide *et al.*, 2001)
IV. Tumor-tumor/tissue specific			
Melan-A/MART-1	Melanoma	Melanocytes, retina, peripheral ganglia	CD8 (Coulie *et al.*, 1994; Kawakami *et al.*, 1994; Castelli *et al.*, 1995; Schneider *et al.*, 1998)
Tyrosinase	Melanoma	Melanocytes, retina, peripheral ganglia	CD8 (Wolfel *et al.*, 1994; Kang *et al.*, 1995; Brichard *et al.*, 1996; Brichard *et al.*, 1996; Corman *et al.*, 1998; Kawakami *et al.*, 1998; Kittlessen *et al.*, 1998; Riley *et al.*, 2001; Scheibenbogen *et al.*, 2002) CD4 (Topalian *et al.*, 1996)
gp100	Melanoma	Melanocytes, retina, peripheral ganglia	CD8 (Bakker *et al.*, 1995; Kawakami *et al.*, 1995; Skipper *et al.*, 1996; Robbins *et al.*, 1997; Tsai *et al.*, 1997; Kawashima *et al.*, 1998; Castelli *et al.*, 1999) CD4 (Kobayashi *et al.*, 2001a)
gp75/TRP-1	Melanoma	Melanocytes, retina, peripheral ganglia	CD8 (Wang *et al.*, 1996b)
Tyrosinase-related protein (TRP-2)	Melanoma	Melanocytes, retina, peripheral ganglia	CD8 (Wang *et al.*, 1996a; Parkhurst *et al.*, 1998; Castelli *et al.*, 1999; Noppen *et al.*, 2000; Harada *et al.*, 2001)
MCIR	Melanoma	Melanocytes, retina, peripheral ganglia	CD8 (Salazar-Onfray *et al.*, 1997)
MG50	Melanoma	Melanocytes, retina, peripheral ganglia	CD8 (Mitchell *et al.*, 2000)
CAMEL	Melanoma	Heart, pancreas, skeletal muscle	CD8 (Rimoldi *et al.*, 2000)
P15	Melanoma	Adrenal, lung, kidney, spleen, lever, thymus, retina	CD8 (Robbins *et al.*, 1995)
PSCA	Prostate	Normal prostate	CD8 (Dannull *et al.*, 2000)
PAP	Prostate	Normal prostate	CD4 (McNeel *et al.*, 2001)
PSA	Prostate	Normal prostate	CD8 (Corman *et al.*, 1998; Correale *et al.*, 1998; Turner *et al.*, 2001) CD4 (Corman *et al.*, 1998)
KLK-4	Prostate	Normal prostate, low in multiple	CD4 Hural *et al.*, 2002
Prostein	Prostate	Normal prostate	CD8 Friedman *et al.*, 2002
a-Fetoprotein	Hepatocellular	None	CD8 (Butterfield *et al.*, 1999)
TGF-β	Colorectal		CD8 (Saeterdal *et al.*, 2001)
Bcr-abl	Leukemia	None	CD8 (Bocchia *et al.*, 1996; Greco *et al.*, 1996; Buzyn *et al.*, 1997; Yotnda *et al.*, 1998; Norbury *et al.*, 2000) CD4 (ten Bosch *et al.*, 1995, 1999; Yasukawa *et al.*, 1998, 2001; Tanaka *et al.*, 2000)
Intestinal carboxyl esterase	Renal	Colon, kidney, liver, small intestine	CD8 (Ronsin *et al.*, 1999)

antigen-specific T cells in cancer patients. In the case of tumor types for which well-characterized tumor antigens have been identified (primarily melanoma), approaches generally involve administration of the antigen to patients in the form of either whole recombinant protein or peptides that have been demonstrated to be immunologically relevant. Defined antigen has been delivered alone (Marchand *et al.*, 1999), in the context of potent adjuvants or cytokines (Jager *et al.*, 1996a; Bendandi *et al.*, 1999; Disis *et al.*, 1999; Wang *et al.*, 1999; Jager *et al.*, 2000; Lee *et al.*, 2001), or in the context of DC (Hsu *et al.*, 1996; Morse *et al.*, 1999; Thurner *et al.*, 1999; Banchereau *et al.*, 2001; Sadanaga *et al.*, 2001; Toungouz *et al.*, 2001). Alternative approaches that do not depend on the previous identification of defined tumor antigens have involved vaccination strategies with allogeneic or autologous whole tumor, irradiated and in some cases modified to express cytokines or co-stimulatory molecules or tumor cell lysates, in adjuvant or loaded ex vivo on to DC (Soiffer *et al.,* 1998; Simons *et al.,* 1999; Geiger *et al.,* 2000; Jaffee *et al.,* 2001). Although encouraging results have been reported from individual patients, results from clinical trials have to date been on the whole disappointing, at least in part because early stage trials are conducted on advanced stage patients with in most cases, severely compromised immune systems as a result of disease or treatment regimens, and large tumor burdens. As discussed above, immune responses have been observed in patients with no tumor remission, and conversely, remissions have been observed in patients with no detectable immune response. It is apparent that a number of variables still need to be optimized in clinical trials. In particular, methodology and route of administration, delivery methodologies, adjuvants, readouts for effective immunization, and clinical endpoints differ widely among clinical trials, and thus the possibility to comparatively assess methodologies has not been possible (see reviews by Hobeika *et al.,* 2001; Simon *et al.,* 2001). The development of objective universally accepted parameters to vaccinate and assess the success of vaccinations is an important consideration to address in future trials.

Future prospects for T-cell therapy

As discussed above, although current T-cell vaccination strategies against cancer have demonstrated efficacy in some cases, overall results to date have not been encouraging. A number of areas can be identified where progress and innovation will be required for the reproducible success of vaccine-based cancer immunotherapy. Primary limitations of current strategies can be identified as (1) Lack of optimal antigens to which a vigorous T-cell response can be generated, (2) the inability to effectively circumvent tumor-induced immunosuppression and T-cell anergy/tolerance for most tumor antigens, (3) lack of appropriate delivery systems for the effective activation of an antitumor immune response.

1. Lack of optimal antigens to which a vigorous T-cell response can be generated. The idea that specific antigens exist that are expressed by tumor cells and could act as targets for T cells extended from the seminal work of Boon and colleagues who demonstrated that CTL responses to the melanoma antigen MAGE-1 could be identified in melanoma patients. Since that discovery, a large number of antigens have been described that could serve as T-cell targets. The majority of these antigens were discovered using serological or molecular expression cloning approaches, both of which require established tumor cell lines and pre-existing immunological reagents (sera and T cells, respectively). Although pre-existing T-cell responses might be considered to be advantageous for tumor eradication, these T-cell responses generally are insufficient to eradicate the corresponding tumors. Thus, it is possible that antigens identified on the basis of pre-existing antitumor T-

cell responses may not be optimal for use as vaccine candidates for tumor immunotherapy.

Recent advances have allowed for the development of high throughput approaches for the identification of genes expressed in tumor or tissue-specific patterns without the requirement for established tumor cell lines or T-cell reagents, thus opening up the potential for identifying novel antigens strictly on the basis of expression profiles. Genes identified by these approaches might be capable of stimulating potent immune responses against tumors upon vaccination. A variety of techniques, including serial analysis of gene expression (SAGE), subtraction hybridization, microarray analysis, and PCR-based differential display or combinations thereof (Lee *et al.,* 1991; Velculescu *et al.,* 1995; Zhang *et al.,* 1997; Lockhart & Winzeler, 2000; Xu *et al.,* 2000) have been described that have resulted in the identification of a large number of novel tumor-specific or overexpressed proteins that are currently being evaluated for their potential as vaccine antigens.

2. The inability to effectively circumvent tumor-induced immunosuppression and T-cell tolerance. As discussed above, as tumors evolve and expand in vivo there are strong selective pressures for the development of tumor-driven mechanisms to evade the host immune response. Furthermore, because the majority of tumor antigens identified are also expressed in some normal tissues, high affinity antigen-specific T cells are deleted and mechanisms are operative in vivo to prevent T-cell activation in response to tumors. Taken together, these issues present a formidable challenge for the development of vaccination strategies to elicit effective tumor-specific T-cell activity.

Since tumors lack co-stimulatory molecules, naïve T cells that can recognize MHC:peptide complexes on the tumor surface either exist in a tolerized state or alternatively remain ignorant to the tumor due to their low affinity for antigen. Strategies have been implemented to overcome the lack of co-stimulation by tumor cells. In a number of mouse models, inhibition of CTLA-4 function (Kwon *et al.,* 1997) or expression of B7 family members in tumors has been shown to improve immunogenicity and enhance the development of prophylactic immunity (Townsend & Allison, 1993; Townsend *et al.,* 1994; Huang *et al.,* 1996; Kwon *et al.,* 1997; Hurwitz *et al.,* 1998). A major limitation with this approach is the requirement for tumor cells that can be cultured and efficiently modified to express co-stimulatory molecules in a stable fashion. The development of culture protocols as well as efficient gene transfer methodologies will have significant impact on the efficacy of such strategies in the future.

An observation that has been made in a number of clinical trials systems is that tumor antigen-specific T cells are physiologically compromised, most likely as a result of encounter with tumor. This observation may reflect the establishment of anergy, or may reflect additional consequences of the tumor:T-cell interaction. Lee *et al.* (1999) examined the status of melanoma antigen-specific CD8$^+$ T cells in patients with advanced metastatic melanoma. Using tetramer assays, these investigators demonstrated that substantial numbers of melanoma antigen-specific T cells could be identified in patients; however, although the T cells had clearly expanded in vivo (reaching up to 2% of the total CD8$^+$ T-cell population in one case) these T cells were functionally inactive since they were neither lytic nor did they produce cytokine in response to tumor. Nielsen *et al.* examined the presence and status of CD8$^+$ T cells specific for a gp100 epitope in eight melanoma patients following peptide vaccination, using HLA-A*0201 tetramers loaded with the gp100 derived epitope, intracellular (ICC)-FACS staining, and quantitative PCR (Nielsen *et al.*, 2000). Despite the absence of clinical responses, enhancement of T-cell precursor frequency and specific production of γ-IFN by antigen-specific T cells were observed postvaccination in the majority of patients. Understanding the mechanisms responsible for T-cell inactivation following immunization is critical to developing methodologies for effective T-cell activation.

A number of transgenic mouse models have been developed to study tumor antigen-specific tolerance. Recently, Ohlen *et al.* (2001) described a transgenic mouse model where the immunodominant CD8$^+$ epitope derived from the Friend Murine Leukemia virus (FmuLV) gag protein was expressed in the liver of mice. Although T cells specific for this epitope could be isolated from animals, the T cells were tolerized in vivo since FmuLV positive tumors grew unimpeded in vivo. T cells could, however, be activated and expanded in vitro and, following re-infusion, could eliminate gag expressing tumors without destruction of host liver tissue (Ohlen *et al.*, 2001). Additionally, in a transgenic mouse model for influenza hemagglutinin, Morgan and colleagues demonstrated that, for a self epitope that was expressed in pancreatic islet β cells and overexpressed in a renal carcinoma cell line, activation of low avidity CTL resulted in tumor rejection with no evidence of autoimmune damage to islet cells (Morgan *et al.*, 1998). These observations demonstrate that if T cells can be activated that are specific for antigens overexpressed by tumors, then, even though the same antigens are expressed at some level in normal tissues, tumor eradication may occur in the absence of autoimmunity.

A promising avenue for T-cell-based immunotherapy of cancer involves adoptive transfer of antigen-specific T cells into cancer patients (Yee *et al.*, 1997). In adoptive transfer, antigen-specific T cells are isolated, expanded ex vivo, and following expansion, re-infused in large numbers into patients at supraphysiologic levels. Adoptive transfer of cloned T cells has been shown to be effective in the setting of CMV, EBV, and HIV (Rooney *et al.*, 1995; Walter *et al.*, 1995; Brodie *et al.*, 1999). The best example of the efficacy of adoptive transfer protocols in the eradication of cancer is illustrated by allogeneic stem cell transplantation. A major complication with allogeneic stem cell transplantation is the development of graft-versus-host disease (GVHD), mediated by donor T cells attacking recipient tissues. The strong corrletion between the development and severity of GVHD and tumor regression has led to the conclusion that adoptively transferred T cells, specific for minor histocompatibility antigens expressed on patient tumor cells are responsible for

tumor eradication (Horowitz *et al.*, 1990). The adoptive transfer of antigen-specific T cells has been applied with limited success in the tumor immunotherapy field. Adoptive transfer of bulk lymphocytes has been shown to be effective in the regression of renal cell carcinoma (Childs *et al.*, 2000), and leukemia (Kolb *et al.*, 1995). Yee *et al.* employed adoptive transfer of MART-1 specific CD8$^+$ T cell clones in a melanoma patient (Yee *et al.*, 2000). While transferred T cells localized and destroyed tissue that expressed the antigen with accompanying vitiligo, residual tumor masses were negative for MART-1 expression, providing evidence that adoptively transferred T cells mediated the elimination of MART-1 expressing tumor cells.

Two major limitations associated with adoptive transfer in the cancer setting are (1) the observation that most tumor antigen-specific T cells identified to date are not particularly effective as effector cells, in part due to their moderate affinity for tumor cells and in part due to their tolerized state, and (2) the difficulty with reproducibly obtaining tumor antigen-specific T cells due to precursor frequency and limitations with in vitro expansion protocols.

One potential approach to overcome the issue of tolerance is derived from the ex vivo activation and adoptive transfer experiments described above. As discussed, ex vivo culture of antigen-specific T cells may allow the re-acquisition of effector functions suppressed in vivo, and re-activated T cells, infused at high numbers, and potentially genetically modified to express gene products to counteract tumor factors, might be very effective at tumor eradication (Ohlen *et al.*, 2001). Further evidence that ex vivo culture can be used to effectively activate T cells and overcome tumor immunosuppressive effects was provided by Cohen *et al.*, who demonstrated that in vitro activation of L-selectin low T cells (4 and 8) and re-infusion resulted in tumor rejection at numerous anatomic sites (Cohen *et al.*, 2001). The demonstration that ex vivo culture of tolerized T cells could result in activation of effector functions and subsequent tumor eradication upon re-infusion supports the development of ex vivo expansion and transfer protocols for the eradication of tumors to which endogenous T-cell responses would be tolerized.

One approach to overcome the difficulty with generating antigen-specific T cells from every patient involves transfer of T-cell specificity via TCR transfer (for a review see Kessels *et al.*, 2001). This approach has been demonstrated to be feasible in viral systems (Clay *et al.*, 1999; Cooper *et al.*, 2000). Methodologies have been developed for the efficient cloning and transfer of TCR into primary T cells. Thus, once a tumor antigen-specific T cell is identified, TCR α and β chains could be cloned and introduced at will into T cells from patients that share the relevant MHC molecule. A number of methodologies are currently under development for generation of tumor antigen-specific T cells with higher affinity for antigen to overcome and to overcome the issue of moderate affinity T cells in vivo. Methodologies with particular promise are the generation of tumor antigen-specific T-cell responses in the context of allogeneic MHC alleles (Wang *et al.*, 1998b; Munz *et al.*, 1999; Yee *et al.*, 1999; Moris *et al.*, 2001), mutagenesis of TCR chains to increase TCR affinity (Kieke *et al.*, 2001) and generation of T-cell response in human HLA-transgenic mice followed by humanization of murine TCR chains. The requirement for antigen processing and presentation of HLA molecules can be bypassed by the genetic modification of T cells to express a chimeric immunoreceptor composed of a single chain immunoglobulin extracellular targeting domain specific for tumor-specific or tumor-associated antigen fused to a CD3-ξ intracellular signaling domain. Such an approach has been taken using CD19 as the target antigen (Cooper *et al.*, 2003).

3. Lack of appropriate delivery systems for the effective activation of an immune response. Although a significant body of research has allowed for the development of methodologies to culture DC ex vivo, much needs to be developed with regard to optimizing DC for use in cancer immunotherapy. Most clinical trials have utilized DC generated from patient PBMC-derived monocytes by differentiation ex vivo in the presence of GM-CSF and IL-4, loaded with recombinant protein or peptide, and subsequently introduced into patients (for review see Lopez & Hart, 2002). However, as discussed above, such immature DC may not be optimal for presenting T-cell epitopes to T cells or for migrating to tumor sites and proximal lymph nodes, and rapidly de-differentiate in the absence of cytokines. The coordination and use of maturation regimens that allow for efficient uptake, processing, and presentation of antigenic epitopes will be a critical area to optimize for the development of successful immunotherapy protocols.

The development of viral gene delivery systems will most certainly be critical for the development of effective tumor vaccine protocols. The potential to genetically modify APC to express vaccine antigens, cytokines, or co-stimulatory factors is likely to allow for more efficient antigen presentation to the immune system. A number of attenuated virus delivery systems (reviewed in Bonnet *et al.*, 2000) have been considered or are in early clinical trials (Scholl *et al.*, 2000; Gomella *et al.*, 2001; Kuball *et al.*, 2002). These viruses, which include vaccinia virus, retroviruses (Lapointe *et al.*, 2001), adenovirus (Wan *et al.*, 1997; Bonnet *et al.*, 2000), canarypox (Engelmayer *et al.*, 2001), and alphavirus (Lundstrom, 2002), have been shown to infect DC with high efficiency, and in early clinical trials have been shown to have some efficacy.

New methodologies for vaccine antigen delivery that include the use of APC such as epidermal Langerhans cells (Kumamoto *et al.*, 2002), heat shock proteins (Menoret & Chandawarkar, 1998; Srivastava & Amato, 2001; Manjili *et al.*, 2002), microsphere encapsulation (Partidos *et al.*, 1997; Egilmez *et al.*, 2000), liposomes (Ignatius *et al.*, 2000; Manjili *et al.*, 2002), or mechanical delivery approaches (Manjili *et al.*, 2002; Mikszta *et al.*, 2002), and the identification of optimal prime-boost strategies (Meng *et al.*, 2001) may allow for efficient delivery and activation of antitumor immunity.

Identification of the optimal routes of administration for vaccine delivery is another critical area for research. Although most clinical trials have involved intravenous administration of vaccines, evidence from both mouse models and clinical trials suggests that intranodal (Lambert *et al.*, 2001) or intradermal (Fong *et al.*, 2001) administration of vaccines is superior in terms of eliciting T-cell responses.

Finally, identification of novel adjuvants that can elicit a potent immune response is likely to be critical for effective antitumor vaccination. In this regard oligonucleotides containing CpG motifs (Davila & Celis, 2000; Miconnet *et al.*, 2002), cationic poly-amino acid complexes (Mattner *et al.*, 2002), and bacterial cell wall components (Miconnet *et al.*, 2001) are being tested in animal model trials for the ability to mediate effective immune system activation.

References

Albert, M.L., Jegathesan, M., & Darnell, R.B. (2001). Dendritic cell maturation is required for the cross-tolerization of CD8+ T cells. *Nature Immunology*, **2**, 1010–17.

Albert, M.L., Sauter, B., & Bhardwaj, N. (1998). Dendritic cells acquire antigen from apoptotic cells and induce class I-restricted CTLs. *Nature*, **392**, 86–9.

Altman, J.D., Moss, P.A., Goulder, P.J. *et al.* (1996). Phenotypic analysis of antigen-specific T lymphocytes. *Science*, **274**, 94–6.

Arienti, F., Belli, F., Napolitano, F. *et al.* (1999). Vaccination of melanoma patients with interleukin 4 gene-transduced allogeneic melanoma cells. *Human Gene Therapy*, **10**, 2907–16.

Atkins, M.B., Lotze, M.T., Dutcher, J.P. *et al.* (1999). High-dose recombinant interleukin 2 therapy for patients with metastatic melanoma: analysis of 270 patients treated between 1985 and 1993. *Journal of Clinical Oncology*, **17**, 2105–16.

Ayyoub, M., Stevanovic, S., Sahin, U. *et al.* (2002). Proteasome-assisted identification of a SSX-2-derived epitope recognized by tumor-reactive CTL infiltrating metastatic melanoma. *Journal of Immunology*, **168**, 1717–22.

Azuma, T., Makita, M., Ninomiya, K. *et al.* (2002). Identification of a novel WT1-derived peptide which induces human leucocyte antigen-A24-restricted anti-leukaemia cytotoxic T lymphocytes. *British Journal of Haematology*, **116**, 601–3.

Bakker, A.B., Schreurs, M.W., Tafazzul, G. *et al.* (1995). Identification of a novel peptide derived from the melanocyte-specific gp 100 antigen as the dominant epitope recognized by an HLA-A2.1-restricted anti-melanoma CTL line. *International Journal of Cancer*, **62**, 97–102.

Banchereau, J., Briere, F., Caux, C. *et al.* (2000). Immunobiology of dendritic cells. *Annual Review of Immunology*, **18**, 767–811.

Banchereau, J., Palucka, A.K., Dhodapkar, M. *et al.* (2001). Immune and clinical responses in patients with metastatic melanoma to CD34(+) progenitor-derived dendritic cell vaccine. *Cancer Research*, **61**, 6451–8.

Barth, R.J., Jr., Mule, J.J., Spiess, P.J., & Rosenberg, S.A. (1991). Interferon gamma and tumor necrosis factor have a role in tumor regressions mediated by murine CD8+ tumor-infiltrating lymphocytes. *Journal of Experimental Medicine*, **173**, 647–58.

Beatty, G. & Paterson, Y. (2001). IFN-gamma-dependent inhibition of tumor angiogenesis by tumor-infiltrating CD4+ T cells requires tumor responsiveness to IFN-gamma. *Journal of Immunology*, **166**, 2276–82.

Beatty, G.L. & Paterson, Y. (2000). IFN-gamma can promote tumor evasion of the immune system in vivo by down-regulating cellular levels of an endogenous tumor antigen. *Journal of Immunology,* **165,** 5502–8.

Beissert, S., Hosoi, J., Grabbe, S. *et al.* (1995). IL-10 inhibits tumor antigen presentation by epidermal antigen-presenting cells. *Journal of Immunology,* **154,** 1280–6.

Bendandi, M., Gocke, C.D., Kobrin, C.B. *et al.* (1999). Complete molecular remissions induced by patient-specific vaccination plus granulocyte-monocyte colony-stimulating factor against lymphoma. *Nature Medicine,* **5,** 1171–7.

Bennett, S.R., Carbone, F.R., Karamalis, F. *et al.* (1998). Help for cytotoxic T-cell responses is mediated by CD40 signalling. *Nature,* **393,** 478–80.

Bennett, S.R., Carbone, F.R., Karamalis, F. *et al.* (1997). Induction of a CD8+ cytotoxic T lymphocyte response by cross-priming requires cognate CD4+ T cell help. *Journal of Experimental Medicine,* **186,** 65–70.

Bennouna, J., Hildesheim, A., Chikamatsu, K. *et al.* (2002). Application of IL-5 ELISPOT assays to quantification of antigen-specific T helper responses. *Journal of Immunological Methods,* **261,** 145–56.

Bevan, M.J. (1976). Cross-priming for a secondary cytotoxic response to minor H antigens with H-2 congenic cells which do not cross-react in the cytotoxic assay. *Journal of Experimental Medicine,* **143,** 1283–8.

Bocchia, M., Korontsvit, T., Xu, Q. *et al.* (1996). Specific human cellular immunity to bcr-abl oncogene-derived peptides. *Blood,* **87,** 3587–92.

Boczkowski, D., Nair, S.K., Snyder, D., & Gilboa, E. (1996). Dendritic cells pulsed with RNA are potent antigen-presenting cells in vitro and in vivo. *Journal of Experimental Medicine,* **184,** 465–72.

Bodey, B., Bodey, B., Jr., Siegel, S.E., & Kaiser, H.E. (2000). Failure of cancer vaccines: the significant limitations of this approach to immunotherapy. *Anticancer Research,* **20,** 2665–76.

Boel, P., Wildmann, C., Sensi, M.L. *et al.* (1995). BAGE: a new gene encoding an antigen recognized on human melanomas by cytolytic T lymphocytes. *Immunity,* **2,** 167–75.

Bohm, C.M., Hanski, M.L., Stefanovic, S. *et al.* (1998). Identification of HLA-A2-restricted epitopes of the tumor-associated antigen MUC2 recognized by human cytotoxic T cells. *International Journal of Cancer,* **75,** 688–93.

Bollard, C.M., Rossig, C., Calonge, M.J. *et al.* (2002). Adapting a transforming growth factor beta-related tumor protection strategy to enhance antitumor immunity. *Blood,* **99,** 3179–87.

Bonnet, M.C., Tartaglia, J., Verdier, F. *et al.* (2000). Recombinant viruses as a tool for therapeutic vaccination against human cancers. *Immunology Letters,* **74,** 11–25.

Bosco, M., Giovarelli, M., Forni, M. *et al.* (1990). Low doses of IL-4 injected perilymphatically in tumor-bearing mice inhibit the growth of poorly and apparently nonimmunogenic tumors and induce a tumor-specific immune memory. *Journal of Immunology,* **145,** 3136–43.

Brichard, V.G., Herman, J., Van Pel, A. *et al.* (1996). A tyrosinase nonapeptide presented by HLA-B44 is recognized on a human melanoma by autologous cytolytic T lymphocytes. *European Journal of Immunology,* **26,** 224–30.

Brodie, S.J., Lewinsohn, D.A., Patterson, B.K. *et al.* (1999). In vivo migration and function of transferred HIV-1-specific cytotoxic T cells. *Nature Medicine,* **5,** 34–41.

Brossart, P., Schneider, A., Dill, P. *et al.* (2001). The epithelial tumor antigen MUC1 is expressed in hematological malignancies and is recognized by MUC1-specific cytotoxic T-lymphocytes. *Cancer Research,* **61,** 6846–50.

Burnet, F.M. (1970). The concept of immunological surveillance. *Progress in Experimental Tumor Research,* **13,** 1–27.

Butterfield, L.H., Jilani, S.M., Chakraborty, N.G. *et al.* (1998). Generation of melanoma-specific cytotoxic T lymphocytes by dendritic cells transduced with a MART-1 adenovirus. *Journal of Immunology,* **161,** 5607–13.

Butterfield, L.H., Koh, A., Meng, W. *et al.* (1999). Generation of human T-cell responses to an HLA-A2.1-restricted peptide epitope derived from alpha-fetoprotein. *Cancer Research,* **59,** 3134–42.

Butterfield, L.H., Meng, W.S., Koh, A. *et al.* (2001). T cell responses to HLA-A*0201-restricted peptides derived from human alpha fetoprotein. *Journal of Immunology,* **166,** 5300–8.

Buzyn, A., Ostankovitch, M., Zerbib, A. *et al.* (1997). Peptides derived from the whole sequence of BCR-ABL bind to several class I molecules allowing specific induction of human cytotoxic T lymphocytes. *European Journal of Immunology,* **27,** 2066–72.

Carbone, J.E. & Ohm, D.P. (2002). Immune dysfunction in cancer patients. *Oncology (Huntington)* **16,** 11–8.

Carreno, B.M. & Collins, M. (2002). The B7 family of ligands and its receptors: new pathways for costimulation and inhibition of immune responses. *Annual Review of Immunology,* **20,** 29–53.

Castelli, C., Storkus, W.J., Maeurer, M.J. *et al.* (1995). Mass spectrometric identification of a naturally processed melanoma peptide recognized by CD8+ cytotoxic T lymphocytes. *Journal of Experimental Medicine,* **181,** 363–8.

Castelli, C., Tarsini, P., Mazzocchi, A. *et al.* (1999). Novel HLA-Cw8-restricted T cell epitopes derived from tyrosinase-related protein-2 and gp100 melanoma antigens. *Journal of Immunology,* **162,** 1739–48.

Caux, C., Massacrier, C., Vanbervliet, B. *et al.* (1994). Activation of human dendritic cells through CD40 cross-linking. *Journal of Experimental Medicine,* **180,** 1263–72.

Cella, M., Sallusto, F., & Lanzavecchia, A. (1997). Origin, maturation and antigen presenting function of dendritic cells. *Current Opinions in Immunology,* **9,** 10–16.

Chang, C.H., Furue, M., & Tamaki, K. (1995). B7-1 expression of Langerhans cells is up-regulated by proinflammatory cytokines, and is down-regulated by interferon-gamma or by interleukin-10. *European Journal of Immunology,* **25,** 394–8.

Chaux, P., Lethe, B., Van Snick, J. *et al.* (2001). A MAGE-1 peptide recognized on HLA-DR15 by CD4(+) T cells. *European Journal of Immunology,* **31,** 1910–16.

Chaux, P., Luiten, R., Demotte, N. *et al.* (1999a). Identification of five MAGE-A1 epitopes recognized by cytolytic T lymphocytes obtained by in vitro stimulation with dendritic cells transduced with MAGE-A1. *Journal of Immunology,* **163,** 2928–36.

Chaux, P., Vantomme, V., Stroobant, V. *et al.* (1999b). Identification of MAGE-3 epitopes presented by HLA-DR molecules to CD4(+) T lymphocytes. *Journal of Experimental Medicine,* **189,** 767–78.

Cheever, M.A., Thompson, J.A., Peace, D.J., & Greenberg, P.D. (1986). Potential uses of interleukin 2 in cancer therapy. *Immunobiology*, **172**, 365–82.

Chen, H.L., Gabrilovich, D., Tampe, R. *et al.* (1996). A functionally defective allele of TAP1 results in loss of MHC class I antigen presentation in a human lung cancer. *Nature Genetics*, **13**, 210–13.

Chen, J.L., Dunbar, P.R., Gileadi, U. *et al.* (2000). Identification of NY-ESO-1 peptide analogues capable of improved stimulation of tumor-reactive CTL. *Journal of Immunology*, **165**, 948–55.

Childs, R., Chernoff, A., Contentin, N. *et al.* (2000). Regression of metastatic renal-cell carcinoma after nonmyeloablative allogeneic peripheral-blood stem-cell transplantation. *New England Journal of Medicine*, **343**, 750–8.

Chouaib, S., Asselin-Paturel, C., Mami-Chouaib, F. *et al.* (1997). The host-tumor immune conflict: from immunosuppression to resistance and destruction. *Immunology Today*, **18**, 493–7.

Clay, T.M., Custer, M.C., Sachs, J. *et al.* (1999). Efficient transfer of a tumor antigen-reactive TCR to human peripheral blood lymphocytes confers anti-tumor reactivity. *Journal of Immunology*, **163**, 507–13.

Clay, T.M., Hobeika, A.C., Mosca, P.J. *et al.* (2001). Assays for monitoring cellular immune responses to active immunotherapy of cancer. *Clinical Cancer Research*, **7**, 1127–35.

Clemente, C.G., Mihm, M.C., Jr., Bufalino, R. *et al.* (1996). Prognostic value of tumor infiltrating lymphocytes in the vertical growth phase of primary cutaneous melanoma. *Cancer*, **77**, 1303–10.

Cohen, P.A., Peng, L., Kjaergaard, J. *et al.* (2001). T-cell adoptive therapy of tumors: mechanisms of improved therapeutic performance. *Critical Reviews in Immunology*, **21**, 215–48.

Cooper, L.J., Kalos, M., Lewinsohn, D.A. *et al.* (2000). Transfer of specificity for human immunodeficiency virus type 1 into primary human T lymphocytes by introduction of T-cell receptor genes. *Journal of Virology*, **74**, 8207–12.

Cooper, L. J. N., Topp, M. S., Serrano, L. M. *et al.* (2003). T-cell clones can be rendered specific for CD19: toward the selective augmentation of the graft-versus-B-lineage leukemia effect. *Blood*, **101**, 1637–44.

Corman, J.M., Sercarz, E.E., & Nanda, N.K. (1998). Recognition of prostate-specific antigenic peptide determinants by human CD4 and CD8 T cells. *Clinical Experimental Immunology*, **114**, 166–72.

Correale, P., Walmsley, K., Nieroda, C. *et al.* (1997). In vitro generation of human cytotoxic T lymphocytes specific for peptides derived from prostate-specific antigen. *Journal of the National Cancer Institute*, **89**, 293–300.

Correale, P., Walmsley, K., Zaremba, S. *et al.* (1998). Generation of human cytolytic T lymphocyte lines directed against prostate-specific antigen (PSA) employing a PSA oligoepitope peptide. *Journal of Immunology*, **161**, 3186–94.

Coulie, P.G., Brichard, V., Van Pel, A. *et al.* (1994). A new gene coding for a differentiation antigen recognized by autologous cytolytic T lymphocytes on HLA-A2 melanomas. *Journal of Experimental Medicine*, **180**, 35–42.

Coulie, P.G., Karanikas, V., Colau, D. *et al.* (2001). A monoclonal cytolytic T-lymphocyte response observed in a melanoma patient vaccinated with a tumor-specific antigenic peptide encoded by gene MAGE-3. *Proceedings of the National Academy of Sciences, USA*, **98**, 10290–5.

Cromme, F.V., van Bommel, P.F., Walboomers, J.M. *et al.* (1994). Differences in MHC and TAP-1 expression in cervical cancer lymph node metastases as compared with the primary tumours. *British Journal of Cancer*, **69**, 1176–81.

Dangles, V., Halberstam, I., Scardino, A. *et al.* (2002). Tumor-associated antigen human chorionic gonadotropin beta contains numerous antigenic determinants recognized by in vitro-induced CD8+ and CD4+ T lymphocytes. *Cancer Immunology and Immunotherapy*, **50**, 673–81.

Dannull, J., Diener, P.A., Prikler, L. *et al.* (2000). Prostate stem cell antigen is a promising candidate for immunotherapy of advanced prostate cancer. *Cancer Research*, **60**, 5522–8.

Davila, E. & Celis, E. (2000). Repeated administration of cytosine-phosphorothiolated guanine-containing oligonucleotides together with peptide/protein immunization results in enhanced CTL responses with anti-tumor activity. *Journal of Immunology*, **165**, 539–47.

De Backer, O., Arden, K.C., Boretti, M. *et al.* (1999). Characterization of the GAGE genes that are expressed in various human cancers and in normal testis. *Cancer Research*, **59**, 3157–65.

De Rosa, S.C., Herzenberg, L.A., Herzenberg, L.A., & Roederer, M. (2001). 11-color, 13-parameter flow cytometry: identification of human naive T cells by phenotype, function, and T-cell receptor diversity. *Nature Medicine*, **7**, 245–8.

Diao, J., Smythe, J.A., Smyth, C. *et al.* (1999). Human PBMC-derived dendritic cells transduced with an adenovirus vector induce cytotoxic T-lymphocyte responses against a vector-encoded antigen in vitor. *Gene Therapy*, **6**, 845–53.

Didenko, V.V., Ngo, H.N., Minchew, C., & Baskin, D.S. (2002). Apoptosis of T lymphocytes invading glioblastomas multiforme: a possible tumor defense mechanism. *Journal of Neurosurgery*, **96**, 580–4.

Dighe, A.S., Richards, E., Old, L.J., & Schreiber, R.D. (1994). Enhanced in vivo growth and resistance to rejection of tumor cells expressing dominant negative IFN gamma receptors. *Immunity*, **1**, 447–56.

Disis, M.L., Grabstein, K.H., Sleath, P.R., & Cheever, M.A. (1999). Generation of immunity to the HER-2/neu oncogeneic protein in patients with breast and ovarian cancer using a peptide-based vaccine. *Clinical Cancer Research*, **5**, 1289–97.

Domenech, N., Henderson, R.A., & Finn, O.J. (1995). Identification of an HLA-A11-restricted epitope from the tandem repeat domain of the epithelial tumor antigen mucin. *Journal of Immunology*, **155**, 4766–74.

Dranoff, G., Jaffee, E., Lazenby, A. *et al.* (1993). Vaccination with irradiated tumor cells engineered to secrete murine granulocyte-macrophage colony-stimulating factor stimulates potent, specific, and long-lasting anti-tumor immunity. *Proceedings of the National Academy of Sciences, USA*, **90**, 3539–43.

Duffour, M.T., Chaux, P., Lurquin, C. *et al.* (1999). A MAGE-A4 peptide presented by HLA-A2 is recognized by cytolytic T lymphocytes. *European Journal of Immunology*, **29**, 3329–37.

Dutoit, V., Rubio-Godoy, V., Dietrich, P.Y. *et al.* (2001). Heterogeneous T-cell response to MAGE-A10(254–262): high avidity-specific cytolytic T lymphocytes show superior antitumor activity. *Cancer Research,* **61,** 5850–6.

Dutton, R.W., Bradley, L.M., & Swain, S.L. (1998). T cell memory. *Annual Review of Immunology,* **16,** 201–23.

Egilmez, N.K., Jong, Y.S., Sabel, M.S. *et al.* (2000). In situ tumor vaccination with interleukin-12-encapsulated biodegradable microspheres: induction of tumor regression and potent antitumor immunity. *Cancer Research,* **60,** 3832–7.

Elgert, K.D., Alleva, D.G., & Mullins, D.W. (1998). Tumor-induced immune dysfunction: the macrophage connection. *Journal of Leukocyte Biology,* **64,** 275–90.

Engelmayer, J., Larsson, M., Lee, A. *et al.* (2001). Mature dendritic cells infected with canarypox virus elicit strong anti-human immunodeficiency virus CD8+ and CD4+ T-cell responses from chronically infected individuals. *Journal of Virology,* **75,** 2142–53.

Esche, C., Shurin, M.R., & Lotze, M.T. (1999). The use of dendritic cells for cancer vaccination. *Current Opinion in Molecular Therapy,* **1,** 72–81.

Espevik, T., Figari, I.S., Shalaby, M.R. *et al.* (1987). Inhibition of cytokine production by cyclosporin A and transforming growth factor beta. *Journal of Experimental Medicine,* **166,** 571–6.

Fallarino, F., Uyttenhove, C., Boon, T., & Gajewski, T.F. (1996). Endogenous IL-12 is necessary for rejection of P815 tumor variants in vivo. *Journal of Immunology,* **156,** 1095–100.

Fallarino, F., Uyttenhove, C., Boon, T., & Gajewski, T.F. (1999). Improved efficacy of dendritic cell vaccines and successful immunization with tumor antigen peptide-pulsed peripheral blood mononuclear cells by coadministration of recombinant murine interleukin-12. *International Journal of Cancer,* **80,** 324–33.

Fanger, N.A., Wardwell, K., Shen, L. *et al.* (1996). Type I (CD64) and type II (CD32) Fc gamma receptor-mediated phagocytosis by human blood dendritic cells. *Journal of Immunology,* **157,** 541–8.

Faulkner, L., Buchan, G., & Baird, M. (2000). Interleukin-10 does not affect phagocytosis of particulate antigen by bone marrow-derived dendritic cells but does impair antigen presentation. *Immunology,* **99,** 523–31.

Ferrone, S. & Marincola, F.M. (1995). Loss of HLA class I antigens by melanoma cells: molecular mechanisms, functional significance and clinical relevance. *Immunology Today,* **16,** 487–94.

Fiorentino, D.F., Zlotnik, A., Mosmann, T.R. *et al.* (1991a). IL-10 inhibits cytokine production by activated macrophages. *Journal of Immunology,* **147,** 3815–22.

Fiorentino, D.F., Zlotnik, A., Vieira, P. *et al.* (1991b). IL-10 acts on the antigen-presenting cell to inhibit cytokine production by Th1 cells. *Journal of Immunology,* **146,** 3444–51.

Fischer, J.R., Schindel, M., Bulzebruck, H. *et al.* (2000). Long-term survival in small cell lung cancer patients is correlated with high interleukin-2 secretion at diagnosis. *Journal of Cancer Research and Clinical Oncology,* **126,** 730–3.

Fisher, R.I., Rosenberg, S.A., & Fyfe, G. (2000). Long-term survival update for high-dose recombinant interleukin-2 in patients with renal cell carcinoma. *Cancer Journal Scientific American,* **6** (Suppl 1), S55–S57.

Fisk, B., Blevins, T.L., Wharton, J.T., & Ioannides, C.G. (1995). Identification of an immunodominant peptide of HER-2/neu pro-tooncogene recognized by ovarian tumor-specific cytotoxic T lymphocyte lines. *Journal of Experimental Medicine,* **181,** 2109–17.

Fleischhauer, K., Gattinoni, L., Dalerba, P. *et al.* (1998). The DAM gene family encodes a new group of tumor-specific antigens recognized by human leukocyte antigen A2-restricted cytotoxic T lymphocytes. *Cancer Research,* **58,** 2969–72.

Fong, L., Brockstedt, D., Benike, C. *et al.* (2001). Dendritic cells injected via different routes induce immunity in cancer patients. *Journal of Immunology,* **166,** 4254–9.

Fransen, L., Van der, H.J., Ruysschaert, R., & Fiers, W. (1986). Recombinant tumor necrosis factor: its effect and its synergism with interferon-gamma on a variety of normal and transformed human cell lines. *European Journal of Cancer Clinical Oncology,* **22,** 419–26.

Friedman, R.S., Spies, A.G., Fling, S.P., & Kalos, M. (2002). Identification of naturally processed CD8+ T cell epitopes from prostein using in vitro stimulation. *Journal of Immunology,* (submitted).

Fujie, T., Tahara, K., Tanaka, F. *et al.* (1999). A MAGE-1-encoded HLA-A24-binding synthetic peptide induces specific anti-tumor cytotoxic T lymphocytes. *International Journal of Cancer,* **80,** 169–72.

Fujii, S., Shimizu, K., Shimizu, T., & Lotze, M.T. (2001). Interleukin-10 promotes the maintenance of antitumor CD8(+) T-cell effector function in situ. *Blood,* **98,** 2143–51.

Gabrilovich, D.I., Chen, H.L., Girgis, K.R. *et al.* (1996). Production of vascular endothelial growth factor by human tumors inhibits the functional maturation of dendritic cells. *Nature Medicine,* **2,** 1096–103.

Garrido, F., Cabrera, T., Concha, A. *et al.* (1993). Natural history of HLA expression during tumor development. *Immunology Today,* **14,** 491–9.

Gastl, G.A., Abrams, J.S., Nanus, D.M. *et al.* (1993). Interleukin-10 production by human carcinoma cell lines and its relationship to interleukin-6 expression. *International Journal of Cancer,* **55,** 96–101.

Gaugler, B., Brouwenstijn, N., Vantomme, V. *et al.* (1996). A new gene coding for an antigen recognized by autologous cytolytic T lymphocytes on a human renal carcinoma. *Immunogenetics,* **44,** 323–30.

Gaugler, B., Van den, E.B., van der, B.P. *et al.* (1994). Human gene MAGE-3 codes for an antigen recognized on a melanoma by autologous cytolytic T lymphocytes. *Journal of Experimental Medicine,* **179,** 921–30.

Geiger, J., Hutchinson, R., Hohenkirk, L. *et al.* (2000). Treatment of solid tumours in children with tumour-lysate-pulsed dendritic cells. *Lancet,* **356,** 1163–5.

Geutskens, S.B., van der Eb, M.M., Plomp, A.C. *et al.* (2000). Recombinant adenoviral vectors have adjuvant activity and stimulate T cell responses against tumor cells. *Gene Therapy,* **7,** 1410–16.

Givan, A.L., Fisher, J.L., Waugh, M. *et al.* (1999). A flow cytometric method to estimate the precursor frequencies of cells proliferating in response to specific antigens. *Journal of Immunological Methods,* **230,** 99–112.

Goedegebuure, P.S. & Eberlein, T.J. (1995). The role of CD4+ tumor-infiltrating lymphocytes in human solid tumors. *Immunology Research,* **14,** 119–31.

Golumbek, P.T., Lazenby, A.J., Levitsky, H.I. *et al.* (1991). Treatment of established renal cancer by tumor cells engineered to secrete interleukin-4. *Science,* **254,** 713–16.

Gomella, L.G., Mastrangelo, M.J., McCue, P.A. *et al.* (2001). Phase I study of intravesical vaccinia virus as a vector for gene therapy of bladder cancer. *Journal of Urology,* **166,** 1291–5.

Gomi, S., Nakao, M., Niiya, F. *et al.* (1999). A cyclophilin B gene encodes antigenic epitopes recognized by HLA-A24-restricted and tumor-specific CTLs. *Journal of Immunology,* **163,** 4994–5004.

Gorelik, L. & Flavell, R.A. (2002). Transforming growth factor-beta in T-cell biology. *Nature Review Immunology,* **2,** 46–53.

Greco, G., Fruci, D., Accapezzato, D. *et al.* (1996). Two brc-abl junction peptides bind HLA-A3 molecules and allow specific induction of human cytotoxic T lymphocytes. *Leukemia,* **10,** 693–9.

Greenberg, P.D. (1986). Therapy of murine leukemia with cyclophosphamide and immune Lyt-2+ cells: cytolytic T cells can mediate eradication of disseminated leukemia. *Journal of Immunology,* **136,** 1917–22.

Greenberg, P.D. (1991). Adoptive T cell therapy of tumors: mechanisms operative in the recognition and elimination of tumor cells. *Advances in Immunology,* **49,** 281–355.

Greenberg, P.D., Kern, D.E., & Cheever, M.A. (1985). Therapy of disseminated murine leukemia with cyclophosphamide and immune Lyt-1+,2- T cells. Tumor eradication does not require participation of cytotoxic T cells. *Journal of Experimental Medicine,* **161,** 1122–34.

Grewal, I.S. & Flavell, R.A. (1996). The role of CD40 ligand in costimulation and T-cell activation. *Immunological Review,* **153,** 85–106.

Groux, H., Bigler, M., de Vries, J.E., & Roncarolo, M.G. (1998). Inhibitory and stimulatory effects of IL-10 on human CD8+ T cells. *Journal of Immunology,* **160,** 3188–93.

Guilloux, Y., Lucas, S., Brichard, V.G. *et al.* (1996). A peptide recognized by human cytolytic T lymphocytes on HLA-A2 melanomas is encoded by an intron sequence of the N-acetylglucosaminyltransferase V gene. *Journal of Experimental Medicine,* **183,** 1173–83.

Gurunathan, S., Wu, C.Y., Freidag, B.L., & Seder, R.A. (2000). DNA vaccines: a key for inducing long-term cellular immunity. *Current Opinions in Immunology,* **12,** 442–7.

Hanson, H.L., Donermeyer, D.L., Ikeda, H. *et al.* (2000). Eradication of established tumors by CD8+ T cell adoptive immunotherapy. *Immunity,* **13,** 265–76.

Harada, M., Li, Y.F., El Gamil, M. *et al.* (2001). Use of an in vitro immunoselected tumor line to identify shared melanoma antigens recognized by HLA-A*0201-restricted T cells. *Cancer Research,* **61,** 1089–94.

Harrison, R.A., Richards, A., Laing, G.D., & Theakston, R.D. (2002). Simultaneous GeneGun immunisation with plasmids encoding antigen and GM-CSF: significant enhancement of murine antivenom IgG1 titres. *Vaccine,* **20,** 1702–6.

Haupt, K., Roggendorf, M., & Mann, K. (2002). The potential of DNA vaccination against tumor-associated antigens for antitumor therapy. *Experimental Biological Medicine,* (Maywood) **227,** 227–37.

Heidecker, L., Brasseur, F., Probst-Kepper, M. *et al.* (2000). Cytolytic T lymphocytes raised against a human bladder carcinoma recognize an antigen encoded by gene MAGE-A12. *Journal of Immunology,* **164,** 6041–5.

Heiser, A., Coleman, D., Dannull, J. *et al.* (2002). Autologous dendritic cells transfected with prostate-specific antigen RNA stimulate CTL responses against metastatic prostate tumors. *Journal of Clinical Investigation,* **109,** 409–17.

Herman, J., van der, B.P., Luescher, I.F. *et al.* (1996). A peptide encoded by the human MAGE3 gene and presented by HLA-B44 induces cytolytic T lymphocytes that recognize tumor cells expressing MAGE3. *Immunogenetics,* **43,** 377–83.

Hobeika, A.C., Clay, T.M., Mosca, P.J. *et al.* (2001). Quantitating therapeutically relevant T-cell responses to cancer vaccines. *Critical Reviews in Immunology,* **21,** 287–97.

Horowitz, M.M., Gale, R.P., Sondel, P.M. *et al.* (1990). Graft-versus-leukemia reactions after bone marrow transplantation. *Blood,* **75,** 555–62.

Hsu, F.J., Benike, C., Fagnoni, F. *et al.* (1996). Vaccination of patients with B-cell lymphoma using autologous antigen-pulsed dendritic cells. *Nature Medicine,* **2,** 52–8.

Huang, A.Y., Bruce, A.T., Pardoll, D.M., & Levitsky, H.I. (1996). Does B7-1 expression confer antigen-presenting cell capacity to tumors in vivo? *Journal of Experimental Medicine,* **183,** 769–76.

Huang, L.Q., Brasseur, F., Serrano, A. *et al.* (1999). Cytolytic T lymphocytes recognize an antigen encoded by MAGE-A10 on a human melanoma. *Journal of Immunology,* **162,** 6849–54.

Huarte, E., Sarobe, P., Lasarte, J.J. *et al.* (2002). Identification of HLA-B27-restricted cytotoxic T lymphocyte epitope from carcinoembryonic antigen. *International Journal of Cancer,* **97,** 58–63.

Hung, K., Hayashi, R., Lafond-Walker, A. *et al.* (1998). The central role of CD4(+) T cells in the antitumor immune response. *Journal of Experimental Medicine,* **188,** 2357–68.

Hural, J.A., Friedman, R.S., McNabb, A. *et al.* (2002). Identification of naturally processed CD4+ T cell epitopes from the prostate specific antigen KLK4 using peptide-based in vitro stimulation. *Journal of Immunology,* **169,** 557–65.

Hurwitz, A.A., Townsend, S.E., Yu, T.F. *et al.* (1998). Enhancement of the anti-tumor immune response using a combination of interferon-gamma and B7 expression in an experimental mammary carcinoma. *International Journal of Cancer,* **77,** 107–13.

Ignatius, R., Mahnke, K., Rivera, M. *et al.* (2000). Presentation of proteins encapsulated in sterically stabilized liposomes by dendritic cells initiates CD8(+) T-cell responses in vivo. *Blood,* **96,** 3505–13.

Ikeda, H., Lethe, B., Lehmann, F. *et al.* (1997). Characterization of an antigen that is recognized on a melanoma showing partial HLA loss by CTL expressing an NK inhibitory receptor. *Immunity,* **6,** 199–208.

Jaffee, E.M., Hruban, R.H., Biedrzycki, B. *et al.* (2001). Novel allogeneic granulocyte-macrophage colony-stimulating factor-secreting tumor vaccine for pancreatic cancer: a phase I trial of safety and immune activation. *Journal of Clinical Oncology,* **19,** 145–56.

Jaffee, E.M., Lazenby, A., Meurer, J. *et al.* (1995). Use of murine models of cytokine-secreting tumor vaccines to study feasibility and toxicity issues critical to designing clinical trials. *Journal of Immunotherapy with Emphasis on Tumor Immunology,* **18,** 1–9.

Jager, E., Chen, Y.T., Drijfhout, J.W. *et al.* (1998). Simultaneous humoral and cellular immune response against cancer-testis antigen NY-ESO-1: definition of human histocompatibility leukocyte antigen (HLA)-A2-binding peptide epitopes. *Journal of Experimental Medicine,* **187,** 265–70.

Jager, E., Maeurer, M., Hohn, H. *et al.* (2000). Clonal expansion of Melan A-specific cytotoxic T lymphocytes in a melanoma patient responding to continued immunization with melanoma-associated peptides. *International Journal of Cancer,* **86,** 538–47.

Jager, E., Ringhoffer, M., Altmannsberger, M. *et al.* (1997). Immunoselection in vivo: independent loss of MHC class I and melanocyte differentiation antigen expression in metastatic melanoma. *International Journal of Cancer,* **71,** 142–7.

Jager, E., Ringhoffer, M., Dienes, H.P. *et al.* (1996a). Granulocyte-macrophage-colony-stimulating factor enhances immune responses to melanoma-associated peptides in vivo. *International Journal of Cancer,* **67,** 54–62.

Jager, E., Ringhoffer, M., Karbach, J. *et al.* (1996b). Inverse relationship of melanocyte differentiation antigen expression in melanoma tissues and CD8+ cytotoxic-T-cell responses: evidence for immunoselection of antigen-loss variants in vivo. *International Journal of Cancer,* **66,** 470–6.

Jenkins, M.K. & Schwartz, R.H. (1987). Antigen presentation by chemically modified splenocytes induces antigen-specific T cell unresponsiveness in vitro and in vivo. *Journal of Experimental Medicine,* **165,** 302–19.

Johnsen, A., France, J., Sy, M.S., & Harding, C.V. (1998). Down-regulation of the transporter for antigen presentation, proteasome subunits, and class I major histocompatibility complex in tumor cell lines. *Cancer Research,* **58,** 3660–7.

Johnsen, A.K., Templeton, D.J., Sy, M., & Harding, C.V. (1999). Deficiency of transporter for antigen presentation (TAP) in tumor cells allows evasion of immune surveillance and increases tumorigenesis. *Journal of Immunology,* **163,** 4224–31.

Kagamu, H. & Shu, S. (1998). Purification of L-selectin(low) cells promotes the generation of highly potent CD4 antitumor effector T lymphocytes. *Journal of Immunology,* **160,** 3444–52.

Kaklamanis, L., Leek, R., Koukourakis, M. *et al.* (1995). Loss of transporter in antigen processing 1 transport protein and major histocompatibility complex class I molecules in metastatic versus primary breast cancer. *Cancer Research,* **55,** 5191–4.

Kang, X., Kawakami, Y., El Gamil, M. *et al.* (1995). Identification of a tyrosinase epitope recognized by HLA-A24-restricted, tumor-infiltrating lymphocytes. *Journal of Immunology,* **155,** 1343–8.

Kaplan, J.M., Yu, Q., Piraino, S.T. *et al.* (1999a). Induction of antitumor immunity with dendritic cells transduced with adenovirus vector-encoding endogeneous tumor-associated antigens. *Journal of Immunology,* **163,** 699–707.

Kaplan, J.M., Yu, Q., Piraino, S.T. *et al.* (1999b). Induction of antitumor immunity with dendritic cells transduced with adenovirus vector-encoding endogenous tumor-associated antigens. *Journal of Immunology,* **163,** 699–707.

Kappler, J.W., Roehm, N., & Marrack, P. (1987). T cell tolerance by clonal elimination in the thymus. *Cell,* **49,** 273–80.

Kawakami, Y., Eliyahu, S., Jennings, C. *et al.* (1995). Recognition of multiple epitopes in the human melanoma antigen gp 100 by tumor-infiltrating T lymphocytes associated with in vivo tumor regression. *Journal of Immunology,* **154,** 3961–68.

Kawakami, Y., Eliyahu, S., Sakaguchi, K. *et al.* (1994). Identification of the immunodominant peptides of the MART-1 human melanoma antigen recognized by the majority of HLA-A2-restricted tumor infiltrating lymphocytes. *Journal of Experimental Medicine,* **180,** 347–52.

Kawakami, Y., Robbins, P.F., Wang, X. *et al.* (1998). Identification of new melanoma epitopes on melanosomal proteins recognized by tumor infiltrating T lymphocytes restricted by HLA-A1, -A2, and -A3 alleles. *Journal of Immunology,* **161,** 6985–92.

Kawano, K., Gomi, S., Tanaka, K. *et al.* (2000). Identification of a new endoplasmic reticulum-resident protein recognized by HLA-A24-restricted tumor-infiltrating lymphocytes of lung cancer. *Cancer Research,* **60,** 3550–8.

Kawashima, I., Hudson, S.J., Tsai, V. *et al.* (1998). The multi-epitope approach for immunotherapy for cancer: identification of several CTL epitopes from various tumor-associated antigens expressed on solid epithelial tumors. *Human Immunology,* **59,** 1–14.

Kawashima, I., Tsai, V., Southwood, S. *et al.* (1999). Identification of HLA-A3-restricted cytotoxic T lymphocyte epitopes from carcinoembryonic antigen and HER-2/neu by primary in vitro immunization with peptide-pulsed dendritic cells. *Cancer Research,* **59,** 431–5.

Kemp, R.A. & Ronchese, F. (2001). Tumor-specific Tc1, but not Tc2, cells deliver protective antitumor immunity. *Journal of Immunology,* **167,** 6497–502.

Keogh, E., Fikes, J., Southwood, S. *et al.* (2001). Identification of new epitopes from four different tumor-associated antigens: recognition of naturally processed epitopes correlates with HLA-A*0201-binding affinity. *Journal of Immunology,* **167,** 787–96.

Kern, D.E., Klarnet, J.P., Cheever, M.A., & Greenberg, P.D. (1990). Requirements for the generation of a Lyt-2+ T-cell proliferative response to a syngeneic tumor in the absence of L3T4+ T-cells. *Cancer Research,* **50,** 6256–63.

Kessels, H.W., de Visser, K.E., Kruisbeek, A.M., & Schumacher, T.N. (2001). Circumventing T-cell tolerance to tumour antigens. *Biologicals,* **29,** 277–83.

Kessler, J.H., Beekman, N.J., Bres-Vloemans, S.A. *et al.* (2001). Efficient identification of novel HLA-A(*)0201-presented cytotoxic T lymphocyte epitopes in the widely expressed tumor antigen PRAME by proteasome-mediated digestion analysis. *Journal of Experimental Medicine,* **193,** 73–88.

Kieke, M.C., Sundberg, E., Shusta, E.V. *et al.* (2001). High affinity T cell receptors from yeast display libraries block T cell activation by superantigens. *Journal of Molecular Biology,* **307,** 1305–15.

Kikuchi, M., Nakao, M., Inoue, Y. *et al.* (1999). Identification of a SART-1-derived peptide capable of inducing HLA-A24-restricted and tumor-specific cytotoxic T lymphocytes. *International Journal of Cancer,* **81,** 459–66.

Kim, C.J., Prevette, T., Cormier, J. *et al.* (1997). Dendritic cells infected with poxviruses encoding MART-1/Melan A sensitize T lymphocytes in vitro. *Journal of Immunotherapy,* **20,** 276–86.

Kinoshita, Y., Kono, T., Yasumoto, R. *et al.* (2001). Antitumor effect on murine renal cell carcinoma by autologous tumor vaccines genetically modified with granulocyte-macrophage colony-stimulating factor and interleukin-6 cells. *Journal of Immunotherapy,* **24**, 205–11.

Kittlesen, D.J., Thompson, L.W., Gulden, P.H. *et al.* (1998). Human melanoma patients recognize an HLA-A1-restricted CTL epitope from tyrosinase containing two cysteine residues: implications for tumor vaccine development. *Journal of Immunology,* **160**, 2099–106.

Klarnet, J.P., Matis, L.A., Kern, D.E. *et al.* (1987). Antigen-driven T cell clones can proliferate in vivo, eradicate disseminated leukemia, and provide specific immunologic memory. *Journal of Immunology,* **138**, 4012–17.

Knipping, E., Debatin, K.M., Stricker, K. *et al.* (1995). Identification of soluble APO-1 in supernatants of human B- and T-cell lines and increased serum levels in B- and T-cell leukemias. *Blood,* **85**, 1562–9.

Kobayashi, H., Lu, J., & Celis, E. (2001a). Identification of helper T-cell epitopes that encompass or lie proximal to cytotoxic T-cell epitopes in the gp100 melanoma tumor antigen. *Cancer Research,* **61**, 7577–84.

Kobayashi, H., Song, Y., Hoon, D.S. *et al.* (2001b). Tumor-reactive T helper lymphocytes recognize a promiscuous MAGE-A3 epitope presented by various major histocompatibility complex class II alleles. *Cancer Research,* **61**, 4773–8.

Kobayashi, H., Wood, M., Song, Y. *et al.* (2000). Defining promiscuous MHC class II helper T-cell epitopes for the HER2/neu tumor antigen. *Cancer Research,* **60**, 5228–36.

Kolb, H.J., Schattenberg, A., Goldman, J.M. *et al.* (1995). Graft-versus-leukemia effect of donor lymphocyte transfusions in marrow grafted patients. European Group for Blood and Marrow Transplantation Working Party Chronic Leukemia. *Blood,* **86**, 2041–50.

Kono, K., Rongcun, Y., Charo, J. *et al.* (1998). Identification of HER2/neu-derived peptide epitopes recognized by gastric cancer-specific cytotoxic T lymphocytes. *International Journal of Cancer,* **78**, 202–8.

Korkolopoulou, P., Kaklamanis, L., Pezzella, F. *et al.* (1996). Loss of antigen-presenting molecules (MHC class I and TAP-1) in lung cancer. *British Journal of Cancer,* **73**, 148–53.

Kuball, J., Wen, S.F., Leissner, J. *et al.* (2002). Successful adenovirus-mediated wild-type p53 gene transfer in patients with bladder cancer by intravesical vector instillation. *Journal of Clinical Oncology,* **20**, 957–65.

Kumamoto, T., Huang, E.K., Paek, H.J. *et al.* (2002). Induction of tumor-specific protective immunity by in situ Langerhans cell vaccine. *Nature Biotechnology,* **20**, 64–9.

Kurokohchi, K., Carrington, M., Mann, D.L. *et al.* (1996). Expression of HLA class I molecules and the transporter associated with antigen processing in hepatocellular carcinoma. *Hepatology,* **23**, 1181–8.

Kwon, E.D., Hurwitz, A.A., Foster, B.A. *et al.* (1997). Manipulation of T cell costimulatory and inhibitory signals for immunotherapy of prostate cancer. *Proceedings of the National Academy of Sciences, USA,* **94**, 8099–103.

Lambert, L.A., Gibson, G.R., Maloney, M. *et al.* (2001). Intranodal immunization with tumor lysate-pulsed dendritic cells enhances protective antitumor immunity. *Cancer Research,* **61**, 641–6.

Lapointe, R., Royal, R.E., Reeves, M.E. *et al.* (2001). Retrovirally transduced human dendritic cells can generate T cells recognizing multiple MHC class I and class II epitopes from the melanoma antigen glycoprotein 100. *Journal of Immunology,* **167**, 4758–64.

Le Naour, F. (2001). Contribution of proteomics to tumor immunology. *Proteomics,* **1**, 1295–302.

Lee, J., Fenton, B.M., Koch, C.J. *et al.* (1998). Interleukin 2 expression by tumor cells alters both the immune response and the tumor microenvironment. *Cancer Research,* **58**, 1478–85.

Lee, P., Wang, F., Kuniyoshi, J. *et al.* (2001). Effects of interleukin-12 on the immune response to a multipeptide vaccine for resected metastatic melanoma. *Journal of Clinical Oncology,* **19**, 3836–47.

Lee, P.P., Yee, C., Savage, P.A. *et al.* (1999). Characterization of circulating T cells specific for tumor-associated antigens in melanoma patients. *Nature Medicine,* **5**, 677–85.

Lee, S.W., Tomasetto, C., & Sager, R. (1991). Positive selection of candidate tumor-suppressor genes by subtractive hybridization. *Proceedings of the National Academy of Sciences, USA,* **88**, 2825–9.

Levitsky, H.I., Lazenby, A., Hayashi, R.J., & Pardoll, D.M. (1994). In vivo priming of two distinct antitumor effector populations: the role of MHC class I expression. *Journal of Experimental Medicine,* **179**, 1215–24.

Lockhart, D.J. & Winzeler, E.A. (2000). Genomics, gene expression and DNA arrays. *Nature,* **405**, 827–36.

Lopez, J.A. & Hart, D.N. (2002). Current issues in dendritic cell cancer immunotherapy. *Current Opinion in Molecular Therapy,* **4**, 54–63.

Lowes, M.A., Bishop, G.A., Crotty, K. *et al.* (1997). T helper 1 cytokine mRNA is increased in spontaneously regressing primary melanomas. *Journal of Investigational Dermatology,* **108**, 914–19.

Luiten, R. & van der, B.P. (2000). A MAGE-A1 peptide is recognized on HLA-B7 human tumors by cytolytic T lymphocytes. *Tissue Antigens,* **55**, 149–52.

Lundstrom, K. (2002). Alphavirus-based vaccines. *Current Opinion in Molecular Therapy,* **4**, 28–34.

Lynch, D.H. (1998). Induction of dendritic cells (DC) by Flt3 ligand (FL) promotes the generation of tumor-specific immune responses in vivo. *Critical Reviews in Immunology,* **18**, 99–107.

Lynch, D.H. & Miller, R.E. (1994). Interleukin 7 promotes long-term in vitro growth of antitumor cytotoxic T lymphocytes with immunotherapeutic efficacy in vivo. *Journal of Experimental Medicine,* **179**, 31–42.

Macatonia, S.E., Doherty, T.M., Knight, S.C., & O'Garra, A. (1993). Differential effect of IL-10 on dendritic cell-induced T cell proliferation and IFN-gamma production. *Journal of Immunology,* **150**, 3755–65.

Manjili, M.H., Wang, X.Y., Park, J. *et al.* (2002). Immunotherapy of cancer using heat shock proteins. *Frontiers in Bioscience,* **7**, d43–d52.

Mannering, S.I., McKenzie, J.L., Fearnley, D.B., & Hart, D.N. (1997). HLA-DR1-restricted bcr-abl (b3a2)-specific CD4+ T lymphocytes respond to dendritic cells pulsed with b3a2 peptide and antigen-presenting cells exposed to b3a2 containing cell lysates. *Blood,* **90**, 290–7.

Marchand, M., van Baren, N., Weynants, P. *et al.* (1999). Tumor regressions observed in patients with metastatic melanoma treated with an antigenic peptide encoded by gene MAGE-3 and presented by HLA-A1. *International Journal of Cancer,* **80,** 219–30.

Marincola, F.M., Jaffee, E.M., Hicklin, D.J., & Ferrone, S. (2000). Escape of human solid tumors from T-cell recognition: molecular mechanisms and functional significance. *Advances in Immunology,* **74,** 181–273.

Marzo, A.L., Kinnear, B.F., Lake, R.A. *et al.* (2000). Tumor-specific CD4+ T cells have a major "post-licensing" role in CTL mediated anti-tumor immunity. *Journal of Immunology,* **165,** 6047–55.

Marzo, A.L., Lake, R.A., Robinson, B.W., & Scott, B. (1999). T-cell receptor transgenic analysis of tumor-specific CD8 and CD4 responses in the eradication of solid tumors. *Cancer Research,* **59,** 1071–9.

Mattner, F., Fleitmann, J.K., Lingnau, K. *et al.* (2002). Vaccination with poly-L-arginine as immunostimulant for peptide vaccines: induction of potent and long-lasting T-cell responses against cancer antigens. *Cancer Research,* **62,** 1477–80.

McKenna, H.J. (1999). Generating a T cell tumor-specific immune response in vivo: can flt3-ligand-generated dendritic cells tip the balance? *Cancer Immunology and Immunotherapy,* **48,** 281–6.

McNeel, D.G., Nguyen, L.D., & Disis, M.L. (2001). Identification of T helper epitopes from prostatic acid phosphatase. *Cancer Research,* **61,** 5161–7.

Meidenbauer, N., Andreesen, R., & Mackensen, A. (2001). Dendritic cells for specific cancer immunotherapy. *Biological Chemistry,* **382,** 507–20.

Mendez, R., Serrano, A., Jager, E. *et al.* (2001). Analysis of HLA class I expression in different metastases from two melanoma patients undergoing peptide immunotherapy. *Tissue Antigens,* **57,** 508–19.

Meng, W.S., Butterfield, L.H., Ribas, A. *et al.* (2001). alpha-Fetoprotein-specific tumor immunity induced by plasmid prime-adenovirus boost genetic vaccination. *Cancer Research,* **61,** 8782–6.

Menoret, A. & Chandawarkar, R. (1998). Heat-shock protein-based anticancer immunotherapy: an idea whose time has come. *Seminars in Oncology,* **25,** 654–60.

Miconnet, I., Coste, I., Beermann, F. *et al.* (2001). Cancer vaccine design: a novel bacterial adjuvant for peptide-specific CTL induction. *Journal of Immunology,* **166,** 4612–19.

Miconnet, I., Koenig, S., Speiser, D. *et al.* (2002). CpG are efficient adjuvants for specific CTL induction against tumor antigen-derived peptide. *Journal of Immunology,* **168,** 1212–18.

Mihm, M.C., Jr., Clemente, C.G., & Cascinelli, N. (1996). Tumor infiltrating lymphocytes in lymph node melanoma metastases: a histopathologic prognostic indicator and an expression of local immune response. *Laboratory Investigation,* **74,** 43–7.

Mikszta, J.A., Alarcon, J.B., Brittingham, J.M. *et al.* (2002). Improved genetic immunization via micromechanical disruption of skin-barrier function and targeted epidermal delivery. *Nature Medicine,* **8,** 415–19.

Mincheff, M., Altankova, I., Zoubak, S. *et al.* (2001). In vivo transfection and/or cross-priming of dendritic cells following DNA and adenoviral immunizations for immunotherapy of cancer—

changes in peripheral mononuclear subsets and intracellular IL-4 and IFN-gamma lymphokine profile. *Critical Reviews in Oncology and Hematology,* **39,** 125–32.

Mitchell, D.A. & Nair, S.K. (2000). RNA transfected dendritic cells as cancer vaccines. *Current Opinion in Molecular Therapy,* **2,** 176–81.

Mitchell, M.S., Kan-Mitchell, J., Minev, B. *et al.* (2000). A novel melanoma gene (MG50) encoding the interleukin 1 receptor antagonist and six epitopes recognized by human cytolytic T lymphocytes. *Cancer Research,* **60,** 6448–56.

Moller, P., Koretz, K., Leithauser, F. *et al.* (1994). Expression of APO-1 (CD95), a member of the NGF/TNF receptor superfamily, in normal and neoplastic colon epithelium. *International Journal of Cancer,* **57,** 371–7.

Moreau-Aubry, A., Le Guiner, S., Labarriere, N. *et al.* (2000). A processed pseudogene codes for a new antigen recognized by a CD8(+) T cell clone on melanoma. *Journal of Experimental Medicine,* **191,** 1617–24.

Morel, S., Levy, F., Burlet-Schiltz, O. *et al.* (2000). Processing of some antigens by the standard proteasome but not by the immunoproteasome results in poor presentation by dendritic cells. *Immunity,* **12,** 107–17.

Morelli, A.E., Larregina, A.T., Ganster, R.W. *et al.* (2000). Recombinant adenovirus induces maturation of dendritic cells via an NF-kappaB-dependent pathway. *Journal of Virology,* **74,** 9617–28.

Morgan, D.J., Kreuwel, H.T., Fleck, S. *et al.* (1998). Activation of low avidity CTL specific for a self epitope results in tumor rejection but not autoimmunity. *Journal of Immunology,* **160,** 643–51.

Moris, A., Teichgraber, V., Gauthier, L. *et al.* (2001). Cutting edge: characterization of allorestricted and peptide-selective alloreactive T cells using HLA-tetramer selection. *Journal of Immunology,* **166,** 4818–21.

Morse, M.A., Deng, Y., Coleman, D. *et al.* (1999). A phase I study of active immunotherapy with carcinoembryonic antigen peptide (CAP-1)-pulsed, autologous human cultured dendritic cells in patients with metastatic malignancies expressing carcinoembryonic antigen. *Clinical Cancer Research,* **5,** 1331–8.

Moses, H.L., Yang, E.Y., & Pietenpol, J.A. (1990). TGF-beta stimulation and inhibition of cell proliferation: new mechanistic insights. *Cell,* **63,** 245–7.

Munz, C., Obst, R., Osen, W. *et al.* (1999). Alloreactivity as a source of high avidity peptide-specific human CTL. *Journal of Immunology,* **162,** 25–34.

Nair, S.K., Morse, M., Boczkowski, D. *et al.* (2002). Induction of tumor-specific cytotoxic T lymphocytes in cancer patients by autologous tumor RNA-transfected dendritic cells. *Annals of Surgery,* **235,** 540–9.

Nakano, O., Sato, M., Naito, Y. *et al.* (2001). Proliferative activity of intratumoral CD8(+) T-lymphocytes as a prognostic factor in human renal cell carcinoma: clinicopathologic demonstration of antitumor immunity. *Cancer Research,* **61,** 5132–6.

Nakao, M., Shichijo, S., Imaizumi, T. *et al.* (2000). Identification of a gene coding for a new squamous cell carcinoma antigen recognized by the CTL. *Journal of Immunology,* **164,** 2565–74.

Natoli, G., Ianni, A., Costanzo, A. *et al.* (1995). Resistance to Fas-mediated apoptosis in human hepatoma cells. *Oncogene,* **11,** 1157–64.

Nestle, F.O. (2000). Dendritic cell vaccination for cancer therapy. *Oncogene*, **19**, 6673–9.

Nestle, F.O., Alijagic, S., Gilliet, M. *et al.* (1998). Vaccination of melanoma patients with peptide- or tumor lysate-pulsed dendritic cells. *Nature Medicine*, **4**, 328–32.

Nielsen, M.B., Monsurro, V., Migueles, S.A. *et al.* (2000). Status of activation of circulating vaccine-elicited CD8+ T cells. *Journal of Immunology*, **165**, 2287–96.

Nishimura, T., Iwakabe, K., Sekimoto, M. *et al.* (1999). Distinct role of antigen-specific T helper type 1 (Th1) and Th2 cells in tumor eradication in vivo. *Journal of Experimental Medicine*, **190**, 617–27.

Noppen, C., Levy, F., Burri, L. *et al.* (2000). Naturally processed and concealed HLA-A2.1-restricted epitopes from tumor-associated antigen tyrosinase-related protein-2. *International Journal of Cancer*, **87**, 241–6.

Norbury, L.C., Clark, R.E., & Christmas, S.E. (2000). b3a2 BCR-ABL fusion peptides as targets for cytotoxic T cells in chronic myeloid leukaemia. *British Journal of Haematology*, **109**, 616–21.

Nouri-Shirazi, M., Banchereau, J., Fay, J., & Palucka, K. (2000). Dendritic cell based tumor vaccines. *Immunology Letters*, **74**, 5–10.

Nukaya, I., Yasumoto, M., Iwasaki, T. *et al.* (1999). Identification of HLA-A24 epitope peptides of carcinoembryonic antigen which induce tumor-reactive cytotoxic T lymphocyte. *International Journal of Cancer*, **80**, 92–7.

O'Connell, J., Bennett, M.W., O'Sullivan, G.C. *et al.* (1999). The Fas counterattack: cancer as a site of immune privilege. *Immunology Today*, **20**, 46–52.

Ohlen, C., Kalos, M., Hong, D.J. *et al.* (2001). Expression of a tolerizing tumor antigen in peripheral tissue does not preclude recovery of high-affinity CD8+ T cells or CTL immunotherapy of tumors expressing the antigen. *Journal of Immunology*, **166**, 2863–70.

Ohnmacht, G.A., Wang, E., Mocellin, S. *et al.* (2001). Short-term kinetics of tumor antigen expression in response to vaccination. *Journal of Immunology*, **167**, 1809–20.

Oiso, M., Eura, M., Katsura, F. *et al.* (1999). A newly identified MAGE-3-derived epitope recognized by HLA-A24-restricted cytotoxic T lymphocytes. *International Journal of Cancer*, **81**, 387–94.

Oka, Y., Elisseeva, O.A., Tsuboi, A. *et al.* (2000). Human cytotoxic T-lymphocyte responses specific for peptides of the wild-type Wilms' tumor gene (WT1) product. *Immunogenetics*, **51**, 99–107.

Osanto, S., Schiphorst, P.P., Weij1, N.I. *et al.* (2000). Vaccination of melanoma patients with an allogeneic, genetically modified interleukin 2-producing melanoma cell line. *Human Gene Therapy*, **11**, 739–50.

Ossendorp, F., Mengede, E., Camps, M. *et al.* (1998). Specific T helper cell requirement for optimal induction of cytotoxic T lymphocytes against major histocompatibility complex class II negative tumors. *Journal of Experimental Medicine*, **187**, 693–702.

Palmer, K., Moore, J., Everard, M. *et al.* (1999). Gene therapy with autologous, interleukin 2-secreting tumor cells in patients with malignant melanoma. *Human Gene Therapy*, **10**, 1261–8.

Panelli, M.C., Bettinotti, M.P., Lally, K. *et al.* (2000). A tumor-infiltrating lymphocyte from a melanoma metastasis with decreased expression of melanoma differentiation antigens recognizes MAGE-12. *Journal of Immunology*, **164**, 4382–92.

Pardoll, D.M. (1995). Paracrine cytokine adjuvants in cancer immunotherapy. *Annual Review of Immunology*, **13**, 399–415.

Parkhurst, M.R., Fitzgerald, E.B., Southwood, S. *et al.* (1998). Identification of a shared HLA-A*0201-restricted T-cell epitope from the melanoma antigen tyrosinase-related protein 2 (TRP2). *Cancer Research*, **58**, 4895–901.

Partidos, C.D., Vohra, P., Jones, D. *et al.* (1997). CTL responses induced by a single immunization with peptide encapsulated in biodegradable microparticles. *Journal of Immunological Methods*, **206**, 143–51.

Pascolo, S., Schirle, M., Guckel, B. *et al.* (2001). A MAGE-A1 HLA-A A*0201 epitope identified by mass spectrometry. *Cancer Research*, **61**, 4072–7.

Pazdrak, K., Justement, L., & Alam, R. (1995). Mechanism of inhibition of eosinophil activation by transforming growth factor-beta. Inhibition of Lyn, MAP, Jak2 kinases and STAT1 nuclear factor. *Journal of Immunology*, **155**, 4454–8.

Peoples, G.E., Goedegebuure, P.S., Smith, R. *et al.* (1995). Breast and ovarian cancer-specific cytotoxic T lymphocytes recognize the same HER2/neu-derived peptide. *Proceedings of the National Academy of Sciences, USA*, **92**, 432–6.

Perez-Diez, A., Butterfield, L.H., Li, L. *et al.* (1998). Generation of CD8+ and CD4+ T-cell response to dendritic cells genetically engineered to express the MART-1/Melan-A gene. *Cancer Research*, **58**, 5305–9.

Perez, S.A., Sotiropoulou, P.A., Sotiriadou, N.N. *et al.* (2002). HER-2/neu-derived peptide 884–899 is expressed by human breast, colorectal and pancreatic adenocarcinomas and is recognized by in-vitro-induced specific CD4(+) T cell clones. *Cancer Immunology and Immunotherapy*, **50**, 615–24.

Peshwa, M.V., Shi, J.D., Ruegg, C. *et al.* (1998). Induction of prostate tumor-specific CD8+ cytotoxic T-lymphocytes in vitro using antigen-presenting cells pulsed with prostatic acid phosphatase peptide. *Prostate*, **36**, 129–38.

Puccetti, P., Bianchi, R., Fioretti, M.C. *et al.* (1994). Use of a skin test assay to determine tumor-specific CD8+ T cell reactivity. *European Journal of Immunology*, **24**, 1446–52.

Qin, Z. & Blankenstein, T. (2000). CD4+ T cell–mediated tumor rejection involves inhibition of angiogenesis that is dependent on IFN gamma receptor expression by nonhematopoietic cells. *Immunity*, **12**, 677–86.

Ranieri, E., Herr, W., Gambotto, A. *et al.* (1999). Dendritic cells transduced with an adenovirus vector encoding Epstein-Barr virus latent membrane protein 2B: a new modality for vaccination. *Journal of Virology*, **73**, 10416–25.

Renkvist, N., Castelli, C., Robbins, P.F., & Parmiani, G. (2001). A listing of human tumor antigens recognized by T cells. *Cancer Immunology and Immunotherapy*, **50**, 3–15.

Ridge, J.P., Di Rosa, F., & Matzinger, P. (1998). A conditioned dendritic cell can be a temporal bridge between a CD4+ T-helper and a T-killer cell. *Nature*, **393**, 474–8.

Riker, A., Cormier, J., Panelli, M. *et al.* (1999). Immune selection after antigen-specific immunotherapy of melanoma. *Surgery*, **126**, 112–20.

Riley, J.P., Rosenberg, S.A., & Parkhurst, M.R. (2001). Identification of a new shared HLA-A2.1 restricted epitope from the melanoma antigen tyrosinase. *Journal of Immunotherapy*, **24**, 212–20.

Rimoldi, D., Rubio-Godoy, V., Dutoit, V. *et al.* (2000). Efficient simultaneous presentation of NY-ESO-1/LAGE-1 primary and nonprimary open reading frame-derived CTL epitopes in melanoma. *Journal of Immunology,* **165,** 7253–61.

Robbins, P.F., El Gamil, M., Li, Y.F. *et al.* (1997). The intronic region of an incompletely spliced gp100 gene transcript encodes an epitope recognized by melanoma-reactive tumor-infiltrating lymphocytes. *Journal of Immunology,* **159,** 303–8.

Robbins, P.F., El Gamil, M., Li, Y.F. *et al.* (1995). Cloning of a new gene encoding an antigen recognized by melanoma-specific HLA-A24-restricted tumor-infiltrating lymphocytes. *Journal of Immunology,* **154,** 5944–50.

Romani, N., Gruner, S., Brang, D. *et al.* (1994). Proliferating dendritic cell progenitors in human blood. *Journal of Experimental Medicine,* **180,** 83–93.

Rongcun, Y., Salazar-Onfray, F., Charo, J. *et al.* (1999). Identification of new HER2/neu-derived peptide epitopes that can elicit specific CTL against autologous and allogeneic carcinomas and melanomas. *Journal of Immunology,* **163,** 1037–44.

Ronsin, C., Chung-Scott, V., Poullion, I. *et al.* (1999). A non-AUG-defined alternative open reading frame of the intestinal carboxyl esterase mRNA generates an epitope recognized by renal cell carcinoma-reactive tumor-infiltrating lymphocytes in situ. *Journal of Immunology,* **163,** 483–90.

Rooney, C.M., Smith, C.A., Ng, C.Y. *et al.* (1995). Use of gene-modified virus-specific T lymphocytes to control Epstein-Barr-virus-related lymphoproliferation. *Lancet,* **345,** 9–13.

Rosenberg, S.A., Spiess, P., & Lafreniere, R. (1986). A new approach to the adoptive immunotherapy of cancer with tumor-infiltrating lymphocytes. *Science,* **233,** 1318–21.

Rouard, H., Leon, A., Klonjkowski, B. *et al.* (2000). Adenoviral transduction of human 'clinical grade' immature dendritic cells enhances costimulatory molecule expression and T-cell stimulatory capacity. *Journal of Immunological Methods,* **241,** 69–81.

Rubartelli, A., Poggi, A., & Zocchi, M.R. (1997). The selective engulfment of apoptotic bodies by dendritic cells is mediated by the alpha(v)beta3 integrin and requires intracellular and extracellular calcium. *European Journal of Immunology,* **27,** 1893–900.

Ruegemer, J.J., Ho, S.N., Augustine, J.A. *et al.* (1990). Regulatory effects of transforming growth factor-beta on IL-2- and IL-4-dependent T cell-cycle progression. *Journal of Immunology,* **144,** 1767–76.

Sadanaga, N., Nagashima, H., Mashino, K. *et al.* (2001). Dendritic cell vaccination with MAGE peptide is a novel therapeutic approach for gastrointestinal carcinomas. *Clinical Cancer Research,* **7,** 2277–84.

Saeterdal, I., Gjertsen, M.K., Straten, P. *et al.* (2001). A TGF betaRII frameshift-mutation-derived CTL epitope recognised by HLA-A2-restricted CD8+ T cells. *Cancer Immunology and Immunotherapy,* **50,** 469–76.

Salazar-Onfray, F., Nakazawa, T., Chhajlani, V. *et al.* (1997). Synthetic peptides derived from the melanocyte-stimulating hormone receptor MC1R can stimulate HLA-A2-restricted cytotoxic T lymphocytes that recognize naturally processed peptides on human melanoma cells. *Cancer Research,* **57,** 4348–55.

Saleh, F.H., Crotty, K.A., Hersey, P., & Menzies, S.W. (2001). Primary melanoma tumour regression associated with an immune response to the tumour-associated antigen melan-A/MART-1. *International Journal of Cancer,* **94,** 551–7.

Scardino, A., Alves, P., Gross, D.A. *et al.* (2001). Identification of HER-2/neu immunogenic epitopes presented by renal cell carcinoma and other human epithelial tumors. *European Journal of Immunology,* **31,** 3261–70.

Scheibenbogen, C., Sun, Y., Keilholz, U. *et al.* (2002). Identification of known and novel immunogenic T-cell epitopes from tumor antigens recognized by peripheral blood T cells from patients responding to IL-2-based treatment. *International Journal of Cancer,* **98,** 409–14.

Schmittel, A., Keilholz, U., Thiel, E., & Scheibenbogen, C. (2000). Quantification of tumor-specific T lymphocytes with the ELISPOT assay. *Journal of Immunotherapy,* **23,** 289–95.

Schneider, J., Brichard, V., Boon, T. *et al.* (1998). Overlapping peptides of melanocyte differentiation antigen Melan-A/MART-1 recognized by autologous cytolytic T lymphocytes in association with HLA-B45.1 and HLA-A2.1. *International Journal of Cancer,* **75,** 451–8.

Schoenberger, S.P., Toes, R.E., van der Voort, E.I. *et al.* (1998). T-cell help for cytotoxic T lymphocytes is mediated by CD40-CD40L interactions. *Nature,* **393,** 480–3.

Scholl, S.M., Balloul, J.M., Le Goc, G. *et al.* (2000). Recombinant vaccinia virus encoding human MUC1 and IL2 as immunotherapy in patients with breast cancer. *Journal of Immunotherapy,* **23,** 570–80.

Schreiber, S., Kampgen, E., Wagner, E. *et al.* (1999). Immunotherapy of metastatic malignant melanoma by a vaccine consisting of autologous interleukin 2-transfected cancer cells: outcome of a phase I study. *Human Gene Therapy,* **10,** 983–93.

Schuler, T., Kammertoens, T., Preiss, S. *et al.* (2001). Generation of tumor-associated cytotoxic T lymphocytes requires interleukin 4 from CD8(+) T cells. *Journal of Experimental Medicine,* **194,** 1767–75.

Schuler, T., Qin, Z., Ibe, S. *et al.* (1999). T helper cell type 1-associated and cytotoxic T lymphocyte-mediated tumor immunity is impaired in interleukin 4-deficient mice. *Journal of Experimental Medicine,* **189,** 803–10.

Schultz, E.S., Lethe, B., Cambiaso, C.L. *et al.* (2000). A MAGE-A3 peptide presented by HLA-DP4 is recognized on tumor cells by CD4+ cytolytic T lymphocytes. *Cancer Research,* **60,** 6272–5.

Schultz, E.S., Zhang, Y., Knowles, R. *et al.* (2001). A MAGE-3 peptide recognized on HLA-B35 and HLA-A1 by cytolytic T lymphocytes. *Tissue Antigens,* **57,** 103–9.

Schultze, J.L. & Vonderheide, R.H. (2001). From cancer genomics to cancer immunotherapy: toward second-generation tumor antigens. *Trends in Immunology,* **22,** 516–23.

Segal, B.M., Glass, D.D., & Shevach, E.M. (2002). Cutting edge: IL-10-producing CD4+ T cells mediate tumor rejection. *Journal of Immunology,* **168,** 1–4.

Serrano, A., Tanzarella, S., Lionello, I. *et al.* (2001). Rexpression of HLA class I antigens and restoration of antigen-specific CTL response in melanoma cells following 5-aza-2'-deoxycytidine treatment. *International Journal of Cancer,* **94,** 243–51.

Simon, R.M., Steinberg, S.M., Hamilton, M. *et al.* (2001). Clinical trial designs for the early clinical development of therapeutic cancer vaccines. *Journal Clinical of Oncology,* **19,** 1848–54.

Simons, J.W., Mikhak, B., Chang, J.F. *et al.* (1999). Induction of immunity to prostate cancer antigens: results of a clinical trial of vaccination with irradiated autologous prostate tumor cells engineered to secrete granulocyte-macrophage colony-stimulating factor using ex vivo gene transfer. *Cancer Research,* **59,** 5160–8.

Singal, D.P., Ye, M., Ni, J., & Snider, D.P. (1996). Markedly decreased expression of TAP1 and LMP2 genes in HLA class I-deficient human tumor cell lines. *Immunology Letters,* **50,** 149–54.

Skipper, J.C., Kittlesen, D.J., Hendrickson, R.C. *et al.* (1996). Shared epitopes for HLA-A3-restricted melanoma-reactive human CTL include a naturally processed epitope from Pmel-17/gp100. *Journal of Immunology,* **157,** 5027–33.

Soiffer, R., Lynch, T., Mihm, M. *et al.* (1998). Vaccination with irradiated autologous melanoma cells engineered to secrete human granulocyte-macrophage colony-stimulating factor generates potent antitumor immunity in patients with metastatic melanoma. *Proceedings of the National Academy of Sciences, USA,* **95,** 13141–6.

Song, E., Chen, J., Ouyang, N. *et al.* (2001). Soluble Fas ligand released by colon adenocarcinoma cells induces host lymphocyte apoptosis: an active mode of immune evasion in colon cancer. *British Journal of Cancer,* **85,** 1047–54.

Sotiriadou, R., Perez, S.A., Gritzapis, A.D. *et al.* (2001). Peptide HER2(776–788) represents a naturally processed broad MHC class II-restricted T cell epitope. *British Journal of Cancer,* **85,** 1527–34.

Speiser, D.E., Lienard, D., Pittet, M.J. *et al.* (2002). In vivo activation of melanoma-specific CD8(+) T cells by endogenous tumor antigen and peptide vaccines. A comparison to virus-specific T cells. *European Journal of Immunology,* **32,** 731–41.

Srivastava, P.K. & Amato, R.J. (2001). Heat shock proteins: the 'Swiss army knife' vaccines against cancers and infectious agents. *Vaccine,* **19,** 2590–7.

Suni, M.A., Picker, L.J., & Maino, V.C. (1998). Detection of antigen-specific T cell cytokine expression in whole blood by flow cytometry. *Journal of Immunological Methods,* **212,** 89–98.

Svane, I.M., Boesen, M., & Engel, A.M. (1999). The role of cytotoxic T-lymphocytes in the prevention and immune surveillance of tumors—lessons from normal and immunodeficient mice. *Medical Oncology,* **16,** 223–38.

Tachibana, O., Nakazawa, H., Lampe, J. *et al.* (1995). Expression of Fas/APO-1 during the progression of astrocytomas. *Cancer Research,* **55,** 5528–30.

Taga, K., Mostowski, H., & Tosato, G. (1993). Human interleukin-10 can directly inhibit T-cell growth. *Blood,* **81,** 2964–71.

Tahara, K., Takesako, K., Sette, A. *et al.* (1999). Identification of a MAGE-2-encoded human leukocyte antigen-A24-binding synthetic peptide that induces specific antitumor cytotoxic T lymphocytes. *Clinical Cancer Research,* **5,** 2236–41.

Tanaka, H., Tsunoda, T., Nukaya, I. *et al.* (2001). Mapping the HLA-A24-restricted T-cell epitope peptide from a tumour-associated antigen HER2/neu: possible immunotherapy for colorectal carcinomas. *British Journal of Cancer,* **84,** 94–99.

Tanaka, Y., Takahashi, T., Nieda, M. *et al.* (2000). Generation of HLA-DRB1*1501-restricted p190 minor bcr-abl (ela2)-specific CD4+ T lymphocytes. *British Journal of Haematology,* **109,** 435–7.

Tanzarella, S., Russo, V., Lionello, I. *et al.* (1999). Identification of a promiscuous T-cell epitope encoded by multiple members of the MAGE family. *Cancer Research,* **59,** 2668–74.

ten Bosch, G.J., Kessler, J.H., Joosten, A.M. *et al.* (1999). A BCR-ABL oncoprotein p210b2a2 fusion region sequence is recognized by HLA-DR2a restricted cytotoxic T lymphocytes and presented by HLA-DR matched cells transfected with an Ii(b2a2) construct. *Blood,* **94,** 1038–45.

ten Bosch, G.J., Toornvliet, A.C., Friede, T. *et al.* (1995). Recognition of peptides corresponding to the joining region of p210BCR-ABL protein by human T cells. *Leukemia,* **9,** 1344–8.

Tepper, R.I., Pattengale, P.K., & Leder, P. (1989). Murine interleukin-4 displays potent anti-tumor activity in vivo. *Cell,* **57,** 503–12.

Thomas, M.C., Greten, T.F., Pardoll, D.M., & Jaffee, E.M. (1998). Enhanced tumor protection by granulocyte-macrophage colony-stimulating factor expression at the site of an allogeneic vaccine. *Human Gene Therapy,* **9,** 835–43.

Thompson, J.A., Peace, D.J., Klarnet, J.P. *et al.* (1986). Eradication of disseminated murine leukemia by treatment with high-dose interleukin 2. *Journal of Immunology,* **137,** 3675–80.

Thurner, B., Haendle, I., Roder, C. *et al.* (1999). Vaccination with mage-3A1 peptide-pulsed mature, monocyte-derived dendritic cells expands specific cytotoxic T cells and induces regression of some metastases in advanced stage IV melanoma. *Journal of Experimental Medicine,* **190,** 1669–78.

Timmerman, J.M. & Levy, R. (1999). Dendritic cell vaccines for cancer immunotherapy. *Annual Review of Medicine,* **50,** 507–29.

Topalian, S.L., Gonzales, M.I., Parkhurst, M. *et al.* (1996). Melanoma-specific CD4+ T cells recognize nonmutated HLA-DR-restricted tyrosinase epitopes. *Journal of Experimental Medicine,* **183,** 1965–71.

Topp, M.S., Papadimitriou, C.A., Eitelbach, F. *et al.* (1995). Recombinant human interleukin 4 has antiproliferative activity on human tumor cell lines derived from epithelial and nonepithelial histologies. *Cancer Research,* **55,** 2173–6.

Toungouz, M., Libin, M., Bulte, F. *et al.* (2001). Transient expansion of peptide-specific lymphocytes producing IFN-gamma after vaccination with dendritic cells pulsed with MAGE peptides in patients with mage-A1/A3-positive tumors. *Journal of Leukocyte Biology,* **69,** 937–43.

Townsend, S.E. & Allison, J.P. (1993). Tumor rejection after direct costimulation of CD8+ T cells by B7-transfected melanoma cells. *Science,* **259,** 368–70.

Townsend, S.E., Su, F.W., Atherton, J.M., & Allison, J.P. (1994). Specificity and longevity of antitumor immune responses induced by B7-transfected tumors. *Cancer Research,* **54,** 6477–83.

Trinchieri, G. (1993). Interleukin-12 and its role in the generation of TH1 cells. *Immunology Today,* **14,** 335–8.

Trinchieri, G. (1994). Interleukin-12: a cytokine produced by antigen-presenting cells with immunoregulatory functions in the generation of T-helper cells type 1 and cytotoxic lymphocytes. *Blood,* **84,** 4008–27.

Tsai, V., Southwood, S., Sidney, J. et al. (1997). Identification of subdominant CTL epitopes of the GP100 melanoma-associated tumor antigen by primary in vitro immunization with peptide-pulsed dendritic cells. Journal of Immunology, 158, 1796–802.

Tsang, K.Y., Zhu, M., Nieroda, C.A. et al. (1997). Phenotypic stability of a cytotoxic T-cell line directed against an immunodominant epitope of human carcinoembryonic antigen. Clinical Cancer Research, 3, 2439–49.

Tureci, O., Sahin, U., & Pfreundschuh, M. (1997). Serological analysis of human tumor antigens: molecular definition and implications. Molecular Medicine Today, 3, 342–9.

Turner, M.J., Abdul-Alim, C.S., Willis, R.A. et al. (2001). T-cell antigen discovery (T-CAD) assay: a novel technique for identifying T cell epitopes. Journal of Immunological Methods, 256, 107–19.

Tuting, T., Storkus, W.J., & Lotze, M.T. (1997). Gene-based strategies for the immunotherapy of cancer. Journal of Molecular Medicine, 75, 478–91.

Valmori, D., Levy, F., Miconnet, I. et al. (2000). Induction of potent antitumor CTL responses by recombinant vaccinia encoding a melan-A peptide analogue. Journal of Immunology, 164, 1125–31.

Van den, E.B., Peeters, O., De Backer, O. et al. (1995). A new family of genes coding for an antigen recognized by autologous cytolytic T lymphocytes on a human melanoma. Journal of Experimental Medicine, 182, 689–98.

van der, B.P., Bastin, J., Gajewski, T. et al. (1994a). A peptide encoded by human gene MAGE-3 and presented by HLA-A2 induces cytolytic T lymphocytes that recognize tumor cells expressing MAGE-3. European Journal of Immunology, 24, 3038–43.

van der, B.P., Szikora, J.P., Boel, P. et al. (1994b). Autologous cytolytic T lymphocytes recognize a MAGE-1 nonapeptide on melanomas expressing HLA-Cw*1601. European Journal of Immunology, 24, 2134–40.

Velculescu, V.E., Zhang, L., Vogelstein, B., & Kinzler, K.W. (1995). Serial analysis of gene expression. Science, 270, 484–7.

Visseren, M.J., van der Burg, S.H., van der Voort, E.I. et al. (1997). Identification of HLA-A*0201-restricted CTL epitopes encoded by the tumor-specific MAGE-2 gene product. International Journal of Cancer, 73, 125–30.

Vissers, J.L., De Vries, I.J., Schreurs, M.W. et al. (1999). The renal cell carcinoma-associated antigen G250 encodes a human leukocyte antigen (HLA)-A2.1-restricted epitope recognized by cytotoxic T lymphocytes. Cancer Research, 59, 5554–9.

Vitale, M., Rezzani, R., Rodella, L. et al. (1998). HLA class I antigen and transporter associated with antigen processing (TAP1 and TAP2) down-regulation in high-grade primary breast carcinoma lesions. Cancer Research, 58, 737–42.

von Boehmer, H. (1994). Positive selection of lymphocytes. Cell, 76, 219–28.

Vonderheide, R.H., Anderson, K.S., Hahn, W.C. et al. (2001). Characterization of HLA-A3-restricted cytotoxic T lymphocytes reactive against the widely expressed tumor antigen telomerase. Clinical Cancer Research, 7, 3343–8.

Walker, P.R., Saas, P., & Dietrich, P.Y. (1998). Tumor expression of Fas ligand (CD95L) and the consequences. Current Opinion in Immunology, 10, 564–72.

Walter, E.A., Greenberg, P.D., Gilbert, M.J. et al. (1995). Reconstitution of cellular immunity against cytomegalovirus in recipients of allogeneic bone marrow by transfer of T-cell clones from the donor. New England Journal of Medicine, 333, 1038–44.

Wan, Y., Bramson, J., Carter, R. et al. (1997). Dendritic cells transduced with an adenoviral vector encoding a model tumor-associated antigen for tumor vaccination. Human Gene Therapy, 8, 1355–63.

Wan, Y., Bramson, J., Pilon, A. et al. (2000). Genetically modified dendritic cells prime autoreactive T cells through a pathway independent of CD40L and interleukin 12: implications for cancer vaccines. Cancer Research, 60, 3247–53.

Wang, F., Bade, E., Kuniyoshi, C. et al. (1999). Phase I trial of a MART-1 peptide vaccine with incomplete Freund's adjuvant for resected high-risk melanoma. Clinical Cancer Research, 5, 2756–65.

Wang, R.F., Appella, E., Kawakami, Y. et al. (1996a). Identification of TRP-2 as a human tumor antigen recognized by cytotoxic T lymphocytes. Journal of Experimental Medicine, 184, 2207–16.

Wang, R.F., Johnston, S.L., Zeng, G. et al. (1998a). A breast and melanoma-shared tumor antigen: T cell responses to antigenic peptides translated from different open reading frames. Journal of Immunology, 161, 3598–606.

Wang, R.F., Parkhurst, M.R., Kawakami, Y. et al. (1996b). Utilization of an alternative open reading frame of a normal gene in generating a novel human cancer antigen. Journal of Experimental Medicine, 183, 1131–40.

Wang, W., Man, S., Gulden, P.H. et al. (1998b). Class I-restricted alloreactive cytotoxic T lymphocytes recognize a complex array of specific MHC-associated peptides. Journal of Immunology, 160, 1091–7.

Watts, C. (1997). Capture and processing of exogenous antigens for presentation on MHC molecules. Annual Review of Immunology, 15, 821–50.

Weiss, A. (1991). Molecular and genetic insights into T cell antigen receptor structure and function. Annual Review of Genetics, 25, 487–510.

Williamson, B.D., Carswell, E.A., Rubin, B.Y. et al. (1983). Human tumor necrosis factor produced by human B-cell lines: synergistic cytotoxic interaction with human interferon. Proceedings of the National Academy of Sciences, USA, 80, 5397–401.

Wolfel, T., Hauer, M., Schneider, J. et al. (1995). A p16INK4a-insensitive CDK4 mutant targeted by cytolytic T lymphocytes in a human melanoma. Science, 269, 1281–4.

Wolfel, T., Van Pel, A., Brichard, V. et al. (1994). Two tyrosinase nonapeptides recognized on HLA-A2 melanomas by autologous cytolytic T lymphocytes. European Journal of Immunology, 24, 759–64.

Wong, D.A., Bishop, G.A., Lowes, M.A. et al. (2000). Cytokine profiles in spontaneously regressing basal cell carcinomas. British Journal of Dermatology, 143, 91–8.

Xu, J., Kalos, M., Stolk, J.A. et al. (2001). Identification and characterization of prostein, a novel prostate-specific protein. Cancer Research, 61, 1563–8.

Xu, J., Stolk, J.A., Zhang, X. et al. (2000). Identification of differentially expressed genes in human prostate cancer using subtraction and microarray. Cancer Research, 60, 1677–82.

Yang, D., Nakao, M., Shichijo, S. *et al.* (1999). Identification of a gene coding for a protein possessing shared tumor epitopes capable of inducing HLA-A24-restricted cytotoxic T lymphocytes in cancer patients. *Cancer Research,* **59,** 4056–63.

Yasukawa, M., Ohminami, H., Kaneko, S. *et al.* (1998). CD4(+) cytotoxic T-cell clones specific for bcr-abl b3a2 fusion peptide augment colony formation by chronic myelogenous leukemia cells in a b3a2-specific and HLA-DR-restricted manner. *Blood,* **92,** 3355–61.

Yasukawa, M., Ohminami, H., Kojima, K. *et al.* (2001). HLA class II-restricted antigen presentation of endogenous bcr-abl fusion protein by chronic myelogenous leukemia-derived dendritic cells to CD4(+) T lymphocytes. *Blood,* **98,** 1498–505.

Yee, C., Gilbert, M.J., Riddell, S.R. *et al.* (1996). Isolation of tyrosinase-specific CD8+ and CD4+ T cell clones from the peripheral blood of melanoma patients following in vitro stimulation with recombinant vaccinia virus. *Journal of Immunology,* **157,** 4079–86.

Yee, C., Riddell, S.R., & Greenberg, P.D. (1997). Prospects for adoptive T cell therapy. *Current Opinion in Immunology,* **9,** 702–8.

Yee, C., Savage, P.A., Lee, P.P. *et al.* (1999). Isolation of high avidity melanoma-reactive CTL from heterogeneous populations using peptide-MHC tetramers. *Journal of Immunology,* **162,** 2227–34.

Yee, C., Thompson, J.A., Roche, P. *et al.* (2000). Melanocyte destruction after antigen-specific immunotherapy of melanoma: direct evidence of T cell-mediated vitiligo. *Journal of Experimental Medicine,* **192,** 1637–44.

York, I.A. & Rock, K.L. (1996). Antigen processing and presentation by the class I major histocompatibility complex. *Annual Review of Immunology,* **14,** 369–96.

Yoshida, H., Enomoto, H., Kawamura, K. *et al.* (1998). Antitumor vaccine effect of irradiated murine neuroblastoma cells producing interleukin-2 or granulocyte macrophage-colony stimulating factor. *International Journal of Oncology,* **13,** 73–8.

Yotnda, P., Firat, H., Garcia-Pons, F. *et al.* (1998). Cytotoxic T cell response against the chimeric p210 BCR-ABL protein in patients with chronic myelogeneous leukemia. *Journal of Clinical Investigation,* **101,** 2290–6.

Zarour, H.M., Storkus, W.J., Brusic, V. *et al.* (2000). NY-ESO-1 encodes DRBI*0401-restricted epitopes recognized by melanoma-reactive CD4+ T cells. *Cancer Research,* **60,** 4946–52.

Zeng, G., Touloukian, C.E., Wang, X. *et al.* (2000). Identification of CD4+ T cell epitopes from NY-ESO-1 presented by HLA-DR molecules. *Journal of Immunology,* **165,** 1153–9.

Zeng, G., Wang, X., Robbins, P.F. *et al.* (2001). CD4(+) T cell recognition of MHC class II-restricted epitopes from NY-ESO-1 presented by a prevalent HLA DP4 allele: association with NY-ESO-1 antibody production. *Proceedings of the National Academy of Sciences, USA,* **98,** 3964–9.

Zhang, L., Zhou, W., Velculescu, V.E. *et al.* (1997). Gene expression profiles in normal and cancer cells. *Science,* **276,** 1268–72.

Zhong, L., Granelli-Piperno, A., Choi, Y., & Steinman, R.M. (1999). Recombinant adenovirus is an efficient and non-perturbing genetic vector for human dendritic cells. *European Journal of Immunology,* **29,** 964–72.

Zorn, E. & Hercend, T. (1999). A MAGE-6-encoded peptide is recognized by expanded lymphocytes infiltrating a spontaneously regressing human primary melanoma lesion. *European Journal of Immunology,* **29,** 602–7.

114 NK-T cells: biology and clinical applications

MICHAEL R. VERNERIS AND ROBERT S. NEGRIN

Stanford University, Stanford, USA

Introduction

Hematopoietic stem cell transplantation (HSCT) has proven successful in the treatment of a variety of malignant hematopoietic disorders. This is due to the combination of both the high-dose chemoirradiation-based conditioning regimens and the immunological reaction of donor lymphocytes toward residual recipient malignant cells, termed the graft-versus-tumor (GVT) effect. Untoward complications of HSCT include graft-versus-host disease (GVHD), which like GVT is mediated by donor lymphocytes, but unlike GVT results in an alloreactive immune response against normal host tissues. While both GVHD and GVT can occur simultaneously, recent animal data and early human studies suggest that GVT and GVHD can exist independently of one another.

Clinical HSCT involves the transfer of complex heterogeneous populations of fully differentiated lymphocytes, and therefore, the occurrence of both GVT and GVHD is not surprising. Inherent in attempts at improving the therapeutic outcome of HSCT (i.e., enhanced GVT effects and limited GVHD) is the need for isolation and likely expansion of phenotypically defined populations of effector cells. Biological activity of such effector cell populations is defined functionally by a number of assays including cytokine production, in vitro cytotoxic activity, and in vivo biological function. Although the cell population(s) responsible for the GVT effect are not known with certainty, both T and natural killer (NK) cell populations of cells are likely candidates. Since the mid-1980s populations of cells that share phenotypic and functional characteristics of both NK and T cells have been defined (Lanier *et al.*, 1986; Schmidt *et al.*, 1986). Studies suggest that such cells may have significant biological activity in tumor models and in limited clinical trials. These cells, collectively termed NK-T cells, are the subject of this chapter.

Types of NK-T cells

NK-T cells are a subset of T cells that have been described in both mouse and humans with immune regulatory and tumor surveillance functions. Three subsets of NK-T cells have been defined based on the expression of the co-receptors CD4 and CD8. These include double negative (DN, CD4$^-$CD8$^-$), CD4$^+$, and CD8$^+$ NK-T cells. There are considerable differences between these different subsets with respect to T-cell receptor (TCR) expression, tissue distribution, thymic dependence, and cytokine production. Most importantly, these different subsets differ in their ability to recognize the nonpolymorphic, major histocompatibility complex (MHC)-I related molecule, CD1. Thus, NK-T cells can be divided into two major groups, those that recognize antigen in the context of CD1 (CD1-restricted) and those that do not (CD1-nonrestricted).

CD1-restricted NK-T cells

CD1-restricted NK-T cells express both the T-cell receptor/CD3 complex and NK1.1 (mice) or CD161 (humans) (Bendelac *et al.*, 1997). CD1-restricted NK-T cells express molecules associated with a memory T-cell phenotype including CD44^{high}, CD69^{high}, CD62L^{low}, IL-2Rβ and CD122^{high} (Bendelac *et al.*, 1997; Watanabe *et al.*, 1993). As well, in rodents other NK-associated markers including DX-5, Ly49 (Eberl *et al.*, 1999; Ortaldo *et al.*, 1998) are variably expressed. Murine studies have demonstrated that the CD4 and the DN subsets are derived from the same (or similar) lineage, since most express a single, invariant TCRα chain (Vα14Jα281) paired with a limited number of Vβ receptors (Vβ8.2 being the most common) (Bendelac *et al.*, 1997; Godfrey *et al.*, 2000). In contrast to classical T cells which recognize peptide in the context of MHC class I or II, the CD4$^+$ and many of the DN NK-T cells recognize glycolipid in the context of the nonclassical MHC molecule CD1d (Benlagha *et al.*, 2000). Synthetic ligands that bind in the groove of CD1d include α-galactosylceramide (α-GalCer) (Benlagha *et al.*, 2000; Kawano *et al.*, 1997). NK-T cells are found in most lymphoid tissues, with CD4$^+$ NK-T cells predominantly in the liver and thymus and DN NK-T cells in the bone marrow and spleen (Eberl *et al.*, 1999).

CD1d restricted NK-T cells are dependent on the thymus for development, since they are markedly reduced in thymectomized mice, nude mice, and arise in Rag$^{-/-}$ β2M$^{-/-}$ mice only after thymus transplantation (Hammond *et al.*, 1998; Coles &

1794

Raulet, 2000). More recently, investigators have addressed the nature of the thymic precursor population that gives rise to CD1-restricted NK-T cells. Such cells are derived from a double positive (CD4+CD8+) precursor population in a manner identical to standard T cells (Gapin et al., 2001). Benlagha and co-workers (Benlagha et al., 2002) elegantly demonstrated that in young mice there are both NK1.1− and NK1.1+ CD1d tetramer reactive populations. They went on to establish that mature NK-T cells arise from this NK1.1− precursor population and that both populations of CD1d tetramer-reactive T cells (NK1.1− and NK1.1+) leave the thymus and migrate into the peripheral tissues. Interestingly, the NK1.1− and NK1.1+ populations differed with regard to proliferative capacity and cytokine secretion. The less mature NK1.1− precursor population had a higher proliferative capacity and secreted large amounts of interleukin (IL)-4 and little interferon-γ (IFN-γ) upon activation, while the more mature NK1.1+ cells had a lower rate of proliferation and secreted minimal IL-4 and high amounts of IFN-γ. Thus, in contrast to previous studies that have demonstrated that mature CD1d tetramer-reactive cells secrete high amounts of both IL-4 and IFN-γ (Bendelac et al., 1997), immature NK-T cells (which leave the thymus and account for some of the peripheral NK-T cells) have cytokine secretion patterns that vary with developmental stage (Fig. 114.1). Such findings may help explain the diverse actions (whether direct or indirect) of NK-T cells in both counterregulatory and antitumor responses.

Human NK-T cells have also been identified in the peripheral blood and liver (Dellabona et al., 1993; Ishihara et al., 2000; Prussin & Foster, 1997). Similar to murine NK-T cells, human NK-T cells express an invariant T-cell receptor (Vα24JαQ, which associates with Vβ11, homologues for the murine receptors Vβ14Jα281 and Vβ8.2, respectively) and three subsets can be identified based on CD4 and CD8 expression. In contrast to the mouse, there is a larger percentage of CD1-restricted CD8+ NK-T cells in humans (Prussin & Foster, 1997). CD1d-tetramer reactive CD8+ NK-T cells express CD8 αβ homodimers and thus differ from conventional peripheral blood CD8+ T cells, which almost exclusively express CD8 αβ heterodimers (Gumperz et al., 2002). Analogous to the above rodent studies, phenotypically distinct lineages of human NK-T cells have been identified. To date these studies have separated human NK-T cell lineages into CD4+ and CD4− and have not distinguished between the CD8 αα and CD4− CD8− populations. These studies show that there are considerable differences between these subpopulations. For example, after activation with PMA/ionomycin, the CD4+ NK-T subset produces IL-2, 4, 5, 6, 10, 13 and GM-CSF, while both the CD4+ and CD4− populations make IFN-γ and TNF-α (Gumperz et al., 2002; Lee et al., 2002). Conversely, freshly isolated CD4− NK-T cells expresses receptors typically found on NK cells (CD94, NKG2A, CD161, and 2B4), while such molecules are rarely found on CD4+ NK-T cells (Lee et al., 2002). The ability to produce effector molecules either after cytokine stimulation or TCR engagement varies between the two subsets such that the

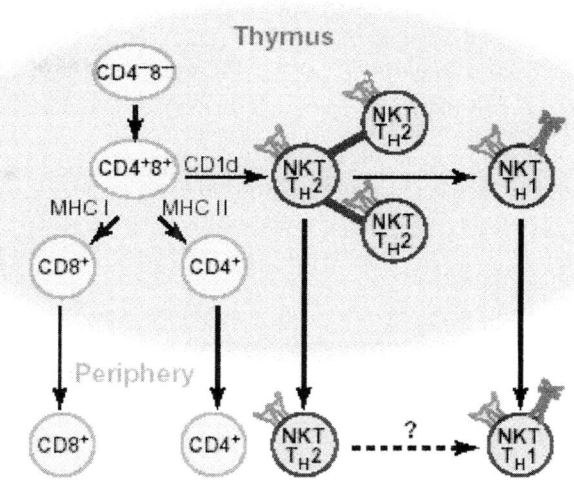

Fig. 114.1. Precursor population that gives rise to NK-T cells. CD4−CD8− thymic precursors are positively selected on either MHC class I, MHC class II, or CD1. The CD1-reactive cells give rise to an early NK-T population that does not express NK1.1 (NK1.1−). These cells have a Th2 cytokine secretion pattern and can migrate to the periphery. As well, CD1d tetramer-reactive, NK1.1− cells can also remain in the thymus, have a high rate of proliferation, and give rise to CD1d tetramer-reactive, NK1.1+ cells, which have a Th1-skewed phenotype. In turn, these slower proliferating NK1.1+ NK-T cells can either remain in the thymus or migrate to the peripheral tissues.

CD4− NK-T subset is more likely to produce perforin and NKG2D while the CD4+ subset produces higher amounts of CD95L (Gumperz et al., 2002). Collectively, these results suggest that the different subsets of CD1-restricted NK-T cells may have differing functions, and the challenge in the coming years will be to further distinguish these functions.

CD1-nonrestricted NK-T cells

Less is known about CD1-nonrestricted NK-T cells. In mice, such cells are known to be CD1-nonrestricted since both CD8+ NK-T and some DN NK-T cells are found in CD1−/− mice (Eberl et al., 1999). In addition, this subset of NK-T cells has a heterogeneous TCR repertoire and does not express the invariant TCR found on CD1-restricted NK-T cells (Eberl et al., 1999; Emoto et al., 2000). As stated above, thymectomy at day 3 of life leads to a significant reduction in CD1-restricted CD4+ and DN NK-T cells in the spleen and thymus (see above), but CD1-nonrestricted splenic CD8+ NK-T cells are relatively unchanged in numbers, suggesting that they are either thymus independent or leave the thymus very early in life. Soon after activation freshly isolated splenic CD8+ NK-T cells produce little IFN-γ or IL-4[10]; however, after prolonged culture they produce large amounts of IFN-γ (Baker et al., 2001).

In humans, populations of T cells that express NK markers (CD56) have been identified for many years (Ortaldo et al., 1991; Baume et al., 1990). Such CD3+CD8+CD56+ cells make up ~4% to 30% of the peripheral blood CD8+ T-cell compartment in healthy donors. Further, the expression of CD56+ on CD8+ T cells is tightly correlated to the presence of intracellular granzyme and perforin, as well as cytotoxic activity (Pittet et al., 2000). Immortalized lines of tumor infiltrating NK-T cells have shown similar phenotype (CD3+CD8+CD56+) and these cells have broad MHC-unrestricted cytotoxicity against a variety of tumor cell lines (Imahayashi et al., 2002). To date, the exact cell surface structures that mediate tumor cell identification are not known, but appear to be independent of the TCR (see below). Moreover, little is known about the specific role of these cells in normal individuals. Some investigators have speculated that CD1-nonrestricted NK-T cells may reflect a population of activated or memory/effector cell types and that these cells may arise in response to chronic antigen stimulation (Tarazona et al., 2000). While this may be the case, it is puzzling why such cells mediate antitumor activity in vitro and it remains to be demonstrated whether such cells mediate tumor surveillance functions in vivo.

Mechanisms of tumor cell killing and immunoregulatory function

Similar mechanisms of tumor cell killing are shared amongst T, NK-T, and NK cells. Upon recognition, adhesion of the effector cell to potential targets occurs through a variety of receptor/counter-receptor pairs such as ICAM/LFA-1 and CD2/LFA-3. Monoclonal antibodies directed against these determinants are capable of blocking cytotoxicity in vitro. Target cell specificity occurs through specific receptor/ligand pairs such as TCR/MHC, TCR/CD1, NK cell receptor/MHC class I, and others. Following target cell engagement, effector cell activation occurs and results in target cell killing through three broad cellular pathways that include granzymes/perforin, tumor necrosis factor (TNF) superfamily molecules, and soluble mediators.

When the effector cell is triggered to kill the target, preformed intracellular granules fuse with the cell membrane and granule exocytosis occurs. Contained within the granules of effector cells are a variety of molecules that induce target cell apoptosis. The best characterized of these molecules are perforin and granzymes. The best evidence for the importance of these molecules is through the development of knock-out mouse strains defective in these key effector molecules. Perforin-deficient mice (pfp$^{-/-}$) are nearly devoid of cell-mediated cytotoxic activity (Kagl et al., 1994). In vitro studies show that purified perforin inserts into the cell membrane and polymerizes in a Ca^{++}-dependent manner to create membrane pores 100 to 200 Å in diameter (Young et al., 1986). While perforin induces target cell necrosis, more recent studies suggest that perforin's true mechanism of action may be to facilitate the entry of other granule contents into the target cell (Trapani et al., 2000). One such family of key proteases include the serine proteases, called granzymes, which induce apoptosis by activating the proteolytic machinery within the target itself (Talanian et al., 1997). The substrates for granzymes include

caspases as well as other cell death pathways (Sarin et al., 1998). Several other molecules contained within the cytoplasmic granules are also capable of inducing target cytolysis. One such molecule, granulysin, induces tumor cytolysis in vitro (Pena & Krensky, 1997), but its in vivo role is not known.

As another class of effector molecules, the TNF superfamily plays an essential role in both cellular activation and proliferation (CD30L, CD40L) as well as cell death [TNF-α, FasL, and TNF-related apoptosis-inducing ligand (TRAIL)] (Gruss et al., 1994; Jumper et al., 1995; Ashkenazi & Dixit, 1999). FasL and TRAIL are expressed on effector cell populations and have specific counter receptors present on a variety of both malignant and nonmalignant cells. For FasL there is a single receptor, CD95 or Fas (Takahashi et al., 1994). There are at least five receptors to which TRAIL can bind to and two are capable of inducing apoptosis (TRAIL-R1 (DR4) and TRAIL-R2 (DR5) (Walczak & Krammer, 2000).

Both FasL and TRAIL induce trimerization of their cognate receptors on the target cells, which in turn activates caspases leading to target cell apoptosis. FasL has been found within cytoplasmic granules and is brought to the effector cell surface upon activation, thereby maintaining target specificity and minimizing injury to surrounding tissues (Bossi & Griffiths, 1999). Once on the cell surface, FasL is rapidly cleaved to a soluble form by matrix metalloproteases (Kayagaki et al., 1995). Most studies suggest that soluble FasL is either inactive or a weak inducer of apoptosis, thus cleavage from the cell surface may be a form of regulation of FasL-mediated immune responses. Whether TRAIL is regulated in the same fashion has not yet been definitively determined. Unlike FasL, TRAIL does not induce apoptosis in normal tissues (Ashkenazi et al., 1999; Walczak et al., 1999). Recent studies have called into question whether normal tissue is truly resistant to the apoptosis-inducing effects of TRAIL (Walczak et al., 1999).

Soluble mediators elaborated by effector cells can also have a variety of either indirect or direct effects on tumor tissue. For example, upon activation NK-T cells secrete large amounts of interferon-γ, which has a variety of actions including the direct activation of NK cells, the upregulation in MHC I and II expression on tumor targets (which in turn increases antigen presentation to conventional T cells), and finally IFN-γ sensitizes some tumor targets to Fas-mediated apoptosis. Similarly, activated NK-T cells can stimulate dendritic cells to elaborate IL-12 (Kitamura et al., 1999), which both activates effector functions of NK and T-cell populations and has direct antiangiogenic properties on tumor vasculature (Majewski et al., 1996).

Function and clinical application of NK-T cells

CD1-restricted NK-T cells

In general, immune responses can be broadly divided into innate or adaptive responses. Innate effector cells are thought to be first line of defense against a variety of insults and hence, are able to respond quickly. NK-T cells are part of this innate immune response given that one of their hallmarks is rapid cytokine secretion upon activation. As mentioned above, this cytokine secretion facilitates significant cross-talk between NK-T cells and other cells of the immune system, including those of the adaptive immune system. Therefore, while NK-T cells act as innate effectors they have an important influence on the adaptive arm of the immune response through cytokine secretion.

Considerable experimental evidence supports the use of NK-T cells for immunotherapy. Treatment of tumor-bearing mice with either Il-12, α-GalCer, or α-GalCer pulsed dendritic cells induces NK-T cell-dependent antitumor activity (Eberl et al., 1999; Toura et al., 1999). In these initial studies it was not determined whether the NK-T cells mediated the antitumor activity directly, since whole splenocytes (and not purified NK-T cells) were used to demonstrate this effect. More recent studies suggest that NK-T cells mediate tumor clearance indirectly, since their activation induces NK cell proliferation and cytotoxicity, which is in part dependent on their prompt IFN-γ production upon activation (Eberl & MacDonald, 2000; Carnaud et al., 1999). Furthermore, the administration of α-GalCer to mice leads to a marked reduction of NK-T cells (Matsuda et al., 2000), supporting the above conclusions that the antitumor activity mediated by murine NK-T cells is indirect. Using a different approach Crowe and co-workers recently established that NK-T cells also play a pivotal role in the surveillance of methylcholanthrene-induced sarcomas. These investigators demonstrated that sarcomas were more likely to grow in animals deficient for CD1-restricted NK-T cells (Jα281$^{-/-}$ mice), and that transfer of NK-T cells to such animals protected them from sarcoma challenge (Smyth et al., 2000; Crowe et al., 2002). Once again, assistance from both NK cells and CD8$^+$ T cells was required for NK-T cell-mediated tumor protection.

Unlike murine NK-T cells, direct antitumor activity has been demonstrated with human NK-T cells. In vitro studies show that α-GalCer-stimulated CD3$^+$ T cells or NK-T cell clones mediate perforin-based cytolysis of tumor targets (Takahashi et al., 2000; Exley et al., 1998; Nicol et al., 2000), and adoptive transfer of NK-T cells inhibits the growth of human esophageal carcinoma cell lines engrafted into SCID mice (Kawano et al., 1999). Direct cytotoxicity can be demonstrated against target cells that are CD1$^+$, but not against those that are CD1$^-$ (Metelitsa et al., 2001). Such CD1$^-$ targets can be rendered sensitive to cytolysis after CD1 gene transfer and pulsing with α-GalCer. The identity of the natural ligands that are presented to NK-T cells are not known with certainty, but phospholipid extracts from tumor cell lines do bind to CD1 and induce NK-T cell activation (Gumperz et al., 2000). Thus, it appears that NK-T cells are able to respond to endogenous antigens presented by tumor cells.

Since only small numbers of NK-T cells are found circulating in human peripheral blood (~0.1–0.01% of peripheral blood T cells) (Gumperz et al., 2002; Lee et al., 2002), methodologies are being developed to expand such cells ex vivo. Culturing NK-T cells with α-GalCer and IL-12 activates NK-T cells (increased intracellular granzyme B), but has little effect

on cell expansion (Van der Vliet et al., 1999). Expansion of human NK-T cells has recently been achieved after culture of peripheral blood T cells with α-GalCer-pulsed dendritic cells and stimulation with IL-7 and/or IL-15 (van der Vliet et al., 2001). Differences between expanded adult and umbilical cord blood (UCB) NK-T cells exist, such that UCB NK-T cells have a more Th2 bias, secreting more IL-4 than adult-derived counterparts (Kadowaki et al., 2001). Such findings may in part account for the reduced GVHD seen after UCB transplantation. UCB-derived NK-T cells appear to have more plasticity than adult NK-T cells and can be skewed to a Th1 cytokine pattern by culturing them in the presence of the DC1 dendritic cells (Kadowaki et al., 2001).Such findings may have important implications for the use of expanded UCB-derived NK-T cells as adoptive immunotherapy after UCB transplantation.

There is mounting evidence for both quantitative and qualitative defects in NK-T cells in cancer patients. Kawano and co-workers noted a reduction in the number of Vα24 cells in melanoma patients (Kawano et al., 1999). A similar decrease in the number of NK-T cells was demonstrated in patients with prostate cancer (Tahir et al., 2001). In a heterogeneous collection of cancer patients there was no decrease noted (Yanagisawa et al., 2002), thus CD1-restricted NK-T cells may be affected differently by various malignancies. Functional NK-T cell defects in cancer patients include a reduced proliferative response to α-GalCer-loaded antigen-presenting cells (Tahir et al., 2001; Yanagisawa et al., 2002). This proliferative defect can be partially rescued by the addition of G-CSF to cultures with α-GalCer-loaded antigen-presenting cells (Yanagisawa et al., 2002). As well, patients who were in remission had improved proliferative NK-T responses compared to those who were not (Tahir et al., 2001). Interestingly, expanded NK-T cells from patients with prostate cancer produced high amounts of IL-4, but not IFN-γ and this was in contrast to normal controls who secreted large amounts of both cytokines (Tahir et al., 2001). This defect in IFN-γ secretion could be corrected by the addition of IL-12 to cultures.

In contrast to the above findings of antitumor activity, NK-T cells have also been implicated in tumor progression and recurrence. In one study, tumor-infiltrating NK-T cells from B16 melanoma-injected mice inhibited antitumor CTL generation, both through the elaboration of TGF-β and cytolysis of cells expressing co-stimulatory molecules (Tamada et al., 1997). In other studies CD4$^+$ NK-T cells played an essential role in the tumor recurrence phase due to the secretion of IL-13 (Terabe et al., 2000). Thus, in certain situations the activation (or adoptive transfer) of NK-T-cell populations might be detrimental and further work is needed to better understand these observations.

Few studies have addressed the role of NK-T cells in GVHD induction. Murine studies have shown that bone marrow NK-T cells transplanted across major histocompatibility barriers actually suppressed GVHD induced by peripheral blood CD4$^+$ and CD8$^+$ cells (Zeng et al., 1999). This protection was lost if cells from IL-4$^{-/-}$ knockout mice were utilized, indicating that in this model IL-4 plays an essential role in GVHD protection.

Similarly, human bone marrow NK-T cells have been shown to have a Th2 bias and are capable of suppressing two-way mixed lymphocyte reactions (Stremmel et al., 2001). However, other investigators have shown that host-derived NK-T cells can be demonstrated in the thymus during acute GVHD (Onoe et al., 1998). Whether these cells actually contribute to GVHD (or arise in response to GVHD) was not determined in these murine studies.

CD1-nonrestricted T cells (CIK cells)

Small numbers of human peripheral blood T cells express the NK cell marker CD56 and these freshly isolated cells have NK-like cytotoxicity against tumor targets (Ortaldo et al., 1991; Baume et al., 1990). Culture conditions have been developed that allow for the expansion of T cells with similar attributes, namely, expression of CD56 and broad MHC-unrestricted cytotoxicity against a variety of tumor targets (Schmidt-Wolf et al., 1991; Schmidt-Wolf et al., 1993; Lu & Negrin, 1994; Ochoa et al., 1987). These ex vivo expanded cells, termed cytokine-induced killer cells (CIK cells) were in fact not derived from either NK cells or $CD3^+CD56^+$ precursor cells, but rather from either $CD3^+CD4^-CD8^-$, $CD3^+CD8^+$, or even $CD3^+CD4^+CD8^+$ cells (Lu & Negrin, 1994).

The culture conditions used to generate CIK cells include prestimulation with IFN-γ, followed by a cross-linking anti-CD3 antibody and intermediate dose IL-2 (300 U/ml). Prestimulation with IFN-γ leads to monocyte activation and IL-12 production, which enhances $CD3^+CD56^+$ expansion through both the secretion of IL-12 and CD58/LFA3 co-stimulation (Lopez et al., 2001). Other studies support these findings, since culture of lymphocytes under identical conditions and IL-12 (as compared to IL-2) leads to higher numbers of $CD3^+CD56^+$ cells (Zoll et al., 2000). Under these culture conditions cells are fed with fresh media every 3 to 4 days and after 14 to 21 days there is a ~100–500 fold expansion of $CD3^+CD56^+$ cells (Lu & Negrin, 1994; Schmidt-Wolf et al., 1994).

Using these conditions CIK cells can be generated from peripheral blood, bone marrow, cord blood (in humans) and spleen, thymus, and liver (in the mouse) (Alvarnas et al., 2001). The ex vivo activated and expanded cells have significant antitumor activity against a broad array of cell lines and fresh autologous leukemic blast cells (Alvarnas et al., 2001). Using a SCID/Hu model of lymphoma, CIK cells were more effective than LAK cells in curing animals, which were rendered free of disease utilizing a sensitive PCR-based assay (Lu & Negrin, 1994). In addition, autologous CIK cells could be generated from patients with chronic phase CML with the majority of samples being Ph-chromosome-negative (Hoyle et al., 1998). These cells were capable of preventing growth of autologous CML in SCID mice (Hoyle et al., 1998). Similarly, CIK cells have been expanded from patients with AML and found to have activity against autologous AML blasts (Alvarnas et al., 2001). CIK cells are more effective in mediating cytotoxicity against cell lines derived from hematopoietic malignancies than solid tumors. Antitumor activity against solid tumor targets could be augmented with bispecific antibodies to redirect CIK cells to target cells that overexpress tumor antigens. CD3xHer2/neu bispecific antibody (bsAb)-redirected CIK cells are significantly more effective in mediating in vitro and in vivo tumor cytolysis when compared to CIK cells or CIK cells and a control bsAb (Sheffold, submitted). Similarly, bsAb-redirected CIK cells are more effective in eradicating residual breast, ovarian, and primitive neural ectodermal tumor (PNET) cell lines engrafted into SCID mice (Verneris, manuscript in preparation).

The cell surface structures involved in CIK cell recognition of tumor targets are not well understood. T-cell-receptor-based identification of targets appear not to be involved, since antibodies against CD3, CD4, CD8, TCR α/β, and MHC I and II are unable to block cytotoxicity (Baker et al., 2001; Schmidt-Wolf et al., 1993; Lu & Negrin, 1994). ICAM and LFA-1 engagement are required for cytotoxicity, since antibodies against these molecules attenuate cytotoxicity. Blocking cytoplasmic granule release inhibits cytotoxicity, suggesting a perforin-based mechanism of cytotoxicity. Further, expanded $CD8^+$ NK-T cells from FasL-deficient mice have cytotoxicity identical to cells from wild-type mice, yet cells derived from the $pfp^{-/-}$ animals were devoid of any cytolytic activity both in vitro and in vivo (Fig. 114.2) (Verneris et al., 2001).

Adoptive transfer of murine CIK cells (expanded $CD8^+$ NK-T) across major histocompatibility barriers shows that such cells have a markedly reduced propensity to induce GVHD compared to naïve splenocytes (Fig. 114.2) (Baker et al., 2001; Verneris et al., 2001). There are many possible explanations as to why the ex vivo expanded $CD8^+$ NK-T cells cause less GVHD than unexpanded cells. Expanded $CD8^+$ NK-T cells have undergone multiple rounds of expansion and the same cellular events that occur in GVHD are not likely to occur (i.e., T-cell activation, proliferation, and "cytokine storm"). Expanded $CD8^+$ NK-T cells express both TGF-β and low levels of IL-10, a combination of cytokines that have been shown by others to prevent alloreactivity (Zeller et al., 1999). Lastly, expanded $CD8^+$ NK-T cells constitutively secrete IFN-γ, which can be protective in murine GVHD (Baker et al., 2001; Yang et al., 2002). In contrast to wild-type expanded $CD8^+$ NK-T cells, those expanded from IFN-$\gamma^{-/-}$ mice induce rapid lethal GVHD (Baker et al., 2001). In this setting of allogeneic transplantation the co-administration of $CD8^+$ NK-T cells with purified hematopoietic stem cells resulted in durable engraftment without GVHD and control of disease recurrence (Fig. 114.2) (Verneris et al., 2001).

Given the above encouraging preclinical results, clinical trials have been performed. We have initiated a dose escalation trial using autologous CIK cells in patients with relapsed/refractory lymphoma (Hodgkin's and non-Hodgkin's) to determine whether sufficient numbers of cells could be generated in a clinical laboratory setting, and to determine the safety of administration of ex vivo expanded and activated cells. The target doses were 1×10^9 to 1×10^{10} cells. Sufficient quantities of cells could be generated from nearly all patients even with relapsed malig-

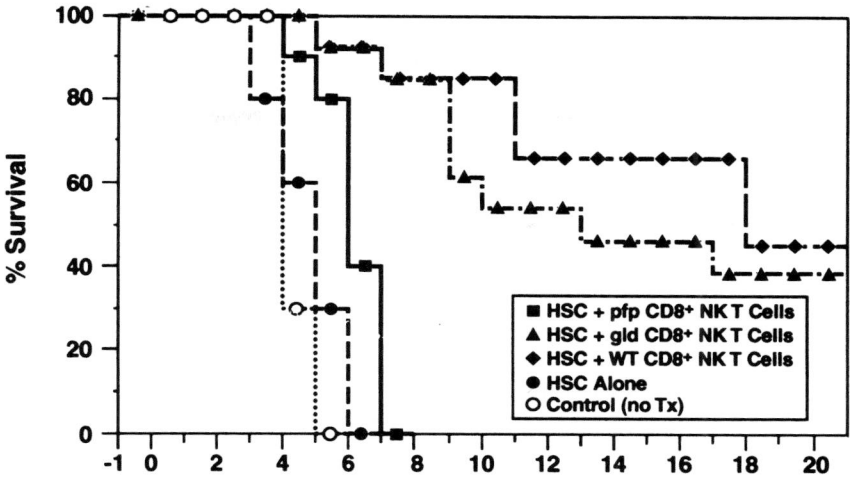

Fig. 114.2. Ex vivo expanded CD8+ NK-T cells can be transplanted across major histocompatibility barriers and mediate perforin-based antitumor activity. CD8+ NK-T cells from C57BL/6 mice (H2^b) [either wild type (WT), or perforin knock out (pfp$^{-/-}$) or FasL deficient (gld)] were generated and co-transplanted with 6,000 purified hematopoietic stem cells (HSCs) into tumor-bearing Balb/c recipient mice (H2^d) that were lethally irradiated (8Gy). Mice that received either no treatment or purified HSCs all died of lymphoma (open and closed circles, respectively; $n = 5$ in both groups). Mice that received 2×10^6 C57BL/6 splenocytes all died of acute GVHD within 14 to 21 days ($n = 5$, not shown). Mice that received 1×10^7 expanded CD8+ NK-T cells did not have signs or symptoms of GVHD (not shown). ~50% of animals that received expanded CD8+ NK-T cells from either WT or gld mice survived (diamonds or triangles, $n = 14$ and 15, respectively). In contrast, animals rescued with expanded CD8+ NK-T cells from pfp$^{-/-}$ animals died of recurrent lymphoma (massive splenomegaly) (squares, $n = 15$).

nancies. The infusion of cells was well tolerated (Leemhuis *et al.*, 2000). Given these results, phase II studies are now underway in autologous and allogeneic settings.

A similar strategy was utilized to treat patients with hepatoma following surgical resection in a prospective, randomized trial. In this study 150 patients who had undergone resection of hepatocellular carcinoma were randomized to receive lymphocyte infusions that were activated ex vivo with anti-CD3 and IL-2 for 14 days, or no further treatment. The patients who received ex vivo activated T cells had a statistically significant reduction in disease recurrence and prolonged disease-free survival (Fig. 114.3) (Takayama *et al.*, 2000).

Overall survival appeared to be improved, although this did not reach statistical significance.

Summary

With the explosion in knowledge of basic immunology and tumor biology, there is renewed interest in exploring immune-based treatment strategies for the treatment of cancer. A number of effector cell populations have been studied that could have important activity in preventing disease growth or relapse. The setting of hematopoietic stem cell transplantation is particularly attractive, since the majority of patients achieve a state of minimal residual disease, and this is likely to be a setting in which immunological mechanisms are effective. NK-T cells represent a novel approach to the immunological treatment of cancer and possibly other conditions such as viral infections.

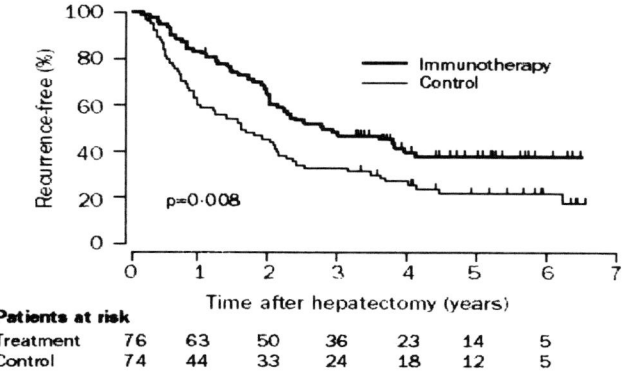

Patients at risk							
Treatment	76	63	50	36	23	14	5
Control	74	44	33	24	18	12	5

Fig. 114.3. Recurrence-free survival for patients with hepatocellular carcinoma who were treated with either adoptive immunotherapy (heavy line) or observation (light line) after surgical resection.[79]

References

Alvarnas, J.C., Linn, Y.C., Hope, E.G., & Negrin, R.S. (2001). Expansion of cytotoxic CD3+ CD56+ cells from peripheral blood progenitor cells of patients undergoing autologous hematopoietic cell transplantation. *Biology of Blood and Marrow Transplantation*, **7**, 216–22.

Ashkenazi, A. & Dixit, V.M. (1999). Apoptosis control by death and decoy receptors. *Current Opinion in Cell Biology*, **11**, 255–60.

Ashkenazi, A., Pai, R.C., Fong, S. *et al.* (1999). Safety and antitumor activity of recombinant soluble Apo2 ligand. *Journal of Clinical Investigation*, **104**, 155–62.

Baker, J., Verneris, M.R., Ito, M. *et al.* (2001). Expansion of cytolytic CD8(+) natural killer T cells with limited capacity for graft-versus-host disease induction due to interferon gamma production. *Blood,* **97,** 2923–31.

Baume, D.M., Caligiuri, M.A., Manley, T.J. *et al.* (1990). Differential expression of CD8 alpha and CD8 beta associated with MHC-restricted and non-MHC-restricted cytolytic effector cells. *Cellular Immunology,* **131,** 352–65.

Bendelac, A., Rivera, M.N., Park, S.H., & Roark, J.H. (1997). Mouse CD1-specific NK1 T cells: development, specificity, and function. *Annual Review of Immunology,* **15,** 535–62.

Benlagha, K., Kyin, T., Beavis, A. *et al.* (2002). A thymic precursor to the NK T cell lineage. *Science,* **296,** 553–5.

Benlagha, K., Weiss, A., Beavis, A. *et al.* (2000). In vivo identification of glycolipid antigen-specific T cells using fluorescent CD1d tetramers. *Journal of Experimental Medicine,* **191,** 1895–903.

Bossi, G. & Griffiths, G.M. (1999). Degranulation plays an essential part in regulating cell surface expression of Fas ligand in T cells and natural killer cells. *Nature Medicine,* **5,** 90–6.

Carnaud, C., Lee, D., Donnars, O. *et al.* (1999). Cutting edge: cross-talk between cells of the innate immune system: NKT cells rapidly activate NK cells. *Journal of Immunology,* **163,** 4647–50.

Coles, M.C. & Raulet, D.H. (2000). NK1.1+ T cells in the liver arise in the thymus and are selected by interactions with class I molecules on CD4+CD8+ cells. *Journal of Immunology,* **164,** 2412–18.

Crowe, N.Y., Smyth, M.J., & Godfrey, D.I. (2002). A critical role for natural killer T cells in immunosurveillance of methylcholanthrene-induced sarcomas. *Journal of Experimental Medicine,* **196,** 119–27.

Dellabona, P., Casorati, G., Friedli, B. *et al.* (1993). In vivo persistence of expanded clones specific for bacterial antigens within the human T cell receptor alpha/beta CD4-8-subset. *Journal of Experimental Medicine,* **177,** 1763–71.

Eberl, G., Lees, R., Smiley, S.T. *et al.* (1999). Tissue-specific segregation of CD1d-dependent and CD1d-independent NK T cells. *Journal of Immunology,* **162,** 6410–9.

Eberl, G., Lowin-Kropf, B., & MacDonald, H.R. (1999). Cutting edge: NKT cell development is selectively impaired in Fyn-deficient mice. *Journal of Immunology,* **163,** 4091–4.

Eberl, G. & MacDonald, H.R. (2000). Selective induction of NK cell proliferation and cytotoxicity by activated NKT cells. *European Journal of Immunology,* **30,** 985–92.

Emoto, M., Zerrahn, J., Miyamoto, M. *et al.* (2000). Phenotypic characterization of CD8(+)NKT cells. *European Journal of Immunology,* **30,** 2300–11.

Exley, M., Porcelli, S., Furman, M. *et al.* (1998). CD161 (NKR-P1A) costimulation of CD1d-dependent activation of human T cells expressing invariant V alpha 24 J alpha Q T cell receptor alpha chains. *Journal of Experimental Medicine,* **188,** 867–76.

Gapin, L., Matsuda, J.L., Surh, C.D., & Kronenberg, M. (2001). NKT cells derive from double-positive thymocytes that are positively selected by CD1d. *Nature Immunology,* **2,** 971–8.

Godfrey, D.I., Hammond, K.J., Poulton, L.D. *et al.* (2000). NKT cells: facts, functions and fallacies. *Immunology Today,* **21,** 573–83.

Gruss, H.J., Boiani, N., Williams, D.E. *et al.* (1994). Pleiotropic effects of the CD30 ligand on CD30-expressing cells and lymphoma cell lines. *Blood,* **83,** 2045–56.

Gumperz, J.E., Miyake, S., Yamamura, T., & Brenner, M.B. (2002). Functionally distinct subsets of CD1d-restricted natural killer T cells revealed by CD1d tetramer staining. *Journal of Experimental Medicine,* **195,** 625–36.

Gumperz, J.E., Roy, C., Makowska, A. (2000). Murine CD1d-restricted T cell recognition of cellular lipids. *Immunity,* **12,** 211–21.

Hammond, K., Cain, W., van Driel, I., & Godfrey, D. (1998). Three day neonatal thymectomy selectively depletes NK1.1+ T cells. *International Immunology,* **10,** 1491–9.

Hoyle, C., Bangs, C.D., Chang, P. *et al.* (1998). Expansion of Philadelphia chromosome-negative CD3+CD56+ cytotoxic cells from chronic myeloid leukemia patients: in vitro and in vivo efficacy in severe combined immunodeficiency disease mice. *Blood,* **92,** 3318–27.

Imahayashi, S., So, T., Sugaya, M. *et al.* (2002). Establishment of an immortalized T-cell line from lung cancer tissue: phenotypic and functional analyses. *International Journal of Clinical Oncology,* **7,** 38–44.

Ishihara, S., Nieda, M., Kitayama, J. *et al.* (2000). Alpha-glycosylceramides enhance the antitumor cytotoxicity of hepatic lymphocytes obtained from cancer patients by activating CD3–CD56+ NK cells in vitro. *Journal of Immunology,* **165,** 1659–64.

Jumper, M.D., Nishioka, Y., Davis, L.S. *et al.* (1995). Regulation of human B cell function by recombinant CD40 ligand and other TNF-related ligands. *Journal of Immunology,* **155,** 2369–78.

Kadowaki, N., Antonenko, S., Ho, S. *et al.* (2001). Distinct cytokine profiles of neonatal natural killer T cells after expansion with subsets of dendritic cells. *Journal of Experimental Medicine,* **193,** 1221–6.

Kagl, D., Ledermann, B., Burki, K. *et al.* (1994). Cytotoxicity mediated by T cells and natural killer cells is greatly impaired in perforin-deficient mice [see comments]. *Nature,* **369,** 31–7.

Kawano, T., Cui, J., Koezuka, Y. *et al.* (1997). CD1d-restricted and TCR-mediated activation of valpha14 NKT cells by glycosylceramides. *Science,* **278,** 1626–9.

Kawano, T., Nakayama, T., Kamada, N. *et al.* (1999). Antitumor cytotoxicity mediated by ligand-activated human V alpha24 NKT cells. *Cancer Research,* **59,** 5102–5.

Kayagaki, N., Kawasaki, A., Ebata, T. *et al.* (1995). Metalloproteinase-mediated release of human Fas ligand. *Journal of Experimental Medicine,* **182,** 1777–83.

Kitamura, H., Iwakabe, K., Yahata, T. *et al.* (1999). The natural killer T (NKT) cell ligand alpha-galactosylceramide demonstrates its immunopotentiating effect by inducing interleukin (IL)-12 production by dendritic cells and IL-12 receptor expression on NKT cells. *Journal of Experimental Medicine,* **189,** 1121–8.

Lanier, L.L., Le, A.M., Civin, C.I. *et al.* (1986). The relationship of CD16 Leu-11 and Leu-19 NKH-1 antigen expression on human peripheral blood NK cells and cytotoxic T lymphocytes. *Journal of Immunology,* **136,** 4480–6.

Lee, P.T., Benlagha, K., Teyton, L., & Bendelac, A. (2002). Distinct functional lineages of human V(alpha)24 natural killer T cells. *Journal of Experimental Medicine,* **195,** 637–41.

Leemhuis, T., Wells, S., Horn, P. *et al.* (2000). Autologous cytokine-induced killer cells for the treatment of relapsed Hodgkin's disease and non-Hodgkin's lymphoma. *Blood,* **96,** 839a.

Lopez, R., Waller, E., Lu, P., & Negrin, R. (2001). CD58/LFA-3 and IL-12 provided by activated monocytes are critical in the in vitro expansion and function of CD56+ T cells. *Cancer Immunology and Immunotherapy,* **49,** 629–40.

Lu, P.H. & Negrin, R.S. (1994). A novel population of expanded human CD3+CD56+ cells derived from T cells with potent in vivo antitumor activity in mice with severe combined immunodeficiency. *Journal of Immunology,* **153,** 1687–96.

MacDonald, H.R. (2002). Immunology. T before NK. *Science,* **296,** 481–2.

Majewski, S., Marczak, M., Szmurlo, A. *et al.* (1996). Interleukin-12 inhibits angiogenesis induced by human tumor cell lines in vivo. *Journal of Investigative Dermatology,* **106,** 1114–18.

Matsuda, J.L., Naidenko, O.V., Gapin, L. *et al.* (2000). Tracking the response of natural killer T cells to a glycolipid antigen using CD1d tetramers. *Journal of Experimental Medicine,* **192,** 741–54.

Metelitsa, L.S., Naidenko, O.V., Kant, A. *et al.* (2001). Human NKT cells mediate antitumor cytotoxicity directly by recognizing target cell CD1d with bound ligand or indirectly by producing IL-2 to activate NK cells. *Journal of Immunology,* **167,** 3114–22.

Nicol, A., Nieda, M., Koezuka, Y. *et al.* (2000). Human invariant valpha24+ natural killer T cells activated by alpha-galactosylceramide (KRN7000) have cytotoxic anti-tumour activity through mechanisms distinct from T cells and natural killer cells. *Immunology,* **99,** 229–34.

Ochoa, A.C., Gromo, G., Alter, B.J. *et al.* (1987). Long-term growth of lymphokine-activated killer LAK cells: role of anti-CD3, beta-IL 1, interferon-gamma and -beta. *Journal of Immunology,* **138,** 2728–33.

Onoe, Y., Harada, M., Tamada, K. *et al.* (1998). Involvement of both donor cytotoxic T lymphocytes and host NK1.1+ T cells in the thymic atrophy of mice suffering from acute graft-versus-host disease. *Immunology,* **95,** 248–56.

Ortaldo, J.R., Winkler-Pickett, R., Mason, A.T., & Mason, L.H. (1998). The Ly-49 family: regulation of cytotoxicity and cytokine production in murine CD3+ cells. *Journal of Immunology,* **160,** 1158–65.

Ortaldo, J.R., Winkler-Pickett, R.T., Yagita, H., & Young, H.A. (1991). Comparative studies of CD3– and CD3+ CD56+ cells: examination of morphology, functions, T cell receptor rearrangement, and pore-forming protein expression. *Cellular Immunology,* **136,** 486–95.

Pena, S.V. & Krensky, A.M. (1997). Granulysin, a new human cytolytic granule-associated protein with possible involvement in cell-mediated cytotoxicity. *Seminars in Immunology,* **9,** 117–25.

Pittet, M.J., Speiser, D.E., Valmori, D. *et al.* (2000). Cutting edge: cytolytic effector function in human circulating CD8+ T cells closely correlates with CD56 surface expression. *Journal of Immunology,* **164,** 1148–52.

Prussin, C. & Foster, B. (1997). TCR V alpha 24 and V beta 11 coexpression defines a human NK1 T cell analog containing a unique Th0 subpopulation. *Journal of Immunology,* **159,** 5862–70.

Sarin, A., Haddad, E.K., & Henkart, P.A. (1998). Caspase dependence of target cell damage induced by cytotoxic lymphocytes. *Journal of Immunology,* **161,** 2810–16.

Schmidt, R.E., Murray, C., Daley, J.F. *et al.* (1986). A subset of natural killer cells in peripheral blood displays a mature T cell phenotype. *Journal of Experimental Medicine,* **164,** 351–6.

Schmidt-Wolf, I.G., Lefterova, P., Johnston, V. *et al.* (1994). Propagation of large numbers of T cells with natural killer cell markers. *British Journal of Haematology,* **87,** 453–8.

Schmidt-Wolf, I.G., Lefterova, P., Mehta, B.A. *et al.* (1993). Phenotypic characterization and identification of effector cells involved in tumor cell recognition of cytokine-induced killer cells. *Experimental Hematology,* **21,** 1673–9.

Schmidt-Wolf, I.G.H., Negrin, R.S., Kiem, H.P. *et al.* (1991). Use of a SCID mouse/human lymphoma model to evaluate cytokine-induced killer cells with potent antitumor cell activity. *Journal of Experimental Medicine,* **174,** 139–49.

Smyth, M.J., Thia, K.Y., Street, S.E. *et al.* (2000). Differential tumor surveillance by natural killer (NK) and NKT cells. *Journal of Experimental Medicine,* **191,** 661–8.

Stremmel, C., Exley, M., Balk, S. *et al.* (2001). Characterization of the phenotype and function of CD8(+), alpha/beta(+) NKT cells from tumor-bearing mice that show a natural killer cell activity and lyse multiple tumor targets. *European Journal of Immunology,* **31,** 2818–28.

Tahir, S.M., Cheng, O., Shaulov, A. *et al.* (2001). Loss of IFN-gamma production by invariant NK T cells in advanced cancer. *Journal of Immunology,* **167,** 4046–50.

Takahashi, T., Nieda, M., Koezuka, Y. *et al.* (2000). Analysis of human V alpha 24+ CD4+ NKT cells activated by alpha-glycosylceramide-pulsed monocyte-derived dendritic cells. *Journal of Immunology,* **164,** 4458–64.

Takahashi, T., Tanaka, M., Brannan, C.I. *et al.* (1994). Generalized lymphoproliferative disease in mice caused by a point mutation in the fas ligand. *Cell,* **76,** 969–76.

Takayama, T., Sekine, T., Makuuchi, M. *et al.* (2000). Adoptive immunotherapy to lower postsurgical recurrence rates of hepatocellular carcinoma: a randomised trial. *Lancet,* **356,** 802–7.

Talanian, R.V., Yang, X., Turbov, J. *et al.* (1997). Granule-mediated killing: pathways for granzyme B-initiated apoptosis. *Journal of Experimental Medicine,* **186,** 1323–31.

Tamada, K., Harada, M., Abe, K. *et al.* Immunosuppressive activity of cloned natural killer (NK1.1+) T cells established from murine tumor-infiltrating lymphocytes. *Journal of Immunology,* **158,** 4846–54.

Tarazona, R., DelaRosa, O., Alonso, C. *et al.* (2000). Increased expression of NK cell markers on T lymphocytes in aging and chronic activation of the immune system reflects the accumulation of effector/senescent T cells. *Mechanisms of Ageing and Development,* **121,** 77–88.

Terabe, M., Matsui, S., Noben-Trauth, N. *et al.* (2000). NKT cell-mediated repression of tumor immunosurveillance by IL-13 and the IL-4R-STAT6 pathway. *Nature Immunology,* **1,** 515–20.

Toura, I., Kawano, T., Akutsu, Y. *et al.* (1999). Cutting edge: inhibition of experimental tumor metastasis by dendritic cells pulsed with alpha-galactosylceramide. *Journal of Immunology,* **163,** 2387–91.

Trapani, J.A., Davis, J., Sutton, V.R., & Smyth, M.J. (2000). Proapoptotic functions of cytotoxic lymphocyte granule constituents in vitro and in vivo. *Current Opinion in Immunology,* **12**, 323–9.

Van Der Vliet, H.J., Nishi, N., Koezuka, Y. *et al.* (1999). Effects of alpha-galactosylceramide (KRN7000), interleukin-12 and interleukin-7 on phenotype and cytokine profile of human Valpha24+ Vbeta11+ T cells. *Immunology,* **98**, 557–63.

van der Vliet, H.J., Nishi, N., Koezuka, Y. *et al.* (2001). Potent expansion of human natural killer T cells using alpha-galactosylceramide (KRN7000)-loaded monocyte-derived dendritic cells, cultured in the presence of IL-7 and IL-15. *Journal of Immunological Methods,* **247**, 61–72.

Verneris, M., Ito, M., Baker, J. *et al.* (2001). Engineering hematopoietic grafts: purified allogeneic hematopoietic stem cells plus expanded CD8+ NK-T cells in the treatment of lymphoma. *Biology of Blood and Marrow Transplantation,* **7**, 532–42.

Walczak, H. & Krammer, P.H. (2000). The CD95 (APO-1/Fas) and the TRAIL (APO-2L) apoptosis systems. *Experimental Cell Research,* **256**, 58–66.

Walczak, H., Miller, R.E., Ariail, K. *et al.* (1999). Tumoricidal activity of tumor necrosis factor-related apoptosis-inducing ligand in vivo. *Nature Medicine,* **5**, 157–63.

Watanabe, H., Iiai, T., Kimura, M. *et al.* (1993). Characterization of intermediate TCR cells in the liver of mice with respect to their unique IL-2R expression. *Cell Immunology,* **149**, 331–42.

Yanagisawa, K., Seino, K., Ishikawa, Y. *et al.* (2002). Impaired proliferative response of V alpha 24 NKT cells from cancer patients against alpha-galactosylceramide. *Journal of Immunology,* **168**, 649–9.

Yang, Y.G., Qi, J., Wang, M.G., & Sykes, M. (2002). Donor-derived interferon gamma separates graft-versus-leukemia effects and graft-versus-host disease induced by donor CD8 T cells. *Blood,* **99**, 4207–15.

Young, J.D., Hengartner, H., Podack, E.R., & Cohn, Z.A. (1986). Purification and characterization of a cytolytic pore-forming protein from granules of cloned lymphocytes with natural killer activity. *Cell,* **44**, 849–59.

Zeller, J.C., Panoskaltsis-Mortari, A., Murphy, W.J. *et al.* (1999). Induction of CD4+ T cell alloantigen-specific hyporesponsiveness by IL-10 and TGF-beta. *Journal of Immunology,* **163**, 3684–91.

Zeng, D., Lewis, D., Dejbakhsh-Jones, S. *et al.* (1999). Bone marrow NK1.1(−) and NK1.1(+) T cells reciprocally regulate acute graft versus host disease. *Journal of Experimental Medicine,* **189**, 1073–81.

Zoll, B., Lefterova, P., Ebert, O. *et al.* (2000). Modulation of cell surface markers on NK-like T lymphocytes by using IL-2, IL-7 or IL-12 in vitro stimulation. *Cytokine,* **12**, 1385–90.

115 Pathophysiologically based strategies to improve reconstitution of thymopoiesis after hematopoietic stem cell transplantation

KENNETH WEINBERG

Childrens Hospital Los Angeles, Los Angeles, USA

Introduction

Although engraftment after hematopoietic stem cell transplantation (HSCT) is conventionally defined by the attainment of sufficient numbers of red blood cells, granulocytes, and platelets, the recovery of the lymphocytes that mediate adaptive immunity is crucial to the outcome of HSCT. Analyses of T lymphocytes after HSCT reconstitution have shown commonly occurring defects in the reconstitution of a broad repertoire of functional T lymphocytes. Therefore, the focus of studies aimed at improving immune function after clinical HSCT has largely been the reconstitution of the T-lymphocyte compartment. While defects in B-lymphocyte function and antibody production exist, these may reflect abnormalities in T-cell help, as well as intrinsic B-lymphocyte defects.

Although unmanipulated marrow or peripheral blood hematopoietic stem cell (HSC) products contain large numbers of preformed donor T lymphocytes, the ability of the adoptively transferred T cells to persist and contribute to immunity in recipients after HSCT is uncertain. Furthermore, many transplant strategies for overcoming either donor-host alloreactivity or the contamination of stem cell products by malignant cells rely on enrichment steps that decrease the number of adoptively transferred T lymphocytes. Long-lasting maintenance of T-lymphocyte function requires production of new donor-derived T lymphocytes in the host thymus. Normally, T lymphopoiesis begins between weeks 7 and 9 in the human fetus, and it has been proposed that the kinetics of T-lymphocyte reconstitution after HSCT follows the same physiologic processes and kinetics (Haynes *et al.*, 1988). A general model of recapitulation of thymic ontogeny in the post-HSCT period has been useful for understanding the physiology of postnatal T-lymphocyte production and the relatively slow production of new T lymphocytes, for example, in uncomplicated HSCT for severe combined immune deficiency (SCID) or in recipients of enzyme replacement therapy for adenosine deaminase deficient SCID (Weinberg *et al.*, 1992; Patel *et al.*, 2000; Myers *et al.*, 2002). However, studies of humans and animal models have demonstrated that thymic function in most HSCT recipients is impaired, leading to defective immune function and abnormali-

ties of immune reconstitution. In most HSCT recipients, other pathophysiologic conditions such as aging, prior chemotherapy, chemoradiotherapy given pre-HSCT as conditioning, and graft-versus-host disease (GVHD) are present, all of which have negative effects on the quality and kinetics of T-lymphocyte reconstitution.

Defective thymopoiesis and immune function has emerged as a major clinical problem. Therapies that might otherwise be effective are limited by the inability of the thymus to generate sufficient numbers of new T lymphocytes to repopulate the mature T-lymphocyte compartment after severe injury. Patients who have received HSCT, high-dose chemotherapy, highly active anti-retroviral therapy (HAART) for HIV infection, or therapy to correct intrinsic defects of lymphohematopoietic differentiation (e.g., severe combined immune deficiency), have all been described as having defective thymopoiesis, abnormally low numbers of naive T lymphocytes, and slow recovery of immune function (Weinberg *et al.*, 1992, 2000; Mackall *et al.*, 1995; Ochs *et al.*, 1995; Storek *et al.*, 1995, 1997; Connors *et al.*, 1997; Small *et al.*, 1997; Aversa *et al.*, 1998). In several studies of HSCT recipients, opportunistic infections due to poor immune reconstitution have either been the major or a leading cause of mortality and morbidity (Ochs *et al.*, 1995; Aversa *et al.*, 1998; Socie *et al.*, 1999). For example, the University of Minnesota group reported that 65% of recipients of allogeneic sibling HSCT developed infections between day 50 and 2 years after transplant (Ochs *et al.*, 1995). The incidence of infection in recipients of unrelated donor grafts was even higher at 85%. The infections seen later after HSCT are mainly viral and fungal, not bacterial, consistent with the increased susceptibility to infection in these patients being due to abnormal T-lymphocyte function, not neutrophil defects. Also consistent with this interpretation is the inability of HSCT recipients to respond to immunization in the first year after transplant (Avigan *et al.*, 2001). Long-term analyses of HSCT recipients have shown abnormally low numbers of T lymphocytes, especially CD4+ cells for over 5 years after HSCT (Storek *et al.*, 1995, 1997, 2001 2002).

The major factors that correlate with poor thymic function after clinical HSCT are age and GVHD. Several studies have demonstrated that older HSCT recipients have lower levels of naive CD45RA+ CD4+ T lymphocytes than younger recipients (Small *et al.*, 1997; Storek *et al.*, 1997). The inflection point for the loss of thymopoietic capacity in studies of normal individuals, chemotherapy and HSCT recipients is adolescence to young adulthood. Beyond this age, thymopoiesis still occurs but reconstitution of peripheral T-lymphocyte compartments is slow and can be incomplete (Small *et al.*, 1997; Jamieson *et al.*, 1999; Mackall *et al.*, 2001). The decreased ability of postpubertal patients to make T lymphocytes after HSCT is also found when populations of patients receiving high-dose chemotherapy or HAART for HIV infection were examined (Douek *et al.*, 1998; Mackall *et al.*, 2001). The etiology of age-related declines in thymopoiesis is unknown, but the association with puberty has raised the possibility that thymic atrophy may normally be mediated by sex hormones (Hirokawa *et al.*, 1994; Utsuyama *et al.*, 1995).

Besides age, the development of GVHD also adversely affects post-HSCT thymopoiesis. GVHD has been shown to correlate with both the levels of naive T lymphocytes and of T-cell receptor excision circles (TREC), a measure of recent thymic emigrants (RTE) (Douek *et al.*, 1998; McFarland *et al.*, 2000; Weinberg *et al.*, 2001). During T-cell receptor-α gene rearrangement, a fragment of the TCR-δ locus is excised but persists in the thymocyte as a circular DNA episome that cannot replicate. During cell division, the TREC is randomly passed to one of the daughter cells. TREC levels are high in populations of RTE, but decline in memory T lymphocytes which represent the products of many cell divisions. In important studies published in the early 1980s, Lapp and Seemayer demonstrated that the thymic microenvironment was the target of alloreactive T lymphocytes, providing a mechanism for the poor thymic function observed in recipients with GVHD (Lapp *et al.*; Seemayer *et al.*). Reagents for characterization of the target cell population within the thymus were not available at that time, nor was there sufficient knowledge of microenvironmental functions to allow understanding of how alloreactive responses against thymic stromal cells could affect thymocyte development.

Besides age and GVHD, other factors that may influence thymopoiesis are damage to the thymus by chemotherapy or chemoradiotherapy given as part of pre-HSCT conditioning. Mackall *et al.* demonstrated that high-dose chemotherapy for cancer patients not receiving HSCT resulted in significant losses of thymopoietic capacity in older patients (Mackall *et al.*, 1995). The effects of conditioning regimens have been difficult to analyze in clinical HSCT because most patients receive intensive therapy and most have received prior chemotherapy. In a murine model of HSCT using graded doses of radiation, loss of thymopoietic capacity was related to the intensity of conditioning (Chung *et al.*, 2001). It is likely that the same phenomenon occurs in humans, but is difficult to analyze given all the other variables associated with clinical HSCT.

The care of patients recovering from diseases or treatments that require regeneration of T lymphocytes has consisted entirely of supportive measures of limited efficacy. Administration of prophylactic and therapeutic antibiotics, and intravenous immunoglobulin (IVIG) are the mainstays of treatment, but opportunistic infections still occur. Unlike B lymphocytes whose function can largely be replaced by administration of IVIG, the functions of T lymphocytes cannot be readily replaced by pharmacologic or cellular products. In this chapter, the pathophysiology of poor thymic function after HSCT will be described and strategies for reconstitution of thymic function will be discussed.

Normal thymopoiesis

Thymic differentiation pathways

Thymopoiesis is a complex process that ultimately results in the generation of large numbers of mature T lymphocytes with diverse antigenic specificities and effector functions from relatively small numbers of T-lymphoid progenitors. Much research in the past 20 years has been focused on the question of how the antigenic and functional repertoire is generated and selected. These efforts have resulted in a great deal of knowledge of how thymocytes and mature T lymphocytes transduce signals, proliferate, differentiate, survive, or undergo apoptosis. Such knowledge has been especially important in HSCT for understanding how graft-versus-host (GVH) reactions occur and how effector T lymphocytes eliminate infectious organisms or malignant cells.

The thymus produces large numbers of intermediate progenitors, most of which undergo apoptosis and do not develop into mature T lymphocytes. Therefore, continued production of new mature T lymphocytes is dependent on the massive expansion and differentiation of immature thymic progenitors into later maturational stages. Like the marrow, the thymic microenvironment provides various signals that are essential for the differentiation of the hematopoietically derived thymocytes. Recently, there has been increased recognition that the interactions between the thymic progenitors and their microenvironment are reciprocal rather than unidirectional from stroma to thymocytes. To address the problem of poor post-HSCT thymopoiesis, it is necessary to understand the microenvironment-derived signals that permit the massive proliferation of thymic progenitors, and the nature of the reciprocal interactions between the thymocytes and their microenvironment, particularly thymic epithelial cells (TEC).

Committed lymphoid progenitors (CLP) have been described immunophenotypically in both mice and humans (Galy *et al.*, 1995; Kondo *et al.*, 1997; Hao *et al.*, 2001; Mebius *et al.*, 2001). CLP have high rates of proliferation but appear to lack self-renewal capacity. As is seen in nonlymphoid lineages, differentiation of lymphoid progenitors occurs via intermediate steps that result in increasingly restricted lineage fates. Thus, CLP give rise to intermediate NK/T progenitors that lack B-lymphoid potential (Rodewald *et al.*, 1992; Moore & Zlotnick, 1995). There continue to be conflicting results on the nature of the hematopoietic cells that colonize the thymus (i.e., whether T-lymphoid commitment occurs before thymic entry or whether the thymus is populated by multipotent cells, or even HSC) (Rodewald et al., 1994; Moore & Zlotnick, 1995). The nature of lymphoid commitment is important as it may be possible to drive cells toward a desired lymphoid lineage. For example, Notch is an extracellular signal that increases the probability of T-lymphoid development from immature multipotent progenitors (Washburn et al., 1997; Radtke et al., 1999; Wilson et al., 2001). Lineage commitment may also involve the down-regulation of cytokine receptors or transcription factors that are associated with non-lymphoid lineages (Kondo et al., 2000).

Thymocytes can be subclassified by immunophenotypic changes that correspond to important biological processes occurring during thymic differentiation. The most immature thymocytes do not expression the T-cell receptor (TCR)-associated invariant complex CD3, nor the CD4 or CD8 co-receptors. During the development of these "triple-negative" (TN) thymocytes, the DNA encoding the variable (V), diversity (D), and joining (J) segments of the TCR genes undergo rearrangements, and transcription of the TCRα and TCR β genes begins. Successful V(D)J recombination is necessary for progression to later stages of differentiation (Rodewald & Frehling, 1998). At the next defined stage, thymocytes express the TCR and CD3, along with both CD4 and CD8 molecules. So-called double-positive (DP) thymocytes are first positively and then negatively selected on the basis of the affinity of the TCR molecules for self-peptides within the major histocompatibility complex (MHC) molecules. Surviving cells then undergo differentiation into either single-positive (SP) CD4+ or CD8+ thymocytes. Further differentiation of SP thymocytes in the thymic medulla occurs, resulting in release of mature CD4+ and CD8+ naive T lymphocytes into the circulation. Such newly released cells are referred to as recent thymic emigrants (RTE). Further expansion of naive T lymphocytes in the periphery can occur, via pathways that depend on self-peptide ligands for the TCR and interleukin-7 (Ernst et al., 1999; Tan et al., 2001; Schluns et al., 2000; Soares et al., 1998; Dardalhon et al., 2001). Naive T lymphocytes also undergo proliferation and differentiation into memory T lymphocytes after activation via TCR and co-stimulatory pathways.

IL-7, the major thymopoietic cytokine

IL-7 is produced by thymic epithelial cells, which in the mouse express MHC class II antigens and are present in both the thymic cortex and medulla (Oosterwegel et al., 1997). IL-7 is also produced by cells in the marrow, fetal liver, and lymph nodes (Napolitano et al., 2001). MHC class II+ TEC can support the proliferation and differentiation of thymic progenitor cells in vitro, using thymic reaggregation assays (Oosterwegel et al., 1997). In these experiments, IL-7 was essential for differentiation of the cultured thymocytes. Progenitors with germline TCR genes undergo TCR gene

rearrangements when cultured with CD45− MHC class II+ stromal cells from normal mice, but not from mice with targeted mutations of the IL-7 gene. The results are consistent with other experiments that have demonstrated that IL-7 signaling induces an open chromatin configuration of the TCR γ gene, which promotes TCR γ gene rearrangements (Durum et al., 1998; Kang, & Raulet, 1999).

IL-7 interacts with the IL-7 receptor (IL-7R), which is expressed by thymic progenitors. The IL-7R is composed of a ligand-specific IL-7R α chain and the common γ chain (γ^c), which besides the IL-7R, is shared with the receptors for IL-2, IL-4, IL-9, IL-15, and IL-21 (Kondo et al., 1993; Noguchi et al., 1993b; Russell et al., 1993; Kimura et al., 1993; Giri et al., 1994; Parrish-Noval et al., 2000). The importance of the IL-7R is illustrated by patients with SCID on the basis of mutations of either of the IL-7R subunits and mice with targeted mutations of the IL-7 or IL-7R genes. Patients with X-linked SCID have mutations of the γ^c chain of the IL-7R (Noguchi et al., 1993a). Because the γ^c chain is a component of multiple receptors, the phenotype of X-SCID is complex with thymopoietic defects due to loss of the IL-7R, NK defects due to the loss of IL-15R, and a defect in class-switching of B lymphocytes because of the IL-4R defect. A less common form of human SCID is an autosomal recessive disease due to mutations of the IL-7R α chain (Puel et al., 1998). Patients with IL-7R α deficient SCID have the same thymopoietic defects as patients with X-SCID, but have NK cells and no defect in class switching. Knockout mice for either γ^c, the IL-7R α, or IL-7, and dogs with naturally occurring X-SCID, have defective thymopoiesis with an apparent block in differentiation at the TN stages of differentiation (Peschon et al., 1994; Somberg et al., 1994; Cao et al., 1995; DiSanto et al., 1995; von Freeden-Jeffry et al., 1995). In mice with targeted mutations of the IL-7R α or γ^c receptor subunits, the presence of a bcl-2 transgene, which promotes cell survival, can overcome some of the abnormalities in thymic development, indicating that the IL-7R transduces signals for cell survival (Akashi et al., 1997; Kondo et al., 1997; Maraskovsky et al., 1997; von Freeden-Jeffry et al., 1997). IL-7 also is important for the survival and proliferation of mature, naive T lymphocytes, a point that will be discussed in more detail below (Mackall et al., 2001; Schluns et al., 2000; Tan et al., 2001). In summary, IL-7 produced by thymic epithelial cells supports the proliferation, survival and differentiation of TN thymocytes and is critical for normal thymopoiesis (Fig. 115.1).

Differentiation pathways for TEC

The thymus is formed from the III-IV pharyngeal pouches, as the result of interactions of endoderm, mesoderm, and ectodermal layers. The TEC are derived from the endoderm, while mesoderm provides the mesenchymal and hematopoietic elements and neuroendocrine cells arise from the ectoderm. Analyses of surface antigens expressed by human TEC have shown that they closely resemble normal skin ker-

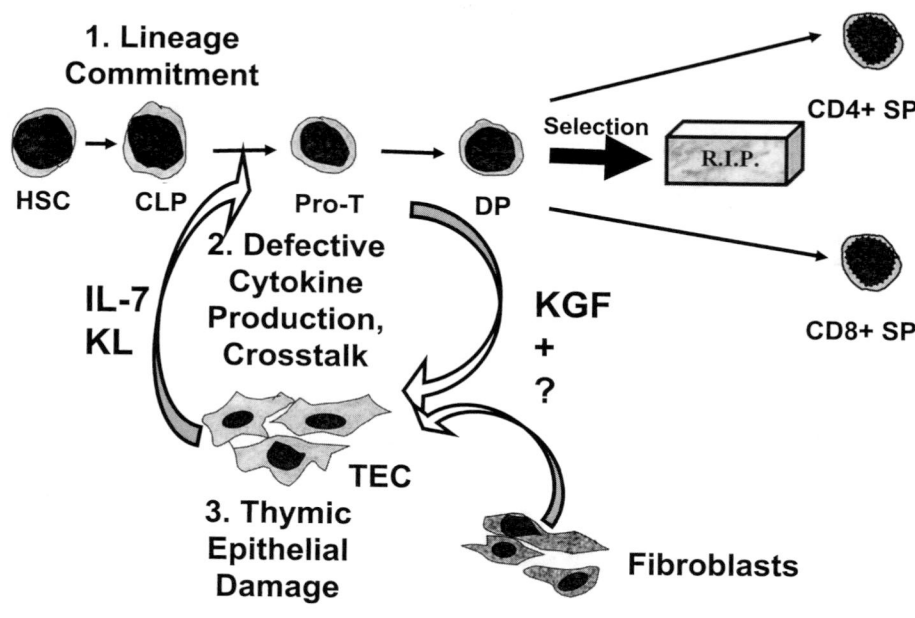

Fig. 115.1. Normal thymic differentiation and potential blocks to post-HSCT thymic recovery. HSC commit to lymphoid differentiation in a stochastic manner, ultimately giving rise to CLP and then T-lymphoid progenitors. The T-lymphoid progenitors undergo differentiation and expansion in the thymus. The immature thymocytes pass through DP, then SP stages of differentiation to generate mature T lymphocytes. Because the majority of thymocytes undergo apoptosis via either neglect or negative selection, maintenance of thymopoiesis depends on expansion of large numbers of input cells, a process that is mediated by IL-7 and KL produced by thymic epithelial cells (TEC). The thymocytes and other cells in the microenvironment supply reciprocal factors, e.g., KGF, that are needed for TEC maintenance. One potential obstacle to post-transplant thymopoiesis is commitment to the T-lymphoid lineage. Another potential bottleneck is decreased intrathymic IL-7 and/or KL production, which could limit the expansion of T-lymphoid progenitors. The lack of intrathymic IL-7 and other factors post-transplant ultimately may reflect damage to the TEC.

atinocytes (Patel *et al.*, 1995). The analogies between the biology of keratinocytes and TEC have led to experiments in which epithelial cell growth factors, such as keratinocyte growth factor, are used to restore thymopoiesis after HSCT (see below)

Although the CD45⁻ MHC class II⁺ thymic stromal cells include TEC, this population is still heterogeneous, and includes both medullary and cortical epithelial cells as well as fibroblasts. Richie's laboratory performed critical studies using cytokeratins to define precursor relationships among TEC (Klug *et al.*, 1998). These studies demonstrated that cytokeratin 5-positive (K5⁺) cytokeratin 8-positive (K8⁺) cells normally lie at the cortical-medullary junction and are the precursors of both K8⁺ TEC, which are cortical, and K5⁺ TEC, which are medullary. Subsequently, medullary regions of the thymus have been shown to arise from single progenitors, although the stage of differentiation at which the medullary TEC pathway diverges from the cortical TEC pathway still needs to be defined. Recently, the MTS24 antibody has been shown to react with a population of intrathymic cells that can give rise to both cortical and medullary TEC (Bennett *et al.*, 2002; Gill *et al.*, 2002). Transplantation of MTS24⁺ cells beneath the kidney capsule of nude mice, which lack an epithelial-specific transcription factor, results in the formation of a normal, albeit ectopic thymus. Thus, MTS24⁺ cells represent a population of

multipotent epithelial progenitors, although degree of heterogeneity within the MTS24⁺ cell population and their self-renewal capacity has yet to be determined.

Several naturally occurring diseases, as well as recombinant mice with loss-of-function mutations, have abnormal TEC differentiation and loss of thymic development. In humans the most well known of these conditions is DiGeorge Syndrome (DGS), which is caused by the loss of contiguous genes on chromosome 22. DGS is complex and very heterogeneous, with differing degrees of thymopoietic defects, cardiac malformations, endocrine defects, and abnormal facial development. No single gene has been established as responsible for the defective thymopoiesis observed in DGS mice, although disruption of the Tbx1 gene in mice results in typical cardiac and thymic abnormalities seen in DGS (Jerome & Papaoiannou, 2001). TEC development is also controlled by a transcription factor, Winged Helix Nude (Whn), which is the allele for the Nude (Nu) mutation. Nude mice, rats, and humans have been shown to have loss-of-function mutations in the Whn gene (Nehls *et al.*, 1994; Frank *et al.*, 1999). As implied by the name, Nu mice have a generalized defect in hair follicle development as well as in development of TEC. Whn is expressed normally by epithelial cells in the skin and thymus; thus, the Nu phenotype is an intrinsic defect of TEC and skin epithelial cell development (Lee *et al.*, 1999).

Manley's laboratory has described mice that are doubly mutated for the Pax 1 and HoxA3 transcription factors (Su *et al.*, 2001). These mice have defective thymopoiesis with decreased numbers of cortical epithelial cells as well as decreased MHC class II expression by TEC. Mice with targeted mutations of the fibroblastic growth factor (FGF) receptor 2-IIIb also have abnormal development of the thymic environment (Revest *et al.*, 2001). The FGFR 2-IIIb- mice are of interest because the receptor is expressed exclusively by epithelial cells and is a receptor for KGF, which will be discussed below. These mutations all illustrate the importance of epithelial cell development in the function of the thymus.

Pathophysiology of abnormal thymopoiesis after HSCT

TEC are damaged by pre-HSCT conditioning regimens

The adverse effects of chemoradiotherapy on epithelial cells comprising mucosal and cutaneous barriers is well known. The finding that T lymphopoiesis is dependent on epithelial cells located in the thymus suggests that TEC might be injured by chemotherapy or radiation, much as other epithelial cells are. The similarities in transcription factor, growth factor receptor, and other surface antigen expression between TEC and skin cells also suggest that the biological responses to chemoradiotherapy might be similar. Using murine HSCT recipients as a model, our laboratory demonstrated that the numbers of phenotypic TEC decline in a dose-dependent manner after radiation (Chung *et al.*, 2001). TEC numbers declined rapidly (<5 days) but took greater than 1 month to recover to normal levels. Furthermore, the decline in TEC numbers was correlated with a fall in intrathymic IL-7 transcript levels (Fig. 115.2). Concomitant with these changes in TEC, the progression from immature TN to DP thymocytes was also inhibited in a dose-dependent manner. Together, the results indicate that TEC damage may be one of the mechanisms by which thymopoiesis is inhibited after HSCT. In experiments that were performed in nontransplanted mice, Aspinall's group has demonstrated a decline in intrathymic IL-7 production during aging (Andrew *et al.*,). However, they did not find a significant decline in the absolute numbers of TEC.

Besides regimen-related toxicity to the thymic microenvironment, the alloreaction occurring in GVHD targets thymic stroma and probably directly kills or injures TEC. As discussed previously, Lapp and Seemayer made the seminal observation over 20 years ago that alloreactive cells could be found within the thymus in mice undergoing experimental GVHD. Consistent with the original observation of GVHD in the thymus, Hollander's laboratory has demonstrated that acute GVHD results in intrathymic production of pro-inflammatory factors (e.g., granzyme B and MIP proteins) (Rossi *et al.*, 1989). In addition the TEC in GVHD express abnormally high levels of the CD80 co-stimulatory molecule. The corticomedullary distinction within the thymus is destroyed during acute GVHD. The injury caused by acute GVHD interferes with cell cycle progression of

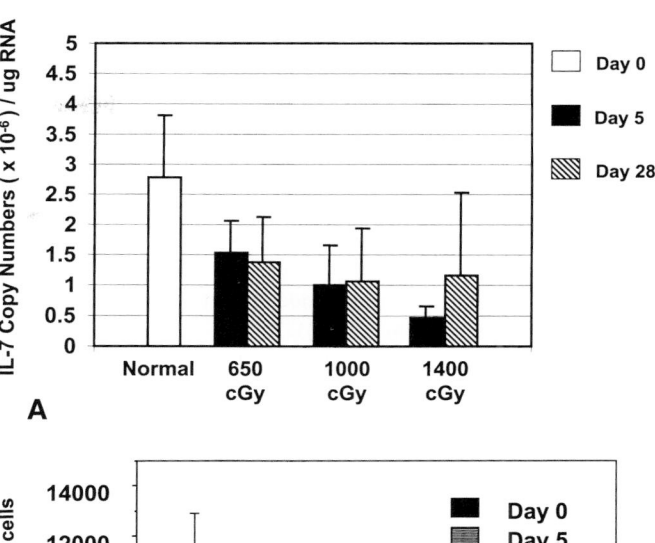

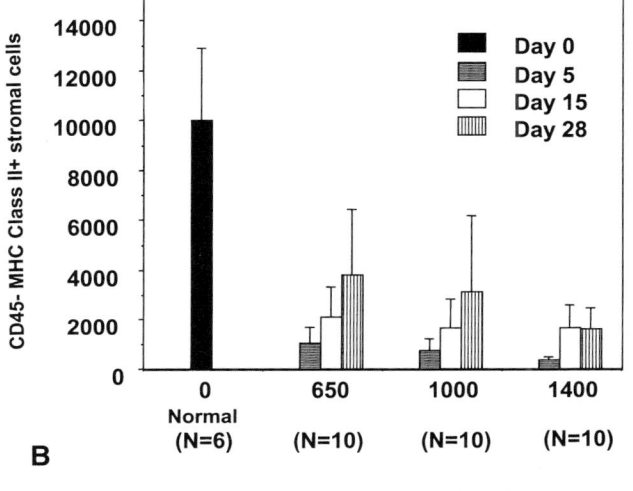

Fig. 115.2. Intrathymic IL-7 production and numbers of TEC are radiosensitive. *A*. Intrathymic IL-7 production was measured by quantitative reverse transcriptase-polymerase chain reaction five days after mice had received graded doses of radiation ranging from 650 to 1400 cGy. *B*. The numbers of TEC were measured in irradiated mice by FACS analysis of MHC Class II+ CD45- cells at 5, 14, and 28 days after irradiation and HSCT. Strategies that either improve TEC function or increase TEC recovery can improve post-HSCT thymopoiesis and immune function. (Reproduced, with permission, from Chung *et al.*, 2001.)

thymocytes (Krenger *et al.*, 2000). A proliferative defect in immature thymocytes was also observed in mice receiving high doses of radiation before HSCT, and was interpreted as related to defective intrathymic IL-7 production (Bolotin *et al.*, 1996; Chung *et al.*, 1989). In contrast, Hollander's laboratory has found elevated IL-7 transcript levels in the thymus of mice with acute GVHD (Rossi *et al.*, 1989). Thus, other aspects of TEC function besides IL-7 production may be adversely affected by GVHD. Despite this difference in results, the observation that TEC dysfunction occurs after HSCT provides important leads in developing clinical strategies to improve thymopoiesis after HSCT by increasing the number or function of TEC.

TEC differentiation depends on input from thymocytes

In addition to intrinsic epithelial cell and mesenchymal signals, maturation of the thymic microenvironment also requires the presence of developing T lymphocytes. Embryonic thymic architecture with fetal vascularization can be detected in patients with severe combined immune deficiency (SCID), but the microenvironment is transformed to an adult architecture after HSC transplantation. The thymic microenvironment is abnormal in mice made immunodeficient by expression of high copy numbers of a human CD3ε transgene (tgε26 strain) (Hollander et al., 1995). Tgε26 mice have defective thymic maturation past the Stage I CD44$^+$ CD25$^+$ prothymocyte stage (Wang et al.,). The thymic architecture is also abnormal in other immunodeficient mice that are double mutated for the IL-7 receptor and c-kit receptor (Rodewald et al., 1995, 1998; Weinberg, unpublished observations) (Fig. 115.3). In such mice, distinct cortical and medullary regions never develop.

Interestingly, the ability of the thymic microenvironment in tgε26 mice to recover after HSCT is limited (Hollander et al., 1995). In utero and early postnatal HSCT will restore thymopoietic capacity, but HSCT at later ages (e.g., 1 month) cannot induce normal thymic architecture or thymopoietic capacity. The ability of the tgε26 mice can be restored by introduction of a cyclin D1 transgene under the control of an epithelial-specific promoter (Klug et al., 2000). The rescue of the postnatal thymopoietic capacity of tgε26 mice by a cell cycle regulatory protein suggests that their defect lies in the ability of the TEC or TEC precursors to proliferate in the absence of a signal from normal thymocytes.

Besides alterations of TEC cell cycle regulation, the tgε26 defect can also be modified by engraftment with T lymphocytes from either normal or other immunodeficient mice with less severe blocks in thymic differentiation (van Ewijk et al., 2000). As noted above, in utero or early postnatal engraftment of tgε26 mice with normal HSC results in restoration of normal thymopoietic capacity, while later HSCT is unsuccessful. Thus, the irreversible damage to the thymic microenvironment is prevented by engraftment with normal hematopoietic cells that can undergo thymic differentiation. The irreversibility of thymic damage in tgε26 mice differs from clinical transplants for SCID, where new thymopoiesis routinely occurs after transplantation of genetically normal hematopoietic progenitors.

The relevance of the tgε26 mice to HSCT is that they illustrate the importance of thymocyte-microenvironmental interactions. Despite the discrepancy regarding the irreversibility of thymic damage from lack of thymocyte occupancy, the human and murine immunodeficiency data indicate that lymphoid progenitors regulate the development of the specialized microenvironment of the thymus. Pre-HSCT chemoradiotherapy usually kills most thymocytes. There are also likely to be thymic effects of posttransplant immunosuppressive drugs, although these have not been demonstrated in clinical HSCT (Weinberg et al., 2001). For example, cyclosporine accelerates involution of the thymus in rats (Beschorner et al., 1991). It is not known whether the lack of thymic occupancy occurring

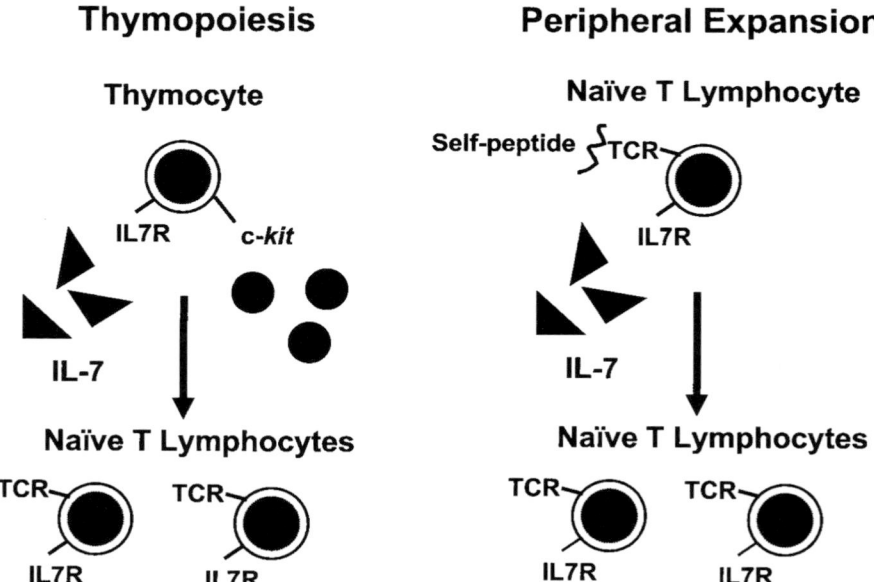

Fig. 115.3. Two roles for IL-7 in T lymphopoiesis. In the thymus, IL-7 produced by thymic epithelial cells, along with c-kit ligand (KL) stimulates immature thymocytes, permitting their development into mature thymocytes. Upon further selection and maturation, the mature thymocytes emigrate from the thymus to generate new naive T lymphocytes. In the periphery, especially under lymphopenic conditions, naive T lymphocytes undergo homeostatic proliferation. The peripheral expansion of naive T lymphocytes is mediated by IL-7 and self ligands binding to the T cell receptor for antigen.

immediately after HSCT induced by pretransplant conditioning or posttransplant immunosuppression results in microenvironmental damage to the thymus. If so, then strategies that rapidly generate new thymocytes after HSCT might help to prevent further injury.

Therapeutic strategies to restore thymopoiesis after HSCT

As discussed above, the production of new T lymphocytes in the thymus is a complex process in which reciprocal interactions between thymocytes and TEC and other microenvironmental cells are essential. A variety of therapeutic strategies to enhance thymopoiesis have been proposed, including stimulation of lymphoid progenitors, stimulation of TEC, transplantation of lymphoid progenitors, and replacement of TEC (Fig. 115.2). One way to understand these therapeutic strategies is to distinguish between those that target lymphoid progenitors and those that are directed at TEC. In some cases, either both thymocytes and TEC are targeted or it is unclear how the biological effect is exerted.

Cytokine therapies

IL-7

With the finding that the development of thymocytes is dependent on IL-7, administration of IL-7 became a logical approach for enhancement of post-HSCT thymopoiesis. In a murine model administration of IL-7 for 14 days after HSCT resulted in significantly increased thymic cellularity after syngeneic HSCT (Bolotin et al., 1996). In these experiments, the number of thymocytes and the distribution of subsets of pro-, DP and SP thymocytes, and TCR Vβ usage normalized in the recipient mice. In the placebo-treated controls, the thymus was hypocellular with evidence of abnormal progression from the CD3⁻ CD4⁻ CD8⁻ prothymocyte to DP stages. Importantly, the IL-7 treatment resulted in increased numbers of T lymphocytes in the periphery. The humoral response of the IL-7-treated recipients to a T-cell-dependent neo-antigen to which they had not been previously exposed increased to near-normal levels within 4 to 6 weeks of transplant. These results clearly demonstrated that IL-7 treatment could enhance the production of T lymphocytes after HSCT.

Additional experiments from Mackall's group have raised a number of questions regarding the effects of IL-7 in the post-HSCT setting (Fry & Mackall, 2002). As previously noted, IL-7 appears to be necessary for the homeostatic proliferation of naive T lymphocytes (Schluns et al., 2000; Tan et al., 2001; Mackall et al., 2001) (Fig. 115.1). IL-7 exerts both proliferative and anti-apoptotic effects on naive T lymphocytes. Mackall's laboratory has demonstrated that besides increasing the numbers of T lymphocytes generated in the host thymus, IL-7 administration also increased the numbers of T lymphocytes that had been generated in a thymus-independent manner from preformed donor T lymphocytes (Mackall et al., 2001). The

effects of pharmacological doses of IL-7 on mature T lymphocytes raises the question of how much of the immune reconstitution seen in IL-7 treated animals is due to increased thymopoiesis versus increased expansion of small numbers of RTE. Other experiments from Mackall's laboratory have demonstrated that IL-7 can even restore immune function to athymic hosts that had been depleted of mature T lymphocytes (Fry et al., 2001). The effects of IL-7 on mature T lymphocytes have raised the question of whether GVHD will be exacerbated by IL-7 treatment. Van den Brink's laboratory found no increase in the frequency or severity of GVHD in several allogeneic models of murine HSCT, using several dose schedules of IL-7 (Alpdogan et al., 2001). However, Mackall's group has observed increased GVHD in a different set of murine HSCT models (Fry et al.,). Although the relevance of murine allogeneic models to clinical GVHD is problematic, the question of enhanced alloreactivity will need to be considered in any clinical trial of IL-7. Furthermore, the dose schedule in humans needed to enhance thymopoiesis may be toxic in the allogeneic setting. Testing in nonhuman primates is under way and may clarify the potential problems. Initial human trials may need to be restricted to either autologous HSCT recipients or to allogeneic recipients of stringently T-cell-depleted grafts.

Keratinocyte growth factor

Based on the evidence that TEC are the target of HSCT conditioning and probably GVHD, agents that would influence the survival, repair, proliferation or differentiation of TEC are an appealing approach to the problem of post-HSCT thymopoiesis. KGF, or FGF7, is a member of the acidic fibroblastic growth factor family. The receptor for KGF is the epithelial cell-specific FGFR 2-IIIb splice variant, deletion of which results in severe thymic atrophy (Miki et al., 1992; Peters et al., 1992; Revest et al., 2001). The FGFR 2-IIIb binds to other FGF species besides KGF so that the specific requirement for KGF in thymopoiesis is not confirmed. KGF was first described as a mesenchyme-derived soluble factor that stimulated the growth of epithelial cells (Mason et al., 1994; Finch et al., 1995; Rubin et al., 1995). A series of experiments in an animal model of chemotherapy-induced gut and skin toxicity demonstrated that KGF administration prevents or reduces the severity of mucosal toxicity (Yi et al., 1996; Farrell et al., 1998). Furthermore, in experimental transplant settings, Blazar's and Ferrara's laboratories demonstrated that KGF treatment before HSCT conditioning significantly reduced regimen-related toxicity and GVHD (Panoskaltsis-Mortari et al., 1998; Krijanovski et al.). The protection from GVHD was independent of KGF-mediated reduction of injury from conditioning, as improvement was also seen in immunodeficient mice that were transplanted with allogeneic cells without cytotoxic conditioning (Panoskaltsis-Mortari et al., 2000).

Based on the above results, the Blazar, Hollander, and Weinberg laboratories have collaboratively investigated whether KGF treatment would also improve post-HSCT thymopoiesis by increasing the survival or function of TEC (Rossi *et al.,* 1989; Min *et al.,* 2002). Initial experiments demonstrated that KGF transcripts were produced by both thymocytes and thymic fibroblasts, while KGF receptors (FGFR 2-IIIb) were expressed by TEC (Min *et al.,* 2002). Thus, an intrathymic KGF signaling pathway probably exists, consistent with the thymic defects seen in FGFR 2-IIIb-deficient mice (Fig. 115.4). Administration of KGF before conditioning in experimental models of congenic HSCT with graded doses of radiation and allogeneic HSCT with two different chemoradiotherapy conditioning regimens demonstrated that KGF-treated mice had normal to increased numbers of thymocytes. Placebo-treated mice had severe thymic hypocellularity. KGF treatment also resulted in rapid (within 4 weeks) reconstitution of peripheral T-lymphocyte populations and improved responses to neo-antigen. The effects of KGF on thymopoiesis and peripheral T cells were persistent, lasting for at least 3 months after transplant. Analyses of the thymic microenvironment also showed increased numbers of IL-7-producing epithelial cells, suggesting that KGF had exerted its effects on thymopoiesis by protecting or increasing the repair or proliferation of TEC. The models described above used T-cell-depleted marrow to prevent overt GVHD.

In a different set of allogeneic experiments, Rossi *et al.* (1989) demonstrated that KGF treatment could preserve thymopoiesis in experimental GVHD. KGF-treated mice had improvements in the architecture of the thymic microenvironment that was abnormal in the control groups. For example, in control animals with acute GVHD, the corticomedullary demarcation disappeared. KGF treatment resulted in normalization of the thymic architecture so that it was indistinguish-

able from syngeneic HSCT recipients. The frequencies of different TEC subtypes were also preserved by KGF treatment, although KGF did not restore a population of minor medullary epithelial cells that may be involved in repertoire selection. Functionally, the TEC from KGF-treated mice had more thymus-expressed chemokine (TECK) production than the untreated controls with GVHD, and there was less expression of pro-inflammatory proteins in the thymus of the KGF-treated mice. Taken together, the murine HSCT experiments indicate that KGF administration can protect the thymus from regimen-related and GVHD-mediated toxicity, resulting in improved thymic function and immunity.

The mechanisms by which KGF enhances thymopoiesis after HSCT are still being determined. It is likely that the effects of KGF are exerted at the level of TEC. At present, it is unclear if KGF exerted proliferative and anti-apoptotic effects on radioresistant mature TEC or whether it stimulated the development of new mature TEC from epithelial progenitors. A concern regarding radioprotective agents is whether they prevent the apoptosis of cells that have undergone severe genomic damage. If so, it is possible that KGF or similar radioprotective cytokines or drugs could increase the frequency of malignancies occurring after chemoradiotherapy. Interestingly, KGF has been shown to increase the expression of Nrf2, a transcription factor that has been linked to activation of a DNA repair program in damaged cells (Braun *et al.,* 2002). Thus, KGF may be able to increase proliferation and survival but enhance the repair and stabilization of the genome of epithelial cells.

KGF is in clinical trial to evaluate its efficacy in prevention of chemoradiotherapy-induced toxicity, regimen-related toxicity in HSCT and GVHD. One approach to study the thymic and immunological effects of KGF is to characterize patients in these other studies for thymopoiesis and immune function. Since many of the radioprotection studies are randomized and placebo-controlled, preliminary data on TREC levels, numbers of naive T lymphocytes, and development of responses to immunization with neo-antigens may generate preliminary data that will justify a trial to determine whether KGF can improve post-HSCT thymopoiesis and immune function.

IGF-1

The size of the thymus in mice is regulated in part by the growth hormone (GH) insulin-like growth factor (IGF) axis (Savino *et al.,* 1995; Welniak *et al.,* 2002). GH is a pituitary hormone that binds to a type I cytokine receptor. IGF-1 produced in response to GH stimulation is the ligand for a receptor tyrosine kinase. If IL-7 is an example of a cytokine that directly stimulates thymocytes and KGF is one that stimulates TEC, the effects of IGF-1 are much more difficult to delineate. IGF-1 receptors have been described on both hematopoietic cells, including thymocytes and on TEC (Kooijman *et al.,* 1995; Kecha *et al.,* 2000; de Mello Coehlo *et al.,* 2002). Experiments in which IGF-1 has been administered to aged or ill mice have demonstrated increased thymopoiesis and T-cell numbers. However, it is unclear if the observed effects of IGF-1 adminis-

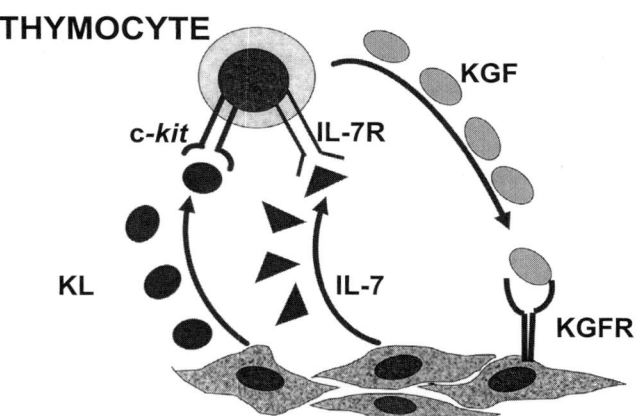

THYMOCYTE

c-kit   IL-7R

KGF

KL   IL-7

KGFR

Thymic Epithelial Cells (TEC)

Fig. 115.4. Reciprocal interactions between thymocytes and thymic epithelial cells (TEC). IL-7 and c-kit ligand produced by TEC interact with the IL-7 receptor and c-kit expressed by thymocytes. The survival, proliferation, and differentiation of the thymocytes are dependent on signals mediated through c-kit and the IL-7R. The thymocytes constitutively produce keratinocyte growth factor (KGF), which supports the survival and proliferation of TEC though interactions with its cognate receptor, the FGF receptor 2-IIIB.

tration are mediated by direct stimulation of thymocytes, or by increasing the number or function of TEC. The combined administration of IGF-1 with transplantation of progenitors from young donor mice could increase thymopoiesis in aged recipients, while each intervention alone had more modest effects (Montecino-Rodriguez et al., 1998). By analogy with the data reviewed above on IL-7 and KGF, a number of questions about the potential role of IL-7 need to be addressed (i.e., whether IGF-1 stimulates proliferation only of thymocytes or mature lymphocytes as well, whether IGF-1 has radioprotective effects on TEC, and the duration of any observed effects).

Other pharmacological manipulations

Endocrine

As noted above, the increase in sex hormone release in puberty has been proposed as a mechanism for the adolescence-associated decline in thymopoiesis. Experiments from rodents have indicated that thymopoiesis can be restored by gonadectomy (Hirokawa et al., 1994; Utsuyama et al., 1995). With the advent of drugs that pharmacologically block the effects of pituitary LHRH, it is feasible to determine whether such blockade can increase thymopoiesis in HSCT recipients or those who are receiving such treatment for hormone-responsive diseases (e.g., prostate cancer).

Cell replacement

The discussion above focused on the use of soluble molecules (e.g., cytokines and hormones), to affect either donor-derived thymic progenitors or host-derived microenvironmental cells. An alternative approach would be to transplant enriched populations of lymphoid progenitors for the purpose of increasing the number of donor-derived cells that can undergo T-lymphoid differentiation. Another approach related to the manipulation of the thymic microenvironment would involve transplantation of thymic tissue or TEC progenitors in an effort to generate a new thymus that was undamaged by cytotoxic agents.

Transplantation of lymphoid progenitors

One possible bottleneck in T-lymphoid development after HSCT could be commitment of limited numbers of HSC to the lymphoid lineages. For example, if lymphoid commitment is a stochastic event that occurred relatively infrequently and the number of transplanted HSC was small, then the generation of T lymphocytes would be expected to be slow. Implicit in such a model is the therapeutic possibility of co-transplantation of common lymphoid progenitors (CLP). Because CLP are already committed to lymphoid differentiation, the likelihood of generating T-lymphoid progeny from a single CLP is likely to be greater than that of generating T-lymphoid cells from a single HSC. CLP are highly proliferative, increasing the likely yield from such a population. Because CLP still have not undergone TCR gene rearrangements, the likelihood of generating a broad repertoire without causing GVHD is much less

than after transplantation of mature T lymphocytes. Thus, CLP transplantation may be a means to rapidly repopulate the thymus and generate a mature population of T lymphocytes.

In a murine model, Brown's laboratory has shown that phenotypically isolated CLP that are co-transplanted with HSC leads to more rapid immune reconstitution than after transplantation of HSC alone (Brown et al.). In these experiments, 500 phenotypic HSC and 3,000 phenotypic CLP were transplanted into each recipient. The sources of HSC and CLP were congenic so that the progeny of each population could be separately tracked. The CLP more rapidly generated T lymphocytes and reconstituted immune function in the recipients. An important novel aspect of the experiments from Brown's group was the demonstration that CLP co-transplantation protected the recipients from experimental challenge with murine cytomegalovirus (MCMV). While the relative contributions of T-lymphoid, NK, and B-lymphoid mechanisms to the observed protection from MCMV still need to be elucidated, the experiments illustrate the potential of such an approach. Two possible limitations of the CLP co-transplantation approach need to be considered. First, the ability of CLP to differentiate into thymocytes and ultimately T lymphocytes, is still dependent on the function of the thymic microenvironment. Thus, the effects of CLP transplantation may depend on other methods that can either augment lost TEC function (e.g., IL-7) or prevent TEC damage (KGF). A second consideration is that the frequency of CLP is low and the ability to isolate human CLP in clinically relevant numbers or to expand them in vitro or in vivo has not been determined. Nevertheless, CLP co-transplantation is a particularly appealing approach to immune reconstitution.

Thymus transplant

Thymus transplantation has been proposed as a strategy to reconstitute the thymic microenvironment after HSCT. The potential advantages of transplantation of normal thymic tissue into HSCT recipients after completion of conditioning is that a new, presumably undamaged thymic microenvironment would be created. Thymic transplantation has been used most extensively in the treatment of DGS. In the pioneering experiments of Hong, cultured fetal thymic tissue was successfully transplanted into children with DGS who had severe T lymphopenia (Hong & Moore, 1996). Markert's group has developed techniques for successful engraftment of postnatally derived thymic tissue and immune reconstitution of DGS patients (Markert et al., 1999). Besides the technical difficulties of thymic transplantation, the major obstacle to application in the post-HSCT setting is likely to be alloreactivity. The success of thymic transplantation in severe DGS is likely to depend in part on the immune incompetence of the host. Indeed, when thymus transplantation was performed for adults with HIV infection, the thymus tissue was rejected (Markert et al., 2000). Whether rejection of transplanted thymic tissue would also occur in the context of HSCT is unknown. The HIV experience with thymic transplantation suggests that its use as a therapeutic modality after HSCT will depend on the ability to overcome alloreactivity.

TEC replacement

The finding by Bennett *et al.* and Gill *et al.* that the MTS24 antibody can be used to identify a multipotent (cortical and medullary) murine TEC progenitor, which can completely induce the formation of a thymic microenvironment in vivo raises the exciting possibility that clinical transplantation of TEC progenitors will be feasible (Bennett *et al.*, 2002; Gill *et al.*, 2002). At present a number of issues must be addressed, including identification of the antigen recognized by MTS24 and determination of its expression pattern and relevance to human TEC. Beyond these issues are a number of important scientific questions, including the progenitor characteristics of MTS24+ cells. Are the MTS24+ cells heterogenous for TEC differentiation or is each MTS24+ cell capable of giving rise to a complete thymic microenvironment? Does MTS24 mark TEC stem cells capable of self-renewal? What are the microenvironmental signals and other cell types required to form a new thymus. Can TEC progenitors be isolated from more accessible sites (e.g., skin) for clinical use? Beyond these questions of stem cell biology, the expression of MHC antigens by TEC raises a number of immunologic issues similar to those seen in thymus transplantation. For example, the outcome of transplantation of allogeneic TEC progenitors might be immunologic rejection or abnormal selection of thymocytes in the host after HSCT. Although these questions will be difficult to answer, the identification of TEC progenitors is an important finding that is likely to translate to clinical HSCT practice.

Clinical trial design

The above discussion of therapeutic strategies has been mainly concerned with methods that are being tested in animal models and are at various stages of preclinical development. Ultimately, these strategies will need to be evaluated in clinical trials that attempt to determine whether thymopoiesis can be safely enhanced after HSCT in a relevant time frame. The murine experiments that have delineated possible solutions to the problem of post-HSCT thymopoiesis have a number of features that will not be possible to replicate in humans. The studies frequently use inbred strains of mice that are congenic rather than allogeneic. The doses of preparative conditioning of the recipient are easy to control, and the dose of HSC or T lymphocytes in the donor inoculum are also tightly controlled. Importantly, the methods of assessing thymic function at predetermined time points after HSCT are generally precise and direct. As the recognition of the clinical relevance of the immune reconstitution problem has increased, the techniques for evaluating clinical responses have become more sophisticated.

A crucial issue that therapeutic studies need to address is the difference between responses to recall antigens and neo-antigens to which neither the donor nor recipient have been previously exposed. While analyses of tetanus or CMV-specific recall responses may be clinically relevant, they are not neces-sarily useful as endpoints for the assessment of thymic function. If the donor has been previously exposed to CMV, for example, then the appearance of CMV-specific T lymphocytes in the recipient soon after HSCT could represent either expansion of existing naive or memory T lymphocytes in the recipient, or the generation de novo of CMV-specific T lymphocytes. This may be especially problematic for strategies that involve the administration of IL-7 or stimulation of IL-7 production, since IL-7 affects both thymopoietic and peripheral expansion via homeostatic proliferation. By using neo-antigen responses as an endpoint, clinical trials will be able to focus on the effects on thymopoiesis or naive cells, not adoptively transferred memory T cells.

The desirable features of clinical trials to address immune reconstitution are easy to elucidate but may be difficult to achieve. Ideally, clinical trials to study immune reconstitution should be stratified by age and restricted to patients who receive the same conditioning regimens. The HSC product should be well characterized for the numbers of phenotypic and clonogenic T lymphocytes. Ideally, the product would have no mature T lymphocytes. The method of GVHD prophylaxis would be consistent. The endpoints would include measures of thymopoiesis, mature T-lymphocyte numbers, and function, as shown in Table 115.1. Thymopoiesis can be measured using TREC as a surrogate (Douek *et al.*, 1998; Weinberg *et al.*, 2000). Immunophenotypic markers of RTE such as CD103 expression may also be useful and reliable (McFarland *et al.*, 2000). Other methods to characterize thymic size or output by imaging or in vivo labeling of thymocytes with nonradioactive isotopes are potentially useful, but are also expensive, time-consuming, and can be cumbersome (Macallan *et al.*). As expected in a progenitor–progeny relationship, the frequency of TREC, number of naive T lymphocytes, and number of total T lymphocytes have generally correlated with each other (Mackall *et al.*, 1995; Weinberg *et al.*, 2001; Storek *et al.*, 2002). The number of cells reacting with MHC tetramers is useful, although studies to correlate the frequency of tetramer-reactive cells with function are still needed. Immunization of the recipients at defined time points with a neoantigen (e.g., KLH) or bacteriophage φX174, will allow determination of the development of antigen-specific function in the recipient after HSCT. Immunity to recall and polysaccharide antigens will also be important determinants of clinical outcome, but large studies will ultimately be needed to address the impact on infectious complications.

Future directions

The rapid advances in the understanding of immune reconstitution have occurred because of increased recognition of the problem by clinical investigators, and improved understanding of progenitor relationships and cytokine signaling in T lymphopoiesis; molecular techniques and immunological reagents for characterizing human lymphocyte development; and recognition of the importance of the thymic microenvironment and

Table 115.1. *Endpoints for clinical trials of T lymphocyte reconstitution after HSCT*

Assay	Rationale
Thymic imaging	Correlation of thymic size with thymic function
Recent thymic emigrant phenotypes	RTE as marker of thymic function; correlation with thymic size; TREC
TREC	Frequency of RTE
Naive and memory T phenotypes	Number and proportion of naive T lymphocytes; correlation with thymic function, RTE
TCR spectratype	Diversity, skewing of TCR repertoire
MHC tetramer	Quantitation and immunophenotype of antigen-specific lymphocytes
Recall antigen immunization	Presence of functional memory T lymphocytes
Neoantigen immunization	Presence of functional, broad repertoire of naive T lymphocytes

its reciprocal relationship with thymocytes. With the improved understanding and the likely clinical evaluation of many individual strategies for reconstitution of thymic function, it is likely that combined modalities of treatment will be more effective than any one of the proposed treatments described in this chapter. An example of a potentially important combination might be the combined use of CLP co-transplantation and cytokines and growth factors that mediate commitment (Notch ligands), expansion (IL-7), or enhanced TEC function (KGF). Multiple manipulations of TEC with KGF and other drugs may be more efficacious than either treatment alone. If the human homologue of MTS24$^+$ TEC progenitors is also capable of differentiation into an entire thymus, then the combinations of TEC progenitor transplantation with epithelial growth factor administration (e.g., KGF) to increase the rate of thymus formation may be possible. It is likely that the next decade of clinical HSCT will be marked by a series of clinical trials that will result in the ability to rapidly produce a broad, durable repertoire of T lymphocytes that will protect recipients from opportunistic infections and normalize their lives.

References

Akashi, K., Kondo, M., von Freeden-Jeffry, U. *et al.* (1997). Bcl-2 rescues T lymphopoiesis in interleukin-7 receptor-deficient mice. *Cell,* **27,** 1033–41.

Alpdogan, O., Schmaltz, C., Muriglan, S.J. *et al.* (2001). Administration of interleukin-7 after allogeneic bone marrow transplantation improves immune reconstitution without aggravating graft-versus-host disease. *Blood,* **98,** 2256–65.

Aversa, F., Tabilio, A., Velardi, A. *et al.* (1998). Treatment of high-risk acute leukemia with T-cell-depleted stem cell from related donor with one fully mismatched HLA haplotype. *New England Journal of Medicine,* **339,** 1186–93.

Avigan, D., Pirofski, L.A., & Lazarus, H.M. (2001). Vaccination against infectious disease following hematopoietic stem cell transplantation. *Biology of Blood and Marrow Transplantation,* **7,** 171–83.

Bennett, A.R., Farley, A., Blair, N.F. *et al.* (2002). Identification and characterization of thymic epithelial progenitor cells. *Immunity,* **16,** 803–14.

Beschorner, W., Divic, J., Pulido, H. *et al.* (1991). Enhancement of thymic recovery after cyclosporine by recombinant human growth hormone and insulin-like growth factor. *Transplantation,* **52,** 879–4.

Bolotin, E., Annett, G., Parkman, R., & Weinberg, K. (1999). Serum levels of IL-7 in bone marrow transplant recipients: relationship to clinical characteristics and lymphocyte count. *Bone Marrow Transplantation,* **23,** 783–8.

Bolotin, E., Smogorzewska, M., Smith, S. *et al.* (1996). Enhancement of thymopoiesis after bone marrow transplant by in vivo interleukin-7. *Blood,* **88,** 1887–94.

Braun, S., Hanselmann, C., Gassmann, M.G. *et al.* (2002). Nrf2 transcription factor, a novel target of keratinocyte growth factor action which regulates gene expression and inflammation in the healing skin wound. *Molecular Cell Biology,* **22,** 5492–505.

Cao, X., Shores, E.W., Hu-Li, J. *et al.* (1995). Defective lymphoid development in mice lacking expression of the common cytokine receptor γ chain. *Immunity,* **2,** 223–38.

Centers for Disease Control and Prevention. (2000). Guidelines for preventing opportunistic infections among hematopoietic stem cell transplant recipients: recommendations of CDC, the Infectious Disease Society of America, and the American Society of Blood and Marrow Transplantation. *Morbidity and Mortality Weekly Report,* **49,** 5–8.

Chung, B., Barbara-Burnham, L., Barsky, L., & Weinberg, K. (2001). Radiosensitivity of thymic IL-7 production and post-bone marrow transplant thymopoiesis. *Blood,* **98,** 1601–6.

Connors, M., Kovacs, J.A., Krevat, S. *et al.* (1997). HIV infection induces changes in CD4+ T-cell phenotype and depletions within the CD4+ T-cell repertoire that are not immediately restored by antiviral or immune-based therapies. *Nature Medicine,* **3,** 533–48.

Dardalhon, V., Jaleco, S., Kinet, S. *et al.* (2001). IL-7 differentially regulates cell cycle progression and HIV-1-based vector infection in neonatal and adult CD4+ T cells. *Proceedings of the National Academy of Sciences USA,* **98,** 9277–82.

de Mello Coelho, V., Villa-Verde, D.M., Farias-de-Oliveira, D.A. *et al.* (2002). Functional insulin-like growth factor-1/insulin-like growth factor-1 receptor-mediated circuit in human and murine thymic epithelial cells. *Neuroendocrinology,* **75,** 139–50.

DiSanto, J.P., Fischer, A., Rajewski, K., & Mulier, W. (1995). Lymphoid development in mice with a targeted deletion of the interleukin 2 receptor γ chain. *Proceedings of the National Academy of Sciences USA,* **92,** 377.

Douek, D.C., McFarland, R.D., Keiser, P.H. *et al.* (1998). Changes in thymic function with age and during the treatment of HIV infection. *Nature,* **396,** 690–5.

Durum, S.K., Candeias, S., Nakajima, H. *et al.* (1998). Interleukin 7 receptor control of T cell receptor γ gene rearrangement: role of receptor-associated chains and locus accessibility. *Journal of Experimental Medicine,* **188,** 2233–41.

Ernst, B., Lee, D.S., Chang, J.M. *et al.* (1999). The peptide ligands mediating positive selection in the thymus control T cell survival and homeostatic proliferation in the periphery. *Immunity,* **11,** 173–81.

Farrell, C.L. *et al.* (1998). Keratinocyte growth factor protects mice from chemotherapy and radiation-induced gastrointestinal injury and mortality. *Cancer Research,* **58,** 933–9.

Finch, P.W., Cunha, G.R., Rubin, J.S. *et al.* (1995). Pattern of keratinocyte growth factor and keratinocyte growth factor receptor expression during mouse fetal development suggests a role mediating morphogenetic mesenchymal-epithelial interactions. *Development Dynamics,* **203,** 223–40.

Frank, J., Pignata, C., Panteleyev, A.A. *et al.* (1999). Exposing the human nude phenotype. *Nature,* **398,** 473–4.

Fry, T.J., Christensen, B.L., Komschlies, K.L. *et al.* (2001a). Interleukin-7 restores immunity in athymic T-cell-depleted hosts. *Blood,* **97,** 1525–33.

Fry, T.J., Connick, E., Falloon, J. *et al.* (2001b). A potential role for interleukin-7 in T-cell homeostasis. *Blood,* **97,** 2983–90.

Fry, T.J. & Mackall, C.L. (2002). Interleukin-7: from bench to clinic. *Blood,* **99,** 3892–904.

Galy, A., Travis, M., Cen, D., & Chen, B. (1995). Human T, B, natural killer, and dendritic cells arise from a common bone marrow progenitor cell subset. *Immunity,* **3,** 459–73.

Gill, J., Malin, M., Hollander, G.A., & Boyd, R. (2002). Generation of a complete thymic microenvironment by MTS24(+) thymic epithelial cells. *Nature Immunology,* **3,** 635–42.

Giri, J.G., Ahdieh, M., Eisenman, J. *et al.* (1994). Utilization of the β and γ chains of the IL-2 receptor by the novel cytokine IL-15. *The Embo Journal,* **13,** 2822–30.

Hao, Q.I., Zhu, J., Price, M.A. *et al.* (2001). Identification of a novel, human multilymphoid progenitor in cord blood. *Blood,* **97,** 3683–90.

Haynes, B.F., Martin, M.E., Kay, H.H., & Kurtzberg, J. (1988). Early events in human T cell ontogeny. Phenotypic characterization and immunohistologic localization of T cell precursors in early human fetal tissues. *Journal of Experimental Medicine,* **168,** 1061–80.

Hirokawa, K., Utsuyama, M., Kasai, M. *et al.* (1994). Understanding the mechanism of the age-change of thymic function to promote T cell differentiation. *Immunology Letter,* **40,** 269–77.

Hollander, G.A. (2002). Keratinocyte growth factor preserves normal thymopoiesis and thymic microenvironment during experimental graft-versus-host disease. *Blood,* **100,** 682–91.

Hollander, G.A., Wang, B., Nichogiannopoulou, A. *et al.* (1995). Developmental control point in induction of thymic cortex regulated by a subpopulation of prothymocytes. *Nature,* **373,** 350–3.

Hong, R. & Moore, A. L. (1996). Organ culture for thymus transplantation. *Transplantation,* **61,** 444–8.

Jamieson, B.D., Douek, D.C., Killian, S. *et al.* (1999). Generation of functional thymocytes in the human adult. *Immunity,* **10,** 569–75.

Jerome, L.A. & Papaioannou, V.E. (2001). DiGeorge syndrome phenotype in mice mutant for the T-box gene, Tbx1. *Nature Genetics,* **27,** 286–91.

Kang, J. & Raulet, D.H. (1999). Defective development of γδ T cells in interleukin 7 receptor-deficient mice is due to impaired expression of T cell receptor γ genes. *Journal of Experimental Medicine,* **190,** 973–82.

Kecha, O., Brilot, F., Martens, H. *et al.* (2000). Involvement of insulin-like growth factors in early T cell development: a study using fetal thymic organ cultures. *Endocrinology,* **141,** 1209–17.

Kimura, Y., Takeshita, T., Kondo, M. *et al.* (1995). Sharing of the IL-2 receptor γ chain with the functional IL-9 receptor complex. *International Immunology,* **7,** 115–20.

Klug, D.B., Carter, C., Crouch, E. *et al.* (1998). Interdependence of cortical thymic epithelial cell differentiation and T-lineage commitment. *Proceedings of the National Academy of Sciences USA,* **95,** 11822–7.

Klug, D.B., Crouch, E., Carter, C. *et al.* (2000). Transgenic expression of Cyclin D1 in thymic epithelial precursors promotes epithelial and T cell development. *Journal of Immunology,* **164,** 1881–8.

Kondo, M., Akashi, K., Domen, J. *et al.* (1997). Bcl-2 rescues T lymphopoiesis, but not B or NK cell development, in common gamma chain-deficient mice. *Immunity,* **7,** 155–62.

Kondo, M., Scherer, D.C., Miyamoto, T. *et al.* (2000). Cell-fate conversion of lymphoid-committed progenitors by instructive actions of cytokines. *Nature,* **407,** 383–6.

Kondo, M., Takeshita, T., Ishii, N. *et al.* (1993). Sharing of the interleukin-2 (IL-2) receptor γ chain between receptors for IL-2 and IL-4. *Science,* **262,** 1874–7.

Kondo, M., Weissman, I.L., & Akashi, K. (1997). Identification of clonogenic common lymphoid progenitors in mouse bone marrow. *Cell,* **91,** 661–72.

Kooijman, R., Scholtens, L.E., Rijkers, G.T., & Zegers, B.J. (1995). Type I insulin-like growth factor receptor expression in different developmental stages of human thymocytes. *Journal of Endocrinology,* **147,** 203–9.

Krenger, W., Rossi, S., Piali, L., & Hollander, G.A. (2000). Thymic atrophy in murine acute graft-versus-host disease is effected by impaired cell cycle progression of host pro-T and pre-T cells. *Blood,* **96,** 347–54.

Lee, D., Prowse, D.M., & Brissette, J.L. (1999). Association between mouse nude gene expression and the initiation of epithelial terminal differentiation. *Developmental Biology,* **208,** 362–74.

Mackall, C.L., Fry, T.J., Bare, C. *et al.* (2001). IL-7 increases both thymic-dependent and thymic-independent T-cell regeneration after bone marrow transplantation. *Blood,* **97,** 1491–7.

Maraskovsky, E., O'Reilly, L.A., Teepe, M. *et al.* (1997). Bcl-2 can rescue T lymphocyte development in interleukin-7 receptor-deficient mice but not in mutant *rag-1⁻/⁻* mice. *Cell,* **89,** 1011–19.

Markert, M.L., Boeck, A., Hale, L.P. *et al.* (1999). Transplantation of thymus tissue in complete DiGeorge syndrome. *New England Journal of Medicine,* **341,** 1180–9.

Markert, M.L., Hicks, C.B., Bartlett, J.A. *et al.* (2000). Effect of highly active antiretroviral therapy and thymic transplantation on immunoreconstitution in HIV infection. *AIDS Research and Human Retroviruses,* **16,** 403–13.

Mason, I.J., Fuller-Pace, F., Smith, R., & Dickson, C. (1994). FGF-7 (keratinocyte growth factor) expression during mouse development suggests roles in myogenesis, forebrain regionalisation and epithelial-mesenchymal interactions. *Mechanisms of Development, 45,* 15–30.

McFarland, R.D., Douek, D.C., Koup, R.A., & Picker, L.J. (2000). Identification of a human recent thymic emigrant phenotype. *Proceedings of the National Academy of Sciences USA, 97,* 4215–20.

Mebius, R.E., Miyamoto, T., Christensen, J. *et al.* (2001). The fetal liver counterpart of adult common lymphoid progenitors gives rise to all lymphoid lineages, CD45+CD4+CD3-cells, as well as macrophages. *Journal of Immunology, 166,* 6593–601.

Miki, T., Bottaro, D.P., Fleming, T.P. *et al.* (1992). Determination of ligand-binding specificity by alternative splicing: two distinct growth factor receptors encoded by a single gene. *Proceedings of the National Academy of Sciences USA, 89,* 246–50.

Min, D., Taylor, P.A., Panoskaltsis-Mortari, A. *et al.* (2002). Protection from thymic epithelial cell injury by keratinocyte growth factor: a new approach to improve thymic and peripheral T-cell reconstitution after bone marrow transplantation. *Blood, 99,* 4592–600.

Montecino-Rodriguez, E., Clark, R., & Dorshkind, K. (1998). Effects of insulin-like growth factor administration and bone marrow transplantation on thymopoiesis in aged mice. *Endocrinology, 139,* 4120–6.

Moore, T.A., von Freeden-Jeffry, U., Murray, R., & Zlotnik, A. (1996). Inhibition of gamma delta T cell development and early thymocyte maturation in IL-7 –/– mice. *Journal of Immunology, 157,* 2366–73.

Moore, T.A. & Zlotnik, A. (1995). T-cell lineage commitment and cytokine responses of thymic progenitors. *Blood, 86,* 1850–60.

Myers, L.A., Patel, D.D., Puck, J.M., & Buckley, R.H. (2002). Hematopoietic stem cell transplantation for severe combined immunodeficiency in the neonatal period leads to superior thymic output and improved survival. *Blood, 99,* 872–8.

Napolitano, L.A., Grant, R.M., Deeks, S.G. *et al.* (2001). Increased production of IL-7 accompanies HIV-1-mediated T-cell depletion: implications for T-cell homeostasis. *Nature Medicine, 7,* 73–9.

Nehls, M., Pfeifer, D., Schorpp, M. *et al.* (1994). New member of the winged-helix protein family disrupted in mouse and rat nude mutations. *Nature, 372,* 103–7.

Noguchi, M., Nakamura, Y., Russell, S.M. *et al.* (1993a). Interleukin-2 receptor γ chain: a functional component of the interleukin-7 receptor. *Science, 262,* 1877–86.

Noguchi, M., Yi, H., Rosenblatt, H.M. *et al.* (1993b). Interleukin 2 receptor γ chain mutation results in X-linked severe combined immunodeficiency in humans. *Cell, 73,* 147–57.

Ochs, L., Shu, X.O., Miller, J. *et al.* (1995). Late infections after allogeneic bone marrow transplantation: comparison of incidence in related and unrelated donor transplant recipients. *Blood, 86,* 3979–86.

Ornitz, D.M., Xu, J.S., Colvin, D.G. *et al.* (1996). Receptor specificity of the fibroblast growth-factor family. *Journal of Biological Chemistry, 271,* 15292–7.

Oosterwegel, M.A., Haks, M.C., Jeffry, U. *et al.* (1997). Induction of TCR gene rearrangements in uncommitted stem cells by a subset of IL-7 producing, MHC class-II-expressing thymic stromal cells. *Immunity, 6,* 351–60.

Panoskaltsis-Mortari, A. *et al.* (2000). Keratinocyte growth factor facilitates alloengraftment and ameliorates graft-versus-host disease in mice by a mechanism independent of repair of conditioning-induced tissue injury. *Blood, 96,* 4350–6.

Panoskaltsis-Mortari, A., Lacey, D.L., Vallera, D.A., & Blazar, B.R. (1998). Keratinocyte growth factor administered before conditioning ameliorates graft-versus-host disease after allogeneic bone marrow transplantation in mice. *Blood, 92,* 3960–7.

Parrish-Novak, J., Dillon, S.R., Nelson, A. *et al.* (2000). Interleukin 21 and its receptor are involved in NK cell expansion and regulation of lymphocyte function. *Nature, 408,* 57–63.

Patel, D.D., Gooding, M.E., Parrott, R.E. *et al.* (2000). Thymic function after hematopoietic stem-cell transplantation for the treatment of severe combined immunodeficiency. *New England Journal of Medicine, 342,* 325–32.

Patel, D.D., Whichard, L.P., Radcliff, G. *et al.* (1995). Characterization of human thymic epithelial cell surface antigens: phenotypic similarity of thymic epithelial cells to epidermal keratinocytes. *Journal of Clinical Immunology, 15,* 80–92.

Peschon, J.J., Morrissey, P.J., Grabstein, K.H. *et al.* (1994). Early lymphocyte expansion is severely impaired in interleukin-7 receptor deficient mice. *Journal of Experimental Medicine, 180,* 1955–60.

Peters, K.G., Werner, S., Chen, G., & Williams, L.T. (1992). Two FGF receptor genes are differentially expressed in epithelial and mesenchymal tissues during limb formation and organogenesis in the mouse. *Development, 114,* 233–43.

Puel, A., Ziegler, S.F., Buckley, R.H., & Leonard, W.J. (1998). Defective IL7R expression in T(–) B(+) NK(+) severe combined immunodeficiency. *Nature Genetics, 20,* 394–7.

Radtke, F., Wilson, A., Stark, G. *et al.* (1999). Deficient T cell fate specification in mice with an induced inactivation of Notch 1. *Immunity, 10,* 547–58.

Revest, J.M., Suniara, R.K., Kerr, K. *et al.* (2001). Development of the thymus requires signaling through the fibroblast growth factor receptor R2-IIIb. *Journal of Immunology, 167,* 1954–61.

Rodewald, H.R. & Fehling, H.J. (1998). Molecular and cellular events in early thymocyte development. *Advanced Immunology, 69,* 1–112.

Rodewald, H.R., Kretzschmar, K., Takeda, S. *et al.* (1994). Identification of pro-thymocytes in murine fetal blood: T lineage commitment can precede thymus colonization. *The Embo Journal, 13,* 4229–40.

Rodewald, H.R., Moingeon, P., Lucich, J.L. *et al.* (1992). A population of early fetal thymocytes expressing Fc gamma RII/III contains precursors of T lymphocytes and natural killer cells. *Cell, 69,* 139–50.

Rodewald, H.-R., Ogawa, M., Haller, C. *et al.* (1997). Pro-thymocyte expansion by c-kit and the common cytokine receptor γ chain is essential for repertoire formation. *Immunity, 6,* 265–72.

Rodewald, H.R., Paul, S., Haller, C. *et al.* (2001). Thymus medulla consisting of epithelial islets each derived from a single progenitor. *Nature, 414,* 763–8.

Rossi, S., Blazar, B.R., Farrell, C.L. *et al.* (1989). Purification and characterization of a newly identified growth factor specific for epithelial cells. *Proceedings of the National Academy of Sciences USA, 86,* 802–6.

Rubin, J.S. *et al.* (1995). Keratinocyte growth factor as a cytokine that mediates mesenchymal-epithelial interaction. In *Epithelial – Mesenchymal Interactions in Cancer,* ed I.D. Goldberg & E.M. Rosen, pp. 191–214. Boston, MA: Birkhauser Verlag.

Russell, S.M., Keegan, A.D., Harada, N. *et al.* (1993). Interleukin-2 receptor γ chain: a functional component of the interleukin-4 receptor. *Science,* **262,** 1880–3.

Savino, W., de Mello Coehlo, & Dardenne, M. (1995). Control of the thymic microenvironment by growth hormone/insulin-like growth factor-I-mediated circuits. *Neuroimmunomodulation,* **2,** 313–8.

Schluns, K.S., Kieper, W.C., Jameson, S.C., & Lefrancois, L. (2000). Interleukin-7 mediates the homeostasis of naive and memory CD8 T cells in vivo. *Nature Immunology,* **1,** 426–32.

Sinha, M.L., Fry, T.J., Fowler, D.H. *et al.* (2002). Interleukin 7 worsens graft versus host disease. *Blood,* **100,** 2642–9.

Small, T.N., Avigan, D., Dupont, B. *et al.* (1997). Immune reconstitution following T-cell depleted bone marrow transplantation: effect of age and posttransplant graft rejection prophylaxis. *Biology of Blood & Marrow Transplantation,* **3,** 65–75.

Soares, M.V., Borthwick, N.J., Maini, M.K. *et al.* (1998). IL-7-dependent extrathymic expansion of CD45RA+ T cells enables preservation of a naive repertoire. *Journal of Immunology,* **161,** 5909–17.

Socie, G., Stone, J.V., Wingard, J.R. *et al.* (1999). Long term survival and late deaths after allogeneic bone marrow transplantation. Late Effects Working Committee of the International Bone Marrow Transplant Registry. *New England Journal of Medicine,* **341,** 14–21.

Somberg, R.L., Robinson, J.P., & Felsburg. (1994). T lymphocyte development and function in dogs with X-linked severe combined immunodeficiency. *Journal of Immunology,* **153,** 4006–15.

Storek, J., Gooley, T., Witherspoon, R.P. *et al.* (1997). Infectious morbidity in long-term survivors of allogeneic marrow transplantation is associated with low CD4 T cell counts. *American Journal of Hematology,* **54,** 131–8.

Storek, J., Joseph, A., Dawson, M.A. *et al.* (2002). Factors influencing T-lymphopoiesis after allogeneic hematopoietic cell transplantation. *Transplantation,* **73,** 1154–8.

Storek, J., Joseph, A., Espino, G. *et al.* (2001). Immunity of patients surviving 20 to 30 years after allogeneic or syngeneic bone transplantation *Blood,* **98,** 3505–12.

Storek, J., Witherspoon, R.P., & Storb, R. (1995). T cell reconstitution after bone marrow transplantation into adult patients does not resemble T cell development in early life. *Bone Marrow Transplantation,* **16,** 413–25.

Su, D., Ellis, S., Napier, A. *et al.* (2001). Hoxa3 and pax1 regulate epithelial cell death and proliferation during thymus and parathyroid organogenesis. *Developmental Biology,* **236,** 316–29.

Tan, J.T., Dudl, E., LeRoy, E. *et al.* (2001). IL-7 is critical for homeostatic proliferation and survival of naive T cells. *Proceedings of the National Academy of Sciences USA,* **98,** 8732–7.

Tan, J.T., Ernst, B., Kieper, W.C. *et al.* (2002). Interleukin (IL)-15 and IL-7 jointly regulate homeostatic proliferation of memory phenotype CD8+ cells but are not required for memory phenotype CD4+ cells. *Journal of Experimental Medicine,* **195,** 1523–32.

Utsuyama, M., Hirokawa, K., Mancini, C. *et al.* (1995). Differential effects of gonadectomy on thymic stromal cells in promoting T cell differentiation in mice. *Mechanisms of Ageing and Development,* **81,** 107–17.

Van Ewijk, W., Hollander, G., Terhorst, C., & Wang, B. (2000). Stepwise development of thymic microenvironments in vivo is regulated by thymocyte subsets. *Development,* **127,** 1583–91.

von Freeden-Jeffry, U., Solvason, N., Howard, M., & Murray, R. (1997). The earliest T lineage-committed cells depend on IL-7 for Bcl-2 expression and normal cell cycle progression. *Immunity,* **7,** 147–54.

Von Freeden-Jeffry, U., Viera, P., Lucian, L.A. *et al.* (1995). Lymphopenia in interleukin (IL)-7 gene-deleted mice identifies IL-7 as a nonredundant cytokine. *Journal of Experimental Medicine,* **181,** 1519–26.

Washburn, T., Schweighoffer, E., Gridley, T. *et al.* (1997). Notch activity influences the α/β versus γ/δ T cell lineage decision. *Cell,* **88,** 833–43.

Weinberg, K., Annett, G., Kashyap, A. *et al.* (1995). The effect of thymic function on immunocompetence following bone marrow transplantation. *Biology of Blood and Marrow Transplantation,* **1,** 18–23.

Welniak, L.A., Sun, R., & Murphy, W.J. (2002). The role of growth hormone in T-cell development and reconstitution. *Journal of Leukocyte Biology,* **71,** 381–7.

Wilson, A., MacDonald, H.R., & Radtke, F. (2001). Notch 1-deficient common lymphoid precursors adopt a B cell fate in the thymus. *Journal of Experimental Medicine,* **194,** 1003–12.

Yamasaki, M., Miyake, A., Tagashira, S., & Itoh, N. (1996). Structure and expression of the rat messenger-RNA encoding a novel member of the fibroblast growth-factor family. *Journal of Biological Chemistry,* **271,** 15918–21.

Yi, E.S. *et al.* (1996). Keratinocyte growth factor ameliorates radiation- and bleomycin-induced lung injury and mortality. *American Journal of Pathology,* **149,** 1963–70.

116 Gene therapy in blood and marrow transplantation

JEFFREY A. MEDIN, MALCOLM BRENNER, AND ARMAND KEATING

Ontario Cancer Institute, Toronto, Canada, Baylor College of Medicine, Houston, USA, and Princess Margaret Hospital/Ontario Cancer Institute, Toronto, Canada

Introduction

Much of the early work on the development of gene therapy protocols has involved the hematopoietic system, partly because of the accessibility of target cells and the relatively well-characterized differentiation pathways and stem cell ontogeny for bone marrow cells. Despite this, single gene disorders of hematopoietic tissue represent only a small proportion of human disease and would suggest that gene therapy may be of limited utility. However, if all disorders with malfunctioning genes are considered, including the malignancies, in which therapy could be achieved by gene transfer into blood or marrow cells, the potentially wide scope of gene therapy becomes readily apparent. Some, but by no means all, of the possible applications considered for gene therapy in the context of blood and marrow transplantation are listed in Table 116.1. Examples of applications to correct single gene disorders include transfer of the ADA gene to correct ADA-severe combined immune deficiency, the beta globin gene to correct beta-thalassemia, and the transfer of the glucocerebrosidase gene to correct the defect in Gaucher's disease (Donahue *et al.*, 1996). Examples of applications to confer drug resistance to normal hematopoietic stem cells (HSC) include the transfer

Table 116.1. *Possible applications of gene therapy*

1. Correct single gene disorders
2. Provide a means of drug or hormone delivery in vivo
3. Confer drug resistance to normal marrow (or other) cells
4. Modify gene regulation to reduce disease phenotype
5. Mark cells to elucidate cell lineage relationships or identify the source of malignant relapse (e.g., after autologous hematopoietic stem cell transplantation)
6. Alter malignant cells to improve or induce immunotherapy
7. Alter normal cells to increase immune responses against malignant cells
8. Introduce genes into autograft cells in order to eliminate the malignant cell
9. Alter normal cells to allow their selective and elective elimination (see Chapter 117)

of the multidrug resistance gene (MDR) and mutations of the dihydrofolate reductase (DHFR) gene to confer resistance to methotrexate or trimetrexate (Flasshove *et al.*, 1995; May *et al.*, 1996; Spencer *et al.*, 1996), along with transfer of the mutant form of the O(6)-methylguanine-DNA methyltransferase to confer resistance to O(6)-benzylguanine (Davis *et al.*, 2000). Examples of applications of the transfer of nontherapeutic genes for gene marking to elucidate hematopoietic cell lineage relationships or to identify the source of malignant relapse after HSC transplantation will be described below. Examples of the alteration of normal cells to allow their selective and elective elimination will be described in Chapter 117 of this volume. Buoyed by some recent successes in this area and provided that major improvements in appropriate long-term expression of transgenes can continue to be achieved, gene therapy is likely to have an important impact on clinical medicine in the twenty-first century.

The appropriate regulatory authorities in the United States and in other countries have approved more than 500 clinical studies of human gene therapy (Rosenberg *et al.*, 2001). Inherited diseases resulting from single gene defects remain an important focus for gene therapy protocols (Keating, 1991). The diseases most likely amenable to genetic intervention in which HSC transplantation could provide a means of delivery of modified cells are identified in Table 116.2. The diverse goals of the approved protocols have ranged from relatively simple gene targeting and marking studies to attempted gene therapy of a range of genetic disorders such as adenosine deaminase (ADA) deficiency and familial hypercholesterolemia. As will be discussed below, in several of the gene marking studies, significant and relatively prolonged expression of the genetic marker could be detected in a proportion of the patients' peripheral blood cells. However, in most cases where gene transfer represented an actual attempt at tangible therapy, although publications reported some degree of successful transfer and, occasionally, prolonged expression of the potentially therapeutic transgene, most cases have failed to demonstrate a significant sustained clinical benefit to the treated patient (for example, Blaese *et al.*, 1995; Bordignon *et al.*, 1995; Hoogerbrugge *et al.*, 1996). One possible exception

Table 116.2. *Some inherited diseases as potential candidates for gene therapy*

Disease	Frequency	Tissue specificity	Stringent regulation of transgene required?
Hemoglobinopathies	1:600 in ethnic groups	Erythroid cells	Yes
Hemophilias	1:10,000 males	Probably none	No
Adenosine deaminase deficiency	Very rare	Bone marrow/peripheral blood cells	No
Leukocyte adhesion deficiency	Rare	Marrow cells	Unknown
Lesch-Nyhan syndrome	Rare	Brain, other?	No
Lysosomal storage disorders, e.g. Gaucher disease, Fabry disease	1:1,000 to 1:12,000	Bone marrow/peripheral blood, brain	No
Phenylketonuria	1:12,000	Liver, other?	No
α-1-antitrypsin deficiency	1:3,500	Liver, lung	No
Familial hypercholesterolemia	1:500	Liver, other?	Unknown
Chronic granulomatous disease	1:250,000	Bone marrow	Unlikely
Cystic fibrosis	1:3,000	Lung, other?	Unlikely
X-linked SCID	Very rare	Peripheral blood cells	Unlikely

Modified from a Keating (1997).

to this may be T-cell "suicide" gene therapy for control of graft-versus-host disease (GVHD) after allogeneic HSC transplantation (Bonini *et al.*, 1997). Overall, progress in treating single gene disorders is likely to be more rapid for the diseases in which the correct transgene need not be stringently regulated, such as factor or enzyme deficiencies (Table 116.2), or where selective advantages exist for transduced cells such as for X-linked SCID (see below). Indeed, clinical experience indicates that, for the hemophilias, low-level constitutive expression of factors VIII or IX may be sufficient to abrogate the disease phenotype. This is also likely true for amelioration of many lysosomal storage disorders, such as Fabry disease.

Another important consideration is that protocols currently consider only additive somatic cell gene therapy. Here, the transgene exists in an extranuclear form or is randomly inserted into the target cell genome and the correct protein expressed. The abnormal gene remains unaffected, and will continue to generate any aberrant product it may encode. A more attractive but long-term strategy is effecting actual corrective gene therapy. This may be done by homologous recombination, for example, in which the abnormal gene undergoes recombination with the corrective gene (Smithies *et al.*, 1985; Capecchi, 1989). At present, however, this method is very inefficient (Capecchi, 1989) and unfortunately, this overall outlook has not really changed in the past decade. Thus, gene therapy protocols remain of the gene augmentative nature rather than seeking to effect true gene correction or replacement.

As mentioned above, until recently current opinion has largely held that true therapeutic efficacy of gene therapy targeting primitive hematopoietic cells has not been convincingly demonstrated in any clinical trials to date. A landmark study by Cavazzana-Calvo *et al.* (2000) has changed this view, however (see below). Notwithstanding this result, though, it is almost universally acknowledged that the apparent previous failures of

gene therapy stemmed primarily from the inadequacies of current technology and the difficulties of achieving efficient gene transfer and of maintaining suitable and prolonged expression of the transgene. Two separate advisory committees to the National Institutes of Health in 1995 concluded that the present tools and techniques are inadequate for therapeutic transfer and expression. Both committees recommended a reduced emphasis on clinical applications with the present methodologies and a greater emphasis on the support of research designed to probe disease mechanisms, and to develop faithful disease models and superior technologies. Many of these recommendations have been implemented either indirectly or directly and, where previously there was a palpable air of frustration about the inability of gene therapy to effect long-term corrective augmentation, there is now renewed optimism in this therapeutic approach generated by numerous incremental technical and conceptual advances that have derived from these studies.

This chapter outlines recent advances in gene transfer studies, how they may apply to the hematopoietic system and blood and marrow transplantation, and how each contributes to the ongoing challenges of gene transfer efficiency and expression.

Gene transfer into hematopoietic cells

Differentiated T cells were among the earliest targets for clinical gene transfer (e.g., ADA deficiency, tumor-infiltrating lymphocytes) and there remains much interest in conferring antigen specificity on T cells for therapeutic purposes, by, for example, introducton of T-cell receptor genes specific for a given antigen. Furthermore, the requirement for antigen processing and presentation by HLA molecules can be bypassed by the genetic modification of T cells to express a chimeric immunoreceptor composed of a single chain immunoglobulin extracellular targeting domain specific for a tumor-specific or tumor-associated antigen fused to a CD3-ξ intracellular signaling domain. Such an approach has been taken using CD19 as the target antigen (Cooper *et al.*, 2003). However, the rapid turnover of most hematopoietic cells (with the exception of true HSCs unfortunately, which are mainly quiescent) suggests that cells with extensive self-renewal capacity should be the target population for applications involving other lineages. Furthermore, while there may be applications where transient expression of factors or enzymes is desirable, in many cases the aim of therapy is to achieve long-term genetic correction. Given these requirements, it is not surprising that most attention has focused on transducing HSC with vectors (for example, retroviruses) that integrate at an appreciable frequency into the host cell genome. The inability to achieve long-term high-level expression in humans has numerous contributing factors that will be discussed further. The specific requirement of retroviral vectors (i.e., onco-retroviral vectors) for target cells to undergo cell division has led to close collaboration with stem cell biologists interested in ex vivo expansion of HSC, and also employment of alternative retroviral-based gene delivery methods such as lenti-retroviruses. In turn, the ability to mark putative stem cells has been instructive in more closely defining the subset of cells with true long-term reconstituting ability in vivo, and enhanced surrogate models have emerged that may better predict gene transfer outcomes into long-term repopulating human hematopoietic cells. While many creative solutions have been, and are being, generated to improve retroviral-mediated gene transfer (Table 116.3), the door has also been opened for alternative methods of gene delivery, including both viral and nonviral systems.

Viral-mediated gene transfer

Retroviral-mediated gene transfer has long been the most efficient means of introducing integrating transgenes into hematopoietic progenitor cells, or indeed into any mammalian cell population, and therefore has been the preferred technique for many human gene therapy protocols. However, side effects are significant (Baum *et al.*, 2003) and the results from early clinical trials have revealed limitations to these "first-generation" retroviral-mediated gene transfer protocols. In addition to retroviruses, a number of other viral-based gene transfer techniques have been developed, and may find a role in future clinical trials. However, in view of the diversity of potential clinical applications and the specific strengths and weaknesses of each viral system (Table 116.4) it is difficult to identify a single method that will gain pre-eminence in the near future. What seems to be emerging is an element of specialization where certain vectors are employed, depending if high infection efficiency is required for the application or if expression in progeny of infected cells, for example, is desired.

Retroviruses

Noncomplex or "simple" recombinant onco-retroviral vectors (as opposed to "complex" retroviruses such as lenti-retroviruses, see below) are engineered such that the therapeutic or

Table 116.3. *Improving gene transfer and expression*

A. Retroviral vector design and transfection methodology
   1. Improving retrovirus vector design
      (i) Identifying optimal regulatory sequences
      (ii) Use of internal promoters with the gene located outside the retrovirus transcriptional unit
      (iii) Increased stability to concentration by ultracentrifugation, e.g., VSV-G pseudotyped
   2. Selecting high titer virus
   3. Enhance retroviral binding to target cells
      (i) Pseudotyped vectors that bind to receptors more highly expressed on hematopoietic cells, e.g., VSV-G, GAL-V
      (ii) Colocalization on bone marrow stroma or fibronectin fragments
      (iii) Stimulate expression of amphotropic retroviral receptors with cytokines
      (iv) Expression of ecotropic retroviral receptors (by transient transfection)
   4. High titer virus supernatant avoids cocultivation with producer lines that may deplete stem cells by adherence
   5. Repeated cycles of infection
   6. Preselection to provide a higher proportion of cells expressing the transgene
B. Manipulation of target cells
   1. Increasing cycling of progenitors:
      (i) Marrow from 5-FU-treated animals
      (ii) Incubation with hematopoietic growth factors IL-3, IL-6, SCF, TPO, flt3 ligand, and others
      (iii) Coculture on bone marrow stroma
   2. Transduction of populations enriched for early cells:
      (i) CD34$^+$ fraction
      (ii) CD34$^+$ CD38$^-$ population
      (iii) Long-term bone marrow culture cells

Abbreviations: 5-FU, 5-fluorouracil; IL, interleukin; SCF, stem cell factor; TPO, thrombopoietin.
Modified from Keating (1991).

marking transgene replaces sequences encoding wild-type retroviral proteins resulting in a "defective" retroviral genome. In order to produce an infectious recombinant virion capable of infecting target cells, the engineered RNA genome and promoter elements must be packaged with structural and other viral proteins. This is achieved with the use of packaging cell lines (lines that constitutively produce supportive retroviral proteins from stably integrated viral sequences), into which the retroviral vector sequence containing the transgene is transfected (often by calcium phosphate transfection or by electroporation). Due to the replication-incompetent nature of the resultant vector, target cells infected with the recombinant virion are unable to produce further infectious virus. Efficient retroviral transduction is also dependent on binding of virus to target cells, entry into the cell, transport to the nucleus, reverse transcription, and integration into the host cell genome.

Retroviral vector design

In recent years, retroviral vectors have become increasingly sophisticated with respect to their inherent safety in in vivo

Table 116.4. *Characteristics of some viral gene transfer vectors*

Virus	Insert size max (kb)	Integration?	Expression (in vivo)	Immunogenicity	Safety concerns
Onco-retrovirus	8–11	Yes	Short/long	No	Insertional mutagenesis
Lenti-retrovirus	>18	Yes	Long	No	Insertional mutagenesis, recombination
Adenovirus	~30	No	Short	Yes	Inflammation, toxicity
AAV	4.5	Low	Long	Yes	Inflammation, toxicity

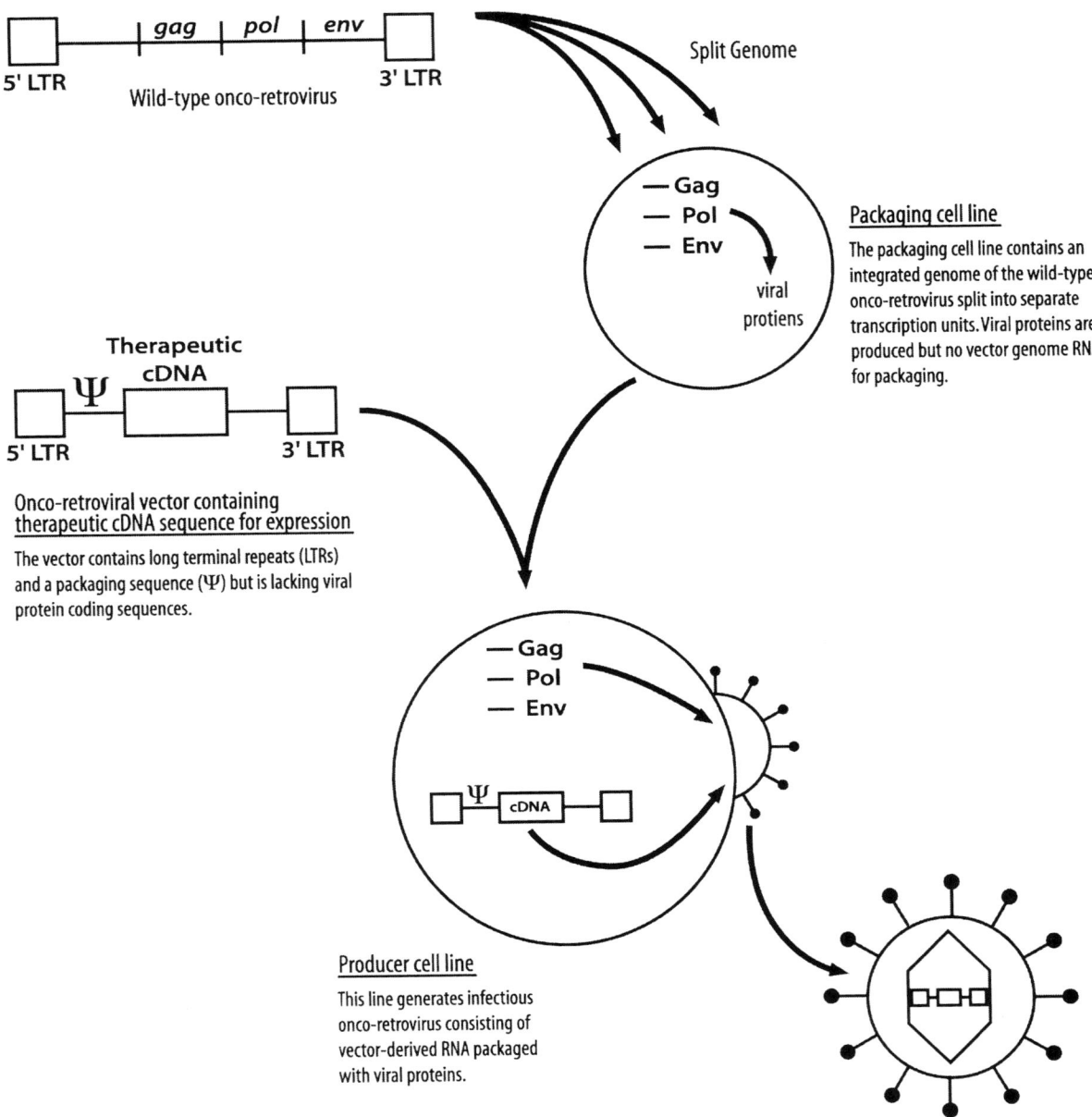

Fig. 116.1. Design of onco-retroviral vectors for gene transfer. The coding sequences of the therapeutic or marking genome are flanked by long terminal repeats (LTR) that contain transcriptional control elements, polyadenylation signals, and sequences required for replication and integration. The encoded genes in the packaging cell line engineer expression of structural proteins *(gag)*, reverse transcriptase *(pol)*, and envelope proteins *(env)*. Incorporation of retroviral RNA into capsids is facilitated by the packaging signal (ψ, psi).

studies, and in the ability to direct infection of specific cell types (Fig. 116.1). An important early limitation of early retrovirus-mediated gene transfer was the possibility of recombination between the retroviral vector and the integrated helper virus of the packaging cell line, resulting in a recombinant replication-competent retrovirus (RCR). In the context of gene therapy, such a recombinant virus could theoretically lead to persistent viremia in a patient receiving the transduced cells, although most murine-based retroviruses are effectively inactivated by human complement. This potential problem has been further circumvented by constructing packaging cell lines containing more effectively crippled helper proviral sequences, thereby reducing the probability of recombination between helper and vector sequences (Miller, 1990). Consequently, replication-competent helper viruses are unlikely to arise. Even so, clinical-grade vector preparations are stringently screened for RCR before use in patients. Compared with the earlier lines, however, the improved packaging lines usually generate lower titers of the defective, transgene-containing retrovirus, thus reducing the efficiency of gene transfer.

Retroviral vectors have been designed to heighten the levels of transgene expression both in vitro and in vivo. Since the promoter/enhancer regions of most somatic genes targeted in gene therapy are incompletely understood with respect to minimum DNA sequence and tissue specificity of expression, or are too large to be efficiently packaged in recombinant retroviruses, the transgene in many retroviral vectors is driven by a constitutively active, moderately tissue-specific, minimal promoter. The choice of promoter in gene therapy often depends on the cell lineage in which optimal expression of the transgene is desired. For example, it has been suggested that in the transcriptional unit of the Moloney murine leukemia virus (MMLV) long terminal repeat (LTR), an endogenous viral promoter often used in retroviral gene transfer vectors (Poznansky et al., 1991; Schuening et al., 1991; Shimada et al., 1991), may be less active in early hematopoietic progenitor cells. This limitation may possibly be overcome by using vectors in which the transgene is placed under the transcriptional control of another viral promoter such as the LTR from the murine stem cell virus (Cheng et al., 1998) or another strong internal promoter (Hantzopoulos et al., 1989). These exogenously added promoters have included, among others, the SV40 early region promoter, the herpes simplex thymidine kinase promoter, and the cytomegalovirus immediate early gene promoter (Schuening et al., 1991; Shimada et al., 1991).

MMLV-based retroviral vectors in common use bind to the amphotropic receptor, Ram-1 (also called Pit-2) on the surface of the target cell. Ram-1 has been characterized as a sodium-dependent phosphate transporter (Kavanaugh et al., 1994). Unfortunately, it has been shown that expression of Ram-1 on human CD34+ cells is quite low, with the lowest levels of all on the critical CD34+ CD38− subset, and that low-level receptor expression correlates with poor transduction efficiency (Orlic et al., 1996). One approach to the problem is to upregulate the level of Ram-1 expression with cytokines (Crooks & Kohn, 1993) or through the use of phosphate-poor culture medium (Kavanaugh et al., 1994). Alternatively, pseudotyped retroviral vectors expressing envelope proteins from other viruses such as the G glycoprotein from vesicular stomatitis virus (VSV-G), the envelope proteins of the gibbon ape leukemia virus (GAL-V which infects through Pit-1), cat endogenous virus RD114, and the 10A1 murine leukemia virus, have been generated (Burns et al., 1993; Von Kalle et al., 1994; Cosset et al., 1995; Miller & Chen, 1996, respectively). Although enhanced gene transfer into CD34+ cells with some of these pseudotyped vectors has been reported (Akkina et al., 1996; Bauer et al., 1998; Movassagh et al., 1998; Gatlin et al., 2001), one group demonstrated that a VSV-G pseudotyped retroviral vector, for example, was incapable of transducing the CD38− subset of CD34+ progenitor cells (Sinclair et al., 1997). An earlier example of pseudotyping involved the use of the env protein of the HIV-1 retrovirus enabling specificity to be conferred upon CD4+ cells (Poznansky et al., 1991; Shimada et al., 1991). A number of other approaches to targeting have been investigated, including modification of retroviral envelope proteins or the coupling of ligands or monoclonal antibodies (Harris & Lemoine, 1996; Benedict et al., 1999). Alternatively, specificity might be conferred at the transcriptional level through the introduction of vectors with tissue-specific promoters (Walther & Stein, 1996). Specific targeting would be particularly attractive in heterogeneous cell populations such as bone marrow or for in vivo applications. Along those lines, "humanized" packaging cell lines have been developed that may allow actual in vivo delivery of recombinant vectors due to their resistance to human complement inactivation (Sheridan et al., 2000) or may provide a supportive microenvironment for hematopoiesis in addition to producing recombinant virions for infections (Dando et al., 2001).

Transgene integration and "cell cycling"

One of the principal difficulties associated with onco-retroviral transduction of HSC is the requirement for the target cells to divide in order for the viral pre-integration complex to enter the nucleus (Miller, Adam, & Miller, 1990) (Table 116.4). Primate HSCs have long been known to be relatively quiescent and therefore efforts have focused on stimulating cells to enter the cell cycle, principally through the use of hematopoietic cytokines. Numerous studies have shown enhanced gene transfer into hematopoietic cells induced to cycle by priming with a variety of cytokines (Laneuville et al., 1988; Bodine, Karlsson, & Nienhuis, 1989) or after treatment in vivo with low-dose chemotherapeutic agents (Bodine et al., 1991). Early murine studies suggested that stem cell factor (SCF) and interleukin (IL)-3 may be an effective combination (Bodine et al., 1992). SCF and IL-3 can increase the efficiency of gene transfer into primate early progenitor cells while a combination of IL-3 and IL-6 is more efficient at promoting the transduction of more mature progenitors (van Beusechem et al., 1995). Other cytokine combinations have been used as well, including an IL-3/GM-CSF fusion protein along with G-CSF (Malech et al., 1997) and megakaryocyte growth and differentiation factor along with SCF and G-CSF (Abonour *et al.*, 2000). While the CD34⁺ CD38⁻ subset, containing cells with long-term repopulating ability, can be stimulated to divide with prolonged stimulation with cytokine combinations (such as IL-3, IL-6, and SCF), this is associated with some loss of clonogenic potential (as measured by in vitro assays), presumably as a result of commitment to differentiation pathways (Reems & Torok-Storb, 1995). Indeed, it may be that any ex vivo manipulation of primitive hematopoietic cells at all leads to some loss of pluripotentcy or a reduction in the capacity for self-renewal.

Culture of primitive hematopoietic cells on supportive stromal monolayers can generate progenitors detectable in standard clonogenic assays for up to 6 weeks. These cells have been operationally defined as long-term culture initiating cells (LT-CIC) and it was speculated that this culture system might serve as an in vitro assay for human HSC (Eaves *et al.*, 1992). Accordingly, these assays have been incorporated into most gene transfer protocols. While successful transduction of colony-forming cells (CFCs) and the more immature LT-CICs has been widely reported, there is a striking lack of correlation with the universally low levels of long-term transduction of hematopoietic cells in clinical studies (Blaese *et al.*, 1995; Emmons *et al.*, 1997). A likely explanation is that neither CFC nor LT-CIC assays measure true stem cells with long-term in vivo reconstituting ability.

Transplantation of primitive hematopoietic cells into immunodeficient NOD/SCID mice has led to the identification of the so-called SCID repopulating cell (SRC) (Larochelle *et al.*, 1996). The SRC is found within the CD34⁺ CD38⁻ fraction of bone marrow or mobilized peripheral blood, is capable of long-term multilineage engraftment, and is thought to represent a more primitive cell than identified in any of the current in vitro assays. Furthermore, poor retroviral transduction of SRCs with conventional protocols has correlated much more closely with the clinical experience of gene transfer into HSC (Larochelle *et al.*, 1996). Thus, it is hoped that the SRC model may be a much more accurate system for assaying HSC and the successful transduction of these cells may predict a successful outcome in future clinical trials. It may be that newer combinations of cytokines and careful timing of stimulation will be able to induce cells to cycle, while maintaining long-term reconstituting ability. Considerable early promise has been shown by the incorporation of flt3 ligand and thrombopoietin into transduction protocols (Shah *et al.*, 1996; Bertolini *et al.*, 1997; Dao *et al.*, 1997). flt3 ligand has been reported to stimulate proliferation of CD34⁺ CD38⁻ cells without induction of differentiation (Bertolini *et al.*, 1997).

An additional consideration is the influence of chemotherapeutic agents or cytokines on hematopoietic progenitors in vivo prior to collection for retroviral transduction. First, since marrows of 5-fluorouracil (5-FU)-treated animals have an increased proportion of very early stem/progenitor cells in cycle, it is not surprising that retroviral infection of marrow cells from 5-FU-treated mice (Bodine *et al.*, 1991) or nonhuman primates (Wieder *et al.*, 1991) leads to an enhanced effi-

ciency of gene transfer. This method, however, is not readily adaptable to human gene therapy, although some investigators have used cyclophosphamide to mobilize peripheral blood CD34⁺ cells (Dunbar *et al.*, 1995).

A second, analogous strategy using bone marrow progenitors from granulocyte colony-stimulating factor (G-CSF)-treated dogs (Schuening *et al.*, 1991) or bone marrow progenitors or peripheral blood cells from SCF and G-CSF-treated Rhesus monkeys (Dunbar *et al.*, 1996) also results in enhanced transduction of long-term repopulating cells. Comparative studies of hematopoietic progenitors derived from bone marrow and mobilized peripheral blood reveals differences in the cell cycling and expression profile of various surface markers (Uchida *et al.*, 1997). Furthermore, clinical differences in engraftment kinetics support the belief that these differences are relevant to stem cell transplantation. Therefore it is likely that the source of progenitors and prior stimulation may influence the efficiency of gene transfer. While retroviral transduction of cytokine-mobilized peripheral blood progenitor cells (PBPCs) has been studied (Emmons *et al.*, 1997), valid comparative data are limited. However, in one study where transduction of PBPCs mobilized with G-CSF or G-CSF and SCF was compared with bone marrow derived progenitors, no difference in efficiency was demonstrated (Elwood *et al.*, 1996). It is interesting that administration of SCF in vivo did not influence efficiency, given its known efficacy in in vitro transduction. This may simply be the result of the overriding influence of the cytokines employed during the transduction course. However, given the low efficiency of retroviral transduction into early progenitors, the observation that a combination of G-CSF and SCF significantly increased the number of harvested PBPCs, still has implications for clinical use. The above findings are in marked contrast to some results where transduced GM-CSF-mobilized peripheral blood and cord blood cells were engrafted in comparative studies into NOD/SCID mice. Pollok *et al.* (2001) demonstrated that recipient animals engrafted with transduced cord blood cells had >10-fold higher levels of marked human cells in bone marrow and spleen. Thus, given current clinically relevant transduction protocols, these cells may be the optimal targets for therapy, if enough can be obtained.

Other factors affecting the efficiency of retroviral gene transfer

In addition to the design of retroviral vectors and the stimulation of cell cycling, several other factors can influence the efficiency of gene transfer. The efficiency of infection may be increased dramatically by repeated cycles of infection (up to five) of the target cells; however, this can dramatically increase the degree of differentiation. Infection can be accomplished either by co-cultivation of target cells with the packaging line (which has been transfected with the defective, transgene-containing retroviral vector), or by culturing the target cells with high titer retrovirus-bearing supernatants from the transfected packaging line. In one early study, a fivefold increase in the frequency of transduced human colony-forming unit—granulocyte-macrophage (CFU-GM) (to over 30%) was documented after repeated cycles of infection (Bordignon et al., 1989). One drawback of co-cultivation with fibroblast packaging lines is the possibility of delayed engraftment after transplantation of the transfected target cells (Kantoff et al., 1987; Bodine et al., 1991), perhaps because of stem cell depletion by adherence to the packaging line (Gordon et al., 1985). While this drawback may be avoided by using high titer cell supernatants, murine studies indicate this latter method to be less effective in transfecting long-term repopulating cells (Bodine et al., 1991). The concentration of supernatant by ultracentrifugation can also enhance transduction but may be associated with loss of vector due to physical instability, although this appears not to be the case with VSV-G or lymphocytic choriomeningitis virus glycoprotein pseudotyped vectors (Burns et al., 1993; Beyer et al., 2002).

After infection of target cells, one approach that has yielded a population highly enriched for the cells actually transduced and suitable for engraftment involves a preselection step. Thus, when the retroviral vector contains both the transgene and an antibiotic resistance gene, for example, cells transduced with the vector may be selected in a medium containing this antibiotic prior to transplantation. Cells may even be selected in vivo (Sorrentino et al., 1992). The use of drug-selectable markers has, however, on one occasion led to induction of a myeloproliferative disorder (Bunting et al., 1998). In addition, this approach will not be useful for recipients unable to tolerate the conditioning regimen. To obviate some of these problems, we (and others) have designed bicistronic recombinant retroviral vectors that also engineer expression of cell surface markers including murine heat-stable antigen, human CD24, and human CD25 (Migita et al., 1995; Medin et al., 1996; Qin et al., 2001). In this way positively transduced hematopoietic cells can be preselected by immunoaffinity enrichment prior to transplantation. Indeed, we have demonstrated significantly enhanced long-term correction in a mouse model of Fabry disease using this approach (Qin et al., 2001). One caution here is that the choice of cell surface marker is important since one group has recently suggested that the sequence for the truncated low affinity nerve growth factor receptor (LNGFR) may itself actually contribute to deleterious proviral integration events (Li et al., 2002).

Another interesting approach to yielding an enriched population of transduced hematopoietic cells, either in vitro or in vivo, is by genetic transfer of fusion protein constructs encoding cytoplasmic domains of cytokine receptor subunits that can be specifically dimerized by unique factors. These unique factors can be nontoxic small molecules that bind to drug-binding domains of the engineered fusion proteins and induce receptor cross-linking. This, in turn, can lead to selective proliferative effects. Synthetic dimerizers have been used for this approach that bind to FKBP12, for example, to induce dimerization and proliferation mediated by the erythropoietin receptor (Blau et al., 1997) and the thrombopoietin receptor (Jin et al., 1998). This approach has also been used to expand transduced

hematopoietic cells in vivo (Jin et al., 2000), and for the synthesis of novel death-inducing fusion genes that can be specifically and selectively activated by the dimerizing agent (Thomis et al., 2001).

In addition to, and possibly distinct from, the effects of hematopoietic growth factors, bone marrow stromal cells have been shown to influence cycling of early hematopoietic progenitors (Cashman, Eaves, & Eaves, 1985) and are capable of sustaining long-term hematopoiesis in vitro (Keating et al., 1984). Since the adherent layer from human long-term bone marrow cultures is a close in vitro counterpart of the hematopoietic microenvironment (Singer, Keating, & Wright, 1985), several groups have investigated the role of marrow stromal cells on transduction efficiency. Not surprisingly, Moore et al. (1992) showed that gene transfer into the human early progenitor population was increased fourfold in the presence of marrow stromal cells and was independent of stimulation with exogenous growth factors. Wells et al. (1995) observed a similar fourfold enhancement of transduction efficiency in the presence of marrow stromal cells.

It is notable that improved results have been reported by transduction on fragments of the fibronectin protein containing integrin-binding domains. Hanenberg et al. (1996) demonstrated that this was dependent on binding of both retroviral particles and target cells to the fragment. However, it is not known whether the beneficial effect of fibronectin is simply the result of co-localization of viral vector with target cell or whether additional signal transduction following integrin engagement is involved. Both seem to be the case, as a recent study by Donahue et al. (2001) demonstrated that apoptosis of CD34+ cells was inhibited, and cell division was actually stimulated, due to transductions done on a fragment of fibronectin.

An intriguing further approach to the release of early hematopoietic progenitor/stem cells from quiescence involves the use in vitro of antisense transforming growth factor (TGF-β) or Rb oligonucleotides (Hatzfield et al., 1991). Antibodies can also be used to effect this ultimate aim of reducing cyclin-dependent kinase inhibitors and allowing cell-cycle progression. For example, Dao et al. (1998) combined anti-TGF-β with antisense oligonucleotides to p27 and demonstrated enhanced transduction of human primitive cells that can engraft mouse models of human hematopoiesis and lead to multilineage gene-marked progeny.

Although retroviral binding and induction of cell division have received the most attention, it should also be noted that there are other steps in retroviral gene transfer that may give rise to problems. Sinclair et al. (1997) demonstrated satisfactory binding of a VSV-G pseudotyped retroviral vector to CD34+ CD38− cells but failed to achieve significant expression of the reporter gene, and concluded that there was a block to reverse transcription. In a separate study, Austin et al. (1997) reported that 46% to 60% of retrovirally transduced CD34+ cells were positive for reverse transcription products by polymerase chain reaction (PCR) at 48 to 72 hours but only 12% to 16% of cells achieved productive expression of integrated vector.

Long-term expression

Early studies of murine transplant recipients showed variable long-term expression of antibiotic resistance genes in cells of the myeloid and lymphoid lineages (Keller *et al.*, 1985). Subsequent studies examined expression of potentially clinically relevant genes such as ADA (Lim *et al.*, 1989), DHFR (Williams *et al.*, 1987), human β-globin (Dzierzak, Papayannopoulou, & Mulligan, 1988), human glucocerebrosidase (Correll *et al.*, 1989), and human argininosuccinate synthetase (Herman *et al.*, 1989). An important goal in the study of in vivo (or indeed, in vitro) models of gene therapy, however, is to demonstrate sustained, long-term expression of the transgene.

Both the level and the durability of expression from a transgene in the target cell can be influenced by a multitude of variables, including the choice of promoter and the exact identity and degree of differentiation of the transduced cell. In some situations, such as human ADA deficiency, it may be sufficient to transduce only lymphocytes and their precursors to reverse the disease phenotype. However, in situations where the aim is durable expression of the transgene in more short-lived, differentiated cells of myeloid and erythroid lineages (such as in thalassemia, for example) transduction of self-renewing pluripotential hematopoietic progenitors is required. The problems associated with transducing this rare and quiescent population have already been discussed. An additional problem that may limit the efficacy of retroviral gene therapy is the phenomenon of transcriptional silencing. When ex vivo transduced cells, which continue to express the transgene in vitro for prolonged periods, are re-infused into animal models, loss of gene expression within days to weeks has been observed (Palmer *et al.*, 1991; Dai *et al.*, 1992). This is not due to loss of transgene or transgene-containing cells, and appears to be an irreversible event. It has been postulated that this event is due to methylation of the proviral LTR (Challita & Kohn, 1994). The extent to which this is likely to be a problem in hematopoietic cell gene therapy is unknown, since issues of low efficiency of gene transfer have been more dominant. However, long-term actual gene expression from retrovirally transduced cells has been demonstrated in animal studies (Kalberer *et al.*, 2000; Takenaka *et al.*, 2000; Goerner *et al.*, 2001) and human clinical trials (Blaese *et al.*, 1995; Bordignon *et al.*, 1995; Cavazzana-Calvo *et al.*, 2000; Aiuti *et al.*, 2002), suggesting that this is not an absolute barrier.

Long-term transgene expression can also be influenced by other phenomena, such as the exact nature of the chromatin at the proviral integration site and by posttranscriptional regulatory elements that can increase the transport or stability of the transcribed gene RNA product. Some investigators have attempted to influence the duration of expression by including chromatin insulator elements, such as the chicken β-globin 5′ constitutive DNAse I hypersensitive site (Emery *et al.*, 2000), and scaffold attachment regions, such as that derived from the human interferon-β locus (Dang *et al.*, 2000) into retroviral vectors. Others have added splice signals to vectors that create artificial introns in the 5′ untranslated regions, and also regulatory elements from the woodchuck hepatitis virus (Schambach

et al., 2000). Since these elements seem to have a contextual bias in vectors themselves, which influences their utility, it remains to be seen which elements optimize expression of key target genes and what the long-term consequences of these approaches are in the hematopoietic system.

Lenti-retroviruses

The principal attraction of these retroviruses, of which the human immunodeficiency virus (HIV) is the best-known example, is an ability to infect nondividing cells. Unlike "simple" or onco-retroviruses, the viral pre-integration complex of lentiviruses appears able to enter the intact nucleus and is not dependent on breakdown of the nuclear membrane during mitosis. Yet even here it appears that cells cannot be completely quiescent as progression into the $G1_b$ phase of the cell cycle is necessary for reverse transcription to occur (Korin & Zack, 1998). By using many of the principles of vector design developed for onco-retroviruses, a number of groups have produced vectors based on HIV-1 (Naldini *et al.*, 1996; Poeschla *et al.*, 1996). Retention of the HIV env gene confers specificity for transducing CD4+ cells (which may be desirable in some instances); however, pseudotyping with the surface G-glycoprotein from VSV extends the potential application to a much broader range of cell types (Akkina *et al.*, 1996). With such a vector, Naldini and colleagues (1996) demonstrated long-term expression of β-galactosidase in rat neurons in vivo. Other investigators have engineered systems that allow for pseudotyping with a variety of env proteins (for example, Hanawa *et al.*, 2002). In that study it was found that RD114- or amphotropic-pseudotyped virions were actually more effective in infecting CD34+ hematopoietic cells than VSV-G pseudotyped virions. Even with these data and these tools, it still remains to be demonstrated conclusively that long-term repopulating HSCs from large animals can be effectively and stably transduced with these vectors.

Another major advantage lentiviruses may have over onco-retroviruses is carrying capacity. Lentiviruses have been shown to be able to be packaged at appreciable titers even when the proviral length is over 18 kbp (Kumar *et al.*, 2001). This has facilitated studies where locus control region elements or introns are added to gene transfer vectors to improve or regulate expression. In one such study it was recently demonstrated in two distinct murine models of sickle cell disease that transduction of murine HSCs with a recombinant lentivirus vector expressing a globin gene variant could lead to long-term expression in circulating erythrocytes and inhibition of sickling (Pawliuk *et al.*, 2001). It also seems possible that lentiviral vectors may not be subject to the transcriptional silencing in vivo that may occur with retroviral vectors. In addition, clinical experience with HIV infection suggests that immunologic responses to these vectors may not be significant. However, both these issues need to be fully tested. This gene transfer approach is likely to be most applicable to tissues in which key cells are predominantly nondividing, including HSCs. While Naldini and co-workers generated a relatively high titer vector, others have not been as successful. In addition, there have been problems with the generation of stable packaging lines (Lever, 1996) that still remain.

Along with production concerns, regulatory and safety issues remain with this delivery system. To date no clinical protocol has been approved that uses this delivery method. Although the development of attenuated vectors, in which the genes thought to encode in vivo virulence factors (vif, vpr, vpu, and nef) have been deleted (Zufferey *et al.,* 1997), will help allay safety concerns, the importance of absolutely preventing the emergence of RCR will mandate highly stringent safety testing. In light of this it may be that lentiviral vectors will find the first clinical applications in the therapy of HIV itself. Alternatively, the lessons learned from HIV may allow development of safer vectors derived from nonpathogenic viruses with similar integrating capabilities. Investigators have also sought to further diminish the chance of deleterious integration events with this vector, such as the activation of cellular oncogenes as it integrates randomly into the genome, by designing "self-inactivating" vectors wherein the viral enhancer and promoter sequences have been deleted (Miyoshi *et al.,* 1998).

Adenovirus

Adenoviruses belong to a family of DNA viruses and are responsible for a proportion of benign upper respiratory tract infections in humans. Adenoviruses have been used in gene therapy applications from early on, as they are capable of infecting a wide variety of cell types, and unlike retroviruses, do not require cell division (Kremer & Perricaudet, 1995). Adenovirus serotype 5 has been used most often in corrective gene transfer studies. Replacement of parts of the EI region of the viral genome allows transfer of up to 7 to 8 kb of a relevant gene, and renders the virus replication deficient (Kremer & Perricaudet, 1995). Following entry into the nucleus, the viral DNA is maintained as a stable episome rather than becoming integrated in the host cell genome. While adenoviral vectors have been shown to achieve long-term expression in some in vitro systems, in vivo expression is usually very short as a result of immunologically mediated clearing of transduced cells expressing viral proteins (Dai *et al.,* 1995) and by dilutions of vector in progeny of infected cells. Prior adenoviral infection may limit clinical efficacy, and the immune response will certainly prevent effective re-administration of adenoviral vectors for in vivo applications. Immunosuppression of the host has been shown to prolong expression in animal models (Fang *et al.,* 1995) but this is a less than elegant approach and is unlikely to be acceptable for long-term clinical use in most patients. Alteration of viral vectors to become less immunogenic may hold some promise for the future.

There have been reports of adenovirus-based vectors for purging malignant cells: Garcia-Sanchez and colleagues (1998) used a replication-incompetent adenoviral vector carrying a CMV-driven transcription unit of the cytosine deaminase gene, allowing the deamination of 5-FC and its conversion to 5-FU. Teoh and colleagues (1998) used adenovirus vectors to deliver the thymidine kinase gene into myeloma cells together with the β-galactosidase gene under the control of the DF3 promoter. (Myeloma cells had previously been shown to express both adenovirus receptors as well as the DF3/MUC1 protein.) In both model systems human hematopoietic cells were largely or completely unaffected by the procedures.

Adenoviral vectors have been reported to transduce human bone marrow $CD34^+$ cells ex vivo with an efficiency of up to 45% (Neering *et al.,* 1996; Watanabe *et al.,* 1996). Furthermore, in that study the $CD34^+38^-$ subset and also cells in G_0 were targeted equally effectively. Another study found high functional transduction efficiencies of $CD34^+$ cells (up to 70%) and also SP cells (up to 80%) when chimeric adenovirus was made from serotype 5 and the short fiber protein from adenovirus serotype 35 (Yotnda *et al.,* 2001). Ex vivo adenovirus-transduced transduced $CD34^+$ cells have not been studied in vivo in detail outside of a few reports (Fan *et al.,* 2000); however, there is no reason to believe that the same problems of short-term expression would not be encountered. Thus, even for potential short-term applications (e.g., transient expression of multidrug resistance, immunological modulation), further basic research is required before adenoviral vectors are likely to become broadly clinically relevant in the hematopoietic system.

Adeno-associated virus

Adeno-associated virus (AAV) is a nonpathogenic, single-stranded DNA virus belonging to the parvovirus family (Kremer & Perricaudet, 1995). The virus has two coding genes, *rep* and *cap,* enclosed between two inverted terminal repeats (ITRs). The *rep* gene is important in replication and integration, while the *cap* gene encodes viral capsid proteins (McKeon & Samulski, 1996). In the absence of helper virus, wild-type AAV becomes integrated in a latent state as a proviral gene, commonly in a site-specific manner on chromosome 19. The properties of nonpathogenicity, integration capability, and a broad specificity of cells that can be infected (including nondividing cells) make AAV an attractive candidate for use in viral-based vectors. As with other viral vectors, viral genes (in this case *rep* and *cap*) are replaced with vector gene(s), and virions are assembled in producer cells. For complete assembly, viral genes are delivered *in trans* on other plasmids, or co-infection of packaging cells with helper virus such as adenovirus or herpesvirus is required. Helper virus-free vectors can be recovered by centrifugation on cesium chloride or by heating. This may be important since, although the presence of adenovirus or adenoviral components may enhance transduction, an increase in immunogenicity may result, potentially shortening the duration of expression (McKeon & Samulski, 1996). AAV vectors have a somewhat limited carrying capacity of foreign DNA (<5 kbp), although recent advances such as trans-splicing vectors may increase this (Yan *et al.,* 2000).

AAV vectors have been reported to transduce a wide variety of cell types and have entered clinical trials in patients with cystic fibrosis, among other disorders. Indeed, the number of reported studies using this delivery system have increased exponentially in the past few years. Several groups have reported transduction of hematopoietic cell lines and early progenitors with AAV vectors, in some cases at high efficiency (Walsh *et al.,* 1992; Zhou *et al.,* 1994). In most initial examples, however, only plasmid entry (measured by PCR) or expression (RT-PCR) in progenitors cultured in vitro for up to 14 days was measured. Several observations suggest that expression from the vector in episomal form may be high and prolonged and that the level of integration (and true long-term expression) may be much lower than initially believed. Malik *et al.* (1997) demonstrated declining expression over more than 2 months in K562 cells expressing nerve growth factor receptor (NGFR) as a reporter gene product after transduction with an AAV vector and showed that reduced levels were due predominantly to continued loss of nonintegrated vector. Similar studies with CD34+ cells showed low levels that were lost after 2 weeks. Fisher-Adams and colleagues (1996) showed expression of an alkaline phosphatase reporter product on 39% to 58% of AAV-transduced cord blood CD34+ cells but were only able to demonstrate integration (by fluorescence in situ hybridization) in 2% to 4%. A higher percentage of transduction and stable integration (as measured by analysis of metaphase spreads) was demonstrated in another study (Chatterjee *et al.,* 1999). Finally, ex vivo AAV-transduced murine hematopoietic progenitors (expressing a human globin gene) have been transplanted into lethally irradiated recipient animals. Analysis of primary recipients after 6 months indicated a human globin gene copy number of 7% to 8% relative to an endogenous murine gene (Ponnazhagan *et al.,* 1997). In this study it was encouraging to note that expression was also maintained, at levels of 4% to 6% relative to murine β^{major} globin as detected by semiquantitative RT-PCR, and contrasts with the possible transcriptional silencing of the transgene observed with retroviral vectors.

AAV vectors have also been used for direct in vivo applications such as direct injection into muscle or liver and are capable of efficiently transducing hepatocytes following intravenous administration in mice (Koeberl *et al.,* 1997). Indeed, their optimal utility may eventually be found to be in intramuscular delivery followed by engineered secretion of corrective factors, for example. A landmark study supporting this was published by Kay *et al.* in 2000. In that study recombinant AAV was injected into the muscle of hemophilia B patients and some factor IX production was observed over time. Further studies are required to develop the direct or selective transduction of hematopoietic progenitors in vivo. Nevertheless, AAV vectors appear to be a promising alternative means of achieving long-term expression of the transgene in vivo.

Nonviral methods of gene transfer

While retroviral-mediated gene transfer into human HSC has numerous drawbacks, all nonviral methods are limited to a greater or lesser extent by low levels of integration of plasmid DNA. Clinical studies involving nonviral gene transfer are under way in conditions in which (1) repeated therapy is practi-

cal and allows maintenance of long-term expression (e.g., cationic lipid gene transfer to airway epithelium in cystic fibrosis) or (2) short-term expression is not a problem or indeed may be desirable (e.g., approaches aimed at killing cancer cells or prevention of arterial restenosis).

The lack of durable expression undoubtedly explains the absence of clinical studies involving targeting of hematopoietic cells using nonviral gene transfer methods. Progress in this area will depend on developments that facilitate integration, maintain stable episomes, incorporate vector DNA in the form of mini-chromosomes, or perhaps on targeted approaches that will permit repeated in vivo administration. Another interesting approach using this type of delivery is to transfect and select cells ex vivo, such as blood outgrowth endothelial cells, that can then be expanded and re-implanted into hosts and secrete corrective factors such as factor VIII (Lin *et al.,* 2002).

Electroporation

Electroporation is a physical method of DNA transfer that relies on an electric field to create transient pores in the outer membrane of target cells through which the vector DNA can enter passively (Toneguzzo, Hayday, & Keating, 1986). Advantages of this method over retrovirus-mediated gene transfer include simplicity, the ability to use vectors lacking retroviral sequences, the lack of size constraints on the transgene (over 30 kb can be transferred), and integration of the transgene in low copy number (Toneguzzo *et al.,* 1988).

In our experience, stable expression of a transgene in transfected human hematopoietic progenitor cells can be detected in up to 5% of progeny with current electroporation methodologies (Toneguzzo & Keating, 1986; A. Keating, unpublished data). Indeed, PCR analyses indicate that up to 40% of hematopoietic colonies arising from electrotransfected, cytokine-stimulated human marrow comprise gene-marked cells (Mathews & Keating, 1994). Earlier studies also showed that marrow stromal cells are readily electrotransfected (Keating *et al,* 1990). Our data showing that gene-marked stromal cells can engraft in murine recipients suggest a potential role for marrow stromal or non-hematopoietic mesenchymal cells as a gene delivery vehicle (Wu & Keating, 1991). A clinical trial of autologous gene-marked stromal cells lends further support to this strategy: gene-marked cells were detected up to 8 months after infusion of electrotransfected stromal cells in unconditioned recipients, and importantly, transcription of the transgene (hFIX cDNA) was detected up to 6 months after infusion (Keating *et al.,* 2002). This inherently attractive approach for use in clinical protocols should be further pursued to improve the efficiency of electrotransfection and enhance engraftment levels of the gene-modified stromal cells.

Cationic liposomes

Positively charged liposomes spontaneously bind negatively charged DNA or RNA and can then deliver the plasmid into the cell cytoplasm. Cationic liposomes have been used for in vitro and in vivo applications. Bulk preparation is relatively easy in addition to the shared advantages of other nonviral methods. Most in vivo applications have been directed toward transduction of airway epithelial cells or blood vessel endothelium. However, at least one group has demonstrated efficacy in transducing murine hematopoietic progenitors both in vitro and in vivo (Aksentijevich et al., 1996).

Other nonviral methods of gene delivery

Two other physical methods of gene transfer are direct injection and particle bombardment. Naked plasmid DNA injected into muscle of mice in vivo can persist for up to 60 days (Wolff et al., 1990). However, the level of expression with direct injection is relatively low. Although the latter can be improved by treatment with bupivicaine or cardiotoxin to induce muscle regeneration, this is unlikely to be clinically applicable. With particle bombardment, DNA is coated onto 1 to 3 μm gold particles, which are then physically propelled into the target tissue. In this way it is possible to simultaneously deliver multiple large DNA constructs to particular cells. The "gene gun" has been used for both in vitro and in vivo approaches, although the latter are limited to accessible tissues such as skin. Expression is transient and efficiency varies depending on the target tissue. Perhaps the greatest potential for these methods lies in the field of DNA vaccine delivery.

Clinical gene therapy studies using human hematopoietic stem/progenitor cells

There are numerous examples in the literature of successful transfer of many clinically relevant genes into murine and human hematopoietic progenitor cells in vitro. Using improved technologies to harvest HSC from bone marrow, peripheral blood, or cord blood, some of these gene transfer protocols have formed the basis for trials aimed at demonstrating quantifiable clinical benefit. While such trials are under way in a wide variety of disease, including many of those listed in Table 116.2, all reported studies, for the most part, are hampered by low gene transfer efficiency and limited transgene expression (Kohn, 1997; Richter, 1997). Yet, as mentioned above, some success in the clinic has recently occurred. In this section we will examine key marking and therapeutic clinical studies focused on gene transfer into hematopoietic stem/progenitor cells.

Gene marking studies

The principle of gene marking is the transfer of a unique DNA sequence (e.g., a nonhuman gene) into a host cell (e.g., T-cell, HSC) allowing the gene or the gene product to be easily detected, thereby serving as a marker for these labeled cells (Brenner et al., 1993). In all these studies gene marking is not intended for direct therapeutic benefit, but rather to obtain information regarding the biology and function of adoptively transferred cells.

Gene marking in autologous stem cell transplantation

By marking HSCs prior to stem cell infusion, it has been possible to determine if contaminating malignant cells in the stem cell harvest contribute to relapse following autologous stem cell transplant (Brenner et al., 1991). The HSC product is marked at the time of harvest with murine retroviral vectors encoding the neomycin resistance gene. Then, at relapse, it is possible to determine whether the marker gene is present in the malignant cells. Since 1991, studies have been initiated using this approach in a variety of malignancies treated by autologous HSC transplantation (Brenner et al., 1991; Deisseroth et al., 1991; Santana et al., 1991; Cornetta et al., 1992) including acute myeloid leukemia (AML), chronic myeloid leukemia (CML), acute lymphoblastic leukemia (ALL), neuroblastoma, and lymphoma.

In pediatric patients receiving autologous bone marrow transplantation (BMT) as part of therapy for AML, 4 of 12 patients who received marked marrow relapsed. In three of the four patients, detection of both the transferred marker and of a tumor-specific marker in the same cells at the time of relapse provided unequivocal evidence that the residual malignant cells in the marrow were a source of leukemic recurrence (Brenner et al., 1991). These marking studies also provided information on the transfer of marker genes to normal hematopoietic cells and showed that marrow autografts contribute to long-term hematopoietic reconstitution after transplant (Brenner et al., 1994). Long-term transfer for more than 10 years has been seen in the mature progeny of marrow precursor cells, including peripheral blood T and B cells and neutrophils (Rill et al., 2000). However, the level of gene transfer has generally been low with levels of 0 to 1% seen in mature peripheral blood cells (Heslop et al., 1999). The data on transfer to normal cells also provide an opportunity to compare different transduction conditions, although other differences between patient groups complicate interpretation. Nevertheless, it appears that long-term gene transfer is higher in children than adults (Brenner et al., 1993; Dunbar et al., 1995). Unfortunately, an approach utilizing transduction in long-term bone marrow culture that improved gene transfer in a canine model did not result in higher gene transfer in a clinical marking study (Stewart et al., 1999).

Gene marking of T cells

Several studies have also shown the feasibility of gene marking cytotoxic T lymphocytes (CTL) to track their expansion, persistence, and homing potential to sites of disease (Heslop et al., 1996; Rooney et al., 1998; Roskrow et al., 1998). For example, gene marking of Epstein Barr virus (EBV)-specific CTL for the prophylaxis and treatment of lymphoproliferative disorder after HSC transplantation demonstrated persistence of gene-marked CTL to 78 months postinfusion. In addition, as described below, gene-marked EBV-CTL given as treatment for relapsed Hodgkin's disease have been shown to traffic to tumor sites (Bollard et al., 2000).

Similarly, studies have been performed in patients with HIV who received peripheral blood lymphocytes from uninfected syngeneic twins transduced with a neomycin phosphotransferase marker gene (Walker et al., 1998). Marked CD4+ T cells persisted in the circulation for 4 to 18 weeks after transfer in all patients, and at 6 months marked cells were found in lymphoid tissues (Walker et al., 1998). Autologous CTL clones specific for the HIV protein gag were administered to patients with HIV. In initial studies the clones were genetically modified with a construct encoding a fusion of the hygromycin phosphotransferase and herpes simplex thymidine kinase (Tk) genes, so that the infused cells could be selected prior to infusion and destroyed in vivo if they induced inflammation (Riddell et al., 1996). This approach was limited by the development of a host CTL response to the hygromycin phosphotransferase and Tk fusion proteins (Riddell et al., 1996). In subsequent studies autologous HIV Gag-specific CD8+ CTL clones genetically marked with the LN retrovirus were infused (Brodie et al., 1999). The infused CTLs accumulated adjacent to HIV-infected cells in lymph nodes and transiently reduced the levels of circulating productively infected CD4+ T cells. However this decline was transient, likely because of a lack of CD4 help, but it did provide some rationale for pursuing this approach in conjunction with strategies to circumvent the requirement for CD4+ cells (Brodie et al., 1999).

Marking to assess clonality of hematopoietic and immune reconstitution

Several studies have used PCR to demonstrate the clonality of the cells recovering after infusion of gene-marked stem cells or T cells (Rill et al., 1994), but this methodology does not permit simultaneous detection of multiple clones. A recently described technique called linear amplification-mediated (LAM) PCR that allows characterization of multiple rare retroviral and lentiviral integration sites in highly complex DNA samples (Schmidt et al., 2001) has already provided additional information about the clonality of reconstitution in primate models (Shi et al., 2002) and human clinical trials. For example, in infants with SCID receiving cord blood cells transduced with a retroviral vector encoding ADA, LAM-PCR has shown that a single transduced progenitor cell has been the predominant source of corrected CD3+ T cells (Carbanaro et al., 2002).

Insertional mutagenesis

One concern with all marking strategies has been the risk of insertional mutagenesis. In a recent murine study (Li et al., 2002) irradiated C57 BL/6J mice were transplanted with bone marrow transduced with the clinically utilized LNGFR marker gene (Bonini et al., 1997) mentioned above. While the primary recipients did not develop any hematopoietic alterations, transplantation of pooled marrow into secondary irradiated recipients was followed by the development of hematologic abnormalities and overt AML (Li et al., 2002). Although all mice had the same leukemic clone with a single vector copy integrated into the murine gene Evil, this is not usually sufficient

as a single event to induce leukemia, and the authors suggested that the LNGFR transgene may have contributed to the oncogenic process. Notwithstanding this result, more than 100 patients who have received gene-marked marrow or T cells have shown no abnormalities attributable to this treatment with more than 10 years of follow-up available for the earliest patients. However, all patients will be followed for 15 years and any malignancies or autoimmune disorders that appear will be carefully studied for a possible contribution from the marker vectors. Disappointingly, T-cell leukemia or a leukemia-like disease has occurred in 2 of 10 patients with SCID given hematopoietic stem cells transduced with a recombinant onco-retroviral vector expressing the common cytokine receptor γ-chain (see below).

Therapeutic studies

One of the most publicized early series of gene therapy clinical studies involved the transfer of the ADA gene into the autologous peripheral blood lymphocytes and HSCs of patients with ADA deficiency. Although transduction of T cells was easier than targeting stem cells, and re-infused cells persisted for greater than 12 months, the frequency of gene transfer varied markedly (Blaese et al., 1995). In the two studies in which cord blood or bone marrow stem/progenitors were targeted, transduced cells could be demonstrated for long periods, but the level of gene transfer was also very low (<1%) (Bordignon et al., 1995; Kohn et al., 1995). However, each of these early trials demonstrated the feasibility and apparent safety of gene therapy with retroviral vectors. Furthermore, some improvement in lymphocyte numbers, T-cell ADA levels, and other indices of T-cell function were demonstrated (Onodera et al., 1998), and the treated patients appeared to obtain some clinical benefit. An important caveat is that in all these studies therapy with exogenous PEG-ADA protein was continued, albeit sometimes at reduced dosage. Kohn et al. (1997) reported the experience of ceasing PEG-ADA in a patient treated with ADA-transduced cord blood CD34+ cells. Unfortunately, a 50% fall in T-cell numbers was noted (although the proportion of transduced T lymphocytes did increase) in addition to a 100-fold fall in circulating B lymphocytes and natural killer (NK) cells. The low levels of long-term expression in the studies targeting ADA deficiency are somewhat disappointing, especially since transduced cells are expected to have a survival advantage over nontransduced cells in vivo and thus might be expected to increase over time, although this selective effect may have been somewhat diminished by the exogenously added PEG-ADA.

In five children with p47phox-deficient chronic granulomatous disease (CGD), Malech and colleagues (1997) collected mobilized peripheral blood stem cells by apheresis, transduced them ex vivo with a retroviral vector containing the p47phox cDNA over a 3-day period, and then re-infused them. Oxidase-positive neutrophils were first detected in the blood after 3 weeks and persisted for the next several months. The maximum percentage of corrected cells, however, represented only 0.004% to 0.05%

of circulating neutrophils. Similarly, in Fanconi anemia, in which transduced hematopoietic progenitors should also have a selective advantage, early results from a clinical trial showed only transient detection of the FANCC gene in peripheral blood and bone marrow cells (Liu *et al.*, 1997).

The above-mentioned studies, targeting a variety of inherited hematopoietic disorders, are tantalizingly close to demonstrating actual lasting clinical benefits from gene therapy. As informative as they were, though, they fall short of establishing an unequivocal lasting benefit from this treatment. In that aspect, the year 2000 was a watershed year for the field. One report (that of Abonour *et al.*, 2000) demonstrated that the incremental advances made in onco-retrovirus–mediated gene transfer efficiency, by using a fibronectin fragment in transduction protocols, for example, could combine to contribute to long-term engraftment of actual transduced HSCs. Indeed, in that study several patients receiving mdr-1 vector-transduced CD34+ cells, originating from mobilized peripheral blood, had 10% of bone marrow progenitor colonies positive for the transgene at 12 months. These levels of marking, if correlated with functional expression, could be curative for many disorders such as a number of lysosomal storage disorders including, for example, Fabry disease. Even more important in 2000, Cavazzana-Calvo and colleagues reported the successful treatment of two boys with X-linked SCID by a gene transfer approach in which HSCs were transduced with a recombinant onco-retroviral vector expressing the common cytokine receptor γ-chain. In that study, cells were transduced again in the presence of a fragment of the fibronectin protein and then infused into nonconditioned recipients. Figure 116.2 shows the results of the analysis of lymphocyte subsets from both patients over time. A clear increase in T-cell numbers occurred, that was accompanied by clinical improvement: both patients had improved immune system func-

tion and were able to leave protective isolation. Clearly a selective growth advantage occurred for these transduced cells; nonetheless, these combined results demonstrate that gene transfer efficiencies are now reaching levels that can impact clinical diseases. This study was expanded to include eight more patients, but unfortunately, at the end of 2002, it was announced that T-cell leukemia or leukemia-like disease had developed in two patients (American Society of Gene Therapy, 2003). The study has been put on hold pending investigation.

Lastly, another study further demonstrates that transduction frequencies are indeed becoming clinically relevant, which is also responsible for some of the current renewed enthusiasm in the field. Aiuti and colleagues (2002) transduced ADA-SCID patient bone marrow-derived CD34+ cells using conditions similar to those described above (Cavazzana-Calvo *et al.*, 2000) and re-infused the autologous, corrected cells into nonconditioned recipients who were not on enzyme replacement therapy. Multilineage gene marking was observed over time, and improved immune function as well as lower concentrations of circulating toxic metabolites were found. Even though these engineered cells likely had a distinct growth advantage in vivo this protocol and its successful outcome opens the door to treatment of a wide variety of inherited disorders that interact with the hematopoietic system in which full myeloablative conditioning of the recipient may not be tolerated.

Conclusions

Therapeutic efficacy of gene therapy has not been consistently demonstrated in many clinical trials to date. These initial studies are nonetheless important since they help identify specific problems to be overcome before gene transfer and delivery becomes effective therapy. Some success has also been

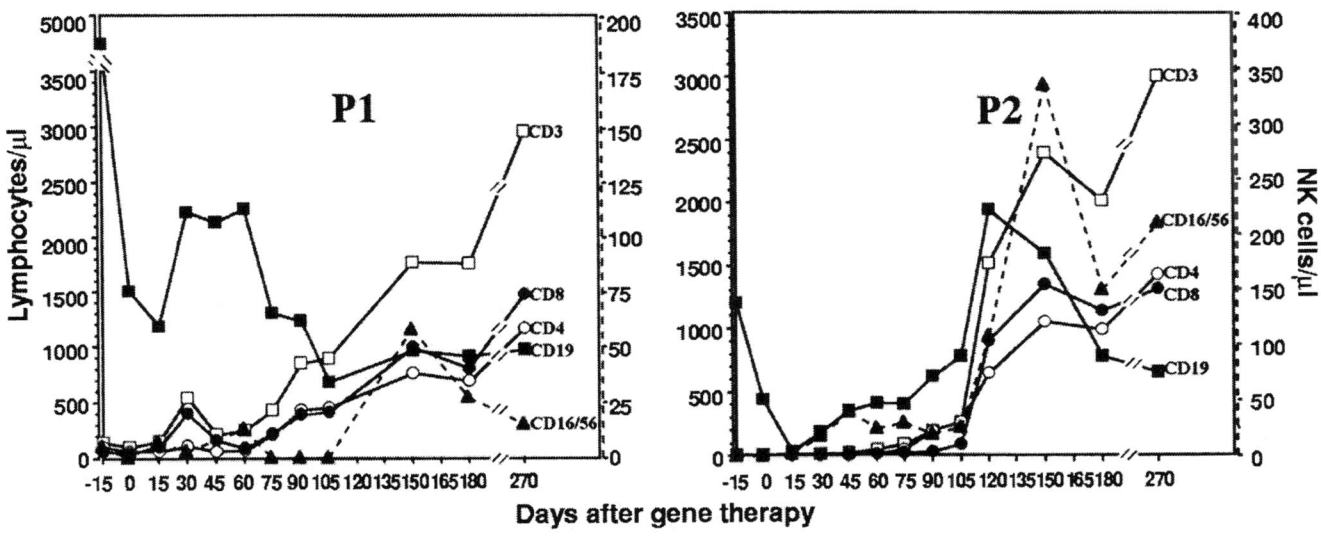

Fig. 116.2. Clinical course before and after gene therapy. Lymphocyte subset delineations from two X-linked SCID patients receiving gene transduced cells. Day 0 is the day of treatment. P1, patient 1; P2, patient 2; T cells (CD3, CD8, CD4), B cells (CD19), NK cells (CD16, CD56). Reproduced, with permission, from Cavazzana-Calvo *et al.* (2000).

observed that has renewed confidence that this therapeutic approach may eventually deliver on early promises. Yet major technical hurdles need to still be overcome before this treatment option is a panacea for all inherited or acquired diseases that interplay with the hematopoietic system.

At least three major issues require attention: the efficiency of gene transfer into pluripotent hematopoietic stem cells must be markedly increased; improvement in long-term expression of the transgene in engrafted cells may be necessary; and reproducible lineage-specific expression is highly desirable. Alternative strategies will also be useful and include the transduction of specific lineage-restricted populations such as lymphocytes (Rosenberg, 1992) or perhaps bone marrow stromal cells (Wu & Keating, 1991). Such cells may have a role as vehicles for delivering the correct gene product to appropriate sites without the necessity of gene transfer into the exact target cell at that site. Furthermore, numerous recent studies demonstrating the plasticity of hematopoietic cells and their utility in remodeling a variety of tissues offer promise that many gene therapy target disorders, whose historical effector cells are often refractory to isolation or transduction, may eventually be corrected.

Selected glossary

Amphotropic viruses

Retroviruses whose coat proteins bind to a receptor found throughout multiple species, including humans, making these vectors suitable for clinical use.

cDNA

A complementary copy of a stretch of DNA produced by recombinant DNA technology. Usually, cDNA represents the mRNA of a given gene of interest.

Calcium phosphate

This method of gene transfer relies on the production of a calcium/phosphate/DNA microprecipitate, which is then taken up by cells by pinocytosis. The method is very effective for a number of commonly used mammalian cell expression systems including COS, BHK, 293, and CHO cells.

Cis-acting factors

These are regions at a gene either upstream, within, or downstream of the coding sequence that contains sites to which transcriptionally important proteins may bind. Sequences that contain 5 to 25 nucleotides are present in a typical cis-acting element.

Ecotropic viruses

Murine retroviruses that contain coat proteins that can only bind to murine cellular receptors

Electroporation

When cells are suspended in buffer between two electrodes, discharge of an electrical impulse momentarily creates pores in the cell membrane. During this time, DNA in solution is free to diffuse into the cells. This method is highly successful in transfecting a large number of cell types, including cells previously thought to be difficult to transfect with other methods, such as endothelial cells and fibroblasts.

Enhancer

An enhancer is a segment of DNA that lies either upstream, within, or downstream of a structural gene that serves to increase transcription initiation from that gene. A classical enhancer element can operate in either orientation and can operate up to 50 kb or more from the gene of interest. Enhancers are cis-acting sequences that function by binding specific proteins, which then interact with the RNA polymerase complex.

Episome

A transient state where the transferred genetic material is not incorporated into the host genome, but exists as an extrachromosomal element that is eventually diluted or lost following cell division.

Expression vector

A plasmid that contains all of the elements necessary to express an inserted cDNA in the host of interest. For a mammalian cell host, such a vector typically contains a powerful promoter coupled to an enhancer, a cloning site, and a polyadenylation signal. In addition, several expression vectors also contain a selectable marker gene such as DHFR or NeoR, which aids in the generation of stable cell lines. The plasmid also requires a bacterial origin of replication and an antibiotic resistance gene (AmpR) to allow propagation and expansion in a bacterial host.

Liposomes

By encapsulating the DNA to be transfected in an artificial lipid carrier, foreign DNA can be introduced into the cell. This method, like electroporation, has been successful in transfecting cells previously thought difficult to manipulate.

Packaging cell

A stable cell line containing an integrated retroviral genome, usually split into multiple transcriptional subunits to minimize the possibility of recombination, and lacking the viral packaging function (ψ) and LTRs.

Polyadenylation

Following transcription of a gene, a specific signal near the 3′ end of the primary transcript (AATAAA) signals that a polyadenine tail be added to the newly formed transcript. The tail may be up to several hundred nucleotides long. The poly A tail seems to play a role in stability of the mRNA and transport through the nuclear membrane.

Polymerase chain reaction (PCR)

This technique finds use in several arenas of recombinant DNA technology. It is based on the ability of sense and antisense DNA primers to hybridize to a cDNA of interest. Following extension from the primers on the cDNA template by a heat-insensitive DNA polymerase, the reaction is heat-denatured and allowed to anneal with the primers once again. Another round of extension leads to a multiplicative increase in DNA products. Therefore, a minute amount of cDNA can be efficiently amplified in an exponential fashion to result in easily detectable and manipulable amounts of cDNA. By including critical controls and new permutations such as "real-time" PCR, the technique can be made fairly quantitative.

Producer cell

A packaging cell line transfected with the appropriate retroviral vector carrying LTR elements, packaging function, and gene(s) of interest. Introduction of the vector allows for recombinant retroviral virus production.

Pseudotyped virus

Alternative env protein components of a recombinant virion to change the tropism of the virus.

Reverse transcriptase

This enzyme, first purified from retrovirus-infected cells, produces a cDNA copy from an mRNA molecule if first provided with an antisense primer (oligo dT or a random primer). This enzyme is critical for converting mRNA into cDNA for purposes of cloning, PCR amplification, or the production of specific probes.

RT-PCR (reverse-transcription PCR)

This technique allows the rapid amplification of cDNA starting with RNA. The first step of the reaction is to reverse-transcribe the RNA into a first strand cDNA copy using the enzyme reverse transcriptase. The primer for the reverse transcription can either be oligo dT, to hybridize to the polyadenylation tail, or the antisense primer that will be used in the subsequent PCR reaction. Following this first step, standard PCR is then performed to rapidly amplify large amounts of cDNA from the reverse transcribed RNA. Often used to detect mRNA for genes that are expressed at low levels or where specific antibodies to detect expressed protein products do not exist.

Trans-acting factors

Proteins that are involved in the transcriptional regulation of a gene of interest.

Transduction

This term is often used to describe the insertion of a retroviral vector into a host that does not result in production of replicating virus because the crippled vector itself cannot initiate synthesis of viral proteins necessary for packaging.

Transfection

Most often referred to introduction of nonviral DNA. Once the expression vector has been assembled, it must be inserted into the host of interest. Several methods are available for such transfections and include calcium/phosphate/DNA complexes, DEAE Dextran, electroporation, and liposomes.

Viral transduction vectors

Onco-retroviral vectors are based on murine retroviruses. They can carry 6 to 7 kb of foreign DNA (promoter + cDNA) but suffer from the drawbacks of requiring the development of high titer packaging lines, requiring that target cells be dividing, and can be subject to host cell down-modulation. Lenti-retroviral vectors are usually based on HIV and, due to expression of numerous associated proteins, can infect nondividing cells. Adenoviral vectors can be produced at high levels and do not require a dividing target cell, but they do not normally integrate, resulting in only transient expression. Adeno-associated viral vectors are defective parvoviruses that can also infect nondividing host cells. Disadvantages are genetic instability, small range of insert size (2–4.5 kb), and production issues.

References

Abonour, R., Williams, D.A., Einhorn, L. *et al.* (2000). Efficient retrovirus-mediated transfer of the multidrug resistance 1 gene into autologous human long-term repopulating hematopoietic stem cells. *Nature Medicine,* **6,** 652–8.

Aiuti, A., Slavin, S., Aker, M. *et al.* (2002). Correction of ADA-SCID by stem cell gene therapy combined with nonmyeloablative conditioning. *Science,* **296,** 2410–3.

Akkina, R.K., Walton, R.M., Chen, M.L. *et al.* (1996). High-efficiency gene transfer into CD34+ cells with a human immunodeficiency virus type 1-based retroviral vector pseudotyped with vesicular stomatitis virus envelope glycoprotein G. *Journal of Virology,* **70,** 2581–5.

Aksentijevich, I., Pastan, I., Lunardi-Iskandar, Y. *et al.* (1996). In vitro and in vivo liposome-mediated gene transfer leads to human

MDR1 expression in mouse bone marrow progenitor cells. *Human Gene Therapy, 7,* 1111–22.

American Society of Gene Therapy (2003). Press release, January 14th, 2003.

Austin, T., Xu, J., Bohnlein, E., & Plavec, I. (1997). Molecular analysis of various stages of retroviral transduction in hematopoietic stem cell populations. *Blood, 90* (Suppl 1), 117a (Abstract).

Baum, C., Düllmann, J., Li, Z. *et al.* (2003). Side effects of retroviral gene transfer into hematopoietic stem cells. *Blood, 101,* 2099–114.

Bauer, Jr., T.R., Shwarz, B.R., Liles, W.C. *et al.* (1998). Retroviral-mediated gene transfer of the leukocyte integrin CD18 into peripheral blood CD34⁺ cells from a patient with leukocyte adhesion deficiency type 1. *Blood, 91,* 1520–6.

Benedict, C.A., Tun, R.Y., Rubinstein, D.B. *et al.* (1999). Targeting retroviral vectors to CD34-expressing cells: binding to CD34 does not catalyze virus-cell fusion. *Human Gene Therapy, 10,* 545–57.

Bertolini, F., Battaglia, M., Lanza, A. *et al.* (1997). Transwell stroma culture in the presence of FLT-ligand and thrombopoietin allows ex vivo expansion and gene transfer in NOD/SCID mice repopulating CD34+CD38– cells. *Blood, 90* (Suppl 1), 365a (Abstract).

Beyer, W.R., Wesphal, M., Ostertag, W., & von Laer, D. (2002). Oncortrovirus and lentivirus vectors pseudotyped with lymphocytic choriomeningitis virus glycoprotein: generation, concentration, and broad host range. *Journal of Virology, 76,* 1488–95.

Blaese, R.M., Culver, K.W., Miller, A.D. *et al.* (1995). T lymphocyte-directed gene therapy for ADA-SCID: initial trial results after 4 years. *Science, 270,* 475–80.

Blau, C.A., Peterson, K.R., Drachman, J.G., & Spencer, D.M. (1997). A proliferation switch for genetically modified cells. *Proceedings of the National Academy of Science USA, 94,* 3076–81.

Bodine, D.M., Karlsson, S., & Nienhuis, A.W. (1989). Combination of interleukins 3 and 6 preserves stem cell function in culture and enhances retrovirus-mediated gene transfer into hematopoietic stem cells. *Proceedings of the National Academy of Sciences USA, 86,* 8897–901.

Bodine, D.M., McDonach, K.T., Seidel, N.E., & Nienhuis, A.W. (1991). Survival and retrovirus infection of murine hemopoietic stem cells in vitro: effects of 5-FU and method of infection. *Experimental Hematology, 19,* 206–12.

Bodine, D.M., Orlic, D., Burkett, N.C. *et al.* (1992). Stem cell factor increases colony-forming unit-spleen number in vitro in synergy with interleukin-6, and in vivo in Sl/Sld mice as a single factor. *Blood, 79,* 913–19.

Bollard, C.M., Rooney, C.M., Huls, M.H. *et al.* (2000). Long term follow-up of patients who received EBV specific CTLs for the prevention or treatment of EBV lymphoma. *Blood, 96,* 478a (Abstract).

Bonini, C., Ferrari, G., Yerzeletti, E. *et al.* (1997). HSV-TK gene transfer into donor lymphocytes for control of graft-versus-leukemia. *Science, 276,* 1719–24.

Bordignon, C., Notarangello, L.D., Nobili, N. *et al.* (1995). Gene therapy in peripheral blood lymphocytes and bone marrow for ADA-immunodeficient patients. *Science, 270,* 470–5.

Bordignon, C., Yu, S.-F., Smith, C.A. *et al.* (1989). Retroviral vector-mediated high-efficiency expression of adenosine deaminase (ADA) in hematopoietic long-term cultures of ADA-deficient marrow cells. *Proceedings of the National Academy of Sciences USA, 86,* 6748–52.

Brenner, M., Mirro, J., Jr., Hurwitz, C. *et al.* (1991). Autologous bone marrow transplant for children with AML in first complete remission: use of marker genes to investigate the biology of marrow reconstitution and the mechanism of relapse. *Human Gene Therapy, 2,* 137.

Brenner, M.K., Rill, D.R., Heslop, H.E. *et al.* (1994). Gene marking after bone marrow transplantation. *European Journal of Cancer, 30A,* 1171–6.

Brenner, M.K., Rill, D.R., Holladay, M.S. *et al.* (1993). Gene marking to determine whether autologous marrow infusion restores long-term haemopoiesis in cancer patients. *Lancet, 342,* 1134–7.

Brodie, S.J., Lewinsohn, D.A., Patterson, B.K. *et al.* (1999). In vivo migration and function of transferred HIV-1 specific cytotoxic T cells. *Nature Medicine, 5,* 34–41.

Bunting, K.D., Galipeau, J., Topham, D. *et al.* (1998). Transduction of murine bone marrow cells with an MDR1 vector enables ex vivo stem cell expansion, but these expanded grafts cause a myeloproliferative syndrome in transplanted mice. *Blood, 92,* 2269–79.

Burns, J.C., Friedmann, T., Driever, W. *et al.* (1993). Vesicular stomatitis virus G glycoprotein pseudotyped retroviral vectors: concentration to very high titer and efficient gene transfer into mammalian and non-mammalian cells. *Proceedings of the National Academy of Sciences USA, 90,* 8033–7.

Carbanaro, D.A., Schmidt, M., Speckmann, C. *et al.* (2002). Clonality analysis after retroviral-mediated gene transfer to umbilical cord blood CD34+ cells from ADA-deficient SCID infants. *Molecular Therapy, 5,* S289 (Abstract).

Capecchi, M.R. (1989). The new mouse genetics: altering the genome by gene targeting. *Trends in Genetics, 5,* 70–6.

Cashman, J., Eaves, A.C., & Eaves, C.J. (1985). Regulation of proliferation of primitive hemopoietic progenitor cells in long-term human marrow cultures. *Blood, 66,* 1002–5.

Cavazzana-Calvo, M., Hacein-Bey, S., de Saint Basile, S. *et al.* (2000). Gene therapy of human severe combined immunodeficiency (SCID) X1 disease. *Science, 288,* 669–72.

Challita, P.M. & Kohn, D.B. (1994). Lack of expression from a retroviral vector after transduction of murine hematopoietic stem cells is associated with methylation in vivo. *Proceedings of the National Academy of Sciences USA, 91,* 2567–71.

Chatterjee, S., Li, W., Wong, C.A. *et al.* (1999). Transduction of primitive human marrow and cord blood-derived hematopoietic progenitor cells with adeno-associated virus vectors. *Blood, 93,* 1882–94.

Cheng, L., Lavau, C., Chen, S. *et al.* (1998). Sustained gene expression in retrovirally transduced, engrafting human hematopoitic stem cells and their lympho-myeloid progeny. *Blood, 92,* 83–92.

Cooper, L.J.N., Topp, M.S., Serrano, L.M. *et al.* (2003). T-cell clones can be rendered specific for CD19; toward the selective augmentation of the graft-versus-B-lineage leukemia effect. *Blood, 101,* 1637–44.

Cornetta, K., Tricot, G., Broun, E.R. *et al.* (1992). Retroviral-mediated gene transfer of bone marrow cells during autologous bone marrow transplantation for acute leukemia. *Human Gene Therapy,* **3,** 305–18.

Correll, P.H., Fink, J.K., Brady, R.O. *et al.* (1989). Production of human glucocerebrosidase in mice after retroviral gene transfer into multipotential hemopoietic progenitor cells. *Proceedings of the National Academy of Sciences USA,* **86,** 8912–16.

Cosset, F.L., Takeuchi, Y., Battini, J.L. *et al.* (1995). High-titer packaging cells producing recombinant retroviruses resistant to human serum. *Journal of Virology,* **69,** 7430–6.

Crooks, G.M. & Kohn, D.B. (1993). Growth factors increase amphotropic retrovirus binding to human CD34+ bone marrow progenitor cells. *Blood,* **82,** 3290–7.

Dai, Y., Roman, M., Naviaux, R.K., & Verma, I.M. (1992). Gene therapy via primary myoblasts: long-term expression of factor IX protein following transplantation in vivo. *Proceedings of the National Academy of Sciences USA,* **89,** 10892–5.

Dai, Y., Schwarz, E.M., Gu, D. *et al.* (1995). Cellular and humoral immune responses to adenoviral vectors containing factor IX gene: tolerization of factor IX and vector antigens allows for long-term expression. *Proceedings of the National Academy of Sciences USA,* **92,** 1401–5.

Dando, J.S., Roncarlo, M.G., Bordignon, C., & Aiuti, A. (2001). A novel human packaging cell line with hematopoietic supportive capacity increases gene transfer into early hematopoietic progenitors. *Human Gene Therapy,* **12,** 1979–88.

Dang, Q., Auten, J., & Plavec, I. (2000). Human beta interferon scaffold attachment region inhibits de novo methylation and confers long-term, copy number-dependent expression to a retroviral vector. *Journal of Virology,* **74,** 2671–8.

Dao, M.A., Hunnum, C.H., Kohn, D.B., & Nolta, J.A. (1997). FLT3 ligand preserves the ability of human CD34+ progenitors to sustain long-term hematopoiesis in immune-deficient mice after ex vivo retroviral-mediated transduction. *Blood,* **89,** 446–56.

Dao, M.A., Taylor, N., & Nolta, J.A. (1998). Reduction in levels of the cyclin-dependent kinase inhibitor p27kip-1 coupled with transforming growth factor β neutralization induces cell-cycle entry and increases retroviral transduction of primitive human hematopoietic cells. *Proceedings of the National Academy of Sciences USA,* **95,** 13006–11.

Davis, B.M., Koc, O.N., & Gerson, S.L. (2000). Limiting numbers of G156A O(6)-methylguanine-DNA methyltransferase-transduced marrow progenitors repopulate nonmyeloablated mice after drug selection. *Blood,* **95,** 3078–84.

Deisseroth, A.B., Kantarjian, H., Talpaz, M. *et al.* (1991). Autologous bone marrow transplantation for CML in which retroviral markers are used to discriminate between relapse which arises from systemic disease remaining after preparative therapy versus relapse due to residual leukemia cells in autologous marrow: A pilot trial. *Human Gene Therapy,* **2,** 359–76.

Donahue, R.E., Byrne, E.R., Thomas, T.E. *et al.* (1996). Transplantation and gene transfer of the human glucocerebrosidase gene into immunoselected primate CD34+ Thy-1+ cells. *Blood,* **88,** 4166–72.

Donahue, R.E., Sorrentino, B.P., Hawley, R.G. *et al.* (2001). Fibronectin fragment CH-296 inhibits apoptosis and enhances ex

vivo gene transfer by murine retrovirus and human lentivirus vectors independent of viral tropism in nonhuman primate CD34+ cells. *Molecular Therapy,* **3,** 359–67.

Dunbar, C.E., Cotter-Fox, M., O'Shaughnessy, J.A. *et al.* (1995). Retrovirally marked CD34-enriched peripheral blood and bone marrow cells contribute to long-term engraftment after autologous transplantation. *Blood,* **85,** 3048–57.

Dunbar, C.E., Seidel, N.E., Doren, S. *et al.* (1996). Improved retroviral gene transfer into murine and Rhesus peripheral blood or bone marrow repopulating cells primed in vivo with stem cell factor and granulocyte colony-stimulating factor. *Proceedings of the National Academy of Sciences USA,* **93,** 11871–6.

Dzierzak, E.A., Papayannopoulou, T., & Mulligan, R.C. (1988). Lineage-specific expression of a human-globin gene in murine bone marrow transplant recipients reconstituted with retrovirus-transduced stem cells. *Nature,* **331,** 35–41.

Eaves, C.J., Sutherland, H.J., Udomsakdi, C. *et al.* (1992). The human hematopoietic stem cell in vitro and in vivo. *Blood Cells,* **18,** 301–7.

Elwood, N.J., Zogos, H., Willson, T., & Begley, C.G. (1996). Retroviral transduction of human progenitor cells: use of granulocyte colony-stimulating factor plus stem cell factor to mobilize progenitor cells in vivo and stimulation by Flt3/Flk-2 ligand in vitro. *Blood,* **88,** 4452–62.

Emery, D.W., Yannaki, E., Tubb, J., & Stamatoyannopoulos, G. (2000). A chromatin insulator protects retrovirus vectors from chromosomal position effects. *Proceedings of the National Academy of Sciences USA,* **97,** 9150–5.

Emmons, R.V.B., Doren, S., Zujewski, J. *et al.* (1997). Retroviral gene transduction of adult peripheral blood or marrow-derived CD34+ cells for six hours without growth factors or on autologous stroma does not improve marking efficiency assessed in vivo. *Blood,* **89,** 4040–6.

Fan, X., Brun, A., Segren, S. *et al.* (2000). Efficient adenoviral vector transduction of human hematopoietic SCID-repopulating and long-term culture-initiating cells. *Human Gene Therapy,* **11,** 1313–27.

Fang, B., Eisensmith, R.C., Wand, H. *et al.* (1995). Gene therapy for hemophilia B: host immunosuppression prolongs the therapeutic effect of adenovirus-mediated factor IX expression. *Human Gene Therapy,* **6,** 1039–44.

Fisher-Adams, G., Wong, Jr., K.K., Podsakoff, G. *et al.* (1996). Integration of adeno-associated virus vectors in CD34+ human hematopoietic progenitor cells after transfection. *Blood,* **88,** 492–504.

Flasshove, M., Banerjee, D., Mineishi, S. *et al.* (1995). Ex vivo expansion and selection of human CD34+ peripheral blood progenitor cells after introduction of a mutated dihydrofolate reductase cDNA via retroviral gene transfer. *Blood,* **85,** 566–74.

Garcia-Sanchez, F., Pizzorno, G., Fu, S.Q. *et al.* (1998). Cytosine deaminase adenoviral vector and 5-fluorocytosine selectively reduce breast cancer cells 1 million–fold when they contaminate hematopoietic cells: a potential purging method for autologous transplantation. *Blood,* **92,** 672–82.

Gatlin, J., Melkus, M.W., Padgett, A. *et al.* (2001). Engraftment of NOD/SCID mice with human CD34(+) cells transduced by concentrated oncoretroviral vector particles pseudotyped with the feline endogenous retrovirus (RD114) envelope protein. *Journal of Virology,* **75,** 9995–9.

Goerner, M., Horn, P.A., Peterson, L. *et al.* (2001). Sustained multilineage gene persistence and expression in dogs transplanted with CD34+ marrow cells transduced by RD114-pseudotype oncoretrovirus vectors. *Blood,* **98,** 2065–70.

Gordon, M.Y., Hibbin, J.A., Dowding, C. *et al.* (1985). Separation of human blast progenitors from granulocytic, erythroid, megakaryocytic and mixed colony-forming cells by 'panning' on cultured marrow-derived stromal layers. *Experimental Hematology,* **13,** 937–40.

Hanawa, H., Kelly, P.F., Nathwani, A.C. *et al.* (2002). Comparison of various envelope proteins for their ability to pseudotype lentiviral vectors and transduce primitive hematopoietic cells from human blood. *Molecular Therapy,* **5,** 242–51.

Hanenberg, H., Xiao, X.L., Dilloo, D. *et al.* (1996). Colocalisation of retrovirus and target cells on specific fibronectin fragments increases genetic transduction of mammalian cells. *Nature Medicine,* **2,** 876–82.

Hantzopoulos, P.A., Sullenger, B.A., Ungers, G., & Gilboa, E. (1989). Improved gene expression upon transfer of the adenosine deaminase minigene outside the transcriptional unit of a retroviral vector. *Proceedings of the National Academy of Sciences USA,* **86,** 3519–23.

Harris, J.D. & Lemoine, N.R. (1996). Strategies for targeted gene therapy. *Trends in Genetics,* **12,** 400–5.

Hatzfield, J., Li, M.-L., Brown, E.L. *et al.* (1991). Release of early human hemopoietic progenitors from quiescence by antisense transforming growth factor b1 or Rb oligonucleotides. *Journal of Experimental Medicine,* **174,** 925–9.

Herman, G.E., Jaskoski, B., Wood, P.A. *et al.* (1989). Expression of human argininosuccinate synthetase in murine hemopoietic cells in vivo. *Somatic Cell Molecular Genetics,* **15,** 289–96.

Heslop, H.E., Ng, C.Y., Li, C. *et al.* (1996). Long-term restoration of immunity against Epstein-Barr virus infection by adoptive transfer of gene-modified virus-specific T lymphocytes. *Nature Medicine,* **2,** 551–5.

Heslop, H.E., Rill, D.R., Horwitz, E.M. *et al.* (1999). Gene marking to assess tumor contamination in stem cell grafts for acute myeloid leukemia. In *Autologous Blood and Marrow Transplantation,* ed. K.A. Dicke & A. Keating, pp. 513–20. Charlottesville, VA: Carden Jennings.

Hoogerbrugge, T.M., van Beusechem, V.W., Fischer, A. *et al.* (1996). Bone marrow gene transfer in three patients with adenosine deaminase deficiency. *Gene Therapy,* **3,** 179–83.

Jin, L., Siritanaratkul, N., Emery, D.W. *et al.* (1998). Targeted expansion of genetically modified bone marrow cells. *Proceedings of the National Academy of Sciences USA,* **95,** 8093–97.

Jin, L., Zeng, H., Chien, S. *et al.* (2000). In vivo selection using a cell-growth switch. *Nature Genetics,* **26,** 64–6.

Kalberer, C.P., Pawliuk, R., Imren, S. *et al.* (2000). Preselection of retrovirally transduced bone marrow avoids subsequent stem cell gene silencing and age-dependent extinction of expression of human beta-globin in engrafted mice. *Proceedings of the National Academy of Sciences USA,* **97,** 5411–5.

Kantoff, P.W., Gillio, A.P., McLachlin, J.R. *et al.* (1987). Expression of human adenosine deaminase in non-human primates after retrovirus-mediated gene transfer. *Journal of Experimental Medicine,* **166,** 219–34.

Kavanaugh, M.P., Miler, D.G., Zhang, W. *et al.* (1994). Cell-surface receptors for gibbon ape leukemia virus and amphotropic murine retrovirus are inducible sodium-dependent phosphate symporters. *Proceedings of the National Academy of Sciences USA,* **91,** 7071–5.

Kay, M.A., Manno, C.S., Ragni, M.V. *et al.* (2000). Evidence for gene transfer and expression of factor IX in haemophilia B patients treated with an AAV vector. *Nature Genetics,* **24,** 257–61.

Keating, A. (1991). New perspectives: gene therapy and autologous bone marrow transplantation. *International Autologous Bone Marrow Transplant Registry Newsletter,* **3,** 1–5.

Keating, A., Filshie, R., Mollee, P., & Wang, X.-H. (2002). Engraftment of gene-marked non-hematopoietic marrow mesenchymal cells: a platform for gene and cell therapy (submitted for publication).

Keating, A., Horsfall, W., Hawley, R., & Toneguzzo, F. (1990). Effect of different promoters on expression of genes introduced into hematopoietic and marrow stromal cells by electroporation *Experimental Hematology,* **18,** 99–102.

Keating, A., Powell, J., Takahashi, M., & Singer, J.W. (1984). The generation of human long-term marrow cultures from marrow depleted of Ia (HLA-DR) positive cells. *Blood,* **64,** 1159–62.

Keller, G., Paige, C., Gilboa, E., & Wangner, E.F. (1985). Expression of a foreign gene in myeloid and lymphoid cells derived from multipotent hematopoietic precursors. *Nature,* **318,** 149–54.

Koeberl, D.D., Alexander, I.E., Halbert, C.L. *et al.* (1997). Persistent expression of human clotting factor IX from mouse liver after intravenous injection of adeno-associated virus vectors. *Proceedings of the National Academy of Sciences USA,* **94,** 1426–31.

Kohn, D.B. (1997). Gene therapy for hematopoietic and lymphoid disorders. *Clinical and Experimental Immunology,* **107,** 54–7.

Kohn, D.B., Weinberg, K.I., Nolta, J.A. *et al.* (1995). Engraftment of gene-modified umbilical cord blood cells in neonates with adenosine deaminase deficiency. *Nature Medicine,* **1,** 1017–23.

Kohn, D.B., Weinberg, K.I., Shiegeoka, A. *et al.* (1997). PEG-ADA reduction in recipients of ADA gene-transduced cord blood CD34⁺ cells. *Blood,* **90** (Suppl 1), 404a (Abstract).

Korin, Y.D. & Zack, J.A. (1998). Progression to the G1b phase of the cell cycle is required for completion of human immunodeficiency virus type 1 reverse transcription in T cells. *Journal of Virology,* **72,** 3161–8.

Kremer, E.J. & Perricaudet, M. (1995). Adenovirus and adeno-associated virus mediated gene transfer. *British Medical Bulletin,* **51,** 31–44.

Kumar, M., Keller, B., Makalou, N., & Sutton, R.E. (2001). Systematic determination of the packaging limit of lentiviral vectors. *Human Gene Therapy,* **12,** 1893–905.

Laneuville, P., Chang, W., Kamel-Reid, S. *et al.* (1988). High-efficiency gene transfer and expression in normal human hemopoietic cells with retrovirus vectors. *Blood,* **71,** 811–14.

Larochelle, A., Vormoor, J., Hanenberg, H. *et al.* (1996). Identification of primitive human hematopoietic cells capable of repopulating NOD/SCID mouse bone marrow: implications for gene therapy. *Nature Medicine,* **2,** 1329–37.

Lever, A.M.L. (1996). HIV and other lentivirus-based vectors. *Gene Therapy,* **3,** 470–1.

Li, Z., Dullmann, J., Schiedlmeier, B. *et al.* (2002). Murine leukemia induced by retroviral gene marking. *Science,* **296,** 497.

Lim, B., Apperley, J.F., Orkin, S.H., & Williams, D.A. (1989). Long-term expression of human adenosine deaminase in mice transplanted with retrovirus-infected hemopoietic stem cells. *Proceedings of the National Academy of Sciences USA,* **86,** 8892–6.

Lin, Y., Chang, L., Solovey, A. *et al.* (2002). Use of blood outgrowth endothelial cells for gene therapy for hemophilia A. *Blood,* **99,** 457–62.

Liu, J.M., Kim, S., Read, E.J. *et al.* (1997). Engraftment of hematopoietic progenitor cells transduced with the Fanconi anemia group C gene (FANCC). *Human Gene Therapy,* **90,** 2337–46.

Malech, H.L., Maples, P.B., Whiting-Theobald, N. *et al.* (1997). Prolonged production of NADPH oxidase-corrected granulocytes after gene therapy of chronic granulomatous disease. *Proceedings of the National Academy of Sciences USA,* **94,** 12133–8.

Malik, P., McQuiston, S.A., Yu, X.-J. *et al.* (1997). Recombinant adeno-associated virus mediates a high level of gene transfer but less efficient integration in the K562 human hematopoietic cell line. *Journal of Virology,* **71,** 1776–83.

Mathews, K.E. & Keating, A. (1994). Gene transfer into IL-3 primed human early hematopoietic progenitors using electroportation: increased cycling improves efficiency. *Experimental Hematology,* **22,** 95 (Abstract).

May, C., James, R.I., Gunther, R., & McIvor, R.S. (1996). Methotrexate dose-escalation studies in transgenic mice and marrow transplant recipients expressing drug-resistant dihydrofolate reductase activity. *Journal of Pharmacology and Experimental Therapeutics,* **278,** 1444–51.

McKeon, C. & Samulski, R.J. (1996). NIDDK workshop on AAV vectors: gene transfer into quiescent cells. *Human Gene Therapy,* **7,** 1615–19.

Medin, J.A., Migita, M., Pawliuk, R. *et al.* (1996). A bicistronic therapeutic retroviral vector enables sorting of transduced CD34+ cells and corrects the enzyme deficiency in cells from Gaucher patients. *Blood,* **87,** 1754–62.

Migita, M., Medin, J.A., Pawliuk, R. *et al.* (1995). Selection of transduced CD34+ progenitors and enzymatic correction of cells from Gaucher patients, with bicistronic vectors. *Proceedings of the National Academy of Sciences USA,* **92,** 12075–9.

Miller, A.D. (1990). Retrovirus packaging cells. *Human Gene Therapy,* **1,** 5–14.

Miller, A.D. & Chen, F. (1996). Retrovirus packaging cells based on 10A1 murine leukemia virus for production of vectors that use multiple receptors for cell entry. *Journal of Virology,* **70,** 5564–71.

Miller, D.G., Adam, M.A., & Miller, A.D. (1990). Gene transfer by retrovirus vectors occurs only in cells that are actively replicating at the time of infection. *Molecular and Cellular Biology,* **10,** 4239–42.

Miyoshi, H., Blomer, U., Takahashi, M. *et al.* (1998). Development of a self-inactivating lentivirus vector. *Journal of Virology,* **72,** 8150–7.

Moore, K.A., Deisseroth, A.B., Reading, C.L. *et al.* (1992). Stromal support enhances cell-free retroviral vector transduction of human bone marrow long-term culture-initiating cells. *Blood,* **79,** 1393–9.

Movassagh, M., Desmyter, C., Baillou, C. *et al.* (1998). High-level gene transfer to cord blood progenitors using gibbon ape leukemia virus pseudotype retroviral vectors and an improved clinically applicable protocol. *Human Gene Therapy,* **9,** 225–34.

Naldini, L., Blomer, U., Gage, F.H. *et al.* (1996). Efficient transfer, integration, and sustained long-term expression of the transgene in adult rat brains injected with a lentiviral vector. *Proceedings of the National Academy of Sciences USA,* **93,** 11382–8.

Neering, S.J., Hardy, S.F., Minamoto, D. *et al.* (1996). Transfection of primitive human hematopoietic cells with recombinant adenovirus vectors. *Blood,* **88,** 1147–55.

Onodera, M., Ariga, T., Kawamure, N. *et al.* (1998). Successful peripheral T-lymphocyte-directed gene transfer for a patient with severe combined immune deficiency caused by adenosine deaminase deficiency. *Blood,* **91,** 30–6.

Orlic, D., Girard, L.J., Jordan, C.T. *et al.* (1996). The level of mRNA encoding the amphotropic retrovirus receptor in mouse and human hematopoietic stem cells is low and correlates with the efficiency of retrovirus transduction. *Proceedings of the National Academy of Sciences USA,* **93,** 11097–102.

Palmer, T.D., Rosman, G.J., Osborne, W.R.A., & Miller, A.D. (1991). Genetically modified skin fibroblasts persist long after transplantation but gradually inactivate introduced genes. *Proceedings of the National Academy of Sciences USA,* **88,** 1330–4.

Pawliuk, R., Westerman, K.A., Fabry, M.E. *et al.* (2001). Correction of sickle cell disease in transgenic mouse models by gene therapy. *Science,* **294,** 2368–71.

Poeschla, E., Corbeau, P., & Wong-Staaal, F. (1996). Development of HIV vectors for anti-HIV gene therapy. *Proceedings of the National Academy of Sciences USA,* **93,** 11395–9.

Pollok, K.E., van Der Loo, J.C., Cooper, R.J. *et al.* (2001). Differential transduction efficiency of SCID-repopulating cells derived from umbilical cord blood and granulocyte colony-stimulating factor-mobilized peripheral blood. *Human Gene Therapy,* **12,** 2095–108.

Ponnazhagan, S., Yoder, M.C., & Srivastava, A. (1997). Adeno-associated virus type 2-mediated transduction of murine hematopoietic cells with long-term repopulating ability and sustained expression of a human globin gene in vivo. *Journal of Virology,* **71,** 3098–104.

Poznansky, M., Lever, A., Bergeron, L. *et al.* (1991). Gene transfer into human lymphocytes by a defective human immunodeficiency virus type 1 vector. *Journal of Virology,* **65,** 532–6.

Qin, G., Takenaka, T., Telsch, K. *et al.* (2001). Preselective gene therapy for Fabry disease. *Proceedings of the National Academy of Sciences USA,* **98,** 3428–33.

Reems, J.A. & Torok-Storb, B. (1995). Cell cycle and functional differences between CD34+/CD38hi and CD34+/38lo human marrow cells after in vitro cytokine exposure. *Blood,* **85,** 1480–7.

Richter, J. (1997). Gene transfer to hematopoietic cells—the clinical experience. *European Journal of Haematology,* **59,** 67–75.

Riddell, S.R., Elliot, M., Lewinsohn, D.A. *et al.* (1996). T-cell mediated rejection of gene-modified HIV-specific cytotoxic T lymphocytes in HIV-infected patients. *Nature Medicine,* **2,** 216–23.

Rill, D.R., Santana, V.M., Roberts, W.M. *et al.* (1994). Direct demonstration that autologous bone marrow transplantation for solid tumors can return a multiplicity of tumorigenic cells. *Blood,* **84,** 380–3.

Rill, D.R., Sycamore, D.L., Smith, S.S. *et al.* (2000). Long term in vivo fate of human hemopoietic cells transduced by moloney-based retroviral vectors. *Blood,* **96,** 844a (Abstract).

Rooney, C.M., Smith, C.A., Ng, C.Y.C. *et al.* (1998). Infusion of cytotoxic T cells for the prevention and treatment of Epstein-Barr virus-induced lymphoma in allogeneic transplant recipients. *Blood,* **92,** 1549–55.

Rosenberg, S.A. (1992). The immunotherapy and gene therapy of cancer. *Journal of Clinical Oncology,* **10,** 180–99.

Rosenberg, S.A., Blaese, R.M., Brenner, M.K. *et al.* (2001). Human gene marker/therapy clinical protocols. *Human Gene Therapy,* **12,** 2251–337.

Roskrow, M.A., Rooney, C.M., Heslop, H.E. *et al.* (1998). Administration of neomycin resistance gene marked EBV specific cytotoxic T-lymphocytes to patients with relapsed EBV-positive Hodgkin disease. *Human Gene Therapy,* **9,** 1237–50.

Santana, V.M., Brenner, M.K., Ihle, J. *et al.* (1991). A phase I trial of high-dose carboplatin and etoposide with autologous marrow support for treatment of stage D neuroblastoma in first remission: use of marker genes to investigate the biology of marrow reconstitution and the mechanism of relapse. *Human Gene Therapy,* **3,** 257–72.

Schambach, A., Wodrich, H., Hildinger, M. *et al.* (2000). Context dependence of different modules for posttranscriptional enhancement of gene expression from retroviral vectors. *Molecular Therapy,* **2,** 435–45.

Schmidt, M., Hoffmann, G., Wissler, M. *et al.* (2001). Detection and direct genomic sequencing of multiple rare unknown flanking DNA in highly complex samples. *Human Gene Therapy,* **12,** 743–9.

Schuening, F.G., Kawahara, K., Miller, D. *et al.* (1991). Retrovirus mediated gene transduction into long-term repopulating marrow cells of dogs. *Blood,* **79,** 2568–76.

Shah, A.J., Smogorzewska, E.M., Hannum, C., & Crooks, G.M. (1996). Flt3 ligand induces proliferation of quiescent human bone marrow CD34+CD38– cells and maintains progenitor cells in vitro. *Blood,* **87,** 3563–70.

Sheridan, P.L., Bodner, M., Lynn, A. *et al.* (2000). Generation of retroviral packaging and producer cell lines for large-scale vector production and clinical application: improved safety and high titer. *Molecular Therapy,* **2,** 262–75.

Shi, P.A., Hematti, P., von Kalle, C., & Dunbar, C.E. (2002). Genetic marking as an approach to studying in vivo hematopoiesis: progress in the non-human primate model. *Oncogene,* **21,** 3274–83.

Shimada, T., Fulii, H., Mitsuya, H., & Neinhuis, A.W. (1991). Targeted and highly efficient gene transfer into CD4+ cells by a recombinant human immunodeficiency virus retroviral vector. *Journal of Clinical Investigation,* **88,** 1043–7.

Sinclair, A.M., Agrawal, Y.P., Elbar, E. *et al.* (1997). Interaction of vesicular stomatitis virus-G pseudotyped retrovirus with CD34+ and CD34+CD38– hematopoietic progenitor cells. *Gene Therapy,* **4,** 918–27.

Singer, J.W., Keating, A., & Wright, T.H. (1985). The human hematopoietic microenvironment. In *Advances in Haematology,* ed. V. Hoffbrand, pp. 1–24. London: Churchill Livingstone.

Smithies, O., Gregg, R.G., Boggs, S.S. *et al.* (1985). Insertion of DNA sequences into the human chromosomal globin locus by homologous recombination. *Nature,* **317,** 2304.

Sorrentino, B.P., Brandt, S.J., Bodine, D. *et al.* (1992). Selection of drug-resistant bone marrow cells in vivo after retroviral transfer of human MDR1. *Science,* **257,** 99–103.

Spencer, H.T., Sleep, S.E., Rehg, J.E. *et al.* (1996). A gene transfer strategy for making bone marrow cells resistant to trimetrexate. *Blood,* **87,** 2579–87.

Stewart, A.K., Sutherland, D.R., Nanji, S. *et al.* (1999). Engraftment of gene-marked hematopoietic progenitors in myeloma patients after transplant of autologous long-term marrow cultures. *Human Gene Therapy,* **10,** 1953–64.

Takenaka, T., Murray, G.J., Qin, G. *et al.* (2000). Long-term enzyme correction and lipid reduction in multiple organs of primary and secondary transplanted Fabry mice receiving transduced bone marrow cells. *Proceedings of the National Academy of Sciences USA,* **97,** 7515–20.

Teoh, G., Chen, L., Urashima, M. *et al.* (1998). Adenovirus vector-based purging of myeloma cells. *Blood,* **92,** 4591–601.

Thomis, D.C., Marktel, S., Bonini, C. *et al.* (2001). A Fas-based suicide switch in human T cells for the treatment of graft-versus-host disease. *Blood,* **97,** 1249–57.

Toneguzzo, F., Hayday, A., & Keating, A. (1986). Electric field mediated DNA transfer: transient and stable gene expression in human and mouse lymphoid cells. *Molecular and Cellular Biology,* **6,** 703–6.

Toneguzzo, F. & Keating, A. (1986). Stable expression of selectable genes introduced into human hematopoietic stem cells by electric field mediated DNA transfer. *Proceedings of the National Academy of Sciences USA,* **83,** 3496–9.

Toneguzzo, F., Keating, A., Glynn, S., & McDonald, K. (1988). Electric field-mediated gene transfer: characterization of DNA transfer and patterns of integration in lymphoid cells. *Nucleic Acids Research,* **16,** 5515–33.

Uchida, N., HE, D., Friera, A.M. *et al.* (1997). The unexpected G0/G1 cell cycle status of mobilized hematopoietic stem cells from peripheral blood. *Blood,* **89,** 465–72.

van Beusechem, V.W., Bart-Baumeister, J.A., Hoogerbrugge, P.M., & Valerio, D. (1995). Influence of interleukin-3, interleukin-6 and stem cell factor on retroviral transduction of rhesus monkey CD34+ hematopoietic progenitor cells measured in vitro and in vivo. *Gene Therapy,* **2,** 245–55.

Von Kalle, C., Kiem, H.P., Goehle, S. *et al.* (1994). Increased gene transfer into human hematopoietic progenitor cells by extended in vitro exposure to a pseudotyped retroviral vector. *Blood,* **84,** 2890–7.

Walker, R.E., Carter, C.S., Muul, L. *et al.* (1998). Peripheral expansion of pre-existing mature T cells is an important means of CD4+ T-cell regeneration HIV-infected adults. *Nature Medicine,* **4,** 852–6.

Walsh, C.E., Liu, J.M., Xiao, X. *et al.* (1992). Regulated high level expression of a human γ-globin gene introduced into erythroid cells by an adeno-associated virus vector. *Proceedings of the National Academy of Sciences USA,* **89,** 7257–61.

Walther, W. & Stein, U. (1996). Cell type specific and inducible promoters for vectors in gene therapy as an approach for cell targeting. *Journal of Molecular Medicine,* **74,** 379–92.

Watanabe, T., Kuszynski, C., Ino, K. *et al.* (1996). Gene transfer into human bone marrow hematopoietic cells mediated by adenoviral vectors. *Blood,* **87,** 5032–9.

Wells, S., Malik, P., Pensiero, M. *et al.* (1995). The presence of an autologous marrow stromal cell layer increases glucocerebrosidase gene transduction of long-term culture initiating cells (LTCICs) from the bone marrow of a patient with Gaucher disease. *Gene Therapy,* **2,** 512–20.

Wieder, R., Cornetta, K., Kessler, S.W., & Anderson, W.F. (1991). Increased efficiency of retroviral-mediated gene transfer and expression in primate bone marrow progenitors after 5-fluorouracil-induced hematopoietic suppression and recovery. *Blood,* **77,** 448–55.

Williams, D.A., Hsiech, K., De Silva, A., & Mulligan, R.C. (1987). Protection of bone marrow transplant recipients from lethal doses of methotrexate by the generation of methotrexate-resistant bone marrow. *Journal of Experimental Medicine,* **166,** 210–18.

Wolff, J.A., Malone, R.W., Williams, P. *et al.* (1990). Direct gene transfer into mouse muscle in vivo. *Science,* **247,** 1465–8.

Wu, D.-D. & Keating, A. (1991). Engraftment of donor-derived bone marrow stromal cells. *Experimental Hematology,* **19,** 485 (Abstract).

Yan, Z., Zhang, Y., Duan, D., & Engelhardt, J.F. (2000). Trans-splicing vectors expand the utility of adeno-associated virus for gene therapy. *Proceedings of the National Academy of Sciences USA,* **97,** 6716–21.

Yotnda, P., Onishi, H., Heslop, H. *et al.* (2001). Efficient infection of primitive hematopoietic cells by modified adenovirus. *Gene Therapy,* **8,** 930–7.

Zhou, S.Z., Cooper, S., Kang, L.Y. *et al.* (1994). Adeno-associated virus 2-mediated high efficiency gene transfer into immature and mature subsets of hematopoietic progenitor cells in human umbilical cord blood. *Journal of Experimental Medicine,* **179,** 1867–75.

Zufferey, R., Nagu, D., Mandel, R.J. *et al.* (1997). Multiply attenuated lentiviral vector achieves efficient gene delivery in vivo. *Nature Biotechnology,* **15,** 871–5.

117 Suicide gene therapy for control of graft-versus-host disease

CHIARA BONINI, FABIO CICERI, AND CLAUDIO BORDIGNON

Cancer Immunotherapy and Gene Therapy Program, Milan, Italy

Introduction

It is now well recognized that the curative potential of allogeneic hematopoietic stem cell transplantation (HSCT) is closely related to the immune advantage conferred by allogeneic T lymphocytes. Although the nature of effector cells is not yet fully elucidated, the allogeneic advantage in minimizing the risk of relapse is well documented by the superior results produced by transplants from allogeneic donors compared to those of autologous or syngeneic transplants. Furthermore, the administration of donor lymphocytes has recently become a new tool for treating relapse of hematologic malignancy postallograft (Kolb *et al.*, 1990, 1995; Collins *et al.*, 1997; Dazzi *et al.*, 2000). Furthermore, other complications related to the severe immunosuppressive status of transplanted patients, such as reactivation of cytomegalovirus (CMV) infection (Riddell *et al.*, 1992; Walter *et al.*, 1995; Einsele *et al.*, 2002) or Epstein-Barr virus-induced B-cell lymphoproliferative disorders (EBV-BLPD) have been successfully prevented and treated with donor lymphocytes (Papadopoulos *et al.*, 1994; Rooney *et al.*, 1995; Heslop *et al.*, 1996; Rooney *et al.*, 1998). However, the therapeutic impact of the allogeneic advantage is limited by the risk of graft-versus-host-disease (GVHD), a potentially life-threatening complication of allogeneic transplantation. The development of GVHD after allografting is mediated by alloreactive donor T lymphocytes infused with the stem cell inoculum. The role of alloreactive T lymphocytes in the induction of GVHD is supported by the impact of both the degree of HLA disparity between donor and recipient and the number of T cells in the graft on the incidence and severity of GVHD. No consistently effective treatment exists for established severe GVHD and the regimens of immunosuppression required to treat acute or chronic GVHD significantly limit the benefit of the transplant by eliminating or reducing the allogeneic attack on leukemic cells and by enhancing the incidence of infectious complications. For these reasons, different strategies have been investigated to prevent GVHD (Storb *et al.*, 1986; Waldman *et al.*, 1994; Ho *et al.*, 2001). Severe GVHD can be efficiently circumvented by the removal of T lymphocytes from the graft (Kernan *et al.*, 1986;

Champlin *et al.*, 2000). However, T-cell depletion increases the incidence of disease relapse and graft rejection, and delays immune reconstitution, resulting in an increased incidence of viral infections. Alternately, pharmacologic immunosuppression following the infusion of a T-replete transplant does not jeopardize marrow engraftment, and allows a significant graft-versus-leukemia (GVL) effect and immune reconstitution, but is only partially successful in preventing GVHD, especially after HLA-matched unrelated or partially HLA-matched related allografts. Thus, the possibility of obtaining all the benefits derived from donor lymphocytes while avoiding the risk of GVHD represents an important goal in the field of allogeneic HSCT. To this end, different strategies have been investigated in recent years.

The clinical application of the adoptive transfer of donor T cells

When the antigenic targets of T cells are known, it is possible to generate and expand antigen-specific cytotoxic T lymphocytes (CTLs) ex vivo. Adoptive transfer of virus-specific T cells has been extensively studied in animal models providing important information on the role of specific effector subsets and demonstrating the therapeutic role of T cells. At the present time, adoptive immunotherapy with T cells specific for viral antigens is being explored as treatment for human diseases caused by CMV and EBV reactivation occurring after allogeneic HSC transplantation (Riddell & Greenberg 1995; Rooney *et al.*, 1998). The transfer of these specific effector cells, rather than a heterogeneous lymphocyte population, should significantly reduce the risk of GVHD.

The first study in human beings investigating adoptive immunotherapy with virus-specific T lymphocytes in the context of allogeneic HSCT was developed by investigators at the Fred Hutchinson Cancer Research Institution, Seattle, as prophylaxis of CMV disease. Experimental animal models and clinical observations had documented that the development of CMV pneumonitis in immunosuppressed transplant recipients (a life-threatening complication) occurred exclusively in individuals without posttransplant CD8+ CMV-specific T-cell responses, and it was predicted that the adoptive recovery transfer of CMV-specific CD8+ T cells should be sufficient to confer protective immunity to this agent. These observations were the basis for the first clinical application that involved the prophylactic infusion of specific anti-CMV CD8+ donor-derived CTL clones to allograft recipients at high risk for developing CMV disease (Riddell et al., 1992; Walter et al., 1995). The adoptive transfer of T cells allowed short-term reconstitution of anti-CMV specific cellular activity and appeared to confer protective immunity, since none of the patients treated with these donor T cells developed CMV viremia or disease. Moreover, no toxicity or GVHD was observed. These studies clearly showed that, although the major effectors of antiviral activity are CD8+ T cells, CD4+ cells have a crucial role in promoting survival of CD8+ lymphocytes and long-term antiviral protection. These observations were then exploited in clinical trials based on the infusion of mixed subpopulations of donor-derived CMV-specific CD4+ and CD8+ T cells to transplanted patients (Einsele et al., 2002).

Another target of specific adoptive immunotherapy in the context of allogeneic HSCT is represented by the Epstein-Barr virus (see also Chapter 88). In allogeneic HSCT recipients, reactivation of EBV results in uncontrolled proliferation of mature B lymphocytes. The transformed B cells have an immunoblastoid or plasmocytoid appearance (Hanto et al., 1985), express virus-encoded latent cycle nuclear antigens, and are positive for most latent membrane proteins and for a number of cell adhesion molecules. All these phenotypic features make them vulnerable to immune effector cells of a normal individual. Normally, in fact, EBV-induced lymphoid proliferation is controlled by EBV-specific and MHC-restricted T lymphocytes that are cytotoxic toward EBV-transformed cells, as well as by MHC-unrestricted cytotoxic T lymphocytes and by antibodies directed toward specific viral antigens (Rickinson, Wallace, & Epstein, 1980). The profound immunosuppressive state of some allograft recipients allows uncontrolled proliferation of EBV-transformed cells. Usually, a lymphoma pattern with lymphadenopathy and hepatosplenomegaly is observed. However, the proliferating lymphoblasts may also infiltrate a variety of other organs including lung, liver, kidney, gut, and bone marrow. The B-cell proliferation may be polyclonal in the early stages, but eventually becomes oligoclonal or monoclonal, and the clinical course is rapidly progressive. In contrast to the drug-induced immune suppression of solid organ transplant recipients, the withdrawal of pharmacologic immunosuppression administered for GVHD to HSCT recipients does not provide fast immunologic reconstitution. For this reason, the prognosis of EBV induced in the setting of HSCT has up to now been very poor. While acyclovir, alpha-interferon, and monoclonal antibodies to CD21 or CD24 were used successfully for some patients with oligoclonal proliferations, they do not significantly modify the growth of EBV-transformed B cells in patients with monoclonal disease. Recently, monoclonal antibodies to CD20 have been used to treat posttransplant EBV-reactivation. Although successful in inducing com-

plete remissions, this approach is still limited by a high rate of relapse (Verschuuren et al., 2002). Since a limited number of specific cytotoxic T lymphocytes is required for controlling EBV-transformed B lymphocytes in normal individuals, it was thought that the administration of donor lymphocytes to treat BLPD in recipients of T-cell-depleted allografts could control this complication by providing donor immunity against EBV. In 1993 a clinical protocol for adoptive immunotherapy of EBV-BLPD was developed at the Memorial-Sloan Kettering Cancer Center, New York. Five patients with EBV-BLPD following T-cell-depleted allogeneic BMT received allogeneic donor lymphocytes. Complete pathologic and clinical response was observed in all patients, indicating the efficacy of the strategy. However, three of the five patients experienced chronic GVHD (Papadopoulos et al., 1994). A different approach was investigated at the St. Jude Children's Research Hospital, Memphis, where a clinical protocol was designed for the prophylactic infusion of genetically modified EBV-specific donor CTLs (Rooney et al., 1995). Although unable to completely eliminate EBV from the body, CTLs seem to be essential in maintaining control of latently infected cells. Specific anti-EBV CTLs can be readily generated in vitro by using autologous lymphoblastoid cell lines as stimulators, since the majority of immunocompetent individuals have a strong immune response to EBV. To determine if adoptive transfer of donor-derived EBV-specific CTLs could reconstitute the immune response to EBV and prevent EBV lymphoma in allograft recipients, both CD4+ and CD8+ anti-EBV CTLs were transduced with a retroviral vector containing a marker gene: the neomycin phosphotransferase (NeoR) gene (conferring resistance to the antibiotic neomycin and to its analog G418). Important information relating to the persistence and immunologic activity of CTLs was obtained from the first 39 patients treated: the transferred cells showed specific anti-EBV cytotoxic activity. EBV-specific T cells bearing NeoR were identified in all but one of the patients. Serial analysis of DNA detected the marker gene for as long as 18 weeks in unmanipulated peripheral blood mononuclear cells and for as long as 38 months in regenerated lines of EBV-specific cytotoxic T cells. The relevance of this phenomenon was indicated in six patients who had greatly increased amounts of EBV-DNA on study entry and showed 2 to 4 log decreases in viral DNA levels within 2 to 3 weeks after infusion. None of these patients developed lymphoma, confirming the antiviral activity of the donor-derived cells. There were no toxic effects that could be attributed to prophylactic T-cell therapy. The efficacy of the strategy was also confirmed in a therapeutic setting: two additional patients who did not receive prophylaxis and developed immunoblastic lymphoma responded fully to T-cell infusion (Rooney et al., 1998). All these observations suggest a wider use of CTL therapy in the future, possibly even for the treatment of solid tumors and leukemia.

The immunologic activity of donor lymphocytes has been successfully used to cure posttransplant relapse of hematologic malignancies. Patients who relapse after allogeneic HSC transplantation usually have a very poor prognosis, unless a second transplant can be performed. Moreover, the organ toxicity due to the transplant and to previous treatments reduces the likelihood of a successful outcome. Since 1989, it has been shown that recurrence of chronic myeloid leukemia (CML), acute myeloid leukemia (AML), lymphoma, or multiple myeloma after allografting can be induced into complete remission with the infusion of donor leukocytes without requiring cytoreductive chemotherapy or radiotherapy (Kolb et al., 1990, 1995; Szer et al., 1993; Drobyski et al., 1993; Van Rhee et al., 1994; Slavin et al., 1996; Tricot et al., 1996; Collins et al., 1997; Porter et al., 1994, 2000; Dazzi et al., 2000).

The use of a heterogeneous T-cell population with a wide range of antigen specificities carries some advantages over the use of antigen-specific CTLs. First, such a population can provide more complete immunologic reconstitution in immunocompromised transplant recipients. Moreover, since the antigen specificity of the GVL effector cells is not completely clear, the use of the entire T-cell repertoire is currently the best option for obtaining a GVL effect. Clinical and experimental studies, and the current concepts of the molecular basis of allorecognition, support the view that GVHD and GVL are mediated by host-specific and leukemia-specific donor T-cell subpopulations, respectively. We cannot yet differentiate, at a clinical level, between GVL and GVHD effector cells. Although the infusion of T lymphocytes long after the HSC transplant is expected to reduce the risk of severe GVHD, this risk is still present at higher doses of donor T cells. This clinical observation has been confirmed by two large studies performed by centers in Europe and the United States. These studies involved the infusion of donor lymphocytes to 135 and 140 patients, respectively, who experienced posttransplant relapse of hematologic malignancies. Acute GVHD of grade II or higher was documented in 41% and 46% of the patients, respectively, and chronic GVHD was observed in 61% of the patients. Moreover, myelosuppression was observed in 34% and 19% of the treated patients (Kolb et al., 1995; Collins et al., 1997). With the aim of obtaining the antitumor and antiviral effects in the absence of GVHD, different strategies have been developed: for example, modulation of the infusion parameters (time and number of administrations, dose of infused lymphocytes), enrichment of the population of infused lymphocytes thought to be responsible for the antitumor or antiviral activities, and depletion of the population responsible for GVHD. Since the number of donor lymphocytes required for a GVL effect is not completely predictable, investigators infused escalating doses of donor lymphocytes, beginning with small number of cells, usually not associated with GVHD, followed by infusions of higher number of donor lymphocytes until complete remission was obtained (Mackinnon et al., 1995). This strategy allows a GVL effect to be obtained, while reducing the risk of GVHD in some patients (Dazzi et al., 2000). However, the efficacy of this strategy is limited by the difficulty in predicting the time (often weeks or even months) required for GVL to occur.

An alternative strategy is enrichment of cells with antigen specificity potentially relevant for GVL. Although the targets of the antileukemic response are still not known, it is possible to isolate donor lymphocyte clones specific for minor histocompatibility antigens with restricted tissue distribution. Some of these antigens are expressed on the hematopoietic cells of the donor and on leukemic blasts (Warren et al., 1998; Mutis et al., 2002). The infusion of donor lymphocytes specific for such antigens could induce a selective GVL effect in the absence of GVHD. This validity of this approach, however, has not yet been confirmed clinically.

Because of these limitations, the possibility of controlling GVHD with an efficient, selective treatment would make both stem cell transplantation and donor lymphocyte infusions safer, more efficacious, and available to a larger number of patients.

The suicide gene strategy

A suicide gene encodes a protein able to convert a nontoxic pro-drug into a toxic product. Therefore, cells expressing the suicide gene become selectively sensitive to the pro-drug. The transfer of a suicide gene into donor lymphocytes could allow the in vivo selective (and elective) elimination of transduced lymphocytes, potentially resulting in a switch-off of the GVHD. Additionally, under appropriate conditions, it may allow in vivo modulation of donor antitumor responses, while eliminating GVHD. Finally, important questions concerning the survival and function of donor lymphocytes could be answered by their being gene-marked.

Different suicide genes have been investigated and described in recent years (Table 117.1), including the herpes simplex virus thymidine kinase (HSV-Tk) (Tiberghien et al., 1994; Bordignon & Bonini, 1995), a chimeric gene based on the death domain of the pro-apoptotic molecule FAS (Thomis et al., 2001) and the human B-cell molecule CD20 (Introna et al., 2000). Up to now, the HSV-Tk seems to be the most effective, and it is the first one to be used in clinical trials (Bordignon & Bonini, 1995; Bonini et al., 1997; Burt et al., 1999; Tiberghien et al., 2001). The HSV-Tk protein converts the pro-drug ganciclovir to its monophosphate intermediate derivative. Cellular kinases phosphorylate it to a triphosphate (GCV-3P) compound, which is the toxic form. GCV-3P can be incorporated into DNA, replacing deoxyguanosine triphosphate, resulting in inhibition of DNA chain elongation (Fig. 117.1). Therefore, gene transfer of the HSV-Tk gene into donor lymphocytes should allow their selective elimination by the administration of ganciclovir.

Safety issues and prelinical data

The safety of gene transfer into peripheral blood lymphocytes has been evaluated both in animal models and in previous clinical protocols of somatic gene therapy (Culver, Anderson, & Blaese, 1991; Bordignon et al., 1995; Blaese et al., 1995). The risk of oncogenic transformation of the cell following transduc-

Table 117.1. *Available suicide gene strategies*

Gene	Source	Pro-drug	Toxic product
Thymidine kinase (HSV-Tk)	Herpes simplex virus	Ganciclovir	Triphosphate-ganciclovir
Cytosine deaminase (CD)	*Escherichia coli*	5-fluorcytosine	5-Fluorouracil
Thymidine kinase (VZV-Tk)	Varicella-zoster virus	6-methoxypurine arabinucleoside (ARA-M)	ARA-ATP
Purine nucleoside phosphorylase (PNP)	*Escherichia coli*	Deoxy-erythropentofuranosyl-6-methylpurine	6-methylpurine
Cytocrome p450 2B1	Hepatocytes	Cyclophosphamide	Phosphoramide
ΔFas	Human cells	AP1903	
CD20	Human B lymphocytes	Anti-CD20 antibodies	

tion with a replication-defective retrovirus is extremely low. A significant number of patients have been treated in several protocols without any reported effect attributable to the gene transfer procedure. Retroviral vectors based on the Moloney murine leukemia virus were the first utilized in clinical trials and remain the most effective approach for the introduction of genes into human T lymphocytes. In fact, such vectors provide some important advantages compared to other gene transfer techniques. These advantages include the ability to incorporate up to 8 kb of cDNA, a high efficiency of gene transfer in replicating cells (more than 50% for human lymphocytes) (Bunnell et al., 1995), and the ability to integrate into the DNA of the target cell, leading to long-term gene expression and avoidance of dilution of the transferred gene by cell replication. The ability of murine amphotropic retroviruses to infect and replicate in primate cells was assessed in vitro, and the safety of gene transfer was extensively tested in monkeys.

The vector utilized in our first clinical study carried two genes: the first encoded the truncated form of the low affinity cell surface receptor of human nerve growth factor (ΔLNGFR); the second encoded a bifunctional protein carrying both the HSV-Tk activity (conferring ganciclovir sensitivity to transduced cells), and NeoR activity (Fig. 117.2). In previous studies, the possibility of using the LNGFR as a cell surface marker had been investigated (Mavilio et al., 1994). The use of a surface molecule for cell marking represents an important advantage over conventional strategies, which typically involve the use of nuclear markers. The cell surface molecule allows a rapid in vitro selection of transduced cells by using magnetic beads conjugated with an antibody directed to LNGFR. This selection

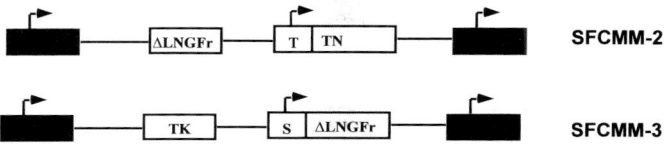

Fig. 117.2. Schematic map of integrated SFCMM-2 and SFCMM-3 proviral genome, indicating the HSV-Tk (T) and the SV40 (S) internal promoters. Solid boxes denote long-terminal repeat sequences. ΔLNGFR, modified form of the low-affinity receptor for nerve growth factor; TN, fusion gene encoding a bifunctional protein carrying both HSV-Tk activity and neomycin resistance; HSV-Tk, wild-type Tk gene. Arrows indicate transcription promoters. Reproduced, with permission, from Bonini et al. (1997).

approach minimizes culture time for the T cells, an important factor for preserving the T cells' immune repertoire. Additionally, a surface marker allows convenient ex vivo detection and characterization of the transduced cells by FACS analysis. To eliminate any possible functional activity of the cell surface marker, a modified form of the LNGFR gene, encoding a protein deleted of its intracellular domain, was utilized. This deletion completely abrogates the signal transduction activity of the receptor. Moreover, since LNGFR is a human protein, it is not expected to be a target of a specific immune response in the recipient of the transduced lymphocytes. The safety of the ΔLNGFR as a surface marker was evaluated both in vitro and in vivo. The addition of the ligand (nerve growth factor) to peripheral blood lymphocytes (PBL) expressing the ΔLNGFR did not change the in vitro pattern of cellular proliferation or of cytotoxic molecule secretion. Additionally, no differences in growth pattern, homing, or ability to metastasize were detected when transduced and nontransduced tumor cells were inoculated into syngeneic mice. The HSV-Tk gene has been successfully transferred into different cell lines to confer ganciclovir sensitivity and its efficacy has been shown both in vitro and in vivo (Moolten et al., 1990; Tiberghien et al., 1994; Munshi et al., 1997) (Figs. 117.3 and 117.4).

Clinical protocols for the treatment of malignant brain tumors through gene therapy with the HSV-Tk ganciclovir strategy have been designed (Culver & Van Gilder, 1994). In order to select an appropriate vector for the clinical study, different suicide retroviral vectors carrying the ΔLNGFR and the

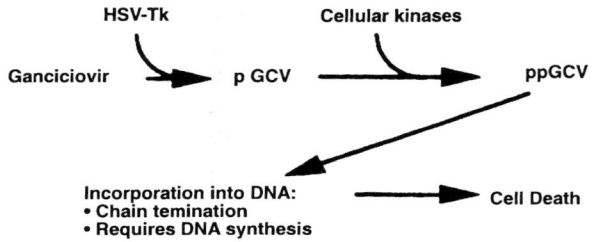

Fig. 117.1. Mechanism of action of ganciclovir.

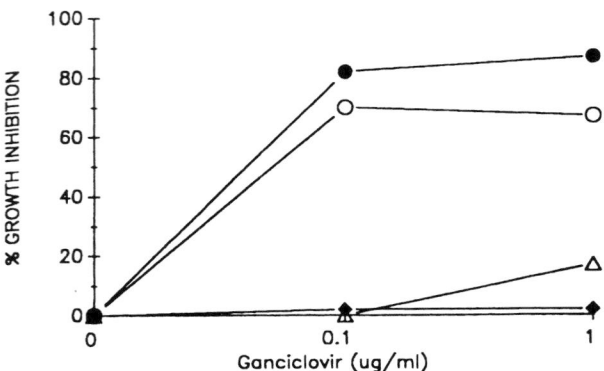

Fig. 117.3. GCV-induced growth inhibition of IL-2-responsive transduced (G1TkSvNa), G318-selected T cells [300 µg/ml G418 (○); 600 µg/ml G418 (•) T cells; transduced, nonselected T cells (△); and nontransduced, nonselected T cells (◆)]. Reproduced, with permission, from Tiberghien *et al.* (1994).

HSV-Tk genes were designed and compared in vitro and in animal models. The Tk activity of the vectors was investigated at different levels:

1. A Tk-deficient murine cell line (LTK) was transduced with the suicide vectors, and then selected in HAT medium in which only Tk positive cells can survive.
2. Interleukin (IL)-2 stimulated lymphocytes, transduced with the suicide vectors, were cultured in the presence of increasing ganciclovir concentrations.
3. Ganciclovir sensitivity conferred by the vectors was confirmed in animal models.

In all models utilized, all the vectors conferred Tk activity and ganciclovir sensitivity to the transduced cells (Bordignon & Bonini, 1995). In addition, animal models have indicated the

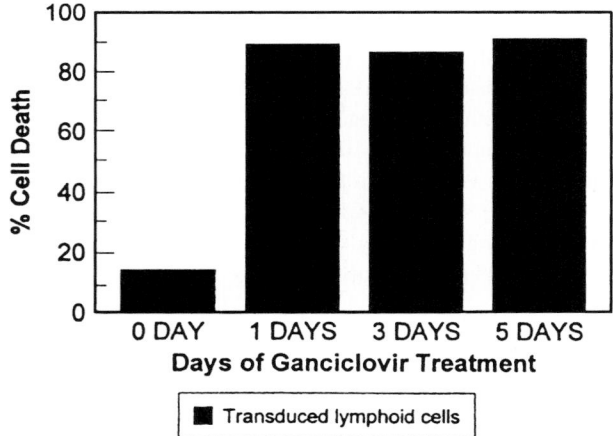

Fig. 117.4. Transduced lymphoid cells were cultured in the presence of 20 µmol/l GCV for 1, 3, or 5 days, at which time cells were resuspended in culture media, and the percentage of dead cells was assessed on day 5. Exposure to GCV for 1 day is sufficient for effective killing. Reproduced, with permission, from Munshi *et al.* (1997).

potential clinical utility of this approach (Cohen *et al.,* 1997; Helene *et al.,* 1997). Both these groups used murine models of BMT with donors transgenic for the HSV-Tk gene. Cohen and colleagues showed that a short (7-day) ganciclovir treatment, initiated at the time of BMT, effectively prevented GVHD in mice receiving Tk-expressing T cells (Fig. 117.5). These mice

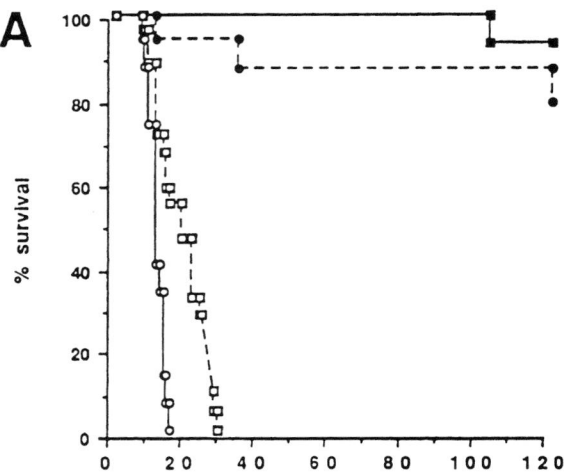

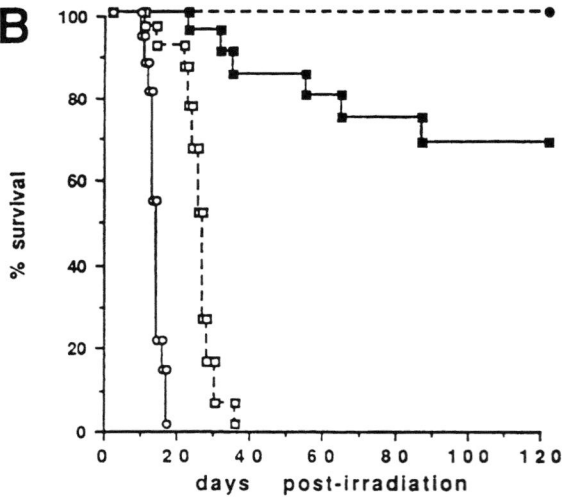

Fig. 117.5. Protective effect of a 7-day GCV treatment on the occurrence of GVHD in mice receiving (**A**) EpTk or (**B**) Ep△Tk transgenic T cells. Irradiation control group (○): Ungrafted irradiated B6 mice [*n* = 15 in both (**A**) and (**B**)]. Reconstitution control group (•): Irradiated B6 mice engrafted with FVB BM [n = *15* (**A**) and 11 (**B**)]. GVHD control group (□): Irradiated B6 mice engrafted with FVB BM plus either FVB nontransgenic T cells and GCV administration or transgenic T cells and PBS administration [*n* = 25 (**A**) and 23 (**B**)]. Experimental group (■): irradiated B6 mice engrafted with FVB BM plus (**A**) EpTk or (**B**) Ep△Tk T cells and treated with GCV [*n* = 13 (**A**) and 19 (**B**)]. Results are presented as Kaplan-Meier survival curves of cumulative data for each set of three independent experiments in both (**A**) and (**B**). Reproduced, with permission, from Cohen *et al.* (1997).

were healthy, had a normal survival, and maintained a T-cell pool of donor origin that responded normally to in vitro stimulation with mitogens or third-party alloantigens, but was tolerant to recipient alloantigens (Fig. 117.6). The same investigators subsequently showed that if the onset of ganciclovir administration is delayed until day 6, the GVL effect is preserved, while GVHD is still controlled (Litvinova et al., 2002). Similar results were obtained in the study by Helene and coworkers. Drobyski and colleagues also showed in a transgenic model that delaying the administration of ganciclovir until 8 to 12 days posttransplant allowed donor T cells that recognized alloantigens enough time to prevent rejection, but not enough time to cause severe GVHD (Drobyski et al., 2001).

A crucial issue raised in preclinical studies relates to the preservation of immune competence after in vitro gene transfer and selection. It has been reported that T-lymphocyte function is impaired by in vitro manipulation: compared to control cells, human T lymphocytes transduced with the HSV-Tk and neomycin resistance genes and selected in G418, had a 2.9 log reduction in clonogenicity (Tabilio et al., 2000). Moreover, Sauce and collaborators (2002) reported that a reduced EBV-specific immune reactivity was observed in genetically modified donor lymphocytes after inappropriate activation and in vitro drug selection. In this study the comparison of genetically modified cells with unmanipulated lymphocytes revealed impairment of immune function after in vitro manipulation. The data suggested that when appropriate activation is associated with immune selection (instead of G418 drug selection), EBV-specific T cells were preserved in the population of genet-

ically modified lymphocytes. Studies in rat and murine models of GVHD confirmed that, after appropriate transduction and immune selection procedures, T cells maintained their alloreactive potential, and that the administration of ganciclovir can control GVHD (Weijtens et al., 2001; Kornblau et al., 2001).

Clinical results

A phase I/II clinical study of the infusion of HSV-Tk transduced donor lymphocytes to patients affected by severe complications after allogeneic BMT began in 1993 at Ospedale S. Raffaele, Milan. This protocol was designed to evaluate:

1. The safety of increasing doses of donor lymphocytes transduced with a suicide retroviral vector
2. The efficacy in terms of survival and immunologic potential of donor lymphocytes after in vitro activation, gene transduction, and immunoselection
3. The possibility of in vivo elimination of GVHD by the administration of ganciclovir to patients treated by Tk-transduced donor lymphocytes

For patients 1 to 8 the SFCMM-2 vector (Fig. 117.2) was used to transduce donor lymphocytes. This vector encodes for the truncated form of the low affinity receptor for human nerve growth factor (ΔNGFR) and for a bifunctional protein carrying both the HSV-TK activity, conferring ganciclovir (GCV) sensitivity to transduced cells, and NeoR activity. For patients 9 to 23 the NeoR gene was removed in order to reduce the immunogenicity of the transgene. The NeoR-less vector, called

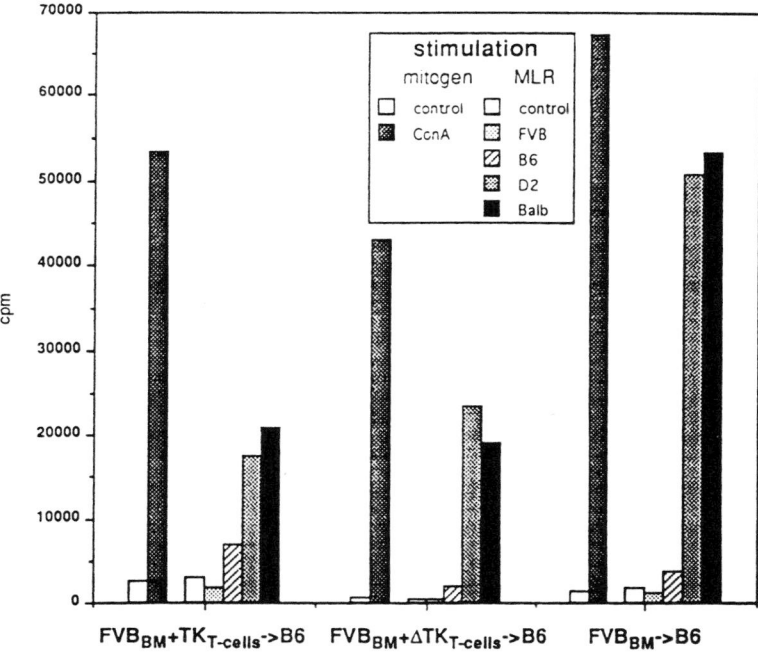

Fig. 117.6. T-cell proliferative responses after GCV treatment. Splenocytes were collected 6 to 8 months post-BMT and cultured in the presence of ConA or in MLR in the presence of donor (FVB), recipient (B6), or third party (D2 or Balb) irradiated splenocytes. Proliferative response of unmanipulated FVB splenocytes to ConA and allogeneic cells were comparable to that obtained with FVB$_{BM}$→B6. Reproduced, with permission, from Cohen et al. (1997).

SFCMM-3, confers higher GCV sensitivity to transduced cells: almost 100% of cells are killed by GCV concentrations reached in vivo. Patients received a mean dose of 4.4×10^7 CD3[+] HSV-Tk cells. More than 95% of transduced cells infused were CD3[+] and ΔLNGFR[+], and most were CD8[+] with an activated phenotype. The in vivo functional properties of transduced lymphocytes were evaluated by assessing immune reconstitution after T-depleted transplants as well as antitumor (GVL) and alloreactive (GVHD) responses; the ganciclovir sensitivity of transduced cells was assessed in vivo. Patients surviving less than 30 days after lymphocyte infusion were excluded from immune response analysis; patients surviving less than 90 days after infusion were excluded from GVHD analysis.

In this study we observed firstly that transduced cells survived in vivo and were detectable at a relatively high level (up to 13.4% of circulating PBL) and long-term (more than 5 years by flow cytometric analysis for the expression of the cell surface marker ΔLNGFR). Secondly, we noted that the infusion of genetically modified donor lymphocytes was followed by an antitumor response in 11 of 16 evaluable patients, with six complete responses. Thirdly, three patients developed GVHD requiring ganciclovir treatment. Ganciclovir-mediated selective elimination of transduced cells resulted in near resolution of all clinical and biochemical signs of acute GVHD in all affected patients (Bonini *et al.*, 1997) (Table 117.2) (Fig. 117.7).

Table 117.2. *Effect of ganciclovir treatment on elimination of genetically modified donor lymphocytes and on GVHD*

| | | Proportion of ΔLNGFR + PBLs (%) | | |
Patient	GVHD (grade)	Pre-ganciclovir	24 hours after ganciclovir	Clinical outcome
1	Acute skin (II–III)	13.4	<10⁻⁴	CR[a]
2	Acute liver (III)	2.0	<10⁻⁴	CR[b]
8	Chronic (extensive) lung, skin, GI	11.9	2.8	PR[c]

[a] Complete remission was revealed by clinical observation of complete regression of all skin GVHD signs.
[b] Complete remission was revealed by the disappearance of all physical and biochemical signs of liver GVHD (Fig. 117.4 and text).
[c] Partial remission of the severe obstructive bronchiolitis was revealed by physical evaluation and spirometric analysis. Amelioration of skin GVHD, but not of oral mucosa, was also observed. In oral mucosa, persistence of chronic GVHD and of genetically modified cells was confirmed histologically and by PCR, respectively. In patients 1 and 2, given the complete elimination of clinical signs of acute GVHD, a biopsy immediately after ganciclovir treatment was considered inappropriate and was not performed. However, follow-up biopsies performed later as part of the patients' monitoring were consistently negative for the presence of the transgene (PCR) and for GVHD.

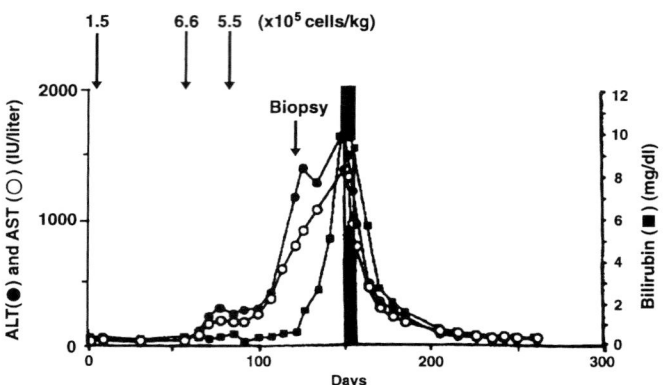

Fig. 117.7. ALT and bilirubin levels in a patient with hepatic GVHD induced by three infusions of HSV-Tk transduced donor lymphocytes (for treatment of relapse of leukemia post–allogeneic transplantation) and the rapid response of the hepatic GVHD to ganciclovir administration (black bar). Reproduced, with permission, from Bonini *et al.* (1997).

The major side effect of the strategy was the development of immunization against the transduced cells in 6 of 15 evaluable patients that resulted in complete disappearance of cells from the circulation. Additional limitations of the HSV-Tk/ganciclovir system include the potential need for ganciclovir to preempt or to treat CMV infection, and cell cycle dependence.

Similar data have been obtained by Tiberghien and colleagues (2001) using the HSV-Tk retroviral construct shown in Figure 117.8. In the latter study, a 3-day culture with IL-2 and an anti-CD3 monoclonal antibody was used to produce maximal proliferation of T cells followed by transduction on day 3 and then selection from days 5 through 12 of culture in G418. Twelve patients received a T-cell-depleted HLA-identical sibling marrow transplant together with HSV-Tk expressing T cells. The first 5 patients received 2×10^5/kg HSV-Tk T cells and the subsequent patients, 6×10^5/kg ($n = 5$) or 20×10^5 ($n = 2$). There was no infusional toxicity. All patients engrafted although 2 developed late graft failure and received a second HSC graft (unmodified). The presence of circulating genetically modified cells was shown in 10 out of 11 evaluable patients. Acute GVHD occurred in 3 patients simultaneously with an increase in the proportion of circulating genetically modified cells. Two patients had grade II (skin) acute GVHD involvement and both had a complete response with 5 to 7 days of ganciclovir treatment. The third had grade III acute GVHD with skin and liver involvement and had a complete response to the combination of ganciclovir and corticosteroids. One patient who developed chronic GVHD had a complete response to ganciclovir. T cells transduced with HSV-Tk were detectable in the circulation early posttransplant and subsequently decreased in number, although long-lasting circulation was documented and these cells were sensitive to in vitro incubation with ganciclovir. Interestingly, in patients treated with ganciclovir for GVHD, there was a progressive increase in the proportion of

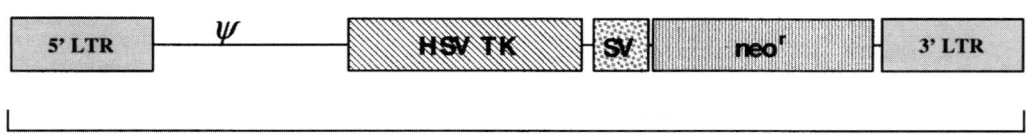

4.5 kb

Fig. 117.8. G1Tk1SvNa vector and preparation of the HS-Tk-expressing T cells. G1Tk1SvNa vector. MSV indicates Moloney sarcoma virus; LTR, long terminal repeat; MLV, Moloney leukemia virus. Reproduced, with permission, from Tiberghien *et al.* (2001).

transduced T cells carrying a deletion due to the presence of cryptic splice donor acceptor sites within the HSV-Tk gene sequence, giving rise to ganciclovir resistance (Garin *et al.*, 2001).

In a study conducted by Link and colleagues (1998), in which lymphocytes expressing HSV-Tk and NeoR were administered for the treatment of posttransplant disease relapse, no adverse reactions attributable to lymphocytes were noted. In treated patients, the percent of circulating transduced lymphocytes ranged from 0 to 3.8%. Three patients responded to the infusion in terms of antitumor activity and 3 did not respond (CML). One patient developed chronic GVHD that did not respond to conventional therapy but did respond to ganciclovir (Link *et al.*, 1998; Burt *et al.*, 1999).

Champlin and colleagues (1999) conducted a Phase I/II study with lymphocytes genetically modified with HSV-Tk for posttransplant relapse. Twenty-three patients were treated with 1 to 4 doses per patient (from 0.7 to 190×10^6 cells/kg). In almost all patients it was possible to document the presence of circulating transduced cells, and there was no adverse reaction to the treatment. Two patients, affected by CML, had a complete remission with a dose of 50 or 85×10^6 cells/kg; 4 remained stable and 17 had disease progression. Only one patient developed grade I GVHD for which no therapy was needed.

Additional novel suicide genes, potentially able to overcome the limitations of HSV-Tk have been proposed. In particular, a Fas-based suicide switch based on chemically induced apoptosis may resolve some or all of these problems (Thomis *et al.*, 2001). In this system a chimeric human protein was expressed comprising an extracellular marker (truncated human LNGFR), the Fas intracellular domain, and two copies of the FK506-binding protein (FKBP). The extracellular marker allowed purification to homogeneity of human T cells transduced with this retroviral construct. These T cells retained the ability to mount a specific allogeneic response. However, they rapidly underwent apoptosis with the addition of subnanomolar concentrations of AP1903, a bivalent dimerizer drug that binds FKBP and induces Fas cross-linking. A single 2-hour treatment eliminated approximately 80% of T cells, and multiple exposures induced further apoptosis. T cells were eliminated regardless of their proliferation status. The technology utilizes a synthetic small molecule to mediate dimerization of proteins leading to activation of a transduced apoptosis gene (Neff & Blau, 2001).

An alternative approach is based on the transduction of human T cells with a retroviral vector coding for the human CD20 cDNA and subsequent destruction by exposure of the T cells to the monoclonal chimeric anti-CD20 monoclonal antibody, Rituxan, in the presence of complement (Introna *et al.*, 2000). If validated in the clinical setting, these genes could permit the full clinical exploitation of the suicide gene strategy in allogeneic HSCT.

The preclinical and clinical data indicate that genetically modified T cells maintain their in vivo potential to mediate both antitumor and GVHD effects, and may represent a potent new tool for exploiting both antitumor and antihost immunity, while providing a selective and elective method for the elimination of acute GVHD, as well as the augmentation of early immune reconstitution (Marktel *et al.*, 2003).

References

Blaese, R.M., Culver, W.K., Miller, A.D. *et al.* (1995). T lymphocyte-directed gene therapy for ADA-SCID: initial trial results after 4 years. *Science*, **270**, 475–80.

Bonini, C., Ferrari, G., Verzeletti, S. *et al.* (1997). HSV-Tk gene transfer into donor lymphocytes for control of allogeneic graft-versus-leukemia. *Science*, **276**, 1719–24.

Bordignon, C. & Bonini, C. (1995). A clinical protocol for gene transfer into peripheral blood lymphocytes for in vivo immunomodulation of donor anti-tumor immunity in patients affected by recurrent disease after allogeneic bone marrow transplantation. *Human Gene Therapy*, **2**, 813–19.

Bordignon, C., Notarangelo, L.D., Nobili, N. *et al.* (1995). Gene therapy in peripheral blood lymphocytes and bone marrow for ADA-immunodeficient patients. *Science*, **270**, 470–5.

Bunnell, B.A., Muul, L.M., Donahue, R.E. *et al.* (1995). High-efficiency retroviral-mediated gene transfer into human and nonhuman primate peripheral blood lymphocytes. *Proceedings of the National Academy of Science USA*, **92**, 7739–43.

Burt, R.K., Drobyski, W.R., Traynor, A.E., & Link, C.J. (1999). Herpes simplex thymidine kinase (HSVTk) transgenic donor lymphocytes. *Bone Marrow Transplantation*, **24**, 1043–51.

Champlin, R., Besinger, W., Henslee-Downey, J. *et al.* (2000). Phase I/II study of thymidine kinase (TK)-transduced donor lymphocyte infusions (DLI) in patients with hematologic malignancies. *Blood*, **94**, 1448a.

Cohen, J.L., Boyer, O., Salomon, B. *et al.* (1997). Prevention of graft-versus-host disease in mice using a suicide gene expressed in T lymphocytes. *Blood*, **89**, 4636–45.

Collins, R.H., Shpilberg, O.J., Drobyski, W.R. *et al.* (1997). Donor leukocyte infusions in 140 patients with relapsed malignancy after allogeneic bone marrow transplantation. *Journal of Clinical Oncology,* **15,** 433.

Culver, K.W., Anderson, W.F., & Blaese, R.M. (1991). Lymphocyte gene therapy. *Human Gene Therapy,* **2,** 107–8.

Culver, K.W. & Van Gilder, J. (1994). Clinical protocol: gene therapy for the treatment of malignant brain tumors with in vivo tumor transduction with herpes simplex thymidine kinase gene/ganciclovir system. *Human Gene Therapy,* **5,** 343–79.

Dazzi, F., Szydlo, R.M., Craddock, C. *et al.* (2000). Comparison of single-dose and escalating-dose regimens of donor lymphocyte infusion for relapse after allografting for chronic myeloid leukemia. *Blood,* **95,** 67.

Drobyski, W.R., Keever, C.A., Roth, M.S. *et al.* (1993). Salvage immunotherapy using donor leukocyte infusions as treatment for relapsed chronic myelogenous leukemia after allogeneic bone marrow transplantation: efficacy and toxicity of a defined T-cell dose. *Blood,* **82,** 2310.

Drobyski, W.R., Morse, H.C., Burns, W.H. *et al.* (2001). Protection from lethal murine graft-versus-host disease without compromise of alloengraftment using transgenic donor T cells expressing a thymidine kinase suicide gene. *Blood,* **97,** 2506.

Einsele, H., Roosnek, E., Rufer, N. *et al.* (2002). Infusion of cytomegalovirus (CMV)-specific T cells for the treatment of CMV infection not responding to antiviral chemotherapy. *Blood,* **99,** 3916.

Garin, M.I., Garrett, E., Tiberghien, P. *et al.* (2001). Molecular mechanism for ganciclovir resistance in human T lymphocytes transduced with retroviral vectors carrying the herpes simplex virus thymidine kinase gene. *Blood,* **97,** 122–9.

Hanto, D.W., Frizzera, G., Gajl-Peczalska, K.J. *et al.* (1985). Epstein-Barr virus, immunodeficiency and B cell lymphoproliferation. *Transplantation,* **39,** 461–72.

Helene, M., Lake-Bullock, V., Bryson, J.C. *et al.* (1997). Inhibition of graft-versus-host disease: use of a T cell-controlled suicide gene. *Journal of Immunology,* **158,** 5079–82.

Heslop, H.E., Ng, C.Y.C., Li, C. *et al.* (1996). Long-term restoration of immunity against Epstein-Barr virus infection by adoptive transfer of gene-modified virus-specific T lymphocytes. *Nature Medicine,* **2,** 551–5.

Ho, V.T. & Soiffer, R.J. (2001). The history and future of T-cell depletion as graft-versus-host disease prophylaxis for allogeneic hematopoietic stem cell transplantation. *Blood,* **98,** 3192.

Introna, M., Bambacioni, F., Barbui, A.M. *et al.* (2000). Genetic modification of human T cells with CD20: a strategy to purify and lyse transduced cells with anti-CD20 antibodies. *Human Gene Therapy,* **11,** 611–20.

Kernan, N.A., Collins, N.H., Juliano, L. *et al.* (1986). Clonable T lymphocytes in T cell-depleted bone marrow transplants correlate with development of graft-versus-host disease. *Blood,* **68,** 770–3.

Kolb, H.J., Mittermtiller, J., Clemm, C.H. *et al.* (1990). Donor leukocyte transfusions for treatment of recurrent chronic myelogenous leukemia in marrow transplant patients. *Blood,* **76,** 2462–5.

Kolb, H.J., Schattenberg, A., Goldman, J.M. *et al.* (1995). Graft-versus-leukemia effect of donor lymphocyte transfusions in marrow grafted patients. *Blood,* **86,** 2041–50.

Kornblau, S.M., Stiouf, I., Snell, V. *et al.* (2001). Preemptive control of graft-versus-host disease in a murine allogeneic transplant model using retrovirally transduced murine suicidal lymphocytes. *Cancer Research,* **61,** 3355.

Link, C.J., Burt, R.K., Traynor, A.E. *et al.* (1998). Adoptive immunotherapy for leukemia: donor lymphocytes transduced with the herpes simplex thymidine kinase gene for remission induction. *Human Gene Therapy,* **9,** 115.

Litvinova, E., Maury, S., Boyer, O. *et al.* (2002). Graft-versus-leukemia effect after suicide-gene-mediated control of graft-versus-host disease. *Blood,* **100,** 2020.

Mackinnon, S., Papadopoulos, E.B., Carabasi, M.H. *et al.* (1995). Adoptive immunotherapy evaluating escalating doses of donor leukocytes for relapse of chronic myeloid leukemia after bone marrow transplantation: separation of graft-versus-leukemia responses from graft-versus-host disease. *Blood,* **86,** 1261.

Marktel, S., Magnani, Z., Ciceri, F. *et al.* (2003). Immunologic potential of donor lymphocytes expressing a suicide gene for early immune reconstitution after hematopoietic T-cell-depleted stem cell transplantation. *Blood,* **101,** 1290–8.

Mavilio, F., Ferrari, G., Rossini, S. *et al.* (1994). Peripheral blood lymphocytes as target cells of retroviral vector-mediated gene transfer. *Blood,* **83,** 1988–97.

Moolten, F.L., Wells, J.M., Heyman, R.A. *et al.* (1990). Lymphoma regression induced by ganciclovir in mice bearing a herpes thymidine kinase transgene. *Human Gene Therapy,* **1,** 125–34.

Munshi, N.C., Govindarajan, R., Drake, R. *et al.* (1997). Thymidine kinase (TK) gene-transduced human lymphocytes can be highly purified, remain fully functional, and are killed efficiently with ganciclovir. *Blood,* **89,** 1334–40.

Mutis, T., Blokland, E., Kester, M. *et al.* (2002). Generation of minor histocompatibility antigen HA-1-specific cytotoxic T cells restricted by nonself HLA molecules: a potential strategy to treat relapsed leukemia after HLA-mismatched stem cell transplantation. *Blood,* **100,** 547.

Neff, T. & Blau, C.A. (2001). Pharmacologically regulated cell therapy. *Blood,* **97,** 2535–40.

Papadopoulos, E.B., Ladanyi, M., Emanuel, D. *et al.* (1994). Infusions of donor leukocytes to treat Epstein-Barr virus-associated lymphoproliferative disorders after allogeneic bone marrow transplantation. *New England Journal of Medicine,* **330,** 1185–91.

Porter, D.L., Collins, R.H.J., Hardy, C. *et al.* (2000). Treatment of relapsed leukemia after unrelated donor marrow transplantation with unrelated donor leukocyte infusions. *Blood,* **95,** 1214.

Porter, D.L., Roth, M.S., Mc Garigle, C. *et al.* (1994). Induction of a graft-versus-host disease as immunotherapy for relapsed chronic myeloid leukemia. *New England Journal of Medicine,* **330,** 100.

Rickinson, A.B., Wallace, L.E., & Epstein, M.A. (1980). HLA restricted T-cell recognition of EBV-infected B cells. *Nature,* **283,** 865–7.

Riddell, S.R. & Greenberg, P.D. (1995). Principles for adoptive T cell therapy of human viral diseases. *Annual Review of Immunology,* **13,** 545–86.

Riddell, S.R., Watanabe, K.S., Goodrich, J.M. *et al.* (1992). Restoration of viral immunity in immunodeficient humans by adoptive transfer of T cell clones. *Science,* **257,** 238–41.

Rooney, C.M., Smith, C.A., Ng, C.Y.C. *et al.* (1995). Use of gene-modified virus-specific T lymphocytes to control Epstein-Barr-virus related lymphoproliferation. *Lancet,* **345,** 9–13.

Rooney, C.M., Smith, C.A., Ng, C.Y.C. *et al.* (1998). Infusion of cytotoxic T cells for the prevention and treatment of Epstein-Barr virus-induced lymphoma in allogeneic transplant recipients. *Blood,* **92,** 1549.

Sauce, D., Bodinier, M., Garin, M. *et al.* (2002). Retrovirus-mediated gene transfer in primary T lymphocytes impairs their anti-Epstein-Barr virus potential through both culture-dependent and selection process-dependent mechanisms. *Blood,* **99,** 1165.

Slavin, S., Naparstek, E., Nagler, A. *et al.* (1996). Allogeneic cell therapy with donor peripheral blood cells and recombinant human interleukin-2 to treat leukemia relapse after allogeneic bone marrow transplantation. *Blood,* **87,** 2195–204.

Storb, R., Deeg, H.J., Whitehead, J, *et al.* (1986). Methotrexate and cyclosporine compared with cyclosporine alone for prophylaxis of acute graft-versus-host disease after marrow transplantation for leukemia. *New England Journal of Medicine,* **314,** 729.

Szer, J., Grigg, A.P., Phillips, G.L., & Sheridan, W.P. (1993). Donor leukocyte infusions after chemotherapy for patients relapsing with acute leukemia following allogeneic BMT. *Bone Marrow Transplantation,* **11,** 109.

Tabilio, A., Di Florio, S., Di Ianni, M. *et al.* (2000). T-lymphocyte function after retroviral-mediated thymidine kinase gene transfer and G418 selection. *Cancer Gene Therapy,* **7,** 920–6.

Theobald, M. (1995). Allo recognition and graft-versus-host disease. *Bone Marrow Transplantation,* **15,** 489–98.

Thomis, D.C., Marktel, S., Bonini, C. *et al.* (2001). A Fas-based suicide switch in human T cells for the treatment of graft-versus-host disease. *Blood,* **97,** 1249–57.

Tiberghien, P., Reynolds, C.W., Keller, J. *et al.* (1994). Ganciclovir treatment of herpes simplex thymidine kinase-transduced primary T lymphocytes: an approach for specific in vivo donor T-cell depletion after bone marrow transplantation? *Blood,* **84,** 1333–41.

Tiberghien, P., Ferrand, C., Lioure, B. *et al.* (2001). Administration of herpes simplex-thymidine kinase-expressing donor T cells with a T-cell-depleted allogeneic marrow graft. *Blood,* **97,** 63–72.

Tricot, G., Vesole, D.H., Jagganath, S. *et al.* (1996). Graft-versus-myeloma effect: proof of principle. *Blood,* **87,** 1196–8.

Van Rhee, F., Lin, F., Cullis, J.O. *et al.* (1994). Relapse of chronic myeloid leukemia after allogeneic bone marrow transplant: the case for giving donor leukocyte transfusions before the onset of hematologic relapse. *Blood,* **83,** 3377.

Verschuuren, E.A., Stevens, S.J., van Imhoff, G.W. *et al.* (2002). Treatment of posttransplant lymphoproliferative disease with rituximab: the remission, the relapse, and the complication. *Transplantation,* **73,** 100.

Waldman, H., Cobbold, S., & Hale, G. (1994). What can be done to prevent graft versus host disease. *Current Opinion in Immunology,* **6,** 777–83.

Walter, E.A., Greenberg, P.D., Gilbert, M.J. *et al.* (1995). Reconstitution of cellular immunity against cytomegalovirus in recipients of allogeneic bone marrow by transfer of T-cell clones from the donor. *New England Journal of Medicine,* **333,** 1038–44.

Warren, E.H., Greenberg, P.D., & Riddell, S.R. (1998). Cytotoxic T-lymphocyte-defined human minor histocompatibility antigens with a restricted tissue distribution. *Blood,* **91,** 2197.

Weijtens, M.E.M., Van Spronsen, M., Martens, A.C.M., & Hagenbeek, A. (2001). Ganciclovir-mediated elimination of HSV-Tk+ T cells and cure of graft-versus-host disease in an allogeneic transplantation model in the rat. *Experimental Hematology,* **29** (Suppl) 1, 6.

118 Novel immunosuppressive agents for the prevention and treatment of graft-versus-host disease

DONNA PRZEPIORKA AND BARBARA E. BIERER

Baylor College of Medicine, Houston, and Dana-Farber Cancer Institute, Boston, USA

Introduction

Graft-versus-host disease (GVHD) is a common and significant complication of allogeneic stem cell transplantation that has limited the general applicability and success of this therapy. Knowledge of the immunobiology of GVHD assists in developing strategies for prevention and treatment. The pathogenesis of GVHD depends on donor T-cell recognition of host antigens. T-cell recognition of foreign antigens expressed on host antigen-presenting cells (e.g., dendritic cells, monocytes, macrophages, activated B cells) initiates the process of T-cell signaling, T-cell cytokine receptor expression, and T-cell cytokine production. In a paracrine and autocrine fashion, cytokine binding to cytokine receptors leads to T-cell proliferation and effector function.

The inflammatory microenvironment and tissue compartments also play a role in the pathogenesis of GVHD, in that inflammatory cytokines [e.g tumor necrosis factor (TNF)-α interleukin (IL)-1, IL-6, endotoxin] promote expression of adhesion molecules on T cells and antigen-presenting cells, enhance T-cell differentiation and activation, dysregulate B-cell activity, and initiate the secretion of secondary waves of inflammatory mediators that contribute further to target-cell damage and stromal proliferation. Under the current paradigm, fever, rash, liver function abnormalities, and diarrhea (clinical manifestations of acute GVHD) are mediated by Th1/Tc1 – type alloreactivity. In contrast, chronic GVHD is thought to be due to dysregulation of Th2 activity dominating over a Th1 response, and as such the clinical signs and symptoms are far more pleiotropic.

The ideal approach to prevention of GVHD would be the induction of donor-specific tolerance to host tissue antigens. In the absence of functioning thymic tissue, central tolerance is not possible. Advances in the understanding of T-cell activation, regulatory T-cells, and soluble mediators enable approaches to peripheral tolerance induction instead. Thus, the current standard of therapy for the prevention and treatment of GVHD is the use of immunosuppressive agents, either singly or in combination.

The history of immunosuppressive agents is a recent one. Glucocorticoids were introduced into clinical practice approximately 50 years ago, followed in 1959 by the introduction of the antiproliferative agents 6-mercaptopurine and azathioprine. The use of polyclonal antithymocyte globulin (ATG), reported in 1968, preceded the first clinical description of the immunosuppressive actions of cyclosporine (CSP) a decade later. Twenty years ago, the murine anti-human CD3 monoclonal antibody (mAb) OKT3 was used to reverse acute organ rejection episodes. Thirteen years ago, the clinical utility of tacrolimus (FK506) in solid organ transplantation was noted, followed in 1991 by mycophenolate mofetil (MMF) and in 1998 by sirolimus (rapamycin). The number and specificity of novel immunosuppressive agents is growing, and thus the choice of agent and of regimen can be tailored more effectively to the clinical setting. Biochemical and genetic methodologies are being used to identify the molecular targets of therapeutic action and thereby enable selection of agents with nonoverlapping spectra of biological action. This chapter will focus on novel agents used in the prevention and treatment of GVHD.

T-cell activation inhibitors

T-cell activation (Fig. 118.1) is initiated by the interaction of the T-cell receptor-CD3 complex with cognate peptide embedded within the groove of major histocompatibility complex proteins expressed on the surface of antigen-presenting cells (APC). Appropriate T-cell activation depends not only on TcR-CD3 engagement but also on co-receptor signaling and/or cytokine action. T-cell signaling results in the activation of a number of early genes, the expression of cytokine receptors, and of cytokines themselves. Cytokine signaling is required for subsequent T-cell differentiation and proliferation. The receptors and mediators important for the early activation of T cells represent appropriate targets for many immunosuppressive agents. For example, binding to the CD3 receptor on the surface of T cells can be mimicked and inhibited by mAbs directed against the monomorphic CD3 proteins, and these agents have been utilized extensively in solid organ transplantation. Co-receptors (e.g., CD2, CD4, CTLA-4), cytokine receptors [e.g, IL-2Rα chain, CD25 or tumor necrosis factor receptor (TNFR)] on the surface of T cells, cytokines them-

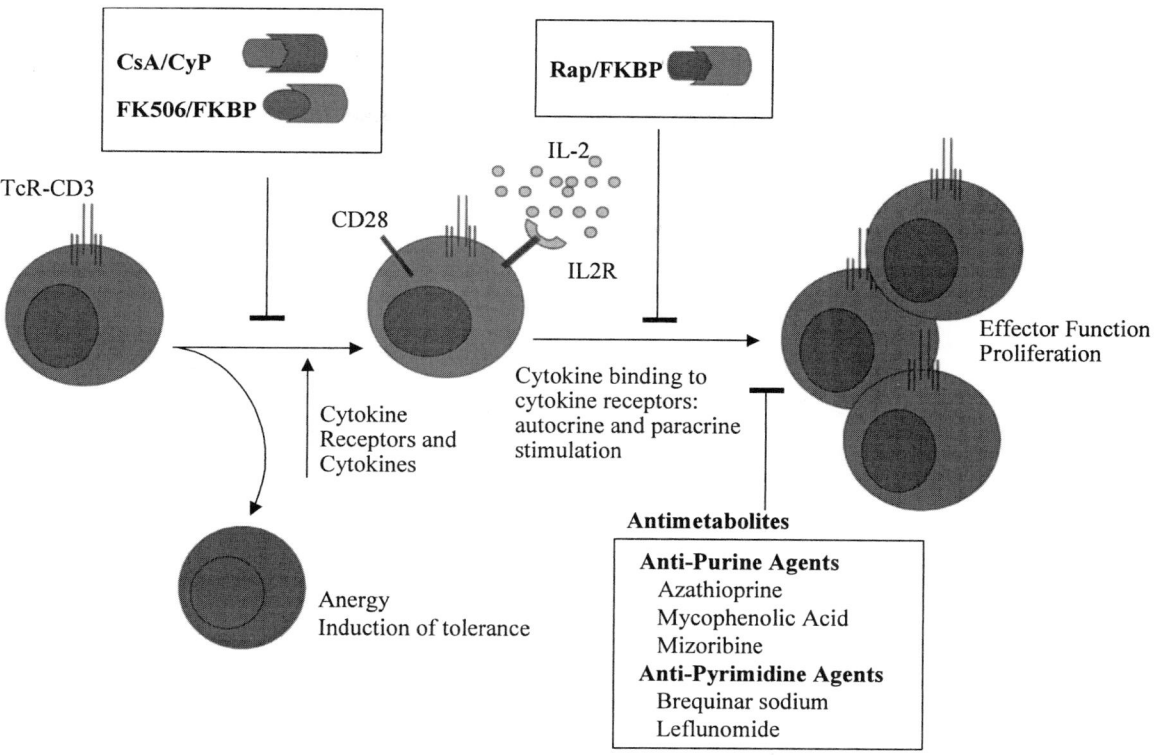

Fig. 118.1. Schematic of T-cell activation. T cells are stimulated following ligation of the TcR-CD3 complex on the cell surface. Binding of ligand to the TcR-CD3 complex in the presence of an appropriate co-stimulatory signal induces the transcription of a number of immediate early genes and cytokine receptor genes. Somewhat later, cytokines themselves are synthesized and secreted; these cytokines then act in a paracrine and autocrine fashion to stimulate T-cell differentiation and proliferation. Cyclosporine binding to its intracellular receptor cyclophilin, and tacrolimus binding to its intracellular binding protein FK506 binding protein (FKBP), inhibit T-cell cytokine production. Sirolimus, also binding to FKBP, acts later in the T-cell activation cascade, inhibiting events subsequent to the production of cytokines. Sirolimus/FKBP inhibits cytokine-dependent signal transduction, thereby also inhibiting T-cell differentiation and proliferation. Antimetabolites inhibit the generation of ribonucleotides that are essential for cell division.

selves, and the intracellular enzymes critical for T-cell signal transmission, are all appropriate molecular targets of immunosuppressant action.

Mechanism of action for cyclosporine, tacrolimus, and rapamycin

Cyclosporine (cyclosporin A, CSP) (Fig. 118.2) was developed for clinical use based on its ability to inhibit a mixed lymphocyte reaction. CSP itself is inert in the absence of its cognate receptor. Highly lipophilic, CSP binds to a family of cytoplasmic immunophilin proteins termed cyclophilins (CyP) and the complex of cyclophilin/CSP binds to and inhibits the activity of calcineurin, a calcium-calmodulin serine-threonine phosphatase. Calcineurin phosphate activity is essential for the dephosphorylation of a number of substrates, including the nuclear factor of activated T-cells (NFAT), a transcription factor. Dephosphorylation of NFAT is required for its translocation from the cytoplasm to the nucleus where it is able to bind DNA recognition sequences. NFAT activity is required for the

transcriptional activation of a number of cytokine and other key early activation genes (Fig. 118.3). It is important to appreciate that NFAT is not the only calcineurin substrate; inhibition or activation of other calcineurin substrates may be important in either the therapeutic or side effect profile of immunophilin-binding reagents (Fig. 118.3)

Cyclosporine has a narrow therapeutic index in that effective concentrations are closely correlated with concentrations associated with toxicity. The bioavailability of cyclosporine is affected by incomplete absorption from the gastrointestinal tract, a property that helps to explain significant interpatient variability in blood levels. A microemulsion preconcentrate formulation of cyclosporine (Neoral) is associated with greater and more consistent bioavailability. Cyclosporine is extensively metabolized by the hepatic cytochrome p450 system and the level of active drug is therefore modified by the co-administration of other compounds that induce or inhibit p450 enzymes. Levels should be monitored carefully and doses adjusted whenever medications are modified and when renal or hepatic function changes. A number of toxicities (Table 118.1), including nephrotoxicity,

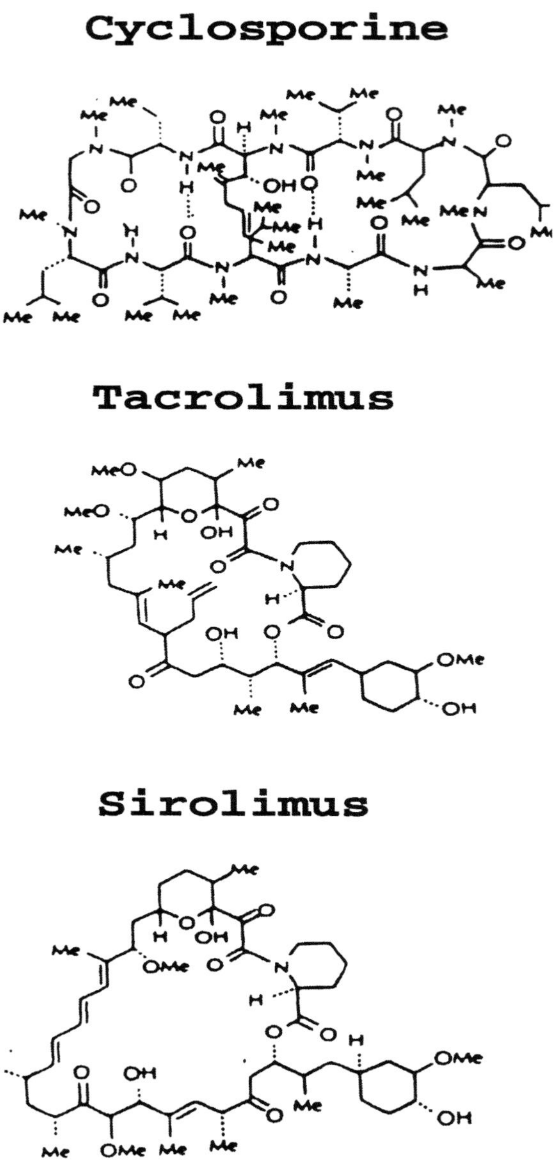

Cyclosporine

Tacrolimus

Sirolimus

Fig. 118.2. Chemical structure of three immunosuppressant drugs: (Top) Cyclosporine (CSP), a cyclic undecapeptide of M, 1203 Da; (middle) tacrolimus (FK506, Prograf), a macrolide antibiotic of M_r 822 Da; and (bottom) sirolimus (rapamycin, Rapamune), another macrolide antibiotic, with M_r 914 Da. ME, methyl group.

neurotoxicity, and hypertension, are common and may relate to substrates of calcineurin activity in tissues and cells other than lymphocytes. A number of the side effects (electrolyte abnormalities) can be reversed with diminution of dose. Some toxicities appear to be idiosyncratic (e.g., severe neurological dysfunction including coma) and may require discontinuation of drug.

Like cyclosporine, tacrolimus (FK506) (Fig. 118.2) functions via intracytoplasmic molecules, these termed FK506 binding proteins (FKBPs), and the complex of tacrolimus/FKBP binds

to and inhibits calcineurin phosphatase activity in a fashion similar to that of CSP/CyP. The consequences of calcineurin inhibition are the same as with cyclosporine (Figs. 118.1 and 118.3). Tacrolimus is also metabolized extensively by the cytochrome p450 system, and therapeutic drug monitoring is important. Like CSP, the common toxicities of tacrolimus include nephrotoxicity, neurotoxicity, and hypertension but, unlike CSP, hirsutism and gingival hyperplasia are rarely observed. Rarely, and more commonly in pediatric transplant recipients, myocardial hypertrophy with ventricular dysfunction has been reported with tacrolimus use.

Sirolimus (RS-61443, rapamycin) is a macrocyclic lactone (Fig. 118.2) isolated from the *Streptomyces hygroscopicus* species. The mechanism of action of sirolimus is distinct from the calcineurin inhibition mediated by CSP and tacrolimus. Like tacrolimus, sirolimus binds to the family of intracytoplasmic FKBP proteins, but its molecular target is a regulatory protein important for progression from the late G1 to S phase of the cell cycle. The complex of sirolimus with FKBP binds to the molecule mammalian target of rapamycin (mTOR) (Fig. 118.4), a protein important for cell cycle progression, mRNA translation, and protein synthesis (Fig. 118.5). In addition to inhibition of cytokine signaling (Fig. 118.1) and T-lymphocyte proliferation, sirolimus also inhibits antibody production. Sirolimus is approved for use for prophylaxis of organ rejection in patients receiving renal transplants, and it is recommended that the immunosuppressive regimen include additional agents such as cyclosporine and corticosteroids.

Currently, sirolimus is administered orally in a fixed dosage schedule. It is lipophilic and extensively bound to plasma proteins in vivo, reaching peak plasma concentrations in most patients within 1 hour. It has a prolonged mean half-life of 62 ± 16 hours, with significant interpatient variability (Yatscoff *et al.,* 1995; Zimmerman & Kahan, 1997). Sirolimus is metabolized principally by hepatic cytochrome P450 III4A (CYP3A4) and excreted in the feces. The effect of renal impairment on its pharmacokinetics is not known. There is a direct relationship between adverse events and blood concentrations, but guidelines for therapeutic drug monitoring have not been established.

While sirolimus is generally well tolerated, certain adverse events such as gastrointestinal complaints (abdominal pain, nausea, vomiting, constipation, etc.) are relatively common. Hyperlipidemia and hypercholesterolemia should be monitored and may require treatment. Leukopenia, thrombocytopenia, and anemia can limit use. Unlike CSP and tacrolimus, however, hypertension, nephrotoxicity, and neurotoxicity are extremely rare. Therefore, immunosuppressive regimens can be designed using drugs that have both distinct molecular targets of action and theoretically nonoverlapping toxicity profiles.

Tacrolimus for prevention of GVHD

The superiority of tacrolimus over cyclosporine for prevention of acute GVHD was demonstrated by randomized trials. For HLA-identical marrow transplant recipients, tacrolimus

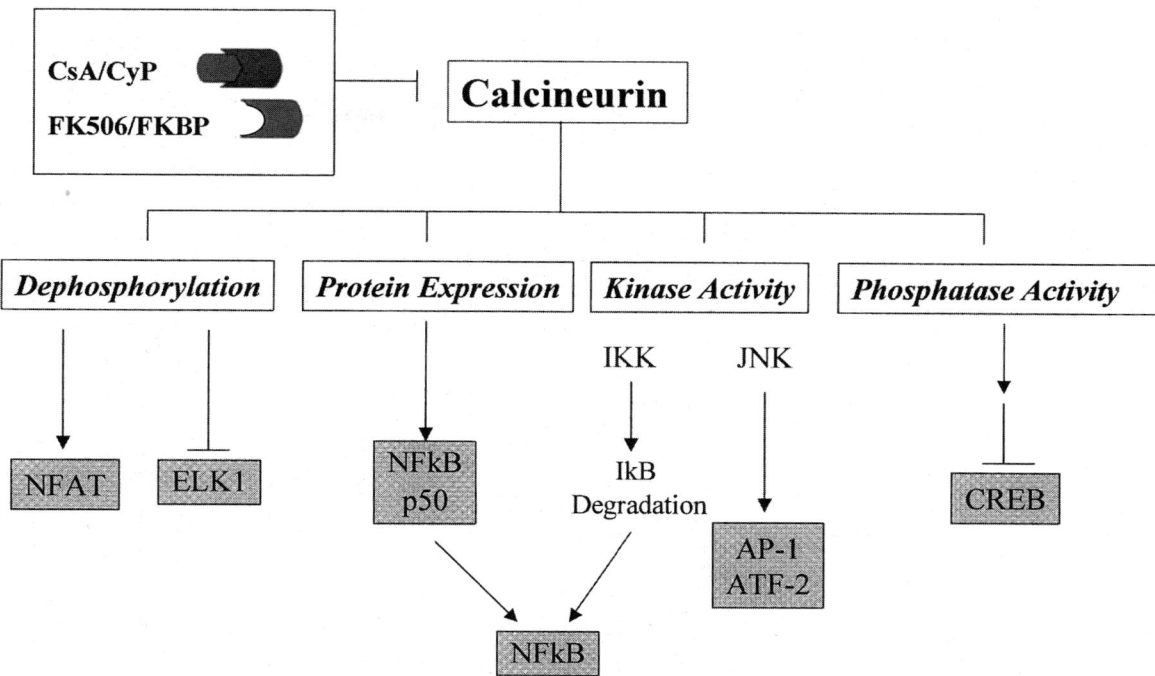

Fig. 118.3. The molecular targets of calcineurin. The complexes CSP/CyP and FK506/FKBP bind to and inhibit the serine-threonine phosphatase calcineurin. While one substrate for calcineurin has been demonstrated to be the transcription factor nuclear factor of activated T cells (NFAT), other substrates exist. It is now appreciated that calcineurin activity plays a role in a number of intracellular functions, including regulating protein translation and subcellular localization and the enzymatic activity of a number of kinases and phosphatases. These, in turn, affect the activity of a number of transcription factors in addition to the NFAT family members, some of which are shown here.

Table 118.1.　*Toxicities of T-cell activation inhibitors*

	Tacrolimus	Cyclosporine	Sirolimus
Renal			
Renal insufficiency	++	++	–
Hypomagnesemia	++	++	–
Metabolic			
Hyperglycemia	++	+	–
Hypertension	+	++	–
Hyperkalemia	++	++	–
Hyperlipidemia	–	+	++
Neurologic			
Tremor	++	++	–
Seizures	++	++	–
Insomnia	++	++	–
Encephalopathy	+	+	–
Headache	+	+	–
Trophic			
Gingival hyperplasia	–	++	–
Hirsutism	–	++	–
Facial dysmorphism	–	++	–
Other			
Anorexia	++	++	+
MAHA	++	++	–
Cytopenias	–	–	++
GI	–	–	+
Capillary leak	+	+	+

Abbreviations: MAHA, microangiopathic hemolytic anemia; GI, gastrointestinal.

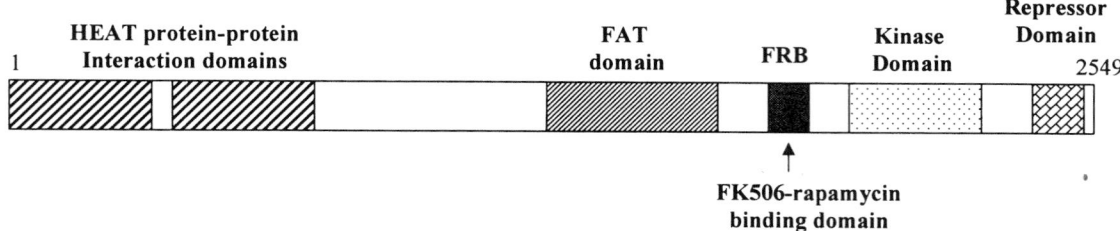

Fig. 118.4. Structure of the mammalian target of rapamycin (mTOR). mTOR is a large protein with multiple domains, including an aminoterminal protein-protein interaction domain, a FAT domain, an FK506 and rapamycin binding (FRB) domain, a kinase domain, and a carboxyterminal repressor domain. The latter domain serves as an autoinhibitory domain to regulate the activity of the enzyme. mTOR is a protein serine-threonine kinase.

reduced the risk of grades II to IV GVHD from 44% to 32% when used with standard methotrexate (Ratanatharathorn *et al.,* 1998), and from 41% to 13% when used with methotrexate or steroids (Hiraoka *et al.,* 2001). For alternative donor marrow transplant recipients, the risk of grades II to IV GVHD was reduced from 74% to 56% (Nash *et al.,* 2000) and from 54% to 21% (Hiraoka *et al.,* 2001) using tacrolimus, respectively. The

groups were not balanced for specific diseases in any of the three trials, and this confounded assessment of long-term outcomes, but a case-control study indicated that use of tacrolimus was not associated with an adverse effect on relapse or survival (Horowitz *et al.,* 1999).

Subsequent reports indicate the safety and activity of tacrolimus for GVHD prevention for unrelated donor cord

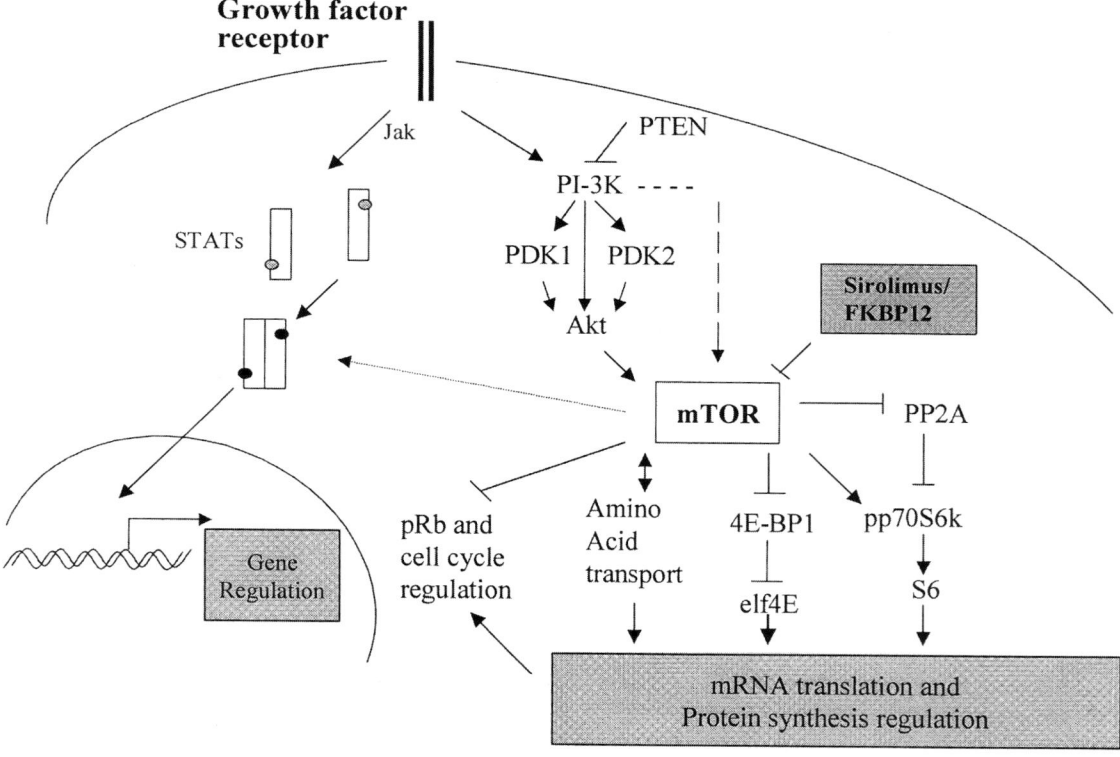

Fig. 118.5. Rapamycin inhibits cell cycle progression in late G1 phase by interacting with the mammalian TOR (mTOR) protein. Binding of growth factor to its cognate receptor initiates early biochemical events such as JAK/STAT activation, protein tyrosine kinase (PTK) activity, and activation of phosphatidyli-nositol (PI)-3 kinase (PI3K) activity. PI3K itself is regulated by the tyrosine phosphatase PTEN and by the serine threonine kinases PDK1 and PDK2. PI3K activates AKT/PKB, and both PI3K and AKT act to regulate mTOR activity. mTOR activity affects the rate of protein biosynthesis by regulating p70 S6 kinase, amino acid transport, and 4E-BP1, among others. Sirolimus/FKBP 12 complexes have been shown to bind to and inhibit the mTOR family of intracellular proteins. Adapted, with permission, from Vander Woude & Bierer (1997).

blood transplantation (Przepiorka *et al.*, 1999d), HLA-identical blood stem cell transplantation (Przepiorka *et al.*, 1999e), HLA-mismatched related donor marrow transplantation (Przepiorka *et al.*, 1999b), and nonmyeloablative transplantation (Khouri *et al.*, 2001). In the phase II studies, tacrolimus has been used safely as a single agent or in combination with standard methotrexate, minidose methotrexate (minimethotrexate), steroids, and mycophenolate mofetil. Tacrolimus has also been used successfully in patients with neurologic complications from cyclosporine (although it also has CNS toxicity), but its value for patients with cyclosporine-induced hemolytic-uremic syndrome (HUS) is unclear (Furlong *et al.*, 2000),

Exploratory analyses showed that toxicities of tacrolimus were associated with elevated blood levels (Wingard *et al.*, 1998; Przepiorka *et al.*, 1999c). Based on these analyses and extensive experience, a consensus panel developed guidelines for use of tacrolimus for GVHD prophylaxis (Przepiorka *et al.*, 1999a) (Table 118.2). The therapeutic range is 10 to 20 ng/ml by whole blood IMx assay, although some have targeted 5 to 15 ng/ml to minimize the chance the patient will have a seriously toxic level (>20 ng/ml). Therapeutic monitoring is imperative, especially in pediatric patients (Przepiorka *et al.*, 2000a), early after transplantation when clearance of tacrolimus changes over the first several weeks of therapy (Woo *et al.*, 1997), and when altering medications that interfere with, or induce, the cytochrome P450 system (Mignat, 1997).

Tacrolimus for treatment of GVHD

Complete responses are seen in fewer than 20% of patients with refractory acute GVHD treated with tacrolimus (Koehler *et al.*, 1995; Furlong *et al.*, 2000). Mollee *et al.* (2001) reported a 40% complete response rate using tacrolimus with antithymocyte globulin for refractory GVHD, but in the absence of controlled trials, it is difficult to know if the combination is better than antithymocyte globulin alone. Chronic GVHD appears to be more amenable to treatment with tacrolimus, especially when therapy is instituted as first salvage for steroid-refractory cases (Kanamaru *et al.*, 1995; Carnevale-Schianca *et al.*, 2000; Nagler *et al.*, 2001). Complete response rates as high as 33% were reported. Topical tacrolimus has been used for cutaneous GVHD, with improvement in local symptoms in more than 70% of patients treated (Narwani *et al.*, 1999; Choi & Nghiem, 2001). Although transcutaneous absorption may occur when the topical ointment is applied, blood levels of tacrolimus are generally not within the therapeutic range using this route, and systemic therapy is still required for concomitant noncutaneous involvement.

Sirolimus for prevention and treatment of GVHD

Only preliminary data are available for the use of sirolimus in the management of GVHD. Antin *et al.* (2001) evaluated

Table 118.2. *Suggested use of tacrolimus*[a]

Dosing	
Initial tacrolimus dose	I.V. 0.03 mg/kg/day (ideal body weight) by continuous infusion starting day −2, and check blood levels 3–5 times per week.
Conversion to oral	Total daily dose orally is 4 times the current daily i.v. dose. The dose is split and given twice daily (i.e., each oral dose is twice the i.v. dose), the blood levels are checked 1–2 times per week until tapering begins.
i.v. dose adjustments[b]	
Serum creatinine	
1.0–1.5 × baseline	75–100% of current dose
1.6–1.9 × baseline	25–50% of current dose
>1.9 × baseline	Hold and resume at 50% of current dose when renal dysfunction is stable.
Tacrolimus blood level[c]	
<5 ng/ml	Increase by 25–50%
5–9 ng/ml	Increase by 0–25%
10–15 ng/ml	No change
16–20 ng/ml	Decrease by 0–25%
21–25 ng/ml	Hold 6 hr and resume at 50% dose
>25 ng/ml	Hold and resume at 25% dose when level is <20
Pharmacokinetic	
	Adjusted dose = *(current dose)* × *(target blood level)*/(current blood level)

[a] Usually used in conjunction with standard dose or minidose methotrexate.

[b] Trough concentrations are not proportional to dose when the drug is given orally. Oral dose modifications should be individualized. Tacrolimus clearance may be excessively prolonged for patients with liver dysfunction or while on medications that inhibit hepatic P450 function. In these patients, hold tacrolimus and follow levels daily to determine when to restart.

[c] Whole blood concentration measured by IMx assay.

From Przepiorka *et al.* (1999a). Consult package insert and literature for updated information.

sirolimus in combination with tacrolimus and mini-methotrexate for prevention of acute GVHD in alternative donor stem cell transplantation. Thirty patients were treated using sirolimus at 4 mg/day orally, and doses were adjusted to maintain blood levels of 2 to 12 ng/ml. The conditional probability of grades II to IV GVHD was 37%. The investigators indicated that compliance with the oral formulation was an issue. An update has been published (Antin *et al.*, 2003).

Sirolimus has also been studied for the treatment of refractory acute and chronic GVHD. Johnston *et al.* (2002) reported a phase II of 16 patients who received sirolimus orally as second or third line therapy for chronic GVHD. Nine (56%) patients were said to have improved using sirolimus, one discontinuing all immunosuppressive therapy and four tapering off steroids. However, six (38%) patients were removed from the study for toxicity. Common adverse events included renal insufficiency, HUS, and thrombocytopenia. Benito *et al.* (2001) found that sirolimus was also active in the treatment of steroid–refractory acute GVHD. Of the 21 patients treated with a 14-day course of the oral formulation, five (24%) achieved a complete response. The most common toxicities were myelosuppression, hyperlipidemia, seizure, and HUS. These data demonstrate that sirolimus is an active therapy for refractory GVHD, but toxicity can be considerable, especially when used in combination with other calcineurin inhibitors.

Cell cycle inhibitors

Since immune cell proliferation is an absolute requirement for acute GVHD, inhibition of cell cycle progression is an effective strategy for prevention and treatment, particularly if the agent used has relative selectivity for the responding cells. Lymphocytes, as other cells, depend on both purine and pyrimidine biosynthesis for the generation of nucleotides, necessary for the later synthesis of DNA, RNA, and proteins (Fig. 118.1). Synthesis of purine nucleotides (adenylic acid, inosinic acid, and guanylic acid) proceeds either by de novo biosynthesis from nonpurine precursors or by the salvage pathway depending on conversion from the purine bases (Fig. 118.6). In both routes of synthesis, inosine monophosphate dehydrogenase (IMPDH) is the common intermediate (Laliberte *et al.*, 1998) and is therefore a good molecular target for immunosuppression. For pyrimidine synthesis, dihydroorotate dehydrogenase (DHO-DH) is a key enzyme. A number of agents currently in use target these enzymes to effect inhibition of cell cycle procession (Fig. 118.6).

Mechanisms of action for mycophenolate mofetil, pentostatin, and leflunomide

Mycophenolate mofetil (MMF) was shown to prolong solid organ allograft survival in animal models over a decade ago

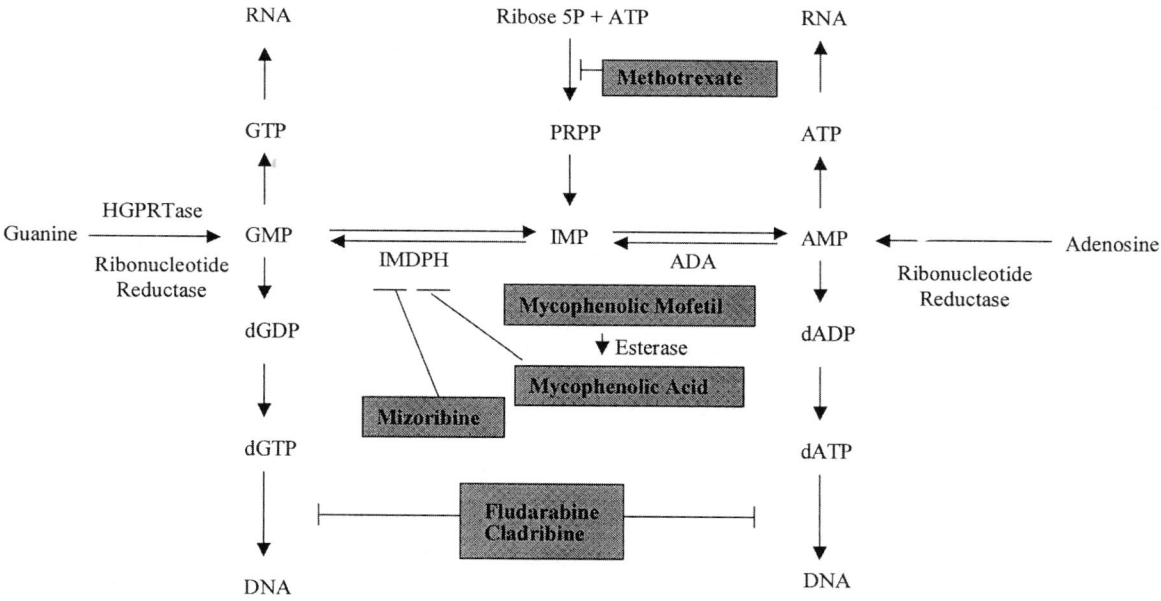

Fig. 118.6. Pathways of purine biosynthesis and sites of action of several antimetabolite agents. Synthesis of the purine nucleotides adenylic acid (AMP), inosinic acid (IMP), and guanylic acid (GMP) occurs via one of two pathways: either directly from the purine bases guanine, hypoxanthine, and adenine or de novo from nonpurine precursors such as ribose 5-phosphate. IMP is a common intermediate in both routes of synthesis. The conversion of IMP to GMP by IMP dehydrogenase (IMPDH) is inhibited by mycophenolic acid and mizoribine. Mycophenolic mofetil (MMF) is rapidly converted to its active agent mycophenolic acid within the cell by an esterase. Both fludarabine and cladribine inhibit the incorporation of dATP and dGTP to DNA. Pentostatin is an inhibitor of adenosine deaminase (ADA), preventing purine synthesis. Methotrexate inhibits the conversion of ribose 5-phosphate to PRPP. By depleting the cell of essential metabolic intermediates required for DNA synthesis, these agents inhibit T-cellular proliferation. Adapted, with permission, from Vander Woude & Bierer (1997).

(Morris, 1989). After initial human trials demonstrating the ability to rescue patients suffering from acute renal rejection (Sollinger et al., 1992), the agent was approved for use in renal and cardiac transplant recipients (Halloran et al., 1997). A prodrug itself, MMF is rapidly and completely metabolized in vivo to mycophenolic acid (MPA), an inhibitor of IMPDH (Fig. 118.6) (Wu, 1994). MPA treatment of human lymphocytes in vitro has been shown to decrease the activity of p27^{Kip1}, resulting in the subsequent inhibition of cyclin D/CDK6 kinase, both correlates of cell proliferation (Laliberte et al., 1998). Predictably, expression of cell surface markers indicative of lymphocyte activation (e.g., CD25, CD134) is also inhibited by MPA (Gummert et al., 1999).

In adult recipients of renal and heart transplants, MMF is administered typically at a dose of 1 to 1.5 g twice daily, at which dosage there is evidence of efficacy. Generally, plasma levels are not monitored, although the MPA trough levels and area under the curve (AUC) have been shown to correlate with prevention of allograft rejection (van Gelder et al., 1999) and with inhibition of lymphocyte proliferation (Gummert et al., 2000). MPA is bound extensively to plasma proteins and its enterohepatic circulation is a major contributor to AUC (Nowak & Shaw, 1995). Its clearance is driven by ADP-glucoronosyltransferase (Nowak & Shaw, 1997). Fixed dosing, independent of body mass, does not account totally for individual variation in pharmacokinetic profiles (Shaw et al., 1998a), and the value of therapeutic monitoring is currently being evaluated. Generally, plasma levels are monitored in patients on multiple immunosuppressants, when doses of interacting drugs are adjusted (Meiser et al., 1999), in patients with renal failure or changing renal or liver function, and in children (Shaw et al., 1998b, 2001).

Another inhibitor of purine biosynthesis, pentostatin (deoxycoformycin), is a transition state inhibitor of the enzyme adenosine deaminase (ADA), and thus, inhibits DNA synthesis (Staubus et al., 1984; Spiers, 1995; Johnson, 2000). RNA synthesis is also inhibited. Thus, treatment with pentostatin results in cytotoxicity and in DNA damage. Pentostatin is approved for use in both untreated and refractory hairy cell leukemia; in this patient population, the drug is relatively well tolerated. The side effects most often reported are nausea and/or vomiting, fever and/or chills, rash, fatigue, dizziness, and shortness of breath.

Leflunomide is a synthetic isoxazole derivative that is an inhibitor of dihydroorotate dehydrogenase (DHO-DH) (Cherwinski et al., 1995). Leflunomide, and its active metabolite, A77 1726, are potent inhibitors of lymphocyte cell cycle progression (Slauson et al., 1999). In addition to inhibition of de novo pyrimidine nucleotide biosynthesis, A77 1726 also appears to inhibit protein tyrosine phosphorylation in vitro (Xu et al., 1996); the mechanism of this action remains obscure.

Leflunomide is biologically active after oral administration. It has a prolonged half-life in humans (11–16 days), potentially posing a safety hazard. Phase II studies in patients with rheumatoid arthritis have demonstrated that the agent is generally well tolerated, with some gastrointestinal symptoms, anemia, rash, and weight loss being the most common adverse effects. Leflunomide has not been evaluated in the prevention or treatment of GVHD.

MMF for prevention of GVHD

MMF has been used in combination with cyclosporine most frequently for prevention of GVHD. Using this combination, the rates of grades II to IV GVHD reported were 38% to 49% for HLA-matched related allograft recipients and 63% to 64% for mismatched or unrelated donor allograft recipients (Table 118.3). How this compares to standard cyclosporine and methotrexate is not clear. In one small retrospective comparison (Bornhauser et al., 1999) and a preliminary report of a prospective randomized trial (Kraut et al., 2002), no significant difference in GVHD was detected comparing patients receiving MMF to those receiving methotrexate with cyclosporine. Preliminary data are also available from studies of tacrolimus and MMF. Although fewer studies have been reported for the tacrolimus combination, the risk of GVHD appears to be lower than with cyclosporine and MMF (Table 118.3).

The optimal dose schedule of MMF for prevention of GVHD has not been determined. The dose schedules used most commonly are 1 g or 15 mg/kg orally or intravenously twice daily. Dosing twice daily may not be sufficient, since the half-life of the active metabolite in hematopoietic allograft recipients is only about 4 hours (Maris et al., 2001), and low trough levels were associated with more severe GVHD (Jenke et al., 2001). The earliest non-myeloablative studies also suggested that a short course (14–28 days) of MMF did not provide sufficient protection against GVHD, especially for patients with mismatched or unrelated donors. Longer courses of MMF, however, are associated with greater expense, the potential for myelosuppression, and a delay in immune reconstitution, so it is not clear whether MMF would truly be an improvement over minidose methotrexate.

MMF for treatment of GVHD

Treatment of acute GVHD with MMF has not proven highly successful (Table 118.4). Few complete responses are induced with MMF. This may be due in part to subtherapeutic drug exposure with oral dosing, especially for patients with gastrointestinal GVHD (Kiehl et al., 1999). In contrast, MMF administered orally appears to be quite active in the treatment of steroid-refractory chronic GVHD (Table 118.4). Prolonged courses are required in order to achieve the maximal benefit, and complete response rates as high as 65% were reported after 1 to 3 years of therapy. Partial responses can be seen with less than a year of therapy, and the majority of patients treated with MMF have had a reduction in dose, or elimination of use, of steroids. Whether MMF is sufficiently active for primary treatment of chronic GVHD and can supercede steroids in this setting remains to be determined.

Table 118.3. *Mycophenolate mofetil for prevention of GVHD*

Reference	Conditioning regimen	Donor	GVHD prophylaxis regimen	Patients	Grade II–IV acute GVHD	Gr III–IV GVHD	Chronic GVHD
CSP-based two-drug							
Bornhauser et al. (1999) (historical controls)	A	Sibling	CSP/MMF 1 g p.o. b.i.d. days 1–14	14	47%[a]	7%[a]	56%[a]
			CSP/MTX	15	60%	13%	50%
Kobbe et al. (2000)	A	Sibling	CSP/MMF 15 mg/kg p.o. b.i.d. (days not stated)	15	38%	–	–
McSweeney et al. (2001)	N	Sibling	CSP/MMF 15 mg/kg p.o. b.i.d. days 0–27	36	47%	11%	74%
Sandmeier et al. (2001)	N	Sibling	CSP/MMF days 0–27	192	49%	16%	–
Maris et al. (2001)	N	Alternative	CSP/MMF (days not stated)	63	63%	13%	50%
Kraut et al. (2002)	A	Mixed	CSP/MMF 1–1.5 g p.o. b.i.d. (days not stated)	22	64%	–	–
(randomized controls)			CSP/MTX	8	38%	–	–
CSP-based multidrug							
Kiehl et al. (1999)	–	Mixed	CSP/MP/MMF 1 g i.v. b.i.d. (days not stated)	16	–	19%	–
Basara et al. (2000)	A	Alternative	CSP/MTX/MP/MMF 1 g p.o. daily days 10–100	13	23%	15%	–
FK506-based two-drug							
LeBlanc et al. (2001)	N	Sibling	FK506/MMF 1 g p.o. b.i.d. days 2–50	19	0%	0%	16%
Rini et al. (2002)	N	Sibling	FK506/MMF 1 g p.o. b.i.d. days 2–60	11	17%	17%	36%
Cairo et al. (2002)	–	Mixed	FK506/MMF 15 mg/kg i.v. b.i.d. (days not stated)	14	28%	9%	0%
McSweeney et al. (2002)	A	Mixed	FK506/MMF 15 mg/kg i.v. b.i.d. days 0–28/56	24	24%	6%	46%

Abbreviations: –, not stated; N, nonmyeloablative or reduced intensity; A, myeloablative; MMF, mycophenolate mofetil; p.o., orally; b.i.d., twice daily; i.v., intravenously; CSP, cyclosporine; MP, methylprednisolone; MTX, methotrexate; FK506, tacrolimus.

[a] Actuarial estimate, cumulative incidence or proportion, depending on the result reported.

Table 118.4. *Mycophenolate mofetil for treatment of GVHD*

Reference	Indication	MMF regimen	Response assessed	Patients	CR	CR + PR
Acute GVHD						
Ihlan *et al.* (1999)	Refractory	1 g p.o. daily	–	2	*a	*
Abhyankar *et al.* (1998)	Refractory	1 g p.o. b.i.d.	–	7	–	29%
Basara *et al.* (2001)	Primary	1 g p.o. b.i.d.	–	36	–	72%
Chronic GVHD						
Basara *et al.* (2001)	Primary	1 g p.o. b.i.d.	–	12	–	(50%)b
Redei *et al.* (1999)	Drug-intolerant	1 g p.o. b.i.d.	–	5	–	(80%)
Roberts *et al.* (1999)	Refractory liver	1 g p.o. b.i.d.	–	11	–	(100%)
Ihlan *et al.* (1999)	Refractory	1 g p.o. daily	–	6	–	(33%)
Redei *et al.* (1999)	Refractory	1 g p.o. b.i.d.	–	9	–	(55%)
Abhyankar *et al.* (1998)	Refractory	1 g p.o. b.i.d.	–	12	–	33%
Pallotta-Filho *et al.* (1998)	Refractory	10 mg/kg p.o. daily	6 weeks	12	17%	83%
Busca *et al.* (2000)	Refractory	15–40 mg/kg p.o. daily	–	15	–	60%
Lopez *et al.* (2001)	Refractory	15 mg/kg p.o. b.i.d.	>6 months	36	39%	81%
Yusuf *et al.* (2001)	Refractory	20 mg/kg p.o. b.i.d.	1–3 years	26	65%	77%
Kalogiannidis *et al.* (2002)	Refractory	10–30 mg/kg p.o. daily	3–22 months	25	64%	80%
Stanzani *et al.* (2002)	Mixed	2 g p.o. daily	3–15 months	21	0%	57%
Mookerjee *et al.* (1999)	Refractory	1 g p.o. b.i.d. + tacrolimus	3 months	26	8%	46%

Abbreviations: –, not stated; CR, complete response; PR, partial response.

[a] Case report of responsive disease indicated by*.

[b] Response rates in parentheses were reported as "improved".

Pentostatin for treatment of GVHD

Pentostatin appears to be a highly potent immunosuppressive agent in the treatment of GVHD. In a preliminary report of 10 patients with chronic GVHD who had failed steroids and one salvage regimen, 5 had a major response when treated with pentostatin 4 mg/m^2 i.v. every other week for 3 months (Jacobsohn *et al.*, 2001). An even lower dose, 1 mg/m^2 i.v. daily for 3 days, was active in the treatment of steroid and/or ATG-refractory intestinal acute GVHD; 7 (64%) of 11 patients achieved a complete response with this therapy (Klein *et al.*, 2002). The immunosuppression induced by pentostatin is quite profound, and infectious complications were a major problem.

TNF inhibitors

The TNF/TNFR-related superfamily of proteins is a large family of molecules important in costimulation, inflammation, migration, proliferation, and cell survival. TNF-α is a homotrimer in its active state. It is synthesized in the cell and transported to the cell surface where it remains membrane-bound until cleaved by a surface metalloproteinase (Fig. 118.7). The secreted form is biologically active and binds with high affinity to both the ubiquitous p55 TNFR1, involved in inflammatory and apoptotic reactions, and the p75 TNFR2 form, expression of which appears to be restricted to inflammatory cells. In addition to TNF-α, both TNFR1 and TNFR2 bind lymphotoxin α, another inducer of apoptosis in T cells.

Binding of TNF-α induces aggregation of the TNFR; the conformational change initiates cell signaling that results in NFkB transcriptional activation, the production of inflammatory proteins (IL-1, IL-6, and chemokines) and, potentially, apoptosis (Fig. 118.7). TNF-α is a key mediator of induction of apoptosis in target tissues in GVHD (Speiser *et al.*, 1997). The central importance of TNF-α and TNFR in inflammation has led to the development of a number of agents to inhibit their actions.

Mechanism of action of infliximab and etanercept

Infliximab is a chimeric murine-human IgG1 mAb directed against TNF-α. Etanercept is a soluble, dimeric p75 TNF receptor fusion protein (sTNFR p75:Fc fusion protein). Conjugation of the soluble receptor to immunoglobulin or a fragment thereof extended the otherwise short biological half-life. Following intravenous or subcutaneous administration, the half-life of these drugs is 5 to 7 days. Both drugs act by neutralizing soluble or surface TNF-α and infliximab may mediate antibody-dependent cellular cytotoxicity (ADCC) of TNF-bearing cells as well.

Infliximab and etanercept have been well tolerated by patients with chronic inflammatory diseases. Initial concerns that the incidence of malignancy (particularly lymphoma) may have been increased were allayed by further experience with greater numbers of patients. An increased incidence of infection remains a real concern, and careful monitoring and appropriate prophylaxis is recommended.

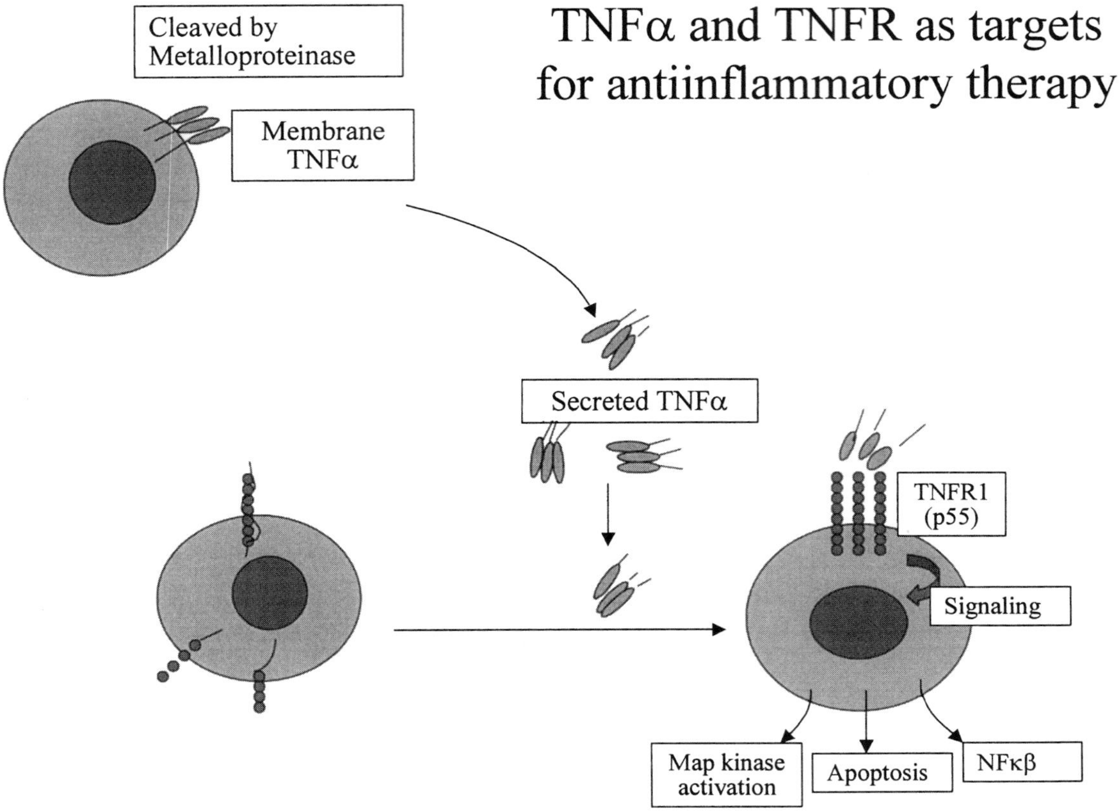

TNFα and TNFR as targets for antiinflammatory therapy

Fig. 118.7. Pathways of TNF-α action on the TNFR. TNF-α is synthesized in the cytoplasm and transported to the cell surface where it remains membrane-bound until cleaved by a surface metalloproteinase. Soluble TNF-α can bind to both the p55 TNFR1 and the p75 TNFR2. TNFR signaling is complex and depends on the cell and receptor type.

TNF inhibitors for treatment of GVHD

The lack of acute toxicities from infliximab and etanercept made them attractive adjuncts for treatment of refractory GVHD. Unfortunately, the ease with which they are used predisposed to rapid incorporation into a polydrug approach without full evaluation of their activity when used as primary or first salvage therapy.

There are a few case reports and case series of infliximab 10 mg/kg weekly for 4 weeks and of etanercept 0.4 mg/kg twice weekly for 8 weeks as treatment of acute GVHD (Andolina *et al.*, 2000; Kobbe *et al.*, 2001; Magalhaes-Silverman *et al.*, 2001; Fuchs *et al.*, 2002; Jacobsohn *et al.*, 2002). These cases demonstrate that the TNF inhibitors are active in this setting. A prolonged time to response (10–14 days) was noted in a number of these cases and probably accounts for the limited use of these drugs as sole therapy for severe GVHD.

Wolff *et al.* (2002) reported that six of seven patients with refractory acute GVHD responded when given etanercept 16 mg/m² twice weekly for 3 weeks in addition to daclizumab and corticosteroids, but other combinations have not been evaluated systematically.

Preliminary data suggest that etanercept may also be useful for steroid-dependent chronic GVHD; after 8 weeks of therapy,

there was 1 complete and 5 partial responses in 10 patients (Chiang *et al.*, 2002). Since there is frequently less imperative for a rapid response with chronic GVHD, this setting may be more amenable to use of the TNF inhibitors.

Mechanism of action of thalidomide

Thalidomide, a 258 Da, *N*-phthaloyl-glutamic acid imide, is a potent immunomodulatory agent (Wendt *et al.*, 1996; Haslett *et al.*, 1998; Corral & Kaplan, 1999). Thalidomide was initially introduced as a sedative and an anti-inflammatory agent in the 1950s, but it was withdrawn from use because of its teratogenic effects. Only recently has the drug enjoyed a resurgence of market distribution for specific indications. It is approved for use, under a specialized distribution agreement, in the treatment of erythema nodosum leprosum, and it is being tested in a variety of malignancies, autoimmune disorders, and GVHD.

Thalidomide has been shown to inhibit TNF-α production both transcriptionally and by accelerating TNF-α mRNA degradation (Moreira *et al.*, 1993; Wendt *et al.*, 1996; Shannon *et al.*, 1997; Tavares *et al.*, 1997; Sampaio *et al.*, 1991, 1993), at concentrations in vitro that are achievable clinically. In addition to

TNF-α, thalidomide inhibits production of the downstream inflammatory cytokines IL-6 (Rowland et al., 1998) and IL-8 (Koch, 1985). The production of a number of cytokines characteristic of Th2 cells (IL-4, IL-5, and IL-10) appears to be enhanced by thalidomide (McHugh & Rowland, 1997; Moreira et al., 1997). Treatment of T lymphocytes and other cells with thalidomide may modulate expression of a number of adhesion molecules (Saitoh et al., 1998). In addition, thalidomide has a variety of anti-angiogenic effects inhibiting the actions of vascular endothelial growth factor (VEGF) and basic fibroblast growth factor (bFGF) (D'Amato et al., 1994; Kruse et al., 1998).

Thalidomide for the treatment of GVHD

The first reports of thalidomide for treatment of GVHD were published in 1988. It was clear that thalidomide was ineffective for refractory acute GVHD (Table 118.5). Others have reported that thalidomide does not improve outcomes when used in addition to standard therapy as primary treatment for chronic GVHD (Arora et al., 2001), and it is not effective for prevention of chronic GVHD (Chao et al., 1996).

For patients with steroid-refractory chronic GVHD, however, complete responses were seen in 3% to 38% of patients treated with thalidomide, and total response rates were 20% to 78% (Table 118.5). Most responses occurred only after several months of treatment. Several dose schedules have been used, and none have been shown to be optimal. Since thalidomide blood assays are not commonly available, most transplant physicians have started with 100 to 200 mg thalidomide daily, doubling the dose every several weeks until drowsiness occurs. The hazard of this approach is the potential for irreversible neuropathies to occur prior to lethargy.

Careful clinical monitoring for other toxicities is required during long-term use. The most common side effects are nausea, constipation, dysesthesias, somnolence, dizziness, liver dysfunction, rash, neutropenia, and teratogenicity. The high rate of toxicity has limited the use of thalidomide as an immunosuppressant agent. In one randomized trial (Koc et al., 2000), toxicity of thalidomide resulted in premature discontinuation of the drug in 92% of the patients.

Monoclonal antibodies

A number of mAbs have been developed and approved for clinical use; additionally, a number of mAbs are currently in development. The highly selective activity against defined and potentially unique molecular targets is a great advantage of mAbs, especially as carriers for therapeutic toxins. Furthermore, while mAb administration is sometimes associated with self-limiting infusional toxicities, mAbs often have little cumulative toxicity on major organs. Genetic approaches to render murine mAbs nonimmunogenic have resulted in a generation of "humanized" mAbs, prolonging half-life, improving bioavailability, and limiting immunogenicity. Major disadvantages of mAbs are their expense, the variable pharmacokinetic profiles, and the requirement for intravenous administration.

Table 118.5. *Thalidomide for treatment of GVHD*

Reference	Indication	Thalidomide regimen	Response assessed	Patients	CR	CR + PR
Acute GVHD						
Lim et al. (1988)	Refractory	400–800 mg p.o. daily	–	1	0%	*a
Ringden et al. (1988)	Refractory	200–1,000 mg p.o. daily	–	3	0%	0%
McCarthy et al. (1988)	Refractory	200–400 mg p.o. daily	–	3	0%	0%
Mehta et al. (1999)	Refractory	12.5–25 mg/kg p.o. daily	–	2	0%	50%
Chronic GVHD						
Arora et al. (2001)	Primary	200–800 mg p.o. daily CSP/MP	6 months	27	17%	88%
(randomized controls)		By blood levels		27	28%	84%
Vogelsang et al. (1992)	High-risk	12–25 mg/kg p.o. daily	6 months	21	33%	8%
Cole et al. (1994)	Dependent	300 mg p.o. daily	–	5	*	*
Saurat et al. (1988)	Refractory	200–400 mg p.o. daily	–	1	0%	*
McCarthy et al. (1988)	Refractory	100–200 mg p.o. daily	–	3	0%	*
Heney et al. (1988)	Refractory		–	2	0%	*
Heney et al. (1991)	Refractory	By blood levels	–	6	–	(83%)b
Vogelsang et al. (1992)	Refractory	100–300 mg p.o. q.i.d.	6 months	23	30%	78%
Parker et al. (1995)	Refractory	3–12 mg/kg p.o. daily	3 months	80	11%	20%
Rovelli et al. (1998)	Refractory	12.5–25 mg/kg p.o. daily	–	13	38%	69%
Mehta et al. (1999)	Refractory	50–200 mg p.o. q.i.d.	1–3 months	4	25%	25%
Brown et al. (2000)	Refractory	200–1,000 mg p.o. daily	–	37	3%	38%
van de Poel et al. (2001)	Refractory		–	12	33%	75%

Abbreviations: –, Not stated; CR, complete response; PR, partial response; CSP, cyclosporine; MP, methylprednisolone.

[a] Case report of responsive disease indicated by *.

[b] Response rates in parentheses were reported as "improved".

The number of potential molecular targets on lymphocytes targeted by mAbs is growing. Certainly, signaling molecules (CD3), co-stimulatory molecules (CD40, CTLA-4), cytokine receptors (CD25, IL-15R), and MHC molecules required for antigen presentation are appropriate targets to test for clinical applicability. In addition, mAbs directed against a number of molecules that promote activation-induced apoptosis of peripheral T cells may help to facilitate transplantation tolerance.

Mechanism of action for anti-CD25 mAb

Daclizumab, basiliximab, and inolimomab (BT-563, B-B10) are mAbs that are directed against CD25, the IL-2 receptor α chain. The α chain is upregulated during T-cell activation, and thus is a potentially selective target for activated T cells specifically. Inhibition of IL-2 binding to the receptor results in inhibition of the cell proliferation and facilitation of activation-induced cell death. Daclizumab is a humanized IgGI mAb and basiliximab is a chimeric IgG1 mAb with half-lives of about 1 week in solid organ transplant recipients following intravenous administration. Inolimomab, a murine mAb, has a much shorter half-life. The drugs are approved for prevention of acute organ rejection in adults following renal transplantation when used in conjunction with other immunosuppressive drugs.

The most frequent adverse reactions reported are gastrointestinal (nausea, vomiting, diarrhea, constipation), although they are very uncommon. There has been no increase in the risk of posttransplant lymphoproliferative disorders or infections compared to appropriate placebo controls, although this susceptible population must be monitored closely.

Anti-CD25 mAb for prevention and treatment of GVHD

Inolimomab was one of the first anti-CD25 antibodies tested for treatment of steroid-refractory GVHD. In a number of small series, complete responses were achieved in 28% to 88% of patients using this antibody (Table 118.6). Daily dosing for an extended period was required in order to achieve the best outcomes. Although this was in part due to the short half-life of this antibody, it was also appreciated that high levels of soluble CD25 in the blood served to neutralize the antibody, reducing the immunosuppressive efficacy.

Cahn et al. (1995) evaluated inolimomab in the primary treatment of acute GVHD. In their randomized trial comparing steroids alone to steroids plus inolimomab, the addition of the mAb did not improve the response rate or survival. It should be noted, however, that the response rates were high in both the inolimomab and placebo arms (70% vs. 63%), and it may have been difficult to detect an effect of the drug in a population that was apparently so steroid-sensitive.

The longer half-life of the humanized anti-CD25 mAbs, daclizumab and basiliximab, allowed for less frequent administration and the potential for less resource utilization in the outpatient setting, although overcoming high levels of soluble CD25 may still require frequent early dosing. With such intensive dose schedules of daclizumab and basiliximab, complete responses of 8% to 47% of patients with refractory acute GVHD were reported (Table 118.6). Responses did not appear to be more frequent when etanercept or sirolimus was added to the therapeutic regimen (Weisser et al., 2002; Wolff et al., 2002), but controlled studies have not been performed.

Table 118.6. *Anti-CD25 monoclonal antibodies for treatment of steroid-refractory acute GVHD*

Reference	Drug	Regimen	Response assessed	Patients	CR	CR + PR
Herve et al. (1990)	InolimomAb	5 mg q 1–2 days × 10	–	32	66%	84%
Cuthbert et al. (1992)	InolimomAb	5 mg q day × 10	–	14	29%	57%
Hertenstein et al. (1994)	InolimomAb	10 mg q day	–	11	45%	55%
Hertenstein et al. (1994)	InolimomAb	5–10 mg q day × 20	–	8	88%	88%
Herbelin et al. (1994)	InolimomAb	0.2 mg/kg q day	–	15	73%	87%
Breucher-Encker et al. (2002)	InolimomAb	0.2 mg/kg q day × 5	–	5	60%	80%
Bay et al. (2002)	InolimomAb	0.3–0.4 mg/kg q day × 28	–	25	28%	80%
Anasetti et al. (1994)	Daclizumab	0.5–1.5 mg/kg × 1	Day 28	20	25%	50%
Przepiorka et al. (2000b)	Daclizumab	1 mg/kg q wk × 5	Day 43	24	29%	33%
Przepiorka et al. (2000b)	Daclizumab	1 mg/kg days 1,4,8,15,21	Day 43	19	47%	74%
Willenbacher et al. (2001)	Daclizumab	1 mg/kg days 1–5,7,14,21	Day 28	12	8%	67%
Wolff et al. (2002)	Daclizumab[a]	1 mg/kg days 1,4,8,15,22	–	7	57%	86%
Weisser et al. (2002)	Daclizumab[b]	1 mg/kg days 1,4,8,15,22,28	–	11	45%	55%
Pasquini et al. (2000)	Basiliximab	10–20 mg q wk × 4	–	12	25%	58%
Massenkeil et al. (2001)	Basiliximab	20 mg q day × 2, then weekly	–	17	47%	(88%)[c]

Abbreviations: –, not stated; CR, complete response; PR, partial response.

[a] In addition to etanercept.

[b] In addition to sirolimus.

[c] Response rates in parentheses were reported as "improved".

Daclizumab was also studied in the prophylaxis setting. In a prospective, randomized trial in unrelated donor marrow transplant recipients, administration of daclizumab weekly from day -1, in addition to standard prophylaxis, delayed the onset of GVHD, but the overall rate of GVHD was unchanged (Anasetti et al., 1995). The lack of efficacy may have been due to blockade of activation-induced cell death resulting from inhibition of the IL-2 signal by early administration of the mAb. A potential alternative involves a pre-emptive strategy, administering the mAb posttransplant after alloactivation has occurred.

Mechanism of action for alemtuzumab

Alemtuzumab (Campath-1H) is a humanized IgG1κ mAb approved for the treatment of refractory B-cell chronic lymphatic leukemia. It binds to, and targets, the 21–28 kDa CD52 antigen, a pan-leukocyte antigen, and promotes death of the cells to which it binds. CD52 is a prominent, nonmodulating cell surface molecule expressed on normal and malignant T and B lymphocytes, natural killer cells, monocytes, and macrophages. It is not expressed on hematopoietic stem cells. Administration of alemtuzumab is thought to induce antibody-dependent lysis of CD52+ cells. Weekly intravenous administration of drug demonstrated marked interpatient variability, relative dose proportionality with alemtuzumab AUC, and an average half-life of 12 days at steady state. In marrow transplant recipients, immunosuppressive levels of alemtuzumab are detectable through 2 to 3 weeks after pretransplant dosing (Rebello et al., 2001).

Infusions of alemtuzumab are relatively well tolerated; infusion-related adverse reactions, including rigors, fever, nausea, vomiting, hypotension, and bronchospasm, have been reported. Many of these immediate reactions are attenuated by premedication with oral antihistamines and acetaminophen prior to dosing, and with gradual escalation of the effective dose. More serious hematologic adverse events include pan- or monocytopenias and marrow hypoplasia. Serious viral, bacterial, fungal, and opportunistic infections have been reported, and concomitant prophylaxis against opportunistic infections is often initiated.

Campath-1H for prevention of GVHD (and see Chapter 109)

There is a growing body of literature supporting the expectation that alemtuzumab would be effective in the prevention of acute GVHD (Table 118.7). Alemtuzumab has been administered in doses of 20 mg for 5 days as part of the conditioning regimen in order to effect ablation of the host immune system, and the prolonged half-life of the mAb allows for continued immunosuppression after transplantation. Alemtuzumab has also been administered in a single dose followed by ex vivo incubation of the allograft "in the bag." Whether other pharmacologic immunosuppression is needed in addition to alemtuzumab is still not clear.

In studies performed using alemtuzumab with cyclosporine, methotrexate or mycophenolate mofetil, the risk of grades II to IV GVHD has generally been less than 10% (Table 118.7), although graft failure is a potential problem, and mixed chimerism is not uncommon. In the absence of additional T-cell activation inhibitors, the risk of GVHD has been higher but still comparable to those achieved with standard pharmacologic interventions (Rizzieri et al., 2001a,b).

The profound immunosuppression induced by alemtuzumab has also resulted in a substantial increase in the risk of infection, especially early cytomegalovirus infections, after allo-

Table 118.7. *Alemtuzumab for prevention of GVHD*

Reference	Conditioning regimen	Donor	GVHD prophylaxis regimen	Patients	Grade II–IV GVHD	Grade III–IV acute GVHD	Graft failure
Hale et al. (2000)	A	Sibling	CAM 10–60 mg ITB +/− CSP/MTX	107	4%[a]	1%	2%
Kottaridis et al. (2000)	A	Sibling	CAM 20 mg i.v. days −8 to −4 + CSP+/−MTX	36	6%	0%	5%
Chakraverty et al. (2001)	A	Sibling	CAM 20 mg i.v. days −9 to −5 + TCD	34	6%	3%	3%
Rizzieri et al. (2001a)	N	Sibling	CAM ITB + 20 mg IV × 5	36	26%	10%	0%[b]
Potter et al. (2000)	M	Mixed	CAM (mixed schedules) +/− CSP	28	7%	0%	7%
Devereux et al. (2001)	N	Mixed	CAM 20 mg i.v. days −5 to −1 + CSP/MMF	6	0%	0%	25%
Rizzieri et al. (2001b)	N	Alternative	CAM ITB + 20 mg i.v. × 5 + MMF	24	29%	21%	0%[b]
Chakraverty et al. (2002)	A	Alternative	CAM 20 mg i.v. days −8 to −4 + CSP	47	21%	0%	5%

Abbreviations: N, non-myeloablative; A, myeloablative or reduced intensity; CAM, Campath-1H, alemtuzumab; ITB, in the bag; MMF, mycophenolate mofetil; i.v., intravenously; CSP, cyclosporine; MTX, methotrexate; TCD, ex vivo T-cell depletion.

[a] Actuarial estimate, cumulative incidence or proportion, depending on the result reported.

[b] Late graft failure reported but not quantitated.

geneic hematopoietic stem cell transplantation (Charkabarti *et al.*, 2002). In addition, early relapse of the primary malignancy has been noted (Devereux *et al.*, 2001). Additional studies are under way to identify a dose schedule that will control GVHD adequately without predisposing patients to prolonged risks of infection and loss of the graft-versus-tumor effect.

Other mAbs for the prevention or treatment of GVHD

A number of clinical manifestations of chronic GVHD are mediated by autoantibodies, and B cells have become a novel target for therapy. Several case reports demonstrate that anti-B-cell therapy using rituximab can be effective in this setting (Ratanatharathorn *et al.*, 2000; Szabolcs *et al.*, 2000; Ackerstein *et al.*, 2002). Prospective studies are lacking.

There are also several mAbs in development that target T-cell antigens. The choice of cell surface antigen targeted is often based on the biology of the molecule, with the aim of inducing apoptosis or interrupting T-cell activation, adhesion, or differentiation. The 50 kDa CD2 molecule, for instance, is known to be important for T and natural killer (NK) adhesion, cell activation, and function. A phase II study of BTI-322, the murine antibody, reported a 30% complete response rate for steroid-refractory acute GVHD with 10 days of therapy (Przepiorka *et al.*, 1998), and preliminary data from a randomized phase I study of siplizumab, the humanized form of this mAb, for primary treatment of acute GVHD suggested that it was more effective than steroids alone (Adkins *et al.*, 2000).

There is promising early experience using visilizumab, a variant of a humanized anti-CD3 IgG2 mAb that does not bind Fc receptors and does not activate complement (Carpenter *et al.*, 2000). This product was evaluated in a phase I study of steroid-refractory severe GVHD (Carpenter *et al.*, 2002). There were no serious immediate or infusional toxicities, and cytokine release syndrome was not a problem. Moreover, 7 (47%) of 15 patients achieved a complete response. Further studies are ongoing.

CD147 is an adhesion molecule expressed on the surface of activated T-cells, B cells, and monocytes. CD147 is found on nonlymphoid tissues as well, including muscle where it is involved in lactate transport. The murine anti-CD147 mAb ABX-CBL was tested in a phase II clinical trial for patients with refractory acute GVHD. Complete responses that lasted at least 14 days occurred in only 16% of the patients treated (Deeg *et al.*, 2001). A randomized trial comparing ABX-CBL to ATG for refractory GVHD has been completed. Systemic toxicities have generally been mild, but myalgias were dose-limiting.

Conclusions

Elucidation of the mechanism of T-cell activation and the mediators of allograft reactions has provided a range of targets for therapeutic immunosuppressive agents. New agents developed over the past decade have targeted specific steps in these pathways, in hopes of producing selective suppression of the allograft reaction while maintaining third party responses and minimizing toxicities. The most potent agents available clearly still have broad rather than selective immunosuppressive activity, but ongoing studies to determine the optimal dose schedule and combinations of immunosuppressive drugs may yet provide a pharmacologic means to facilitate peripheral tolerance for allogeneic hematopoietic stem cell transplant recipients without inducing paralysis of the immune system.

References

Abhyankar, S., Godder, K., Christiansen, N. *et al.* (1998). Treatment of resistant acute and chronic graft versus host disease with mycophenolate mofetil. *Blood*, **92**, 340b.

Ackerstein, A., Slavin, S., Shapira, M. *et al.* (2002). MAbThera: an optional treatment for chronic graft-vs-host disease (GVHD). *Bone Marrow Transplantation*, **29**, S188.

Adkins, D., Ratanatharathorn, V., & Dingivan, C. (2000). A Phase I placebo-controlled, randomized, dose-escalation safety study of MEDI-507, a humanized anti-CD2 monoclonal antibody, in the initial treatment of at least grade II acute graft-versus-host disease (GVHD). *Blood*, **96**, 476a.

Anasetti, C., Hansen, J.A., Walsmann, T.A. *et al.* (1994). Treatment of acute graft-versus-host disease with humanized anti-Tac, an antibody that binds to the interleukin-2 receptor. *Blood*, **84**, 1320–7.

Anasetti, C., Lin, A., Nademanee, A. *et al.* (1995). A phase II/III randomized, double-blind, placebo-controlled multicenter trial of humanized anti-Tac for prevention of acute graft-versus-host disease (GVHD) in recipients of marrow transplants from unrelated donors. *Blood*, **86**, 621a.

Andolina, M., Rabusin, M., Maximova, N. *et al.* (2000). Etanercept in graft-versus-host disease. *Bone Marrow Transplantation*, **26**, 929.

Antin, J.H., Lee, S.J., Neuberg, D. *et al.* (2001). Sirolimus (RAP), tacrolimus (FK), and low dose methotrexate (MTX) for GVHD prophylaxis in mismatched related donor or unrelated donor transplantation. *Blood*, **98**, 857a.

Antin, J.H., Kim, H. T., Cutler, C. *et al.* (2003). Sirolimus, tacrolimus, and low-dose methotrexate for graft-versus-host disease prophylaxis in mismatched related donor or unrelated donor transplantation. *Blood*, in press.

Arora, M., Wagner, J.E., Davies, S.M. *et al.* (2001). Randomized clinical trial of thalidomide, cyclosporine and prednisone versus cyclosporine and prednisone as initial therapy for chronic graft-versus-host disease. *Biology of Blood and Marrow Transplantation*, **7**, 265–73.

Basara, N., Blau, W.I., Kiehl, M.G. *et al.* (2000). Mycophenolate mofetil for the prophylaxis of acute GVHD in HLA-mismatched bone marrow transplant patients. *Clinical Transplantation*, **14**, 121–6.

Basara, N., Kiehl, M.G., Blau, W. *et al.* (2001). Mycophenolate mofetil in the treatment of acute and chronic GVHD in hematopoietic stem cell transplant patients: four years of experience. *Transplantation Proceedings*, **33**, 2121–3.

Bay, J., Sutton, L., Vannier, J. *et al.* (2002). InolimomAb (Leukotac) in the treatment of acute graft versus host disease following allogeneic hematopoietic stem cell transplantation. *Bone Marrow Transplantation,* **29,** S183.

Benito, A.I., Furlong, T., Martin, P.J. *et al.* (2001). Sirolimus (rapamycin) for the treatment of steroid-refractory acute graft-versus-host disease. *Transplantation,* **72,** 1924–9.

Bornhauser, M., Schuler, U., Porksen, G. *et al.* (1999). Mycophenolate mofetil and cyclosporine as graft-versus-host disease prophylaxis after allogeneic blood stem cell transplantation. *Transplantation,* **67,** 499–504.

Browne, P.V., Weisdorf, D.J., DeFor, T. *et al.* (2000). Response to thalidomide therapy in refractory chronic graft-versus-host disease. *Bone Marrow Transplantation,* **26,** 865–9.

Bruecher-Encke, B., Hoepfner, S., Luft, T. *et al.* (2002). InolimomAb treatment of steroid refractory acute GVHD—association with invasive aspergillosis? *Bone Marrow Transplantation,* **29,** S182.

Busca, A., Saroglia, E.M., Lanino, E. *et al.* (2000). Mycophenolate mofetil (MMF) as therapy for refractory chronic GVHD (cGVHD) in children receiving bone marrow transplantation. *Bone Marrow Transplantation,* **25,** 1067–71.

Cahn, J.Y., Bordigoni, P., Tiberghein, P. *et al.* (1995). Treatment of acute graft-versus-host disease with methylprednisolone and cyclosporine with or without an anti-interleukin-2 receptor monoclonal antibody. A multicenter phase III study. *Transplantation,* **60,** 939–42.

Cairo, M.S., Harrison, L., Bessmertny, O. *et al.* (2002). A pilot study of tacrolimus (FK506) and mycophenolate mofetil (MMF) for GVHD prophylaxis in allogeneic related and unrelated SCT (allo SCT). *Biology of Blood and Marrow Transplantation,* **8,** 84.

Carnevale-Schianca, F., Martin, P., Sullivan, K. *et al.* (2000). Changing from cyclosporine to tacrolimus as salvage therapy for chronic graft-versus-host disease. *Biology of Blood and Marrow Transplantation,* **6,** 613–20.

Carpenter, P.A., Appelbaum, F.R., Corey, L. *et al.* (2002). A humanized non-FcR-binding anti-CD3 antibody, visilizumAb for treatment of steroid-refractory acute graft-versus-host disease. *Blood,* **99,** 2712–9.

Carpenter, P.A., Pavlovic, S., Tso, *et al.* (2000). Non-Fc receptor-binding humanized anti-CD3 antibodies induce apoptosis of activated human T-cells. *Journal of Immunology,* **165,** 6205–13.

Chakrabarti, S., Mackinnon, S., Chopra, R. *et al.* (2002). High incidence of cytomegalovirus infection after nonmyeloablative stem cell transplantation: potential role of Campath-1H in delaying immune reconstitution. *Blood,* **99,** 4357–63.

Chakraverty, R., Peggs, K., Chopra, R. *et al.* (2002). Limiting transplantation-related mortality following unrelated donor stem cell transplantation by using a nonmyeloablative conditioning regimen. *Blood,* **99,** 1071–8.

Chakraverty, R., Robinson, S., Peggs, K. *et al.* (2001). Excessive T-cell depletion of peripheral blood stem cells has an adverse effect upon outcome following allogeneic stem cell transplantation. *Bone Marrow Transplantation,* **28,** 827–34.

Chao, N.J., Parker, P.M., Niland, J.C. *et al.* (1996). Paradoxical effect of thalidomide prophylaxis on chronic graft-vs-host disease. *Biology of Blood and Marrow Transplantation,* **2,** 86–92.

Cherwinski, H.M., McCarley, D., Schatzman, R. *et al.* (1995). The immunosuppressant leflunomide inhibits lymphocyte progression through cell cycle by a novel mechanism. *Journal of Pharmacology and Experimental Therapeutics,* **272,** 460–8.

Chiang, K.Y., Abhyankar, S., Bridges, K. *et al.* (2002). Recombinant human tumor necrosis factor receptor fusion protein as complementary treatment for chronic graft-versus-host disease. *Transplantation,* **73,** 665–7.

Choi, C.J. & Nghiem, P. (2001). Tacrolimus ointment in the treatment of chronic cutaneous graft-vs-host disease: a case series of 18 patients. *Archives of Dermatology,* **137,** 1202–6.

Cole, C.H., Rogers, P.C., Pritchard, S. *et al.* (1994). Thalidomide in the management of chronic graft-versus-host disease in children following bone marrow transplantation. *Bone Marrow Transplantation,* **14,** 937–42.

Corral, L.G. & Kaplan, G. (1999). Immunomodulation by thalidomide and thalidomide analogues. *Annals of Rheumatic Diseases,* **58,** 107–13.

Cuthbert, R.J., Phillips, G.L., Barnett, M.J. *et al.* (1992). Anti-interleukin-2 receptor monoclonal antibody (BT563) in the treatment of severe acute GVHD refractory to systemic corticosteroid therapy. *Bone Marrow Transplantation,* **10,** 451–5.

D'Amato, R.J., Loughnan, M.S., Flynn, E. *et al.* (1994). Thalidomide is an inhibitor of angiogenesis. *Proceedings of the National Academy of Sciences, USA,* **91,** 4082–5.

Deeg, H.J., Blazar, B.R., Bolwell, B.J. *et al.* (2001). Treatment of steroid-refractory acute graft-versus-host disease with anti-C147 monoclonal antibody ABX-CBL. *Blood,* **98,** 2052–8.

Devereux, S., Parker, J.E., Shafi, T. *et al.* (2001). CAMPATH-1H reduces the risk of graft versus host disease following allogeneic hematopoietic stem cell transplantation and minimally myelosuppressive conditioning treatment with low dose total body irradiation and cyclosporine/mycophenolate mofetil immunosuppression. *Blood,* **98,** 355b.

Fuchs, M., Waldschmidt, D., Scheid, C. *et al.* (2002). Anti-TNF-alpha antibody in the treatment of severe acute graft versus host disease. *Bone Marrow Transplantation,* **29,** S182.

Furlong, T., Storb, R., Anasetti, C. *et al.* (2000). Clinical outcome after conversion to FK506 (tacrolimus) therapy for acute graft-versus-host disease resistant to cyclosporine or for cyclosporine-associated toxicities. *Bone Marrow Transplantation,* **26,** 985–91.

Gummert, J.F., Barten, M.J., Sherwood, S.W. *et al.* (1999). Pharmacodynamics of immunosuppression by mycophenolic acid: inhibition of both lymphocyte proliferation and activation correlates with pharmacokinetics. *Journal of Pharmacology and Experimental Therapeutics,* **291,** 1100–12.

Gummert, J.F., Barten, M.J., van Gelder, T. *et al.* (2000). Pharmacodynamics of mycophenolic acid in heart allograft recipients: correlation of lymphocyte proliferation and activation with pharmacokinetics and graft histology. *Transplantation,* **70,** 1038–49.

Hale, G., Jacobs, P., Wood, L. *et al.* (2000). CD52 antibodies for prevention of graft-versus-host disease and graft rejection following transplantation of allogeneic peripheral blood stem cells. *Bone Marrow Transplantation,* **26,** 69–76.

Halloran, P., Mathew, T., Tomlanovich, S. *et al.* (1997). Mycophenolate mofetil in renal allograft recipients: a pooled efficacy analysis of three randomized, double-blind, clinical studies in prevention of rejection. The International Mycophenolate Mofetil Renal Transplant Study Groups. *Transplantation*, **63**, 39–47.

Haslett, P.A., Corral, L.G., Albert, M. *et al.* (1998). Thalidomide costimulates primary human T lymphocytes, preferentially inducing proliferation, cytokine production, and cytotoxic responses in the CD8+ subset. *Journal of Experimental Medicine*, **187**, 1885–92.

Heney, D., Lewis, I.J., & Bailey, C.C. (1988). Thalidomide for chronic graft-versus-host disease in children. *Lancet*, **2**, 1317.

Heney, D., Norfolk, D.R., Wheeldon, J. *et al.* (1991). Thalidomide treatment for chronic graft-versus-host disease. *British Journal of Haematology*, **78**, 23–7.

Herbelin, C., Stephan, J.-L., Donadieu, J. *et al.* (1994). Treatment of steroid-resistant acute graft-versus-host disease with an anti-IL-2-receptor monoclonal antibody (BT563) in children who received T-cell depleted, partially matched, related bone marrow transplants. *Bone Marrow Transplantation*, **13**, 563–9.

Hertenstein, B., Stefanic, M., Sandherr, M. *et al.* (1994). Treatment of steroid-resistant acute graft-vs-host disease after allogeneic marrow transplantation with anti-interleukin-2 receptor antibody (BT563). *Transplantation Proceedings*, **26**, 3114–6.

Herve, P., Wijdenes, J., Bergerat, J.P. *et al.* (1990). Treatment of corticosteroid resistant acute graft-versus-host disease by in vivo administration of anti-interleukin-2 receptor monoclonal antibody (B-B10). *Blood*, **75**, 1017–23.

Hiraoka, A., Ohashi, Y., Okamoto, S. *et al.* (2001). Phase III study comparing tacrolimus (FK506) with cyclosporine for graft-versus-host disease prophylaxis after allogeneic bone marrow transplantation. *Bone Marrow Transplantation*, **28**, 181–5.

Horowitz, M.M., Przepiorka, D., Bartels, P. *et al.* (1999). Tacrolimus versus cyclosporine immunosuppression: results in advanced stage disease patients with comparison to historical controls treated exclusively with cyclosporine. *Biology of Blood and Marrow Transplantation*, **5**, 180–6.

Ihlan, O., Celebi, H., Arat, O. *et al.* (1999). Treatment of acute and chronic graft versus host disease with mycophenolate mofetil. *Blood*, **94**, 368b.

Jacobsohn, D.A., Hallick, J., Anders, V. *et al.* (2002). Infliximab for the treatment of steroid-refractory acute GVHD. *Biology of Blood and Marrow Transplantation*, **8**, 87.

Jacobsohn, D.A., Margolis, J., Chen, A.R. *et al.* (2001). Pentostatin: a promising treatment for refractory chronic GVHD. *Blood*, **98**, 399a.

Jenke, A., Renner, U., Richte, M. *et al.* (2001). Pharmacokinetics of intravenous mycophenolate mofetil after allogeneic blood stem cell transplantation. *Clinical Transplantation*, **15**, 176–84.

Johnson, S.A. (2000). Clinical pharmacokinetics of nucleoside analogues: focus on haematological malignancies. *Clinical Pharmacokinetics*, **39**, 5–26.

Johnston, L.J., Shizuru, J.S., & Stockerl-Goldstein, K.E. (2002). Rapamycin for treatment of chronic graft versus host disease. *Biology of Blood and Marrow Transplantation*, **8**, 87.

Kalogiannidis, P., Papadakis, E., Sakellari, I. *et al.* (2002). Treatment of refractory chronic graft versus host disease (cGVHD) with MMF: preliminary results. *Bone Marrow Transplantation*, **29**, S185.

Kanamaru, A., Takemoto, Y., Kakishita, E. *et al.* (1995). FK506 treatment of graft-versus-host disease developing or exacerbating during prophylaxis with cyclosporin and/or other immunosuppressants. *Bone Marrow Transplantation*, **15**, 885–9.

Khouri, I.F., Saliba, R.M., Giralt, S.A. *et al.* (2001). Nonablative allogeneic hematopoietic transplantation as adoptive immunotherapy for indolent lymphoma: low incidence of toxicity, acute graft-versus-host disease, and treatment-related mortality. *Blood*, **98**, 3595–9.

Kiehl, M.G., Armstrong, V., Basara, N. *et al.* (1999). Intravenous mycophenolate mofetil plus prednisolone and cyclosporine in the prophylaxis of GVHD after stem cell transplantation. *Blood*, **94**, 153a.

Klein, S.A., Dietrich, C.F., Wassman, B. *et al.* (2002). Treatment of steroid refractory acute intestinal graft versus host disease with pentostatin. *Bone Marrow Transplantation*, **29**, S187.

Kobbe, G., Aivado, M., Huenerlituerkoglu, A. *et al.* (2000). High incidence of acute GVHD after allogeneic blood stem cell transplantation following minimal intensive conditioning. *Blood*, **96**, 784a.

Kobbe, G., Schneider, P., Rohr, U. *et al.* (2001). Treatment of severe steroid refractory acute graft-versus-host disease with infliximab, a chimeric human/mouse anti-TNF alpha antibody. *Bone Marrow Transplantation*, **28**, 47–9.

Koc, S., Leisenring, W., Flowers, M.E. *et al.* (2000). Thalidomide for treatment of patients with chronic graft-versus-host disease. *Blood*, **96**, 3995–6.

Koch, H.P. (1985). Thalidomide and congeners as anti-inflammatory agents. *Progress in Medicinal Chemistry*, **22**, 165–242.

Koehler, M.T., Howrie, D., Mirro, J. *et al.* (1995). FK506 (tacrolimus) in the treatment of steroid-resistant acute graft-versus-host disease in children undergoing bone marrow transplantation. *Bone Marrow Transplantation*, **15**, 895–9.

Kottaridis, P.D., Milligan, D.W., Chopra, R. *et al.* (2000). In vivo CAMPATH-1H prevents graft-versus-host disease following non-myeloablative stem cell transplantation. *Blood*, **96**, 2419–25.

Kraut, L., Guenzelmann, S., Shipkova, M. *et al.* (2002). Randomized multicenter prospective clinical trial on the efficacy of mycophenolate mofetil in comparison to methotrexate for the prophylaxis of acute GVHD in stem cell transplant recipients. *Bone Marrow Transplantation*, **29**, S177.

Kruse, F.E., Joussen, A.M., Rohrschneider, K. *et al.* (1998). Thalidomide inhibits corneal angiogenesis induced by vascular endothelial growth factor. *Graefes Archive for Clinical and Experimental Ophthalmology*, **236**, 461–6.

Laliberte, J., Yee, A., Xiong, Y. *et al.* (1998). Effects of guanine nucleotide depletion on cell cycle progression in human T lymphocytes. *Blood*, **91**, 2896–904.

LeBlanc, R., Belanger, R., Busque, L. *et al.* (2001). Early introduction of FK506 followed by MMF in non-myeloablative hematopoietic stem cell allotransplantation (NMA-HSCAT) leads to prompt engraftment without acute GVHD. *Blood*, **98**, 186a.

Lim, S.H., McWhannell, A., Vora, A.J. *et al.* (1988). Successful treatment with thalidomide of acute graft-versus-host disease after bone-marrow transplantation. *Lancet*, **1**, 117.

Lopez, F., Parker, P., Rodriguez, R. *et al.* (2001). Efficacy of mycophenolate mofetil (MMF) in the treatment of chronic graft versus host disease. *Blood*, **98**, 398a.

Magalhaes-Silverman, M., Lee, C-K., Hohl, R. et al. (2001). Treatment of severe steroid refractory acute graft versus host disease with infliximab. Blood, 98, 359b.

Maris, M., Niederwieser, D., Sandmaier, B. et al. (2001). Nonmyeloabltaive hematopoietic stem cell transplants (HSCT) using 10/10 HLA antigen matched unrelated donors (URDs) for patients with advanced hematologic malignancies ineligible for conventional HCT. Blood, 98, 858a.

Massenkeil, G., Genvresse, I., Rackwitz, S. et al. (2001). The interleukin 2 receptor antagonist basiliximab is well tolerated and effective in the therapy of steroid-resistant acute graft-versus-host disease (GVHD) after allogeneic stem cell transplantation. Blood, 98, 663a.

McCarthy, D.M., Kanfer, E., Taylor, J. et al. (1988). Thalidomide for graft-versus-host disease. Lancet, 2, 1135.

McHugh, S.M. & Rowland, T.L. (1997). Thalidomide and derivatives: immunological investigations of tumor necrosis factor-alpha (TNF-alpha) inhibition suggest drugs capable of selective gene regulation. Clinical and Experimental Immunology, 110, 151–4.

McSweeney, P., Abhyankar, S., Blunk, B. et al. (2002). Tacrolimus and mycophenolate mofetil for GVHD prevention in adult hematopoietic allograft recipients. Experimental Hematology, 30, 119.

McSweeney, P.A., Niederweiser, D., Shizuru, J.A. et al. (2001). Hematopoietic cell transplantation in older patients with hematologic malignancies: replacing high-dose cytotoxic therapy with graft-versus-tumor effects. Blood, 97, 3390–400.

Mehta, P., Kedar, A., Graham-Pole, J. et al. (1999). Thalidomide in children undergoing bone marrow transplantation: series at a single institution and review of the literature. Pediatrics, 103, e44.

Meiser, B.M., Pfeiffer, M., Schmidt, D. et al. (1999). Combination therapy with tacrolimus and mycophenolate mofetil following cardiac transplantation: importance of mycophenolic acid therapeutic drug monitoring. Journal of Heart and Lung Transplantation, 18, 143–9.

Mignat, C. (1997). Clinically significant drug interactions with new immunosuppressive agents. Drug Safety, 16, 267–78.

Mollee, P., Morton, A.J., Irving, I. et al. (2001). Combination therapy with tacrolimus and anti-thymocyte globulin for the treatment of steroid-resistant acute graft-versus-host disease developing during cyclosporine prophylaxis. British Journal of Haematology, 113, 217–23.

Mookerjee, B., Altomonte, V., & Vogelsang, G. (1999). Salvage therapy for refractory chronic graft-versus-host disease with mycophenolate mofetil and tacrolimus. Bone Marrow Transplantation, 24, 517–20.

Moreira, A.L., Sampaio, E.P., Zmuidzinas, A. et al. (1993). Thalidomide exerts its inhibitory action on tumor necrosis factor alpha by enhancing mRNA degradation. Journal of Experimental Medicine, 177, 1675–80.

Moreira, A.L., Tsenova-Berkova, L., Wang, J. et al. (1997). Effect of cytokine modulation by thalidomide on the granulomatous response in murine tuberculosis. Tubercle and Lung Disease, 78, 47–55.

Morris, J.A. (1989). A mutational theory of leukaemogenesis. Journal of Clinical Pathology, 42, 337–40.

Nagler, A., Menachem, Y., & Ilan, Y. (2001). Amelioration of steroid-resistant chronic graft-versus-host mediated liver disease via tacrolimus treatment. Journal of Hematotherapy and Stem Cell Research, 10, 411–7.

Narwani, R.R., Reddy, V., Wingard, J.R. et al. (1999). Topical tacrolimus may be useful for skin manifestations of acute and chronic graft-versus-host disease (GVHD) after bone marrow transplantation (BMT). Blood, 94, 370b.

Nash, R.A., Antin, J.H., Karanes, C. et al. (2000). A phase III study comparing methotrexate and tacrolimus with methotrexate and cyclosporine for prophylaxis of acute graft-versus-host disease after marrow transplantation from unrelated donors. Blood, 96, 2062–8.

Nowak, I. & Shaw, L.M. (1995). Mycophenolic acid binding to human serum albumin: characterization and relation to pharmacodynamics. Clinical Chemistry, 41, 1011–7.

Nowak, I. & Shaw, L.M. (1997). Effect of mycophenolic acid glucuronide on inosine monophosphate dehydrogenase activity. Therapeutic Drug Monitoring, 19, 358–60.

Pallotta-Filho, R.S., Barbosa, J.A.L., Macedo, M.C.M.A. et al. (1998). The use of mycophenolate mofetil in the treatment of refractory chronic graft versus host disease. Blood, 92, 346b.

Parker, P.M., Chao, N., Nademanee, A. et al. (1995). Thalidomide as salvage therapy for chronic graft-versus-host disease. Blood, 86, 3604–9.

Pasquini, R., Moreira, V.A., de Medeiros, C.R. et al. (2000). Basiliximab (BaMAb)—a selective interleukin-2 receptor (IL-2R) antagonist—as therapy for refractory acute graft versus host disease (a-GVHD) following bone marrow transplantation (BMT). Blood, 96, 177a.

Potter, M.N., Grace, S.C., Teehan, C. et al. (2000). Campath 1 H "in the bag" is an effective method of GVHD prevention in allogeneic stem cell transplantation. Blood, 96, 476a.

Przepiorka, D., Blamble, D., Hilsenbeck, S. et al. (2000a). Tacrolimus clearance is age-dependent within the pediatric population. Bone Marrow Transplantation, 26, 601–5.

Przepiorka, D., Devine, S.M., Fay, J.W. et al. (1999a). Practical considerations in the use of tacrolimus for allogeneic marrow transplantation. Bone Marrow Transplantation, 24, 1053–6.

Przepiorka, D., Kernan, N.A., Ippoliti, C. et al. (2000b). Daclizumab, a humanized anti-interleukin-2 receptor alpha chain antibody, for treatment of acute graft-versus-host disease. Blood, 95, 83–9.

Przepiorka, D., Khouri, I., Ippoliti, C. et al. (1999b). Tacrolimus and minidose methotrexate for prevention of acute graft-vs-host disease after HLA-mismatched marrow or blood stem cell transplantation. Bone Marrow Transplantation, 24, 763–8.

Przepiorka, D., Nash, R.A., Wingard, J.R. et al. (1999c). Relationship of tacrolimus whole blood levels to efficacy and safety outcomes after unrelated donor marrow transplantation. Biology of Blood and Marrow Transplantation, 5, 94–7.

Przepiorka, D., Petropoulos, D., Mullen, C. et al. (1999d). Tacrolimus for prevention of graft-vs-host disease after mismatched unrelated donor cord blood transplantation. Bone Marrow Transplantation, 23, 1291–5.

Przepiorka, D., Phillips, G.L., Ratanatharathorn, V. et al. (1998). A phase II study of BTI-322, a monoclonal anti-CD2 antibody, for treatment of steroid-resistant acute graft-versus-host disease. Blood, 92, 4066–71.

Przepiorka, D., Smith, T., Folloder, J. et al. (1999e). Risk factors for acute graft-versus-host disease after allogeneic blood stem cell transplantation. *Blood*, **94**, 1465–70.

Ratanatharathorn, V., Carson, E., Reynolds, C. et al. (2000). Anti-CD20 chimeric monoclonal antibody treatment of refractory immune-mediated thrombocytopenia in a patient with chronic graft-versus-host disease. *Annals of Internal Medicine*, **15**, 275–9.

Ratanatharathorn, V., Nash, R.A., Przepiorka, D. et al. (1998). Phase III study comparing methotrexate and tacrolimus (Prograf, FK506) with methotrexate and cyclosporine for graft-versus-host disease prophylaxis after HLA-identical sibling bone marrow transplantation. *Blood*, **92**, 2303–14.

Rebello, P., Cwynarski, K., Varughese, M. et al. (2001). Pharmacokinetics of CAMPATH-1H in BMT patients. *Cytotherapy*, **3**, 261–7.

Redei, I., Langston, A.A., Cherry, J.K. et al. (1999). Salvage therapy with mycophenolate mofetil (MMF) for patients with severe chronic GVHD. *Blood*, **94**, 159a.

Ringden, O., Aschan, J., & Westerberg, L. (1988). Thalidomide for severe acute graft-versus-host disease. *Lancet*, **2**, 568.

Rini, B.I., Zimmerman, T., Stadler, W.M. et al. (2002). Allogeneic stem-cell transplantation of renal cell cancer after nonmyeloablative chemotherapy: feasibility, engraftment, and clinical results. *Journal of Clinical Oncology*, **20**, 2017–24.

Rizzieri, D.A., Long, G.D., Vredenburgh, J.J. et al. (2001a). Nonmyeloablative allogeneic transplantation using T depleted matched sibling peripheral blood stem cells. *Blood*, **98**, 420a.

Rizzieri, D.A., Long, G.D., Vredenburgh, J.J. et al. (2001b). Nonmyeloablative allogeneic transplantation using CAMPATH 1H for T depletion of mismatched related donor peripheral blood stem cells. *Blood*, **98**, 669a.

Roberts, T., Koc, Y., Sprague, K. et al. (1999). Mycophenolate mofetil (MMF) for the treatment of chronic graft versus host disease (cGVHD) of the liver. *Blood*, **94**, 159a.

Rovelli, A., Arrigo, C., Nesi, F. et al. (1998). The role of thalidomide in the treatment of refractory chronic graft-versus-host disease following bone marrow transplantation in children. *Bone Marrow Transplantation*, **21**, 577–81.

Rowland, T.L., McHugh, S.M., Deighton, J. et al. (1998). Differential regulation by thalidomide and dexamethasone of cytokine expression in human peripheral blood mononuclear cells. *Immunopharmacology*, **40**, 11–20.

Saitoh, O., Nakagawa, K., Sugi, K. et al. (1998). Bile acids inhibit tumour necrosis factor alpha-induced interleukin-8 production in human colon epithelial cells. *Journal of Gastroenterology and Hepatology*, **13**, 1212–7.

Sampaio, E.P., Kaplan, G., Miranda, A. et al. (1993). The influence of thalidomide on the clinical and immunologic manifestation of erythema nodosum leprosum. *Journal of Infections Diseases*, **168**, 408–14.

Sampaio, E.P., Sarno, E.N., Galilly, R. et al. (1991). Thalidomide selectively inhibits tumor necrosis factor alpha production by stimulated human monocytes. *Journal of Experimental Medicine*, **173**, 699–703.

Sandmaier, B.M., Maloney, D.G., Gooley, T. et al. (2001). Nonmyeloablative hematopoietic stem cell transplant (HSCT) from HLA-matched related donors for patients with hematologic malignancies: Clinical results of a TBI-based conditioning regimen. *Blood*, **98**, 742a.

Saurat, J-H., Camenzind, M., Helg, C. et al. (1988). Thalidomide for graft-versus-host disease after bone marrow transplantation. *Lancet*, **1**, 359.

Shannon, E.J., Morales, M.J., & Sandoval, F. (1997). Immunomodulatory assays to study structure-activity relationships of thalidomide. *Immunopharmacology*, **35**, 203–12.

Shaw, L.M., Nicholls, A., Hale, M. et al. (1998a). Therapeutic monitoring of mycophenolic acid. A consensus panel report. *Clinical Biochemistry*, **31**, 317–22.

Shaw, L.M., Kaplan, B., & Brayman, K.L. (1998b). Prospective investigations of concentration-clinical response for immunosuppressive drugs provide the scientific basis for therapeutic drug monitoring. *Clinical Chemistry*, **44**, 381–7.

Shaw, L.M., Korecka, M., DeNofrio, D. et al. (2001). Pharmacokinetic, pharmacodynamic, and outcome investigations as the basis for mycophenolic acid therapeutic drug monitoring in renal and heart transplant patients. *Clinical Biochemistry*, **34**, 17–22.

Slauson, S.D., Silva, H.T., Sherwood, S.W. et al. (1999). Flow cytometric analysis of the molecular mechanisms of immunosuppressive action of the active metabolite of leflunomide and its malononitrilamide analogues in a novel whole blood assay. *Immunology Letters*, **67**, 179–83.

Sollinger, H.W., Deierhoi, M.H., Belzer, F.O. et al. (1992). RS-61443—a phase I clinical trial and pilot rescue study. *Transplantation*, **53**, 428–32.

Speiser, D.E., Bachmann, M.F., Frick, T.W. et al. (1997). TNF receptor p55 controls early acute graft-versus-host disease. *Journal of Immunology*, **158**, 5185–90.

Spiers, A.S. (1995). Pentostatin (2'-deoxycoformycin): clinical pharmacology, role in cancer chemotherapy, and future prospects. *American Journal of Therapy*, **2**, 196–216.

Stanzani, M., Rondelli, D., Bandini, G. et al. (2002). Role of micophenolate mofetil (MMF) in the treatment of cGVHD. *Bone Marrow Transplantation*, **29**, S183.

Staubus, A.E., Weinrib, A.B., Malspeis, L. (1984). An enzymatic kinetic method for the determination of 2'-deoxycoformycin in biological fluids. *Biochemical Pharmacology*, **33**, 1633–7.

Szabolcs, P., Reese, M., Yancey, K. et al. (2000). Combination treatment of bullous skin GVHD and anti-CD20 and anti-CD25 antibodies. *Blood*, **96**, 350b.

Tavares, J.L., Wangoo, A., Dilworth, P. et al. (1997). Thalidomide reduces tumour necrosis factor-alpha production by human alveolar macrophages. *Respiratory Medicine*, **91**, 31–9.

van de Poel, M.H., Pasman, P.C., & Schouten, H.C. (2001). The use of thalidomide in chronic refractory graft versus host disease. *Netherlands Journal of Medicine*, **59**, 45–9.

van Gelder, T., Hilbrands, L.B., Vanrenterghem, Y. et al. (1999). A randomized double-blind, multicenter plasma concentration controlled study of the safety and efficacy of oral mycophenolate mofetil for the prevention of acute rejection after kidney transplantation. *Transplantation*, **68**, 261–6.

Vander Woude, A., & Bierer, B. (1997). Immunosuppression and immunophilin ligands: Cyclosporin A, FK506, and rapamycin. In *Graft-versus-Host Disease*, ed. J. Ferrara, J. Deeg, & S. Burakoff, p.111. New York: Marcel Dekker, Inc.

Vogelsang, G.B., Farmer, E.R., Hess, A.D. *et al.* (1992). Thalidomide for the treatment of chronic graft-versus-host disease. *New England Journal of Medicine,* **326,** 1055–8.

Weisser, M., Stoetzer, O., Schleuning, M. *et al.* (2002). Combination therapy using daclizumab (anti-CD25) and sirolimus in steroid refractory acute GVHD. *Bone Marrow Transplantation,* **29,** S184.

Wendt, S., Finkam, M., Winter, W. *et al.* (1996). Enantioselective inhibition of TNF-alpha release by thalidomide and thalidomide-analogues. *Chirality,* **8,** 390–6.

Willenbacher, W., Basara, N., Blau, I.W. *et al.* (2001). Treatment of steroid refractory acute and chronic graft-versus-host disease with daclizumab. *British Journal of Haematology,* **112,** 820–3.

Wingard, J.R., Nash, R.A., Przepiorka, D. *et al.* (1998). Relationship of tacrolimus (FK506) whole blood concentrations to efficacy and safety after HLA-identical sibling bone marrow transplantation. *Biology of Blood and Marrow Transplantation,* **4,** 157–63.

Wolff, D., Casper, J., Steiner, B. *et al.* (2002). Treatment of steroid resistant acute GVHD with daclizumab and etanercept. *Bone Marrow Transplantation,* **29,** S184.

Woo, M.H., Przepiorka, D., Ippoliti, C. *et al.* (1997). Toxicities of tacrolimus and cyclosporine after allogeneic blood stem cell transplantation. *Bone Marrow Transplantation,* **20,** 1095–8.

Wu, J. (1994). Mycophenolate mofetil: molecular mechanism of action. *Perspectives in Drug Discovery and Design,* **2,** 185.

Xu, X., Williams, J.W., Gong, H. *et al.* (1996). Two activities of the immunosuppressive metabolite of leflunomide, A77 1726. Inhibition of pyrimidine nucleotide synthesis and protein tyrosine phosphorylation. *Biochemical Pharmacology,* **52,** 527–34.

Yatscoff, R.W., Wang, P., Chan, K. *et al.* (1995). Rapamycin: distribution, pharmacokinetics, and therapeutic range investigations. *Therapeutic Drug Monitoring,* **17,** 666–71.

Yusuf, U., Sanders, J.E., & Stephan, V. (2001). Mycophenolate mofetil (MMF) as salvage treatment for steroid-refractory chronic graft-versus-host disease (GVHD) in children. *Blood,* **98,** 398a.

Zimmerman, J.J. & Kahan, B.D. (1997). Pharmacokinetics of sirolimus in stable renal transplant patients after multiple oral dose administration. *Journal of Clinical Pharmacology,* **37,** 405–15.

119 Transplantation for autoimmune diseases

ALAN TYNDALL, PETER McSWEENEY, AND ALOIS GRATWOHL

University Hospital, Basle, Switzerland and University of Colorado Health Sciences Center, Denver, USA

Introduction

The use of autologous and allogeneic hematopoietic stem cell transplantation (HSCT) for the treatment of various hematologic, immunologic, and metabolic disorders is now well established. The primary objectives of high-dose chemotherapy or chemoradiotherapy are first to eradicate disease in the recipient and second to ablate the recipient's immune system to permit engraftment of donor marrow. Following allogeneic HSCT, the engrafted immune and hematopoietic systems can be shown to be of donor origin in most patients (Atkinson, 1990), and the donor stem cells contribute cells to other tissues as well, including hepatocytes and epithelium (Korbling et al., 2002). A minority of patients are, however, mixed chimeras with residual cells of host origin present. Humoral and cellular immunity is usually restored by 12 months posttransplant, although in some cases cell-mediated immunity may remain impaired for years, especially in the presence of chronic graft-versus-host disease (GVHD). With the eradication of the host's lymphoid system, one might anticipate that any abnormal immune process present in the host would simultaneously disappear. Thus, following an allogeneic HSC grafting with establishment of complete donor chimerism, any pre-existing autoimmune disease in the host might be expected to remit (Marmont et al., 1995; Marmont, 1997). At least these were the concepts before a wider experience of HSCT in autoimmune disease was obtained.

Evidence that allogeneic HSCT can indeed cure or alter the course of systemic and organ-specific autoimmune diseases comes from experimental work in animal models and clinical experience in humans. Furthermore, there are experimental data to suggest that autologous HSCT can also be beneficial in autoimmune disorders, and this paved the way for investigating the use of autologous transplants in severe human autoimmune disease (reviewed in Openshaw, Nash, and McSweeney, 2002). With the advent of immunosuppressive therapy, the prognosis in autoimmune disease has improved, although the outcome, in terms of both morbidity and mortality, in some patients remains poor. The epidemiology and prognosis of some autoimmune diseases are shown in Table 119.1.

Adoptive immunity

The effects of the transfer of both normal and abnormal (for example, autoimmune) donor immunity to the recipient by the transplant procedure will first be discussed (adoptive immunity). The transfer of normal donor immunity is well estab-

Table 119.1.   *Epidemiology and prognosis of common autoimmune diseases*

	Incidence (per 10^6 population)	Prevalence (per 10^6 population)	Prognosis (survival) 5 year	Prognosis (survival) 10 year
SLE	40 (18–76)	250 (50–500)	95% (all) 88% (end-stage renal failure)	88% (all) 75%
SSc	6–19	126–250	60%	50%
RA	360	10,000	45% (severe, destructive disease)	35%
MS	30–50	50–200	Life span reduced by 10 years, 60% disabled at 10 years	

Abbreviations: SLE, systemic lupus erythematosus; SSc, sytemic sclerosis (scleroderma); RA, rheumatoid arthritis; MS, multiple sclerosis.

lished and has been demonstrated in a number of studies. Transfer of specific immunity to tetanus and diphtheria toxoids and of allergen-specific donor-derived IgE have been described (Agosti *et al.*, 1988; Lum *et al.*, 1988). The transfer of abnormal donor immunity, resulting in the appearance of disease states in the recipient, is also well recognized, although it is impossible to exclude de novo disease in a graft from a genetically predisposed, HLA-matched sibling. Thus, it has been shown that clinical illnesses such as allergic rhinitis and asthma (Agosti *et al.*, 1988), papular urticaria (Smith *et al.*, 1988), and contact dermatitis (Olagguibel *et al.*, 1989) can be transferred from donors to previously symptomless recipients.

Additionally, numerous cases of acquired autoimmune thrombocytopenia (AITP) following allogeneic bone marrow transplantation (BMT) have been reported in the literature. These represent the most frequent examples of clinical adoptive autoimmunity following BMT. Minchinton *et al.* (1982) described a female patient who developed AITP after receiving a bone marrow transplant from a matched unrelated male donor. The donor was shown to have an identical IgM antiplatelet autoantibody, although his platelet count was normal. The recipient's AITP responded to high-dose intravenous immunoglobulin. It is suggested that, in the donor, there was compensation of antibody-mediated platelet destruction, whereas thrombocytopenia occurred in the recipient, presumably through the same mechanism, owing to reduced megakaryocyte production in the engrafted marrow. This interesting case is different from the many cases of immune mediated thrombocytopenia reported following HSCT. Many of these are most likely autoimmune in origin, but other potential factors such as GVHD and cytomegalovirus infection need to be considered as well. It is also worth noting that immune-mediated thrombocytopenia may occur after both autologous and syngeneic BMT (Plouvier *et al.*, 1983; Cahn *et al.*, 1989).

The reverse has been observed in a case report of two brothers, one of whom required HSCT for acute myeloid leukemia, with the HLA-identical donor brother having inactive systemic lupus erythematosus (SLE), including antibody to Clq (Sturfelt *et al.*, 1996). The recipient did not have this autoantibody, considered highly specific for SLE, pretransplant, but did develop it 3 months posttransplant during the period of B-cell immune reconstitution. However, it disappeared after 2 months and at no stage did he develop symptoms or signs of SLE. This indicates that in the new host, an autoaggressive clone of cells may be controlled or suppressed.

Another example of adoptive autoimmunity after BMT resulting in clinical illness is the case of a 12-year-old girl with aplastic anemia who developed GVHD, and subsequently severe myasthenia gravis, 27 months after receiving a marrow graft from her histocompatible brother. She was shown to have high levels of acetylcholine receptor IgG antibodies. The donor had no symptoms of myasthenia and no detectable acetylcholine receptor antibody. However, when he was examined with single fiber electromyography, he was found to have changes indicative of a predisposition to myasthenia gravis. It

is postulated that the myasthenia was of donor origin; it should be remembered, however, that myasthenia gravis has been described in association with chronic GVHD in other patients (Bolger *et al.*, 1986).

Finally, cases of adoptive transfer of autoimmune thyroiditis (Aldouri *et al.*, 1990; Wyatt *et al.*, 1990; Thomson *et al.*, 1995; Karthaus *et al.*, 1997; Kishimoto *et al.*, 1997; Berisso *et al.*, 1999), autoimmune hypothyroidism (from a donor with Graves' disease) (Marazuela *et al.*, 2000), insulin-dependent diabetes mellitus (Lampeter *et al.*, 1993, 1998), polyendocrine failure (Vialettes *et al.*, 1993), celiac disease (Bargetzi *et al.*, 1997), ulcerative colitis (Baron *et al.*, 1998), sarcoidosis (Heyll *et al.*, 1994), and psoriasis (Gardempas-Pain *et al.*, 1990; Snowden *et al.*, 1997a), following HSCT have also been reported. However, it is interesting to note that there have been no reports of adoptive transfer of rheumatoid arthritis (RA), SLE, or other systemic autoimmune disease to recipients transplanted from donors with these diseases (Snowden *et al.*, 1997, 1997a). Whether this reflects specific aspects of autoimmune diseases, or merely reflects the fact that such autoimmune disease patients are rarely selected as donors, remains to be seen. This is probably because some organ-specific autoreactive clones of T cells escape thymic deletion and are controlled in the periphery by, among other mechanisms, suppressor or regulatory T cells (Shevach, 2001). During HSCT, especially if T-cell purging is performed, a loss of these regulatory cells could result in differentiation and proliferation of such organ-specific T cells with disease expression. A cohort of 160 patients receiving T-cell-depleted allogeneic HSCT for various malignancies showed a 15% incidence of autoimmune disease posttransplant: 14 with thyroid involvement, 4 with autoimmune hemolytic anemia (AIHA), and 4 with idiopathic thrombocytopenic purpura (ITP) (Wiesneth *et al.*, 2002). This has also been observed following other severe immunosuppressive strategies. One third of patients receiving CAMPATH 1H for multiple sclerosis developed autoimmune thyroid disease (Coles *et al.*, 1999). Overall these observations suggest that patients exposed to intensive immunosuppressive treatments may, counterintuitively, be exposed to a risk of autoimmunity through dysregulation of previously intact immunoregulatory networks.

Autoimmune disease

Autoimmune diseases affect around 5% of the world population and, apart from RA, autoimmune thyroid diseases are rather rare. No perfect definition exists, but one such is "a clinical syndrome caused by the activation of T cells or B cells, or both, in the absence of an ongoing infection or other discernible cause" (Davidson & Diamond, 2001). Concepts of these poorly understood disorders have changed recently from the dogma of a clonal, autoaggressive process that was not deleted in the thymus; a degree of autoreactivity is now thought necessary for maintaining normal immunity (Dighiero & Rose, 1999), with continuous exposure to autoantigen being physiological for the development of the mature T-cell repertoire and naïve T-cell

(Goldrath & Bevan, 1999) and B-cell survival (Manis *et al.*, 1998). As self and foreign antigen are fundamentally not structurally different, the control of auto versus foreign antigen response is probably dependent on the balance between stimulatory and inhibitory factors of cellular (e.g., activated T cells) or humoral (cytokine) origin. Endogenous as well as exogenous factors influence antigen presentation, antigen recognition, and immune response. This implies that the innate immune system may have a more important role in determining self and non-self reactions (Medzhitov & Janeway, 2002).

Rationale for the treatment of autoimmune diseases by blood and marrow transplantation

Animal models

Experimental work in animal models has provided considerable insight into the pathogenesis of autoimmune disease. The availability of several murine strains that develop systemic or organ-specific autoimmune diseases has allowed extensive studies of the immunologic abnormalities in these mice. MRLIMP-lpr/lpr (MRLII) and BXSB mice as well as (NZB × NZW) F_1 hybrids spontaneously develop systemic autoimmune diseases characterized by anti-double-stranded DNA antibodies, immune complex glomerulonephritis, and renal failure. In contrast, nonobese diabetic (NOD) mice spontaneously develop organ-specific autoimmune disease characterized by a striking infiltration of T cells in the pancreatic islets and selective destruction of islet cells leading to overt diabetes.

In the mice that develop the lupus-like syndrome, abnormalities have been demonstrated in, or attributed to, T cells, the thymus, B cells, macrophages, and environmental factors such as hormones and viruses. However, research has revealed that murine lupus is caused by defects at the level of the HSC or lymphoid precursor cell (Theophilopoulos & Dixon, 1987). It thus appeared logical to examine whether transfer of normal stem cells to these strains of mice could prevent or treat autoimmune diseases. Allogeneic marrow transplantation offered a practical way to test this hypothesis.

In 1983, Shikari, Fujiwara, and Kano published results of BMT in MLR/I mice. The MLR/I strain of mice, which develop severe lupus nephritis early in life, were given total body irradiation (TBI) and received marrow grafts from the MRL/n strain. The latter strain lacks the lpr gene responsible for lymphoproliferation and the development of autoimmune disease. The transplanted mice did not show the early onset of severe lupus nephritis, as seen in the MRL/I strain. There was reduced proteinuria, decreased immune complex deposition in glomeruli, and milder histologic changes in the kidneys.

Similarly, Ikehara *et al.* (1985a) showed that when MRL/I and BXSB mice with autoimmune diseases were lethally irradiated and then reconstituted with T-cell-depleted bone marrow from young mice carrying the nu/nu genes (BALB/c nu/nu) (athymic nude mice), the recipients survived for more than 3 months posttransplant with no evidence of GVHD. This was accompanied by resolution of lymphadenopathy and marked correction of autoimmune disease activity in the kidneys. Moreover, normal T cells, B cells, and macrophages had developed by 3 months posttransplant.

Having demonstrated that BMT could be used to treat systemic autoimmune disease in specific strains of mice, Ikehara and colleagues went on to treat NOD mice (which develop organ-specific insulitis and type I diabetes mellitus) with marrow transplantation (Ikehara *et al.*, 1985b). When NOD mice were irradiated and received marrow grafts from young BALB/c nu/nu mice, they exhibited neither insulitis nor diabetes. In addition, immunoglobulin deposits in the mesangial areas of the glomeruli disappeared within 3 months of transplant. Transplanted mice displayed normal T- and B-cell function. On the basis of their experimental work, these workers have proposed that allogeneic BMT is a strategy that could be considered for the treatment of systemic and organ-specific autoimmune disease in humans.

In 1991 Van Bekkum's group unexpectedly showed a protective and curative effect of syngeneic (and later autologous) BMT in the Buffalo rat arthritis model (Knaan-Shanzer *et al.*, 1991). In addition, the rats were tolerant to the inciting agent, Freund's adjuvant following transplant, and adding back lymphocytes from diseased animals did not cause disease at any of the doses tested (van Bekkum, 2000). This model is close to human RA in that a predisposing genetic factor plus a trigger are required for full disease expression, and gives some hope that autologous BMT may not just treat the disease but also induce tolerance. Similar results were seen in MRL/lpr lupus prone mice in a syngeneic system (Karussis *et al.*, 1995).

Similar but less complete results were reported by the same group in experimental allergic encephalomyelitis (EAE), the model for multiple sclerosis (MS) in humans (van Gelder *et al.*, 1993, 1995). Kirzner and colleagues (2000) have shown that coronary vascular disease can be prevented in autoimmune disease-prone W/BF1 mice transplanted with haploidentical T-cell-depleted HSC preparations. This is especially important in regards to newly emerging data concerning the relationship between chronic inflammatory autoimmune disease and early coronary artery disease-related death (Sherer *et al.*, 2002). When interpreting animal model data, it is, however, essential to distinguish between prevention of disease and modification of established clinical disease. In this regard, as might be anticipated in human clinical applications, that prevention of permanent organ damage is highly dependent on the timing of transplantation in relationship to development of autoimmune disease and its organ-specific manifestations.

Clinical experience

Allogeneic transplantation and coincidental autoimmune disease

There have been many case reports over the past years of patients who received HSC for a conventional indication (e.g., aplastic anemia or leukemia) and in whom a coincidental

Table 119.2. *Coincidental autoimmune disease and allogeneic HSC transplantation*

Disease for which transplant performed	AD present	Outcome of autoimmune disease	Patient outcome	Reference
SAA	RA	Remission	Died	Baldwin *et al.* (1977)
SAA	RA	Remission	Died	Baldwin *et al.* (1977)
SAA	RA	Remission	Died	Baldwin *et al.* (1977)
SAA	RA	Remission	Well	Baldwin *et al.* (1977)
SAA	RA	Partial remission	Well	Jacobs *et al.* (1986)
SAA	RA	Remission	Well	Lowenthal *et al.* (1993)
SAA	RA	Remission	Well	Lowenthal *et al.* (1993)
AML	Psoriasis	Remission	Well	Eedy *et al.* (1990)
CML	Psoriasis	Remission	Well	Liu Yin & Jowitt (1992)
AML	Ulcerative colitis	Remission	Well	Liu Yin & Jowitt (1992)
ALL	Autoimmune hepatitis	Remission	Well	Vento *et al.* (1996)
CML	Multiple Sclerosis	Remission	Well	McAllister *et al.* (1997)
Various	Multiple sclerosis Hyperthyroidism IDDM SLE, RA Crohn's disease Vasculitis Dermatitis herpetiformis Sjögren's	No recurrence No effect	Alive	Nelson *et al.* (1997)
MALT lymphoma			Alive	Ferraccioli *et al.* (2001)

Abbreviations: SAA, severe aplastic anemia; AML, acute myeloid leukemia; CML, chronic myeloid leukemia; ALL, acute lymphoblastic leukemia; RA, rheumatoid arthritis; IDDM, insulin-dependent diabetes mellitus; SLE, systemic lupus erythematosus; MALT, mucosa-associated lymphoid tissue; AD, autoimmune disease.

autoimmune disorder was present. In most cases the HSC transplant had a beneficial effect on the course of the pre-existing autoimmune or immune-mediated disease in the transplanted recipients (Table 119.2).

Rheumatoid arthritis

Important data pointing to an effect of allografting in autoimmune disease has come from patients with RA. Long follow-ups are available on several patients, all of whom were transplanted for a concurrent autoimmune disorder, aplastic anemia. Most were conditioned with a regimen of high-dose cyclophosphamide (CY) 200 mg/kg. In an early publication from Seattle on the outcome of marrow allografting in patients with gold-induced marrow aplasia, one successfully treated patient with severe RA was reported to be alive and free of arthritis, both serologically and clinically, 2 years posttransplant (Baldwin *et al.*, 1977). In a follow-up report the patient remained in remission of RA at 20 years after transplant (Nelson *et al.*, 1997). Lowenthal *et al.* (1993) also reported apparent cure (6 years follow-up) of active, nodular RA in two women transplanted for gold-induced and penicillamine-induced aplastic anemia, respectively. Similarly, Jacobs, Vincent, and Martell (1986) described a 33-year-old woman who went into prolonged remission of her refractory RA after receiving a marrow transplant for drug-induced aplastic anemia. The patient was conditioned with cyclophosphamide 200 mg/kg. However, 2 years later, her joint symptoms reappeared, as did her rheumatoid

factor. This raised the possibility of the re-emergence of autoreactive host lymphocytes, but cytogenetic studies apparently failed to show autologous marrow recovery. In a follow-up report the patient had entered remission of RA for 11 years and two other patients had RA-free intervals after transplant of 10 and 11 years (Snowden *et al.*, 1998b). McKendry *et al.* (1996) also reported a patient whose RA, 2 years post-BMT, relapsed and became progressive, in spite of continuing donor-origin-lymphohematopoietic chimerism. Whether this case represented recurrence of the original disease, or de novo disease in cells of donor origin, remains unclear. Thus, not all patients with RA have had sustained remission after allogeneic HSC transplantation. Additionally, there is a case report of disappearance of lupus anticoagulant (in a patient without evidence of SLE) after allogeneic transplantation for chronic myeloid leukemia (Olalla *et al.*, 1999).

Psoriasis, ulcerative colitis, and Crohn's disease

Further evidence that allogeneic BMT can cure pre-existing immune disorders comes from case reports on patients with psoriasis and ulcerative colitis (UC), who received an allograft for leukemia. There is now a substantial body of evidence to suggest that both psoriasis and UC are disorders that are mediated by abnormal immunologic mechanisms. The role of cellular immunity in the pathogenesis of psoriasis is not in doubt. Similarly, while it is not generally agreed that UC is an autoimmune disease, the consensus is that immunologic mechanisms play an important role in its pathogenesis. Eedy et al. (1990) reported sustained clearance of severe psoriasis in a patient transplanted twice for acute myeloid leukemia (AML). Five years later, the patient remained completely free of psoriasis and off immune suppression. A second patient transplanted from his histocompatible brother for Philadelphia chromosome-positive chronic myeloid leukemia (CML) also had complete resolution of pre-existing psoriasis and arthropathy 10 years after marrow transplantation (Liu Yin & Jowitt, 1992). Kishimoto and colleagues (1997) and Adkins et al. (2000) described additional cases. It is unlikely that the long-lasting remission of psoriasis achieved in these patients could be ascribed to the immune suppressive pretransplant conditioning regimen or to the posttransplant cyclosporine, since relapse of psoriasis after withdrawing cyclosporine is almost universal. However, relapse of psoriasis with arthropathy has recently been described in a patient 1 year after undergoing BMT for CML (Snowden et al., 1998b).

Resolution of UC after BMT has also been described (Liu Yin & Jowitt, 1992). In this case, the patient had suffered from UC for 12 years and was still receiving treatment for it at the time of her transplant for AML. The donor was her histocompatible brother. Ten years posttransplant, she remains in complete remission of both the UC and the leukemia. Lopez-Cubero, Sullivan, and McDonald (1998) described 4 of 5 patients followed up for 4.5 to 15.3 years after allogeneic HSCT for CML or AML who remained free of recurrent Crohn's disease[1] in the period of follow-up. All 5 had active Crohn's disease pretransplant and 3 had clinical evidence of sclerosing cholangitis. One patient who had mixed donor-host hematopoietic chimerism had a relapse of Crohn's disease 1.5 years posttransplant. In addition there are several reports of patients with active Crohn's disease who underwent autologous marrow transplantation with no evidence of bowel disease activity 6 months and 6 years posttransplant (Drakos et al., 1993; Kashyap & Forman, 1998; Musso et al., 2000).

Additionally, there are two cases of remission posttransplant of Hashimoto's thyroiditis[2] in patients allografted for aplastic anemia (Lee et al., 2001), two case reports of remission of Graves' disease[3] (hyperthyroidism and ophthalmopathy) in patients also allografted for severe aplastic anemia (Diez et al., 1999; Lee et al., 2001), a case of marrow sarcoidosis diagnosed posttransplant at the time of hematologic relapse of CML, which resolved completely with donor lymphocyte infusions, as did the CML (Tauro et al., 2001), and a case of pure red cell aplasia associated with chronic lymphatic leukemia that resolved after HLA-identical sibling BMT (de Vetten et al., 2001). In this setting, pure red cell aplasia is thought to be a T-cell-mediated autoimmune phenomenon. More recently, hair regrowth has been reported in a patient with alopecia totalis

following his successful allogeneic transplantation for CML. The hair follicles were of donor origin (Sieffert et al., 2002).

Hinterberger, Hinterberger-Fischer, and Marmont (2002) reviewed the literature from 1977 to 2001 for case reports in which an allogeneic or autologous transplant was performed for a hematological disorder in a patient with a concomitant autoimmune disease (AID). Disease-free survival (DFS) after allogeneic HSC transplantation for 23 patients with severe aplastic anemia was 78% at 16 years and survival in unmaintained remission of concomitant AID was 64% at 13 years. DFS after allogeneic transplantation for 24 patients with hematologic malignancies was 87% at 15 years and survival in unmaintained remission for concomitant AID was 70% at 11 years. DFS after autologous HSC transplantation for 24 patients with hematologic malignancies and concomitant AID was 48% at 6 years and survival in unmaintained remission for concomitant AID was 29% at 3 years. After allogeneic transplantation, 3 of 11 patients without GVHD experienced a relapse of their concomitant AID, whereas none of 19 with GVHD did so. These data suggest that a graft-versus-autoimmunity effect after allogeneic HSC transplantation at least partially mediates elimination of autoimmunity.

These case reports, together with the animal data, provide evidence that, by eradication of the host's immune system using chemoradiotherapy or high-dose chemotherapy, it is possible to eradicate pre-existing autoimmunity or immune dysregulation causing clinical disease in the host. Allogeneic HSCT by providing a genetically different immune system to the recipient, thus appears to be a strategy that could be applied to the treatment of serious and life-threatening autoimmune disorders in humans. However, the fact that not all animal models and patients respond and that some relapses of autoimmunity in a setting of complete donor hematopoietic chimerism have been described, suggests that allogeneic HSCT will not invariably result in cure.

Autologous transplantation and coincidental autoimmune disease

There have also been reports of patients with coincidental autoimmune disease, treated by autologous transplantation, mainly for malignancy (Table 119.3). Both remission and relapse after autotransplantation have been described. A definite selection and publication bias exists toward a positive outcome, although some reports stress the relapse of the autoimmune disease after a period of apparent remission. More recently negative responses have been also reported, as in the case of a MALT lymphoma, but not the concurrent Sjögren's syndome, responding to autologous HSCT (Ferraccioli et al., 2001). Often details concerning autoimmune features and severity are lacking.

Autoimmune disease as the primary indication for HSCT

The past 10 years have seen a shift in attitude toward the treatment of autoimmune disease with a trend for earlier, aggressive

---

[1] Burrill B. Crohn, U. S. physician, 1884–1993.

[2] Hakaru Hashimoto, Japanese surgeon, 1881–1934.

[3] Robert James Graves, Irish Physician, 1796–1853.

Table 119.3.   *Coincidental autoimmune disease and autologous HSC transplantation*

Disease for which transplant performed	Autoimmune disease present	Outcome of autoimmune disease	Patient outcome	Reference
NHL	Myasthenia gravis	Remission	Well	Salzmann *et al.* (1994)
Ovarian cancer	Thyroiditis myasthenia	Relapse	Alive	Euler *et al.* (1996)
NHL	SLE	Relapse	Died	Euler *et al.* (1996)
NHL	Atopic dermatitis	Relapse	Alive	Euler *et al.* (1996)
NHL	RA	Relapse	Alive	Euler *et al.* (1996)
NHL	SLE	Remission	Alive	Snowden *et al.,* 1997
CML	SLE	Remission	Alive	Meloni *et al.* (1997)
NHL	RA	Remission	Alive	Jondeau *et al.* (1997)
NHL	RA	Relapse	Alive	Cooley *et al.* (1997)
NHL	Psoriasis	Relapse	Alive	Cooley *et al.* (1997)
AML	Psoriasis	Relapse	Alive	Cooley *et al.* (1997)
Plasma cell leukemia	Psoriasis	Relapse	Alive	Cooley *et al.* (1997)
NHL	Crohn's disease	Remission	Alive	Kashyap *et al.* (1998)
Hodgkin's disease	Crohn's disease	Remission	Alive	Musso *et al.* (2000)

Abbreviations: NHL, non-Hodgkin's lymphoma. Others as for Table 119.2.

induction treatment, followed by less toxic maintenance therapy. Typical examples are SLE with renal involvement (Lewis, 1992) and Wegener's granulomatosis and other systemic necrotizing vasculitic crises (Fauci *et al.,* 1983). This has arisen through a better understanding of the natural history, differentiation between active inflammation (and hence potential reversibility) and permanent scarring, and an appreciation of the long-term cumulative toxicity of corticosteroids and immunosuppressive agents in these disorders. However, despite improved prognosis over the past 40 years, some patients still have a poor outcome with loss of life or vital organ function and the search for more effective, less toxic therapies continues. There is a striking similarity in these activities, whether it applies to, for example, RA or MS: combination drug therapy, antilymphocyte monoclonal antibody treatment, anticytokine strategies, novel immunosuppressive agents such as mycophenolate mofetil, and oral vaccination.

Until now there has been no effective induction of tolerance, and some attempts have resulted in exacerbation of disease, such as the MS IV vaccination with altered myelin basic protein sequence (Bielekova *et al.,* 2000).

HSCT has now joined this panel of options with the first case of a patient receiving HSCT for an autoimmune disease alone published in 1996 (Tamm *et al.,* 1996) (pulmonary hypertension complicating a connective tissue disease). This was followed by a succession of other case reports or small series [Euler *et al.,* 1996; Joske, 1997 (rheumatoid arthritis); Lim *et al.,* 1997 (ITP); Raetz, Beatty, & Adams, 1997 (Evans' syndrome); Tyndall *et al.,* 1997 (diffuse skin systemic sclerosis); Wulffraat *et al.,* 1999 (juvenile chronic arthritis); Baron *et al.,* 2000 (Jo-1-antibody-associated polymyositis); Paillard *et al.,* 2000 (autoimmune hemolytic anemia); Fassas *et al.,* 1997 (multiple sclerosis), and Traynor *et al.,* 2002 (SLE)].

An international collaboration was established early and a consensus statement was produced to deal with unclear aspects

Table 119.4.   *Main indications for autologous HSCT in autoimmune diseases*

Disease and disease category	N
Neurological disorders	
Multiple sclerosis	122
Myasthenia gravis	1
Polyneuropathy	1
Cerebellar degeneration	1
Amyotrophic lateral sclerosis	2
Rheumatological disorders	
Systemic sclerosis	63
Rheumatoid arthritis	69
Juvenile idiopathic arthritis	43
Systemic lupus erythematosus	51
Dermatomyositis	7
Mixed connective tissue disorders	3
Behcet's disease[a]	3
Psoriatic arthritis	2
Ankylosing spondylitis	1
Sjogren's[b]	1
Vasculitides	
Wegener's[c]	3
Cryoglobulinemia	3
Classical polyarteritis nodosa	1
Not classified	1
Hematological immuncytopenias	
Immune thrombocytopenia	10
Pure red cell aplasia	4
Autoimmune hemolytic anemia	3
Thrombotic thrombocytopenic anemia	2
Evans' syndrome[d]	1
Gastrointestinal	
Enteropathy	1
Inflammatory bowel disease	1

Data from the EBMT/EULAR combined database.
[a] Hulusi Behcet, Turkish dermatologist, 1889–1948.
[b] Henrik Sjögren, Swedish opthalmologist, 1896–1976.
[c] Friedrich Wegener, German pathologist, 1909–1990.
[d] Robert Evans, U.S. physician, 1912–1974.

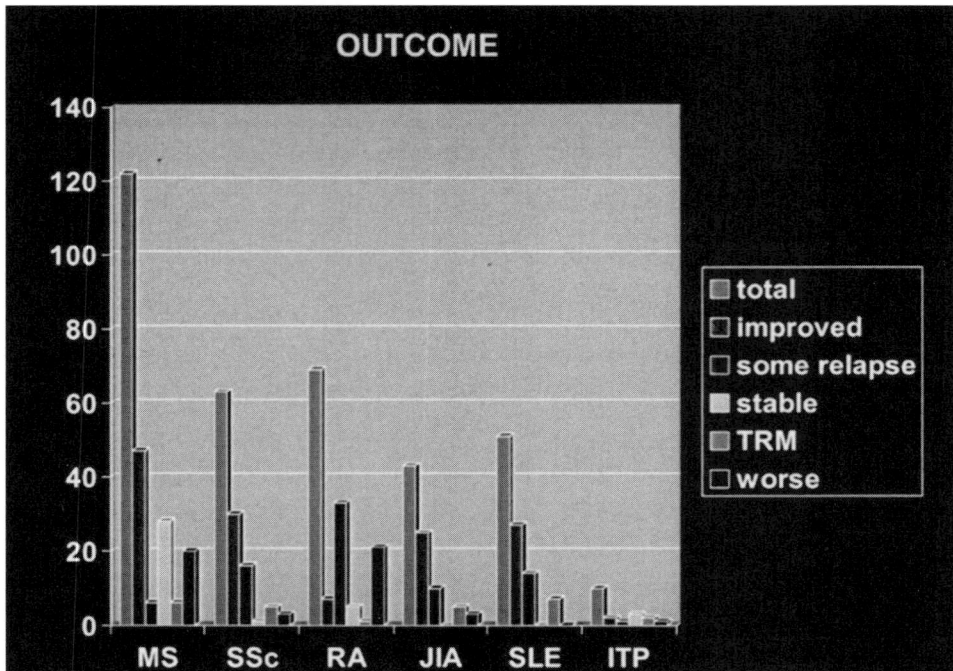

Fig. 119.1. Responses and outcomes in patients receiving an autologous HSCT for autoimmune disease. Each autoimmune disease shows a different response pattern and toxicity profile to the transplant procedure (mobilization toxicity included in TRM). MS, multiple sclerosis; SSc, systemic sclerosis; RA, rheumatoid arthritis; JIA, juvenile idiopathic arthritis; SLE; systemic lupus erythematosus; ITP, idiopathic thrombocytopenic purpura; TRM, transplant-related mortality. Reproduced, with permission, from the EBMT/EULAR Autoimmune Disease Working Party database.\

(Tyndall & Gratwohl, 1997). Indications for high-dose immune-ablative therapy and autologous HSCT were proposed and as of June 2002, approximately 500 patients transplanted for an autoimmune disease have been registered in either the EBMT or IBMTR registries. The most common autoimmune diseases transplanted are MS, RA, systemic sclerosis (SSc), juvenile idiopathic arthritis (JIA), and SLE (Table 119.4).

Although each autoimmune disease reacts differently in terms of response and toxicity, the phase I and II studies allow some conclusions to be drawn. In the EBMT/EULAR registry of 470 patients, the overall transplant-related mortality is 7% to 8% (actuarially adjusted), with marked interdisease differences: 1 death only in RA and 12.5% in SSc. This variation probably reflects the differing general state of illness and differing degrees of intensity of the conditioning regimens in the different groups, and, in particular, differential effects of the diseases and prior therapy on internal organ function and infection risks. Responses have been mostly positive, with some degree of relapse in each group mostly responding to agents that had been ineffective pretransplant (Fig. 119.1). A summary and phase III randomized trial plans have been published (Tyndall et al., 2001).

Multiple sclerosis

In MS 78% of patients with nonprimary progressive disease experienced a 3-year progression-free survival, and in those studied, the gadolinium enhancing lesions were markedly reduced (Fassas et al., 2002). It remains to be seen whether these results will be maintained over longer periods, given that this is a slowly progressive disease with a component of neuronal degeneration following the inflammation. A phase III randomized trial will soon start comparing BEAM (carmustine, etoposide, cytosine arabinoside, and melphalan) and ATG and an unmanipulated graft versus mitoxanthrone, and is called the Autologous Stem Cell Transplantation International Multiple Sclerosis (ASTIMS) trial.

Systemic sclerosis (SSc)

The analysis of the first 41 patients with SSc showed an improvement of greater than 25% in the baseline skin score in nearly 70% of patients (Binks, 2001). Lung function tended to stabilize, as did pulmonary hypertension if initial values were below a mean pulmonary artery pressure (PAP) of 50 mm Hg. The initial treatment-related mortality (TRM) rate was 17%, which dropped to 10% in a later follow-up analysis of 72 patients (EBMT registry). Most patients who responded experienced a durable remission with respect to skin score improvement, and some of the relapses responded to simple immunosuppressive agents such as methotrexate weekly or cyclosporine. A phase II randomized trial is ongoing (ASTIS trial) comparing transplantation (mobilization with cyclophosphamide and G-CSF) followed by cyclophosphamide/ATG conditioning with a CD34-selected graft versus monthly pulse i.v. cyclophosphamide 750 mg/m² for 12 months. The primary endpoint is 2-year event-free survival, events being death or permanent end-stage organ failure. So far 17 patients have been randomized and there have been no deaths in the trial. In the United States, a Seattle-based collaborative group reported outcomes on 19 SSc patients treated with a protocol of TBI 8 Gy, CY 120 mg/kg, and equine ATG 90 mg/kg followed by an infusion of CD34-selected, G-CSF mobilized peripheral blood stem cells (McSweeney *et al.*, 2002). Three patients died of treatment-related causes (two of pulmonary toxicity and one of EBV-related lymphoproliferative disease) and one patient died of disease progression. Modified Rodnan skin scores at 1 year were greater than 25% improved in 12 of 12 patients with a median reduction of 39% (32–93%) (*P* = .0005). Functional index evaluations, using a modified Health Assessment Questionnaire–Disability Index scores, were also markedly improved. Internal organ functions remained stable overall. Decrements in DLCO were found at 3 months but were not different from baseline 1 year after treatment. With a median follow-up of 14 months, projected 2-year survival was 79%. With accrual increased to 28 patients, there were no further deaths as of May 2002. Based on these results, a U.S. randomized study is planned that will randomize patients to either the high-dose therapy with TBI/CY/ATG as described or monthly intravenous CY 750 mg/m².

Rheumatoid arthritis

More than 70 RA patients have received autologous HSCT, mostly with cyclophosphamide conditioning. The majority responded, having failed on average three disease-modifying antirheumatic drugs (DMARDs), including in the later series anti-TNF-α treatment. There was some degree of relapse in 50%, easily controlled on DMARDs that had been ineffective pretransplant. Only one death occurred and none in the cyclophosphamide-only conditioning group. There was no clear evidence that CD34 selection gave more lasting remissions. Based on the phase I and II data, a prospective randomized trial has begun (ASTIRA), all patients being mobilized with CY 4 g/m² and G-CSF, harvested, then randomized to HSCT with CY 200 g/mg body weight or continued methotrexate (MTX) or leflunamide. Entry criteria include having failed at least three DMARDs, as well as a combination and anti-TNF-α therapy. The primary endpoint is response at 6 months, as measured by the composite ACR 20 or moderate/good EULAR response index.

Systemic lupus erythematosus

In the EBMT/EULAR database, 51 SLE patients are registered with the majority receiving a peripheral blood, CY and G-CSF-mobilized transplant following conditioning with CY plus ATG (*n* = 23). Eleven were conditioned with CY plus TBI, with particular advantage being noted. An overall TRM of 11% was observed. All patients responded in terms of SLE disease activity index (SLEDAI), with a disease activity-free survival of 58% +/– 17%. Again, as with other autoimmune diseases, responsiveness to previous treatment was observed in many. Given that many patients with SLE responded to CY 4 g/m² mobilization alone, and that relapse was a problem, a phase II study (ASTIL) is planned with four arms: mobilization alone, mobilization and HSCT, and both followed by maintenance with mycophenolate mofetil.

In the United States, Traynor and colleagues (2000) reported on seven patients with severe SLE, who, at a median follow-up of 25 months posttransplant, were free of signs of active lupus. The high-dose chemotherapy consisted of cyclophosphamide 200 mg/kg, methylprednisolone 1 g, and equine ATG 90 mg/kg. Eligible patients had WHO class III to IV glomerulonephritis, or lupus cerebritis or transverse myelitis, or lupus vasculitis involving the heart or lung parenchyma—all unresponsive to at least six cycles of intravenous cyclophosphamide; or lupus-associated, life-threatening, severe cytopenias unresponsive to standard-dose cyclophosphamide; or catastrophic anti-phospholipid syndrome. Of the seven patients, two were referred because of progressive lung disease and hypoxia at rest, but were not ventilator-dependent. One patient with alveolar hemorrhage was oxygen-dependent and required intermittent ventilator support. Four had WHO class III to IV glomerulonephritis and nephrotic syndrome. Five had a creatine clearance rate below the normal range. All had uncontrolled hypertension requiring four antihypertensive agents. Two had myocardial hypokinesis. Two had seizures immediately pretransplant. All patients had been diagnosed with chronic fatigue and depression and four had severe and recurrent headaches requiring narcotic analgesics.

Fluid retention (5–30 kg) occurred in all patients during mobilization and conditioning. Volume overload required dialysis or continuous veno-venous hyperfiltration in three patients, and two required mechanical ventilation for this.

Lupus remained in clinical remission in all patients posttransplant. Serum complement and sedimentation rates stayed normal and there was no evidence of active disease as defined by symptoms or findings of serositis, synovitis, cerebritis, or glomerulonephritis. SLE disease activity (SLEDAI) scores ranged from 0 to 5 in all patients and improved with time (Fig. 119.2). ANA, anti-ds DNA antibody, C3 and C4 normalized posttransplant (Fig. 119.2). Creatinine clearance in three of the five affected improved substantially by 270 days posttransplant, and 24-hour urinary protein excretion declined significantly in 6 patients in the first year (Fig. 119.3). Two patients with predominantly pulmonary symptoms had normal lung function in the 12 months after transplantation, and remained free of supplemental oxygen. In two patients with abnormal cardiac function pretransplant, ventricular motility and fractional shortening normalized posttransplant. Additionally, T-cell receptor diversity and responsiveness to mitogenic stimulation was restored. The durability of these striking results remains to be determined.

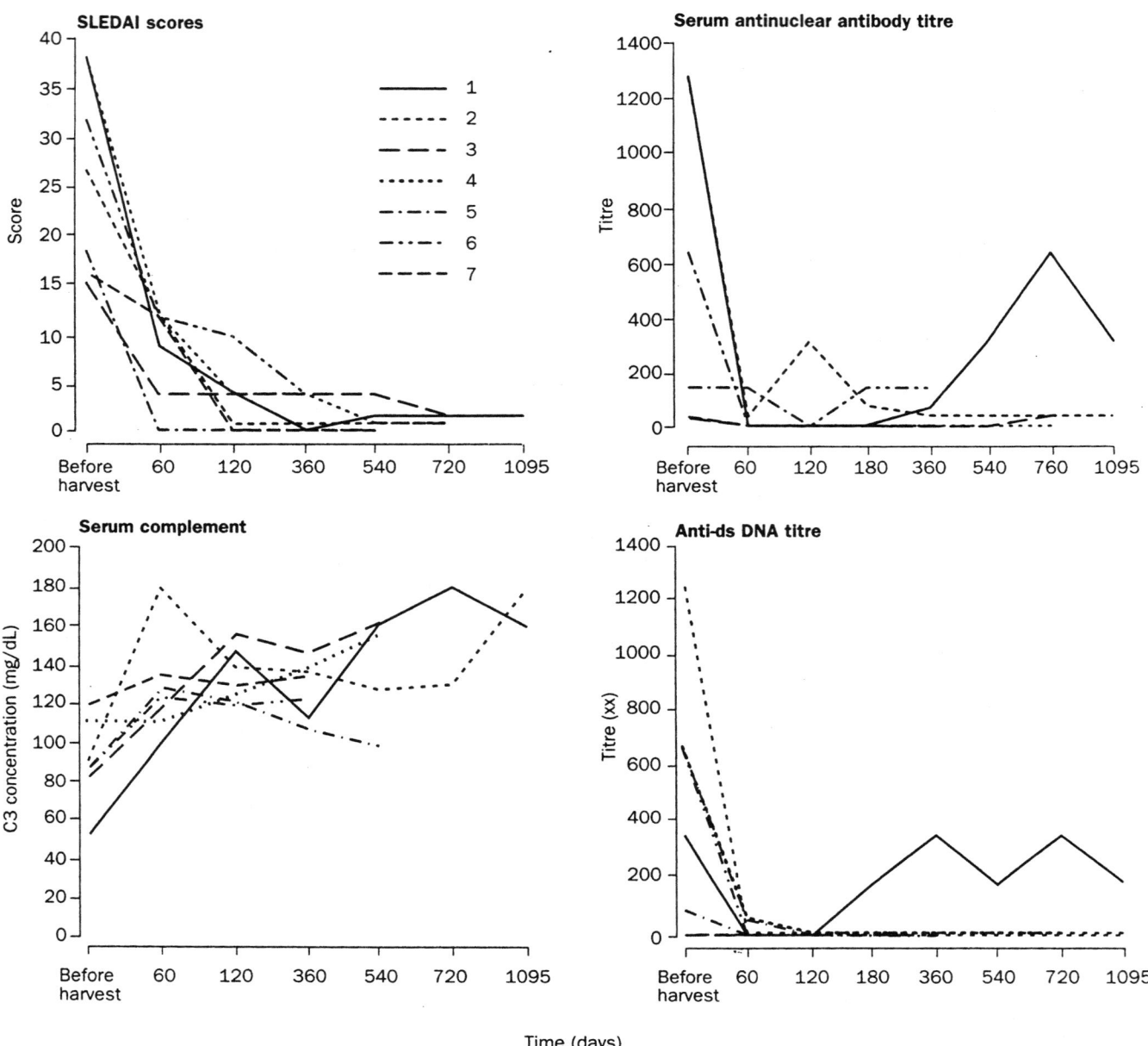

Fig. 119.2. Systemic lupus erythematosus disease activity index scores and pertinent serological values for each patient before and after transplant. Reproduced, with permission, from Traynor *et al.* (2000).

Juvenile idiopathic arthritis

A total of 43 children with juvenile idiopathic arthritis, mostly the systemic form called Still's disease[4], have been registered. Most of these cases were treated in two Dutch centers using bone marrow stem cells and a conditioning protocol of CY 200 mg/kg body weight, TBI 4 Gy, and ATG (N. Wulffraat, personal communication).

[4] Sir Frederrick Still, English pediatrician, 1868–1941.

In the whole group there were 15 complete remissions and 3 partial remissions reported. In those attaining remission, the corticosteroid dose could be reduced and some patients experienced puberty and catch-up growth. Three patients died of macrophage activation syndrome, thought to be related to intercurrent infection or uncontrolled systemic activity of the disease at the time of transplantation. Protocols were modified accordingly such that systemic activity was controlled before the transplant with methylprednisolone intravenously. Since this modification, no further such deaths have occurred. Further

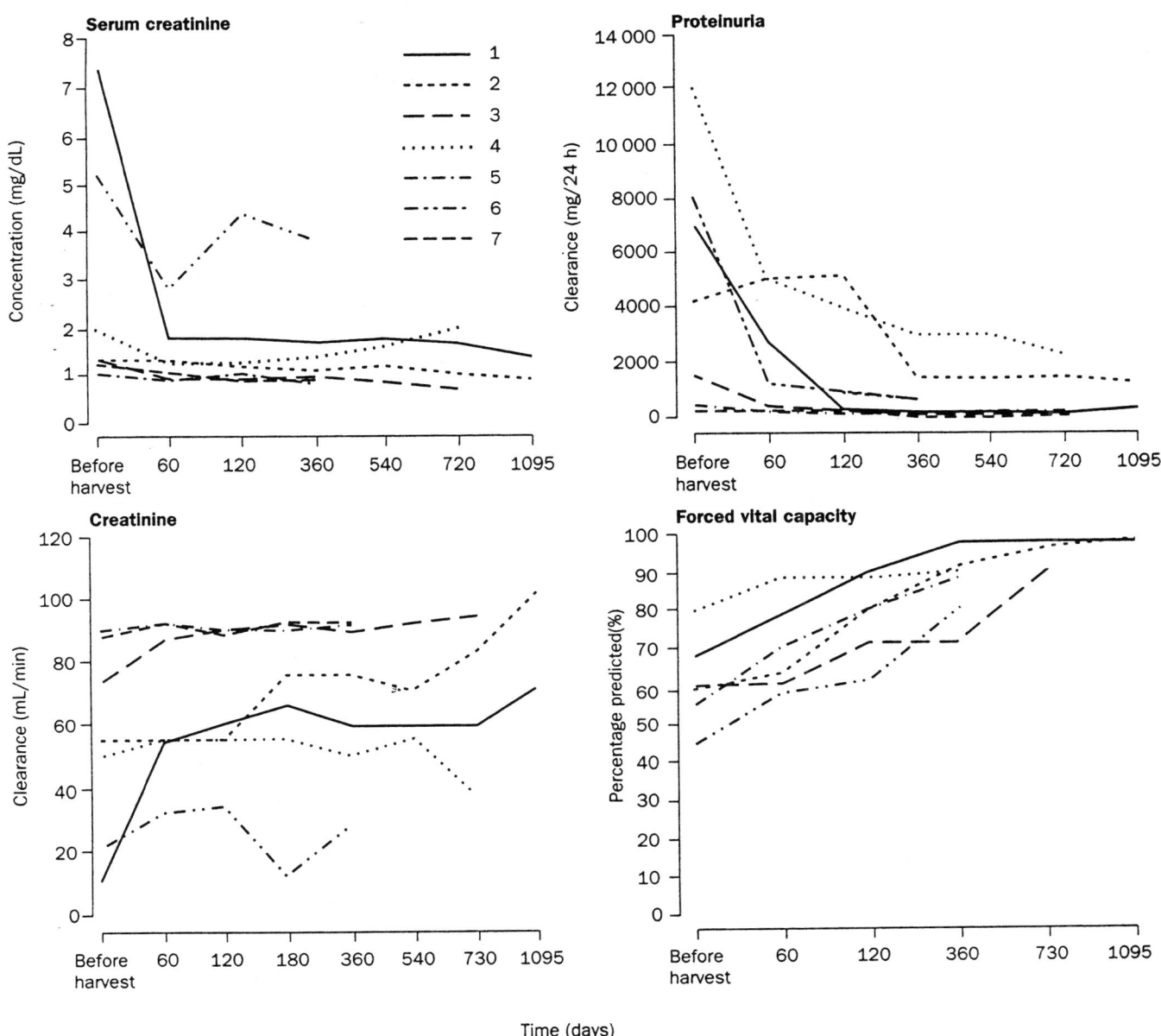

Fig. 119.3. Kidney and lung function before and after transplantation. Reproduced, with permission, from Traynor *et al.* (2000).

phase I and II pilot studies will be undertaken before the optimal phase III randomized study is proposed.

Refractory autoimmune cytopenias

A preliminary review of 16 cases from the EBMT/EULAR registry has been reported (Passweg *et al.*, 2002) consisting of the following diseases: idiopathic thrombocytopenic purpura (*n* = 9), pure red cell aplasia (*n* = 4), autoimmune hemolytic anemia (*n* = 2), and Evans' syndrome (*n* = 1). Median age was 31 (4–45) years and median time to transplantation was 93 (12–236) months. Most received stem cells from blood mobi-

lized with either growth factors (*n* = 7) or CY plus growth factors (*n* = 6). There were two bone marrow harvests. Conditioning regimens included CY alone (*n* = 3), CY with other drugs or ATG (*n* = 9), melphalan (*n* = 2), or were fludarabine-based (*n* = 2). Most (*n* = 12) had purging of immune cells from the graft product.

Median follow-up of surviving patients is 30 (5–53) months. Three patients died within 100 days posttransplant, two of hemorrhage and one of progressive hemolysis. Eight patients showed a response to treatment, with 4 complete remissions [2 ITP, 1 Evan's syndrome, and 1 pure red cell aplasia (PRCA)], sustained in 3 patients. Huhn and colleagues (2003) reported on 14 patients with chronic autoimmune thrombocytopenia, all of whom had failed multiple prior therapies. They received cyclophosphamide 50 mg/kg/day for 4 days prior to a G-CSF-mobilized PBSC transplant depleted of lymphocytes by CD34 selection. Six obtained a durable complete response (platelet counts > 100,000/μl), with a maximum follow-up of 42 months. Two additional patients obtained durable partial responses (cessation of bleeding complications). Some patients, however, failed to show a response, as did patients reported by Skoda et al. (1997) and Marmont et al. (1998). Randomized trials are under discussion for ITP.

Vasculitides

The numbers of cases with vasculitis, inflammatory bowel disease, Bechet's disease, relapsing polychondritis, and other autoimmune diseases are too small to draw meaningful conclusions, with further phase I and II standardized protocol pilot studies proceeding.

Crohn's disease

Two patients with severe Crohn's disease refractory to conventional therapy, including anti-TNF-α treatment, received conditioning with cyclophosphamide 200 mg/kg and equine ATG 90 mg/kg prior to CD34-selected autologous PBSC transplantation. Both patients remained in remission 1 year posttransplant at the time of the report (Burt et al., 2003).

Autologous blood stem cell mobilization

The consensus guidelines recommended the use of granulocyte colony-stimulating factor (G-CSF) 10 μg/kg or cyclophosphamide 4 g/m^2 and G-CSF 10 μg/kg as the mobilization regimen for autoimmune disease patients. A prospective randomized study of filgrastim in 16 patients with RA also recommended this dose; a flare of the RA was seen in 1 of 8 patients receiving 5 μg/kg and in 2 of 8 receiving 10 μg/kg (Snowden et al., 1998b). Flare of disease has also been seen in patients with MS mobilized by G-CSF (Openshaw et al., 2000). Disease flare was not reported in two other studies utilizing G-CSF for PBSC mobilization—one in patients with systemic sclerosis (Locatelli et al., 1999) and one in patients with RA (McGonagle et al., 1997). In another study of 19 patients with SSc, minor reactivations were observed in four patients during mobilization with G-CSF (McSweeney et al., 2002).

A retrospective survey found G-CSF to be associated with a flare in 5 of 56 patients (but restricted to those with RA and MS) versus none of 117 patients mobilized by G-CSF and cyclophosphamide (although 3 patients in the latter group died as a result of mobilization versus none of the G-CSF recipients) (Burt et al., 2001). Mobilized blood stem cells from RA patients contained fewer CD34$^+$ cells but more monocytes than those from normal donors. There were no differences in colony counts [colony-forming units–granulocyte-macrophage (CFU-GM), CFU-GEMM, burst-forming units–erythroid (BFU-E)] between the two groups, and long-term culture-initiating cells were successfully grown. In fact, with, few exceptions, there was no indication that mobilization of hematopoietic precursor cells with G-CSF in patients with autoimmune diseases differs from mobilization in patients with hematological malignancies or normal donors.

To date, the optimal approaches to PBSC mobilization have not been established through prospective studies. The optimal strategies may differ and will need to be determined by appropriately designed studies.

T-cell depletion of the autologous stem cell inoculum

With the advent of technology that will allow for positive and negative selection of cells, graft manipulation as part of the transplant strategy can now be readily carried out (Durez et al., 1998; Munro & Madhok, 1998; Wulffraat et al., 1999) (and see Chapters 26 and 27). The question is whether residual autoreactive (T and/or B cells) present in the autologous stem cell inoculum can cause recurrence of disease posttransplant. There are some animal data suggesting that this is possible. However, the clinical benefit of graft manipulation in HSCT of autoimmune disease in humans remains to be established. Certainly, an intense graft purging of immune competent cells without a similar attempt in the patient is illogical, as is the reverse. The currently confirmed higher risk of infectious complications in patients undergoing stringent graft purging, without a concomitant better outcome concerning the autoimmune disease, needs to be considered. This may differ among the different autoimmune diseases.

Pretransplant conditioning

So far there is no clear indication that the more intense the conditioning, the more frequent or prolonged will be the remission of the autoimmune disease. Preliminary analysis suggests that only toxicity correlated with conditioning severity (Kashyap & Passweg, EBMT/EULAR data base, 2000). Also, the degree of clinical response does not directly correlate with degree and duration of suppression of CD4$^+$ or other immune competent cells. Similar data have been reported recently in long-term follow up of RA patients following total lymph node irradiation (Uhrin et al., 2001) and CAMPATH 1 (Isaacs et al., 2001) in RA patients. This further supports the concept of a complex network failure resulting in autoimmune disease rather than a single clonal defect.

Posttransplant therapies

While autologous transplants appear to reliably provide short-term disease remissions and could be used for this purpose, recurrences have been recorded in all disease categories. This has raised the question of using immunosuppressive therapies as consolidation therapies after autografting in order to sustain the initial response, particularly in RA and SLE in which relapses were especially responsive to further conventional therapy. Such a maintenance strategy is being tested in the ASTIRA (RA) and ASTIL (lupus) randomized trials.

Allogeneic HSCT

A major unresolved question is whether there is a role for allogeneic HSCT in severe autoimmune disease treatment. The lower mortality of autologous blood stem cell transplantation made it an attractive and immediate option for autoimmune disease treatment. Data to date have shown that even with relatively short follow-ups, relapses occur at variable frequencies among the different diseases and this suggests that cures may be infrequent, although that does not exclude meaningful clinical benefit. Limitations for autologous transplants have been several factors:

1. Regimens generally have been less than maximally intensive and thus eradication of immunologic memory may not be possible with currently tolerable regimens.
2. There may be a risk of relapse if autoimmune-disease–mediating T or B cells are reinfused with the stem cell inoculum. If cure is to be achieved, then allogeneic transplantation may be necessary, with its attendant higher risks (10%–30% mortality), mainly relating to GVHD. (In this regard, it is of interest that a child with autoimmune hemolytic anemia that was refractory to immunosuppression and splenectomy had only a 7-week remission after autologous transplantation, but was still in remission at the time of report 18 months after an HLA-identical unrelated donor transplant [De Stefano et al., 1999]. Additionally, a graft-versus-autoimmunity effect has been proposed in a patient given an allogeneic stem cell transplant for CML who also had severe psoriasis [Slavin et al., 2000]. This effect is suggested also by observations in RA where long-term control has been achieved in a small number of allograft recipients. These patients received conditioning therapy very similar to that given in trials of autografting in RA [i.e., CY 200 mg/kg] in which early relapses of RA have occurred, thus suggesting that the allografts rather than the conditioning mediated long-term control.) However, both long-term remissions with autologous HSCT and relapses following allogeneic HSCT (with full donor chimerism) have been observed in autoimmune disease posttransplant.

The application of allogeneic HSCT for the treatment of severe autoimmune disease must await further refinement of the transplant procedure and, in particular, the prevention of GVHD.

Novel concepts with non-myeloablative (reduced intensity) conditioning regimens generate hopes that early transplant-related mortality might be reduced to less than 10% and allogeneic transplant for autoimmune disease patients may become a reality. Still, the risk of GVHD will remain (McSweeney et al., 2001), and it is unclear if the disease target for HSCT in autoimmune disease can be defined as well as in malignant and inherited disorders. Clearly, carefully selected cases with early but high-risk disease and low risk for transplant-related mortality (young age, HLA identical siblings) should provide an answer within the next few years.

Autoimmunity and GVHD

The development of immunity after allogeneic HSCT is complex and can be significantly impaired in the presence of chronic GVHD. Furthermore, chronic GVHD itself can manifest as a disorder very similar to autoimmune connective tissue disorders and remains a significant cause of posttransplant morbidity. The clinical features of chronic GVHD (see Chapter 72) mimic those of connective tissue disorders, especially scleroderma and Sjögren's syndrome. Anti-nuclear, anti-smooth muscle, anti-mitochondrial, and anti-epidermal autoantibodies are frequently present, but their precise role in the pathogenesis of GVHD remains unknown (Rouquette-Gally et al., 1988). In this respect it would seem ironic and perverse if patients undergoing allogeneic HSC transplantation to rid themselves of their autoimmune disease were to end up with a similar disabling disorder, albeit with a different pathogenesis.

Current status and future directions

At the present time due to the risks associated with any HSCT procedure and the uncertainty of the long-term efficacy in autoimmune disease, it is recommended that this treatment be offered only in the context of controlled clinical trials. Several basic questions should be answered before it is routinely applied in the clinic:

1. Will long-term remission (drug-free or with minimal drug maintenance) be possible?
2. What is the risk of malignancy developing due to the conditioning regimens?
3. What degree of immune compromise will persist following hematopoietic reconstitution, if successful remission and tolerance are induced?

These and other questions will only be answered by properly designed and executed prospective comparative studies. Such studies are currently being planned on an international, multicenter basis and should form the basis for rational decision-making on the future of this strategy.

References

Adkins, D.R., Abidi, M.H., Brown, R.A. et al. (2000). Resolution of psoriasis after allogeneic bone marrow transplantation for chronic myelogenous leukemia: late complications of therapy. Bone Marrow Transplantation, 26, 1239–41.

Agosti, J.M., Sprenger, J.D., Lum, L.G. et al. (1988). Transfer of allergen-specific IgE-mediated hypersensitivity with allogeneic bone marrow transplantation. *New England Journal of Medicine,* **319,** 1623–8.

Aldouri, M.A., Ruggier, R., Epstein, O., & Prentice, H.G. (1990). Adoptive transfer of hyperthyroidism and autoimmune thyroiditis following allogeneic bone marrow transplantation for chronic myeloid leukaemia. *British Journal of Haematology,* **74,** 118–19.

Atkinson, K. (1990). Reconstitution of the haemopoietic and immune systems after bone marrow transplantation. *Bone Marrow Transplantation,* **5,** 209–26.

Baldwin, J.L., Storb, R., Thomas, E.D., & Mannick, M. (1977). Bone marrow transplantation in patients with gold-induced marrow aplasia. *Arthritis and Rheumatism,* **20,** 1043–8.

Bargetzi, M.J., Schonenberger, A., Tichelli, A. *et al.* (1997). Coeliac disease transmitted by allogeneic non-T-cell-depleted bone marrow transplantation. *Bone Marrow Transplantation,* **20,** 607–9.

Baron, F.A., Hermanne, J-P., Dowlati, A. *et al.* (1998). Case report. Bronchiolitis obliterans organizing pneumonia and ulcerative colitis after allogeneic bone marrow transplantation. *Bone Marrow Transplantation,* **21,** 951–4.

Baron, F., Ribbens, C., Kaye, O. *et al.* (2000). Effective treatment of Jo-1-associated polymyositis with T-cell-depleted autologous peripheral blood stem cell transplantation. *British Journal of Haematology,* **110,** 339–42.

Berisso, G.A., Lint, M.T., Bacigalupo, A., & Marmont, A.M. (1999). Adoptive autoimmune hyperthyroidism following allogeneic stem cell transplantation from an HLA-identical sibling with Graves' disease. *Bone Marrow Transplantation,* **23,** 1091–2.

Bielekova, B., Goodwin, B., Richert, N. *et al.* (2000). Encephalitogenic potential of the myelin basic protein peptide (amino acids 83–99) in multiple sclerosis: results of a phase II clinical trial with an altered peptide ligand. *Nature Medicine,* **6,** 1167–75.

Blinks, M., Passweg, J. R., Furst, D. *et al.* (2001). Phase I/II trial of autologous stem cell transplantation in systemc sclerosis: procedure related mortality and impact on skin disease. *Annals of Rheumatic Diseases,* **60,** 577–84.

Bolger, G.B., Sullivan, K.M., Spence, M.A. *et al.* (1986). Myasthenia gravis after allogeneic bone marrow transplantation: relationship to chronic graft versus host disease. *Neurology,* **36,** 1087–91.

Burt, R.K. (1997). BMT for severe autoimmune diseases: an idea whose time has come. *Oncology,* **11,** 1001–22.

Burt, R.K., Burns, W., & Hess, A. (1995). Bone marrow transplantation for multiple sclerosis. *Bone Marrow Transplantation,* **16,** 1–6.

Burt, R.K., Fassas, A., Snowden, J.A. *et al.* (2001). Collection of hematopoietic stem cells from patients with autoimmune diseases. *Bone Marrow Transplantation,* **28,** 1–12.

Burt, R.K., Padilla, J., Begolka, W.S. *et al.* (1998). Effect of disease stage on clinical outcome after syngeneic bone marrow transplantation for relapsing experimental autoimmune encephalomyelitis. *Blood,* **91,** 2609–16.

Burt, R. K., Traynor, A., Oyama, Y., & Craig, R. (2003). High-dose immune suppression and autologous hematopoietic stem cell transplantation in refractory Crohn's disease. *Blood,* **101,** 2064–6.

Cahn, J.Y., Chabot, J., Esperou, H. *et al.* (1989). Autoimmune-like thrombocytopenia after bone marrow transplantation. *Blood,* **74,** 2771.

Coles, A.J., Wing, M., & Smith, S. (1999). Pulsed monoclonal antibody treatment and autoimmune thyroid disease in multiple sclerosis. *Lancet,* **354,** 1691–5.

Cooley, H.M., Suarden, J.A., Grigg, A.P. & Wicks, I.P. (1997). Outcome of rheumatoid arthritis and psoriasis following autologous stem cell transplantation for hematologic malignancy. *Arthritis and Rheumatism,* **40,** 1712–5.

Davidson, A. & Diamond, B. (2001). Autoimmune diseases. *New England Journal of Medicine,* **345,** 340–50.

De Stefano, P., Zecca, M., Giorgiani, C. *et al.* (1999). Resolution of immune haemolytic anaemia with allogeneic bone marrow transplantation after an unsuccessful autograft. *British Journal of Haematology,* **106,** 1063–4.

de Vetten, M.P., van Gelder, M., & de Greef, G.E. (2001). Recovery of erythropoiesis following allogeneic bone marrow transplantation for chronic lymphoytic leukaemia-associated pure red cell aplasia. *Bone Marrow Transplantation,* **27,** 771–3.

Diez, S., Banias, H., Diez-Martin, J.L. *et al.* (1999). Apparent cure of Graves-Basedow disease after sibling allogeneic bone marrow transplantation. *Clinical Endocrinology,* **50,** 267–70.

Dighiero, G. & Rose, N.R. (1999). Critical self-epitopes are key to the understanding of self-tolerance and autoimmunity. *Immunology Today,* **20,** 423–8.

Drakos, P.E., Nagler, A., & Or, R. (1993). Case of Crohn's disease in bone marrow transplantation. *American Journal of Hematology,* **43,** 157–8 (Letter).

Durez, P., Toungouz, M., Schandene, L. *et al.* (1998). Remission and immune reconstitution after T-cell depleted stem cell transplantation for rheumatoid arthritis. *Lancet,* **352,** 881 (Letter).

Eedy, D.J., Burrows, D., Bridges, J.M., & Jones, F.G.C. (1990). Clearance of severe psoriasis after allogeneic bone marrow transplantation. *British Medical Journal,* **300,** 908–9.

Euler, H.H., Marmont, A.M., Bacigalupo, A. *et al.* (1996). Early recurrence of or persistence of autoimmune disease after unmanipulated autologous stem cell transplantation. *Blood,* **88,** 3621–5.

Fassas, A., Anagnostopoulos, A., Kazis, A. *et al.* (1997). Peripheral blood stem cell transplantation in the treatment of progressive multiple sclerosis—first results from a pilot study. *Bone Marrow Transplantation,* **20,** 631–8.

Fassas, A., Passweg, J.R., Anagnostopoulos, A. *et al.* (2002). Hematopoietic stem cell transplantation for multiple sclerosis: a retrospective multicenter study. *Journal of Neurology,* **249,** 1088–97.

Fauci, A.S., Hayes, B.F., Katz, P. *et al.* (1983). Wegener's granulomatosis: prospective clinical and therapeutic experience with 85 patients for 21 years. *Annals of Internal Medicine,* **98,** 76–85.

Ferraccioli, G., Damato, R., De Vita, S. *et al.* (2001). Haematopoietic stem cell transplantation (HSCT) in a patient with Sjogren's syndrome and lung MALT lymphoma cured lymphoma not the autoimmune disease. *Annals of the Rheumatic Diseases,* **60,** 174–6.

Gardembas-Pain, M., Ifrah, N., Foussard, C. *et al.* (1990). Psoriasis after allogeneic bone marrow transplantation. *Archives of Dermatology,* **1326,** 1523.

Goldrath, A.W. & Bevan, M.J. (1999). Selecting and maintaining a diverse T-cell repertoire. *Nature,* **402,** 255–62.

Heyll, A., Meckenstock, G., Aul, C. *et al.* (1994). Possible transmission of sarcoidosis via allogeneic bone marrow transplantation. *Bone Marrow Transplantation,* **14,** 161–4.

Hinterberger, W., Hinterberger-Fischer, M., & Marmont, A. (2002). Clinically demonstrable anti-autoimmunity mediated by allogeneic immune cells favorably affects outcome after stem cell transplantation in human autoimmune diseases. *Bone Marrow Transplantation,* **30,** 753–9.

Huhn, R.D., Fogarty, P.F. , Nakamura, R. *et al.* (2003). High-dose cyclophosphamide with autologous lymphocyte-depleted peripheral blood cell (BPSC) support for treament of refractory chronic autoimmune thrombocytopenia. *Blood,* **101,** 71–7.

Ikehara, S., Good, R.A., Nakamura, T. *et al.* (1985a). Rationale for bone marrow transplantation in the treatment of autoimmune diseases. *Proceedings of the National Academy of Sciences USA,* **82,** 2483–7.

Ikehara, S., Ohtsuki, H., Good, R.A. *et al.* (1985b). Prevention of type 1 diabetes in non-obese diabetic mice by allogeneic bone marrow transplantation. *Proceedings of the National Academy of Sciences USA,* **82,** 7743–7.

Isaacs, J.D., Greer, S., Sharma, S. *et al.* (2001). Morbidity and mortality in rheumatoid arthritis patients with prolonged and profound therapy-induced lymphopenia. *Arthritis and Rheumatism,* **44,** 1998–2008.

Jacobs, P., Vincent, M.D., & Martell, R.W. (1986). Prolonged remission of severe refractory rheumatoid arthritis following allogeneic bone marrow transplantation for drug-induced aplastic anaemia. *Bone Marrow Transplantation,* **1,** 237–9.

Jondeau, K., Job-Deslandre, C., Bouscary, D. *et al.* (1997). Remission of nonerosive polyarthritis associated with Sjögren's syndrome after autologous hematopoietic stem cell transplantation for lymphoma. *Journal of Rheumatology,* **24,** 2466–8.

Joske, D.J.L. (1997). Autologous bone marrow transplantation for rheumatoid arthritis. *Lancet,* **350,** 337–8.

Karthaus, M., Gabrysiak, T., Brabant, G. *et al.* (1997). Immune thyroiditis after transplantation of allogeneic CD34⁺-selected peripheral blood cells. *Bone Marrow Transplantation,* **20,** 697–9.

Karussis, D.M., Vourka-Karussis, U., Lehmann, D. *et al.* (1995). Immunomodulation of autoimmunity in MRL/lpr mice with syngeneic bone marrow transplantation (SBMT). *Clinical and Experimental Immunology,* **100,** 111–7.

Kashyap, A. & Forman, S.J. (1998). Autologous bone marrow transplantation for non-Hodgkin's lymphoma resulting in long-term remission of coincidental Crohn's disease. *British Journal of Hematology,* **103,** 651–2.

Kirzner, R.P., Engelman, R.W., Mizutani, H. *et al.* (2000). Prevention of coronary vascular disease by transplantation of T-cell-depleted bone marrow and hematopoietic stem cell preparation in autoimmune-prone W/BF₁ mice. *Biology of Blood and Marrow Transplantation,* **6,** 513–22.

Kishimoto, Y., Yamamoto, Y., Ito, T. *et al.* (1997). Case report. Transfer of autoimmune thyroiditis and resolution of palmoplantar pustular psoriasis following allogeneic bone marrow transplantation. *Bone Marrow Transplantation,* **19,** 1041–3.

Knaan-Shanzer, S., Houben, P.F.J., Kinwelbohre, E.P.M. *et al.* (1991). Remission induction of adjuvant arthritis in rats by total

body irradiation and autologous bone marrow transplantation. *Bone Marrow Transplantation,* **8,** 333–8.

Korbling, M., Katz, R.L., Khanna, A. *et al.* (2002). Hepatocytes and epithelial cells of donor origin in recipients of peripheral-blood stem cells. *New England Journal of Medicine,* **346,** 738–46.

Lampeter, E.F., Homberg, M., Qunbeck, K. *et al.* (1993). Transfer of insulin-dependent diabetes between HLA-identical siblings by bone marrow transplantation. *Lancet,* **341,** 1243–4.

Lampeter, E.F., McCann, S.R., & Kolb, H. (1998). Transfer of diabetes type 1 by bone marrow transplantation. *Lancet,* **351,** 568–9.

Lee, W.Y., Oh, E.S., Min, C.K. *et al.* (2001). Changes in autoimmune thyroiditis following allogeneic bone marrow transplantation. *Bone Marrow Transplantation,* **28,** 63–6.

Lewis, E.J. (1992). Plasmapheresis for lupus nephritis. *New England Journal of Medicine,* **14,** 1029–30 (Letter).

Lim, H.S., Kell, J., Al-Sabah, A. *et al.* (1997). Peripheral blood stem cell transplantation for refractory autoimmune thrombocytopenic purpura. *Lancet,* **349,** 475.

Liu Yin, J.A. & Jowitt, S.N. (1992). Resolution of immune-mediated diseases following bone marrow transplantation for leukaemia. *Bone Marrow Transplantation,* **9,** 31–3.

Locatelli, F., Perotti, C., Torretta, L. *et al.* (1999). Mobilization and selection of peripheral blood hematopoietic progenitors in children with systemic sclerosis. *Haematologica,* **84,** 839–43.

Lopez-Cubero, S.O., Sullivan, K.M., & McDonald, G.B. (1998). Course of Crohn's disease after allogeneic bone marrow transplantation. *Gastroenterology,* **114,** 433–40.

Lowenthal, R., Cohen, M., Atkinson, K., & Biggs, J. (1993). Apparent cure of rheumatoid arthritis following bone marrow transplantation. *Journal of Rheumatology,* **20,** 137–40.

Lum, I.G., Noges, J.E., Beatty, P. *et al.* (1988). Transfer of specific immunity in recipients given HLA mismatched, T cell-depleted or HLA-identical marrow grafts. *Bone Marrow Transplantation,* **3,** 399–406.

Manis, J.P., Gu, Y., Lansford, R. *et al.* (1998). Ku70 is required for late B cell development and immunoglobulin heavy chain class switching. *Journal of Experimental Medicine,* **187,** 2081–9.

Marazuela, M. & Steegman, J.L. (2000). Transfer of autoimmune hypothyroidism following bone marrow transplantation from a donor with Graves' disease. *Bone Marrow Transplantation,* **26,** 1217–20.

Marmont, A.M. (1997). Stem cell transplantation for severe autoimmune disorders, with special reference to rheumatic diseases. *Journal of Rheumatology,* **24** (Suppl 48), 13–18.

Marmont, A.M. & Van Bekkum, D.W. (1995). Stem cell transplantation for severe autoimmune diseases: new proposals but still unanswered questions. *Bone Marrow Transplantation,* **16,** 497–8.

Marmont, A.M., Van Lint, M.T., Occhini, D. *et al.* (1998). Failure of autologous stem cell transplantation in refractory thrombocytopenic purpura. *Bone Marrow Transplantation,* **22,** 827–8.

McAllister, L.D., Beatty, P.G., & Rose, J. (1997). Allogeneic bone marrow transplant for chronic myelogenous leukaemia in a patient with multiple sclerosis. *Bone Marrow Transplantation,* **19,** 395–7.

McGonagle, D., Rawstron, A., Richards, S. *et al.* (1997). A phase I study to address the safety and efficacy of granulocyte colony-stimulating factor for the mobilization of hematopoietic progenitor cells in active rheumatoid arthritis. *Arthritis and Rheumatism*, **40**, 1838–42.

McKendry, R.J.R., Huebsch, L., & Le Clair, B. (1996). Progression of rheumatoid arthritis following bone marrow transplantation: a case report with a 13 year follow up. *Arthritis and Rheumatism*, **39**, 1246–53.

McSweeney, P.A., Niederwieser, D., Shizuru, J.A. *et al.* (2001). Hematopoietic cell transplantation in older patients with hematologic malignancies: replacing high-dose cytotoxic therapy with graft-versus-tumor effects. *Blood*, **97**, 3390–400.

McSweeney, P.A., Nash, R.A., Sullivan, K.M. *et al.* (2002). High-dose immunosuppressive therapy for severe systemic sclerosis: initial outcomes. *Blood*, **100**, 1602–10.

Medzhitov, R. & Janeway, C.A. Jr. (2002). Decoding the patterns of self and nonself by the innate immune system. *Science*, **296**, 298–300.

Meloni, G., Capria, S., Vignetti, M. *et al.* (1997). Blast crisis of chronic myelogenous leukaemia in long-lasting systemic lupus erythematosus: regression of both diseases after autologous bone marrow transplantation. *Blood*, **89**, 4659.

Minchinton, R.M., Waters, A.H., Kendra, J., & Barrett, A.J. (1982). Autoimmune thrombocytopenia acquired from an allogeneic bone marrow graft. *Lancet*, **2**, 627–9.

Munro, R. & Madhok, R. (1998). T-cell depleted stem-cell transplantation for rheumatoid arthritis. *Lancet*, **352**, 1628–9 (Letter).

Musso, M., Porretto, F., Crescimanno, A. *et al.* (2000). Crohn's disease complicated by relapsed extranodal Hodgkin's lymphoma: prolonged complete remission after unmanipulated PBPC autotransplant. *Bone Marrow Transplantation*, **26**, 921–3.

Nelson, J.L., Torrez, R., Louie, F.M. *et al.* (1997). Pre-existing autoimmune disease in patients with long term survival after allogeneic bone marrow transplantation. *Journal of Rheumatology*, **24** (Suppl 48), 23.

Olagguibel, J., Almodovar, A., Giner, A. *et al.* (1989). Passive transfer of contact sensitivity to colophony as a complication of an allogeneic bone marrow transplant. *Contact Dermatitis*, **20**, 1824.

Olalla, J.I., Ortin, M., Hermida, G. *et al.* (1999). Disappearance of lupus anticoagulant after allogeneic bone marrow transplantation. *Bone Marrow Transplantation*, **23**, 83–5.

Openshaw, H., Nash, R.A., & McSweeny, P.A. (2002). High-dose immunosuppression and hematopoietic stem cell transplantation in autoimmune disease: clinical review. *Biology of Blood and Marrow Transplantation*, **8**, 233–48.

Openshaw, H., Stuve, O., Antel, J.P. *et al.* (2000). Multiple sclerosis flares associated with recombinant granulocyte colony-stimulating factor. *Neurology*, **54**, 2147–50.

Paillard, C., Kanold, J. Halle, P. *et al.* (2000). Two-step immunoablative treatment with autologous peripheral blood CD34⁺ cell transplantation in an 8-year-old boy with autoimmune haemolytic anaemia. *British Journal of Haematology*, **110**, 900–2.

Passweg, J., Rabusin, M., Musso, M. *et al.* (2002). Autologous transplantation for refractory autoimmune cytopenias. *Bone Marrow Transplantation*, **29** (Suppl), S107.

Plouvier, E., Herre, P., Faivre, L., & Noir, A. (1983). Refractory autoimmune thrombocytopenia following autologous stem cell grafting. *British Journal of Haematology*, **II** (Suppl 13), 172 (Abstract).

Raetz, E., Beatty, P.G., & Adams, R.H. (1997). Case report. Treatment of severe Evans syndrome with an allogeneic cord blood transplant. *Bone Marrow Transplantation*, **20**, 427–9.

Rouquette-Gally, A.M., Boyeldieu, D., Prost, A.C., & Gluckman, E. (1988). Autoimmunity after allogeneic bone marrow transplantation. A study of 53 long-term-surviving patients. *Transplantation*, **46**, 238–40.

Salzman, D., Tam, J., Jackson, C. *et al.* (1994). Clinical remission of myasthenia gravis (MG) in a patient (PT) after high dose therapy and autologous transplantation with CD34+ stem cells (SC). *Blood*, **84** (Suppl 1), 206a (Abstract).

Seiffert, B., Passweg, J., Gregor, M. *et al.* (2002). Total alopecia cured by PBSCT. Proof of principle of autoimmune pathogenesis? *Bone Marrow Transplantation*, **29** (Suppl), S107.

Sherer, Y. & Shoenfeld, Y. (2002). Atherosclerosis. *Annals of Rheumatic Diseases*, **61**, 97–9.

Shevach, E.M. (2001). Certified professionals: CD4(+)CD25(+) suppressor T cells. *Journal of Experimental Medicine*, **193**, F41–6.

Shikari, M., Fujiwara, M., & Kano, K. (1983). Rectification of immunological abnormalities and lupus nephritis by the transfer of bone marrow cells. *Annals of New York Academy of Sciences*, **420**, 309–14.

Skoda, R.C., Tichelli, A., Tyndall, A. *et al.* (1997). Autologous peripheral blood stem cell transplantation in a patient with chronic autoimmune thrombocytopenia. *British Journal of Haematology*, **99**, 56–7.

Slavin, S., Nagler, A., Varadi, G., & Or, R. (2000). Graft vs autoimmunity following allogeneic non-myeloablative blood stem cell transplantation in a patient with chronic myelogenous leukemia and severe systemic psoriasis and psoriatic polyarthritis. *Experimental Hematology*, **28**, 853–7.

Smith, S.R., MacFarlane, A.W., & Lewis-Jones, M.S. (1988). Papular urticaria and transfer of allergy following bone marrow transplantation. *Clinical and Experimental Dermatology*, **13**, 260–2.

Snowden, J.A., Atkinson, K., Kearney, J.C. *et al.* (1997). Allogeneic bone marrow transplantation from a donor with severe active rheumatold arthritis not resulting in adoptive transfer of disease to recipient. *Bone Marrow Transplantation*, **20**, 71–3.

Snowden, J.A., Biggs, J.C., Milliken, S.T. *et al.* (1998a). A randomized, blinded, placebo-controlled, dose-escalation study of the tolerability and efficacy of filgrastim for haemopoietic stem cell mobilization in patients with severe rheumatoid arthritis. *Bone Marrow Transplantation*, **22**, 1035–41.

Snowden, J.A., Brooks, P.M., & Biggs, S.J.C. (1997). Haemopoietic stem cell transplantation for autoimmune disease. *British Journal of Haematology*, **99**, 9–22.

Snowden, J.A. & Heaton, D.C. (1997). Development of psoriasis after syngeneic bone marrow transplantation from psoriatic donor: further evidence for adoptive autoimmunity. *British Journal of Dermatology*, **137**, 130–2.

Snowden, J.A., Kearney, P., Kearney, A. *et al.* (1998b). Long term follow up of autoimmune disease following allogeneic bone marrow transplantation. *Arthritis and Rheumatism*, **41**, 453–9.

Snowden, J.A., Patton, W.N., O'Donnell, J.L. *et al.* (1997). Prolonged remission of longstanding systemic lupus erythematosus after autologous bone marrow transplant for non-Hodgkin's lymphoma. *Bone Marrow Transplantation*, **19**, 1247–50.

Sturfelt, G., Lenhoff, S., Sallerfors, B. *et al.* (1996). Transplantation with allogenic bone marrow from a donor with systemic lupus erythematosus (SLE): successful outcome in the recipient and induction of an SLE flare in the donor. *Annals of the Rheumatic Diseases,* **55,** 638–41.

Tamm, A., Gratwohl, A., Tichelli, A. *et al.* (1996). Autologous haemopoietic stem cell transplantation in a patient with severe pulmonary hypertension complicating connective tissue disease. *Annals of Rheumatic Diseases,* **55,** 779–80.

Tauro, S. & Mahendra, P. (2001). Resolution of sarcoidosis after allogeneic bone marrow transplantation with donor lymphocyte infusions. *Bone Marrow Transplantation,* **27,** 757–9.

Theophilopoulos, A.N. & Dixon, F.J. (1987). Experimental murine systemic lupus erythematosus. In *Systemic Lupus Erythematosus,* ed. R.G. Lahita, pp. 121–202. Lahita, York, Singapore: Wiley.

Thomson, J.A., Wilson, R.M., Franklin, I.M. *et al.* (1995). Transmission of thyrotoxicosis of autoimmune type by sibling allogeneic bone marrow transplant. *European Journal of Endocrinology,* **133,** 564–6.

Traynor, A.E., Schroeder, J., Rosa, R.M. *et al.* (2000). Treatment of severe systemic lupus erythematosus with high-dose chemotherapy and haemopoietic stem-cell transplantation: a phase I study. *Lancet,* **356,** 701–7.

Tyndall, A., Black, C., Finke, J. *et al.* (1997). Treatment of systemic sclerosis with autologous haemopoietic stem cell transplantation. *Lancet,* **349,** 254.

Tyndall, A. & Gratwohl, A. (1997). Blood and marrow stem cell transplants in autoimmune disease: a consensus report written on behalf of the European League Against Rheumatism (EULAR) and the European Group for Blood and Marrow Transplant (EBMT). *Bone Marrow Transplantation,* **19,** 643–5.

Tyndall, A., Passweg, J., & Gratwohl, A. (2001). Haemopoietic stem cell transplantation in the treatment of severe autoimmune diseases 2000. *Annals of the Rheumatic Diseases,* **60,** 702–7.

Uhrin, Z., Wang, B.W., Matsuda, Y. *et al.* (2001). Treatment of rheumatoid arthritis with total lymphoid irradiation: long-term survival. *Arthritis and Rheumatism,* **44,** 1525–8.

van Bekkum, D.W. (2000). Conditioning regimens for the treatment of experimental arthritis with autologous bone marrow transplantation. *Bone Marrow Transplantation,* **25,** 357–64.

van Gelder, M., Kinwel-Bohre, E.P.M., & van Bekkum, D.W. (1993). Treatment of experimental allergic encephalomyelitis in rats with total body irradiation and syngeneic BMT. *Bone Marrow Transplantation,* **11,** 233–41.

van Gelder, M. & van Bekkum, D.W. (1995). Treatment of relapsing experimental autoimmune encephalomyelitis in rats with allogeneic bone marrow transplantation from a resistant strain. *Bone Marrow Transplantation,* **16,** 343–51.

Vento, S., Cainelli, F., Renzini, C. *et al.* (1996). Resolution of autoimmune hepatitis after bone marrow transplantation. *Lancet,* **348,** 544–5.

Vialettes, B., Maraninchi, D., San Marco, M.P. *et al.* (1993). Autoimmune polyendocrine failure type 1 (insulin dependent) diabetes mellitus and hypothyroidism after allogeneic bone marrow transplantation in a patient with lymphoblastic leukaemia. *Diabetologica,* **36,** 541–6.

Wiesneth, M., Duncker, C., Stefanic, W. *et al.* (2002). A high incidence of autoimmune thyroid disease and autoimmune cytopenia after T-cell depleted allogeneic peripheral blood progenitor cell transplants: clinical features and analysis of risk factors. *Bone Marrow Transplantation,* **29** (Suppl), S14.

Wyatt, D.T., Lum, L., Caper, J. *et al.* (1990). Autoimmune thyroiditis after bone marrow transplantation. *Bone Marrow Transplantation,* **5,** 357–61.

Wulffraat, N., van Royen, A., Bierings, M. *et al.* (1999). Autologous haemopoietic stem-cell transplantation in four patients with refractory juvenile chronic arthritis. *Lancet,* **353,** 550–3.

120 Allogeneic hematopoietic stem cell transplantation for solid tumors

RAM SRINIVASAN AND RICHARD CHILDS

National Heart, Lung and Blood Institute, Bethesda, USA

Introduction

The vast majority of patients with metastatic solid tumors will ultimately succumb to complications related to disease progression. Advances in the areas of chemotherapy and biologic therapy over the last two to three decades have largely resulted in providing palliation with minimal to modest prolongations of survival. Given the dismal prognosis of most patients with metastatic cancer, there exists a need to explore novel therapeutic options.

Allogeneic hematopoietic stem cell transplantation (allo-HSCT) is an effective therapeutic option for patients with a variety of hematologic malignancies. Awareness that the alloimmune graft-vs-leukemia (GVL) effect is largely responsible for providing long-term remission of hematologic malignancies has kindled interest in studying this modality as a treatment for solid tumors. Based on the promising results seen in several pilot trials of non-myeloablative allogeneic blood stem cell transplantation (NST) in metastatic renal cell carcinoma (RCC), the therapeutic potential of the graft-vs-tumor (GVT) effect in other solid tumors is now being explored.

This chapter will describe the development of NST as a form of immunotherapy for metastatic solid tumors and will review the clinical results of pilot allo-HSCT trials in solid tumors.

Immune-based therapy for solid tumors

The limited efficacy of conventional therapeutic approaches in combating advanced cancer, and the recognition that malignancies may occur in part as a result of failed "immune surveillance," has led to considerable interest in investigating the therapeutic potential of immuno-modulatory agents in refractory solid tumors. Early immunotherapy trials utilized cytokines such as interferons and interleukin-2 primarily with the intent of enhancing innate host immune responses against tumor. Pioneering studies by Rosenberg and others in the 1980s defined for the first time the utility of immune manipulations in the management of metastatic melanoma and renal

cell carcinoma (Quesada, Swanson, & Trindade, 1983; Rosenberg *et al.*, 1994; Negrier *et al.*, 1998). Although some patients enjoyed a direct therapeutic effect, the principal contribution of these early trials was to establish proof-of-principle of the efficacy of immunotherapy for cancer and provide the foundation for the development of novel immunotherapeutic approaches. Unfortunately, the use of cytokine-based therapy has been constrained by limited clinical responses with a less than desirable toxicity profile. More recently, a number of tumor-associated antigens have been identified which has led to the development of vaccine strategies aimed at generating immune responses specifically targeted to cancer antigens (Boon, Coulie, & Van den Eynde, 1997; Ada, 1999; Rosenberg, 1999). Vaccine-based strategies hold tremendous promise and have already been shown in some circumstances to result in significant expansions of tumor-specific cytotoxic lymphocytes. However, at present, only a minority of humans with cancer have benefited from such vaccine-based approaches.

Limitations of autologous immunotherapy

Although cytokine and vaccine-based trials have demonstrated the feasibility of generating tumor-specific T-cell responses in patients with cancer (Stevens *et al.*, 1995; Gilboa, Nair, & Lyerly, 1998; Timmerman & Levy, 1999), at least two factors limit the efficacy and broader applicability of this response. First, since the vast majority of patients with solid tumors have received prior chemotherapeutic agents, physicians are often confronted with an immune system that has been crippled to the point where a vigorous response to an antigenic stimulus is no longer possible. Second, it is likely that progression of the neoplasm occurs in association with the development of "immune tolerance" to tumor cells. It is reasonable to assume that only after tolerance to tumor antigens has been broken that an adequate immune response can be mounted. Both these hurdles could theoretically be overcome by providing an allogeneic immune system that is both "intact" and in a "non-tolerized" state. Furthermore, an allogeneic immune system, even in the context of complete HLA compatibility, is capable of mounting immune responses to polymorphic variants of tumor-specific or broadly expressed minor histocompatibility antigens (De Buerger *et al.*, 1992; Goulmy, 1996; Warren, Greenberg, & Riddell, 1998). These potential advantages make allogeneic immunotherapy an attractive alternative to autologous immunotherapeutic approaches.

The graft-vs-tumor (GVT) effect

Recognition of GVT in hematologic malignancies

The use of dose-intensive HSCT is based on the concept that malignancies can be completely eradicated by conditioning agents when administered in sufficiently high doses. The ability to administer high doses of chemotherapy was, however, limited by the accompanying annihilation of hematopoietic stem cells. This problem could be circumvented by the infusion of normal bone marrow cells from a healthy donor, with the sole intended purpose of this procedure being to provide host hematopoietic reconstitution (Thomas & Blume, 1999). Over the last two decades, several lines of evidence have emerged showing the anti-neoplastic component of allo-HSCT resides not only in high-dose chemotherapy, but a more prolonged and durable anti-tumor effect mediated by donor immune cells. The earliest suggestion of the existence of an alloimmune graft-versus-leukemia effect came from the work of Weiden *et al.* (1979), who noted that the occurrence of acute and chronic graft-versus-host disease (GVHD) in leukemic patients who had undergone allogeneic bone marrow transplantation was associated with a reduced risk of relapse. Several subsequent observations further led to the conclusion that the conditioning regimen itself, no matter how dose-escalated, was by itself insufficient to cure the vast majority of hematological malignancies. The observation that the risk of CML relapse was higher in recipients of a T-cell depleted allograft, as well as in those receiving a syngeneic transplant versus an HLA-matched, allogeneic donor graft lent credence to this concept (Apperley *et al.*, 1986; Goldman *et al.*, 1988; Horowitz *et al.*, 1990; Marmont *et al.*, 1991). Perhaps most importantly, the demonstration that patients with CML which had relapsed following an allo-transplant could be induced back into a durable remission by the single act of infusing donor lymphocytes established conclusively both the existence and curative potential of the graft-versus-leukemia effect (GVL) (Kolb *et al.*, 1990). Similar GVL effects have since been demonstrated in other hematological cancers including acute leukemia (Kolb *et al.*, 1995), posttransplant Epstein Barr virus-associated lymphoproliferative disorder (Heslop *et al.*, 1994; Papadopoulos *et al.*, 1994, chronic lymphatic leukemia (Mehta *et al.*, 1996), Hodgkin's and non-Hodgkin's lymphoma (Jones *et al.*, 1991; van Besien *et al.*, 1997), and multiple myeloma (Tricot *et al.*, 1996; Verdonck *et al.*, 1996; Lokhorst *et al.*, 1997).

Harnessing GVT against metastatic solid tumors

Studies exploring the ability to generate a graft-versus-solid tumor response following allogeneic HSCT were first pursued in murine models. Moscovitch and Slavin (1984) demonstrated that allogeneic transplantation could confer resistance to spontaneous development of lymphosarcoma in NZB/WF1 mice. The same group also demonstrated that allogeneic T-cells could induce GVT effects against minor histocompatibility antigens expressed on murine mammary adenocarcinoma which were polymorphic between recipient and donor (Morecki *et al.*, 1997, 1998). These experiments provided preliminary evidence that minor histocompatibility antigens are expressed on tumors of epithelial origin, and in the setting of an allogeneic transplant, might indeed serve as targets for the induction of a GVT effect.

The existence of clinically meaningful graft-versus-solid tumor effects in humans is a topic of ongoing investigation. Early evidence affirming the existence of graft-versus-solid tumor effects took the form of case reports and small case series. Eibl *et al.* (1996) reported a case of a woman with breast cancer treated with an allogeneic stem cell transplant from an HLA-identical sibling following conventional myeloablative conditioning. Regression of a liver metastasis coincident with acute GVHD led investigators to infer a graft-versus-breast carcinoma effect had occurred. The isolation of minor histocompatibility antigen-reactive cytotoxic T lymphocytes from patient blood which were capable of lysing breast cancer cell lines provided in vitro evidence supporting such a phenomenon. Ueno *et al.* (1998) reported on a series of ten patients with metastatic breast cancer treated at the M.D. Anderson Cancer Center with a conventional myeloablative allogeneic transplant. Six out of ten patients were reported to have achieved partial (5 of 10) or complete remission (1 of 10). Two of these responses occurred in the context of acute skin GVHD and withdrawal of immunosuppression, suggesting that these responses may have been induced as a consequence of a GVT effect. Exciting as these results were, the significant and often fatal toxicities associated with myeloablative conditioning discouraged investigators from pursuing similar studies in patients with other types of solid tumors.

Conventional versus non-myeloablative conditioning

Allo-HSCT is far from a benign procedure, with treatment-related mortality (TRM) rates in the range of 20%–35%. Several factors including patient age, co-morbid medical illness, and HLA compatibility directly impact outcome following transplantation. As a consequence, many patients who might derive benefit from an allogeneic transplant are denied this approach due to the presence of one or more factors which make the risk of TRM prohibitive. In the mid-1990s, investigators first studied the effects of "de-intensifying" transplant conditioning in the hope that this would help reduce the risk of TRM (Giralt *et al.*, 1997; Khouri *et al.*, 1998; Slavin *et al.*, 1998). A number of important observations led to the development of transplant regimens which utilized reduced intensity conditioning. First, TRM was at least partly related to the intensity of the conditioning regimen, with early morbidity and mortality following HSCT being largely a consequence of regimen-related toxicity. Second, an increased understanding of the power of the GVL effect and an appreciation that GVL alone, for some hematological malignancies, could be curative. Third, the perception that the major role of the conditioning regimen is to induce sufficient host immunosuppression to enable engraftment of the donor immune system for the subsequent generation of a GVT effect. As a consequence, NST conditioning regimens were designed to be highly immunosuppressive, while causing only transient myelosuppression leading to autologous marrow recovery sufficient to support hematopoiesis even in the event of graft failure (Giralt *et al.*, 1997; Khouri *et al.*, 1998; Slavin *et al.*, 1998; Childs *et al.*, 2000; McSweeney, Niederwieser, & Shiruzu, 2001). These reduced intensity, non-myeloablative regimens were initially evaluated in hematologic malignancies known to be responsive to a GVL effect. Although randomized studies comparing NST versus myeloablative allo-HSCT have not yet been published, preliminary results from several trials investigating NST would suggest this approach is indeed safer than conventional high dose regimens. More importantly, powerful and curative GVT effects have been induced against a number of hematologic malignancies following NST (Giralt *et al.*, 1997; Khouri *et al.*, 1998; Slavin *et al.*, 1998; McSweeney, Niederwieser, & Shiruzu, 2001). Older patients with hematologic malignancies (up to 65–70 years of age) and those with co-morbid medical conditions can now undergo allogeneic transplantation with more acceptable transplant-related risks. Importantly, the reduced risk of TRM associated with NST conditioning has opened the door for investigating graft-versus-tumor effects in patients with advanced and incurable metastatic solid tumors.

Results

Allogeneic hematopoietic stem cell transplantation in renal cell carcinoma

The advent of non-myeloablative conditioning has made possible systematic evaluations for graft-versus-solid tumor effects in a variety of solid tumors. It is speculated that several factors related to the tumor might predict for susceptibility to a GVT effect (Table 120.1). Based on these criteria, metastatic RCC would appear to be a reasonable candidate tumor to investigate for susceptibility to an allo-immune effect (Fairlamb, 1981; Quesada *et al.*, 1983; Rosenberg *et al.*, 1984; Figlin *et al.*, 1997; van den Eynde *et al.*, 1999). Furthermore, the dismal prognosis associated with metastatic RCC (Motzer, Bander, & Nanus, 1996) and the limited therapeutic options available to

Table 120.1. *Solid tumor characteristics that might be associated with susceptibility to allogeneic immune attack*

Documented response to other immune manipulations (cytokines, vaccines)
Associated with spontaneous remission
High degrees of MHC class I expression
Expression of immunogenic tumor-associated antigen(s)
Data showing in vitro susceptibility of tumor to T-cell attack
Slow to moderate proliferative capacity
Tissue of origin a target for acute or chronic GVHD

Abbreviations: MHC, major histocompatibility complex; GVHD, graft-versus-host disease.

these patients justifies the risks of morbidity and mortality associated with an allogeneic transplant.

We and others first began exploring for GVT effects in metastatic RCC in the late 1990s. The experimental nature of NST mandated that selection criteria for patients enrolled on such studies be rigorous. Accordingly, only those patients with evaluable metastatic disease who had failed cytokine-based therapy and who had an excellent performance status (ECOG 0–1) with a life expectancy of at least 3 months were considered eligible. The treatment scheme we evaluated is outlined in Figure 120.1 The dual goals of achieving maximal immunosuppression to ensure engraftment with minimal myelosuppression to improve safety were accomplished by pretransplant conditioning with fludarabine (125 mg/m^2 and cyclophosphamide (120 mg/kg). Acute graft-versus-host disease prophylaxis initially consisted of single agent cyclosporine (CSP). However, an unacceptably high incidence of GVHD-related mortality in the first 25 patients prompted the addition of mycophenolate mofetil (MMF) to the GVHD prophylactic regimen for subsequent patients. An unmanipulated peripheral blood stem cell graft collected from a 6 of 6 or 5 of 6 HLA-matched sibling donor following granulocyte-colony stimulating factor (G-CSF) mobilization was infused following conditioning. Immunosuppression withdrawal and donor lymphocyte infusion (DLI) schemes were designed to promote rapid donor T-cell engraftment, a factor shown previously to be important for the generation of a clinically meaningful GVT effect.

The clinical results from the first 19 patients with RCC undergoing NST have been reported (Childs *et al.*, 2000). Ten of 19 (53%) patients responded to therapy, including 3 complete remissions (CR) and 7 partial remissions (PR). More than 50 patients with metastatic RCC have now undergone NST at the National Institutes of Health (NIH). Twenty-two (44%) of 50 patients evaluable for a response have had evidence for a GVT effect, including 4 who have had a CR and 18 who have had a PR. Five patients experienced a mixed response. Many of these responses have been durable with the first complete responder still remaining disease-free over 50 months after transplantation. The most dramatic responses have involved regression of pulmonary metastatic disease,

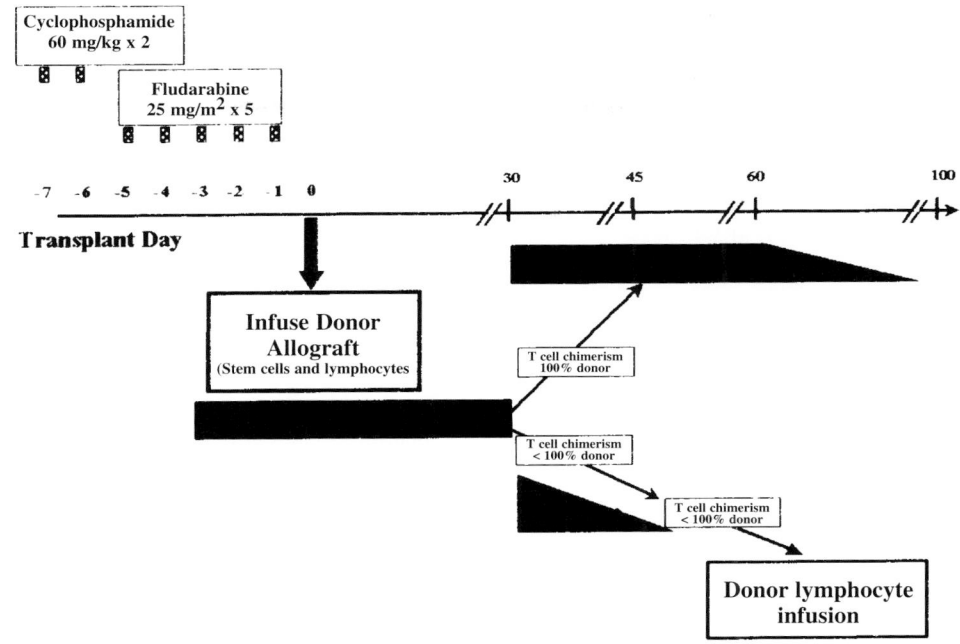

Fig. 120.1. Non-myeloablative HSC transplant strategy: patients with metastatic RCC received pretransplant conditioning with cyclophosphamide (120 mg/kg) and fludarabine 125 mg/m^2) followed by infusion of a G-CSF-mobilized peripheral blood stem cell allograft on day 0. Cyclosporine (CSP) was started on day −4 to prevent graft rejection and continued thereafter as graft-vs-host disease (GVHD) prophylaxis. Patients with mixed T-cell chimerism on day 30 were tapered off CSP, and if necessary, received incremental doses of donor lymphocyte infusions monthly until GVHD, or disease regression, occurred. Patients with 100% donor T-cell chimerism by day 30 continued on CSP until day 60 at which point it was tapered off over the following 40 days. (MMF was added to CSP as GVHD prophylaxis after RCC patient #25 and was discontinued in conjunction with CSP.)

although impressive disease regression in other metastatic sites has been observed (Fig. 120.2). Regression of metastatic disease appeared to make a clinically meaningful impact with survival in responders being prolonged relative to nonresponders (Fig. 120.3) (Childs *et al.*, 2000). About two-thirds of patients have developed grade II–IV acute GVHD, with slightly less than a third developing chronic GVHD. Six patients (12%) have died from transplant-related causes, including 4 who died from complications related to GVHD. No decline in the incidence of acute GVHD was observed following the addition of MMF to CSP as GVHD prophylaxis. As a consequence, we are presently evaluating the impact of adding low-dose methotrexate (5 mg/m^2 days +1, +3, +6) to CSP on the incidence and severity of acute GVHD following our NST approach.

Since alloimmune effects depend largely on donor-derived T cell responses, the degree and rapidity of donor T-cell engraftment is likely a factor that ultimately impacts on the ability to generate a GVT effect. The fludarabine/cyclophosphamide regimen that we have used predictably results in an early transition to complete donor T-cell chimerism, while donor myeloid engraftment occurs more gradually (Childs *et al*, 1999). Our transplant strategy also calls for expeditious withdrawal of immunosuppression and DLI administration to enhance GVT effects in a timely fashion.

The pattern of engraftment observed in RCC patients following NST may vary considerably depending on a number of factors including the immunosuppressive versus myelosuppressive potential of the conditioning regimen, CD34$^+$ cell dose, and the pretransplant immune status of the patient, which is frequently weakened as a consequence of prior chemotherapy exposure. For instance, conditioning with 200 cGy TBI in combination with fludarabine (90 mg/m^2) for hematologic malignancies (McSweeney, Niederwieser, & Shiruzu, 2001) typically results in rapid myeloid engraftment in contrast to T cell engraftment, which occurs more slowly.

Several instructive observations have emerged from the analysis of responding RCC patients. The majority of patients who ultimately had a disease response had tumor growth in the first few months following the procedure. Tumor regression occurred late in the course of the transplant (median 5 months, range 1–15 months), leading one to infer these responses were the consequence of an immune effect. The role of a graft-versus-tumor effect is further supported by the observation that disease regressions typically occurred following withdrawal of immunosuppression and only after lymphoid cells had transitioned from mixed to predominantly donor T-cell chimerism. It is important to note in this regard that the vast majority of our patients had achieved complete donor T-cell chimerism by day 100. Acute GVHD was favorably associated with disease

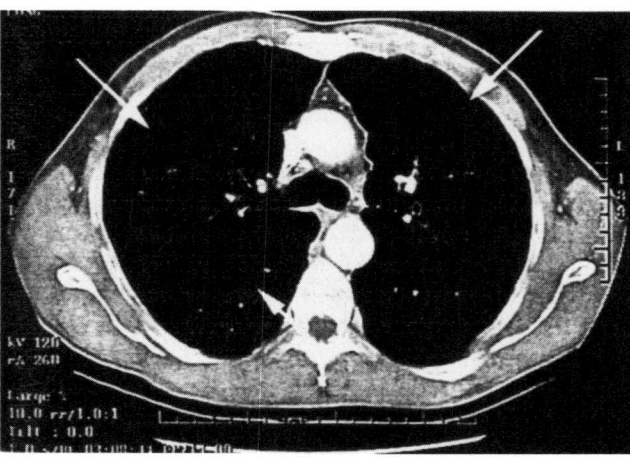

A

B

Fig. 120.2. CT images of pulmonary metastases (arrows) 60 days (panel A) and 285 days (panel B) after transplantation in Patient 19.

response (Fig. 120.4), although it was not required, as evidenced by delayed disease responses that occurred temporally distant from periods of active GVHD. The separation of GVHD from GVT is illustrated in a patient who had a disease response several weeks after acute GVHD had resolved (Fig. 120.5). Figure 120.6 illustrates the time course of common posttransplant events observed following NST using our transplant approach.

Several other investigators have reported GVT effects in RCC following NST (Table 120.2). Rini *et al.* (2002) transplanted 15 patients with a fludarabine/cyclophosphamide-based regimen. The initial cohort received fludarabine (90 mg/m^2) and cyclophosphamide (2 g/m^2) at doses that were insufficient to produce adequate host immunosuppression. Consequently, three of the first four (75%) patients treated ultimately rejected the allograft. Subsequent patients received higher doses of these conditioning agents (fludarabine 150 mg/m^2 and cyclophosphamide 4 g/m^2) with suc-

cessful engraftment. Four of the 12 patients who engrafted had a partial response consistent with a GVT effect. Predictably, none of the patients who failed to engraft had evidence for a disease response. However, one patient with graft rejection underwent a second transplant with the intensified conditioning regimen, achieved complete donor engraftment, and subsequently had a partial response. Only 2 of 12 patients experienced grade ≥2 acute GVHD, probably the consequence of withdrawing post transplant immunosuppression more gradually.

Bregni *et al.* (2002) reported their experience in 7 patients with metastatic RCC undergoing NST with a thiotepa based conditioning regimen (Table 120.2). This regimen was well tolerated and resulted in fairly rapid donor immune and hematopoetic engraftment without the occurrence of graft rejection. CSP withdrawal and/or DLI administration was followed by partial responses in 4 of 7 compatible with donor immune-mediated disease regression.

There now seems to be sufficient evidence to suggest that an alloimmune GVT effect can be induced against metastatic RCC. However, several problems still remain that limit the broader applicability of this procedure. First, less than a third of all patients with metastatic RCC can be expected to have an HLA-matched sibling. To address this limitation, several groups are currently investigating the safety and efficacy of HLA-matched unrelated donor NST in patients with metastatic RCC who lack sibling donors. Second, patients with rapidly progressive disease are unlikely to benefit from this intervention, as GVT effects typically do not occur until several months following transplant. These two issues were highlighted by Rini *et al.* (2002); 284 patients with metastatic RCC were screened over a 2-year period, 18 of whom were ultimately transplanted. A third important consideration in pursuing NST as a treatment option is the risk the procedure will lead to significant morbidity or result in transplant-related mortality. Although retrospective data suggest the risk of early TRM is less with reduced intensity conditioning, overall TRM remains around 5–20%, largely as a consequence of acute GVHD and/or infection related complications (Giralt *et al.*, 1997; Khouri *et al.*, 1998; Slavin *et al.*, 1998; Childs *et al.*, 2000; McSweeney, Niederwieser, & Shiruzu, 2001). In fact, 3 of the first 25 patients with RCC transplanted at the NIH died from GVHD-related causes. Treatment with drugs such as daclizumab and infliximab for steroid-refractory GVHD might ultimately decrease the incidence of GVHD-related TRM (Anderlini *et al.*, 2000; Przepiorka *et al.*, 2000), although the immunosuppressive effects of these agents could negate beneficial GVT effects. Careful patient selection, with particular attention to performance status and co-existing medical conditions may further improve transplant-related outcome. The importance of patient selection is highlighted in a recent study of NST in patients with a variety of treatment-refractory malignancies, including 8 patients with metastatic RCC (Pedrazzoli *et al.*, 2002). All six study patients with an ECOG performance sta-

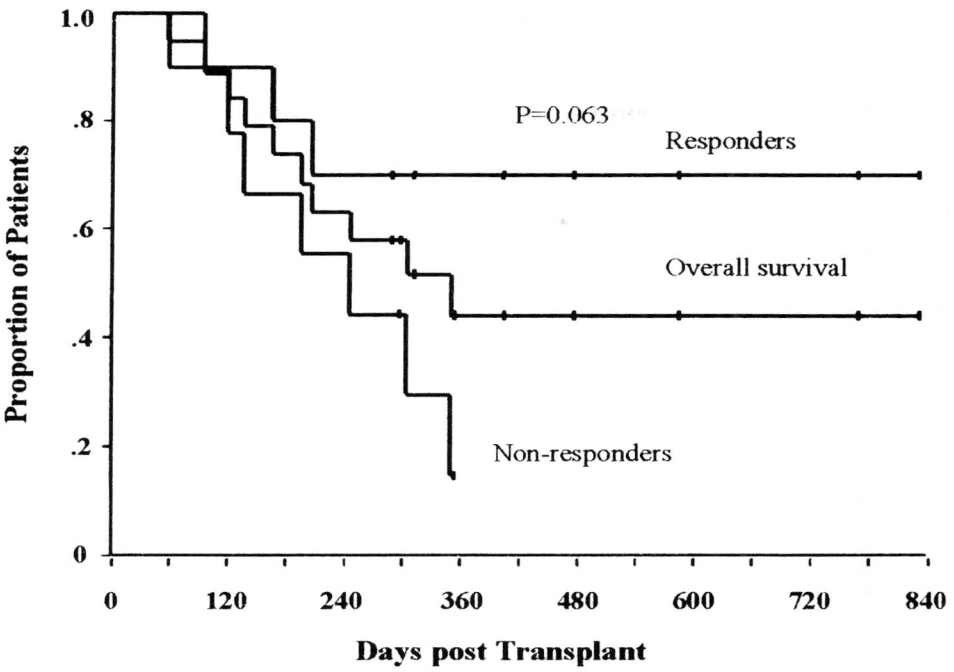

Fig. 120.3. Disease response and survival in patients with metastatic RCC undergoing NST. A Kaplan-Meier estimate of survival in the first 19 patients with metastatic RCC undergoing NST showed a trend towards a survival advantage among patients with a response.

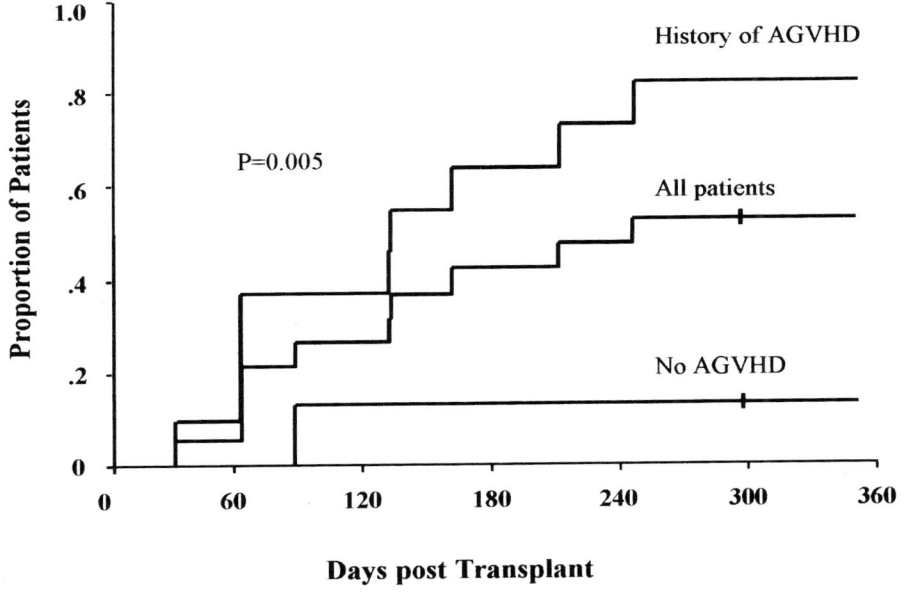

Days post Transplant

Figure 120.4. Association of disease response with acute GVHD in patients with metastatic RCC undergoing NST. A Kaplan-Meier estimate of the cumulative probability of response in the first 19 patients with metastatic RCC undergoing NST at The National Institutes of Health. Patients who had grade ? 2 acute GVHD had a higher probability of response (P = .005).

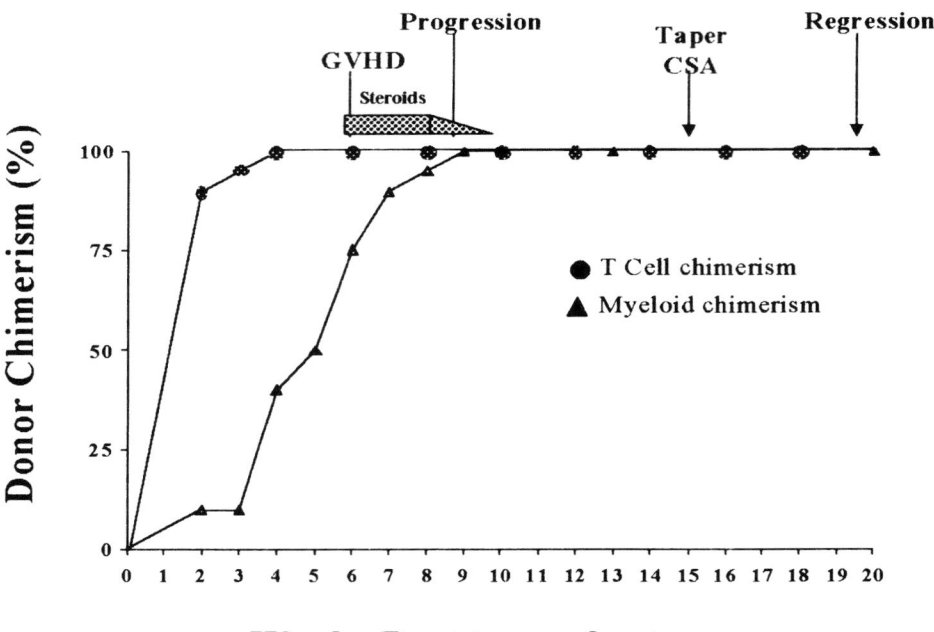

Fig. 120.5. Engraftment profile and clinical outcome in a RCC patient undergoing non-myeloablative transplantation. T-cell engraftment (circles), and myeloid engraftment (triangles), shown as percentage donor, were initially mixed, with donor T-cell engraftment preceding donor myeloid engraftment. Acute GVHD occurred early in the course of transplantation and resolved with oral corticosteroids. Initial disease progression was followed by disease regression at multiple metastatic sites once CSP was withdrawn.

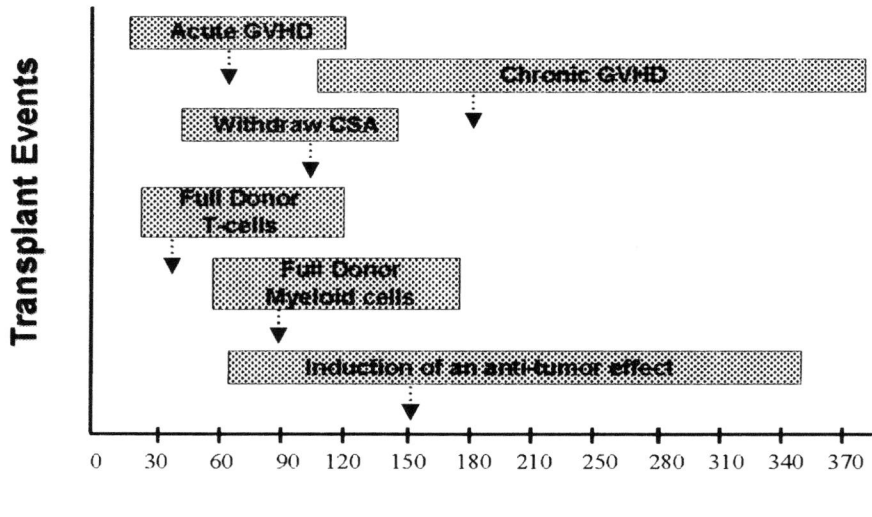

Fig. 120.6. Time course of events occurring in patients with metastatic RCC following NST using cyclophosphamide/fludarabine conditioning. Boxes show time range of events and arrows represent median time point of individual event occurrence.

Table 120.2. *Summary of clinical trials of NST in metastatic renal cell carcinoma*

Investigators	Conditioning agents	GVHD prophylaxis	Comment	Response	Median time to response	GVHD
Childs *et al.* (2000)	Cyclophosphamide 120 mg/kg Fludarabine 125mg/m^2	CSP	Decisions regarding CSP taper/DLI infusion based on T-cell chimerism MMF subsequently added to CSP, given high incidence of acute GVHD	Overall RR 53% (10/19) CR 16% (3/19) PR 37% (7/10)	5 months	Acute II–IV GVHD 53% (10/19) Chronic GVHD 21% (4/19)
Rini *et al.* (2002)	Cyclophosphamide 2 g/m^2 Fludarabine 90 mg/m^2	Tacrolimus and MMF	High incidence of graft rejection (3/4 patients treated) Cyclophosphamide subsequently increased to 4 g/m^2 Fludarabine increased to 150 mg/m^2 Response in renal primary observed	Overall RR 33% (4/12) All PRs	>100 days	Acute II–IV GVHD 17% (2/12) Chronic GVHD 50% (6/12)
Bregni *et al.* (2002)	Thiotepa 5 mg/kg Fludarabine 60 mg/m^2 Cyclophosphamide 60 mg/kg	CSP + methotrexate	Decisions regarding CSP tapering based on disease status Delayed disease regression observed in 4 of 7 treated RCC patients	Overall RR 57% (4/7)	>100 days	Acute II–IV GVHD 86% (6/7)
Pedrazzoli *et al.* (2002)	Cyclophosphamide 60 mg/kg Fludarabine 120 mg/m^2	CSP + methotrexate	8 of 8 RCC patients died by day 110 as a consequence of disease progression or TRM Poor PS and rapidly advancing disease may have contributed to poor patient outcome	Overall RR 0% (0/8)	NA	Acute GVHD-0% (0/7 evaluable) Chronic GVHD (0/1 evaluable)

Abbreviations: CSP, cyclosporine; DLI, donor lymphocyte infusion; MMF, mycophenolate mofetil; RR, response rate; CR, complete response; PR, partial response; PS, performance status; TRM, treatment related mortality; GVHD, graft-versus-host disease.

tus of 2–3 experienced severe transplant-related toxicities and succumbed to either transplant-related causes or rapidly progressive disease by day 100 posttransplant. In contrast, 11 patients with a performance status of ECOG 0–1 did relatively well, with only one death before day 100 attributable to transplant-related causes.

Allogeneic hematopoietic stem cell transplantation in melanoma

Malignant melanoma shares several biologic features with RCC that would lead one to speculate it too might make an attractive target for a GVT effect. However, the preliminary outcome of several groups investigating NST in this tumor has been surprisingly poor (unpublished data). We have transplanted 12 patients with metastatic melanoma with a fludarabine/cyclophosphamide based conditioning regimen. Five patients died as a result of rapid disease progression before day 100. Three partial responses were seen, 2 that occurred in the immediate posttransplant period (likely a chemotherapy effect), and 1 delayed

regression of metastatic disease (day +130) compatible with a GVT effect. Unfortunately disease regression was not durable with subsequent progression occurring within 1–3 months of the initial response. Median survival of the entire cohort was only 100 days with disease progression (typically rapid) being the major cause death. Similar poor outcome and short survival has been observed by other groups investigating NST in melanoma (personal communications—K. Bradstock, Sydney, Australia; D. Blaise, Marseille, France; D. Niederwieser, Leipzig, Germany). These data suggest that durable, clinically meaningful responses may be difficult to obtain in melanoma. The reasons accounting for a paucity of GVT effects against what is traditionally considered an "immunoresponsive" tumor remain unclear. It is reasonable to speculate that unfavorable tumor kinetics and extensive pretransplant disease probably contributed at least in part to these poor results. Although transient conditioning-related regression of metastatic melanoma may occur following NST, the likelihood of a clinically meaningful GVT effect appears low. The high risk of death from rapid disease progression discourages the present approach and highlights the need for alternative investigational immune based strategies for treatment-refractory melanoma.

Allogeneic hematopoietic stem cell transplantation in other solid tumors

The early favorable outcome of NST in RCC has emboldened investigators to extend this investigational approach to other types of solid tumors. However, only a handful of reports attesting to the efficacy of HSCT in tumors other than RCC exist. The limited experience with myeloablative allo-HSCT in breast cancer (Eibl *et al.*, 1996; Ueno *et al.*, 1998) has already been described. Bregni *et al.* (2002) have reported their experience in 6 patients with metastatic breast cancer undergoing a matched related nonmyeloablative transplant. Two of six patients in their series had a partial response, both approximately 7–8 months posttransplant. In both cases, responses followed DLI administration and GVHD consistent with a GVT effect. Another short case series reported the use of nonmyeloablative conditioning with cladribine/fludarabine in combination with busulfan and ATG prior to transplantation in seven patients with an assortment of metastatic solid tumors (Makimoto *et al.*, 2001). One patient with osteosarcoma was reported to have a partial response that was attributed to a GVT effect.

The outcome of five patients with chemotherapy-resistant metastatic ovarian cancer undergoing an allo-HSCT (Bay *et al.*, 2002) has been reported. One patient underwent a conventional "myeloablative" transplant from an HLA-matched sibling following conditioning with busulfan and cyclophosphamide. This patient experienced an early partial response, probably chemotherapy-related, which then progressed to complete response several months later in the context of ongoing chronic liver GVHD. The patient had a prolonged remission, relapsing 2 years posttransplant with slowly evolving disease. The four other patients in this series underwent nonmyeloablative conditioning with fludarabine, busulfan, and antithymocyte globulin (Slavin *et al.*, 1998). Three had a brief chemotherapy-induced partial remission in the first two months posttransplant, including one patient who was reported to have an ongoing PR 4 months following the procedure. Further follow-up and larger studies will be required to delineate whether clinically meaningful GVT effects can be induced against this malignancy. This case series highlights an important aspect of solid tumors, namely that responses to agents used in the conditioning regimen may occur even in tumors deemed "treatment-refractory." Therefore, in terms of etiology, disease regression seen in the immediate posttransplant period should be interpreted with caution. Tumor regression which occurs temporally removed from chemotherapy, in association with GVHD or following immunosuppression withdrawal is much more classic of a GVT effect.

To identify other solid tumors that might be susceptible to a GVT effect, we initiated studies of NST in a variety of different tumors using a conditioning regimen identical to that used in our RCC patients. Eligible patients are required to have incurable metastatic solid tumors that have progressed following treatment with all agents known to prolong survival. The initial phase of this study is intended to treat 10 patients each with a particular tumor type. Although these trials are ongoing, disease regression compatible with a GVT effect has been seen in one patient with pancreatic cancer and in one with metastatic colon cancer.

Immune mediators of graft-versus-malignancy effects

The mediators as well as the target antigens of the GVT effect remain incompletely characterized. Both CD4+ and CD8+ T-cells have been implicated as contributors to the anti-tumor effects seen following allogeneic stem cell transplantation for hematological malignancies (Truitt & Atasoylu, 1991; Faber *et al.*, 1992). While MHC class I restricted CD8+ T cells are believed to be the principal mediators of tumor lysis, reports of CD4+ T-cells that kill leukemia cells via HLA class II restricted molecules exist (Jiang & Barrett, 1995; Jiang *et al.*, 1996). NK cells have also been implicated in some studies as mediating both GVL and GVHD (Jiang *et al.*, 1997). A recent analysis in patients receiving haploidentical transplants with KIR ligand incompatibility has implicated donor NK cells as having activity against AML (Ruggeri *et al.*, 2001, 2002). Whether a similar beneficial NK cell effect could occur against some solid tumors is currently an area of investigation.

Tumor-associated antigens and minor histocompatibility antigens (both lineage-restricted and those with broad tissue distribution) have been postulated as targets for alloimmune reactions. Preliminary data from RCC patients responding after allogeneic transplantation suggests that the target antigens may differ in those who experience tumor regression in the context of GVHD as opposed to those without. T-cell clones that specifically lysed renal carcinoma cells or both renal carcinoma cells and patient hematopoetic cells were expanded from a patient who had a disease response in the absence of GVHD (Mena *et al.*, 2001). In contrast, we could only isolate T-cell clones that reacted against both tumor and hematopoetic cells from a patient who had disease regression that occurred in the setting of active GVHD. It is conceivable, therefore, that cellular immune responses directed against antigens shared by tumor and normal tissues could result in both GVHD as well as GVT, while GVT without GVHD might be expected to occur in those having a cellular immune response against tumor-restricted antigens. The identity of antigens serving as potential targets is an area of active enquiry, one that is likely to aid in the development of tumor targeted immunotherapeutic approaches.

Conclusions and future developments

These preliminary studies have provided proof of the principle that GVT effects can be induced against some solid tumors.

The clinical responses observed in RCC patients refractory to cytokine therapy highlights the power of the alloimmune response that occurs following allogeneic stem cell transplantation. Future investigations will focus on limiting toxicity related to the procedure, and directing the immune response specifically to the tumor. Such tumor-specific immune responses might be enhanced by vaccination strategies employing a variety of platforms. Ex vivo generation of tumor-reactive T cells followed by their adoptive transfer, or "targeted DLI" could also enhance antitumor responses without increasing the risk of GVHD. Immuno-modulatory cytokines such as GM-CSF (Schmid *et al.*, 1999), interferons and IL-2 may also be useful in the posttransplant period to enhance or expedite GVT effects. A major challenge will be the development of transplant strategies that obtain blockade of GVHD without compromising GVT effects. A better understanding of the mediators of GVHD and GVT and means for separating the two are needed to further advance this new and promising field of solid tumor immunotherapy.

References

Ada, G. (1999). The coming of age of tumour immunotherapy. *Immunology and Cell Biology*, **77**, 180–185.

Anderlini, P., Andersson, B., Champlin, R. *et al.* (1999). Infliximab for the treatment of graft-versus-host disease in allogeneic transplant recipients. *Proceedings of the American Society of Hematology*, **52a**, 200.

Apperley, J. E., Jones, L., Hale, G. *et al.* (1986). Bone marrow transplantation for patients with chronic myeloid leukemia: T cell depletion with Campath-1 reduces the incidence of graft-versus-host disease but may increase the risk of leukemic relapse. *Bone Marrow Transplantation*, **1**, 53–68.

Bay, J. O., Fleury, J., Choufi, B. *et al.* (2002). Allogeneic hematopoietic stem cell transplantation in ovarian carcinoma: results of five patients. *Bone Marrow Transplantation*, **30**, 95–102.

Boon, T., Coulie, P. G., & Van den Eynde, B. (1997). Tumor antigens recognized by T cells. *Immunology Today*, **18**, 267–268.

Bregni, M., Dodero, A., Peccatori, J. *et al.* (2002). Nonmyeloablative conditioning followed by hematopoietic cell allografting and donor lymphocyte infusions for patients with metastatic renal and breast cancer. *Blood*, **99**, 4234–6.

Childs, R., Chernoff, A., Contentin, N. *et al.* (2000). Regression of metastatic renal-cell carcinoma after nonmyeloablative allogeneic peripheral-blood stem-cell transplantation. *New England Journal of Medicine*, **343**, 750–8.

Childs, R., Clave, E., Contentin, N. *et al.* (1999). Engraftment kinetics after nonmyeloablative allogeneic peripheral blood stem cell transplantation: full donor T-cell chimerism preceded alloimmune responses. *Blood*, **94**, 3234–3241.

De Buerger, M., Bakker, A., Van Rood, J. J., Van der Woude, F., & Goulmy, E. (1992). Tissue distribution of minor histocompatibility antigens. *Journal of Immunology*, **149**, 1788–1794.

Eibl, B., Schwaighofer, H., Nachbaur, D. *et al.* (1996). Evidence of a graft-versus-tumor effect in a patient treated with marrow abla-tive chemotherapy and allogeneic bone marrow transplantation for breast cancer. *Blood*, **88**, 1501–1508.

Faber, L. M., Van Luxemburg-Heijs, S.A.P., Willemze, R. *et al.* (1992). Generation of leukemia-reactive cytotoxic T lymphocyte clones from the HLA-identical bone marrow donor of a patient with leukemia. *Journal of Experimental Medicine*, **176**, 1283–1289.

Fairlamb, D. J. (1981). Spontaneous regression of metastases of renal cancer: a report of two cases including the first recorded regression following irradiation of a dominant metastasis and review of the world literature. *Cancer*, **47**, 2102–6.

Figlin, R. A., Pierce, W. C., Kaboo, R. *et al.* (1997). Treatment of metastatic renal cell carcinoma with nephrectomy, interleukin-2 and cytokine-primed or CD8(+) selected tumor infiltrating lymphocytes from primary tumor. *Journal of Urology*, **158**, 740–745.

Gilboa, E., Nair, S. K., & Lyerly, H. K. (1998). Immunotherapy of cancer with dendritic-cell-based vaccines. *Cancer Immunology, Immunotherapy: CII*, **46**, 82–87.

Giralt, S., Estey, E., Albitar, M. *et al.* (1997). Engraftment of allogeneic hematopoietic progenitor cells with purine analog-containing chemotherapy: harnessing graft versus leukemia without myeloablative therapy. *Blood*, **89**, 4531–4536.

Goldman, J. M., Gale, R. P., Bortin, M. M. *et al.* (1988). Bone marrow transplantation for chronic myelogenous leukemia in chronic phase: increased risk of relapse associated with T-cell depletion. *Annals of Internal Medicine*, **108**, 806–814.

Goulmy, E. (1996). Human minor histocompatibility antigens. *Current Opinion in Immunology*, **8**, 75–81.

Heslop, H. E., Brenner, M. K., Rooney, C. M. *et al.* (1994). Donor T cells to treat EBV-associated lymphoma. *New England Journal of Medicine*, **331**, 679–680.

Horowitz, M., Gale, R. P., Sondel, P. *et al.* (1990). Graft-versus-leukemia reactions after bone marrow transplantation. *Blood*, **75**, 552–562.

Jiang, Y.-Z. & Barrett, A. J. (1995). Cellular and cytokine mediated effects of CD4-positive lymphocyte lines generated in vitro against chronic myelogenous leukemia. *Experimental Hematology*, **23**, 1167–1172.

Jiang, Y.-Z., Barrett, A. J., Goldman, J. M. *et al.* (1997). Association of natural killer cell immune recovery with a graft versus leukemia effect independent of graft versus host disease following allogeneic bone marrow transplantation. *Annals of Hematology*, **74**, 1–6.

Jiang, Y.-Z., Mavroudis, D., Dermime, S. *et al.* (1996). Alloreactive CD4+ T lymphocytes can exert cytotoxicity to chronic myeloid leukemia cells processing and presenting exogenous antigen. *British Journal of Haematology*, **93**, 606–612.

Jones, R. J., Ambinder, R. F., Piantadosi, S., & Santos, G. W. (1991). Evidence of a graft-versus lymphoma effect associated with allogeneic bone marrow transplantation. *Blood*, **77**, 649–53.

Khouri, I. F., Keating, M., Korbling, M. *et al.* (1998). Transplant-lite: Induction of graft versus malignancy using fludarabine-based nonablative chemotherapy and allogeneic blood progenitor-cell transplantation as treatment for lymphoid malignancies. *Journal of Clinical Oncology*, **16**, 2817–2824.

Kolb, H. J., Mittermueller, J., Clemm, C. *et al.* (1990). Donor leuko-cyte transfusions for treatment of recurrent chronic myelogenous leukemia in marrow transplant patients. *Blood,* **76,** 2462–2465.

Kolb, H.-J., Schattenberg, A., Goldman, J. M. *et al.* (1995). Graft-versus-leukemia effect of donor lymphocyte transfusions in mar-row grafted patients. *Blood,* **86,** 2041–2047.

Lokhorst, H. M., Schattenberg, A., Cornelissen, J. J., Thomas, L.L.M., & Verdonck, L. F. (1997). Donor leukocyte infusions are effective in relapsed multiple myeloma after allogeneic bone marrow transplantation. *Blood,* **90,** 4206–4211.

Makimoto, A., Mineishi, S., Tanosaki, R. *et al.* (2001). Nonmyeloablative stem cell transplantation (NST) for refractory solid tumors. *Proceedings of The American Society of Clinical Oncology,* **20,** 44.

Marmont, A. M., Horowitz, M. M., Gale, R. P. *et al.* (1991). T cell depletion of HLA_identical transplants in leukemia. *Blood,* **78,** 2120–2130.

McSweeney, P. A., Niederwieser, D., & Shiruzu, J. A. (2001). Hematopoietic cell transplantation in older patients with hemato-logic malignancies: replacing high-dose cytotoxic therapy with graft-versus-tumor effects. *Blood,* **97,** 3390–400.

Mehta, J., Powles, R., Singhal, S., Iveson, T., Treleaven, J., & Catovsky, D. (1996). Clinical and hematologic response of chronic lymphocytic and prolymphocytic leukemia persisting after allogeneic bone marrow transplantation with the onset of acute graft-versus-host disease: possible role of graft-versus-leukemia. *Bone Marrow Transplantation,* **17,** 371–375.

Mena, O., Igarashi, T., Srinivasan, R. *et al.* (2001). Immunologic mechanisms involved in the graft versus tumor effect in renal cell carcinoma (RCC) following nonmyeloablative allogeneic periph-eral blood stem cell transplantation. *Blood,* **98,** 356a.

Morecki, S., Moshel, Y., Gelfand, Y., Pugatsch, T., & Slavin, S. (1997). Induction of graft vs. tumor effect in a murine model of mammary carcinoma. *International Journal of Cancer,* **71,** 59–63.

Morecki, S., Yacovlev, E., Diab, A., & Slavin, S. (1998). Allogeneic cell therapy for murine mammary carcinoma. *Cancer Research,* **58,** 3891–3895.

Moscovitch, M. & Slavin, S. (1984). Antitumor effects of allogeneic bone marrow transplantation in (NZB X NZW) F1 hybrids with spontaneous lymphosarcoma. *Journal of Immunology,* **132,** 997–1003.

Motzer, R. J., Bander, N. H., & Nanus, D. M. (1996). Renal-cell car-cinoma. *New England Journal of Medicine,* **335,** 865–75.

Negrier, S., Escudier, B., Lasset, C. *et al.* (1998). Recombinant human interleukin-2, recombinant human interferon alfa 2a, or both in metastatic renal-cell carcinoma. *New England Journal of Medicine,* **338,** 1272–1278.

Papadopoulos, E. B., Ladanyi, M., Emanuel, D. *et al.* (1994). Infusions of donor leukocytes to treat EBV associated lympho-proliferative disorders after allogeneic bone marrow transplanta-tion. *New England Journal of Medicine,* **330,** 1185–1191.

Pedrazzoli, P., Da Prada, G. A., Giogiani, G. *et al.* (2002). Allogeneic blood stem cell transplantation after a reduced-inten-sity, preparative regimen: a pilot study in patients with refractory malignancies. *Cancer,* **94,** 2409–15.

Przepiorka, P., Kernan, N. A., Ippoliti, C. *et al.* (2000). Daclizumab, a humanized anti-interleukin-2 receptor alpha chain antibody, for treatment of acute graft-versus-host disease. *Blood,* **95,** 83–9.

Quesada, J. R., Swanson, D. A., & Trindade, A. (1983). Renal cell carcinoma: Anti-tumor effects of leukocyte interferon. *Cancer Research,* **43,** 940.

Rini, B. I., Zimmerman, T., Stadtler, W. M. *et al.* (2002). Allogeneic stem-cell transplantation of renal cell cancer after nonmyeloabla-tive chemotherapy: feasibility, engraftment, and clinical results. *Journal of Clinical Oncology,* **20,** 2017–24.

Rosenberg, S. A. (1999). A new era for cancer immunotherapy based on the genes that encode cancer antigens. *Immunity,* **10,** 281–287.

Rosenberg, S. A., Yang, J. C., Topalian, S. L. *et al.* (1994). Treatment of 283 consecutive patients with metastatic melanoma or renal cell carcinoma using high-dose bolus inter-leukin-2. *JAMA: The Journal of the American Medical Association,* **271,** 907–913.

Ruggeri, L., Capanni, M., Martelli, M. F., & Velardi, A. (2001). Cellular therapy: exploiting NK cell alloreactivity in transplanta-tion. *Current Opinion in Hematology,* **8,** 355–9.

Ruggeri, L., Capanni, M., Urbani, E. *et al.* (2002). Effectiveness of donor natural killer cell alloreactivity in mismatched hematopoi-etic transplants. *Science,* **295,** 2097–100.

Schmid, C., Lange, C., Salat, C. *et al.* (1999). Treatment of recurrent acute leukemia after marrow transplantation with donor cells and GM-CSF. *Proceedings of the American Society of Hematology,* **668a,** 2965.

Slavin, S., Nagler, A., Naparastak, E. *et al.* (1998). Nonmye-loablative stem cell transplantation and cell therapy as an alterna-tive to conventional bone marrow transplantation with lethal cytoreduction for the treatment of malignant and nonmalignant hematologic diseases. *Blood,* **91,** 756–63.

Stevens, E. J., Jacklin, L., Robbins, P. F. *et al.* (1995). Generation of tumor-specific CTLs from melanoma patients by using peripheral blood stimulated with allogeneic melanoma tumor cell lines. Fine specificity and MART-1 melanoma antigen recognition. *Journal of Immunology,* **154,** 762–771.

Thomas, E. D. & Blume, K. G. (1999). Historical markers in the development of allogeneic hematopoietic cell transplantation. *Biology of Blood and Marrow Transplantation,* **5,** 341–6.

Timmerman, J. M. & Levy, R. (1999). Dendritic cell vaccines for cancer immunotherapy. *Annual Review of Medicine,* **50,** 507–529.

Tricot, G., Vesole, D., Jagannath, S., Hilton, J., Munshi, N., & Barlogie, B. (1996). Graft-versus myeloma effect: proof of prin-ciple. *Blood,* **87,** 1196–8.

Truitt, R. L. & Atasoylu, A. A. (1991). Contribution of CD4+ and CD8+ T cells to graft versus host disease and graft versus leukemia reactivity after transplantation of MHC-compatible bone marrow. *Bone Marrow Transplantation,* **8,** 51–58.

Ueno, N. T., Rondon, G., Mirza, N. Q. *et al.* (1998). Allogeneic peripheral-blood progenitor-cell transplantation for poor-risk patients with metastatic breast cancer. *Journal of Clinical Oncology,* **16,** 986–93.

van Besien, K. W., de Lima, M., Giralt, S. A. *et al.* (1997). Management of lymphoma recurrence after allogeneic transplantation: the relevance of graft-versus-lymphoma effect. *Bone Marrow Transplantation,* **19,** 977–982.

van den Eynde, B. J., Gaugler, B., Probst-Kepper, M. *et al.* (1999). A new antigen recognized by cytolytic T lymphocytes on a human kidney tumor results from reverse strand transcription. *The Journal of Experimental Medicine,* **190,** 1793–800.

Verdonck, L., Lokhorst, H., Dekker, A. *et al.* (1996). Graft-versus-myeloma effect in 2 cases. *Lancet,* **347,** 800–801.

Warren, E. H., Greenberg, P. D., & Riddell, S. R. (1998). Cytotoxic T-lymphocyte–defined human minor histocompatibility antigens with a restricted tissue distribution. *Blood,* **91,** 2197–2207.

Weiden, P., Flournoy, N., Thomas, E. *et al.* (1979). Antileukemic effects of graft-versus-host disease in human recipients of allogeneic marrow grafts. *New England Journal of Medicine,* **300,** 1068–1073.

121 Hematopoietic stem cell transplantation for HIV infection

SAM MILLIKEN

St. Vincent's Hospital, Sydney, Australia

Introduction

Since the mid 1990s prognosis and survival from HIV infection has improved dramatically mainly due to the introduction of highly active anti-retroviral therapy (HAART). The introduction of new classes of anti-retroviral drugs used in combination has seen significant improvements in many patients' immune function, parallelled by marked reductions in the incidence of opportunistic infections (Flexner, 1998; Palella *et al.*, 1998). The incidence of non-Hodgkin's lymphoma (NHL), however, has not decreased nearly as dramatically. Most of the fall in incidence is accounted for by a dramatic drop in the incidence of primary central nervous system lymphoma (PCNSL), a disease associated with severe immunodeficiency and not systemic NHL, which may occur at more modest degrees of immunodeficiency (Grulich, 1999; Levine *et al.*, 2000). In the era of HAART, patients with NHL are presenting with a longer history of HIV infection and higher CD4+ cell counts than previously reported, and survival has also improved from a median of 6 to 20 months in one study of 145 patients (Besson *et al.*, 2001).

NHL is well established as an AIDS-defining condition with PCNSL reported with the initial descriptions of the syndrome in the early 1980s and systemic NHL becoming recognized by the Centers for Disease Control in 1987 (Centers for Disease Control, 1987). Early treatment results were poor with high levels of morbidity and mortality with standard forms of chemotherapy, leading investigators to focus on strategies to minimize toxicity (Kaplan *et al.*, 1997). However, HAART together with improvements in supportive care has led to better results with standard therapy and to more aggressive protocols of the treatment for AIDS-NHL (Tirelli *et al.*, 1999). The recognition in HIV-seronegative patients that high-dose chemotherapy and hematopoietic stem cell transplantation (HSCT) is the optimal treatment of relapsed aggressive NHL (Philip *et al.*, 1995), and may be appropriate for high-risk first remission patients (Haioun *et al.*, 2000), led to investigation of the feasibility of HSCT in HIV-seropositive patients with lymphoma. Other cancers where HSCT may be of benefit, such as Hodgkin's disease (HD) and testicular carcinoma, appear to have an increased incidence in HIV infection (Dal Maso, Serraino, & Franceschi, 2001), and there have been reports of acute leukemia and multiple myeloma (Monfardini *et al.*, 1989; Pulik *et al.*, 1998) in HIV-seropositive patients—all tumor types that may respond well to HSCT. Acute myeloid leukemia (AML) has a better prognosis when treated in selected HIV-seropositive patients and intensive remission-induction therapy can be given safely (Pulik *et al.*, 1998; Sutton *et al.*, 2001). Most cases of acute lymphoblastic leukemia are of Burkitt's type and probably represent advanced presentations of lymphoma (Geriniere *et al.*, 1994). These patients can be safely and successfully treated with intensive remission-induction protocols (Milpied *et al.*, 1988; Geriniere *et al.*, 1994; Greenberg & Droller, 1994). Solid organ transplantation has also been performed in an HIV-seropositive patient (Ragni *et al.*, 2000).

Early reports of syngeneic and allogeneic transplants to treat HIV infection were disappointing, with either poor results or excessive mortality. However, they did demonstrate that engraftment was possible in an HIV-seropositive patient (Holland *et al.*, 1989; Contu *et al.*, 1993). Improvements in the overall survival and well-being of persons living with HIV infection and AIDS (PLWHA), and scientific developments in our understanding and manipulation of stem cells has led to a resurgence of interest in HSCT, not only in the therapy of malignancy but also as a means of "delivering" genetically modified stem cells to PLWHA in an effort to treat their HIV infection.

HIV infection necessitates a number of special considerations if HSCT is to be undertaken, including issues related to collection and storage of stem cells, concomitant HAART and supportive therapy.

Treatment of HIV infection

Despite the major improvements in reduction of morbidity and mortality of HIV/AIDS brought about by HAART, problems with this therapy persist. HIV infection is not completely eradicated and perhaps all infected individuals will develop therapy-resistant virus with time (Natarajan *et al.*, 1999). HIV infection persists for life and individuals remain infective to others (Zhang et al., 1998). There may be significant toxic effects of therapy such as hyperlipidemia and lipodystrophy syndrome. Treatment is expensive and unavailable to the majority of PLWHA residing in the third world. Consequently research continues looking for more effective, less expensive therapy. Major new strategies in development have been in the area of vaccine development and gene transfer into stem cells, with the latter approach employing HSCT. Recent studies suggest that adult human stem cells are resistant to infection with HIV. This finding is fundamental to the development of treatment protocols involving HSCT.

Lymphocyte transfer

Early attempts to induce cell-mediated immune function against HIV by adoptive transfer of lymphocytes from HIV-seronegative syngeneic donors were unsuccessful. An NIH study (Lane et al., 1990) of 16 patients treated with either zidovudine or placebo were given peripheral blood lymphocyte infusions or bone marrow transplants with cells from HIV-seronegative identical twin donors. The procedure was well tolerated, but there was no significant clinical or immunological improvement. A later study in a single patient (Bex et al., 1994) used primed lymphocytes from an HIV-seronegative identical twin brother vaccinated with a recombinant vaccinia virus construct expressing gp160. There was a temporary increase in CD4+ and CD8+ cells with enhanced in vitro lymphoproliferation and cytotoxicity. However a 3-log increase in HIV viral load (VL) occurred, thought related to infection of passively transfused CD4+ cells and the use of only a single antiretroviral drug.

Allogeneic HSC transplantation

In the first case report of an elective allogeneic bone marrow transplant for a patient with lymphoma and HIV infection, the patient died from relapse of their lymphoma at 47 days posttransplant without any evidence for HIV infection on examination of post-mortem material (Holland et al., 1989). However it seems likely the virus would have re-emerged given subsequent cases have not demonstrated HIV eradication (Vilmer et al., 1987; Hassett et al., 1983; Bowden et al., 1990; Bardini et al., 1991; Giri, Vowels, & Zeigler, 1992; Torlontano et al., 1992; Contu et al., 1993) and more sensitive techniques for detecting low levels of HIV infection are now available.

Genetic manipulation

A number of researchers are investigating gene transfer into hematopoietic stem cells as a means of treating HIV infection and many of the necessary tools for such therapy are well developed. There are a number of limitations to HAART therapy, with many patients not achieving complete suppression of HIV viral load (VL), and all that do still harboring persistent

infection for life (Natarajan et al., 1999; Finzi et al., 1999) which may be transmissable (Zhang et al., 1998) and with an increasing risk over time of developing resistant and hence progressive infection (Loveday et al., 1999). Regimens may be complex with unpleasant effects not uncommon, making compliance difficult. Treatment is costly and not readily available on a global scale.

Two basic types of transgenes have been developed to suppress HIV infection or replication: RNA based suppressors such as antisense molecules and RNA homologues, and ribozymes (Levine et al., 2001). A number of protein structures have been identified for targeting HIV and a number of intracellular toxins designed for anti-HIV activity have been developed. Hematopoietic stem cells allow a self-renewing population for manipulation in this way to create HIV-resistant progeny and a reservoir of HIV-resistant cells. Persisting problems with these techniques are the inability to transduce a sufficiently large number of pluripotent stem cells, as most currently effective techniques cause these cells to commit to lineage and not persist, and loss of transgene activation with time. These problems continue to hamper clinical progress.

The City of Hope group treated 5 lymphoma patients with CD34+ cells transduced with a retrovirus encoding ribozymes targeted against the tat and rev genes of HIV, together with unmanipulated CD34+ cells (Levine et al., 2001). No improvement in immune function was demonstrable with the procedure appearing safe and without any long-term adverse effects. Gene marking demonstrated transduced cells persisted for up to 6 months posttransplant, then fell to minimal levels of detection at one year. The use of myeloablative conditioning in these patients was associated with a 10- to 50-fold increase in gene-marked cells compared to previously treated HIV patients without lymphoma (Zaia et al., 1999).

There has been a case report of an HIV-seropositive patient undergoing a genetically modified peripheral blood allogeneic stem cell transplant following non-myeloablative conditioning for secondary acute leukemia. Detectable transduced cells remained at low levels over 2 years of follow-up and the patient remained in remission. The impact of these cells is unknown, but likely did not contribute to the remission as HIV VL increased in the posttransplant period (Kang et al., 2002).

Treatment of malignancy

Autologous HSC transplantation

There have been two small pilot studies that have established the safety and utility of HSCT in AIDS-NHL patients (Table 121.1).

Gabarre et al. (2000) reported on 8 patients, 4 with NHL and 4 with HD, all with either primary refractory disease (2 patients) or in first (5 patients) or second relapse (1 patient). Three patients had conditioning with chemotherapy alone (protocol not specified) and 5 with chemotherapy plus total body

Table 121.1. *Results of studies investigating autologous HSCT for HIV lymphoma*

Study	Number (pts)	HAART (pts)	Conditioning	Engraftment (days) Granulocytes >0.5	Platelets >20	Results	Survival in CR	TRM
Gabarre et al., 2000	8 (4 NHL; 4HD)	7	5 chemo/TBI 3 chemo	12 (9–23)	12 (9–23)	5 CR 1 death, OI at 2 yrs 3 deaths, rel. 1–3 mo	18.5 mo median	0
Krishan et al., 2001 Levine et al., 2001	12 (10 NHL; 2 HD)	12	1 cyclo/TBI 11 CBV	10.5 (9–12)	10 (7–15)	9 CR (3 CCR) 2 deaths, rel. 4 mo	4–24 mo	1 (day 22)

Abbreviations: HSCT, hematopoietic stem cell transplantation; HIV, human immunodeficiency virus; pts, patients; HAART, highly active anti-retroviral therapy; CR, complete remission; TRM, transplant-related mortality; NHL, non Hodgkin's lymphoma; HD, Hodgkin's disease; chemo, chemotherapy; TBI, total body irradiation; CBV, cyclophosphamide, carmustine, etoposide; CCR, continuous complete remission; OI, opportunistic infection; rel, relapse.

irradiation (TBI). Five patients achieved a complete response with follow-up reported from four months to two years. One of these patients died at two years from opportunistic infection. Interestingly, this patient was the only one not to receive anti-retroviral therapy at transplantation. Three patients died from relapsed lymphoma between one and three months posttransplant. All of these 3 patients were assessed as having resistant disease prior to HSCT.

The City of Hope group (Krishnan et al., 2001) initially reported on 9 patients undergoing HSCT for AIDS-NHL and HD and subsequently gave an updated report on 12 patients (Levine et al., 2001). Ten patients with NHL and 2 patients with HD were conditioned using the CBV (cyclophosphamide, carmustine, etoposide) protocol (Philip et al., 1987), with one patient given cyclophosphamide and TBI. Nine patients had relapsed disease or only achieved partial remission and 3 patients were in first remission but with high-risk features defined by the International Prognostic Index (Shipp, 1994). Five patients were also part of a gene therapy trial and received genetically modified stem cells following an unmanipulated stem cell infusion. Nine of these 12 patients achieved CR (3 continuous CR) with follow-up between seven months and three years. Two patients died from lymphoma four months posttransplant. There was one treatment-related death due to cardiomyopathy and multi-organ failure in the oldest patient (69 years) in the study. All of the CR patients remained alive at the time of the report with a median survival of 18.5 months. The first 2 patients reported (Molina et al., 2000) continue in remission beyond two years.

In both of these studies stem cells were collected using granulocyte colony-stimulating factor (G-CSF) after conventional dose chemotherapy. The median dose of CD34+ cells/kg collected was 7.17×10^6 (Gabarre et al., 2000) and 10.9×10^6 (Krishnan et al., 2001; Levine et al., 2001). In both studies engraftment times were similar to that expected for an HIV-seronegative patient population. The median times for granulocyte counts to reach 0.5×10^9/l were 12 (9–23) and 10.5 (9–12)

days respectively. The number of days to platelet counts of 20×10^9/l were 12 (9–23) and 10 (7–15) respectively.

Posttransplant infections were not detailed in the report by Gabarre et al., with only one patient described dying of opportunistic infection, presumably AIDS-related, and in remission of lymphoma, 2 years after transplant. In the City of Hope study 6 pre-engraftment infections occurred in the first 9 patients. Four of these infections were proven due to bacteria. One of these was severe, causing culture-negative fever of unknown origin, hypotension and gastrointestinal bleeding, with the patient surviving after a period of intensive care. Post-engraftment opportunistic infections were seen in 3 patients and all responded to treatment. Two patients developed interstitial pneumonia 40 and 60 days posttransplant and there were 2 cases of lobar pneumonia in the second posttransplant year. All of these cases responded to therapy.

In both studies patients were started or maintained on HAART. Immune function was monitored by CD4+ lymphocyte count and HIV viral load. In the Gabarre study, CD4+ counts fell for 8 evaluable patients by 3 months. In 2 evaluable patients the drop in CD4+ cells had returned to pretransplant levels at 6 months and improved by one year. However, 3 patients were noted to have an increased HIV VL post HSCT and in 3 patients the VL was undetectable. In the City of Hope study 8 patients were evaluable, with the CD4+ count nadir at 4.5 months and recovery to pretransplant levels by 9 months. One patient with a very high pretransplant CD4+ count did not return to such a high level. VL was evaluable in 9 patients with 7 having a transient rise within the first 2 years posttransplant. The authors concluded these changes were predominantly due to non-adherence to HAART by 6 patients.

At St. Vincent's Hospital we have treated 2 patients with HSCT, one with AML and one with multiple myeloma. The AML patient declined HAART and it was discontinued in the other patient at the time of HSCT and recommenced after engraftment. In both patients engraftment was slow with neutrophils reaching 0.5×10^9/l taking 42 days for the AML patient and 40 days for the myeloma patient. Platelet recovery to $20 \times 10^9/l$ was 150 and 40 days respectively. The first patient had an episode of herpes retinitis that improved with acyclovir therapy. This patient commenced HAART and has had a significant improvement in immune function. Both patients remain alive with the AML patient in remission beyond 20 months. The myeloma patient relapsed at 11 months, but has remained well at 18 months in a partial remission on thalidomide. These slow engraftment rates contrast with the results seen in the above studies. In both patients blood counts have fully recovered since commencing HAART, implying that its use may be important in allowing stem cell recovery in the posttransplant period, perhaps by preventing HIV-related marrow suppression.

Syngeneic HSC transplantation

There have been case reports of successful syngeneic hematopoietic stem cell transplantation for HIV-NHL (Campbell *et al.,* 1999) and ALL (Turner *et al.,* 1992). A 33-year-old male with chemosensitive relapsed immunoblastic lymphoma was conditioned with CBV and given G-CSF mobilized peripheral blood stem cells from his twin. Engraftment was rapid with neutrophil count $>0.5 \times 10^9/l$ at day 9 and platelet count $>20 \times 10^9/l$ at day 10. Anti-retroviral therapy was continued through therapy except for a short period in the immediate posttransplant course. There were no major toxicities and he remained in CR at one year. $CD4^+$ cell count remained above pretransplant levels with undetectable VL till 13 months, when low level viremia was detected. A 26-year-old hemophiliac with ALL was transplanted from an identical twin who was also HIV-seropositive. The patient died 18 months posttransplant with isolated intracranial relapse.

The first 6 patients (ALL, AML, NHL, severe combined immunodeficiency [SCID] (two), severe aplastic anemia [SAA]) reported to the International Bone Marrow Transplant Registry treated by syngeneic transplants all died from progressive disease, 5 of them within 6 months (Campbell *et al.,* 1999).

Allogeneic HSC transplantation

There have only been a few reports of allogeneic transplantation in HIV-seropositive patients, with disappointing results (Hassett *et al.,* 1983; Vilmer *et al.,* 1987; Holland *et al.,* 1989; Bowden *et al.,* 1990; Bardini *et al.,* 1991; Giri, Vowels, & Zeigler, 1992; Torlontano *et al.,* 1992; Contu *et al.,* 1993). Generally patients engraft but develop opportunistic infection and die of HIV/AIDS or progressive malignancy. Vilmer *et al.* (1987) first reported on 2 patients who developed transfusion-related HIV infection 22 and 56 months after allogeneic transplantation for aplastic anemia, and a third patient who was HIV-seropositive at allogeneic transplantation for acute leukemia. This last patient had impaired engraftment attributed to the HIV infection. They treated these patients with donor lymphocyte infusions and low dose alpha-interferon. Immune function improved transiently, with HIV persisting in all follow-up blood samples. The second patient died 2 years after the diagnosis of AIDS from neurologic disease. The first case report of an elective allogeneic transplant in a patient with lymphoma known to be HIV-seropositive was reported in 1989. The patient died from relapsed lymphoma 47 days post marrow transplant, but without evidence of HIV disease as measured by viral culture and polymerase chain reaction for HIV-1 RNA on multiple tissues (Holland *et al.,* 1989).

Sora *et al.* (2002), reported a successful allogeneic peripheral blood stem cell transplant for AML in a 33-year-old woman with HIV and hepatitis C co-infection. HAART was commenced prior to transplant and engraftment was prompt and durable. Grade II acute GVHD was controlled with corticosteroids, and CMV prophylaxis was prolonged, with the patient remaining well and in remission with an improved $CD4^+$ cell count beyond three years.

Non-myeloablative allogeneic HSC transplantation

In recent years there has been increasing interest in the use of non-myeloablative allogeneic transplantation for hematological malignancy, particularly in poorer risk patients such as those greater than 50 years of age. HIV-seropositive patients might be considered another poor-risk group and considered for trials of such an approach. To date there has been a single report of 2 HIV-seropositive patients undergoing non-myeloablative allogeneic transplantation for hematological malignancy (Kang *et al.,* 2002). One patient was a 42-year-old with AML secondary to cytotoxic therapy of NHL and the other a 31-year-old with primary refractory Hodgkin's disease. Both were conditioned with cyclophosphamide 120 mg/kg, fludarabine 125 mg/m^2, and cyclosporine, and both received HAART. The patients were discharged at 9 and 11 days posttransplant respectively and engraftment was reported similar to that expected for HIV-seronegative patients. Both developed 100% donor chimerism by day 96 and achieved complete remission, with the Hodgkin's disease patient dying of relapse at one year. GVHD of the skin occurred beyond day 100, necessitating prednisone therapy and continued cyclosporine. Both regained $CD4^+$ cell counts to better than pretransplant levels and VL was controlled as long as the patients remained on HAART. CMV antigenemia occurred in both (who were given pre-emptive therapy) without the occurrence of clinical disease. Cerebral toxoplasmosis occurred in the Hodgkin's disease patient and responded to treatment. The secondary AML patient remained in remission beyond 2 years with ongoing limited chronic GVHD. This patient also received genetically modified cells with the percentage of these cells remaining low but still detectable at 2 years.

Procedural issues

Particular attention needs to be given to supportive therapy in this group of patients. As well as the standard infection prophylaxis given to HIV-seronegative patients, consideration needs to be given to issues of recognition and prompt treatment of opportunistic infection, management of antiretroviral therapy, and avoidance of drug-drug interactions (Sparano & Kalkut, 2001). The United States Public Health Service and the Infectious Diseases Society of America (1999) have established clear guidelines for infection prophylaxis in the HIV-seropositve population based on level of immunosuppression, incidence of infection, severity of disease, efficacy of intervention including impact on quality of life and drug toxicity and resistance risks.

Common opportunistic infections are *Pneumocystis carinii* pneumonia (PCP), *Toxoplasma gondii*, *Cryptococcus neoformans,* and atypical mycobacterial infections. These occur with high frequency when $CD4^+$ counts fall below 200 cells/µl for PCP and 100 cells/µl for the latter infections. Prophylaxis with cotrimoxazole is effective for PCP and *Toxoplasma* infections. Azole antifungal agents will protect against cryptococcal infection. These patients are also at increased risk for *Mycobacterium tuberculosis* and consideration should be given to pre-emptive therapy if there are any suspicious lesions on chest x-rays or skin testing is positive.

Anti-retroviral therapy

To date there have been only preliminary studies of the interaction of standard-dose chemotherapy and HAART. One randomized study demonstrated that didanosine used with chemotherapy was associated with reduced hematological toxicity (Sparano *et al.,* 1996). The AIDS Malignancy Consortium studied the HAART combination of stavudine, lamivudine, and indinavir with either low- or standard-dose CHOP and found no increase in toxic side effects (Straus *et al.,* 1998). Cyclophosphamide clearance was reduced by 50% compared to historical controls, with no difference in expected clearance of doxorubicin or indinavir. This reduction in cyclophosphamide clearance may influence results of high-dose therapy and deserves investigation in the HSCT setting. Zidovudine should be avoided because of its well-recognized hematological toxicity (Sparano & Kalkut, 2001). Given that HAART substantially reduces morbidity and mortality of AIDS complications and that pre-HAART studies of chemotherapy for HIV-related NHL demonstrated as many as 25% of complete remission patients dying of these complications, it is sensible to recommend HAART be given either during or after completion of chemotherapy. Those patients reported to date have not experience delayed engraftment. One non-randomized study has reported an improvement in median survival from 8.2 months to 17.8 months for patients with HIV-related NHL treated with conventional-dose therapy in the post-HAART era (Sparano *et al.,* 2000).

Collection, cryopreservation, and storage of stem cells

A number of reports have established that adequate numbers of peripheral blood stem cells can be mobilized from asympto-matic HIV-seropositive patients without lymphoma, and that $CD34^+$ Thy 1^+ cells collected demonstrate clonogenic potential (Junker *et al.,* 1996). Administration of G-CSF does not effect HIV viral load.

The majority of HSCT case reports have used G-CSF and chemotherapy for stem cell mobilization and have not reported any difficulty in stem cell collection or engraftment. In view of the report of transmission of hepatitis B in liquid nitrogen storage (Tedder *et al.,* 1995) it is important that cryopreserved stem cell collections be stored in dedicated freezers to minimize any potential risk of cross-infection. Collections may be adequately stored by direct immersion at $-130°$ to $-150°$ C in a dedicated freezer or maintained in the vapor phase of liquid nitrogen (Molina *et al.,* 2000).

Conclusions

The last decade has seen major advances in the management of HIV infection predominantly due to the development and application of HAART. Improved morbidity and mortality of HIV-seropositive patients has largely been due to a reduction in opportunistic infections, with malignancy, especially lymphoma, remaining a common problem. Early pre-HAART studies demonstrated that in selected patients, without severe immunosuppression, intensive therapy, including myeloablative regimens for transplantation, could be given with acceptable risk. More recent studies, although only with small patient numbers, have confirmed this finding, particularly for autologous transplantation. An added benefit of HAART may be to allow better protection against opportunistic infection and possibly improve engraftment times, thus providing an acceptable risk/benefit for intensive therapy and HSCT. HSCT also offers the potential to deliver effective gene therapy to treat HIV infection itself. Studies to date have demonstrated the safety and feasibility of these approaches but a great deal more work needs to be done to determine the effectiveness of such therapies, particularly in the setting of allogeneic transplantation.

References

Bardini, G., Re, M. C., Rosti, G. *et al.* (1991). HIV infection and bone marrow transplantation. *Lancet,* **337,** 1163–1164 (Letter; comment).

Besson, C., Goubar, A., Gabarre, J. *et al.* (2001). Changes in AIDS-related lymphoma since the era of highly active antiretroviral therapy. *Blood,* **98,** 2339–2344.

Bex, F., Hermans, P., Sprecher, S. *et al.* (1994). Syngeneic adoptive transfer of anti-human immunodeficiency virus-1 (HIV-1)–primed lymphocytes from a vaccinated HIV-seronegative individual to his HIV-1 infected identical twin. *Blood,* **84,** 3317–3326.

Bowden, R. A., Coombs, R. W., Nikora, B. H. *et al.* (1990). Progression of human immunodeficiency virus type-1 infection after allogeneic marrow transplantation. *The American Journal of Medicine,* **88,** 49–52.

Campbell, P., Iland, H., Gibson, J., & Joshua, D. (1999). Syngeneic stem cell transplantation for HIV-related lymphoma. *British Journal of Haematology, 105,* 795–798.

Centers for Disease Control (1987). Revision of the CDC surveillance case definition for acquired immunodeficiency syndrome. MMWR. *Morbidity and Mortality Weekly Report, 36,* (Suppl), 1S–15S.

Contu, L., LaNasa, G., Arras, M. *et al.* (1993). Allogeneic bone marrow transplantation combined with multiple anti-HIV treatment in a case of AIDS. *Bone Marrow Transplantation, 12,* 669–671.

Dal Maso, L., Serraino, D., & Franceschi, S. (2001). Epidemiology of HIV-associated malignancies. In *HIV and HTLV-1 Associated Malignancies,* ed. J. A. Sparano. Kluwer Academic Publishers, 1–18.

Finzi, D., Blankson, J., Siliciano, J. D. *et al.* (1999). Latent infection of CD4+ T cells provides a mechanism for lifelong persistance of HIV-1, even in patients on effective combination therapy. *Nature Medicine, 5,* 512–517.

Flexner, C. (1998). HIV protease inhibitors. *New England Journal of Medicine, 338,* 1281–1292.

Gabarre, J., Azar, N., Autran, B., Katlama, C., & Leblond, V. (2000). High-dose therapy and haematopoietic stem-cell transplantation for HIV-1 associated lymphoma. *Lancet, 355,* 1071–1072.

Gabarre, J., Leblond, V., Sutton, L. *et al.* (1996). Autologous bone marrow transplantation in relapsed HIV-related non-Hodgkin's lymphoma. *Bone Marrow Transplantation, 18,* 1195–1197.

Geriniere, L., Bastion, B., Dumontet, C. *et al.* (1994). Heterogeneity of acute lymphoblastic leukemia in HIV-seropositive patients. *Annals of Oncology, 5,* 437–440.

Giri, N., Vowels, M. R., & Zeigler, J. B. (1992). Failure of allogeneic bone marrow transplantation to benefit HIV infection. *Journal of Paediatrics and Child Health, 28,* 331–333.

Greenberg, A. L. & Droller, D. G. (1994). Successful treatment of a patient with seropositive human immunodeficiency virus with high risk Burkitt's leukemia. *Cancer, 74,* 1261–1264.

Grulich, A. E. (1999). AIDS-associated non-Hodgkin's lymphoma in the era of highly active antiretroviral therapy. *Journal of Acquired Immune Deficiency Syndromes, 21,* S27.

Haioun, C., Lepage, E., Gisselbrecht, C. *et al.* (2000). Survival benefit of high-dose therapy in poor-risk aggressive non-Hodgkin's lymphoma: final analysis of the prospective LNH87-2 protocol-a Groupe d'Etude des Lymphomes de I'Adulte Study. *Journal of Clinical Oncology, 18,* 3025–3030.

Hassett, J. M., Zaroulis, C. G., Greenberg, M. L. *et al.* (1983). Bone marrow transplantation in AIDS. *New England Journal of Medicine, 309,* 665 (Letter).

Holland, H. K., Saral, R., Rossi, J. J. *et al.* (1989). Allogeneic bone marrow transplantation, zidovudine and human immunodeficiency virus type 1 (HIV-1) infection. Studies in a patient with non-Hodgkin lymphoma. *Annals of Internal Medicine, 111,* 973–981.

Junker, U., Moon, J. J., Sniecinski, I., Zaia, J. A., Bohnlein, E., & Kaneshima, H. (1996). HIV status and function of G-CSF mobilized peripheral blood stem cells from asymptomatic HIV-1 infected individuals, implications for anti-HIV gene therapy. *Blood, 88,* 271a.

Kang, E., de Witte, M., Malech, H. *et al.* (2002). Nonmyeloablative conditioning followed by transplantation of genetically modified HLA-matched peripheral blood progenitor cells for hematologic malignancies in patients with acquired immunodeficiency syndrome. *Blood, 99,* 698–701.

Kaplan, L. D., Straus, D. J., Stellini, R. *et al.* (1997). Low-dose compared with standard dose m-BACOD chemotherapy for non-Hodgkin's lymphoma associated with human immunodeficiency virus infection. *New England Journal of Medicine, 336,* 1641–1648.

Krishnan, A., Molina, A., Zaia, J. *et al.* (2001). Autologous stem cell transplantation for HIV-associated lymphoma. *Blood, 98,* 3857–3859.

Lane, H. C., Zunich, K. M., Wilson, W. *et al.* (1990). Syngeneic bone marrow transplantation and adoptive transfer of peripheral blood lymphocytes combined with zidovudine in human immunodeficiency virus (HIV) infection. *Annals of Internal Medicine, 113,* 512–519.

Levine, A., Seneviratne, L., Espina, B. M. *et al.* (2000). Evolving characteristics of AIDS-related lymphoma. *Blood, 96,* 4084–4090.

Levine, A. M., Scadden, D. T., Zaia, J. A., & Krishnan, A. (2001). Hematologic aspects of HIV/AIDS. Hematology/the Education Program of the American Society of Hematology. American Society of Hematology. Education Program, 2001, 463–478.

Loveday, C., Devereux, H., Huckett, L., & Johnson, J. (1999). High prevalence of multiple drug resistance mutations in a UK HIV/AIDS patient population. *AIDS, 13,* 627–628.

Milpied, N., Bourhis, J. H., Garand, R., & Harousseau, J. L. (1988). B cell ALL in an anti-HIV positive patient: achievement of a complete response with aggressive chemotherapy. *British Journal of Haematology, 70,* 501–502.

Molina, A., Krishnan, A. Y., Nademanee, A. *et al.* (2000). High dose therapy and autologous stem cell transplantation for human immunodeficiency virus-associated non-Hodgkin lymphoma in the era of highly active antiretroviral therapy. *Cancer, 89,* 680–689.

Monfardini, S., Vaccher, E., Pizzocaro, G. *et al.* (1989). Unusual malignant tumours in 49 patients with HIV infection. *AIDS, 3,* 449–452.

Natarajan, V., Bosche, M., Metcalf, J. A. *et al.* (1999). HIV-1 replication in patients with undetectable plasma virus receiving HAART, highly active antiretroviral therapy. *Lancet, 353,* 119–120.

Palella, F. Jr., Delaney, K. M., Moorman, A. C. *et al.* (1998). Declining morbidity and mortality among patients with advanced human immunodeficiency virus infection. *New England Journal of Medicine, 338,* 853–860.

Philip, T., Armitage, O., Spitzer, G. *et al.* (1987). High dose therapy and autologous bone marrow transplantation after failure of conventional chemotherapy in adults with intermediate-grade non Hodgkin's lymphoma. *New England Journal of Medicine, 316,* 1493–1498.

Philip, T., Gugliermi, C., Hagenbeek, A. *et al.* (1995). Autologous bone marrow transplantation as compared with salvage chemotherapy in relapses of chemotherapy sensitive non-Hodgkin's lymphoma. *New England Journal of Medicine, 333,* 1540–1545.

Pulik, M., Genet, P., Jary, L., Lionnet, F., & Jondeau, K. (1998). Acute myeloid leukemias, multiple myelomas, and chronic leukemias in the setting of HIV infection. *AIDS Patient Care and STDs*, **12**, 913–919.

Ragni, M., Dodson, S. F., Hunt, S., Bontempo, F., & Fung, J. (2000). Liver transplantation in a hemophilia patient with acquired immunodeficiency syndrome. *Blood*, **94**, 1113–1114.

Shipp, M. A. (1994). Prognostic factors in aggressive non-Hodgkin's lymphoma: who has "high-risk" disease? *Blood*, **83**, 1165–1173.

Sora, F., Antinori, A., Piccirillo, N. *et al.* (2002). Highly active anti-retroviral therapy and allogeneic CD34(+) peripheral progenitor cells transplantation in an HIV/HCV coinfected patient with acute myeloid leukemia. *Experimental Hematology*, **30**, 279–284.

Sparano, J. A. & Kalkut, G. (2001). Special considerations regarding antiretroviral therapy and infection prophylaxis in the HIV-infected individual with cancer. In *HIV and HTLV-1 Associated Malignancies*, ed. J. A. Sparano, pp. 347–366. Boston Kluwer Academic Publishers.

Sparano, J. A., Tirelli, U. *et al.* (2000). Infusional cyclophosphamide, doxorubicin and etoposide in HIV-associated non-Hodgkin's lymphoma: a review of the Einstein, Aviano and ECOG experience in 182 patients. *Journal of Acquired Immune Deficiency Syndrome*, **23**, A12, (Abstract).

Sparano, J. A., Wiernik, P. H., Hu, X. *et al.* (1996). Pilot trial of infusional cyclophosphamide, doxorubicin and etoposide plus didanosine and filgrastim in patients with human immunodeficiency virus-associated non-Hodgkin's lymphoma. *Journal of Clinical Oncology*, **14**, 3026–3035.

Straus, D., Redden, D., Hamzeh, F. *et al.* (1998). Excessive toxicity is not seen with low-dose chemotherapy for HIV-associated non-Hodgin's lymphoma (HIV-NHL) in combination with highly active antiretroviral therapy (HAART). *Blood*, **92**, 624a.

Sutton, L., Guenel, P., Tanguy, M. L. *et al.* (2001). Acute myeloid leukemia in human immunodeficiency virus-infected adults: epidemiology, treatment feasibility and outcome. *British Journal of Haematology*, **12**, 900–908.

Tedder, R. S., Zuckerman, M. A., Goldstone, A. H. *et al.* (1995). Hepatitis B transmission from contaminated cryopreservation tank. *Lancet*, **346**, 137–140.

Tirelli, U., Spina, M., Gabarre, J. *et al.* (1999). Treatment of HIV-related non-Hodgkin's lymphoma adapted to prognostic factors. *Journal of Acquired Immune Deficiency Syndromes*, **21**, A32, (Abstract).

Torlontano, G., DiBartolomeo, P., DiGirolamo, G. *et al.* (1992). AIDS-related complex treated by antiviral drugs and allogeneic bone marrow transplantation following conditioning protocol with busulphan, cyclophosphamide and cyclosporin. *Haematologica*, **77**, 287–290.

Turner, M. L., Watson, H. G., Russell, L. *et al.* (1992). An HIV positive haemophiliac with acute lymphoblastic leukemia successfully treated with intensive chemotherapy and syngeneic bone marrow transplantation. *Bone Marrow Transplantation*, **9**, 387–389.

United States Public Health Service and the Infectious Diseases Society of America (USPHS/IDSA) (1999). Guidelines for the prevention of opportunistic infections in persons infected with human immunodeficiency virus. **48**, 1–82.

Vilmer, E., Rhodes-Feuillette, A., Rabian, C. *et al.* (1987). Clinical and immunological restoration in patients with AIDS after marrow transplantation, using lymphocyte transfusions from the marrow donor. *Transplantation*, **44**, 25–29.

Zaia, J. A., Rossi, J. J., Krishnan, A. *et al.* (1999). Autologous stem cell transplantation using retrovirus-transduced peripheral blood progenitor cells in HIV-infected persons: comparison of gene marking post-engraftment with and without myeloablative therapy. *Blood*, **94**, 642a.

Zhang, H., Dornadula, G., Beaumont, M. *et al.* (1998). Human immunodeficiency virus type 1 in the semen of men receiving highly active antiretroviral therapy. *New England Journal of Medicine*, **339**, 1803–1809.

122 Donor-specific infusion of hematopoietic cells for tolerance induction in solid organ transplantation

KIMBERLY L. GANDY

Duke University Medical Center, Durham, USA

Introduction

The use of hematopoietic stem cell (HSC) inocula in solid organ tolerance induction has a long history. The theoretical groundwork for this field was established in the 1950s in the laboratory of Sir Peter Medawar where it was determined that infusion of various donor-specific tissues under certain conditions in fetal and neonatal recipients led to donor-specific tolerance. Extrapolation of these findings to the clinical arena, however, has been limited. Infusion of hematopoietic cells from one individual to another has associated complications which have prevented widespread utilization of hematopoietic cell infusion in tolerance induction. Similarly, over the same period of time, advances in immunosuppressive pharmacology have resulted in high short-term graft survival rates. The resulting transplantation environment is that in which clinical improvement will necessarily be demonstrated by improvements in long-term graft survival or decreased toxicity profiles, making it more difficult to demonstrate benefits of novel therapeutic modalities. Even so, developments in the field of hematopoietic cell transplantation within the last several years may have altered clinical potential to the point that useful tolerance induction protocols through hematopoietic cell infusion may be on the horizon.

Laboratory models of hematopoeitic cell infusion and tolerance induction

The fundamental principles involved in tolerance induction with hematopoietic cell infusion were established in the 1950s. Medawar's group performed a series of experiments in which they unexpectedly found skin grafts could be accepted between genetically disparate twin cattle (Anderson *et al.*, 1951). The link to hematopoietic mosaicism was provided by H. P. Donald who recommended that the investigators consult the work of Owen. Owen had noted the high rate of hematopoietic mosaicism in adult cattle and proposed that it could be explained by the exchange of hematopoietic cells in utero (Owen, 1945) through vascular anastomoses in fused placentas previously documented by Lillie (Lillie, 1916). This fortuitous combination of experimentation, observation, and insight established the potential linkage between the exchange of hematopoietic cells and tolerance induction and provided the foundation for the decades of work to follow.

The team led by Medawar went on to perform a series of landmark studies in the 1950s. They determined that when donor-specific cells were injected into fetal or neonatal mice, the recipients were tolerant of subsequently placed donor-specific grafts (Billingham, Brent, & Medawar, 1953, 1956). These studies were extensively expanded in the ensuing years with marked success. Additional models of donor-specific tolerance after hematopoietic cell infusion have been developed in fetal (Hasek, 1953; Kline *et al.*, 1994; Yuh *et al.*, 1996), neonatal (Cannon & Longmire, 1952; Streilein & Klein, 1977; West, Morris, & Wood, 1994), and adult recipients (Lindsley *et al.*, 1955; Main & Prehn, 1955; Wilson, Dealy, & Sadowsky, 1959; Thomas *et al.*, 1969, 1983a and b; Monaco & Wood, 1970; Rapaport *et al.*, 1977; Slavin *et al.*, 1977; Myburgh *et al.*, 1980; Gratwohl, Forster, & Speck, 1982; Ildstad & Sachs, 1984; Nakamura *et al.*, 1986; Gammie *et al.*, 1996; Pearson *et al.*, 1996; Sykes, 1996; Tomita *et al.*, 1996). These studies have evaluated tolerance in a number of animal species including mouse, rat, chicken, rabbit, dog, and the nonhuman primate, further illustrating the enormous potential contained within this seemingly simple principle.

Though tolerance induction appeared to be more likely with the intensive conditioning regimens used immediately prior to standard HSC transplantation, the toxicity associated with these regimens precluded widespread use in clinical solid organ transplantation. Some regimens employed total lymphatic irradiation (TLI) as opposed to total body irradiation (TBI), as a means by which to ensure that hematopoietic tissue was shielded from the radiation dose. When mice were exposed to 3,400 rads TLI and given 10^7 semi-allogeneic whole bone marrow cells, 87.5% accepted donor-specific skin grafts at more than 250 days posttransplant. Such levels dropped to 53% in recipients of fully allogeneic marrow (Slavin *et al.*, 1977). A long series of studies has continued to pursue sublethal conditioning regimens. Some of the most promising of these results involve perioperative antithymocyte globulin (ATG), TBI 3 Gy,

1903

thymic irradiation 7 Gy, splenectomy, and donor-specific bone marrow infusion (Kawai *et al.,* 1995, 1999). In the first such study five of six monkeys so conditioned had long-term graft acceptance of donor-specific kidney grafts (Kimikawa *et al.,* 1997). Further analysis was impaired by technical complications related to transplantation. The success of these induction protocols must await further long-term analysis to answer several pertinent questions: does the thymic irradiation required in this protocol induce lymphoproliferative disease, one of the complications that precipitated the search for this sublethal induction protocol? Will the low levels of donor chimerism detected in these recipients remain stable over time? Will the low-level chimerism remain stable in the face of hematologic challenges to the recipient such as infection?

With continued improvements in solid organ graft survival, the search heightened for sublethal preconditioning regimens which would allow significant levels of donor-derived engraftment. Such a search was given direction by the findings that hematopoietic stem cells and multipotent progenitors could be mobilized into the peripheral blood by G-CSF treatment, and that infusion of large numbers of such mobilized cells could overcome the allogeneic transplantation barrier with lower levels of immunosuppression.

Experimental models in which hematopoietic chimerism has been of low levels or temporary in nature have resulted in unpredictable and often unstable "tolerance" induction. Experimental models in which hematopoietic reconstitution has been at high levels have resulted in sustained stable tolerance induction. For example, success utilizing the antilymphocyte serum (ALS) bone marrow protocol was never greater than 80% at 400 days in rabbits, mice, or dogs. In fact, in a study in which dogs were given ALS, varying dosages of cyclosporine (CSP) and 50 to 100 × 10^6 cells/kg from a bone marrow density gradient separation, survival at 6 months was never greater than 30% in any group studied (Hartner *et al.,* 1991). Conversely, recipients that received high dosages of irradiation and cellular preparations containing HSC (a regimen known to result in high levels of donor-derived hematopoietic reconstitution) invariably had graft survival rates of greater than 80% (Main & Prehn, 1955; Ildstad & Sachs, 1984; Ildstad *et al.,* 1985; Gandy & Weissman, 1998). As will be described below, these findings were extremely predictive of the results to come in the clinical arena.

Success and complications in solid organ transplantation

The current short-term success rates in solid organ transplantation are remarkable. The 1-year graft survival rates in kidney transplantation from cadaveric and living-related donors are 87.7% and 93.9%, respectively (Hariharan *et al.,* 2000). The 1-year graft survival rate in pancreatic transplantation is 75% (Sutherland, Gruessner, & Gores, 1995), while the 1-year patient survival rates for heart, lung, and liver transplantation are 83.5%, 74.1%, and 83% (Keck *et al.,* 1996), respectively (Fig. 122.1). Success in small bowel transplantation is more

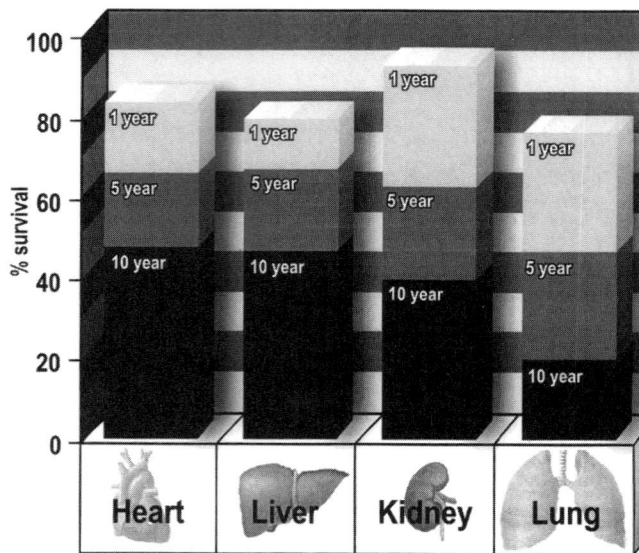

Fig. 121.1. Patient survival rates.

limited. Although 1-year graft survival rates are 60% (Grant, 1996), postoperative stay is long and complicated, and bowel function is slow to recover. The early success rates of all grafts, however, are somewhat misleading as long-term graft survival is much less favorable: the 10-year graft survival in kidney transplantation is 39% (Cecka & Terasaki, 1996), while the 10-year patient survival in heart transplantation is 37% (Keck *et al.,* 1996). Although early success rates are improving, long-term improvement is yet to be determined. Though recent reports suggest a trend in long-term graft survival in kidney transplantation (Hariharan *et al.,* 2000), such data is predominantly actuarial and long-term improvement is yet to be demonstrated. On a similar note, reports have suggested that the complication rates may be increased with the new immunosuppressive regimens which result in improved graft survival. There have been reports of isolated kidney and liver transplant recipients being withdrawn from immunosuppression with continued survival of their organ graft, but such reports are rare, and it has been difficult to predict which patients will tolerate such immunosuppressive withdrawal. Thus, donor-specific tolerance has yet to be reliably accomplished in the clinic.

As very few patients and/or experimental animal recipients can have all immune suppression withdrawn after current solid organ transplantation regimens, the majority of patients are subjected to the complications of long-term immunosuppression. The frequency of such complications is often underestimated. For example, infectious complications are still reported in 15%–44% of renal transplant recipients, though the severity of such infectious complications has declined in recent years with only a 5% resultant mortality rate (Sia, 1998). Infectious complications are linked to the degree of immunosuppression, with patients being treated for multiple rejection episodes and those undergoing more aggressive regimens at higher risk. Similarly, patients undergoing immunosuppression are at a significantly increased risk for other malignancies. Skin malignancies are the most common malignancy seen in patients after renal transplantation though posttransplant lymphoproliferative disorder (PTLD) is probably the most feared of the posttransplant malignancies. PTLD is seen in 1%–20% of solid organ transplant recipients and the incidence is 25- to 100-fold greater than that found in age-matched controls. Complications can be directly attributed to specific immunosuppressive agents. The complications associated with cyclosporine treatment include hepatotoxicity, nephrotoxicity, neurotoxicity, hypertension, gingival hypertrophy, and lymphoid malignancies (Bennett & Pulliam, 1983; Kahan et al., 1986). Long-term corticosteroid therapy can lead to a similarly long list: hypertension, diabetes, osteoporosis, aseptic necrosis of bone, and fluid retention (Newman, 1964; de Lange & Doorenbos, 1975). Newer agents such as tacrolimus (FK-506) may be more effective for prevention of rejection, though the toxicity profile may not be less. One of the founding principles behind the attempt to achieve tolerance induction is the hope of removal of such long-term immunosuppresion with resulting reduction in such toxicities.

Historical clinical experience with hematopoietic cell transplantation in solid organ transplantation

Clinical experience with HSC transplantation in solid organ transplantation has involved the use of whole bone marrow or T-cell–depleted whole bone marrow and dates back to 1976 (Monaco et al., 1976). Results of more recent studies will be discussed. For the most part, the approaches can be divided into two categories: those that administer donor-specific hematopoietic cells in regimens which result in low levels of donor-derived hematopoietic reconstitution and those which administer hematopoietic cells in regimens which result in high levels of donor-derived hematopoietic reconstitution.

A series of studies have involved protocols which resulted in low levels of donor-derived hematopoietic reconstitution. Several studies have been published from the University of Alabama at Birmingham that evaluated the use of cadaveric bone marrow for the induction of tolerance in kidney transplantation (Barber et al., 1989, 1991; McDaniel et al., 1994). These studies were modeled after the protocols pioneered by Monaco and Wood in rabbits (Monaco & Wood, 1970), mice (Monaco et al., 1971; Wood et al., 1971), and dogs (Caridis et al., 1973; Hartner et al., 1991) and subsequently extended to nonhuman primates by Thomas (Thomas et al., 1983, 1987, 1989, 1991a, 1991b). Recipients in these studies received antilymphocyte serum (ALS) or antilymphocyte globulin (ALG) and bone marrow transplantation in the period surrounding solid organ transplantation. In the first clinical study from this center (Barber et al., 1989), patients were given ALG for the first 10 to 14 days after renal transplant followed by the infusion of 2 to 3×10^8 nucleated bone marrow cells/kg on day 21 (or 7 days after ALG cessation). Additionally, patients received prednisone, azathioprine (AZA), cyclophosphamide, and cyclosporine (CSP) (Table 122.1). This study reported 11

acute rejection episodes in 9 patients within the first 3 to 6 months after transplant. The second study extended the scope and chronologic follow-up of these patients and reported a graft survival at 18 months of 85% versus 67% in control subjects that received the same immunosuppressive regimen without whole bone marrow infusion (Barber et al., 1991). This difference in graft survival was not statistically significant. In the last study the incidence of chronic rejection was assessed and was found not to differ from that found in control patients not receiving bone marrow infusion. However, when the presence of donor-derived cells was evaluated in the circulation, an interesting phenomenon was noted: 91% of recipients that had demonstrable donor-derived peripheral blood lymphocytes (PBL) were rejection-free at the end of the study, a percentage significantly higher than that found in comparative controls (14.3%) (McDaniel et al., 1994). Therefore, while none of these published studies demonstrated a significant improvement in acute or chronic rejection rates of the solid organ grafts with bone marrow infusion, they were able to lend further support to the finding that the presence of donor-derived cells in recipients of solid organ grafts correlated with high success rates of solid organ engraftment.

A similar protocol was used by Rolles et al. (1994) for liver transplantation. Patients received a 10-day course of ATG beginning on the day of liver transplantation followed 5 days later by the infusion of 2 to 3×10^8 cadaveric nucleated whole bone marrow cells/kg. Cyclosporine was begun on day 5 but no posttransplant AZA or prednisone was given. No donor-derived cells were detected in the blood at 6 months and no improvement in patient or graft survival was noted.

A large body of work from the University of Pittsburgh has further substantiated the idea that hematopoietic chimerism is instrumental in tolerance induction (reviewed in Starzl et al., 1993a, 1993b). This work focused on the recognition that hematopoietic cells from a variety of transplanted organs (liver, kidney, small bowel) seem to migrate from the transplanted organ into the tissues of the recipient and engraft (Starzl et al., 1992a, 1992b, 1992c, 1993; Demetris et al., 1993), with donor-derived cells being detected as late as 13 years after organ transplantation. Data from this group have again suggested that the presence of donor-derived cells has a strong correlation with tolerance of the solid organ graft. Indeed, in several patients in whom donor-derived hematopoietic cells were detected long after the transplant, the recipients could be removed from immunosuppression with no deleterious consequences to their grafts (Starzl et al., 1993). Using these data as a guide, the group embarked on a study attempting to augment the degree of donor-derived chimerism in solid organ recipients with perioperative bone marrow infusions (Fontes et al., 1994). Forty-four subjects were given a standard perioperative regimen of tacrolimus and prednisone. The eighteen experimental subjects received an additional 3×10^8 unmodified donor bone marrow cells/kg within 2 to 12 hours after revascularization of the transplanted organ. Although donor-derived cells were detected in the blood of all recipients in whom donor-derived

Table 122.1. *Outcome with current BMT regimens in solid organ transplantation*

Organ, Center, Date Reported	n Exp/Ctrl	Hematopoietic Inoculum and Day of Infusion	Barrier, Dose	Pre-conditioning	Post-solid organ transplant Immuno-suppression	Tolerance/ Rejection	Engraftment	Complications	Reference
Kidney, Birmingham, 1989	20/20	Cadaveric marrow, day 21	$2-3 \times 10^8$/kg		MALG 20 mg/kg × 14 days, AZA 25 mg day Prednisone 30→20 mg/day, 14 day course of cyclophosphamide after marrow infusion	Rejection at 3–6 months, 11 episodes in 9 exp patients; 17 in 12 controls	NA	No GVHD at 2 months	Barber et al., 1989
1991	57/54	Cadaveric marrow, day 14 or 21	$2-3 \times 10^8$/kg	None		87% grafts survival after 18 months vs. 67% in controls	NA	NA	Barber et al., 1991
1994	30/20	Cadaveric marrow, day 14 or 21	$2-3 \times 10^8$/kg			Incidence of chronic rejection unchanged	92% with peripheral chimerism rejection free at 18 months		McDaniel et al., 1994
Liver, Miami, 1994	9/16	Cadaveric marrow, day 15	$2-3 \times 10^8$/kg		ATG (2.5 mg/kg) × 10 days CSP 2.5 mg/day	89% at 6 months vs. 75% controls	None in PBL by FACS/PCR	GVHD in 5/9 exp subjects	Rolles et al., 1994
Kidney, liver, heart, pancreas, Pittsburgh, 1994	18/26	WBM, 2–12 hours postoperatively	3×10^8/kg	None	Tacrolimus Prednisone	50% between day 7 and 263, not different from controls		2/18 GVHD	Fontes et al., 1994
Lung, Pittsburgh, 2000	26/13	WBM, day 0	$3-6 \times 10^8$/kg	None	Tacrolimus Methylprednisolone Prednisone	None/Less BO at early time points (9% vs. 42%)	Minimal, <3% in all recipients at the highest point	No GVHD	Pham et al., 2000
Kidney, Brigham, 1991	2	BMT, −7 yrs, 3 yrs	HLA identical siblings	NA	NA	Off immuno-suppression	NA	Renal failure after BMT requiring kidney transplant	Sayegh et al., 1991
Kidney, Denmark, 1994	1	Non-T-cell depleted bone marrow, −1 year	HLA B/DR Mismatch	fractionated TBI Cyclophosphamide ATG	Prednisolone CSP Methotrexate	Off immuno-suppression after 4.5 years	100% in lymphoid and myeloid lineages	Transient oliguria	Jacobsen et al., 1994
Kidney, UCSF, 1995	1	T-cell depleted bone marrow	Haploidentical 0.3 × 10^8/kg	TBI 12 Gy ARA-c, ATG Cyclophosphamide	CSP Methylprednisolone/ Prednisone	All immunosuppression withdrawn at 1 year	All Donor	Renal failure after BMT requiring kidney transplant	Sorof et al., 1995
Lobar lung, Copenhagen, 1999	1	Maternal BM, several years	1 HLA-DR mismatch	Busulfan Cyclophosphamide ATG	Methylprednisolone/ Prednisone	Off immuno-suppression after 16 weeks	All Donor	None	Svendsen et al., 1999
Lobar Lung, Children's Hospital in Boston, 1998	1	Paternal BMT	NA	NA	NA	Off immuno-suppression	NA	NA	Lillehei et al., 1999
Kidney, Mass. General, 1999	1	WBM, day 0	HLA identical Sister, 2×10^8 WBM	Cyclophosphamide ATG, 700 cGy thymic irradiation	100 mg po CSP b.i.d., day 0–23	Off immuno-suppression after 147 days	Early engraftment, <1% donor T cells at 147 days	None	Spitzer et al., 1999

Abbreviations: MALG, Minnesota antilymphocyte globulin; AZA, azathioprine; GVHD, graft-versus-host disease; ATG, antithymocyte globulin; CSP, cyclosporines; PBL, peripheral blood lymphocytes; FACS, fluorescence activated cell sorter; PCR, polymerase chain reaction; WBM, whole bone marrow; BO, brionchiolitis obliterans; BMT, bone marrow transplantation; HLA, human leukocyte antigen; TBI, total body irradiation; ARA-c, cytosine arabinoside; BM, bone marrow.

cells could be monitored, 50% of the patients had episodes of rejection between postoperative days 7 and 263. The median time to first rejection, the rejection-free interval, and the cumulative incidence of rejection were not different between control and experimental individuals. Thus, while persistent donor-derived hematopoietic microchimerism was detected in these recipients, no improvement in overall clinical outcome was found. Two follow-up studies of these patients confirmed these findings (Rao *et al.*, 1997).

Results from a regimen utilized at the University of Miami, however, continue to suggest the potential for tolerance induction with hematopoietic cell infusion. Cadaveric renal transplantation was performed in 63 recipients with a perioperative infusion of 7.01 ($\pm$ 1.9) $\times 10^8$ nucleated cells/kg of donor-specific unmodified marrow. Controls were 219 cadaveric transplant recipients transplanted during the same time interval. Both groups were given OKT3, tacrolimus, mycophenolate mofetil, and methylprednisolone as pharmacological immunosuppresion (Ciancio, 2001). Though patient and graft survival appeared to be similar in the two groups, chronic rejection was detectably less in the group treated with bone marrow when compared to controls (5% vs. 16%) (Ciancio, 1999). It is of note, however, that most of these patients remained on immunosuppresion. Therefore, though these studies and others from the same group suggest that bone marrow may have an immunoregulatory role, they do not demonstrate true tolerance induction.

The most promising results originate from isolated case reports. There have been a number of case reports where kidney transplantation followed bone marrow transplantation (BMT) from the same donor: two in HLA-identical siblings (Sayegh *et al.*, 1991), one in an HLA-B/DR mismatch (Jacobsen *et al.*, 1994), and one in a haploidentical family member (Sorof *et al.*, 1995). In each of these cases, the recipients have permanently accepted their grafts and have eventually been withdrawn from all immunosuppression. It is of note that all of these patients received intensive preconditioning treatment prior to their BMT; these regimens included total body irradiation (TBI) and the patients were reconstituted predominantly with donor-derived cells at subsequent analysis. Additional cases have been reported by Heig *et al.* (1994), Butcher *et al.* (1999), and Spitzer *et al.* (1999). There have also been two case reports of living-related donor lobar lung transplantation following donor-specific bone marrow transplantation where tolerance to donor antigens was achieved (Lillehei, 1999; Svendsen, 1999). Additionally, a patient given a cadaveric liver transplant was subsequently given 4 × 2 Gy total lymphoid irradiation, 120 mg/kg cyclophoshamide, and 7.5 Gy total body irradiation prior to the intravenous infusion, 12 days after the liver transplant, of a T-cell–depleted combined autologous and cadaveric bone marrow transplant (Ringden, 2000). The donor differed from the recipient for 1 HLA antigen. Hematopoietic engraftment of both donor and recipient origin was prompt. Due to a reduction in donor T cells at one month posttransplant, an infusion of donor T cells was given and at 3 months posttransplant the recipient was a complete donor chimera. This patient was never withdrawn completely from immunosuppression, continuing on FK-506 and steriods postoperatively. Unfortunately, the patient died at 5 months posttransplant from *Aspergillus* pneumonia. It is difficult to determine if this individual would have been tolerant of his transplanted organ and/or the degree to which his immunocompetence would have been improved after transplantation. Therefore, to date, no clinical trials have demonstrated donor-specific tolerance after hematopoietic cell infusion and tolerance has only been demonstrated in isolated case reports.

The current clinical environment: specific considerations of hematopoietic reconstitution in the solid organ transplant recipient

The reported high short-term success in clinical solid organ transplantation constrains the parameters by which improvement can be demonstrated. With graft survival in living related donor (LRD) kidney transplantation in the 90% range at one year, it would take a large trial to demonstrate improved outcome within one year in kidney transplantation.

Cadaveric versus living donors

Cadaveric and living-related tissue sources can be utilized in solid organ transplantation. There is a reasonable amount of experience in living related kidney transplantation. Many donor nephrectomies are now performed laparoscopically, a process which seems to have increased the willingness of individuals to donate kidneys, though the potential clinical benefits are somewhat more difficult to prove. Living-related lobar transplantation is possible in lung and liver transplantation, Most protocols of lobar lung transplantation, however, require two lobar lung donors in order to achieve sufficient recipient lung parenchyma for functional recovery, a factor which obviously restricts the number of individuals eligible for the procedure, as well as complicating the issues regarding the source of the hematopoietic donor. Living related heart transplantation is not a part of the current clinical armamentarium.

There are potential benefits to living-related procedures in tolerance induction protocols. First of all, use of living-related donors allows for the identification of suitable donors with less genetic disparity, with an attendant reduction in GVHD induction potential. Similarly, use of living-related donors facilitates a system in which the hematopoietic cell infusion can be performed far in advance of the solid organ transplant. Hematopoietic engraftment and freedom from treatment-related toxicity can be established before the solid organ transplant is performed. Similarly, additional hematopoietic cell infusions can be performed if it appears that the individual is losing a first hematopoietic graft. Such repeated infusions are more difficult in cadaveric transplantation protocols, since the numbers of cells obtained from the vertebral marrow harvest are just in the realm of those needed for high-dose hematopoietic reconstitution.

Critical issues of HLA disparity in solid organ transplantation

HLA compatibility is critical in hematopoietic cell transplantation. HLA compatibility has a more controversial role in solid organ transplantation. Most solid organ donors continue to be cadaveric and ischemic time is critical. Historically, tissue typing has taken longer than 6 hours and it has not always been possible to obtain prospective tissue typing in solid organ transplantation such as heart transplantation when ischemic times are ideally limited to less than 6 hours. Currently, tissue typing techniques are available which will allow low resolution typing of MHC class I antigens within 6 hours, but high resolution typing of class I antigens may take longer and thus exceed the allotted timing for organ transplantation. Living-related organ donation would allow typing of such organ transplants to be performed prospectively, and living related donation has been performed for such organs as pancreas, small bowel (Fortner *et al.*, 1972; Deltz *et al.*, 1989; Morris *et al.*, 1995; Pollard *et al.*, 1996; Tesi *et al.*, 1996; Gruessner & Sharp, 1997), liver (Haberal *et al.*, 1992; Makuuchi *et al.*, 1992; Nagasue *et al.*, 1992; Broelsch & Lloyd, 1993), lung, and kidney. The frequency of LRD transplantation, however, in all but the latter types of transplantation is low. Therefore, the option of utilizing HLA typing for improvement in donor-recipient pairing is not always possible. In renal transplantation, where ischemic time is less critical, the significance of HLA compatibility remains controversial. Whereas some studies show an association of HLA match with graft outcome (Opelz, 1997), others do not (Ferguson, 1988; Matas *et al.*, 1990). Opelz (1997) published an analysis of the largest database available to date of unrelated living donor kidney transplantation and found a definite association between outcome and HLA class I (HLA-A and HLA-B) and class II (HLA-DR) compatibility. Although this finding is disputed by others, the possible importance of histocompatibility in solid organ grafting is overshadowed by the undisputed importance of HLA compatibility in HSC transplantation. As discussed, the likelihood of long-term tolerance induction is probably dependent on the success of the hematopoietic graft. Most solid organ transplants are performed in HLA disparate individuals. The relatively low success of HLA disparate grafts in HSC transplantation, therefore, poses a problem. Recent data, however, suggest that even high levels of HLA disparity may be crossed with appropriate preconditioning. The critical issues will be the degree of GVHD that is associated with crossing such barriers.

Sources of HSC

The implications of mobilized peripheral blood

HSC can also be harvested from mobilized peripheral blood. When living related donors are utilized, the situation will be relatively simple. Efforts should be made, however, to mobilize the stem cells at least 3 weeks prior to the solid organ donation in order to minimize the associated morbidity to the donor. The potential for mobilization of blood HSC in cadaveric donors will be important to evaluate, since it may increase the total number of HSC available for harvest. This scenario will be restricted, however. Firstly, there will be time constraints for mobilization; it will be a rare circumstance where the opportunity will be afforded to administer a 3- to 5-day course of granulocyte colony-stimulating factor (G-CSF) prior to cadaveric organ procurement. In this regard, it should be noted that some agents, for example, interleukin-8, mobilize HSC from the marrow into the blood within hours of administration. Secondly, the stressful situation of the death of the donor may have resulted in mobilization of HSC into the periphery prior to the declaration of brain death, and the kinetics of HSC mobilization may be significantly altered. It will also be necessary to evaluate the potential adverse effects of such mobilization on the immunogenicity of the harvested organ. Mobilization increases the efflux of mature T cells into the periphery. G-CSF has been shown to alter the function of T cells, with polarization toward a Th2 rather than a Th1 phenotype. It is likely that there will be an accumulation of T cells in prospective solid organs and that the resultant increase in the passenger leukocyte load of such tissues may have detrimental effects on graft outcome. All of these complex issues warrant further study.

Another source of HSC that should be a part of the clinical protocol is the recipient's own HSC, which can be collected in case there is a need for an autologous rescue transplant. Two to four weeks prior to the solid organ transplant, an effort should be made to harvest blood HSC from the recipient. Again, it is advisable that such a procedure be undertaken as soon as the critical condition of the recipient is identified, in order to reduce the risk of the recipient being thrombocytopenic at the time of solid organ transplant.

Continued importance of whole bone marrow

Until recently, the majority of hematopoietic cell inocula for clinical HSC transplantation was obtained from the marrow. Almost all such donors have been living donors, from whom the marrow was harvested in an operating suite. The common requirement for a cadaveric donor in solid organ transplantation results in marrow being harvested from the pelvis, ribs, and/or vertebral bodies of the prospective solid organ donor at the time of the solid organ harvest. This marrow source has been found to be more readily depleted of T cells (Lucas *et al.*, 1988) and, indeed, many of the clinical trials using HSC transplantation in solid organ transplantation have utilized this source of HSC. Additionally, several studies have suggested that hematopoietic cell infusion from whole bone marrow sources may have less potential for GVHD induction (Cutler, 2001).

Purified HSC infusion

The HSC has been well characterized in both the mouse and human (see Chapter 2). Such characterization potentially allows the infusion of purified populations of cells with reconstitution capacity without cell populations with GVHD-inducing potential. Studies in mice suggest that even the greatest degree of histocompatibility disparity can be crossed using purified HSC alone (Shizuru *et al.*, 1996; Gandy & Weissman, 1998; Uchida, 1998), although the number of cells required increases with the degree of histocompatibility disparity (Shizuru *et al.*, 1996). Studies in the mouse have also shown that this purified population does not induce graft-versus-host disease (GVHD) (Shizuru *et al.*, 1996) and that the numbers necessary for allogeneic reconstitution of at least three mice can be obtained from the long bones of a single donor. Similar extrapolations can be made in the human. Current technologies, which allow for the isolation of an HSC inoculum that is 4- to 5-log depleted of T cells, should allow high-dose HSC therapy to safely and effectively enter the clinical arena and enable an assessment of the dosage requirements for the engraftment of hematopoieic cells across allogeneic barriers to be made. Studies using bone marrow or blood stem cells selected (and thus purified) on the basis of cell surface expression of the CD34 antigen have evaluated their allogeneic engraftment potential in patients with a variety of hematologic diseases (see Chapter 27) and appear promising. Harvest of whole bone marrow from prospective cadaveric donors may make it possible to obtain enough purified HSC for reconstitution of at least up to three recipients and probably up to six if myeloablative preconditioning is utilized. Quantification of the number of purified HSC needed after sublethal or non-myeloablative conditioning regimens is forthcoming. The field of solid organ transplantation currently enjoys a fortunate vantage point: the results of these studies in HSC transplantation can be used in the future to tailor the selection of cellular isolates for use in solid organ transplantation.

Optimizing engraftment while avoiding GVHD: the role of facilitator cells and donor lymphocyte infusions (DLI) in HSC therapy for solid organ transplantation

The ability of populations of T cells and cells with T-cell-associated markers to enhance the engraftment of hematopoietic cells across allogeneic barriers has been recognized for several decades (Storb *et al.*, 1968; Deeg *et al.*, 1979; Ildstad *et al.*, 1986; Sykes, Sheard, & Sachs, 1988, 1989; Lapidot *et al.*, 1992; Martin, 1993; Kaufman *et al.*, 1994). Previous studies also evaluated the potential of cellular populations expressing the CD8+ cell surface marker to facilitate the engraftment of hematopoietic progenitors or purified HSC across allogeneic barriers (Kaufman *et al.*, 1994; Gandy & Weissman, 1996). When HSC transplantation is performed to treat leukemia or other hematologic malignancies, T cells are necessary to mediate facilitation of HSC engraftment and a graft-versus-leukemia effect, as well as to optimize recovery of immune competence. However, T cells also cause GVHD. The role of such cellular populations in solid organ transplantation, however, has yet to be determined. If only two elements, GVHD and engraftment, are considered,

the balance in solid organ transplantation might be shifted away from the use of facilitator cells.

Current protocols

The group at Massachusetts General Hospital has designed a protocol which addresses these issues by performing kidney transplantation in patients with concurrent renal failure and myeloma. One patient has been reported to date: a 55-year-old female with myeloma and resulting renal failure. An HLA-identical sibling was identified and the patient underwent a protocol consisting of cyclophosphamide 60 mg/m^2 on day −5 and −4; ATG 15 mg/kg on days −1, +1, +3 and +5; 700 cGy of thymic irradiation on day −1; and CSP 5 mg/kg on day −1 followed by 6 mg/kg b.i.d. thereafter. On day 0, the recipient received the kidney graft followed by the immediate infusion of 2.7 × 10^8 unmanipulated nucleated marrow cells/kg obtained form the iliac crests of the donor on the same day. The patient had an unremarkable post-procedure course except for a brief period of febrile neutropenia and recurrent episodes of atrial fibrillation and was discharged 23 days after the procedure. Cyclosporine was tapered and finally discontinued on day +73 posttransplant. Renal function remained normal at the time of the clinical report, 170 days post-procedure. It is of note, however, that the donor-derived hematopoietic reconstitution was again only transient. Though stable mixed hematopoietic chimerism was detected during the first nine weeks posttransplant, these values declined, first in the CD3+ fraction followed shortly thereafter by the CD3− fraction. Though two separate DLIs were given, the percentage of donor-derived cells in both the CD3+ and CD3− fraction was less than 1% by 147 days after the procedure.

Results of a different sublethal preconditioning protocol have been reported by Millan and Strober (Millan, 2002). Four patients were entered into a trial in which they were given CD34-enriched cells from mobilized peripheral blood after a preconditioning regimen utilizing TLI. All donor-recipient pairs were mismatched for at least one HLA antigen. Eight hundred cGy of TLI was administered in 80 cGy dosages on days 1–18 in two differing schedules. CD34-enriched cells were collected after leukapheresis by isolation on Isolex columns and 3–5 × 10^6 cells/kg were given after the last dose of TLI. ATG (1.5 mg/kg) was administered on days 1, 3, 5, 9, and 14 in three patients and on days 1 and 2 in one patient. Patients were placed on cyclosporine and prednisone after the hematopoietic cell infusion. Candidacy for withdrawal from immunosuppresion was defined as donor-specific unresponsiveness in MLR at monthly intervals after 7 months, and two graft biopsies without graft rejection. All immunosuppression was withdrawn from one patient at the end of 12 months and prednisone has been withdrawn from another at 8 months and candidacy for cyclosporine withdrawal was being further evaluated. One patient did not have immunosuppresion tapered due to anti-donor responsiveness in MLR and an early rejection episode. Three of the four patients had peripheral blood microchimerism ranging from 2%–18% though all patients had undetectable levels of donor-derived cells in the peripheral blood by 143 days after hematopoietic cell infusion. Importantly, none of the patients developed systemic viral or bacterial infections or GVHD during the period of evaluation. Though the results in the first patient are promising, the ultimate success of this protocol will have to be evaluated when more data are available in the other three patients, and when long-term follow-up data are available on the patient in whom immunosuppressive therapy has been withdrawn.

A protocol has been initiated at Duke University Medical Center in which high levels of donor-derived hematopoietic reconstitution is used to achieve tolerance induction. A sublethal preconditioning protocol has been used in the treatment of patients with hematological malignancies and hematopoietic failure, which results in greater than 80% donor-derived reconstitution in over 80% of recipients by 6 weeks. The preconditioning protocol consists of administration of fludarabine (30 mg/kg), cyclophosphamide (500 mg/kg), and Campath-1H over a 5 day period prior to the infusion of Campath-1H–treated hematopoietic cells. Six patients who have received this protocol have been given donor-specific skin grafts and each have accepted these grafts. Four have been withdrawn from all immunosuppresion with continued survival of the graft. These findings have been used to extend this protocol to tolerance induction for kidney transplantation. The clinical protocol involves patients with concurrent hematopoietic failure/malignancy and renal failure and proposes to give recipients of such hematopoietic grafts donor-specific kidney grafts. This protocol utilizes living-related donors for tissue transplantation and is based upon the establishment of hematopoietic engraftment prior to solid organ transplantation.

Immunocompetence: a critical issue

As clinical success in a field is realized, focus shifts. Now that full donor-derived reconstitution appears to be a realistic clinical expectation, concern is shifting to the immunocompetence of the resultant chimeras. The issue is critical and complex and can be analyzed from different vantage points: 1) comparison of immune competence to that of unmanipulated, healthy individuals; 2) comparison to individuals with similar disease processes undergoing other treatment regimens.

Studies from Zinkernagel's group in the 1980s demonstrated that mice reconstituted across allogeneic barriers were deficient in their responses to viral antigens (Zinkernagel et al., 1978, 1980, 1984). These and other similar studies provided the foundation of thought in the field that posited that immune competence of T cells in these animals was compromised because the T cells necessarily matured on thymic epithelium that was not histocompatible to that which would subsequently be used for antigen presentation. Other studies have presented seemingly conflicting data. Immune competence does seem to be eventually attained, though with delayed kinetics, in a series of animal models. In a large series of BMT studies in dogs, it was found that chimeric animals early posttransplant were deficient in many immunologic responses. However, at later time points,

these animals seemed to attain competence to respond to both T- and B-cell dependent antigens and to be capable of living in normal environments without an increased incidence of infection (Ochs et al., 1974). Kitagawa et al. (1993, 1994) performed studies of immunocompetence in chimeric mice and found that hematopoietic chimeras were able to respond normally to viral stimuli. Several factors may be important in understanding the observed differences between these studies. As noted by Ochs et al. (1974) large numbers of unmodified bone marrow cells were used for reconstitution in their study in dogs and the animals engrafted well. In the studies by Zinkernagel et al. (1978, 1980), engraftment was poor, as the survival rate was only 5% in the first group of animals studied.

The most relevant question is whether immunocompetence in optimally reconstituted recipients approaches a level that is clinically acceptable. Current solid organ transplant protocols still render recipients susceptible to infection.

The use of facilitator cells for potentially improving immunocompetence has been mentioned. Another area that has received renewed interest recently involves the common lymphoid progenitor. A population was identified in the human characterized by the phenotype $CD10^+$, $CD34^+$, Lin^-, $c-kit^-$, $Thy-1^-$ that gave rise to T, B, natural killer (NK), and lymphoid dendritic cells (Galy et al., 1995). The proliferative capacity, however, of this population was questionable, and as a result, clinical interest in utilizing this population for immune recovery waned. Recently, however, a common lymphoid progenitor has been identified in the mouse with marked proliferative capacity, stimulating renewed interest in the ability of these populations to confer immune competence in the peritransplant period (Kondo, Weissman, & Akashi, 1997). This population markedly enhanced the kinetics of lymphocyte recovery in congenic animals; the immunocompetence of this population in allogeneic reconstitution is yet to be demonstrated. This represents an important area in evaluating the potential of HSC therapy in solid organ transplantation.

Conclusions

Clinical protocols utilizing hematopoietic cell infusion for tolerance induction continue to remain elusive. Small steps, however, towards successful protocol development are being made. Current protocols necessarily require the cooperation of multidisciplinary teams. It is likely that the ideal protocol at a given institution will utilize the expertise at that institution resulting in an environment in which different protocols should be evaluated at different institutions. Indeed, it will most likely be from a coordinated evaluation of the successes and failures of these different protocols that the ideal protocol will be discovered.

References

Advisory Committee to the Renal Transplant Registry (1975). The Twelfth Report of the Human Transplant Registry. *Journal of the American Medical Association, **233**, 787–96.*

Anderson, A., Billingham, R., Lampkin, G., & Medawar, P. B. (1951). Use of skin grafting to distinguish between monozygotic and dizygotic twins in cattle. *Heredity*, **5**, 379–97.

Barber, W. H., Diethelm, A. G., Laskow, D. A. *et al.* (1989). Use of cryopreserved donor bone marrow in cadaver kidney allograft recipients. *Transplantation*, **47**, 66–71.

Barber, W. H., Mankin, J. A., Laskow, D. A. *et al.* (1991). Long-term results of a controlled prospective study with transfusion of donor-specific bone marrow in 57 cadaveric renal allograft recipients. *Transplantation*, **51**, 70–5.

Bennett, W. M. & Pulliam, J. P. (1983). Cyclosporine nephrotoxicity. *Annals of Internal Medicine*, **99**, 851–4.

Billingham, R., Brent, L., & Medawar, P. (1953). Actively acquired tolerance of foreign cells. *Nature*, **172**, 603–6.

Billingham, R. E., Brent, L., & Medawar, P. B. (1956). Quantitative studies on tissue transplantation immunity. III. Actively acquired tolerance. Philosophical Transactions of the Royal Society of London. *Biology*, **239**, 357.

Brent, L. A. (1997). *History of Transplantation Immunology*. San Diego, CA: Academic Press.

Broelsch, C. E. & Lloyd, D. M. (1993). Living related donors for liver transplants. *Advances in Surgery*, **26**, 209–31.

Burlinham, W. J., Grailer, A. P., Heisey, D. M. *et al.* (1998). The effect of tolerance to noninherited maternal HLA antigens on the survival of renal transplants from sibling donors. *New England Journal of Medicine*, **339**, 1657–64.

Butcher, J. A., Hariharan, S., Adams, M. B. *et al.* (1999). Renal transplantation for end-stage renal disease following bone marrow transplantation: a report of six cases, with and without immunosuppression. *Clinical Transplantation*, **13**, 330–5.

Cannon, J. & Longmire, W. (1952). Studies of successful skin homografts in the chicken. *Annals of Surgery*, **135**, 60–8.

Caridis, D. T., Liegeois, A., Barrett, I., & Monaco, A. P. (1973). Enhanced survival of canine renal allografts of ALS-treated dogs given bone marrow. *Transplantation Proceedings*, **5**, 671.

Cecka, J. M. & Terasaki, P. I. (1996). The UNOS Scientific Renal Transplant Registry. In *Clinical Transplants 1995*, eds. J. M. Cecka & P. I. Terasaki, pp. 1–18. Los Angeles, California: UCLA Tissue Typing Laboratory.

Ciancio, G., Garcia-Morales, R., Burke, G. W. *et al.*, (1999). Donor bone marrow, chimerism, histocompatibility and renal allograft rejection. *Transplantation Proceedings*, **31**, 679.

Ciancio G., Miller, J., Garcia-Morales, R. O. *et al.* (2001). Six-year clinical effect of donor bone marrow infusions in renal transplant patients. *Transplantation*, **71**, 827–35.

Cutler, C., Giri, S., Jeyapalan, S. *et al.* (2001). Acute and chronic graft-versus-host disease after allogeneic peripheral-blood stem-cell and bone marrow transplantation: a meta-analysis. *Journal of Clinical Oncology*, **19**, 3685–91.

de Lange, W. E. & Doorenbos, H. (1975). Corticotrophins and corticosteroids. In *Meyler's Side Effects of Drugs: A Survey of Unwanted Effects of Drugs Reported in 1972–1975*, ed. M.N.G. Dukes, pp. 812–40, vol. 8. Amsterdam: Excerpta Medica.

Deeg, H. J., Storb, R., Weiden, P. L. *et al.* (1979). Abrogation of resistance to and enhancement of DLA-nonidentical unrelated marrow grafts in lethally irradiated dogs by thoracic duct lymphocytes. *Blood*, **53**, 552–7.

Deltz, E., Schroeder, P., Gebhardt, H. *et al.* (1989). Successful clinical bowel transplantation: report of a case. *Clinical Transplantation*, **3**, 89.

Demetris, A. J., Murase, N., Fujisaki, S. *et al.* (1993). Hematolymphoid cell trafficking, microchimerism, and GVH reactions after liver, bone marrow, and heart transplantation. *Transplantation Proceedings*, **25**, 3337–44.

Ferguson, R. M. (1988). Treatment protocols: is there a role for tissue typing in renal transplantation? *Transplantation Proceedings*, **6**, 42–5.

Fontes, P., Rao, A. S., Demetris, A. J. *et al.* (1994). Bone marrow augmentation of donor-cell chimerism in kidney, liver, heart, and pancreas islet transplantation. *Lancet*, **344**, 151–5.

Fortner, J. G., Sichuk, G., Litwin, S. D., & Beattie, E. J., Jr. (1972). Immunological responses to an intestinal allograft with HLA-identical donor-recipient. *Transplantation*, **14**, 531–5.

Galy, A., Travis, M., Cen, D., & Chen, B. (1995). Human T, B, natural killer, and dendritic cells arise from a common bone marrow progenitor cell subset. *Immunity*, **3**, 459–73.

Gammie, J. S., Colson, Y. L., Griffith, B. P., & Pham, S. M. (1996). Chimerism and thoracic organ transplantation. *Seminars in Thoracic and Cardiovascular Surgery*, **8**, 149–55.

Gandy, K. L. & Weissman, I. L. (1996). Characterization of the CD8+ subpopulations of whole bone marrow that facilitate hematopoietic stem cell engraftment across allogeneic barriers. *Blood*, **88** (Suppl 1), 594a (Abstract).

Gandy, K. L. & Weissman, I. L. (1997). Characterization of the mechanism of CD8+ facilitation of HSC engraftment across allogeneic barriers. *Blood*, **90**, 253a(Abstract).

Gandy, K. L. & Weissman, I. L. (1998). Tolerance of allogeneic heart graft in mice simultaneously reconstituted with purified allogeneic hematopoietic stem cells. *Transplantation*, **65**, 295–304.

Grant, D. (1996). Current results of intestinal transplantation. *Lancet*, **347**, 1801–3.

Gratwohl, A., Forster, I., & Speck, B. (1982). Histoincompatible skin and marrow grafts in rabbits on cyclosporine-A. *Transplantation*, **4**, 361–4.

Gruessner, R.W.G. & Sharp, H. L. (1997). Living-related intestinal transplantation. *Transplantation*, **64**, 1605–7.

Haberal, M., Tokyay, H., Buyukpamukcu, N. *et al.* (1992). Living related and cadaver donor liver transplantation. *Transplantation Proceedings*, **24**, 1967–9.

Hariharan, S., Johnson, C. P., Bresnahan, B. A. *et al.* (2000). Improved graft survival after renal transplantation in the United States, 1988 to 1996. *New England Journal of Medicine*, **342**, 605–12.

Hartner, W. C., Markees, T. G., De Fazio, S. R. *et al.* (1991). The effect of antilymphocyte serum, fractionated donor bone marrow, and cyclosporine on renal allograft survival in mongrel dogs. *Transplantation*, **52**, 784–9.

Hasek, M. (1953). Parabiosis of birds during embryonic development. *Czechoslovakian Biology*, **2**, 265.

Helg, C. Chapuis, B., Bolle, J. F. *et al.* (1999). Renal transplantation without immunosuppression in a host with tolerance induced by allogeneic bone marrow transplantation. *Transplantation*, **58**, 1420–22.

Ildstad, S. T. & Sachs, D. H. (1984). Reconstitution with syngeneic plus allogeneic or xenogeneic bone marrow leads to specific acceptance of allografts or xenografts. *Nature*, **307**, 168–70.

Ildstad, S. T., Wren, S. M., Bluestone, J. A. *et al.* (1985). Characterization of mixed allogeneic chimeras: immunocompetence, in vitro reactivity, and genetic specificity of tolerance. *Journal of Experimental Medicine, 162,* 231–44.

Ildstad, S. T., Wren, S. M., Bluestone, J. A. *et al.* (1986). Effect of selective T cell depletion of host and/or donor bone marrow on lymphopoietic repopulation, tolerance, and graft-vs-host disease in mixed allogeneic chimeras (B10 + B10.D2→B10). *Journal of Immunology, 136,* 28–33.

Jacobsen, N., Taaning, E., Ladefoged, J. *et al.* (1994). Tolerance to an HLA-B, DR disparate kidney allograft after bone-marrow transplantation from the same donor. *Lancet, 343,* 800.

Kahan, B. D., Flechner, S. M., Lorber, M. I. *et al.* (1986). Complications of cyclosporine therapy. *World Journal of Surgery, 99,* 851–4.

Kapelushnik, J., Aker, M., Pugatsch, T. *et al.* (1998). Case report. Bone marrow transplantation from a cadaveric donor. *Bone Marrow Transplantation, 21,* 857–8.

Kaufman, C. L., Colson, Y. L., Wren, S. M. *et al.* (1994). Phenotypic characterization of a novel bone marrow-derived cell that facilitates engraftment of allogeneic bone marrow stem cells. *Blood, 84,* 2436–46.

Kawai, T., Cosimi, A. B., Colvin, R. B. *et al.* (1995). Mixed allogeneic chimerism and renal allograft tolerance in cynomolgus monkeys. *Transplantation, 59,* 256–62.

Kawai, T., Poncelet, A., Sachs *et al.* (1999). Long-term outcome and alloantibody production in a non-myeloablative regimen for induction of renal allograft tolerance. *Transplantation, 68,* 1767–75.

Keck, B. M., Bennett, L. E., Fiol, B. S. *et al.* (1995, 1996). Worldwide thoracic organ transplantation: a report from the UNOS/ISHLT International Registry for Thoracic Organ Transplantation. In *Clinical Transplants,* eds. M. J. Cecka & P. I. Terasaki, pp. 35–48.

Kimikawa, M., Kawai, T., Sachs, D. H. *et al.* (1997). Mixed chimerism and transplantation tolerance induced by a nonlethal preparative regimen in cynomolgus monkeys. *Transplantation Proceedings, 29,* 1218.

Kitagawa, M., Kamisaku, H., Aizawa, S., & Sado, T. (1994). Bone marrow transplantation from Fv-4–resistant donors rescues friend leukemia virus-infected mice from leukemia: a model of bone marrow transplantation therapy against retroviral infection. *Leukemia, 8,* 2200–6.

Kitagawa, M., Kamisaku, H., Sado, T., & Kasugo, T. (1993). Friend leukemia virus-induced leukemogenesis in fully H-2 incompatible C57B1/6→ C3H radiation bone marrow chimeras. *Leukemia, 7,* 1041–6.

Kline, G., Shen, Z., Mohiuddin, M. *et al.* (1994). Development of tolerance to experimental cardiac allografts in utero. *Annals of Thoracic Surgery, 57,* 72–5.

Kondo, M., Weissman, I. L., & Akashi, A. (1997). Identification of clonogenic common lymphoid progenitors in mouse bone marrow. *Cell, 91,* 661–72.

Lapidot, T., Faktorowich, T., Lubin, I., & Reisner, Y. (1992). Enhancement of T cell depleted bone marrow allografts in the absence of GVHD is mediated by CD8+CD4– and not by CD8–CD4+ thymocytes. *Blood, 80,* 2046–11.

Lillie, F. R. (1916). *Science, 43,* 611.

Lillehei, C. W., Mayer, J. E., Jr., Shamberger, R. C. *et al.* (1999). Pediatric lung transplantation and "lessons from Green Surgery." *Annals of Thoracic Surgery, 68,* (3 Suppl), 525–7.

Lindsley, D. L., Odell, T. T., & Tausche, F. G. (1955). Implantation of functional erythropoietic elements following total body irradiation. *Proceedings of the Society of Experimental Biology and Medicine, 90,* 512–15.

Lucas, P. J., Quinones, R. R., Moses, R. D. *et al.* (1988). Alternative donor sources in HLA-mismatched marrow transplantation: T cell depletion of surgically resected cadaveric marrow. *Bone Marrow Transplantation, 3,* 211–20.

Main, J. M. & Prehn, R. T. (1955). Successful skin homografts after the administration of high dosage X radiation and homologous bone marrow. *Journal of the National Cancer Institute, 15,* 1023–9.

Makuuchi, M., Kawarazaki, H., Iwanaka, T. *et al.* (1992). Living related liver transplantation. *Surgery Today, 22,* 297–300.

Martin, P. J. (1993). Donor CD8 cells prevent allogeneic marrow graft rejection in mice: potential implications for marrow transplantation in humans. *Journal of Experimental Medicine, 178,* 703–12.

Matas, A. J., Frey, D. J., Gillingham, K. J. *et al.* (1990). The impact of HLA matching on graft survival and on sensitization after a failed transplant: evidence that failure of poorly matched renal transplants does not result in increased sensitization. *Transplantation, 50,* 599–607.

Mathew, J. M. & Miller, J. (2001). Immunoregulatory role of chimerism in clinical organ transplantation. *Bone Marrow Transplantation, 28,* 115–20.

McDaniel, D. O., Naftilan, J., Hulvey, K. *et al.* (1994). Peripheral blood chimerism in renal allograft recipients transfused with donor bone marrow. *Transplantation, 57,* 852–6.

Millan, M. T., Shizuru, J. A., Hoffmann, P. *et al.* (2002). Mixed chimerism and immunosuppressive drug withdrawal after HLA-mismatched kidney and hematopoietic progenitor transplantation. *Transplantation, 73,* 1386–91.

Monaco, A. P., Clark, A. W., Wood, M. L. *et al.* (1976). Possible active enhancement of a human cadaver renal allograft with anti-lymphocyte serum (ALS) and donor bone marrow: case report of an initial attempt. *Surgery, 79,* 384–92.

Monaco, A. P., Gozzo, J. J., Wood, M. L., & Liegeois, A. (1971). Use of low doses of homozygous allogeneic bone marrow cells to induce tolerance with antilymphocyte serum (ALS): tolerance by intraorgan injection. *Transplantation Proceedings, 3,* 680–3.

Monaco, A. P. & Wood, M. L. (1970). Studies on heterologous ALS in mice: VII. optimal cellular antigen for induction of immunological tolerance with ALS. *Transplantation Proceedings, 2,* 489.

Morris, J. A., Johnson, D. L., Rimmer, J. A. *et al.* (1995). Identical-twin small-bowel transplant for desmoid tumor. *Lancet, 345,* 1577–8.

Myburgh, J. A., Smit, J. A., Browde, S., & Hill, R.R.H. (1980). Transplantation tolerance in primates following total lymphoid irradiation and allogeneic marrow injection. *Transplantation, 29,* 401–4.

Nagasue, N., Kohno, H., Matsuo, S. *et al.* (1992). Segmental (partial) liver transplantation from a living donor. *Transplantation Proceedings, 24,* 1958–9.

Nakamura, T., Good, R. A., Yasumizu, R. *et al.* (1986). Successful liver allografts in mice by combination with allogeneic bone marrow transplantation. *Proceedings of the National Academy of Sciences of the USA*, **83**, 4529–32.

Newman, S. (1964). Hormone induced diseases. In *Diseases of Medical Progress: A Contemporary Analysis of Illness Produced by Drugs and Other Therapeutic Procedures*, ed. R. H. Moser, pp. 190–232. Springfield, IL: Charles C Thomas.

Ochs, H. D., Storb, R., Thomas, E. D. *et al.* (1974). Immunologic reactivity in canine marrow graft recipients. *Journal of Immunology*, **113**, 1039–57.

Opelz, G. (1997). Impact of HLA compatibility on survival of kidney transplants from unrelated live donors. *Transplantation*, **64**, 1473–5.

Owen, R. (1945). Immunogenetic consequences of vascular anastomoses between bovine twins. *Science*, **102**, 400–1.

Pearson, T. C., Alexander, D. Z., Hendrix, R. *et al.* (1996). CTLA4-Ig plus bone marrow induces long term allograft survival and donor specific unresponsiveness in the murine model. Evidence for hematopoietic chimerism. *Transplantation*, **61**, 997–1004.

Pham, S. M., Rao, A. S., Zeevi, A. *et al.* (2000). Effects of donor bone marrow infusion in clinical lung transplantation. *Annals of Thoracic Surgery*, **69**, 345–50.

Pollard, S. G., Lodge, P., Selvakumar, S. *et al.* (1996). Living related small bowel transplantation: the first United Kingdom case. *Transplantation Proceedings*, **28**, 2733.

Rao, A. S., Fontes, P., Lyengar, A. *et al.* (1997). Augmentation of chimerism with perioperative donor bone marrow infusion in organ transplant recipients: a 44 month follow-up. *Transplantation Proceedings*, **29**, 1184–5.

Rapaport, F. T., Bachvaroff, R. J., Watanabe, K. *et al.* (1977). Immunologic tolerance: irradiation and bone marrow transplantation in induction of canine allogeneic unresponsiveness. *Transplantation Proceedings*, **9**, 891–4.

Ringden, O., Duraj, F., Elmhorn-Rosenborg, A. *et al.* (2000). Transplantation of autologous and allogeneic bone marrow with liver from a cadaveric donor for primary liver cancer. *Transplantation*, **69**, 2043–8.

Rolles, K., Burroughs, A. K., Davidson, B. R. *et al.* (1994). Donor-specific bone marrow infusion after orthotopic liver transplantation. *Lancet*, **343**, 263–5.

Sayegh, M. H., Fine, N. A., Smith, J. L. *et al.* (1991). Immunological tolerance to renal grafts after bone marrow transplants from the same donors. *Annals of Internal Medicine*, **114**, 954.

Shizuru, J. A., Jerabek, L., Edwards, C. T., & Weissman, I. L. (1996). Transplantation of purified hematopoietic stem cells: requirements for overcoming the barriers of allogeneic engraftment. *Biology of Blood and Marrow Transplantation*, **2**, 3–14.

Slavin, S., Strober, S., Fuks, Z., & Kaplan, H. S. (1977). Induction of specific tissue transplantation tolerance using fractionated total lymphoid irradiation in adult mice: long-term survival of allogeneic bone marrow and skin grafts. *The Journal of Experimental Medicine*, **146**, 34–48.

Söderdahl, G., Tammik, C., Remberger, M., & Ringdén, O. (1998). Cadaveric bone marrow and spleen cells for transplantation. *Bone Marrow Transplantation*, **21**, 79–84.

Sorof, J. M., Koerper, M. A., Portale, A. A. *et al.* (1995). Renal transplantation without chronic immunosuppression after T cell-depleted HLA-mismatched bone marrow transplantation. *Transplantation*, **59**, 1633–5.

Spitzer, T., Delmonico, F., Tolkoff-Rubin, N. *et al.* (1999). Combined histocompatibility leukocyte antigen matched donor bone marrow and renal transplant for multiple myeloma with end stage renal disease; the induction of allograft tolerance through mixed lymphohematopoietic chimerism. *Transplantation*, **68**, 480–4.

Starzl, T. E., Demetris, A. J., & Murase, N. (1992a). Cell migration, chimerism, and graft acceptance. *Lancet*, **339**, 1579–82.

Starzl, T. E., Demetris, A. J., Trucco, M. *et al.* (1992b). Systemic chimerism in human female recipients of male livers. *Lancet*, **340**, 876–7.

Starzl, T. E., Demetris, A. J., Trucco, M. *et al.* (1992c). Chimerism after liver transplantation for type IV glycogen storage disease and type 1 Gaucher's disease. *New England Journal of Medicine*, **348**, 745–9.

Starzl, T. E., Demetris, A. J., Trucco, M. *et al.* (1993a). Cell migration and chimerism after whole-organ transplantation: the bases of graft acceptance. *Hepatology*, **17**, 1127–52.

Starzl, T. E., Demetris, A. J., Trucco, M. *et al.* (1993b). Chimerism and donor-specific nonreactivity 27 to 29 years after kidney allotransplantation. *Transplantation*, **55**, 1272–7.

Storb, R., Epstein, R. B., Bryant, J. *et al.* (1968). Marrow grafts by combined marrow and leukocyte infusions in unrelated dogs selected by histocompatibility typing. *Transplantation*, **6**, 587–93.

Streilein, J. & Klein, J. (1977). Neonatal tolerance induction across regions of H-2 complex. *Journal of Immunology*, **119**, 2147–50.

Sutherland, D., Gruessner, R., & Gores, P. (1995). Pancreas and islet cell transplantation. In *Transplantation Immunology*, ed. F. H. Bach & H. Auchincloss, Jr., pp. 147–60. New York: Wiley-Liss.

Svendsen, U. G., Aggestrup, S., Heilmann, C. *et al.* (1999). Transplantation of a lobe of lung from mother to child following previous transplantation with maternal bone marrow. *Journal of Heart and Lung Transplantation*, **18**, 388–90.

Sykes, M. (1996). Hematopoietic cell transplantation for the induction of allo- and xenotolerance. *Clinical Transplantation*, **10**, 357–63.

Sykes, M., Chester, C. H., Sundt, T. M. *et al.* (1989). Effects of T cell depletion in radiation bone marrow chimeras. III. Characterization of allogeneic bone marrow cell populations that increase allogeneic chimerism independently of graft-vs-host disease in mixed marrow recipients. *Journal of Immunology*, **143**, 3503–11.

Sykes, M., Sheard, M., & Sachs, D. H. (1988). Effects of T cell depletion in radiation bone marrow chimeras. I. Evidence for a donor cell population which increases allogeneic chimerism but which lacks the potential to produce GVHD. *Journal of Immunology*, **141**, 2282–8.

Tesi, R., Beck, R., Lambiase, L. *et al.* (1996). Living related small bowel transplantation: donor evaluation and outcome. *Proceedings of the XVI International Congress of the Transplantation Society*, **22**, 40 (Abstract).

Thomas, E. D., Storb, R., Epstein, R. B., & Rudolph, R. H. (1969). Symposium on bone marrow transplantation: experimental aspects in canines. *Transplantation Proceedings*, **1**, 31–3.

Thomas, F. T., Carver, F. M., Foil, M. B. *et al.* (1983a). Long-term incompatible kidney survival in outbred higher primates without chronic immunosuppression. *Annals of Surgery,* **198,** 370–8.

Thomas, J. M., Carver, M., Cunningham, P. *et al.* (1987). Promotion of incompatible allograft acceptance in rhesus monkeys given posttransplant antithymocyte globulin and donor bone marrow: I. In vivo parameters and immunohistologic evidence suggesting microchimerism. *Transplantation,* **47,** 209–15.

Thomas, J. M., Carver, M., Cunningham, P. *et al.* (1989). Promotion of incompatible allograft acceptance in rhesus monkeys given posttransplant antithymocyte globulin and donor bone marrow: II. Effects of adjuvant immunosuppressive drugs. *Transplantation,* **47,** 209.

Thomas, J., Carver, M., Cunningham, P. *et al.* (1991a). The effect of antilymphocyte serum, fractionated donor bone marrow, and cyclosporine on renal allograft survival in mongrel dogs. *Transplantation,* **52,** 784–9.

Thomas, J. M., Carver, F. M., Cunningham, P.R.G. *et al.* (1991b). Kidney allograft tolerance in primates without chronic immunosuppression—the role of veto cells. *Transplantation,* **51,** 198–207.

Thomas, J. M., Carver, F. M., Foil, M. B. *et al.* (1983b). Renal allograft tolerance induced with ATG and donor bone marrow in outbred rhesus monkeys. *Transplantation,* **36,** 104–6.

Tomita, Y., Sachs, D. H., Khan, A., & Sykes, M. (1996). Additional monoclonal antibody (mAB) injections can replace thymic irradiation to allow induction of mixed chimerism and tolerance in mice receiving bone marrow transplantation after conditioning with anti T cell mABs and 3-Gy whole body irradiation. *Transplantation,* **61,** 469–77.

Uchida, N. (1998). High doses of purified stem cells cause early hematopoietic recovery in syngeneic and allogeneic hosts. *Journal of Clinical Investigation,* **101,** 961–6.

West, L. J., Morris, P. J., & Wood, K. J. (1994). Fetal liver hematopoietic cells and tolerance to organ allografts. *Lancet,* **343,** 148–9.

Wilson, R., Dealy, J., & Sadowsky, N. (1959). Transplantation of homologous bone marrow and skin from common multiple donors following total body irradiation. *Surgery,* **46,** 261–76.

Wood, M. L., Monaco, A. P., Gozzo, J. J., & Liegeois, A. (1971). Use of homozygous allogeneic bone marrow for induction of tolerance with antilymphocyte serum: dose and timing. *Transplantation Proceedings,* **3,** 676–9.

Yuh, D. D., Gandy, K. L., Hoyt, G. *et al.* (1996). Tolerance to cardiac allografts induced in utero with fetal liver cells. *Circulation,* **94,** 304–7.

Zinkernagel, R. M., Althage, A., Callahan, G., & Welsh, R. M. (1980). On the immunocompetence of H-2 incompatible irradiation bone marrow chimeras. *Journal of Immunology,* **124,** 2356–65.

Zinkernagel, R. M., Callahan, G. N., Althage, A. *et al.* (1978). On the thymus in the differentiation of "H-2 self-recognition" by T cells: evidence for dual recognition? *Journal of Experimental Medicine,* **147,** 882–96.

Zinkernagel, R. M., Sado, T., Althage, A., & Kamisaku, H. (1984). Anti-viral immune response of allogeneic irradiation bone marrow chimeras: cytotoxic T cell responsiveness depends upon H-2 combination and infectious agent. *European Journal of Immunology,* **14,** 14–23.

PART XIV   THE FUTURE

123 The future of blood and bone marrow transplantation

JAYESH MEHTA AND RAY POWLES

Northwestern University, Chicago, USA and Royal Marsden Hospital, Sutton, UK

Introduction

Despite a history that now approaches two decades of reasonably widespread practice, hematopoietic stem cell transplantation (HSCT) has remained a relatively crude and toxic procedure (Mehta & Powles, 2000), and concrete clinical developments have markedly lagged imaginative attempts at peering into the future (Powles & Mehta, 1994; Mehta & Powles, 2000).

While the lack of fruition of our desires has been somewhat disappointing, it has not deterred us from extending our wish list further. This most recent attempt at looking into the future of HSCT complements our chapters from the previous editions of this book rather than replacing them.

Recent developments

Since the second edition of this book, two major trends have become obvious. Firstly, the use of blood-derived hematopoietic stem cells for allogeneic transplantation has become even more widespread. The impetus for this has been the demonstration that blood cell transplantation not only results in faster hematopoietic reconstitution in comparison with marrow grafts, but also probably results in reduced relapse and improved survival (Powles *et al.*, 2000; Bensinger *et al.*, 2001).

Secondly, and related at least in part to the use of blood-derived stem cells, there has been a sizeable increase in the number of reduced-intensity or non-myeloablative transplants (Feinstein & Storb, 2001). The increase has been partly due to transplantation being performed in patients who would never have been subjected to an allograft in the past because of age or performance status, and partly due to a shift away from conventional-intensity allografts even in patients who are eligible for them based upon standard criteria.

Development of newer anti-cancer agents

At the risk of making HSCT obsolete, it is necessary to have specific antimalignancy drugs that could control, if not eliminate, cancer long-term, easily and safely. Based on past experience with conventional cytotoxic agents, these agents are more likely to be monoclonal antibodies, angiogenesis-inhibiting agents, antisense molecules, immunomodulators, and other biological agents.

There was excitement when thalidomide was found to be active in patients with myeloma (Singhal *et al.*, 1999). However, it became obvious rapidly that thalidomide-induced responses were not sustained indefinitely and relapse was inevitable. Thus, rather than replacing HSCT, thalidomide has found a place as induction therapy (pre-autograft cytoreduction), as salvage therapy (for relapse after HSCT), or as maintenance therapy (after autograft) (Singhal & Mehta, 2002) – i.e., as adjunctive therapy to be used with HSCT.

Even the drug that has set a benchmark for targeted therapy, imatinib mesylate (STI 571, Gleevec), is not effective at inducing molecular remissions in all patients with chronic myeloid leukemia (CML) and nor are such responses sustained indefinitely (Druker *et al.*, 2001). Imatinib, therefore, does not replace allogeneic HSCT in patients with HLA-identical sibling donors who are in a suitable age group. It has clearly had a negative impact on the trend towards early allografts from HLA-matched unrelated donors in patients who lack an HLA-matched sibling. It is somewhat difficult to justify an early alternative-donor transplant in CML at the moment; it may be prudent to use imatinib and wait for long-term follow-up data to decide about the best timing for the allograft.

Thus, while newer drugs will continue to improve the outcome of patients with malignant diseases, it is unlikely that they will replace HSCT. It is far likelier that they will be used in conjunction with HSCT in suitable patients to improve the overall outcome significantly.

Microarrays

DNA or gene chips and protein arrays (Friend & Stoughton, 2002) have the potential to affect every stage of HSCT profoundly within the foreseeable future. This technology will provide critical and specific information needed to individualize each stage of therapy for a given patient – and optimize outcome. Already, polymorphisms of genes encoding proteins involved in innate immunity and inflammation influence transplant outcomes in HSC allograft recipients, including engraftment rate, infection, GVHD, and transplant-related mortality (Rocha *et al.*, 2002).

This approach will determine selection of appropriate patients (transplant or no transplant) and choice of procedure (autograft or allograft) based upon prognosis (Alizadeh *et al.*, 2000) and minimal residual disease status. The choice of donor will be based upon patient and donor profiles. Comparison of profiles will allow selection of donors whose cells may have favorable profiles from the perspective of maximizing anti-tumor effects and minimizing undesirable complications such as graft-versus-host disease (GVHD). While this will not replace HLA typing, it will probably replace the search for minor histocompatibility loci.

After the transplant, protein arrays will serve as an early indicator of infections and impending relapse; permitting early and specific pharmacologic or cellular therapy.

Donor selection

Most factors related to the patient (e.g., age, performance status, organ function) are not modifiable. Donor factors are potentially modifiable, particularly if multiple donors are available. An adequate cell dose is already known to be an important variable (Singhal *et al.*, 2000).

There will be increased investigation into donor factors that could improve outcome of HSCT so that the best donor is selected when more than one donor is available. Donor factors that will be considered may be based upon complex microarray studies as discussed above or relatively simple parameters such as age (Kollman *et al.*, 2001) and blood group (Mehta *et al.*, 2002). Killer inhibitory receptor (KIR) epitope mismatches in the graft-versus-host direction—which can result in NK-cell–mediated graft-versus-leukemia reactions—have been shown to result in lower relapse and better outcome of acute myeloid leukemia patients undergoing haploidentical HSCT (Ruggeri *et al.*, 2002). This information may well prove to be relevant for other types of donors too.

Allele-level matching for HLA A, B, C, DRB1 and DQB1 is associated with better outcome after HSCT from unrelated donors (Petersdorf *et al.*, 1998, 2001). However, ancestral or extended haplotypes can improve on the matching further in selected patients (those who happen to have inherited one or two extended haplotypes). This has been shown to result in improved outcome of patients with thalassemia allografted from unrelated donors (La Nasa *et al.*, 2002).

In addition to selecting the best donor when multiple donors are available, patients considered to be at a higher-than-average risk of treatment-related toxicity (e.g., older or poorer performance status) will be accepted for a transplant procedure if an extended-haplotype–matched donor is available.

Blood or marrow?

It is fairly clear that the use of blood rather than marrow for HSCT is more convenient and almost certainly results in superior outcome of allogeneic as well as autologous grafts. However, the issue of possibly increased chronic GVHD with blood-derived stem cells still remains unsettled. Interestingly, those who have not seen a substantial increase in chronic GVHD are mostly those who have continued to use methotrexate-based GVHD prophylaxis—usually conventional cyclosporine-methotrexate prophylaxis (Mehta & Singhal, 2002). While it is important to ensure that a minimum dose of stem cells is used to decrease treatment-related mortality (Singhal *et al.*, 2000), there is evidence to suggest that use of very high doses of CD34[+] cell results in an increased risk of GVHD (Przepiorka *et al.*, 2001; Zaucha *et al.*, 2001).

The question for the future is not whether there is a significantly higher incidence of chronic GVHD with blood-derived stem cells but what strategies can be adopted to decrease the incidence of GVHD to improve overall outcome. This may be something as simple as using methotrexate-containing combinations for GVHD prophylaxis and infusing a controlled number of CD34[+] cells, continuing full-dose GVHD prophylaxis for longer than usual, or the addition of other immunosuppressive agents to the standard combinations. Whatever approach is chosen, it is very likely that blood will replace marrow as the source of hematopoietic stem cells completely within the foreseeable future.

Non-myeloablative conditioning regimens

The demonstration that non-myeloablative conditioning permits alloengraftment, as long as adequate immunosuppression is provided, has proved an old dogma wrong—the long-held belief that adequate "space" had to be created through destruction of recipient hematopoiesis to allow donor hematopoiesis to become established. This is a major advance from the perspective of understanding the immunobiology of HSCT.

While conventional conditioning regimens relied on the brute, non-specific force of high-dose therapy to eliminate disease, reduced intensity conditioning regimens (mini-allografts) rely on an immunologically-mediated graft-versus-tumor reaction to eliminate cancer.

Mini-allografts are certainly much safer than conventional allografts in the short term, but because of GVHD, toxicity will still occur over an extended period of time. Long-term data are not yet available to predict eventual outcome, but it is possible that longer follow-up will show a continuing, albeit modest, decline in survival in a pattern somewhat different from what has been seen with conventional allografts. Deaths occurring 2–3 years beyond mini-transplantation will be from recurrent disease in a proportion of those without GVHD (no ongoing graft-versus-tumor reactions) or from complications of GVHD in those who have severe chronic GVHD.

The answer to the morbidity resulting from crude, non-specific, and toxic conditioning regimens will not be their elimination or marked attenuation of their intensity, but the development of cytotoxic agents that specifically target tumor cells.

Repairing and replacing non-hematopoietic tissue

The ethical debate surrounding the use of embryonic stem cells will be laid to rest when the right cytokine and environmental stimuli are discovered which will make marrow-resident totipotent stem cells develop into other cell types. The presence of such cells will be exploited by isolating them and placing/transplanting them into appropriate areas of the body such as the myocardium in patients with ischemic heart disease or the spinal cord in patients with trauma. Eventually, it will be possible to simply administer cytokines systemically that will direct the appropriate cell subpopulations to migrate to a site requiring repair and develop and differentiate as needed.

This procedure, probably a manipulation of stem cells that are different from what we know as hematopoietic stem cells today but done much the way HSCT is performed, holds a great deal of promise for many diseases for which regenerative therapy is simply not yet available.

Nanotechnology

Nanotechnology—the use of miniature/microscopic robots to perform all sorts of tasks—is supposed to be the next major advance in technology. Time will tell whether nanotechnology is of real benefit or is mere hype.

Some of its possible medical applications, the use of microscopic structures such as fullerenes and nanoshells to deliver drugs directly to selected cells, appear considerably less far-fetched than some of the other hypothetical applications in industry. However, it is difficult to imagine nanoparticles with computing and mechanical capabilities forming an artificial immune system (*Nano Technology Magazine*, 2002). The day that this comes true, HSCT will not exist as we know it because there will be no place for it.

Evaluation of HSCT as a therapeutic tool

HSCT is a very expensive procedure. However, it can also potentially be a lucrative business. This often underlies, at least in part, development of treatment strategies that maximize use of HSCT (broadening indications and/or multiple transplant procedures in the same patient). Unfortunately, few studies have measured the benefits of HSCT in terms of cost per quality-adjusted life years.

High-profile (and thus by definition expensive) medical interventions eventually attract close external scrutiny. This is beneficial because it ensures appropriateness of the intervention. Autotransplantation for breast cancer is an example. An exponential growth in the number of autografts being performed for breast cancer led to controlled studies which failed to show efficacy (Bergh *et al.*, 2000; Stadtmauer *et al.*, 2000). That coupled with discovery of fraud in studies apparently showing benefit from autotransplantation (Weiss *et al.*, 2000; Weiss, Gill, & Hudis, 2001) has resulted in an implosion in the number of autografts for breast cancer.

With health care costs skyrocketing, it is inevitable that HSCT for other diseases is going to be evaluated stringently by insurance companies (who are responsible for paying for the procedure) and government agencies (who are responsible either for paying, or for determining policy, or for ensuring that clinical research is done in an appropriate fashion) (Kalb & Koehler, 2002). In fact, payments made by insurance companies in the United States for HSCT procedures are declining, even without adjustment for cost of living or inflation. The way to ensure that patients who require HSCT receive it in a way that is economically feasible for all concerned is to eliminate HSCT for indications that are unproven or unnecessary.

A case in point is tandem transplantation for myeloma. While some centers have strongly advocated double autografts (Desikan *et al.*, 2000), it is appears that two transplants are not better than a single one that is performed optimally (Attal, Harousseau, & Facon, 2001; Cavo *et al.*, 2001; Sirohi *et al.*, 2002). The cost implications of the usefulness for one versus two autografts in myeloma are enormous. If 4,000–6,000 of the 14,000 new cases of myeloma diagnosed in the United States every year are autografted, at $60,000–90,000 per procedure, the increased annual cost of therapy with tandem transplantation (compared with single) would be in the region of $200–500 million in the United States alone.

If it is not possible or practical to perform prospective studies to answer important scientific questions with economic implications, the only alternative may be for detailed data from large centers to be pooled and analyzed (Powles *et al.*, 2001). Analyses from group databases such as the International Bone Marrow Transplant Registry, Autologous Blood and Marrow Transplant Registry, or European Bone Marrow Transplant Group (BMTR, ABMTR, or EBMT) will not suffice for this because of lack of sufficiently detailed information. The centers contributing data for such analyses will be large centers with detailed patient information, and the analyses will be carried out under the auspices of independent organizations such as the National Cancer Institute (USA) or the Medical Research Cancer (UK).

The future

The art and science of HSCT continues to make steady progress. Dramatic improvements, such as that seen with the introduction of ganciclovir, are infrequent. We envisage that improvements will continue to occur. The ultimate success of targeted and specific therapy for cancer and other serious diseases will result in the elimination of HSCT as a treatment modality. While it is difficult to predict when this will happen, we do expect to be thinking about it for at least the next couple of editions of this book.

References

Alizadeh, A. A., Eisen, M. B., Davis, R. E. *et al.* (2000). Distinct types of diffuse large B-cell lymphoma identified by gene expression profiling. *Nature,* **403,** 503–511.

Attal, M., Harousseau, J. L., & Facon, T. (2001). Single versus double transplant in myeloma: a randomized trial of the Inter Groupe Français Du Myélome (IFM). *Abstract Book of the VIIIth International Myeloma Workshop,* Banff, Alberta, Canada, 4–8 May 2001, p. 28 (S15).

Bensinger, W. I., Martin, P. J., Storer, B. et al. (2000). Transplantation of bone marrow as compared with peripheral-blood cells from HLA-identical relatives in patients with hematologic cancers. New England Journal of Medicine, 344, 175–181.

Bergh, J., Wiklund, T., Erikstein, B. et al. (2000). Tailored fluorouracil, epirubicin, and cyclophosphamide compared with marrow-supported high-dose chemotherapy as adjuvant treatment for high-risk breast cancer: a randomised trial. Lancet, 356, 1384–1391.

Cavo, M., Tosi, P., Zamagni, E. et al. (2001). The "Bologna 96" clinical trial of single vs. double PBSC transplantation for previously untreated MM: results of an interim analysis. Abstract Book of the VIIIth International Myeloma Workshop, Banff, Alberta, Canada, 4–8 May 2001, p. 29–30 (S16).

Desikan, R., Barlogie, B., Sawyer, J. et al. (2000). Results of high-dose therapy for 1000 patients with multiple myeloma: durable complete remissions and superior survival in the absence of chromosome 13 abnormalities. Blood, 95, 4008–4010.

Druker, B. J., Talpaz, M., Resta, D. J. et al. (2001). Efficacy and safety of a specific inhibitor of the BCR-ABL tyrosine kinase in chronic myeloid leukemia. New England Journal of Medicine, 344, 1031–1037.

Feinstein, L. & Storb, R. (2001). Reducing transplant toxicity. Current Opinion in Hematology, 8, 342–348.

Friend, S. H., & Stoughton, R. B. (2002). The magic of microarrays. Scientific American, 282, 44–53.

Kalb, P. E. & Koehler, K. G. (2002). Legal issues in scientific research. JAMA: The Journal of the American Medical Association, 287, 85–91.

Kollman, C., Howe, C.W.S., Anasetti, C. et al. (2001). Donor characteristics as risk factors in recipients after transplantation of bone marrow from unrelated donors: the effect of donor age. Blood, 98, 2043–2051.

La Nasa, G., Giardini, C., Argiolu, F. et al. (2002). Unrelated donor bone marrow transplantation for thalassemia: the effect of extended haplotypes. Blood, 99, 4350–4356.

Mehta, J. & Powles, R. (2000). The future of bone marrow transplantation. In Clinical Bone Marrow and Blood Stem Cell Transplantation, Second Edition, ed. K. Atkinson, pp. 1457–1465. Cambridge, Cambridge University Press.

Mehta, J., Powles, R., Sirohi, B. et al. (2002). Does donor-recipient ABO-incompatibility protect against relapse after allogeneic bone marrow transplantation in first remission acute myeloid leukemia? Bone Marrow Transplantation, 29, 853–859.

Mehta, J. & Singhal, S. (2002). Chronic graft-versus-host disease after allogeneic peripheral-blood stem-cell transplantation: a little methotrexate goes a long way. Journal of Clinical Oncology, 20, 603–604.

Nano Technology Magazine. Nanotechnology health. www.nanozine.com/nanomed.htm (accessed 1 July 2002).

Petersdorf, E. W., Gooley, T. A., Anasetti, C. et al. (1998). Optimizing outcome after unrelated marrow transplantation by comprehensive matching of HLA class I and II alleles in the donor and recipient. Blood, 92, 3515–3520.

Petersdorf, E. W., Hansen, J. A., Martin, P. J. et al. (2001). Major-histocompatibility-complex class I alleles and antigens in hematopoietic-cell transplantation. New England Journal of Medicine, 345, 1794–1800.

Powles, R. L. & Mehta, J. (1994). The future of bone marrow transplantation. In: Clinical Bone Marrow Transplantation: A Reference Textbook, ed. K. Atkinson, pp. 736–740. Cambridge, Cambridge University Press.

Powles, R., Mehta, J., Kulkarni, S. et al. (2000). Allogeneic blood and bone-marrow stem-cell transplantation in haematological malignant diseases: a randomised trial. Lancet, 355, 1231–1237.

Powles, R., Milan, S., Horton, C. et al. (2001). The Royal Marsden Hospital leukemia-myeloma database: an "operations research" resource for assessing clinical outcomes and planning new drug trials. Blood, 98 (Suppl), 426a.

Przepiorka, D., Anderlini, P., Saliba, R. et al. (2001). Chronic graft-versus-host disease after allogeneic blood stem cell transplantation. Blood, 98, 1695–1700.

Rocha, V., Franco, R. F., Porcher, R. et al. (2002). Host defense and inflammatory gene polymorphisms are associated with outcomes after HLA-identical sibling bone marrow transplantation. Blood, 100, 3908–18.

Ruggeri, L., Capanni, M., Urbani, E. et al. (2002). Striking survival advantage of bad-risk acute myeloid leukemia patients transplanted from haploidentical donors with KIR epitope incompatibility in the GVH direction. Bone Marrow Transplantation, 29 (Suppl 2), S1.

Singhal, S. & Mehta, J. (2002). Thalidomide in cancer. Biomedicine & Pharmacotherapy-Biomedicine & Pharmacotherapie, 56, 4–12.

Singhal, S., Mehta, J., Desikan, R. et al. (1999). Antitumor activity of thalidomide in refractory multiple myeloma. New England Journal of Medicine, 341, 1565–1571.

Singhal, S., Powles, R., Treleaven, J. et al. (2000). A low CD34+ cell dose results in higher mortality and poorer survival after blood or marrow stem cell transplantation from HLA-identical siblings: should 2×10^6 CD34+ cells/kg be considered the minimum threshold? Bone Marrow Transplantation, 26, 489–496.

Sirohi, B., Powles, R., Mehta, J. et al. (2002). Single-center results of 200 mg/m² melphalan (HDM200) and autograft (tx) in 451 myeloma (MM) patients: identifying patients with prolonged survival based upon albumin (ALB) and β_2-microglobulin (β_2M) at transplant. Proceedings of the American Society of Clinical Oncology, 269a (Abstract).

Stadtmauer, E. A., O'Neill, A., Goldstein, L. J. et al. (2000). Conventional-dose chemotherapy compared with high-dose chemotherapy plus autologous hematopoietic stem-cell transplantation for metastatic breast cancer. New England Journal of Medicine, 342, 1069–1076.

Weiss, R. B., Gill, G. G., & Hudis, C. A. (2001). An on-site audit of the South African trial of high-dose chemotherapy for metastatic breast cancer and associated publications. Journal of Clinical Oncology, 19, 2771–2777.

Weiss, R. B., Rifkin, R. M., Stewart, F. M. et al. (2000). High-dose chemotherapy for high-risk primary breast cancer: an on-site review of the Bezwoda study. Lancet, 355, 999–1003.

Zaucha, J. M., Gooley, T., Bensinger, W. J. et al. (2001). CD34 cell dose in granulocyte colony-stimulating factor-mobilized peripheral blood mononuclear cell grafts affects engraftment kinetics and development of extensive chronic graft-versus-host disease after human leukocyte antigen-identical sibling transplantation. Blood, 98, 3221–3227.

124 Breaking News . . .

KERRY ATKINSON, RICHARD CHAMPLIN, JEROME RITZ, WILLEM FIBBE, PER LJUNGMAN, AND MALCOM BRENNER

Introduction

A textbook of this size takes considerable time to produce and this allows potential for the book to be partially outdated by the time it is published. We have tried to minimize this by updating the manuscript throughout production, and indeed it is referenced through July 2003.

Additionally, in this chapter, the editors highlight specific areas of interest presenting in the literature that have emerged or have been re-emphasized in the 12 months prior to publication.

Current trends in HSC transplantation

Major changes have occurred in the transplantation of hematopoietic stem cells in the last decade. These changes are well illustrated in data reported on 132,963 patients transplanted in 619 centers in 35 European countries between 1990 (4234 HSC transplants) and 2000 (19, 136 transplants) (Gratwohl *et al.*, 2002). There were 44,165 allografts (33%) and 88,798 autografts (67%). During this decade the rate of allogeneic transplantation (Fig. 124.1) increased continuously for all indications except CML and inborn errors, for which the maximum number of transplants was reached in 1999. For CML, the likely explanation is the advent of imatinib mesylate. For autologous transplantation, the changes in transplantation rate differed from the pattern seen in allogeneic grafting (Fig. 124.1). For some indications including non-Hodgkin's lymphoma, Hodgkin's disease, myeloma, CLL, MDS, and AML there was a continuous increase. For others, most notably breast cancer, there was a peak between 1997 and 1998, followed by a rapid decline. Transplantation rates for selected diseases are shown in Fig. 124.2. Based on this analysis it was predicted that allogeneic transplantation rates for all indications except CML will continue at the same, or a higher, level in the medium term. Rates for autologous transplantation for NHL, HD, myeloma, and AML will also continue to increase in the medium term.

The EBMT has also published reports on current practice of HSC transplantation for specific diseases in Europe (Urbano-Ispizua et al., 2002) (Tables 124.1 and 124.2).

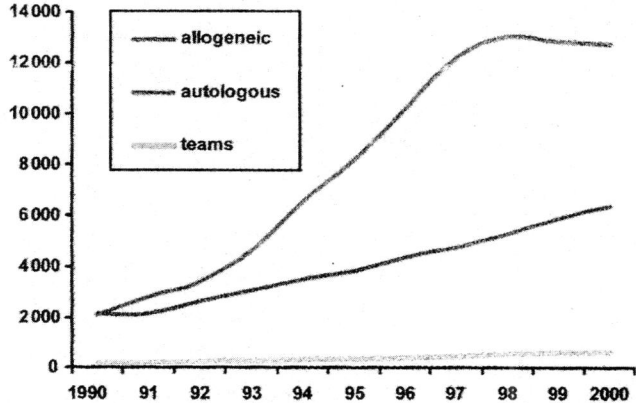

Fig. 124.1. Evolution of HSCT in Europe from 1990 to 2000. Annual numbers of allogeneic and autologous HSCT and of participating teams. Reproduced, with permission, from Gratwohl *et al.* (2002).

CD34+ and CD3+ cell dose as risk factors for acute graft-versus-host disease in T cell-depleted transplantation

Both increasing CD34+ cell dose and increasing CD3+ cell dose were risk factors for acute GVHD in a study of 315 patients given CD34-selected HLA-identical sibling PBSC grafts (Urbano-Ispizua *et al.*, 2002) (Fig. 124.3). All but 6 patients received posttransplant GVHD prophylaxis of cyclosporine or cyclosporine plus prednisolone or methotrexate.

Home care for allogeneic HSC transplantation utilizing myeloablative conditioning

Initial results in one study using both family member and unrelated donors have been encouraging: 36 patients, 30 of whom received a full myeloablative conditioning regimen prior to an allograft, elected to be treated at home after the graft was infused. Compared to patients who chose to be treated in the hospital and to a matched control group of patients, those electing home care had fewer days on TPN,

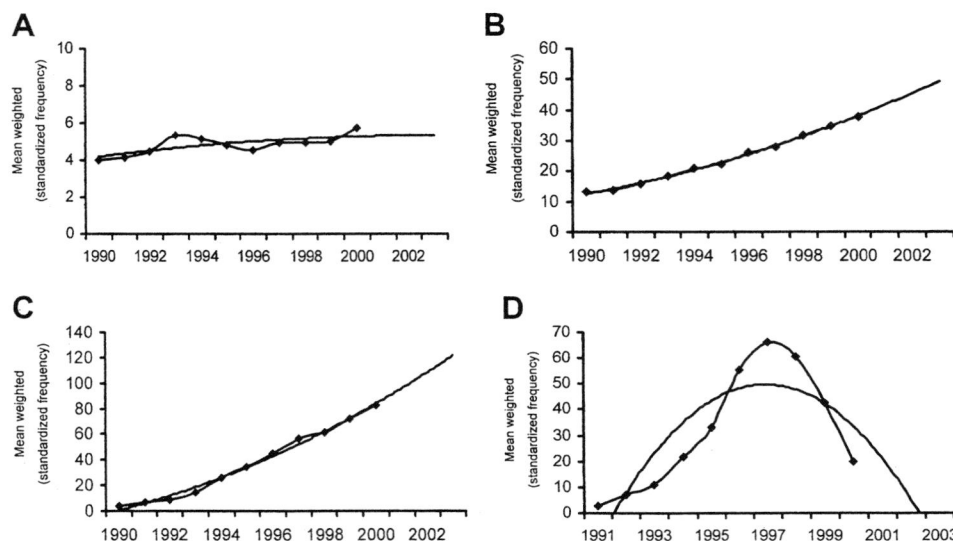

Fig. 124.2. Transplantaion rates for selected indications in nine European countries from 1990 to 2000. Weighted transplantation rates (per 10 million inhabitants) are given (♦) and best fitting curves (lines). (**A**) Aplastic anemia, allogeneic HSCT. (**B**) Acute myeloid leukemia, allogeneic HSCT. (**C**) Multiple myeloma, autologous HSCT. (**D**) Breast cancer, autologous HSCT. Reproduced, with permission, from Gratwohl et al. (2002).

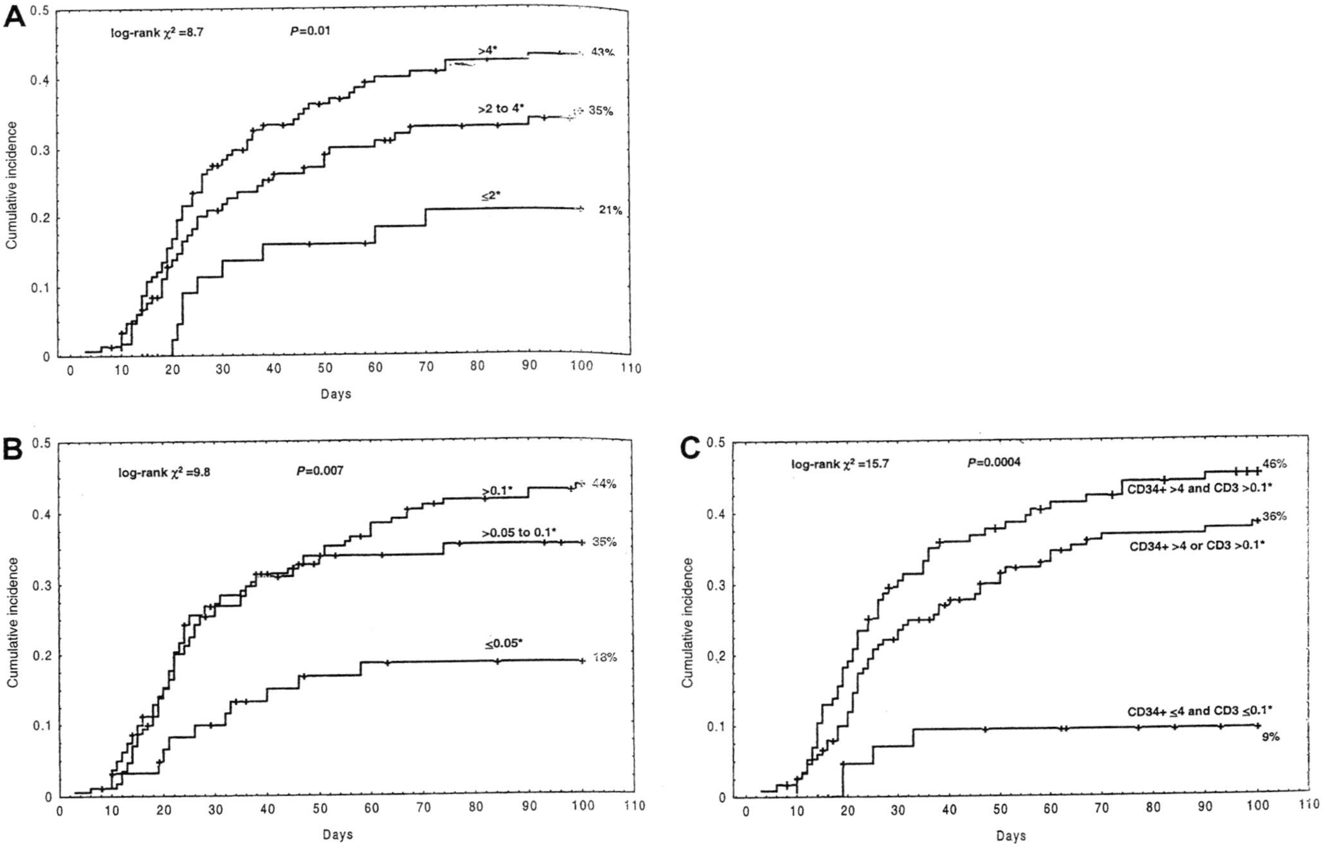

Fig. 124.3. Cumulative incidence of acute GVHD grades I-IV depending on the quantity of infused cells. (**A**) CD34+ cells infused. (**B**) CD3+ cells infused. (**C**) The combination of CD34+ and CD3+ cells infused. * Indicates x 10⁶/kg. Reproduced, with permission, from Urbano-Ispizua *et al.* (2002).

Table 124.1. *Proposed classification of transplant procedures for adults – 2001.*

Disease	Disease status	Allo		Auto
		Sibling donor	Alternative donor	
AML	CR1, CR2	S	CP	S
	CR3, incipient relapse	S	CP	CP
	M3 Molecular persistence[a]	S	CP	NR
	M3 2nd Molecular remission	S	CP	S
	Relapse or refractory	CP	NR	NR
ALL	CR1 (high risk), CR2, incipient relapse	S	S	CP
	Relapse or refractory	CP	NR	NR
CML	Chronic phase	S	S	CP
	Accelerated phase	S	S	NR
	Blast crisis	D	NR	NR
Myeloproliferative disorders (non-CML)		CP	D	D
Myelodysplastic syndrome	RA, RAEB	S	S	CP
	RAEBt, sAML in CR1 or CR2	S	CP	CP
	More advanced stages	S	CP	NR
CLL		S	D	CP
NHL				
High and intermediate grade	CR1	NR	NR	S
	Relapse, CR2, CR3	CP	CP	S
	Refractory	CP	NR	NR
Low grade	CR1	NR	NR	CP
	Relapse, CR2, CR3	CP	D	S
Hodgkin's disease	CR1	NR	NR	CP
	1st relapse, CR2, CR3	CP	NR	S
	Refractory	CP	NR	CP
Myeloma		CP	D	S
Severe aplastic anaemia	Patient <45 years	S	D	NR
Paroxysmal nocturnal hemoglobinuria		CP	D	
Solid tumours				
Breast cancer	Adjuvant and inflammatory	NR	NR	CP
Breast cancer	Metastatic responding	D	NR	CP
Germ cell tumours	Sensitive relapses	NR	NR	S
Germ cell tumours	Refractory	NR	NR	CP
Ovarian cancer	MRD	NR	NR	CP
Ovarian cancer	Refractory	D	NR	NR
Glioma	Post-surgery	NR	NR	D
Small cell lung cancer (limited/'good')	Upfront	NR	NR	CP
Renal cell carcinoma	Metastatic	D	NR	NR
Autoimmune disorders				
ITP with bleeding		—	—	D
Systemic sclerosis		—	—	D
Rheumatoid arthritis		—	—	D
Multiple sclerosis		—	—	D
SLE		—	—	D
Amyloidosis (AL)		D	NR	D

S = in standard use for selected patients; CP = to be undertaken in approved Clinical Protocols; D = developmental or pilot studies can be approved in specialist units; NR = not generally recommended; MRD = minimal residual disease; CR1, 2, 3 = first, second, third complete remission; RA = refractory anaemia; RAEB = refractory anaemia with excess blasts; sAML = secondary acute myeloid leukaemia. This classification does not cover patients for whom a syngeneic donor is available. Haemopoietic transplant is not recommended for either breast cancer with refractory metastasis and for non-small cell lung cancer.

[a]After consolidation or salvage treatment.

Reproduced, with permission, from Urbano-Ispizua *et al.* (2002a)

Table 124.2. *Proposed classification of transplant procedures for children – 2001.*

Disease	Disease status	Allo		Auto
		Sibling donor	Alternative donor	
AML	CR1 (low risk)	NR	NR	NR
	CR1 (high risk)	S	NR	S
	CR2	S	S	S
ALL	CR1 (low risk)	NR	NR	NR
	CR1 (high risk)	CP	CP	NR
	CR2 (see text)	S	S	CP
	> CR2	S	S	CP
CML	Chronic phase	S	S	CP
	Advanced phase	S	S	NR
NHL	CR1 (low risk)	NR	NR	NR
	CR2 (high risk)	CP	CP	CP
	CR2 (see text)	S	S	CP
Hodgkin's disease	CR1	NR	NR	NR
	1st relapse, CR2	CP	D	S
Myelodysplastic syndrome	See text	S	S	NR
Immunodeficiency		S	S	—
Thalassaemia	See text	S	D	—
Sickle cell disease	See text	S	D	—
Aplastic anaemia		S	CP	—
Blackfan–Diamond anaemia		S	CP	—
Inborn errors of metabolism		CP	CP	—
Solid Tumours	Germ cell tumour	NR	NR	CP
	Ewing's sarcoma	NR	NR	CP
	Soft tissue sarcoma	D	D	CP
	Neuroblastoma	NR	NR	CP
	Wilms tumour	NR	NR	CP
	Osteogenic sarcoma	NR	NR	D
	Brain tumours	NR	NR	CP
Autoimmune diseases		NR	NR	D

S = in standard use for selected patients; CP = to be undertaken in approved Clinical Protocols; D = developmental or pilot studies can be approved in specialist units; NR = not generally recommended;
Reproduced, with permission, from Urbano-Ispizua et al. (2002b).

less acute GVHD grades II-IV, lower transplant-related mortality and lower costs. The 2 year survival rates were 70% in the home care group versus 51% and 57% (NS) in the control groups (Svahn *et al.*, 2002).

A new approach to haploidentical family member transplantation

This involves the selection of haploidentical family donors based on the presence of feto-maternal microchimerism. Feto-maternal microchimerism is the presence of fetal hematopoietic cells in the maternal blood and maternal hematopoietic cells in the fetal circulation. This may be a mechanism of the immunologic tolerance that exists between mother and offspring. Van Rood and colleagues (2002) showed that recipients of non-T-cell-depleted maternal transplants had a significantly lower incidence of chronic GVHD than recipients of paternal transplants; they also demonstrated a lower rate of acute GVHD in sibling transplants mismatched for noninherited maternal antigens (NIMAs) compared to those mismatched for noninherited paternal antigens. These observations support the hypothesis that recipients may be tolerant to haploidentical-related donors expressing NIMAs (mother or NIMA-mismatched siblings), and that the microchimeric mother may be hyporesponsive to inherited paternal antigens in the offspring. Shimazaki et al. (2003) performed five non-T cell-depleted haploidentical family member transplants based on this hypothesis. At the time of the report, three patients were alive at 105+, 390+, and 467+ days posttransplant respectively.

Reduced intensity conditioning regimens

Non-Hodgkin's lymphoma

An EBMT Registry series of 188 patients, 48% of whom had received a prior autologous transplant, described an overall progression-free survival rate of 46%, but the rate was significantly better than this in patients with low-grade NHL, Hodgkin's disease, and in those with chemosensitive disease (Robinson et al., 2002). Patients with high-grade lymphoma, mantle cell lymphoma, and those with chemoresistant lymphoma had a poor outcome.

Myeloma

Autologous HSC transplantation followed by elective reduced intensity conditioning and allografting. A new approach involves the use of a standard autograft for tumor debulking purposes followed by an elective allograft (using reduced intensity conditioning) and an allograft to exploit the graft-versus-myeloma effect (Maloney et al., 2001; Kröger et al., 2002). Kröger and colleagues (2002) treated 17 patients with advanced stage II/III myeloma with melphalan 200 mg/m^2 and an autologous transplant. After a median interval of 119 days, a reduced intensity conditioniong regimen of fludarabine 180 mg/m^2, melphalan 100mg/m^2, and ATG 10 mg/kg for 3 doses was administered prior to an allogeneic transplant from an HLA-matched related donor in 7 patients, an HLA-mismatched related donor in 2 patients, and an unrelated donor in 8 patients. Complete donor chimerism was detected after a median of 30 days. The 100 day mortality rate post-allograft was 11%. The complete remission rate with negative immunofixation increased from 0% after induction or salvage chemotherapy to 18% after autologous transplantation to 73% after allografting. At a median follow-up of 13 months post allografting, the 2-year estimated overall survival was 74% and event-free survival was 56% (Figs. 124.4 and 124.5).

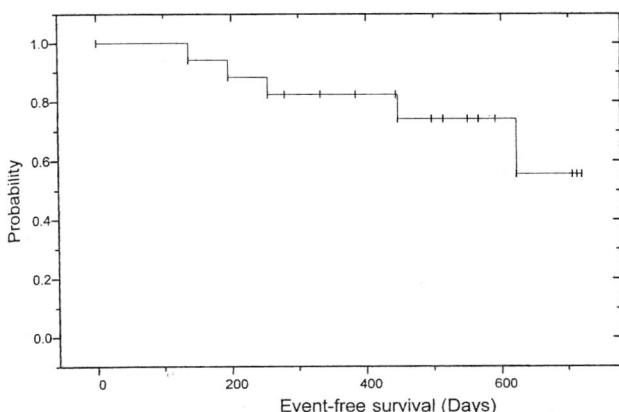

Fig.124.5. Event-free survival. Reproduced, with permission, from Kröger et al. (2002).

Use of imatinib to treat relapse after allografting for CML

The M.D. Anderson group reported on 28 patients given 400–1000 mg/day for relapse occurring a median of 9 (range 1-137) months posttransplant. Thirteen patients had undergone salvage DLI. Complete hematologic responses occurred in 100% of those in chronic phase, 83% for accelerated phase, and 43% for blast phase. Cytogenetic response rates were 63% for chronic or accelerated phase and 43% for blast phase. The 1 year estimated survival was 74%. Recurrence of GVHD occurred in 5 patients. Severe granulocytopenia occurred in 43% and thrombocytopenia in 27% (Kantarjian et al., 2002).

Graft-versus-autoimmune cells after allogeneic HSC transplantation

Hinterberger, Hinterrberger-Fischer, & Marmont (2002) reviewed the literature from 1977 to 2001 for case reports in which an allogeneic or autologous transplant was performed for a hematological disorder in a patient with a concomitant autoimmune disease (AID). Disease-free survival (DFS) after allogeneic HSC transplantation for 23 patients with severe aplastic anemia was 78% at 16 years and survival in unmaintained remission of concomitant AID was 64% at 13 years (Fig. 124.6). DFS after allogeneic transplantation for 24 patients with hematologic malignancies was 87% at 15 years and survival in unmaintained remission for concomitant AID was 70% at 11 years (Fig. 124.7). DFS after autologous HSC transplantation for 24 patients with hematologic malignancies and concomitant AID was 48% at 6 years and survival in unmaintained remission for concomitant AID was 29% at 3 years (Fig. 124.8). After allogeneic transplantation, 3 of 11 patients without GVHD experienced a relapse of their concomitant AID, whereas none of 19 with GVHD did so (Fig. 124.9). These data suggest that a graft-versus-autoimmunity effect after allogeneic HSC transplantation at least partially mediates elimination of autoimmunity.

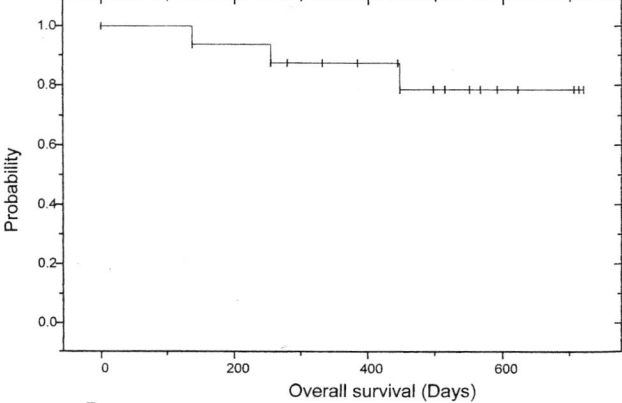

Fig. 124.4. Overall survival. Reproduced, with permission, from Kröger et al. (2002).

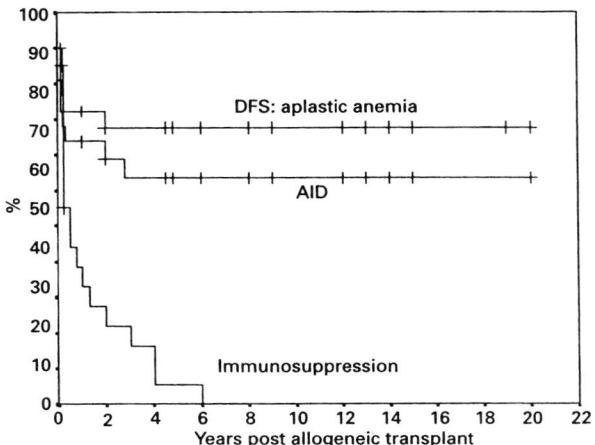

Fig. 124.6. Disease-free survival (DFS), survival in unmaintained remission of a concomitant autoimmune disease (AID), and duration of immunosuppression (GVHD prophylaxis/therapy) in 23 patients after allogeneic stem cell transplantaion for severe aplastic anemia (SAA). Reproduced, with permission, from Hinterberger *et al.* (2002).

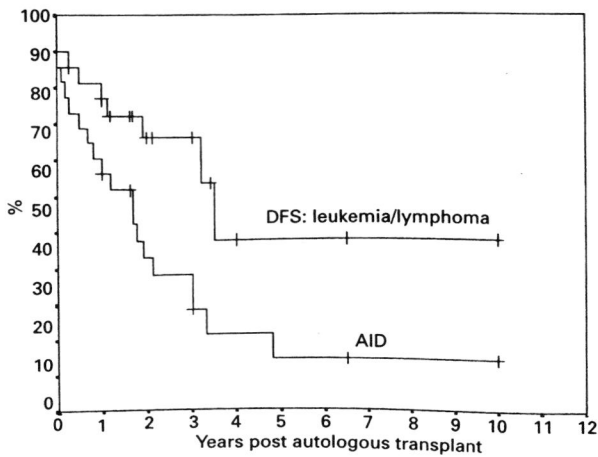

Fig. 124.8. Disease-free survival (DFS) and survival in unmaintained remission of a concomitant autoimmune disease (AID) after autologous hematopoietic stem cell transplantation of 24 patients with leukemia/lymphoma. Reproduced, with permission, from Hinterberger *et al.* (2002).

Mechanism of action of extracorporeal photo-chemotherapy (ECP) in graft-versus-host disease

ECP involves ex vivo exposure of leukapheresed peripheral blood mononuclear cells to ultraviolet A light in the presence of the DNA-intercalating agent 8-methoxypsoralen (8-MOP), with subsequent reinfusion of the cells. Clinical responses to ECP have been demonstrated in chronic GVHD, and the approach may be useful in the prevention of acute GVHD. ECP has been shown to reduce type 1 dendritic cells (DC1) preferentially. An

increase in DC2 numbers (CD83+/CD86+) stimulated Th2 helper T cells to secrete Th2 cytokines, which indirectly inhibited Th1-mediated alloreactivity (Gorgun *et al.*, 2002).

Advances in cellular immunotherapy

Adoptive cellular immunotherapy with antigen-specific T cells

There remains much interest in conferring antigen specificity on T cells for therapeutic purposes, by, for example, introduction of

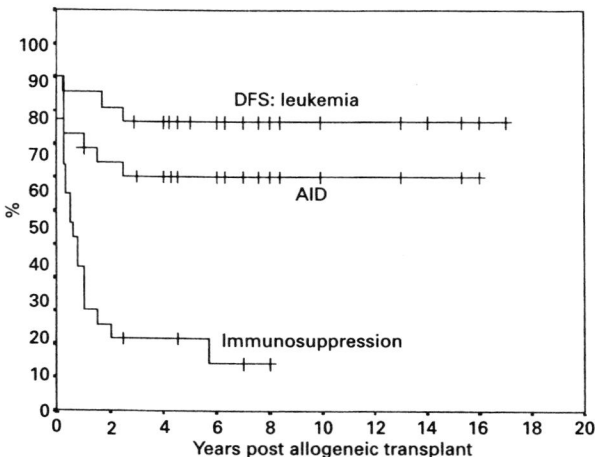

Fig. 124.7. Disease-free survival (DFS), survival in unmaintained remission of a concomitant autoimmune disease (AID) and duration of immunosuppression (GVHD prophylaxis/therapy) in 24 patients after allogeneic stem cell transplantation for leukemia. Reproduced, with permission, from Hinterberger *et al.* (2002).

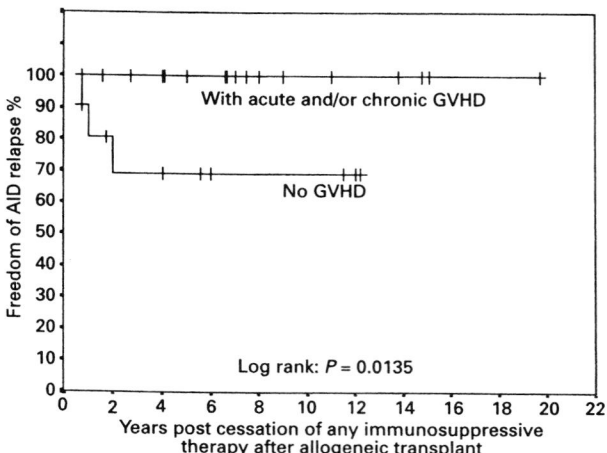

Fig. 124.9. Freedom from relapse of concomitant autoimmune disease (AID) in 30 patients suffering from leukemia/lymphoma/aplastic anemia in relation to GVHD (graft-versus-host disease) manifestation post transplant. Immunosuppression discontinued (= day 0). Reproduced, with permission, from Hinterberger *et al.* (2002).

T-cell receptor genes specific for a given antigen. HLA restriction represents a significant hurdle to the wide applicability of this approach. However, the requirement for antigen processing and presentation by HLA molecules can be bypassed by the genetic modification of T cells to express a chimeric immunoreceptor composed of a single chain immunoglobulin extracellular targeting domain specific for a tumor-specific or tumor-associated antigen fused to a CD3-ζ intracellular signaling domain. Such an approach has been taken using CD19 as the target antigen (Cooper et al., 2003). Both CD4+ and CD8+ cells modified in this way displayed potent CD19-specific lytic activity including activity against primary B-ALL blast cells. They also demonstrated chimeric immunoreceptor-regulated cytokine production and proliferation. These preclinical observations form a basis for clinical trials using donor-derived CD19-specific T-cell clones to treat or prevent relapse of B-ALL after allogeneic HSC transplantation.

Use of CD4+ CD25+ T cells to inhibit GVHD

In murine models, depletion of CD4+ CD25+ T cells from the donor T-cell inoculum, or in vivo CD25 depletion of the recipient pretransplant, resulted in increased GVHD mediated by CD4+ T cells or whole T cells (Taylor et al., 2002). Administration of ex vivo activated and expanded CD4+ CD25+ cells administered in equal numbers with CD4+ T cells resulted in significant inhibition of rapidly lethal GVHD, raising the possibility of a new modality of cellular therapy for the inhibition of undesirable allogeneic responses.

WT1 as a panleukemic marker of minimal residual disease posttransplant

Measurement of WT1 gene transcripts by reverse transcriptase PCR appears useful as "panleukemic MRD marker" for predicting and managing relapse following allogeneic HSC transplantation for a variety of acute leukemias and chronic myeloid leukemia (Ogawa et al., 2003). The probability of relapse occurring within 40 days significantly increased step-wise according to the increase in WT1 expression level. WT1 levels in patients with relapse increased exponentially with a constant doubling time. Additionally, the doubling time of the WT1 level in patients for whom the discontinuation of immunosuppressive agents, or administration of donor leukocyte infusion, was effective, was significantly longer than that for patients in whom such approaches were ineffective.

Risk-adapted conditioning regimen prior to autologous HSC transplantation for systemic amyloidosis

Because the toxicity of melphalan is dose-related and survival with amyloidosis may be age-related, patient age and the extent of organ involvement can provide the basis for a risk-adapted approach to melphalan dosing for the conditioning regimen (Commenzo & Gertz, 2002) (Fig. 124.10).

Good risk (Any age; all criteria met)
- 1 or 2 organs involved
- No cardiac involvement
- Creatinine clearance ≥ 51 mL/min

Intermediate risk (Age < 71; either criteria)
- 1 or 2 organs involved (must include cardiac or renal with creatinine clearance < 51 mL/min)
- Asymptomatic or compensated cardiac

Poor risk (either criteria)
- 3 organs involved
- Advanced cardiac involvement

Melphalan dosing: based on risk group and age

Good risk	Intermediate risk	Poor risk
200 mg/m² if ≤ 60	140 mg/m² if ≤ 60	Standard therapy
140 mg/m² if 61-70	100 mg/m² if 61-70	Clinical trials
100 mg/m² if ≥ 71		

Fig. 124.10. A risk-adapted approach to assessing suitability of amyloidosis patients for stem cell transplantation. Reproduced, with permission, from Commenzo & Gertz (2002).

Encouraging results in autologous transplantation for autoimmune disorders

Systemic sclerosis

A Seattle-based collaborative group reported outcomes on 19 SSc patients treated with a protocol of TBI 8Gy, CY 120mg/kg, and equine ATG 90 mg/kg followed by an infusion of CD34-selected, G-CSF mobilized PBSC (McSweeney et al., 2002). Three patients died of treatment-related causes (two of pulmonary toxicity and one of EBV-related lymphoproliferative disease) and one patient died from disease progression. Modified Rodnan skin scores at 1 year were >25% improved in 12/12 patients with a median reduction of 39% (32-93%) ($p = 0.0005$). Functional index evaluations, using a modified Health Assessment Questionnaire – disability index scores, were also markedly improved. Internal organ functions remained stable overall. Decrements in DLCO were found at 3 months but were not different from baseline 1 year after treatment. With a median follow-up of 14 months, projected 2-year survival was 79%. With accrual increased to 28 patients, there were no further deaths as of May 2002. Based on these results, a USA randomized study is planned which will randomize patients to either the high-dose therapy with TBI/CY/ATG as described or monthly intravenous CY 750mg/m².

Chronic autoimmune thrombocytopenia

Huhn and colleagues (2003) reported on 14 patients with chronic autoimmune thrombocytopenia, all of whom had failed multiple prior therapies. They received cyclophosphamide 50 mg/kg/day for 4 days prior to a G-CSF-mobilized PBSC transplant depleted of lymphocytes by CD34 selection. Six obtained a durable complete response (platelet counts >100,000/µl), with a maximum follow-up of 42 months Two additional patients obtained durable partial responses (cessation of bleeding complications). Some patients, however, failed to show a response, as did patients reported by Skoda *et al.* (1997) and Marmont et al. (1998). Randomized trials are under discussion for ITP.

Crohn's disease

Two patients with severe Crohn's disease refractory to conventional therapy, including anti-TNF-α treatment, received conditioning with cyclophosphamide 200 mg/kg and equine ATG 90 mg/kg prior to CD34-selected autologous PBSC transplantation. Both patients remained in remission 1-year posttransplant at the time of the report (Burt et al., 2003).

Prospective randomized controlled trials of high-dose chemotherapy and autologous transplantation for high-risk breast cancer

In July 2003, two large prospective randomized controlled trials of high-dose chemotherapy and autologous HSC transplantation in women with stage II or III breast cancer and 10 or more axillary lymph nodes involved by tumor were reported (Rodenhuis *et al.*, 2003; Tallman *et al.*, 2003). The studies were large, enrolling 885 and 540 patients, respectively, and the median duration of follow up was 4.8 and 6.1 years, respectively. Both studies had similar designs: women were randomized to receive conventional adjuvant therapy or conventional adjuvant therapy followed by high-dose chemotherapy and autologous HSC transplantation. The Dutch study concluded that "high-dose alkylating therapy improves relapse-free survival among patients with stage II or III breast cancer and 10 or more positive axillary lymph nodes" (Rodenhuis *et al.*, 2003). The U.S. study concluded that "the addition of high-dose chemotherapy and autologous hematopoietic stem cell transplantation to six cycles of adjuvant chemotherapy . . . may reduce the risk of relapse but does not improve the outcome among patients with primary breast cancer and at least 10 involved axillary lymph nodes". While neither trial showed a significant difference in overall survival, both trials showed a significant reduction in the relapse rate in the group assigned to high-dose chemotherapy. As indicated in an accompanying editorial, such an effect provided by high-dose therapy and autografting may provide the best launching pad from which to explore new or additional methods of reducing relapse further (Elfenbein, 2003).

References

Burt, R.K., Traynor, A., Oyama, Y. & Craig, R. (2003). High-dose immune suppression and autologous hematopoietic stem cell transplantation in refractory Crohn disease. *Blood*, **101**, 2064–6.

Commenzo, R.L. & Gertz, M.A. (2002). Autologous stem cell transplantation for primary systemic amyloidosis. *Blood*, **99**, 4276–82.

Cooper, L.J.N., Topp, M.S., Serrano, L.M. et al. (2003). T-cell clones can be rendered specific for CD19: toward the selective augmentation of the graft-versus-B-lineage leukemia effect. *Blood*, **101**, 1637–44.

Elfenbein, G. (2003). Stem-cell transplantation for high-risk breast cancer (Editorial). *New England Journal of Medicine*, **349**, 80–82.

Gorgun, G., Miller, K.B. & Foss, F.M, (2002). Immunologic mechanisms of extracorporeal photochemotherapy in chronic graft-versus-host disease. *Blood*, **100**, 941–7.

Gratwohl, A., Baldomero, H., Horisberger, B. et al. (2002). Current trends in hematopoietic stem cell transplantation in Europe. *Blood*, **100**, 2374–86.

Hinterberger, W., Hinterberger-Fischer, M. & Marmont, A. (2002). Clinically demonstrable anti-autoimmunity mediated by allogeneic immune cells favorably affects outcome after stem cell transplantation in human autoimmune diseases. *Bone Marrow Transplantation*, **30**, 753–9.

Huhn, R.D., Fogarty, P.F., Nakamura, R. et al. (2003). High-dose cyclophosphamide with autologous lymphocyte-depleted peripheral blood cell (PBSC) support for treatment of refractory chronic autoimmune thrombocytopenia. *Blood*, **101**, 71–7.

Kantarjian, H.M., O'Brien, S., Cortes, J.E. et al. (2002). Imatinib mesylate therapy for relapse after allogeneic stem cell transplantation for chronic myelogenous leukemia. *Blood*, **100**, 1590–5.

Kröger, N., Schwerdtfeger, R., Kiehl, M. et al. (2002). Autologous stem cell transplantation followed by a reduced-dose allograft induces high complete remission rate in multiple myeloma. *Blood*, **100**, 755–60.

Maloney, D.G., Sahebi, F., Stockerl-Goldstein, K. E., et al (2001). Combining an allogeneic graft -vs- myeloma effect with high-dose autologous stem cell rescue in the treatment of multiple myeloma. *Blood*, **98**, 434–5a (abstract).

McSweeney P. A., Nash, R.A., Sullivan, K.M. et al. (2002). High-dose immunosuppressive therapy for severe systemic sclerosis: initial outcomes. *Blood*, **100**, 1602–10.

Ogawa, H., Tamaki, H., Ikegame, K. et al. (2002). The usefulness of monitoring WT1 gene transcripts for the prediction and management of relapse following allogeneic stem cell transplantation in acute type leukemia. *Blood*, **101**, 1698–1704.

Robinson, S.P., Goldstone, A.H., Mackinnon, S. et al. (2002). Chemoresistant or aggressive lymphoma predicts for a poor outcome following reduced-intensity allogeneic progenitor cell transplantation: an analysis from the Lymphoma Working Party of the European Group for Blood and Marrow Transplantation. *Blood*, **100**, 4310–6.

Rodenhuis S., Bontenbal M., Beex L.V. et al. (2003). High-dose chemotherapy with hematopoietic stem-cell rescue for high-risk breast cancer. *New England Journal of Medicine*, **349**, 7–16.

Shimazaki, C., Ochiai, N., Uchida, R. et al. (2003). Non-T-cell-depleted HLA-haploidentical stem cell transplantation in advanced hematologic malignancies based on the feto-maternal microchimerism. *Blood*, **101**, 3334–6.

Svahn, B-M, Remberger, M., Myrbäck, K.-E. et al. (2002). Home care during the pancytopenic phase after allogeneic hematopoietic stem cell transplantation is advantageous compared with hospital care. *Blood*, **100**, 4317–24.

Tallman, M.S., Grat, R., Robert, N.J. et al. (2003). Conventional adjuvant chemotherapy with or without high-dose chemotherapy and autologous stem-cell transplantation in high-risk breast cancer. *New England Journal of Medicine*, **349**, 17–26.

Taylor, P.A., Lees, C.J. & Blazar, B.R. (2002). The infusion of ex vivo activated and expanded CD4$^+$ CD25$^+$ immune regulatory cells inhibits graft-versus-host diseae lethality. *Blood*, **99**, 3493–9.

Urbano-Ispizua, A., Rozman, C. Pimentel, P. et al. (2002). Risk factors for acute graft-versus-host disease in patients undergoing transplantation with CD34$^+$ selected blood cells from HLA-identical siblings. *Blood*, **100**, 724–7.

Urbano-Ispizua, A., Schmitz, N., de Witte, T. et al. (2002). Allogeneic and autologous transplantation for haematological diseases, solid tumors and immune disorders: definition and current practice in Europe. *Bone Marrow Transplantation*, **29**, 639–46.

van Rood, J.J., Loberiza, F.R., Zhang, M.J. et al. (2002). Effect of tolerance to noninherited maternal antigens on the occurrence of graft-versus-host disease after bone marrow transplantation from a parent or an HLA-haploidentical sibling. *Blood*, **96**, 1572–7.

Index